21ST EDITION

SABISTON TEXTBOOK of SURGERY

The BIOLOGICAL BASIS of MODERN SURGICAL PRACTICE

COURTNEY M. TOWNSEND, JR., MD
Professor
Robertson-Poth Distinguished Chair in General Surgery
Department of Surgery
The University of Texas Medical Branch
Galveston, Texas

R. DANIEL BEAUCHAMP, MD
J.C. Foshee Distinguished Professor of Surgery
Professor of Cell and Developmental Biology
Deputy Director, Vanderbilt-Ingram Cancer Center
Vice President Cancer Center Network Affairs
Vanderbilt University Medical Center
Nashville, Tennessee

B. MARK EVERS, MD
Professor and Vice-Chair for Research
Department of Surgery
Director, Lucille P. Markey Cancer Center
Markey Cancer Foundation Endowed Chair
Physician-in-Chief, Oncology Service Line UK Healthcare
University of Kentucky
Lexington, Kentucky

KENNETH L. MATTOX, MD
Distinguished Service Professor
Michael E. DeBakey Department of Surgery
Baylor College of Medicine
Chief of Staff and Surgeon-in-Chief
Ben Taub General Hospital
Houston, Texas

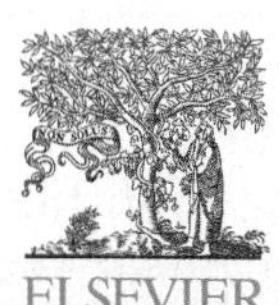

ELSEVIER

Elsevier
3251 Riverport Lane
St. Louis, Missouri 63043

SABISTON: TEXTBOOK OF SURGERY: THE BIOLOGICAL BASIS OF MODERN SURGICAL PRACTICE, TWENTY FIRST EDITION
Standard Edition: 978-0-323-64062-6
International Edition: 978-0-323-64063-3

Notices

Practitioners and researchers must always rely on their own experience and knowledge in evaluating and using any information, methods, compounds or experiments described herein. Because of rapid advances in the medical sciences, in particular, independent verification of diagnoses and drug dosages should be made. To the fullest extent of the law, no responsibility is assumed by Elsevier, authors, editors or contributors for any injury and/or damage to persons or property as a matter of products liability, negligence or otherwise, or from any use or operation of any methods, products, instructions, or ideas contained in the material herein.

Library of Congress Control Number: 2020936664

Content Strategist: Jessica L. McCool
Senior Content Development Specialist: Joanie Milnes
Content Development Manager: Kathryn DeFrancesco
Publishing Services Manager: Shereen Jameel
Senior Project Manager: Umarani Natarajan
Design Direction: Margaret Reid

Printed in Canada

Last digit is the print number: 9 8 7 6 5 4 3 2 1

To our patients, who grant us the privilege of practicing our craft; to our students, residents, and colleagues, from whom we learn; and to our wives—Mary, Shannon, Karen, and June—without whose support this would not have been possible.

CONTRIBUTORS

Corinne M. Aberle, MD
Assistant Professor
Division of Cardiothoracic Surgery
University of Miami
Miami, Florida
United States

Naim Abu-Freha, MD, MHA
Department of Gastroenterology and Hepatology
Soroka University Medical Center
Faculty of Health Sciences
Ben-Gurion University of the Negev
Director, Department of Gastroenterology
Assuta Medical Center—Beer Sheva
Beer Sheva, Israel

Andrew B. Adams, MD, PhD
Associate Professor
Surgery
Emory University School of Medicine
Atlanta, Georgia
United States

Reid B. Adams, MD
Chair, Department of Surgery
Claude A. Jessup Professor of Surgery
University of Virginia
Charlottesville, Virginia
United States

Nikhil Agrawal, MD
Resident
Surgery
Baylor College of Medicine
Houston, Texas
United States

Vanita Ahuja, MPH, MBA, MD
Associate Professor of Surgery
Yale University School of Medicine
New Haven, Connecticut
United States
Chief, General Surgery
VA Connecticut HealthCare System
West Haven, Connecticut
United States

Sophoclis Alexopoulos, MD
Associate Professor
Section of Surgical Sciences
Chief, Division of Liver Transplantation and Hepatobiliary Surgery
Vanderbilt University Medical Center
Nashville, Tennessee
United States

Kristen A. Aliano, MD
Plastic Surgeon
Private Practice
McGuiness Dermatology and Aesthetics
Dallas-Fort Worth, Texas
United States

Ronald D. Alvarez, MD, MBA
Professor and Chair
Obstetrics and Gynecology
Vanderbilt University Medical Center
Nashville, Tennessee
United States

Vamsi Aribindi, MD
Surgical Resident
Department of Surgery
Baylor College of Medicine
Houston, Texas
United States

Amanda K. Arrington, MD
Associate Professor
Department of Surgery
University of Arizona
Tucson, Arizona
United States

Omar Atassi, MD
Assistant Professor of Orthopedic Trauma
Ben Taub General Hospital
Department of Orthopedic Surgery
Baylor College of Medicine
Houston, Texas
United States

I. Raul Badell, MD
Assistant Professor
Surgery
Emory University School of Medicine
Atlanta, Georgia
United States

Faisel G. Bakaeen, MD
Professor
Thoracic and Cardiovascular Surgery
Cleveland Clinic
Cleveland, Ohio
United States

Juan Camilo Barreto, MD
Assistant Professor of Surgery
Division of Surgical Oncology
University of Arkansas for Medical Sciences
Little Rock, Arkansas
United States

R. Daniel Beauchamp, MD, FACS
J.C. Foshee Distinguished Professor of Surgery
Professor of Cell and Developmental Biology
Deputy Director, Vanderbilt-Ingram Cancer Center
Vice President Cancer Center Network Affairs
Vanderbilt University Medical Center
Nashville, Tennessee
United States

Yolanda Becker, MD, FACS, FAST
Professor of Surgery
Director of Kidney and Pancreas Transplant
University of Chicago
Chicago, Illinois
United States

Elizabeth E. Blears, MS
General Surgery Resident
Allegheny Health Network
Pittsburgh, Pennsylvania
United States

Iuliana Bobanga, MD
Case Western Reserve University School of Medicine
Clinical Assistant Professor
Department of Surgery
University Hospitals Cleveland Medical Center
Cleveland, Ohio
United States

Morgan Bonds, MD
Fellow
General, Vascular, and Thoracic Surgery
Virginia Mason Medical Center
Seattle, Washington
United States

Mimi R. Borrelli, MBBS, MSc
Research Fellow
Surgery
Stanford University
Palo Alto, California
United States
Resident
Department of Plastic Surgery
Brown University
Providence, Rhode Island
United States

Stefanos Boukovalas, MD
Microvascular Reconstructive Fellow
Department of Plastic Surgery
The University of Texas MD Anderson Cancer Center
Houston, Texas
United States

Benjamin S. Brooke, MD, PhD
Associate Professor of Surgery & Population Health Sciences
Chief, Division of Vascular Surgery
Section Chief, Health Services Research
Department of Surgery
University of Utah
Salt Lake City, Utah
United States

Carlos V.R. Brown, MD, FACS
Chief, Division of Acute Care Surgery
Department of Surgery
Dell Medical School, University of Texas at Austin
Austin, Texas
United States

Alfredo Maximiliano Carbonell, DO
Vice Chairman of Academic Affairs
Department of Surgery
Prisma Health -Upstate
Professor of Surgery
University of South Carolina School of Medicine - Greenville
Greenville, South Carolina
United States

Samuel P. Carmichael II, MD MS
Assistant Professor of Surgery
Department of Surgery
Wake Forest University School of Medicine
Wake Forest Baptist Health
Winston-Salem, North Carolina
United States

Joshua S. Carson, MD
Assistant Professor of Surgery
Department of Surgery
University of Florida College of Medicine
Gainseville, Florida
United States

Howard C. Champion, MD, FACS
Professor of Surgery
F. Edward Hébert School of Medicine
Uniformed Service University of the Health Sciences
Bethesda, Maryland
United States

Kevin J. Chiang, BA, MD
Acute Care Surgery Fellow
Division of Trauma, Emergency Surgery, and Surgical Critical Care
Massachusetts General Hospital
Harvard Medical School
Cambridge, Massachusetts
United States

Dai H. Chung, MD, FACS
Professor and Strauss Chair in Pediatric Surgery
UT Southwestern Medical Center
Dallas, Texas
United States

Michael Coburn, MD
Professor and Chairman
Scott Department of Urology
Baylor College of Medicine
Houston, Texas
United States

Eric L. Cole, MD
Assistant Professor
Division of Plastic Surgery
The University of Texas Medical Branch
Galveston, Texas
United States

Carlo M. Contreras, MD
Associate Professor
Surgery
The Ohio State University
Columbus, Ohio
United States

Robert N. Cooney, MD, FACS, FCCM
Professor and Chairman
Surgery
SUNY Upstate Medical University
Syracuse, New York
United States

Jack Dawson, MD
Associate Professor of Orthopedic Trauma
Chief of Orthopedic Surgery
Ben Taub General Hospital
Department of Orthopedic Surgery
Baylor College of Medicine
Houston, Texas
United States

Abe DeAnda Jr., MD
Professor and Chief
Division of Cardiovascular and Thoracic Surgery
University of Texas Medical Branch
Galveston, Texas
United States

Bradley M. Dennis, MD, FACS
Associate Professor of Surgery
Division of Trauma and Surgical Critical Care
Vanderbilt University Medical Center
Nashville, Tennessee
United States

Rajeev Dhupar, MD, MBA, FACS
Chief of Thoracic Surgery
Surgical Services Division
VA Pittsburgh Healthcare System
Assistant Professor
Cardiothoracic Surgery
University of Pittsburgh School of Medicine
Pittsburgh, Pennsylvania
United States

Jose J. Diaz, MD, CNS, FACS, FCCM
Professor of Surgery
Vice Chair Quality & Safety
Chief, Division of Acute Care Surgery
Program Director Acute Care Surgery
Fellowship Program in Trauma
R. Adams Cowley Shock Trauma Center
University of Maryland School of Medicine
Baltimore, Maryland
United States

Sharmila Dissanaike, MD, FACS, FCCM
Peter C. Canizaro Chair and Professor
Department of Surgery
Texas Tech University Health Sciences Center
Lubbock, Texas
United States

Roger R. Dmochowski, MD, MMHC
Professor
Department of Urologic Surgery
Vice Chair for Faculty Affairs and Professionalism
Section of Surgical Sciences
Associate Surgeon-in-Chief
Vanderbilt University Medical Center
Nashville, Tennessee
United States

Vikas Dudeja, MBBS, FACS
Selwyn M. Vickers Endowed Scholar
Director and Associate Professor
Division of Surgical Oncology
University of Alabama
Department of Surgery
Birmingham, Alabama
United States

Quan-Yang Duh, MD
Professor, Chief Section of Endocrine Surgery
Surgery
University of California, San Francisco
Attending Surgeon
Surgery
Veterans Affairs Medical Center
San Francisco, California
United States

James S. Economou, MD, PhD
Beaumont Distinguished Professor of Surgery
Distinguished Professor of Microbiology, Immunology, and Molecular Genetics
Distinguished Professor of Molecule and Medical Pharmacology
University of California-Los Angeles David Geffen School of Medicine
Los Angeles, California
United States

Michael E. Egger, MD, MPH
Assistant Professor
Hiram C. Polk Jr, MD, Department of Surgery
University of Louisville
James Graham Brown Cancer Center
Louisville, Kentucky
United States

C. Tyler Ellis, MD, MSCR
Instructor of Surgery
Surgery
University of Louisville
Louisville, Kentucky
United States

B. Mark Evers, MD, FACS
Professor and Vice-Chair for Research
Department of Surgery
Director, Lucille P. Markey Cancer Center
Markey Cancer Foundation Endowed Chair
Physician-in-Chief, Oncology Service Line UK Healthcare
University of Kentucky
Lexington, Kentucky
United States

Diana L. Farmer, MD, FACS, FRCS
Chair and Professor
Surgery
University of California, Davis
Sacramento, California
United States

Jeffrey S. Farroni, PhD, JD
Associate Professor
Institute for the Medical Humanities
The University of Texas Medical Branch
Galveston, Texas
United States

Anthony Ferrantella, MD
General Surgery Resident
Department of Surgery
University of Miami Miller School of Medicine
Miami, Florida
United States

Ryan Fields, MD
Chief, Surgical Oncology; Professor of Surgery
Surgery
Barnes-Jewish Hospital & The Alvin J. Siteman Comprehensive Cancer Center at Washington University School of Medicine
St. Louis, Missouri
United States

Samuel R.G. Finlayson, MD, MPH, MBA, FACS
Professor of Surgery
Claudius Y. Gates, MD, and Catherine B. Gates Presidential Endowed Chair in Surgery
Department of Surgery
University of Utah School of Medicine
Salt Lake City, Utah
United States

Celeste C. Finnerty, PhD
Professor
Surgery
The University of Texas Medical Branch
Galveston, Texas
United States

Nicholas A. Fiore II,
Private Practice
Fiore Hand and Wrist
Houston, Texas
United States

Thomas Fishbein, MD
Executive Director
MedStar Georgetown Transplant Institute
MedStar Georgetown University Hospital
Professor of Surgery
Georgetown University School of Medicine
Washington, DC
United States

Yuman Fong, MD
Sangiacomo Chair and Chairman
Department of Surgery
City of Hope Medical Center
Duarte, California
United States

Chuck D. Fraser Jr., MD, FACS
Professor of Surgery and Perioperative Care
Department of Surgery and Perioperative Care
The University of Texas at Austin - Dell Medical School
Section Chief for Pediatric and Congenital Cardiothoracic Surgery
Texas Center for Pediatric and Congenital Heart Disease
Austin, Texas
United States

Gerald M. Fried, MD, CM, FRCSC, FACS
Edward W. Archibald Professor and Chairman
Department of Surgery
McGill University
Surgeon-in-Chief, McGill University Health Centre
Montreal, Quebec
Canada

Susan Galandiuk, MD
Professor of Surgery, Program Director, Section of Colon & Rectal Surgery
Hiram C. Polk Jr, MD, Department of Surgery
University of Louisville
Director
Price Institute of Surgical Research
University of Louisville
Louisville, Kentucky
United States

Tong Gan, MD, MS
Resident Physician
Surgery
University of Kentucky
Lexington, Kentucky
United States

S. Peter Goedegebuure, PhD
Associate Professor
Surgery
Washington University School of Medicine
Saint Louis, Missouri
United States

Oliver L. Gunter, MD, FACS
Associate Professor
Director of Emergency General Surgery
Division of Trauma & Surgical Critical Care
Vanderbilt University Medical Center
Nashville, Tennessee
United States

Jennifer M. Gurney, MD, FACS
Chief Defense Committee on Trauma
Joint Trauma System
Falls Church, Virginia
Surgeon
United States Army Institute of Surgical Research
San Antonio, Texas
United States

Jennifer L. Halpern, MD
Assistant Professor
Department of Orthopedics
Vanderbilt University Medical Center
Nashville, Tennessee
United States

Jason Hawksworth, MD
Transplant Surgeon
Hepatopancreatobiliary and Transplant Surgeon
Assistant Professor of Surgery
MedStar Georgetown Transplant Institute
MedStar Georgetown University Hospital
Washington, DC
United States

Mary Hawn, MD, MPH
Professor and Chair
Surgery
Stanford University
Stanford, California
United States

Antonio Hernandez, MSc, MD
Associate Professor
Anesthesiology
Vanderbilt University Medical Center
Nashville, Tennessee
United States

David N. Herndon, MD
Retired
Kelleys Island, Ohio
United States

Marty J. Heslin, MD, MSHA
Professor and Vice Chair
Surgery
The University of Alabama at Birmingham
Birmingham, Alabama
United States

Shinjiro Hirose, MD
Professor of Pediatric Surgery
University of California, Davis
Sacramento, California
United States

Trung Ho, MD
Staff Physician
Surgery
Baylor College of Medicine
Houston, Texas
United States

Richard Hodin, MD
Professor of Surgery
Chief of Academic Affairs
Massachusetts General Hospital
Harvard Medical School
Boston, Massachusetts
United States

Wayne L. Hofstetter, MD
Professor of Surgery and Deputy Chair
Thoracic and Cardiovascular Surgery
The University of Texas MD Anderson Cancer Center
Houston, Texas
United States

Ginger E. Holt, MD
Professor and Vice Chair of Education
Orthopaedic Surgery and Rehabilitation
Adult Reconstruction Surgery and Musculoskeletal Oncology
Director, Musculoskeletal Oncology
Program Director, Orthopaedic Residency Program, Musculoskeletal Oncology Fellowship
Division of Pediatric Orthopaedics
Vanderbilt University Medical Center
Nashville, Tennessee
United States

Michael S. Hu, MD, MPH, MS
Post-Doctoral Fellow
Surgery
Stanford University
Stanford, California
United States
Resident Physician
Plastic Surgery
University of Pittsburgh Medical Center
Pittsburgh, Pennsylvania
United States

Yinnin Hu, MD
Fellow, Complex General Surgical Oncology, Department of Surgery
Memorial Sloan-Kettering Cancer Center
New York, New York
United States

Kelly K. Hunt, MD, FACS
Professor and Chair
Breast Surgical Oncology
The University of Texas MD Anderson Cancer Center
Houston, Texas
United States

Neil Hyman, MD
Chief, Section of Colon and Rectal Surgery, Codirector Digestive Disease Center
Department of Surgery
University of Chicago Medicine
Chicago, Illinois
United States

Uzi Izhar, MD
Professor of Cardiothoracic Surgery
Head - General Thoracic Surgery Unit
Cardiothoracic Surgery
Hadassah University Medical Center
Jerusalem, Israel

Eric H. Jensen, MD, FACS
Professor and Chief of Surgical Oncology
Department of Surgery
University of Minnesota Medical Center
Minneapolis, Minnesota
United States

Gregory J. Jurkovich, MD
Professor and Vice-Chairman
Department of Surgery
University of California, Davis
Sacramento, California
United States

Shana S. Kalaria, MD, MBA
Resident Physician
Division of Plastic Surgery
University of Texas Medical Branch
Galveston, Texas
United States

Seth J. Karp, MD
Chairman
Section of Surgical Sciences
Surgeon-in-Chief
Director
Vanderbilt Transplant Center
Vanderbilt University Medical Center
Nashville, Tennessee
United States

Samuel J. Kesseli, MD
Resident Physician
General Surgery
Duke University Medical Center
Durham, North Carolina
United States

Leena Khaitan, MD, MPH
Professor of Surgery
Department of Surgery
Director, Metabolic and Bariatric Surgery Center
Director, Esophageal and Swallowing Center
Digestive Health Institute
University Hospitals, Cleveland Medical Center
Cleveland, Ohio
United States

Kimberly H. Khoo, BS
Medical Student
School of Medicine
The University of Texas Medical Branch
Galveston, Texas
United States

Jae Y. Kim, MD
Chief, Division of Thoracic Surgery
Surgery
City of Hope Cancer Center
Duarte, California
United States

V. Suzanne Klimberg, MD, PhD, MSHCT, FACS
Courtney M. Townsend, Jr., MD Distinguished Chair in General Surgery
Department of Surgery
The University of Texas Medical Branch
Galveston, Texas
Adjunct Professor
The University of Texas MD Anderson Cancer Center
Houston, Texas
United States

Patrick H. Knight, MD
Resident
Department of Surgery
Western Michigan University
Homer Stryker MD School of Medicine
Kalamazoo, Michigan
United States

Katherine E. Kramme, DO
Resident
Department of Surgery
Western Michigan University
Homer Stryker MD School of Medicine
Kalamazoo, Michigan
United States

Bradley A. Krasnick, MD
Resident
Surgery
Washington University School of Medicine
St. Louis, Missouri
United States

Amanda M. Laird, MD
Chief, Section of Endocrine Surgery
Surgical Oncology
Rutgers Cancer Institute of New Jersey
Associate Professor of Surgery
Surgery
Rutgers Robert Wood Johnson Medical School
New Brunswick, New Jersey
United States

Alessandra Landmann, MD
Pediatric Surgery Fellow
Surgery
University of Oklahoma Health Sciences Center
Oklahoma City, Oklahoma
United States

Christian P. Larsen, MD, DPhil
Professor of Surgery
Mason Professor of Transplantation
Emory University School of Medicine
Atlanta, Georgia
United States

Lillian Liao, MD, MPH
Associate Professor of Surgery
Pediatric Trauma Medical Director
UT Health San Antonio
San Antonio, Texas
United States

Steven K. Libutti, MD
Director
Rutgers Cancer Institute of New Jersey
New Brunswick, New Jersey
United States

Masha Livhits, MD
Assistant Professor of Surgery
Surgery
University of California-Los Angeles David Geffen School of Medicine
Los Angeles, California
United States

Michael T. Longaker, MD, MBA
Deane P. and Louise Mitchell Professor
Surgery
Stanford University
Stanford, California
United States

H. Peter Lorenz, MD
Pediatric Plastic Surgery Service Chief and Professor
Plastic and Reconstructive Surgery
Stanford University School of Medicine
Palo Alto, California
United States

Amin Madani, MD, PhD, FRCSC, DABS
Resident
Department of Surgery University Health Network
Toronto General Hospital
Toronto, Ontario
Canada

David A. Mahvi, MD
Surgical Resident
Surgery
Brigham and Women's Hospital
Boston, Massachusetts
United States

David M. Mahvi, MD
Professor of Surgery
Surgery
Medical University of South Carolina
Charleston, South Carolina
United States

William Marston, MD
Professor
Division of Vascular Surgery
University of North Carolina School of Medicine
Chapel Hill, North Carolina
United States

Matthew J. Martin, MD, FACS, FASMBS
Director of Trauma Research
Scripps Mercy Hospital
San Diego, California
United States

R. Shayn Martin, MD, MBA, FACS
Associate Professor of Surgery
Department of Surgery
Wake Forest University School of Medicine
Executive Director, Critical Care Services
Wake Forest Baptist Health
Winston-Salem, North Carolina
United States

Christopher R. McHenry, MD, FACS
Professor of Surgery
Case Western Reserve University School of Medicine
Vice Chair
Department of Surgery
MetroHealth Medical Center
Cleveland, Ohio
United States

Kelly M. McMasters, MD, PhD
Chairman
Surgery
University of Louisville
Louisville, Kentucky
United States

Saral Mehra, MD, MBA, FACS
Associate Professor
Surgery
Yale University School of Medicine
New Haven, Connecticut
United States

Matthew Mell, MD, MS
Professor and Chief, Division of Vascular Surgery
Surgery
University of California, Davis
Sacramento, California
United States

J. Wayne Meredith, MD, FACS
Richard T. Myers Professor and Chair
Department of Surgery
Wake Forest University School of Medicine
Chief of Clinical Chairs
Chief of Surgery
Wake Forest Baptist Health
Winston-Salem, North Carolina
United States

Richard S. Miller, MD, FACS
Professor of Surgery, Chief, Division of Trauma and Surgical Critical Care
Carol Ann Galvin Directorship in Trauma and Surgical Care Surgery, Section of Surgical Sciences
Vanderbilt University Medical Center
Nashville, Tennessee
United States

Joseph L. Mills Sr., MD
Reid Professor and Chief of Vascular Surgery and Endovascular Therapy
Michael E. DeBakey Department of Surgery
Baylor College of Medicine
Houston, Texas
United States

Emilio Morpurgo, MD, FASCRS
Chairman
Department of Surgery
Regional Center for Videolaparoscopic Robotic Surgery
Hospital Camposampiero
Chief ad interim Department of Surgery
Hospital Sant Antonio
Padova, Italy

Nathan T. Mowery, MD, FACS
Associate Professor of Surgery
Department of Surgery
Wake Forest University School of Medicine
Wake Forest Baptist Health
Winston-Salem, North Carolina
United States

Carmen L. Mueller, BSc(H), MD, MEd, FRCSC, FACS
Associate Professor
Department of Surgery
McGill University
Montreal, Quebec
Canada

Aussama K. Nassar, MD, MSc, FACS, FRCSC
Clinical Assistant Professor
Surgery
Stanford University
Stanford, California
United States

Elaine E. Nelson, MD
Medical Director of the Emergency Department
Regional Medical Center of San Jose
San Jose, California
United States

David Netscher, MD
Professor
Division of Plastic Surgery, Department of Orthopedic Surgery
Baylor College of Medicine
Houston, Texas
United States

Uri Netz, MD
Vice Chairman
Department of Surgery A
Soroka University Medical Center
Faculty of Health Sciences
Ben-Gurion University of the Negev
Beer Sheva, Israel

William B. Norbury, MD, FRCS (Plast)
Assistant Professor
Division of Plastic Surgery
The University of Texas Medical Branch
Staff Surgeon
Critical Care and Burns Reconstruction
Shriners Hospital for Children
Galveston, Texas
United States

Robert L. Norris, MD
Emeritus Professor of Emergency Medicine
Stanford University Medical Center
Stanford, California
United States

Brant K. Oelschlager, MD
Professor and Chief; Byers Endowed Professor of Esophageal Research
Division of General Surgery
University of Washington Medical Center
Seattle, Washington
United States

Shuab Omer, MD
Associate Professor
Advanced Cardiopulmonary Therapies and Transplantation
University of Texas Health Science Center Houston
Houston, Texas
United States

Edwin OnKendi, MBChB, FACS
Assistant Professor
Department of Surgery
Texas Tech University Health Sciences Center
Lubbock, Texas
United States

Pablo L. Padilla, MD
Plastic Surgery Resident
Division of Plastic and Reconstructive Surgery
The University of Texas Medical Branch
Galveston, Texas
United States

Zachary S. Pallister, MD
Assistant Professor of Surgery
Michael E. DeBakey Department of Surgery
Baylor College of Medicine
Houston, Texas
United States

Julie E. Park, MD, FACS
Stephen R. Lewis Professor and Program Director
Division of Plastic Surgery
Department of Surgery
The University of Texas Medical Branch
Galveston, Texas
United States

Luigi Pascarella, MD, FACS
Associate Professor of Surgery
University of North Carolina School of Medicine
Chapel Hill, North Carolina
United States

Samip Patel, MD, FACS
Associate Professor
Otolaryngology/Head and Neck Surgery
University of North Carolina School of Medicine
Chapel Hill, North Carolina
United States

Joel T. Patterson, MD, FACS
Associate Professor
Department of Neurosurgery
The University of Texas Medical Branch
Galveston, Texas
United States

Linda G. Phillips, MD
Truman G. Blocker Distinguished Professor and Chief
Division of Plastic Surgery
Surgery
University of Texas Medical Branch
Galveston, Texas
United States

Iraklis I. Pipinos, MD, PhD
Professor
Surgery
University of Nebraska Medical Center
Chief
Vascular Surgery
VA Nebraska and Western Iowa Medical Center
Omaha, Nebraska
United States

Russell Postier, MD
Dean Emeritus
College of Medicine
University of Oklahoma
Oklahoma City, Oklahoma
United States

Benjamin K. Poulose, MD, MPH
Robert M. Zollinger Lecrone-Baxter Chair
Chief, Division of General and Gastrointestinal Surgery
Center for Abdominal Core Health
The Ohio State University Wexner Medical Center
Columbus, Ohio
United States

Lauren S. Prescott, MD, MPH
Assistant Professor
Obstetrics and Gynecology, Division of Gynecologic Oncology
Vanderbilt University Medical Center
Nashille, Tennessee
United States

Anna M. Privratsky, DO
Assistant Professor of Surgery
Division of Trauma, Critical Care, and Acute Care Surgery
University of Arkansas for Medical Sciences
Little Rock, Arkansas
United States

Napat Pruekprasert, MD
Resident
General Surgery
SUNY Upstate Medical University
Syracuse, New York
United States

Pejman Radkani, MD, MSPH
Assistant Professor of Surgery, Hepatopancreatobiliary, and Liver Transplant Surgeon
Transplant Institute
Medstar Georgetown University Hospital
Assistant Professor of Surgery
Surgery
Georgetown University School of Medicine
Washington, DC
United States

Ravi Rajaram, MD, MSc
Assistant Professor of Surgery
Thoracic and Cardiovascular Surgery
The University of Texas MD Anderson Cancer Center
Houston, Texas
United States

Taylor S. Riall, MD, PhD
Professor
Department of Surgery
University of Arizona
Tucson, Arizona
United States

William O. Richards, MD
Professor and Chair
Department of Surgery
University of South Alabama College of Medicine
Mobile, Alabama
United States

Bryan Richmond, MD, MBA
The Bert Bradford Chairman and Professor of Surgery and Section Chief-General Surgery
Department of Surgery
West Virginia University/Charleston Division
Charleston, West Virginia
United States

J. Bart Rose, MD, MAS, FACS
Director of Pancreatobiliary Disease Center
Assistant Professor
Division of Surgical Oncology
University of Alabama
Department of Surgery
Birmingham, Alabama
United States

Michael J. Rosen, MD
Professor of Surgery
Lerner College of Medicine
Cleveland Clinic Foundation
Cleveland, Ohio
United States

Todd K. Rosengart, MD
Professor and Chairman
Michael E. DeBakey Department of Surgery
Baylor College of Medicine
Professor
Texas Heart Institute
Houston, Texas
United States

Ronnie A. Rosenthal, MS, MD
Professor of Surgery and Geriatrics
Yale University School of Medicine
New Haven, Connecticut
United States
Chief
Surgical Service
VA Connecticut Health Care System
West Haven, Connecticut
United States

Evan Ross, MD
Postdoctoral Fellow
Department of Surgery
The University of Texas Medical Branch
Galveston, Texas
United States

Rachel M. Russo, MD, MS
Assistant Professor
Department of Surgery
University of California, Davis
Sacramento, California
United States
Major
United States Air Force Medical Corps
Travis Air Force Base, California
United States

Ira Rutkow, MD, DrPH
Independent Scholar
New York
United States

Christopher Ryan, MD
Resident
General Surgery
Baylor College of Medicine
Houston, Texas
United States

Payam Saadai, MD, FACS, FAAP
Assistant Professor
Pediatric Surgery
University of California, Davis
Assistant Professor
Pediatric Surgery
Shriners Hospitals Northern California
Sacramento, California
United States

Noelle N. Saillant, MD, FACS
Instructor of Surgery
Division of Trauma, Emergency Surgery, and Surgical Critical Care
Massachusetts General Hospital
Harvard Medical School
Boston, Massachusetts
United States

Warren Sandberg, MD, PhD
Professor and Chair
Department of Anesthesiology
Chief of Staff for Perioperative and Critical Care Services
Vanderbilt University Medical Center
Nashville, Tennessee
United States

Ariel P. Santos, MD, MPH, FRCSC, FACS, FCCM
Associate Professor and Director of Telemedicine
Department of Surgery
Texas Tech University Health Sciences Center
Lubbock, Texas
United States

Robert G. Sawyer, MD, FACS, FCCM
Professor and Chair of Surgery
Surgery
Western Michigan University Homer Stryker MD School of Medicine
Kalamazoo, Michigan
Adjunct Professor of Surgery
Surgery
University of Virginia
Charlottesville, Virginia
Adjunct Professor of Engineering and Applied Sciences
Engineering and Applied Sciences
Western Michigan University
Kalamazoo, Michigan
United States

John P. Saydi, MD
Surgical Resident
Michael E. DeBakey Department of Surgery
Baylor College of Medicine
Houston, Texas
United States

Martin Allan Schreiber, MD
Professor of Surgery and Chief, Division of Trauma, Critical Care & Acute Care Surgery
Oregon Health & Science University
Portland, Oregon
United States

Herbert S. Schwartz, MD
Professor of Orthopaedic Surgery and Rehabilitation
Professor of Pathology, Microbiology, and Immunology
Vanderbilt University
Medical Center
Nashville, Tennessee
United States

Boris Sepesi, MD
Associate Professor
Thoracic and Cardiovascular Surgery
The University of Texas MD Anderson Cancer Center
Houston, Texas
United States

Edward R. Sherwood, MD, PhD
Professor and Vice Chair for Research
Department of Anesthesiology
Vanderbilt University Medical Center
Nashville, Tennessee
United States

Mihir Sheth, MD
Orthopedic Surgery Resident
Department of Orthopedic Surgery
Baylor College of Medicine
Houston, Texas
United States

Michael J. Sise, MD, FACS
Clinical Professor of Surgery
University of California-San Diego School of Medicine
Senior Vascular and Trauma Surgeon
Scripps Mercy Hospital
San Diego, California
United States

Michael C. Smith, MD
Assistant Professor
Surgery
Vanderbilt University Medical Center
Nashville, Tennessee
United States

Sawyer Gordon Smith, MD
Surgery Resident
Department of Surgery
Oregon Health & Science University
Portland, Oregon
United States

Thomas G. Smith III, MD
Associate Professor
Department of Urology, Division of Surgery
The University of Texas MD Anderson Cancer Center
Houston, Texas
United States

Christian Sommerhalder, MD, MMS
Surgical Resident
Surgery
The University of Texas Medical Branch
Galveston, Texas
United States

Julie Ann Sosa, MD, MA
Leon Goldman MD Distinguished Professor of Surgery and Chair
Department of Surgery
Professor
Department of Medicine
University of California San Francisco
Affiliated faculty
Philip R. Lee Institute for Health Policy Studies
University of California-San Francisco
San Francisco, California
United States

Jonathan D. Spicer, MD, PhD
Assistant Professor of Surgery
Department of Surgery
McGill University
Montreal, Canada

Ronald M. Stewart, MD
Professor and Chair of Surgery
Dr. Witten B. Russ Endowed Chair in Surgery
Department of Surgery
University of Texas Health Science Center at San Antonio
San Antonio, Texas
United States

Debra L. Sudan, MD
Professor of Surgery
Chief, Division of Abdominal Transplant Surgery
Duke University Medical Center
Durham, North Carolina
United States

David J. Sugarbaker
Chief of Division of Thoracic Surgery
Baylor College of Medicine
Houston, Texas
United States

Insoo Suh, MD
Associate Professor
Section of Endocrine Surgery
Department of Surgery
University of California, San Francisco
Staff Surgeon, Endocrine and General Surgery
San Francisco Veterans Affairs Health Care System
San Francisco, California
United States

Daniel Sun, MD
Orthopedic Surgery Resident
Department of Orthopedic Surgery
Baylor College of Medicine
Houston, Texas
United States

Jennifer M. Taylor, MD, MPH
Assistant Professor
Scott Department of Urology
Baylor College of Medicine
Houston, Texas
United States

Jonathan R. Thompson, MD, RPVI
Assistant Professor of Surgery
Surgery
University of Nebraska Medical Center
Omaha, Nebraska
United States

S. Rob Todd, MD, FACS, FCCM
Senior Vice President
Chief, Acute Care Surgery
Grady Health System
Atlanta, Georgia
United States

James S. Tomlinson, MD, PhD
Professor of Surgery
University of California-Los Angeles David Geffen School of Medicine
Los Angeles, California
United States

Alfonso Torquati, MD, MSCI
Helen Sheddd Keith Professor and Chairman
Department of Surgery
Rush University
Chicago, Illinois
United States

Sara Maria Tosato, MD
General Surgeon
Department of Surgery
Regional Center for Videolaparoscopic Robotic Surgery
Hostpital of Camposampiero, Padova, Italy

Richard H. Turnage, MD
Professor of Surgery
Department of Surgery
University of Arkansas for Medical Sciences Little Rock, Arkansas
Executive Associate Dean for Clinical Affairs
College of Medicine
University of Arkansas for Medical Sciences Medical Center
Little Rock, Arkansas
United States

Douglas S. Tyler, MD, MSHCT, FACS
John Woods Harris Distinguished Chair in Surgery, Professor and Chairman
Department of Surgery
The University of Texas Medical Branch
Galveston, Texas
United States

Konstantin Umanskiy, MD
Associate Professor of Surgery
Department of Surgery
University of Chicago Medicine
Chicago, Illinois
United States

Selwyn M. Vickers, MD, FACS
James C. Lee, Jr. Endowed Chair and Professor
Senior Vice President and Dean
School of Medicine
University of Alabama Birmingham
Birmingham, Alabama
United States

Ori Wald, MD, PhD
Attending Thoracic Surgeon
Cardiothoracic Surgery
Hadassah Hebrew University Hospital
Jerusalem, Israel

Andrew Well, MD, MPH, MSHCT
Health Transformation Fellow
Congenital Heart Surgery
Texas Center for Pediatric and Congenital Heart Disease at Dell Medical School
University of Texas
Austin, Texas
United States

William J. Winslade, PhD, JD, PhD
James Wade Rockwell Professor of Philosophy in Medicine
Institute for the Medical Humanities and Department of Preventive Medicine and Community Health
The University of Texas Medical Branch
Galveston, Texas
United States

Steven E. Wolf, MD
Joseph D. and Lee Hage Jamail Chari in Surgery
Professor and Vice-Chair for Finance
Division Chief - Trauma, Burns, and Acute Care Surgery
Surgery
The University of Texas Medical Branch
Chief of Staff
Shriners Hospital for Children - Texas
Galveston, Texas
United States

Yanghee Woo, MD, FACS
Associate Professor
Director of Gastrointestinal Minimally Invasive Therapies
Vice Chair of International Affairs
City of Hope National Medical Center
Duarte, California
United States

Jennifer Worsham, MD
Assistant Professor
Surgery - Vascular Surgery
The University of Texas Medical Branch
Galveston, Texas
United States

James C. Yang, MD
Senior Investigator
Surgery Branch
National Cancer Institute
Bethesda, Maryland
United States

Wendell G. Yarbrough, MD, MMHC, FACS
Thomas J. Dark Distinguished Chair
Otolaryngology/Head and Neck Surgery
University of North Carolina School of Medicine
Chapel Hill, North Carolina
United States

Robert B. Yates, MD
Clinical Assistant Professor
Center for Esophageal and Gastric Surgery
University of Washington Medical Center
Montlake, Washington
United States

Michael W. Yeh, MD
Professor, Chief Section of Endocrine Surgery
University of California-Los Angeles David Geffen School of Medicine
Los Angeles, California
United States

Natesh Yepuri, MBBS
Resident
Anesthesiology
The Guthrie Clinic
Sayve, Pennsylvania
United States

Amanda C. Yunker, DO, MSCR
Associate Professor
Obstetrics and Gynecology
Vanderbilt University Medical Center
Nashville, Tennessee
United States

Adam Zanation, MD, FACS
Harold C. Pillsbury Distinguished Professor
Executive Vice Chair
Otolaryngology/Head and Neck Surgery
University of North Carolina School of Medicine
Chapel Hill, North Carolina
United States

Ramón Zapata Sirvent, MD, FACS
Associate Professor
Department of Surgery, Division of Plastic Surgery
The University of Texas Medical Branch
Galveston, Texas
United States

Victor M. Zaydfudim, MD, MPH
Associate Professor of Surgery
Section of Hepatobiliary and Pancreatic Surgery, Division of Surgical Oncology
University of Virginia
Charlottesville, Virginia
United States

PREFACE

Surgery continues to evolve as new technology, techniques, and knowledge are incorporated into the care of surgical patients. The 21st edition of the *Sabiston Textbook of Surgery* reflects these exciting changes and new knowledge. We have incorporated two new chapters (Robotic Surgery and Fetal Surgery) and more than 119 new authors to ensure that the most current information is presented. This new edition has been revised and the current chapters have been enhanced to reflect these changes.

The primary goal of this new edition is to remain the most thorough, useful, readable, and understandable textbook presenting the principles and techniques of surgery. It is designed to be equally useful to students, trainees, and experts in the field. We are committed to maintaining this tradition of excellence begun in 1936. Surgery, after all, remains a discipline in which the knowledge and skill of a surgeon combine for the welfare of our patients.

COURTNEY M. TOWNSEND, JR., MD

FOREWORD

This is the 21st edition of *Sabiston's Textbook of Surgery*. It continues the strong tradition of being *the* definitive text for our discipline. Each chapter provides evidence-based references, and each has special references that will be of particular interest to the reader. The majority of authors are new and are recognized experts or "rising stars" in their respective fields. Each chapter provides the most up-to-date information on surgical innovations and techniques, as well as the latest in multidisciplinary treatments. This edition begins with an historical overview as well as a newly designed chapter on ethics and professionalism. The book then continues with knowledge needed to care for the surgical patient. The chapters on inflammatory response to surgical illness, shock, metabolism, and wound healing provide practical suggestions for the management of otherwise complex conditions in the surgical patient. There is a completely new chapter on assessment of surgical outcomes and an overview of health services research. This edition emphasizes the practical support of an actively practicing surgeon, as seen in emergency care of musculoskeletal injuries and the surgeon's role in mass casualty incidents. Similarly, there is a new chapter on robotic surgery, which balances the need for innovation and technical advancement with an obligation for additional training and increased cost. Many chapters provide detailed descriptions of the most innovative surgical approaches, such as the chapter on breast reconstruction detailing not only reconstructive techniques following mastectomy, but oncoplastic reconstructive interventions as well. There are superb chapters dealing with various disciplines within surgery, such as the pathophysiology and underlying biologic principals of transplantation and tumor immunology and immunotherapy. Each anatomic area is presented by a disease expert. For example, the chapter on melanoma not only provides the most recent recommendations for surgical intervention, but also details the multidisciplinary approaches of novel immunotherapies and targeted therapies. The chapter on the liver is particularly comprehensive, detailing new nonoperative interventions, advances in the medical management of hepatitis and fatty liver, and new minimally invasive surgical techniques. Each chapter is concise, focused, and provides the reader with the evidence-based information to provide contemporary surgical management for any clinical problem.

This new edition is available in both print and electronic format. Enhanced content, consisting of interactive images with magnification, and specific details, is available through Expert Consult (https://expertconsult.inkling.com/). There is also annotated self-testing material available through this feature.

Frederick Christopher first published this *Textbook of Surgery* in 1936. Dr. Townsend and his coeditors have once again done a masterful job in balancing the comprehensiveness of this text with a prioritization for information most needed by the practicing surgeon as well as the surgeon-in-training. The emphasis is on understanding the biologic basis of disease and presenting the most precise, state-of-the-art approach to treatment. This edition sets the standard for what a comprehensive textbook of surgery should be. It is a mandatory, efficient reference for any surgeon intent on expanding their knowledge.

Timothy J. Eberlein, MD, FACS, FRCSEd (Hon), FRCS, Glasg (Hon)
Bixby Professor and Chair, Department of Surgery
Spencer T. and Ann W. Olin Distinguished Professor
Director, Alvin J. Siteman Cancer Center
Senior Associate Dean for Cancer Programs
Washington University School of Medicine in St. Louis

ACKNOWLEDGMENTS

We would like to recognize the invaluable contributions of Karen Martin, Steve Schuenke, Eileen Figueroa, David Chavarria, and administrator Barbara Petit. Their dedicated professionalism, tenacious efforts, and cheerful cooperation are without parallel. They accomplished whatever was necessary, often on short or instantaneous deadlines, and were vital for the successful completion of the endeavor.

Our authors, respected authorities in their fields and busy physicians and surgeons, all did an outstanding job in sharing their wealth of knowledge.

We would also like to acknowledge the professionalism of our colleagues at Elsevier: Jessica McCool, Content Strategist; Joanie Milnes, Senior Content Development Specialist; Kathryn DeFrancisco, Content Development Manager; Shereen Jameel, Publishing Services Manager; Umarani Natarajan, Senior Project Manager and Margaret Reid, Senior Book Designer.

CONTENTS

VIDEO CONTENTS

SECTION I

Surgical Basis Principles

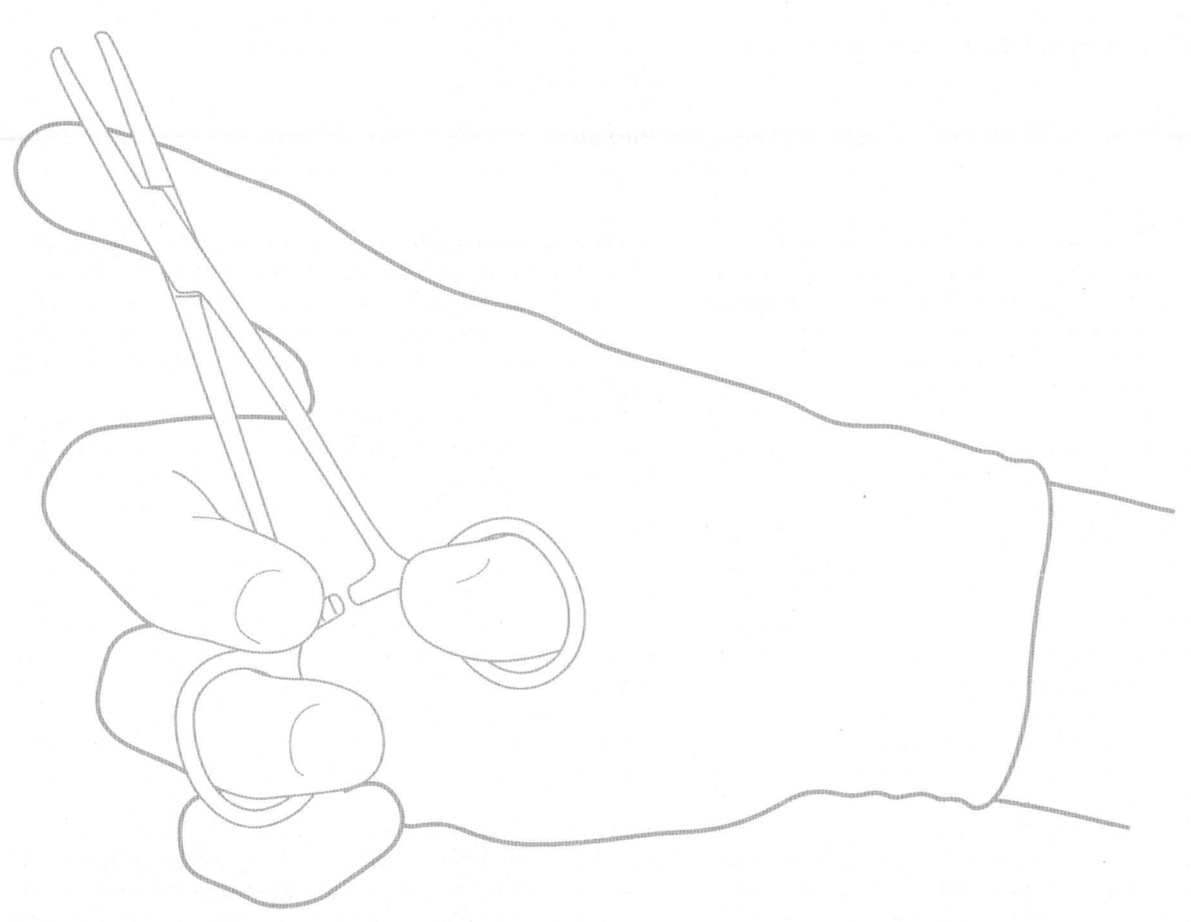

1 CHAPTER

The Rise of Modern Surgery: An Overview

Ira Rutkow

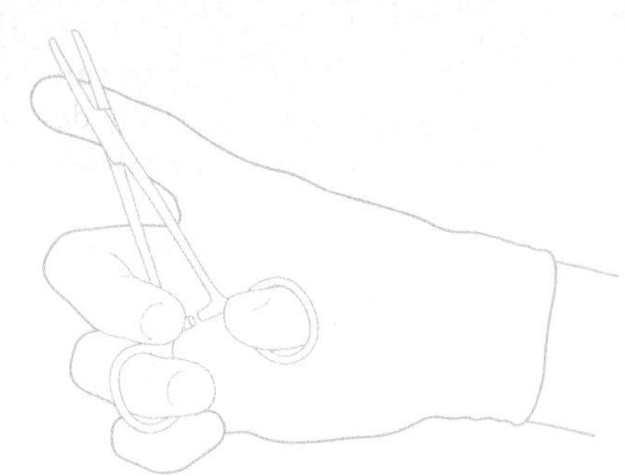

"If there were no past, science would be a myth; the human mind a desert. Evil would preponderate over good, and darkness would overspread the face of the moral and scientific world."

Samuel D. Gross (Louisville Review 1:26–27, 1856)

OUTLINE

THE BEGINNINGS

From earliest recorded history through late in the 19th century, the manner of surgery changed little. During those thousands of years, surgical operations were always frightening, often fatal, and frequently infected. In this prescientific, preanesthetic, and preantiseptic time, procedures were performed only for the direst of necessities and were unlike anything seen today; fully conscious patients were held or tied down to prevent their fleeing the surgeon's unsparing knife. When the surgeon, or at least those persons who used the sobriquet "surgeon," performed an operation, it was inevitably for an ailment that could be visualized (i.e., on the skin and just below the surface, on the extremities, or in the mouth).

Through the 14th century, most surgical therapy was delivered by minimally educated barber-surgeons and other itinerant adherents of the surgical cause. These faithful but obscure followers of the craft of surgery, although ostracized by aristocratic, university-educated physicians who eschewed the notion of working with one's hands, ensured the ultimate survival of what was then a vocation passed on from father to son. The roving "surgeons" mainly lanced abscesses; fixed simple fractures; dressed wounds; extracted teeth; and, on rare occasions, amputated a digit, limb, or breast. Around the 15th century, the highborn physicians began to show an interest in the art of surgery. As surgical techniques evolved, knife bearers, whether privileged physicians or wandering vagabonds, ligated arteries for readily accessible aneurysms, excised large visible tumors, performed trephinations, devised ingenious methods to reduce incarcerated and strangulated hernias, and created rudimentary colostomies and ileostomies by simply incising the skin over an expanding intraabdominal mass that represented the end stage of an intestinal blockage. The more entrepreneurial scalpel wielders widened the scope of their activities by focusing on the care of anal fistulas, bladder stones, and cataracts. Notwithstanding the growing boldness and ingenuity of "surgeons," surgical operations on the cavities of the body (i.e., abdomen, cranium, joints, and thorax) were generally unknown and, if attempted, fraught with danger.

Despite the terrifying nature of surgical intervention, operative surgery in the prescientific era was regarded as an important therapy within the whole of Medicine. (In this chapter, "Medicine" signifies the totality of the profession, and "medicine" indicates internal medicine as differentiated from surgery, obstetrics, pediatrics, and other specialties.) This seeming paradox, in view of the limited technical appeal of surgery, is explained by the fact that surgical procedures were performed for disorders observable on the surface of the body: There was an "objective" anatomic diagnosis. The men who performed surgical operations saw what needed to be fixed (e.g., inflamed boils, broken bones, bulging tumors, grievous wounds, necrotic digits and limbs, rotten teeth) and treated the problem in as rational a manner as the times permitted.

For individuals who practiced medicine, care was rendered in a more "subjective" manner involving diseases whose etiologies were neither seen nor understood. It is difficult to treat the symptoms of illnesses such as arthritis, asthma, diabetes, and heart failure when there is no scientific understanding as to what constitutes their pathologic and physiologic underpinnings. It was not until the 19th century and advances in pathologic anatomy and experimental physiology that practitioners of medicine were able to embrace a therapeutic viewpoint more closely, approximating that of surgeons. There was no longer a question of treating signs and symptoms in a blind manner. Similar to surgeons who operated on maladies that could be physically described, physicians now cared for patients using clinical details based on "objective" pathophysiologic findings.

Surgeons never needed a diagnostic and pathologic/physiologic revolution in the style of the physician. Despite the imperfection of their knowledge, prescientific surgeons with their unwavering amputation/extirpation approach to treatment sometimes did cure with technical confidence. Notwithstanding their dexterity, it required the spread of the revolution in Medicine during the 1880s and 1890s and the implementation of aseptic techniques along with other soon-to-come discoveries, including the x-ray, blood transfusion, and frozen section, to allow surgeons to emerge as specialists. It would take several more decades, well into the 20th century, for administrative and organizational events to occur before surgery could be considered a bona fide profession.

The explanation for the slow rise of surgery was the protracted elaboration of four key elements (knowledge of anatomy, control of bleeding, control of pain, and control of infection) that were more critical than technical skills when it came to the performance of a surgical procedure. These prerequisites had to be understood and accepted before a surgical operation could be considered a viable therapeutic option. The first two elements started to be addressed in the 16th century, and, although surgery greatly benefited from the breakthroughs, its reach was not extended beyond the exterior of the body, and pain and infection continued to be issues for the patient and the surgical operation. Over the ensuing 300 years, there was little further improvement until the discovery of anesthesia in the 1840s and recognition of surgical antisepsis during the 1870s and 1880s. The subsequent blossoming of scientific surgery brought about managerial and socioeconomic initiatives (standardized postgraduate surgical education and training programs; experimental surgical research laboratories; specialty journals, textbooks, monographs, and treatises; and professional societies and licensing organizations) that fostered the concept of professionalism. By the 1950s, the result was a unified profession that was practical and scholarly in nature. Some of the details of the rise of modern surgery follow—specifically how the four key elements that allowed a surgical operation to be viewed as a practical therapeutic choice came to be acknowledged.

KNOWLEDGE OF ANATOMY

Although knowledge of anatomy is the primary requirement of surgery, it was not until the mid-1500s and the height of the European Renaissance that the first great contribution to an understanding of the structure of the human body occurred. This came about when Popes Sixtus IV (1414–1484) and Clement VII (1478–1534) reversed the church's long-standing ban of human dissection and sanctioned the study of anatomy from the cadaver. Andreas Vesalius (1514–1564) (Fig. 1.1) stepped to the forefront of anatomic studies along with his celebrated treatise, *De Humani Corporis Fabrica Libri Septem* (1543). The *Fabrica* broke with the past and provided more detailed descriptions of the human body than any of its predecessors. It corrected errors in anatomy that were propagated thousands of years earlier by Greek and Roman authorities, especially Claudius Galen (129–199 AD), whose misleading and later church-supported views were based on animal rather than human dissection. Just as groundbreaking as his anatomic observations was Vesalius' blunt assertion that dissection

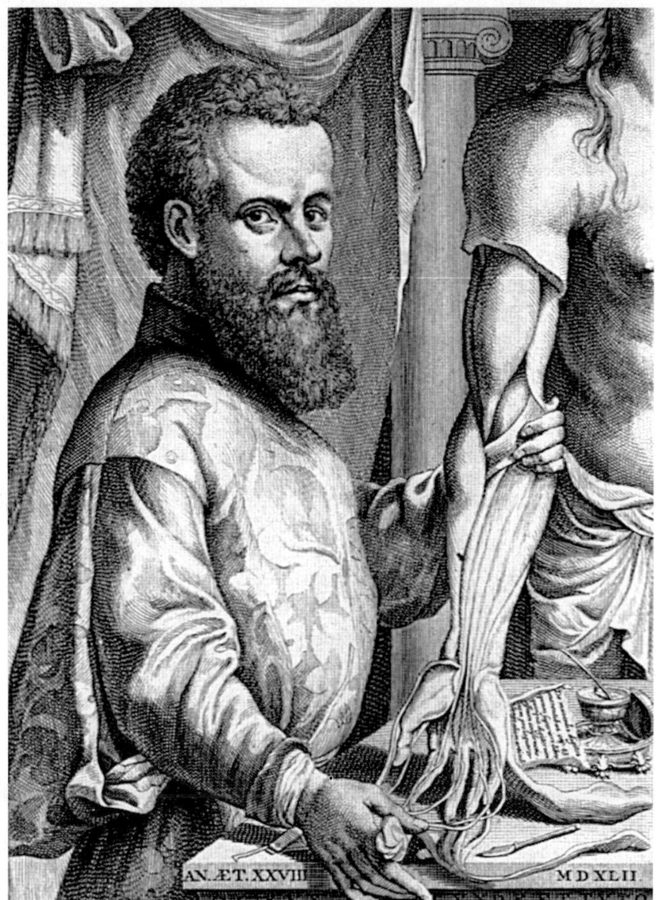

FIG. 1.1 Andreas Vesalius (1514–1564).

had to be completed hands-on by physicians themselves. This was a direct repudiation of the long-standing tradition that dissection was a loathsome task to be performed only by individuals in the lower class while the patrician physician sat on high reading out loud from a centuries-old anatomic text.

Vesalius was born in Brussels to a family with extensive ties to the court of the Holy Roman Emperors. He received his medical education in France at universities in Montpellier and Paris and for a short time taught anatomy near his home in Louvain. Following several months' service as a surgeon in the army of Charles V (1500–1558), the 23-year-old Vesalius accepted an appointment as professor of anatomy at the University of Padua in Italy. He remained there until 1544, when he resigned his post to become court physician to Charles V and later to Charles' son, Philip II (1527–1598). Vesalius was eventually transferred to Madrid, but for various reasons, including supposed trouble with authorities of the Spanish Inquisition, he planned a return to his academic pursuits. However, first, in 1563, Vesalius set sail for a year-long pilgrimage to the Holy Land. On his return voyage, Vesalius' ship was wrecked, and he and others were stranded on the small Peloponnesian island of Zakynthos. Vesalius died there as a result of exposure, starvation, and the effects of a severe illness, probably typhoid.

The 7 years that Vesalius spent in Padua left an indelible mark on the evolution of Medicine and especially surgery. His well-publicized human dissections drew large crowds, and Vesalius was in constant demand to provide anatomic demonstrations in other Italian cities, all of which culminated in the publication of the

Fabrica. Similar to most revolutionary works, the book attracted critics and sympathizers, and the youthful Vesalius was subjected to vitriolic attacks by some of the most renowned anatomists of that era. To his many detractors, the impassioned Vesalius often responded with intemperate counterattacks that did little to further his cause. In one fit of anger, Vesalius burned a trove of his own manuscripts and drawings.

The popularity of Vesalius' *Fabrica* rested on its outstanding illustrations. For the first time, detailed drawings of the human body were closely integrated with an accurate written text. Artists, believed to be from the school of Titian (1477–1576) in Venice, produced pictures that were scientifically accurate and creatively beautiful. The woodcuts, with their majestic skeletons and flayed muscled men set against backgrounds of rural and urban landscapes, became the standard for anatomic texts for several centuries.

The work of Vesalius paved the way for wide-ranging research into human anatomy, highlighted by a fuller understanding of the circulation of blood. In 1628, William Harvey (1578–1657) showed that the heart acts as a pump and forces blood along the arteries and back via veins, forming a closed loop. Although not a surgeon, Harvey's research had enormous implications for the evolution of surgery, particularly its relationship with anatomy and the conduct of surgical operations. As a result, in the 17th century, links between anatomy and surgery intensified as skilled surgeon-anatomists arose.

During the 18th century and first half of the 19th century, surgeon-anatomists made some of their most remarkable observations. Each country had its renowned individuals: In The Netherlands were Govard Bidloo (1649–1713), Bernhard Siegfried Albinus (1697–1770), and Pieter Camper (1722–1789); Albrecht von Haller (1708–1777), August Richter (1742–1812), and Johann Friedrich Meckel (1781–1833) worked in Germany; Antonio Scarpa (1752–1832) worked in Italy; and in France, Pierre-Joseph Desault (1744–1795), Jules Cloquet (1790–1883), and Alfred Armand Louis Marie Velpeau (1795–1867) were the most well-known. Above all, however, were the efforts of numerous British surgeon-anatomists who established a well-deserved tradition of excellence in research and teaching.

William Cowper (1666–1709) was one of the earliest and best known of the English surgeon-anatomists, and his student, William Cheselden (1688–1752), established the first formal course of instruction in surgical anatomy in London in 1711. In 1713, *Anatomy of the Human Body* by Cheselden was published and became so popular that it went through at least 13 editions. Alexander Monro *(primus)* (1697–1767) was Cheselden's mentee and later established a center of surgical-anatomic teaching in Edinburgh, which was eventually led by his son Alexander *(secundus)* (1737–1817) and grandson Alexander *(tertius)* (1773–1859). In London, John Hunter (1728–1793) (Fig. 1.2), who is considered among the greatest surgeons of all time, gained fame as a comparative anatomist-surgeon, while his brother, William Hunter (1718–1783), was a successful obstetrician who authored the acclaimed atlas, *Anatomy of the Human Gravid Uterus* (1774). Another brother duo, John Bell (1763–1820) and Charles Bell (1774–1842), worked in Edinburgh and London, where their exquisite anatomic engravings exerted a lasting influence. By the middle of the 19th century, surgical anatomy as a scientific discipline was well established. However, as surgery evolved into a more demanding profession, the anatomic atlases and illustrated surgical textbooks were less likely to be written by the surgeon-anatomist and instead were written by the full-time anatomist.

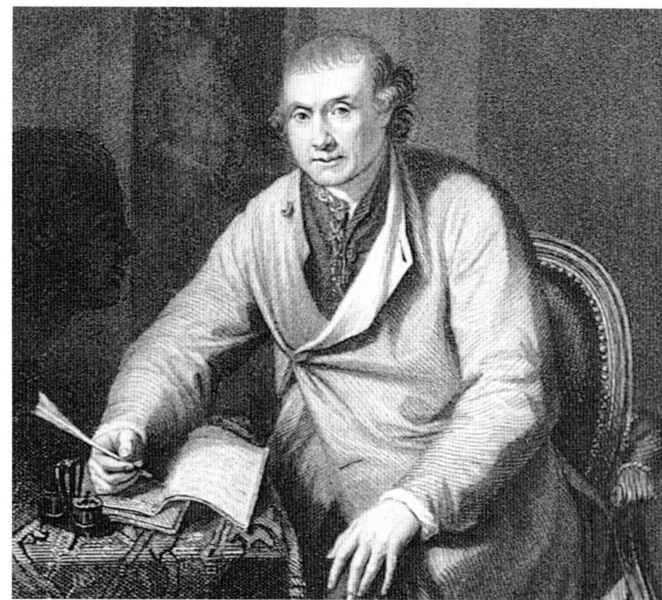

FIG. 1.2 John Hunter (1728–1793).

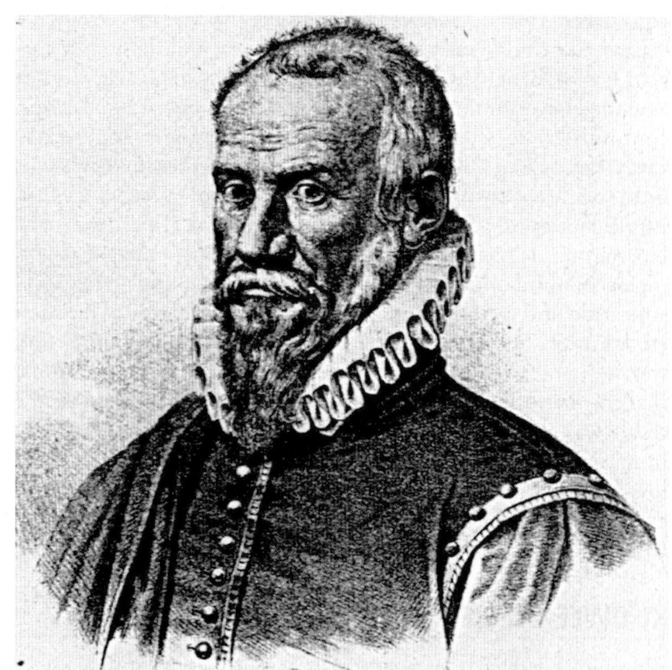

FIG. 1.3 Ambroise Paré (1510–1590).

CONTROL OF BLEEDING

Although Vesalius brought about a greater understanding of human anatomy, one of his contemporaries, Ambroise Paré (1510–1590) (Fig. 1.3), proposed a method to control hemorrhage during a surgical operation. Similar to Vesalius, Paré is important to the history of surgery because he also represents a severing of the final link between the surgical thoughts and techniques of the ancients and the push toward a more modern era. The two men were acquaintances, both having been summoned to treat Henry II (1519–1559), who sustained what proved to be a fatal lance blow to his head during a jousting match.

Paré was born in France and, at an early age, apprenticed to a series of itinerant barber-surgeons. He completed his indentured education in Paris, where he served as a surgeon's assistant/wound dresser in the famed Hôtel Dieu. From 1536 until just before his death, Paré worked as an army surgeon (he accompanied French armies on their military expeditions) while also maintaining a civilian practice in Paris. Paré's reputation was so great that four French kings, Henry II, Francis II (1544–1560), Charles IX (1550–1574), and Henry III (1551–1589) selected him as their surgeon-in-chief. Despite being a barber-surgeon, Paré was eventually made a member of the Paris-based College of St. Côme, a self-important fraternity of university-educated physician/surgeon. On the strength of Paré's personality and enormity of his clinical triumphs, a rapprochement between the two groups ensued, which set a course for the rise of surgery in France.

In Paré's time, applications of a cautery or boiling oil or both were the most commonly employed methods to treat a wound and control hemorrhage. Their use reflected belief in a medical adage dating back to the age of Hippocrates: Those diseases that medicines do not cure, iron cures; those that iron cannot cure, fire cures; and those that fire cannot cure are considered incurable. Paré changed such thinking when, on a battlefield near Turin, his supply of boiling oil ran out. Not knowing what to do, Paré blended a concoction of egg yolk, rose oil (a combination of ground-up rose petals and olive oil), and turpentine and treated the remaining injured. Over the next several days, he observed that the wounds of the soldiers dressed with the new mixture were neither as inflamed nor as tender as the wounds treated with hot oil. Paré abandoned the use of boiling oil not long afterward.

Paré sought other approaches to treat wounds and staunch hemorrhage. His decisive answer was the ligature, and its introduction proved a turning point in the evolution of surgery. The early history of ligation of blood vessels is shrouded in uncertainty, and whether it was the Chinese and Egyptians or the Greeks and Romans who first suggested the practice is a matter of historical conjecture. One thing is certain: The technique was long forgotten, and Paré considered his method of ligation during an amputation to be original and nothing short of divine inspiration. He even designed a predecessor to the modern hemostat, a pinching instrument called the bec de corbin, or "crow's beak," to control bleeding while the vessel was handled.

As with many groundbreaking ideas, Paré's suggestions regarding ligatures were not readily accepted. The reasons given for the slow embrace range from a lack of skilled assistants to help expose blood vessels to the large number of instruments needed to achieve hemostasis—in preindustrial times, surgical tools were hand-made and expensive to produce. The result was that ligatures were not commonly used to control bleeding, especially during an amputation, until other devices were available to provide temporary hemostasis. This did not occur until the early 18th century when Jean-Louis Petit (1674–1750) invented the screw compressor tourniquet. Petit's device placed direct pressure over the main artery of the extremity to be amputated and provided the short-term control of bleeding necessary to allow the accurate placement of ligatures. Throughout the remainder of the 18th and 19th centuries, the use of new types of sutures and tourniquets increased in tandem as surgeons attempted to ligate practically every blood vessel in the body. Nonetheless, despite the abundance of elegant instruments and novel suture materials (ranging from buckskin to horsehair), the satisfactory control of bleeding, especially in delicate surgical operations, remained problematic.

Starting in the 1880s, surgeons began to experiment with electrified devices that could cauterize. These first-generation electrocauteries were ungainly machines, but they did quicken the conduct of a surgical operation. In 1926, Harvey Cushing (1869–1939), professor of surgery at Harvard, experimented with a less cumbersome surgical device that contained two separate electric circuits, one to incise tissue without bleeding and the other simply to coagulate. The apparatus was designed by a physicist, William Bovie (1881–1958), and the two men collaborated to develop interchangeable metal tips, steel points, and wire loops that could be attached to a sterilizable pistol-like grip used to direct the electric current. As the electrical and engineering snags were sorted out, the Bovie electroscalpel became an instrument of trailblazing promise; almost a century later, it remains a fundamental tool in the surgeon's armamentarium.

CONTROL OF PAIN

In the prescientific era, the inability of surgeons to perform pain-free operations was among the most terrifying dilemmas of Medicine. To avoid the horror of the surgeon's merciless knife, patients often refused to undergo a needed surgical operation or repeatedly delayed the event. That is why a scalpel wielder was more concerned about the speed with which he could complete a procedure than the effectiveness of the dissection. Narcotic and soporific agents, such as hashish, mandrake, and opium, had been used for thousands of years, but all were for naught. Nothing provided any semblance of freedom from the misery of a surgical operation. This was among the reasons why the systematic surgical exploration of the abdomen, cranium, joints, and thorax had to wait.

As anatomic knowledge and surgical techniques improved, the search for safe methods to render a patient insensitive to pain became more pressing. By the mid-1830s, nitrous oxide had been discovered, and so-called laughing gas frolics were coming into vogue as young people amused themselves with the pleasant side effects of this compound. After several sniffs, individuals lost their sense of equilibrium, carried on without inhibition, and felt little discomfort as they clumsily knocked into nearby objects. Some physicians and dentists realized that the pain-relieving qualities of nitrous oxide might be applicable to surgical operations and tooth extractions.

A decade later, Horace Wells (1815–1848), a dentist from Connecticut, had fully grasped the concept of using nitrous oxide for inhalational anesthesia. In early 1845, he traveled to Boston to share his findings with a dental colleague, William T.G. Morton (1819–1868), in the hopes that Morton's familiarity with the city's medical elite would lead to a public demonstration of painless tooth-pulling. Morton introduced Wells to John Collins Warren (1778–1856), professor of surgery at Harvard, who invited the latter to show his discovery before a class of medical students, one of whom volunteered to have his tooth extracted. Wells administered the gas and grasped the tooth. Suddenly, the supposedly anesthetized student screamed in pain. An uproar ensued as catcalls and laughter broke out. A disgraced Wells fled the room followed by several bystanders who hollered at him that the entire spectacle was a "humbug affair." For Wells, it was too much to bear. He returned to Hartford and sold his house and dental practice.

However, Morton understood the practical potential of Wells' idea and took up the cause of pain-free surgery. Uncertain about the reliability of nitrous oxide, Morton began to test a compound that one of his medical colleagues, Charles T. Jackson (1805–1880), suggested would work better as an inhalational anesthetic—sulfuric ether. Armed with this advice, Morton studied the properties of the substance while perfecting his inhalational techniques. In fall 1846, Morton was ready to demonstrate the results of his experiments to the world and implored Warren to provide him a public venue. On October 16, with the seats of the operating amphitheater of Massachusetts General Hospital filled to capacity, a tense Morton, having anesthetized a 20-year-old man, turned to Warren and told him that all was ready. The crowd was silent and set their gaze on the surgeon's every move. Warren grabbed a scalpel, made a 3-inch incision, and excised a small vascular tumor on the patient's neck. For 25 minutes, the spectators watched in stunned disbelief as the surgeon performed a painless surgical operation.

Whether the men in the room realized that they had just witnessed one of the most important events in Medical history is unknown. An impressed Warren, however, slowly uttered the five most famous words in American surgery: "Gentlemen, this is no humbug." No one knew what to do or say. Warren turned to his patient and repeatedly asked him whether he felt anything. The answer was a definitive no—no pain, no discomfort, nothing at all. Few medical discoveries have been so readily accepted as inhalational anesthesia. News of the momentous event spread swiftly as a new era in the history of surgery began. Within months, sulfuric ether and another inhalational agent, chloroform, were used in hospitals worldwide.

The acceptance of inhalational anesthesia fostered research on other techniques to achieve pain-free surgery. In 1885, William Halsted (1852–1922) (Fig. 1.4), professor of surgery at the Johns Hopkins Hospital in Baltimore, announced that he had used cocaine and infiltration anesthesia (nerve-blocking) with great success in more than 1000 surgical cases. At the same time, James Corning (1855–1923) of New York carried out the earliest experiments on spinal anesthesia, which were soon expanded on by August Bier (1861–1939) of Germany. By the late 1920s, spinal anesthesia and epidural anesthesia were widely used in the United States and Europe. The next great advance in pain-free surgery occurred in 1934, when the introduction of an intravenous anesthetic agent (sodium thiopental [Sodium Pentothal]) proved tolerable to patients, avoiding the sensitivity of the tracheobronchial tree to anesthetic vapors.

CONTROL OF INFECTION

Anesthesia helped make the potential for surgical cures more seductive. Haste was no longer of prime concern. However, no matter how much the discovery of anesthesia contributed to the relief of pain during surgical operations, the evolution of surgery could not proceed until the problem of postoperative infection was resolved. If ways to deaden pain had never been conceived, a surgical procedure could still be performed, although with much difficulty. Such was not the case with infection. Absent antisepsis and asepsis, surgical procedures were more likely to end in death rather than just pain.

In the rise of modern surgery, several individuals and their contributions stand out as paramount. Joseph Lister (1827–1912) (Fig. 1.5), an English surgeon, belongs on this select list for his efforts to control surgical infection through antisepsis. Lister's research was based on the findings of the French chemist Louis Pasteur (1822–1895), who studied the process of fermentation and showed that it was caused by the growth of living microorganisms. In the mid-1860s, Lister hypothesized that these invisible "germs," or, as they became known, bacteria, were the cause of wound healing difficulties in surgical patients. He proposed that it was feasible to prevent suppuration by applying an antibacterial solution to a wound and covering the site in a dressing saturated with the same germicidal liquid.

Lister was born into a well-to-do Quaker family from London. In 1848, he received his medical degree from University College. Lister was appointed a fellow of the Royal College of Surgeons 4 years later. He shortly moved to Edinburgh, where he became an assistant to James Syme (1799–1870). Their mentor/mentee

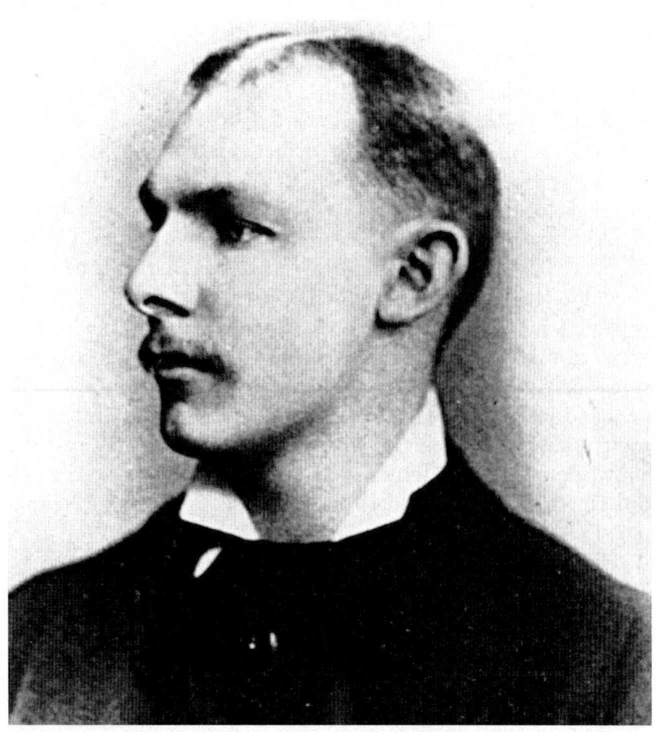

FIG. 1.4 William Halsted (1852–1922).

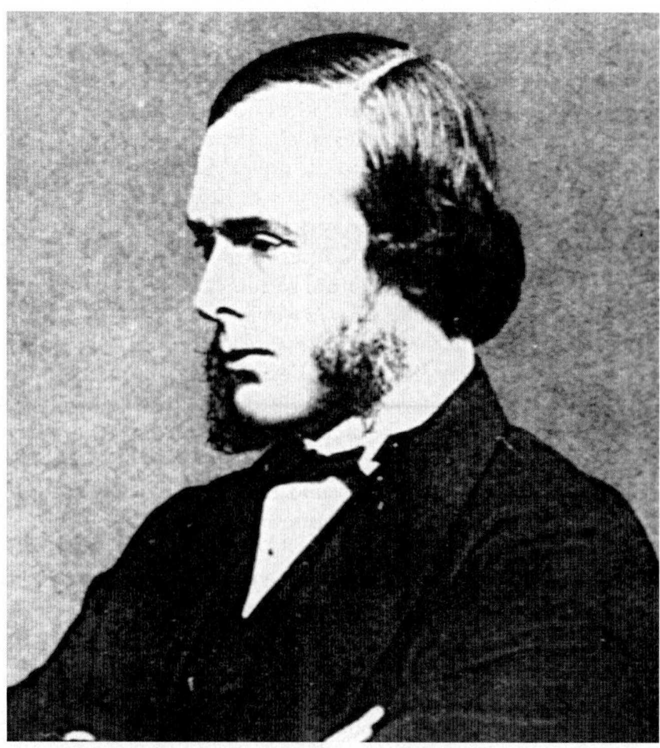

FIG. 1.5 Joseph Lister (1827–1912).

relationship was strengthened when Lister married Syme's daughter Agnes (1835–1896). At the urging of his father-in-law, Lister applied for the position of professor of surgery in Glasgow. The 9 years that he spent there were the most important period in Lister's career as a surgeon-scientist.

In spring 1865, a colleague told Lister about Pasteur's research on fermentation and putrefaction. Lister was one of the few surgeons of his day who, because of his familiarity with the microscope (his father designed the achromatic lens and was one of the founders of modern microscopy), had the ability to understand Pasteur's findings about microorganisms on a first-hand basis. Armed with this knowledge, Lister showed that an injury was already full of bacteria by the time the patient arrived at the hospital.

Lister recognized that the elimination of bacteria by excessive heat could not be applied to a patient. Instead, he turned to chemical antisepsis and, after experimenting with zinc chloride and sulfites, settled on carbolic acid (phenol). By 1866, Lister was instilling pure carbolic acid into wounds and onto dressings and spraying it into the atmosphere around the operative field and table. The following year, he authored a series of papers on his experience in which he explained that pus in a wound (these were the days of "laudable pus," when it was mistakenly believed the more suppuration the better) was not a normal part of the healing process. Lister went on to make numerous modifications in his technique of dressings, manner of applying them, and choice of antiseptic solutions—carbolic acid was eventually abandoned in favor of other germicidal substances. He did not emphasize hand scrubbing but merely dipped his fingers into a solution of phenol and corrosive sublimate. Lister was incorrectly convinced that scrubbing created crevices in the palms of the hands where bacteria would proliferate.

A second major advance by Lister was the development of sterile absorbable sutures. Lister believed that much of the suppuration found in wounds was created by contaminated ligatures. To prevent the problem, Lister devised an absorbable suture impregnated with phenol. Because it was not a permanent ligature, he was able to cut it short, closing the wound tightly and eliminating the necessity of bringing the ends of the suture out through the incision, a surgical practice that had persisted since the days of Paré.

For many reasons, the acceptance of Lister's ideas about infection and antisepsis was an uneven and slow process. First, the various procedural changes that Lister made during the evolution of his method created confusion. Second, listerism, as a technical exercise, was complicated and time-consuming. Third, early attempts by other surgeons to use antisepsis were abject failures. Finally, and most importantly, acceptance of listerism depended on an understanding of the germ theory, a hypothesis that many practical-minded scalpel wielders were loathed to recognize.

As a professional group, German-speaking surgeons were the earliest to grasp the importance of bacteriology and Lister's ideas. In 1875, Richard von Volkmann (1830–1889) and Johann Nussbaum (1829–1890) commented favorably on their treatment of compound fractures with antiseptic methods. In France, Just Lucas-Championière (1843–1913) was not far behind. The following year, Lister traveled to the United States, where he spoke at the International Medical Congress held in Philadelphia and gave additional lectures in Boston and New York. Lister's presentations were memorable, sometimes lasting more than three hours, but American surgeons remained unconvinced about his message. American surgeons did not begin to embrace the principles of antisepsis until the mid-1880s. The same was also true in Lister's home country, where he initially encountered strong opposition led by the renowned gynecologist Lawson Tait (1845–1899).

Over the years, Lister's principles of antisepsis gave way to principles of asepsis, or the complete elimination of bacteria. The concept of asepsis was forcefully advanced by Ernst von Bergmann (1836–1907), professor of surgery in Berlin, who recommended steam sterilization (1886) as the ideal method to eradicate germs. By the mid-1890s, less clumsy antiseptic and aseptic techniques had found their way into most American and European surgical amphitheaters. Any lingering doubts about the validity of Lister's concepts of wound infection were eliminated on the battlefields of World War I. Aseptic technique was virtually impossible to attain on the battlefield, but the invaluable principle of wound treatment by means of surgical debridement and mechanical irrigation with an antiseptic solution was developed by Alexis Carrel (1873–1944) (Fig. 1.6), the Nobel prize-winning French-American surgeon, and Henry Dakin (1880–1952), an English chemist.

Once antiseptic and aseptic techniques had been accepted as routine elements of surgical practice, it was inevitable that other antibacterial rituals would take hold, in particular, the use of caps, hats, masks, drapes, gowns, and rubber gloves. Until the 1870s, surgeons did not use gloves because the concept of bacteria on the hands was not recognized. In addition, no truly functional glove had ever been designed. This situation changed in 1878, when an employee of the India-Rubber Works in Surrey, England, received British and U.S. patents for the manufacture of a surgical glove that had a "delicacy of touch." The identity of the first surgeon who required that flexible rubber gloves be consistently worn for every surgical operation is uncertain. Halsted is regarded as the individual who popularized their use, although the idea of rubber gloves was not fully accepted until the 1920s.

In 1897, Jan Mikulicz-Radecki (1850–1905), a Polish-Austrian surgeon, devised a single-layer gauze mask to be worn during a surgical operation. An assistant modified the mask by placing two layers of cotton-muslin onto a large wire frame to keep the gauze away from the surgeon's lips and nose. This modification was crucial because a German microbiologist showed that bacteria-laden droplets from the mouth and nose enhanced the likelihood of wound infection. Silence in the operating room became a cardinal feature of surgery in the early 20th century. At approximately

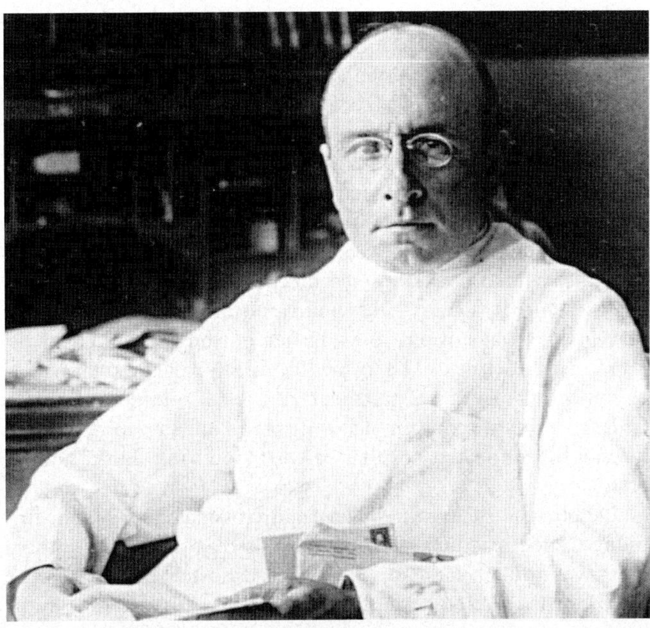

FIG.1.6 Alexis Carrel (1873–1944).

the same time, when it was also determined that masks provided less protection if an individual was bearded, the days of surgeons sporting bushy beards and droopy mustaches went by the wayside.

OTHER ADVANCES THAT FURTHERED THE RISE OF MODERN SURGERY

X-Rays

Most prominent among other advances that furthered the rise of modern surgery was the discovery by Wilhelm Roentgen (1845–1923) of x-rays. He was professor of physics at Würzburg University in Germany, and in late December 1895, he presented to that city's medical society a paper on electromagnetic radiation. Roentgen was investigating the photoluminescence from metallic salts that had been exposed to light when he noticed a greenish glow coming from a screen painted with a phosphorescent substance located on a shelf over 9 feet away. He came to realize there were invisible rays (he termed them *x-rays*) capable of passing through objects made of wood, metal, and other materials. Significantly, these rays also penetrated the soft tissues of the body in such a way that more dense bones were revealed on a specially treated photographic plate. Similar to the discovery of inhalational anesthesia, the importance of x-rays was realized immediately. By March 1896, the first contributions regarding the use of roentgenography in the practice of Medicine in the United States were reported. In short order, numerous applications were developed as surgeons rapidly applied the new finding to the diagnosis and location of dislocations and fractures, the removal of foreign bodies, and the treatment of malignant tumors.

Blood Transfusion

Throughout the late 19th century, there were scattered reports of blood transfusions, including one by Halsted on his sister for postpartum hemorrhage with blood drawn from his own veins. However, it was not until 1901, when Karl Landsteiner (1868–1943), an Austrian physician, discovered the major human blood groups, that blood transfusion became a less risky practice. George Crile (1864–1943), a noted surgeon from Cleveland, performed the first surgical operation during which a blood transfusion was used, and the patient survived 5 years later.

The development of a method to make blood noncoagulable was the final step needed to ensure that transfusions were readily available. This method was developed in the years leading up to World War I when Richard Lewisohn (1875–1962) of New York and others showed that by adding sodium citrate and glucose as an anticoagulant and refrigerating the blood, it could be stored for several days. Once this was known, blood banking became feasible as demonstrated by Geoffrey Keynes (1887–1982), a noted British surgeon (and younger brother of the famed economist John Maynard Keynes), who built a portable cold-storage unit that enabled transfusions to be carried out on the battlefield. In 1937, Bernard Fantus (1874–1940), director of the pharmacology and therapeutics department at Cook County Hospital in Chicago, took the concept of storing blood one step further when he established the first hospital-based "blood bank" in the United States.

Despite the success in storing and crossmatching blood, immune-related reactions persisted. In this regard, another important breakthrough came in 1939, when Landsteiner identified the Rh factor (so named because of its presence in the rhesus monkey). At the same time, Charles Drew (1904–1950) (Fig. 1.7), a surgeon working at Columbia University, showed how blood could be separated into two main components, red blood cells and plasma, and that the plasma could be frozen for long-term storage. His discovery led to the creation of large-scale blood banking, especially for use by the military during World War II. The storing of blood underwent further refinement in the early 1950s when breakable glass bottles were replaced with durable plastic bags.

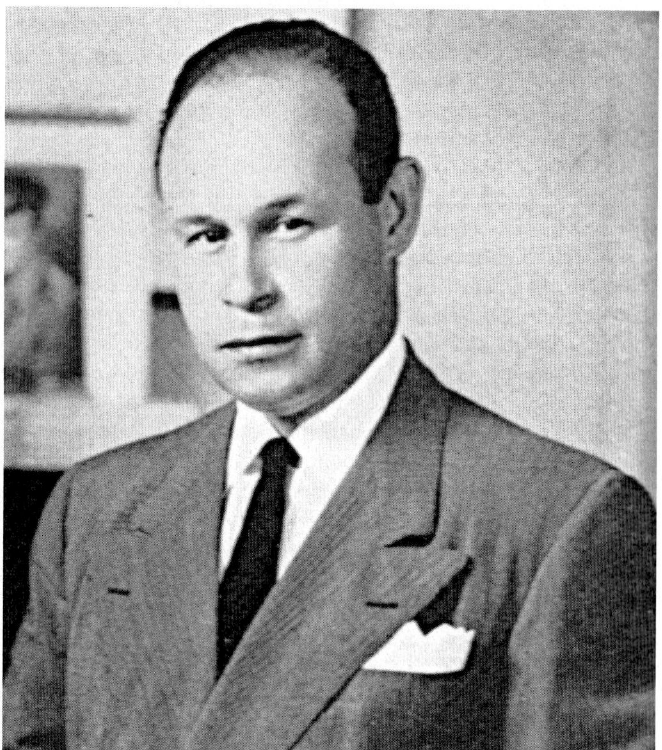

FIG. 1.7 Charles Drew (1904–1950).

Frozen Section

The introduction of anesthesia and asepsis allowed surgeons to perform more technically demanding surgical operations. It also meant that surgeons had to refine their diagnostic capabilities. Among the key additions to their problem-solving skills was the technique of frozen section, an innovation that came to be regarded as one of the benchmarks of scientific surgery. In the late 19th century and early years of the 20th century, "surgical pathology" consisted of little more than a surgeon's knowledge of gross pathology and his ability to recognize lesions on the surface of the body. Similar to the notion of the surgeon-anatomist, the surgeon-pathologist, exemplified by James Paget (1814–1899) of London and the renowned Theodor Billroth (1829–1894) (Fig. 1.8) of Vienna, authored the major textbooks and guided the field.

In 1895, Nicholas Senn (1844–1908), professor of pathology and surgery at Rush Medical College in Chicago, recommended that a "freezing microtome" be used as an aid in diagnosis during a surgical operation. However, the early microtomes were crude devices, and freezing led to unacceptable distortions in cellular morphology. This situation was remedied as more sophisticated methods for hardening tissue evolved, particularly systems devised by Thomas Cullen (1868–1953), a gynecologist at the Johns Hopkins Hospital, and Leonard Wilson (1866–1943), chief of pathology at the Mayo Clinic. During the late 1920s and early 1930s, a time when pathology was receiving recognition as a specialty within Medicine and the influence of the surgeon-pathologist was

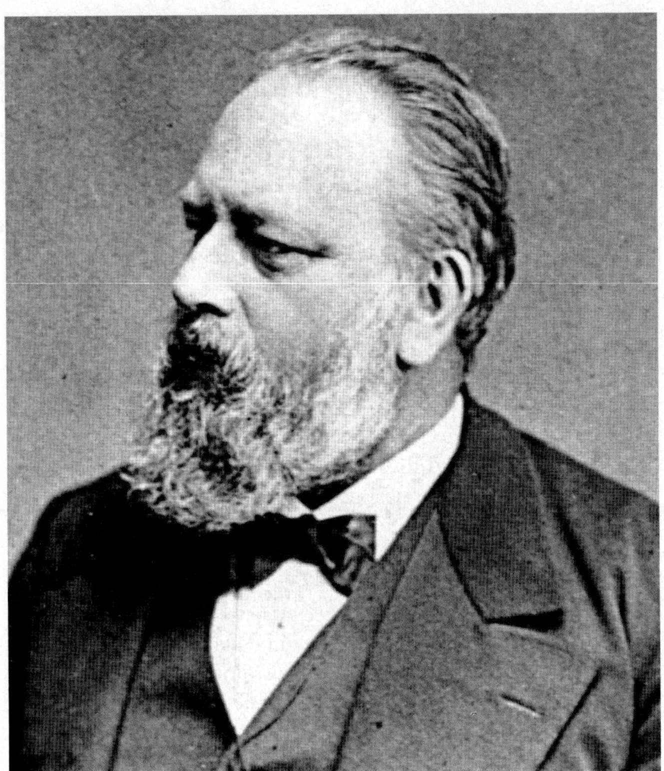

FIG. 1.8 Theodor Billroth (1829–1894).

on the decline, the backing by Joseph Bloodgood (1867–1935), a distinguished surgeon from Baltimore and one of Halsted's earliest trainees, led to the routine use of frozen section during a surgical operation.

ASCENT OF SCIENTIFIC SURGERY

By the first decades of the 20th century, the interactions of politics, science, socioeconomics, and technical advances set the stage for what would become a spectacular showcasing of the progress of surgery. Surgeons wore antiseptic-appearing white caps, gowns, and masks. Patients donned white robes, operating tables were draped in white cloth, and instruments were bathed in white metal basins that contained new and improved antiseptic solutions. All was clean and tidy, with the conduct of the surgical operation no longer a haphazard affair. So great were the innovations that the foundation of basic surgical procedures, including procedures involving the abdomen, cranium, joints, and thorax, was completed by the end of World War I (1918). This transformation was successful not only because surgeons had fundamentally changed, but also because Medicine and its relationship to science had been irrevocably altered. Sectarianism and quackery, the consequences of earlier medical dogmatism, were no longer tenable within the confines of scientific inquiry.

Nonetheless, surgeons retained a lingering sense of professional and social discomfort and continued to be pejoratively described by some physicians as nonthinkers who worked in an inferior manual craft. The result was that scalpel bearers had no choice but to allay the fear and misunderstanding of the surgical unknown of their colleagues and the public by promoting surgical procedures as an acceptable part of the new armamentarium of Medicine. This was not an easy task, particularly because the negative consequences of surgical operations, such as discomfort and complications, were often of more concern to patients than the positive knowledge that devastating disease processes could be thwarted.

It was evident that theoretical concepts, research models, and clinical applications were necessary to demonstrate the scientific basis of surgery. The effort to devise new surgical operations came to rely on experimental surgery and the establishment of surgical research laboratories. In addition, an unimpeachable scientific basis for surgical recommendations, consisting of empirical data collected and analyzed according to nationally and internationally accepted standards and set apart from individual assumptions, had to be developed. Surgeons also needed to demonstrate managerial and organizational unity, while conforming to contemporary cultural and professional norms.

These many challenges involved new administrative initiatives, including the establishment of self-regulatory and licensing bodies. Surgeons showed the seriousness of their intent to be viewed as specialists within the mainstream of Medicine by establishing standardized postgraduate surgical education and training programs and professional societies. In addition, a new type of dedicated surgical literature appeared: specialty journals to disseminate news of surgical research and technical innovations promptly. The result of these measures was that the most consequential achievement of surgeons during the mid-20th century was ensuring the social acceptability of surgery as a legitimate scientific endeavor and the surgical operation as a bona fide therapeutic necessity.

The history of the socioeconomic transformation and professionalization of modern surgery varied from country to country. In Germany, the process of economic and political unification under Prussian dominance presented new and unlimited opportunities for physicians and surgeons, particularly when government officials decreed that more than a simple medical degree was necessary for the right to practice. A remarkable scholastic achievement occurred in the form of the richly endowed state-sponsored university where celebrated professors of surgery administered an impressive array of surgical training programs (other medical disciplines enjoyed the same opportunities). The national achievements of German-speaking surgeons soon became international, and from the 1870s through World War I, German universities were the center of world-recognized surgical excellence.

The demise of the status of Austria-Hungary and Germany as the global leader in surgery occurred with the end of the World War I. The conflict destroyed much of Europe—if not its physical features, then a large measure of its passion for intellectual and scientific pursuits. The result was that a vacuum existed internationally in surgical education, research, and therapeutics. It was only natural that surgeons from the United States, the industrialized nation least affected psychologically and physically by the outcome of the war, would fill this void. So began the ascent of American surgery to its current position of worldwide leadership. Some details about the transformation and professionalization of modern American surgery follow.

Standardized Postgraduate Surgical Education and Training Programs

For the American surgeon of the late 19th century, any attempt at formal learning was a matter of personal will with limited practical opportunities. There were a few so-called teaching hospitals but no full-time academic surgeons. To study surgery in these institutions consisted of assisting surgeons in their daily rounds and observing the performance of surgical operations; there was minimal hands-on operative experience. Little, if any, integration of the basic sciences with surgical diagnosis and treatment took place. In the end, most American surgeons were self-taught and, consequently, not eager to hand down hard-earned and valuable skills to younger men who were certain to become competitors.

Conversely, the German system of surgical education and training brought the basic sciences together with practical clinical teaching coordinated by full-time academicians. There was a competitiveness among the young surgeons-in-training that began in medical school with only the smartest and strongest willed being rewarded. At the completion of an internship, which usually included a stint in a basic science laboratory, the young physician would, if fortunate, be asked to become an assistant to a professor of surgery. At this point, the surgeon-to-be was thrust into the thick of an intense contest to become the first assistant (called the chief resident today). There was no regular advancement from the bottom to the top of the staff, and only a small number ever became the first assistant. The first assistant would hold his position until called to a university's chair of surgery or until he tired of waiting and went into practice. From this labyrinth of education and training programs, great surgeons produced more great surgeons, and these men and their schools of surgery offered Halsted the inspiration and philosophies he needed to establish an American system of education and training in surgery.

Halsted was born into a well-to-do New York family and received the finest educational opportunities possible. He had private elementary school tutors, attended boarding school at Phillips Andover Academy, and graduated from Yale in 1874. Halsted received his medical degree three years later from the College of Physicians and Surgeons in New York (now Columbia University) and went on to serve an 18-month internship at Bellevue Hospital. With the accomplishments of the German-speaking medical world attracting tens of thousands of American physicians to study abroad, Halsted joined the pilgrimage and spent 1878 through 1880 at universities in Berlin, Hamburg, Kiel, Leipzig, Vienna, and Würzburg. He could not help but notice the stark difference between the German and American manner of surgical education and training.

The surgical residency system that Halsted implemented at the Johns Hopkins Hospital in 1889 was a consolidation of the German approach. In his program, the first of its kind in the United States, Halsted insisted on a more clearly defined pattern of organization and division of duties. The residents had a larger volume of operative material at their disposal, a more intimate contact with practical clinical problems, and a graduated concentration of clinical authority and responsibility in themselves rather than the professor. Halsted's aim was to train outstanding surgical teachers, not merely competent operating surgeons. He showed his residents that research based on anatomic, pathologic, and physiologic principles, along with animal experimentation, made it possible to develop sophisticated operative procedures.

Halsted proved to an often leery profession and public that an unambiguous sequence of discovery to implementation could be observed between the experimental research laboratory and the clinical operating room. In so doing, he developed a system of surgery so characteristic that it was termed a "school of surgery." More to the point, Halsted's principles of surgery became a widely acknowledged and accepted scientific imprimatur. More than any other surgeon, it was the aloof and taciturn Halsted who moved surgery from the melodramatics and grime of the 19th century surgical theater to the silence and cleanliness of the 20th century operating room.

Halsted is regarded as "Adam" in American surgery, but he trained only 17 chief residents. The reason for this was that among the defining features of Halsted's program was an indefinite time of tenure for his first assistant. Halsted insisted that just one individual should survive the steep slope of the residency pyramid and only every few years. Of these men, several became professors of surgery at other institutions where they began residency programs of their own, including Harvey Cushing at Harvard, Stephen Watts (1877–1953) at Virginia, George Heuer (1882–1950) and Mont Reid (1889–1943) at Cincinnati, and Roy McClure (1882–1951) at Henry Ford Hospital in Detroit. By the 1920s, there were a dozen or so Halsted-style surgical residencies in the United States. However, the strict pyramidal aspect of the Halsted plan was so self-limiting (i.e., one first assistant/chief resident with an indefinite length of appointment) that in an era when thousands of physicians clamored to be recognized as specialists in surgery, his restrictive style of surgical residency was not widely embraced. For that reason, his day-to-day impact on the number of trained surgeons was less significant than might be thought.

There is no denying that Halsted's triad of educational principles—knowledge of the basic sciences, experimental research, and graduated patient responsibility—became a preeminent and permanent feature of surgical training programs in the United States. However, by the end of World War II, most surgical residencies were organized around the less severe rectangular structure of advancement employed by Edward Churchill (1895–1972) at the Massachusetts General Hospital beginning in the 1930s. This style of surgical education and training was a response to newly established national standards set forth by the American Medical Association (AMA) and the American Board of Surgery.

In 1920, for the first time, the AMA Council on Medical Education published a list of 469 general hospitals with 3000 "approved" internships. The annual updating of this directory became one of the most important and well-publicized activities of the AMA and provided health care planners with their earliest detailed national database. The AMA expanded its involvement in postgraduate education and training 7 years later when it issued a registry of 1700 approved residencies in various medical and surgical specialties, including anesthesia, dermatology, gynecology and obstetrics, medicine, neuropsychiatry, ophthalmology, orthopedics, otolaryngology, pathology, pediatrics, radiology, surgery, tuberculosis, and urology. By this last action, the AMA publicly declared support for the concept of specialization, a key policy decision that profoundly affected the professional future of physicians in the United States and the delivery of health care.

Experimental Surgical Research Laboratories

Halsted believed that experimental research provided residents with opportunities to evaluate surgical problems in an analytic fashion, an educational goal that could not be achieved solely by treating patients. In 1895, he organized an operative course on animals to teach medical students how to handle surgical wounds and use antiseptic and aseptic techniques. The classes were popular, and, several years later, Halsted asked Cushing, who had recently completed his residency at Hopkins and then spent time in Europe sharpening his experimental research skills with the future Nobel laureates Theodor Kocher (1841–1917) (Fig. 1.9) and Charles Sherrington (1857–1952), to assume responsibility for managing the operative surgery course as well as his experimental laboratory.

Cushing, the most renowned of Halsted's assistants, was a graduate of Yale College and Harvard Medical School. He would go

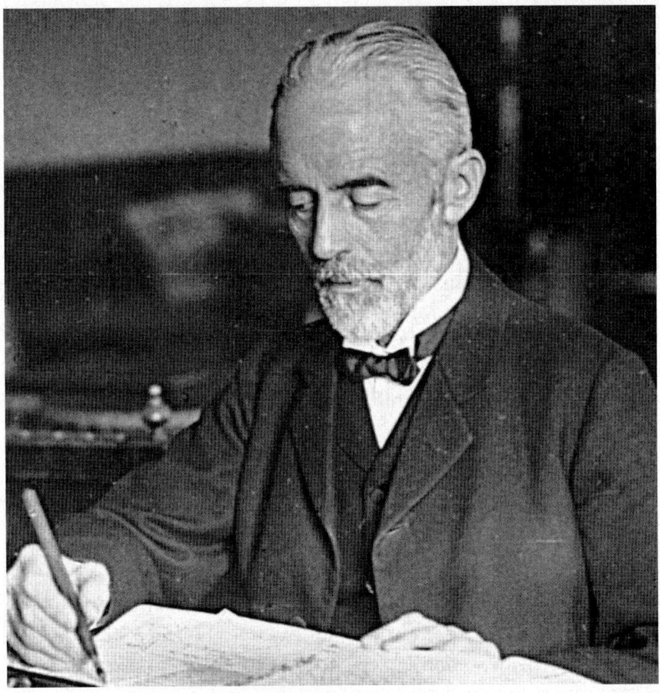

FIG. 1.9 Theodor Kocher (1841–1917).

on to become professor of surgery at Harvard and first surgeon-in-chief of the newly built Peter Bent Brigham Hospital. Cushing's clinical accomplishments are legendary and include describing basophil adenomas of the pituitary gland, discovering the rise in systemic blood pressure that resulted from an increase in intracranial pressure, and devising ether charts for the surgical operating room. Just as impressive are Cushing's many achievements outside the world of medical science, the foremost being a Pulitzer Prize in Biography or Autobiography in 1926 for his two-volume work *Life of Sir William Osler*.

Cushing found the operative surgery classroom space to be limited, and he persuaded university trustees to authorize funds to construct the first animal laboratory for surgical research in the United States, the Hunterian Laboratory of Experimental Medicine, named after the famed Hunter. Halsted demanded the same excellence of performance in his laboratory as in the hospital's operating room, and Cushing assured his mentor that this request would be respected. Similar to Halsted, Cushing was an exacting and demanding taskmaster, and he made certain that the Hunterian, which included indoor and outdoor cages for animals, cordoned-off areas for research projects, and a large central room with multiple operating tables, maintained a rigorous scholarly environment where students learned to think like surgical investigators while acquiring thc basics of surgical technique. As for the residents in Halsted's program, time in the Hunterian became an integral part of their surgical education and training.

Other American surgeons at the turn of the century demonstrated an interest in experimental surgical research (Senn's book, *Experimental Surgery*, the first American book on the subject, was published in 1889, and Crile's renowned treatise, *An Experimental Research into Surgical Shock*, was published in 1899), but their scientific investigations were not conducted in as formal a setting as the Hunterian. Cushing went on to use the Hunterian for his own neurosurgical research and later took the concept of a surgical research laboratory to Boston where, several surgical generations later, Joseph Murray (1919–2012), working alongside the Brigham's

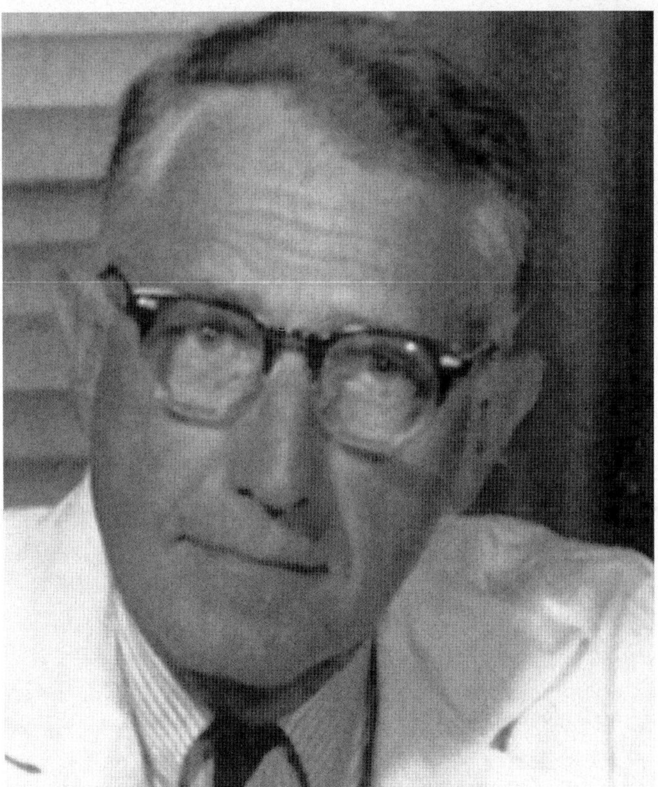

FIG. 1.10 Francis D. Moore (1913–2001).

Moseley Professor of Surgery, Francis D. Moore (1913–2001) (Fig. 1.10), won the 1990 Nobel Prize in Physiology or Medicine for his work on organ and cell transplantation in the treatment of human disease, specifically kidney transplant.

One other American surgeon has been named a Nobel laureate. Charles Huggins (1901–1997) (Fig. 1.11) was born in Canada but graduated from Harvard Medical School and received his surgical training at the University of Michigan. While working at the surgical research laboratory of the University of Chicago, Huggins found that antiandrogenic treatment, consisting of orchiectomy or the administration of estrogens, could produce long-term regression in patients with advanced prostatic cancer. These observations formed the basis for the treatment of malignant tumors by hormonal manipulation and led to his receiving the Nobel Prize in Physiology or Medicine in 1966.

Regarding the long-term influence of the Hunterian, it served as a model that was widely embraced by many university hospital officials and surgical residency directors. Thus began a tradition of experimental research that remains a feature of modern American surgical education and training programs, the results of which continue to be seen and heard at the American College of Surgeons Owen H. Wangensteen Forum on Fundamental Surgical Problems, held during the annual Clinical Congress. Owen H. Wangensteen (1898–1981) (Fig. 1.12) was the long-time professor of surgery at the University of Minnesota where he brought his department to prominence as a center for innovative experimental and clinical surgical research.

Specialty Journals, Textbooks, Monographs, and Treatises

Progress in science brought about an authoritative and rapidly growing body of medical and surgical knowledge. The timely

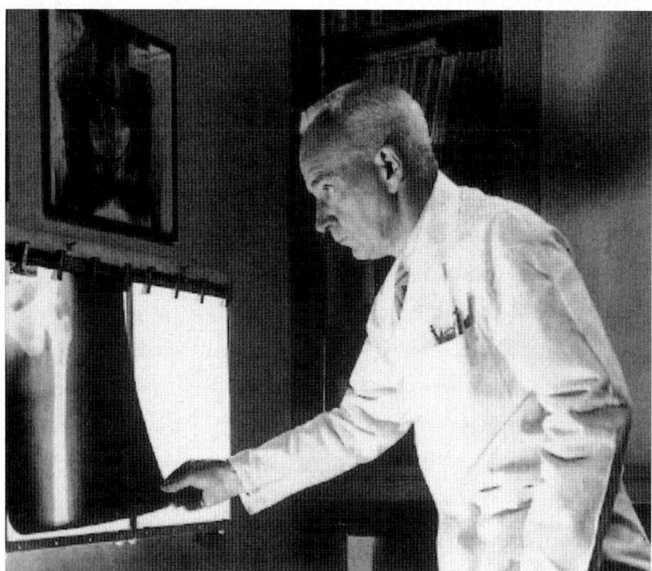

FIG. 1.11 Charles Huggins (1901–1997).

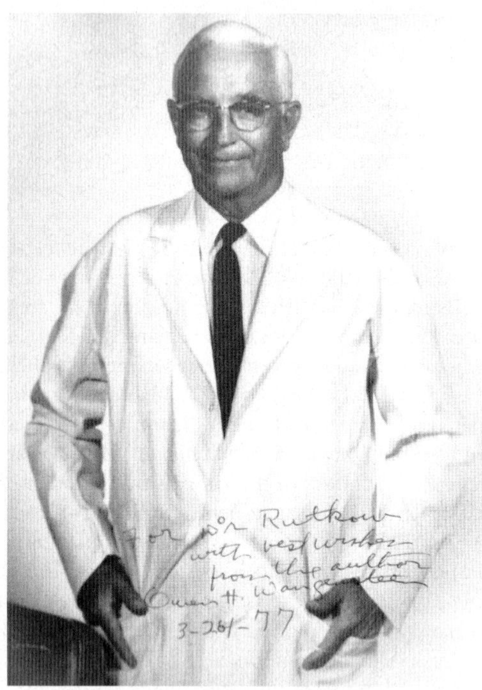

FIG. 1.12 Owen H. Wangensteen (1898–1981).

dissemination of this information into the clinical practice of surgery became dependent on weekly and monthly medical journals. Physicians in the United States proved adept at promoting this new style of journalism, and by the late 1870s, more health-related periodicals were published in the United States than in almost all of Europe. However, most medical magazines were doomed to early failure because of limited budgets and a small number of readers. Despite incorporating the words "Surgery," "Surgical," or "Surgical Sciences" in their masthead, none of these journals treated surgery as a specialty. There were simply not enough physicians who wanted to or could afford to practice surgery around the clock. Physicians were unable to operate with any reasonable anticipation of success, until the mid to late 1880s, and the acceptance of the germ theory and Lister's concepts of antisepsis. Once this occurred, the push toward specialization gathered speed as numbers of surgical operations increased along with a cadre of full-time surgeons.

For surgeons in the United States, the publication of the *Annals of Surgery* in 1885 marked the beginning of a new era, one guided in many ways by the content of the specialty journal. The *Annals* became intimately involved with the advancement of the surgical sciences, and its pages record the story of surgery in the United States more accurately than any other written source. The magazine remains the oldest continuously published periodical in English devoted exclusively to surgery. Other surgical specialty journals soon appeared, and they, along with the published proceedings and transactions of emerging surgical specialty societies, proved crucial in establishing scientific and ethical guidelines for the profession.

As important as periodicals were to the spread of surgical knowledge, American surgeons also communicated their know-how in textbooks, monographs, and treatises. Similar to the rise of the specialty journal, these massive, occasionally multivolume works first appeared in the 1880s. When David Hayes Agnew (1818–1892), professor of surgery at the University of Pennsylvania, wrote his three-volume, 3000-page *Principles and Practice of Surgery,* he was telling the international surgical world that American surgeons had something to say and were willing to stand behind their words. At almost the same time, John Ashhurst (1839–1900), soon-to-be successor to Agnew at the University of Pennsylvania, was organizing his six-volume *International Encyclopedia of Surgery* (1881–1886), which introduced the concept of a multiauthored surgical textbook. The *Encyclopedia* was an instant publishing success and marked the first time that American and European surgeons worked together as contributors to a surgical text. Ashhurst's effort was shortly joined by Keen's *An American Text-Book of Surgery* (1892), which was the first surgical treatise written by various authorities all of whom were American.

These tomes are the forebears of the present book. In 1936, Frederick Christopher (1889–1967), an associate professor of surgery at Northwestern University and chief surgeon to the Evanston Hospital in Evanston, IL, organized a *Textbook of Surgery.* The *Textbook,* which Christopher described as a "cross-sectional presentation of the best in American surgery," quickly became one of the most popular of the surgical primers in the United States. He remained in charge for four more editions and, in 1956, was succeeded by Loyal Davis (1896–1982) (Fig. 1.13), professor of surgery at Northwestern University. Davis, who also held a Ph.D. in the neurologic sciences and had studied with Cushing in Boston, was an indefatigable surgical researcher and prolific author. Not only did he edit the sixth, seventh, eighth, and ninth editions of what became known as *Christopher's Textbook of Surgery,* but from 1938 to 1981, Davis also was editor-in-chief of the renowned journal, *Surgery, Gynecology and Obstetrics.* (In the last years of his life, Davis gained further recognition as the father-in-law of President Ronald Reagan.) In 1972, David Sabiston (1924–2009) (Fig. 1.14), professor of surgery at Duke, assumed editorial control of the renamed *Davis-Christopher Textbook of Surgery.* Sabiston was an innovative vascular and cardiac surgeon who held numerous leadership roles throughout his career, including President of the American College of Surgeons, the American Surgical Association, the Southern Surgical Association, and the American Association for Thoracic Surgery. Not only did Sabiston guide editions 10 through 15 of the *Davis-Christopher Textbook,* but he also served as editor-in-chief of the *Annals of Surgery* for 25 years. Starting in 2000 with the 16th edition, Courtney M. Townsend, Jr. (1943-),

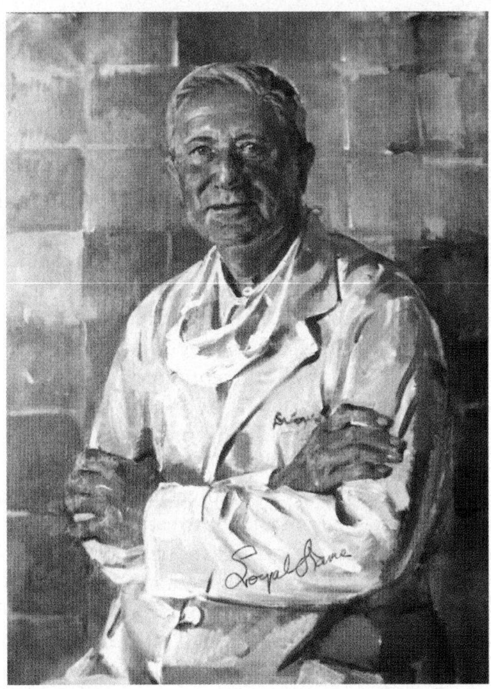
FIG. 1.13 Loyal Davis (1896–1982).

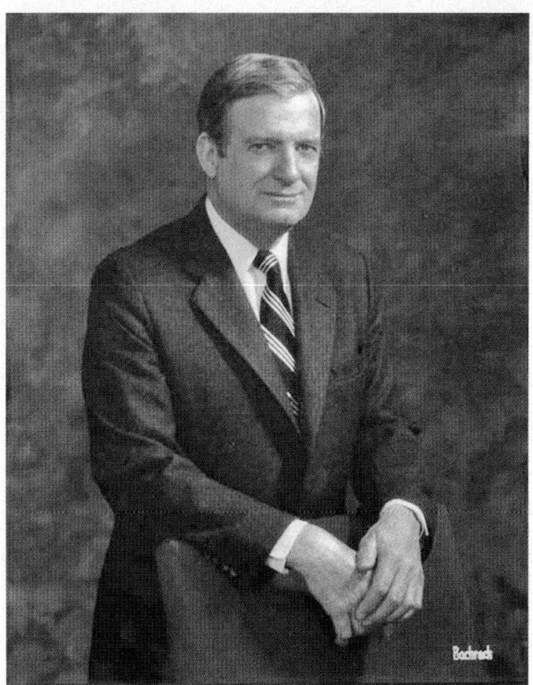
FIG. 1.14 David Sabiston (1924–2009).

professor of surgery at the University of Texas Medical Branch in Galveston, took over editorial responsibility for the retitled *Sabiston Textbook of Surgery: The Biological Basis of Modern Surgical Practice*. He has remained in charge through the current 21st edition, and the now legendary work, which Christopher first organized more than 8 decades ago, holds the record for having been updated more times and being the longest lived of any American surgical textbook.

Professional Societies and Licensing Organizations

By the 1920s, surgery was at a point in American society where it was becoming "professionalized." The ascent of scientific surgery had led to technical expertise that gave rise to specialization. However, competence in the surgical operating room alone was not sufficient to distinguish surgery as a profession. Any discipline that looks to be regarded as a profession must assert exclusive control over the expertise of its members and convince the public that these skills are unique and dependable (i.e., act as a monopoly). For the community at large, the notion of trustworthiness is regarded as a fundamental criterion of professional status. To gain and maintain that trust, the professional group has to have complete jurisdiction over its admission policies and be able to discipline and force the resignation of any associate who does not meet rules of acceptable behavior. In their quest for professionalization and specialization, American surgeons created self-regulating professional societies and licensing organizations during the first half of the 20th century.

Around 1910, conflicts between general practitioners and specialists in surgery reached a fever pitch. As surgical operations became more technically sophisticated, inadequately trained or incompetent physicians cum surgeons were viewed as endangering patients' lives as well as the reputation of surgery as a whole. That year, Abraham Flexner (1866–1959) issued his now famous report that reformed medical education in the United States. Much as Flexner's manifesto left an indelible mark on more progressive and trustworthy medical schooling, the establishment of the American College of Surgeons three years later was meant to impress on general practitioners the limits of their surgical abilities and to show the public that a well-organized group of specialist surgeons could provide dependable and safe operations.

The founding of the American College of Surgeons fundamentally altered the course of surgery in the United States. Patterned after the Royal Colleges of Surgeons of England, Ireland, and Scotland, the American College of Surgeons established professional, ethical, and moral guidelines for every physician who practiced surgery and conferred the designation Fellow of the American College of Surgeons (FACS) on its members. For the first time, there was a national organization that united surgeons by exclusive membership in common educational, socioeconomic, and political causes. Although the American Surgical Association had been founded more than three decades earlier, it was composed of a small group of elite senior surgeons and was not meant to serve as a national lobbying front. There were also regional surgical societies, including the Southern Surgical Association (1887) and the Western Surgical Association (1891), but they had less restrictive membership guidelines than the American College of Surgeons, and their geographic differences never brought about national unity.

Because the integrity of the medical profession is largely assured by the control it exercises over the competency of its members, the question of physician licensing and limits of specialization, whether mandated by the government or by voluntary self-regulation, became one of crucial importance. State governments had begun to establish stricter licensing standards, but their statutes did not adequately delineate generalist from specialist. This lack of rules and regulations for specialty practice was a serious concern. Leaders in Medicine realized that if the discipline did not move to regulate specialists, either federal or state agencies would be forced to fill this role, a situation that few physicians wanted. There was also lay pressure. Patients, increasingly dependent on physicians for scientific-based medical and surgical care, could not determine who was qualified to do what—state licensure only established a minimum standard, and membership in loosely managed professional societies revealed little about competency.

By the end of World War I, most surgical (and medical) specialties had established nationally recognized fraternal organizations, such as the American College of Surgeons. In the case of the American College of Surgeons, although its founders hoped to distinguish full-time surgeons from general practitioners, the organization initially set membership guidelines low in its haste to expand enrollment—10 years after its creation, there were more than 7000 Fellows. The American College of Surgeons emphasized an applicant's ability to perform a surgical operation and was less concerned about the depth of overall medical knowledge that sustained an individual's surgical judgment. Furthermore, membership did not depend on examinations or personal interviews. Despite these flaws, the American College of Surgeons did begin to clarify the concept of a surgical specialist to the public. The sheer presence of the American College of Surgeons implied that full-time surgeons outperformed general practitioners and their part-time approach to surgery, while reinforcing the professional authority and clinical expertise of the surgical specialist.

Even with the presence of organizations such as the American College of Surgeons, without a powerful centralized body to coordinate activities, attempts to regulate the push toward specialization in Medicine progressed in a confused and desultory manner. In response to this haphazard approach as well as mounting external pressures and internal power struggles, specialties began to form their own organizations to determine who was a bona fide specialist. These self-governed and self-regulated groups became known as "boards," and they went about evaluating candidates with written and oral examinations as well as face-to-face interviews.

The first board was created in 1917 for ophthalmology and was followed by boards for otolaryngology (1924), obstetrics and gynecology (1930), pediatrics (1933), psychiatry and neurology (1934), radiology (1934), and pathology (1936). Certification by a board indicated a practitioner's level of expertise; thus the limits of specialization set by the board delineated the clinical boundaries of the specialty. For example, in 1936, practitioners of medicine organized a board to cover the whole of internal medicine. In doing so, the specialty exerted firm control over its budding subspecialties, including cardiology, endocrinology, gastroenterology, hematology, and infectious disease. Surgery took a more difficult and divisive path. Before surgeons were able to establish a board for the overall practice of surgery, surgical subspecialists had organized separate boards in otolaryngology, colon and rectal (1935), ophthalmology, orthopedics (1935), and urology (1935). The presence of these surgical subspecialty boards left an open and troubling question: What was to become of the general surgeon?

In the mid-1930s, a faction of younger general surgeons, led by Evarts Graham (1883–1957), decided to set themselves apart from what they considered the less than exacting admission standards of the American College of Surgeons. Graham was professor of surgery at Washington University in St. Louis and the famed discoverer of cholecystography. He demonstrated the link between cigarettes and cancer and performed the first successful one-stage pneumonectomy (as fate would have it, the chain-smoking Graham died of lung cancer). Graham would go on to dominate the politics of American surgery from the 1930s through the 1950s. For now, Graham and his supporters told the leaders of the American College of Surgeons about their plans to organize a certifying board for general surgeons. Representatives of the American College of Surgeons reluctantly agreed to cooperate, and the American Board of Surgery was organized in 1937.

Despite optimism that the American Board of Surgery could formulate a certification procedure for the whole of surgery, its actual effect was limited. Graham attempted to restrain the surgical subspecialties by brokering a relationship between the American Board of Surgery and the subspecialty boards. It was a futile effort. The surgical subspecialty boards pointed to the educational and financial rewards that their own certification represented as reason enough to remain apart from general surgeons. The American Board of Surgery never gained control of the surgical subspecialties and was unable to establish a governing position within the whole of surgery. To this day, little economic or political commonality exists between general surgery and the various subspecialties. The consequence is a surgical lobby that functions in a divided and inefficient manner.

Although the beginning of board certification was a muddled and contentious process, the establishment of the various boards did bring about important organizational changes to Medicine in the United States. The professional status and clinical authority that board certification afforded helped distinguish branches and sub-branches of Medicine and facilitated the rapid growth of specialization. By 1950, almost 40% of physicians in the United States identified themselves as full-time specialists, and of this group, greater than 50% were board certified. It was not long before hospitals began to require board certification as a qualification for staff membership and admitting privileges.

THE MODERN ERA

The three decades of economic expansion after World War II had a dramatic impact on the scale of surgery, particularly in the United States. Seemingly overnight, Medicine became big business with health care rapidly transformed into society's largest growth industry. Spacious hospital complexes were built that epitomized not only the scientific advancement of the healing arts but also demonstrated the strength of America's postwar boom. Society gave surgical science unprecedented recognition as a prized national asset, noted by the vast expansion of the profession and the extensive distribution of surgeons throughout the United States. Large urban and community hospitals established surgical education and training programs and found it relatively easy to attract residents. Not only would surgeons command the highest salaries, but also Americans were enamored with the drama of the operating room. Television series, movies, novels, and the more than occasional live performance of a heart operation on television beckoned the lay individual.

It was an exciting time for American surgeons, with important advances made in the operating room and the basic science laboratory. This progress followed several celebrated general surgical firsts from the 1930s and 1940s, including work on surgical shock by Alfred Blalock (1899–1964) (Fig. 1.15), the introduction of pancreaticoduodenectomy for cancer of the pancreas by Allen Oldfather Whipple (1881–1963), and decompression of mechanical bowel obstruction by a suction apparatus by Owen Wangensteen. Among the difficulties in identifying the contributions to surgery after World War II is a surfeit of famous names—so much so that it becomes a difficult and invidious task to attempt any rational selection of representative personalities along with their significant writings. This dilemma was remedied in the early 1970s, when the American College of Surgeons and the American Surgical Association jointly sponsored Study on Surgical Services for the United

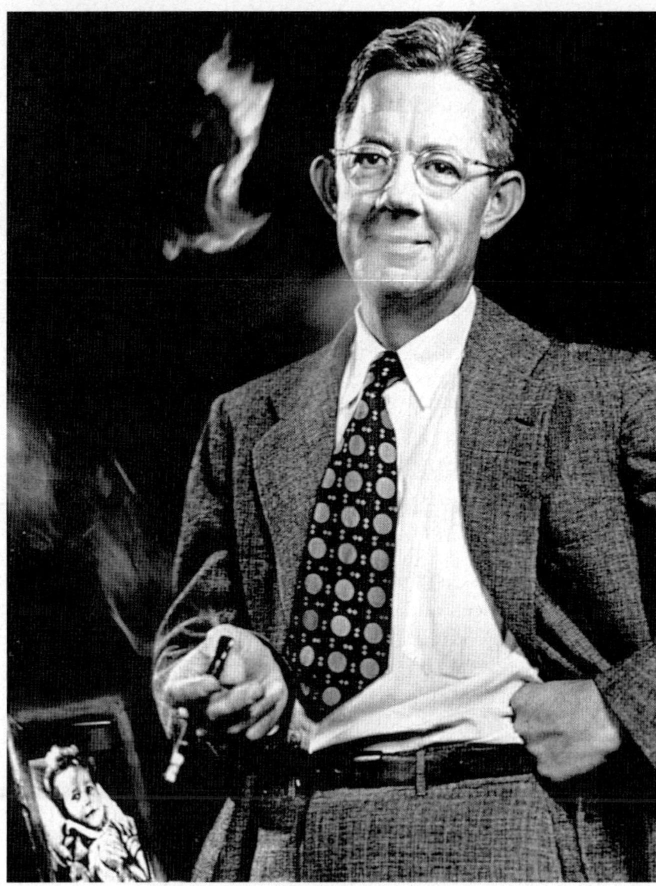

FIG. 1.15 Alfred Blalock (1899–1964).

States (SOSSUS). It was a unique and vast undertaking by the surgical profession to examine itself and its role in the future of health care in the United States. Within the study's three-volume report (1975) is an account from the surgical research subcommittee that named the most important surgical advances in the 1945 to 1970 era.

In this effort, a group of American surgeons from all specialties and academic and private practice attempted to appraise the relative importance of advances in their area of expertise. General surgeons considered kidney transplantation, the replacement of arteries by grafts, intravenous hyperalimentation, hemodialysis, vagotomy and antrectomy for peptic ulcer disease, closed chest resuscitation for cardiac arrest, the effect of hormones on cancer, and topical chemotherapy of burns to be of first-order importance. Of second-order importance were chemotherapy for cancer, identification and treatment of Zollinger-Ellison syndrome, the technique of portacaval shunt, research into the metabolic response to trauma, and endocrine surgery. Colectomy for ulcerative colitis, endarterectomy, the Fogarty balloon catheter, continuous suction drainage of wounds, and development of indwelling intravenous catheters were of third-order importance.

Among the other surgical specialties, research contributions deemed of first-order importance were as follows: Pediatric surgeons chose combined therapy for Wilms tumor; neurosurgeons chose shunts for hydrocephalus, stereotactic surgery and microneurosurgery, and the use of corticosteroids and osmotic diuretics for cerebral edema; orthopedists chose total hip replacement; urologists chose ileal conduits and the use of hormones to treat prostate cancer; otorhinolaryngologists selected surgery for conductive deafness; ophthalmologists selected photocoagulation and retinal surgery; and anesthesiologists selected the development of nonflammable anesthetics, skeletal muscle relaxants, and the use of arterial blood gas and pH measurements.

Additional innovations of second-order and third-order value consisted of the following: Pediatric surgeons chose understanding the pathogenesis and treatment of Hirschsprung disease, the development of abdominal wall prostheses for omphalocele and gastroschisis, and surgery for imperforate anus; plastic surgeons chose silicone and Silastic implants, surgery of cleft lip and palate, and surgery of craniofacial anomalies; neurosurgeons chose percutaneous cordotomy and dorsal column stimulation for treatment of chronic pain and surgery for aneurysms of the brain; orthopedic surgeons chose Harrington rod instrumentation, compression plating, pelvic osteotomy for congenital dislocation of the hip, and synovectomy for rheumatoid arthritis; urologists selected the treatment of vesicoureteral reflux, diagnosis and treatment of renovascular hypertension, and surgery for urinary incontinence; otorhinolaryngologists selected translabyrinthine removal of acoustic neuroma, conservation surgery for laryngeal cancer, nasal septoplasty, and myringotomy and ventilation tube for serous otitis media; ophthalmologists selected fluorescein fundus angiography, intraocular microsurgery, binocular indirect ophthalmoscopy, cryoextraction of lens, corneal transplantation, and the development of contact lenses; and anesthesiologists chose progress in obstetric anesthesia and an understanding of the metabolism of volatile anesthetics.

All these advances were important to the rise of surgery, but the clinical developments that most captivated the public imagination and showcased the brilliance of post–World War II surgery were the growth of cardiac surgery and organ transplantation. Together, these two fields stand as signposts along the new surgical highway. Fascination with the heart goes far beyond that of clinical medicine. From the historical perspective of art, customs, literature, philosophy, religion, and science, the heart has represented the seat of the soul and the wellspring of life itself. Such reverence also meant that this noble organ was long considered a surgical untouchable.

Although suturing of a stab wound to the pericardium in 1893 by Daniel Hale Williams (1856–1931) and successful treatment of an injury that penetrated a cardiac chamber in 1902 by Luther Hill (1862–1946) were significant triumphs, the development of safe cardiothoracic surgery that could be counted on as something other than an occasional event did not occur until the 1940s. During World War II, Dwight Harken (1910–1993) gained extensive battlefield experience in removing bullets and shrapnel in or near the heart and great vessels. Building on his wartime experience, Harken and other pioneering surgeons, including Charles Bailey (1910–1993), expanded intracardiac surgery by developing operations for the relief of mitral valve stenosis. In 1951, Charles Hufnagel (1916–1989), working at Georgetown University Medical Center, designed and inserted the first workable prosthetic heart valve in a man. The following year, Donald Murray (1894–1976) completed the first successful aortic valve homograft.

At approximately the same time, Alfred Blalock, professor of surgery at Johns Hopkins, working with Helen Taussig (1898–1986), a pediatrician, and Vivien Thomas (1910–1985), director of the hospital's surgical research laboratories, developed an operation for the relief of congenital defects of the pulmonary artery. The Blalock-Taussig-Thomas subclavian artery–pulmonary artery shunt for increasing blood flow to the lungs of a "blue baby" proved to be an important event in the rise of modern surgery. Not only was it a pioneering technical accomplishment, but it

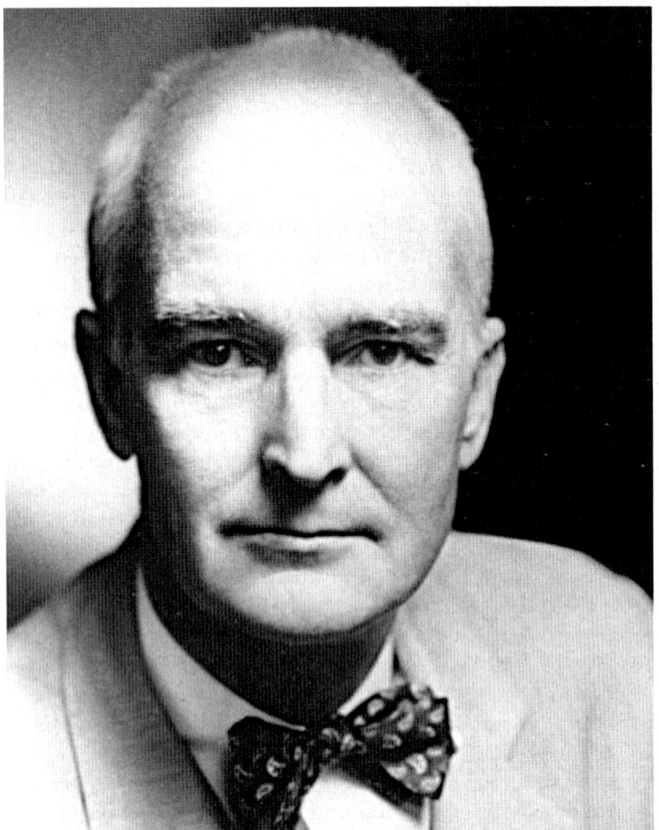

FIG. 1.16 John H. Gibbon, Jr. (1903–1973).

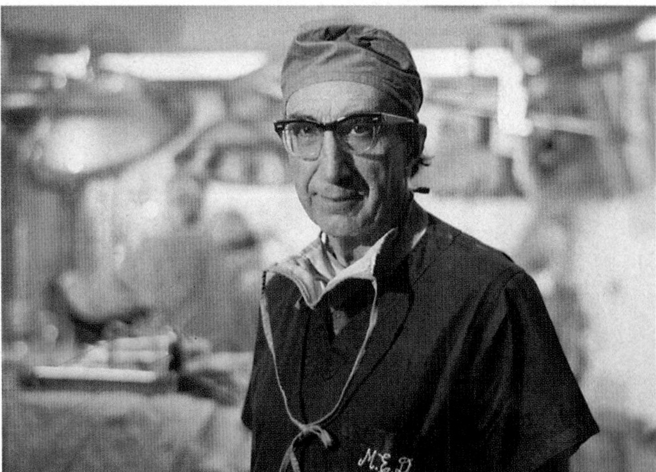

FIG. 1.17 Michael DeBakey (1908–2008).

also managed to give many very ill children a relatively normal existence. The salutary effect of such a surgical feat, particularly its public relations value, on the growth of American surgery cannot be overstated.

Despite mounting successes, surgeons who operated on the heart had to contend not only with the quagmire of blood flowing through the area of dissection but also with the unrelenting to-and-fro motion of a beating heart. Technically complex cardiac repair procedures could not be developed further until these problems were solved. John H. Gibbon, Jr. (1903–1973) (Fig. 1.16), addressed this problem by devising a machine that would take on the work of the heart and lungs while the patient was under anesthesia, in essence pumping oxygen-rich blood through the circulatory system while bypassing the heart so that the organ could be more easily operated on. The first successful open-heart operation in 1953, conducted with the use of a heart-lung machine, was a momentous surgical contribution.

The surgical treatment of coronary artery disease gained momentum during the 1960s, and by 1980, more cardiac operations were completed annually for coronary artery insufficiency than for all other types of cardiac disease. Although the performance of a coronary artery bypass procedure at the Cleveland Clinic in 1967 by René Favaloro (1923–2000) is commonly regarded as the first successful surgical approach to coronary artery disease, Michael DeBakey (1908–2008) (Fig. 1.17) had completed a similar procedure three years earlier but did not report the case until 1973. DeBakey is probably the best-known American surgeon of the modern era. He was a renowned cardiac and vascular surgeon, clinical researcher, medical educator, and international medical statesman as well as the long-time Chancellor of Baylor College of Medicine. He pioneered the use of Dacron grafts to replace or repair blood vessels, invented the roller pump, developed ventricular assist devices, and created an early version of what became the Mobile Army Surgical Hospital (MASH) unit. DeBakey was an influential advisor to the federal government about health care policy and served as chairman of the President's Commission on Heart Disease, Cancer, and Stroke during the Lyndon Johnson administration.

As reported in SOSSUS, when cardiothoracic surgeons were queried about first-order advances in their specialty for the 1945 to 1970 time period, they selected cardiopulmonary bypass, open and closed correction of congenital cardiovascular disease, the development of prosthetic heart valves, and the use of cardiac pacemakers. Of second-order significance was coronary bypass for coronary artery disease.

What about the replacement of damaged or diseased organs? Even in the mid-20th century, the thought of successfully transplanting worn-out or unhealthy body parts verged on scientific fantasy. At the beginning of the 20th century, Alexis Carrel had developed revolutionary new suturing techniques to anastomose the smallest blood vessels. Using his surgical élan on experimental animals, Carrel began to transplant kidneys, hearts, and spleens. His research was a technical success, but some unknown biologic process always led to rejection of the transplanted organ and death of the animal. By the middle of the 20th century, medical researchers began to clarify the presence of underlying defensive immune reactions and the necessity of creating immunosuppression as a method to allow the host to accept the foreign transplant. In the 1950s, using high-powered immunosuppressant drugs and other modern modalities, David Hume (1917–1973), John Merrill (1917–1986), Francis Moore, and Joseph Murray blazed the way with kidney transplants. In 1963, the first human liver transplant occurred; four years later, Christiaan Barnard (1922–2001) successfully completed a human heart transplant.

DIVERSITY

The evolution of surgery has been influenced by ethnic, gender, racial, and religious bias. Every segment of society is affected by such discrimination, particularly African Americans, women, and certain immigrant groups, who were victims of injustices that forced them into struggles to attain competency in surgery. In the 1930s, Arthur Dean Bevan (1861–1943), professor of surgery at Rush Medical College and an important voice in American surgery, urged that restrictive measures be taken against individuals with Jewish-sounding surnames to decrease their presence in Medicine. It would be historically wrong to deny the long-whispered belief held by the Jewish medical community that anti-Semitism was particularly rife in general surgery before the 1950s compared with the other surgical specialties.

In 1868, a department of surgery was established at Howard University. However, the first three chairmen all were white Anglo-Saxon Protestants. Not until 1928, when Austin Curtis (1868–1939) was appointed professor of surgery, did the department have its first African American head. Similar to all black physicians of his era, Curtis was forced to train at a so-called Negro hospital, Provident Hospital in Chicago, where he came under the tutelage of Daniel Hale Williams, the most influential and highly regarded of that era's African American surgeons.

With little likelihood of obtaining membership in the AMA or its related societies, African American physicians joined together in 1895 to form the National Medical Association. Black surgeons identified an even more specific need when the Surgical Section of the National Medical Association was created in 1906. From its start, the Surgical Section held "hands-on" surgical clinics, which represented the earliest example of organized, so-called "show me" surgical education in the United States. When Williams was named a Fellow of the American College of Surgeons in 1913, the news spread rapidly throughout the African American surgical community. Still, applications of African American surgeons for the American College of Surgeons were often acted on slowly, which suggests that denials based on race were clandestinely conducted throughout much of the United States.

In the mid-1940s, Charles Drew, chairman of the Department of Surgery at Howard University School of Medicine, acknowledged that he refused to accept membership in the American College of Surgeons because this supposedly representative surgical society had, in his opinion, not yet begun to accept routinely capable and well-qualified African American surgeons. Strides toward more racial equality within the profession have been taken since that time, as noted in the career of Claude H. Organ, Jr. (1926–2005) (Fig. 1.18), a distinguished editor, educator, and historian. Among his books, the two-volume *A Century of Black Surgeons: The U.S.A. Experience* and the authoritative *Noteworthy Publications by African-American Surgeons* underscored the numerous contributions made by African American surgeons to the U.S. health care system. In addition, as the long-standing editor-in-chief of the *Archives of Surgery* as well as serving as president of the American College of Surgeons and chairman of the American Board of Surgery, Organ wielded enormous influence over the direction of American surgery.

One of the many overlooked areas of surgical history concerns the involvement of women. Until more recent times, options for women to obtain advanced surgical training were severely restricted. The major reason was that through the mid-20th century, only a handful of women had performed enough operative surgery to become skilled mentors. Without role models and with limited access to hospital positions, the ability of the few practicing female physicians to specialize in surgery seemed an impossibility. Consequently, women surgeons were forced to use different career strategies than men and to have more divergent goals of personal success to achieve professional satisfaction.

Through it all and with the aid of several enlightened male surgeons, most notably William Williams Keen of Philadelphia and William Byford (1817–1890) of Chicago, a small cadre of female surgeons did exist in turn-of-the-century America, including

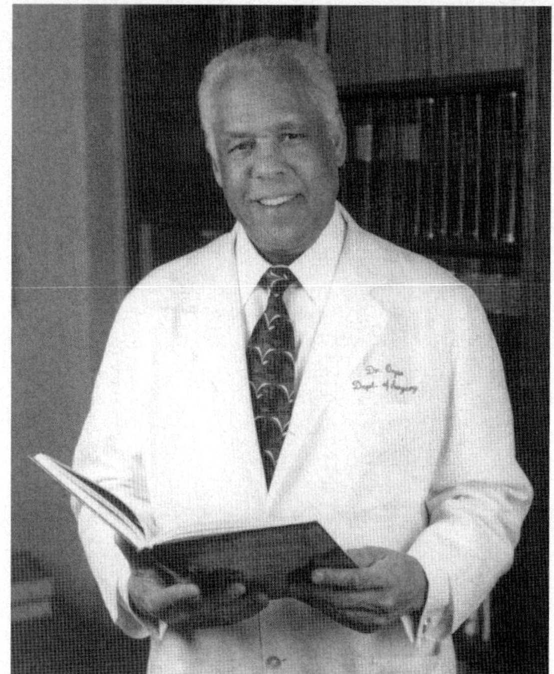

FIG. 1.18 Claude H. Organ, Jr. (1926–2005).

Mary Dixon Jones (1828–1908), Emmeline Horton Cleveland (1829–1878), Mary Harris Thompson (1829–1895), Anna Elizabeth Broomall (1847–1931), and Marie Mergler (1851–1901). The move toward full gender equality is seen in the role that Olga Jonasson (1934–2006) (Fig. 1.19), a pioneer in clinical transplantation, played in encouraging women to enter the modern, male-dominated world of surgery. In 1987, when she was named chair of the Department of Surgery at Ohio State University College of Medicine, Jonasson became the first woman in the United States to head an academic surgery department at a coeducational medical school.

THE FUTURE

History is easiest to write and understand when the principal story has already finished. However, surgery continues to evolve. As a result, drawing neat and tidy conclusions about the future of the profession is a difficult task fraught with ill-conceived conclusions and incomplete answers. Nonetheless, several millennia of history provide plentiful insights on where surgery has been and where it might be going.

Throughout its rise, the practice of surgery has been largely defined by its tools and the manual aspects of the craft. The last decades of the 20th century and beginning years of the 21st century saw unprecedented progress in the development of new instrumentation and imaging techniques. Advancement will assuredly continue; if the study of surgical history offers any lesson, it is that progress can always be expected, at least relative to technology. There will be more sophisticated surgical operations with better results. Automation will robotize the surgeon's hand for certain procedures. Still, the surgical sciences will always retain their historical roots as, fundamentally, a manually based art and craft.

Despite the many advances, these refinements have not come without noticeable social, economic, and political costs. These dilemmas frequently overshadow clinical triumphs, and this suggests that going forward, the most difficult challenges of surgeons may

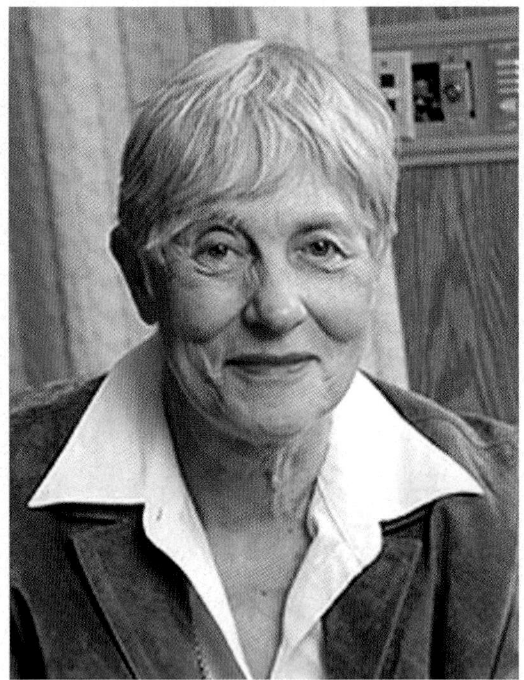

FIG. 1.19 Olga Jonasson (1934–2006).

not be in the clinical realm but, instead, in better understanding the sociologic forces that affect the practice of surgery. The most recent years can be seen as the beginnings of a schizophrenic existence for surgeons in that newly devised complex and lifesaving operations are met with innumerable accolades, whereas criticism of the economics of surgery portrays the surgeon as a financially driven selfish individual.

Although they are philosophically inconsistent, the very dramatic and theatrical features of surgery, which make surgeons heroes from one perspective and symbols of mendacity and greed from the opposite point of view, are the very reasons why society demands so much of surgeons. There is the precise and definitive nature of surgical intervention, the expectation of success that surrounds every operation, the short time frame in which outcomes are realized, the high income levels of most surgeons, and the insatiable inquisitiveness of lay individuals about every aspect of consensually cutting into another human's flesh. These phenomena, ever more sensitized in this age of mass media and instantaneous communication, make surgeons seem more accountable than their medical colleagues and, simultaneously, symbolic of the best and worst in Medicine. In ways that were previously unimaginable, this vast economic, political, and social transformation of surgery controls the fate of the individual surgeon to a much greater extent than surgeons as a collective force can manage through their own profession.

National political aims have become overwhelming factors in securing and shepherding the future growth of surgery. Modern surgery is an arena of tradeoffs, a balance between costs, organization, technical advances, and expectations. Patients will be forced to confront the reality that no matter how advanced surgery becomes, it cannot solve all the health-related problems in life. Society will need to come to terms with where the ethical lines should be drawn on everything from face transplants to robotized surgery to gene therapy for surgical diseases. The ultimate question remains: How can the advance of science, technology, and ethics be brought together in the gray area between private and public good?

Studying the fascinating history of our profession, with its many magnificent personalities and outstanding scientific achievements, may not help us predict the future of surgery. Recall Theodor Billroth's remark at the end of the 19th century, "A surgeon who tries to suture a heart wound deserves to lose the esteem of his colleagues." The surgical crystal ball is a cloudy one at best. However, to understand our past does shed some light on current and future clinical practices. Still, if history teaches us anything, it is that surgery will advance and grow inexorably. If surgeons in the future wish to be regarded as more than mere technicians, members of the profession need to appreciate the value of its past glories better. Study our history. Understand our past. Do not allow the rich heritage of surgery to be forgotten.

SELECTED REFERENCES

Bishop WJ. *The Early History of Surgery*. London: Robert Hale; 1960.

Bishop, a distinguished medical bibliophile, describes surgery from the Middle Ages through the 18th century.

Cartwright FF. *The Development of Modern Surgery From 1830*. London: Arthur Barker; 1967.

An anesthetist at King's College Hospital in London, Cartwright's book is rich in detail and interpretation.

Earle AS. *Surgery in America: From the Colonial Era to the Twentieth Century*. New York, NY: Praeger; 1983.

A fascinating compilation of journal articles by well-known surgeons that trace the development of surgery in America.

Ellis H. *A History of Surgery*. London: Greenwich Medical; 2001.

Ellis is one of modern day's most prominent surgeon/historians. Renowned for his elegant prose, this book educates and entertains the reader.

Hollingham R. *Blood and Guts, a History of Surgery*. New York, NY: Thomas Dunne; 2008.

Hollingham is a science journalist who weaves a compelling narrative of the key moments in surgical history.

Hurwitz A, Degenshein GA. *Milestones in Modern Surgery*. New York, NY: Hoeber-Harper; 1958.

The numerous chapters contain a short biography and a reprinted or translated excerpt of each surgeon's most important clinical contribution.

Lawrence C, ed. *Medical Theory, Surgical Practice: Studies in the History of Surgery*. London: Routledge; 1992.

This short book looks critically at orthodox surgical history and discusses how the act of surgery became increasingly possible from the mid-17th century onward.

Leonardo RA. *History of Surgery*. New York, NY: Froben; 1943.

Leonardo RA. *Lives of Master Surgeons.* New York, NY: Froben; 1948.

Leonardo RA. *Lives of Master Surgeons*; supplement 1. New York, NY: Froben; 1949.

These texts by the eminent Rochester, New York, surgeon and historian provide an in-depth description of the whole of surgery, from ancient times to the mid-20th century. Especially valuable are the countless biographies of famous and near-famous scalpel bearers.

Meade RH. *An Introduction to the History of General Surgery.* Philadelphia, PA: WB Saunders; 1968.

Meade, an indefatigable researcher of historical topics, proacticed surgery in Grand Rapids, Michigan. With an extensive bibliography, this book is among the most ambitious of such systematic works.

Nuland SB. *Doctors, The Biography of Medicine.* New York, NY: Knopf; 1988.

Nuland, a general surgeon, was the author of "How We Die: Reflections on Life's Final Chapter," winner of the 1994 National Book Award for Nonfiction. "Doctors" is the fascinating story of the development of modern medicine but with a slant towards the surgical side.

Porter R. *The Greatest Benefit to Mankind, A Medical History of Humanity.* New York, NY: WW Norton; 1997.

A wonderful literary tour de force by one of the most erudite and entertaining of modern medical historians. Although more a history of the whole of medicine than of surgery, this text has become an instantaneous classic and should be required reading for all physicians and surgeons.

Ravitch MM. *A Century of Surgery: 1880–1980, the History of the American Surgical Association.* Philadelphia, PA: JB Lippincott; 1981.

Ravitch's text provides a year-by-year account of the meetings of the American Surgical Association, once the most influential of America's surgical organizations.

Richardson R. *The Story of Surgery: An Historical Commentary. Shrewsbury.* London, GB: Quiller Press; 2004.

An absorbing account of surgical triumphs written by a physician turned medical historian.

Rutkow IM. *The History of Surgery in The United States, 1775–1900.* San Francisco, CA: Norman Publishing; 1988. 1992.

Rutkow IM. *Surgery, An Illustrated History.* St. Louis, MO: Mosby–Year Book; 1993.

Rutkow IM. *American Surgery, An Illustrated History.* Philadelphia, PA: Lippincott-Raven; 1998.

Rutkow IM. *Bleeding Blue and Gray: Civil War Surgery and The Evolution of American Medicine.* New York, NY: Random House; 2005.

Rutkow IM. *Seeking The Cure: A History of Medicine in America.* New York, NY: Scribner; 2010.

Using biographic compilations, colored illustrations, and detailed narratives, these books explore the evolution of surgery, internationally and in the United States.

Schlich T, ed. *The Palgrave Handbook of the History of Surgery.* London, GB: Palgrave; 2018.

An important and scholarly work that covers the cultural, social, and technical history of surgery with special attention to the established historiography.

Thorwald J. *The Century of The Surgeon.* New York, NY: Pantheon; 1956.

Thorwald J. *The Triumph of Surgery.* New York, NY: Pantheon; 1960.

In a most dramatic literary fashion, Thorwald uses a fictional eyewitness narrator to create continuity in the story of the development of surgery during its most important decades of growth, the late 19th and early 20th centuries.

Van de Laar A. *Under The Knife: A History of Surgery In 28 Remarkable Operations.* New York, NY: St.: Martin's Press; 2018.

Van de Laar, a surgeon, provides a deft and incisive look into the history of his profession.

Wangensteen OH, Wangensteen SD. *The Rise of Surgery, From Empiric Craft to Scientific Discipline.* Minneapolis, MN: University of Minnesota Press; 1978.

Not a systematic history but an assessment of various operative techniques and technical achievements that contributed to or retarded the evolution of surgery. Wangensteen was a noted professor of experimental and clinical surgery at the University of Minnesota; his wife was an esteemed medical historian.

Young A. *Scalpel, Men Who Made Surgery.* New York, NY: Random House; 1956.

This easy-to-read book tells surgery's story through the lives of the men who brought about advances in surgical knowledge, specifically, the control of hemorrhage, the control of pain, the control of infection, and the control of shock.

Zimmerman LM, Veith I. *Great Ideas in the History of Surgery.* Baltimore, MD: Williams & Wilkins; 1961.

A unique book that provides well-written biographic narratives to accompany numerous readings and translations from the works of almost fifty renowned surgeons of varying eras.

2 CHAPTER

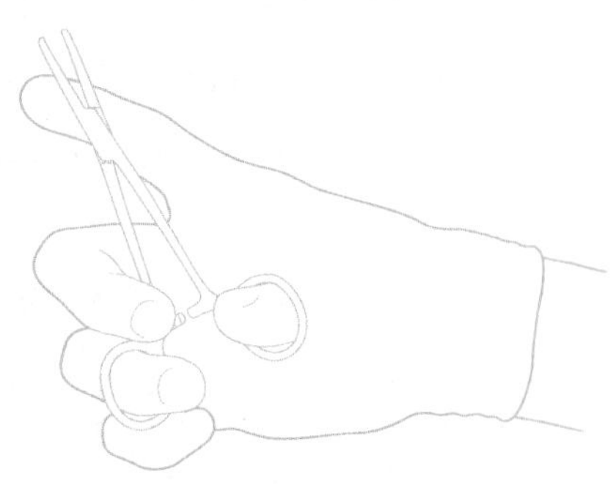

Ethics and Professionalism in Surgery

Jeffrey S. Farroni, William J. Winslade

OUTLINE

"The intimacy between patient and surgeon is short-lived, but closer than between a son and his own father."

Aleksandr Solzhenitsyn, **Cancer Ward**

The privilege of opening the body of another to manipulate, remove, repair, or implant is a profound endeavor for both the surgeon and patient. The medical team viscerally bears witness to parts of the body the patient never sees. The surgeon's practice, a culmination of extensive technical training, skill, and technology, renders the patient better off for the experience of being pierced, cut, and violated. High expectations and responsibilities are imposed upon the surgeon due, in part, to the rich history and current elevation in social standing of medical practice. Physician and author Brian Goldman analogizes these expectations to baseball. While referring to a legendary hitter as one with a batting average of 0.400, he poses the question: "What do you think a batting average for a cardiac surgeon or a nurse practitioner or an orthopedic surgeon, an OBGYN, or a paramedic is supposed to be?"[1] The purpose of his inquiry is to highlight the high expectations of perfection; of batting 1.000. Patients do not want to be the exception, the mistake, or the error.

These pressures are not new, in fact, accountability in medical practice has existed since the dawn of recorded history. The ~4,200 year-old Persian Code of Hammurabi includes schedules of income-based payment and penalties for unsuccessful treatments.[2] Documents from the Ottoman Empire in the sixteenth and seventeenth centuries indicate expectations for treatment, fees, and provision of postoperative care.[3,4] Threads that connect ancient wisdom and modern practice include trust, vulnerability, and responsibility. Values such as elevating the patient's benefit above one's own interest, fidelity to one's profession, and commitment to training echo through time, from the Hippocratic Oath to codification into professional standards such as the American College of Surgeons' Code of Professional Conduct. In the latter, more contemporary notions of disclosure and informed consent arise.[5] Entering the surgical profession means that one becomes part of its history, participates in its value-laden decisions that profoundly impacts people's lives, and contributes to its future innovation. Medicine is as much a moral endeavor as it is a technical one and, as such, we need to reflect upon ways to analyze ethical dilemmas during the course of practice.

ETHICAL FRAMEWORKS

The focus on ethical issues and moral ambiguity in healthcare is due to the increase in technology, our ability to keep bodies alive, and the need to have a reflective and systematic way for us to navigate these dilemmas. One of the most popular conceptions of clinical ethics is that practice should be guided by principles (i.e., autonomy, beneficence/nonmaleficence, and justice).[6] These terms have become familiar to many clinicians and provide a foundational framework to consider when contemplating appropriate medical care. An example of honoring a patient's autonomy is through the informed consent process by which the team bears the responsibility to provide sufficient information on treatment (or research) options so that the patient himself/herself can decide what is best for him/her based upon his/her values, preferences, and goals. Autonomy, or right to self-determination, is often recognized as a dominant principle in Western culture. However, we must appreciate that we live in an increasingly mobile and diverse global community. Sensitivity to cultural practices and traditions may require us to not necessarily place the individual at the center of concern. While striving for proficiency in cultural competence is a worthwhile endeavor, we cannot not forget to engage with the individual.[7] Having direct conversations and inviting the patient to indicate how best they wish to be informed is a good way to ensure their autonomy is respected.

Beneficence and nonmaleficence are often contemplated together in the form of balancing the provision of benefit with mitigating risks/harms to the patient. The Hippocratic notion of *primum non nocere* is often invoked as a maxim to convey our commitment to the care and healing of the patient. Clinical risk:benefit analyses should be contextualized to the patient's goals of care (e.g., the therapeutic options that may offer the "best" clinical outcomes may not be what the patient prefers based upon other considerations).

The final principle is justice, or fairness. We typically think of justice in terms of equitable access to care, even distribution of health benefits and outcomes across society, and nondiscriminatory treatment.[8] At a patient level, an appeal to justice would have the individual practitioner not succumb to the judgments of social worth, to consciously or unconsciously impose stigma based upon race, gender, socioeconomic, mental health status, addiction, country of origin, etc. Taken together, the principles of autonomy, beneficence, nonmaleficence, and justice are the foundational elements by which we view ethical issues.

TABLE 2.1 Examples of moral frameworks.

MORAL FRAMEWORK	GUIDING PRINCIPLES
Consequentialism	**Results of Action**
Utilitarian	Maximize the good with the least harm
Common good	Maximize the good of the whole; mindful of the vulnerable
Nonconsequentialism	**Intentions of the Agents**
Duty-based	Moral obligations are binding irrespective of consequences; the categorical imperative
Rights	The best action is the one that protects the rights of those affected by the action
Fairness	Social contract, equity
Agent-Centered	**Overall Status of the Individual**
Virtue	Good ethical decision-making is based upon good character
Feminist	Particularly focused on gender-related oppression and the perspectives of the vulnerable and marginalized; ethics of care

However, principlism is only one framework within which we can analyze ethical questions in medicine. There are a number of moral traditions one may employ to broaden and enrich reflection on an ethical dilemma. Changing one's perspective can provide different insights into the resolution of a quandary whether it be from the character of each agent (virtue), the act or duty (deontology), or the results (consequentialism) (see Table 2.1). Each framework will have its utility and caveats, but deeper reflection may provide a more robust understanding of the issue at hand. Some have argued ethical inquiry should be "a synthesis of theory and experience, reason and emotion, and philosophy and rhetoric."[9] What we may strive for is "getting beyond an overreliance upon a single approach…to remind us that ethical problems do not simply have a logic—they have a history; they have narrative meaning; and they occur within a social and cultural context."[10]

With respect to qualities of character, renowned physician bioethicist, Edmond Pellegrino, indicated that essential virtues of medical practice include fidelity to trust, suppression of self-interest, intellectual honesty, compassion, courage, and prudence.[11] The recognition of qualities that are inherent to the practice of medicine underscores the privileged space by which the physician is allowed to enter and the responsibility bestowed upon them.[12]

Another mechanism for ethical inquiry is casuistry or case-based analysis. In this method, one would attempt to derive principles from previously resolved cases and apply them to the issues or conflicts at hand.[13,14] Problems may arise when attempting to abstract grand notions from a single or handful of instances; however, an advantage of a casuistic approach is that it is steeped in clinical reality, which may offer concrete, pragmatic solutions to ethical dilemmas.[14] Whichever moral framework resonates with the physician, it can be helpful to have a general approach to ethical dilemmas which encourages practical thinking and reflection.

A GENERAL APPROACH FOR ETHICAL ISSUE RESOLUTION

1. ***Recognizing a Need for Ethical Inquiry***

We are constantly making judgments, often unconsciously, ranging from the mundane, for example, deciding what to eat for lunch, to the life-changing, for example, what treatment modality am I going to recommend to my patient? The foundation of our practice is built upon judgement through training, knowledge, and experience as well as our own agency, values, and principles. Most of the time we do not even think about the ethical milieu that underpins our actions; for example, the patient comes to you with a problem, you offer a solution, the patient agrees, and hopefully all goes well. However, there are times when real conflicts arise and it may be unclear as to the preferred course of action, where technical training or experience fails to provide a concrete solution to an issue. Examples include when to consider the transition from curative intervention to palliative, encountering a colleague whose ability/judgment appears compromised, or a patient, who by your estimation, is making decisions that seem irrational or imprudent. These are all situations in which uncertainty can impose significant moral distress.

It may seem an obvious point, but the initial step in analyzing an ethical dilemma is the recognition that there exists value conflict or moral ambiguity either in the patient's care, within/between the care team(s), or in the organization/operation of the health care facility. The next step is to then take action in gathering the necessary information to resolve the issue.

2. ***Collecting Significant Facts and Understanding the Perspectives of Relevant Stakeholders***

One useful, and most commonly used, tool to collect relevant information to analyze an ethical dilemma is the four topics method, which captures information within the domains of medical indications, patient preferences, quality-of-life factors, and contextual features (Table 2.2).[15] Sometimes we may focus on the clinical disposition of the patient when there are other externalities that may be impacting the patient's decision-making process. What we may identify as the clear medical recommendation may not be greeted with enthusiasm by the patient due to other circumstances. A conversation with the patient that delves into illuminating their values, preferences, motivations, etc. may reveal key insights that will aid in facilitating a solution to the dilemma. The four topics method includes prompts to consider within each domain that may evoke pertinent information. It is important to speak with all relevant parties involved in the dilemma, including other team members, other services, and significant family and loved ones, if appropriate. Reflecting upon a diversity of perspectives and opinions is a thorough approach to complex, value-laden issues.

3. ***Identify the Ethical Issues/Values at Conflict***

After pertinent information has been gathered, the next step is to identify which principles or values may be in conflict. The four topics method mentioned above maps each category of information to the ethical principles. Itemizing conflicting principles or competing obligations/duties will help formulate a spectrum of ethically appropriate options. Those options can then be prioritized into those that are ethically obligatory, ethically permissible, and ethically prohibitive. For example, abandoning the patient would clearly be ethically prohibitive, and ensuring the patient's voice is heard or not denying basic care and hygiene would be things that are ethically obligatory. Often, the challenge is selecting options that are ethically permissible as there may be disagreement as to which option(s) is(are) the "right" one(s) with which to move forward.

4. ***Discuss Options and Develop a Plan***

Emerging from the previous step with a selected set of options, stakeholders are reengaged when the plan to move forward is realized. Generally, it would be advisable for the team to be on the

TABLE 2.2 The four topics commonly used to analyze ethical dilemmas in health care.

TOPIC	ETHICAL PRINCIPLE(S)	CONSIDERATIONS
Medical Indications	Beneficence Nonmaleficence	• What is the patient's medical problem? Is the problem acute? Chronic? Critical? Reversible? Emergent? Terminal? • What are the goals of treatment? • In what circumstances are medical treatments not indicated? • What are the probabilities of success of various treatment options? • In sum, how can this patient be benefited by medical and nursing care, and how can harm be avoided?
Patient Preferences	Respect for Autonomy	• Has the patient been informed of benefits and risks of diagnostic and treatment recommendations, understood this information, and given consent? • Is the patient mentally capable and legally competent, and is there evidence of incapacity? • If mentally capable, what preferences about treatment is the patient stating? • If incapacitated, has the patient expressed prior preferences? • Who is the appropriate surrogate to make decisions for the incapacitated patient? What standards should govern the surrogate's decisions? • Is the patient unwilling or unable to cooperate with medical treatment? If so, why?
Quality of Life	Beneficence Nonmaleficence Respect for Autonomy	• What are the prospects, with or without treatment, for a return to normal life, and what physical, mental, and social deficits might the patient experience even if treatment succeeds? • On what grounds can anyone judge that some quality of life would be undesirable for a patient who cannot make or express such a judgment? • Are there biases that might prejudice the provider's evaluation of the patient's quality of life? • What ethical issues arise concerning improving or enhancing a patient's quality of life? • Do quality-of-life assessments raise any questions regarding changes in treatment plans, such as forgoing life-sustaining treatment? • Are there plans to provide pain relief and provide comfort after a decision has been made to forgo life-sustaining treatment? • Is medically assisted dying ethically or legally permitted? • What is the legal and ethical status of suicide?
Contextual Features	Justice (Fairness)	• Are there professional, interprofessional, or business interests that might create conflicts of interest in the clinical treatment of patients? • Are there parties other than clinicians and patients, such as family members, who have an interest in clinical decisions? • What are the limits imposed on patient confidentiality by the legitimate interests of third parties? • Are there financial factors that create conflicts of interest in clinical decisions? • Are there problems of allocation of scarce health resources that might affect clinical decisions? • Are there religious issues that might affect clinical decisions? • What are the legal issues that might affect clinical decisions? • Are there considerations of clinical research and education that might affect clinical decisions? • Are there issues of public health and safety that affect clinical decisions? • Does institutional affiliation create conflicts of interest that might influence clinical decisions?

From Jonsen AR, Siegler M, Winslade WJ. *Clinical ethics: a practical approach to ethical decisions in clinical medicine.* 8th ed. New York: McGraw-Hill Education; 2015.

same page with regard to a treatment plan (if that is the issue) prior to sitting down with the patient and/or family. Having a unified presentation typically provides for a more productive meeting than if the team(s) are debating issues in front of the family.

5. ***Implement Decisions and Reflect Upon Outcomes***

The final step is to realize the plan of action. An important consideration here is to have the tolerance for uncertainty. "The best laid schemes of mice and men, go often askew…"[16] Words from an old Scottish poem ring true here as even despite careful reflection, consideration, and planning, things may not proceed as envisioned. Taking the time to contemplate how events could have been better planned, thinking about alternative scenarios, or contingency planning may better prepare for future care needs of the patients and/or refine one's thinking should a similar case present itself in the future. See Box 2.1 for a scenario that highlights this process.[17]

PHYSICIAN–PATIENT RELATIONSHIP

The vulnerability of illness and injury, the potential impact of interventions, and the inherent power disparity of the physician–patient relationship imposes mindfulness of one's moral agency in the practice of medicine. Patient care is as much a moral enterprise as it is a technical one. The relationship between a physician and the patient has changed over the course of the last 50 years since the dawn of the patient's rights movement. Our jurisprudence has recognized a right to refuse treatment[18] as well as to allow others to consent or refuse treatment on behalf of an incapacitated patient.[19] As the pendulum has swung away from paternalistic medicine toward respecting the right of patients to do with their bodies as they see fit, a model of shared decision-making has emerged. This model incorporates the delivery of relevant medical information;

BOX 2.1 Ethics scenario—palliative surgery.

Ms. Smith is a 78-year-old woman with advanced breast cancer who presents with a fungating malodorous lesion. The cancer is treatment-refractory and her current goals of care, in coordination with the palliative care team, include a focus on quality of life and comfort. She was referred to surgery for lesion resection. She is currently not receiving therapeutic interventions and has an Out-of-Hospital Do Not Resuscitate (DNR) order. Ms. Smith informs the team that someone told her the DNR order *must* be rescinded or she cannot have the procedure. Ms. Smith is unsure if she is willing to agree.

Case Analysis:

1. ***Recognition***

The decision to offer Ms. Smith a surgical intervention may be complicated by reluctance to perform the procedure if she is imposing unreasonable restraints on its proper outcomes.

2. ***Facts***

Using the four topics method, we would consider whether or not the intervention is appropriate from a medical perspective. Clearly, Ms. Smith's preference is to undergo the procedure to improve the quality of her life. Perhaps she wishes to comfortably interact with her family during her remaining time or maybe she is embarrassed by the smell and feels family will not attend to her. Contextual features could include liability exposure if the team agrees to not resuscitate her and she dies during the procedure. Important perspectives to understand are those of Ms. Smith, the palliative team, the surgical team, and her family (if she consents).

3. ***Issue Conflict***

There is an obvious risk:benefit (nonmaleficence:beneficence) conflict in that the procedure may not be safe to perform or the team may feel unduly constrained by Ms. Smith's DNR order. Ms. Smith's autonomy interest is at stake in that she is willing to accept potential risks for the prospect of reducing her illness burden and, hopefully, enjoy a better quality of life. A team's denial of this intervention is denying her that prospect.

4. ***Discuss/Plan***

The possible options include: do not offer surgery unless Ms. Smith agrees to full resuscitation; offer surgery with the explicit agreement and Ms. Smith's consent that no attempts at resuscitation will be made during the procedure; reach an agreement with Ms. Smith that limited attempts at resuscitation can be made, if appropriate. The first option seeks to maximize outcomes by offering the most flexibility to the team but may impose interventions that are contrary to Ms. Smith's goals of care. What if she would not want prolonged intubation because that would negate her desire to spend what time she has interacting with family? Then again, not having the procedure may also compromise her goals. The second option may best honor her preferences, but the team may be unwilling to agree to such a plan, particularly if a transient, relatively easily correctable condition manifests. A risk of requiring resuscitation is always present under anesthesia, and it may be reasonable for the team to not offer the intervention rather than allowing a patient to die on the table, even if the patient agreed to such risk. The third option offers a compromise in having a more nuanced conversation with Ms. Smith. Instead of an all-or-nothing approach, the team may offer limited interventions during the perioperative period that are defined by her goals and expectations.* After discussions with all relevant stakeholders, it was decided that Ms. Smith would rescind her DNR order allowing limited interventions during the time of the procedure and recovery. The order would then be reinstated.

5. ***Act/Reflect***

How did the case turn out? What could have been done differently, if anything?

For Further Consideration:

- What if Ms. Smith is adamantly opposed to rescinding the DNR during the procedure?
- Is there a policy solution for this dilemma and, if so, what would that policy be?
- Would the intervention be appropriate if Ms. Smith did not have capacity and the family is asking for the surgery on her behalf? What if the family wants Ms. Smith to have surgery because it will make it easier for them to care for her?

*Sumrall WD, Mahanna E, Sabharwal V, et al. Do not resuscitate, anesthesia, and perioperative care: a not so clear order. *Ochsner J.* 2016;16:176–179.

an explanation of treatment options (including no treatment); an exploration of the patient's values, preferences, and goals; and, finally, the decision-making process.[20] With shared decision-making, the physician is not imposing treatment upon the patient nor is the patient demanding interventions; rather, it is patient-driven care facilitated through mutual understanding (Box 2.2).

A question may arise as to whether or not ethics in surgery offers unique issues for consideration. One perspective answers this question affirmatively based upon the "moral domain of the surgeon–patient relationship" and categorizes five distinctive features of surgical practice: rescue, proximity, ordeal, aftermath, and presence.[21] These five domains exemplify a surgeon's power and the intimacy by which he/she participates in the destruction and rebuilding of a person. The patient is aware of, and the surgeon is accountable to, the immediate aftermath of the procedure. As such, ethical issues and moral ambiguity are worthwhile topics for reflection and consideration.

SURGICAL TRAINING AND INNOVATION

Surgical training is rooted in antiquity, adopting an apprenticeship model of experiential learning. There have been concerns that this training modality may be compromised with residency hour restrictions and increased demands on operating room throughput and outcomes.[22] An ethical tension may arise when patient expectations demand the "best" care or the most competent and skilled surgeon with the fact that no one begins practice as "the best." There always exists the first cut, the first mistake, and the first complication.

The same is true for innovative practice and advancing the profession; we have an essential need to refine and improve techniques and approaches. However, surgical intervention does not necessarily lend itself to randomized controlled trials as, say, a pharmaceutical agent. Surgical innovation relies upon not only technology, but also new techniques, approaches, and strategies. One ethical justification for surgical innovation involves the prudent balancing of laboratory background (animal experience), field strength, and institutional stability.[23] For example, while technology involved in routine neurosurgical practice would not be possible without innovation, development of new techniques does not always follow a systematic framework.[24] One approach is innovation, development, exploration, assessment, and long-term study.[25,26] Innovation may also be facilitated through varying degrees of oversight based upon the purpose, risk, ethical issues, and safety.[27] An ethical approach to surgery including the imperative to

BOX 2.2 Ethics scenario—level of appropriate treatment.

Mr. Johnson, 27 years -old, was involved in a highspeed motorcycle accident while not wearing a helmet. He suffered numerous broken bones and severe head trauma. He is on ventilator support, and there is no evidence of awareness of self or environment. He shows no evidence of sustained, reproducible, purposeful, or voluntary behavioral responses to visual, auditory, tactile, or noxious stimuli. His acetabulum has been shattered and, from a medical perspective, in need of repair. At the bedside, both his wife and brother indicate that Mr. Johnson would not want to live like this, that the surgery should not be done, and they would like the team to "pull the plug." Mr. Johnson's parents vigorously disagree, informing the team that he had a passion for life, he has a 5-year-old daughter to live for, and they cannot "give up" on him. The parents feel he would want everything done to preserve his life, including the surgery.

Case Analysis:

1. ***Recognition***

   There is much uncertainty if Mr. Johnson should undergo surgery.

2. ***Facts***

   The clinical picture may not be clear as there may be reasonable differences in practice as to whether or not surgery is appropriate for Mr. Johnson. Typically, this type of injury would need to be repaired as soon as possible but his prognosis and prospect for recovery is uncertain. Perhaps a formal consult with Neurology would be helpful. Since we cannot ask Mr. Johnson's preferences, it is important to speak with all relevant stakeholders. Here, it will be Mr. Johnson's spouse, parents and brother. All of them know Mr. Johnson through very different perspectives. We presume they all have his best interests in mind, and they each articulate different aspects of his personality that may all be true. The challenge from the team will be to discern how much each member of his family are projecting their own preferences into the conversation. We must try to understand what Mr. Johnson would find to be either an acceptable or unacceptable quality of life. [2,3]

3. ***Issue Conflict***

   The primary conflict here is discerning Mr. Johnson's treatment preferences, i.e., honoring his right to self-determination, with what others may feel are his best medical interests, i.e., balancing beneficence versus nonmaleficence. This conflict is embodied by two central issues:

   a) Who gets to serve as health care agent for Mr. Johnson?

   Without a directive, most States define a prioritized list of people who may serve as surrogate decision-maker. The policy behind these laws is that the people who are closest to the patient, know them best and are in a position to help guide the team in making treatment decisions. For example, in most jurisdictions, the spouse would be the decision-maker.

   b) Should he have the surgery?

   Shared decision-making does not mean total acquiescence to the spouse. As noted in the chapter, we would discuss treatment options within the context of the patient's preferences, values, and beliefs to reach a mutual understanding in the goals of care and the treatment plan. Everyone in the family is in a position to illuminate the team in this regard despite acknowledging that the spouse holds decision-making authority.

4. ***Discuss/Plan***

   Possible options include proceeding with the surgery despite the surrogate indicating otherwise, deferring the surgical option while gathering more facts or refusing to consider surgery, which will satisfy the spouse and brother but marginalize the parents input. The first option would be difficult to justify on the basis of the facts. The second option offers a measured approach with a couple of advantages, namely, it may provide more information that may clarify the course of action (e.g., screen for death by neurological criteria) and it affords more time to engage the family. It may be asking too much during the immediacy of this tragedy for the family to entertain end-of-life decisions. The tincture of time may be necessary to facilitate goals of care with active listening, empathy, and trust building. For this reason, the third option may not be ideal either. The outright rejection may be misinterpreted as abandonment.

5. ***Act/Reflect***

   How did the case turn out? What could have been done differently?

For Further Consideration:

- Would this case have been easier if Mr. Johnson had a directive to physicians? What if Mr. Johnson's surrogate decision-maker was requesting interventions that his directives clearly indicated he did not want?
- How important is the concept of dignity in cases like this, if at all?
- Would your perspective on this case change if the parents were malpractice attorneys?
- Would it be acceptable to attempt surgical intervention, in part, because it offers a good training opportunity?

From Schneiderman LJ, Jecker NS, Jonsen AR. Medical futility: its meaning and ethical implications. *Ann Intern Med.* 1990;112:949–954; and Jox RJ, Schaider A, Marckmann G, et al. Medical futility at the end of life: the perspectives of intensive care and palliative care clinicians. *J Med Ethics.* 2012;38:540–545.

improve practice yet progress for its own sake is an insufficient rationale. It must be conducted in a way that protects patients, offers the prospect of benefit, and is conducted with the proper checks and balances.

CONCLUSION

It has been two decades since the Institute of Medicine (now the National Academy of Medicine) released their report identifying causes of patient deaths related to medical error and proposed solutions to creating safer health care systems.[28] The increasing emphasis on patient safety and satisfaction in the service of not just better outcomes, but also increasingly slim profit margins, has culminated in higher demands on the health care team. Increasing focus on revenue value units, quality metrics, and resource allocation have driven a corporatization of medical care that has arguably dehumanized medical practice to an extent. Consequences of this expanded professional distance includes a rise in provider stress, burnout, substance abuse, suicide, and compassion fatigue.

Amongst all these performance and institutional pressures, the surgeon is left to care for his/her patient, as mentioned previously, without failure. Fallibility almost seems to be something that is impermissible to discuss openly. Additionally, surgery is a discipline that can carry negative stereotypes with the public that are not representative of its increasing diversity and inclusivity.[29] Again, we return to the idea that the challenges facing physicians today have reverberated through history and are not insurmountable. What it may mean is that becoming a "complete surgeon" will be through not only technical mastery but also by the embodiment of the "great doctor" who is an effective communicator, worthy of a patient's trust.[30]

SELECTED REFERENCES

Bosk CL. *Forgive and Remember: Managing Medical Failure*. 2nd ed. Chicago, IL: University of Chicago Press; 2003.

A sociologist's classic examination on the training and professionalization of surgeons.

Cassel EJ. The nature of suffering and the goals of medicine. *N Engl J Med*. 1982;306:639–645.

A seminal article on the definition of suffering, its distinction from pain, and how we can broaden how we view our patients and increase our capacity for empathy.

Farmer P. *Pathologies of Power: Health, Human Rights, and the New War on the Poor*. Berkeley: University of California Press; 2004.

A physician/medical anthropologist's personal perspective on global health, human rights, and social justice.

Ferreres AR, Angelos P, Singer EA. *Ethical Issues in Surgical Care*. Chicago, IL: American College of Surgeons; 2017.

An excellent resource for further information on the topics discussed in this chapter.

Jonsen AR, Siegler M, Winslade WJ. *Clinical Ethics: A Practical Approach to Ethical Decisions in Clinical Medicine*. 8th ed. New York, NY: McGraw-Hill Education; 2015.

This book sets the standard for how to approach ethical dilemmas and their resolution.

Kalanithi P. *When Breath Becomes Air*. New York, NY: Random House; 2016.

A neurosurgical resident's posthumously published account of his illness journey with metastatic lung cancer.

Selzer R. *Letters to a Young Doctor*. New York, NY: Simon & Schuster; 1982.

Insightful musings from an accomplished surgeon–writer.

Solzhenitsyn A. *Cancer Ward*. New York, NY: Farrar, Straus and Giroux; 1968.

Literature Nobel laureate's depiction of a provincial Soviet hospital. Although a complex sociopolitical polemic, the novel offers stirring perspectives of patient care through the lenses of surgeons, radiologists, nurses, and patients.

REFERENCES

1. Goldman B. Doctors make mistakes, can we talk about that? TED (TEDxToronto2010) website. https://www.ted.com/talks/brian_goldman_doctors_make_mistakes_can_we_talk_about_that. Accessed February 6, 2019.
2. Holmes B. The most ancient medical practice laws. The code of Hammurabi, 2200 B. C. *JAMA*. 1905;XLIV:293–294.
3. Ajlouni KM. History of informed medical consent. *Lancet*. 1995;346:980.
4. Selek S. A written consent five centuries ago. *J Med Ethics*. 2010;36:639.
5. American College of Surgeons. *Statements on Principles*. American College of Surgeons; 2016:19–34.
6. Beauchamp TL, Childress JF. *Principles of Biomedical Ethics*. 7th ed. New York, NY: Oxford University Press; 2013.
7. Epner DE, Baile WF. Patient-centered care: the key to cultural competence. *Ann Oncol*. 2012;23(suppl 3):33–42.
8. Rawls J. *A Theory of Justice*. Cambridge, MA: Belknap Press; 1971.
9. Carter MA. A synthetic approach to bioethical inquiry. *Theor Med Bioeth*. 2000;21:217–234.
10. Brody H. Literature and bioethics: different approaches? *Lit Med*. 1991;10:98–110.
11. Pellegrino ED. The internal morality of clinical medicine: a paradigm for the ethics of the helping and healing professions. *J Med Philos*. 2001;26:559–579.
12. MacIntyre AC. *After Virtue : A Study in Moral Theory*. 3rd ed. Notre Dame: University of Notre Dame Press; 2007.
13. Jonsen AR, Toulmin S. *The Abuse of Casuistry : A History of Moral Reasoning*. Berkeley: University of California Press; 1988.
14. Arras JD. Getting down to cases: the revival of casuistry in bioethics. *J Med Philos*. 1991;16:29–51.
15. Jonsen AR, Siegler M, Winslade WJ. *Clinical Ethics : A Practical Approach to Ethical Decisions in Clinical Medicine*. 8th ed. New York: McGraw-Hill Education; 2015.
16. Burns R. *Poems, Chiefly in the Scottish Dialect*. 1st ed. Edinburgh: William Creech of Edinburgh 1787.
17. Deleted in review.
18. In the matter of Karen Quinlan. *Atl Report*. 1976;355:647–672.
19. Director Cruzan v. *Missouri Department of Health*: US: U.S. Supreme Court. *U.S. Reports*. 1990;497:261–357.
20. Beers E, Lee Nilsen M, Johnson JT. The role of patients: shared decision-making. *Otolaryngol Clin North Am*. 2017;50:689–708.
21. Little M. Invited commentary: is there a distinctively surgical ethics? *Surgery*. 2001;129:668–671.
22. Holt G, Nunn T, Gregori A. Ethical dilemmas in orthopaedic surgical training. *J Bone Joint Surg Am*. 2008;90:2798–2803.
23. Moore FD. Ethical problems special to surgery: surgical teaching, surgical innovation, and the surgeon in managed care. *Arch Surg*. 2000;135:14–16.
24. Muskens IS, Diederen SJH, Senders JT, et al. Innovation in neurosurgery: less than IDEAL? A systematic review. *Acta Neurochir (Wien)*. 2017;159:1957–1966.
25. McCulloch P, Cook JA, Altman DG, et al. IDEAL framework for surgical innovation 1: the idea and development stages. *BMJ*. 2013;346:f3012.
26. McCulloch P, Altman DG, Campbell WB, et al. No surgical innovation without evaluation: the IDEAL recommendations. *Lancet*. 374:1105–1112.
27. Gupta S, Muskens IS, Fandino LB, et al. Oversight in surgical innovation: a response to ethical challenges. *World J Surg*. 2018;42:2773–2780.
28. Kohn LT, Corrigan JM, Donaldson MS. *To Err is Human: Building a Safer Health System*. Washington, DC: National Academy Press; 2000.
29. Logghe HJ, Rouse T, Beekley A, et al. The Evolving Surgeon Image. *AMA J Ethics*. 2018;20:492–500.
30. Angelos P. Surgical ethics and the future of surgical practice. *Surgery*. 2018;163:1–5.

3 CHAPTER

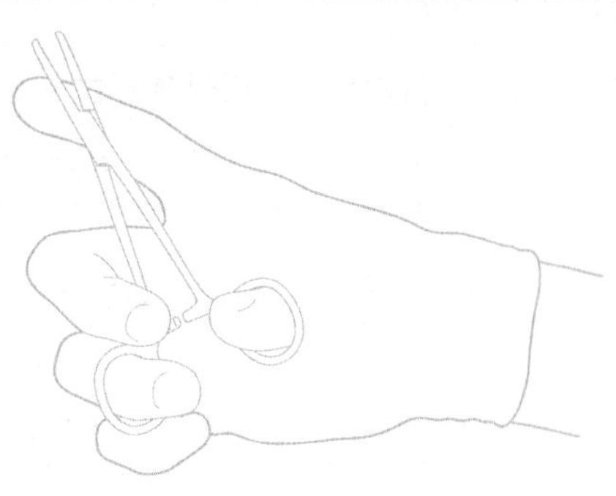

The Inflammatory Response

Katherine E. Kramme, Patrick H. Knight, Robert G. Sawyer

OUTLINE

The inflammatory response occurs following invasion by foreign microbes with direct tissue injury or in response to systemic stress such as hypothermia or hypotension. Multiple cellular pathways function simultaneously in an attempt to limit further injury and spur healing. While localized inflammatory response can be beneficial, major bodily insult can result in a dysregulated, inappropriate inflammatory response. The outcome can be catastrophic. It has become evident that the body's response to injury is often as important a determinant in patient outcomes as the initial injury itself.

Surgeons exist in a world of acute and chronic inflammatory response. The mechanisms regulating initiation, mitigation, and potentiation of the inflammatory response are critical to understanding the many phenotypes of a patient with a local reaction to surgery, systemic inflammatory response syndrome (SIRS), multisystem organ failure, and chronic critical illness.

COMPONENTS OF THE INFLAMMATORY RESPONSE

The immune system is comprised of multiple cellular lineages, hormones, and signaling molecules functioning simultaneously. The balance between pro- and antiinflammatory pathways is essential for healing.

Cells of the Immune System

Neutrophils

The neutrophil, a type of polymorphonuclear (PMN) leukocyte, is a potent mediator of acute inflammation and often the first cell type recruited in response to injury and infection. As a circulating PMN leukocyte, neutrophils have a short half-life of approximately 8 hours; the longevity of the neutrophil is increased in response to inflammatory signals, although the exact duration is a topic of debate. Neutrophils are continuously produced in the bone marrow in response to granulocyte colony-stimulating factor (G-CSF), and their production is regulated by interleukin (IL)-17 from T-cells and IL-23 from macrophages. The neutrophil undergoes a process of tethering, rolling, adhesion, crawling, and transmigration to move from the bloodstream to the tissue (Fig. 3.1). Neutrophils contain three types of proinflammatory granules – azurophilic (primary) granules, specific (secondary) granules, and gelatinase (tertiary) granules. Proteolytic contents of these granules can be released extracellularly or into the intracellular phagosome to aid elimination of invading microbes. Neutrophils also release fiber meshwork to which histones, proteins, and enzymes adhere; this is the neutrophil extracellular trap (NET). Extracellular pathogens are trapped within the NET to prevent spread of the pathogen and aid phagocytosis.[1]

Although classically considered a key mediator of the initial inflammatory response, the functions of the neutrophil have been shown to extend beyond the acute inflammatory period. The neutrophil granules contain a number of proteases that are essential for tissue remodeling and wound healing. They directly stimulate angiogenesis via release of vascular endothelial growth factors (VEGFs). In addition, neutrophils display plasticity, and, although typically proinflammatory, antiinflammatory subsets of neutrophils have been identified in certain pathologic states.[1]

Macrophages

Named for its ability to consume and degrade extracellular debris, the macrophage is a key player in innate immunity. Monocytes, the precursor to the macrophage, differentiate into macrophages in response to infection and tissue injury. Not displayed on immature monocytes, the macrophage expresses a large array of pattern

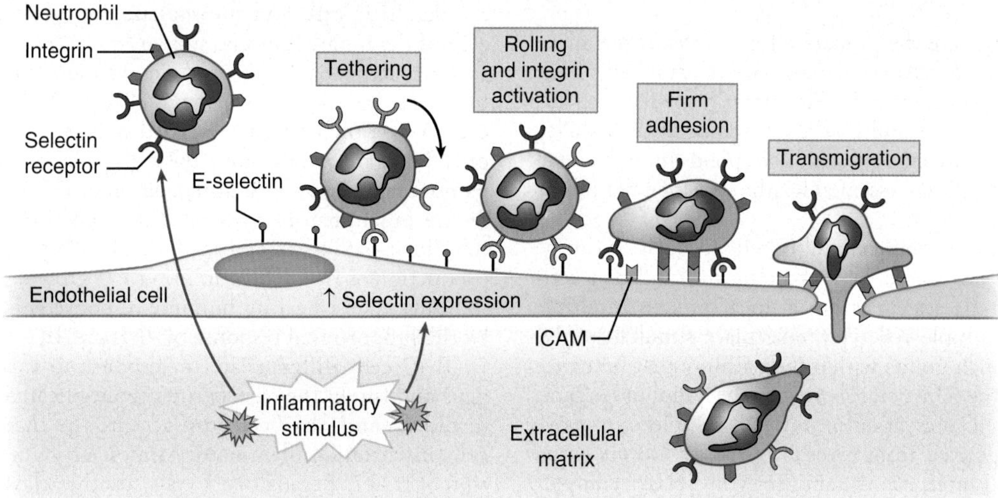

FIG. 3.1 Neutrophil recruitment and migration from the blood to the peripheral tissue. Once activated by an inflammatory signal, endothelial cells upregulate expression of adhesion molecules or selectins. Neutrophils bind selectins and roll along the endothelial cell. Integrins on the neutrophil surface interact tightly with intracellular adhesion molecules *(ICAM)* on the endothelial cell. Expression of molecules such as cadherin and platelet endothelial cell adhesion molecule (PECAM) facilitate transmigration into the periphery. (Adapted from Ouellete Y. *Pediatric Critical Care*. Philadelphia, PA: Elsevier, Inc; 2017.)

recognition receptors (PRRs) – receptors that recognize a variety of intracellular and extracellular danger signals. In response to PRR stimulation, macrophages neutralize, invading pathogens via phagocytosis and lysosomal degradation; they additionally secrete proinflammatory mediators, including IL-1β and tumor necrosis factor-α (TNF-α) that recruit other immune cells to the damaged tissue. Macrophages also process antigenic substances and present them on their surface to help stimulate the differentiation of helper T cells; thus, macrophages are professional antigen-presenting cells (APCs).[2]

Similar to neutrophils, once thought to be a single cell type, the macrophage demonstrates plasticity and phenotypic variance depending upon its environment. M1 macrophages express proinflammatory cytokines and proteolytic substances; they are predominant in viral and bacterial infection. M1 macrophages stimulate proinflammatory helper T cells. While M1 macrophage products facilitate a beneficial inflammatory response against invading microbes, they can result in a dangerous inflammatory state for the human host. High concentrations of M1-type cytokines correlate with mortality in sepsis models. M2 macrophages are essential for tissue remodeling and wound healing; they express a variety of antiinflammatory markers, including IL-10.[2] Macrophages are abundant throughout the body. Their functions vary depending on the tissue in which they reside. For example, Kupffer cells of the liver and microglia of the central nervous system are macrophages.

Dendritic Cells

Dendritic cells bridge the innate and adaptive immune response as the major professional APC. Upon encountering foreign material, the dendritic cell will engulf and degrade pathogen-derived proteins. These antigenic proteins are loaded onto a major histocompatibility (MHC) complex class I or class II molecule. The antigen-MHC complex is transported to the surface of the dendritic cell, and the dendritic cell travels from the tissue to the lymphoid organs, primarily the lymph nodes, and the spleen. Within the lymphoid organs, it stimulates naïve, resting T cells to differentiate into either cytotoxic T cells or helper T cells.[3] Extracellular proteins are processed within the dendritic cell lysosome, and they are presented in conjunction with the MHC class II molecule to activate CD4+ helper T cells. In contrast, intracellular proteins are processed within the cytosol by the proteasome, and they are presented via the MHC class I molecule to CD8+ cytotoxic T cells. Certain subsets of dendritic cells, however, process extracellular proteins through a process called cross-presentation and allow for presentation of these molecules via MHC class I. Through the process of MHC-antigen presentation, the adaptive immune response begins.[4]

Dendritic cells additionally stimulate T cell activity via surface ligands, such as CD80 and CD86, and via production of proinflammatory cytokines, such as IL-12. As a result of its many costimulatory mechanisms, dendritic cells are highly efficient at provoking the adaptive immune response. While macrophages and B cells are also considered APCs, they do not function at this level of efficiency for adaptive immune stimulation.[3]

Dendritic cells also process self-antigens and nonpathogenic antigens. Presentation of this antigen type to a naïve T cell induces the regulatory T cell – an immunosuppressive type cell essential for tolerance and immune homeostasis. Disorders of this pathway result in autoimmunity to self-antigens and allergy response against nonpathogenic environmental material. The fact that dendritic cells use similar machinery both to induce an active immune response to foreign pathogens and to induce a tolerant response toward self-antigens is an interesting paradox and an area of interest in cancer immunobiology. Tumor cells can be considered master evaders of the immune system. One of their many and only partially understood mechanisms of immune evasion is via inhibition of dendritic cell function.[3]

T Cell

T and B lymphocytes are the primary effector cells of the adaptive immune system; T cells are the primary effector cell of the cellular immune response, while B cells primarily mediate the humoral immune response. T and B cells are unique in their ability to recognize specific antigens and rapidly respond through clonal expansion. T and B cells are essential for the development of immune memory.

T cell activation is a complex, multifaceted process. It can be simplified to three key steps. While keeping in mind that activation of the immune system is not a linear process (multiple events involving multiple cell types take place simultaneously) there are many branch points within the pathway that influence the ultimate outcome. Once transported to the lymphoid organs, mature dendritic cells present antigen-MHC complexes to naïve T cells. Antigens derived from cytosolic proteins are presented via the MHC class I molecule; the antigen-MHC class I complex activates CD8+ cytotoxic T cells. Antigens derived from extracellular proteins are presented via the MHC class II molecule; the antigen-MHC class II complex activates CD4+ helper T cells. Whereas MHC class I molecules can be found on all nucleated cells, MHC class II is confined to APCs. Although consistent with classic teaching, emerging research indicates that the formation of antigen-MHC complexes is not so straight forward. Recent studies have shown that activation of certain PRRs can alter whether a protein is loaded onto an MHC class I or MHC class II receptor following uptake. For example, toll-like receptor 4 (TLR4) is a PRR most famous for its role in recognizing lipopolysaccharide, a key component of the cell wall of extracellular gram-negative bacteria. Activation of TLR4 at the cell surface transiently results in an increase in cross-presentation and thus an increase in loading of antigenic peptides onto MHC class I molecules with activation of CD8+ cytotoxic T cells. However, once engulfed within the endosome, TLR4 switches to promote loading of antigenic peptides onto MHC class II molecules; this ultimately promotes a CD4+ helper T cell predominant immune response.[4]

As self-antigens and benign environmental antigens are able to be loaded on to MHC molecules, presentation of the antigen-MHC complex alone is not sufficient to activate the adaptive immune pathway. Costimulatory molecules are additionally necessary for full T cell activation, most notably, CD80 and CD86, located on the activated dendritic cell and its interaction with CD28 upon T cells (Fig. 3.2). Stimulation of CD28 pathways results in a lower threshold for T cell activation and production of IL-2.[4]

Cytokines are also essential for full T cell activation, and the innate cytokine milieu varies based upon the type of PRR that has been stimulated. IL-12, IL-6, and TNF-α potentiate acute inflammation and influence T cell differentiation. IL-1 is essential for upregulating the acute-phase response. Interferon (IFN) type 1 drives an antiviral predominant response and drives activation of CD8+ cytotoxic T cells. In the context of CD4+ helper T cells, IL-12 promotes differentiation of helper T cell type 1 (Th1) cells. IL-4 promotes differentiation to Th2 cells. IL-6 and transforming growth factor-β (TGF-β) promote differentiation of Th17 cells. TGF-β can also promote differentiation to regulatory-type T cells in the absence of infection. In summary, T cell activation is achieved by three key steps: presentation of an antigen-MHC complex to a naïve T cell by a mature dendritic cell, costimulation of the T cell by surface molecules located on the dendritic cell, and the presence of cytokines produced by cells of the innate immune system.[4]

Each activated T cell produces a unique profile of cytokines to elicit a variety of downstream effects. Of the CD4+ helper T cell lineage, the best-characterized cells are Th1, Th2, and Th17 cells. In regard to infection, Th1 cells primarily fight intracellular pathogens and do so via upregulation of IFN-γ and propagation of the inflammatory response. Th2 cells function to clear extracellular pathogens and mediate the allergic response through production of IL-4, IL-5, and IL-13. A growing body of research indicates that a healthy immune response is heavily influenced by the proportional response of Th1 and Th2 cells.[5]

Th17 cells differentiate in response to extracellular pathogens and fungi; they are frequently implicated in autoimmune disorders, and Th17 cells can acquire the characteristic of Th1 cells in chronic inflammatory states. Th17 cells drive production of IL-17. Regulatory T cells, another class of CD4+ helper T cells, are essential for the development of memory and tolerance to self-antigens; they produce potent antiinflammatory cytokines such as IL-10 and TGF-β. CD8+ cytotoxic T cells target cells that have been infected with a virus for destruction, and they produce the potent proinflammatory cytokine IFN-γ.[5]

In general, studies have shown that the adaptive T cell–dependent inflammatory response is dampened following general anesthesia, surgical stress, blood transfusion, hypothermia, hyperglycemia, and postoperative pain; this occurs with a simultaneous increase in adrenocorticotropic hormone (ACTH) and glucocorticoids. As T cells play a role in the destruction of circulating tumor cells and the prevention of micrometastasis, this observation has particular importance within the realm of surgical oncology. A recent study compared the postoperative T cell profile of patients undergoing surgery for invasive breast cancer and for benign fibroadenomas. Postoperatively, no change in the T cell profile was exhibited in patients within the fibroadenoma group, whereas patients within the invasive breast cancer group exhibited an increase in regulatory T cells. The regulatory T cells increase at 72 hours postoperatively correlated with a larger tumor size, human epidermal growth factor receptor-2 (HER2) positivity, and decrease in the length of disease-free survival. A lower burden of Th1 cells was correlated with a greater tumor burden and HER2 positivity. This suggests that postoperative immunosuppression may leave patients vulnerable to metastases and invites opportunity for research into immunomodulation in the postoperative immunosuppressed state.[6]

B Cell

B cells, the primary effector cell of the humoral immune response, produce antibodies or immunoglobulins (Ig) and function as professional APCs. B cells initially develop in the bone marrow, where their cellular maturation can be correlated to the structural rearrangement of the immunoglobulin gene segments. B cells undergo a process termed V(D)J recombination in which a number of genetic recombinant events among gene segments V, D, and J of the immunoglobulin light and heavy chains ultimately allow for the production of different immunoglobulins; immunoglobulins have the capacity to recognize more than 5×10^{13} different antibodies. During the process of V(D)J recombination, the B cell progresses through the pro-B and pre-B cell phases. Following V(D)J recombination, surface-bound IgM marks the entrance of the B cell into the immature B cell state; it is at this point in its life

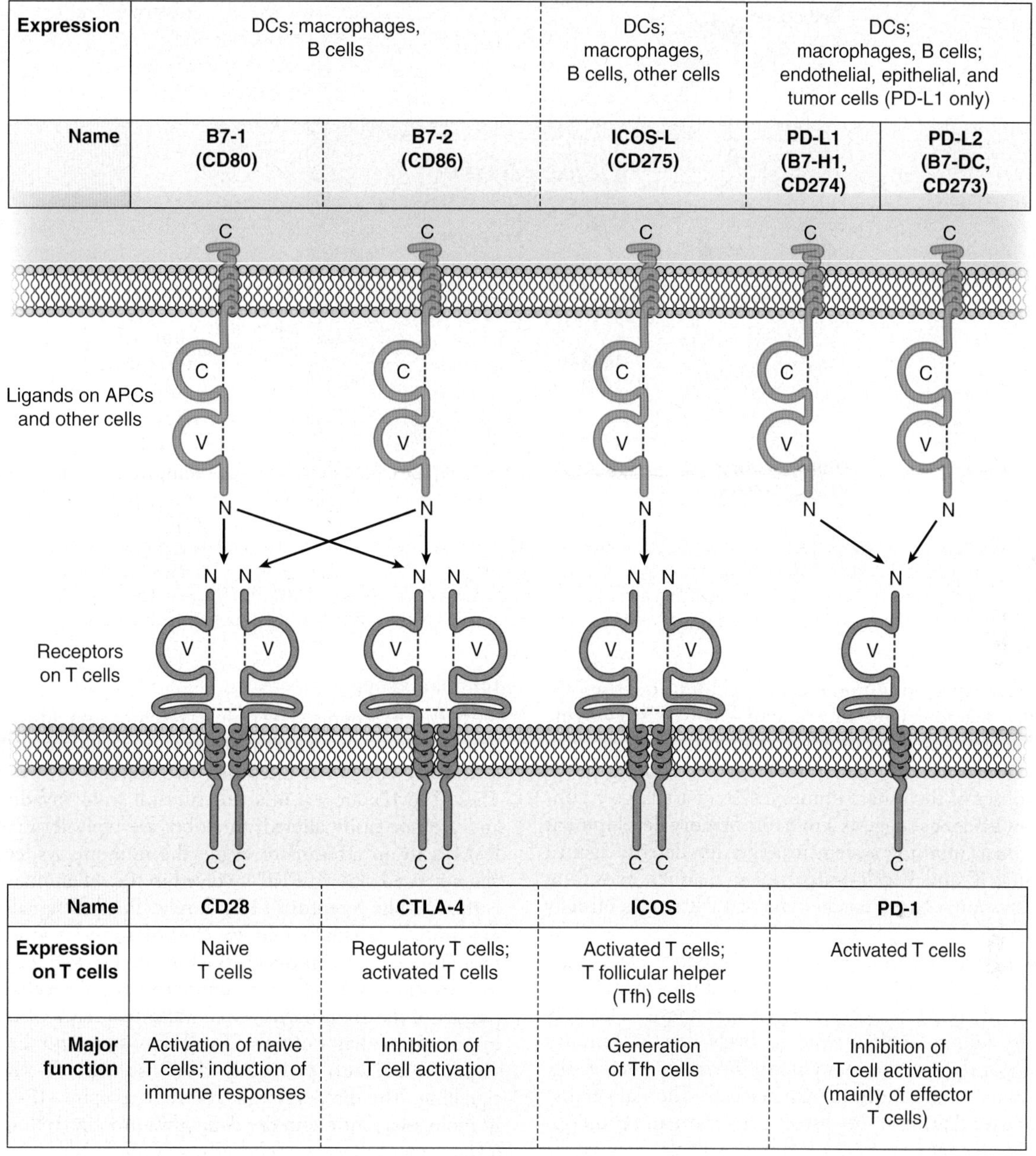

FIG. 3.2 Costimulatory molecules of the B7 family, including CD80/CD86, are expressed on antigen-presenting cells *(APCs)*. CD28 receptors are expressed primarily on naïve T cells. The ligand-receptor binding produces a different effect depending upon the type of T cells being stimulated. (Adapted from Abbas AK, Lichtman AH, Pillai S. *Cellular and Molecular Immunology*. Philadelphia, PA: Elsevier, Inc; 2018.)

cycle that it leaves the bone marrow and migrates to the spleen. Within the spleen, immature B cells will become naïve follicular or marginal zone B cells.[7]

Marginal zone B cells function in the spleen as the first line of defense against blood borne invaders. Independent of T cells, these B cells can rapidly produce soluble IgM during the early stages of infection. Naïve follicular B cells can be found within the lymph nodes or as circulating B cells. Their activation is T cell–dependent. Activation of follicular B cells results in a process termed class switching in which B cells transition from the production of IgM antibodies to the production of other classes of immunoglobulin, primarily IgG, IgA, and IgE, during times of infection. During the transition from IgM to other types of immunoglobulins, further genetic rearrangements occur that result in immunoglobulins with a higher affinity for the antigen recognized by the B cell. Memory B cells are B cells that are maintained following an immune response. These memory cells retain the capacity to produce high-affinity immunoglobulins toward a certain antigen and, should that antigen ever be introduced again, these B cells can rapidly mount a robust immunologic response.[7]

Innate Immunity

Innate immunity represents the first line of cellular defense, as well as a key activator of the adaptive immune system. The innate components include physical barriers, such as epithelial

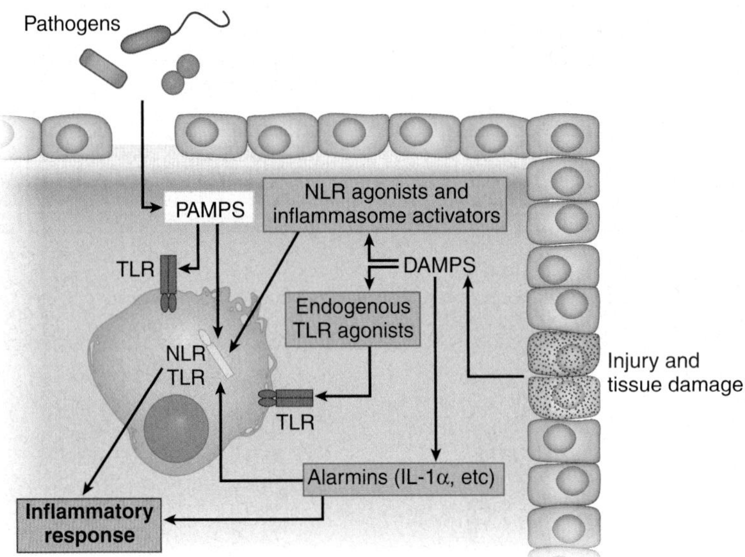

FIG. 3.3 Pathogen-associated molecular patterns *(PAMPs)* present on foreign invaders and danger-associated molecular patterns *(DAMPs)* prompted by cellular damage trigger multiple cellular signaling pathways via toll-like receptors *(TLRs)* and nucleotide-binding and oligomerization domain–like receptors *(NLRs)*. The result is the production of pro- and antiinflammatory cytokines and the propagation of the inflammatory response. *IL*, Interleukin.

cells and mucus; specific immune cells including neutrophils, dendritic cells, macrophages, and natural killer cells; cytokine proteins that regulate an array of immunologic activity; and proteins of the complement system. While classic teaching posits that the responses of the innate immune system are largely nonspecific, recent evidence suggests a role for memory development within the innate immune system to allow for defense against reinfection in a T and B cell–independent manner, as well as specificity of response based on the type of PRR that is initially stimulated.[8]

The immunologic self/nonself theory – a theory that hinges on immune system activation by foreign stimuli – has largely been supplanted by Matzinger's danger hypothesis. The self/nonself theory fails to explain why the body does not mount an immunologic response to many nonself stimuli, such as the developing fetus or the mutating cancer cell. The danger hypothesis proposes that immune system activation and propagation is more dependent on cellular damage signals than on the presence of foreign substance.[9] Cellular damage is communicated by danger signals known as danger-associated molecular patterns (DAMPs), also termed alarmins (Fig. 3.3). Danger signals specific to foreign pathogens are termed pathogen-associated molecular patterns (PAMPs). The initial danger hypothesis suggests that cellular necrosis and decompartmentalization occur during times of severe cellular stress, leading to a passive release of alarmins. These alarmins are typically confined to the intracellular space and, furthermore, are not typically released during programmed cellular death, or apoptosis. Newer theories suggest that severely stressed cells that are not undergoing necrosis are also capable of releasing alarmins in a more active manner by upregulation and overexpression.[10] For example, IL-1α, a well-studied alarmin, can sense chromatin damage and actively report this finding to neighboring tissue via increased IL-1α secretion. In this instance, IL-1α can report genotoxic stress taking place in a cell that has not yet lost plasma membrane integrity.[11]

Toll-Like Receptors

DAMPs are recognized by cellular receptors, broadly termed PRR, that are found on the cell surface or intracellularly. PRRs are evolutionarily conserved receptors that respond to specific PAMPs. These PAMPs are essential for survival from invading microbes and are not easily altered; microbes are typically unable to alter PAMPs in an attempt to evade the immune system. The best-characterized class of PRR involved in the inflammatory response is the toll-like receptor (TLR) family. The Toll signaling pathway was initially characterized in *Drosophila melanogaster*. The Toll protein had a known nuclear factor-κB (NF-κB)–dependent role in activation of B cells in response to lipopolysaccharide, a component of the gram-negative cell wall and a classic PAMP. IL-1, an important mediator of fever, T-cell activation, and the acute phase response had also previously demonstrated NF-κB–dependent signaling. The discovery that the IL-1 receptor (IL-1R) shared a homologous motif with the *Drosophila* protein, Toll, marked a key advancement in the understanding of intracellular signaling pathways of the innate immune system.[12]

The TLR is a transmembrane protein with an extracellular ligand-binding domain and an intracellular signaling domain. TLRs are expressed on the cell surface or within the endosome. Binding of a DAMP prompts dimerization of the TLR and subsequent intracellular activation of multiple signaling pathways. Ten human TLRs have been identified, each recognizing various PAMPs and triggering a variety of downstream cellular responses. TLR4 plays a key role in recognition of bacterial LPS, while TLR1, TLR2, and TLR6 recognize other common bacterial lipoproteins. TLR4 additionally plays a role in recognition of high-mobility group box protein 1 (HMGB1) and heat shock protein 70, two common alarmins, as well as mediation of sterile inflammation in the setting of ischemia-reperfusion injury. TLR3 recognizes double-stranded ribonucleic acid (RNA), and TLR7 and TLR8 recognize single-stranded RNA specific to viral invaders.[12]

TLRs function through NF-κB and mitogen-activated protein kinase intracellular pathways to upregulate a number of proinflammatory cytokines, including IL-1 and TNF-α. This allows for activation of neighboring innate immune cells, and for activation of cell lines involved in adaptive immunity, including helper T cells, cytotoxic T cells, regulatory T cells, and B cells.[12]

Inflammasome

Another well-characterized family of PRR is the nucleotide-binding and oligomerization domain (NOD)–like receptor (NLR) family. NLRs are assembled in the cytoplasm to form a key intracellular structure known as the inflammasome – an essential intracellular PRR. NLRs complex with apoptosis-associated speck-like protein containing a caspase recruitment domain to form the inflammasome. The inflammasome plays an essential role in regulating sterile inflammation via recognition of endogenous alarmins, as well as activating the innate immune response via recognition of foreign PAMPs.[13]

The best studied NLR is NLRP3. Once an NLRP3 inflammasome has been primed, it activates protease caspase 1. Caspase 1 is essential in the cleaving and subsequent secretion of proinflammatory cytokines IL-1β and IL-18 by macrophages in addition to the proinflammatory alarmin HMGB1. Endogenous factors capable of priming the NLRP3 inflammasome include hypoxia, complement, reactive oxygen species, oxidized low-density lipoproteins, amyloids, and misfolded proteins. The inflammasome plays a key role in the sterile inflammatory process that accompanies metabolic diseases, atherosclerosis, and neuroinflammatory disorders. Emerging evidence suggests that the NLRP3 inflammasome also plays a role in cardiomyopathy associated with sepsis.[14]

High-Mobility Group Box Protein 1

HMGB1 is an endogenous DAMP that mediates a plethora of downstream effects within the inflammatory cascade. It is highly conserved across multiple species, and it can be found in all human cell lines. The function of the molecule varies based on its location, the receptor it binds, and its reduction-oxidation state. Although initially identified as a deoxyribonucleic acid–binding protein in 1973, in 1999 it was found to additionally be an extracellular secretory product of macrophages in response to LPS and a key mediator of lethal endotoxemia.[15]

Within the nucleus, HMGB1 plays a role in regulation of gene transcription. In response to cellular injury or PAMPs such as LPS, HMGB1 is shuttled into the cytoplasm. HMGB1 makes its way to the extracellular space via both active and passive pathways. In cells undergoing necrotic death, the release of nonacetylated HMGB1 is nearly instantaneous. In stressed cells, pyropoptosis – or programmed, proinflammatory cellular death – facilitates release of hyperacetylated HMGB1 into the extracellular environment in a slower fashion. Pyropoptosis requires a functioning inflammasome and activated caspase 1. Extracellular HMGB1 stimulates release of proinflammatory cytokines TNF-α, IL-1, IL-6, and IL-18, and macrophage inflammatory protein 1 (MIP-1). It also serves as a chemoattractant for macrophages and neutrophils. In mouse models, neutralization via administration of anti-HMGB1 antibodies has been shown to significantly reduce the lethality associated with endotoxemia.[15]

HMGB1 is a rapidly growing target of molecular and clinical research, both as a predictor of morbidity and mortality, and an immunologic therapeutic target. It has clinical implications in many acute conditions, including sepsis and hemorrhagic shock, as well as conditions of chronic inflammation, such as atherosclerosis and inflammatory bowel disease, and displays a key role in both pathogen-associated immune response and sterile immunity.[15]

Cytokines

Cytokines are small proteins that direct the inflammatory response through a variety of local and systemic effects. Individual cytokines typically achieve either proinflammatory or antiinflammatory downstream effects via induction of intracellular signaling pathways that influence gene expression. They can participate in autocrine, paracrine, or endocrine signaling.[16] Historically, in regard to sepsis, it was thought that deaths occurring in early sepsis were primarily due to an overwhelming proinflammatory response rather than the infection itself. Late deaths were attributed to a diminished immune response secondary to the upregulation of antiinflammatory mediators that allowed the infection to overwhelm the host.[17] Many studies have since shown that the acute inflammatory response is a complex balance between proinflammatory and antiinflammatory mediators coexisting and working in tandem. The following is a selection of important cytokines and their functions. An expanded list of cytokines, including their cellular origin and biologic effect, can be found in Tables 3.1 and 3.2.

Key cytokines involved in the acute proinflammatory response include TNF-α, IL-1, IL-6, IL-8, IL-12, and IFN-γ.[16,18,19] TNF-α and IL-1β are considered hyperacute mediators of the acute inflammatory response, exhibiting effects within 1 to 2 hours of injury, whereas IL-6 and IL-8 function in a subacute fashion with a peak at 1 to 4 hours postinjury and a more sustained plasma concentration as compared to the hyperacute mediators.[18] Of the mediators of the antiinflammatory response, perhaps the best studied are TGF-β, IL-4, and IL-10.[19] Within the first few hours of the acute inflammatory response, cytokines mediate recruitment of PMN leukocytes and stimulate the production of reactive oxygen species. Proinflammatory cytokines are intricately involved in the procoagulant state seen in trauma and infection.

TNF-α is a 17-kDa protein secreted by both innate and adaptive immune cells, as well as nonimmune cells, such as fibroblasts. Along with IL-1, it is released rapidly in response to foreign invaders and tissue injury; in fact, TNF-α begins to elevate within 30 minutes of an inciting event.[19] The half-life of TNF-α is a brief 14 to 18 minutes, and peak levels are reached within 1 to 2 hours of host tissue injury.[18] TNF-α and IL-1 are two of the most extensively studied cytokines, as they play a role in nearly all inflammatory responses from sepsis and trauma to autoimmune disease and Alzheimer disease. TNF-α prompts cell signaling by binding to TNF receptor 1 (TNFR1) or TNFR2 – two transmembrane receptors found on a large variety of cells. The soluble TNF-α receptor (sTNFR) modulates the function of circulating TNF-α.[19]

IL-1 is released primarily from macrophages, although cells of the adaptive immune system and nonimmune cells secrete IL-1. IL-1 signals via two transmembrane receptors, IL-1 receptor type 1 (IL-1R1) and IL-1R2. Soluble IL-1R2 and IL-1R antagonist (IL1-Ra) modulate IL-1.[19] Along with TNF-α, IL-1 is a hyperacute proinflammatory cytokine with a half-life of approximately 10 minutes. As the half-life and peak concentration of TNF-α and IL-1 are so brief, neither has proven to be a valuable prognosticator for injury severity or to predict development of organ dysfunction.[18]

TNF-α and IL-1 have many overlapping functions and act synergistically. Both mediate the fever response and are thus pyrogens. In addition to being secreted by macrophages, TNF-α and IL-1 act on macrophages in an autocrine and paracrine fashion to promote increased macrophage production, activity, and survival. In response to stimulation by TNF-α and IL-1, macrophages secrete other proinflammatory cytokines (including IL-6, IL-8, and macrophage migration inhibitory factor), lipid mediators, and

TABLE 3.1 **Cellular sources and important biologic effects of selected cytokines**

CYTOKINE	ABBREVIATION	MAIN SOURCES	IMPORTANT BIOLOGIC EFFECTS
Tumor necrosis factor	TNF	Mφ, others	See Table 3.2
Lymphotoxin-α	LT-α	Th1 cells, NK cells	Same as TNF
Interferon-α	IFN-α	Leukocytes	Increases expression of cell surface class I MHC molecules; inhibits viral replication
Interferon-β	IFN-β	Fibroblasts	Same as IFN-α
Interferon-γ	IFN-γ	Th1 cells	Activates Mφ; promotes differentiation of CD4+ T cells into Th1 cells; inhibits differentiation of CD4+ T cells into Th2 cells
Interleukin-1α	IL-1α	Keratinocytes, others	See Table 3.2
Interleukin-1β	IL-1β	Mφ, NK cells, DC	See Table 3.2
Interleukin-2	IL-2	Th1 cells	In combination with other stimuli, promotes proliferation of T cells; promotes proliferation of activated B cells; stimulates secretion of cytokines by T cells; increases cytotoxicity of NK cells
Interleukin-3	IL-3	T cells, NK cells	Stimulates pluripotent bone marrow stem cells to increase production of leukocytes, erythrocytes, and platelets
Interleukin-4	IL-4	Th2 cells	Promotes growth and differentiation of B cells; promotes differentiation of CD4+ T cells into Th2 cells; inhibits secretion of proinflammatory cytokines by Mφ
Interleukin-5	IL-5	T cells, mast cells, Mφ	Induces production of eosinophils from myeloid precursor cells
Interleukin-6	IL-6	Mφ, Th2 cells, EC, enterocytes	Induces fever; promotes B cell maturation and differentiation; stimulates hypothalamic-pituitary-adrenal axis; induces hepatic synthesis of acute-phase proteins
Interleukin-8	IL-8	Mφ, EC, enterocytes	Stimulates chemotaxis by PMN neutrophils; stimulates oxidative burst by PMN neutrophils
Interleukin-9	IL-9	Th2 cells	Promotes proliferation of activated T cells; promotes immunoglobulin secretion by B cells
Interleukin-10	IL-10	Th2 cells, Mφ	Inhibits secretion of proinflammatory cytokines by Mφ
Interleukin-11	IL-11	DC, bone marrow	Increases production of platelets; inhibits proliferation of fibroblasts
Interleukin-12	IL-12	Mφ, DC	Promotes differentiation of CD4+ T cells into Th1 cells; enhances IFN-γ secretion by Th1 cells
Interleukin-13	IL-13	Th2 cells, others	Inhibits secretion of proinflammatory cytokines by Mφ
Interleukin-17A	IL-17A	Th17 cells	Stimulates production of proinflammatory cytokines by Mφ and many other cell types
Interleukin-18	IL-18	Mφ, others	Costimulation with IL-12 of IFN-γ secretion by Th1 cells and NK cells
Interleukin-21	IL-21	Th2 cells, Th17 cells	Modulation of B cell survival; inhibition of IgE synthesis; inhibition of proinflammatory cytokine production by Mφ
Interleukin-23	IL-23	Mφ, DC	In conjunction with TGF-β, promotes differentiation of naïve T cells into Th17 cells
Interleukin-27	IL-27	Mφ, DC	Suppresses effector functions of lymphocytes and Mφ
Monocyte chemotactic protein-1	MCP-1	EC, others	Stimulates chemotaxis by monocytes; stimulates oxidative burst by Mφ
Granulocyte-macrophage colony-stimulating factor	GM-CSF	T cells, Mφ, EC, others	Enhances production of granulocytes and monocytes by bone marrow; primes Mφ to produce proinflammatory mediators after activation by another stimulus
Granulocyte colony-stimulating factor	G-CSF	Mφ, fibroblasts	Enhances production of granulocytes by bone marrow
Erythropoietin	EPO	Kidney cells	Enhances production of erythrocytes by bone marrow
Transforming growth factor-β	TGF-β	T cells, Mφ, platelets, others	Stimulates chemotaxis by monocytes and induces synthesis of extracellular proteins by fibroblasts; promotes differentiation of naïve T cells into Treg cells; with IL-6 or IL-23, promotes differentiation of naïve T cells into Th17 cells; inhibits immunoglobulin secretion by B cells; downregulates activation of NK cells

DC, Dendritic cells; *EC*, endothelial cells; *IgE*, immunoglobulin E; *Mφ*, cells of the monocyte-macrophage lineage; *MHC*, major histocompatibility complex; *NK*, natural killer; *PMN*, polymorphonuclear neutrophils; *Th1, Th2, Th17*, subsets of differentiated CD4+ helper T cells; *Treg*, T-regulatory.

reactive oxygen species and thus propagate the inflammatory cascade. TNF-α upregulates the expression of adhesion molecules in endothelial cells, increases production of multiple chemokines, and promotes increased adhesive integrin molecule expression on neutrophils, thereby facilitating immune cell transmigration into the tissue. Together, IL-1 and TNF-α, along with the complement system, are the primary culprits implicated in the procoagulant state seen with acute inflammation, in part by inducing expression of procoagulant on endothelial cells. IL-1, TNF-α, and the various cytokines they induce also activate the hypothalamic-pituitary-adrenal (HPA) axis and increase cortisol production. On its own, TNF-α infusion into experimental animals produces an inflammatory state that is nearly indistinguishable from septic shock; a similar state is provoked by isolated infusion of IL-1.[19]

Interleukin-6. IL-6 is a 21-kDa protein that is considered a secondary cytokine – that is, it is induced by the primary cytokines IL-1 and TNF-α, as well an array of other stimuli, including bacterial endotoxin LPS. IL-6 is secreted from multiple cell types, primarily macrophages, dendritic cells, lymphocytes, endothelial cells, fibroblasts, and smooth muscle cells. It is a pyrogen similar to IL-1 and TNF-α. In fact, the key function of IL-6 is to mediate the acute phase response, a stage of the inflammatory cascade characterized by

TABLE 3.2 Partial list of physiologic effects induced by infusing interleukin-1 or tumor necrosis factor into human subjects

EFFECT	IL-1	TNF
Fever	+	+
Headache	+	+
Anorexia	+	+
Increased plasma adrenocorticotropic hormone level	+	+
Hypercortisolemia	+	+
Increased plasma nitrite-nitrate levels	+	+
Systemic arterial hypotension	+	+
Neutrophilia	+	+
Transient neutropenia	+	+
Increased plasma acute-phase protein levels	+	+
Hypoferremia	+	+
Hypozincemia	–	+
Increased plasma level of IL-1Ra	+	+
Increased plasma level of TNFR1 and TNFR2	+	+
Increased plasma level of IL-6	+	+
Increased plasma level of IL-8	+	+
Activation of coagulation cascades	–	+
Increased platelet count	+	–
Pulmonary edema	–	+
Hepatocellular injury	–	+

IL-1, Interleukin-1; *IL-1Ra,* interleukin-1 receptor antagonist; *IL-6,* interleukin-6; *IL-8,* interleukin-8; *TNF,* tumor necrosis factor; *TNFR1,* tumor necrosis factor type 1 receptor; *TNFR2,* tumor necrosis factor type 2 receptor.

fever, leukocytosis, and an increase in serum concentration of acute phase reactants.[19] Acute phase reactants such as C-reactive protein (CRP), complement proteins, fibrinogen, and ferritin are produced by the liver.[18,19] In trauma, CRP elevations begin around 8 hours postinjury and peak within 48 hours; as opposed to TNF-α and IL-1, IL-6 is a subacute mediator of the proinflammatory response.[18] In trauma patients with SIRS, sepsis, or multiorgan dysfunction syndrome (MODS), IL-6 is currently considered the most accurate prognosticator of outcome with increased and sustained levels of IL-6 directly correlating with a poorer prognosis.[18,19]

IL-6 is also implicated in the procoagulant state of the acute inflammatory response. IL-6 not only influences the innate immune response, but it also it has direct influence on the adaptive immune response by facilitating the activation and the differentiation of T and B cells and the production of new T and B cells from myeloid precursors. Evidence suggests that the myocardial dysfunction that accompanies septic shock is strongly mediated by IL-6.[19]

Interestingly, IL-6 also has antiinflammatory effects. Although its release is stimulated by IL-1 and TNF-α, IL-6 inhibits the release of subsequent TNF-α and IL-1 and upregulates the secretion of the modulatory IL-1Ra. Other antiinflammatory cytokines such as IL-10 and TGB-β are also produced in response to IL-6 stimulation.[19] Prostaglandin E2, a potent endogenous immunosuppressant, is released from macrophages following IL-6 signaling. IL-6 and its downstream antiinflammatory products have been heavily implicated in the development of the compensatory antiinflammatory response syndrome (CARS) – an immunosuppressed state that occurs in parallel with SIRS.[18]

Interleukin-4. The antiinflammatory cytokine IL-4 is secreted by innate immune cells common to the inflammatory response directed against extracellular pathogens, including mast cells, basophils, and eosinophils, as well as the adaptive immunity Th2 cell. It can act in both autocrine and paracrine pathways to increase release of IL-4, TGF-β, and IL-10. The most well characterized role of IL-4 is the promotion of Th2 cell differentiation and simultaneous inhibition of Th1 cell differentiation. Thus, IL-4 promotes the humoral, B-cell mediated immune response and antagonizes the cell mediated cytotoxic immune response.[19] Following central nervous system injury, a population of IL-4–producing T cells appears. The presence of these IL-4–producing T cells appears to have a highly neuroprotective role and induces recovery in injured neurons. In mice models, IL-4–deficient mice with induced central nervous system injury exhibit a decreased functional recovery.[20]

Interleukin-10. IL-10 is a 35-kDa protein produced by cells of the innate and adaptive immune systems, including monocytes, macrophages, natural killer cells, and lymphocytes. IL-10 downregulates the expression of proinflammatory TNF-α, IL-1, IL-6, and IFN-γ while simultaneously upregulating the expression of proinflammatory cytokine modulators IL-1Ra and sTNFR to neutralize circulating TNF-α and IL-1. IL-10 impair phagocytosis among cells of the innate immune system and prevents efficient antigen presentation among APCs. In mouse models, infusion of recombinant IL-10 has shown protective effects in LPS endotoxemia, and immunoneutralization of IL-10 in these same models exhibits reversal of the protective effect. Interestingly, however, in models of polymicrobial sepsis induced by cecal ligation and puncture, this protective effect of IL-10 was not seen; in fact, inhibition of IL-10 12 hours after cecal ligation and puncture markedly increased survival. Taken together, this indicates that IL-10 can have both protective and injurious effects within the septic inflammatory response. It has been proposed that IL-10 plays a role in the transition from early reversible sepsis to late irreversible sepsis.[19]

Transforming growth factor-β. TGF-β is a 25-kDa dimeric cytokine with an array of functions that overall exert an antiinflammatory effect. It has three isoforms – TGF-β1, -β2, and -β3 – that exhibit overlapping functions. TGF-β1 is found within the bone, cartilage, and skin; TGF-β2 is expressed in neurons and astroglial cells; and TGF-β3 is localized to the palate and lung tissue. TGF-β regulates the epithelial-to-mesenchymal transition (EMT), a process essential for embryonic development, tissue remodeling, and wound repair. TGF-β upregulates VEGF on endothelial cells and is intricately involved in angiogenesis. Notably, TGF-β is involved in the development of all T cell types within the thymus, and it inhibits the survival of autoreactive T cells in the periphery.[21] TGF-β inhibits various T cells functions, including IL-2 secretion and T cell proliferation; the presence of TGF-β promotes development of immunosuppressive regulatory T cells. Proinflammatory mediators from monocytes and macrophages including IL-1, TNF-α, and HMGB1 are suppressed by TGF-β, whereas immunosuppressive sTNFR and IL-1Ra are upregulated by TGF-β.[19]

TGF-β has an interesting paradoxical effect on malignant cells. In early malignancy, TGF-β functions as a tumor suppressor. In

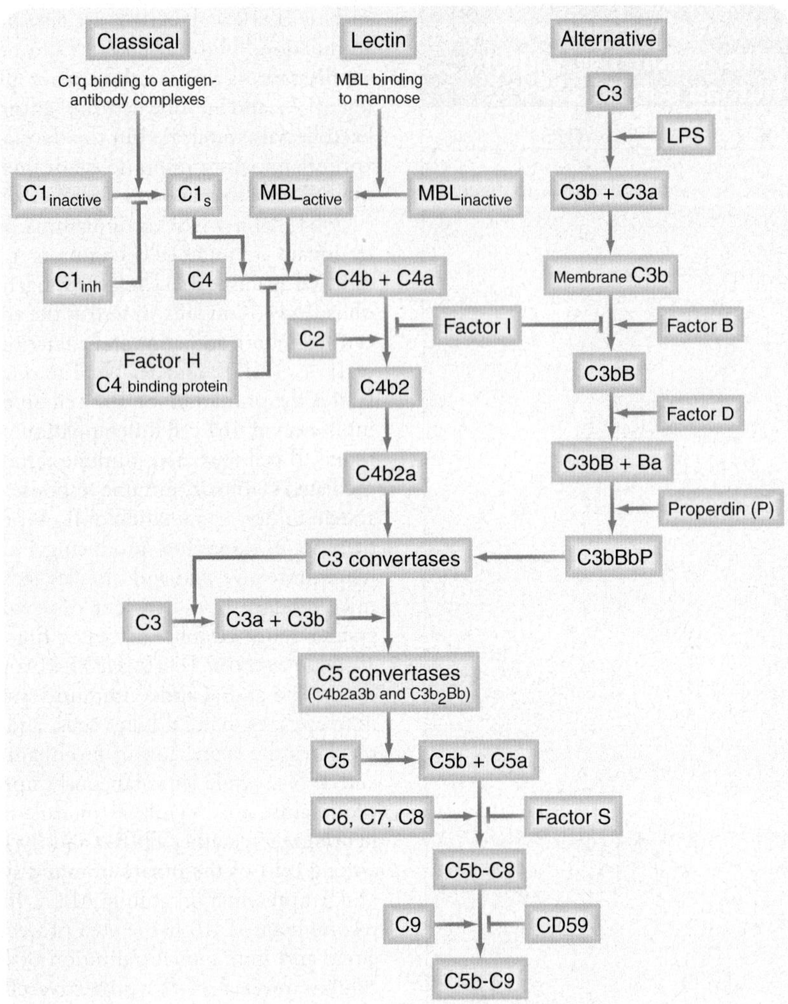

FIG. 3.4 Activation of the complement cascade via the classical, lectin, or alternative pathway. The common end result is formation of the membrane attack complex, or C5b-C9 complex. Inhibitors of the complement pathway include C1 inhibitor ($C1_{inh}$), factor I, factor H, C4-binding protein, factor S, and CD59, among others not pictured.

healthy cells, TGF-β arrests the cell in the G1 phase of mitosis and thus limits cell division. This process also takes place in malignant cells early on. However, as malignancy progresses and the malignant cells acquire various mutations and adaptations, malignant cells can turn TGF-β to their advantage and use it to promote tumor cell proliferation, invasion, and metastasis. Through EMT, angiogenesis, and downregulation of the proinflammatory response, malignant cells can use TGF-β to proliferate, metastasize, and evade phagocytic and chemotoxic cells of the immune response.[21]

Complement System

Although classically recognized under the umbrella of the innate immune system, the complement system has now been distinguished as a major mediator of the inflammatory response with influence throughout both the innate and the adaptive immune system. As a common theme within the immune system, complement proteins assemble and activate in response to a number of DAMPs. There are three activation pathways for the complement pathway – termed the classical pathway, the lectin pathway, and the alternative pathway – that ultimately result in destruction of a targeted cell (Fig. 3.4).

In the classical pathway, an antigen-antibody complex (mediated by either IgM or IgG) binds with complement component 1q (C1q). C1q can also be bound by CRP or serum amyloid P within the classical activation pathway. From this point, the lectin pathway proceeds identically to the classical pathway, however, the lectin pathway initially activates C1q via mannan-binding lectin, ficolins, and collectins. C1q complexes with several other C1 proteins to form the C1q complex; the C1q complex further cleaves complement proteins C4 and C2, resulting in the C3 convertase (C4b2b complex). C3 convertase splits C3 into C3a and C3b. C3b complexes with C4b2b to form the C5 convertase and allows production of C5a and C5b. The primary function of C5b is to initiate the formation of the membrane-attack complex (MAC). The alternative pathway relies on a baseline spontaneous hydrolysis of C3 proteins. The resultant C3b can covalently bond with several components of the bacterial cell wall. Upon binding, factor B is recruited; the result is a C3bBb complex that also functions as a C3 convertase. From this point, the alternative pathway can proceed in a similar manner to the classical and lectin pathways.[22]

Over 30 mediators of the complement pathway have been identified, each with its own function. The end goal of the complement pathway, regardless of route of activation, is formation of the MAC. The MAC exists in two forms. It inserts into the membrane of targeted cells – including bacteria, cells invaded by a pathogen, or stressed cells expressing damage signals – where it promotes leakage of intracellular contents, cell lysis, and destruction. In its soluble form, the MAC, or sC5b-9, is a potent proinflammatory mediator.[22]

In addition to direct cell death, many components of the complement system also function as chemoattractants for other cells of the immune system. Complement proteins are recognized by professional APCs and promote phagocytosis. They also mediate T cell activity and lower the activation threshold of B cells.

Host cells contain complement regulating proteins that function to prevent aberrant activation of the complement system against self. However, massive cellular damage and release of DAMPs, such as occurs with sepsis or trauma, can overwhelm the regulatory functions of the complement system and result in overactivation. This is one of the many mediators in systemic inflammation and thrombosis seen in traumatic injury. First in its class, the therapeutic agent eculizumab is an anti-C5 antibody that is approved by the U.S. Food and Drug Administration (FDA) in the treatment of paroxysmal nocturnal hemoglobinuria and atypical hemolytic uremic syndrome (aHUS). Eculizumab has off-label uses in many processes, ranging from nephropathies to transplant medicine. A large number of clinical trials are underway to assess its efficacy in various disease states; notably, sepsis is a focus of several of these trials. Multiple other immunobiologic medications targeting the complement system are in development. An understanding of the pathophysiology of the complement system is key to expanding knowledge in this field.[22]

Adaptive Immunity

Historically, the terms innate and adaptive immunity were used to broadly categorize the immune response into nonspecific and specific phases of cellular response. The innate immune system, by its classic definition, is comprised of cells and cellular mediators that are conserved evolutionarily and are present within the host prior to introduction of a pathogen or tissue injury. In classic theory, the innate immune system responds essentially the same to repeated instances of tissue damage or infection. This classic definition falls short; more recent evidence suggests many innate immune cell types have some capacity for memory development. For example, epigenetic changes, primarily via methylation and acetylation, within macrophages and natural killer cells following exposure to various danger molecules induce a functional cellular reprogramming. Upon secondary stimulation, these cells can reactivate and function more efficiently and in a manner that is independent of either B or T cell stimulation.[23] The line between innate and adaptive immunity has become less distinct.[8,23,24]

Adaptive immunity, in contrast, is historically characterized by the development of an efficient, targeted immune response to an invading pathogen and the subsequent development of memory cells. If the inciting antigen is reintroduced in a second encounter, memory cells mediate a vigorous, specific immune response to clear the invader. Although the classic separation of innate and adaptive immunity on the basis of specificity may no longer be entirely accurate, the adaptive immune system retains one critical, unique function – that is, the ability to undergo clonal expansion and the clonal expression of highly diversified antigen receptors, including T cell receptors (TCRs) and immunoglobulins.[24]

Adaptive immunity is further categorized into the humoral immune response and the cell-mediated immune response. The cell-mediated immune response is driven by activated T lymphocytes; the effects of T cells are largely driven by cytokines. The humoral immune response is directed by activated B cells; immunoglobulins and cytokines carry out the end effects of the humoral immune system.

Cellular immunity is dependent on activated T cells. When the TCR recognizes its corresponding antigen-MHC complex, the T cell undergoes maturation and differentiation as previously discussed. Essential in this process is IL-2 – a potent T cell growth factor. IL-2 is produced by CD4+ helper T cells in both autocrine and paracrine fashion and results in accelerated T lymphocyte differentiation and clonal expansion. IL-2 also promotes survival of regulatory T cells. In a secondary response to a repeat provocation of the immune system, IL-2 can be produced by CD8+ cytotoxic T cells directly. This drives rapid CD8+ cytotoxic T cell expansion and activation, rather than CD8+ cells depending on CD4+ cells for stimulation by IL-2.[25]

The humoral immune response is driven by activated B lymphocytes. In contrast to T cells, which require the MHC molecule to be present in order to recognize an antigen, B cells are able to recognize lone soluble and membrane-bound antigens via the B cell receptor (BCR). Once an antigen is recognized by the BCR, the B cell requires costimulatory signals for full activation. The costimulatory signals are provided by CD4+ helper T cells. The result is B cell maturation, class switching to IgG, IgA, and IgE production, and B cell clonal expansion. B cells can also recognize antigens and subsequently mature in a process that is facilitated by complement proteins and is independent of T cells.[25]

The Nervous System and Immunity

It has become increasingly clear that inflammation is a not a linear process mediated only by cells and proteins strictly associated with the immune system. Extensive crosstalk between the nervous system and the immune system is demonstrated in both chronic and acute inflammatory processes. Multiple neural circuits have been characterized in both the proinflammatory and antiinflammatory response. Multiple PRRs have been shown to be expressed directly on neurons, including TLRs (notably this includes TLR4), TNFR1, and IL-1R. Likewise, peripheral immune cells including macrophages, dendritic cells, and T cells express receptors for common neurotransmitters such as acetylcholine. Peripheral immune cells additionally produce and secrete acetylcholine, catecholamines, and other common neurotransmitters. The nervous system functions to suppress the inflammatory response by two key pathways: (1) the inflammatory reflex arc and cholinergic antiinflammatory pathway and (2) the HPA axis and glucocorticoid secretion.[26–28]

The Inflammatory Reflex Arc

A neural reflex arc is characterized by peripheral afferent sensory input that is transmitted to the central nervous system and processed; the resultant action is carried by efferent motor neurons to the periphery. Thus, at least two synaptic connections are involved in every reflex arc. The vagus nerve mediates multiple reflex arcs across the cardiovascular, gastrointestinal, and endocrine systems. As the primary parasympathetic nerve, it is no surprise that it also plays a role in mediating the immune response. It is composed of 80% sensory fibers. Afferent sensory vagus neurons transmit peripheral signals to brainstem nuclei; efferent motor vagus neurons project to the periphery and signal primarily via acetylcholinesterase both at pre- and postganglionic neurons. Vagal neural arcs are integrated in the brain within the dorsal vagal complex, which is comprised of the nucleus tractus solitarius, dorsal motor nucleus of the vagus, and the area postrema.[26] In addition to vagally mediated reflex arcs, the inflammatory signals carried via the afferent vagal fibers also play a role in mediating the fever response and regulating the HPA axis and subsequent glucocorticoid secretion.[27]

Neural regulation of the innate immune system. Sensory neurons in the periphery express several types of PRRs, including multiple subsets of TLRs and receptors for IL-1 and TNF-α, that can directly communicate the presence of inflammation to the nervous system.[27] Vagal paraganglia also contain chemosensory cells that serve as mediators between the cells of the immune system and the neurons.[26] The vagus participates in the cholinergic antiinflammatory pathway. Peripheral vagal nerve stimulation by proinflammatory mediators results in an increase in efferent vagal nerve signals that lead to a downregulation of TNF-α and other proinflammatory cytokines. This pathway has been demonstrated in the liver, heart, pancreas, and gastrointestinal tract to suppresses excess inflammation.[26]

Many efferent motor vagal nerve fibers travel to the spleen via the splenic nerve. The catecholaminergic nerve endings of the splenic nerve are in close association with splenic lymphocytes, particularly T cells, that express choline acetyltransferase (ChAT), the enzyme that catalyzes synthesis of acetylcholine. Acetylcholine produced by ChAT-expressing T lymphocytes acts upon the α7 nicotinic receptor expressed on macrophages; the result is an inhibition of NF-κB signaling pathways and an upregulation of Janus Kinase 2-Signal Transducer and Activator of Transcription Protein 3 (JAK2-STAT3) signaling pathways. This impairs the function of the inflammasome and overall decreases transcription of proinflammatory cytokines.[26]

In the rodent model, approximately 90% of TNF released systemically in the early stages of LPS-mediated endotoxemia originates from the spleen; in fact, splenectomy in this model is protective against lethality in endotoxemia. Efferent vagal signaling through the splenic nerve dramatically decreases systemic levels of TNF and is protective in the septic response. Thus, the spleen is a key site of vagally-mediated mitigation of the proinflammatory state within the inflammatory reflex.[27]

Neural regulation of the adaptive immune system. The inflammatory reflex arc has been linked to antibody production in B cells following exposure to blood borne antigens. In response to *Streptococcus pneumoniae* infection, vagus nerve signaling has been shown to promote retention of B cells within the marginal zone of the spleen. B cells retained within the marginal zone fail to migrate to the red pulp – the typical site of antibody production within the spleen.[26,27] Daily treatment of the α7 nicotinic receptor with an agonist results in a 50% reduction of antibody production within the spleen during times of infection.[27] Thus, by modulating cell trafficking, lymphoid architecture, and antibody production, the neural inflammatory reflex arc downregulates the humoral immune response to infection.

The Neuroendocrine System and Inflammation

The HPA axis is activated in response to a large variety of stress signals and is responsible for the increase in glucocorticoids associated with injury and inflammation, as well as multiple other hormones that elevate with the inflammatory response. The protective role of glucocorticoids, primarily cortisol, in the stress response is well established. Proinflammatory cytokines TNF-α, IL-1, and IL-6 exert effects at all three levels of the HPA axis – at the paraventricular nucleus within the hypothalamus, they upregulate corticotropic release hormone (CRH); at the anterior pituitary, they upregulate ACTH; and at the adrenal gland, they directly stimulate release of cortisol.[28] Direct input from afferent vagal fibers also signals the hypothalamus and prompts CRH release.[27] Cortisol negatively feedbacks on the hypothalamus and pituitary to decrease release of CRH and ACTH, respectively. Additionally, cortisol exerts negative feedback on immune cells, resulting in a decrease in the production of proinflammatory TNF-α, IL-1, and IL-6.[28]

As a lipophilic molecule, cortisol is able to cross the cell membrane. Glucocorticoids exert their effects by binding the glucocorticoid receptor (GR) – a receptor found in nearly all cell types. The ubiquity of the GR allows glucocorticoids to influence nearly every cell type in the body, and it explains the incredible array of functions that are modulated by glucocorticoids. Upon binding cortisol, the GR is freed from its complex with heat shock proteins, and the new glucocorticoid–GR complex enters the nucleus and promotes or suppresses transcription of many target genes. The production of IL-1, TNF-α, and IL-6 notably decreases following glucocorticoid administration as does the production of key chemokines, adhesion molecules, inflammatory enzymes, and proinflammatory receptors. The GR also directly interacts with the NF-κB transcription factor to inhibit its function and thus limits the proinflammatory signaling pathway of the TLR system. These effects of glucocorticoids are, overall, antiinflammatory and are seen throughout the innate and adaptive immune systems.[29]

At the cellular level, glucocorticoids promote apoptosis of basophils, eosinophils, and neutrophils. They additionally promote apoptosis among Th1 and Th2 lymphocytes. Chronic exposure to glucocorticoids promotes a transition in the cytokine profile of the macrophage from proinflammatory to antiinflammatory and increases phagocytotic activity of the macrophage.[29]

As is a common theme throughout the immune system, once thought to be purely an antiinflammatory mediator, glucocorticoids also display some proinflammatory effects. Whether glucocorticoids exhibit a pro- or antiinflammatory effect is dependent upon the basal state of the immune system and the type of exposure to glucocorticoids. For example, chronic exposure to glucocorticoids certainly exemplifies an antiinflammatory response; however, acute exposure to high levels of glucocorticoids (as can be seen with infection, ischemia, and trauma) temporarily enhances the peripheral immune system. Studies suggest glucocorticoids play a role in transient expression of several genes of the innate immune response, including TLRs. Cytokines produced in response to stimulation of these TLRs by DAMPs are responsible for mediating the increase in proinflammatory IL-1, IL-6, and IL-8. Paradoxically, it is within these same cells that glucocorticoids downregulate the expression of proinflammatory cytokines. Genome microarray studies have suggested that dexamethasone and TNF-α may have a synergistic function; cells cotreated with dexamethasone and TNF-α exhibited a more robust secretion of the proinflammatory, acute phase protein SerpinA3. Expression of NLRP3, a key component of the proinflammatory inflammasome, in macrophages is also upregulated in response to glucocorticoids.[29]

The initial actions of glucocorticoid within the innate immune system suggest that it is an essential mediator for the acute inflammatory response. Mice that have undergone bilateral adrenalectomy are more susceptible to LPS endotoxemia, and humans with pathologic deficiencies of glucocorticoids are known for their tendency to develop recurrent infections.[29] The extensive pro- and antiinflammatory effects of glucocorticoids, several of which appear to be mediated simultaneously, are prime examples of the complexity and nonlinearity of the immune system.

An overwhelming inflammatory response can impair the HPA axis. A state of true or relative hypocortisolism can result from increased levels of cortisol-binding globulin, alterations in function of the enzymes involved in glucocorticoid metabolism, or impairment of the cytosolic GR through mechanisms such as decreased binding affinity, receptor expression downregulation, or decreased translocation to the nucleus. In addition, glucocorticoid signaling at the level of CRH and ACTH can also occur. Taken together, there are a variety of ways that a state of hypocortisolism can result during the inflammatory response.[28]

In 2008, the Society for Critical Care Medicine introduced a term to describe the impaired function of the HPA axis seen with critical illness – critical illness–related corticosteroid insufficiency (CIRCI). It is characterized by a dysregulated systemic inflammatory state in the face of inadequate glucocorticoids and their antiinflammatory effects. The effects of CIRCI are seen throughout the neurologic, gastrointestinal, pulmonary, and cardiovascular systems and include signs and symptoms such as delirium, refractory hypotension, elevated cardiac index, intolerance of enteral nutrition, electrolyte imbalances, and persistent hypoxia. Updated guidelines for the management of CIRCI were published by the Society of Critical Care Medicine (SCCM) in conjunction with the European Society of Intensive Care Medicine (ESICM) in 2017; these guidelines highlight the patient-centered outcomes that have been published regarding CIRCI and provide recommendations for management of a clinical condition that appears to be much more prevalent than previously recognized.[30]

INFLAMMATION AND THE CRITICALLY ILL

Historical Perspective

Historically, sepsis was characterized as the inflammatory response that resulted from a local infection transitioning to a systemic insult. It was manifested by systemic symptoms such as fever, tachycardia, and tachypnea. In the 1970s and 1980s, multiple clinical studies and case reports observed that the symptoms of sepsis could be present in patients without an infectious source. Major physiologic insults such as trauma, burns, and surgery were noted to evoke a clinical picture that suspiciously mimicked sepsis and often responded to similar therapies as sepsis – hence the term "sepsis syndrome" emerged. Multiple theories to explain this sepsis syndrome were put forth, including severe direct cellular injury and necrosis, bacterial translocation in the gut, cytokine storming, and ischemia-reperfusion injury. As understanding progressed, the term "sepsis syndrome" was gradually replaced by the SIRS.[31] In 1992, Bone and colleagues defined SIRS as at least two of the following four criteria: temperature >38.0° Celsius (C) or <36.0°C; heart rate >90 beats/minute; respiratory rate >20 breaths/min; and white blood count (WBC) >12,000 cells/mm,^{3} <4000 cells/mm^3, or >10% immature (band) forms.[32,33] Today, clinicians accept that SIRS is intricately involved in the inflammatory response of patients with infectious and noninfectious insult.

As a deeper understanding of SIRS developed, it became clear that systemic response to infection and trauma was not only driven by proinflammatory mediators, but that antiinflammatory mediators additionally complicated the picture. In the 1990s, the term CARS was introduced to describe the immunosuppressed state that accompanies the critically ill patient. SIRS was implicated in the overwhelming proinflammatory response propagated by the innate immune system while CARS was primarily associated with the adaptive immune system and an attempt to return to immune homeostasis. The SIRS/CARS paradigm proposed that the early deaths following a large systemic insult (be it infectious or noninfectious) were the result of a vigorous SIRS response and that late deaths could be attributed to the immunosuppressed state driven by CARS. The paradigm has shifted over the last fifteen years, however, and it is now understood that a systemic insult appears to simultaneously trigger SIRS and CARS.[33]

The concept of an intensive care unit (ICU) dedicated to caring for the most critically ill of patients was first introduced in the 1970s. This, along with advancing clinical knowledge, facilitated an increase in survival of patients with single organ failure. Through the 1980s, as single organ failure survival improved, a new subset of organ failure patients emerged – the multiple organ failure (MOF) patients. Carrying a mortality of 40% to 80%, MOF rapidly became a topic of academic and clinical interest.[33,34]

Epidemiological studies suggest that MOF is a bimodal phenomenon with early and late mortality. Early mortality in MOF can occur following a single severe insult or a series of amplifying insults, termed the one-hit and two-hit models, respectively. Late mortality in MOF was attributed to secondary nosocomial infections (Fig. 3.5). Based on the previous understanding of the SIRS/CARS paradigm, early mortality in MOF was attributed to the overwhelming SIRS response, and late mortality in MOF was attributed to the immunosuppression of CARS, leaving patients vulnerable to develop secondary nosocomial infections.[33] The changing SIRS/CARS paradigm complicates this initial theory.

As clinical knowledge continues to move forward, early MOF deaths have declined due in large part to a better understanding of the pathophysiology of MOF, improved treatment strategies for shock and organ damage, and the increasing implementation of evidence-based, consensus protocols within the ICU, such as the Surviving Sepsis Campaign, ARDSnet, and ABCDEF Bundle for pain and delirium. Increasing compliance with these protocolized strategies correlates with a decrease in mortality.[35] As overall deaths from MOF decline, more patients are moving into a state of chronic critical illness. Patients who do not succumb to early MOF enter one of two pathways: one of rapid restoration of immunologic homeostasis or one of continued immune dysregulation and the transition from acute critical illness to chronic critical illness. While the pathophysiology of this latter state is not completely understood, attempts to understand this increasing phenomenon have resulted in a new clinical entity: the persistent inflammation, immunosuppression, and catabolism syndrome (PICS).[34]

Systemic Inflammatory Response Syndrome

SIRS is primarily governed by the innate immune system. Tissue injury and cellular necrosis, ischemia-reperfusion injury, and invasive pathogens signal host danger locally via interaction with PRRs. These inciting signals trigger an array of systemic events including thrombosis, loss of cellular polarity, leakage of intracellular content, and leakage of fluid from the capillary system. Vasodilatation occurs secondary to mediators such as histamine and bradykinin; this, along with the upregulation of chemokines, allows extravasation of immune cells, notably phagocytic immune cells, into the periphery. Edema ensues. As described previously, an array of cytokines and other inflammatory proteins flood the area to direct cell signaling. This influx of cytokines and the ongoing inflammatory stimulus prompts the production of more

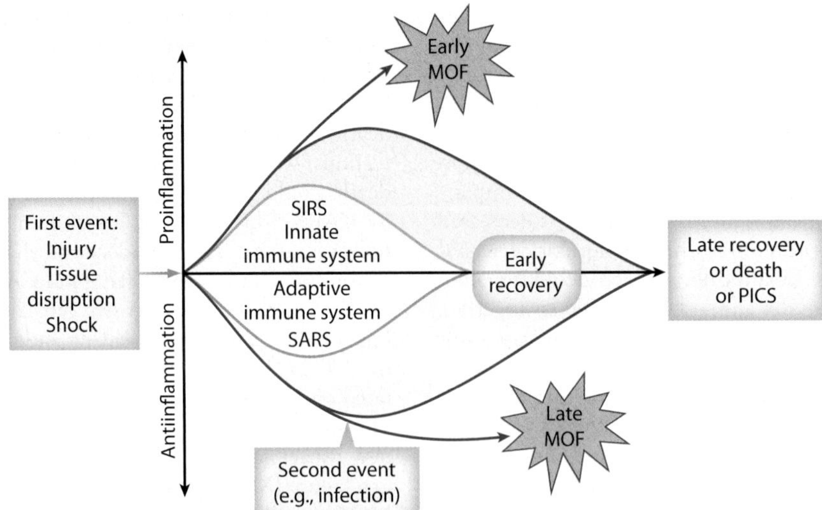

FIG. 3.5 The proposed framework of early and late mortality in multisystem organ failure, including the simultaneous functioning of the systemic inflammatory and systemic antiinflammatory response syndromes (*SIRS and SARS*, respectively). (Adapted from Sauaia A, Moore FA, Moore EE. Postinjury inflammation and organ dysfunction. *Critical Care Clinics*. 2017;33(1):167-91.)

cytokines through a series of positive feedback loops – this is the cytokine storm.[16] When a critical threshold of inflammatory signaling is reached, microthrombi begin to form in the vessels about the inflamed area in an attempt to limit bacteria and injurious proinflammatory cytokines from accessing the systemic circulation.[31]

When local inflammatory responses fail to control a local insult or the inciting event is substantial enough to provoke an initial systemic response, the systemic effects of the inflammatory cascade become rapidly apparent. It is important to consider that, in addition to the magnitude of the inciting event, baseline patient factors such as chronic corticosteroid use, malnutrition, and age play a key role in determining the adequacy of the initial inflammatory response. Many of the local inflammatory actions that are viewed as beneficial, such thrombosis, vasodilation, and release of cytotoxic substances, have a detrimental effect when applied systemically.[31] These events manifest as a decrease in systemic vascular resistance and an increase in venous capacitance. The cardiac index increases in response to a reduced afterload. Leakage from the vasculature leads to pulmonary edema. Cytotoxic mediators directly injure peripheral and central neurons and predispose toward ICU myopathy syndromes and delirium. The host is thus left vulnerable to subsequent development of multisystem organ dysfunction.

Many therapies that target the cytokines and inflammatory mediators of the innate immune response have been proposed, including anti-TNF antibody, recombinant IL-1Ra, and recombinant activated protein C. Unfortunately, these have not shown a significant impact on decreasing mortality associated with sepsis and SIRS.[31,36]

Compensatory Antiinflammatory Response

The CARS was initially named as such under the assumption that it followed the SIRS response in a stepwise, compensatory fashion. This has proven to be a misnomer; it is now widely accepted that SIRS and CARS mediate simultaneous, opposing, inflammatory responses. If SIRS represents the overwhelming activation of the innate immune system, CARS can be succinctly described as suppression of the adaptive immune system. CARS functions to limit the adaptive immune system and to prompt a return to a state of immunologic homeostasis, as well hasten the healing process. When the local proinflammatory response is overwhelmed, the SIRS response is seen. The same can be said for CARS – when the local antiinflammatory response is overwhelmed, the antiinflammatory effects begin to be seen systemically, leaving the host vulnerable to immunoparalysis, impaired healing, nosocomial infection, and potential for multisystem organ dysfunction.[36,37]

CARS has been tied to an increase in antiinflammatory IL-10 and IL-6 and a downregulation of the human leukocyte antigen-DR (HLA-DR); HLA-DR is one of several molecules that can make up the MHC class II surface complex and is critical in presentation of antigens to the lymphocytes of the adaptive immune system. Without proper expression of HLA-DR on monocytes, CD4+ helper T cells are unable to properly differentiate into an effector cell in response to antigen stimulation, and a state of immunosuppression ensues.[38,39] Lymphocytes, particularly T lymphocytes, undergo apoptosis, and a state of lymphopenia develops. Regulatory T cells appear and mediate the suppression of both APCs and effector T cells. Between the appearance of regulatory T cells and the decrease in activated CD4+ helper T cells, CD8+ cytotoxic T cell function fails. In both CD4+ and CD8+ populations, memory T cells fail to develop. As a result of the poor induction of the memory class cells and antiinflammatory genomic changes, immunoparalysis can extend beyond the acute inflammatory period and leave the host vulnerable to development of subsequent infection.[40]

Genomics and Understanding Inflammation

The previous SIRS/CARS paradigm – that the acute inflammatory response is initially governed by a proinflammatory response and then an antiinflammatory response subsequently follows over a period of days – is a tempting one. It takes the complex immune system, in addition to the neurohormonal system, and compartmentalizes it in a way that is academically easier to digest. However, multiple studies have debunked this previous line of thought. It has become evident that the systemic proinflammatory and the systemic antiinflammatory response to infectious and noninfectious inciting events occur simultaneously.

The first-SIRS-then-CARS paradigm was challenged in 2011 by Xiao and colleagues as part of the Glue Grant consortium, which endeavored to study the human response to injury at the genomic level.[41] The group performed genome-wide expression analysis of whole blood leukocytes in patients with severe burn injury or severe blunt trauma and a small number of healthy patients following the administration of a low dose of bacterial endotoxin. The results were impressive. In patients with severe blunt trauma, 80% of the leukocyte genome exhibited changes in gene expression within the first 28 days following injury; this extreme reorganization and reprioritization of the leukocyte transcriptome in response to severe blunt trauma was termed the genomic storm. The expression of some leukocyte genes increased, including those genes involved in the innate response such as the TLRs, NOD receptors, and haptoglobin. The expression of leukocyte genes that decreased included genes for antigen presentation and T cell activation. Results were extraordinarily similar among burn patients, and remarkably similar among the healthy subjects receiving bacterial endotoxin. Interestingly, common clinical parameters that typically correlate with a poor outcome, such as volume of blood transfused, base deficit, and injury severity scores, had a very limited effect on gene expression.[35,41]

Importantly, Xiao and colleagues also demonstrated that levels of altered gene expression remain elevated in the postinjury period.[41] At 28 days in the severe blunt trauma patients and at 90 days in the severe burn patients, messenger RNA of the leukocyte genes had not returned to baseline levels.[41] They demonstrated that the posttraumatic outcomes are largely dependent on quantitative and not qualitative gene expression. In patients with an uncomplicated recovery, levels of gene expression had returned to or were in the process of returning to baseline by 7 to 14 days postinjury. This was seen for both upregulated and downregulated genes. In patients who experienced a more complicated hospital course, changes in gene expression largely did not return to baseline by 28 days; it was additionally noted in this subset that the early changes in gene expression were of a greater magnitude.[41]

Given the numerous changes in gene expression that occur with systemic inflammation, it can be logically assumed that genetic variants may alter the severity of an individual's response to systemic inflammation and may subsequently alter clinical outcome. Certain single nucleotide polymorphisms (SNP) within the NF-κB signaling pathway have been tied to an increased risk of sepsis and multisystem organ failure following severe trauma.[42] Persistent downregulation of HLA-DR, associated with the MHC-II receptor, has been shown to increase the risk of development of infected pancreatic necrosis following an episode of severe acute pancreatitis.[38] The expanding field of genomics offers new insights into the pathophysiology of systemic inflammation and those patients most at risk for a complicated clinical course, as well as opens many doors for the development of clinical prognosticators and targeted therapeutics.

Diagnosis and Immunotherapy in Sepsis

Decades of research have attempted to develop an immunomodulatory therapy that alters the outcomes of sepsis. Unfortunately, immunomodulatory therapies for sepsis and systemic inflammation have shown variable, often unreproducible results. Targeted antibodies or recombinant formulations have been tested for IL-1, TNF-α, IL-10, activated protein C, bradykinin, antithrombin III, and TLR4, among many others, without encouraging results.[37] Considering the results of the Glue Grant consortium, which strongly suggest that the changes in the leukocyte transcriptome begin almost immediately postinjury and that multiple pro- and antiinflammatory genomic changes occur simultaneously, if an intervention is intended to alter the trajectory of the innate or the adaptive immune response, it is conceivable that a benefit will be seen only if the intervention can be implemented almost immediately postinjury or post infection.

One target that shows promise is IFN-γ. As described, HLA-DR downregulation accompanies the acute inflammatory response and has been implicated in CARS as one of the contributors to impaired T cell function. The loss of HLA-DR in the acute postoperative period has been linked to increased postoperative infection. Recent data suggest that soluble mediators that remain present in the serum 24 hours postoperatively are responsible for this downregulation of HLA-DR rather than direct tissue injury or anesthesia. Treatment in vitro with IFN-γ, however, improved antigen presentation among monocytes postoperatively.[43] Other work has suggested that granulocyte-macrophage colony-stimulating factor (GM-CSF) may also improve expression of HLA-DR among critically ill patients.[44]

As immune-targeted therapeutic approaches for SIRS and sepsis remain limited, the importance of prevention and early recognition cannot be understated. Emphasis has been placed on the missed diagnosis of sepsis, as no standard test exists to determine whether a patient with systemic inflammation also has an underlying infection; the consequences of a missed diagnosis of sepsis include an increase in mortality, improper usage of antibiotics, and an increase in healthcare spending. A relatively new approach to this problem is the use of gene expression microarrays to better delineate patients with systemic inflammation. At the time of this review, three diagnostic gene expression microarrays – Sepsis MetaScore, FAIM3:PLAC8 ratio, and the Septicyte Lab – have been introduced with the aim to distinguish septic patients from patients with noninfectious inflammation. While all three scores require further testing and validation before widespread application, early data are promising for the performance of these microprofiling tests in distinguishing infectious from noninfectious systemic inflammation.[45]

Multiple Organ Failure

Sustained activation of SIRS and CARS results in systemic injury that can progress to a point of MOF. Innate immune effector cells extravasate from the vasculature systemically into the tissues; however, without adequate local levels of chemoattractant signals, these cells fail to migrate further than the tissue surrounding the microvasculature.[31] While postinjury patients who do not develop MOF and those who do both exhibit an initial neutrophilia (within 3 hours postinjury), those patients who develop MOF exhibit a profound neutropenia within 6 to 12 hours postinjury; this suggests sequestration of neutrophils in the peripheral tissues. As activated immune cells, though, they continue to degranulate and release cytotoxic mediators. These cytotoxic substances directly injure the surrounding parenchyma. They additionally damage the microvasculature and severely limit the transport of nutrients into the tissue.[31]

Complement activation not only contributes to the hypercoagulable state, but also to the production of the lytic MAC, multiple inflammatory cytokines, and harmful reactive oxygen species.[37] Prolonged exposure to inflammatory cytokines and prolonged alterations in leukocyte gene expression prompt the production of the powerfully immunosuppressive myeloid-derived suppressor cell (MDSC). MDSCs, unlike typical myeloid-derived cells, do not differentiate into immune cells with effector function. The result is immature immune cells that are unable to propagate inflammatory pathways implicated in the resolution of inflammation.[36]

Risk factors for the development of MOF include abdominal compartment syndrome, early requirement for blood product transfusion, and infection, among many others. Although resuscitation with blood products versus excessive crystalloid has been shown to lower the incidence of MOF, early transfusion requirement remains one of the strongest MOF risk factors. Blood products contain numerous immunoactive substances, including proinflammatory lipids and cytokines within the red blood cells that remain despite leukodepletion of blood products.[36] Other risk factors include advanced age, increased body mass index (BMI), male sex, injury severity score, and base deficit on admission. Interestingly, while male sex confers a greater risk of developing MOF, female sex confers a greater risk of death.[46] Additionally, orthopedic literature has indicated that damage control with external fixation is associated with a more controlled postoperative inflammatory response than in patients who undergo primary intramedullary nailing, despite more severe injuries in the damage control group.[36]

At this point, it is worth noting that the nomenclature surrounding multiple organ dysfunction and failure (as well as the nomenclature surrounding SIRS, CARS, and sepsis) is vast. Multiple definitions of MOF have been proposed, and multiple scoring systems exist in the literature. The most widely accepted scoring systems are the Denver Postinjury Multiple Organ Failure Score, the Sequential Organ Failure Assessment (SOFA), and the Marshall Multiple Organ Dysfunction Score (MODS). A recent study published in the *Journal of Trauma and Acute Care Surgery* advocates the use of the Denver scoring system based on its simplicity and ability to identify high-risk patients and its strongest association with early trauma mortality. The Denver scoring system uses laboratory values representing the respiratory, renal, hepatic, and cardiac systems to assign a score in patients with an injury severity score >15 who have survived more than 48 hours from injury to predict various outcomes.[47] Another recently published study suggests that, in patients with traumatic hemorrhagic shock, a better prognostic indicator may be measurement of microcirculatory perfusion as an endpoint in resuscitation. This underscores the critical role of the hypercoagulable state in the pathophysiology of MOF.[48]

With improvements in understanding of disease and early implementation of protocolized ICU bundles, outcomes in MOF mortality have improved over time. For the patients who survive MOF, they enter into one of two clinical phenotypes. In the first phenotype, immunologic homeostasis is restored within 14 days of the clinical insult. In the second phenotype, immunologic dysfunction and organ dysfunction persist; these patients enter a state of chronic critical illness. This chronic critical illness is underpinned by persistent inflammation, immunosuppression, and catabolism.[34]

Persistent Inflammation, Immunosuppression, and Catabolism Syndrome

The physiologic effect on patients with chronic critical illness requiring prolonged intensive care has been a notable area of interest and study over the last 20 years. Within this group, a subset of patients exists that maintains a state of lingering, simultaneous immunosuppression, and inflammation associated with a persistent acute phase response that drives a baseline catabolic state. The mechanism of this – (PICS) – is based on a pathophysiologic maintenance of low-grade inflammation with increased serum levels of IL-6 and neutrophils in conjunction with immunosuppression through lymphocyte depletion and dysfunction. Multiple organ injury and failure further reinforced the baseline immune dysfunction in a cycle that can prove extraordinarily hard to break.[34]

Although typically relatively quiescent, one of the functions of the innate immune system is activation and differentiation of hematopoietic stem cells. With activation of hematopoietic stem cells through multiple redundant pathways utilizing growth factors and cytokines as ligands, including IL-1, IL-6, and IL-17, the body attempts to replenish cells of the innate immune system. Severe cellular stress creates a state of "emergency myelopoiesis" at the expense of lymphopoiesis and erythropoiesis. It is through this process that MDSCs are formed. Although their function is incompletely understood, these cells prevent the toxic effects of persistent T cell proliferation and cytokine production. However, their action in chronic critical illness allows for continued immunosuppression, and the expansion of MDSCs after sepsis correlates with poor clinical outcomes.[34]

The chronicity of these pathways in critical illness is based upon the continual presence of DAMPs and PAMPs. PAMPs and DAMPs act on a number of receptors, such as TLRs, NLRs, retinoic acid-inducible gene-like receptors, and scavenger receptors with the resultant activation of the proinflammatory pathways and cytokine release. Neutrophilia occurs, although these immature myeloid cells lack full functionality for antigen presentation, expression of adhesion molecules, and formation of NETs. Simultaneously, the antiinflammatory IL-10 and TGF-β appear, MDSCs begin to form, and T lymphocytes fail to properly develop, leading to an immunosuppressed state. This immunosuppressed state is characterized by an overall lymphopenia, the appearance of regulatory T cells, Th2 polarization, and impaired functioning of dendritic cells. In addition to this myelodysplastic effect, lymphopenia is also induced by apoptosis of effector T and B lymphocytes (Fig. 3.6). Additionally, the ongoing physiologic stress perpetuates a state of catabolism, manifested by derangements in carbohydrate, lipid, and protein metabolism.[34]

Also problematic in chronic critical illness is the kidney. There is a strong correlation between acute kidney injury and the development of sepsis, and acute kidney injury progressing to chronic kidney disease has proven to be a risk factor for development of chronic critical illness. The epithelial cells that line the renal tubules are exquisitely sensitive to oxidative stress; necrosis of these cells provides a wide array of DAMPs to perpetuate the inflammatory process. An upregulation of TLRs occurs in the kidneys in response to stress, too. The overall result is direct toxicity to the kidney and release of DAMPs, a decrease in glomerular filtration, and an upregulation of one of the key receptor types responsible for the perpetuation of the innate immune response.[49]

Within skeletal muscle, sepsis and severe cellular stress induce dysfunction in the mitochondria, decrease in protein synthesis, and breakdown of myofibrillar proteins. The breakdown of skeletal muscle mitochondria releases proinflammatory substances and, given the size of the skeletal muscle system, provides an ample source of DAMPs. Clinically, this manifests as severe muscle wasting and cachexia; in a matter of weeks, patients can lose up to 30% of their lean muscle mass.[49]

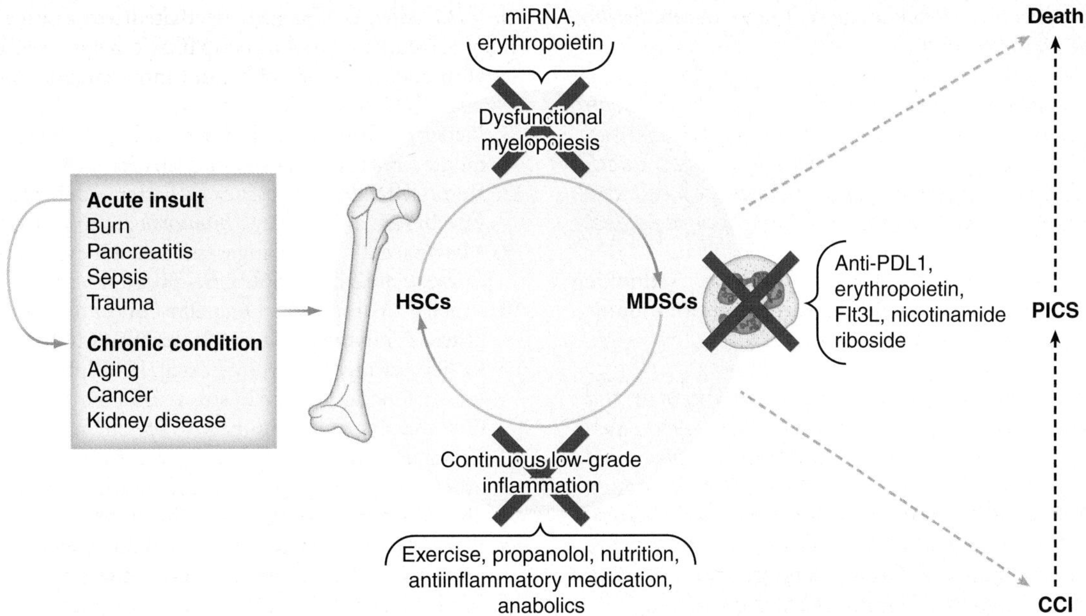

FIG. 3.6 Myelodysplasia and continuous inflammatory stimulus results in a vicious cycle associated with persistent inflammation, immunosuppression, and catabolism syndrome *(PICS)*. Certain chronic conditions or aging increases the risk of PICS. *CCI,* Chronic critical illness; *Flt3L,* XXX. *HSCs,* hematopoietic stem cells; *MDSCs,* myeloid-derived suppressor cells; *miRNA,* microRNA; *PDL1,* XXX. (Adapted from Efron PA, Mohr AM, Bihorac A, et al. Persistent inflammation, immunosuppression, and catabolism and the development of chronic critical illness after surgery. *Surgery.* 2018;164(2):178-84.)

Specific therapies for sepsis and inflammation remain relatively elusive. Current recommendations continue to underscore the importance of optimal ICU care, including early recognition of sepsis; utilization of validated, protocolized bundles (such as those to treat pain and delirium); and early, aggressive patient mobilization. Several immunotherapies that have shown promise in the treatment of oncologic disease are under investigation for their potential role in treating sepsis, as these patients share certain characteristics of their immunosuppressed states.[34] Adequate nutrition administration is emphasized, although septic patients demonstrate a dysfunctional utilization and metabolism of nutrients even in the presence of normal levels of key nutrients. The recommended daily protein supplementation for critically ill patients has recently been increased to >1.5 g/kg/day, with some top researchers continuing to recommend supplementation with 2.0 g/kg/day for the most critically ill patients.[50] Although not yet studied in the chronically critically ill patient, administration of propranolol and oxandrolone, with the intent to decrease catabolic requirements, has shown good outcomes in the pediatric burn population, and the same principles may apply to critically ill adults.[34,50]

The end result of these processes is a chronic dysregulated inflammatory state that leaves the host vulnerable to opportunistic infection; this can have a particularly devastating effect in the critical care setting with multi–drug-resistant pathogens. With the onset of such infections, additional critical care measures are required and further PAMPs and DAMPs are provided for proliferation of this vicious cycle. For those patients who survive their ICU stay, chronic critical illness confers an increased risk of death following hospital discharge. Discharge to a skilled nursing facility remains one of the strongest predictors of mortality in this patient group. With such a profound effect on the patient, poor clinical outcomes in terms of mortality and functional status following discharge from the ICU are unfortunately commonplace.[34,49] As the elderly population continues to grow, the incidence of chronic critical illness and PICS will likely increase as well.[50]

SELECTED REFERENCES

Cruz-Topete D, Cidlowski JA. One hormone, two actions: anti- and pro-inflammatory effects of glucocorticoids. *Neuroimmunomodulation.* 2015;22(1-2):20–32.

Historically thought to be primarily antiinflammatory, the proinflammatory role of glucocorticoids has proven to be important in a functional immune response. With the glucocorticoid receptor residing within nearly every cell in the human body, the proinflammatory and antiinflammatory effects and clinical implications of glucocorticoids are vast.

Efron PA, Mohr AM, Bihorac A, et al. Persistent inflammation, immunosuppression, and catabolism and the development of chronic critical illness after surgery. *Surgery.* 2018;164(2):178–184.

As clinical care improves, in-hospital mortality of critically ill has declined. As more critically ill patients are surviving the early stages of multiple organ dysfunction, a new phenotype of multiple organ dysfunction and chronic critical illness has appeared: the persistent inflammation, immunosuppression, and catabolism syndrome. In this review, the pathophysiology and long-term clinical implications of this entity is reviewed.

Jain A, Pasare C. Innate control of adaptive immunity: beyond the three-signal paradigm. *J Immunol.* 2017;198(10):3791–3800.

T cell activation within the adaptive immune system requires multiple signaling events from cells within the innate immune system. The complex process of T cell receptor engagement, presentation of costimulatory molecules, and essential priming cytokines is reviewed.

Matzinger P. The danger model: a renewed sense of self. *Science.* 2002;296(5566):301–305.

Matzinger's danger hypothesis postulated that the immune response is more concerned with the presence of danger signals that are intrinsic to the host and to foreign invaders, as opposed to self versus nonself antigens. This represented a pivotal shift in understanding how the immune response begins.

Olofsson PS, Rosas-Ballina M, Levine YA, et al. Rethinking inflammation: neural circuits in the regulation of immunity. *Immunol Rev.* 2012;248(1):188–204.

Recent advances in molecular genetics have improved the understanding of the complex interplay of the nervous system and the immune system. Many of the same signals that activate the immune response also stimulate afferent sensory fibers of the vagus nerve; information is integrated centrally and relayed via efferent fibers that return to the periphery to complete the inflammatory reflex arc. A review of the physiology and potential therapeutic interventions is presented.

Rider P, Voronov E, Dinarello CA, et al. Alarmins: feel the stress. *J Immunol.* 2017;198(4):1395–1402.

Danger-associated molecular patterns (DAMPs) propagate the noninfectious inflammatory response. Release of DAMPs has long been thought to be a passive process that occurs secondary to cell necrosis and release of intracellular products. Here, the authors demonstrate that DAMP release can be an active process that can occur without loss of subcellular compartmentalization.

Xiao W, Mindrinos MN, Seok J, et al. A genomic storm in critically injured humans. *J Exp Med.* 2011;208(13):2581–2590.

The human response to injury was historically thought to occur in a stepwise fashion: the initial proinflammatory response and the subsequent antiinflammatory response. In this study, the authors propose a new paradigm of simultaneous activation of the pro- and antiinflammatory components of the immune system based on genomic wide expression from leukocytes. They show that 80% of the leukocyte transcriptome expression is altered in the event of injury, a true genomic storm.

REFERENCES

1. Kolaczkowska E, Kubes P. Neutrophil recruitment and function in health and inflammation. *Nat Rev Immunol.* 2013;13(3):159–175.
2. Franken L, Schiwon M, Kurts C. Macrophages: sentinels and regulators of the immune system. *Cell Microbiol.* 2016;18(4):475–487.
3. Mellman I. Dendritic cells: master regulators of the immune response. *Cancer Immunol Res.* 2013;1(3):145–149.
4. Jain A, Pasare C. Innate control of adaptive immunity: beyond the three-signal paradigm. *J Immunol.* 2017;198(10):3791–3800.
5. Geginat J, Paroni M, Facciotti F, et al. The CD4-centered universe of human T cell subsets. *Semin Immunol.* 2013;25(4):252–262.
6. Fu G, Miao L, Wang M, et al. The postoperative immunosuppressive phenotypes of peripheral T helper cells are associated with poor prognosis of breast cancer patients. *Immunol Invest.* 2017;46(7):647–662.
7. Pieper K, Grimbacher B, Eibel H. B-cell biology and development. *J Allergy Clin Immunol.* 2013;131(4):959–971.
8. Romo MR, Perez-Martinez D, Ferrer CC. Innate immunity in vertebrates: an overview. *Immunology.* 2016;148(2):125–139.
9. Matzinger P. The danger model: a renewed sense of self. *Science.* 2002;296(5566):301–305.
10. Rider P, Voronov E, Dinarello CA, et al. Alarmins: feel the Stress. *J Immunol.* 2017;198(4):1395–1402.
11. Cohen I, Rider P, Vornov E, et al. IL-1alpha is a DNA damage sensor linking genotoxic stress signaling to sterile inflammation and innate immunity. *Sci Rep.* 2015;5:14756.
12. Kawai T, Akira S. Toll-like receptors and their crosstalk with other innate receptors in infection and immunity. *Immunity.* 2011;34(5):637–650.
13. Patel MN, Carroll RG, Galvan-Pena S, et al. Inflammasome priming in sterile inflammatory disease. *Trends Mol Med.* 2017;23(2):165–180.
14. Kalbitz M, Fattahi F, Grailer JJ, et al. Complement-induced activation of the cardiac NLRP3 inflammasome in sepsis. *FASEB J.* 2016;30(12):3997–4006.
15. Yang H, Wang H, Chavan SS, et al. High mobility group box protein 1 (HMGB1): the prototypical endogenous danger molecule. *Mol Med.* 2015;21(suppl 1):S6–S12.
16. Chousterman BG, Swirski FK, Weber GF. Cytokine storm and sepsis disease pathogenesis. *Semin Immunopathol.* 2017;39(5):517–528.
17. King EG, Bauza GJ, Mella JR, et al. Pathophysiologic mechanisms in septic shock. *Lab Invest.* 2014;94(1):4–12.
18. Guisasola MC, Alonso B, Bravo B, et al. An overview of cytokines and heat shock response in polytraumatized patients. *Cell Stress Chaperones.* 2018;23(4):483–489.
19. Schulte W, Bernhagen J, Bucala R. Cytokines in sepsis: potent immunoregulators and potential therapeutic targets-an updated view. *Mediators of Inflammation.* 2013;2013:165974.
20. Walsh JT, Hendrix S, Boato F, et al. MHCII-independent CD4+ T cells protect injured CNS neurons via IL-4. *J Clin Invest.* 2015;125(2):699–714.
21. Haque S, Morris JC. Transforming growth factor-β: a therapeutic target for cancer. *Hum Vaccin Immunother.* 2017;13(8):1741–1750.
22. Ricklin D, Barratt-Due A, Mollnes TE. Complement in clinical medicine: clinical trials, case reports and therapy monitoring. *Mol Immunol.* 2017;89:10–21.
23. Netea MG, Latz E, Mills KH, et al. Innate immune memory: a paradigm shift in understanding host defense. *Nat Immunol.* 2015;16(7):675–679.
24. Boehm T, Swann JB. Origin and evolution of adaptive immunity. *Annu Rev Anim Biosci.* 2014;2:259–283.
25. den Haan JM, Arens R, van Zelm MC. The activation of the adaptive immune system: cross-talk between antigen-presenting cells, T cells and B cells. *Immunol Lett.* 2014;162(2 Pt B):103–112.
26. Pavlov VA, Tracey KJ. Neural regulation of immunity: molecular mechanisms and clinical translation. *Nat Neurosci.* 2017;20(2):156–166.
27. Olofsson PS, Rosas-Ballina M, Levine YA, et al. Rethinking inflammation: neural circuits in the regulation of immunity. *Immunol Rev.* 2012;248(1):188–204.

28. Silverman MN, Sternberg EM. Glucocorticoid regulation of inflammation and its functional correlates: from HPA axis to glucocorticoid receptor dysfunction. *Ann N Y Acad Sci.* 2012;1261:55–63.
29. Cruz-Topete D, Cidlowski JA. One hormone, two actions: anti- and pro-inflammatory effects of glucocorticoids. *Neuroimmunomodulation.* 2015;22(1-2):20–32.
30. Annane D, Pastores SM, Rochwerg B, et al. Guidelines for the Diagnosis and Management of Critical Illness-Related Corticosteroid Insufficiency (CIRCI) in critically ill patients (Part I): Society of Critical Care Medicine (SCCM) and European Society of Intensive Care Medicine (ESICM) 2017. *Crit Care Med.* 2017;45(12):2078–2088.
31. Fry DE. Sepsis, systemic inflammatory response, and multiple organ dysfunction: the mystery continues. *Am Surg.* 2012;78(1):1–8.
32. Bone RC, Balk RA, Cerra FB, et al. Definitions for sepsis and organ failure and guidelines for the use of innovative therapies in sepsis. The ACCP/SCCM Consensus Conference Committee. American College of Chest Physicians/Society of Critical Care Medicine. *Chest.* 1992;101(6):1644–1655.
33. Rosenthal MD, Moore FA. Persistent inflammatory, immunosuppressed, catabolic syndrome (PICS): a new phenotype of multiple organ failure. *J Adv Nutr Hum Metab.* 2015;1(1):e784.
34. Efron PA, Mohr AM, Bihorac A, et al. Persistent inflammation, immunosuppression, and catabolism and the development of chronic critical illness after surgery. *Surgery.* 2018;164(2):178–184.
35. Tompkins RG. Genomics of injury: the glue grant experience. *J Trauma Acute Care Surg.* 2015;78(4):671–686.
36. Binkowska AM, Michalak G, Slotwinski R. Current views on the mechanisms of immune responses to trauma and infection. *Cent Eur J Immunol.* 2015;40(2):206–216.
37. Sauaia A, Moore FA, Moore EE. Postinjury inflammation and organ dysfunction. *Crit Care Clin.* 2017;33(1):167–191.
38. Sharma D, Jakkampudi A, Reddy R, et al. Association of systemic inflammatory and anti-inflammatory responses with adverse outcomes in acute pancreatitis: preliminary results of an ongoing study. *Dig Dis Sci.* 2017;62(12):3468–3478.
39. Doughty L. Adaptive immune function in critical illness. *Curr Opin Pediatr.* 2016;28(3):274–280.
40. Jensen IJ, Sjaastad FV, Griffith TS, et al. Sepsis-induced T cell immunoparalysis: the ins and outs of impaired T cell immunity. *J Immunol.* 2018;200(5):1543–1553.
41. Xiao W, Mindrinos MN, Seok J, et al. A genomic storm in critically injured humans. *J Exp Med.* 2011;208(13):2581–2590.
42. Pan W, Zhang AQ, Gu W, et al. Identification of haplotype tag single nucleotide polymorphisms within the nuclear factor-κB family genes and their clinical relevance in patients with major trauma. *Crit Care.* 2015;19(1):95.
43. Longbottom ER, Torrance HD, Owen HC, et al. Features of postoperative immune suppression are reversible with interferon gamma and independent of interleukin-6 pathways. *Ann Surg.* 2016;264(2):370–377.
44. Shankar Hari M, Summers C. Major surgery and the immune system: from pathophysiology to treatment. *Curr Opin Crit Care.* 2018;24(6):588–593.
45. Sweeney TE, Khatri P. Benchmarking sepsis gene expression diagnostics using public data. *Crit Care Med.* 2017;45(1):1–10.
46. Sauaia A, Moore EE, Johnson JL, et al. Temporal trends of postinjury multiple-organ failure: still resource intensive, morbid, and lethal. *J Trauma Acute Care Surg.* 2014;76(3):582–592; discussion 592–583.
47. Hutchings L, Watkinson P, Young JD, et al. Defining multiple organ failure after major trauma: a comparison of the denver, sequential organ failure assessment, and marshall scoring systems. *J Trauma Acute Care Surg.* 2017;82(3):534–541.
48. Hutchings SD, Naumann DN, Hopkins P, et al. Microcirculatory impairment is associated with multiple organ dysfunction following traumatic hemorrhagic shock: the MICROSHOCK study. *Crit Care Med.* 2018;46(9):e889–e896.
49. Hawkins RB, Raymond SL, Stortz JA, et al. Chronic critical illness and the persistent inflammation, immunosuppression, and catabolism syndrome. *Front Immunol.* 2018;9:1511.
50. Rosenthal MD, Kamel AY, Rosenthal CM, et al. Chronic critical illness: application of what we know. *Nutr Clin Pract.* 2018;33(1):39–45.

4 CHAPTER

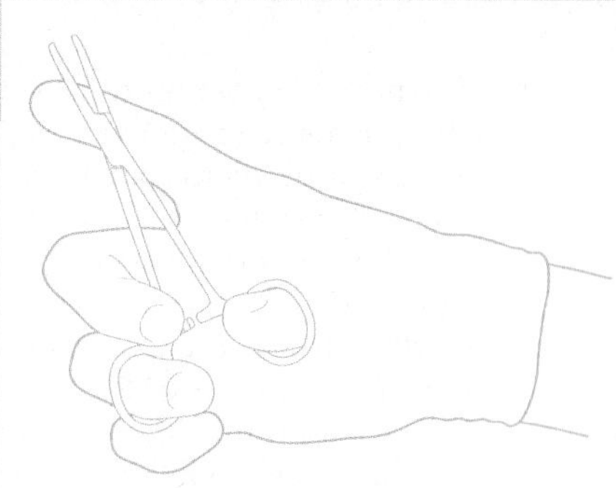

Shock, Electrolytes, and Fluid

Sawyer Gordon Smith, Martin Allan Schreiber

OUTLINE

Surgeons are the masters of fluids because they need to be. They care for patients who cannot eat or drink for various reasons; for example, they have hemorrhaged, undergone surgery, or lost fluids from tubes, drains, or wounds. Surgeons are obligated to know how to care for these patients, who put their lives in their hands. This topic might appear simple only for those who do not understand the complexities of the human body and its ability to regulate and compensate fluids. In reality, the task of managing patients' blood volume is one of the most challenging burdens surgeons face, often requiring complete control of the intake and output of fluids and electrolytes and often in the presence of blood loss. Surgeons do not yet completely understand the physiology of shock and resuscitation, and their knowledge is superficial. Given the nature of the profession, they have studied those topics and dealt with patients who bleed and exsanguinate. Historically, wartime experience has always helped them move ahead in their knowledge of the management of fluids and how to better resuscitate. The recent wars in Iraq and Afghanistan are no exception as we have learned much from these wars.

Constant attention to and titration of fluid loss therapy is required because the human body is dynamic. The key to treatment is to realize what an individual patient's initial condition is and to understand that their fluid status is constantly changing. Bleeding, sepsis, neuroendocrine disturbances, and dysfunctional regulatory systems can all affect patients who are undergoing the dynamic changes of illness and healing. The correct management of blood volume is highly time-dependent. If it is managed well, surgeons are afforded the chance to manage other aspects of surgery, such as nutrition, administration of antibiotics, drainage of abscesses, relief of obstruction and of incarceration, treatment of ischemia, and resection of tumors. Knowing the difference between dehydration, anemia, hemorrhage, and overresuscitation is vital.

The human body is predominantly water, which resides in the intravascular, intracellular, and interstitial (or third) space. Water movement between these spaces is dependent on many variables. This chapter focuses on the management of the intravascular space because it is the only space surgeons have direct access to, and managing the intravascular space is the only way to impact the other two fluid compartments.

This chapter also examines historical aspects of shock, fluids, and electrolytes—not just to note interesting facts or to pay tribute to deserving physicians, but also to try to understand how knowledge evolved over time. Doing so is vital to understanding past changes in management as well as to accept future changes. We are often awed at the discoveries of the past yet also astounded by how wrong we often were and why. Certainly, in turn, future surgeons will look back at our current body of knowledge and be amazed at how little we knew and how frequently we were wrong. A consequence of not studying the past is to repeat its errors.

After the historical highlights, this chapter discusses various fluids that are now used along with potential fluids under development. Finally, caring for perioperative patients is explored from a daily needs perspective.

HISTORY

History is disliked by those who are in a hurry to just learn the bottom line. Learning from the past, however, is essential to know which treatments have worked and which have not. Dogma must always be challenged and questioned. Were the current treatments based on science? Studying the history of shock is important for at least three reasons. First, physicians and physiologists have been fascinated with blood loss out of necessity. Second, we need to assess what experiments have or have not been done. Third, we need to know more, because our current understanding of shock is elementary.

Resuscitation

One of the earliest authenticated resuscitations in the medical literature is the "miraculous deliverance of Anne Green," who was executed by hanging on December 14, 1650.[1] Green was executed in the customary way by "being turned off a ladder to hang by the neck." She hanged for half an hour, during which time some of her friends pulled "with all their weight upon her legs, sometimes lifting her up, and then pulling her down again with a sudden jerk, thereby the sooner to dispatch her out of her pain" (Fig. 4.1). When everyone thought she was dead, the body was taken down, put in a coffin, and taken to the private house of Dr. William Petty, who, by the King's orders, was allowed to perform autopsies on the bodies of all persons who had been executed.

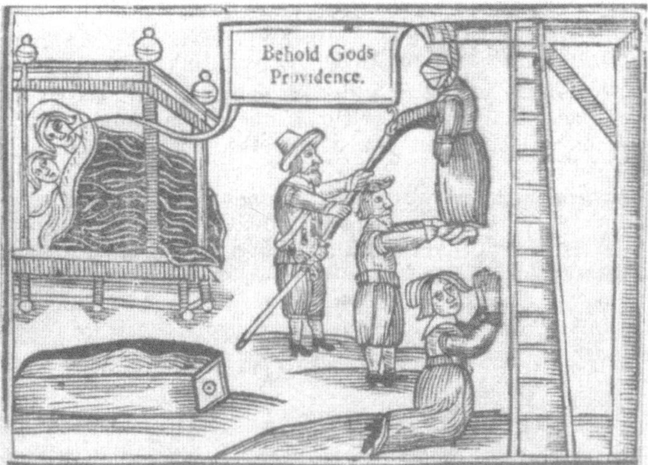

FIG. 4.1 Miraculous deliverance of Anne Green, who was executed in 1650. (From Hughes JT. Miraculous deliverance of Anne Green: an Oxford case of resuscitation in the seventeenth century. *Br Med J (Clin Res Ed)*. 1982;285:1792–1793; by kind permission of the Bodleian Library, Oxford.)

When the coffin was opened, Green was observed to take a breath, and a rattle was heard in her throat. Petty and his colleague, Thomas Willis, abandoned all thoughts of dissection and proceeded to revive their patient. They held her up in the coffin and then, by wrenching her teeth apart, poured hot cordial into her mouth, which caused her to cough. They rubbed and chafed her fingers, hands, arms, and feet; after a quarter of an hour of such effort, they put more cordial into her mouth. Then, after tickling her throat with a feather, she opened her eyes momentarily.

At that stage, they opened a vein and bled her of 5 ounces of blood. They continued administering the cordial and rubbing her arms and legs. Next, they applied compressing bandages to her arms and legs. Heating plasters were put to her chest, and another plaster was inserted as an enema "to give heat and warmth to her bowels." They then placed Green in a warm bed with another woman to lie with her to keep her warm. After 12 hours, Green began to speak; 24 hours after her revival, she was answering questions freely. At 2 days, her memory was normal, apart from her recollection of her execution and the resuscitation.

Shock

Hemorrhagic shock has been extensively studied and written about for many centuries. Injuries, whether intentional or not, have occurred so frequently that much of the understanding of shock has been learned by surgeons taking care of the injured.

What is shock? The current widely accepted definition is inadequate perfusion of tissue. However, many subtleties lie behind this statement. Nutrients for cells are required, but which nutrients are not currently well defined. Undoubtedly, the most critical nutrient is oxygen, but concentrating on just oxygenation alone probably represents very elemental thinking. Blood is highly complex and carries countless nutrients, buffers, cells, antibodies, hormones, chemicals, electrolytes, and antitoxins. Even if we think in an elemental fashion and try to optimize the perfusion of tissue, the delivery side of the equation is affected by blood volume, anemia, and cardiac output (CO). Moreover, the use of nutrients is affected by infection and drugs. The vascular tone plays a role as well; for example, in neurogenic shock, the sympathetic tone is lost, and in sepsis, systemic vascular resistance decreases because of a broken homeostatic process or possibly because of evolutionary factors.

The term *shock* appears to have been first employed in 1743 in a translation of the French treatise of Henri Francois Le Dran regarding battlefield wounds. He used the term to designate the act of impact or collision, rather than the resulting functional and physiologic damage. However, the term can be found in the book *Gunshot Wounds of the Extremities*, published in 1815 by Guthrie, who used it to describe physiologic instability.

Humoral theories persisted until the late nineteenth century, but in 1830, Herman provided one of the first clear descriptions of intravenous (IV) fluid therapy. In response to a cholera epidemic, he attempted to rehydrate patients by injecting 6 ounces of water into the vein. In 1831, O'Shaughnessy also treated cholera patients by administering large volumes of salt solutions intravenously and published his results in *Lancet*.[2] Those were the first documented attempts to replace and to maintain the extracellular internal environment or the intravascular volume. Note, however, that the treatment of cholera and dehydration is not the ideal treatment of hemorrhagic shock.

In 1872, Gross defined shock as "a manifestation of the rude unhinging of the machinery of life." His definition, given its accuracy and descriptiveness, has been repeatedly quoted in the literature.

Theories on the cause of shock persisted through the late nineteenth century; although it was unexplainable, it was often observed. George Washington Crile concluded that the lowering of the central venous pressure in the shock state in animal experiments was due to a failure of the autonomic nervous system.[3] Surgeons witnessed a marked change in ideas about shock between 1888 and 1918. In the late 1880s, there were no all-encompassing theories, but most surgeons accepted the generalization that shock resulted from a malfunctioning of some part of the nervous system. Such a malfunctioning has now been shown to *not* be the main reason—but surgeons are still perplexed by the mechanisms of hemorrhagic shock, especially regarding the complete breakdown of the circulatory system that occurs in the later stages of shock.

In 1899, using contemporary advances with sphygmomanometers, Crile proposed that a profound decline in blood pressure (BP) could account for all symptoms of shock. He also helped alter the way physicians diagnosed shock and followed its course. Before Crile, most surgeons relied on respiration, pulse, or a declining mental status when evaluating the condition of patients. After Crile's first books were published, many surgeons began measuring BP. In addition to changing how surgeons thought about shock, Crile was a part of the therapeutic revolution. His theories remained generally accepted for nearly two decades, predominantly in surgical circles. Crile's work persuaded Harvey Cushing to measure BP in all operations, which in part led to the general acceptance of BP measurement in clinical medicine. Crile also concluded that shock was not a process of dying but rather a marshaling of the body's defenses in patients struggling to live. He later deduced that the reduced volume of circulating blood, rather than the diminished BP, was the most critical factor in shock.

Crile's theories evolved as he continued his experimentations; in 1913, he proposed the kinetic system theory. He was interested in thyroid hormone and its response to wounds but realized that epinephrine was a key component of the response to shock. He relied on experiments by Walter B. Cannon, who found that epinephrine was released in response to pain or emotion, shifting blood from the intestines to the brain and extremities. Epinephrine release also stimulated the liver to convert glycogen to sugar for release into the circulation. Cannon argued that all the actions of epinephrine aided the animal in its effort to defend itself.[4]

Crile incorporated Cannon's study into his theory. He proposed that impulses from the brain after injury stimulated glands to secrete their hormones, which, in turn, effected sweeping changes throughout the body. Crile's kinetic system included a complex interrelationship among the brain, heart, lungs, blood vessels, muscles, thyroid gland, and liver. He also noted that if the body received too much stress, the adrenal glands would run out of epinephrine, the liver of glycogen, the thyroid of its hormone, and the brain itself of energy, accounting for autonomic changes. Once the kinetic system ran out of energy, BP would fall, and the organism would go into shock.

Henderson recognized the importance of decreased venous return and its effect on cardiac output and arterial pressure. His work was aided by advances in techniques that allowed careful recording of the volume curves of the ventricles. Fat embolism also led to a shock-like state, but its possible contribution was questioned because study results were difficult to reproduce. The vasomotor center and its contributions in shock were heavily studied in the early 1900s. In 1914, Mann noted that unilaterally innervated vessels of the tongues of dogs, ears of rabbits, and paws of kittens appeared constricted during shock compared with contralaterally denervated vessels.

Battlefield experiences continued to intensify research on shock. During the World War I era, Cannon used clinical data from the war as well as data from animal experiments to examine the shock state carefully. He theorized that toxins and acidosis contributed to the previously described lowering of vascular tone. He and others then focused on acidosis and the role of alkali in preventing and prolonging shock. The adrenal gland and the effect of cortical extracts on adrenalectomized animals were of fascination during this period.

Then, in the 1930s, a unique set of experiments by Blalock[5] determined that almost all acute injuries are associated with changes in fluid and electrolyte metabolism. Such changes were primarily the result of reductions in the effective circulating blood volume. Blalock showed that those reductions after injury could be the result of several mechanisms (Box 4.1). He clearly showed that fluid loss in injured tissues was loss of extracellular fluid (ECF) that was unavailable to the intravascular space for maintaining circulation. The original concept of a "third space," in which fluid is sequestered and therefore unavailable to the intravascular space, evolved from Blalock's studies.

Carl John Wiggers first described the concept of "irreversible shock."[6] His 1950 textbook, *Physiology of Shock,* represented the attitudes toward shock at that time. In an exceptionally brilliant summation, Wiggers assembled the various signs and symptoms of shock from various authors in that textbook (Fig. 4.2), along with his own findings.

His experiments used what is now known as the Wiggers prep. In his most common experiments, he used previously splenectomized dogs and cannulated the arterial system. He took advantage of an evolving technology that allowed him to measure the pressure within the arterial system, and he studied the effects of lowering BP through blood withdrawal. After removing the dogs' blood to an arbitrary set point (typically, 40 mm Hg), he noted that their BP soon spontaneously rose as fluid was spontaneously recruited into the intravascular space.

To keep the dogs' BP at 40 mm Hg, Wiggers had to continually withdraw additional blood. During this compensated phase of shock, the dogs could use their reserves to survive. Water was recruited from the intracellular compartment as well as from the extracellular space. The body tried to maintain the vascular flow necessary to survive. However, after a certain period, he found that to keep the dogs' BP at the arbitrary set point of 40 mm Hg, he had to reinfuse shed blood; he termed this phase *uncompensated,* or *irreversible, shock*. Eventually, after a period of irreversible shock, the dogs died.

BOX 4.1 Causes of shock according to Blalock in 1930.

- Hematogenic (oligemia)
- Neurogenic (caused primarily by nervous influences)
- Vasogenic (initially decreased vascular resistance and increased vascular capacity, as in sepsis)
- Cardiogenic (failure of the heart as a pump as in cardiac tamponade or myocardial infarction)
- Large volume loss (extracellular fluid, as occurs in patients with diarrhea, vomiting, and fistula drainage)

Data from Blalock A. *Principles of surgical care: Shock and other problems*. St. Louis, MO: CV Mosby; 1940.

The ideal model is uncontrolled hemorrhage, but its main problem is that the volume of hemorrhage is uncontrolled by the nature of the experiment. Variability is the highest in this model even though it is the most realistic. Computer-assisted pressure models that mimic the pressures during uncontrolled shock can be used to reduce the artificiality of the pressure-controlled model. Smith and colleagues[7] developed a hybrid model of controlled, uncontrolled hemorrhage whereby a standardized grade V liver laceration is made in swine. The swine bleed to either a specified pressure or fixed volume, and bleeding is controlled with packing. This removes the variability classically associated with uncontrolled hemorrhage.[7]

Fluids

How did the commonly used IV fluids, such as normal saline, enter medical practice? It is often taken for granted, given the vast body of knowledge in medicine, that they were adopted through a rigorous scientific process, but that was not the case.

Normal saline has a long track record and is extremely useful, but we now know that it also can be harmful. Hartog Jakob Hamburger, in his in vitro studies of red cell lysis in 1882, incorrectly suggested that 0.9% saline was the concentration of salt in human blood. He chose 0.9% saline because it has the same freezing point as human serum. This fluid is often referred to as physiologic or normal saline, but it is neither physiologic nor normal.

In 1831, O'Shaughnessy described his experience in the treatment of cholera:

> *Universal stagnation of the venous system, and rapid cessation of the arterialization of the blood, are the earliest, as well as the most characteristic effects. Hence the skin becomes blue—hence animal heat is no longer generated—hence the secretions are suspended; the arteries contain black blood, no carbonic acid is evolved from the lungs, and the returned air of expiration is cold as when it enters these organs.*[8]

SYMPTOM COMPLEX OF SHOCK

General appearance and reactions	Skin and mucous membranes	Circulation and blood
Mental state	*Skin*	*Superficial veins*
Apathy	Pale, livid, ashen gray	Collapsed and invisible
Delayed responses	Slightly cyanotic	Failure to fill on compression or massage
Depressed cerebration	Moist, clammy	Inconspicuous jugular pulsations
Weak voice	Mottling of dependent parts	*Heart*
Listless or restlessness	Loose, dry, inelastic, cold	Apex sounds feeble
Countenance	*Mucous membranes*	Rate usually rapid
Drawn–anxious	Pale, livid, slightly cyanotic	*Radial pulse*
Lusterless eyes	*Conjunctiva*	Usually rapid
Sunken eyeballs	Glazed, lusterless	Small volume "feeble," "thready"
Ptosis of upper lids (slight)	*Tongue*	*Brachial blood pressures*
Upward rotation of eyeballs (slight)	Dry, pale, parched, shriveled	Lowered
Neuromuscular state	Respiration and metabolism	Pulse pressure small
Hypotonia	*Respiration*	*Retinal vessels*
Muscular weakness	Variable but not dyspneic	Narrowed
Tremors and twitchings	Usually increased rate	*Blood volume*
Involuntary muscular movements	Variable depth	Reduced
Difficulty in swallowing	Occasional deep sighs	*Blood chemistry*
Neuromuscular tests	Sometimes irregular or phasic	Hemoconcentration or hemodilution
Depressed tendon reflexes	*Temperature*	Venous O_2 decreased
Depressed sensibilities	Subnormal, normal, supernormal	A-V O_2 difference increased
Depressed visual and auditory reflexes	*Basal metabolic rate*	Arterial CO_2 reduced
General but variable symptoms	reduced (?)	Alkali reserve reduced
Thirst		
Vomiting		
Diarrhea		
Oliguria		
Visible or occult blood in vomitus and stools		

FIG. 4.2 Wiggers' description of symptom complex of shock. (From Wiggers CJ. The present status of shock problem. *Physiol Rev.* 1942;22:74–123.)

O'Shaughnessy wrote those words at the age of 22, having just graduated from Edinburgh Medical School. He tested his new method of infusing IV fluids on a dog and observed no ill effects. Eventually, he reported that the aim of his method was to restore blood to its natural specific gravity and to restore its deficient saline matters. His experience with human cholera patients taught him that the practice of bloodletting, then highly common, was good for "diminishing the venous congestion" and that nitrous oxide (laughing gas) was not useful for oxygenation.

In 1832, Robert Lewins reported that he witnessed Thomas Latta injecting extraordinary quantities of saline into veins, with the immediate effects of "restoring the natural current in the veins and arteries, of improving the color of the blood, and [of] recovering the functions of the lungs." Lewins described Latta's saline solution as consisting of "two drachms of muriate, and two scruples of carbonate, of soda, to sixty ounces of water." Later, however, Latta's solution was found to equate to having 134 mmol per liter of Na^+, 118 mmol per liter of Cl^-, and 16 mmol per liter of bicarbonate (HCO_3^-).

During the next 50 years, many reports cited various recipes used to treat cholera, but none resembled 0.9% saline. In 1883, Sydney Ringer reported on the influence exerted by the constituents of the blood on the contractions of the ventricle (Fig. 4.3). Studying an isolated heart model from frogs, he used 0.75% saline and a blood mixture made from dried bullocks' blood.[9] In his attempts to identify which aspect of blood caused better results, he found that a "small quantity of white of egg completely obviates the changes occurring with saline solution." He concluded that the benefit of "white of egg" was because of the albumin or the potassium chloride. To show what worked and what did not, he described endless experiments with alterations of multiple variables.

However, Ringer later published another article stating that his previously reported findings could not be repeated; through careful study, he realized that the water used in his first article was actually not distilled water, as reported, but rather tap water from the New River Water Company. It turned out that his laboratory technician, who was paid to distill the water, took shortcuts and used tap water instead. Ringer analyzed the water and found that it contained many trace minerals (Fig. 4.4). Through careful and diligent experimentation, he found that calcium bicarbonate or calcium chloride—in doses even smaller than in blood—restored good contractions of the frog ventricles. The third component that he found essential to good contractions was sodium bicarbonate. Thus, the three ingredients that he found essential were potassium, calcium, and bicarbonate. Ringer solution soon became ubiquitous in physiologic laboratory experiments.

In the early twentieth century, fluid therapy by injection under the skin (hypodermoclysis) and infusion into the rectum (proctoclysis) became routine. Hartwell and Hoguet reported its use in intestinal obstruction in dogs, laying the foundation for saline therapy in human patients with intestinal obstruction.

As IV crystalloid solutions were developed, Ringer solution was modified, most notably by pediatrician Alexis Hartmann. In 1932, wanting to develop an alkalinizing solution to administer to his acidotic patients, Hartmann modified Ringer solution by adding sodium lactate. The result was lactated Ringer (LR) or Hartmann solution. He used sodium lactate (instead of sodium bicarbonate); the conversion of lactate into sodium bicarbonate was sufficiently slow to lessen the danger posed by sodium bicarbonate, which could rapidly shift patients from compensated acidosis to uncompensated alkalosis.

In 1924, Rudolph Matas, regarded as the originator of modern fluid treatment, introduced the concept of the continued IV drip but also warned of potential dangers of saline infusions. He stated, "Normal saline has continued to gain popularity but the problems with metabolic derangements have been repeatedly shown but seem to have fallen on deaf ears." In healthy volunteers, modern-day experiments have shown that normal saline can cause abdominal discomfort and pain, nausea, drowsiness, and decreased mental capacity to perform complex tasks.

The point is that normal saline and LR solution have been formulated for conditions other than the replacement of blood, and the reasons for the formulation are archaic. Such solutions have been useful for dehydration; when they are used in relatively small volumes (1–3 L/day), they are well tolerated and relatively harmless; they provide water, and the human body can tolerate the amounts of electrolytes they contain. Over the years, LR solution has attained widespread use for treatment of hemorrhagic shock. However, normal saline and LR solution are mostly permeable through

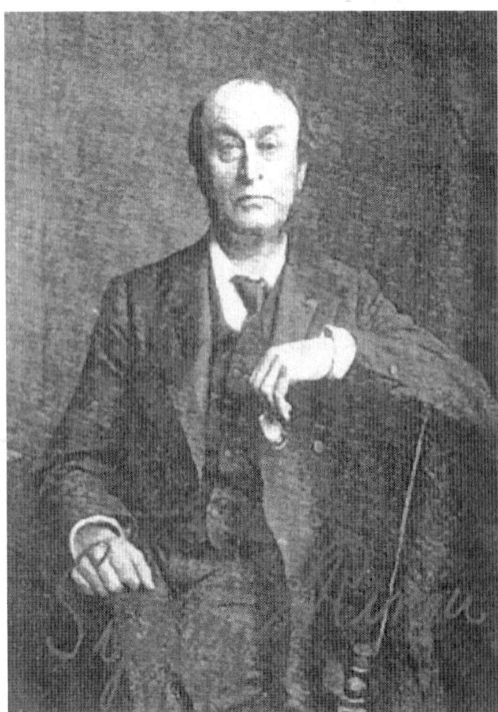

FIG. 4.3 Sydney Ringer, credited for the development of lactated Ringer solution. (From Baskett TF. Sydney Ringer and lactated Ringer's solution. *Resuscitation.* 2003;58:5–7.)

They consist of:		
Calcium	38.3	per million.
Magnesium	4.5	"
Sodium	23.3	"
Potassium	7.1	"
Combined carbonic acid	78.2	"
Sulfuric acid	55.8	"
Chlorine	15	"
Silicates	7.1	"
Free carbonic acid	54.2	"

FIG. 4.4 Sidney Ringer's report of contents in water from the New River Water Company. (From Baskett TF. Sydney Ringer and lactated Ringer's solution. *Resuscitation.* 2003;58:5–7.)

the vascular membrane, but they are poorly retained in the vascular space. After a few hours, only about 175 to 200 mL of a 1-L infusion remains in the intravascular space. In countries other than the United States, LR solution is often referred to as Hartmann solution, and normal saline is referred to as physiologic (sometimes even spelled *fisiologic*) solution. With the advances in science in the last 50 years, it is difficult to understand why advances in resuscitation fluids have not been made.

Blood Transfusions

Concerned about the blood that injured patients lost, Crile began to experiment with blood transfusions. As he stated, "After many accidents, profuse hemorrhage often led to shock before the patient reached the hospital. Saline solutions, adrenalin, and precise surgical technique could substitute only up to a point for the lost blood." At the turn of the nineteenth century, transfusions were seldom used. Their use waxed and waned in popularity because of transfusion reactions and difficulties in preventing clotting in donated blood. Through his experiments in dogs, Crile showed that blood was interchangeable: he transfused blood without blood group matching. Alexis Carrel was able to sew blood vessels together with his triangulation technique, using it to connect blood vessels from one person to another for the purpose of transfusions. However, Crile found Carrel's technique too slow and cumbersome in humans, so he developed a short cannula to facilitate transfusions.

By the time World War II occurred, shock was recognized as the single most common cause of treatable morbidity and mortality. At the time of the Japanese attack on Pearl Harbor on December 7, 1941, no blood banks or effectual blood transfusion facilities were available. Most military locations had no stocks of dried pooled plasma. Although the wounded of that era were evacuated quickly to a hospital, the mortality rate was still high. IV fluids of any kind were essentially unavailable, except for a few liters of saline manufactured by means of a still in the operating room. IV fluid was usually administered by an old Salvesen flask and a reused rubber tube. Often, a severe febrile reaction resulted from the use of that tubing.

The first written documentation of resuscitation in World War II patients was 1 year after Pearl Harbor, in December 1942, in notes from the 77th Evacuation Hospital in North Africa. E. D. Churchill stated, "The wounded in action had for the most part either succumbed or recovered from any existing shock before we saw them. However, later cases came to us in shock, and some of the early cases were found to be in need of whole blood transfusion. There was plenty of reconstituted blood plasma available. However, some cases were in dire need of whole blood. We had no transfusion sets, although such are available in the United States: no sodium citrate; no sterile distilled water; and no blood donors."

The initial decision to rely on plasma rather than on blood appears to have been based in part on the view held in the Office of the Surgeon General of the Army and in part on the opinion of the civilian investigators of the National Research Council. Those civilian investigators thought that, in shock, the blood was thick and the hematocrit level was high. On April 8, 1943, the Surgeon General stated that no blood would be sent to the combat zone. Seven months later, he again refused to send blood overseas because of the following: (1) his observation of overseas theaters had convinced him that plasma was adequate for resuscitation of wounded men; (2) from a logistics standpoint, it was impractical to make locally collected blood available farther forward than general hospitals in the combat zone; and (3) shipping space was too sparse. Vasoconstricting drugs such as epinephrine were condemned because they were thought to decrease blood flow and tissue perfusion as they dammed the blood in the arterial portion of the circulatory system.

During World War II, out of necessity, efforts to make blood transfusions available heightened and led to the institution of blood banking for transfusions. Better understanding of hypovolemia and inadequate circulation led to the use of plasma as a favored resuscitative solution, in addition to whole blood replacement. Thus, the treatment of traumatic shock greatly improved. The administration of whole blood was thought to be extremely effective, so it was widely used. Mixing whole blood with sodium citrate in a 6:1 ratio to bind the calcium in the blood, which prevented clotting, worked well.

However, no matter what solution was used—blood, colloids, or crystalloids—the blood volume seemed to increase by only a fraction of what was lost. In the Korean War era, it was recognized that more blood had to be infused for the blood volume lost to be adequately regained. The reason for the need for more blood was unclear, but it was thought to be due to hemolysis, pooling of blood in certain capillary beds, and loss of fluid into tissues. Considerable attention was given to elevating the feet of patients in shock.

PHYSIOLOGY OF SHOCK

Bleeding

Research and experience have both taught us much about the physiologic responses to bleeding. The advanced trauma life support (ATLS) course defines four classes of shock (Table 4.1). In general, that categorization has helped point out the physiologic responses to hemorrhagic shock, emphasizing the identification of blood loss and guiding treatment. Conceptually, shock occurs at three anatomical areas of the cardiovascular system (Fig. 4.5). The first level occurs at the heart where cardiogenic abnormalities can be either extrinsic (tension pneumothorax, hemothorax, or cardiac tamponade) or intrinsic (myocardial infarction causing pump failure, cardiac contusion or laceration, or cardiac failure). The second level occurs at the large or medium vessel level in which hemorrhage and loss of blood volume leads to shock. The last level occurs with the small vessels in which either neurologic dysfunction or sepsis leads to vasodilatation and maldistribution of the blood volume leading to shock.

The four classes of shock according to the ATLS course are problematic as they were not rigorously tested or proven and were

TABLE 4.1 ATLS classes of hemorrhagic shock.

	CLASS I	CLASS II	CLASS III	CLASS IV
Blood loss (%)	0–15	15–30	30–40	>40
Central nervous system	Slightly anxious	Mildly anxious	Anxious or confused	Confused or lethargic
Pulse (beats/min)	<100	>100	>120	>140
Blood pressure	Normal	Normal	Decreased	Decreased
Pulse pressure	Normal	Decreased	Decreased	Decreased
Respiratory rate	14–20/min	20–30/min	30–40/min	>35/min
Urine (mL/hr)	>30	20–30	5–15	Negligible
Fluid	Crystalloid	Crystalloid	Crystalloid + blood	Crystalloid + blood

ATLS, Advanced trauma life support.

admittedly arbitrarily generated. Patients often do not exhibit all of the physiologic changes described by this table, particularly those at age extremes. Due to higher water composition of their bodies, children are able to compensate with large volumes of blood loss, often exhibiting only tachycardia until they reach a tipping point where they are no longer able to compensate, at which point they have a rapid clinical decline. Elderly patients show almost an opposite physiology, as they are less equipped to compensate for blood loss and will show signs of a higher level of shock at a lower volume of blood loss. This is due to a reduced ability of cardiac compensation and fluid reserve recruitment.

The problem with the signs and symptoms classically taught in ATLS classes is that, in reality, the manifestations of shock can be confusing and difficult to assess, particularly in trauma patients. For example, changes in mental status can be caused by blood loss, traumatic brain injury (TBI), pain, or illicit drugs. The same dilemma applies for respiratory rate and skin changes. Are alterations in a patient's respiratory rate or skin color caused by pneumothorax, rib fracture pain, or inhalation injury?

Although there are various methods that have been developed for monitoring patients in shock, BP continues to be the most clinically useful measure. When caring for a patient in shock, goals of resuscitation need to be established, remembering that baseline BP and blood volume are extremely variable and often unknown while initiating treatment. Although there is no single universally applicable endpoint of resuscitation, a combination of normalization of serum lactate, base deficit, pH, and hemorrhage control, if applicable, are markers that can be considered along with the rest of the patient's overall clinical status.[10]

Clinical symptoms are relatively few in patients who are in class I shock with the exception of anxiety. Is the anxiety after injury from blood loss, pain, trauma, or drugs? A heart rate higher than 100 beats/min has been used as a physical sign of bleeding, but evidence of its significance is minimal. Brasel and collegues[11] have shown that heart rate was neither sensitive nor specific in determining the need for emergent intervention, the need for packed red blood cell (PRBC) transfusions in the first 2 hours after an injury, or the severity of the injury. Heart rate was not altered by the presence of hypotension (systolic BP <90 mm Hg).

In patients who are in class II shock, we are taught that their heart rate is increased, but, as previously mentioned, this is a highly unreliable marker; pain and mere nervousness can also increase heart rate. The change in pulse pressure, the difference between systolic and diastolic pressure, is also difficult to identify because the baseline BP of patients is not always known. The change in pulse pressure is thought to be caused by an epinephrine response constricting vessels, resulting in higher diastolic pressures.

Not until patients are in class III shock does BP theoretically decrease. At this stage, patients have lost 30% to 40% of their blood volume; for an average man weighing 75 kg (168 pounds), this equates to 2 L of blood loss (Fig. 4.6). It is helpful to remember that a can of soda or beer is 355 mL; a six-pack is 2130 mL. Theoretically, if a patient is hypotensive from blood loss, they have loss the equivalent of a six-pack of blood. The first and most

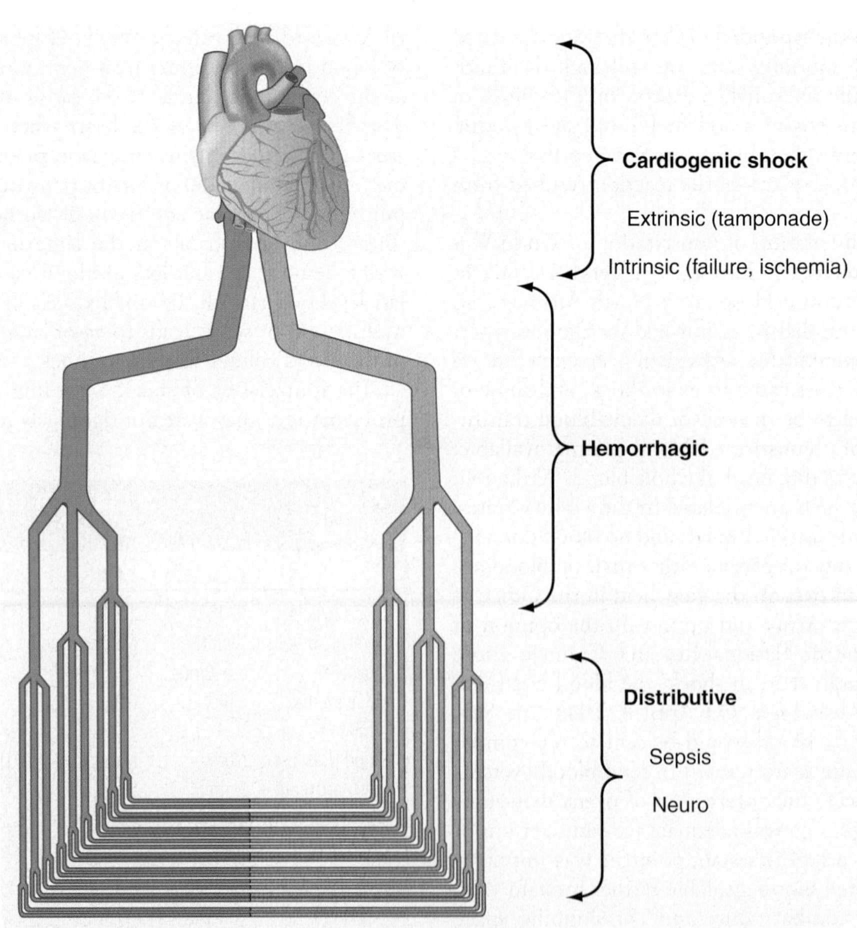

FIG. 4.5 Types of shock.

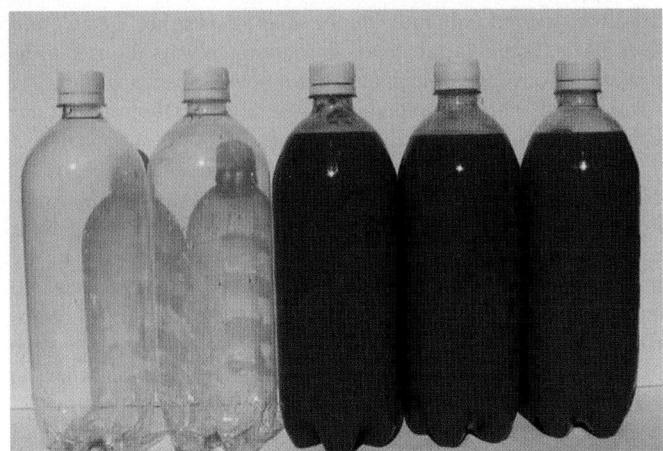

FIG. 4.6 Liters of blood lost for class III shock, or 40% of 5 L, according to the advanced trauma life support (ATLS).

important key when a patient is in shock due to hemorrhage is recognizing that blood loss is the cause of their shock and identify the source of bleeding and treat it. Resuscitation occurs simultaneously as needed.

Since ATLS is designed for physicians who are not surgeons, many subtleties around the physiology of a bleeding patient are missing. However, surgeons know that there are some nuances of the varied responses to injuries in both animals and humans. In the case of arterial hemorrhage, for example, animals do not necessarily manifest tachycardia as their first response when bleeding, but actually become bradycardic. It is speculated that this is a teleological mechanism as a bradycardic response reduces cardiac output and minimizes uncontrolled exsanguination. A bradycardic response to bleeding is not consistently shown in all animals, including humans. Some evidence shows that this response, termed relative bradycardia, does occur in humans. Relative bradycardia is defined as a heart rate less than 100 beats/min while simultaneously having a systolic BP below 90 mm Hg. When bleeding patients have relative bradycardia, their mortality rate is lower. Up to 44% of hypotensive patients who are not bleeding have relative bradycardia. However, this lower heart rate is only protective to a certain level as patients with a heart rate below 60 beats/min are usually moribund. Bleeding patients with a heart rate of 60 to 90 beats/min have the highest survival rate compared with patients with tachycardia (a heart rate of more than 90 beats/min).[12]

The physiologic response to bleeding also subtly differs according to whether the source of bleeding is arterial or venous. Arterial bleeding is an obvious problem, but it often stops temporarily on its own; the human body has evolved to trap the blood loss in adventitial tissues, and the transected artery will spasm and thrombose. A lacerated artery can actually bleed more than a transected artery as the spasm of the lacerated artery can enlarge the hole in the vessel. Thrombosis of the artery sometimes does *not* occur in transected or lacerated vessels. Also, since the arterial system does not have valves, the recorded BP can drop early even before large-volume loss has occurred. In these patients with arterial bleeding, hypotension may occur soon, but because ischemia has not yet had a chance to occur, measurements of lactate or base deficit can yield normal results.

In contrast, venous bleeding is typically slower, allowing the human body time to compensate. This slower progression provides the time necessary for recruitment of water from the intracellular and interstitial spaces. This leads to large volumes of blood that can be lost before hypotension ensues. Since venous or capillary bed bleeding is slower and the body has a chance to compensate, this allows for tissue ischemia to develop during the process and thus there is time for lactate and base deficit results to be abnormal. Venous blood loss can be massive before hypotension occurs.

It is generally taught that the hematocrit or hemoglobin (Hgb) level is not reliable in predicting blood loss. This can be true in patients who have not been resuscitated, but in patients who have received crystalloids, a rapid drop in the hematocrit and hemoglobin levels can occur. Bruns and associates[13] have shown that the hemoglobin level can be low within the first 30 minutes after patients arrive at trauma centers. Therefore, high or normal hemoglobin levels do not rule out significant bleeding. But, a low hemoglobin level, because it occurs rapidly, generally reflects severe blood loss.

The lack of good indicators to distinguish which patients are bleeding has led many investigators to examine heart rate variability or complexity as a potential new vital sign. Many clinical studies have shown that heart rate variability or complexity is associated with poor outcome. Heart rate variability or complexity would have to be calculated using software, with a resulting index on which clinicians would have to rely. This information would not be available by merely examining patients. Another issue with heart rate variability or complexity is that the exact physiologic mechanism for its association with poor outcome has yet to be elucidated.[14] This new vital sign may be programmable into currently used monitors, but its usefulness has yet to be confirmed.

Hypotension has been traditionally set, arbitrarily, at 90 mm Hg and below. But this level can be variable from patient to patient, especially depending on age. Eastridge and coworkers[15] have suggested that hypotension be redefined as below 110 mm Hg. In 2008, Bruns and colleagues[16] confirmed the concept, showing that a prehospital BP below 110 mm Hg was associated with a sharp increase in mortality and that 15% of patients with BP below 110 mm Hg would eventually die in the hospital. As a result, they recommended redefining prehospital trauma triage criteria. In older patients, normal vital signs may miss occult hypoperfusion as geriatric patients often have increased lactate and base deficit levels.

Shock Index

Since heart rate and systolic BP individually are not accurate at identifying hemorrhagic shock and because the traditionally taught combination of tachycardia and decreased systolic BP does not always occur together, the shock index (SI), which uses these two variables together, was developed. SI is defined as heart rate divided by systolic BP. It has been shown to be a better marker for assessing severity of shock than heart rate and BP alone. It has utility not only in trauma patients often in hemorrhagic shock, but also in patients who are in shock from other causes such as sepsis, obstetrics, myocardial infarction, stroke, and other acute illnesses. In the trauma population, SI has been shown to be more useful than heart rate and BP alone, and it has also been shown to be of benefit specifically in the pediatric and geriatric populations. It has been correlated with need for interventions such as blood transfusion and invasive procedures including operations. SI is known as a hemodynamic stability indicator. However, SI does not consider the diastolic BP, and thus a modified SI (MSI) was created. MSI is defined as heart rate divided by mean arterial pressure. As MSI rises, this indicates a low stroke volume and low systemic vascular resistance, a sign of hypodynamic circulation. In contrast, low MSI indicates a hyperdynamic state. MSI has been considered a better marker than SI for mortality rate prediction. Although SI or

MSI is better than heart rate and systolic BP alone, the combination of one of these variables with heart rate and systolic BP will undoubtedly be more useful. There are additional studies showing that more complex calculations with more variables are more useful than simpler ones. For example, taking into account the age, mechanism of injury, Glasgow Coma Scale (GCS) score, lactate levels, hemoglobin levels, and other physiologic parameters will result in statistically better prediction than with one individual vital sign. It is intuitive that the addition of variables would be more predictive of outcome. That is why the presence of an experienced surgeon is critical; in a few seconds, the astute clinician will quickly consider multiple variables, including gender, age, GCS score, mechanism of injury, and other parameters. Whereas SI and MSI are statistically more accurate than one individual parameter, there is no substitute for the experienced clinician at the bedside. This may be the reason that SI and MSI have not been widely adopted.

Lactate and Base Deficit

Lactate has stood the test of time as an associated marker of injury and possibly ischemia.[17] However, new data question the etiology and role of lactate. The emerging information is confusing; it suggests that we may not understand lactate for what it truly implies. Lactate has long been thought to be a byproduct of anaerobic metabolism and is routinely perceived to be an end waste product that is completely unfavorable. Physiologists are now questioning this paradigm and have found that lactate behaves more advantageously than not. An analogy would be that firefighters are associated with fires, but that does not mean that firefighters are bad nor does it mean that they caused the fires.

Research has shown that lactate increases in muscle and blood during exercise. It is at its highest level at or just after exhaustion, which led to the assumption that lactate was a waste product. In addition, we also know that lactic acid appears in response to muscle contraction and continues in the absence of oxygen. Furthermore, accumulated lactate disappears when an adequate supply of oxygen is present in tissues.

Recent evidence indicates that lactate is an active metabolite, capable of moving between cells, tissues, and organs where it may be oxidized as fuel or reconverted to form pyruvate or glucose. It now appears that increased lactate production and concentration, as a result of anoxia or dysoxia, are often the exception rather than the rule. Lactate seems to be a shuttle for energy; the lactate shuttle is now the subject of much debate. The end product of glycolysis is pyruvic acid. Lack of oxygen is thought to convert pyruvate into lactate. However, lactate formation may allow carbohydrate metabolism to continue through glycolysis. It is postulated that lactate is transferred from its site of production in the cytosol to neighboring cells and to a variety of organs (e.g., heart, liver, and kidney), where its oxidation and continued metabolism can occur.

Lactate is also being studied as a pseudohormone as it seems to regulate the cellular redox state through exchange and conversion into pyruvate and through its effects on the ratio of nicotinamide adenine dinucleotide to nicotinamide adenine dinucleotide (reduced)—the NAD^+/NADH ratio. It is released into the systemic circulation and taken up by distal tissues and organs, where it also affects the redox state in those cells. Further evidence has shown that it affects wound regeneration with promotion of increased collagen deposition and neovascularization. Lactate may also induce vasodilatation and catecholamine release and stimulate fat and carbohydrate oxidation.

Lactate levels in blood are highly dependent on the equilibrium between production and elimination from the bloodstream. The liver is predominantly responsible for clearing lactate, and liver disease affects lactate levels. Lactate was always thought to be produced from anaerobic tissues, but it now seems that a variety of tissue beds that are not undergoing anaerobic metabolism produce lactate when they are signaled with distress.

In canine muscle, lactate is produced by moderate-intensity exercise when the oxygen supply is ample. A high adrenergic stimulus also causes a rise in lactate as the body prepares for or responds to stress. A study of climbers of Mount Everest showed that the resting PO_2 on the summit was about 28 mm Hg and decreased even more during exercise. The blood lactate level in those climbers was essentially the same as at sea level even though they were in a state of hypoxia.[18] These facts lead us to question what we believed we knew about lactate and its true role.

In humans, lactate may be the preferred fuel in the brain and heart; in these tissues, infused lactate is used before glucose at rest and during exercise. Since lactate is glucose sparing, it allows glucose and glycogen levels to be maintained. In addition to lactate's being preferred in the brain, evidence seems to indicate that lactate is protective to brain tissues in TBI and acts as fuel during exercise for the brain.[19] The level of lactate, whether it is a waste product or a source of energy, seems to signify tissue distress whether it is from anaerobic conditions or other factors.[20] During times of stress, there is a release of epinephrine and other catecholamines, which also causes a release of lactate.

Base deficit, a measure of the number of millimoles of base required to correct the pH of a liter of whole blood to 7.4, seems to correlate well with lactate level, at least in the first 24 hours after a physiologic insult. Rutherford, in 1992, showed that a base deficit of 8 was associated with a 25% mortality rate in patients older than 55 years without a head injury or in patients younger than 55 years with a head injury. When base deficit remains elevated, most clinicians believe that it is an indication of ongoing shock.[21]

One problem with base deficit is that it is commonly influenced by the chloride in various resuscitation fluids, resulting in a hyperchloremic nongap acidosis. In patients with renal failure, base deficit can also be a poor predictor of outcome; in the acute stage of renal failure, a base deficit of less than 6 mmol/L is associated with poor outcome.[22] With the use of hypertonic saline (HTS), which has three to eight times the sodium chloride concentration of normal saline, the hyperchloremic acidosis has been shown to be relatively harmless. However, when HTS is used, base deficit should be interpreted with caution.

Compensatory Mechanisms

When shock occurs, blood flow is diverted from less critical to more critical tissues. The earliest compensatory mechanism in response to a decrease in intravascular volume is an increase in sympathetic activity. Such an increase is mediated by pressure receptors or baroreceptors in the aortic arch, atria, and carotid bodies. A decrease in pressure inhibits parasympathetic discharge while norepinephrine and epinephrine are liberated and cause adrenergic receptors in the myocardium and vascular smooth muscle to be activated. Heart rate, contractility, and peripheral vascular resistance are increased, resulting in increased BP. However, the various tissue beds are not affected equally; blood is shunted from less critical organs (e.g., skin, skeletal muscle, and splanchnic circulation) to more critical organs (e.g., brain, liver, and kidneys).

The juxtaglomerular apparatus in the kidney, in response to the vasoconstriction and decrease in blood flow, produces the enzyme renin, which leads to the generation of angiotensin I. The angiotensin-converting enzyme located on the endothelial cells of the pulmonary arteries converts angiotensin I to angiotensin II. In turn, angiotensin II stimulates an increased sympathetic drive at the level of the nerve terminal by releasing hormones from the adrenal medulla. In response, the adrenal medulla affects intravascular volume during shock by secreting catechol hormones—epinephrine, norepinephrine, and dopamine—which are all produced from phenylalanine and tyrosine. They are called *catecholamines* because they contain a catechol group derived from the amino acid tyrosine. The release of catecholamines is thought to be responsible for the elevated glucose level in hemorrhagic shock. Although the role of glucose elevation in hemorrhagic shock is not fully understood, it does not seem to affect outcome.[23]

Cortisol, also released from the adrenal cortex, plays a major role in fluid equilibrium. In the adrenal cortex, the zona glomerulosa produces aldosterone in response to stimulation by angiotensin II. Aldosterone is a mineralocorticoid that modulates renal function by increasing recovery of sodium and excretion of potassium. Angiotensin II also causes the reabsorption of sodium through a direct action on the renal tubules. Sodium is the primary osmotic ion in the human body in the regulation of water balance, with the reabsorption of sodium leading to the reabsorption of water, which subsequently leads to intravascular volume expansion in response to shock. One problem is that the release of these hormones is not infinite, thus the supply can be exhausted in a state of ongoing shock.

This regulation of intravascular fluid status is further affected by the carotid baroreceptors and the atrial natriuretic peptides. Signals are sent to the supraoptic and paraventricular nuclei in the brain. Antidiuretic hormone (ADH) is released from the pituitary, causing retention of free water at the level of the kidney. Simultaneously, volume is recruited from the extravascular and cellular spaces. A shift of water occurs as hydrostatic pressures fall in the intravascular compartment. At the capillary level, hydrostatic pressures also are reduced because the precapillary sphincters are vasoconstricted more than the postcapillary sphincters.

Lethal Triad

The lethal triad of acidosis, hypothermia, and coagulopathy is common in resuscitated patients who are bleeding or in shock from various factors. Our basic understanding is that inadequate tissue perfusion results in acidosis caused by lactate production. In the shock state, the delivery of nutrients to the cells is thought to be inadequate, leading to a decrease in the body's main energy storage molecule, adenosine triphosphate (ATP). The human body relies on ATP production to maintain homeostatic temperatures, like all homeothermic (warm-blooded) animals do. Thus, if ATP production is inadequate to maintain body temperature, the body will trend toward the ambient temperature. For most human patients, this is 22°C (72°F), the temperature inside typical hospitals. The resulting hypothermia and acidosis then affect the efficiency of enzymes, which work best at 37°C and a pH of 7.4. For surgeons, the critical issue with hypothermia is the coagulation cascade dependence on enzymes that are affected by hypothermia. If enzymes are not functioning optimally due to hypothermia, coagulopathy worsens, which can contribute to uncontrolled bleeding from injuries or the surgery itself. Further bleeding continues to fuel the triad. The optimal method to break the "vicious circle of death" is to stop the bleeding and the causes of hypothermia. In most typical scenarios, hypothermia is not spontaneous from ischemia but is induced because of use of room temperature fluid or cold blood products.

Acidosis

Bleeding causes a host of responses. During the resuscitative phase, the lethal triad (acidosis, hypothermia, and coagulopathy) is frequent in severely bleeding patients, most likely because of two major factors. First, decreased perfusion causes lactic acidosis and consumptive coagulopathy. Second, room temperature and large volume fluids lead to worsening hypothermia and dilutional coagulopathy, creating a resuscitation injury. Some believe that the acidotic state is not necessarily undesirable because the body tolerates acidosis better than alkalosis. Oxygen is more easily offloaded from hemoglobin in the acidotic environment. Basic scientists who try to preserve tissue ex vivo find that cells live longer in an acidotic environment. Correcting acidosis with sodium bicarbonate has classically been avoided as it is treating a laboratory value or symptom. The focus should be to correct the cause of the acidosis. Treating the pH alone has shown no benefit, but it can lead to complacency. It is also argued that rapidly injecting sodium bicarbonate can worsen intracellular acidosis from the diffusion of the converted CO_2 into the cells.

The best fundamental approach to metabolic acidosis from shock is to treat the underlying cause of shock. In the surgeon's case, this is due to blood loss or ischemic tissue. However, some clinicians believe that treating the pH has advantages because the enzymes necessary for clotting function better at an optimal temperature and optimal pH. Coagulopathy can contribute to uncontrolled bleeding, so some have recommended treating acidosis with bicarbonate infusion for patients in dire scenarios. Treating acidosis with sodium bicarbonate may have a benefit in an unintended and unrecognized way. Rapid infusion of bicarbonate is usually accompanied by a rise in BP in hypotensive patients. This rise is usually attributed to correcting the pH; however, sodium bicarbonate in most urgent scenarios is given in ampules. The 50-mL ampule of sodium bicarbonate has 1 mEq/mL—in essence, similar to giving a hypertonic concentration of sodium, which quickly draws fluid into the vascular space. Given its high sodium concentration, a 50-mL bolus of sodium bicarbonate has physiologic results similar to 325 mL of normal saline or 385 mL of LR solution. Essentially, it is like giving small doses of HTS. Sodium bicarbonate quickly increases CO_2 levels by its conversion in the liver, so if the minute ventilation is not increased, respiratory acidosis can result.

THAM (tromethamine; tris[hydroxymethyl] aminomethane) is a biologically inert amino alcohol of low toxicity that buffers CO_2 and acids. It is sodium free and limits the generation of CO_2 in the process of buffering. At 37°C, the pK_a of THAM is 7.8, making it a more effective buffer than sodium bicarbonate in the physiologic range of blood pH. In vivo, THAM supplements the buffering capacity of the blood bicarbonate system by generating sodium bicarbonate and decreasing the partial pressure of CO_2. It rapidly distributes to the extracellular space and slowly penetrates the intracellular space, except in the case of erythrocytes and hepatocytes, and it is excreted by the kidney. Unlike sodium bicarbonate, which requires an open system to eliminate CO_2 to exert its buffering effect, THAM is effective in a closed or semiclosed system, and it maintains its buffering ability during hypothermia. THAM acetate (0.3 M, pH 8.6) is well tolerated, does not cause tissue or venous irritation, and is the only formulation available in the United States. THAM may induce respiratory depression and hypoglycemia, which may require ventilatory assistance and the administration of glucose.

The initial loading dose of THAM acetate (0.3 M) for the treatment of acidemia may be estimated as follows:

$$\text{THAM (in milliliters of 0.3-M solution)} = \text{Lean body weight (in kilograms)} \times \text{Base deficit (in millimoles per liter)}$$

The maximal daily dose is 15 mmol/kilogram/day for an adult (3.5 L of a 0.3-M solution in a patient weighing 70 kg). It is indicated in the treatment of respiratory failure (acute respiratory distress syndrome [ARDS] and infant respiratory distress syndrome) and has been associated with the use of hypothermia and permissive hypercapnia (controlled hypoventilation). Other indications are diabetic and renal acidosis, salicylate and barbiturate intoxication, and increased intracranial pressure (ICP) associated with brain trauma. It is used in cardioplegic solutions and during liver transplantation. Despite these attributes, THAM has not been documented clinically to be more efficacious than sodium bicarbonate.

Hypothermia

Hypothermia can be both beneficial and detrimental. A fundamental knowledge of hypothermia is of vital importance in the care of surgical patients. The beneficial aspects of hypothermia are mainly a result of decreased metabolism. Injury sites are often iced, creating vasoconstriction and decreasing inflammation through decreased metabolism. This concept of cooling to slow metabolism is also the rationale behind using hypothermia to decrease ischemia during cardiac, transplant, pediatric, and neurologic surgery. Also, amputated extremities are iced before reimplantation. Cold water near-drowning victims have higher survival rates, thanks to preservation of the brain and other vital organs. The Advanced Life Support Task Force of the International Liaison Committee of Resuscitation now recommends cooling (to 32°C–34°C for 12–24 hours) of unconscious adults who have spontaneous circulation after out-of-hospital cardiac arrest caused by ventricular fibrillation. Induced hypothermia is vastly different from spontaneous hypothermia, which is typically from shock, inadequate tissue perfusion, or cold fluid infusion.

Medical or accidental hypothermia is vastly different from trauma-associated hypothermia (Table 4.2). The survival rates after accidental hypothermia range from about 12% to 39%. The average temperature drop is to about 30°C (range, 13.7°C–35.0°C). That lowest recorded temperature in a survivor of accidental hypothermia (13.7°C, or 56.7°F) was in an extreme skier in Norway; she was trapped under the ice and eventually fully recovered neurologically.

The data in patients with trauma-associated hypothermia differ. Their survival rate falls dramatically with their core temperature, reaching 100% mortality when it reaches 32°C at any point—whether it is in the emergency department, operating room, or intensive care unit (ICU). In trauma patients, hypothermia is due to shock and is thought to perpetuate uncontrolled bleeding because of the associated coagulopathy. Trauma patients with a postoperative core temperature below 35°C have a fourfold increase in death; below 33°C, a sevenfold increase in death. Hypothermic trauma patients tend to be more severely injured, older, and have increased blood loss requiring increased number of transfusions.[24]

Surprisingly, in a study using the National Trauma Data Base, Shafi and colleagues showed that hypothermia and its associated poor outcome were not related to the state of shock. It was previously thought that a core temperature below 32°C was uniformly fatal in trauma patients who have the additional insult of tissue injury and bleeding. However, a small number of trauma patients have now survived, despite a recorded core temperature below 32°C. Beilman and coworkers demonstrated that hypothermia was associated with more severe injuries, bleeding, and a higher rate of multiple-organ dysfunction in the ICU, but not with death on multivariate analysis.[25]

To understand hypothermia, we have to remember that humans are homeothermic (warm-blooded) animals, in contrast to poikilothermic (cold-blooded) animals such as snakes and fish. To maintain a body temperature of 37°C, our hypothalamus uses a variety of mechanisms to tightly control core body temperature. We use oxygen as the key ingredient or fuel to generate heat in the mitochondria in the form of ATP. When ATP production is below its lowest threshold, one of the side effects is the lowering of body temperature to the ambient temperature, which typically is less than core body temperature. In contrast, during exercise, we use more oxygen as more ATP is required, and we produce excess heat. In an attempt to modulate core temperature, we start perspiring to use the cooling properties of evaporation.

Hypothermia, although potentially beneficial, is detrimental in trauma patients mainly because it causes coagulopathy. Cold affects the coagulation cascade by decreasing enzyme activity, enhancing fibrinolytic activity, and causing platelet dysfunction. Platelets are affected by the inhibition of thromboxane B_2 production, resulting in decreased aggregation. A heparin-like substance is released, causing diffuse intravascular coagulation–like syndrome. Hageman factor and thromboplastin are some of the enzymes most affected. Even a drop in core temperature of just a few degrees results in 40% inefficiency in some of the enzymes.

Heat affects the coagulation cascade so much that when blood is drawn in cold patients and sent to the laboratory, the sample is heated to 37°C, because even 1 or 2 degrees of cold delays clotting and renders test results inaccurate. Thus, in a cold and coagulopathic patient, if the coagulation profile obtained from the laboratory shows an abnormality, the result represents the level of coagulopathy if the patient (and not just the sample) had been warmed to 37°C. Therefore, a cold patient is always more coagulopathic than indicated by the coagulation profile. A normal coagulation profile does not necessarily represent what is going on in the body.

Heat is measured in calories. One calorie is the amount of energy required to raise the temperature of 1 mL of water (which has, by definition, a specific heat of 1.0). It takes 1 kcal to raise the temperature of 1 L of water by 1°C. If an average man (weight, 75 kg) consisted of pure water, it would take 75 kcal to raise his temperature by 1°C. However, we are not made of pure water, and blood has a specific heat coefficient of 0.87. Thus, the human body as a whole has a specific heat coefficient of 0.83. Therefore, it actually takes 62.25 kcal (75 kg × 0.83) to raise body temperature by 1°C. If a patient were to lose 62.25 kcal, body temperature would drop by 1°C. This basic science is important in choosing methods to retain heat or to treat hypothermia or hyperthermia. It allows one to compare the efficacy of one method with another.

The normal basal metabolic heat generation is about 70 kcal/hr. Shivering can increase this to 250 kcal/hr. Heat is transferred to and from the body by contact or conduction (as in a frying pan

TABLE 4.2 Classification of hypothermia.

	TRAUMA	ACCIDENTAL
Mild	36–34°C	35–32°C
Moderate	34–32°C	32–28°C
Severe	<32°C (<90°F)	<28°C (<82°F)

and Jacuzzi), air or convection (as in an oven and sauna), radiation, and evaporation. Convection is an extremely inefficient way to transfer heat as the air molecules are so far apart compared with liquids and solids. Conduction and radiation are the most efficient ways to transfer heat. However, heating the patient with radiation is fraught with inconsistencies and technical challenges, and thus it is difficult to apply clinically, so we are left with conduction to transfer energy efficiently.

Warming or cooling through manipulation of the temperature of IV fluids is useful as it uses conduction to transfer heat. Although IV fluids can be warmed, the U.S. Food and Drug Administration (FDA) allows fluid warmers to be set at a maximum of 40°C. Therefore, the differential between a cold trauma patient (34°C) and warmed fluid is only 6°C. Thus, 1 L of warmed fluids can transfer only 6 kcal to the patient. As previously calculated, one needs about 62 kcal to raise the core temperature by 1°C. Therefore, we need 10.4 L of warmed fluids to raise the core temperature by 1°C to 35°C. Once that has been achieved, the differential is now only 5°C between the patient and the warmed fluid, so it actually takes 12.5 L of warmed fluids to raise the patient from 35°C to 36°C. A cold patient at 32°C needs to be given 311 kcal (75 kg × 0.83) to be warmed to 37°C. Note that a liter of fluid must be given at the highest rate possible because, if the infusion rate is slow, it cools to room temperature as the IV line is exposed to ambient room temperature. To avoid IV-line cooling, devices that warm fluids up to the point of insertion into the body should be used.

Warming of patients by infusion of warmed fluids is difficult, but fluid warmers are still critically important; the main reason to warm fluids is to prevent patients from being cooled further. Cold fluids can cool patients quickly. The fluids that are typically infused are at either room temperature (22°C) or 4°C if the fluids were refrigerated. The internal temperature of a refrigerator is 4°C, and this is where PRBCs are stored. Therefore, it takes 5 L of 22°C fluid or 2 L of cold blood products to cool a patient by 1°C. Again, the main reason for using fluid warmers is not necessarily to warm patients but to prevent cooling them during resuscitation.

Rewarming techniques are classified as passive or active. Active warming is further classified as external or internal (Table 4.3). Passive warming involves *preventing* heat loss. An example of passive warming is drying the patient to minimize evaporative cooling, giving warm fluids to prevent cooling, or covering the patient so that the ambient air temperature immediately around the patient can be higher than the room temperature. Covering the patient's head helps reduce a tremendous amount of heat loss. Aluminum-lined head covers are preferred; they reflect back the heat that is normally lost through the scalp. Warming of the room technically helps reduce the heat loss gradient, but the surgical staff is usually unable to work in a humidified room of 37°C. Preventing evaporative heat loss also includes closing an open body cavity, such as the chest or abdomen. The most important way to prevent heat loss is to treat hemorrhagic shock by controlling bleeding. Once shock has been treated, metabolism will heat the patient from his or her core. This point cannot be overemphasized.

Active warming is the act of transferring calories to the patient, either externally through the skin or internally. Skin and fat are designed to be highly efficient in preventing heat transfer. Whereas the fat is insulating against loss of heat, it is also the reason that transfer of heat past the skin is difficult. Active external warming is thus inefficient because of our built-in insulation compared with internal warming. The first and most important step for active rewarming is to remove any wet clothes or bedding that is present and dry the patient prior to starting any active warming technique. Without this step, the efficiency of all methods will drop dramatically, and the importance of this step cannot be overstated. External active warming with forced-air heating, such as with Bair Hugger temperature management therapy (Arizant Healthcare Inc., Eden Prairie, MN), is technically classified as active warming, but since air is a terribly inefficient medium, so few calories are provided to patients. Forced-air heating increases only the patient's ambient temperature, but it can actually cool the patient initially because it increases evaporative heat loss if the patient is wet from blood, fluids, clothes, or sweat. Warming the skin may feel good to the patient and the surgeon, but it actually decreases shivering (a highly efficient method of internal warming that tricks the thermoregulatory nerve input on the skin). Because forced-air heating uses convection, the actual amount of active warming is estimated to be only 10 kcal/hr.

Active external warming is more efficiently performed by placing patients on heating pads, which use conduction to transfer heat. Beds are available that can warm patients faster, such as the Clinitron bed (Hill-Rom, Batesville, IN), which uses heated air-fluidized beads. Such beds are not practical in the operating room but are applicable in the ICU. Another option is the use of heating pads, which use heated water for countercurrent heat exchange. These can be placed under the patient during surgery and can be effective in minimizing mild hypothermia. The number of kilocalories per hour depends on the extent of dilatation or vasoconstriction of the blood vessels in the skin. This countercurrent heat exchange system can also be used to cool the patient if necessary.

The best method to warm patients is to deliver calories internally (Table 4.4). Heating the air used for ventilators is technically a form of internal active warming, but, again, is an inefficient method as this transfers heat via convection. The surface area of the lungs is massive, but the energy is mainly transferred through

TABLE 4.3 Classification of warming techniques.

PASSIVE	ACTIVE EXTERNAL	ACTIVE INTERNAL
Dry the patient	Bair hugger	Warmed fluids
Warm fluids	Heated warmers	Heat ventilator
Warm blankets and sheets	Lamps	Cavity lavage, chest tube, abdomen, bladder
Provide head covers	Radiant warmers	Continuous arterial or venous rewarming
Warm the room	Clinitron bed	Full or partial bypass

TABLE 4.4 Calories delivered by active warming.

METHOD	Kcal/hr
Airway from vent	9
Overhead radiant warmers	17
Heating blankets	20
Convective warmers	15–26
Body cavity lavages	35
Continuous arteriovenous rewarming	92–140
Cardiopulmonary bypass	710

humidified water droplets, mostly by convection and not conduction. The amount of heat transferred through warmed humidified air is also minimal by comparison to methods that use conduction. One method by which this can be done is the lavage of warmed fluids into body cavities via nasogastric tubes, Foley catheters, chest tubes, or lavage of the peritoneal cavity. If gastric lavage is desired, one method is continuous lavage by infusion of warmed fluids through the sump port while the fluid is sucked out of the main tube. Instruments to warm the hand through conduction show much promise but are not yet readily available.

A method that can actively rewarm a patient and also assist in the treatment of shock is extracorporeal membrane oxygenation (ECMO). With ECMO, the patient's blood is pumped through an artificial lung and then back into the bloodstream, which can support either a failing pulmonary or cardiac system. Along with oxygenation in the artificial lung, the blood can also be warmed and then returned to the patient. Recent literature also shows promise in using ECMO for rewarming after accidental hypothermia through case reports and cost-effectiveness analysis.[26,27] Cardiopulmonary bypass can also be used as it delivers heated blood at a rate of more than 5 L/min to every place in the body where there are capillaries. If full cardiopulmonary bypass is not available or not desired, alternatives include continuous venous or arterial rewarming. Venous-venous rewarming can also be accomplished using the roller pump of a dialysis machine (which is often more available to the average surgeon). A prospective study showed arterial-venous rewarming to be highly effective. It can warm patients to 37°C in about 39 minutes compared with an average warming time of 3.2 hours with standard techniques. Special Gentilello arterial warming catheters are inserted into the femoral artery, and a second line is inserted into the opposite femoral vein. The pressure from the artery produces flow, which is then directed to a fluid warmer and back into the vein. This method depends highly on the patient's BP as flow is directly related to BP. There are also commercially available central line catheters that directly heat the blood; a countercurrent exchange system heats the tip of the catheter with warmed fluids, and as blood passes over this warmed catheter, heat is directly transferred.

During recent decades, with the changes in resuscitation methods, the incidence of hypothermia has decreased. Dilutional coagulopathy also occurs less frequently as the volume of crystalloids has been minimized and particular attention has been paid to ensure that all resuscitation fluids and blood are warmed before infusion.

Coagulopathy

Coagulopathy in surgical patients is multifactorial. In addition to acidosis and hypothermia, the other usual cause of coagulopathy is decreased clotting factors. This decrease can be caused by consumption (from the innate attempt to stop bleeding), dilution (from infused fluids devoid of clotting factors), and genetic (hemophilia) factors.

Coagulopathy often needs to be corrected. The most commonly used tests for coagulopathy are prothrombin time, partial thromboplastin time, and international normalized ratio. However, these tests have been shown to be inaccurate in detecting coagulopathy in surgical patients. One of the major reasons is that coagulopathy is a dynamic state that evolves through different stages of hypocoagulability, hypercoagulability, and fibrinolysis. The traditional tests of blood clotting lack the ability to detect the evolution of coagulopathy through these stages as they only depict the coagulation state at a snapshot in time. Moreover, the traditional tests are performed at normal pH and temperature, so they do not consider the effects of hypothermia and acidosis on coagulation. These traditional tests are also performed on serum and not on whole blood and do not have the ability to measure the interaction of coagulation factors and platelets.

More recently, thromboelastography (TEG) and rotational thromboelastometry have emerged as dynamic measures of coagulation that provide a more sensitive and accurate measure of the coagulation changes seen in surgical patients. TEG and thromboelastometry are based on similar principles of detecting clot strength, which is the final product of the coagulation cascade. They are also performed on whole blood, so they consider the functional interaction of coagulation factors and platelets.

TEG parameters include R-time, reaction time; α, alpha angle; and MA, maximum amplitude. The R-time reflects the latent time until fibrin formation begins. An increase in this time may result from either decreased activity or deficiencies of coagulation factors, whereas a decrease in R-time reflects a hypercoagulable state. The steepness of the α-angle reflects the rate of fibrin formation and cross-linking with a sharper angle indicating increased fibrin formation and a flatter angle indicating slower formation. The measure of clot strength is MA, which reflects clot elasticity. The value of MA is a measure of the strength of interaction between the coagulation factors, fibrin, and platelets. Qualitative or quantitative defects in either of these would result in decreased MA. TEG provides the additional ability to measure the fibrinolytic arm of the coagulation cascade. LY30 and LY60 indices provide a measure of the fibrinolysis rate by calculating the decrease in clot strength at 30 and 60 minutes, respectively. A large lysis index reflects rapid fibrinolysis and may help guide the use of antifibrinolytic therapy, which has been shown to reduce mortality if it is used within 3 hours of injury, in these patients. Components of a TEG can help guide treatment of a bleeding patient as they can give the surgeon information regarding what part of the clotting cascade is defective. These tests are routinely used in cardiac surgery and are becoming more popular in trauma and liver transplant surgery in the form of point-of-care testing, but they are not widely available in most hospitals (Fig. 4.7).

The methods to define and to treat coagulopathy are still varied. As discussed earlier, stopping the lethal triad is the most important step to stop the vicious cycle of hemorrhage. Prothrombin complex concentrate (PCC) has become popular for the treatment of surgical coagulopathy. PCC actually has many factors (factors II, VII, IX, X) in it, including variable amounts of factor VIIa, depending on the brand of PCC used. For patients taking warfarin, PCC is the recommended treatment of choice as this treatment replaces the factors lost with warfarin. This is of particular benefit in elderly patients with TBI, in whom treatment with fresh frozen plasma (FFP) can potentially be a problem if the patient has comorbid cardiac

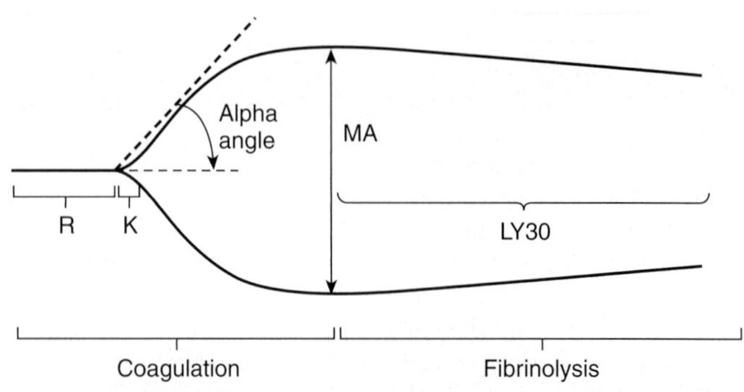

FIG. 4.7 Coagulation and fibrinolysis testing.

disease and could induce cardiac heart failure from volume overload. Additional benefit of using PCC is that the time to reversal of coagulopathy is shorter than when FFP is used. The use of blood-based component therapy is paramount in treating coagulopathy (see later, "Evolution of Modern Resuscitation"). PCC has been studied in trauma patients at risk for bleeding with promising results, but the studies are not randomized and require further confirmation.[28] If there were a drug that would stop or reduce bleeding, treat coagulopathy at a low cost, and not cause serious complications, it would be a landmark contribution to medicine. Again, the problem is that current candidates are expensive, and the adverse events from administering such a drug are still not fully elucidated.

Another target of the coagulation cascade for medications is modulating the fibrinolytic pathways. Tranexamic acid (TXA) is a synthetic analogue of the amino acid lysine and is an antifibrinolytic medication that competitively inhibits the activation of plasminogen to plasmin. It prevents degradation of fibrin, which is a protein that forms the framework of blood clots. TXA has about eight times the antifibrinolytic activity of an older analogue, ε-aminocaproic acid. It is used to treat or to prevent excessive blood loss during cardiac, liver, vascular, and orthopedic surgical procedures. It seems that topical TXA is effective and safe after total knee and hip replacement surgery along with mucosal oropharyngeal bleeding in patients who are thrombocytopenic, reducing bleeding and the need for blood transfusions. Studies have shown similar results in children undergoing craniofacial surgery, spinal surgery, and others. It is even used for heavy menstrual bleeding in oral tablet form and in dentistry as a 5% mouthwash. It has been advocated for use in trauma. It seems to be effective in reducing rebleeding in spontaneous intracranial bleeding. A small double-blinded, placebo-controlled, randomized study of 238 patients showed a reduction in progression of intracranial bleeding after trauma, but, because of the small sample size, it was not statistically significant. TXA is used to treat primary fibrinolysis, which is integral in the pathogenesis of the acute coagulopathy of trauma.

The Clinical Randomization of an Antifibrinolytic in Significant Hemorrhage (CRASH-2) trial, a multicenter randomized controlled civilian trial of 20,211 patients, showed that TXA reduced all-cause mortality versus placebo (14.5% vs. 16.0%).[29] The risk of death caused by bleeding was also reduced (4.9% vs. 5.7%). CRASH-2 also suggested that TXA was less effective and could even be harmful if treatment was delayed more than 3 hours after admission. This was confirmed in the retrospective Military Application of Tranexamic Acid in Trauma Emergency Resuscitation (MATTER) study and rapidly incorporated into military practice guidelines and subsequently for civilians worldwide.[30] The PED-TRAX study demonstrated that in children treated at a military hospital in Afghanistan, TXA administration to 66 of the 766 children was independently associated with decreased mortality and improved neurologic and pulmonary outcomes. Although the CRASH-2 trial was a randomized study with placebo, the critics of the study point out that it was performed in 270 hospitals in 40 countries, and the large sample size may result in a beta 1 error, meaning that the study was statistically significant because of the large number of patients in the study, but the small differences in outcome may not necessarily be clinically relevant. The absolute risk reduction was approximately 1.5% with an estimated number needed to treat of 68. The CRASH-3 trial is currently being conducted to assess the effect of TXA on risk of death or disability in patients with TBI. The key will be dosing, timing, and patient selection. The drug is attractive because it is inexpensive ($5.70 per dose) and easy to use with seemingly minimal side effects.

Oxygen Delivery

The definition of shock is inadequate tissue perfusion, but many clinicians have incorrectly simplified it to inadequate tissue oxygenation. Much of what we know about oxygen delivery and consumption started with a physiologist named Archibald V. Hill. He was an avid runner who measured the oxygen consumption of four runners running around an 88-m grass track (Fig. 4.8). In the process of his work, Hill defined the terms *maximum O_2 intake*, *O_2 requirement*, and *O_2 debt*. He is mostly known for his work with Otto Meyerhof, who unraveled the distinction between aerobic and anaerobic metabolism, for which they were awarded the Nobel Prize in 1922.

Blood delivers oxygen by red cells, which contain hemoglobin. The simple calculation of oxygen delivery (Do_2) is the cardiac output (CO) multiplied by the content of oxygen carried by a volume of blood (Cao_2):

$$Do_2 = CO \times Cao_2$$

The average hemoglobin molecule carries 1.34 mL of oxygen per gram, depending on the arterial hemoglobin (Hgb) oxygen saturation (Sao_2) of the red cell. In addition, a minor amount of oxygen is dissolved in plasma. This amount is calculated by multiplying the solubility constant 0.003 times the partial pressure of oxygen in the arterial blood (Pao_2). The Cao_2 of arterial blood is calculated as follows:

$$Cao_2 = (1.34 \times Hgb \times Sao_2) + (0.003 \times Pao_2)$$

where hemoglobin is in grams per deciliter. Cardiac output is heart rate multiplied by the stroke volume. In a normal state, the stroke volume can be increased by shunting blood from one tissue

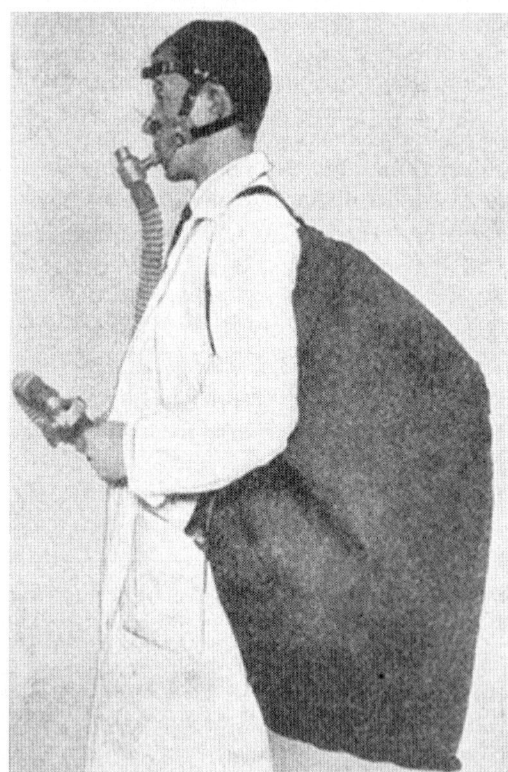

FIG. 4.8 Bag with side tube, low on the left-hand side, for use while running. The tap is carried in the left hand. (From Hill AV, Lupton H. Muscular exercise, lactic acid, and the supply and utilization of oxygen. *Q J Med.* 1923;16:135–171.)

bed to the central vasculature, but most of the change in cardiac output is due to increased heart rate. In states of hemorrhage and resuscitation, the stroke volume is affected by infusion of fluids. As blood volume is decreased, it will ultimately affect stroke volume and is compensated by an increase in heart rate.

Oxygen consumption (Vo_2) by cells is calculated by subtracting the content of oxygen in the venous system (Cvo_2) from delivered oxygen content in the arterial blood (Cao_2):

$$Vo_2 = CO \times (Cao_2 - Cvo_2)$$

After simplifying the terms and converting the units, the result is as follows:

$$Vo_2 = CO \times 1.34 \times Hgb \times (Sao_2 - Svo_2)$$

The most conventional method of sampling the venous oxygen content is by drawing blood from the most distal port of a pulmonary artery catheter. The sample is taken from the pulmonary artery because venous blood is mixed there from all parts of the body. Oxygen content in the inferior vena cava is typically higher than in the superior vena cava, which is higher than in the coronary sinus. The average mixed venous sample is 75% saturated, so the oxygen consumption is thought to be, on average, 25% of the oxygen delivered (Fig. 4.9). Thus, teleologically, there is ample reserve of oxygen delivered.

With advancements in technology, catheters are now available that can continuously measure the venous saturation in the pulmonary artery. These use technology similar to the pulse oximeter built into the tip of a pulmonary artery catheter, which uses near-infrared (NIR) light waves to measure the oxygen saturation state of hemoglobin. These advanced catheters can also provide cardiac output continuously. In the past, cardiac output was inferred by measuring the rate of change in temperature in the heart at the distal aspect of a pulmonary artery catheter by infusing a standard volume of iced or room temperature water into the proximal port and measuring the change in temperature. In recent years, pulmonary artery catheters are no longer commonly used. Venous oxygenation can still be measured from central lines, but these assessments are no longer mixed venous in nature.

Cardiac output and oxygen delivery are also affected by the end-diastolic volume of the left ventricle. As described by Starling in 1915, cardiac output increases when the ventricular fibers increase in length. There is a maximum filling point, then cardiac output no longer increases (Fig. 4.10). Left ventricular end-diastolic (LVED) volume can be inferred by using a pulmonary artery catheter and measuring the wedge pressure, which represents preload. This reflects the pressure in the left ventricle because the vessels from the pulmonary artery to the left ventricle have no valves. Alternative approaches can help optimize the filling volume in the left ventricle. Pulmonary artery catheters for calculating the right ventricular end-diastolic volume are available but are rarely used. Echocardiography using transthoracic or esophageal probes can directly estimate filling volumes in the heart. However, variations in volume

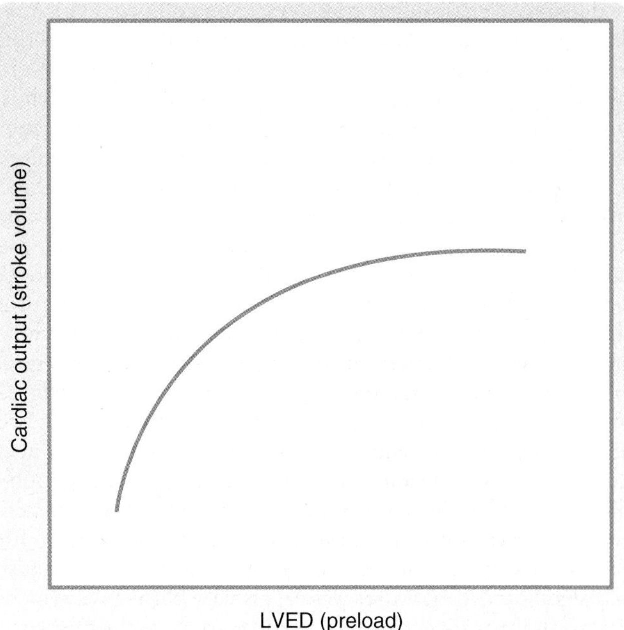

FIG. 4.10 Starling curve. As left ventricular end-diastolic *(LVED)* pressure is increased, the fibers of the heart muscle are lengthened, resulting in increased contraction and increased cardiac output. This occurs to a certain point, at which increases in volume and length do not result in increases in cardiac output.

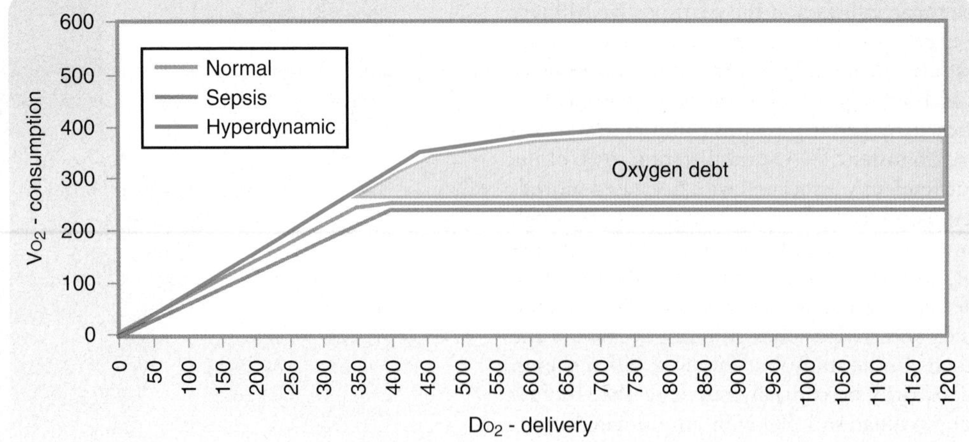

FIG. 4.9 Oxygen delivery *(Do_2)* and consumption *(Vo_2)*. During normal states, oxygen delivery is approximately 1000 mL/min of O_2. The oxygen consumption in a normal state is 25% of delivery and is approximately 250 mL/min. At very low oxygen delivery, it is believed that consumption is delivery dependent and occurs in shock. There is oxygen debt during shock and during recovery, and there is a hyperdynamic stage during which the circulatory system is paying back its oxygen debt.

and heart size can distort results. Heart size is also affected by medical conditions that can stress and dilate the heart. The interpretation of heart size and adequate resuscitation data is thus subjective.

Optimization (Supernormalization)

During the late 1980s, surgical critical care evolved into a specialty, focusing heavily on ventilator support and optimizing oxygen delivery to tissues. One of the pioneers of modern surgical critical care, William Shoemaker, theorized that during shock, because of a lack of oxygen delivery, there was anaerobic metabolism and an oxygen debt that needed to be repaid. He showed that after volume loading, if oxygen delivery increased, consumption would also increase—until a certain point, when an additional increase in oxygen delivery did not result in increased consumption. This increased oxygen consumption was thought to be the process of paying back the oxygen debt that occurred during ischemia throughout the body. Patients in shock were found to have a hyperdynamic stage in which increased oxygen delivery resulted in increased consumption. The assumption was that increased consumption was replenishing the oxygen debt that the body had incurred.

Shoemaker popularized the concept of optimization or supernormalization of oxygen delivery, which means that oxygen delivery is maximized or increased until its consumption no longer increases but instead levels off (flow independence). The optimization process involved administering a rapid bolus of fluid and confirming that it raised wedge pressure. Because the response to fluid infusion was dynamic, the infusion process had to occur during a short period, such as 20 minutes. If it took longer, changes in the vascular space and specifically the heart may be due to other variables in addition to the fluids used. Also, if the response was not measured immediately after infusion, the effect of the infusion was known to degrade quickly as fluids moved out of the vascular space. Wedge pressure and cardiac output must be measured minutes before fluid infusion to determine whether it is effective. If cardiac output increases with the wedge pressure increase, it is assumed that oxygen delivery increases. By sampling the central venous oxygen content when measuring cardiac output, clinicians can determine whether oxygen consumption also increases. This process was originally repeated until it was demonstrated that the fluid bolus did not increase cardiac output. The goal was to optimize oxygen delivery from the delivery-dependent portion of the curve to the portion that was not delivery dependent (Fig. 4.9).

The preferred fluid during the optimization process was LR solution as it was inexpensive and thought to be innocuous. Once the Starling curve was optimized, in that LVED volume could no longer be increased with increases in wedge pressure (preload), wedge pressure would be kept at that maximal level. Further increases in wedge pressure without increasing LVED volume meant that patients might suffer from unnecessary pulmonary edema.

Once fluid infusion maximized cardiac output and oxygen delivery, an inotropic agent would be added to further push cardiac output to a higher level. The agent recommended at that time was dobutamine. The dose was increased, and its effect on cardiac output was documented. With each maneuver, oxygen consumption was measured and cardiac output "optimized" to meet the consumption demands. This optimizing process maximized oxygen delivery to ensure that all tissue beds were being fed adequately. Shoemaker's earlier clinical trials had shown that patients resuscitated in this manner had a lower incidence of multiple-organ dysfunction syndrome (MODS) and death. During this optimizing era, ARDS and MODS were the leading causes of late death in trauma patients.

However, subsequent clinical studies failed to repeat Shoemaker's success. Randomized prospective trials showed that the optimization of oxygen delivery and consumption did not improve outcome. In general, patients who responded to the optimization process did well, but those who could not have their oxygen delivery augmented to a higher level did poorly. Thus, although response to optimization was prognostic of outcome, the process itself did not seem to change outcome. One of the reasons that the earlier studies succeeded may have been because the control patients were not adequately resuscitated. With the later trials, when patients were adequately resuscitated, the optimization process did not improve outcome. In fact, the aggressive use of fluids to achieve supranormal oxygen delivery could cause increased multiple-organ failure, abdominal compartment syndrome, and increased mortality from excessive crystalloid infusions.[31] Over time, the widely used pulmonary artery catheter fell out of favor. Studies have shown that the discontinued use of the pulmonary artery catheter has not adversely affected outcome. Due to the invasive nature of the pulmonary artery catheter and concern that the data derived from the catheter were often misinterpreted, its use has virtually disappeared from the modern-day surgical ICU aside from the use in cardiac surgery patients.

Moreover, oxygen delivery in hyperdynamic patients could not be driven to a point at which consumption seemed to level off. One theory was that as the heart was being pushed with the supernormalization process, the heart's metabolism increased such that it was the major organ seemingly consuming all of the excess oxygen being delivered. The harder the heart worked to deliver the oxygen, the more it had to use. Normal cardiac output for an average man is about 5 L/min, yet patients were often driven to a cardiac output of 15 L/min or more for days at a time.

The critics of the optimization process asserted that there was a point during oxygen delivery when it was flow dependent, but the coupling of consumption and delivery made it seem like increased delivery was the factor that increased consumption. Furthermore, optimization advocates neglected the fact that the body was usually already at the flat part of the oxygen consumption curve. Rarely was oxygen delivered when it was critical or when the body was consuming all that was being delivered. The result of the optimization process usually meant that patients were flooded with fluids. The hyperdynamic response and MODS may have resulted from the fluids used, which may have caused an inflammatory response at excessive volumes.

The concept of oxygen debt, introduced by the physiologist Archibald Hill almost 100 years ago, may have some vital flaws in it. His original work on aerobic and anaerobic metabolism in just four patients has now been propagated for a century. However, modern exercise physiology studies have shown that oxygen debt is repaid during a short period; it does not take days. In contrast, the optimization process showed oxygen debt for long periods.

During massive hemorrhage, ischemia to some tissues is theoretically possible. However, in acute hemorrhage, when the BP falls to 40 mm Hg, cardiac output and thus oxygen delivery are typically reduced by only 50%. Before resuscitation with acellular fluids, the hemoglobin level does not fall significantly. In this state, oxygen delivery is cut by only half, and the body is designed to have plenty of reserves (cells consume only 25% of the delivered oxygen in the normal state). Whether any ongoing anaerobic metabolism is actually occurring is questionable, as the oxygen delivery has to fall to 25% of baseline to theoretically be anaerobic. When resuscitation takes place without blood to restore the intravascular volume, the hemoglobin level theoretically may fall by 50%, but cardiac output is generally restored to the original state. Again, oxygen delivery is only halved, with plenty of oxygen still being delivered to avoid ongoing anaerobic metabolism. It is difficult to reduce cardiac output and hemoglobin level to a level at which oxygen delivery is reduced by 75%, that is, to below the anaerobic threshold.

In hypovolemic shock states, it was thought that, even though global oxygen delivery may be adequate, regional hypoxia is ongoing. Different organs and tissue beds are not similar in their oxygen needs or consumption. Hypoxic insult may be experienced by the critical organs, whose flow is usually preserved, whereas nonessential organs are sacrificed in terms of oxygen delivery. Yet, such patients are not actively moving, and their oxygen demand is minimal. Thus, the theory of oxygen debt is in question. In exercise states, even if there is oxygen debt, it is paid back quickly and does not take days.

To optimize oxygen delivery, one of the most efficient ways, according to past calculations, was to add hemoglobin. If the hemoglobin level increased from 8.0 to 10 g/dL, by transfusing two units of blood, oxygen delivery would increase by 25%. Blood transfusions were part of the optimization process because they also increased wedge pressure and LVED volume and thus cardiac output, but it was rarely noted that transfusions placed patients on the flat part of the consumption curve (Fig. 4.9).

Decades ago it was also thought that an increased hematocrit would reduce flow in the capillaries, so clinicians had reservations about transfusing too much blood. Studies in the 1950s demonstrated better flow at the capillary level with diluted blood. However, the small amount of decreased flow with the higher viscosity was in the range of a few percentage points and did not compare to the 25% increase in oxygen delivery with a transfusion of a couple of units of PRBCs. Blood transfusions by calculations would be the most efficient way of increasing oxygen delivery, if that were the goal.

Current exercise physiology studies have shown that professional athletes perform better when their hemoglobin levels are above normal. The athletes who blood dope, by undergoing autologous blood transfusions or by taking red cell production enhancers such as erythropoietin or testosterone, are now banned for illegal performance enhancement. Such athletes have cardiac outputs of more than 20 to 50 L/min. They do not seem to have any problems with blood sludging from the higher flow and more viscous blood than normal. The argument against this analogy of athletes and their capability to deliver oxygen despite a high hematocrit level is that injured patients have capillaries that are not vasodilated and are often plugged with white and red cells.

Global Perfusion Versus Regional Perfusion

Gaining the ability to measure BP was revolutionary. However, because the main functions of the vascular system are to deliver needed nutrients and to carry out excreted substances from the cells, clinicians constantly ask whether BP or flow is more important. During sepsis, systemic vascular resistance is low. A malfunction somewhere in the autoregulatory system is assumed.

A teleologic explanation, however, is possible. Lower systemic vascular resistance could be a way our body evolved so that cardiac output can be easily increased as afterload is reduced. Some shunting is believed to occur at the capillary level; however, an important question is, "Should BP be augmented with exogenous administration of pressor agents, normalizing BP at the expense of capillary flow?" High doses of pressor agents most likely worsen flow because lactate levels rise if the pressor dose is too high. That rise in lactate levels could be caused by a stress response as catecholamines are known to increase lactate levels, or it could also be caused by decreased flow at the capillary bed.

Purists would prefer to have lower pressure as long as flow is adequate, but some organs are somewhat sensitive to pressure. For example, the brain and kidneys are traditionally thought to be pressure dependent; however, when early experiments were done, it was difficult to isolate flow from pressure due to the interrelation of those two values. With the concept that flow might be more important than just pressure, technology developed to focus on measuring flow of nutrients rather than pressure.

During hemorrhage or hypovolemia, blood is redirected to organs such as the brain, liver, heart, and kidneys—at the expense of tissue beds such as the skin, muscle, and gut. Thus, the search ensued to find the consequences of this shunting process. The gastrointestinal (GI) tract became the focus of much of this research. Two main methods were developed, gastric tonometry and NIR technology.

Gastric tonometry measures the adequacy of blood flow in the GI tract through placement of a CO_2-permeable balloon filled with saline in the stomach of a patient after gastric acid suppression. The balloon is left in contact with the mucosa of the stomach for 30 minutes, allowing the CO_2 of the gastric mucosa to pass into the balloon and equilibrate. The saline and gas are then withdrawn from the balloon, and the partial pressure of the CO_2 is measured. That value, in conjunction with the arterial HCO_3^-, is used in the Henderson-Hasselbalch equation to calculate the pH of the gastric mucosa and, by inference, to determine the adequacy of blood flow to the splanchnic circulation.

The logistic difficulties of gastric tonometry are concerning. Data on its use have suggested that even though it can help predict survival, resuscitating patients to an improved value had no survival benefit. Most clinicians have now abandoned gastric tonometry. A multicenter trial showed that in patients with septic shock, gastric tonometry was predictive of outcome, but implementing this technology was no better than using the cardiac index as a resuscitation goal.[32] Regional variables of organ dysfunction are thought to be better monitoring variables than global pressure-related hemodynamic variables. However, the data seem to consistently indicate that initial resuscitation of critically ill patients with shock does not require monitoring of regional variables. After stabilization, regional variables are, at best, merely predictors of outcome rather than goals that should be targeted.

The optimal device for monitoring the adequacy of resuscitation should be noninvasive, simple, cheap, and portable. NIR spectroscopy uses the NIR region of the electromagnetic spectrum from about 800 nm to 2500 nm. Typical applications are wide ranging: physics, astronomy, chemistry, pharmaceuticals, medical diagnostics, and food and agrochemical quality control. The main attraction of NIR is that light at those wavelengths can penetrate skin and bone. This is why your hand looks red when it is placed over a flashlight; the other visible light waves are absorbed or reflected, but red light and infrared light pass through skin and bone readily.

A common device using NIR technology that has now become standard in the medical industry is the pulse oximeter. Using slightly different light waves, it yielded correlations with such variables as the cytochrome aa_3 status by adding a third light wave in the 800-nm region. When the oxygen supply is less than adequate, the rate of electron transport is reduced and oxidative phosphorylation decreases, leading ultimately to anaerobic metabolism. Optical devices that use NIR wavelengths can determine the redox potential of copper atoms on cytochrome aa_3 and have been used to study intracellular oxidative processes noninvasively. Thus, with NIR technology, the metabolic rate of tissue can be directly determined to assess whether it is being adequately perfused. Animal models of hemorrhagic shock have validated the potential use of NIR technology in that they showed changes in regional tissue beds (Fig. 4.11). The superiority of NIR results over conventional measurements of shock has been shown in animal and human studies.

To test the utility of this potentially ideal monitoring device, a multicenter prospective study was conducted to determine whether NIR technology could detect patients at risk of hemorrhagic shock and its sequelae. Performed in seven level I trauma centers, the study enrolled 383 patients who were in severe traumatic shock with hypotension and who required blood transfusions. A probe similar to a pulse oximeter was placed on the thenar muscle of patients' hands, continuously gathering NIR values. The NIR probe was found to be as sensitive as base deficit in predicting death and MODS in hypotensive trauma patients.[33] The receiver operating characteristic curves shows that it also may be somewhat better than BP in predicting outcome. More importantly, the negative predictive value was 90% (Fig. 4.12). The noninvasive and continuous NIR probe was able to demonstrate perfusion status. Note, however, that MODS developed in only 50 patients in that study. This was probably because the method of resuscitating trauma patients changed during this period, and this reduced MODS and death rates. The changes that took place are discussed later in this chapter but, in brief, were due to damage control resuscitation.

NIR technology may be able to show when a patient is in shock or even when a patient is doing well. Occult hypoperfusion can be detected or even ruled out reliably with NIR. In the trauma setting, a noninvasive method that can continuously detect trends in parameters such as regional oxygenation status, base deficit, or BP will surely find a role. Will this technology change how patients are treated? The debate now centers on this issue and raises some questions. Once a patient's hypoperfusion status has been determined, whether by BP, NIR technology, or some other device, what should we do with that information? Is it necessary to increase oxygen delivery to regional tissue beds that are inadequately oxygenated? Previous studies have shown that optimizing global oxygen delivery is not useful and that regional tissue monitoring with gastric tonometry has also failed to show benefit, so will NIR technology be helpful or harmful? An example of harm is over resuscitating a patient to fix an abnormal value that may or may not be clinically relevant. The end point of resuscitation is constantly being debated. Since NIR results correlate well with base deficit, we may one day use NIR technology to infer the base deficit value indirectly.

NIR technology has other promising uses in surgery, such as direct monitoring of flow and tissue oxygenation in high-risk patients (e.g., in those undergoing organ transplantation; for free flap perfusion; for classification of burn injuries; in intraoperative assessment of bowel ischemia; with compartment syndrome; or even subdural and epidural hematomas). Perhaps the most useful application will be in the ICU in septic shock patients at risk for multiple-organ failure.

Septic Shock

In 2001, Rivers and colleagues reported that among patients with severe sepsis or septic shock in a single urban emergency department, mortality was significantly lower among those who were

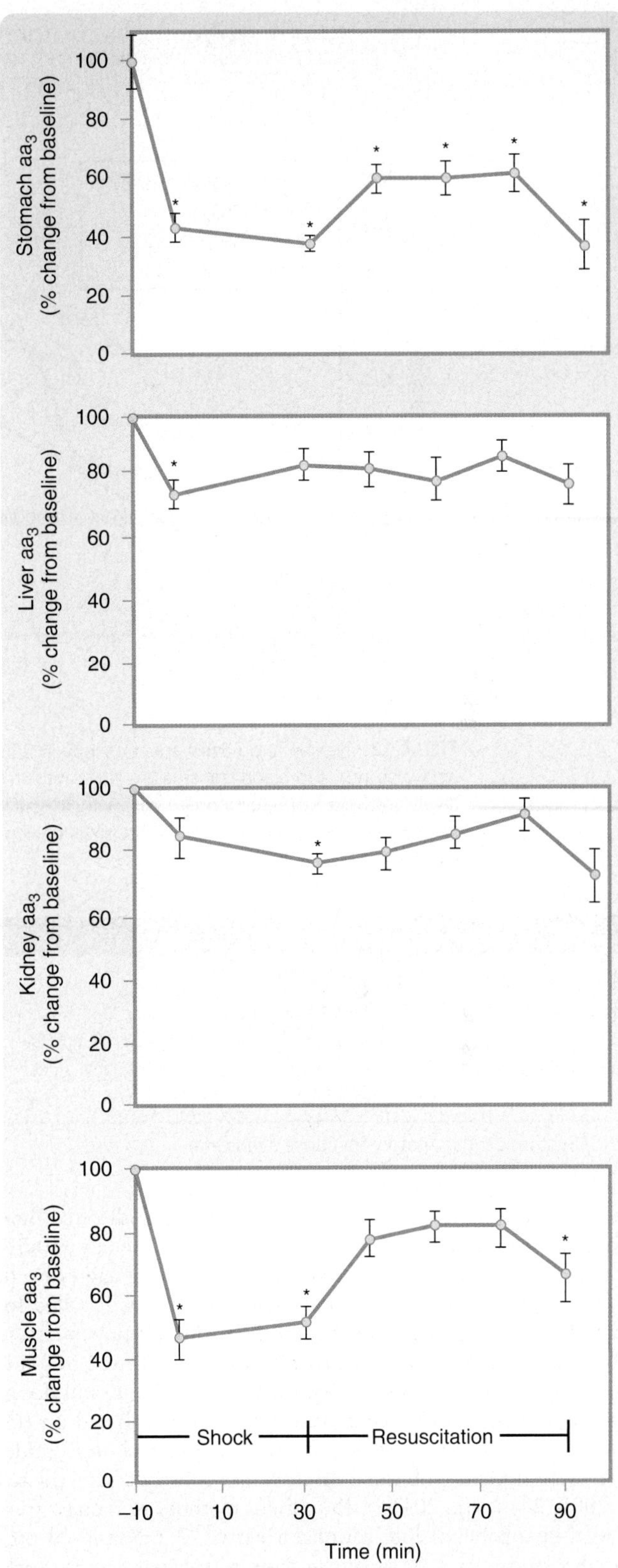

FIG. 4.11 Cytochrome aa_3 measurements in rabbits during hemorrhagic shock. Shown are regional tissue beds and implied tissue oxygenation. Oxygenation at the mitochondrial level is preserved in kidney and liver compared with muscle and stomach. (From Rhee P, Langdale L, Mock C, et al. Near-infrared spectroscopy: continuous measurement of cytochrome oxidation during hemorrhagic shock. *Crit Care Med.* 1997;25:166–170.)

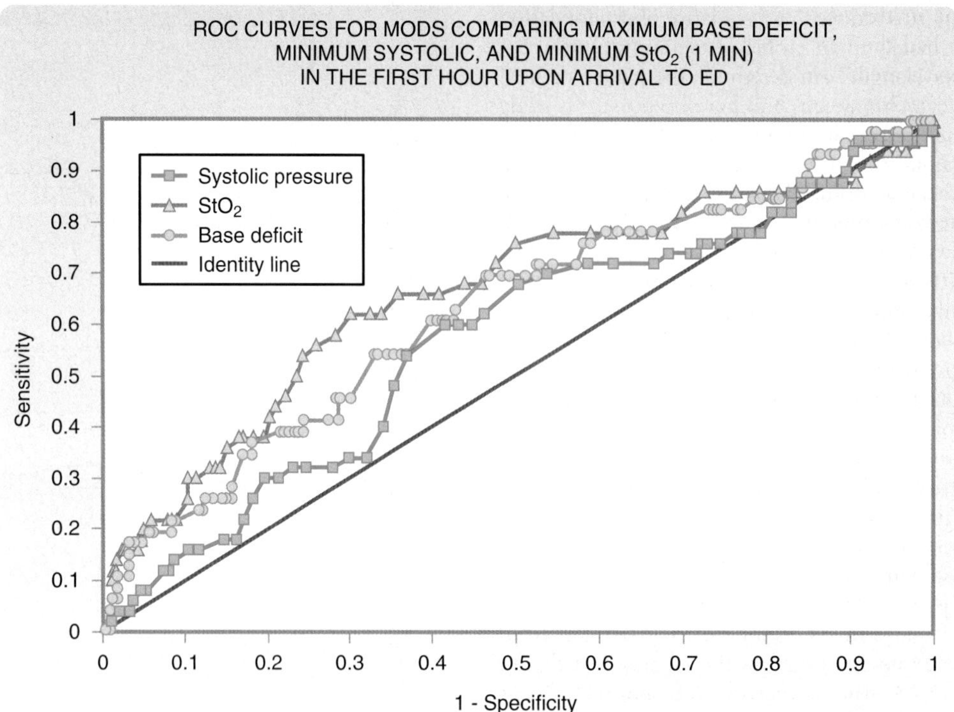

FIG. 4.12 Near-infrared (NIR) spectroscopy in 383 patients with traumatic hemorrhagic shock with hypotension who required blood transfusion. NIR measured tissue oxygenation levels in the thenar muscle noninvasively and was found to correlate well with arterial base deficit. (From Cohn SM, Nathens AB, Moore FA, et al. Tissue oxygen saturation predicts the development of organ dysfunction during traumatic shock resuscitation. *J Trauma.* 2007;62:44–54.)

TABLE 4.5 SIRS criteria.

Body Temperature	>38°C or <36°C
Heart Rate	> 90 Beats per min
Tachypnea	Respiratory rate >20/min or $PaCO_2$ <32 mm Hg
White Blood Cell Count	>12,000/mm^3, <4000/mm^3, or >10% immature neutrophils

SIRS, Systemic inflammatory response syndrome.

treated according to a 6-hour protocol of early goal-directed therapy than among those who were given standard therapy (30.5% vs. 46.5%). The premise was that usual care was not aggressive or timely. Early goal-directed therapy addressed this as it called for central venous catheterization to monitor central venous pressure and central venous oxygen saturation, which were used to guide the use of IV fluids, vasopressors, PRBC transfusions, and dobutamine to achieve prespecified physiologic targets. Based on this type of research, the Surviving Sepsis Campaign clinical guidelines were initially published in 2004 and subsequently updated in 2008, 2014, and 2016.[34] The various methods of therapy were graded by a panel of international experts.[35] A randomized prospective study has now shown that protocol-based care for early septic shock does not improve outcome.[36] The newer study was not identical to the original Rivers study as the survival rates were much higher, but this study may just show that the usual therapy may have already adopted many of the principles of early goal-directed therapy, and thus the difference is negligible. This study also found no significant benefit of the mandated use of central venous catheterization and central hemodynamic monitoring in all patients.

In the most recent update of the Surviving Sepsis campaign clinical guidelines published in 2016 there was a major transition in the way that sepsis was defined. Previous iterations of the campaign used SIRS criteria (Table 4.5) to define sepsis in which the patient needed to have two out of four of the criteria present and a source of infection to be deemed to have sepsis. This definition was fraught with problems as any noninfectious process that activated the inflammatory cascade could lead to a similar physiologic picture. Instead of using SIRS criteria, sepsis was now defined as an increase in a patient's sequential organ failure assessment (SOFA) score by 2 points from baseline (Table 4.6). Since the SOFA score can be cumbersome to calculate at bedside and requires laboratory test results, a simpler version was developed. The qSOFA (Table 4.7) can be calculated at a patient bedside by identifying tachypnea, altered mental status, and hypotension. If the patient meets two of these criteria and they are at risk for sepsis, further workup for an infectious source should be conducted.[37]

PROBLEMS WITH RESUSCITATION

Lessons learned from the Korean War showed that resuscitation with blood and blood products was useful. Throughout that war, the concept prevailed that a limited amount of salt and water should be given to patients after injuries. By the time of the Vietnam War, volume resuscitation in excess of replacement of shed blood became an acceptable practice. That practice may have been influenced by studies of hemorrhagic shock performed by Tom Shires. In his classic study, Shires used the Wiggers model and bled 30 dogs to a mean BP of 50 mm Hg for 90 minutes. He then infused LR solution (5% of body weight) followed by blood in 10 dogs, plasma (10 mL/kg) followed by blood in another 10 dogs and shed blood alone in the remaining 10 dogs. The dogs that received LR solution had the best survival rate. Shires concluded that, although the replacement of lost blood with whole blood remains the primary treatment of shock, adjunctive replacement of the coexisting functional volume deficit in the interstitium with a balanced salt solution appears to be beneficial. Shires concluded that resuscitation with LR solution should be initiated while whole blood transfusions are being mobilized.

Soon the surgical community went from being judicious with crystalloid solutions to being aggressive. Surgeons returning from the Vietnam War advocated the use of crystalloids, a seemingly cheap and easy method of resuscitating patients, touting that it saved lives. However, what evolved from this method of resuscitation was the so-called Da Nang lung, also known as Shock Lung and eventually ARDS. (The U.S. Navy had its field hospital in Da Nang, Vietnam.) The explanation for the evolution of the new condition was that battlefield patients were now living long enough to develop ARDS because their lives were saved with aggressive resuscitation and better critical care, including a greater capability to treat renal failure.

However, that explanation had no supporting evidence. The killed in action rate (the number of wounded patients who died before reaching a facility that had a surgeon) had not changed for more than a century (Table 4.8). The died-of-wounds rate (the number of wounded patients who died after reaching a facility that had a physician) had decreased during World War II, thanks to the use of antibiotics, but it was slightly higher during the Vietnam War. The perceived reason for slightly higher died-of-wounds rates was that patients in Vietnam were transported to medical facilities much more quickly by helicopters. Transport times did indeed decrease from an average of 4 hours to 40 minutes, but if the sicker patients who would have normally died in the field were transported more quickly to die in the medical facility, then the killed-in-action rate should have fallen—and it did not.

Moreover, the renal failure rate and the cause of renal failure did not significantly change between the Korean War and the Vietnam War. Another false argument was that the wounds seen during the Vietnam War were worse because of the enemy's high-velocity AK-47 rifles. Actually, the rounds or bullets used by the AK-47 were similar to those used by the enemy in the Russo-Japanese War, World War I, and World War II. The 7.62-mm round used in the AK-47 rifle was invented by the Japanese in the 1890s.

In the early 1970s, the prehospital system in the United States started to evolve. Previously, ambulances were usually hearses driven by morticians. That is why the early ambulances had a station wagon configuration. As the career paths of emergency medical technicians and paramedics grew, they started resuscitation in the field and continued it to the hospital. In 1978, the first ATLS course was given. To prevent shock, the ATLS course recommended that all trauma patients have two large-bore IV lines placed and receive 2 L of LR solution. The actual recommendation in the ATLS text specifically states that patients in class III shock should receive 2 L of LR solution followed by blood products. However, clinicians learned that crystalloid solutions seemed innocuous and improved BP in hypotensive patients.

In the 1980s and early 1990s, aggressive resuscitation was taught and endorsed. The two large-bore IV lines started in the field were converted to larger IV lines through a wire-guided exchange system. Central venous lines were placed early for aggressive fluid resuscitation. In fact, some trauma centers routinely performed cut-downs on the saphenous vein at the ankle to place IV tubing directly into the vein and thereby maximize flow during resuscitation.

Technology soon caught up, and machines were built to rapidly infuse crystalloid solutions. The literature was filled with data showing that ischemia to tissues resulted in disturbances of all types. Optimization of oxygen delivery was the goal. As a result, massive volumes of crystalloids were infused into patients.

TABLE 4.7 qSOFA.

Respiratory rate ≥22
Altered mental status
Systolic blood pressure ≤100 mm Hg

SOFA, Sequential organ failure assessment.

TABLE 4.8 Mortality rates.

	KILLED IN ACTION (%)	DIED OF WOUNDS (%)
Civil War	16.0	13.0
Russo-Japanese War	20.0	9.0
World War I	19.6	8.1
World War II	19.8	3.0
Korean War	19.5	2.4
Vietnam War	20.2	3.5

TABLE 4.6 Sequential organ failure assessment (SOFA) score.

		SCORE				
System		0	1	2	3	4
Respiratory	PaO_2/FiO_2, mm Hg	≥400	<400	<300	<200 With respiratory support	<100 With respiratory support
Coagulation	Platelets, x10>3/μL	≥150	<150	<100	<50	<20
Liver	Bilirubin, mg/dL	<1.2	1.2–1.9	2.0–5.9	6.0–11.9	>12.0
Cardiovascular		MAP ≥70 mm Hg	MAP <70 mm Hg	Dopamine <5 or dobutamine (any dose)	Dopamine 5.1–15 or epinephrine ≤0.1 or norepinephrine ≤0.1	Dopamine >15 or epinephrine >0.1 or norepinephrine >0.1
Central Nervous System	Glasgow coma scale score	15	13–14	10–12	6–9	<6
Renal	Creatinine, mg/dL	<1.2	1.2–1.9	2.0–3.4	3.5–4.9	>5.0
	Urine output, mL/day				<500	<200

FiO_2, Percentage of inspired oxygen; *MAP*, mean arterial pressure; *PaO_2*, partial pressure of arterial oxygen.

Residents were encouraged to "pound" patients with fluids. If trauma patients did not develop ARDS, it was taught that the patients were not adequately resuscitated, but many clinical trials eventually showed that prehospital fluids did not improve outcome (Table 4.9).

Bleeding

One of the most influential studies on hemorrhagic shock was performed by Ken Mattox, and in 1994, the results were reported by Bickell and coworkers.[38] The aim of Mattox's study, a prospective clinical trial, was to determine whether withholding of prehospital fluids affected outcomes in hypotensive patients after a penetrating torso injury. IV lines were started in patients with penetrating torso trauma with BP lower than 90 mm Hg. On alternating days, patients received standard fluid therapy in the field or had fluids withheld until hemorrhage control was achieved. Withholding of prehospital fluids conferred a statistically significant survival advantage—a revolutionary, counterintuitive finding that shocked surgeons.

That 1994 article popularized the concept of permissive hypotension, that is, allowing hypotension during uncontrolled hemorrhage. The fundamental rationale for permissive hypotension was that restoration of BP with fluids would increase bleeding from uncontrolled sources. In fact, Cannon in 1918 had stated that "inaccessible or uncontrolled sources of blood loss should not be treated with IV fluids until the time of surgical control."

Animal studies have validated the idea of permissive hypotension. Burris and colleagues have shown that moderate resuscitation results in a better outcome compared with no resuscitation or aggressive resuscitation. In a swine model of uncontrolled hemorrhage, Sondeen showed that raising BP with either fluids or pressors could lead to increased bleeding. The theory was that increasing BP would dislodge the clot that had formed. The study also found that the pressure that would cause rebleeding was a mean arterial pressure of 64 ± 2 mm Hg, with a systolic pressure of 94 ± 3 mm Hg and diastolic pressure of 45 ± 2 mm Hg. Other animal studies have confirmed these concepts.

The next question was whether the continued strategy of permissive hypotension in the operating room would result in improved survival. Dutton and associates randomized one group of patients to a target systolic BP of higher than 100 mm Hg and another group to a target systolic BP of 70 mm Hg. Fluid therapy was titrated until definitive hemorrhage control was achieved. However, despite attempts to maintain BP at 70 mm Hg, the average BP was 100 mm Hg in the low-pressure group and 114 mm Hg in the high-pressure group. Patients' BP rose spontaneously. Titrating patients' BP to the low target was difficult, even with less use of fluids. The survival rate did not differ between the two groups.

The idea of permissive hypotension was slow to catch on. The argument against allowing anything besides aggressive resuscitation was dismissed. Critics continued to emphasize that the Mattox trial focused only on penetrating injuries and should not be extrapolated to blunt trauma. Clinicians feared that patients with traumatic blunt head injuries would be harmed without a normalized BP. However, Shafi and Gentilello examined the National Trauma Data Bank and found that hypotension was an independent risk factor for death, but it did not increase the mortality rate in patients with TBIs any more than in patients without TBIs. The risk of death quadrupled in patients with hypotension, in both the TBI group (odds ratio, 4.1; 95% confidence interval, 3.5–4.9) and the nonTBI group (odds ratio, 4.6; 95% confidence interval, 3.4–6.0). Furthermore, in 2006, Plurad and coworkers showed that emergency department hypotension was not an independent risk factor for acute renal dysfunction or failure.

Trauma Immunology and Inflammation

The 1990s witnessed an explosion of information regarding alterations of homeostasis and cellular physiochemistry during shock. The scientific investigations of Shires, Carrico, Baue, and countless others shed light on the basic mechanisms underlying resuscitation of patients in shock. The pathophysiologic process has been identified as having an aberrant inflammatory status, resulting in the body's immune system damaging the endothelial tissues and ultimately the end organ. This inflammatory state leads to a spectrum of conditions, including fluid sequestration, which leads to edema and progresses to acute lung injury, systemic inflammatory response syndrome, ARDS, and MODS. Such conditions were in every surgical ICU. Attention focused on biochemical perturbations and altered mediators as sites for possible interventions. The fundamental cause

TABLE 4.9 Prehospital fluid studies in trauma patients.

ARTICLE	SUMMARY OF FINDINGS
Aprahamian C, Thompson BM, Towne JB, et al. The effect of a paramedic system on mortality of major open intraabdominal vascular trauma. *J Trauma.* 1983;23:687–690.	Paramedic system Open intraabdominal vascular trauma
Kaweski SM, Sise MJ, Virgilio RW. The effect of prehospital fluids on survival in trauma patients. *J Trauma.* 1990;30:1215–1218.	Prehospital fluids Trauma patients
Bickell WH, Wall MJ Jr, Pepe PE, et al. Immediate versus delayed fluid resuscitation for hypotensive patients with penetrating torso injuries. *N Engl J Med.* 1994;331:1105–1109.	Presurgery fluids Hypotensive penetrating torso injuries
Turner J, Nicholl J, Webber L, et al. A randomised controlled trial of prehospital intravenous fluid replacement therapy in serious trauma. *Health Technol Assess.* 2000;4:1–57.	Prehospital 1309 Serious trauma patients
Kwan I, Bunn F, Roberts I. Timing and volume of fluid administration for patients with bleeding following trauma. *Cochrane Database Syst Rev.* 2001;1:CD002245.	Prehospital Bleeding trauma patients
Dula DJ, Wood GC, Rejmer AR, et al. Use of prehospital fluids in hypotensive blunt trauma patients. *Prehosp Emerg Care.* 2002;6:417–420, 2002.	Prehospital Hypotensive blunt trauma patients
Greaves I, Porter KM, Revell MP. Fluid resuscitation in pre-hospital trauma care: a consensus view. *J R Coll Surg Edinb.* 2002;47:451–457.	Prehospital A consensus view
Dutton RP, Mackenzie CF, Scalea TM. Hypotensive resuscitation during active hemorrhage: impact on in-hospital mortality. *J Trauma.* 2002;52:1141–1146.	Presurgery fluids Hypotensive active hemorrhage
Dula DJ, Wood GC, Rejmer AR, et al. Use of prehospital fluids in hypotensive blunt trauma patients. *Prehosp Emerg Care.* 2002;6:417–420.	Prehospital fluids Hypotensive patients

was thought to be that ischemia and reperfusion as shown in animal models would create a state of damage to the capillary endothelium and subsequent changes to the end organ. It was generally accepted that the reason for the reperfusion injury was mediated by activated neutrophils that emitted deleterious cytokines and released free oxygen radicals. The animal models used to study these concepts were actually ischemia-reperfusion models in which the superior mesenteric artery that supplied blood to the intestines was clamped for a prolonged time before the clamp was removed. Later it was thought that this was not an appropriate model to study hemorrhagic shock. It was found that there was a difference in pathophysiologic mechanisms between ischemia-reperfusion injury and resuscitation injury.

Death after traumatic injury was described as trimodal. Some patients died within a short time after injury, some died in the hospital within a few hours, and many died late in the hospital course. However, a more recent trial in trauma patients has shown that deaths occur in a logarithmic decay fashion and follow the rule of biology; no grouping of deaths can be seen, unless the data are represented or lumped together as immediate, early, or late. The only reason for the initial trimodal distribution was that patients who died after 24 hours were labeled under late deaths.[39]

According to the traditional (although now discredited) trimodal pattern, the patients who typically died first could be aided by a better prehospital system and, more important, by injury prevention. For the second group of patients, better resuscitation and hemorrhage control was thought to be a potentially lifesaving intervention. For the third group (the late deaths), immunomodulation was considered to be key. The cause was thought to be the inflammatory adaptive aberrancy after successful resuscitation. When there is prolonged end-arteriole cessation of flow producing tissue ischemia for a time, followed by reperfusion, it is termed *reperfusion injury*. For example, with an injury to the femoral artery that requires 4 to 6 hours for circulation to be restored, muscle cells undergo ischemia and reperfusion in which the cells will start to swell, which can result in compartment syndrome in the lower leg. This ischemia and reperfusion were thought to occur after a period of hypotension. However, it is now known that the pathophysiologic change is due to resuscitation injury rather than to reperfusion injury.

With improved technology, the immunologic response after trauma was heavily researched. In the past, we were limited to studying physiology. A theory started to evolve that shock caused an aberrant inflammatory response that then needed to be modulated and suppressed. Many studies during this era showed that the inflammatory system was upregulated or activated after shock. The white cells in the blood became activated. Neutrophils were identified as the key mediators in the acute phase of shock, whereas lymphocytes are typically key players in chronic diseases (e.g., cancer and viral infections). Shock, caused by various mechanisms, was thought to induce ischemia to tissues and, after reperfusion, to set off an inflammatory response, which primarily affected the microcirculation and caused leaks (Fig. 4.13).

Typically, neutrophils are rapidly transported through capillaries. However, when they are signaled by chemokines, neutrophils will start to roll, firmly adhere to the endothelium, and migrate out of the capillaries to find the body's foes and initiate healing. Early researchers thought that neutrophils would battle invaders (e.g., bacteria) through phagocytic activity and the release of oxygen-free radicals; this was thought to be the reason for the leak in the capillary system (Fig. 4.14). Since neutrophils can be primed to have an enhanced response, a massive search took place to identify causes of neutrophil priming and downregulation. The

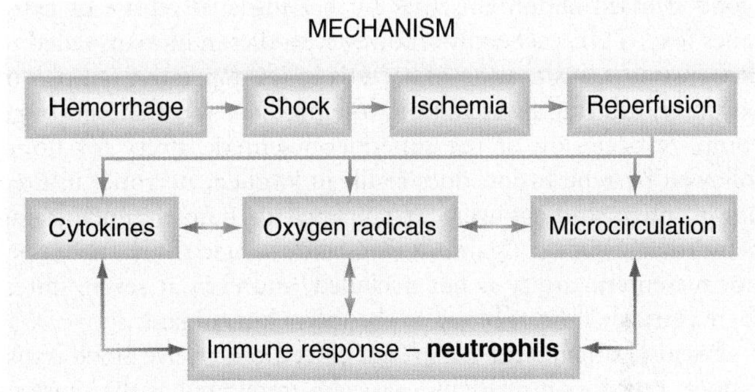

FIG. 4.13 Hemorrhage causing neutrophil activation.

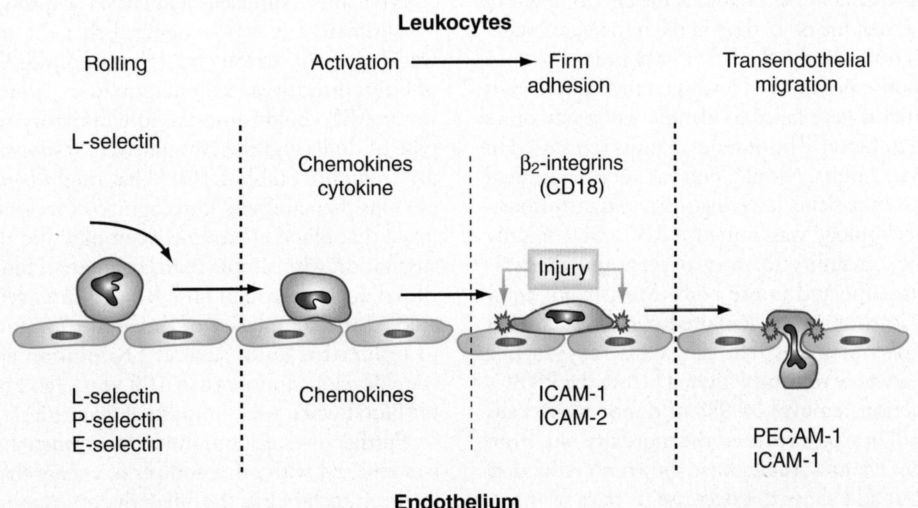

FIG. 4.14 Intravascular neutrophils that are activated will adhere and roll until another set of mechanisms causes firm adherence and transendothelial migration out of the vascular system occurs. It is believed that this transmigration process injures the endothelium with the release of an oxygen free radical. This could result in fluid leaks out of the vascular system. *ICAM,* Intercellular adhesion molecules; *PECAM,* platelet–endothelial cell adhesion molecule.

many cytokines targeted included interleukin types 1 through 18, tumor necrosis factor (TNF), and adhesion molecules, such as intercellular adhesion molecules, vascular cell adhesion molecules, E-selectin, L-selectin, P-selectin, and platelet-activating factor.

That research had much overlap with the research being performed in the arenas of reimplantation, vascular ischemia, and reperfusion. Clinically, it was already known that the implantation of severed extremities would have pathophysiologic results similar to those from ischemia, reperfusion, and swelling caused by leaky capillaries. The immune response was described as bimodal. The first response was the priming by trauma or shock, followed by an exaggerated response when hit with a second insult (e.g., infection).

In the late 1990s, other researchers focused on the role of the alimentary tract. They knew that the splanchnic circulation was shunted of blood by vasoconstriction during hemorrhagic shock, so the gut suffers the most ischemia during shock and is the most susceptible to reperfusion injury. The animal model most often used to study the gut's role in inflammation was a rat model of superior mesenteric artery occlusion and reperfusion. Because systemic inflammatory response syndrome is a sterile phenomenon, the gut was implicated as a potential player in the development of MODS. Animals were shown to have a translocation of bacteria into the portal system, and this initiation of the inflammatory cascade was investigated as the source of MODS. Investigators also knew that the release of *Escherichia coli* bacteria in the blood released endotoxins that further initiated release of cytokines (e.g., TNF, cachectin). However, studies in humans failed to demonstrate translocation of bacteria in intraoperative samples of portal vein during resuscitation. The problem was that, although complete occlusion of the superior mesenteric artery for hours followed by reperfusion does result in swollen, necrotic, injured bowel, these findings were extrapolated to humans undergoing hemorrhagic shock. Again, during hemorrhagic shock, the superior mesenteric artery is not occluded, and even at severe states, there is trickle flow of blood to the splanchnic organs.

Because patients who are in shock bleed and receive blood transfusions, transfusion of PRBCs was also implicated as the cause of MODS. Patients who required massive amounts of PRBCs were most likely to develop MODS. Researchers found that the use of older PRBCs was an independent risk factor for the development of MODS. PRBCs have a shelf life of 42 days in the refrigerated state. As blood ages, changes occur in the fluid that have been shown to affect the immune response negatively. However, randomized trials in cardiac and ICU patients have failed to identify worse outcomes in patients receiving older blood. The number of units transfused in these studies averages 3 to 4 units. Age of blood has not been studied in a randomized fashion in patients receiving massive transfusions.

In the past, when technology was limited, PRBCs were mainly tested for the red cells' capability to carry oxygen and their viability under the microscope and in the body. Most major trauma centers now have learned to use leukoreduced PRBCs, that is, the small number of white cells that can release oxygen-free radicals and cytokines are now routinely filtered before the PRBCs are stored. Leukoreduction removes 99.9% of donor white cells and, in one large Canadian study, reduced the mortality rate from 7.03% to 6.19%. Other trauma studies have shown no reduction in the mortality rate but still showed a decrease in rates of infection, infectious complications, and late ARDS. To date, the largest study of leukoreduction in trauma patients has not shown any reduction in the rates of infection, organ failure, or mortality.[40]

Numerous trials have examined the blockage of cytokines to treat septic patients. Two prospective, randomized, multicenter, double-blinded trials, the North American Sepsis Trial (NORASEPT) and the International Sepsis Trial (INTERSEPT), studied the 28-day mortality rate of critically ill patients who received anti-TNF antibody. Neither trial showed any benefit. Other trials testing other potential cytokines were disappointing as well. The cytokines tested included CD11/CD18,[41] antiinterleukin 1 receptor, antiendotoxin antibodies, bradykinin antagonists, and platelet-activating factor receptor antagonists. The search continues for one key mediator that could be manipulated to solve the "toxemia" of shock.[42] However, such attempts to simplify the events and to find one solution may be the main problem because there is no simple answer and no simple solution. The answer may lie in cocktails of substances. The humoral and endocrine systems, which are always mediated by blood, are exceedingly complex. Shock has many causes and mechanisms. Understanding this is crucial as we look for solutions.

EVOLUTION OF MODERN RESUSCITATION

Detrimental Impact of Fluids

As early as 1996, the U.S. Navy used a swine model to study the effects of fluids on neutrophil activation after hemorrhagic shock and resuscitation. It was shown that neutrophils are activated after a 40% blood volume hemorrhage when followed by resuscitation with LR solution. That finding was not surprising. What was enlightening was that the level of neutrophil activation was similar in control animals that did not undergo hemorrhagic shock but merely received LR solution (Fig. 4.15). In other control animals that did not receive LR solution but instead were resuscitated with shed blood or HTS after hemorrhagic shock, the neutrophils were not activated. The implication was that the inflammatory process was not caused by shock and resuscitation but by LR solution itself.

Those findings were repeated over several years in a series of experiments using human blood as well as in experiments in small and large animal models of hemorrhagic shock. When the blood was diluted with various resuscitation fluids, the inflammatory changes depended on the fluid used; despite similar physiologic results in vivo, the immunologic results were different (Fig. 4.16). The response was ubiquitous throughout the entire inflammatory response system, including at the levels of deoxyribonucleic acid (DNA) and ribonucleic acid (RNA) expression.

Ultimately, it was recognized that the inflammatory response was due to the various resuscitation fluids. The type and amount of fluids directly caused inflammation. All the artificial fluids used to raise BP could cause the inflammatory sequelae of shock. The type of fluids and the amount were responsible for the inflammatory response (Table 4.10). What might be obvious today was not obvious then and was unrecognized for decades. It was not recognized that blood is extremely complex and that replacement or resuscitation with simple fluids other than blood had consequences. Blood does more than raise BP and carry red cells. In the past, we studied the complexity of the body's immune response but failed to realize that fluids such as LR solution and normal saline that were developed more than 100 years ago are not ideal substitutes for blood when used in massive quantities.

Further investigations showed that when the lactate in LR solution was replaced with other sources of energy that could be better used by the mitochondria, the inflammatory aspects were attenuated. One such novel fluid was ketone Ringer solution (Table 4.11). Lactic acid occurs in two stereoisomeric forms as well as in a true racemic mixture of the isomers. In biologic systems, the true racemic mixture or equal molarity of the isomers rarely occurs. Usually, one or the other isomer predominates. The stereoisomers are named L(+) and D(−) lactic acid.

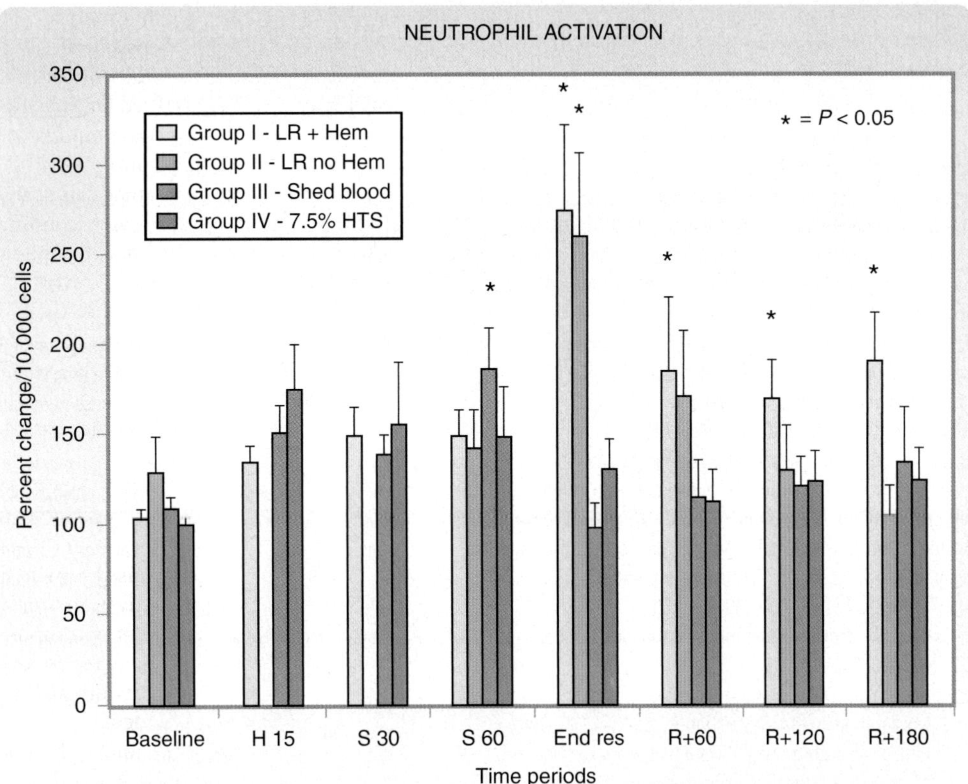

FIG. 4.15 Neutrophil activation in whole blood of swine measured by flow cytometry. The highest neutrophil activation followed hemorrhagic shock *(Hem)* and resuscitation *(res)* using lactated Ringer *(LR)* solution. Similar neutrophil activation occurred when the animal was not resuscitated but was infused with LR solution. No activation occurred when shocked animals were resuscitated with whole blood or 7.5% hypertonic saline *(HTS)*. (From Rhee P, Burris D, Kaufmann C, et al. Lactated Ringer's resuscitation causes neutrophil activation after hemorrhagic shock. *J Trauma.* 1998;44:313–319.)

L(+)-lactate is a normal intermediary of mammalian metabolism. The isomer D(−)-lactate is produced when tissue glyoxalase converts methylglyoxal into a lactic acid of the D form, such as in lactose-fermenting bacteria. L(+)-lactate has low toxicity as a consequence of the rapid metabolism. D(−)-lactate, however, has higher toxic potential. Psychoneurotic disturbances have been described with pure D(−)-lactate. Increasing evidence has indicated a connection between high plasma concentration of racemic lactate and anxiety and panic disorders. Racemic dialysis fluids have reportedly been associated with clinical cases of D-lactate toxicity. Experiments with the isomers have shown that D(−)-lactate causes significant inflammatory changes in rats and swine as well as activation of human neutrophils.

In 1999, with the new information implicating LR solution as the cause of ARDS and MODS, the U.S. Navy contracted with the Institute of Medicine to review the topic of the optimal resuscitation fluid.[43] The report made many recommendations; key recommendations were that LR solution be manufactured with only the L(+) isomer of lactate and that researchers continue to search for alternative resuscitation fluids that do not contain lactate but rather other nutrients, such as ketones. It stated that the optimal resuscitation fluid is 7.5% HTS because of the decreased inflammation associated with it as well as its logistic advantage in terms of weight and size. Although the Institute of Medicine had been asked to make recommendations for the military, the report's authors thought that the evidence was applicable to civilian injuries as well. The U.S. military also requested Baxter, among other manufacturers of LR solution, to eliminate D(−)-lactate in LR solution, which it has done. The LR solution from Baxter currently contains only the L(+)-lactate isomer.

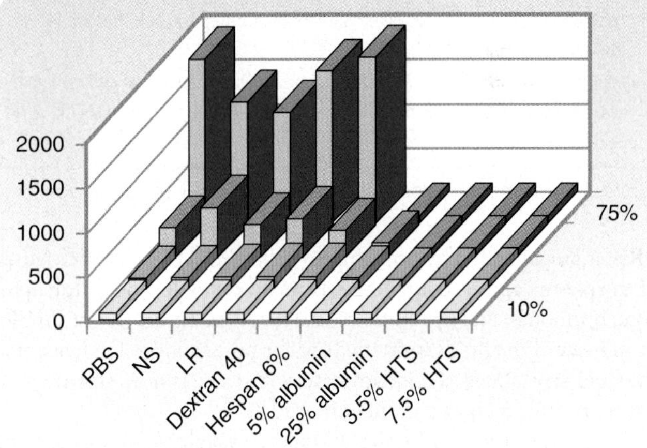

FIG. 4.16 Human neutrophil activation using whole blood diluted with various resuscitation fluids, as measured by flow cytometry. Phosphate-buffered saline *(PBS)* was used because it has a pH of 7.4. (From Rhee P, Wang D, Ruff P, et al. Human neutrophil activation and increased adhesion by various resuscitation fluids. *Crit Care Med.* 2000;28:74–78.)

HTS has a long record of research and development. It has been used in humans for decades and has been consistently shown to be less inflammatory than LR solution. This represented a paradigm shift in recognizing that LR solution and normal saline may be detrimental. Again, blood is complex, and the fluids used in the past were a poor replacement.

It was also being recognized that PRBCs are different from whole blood and a poor replacement of whole blood lost during hemorrhage.

TABLE 4.10 Summary of studies by U.S. Navy demonstrating fluids causing inflammation after resuscitation.

ARTICLE	MODEL	SUMMARY OF FINDINGS
Rhee P, Burris D, Kaufmann C, et al. Lactated Ringer's solution resuscitation causes neutrophil activation after hemorrhagic shock. *J Trauma.* 1998;44:313–319.	Swine	LR causes neutrophil activation; blood HTS does not.
Deb S, Martin B, Sun L, et al. Resuscitation with lactated Ringer's solution in rats with hemorrhagic shock induces immediate apoptosis. *J Trauma.* 1999;46:582–588.	Rats	LR causes apoptosis in liver and gut more than HTS does.
Sun LL, Ruff P, Austin B, et al. Early up-regulation of intercellular adhesion molecule-1 and vascular cell adhesion molecule-1 expression in rats with hemorrhagic shock and resuscitation. *Shock.* 1999;11:416–422.	Rats	LR causes cytokine release more than HTS does.
Alam HB, Sun L, Ruff P, et al. E- and P-selectin expression depends on the resuscitation fluid used in hemorrhaged rats. *J Surg Res.* 2000;94:145–152.	Rats	LR causes increased E- and P-selectin expression more than HTS does.
Rhee P, Wang D, Ruff P, et al. Human neutrophil activation and increased adhesion by various resuscitation fluids. *Crit Care Med.* 2000;28:74–78.	Human cells	Artificial fluids cause neutrophil activation more than HTS and albumin do.
Deb S, Sun L, Martin B, et al. Lactated Ringer's solution and hetastarch but not plasma resuscitation after rat hemorrhagic shock is associated with immediate lung apoptosis by the up-regulation of the Bax protein. *J Trauma.* 2000;49:47–53.	Rats	LR and hetastarch increase lung apoptosis compared with plasma whole blood, plasma, and albumin.
Alam HB, Austin B, Koustova E, et al. Resuscitation-induced pulmonary apoptosis and intracellular adhesion molecule-1 expression in rats are attenuated by the use of ketone Ringer's solution. *J Am Coll Surg.* 2001;193:255–263.	Rats	Substituting ketones for lactate reduces pulmonary apoptosis and release of intercellular adhesion molecules.
Koustova E, Stanton K, Gushchin V, et al. Effects of lactated Ringer's solutions on human leukocytes. *J Trauma.* 2002;52:872–878.	Human cells	D-LR causes inflammation more than L-LR does.
Alam HB, Stegalkina S, Rhee P, et al. cDNA array analysis of gene expression following hemorrhagic shock and resuscitation in rats. *Resuscitation.* 2002;54:195–206.	Rats	Different fluids cause gene expression at different levels.
Koustova E, Rhee P, Hancock T, et al. Ketone and pyruvate Ringer's solutions decrease pulmonary apoptosis in a rat model of severe hemorrhagic shock and resuscitation. *Surgery.* 2003;134:267–274.	Rats	Ketone and pyruvate Ringer solutions protect against apoptosis compared with LR.
Stanton K, Alam HB, Rhee P, et al. Human polymorphonuclear cell death after exposure to resuscitation fluids in vitro: apoptosis versus necrosis. *J Trauma.* 2003;54:1065–1074.	Human cells	Artificial fluids cause apoptosis and necrosis.
Gushchin V, Alam HB, Rhee P, et al. cDNA profiling in leukocytes exposed to hypertonic resuscitation fluids. *J Am Coll Surg.* 2003;197:426–432.	Human cells	LR causes more cytokine release by gene expression than HTS does.
Alam HB, Stanton K, Koustova E, et al. Effect of different resuscitation strategies on neutrophil activation in a swine model of hemorrhagic shock. *Resuscitation.* 2004;60:91–99.	Swine	Artificial fluids cause neutrophil activation despite resuscitation rates.
Jaskille A, Alam HB, Rhee P, et al. D-Lactate increases pulmonary apoptosis by restricting phosphorylation of bad and eNOS in a rat model of hemorrhagic shock. *J Trauma.* 2004;57:262–269.	Rats	D-Lactate in fluids causes more apoptosis than L-lactate does.

cDNA; Complementary deoxyribonucleic acid; *HTS*, hypertonic saline; *LR*, lactated Ringer solution.

PRBCs are separated by centrifuge, washed, and then filtered. Much of the plasma and its content are decanted out. Clotting factors, glucose, hormones, and cytokines crucial for signaling are not in PRBCs or in most of the fluids formerly used for resuscitation. Evidence that the fluid type affects the inflammatory response is now growing and has been confirmed in a number of studies.[44]

The Committee on Tactical Combat Casualty Care was formed in 2000 by the U.S. Navy and now sets policy on the prehospital management of combat casualties. Their recommendations and algorithm for resuscitation were revolutionary compared with the civilian recommendations (Fig. 4.17). The algorithm was formed with the following points in mind:

1. Most combat casualties do not require fluid resuscitation.
2. Oral hydration is an underused option as most combat casualties require resuscitation.
3. Aggressive resuscitation has not been shown to be beneficial in civilian victims of penetrating trauma.
4. Moderate resuscitation in animal models of uncontrolled hemorrhage offers the best outcome.
5. Large volumes of LR solution are not safe.
6. Colloid or HTS offers a significant advantage in terms of less weight and cube for the military medic or corpsman.

TABLE 4.11 Components of ketone Ringer solution.

COMPONENT	NORMAL SALINE (mEq/L)	D-LR (mEq/L)	L-LR (mEq/L)	KETONE RINGER (mEq/L)
D-Lactate	–	14	–	–
L-Lactate	–	14	28	–
3-D-β-Hydroxybutyrate	–	–	–	28
Sodium	154	130	130	130
Potassium	–	4	4	4
Calcium	–	3	3	3
Chloride	154	109	109	109

Replacing lactate with an alternative fuel source such as ketone affected the immunologic response after resuscitation. *LR*, Lactated Ringer solution.

The resuscitation fluids of choice for casualties in hemorrhagic shock, listed from most to least preferred are whole blood; plasma, RBCs, and platelets in a 1:1:1 ratio; plasma and RBCs, in a 1:1 ratio; plasma or RBCs alone; and Hextend and crystalloid (LR solution or Plasma-Lyte A).

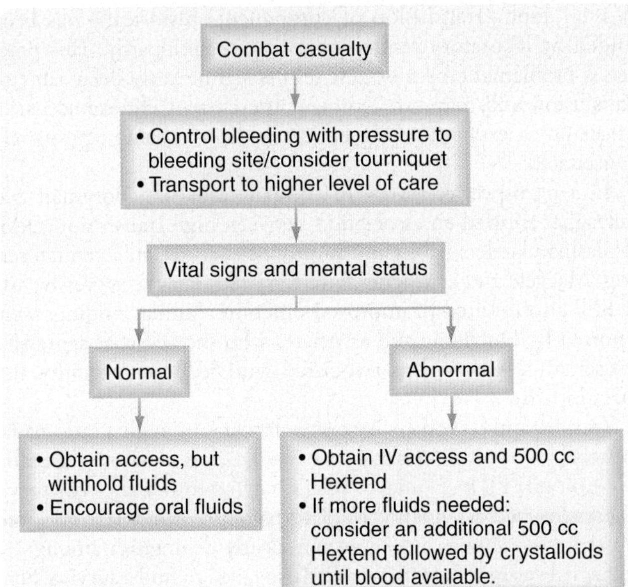

FIG. 4.17 New recommendation for fluid resuscitation from the U.S. military by the Committee on Tactical Combat Casualty Care. (From Rhee P, Koustova E, Alam H. Searching for the optimal resuscitation method: recommendations for the initial fluid resuscitation in combat casualties. *J Trauma.* 2003;54:S52–S62.)

As crystalloids were being recognized as potentially harmful to bleeding patients, a consensus panel of military experts recommended that a plasma volume expander, 6% hetastarch (Hextend), should be the nonblood fluid of choice for the military.[45] The rationale was that even though the Institute of Medicine recommended 7.5% HTS, it was not commercially available and it was not approved by the FDA for use in bleeding patients. The panel believed that a colloid offered the benefit of less weight and cube, meaning that the average medic could resuscitate patients with one-third of the volume (compared with HTS) and would not have to carry large bags of LR solution or normal saline in the field. It was recognized that most casualties were not undergoing hemorrhagic shock and were not in any jeopardy of bleeding to death. Only a minority of patients required fluid resuscitation in the field. Surgeons and anesthesiologists generally would prefer all patients to be nil per os (NPO; nothing by mouth) to avoid aspiration during induction of anesthesia and surgery, but trauma patients are never NPO. With the rapid sequence induction of anesthesia, aspiration is a minimal risk. The committee recommended placing an IV line, but not administering IV fluid, in casualties with normal mentation and normal radial pulse character. Instead, oral hydration was advised. In those undergoing hemorrhagic shock manifested by altered mental status and decreased pulse amplitude, they recommended administering 500 mL of Hextend. The use of Hextend was limited to 1 L, given its potential for exacerbating coagulopathy.

Damage Control Resuscitation

Once crystalloid solutions were recognized as possibly being the primary cause of the inflammatory process after traumatic hemorrhagic shock, efforts were made to reduce their use in the battlefield. Abdominal compartment syndrome (Fig. 4.18), which had been described after aggressive resuscitation, was also found to be directly associated with the volume of crystalloid infused. Thus, the concept of damage control resuscitation or hemostatic resuscitation was developed.[46] It involved concentrating on rapid control of bleeding as the highest priority; using permissive hypotension because this would minimize the use of acellular fluids as well as potential disruption of natural clot formation; minimizing the use of crystalloid solutions; using HTS to reduce the total volume of crystalloid necessary; using blood products early; and considering the use of drugs, such as PCC and TXA, to stop bleeding and to reduce coagulopathy (Box 4.2). The rationale for the early use of blood products was that large volumes of crystalloids were detrimental; if whole blood is available, this should be used first, followed by component therapy with PRBCs, thawed plasma, and platelets in a 1:1:1 ratio that would approximate whole blood and minimize the use of acellular fluids. Component therapy is not as ideal compared with fresh whole blood, but due to logistic problems, it was not always readily available, and component therapy was used empirically for massively bleeding patients with ongoing uncontrolled hemorrhage. Mental status was thought to be a useful guide to determine who needed care; the use of the radial pulse was preferred to BP cuffs, which are not practical when personnel are under fire in the combat setting.

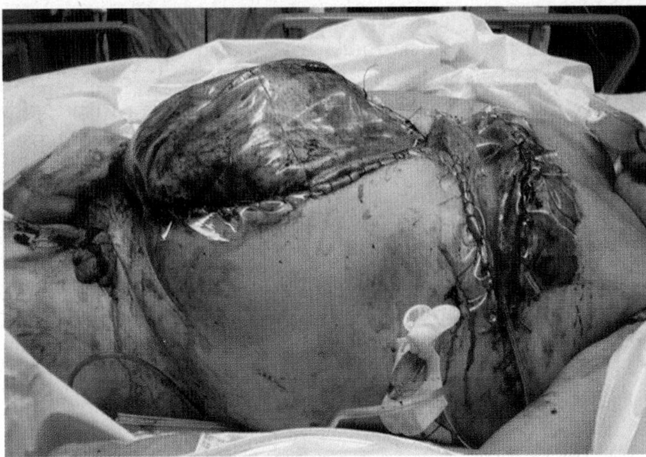

FIG. 4.18 Patient after damage control surgery with abdominal and thoracic compartment syndrome caused by massive fluid resuscitation. (Courtesy Dr. Demetri Demetriades, Trauma Recovery Surgical Critical Care Program, USC University Hospital, Los Angeles.)

BOX 4.2 Components of damage control or hemostatic resuscitation.

- Permissive hypotension until definitive surgical control
- Minimize crystalloid use
- Initial use of 5% hypertonic saline
- Early use of blood products (PRBCs, FFP, platelets, cryoprecipitates)
- Consider drugs to treat coagulopathy (rFVIIa, prothrombin complex concentrate, TXA)

From Dellinger RP, Levy MM, Carlet JM, et al. Surviving Sepsis Campaign: International guidelines for management of severe sepsis and septic shock: 2008. *Crit Care Med.* 2008;36:296–327.

FFP, Fresh frozen plasma; *PRBCs*, packed red blood cells; *TXA*, tranexamic acid.

With the promotion of damage control resuscitation, clinical studies indicated that aggressive early use of blood products, such as PRBCs and FFP, actually reduced the total volume of PRBCs used by 25%.[47] These studies also used permissive hypotension and focused on surgical control of hemorrhage rather than on resuscitation first. Other studies have shown that, with damage control resuscitation, the incidence of ARDS decreased from 25% of ICU admissions to 9%.[48] ARDS now occurs in patients with pulmonary contusion, long bone fractures, pneumonia, or sepsis, but it is no longer a routine complication in trauma patients who undergo damage control resuscitation.

Whole Blood Resuscitation

Damage control resuscitation was developed because surgeons in the war in Iraq recognized that fresh whole blood was useful for massively bleeding soldiers. Although early in this war the surgeons were hesitant and reluctant to try the walking blood bank (see later) that was used to obtain fresh whole blood from noncombat soldiers, eventually they tried it and found it to be highly successful. Returning military surgeons repeatedly noted that patients resuscitated with whole blood did not seem to have the coagulation or pulmonary problems seen previously. After operative procedures, even patients who underwent several blood volume replacement procedures were warm, not acidotic, and not coagulopathic. Trauma surgeons were starting to recognize that crystalloid resuscitation should and could be avoided by using damage control resuscitation. Since it was only recently recognized that the use of excessive fluids had an impact on outcome, they had not yet had a chance to develop the optimal resuscitation fluid to replace blood. As a result, military surgeons advocated the aggressive use of FFP, not because it was ideal, but because it was likely better than crystalloid or colloidal solutions.

The military has a logistic advantage that the civilian sector does not yet have. When casualties arrive, military surgeons activate the walking blood bank, resulting in warfighters reporting to donate their blood. Given the relative safety of these donors from an infectious aspect as they were all prescreened and they had been previously blood typed, fresh whole blood is readily available. Donated blood undergoes rapid testing for human immunodeficiency virus (HIV) and hepatitis C. These tests are around 85% sensitive. Bleeding patients are transfused with PRBCs and plasma in a 1:1 ratio until fresh whole blood is available, usually within 60 minutes of activating the walking blood bank.

Retrospective studies performed by Nessen and Spinella showed that, in combat, scenarios controlling for injury severity reveal that fresh whole blood transfusion is associated with improved survival. As the operational tempo in Afghanistan has decreased and medical treatment facilities have closed, austere surgical teams that provide care at the site of injury have been developed. These teams utilize liquid cold stored whole blood. The whole blood is stored at 4°C in citrate-phosphate-dextrose for up to 21 days, and if adenosine is added to the storage solution, it can be stored for 35 days. Select centers in the United States are now using liquid cold stored whole blood for resuscitation. Type O whole blood with low antibody titers to A and B antigens is utilized. Although most sites that utilize liquid cold stored whole blood have limited transfusion to up to 4 units, a case report of a massive transfusion of 38 units has been reported in the civilian literature.[49]

Resuscitation With 1:1:1

As news of these successful battlefield practices spread, the civilian literature started to echo the benefits of surgical hemorrhage control before resuscitation and the aggressive use of PRBCs and FFP, summarized in Table 4.12. Because whole blood is only now becoming available in the civilian sector, efforts are focused on trying to replicate whole blood by transfusing components of blood in 1:1:1 ratio. Transfusion of components historically has been guided by laboratory results indicating coagulopathy. This practice is problematic because test results significantly delay time to transfusion and may not represent the current clinical scenario, especially in exsanguinating patients who are being aggressively resuscitated.

In a retrospective review of combat casualties, Borgman and colleagues showed an association between high transfusion ratios of plasma:platelets:RBCs and improved survival. In a civilian setting, Maegele and colleagues have reported that the aggressive use of FFP also resulted in improved outcome. Similar findings were reported by Duchesne and associates who showed that aggressive resuscitation with FFP is associated with reduced mortality and coagulopathy.

Tiexaira and coworkers have shown that, although a ratio-based approach to transfusion is associated with better outcomes, the ratio of 1 unit of FFP to 2 units of RBCs may be equivalent. The previous studies had a tendency to place patients with a 1:2 ratio into the aggressive group and could not clearly distinguish among 1:1 versus 1:2 versus 1:3. Other studies also failed to find a survival benefit with FFP but showed that it reduces coagulopathy. Aggressive use of platelets[50] and fibrinogen[51] have also been associated with improved outcome. In a six-center retrospective study, Zink and associates[52] showed an association between early administration of a high ratio of FFP and platelets improved survival and decreased overall need for RBCs in massively transfused patients. The largest difference in mortality occurred during the first 6 hours after admission, suggesting that the early administration of FFP and platelets is critical. Most hospitals use apheresis platelets, which are pooled platelets; 1 unit is equivalent to what was previously called a six-pack of platelets. Hence, to achieve a 1:1:1 ratio, 1 unit of apheresis platelets should be given for every 6 units of PRBCs and FFP.

There have been multiple studies using large databases and prospective studies trying to determine if aggressive use of FFP and platelets can lead to improved outcome. It was argued that the studies showing an advantage were flawed in that they suffered from selection bias, whereby early survivors lived long enough to achieve high ratios. The prospective, observational, multicenter, major trauma transfusion (PROMMTT) study demonstrated that clinicians were transfusing patients with a blood product ratio of 1:1:1 or 1:1:2 and that early transfusion of plasma was associated with improved 6-hour survival.[53]

To settle this debate, the (PROPPR) trial was designed. This study was a prospective randomized multicenter clinical trial designed as an effectiveness and safety study in severe bleeding trauma patients comparing plasma, platelets, and red blood cells (RBCs) transfused in a 1:1:1 ratio to a 1:1:2 ratio.[54] The primary outcomes were 24-hour and 30-day all-cause mortality. It showed that there was no significant difference in mortality at 24 hours ($P = 0.12$) or at 30 days ($P = 0.26$). However, more patients in the 1:1:1 group achieved hemostasis, and fewer experienced death as a result of exsanguination by 24 hours. There were no safety differences between the two groups. The 1:1:1 group received more blood product but did not experience high rates of ARDS or MODS, infection, venous thromboembolism, or sepsis. Holcomb and colleagues[54] suggested that clinicians should consider using a 1:1:1 transfusion protocol starting with the initial units transfused while patients are actively bleeding and then transition to laboratory-guided treatment once hemorrhage control is achieved. The authors also noted that the 1:1:2 group approached a cumulative ratio of 1:1:1 after the initial ratio-driven protocol ended as they used laboratory-guided treatment, which caused them to catch up to the 1:1:1 group.[54]

TABLE 4.12 **Summaries of recent retrospective studies on the use of FFP.**

ARTICLE	SUMMARY OF FINDINGS
Borgman MA, Spinella PC, Perkins JG, et al. The ratio of blood products transfused affects mortality in patients receiving massive transfusions at a combat support hospital. *J Trauma.* 2007;63:805–813.	Retrospective study of 246 patients; PRBC: FFP ratio group of 1:1.4 had better survival rates.
Gonzalez EA, Moore FA, Holcomb JB, et al. Fresh frozen plasma should be given earlier to patients requiring massive transfusion. *J Trauma.* 2007;62:112–119.	Retrospective study of 97 patients; they recommended early use of FFP before ICU admission.
Kashuk JL, Moore EE, Johnson JL, et al. Postinjury life threatening coagulopathy: Is 1:1 fresh frozen plasma:packed red blood cells the answer? *J Trauma.* 2008;65:261–270.	Retrospective study of 133 patients; logistic regression showed improved coagulopathy but no improvement in survival.
Gunter OL, Jr, Au BK, Isbell JM, et al. Optimizing outcomes in damage control resuscitation: Identifying blood product ratios associated with improved survival. *J Trauma.* 2008;65:527–534.	Retrospective study of 259 patients; increased use of FFP and platelets improved survival after major trauma.
Holcomb JB, Wade CE, Michalek JE, et al. Increased plasma and platelet to red blood cell ratios improves outcome in 466 massively transfused civilian trauma patients. *Ann Surg.* 2008;248:447–458.	Retrospective study of 467 patients undergoing transfusion of 10 units of PRBCs or more; survival was better with increased use of FFP and platelets.
Spinella PC, Perkins JG, Grathwohl KW, et al. Effect of plasma and red blood cell transfusions on survival in patients with combat related traumatic injuries. *J Trauma.* 2008;64:S69–S77.	708 Patients undergoing transfusion showed that FFP use was associated with improved survival.
Maegele M, Lefering R, Paffrath T, et al. Red-blood-cell to plasma ratios transfused during massive transfusion are associated with mortality in severe multiple injury: A retrospective analysis from the Trauma Registry of the Deutsche Gesellschaft für Unfallchirurgie. *Vox Sang.* 2008;95:112–119.	Retrospective study of 713 patients showed improved survival with increased aggressive use of FFP in patients undergoing massive transfusion.
Duchesne JC, Hunt JP, Wahl G, et al. Review of current blood transfusions strategies in a mature level I trauma center: Were we wrong for the last 60 years? *J Trauma.* 2008;65:272–276.	Retrospective study of 135 patients with massive transfusions who had better outcome with 1:1.
Sperry JL, Ochoa JB, Gunn SR, et al. An FFP: PRBC transfusion ratio ≥1:1.5 is associated with a lower risk of mortality after massive transfusion. *J Trauma.* 2008;65:986–993.	Multicenter prospective cohort study with 415 patients showed that higher FFP use was associated with less mortality.
Moore FA, Nelson T, McKinley BA, et al. Is there a role for aggressive use of fresh frozen plasma in massive transfusion of civilian trauma patients? *Am J Surg.* 2008;196:948–958.	Retrospective study of 93 patients; concluded that damage control resuscitation with FFP may have a role in civilian trauma.
Teixeira PG, Inaba K, Shulman I, et al. Impact of plasma transfusion in massively transfused trauma patients. *J Trauma.* 2009;66:693–697.	Retrospective study of 383 patients showing that high FFP use was associated with better survival.
Duchesne JC, Islam TM, Stuke L, et al. Hemostatic resuscitation during surgery improves survival in patients with traumatic-induced coagulopathy. *J Trauma.* 2009;67:33–37.	Seven-year retrospective study with 435 patients showed survival advantage in patients receiving FFP: RBC ratio of 1:1 compared with 1:4.
Snyder CW, Weinberg JA, McGwin G Jr, et al. The relationship of blood product ratio to mortality: Survival benefit or survival bias? *J Trauma.* 2009;66:358–362.	Retrospective study of 134 patients showed improved survival with higher use of FFP, but the advantage was not persistent when adjusted for survival bias.
Watson GA, Sperry JL, Rosengart MR, et al. Fresh frozen plasma is independently associated with a higher risk of multiple organ failure and acute respiratory distress syndrome. *J Trauma.* 2009;67:221–227.	Prospective multicenter cohort study of blunt trauma patients showed that FFP was associated with increased risk of multiple-organ failure and ARDS.
Zink KA, Sambasivan CN, Holcomb JB, et al. A high ratio of plasma and platelets to packed red blood cells in the first 6 hours of massive transfusion improves outcomes in a large multicenter study. *Am J Surg.* 2009;197:565–570.	Retrospective multicenter (16) study with 466 patients who had lower mortality if FFP and platelets were used early and as 1:1.
Riskin DJ, Tsai TC, Riskin L, et al. Massive transfusion protocols: The role of aggressive resuscitation versus product ratio in mortality reduction. *J Am Coll Surg.* 2009;209:198–205.	Retrospective study of 77 patients; concluded that massive transfusion protocol was associated with improved survival.

ARDS, Acute respiratory distress syndrome; *FFP*, fresh frozen plasma; *ICU*, intensive care unit; *PRBC*, packed red blood cell; *RBC*, red blood cell.

The delivery of increased clotting factors to exsanguinating patients may explain part of the benefit of a high-ratio approach in massive transfusion. Plasma is composed of over a thousand proteins, some of which may have beneficial effects. Trauma and shock result in degradation of the vascular glycocalyx and increased endothelial permeability. This process is known as the *endotheliopathy of trauma*. Resuscitation with LR solution exacerbates this process while resuscitation with plasma rebuilds the glycocalyx and reduces vascular permeability.[55] This phenomenon likely explains the development of ARDS and abdominal compartment syndrome that occurs with massive crystalloid reduction and the reduction in multiple-organ dysfunction that has occurred as crystalloid resuscitation after trauma has been deemphasized.

Massive Transfusion Protocol

Studies have led to the development of the massive transfusion protocol (MTP), which calls for the aggressive use of component therapy or liquid cold stored, low titer O whole blood. The

TABLE 4.13 **Commercially available crystalloids and their composition.**

	NORMAL SALINE	LACTATED RINGER	PLASMA-LYTE A	NORMOSOL	PLASMA
Positive Ions					
Sodium	154	130	140	140	134–145
Potassium		4	5	5	3.4–5
Calcium		3			2.25–2.65
Magnesium			3	3	0.7–1.1
Negative Ions					
Chloride	154	109	98	98	98–108
Lactate		28	27	27	
Bicarbonate					22–32
Gluconate			23	23	
pH	5.4–7.0	6.5	7.4	7.4	7.4
Osmolarity	308	273	294	295	280–295

protocol was designed to enable a hospital's blood bank to improve logistic systems for the empirical use of blood components. A number of studies have shown that implementing an MTP improves survival in trauma patients.[56] To qualify as a trauma center, the American College of Surgeons Verification Review Committee requires that all trauma centers have an MTP in place.

An example of an MTP directive is that for severely injured patients, the blood bank should provide a cooler containing 4 units of type O RBCs and 4 units of AB or A plasma. If possible, a patient's blood sample should be drawn before the uncrossmatched blood is transfused; even 1 unit of RBCs can sometimes interfere with crossmatching. O negative blood is reserved for transfusing females of childbearing age when their blood type is unknown or when they are known to be Rh-. If the initial cooler of blood is utilized, the blood bank sends additional coolers containing plasma, platelets, and RBCs in a 1:1:1 ratio or coolers of whole blood.

CURRENT STATUS OF FLUID TYPES

Crystalloids

Large volume normal saline resuscitation produces acidosis by dilution of serum HCO_3^-. Normally, chloride and bicarbonate ions are reciprocated up or down with each other maintaining electrical neutrality. Often, the result of massive normal saline infusion is a hyperchloremic nonanion gap metabolic acidosis. At extreme levels, acidosis can impair cardiac performance, decrease responsiveness to cardiac inotropic drugs, affect cellular metabolism, change enzyme activity, and alter the coagulation cascade. Many would argue that, for cellular protection, the human body offloads oxygen more easily from hemoglobin in the acidotic state and that acidosis, at least to a degree, is actually better for a patient than alkalosis.

Regardless of the theoretical advantages and disadvantages of induced metabolic acidosis, no clinical evidence exists that it makes a difference. Surgeons with experience using HTS sometimes encounter induced metabolic acidosis but have found it to be of minimal clinical consequence. Induced metabolic hyperchloremic acidosis is different from spontaneous metabolic acidosis and from hypovolemic lactic acidosis. No evidence exists that hyperchloremic acidosis does anything more than confuse the interpretation of the metabolic state. Given the lack of any significant proven benefit of one crystalloid over another, many trauma systems use normal saline in the prehospital setting. This is because stocking just one form of fluid is convenient. Another reason is that when transfusion is required, the LR solution has to be switched to normal saline as LR solution contains calcium, which binds citrate, theoretically producing clotting. This is a regulatory policy even though studies have shown that the use of LR solution as a carrier in the same IV line as blood has no relevant side effects.

Plasma-Lyte (Baxter, Deerfield, IL), a balanced crystalloid solution, was developed more than 20 years ago and contains additional electrolytes, such as acetate and gluconate. The overall chloride level is also lower. Plasma-Lyte also contains magnesium, so this should be considered in patients with renal failure. It may also affect peripheral vascular resistance and heart rate, and it may worsen organ ischemia. It is similar to other crystalloids in that it can cause lung edema and increase ICP and generalized edema. The numerous reports of its use have addressed its safety during the priming of extracorporeal circulation pumps and its use in cold ischemia, circulatory arrest, organ transplantation, and organ preservation.

In a study examining the use of HTS with dextran, patients were randomized to receive 7.5% HTS with dextran or Plasma-Lyte A. The 2-hour sodium, bicarbonate, CO_2, and pH values were comparable. The HTS with dextran group required less crystalloid. However, the volumes infused were also different. In a study by McFarlane, 30 patients undergoing hepatobiliary or pancreatic surgery were randomized to 0.9% normal saline or Plasma-Lyte 148 at 15 mL/kg/hr. During surgery, Plasma-Lyte was found to be more efficacious, also producing less hyperchloremia and acidosis. However, no significant difference in sodium, potassium, or blood lactate level was found. In a kidney transplantation study, Plasma-Lyte A did not increase lactate levels (like LR solution) and did not cause acidosis (like normal saline); the best metabolic profile was maintained in patients receiving Plasma-Lyte. Plasma-Lyte is also favored in various cell preparations and as a storage medium for platelets. Compared with LR solution and normal saline, Plasma-Lyte may be a superior balanced solution, but no studies exist that show it is safer or more efficacious in large volumes. It may be an ideal solution for daily maintenance fluid, but it does not offer a significant benefit for resuscitation over other crystalloids. A randomized trial by Young and colleagues[57] showed that, compared with normal saline, patients resuscitated with Plasma-Lyte A had improved acid-base status and less hyperchloremia at 24 hours after injury. The components of the various crystalloids are shown in Table 4.13. In summary, there are advantages and disadvantages for various crystalloids. Plasma-Lyte has the advantage in that it has magnesium, and studies have shown that this reduces the need for magnesium replacement, although there are concerns of infusing large volumes of Plasma-Lyte due to too much magnesium.

From the chloride point of view, LR solution may be better than Plasma-Lyte, which may be better than normal saline. In a large volume, there may be an advantage of resuscitating with LR solution as it has the least amount of chloride. There are no studies showing survival advantage with any crystalloids. In short-term hemorrhagic shock studies in swine using large volumes of crystalloids, LR solution was shown to be better than normal saline and Plasma-Lyte solution. In most institutions, the costs of normal saline and LR and Plasma-Lyte solutions are similar, which is about $3.00/L. In a pragmatic, randomized trial of 15,802 ICU patients, LR and Plasma-Lyte solutions were compared with normal saline as primary resuscitation fluids. Patients who received balanced crystalloids had a lower rate of the composite outcome of death, new renal-replacement therapy, and persistent renal dysfunction compared with patients who received normal saline.[58]

Hypertonic Saline

HTS has been extensively studied. In summary, the studies have shown that sodium is the main electrolyte that controls intravascular volume. Investigators who have worked with HTS in bleeding animals have learned that resuscitation goals can be achieved with much smaller volumes as long as the sodium load is the same. For example, in an animal model of hemorrhagic shock, if 1 L of normal saline is required to achieve a BP of 120 mm Hg, the same result can be obtained with an infusion of 120 mL of 7.5% normal saline. For 5% HTS, only 182 mL would be needed. In animal studies, HTS draws water into the intravascular space from the intracellular and interstitial spaces.

HTS has consistently been shown to reduce the inflammatory response and is thus considered to be immunomodulatory (Fig. 4.19). Immunosuppression from HTS may thus be beneficial and detrimental, depending on when and how it is used. In randomized prospective studies with HTS alone or with a colloid such as hetastarch or dextran, results show that HTS is equivalent to crystalloid solutions in terms of mortality. The concentration that has been studied the most is 7.5% HTS. From 1995 to 2005, when inflammation was being extensively studied, the theoretical advantages of HTS were a decrease in the inflammatory response and potentially a reduction in ARDS and MODS. Thus, it was thought to be potentially the ideal fluid of choice in hemorrhagic shock resuscitation. One of the main problems with 7.5% HTS is that there is no manufacturer that makes and sells it. This is because it is extremely difficult and expensive to obtain FDA approval, and there is little profit in selling salt water. In Europe, 7.5% HTS with dextran is available.

The Resuscitation Outcomes Consortium (ROC), which is composed of 10 trauma centers in the United States and Canada, has been funded to participate in trauma and emergency medicine trials. ROC is a federally funded organization to examine potential prehospital interventions.

The first trauma trial by ROC examined HTS. This prospective randomized trial enrolled hypotensive patients with blunt or penetrating trauma, with and without traumatic head injury. Patients were randomized into one of three arms by dose and fluid: (1) 250-mL bolus of normal saline; (2) 250-mL bolus of 7.5% HTS; and (3) 250-mL of 7.5% HTS with 6% dextran 70. The HTS trial enrolled 2221 patients using exception from informed consent. There were two studies in this trial. The hemorrhagic shock study enrolled 894 patients, and 1327 patients were enrolled into the TBI study. The TBI trial enrolled patients with or without hypotension; the main enrollment criterion was a GCS score of 8 or less.

The HTS shock trial showed that patients receiving HTS had only a mild elevation in their sodium level (147 mEq/L vs. 140 mEq/L in the normal saline group) as the infusion volume was small and only in the prehospital setting. The admission hemoglobin level was also significantly lower. The patients who received HTS with or without dextran had a hemoglobin level of 10.2 g/dL compared with 11.1 g/dL in the normal saline group. This may reflect the amount of intravascular resuscitation from HTS versus normal saline. The overall 28-day survival rates were almost identical: HTS patients, 73%; HTS with dextran patients, 74.5%; and normal saline patients, 74.4% ($P = 0.91$).

However, the HTS trial was stopped before the end of its planned enrollment by the Data Safety and Monitoring Board for two main reasons. First, interim analysis showed futility because the outcomes were so similar. Second, a detailed subgroup analysis found a potential for harm in a subgroup of patients who did not receive RBC transfusion in the first 24 hours. For unexplained reasons, their mortality rate was significantly higher if they received HTS or HTS with dextran. HTS and HTS with dextran patients who received more than 10 units of RBCs within the first 24 hours had a lower mortality rate, although the difference was not statistically significant.

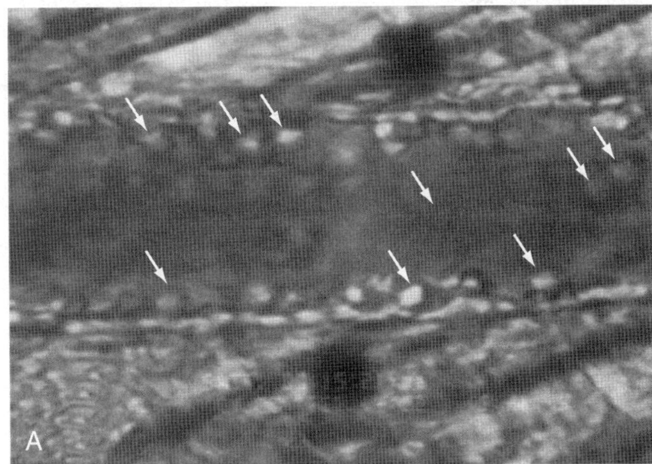

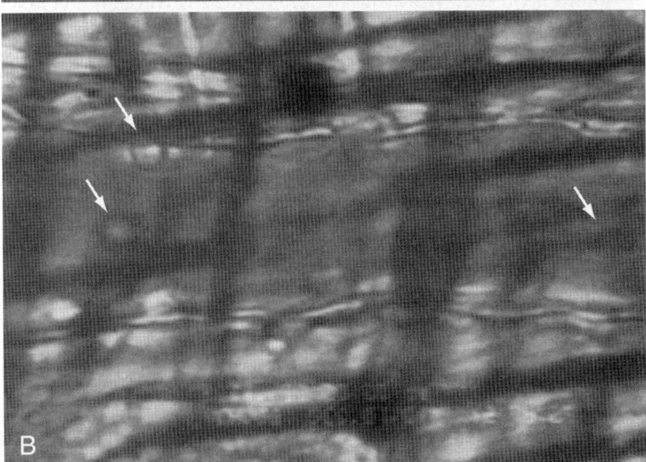

FIG. 4.19 Immunologic response from hypertonic resuscitation is less than that after lactated Ringer solution has been given. (From Pascual JL, Khwaja KA, Ferri LE, et al. Hypertonic saline resuscitation attenuates neutrophil lung sequestration and transmigration by diminishing leukocyte-endothelial interactions in a two-hit model of hemorrhagic shock and infection. *J Trauma.* 2003;54:121–132.)

The main criticism of this study was that it allowed only a small dose in the prehospital phase, and HTS infusion did not continue in the hospital. Additional resuscitation was not regulated in this study and all patients received about the same amount of prehospital fluid. Also, the sodium level was raised to only 147 mEq/L, signifying that not enough HTS was used to affect the immunomodulatory capability of HTS as some feel that the sodium level needs to be much higher to achieve that affect. In hypotensive patients, 250 mL of normal saline is clinically irrelevant, but because 250 mL of HTS with dextran 0 or HTS is approximately equivalent to 2 L of normal saline, the group of patients who received HTS were being resuscitated more, whereas the normal saline group was not. Thus, the trial seemed to compare 250 mL of normal saline to the equivalent of 2 L of normal saline. Support for this theory is that the hemoglobin level was lower in the group of patients who received HTS. The trial of HTS in patients with TBI was also halted; the interim analysis also showed futility, meaning that the primary outcome was almost identical between the normal saline and HTS groups. Such an outcome can also be interpreted as showing that HTS is safe, but technically the trial was not powered to show noninferiority.

HTS was studied in TBI because preliminary studies had shown promise. HTS infusion is highly effective in decreasing ICP and can do this while increasing blood volume, BP, and blood flow to the brain. Compared with mannitol, which is customarily used for lowering ICP, HTS might do this without dehydrating patients or putting them at further risk for secondary brain injury caused by hypotension or renal failure from mannitol. Patients receiving high-dose mannitol drips are also susceptible to pulmonary insufficiency, causing longer ICU stays. Infusion of mannitol requires high daily volumes. Mannitol is safe if it is used carefully in patients with isolated TBIs, but in hypotensive polytrauma patients, it can be detrimental and might exacerbate hypotension.

Commercially, HTS comes in 23%, 5%, and 3% concentrations in the United States. Curiously, all the human studies used 7.5% HTS, but this formulation is not commercially available. This could be the main strategic mistake of the HTS studies. Most animal and human studies have used 7.5% HTS, an arbitrary concentration as 10% HTS was found to be highly irritating to peripheral veins. HTS injected rapidly into human volunteers causes pain at the infusion site. Thus, the preferred route is through a central vein. In animal studies, if 7.5% HTS is given through the interosseous route, osteomyonecrosis and compartment syndrome can ensue. Some nontrauma studies have used 3% and 23% concentrations, but minimal clinical experience has been reported with 5%. There are two studies reporting their experience using 5% HTS in trauma patients, with or without TBI, and it has been found to be safe.[59] This finding is logical because the 7.5% HTS studies have also shown safety. Using 5% HTS may be the best strategy to recruit intravascular volume compared with crystalloid resuscitation. The method used in trauma patients is to give 5% HTS in 250-mL infusions and, if more than 500 mL is needed, to check sodium levels. The sodium content of 250 mL of 5% HTS is equivalent to 1645 mL of LR solution. Thus, a bolus can be given quickly, without having to use hypotonic solutions such as LR solution.

Colloids

Human albumin (4%–5%) in saline is considered to be the reference colloidal solution. It is fractionated from blood and heat treated to prevent transmission of viruses. It has many theoretical advantages, especially in animal studies, but clinical studies have not shown outcome differences. Its main theoretical advantage is that, compared with crystalloids, it is less inflammatory. This may be because it is a natural molecule. Other than its dilutional effect, albumin is associated with minimal coagulopathy. No clinical evidence has shown that albumin is better than other colloids, but the (SAFE) study in Australia has shown 4% albumin to be safe, compared with normal saline, in ICU patients.[60] The SAFE study, whose main intent was to show equivalency, found no difference in the primary outcome (28-day mortality rate) or in any secondary outcome. The Committee on Tactical Combat Casualty Care has recommended a low-volume resuscitation fluid using 500 mL of Hextend for tactical reasons. The reason for that choice was that 7.5% HTS is not commercially available. The adoption of damage control or hemostatic resuscitation has been thought to result in improved outcome, decreased blood use, and decreased incidence of ARDS.[61] ARDS and MODS still occur, but at a much lower rate than previously seen.

There are still other advantages of 25% albumin over artificial colloids. Albumin has a proven immunologic antiinflammatory effect and five times less volume than current artificial colloids. Unlike artificial colloids, it does not potentially lead to coagulopathic side effects. It has been proven to be safe from infectious and clinical standpoints. The volume of fluid that has to be carried is obviously much less (Fig. 4.20). Albumin costs approximately 30 times more than crystalloids and three times more than dextran or Hextend, but those comparisons were made against 5% human albumin. The cost of 100 mL of 25% albumin, compared with 500 mL of Hextend on a physiologic basis, is only approximately three times as much. During the Vietnam War, 25% albumin was first made available, and it seemed to have worked well. It was packaged in a green can that could be transported without damage, had a long shelf life, and was easy to use.

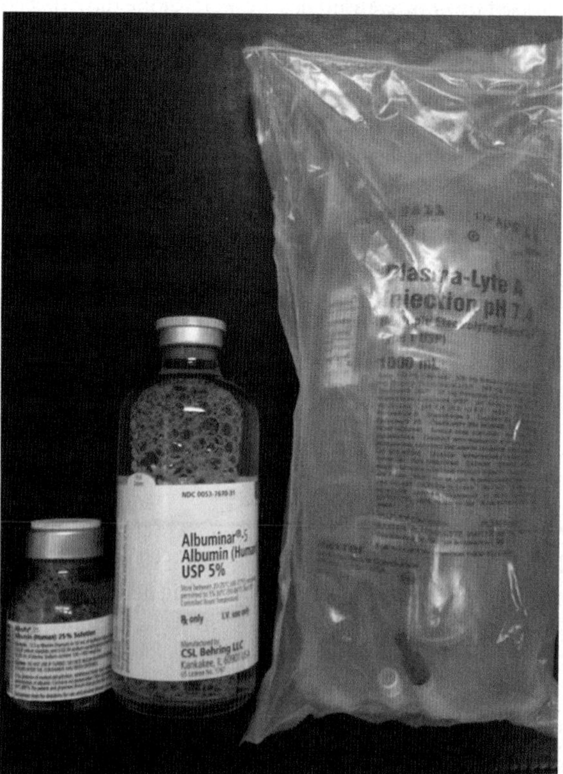

FIG. 4.20 Comparison of container sizes: 50 mL of 25% albumin, 500 mL of 5% albumin, and 1 L of lactated Ringer solution. The 50 mL of 25% albumin is physiologically equivalent to approximately 2000–2500 mL of crystalloids.

The commonly used synthetic colloids are plasma, albumin, dextran, gelatin, and starch-based colloids. Hetastarch solutions are produced from amylopectin obtained from sorghum, maize, or potatoes. Extensive randomized controlled trials have examined the safety and efficacy of 5% albumin, 6% hetastarch, and 6% dextran. However, no evidence has shown that one colloid is superior to another or that colloids are better or worse than crystalloids.[62] Colloids such as hetastarch can have proinflammatory effects similar to those of crystalloids. In some cases, colloids will do more harm in large volumes than crystalloids, but not all colloids should be considered the same. It is well known that artificial colloids can perpetuate coagulopathy; dextran is used specifically to help prevent clotting after vascular surgery. The inflammatory system is tightly interwoven with the coagulation process. Hetastarch, particularly the high–molecular-weight preparations, is associated with alterations in coagulation, specifically resulting in changes in the viscoclastic measurements and fibrinolysis. Studies have questioned the safety of concentrated (10%) hetastarch solutions with a molecular weight of more than 200 and a molar substitution ratio of more than 0.5 in patients with severe sepsis, citing increased rates of death, acute kidney injury, and use of renal replacement therapy. To prolong intravascular expansion, a high degree of substitution on glucose molecules protects against hydrolysis by nonspecific amylases in the blood. However, this results in accumulation in reticuloendothelial tissues such as skin, liver, and kidneys. Because of the potential for accumulation in tissues, the recommended maximal daily dose of hetastarch is 33 to 55 mL/kg/day. Thus, it would be prudent to limit the use of Hextend to 1 L in trauma patients who are often harmed if they have coagulopathy from increased bleeding. Studies in trauma patients have shown an association between acute kidney injury and death after blunt trauma. Patients with severe sepsis assigned to fluid resuscitation with hydroxyethyl starch 130/0.4 had an increased risk of death at day 90 and were more likely to require renal replacement therapy compared with those receiving Ringer acetate. In animal models, albumin seems to be better for preventing inflammation, whereas hetastarch and dextran in high doses appear to cause inflammation and coagulopathy.

FUTURE RESUSCITATION RESEARCH

Blood Substitutes

In contrast to volume expanders, blood substitutes refer to fluids that can carry oxygen. Each year in the United States, 15 million units of RBCs are transfused. Methods to decrease the need for blood transfusions include preoperative autologous donation, intraoperative blood retrieval with reinfusion, and isovolemic hemodilution. Such methods allow withdrawing of a patient's blood at the start of surgery, replacing it with volume expanders, and then, at the end of surgery, retransfusing the patient with his or her donated blood. Because of blood supply limitations, infectious and transfusion complications, and storage limitations, the need for blood substitutes remains. The ideal blood substitute would do the following:

- Deliver oxygen
- Be compatible with all blood types
- Have few side effects
- Have prolonged storage capabilities
- Persist in the circulation
- Be cost-effective.

Currently, blood substitutes are either hemoglobin based or nonhemoglobin based. Research on hemoglobin-based fluids dates back to the 1920s when the stroma of the cells was lysed to obtain hemoglobin. Purification and sterilization were hurdles that took decades to overcome, but it was soon realized that free hemoglobin had toxic effects (because of the breakdown products). Problems with free hemoglobin include osmotic diuretic effects, renal toxicity, coagulation abnormalities, short half-life, and vasoconstrictive effects (which are known to be caused by hemoglobin solutions scavenging nitric oxide).

During the next three decades (the 1930s, 1940s, and 1950s), efforts concentrated on stabilizing the hemoglobin molecule to increase its persistence in the circulation and to prevent toxic effects. Such strategies included cross-linking the molecule between the tetramer subunits, polymerizing it, encapsulating it in an artificial red cell or in liposomes, and using microsphere technology to form a million stable micromolecules. Development of some hemoglobin substitutes advanced to clinical trials.

Blood substitutes are referred to as hemoglobin oxygen carriers (HBOCs). Current second-generation HBOCs are pasteurized and thus free of communicable pathogens; they also have no ABO/Rh or other blood antigens. They are universally compatible and require no blood banking. They can be easily administered without special training or expertise. The problems of a short half-life and renal toxicity have now been overcome, but some troublesome side effects remain: ree radical generation and exacerbation of reperfusion injury, methemoglobin production, and immunologic effects (including immunosuppression and potentiation of endotoxin-related pathogenicity).

The hemoglobin for blood substitutes comes from a variety of sources, such as outdated donated human blood, bovine or swine blood, and transgenic *E. coli*. Each source has its benefits (availability, cost) as well as its side effects (infections, other complications). Human hemoglobin has the advantage of being a naturally occurring product that has been extensively studied. Its obvious disadvantage is lack of availability. About 2 units of discarded blood are required to make 1 unit of the HBOC. Even if we were to capture all of the discarded human blood, the numbers of units made would only be half of what was discarded.

The potential advantages of animals as a source of hemoglobin are tremendous; they are a relatively cheap source, and their supply is ample. Yet despite efforts at controlling a herd, problems such as bovine spongiform encephalitis will inevitably surface. Recombinant hemoglobin has problems as well. Volumes of bacterial culture and the stringent processing methods are costly. It is estimated that only 0.1 g of hemoglobin can be generated from 1 L of *E. coli* culture. This equates to 750 L to make 1 unit. Production of 3 million units would require more than 1.125 billion liters of culture.

One of the first HBOC products tested was manufactured by Baxter in 1999. Diaspirin cross-linked hemoglobin (DCLHb), known as HemAssist, was tested. This chemically modified human hemoglobin solution was used in a highly publicized trial in patients with traumatic hemorrhagic shock, one of the first trials to use except from informed consent (instead of individual patient consent). Baxter terminated the trial early because the patients who received the test product had a higher 28-day mortality rate (47%) than those who received normal saline (25%) ($P < 0.015$). The trial brought disappointment to investigators anticipating the success of the first red cell substitute.

A recent analysis compared data from the Baxter trial with the 17 U.S. emergency departments and the parallel 27 European

Union prehospital systems now using DCLHb. This analysis did not show any difference in outcome. The authors reported that neither mean BP readings nor elevated BP readings correlated with DCLHb treatment of traumatic hemorrhagic shock patients. As such, no clinically demonstrable DCLHb pressor effect could be directly related to the adverse mortality outcome observed in the Baxter trial.

Two other products currently have potential for clinical use. Both are polymerized rather than tetramerized. Polymerization is thought to be better because the molecular masses are higher (130 kDa) than with tetramerization (65 kDa), resulting in longer intravascular presence. Some investigators have proposed that polymerization avoids contact with nitric oxide, attenuating the vasoconstriction seen with previous products.

One of those products is HBOC-201 (Hemopure; Biopure Corporation), made from bovine blood. It is universally compatible and is stable at room temperature for up to 3 years. Animal studies showed great promise. Human trials involving orthopedic patients also showed promise, but safety issues were a concern; patients who received Hemopure had an increased number of serious adverse events. The vasoconstrictive properties of Hemopure may have caused myocardial infarction in susceptible patients. Biopure Corporation went bankrupt and was taken over by OPK Biotech, which has a product called Oxyglobin (HBOC-301) for veterinary use. FDA approval for Hemopure is still pending. OPK Biotech has continued to develop Hemopure for human use; the U.S. Navy is supporting research for potential use in the military setting. Studies have been proposed to coinfuse a nitric oxide donor such as nitroglycerin in a fixed ratio, in a single-bag compound, or as separate infusions. However, there is little likelihood that surgeons will accept a product to treat shock that requires coinfusion of a vasodilator.

The more promising hemoglobin-based product is PolyHeme. The way it is produced removes nearly all of the cross-linked tetrameric hemoglobin (<1% residual). PolyHeme is made from outdated human donated blood and has a shelf life of about a year at room temperature. Of several human trials, the most recent was a multicenter study in trauma patients with the need for informed consent waived. Patients were randomized to receive PolyHeme or to receive crystalloids and RBCs. A total of 29 trauma centers enrolled 714 patients. They reported that patients can be resuscitated with up to 6 units of PolyHeme within 12 hours of injury, without using stored blood; outcomes between the two groups were comparable (30-day mortality rate: 13.4%, PolyHeme group; 9.6%, control group). However, the PolyHeme group had more serious adverse events, specifically, an increased number of myocardial infarctions. Nonetheless, the benefit-risk ratio of PolyHeme may be favorable when blood is needed but not available. PolyHeme is not currently being used due to the increased incidence of serious adverse events.

A metaanalysis of 16 HBOC trials, including 4 trauma trials involving HemAssist or PolyHeme, showed that HBOC patients had a significantly increased risk of myocardial infarctions and death compared with controls. The problem of vasoconstriction remains. Vasodilators can be added to mitigate vasoconstriction, but whether enthusiasm for HBOCs persists remains to be seen. Without doubt, however, they have a real potential benefit for patients who do not have access to RBCs, such as in rural areas or austere combat conditions.

Third-generation hemoglobin substitutes have begun to address the deficiencies of earlier formulations. The encapsulation of hemoglobin in liposomes is an innovation, but efforts to optimize these continue. The mixing of phospholipids and cholesterol in the presence of free hemoglobin forms a sphere with hemoglobin in the center. These liposomes have oxygen dissociation curves similar to red cells, and administration can transiently achieve high circulating levels of hemoglobin and oxygen delivery. Research is still in the preclinical testing stage; progress in prolonging the half-life and elucidating the effects on the immune system, particularly reticuloendothelial sequestration, is crucial before clinical testing can begin.

Perfluorocarbons

Perfluorocarbons (PFCs) are completely inert biologically and similar to Teflon or Gore-Tex. Altering the molecule (by fluoridating the ring structure) lowers the melting point and thus makes it a liquid at room temperature. PFCs captured the imagination of many in 1966, when photographs were introduced of a mouse completely submerged in the liquid form but breathing and surviving in it (Fig. 4.21). PFCs dissolve larger quantities of oxygen and CO_2 than plasma. They have yet to find a purpose in liquid form, but enthusiasm has increased for their use in partial liquid ventilation. Trials in adults with ARDS have shown no benefit, but trials are still ongoing in children with hyaline membrane disease.

PFCs have two challenges to overcome for use as blood substitutes. The first is that the liquid form is immiscible in water; thus, PFCs must be suspended as microdroplets with the use of emulsifying agents. The second is that unlike hemoglobin, the oxygen that is dissolved in PFCs has a linear relationship to the Po_2, whereas hemoglobin has a sigmoidal disassociation curve favoring

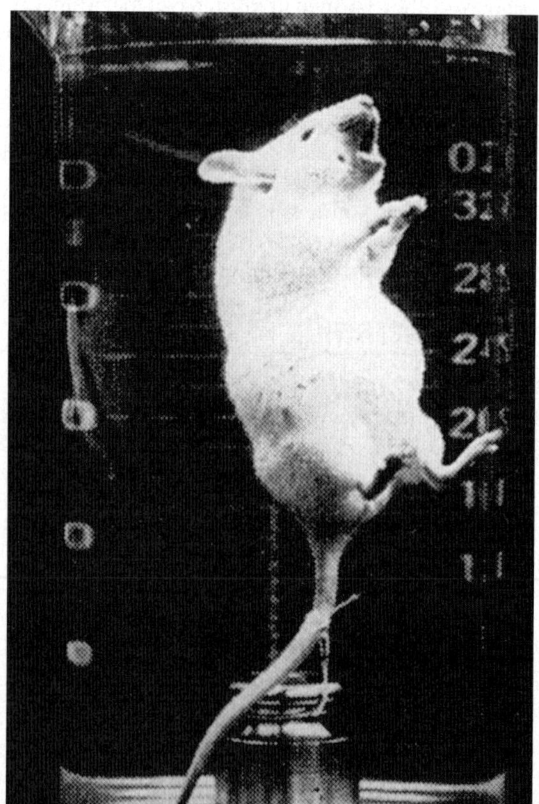

FIG. 4.21 Mouse surviving while submerged in perfluorocarbons. (From Shaffer TH, Wolfson MR. Liquid ventilation. In: Polin RA, Fox WW, Abman SH, eds. *Fetal and Neonatal Physiology*, 3rd ed. Philadelphia, PA: WB Saunders; 2003.)

full loading at normal atmospheric oxygen levels. Thus, the percentage of inspired oxygen (FIO_2) that is required to be applied for PFCs is high.

Second-generation PFCs have been formulated to allow more oxygen-carrying capacity, with alterations in the emulsion properties. Such new compounds can also be stored at 4°C, whereas previous solutions had to be frozen. Oxygent (Alliance Pharmaceutical Corp./Baxter Healthcare Corp.) is a 60% perflubron emulsion with a median particle diameter of less than 0.2 μm. The use of lecithin as an emulsifier eliminated the adverse effects of complement activation observed in earlier studies of PFCs. Possible current scenarios for its use include cardiopulmonary bypass with normovolemic hemodilution and balloon angioplasty (to provide oxygenated blood past the catheter while it is inflated). In a phase 3 study, Oxygent was shown to reduce the need for RBC transfusion in patients undergoing noncardiac surgery (16%, Oxygent group; 26%, control group; $P < 0.05$). Oxygent patients, however, had more serious adverse events (32% in the Oxygent group vs. 21% in the control group; $P < 0.05$). In another phase 3 study, in patients undergoing cardiac bypass, Oxygent possibly increased the incidence of strokes. All further studies were halted.

Two other PFC products have been introduced. In early-phase clinical trials, OxyFluor (HemaGen) produced mild thrombocytopenia and influenza-like symptoms in healthy volunteers. Baxter International has withdrawn support for further development. Phase 2 trials of Oxycyte (Synthetic Blood International) have been suspended; it has been taken over by Oxygen Biotherapeutics, Inc., and is being sold over the counter as a cosmetic product known as Dermacyte, an oxygen concentrate gel for wound healing. Dermacyte is also being investigated for the treatment of cancer during chemotherapy or radiation therapy because oxygen-free radicals are thought to kill cancer cells. PFCs are not free of side effects and are not efficacious for oxygen delivery and use.

Novel Fluids

The recognition that currently available fluids are not a replacement for blood and that they in fact can be harmful if used in large amounts to expand blood volume has initiated exciting research for better fluids. Blood is so highly complex that the ultimate goal is to develop artificial whole blood, but doing so will take much time. The ideal method would be to manufacture whole blood with a bioreactor using stem cells, but the development of this would take decades.

The permutations of future fluid development are endless. Novel crystalloids are being tested, as are hypertonic solutions with and without oxygen carriers, hypertonic colloids, freeze-dried plasma (FDP), and drug therapy.

The Institute of Medicine in 1999 recommended research to eliminate lactate in LR solution and to investigate the use of alternative energy substrates in resuscitation fluids. It recognized that, although reperfusion injury can occur in shock resuscitation, a separate entity called *resuscitation injury* is a result of the method of resuscitation and the fluids used.

Two substances have since been identified that may alter the inflammatory response after resuscitation. In small and large animal models, studies found that simply replacing the lactate in LR solution with either ketones or pyruvate reduced the inflammatory response after hemorrhagic shock resuscitation. Other investigators have concentrated on various forms of pyruvate to minimize resuscitation injury; ethyl pyruvate seems promising. Studies in animals show that pyruvate Ringer solution corrects lactic acidosis and prolongs survival during hemorrhagic shock in rats. From a cellular level, a combination of antiinflammatory constituents in fluids seems more efficacious.

Studies of the mechanisms behind such improved results found that monocarboxylate-supplemented resuscitation provides energy substrates, with minimal alteration in the conventionally used fluids such as LR solution. Replacing the lactate in LR solution with either pyruvate or ketones protected the brain and other tissues after shock. That finding led to research on the reasons for this protective effect and on the potential of using drugs alone to treat hemorrhagic shock.

Dried Plasma

Dried plasma was utilized during World War II, when the U.S. Army initially believed that plasma was adequate to resuscitate hemorrhagic shock (Fig. 4.22). Dried plasma utilized in WWII came from multiple donors and was not screened for viral pathogens. Hepatitis transmission in injured warfighters was common. There has been no dried plasma product available in the United States since WWII. However, the capability of removing potential infectious agents along with the improved technology for manufacturing of dried plasma resurrected research in this field. Dried plasma is prepared in one of two ways. It can be FDP or lyophilized with a combination of low-temperature, low-pressure, and low-moisture circulating air. It can also be spray dried in a high-temperature chamber, where it is aerosolized. The product can be stored in either of these forms with minimal protein degradation until it is reconstituted, pH adjusted, and then administered. The advantages of dried plasma are the long shelf life and that it does not need refrigeration and tight temperature control. It avoids the difficult logistics of storing fresh frozen products and the preparation time of thawing FFP. Modern-day dried plasma has been

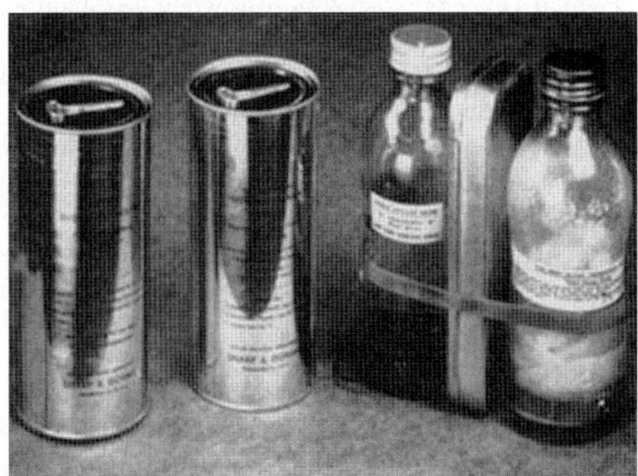

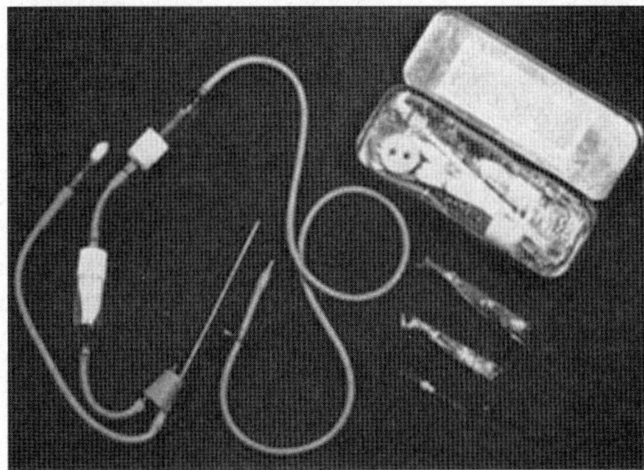

FIG. 4.22 Freeze-dried plasma used during World War II. (Courtesy Office of Medical History, U.S. Army Medical Department, Center of History and Heritage, Washington, DC.)

pathogen reduced so that the historical concerns of transmitting viruses are minimized.

Through funding by the U.S. Navy, plasma separated from fresh porcine blood was lyophilized to produce FDP and then compared with FFP. After a 60% blood volume hemorrhage, pigs were resuscitated with reconstituted FDP, which was just as efficacious as thawed plasma and had an identical coagulation profile. A multiinstitutional polytrauma animal trial found that FDP was better than Hextend (which led to anemia and coagulopathy).[63] Currently, this area of research and development is exciting and promising. FDP is currently available in Europe and Africa but not in the United States.

The French Army has been using freeze-dried and plasma (FLyP) since 1994. It is made from fresh leukodepleted blood of up to 10 volunteers. Blood type selection allows the dilution and neutralization of natural anti-A and anti-B hemagglutinins. This FDSP is thus compatible with any blood type. It is also shelf stable in ambient temperatures for 2 years and is easily rehydrated with 200 mL of water for use in less than 3 minutes. FLyP contains all clotting factors and proteins. The fibrinogen and clotting factor levels of FDSP are equivalent to FFP. Early reports of using FLyP in 87 battlefield casualties show that it is effective for preventing or treating coagulopathy in a French ICU in Afghanistan. FLyP has been studied in the civilian setting revealing that it is effective compared with FFP and results in increased fibrinogen levels early after trauma. (Garrigue D, Coagulation) This French product is carried by U.S. Special Forces medics for use in austere conditions under an Institutional Review Board (IRB) protocol.

Germany also has FDP (LyoPlas N-w), which comes from a single donor screened for blood-borne pathogens. Unlike FFP, LyoPlas N-w undergoes filtration to further remove cellular remnants to reduce the risk of infection or transfusion immune reactions. It remains effective for 12 months when it is maintained at a temperature range of 4°C to 25°C. Germany has fielded more than 500,000 units of LyoPlas N-w without unusual or significant adverse effects compared with FFP. In addition to the ability to prevent or to treat coagulopathy, it is an excellent way to restore volume as it is a colloid. The Israeli Defense Forces Medical Corps policy is that plasma is the fluid of choice for selected, severely wounded patients, and thus it included LyoPlasN-w as part of its armamentarium for use at the point of injury by advanced lifesavers across the entire military. Several companies are developing dried plasma in the United States, but, to date, there is no FDA-approved product.

There has been research to develop freeze-dried red blood cells, but the challenge has been to overcome the freezing, drying, and rehydration process without stressful injury to the RBCs. Although freeze-dried red blood cells have been shown to have acceptable viscoelastic deformability properties, with storage times of about 1 week by adding trehalose, a sugar molecule, this product is still in very early stages of development. Freeze-dried platelets and platelet-derived particles are also being developed. Frozen platelets are cryopreserved in 6% dimethyl sulfoxide and can be stored for up to 10 years at −80°C. Freeze-dried platelets have been in development for more than 50 years but preserving functionality has been a challenge. Modern preparations, which are treated with 1.8% paraformaldehyde, frozen in 5% albumin, and then lyophilized, have been more encouraging. Once rehydrated, they seem structurally intact, contain most of the glycoproteins, and are capable of supporting thrombin generation and fibrin deposition. However, in vivo testing shows that the duration of hemostatic activity is brief, approximately 4 to 6 hours, and sometimes limited to 15 minutes. Recent studies of human freeze-dried platelets in a swine liver injury model have demonstrated improved survival and reduced blood loss, but 13% of the surviving animals were found to have thrombotic complications. The idea of FDP, red blood cells, and platelets would mean reconstitutable whole blood.

Pharmacologic Agents

Resuscitation fluids simply replace the lost intravascular volume but have no inherent prosurvival properties. Therefore, a body of work is investigating whether it would be logical to design therapies promoting a prosurvival phenotype. Among patients resuscitated from hemorrhagic shock, a wide spectrum of responses is observed. Although some patients recover without any complications, others develop multiple-organ failure. This unpredictable response is not caused by a widespread variation in the human genome. Since the decoding of the human genome, it has become apparent that only 20,000 to 35,000 protein-coding genes are responsible for millions of different phenotypes. The rapidly expanding field of epigenetics focuses on mechanisms and phenomena that affect the phenotype of a cell or an organism without affecting the genotype. Over the years, many pharmacologic agents have been tested as possible adjuncts (or substitutes) to conventional fluid resuscitation. These drugs cover a wide spectrum, including neuroendocrine agents, calcium channel blockers, ATP pathway modifiers, prostaglandins, sex steroids, antioxidants, antiinflammatory agents, and immune modulators. Although there is strong laboratory evidence of their beneficial effects on tissue perfusion, myocardial contractility, reticuloendothelial function, cell survival, oxidative injury, and immune activation, most of these agents are not yet in clinical use as resuscitative agents.

This area of work is an example of translational research that is novel and could be revolutionary. DNA transcription is regulated, in part, by acetylation of nuclear histones that are controlled by two groups of enzymes: histone deacetylases (HDACs) and histone acetyltransferases. Animal experiments showed that hemorrhagic shock and resuscitation were associated with HDAC/histone acetyltransferase activity misbalance and that the acetylation status of cardiac histones is influenced by the choice of resuscitation strategy. Shock-induced changes can be reversed through the infusion of a pharmacologic HDAC inhibitor, even when it is administered for only a limited period after the insult. Animal experiments have shown tremendous promise in elucidating mechanisms behind the success of using an HDAC inhibitor to prolong life after shock.[64]

Alam and colleagues have been investigating the role of HDAC inhibitors, such as valproic acid (VPA, an anticonvulsant) and suberoylanilide hydroxamic acid. They hypothesized that they may be useful in the treatment of shock through restoration of normal cellular acetylation. In their experiments, large swine subjected to trauma (femur and liver injury) and to severe hemorrhage (60% blood loss) were randomized into one of three groups: no treatment (control group), treatment with fresh whole blood, or treatment with VPA (400 mg/kg) without resuscitation. The early survival rate was 100% in the fresh whole blood group, 86% in the VPA group, and 25% in the control group.[65] Impressively, this survival improvement was achieved without conventional fluid resuscitation or blood transfusion, which makes this approach appealing for the logistically constrained prehospital and battlefield environments. It appears that HDAC inhibitors rapidly activate nuclear histones as well as numerous cellular proteins to create a prosurvival phenotype in hemorrhagic and septic shock. This group has also reported that VPA is neuroprotective and is promising for the treatment of TBI. It has also been shown to be beneficial in sepsis. A number of these HDAC inhibitors are being tested in phase 1 and 2 clinical trials (nontraumatic situations).

Given concerns that inflammation after trauma might be a pathologic event, another unique approach is to use estrogen and progesterone to treat patients after traumatic hemorrhagic shock. A number of independent laboratory studies have pointed to the use of estrogen and progesterone as a promising method to reduce secondary injury in hemorrhagic shock and other similar processes. Those studies have shown that the early administration of estrogen (a strong antioxidant, antiinflammatory, and mitochondrial stabilizer as well as an antiapoptotic agent) significantly decreased the severity of injury caused by early, devastating cell death. The use of estrogen has now been tested in 60 clinical trials, mostly in the fields of prostate cancer, uremic bleeding, liver transplantation, spine surgery, cardiology, cardiac surgery, and TBI. Its safety record is good. However, human trials in TBI have failed to show any efficacy.

Suspended Animation

The military has supported research to develop a technique to prevent patients from dying of exsanguination. Repairable torso hemorrhage is still a major cause of potentially preventable death in the battlefield, so research is being conducted to identify a method of preserving a patient's life long enough to later repair the sources of hemorrhage. This concept is termed suspended animation. Rather than resuscitation, the goal is to stop cellular death, either with induced hypothermia or by chemical means.

Initially, animal studies focused on identifying hibernation inducers that chemically signal cells to decrease metabolism. Serum from hibernating squirrels can be injected into nonhibernating squirrels and induce hibernation. Metabolism slows, heart rate decreases, and life seems to be suspended. Many mammals are highly tolerant of ischemia, such as diving seals, which can remain underwater for 45 minutes at a time. Bears hibernate in the cold, and turtles can bury themselves in mud without dying. The search continues for the answer to this question: How can human life persist without oxygenation at the rate we are accustomed to? This fascinating area of research should help us understand the meaning of life at the cellular level, but the clinical use of hibernating inducers is many years away.

Hypothermia or cooling reduces the metabolic needs of cells. Thus, induced hypothermia has been studied to determine whether it can put life on hold. Once metabolic demands are decreased, life can be slowed or "suspended." This metabolic suspension can be effectively achieved with hypothermia as well as with various chemical infusions. Interestingly, life or metabolism does not seem to end with the cessation of perfusion; rather, it actually ends during reperfusion, when irreversible cellular damage is done. Reperfusion of cells that have exhausted their supply of nutrients can damage cells and thus end life. The mechanisms are complex, but calcium exchange may be a key component.

Because exsanguination is a major cause of death both in the battlefield and in civilian trauma, the suspension of life with hypothermia or chemical cellular arrest could buy time to transport patients to a hospital where their vascular injuries can be repaired and their life restored. Animal work has been performed to perfect a method of inducing suspended animation and then successfully restoring life without neurologic injury. Clinically induced hypothermic arrest is actually already being used in cardiothoracic surgery and neurosurgery, but the current length of time that flow to the brain can be halted is only about 45 minutes. In cardiac surgery, the heart is arrested and cooled while the rest of the body is perfused with a pump. The idea is to take the methods that are used to preserve the heart and apply them to the whole body, including the brain. However, such methods are complex and require extensive preparation and immense teamwork; whether they can be simplified for emergencies, such as unexpected exsanguination, is unknown.

Animal work on this topic has been performed for 60 years. The late Peter Safar, the father of modern-day cardiopulmonary resuscitation, studied induced profound hypothermic arrest in dogs and rats under controlled conditions. Research funded by the U.S. Navy involved a series of experiments showing that profound hypothermia to 10°C can be induced by infusing cold fluids containing massive doses of potassium. Essentially, the process is similar to achieving cardioplegia except that a solution is infused to arrest not only the heart but the entire body. The solution used to induce such massive hypothermic and chemical arrest is an organ preservation fluid (HypoThermosol) that contains potassium in levels of 70 mEq/L.

Patients who have in effect died of exsanguinating traumatic hemorrhage typically undergo a resuscitative thoracotomy in the emergency department to stop their bleeding and to attempt to resuscitate them. However, this is a desperate maneuver with dismal results; only 7.4% of such patients survive. The U.S. Navy developed a new method; once the chest is opened, instead of trying to resuscitate patients, they are infused with cold HypoThermosol.

Large animal (swine) models have been used to develop the techniques that induce suspended animation in the emergent setting; studies have repeatedly shown that swine could be put into whole body arrest and then rapidly (within 20 to 30 minutes) made hypothermic to 10°C. During this process, all the blood is removed from the swine; they are left in that state for about 1 to 3 hours. This, by clinical definition, "kills" the swine; no metabolism occurs during that state, no brain or heart activity can be detected, and no blood is in the body. These animal studies have shown feasibility of this approach in a clinically realistic model with a variety of injuries including hemorrhagic shock with soft tissue injuries, vascular injuries below the diaphragm, and solid organ injuries. The survival is better than 75% long term, and the animals recover neurologically intact with normal cognitive function.

Theoretically, this is the period during which human patients could be taken to the operating room for vascular repairs; such patients almost always have suffered major vascular injury causing exsanguination. Because the vascular repairs would be done in an asanguineous state, no blood loss during the repairs would occur. Such repairs have been accomplished with portable pumps that are smaller than a can of soda.[65] This is also the period during which human patients could be put on a standard bypass machine by a second team of surgeons; that machine would be used to revive patients by flushing out the potassium and warming them while blood is infused. In the swine model, this entire process has been shown to be feasible, even after extended periods of shock and even with associated vascular, solid organ, and hollow viscus injuries.

Research on this concept by the military has advanced to a point at which a multicenter clinical trial is now planned. The mechanisms and methods to suspend life and then to restart it have clearly been identified. The traditional teaching has been that hypothermia during trauma care is bad, but there is a difference between spontaneous hypothermia and induced hypothermia. Spontaneous hypothermia indicates hemorrhagic shock and is often associated with massive resuscitation with cold or room temperature fluids. Such severely injured patients will do poorly, given their blood loss and the dilutional coagulopathy (which is obviously detrimental when patients have uncontrolled bleeding). Appropriately induced hypothermia, however, can be beneficial.

PERIOPERATIVE FLUID MANAGEMENT

Body Water

Humans are made predominantly of water (50%–70% of body weight). The precise percentage is affected by gender, body fat, and age with an increase in water percentage in males, increase in lean body mass, and extremes of age. The human body can do without many things for long periods, but water is not one of them. In the body, water resides in three compartments or spaces: (1) intracellular, (2) intravascular, and (3) interstitial. The intracellular compartment has the largest volume of water, constituting about 30% to 40% of body weight (two thirds of the body's total water). The intravascular volume is usually calculated as 5% to 7% of body weight (one sixth of the body's total water). Water shifts rapidly between the three compartments. Large resources of water can be pulled from the intracellular compartment into the intravascular compartment; large volumes of water can be stored in the interstitial compartment. Water in the interstitial compartment is recirculated by the lymphatics and eventually returns into the intravascular compartment.

A fixed amount of water is in bones and dense connective tissue, but this water is relatively stable and not considered to be in circulation. Water is secreted by various cells in the skin, cerebrospinal fluid, and intraocular, synovial, renal, and GI systems; this water is also not considered to be in circulation.

Clinical tools are available to accurately measure the volume of water in the body. One method is bioimpedance spectroscopy, which measures electrical current impedance that is imperceptible to the person to estimate total body water. The method is best used to calculate body fat.

Methods to measure intravascular volume are also commercially available. They usually involve injecting a known concentration of tagged molecules (such as potassium-40 or albumin) that remain intravascular for a known time period. Potassium is predominantly an intracellular solute, and albumin is predominantly extracellular. Sampling the blood and calculating the volume based on the decreased concentration of the injected tracer is fairly accurate. This method has not caught on for clinical use because the baseline volume is not known; even if it were known, the intravascular volume is contractible and expandable, so the desired intravascular target volume is not yet known. During injuries and illnesses, when homeostasis has not been maintained, normal values may not be applicable or desirable during resuscitation. The practicality of measuring these spaces has not been identified, yet research has shown that a person's extracellular volume can be expanded even if they are dehydrated intracellularly.

The main intracellular electrolytes are potassium and magnesium. Intracellularly, they are the principal cations; phosphates and proteins are the principal anions. Extracellularly, in contrast, sodium is the predominant cation; chloride and bicarbonate are the predominant anions. In plasma (given its higher protein content, which is due to organic anions), the total concentrations of cations are higher, whereas the concentrations of inorganic anions are lower than in the interstitial fluids. The Gibbs-Donnan equilibrium equation states that the product of the concentrations of any pair of diffusible cations and anions on one side of a semipermeable membrane will equal the product of the same pair of ions on the other side. Cell walls are semipermeable membranes; the flow of water is determined by the osmotically active particles (about 290–310 mOsm). The effective osmotic pressure depends on those substances that fail to pass through the pores of the semipermeable membrane.

The unit of milliequivalents per liter (mEq/L) refers to the number of electrical charges; milliosmoles per liter (mOsm/L), to the number of osmotically active particles or ions. A milliequivalent in a solution must be precisely balanced by the same number of milliequivalents of a cation and anion. The balance affects the direction of water as it equilibrates. The osmotic pressure of a solution refers to the actual number of osmotically active particles present in the solution, but it does not depend on the chemical-combining capacities of the substances. For example, sodium chloride dissociates to 2 mOsm, whereas sodium sulfate (Na_2SO_4) dissociates into three particles: 2 mOsm of sodium and 1 mOsm of sulfate. However, 1 mOsm of an un-ionized substance such as glucose is equal to 1 mOsm of the substance.

The dissolved proteins in the plasma are responsible for the effective osmotic pressure between the plasma and the interstitial fluid, frequently referred to as the colloid osmotic pressure. Sodium is pumped outside the cell and potassium inside the cell. Thus, sodium is the major electrolyte responsible for the osmotic pressure, but glucose and urea (which do not easily penetrate the cell membrane) also increase the effective osmotic pressure. Water passes across the cell membrane freely, so sodium has a highly important impact on the movement of water. However, the concentration of sodium is not necessarily related to the volume status of ECF. A severe extracellular volume deficit can occur with a low or high sodium concentration over time.

The osmotic gradient is also important in controlling water. The number of osmotic particles is the key. The size of the osmotic particle does not matter. For example, transfusion of PRBCs will actually cause water to pass from the intravascular space to the interstitial space. Immediately after transfusion of PRBCs, hydrostatic pressure increases inside the vascular space, and water is pushed out. Although the hematocrit level of PRBCs is 60% to 70%, the red cells act as one osmotic particle. Due to the size difference between red cells and proteins in the blood, fewer osmotic particles are in a given volume of PRBCs compared with whole blood. Therefore, the osmotic pressure intravascularly is actually reduced after transfusion of PRBCs.

The size difference between a red cell and albumin is large (like a soccer ball versus a grain of sand), but each will act as one osmotic particle. The number of soccer balls that can fit into a stadium is limited, but the number of grains of sand that can fit is many orders of magnitude higher. Similarly, with a transfusion of PRBCs, water is pushed out of the intravascular space into either the interstitial or the intercellular space because of the decrease in the number of osmotic particles per volume.

Maintenance Fluids

In surgical patients, assessing the intravascular status is a pivotal task but also one of the most difficult. Surgical patients have blood loss from trauma, operations, and diseases. In addition, volume deficits occur from losses of GI fluids because of vomiting, diarrhea, nasogastric suctioning, fistulas, and drains. Fluid also shifts out of the intravascular space because of burns, inflammation (as in pancreatitis), intestinal obstruction, infection, and sepsis.

Nonetheless, the main daily task of perioperative patient care is assessing the intravascular status. Is it where it needs to be? It is safer for surgeons to assume that a patient is hypovolemic or hypervolemic than normal; the normovolemic band is very small. The maintenance fluid should constantly be adjusted, depending on the individual patient's current status. Surgeons must pay attention to each patient's fluid status and body needs rather than infuse maintenance fluid at a fixed rate.

For the routine preoperative care of patients about to undergo elective surgery, the customary approach is to start a maintenance drip of crystalloids. Note, however, that patients who undergo same-day surgery have little need for preoperative fluids. All preoperative patients are asked to not take in any fluids by mouth starting the night before surgery, a directive that typically does not result in any problems. Remember that all of us (whether or not we are surgical patients) are NPO (Latin for *nil per os* or nothing by mouth) when we go to sleep; we do not normally wake up hypotensive or in renal failure. Thus, for patients about to undergo major surgery requiring inpatient hospitalization after surgery, IV fluids the night before are not necessary; they typically will receive plenty of fluids from the anesthesiologist during the operation.

In patients who underwent a colectomy, a small prospective randomized study showed that minimizing crystalloids during surgery led to a better outcome; such patients had less nausea and vomiting, decreased hospital length of stay, and faster return of GI function. However, starting such patients on a maintenance fluid is safe, mainly to provide water (Box 4.3). In adult patients weighing more than 40 kg, the simple rule for calculating the fluid rate in ml/hr is 40 plus the weight in kilograms; that is, a 73-kg patient's maintenance rate would be 113 ml/hr (73 + 40).

Maintenance fluids have not been rigorously tested, so the ideal fluid is unknown. The current standard is to use 5% dextrose in half-normal saline with 20 mEq per liter of potassium. The source of the standard's formulation remains unclear. For a 70-kg NPO man, it would provide sodium and potassium, yet it is not what the average person requires (Table 4.14). The average 70-kg man's requirements are listed in Table 4.15.

The average salt intake per day in American men has been difficult to assess; the median is an estimated 7.8 to 11.8 g/day. Since that range does not include salt added at the table, it is probably an underestimate. The U.S. Department of Agriculture recommends a salt intake of less than 2.3 g/day. Normal saline contains 9 g of sodium chloride in 1 L of water. The amount of fluids and electrolytes infused into patients with the standard formulation is highly inaccurate. The decision to give 5% dextrose in maintenance fluid is thought to derive from fasting studies of Harvard medical students in the 1920s. Those studies found that providing about 100 g of glucose decreased protein spillage in the urine. The rationale for the use of half-normal saline and 20 mEq per liter of potassium is unknown. A survey of critical care intensivists showed that most did not know the daily-recommended intake of sodium or potassium.

Surgeons fear that an insufficient volume of fluid will lead to renal failure. Oliguria in a 70-kg man is defined by less than 400 mL of urine produced and excreted in a 24-hour period. That is the minimum volume required to maintain normal serum blood urea nitrogen and creatinine levels so that the kidney is able to maximally function. That volume equates to 0.24 mL/kg/hr. Historically, surgical residents were mandated to give patients enough IV maintenance fluid to produce 0.5 mL/kg/hr, probably to build in a safety margin to ensure enough volume. Today, it is not uncommon to see residents give patients a 1-L fluid bolus of crystalloids for urine output of less than 50 mL/kg/hr, a practice that will usually lead to overhydration. The kidneys are marvelous at protecting the body from physicians who have not studied physiology. In general, overhydration has not been typically seen as a problem, and anasarca has been seen as harmless; however, that view is inaccurate as it can lead to issues with ventilation and intraabdominal hypertension.

Postoperatively, patients are more often hypervolemic initially due to higher than necessary IV fluid infusions. Due to bleeding from surgery and the need for IV infusion, patients often receive too much blood and fluid during surgery due to fears of hypotension. Giving a few liters of blood and fluid is probably inconsequential. For patients who have lost liters of blood, however, accurate measurement is impossible; inferences have to be made as to what the volume status is. Patients who have lost a minimal amount of blood during elective surgery, who have received liters of crystalloids, and who have adequate urine output do not necessarily need IV maintenance fluids. For typical patients on the surgical ward, normal functioning kidneys will generally make up

BOX 4.3 Maintenance fluid calculation.

Maintenance Intravenous Fluid Calculation

- 4 mL/kg/hr for first 10 kg
- 2 mL/kg/hr for next 10 kg
- 1 mL/kg/hr for every kilogram over 20 kg

Sample Calculation for 45-kg Patient

- 10 kg × 4 mL/kg/hr = 40 mL/hr
- 10 kg × 2 mL/kg/hr = 20 mL/hr
- 25 kg × 1 mL/kg/hr = 25 mL/hr
- Maintenance rate = 85 mL/hr

Sample Calculation for 73-kg Patient

- 10 kg × 4 mL/kg/hr = 40 mL/hr
- 10 kg × 2 mL/kg/hr = 20 mL/hr
- 53 kg × 1 mL/kg/hr = 53 mL/hr
- Maintenance rate = 113 mL/hr

TABLE 4.14 Contents of maintenance solution.*

	TOTAL IN 24 HOURS
Water	2760 mL
Dextrose	132 g
Sodium	11.8 g (203 mEq)
Potassium	1.9 g (53 mEq)

*With 5% dextrose in half-normal saline with 40 mEq per liter of potassium in a 70-kg patient for 24 hours.

TABLE 4.15 Normal needs for a 70-kg man per day.

	TOTAL IN 24 HOURS
Water	2000 mL
Urine	1500 mL
Sodium	2–4 g
Potassium	100 mEq

for any errors in the amount of blood and fluid given. However, for ICU patients on a ventilator who have severe traumatic injuries, sepsis, other comorbid conditions, or blood loss, there is less room for error.

For ICU patients, in general, too much intravascular volume is better than too little. Too much volume equates to increased time on the ventilator, too little equates to renal insufficiency or renal failure. Pulmonary failure has an associated mortality rate of 20% to 25%, whereas renal failure has an associated mortality rate of 48%. Managing volume correctly would equate to a perfect number of days on the ventilator and to no days on dialysis.

Immediately after surgery, volume requirements are vastly different than during the next day. Again, for ICU patients, it is generally better to err on the conservative side with increased IV volume postoperatively for a predetermined period. Most surgeons do not have an issue with giving several 1-L boluses of fluids but are terribly afraid of having an IV rate of 500 mL for 4 hours even though the total volume of fluid may be the same. When fluids are given as a bolus, the body tends to be confused; hormone releases will wildly fluctuate as it tries to compensate for such wide swings in pressure and volume in the vascular system.

Surgical patients are often hypovolemic intravascularly, despite being overhydrated during the operation. The body can be dramatically overloaded by many liters (at least per calculations of how much fluid has been infused) yet still be hypovolemic intravascularly. This is due to an inflammatory response that leads to increase permeability of the vasculature and increasing fluid in the interstitial space. The total daily water input in such patients may be up, but determining the current intravascular volume is vital to try to predict volume status over time as the water shifts from the interstitial space to the intravascular space.

Especially for ICU patients, the same maintenance rate over days can be a problem. Again, determining their fluid status is difficult. Surgeons need to gather as much information as possible to estimate what the IV maintenance rate should be. Knowing the blood urea nitrogen to creatinine ratio is helpful. A ratio higher than 20 is generally thought to be prerenal; a ratio lower than 10 suggests a volume replete state. Such generalizations are true only for patients with normal renal function. Urine output is an excellent way to determine volume states. High output generally will mean that the body is trying to rid itself of water; surgeons should assist it by decreasing the maintenance fluid rate. Anasarca is another helpful clue, as are the customary vital signs.

In older patients with heart failure or sepsis who are intravascularly hypovolemic, anasarca can be profound. Many such patients will need more IV fluids despite having anasarca. To help estimate vascular volume, central venous pressure and data from pulmonary artery catheters (if available) may be useful. However, caution should be taken in interpreting heart rate. Central venous pressure, wedge pressure from pulmonary artery catheter, stroke volume, cardiac output, and volume status all roughly correlate, but heart rate and intravascular volume are difficult to correlate. Heart rate is affected by many known and unknown variables, including pain, anxiety, hormone levels, and temperature.

For patients with arterial blood gases, the PaO_2 to FiO_2 (P/F) ratio is extremely helpful. The P/F ratio is the arterial oxygen concentration divided by the inspired percentage of oxygen. In a healthy young patient without heart disease, the arterial oxygen content is about 100; because room air is 0.21% oxygen, the P/F ratio is about 500 (100/0.21). If that same patient is placed on 100% oxygen, arterial oxygen content would be 500 with a P/F ratio of 500. In a healthy patient who does not have pneumonia, sepsis, or pulmonary contusion, the P/F ratio can reflect interstitial or lung water status; it will help direct what the maintenance rate should be.

If patients have a calculated maintenance IV rate, the surgeon evidently thinks that the intravascular volume rate is ideal and that the water shifts that occur all the time are not expected to be an issue (because the total water content is deemed ideal).

In surgical patients with low urine output, the most common error is to provide furosemide as an IV bolus. In most, if not all such patients, low urine output postoperatively means that they have deceased renal blood flow from insufficient intravascular volume. When blood flow to the kidneys is decreased, the kidneys sense inadequate intravascular volume; therefore, the renin-angiotensin system, ADH, atrial natriuretic peptide, carotid baroreceptors, and other mechanisms function in an effort to preserve water. If furosemide is injected as a bolus, it prevents the distal Henle loop from reabsorbing water thus increasing urine output. Increased urine output in patients with an intravascular volume deficit exacerbates the problem. An entire set of compensatory mechanisms will kick in again in an effort to preserve more water.

Low urine output is a signal that the maintenance rate should be higher; high urine output is usually a signal that the maintenance rate should be lower. If surgeons are forced to pull water out of a patient's body because of life-threatening hypoxia, diuretics such as furosemide can be used in a drip form, which does not result in the toxic side effects seen with a bolus of furosemide. Still, decreasing intravascular volume status will have multiple effects on many organs.

For resuscitation of patients, our knowledge of biochemistry and physiology might suggest that one particular fluid would make much more sense than another. For example, fluids such as Plasma-Lyte and Normosol-R resemble the contents of the electrolytes in blood more than solutions such as LR solution or normal saline. Solutions resembling serum may be optimal in that they lessen the chance of hyperchloremic acidosis caused by the higher concentrations of chloride in normal saline. In the body, chloride and bicarbonate are in equilibrium; in the presence of high levels of chloride, a nonanion gap acidosis will result. However, advocates of normal saline argue that even though acidosis due to anaerobic metabolism is not generally desired, hyperchloremic acidosis is not necessarily harmful. It may help offload oxygen at the tissue level from the hemoglobin molecule. As noted above, balanced crystalloid solutions have been shown to result in improved outcomes compared with normal saline in ICU patients.

The costs of monitoring and replacing electrolytes can be significant. Normal saline is problematic due to the chloride load, and the balanced fluids like Plasma-Lyte reduce the need for frequent replacement of electrolytes such as calcium, potassium, and magnesium. None of the crystalloids are truly balanced, and they all have some advantages and disadvantages. These solutions can also be problematic when the patient is in renal failure. High doses of magnesium are also a potential issue in certain circumstances. Because surgical patients often require blood transfusions, purists will urge the use of crystalloids as carriers without calcium because there is fear that calcium will cause blood to clot in the IV lines. Whole blood or PRBCs mixed with an equal volume of LR solution has not increased clot formation in vitro compared with saline reconstitution. These are tools in the armamentarium, and there are times for all of them. For daily maintenance needs of a few liters a day in a patient without renal failure, Plasma-Lyte or Normosol may be better than LR or saline solutions.

Adrenal Gland

The adrenal medulla affects intravascular volume during shock by secreting catechol hormones. They are called catecholamines because they contain a catechol group derived from the amino acid tyrosine. The most abundant catecholamines are epinephrine, norepinephrine, and dopamine, all of which are produced from phenylalanine and tyrosine. Cortisol is also released from the adrenal cortex and plays a major role in that it controls fluid equilibrium. From the adrenal cortex and the zona glomerulosa, aldosterone is produced in response to stimulation by angiotensin II and hyperkalemia. Aldosterone is a mineralocorticoid that modulates renal function by increasing recovery of sodium and excretion of potassium.

Many other organs are involved in the control of hormones, including the hypothalamic-pituitary interface, which leads to the release of adrenocorticotropic hormone from the anterior pituitary gland. This system is affected by a variety of circumstances, including intravascular pressure, intravascular volume, and electrolytes such as sodium. The juxtaglomerular apparatus of the kidney produces the enzyme renin, which generates angiotensin I. Angiotensin I is converted to angiotensin II by the angiotensin-converting enzyme located on the endothelial cells of the pulmonary arteries. This regulation of intravascular fluid status is further affected by the carotid baroreceptors and the atrial natriuretic peptides. To infuse any of these hormones or to block them leads to compensatory mechanisms and perturbations within this complicated system.

The system is also affected by many other factors that we have recently discovered—and is likely affected by others that we have yet to elucidated. For example, TBI has been shown to affect the hypothalamic-pituitary interface directly by mechanical trauma or by elevated ICP. For such patients, treatment becomes difficult to control as they go through a wide range of physiologic responses. Patients undergoing brain herniation will go from a bradycardic hypertensive state to a profoundly tachycardic and hypotensive state. During that roller coaster ride, urine output is also affected, and diabetes insipidus (DI) or syndrome of inappropriate ADH (SIADH) can occur. Most likely, the human body has teleologically evolved to try to reduce brain edema at all costs; high-volume urine output often results, requiring vasopressin infusions. Patients whose regulatory system is malfunctioning or whose adrenal glands have been exhausted also have a need for high dose pressors. However, studies have shown that the infusion of cortisol and thyroid hormone in drip form can decrease such instability and minimize the need for fluid infusion and pressors. Patients undergoing brain herniation illustrate how complex the regulatory system is; surgeons must be cognizant of the minute-to-minute changes that can occur.

Adrenal glucocorticoid insufficiency, but not complete failure, occurs in patients with impaired function of the hypothalamic-pituitary-adrenal axis. Such patients produce limited amounts of corticosteroids. Clinical problems develop when patients are stressed by hypovolemia from hemorrhage, onset of an infection, fear, or hypothermia. In evaluating patients during a surgical emergency, chronic adrenal insufficiency may be initially diagnosed after intractable hypotension is found. Pathologic causes of chronic adrenal insufficiency include autoimmune destruction of the adrenal gland in which cytotoxic lymphocytes gradually destroy cortisol-synthesizing cells in the adrenal cortex. Patients can also develop adrenalitis where symptoms of fatigue, inanition, weight loss, and postural dizziness occur gradually. Their chief complaint may be vague cramping abdominal pain, nausea, and a change in bowel habits. Laboratory findings suggesting adrenal insufficiency are hyperkalemia, acidemia, hyponatremia, and elevated serum creatinine levels due to a deficiency in aldosterone. The diagnosis of adrenal insufficiency secondary to end-organ failure is established by disproportionately elevated adrenocorticotropic hormone levels (compared with cortisol levels).

Clinical findings in patients with sudden acute adrenal insufficiency can be nonspecific. If plasma cortisol levels precipitously decline to nil, patients will have abdominal pain syndrome, vomiting, and a tender abdomen and then will progress to prostration, coma, and hypotension unresponsive to catecholamine infusion. Signs and symptoms of a gradual reduction in cortisol function include malaise, fatigue, and hyponatremia with hyperkalemia. Patients with a complete loss of circulating glucocorticoids can die within hours after irreversible hypotension.

In critically ill patients, quickly establishing the diagnosis of adrenal insufficiency is difficult. Laboratory tests can confirm that plasma levels of the hormones are depressed, but test results take hours to obtain. Pending the laboratory test results, surgeons treat such patients empirically with hormone replacement therapy. Treatment of glucocorticoid deficiency in adults consists of an IV infusion of dexamethasone, methylprednisolone, or hydrocortisone. Using dexamethasone is preferred if sending simultaneous laboratory tests to confirm the diagnosis of acute hypercortisolism as this medication does not interfere with the cosyntropin test. Once test results have returned, the exogenous steroids can be rapidly tapered during the subsequent days as the patient's condition stabilizes.

Methylprednisolone has an antiinflammatory milligram-per-milligram potency of 5; dexamethasone, of 25 (relative to 1.0 for hydrocortisone). Patients whose adrenal glands are nonfunctional may also require replacement of mineralocorticoids. Patients with primary adrenal failure should be treated with 50 to 200 μg/day of fludrocortisone for mineralocorticoid replacement.

Antidiuretic Hormone and Water

ADH causes water to be reabsorbed and thus reduces urine output. Synthesized in the hypothalamic region, ADH is stored in the pituitary from where it is released into the circulation. Excess production or release of ADH causes overhydration; water is retained and thus sodium levels are lowered. Because serum osmolality is predominantly related to sodium, it will be lower than normal (285 mmol/kg) with excess ADH.

One example of overhydration is SIADH. Despite being overhydrated due to excess ADH production, the kidneys are signaled to hold onto water. Therefore, urine osmolality will be high (>300 mmol/kg) even though serum osmolality is low.

Yet if ADH is not synthesized or released, such as in patients with TBI, the kidneys will start to put out high volumes of water; urine osmolality will be as low as 100 mmol/kg. The resulting dehydration will lead to elevated serum sodium levels. In patients with TBI, the development of DI is associated with significant brain injury and poor prognosis. In patients with DI or SIADH, the body's water thermostat or regulator is dysfunctional; close attention needs to be paid to maintain volume control. Treatment of patients with DI should include desmopressin (1-desamino-8-D-arginine vasopressin, or DDAVP); of patients with SIADH, water restriction.

ELECTROLYTES

Sodium

Sodium is vital for homeostasis and the action potential in the body. It is the predominant molecule that controls water movement in and out of the vascular system. The normal range of serum sodium concentration is 135 to 145 mEq/L. Hyponatremia and hypernatremia, heavily controlled by ADH, are common problems in surgical patients. In general, mild forms of hyponatremia and hypernatremia are not a problem, but hyponatremia is more concerning than hypernatremia. Of the many signs and symptoms associated with each, none of them is specific; none of the signs or symptoms alone would lead a clinician to diagnose a sodium abnormality. A blood test is always required.

Hyponatremia

Hyponatremia can be mild (130–138 mEq/L), moderate (120–130 mEq/L), or severe (<120 mEq/L). Both mild hyponatremia and moderate hyponatremia are common but only rarely symptomatic. Severe hyponatremia, however, can cause headaches and lethargy; patients can even become comatose or have seizures. Typically, acute hyponatremia is symptomatic while chronic severe hyponatremia can often be asymptomatic. Hyponatremia is a problem when cells swell as a result of the body's decreased ability to maintain homeostatic osmolality. The most common reason for hyponatremia is iatrogenic with excess water given via IV fluids, but it can also be commonly caused by pathologic processes in the brain or lungs.

Assessing the cause of hyponatremia is important as patients are usually classified on the basis of their volume status. Patients with hyponatremia are usually hypotonic; on occasion, they may be hypertonic, with high serum glucose or mannitol levels. In severe hyperglycemia, osmolality of the ECF rises and exceeds that of the intracellular fluid. The cause of this is that glucose penetrates cell membranes slowly when insulin is absent, so hyperglycemia draws water out of the cells into the ECF. Serum sodium concentrations fall in proportion to the dilution caused by the hyperglycemia. The measured sodium level is lowered by 1.6 mEq/L for every 100 mg/dL of glucose above 100. That phenomenon is referred to as transitional hyponatremia because no net change in body water occurs. No specific therapy is required other than treating the hyperglycemia; artificially lowered sodium concentrations will return to normal once the plasma glucose level is normalized. The most common formulas for sodium are shown in Box 4.4.

The patient's fluid volume status is critical in assessing hyponatremia. In general, hyponatremia is thought of as either renal or extrarenal. Impaired excretion of sodium by the kidneys is due to renal failure or to problems with ADH or diuretics. Extrarenal causes include sodium loss due to wounds, burns, sweating, congestive heart failure, cirrhosis, hypothyroidism, GI losses, and cerebral salt-wasting syndrome. Acute hyponatremia can also occur if dehydrated patients are infused with fluids free of sodium. In patients who have bled or who are intravascularly depleted of water (e.g., because of vomiting, diarrhea, pancreatitis, or burns), IV infusion of 5% dextrose in water can rapidly cause hyponatremia. As the normal response to hyponatremia is the suppression of ADH release in the pituitary leading to the secretion of water to increase the sodium concentration in the serum, the problem is exacerbated in hypovolemic patients because the hypothalamus is secreting ADH in an effort to preserve water. Thus, hyponatremic patients should have undetectable levels of ADH. However, ADH release can be stimulated both by elevated ECF osmolality and by reduced ECF volume. ADH secretion commonly occurs transiently after trauma or burns and even in the early postoperative period, causing euvolemic hyponatremia. In hypovolemic patients, baroreceptors also stimulate the hypothalamus to retain water through ADH release since the homeostatic mechanism for maintaining intravascular volume is stronger than maintaining proper sodium concentration.

Diuresis with furosemide or mannitol, in addition to causing intravascular fluid loss, can cause hyponatremia. It also increases sodium loss by the kidneys and increases ADH release as the body tries to counteract the rapid fluid loss by preserving water. Hyperglycemia, if it is high enough for glucose to be spilled in the urine, will also induce an osmotic diuresis that depletes extracellular water and also leads to hyponatremia. Along with diuresis, hyperglycemia can lead to a variety of electrolyte imbalances (many regulatory mechanisms are involved) and can cause wild hormonal swings and imbalances.

Renal loss of sodium can lead to hyponatremia and to excessive release of natriuretic peptides related to brain injury or disease. One particularly difficult condition to treat is cerebral salt-wasting syndrome. Even when such patients are treated with salt, the regulatory mechanisms cause high urine output (up to 4–6 L/day) with consequent urine sodium losses. Those losses correlate with elevated brain natriuretic peptide levels in plasma. The lost sodium must be replaced either through an IV line or by enteral intake.

In patients with a brain injury, hyponatremia that is normally well tolerated may be devastating; it is thought to cause cerebral intracellular swelling as osmolality is reduced. In such patients, infusion of HTS may be required. Depending on the electrolyte imbalances, salt infusions can take a variety of forms; sodium can be provided as sodium chloride, sodium acetate, or sodium bicarbonate or in combinations.

If urologic or gynecologic surgery is performed with hypoosmotic irrigation, acute hyponatremia can occur. During endometrial resection as well as in transurethral resection of the prostate, acute water intoxication has been reported as a complication.

In surgical ICU patients, a frequent cause of hyponatremia is SIADH. This syndrome can be acute or chronic. In hypovolemic patients, the body's natural response is to release ADH; however, if the body is euvolemic and yet releases ADH inappropriately, the diagnosis of SIADH can be made. Therefore, the diagnosis of SIADH should be made only in euvolemic patients. In addition, the urine osmolarity is usually above 150 mmol/kg and the urine sodium above 20 mmol/L. Given the aberrant release of ADH, the serum osmolality is often less than 270 mmol, and yet

BOX 4.4 Sodium equations for clinical use.

Sodium Deficit

Sodium deficit (mEq) = ([Na] goal – [Na] plasma) × TBW

TBW = (Weight × 60%)

Free Water Deficit

Free water deficit = (([Na]/140) – 1) × TBW

Corrected Sodium

Corrected sodium = [Na] + 0.016 × (Glucose – 100)

Serum Osmolality (Calculated)

2 × [Na] + BUN/2.8 + Glucose/18

Fractional Excretion of Sodium

FeNa = [Na] urine + Creatinine plasma /[Na] plasma + Creatinine urine

<1% = ?Prerenal (hypovolemia)

>2% = Intrinsic renal disorder

BUN, Blood urea nitrogen; *TBW*, total body water.

the kidneys still excrete concentrated urine. It is usually managed with fluid restrictions. Furthermore, it is important to differentiate SIADH from adrenal insufficiency, in which hypokalemia also does occur.

A hyponatremic patient with a urine osmolality of 350 mmol is producing ADH, and the kidneys are concentrating it as they should; the source of hyponatremia is usually extrarenal. ADH-secreting tumors (such as carcinoid tumors or small cell carcinomas of the lung) can cause chronic SIADH. These lung tumors usually cause euvolemic hyponatremia. Up to 35% of patients with active acquired immunodeficiency syndrome (AIDS) who are admitted for hospitalization have SIADH. Hyponatremia can also be caused by renal dysfunction in patients with conditions that impair the capability to retain sodium, such as medullary cystic disease, polycystic kidney disease, analgesic nephropathy, chronic pyelonephritis, and obstructive uropathy after decompression syndrome.

Hypernatremia

Hypernatremia is usually defined as serum sodium concentration above 145 mEq/L. Moderate hypernatremia (146–59 mEq/L) is fairly well tolerated, whereas severe hypernatremia (>160 mEq/L) can be detrimental. Hypernatremia is associated with muscle weakness, restlessness, lethargy, insomnia, and, in severe cases, central pontine myelinolysis or coma. The common causes of hypernatremia include endocrine syndromes (in which ADH synthesis or release fails), failure of renal tubular cells to respond to ADH, increased salt intake or infusion, and loss of water. Hypernatremia can be a problem since osmosis will pull water out of the cells; the primary concern is that it is thought to contract the cerebral cells. However, recent experience with HTS has shown that acutely elevated sodium levels are relatively safe. HTS is used to contract cerebral intracellular volume in patients with TBI to reduce the total brain volume when intracranial swelling or mass effect is a factor. The normal response to hypernatremia is for the kidneys to generate hyperosmolar urine and to retain water. Renal correction of hypernatremia depends on the patient's having access to water.

Hypernatremia is associated with hypertonicity and should be classified in the context of hypovolemia, euvolemia, or hypervolemia. Hypovolemic hypernatremia commonly occurs in dehydrated patients with low water intake, high fluid losses such as vomiting, nasogastric tube loss, or diarrhea. Euvolemic hypernatremia is seen in patients with DI (nephrogenic or neurogenic) because of excess loss of urinary free water. Hypervolemic hypernatremia is usually iatrogenic caused by resuscitation with hypertonic solutions or a result of excess mineralocorticoids in Conn or Cushing syndrome.

Hypernatremia (like hyponatremia) is thought of as either renal or extrarenal. Renal fluid losses are due to diuretics, the polyuric phase of acute tubular necrosis, or postobstructive diuresis of the kidney. After decompression of a chronically obstructed ureter, renal tubular cells seem to respond less to ADH. Nephrogenic DI is defined as an impaired capacity of the renal tubules to respond to ADH and to concentrate urine. Moderate hypernatremia develops in patients with nephrogenic DI when they lose water in dilute urine, despite elevated plasma levels of ADH. If an infusion of ADH does not increase urine osmolality, nephrogenic DI is the likely diagnosis. Drugs such as lithium, glyburide, demeclocycline, and amphotericin B can induce DI. The treatment of patients with lithium-induced nephrogenic DI is amiloride (5–10 mg daily).

Hypercalcemia or severe hypokalemia also impairs the capacity of renal tubular cells to absorb sodium. Patients with end-stage renal dysfunction and low glomerular filtration rates may produce a fixed volume of 2 to 4 L/day of isoosmotic urine. In hot and arid environments, such patients are particularly susceptible to dehydration and hypernatremia.

The extrarenal causes of hypernatremia include loss of water from vomiting, diarrhea, nasogastric tube suctioning, burns, sweating, fever, or problems with insufficient ADH levels. Infusion of sodium (like HTS) can also cause hypernatremia; the duration depends on the volume of crystalloids infused for resuscitation during 24 hours. A study on the use of 5% HTS in trauma patients showed that sodium levels rose above 150 mEq/L and stayed elevated for days. In contrast, previous studies on the use of 7.5% HTS infusions found that the hypernatremia was brief. The transient hypernatremia was probably caused by aggressive use of other crystalloids for resuscitation after the HTS infusion, which quickly diluted the hypernatremia.

In dealing with hypernatremia, it is again important to first assess volume status. Correcting the hypernatremia depends on volume status. In hypovolemic patients, offsetting the volume deficit with isotonic fluids is sufficient. However, nonhypovolemic patients need free water replacement with hypotonic solutions. In hypervolemic patients, diuretics may be used—carefully. In general, in asymptomatic patients, sodium levels should not be corrected too rapidly; doing so could cause cerebral edema. In patients with acute hypernatremia, the rate is usually no more than 1 to 2 mEq/hr; with chronic hyponatremia, no more than 0.5 mEq/hr. Sodium levels should not be corrected at a rate of more than 8 mEq/day. Careful and frequent sodium monitoring is often required.

Patients with DI are producing dilute urine at rates of hundreds of milliliters per hour. They should be treated with desmopressin (DDAVP), a synthetic analogue of ADH that has a half-life of several hours. DDAVP increases water movement out of the collecting duct, but it does not have the vasoconstrictive properties of ADH. Patients with mild DI can be treated with intranasal DDAVP and water intake. DDAVP can be administered orally, intranasally, subcutaneously, or intravenously. The intranasal dose is 10 μg once or twice daily. In ICU patients, IV administration is preferred for control and accuracy.

Potassium

Potassium is the main intracellular ion; sodium, the main extracellular ion. The normal potassium concentration in serum is 4.5 mmol/L. Small changes in serum reflect large intracellular changes that may cause significant morbidity and mortality. The daily average intake of potassium is 50 to 100 mmol/day. The kidneys control the daily excretion, which ranges widely from 20 to 400 mmol. The renin-angiotensin-aldosterone hormone axis is the key regulator of potassium clearance. As aldosterone increases in plasma, so does potassium excretion.

Hypokalemia

Patients with hypokalemia have a $[K^+]$ lower than 3.5 mmol/L. Hypokalemia is commonly a result of hyperpolarization of the resting potential of the cell. Hyperpolarization interferes with neuromuscular function. Hypokalemia is associated with generalized fatigue and weakness, ileus, atrial arrhythmia, and acute renal insufficiency. On occasion, rhabdomyolysis occurs in patients whose $[K^+]$ drops below 2.5 mmol/L. Flaccid paralysis with respiratory compromise can occur as $[K^+]$ decreases to less than 2 mmol/L.

Hypokalemia is caused by renal losses, extrarenal losses, intracellular shifts from medications, or hyperthyroidism. Extrarenal losses can be caused by persistent vomiting, gastric tubes, diarrhea, alkalosis, catecholamine secretion, insulin administration, or high-output enteric or pancreatic fistulas. Hypokalemia is a common problem in patients with congestive heart failure who are receiving multiple drugs. It can also develop in patients treated with diuretics that force renal function to excrete urine with an elevated potassium concentration. Long-term diuretic therapy can produce a sustained negative potassium balance. Patients with a chronic potassium deficiency can develop a cardiac rhythm disturbance. The electrocardiogram of patients with hypokalemia will show depressed T waves and development of U waves. Hypokalemia leads to cardiac arrhythmia, particularly atrial tachycardia with or without block, atrioventricular dissociation, ventricular tachycardia, and ventricular fibrillation. The risk for hypokalemia-associated arrhythmia is higher in patients treated with digoxin, even when potassium concentrations are in the low-normal range. Hypokalemia not caused by diuretics may be due to a rare endocrine disorder, including primary hyperaldosteronism and renin-secreting tumors. Hypokalemia is also frequently associated with hypomagnesemia and acidemia.

Treatment of acute hypokalemia. Hypokalemic patients require potassium replacement, which can be achieved by oral or IV routes. Oral supplementation is generally 40 to 100 mEq/day, in two to four doses. The IV rate is 10 to 20 mEq/hr; if potassium is infused at rates of more than 10 mEq/hr, cardiac monitoring is required. In emergency situations, the rate can be as high as 40 mEq/hr, but it should be infused through a central vein; high concentrations of potassium in IV fluids can be irritating to peripheral veins. In patients with renal dysfunction, whose potassium excretion is reduced, both the IV rate of potassium replacement and the total dose should be lower.

After treatment, frequent monitoring of potassium levels is necessary. Since hypokalemia represents large intracellular deficits, replenishing total body levels may take days. Potassium therapy is given as the chloride salt because hypokalemia is commonly associated with a contraction in the extracellular water, in which chloride is the predominant anion. Potassium in foods is linked to phosphate. Potassium phosphate salts may need to be given by the IV route, particularly when expansion of intracellular water is anticipated. To reduce the risk of serious cardiac arrhythmia with cardiac disease or after cardiac surgery in patients who have a serum value below 3.5 mmol/L, serum [K^+] should be promptly corrected to a level higher than 4.0 mmol/L. Patients with substantial and continuing GI loss of potassium require extraordinary potassium replacement to achieve correction of hypokalemia.

Magnesium levels should be concomitantly monitored; hypomagnesemia can produce refractory hypokalemia. Magnesium is an important cofactor for potassium uptake and for maintenance of intracellular potassium levels and magnesium levels must be replete prior to repletion of potassium. In addition, supplemental magnesium reduces the risk of arrhythmia.

Hypokalemic patients with concurrent acidemia are treated with potassium replacement before their pH is corrected by bicarbonate administration. Diabetic patients with ketoacidosis may initially have normal [K^+], but hypokalemia rapidly develops as insulin is administered and as glucose shifts into cells; for such patients, potassium supplements should be added to the resuscitation fluid, once the physician is confident that renal function is adequate. If hypokalemia develops while patients are undergoing diuretic therapy, additional drugs can reduce the renal loss of potassium. For example, triamterene or spironolactone blocks the effect of aldosterone and reduces potassium loss in urine.

Hyperkalemia

Hyperkalemia is defined as [K^+] of more than 5.0 mmol/L. If levels exceed 6 mmol/L, perturbations in the resting cell membrane potential occur, and normal depolarization and repolarization are impaired. The most common cause of hyperkalemia is renal failure in hospitalized patients. The transport of potassium is passive, but the transport of sodium requires energy. This difference across the cell is maintained by Na^+,K^+-adenosine triphosphatase (ATPase) activity, which requires energy. This energy is supplied in the form of cellular ATP. Its levels are highly variable in different stages of shock when nutrients are not available (whether carbohydrates or oxygen). When cellular ATP levels fall, the sodium pump is impaired. If either sodium or potassium levels are severely high or low, the membrane potential will be affected. Eventually, without energy, cell death occurs, and the sodium-potassium gradient cannot be maintained; the sodium gradient is needed to maintain the membrane potential.

The primary clinical problem with hyperkalemia is cardiac arrhythmia, which can be lethal. Hyperkalemia is associated with peaked T waves; dangerous hyperkalemia (6–7 mmol/L) is indicated by T waves higher than R waves (Fig. 4.23).

The most common cause of hyperkalemia is acute onset of renal dysfunction or failure. Cellular injury (such as sepsis or ischemia-reperfusion) can also release potassium from its intracellular source, which can overwhelm the kidneys' ability to clear potassium. At least 20% of normal renal function is required to respond to aldosterone and to maintain normal potassium levels. The reperfusion of ischemic tissues resulting in rhabdomyolysis causes high potassium levels; to prevent cardiac arrest, a bolus of IV sodium bicarbonate may be of some benefit. The bicarbonate shifts potassium intracellularly.

Drugs can have a direct effect on the renal tubules and on potassium excretion; examples include triamterene, spironolactone, beta blockers, cyclosporine, and tacrolimus. They are usually a contributing factor but not a primary cause. Succinylcholine, a depolarizing paralytic agent, is used in patients with muscle atrophy from disuse, prolonged bed rest, neurologic denervation syndromes, severe burns, direct muscle trauma, or rhabdomyolysis; it can cause severe hyperkalemia, resulting in cardiac arrest. When

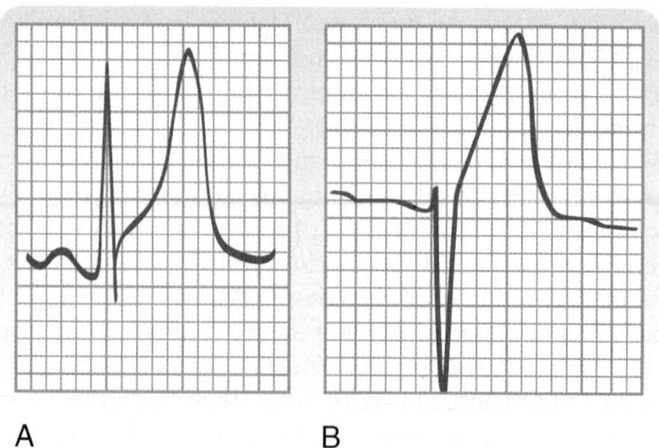

FIG. 4.23 Electrocardiographic changes. (A) Indicating hyperkalemia. The T wave is tall, narrow, and symmetrical. (B) Indicating acute myocardial infarction. The T wave is tall but broad based and asymmetrical. (From Somers MP, Brady WJ, Perron AD, et al. The prominent T wave: electrocardiographic differential diagnosis. *Am J Emerg Med.* 2002;20:243–251.)

drawing blood samples from patients, clinicians must recognize that sample hemolysis can release potassium, so laboratory test results could be spurious. If the sample or test results are suspect, another sample should be taken before drastic efforts are made to treat hyperkalemia.

In addition, ischemia-reperfusion injury is associated with hyperkalemia. Revascularization after an ischemic injury may cause severe hyperkalemia based on duration of the ischemic episode, ranging from 4 to 6 hours. As a result, it is usually recommended to administer bicarbonate before reperfusion.

Treatment of hyperkalemia. In patients at risk for development of cardiac arrhythmia from hyperkalemia, several interventions are useful. Calcium administered via IV can immediately reduce the risk of arrhythmia, and this should be the first therapy administered; it antagonizes the depolarization effect of elevated [K^+]. Sodium bicarbonate infusion buffers extracellular protons and allows net transfer of cytosolic protons across the cell membrane through carbonic acid. The shift of protons out of the cell is associated with a shift of potassium into the cells. Bicarbonate therapy is most effective in hyperkalemic patients with metabolic acidemia. Insulin and glucose infusions prompt an increase in Na^+,K^+-ATPase activity and a decline in extracellular water potassium concentration as the extracellular water potassium is driven into the cell.

In patients with both aldosterone deficiency and hyperkalemia, a mineralocorticoid drug such as 9α-fludrocortisone will increase renal excretion of potassium. In patients with acute renal failure, hemodialysis is the most reliable method to control hyperkalemia. Continuous filtration methods clear potassium at a slower rate than hemodialysis does. Chronic hyperkalemia associated with renal dysfunction can be managed by oral or rectal administration of sodium polystyrene sulfonate, a cation exchange resin that binds potassium in the gut lumen. Rectally administered binding resins are particularly effective because the colonic mucosa can excrete mucus with large amounts of potassium. Surgeons should clearly establish a process for managing hyperkalemia as rapidly escalating potassium levels pose an immediate threat and require prompt therapy (Box 4.5). Dysfunctional renal handling of potassium from mineralocorticoid deficiency or resistance leads to hyperkalemia. Renal failure is commonly associated with tubular defects and potassium management problems along with hyperaldosteronism. However, in patients with normal renal function, assessing levels of aldosterone, renin, and cortisol can help differentiate between mineralocorticoid deficiency and resistance. In patients with aldosterone deficiency, fludrocortisone is useful.

BOX 4.5 Guidelines for treatment of adult patients with hyperkalemia.

First: Stop all infusion of potassium.

Electrocardiographic Evidence of Pending Arrest

Loss of P wave and broad slurring of QRS; immediate effective therapy indicated

1. Intravenous (IV) infusion of calcium salts
   10 mL of 10% calcium chloride during a 10-minute period *or* 10 mL of 10% calcium gluconate during a 3- to 5-minute period
2. IV infusion of sodium bicarbonate
   50-100 mEq during a 10- to 20-minute period; benefit proportional to extent of pretherapy acidemia

Electrocardiographic Evidence of Potassium Effect

Peaked T waves; prompt therapy needed

1. Glucose and insulin infusion
   IV infusion of 50 mL of $D_{50}W$ and 10 units of regular insulin; monitor glucose
2. Immediate hemodialysis

Biochemical Evidence of Hyperkalemia and No Electrocardiographic Changes

Effective therapy needed within hours

1. Potassium-binding resins into the gastrointestinal tract with 20% sorbitol
2. Promotion of renal kaliuresis by loop diuretic

$D_{50}W$, 50% Dextrose in water.

Calcium

Calcium, a divalent cation, is a critical component of many extracellular and intracellular reactions. It is the most abundant electrolyte in the body overall. About 99% of it is found in the bones; the remaining 1% circulates in the blood. For surgeons, it is of particular interest; it is an essential cofactor in the coagulation cascade, and intracellular ionized calcium (iCa^{2+}) participates in the regulation of neuronal, hormonal, muscular, and renal cellular function. Total serum calcium concentration (normally, 8.5 to 10.5 mg/dL) is present in three molecular forms: protein-bound calcium, diffusible calcium bound to anions (bicarbonate, phosphate, and acetate), and freely diffusible calcium as iCa^{2+}.

The biochemically active species is iCa^{2+}, which constitutes about 45% of total serum calcium. More than 80% of protein-bound calcium is attached to albumin, so the total calcium concentration in serum will decrease in patients with hypoalbuminemia. Physiologically, the total plasma calcium level must be corrected relative to the albumin level. Normal calcium levels may range from 8.5 to 10.5 mg/day, assuming an albumin level of 4.5 g/dL. The calcium concentration [Ca] usually changes by 0.8 mg/dL for every change of 1.0 g/dL in plasma albumin concentration. This formula estimates the actual total plasma calcium level:

$$\text{Corrected }[iCa^{2+}] = \text{Total }[Ca] + (0.8 \times [4.5 - \text{Albumin level}])$$

Acidosis decreases the amount of calcium bound to albumin, whereas alkalosis increases the bound fraction of calcium. A small amount of calcium (about 6%) is bound to anions such as citrate and sulfate. The remainder is [iCa^{2+}] that is biologically active.

The increase in [iCa^{2+}] is controlled by cell membrane enzymes that transport calcium out of the cell. In muscle cells, [iCa^{2+}] is stored in the sarcoplasmic reticulum. It can be quickly released into intracellular fluid, in which it has a key role in the molecular events that cause muscle contraction. Tight control of [iCa^{2+}] in ECF is essential. The serum calcium concentration is controlled by the interaction of parathyroid hormone (PTH), calcitonin, and vitamin D. PTH and calcitonin are hormones subject to regulatory release by endocrine cells, whereas vitamin D is either consumed in the diet or formed in the skin as cholecalciferol in response to ultraviolet irradiation. Bone contains an enormous reservoir of calcium in the form of a matrix of calcium and other molecules. Turnover of calcium salts in bone is constant and integral to maintaining a stable [iCa^{2+}] in ECF. Receptors in the membranes of parathyroid cells release PTH when [iCa^{2+}] in ECF declines. PTH activates osteoclasts in bones, which release calcium from the structural matrix of bone. PTH stimulates tubule cells in the proximal nephron both to absorb calcium from the filtrate and to excrete phosphates. PTH with vitamin D enhances calcium absorption from the lumen of the gut.

Calcitonin has the opposite effects on calcium metabolism (compared with PTH). As calcitonin levels in the ECF increase because of its excretion from type C cells of the thyroid, [iCa^{2+}] declines and more calcium becomes bound to the bone matrix. Vitamin D circulating in blood is converted in the liver to 25-hydroxycholecalciferol. Then, 25-hydroxycholecalciferol circulating in blood encounters kidney cells that further hydroxylate the sterol to 1,25-dihydroxycholecalciferol, which is the most potent calcium-modulating hormone. Next, 1,25-dihydroxycholecalciferol increases the transport of calcium and phosphate from the lumen of the bowel into the ECF of the intestine. Furthermore, in conjunction with PTH, 1,25-dihydroxycholecalciferol increases bone resorption, increasing the calcium concentration in ECF. In summary, multiple hormonal mechanisms produce a balance of influences on the concentration of calcium in ECF.

Hypocalcemia

Hypocalcemia is defined as total serum concentration below 8.4 mg/dL or ionized calcium concentration below 4.5 mg/dL. It varies from an asymptomatic biochemical abnormality to a life-threatening disorder, depending on its duration, severity, and rapidity of development. It is caused by loss of calcium from the circulation or by insufficient entry of calcium into the circulation.

Acute hypocalcemia can be life-threatening. It impairs transmembrane depolarization; [iCa^{2+}] below 0.8 mEq/L can lead to central nervous system dysfunction. Hypocalcemic patients can have paresthesias, muscle spasms (including tetany), and seizures. If patients hyperventilate, a respiratory alkalosis may exacerbate their condition and further reduce [iCa^{2+}]. Cardiac dysfunction is also common. Patients with low [iCa^{2+}] may require IV infusion of calcium to restore cardiac function. Hypocalcemic patients have a prolonged QT interval on electrocardiograms that may progress to complete heart block or ventricular fibrillation.

Hypoparathyroidism, the most common cause of hypocalcemia, often develops because of surgery in the central neck, such as radical resection of head and neck cancers or incidentally after thyroidectomy. Hypocalcemia develops in 1% to 2% of patients after a total thyroidectomy. The hypocalcemia may be transient, permanent, or intermittent, as with vitamin D deficiency during the winter. Autoimmune hypoparathyroidism can be an isolated defect or part of polyglandular autoimmune syndrome type I in association with adrenal insufficiency and mucocutaneous candidiasis; most of these patients have autoantibodies directed against the calcium-sensing receptor. Congenital causes of hypocalcemia include activation of mutations of the calcium-sensing receptor, which resets the calcium-PTH relation to a lower serum calcium level. Mutations affecting intracellular processing of the pre-pro-PTH molecule can lead to hypoparathyroidism, hypocalcemia, or both. Finally, some cases of hypoparathyroidism are associated with hypoplasia or aplasia of the parathyroid glands; the best known is DiGeorge syndrome.

Pseudohypoparathyroidism is a group of disorders characterized by postreceptor resistance to PTH. One classic variant is Albright hereditary osteodystrophy, associated with low stature, round facies, short digits, and mental retardation. Hypomagnesemia induces PTH resistance and also affects PTH production. Severe hypermagnesemia (>6 mg/dL) can lead to hypocalcemia by inhibiting PTH secretion. When it is associated with decreased dietary calcium intake, vitamin D deficiency leads to hypocalcemia. The low calcium level stimulates PTH secretion (secondary hyperparathyroidism), leading to hypophosphatemia.

Rhabdomyolysis and tumor lysis syndrome cause loss of calcium from the circulation when large amounts of intracellular phosphate are released, thereby increasing calcium levels in bone and extraskeletal tissues. A similar mechanism causes hypocalcemia with phosphate administration.

Acute pancreatitis results in calcium sequestration in the abdomen, causing hypocalcemia. After surgery for hyperparathyroidism, patients with severe prolonged disease (such as those with secondary or tertiary hyperparathyroidism who are in renal failure) can develop a form of hypocalcemia known as hungry bone syndrome, in which serum calcium is rapidly deposited into the bone. The syndrome is also rarely seen after correction of long-standing metabolic acidosis or after thyroidectomy for hyperthyroidism.

Several medications (such as ethylenediaminetetraacetic acid [EDTA], citrate present in transfused blood, lactate, and foscarnet) chelate calcium in the circulation, sometimes producing hypocalcemia in which the iCa^{2+} level is decreased even though the total calcium level may be normal. Acute hypocalcemia in the postoperative period can occur in response to rapid blood transfusions. In the past, stored blood contained a higher concentration of citrate, which binds to and chelates serum calcium. Now that citrate has been eliminated from blood-banking techniques, this is rarely seen. Extensive osteoblastic skeletal metastases (such as from prostate and breast cancers) may also cause hypocalcemia. Chemotherapy, including cisplatin, 5-fluorouracil, and leucovorin, causes hypocalcemia mediated through hypomagnesemia. In patients with sepsis, hypocalcemia is usually associated with hypoalbuminemia.

Tumor lysis syndrome is a constellation of electrolyte abnormalities that include hypocalcemia, hyperphosphatemia, hyperuricemia, and hyperkalemia. Such abnormalities occur when antineoplastic therapy causes a sudden surge in tumor cell death and a release of cytosolic contents. Solid tumors and lymphomas have been implicated. Acute renal failure occurs in patients with tumor lysis syndrome and prevents spontaneous correction of the electrolyte abnormalities; emergency dialysis may be the only way to comprehensively correct the abnormalities.

Acute hypocalcemia is frequent after resuscitation from shock. In a study of patients in burn shock, Wray and associates hypothesized that a major factor contributing to the development of hypocalcemia was depressed levels of 1,25-dihydroxycholecalciferol, perhaps caused by a sudden lack of vitamin D in the diet. In patients with severe pancreatitis, the fall in calcium is speculated to be the consequence of ionized extracellular calcium becoming linked to fats in the peripancreatic inflammatory phlegmon. Rapid infusion of a citrate load during the transfusion of blood products (particularly platelet concentrates and FFP) may also lead to acute severe hypocalcemia ([iCa^{2+}] <0.62 mmol/L) and to hypotension. Rapid increases in serum phosphate can occur after improper administration or excessive dosing of phosphate-containing cathartics; as the phosphate concentration increases, severe hypocalcemia ensues.

Treatment of hypocalcemia. Patients with acute symptomatic hypocalcemia (calcium level <7.0 mg/dL, iCa^{2+} level <0.8 mmol/L) should be treated promptly with an IV calcium infusion. Calcium may be given orally or intravenously in the form of calcium gluconate or calcium chloride. Calcium gluconate is preferred to calcium chloride as it causes less tissue necrosis if it extravasates. The first 100 to 200 mg of elemental calcium (1–2 g calcium gluconate) should be given over 10 to 20 minutes. Faster administration may result in cardiac dysfunction and even arrest. Those first 100 to 200 mg should then be followed by a slow calcium infusion at 0.5 to 1.5 mg/kg/hr. Calcium infusion should continue until the patient is receiving effective doses of oral calcium and vitamin D. Calcium for infusion should be diluted in saline or dextrose solution to avoid vein irritation. The infusion should not contain bicarbonate or phosphate, either of which can form an insoluble calcium salt. If bicarbonate or phosphate administration is necessary, a separate IV line should be used.

Coexisting hypomagnesemia should be corrected in every patient. Care should be taken in patients with renal insufficiency because they cannot excrete excess magnesium. Magnesium is given by infusion, initiated with 2 g of magnesium sulfate during 10 to 15 minutes, followed by 1 g/hr. In patients with severe hyperphosphatemia (such as those with tumor lysis syndrome, rhabdomyolysis, or chronic renal failure), treatment is focused on correcting the hyperphosphatemia.

Acute hyperphosphatemia usually resolves in patients with intact renal function. Phosphate excretion may be aided by saline infusion (this can lead to worsening of hypocalcemia); in addition, acetazolamide, a carbonic anhydrase inhibitor, can be given at 10 to 15 mg/kg every 3 to 4 hours. Hemodialysis may be necessary for patients with symptomatic hypocalcemia and hyperphosphatemia, especially if renal function is impaired. Chronic hyperphosphatemia is managed by a low-phosphate diet and by use of phosphate binders with meals.

Chronic hypocalcemia (hypoparathyroidism) is treated by oral calcium administration and, if that is insufficient, vitamin D supplementation. The serum calcium level should be targeted to about 8.0 mg/dL. Most patients will be entirely asymptomatic at that level. Further elevation will lead to hypercalciuria because of the lack of PTH effect on the renal tubules. Chronic hypercalciuria carries the risks of nephrocalcinosis, nephrolithiasis, and renal impairment.

Several oral calcium preparations are available. Calcium carbonate is the cheapest form, but it may be poorly absorbed, especially in older patients and those with achlorhydria. Similarly, various forms of vitamin D are available. If oral calcium preparations cannot achieve adequate calcium repletion, vitamin D should be added. The usual initial daily dose is 50,000 IU of 25-hydroxyvitamin D (or 0.25 to 0.5 mg of 1,25-hydroxyvitamin D). Calcium and vitamin D doses are established by gradual titration. When adequate calcium levels are achieved, urinary calcium excretion is measured. If hypercalciuria is detected, a thiazide diuretic may be added to diminish calciuria and to further increase the serum calcium level. If the phosphorus level is higher than 6.0 mg/dL when the calcium level is satisfactory, an unabsorbable phosphate binder should be added. Once calcium and phosphorus levels are controlled, the patient should be monitored every 3 to 6 months for both levels and for urinary calcium excretion.

Special consideration is necessary for the treatment of women with hypoparathyroidism who are pregnant or nursing. During pregnancy, vitamin D requirements gradually increase, up to three times as high as the prepregnancy requirements. Supplementary doses of vitamin D should be titrated, using frequent serum calcium level measurements. After delivery, if the baby is to be bottle fed, the dose should be decreased to the prepregnancy dose. If the baby is to be nursed, the dose of calcitriol should be decreased to 50% of the prepregnancy dose[4] because endogenous calcitriol production is stimulated by prolactin and by increased production of PTH-related peptide (PTHrP), which is also stimulated by prolactin.

Several reports have described successful control of hypocalcemia with synthetic PTH (1,34-PTH, teriparatide) by twice-daily subcutaneous administration, with a lower risk of hypercalciuria.

Hypercalcemia

Mild hypercalcemia is suspected when total serum calcium levels are in the range of 10.5 to 12 mg/dL. Patients with a serum calcium concentration of 12 to 14.5 mg/dL have moderate hypercalcemia. Patients with transient hypercalcemia are generally asymptomatic. Those with sustained elevations in renal calcium excretion are susceptible to the development of renal lithiasis, abdominal pain, and bone pain. Patients have severe hypercalcemia when serum calcium levels exceed 15 mg/dL; such patients have symptoms of weakness, stupor, and central nervous system dysfunction. In hypercalcemic patients, a renal concentrating defect also occurs, leading to polyuria and to loss of sodium and water. Indeed, many hypercalcemic patients are dehydrated. Hypercalcemic crisis is a syndrome in which total serum calcium levels exceed 17 mg/dL; such patients are subject to life-threatening cardiac tachyarrhythmia, coma, acute renal failure, and ileus with abdominal distention.

The most common cause of hypercalcemia (in fact, in 90% of all patients) is primary hyperparathyroidism; other causes include unregulated PTH secretion and malignant disease. It occurs most commonly with malignant diseases in hospitalized patients and with hyperparathyroidism in the general population. Breast cancer is the most common malignant cause. Other rare causes include thyrotoxicosis, vitamin A and D overdose, granulomatous diseases, and commonly used drugs like thiazide diuretics and lithium. Another rare cause of hypercalcemia is familial hypocalciuric hypercalcemia, which is due to an autosomal dominant mutation in the calcium-sensing receptor causing increased calcium and magnesium retention by the kidneys. Signs and symptoms of hypercalcemia are nonspecific and include nausea, vomiting, altered mental status, constipation, depression, lethargy, myalgias, arthralgias, polyuria, headache, abdominal and flank pain (renal stones), and coma. They are sometimes described as abdominal groans, psychic moans, and renal stones. However, most of these symptoms are manifested after chronic hypercalcemia and not after acute hypercalcemia. Usually, a patient's clinical presentation is recognized as related to hypercalcemia only after it has been diagnosed by blood test results. It is extremely difficult to diagnose hypercalcemia by a patient's history alone.

Bone demineralization is found in patients with severe and prolonged hyperparathyroidism. The majority (85%) of such patients have a solitary hyperfunctioning adenoma in one parathyroid gland; the remaining 15% have excessive PTH release as a result of hyperplasia of all four glands. PTH induces phosphaturia and depresses serum phosphate concentrations; such a laboratory finding corroborates the diagnosis of primary hyperparathyroidism. Secondary hyperparathyroidism, an endocrine disease characterized by hyperplasia of the parathyroid glands, develops in patients with chronic renal failure. Decreased renal function results in impaired synthesis of 1,25-dihydroxycholecalciferol. Although patients have low serum calcium levels, their osteomalacia indicates excessive PTH secretion. To control elevated PTH levels in patients with secondary hyperparathyroidism, surgical removal of most of the parathyroid tissue may be required.

Humoral hypercalcemia of malignancy (HHM) is a clinical syndrome in which elevated calcium levels are caused by synthesis of the humoral factor by the tumoral process. Usually, HHM is applied to patients with excessive tumoral production of PTHrP. However, rare cases characterized by excessive production of PTH and calcitriol have also been described. Patients with HHM constitute about 80% of all patients with hypercalcemia associated with malignant disease. PTHrP and PTH share the same receptor, but the clinical presentation differs. HHM patients have a markedly larger degree of renal calcium excretion; PTH potently stimulates tubular calcium resorption, and hypercalciuria is less pronounced. HHM is usually associated with low serum calcitriol levels; PTH stimulates calcitriol production, and its level is usually elevated. PTHrP stimulates only bone resorption, with very low osteoblastic activity and therefore usually normal alkaline phosphatase levels; PTH stimulates bone resorption and formation.

HHM patients usually have a clinically obvious malignant disease and a poor prognosis. The only exceptions to this rule are patients with small, well-differentiated endocrine tumors (such as pheochromocytomas or islet cell tumors). However, such tumors constitute a minority of cases. HHM is most commonly seen with squamous cell carcinomas (e.g., of the lung, esophagus, cervix, or head and neck) and with renal, bladder, and ovarian cancers. Treatment of HHM patients is aimed at reducing the tumor burden, reducing osteoclastic resorption of the bone, and increasing calcium excretion through the urine.

Most cases of hypercalcemia are associated with Hodgkin disease. The other third of cases are associated with non-Hodgkin lymphoma and are caused by increased production of calcitriol by the malignant cells. Hypercalcemia usually responds well to treatment with corticosteroids. Multiple myeloma, lymphoma, and solid tumors metastatic to bone (particularly breast, lung, and prostate cancer) cause hypercalcemia by excessive osteoclastic activity. Drugs can also cause hypercalcemia, including theophylline, lithium, thiazide diuretics, and extraordinarily high doses of vitamin A and D. In addition, hypercalcemia can develop in young, normally active patients with high bone turnover rates who are suddenly forced into immobility, such as during forced bed rest after injury or major illness. This hypercalcemia of immobilization resolves with return to normal activity.

Another cause of hypercalcemia is milk-alkali syndrome, a rare condition caused by ingestion of large amounts of calcium together with sodium bicarbonate. It is currently associated with ingestion of calcium carbonate in over-the-counter antacid preparations and in drugs used to prevent and to treat osteoporosis. Features of the syndrome include hypercalcemia, renal failure, and metabolic alkalosis. The exact pathophysiologic mechanism is unknown. In rare cases, the amount of calcium ingested may be as low as 2000 to 3000 mg/day, but in most patients, the amount is between 6000 and 15,000 mg/day. Treatment consists of rehydration, diuresis, and cessation of calcium and antacid ingestion. If diuresis is impossible because of renal failure, dialysis using a dialysate with a low calcium concentration is effective. Renal failure usually resolves in patients with short-term hypercalcemia but may persist in those with chronic hypercalcemia.

Treatment of hypercalcemia. Definitive management of hypercalcemia depends on correction of the primary problem. Thus, patients with hyperparathyroidism secondary to a parathyroid adenoma or hyperplasia are cured of hypercalcemia by excision of the diseased parathyroid tissue. Hypercalcemic patients taking thiazide drugs should be converted to alternative therapies. Patients with a malignant neoplasm and hypercalcemia may respond to surgical excision, radiation therapy, or chemotherapy. Symptomatic patients with severe hypercalcemia related to malignant disease can be quickly and effectively treated by saline infusion to expand intravascular volume, followed by the administration of a loop diuretic (i.e., furosemide) to induce saline diuresis with associated urinary calcium clearance. Patients with severe hypercalcemia frequently have a contracted extracellular volume, so isotonic saline infusion is essential. Hypercalcemic patients in renal failure who cannot benefit from drug-induced diuresis can be treated by hemodialysis.

Severe hypercalcemia referred to as hypercalcemic crisis occurs with serum calcium concentration above 14 mg/dL and is related to release of calcium from bone by tumor; it can be managed by administration of bisphosphonates. Such drugs have a potent capacity to reduce osteoclast-mediated release of calcium from bone. Several formulations of bisphosphonates are available (in order of preference, zoledronic acid, pamidronate disodium, and etidronate disodium), all of which produce a slow decline in [iCa^{2+}] during several days. In patients with metastatic breast cancer, bisphosphonates given as long-term prophylactic agents at a regular dosage have been shown to effectively prevent hypercalcemia.

Administration of exogenous calcitonin is often initially effective in patients with hypercalcemia. Calcitonin (4 U/kg subcutaneously every 12 hours) inhibits bone resorption and decreases renal tubular resorption of calcium, with a shorter onset of action than bisphosphonates; therefore, it is the better choice for short-term control of calcium. However, long-term treatment frequently leads to tachyphylaxis, possibly related to the development of antibodies to the exogenous calcitonin. Chelating agents (EDTA or phosphate salts) that bind and neutralize [iCa^{2+}] are rarely indicated. Such agents are associated with the complications of metastatic calcification, acute renal failure, and with the risk of depressing [iCa^{2+}] to hypocalcemic levels.

Magnesium

Magnesium, an essential cation in the cell, is the second most prevalent cation. It is a critical cofactor in any reaction powered by ATP, so deficiencies can affect metabolism. It also acts as a calcium channel antagonist and plays a key role in the modulation of any activity involving calcium, such as muscle contraction and insulin release. The normal concentration of magnesium [Mg^{2+}] in plasma ranges between 1.5 and 2.0 mEq/L. Like calcium, it exists in three states: protein bound (30%, bound mostly to albumin), bound to anions (10%), and ionized (60%).

Magnesium is primarily intracellular, with less than 1% of body stores in the ECF. Measured plasma magnesium levels often do not reflect total body magnesium content. Clinical sequelae of altered magnesium content depend more on tissue magnesium levels than on the blood magnesium concentration. Consequently, it is often difficult to consistently correlate symptoms to specific plasma magnesium levels. One method to infer the tissue magnesium level is a physiologic test that measures the renal response to a magnesium load. Patients who retain more than 30% of an 800-mg load of magnesium via IV are thought to be magnesium depleted, whereas those who retain less than 20% are said to be magnesium replete.

The kidneys are responsible for maintaining magnesium balance by excreting the absorbed magnesium. The ionized and bound forms of magnesium are freely filtered by the glomerulus. The distal tubule resorbs 10% of the filtered magnesium and plays an important role in calcium-independent magnesium homeostasis. The hormonal regulation of magnesium homeostasis has not been completely determined. PTH, glucagon, and ADH increase the resorption of magnesium in the Henle loop. In the distal convoluted tubule, aldosterone, ADH, and glucagon are thought to increase magnesium resorption. To maintain magnesium homeostasis, renal resorption of magnesium varies widely. Fractional resorption of filtered magnesium can decline to nearly zero in the presence of hypermagnesemia or reduced glomerular filtration rate. In contrast, in response to magnesium depletion or decreased intake, the fractional resorption of magnesium can rise to 99.5% to minimize urinary losses.

Hypomagnesemia

In ICU patients, the prevalence of hypomagnesemia ranges from 11% to 65%, but it is usually asymptomatic. Some studies have shown little significance to hypomagnesemia; other studies have shown an association with mortality. Any association with mortality is not necessarily causal, of course, and may merely reflect the patient's state of health. Symptoms of hypomagnesemia have been reported at modest degrees of depletion, but in general, symptoms become more common as the serum magnesium level falls below 1.2 mg/dL. Associating specific symptoms with hypomagnesemia is difficult. However, severe hypomagnesemia in postsurgical patients can lead to life-threatening ventricular arrhythmias such as torsades de pointes.

Hypokalemia is commonly associated with hypomagnesemia and reportedly occurs in 40% of patients with hypomagnesemia. The converse is also true; 60% of patients with hypokalemia have concurrent hypomagnesemia. The causes of hypomagnesemia are multiple, including renal, GI, and skin losses as well as hungry bone syndrome. Skin losses can be due to burns or toxic epidermal necrolysis. Renal losses can be due to a long list of drugs, but the most common are diuretics.

Hypomagnesemia also causes a specific disorder of renal potassium wasting that is refractory to potassium supplementation until magnesium is adequately replete. Recently, the mechanism whereby magnesium depletion results in renal potassium loss has been elucidated. Decreased intracellular magnesium slows ATP production. Throughout the body, such slowed ATP production has a negative effect on Na^+,K^+-ATPase activity. The result is loss of intracellular potassium, which flows downs its concentration gradient into the tubule and is lost in the urine.

Hypocalcemia, hyponatremia, and hypophosphatemia are also common in patients with hypomagnesemia. Intracellular hypomagnesemia can develop in patients with chronic diarrhea syndrome or in those who undergo prolonged aggressive diuretic therapy. Magnesium deficiency is also common in patients with heavy ethanol intake. Diabetic patients with persistent osmotic diuresis from glycosuria commonly have hypomagnesemia.

Treatment of hypomagnesemia. Patients with mild hypomagnesemia can be treated with oral replacement; symptomatic hypomagnesemia should be treated with an IV magnesium infusion. The most common formulation is magnesium sulfate; 1 g of magnesium sulfate contains 0.1 g of elemental magnesium. No trials have been done to determine the optimal regimen for magnesium replacement, but consensus statements suggest 8 to 12 g of magnesium sulfate in the first 24 hours followed by 4 to 6 g/day for 3 or 4 days to replete body stores. IV magnesium therapy is advocated in some acutely ill patients without documented magnesium depletion. The American College of Cardiology and the American Heart Association recommend 1 to 2 g of magnesium sulfate as an IV bolus during 5 minutes for torsades de pointes therapy. Emerging data have suggested that magnesium may also play a role in reducing reperfusion injury and decreasing infarct size in patients with acute myocardial infarction. Currently, the American Heart Association recommends 2 g of magnesium sulfate for 15 minutes, followed by 18 g during 24 hours in patients with suspected myocardial infarction who have hypomagnesemia.

Magnesium replacement should be done cautiously in patients with renal insufficiency, and recommendations call for dose reductions of 50% to 75% of baseline. During infusions, patients should be monitored closely for decreased deep tendon reflexes. Magnesium levels should be checked at regular intervals. Oral supplementation has been shown to successfully correct increased magnesium retention. Potassium-sparing diuretics may be helpful in patients with chronic renal magnesium wasting. Diuretics that block the sodium channel in the distal convoluted tubule, such as amiloride and triamterene, reduce magnesium wasting in some patients. Severe hypomagnesemia (<1.0 mEq/L) requires sustained therapy because of the slow equilibration of extracellular magnesium with intracellular stores. Correction of hypomagnesemia can also reduce the risk of cardiac arrhythmia. The magnitude of magnesium deficiency frequently parallels the magnitude of hypocalcemia. Hypocalcemia in patients with magnesium deficiency is resistant to calcium replacement alone, so such patients should receive magnesium concurrently.

Hypermagnesemia

Hypermagnesemia is a common abnormality in patients with renal failure but is otherwise uncommon among other patients. Theophylline toxicity, now rare, was associated with hypermagnesemia in the past. Hypermagnesemia can be exacerbated by the ingestion of magnesium-containing drugs, particularly antacids; Epsom salts also contain magnesium, as does magnesium citrate, which is often used in surgical care. High levels of magnesium seem to be tolerated well and, in general, without sequelae. In one report, a patient in diabetic ketoacidosis with hypomagnesemia received 50 g of magnesium sulfate for 6 hours, rather than the intended 2 g. Despite a documented magnesium level of 24 mg/dL and significant short-term morbidity, the patient completely recovered.

Magnesium overdoses given via IV may be better tolerated than oral overdoses. Hypermagnesemia due to oral ingestion of magnesium is unusual in the absence of renal insufficiency. A fatal case of hypermagnesemia was documented in a developmentally disabled child who was given magnesium to relieve constipation. Despite calcium infusions and dialysis, the child died. The chronic ingestion of magnesium likely made the child's condition refractory to treatment, perhaps because of greater total body magnesium burden from chronic overload. Hypermagnesemia has also been repeatedly reported after the use of magnesium-containing enemas. In postsurgical patients who are oliguric, hypermagnesemia may occur because of magnesium retention, particularly if the patient is acidotic.

Magnesium can block synaptic transmission of nerve impulses. It also causes the initial loss of deep tendon reflexes and may lead to flaccid paralysis and apnea. Neuromuscular toxicity also affects smooth muscle, resulting in ileus and urinary retention. In cases of oral intoxication, the development of ileus can slow intestinal transit times, further increasing absorption of magnesium. Hypermagnesemia has also been reported to cause a parasympathetic blockade resulting in fixed and dilated pupils, mimicking brainstem herniation. Other neurologic signs include lethargy, confusion, and coma.

Magnesium blocks the shift of calcium into myocardial cells and can act as a calcium channel blocker. In cardiac tissue, it also blocks potassium channels needed for repolarization. Patients with severe hypermagnesemia can show evidence of heart failure. Other cardiac manifestations of hypermagnesemia, at least initially, include bradycardia and hypotension. Higher magnesium levels cause a prolonged PR interval, increased QRS duration, and prolonged QT interval. Extreme cases can result in complete heart block or cardiac arrest.

Metabolic disturbances due to hypermagnesemia have been less recognized than those due to hypomagnesemia. Hypocalcemia can occur, although it is typically mild and asymptomatic. Symptomatic hypermagnesemia (despite normal renal function) has been reported with magnesium infusions, typically during treatment of patients who are in preterm labor or who have preeclampsia or eclampsia. Routine magnesium measurements are often not performed, although the infusion protocols (a load of 4–6 g, followed by 1–2 g/hr) result in serum magnesium levels of 4 to 8 mg/dL. Obstetric patients who experience accidental overdoses of magnesium usually have good outcomes, despite magnesium levels as high as 19 mg/dL.

Treatment of hypermagnesemia. The principles for treatment of hypermagnesemia are similar to those for treatment of hypercalcemia. Calcium is given to stabilize the heart, normal saline is given for fluid expansion, and diuretics are given to hasten renal excretion. In patients with hypermagnesemia and intact renal function, stopping the infusion or supply of magnesium will allow them to recover. Severe hypermagnesemia is treated calcium gluconate 10% (10–20 mL for 10 minutes) administered via IV. Patients are typically given 100 to 200 mg IV of elemental calcium during 5 to 10 minutes. To speed the renal clearance of magnesium, loop diuretics and saline diuresis are intuitive options, but no literature explicitly supports this use.

In critically ill patients, disorders of magnesium homeostasis can have dramatic effects. Yet such disorders often go unrecognized. In ICU patients, hypomagnesemia is common and associated with poor outcomes, so measurement of serum magnesium should be routine. Unlike magnesium depletion, hypermagnesemia is a rare but frequently iatrogenic and fatal problem.

In patients with renal insufficiency, dialysis rapidly corrects hypermagnesemia and is the only way to acutely lower magnesium levels. Aggressive use of dialysis may improve survival. In patients with severe renal dysfunction, dialysis offers a way to rapidly clear magnesium. Both peritoneal dialysis and hemodialysis are effective at lowering magnesium levels. Intermittent hemodialysis corrects hypermagnesemia more rapidly than peritoneal dialysis or continuous renal replacement therapy.

SELECTED REFERENCES

Dellinger RP, Levy MM, Carlet JM, et al. Surviving sepsis campaign: international guidelines for management of severe sepsis and septic shock; 2008. *Crit Care Med.* 2008;36:296–327.

Most recent update on conscious guidelines on the definition, diagnosis, and management of patients in sepsis and septic shock.

Bickell WH, Wall Jr MJ, Pepe PE, et al. Immediate versus delayed fluid resuscitation for hypotensive patients with penetrating torso injuries. *N Engl J Med.* 1994;331:1105–1109.

Classic study, probably the most referenced paper in trauma, showing that despite their being hypotensive in the field after penetrating torso injury, treating these patients with crystalloid solutions resulted in worse outcome and not infusing fluids improved outcome.

Committee on Fluid Resuscitation for Combat Casualties. *Fluid Resuscitation: State of the Science for Treating Combat Casualties and Civilian Injuries. Report of the Institute of Medicine.* Washington, DC: National Academy Press; 1999.

Considered a white paper by the Institute of Medicine, it was considered radical in that it did not recommend lactated Ringer solution as the fluid of choice for civilians and the military. It recommended hypertonic saline and additional research to eliminate d-isomer lactate from lactated Ringer solution and to investigate other metabolites, such as ketones, as an alternative.

Finfer S, Bellomo R, Boyce N, et al. A comparison of albumin and saline for fluid resuscitation in the intensive care unit. *N Engl J Med.* 2004;350:2247–2256.

Prospective multicenter study designed to show that albumin is safe in the intensive care unit. However, it used 4% albumin and showed that the outcome was no different.

Fluid resuscitation of combat casualties: conference proceedings. June 2001 and October 2001. *J Trauma.* 2003;54(suppl):S1–S234.

This entire supplement summarizes the rationale for the changes recommended for the treatment of combat casualties.

Holcomb JB, Jenkins D, Rhee P, et al. Damage control resuscitation: directly addressing the early coagulopathy of trauma. *J Trauma.* 2007;62:307–310.

This paper describes the evolution of damage control resuscitation and rationale behind the recommendation of permissive hypotension, reduction of crystalloid use, use of hypertonic saline, and aggressive use of blood products early and often for best results.

Moore EE, Moore FA, Fabian TC, et al. PolyHeme study group: human polymerized hemoglobin for the treatment of hemorrhagic shock when blood is unavailable: the USA Multicenter trial. *J Am Coll Surg.* 2009;208:1–13.

Study showing that artificial hemoglobin made from expired human blood could be used safely and as a replacement of blood in the field and in the hospital.

Plurad D, Martin M, Green D, et al. The decreasing incidence of late post-traumatic acute respiratory distress syndrome: the potential role of lung protective ventilation and conservative transfusion practice. *J Trauma.* 2007;63:1–7.

This paper shows the decreasing incidence of acute respiratory distress syndrome (ARDS) in trauma and its association with decreased crystalloid use.

Spinella PC, Perkins JG, Grathwohl KW, et al. Warm fresh whole blood is independently associated with improved survival for patients with combat-related traumatic injuries. *J Trauma.* 2009;66:S69–S76.

Describes the usefulness of whole blood transfusion practice found by the military.

REFERENCES

1. Hughes JT. Miraculous deliverance of Anne Green: an Oxford case of resuscitation in the seventeenth century. *Br Med J (Clin Res Ed)*. 1982;285:1792–1793.
2. O'Shaughnassy WB. Experiments on the blood in cholera. *Lancet*. 1831;32:490–495.
3. Crile GW. *An Experimental Research into Surgical Shock*. Philadelphia, PA: JB Lippincott; 1899.
4. Cannon WB. The emergency function of the adrenal medulla in pain and the major emotions. *Am J Physiol*. 1914;33:356–372.
5. Blalock A. Experimental shock: the cause of low blood pressure caused by muscle injury. *Arch Surg*. 1930;20:959–996.
6. Wiggers CJ. The present status of shock problem. *Physiol Rev*. 1942;22:74–123.
7. Smith S, McCully B, Bommiasamy A, et al. A combat relevant model for the creation of acute lung injury in swine. *J Trauma Acute Care Surg*. 2018;85:S39–S43.
8. O'Shaughnessy WB. Proposal of a new method of treating the blue epidemic cholera by the injection of highly-oxygenated salts into the venous system. *Lancet*. 1831;17:366–371.
9. Ringer S. Concerning the influence exerted by each of the constituents of the blood on the contraction of the ventricle. *J Physiol*. 1882;3:380–393.
10. Connelly CR, Schreiber MA. Endpoints in resuscitation. *Curr Opin Crit Care*. 2015;21:512–519.
11. Brasel KJ, Guse C, Gentilello LM, et al. Heart rate: is it truly a vital sign? *J Trauma*. 2007;62:812–817.
12. Ley EJ, Salim A, Kohanzadeh S, et al. Relative bradycardia in hypotensive trauma patients: a reappraisal. *J Trauma*. 2009;67:1051–1054.
13. Bruns B, Lindsey M, Rowe K, et al. Hemoglobin drops within minutes of injuries and predicts need for an intervention to stop hemorrhage. *J Trauma*. 2007;63:312–315.
14. Riordan Jr WP, Norris PR, Jenkins JM, et al. Early loss of heart rate complexity predicts mortality regardless of mechanism, anatomic location, or severity of injury in 2178 trauma patients. *J Surg Res*. 2009;156:283–289.
15. Eastridge BJ, Salinas J, McManus JG, et al. Hypotension begins at 110 mm Hg: redefining "hypotension" with data. *J Trauma*. 2007;63:291–297.
16. Bruns B, Gentilello L, Elliott A, et al: Prehospital hypotension redefined. *J Trauma*. 65:1217-1221.
17. Krishna U, Joshi SP, Modh M. An evaluation of serial blood lactate measurement as an early predictor of shock and its outcome in patients of trauma or sepsis. *Indian J Crit Care Med*. 2009;13:66–73.
18. Grocott MP, Martin DS, Levett DZ, et al. Arterial blood gases and oxygen content in climbers on Mount Everest. *N Engl J Med*. 2009;360:140–149.
19. Cureton EL, Kwan RO, Dozier KC, et al. A different view of lactate in trauma patients: protecting the injured brain. *J Surg Res*. 2010;159:468–473.
20. Reynolds PS, Barbee RW, Ward KR. Lactate profiles as a resuscitation assessment tool in a rat model of battlefield hemorrhage resuscitation. *Shock*. 2008;30:48–54.
21. Rutherford EJ, Morris Jr JA, Reed GW, et al. Base deficit stratifies mortality and determines therapy. *J Trauma*. 1992;33:417–423.
22. Bilello JF, Davis JW, Lemaster D, et al. Prehospital hypotension in blunt trauma: identifying the "crump factor. *J Trauma*. 2011;70:1038–1042.
23. Sperry JL, Frankel HL, Nathens AB, et al. Characterization of persistent hyperglycemia: what does it mean postinjury? *J Trauma*. 2009;66:1076–1082.
24. Inaba K, Teixeira PG, Rhee P, et al. Mortality impact of hypothermia after cavitary explorations in trauma. *World J Surg*. 2009;33:864–869.
25. Beilman GJ, Blondet JJ, Nelson TR, et al. Early hypothermia in severely injured trauma patients is a significant risk factor for multiple organ dysfunction syndrome but not mortality. *Ann Surg*. 2009;249:845–850.
26. Kosinski S, Darocha T, Czerw A, et al. Cost-utility of extracorporeal membrane oxygenation rewarming in accidentally hypothermic patients: a single-centre retrospective study. *Acta Anaesthesiol Scand*. 2018;62:1105–1111.
27. Morley D, Yamane K, O'Malley R, et al. Rewarming for accidental hypothermia in an urban medical center using extracorporeal membrane oxygenation. *Am J Case Rep*. 2013;14:6–9.
28. Joseph B, Aziz H, Pandit V, et al: Prothrombin complex concentrate versus fresh-frozen plasma for reversal of coagulopathy of trauma: is there a difference? *World J Surg*. 38:1875-1881.
29. Shakur H, Roberts I, Bautista R, et al. Effects of tranexamic acid on death, vascular occlusive events, and blood transfusion in trauma patients with significant haemorrhage (CRASH-2): a randomised, placebo-controlled trial. *Lancet*. 2010;376:23–32.
30. Morrison JJ, Dubose JJ, Rasmussen TE, et al. Military Application of Tranexamic Acid in Trauma Emergency Resuscitation (MATTERs) Study. *Arch Surg*. 2012;147:113–119.
31. Madigan MC, Kemp CD, Johnson JC, et al. Secondary abdominal compartment syndrome after severe extremity injury: Are early, aggressive fluid resuscitation strategies to blame? *J Trauma*. 2008;64:280–285.
32. Palizas F, Dubin A, Regueira T, et al. Gastric tonometry versus cardiac index as resuscitation goals in septic shock: a multicenter, randomized, controlled trial. *Crit Care*. 2009;13:R44.
33. Cohn SM, Nathens AB, Moore FA, et al. Tissue oxygen saturation predicts the development of organ dysfunction during traumatic shock resuscitation. *J Trauma*. 2007;62:44–54; discussion 54–45.
34. Dellinger RP, Levy MM, Rhodes A, et al. Surviving sepsis campaign: international guidelines for management of severe sepsis and septic shock: 2012. *Crit Care Med*. 2013;41:580–637.
35. Singer M, Deutschman CS, Seymour CW, et al. The third international consensus definitions for sepsis and septic shock (Sepsis-3). *JAMA*. 2016;315:801–810.
36. Dellinger RP, Levy MM, Carlet JM, et al. Surviving sepsis campaign: International guidelines for management of severe sepsis and septic shock: 2008. *Crit Care Med*. 2008;36:296–327.
37. Yealy DM, Kellum JA, Huang DT, et al. A randomized trial of protocol-based care for early septic shock. *N Engl J Med*. 2014;370:1683–1693.
38. Bickell WH, Wall Jr MJ, Pepe PE, et al. Immediate versus delayed fluid resuscitation for hypotensive patients with penetrating torso injuries. *N Engl J Med*. 1994;331:1105–1109.
39. Demetriades D, Kimbrell B, Salim A, et al. Trauma deaths in a mature urban trauma system: is "trimodal" distribution a valid concept? *J Am Coll Surg*. 2005;201:343–348.
40. Englehart MS, Cho SD, Morris MS, et al. Use of leukoreduced blood does not reduce infection, organ failure, or mortality following trauma. *World J Surg*. 2009;33:1626–1632.
41. Rhee P, Morris J, Durham R, et al. Recombinant humanized monoclonal antibody against CD18 (rhuMAb CD18)

in traumatic hemorrhagic shock: results of a phase II clinical trial. Traumatic Shock Group. *J Trauma*. 2000;49:611–619.
42. Todd SR, Kao LS, Catania A, et al. Alpha-melanocyte stimulating hormone in critically injured trauma patients. *J Trauma*. 2009;66:465–469.
43. *Committee on Fluid Resuscitation for Combat Casualties: Fluid Resuscitation: State of the Science for Treating Combat Casualties and Civilian Injuries. Report of the Institute of Medicine*. Washington, DC: National Academy Press; 1999.
44. Gao J, Zhao WX, Xue FS, et al. Effects of different resuscitation fluids on acute lung injury in a rat model of uncontrolled hemorrhagic shock and infection. *J Trauma*. 2009;67:1213–1219.
45. Fluid resuscitation of combat casualties. Conference proceedings. June 2001 and October 2001. *J Trauma*. 2003;54:S1–S234.
46. Holcomb JB, Jenkins D, Rhee P, et al. Damage control resuscitation: directly addressing the early coagulopathy of trauma. *J Trauma*. 2007;62:307–310.
47. Teixeira PG, Oncel D, Demetriades D, et al. Blood transfusions in trauma: six-year analysis of the transfusion practices at a Level I trauma center. *Am Surg*. 2008;74:953–957.
48. Plurad D, Martin M, Green D, et al. The decreasing incidence of late posttraumatic acute respiratory distress syndrome: the potential role of lung protective ventilation and conservative transfusion practice. *J Trauma*. 2007;63:1–7.
49. Condron M, Scanlan M, Schreiber M. Massive transfusion of low-titer cold-stored O-positive whole blood in a civilian trauma setting. *Transfusion*. 2019;59:927–930.
50. Perkins JG, Cap AP, Spinella PC, et al. An evaluation of the impact of apheresis platelets used in the setting of massively transfused trauma patients. *J Trauma*. 2009;66:S77–S84.
51. Stinger HK, Spinella PC, Perkins JG, et al. The ratio of fibrinogen to red cells transfused affects survival in casualties receiving massive transfusions at an army combat support hospital. *J Trauma*. 2008;64:S79–S85; discussion S85.
52. Zink KA, Sambasivan CN, Holcomb JB, et al. A high ratio of plasma and platelets to packed red blood cells in the first 6 hours of massive transfusion improves outcomes in a large multicenter study. *Am J Surg*. 2009;197:565–570.
53. Holcomb JB, del Junco DJ, Fox EE, et al. The prospective, observational, multicenter, major trauma transfusion (PROMMTT) study: comparative effectiveness of a time-varying treatment with competing risks. *JAMA Surg*. 2013;148:127–136.
54. Holcomb JB, Tilley BC, Baraniuk S, et al. Transfusion of plasma, platelets, and red blood cells in a 1:1:1 vs a 1:1:2 ratio and mortality in patients with severe trauma: the PROPPR randomized clinical trial. *JAMA*. 2015;313:471–482.
55. Pati S, Peng Z, Wataha K, et al. Lyophilized plasma attenuates vascular permeability, inflammation and lung injury in hemorrhagic shock. *PLoS One*. 2018;13:e0192363.
56. Dente CJ, Shaz BH, Nicholas JM, et al. Improvements in early mortality and coagulopathy are sustained better in patients with blunt trauma after institution of a massive transfusion protocol in a civilian level I trauma center. *J Trauma*. 2009;66:1616–1624.
57. Young JB, Utter GH, Schermer CR, et al. Saline versus Plasma-Lyte A in initial resuscitation of trauma patients: a randomized trial. *Ann Surg*. 2014;259:255–262.
58. Semler MW, Self WH, Rice TW. Balanced crystalloids versus saline in critically Ill adults. *N Engl J Med*. 2018;378:1951.
59. Joseph B, Aziz H, Snell M, et al. The physiological effects of hyperosmolar resuscitation: 5% vs 3% hypertonic saline. *Am J Surg*. 2014;208:697–702.
60. Finfer S, Bellomo R, Boyce N, et al. A comparison of albumin and saline for fluid resuscitation in the intensive care unit. *N Engl J Med*. 2004;350:2247–2256.
61. Martin M, Salim A, Murray J, et al. The decreasing incidence and mortality of acute respiratory distress syndrome after injury: a 5-year observational study. *J Trauma*. 2005;59:1107–1113.
62. Annane D, Siami S, Jaber S, et al. Effects of fluid resuscitation with colloids vs crystalloids on mortality in critically ill patients presenting with hypovolemic shock: the CRISTAL randomized trial. *JAMA*. 2013;310:1809–1817.
63. Alam HB, Bice LM, Butt MU, et al. Effects of fluid resuscitation with colloids vs crystalloids on mortality in critically ill patients presenting with hypovolemic shock: the CRISTAL randomized trial. *JAMA*. 2013;210:1809–1817.
64. Lin T, Chen H, Koustova E, et al. Histone deacetylase as therapeutic target in a rodent model of hemorrhagic shock: effect of different resuscitation strategies on lung and liver. *Surgery*. 2007;141:784–794.
65. Alam HB, Casas F, Chen Z, et al. Development and testing of portable pump for the induction of profound hypothermia in a Swine model of lethal vascular injuries. *J Trauma*. 2006;61:1321–1329.
66. Baskett TF. Syndey Ringer and lactated Ringer's solution. *Resuscitation*. 2003;58:5–7.
67. Hill AV, Lupton H. Muscular exercise, lactic acid, and the supply and utilization of oxygen. *Q J Med*. 1923;16:135–171.
68. Rhee P, Langdale L, Mock C, et al. Near-infrared spectroscopy: continuous measurement of cytochrome oxidation during hemorrhagic shock. *Crit Care Med*. 1997;25:166–170.
70. Rhee P, Burris D, Kaufmann C, et al. Lactated Ringer's resuscitation causes neutrophil activation after hemorrhagic shock. *J Trauma*. 1998;44:313–319.
71. Rhee P, Koustova E, Alam H. Searching for the optimal resuscitation method: recommendations for the initial fluid resuscitation in combat casualties. *J Trauma*. 2003;54:S52–S62.
72. Pascual JL, Khwaja KA, Ferri LE, et al. Hypertonic saline resuscitation attenuates neutrophil lung sequestration and transmigration by diminishing leukocyte-endothelial interactions in a two-hit model of hemorrhagic shock and infection. *J Trauma*. 2003;54:121–132.
73. Shaffer TH, Wolfson MR. Liquid ventilation. In: Polin RA, Fox WW, Abman SH, eds. *Fetal and Neonatal Physiology*. 3rd ed. Philadelphia, PA: WB Saunders; 2003.
74. Somers MP, Brady WJ, Perron AD, et al. The prominent T wave: electrocadiographic differential diagnosis. *Am J Emerg Med*. 2002;20:243–251.

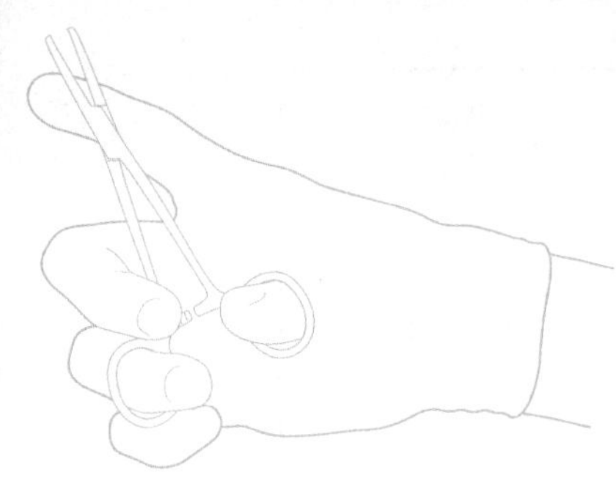

CHAPTER 5

Metabolism in Surgical Patients

Elizabeth E. Blears, Joshua S. Carson, Celeste C. Finnerty, Evan Ross, Christian Sommerhalder, David N. Herndon

OUTLINE

Please access Elsevier eBooks for Practicing Clinicians to view the videos for this chapter https://expertconsult.inkling.com/.

METABOLIC SCIENCE

Metabolism encompasses all of the biochemical and biophysical reactions that maintain the organism-level energy homeostasis necessary for continued cellular life in response to ever-shifting environmental conditions.[1,2] Fully understanding the metabolic processes at work in living systems requires exploring the overlap between chemistry, physics, and biology.[2] Conceptually, these processes are organized into pathways in which enzymes and substrates interact in a stepwise manner to achieve certain outputs that are critical to life.[2] These pathways are interlinked and influenced, such that the output of one pathway can serve as either the input or a regulator of another pathway.[2] Metabolic pathways therefore have the capacity to influence and be influenced by one another.[2] These are characterized as either anabolic, serving to build and develop the organism, or catabolic, breaking down components of the organism.[1,2] Processes from both of these categories work in concert under tight regulation to achieve the major goals of metabolism: the maintenance of life through a positive energetic and structural balance alongside a negative waste balance.[1–3]

History of Metabolism Research

Formal research into metabolism essentially began in the laboratory of French chemist Antone-Laurent de Lavoisier in the late 1700s.[2,3] A contemporary of Lavoisier's, Joseph Priestly, had previously demonstrated that a mouse could not survive in a sealed flask if a flame had first burned in it; likewise, a flame could not burn in a flask in which a mouse had first breathed (and suffocated).[2,3] Lavoisier soon established that oxygen was the common limiting factor for both the survival of a burning flame and the survival of a breathing mouse.[2,3] By making this connection, Lavoisier discovered the fundamental overlap between chemistry and biology that sits at the core of bioenergetics: oxidation.[2,3]

Prior to the use of ether as a surgical anesthetic in the mid-1800s, surgical procedures were performed on awake patients.[4] By rendering patients unconscious, etherization allowed for a slower, more measured approach to operating.[4] At around the same time, Joseph Lister pioneered the use of carbolic acid to prevent infection, and surgical mortality predictably began to decline.[4] As surgical survival increased, the consequences of operations became more observable, leading to an increase in the understanding of recovery from tissue trauma and the surgical resection of organs.[4] By the 1930s, David Cuthbertson had described the phenomenon of negative nitrogen balance after tissue trauma and argued that the losses were mostly due to muscle wasting.[5]

Since then, it has become clear that tissue trauma, whether from surgical intervention or injury, induces a catabolic state driven by stress signaling (Fig. 5.1).[2,3,5] From the cell to the organism as a whole, the surgeon encounters severe responses to stress.[4] Accordingly, the informed surgeon is well versed in the metabolic consequences of injury and illness, as well as in techniques for ameliorating those disruptions for the benefit of his or her patients.[4]

Cellular Bioenergetics

Adenosine triphosphate (ATP) is the most common currency of cellular bioenergetics by virtue of the chemical energy stored within the terminal phosphate bond.[3] Rather than allowing the hydrolysis of ATP's phosphate bond to occur spontaneously, the cell pairs the reaction with others, requiring large amounts of free energy in order to proceed, such as the activation and inactivation of enzymes.[2,3] ATP is synthesized from adenosine diphosphate (ADP) and phosphate via a reaction known as phosphorylation.[2,3] Multiple enzymes are capable of phosphorylating ADP to create ATP, with the most relevant to bioenergetics being ATP synthase, phosphoglycerate kinase, and pyruvate kinase.[2,3]

Phosphorylation occurs under anaerobic conditions as part of glycolysis and in the presence of oxygen via oxidative phosphorylation.[2,3] A number of metabolic processes are linked together in order to support the process of oxidative phosphorylation, including glycolysis, amino acid catabolism, lipolysis, and the citric acid cycle (Fig. 5.2).[2,3]

The Citric Acid Cycle

The citric acid cycle, also called the tricarboxylic acid (TCA) cycle or the Krebs cycle, is an evolutionarily conserved series of enzymatic reactions that occur almost exclusively in the mitochondrial

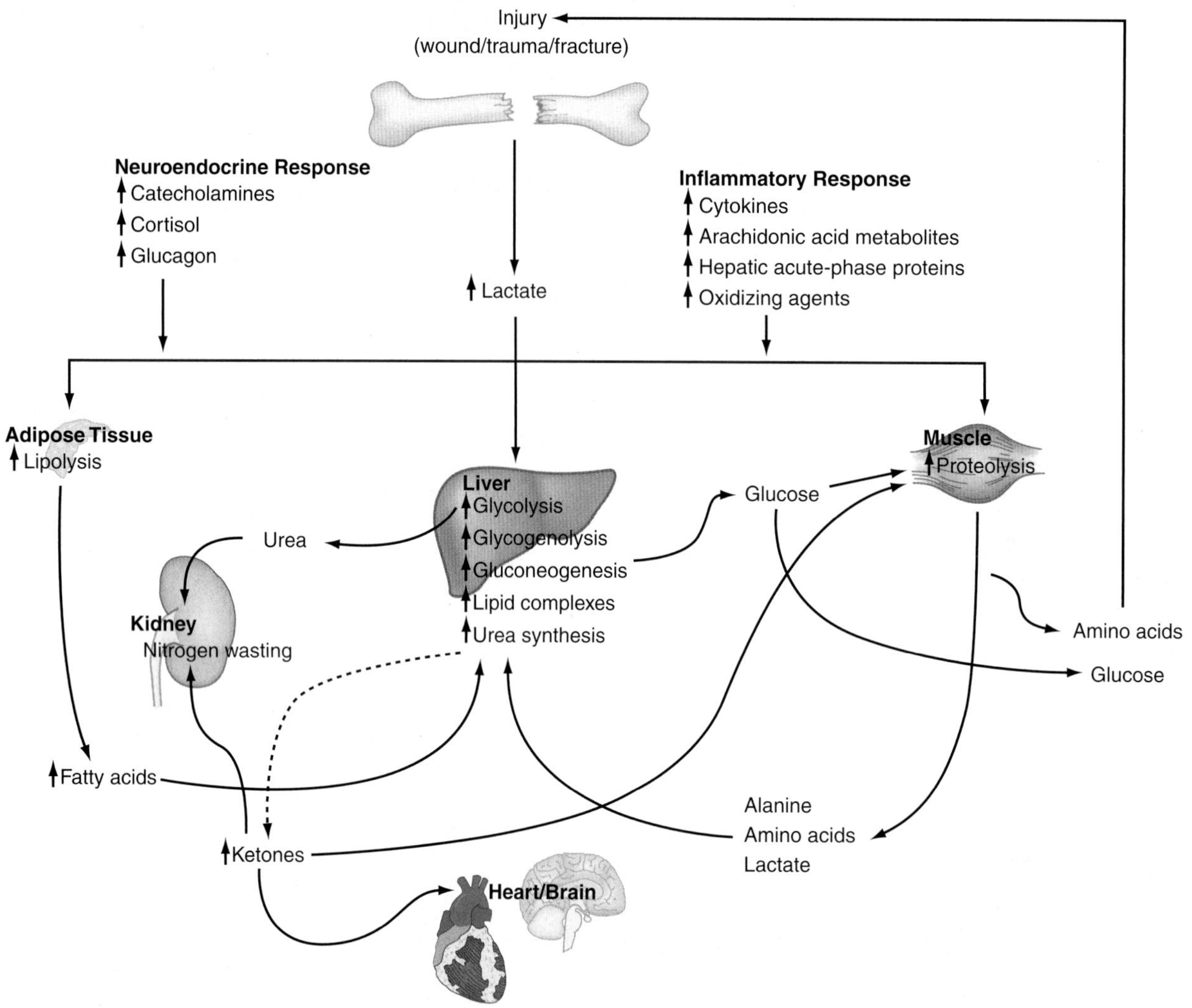

Injury
(wound/trauma/fracture)
Neuroendocrine Response
↑ Catecholamines
↑ Cortisol
↑ Glucagon
↑ Lactate
Inflammatory Response
↑ Cytokines
↑ Arachidonic acid metabolites
↑ Hepatic acute-phase proteins
↑ Oxidizing agents
Adipose Tissue
↑ Lipolysis
Muscle
↑ Proteolysis
Liver
↑ Glycolysis
↑ Glycogenolysis
↑ Gluconeogenesis
↑ Lipid complexes
↑ Urea synthesis
Urea
Glucose
Kidney
Nitrogen wasting
Amino acids
Glucose
↑ Fatty acids
Alanine
Amino acids
Lactate
↑ Ketones
Heart/Brain

FIG. 5.1 Simplified overview of metabolic pathways.

Glucose
Glycerol
Lipids
Lactate
Pyruvate
Amino acids
Acetoacetate
Acetyl-CoA
Fatty acids
Acyl-CoA
TCA
cycle
Amino acids

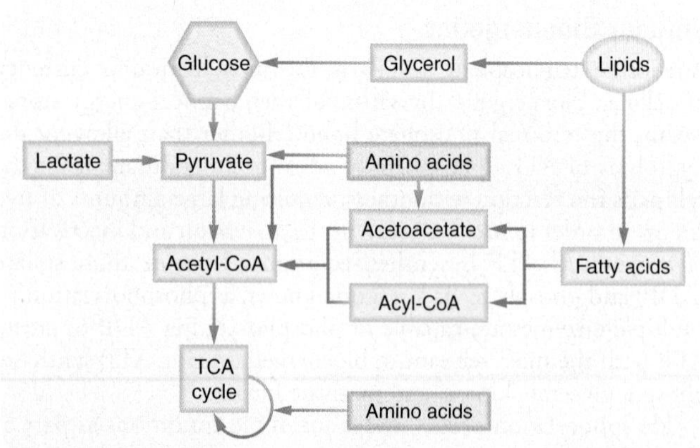

FIG. 5.2 Overview of basic fuel substrate pathways. *CoA*, Coenzyme A; *TCA*, tricarboxylic acid.

matrix (Fig. 5.3).[2,3,6] The proton motive force required to drive ATP synthesis is derived from the reducing capacity of flavin adenine dinucleotide ($FADH_2$) and nicotine adenine dinucleotide (NADH). These carriers donate the high-energy electrons that power the electron transport chain.[2,3,6] Importantly, the TCA cycle only proceeds when oxygen delivery is high. When cellular oxygen availability is low, the cell instead ferments pyruvate to lactate, making pyruvate unavailable for conversion to acetyl-coenzyme A (CoA) and initiation of the TCA cycle.[2,3,6] As not all cells contain mitochondria (e.g., red blood cells), a baseline concentration of lactate production is present at all times in the human body.[2,3,6]

Acetyl-CoA, derived from fatty acid oxidation, amino acid degradation, or glycolysis, provides the starting carbons in the form of an acetyl group attached to CoA.[2,3,6] At the start of the cycle, citrate is synthesized by the enzyme citrate synthase from oxaloacetate and acetyl-CoA.[2,3,6] Citrate is then converted to isocitrate by the enzyme aconitase.[2,3,6] In the next step, NADH is regenerated from oxidized nicotinamide adenine dinucleotide (NAD+) and a molecule of CO_2 is released following the conversion of isocitrate to α-ketoglutarate by the enzyme isocitrate dehydrogenase.[2,3,6] Next, α-ketoglutarate is converted to succinyl-CoA via the addition of a CoA and the removal of CO_2 by α-ketoglutarate dehydrogenase, regenerating another molecule of NADH.[2,3,6] Succinyl-CoA becomes succinate via the action of succinyl-CoA synthetase.[2,3,6]

Succinate then is converted to fumarate via the action of succinic dehydrogenase, a reaction that also regenerates $FADH_2$ from FADH, which in turn reduces coenzyme Q.[2,3,6] Importantly, succinate dehydrogenase is also Complex II in the electron transport chain and so marks a critical intersection between the TCA and

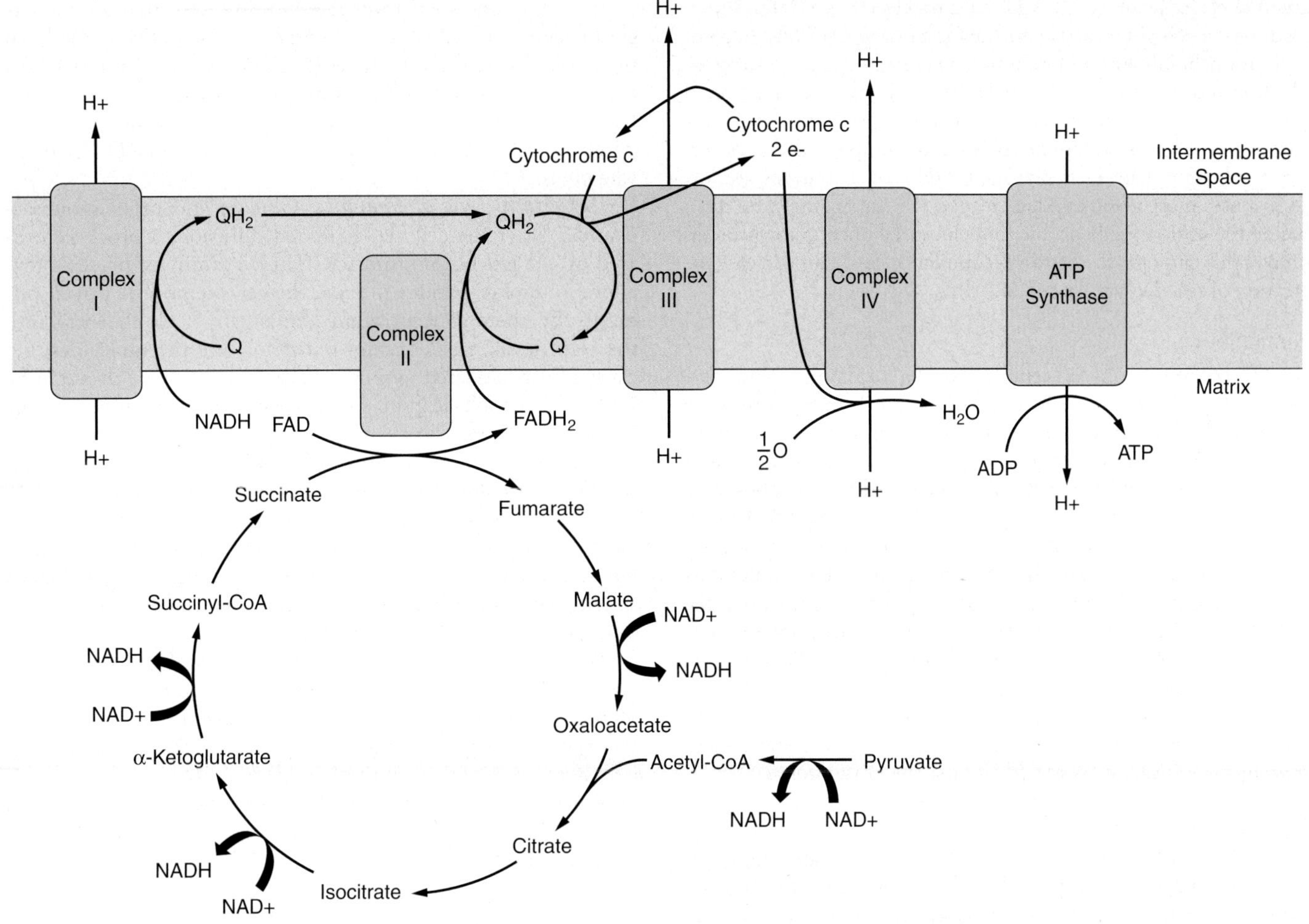

FIG. 5.3 The citric acid (TCA/tricarboxylic acid/Krebs) cycle harnesses high energy electrons via the oxidation of pyruvate to power the electron transport chain, which generates the proton gradient that is used by ATP synthase to synthesize ATP. (Adapted from Berg JM, Tymoczko JL, Stryer L. *Biochemistry.* 7th ed. New York: W. H. Freeman & Co; 2012; and Sazanov LA. A giant molecular proton pump: structure and mechanism of respiratory complex I. *Nat Rev Mol Cell Biol.* 2015;16:375–388.) *ADP*, Adenosine diphosphate; *ATP*, adenosine triphosphate; *CoA*, coenzyme A; *FADH₂*, flavin adenine dinucleotide; *NAD+*, oxidized nicotine adenine dinucleotide; *NADH*, nicotinamide adenine dinucleotide; *TCA*, tricarboxylic acid.

the electron transport chain.[2,3,6] Fumarate is converted to malate by the addition of water by fumarase, and malate is converted to oxaloacetate by malate dehydrogenase, regenerating a final molecule of NADH and resetting the cycle to begin again.[2,3,6]

Oxidative Phosphorylation

Oxidative phosphorylation is the process by which ATP synthesis is coupled to the movement of electrons through the mitochondrial electron transport chain and the associated consumption of oxygen.[2,3,6] This process is the most efficient for ATP synthesis, generating approximately 36 ATP molecules per glucose molecule, compared to the two molecules of ATP generated during glycolysis.[2,3,6]

The free energy released by stepwise oxidation reactions between NADH, $FADH_2$, and ubiquinol pumps protons from the mitochondrial matrix, across the mitochondrial inner membrane, and into the intermembrane space.[2,3,6] This pumping action creates a tremendous proton concentration imbalance between the intermembrane space and the matrix.[2,3,6] The potential energy stored in this proton gradient is then used to power ATP synthase phosphorylating ADP to generate ATP.[2,3,6]

The electron transport chain (Fig. 5.3) involves the transfer of electrons from NADH and $FADH_2$ to ubiquinone (also called Coenzyme Q) through a series of four large protein complexes that reside in the mitochondrial inner membrane.[2,3,6] Because the electrons begin the process at a high energy state and end the process in a low energy state, the electron transport chain entails the stepwise release of energy, which the protein complexes harness in order to pump protons from the mitochondrial matrix into the intermembrane space; each reaction in the electron transport chain represents a slight decrease in the energy of the electrons as they pass from complex to complex.[2,3,6] An oxygen molecule sits at the end of the electron transport chain as the final electron acceptor, where it joins with two free protons to become water in a highly exothermic reaction.[2,3,6] Without oxygen, the electrons in the electron transport chain cannot continue to fall down their potential energy gradient, and progression of electrons through the transport chain stops.[2,3,6]

In addition to the controlled transfer of electrons from complex to complex in the electron transport chain, thermodynamic factors at work within the mitochondria sometimes also favor the unintentional creation of reactive oxygen species, especially the superoxide anion (a molecule of oxygen with an extra electron).[2,3,6] The superoxide anion is highly reactive, making it damaging to cells. Accordingly, mitochondria have an inbuilt manganese-dependent superoxide dismutase enzyme that immediately catalyzes the conversion of superoxide to the more manageable hydrogen peroxide.[2,3,6] The accumulation of electrons at Complex I and Complex III that occurs when substrate delivery is high and ADP concentrations are low contributes most to superoxide creation.[2,3,6] Intriguingly, by dissipating the proton gradient, the mitochondrial uncoupling proteins offload this pathogenic electron accumulation and thus decrease the creation of reactive oxygen species.[7,8]

Fermentation

At low concentrations of cellular oxygen, oxidative phosphorylation ceases to function efficiently, yet the cell must continue to create ATP.[2,3,6] Because ATP can be produced without oxygen via glycolysis, the cell must rely on the glycolytic pathway to support its energy needs.[2,3,6] During glycolysis, glyceraldehyde-3-phosphate dehydrogenase reduces NAD+ to NADH when glyceraldehyde-3-phosphate is converted into 1,3-bisphosphoglycerate.[2,3,6] Because NADH is not consumed by the electron transport chain under low-oxygen conditions, NADH concentrations begin to increase in the cell.[2,3,6] In order to offload the accumulating NADH and regenerate NAD+ for use in the glycolytic pathway, the cell relies upon the fermentation of pyruvate into lactate by the lactate dehydrogenase enzyme, leading to the cellular accumulation of lactate.[2,3,6] This process underlies blood lactate elevation observed with hypoperfusion during critical illness or with compartment syndrome.[2,3,5,6]

The Lactic Acid (Cori) Cycle

In the first step of the Cori cycle (Fig. 5.4), lactate created in peripheral tissues is transported in the bloodstream to the liver, where lactate dehydrogenase converts lactate into pyruvate for gluconeogenesis.[2,3,6] The glucose thus produced is transported back into the bloodstream, where it can be delivered to cells in need of fuel substrates.[2,3,6] If oxygen delivery has returned to normal, the pyruvate created by glycolysis will enter the TCA cycle—if oxygen delivery remains low, the cells will continue to ferment the pyruvate into lactate, causing the Cori cycle to repeat.[2,3,6]

Glycolysis

In the process of glycolysis (Fig. 5.5), glucose is converted to pyruvate via the sequential action of 10 enzymes at the cost of two molecules of ATP but with the generation of four molecules of ATP.[2,3,6] Glycolysis has three rate-limiting steps that are the target of regulatory processes: (1) entry into the pathway catalyzed by hexokinase and glucokinase, (2) the irreversible conversion of fructose-6-phosphate into fructose-1,6-bisphosphate by phosphofructokinase, and (3) the final step in the pathway, the creation of pyruvate and ATP from phosphoenolpyruvate and ADP by pyruvate kinase.[2,3,6]

Hexokinase and glucokinase. Glucose and other monosaccharides enter the cell via facilitated diffusion, a process mediated by the glucose transporter (GLUT) family of proteins that allows monosaccharides to cross the cell membrane driven primarily by their concentration gradients.[2,3,6] Upon entry into the cell, hexokinase enzymes phosphorylate the molecules; because phosphorylated monosaccharides cannot pass through the GLUT, this modification effectively traps the monosaccharide inside the cell.[2,3,6]

Glucokinase is an isoform of hexokinase with two peculiarities: first, in contrast to hexokinase, the product of its reaction, glucose-6-phosphate, does not inhibit glucokinase, and second, it has a low binding affinity for glucose compared to the other hexokinase enzymes.[2,3,6] These two differences mean that glucokinase activity varies only in response to glucose availability, allowing it to act as a sensor of fuel availability.[2,3,6]

Phosphofructokinase. Of the 10 reactions that comprise the glycolytic pathway, the first irreversible reaction is the conversion of fructose-6-phosphate to fructose-1,6-bisphosphate by phosphofructokinase.[2,3,6] Because this step in the pathway is irreversible, it acts as a critical point of regulation—the activity of phosphofructokinase is sensitive to changes in energy availability due to inhibition by products of the glycolytic process and facilitation by excess glucose.[2,3,6]

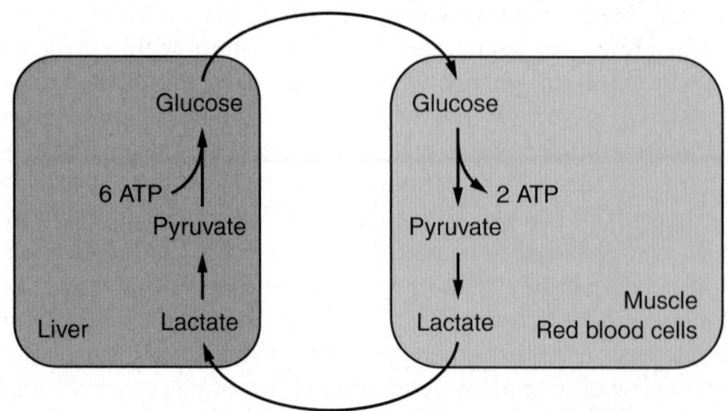

FIG. 5.4 In the lactic acid (Cori) cycle, the lactate that is produced in peripheral tissues is converted back to glucose by the liver, then released into the circulation to support ongoing glycolysis in the periphery. (Adapted from Berg JM, Tymoczko JL, Stryer L. *Biochemistry.* 7th ed. New York: W. H. Freeman & Co; 2012. *ATP,* Adenosine triphosphate.)

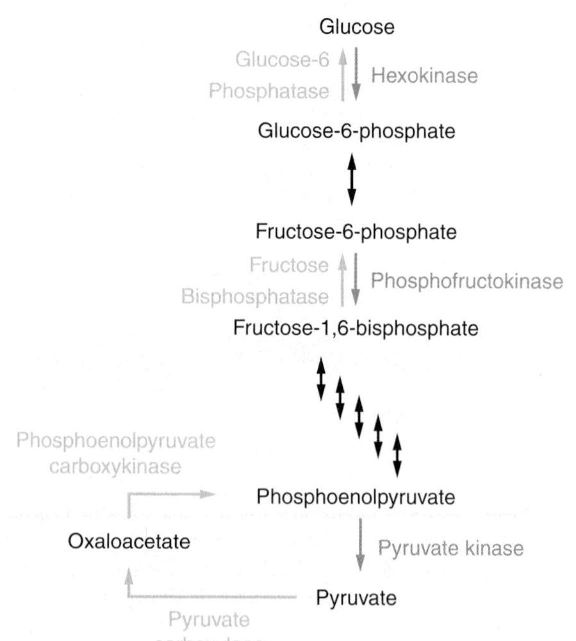

FIG. 5.5 Glycolysis and gluconeogenesis are the two opposing processes that sit at the core of glucose metabolism; where glycolysis makes energy available to the cell, gluconeogenesis can be used to export glucose into the circulation to make energy available to the body. Highlighted in *gold* are the points of regulation in gluconeogenesis, while the points of regulation in glycolysis are highlighted in *blue*. (Adapted from Berg JM, Tymoczko JL, Stryer L. *Biochemistry.* 7th ed. New York: W. H. Freeman & Co; 2012.)

Pyruvate kinase. The final step of glycolysis entails the removal of a phosphate from phosphoenolpyruvate and the subsequent phosphorylation of ADP to regenerate ATP.[2,3,6] This irreversible reaction is catalyzed by pyruvate kinase.[2,3,6] Pyruvate kinase is inhibited by its products and by signals from stress hormones like epinephrine and glucagon.[4,5] On the other hand, insulin drives pyruvate kinase activity, and thus glycolysis, forward.[2,3,6]

Gluconeogenesis

As with all processes in bioenergetics, glycolysis has an opposing process that essentially runs all of the glycolytic reactions in reverse—gluconeogenesis (Fig. 5.5).[2,3,6] Where as glycolysis breaks glucose and other monosaccharides down into pyruvate, gluconeogenesis takes various starting substrates, converts them to pyruvate or oxaloacetate, and then converts those substrates into glucose.[2,3,6] While all cells in the human body can perform gluconeogenesis, only when the process occurs in the liver and kidneys can the resulting glucose be transported back into the bloodstream in order to defend against hypoglycemia.[2,3,6] This is due to the tissue-specific expression of the glucose-6-phosphatase enzyme that dephosphorylates glucose-6-phosphate, allowing it to pass through the GLUT.[2,3,6]

The most important of the starting substrates for gluconeogenesis are lactate, fatty acids, and amino acids.[2,3,6] Lactate enters the gluconeogenic pathway via the action of lactate dehydrogenase, an enzyme that converts lactate into pyruvate.[2,3,6] Fatty acids that contain an odd number of carbons can be converted to pyruvate from propionyl-CoA via the combined action of propionyl-CoA carboxylase and the enzymes of the TCA cycle. Finally, some (but not all) amino acids can be converted into glucose and/or oxaloacetate.[2,3,6]

Glycogen

Glycogen is a large polysaccharide molecule composed of long chains of glucose molecules; it is found primarily in liver and skeletal muscle cells, where it serves as a storage form of glucose.[2,3,6] Glycogen is synthesized by glycogen synthase, an enzyme that essentially polymerizes glucose in response to signals of increased energy availability, such as cellular concentrations of glucose-6-phoshpate and insulin.[2,3,6] Glycogen can be broken down by glycogen phosphorylase, an enzyme that releases glucose-1-phosphate from the glycogen molecule—glycogen phosphorylase is activated by stress signals like epinephrine and glucagon.[2,3,6]

Glycogen is stored primarily in the liver and skeletal muscle cells.[2,3,6] When a glucose-1-phosphate molecule is released from the glycogen molecule, it can be converted to glucose-6-phosphate by phosphoglucomutase.[2,3,6] Glucose-6-phosphate can then be stripped of its phosphate by glucose-6-phosphatase and exported into the circulation in order to defend against hypoglycemia for approximately the first 24 hours after starvation.[2,3,6] Where as liver cells possess high concentrations of the glucose-6-phosphatase enzyme and can release glucose molecules into the circulation, other glycogen-rich tissues like skeletal muscles have very low concentrations and cannot export meaningful amounts of glucose into the bloodstream.[2,3,6]

Fatty Acid Oxidation

In addition to monosaccharides, cells can use lipids as fuel substrates via the process of fatty acid oxidation, also called beta-oxidation.[2,3,6] Although peroxisomes can degrade lipids via beta-oxidation, when the process is intended to fuel ATP synthesis, it takes place in the mitochondria.[2,3,6] The long carbon chains of fatty acids are degraded two carbons at a time into acetyl groups, which are then attached to CoA, forming acetyl-CoA for entry into the TCA cycle.[2,3,6] This process also regenerates $FADH_2$ and NADH in its own right, rendering the process of fatty acid oxidation very bioenergetically rewarding for the cell.[2,3,6]

Ketogenesis

The term *ketone body* generally refers to three substances: β-hydroxybutyrate, acetoacetate, and acetone.[2,3,6] When carbohydrate availability is extremely low, such as during fasting or starvation when gluconeogenesis and glycogenolysis have been exhausted, the body will switch to a reliance on ketone bodies as fuel substrates.[2,3,6] For example, while the brain normally uses glucose for energy, by the fourth day of fasting, the brain obtains about 70% of its energy from ketone bodies.[2,3,6] Acetyl-CoA generated via fatty acid degradation would normally enter the TCA cycle; however, because oxaloacetate is depleted by ongoing gluconeogenesis during starvation, acetyl-CoA is instead used to form ketone bodies.[2,3,6] The ketone bodies, in turn, can be broken down into pyruvate for use as fuel by the brain, heart, and muscles.[2,3,6]

Mitochondria

Mitochondria are double-membrane enveloped, energy-producing organelles that sit at the nexus of cellular energy homeostasis.[2] Mitochondria generate ATP, the body's main source of fuel, through oxidative phosphorylation and act as critical components of the cellular and organismal response to severe stress; in times of survivable cellular stress, the mitochondria are capable of buffering cellular calcium concentrations, while in times of lethal stress, they release cytochrome c into the cytoplasm, activating the caspase cascade, which leads to programmed cell death.[2] On the organism level, mitochondria within the adrenal cortex synthesize the glucocorticoid and mineralocorticoid hormones that assist in adaptation to stress.[2]

The mitochondria are of ancient and intriguing evolutionary origin: Although the details of the process are still debated, it is clear that, at some point in the distant past, a single-celled organism engulfed a mitochondrion-like cell and, rather than digest the protomitochondrion for food, established an endosymbiotic relationship.[2] Since that time, the host and mitochondrion have peacefully coexisted, with each becoming ever-more dependent upon the other for survival.[2] The evolutionary history of the mitochondrion is clear in its structure: it is the only organelle in eukaryotic cells that contains its own deoxyribonucleic acid (DNA), labeled mitochondrial DNA (mtDNA) to distinguish it from nuclear DNA.[2] Furthermore, mitochondria undergo their own processes of fission and fusion independently of the cellular mitotic process.[2]

Mitochondrial coupling control. When a mitochondrion is able to fully convert the potential energy of the proton gradient into ATP phosphorylation, it is said to be fully "coupled"—in other words, the synthesis of ATP is *coupled* to the proton motive force.[2,3] Various chemicals and proteins are able to interfere with mitochondrial electron transport chain coupling, leading to the proton-motive force dissipating as heat energy rather than the phosphorylation of ADP—these mitochondria are often referred to as "leaky."[2,3,7] Several proteins have recently been described that are capable of dissipating the proton gradient without ATP synthesis by allowing protons to bypass ATP synthase and diffuse directly into the mitochondrial matrix.[7] The best understood of these proteins is called uncoupling protein 1, which serves to uncouple the diffusion of protons from the synthesis of ATP, thereby causing the mitochondria to become thermogenic and inefficient in times of stress or inflammation.[7]

Brown Adipose Tissue

Brown adipose tissue (BAT) is a thermogenic tissue of mesenchymal lineage, named due to its characteristically dark appearance in histologic section due to abundant mitochondrial content and limited lipid droplets.[8] Because BAT contains highly uncoupled and therefore inefficient mitochondria, each cell acts as an energy sink and therefore may be useful in humans as a potential treatment for obesity and diabetes.[8]

Adult humans have very small depots of BAT, generally located above the clavicle, near the vertebrae, in the mediastinum, and around the kidney.[8] BAT is characterized by abundant uncoupling protein expression, leading to mitochondria that are highly thermogenic due to elevated expression of uncoupling protein-1.[8] Although the exact mechanism of mitochondrial thermogenesis is unclear, it is clearly linked to the dissipation of the proton gradient.[8] For example, loss of the proton gradient causes the ATP synthase molecule to run in reverse, acting instead as a proton pump that attempts to restore the proton gradient at the expense of the highly exothermic hydrolysis of ATP.[2,8] Additionally, the dissipation of the proton gradient allows the electron transport chain to proceed at its maximal rate, resulting in increased consumption of oxygen by combustion with H_2 to yield H_2O.[2,8]

The BAT moniker is somewhat misleading, as BAT cells are thought to be derived from cells positive for the myogenic factor 5 surface marker, making them more closely related to muscle cells than white adipose tissue cells.[8] Intriguingly, white adipose tissue cells are capable of acquiring BAT characteristics in response to stress in a process called "beiging" or "browning" that appears to be driven by peroxisome proliferator-activated receptor gamma coactivator 1α, the "master regulator" of mitochondrial biogenesis.[8] For example, evidence of white adipose tissue browning can be found in patients after severe burns, which suggests that this process may contribute to the increase in nutritional needs during severe stress.[7]

Maintenance of Cell Structure and Function

The structural and functional aspects of cells are composed of various combinations of proteins, lipids, carbohydrates, and nucleic acids.[2] The synthesis and degradation of these cell components are under tight regulation, the loss of which can lead to severe cellular dysfunction.[2]

Amino Acid Metabolism

Amino acids (also called peptides) are small organic molecules that consist of a carboxyl group, an amino group, and various side chains, the identity of which determines the behavior of the amino acid.[2,3] Although more than 500 amino acids can be found in nature, only 21 amino acids appear in human proteins.[2,3] There are a number of purposes in the body for amino acids beyond protein synthesis, including their use as precursors to neurotransmitters and nucleic acids or as fuel substrates (both as glucose and as ketones).[2,3]

Proteinogenic amino acids. Human proteins are formed from long chains of amino acids that are sequentially linked via covalent peptide bonds between the carboxyl and amino groups; chains of amino acids are therefore called *polypeptides*.[2,3] Of the 21 amino acids that appear in human proteins (Table 5.1), only 20 are directly coded for in the genetic code, with the 21st—selenocysteine—encoded by a stop codon that is differentially translated under specific circumstances.[2,3]

TABLE 5.1 The proteinogenic amino acids.

	NAME	ABBREVIATION	
Essential amino acids	Histidine	HIS	H
	Isoleucine	ILE	I
	Leucine	LEU	L
	Lysine	LYS	K
	Methionine	MET	M
	Phenylalanine	PHE	F
	Threonine	THR	T
	Tryptophan	TRP	W
	Valine	VAL	V
Conditionally essential amino acids	Arginine	ARG	R
	Cysteine	CYS	C
	Glutamine	GLN	Q
	Glycine	GLY	G
	Proline	PRO	P
	Tyrosine	TYR	Y
Nonessential amino acids	Alanine	ALA	A
	Asparagine	ASN	N
	Aspartate	ASP	D
	Glutamate	GLU	E
	Selenocysteine	SEC	U
	Serine	SER	S

Sources of amino acids. Of the 21 amino acids that are used to build human proteins, 12 can be synthesized by the body from various other substrates, while the remaining 9 must be consumed in the diet—these amino acids that must be taken in from external sources are called the "essential" amino acids.[2,3,9] In addition to being classified by their source, amino acids can be classified by their structure, as in the case of the three branched-chain amino acids (BCAAs) that contain an aliphatic side chain: isoleucine, leucine, and valine.[2,3,9] The BCAAs, leucine in particular, are an important component of nutritional status signaling in skeletal muscle; BCAAs in isolation stimulate muscle protein synthesis to the same degree that a complete mixture of all amino acids does, suggesting that the BCAAs signal the availability of amino acids for protein synthesis.[2,3,9]

Amino acids as fuel. Thirteen amino acids can be oxidized into glucose and as such are termed the "glucogenic" amino acids (alanine, arginine, asparagine, aspartate, cysteine, glutamate, glycine, histidine, methionine, proline, serine, valine, and glutamine), while five (isoleucine, phenylalanine, threonine, tryptophan, and tyrosine) can be converted to either ketones or glucose, and the final two (leucine and lysine) can only be converted into ketones.[2,3,9]

Alanine is converted to pyruvate and then glucose in the liver as part of the glucose-alanine cycle, a process with close similarity to the Cori cycle.[3] The catabolism of BCAAs in skeletal muscle leads to the creation of toxic ammonium ions.[3] In order to offload the accumulating ammonium ions, skeletal muscle cells synthesize alanine, which is transported to the liver for conversion back to glucose.[3]

Amino acids as precursors to neurotransmitters. The human body uses the amino acids tryptophan, tyrosine, and phenylalanine as precursors to neurotransmitters.[3,9] Tryptophan is converted into serotonin, while tyrosine (itself a product of phenylalanine) is converted to all of the catecholamine neurotransmitters, including dopamine, epinephrine, and norepinephrine. Phenylalanine can be converted to tyrosine as well as phenylethylamine.[3,9]

Toxic by-products of amino acid metabolism. Toxic ammonia, the ultimate result of amino acid and nucleotide breakdown, must be converted into water-soluble urea for excretion in the urine.[3]

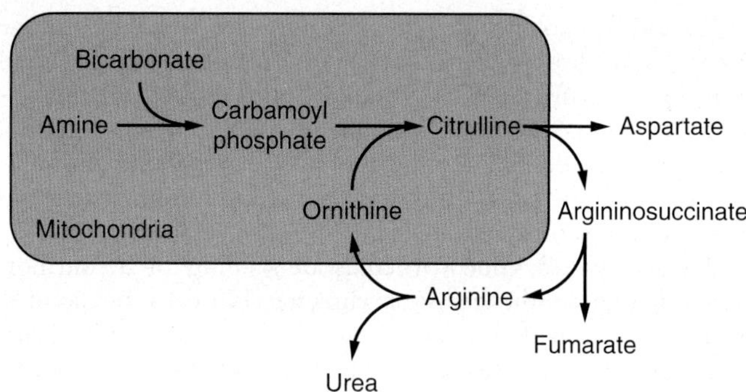

FIG. 5.6 The urea cycle serves to convert potentially harmful amines to water soluble urea for excretion in the urine. (From Blair NF, Cremer PD, Tchan MC. Urea cycle disorders: a life-threatening yet treatable cause of metabolic encephalopathy in adults. *Pract Neurol.* 2015;15:45–48.)

While nitrogenous waste is formed throughout the body, the liver is the principal organ that converts wastes into urea.[3] Because the body can ill afford to have the highly reactive ammonium ion freely circulating, the nitrogenous waste products are packaged into the amino acids glutamine and alanine for transport in the blood to the liver, where the amine group can be removed and converted into urea by the enzymes of the urea cycle.[3] Patients with liver failure are at risk for developing hepatic encephalopathy, an accumulation of urea and other toxins in the bloodstream that interferes with normal neural function.[10] Accordingly, caution must be exercised when managing the protein nutrition of liver failure patients.[10]

The Urea Cycle

In the liver, mitochondrial and cytosolic enzymes work together to produce urea from ammonia in a process called the *urea cycle* (Fig. 5.6).[3] The urea cycle begins in the mitochondria with the transfer of ammonia from either glutamate or glutamine to a phosphorylated molecule of bicarbonate by the enzyme carbamoyl phosphate synthetase 1, creating carbamoyl phosphate.[3] Carbamoyl phosphate then reacts with ornithine to form citrulline via the action of ornithine transcarbamylase, also in the mitochondria.[3] Then, citrulline is transported out of the mitochondria and into the cytoplasm via the ornithine-citrulline transporter, where it reacts with aspartate to form argininosuccinate via the enzyme argininosuccinate synthetase.[3] In turn, argininosuccinate is broken down to arginine and fumarate via the action of argininosuccinate lyase.[3] Fumarate is then free to join the citric acid cycle, while arginine is degraded to urea and ornithine via the arginase enzyme.[3] Ornithine is then transported back into the mitochondria via the ornithine-citrulline transporter, where the cycle can begin again.[3]

Lipid Metabolism

Cholesterol. Along with phospholipids, cholesterol is a critical element of cell membranes.[3] Cholesterol is a steroid alcohol that consists of three cyclohexanes and a single cyclopentane.[3] The starting substrate of the cholesterol biosynthesis pathway is acetyl-CoA and the key rate-limiting enzyme, β-hydroxy β-methylglutaryl-CoA.[3] β-hydroxy β-methylglutaryl-CoA reductase is targeted by the statin class of cholesterol-lowering drugs.[3] Because cholesterol can be fully synthesized by the human body, it has no dietary requirement.[3]

The cholesterol molecule is the backbone of all steroid hormones in human physiology.[3] The first (and rate-limiting) reaction to synthesize all steroid hormones is the conversion of cholesterol to pregnenolone by a cholesterol side chain cleavage enzyme.[3] Additionally, while the sex steroids are synthesized in the endoplasmic reticulum, the final reactions of aldosterone, corticosterone, and cortisol biosynthesis also take place in the mitochondria.[3] Where female sex steroid hormones are exclusively derived from the gonadal tissues, some intermediate androgens are synthesized within the adrenal glands and sent to the gonads for further processing.[3] All mineralocorticoids and glucocorticoids are derived from the adrenal glands.[3]

Fatty acids. Fatty acids are hydrophobic organic molecules that consist of aliphatic (hydrocarbon) chains bound to a carboxylic acid group.[3] The length of their aliphatic chain and the location (if any) of double and/or triple carbon-carbon bonds are used to categorize fatty acids.[3] Fatty acids that do not contain multiple bonds are termed "saturated" fatty acids, while those that contain at least one multiple bond are termed "unsaturated."[3] A fatty acid that has a single multiple bond is termed a "monounsaturated" fatty acid, while one that contains more than one multiple bond is termed a "polyunsaturated" fatty acid.[3] When the first saturated bond occurs at the third carbon-carbon bond when counted from the tail (or "omega" end) of the aliphatic chain, the fatty acid is called an "omega-3" fatty acid.[3] When the bond is at the sixth carbon-carbon bond when counted from the tail, the fatty acid is called an "omega-6" fatty acid.[3] Notably, the omega-3 and omega-6 fatty acids cannot be synthesized in the human body, making them essential nutrients.[3,11]

Omega-3 and omega-6 fatty acids are converted into eicosanoids, powerful but short-lived 20-carbon molecules that are synthesized in response to tissue injury and stress.[11,12] Cyclooxygenase (COX) and lipoxygenase are the best understood of the enzyme families that participate in these reactions.[3] The prostaglandins, powerful and pleiotropic injury signaling molecules, are synthesized from arachidonic acid by COX-1 and COX-2 enzymes.[3] The inhibition of COX-1 and COX-2 enzymes by nonsteroidal antiinflammatory medications leads to a reduction in pain and inflammation due to the decrease in prostaglandin synthesis at the site of injury.[3] The lipoxygenase enzymes synthesize the pro-inflammatory leukotrienes, which are implicated in asthma.[3,11,12]

Phospholipids. Phospholipids are polar molecules that consist of a hydrophilic phosphorylated head group and a pair of hydrophobic fatty-acid tails, with one tail being fully saturated and the other tail being unsaturated.[3] Because of their polarity, phospholipids spontaneously form lipid bilayers in water; accordingly, they serve as the primary component of the cell membrane.[2] The common backbone of all phospholipids, phosphatidic acid, is synthesized in the cell from diacylglycerol, which in turn is synthesized from glycerol-6-phosphate and acyl-CoA by the sequential actions of glycerol-3-phosphate acyltransferase and acylglycerol-3-phosphate acyltransferase.[3]

Triglycerides. Human body fat is primarily made up of triglycerides, the storage and transport form of lipids that consists of a glycerol molecule bound to three fatty acid tails.[2] Triglycerides are stored in lipid droplets in adipose tissue—when the body needs to release the energy stored in the triglyceride, hormonal signals like epinephrine or glucagon activate hormone sensitive lipase in adipose tissue to hydrolyze the ester bond and release free fatty acids into the circulation.[3] Because hormone-sensitive lipase responds to many of the stress hormones, transient elevations in blood-free fatty acid concentrations are normal in the perioperative period, although the clinical significance of this elevation is unclear.[3,4]

Nucleic Acid Metabolism

Nucleotide synthesis and degradation. Nucleotides are small organic molecules composed of a five-carbon sugar, a nitrogenous base, and a phosphate group.[2] Nucleotides fall into two categories based on their structure: pyrimidines and purines.[2] In pyrimidine nucleotides, the nitrogenous base is a pyrimidine ring, while purine nucleotides contain a purine ring (a pyrimidine ring joined with an imidazole ring).[2,3] Adenine and guanine are purine nucleotides, while cytosine, uracil, and thymine are pyrimidine nucleotides.[2,3] Nucleic acids, long polymers of nucleotides, form the DNA and ribonucleic acid (RNA) molecules that form the information storage system of all cellular life; when the nucleotide sugar is a ribose, the molecule is designated RNA, and when the sugar is a deoxyribose, the molecule is known as a DNA.[2,3]

Nucleotide synthesis largely takes place in the liver, where amino acids serve as structural substrates.[3] Aspartate, glycine, and glutamine are required to synthesize the purine nucleotides, while aspartate and glutamine are required to build the pyrimidine nucleotides.[3] Due to their nitrogenous content, nucleotide degradation generates ammonia that the body must excrete as urea.[3,10]

Anabolic and Catabolic Hormones

Insulin. Insulin is a powerful anabolic peptide hormone that facilitates the cellular uptake of structural and fuel substrates.[3] In bioenergetic terms, insulin drives the cellular uptake of fuel substrates from the bloodstream, promotes the use of glucose for fuel, and enhances glycogen synthesis while suppressing glycogenolysis.[3]

Insulin is synthesized by the pancreas and secreted into the bloodstream in response to elevations in blood glucose.[3] Endogenous insulin is degraded primarily by the liver and kidneys and has a half-life of between 5 and 15 minutes.[3] The insulin receptor is a tyrosine kinase that signals through the phosphatidylinositol-3,4,5-triphosphate secondary messenger system to activate protein kinase B.[3] Insulin drives the uptake of glucose from the bloodstream via stimulating the trafficking of presynthesized GLUT-4 to the membrane of skeletal muscle and adipose tissue cells.[3] This mechanism accounts for the rapid decrease in blood glucose concentrations induced by the exogenous administration of insulin.[3] Although the exact mechanism is not clear, insulin also increases the activity of the Na-K ATPase pumps on cell membranes, leading to a decrease in blood potassium.[3]

Glucagon. Glucagon is a peptide hormone that defends the body against hypoglycemia by stimulating gluconeogenesis and the breakdown of glycogen in the liver.[3] Simultaneously, glucagon suppresses fatty acid synthesis and promotes fatty acid release into the bloodstream via a stimulatory effect on hormone sensitive lipase in adipose tissue.[3] While glucagon is largely known for its effects on glucose and fatty acid metabolism, recent evidence suggests that glucagon also influences amino acid turnover, although the exact mechanisms behind this effect are not well understood.[3]

Like insulin, glucagon is synthesized in the pancreas and released in response to changes in blood glucose concentrations.[3] However, where insulin is secreted from beta cells in response to rising blood glucose, glucagon is secreted from alpha cells in response to falling blood glucose concentrations.[3] Importantly, glucagon secretion can also be driven by epinephrine.[3] Glucagon binds to G-protein–coupled receptors that signal through the cyclic adenosine monophosphate second messenger system.[2,3]

Thyroid hormone. The thyroid gland plays an important role in energy homeostasis through the actions of the two peptide hormones it secretes: triiodothyronine (T3) and thyroxine (T4).[3] The thyroid hormones are synthesized from tyrosine and iodine in the thyroid gland and are metabolized via selenium containing enzymes in target tissues—thus, iodine and selenium are essential minerals for the function of the thyroid gland.[3] The hypothalamus drives secretion of thyroid hormone through its regulation of the pituitary gland, thus making the thyroid a component of the hypothalamic-pituitary axis.[3]

Thyroid hormones function by binding the thyroid hormone receptor, a nuclear receptor that targets metabolic and structural genes for upregulation.[3] The thyroid hormone receptor upregulates many genes associated with glucose and lipid consumption, leading to increased lipid and carbohydrate availability and utilization as fuel substrates.[3] Additionally, thyroid hormone increases heart rate and cardiac output.[3]

Glucocorticoids. Glucocorticoids are a family of steroid hormones that are synthesized from cholesterol in the mitochondria of cells in the zona fasciculata of the adrenal cortex.[2,3] Glucocorticoid synthesis and release are under the control of adrenocorticotropic hormone secreted by the pituitary gland in response to stress.[2,3] The glucocorticoids are remarkably powerful with pleiotropic effects that increase fuel substrate availability and utilization.[2,3] The glucocorticoids promote gluconeogenesis and any catabolic process that liberates gluconeogenic substrates; accordingly, the glucocorticoids promote amino acid degradation and lipolysis.[2,3] Cortisol is considered to be the most significant of the glucocorticoids in human physiology.[2–5] The high concentrations of glucocorticoids and catecholamines in times of stress are thought to be the cause of stress hyperglycemia.[2–5]

According to the classical understanding of their function, glucocorticoids bind to the glucocorticoid receptor, a cytoplasmic receptor that translocates to the nucleus upon binding.[2] In the nucleus, the glucocorticoid receptor upregulates and suppresses various genes.[2] Although they are much less well understood, a subclass of glucocorticoid receptors found on the cell membrane mediate rapid, nongenomic cellular responses to glucocorticoid administration.[2]

Sex hormones. The sex hormones are steroid hormones that determine secondary sexual characteristics via altering gene transcription.[3] The sex hormones encompass the androgens (responsible for male secondary sexual characteristics) and estrogens (responsible for female secondary sexual characteristics).[3] The androgens drive structural and bioenergetic changes in cells, especially in skeletal muscle, that promote protein accretion as well as glucose uptake and oxidation.[3] Androgenic hormones, and especially their synthetic analogues, can have different degrees of androgenic activities relative to their anabolic effects—for instance, the synthetic testosterone analogue oxandrolone has about 25% of the androgenic potential of testosterone but more than 300% of its anabolic activity.[3] Although the role of estrogens in energy metabolism remains unclear, estrogens are known to decrease lipogenesis and promote overall glucose homeostasis.[3]

SURGICAL METABOLISM

Assessment of Nutritional Status

Nutrient availability plays an important role in determining the likelihood of successful recovery from operation, making the assessment of nutritional status one of the quintessential aspects of care for the surgical patient.[9] Patients with surgical needs can present anywhere on the spectrum of nutritional status, from underfed to overfed; both can cause serious detriment to patients as evidenced by increases in surgical morbidity and mortality.[9,13] The appropriate assessment and diagnosis of malnutrition is important for normalizing outcomes and should be noted in the medical record according to the following.

History and Physical

During assessment, the clinician must first determine if any historical factors may affect the patient's current nutritional status: an exploration of potential causes of poor food intake, malabsorption, or poor nutrient utilization must be included in the history. Common

TABLE 5.2 **ICD-9 and ICD-10 codes for malnutrition.**

ICD-9 CODE	ICD-9 TITLE	ICD-10 CODE	ICD-10 TITLE	CRITERIA/DESCRIPTION
260	Kwashiorkor*	E40	Kwashiorkor*	Nutritional edema with dyspigmentation of skin and hair
260	Kwashiorkor*	E42	Marasmic kwashiorkor*	Intermediate form of severe protein-calorie malnutrition with signs of both kwashiorkor and marasmus.
261	Nutritional marasmus*	E41	Nutritional marasmus*	Nutritional atrophy/cachexia; severe malnutrition otherwise stated; severe energy deficiency
262	Other severe protein calorie malnutrition	E43	Unspecified severe protein-calorie malnutrition	Nutritional edema without mention of dyspigmentation of skin and hair
263	Malnutrition of moderate degree	E44.0	Moderate protein-calorie malnutrition	†
263.1	Malnutrition of mild degree	E44.1	Mild protein-calorie malnutrition	†
263.2	Arrested development following protein-calorie malnutrition	E45	Retarded development following protein-calorie malnutrition	†
263.8	Other protein-calorie malnutrition	E46	Unspecified protein calorie malnutrition	Disorder due to lack of proper nutrition or inability to absorb nutrients from food; poor nutritional status due to insufficient intake, malabsorption, or abnormal nutrient distribution; lack of sufficient energy/protein to meet functional demands as a result of either inadequate dietary protein, poor quality protein, or increased demands due to disease
263.9	Unspecified protein-calorie malnutrition	E46	Unspecified protein calorie malnutrition	See 263.8
263.9	Unspecified protein-calorie malnutrition	E64	Sequelae of protein-calorie malnutrition	See 263.8

Adapted from Centers for Medicare and Medicaid Services. ICD-10 Medicare & Medicaid services. 2018. https://www.cms.gov/Medicare/Coding/ICD10/index.html?redirect=/icd10. Accessed February 22, 2019.

ICD-9, International Classification of Diseases, 9th revision; *ICD-10, International Classification of Diseases*, 10th revision.

ICD-9 and -10 both have many more specific diagnoses such as niacin deficiency (E52), failure to thrive—adult (R62.7), failure to thrive—child (R62.51), obesity (E66), etc.

*Should rarely be used in the United States.

†Not listed in the ICD-10 description but description added for completeness.

factors include poverty or geographic location, previous gastrointestinal (GI) operations, drug or alcohol abuse, as well as congenital or pathologic causes of malabsorption.[9] Second, the clinician must decide which specific subtype of malnutrition the patient is suffering from (i.e., protein deficiency, micronutrient deficiency, overall caloric deficit, etc.).[13,14] Categorization should further continue by specific pathology: starvation related, disease related, or injury related.[9,13–15] Lastly, whichever pathologic cause is found should be categorized into acute versus chronic symptoms.[9,13–15] In pediatric patients, overt signs of acute malnutrition include pitting edema, sunken eyes, and poor skin turgor, while experiencing chronic malnutrition could cause symptoms such as kwashiorkor signs and growth stunting (Table 5.2).[9,13–15] For adults, ascertaining timelines from the patient or family are more useful since severe cancers or malabsorptive syndromes can cause rapid- or slow-onset weight loss leading to a cachectic-appearing patient in a matter of weeks or over years with no other major phenotypic differences between the two.[9,13–15] Lastly, it should be noted that phenotypic changes may be deceiving, as obese patients can be malnourished despite a surplus of caloric energy due to hormonal resistances and poor lean body mass.[16]

Nutritional Assessment Scores

Many different nutritional assessment scores have been developed to complement the history and physical examination. The Nutrition Risk Screening (NRS 2002) and the Nutrition Assessment in Critically Ill (NUTRIC) scores (Table 5.3) are currently the only two scores that take into account the severity of disease as well as nutritional factors.[9,13,15] Other scores such as the Malnutrition Universal Screening Tool, the Mini Nutritional Assessment, and the newer Perioperative Nutrition Screen (Fig. 5.7) only take into account current nutritional status.[9,13,15] Because serum markers have been found to be ineffective for stratifying risk of malnutrition postoperatively due to potential confounding by the acute stress response, any patient admitted to the intensive care unit (ICU) as well as any patient with a suspected risk of malnutrition should be screened at least with a general assessment.[9,13,15] If malnutrition is considered, a nutrition risk score should also be utilized.[9,13,15]

Serum Markers

While previously advocated as reliable measures of nutritional status, the utility of serum markers such as albumin, prealbumin, retinol binding protein, and transferrin has come into question.[17,18] In a recent metaanalysis with otherwise healthy nutrient-deprived patients, albumin and prealbumin remained normal until severe malnutrition (body mass index [BMI] <12 or 6 weeks of starvation) had already occurred.[17] It also appears that during inflammatory stress, the body may transfer amino acid resources to the

TABLE 5.3 The Nutrition Assessment in Critically Ill (NUTRIC) score.

VARIABLE	CRITERIA	POINTS
Age	<50 years	0
	50 to <70 years	1
	≥75 years	2
APACHE II	<15 points	0
	15 to <20 points	1
	20 to 28 points	2
	≥28 points	3
SOFA	<6 points	0
	6 to <10 points	1
	≥10 points	2
Number of comorbidities	0 to 1	0
	≥2	1
Days from hospital admission to ICU admit	0 to <1	0
	≥1	1
Total	0 to 4	Low malnutrition risk
	5 to 9	High malnutrition risk, need nutritional plan

Adapted from Heyland DK, Dhaliwal R, Jiang X, et al. Identifying critically ill patients who benefit the most from nutrition therapy: the development and initial validation of a novel risk assessment tool. *Crit Care.* 2011;15:R268.
APACHE II, Acute Physiology and Chronic Health Evaluation; *ICU*, intensive care unit; *IL-6*, interleukin-6; *SOFA*, sequential organs failure assessment.
A score of 5 or greater signifies a high risk of malnutrition. The NUTRIC score can also include IL-6 concentrations, with ≥400 adding 1 point. If IL-6 concentrations are obtained, a score of 6 or greater is then considered high risk.

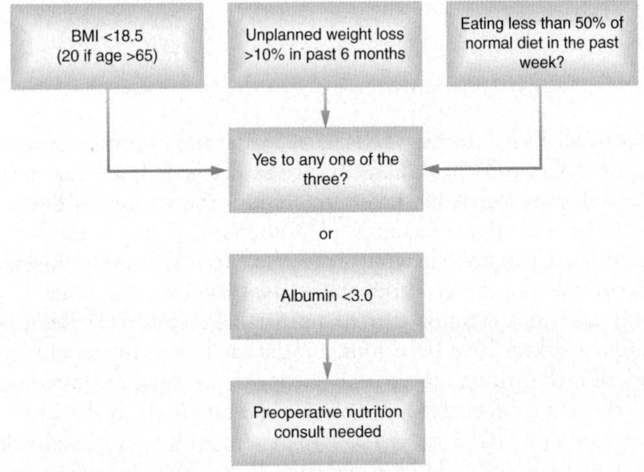

FIG. 5.7 The Perioperative Nutrition Screen (PONS) is a simple tool to assess the need for dietician/nutrition consultation in order to optimize preoperative nutritional status. (Adapted from Nygren J, Thacker J, Carli F, et al. Guidelines for perioperative care in elective rectal/pelvic surgery: Enhanced Recovery After Surgery (ERAS®) Society recommendations. *World J Surg.* 2013;37:285–305.) *BMI*, Body mass index.

creation of inflammatory proteins, thus decreasing concentrations of nutritional markers even when the patient is adequately nourished.[17,19] More specifically, the fractional synthesis of albumin is unchanged after abdominal surgery (and possibly other inflammatory processes), while the albumin capillary leak positively correlates with inflammation, creating a net decrease in intravascular

TABLE 5.4 Association between preoperative serum albumin and surgical outcome.

SERUM ALBUMIN (g/dL)	30-DAY MORTALITY RATE (%)	30-DAY MORBIDITY RATE (%)
>4.5	≤1	≤10
3.5	5	25
3	9	35
2.5	15	45
<2.1	≈30	65

Adapted from Gibbs J, Cull W, Henderson W, et al. Preoperative serum albumin level as a predictor of operative mortality and morbidity: results from the National VA Surgical Risk Study. *Arch Surg.* 1999;134:36–42.

albumin/prealbumin.[17,20] The relationship between albumin and outcome is unlikely to be causal; in several clinical studies, the administration of albumin secondary to low serum concentrations showed no improvement in clinical outcomes.[21]

Despite these limitations with the use of nutritional serum markers in the postoperative state, studies have shown good or excellent correlation between preoperative albumin and/or prealbumin concentrations with patient outcomes (Table 5.4).[15,20] Serum markers can therefore be considered as preoperative prognostic factors but not necessarily as nutritional status indicators.[15,20]

Although none of the above assessment methods is perfect, the combination of screening to identify at-risk patients and a recognition of phenotypic as well as potential etiologic factors can reliably establish a patient's nutritional state.

Imaging

Imaging techniques can be used as an adjunct to the history and physical exam. Multiple imaging techniques are available for monitoring trends in lean body mass, bone mineral/density, and adiposity in patients, further assisting in nutritional assessment, especially for the long term.[9,15]

Dual emission x-ray absorptiometry (DXA, previously DEXA) scans are considered the gold standard, capable of providing highly accurate measures of bone and soft tissues.[9,22,23] DXA uses low-dose ionizing radiation at two different energies in order to differentiate soft tissues and bone.[9,22,23] The amount of each type of tissue can be isolated based on its calculated density, allowing for calculations of body fat, lean body mass, and bone mineral density/content.[9,22,23] Unfortunately, the precision and reproducibility of the scans can drop rapidly if a standard protocol is not maintained across measurements.[9,22,23] For example, variables such as clothing, nasogastric tubes, or prosthetics can potentially alter the results.[9,22,23]

Ultrasound has become a rapid and reliable bedside method to assess muscle mass, especially when the age and sex of the patient are incorporated into the assessment.[9,22,23] By comparison to DXA scanning, ultrasound is advantageous because it involves no radiation, can be performed at the bedside, and individual muscles can be measured.[9,22,23] Additionally, ultrasound can give both quantitative and qualitative measurements of muscle mass by combining the measurement of muscle dimension with muscular density.[9,22,23] In a recent study, ultrasound measurements correlated well with DXA scans; however, standardized measurement protocols are required due to the operator dependency of ultrasound examination.[9,22,23] A simple measurement can be done using B-mode ultrasound to determine the cross-sectional dimensions of the rectus femoris at the midpoint of the femur between the anterior iliac spine and the upper lateral epicondyle of the femur.[9,22,23]

Computed tomography (CT) scan can be used to calculate lean body mass with the help of computer algorithms. For example, at the L3 vertebrae, the psoas muscles can be used to calculate whole body lean mass.[9,22,23] Additionally, CT scan has the advantage of being able to measure Hounsfield density units, which can be used as a proxy of muscle quality in addition to quantitative measurements of muscular dimensions.[9,22,23] The major limitations of the use of CT scanning for anthropometric analysis are the high cost and exposure to ionizing radiation; therefore, measurements of lean mass should only be done on CT scans ordered for other reasons.[9,22,23]

Anthropometric Assessment

Anthropometry consists of any physical measurement of the human body. In medicine, whichever anthropometric measurement is used, whether for clinical or research purposes, the most important factor is that the methods are standardized from measurement to measurement. The Centers for Disease Control and Prevention has published the National Health and Nutrition Examination Survey (NHANES) anthropometry procedures manual in order to assist in national standardization of anthropometric measures for this very reason.[24]

Weight

Accurate and precise weight measurements in hospitalized patients allow for improved fluid resuscitation and monitoring of patient's nutrition.[9,15] Daily weights in intensive care patients allow for monitoring both long-term trends as well as smaller fluctuations that occur with boluses of nutrients or other fluids.[9,15] Body weight increases early in a patient's ICU stay, likely due to fluid overload, are associated with an increased risk of mortality, making close monitoring of body weight a vital component of ICU care.[9,15] Current weight minus historical dry weight (if available) along with intake and output recordings and physical exam finding should be used to assess for fluid overload.[9,15] Because no verified method for calculating or estimating dry weight exists, it is considered a clinically determined variable using either the initial admit weight of the patient or extrapolation from previous heights and weights in the medical record prior to admission.[9,15] As with nutritional assessment, the fluid status of a patient is always best determined using a combination of factors, creating a larger clinical picture.

Ideal body weight. For patients at the extremes of body size, the calculated ideal body weight is a more clinically useful value for body weight than the measured weight. One common method is:

$$\text{Males}: 50\text{ kg} + 2.3\text{ kg for every } 2.54\text{ cm over } 152.4\text{ cm}$$
$$\text{Females}: 45\text{ kg} + 2.3\text{ kg for every } 2.54\text{ cm over } 152.4\text{ cm}$$

As this method is limited to patients over 5 feet tall and is known to underestimate ideal body weight for women, the BMI method can also be used by taking patient height and calculating the 19 to 21 BMI range (21–23 for women), giving an ideal weight range.[9,15] In obese patients, the adjusted body weight provides another alternative,[25,26] which may be beneficial:

$$\text{Adjusted body weight} = \text{Ideal body weight} + 0.4\,(\text{Current body weight} - \text{Ideal Body Weight})$$

Adjusted body weight is often used by nutritionists for energy calculations in bariatric surgery.[25,26]

Height. Since height is generally not anticipated to change during hospitalization, an initial height measurement is usually sufficient for medical purposes with the exception of pediatric patients with extended hospital stays.[4,9,15] It should be noted that, often, intensive care and infant heights are measured while the patient is supine, while outpatient measurements are taken standing; this can lead to false diagnoses of growth stunting in pediatric patients if not taken into account.[4,9,15]

Body mass index. The BMI is calculated by dividing weight in kilograms by height in meters, squared. Although generally a good estimate of body size, BMI is limited by the fact that one cannot determine the proportions of fat, muscle, and bone that comprise the body mass.[15] Therefore, the use of BMI as the sole indicator of health and/or nutritional status can be misleading.[27,28]

Lean body mass. The determination of total lean body mass can be an important adjunct to BMI. The loss of lean body mass that occurs in response to the catabolic milieu of critical illness and after operation is thought to contribute to worse outcomes, including higher mortality rates, increased ventilator reliance, and longer ICU stays.[19,29,30]

Predicted Nutritional Needs

Once the patient has been assessed for clinical risk of malnutrition, the amount of nutritional supplementation must then be considered. Not only is the amount of caloric intake important, but the contents of these calories must also be determined.[31] For example, burned patients are thought to benefit from high-protein and high-carbohydrate diets with a low-fat content, while diabetic patients should have limited carbohydrates provided in their diet.[23,32] In general, critically ill adult patients are thought to benefit from high-protein diets, while this approach would be prohibitive in patients with renal failure who require low-protein diets that are highly concentrated so as to avoid urea toxicity and fluid overload.[9,33]

Energy Expenditure

Correctly estimating a patient's energy expenditure remains a challenge in clinical practice. Although indirect calorimetry remains the gold standard for estimating nutritional needs, large variation occurs during the process of obtaining resting energy expenditure (REE) clinically.[22,28] Errors between two tests even on the same day can be up to 13%, while errors within the same week can be up to 23%.[22,28] Additionally, using REE to supplement caloric goals has been shown to have no significant benefits in outcomes.[22,28] Therefore, if indirectly calorimetry is to be used, strict protocols must be in place to standardize the measurements.[22,28] If an indirect calorimeter is not available, the REE may be estimated using equations like the Harris-Benedict:

$$\text{Men}: \text{REE} = 66.5 + (13.75 \times \text{Weight [kg]}) + (5.003 \times \text{Height [cm]}) - (6.755 \times \text{Age [years]})$$

$$\text{Women}: \text{REE} = 655.1 + (9.563 \times \text{Weight [kg]}) + (1.85 \times \text{Height [cm]}) - (4.676 \times \text{Age [years]})$$

Other equations exist, including the Korth and World Health Organization equations, both of which have higher accuracy in normal-weight patients, while the Harris-Benedict equation predicts better in obese patients.[15,16] It is important to note that the REE is estimated for a patient at rest, while the critically ill and postsurgical patients have elevated metabolic rates.[22,28] Accordingly, stress and activity factor multipliers (ranging from 1.2 for light activity to 2 for thermal injury) should be used to adjust for the clinical scenario, creating an estimate for the total energy expenditure (Table 5.5).[22,28,32]

Using a combination of parameters is important to ensure that the patient is not being underfed or overfed since any single assessment method can consistently underestimate or overestimate

TABLE 5.5 Harris-Benedict energy expenditure multipliers.

SCENARIO	ENERGY EXPENDITURE MULTIPLIER
Resting (AF)	1.1
Confined to bed (AF)	1.2
Out of bed (AF)	1.3
Minor operation (IF)	1.2
Skeletal trauma (IF)	1.35
Cancer cachexia (IF)	1.3–1.5
Major sepsis (IF)	1.6
Severe thermal injury (IF)	2.1
Febrile (IF)	1 + 0.09 per 0.5°C >38.5

Adapted from Long CL, Schaffel N, Geiger JW, et al. Metabolic response to injury and illness: estimation of energy and protein needs from indirect calorimetry and nitrogen balance. *JPEN J Parenter Enteral Nutr.* 1979;3:452–456; and Reeves MM, Capra S. Predicting energy requirements in the clinical setting: are current methods evidence based? *Nutr Rev.* 2003;61:143–151.
AF, Activity factor; *IF*, injury factor.

TABLE 5.6 Varying caloric needs based on BMI classification.

BMI	CLASSIFICATION	BASELINE DAILY CALORIC INTAKE
<18.5	Underweight	30–40 kcal/kg actual body weight
18.5–24.9	Normal weight	25–30 kcal/kg actual body weight
25.0–29.9	Overweight	11–14 kcal/kg actual body weight
30.0–34.9	Obesity class I	11–14 kcal/kg actual body weight
35.0–39.9	Obesity class II	11–14 kcal/kg actual body weight
≥40.0	Obesity class III	11–14 kcal/kg actual body weight
>50	Obesity class III*	22–25 kcal/kg ideal body weight

Adapted from Dickerson RN, Boschert KJ, Kudsk KA, et al. Hypocaloric enteral tube feeding in critically ill obese patients. *Nutrition.* 2002;18:241–246; Dickerson RN. Hypocaloric, high-protein nutrition therapy for critically ill patients with obesity. *Nutr Clin Pract.* 2014;29:786–791; and Choban PS, Burge JC, Scales D, et al. Hypoenergetic nutrition support in hospitalized obese patients: a simplified method for clinical application. *Am J Clin Nutr.* 1997;66:546–550.
BMI, Body mass index.
*Subdivision created solely for caloric intake; obesity class III consists of any BMI greater than 40.0.

caloric needs.[22,28] Underfeeding below 70% of the true REE can increase mortality, while overfeeding can cause both increased mortality, ventilator days, and increased length of stay.[15,34–36]

Other factors that should be taken into account when estimating nutritional needs are fluid and protein losses secondary to the clinical condition. For example, a burn patient's protein needs are 1.5 to 2.5 g/kg/day to compensate for increased losses.[15,32] In a similar vein, critically ill surgical patients with an open abdomen have protein needs that are approximately equivalent to a patient with 40% total body surface area burn and require about 15 to 30 g of extra protein per liter of intraperitoneal fluid lost in order to compensate for protein losses.[9,15,32]

Nutritional Support of the Surgical Patient

Nutritional support before and after surgery are critical for increasing the likelihood of positive outcomes.[9] When planning nutritional support, it is important to take into account the differences between prescribed and actual administration of feeding.[9,37,38] Surgical patients can have 12% to 20% of their feeding time interrupted, with the majority of this interruption time due to avoidable causes as opposed to feeding intolerance.[39] Wherever possible, hospitals should have strict protocols in place to minimize the time where feeds are stopped (for instance, a recent study suggests that 65% of the missed feeding time can be avoided by appropriate planning).[39] To meet predicted nutritional needs, one possible solution is nurse-directed feeding with 24-hour goals as opposed to hourly rates.[38,40]

Optimizing preoperative nutrition. In chronically ill patients, preoperative nutrition is vital to improving postoperative outcomes. The important proven aspects of preoperative nutrition for underweight surgical patients appears to be both omega-3 fatty acids and arginine, which independently show reduced hospital stays and infection rates postoperatively.[11,12] Omega-3 fatty acids have a beneficial antiinflammatory effect because they can compete with the proinflammatory omega-6 fatty acids, which assist in minimizing the inflammatory response secondary to surgery via shunting of arachidonic acid away from inflammatory prostaglandins/leukotrienes PGE2 and LTB2 and toward PGE3 and LTB5; they may also decrease local inflammation by preventing neutrophil translocation.[11,12] During the stress response, synthesis of nitric oxide via arginine and decreased uptake of arginine lead to overall arginine deficits, suggesting that supplementation may allow for return-to-normal concentrations, improved T-cell function, and improved collagen synthesis.[11,12] Omega-3 and omega-6 fatty acids in approximately 1:1 or "immune neutral" ratios have demonstrated the most benefit in surgical patients, but metaanalyses fail to demonstrate any superiority of one formulation or ratio over another.[11,12] If oral tolerance is not possible, then parental supplementation can be used.[40]

At the other end of the spectrum, just under 50% of adult ICU patients are obese, while about 19% of pediatric patients are obese.[16] It is important to categorize obese patients separately as their nutritional needs differ from normal sized individuals.[16] Obese patients are at high risk of malnutrition even if the phenotype is not as obvious as with underweight patients; patients with a BMI greater than 30 are 1.5 times more likely to be in a state of malnutrition than normal BMI patients.[16] Obese individuals are more resistant to nutrient mobilization at baseline, making it difficult for their bodies to respond to surgical stress.[16] Obese surgical patients should receive high-protein, low-fat, low-carbohydrate diets in order to best preserve lean body mass and mobilize unnecessary triglycerides.[16] In these patients, caloric intake should be scaled back toward their ideal body weight by using 65% to 70% of their REE or 11 to 14 kcal/kg actual body weight per day while maintaining 2.0 to 2.5 g/kg /ideal body weight per day of protein to prevent the catabolism of lean body mass (Table 5.6).[16] Outside of more specific caloric needs, obese patients are at higher risk of complications such as hyperlipidemia, hyperglycemia secondary to increased gluconeogenesis, and others; therefore, they should be monitored closely during hospital stay for complications related to both overfeeding and underfeeding.[16]

Enhanced recovery after surgery (ERAS) protocols that include attention to preoperative and postoperative nutrition have proven useful in promoting successful outcomes.[41] Preoperatively, these protocols often include proper nutrition through the day prior to surgery and carbohydrate loading via clear liquids up to 2 hours prior to surgery (Table 5.7).[41] Postoperatively, ERAS protocols attempt to minimize the use of opioid medications that slow gastric/intestinal transit while balancing this against the requirement to

TABLE 5.7 American Society of Anesthesiologist Task Force guidelines for preoperative fasting.

TYPE OF FOOD	TIMING	NOTES
Solids	Up to 6 hours prior to procedure with general or regional anesthesia	Large or fat/carbohydrate meals may need to be delayed further.
Clear liquids	2 Hours prior to procedure with general or regional anesthesia	This includes carbohydrate/protein shakes. Breast milk for infant should be delayed to 4 hours. This does not include alcohol.

Adapted from Practice guidelines for preoperative fasting and the use of pharmacologic agents to reduce the risk of pulmonary aspiration: application to healthy patients undergoing elective procedures: an updated report by the American Society of Anesthesiologists Committee on Standards and Practice Parameters. *Anesthesiology.* 2011;114:495–511.

provide appropriate pain control and to initiate a regular diet as soon as a few hours postoperatively as opposed to waiting for clear signs of a return of bowel function.[41] These recommendations can both shorten hospital stay and improve outcomes from surgery.[41]

Safe initiation of postoperative nutrition. Appropriate postoperative nutrition depends on the clinical scenario, including swallowing ability and intestinal continuity, among others.[42] In the absence of hard contraindications for enteral feeding, such as intestinal discontinuity, enteral nutrition (EN) can safely begin within 24 hours postoperatively.[40,42] Early postoperative nutrition decreases mortality as compared to intravenous fluids alone and additionally may decrease nausea and vomiting.[36,40] Although it has historically been standard practice, no evidence supports starting oral feeding with a clear liquid diet after operation as opposed to a regular, solid diet.[37,42] In the absence of contraindications to solid food, clear liquid diets have been found to have no physiologic advantage over solids.[37,42] Immediate nutrition of the appropriate consistency has been shown to be beneficial in various fields, including after colorectal anastomosis and esophagectomy by decreasing hospital stay and postoperative complications.[36,40] The American Society for Parenteral and Enteral Nutrition (ASPEN) guidelines recommend early EN despite possible lack of bowel function in the patient.[9] As lack of bowel function may be due to atrophy of mucosa and immune barrier dysfunction, initiating enteral feeds may actually improve postoperative GI dysfunction and decrease ileus.[15] This EN or parenteral nutrition should be continued in surgical patients until at least 60% of their caloric needs can be met by oral intake.[15] Lastly, it is vital to remember that a patient's nutrition supplementation should not stop at discharge since patients with malnutrition are twice as likely to be readmitted.[15] Therefore, instructions or even prescriptions should be given to patients as needed.[15]

Gastrointestinal anastomoses. It was previously thought that *nil per os* status must be maintained for several days after intestinal anastomosis out of concern for perforation.[15,42] However, recent literature has demonstrated that EN is beneficial to anastomotic healing.[9,15] Alternatively, in cases where oral intake is truly not feasible and insertion of nasogastric feeding tube may cause perforation, parenteral nutrition is indicated after 5 to 7 days for low-risk patients and earlier for high-risk patients if it is expected to be necessary for ≥7 days.[15,42] Because the majority of improvement was found in patients who started parenteral nutrition 7 days prior to surgery, preoperative planning is essential if postoperative enteral feeding is not expected to be possible.[15,40,42]

BOX 5.1 ASPEN recommended intensive care unit (ICU) nutrition bundle.

- Assess patients on admission to the ICU for nutrition risk, and calculate both energy and protein requirements to determine goals of nutrition therapy.
- Initiate enteral nutrition (EN) within 24–48 hours following the onset of critical illness and admission to the ICU, and increase to goals over the first week of ICU stay.
- Take steps as needed to reduce risk of aspiration or improve tolerance to gastric feeding (use prokinetic agent, continuous infusion, and chlorhexidine mouthwash; elevate the head of bed; and divert level of feeding in the gastrointestinal tract).
- Implement enteral feeding protocols with institution-specific strategies to promote delivery of EN.
- Do not use gastric residual volumes as part of routine care to monitor ICU patients receiving EN.
- Start parenteral nutrition early when EN is not feasible or sufficient in high-risk or poorly nourished patients (recommend holding for up to 7 days for low-risk patients).

From McClave SA, Taylor BE, Martindale RG, et al. Guidelines for the provision and assessment of nutrition support therapy in the adult critically Ill patient: Society of Critical Care Medicine (SCCM) and American Society for Parenteral and Enteral Nutrition (A.S.P.E.N.). *JPEN J Parenter Enteral Nutr.* 2016;40:159–211.
ASPEN, American Society for Parenteral and Enteral Nutrition.

Hemodynamic instability/vasopressor infusion. During times of hemodynamic instability and vasopressor initiation and escalation, EN should be held due to lack of perfusion to the gut and possible intestinal necrosis.[15] However, if a patient is beginning to recover their hemodynamic stability and is being weaned off of vasopressor support, enteral feeding can be considered—this practice has been found to be associated with decreased hospital mortality.[9,15] If early EN during vasopressor withdrawal is considered, close monitoring for potential intestinal ischemia should be performed.[15]

Enteral Versus Parenteral Nutrition

ASPEN guidelines currently recommend enteral feeding over parenteral nutrition based on best available evidence (Box 5.1).[9] Although a recent metaanalysis showed no differences in rates of mortality between early EN and early parenteral nutrition, the EN group experienced reduced infectious complications, including catheter-related blood stream infections and reduced hospital length of stay.[36] Total parenteral nutrition (TPN) may be beneficial for critically ill patients who have a baseline malnutrition: the current Society for Critical Care Medicine guidelines recommend early TPN for any patient with an NRS 2002 or NUTRIC score ≥5 or severe malnourishment *and* intolerance to EN.[9] Biochemically, patients with adequate nutritional status as evidenced by low risk nutrition scores (NRS score ≤3 or NUTRIC score ≤5) can tolerate starvation for up to 7 days without major detrimental effects if clinical improvement and the resumption of nutritional support is expected within this time.[9]

EN has been shown to improve intestinal blood flow, cause release of bile salts and gastrin, and assist in tight junction maintenance in the gut.[33,40,43] Lack of enteral feeding can lead to dysbiosis of the gut microbiome, allowing bacteria to traverse the intestinal wall, leading to sepsis and multisystem organ failure.[40,44] The net effect of enteral feeding on the gut and immune response is still an area of active debate, with existing literature demonstrating both benefit (intestinal villi and structural integrity) and harm (possible worsening of the inflammatory response by providing precursors for leukotrienes and prostaglandins).[29,45]

In terms of location of enteral feeding, studies have shown no differences in pneumonia, length of stay, and mortality, while some have shown improved nutrient delivery with small bowel feeding when compared to gastric feeding.[36,37,40] Current evidence suggests that gastric feeding is safe unless there is a high risk for aspiration, in which postpyloric feeding can reduce aspiration and pneumonia.[42]

Types of Formulas

EN comes in many different formulas to meet different clinical needs. The majority of patients do well with standard formulas (which have the advantage of being less expensive), but specialized formulas may be required, depending on the situation. Importantly, the majority of specialty formulas have no large clinical trials demonstrating any benefit over standard formulations.[31] Specifically modified formulas exist for patients with allergies, including gluten, egg, whey, casein, and soy-free formulas.[31]

Fiber

Fiber can augment enteral feeding in various ways depending on the type of fiber used. Soluble fiber can be fermented by gut bacteria, allowing for slower transit especially in the case of diarrhea.[31] Despite this theoretical advantage, few studies have shown decreased incidence of diarrhea with soluble fiber. Soluble fiber is also able to be used as an energy source for colonocytes by bacterial fermentation of disaccharides and oligosaccharides into short chain fatty acids, specifically butyrate, propionate, and acetate.[9,15,31] Insoluble fiber, on the other hand, increases nutrient transit through the gut via increased peristalsis and increased fecal bulk.[9,31] Recommendations of soluble fiber are usually for 10 to 20 g/day in normal patients, especially with patients suffering from diarrhea with no other identifiable cause.[9,31] Prebiotics, or fibers digested only in the colon after bacterial fermentation, have been shown to improve the composition of the gut microbiota.[15,31,45]

Trophic Feeds

Trophic feeding is generally advocated in scenarios in which a patient may not tolerate full feeding. In these situations, the appeal of trophic feeding is that it may still help to maintain intestinal integrity while avoiding the complications of feeding intolerance.[36,40,44] However, major outcomes including mortality, infection, and ventilator days showed no significant difference between\ full and trophic feeding several multicenter trials.[9,15,42]

Continuous and Bolus Feeding

Continuous feeds are still often used in hospitals in the United States.[36,40] An hourly rate or daily total will be estimated for a patient, with the goal rate held steady throughout the day.[36,40] To assess tolerance, hospitals often still use gastric residuals, although it has been proven to be a poor predictor of complications: several randomized controlled trials demonstrated no increases in aspiration incidence in patients where the gastric residual to hold feeds was increased from 50 to 150 mL to 250 to 500 mL.[36,40] As an alternative, hospital protocols should include screening for and protection against aspiration (raising the head of bed, etc.) and physical exam for distention or abdominal pain of the patient.[36,40] Prokinetic agents such as erythromycin (3–7 mg/kg/day) or metoclopramide (10 mg 4 times daily) can be used; however, no clinical outcome changes have been demonstrated with these therapies.[36,40]

Bolus feeding has the theoretical advantage of replicating the more normal physiology of meals, although no evidence currently exists to guide the decision between continuous and bolus feeding.[36,40] When bolus feeding, formulas with a higher caloric density should be used to reduce the risk of fluid overload.[36,40] Water, one half normal saline or normal saline boluses may be given via the enteral tube when necessary for hydration between feeds, depending on the sodium concentrations of the patient.[36,40]

Caloric Concentration

The concentration of formula can be modified depending on the patient's age and reason for hospitalization.[31] Certain pathologies that may require higher concentration formulas include renal failure, congestive heart failure, liver failure, and the syndrome of inappropriate diuretic hormone release.[31] It is important to note that increasing the caloric concentration does not necessarily correlate with the same change in volume as seen in the example below for a patient who needs 1200 kcal/mL[15,31]:

1.0 kcal/mL formula = 1200 mL/day
} 400 mL change
1.5 kcal/mL formula = 800 mL/day
} 200 mL change
2.0 kcal/mL formula = 600 mL/day

Metabolism in Critical Illness

Understanding metabolism in critical illness is traditionally traced to Cuthbertson's description of "ebb and flow," whereby the immediate, "ebb" phase of low energy expenditure is replaced by the high rate of energy expenditure, or "flow" phase, several days after injury.[5] The initial "ebb" phase occurs approximately 12 hours after trauma or surgical stress.[5] In this phase, decreased oxygen consumption and reduced temperatures lower the body's total energy needs and shunt energy toward immune responses.[4,5,19] Thereafter, the "flow" phase is marked by an increase in baseline energy expenditure that can progress to a chronic "hypermetabolism," a catabolic state that does not respond to adequate nutrient provision if the primary injury is severe enough.[4,5,19] These two phases combine to produce the first inflammatory response to injury, known as "systemic inflammatory response syndrome" or the "acute phase reaction."[19]

One of the primary mechanisms underlying this hypermetabolism is the activation of toll-like receptors on innate immune cells by damage-associated molecular pattern molecules—intracellular contents that the immune cells recognize as antigens from contaminating microorganisms, such as endotoxin.[19] These activated leukocytes produce proinflammatory cytokines that cause the body to shunt amino acids in lean body mass and peripheral fat to the liver to make acute phase proteins such as C-reactive protein instead of transport proteins such as albumin and transferrin.[17–19] These proteins can then play additional roles as antiproteases, opsonins, coagulation factors, and structural components for wound healing.[17–19] While many different types of amino acids are used as acute phase proteins, glutamine becomes the preferred energy source for immune cells since it is used to synthesize the antioxidant glutathione.[17–19]

While the immune system has abundant self-regulatory antiinflammatory responses, if the primary injury is severe enough, these counterregulatory responses can drive an overcompensation into immunosuppression, which has become known as compensatory antiinflammatory response syndrome ("CARS").[46]

While the hyperimmune and immunosuppressive effects are necessary for maintaining the balance between fighting infection and limiting collateral host injury, these effects can lead to chronic immunosuppression.[19,46] As more patients survive their initial injuries, a condition called *persistent inflammation, immunosuppression*, and *catabolism syndrome* has been well described, occurring in 30% to 50% of patients who survive prolonged ICU stays with organ dysfunction.[46] This catabolic state is particularly challenging to manage, as it is refractory to nutrition replacement.[46] This nutrient deficit contributes to global immunosuppression of the host as less fuel is available for protective immune and sympathetic responses.[19,46]

Treatments aimed at reducing the "flow" phase by blocking inflammatory cytokines, such as tumor necrosis factor-α (TNF-α), interleukin-1 (IL-1), and interleukin-6 (IL-6), have not conveyed benefits to ICU patients in prospective clinical trials.[29,47] While other drugs that aim to reduce hyperstimulated stress responses through β-adrenergic receptor blockade have shown positive effects, their efficacies are limited to particular populations, such as the severely burned.[32] Additionally, trials aimed at boosting immune function have been attempted with antioxidants and amino acid supplementation such as glutamine and arginine; but many of these efforts have not improved outcomes and some have actually contributed to harm in the ICU population.[11,12,29,47,48] These challenges have highlighted how changes in metabolism drive complex alterations of the immune system.

Biology of Acute Catabolism: Protein Wasting and Nitrogen Balance

The most obvious change in critical illness is the breakdown of protein within lean body mass.[29,30] Unlike fats and carbohydrates, the body does not have a mechanism for the long-term storage of free amino acids and instead liberates them from structural proteins throughout the skeletal muscle.[3] The degree of protein turnover can be understood in its most raw form as a daily nitrogen balance:

$$\text{Nitrogen balance} = [\text{Nitrogen}]^{(\text{Intake})} - [\text{Nitrogen}]^{(\text{Output})}$$

$$[\text{Nitrogen}]^{(\text{Intake})} = \frac{\text{g Protein}}{(6.25\text{ g Protein})/\text{g Nitrogen}} \quad [\text{Nitrogen}]^{(\text{Output})}$$

$$= \left[\text{UUN}^{*} \times \frac{1000\text{ mL}}{\text{Liter}} \times 24-\text{hour Urine (Liters)}\right.$$

$$\left. \times \frac{\text{g Protein}}{(6.25\text{ g Protein})/\text{g Nitrogen}} + 3\right]$$

After the depletion of liver glycogen stores during starvation, the body switches over to the use of fatty acids as a fuel substrate, generating ketone bodies in the process.[3] As the body transitions from the fed state to the starved state, proteolysis supports gluconeogenesis until critical tissues can primarily use ketone bodies for fuel.[3] Even early in starvation, the body degrades approximately 75 g of muscle protein per day for an average adult.[3,9,14] This catabolism is caused primarily by glucagon, catecholamines, and glucocorticoids and contributes to the loss of muscle mass observed in the critically ill.[3,9,14]

Biology of Acute Catabolism: Mineral and Antioxidant Alterations

Along with changes in macronutrients, inflammatory responses cause alterations in micronutrients (vitamins and minerals) from baseline physiology (Table 5.8).[9,19] The most prominent of these responses is anemia, as IL-1 and TNF cause reduction in blood iron and zinc content.[9,15,30] Since many microorganisms use iron and zinc as growth factors, it is speculated that these acute decreases in serum concentrations are part of protective immune responses against invading microorganisms.[9,15,30] Moreover, these elements are decreased in serum, but they are not excreted from the body; they are stored in the liver and can be used again in cellular metabolism for the host after infection has resolved.[9,15,30] While serum concentrations of both zinc and iron decrease, plasma copper concentrations rise because of the significant increase in ceruloplasmin, an additional acute phase protein.[9,15,30] Deficiencies of water-soluble vitamins may also be identified, as diuresis begins during the resolution of the acute phase of stress.[9,15,30]

Anabolic Resistance

Stress responses that endure beyond the timeframe in which they are adaptive coincide with cachexia that is refractory to feeding and no longer contributes to homeostasis.[19] In this metabolic state, not only is there increased muscle breakdown, but there is also increased resistance to building lean body mass.[19,46] The term "anabolic resistance" is used to describe the failure of normal anabolic stimuli to induce translation of cellular proteins that frequently occurs in critical illness: The amount of protein needed to overcome anabolic resistance in severe illness is estimated to be at least 1.2 to 2.0 g/kg/day depending on age and illness severity.[19,46] Anabolic hormones are decreased in critical stress, and the patients are often bedridden, both of which amplify anabolic resistance.[19,46] However, immobility-induced anabolic resistance may be a reversible phenomenon, as early mobilization and physical therapy have been correlated with earlier ICU and hospital discharges.[19,46]

Nutritional Support of Refeeding Syndrome

Refeeding syndrome is a potentially fatal condition that occurs in patients who have experienced prolonged periods of starvation.[9,13,15] Upon initiation of nutritional support, either enterally or parenterally, patients can experience dramatic shifts of fluids and electrolytes (early) or hypoglycemic episodes (late).[9,13,15] The hallmark feature is hypophosphatemia but often also includes cachexic habitus, thiamine deficiency, hypomagnesemia, and hypokalemia.[9,13,15] As phosphate is shifted to the intracellular compartment for the production of ATP for energy, there are profound decreases in extracellular phosphate concentrations.[9,13,15] This hypophosphatemia can cause cardiac arrhythmias, infarctions, and even arrest.[13,15] Before initiating nutritional support for the severely starved patient, electrolyte abnormalities or deficiencies must be determined and corrected.[9] If refeeding syndrome is anticipated, high-potency B vitamins and daily vitamin supplementation is recommended prior to starting EN.[9] Feedings should commence at 10 kcal/kg/day with slow increases over 4 to 7 days.[15] Rehydration should proceed with replacement of potassium, phosphate, calcium, and magnesium and monitored until restoration of body habitus to a healthy state.[15]

Inflammatory Diseases Without Hypermetabolism

Transplant Patients

The number of transplant operations is increasing as donor systems and hospitals become more equipped to address the increases in chronic, treatment refractory diseases. Developments in surgical techniques and immunosuppressive drugs have led to significant improvements in survival rates.[49] In aggregate, transplant patients have been noted to have elevated REEs for up to 1 year

TABLE 5.8 **Micronutrients.**			
MICRONUTRIENT	**FUNCTION**	**DEFICIENCY**	**RELEVANCE**
Vitamin A	Cofactor in collagen synthesis and cross linking; antioxidant; immune stimulation; macrophage extravasation; mucosal integrity; regulation of glycoprotein synthesis	Dermatitis, night blindness, xerophthalmia, respiratory ailments (pneumonia, bronchopulmonary dysplasia), impaired gut epithelial integrity	Wound healing and epithelial regeneration; deficiency can result in diminished activity of helper T cells, impaired mucous secretion; retinol-binding protein sensitive to nutritional status of individuals
Vitamin D	Promotes absorption of calcium and phosphorus (by intestine and kidney), bone growth, and bone remodeling (by osteoblasts and osteoclasts); regulates synthesis of several structural proteins, including type I collagen	Bone demineralization	Deficiency and impairment causing bone demineralization and osteopenia
Vitamin E	Antioxidant properties promote cell membrane integrity	Increased platelet aggregation, decreased red blood cell survival, hemolytic anemia, neurologic abnormalities, decreased serum creatinine level, excessive creatinuria	Prolonged steatorrhea and neuronal degeneration
Vitamin K	Essential for coagulation; prerequisite for wound healing	Bruising, hemorrhage	Deficiency reported in long-term antibiotic therapy, TPN lacking fat emulsions, malabsorption
Vitamin B_1 (thiamine)	Cofactor in collagen cross linking; facilitates entry of glucose into TCA cycle	Beriberi, lactic acidosis, anorexia, fatigue, peripheral neuropathy, Wernicke-Korsakoff syndrome, cardiomegaly	Deficiency reported in depleted patients who receive sudden load of carbohydrates; wound healing; treated with thiamine 25–100 mg/day
Vitamin B_5 (pantothenic acid)	Component of coenzymes involved in energy release from macronutrients and synthesis of heme and fat	Fatigue, sleep disturbances, nausea, abdominal cramps, vomiting, diarrhea, muscle cramps, mental depression, hypoglycemia	Deficiency leading to poor wound healing and skin graft take
Biotin	Coenzyme in carboxylation reactions (gluconeogenesis, fatty acid, propionate synthesis)	Glossitis, dermatitis, pallor, hair loss	Long-term TPN, alcoholism, postgastrectomy
Vitamin C	Antioxidant, protects against free radical damage; collagen cross linking and hydroxylation of lysine and proline during collagen formation; immune-mediated and antibacterial functions of white blood cells; DNA and RNA replication; lymphocyte function	Fatigue, anorexia, muscular pain, scurvy (anemia, hemorrhagic disorders, defective collagen in bone, cartilage, teeth, connective tissues, muscle degeneration, gingivitis, capillary weakness, impaired wound healing)	Crucial in wound healing; facilitates tissue regeneration and collagen formation in bone, teeth, connective tissue
Calcium	Remodeling and degradation of collagen rely on calcium-dependent collagenases	Osteoporosis	Important in reducing osteopenia and function of collagenases; deficiency leading to hypotension, cardiovascular collapse, unresponsiveness to fluids and pressors, PTH end-organ resistance, arrhythmias
Copper	Promotes cross-linking of collagen and elastin synthesis; scavenges free radicals	Skeletal demineralization, impaired glucose tolerance, anemia, neutropenia, leukopenia, changes in skin and hair pigmentation; linked to fatal arrhythmias and poorer outcomes	Significant wound exudate; losses of copper and zinc known to occur in pediatric burn patients
Iron	Essential in heme-containing molecules for oxygen transport (hemoglobin) and storage (myoglobin), electron transport, and redox reactions (cytochromes)	Anemia, cheilosis, glossitis, hair loss, brittle fingernails, koilonychias, pallor, tissue hypoxia, exertional dyspnea, heart enlargement	Deficiency may occur because of anemia and blood loss; inadequacy leading to reduced resistance to infection and cold intolerance
Magnesium	Cofactor in protein and collagen synthesis	Nausea, muscle weakness, irritability, mental derangement	Deficiency can lead to cardiac arrhythmia, increased nervous system irritability, tetany
Selenium	Reduces intracellular hydroperoxides; protects membrane lipids from oxidative damage; may reduce mortality in critically ill patients	Growth retardation, muscle pain and weakness, myopathy, cardiomyopathy	Important in cell-mediated immune function; deficiency can lead to altered thyroid hormone metabolism, increased plasma glutathione concentrations
Zinc	Essential cofactor in a wide range of enzyme systems involved in protein synthesis, metalloenzymes, DNA replication, immune function, collagen formation, cross-linking	Hair loss, dermatitis, growth retardation, delayed sexual maturation, testicular atrophy, decreased appetite, depressed smell and taste acuity, depression, diarrhea	Deficiency can cause impaired wound healing; may affect bone formation; wound exudate losses

Adapted from Norbury WB, Situ E, Herndon DN. Nutritional support in the critically ill. In: Cameron JL, ed. *Current Surgical Therapy*. 9th ed. Philadelphia: Mosby; 2007:1234–1245.

DNA, Deoxyribonucleic acid; *PTH*, parathyroid hormone; *RNA*, ribonucleic acid; *TCA*, tricarboxylic acid; *TPN*, total parenteral nutrition.

posttransplant, compounding nutritional deficits created by surgical stress and inflammation.[49] Moreover, side effects of immunosuppressive medications include nausea, vomiting, dyspepsia, pancreatitis, and diarrhea, leading to poor food intake.[49] Postoperatively, nutritional support helps to prevent protein-calorie malnutrition–induced immunosuppression, which can arise from the side effects of immunomodulatory medications from the inflammatory response associated with surgical stress or allogenic immune reactions.[49] Thus, current recommendations for caloric and protein intake are currently 30 to 35 kcal/kg and 1.3 to 1.5 g/kg/day, respectively.[49]

Opportunistic infections are an important cause of death for all major organ transplant patients, and nutritional optimization helps to reduce the immunosuppression underlying these infections.[29,49] Because the physiologic consequences of organ transplantation are different for each organ, the specific nutritional guidelines vary based on type of organ system for which a transplant is being considered. For patients undergoing evaluation for kidney transplantation, end-stage renal disease is associated with alterations in protein turnover, as some patients can have accumulation of toxic ammonia-containing compounds and thus need protein restriction.[49] Similarly, hepatic transplantation patients experience a hypermetabolic response similar to severe burns or cancer, as the liver is the source of most circulating proteins and its failure heralds lack of protein processing for important physiologic roles, such as coagulation or glucose usage, which results in higher protein needs.[49]

Overall, transplant patients present with a wide range of preoperative metabolic challenges and postoperative immunosuppression patterns. While the specific regimens for a given type of transplant patient and specific malnutrition issues with immune suppressive drug regimens are beyond the scope of this chapter, the American Society of Transplantation (www.myast.org) and The Transplantation Society (www.tts.org) provide resources for further study.

Nutrition Support in Inflammatory Bowel Disease and Short Bowel Syndrome

Patients with inflammatory bowel disease, which includes Crohn disease and ulcerative colitis, frequently experience abdominal pain, diarrhea, and constipation. Whether due to decreased caloric intake or destruction of absorptive mucosa by the autoimmune disease itself, these patients are prone to protein-calorie malnutrition and micronutrient deficiencies.[45] Common examples include selenium and glutathione deficiencies and osteoporosis due to vitamin D deficiency, particularly in children and the elderly.[45] This form of malnutrition, in combination with the tissue destruction from the disease itself, can lead to reciprocal protein wasting and tissue injury with complications such as GI bleeding, fistulas, and steatorrhea.[45]

The dysbiosis of the microbiota caused by these pathologies is marked by a reduction in bacterial diversity and higher amounts of more virulent *Escherichia coli* strains, *Bacteroides* species, and *Mycobacterium avium* subspecies, which can lead to further malabsorption of nutrients.[45] While current strategies center around restoring a healthy gut microbiome with dietary changes, additional strategies under investigation include prebiotics (foods that are typically high in fiber that are used with the intention of improving the balance of the gut microbiome), probiotics (foods or supplements that contain live microorganisms), antibiotics, and fecal transplantation.[45]

The most successful regimens to improve oral food intake in inflammatory bowel disease patients include high-protein, low-fat, low-carbohydrate diets.[45] Diets high in sucrose, refined carbohydrates, and omega-6 fatty acids and diets low in fruit and vegetables increase the risk of inflammatory bowel disease, especially Crohn disease.[45] It remains unclear if the symptoms are due to increased simple sugars or if people consume simple sugars in a failed attempt to alleviate their symptoms, as restriction of these foods has led to little improvement.[45] Identifying key trigger foods can be done by fasting for 1 week followed by gradual reintroduction of individual foods while assessing improvement or worsening of symptoms with each food.[45] These dietary modifications can lead to significant improvement in symptoms over the long-term.[45] Importantly, diets high in meat and alcohol increase the likelihood of ulcerative colitis relapse.[45] Since many regimens tend to be highly individualized, work on detection of single-nucleotide polymorphism genotyping may provide an avenue for improving symptoms with personalized medical approaches.[45]

Nutritional Support in Patients With Enterocutaneous Fistula

For patients who have developed primary or iatrogenic enterocutaneous fistulas, TPN is preferred because it has been proven to increase the spontaneous closure rate of fistulas without increasing mortality.[15] Moreover, improvements in surgical care and safety of parenteral nutrition have significantly decreased mortality in this population.[15] For patients with irradiated bowel and other types of fistulae that are associated with a low likelihood of closure, aggressive surgical treatment should follow only after preoperative sepsis control, diagnostic studies to identify the path of the fistula, and aggressive TPN support.[15,29] An exception to this rule is if a fistula is located in the distal bowel or has very low output (less than 200 mL/day): then EN can be attempted with vigilant monitoring for increases in fistula output.[29,30] Parenteral nutrition should be administered for as limited time as possible and can also be supplemented with antibiotics, such as ciprofloxacin, metronidazole, or rifaximin, that provide coverage of aerobic and anaerobic gut flora as home therapy.[15,29]

Short Gut/Bowel Syndrome

After resection of the small bowel, the endothelial lining of remaining bowel hypertrophies within 48 hours, providing adequate nutrient absorption despite significant resection.[15,29] However, if resection of the gut occurs and there is a lack of hypertrophy or if sufficient gut is resected (approximately less than 100 cm of gut remaining without the ileocecal valve or 50 to 75 cm with the ileocecal valve), chronic nutrient deficiencies can occur.[15,29] The most common causes of short bowel syndrome in adults is Crohn disease, followed by mesenteric thrombosis and gut volvulus.[15,29,45] In children, the most common cause of short gut/bowel syndrome (SBS) is necrotizing enterocolitis.[45] Treatment recommendations for SBS revolve around aggressive enteral support to stimulate hypertrophy of the villi.[45]

As a last resort, the treatment is home TPN, which has been shown to increase life expectancy between 10 and 20 years and promote survival.[15] Additionally, a combination of growth hormone, glutamine, and diet optimization reduces the amount of TPN needed or eliminates the need altogether in trials of patients with SBS.[45] Growth hormone has shown positive effects on weight gain and energy absorption, but the majority of these trials are short term with patients returning to baseline undernourishment after stopping the treatment.[45] At present, evidence is inconclusive regarding human growth hormone and glutamine for patients with SBS.[45] Fiber supplementation and elemental feeds may help in optimizing nutrient uptake, although the evidence for these practices is poor.[31,45]

Nutrition Support in Acute and Chronic Pancreatitis

Patients with complicated pancreatitis were historically fasted until the episode of inflammation "cooled off."[50] However, a meta-analysis of clinical trials has shown that low-fat diets started within

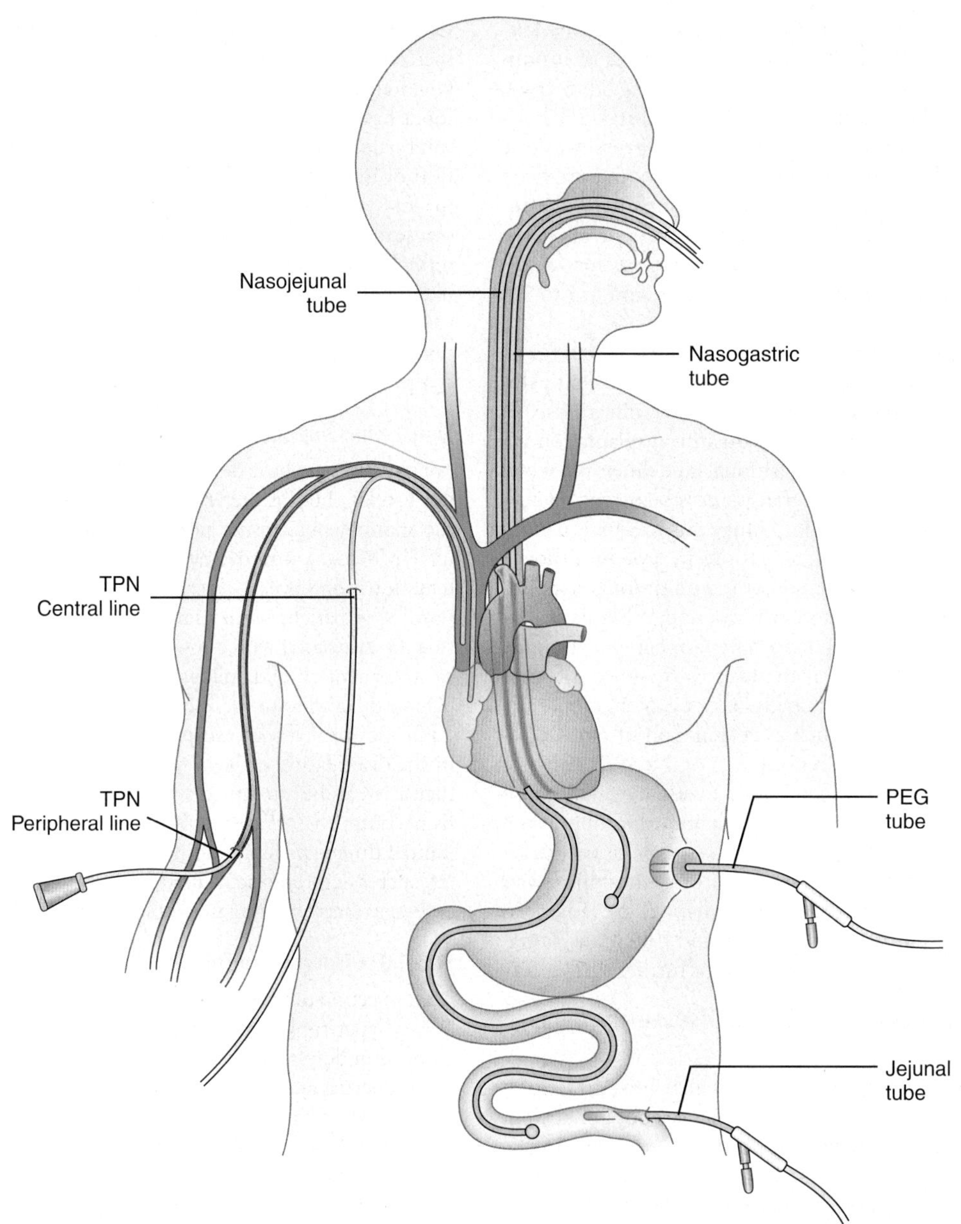

FIG. 5.8 Nasogastric and nasojejunal tube positions. (From Norbury WB, Herndon DN. Modulation of the hypermetabolic response after burn injury. In: Herndon DN, ed. *Total Burn Care.* 3rd ed. Edinburgh: Saunders; 2007:423.) *PEG,* Percutaneous endoscopic gastrostomy; *TPN,* total parenteral nutrition.

48 hours of admission are safe in patients with severe acute or predicted severe acute pancreatitis, reducing rates of multiple organ failure, but not mortality when compared to EN that was delayed beyond 48 hours.[50] Optimal enteral feeding regimens include peptide-based formulas, low long-chain fatty acid, medium-chain fatty acid enriched, and hypertonic solutions given to the jejunum.[50] If enteral feedings are not tolerated, parenteral options include crystalline amino acids and hypertonic glucose–containing solution with just enough lipid to meet essential fatty acid requirements.[50]

The surgical care of patients with chronic pancreatitis can prove exceptionally challenging. The symptoms of exocrine pancreatic failure, such as steatorrhea, are only apparent when approximately 80% to 90% of exocrine tissue is lost.[50] Due to the inability to process fats, these patients respond best to diets that are low in fat, low in carbohydrate, and high in protein (0.8–1.0 g/kg/day).[50] Dietary optimization with reduction in fat intake and pancreatic enzyme supplementation is sufficient treatment in 80% of patients with chronic pancreatitis–induced malnutrition.[50]

However, if alterations in diet fail to restore nutritional status, alternative routes for enteral feeding should be considered (Fig. 5.8, Table 5.9).[50] A trial with a nasojejunal tube feeding with a low-fat formula can be performed, and if this is tolerated, a jejunostomy for home EN can be considered.[50] Jejunal EN may improve nutritional status without worsening abdominal pain and enable definitive surgery to be delayed until nutritional status is improved; in some cases, surgery can be avoided altogether.[50] Additionally, supplementation with calcium, vitamin B, and fat-soluble vitamins is recommended due to the common deficiencies of these micronutrients.[50]

Many pancreatic enzyme supplements have been proposed as a means of restoring exocrine function to the gut; however, no studies have provided reliable enough evidence to recommend their use in acute or chronic pancreatitis patients routinely.[50] Prolonged

TABLE 5.9 **Routes for tube feeding.**

ROUTE	SUITABILITY	INSERTION METHOD, CONFIRMATION	ADVANTAGES	DISADVANTAGES
Nasogastric	Short term—functional GI tract	Blind at bedside; fluoroscopy guided	Easy to insert, replace; can monitor gastric pH and residual volume; capable of bolus feeding	Misplacement complications, sinusitis, epistaxis, nasal necrosis, esophageal strictures, erosive esophagitis
Nasoduodenal, nasojejunal	Short term—functional GI tract but poor gastric emptying, reflux, aspiration risk; begin feed only when volume resuscitated and hemodynamically stable	Blind at bedside; fluoroscopy guided, endoscopy guided	Reduced aspiration risk; some tubes enable decompression of stomach while feeding into jejunum	Easily clogged or displaced, aspiration risk, misplacement complications, displacement and reflux into stomach, sinusitis, epistaxis, nasal necrosis; requires continuous infusion; cannot check gastric residuals except with specialized gastric port
Gastrostomy	Long term—good gastric emptying; avoid if significant reflux or aspiration problem	Surgical, percutaneous, endoscopic, radiologic	Bolus feeding; large-bore tube less likely to block	Procedure risks include bleeding, perforation, aspiration risk, dislodgment with peritoneal contamination, wound site infection, granulation
Jejunostomy	Long term—functional GI tract but poor gastric emptying, reflux, aspiration risk, gastroparesis, gastric dysfunction	Surgical, percutaneous, endoscopic, radiologic	Theoretical reduced aspiration risk	Bleeding, infection, perforation, migration, aspiration, dislodgment and leakage into peritoneal cavity, occlusion, pneumatosis, intestinal ischemia or infarction, bowel obstruction; difficult to replace; cannot check residuals; requires continuous infusion

Adapted from Al-Mousawi A, Branski LK, Andel HL, et al. Ernährungstherapie bei brandverletzten. In: Kamolz LP, Herndon DN, Jeschke MG, eds. *Verbrennungen: Diagnose, therapie und rehabilitation des thermischen traumas* [German]. New York: Springer-Verlag; 2009:183–194.
GI, Gastrointestinal.

preoperative nutritional supplementation to raise albumin to >1.5 g/dL has been linked to decreased rates of mortality and infectious complications after surgery for chronic pancreatitis.[50]

Inflammatory Diseases With Hypermetabolism

Burn Injury and the Metabolic Stress Response

A massive burn is as much a metabolic injury as it is a physical trauma. Following all forms of major trauma, inflammatory and hormonal responses are activated and influence the use of macronutrients.[32] Burned tissue is a uniquely potent stimulant of the systemic immune response.[32] As such, the metabolic response to burn injury is an instructive example of the metabolic response to stress and trauma.[32] The study of the body's recovery after thermal injury has brought great insights to the broader field of surgical nutrition.[5]

Burn injury represents the ultimate example of stress-induced changes in metabolism. The stress response incited by thermal injury leads to activation of an array of physiologic processes that respond to altered nutritional requirements and attempt to restore homeostasis.[23] Nutrient intake, absorption, and substrate usage are all altered by the systemic response. While they may offer transient physiologic benefits in the evolutionary context of the immediate fight-or-flight response to injury, in the context of prolonged critical illness, these changes are often exaggerated and prolonged.[32] The metabolic dysregulation associated with massive thermal injury directly contributes to clinical complications, delayed recovery, and increased mortality.[4]

The inflammatory and hormonal mechanisms underlying this response are complex but are known to include a prolonged rise in circulating catecholamine, glucocorticoid, and glucagon concentrations, leading to elevated rates of gluconeogenesis, glycogenolysis, and protein catabolism.[23,32] Other features of altered macronutrient usage include insulin resistance and increased peripheral lipolysis.[4] While nutrient requirements will become more difficult to predict, additional enteral or parenteral feeding will often be necessary to augment profound deficits.[32] Even in the context of aggressive delivery of nutrition, significant lean-body-mass loss over the course of acute burn treatment is inevitable with the current standard of care.[32] Outside of the acute phase of burn injury, elements of catabolic pathology persist in pediatric survivors of massive thermal injury.[4] Negative nitrogen balance, insulin resistance, lipolysis, and protein wasting may persist for as long as 2 years following severe injuries, leading to a significant delay in rehabilitation.[4] Identifying a therapy or (more likely) a constellation of interventions capable of arresting or even reversing this protein catabolism remains an active pursuit in burn research.[4]

A review of advances in burn center nutrition literature reveals a microcosm of the developing discipline of surgical nutrition. In the pre-early–excision era, studies of burn patients yielded the first concrete data demonstrating a catecholamine surge and increased REEs in response to trauma.[4] After documenting the concept of a proportionate metabolic response to traumatic injury, the burn nutrition literature was crucial in recognizing the variability of this response between patients.[4] Burn surgery led the way in the movement away from empiric calorie prescriptions by showing that even in the context of a population with homogenous injuries (when controlling for burn size), none of the equations commonly utilized to predict caloric needs were capable of predicting a patient's REE.[4] The burn literature clearly established the value and safety of early initiation of enteral feeds in critically ill burn patients.[32] Other tenants of modern surgical nutrition with roots in burn research include the concept of enteric bacterial translocation and the value of trophic feeding, the safety of uninterrupted perioperative postpyloric feeding, and the inflammatory side effects of high-fat nutrition therapy.[4]

Perhaps most importantly, burn nutrition research was critical in one of the fundamental paradigm shifts in surgical nutrition: in both animal models and human studies of thermal injury, the refractory protein-calorie deficits seen with this injury were shown to be directly tied to fundamental links between systemic inflammation and catabolic pathways.[4,46] Furthermore, through rigorous analysis of the impact of various nutritional regimens on body mass and composition in burn patients, Hart and colleagues established that after a certain threshold, increasing calorie delivery to severely burned patients ultimately resulted in fat accretion rather than restoration of muscle mass.[23] Together, these insights laid the groundwork for a fundamental shift in contemporary surgical nutrition—the concept that malnutrition is not simply a state of starvation, but rather a global state of metabolic dysfunction.[4]

Burn surgery has also served as a foundation for efforts to integrate therapies that improve energy wasting into treatment of the acutely stressed surgical patient. Thermal injury patients have been the testing ground for a wide range of interventions designed to mitigate the catabolic response to trauma.[4] In terms of pharmaceutical interventions, recombinant human growth hormone in children, oxandrolone, insulin, insulin-like growth factor (IGF-1), and beta-adrenergic receptor (β-AR) blockers such as propranolol have all been used to mitigate the overwhelming catabolic response to thermal injury—with propranolol and oxandrolone showing the most significant impact.[4] Propranolol is a nonselective β-AR antagonist that has been shown to reduce thermogenesis, tachycardia, and REE in burn patients.[4] It also appears to reduce the prolipolytic effect of excessive circulating catecholamines and substantially decreases fatty infiltration of the liver.[4] These findings have prompted investigators in other areas to begin exploring beta blockade as a strategy for countering the metabolic consequences of a wide range of injuries, including brain injury, mechanical trauma, and sepsis.

Along with cardiac surgery, burn surgery has been among the first areas to demonstrate the decidedly anabolic effect of structured exercise programs in patients recovering from traumatic injury.[4] Modulation of the stress response also includes pain and anxiety control through the administration of analgesics and anxiolytics as well as psychological therapy.[4]

Of all the interventions used to mitigate the stress-associated response to thermal injury, early excision of burn eschar is by far the most effective in terms of reducing total energy demand.[4] While burn excision is obviously uniquely relevant to thermally injured patients, there is a much broader lesson here that applies to nearly all surgical patients. The salutary impact of early excision on the recovery of burn patients demonstrates the importance of "source control" in managing the inflammatory response to trauma.[4] We have long appreciated the value of early surgical intervention as a means to preempting the vicious sequelae of cancers and infections.[4] Over the past 25 years, a generation of burn surgeons has taught us that this same principle of early, aggressive control of the inflammatory nidus in the acutely injured patient is ultimately our most effective tool to address the physiologic derangements associated with traumatic disease.[4]

Nutritional support of severe burn injury. Burn studies were among the first to show the molecular mechanisms behind improved immune responses with dietary modifications.[4] In one animal model of severe burn injury, altering nutrition demonstrated reductions in cytokine releases.[4] Moreover, REE decreased when early enteral feeding was administered in humans as compared to delayed enteral feedings.[32] However, the additions of immunonutrients (such as glutamine and the omega-3 fatty acids) have not been shown to provide benefits in this population.[32] Established recommendations for the care of severely burned patients include starting feeding as soon as possible; giving high-protein, high-carbohydrate, low-fat feeds to offset hypermetabolism; feeding the gut whenever possible; and supplementing micronutrients even if not identified as deficient.[32] While early nutrition is clearly important, the data are insufficient at this time to recommend specific feeding formulas or nutritional supplements.[32]

Nutrition Support in Sepsis

The treatment of septic patients begins with prevention. Many tools in the armamentarium of the critical care physician, such as blood transfusions and invasive venous, arterial, or urinary catheters, are associated with increased infections.[29] Preventing infections therefore involves minimizing these interventions as well as optimizing infection prevention. These measures can be supplemented with early mobilization and deep vein thrombosis prophylaxis to prevent thrombosis and other aggravating factors of critical illness that can contribute to immune suppression and secondary sepsis.[29,30]

In contrast to the clear benefits of preventative measures, nutritional support of a patient who has developed sepsis is still somewhat controversial. While some advocate the administration of immediate and aggressive nutritional support, trophic EN is more commonly recommended.[36,37,40] EN is believed to provide benefits in septic patients by maintaining the epithelial lining of the gut, thus preventing translocation of bacteria and further microbial burden.[45] The recommended amount of protein for septic patients during acute resuscitation is approximately 1.0 g/kg/day, and the recommended amount of nonprotein calories is approximately 15 kcal/kg/day.[36,37,40] Additionally, immunonutrition with glutamine or arginine is not recommended since each has been shown to have unwanted effects in ICU patients, especially those with preexisting infections.[29,47] The overall dogma of nutritional support in septic patients remains close monitoring of the patient's tolerance or intolerance to feeds during the acute phase of critical illness with prolonged protein calorie support (>1.5 g/kg/day) during the convalescent phase of care.[36,37,40]

During severe sepsis, oxygen consumption may rise 50% to 60% above baseline.[29] If a septic patient develops compromised pulmonary function from edema, pneumonia, or weakness of respiratory muscles, the patient may not be able to meet the body's oxygen needs, a condition that can be further exacerbated by certain diets.[29,30] The ratio of carbon dioxide produced to oxygen consumed (VCO_2/VO_2) during the metabolism of fuel substrates is known as the respiratory quotient (RQ).[29,30] Because different processes are involved in the use of fats and carbohydrates, their RQs differ: pure carbohydrate consumption results in an RQ of 1.0, whereas the consumption of lipid results in an RQ of 0.7.[29,30] Normally, pulmonary reserve is substantial enough to provide adequate elimination of CO_2, regardless of dietary composition; however, in critically ill patients, overfeeding with carbohydrate can compound this problem, making it harder for patients to wean from ventilator support.[31] However, lowering carbohydrate intake must be considered in light of studies that point to the potential for lung injury with diets higher in fat, particularly omega-6 fatty acids.[11,12] Tailoring the correct ratio of macronutrients and supplementing with micronutrients when in deficiency may help optimize survival and facilitate return to activities of daily living after an acute ICU stay and healing of chronic wounds, but further study in this population is needed.[9]

Nutrition Support AIDS and Cancer: Disorders of Severe Cachexia

An attempt to discover the mechanism behind protein wasting refractory to nutrition supplementation led to the identification of TNF-α, or "cachexin."[15,46] Later, this cytokine was found to contribute to cachexic effects in the acute inflammation of sepsis and in a variety of other pathologies.[15,46] The cachexia of cancer is almost identical to that of acquired immunodeficiency syndrome (AIDS), as the mechanism of chronic inflammation and cytokine profiles are similar (high in proinflammatory cytokines TNF-a, IL-1, and IL-6).[15,46] These cytokines can be released by the host immune system or directly from the tumor.[46] Whether because of a virus or chemotherapy, both of these patient populations can become profoundly immunosuppressed in conjunction with severe cachexia.[46]

Patients with AIDS and patients suffering from cancer face opportunistic infections that affect the aerodigestive tract, candida overgrowth, or viral ulcers.[46] Moreover, the side effects of highly active antiretroviral therapy or chemotherapy most often have digestive side effects that reduce a patient's ability to stay nourished.[46] Whether due to primary cancer or ulcerative lesions, many patients have nutrient deficiencies secondary to defects of the oral cavity, esophagus or neuromuscular mechanisms of the swallowing mechanism.[46] General strategies for optimizing nutrient support in these challenging pathologies include the provision of nutrition by enteral or parenteral routes when symptoms of disease or side effects of medications preclude sufficient nutrient intake.[31,46] If the reason for caloric restriction is partial obstruction of the oropharynx or esophagus, high nutrient liquid or puree drinks can be prepared as an alternative to enteral feeding if the obstruction is only partial.[31]

TPN plays an important role in the treatment of malnutrition after abdominal or pelvic radiation and secondary epithelial inflammation that prevents nutrient absorption until enteritis resolves, when enteral feeding can resume.[9,37] Often, dysgeusia can arise from underlying mineral deficiencies, such as iron, zinc, and B vitamins; correcting these underlying deficiencies can help restore normal nutritional intake.[9] Finally, medications that help reduce nausea or improve gut motility can help address the associated nausea, constipation, or diarrhea that exacerbates lack of appetite.[9] Other novel strategies have been trialed to decrease the underlying immune response causing cachexia, such as giving nonsteroidal antiinflammatory medications, anticytokine medications, amino acids, and omega-3 fatty acid supplements.[19,29,46] Finally, coinciding depression or pain contributes to appetite suppression as well as inflammation from the stress response.[15]

Significant controversies exist about how best to use nutritional support to improve outcomes in cancer and immunocompromised patients.[15,19,29] Low-protein diets are associated with lower cancer rates by inhibiting tumor growth via engaging the molecular target of rapamycin pathway and IGF-1 as well as fibroblastic growth factor-21. In patients, omega-3 fish oil supplements, high-dose vitamin D, increasing dietary fiber, and coffee have all been found to lower risk of recurrence of colorectal cancer, lengthen survival, and decrease mortality. Omega-3 fatty acid supplements improve cancer cachexia in bile duct and pancreatic cancer.[11,12]

Nutrition Support in Hepatic Insufficiency

Up to 90% hepatocyte destruction is required for clinical features of cirrhosis, such as ascites, caput medusa, or jaundice, to appear. Laboratory values of patients with hepatic insufficiency will reveal elevation of alanine aminotransferase, aspartate aminotransferase, decreased albumin, and prolonged prothrombin time, as the liver produces all of the coagulation factors with the exception of von Willebrand factor (vWF)/factor VIII, which is produced by the endothelium.[49] Therefore, the most consistent markers of decreased intrinsic liver function are prolonged prothrombin time and hypoalbuminemia.[49] While partial thromboplastin is almost always normal in hepatic insufficiency, bleeding time can either be prolonged or normal.[49]

With the loss of the glycemic control typically provided by the liver through glycogenesis, glycogenolysis, and gluconeogenesis, glycogen stores within the muscle are rapidly depleted and insulin resistance develops.[49] Proteins and lipids become sources of energy, causing decreases in peripheral reserves.[49] A catabolic condition closely resembling burn hypermetabolism or sepsis develops during hepatic insufficiency; increased concentrations of TNF-α, IL-1, and IL-6 have been demonstrated and are implicated as a potential causal mechanism behind the associated protein-calorie malnutrition.[49] Diets high in BCAAs have been suggested as ways to reduce protein wasting, but these approaches are not well established.[49] Patients with hepatic insufficiency often have related nutrient deficiencies that may require supplementation, such as low serum concentrations of potassium, magnesium, and zinc.[49]

The treatment of patients with hepatic insufficiency centers around meeting the caloric intake required to maintain lean body mass while maintaining low fluid intake.[49] However, the optimization of specific regimens, timing, and routes of supplementation are not well studied in this population.[49] Methods to improve oral intake include techniques aimed at improving meal sensory perception, encouraging uninterrupted meals, increasing meal frequency, decreasing meal sizes, fortifying meals with high-protein or high-calorie products, and increasing support from healthcare staff.[49] Because encephalopathy is likely a result of the accumulation of ammonia, protein restriction to <40 g/day is indicated before more invasive measures such as hepatorenal shunts are attempted.[49] If ascites is present, treatment involves sodium restriction and diuresis or paracentesis if necessary.[49]

Nutrient Deficiencies in Bariatric Patients

Much work has been done to understand the pathways that drive appetite and how to treat those who experience it in excess. Whenever fewer calories are consumed as part of a planned diet or undesired starvation, the main orexigenic hormone, ghrelin, is released. Part of the success of bariatric surgery in reducing appetite is theorized to come from removing the parts of the stomach that secrete the majority of ghrelin, thus decreasing appetite signals.[16,25,26]

Operative procedures aimed at inducing weight loss fall into two broad categories: restrictive and malabsorptive. Restrictive procedures reduce the gastric volume, thus triggering neurohumoral responses of satiety with smaller food portions. Restrictive procedures include banding procedures, vertical banded gastroplasty, and sleeve gastrectomy. Unlike restrictive procedures, malabsorptive procedures reroute the track of normal absorption, often removing a significant length of the gut, to induce weight loss by decreased nutrient absorption. Malabsorptive procedures include jejunoileal bypass (JIB), biliary-pancreatic diversion (BPD), BPD with duodenal switch (BPD-DS), and Roux-en-Y gastric bypass (RYGB). Of these, JIB functions solely via a malabsorptive mechanism, while BPD/BPD-DS and RYGB involve the resection of sections of the stomach to provide both a restrictive and malabsorptive mechanism to maximize weight loss. Each of these procedures is associated with predictable postoperative complications that include specific nutrient deficiencies.

Despite a clear understanding of the risks of deficiencies associated with each operation, the rate of nutrient deficiencies in bariatric patients remains high.[26] Of the macronutrients, patients are at greatest risk of developing a protein deficiency, as they are unable to meet their daily requirement due to diminished overall food intake.[26] Dietary deficiencies in the postoperative bariatric patient are speculated to be due to poor adherence with prescribed dietary supplementation or undiagnosed preoperative deficiencies.[26] For example, iron deficiency was found in 44% of adults prior to bariatric surgery, making it one of the most common deficiencies in bariatric patients.[25] Additionally, most studies of bariatric procedures only follow patients for 1 to 2 years postoperatively, so the long-term metabolic consequences remain unknown.

Adjustable gastric band. The most common nutrient deficiency after the adjustable gastric band procedure is iron deficiency, and clinicians should maintain a low threshold to perform a workup for iron deficiency anemia.[26] Of all bariatric procedures, the lap band has the lowest rate of nutrient deficiencies, but the highest rate of reoperation and failure for weight loss.[26]

Sleeve gastrectomy. The fundus of the stomach is the primary source of intrinsic factor, a cofactor of vitamin B_{12} necessary for its absorption in the ileum.[25] When the greater curvature is stapled/resected in a sleeve gastrectomy, there are decreased amounts of intrinsic factor and less absorption of vitamin B_{12} in the ileum.[25] Thus, vitamin B_{12} deficiency is the most common nutrient deficiency associated with sleeve gastrectomy.[25] This vitamin deficiency becomes clinically apparent as pallor, fatigue, and megaloblastic anemia on blood smear.[25]

RYGB surgery. Open RYGB surgery, laparoscopic RYGB, and laparoscopic sleeve gastrectomy all have been shown to provide significant weight loss and all were superior to adjustable gastric banding.[26] RYGB is able to provide sustained weight loss not seen in restrictive procedures while simultaneously avoiding severe complications associated with other malabsorptive procedures.[16] After RYGB, patients have increased glucagon like peptide-1 (also known as "incretin"), which has been shown to contribute to decreases in appetite.[16] There are also sustained improvements in obstructive sleep apnea, diabetes, hypertension, and other features of metabolic syndrome.[16]

The most common nutrient deficiency associated with RYGB is iron deficiency anemia.[25] If portions of the stomach are bypassed or resected, patients are at risk of incomplete protein digestion and protein bound nutrients, such as iron, intrinsic factor, and vitamin B_{12}.[25] If the proximal small bowel is bypassed, as is the case for JIB, BPD and BPD-DS, and RYGB, then patients are at increased risk of deficiencies in nutrients primarily absorbed early, principally iron, vitamin D, copper, and calcium.[25] The risk of nutrient deficiencies is proportional to the amount of small bowel bypassed, which is greatest in JIB and BPD.[25]

BPD and BPD-DS. BPD and BPD-DS are only undertaken after extremely careful patient selection because they are associated with the highest rates of nutritional deficiencies.[25] The most common nutrient deficiency in BPD and BPD-DS is protein malnutrition, represented by hypoalbuminemia, with an incidence that ranges from 3% to 11%.[25] Iron deficiency anemia is also common, with an incidence of approximately 5% of cases, although the incidence could be as high as 12% to 47%.[25] In long-term follow-up of these patients, deficiencies of other vitamins and minerals have been identified, particularly calcium and zinc.[25] Moreover, this procedure reduces absorption of fat by 70% and is associated with high rates of fat-soluble vitamin deficiencies.[25]

General recommendations for nutritional optimization in bariatric patients. Bariatric patients can present with altered nutrient concentrations and nutrient usage that range from mild to life threatening.[25] Moreover, postoperative complications can cause considerable challenges in helping these patients recover from severe surgical challenges or nutrient derangements. In general, nutritional counseling should be started months prior to bariatric or other reconstructive surgery.[25] Most providers trial a time of preoperative weight loss to see if the patient can be compliant with simulated postoperative dietary restrictions.[26] Even a weight loss of 10% for severely obese patients will provide significant improvements in visualization during the surgery by minimizing the size of liver, omentum, and peritoneal fat.[25] Moreover, it will decrease rates of postoperative complications involving the cardiopulmonary and vascular systems.[16] These patients also require close follow-up in outpatient clinic settings. Multivitamins should be taken daily by all patients after any bariatric procedure, with additional supplementation of iron and vitamin B_{12} to prevent anemia after restrictive-malabsorptive procedures.[25] Recommended screening procedures as well as specific recommendations for which supplements should be provided due to higher risks of nutrient deficiencies based on the bariatric surgical procedure are detailed by the American Society for Metabolic and Bariatric Surgery.[25]

CONCLUSION

The surgeon has experience with the causes and consequences of disordered metabolism in the most extreme cases seen by medical specialists. Accordingly, the well-informed surgeon is well versed in the interconnectedness of metabolic pathways and the means of modulating these for the benefit of their patients. As the field of bioenergetics continues to expand, we are likely to discover better therapies that can optimize the body's metabolic responses to illness and injury, both within and outside the operating theater. Nutritional pathologies have never been more challenging, and thoughtful and hard-working surgeon-scientists will continue to contribute to breakthroughs that address them.

SELECTED REFERENCES

Alberts B, Johnson A, Lewis J, et al. *Molecular Biology of the Cell.* 6th ed. New York: W. W. Norton & Company; 2015.

An additional core reference text for the molecular biologic processes governing cellular biology.

Berg JM, Tymoczko JL, Gatto Jr GJ, et al. *Biochemistry.* 7th ed. New York: WH Freeman; 2015.

A core reference text for the biochemical sections—extensive detail regarding the interrelatedness of metabolic processes.

Cuthbertson DP. Post-shock metabolic response. *Lancet.* 1942;239:433–437.

A classic work highlighting the role of trauma in stimulating changes in metabolism.

Herndon DN. *Total Burn Care.* 5th ed. Philadelphia: Elsevier; 2018.

A comprehensive text, written by a diverse multidisciplinary team, aimed at covering all issues relevant to modern surgical care of the severely burned.

McClave SA, Taylor BE, Martindale RG, et al. Guidelines for the provision and assessment of nutrition support therapy in the adult critically ill patient: Society of Critical Care Medicine (SCCM) and American Society for Parenteral and Enteral Nutrition (A.S.P.E.N.). *JPEN J Parenter Enteral Nutr.* 2016;40:159–211.

The most recent comprehensive guidelines for nutritional support for the critically ill endorsed by the most prominent professional societies in medical nutrition.

REFERENCES

1. Kleiber M, Rogers TA. Energy metabolism. *Annu Rev Physiol.* 1961;23:5–36.
2. Alberts B, Johnson A, Lewis J, et al. *Molecular Biology of the Cell.* 6th ed. New York: W. W. Norton & Company; 2015.
3. Berg JM, Tymoczko JL, Gatto Jr GJ, et al. *Biochemistry.* 7th ed. New York: WH Freeman; 2015.
4. Herndon DN. *Total Burn Care.* 5th ed. Philadelphia: Elsevier; 2018.
5. Cuthbertson DP. The disturbance of metabolism produced by bony and non-bony injury, with notes on certain abnormal conditions of bone. *Biochem J.* 1930;24:1244–1263.
6. Sazanov LA. A giant molecular proton pump: structure and mechanism of respiratory complex I. *Nat Rev Mol Cell Biol.* 2015;16:375–388.
7. Porter C, Herndon DN, Borsheim E, et al. Uncoupled skeletal muscle mitochondria contribute to hypermetabolism in severely burned adults. *Am J Physiol Endocrinol Metab.* 2014;307:E462–E467.
8. Lidell ME, Enerback S. Brown adipose tissue—a new role in humans? *Nat Rev Endocrinol.* 2010;6:319–325.
9. McClave SA, Taylor BE, Martindale RG, et al. Guidelines for the provision and assessment of nutrition support therapy in the adult critically Ill patient: Society of Critical Care Medicine (SCCM) and American Society for Parenteral and Enteral Nutrition (A.S.P.E.N.). *JPEN J Parenter Enteral Nutr.* 2016;40:159–211.
10. Blair NF, Cremer PD, Tchan MC. Urea cycle disorders: a life-threatening yet treatable cause of metabolic encephalopathy in adults. *Pract Neurol.* 2015;15:45–48.
11. Kristine Koekkoek W, Panteleon V, van Zanten AR. Current evidence on omega-3 fatty acids in enteral nutrition in the critically ill: a systematic review and meta-analysis. *Nutrition.* 2019;59:56–68.
12. Kreymann KG, Heyland DK, de Heer G, et al. Intravenous fish oil in critically ill and surgical patients—historical remarks and critical appraisal. *Clin Nutr.* 2018;37:1075–1081.
13. Cederholm T, Jensen GL, Correia M, et al. GLIM criteria for the diagnosis of malnutrition—a consensus report from the global clinical nutrition community. *Clin Nutr.* 2019;38:1–9.
14. Long CL, Schaffel N, Geiger JW, et al. Metabolic response to injury and illness: estimation of energy and protein needs from indirect calorimetry and nitrogen balance. *JPEN J Parenter Enteral Nutr.* 1979;3:452–456.
15. Norbury WB, Situ E, Herndon DN. Nutritional support in the critically ill. In: Cameron JL, ed. *Current Surgical Therapy.* 9th ed. Philadelphia: Mosby; 2007:1234–1245.
16. Mauldin K, O'Leary-Kelley C. New guidelines for assessment of malnutrition in adults: obese critically ill patients. *Crit Care Nurse.* 2015;35:24–30.
17. Lee JL, Oh ES, Lee RW, et al. Serum albumin and prealbumin in calorically restricted, nondiseased individuals: a systematic review. *Am J Med.* 2015;128:1023. e1021–e1022.
18. Davis CJ, Sowa D, Keim KS, et al. The use of prealbumin and C-reactive protein for monitoring nutrition support in adult patients receiving enteral nutrition in an urban medical center. *JPEN J Parenter Enteral Nutr.* 2012;36:197–204.
19. Gentile LF, Cuenca AG, Efron PA, et al. Persistent inflammation and immunosuppression: a common syndrome and new horizon for surgical intensive care. *J Trauma Acute Care Surg.* 2012;72:1491–1501.
20. Gibbs J, Cull W, Henderson W, et al. Preoperative serum albumin level as a predictor of operative mortality and morbidity: results from the National VA Surgical Risk Study. *Arch Surg.* 1999;134:36–42.
21. Caraceni P, Tufoni M, Bonavita ME. Clinical use of albumin. *Blood Transfus.* 2012;11(suppl 4):s18–s25.
22. Reeves MM, Capra S. Predicting energy requirements in the clinical setting: are current methods evidence based? *Nutr Rev.* 2003;61:143–151.
23. Hart DW, Wolf SE, Herndon DN, et al. Energy expenditure and caloric balance after burn: increased feeding leads to fat rather than lean mass accretion. *Ann Surg.* 2002;235:152–161.
24. Center for Health Statistics. National Health and Nutrition Examination Survey: analytic guidelines, 2011–2014 and 2015–2016. https://wwwn.cdc.gov/nchs/data/nhanes/2011-2012/analyticguidelines/analytic_guidelines_11_16.pdf. Accessed April 22, 2019.
25. Parrott J, Frank L, Rabena R, et al. American Society for Metabolic and Bariatric Surgery integrated health nutritional guidelines for the surgical weight loss patient 2016 update: micronutrients. *Surg Obes Relat Dis.* 2017;13:727–741.
26. Xanthakos SA. Nutritional deficiencies in obesity and after bariatric surgery. *Pediatr Clin North Am.* 2009;56:1105–1121.
27. Norbury W, Herndon DN, Tanksley J, et al. Infection in burns. *Surg Infect (Larchmt).* 2016;17:250–255.
28. Gasic S, Schneider B, Waldhausl W. Indirect calorimetry: variability of consecutive baseline determinations of carbohydrate and fat utilization from gas exchange measurements. *Horm Metab Res.* 1997;29:12–15.
29. Wischmeyer PE. Nutrition therapy in sepsis. *Crit Care Clin.* 2018;34:107–125.
30. Ingels C, Vanhorebeek I, Van den Berghe G. Glucose homeostasis, nutrition and infections during critical illness. *Clin Microbiol Infect.* 2018;24:10–15.
31. Brown B, Roehl K, Betz M. Enteral nutrition formula selection: current evidence and implications for practice. *Nutr Clin Pract.* 2015;30:72–85.
32. Rousseau AF, Losser MR, Ichai C, et al. ESPEN endorsed recommendations: nutritional therapy in major burns. *Clin Nutr.* 2013;32:497–502.
33. Simpson F, Doig GS. Parenteral vs. enteral nutrition in the critically ill patient: a meta-analysis of trials using the intention to treat principle. *Intensive Care Med.* 2005;31:12–23.
34. Peter JV, Moran JL, Phillips-Hughes J. A metaanalysis of treatment outcomes of early enteral versus early parenteral nutrition in hospitalized patients. *Crit Care Med.* 2005;33:213–220; discussion 260–211.
35. Reignier J, Boisrame-Helms J, Brisard L, et al. Enteral versus parenteral early nutrition in ventilated adults with shock: a randomised, controlled, multicentre, open-label, parallel-group study (NUTRIREA-2). *Lancet.* 2018;391:133–143.
36. Lewis SR, Schofield-Robinson OJ, Alderson P, et al. Enteral versus parenteral nutrition and enteral versus a combination

of enteral and parenteral nutrition for adults in the intensive care unit. *Cochrane Database Syst Rev*. 2018;6:CD012276.

37. Elke G, van Zanten AR, Lemieux M, et al. Enteral versus parenteral nutrition in critically ill patients: an updated systematic review and meta-analysis of randomized controlled trials. *Crit Care*. 2016;20:117.
38. Harvey SE, Parrott F, Harrison DA, et al. Trial of the route of early nutritional support in critically ill adults. *N Engl J Med*. 2014;371:1673–1684.
39. Montejo JC, Minambres E, Bordeje L, et al. Gastric residual volume during enteral nutrition in ICU patients: the regane study. *Intensive Care Med*. 2010;36:1386–1393.
40. Casaer MP, Mesotten D, Hermans G, et al. Early versus late parenteral nutrition in critically ill adults. *N Engl J Med*. 2011;365:506–517.
41. Nygren J, Thacker J, Carli F, et al. Guidelines for perioperative care in elective rectal/pelvic surgery: Enhanced Recovery After Surgery (ERAS((R))) society recommendations. *World J Surg*. 2013;37:285–305.
42. Practice guidelines for preoperative fasting and the use of pharmacologic agents to reduce the risk of pulmonary aspiration: application to healthy patients undergoing elective procedures: an updated report by the American Society of Anesthesiologists Committee on Standards and Practice Parameters. *Anesthesiology*. 2011;114:495511.
43. D'Amico DF, Parimbelli P, Ruffolo C. Antibiotic prophylaxis in clean surgery: breast surgery and hernia repair. *J Chemother*. 2001;13(spec no 1):108–111.
44. Heyland D, Muscedere J, Wischmeyer PE, et al. A randomized trial of glutamine and antioxidants in critically ill patients. *N Engl J Med*. 2013;368:1489–1497.
45. Neuman MG, Nanau RM. Inflammatory bowel disease: role of diet, microbiota, life style. *Transl Res*. 2012;160:29–44.
46. Ward NS, Casserly B, Ayala A. The compensatory anti-inflammatory response syndrome (CARS) in critically ill patients. *Clin Chest Med*. 2008;29:617–625, viii.
47. van Zanten AR, Dhaliwal R, Garrel D, et al. Enteral glutamine supplementation in critically ill patients: a systematic review and meta-analysis. *Crit Care*. 2015;19:294.
48. Drover JW, Dhaliwal R, Weitzel L, et al. Perioperative use of arginine-supplemented diets: a systematic review of the evidence. *J Am Coll Surg*. 2011;212:385–399, 399 e381.
49. Hammad A, Kaido T, Aliyev V, et al. Nutritional therapy in liver transplantation. *Nutrients*. 2017;9:e1126.
50. Song J, Zhong Y, Lu X, et al. Enteral nutrition provided within 48 hours after admission in severe acute pancreatitis: a systematic review and meta-analysis. *Medicine (Baltimore)*. 2018;97:e11871.

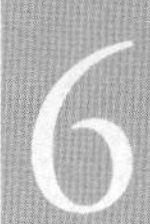

CHAPTER 6

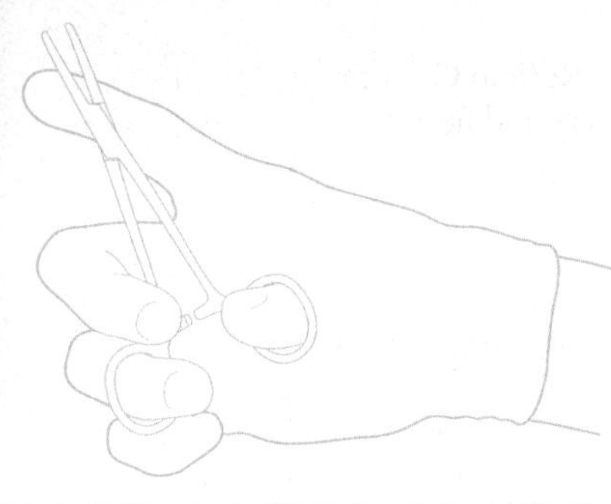

Wound Healing

Stefanos Boukovalas, Kristen A. Aliano, Linda G. Phillips, William B. Norbury

OUTLINE

Although the treatment and healing of wounds are some of the oldest subjects discussed in the medical literature, and although there have been numerous advances in understanding the steps involved in wound healing, the exact mechanisms underlying wound healing remain unclear.

TISSUE INJURY AND RESPONSE

Attempts to restore mechanical integrity, to repair barriers to fluid loss and infection, and to reestablish normal blood and lymphatic flow patterns are termed *wound repair*. During wound repair, flawless reconstruction is sacrificed in order to speed up the return to function. In contrast, regeneration, which is the goal of wound healing, is the perfect restoration of the preexisting tissue architecture without scar formation; regeneration is achievable only during embryonic development, in lower organisms, or in certain tissues such as bone and liver.

All wounds undergo the same basic steps of repair. Acute wounds proceed in an orderly and timely reparative process to achieve sustained restoration of structure and function. A chronic wound stalls during a sustained inflammatory phase and fails to heal.

WOUND-HEALING PHASES

The three phases of wound healing are inflammation, proliferation, and maturation. In a large wound such as a pressure sore, the eschar or fibrinous exudate reflects the inflammatory phase, the granulation tissue is part of the proliferative phase, and the contracting or advancing edge is part of the maturational phase. All three phases may occur simultaneously, and the phases may overlap with their individual processes (Fig. 6.1).

Inflammatory Phase

During the immediate reaction of the tissue to injury, hemostasis occurs quickly and is rapidly followed by inflammation. This phase represents an attempt to limit damage by stopping bleeding; sealing the wound surface; and removing necrotic tissue, foreign debris, and bacteria. The inflammatory phase is characterized by increased vascular permeability, migration of cells into the wound by chemotaxis, secretion of cytokines and growth factors into the wound, and activation of the migrating cells.

Hemostasis and Inflammation

Blood vessel injury results in intense local arteriolar and capillary vasoconstriction followed by vasodilatation and increased vascular permeability (Fig. 6.2). Erythrocytes and platelets adhere to the damaged capillary endothelium, resulting in plugging of capillaries and leading to cessation of hemorrhage. Platelet adhesion to the endothelium is primarily mediated through the interaction between high-affinity glycoprotein receptors and the integrin receptor GPIIb-IIIa ($\alpha_{IIb}\beta_3$). Platelets also express other integrin receptors that mediate direct binding to collagen ($\alpha_2\beta_1$) and laminin ($\alpha_6\beta_1$) or indirect binding to subendothelial matrix-bound fibronectin ($\alpha_5\beta_1$), vitronectin ($\alpha_v\beta_3$), and other ligands. Platelet activation occurs by binding to exposed type IV and type V collagen from the damaged endothelium, resulting in platelet aggregation. The initial contact between platelets and collagen requires von Willebrand factor VIII, a heterodimeric protein synthesized by megakaryocytes and endothelial cells.

Increased Vascular Permeability

Platelet binding results in conformational changes in platelets that trigger intracellular signal transduction pathways that lead to platelet activation and the release of biologically active proteins.

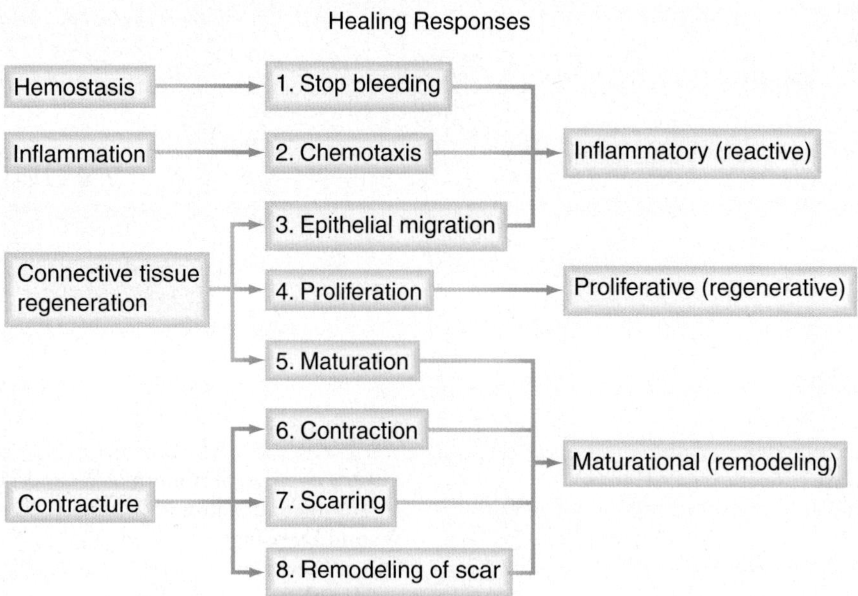

FIG. 6.1 Schematic diagram of the wound-healing continuum.

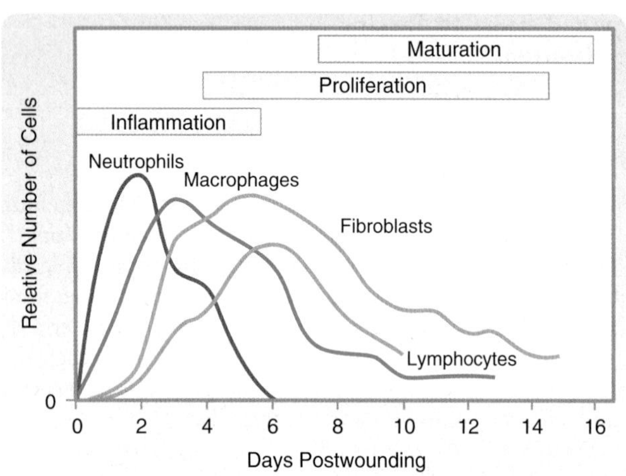

FIG. 6.2 Time course of the appearance of different cells in the wound during healing. Macrophages and neutrophils are predominant during the inflammatory phase (peak at days 3 and 2, respectively). Lymphocytes appear later and peak at day 7. Fibroblasts are the predominant cells during the proliferative phase. (Adapted from Witte MB, Barbul A. General principles of wound healing. *Surg Clin North Am.* 1997;77:509–528.)

Platelets release factors from two different sources: alpha granules and dense bodies. Platelet alpha granules are storage organelles that contain platelet-derived growth factor (PDGF), transforming growth factor-β (TGF-β), insulin-like growth factor 1 (IGF-1), fibronectin, fibrinogen, thrombospondin, and von Willebrand factor. The dense bodies contain vasoactive amines, such as serotonin, that cause vasodilatation and increased vascular permeability. Mast cells adherent to the endothelial surface release histamine and serotonin, resulting in increased permeability of endothelial cells and causing leakage of plasma from the intravascular space to the extracellular compartment.

The platelets become activated, and the membrane phospholipids bind factor V, which allows interaction with factor X. Membrane-bound prothrombinase activity is generated and potentiates thrombin production exponentially. The thrombin itself activates platelets and catalyzes the conversion of fibrinogen to fibrin. The fibrin strands trap red blood cells to form the clot and seal the wound. The resulting lattice framework is the scaffold for endothelial cells, inflammatory cells, and fibroblasts to repair the damaged vessel.

Thromboxane A2 and prostaglandin F2α, formed from the degradation of cell membranes in the arachidonic acid cascade, also assist in platelet aggregation and vasoconstriction. Although these activities serve to limit the amount of injury, they can also cause localized ischemia, resulting in further damage to cell membranes and the release of more prostaglandin F2α and thromboxane A2.

Chemokines

Chemokines stimulate the migration of different cell types, particularly inflammatory cells, into the wound and are active participants in the regulation of the different phases of wound healing. The CXC, CC, and C ligand families bind to G protein–coupled surface receptors called CXC receptors and CC receptors.

Macrophage chemoattractant protein (MCP-1 or CCL2) is induced in keratinocytes after injury. It is a potent chemoattractant for monocytes/macrophages, T lymphocytes, and mast cells. Expression of this chemokine is sustained in chronic wounds and results in the prolonged presence of polymorphonuclear cells (PMNs) and macrophages, leading to the prolonged inflammatory response. Chemokine (C-X-C motif) ligand 1 (CXCL1; previously called GRO-α) is a potent PMN chemotactic regulator and is increased in acute wounds. It is also involved in reepithelialization. Interleukin-8 (IL-8; also known as CXCL8) expression is increased in acute and chronic wounds. It is involved in reepithelialization and induces the leukocyte expression of matrix metalloproteinases (MMPs), which stimulates remodeling. It is also a strong chemoattractant for PMNs and participates in inflammation. Relatively low levels of IL-8 are found in fetal wounds and may be why fetal wounds have decreased inflammation and heal without scars. Expression of the keratinocyte-produced CXCL10 is elevated in acute wounds and chronic inflammatory conditions in response to interferon-γ (IFN-γ). It impairs wound healing by increasing inflammation and recruiting lymphocytes to the wound. It also inhibits proliferation by decreasing reepithelialization and angiogenesis and preventing fibroblast migration. Stromal cell–derived factor-1 (SDF-1, also known as CXCL12) is expressed by endothelial cells, myofibroblasts, and keratinocytes and is involved in inflammation by recruiting lymphocytes to the wound and promoting angiogenesis. It is a potent chemoattractant for endothelial cells and bone marrow progenitors from the circulation to peripheral tissues. It also enhances keratinocyte proliferation, resulting in reepithelialization.

Polymorphonuclear Cells

The release of histamine and serotonin leads to vascular permeability of the capillary bed. Complement factors such as C5a and leukotriene B4 promote neutrophil adherence and chemoattraction. In the presence of thrombin, endothelial cells exposed to leukotriene C4 and D4 release platelet-aggregating factor, which further enhances neutrophil adhesion. Monocytes and endothelial cells produce the inflammatory mediators IL-1 and tumor necrosis factor-α (TNF-α), and these mediators further promote endothelial-neutrophil adherence. Increased capillary permeability and chemotactic factors facilitate diapedesis of neutrophils into the inflammatory site. As the neutrophils begin their migration, they release the contents of their lysosomes and enzymes such as elastase and other proteases into the extracellular matrix (ECM), which further facilitates neutrophil migration. The combination of intense vasodilatation and increased vascular permeability leads to clinical findings of inflammation, rubor (redness), tumor (swelling), calor (heat), and dolor (pain). Local tissue swelling is further promoted by the deposition of fibrin, a protein end product of coagulation that becomes entrapped in lymphatic vessels.

Evidence suggests that the migration of PMNs requires sequential adhesive and deadhesive interactions between β_1 and β_2 integrins and ECM components. Integrin molecules are a family of cell surface receptors that are closely coupled with the cell's cytoskeleton. These molecules interact with components of the ECM, such as fibronectin, to provide adhesion and to transduce signals to the interior of the cell.

Integrins are crucial for cell motility and are required in inflammation and normal wound healing as well as in embryonic development and tumor metastases. After extravasation, PMNs, attracted by chemotaxins, migrate through the ECM via transient interactions between integrin receptors and their ligands. Four phases of integrin-mediated cell motility have been described: adhesion, spreading, contractility or traction, and retraction. Activation of specific integrins through ligand binding has been shown to increase cell adhesion and activate reorganization of the cell's actin cytoskeleton. Spreading is characterized by the development of lamellipodia and filopodia. Traction at the leading edge of the cell develops through binding of integrin followed by translocation of the cell over the adherent segment of the plasma membrane. The integrin is shifted to the rear of the cell and releases its substrate, permitting cell advancement. Regulation of integrin function by adhesive substrates offers a mechanism for local control of migrant cells. Within the assembled framework of the ECM, binding sites for integrins have been identified on collagen, laminin, and fibronectin.

The chemotactic agent mediates the PMN response through signal transduction as the chemotaxin binds to receptors on the cell surface. Bacterial products such as *N*-formyl-methionyl-leucyl-phenylalanine bind to induce cyclic adenosine monophosphate (AMP), but if there is maximal receptor occupancy, superoxide is produced at peak rates. Neutrophils also possess receptors for immunoglobulin G (IgG; Fc receptor) and the complement proteins C3b and C3bi. As the complement cascade is released and bacteria are opsonized, binding of these proteins to cell receptors on neutrophils allows recognition by the neutrophils and phagocytosis of the bacteria. When neutrophils are stimulated, they express more CR1 and CR3 receptors, permitting more efficient binding and phagocytosis of these bacteria.

Functional activation occurs after migration of PMNs into the wound site, which may induce new cell surface antigen expression, increased cytotoxicity, or enhanced production and release of cytokines. These activated neutrophils scavenge for necrotic debris, foreign material, and bacteria and generate free oxygen radicals with electrons donated by the reduced form of nicotinamide adenine dinucleotide phosphate. The electrons are transported across the membrane into lysosomes, where superoxide anion (O_2^-) is formed. Superoxide dismutase catalyzes the formation of hydrogen peroxide (H_2O_2), which is then degraded by myeloperoxidase in the azurophilic granules of neutrophils. This interaction oxidizes halides with the formation of byproducts such as hypochlorous acid. The iron-catalyzed reaction between H_2O_2 and O_2^- forms hydroxyl radicals (OH·). This potent-free radical is bactericidal as well as toxic to neutrophils and surrounding viable tissues.

Migration of PMNs stops after several days or when wound contamination has been controlled. Individual PMNs survive no longer than 24 hours and are replaced predominantly by mononuclear cells. Continuing wound contamination or secondary infection causes complement system activation that provides a steady supply of chemotactic factors and a sustained influx of PMNs into the wound. A prolonged inflammatory phase delays wound healing, destroys normal tissue, and results in abscess formation and possibly systemic infection. PMNs are not essential for wound healing because their phagocytosis and antimicrobial role can be taken over by macrophages. Sterile incisions heal normally without the presence of PMNs.

Macrophages

The macrophage is the one cell that is truly crucial to wound healing by orchestrating the release of cytokines and stimulating many subsequent processes in wound healing (Fig. 6.3). Tissue macrophages are derived from chemotaxis of migrating monocytes and appear within 24 to 48 hours of injury. When neutrophils start to disappear, macrophages appear and induce PMN apoptosis. Monocyte chemotactic factors include bacterial products, complement degradation products (C5a), thrombin, fibronectin, collagen, TGF-β, and PDGF-BB. Monocyte chemotaxis occurs as a result of the interaction of integrin receptors on the monocyte surface with ECM fibrin and fibronectin. The β integrin receptor also transduces the signal to initiate macrophage phagocytic activity. Activated integrin expression mediates monocyte transformation into wound macrophages. Transformation results in increased phagocytic activity and selective expression of cytokines and signal transduction elements by messenger RNA (mRNA), including the early growth response (EGR) genes, *EGR2* and *c-fos*. Macrophages have specific receptors for IgG, C3b (CR1 and CR3), and fibronectin (integrin receptors) that permit surface recognition and phagocytosis of opsonized pathogens.

Bacterial debris, such as lipopolysaccharide, activates monocytes to release free radicals and cytokines that mediate angiogenesis and fibroplasia. The presence of IL-2 increases free radical release and enhances bactericidal activity. The activity of the free radicals is potentiated by IL-2. Free radicals generate bacterial debris, which further potentiates the activation of monocytes.

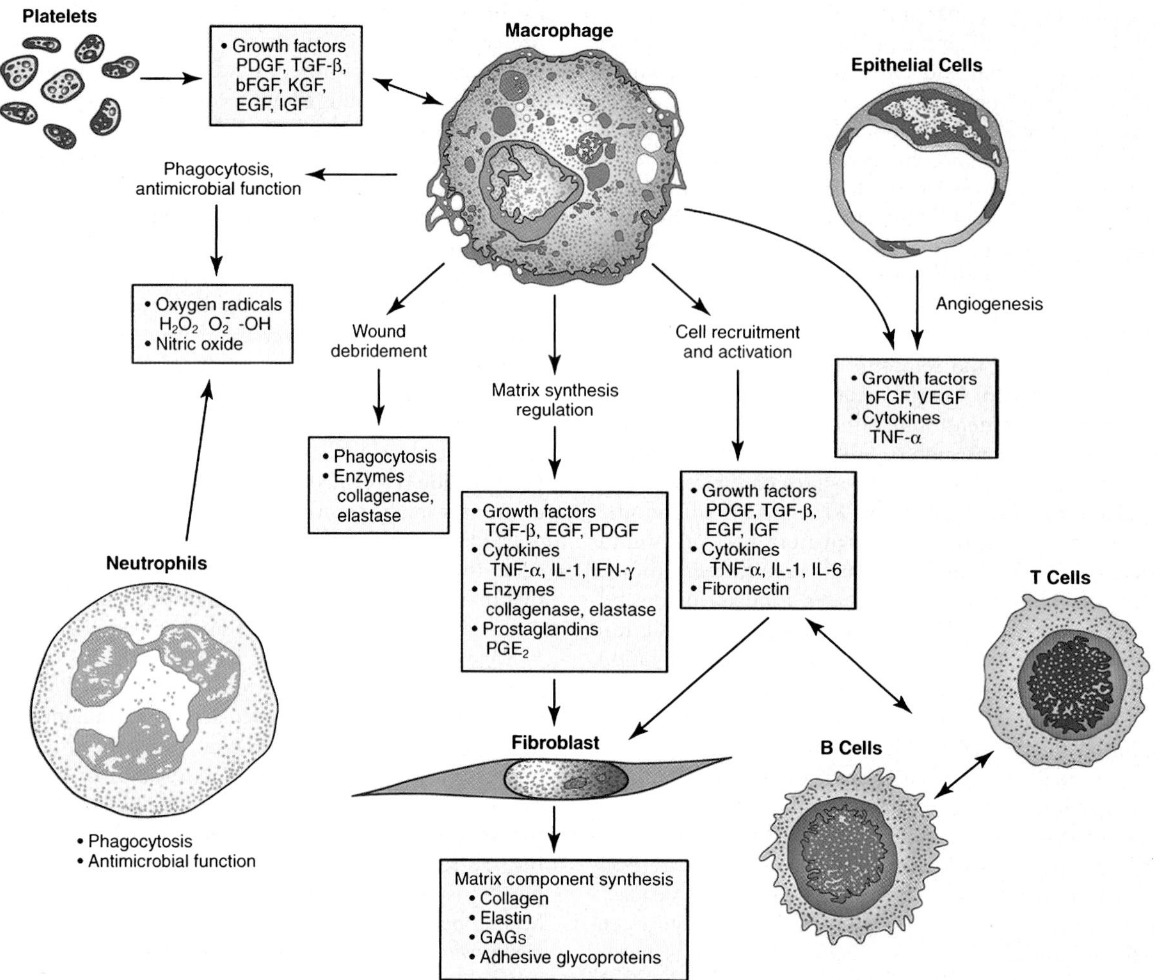

FIG. 6.3 Interaction of cellular and humoral factors in wound healing. Note the key role of the macrophage. *bFGF*, Basic fibroblast growth factor; *EGF*, epidermal growth factor; *GAGs*, glycosaminoglycans; *H_2O_2*, hydrogen peroxide; *IFN-γ*, interferon-γ; *IGF*, insulin-like growth factor; *IL-1*, interleukin-1; *IL-6*, interleukin-6; *KGF*, keratinocyte growth factor; *O_2^-*, superoxide; *–OH*, hydroxyl radical; *PDGF*, platelet-derived growth factor; *PGE_2*, prostaglandin E2; *TGF-β*, transforming growth factor-β; *TNF-α*, tumor necrosis factor-α; *VEGF*, vascular endothelial growth factor. (Adapted from Witte MB, Barbul A. General principles of wound healing. *Surg Clin North Am.* 1997;77:509–528.)

Activated wound macrophages also produce nitric oxide (NO), a substance that has been demonstrated to have many functions other than antimicrobial properties.

As the monocyte or macrophage is activated, phospholipase is induced, cell membrane phospholipids are enzymatically degraded, and thromboxane A2 and prostaglandin F2α are released. The macrophage also releases leukotrienes B4 and C4 and 15-hydroxyeicosatetraenoic acid and 5-hydroxyeicosatetraenoic acid. Leukotriene B4 is a potent chemotaxin for neutrophils and increases their adherence to endothelial cells.

Wound macrophages release proteinases, including MMPs (MMP-1, MMP-2, MMP-3, and MMP-9), which degrade the ECM and are crucial for removing foreign material, promoting cell movement through tissue spaces and regulating ECM turnover. This activity is dependent on the cyclic AMP pathway and can be blocked by nonsteroidal antiinflammatory drugs or glucocorticoid drugs. Colchicine and retinoic acid appear to decrease collagenase production as well.

Macrophages secrete numerous cytokines and growth factors (Tables 6.1 and 6.2). IL-1, a proinflammatory cytokine, is an acute-phase response cytokine. This endogenous pyrogen causes lymphocyte activation and stimulation of the hypothalamus, inducing the febrile response. It also directly affects hemostasis by inducing the release of vasodilators and stimulating coagulation. Its effect is further amplified as endothelial cells produce it in the presence of TNF-α and endotoxin. IL-1 has numerous effects, such as enhancement of collagenase production, stimulation of cartilage degradation and bone reabsorption, activation of neutrophils, regulation of adhesion molecules, and promotion of chemotaxis. It stimulates other cells to secrete proinflammatory cytokines. Its effects extend into the proliferative phase during which it increases fibroblast and keratinocyte growth and collagen synthesis. Studies have demonstrated increased levels of IL-1 in chronic nonhealing wounds, suggesting its role in the pathogenesis of poor wound healing. The early beneficial responses of IL-1 in wound healing appear to be maladaptive if elevated levels last beyond the first week after injury.

Microbial byproducts induce macrophages to release TNF. TNF-α is crucial in initiating the response to injury or bacteria. It upregulates cell surface adhesion molecules that promote the interaction of immune

TABLE 6.1 **Cytokine activity in wound healing.**

CYTOKINE	CELL SOURCE	FUNCTION	TYPE OF WOUND	
			ACUTE	CHRONIC
Proinflammatory Cytokines				
TNF-α	PMNs, macrophages	Inflammation, reepithelialization, PMN margination and cytotoxicity, with or without collagen synthesis; provides metabolic substrate	Increased levels	Increased levels
IL-1	PMNs, monocytes, macrophages, keratinocytes	Inflammation, reepithelialization, fibroblast and keratinocyte chemotaxis, collagen synthesis	Increased levels	Increased levels
IL-2	T lymphocytes	Increases fibroblast infiltration and metabolism		
IL-6	PMNs, macrophages, fibroblasts	Inflammation, reepithelialization, fibroblast proliferation, hepatic acute phase protein synthesis	Increased levels	Increased levels
IL-8	Macrophages, fibroblasts	Inflammation, macrophage and PMN chemotaxis; reepithelialization, keratinocyte maturation and proliferation	Increased levels	Increased levels
IFN-γ	T lymphocytes, macrophages	Activates macrophages and PMNs, retards collagen synthesis and cross-linking, stimulates collagenase activity		
Antiinflammatory Cytokines				
IL-4	T lymphocytes, basophils, mast cells	Inhibition of TNF-α, IL-1, IL-6 production; fibroblast proliferation, collagen synthesis		
IL-10	T lymphocytes, macrophages, keratinocytes	Inhibition of TNF-α, IL-1, IL-6 production, inhibition of macrophage and PMN activation		

Adapted from Rumalla VK, Borah GL. Cytokines, growth factors, and plastic surgery. *Plast Reconstr Surg.* 2001;108:719–733; and Barrientos S, Stojadinovic O, Golinko MS, etal. Growth factors and cytokines in wound healing. *Wound Repair Regen.* 2008;16:585–601.
IFN-γ, Interferon-γ; *IL-1, -2, -4, -6, -8, -10,* interleukin-1, -2, -4, -6, -8, -10; *PMNs,* polymorphonuclear cells; *TNF-α,* tumor necrosis factor-α.

cells and endothelium. TNF-α is detected in a wound within 12 hours and peaks after 72 hours. Its effects include hemostasis, increased vascular permeability, and enhanced endothelial proliferation. Similar to IL-1, TNF-α induces fever, increased collagenase production, resorption of cartilage and bone, and release of PDGF as well as the production of more IL-1. However, excessive production of TNF-α has been associated with multisystem organ failure and increased morbidity and mortality in inflammatory disease states, partly through its effects on activating macrophages and neutrophils. Studies have noted elevated levels of TNF-α in nonhealing versus healing chronic venous ulcers. As in the case of IL-1, TNF-α appears to be essential in the early inflammatory response required for wound healing, but local and systemic persistence of this cytokine may lead to impaired wound maturation.

IL-6, which is produced by monocytes and macrophages, is involved in stem cell growth, activation of B cells and T cells, and regulation of the synthesis of hepatic acute-phase proteins. Within acute wounds, IL-6 is also secreted by PMNs and fibroblasts; an increase in IL-6 parallels the increase in the PMN count locally. IL-6 is detectable within 12 hours of experimental wounding and may persist at high concentrations for longer than 1 week. It also works synergistically with IL-1, TNF-α, and endotoxins. It is a potent stimulator of fibroblast proliferation and is decreased in aging fibroblasts and fetal wounds.

IL-8 is secreted primarily by macrophages and fibroblasts in the acute wound with peak expression within the first 24 hours. Its major effects have already been discussed and include increased PMN and monocyte chemotaxis, PMN degranulation, and expression of endothelial cell adhesion molecules.

IFN-γ, another proinflammatory cytokine, is secreted by T lymphocytes and macrophages. Its major effects are macrophage and PMN activation and increased cytotoxicity. It has also been shown to reduce local wound contraction and aid in tissue remodeling. IFN-γ has been used in the treatment of hypertrophic and keloid scars, possibly by its effect in slowing collagen production and cross-linking, whereas collagenase (MMP-1) production increases. Experimentally, it has been shown to impair reepithelialization and wound strength in a dose-dependent manner when applied locally or systemically. These findings suggest that administration of IFN-γ may improve scar hypertrophy by decreasing the strength of the wound.

Macrophages also release growth factors that stimulate fibroblast, endothelial cell, and keratinocyte proliferation and are important in the proliferative phase (see Table 6.2). Macrophage-secreted PDGF stimulates collagen and proteoglycan synthesis. PDGF exists as three isomers—PDGF-AA, PDGF-AB, and PDGF-BB. The PDGF-BB isomer is the only growth factor preparation approved by the U.S. Food and Drug Administration and is the most widely studied clinically.

TGF-α and TGF-β are released by activated monocytes. TGF-α stimulates epidermal growth and angiogenesis. TGF-β itself stimulates monocytes to express other peptides, such as TGF-α, IL-1, and PDGF. TGF-β, which is also released by platelets and fibroblasts within wounds, exists as at least three isomers—β_1, β_2, and β_3—and its effects include fibroblast migration and maturation and ECM synthesis. TGF-β_1 has been shown to play an important role in collagen metabolism and healing of gastrointestinal injuries and anastomoses. In experimental models, TGF-β_1 accelerates wound healing in normal, steroid-impaired, and irradiated animals.

TGF-β is the most potent stimulant of fibroplasia, and its strong mitogenic effects have been implicated in the fibrogenesis

TABLE 6.2 Growth factors that affect wound healing.

GROWTH FACTOR	CELL SOURCE	FUNCTION	TYPE OF WOUND: ACUTE	TYPE OF WOUND: CHRONIC
PDGF	Platelets, macrophages, endothelial cells, keratinocytes, fibroblasts	Inflammation; granulation tissue formation; reepithelialization; matrix formation and remodeling; chemotactic for PMNs, macrophages, fibroblasts, and smooth muscle cells; activates PMNs, macrophages, and fibroblasts; mitogenic for fibroblasts and endothelial cells; stimulates production of MMPs, fibronectin, and HA; stimulates angiogenesis and wound contraction	Increased levels	Decreased levels
TGF-β (including isoforms β_1, β_2, and β_3)	Platelets, T lymphocytes, macrophages, endothelial cells, keratinocytes, fibroblasts	Inflammation; granulation tissue formation; reepithelialization; matrix formation and remodeling; chemotactic for PMNs, macrophages, lymphocytes, and fibroblasts; stimulates TIMP synthesis, keratinocyte migration, angiogenesis, and fibroplasia; inhibits production of MMPs and keratinocyte proliferation; induces TGF-β production	Increased levels	Decreased levels
EGF	Platelets, macrophages, fibroblasts	Mitogenic for keratinocytes and fibroblasts; stimulates keratinocyte migration	Increased levels	Decreased levels
FGF-1 and FGF-2 family	Macrophages, mast cells, T lymphocytes, endothelial cells, fibroblasts, keratinocytes, smooth muscle cells, chondrocytes	Granulation tissue formation; reepithelialization; matrix formation and remodeling; chemotactic for fibroblasts; mitogenic for fibroblasts and keratinocytes; stimulates keratinocyte migration; angiogenesis; wound contraction and matrix deposition	Increased levels	Decreased levels
KGF (also called FGF-7)	Fibroblasts, keratinocytes, smooth muscle cells, chondrocytes, endothelial cells, mast cells	Stimulate proliferation and migration of keratinocytes, increase transcription of factors involved in detoxification of ROS; potent mitogen for vascular endothelial cells; upregulates VEGF; stimulates endothelial cell production of UPA	Increased levels	Decreased levels
VEGF	Keratinocytes, platelets, PMNs, macrophages, endothelial cells, smooth muscle cells, fibroblasts	Granulation tissue formation; increases vasopermeability; mitogenic for endothelial cells	Increased levels	Decreased levels
TGF-α	Macrophages, T lymphocytes, keratinocytes, platelets, fibroblasts, lymphocytes	Reepithelialization; increase keratinocyte migration and proliferation		
IGF-1	Macrophages, fibroblasts	Stimulates elastin production and collagen synthesis, fibroblast proliferation		

Adapted from Schwartz SI, ed. *Principles of Surgery*. 7th ed. New York: McGraw-Hill; 1999:269; and Barrientos S, Stojadinovic O, Golinko MS, et al. Growth factors and cytokines in wound healing. *Wound Repair Regen*. 2008;16:585–601.

EGF, Epidermal growth factor; *FGF-1, -2, -7*, fibroblast growth factor-1, -2, -7; *HA*, hyaluronic acid; *IGF-1*, insulin-like growth factor-1; *KGF*, keratinocyte growth factor; *MMP*, matrix metalloproteinase; *PDGF*, platelet-derived growth factor; *PMNs*, polymorphonuclear cells; *ROS*, reactive oxygen species; *TGF-α,-β*, transforming growth factor-α, -β; *TIMP*, tissue inhibitors of metalloproteinase; *UPA*, urokinase-type plasminogen activator; *VEGF*, vascular endothelial growth factor.

seen in disease states such as scleroderma and interstitial pulmonary fibrosis. Enhanced expression of TGF-β_1 mRNA is found in keloid and hypertrophic scars. In contrast, fetal wounds have been demonstrated to have a paucity of TGF-β, suggesting that the scarless repair seen in utero occurs because of low or absent amounts of TGF-β. Studies of the three isomers have suggested that although TGF-β_1 and TGF-β_2 play an important role in tissue fibrosis and postinjury scarring, TGF-β_3 may limit scarring. As the concentration of TGF-β increases in the inflammatory site, fibroblasts are directly stimulated to produce collagen and fibronectin, leading to the proliferative phase.

Wound macrophages exhibit different functional phenotypes—M1 (classically activated) and M2 (alternatively activated)—that are at the extremes of a continuum of macrophage function. Lipopolysaccharide and IFN-γ stimulate the differentiation into M1 macrophages that release TNF-α, NO, and IL-6. These mediators are responsible for host defense but at the expense of significant collateral tissue damage. M2 macrophages are activated by IL-4 and IL-13; suppress inflammatory reactions and adaptive immune responses; and play an important role in wound healing, angiogenesis, and defense against parasitic infections. However, despite their beneficial functions, M2 macrophages can also be involved in different diseases, such as allergy, asthma, and fibrosis, which is the result of a helper T-cell (Th2) response predominated by IL-4 or IL-10. Both phenotypes are important when correctly balanced during the different phases of wound healing. In the inflammatory phase, greater M1 macrophage activity is required for macrophage debris scavenging and invading pathogen destruction. In the proliferative phase, M2 macrophages predominate. The balance between M1 and M2 macrophages is likely disturbed during abnormal wound-healing responses.

Several studies have demonstrated the importance of macrophages in wound healing by macrophage depletion. Macrophage depletion delays wound infiltration by fibroblasts and decreased wound fibrosis. Newborn animals that lacked macrophages, mast cells, and functional neutrophils as a result of defective myelopoiesis healed without scarring at the same speed as wild-type animals if their wounds were protected by antibiotic coverage, suggesting that inflammatory cells are not essential for wound closure. However, several models of specific inducible macrophage depletion based on genetically modified mice resulted in a detrimental effect of preinjury depletion of macrophages. Mice depleted before injury typically showed a defect in reepithelialization, granulation tissue formation, angiogenesis, wound cytokine production, and myofibroblast-associated wound contraction. Macrophage depletion 9 days after injury did not result in any morphologic or biologic differences between control and treatment mice, suggesting that macrophages may not be required at later stages of wound healing.

Lymphocytes

Significant numbers of T lymphocytes appear by day 5 after injury and peak on day 7. B lymphocytes appear to be principally involved in downregulating healing as the wound closes. Lymphocytes stimulate fibroblasts with cytokines (IL-2 and fibroblast-activating factor). Lymphocytes also secrete inhibitory cytokines (TGF-β, TNF-α, and IFN-γ). Antigen-presenting macrophages present bacterial "debris" or enzymatically degraded host proteins to lymphocytes, stimulating lymphocyte proliferation and cytokine release. T cells produce IFN-γ, which stimulates the macrophage to release TNF-α and IL-1. IFN-γ decreases prostaglandin synthesis, enhancing the effect of inflammatory mediators, suppressing collagen synthesis, and inhibiting macrophage exodus. IFN-γ appears to be an important mediator of chronic nonhealing wounds, and its presence suggests that T lymphocytes are primarily involved in chronic wound healing.

Drugs that suppress T-lymphocyte function and proliferation (steroids, cyclosporine, and tacrolimus) result in impaired wound healing in experimental wound models, possibly through decreased NO synthesis. In vivo lymphocyte depletion suggests the existence of an incompletely characterized T-cell lymphocyte population that is neither CD4+ nor CD8+ that seems to be responsible for the promotion of wound healing.

Proliferative Phase

As the acute responses of hemostasis and inflammation begin to resolve, the scaffolding is laid for repair of the wound through angiogenesis, fibroplasia, and epithelialization. This stage is characterized by the formation of granulation tissue, which consists of a capillary bed; fibroblasts; macrophages; and a loose arrangement of collagen, fibronectin, and hyaluronic acid. Numerous studies have used growth factors to modify granulation tissue, particularly fibroplasia. Adenoviral transfer, topical application, and subcutaneous injection of PDGF, TGF-β, keratinocyte growth factor (KGF), vascular endothelial growth factor (VEGF), and epidermal growth factor (EGF) have been shown to increase the proliferation of granulation tissue.

Angiogenesis

Angiogenesis is the process of new blood vessel formation and is necessary to support a healing wound environment. After injury, activated endothelial cells degrade the basement membrane of postcapillary venules, allowing the migration of cells through this gap. Division of these migrating endothelial cells results in tubule or lumen formation. Eventually, deposition of the basement membrane occurs and results in capillary maturation.

After injury, the endothelium is exposed to numerous soluble factors and comes in contact with adhering blood cells. These interactions result in upregulation of the expression of cell surface adhesion molecules, such as vascular cell surface adhesion molecule-1. Matrix-degrading enzymes, such as plasmin and the metalloproteinases, are released and activated and degrade the endothelial basement membrane. Fragmentation of the basement membrane allows migration of endothelial cells into the wound, promoted by fibroblast growth factor (FGF), PDGF, and TGF-β. Injured endothelial cells express adhesion molecules, such as the integrin $\alpha_v\beta_3$, which facilitates attachment to fibrin, fibronectin, and fibrinogen and facilitates endothelial cell migration along the provisional matrix scaffold. Platelet endothelial cell adhesion molecule-1 (PECAM-1), also found on endothelial cells, modulates their interaction with each other as they migrate into the wound.

Capillary tube formation is a complex process that involves cell-cell and cell-matrix interactions, modulated by adhesion molecules on endothelial cell surfaces. PECAM-1 has been observed to mediate cell-cell contact, whereas β_1 integrin receptors may aid in stabilizing these contacts and forming tight junctions between endothelial cells. Some of the new capillaries differentiate into arterioles and venules, whereas others undergo involution and apoptosis with subsequent ingestion by macrophages. Regulation of endothelial apoptosis is not well understood.

Angiogenesis appears to be stimulated and manipulated by various cytokines predominantly produced by macrophages and platelets. As the macrophage produces TNF-α, it orchestrates angiogenesis during the inflammatory phase. Heparin, which can stimulate the migration of capillary endothelial cells, binds with high affinity to a group of angiogenic factors.

VEGF, a member of the PDGF family of growth factors, has potent angiogenic activity. It is produced in large amounts by keratinocytes, macrophages, endothelial cells, platelets, and fibroblasts during wound healing. Cell disruption and hypoxia, hallmarks of tissue injury, appear to be strong initial inducers of potent angiogenic factors at the wound site, such as VEGF and its receptor. VEGF family members include VEGF-A, VEGF-B, VEGF-C, VEGF-D, VEGF-E, and placental growth factor. VEGF-A promotes early events in angiogenesis and subsequently is crucial to wound healing. It binds to tyrosine kinase surface receptors Flt-1 (VEGF receptor-1) and kinase insert domain receptor (VEGF receptor-2). Flt-1 is required for blood vessel organization, whereas kinase insert domain receptor is important for endothelial cell chemotaxis, proliferation, and differentiation. Animal studies have shown that VEGF-A administration restores impaired angiogenesis found in diabetic ischemic limbs; however, other studies have shown that exogenous VEGF results in vascular leakage and disorganized blood vessel formation. VEGF-C, which is also elevated during wound healing, is primarily released by macrophages and is important during the inflammatory phase of wound healing. Although it works primarily through VEGF receptor-3, which is expressed in macrophages and lymphatic endothelium, it can also activate VEGF receptor-2, increasing vascular permeability. In vivo administration of VEGF-C in an animal model using an adenoviral vector to genetically diabetic mice resulted in accelerated healing. Placental growth factor is another proangiogenic factor that is elevated after wounding. It is involved in inflammation and expressed by keratinocytes and endothelial cells. It is believed to work synergistically with VEGF, potentiating its proangiogenic function.

Both acidic and basic FGFs (FGF-1 and FGF-2) are released from disrupted parenchymal cells and are early stimulants of angiogenesis. FGF-2 provides the initial angiogenic stimulus within the first 3 days of wound repair followed by a subsequent prolonged stimulus mediated by VEGF from day 4 through day 7. There is a dose-dependent effect of VEGF and FGF-2 on angiogenesis. Both TGF-α and EGF stimulate endothelial cell proliferation. TNF-α is chemotactic for endothelial cells; it promotes formation of the capillary tube and may mediate angiogenesis through its induction of hypoxia-inducible factor 1 (HIF-1). It regulates the expression of other hypoxia-responsive genes, including inducible NO synthase and VEGF. HIF-1α mRNA is prominently present in wound inflammatory cells during the initial 24 hours, and HIF-1α protein is present in cells isolated from the wound 1 and 5 days after injury in vitro. Data also suggest that there is a positive interaction between endogenous NO and VEGF, with endogenous NO enhancing VEGF synthesis. Similarly, VEGF has been shown to promote NO synthesis in angiogenesis, suggesting that NO mediates aspects of VEGF signaling required for endothelial cell proliferation and organization.

TGF-β is a chemoattractant for fibroblasts and probably assists in angiogenesis by signaling the fibroblast to produce FGFs. Other factors that have been shown to induce angiogenesis include angiogenin, IL-8, and lactic acid. Several of the matrix materials, such as fibronectin and hyaluronic acid from the wound site, are angiogenic. Fibronectin and fibrin are produced by macrophages and damaged endothelial cells. Collagen appears to interact by causing the tubular formation of endothelial cells in vitro. Angiogenesis results from the complex interaction of ECM material and cytokines.

Fibroplasia

Fibroblasts are specialized cells that differentiate from resting mesenchymal cells in connective tissue; they do not arrive in the wound cleft by diapedesis from circulating cells. After injury, the normally quiescent and sparse fibroblasts are chemoattracted to the inflammatory site; they divide and produce the components of the ECM. After stimulation by macrophage-derived and platelet-derived cytokines and growth factors, the fibroblast, which is normally arrested in the G_0 phase, undergoes replication and proliferation. Platelet-derived TGF-β stimulates fibroblast proliferation indirectly by releasing PDGF. The fibroblast can also stimulate replication in an autocrine manner by releasing FGF-2. To continue proliferating, fibroblasts require further stimulation by factors such as EGF or IGF-1. Although fibroblasts require growth factors for proliferation, they do not need growth factors to survive. Fibroblasts can live quiescently in growth factor–free media in monolayers or three-dimensional cultures.

The primary function of fibroblasts is to synthesize collagen, which they begin to produce during the cellular phase of inflammation. The time required for undifferentiated mesenchymal cells to differentiate into highly specialized fibroblasts accounts for the delay between injury and the appearance of collagen in a healing wound. This period, generally 3 to 5 days depending on the type of tissue injured, is termed the *lag phase* of wound healing. Fibroblasts begin to migrate in response to chemotactic substances such as growth factors (PDGF, TGF-β), C5 fragments, thrombin, TNF-α, eicosanoids, elastin fragments, leukotriene B4, and fragments of collagen and fibronectin.

The rate of collagen synthesis declines after 4 weeks and eventually balances the rate of collagen destruction by collagenase (MMP-1). At this point, the wound enters a phase of collagen maturation. The maturation phase continues for months or years. Glycoprotein and mucopolysaccharide levels decrease during the maturation phase, and new capillaries regress and disappear. These changes alter the appearance of the wound and increase its strength.

Epithelialization

The epidermis serves as a physical barrier to prevent fluid loss and bacterial invasion. Tight cell junctions within the epithelium contribute to its impermeability, and the basement membrane zone gives structural support and provides attachment between the epidermis and the dermis. The basement membrane zone consists of several layers that secure the epidermodermal interface and connect the lamina densa to the dermis: (1) lamina lucida (electron clear), consisting of laminin and heparan sulfate; (2) lamina densa (electron dense), containing type IV collagen; and (3) anchoring fibrils, consisting of type IV collagen.

The basal layer of the epidermis attaches to the basement membrane zone by hemidesmosomes. Reepithelialization of wounds begins within hours after injury. Initially, the wound is rapidly sealed by clot formation and then by epithelial (epidermal) cell migration across the defect. Keratinocytes located at the basal layer of the residual epidermis or in the depths of epithelium-lined dermal appendages migrate to resurface the wound. Epithelialization involves a sequence of changes in wound keratinocytes—detachment, migration, proliferation, differentiation, and stratification. If the basement membrane zone is intact, epithelialization proceeds more rapidly. The cells are stimulated to migrate. Attachments to neighboring and adjoining cells and to the dermis are loosened, as demonstrated by intracellular tonofilament retraction, dissolution of intercellular desmosomes and hemidesmosomes linking the epidermis to the basement membrane, and formation of cytoplasmic actin filaments.

Epidermal cells express integrin receptors that allow them to interact with ECM proteins such as fibronectin. The migrating cells dissect the wound by separating the desiccated eschar from viable tissue. This path of dissection is determined by the integrins that the epidermal cells express on their cell membranes. Degradation of the ECM, required if epidermal cells are to migrate between the collagenous dermis and fibrin eschar, is driven by epidermal cell production of collagenase (MMP-1) and plasminogen activator, which activates collagenase and plasmin. The migrating cells are also phagocytic and remove debris in their path. Cells behind the leading edge of migrating cells begin to proliferate. The epithelial cells move in a leapfrog and tumbling fashion until the edges establish contact. If the basement membrane zone is not intact, it will be repaired first. The absence of neighboring cells at the wound margin may be a signal for the migration and proliferation of epidermal cells. Local release of EGF, TGF-α, and KGF and increased expression of their receptors may also stimulate these processes. Topical application of keratinocyte growth factor-2 (KGF-2) in young and aged animals accelerates reepithelialization. Basement membrane proteins, such as laminin, reappear in a highly ordered sequence from the margin of the wound inward. After the wound is completely reepithelialized, the cells become columnar and stratified again while firmly attaching to the reestablished basement membrane and underlying dermis.

Extracellular Matrix

The ECM exists as a scaffold to stabilize the physical structure of tissues, but it also plays an active and complex role by regulating the behavior of cells that contact it. Cells within it produce the macromolecular constituents, including (1) glycosaminoglycans (GAGs), or polysaccharide chains, usually found covalently linked to protein in the form of proteoglycans and (2) fibrous proteins such as collagen, elastin, fibronectin, and laminin.

In connective tissue, proteoglycan molecules form a gel-like ground substance. This highly hydrated gel allows the matrix to withstand compressive force while permitting rapid diffusion of nutrients, metabolites, and hormones between blood and tissue cells. Collagen fibers within the matrix serve to organize and strengthen the matrix, whereas elastin fibers give it resilience (matrix proteins have adhesive functions).

The wound matrix accumulates and changes in composition as healing progresses, balanced between new deposition and degradation (Fig. 6.4). The provisional matrix is a scaffold for cellular migration and is composed of fibrin, fibrinogen, fibronectin, and vitronectin. GAGs and proteoglycans are synthesized next and support further matrix deposition and remodeling. Collagens, which are the predominant scar proteins, are the end result. Attachment proteins, such as fibrin and fibronectin, provide linkage to the ECM through binding to cell surface integrin receptors.

Stimulation of fibroblasts by growth factors induces upregulated expression of integrin receptors, facilitating cell-matrix interactions. Ligand binding induces clustering of integrin into focal adhesion sites. Regulation of integrin-mediated cell signaling by the extracellular divalent cations Mg^{2+}, Mn^{2+}, and Ca^{2+} perhaps is caused by induction of conformational changes in the integrins.

A dynamic and reciprocal relationship exists between fibroblasts and the ECM. Cytokine regulation of fibroblast responses is altered by variations in the composition of the ECM. For example, expression of matrix-degrading enzymes, such as the MMPs, is upregulated after cytokine stimulation of fibroblasts. Collagenolytic MMP-1 is induced by IL-1 and downregulated by TGF-β. Activation of plasminogen to plasmin by plasminogen activator and procollagenase to collagenase by plasmin results in matrix degradation and facilitates cell migration. Modulation of these processes provides additional mechanisms whereby the cell-matrix interaction can be regulated during wound healing. Matrix modulation is also seen in tumor metastasis. Neoplastic cells lose their dependence on anchorage, mediated mainly by integrins; this is probably caused by decreased production of fibronectin and subsequent decreased adhesion, and, as a result, these cells can break away from the primary tumor and metastasize.

An example of the necessary dynamic interactions occurring in the provisional matrix during wound healing is the effect of TGF-β on incisional wounds sealed with fibrin sealant. Fibrin sealant is a derivative of plasma components that mimics the last step in the coagulation cascade. Commercially available fibrin sealant has an approximately ten fold greater concentration of fibrin than plasma and consequently provides a more airtight, waterproof seal. Fibrin sealant may serve as a mechanical barrier to the early cell-mediated events occurring in wound healing. Supplementation of fibrin sealant with TGF-β has been demonstrated to reverse the

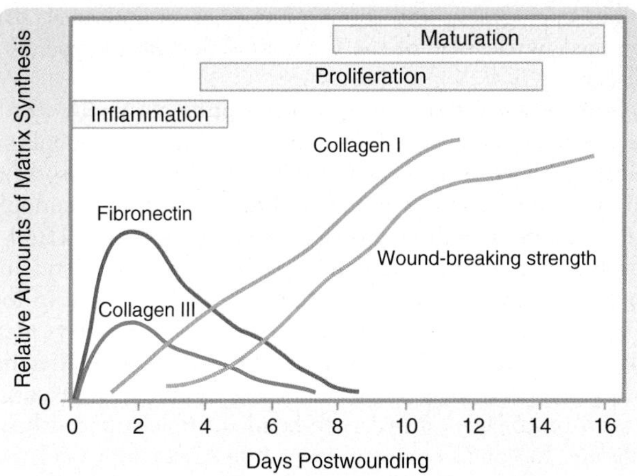

FIG. 6.4 Wound matrix deposition over time. Fibronectin and type III collagen constitute the early matrix. Type I collagen accumulates later and corresponds to the increase in wound-breaking strength. (Adapted from Witte MB, Barbul A. General principles of wound healing. *Surg Clin North Am.* 1997;77:509–528.)

inhibitory effects of fibrin sealant on wound healing and increase tensile strength compared with sutured wounds. The increased tensile strength may be a result of improved cell migration into the wound site, more rapid clearance of fibrin sealant, suppression of gelatinase (MMP-9), and enhancement of ECM synthesis in TGF-β–supplemented wounds.

Collagen structure. Collagens are found in all multicellular animals and are secreted by various cell types. They are a major component of skin and bone and constitute 25% of the total protein mass in mammals. The proline-rich and glycine-rich collagen molecule is a long, stiff, triple-stranded helical structure that consists of three collagen polypeptide α chains wound around one another in a ropelike superhelix. With its ringlike structure, proline provides stability to the helical conformation in each α chain, whereas glycine, because of its small size, allows tight packing of the three α chains to form the final superhelix. There are at least 20 types of collagen, the main constituents of connective tissue being types I, II, III, V, and XI. Type I is the principal collagen of skin and bone and is the most common. In adults, the skin is approximately 80% type I and 20% type III. In newborns, the content of type III collagen is greater than that found in adults. In early wound healing, there is also increased expression of type III collagen. Type I collagens are the fibrillar, or fibril-forming, collagens. They are secreted into the extracellular space, where they assemble into collagen fibrils (10–300 nm in diameter), which then aggregate into larger, cable-like bundles called collagen fibers (several micrometers in diameter).

Other types of collagens include types IX and XII (fibril-associated collagens) and types IV and VII (network-forming collagens). Types IX and XII are found on the surface of collagen fibrils and serve to link the fibrils to one another and to other components in the ECM. Type IV molecules assemble into a meshlike pattern and are a major part of the mature basal lamina. Dimers of type VII form anchoring fibrils that help attach the basal lamina to the underlying connective tissue and are especially abundant in the skin.

Type XVII and type XVIII collagens are two of a number of collagen-like proteins. Type XVII has a transmembrane domain and is found in hemidesmosomes. Type XVIII is located in the basal laminae of blood vessels. The peptide endostatin, which inhibits angiogenesis and shows promise as an anticancer drug, is formed by cleavage of the C-terminal domain of type XVIII collagen.

Collagen synthesis. Collagen polypeptide chains are synthesized on membrane-bound ribosomes and enter the endoplasmic reticulum lumen as pro-α chains (Fig. 6.5). These precursors have amino-terminal signal peptides to direct them to the endoplasmic reticulum as well as propeptides at the N-terminal and C-terminal ends. Within the lumen of the endoplasmic reticulum, some of the prolines and lysines undergo hydroxylation to form hydroxyproline and hydroxylysine. Hydroxylation results in the stable triple-stranded helix through the formation of interchain hydrogen bonds. The pro-α chain then combines with two others to form procollagen, a hydrogen-bonded, triple-stranded helical molecule. In conditions such as vitamin C (ascorbic acid) deficiency (scurvy), proline hydroxylation is prevented, resulting in the formation of unstable triple helices secondary to the synthesis of defective pro-α chains. Vitamin C deficiency is characterized by the gradual loss of preexisting normal collagen, which leads to fragile blood vessels and loose teeth.

After secretion into the ECM, specific proteases cleave the propeptides of the procollagen molecules to form collagen monomers. These monomers assemble to form collagen fibrils in the ECM, driven by the tendency of collagen to self-assemble. Covalent cross-linking of the lysine residues provides tensile strength. The extent and type of cross-linking vary from tissue to tissue. In tissues such as tendons in which tensile strength is crucial, collagen cross-linking is extremely high. In mammalian skin, the fibrils are organized in a basketweave pattern to resist multidirectional tensile stress. In tendons, fibrils are in parallel bundles aligned along the major axis of tension.

Numerous factors can affect collagen synthesis. Vitamin C (ascorbic acid), TGF-β, IGF-1, and IGF-2 increase collagen synthesis. IFN-γ decreases type I procollagen mRNA synthesis, and glucocorticoids inhibit procollagen gene transcription, leading to decreased collagen synthesis.

Several genetic disorders are caused by abnormalities in collagen fibril formation. In osteogenesis imperfecta, deletion of one procollagen α_1 allele results in weak, easily fractured bones. Ehlers-Danlos syndrome is a result of mutations affecting type III collagen and is characterized by fragile skin and blood vessels and hypermobile joints.

Elastic fibers. Tissues such as skin, blood vessels, and lungs require strength and elasticity to function. Elastic fibers in the ECM of these tissues provide the resilience to allow recoil after transient stretching.

Elastic fibers are predominantly composed of elastin, a highly hydrophobic protein (≈750 amino acids long). Soluble tropoelastin is secreted into the extracellular space, where it forms lysine cross-links to other tropoelastin molecules to generate a large network of elastin fibers and sheets. Elastin is composed of hydrophobic and alanine-rich and lysine-rich α-helical segments that alternate along the polypeptide chain. The hydrophobic segments are responsible for the elastic properties of the molecule. The alanine-rich and lysine-rich α-helical segments form cross-links between adjacent molecules. Although the proposed conformation of elastin molecules is controversial, the predominant theory is that the elastin polypeptide chain adopts a random coil conformation that allows the network to stretch and recoil like a rubber band. Elastic fibers consist of an elastin core covered by a sheath of microfibrils, which are composed of several distinct glycoproteins such as fibrillin. Elastin-binding fibrillin is essential for the integrity of the elastic fibers.

Microfibrils appear before elastin in developing tissues and seem to form a scaffold on which the secreted elastin molecules are deposited. Elastin is produced early in life, stabilizes, and does not

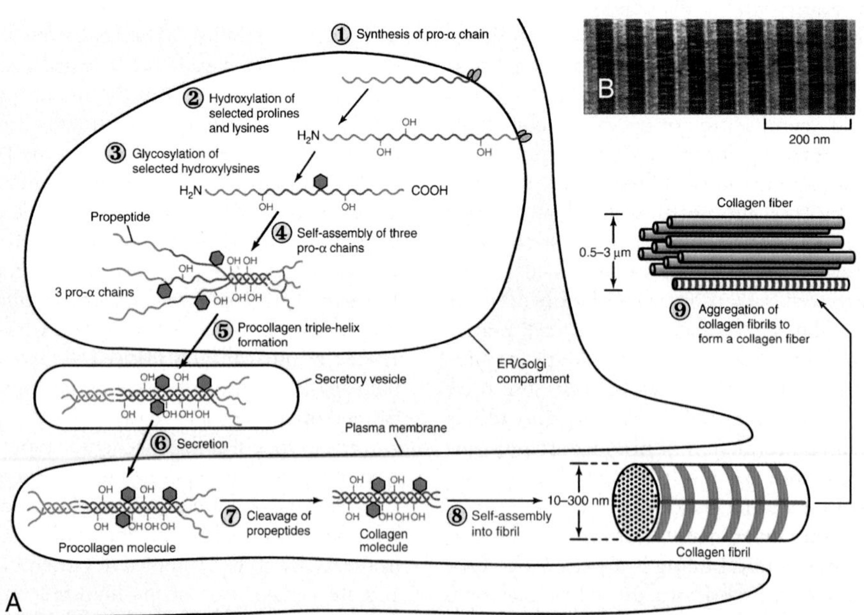

FIG. 6.5 Intracellular and extracellular events in the formation of a collagen fibril. (A) Collagen fibrils are shown assembling in the extracellular space contained within a large infolding in the plasma membrane. As one example of how collagen fibrils can form ordered arrays in the extracellular space, they are shown further assembling into large collagen fibers, which are visible with a light microscope. The covalent cross-links that stabilize the extracellular assemblies are not shown. (B) Electron micrograph of a negatively stained collagen fibril revealing its typical striated appearance. *ER,* Endoplasmic reticulum. (A, From Alberts B, Johnson A, Lewis J, et al, eds. *Molecular Biology of the Cell.* 4th ed. New York: Garland; 2002:1100; B, Courtesy Robert Horne.)

undergo much further synthesis or degradation, with a turnover that approaches the life span. Age-related modification is a result of progressive degradation as the elastic fibers gradually become tortuous, frayed, and porous. Scanning electron microscopy shows that, in humans, the elastic meshwork grows largely undistorted during postnatal growth, during which fibers seem to enlarge in synchrony with growth of the tissue. In circumstances not involving a wound, there is little elastin degradation probably because of the hydrophobic nature of elastin, which makes the interior of this highly folded protein inaccessible. As a result of this high degree of three dimensionality and extensive cross-linking, cleavage must be considerable before there is much loss of elasticity. IGF-1 and TGF-β stimulate the production of elastin. Glucocorticoids and basic FGF reduce the production of elastin in adult skin cells.

Mutations causing a deficiency of elastin protein result in arterial narrowing as a consequence of excessive smooth muscle cell proliferation in the arterial wall (intimal hyperplasia). These findings suggest that the normal elasticity of an artery is needed to prevent the proliferation of these cells. Gene mutations in fibrillin result in Marfan syndrome; severely affected individuals are prone to aortic rupture.

Glycosaminoglycans and proteoglycans. GAGs are unbranched polysaccharide chains composed of repeating disaccharide units, a sulfated amino sugar (*N*-acetylglucosamine or *N*-acetylgalactosamine), and uronic acid (glucuronic or iduronic). GAGs are highly negatively charged because of the sulfate or carboxyl groups on most of their sugars. Four types of GAGs exist: (1) hyaluronan, (2) chondroitin sulfate and dermatan sulfate, (3) heparan sulfate, and (4) keratan sulfate.

GAGs in connective tissue usually constitute less than 10% of the weight of fibrous proteins. Their highly negative charge attracts osmotically active cations, such as Na^+, which causes large amounts of water to be incorporated into the matrix. This results in porous hydrated gels and is responsible for the turgor that enables the matrix to withstand compressive force.

Hyaluronan is the simplest GAG. It is composed of repeating nonsulfated disaccharide units and is found in adult tissues, but it is especially prevalent in fetal tissues. Its abundance in fetal wounds is believed to be a factor in the scarless wound healing seen in fetal tissues. In contrast to the other GAGs, hyaluronan is not covalently attached to any protein and is synthesized directly from the cell surface by an enzyme complex embedded in the plasma membrane.

Hyaluronan plays several different roles because of its large hydration shell. It is produced in large quantities during wound healing, during which it facilitates cell migration by physically expanding the ECM and allowing cells additional space for migration; it also reduces the strength of adhesion of migrating cells to matrix fibers. Hyaluronan synthesized from the basal side of epithelium creates a cell-free space for cell migration, such as during embryogenesis and formation of the heart and other organs. When cell migration is finished, the excess hyaluronan is degraded by hyaluronidase. Studies using hyaluronic acid derivative have suggested that these derivatives can accelerate wound healing in burns, surgical wounds, and chronic wounds.

Proteoglycans are a diverse group of glycoproteins with functions mediated by their core proteins and GAG chains. The number and types of GAGs attached to the core protein can vary greatly, and the GAGs themselves can be modified by sulfonation. Because of their GAGs, proteoglycans provide hydrated space around and between cells. They also form gels of different pore size and charge density to regulate the movement of cells and molecules. Perlecan, a heparan sulfate proteoglycan, plays this role in the basal lamina of the kidney glomerulus. Decreased levels of perlecan are believed to play a role in diabetic albuminuria.

Proteoglycans function in chemical signaling by binding various secreted signal molecules, such as growth factors, and modulating their signaling activity. Proteoglycans also can bind other secreted proteins, such as proteases and protease inhibitors. This binding allows proteoglycans to regulate proteins by (1) immobilizing the protein and restricting its range of action, (2) providing a reservoir of the protein for delayed release, (3) altering the protein to allow more effective presentation to cell surface receptors, (4) prolonging the action of the protein by protecting it from degradation, or (5) blocking the activity of the protein.

Proteoglycans can be components of plasma membranes and have a transmembrane core protein or are attached to the lipid bilayer by a glycosylphosphatidylinositol anchor. These proteoglycans act as coreceptors that work with other cell surface receptor proteins in binding cells to the ECM and initiating the response of cells to extracellular signaling proteins. For example, the syndecans are transmembrane proteoglycans located on the surface of many cells, including fibroblasts and epithelial cells. In fibroblasts, syndecans are found in focal adhesions, where they interact with fibronectin on the cell surface and with cytoskeletal and signaling proteins inside the cell. Mutations leading to inactivation of these coreceptor proteoglycans result in severe developmental defects.

The ECM has other noncollagen proteins, such as the fibronectins, that have multiple domains and can bind to other matrix macromolecules and cell surface receptors. These interactions help organize the matrix and facilitate cell attachment.

Fibronectin exists as soluble and fibrillar isoforms. Soluble plasma fibronectin circulates in various body fluids and enhances blood clotting, wound healing, and phagocytosis. The highly insoluble fibrillar forms assemble on cell surfaces and are deposited in the ECM. The fibronectin fibrils that form on the surface of fibroblasts are usually coupled with neighboring intracellular actin stress fibers. The actin filaments promote assembly of the fibronectin fibril and influence fibril orientation. Integrin transmembrane adhesion proteins mediate these interactions. The contractile actin and myosin cytoskeleton pulls on the fibronectin matrix and generates tension.

Basal lamina. Basal laminae are flexible, thin (40–120 nm) mats of specialized ECM that separate cells and epithelia from the underlying or surrounding connective tissue. In skin, the basal lamina is tethered to the underlying connective tissue by specialized anchoring fibrils. This composite of basal lamina and collagen is the basement membrane.

The basal lamina acts in numerous ways: (1) as a molecular filter to prevent the passage of macromolecules (i.e., in the kidney glomerulus), (2) as a selective barrier to certain cells (i.e., the lamina beneath the epithelium prevents fibroblasts from contacting epithelial cells but does not stop macrophages or lymphocytes), (3) as a scaffold for regenerating cells to migrate, and (4) as an important element in tissue regeneration in locations where the basal lamina survives.

Although composition may vary from tissue to tissue, most mature basal laminae contain type IV collagen, perlecan, and the glycoproteins laminin and nidogen. Type IV collagen has a more flexible structure than the fibrillar collagens; its triple-stranded helix is interrupted, allowing multiple bends.

Laminins generally consist of three long polypeptide chains (α, β, and γ). Mice lacking the laminin γ_1 chain die during embryogenesis because they cannot make a basal lamina. The laminin in basement membranes consists of several domains that bind to perlecan, nidogen, and laminin receptor proteins found on cell surfaces. The type IV collagen and laminin networks are connected by nidogen and perlecan, which act as stabilizing bridges. Many of the cell surface receptors for type IV collagen and laminin are members of the integrin family. Another important type of laminin receptor is dystroglycan, a transmembrane protein that, together with integrins, may organize assembly of the basal lamina.

Degradation of the extracellular matrix. Regulated turnover of the ECM is crucial to many biologic processes. ECM degradation occurs during metastasis when neoplastic cells migrate from their site of origin to distant organs via the bloodstream or lymphatics. In injury or infection, localized degradation of the ECM occurs so that cells can migrate across the basal lamina to reach the site of injury or infection. Locally secreted cellular proteases, such as MMPs or serine proteases, degrade the ECM components. Matrix proteolysis helps the cell migrate by (1) clearing a path through the matrix; (2) exposing binding sites, promoting cell binding or migration; (3) facilitating cell detachment so that a cell can move forward; and (4) releasing signal proteins that promote cell migration.

Proteolysis is tightly regulated. Many proteases are secreted as inactive precursors that are activated when required. In addition, cell surface receptors bind these proteases to ensure that they act only on sites where they are needed. Finally, protease inhibitors, such as tissue inhibitors of metalloproteinase (TIMP), can bind these enzymes and block their activity.

Maturational Phase

Wound contraction occurs by centripetal movement of the whole thickness of the surrounding skin and reduces the amount of disorganized scar. In contrast, wound contracture is a physical constriction or limitation of function and is a result of the process of wound contraction. Contractures occur when excessive scar exceeds normal wound contraction, and it results in a functional disability. Examples of contractures are scars that traverse joints and prevent extension and scars that involve the eyelid or mouth and cause an ectropion.

Wound contraction appears to take place as a result of a complex interaction of the extracellular materials and fibroblasts that is not completely understood. Using a fibroblast-populated collagen lattice, Ehrlich demonstrated that aborted cell locomotion appears to cause bunching and contraction of the collagen fibers. In this in vitro model, trypsinized collagen is populated by fibroblasts that adhere to it in culture. If normal dermal fibroblasts are cultured, they attempt to move but are trapped by the collagen fibers. The tractional forces cause the lattice to bunch and contract.

Numerous studies have shown that fibroblasts in a contracting wound undergo change to stimulated cells, termed *myofibroblasts*. These cells have function and structure in common with fibroblasts and smooth muscle cells and express alpha smooth muscle actin in bundles termed *stress fibers*. The actin appears at day 6 after wounding, persists at high levels for 15 days, and is gone by 4 weeks, when the cell undergoes apoptosis. It appears that a stimulated fibroblast develops contractile ability related to the formation of cytoplasmic actin-myosin complexes. When this stimulated cell is placed in the fibroblast-populated collagen lattice, contraction occurs even more quickly. The tension that is exerted by the fibroblasts' attempt at contraction appears to stimulate the actin-myosin structures in their cytoplasm. If colchicine, which inhibits microtubules, or cytochalasin D, which inhibits microfilaments, is added to the tissue culture, the result is minimal contraction of the collagen gels. Fibroblasts develop a linear arrangement in the line of tension that, when removed, causes the cells to round up.

Stimulated fibroblasts, or myofibroblasts, are found to be a constant feature present in abundance in diseases involving excessive fibrosis, including hepatic cirrhosis, renal and pulmonary fibrosis, Dupuytren contracture, and desmoplastic reactions induced by neoplasia. The actin microfilaments are arranged linearly along the long axis of the fibroblast. They are associated with dense bodies that allow attachment to the surrounding ECM. Fibronexus is the attachment entity that connects the cytoskeleton to the ECM and spans the cell membrane in doing so.

MMPs also appear to be important for wound contraction. It has been demonstrated that stromelysin-1 (MMP-3) strongly affects wound contraction. MMPs may be necessary to allow cleavage of the attachment between the fibroblast and the collagen so that the lattice can be made to contract. Different populations of fibroblasts from different organs respond to the contraction stimulus in a heterogeneous fashion. It is likely that the stromelysin-1, with the participation of β_1 integrins, allows modification of attachment sites between fibroblasts and the collagen fibrils. Similarly, cytokines such as TGF-β_1 affect contraction by increasing the expression of β_1 integrin.

Remodeling

The fibroblast population decreases, and the dense capillary network regresses. Wound strength increases rapidly within 1 to 6 weeks and then appears to plateau up to 1 year after the injury (see Fig. 6.5). Compared with nonwounded skin, tensile strength is only 30% in the scar. An increase in breaking strength occurs after approximately 21 days, mostly as a result of cross-linking. Although collagen cross-linking causes further wound contraction and an increase in strength, it also results in a scar that is more brittle and less elastic than normal skin. In contrast to normal skin, the epidermodermal interface in a healed wound is devoid of rete pegs, the undulating projections of epidermis that penetrate into the papillary dermis. Loss of this anchorage results in increased fragility and predisposes the neoepidermis to avulsion after minor trauma.

ABNORMAL WOUND HEALING

In such a complex series of interweaving events as wound healing, many factors can impede the outcome (Box 6.1). The amount of tissue lost or damaged, the amount of foreign material or bacterial inoculation, and the length of exposure to toxic factors can affect the time to recovery. Intrinsic factors such as age, chemotherapeutic agents, atherosclerosis, cardiac or renal failure, and location on the body all affect wound healing. Ultimately, the type of scar—whether it is adequate, inadequate, or proliferative—is dictated by the amount of collagen deposition and balanced by the amount of collagen degradation. If the balance is tipped in either direction, the result is poor.

Hypertrophic Scars and Keloids

Hypertrophic scars and keloids are proliferative scars characterized by excessive net collagen deposition (Fig. 6.6). Hypertrophic scars are raised scars within the confines of the original wound and frequently regress spontaneously. Keloids, by definition, grow beyond the borders of the original wounds and rarely regress with time; they are more prevalent in darkly pigmented skin, developing in 15% to 20% of African Americans, Asians, and Hispanics. There is strong evidence suggesting a genetic susceptibility, including familial heritability, common occurrence in twins, and high prevalence in certain ethnic populations. Recent studies have suggested a strong multigenetic disposition to keloid formation and differential

BOX 6.1 Factors that inhibit wound healing.

Infection
Ischemia
  Circulation
  Respiration
  Local tension
Diabetes mellitus
Ionizing radiation
Advanced age
Malnutrition
Vitamin deficiencies
  Vitamin C
  Vitamin A
Mineral deficiencies
  Zinc
  Iron
Exogenous drugs
  Doxorubicin (Adriamycin)
  Glucocorticosteroids

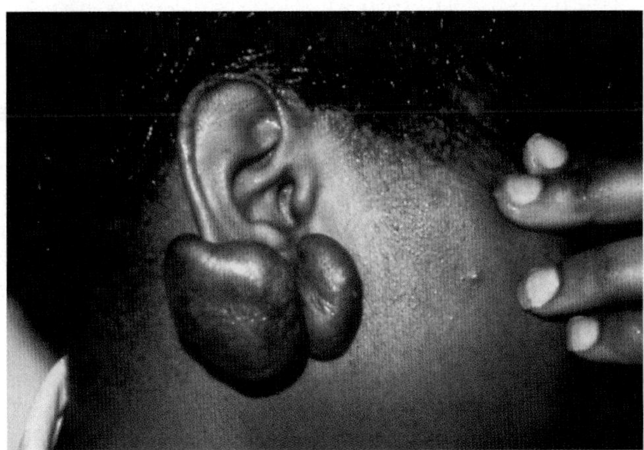

FIG. 6.6 Keloids caused by ear piercing.

expression with a varied inheritance. Proposed pathways include apoptosis, endocytosis, cytokine-cytokine receptor interaction, mitogen-activated protein kinase signaling pathway, tenascin C, jun proto-oncogene, and growth factors such as TGF-β and VEGF.[1,2]

Keloids often occur above the clavicles, on the trunk, on the upper extremities, and on the face. Their occurrence cannot be predicted and are frequently refractory to medical and surgical intervention. To date, there is no known effective prevention method for keloid formation. Zhang and colleagues[2] have identified potential molecular and genetic targets that could allow for prevention of keloids and scarring, such as Fos proto-oncogene (FOS) and EGR1 transcriptional factors.

Keloids and hypertrophic scars differ histologically from normal scars. Hypertrophic scars primarily contain well-organized type III collagen, whereas keloids contain disorganized type I and type III collagen bundles. Keloids and hypertrophic scars have stretched collagen bundles aligned in the same plane as the epidermis, whereas collagen bundles are randomly arrayed and relaxed in normal scars. Keloid scars have thicker, abundant collagen bundles that form acellular nodelike structures in the deep dermis with a paucity of cells centrally. Hypertrophic scars, in contrast, contain islands composed of aggregates of fibroblasts, small vessels, and collagen fibers throughout the dermis.

Hypertrophic scars are often preventable. Prolonged inflammation and insufficient resurfacing (e.g., burn wounds) promote hypertrophic scarring. Scars perpendicular to the underlying muscle fibers tend to be flatter and narrower, with less collagen formation than when they are parallel to the underlying muscle fibers. Tension appears to signal the formation of activated fibroblasts resulting in excessive collagen deposition. The position of an elective scar can be chosen to induce a narrower, less obvious healed scar. As muscle fibers contract, the wound edges become reapproximated when they are perpendicular to the underlying muscle and tend to gape if placed parallel to it, leading to greater wound tension and scar formation.

Hypertrophic scars represent a reversible hyperproliferative scar phenotype that tends to regress when the original stimuli (skin tension, stimulatory growth factors) are removed. Keloids appear to be genetically predisposed and switched on irreversibly by factors such as TGF-β. In addition, in these scars, collagen synthesis is elevated, whereas collagen degradation is low. MMPs are also affected in these scars: MMP-1 (collagenase) and MMP-9 (gelatinase, early tissue repair) are decreased, whereas MMP-2 (gelatinase, late tissue remodeling) is significantly elevated. Blocking TGF-β activity with antibodies decreases scar fibrosis. Barnes and colleagues[3] demonstrated that increased mechanical stress at the wound bed promotes hypertrophic scaring by activating mechanotransduction pathways. Targeting these pathways may reduce excessive scarring and fibrosis, and new prevention therapies at the molecular and genetic level may soon be available.[3]

Prevention of Hypertrophic or Keloid Scars

The three strategies that reduce adverse scarring immediately after wound closure are tension relief, hydration/occlusion, and use of taping/pressure garments. Wounds with greater tension (perpendicular to Langer lines) with excessive tension on closure and in certain anatomic locations (deltoid and sternal) are at a higher risk of adverse scarring. Scarring can be reduced by postsurgical taping of the wound for 3 months. Moisturizing lotions and moisture-retentive dressings (silicone sheets and gels) can reduce the thickness, discomfort, and itching and improve the appearance of the scar. After wound healing, water still evaporates more rapidly through scar tissue and may take more than a year to recover to preinjury levels. Silicone products may ameliorate evaporative losses and assist hydration of the stratum corneum. These strategies need to be employed soon after initial wound healing. Pressure garments should be used prophylactically in wounds that are wide (e.g., burns); these wounds may take more than 2 or 3 weeks to heal. Garments should be applied as soon as the wound is closed and the patient can tolerate the pressure.[4] Tejiram and colleagues[4] noted a significant decrease in collagen I and III levels as early as 1 week after initiation of pressure treatment. Avoidance of sun exposure and use of SPF 50+ sunscreens for 1 year postoperatively reduce scar hyperpigmentation and improve clinical appearance.

Linear Hypertrophic Scars

Early linear scar hypertrophy (e.g., after trauma or surgery) at 6 weeks to 3 months should be treated with pressure therapy. After 6 months, silicone therapy should be continued for as long as necessary if there is further scar maturation. Ongoing hypertrophy may be treated with intralesional corticosteroids (triamcinolone acetonide, 10–40 mg/mL) injected into the papillary dermis every 2 to

4 weeks until flat. This is the only noninvasive management option that has enough supporting evidence to be recommended in evidence-based guidelines. Approximately 50% to 100% of patients respond, and up to 50% experience recurrence. Adverse steroid effects include skin atrophy, hypopigmentation, telangiectasias, and excessive pain during injections. Injections should be limited to the scar itself to minimize adjacent fat atrophy.

Surgical scar revision may be considered for permanent linear hypertrophic scars present after 1 year. Simple resection and primary closure may be combined with adjacent tissue undermining, subcutaneous sutures, adjunctive Z-plasty, and postsurgical taping and silicone therapy.

Hypertrophic scars also can be seen in conjunction with a scar contracture. Scar contractures are abnormal shortening of nonmatured scars resulting in functional impairment, particularly if the scar is across a joint. Correction of a scar contracture generally requires surgery with Z-plasty, skin graft, or flap to release tension in the scar to restore function and reduce scar hypertrophy.

Widespread Hypertrophic Scars

Severe burns, mechanical trauma, necrotizing infections, wounds requiring more than 2 to 3 weeks to heal, or wounds healed with skin grafting require early application of silicone and compression therapy.[4] This therapy should be initiated as soon as the wound is closed and the patient can tolerate the pressure.

The mechanism of action of pressure therapy is poorly understood but may involve reduction of wound oxygen tension by occlusion of small blood vessels resulting in a decrease in myofibroblast proliferation and collagen synthesis. Pressure therapy is believed to act on cellular mechanoreceptors that are involved in cellular apoptosis and linked to the ECM. The increased pressure regulates apoptosis of dermal fibroblasts and diminishes hypertrophic scarring. In addition, sensory nerve cells transduce mechanical pressure into intracellular biochemical and gene expression, synthesizing and releasing different cytokines involved in the physiopathogenesis of proliferative scarring.[2,4]

Pressure and silicone therapy should be continued or intensified and combined with selective localized corticosteroid injections in resistant areas. Bleomycin, 5-fluorouracil (5-FU), and verapamil have been used as adjuncts to corticosteroid therapy. In a small pilot study, Losartan ointment (5%) was found to significantly decrease vascularity and pliability and improve scar quality after 3 months of treatment, with no recurrences in a 6-month follow-up.[5] More therapies are being investigated alone or in combination with conventional modalities.

Laser therapy, although invasive, is another useful adjunct to reduce scar thickness; resurface scar texture; and treat residual redness, telangiectasias, or hyperpigmentation. Hultman and colleagues[6] performed the first large-scale prospective study demonstrating remarkable improvement in signs and symptoms of hypertrophic burn scars after treatment with pulsed dye laser and CO_2 laser.

Early surgery is indicated for functional impairment. Burn scar contracture release procedures in the neck and axilla are best performed with flaps to improve functional and cosmetic outcomes further that may not be achievable with skin grafts. Widespread large hypertrophic scars may require serial excision or tissue expansion.

Keloids

First-line treatments include intralesional corticosteroid injections in combination with silicone dressings and pressure therapy. Intralesional 5-FU, bleomycin, and verapamil should be used in accordance with established treatment protocols. One study showed improved results when intralesional triamcinolone acetonide and 5-FU were used in combination compared with individual treatments.[7] Refractory cases after 12 months of therapy should be considered for surgical excision in combination with adjuvant therapy. Excision alone results in a high recurrence rate of 50% to 100% and potential enlargement of the keloid. Immediate postoperative electron beam irradiation or brachytherapy reduces recurrence rates by 50% to 95%. Hypothetically, it may be associated with radiation damage to adjacent tissues or induction of malignancy; however, literature has failed to prove significant association. Shin and colleagues[8] compared surgical excision with triamcinolone versus radiation therapy, and recurrence rates were found to be 15.4% and 14%, respectively. Another study demonstrated that surgical excision combined with intraoperative autologous platelet-rich plasma and postoperative radiation therapy lead to effective treatment of ear keloids with 6% recurrence rates.[9] Other potential therapies include cryotherapy, imiquimod, tacrolimus, sirolimus, bleomycin, doxorubicin, TGF-β, EGF, losartan,[5] verapamil, retinoic acid, tamoxifen, botulinum toxin A, onion extract, and skin tension-offloading devices, with limited evidence to date.

Although existing strategies for the management of hypertrophic scars and keloids are broadly similar, the histologic differences between the two scars suggest that, in the future, therapeutic approaches could be developed that are specifically tailored for these different types of scars. However, at the present time, there is no single proven best therapy for the management of these excessive healing scars, and the large number of treatment options reflects this (Table 6.3).

Chronic Nonhealing Wounds

By definition, chronic wounds are wounds that have failed to proceed through an orderly and timely reparative process to produce anatomic and functional integrity over a period of 3 months. In the United States, it is estimated that 3 to 4 million patients per year are at risk of developing diabetic ulcers, up to 2 million patients per year develop chronic leg ulcers secondary to venous insufficiency, and 2 to 3 million patients per year develop pressure ulcers secondary to immobility. These numbers have been increasing as a result of an aging population and the rising incidence of risk factors for atherosclerotic disease, such as diabetes mellitus and smoking. These wounds are a significant challenge to health care professionals and an immense burden on health care systems and the economy. Patients also report reduced quality of life and social isolation.

Numerous common factors promote adverse wound healing conditions (see Fig. 6.1). Systemic factors, such as malnutrition, aging, tissue hypoxia, and diabetes, contribute significantly to the pathogenesis of chronic wounds. A combination of systemic and localized adverse wound factors collectively overwhelms the normal healing processes, resulting in a hostile wound healing environment (Fig. 6.7).

Chronic wounds have derangements in the various stages of wound healing and have unusually elevated or depressed levels of cytokines, growth factors, or proteinases. Chronic wound fluid, in contrast to acute wound fluid, has been shown to have greater levels of IL-1, IL-6, and TNF-α; levels of these proinflammatory cytokines decreased as the wound healed. An inverse relationship between TNF-α and essential growth factors, such as EGF and PDGF, has been demonstrated.

Chronic wounds typically exhibit powerful proinflammatory stimuli, including bacterial colonization, necrotic tissue, foreign bodies, and localized tissue hypoxia. Tissue edema is significant, and the distance between capillaries is increased, reducing oxygen diffusion to individual cells. Chronic wounds typically have high bacterial counts, which stimulates an inflammatory host response

TABLE 6.3 Prevention and treatment options for keloids and hypertrophic scars.

MODALITY OR TREATMENT OPTION	RESPONSE RATE (%)	RECURRENCE RATE (%)	COMMENTS	STUDY DESIGN
Prevention				
Preventive silicone sheeting (postsurgery)	0–75	25–36	Multiple preparations available; tolerated by children; expensive; avoid on open wounds; poor study design	Review of multiple case studies
Postsurgical intralesional corticosteroid injection (triamcinolone acetonide [Kenalog], 10–40 mg/mL at 6-week intervals)	NA	0–100 (mean, 50)	Patient acceptance and safety; may cause hypopigmentation, skin atrophy, telangiectasia	Review of multiple case studies
Postsurgical topical imiquimod, 5% cream (Aldara)	NA	28	May cause hyperpigmentation, irritation	Case study
Postsurgical fluorouracil, triamcinolone acetonide, and pulsed dye lasers (best outcomes)	70 at 12 weeks	NA	Effective; may cause hyperpigmentation, wound ulceration	Clinical trial
First-Line Treatment				
Cryotherapy	50–76	NA	Useful on small lesions; easy to perform; may cause hypopigmentation, pain	Review of multiple case studies
Intralesional corticosteroid injection (triamcinolone acetonide [Kenalog], 10–40 mg/mL at 6-week intervals)	50–100	9–50	Inexpensive, requires multiple injections; may cause discomfort, skin atrophy, telangiectasia	Review of multiple case studies
Silicone elastomer sheeting	50–100	NA	Multiple preparations available; tolerated by children; expensive; poor study design	Review of multiple case studies
Pressure dressing (24–30 mm Hg) worn for 6–12 months	90–100	NA	Inexpensive; difficult schedule; poor adherence	Review of multiple case studies
Surgical excision	NA	50–100	Z-plasty option for burns; immediate postsurgical treatment needed to prevent regrowth	Review of multiple case studies
Combined cryotherapy and intralesional corticosteroid injection	84	NA	See benefits of individual treatments; may cause hypopigmentation	Case study
Triple-keloid therapy (surgery, corticosteroids, silicone sheeting)	88 at 13 months	12.5 at 13 months	Tedious; time-intensive; expensive	Case study
Pulsed dye laser	NA	NA	Specialist referral needed; expensive; variable results depending on trial (controversial)	Case studies
Second-Line and Alternative Treatment				
Verapamil, 2.5 mg/mL, intralesional injection combined with perilesional excision and silicone sheeting	54 at 18 months	NA	Repeated injections; limited experience; may cause discomfort	Clinical trial
Fluorouracil, 50 mg/mL, intralesional injection two to three times a week	88	0	Effective; may cause hyperpigmentation, wound ulceration	Review of multiple case studies
Bleomycin tattooing, 1.5 IU/mL	92, 88	NA	Effective; may cause pulmonary fibrosis, cutaneous reactions	Review of case study; control trial
Postsurgical interferon-α2b, 1.5 million IU, intralesional injection bid for 4 days	30–50	8–19	Expensive; may cause pruritus, altered pigmentation, pain	Review of multiple case studies
Radiation therapy alone	56 (mean)	NA	Local growth inhibition; may cause cancer, hyperpigmentation, paresthesias	Review of multiple case studies
Postsurgical radiation therapy	76	NA	Local growth inhibition; may cause cancer	Review of multiple case studies
Onion extract topical gels (Mederma)	NA	NA	Limited effect alone, better in combination with silicone sheeting	Prospective case study

Adapted from Juckett G, Hartman-Adams H. Management of keloids and hypertrophic scars. *Am Fam Physician.* 2009;80:253–260.
bid, Twice daily; *NA,* not available.

with PMNs expressing reactive oxygen species and proteases, resulting in a highly pro-oxidant environment. Disturbed oxidant balance is the likely key factor in the amplification and persistence of the inflammatory state in chronic wounds. In addition to direct cell membrane and ECM protein damage, PMN-derived reactive oxygen species, such as superoxide, hydroxyl radicals, and hydrogen peroxide, can selectively activate signaling pathways leading to the activation of transcription factors that control the expression of proinflammatory chemokines and cytokines such as IL-1, IL-6, and TNF-α and proteolytic enzymes such as MMPs and serine

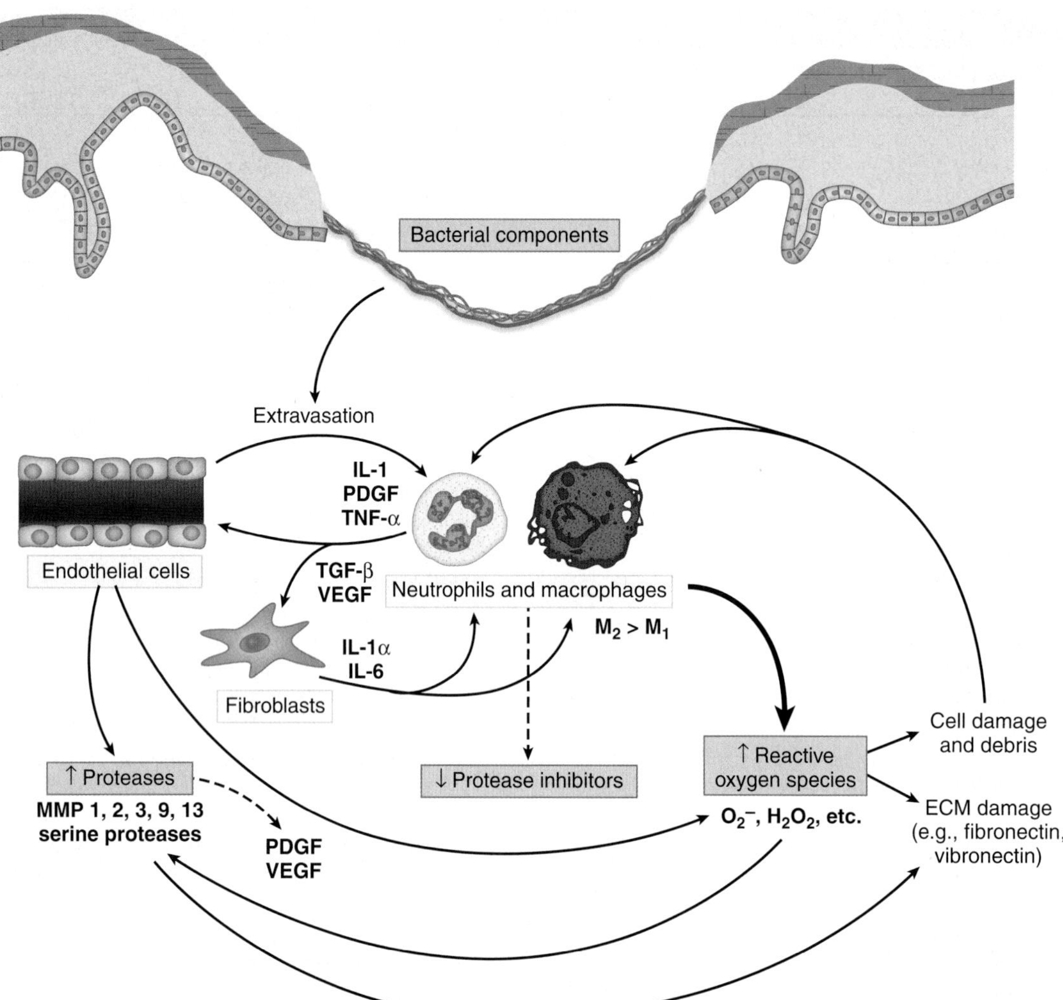

FIG. 6.7 Mechanisms involved in the development and persistence of chronic wounds. Chronic wounds do not adequately complete the "normal" phases of wound healing. A state of chronic inflammation develops as many of the cells recruited to the wound in the proliferative phase of healing adopt a proinflammatory secretory profile. Inflammatory cells, particularly neutrophils and macrophages (M_1 phenotype > M_2 phenotype), persist in the wound, creating a highly pro-oxidant, protease-rich environment with an abundance of proinflammatory cytokines such as interleukin-1 (*IL-1*), interleukin-6 (*IL-6*), and tumor necrosis factor-α (*TNF-α*). The result is a hostile environment with downregulation of protease inhibitors and direct damage to extracellular matrix (*ECM*), cellular components, and protective growth factors such as platelet-derived growth factor (*PDGF*) and vascular endothelial growth factor (*VEGF*). Reactive oxygen species and proteases, such as matrix metalloproteinases (*MMP-1, -2, -3, -9, -13*), are the most significant deleterious influences. *Solid lines* indicate upregulation, and *dashed lines* indicate downregulation. Width of the line is proportional to the effect of the influence. H_2O_2, Hydrogen peroxide; O_2^-, superoxide; *TGF-β*, transforming growth factor-β. (From Greaves NS, Iqbal SA, Baguneid M, et al. The role of skin substitutes in the management of chronic cutaneous wounds. *Wound Repair Regen.* 2013;21:194–210.)

proteases. Bacterial components, including formyl methionyl peptides and extracellular adherence proteins, may also contribute to the upregulation of the inflammatory response.

The amount of normal wound ECM is determined by a dynamic balance among overall matrix synthesis, deposition, and degradation. A defining feature of chronic wounds is unbalanced activity that overwhelms tissue protective mechanisms. Although activated keratinocytes, fibroblasts, and endothelial cells have been shown to increase the expression of proteases, incoming neutrophils and macrophages are considered to be the source of proteases, particularly cathepsin G, urokinase-type plasminogen activator, and neutrophil elastase. The expression and activity of gelatinases (MMP-2, MMP-9), collagenases (MMP-1, MMP-8), stromelysins (MMP-3, MMP-10, MMP-11), and membrane-type MMP (MT1-MMP) are upregulated in chronic venous ulcers.

Proinflammatory cytokines are potent inducers of MMP expression in chronic wounds, also reducing TIMP expression, resulting in a relative excess of MMP activity. For example, α_1-proteinase inhibitor, α_2-macroglobulin, and components of the ECM, such as fibronectin and vibronectin, are downgraded or inactivated within chronic wounds. Growth factors, such as PDGF and VEGF, are also targeted when there is excess protease activity.

Other proposed causes for wound chronicity include keratinocyte hyperproliferation at the periphery resulting in inhibition of fibroblast and keratinocyte migration and apoptosis. Fibroblasts have altered morphologies, slower rates of proliferation, and less

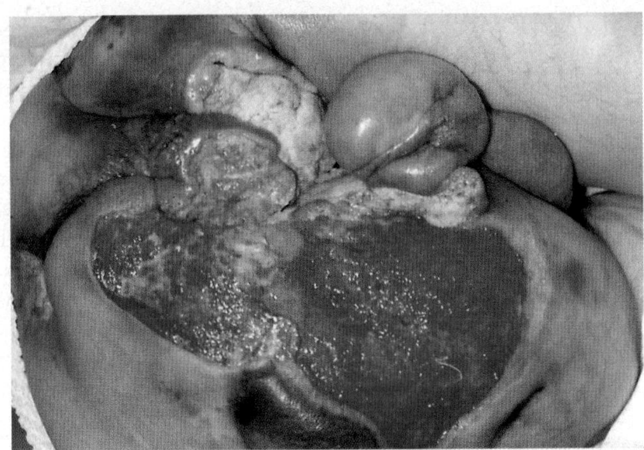

FIG. 6.8 Squamous cell carcinoma in a chronic pressure sore.

responsiveness to applied growth factors. The CD4/CD8 cell ratio is significantly lower in chronic wounds and is likely to be important in the pathogenesis of diabetic ulcers. Finally, chronic wounds have reduced levels of important growth factors (FGF, EGF, and TGF-β) likely secondary to degradation by excessive proteases or trapping by ECM molecules.

Chronically inflamed wounds are susceptible to neoplastic transformation. Squamous cell carcinoma (Fig. 6.8) was originally reported in chronic burn scars by Marjolin. Chronic osteomyelitis, pressure sores, venous stasis ulcers, and hidradenitis may also develop neoplastic change. Biopsies should be performed in cases of chronic wounds that appear clinically atypical. Cutaneous wounds may first exhibit pseudoepitheliomatous hyperplasia—a premalignant condition. Such a diagnosis on biopsy should prompt additional biopsies to exclude squamous cell carcinoma, which may already be present in other areas of the wound.

Other Causes of Abnormal Wound Healing

Hypoxia

Molecular oxygen is essential for collagen formation. Ischemia secondary to cardiac failure, arterial disease, or simple wound tension prevents adequate local tissue perfusion. Under hypoxic conditions, energy derived from glycolysis may be sufficient to initiate collagen synthesis, but the presence of molecular oxygen is critical for posttranslational hydroxylation of the prolyl and lysyl residues required for triple-helix formation and cross-linking of collagen fibrils. Although mild hypoxia stimulates angiogenesis, this essential step in collagen fibril assembly proceeds poorly when partial pressure of oxygen (Po_2) becomes less than 40 mm Hg. Optimal Po_2 for collagen synthesis may be present at the periphery of the wound, but the center may remain hypoxic.

The role of anemia in wound healing has long been attributed to be predominantly secondary to hypoperfusion. However, studies evaluating colonic anastomoses in a crystalloid-resuscitated hemorrhagic shock model demonstrated altered histologic parameters—decreased white blood cell infiltration, angiogenesis, fibroblast production, and collagen production, all contributing to delayed wound healing.

Tobacco smoking and consumption of tobacco products causes peripheral vasoconstriction and a 30% to 40% reduction in wound blood flow. Elevated levels of serum carbon monoxide inhibit enzyme systems necessary for oxidative cellular metabolism. Nicotine also inhibits platelet prostacyclin, promoting platelet adhesiveness, thrombotic microvascular occlusion, and tissue ischemia. Tobacco use inhibits endothelial cell and fibroblast function, NO synthase activity, VEGF production, fibroblast proliferation, collagen synthesis, and vitamin C levels. Studies in animals suggested that nicotine cessation for 14 days before flap surgery resulted in similar outcomes to controls, although most clinicians recommend complete smoking cessation in human patients for 4 to 6 weeks before elective procedures.

Diabetes

Diabetes mellitus impairs wound healing in several ways.[10] Diabetes-associated large vessel occlusion and end-organ microangiopathy each lead to tissue ischemia and infection. Diabetic sensory neuropathy leads to repeated trauma and unrelieved wound pressure. Tissue hypoxia can be demonstrated by reduced dorsal foot transcutaneous oxygen tension. The thickened capillary basement membrane decreases perfusion in the microenvironment, and elevated perivascular localization of albumin suggests increased capillary leak.[11] VEGF upregulation in patients with diabetes is also impaired. Hypoxia is normally a potent upregulator of VEGF, but cells from patients with diabetes do not upregulate VEGF expression in response to hypoxia.

Sensory neuropathy in patients with diabetes predisposes them to repeated trauma. They are susceptible to infection because of an attenuated inflammatory response, impaired chemotaxis, and inefficient bacterial killing. Infection further increases local tissue metabolism, placing an additional burden on the tenuous blood supply, amplifying the risk for tissue necrosis. Lymphocyte and leukocyte function are impaired. Collagen degradation is increased, whereas collagen deposition is impaired. Collagen is brittle secondary to glycosylation in the ECM. In addition, collagen glycation diminishes focal adhesion formation between fibroblast and matrix resulting in decreased fibroblast migration.

Hyperglycemia causes increased advanced glycation end-products, which induce the production of inflammatory molecules (TNF-α, IL-1) and interfere with collagen synthesis. High glucose exposure also results in changes in cellular morphology, decreased proliferation, and abnormal differentiation of keratinocytes. Decreased chemotaxis, phagocytosis, bacterial killing, and reduced heat shock protein expression impair the early phase of wound healing in patients with diabetes. Altered leukocyte infiltration and wound fluid IL-6 characterize the late inflammatory phases of wound healing in these patients. Growth factors are abnormally expressed and degraded rapidly in wound fluids as a result of increased insulin degrading enzyme activity. Insulin degrading enzyme activity in wound fluid is positively correlated with hemoglobin A_{1c} levels. Elevated MMP and reduced TIMP levels are seen in diabetic wounds in a pattern similar to chronic wounds. Finally, there is increasing evidence that resident cells in chronic wounds undergo phenotypic changes that render them senescent and impair their capacity for proliferation and movement.

Recent literature suggests genetic pathways that may play a role in the pathophysiology of diabetic ulcers and chronic nonhealing wounds.[11] Epigenetic alterations, including micro-RNA expression patterns, impair normal inflammatory mediators release; modulate macrophage, monocyte, and fibroblast function; and derange inflammatory response in diabetic wounds.[11]

Ionizing Radiation

Ionizing radiation has its greatest effect on rapidly dividing cells in phases G_2 through M of the cell cycle. Injury to keratinocytes and fibroblasts impairs epithelialization and formation of granulation tissue during wound healing. Radiation injury in endothelial cells results in endarteritis, atrophy, fibrosis, and delayed tissue repair. Repetitive radiation injury results in repetitive inflammatory responses

TABLE 6.4 Possible key wound-healing factors affected by radiotherapy with respect to the phases of wound healing.

PHASE OF WOUND HEALING	FACTORS AFFECTED BY RADIATION THERAPY
Inflammation	TGF-β, VEGF, IL-1, IL-8, TNF-α, IFN-γ
Proliferation	TGF-β, VEGF, EGF, FGF, PDGF, NO
Remodeling	MMP-1, MMP-2, MMP-12, MMP-13, TIMP

From Haubner F, Ohmann E, Pohl F, et al: Wound healing after radiation therapy: Review of the literature. *Radiat Oncol.* 2012;7:162. *EGF*, Epidermal growth factor; *FGF*, fibroblast growth factor; *IFN-γ*, interferon-γ; *IL-1, -8*, interleukin-1, -8; *MMP-1, -2, -12, -13*, matri 18 x metalloproteinase-1, -2, -12, -13; *NO*, nitric oxide; *PDGF*, platelet-derived growth factor; *TGF-β*, transforming growth factor-β; *TIMP*, tissue inhibitors of metalloproteinase; *TNF-α*, tumor necrosis factor-α; *VEGF*, vascular endothelial growth factor.

and ongoing cellular regeneration. Early side effects include erythema, dry desquamation, skin hyperpigmentation, and local hair loss. Late effects include skin atrophy, dryness, telangiectasia, dyschromia, dyspigmentation, fibrosis, and ulceration.[12–14] The inflammatory and proliferative phases may be disrupted by the early effects of radiation. Affected factors include TGF-β, VEGF, TNF-α, IFN-γ, and cytokines such as IL-1 and IL-8. These cytokines are overexpressed after the radiation injury, leading to uncontrolled matrix accumulation and fibrosis. NO, which induces collagen deposition, is decreased in irradiated wounds; this may explain the impaired wound strength seen in irradiated wounds. Decreased MMP-1 may contribute to inadequate soft tissue reconstitution (Table 6.4).

Keratinocytes, which are crucial for wound epithelialization, demonstrate a shift in expression from the high molecular keratins 1 and 10 to the low molecular keratins 5 and 14 after radiation injury. In nonhealing ulcers, these cells display decreased expression of TGF-α, TGF-β_1 FGF-1, FGF-2, KGF, VEGF, and hepatocyte growth factor (HGF). Expression of MMP-2, MMP-12, and MMP-13 has been shown to be elevated in irradiated human keratinocytes and fibroblasts. Fibroblasts play a central role in wound healing through deposition and remodeling of collagen fibers. However, in irradiated tissue, fibroblasts generate disorganized collagen bundles from dysregulation of MMP and TIMP. Because TGF-β regulates MMPs and TIMP, it may be of particular relevance to radiogenic ulcers (see Table 6.4).

Strategies for treating problematic radiogenic ulcers include standard wound care, negative pressure wound therapy, nutritional optimization, and optimized blood and oxygen delivery. Hyperbaric oxygen (HBO) therapy may improve tissue oxygen partial pressure in the treatment of osteoradionecrosis via increased capillary density and more complete neovascularization.[12,15,16] HBO therapy is used clinically in patients with chronic diabetic ulcers and wound-healing complications after radiotherapy, and randomized clinical trials have demonstrated efficacy when HBO therapy was used in conjunction with standard wound care in cases of recalcitrant, diabetic, and potentially radiation-induced wounds.[16,17] In recent years, we have seen further investigation in this area. For example, Wu and colleagues[14] demonstrated improved wound healing with injection of adipose-derived stem cells, centrifuged adipose cells, and other products extracted from adipose matrix in an irradiated mouse model.

Aging

Older patients are more likely to experience delayed healing and surgical wound dehiscence. The aging epidermis has fewer Langerhans cells and melanocytes and flattening of the dermal-epidermal junction. Keratinocyte proliferation is reduced, and the turnover time is increased by 50%. The dermis has fewer fibroblasts, macrophages, and mast cells; reduced vascularity; and less collagen and GAGs. There is a quantitative imbalance between collagen production and degradation and a qualitative alteration of the remaining collagen, which has fewer ropelike bundles and shows greater disorganization. Skin elasticity is decreased because of altered elastin morphology. Diminished light touch and pressure reduced nociceptive receptors together with dermal atrophy increase susceptibility to injury by mechanical forces. Immunosenescence (reduced Langerhans cells and fibroblast activity) impairs wound healing and increases the likelihood of chronic wounds. Microvascular disturbances predispose to ischemic ulcers. Finally, there is reduced sebum secretion and vitamin D_3 production.

Dysregulation of ECM components, including MMPs, decreased reepithelialization, depressed collagen synthesis, impaired angiogenesis, and decreased growth factors (especially proangiogenic FGF-2 and VEGF) have been seen in elderly animal studies. Impaired macrophage activity (reduced phagocytosis and delayed infiltration) and impaired B lymphocyte activity also have been demonstrated in animal studies. Zhao and colleagues[18] recently demonstrated the potential benefit in chronic application of antiaging agents, including metformin and resveratrol, via activation of AMP-activated protein kinase pathway in an elderly animal study.

Malnutrition

Protein catabolism delays wound healing and promotes wound dehiscence, particularly when serum albumin levels are less than 2.0 g/dL. Protein supplements can reverse this deficiency.

Vitamin deficiencies affect wound healing primarily as a result of their effect as cofactors. Delayed healing can occur 3 months after vitamin C deprivation and can be reversed by supplements of 10 mg/day and no more than 2000 mg/day. Deficiency of vitamin A impedes monocyte activation and deposition of fibronectin, affecting cellular adhesion, and impairs TGF-β receptors. Vitamin A contributes to lysosomal membrane destabilization and directly counteracts the effect of glucocorticoids. Vitamin K deficiency limits the synthesis of prothrombin and factors VII, IX, and X. Vitamin K metabolism is impeded by antibiotics; patients who have chronic or recurrent infections need to have clotting parameters checked before surgical procedures are performed.

Zinc is a necessary cofactor for RNA polymerase and deoxyribonucleic acid (DNA) polymerase. Zinc deficiency impairs early wound healing, but it is rare except with large burns, severe polytrauma, and hepatic cirrhosis. Iron deficiency anemia is a debatable cause of delayed wound healing. Although ferrous ion is a cofactor needed to convert proline to hydroxyproline, reports are conflicting regarding the effects of acute and chronic anemia on wound healing. In general, patients should have a well-rounded diet consisting of adequate protein intake and caloric value plus vitamin and mineral supplementation.

Drugs

Some exogenously administered drugs directly impair wound healing. Chemotherapeutic agents, such as doxorubicin (Adriamycin), nitrogen mustard, cyclophosphamide, methotrexate, and bis-chloroethylnitrosourea, are potent wound inhibitors in animal models and interfere with uncomplicated wound healing clinically. They reduce mesenchymal cell proliferation, platelet and inflammatory cell counts, and availability of growth factors, particularly if given preoperatively. Tamoxifen, an antiestrogen, decreases cellular proliferation, with a decrease in wound-breaking strength that is dose dependent and may be secondary to decreased TGF-β production. Glucocorticosteroids impair fibroblast proliferation and collagen synthesis, resulting in decreased granulation tissue formation. Furthermore, steroids stabilize lysosomal membranes. More recently, Jozic and colleagues[19] demonstrated that steroids inhibit keratinocyte migration and proper wound healing by activating a Wnt-like phospholipase/protein kinase C signaling cascade, which is present in several types of cells, including the skin. This mechanism may shed more light in stress-induced cellular dysfunction and impaired wound healing, providing potential for future targeted therapies.

Administration of vitamin A can reverse this particular effect. Diminished wound-breaking strength caused by exogenous steroids is time and dose related. High doses of nonsteroidal antiinflammatory drugs have been reported to delay healing, but doses in the therapeutic range are unlikely to have an effect.

Treatment of Chronic Wounds

The management of a chronic wound depends on its etiology.[20,21] Currently available therapies are slow, labor-intensive, and expensive without any guarantee of healing if all local and systemic factors are not addressed. Wound-healing research identified key structural proteins and molecules in normal and disordered wound healing as possible targets for future interventions. This research led to the application of topical growth factors to chronic wounds, which, although initially promising, almost universally failed to produce clinically significant improvements in wound healing. The reason for the failure is presumed to be a result of degradation of the growth factors by proteases in the wound fluid. This failure highlighted the complex nature of wound healing in which simply replacing one element is not enough.

Skin substitutes (discussed later) provide multiple factors that may alter the nature of the wound microenvironment in favor of and allowing healing to occur. Split-thickness skin grafting is the surgical substitution of native epidermis and partial dermis to assist wound closure, and it has a strong evidence base from treatment of acute burn wounds and chronic nonhealing wounds. Skin is harvested from the patient and transferred to an adequately prepared wound bed. The graft provides wound coverage by providing a favorable healing environment through exclusion of pathogenic bacteria and provision of ECM, cells (keratinocytes and fibroblasts), and bioactive molecules (cytokines, chemokines, and growth factors) that facilitate wound repair through a process of "dynamic reciprocity" (Fig. 6.9). However, autologous skin grafts occasionally are limited or unavailable. Biologic skin substitutes have been used for many years and include cadaveric skin allografts and porcine and bovine xenografts. These grafts are not durable because they do not integrate into the host, and they are associated with rejection and disease transfer. However, they provide adequate temporary wound cover, limiting complications until autologous grafts or other definitive management strategies are available.

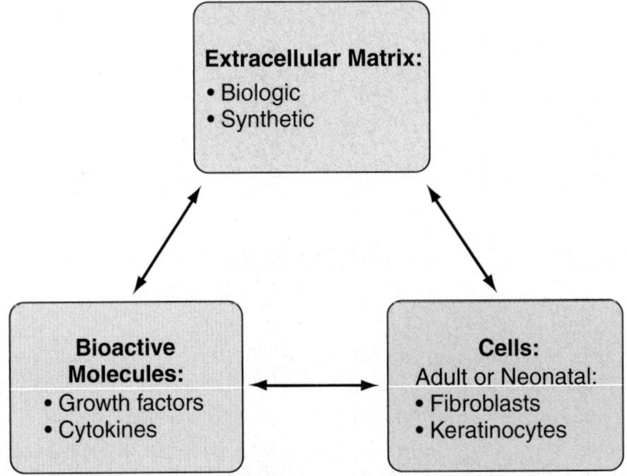

FIG. 6.9 The "dynamic reciprocity" model of wound healing. Interactions are dynamic as they vary with time and location within the wound site. Products of any one element influence the actions of the others. Inappropriate downregulation of any one element can result in conversion from an acute to a chronic wound. (From Greaves NS, Iqbal SA, Baguneid M, et al. The role of skin substitutes in the management of chronic cutaneous wounds. *Wound Repair Regen.* 2013;21:194–210.)

WOUND DRESSINGS

Wound dressings—present since antiquity—evolved very little for many years until 1867, when Lister introduced antiseptic dressings by soaking lint and gauze in carbolic acid. Since then, numerous more sophisticated products have become available; however, certain characteristics in wound dressings should be considered in the nonsurgical treatment of a wound (Box 6.2). Wound healing is most successful in a moist, clean, and warm environment. Not all dressings can provide all of these characteristics, and not all wounds require all of them; hence, the choice of dressing should match the prevailing wound conditions.[20,21]

Two concepts that are critical when selecting appropriate dressings for wounds are occlusion and absorption. Studies have demonstrated that the rate of epithelialization under a moist occlusive dressing is twice that of a wound that is left uncovered and allowed to dry. An occlusive dressing provides a mildly acidic pH and low oxygen tension on the wound surface, which is conducive for fibroblast proliferation and formation of granulation tissue. However, wounds that produce significant amounts of exudate or have high bacterial counts require a dressing that is absorptive and prevents maceration of the surrounding skin. These dressings also need to reduce the bacterial load while absorbing the exudate produced. Placement of a pure occlusive dressing without bactericidal properties would allow bacterial overgrowth and worsen the infection.

Dressings can be categorized into four classes: (1) nonadherent fabrics; (2) occlusive dressings; (3) absorptive dressings; and (4) creams, ointments, and solutions (Table 6.5). Briefly, nonadherent fabrics are fine-mesh gauze supplemented with a substance to augment their occlusive properties or antibacterial abilities, such as Scarlet Red, a relatively nonocclusive dressing that is impregnated with *O*-tolylazo-*O*-tolylazo-β-naphthol that is used on skin graft harvest sites in burn care. Xeroform is a relatively occlusive, hydrophobic dressing containing 3% bismuth tribromophenate in a petrolatum base, which helps mask wound odors and has antimicrobial activity against *Staphylococcus aureus* and *Escherichia coli.*

BOX 6.2 Characteristics of ideal dressing.

Creates a moist environment
Removes excess exudate
Prevents desiccation
Allows for gaseous exchange
Impermeable to microorganisms
Thermally insulating
Prevents particulate contamination
Nontoxic to beneficial host cells
Provides mechanical protection
Nontraumatic
Easy to use
Cost-effective

Adapted from Morin RJ, Tomaselli NL. Interactive dressings and topical agents. *Clin Plast Surg.* 2007;34:643–658.

TABLE 6.5 Types of dressings.

CATEGORY	COMPOSITION AND CHARACTERISTICS	FUNCTION	EXAMPLES	COMMENTS
Nonadherent fabrics	Fine mesh gauze with supplement to augment occlusive and nonadherent properties, healing-facilitating capabilities, and antibacterial characteristics	Protection, moist environment	Scarlet Red, Vaseline gauze, Xeroform, Xeroflo, Mepitel, Adaptic, Telfa	Scarlet Red, Xeroform, Telfa, Vaseline gauze—hydrophobic, more occlusive; Xeroflo, Mepitel, Adaptic—less occlusive, allow drainage of fluid into overlying dressing layers
Absorptive				
Gauze	Wide mesh gauze	Removal of exudates, prevention of maceration	Wide mesh gauze	Not effective when saturated; can be used for wound debridement if in contact with wound
Foams	Hydrophobic polyurethane sheets	Protection, absorption of exudate	Lyofoam, Allevyn, Curafoam, Flexzan, Vigifoam	Advantages—comfortable, can expand and conform to wound, easily removed for cleansing Disadvantages—need to be replaced as wounds heal, custom shapes are labor-intensive to make, limited protection from bacteria, cannot be used while bathing
Occlusive				
Nonbiologic		Insulation, moisture retention, protective barrier acts against bacteria		
Films	Clear polyurethane membranes with acrylic adhesive on one side	See above	Tegaderm, Mefilm, Carrafilm, Bioclusive, Transeal, Opsite	Waterproof; permeable to oxygen, carbon dioxide, and water vapor; do not interfere with patient function; allow visualization of wound; nonabsorptive, can leak; require intact skin around wound area; wound contraction may be slowed; removal may disrupt new epithelium
Hydrocolloids	Hydrocolloid matrix (gelatin, pectin, carboxymethylcellulose)	As above; absorbs water from wound exudates, swells, liquefies to form moist gel	Duoderm, NuDerm, Comfeel, Hydrocol, Cutinova, Tegasorb	Available as adhesive wafers, paste, powders; similar features as films, but bulkier; more protection, but may interfere more with function
Alginates	Cellulose-like polysaccharide fibers derived from calcium salt of alginate (seaweed)	As above; calcium alginate conversion to soluble sodium salt after contact with wound exudates results in hydrophilic gel	Algiderm, Algosteril, Kaltostat, Curasorb, Carasorb, Melgisorb, SeaSorb, Kalginate, Sorbsan	Occlusive environment; various forms—ropes, ribbons, pads
Hydrogels	Polyethylene oxide or carboxymethylcellulose polymer and water (80%)	As above; rehydrating agents for dry wounds; little water absorption (high water content)	Vigilon, Nu-gel, Tegagel, FlexiGel, Curagel, Flexderm	Available as gels, sheets, impregnated gauze; occlusive environment
Biologic		Similar to nonbiologics		
Homograft	Derived from genetically unique humans		Cadaver skin	Temporary dressing; is rejected if left on wound for extended period
Xenograft	Interspecies graft (e.g., pig)		Pigskin	Same as above
Amnion	Human placenta			Good biologic dressing
Skin substitutes	Different compositions		Integra, Alloderm, Apligraf, Biobrane, Transcyte	Integra—bilayered membrane skin substitute; AlloDerm—acellular cadaveric dermis; Apligraf—living, bilayered, biologic dressing composed of neonatal dermal fibroblasts on collagen matrix

Continued

TABLE 6.5 Types of dressings.—cont'd

CATEGORY	COMPOSITION AND CHARACTERISTICS	FUNCTION	EXAMPLES	COMMENTS
Creams, Ointments, and Solutions				
Antibacterial	Different compositions	Used to treat infected wounds	Acetic acid (gram-negative, *Pseudomonas*); Dakin's solution (broad antibacterial spectrum); iodine-containing antibacterials (Iodosorb, Iodoflex, Betadine; broad antibacterial and antifungal spectrum); silver nitrate (broad antibacterial spectrum); mafenide acetate (Sulfamylon; broad antibacterial spectrum); silver sulfadiazine (Silvadene; broad antibacterial, antifungal, and antiviral spectrum); Acticoat (broad antibacterial spectrum)	Acetic acid—impairs wound healing; Dakin's—toxic to fibroblasts; iodine-containing solutions—toxic to fibroblasts, impairs wound healing; silver nitrate—treats burns, slows epithelialization, hyponatremia, stains clothes black; mafenide acetate—penetrates eschar, painful application, inhibits reepithelialization, carbonic anhydrase inhibitor; silver sulfadiazine—transient neutropenia, accelerates epithelialization of partial-thickness burns, neovascularization, commonly used for burns; Acticoat—silver-impregnated occlusive dressing, antibacterial activity lasts 3 days
Antibacterial ointments	Different compositions	Used to treat infected wounds; soothing to apply; lubricates wound surface; occlusive; antibacterial activity lasts 12 hours	Bacitracin (gram-positive cocci and bacilli); neomycin (gram-negative) polymyxin B sulfate (gram-negative); Polysporin (polymyxin B, bacitracin); Neosporin (polymyxin B, bacitracin, neomycin); triple antibiotic ointment (polymyxin B, bacitracin, neomycin)	Neosporin—increased reepithelialization in experimental wounds by 25% compared with wounds with no dressing
Enzymatic	Different compositions; uses naturally occurring enzymes	Removal of necrotic tissue	Sutilains (derived from *Bacillus subtilis*); collagenase (Santyl; derived from *Clostridium histolyticum*); papain (derived from vegetable pepsin)	Sutilains—digests denatured collagen; collagenase—digests denatured and native collagen; papain—effective against collagen in presence of cofactor containing sulfhydryl group; addition of urea doubles enzymatic action of papain
Other	Normal saline wet to dry gauze dressing	Removal of necrotic tissue		Nondiscriminating—necrotic and newly formed granulation tissue and epithelium removed; can be painful

Adapted from Lionelli GT, Lawrence WT. Wound dressings. *Surg Clin North Am.* 2003;83:617–638.

Occlusive dressings provide moisture retention, mechanical protection, and a barrier to bacteria. These dressings can be divided into biologic and nonbiologic dressings. Examples of biologic dressings are allograft, xenograft, amnion, and skin substitutes. An allograft is a graft transplanted between genetically unique humans, whereas a xenograft is a graft, such as pigskin, transplanted between species. Allografts and xenografts are temporary dressings; both will be rejected if left on a wound for an extended period. Amnion is derived from human placentas and is another effective biologic wound dressing. Initially, these dressings were most often used in the treatment of burn wounds; however, they can be used as a temporary measure in other wounds.

Absorptive dressings are useful for wounds with a significant amount of exudate. Leg ulcers can produce 12 g/10 cm^2/24 hours of exudate. Examples include wide-mesh gauze, the oldest of this type of dressing, which loses its effectiveness when saturated and newer materials such as foam dressings, which provide the absorbent qualities for removing large quantities of exudate and have a nonadherent quality to prevent disruption of newly formed granulation tissue on removal. Examples include Lyofoam (ConvaTec, Skillman, NJ), Allevyn (Smith & Nephew, Largo, FL), and Curafoam (Kendall Company, Mansfield, MA). Wound healing beneath absorptive dressings appears to be slower than under occlusive dressings, possibly because of wicking of cytokines from the wound bed or decreased keratinocyte migration.

The final class of wound dressings consists of creams, ointments, and solutions. This is a broad category that extends from traditional materials, such as zinc oxide paste to preparations containing growth factors. Various categories include dressings with antibacterial properties such as acetic acid, Dakin solution, silver nitrate, mafenide (Sulfamylon), silver sulfadiazine (Silvadene), iodine-containing ointments (Iodosorb), and bacitracin. Application of these products is indicated when clinical signs of infection are present or if quantitative culture demonstrates more than 10^5 organisms per gram of tissue.

The number of available wound products is constantly growing so that the surgeon must have information about available dressings to allow effective wound management (Box 6.3).

OTHER THERAPIES

Hyperbaric Oxygen Therapy

Wound ischemia is the most common cause of wound-healing failure. HBO therapy uses oxygen as a drug and the hyperbaric chamber

BOX 6.3 Dressing options for noninfected clean wounds.

Incisional wound
- Three-layer dressings
- Ointments
- Occlusive dressings

Partial-thickness wounds (e.g., abrasions, donor sites)
- No dressing (scab)
- Impregnated gauze
- Creams, ointments
- Occlusive dressings

Full-thickness wounds (e.g., pressure sores)
- Alginates or hydrogels—rarely applicable
- Creams, gels (e.g., Silvadene)
- Wet to dry dressing changes
- Vacuum-assisted closure device

as a delivery system to increase PO_2 at the target area. HBO therapy is used for myriad disease processes, including bacterial infections, decompression sickness, improvement of split-thickness skin graft take, flap survival and salvage, acute thermal burns, necrotizing fasciitis, chronic wounds, hypoxic wounds, osteoradionecrosis, and radiation injuries. There is evidence for treatment of chronic diabetic ulcers and radiation-induced wounds.[20,21] Ischemia or tissue hypoxia (PO_2 <30 mm Hg) significantly impairs normal metabolic activity and decreases wound healing by impairing fibroblast proliferation, collagen synthesis, and epithelialization. HBO therapy involves inhalation of 100% oxygen at 1.9 to 2.5 atm, which can increase tissue PO_2 10 times higher than usual. A higher PaO_2 is sufficient to supply the tissue with all its metabolic requirements, even in the absence of hemoglobin; this elevated level lasts for 2 to 4 hours after termination of HBO therapy and induces synthesis of endothelial cell NO synthase as well as angiogenesis. Oxygen has been reported to stimulate angiogenesis, enhance fibroblast and leukocyte function, and normalize cutaneous microvascular reflexes.

A recent animal study analyzed the effects of HBO therapy on rodent cells metabolism, angiogenesis, and wound healing in diabetic wounds.[22] Experiments showed increased proliferation of stem cells, upregulated angiogenesis, and improved wound healing capacity. Additionally, this study demonstrates that a combination of HBO treatment and stem cell therapy has a synergistic effect and may open new horizons in treatment of nonhealing wounds.[22]

Evaluation of the vascular supply to the target area is essential, and revascularization before HBO therapy is an essential prerequisite to HBO therapy. Patients will likely benefit from adjuvant HBO therapy if improvement in tissue oxygenation can be demonstrated in a hypoxic wound while breathing oxygen under hyperbaric conditions. Transcutaneous oxygen pressure ($tcpO_2$) is used to assess wound perfusion and oxygenation. A wound $tcpO_2$ less than 35 mm Hg in room air indicates a hypoxic wound. An in-chamber $tcpO_2$ of 200 mm Hg or more suggests potential benefit from HBO therapy.

HBO treatments for hypoxic wounds are usually delivered at 1.9 to 2.5 atm for sessions of 90 to 120 minutes each, with the patient breathing 100% oxygen during the treatment. Treatments are given once daily, five to six times per week, and should be given as an adjunct to surgical or medical therapies. Clinical evidence of wound improvement should be noted after 15 to 20 treatments.

Complications of HBO therapy are caused by changes in atmospheric pressure and elevated PO_2. Middle ear barotrauma, ranging from tympanic membrane hyperemia to eardrum perforation, is the most common complication. Pneumothorax (particularly tension pneumothorax) is far less common but potentially life-threatening. Other complications associated with increased PO_2 include brain oxygen toxicity, manifested by convulsions resembling grand mal seizures; oxygen lung toxicity, resulting from damage from oxygen free radicals to lung parenchyma and airways and ranging from tracheobronchitis to full-blown respiratory distress syndrome; and transient myopia. Absolute contraindications to HBO therapy are (1) uncontrolled pneumothorax, (2) current or recent treatment with bleomycin or doxorubicin (potential aggravation of cardiac and pulmonary toxicity), and (3) treatment with disulfiram (increases risk of developing oxygen toxicity).

Older small-scale randomized clinical trials had demonstrated that HBO is a useful adjunctive therapy for diabetic ischemic foot ulcers and reduces the rate of extremity amputation. Thistlethwaite and colleagues[23] performed a double-blinded randomized study in patients with chronic venous ulcers that demonstrated that HBO therapy can improve refractory healing but that patient selection is important. Patients with hypoxic periwound margins should have 4 weeks of high-quality wound care to achieve healthy wound bed and establish their wound healing trajectory.[23] A more recent multicenter randomized clinical trial (DAMO2CLES study) in Europe showed improved rates of limb salvage and wound healing 12 months after initiation of treatment and amputation-free survival, but the results were not statistically significant.[24] A systematic review of Cochrane Database in 2016 reviewed HBO therapy for chronic irradiated wounds and concluded that HBO therapy improves outcomes in patients that had undergone radiation in the head, neck, and anus and rectum area and reduces rates of osteoradionecrosis after teeth extractions.[16] However, the recommendations were based on small, underpowered studies, and further randomized studies were greatly needed to clarify the benefits of this costly therapy. These results, which concluded that HBO therapy may have promising results in chronic radiation-induced wounds, are consistent with a different systematic review by Borab and colleagues.[17] however, further evidence is required.

The European Consensus Conference on Hyperbaric Medicine in 2016 reviewed the available evidence in the effects of HBO therapy and concluded that it is indicated in open fractures with crush injury, prevention or treatment of osteoradionecrosis of the mandible, soft tissue radionecrosis (cystitis, proctitis), diabetic foot ulcers, and femoral head necrosis.[25] Additionally, the consensus agreed that there is weak evidence supporting the beneficial effects of HBO therapy in compromised skin grafts and flaps, ischemic ulcers, refractory osteomyelitis, extensive second-degree burns, and osteoradionecrosis to bones other than the mandible.[25]

Despite evidence suggesting potential benefit of HBO therapy on healing chronic wounds, its cost is high. Patients often travel long distances for daily treatments at great cost to themselves and their families. Although reported protocols for treatment of ischemic limb ulcers vary significantly, most involve a total cost of $15,000 to $40,000. HBO therapy is not recommended as a primary treatment for patients with uncomplicated diabetic or ischemic ulcers; however, in selected more complicated cases, HBO therapy may have a role.

Negative Pressure–Assisted Wound Therapy

One of the most significant discoveries in wound management in recent decades was the improvement in wounds with negative pressure–assisted wound therapy (NPWT) (Fig. 6.10). With this technology, the surgeon has options in addition to immediate

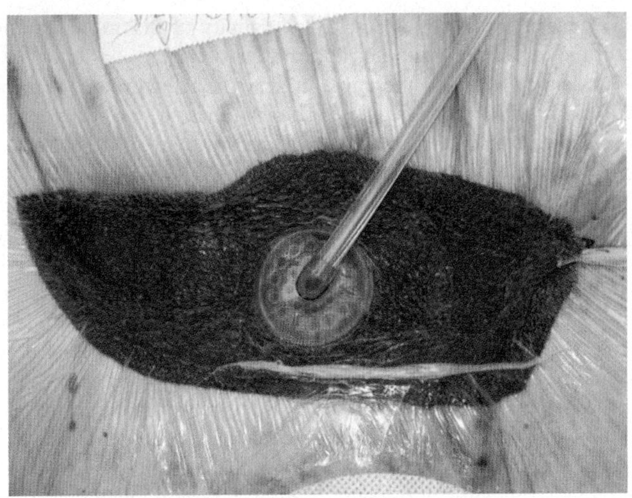

FIG. 6.10 Negative pressure–assisted wound closure sponge in place on a patient's abdomen.

closure of wounds (i.e., adjunctive therapy before or after surgery or an alternative to surgery in extremely ill patients).

Argenta and associates[26] originally described the use of negative pressure to assist in wound closure in 1997. By applying subatmospheric pressure to wounds, they demonstrated removal of chronic edema, an increase in local blood flow, and stimulation of granulation tissue. This technique may be used on acute, subacute, and chronic wounds. Additional studies demonstrated significant improvement in wound depth in chronic wounds treated with NPWT compared with wounds treated with saline wet to moist dressings. In addition, treatment with negative pressure results in faster healing times with fewer associated complications.[20,21,27]

The exact mechanism of the improvement in healing with NPWT has yet to be determined. Many investigators initially believed that the reason for increased wound healing is the removal of wound exudates while keeping the wound moist. As originally hypothesized by Argenta and associates,[26] with NPWT, there is a fivefold increase in blood flow to cutaneous tissues. Further studies showed an increase in capillary caliber and stimulated endothelial proliferation and angiogenesis. It is well known that increased bacterial loads result in slowed wound healing; however, despite increased wound healing with NPWT, it has been shown to result in increased bacterial counts. Other studies suggested that NPWT produces three-dimensional stress within the cells (microstrain) and across the whole area of the wound (macrostrain), resulting in changes such as increased cellular proliferation and higher microvessel density. Evidence suggests that NPWT alters wound fluid composition by removing potentially deleterious proteinases and inflammatory cytokines, such as MMP-1, MMP-2, MMP-9, and TNF-α.[27]

Clinical benefits of NPWT have been demonstrated in randomized controlled trials and include a decrease in wound volume or size, accelerated wound bed preparation and granulation tissue formation, accelerated wound healing, improved rate of graft take, decreased drainage time for acute wounds, reduction of complications, enhancement of response to first-line treatment, increased patient survival, and decreased cost. More recent data have demonstrated improved outcomes in patients with diabetic wounds, ischemic ulcers, and complex vascular, abdominal, gynecologic, and other oncologic surgical wounds with or without contamination. Karam and colleagues[27] performed a randomized controlled trial including a total of 40 patients with diabetic nonhealing ulcers. Pretreatment and posttreatment biopsies were obtained after 10 days of continuous therapy, and molecular analysis was performed. Results demonstrated that NPWT led to significant downregulation of IL-1β, TNF-α, MMP-1, and MMP-9 and significant upregulation of VEGF, TGF-β1, and TIMP-1 compared with advanced wound care with dressing changes. The authors concluded that NPWT significantly increased growth factors, decreased inflammatory cytokines, and normalized MMP activity, enhancing wound healing.

Additional to the improved outcomes, this treatment represents a significant improvement in cost-effectiveness and has decreased length of stay after acute and chronic wounds. There have been reports of a 78% decrease in hospital stay and a 76% decrease in cost with NPWT. This cost decrease and effectiveness of wound treatment with NPWT have translated to home health care treatment of Medicare patients.

NPWT with instillation has been another recent development. Evolution of the technology of this novel treatment method has allowed for creation and use of open-cell foam sponge that allows for periodic instillation of the wound bed with sterile fluid, facilitating removal of thick exudate and infectious products. The duration as well as time interval between each instillation can be adjusted based on the requirements of the wound. Different solutions have been used for instillation, including normal saline and dilute Dakin solution. Kim and colleagues[28] performed a prospective randomized study and concluded that there was no difference in the effectiveness of normal saline and an antiseptic solution (0.1% polyhexanide plus 0.1% betaine) in the treatment of infected wounds. Another technological improvement is the implementation of portable wound vacuum-assisted closure devices that are suitable for outpatient treatment. Additionally, the utilization of one-use disposable devices has become more popular recently. These devices do not require replacement of the dressing, typically last for a few days, and are particularly useful in the setting of incisional NPWT or treatment of relatively superficial wounds with low exudative fluid output.

FETAL WOUND HEALING

Fetal skin wounds heal rapidly without the scarring and inflammation characteristic of adult skin wounds. In adult cutaneous healing, dermal appendages (hair follicles, sweat and sebaceous glands) fail to regenerate. In addition, healed adult wounds have densely packed collagen bundles oriented perpendicularly to the wound surface, whereas collagen in uninjured and fetal skin retains a reticular pattern. Fetal wounds reepithelialize faster, with less neovascularization and a faster increase in strength. Fetal wounds differ in inflammatory responses, ECM components, growth factor expression, and biologic responses to growth factor expression. It was thought that fetal wound healing represented ideal tissue repair and that understanding fetal wound healing would provide surgeons the tools to regulate and control the different steps in adult wound healing.[29,30]

Fetal repair depends on gestational age and wound size. The wound size threshold (diameter of excised skin at which 50% of wounds heal without scarring at a given gestational age) appears to be 6 to 10 mm for 60-day-gestation and 70-day-gestation animals and 4 to 6 mm for 80-day-gestation and 90-day-gestation animals. Larger wounds may extend the time to healing and expose wound tissue to a different ECM and growth factor profile. Larger excisional wounds may also stimulate the formation of myofibroblasts resulting in scar formation. The transition from scarless to scarring repair occurs at the beginning of the third trimester. Wounds heal faster in a fetus than in a neonate, and they heal more slowly in adults compared with neonates.

Skin appendages are formed when dermal fibroblasts induce the epithelium to form hair follicles or glands. Wounds created early in gestation heal without scarring and with dermal appendages, suggesting tissue regeneration versus repair. In contrast, late-gestation wounds heal with scarring and without dermal appendages. The transition from scarless healing to healing without dermal appendages suggests that fetal fibroblasts lose their ability to induce the epithelium to form dermal appendages with advancing gestational age.

Extrinsic (amniotic fluid environment) and intrinsic (i.e., oxygen tension of the human fetus, differences in cellular receptors and growth hormones expression) properties between fetal and adult wound healing explain the difference in wound healing and scar formation.[30]

The fetal environment, an extrinsic difference between fetal and adult wounds, is characterized by a sterile hyaluronic acid–rich amniotic fluid with concomitant decreased inflammatory response. Additionally, the increased number of hyaluronic acid receptors and increased amount of hyaluronic acid may create a permissive environment in which fibroblast movement is facilitated, resulting in the increased rate and efficiency of fetal healing.

Much of fetal wound-healing research has recently focused on fetal fibroblasts and other intrinsic factors that are thought to play a more critical role. Fetal fibroblasts appear to have characteristics quite different from adult fibroblasts. Proline hydroxylation is a rate-limiting step in collagen synthesis by dermal cells. Early-gestation fetal human fibroblasts have increased prolyl hydroxylase activity that gradually decreases to adult levels after 20 weeks' gestation. Collagen types I, III, V, and VI appear earlier, and the ratio of type III to type I is greater in fetal wounds, which is consistent with the higher prevalence of type III collagen in normal fetal tissue. Fetal fibroblasts in vitro have higher collagen production than their adult counterparts. This higher collagen production may be secondary to the unique regulatory mechanism for prolyl hydroxylase and may explain why there is higher fibroblast activity in fetuses younger than 20 weeks' gestation.

Collagen synthesis decreases to adult levels after 20 weeks' gestation, and collagen degradation increases with gestational age. Increased gene expression of MMP-1, MMP-3, and MMP-9 correlates with the onset of scar formation in nonwounded fetal skin. These findings suggest that late-gestation fetal rat skin undergoes an adult type of tissue remodeling after wounding that leads to the scarring seen in adult skin.

There are also differences in the components of the ECM of fetal and adult wounds. After injury, fibronectin levels are similar in adults and fetuses, but tenascin, an inhibitor of fibronectin, increases earlier and returns to normal more rapidly in the fetus. Larger amounts of fibronectin in fetal wounds stimulate immediate cell attachment, whereas the more rapid deposition of tenascin in the fetus allows cells to migrate and fully epithelialize the wound more rapidly and decrease wound-healing time.

Hyaluronic acid is persistently elevated in fetal wounds. During gestation, decreasing levels of hyaluronic acid correlate with increasing scarring potential. The unique ECM composition of fetal tissues may influence collagen fibril deposition by facilitating cell mobility and migration, leading to the loose collagen pattern seen in healed fetal wounds as opposed to the dense collagenous pattern seen in adult scars. However, few studies have examined the effect of modifying the ECM components.

In addition, the fetus exhibits a reduced inflammatory response with a lack of neutrophil infiltration and decreased infiltration of endogenous immunoglobulins. The paucity of macrophages and a difference in the temporal appearance of macrophages in fetal wounds may explain differences in growth factor profiles and the reduced inflammatory response. These studies cite a direct correlation between increased macrophage recruitment in older fetuses and the development of increased scarring.

Fetal wounds have decreased levels of TGF-β and FGF-2. TGF-β is the growth factor that has been most extensively studied in fetal wound repair. Its production may be blunted in hypoxemic conditions, leading to the theory that the decreased oxygen tension in the fetal environment inhibits TGF-β production and results in decreased scar formation. It has been suggested that differential expression of the different TGF-β isoforms, rather than the presence of TGF-β, may be important in explaining the differences in repair.

Wnt signaling plays a significant role in embryogenesis as well as in multiple phases of wound healing.[29] This pathway is involved in tissue remodeling and repair, leading to scarring when dysfunctional. Several studies have also identified a link between Wnt signaling and TGF-β expression and function. Further insight into its mechanism of action and interaction with other pathways involved in wound healing may allow for therapeutic interventions toward decreased scarring and fibrosis.[29]

PDGF also disappears more rapidly in fetal wounds. The paucity of growth factors may be explained by decreased inflammatory cell recruitment. Normal inflammatory (adult-type) wound healing may have evolved to reduce the risk of infection at the expense of healing quality. Growth factor manipulation to make wounds more fetal-like has failed to result in completely scarless healing and has failed to regenerate dermal appendages. Other growth factors and cytokines have been proposed to play a role in fetal healing, including IGF, EGF, migration stimulation factor, TNF-α, and IL-1β.

The presence of myofibroblasts and concurrent scar formation suggests that a transition in fibroblast phenotype may contribute to scarring. Excisional wounds in 75-day-gestation fetal lambs showed an absence of scar formation and alpha smooth muscle actin expression. Alpha smooth muscle actin appears after 100 days of gestation along with scar formation.

Additional recent findings have highlighted the role of multiple pluripotent stem cells, such as epithelial stem cells, mesenchymal stem cells (MSCs), and "small dot" cells, in fetal wound healing. The slowly proliferating epithelial stem cells, which are interspersed throughout the basal layers, are surrounded by more quickly proliferating basal cells and their suprabasal progeny to form epidermal proliferative units. Epithelial stem cells are also found within the bulge area of hair follicles and are believed to migrate to the epidermis after injury and differentiate into dermal, vascular, and neural components.

MSCs play a role in regenerative healing, including immunomodulation, antifibrosis, antiapoptosis, and angiogenesis, as well as preventing excessive inflammation. They immunoregulate through multiple independent pathways, including the induction of IL-10 secretion by macrophages. "Small dot" cells also have been identified to play a role in fetal wound healing. There is a twenty fold greater increase of these cells in fetal blood than postnatal blood. Fluorescence-labeled "small dot" cells transplanted into a postnatal murine incisional wound model migrated to the wound bed and decreased scarring. Further investigations should help to elucidate the importance of these stem cell populations in fetal wound healing and in treating abnormal wound healing.

Finally, it has been shown that cells may lose their ability to replicate after certain stimuli, such as multiple cycles of duplication, exposure to subcytotoxic doses of exogenous stresses (ionizing radiation, oxidative agents, chemotherapeutic drugs, inflammatory cytokines, etc.), even though they remain metabolically active. This phenomenon is described as cellular senescence. Even though its role was initially identified to contribute to delayed wound healing in venous or diabetic ulcers, it is now believed that it may influence wound healing and tissue remodeling and potentially explain the differences between fetal and adult wound healing.[30]

Further investigations should help to elucidate the importance of these mechanisms and pathways in fetal wound healing and will allow for clinical application aiming to improve wound healing with decreased scarring (Table 6.6).[29,30]

TABLE 6.6 Comparison of fetal regenerative wound healing profile with postnatal wound healing.

	FETAL	POSTNATAL
Phenotype	Regenerative	Scar formation
Growth Factors		
bFGF	Lower	Higher
PDGF	Lower	Higher
VEGF	Higher	Lower
TGF-β		
$TGF\text{-}\beta_1$	Low levels	High levels
$TGF\text{-}\beta_2$	Low levels	High levels
$TGF\text{-}\beta_3$	High levels	Low levels
Inflammatory Response		
Inflammatory cell	Minimal	High levels leukocytes, macrophages, mast cells infiltrate
Cytokines		
Proinflammatory: IL-6, IL-8	Low levels	High levels
Antiinflammatory: IL-10	High levels	Low levels
Extracellular Matrix		
Collagen		
Histology	Fine, reticular weave	Thick, ropelike bundles
Type III collagen	High levels	Low levels
Deposition	Immediate	Delayed
Cross-linking	Low levels	High levels
$TGF\text{-}\beta_1$-stimulated deposition	Absent	Present
Hyaluronan		
Expression	High levels Persistent expression	Low levels Transient expression
Molecular weight	High	Low
HA receptors (fibroblast)	High levels	Low levels
Mechanical Force		
Myofibroblast (day 14)	Absent	Present
Stem Cells		
MSC	High levels	Lower levels
Dot cells	Present	Absent

From Leung A, Crombleholme TM, Keswani SG. Fetal wound healing: Implications for minimal scar formation. *Curr Opin Pediatr.* 2012;24:371–378.

bFGF, Basic fibroblast growth factor; *HA*, hyaluronan; *IL-6, -8, -10*, interleukin-6, -8, -10; *MSC*, mesenchymal stem cell; *PDGF*, platelet-derived growth factor; *TGF-β*, transforming growth factor-β; *VEGF*, vascular endothelial growth factor.

TISSUE ENGINEERING

In 1987, the National Science Foundation bioengineering panel defined tissue engineering as "the application of the principles and methods of engineering and the life sciences toward the development of biologic substitutes to restore, maintain, or improve function." These principles and methods have been used toward the creation of skin products made of cells, ECM components, or combinations of the two. This tissue-engineered skin has developed and progressed rapidly over the past 25 years, mainly driven by the limitations associated with autografts, and may function by providing the cellular or matrix components that could be necessary for wounds to heal. These new skin substitutes more accurately mimic native tissues to promote sustained healing without rejection. The use of biologic dressings, scaffolds, stem cell therapy, and gene therapy is an example of tissue engineering in which new tissues are created rather than transferred.

Bioengineered skin substitutes can potentially save millions of dollars a year for health care delivery services through reduced spending on dressings and treatment of wound-induced complications, particularly in the treatment of venous, diabetic, and pressure ulcers that form 90% of all chronic wounds. Bioengineered skin substitutes act as protective dressings by limiting bacterial colonization and fluid loss, but they also stimulate healing (Fig. 6.11). Their design is variable and dependent on the layer of skin they are designed to replace.

There are epidermal, dermal, and bilayer skin substitutes. Epidermal replacements are created by expansion of patient-derived keratinocytes in the laboratory.[31] These are fragile constructs that are attached to a carrier material to facilitate application to the wound. Dermal substitutes are based on a structural three-dimensional matrix material that behaves similar to ECM and may incorporate cells or bioactive molecules. Provision of these key factors to the wound bed may provide the necessary stimulus to rebalance the wound microenvironment in favor of healing. Bilayer materials represent a combination of features seen in epidermal and dermal models.

Skin substitutes can be utilized in the treatment of both acute and chronic wounds. This wide array of products have advantages and disadvantages. Some, such as Apligraf, are temporary, while others offer permanent wound coverage. However, like any medical device, a high cost is often involved. There is no one ideal skin substitute, making this an active realm of research.[31,32]

Although skin grafts can provide adequate permanent wound coverage, donor site morbidity, pain, scarring, and limitations in donor site locations have pushed researchers into the development of skin substitutes. One of the first major breakthroughs in tissue engineering for wound coverage was the development of Integra™. Integra™ is a bilayer substitute containing a silicone outer layer and a deeper layer consisting of bovine cartilage and GAGs. The outer layer can be removed after 2 to 3 weeks of application, and a split-thickness skin graft can be applied over the dermal component. It can be utilized for burn wound coverage and can be directly applied to tendon and bone.[32]

Regenerative medicine is playing a key role in new advances in wound care and has provided for the development of many other skin substitutes; these products have been found to advance reconstructive outcomes. These substitutes may be epidermal only or dermal only or may replace full-thickness skin. They also differ on how they are processed and whether they are animal or synthetically derived.[33] Many classification systems have been devised in the past in order to categorize the array of products available. Davison-Kotler and colleagues[34] proposed an updated system in 2018. Their system is based on five different characteristics: cellularity, layering, replaced

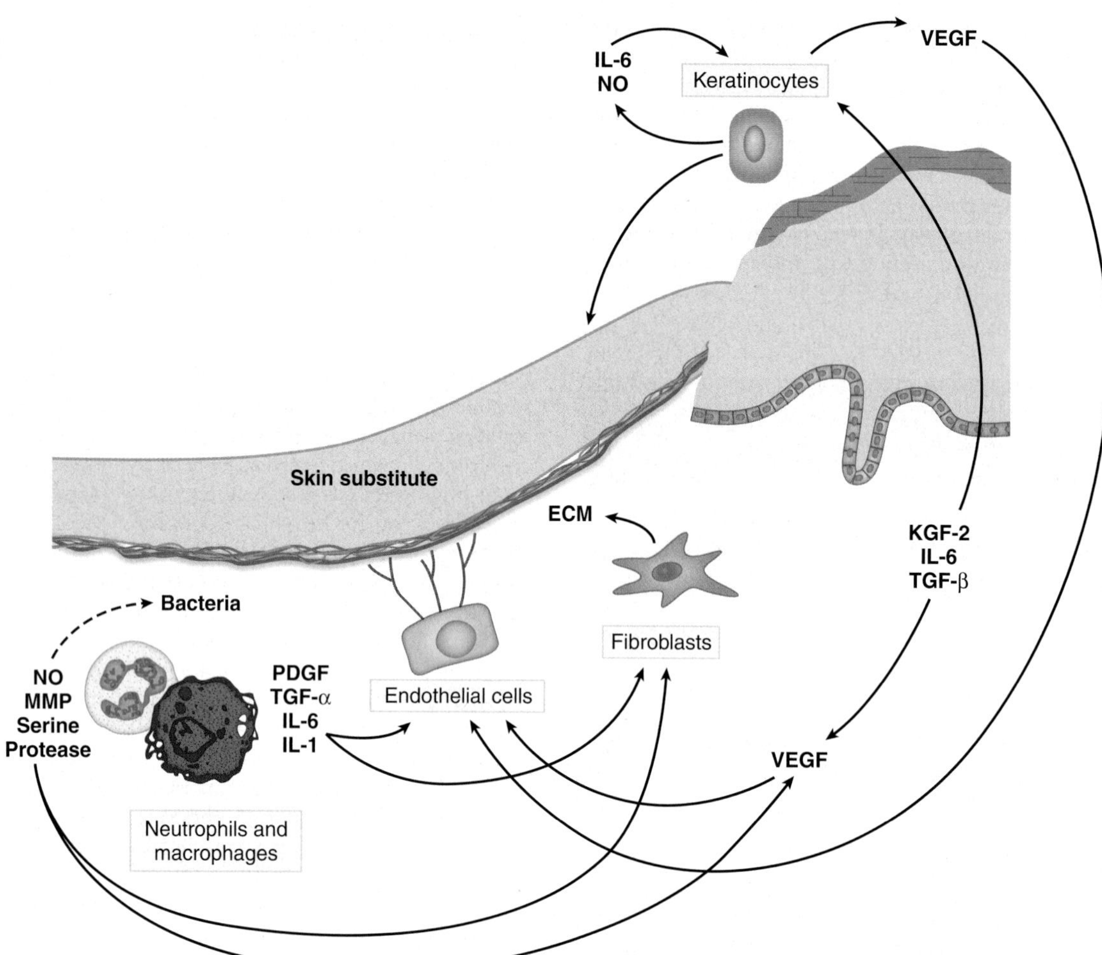

FIG. 6.11 The effect of skin substitutes in the wound bed. Skin substitutes have variable structures and cellular content. They may be cellular or acellular, but both forms induce the influx of endogenous cells, including fibroblasts, keratinocytes, endothelial cells, macrophages, and neutrophils into the wound bed. These cells secrete various cytokines and growth factors that stimulate angiogenesis, extracellular matrix (*ECM*) deposition, and reepithelialization via the process of dynamic reciprocity. The skin substitute is replaced by native tissues eventually resulting in a healed wound. *Solid lines* indicate upregulation, and *dashed lines* indicate downregulation. *IL-1*, Interleukin-1; *IL-6*, interleukin-6; *KGF-2*, keratinocyte growth factor-2; *MMP*, matrix metalloproteinase; *NO*, nitric oxide; *PDGF*, platelet-derived growth factor; *TGF-α*, transforming growth factor-α; *TGF-β*, transforming growth factor-β; *VEGF*, vascular endothelial growth factor. (From Greaves NS, Iqbal SA, Baguneid M, et al. The role of skin substitutes in the management of chronic cutaneous wounds. *Wound Repair Regen.* 2013;21:194–210.)

region, material, and permanence. Each product is described using these terms so that their exact nature is easily understood by clinicians. For example, Alloderm is an acellular, single-layer, temporary dermal substitute derived from cadavers; it has been used a great deal in breast reconstruction. On the other hand, Biobrane is an acellular bilayer that replaces full-thickness skin and is comprised of silicone, nylon mesh, and porcine collagen. It is placed on wounds until they have fully healed, at which point it is removed. EpiCel is an example of an epidermal-only substitute. It is a cellular product derived from autogenic keratinocytes.[34] One of the major drawbacks of cultured autografts is that they are extremely thin, susceptible to shearing forces, and experience a great deal of contraction.

Recent advances have been made with regard to epidermal-dermal substitutes and stem cells in the realm of burn treatment. Researchers found that skin debrided from burn patients contain living cells that can be cultured; cell lines with characteristics of MSCs can be created. Amini-Nik and colleagues[35] embedded these cells in a skin scaffold that was then used to treat wounds in immunocompromised mice and Yorkshire pigs. The experiment did not demonstrate any negative sequelae, and the cells promoted angiogenesis and reepithelialization.[35] Combining stem cell therapy with skin substitutes may pave the way for more individually tailored wound care treatments in the future

GENE AND STEM CELL THERAPY

Gene therapy has applications in wound healing, as well. The clustered regularly interspersed short palindromic repeats (CRISPR) system is utilized for gene editing. Originally a prokaryotic cell defense mechanism, this system has the potential to target human genes that encode growth factors and cytokines involved in the wound healing process. CRISPR can be utilized to upregulate these genes in an inducible manner.[36]

MSCs are multipotent undifferentiated cells that play major roles in wound healing. They are found in a variety of tissues, including the placenta, bone marrow, and fat. They have been found

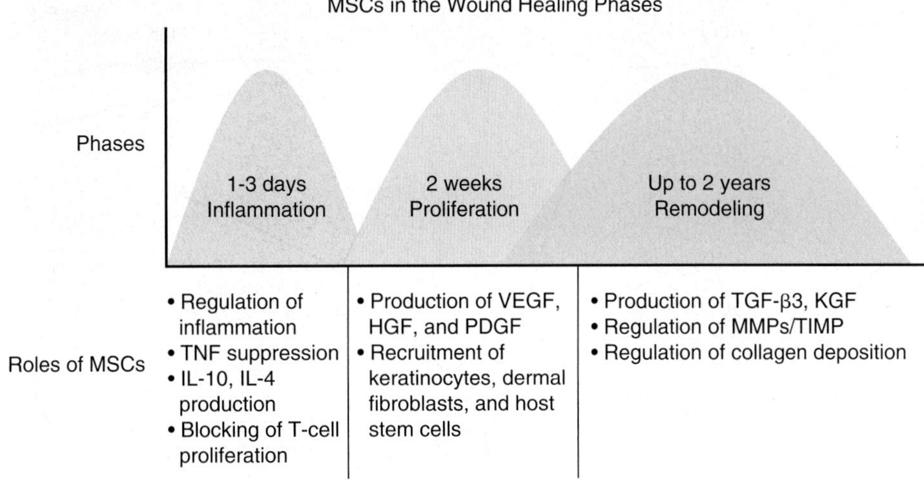

FIG. 6.12 Mesenchymal stem cell (*MSC*) roles in each phase of the wound-healing process. *HGF*, Hepatocyte growth factor; *IL-4*, interleukin-4; *IL-10*, interleukin-10; *KGF*, keratinocyte growth factor; *MMPs*, matrix metalloproteinases; *PDGF*, platelet-derived growth factor; *TGF-β3*, transforming growth factor-β3; *TIMP*, tissue inhibitors of metalloproteinase; *TNF*, tumor necrosis factor; *VEGF*, vascular endothelial growth factor. (From Maxson S, Lopez EA, Yoo D, et al. Concise review: role of mesenchymal stem cells in wound repair. *Stem Cells Transl Med.* 2012;1:142–149.)

TABLE 6.7 Functional classes of wound-healing proteins in human mesenchymal stem cell–containing skin substitutes.

SPECIFIC PROTEINS	PRIMARY FUNCTION
MMP-1, MMP-2, MMP-3, MMP-7, MMP-8, MMP-9, MMP-10, MMP-13	Matrix and growth factor degradation, facilitate cell migration
TIMP-1 and TIMP-2	Inhibit activity of MMPs, angiogenic
Ang-2, HB-EGF, EGF, FGF-7 (also known as KGF), PIGF, PEDF, TPO, TGF-α, IGF	Stimulate growth and migration
bFGF, PDGF-AA, PDGF-AB, PDGF-BB, VEGF, VEGF-C, VEGF-D	Promote angiogenesis, also proliferative and migration stimulatory effects
TGF-β3, HGF	Inhibit scar and contracture formation
IFN-α2	Prevent fibrosis by decreasing TGF-β1 and TGF-β2
α2-Macroglobulin	Inhibit protease activity, coordinate growth factor bioavailability
Acrp-30	Regulate growth and activity of keratinocytes
IL-1Ra	Antiinflammatory
N-GAL	Antibacterial
LIF	Support of angiogenic growth factors
SDF-1β	Recruit cells to site of tissue damage
IGFBP-1, IGFBP-2, IGFBP-3	Regulate IGF and its proliferative effects

From Maxson S, Lopez EA, Yoo D, et al. Concise review: role of mesenchymal stem cells in wound repair. *Stem Cells Transl Med.* 2012;1:142–149.
Acrp-30, Adiponectin; *Ang-2*, angiotensin-2; *bFGF*, basic fibroblast growth factor; *EGF*, epidermal growth factor; *FGF-7*, fibroblast growth factor-7; *HB-EGF*, heparin-bound epidermal growth factor; *HGF*, hepatocyte growth factor; *IFN-α2*, interferon-α2; *IGF*, insulin-like growth factor; *IGFBP-1, -2, -3*, insulin-like growth factor binding protein-1, -2, -3; *IL-1Ra*, interleukin-1 receptor antagonist; *KGF*, keratinocyte growth factor; *LIF*, leukemia inhibitory factor; *MMP-1, -2, -3, -7, -8, -9, 10, -13*, matrix metalloproteinase-1, -2, -3, -7, -8, -9, 10, -13; *N-GAL*, neutrophil gelatinase–associated lipocalin; *PDGF*, platelet-derived growth factor; *PEDF*, pigment epithelium-derived factor; *PlGF*, placenta growth factor; *SDF-1β*, stromal cell–derived factor-1β; *TGF-α*, transforming growth factor-α; *TIMP-1, -2*, tissue inhibitors of matrix metalloproteinase-1, -2; *TPO*, thrombopoietin; *VEGF*, vascular endothelial growth factor.

to mediate each phase of the wound-healing process (Fig. 6.12).[37] These cells coordinate inflammatory cell activity, inhibit the effects of proinflammatory cytokines, stimulate phagocytosis, and promote organized ECM deposition. Skin substitutes containing MSCs have been used to characterize the array of cytokines, growth factors, and chemokines needed to carry out normal wound healing (Table 6.7).[37] Epithelial cell stimulatory proteins (EGF, KGF), angiogenic proteins (VEGF), and antiscarring proteins (HGF) are among the signaling molecules produced by these cells. MSCs have the potential to be utilized as a therapy in the treatment of wounds because of their ability to interact with the cells surrounding the wound. They can express the trophic factors required for dermal wound healing in a regulated manner, thus reducing the fibrotic burden of the wound and improving scarring (Fig. 6.13).[38]

NEW HORIZONS

With advances in tissue engineering, there has been the development of a plethora of innovative wound care treatments aimed at stimulating the cells and chemical mediators needed for wound healing. These treatments include electrical stimulation, therapeutic ultrasound, and vibration therapy.[39]

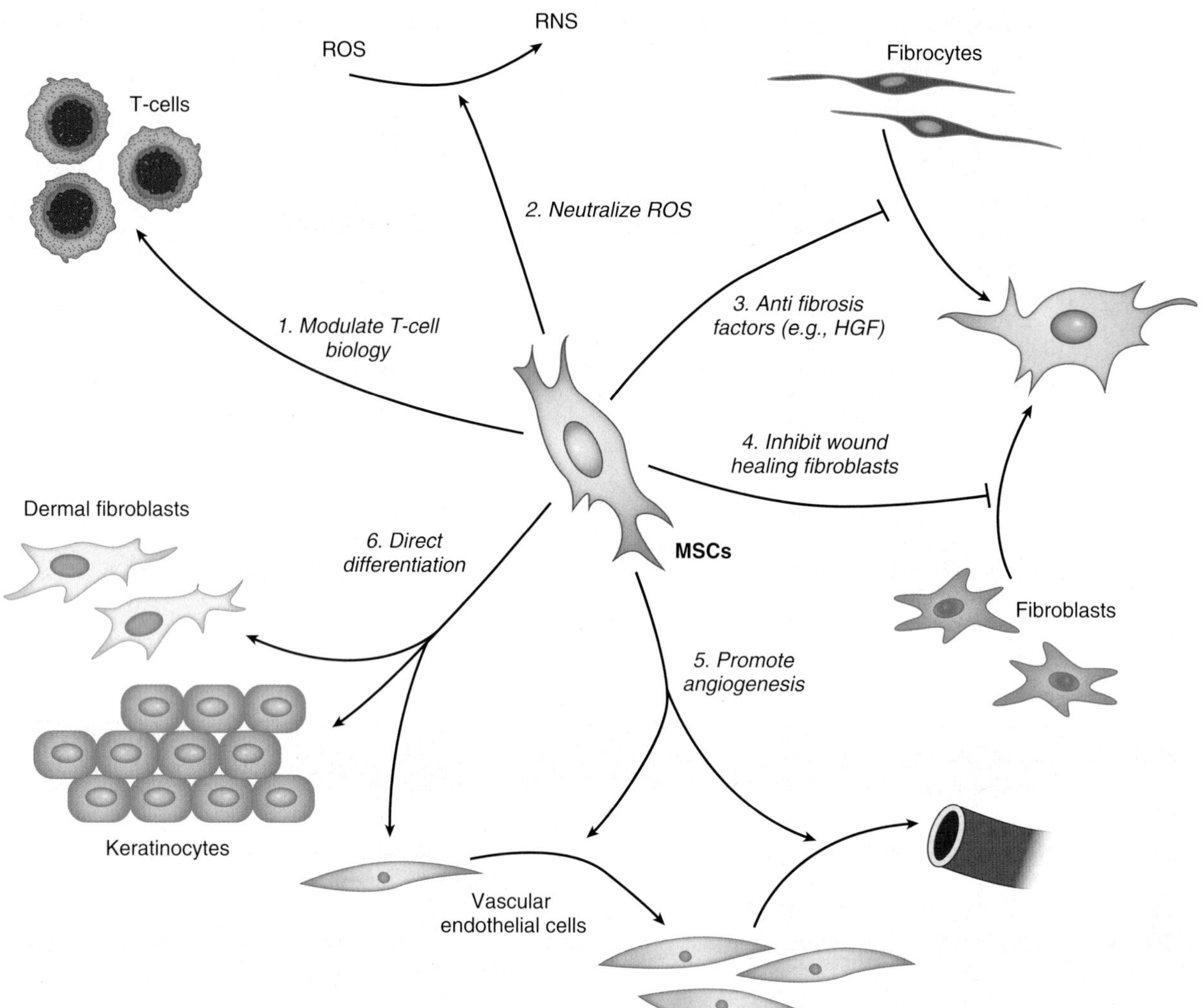

FIG. 6.13 Mesenchymal stem cells (*MSCs*) can influence cutaneous regeneration by multiple distinct mechanisms acting on multiple cell types. *HGF*, Hepatocyte growth factor; *RNS*, reactive nitrogen species; *ROS*, reactive oxygen species. (From Jackson WM, Nesti LJ, Tuan RS. Mesenchymal stem cell therapy for attenuation of scar formation during wound healing. *Stem Cell Res Ther.* 2012;3:20.)

Wounds carry a direct current electrical gradient that can be utilized to hasten the healing process. Biochemical studies have found that electrical stimulation alters gene expression; this then affects the production of chemokines, cytokines, and collagen, promoting an environment favorable for healing.[39] Pathways activated by electrical energy include those of intracellular polyamines, the PI3K/PTEN pathway, and the KCNJ15/Kir4.2 membrane channel.[40] Nguyen and colleagues[41] found that when human dermal fibroblasts are stimulated with electrical current in a bioreactor, collagen and MMP-1 levels increased within the cells.

Studies in humans have found that monophasic and biphasic pulsed currents have been effective, but microcurrents impregnated in dressings have not.[39] A pilot study conducted in a small sample of older adults with lower extremity pressure wounds found that patients treated with transcutaneous electrical nerve stimulation treatment plus standard wound care had significant improvements in pain and wound size, among other outcome measures, than standard wound care alone.[42] It is likely that electrical stimulation affects gene expression. When healthy volunteers were exposed to electrical stimulation via a small medical device over 2 days, the levels of expression of 105 genes were found to be changed; the majority had decreased protein production than prior to the treatment.[43]

Ultrasound, particularly kilohertz ultrasound, causes microstreaming and cavitation, which produces mechanical energy and alters the cell membrane through conformational changes in proteins and activation of signaling pathways in cells. It is believed that ultrasound therapy affects the proliferative phase of wound healing; among other effects, it increases macrophage activity and increases collagen production. Low-frequency ultrasound has been shown to decrease venous leg ulcer size in 4 weeks.[39]

Noncontact low-frequency ultrasound has been used in the treatment of venous, diabetic, and pressure wounds. When this modality was used in comparison to standard of care methods, bacterial burden was reduced and proinflammatory mediators were found to be decreased in the wounds, indicating that the treatment affects the body at a cellular level.[44]

On a clinical level, in a small study, sternal wound patients who underwent debridement with low-frequency ultrasound and vacuum-assisted closure had improved outcomes compared with those individuals who underwent vacuum-assisted closure alone. The patients who received the ultrasound debridement had shorter hospitalization stays, a shorter duration of time until they had negative cultures, a shorter length of antibiotic treatment, and a shorter amount of time between eradication and wound closure.[45] Unfortunately, there are few studies in the literature of higher level evidence that demonstrate clinical improvements with ultrasound therapy. For example, a randomized clinical trial comparing nonsurgical sharp debridement and low-frequency ultrasonic debridement in diabetic foot ulcers was ended early due to recruitment issues, and the results of their 10-patient study were not applicable to other, larger populations.[46]

Vibration therapy is another modality that may improve wound healing. It previously has been found to play a role in promoting angiogenesis in bone.[47] Low-magnitude, high-frequency vibration therapy was also found to recruit mesenchymal cells to fracture sites in rats with osteoporosis.[48] Mechanical stimulation in the form of high frequency acceleration has been found in a rat model to preserve alveolar bone after tooth extraction.[49] In a mouse model, low-intensity vibration was found to increase angiogenesis and granulation tissue 1 week after wound creation. The mice treated with the vibration therapy also had higher levels of IGF-1 and VEGF.[47] In humans, whole-body vibration may play a role in reducing pain of extremity burn patients. Ray and colleagues[50] conducted a randomized pilot study in which patients with 1% or greater burns to at least one extremity were randomized to receive whole body vibration therapy or standard of care treatment during rehabilitation. The researchers found that patients who received the therapy had less pain during and after their therapy sessions.[50] Although this study did not demonstrate an impact of vibration therapy on wound healing directly, it did demonstrate a potential benefit in the overall well-being of patients with burn wounds. Whole-body vibration therapy was also found, in a small-randomized study, to mitigate bone loss in pediatric burn patients.[51]

In 2016, Ennis and colleagues[39] published a review of the current literature regarding these treatment modalities and found that most studies were underpowered and inconclusive. There is a paucity of Level I data for electrical stimulation and ultrasound-guided therapy. However, the strongest evidence exists for the use of electrical stimulation therapy. It is often used as an alternative treatment once others fail, but the evidence is mounting to indicate its use more readily. Much more work needs to be done regarding the efficaciousness of these treatments and how to utilize them in clinical practice, but this is an area of active research.[39]

As the twenty-first century continues to unfold, wound healing will continue to be a major area of innovation and discovery. The field provides for the intersection of genetics, molecular biology, stem cell therapy, bioengineering, and complementary/alternative medicine modalities. Advances in these fields will ultimately translate to improved patient outcomes, a wider array of effective treatments, and the mitigation of chronic, recalcitrant wounds.

SELECTED REFERENCES

Davison-Kotler E, Sharma V, Kang NV, et al. A universal classification system of skin substitutes inspired by factorial design. *Tissue Eng Part B Rev*. 2018;24:279–288.

This article discusses a new classification system for the wide variety of dermal and epidermal substitutes.

Ennis WJ, Lee C, Gellada K, et al. Advanced technologies to improve wound healing: electrical stimulation, vibration therapy, and ultrasound—what is the evidence? *Plast Reconstr Surg*. 2016;138:94S–104S.

This article provides a review of the current literature regarding alternative modalities in wound healing treatment.

Hultman CS, Friedstat JS, Edkins RE, et al. Laser resurfacing and remodeling of hypertrophic burn scars: the results of a large, prospective, before-after cohort study, with long-term follow-up. *Ann Surg*. 2014;260:519–529; discussion 529–532.

This article describes a large, prospective trial in which laser therapy was used to treat hypertrophic burn scarring with extremely promising results.

Jones CM, Rothermel AT, Mackay DR. Evidence-based medicine: wound management. *Plast Reconstr Surg*. 2017;140:201e–216e.

This article from the plastic surgery literature discusses the basic science of chronic wounds, methods of wound preparation, dressings, and other modalities in wound care treatment, such as hyperbaric oxygen therapy and ultrasound.

Lucich EA, Rendon JL, Valerio IL. Advances in addressing full-thickness skin defects: a review of dermal and epidermal substitutes. *Regen Med*. 2018;13:443–456.

This article provides an up-to-date description of a variety of skin substitutes used in wound care treatment.

REFERENCES

1. Zhang L, Qin H, Wu Z, et al. Gene expression profiling analysis: the effect of hydrocortisone on keloid fibroblasts by bioinformatics. *J Dermatolog Treat*. 2019 Mar;30(2)200–205.
2. Zhang L, Qin H, Wu Z, et al. Identification of the potential targets for keloid and hypertrophic scar prevention. *J Dermatolog Treat*. 2018;29:600–605.
3. Barnes LA, Marshall CD, Leavitt T, et al. Mechanical forces in cutaneous wound healing: emerging therapies to minimize scar formation. *Adv Wound Care (New Rochelle)*. 2018;7:47–56.
4. Tejiram S, Zhang J, Travis TE, et al. Compression therapy affects collagen type balance in hypertrophic scar. *J Surg Res*. 2016;201:299–305.
5. Hedayatyanfard K, Ziai SA, Niazi F, et al. Losartan ointment relieves hypertrophic scars and keloid: a pilot study. *Wound Repair Regen*. 2018;26:340–343.
6. Hultman CS, Friedstat JS, Edkins RE, et al. Laser resurfacing and remodeling of hypertrophic burn scars: the results of a large, prospective, before-after cohort study, with long-term follow-up. *Ann Surg*. 2014;260:519–529; discussion 529–532.
7. Srivastava S, Patil A, Prakash C, et al. Comparison of intralesional triamcinolone acetonide, 5-fluorouracil, and their combination in treatment of keloids. *World J Plast Surg*. 2018;7:212–219.
8. Shin JY, Lee JW, Roh SG, et al. A comparison of the effectiveness of triamcinolone and radiation therapy for ear keloids after surgical excision: a systematic review and meta-analysis. *Plast Reconstr Surg*. 2016;137:1718–1725.
9. Jones ME, McLane J, Adenegan R, et al. Advancing keloid treatment: a novel multimodal approach to ear keloids. *Dermatol Surg*. 2017;43:1164–1169.
10. Armstrong DG, Boulton AJM, Bus SA. Diabetic foot ulcers and their recurrence. *N Engl J Med*. 2017;376:2367–2375.

11. Davis FM, Kimball A, Boniakowski A, et al. Dysfunctional wound healing in diabetic foot ulcers: new crossroads. *Curr Diab Rep*. 2018;18:2.
12. Oscarsson N, Ny L, Molne J, et al. Hyperbaric oxygen treatment reverses radiation induced pro-fibrotic and oxidative stress responses in a rat model. *Free Radic Biol Med*. 2017;103:248–255.
13. Fujita K, Nishimoto S, Fujiwara T, et al. A new rabbit model of impaired wound healing in an X-ray-irradiated field. *PLoS One*. 2017;12:e0184534.
14. Wu SH, Shirado T, Mashiko T, et al. Therapeutic effects of human adipose-derived products on impaired wound healing in irradiated tissue. *Plast Reconstr Surg*. 2018;142:383–391.
15. Ceponis P, Keilman C, Guerry C, et al. Hyperbaric oxygen therapy and osteonecrosis. *Oral Dis*. 2017;23:141–151.
16. Bennett MH, Feldmeier J, Hampson NB, et al. Hyperbaric oxygen therapy for late radiation tissue injury. *Cochrane Database Syst Rev*. 2016;4:CD005005.
17. Borab Z, Mirmanesh MD, Gantz M, et al. Systematic review of hyperbaric oxygen therapy for the treatment of radiation-induced skin necrosis. *J Plast Reconstr Aesthet Surg*. 2017;70:529–538.
18. Zhao P, Sui BD, Liu N, et al. Anti-aging pharmacology in cutaneous wound healing: effects of metformin, resveratrol, and rapamycin by local application. *Aging Cell*. 2017;16:1083–1093.
19. Jozic I, Vukelic S, Stojadinovic O, et al. Stress signals, mediated by membranous glucocorticoid receptor, activate PLC/PKC/GSK-3beta/beta-catenin pathway to inhibit wound closure. *J Invest Dermatol*. 2017;137:1144–1154.
20. Frykberg RG, Banks J. Challenges in the treatment of chronic wounds. *Adv Wound Care (New Rochelle)*. 2015;4:560–582.
21. Jones CM, Rothermel AT, Mackay DR. Evidence-based medicine: wound management. *Plast Reconstr Surg*. 2017;140:201e–216e.
22. Pena-Villalobos I, Casanova-Maldonado I, Lois P, et al. Hyperbaric Oxygen increases stem cell proliferation, angiogenesis and wound-healing ability of WJ-MSCs in diabetic mice. *Front Physiol*. 2018;9:995.
23. Thistlethwaite KR, Finlayson KJ, Cooper PD, et al. The effectiveness of hyperbaric oxygen therapy for healing chronic venous leg ulcers: a randomized, double-blind, placebo-controlled trial. *Wound Repair Regen*. 2018;26:324–331.
24. Santema KTB, Stoekenbroek RM, Koelemay MJW, et al. Hyperbaric oxygen therapy in the treatment of ischemic lower-extremity ulcers in patients with diabetes: results of the DAMO2CLES multicenter randomized clinical trial. *Diabetes Care*. 2018;41:112–119.
25. Mathieu D, Marroni A, Kot J. Tenth European Consensus Conference on Hyperbaric Medicine: recommendations for accepted and non-accepted clinical indications and practice of hyperbaric oxygen treatment. *Diving Hyperb Med*. 2017;47:24–32.
26. Argenta LC, Morykwas MJ. Vacuum-assisted closure: a new method for wound control and treatment: clinical experience. *Ann Plast Surg*. 1997;38:563–576; discussion 577.
27. Karam RA, Rezk NA, Abdel Rahman TM, et al. Effect of negative pressure wound therapy on molecular markers in diabetic foot ulcers. *Gene*. 2018;667:56–61.
28. Kim PJ, Attinger CE, Oliver N, et al. Comparison of outcomes for normal saline and an antiseptic solution for negative-pressure wound therapy with instillation. *Plast Reconstr Surg*. 2015;136:657e–664e.
29. Leavitt T, Hu MS, Marshall CD, et al. Scarless wound healing: finding the right cells and signals. *Cell Tissue Res*. 2016;365:483–493.
30. Pratsinis H, Mavrogonatou E, Kletsas D. Scarless wound healing: from development to senescence. *Adv Drug Deliv Rev*. 2019 Jun;146:325–343.
31. Dai C, Shih S, Khachemoune A. Skin substitutes for acute and chronic wound healing: an updated review. *J Dermatolog Treat*. 2020 Jan;30:1–10.
32. Haddad AG, Giatsidis G, Orgill DP, et al. Skin substitutes and bioscaffolds: temporary and permanent coverage. *Clin Plast Surg*. 2017;44:627–634.
33. Lucich EA, Rendon JL, Valerio IL. Advances in addressing full-thickness skin defects: a review of dermal and epidermal substitutes. *Regen Med*. 2018;13:443–456.
34. Davison-Kotler E, Sharma V, Kang NV, et al. A universal classification system of skin substitutes inspired by factorial design. *Tissue Eng Part B Rev*. 2018;24:279–288.
35. Amini-Nik S, Dolp R, Eylert G, et al. Stem cells derived from burned skin—the future of burn care. *EBioMedicine*. 2018;37:509–520.
36. Roh DS, Li EBH, Liao EC. CRISPR craft: DNA editing the reconstructive ladder. *Plast Reconstr Surg*. 2018;142:1355–1364.
37. Maxson S, Lopez EA, Yoo D, et al. Concise review: role of mesenchymal stem cells in wound repair. *Stem Cells Transl Med*. 2012;1:142–149.
38. Jackson WM, Nesti LJ, Tuan RS. Mesenchymal stem cell therapy for attenuation of scar formation during wound healing. *Stem Cell Res Ther*. 2012;3:20.
39. Ennis WJ, Lee C, Gellada K, et al. Advanced technologies to improve wound healing: electrical stimulation, vibration therapy, and ultrasound—what is the evidence? *Plast Reconstr Surg*. 2016;138:94S–104S.
40. Tai G, Tai M, Zhao M. Electrically stimulated cell migration and its contribution to wound healing. *Burns Trauma*. 2018;6:20.
41. Nguyen EB, Wishner J, Slowinska K. The effect of pulsed electric field on expression of ECM proteins: collagen, elastin, and MMP1 in human dermal fibroblasts. *J Electroanal Chem (Lausanne)*. 2018;812:265–272.
42. Garcia-Perez S, Garcia-Rios MC, Perez-Marmol JM, et al. Effectiveness of transcutaneous electrical nerve stimulation energy in older adults: a pilot clinical trial. *Adv Skin Wound Care*. 2018;31:462–469.
43. Lallyett C, Yeung CC, Nielson RH, et al. Changes in S100 proteins identified in healthy skin following electrical stimulation: relevance for wound healing. *Adv Skin Wound Care*. 2018;31:322–327.
44. Wiegand C, Bittenger K, Galiano RD, et al. Does non-contact low-frequency ultrasound therapy contribute to wound healing at the molecular level? *Wound Repair Regen*. 2017;25:871–882.
45. Tewarie L, Chernigov N, Goetzenich A, et al. The effect of ultrasound-assisted debridement combined with vacuum pump therapy in deep sternal wound infections. *Ann Thorac Cardiovasc Surg*. 2018;24:139–146.
46. Michailidis L, Bergin SM, Haines TP, et al. Healing rates in diabetes-related foot ulcers using low frequency ultrasonic debridement versus non-surgical sharps debridement: a randomised controlled trial. *BMC Res Notes*. 2018; 11:732.

47. Weinheimer-Haus EM, Judex S, Ennis WJ, et al. Low-intensity vibration improves angiogenesis and wound healing in diabetic mice. *PLoS One*. 2014;9:e91355.
48. Wei FY, Chow SK, Leung KS, et al. Low-magnitude high-frequency vibration enhanced mesenchymal stem cell recruitment in osteoporotic fracture healing through the SDF-1/CXCR4 pathway. *Eur Cell Mater*. 2016;31:341–354.
49. Alikhani M, Lopez JA, Alabdullah H, et al. High-frequency acceleration: therapeutic tool to preserve bone following tooth extractions. *J Dent Res*. 2016;95:311–318.
50. Ray JJ, Alvarez AD, Ulbrich SL, et al. Shake It Off: a randomized pilot study of the effect of whole body vibration on pain in healing burn wounds. *J Burn Care Res*. 2017;38:e756–e764.
51. Edionwe J, Hess C, Fernandez-Rio J, et al. Effects of whole-body vibration exercise on bone mineral content and density in thermally injured children. *Burns*. 2016;42:605–613.

7 CHAPTER

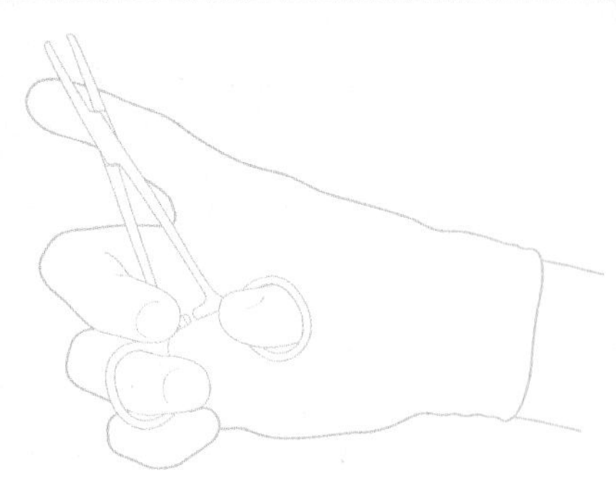

Regenerative Medicine

Mimi R. Borrelli, Michael S. Hu, Michael T. Longaker, H. Peter Lorenz

OUTLINE

Regenerative medicine is a continually developing field that combines the diverse disciplines of cellular and molecular biology, tissue engineering, and biomaterial science in order to design therapies to restore or maintain cells, tissue, and organs. While many other complex organisms retain the capacity to regrow limbs and repair organs throughout adult life, humans have traded in this regenerative potential for speed and strength of repair, which increases our vulnerability to scarring and its associated loss of functionality and aesthetic appeal. However, over the past decade, there has been tremendous progress toward the scientific underlying of stem cell biology and the clinical use of cell-based regenerative medicine to restore normal tissue and organ architecture and function. With continued success in clinical trials, tissue engineering has the potential to reduce the impact of organ shortages, donor site morbidity, and immune rejection, all of which are current limits to transplant surgeries. Developing technologies able to induce true tissue regeneration will enhance normal wound healing and minimize problematic repair through scarring. This chapter provides an overview of the current status of stem cell biology, tissue engineering, and clinical applications and describes the actions required to incorporate regenerative medicine into routine clinical practice.

STEM CELL SOURCES

Stem cells are undifferentiated cells characterized by their unique capacity for long-term self-renewal and the ability to differentiate into multiple specialized cell types under the appropriate conditions (Table 7.1). This potential to enter any desired differentiation program has made stem cells a strong focus of investigation within regenerative medicine. Traditionally, stem cells are classified as either pluripotent cells, which can differentiate into all three embryonic lineages (the ectoderm, mesoderm, and endoderm), or multipotent cells ("postnatal" or "tissue-specific"), which are more limited in their differentiation capacity and can only give rise to specialized cells of a specific tissue type (Fig. 7.1). Multiple stem cells have been investigated within regenerative medicine.

Embryonic Stem Cells

Embryonic stem cells (ESCs) are cells derived from the inner cell mass of the blastocyst prior to implantation. They are pluripotent and have an unlimited capacity for self-renewal and the ability to differentiate into any somatic cell type. In the past, ESCs were cultured with animal material (e.g., mouse fibroblast "feeder" layers), which supplied the necessary growth factors to maintain ESCs in an undifferentiated state. Recently, human ESCs, developed for clinical use, are cultured and maintained in serum- and feeder-free conditions and undergo extensive microbiologic testing as per recommendations from the International Stem Cell Banking Initiative. The U.S. Food and Drug Administration also requires documentation of the source, potential genetically modified components, and any pathogenic agents used for all ESC-derived cells intended for therapeutic use.

A number of human ESC cell lines have been derived from embryos carrying monogenic inherited diseases or chromosomal abnormalities, including Huntington disease and cystic fibrosis. These cell lines are used to model diseases, thus providing a better understanding of their etiology and pathophysiology.[1]

TABLE 7.1 Definitions of the different types of stem cells.

TERM	DEFINITION	EXAMPLES
Totipotent	Ability to form all differentiated cells in the embryo and extraembryonic tissue (e.g., placenta)	Zygote, morula
Pluripotent	Ability to form all lineages of the body but not extraembryonic tissue (e.g., placenta)	Embryonic stem cells (ESCs)—derived from the blastocyst inner cell mass
Multipotent	Adult stem cells that can form multiple cells in a particular cell lineage	Skeletal stem cells (SSCs)
Unipotent	Cells from one cell type	Osteocytes, chondrocytes

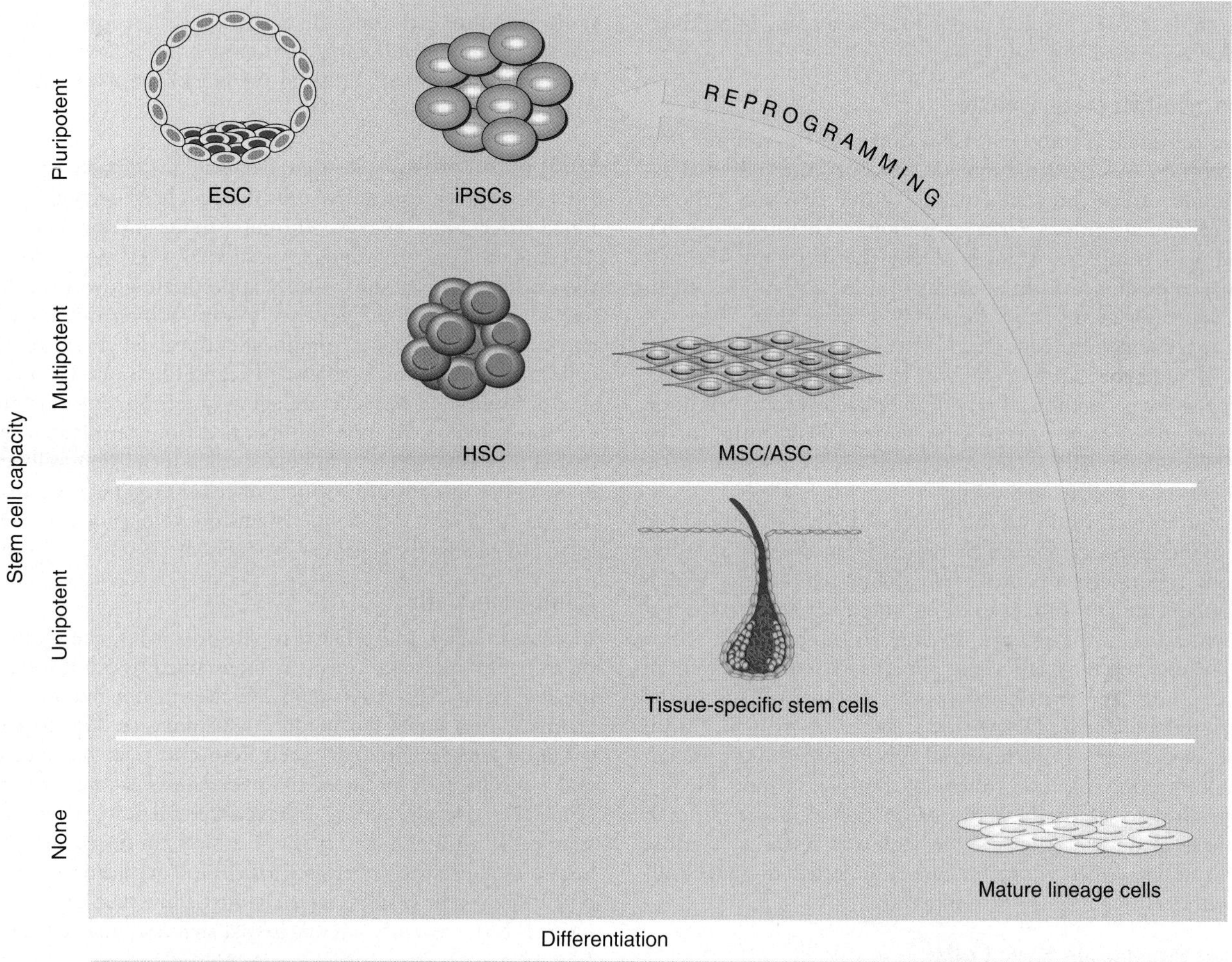

FIG. 7.1 Schematic of stem cell organization. Embryonic stem cells *(ESCs),* derived from the inner cell mass of the blastocyst, have the highest stem cell capacity (pluripotent) and are the least committed to any tissue lineage. Adult stem cells, such as hematopoietic stem cells *(HSCs)* and mesenchymal stem cells *(MSCs)*, have differentiation fates limited to certain tissue lineages (multipotent) and remain in a relatively undifferentiated state at rest but become activated upon injury. Tissue-specific stem cells, such as skin follicular bulge cells, are limited to producing a single cell and tissue type (unipotent) and retain considerable proliferative capacity to regenerate their specific tissue. Mature lineage cells, such as epithelial cells, do not have regenerative potential. Induced pluripotent stem cells (iPSCs) are mature lineage cells or adult stem cells that have been reprogrammed to a state of relative pluripotency and have much of the same regenerative potential as ESCs. *ASC,* Adipose stem cell.

Healthy human ESC lines have also been established in order to build cell banks that can differentiate into specific cells and tissues for reconstruction following congenital, traumatic, infective, or malignant lesions. Human ESCs are currently being investigated for the treatment of macular degeneration, cardiac diseases, and cancer.[1]

Research into the use of human ESCs for regenerative medicine has been met with significant technical, political, and ethical hurdles.[2] Despite a large number of human ESC lines established, only few peer-reviewed publications and a limited number of clinical trials have been conducted to date.[1] Blastomere harvesting has raised concerns that this process damages potentially viable embryos. Although there are now techniques to isolate single cells from cleaved-stage embryos, at which point there are sufficient remaining cells for embryogenesis to proceed unperturbed, these processes have failed to satisfy those in opposition.[1] Furthermore, the extensive pluripotentiality and capacity for unlimited self-renewal of ESCs put them at risk for dysregulated growth and tumorigenesis. In addition, the in vitro expansion of blastomeres required to transition to ESCs can profoundly alter their cellular and genetic biology and further predispose to tumor formation.[3] While undifferentiated ESCs do not provoke an immune response upon transplantation, this is not true for more differentiated cells derived from ESCs, which begin to express major histocompatibility complex (MHC) types 1 and 2. MHC matching is indicated when ESCs are used clinically.[4]

Somatic Cell Nuclear Transfer

Somatic cell nuclear transfer (SCNT) involves the transfer of a nucleus from a differentiated somatic cell containing a desired genetic profile into an enucleated ovum. Mitotic divisions of the resultant cell in culture lead to the generation of a blastocyst capable of yielding a complete organism. Dolly the sheep was the first mammal to be cloned from a somatic cell in 1997.[5] Since then, SCNT has been used to successfully clone more than 20 mammalian species, including monkeys. After significant optimization of SCNT protocols, human embryos have also been generated.[6] SCNT enables generation of genetically matched stem cell lines, which provides a huge potential for human therapeutics in the screening of potentially useful treatments and as a source of replacement cells for damaged organs.

Numerous technical hurdles, however, have also limited the use of SCNT for regenerative therapies. First, the resultant hybrid cells are imperfect copies of the donor cell nucleus, which may explain the abnormalities often noted in the extraembryonic tissues and, if the embryo is viable, in cloned animals after birth. Second, cloning efficiency remains extremely low in all species.[6] Third, the enucleated ovum contains mitochondrial deoxyribonucleic acid (DNA) that is genetically distinct from the nucleus donor's mitochondrial DNA, and this mismatch may risk immune rejection following transplantation.[7] Finally, there is also a scarcity of high-quality donor mature human metaphase II oocytes that are available for research.[8] Before SCNT can be applied widely in clinical practice, these technological limitations need to be addressed.

Induced Pluripotent Stem Cells

In 2006, Takahashi and Yamanaka made a major scientific breakthrough and identified a set of four transcription factors (Oct4, Sox2, KLF4, and cMyc—the "Yamanaka factors") able to reprogram mouse somatic cells (e.g., fibroblasts) back into ESC-like induced pluripotent stem cells (iPSCs).[9] Shortly after this discovery, in 2007, the first human iPSCs were generated from human fibroblasts.[10,11] iPSCs sparked a huge interest in the field of regenerative medicine given the ease and reproducibility with which they can be generated and the relative lack of ethical or political concerns. Autologous iPSCs can theoretically reduce the need for immunosuppression posttransplantation. iPSCs are also reported to be more tolerance-inducing than other transplanted cells (such as ESCs). This may permit extensive cell banking and the use of allogenic cells without the need for long-term immune suppression.[12] Since 2007, human iPSC technology has rapidly evolved, and human iPSCs are being used to model a variety of human diseases, develop cell therapies, and discover candidate drugs.[12] CRISPR-Cas9 technology has helped advance iPSC-based disease modeling by introducing disease-causing mutations to wild-type iPSCs and eliminating the same mutations in patient iPSCs.[12]

Although the first clinical trial using human iPSC products was launched in 2014,[13] the translation of human iPSCs to clinical trials has not been straightforward. The risk of tumorigenicity is a major concern, and genetic mutations in iPSCs in the first human iPSC-mandated trial suspension.[14] iPSCs, like ESCs, are maintained in culture for prolonged periods of time, which increases the risk of accumulating karyotypic abnormalities and of losing heterozygosity.[15] Methods to rigorously test and purify iPSC-derived products and to monitor the tumor formation following transplantation are topics of current investigation.[12] Preserving the self-renewing and pluripotent nature of iPSCs while eliminating tumorigenesis and directing the fate of these cells in vivo is a continuous challenge.

Fetal Stem Cells

Fetal stem cells are primitive cells that can been derived from fetal blood, liver, bone marrow, amniotic fluid, and placental tissue. They are similar in immunogenicity to ESCs but more restricted in their differentiation fates. Under appropriate growth conditions, fetal stem cells can differentiate toward adipogenic, osteogenic, and chondrogenic fates.[16] Significant ethical debate surrounds the collection and use of fetal tissue because the intrauterine collection of fetal blood can risk damaging or terminating a pregnancy. Currently, fetal stem cells are obtained from terminated fetuses, tissues that otherwise would be discarded. Fetal stem cells are unlikely to become a routine source of cells in regenerative medicine but may provide a means whereby future autogenous in utero cellular and genetic therapies can be devised.

Adult Stem Cells

In adult humans and other complex organisms, the regenerative capacity of tissues and organs is maintained by adult (or "tissue-specific") stem cells. Adult stem cells are multipotent and can differentiate into some, but not all, tissue lineages. Typically, differentiation fates are limited to cells found in their tissue of origin and are influenced by the microenvironment or "stem cell niche" (Fig. 7.2).[17] Despite a more limited differentiation, potential adult stem cells can be isolated without ethical concerns, and this has helped establish their relevance for clinical applications. Hematopoietic stem cells (HSCs) were the first adult stem cells to be described. More recently, mesenchymal stem/stromal cells (MSCs), adipose-derived stem/stromal cells (ASCs), and skeletal stem cells (SSCs) also have become the focus of research in the field of regenerative medicine. It is likely that many additional tissue resident stem cells soon will be discovered.

Hematopoietic Stem Cells

HSCs have been the most studied and best characterized adult multipotent stem cell since their definitive isolation in mice several decades ago. HSCs have subsequently served as the experimental paradigm for basic studies into the biology of all adult stem cells. HSCs are blood-forming cell that reside in specialized niches within adult bone marrow and function to maintain homeostasis of all lineages of hematopoietic cells throughout adult life. Transplantation of HSCs for hematologic diseases and malignancies remains the most widely used stem cell therapy to date. HSCs transplanted into patients with cleared bone marrow niches engraft and function to repopulate all lineages of the hematopoietic system.[18]

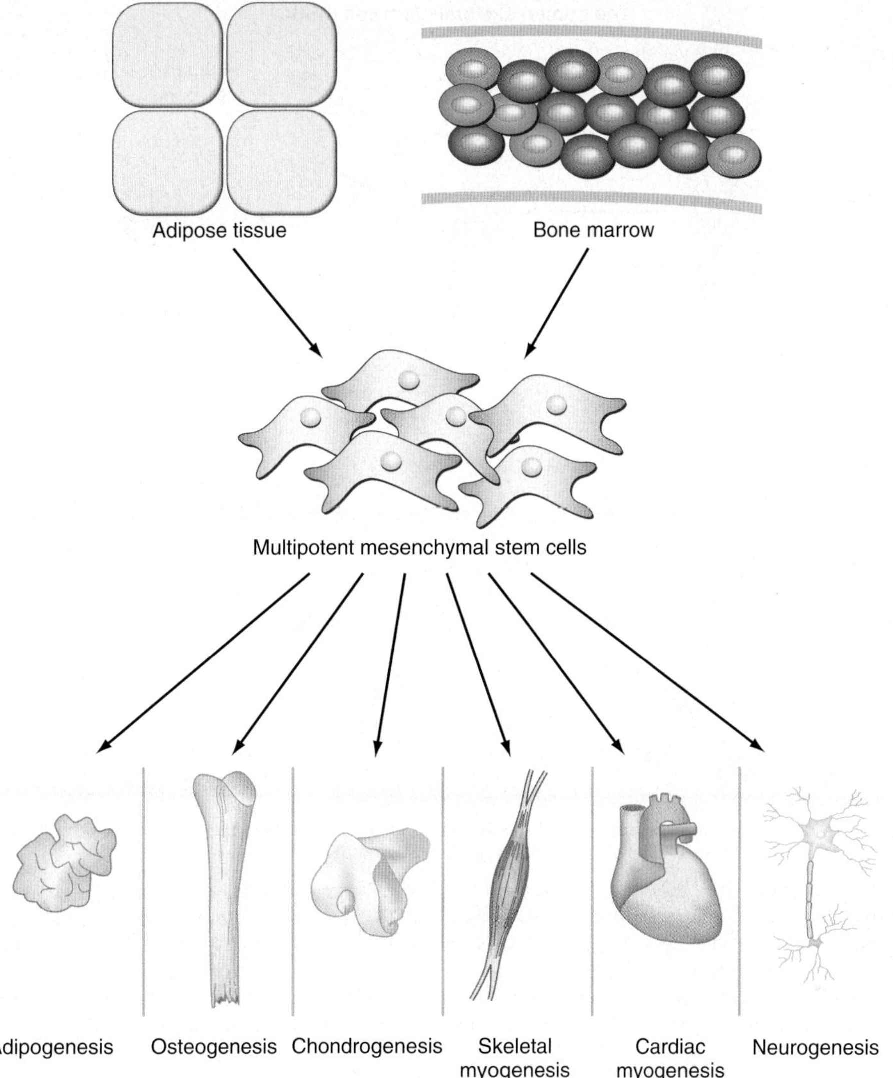

FIG. 7.2 Adult multipotent mesenchymal stem cells (MSCs) can be isolated from adipose tissue (adipose stem cells [ASCs]) or from bone marrow (MSCs). These cells have been shown to differentiate into multiple tissue types in vitro, including adipose (adipogenesis), bone (osteogenesis), cartilage (chondrogenesis), skeletal and cardiac muscle (skeletal and cardiac myogenesis), and nerve (neurogenesis) tissues. There has been varying success in experimentally differentiating these cells into these tissue types in vivo, a necessary step before adult multipotent stem cells can be used clinically for regenerative medicine applications.

Mesenchymal Stem/Stromal Cells

MSCs represent the collection of nonhematopoietic progenitor cells of mesodermal origin that have characteristic spindle shapes and can derive colonies from single cells ("colony-forming units-fibroblastic"). MSCs are considered immune-privileged[19] and able to generate various types of connective tissue cells, including osteoblasts, adipocytes, chondroblasts, fibroblasts, and pericytes,[20] which has made them attractive candidates for cell-based therapy. MSCs are thought to mediate their regenerative effects primarily through paracrine signaling, specifically the release of immunomodulators, antioxidant, antiapoptotic, angiogenic, and chemotactic agents.[21]

However, there have been substantial inconsistencies in the definition of MSCs and the methods of isolation. Because there are no well-defined universal surface markers to prospectively isolate MSCs, they have been typically isolated by their inherent ability to adhere to polystyrene tissue culture plastic, a nonspecific technique. The development of standardized definitions and isolation techniques is essential in the continued use of MSCs for regenerative medicine. Because of this heterogeneity, there is a growing trend toward using the term "MSC" as an umbrella for many tissue-specific multipotent stem cells with unique differentiation abilities.[22]

Bone Marrow–Derived Stromal Cells

Bone marrow–derived stromal cells (BMSCs), first isolated from the bone marrow in the 1970s, are a rare percentage (1 in 10,000) of the heterogeneous stromal fraction of adult bone marrow. Since this discovery, BMSCs have been a strong focus of research, but the relatively invasive methods of isolation and their low proliferation potential makes BMSCs not an attractive cell source for widespread clinical applications. Alternate sources of MSCs in different tissue types have therefore been investigated.

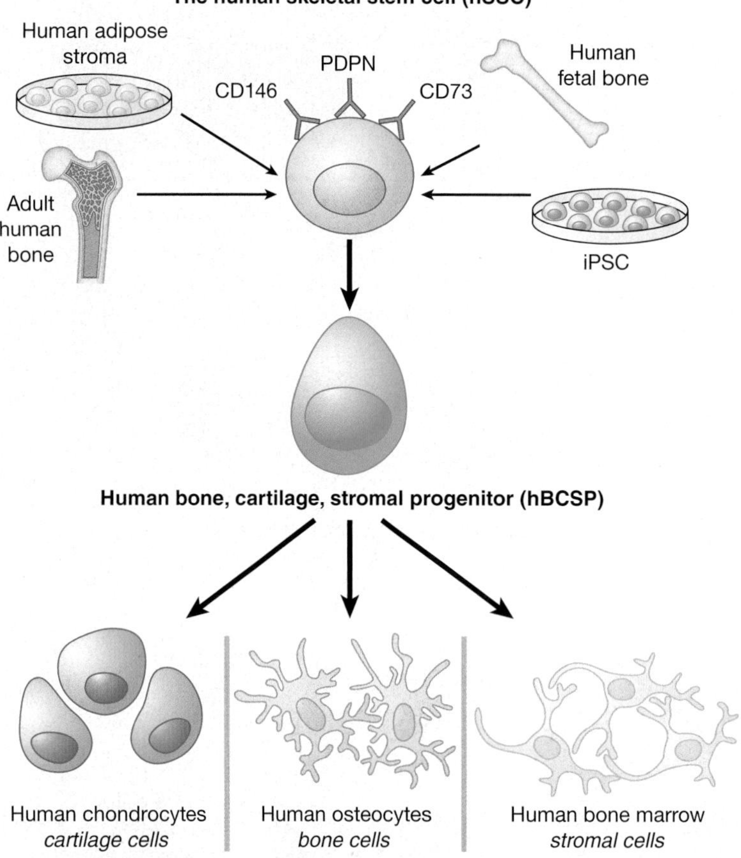

FIG. 7.3 Lineage map of the human skeletal stem cell *(hSSC)* and its downstream skeletal progenitor, the human bone cartilage stromal progenitor *(hBCSP)* cells. The hSSC can differentiate into chondrocytes, osteocytes, and bone marrow stromal cells. To date, the hSSC has been isolated from human fetal bones, human adult bones, induced pluripotent stem cells *(iPSCs)*, and adult human adipose stroma. hSSCs are identified by the presence of three surface antigens: cluster differentiation (CD)73, CD164, and PDPN (podoplanin). (From Chan CKF, Gulati GS, Sinha R, et al. Identification of the human skeletal stem cell. *Cell.* 2018;175:43–56 e21.)

Adipose Tissue–Derived Stem/Stromal Cells

ASCs are located within the stromal vascular fraction of adipose tissue and are attractive as stem cell candidates given their abundance and the ease with which they can be harvested. Furthermore, ASCs can differentiate into bone, adipose tissue, cartilage, and muscle in vitro[23] and have potent angiogenic, adipogenic, antifibrotic, and antiapoptotic potential in vivo.[24] Recent research indicates that ASCs are a heterogeneous mix of multiple stem and pluripotent stem cells, which remain to be further characterized.

Endothelial Progenitor Cells

Endothelial progenitor cells (EPCs) are cells expressing hematopoietic and endothelial surface markers found in the peripheral blood. Evidence indicates that EPCs enter the circulation in response to vascular injury and ischemia to participate in vasculogenesis. EPCs are thought to be mesenchymal in origin, but there are no widely agreed upon methods of isolation nor defining surface antigens to enable their prospective isolation.[25] Recent research has subcategorized EPCs into (1) myeloid angiogenic cells, which are hematopoietic derived and are unable to differentiate into endothelial cells, and (2) endothelial colony-forming cells, which can self-assemble into blood vessels and express vascular endothelial growth factor receptor 2, cluster differentiation (CD)146, CD31, E-cadherin, and von Willebrand factor (vWF).[26]

Skeletal Stem Cells

In the skeleton, a population of postnatal SSCs has been identified in both mice (mSSC)[27] and humans (hSSC).[28] These are self-renewing cells, which are up-regulated following fracture and are able to differentiate into bone, cartilage, and bone marrow stroma but not fat (Fig. 7.3). Specific combinations of niche factors can activate SSC programs in situ to form cartilage or bone and bone marrow stroma. These recent discoveries have huge implications in the future of cell-based therapies and their use in skeletal disorders such as osteosarcoma, fractures, and damaged cartilage.

Miscellaneous Adult Stem Cells

In recent years, resident pools of tissue-specific stem cells have been identified in a number of other organ systems, especially those with a high cell turnover and significant regenerative capacity. In the skin, epidermal stem cells are reported to reside in two general niches along the hair follicles in the bulge region deep to the sebaceous glands and in the deep interfollicular epidermis.[29] These multipotent epidermal stem cells are believed to maintain normal homeostasis of the epidermis and to regenerate the epidermis following trauma or injury. In the small intestine, a group of proliferative cells has been identified at the base of the crypts. These stem cells give rise to more differentiated cells, which migrate upward to repopulate the mature gut epithelium.[30] Other adult stem cells have also been isolated from organ systems that

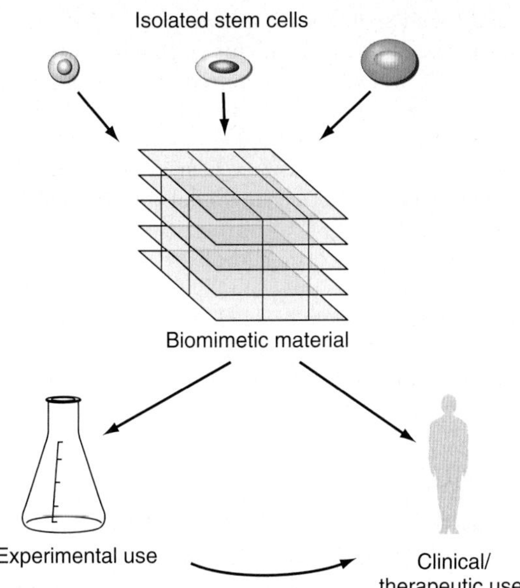

FIG. 7.4 Biomimetic materials are engineered to create favorable stem cell niches for in vitro experimental stem cell biology studies and for clinical use in regenerative medicine applications. All stem cells are exquisitely sensitive to environmental cues, and consequently, the bioengineering component of regenerative medicine is crucial in modulating and controlling stem cell behavior.

were previously thought to have little or no regenerative capacity, including cardiac,[31] muscle,[32] and neural tissue.[33] The role of these adult stem cell populations in local tissue homeostasis and organ regeneration remains to be investigated.

Stem Cells and Cancer

Mutations and dysregulation of endogenous stem cells is thought to underlie cancer biology.[34] Indeed, as stem cell–based therapy is adapted for clinical use, minimizing the risk of potential stem cell dysregulation and malignant transformation of therapeutic stem cells must be prioritized.

BIOENGINEERING FOR REGENERATIVE MEDICINE

Understanding the biochemical and biophysical factors that contribute to the success of regenerative medicine is essential for its widespread clinical application. Stem cells are exquisitely sensitive to their surrounding niche, which comprises surrounding cells (biochemical as well as biophysical processes like mechanotransduction, electrical fields, and temperature gradients).[17] Specific biochemical and biophysical factors likely affect specific stem cells and bias their differentiation fate. Substantial progress has been made in engineering to create a biomimetic microenvironment able to support engraftment, survival, and therapeutic function and to help direct stem cell fate (Fig. 7.4). "Regenerative rehabilitation" is an emerging field that combines regenerative medicine with rehabilitative principles, such as physiotherapy, to enhance the success of cell-based therapies.[35]

Biomaterials as Constructs for Cell Delivery and Cell Differentiation

Biomaterials have been designed as synthetic scaffolds that can facilitate stem cell survival, engraftment, proliferation, and retention.[35] Commonly used biomaterials include collagen polymers, polyglycolic acid, poly (lactic-co-glycolic acid), and polyethylene glycol hydrogels. These materials are porous to allow cell ingress and can be easily molded and shaped to a desired configuration. Three-dimensional (3D) bioprinting technology has helped to create versatile scaffolds with precisely defined biomimetic properties for cellular support and growth factor delivery, which has helped to bridge the disparity between artificially engineered constructs and native tissues.[36] While more effective delivery systems theoretically enable implantation of a relatively small number of stem cells, the development of stem cell–specific delivery systems able to mimic tissue physiologic extracellular matrix and promote directed proliferation and differentiation following delivery requires an in-depth understanding of the complex and idiosyncratic cell–cell and cell–matrix interactions and how they are modified in vivo by physical stimuli.[35] This research is in its early stages, but future developments hold enormous promise for their ability to augment stem cell–based therapies for regenerative medicine applications.

Organ-Level Tissue Engineering

In organ-level engineering, biomaterial science and tissue engineering are used to create synthetic or partially engineered organs for transplantation. This is a promising solution to the limited supply of donor organs.

Hollow structures, such as blood vessels and urethral structures, are simpler in design and have quickly reached clinical trials. Bioengineered human acellular vessels provided safe and functional hemodialysis access in a phase II clinical study (NCT01744418 and NCT01840956).[37] In contrast, despite early clinical success, autologous cell-seeded biodegradable scaffold for bladder augmentation in patients with spina bifida did not improve bladder compliance or capacity in a recent phase II clinical trial, and most individuals needed additional surgeries due to bladder rupture and bowel obstruction.[38] Diseased host tissues may provide poor environments for transplanted cells, and substantial optimization is required before engineered bladders may be translated into the clinic.

Engineering of solid 3D organs with complex internal physiology, such as the liver and kidney, is extremely challenging given the additional cellular and material requirements, the tissue maturation, and functionality considerations. Although progress has lagged behind that of hollow structures, recent advances in bioengineering technologies have been impressive in preclinical work.[39]

Organoids, a form of a 3D in vitro culture system derived from stem cells, are able to recapitulate the architecture, function, and genetic identity of a number of solid organs. Organoids, established from a number of organs including the brain, liver, kidney, stomach, pancreas, ovary, intestine, skin, and lung, have been used to model diseases, screen drugs, and simulate regenerative medicine therapies. Recently, patient-derived organoids have also been developed, which has tremendous potential in personalized therapy.[40]

CLINICAL APPLICATIONS OF STEM CELLS

Stem cell–mediated therapies have transformed the field of regenerative medicine, and a number of therapies are currently under careful scrutiny in clinical trials to evaluate their safety and efficacy in the treatment of a range of diseases.

Embryonic Stem Cells

A phase I clinical trial engineered monolayers of human ESC–derived retinal pigment epithelium (RPE) cells and found them to improve visual acuity when delivered to the subretinal space of patients with severe age-related macular degeneration (ARMD).[41] ESCs are also currently being tested for their ability to generate insulin - producing pancreatic cells to help correct type 1 diabetes.[42]

Somatic Cell Nuclear Transfer

A landmark study combined the nucleus from a type 1 diabetic patient with donated enucleated oocyte to produce stem cells that were capable of being differentiated into beta pancreatic cells capable of producing insulin.[42] Although SCNT research is promising, regulatory and funding considerations have hindered translational progress.

Induced Pluripotent Stem Cells

The first clinical study on iPSCs was launched in 2013 and involved transplanting autologous iPSC-derived RPE cells reprogrammed from skin cells into eyes damaged by ARMD. The first patient received autologous cells and had no signs of immune rejection or teratoma formation in the absence of immunosuppressants, but visual acuity neither improved nor declined at 1-year follow-up.[43] Unfortunately, the trial was halted due to the discovery of undisclosed mutations found in the iPSCs intended for the second patient.[14]

Bone Marrow Transplant

Bone marrow transplantation has been used successfully for over 50 years and is a spectacular example of the potential of cell-based therapies. HSC transplantation provides the best chance for cure for a range of malignant and nonmalignant diseases and has the potential to induce tolerance in the setting of organ transplantation.[44] Currently, however, the myeloablative regimens required to ensure HSCs engraft and survive are highly toxic, and the use of HSCs for nonmalignant patients is currently unjustified.

Multipotent Adult Stem Cells

Following encouraging preliminary results, autologous BMSCs were used to treat chronic advanced ischemic heart failure in a phase III trial (NCT01768702). The outcomes, however, failed to show any benefit in the treated versus placebo group in any outcome measures up to 39 weeks posttransplantation. A post hoc analysis of ventricular remodeling at 52 weeks suggested a U-shaped response curve with patients receiving the medium dose showing most benefit.[45] More studies are needed to determine the role of MSC-based treatments in ischemic myocardial pathologies.

A recent phase III clinical study (NCT00475410) delivered harvested autologous ASCs in multiple local injections (up to 60 million ASCs), with or without fibrin glue, into complex perianal fistulas of patients without inflammatory bowel disease. There was no greater benefit found in using transplanted cells compared to glue alone with regard to fistula closure at 6 months.[46] In contrast, a phase III clinical trial (NCT01541579) found that injection of 120 million allogeneic ASCs, without glue, to be superior compared to placebo in providing closure of chronic perianal fistulas associated with Crohn disease. Benefits were present at 24 weeks[47] and remained evident at least 1 year after treatment.[48]

MSCs have also reached phase III clinical studies for the treatment of graft-versus-host disease (GVHD) due to their immunomodulatory properties. In one trial, MSCs were used to treat GVHD refractory to steroid treatment (NCT00366145) but demonstrated no benefit over placebo 28 days after infusion.[49] The second trial (NCT02336230) used a select pediatric patient group with severe steroid-resistant GVHD and strict outcome criteria and found significant improvements of MSC-treated patients versus placebo-treated patients at 28 days. A recent phase I clinical trial (NCT02923375) reported encouraging early results using iPSC-derived cells to MSCs for adult with GVHDs.[50]

EPCs have been used in a number of randomized and nonrandomized clinical studies to treat vascular injury. However, significant heterogeneity in reported methodology makes it difficult to draw firm conclusions.[25]

A number of phase III clinical trials are currently underway exploring the use of MSCs for Crohn disease (NCT004829092), chronic heart failure (NCT02032004), back pain (NCT02412735), and pediatric GVHD (NCT02336230), mostly sponsored by industry and focused on demonstrating the efficacy of banked and thawed allogeneic MSCs.

CONCLUSION

Regenerative medicine and stem cell–based therapies are promising, but their full clinical potential remains to be fully realized. Considerable groundwork is required to confirm the safety, efficiency, and effectiveness of currently engineered tissues and cells before more widespread application is possible. However, exciting advances in biomedical sciences and engineering approaches are helping to significantly expedite this process, and it is likely that many important milestones will be met in the upcoming years.

SELECTED REFERENCES

Campbell KH, McWhir J, Ritchie WA, et al. Sheep cloned by nuclear transfer from a cultured cell line. *Nature.* 1996;380:64–66.

This is a landmark paper describing how somatic cell nuclear transfer technology was used to successfully clone a viable mammal—Dolly the sheep—for the very first time.

Cossu G, Birchall M, Brown T, et al. Lancet commission: stem cells and regenerative medicine. *Lancet.* 2018;391:883–910.

This commissioned article describes the threats to regenerative medicine in its transition from preclinical studies to clinical applications. There is discussion of the unconventional routes to market poorly regulated clinics, the high cost of research, and high public expectation, which pose ethical and governance issues. The authors recommend better science, funding models, governance, and engagement with the public to help ensure the success of regenerative medicine license to practice.

Gonzales KAU, Fuchs E. Skin and its regenerative powers: an alliance between stem cells and their niche. *Dev Cell.* 2017;43:387–401.

This is an excellent review that outlines the current understanding of epidermal stem cells in the skin and how they maintain homeostasis and repair following wounding. The authors discuss how this plasticity can be harnessed for wound therapeutics and emphasize the need for greater understanding of the influence of the niche on stem cell behavior.

Ilic D, Ogilvie C. Concise review: human embryonic stem cells-what have we done? What are we doing? Where are we going? *Stem Cells.* 2017;35:17–25.

This succinct review provides a broad overview of the progress made using human embryonic stem cells for regenerative medicine. The authors discuss the encouraging success to date and the major challenges and obstacles encountered.

Kaushik G, Leijten J, Khademhosseini A. concise review: organ engineering: design, technology, and integration. *Stem Cells.* 2017;35:51–60.

This article outlines the current progress made in organ engineering and discusses the key design principles, technological advances, and engineering approaches needed to help deliver the complex array of necessary cues and thus achieve the desired regeneration of stem cells.

Shi Y, Inoue H, Wu JC, et al. Induced pluripotent stem cell technology: a decade of progress. *Nat Rev Drug Discov.* 2017;16:115–130.

This review discusses the progress in applications of iPSC technology that are particularly relevant to disease modeling, drug discovery, and regenerative medicine. The authors describe the current challenges and emerging opportunities in the field.

Takahashi K, Yamanaka S. Induction of pluripotent stem cells from mouse embryonic and adult fibroblast cultures by defined factors. *Cell.* 2006;126:663–676.

This was the original description of the creation of induced pluripotent stem cells by viral transfection with four genes. Subsequent studies have generated iPSCs from human skin cells and ASCs. Because the original transfection methods involved genomic integration of viral particles, much work is ongoing to allow for the safe induction of pluripotency in cells using techniques that would allow clinical applications.

Zuk PA, Zhu M, Ashjian P, et al. Human adipose tissue is a source of multipotent stem cells. *Mol Biol Cell.* 2002;13:4279–4295.

In this seminal description of adipose stromal cells, the authors demonstrated that multipotent mesenchymal stem cells could be isolated from the stromal vascular fraction of human adipose tissue. This was the first account of an adult stem cell population isolated from a tissue other than the bone marrow.

REFERENCES

1. Ilic D, Ogilvie C. Concise review: human embryonic stem cells—what have we done? What are we doing? Where are we going? *Stem Cells.* 2017;35:17–25.
2. Trounson A, DeWitt ND. Pluripotent stem cells progressing to the clinic. *Nat Rev Mol Cell Biol.* 2016;17:194–200.
3. Merkle FT, Ghosh S, Kamitaki N, et al. Human pluripotent stem cells recurrently acquire and expand dominant negative P53 mutations. *Nature.* 2017;545:229–233.
4. Rameshwar P, Moore CA, Shah NN, et al. An update on the therapeutic potential of stem cells. In: Singh SR, Rameshwar P, eds. *Somatic Stem Cells: Methods and Protocols (Methods in Molecular Biology).* 2nd ed. New York: Humana Press; 2018:3–27.
5. Campbell KH, McWhir J, Ritchie WA, et al. Sheep cloned by nuclear transfer from a cultured cell line. *Nature.* 1996;380:64–66.
6. Matoba S, Zhang Y. Somatic cell nuclear transfer reprogramming: mechanisms and applications. *Cell Stem Cell.* 2018;23:471–485.
7. Deuse T, Wang D, Stubbendorff M, et al. SCNT-derived ESCs with mismatched mitochondria trigger an immune response in allogeneic hosts. *Cell Stem Cell.* 2015;16:33–38.
8. Armstrong L, Lako M. The future of human nuclear transfer? *Stem Cell Rev.* 2006;2:351–358.
9. Takahashi K, Yamanaka S. Induction of pluripotent stem cells from mouse embryonic and adult fibroblast cultures by defined factors. *Cell.* 2006;126:663–676.
10. Yu J, Vodyanik MA, Smuga-Otto K, et al. Induced pluripotent stem cell lines derived from human somatic cells. *Science.* 2007;318:1917–1920.
11. Takahashi K, Tanabe K, Ohnuki M, et al. Induction of pluripotent stem cells from adult human fibroblasts by defined factors. *Cell.* 2007;131:861–872.
12. Shi Y, Inoue H, Wu JC, et al. Induced pluripotent stem cell technology: a decade of progress. *Nat Rev Drug Discov.* 2017;16:115–130.
13. Kimbrel EA, Lanza R. Current status of pluripotent stem cells: moving the first therapies to the clinic. *Nat Rev Drug Discov.* 2015;14:681–692.
14. Garber K. RIKEN suspends first clinical trial involving induced pluripotent stem cells. *Nat Biotechnol.* 2015;33:890–891.
15. Yoshihara M, Hayashizaki Y, Murakawa Y. Genomic instability of iPSCs: challenges towards their clinical applications. *Stem Cell Rev.* 2017;13:7–16.
16. Gotherstrom C, Ringden O, Tammik C, et al. Immunologic properties of human fetal mesenchymal stem cells. *Am J Obstet Gynecol.* 2004;190:239–245.
17. So W-K, Cheung TH. Molecular regulation of cellular quiescence: a perspective from adult stem cells and its niches. In: Locorazza HD, ed. *Cellular Quiescence.* New York: Humana Press; 2018:1–25.
18. Crane GM, Jeffery E, Morrison SJ. Adult haematopoietic stem cell niches. *Nat Rev Immunol.* 2017;17:573–590.
19. Gao F, Chiu SM, Motan DA, et al. Mesenchymal stem cells and immunomodulation: current status and future prospects. *Cell Death & Disease.* 2016;7:e2062.
20. Budd E, Waddell S, de Andres MC, et al. The potential of microRNAs for stem cell-based therapy for degenerative skeletal diseases. *Curr Mol Biol Rep.* 2017;3:263–275.
21. Merino-Gonzalez C, Zuniga FA, Escudero C, et al. Mesenchymal stem cell–derived extracellular vesicles promote angiogenesis: potential clinical application. *Front Physiol.* 2016;7:24.
22. Bianco P, Robey PG. Skeletal stem cells. *Development.* 2015;142:1023–1027.
23. Zuk PA, Zhu M, Ashjian P, et al. Human adipose tissue is a source of multipotent stem cells. *Mol Biol Cell.* 2002;13:4279–4295.
24. Spiekman M, van Dongen JA, Willemsen JC, et al. The power of fat and its adipose-derived stromal cells: emerging

concepts for fibrotic scar treatment. *J Tissue Eng Regen Med.* 2017;11:3220–3235.
25. Pysna A, Bem R, Nemcova A, et al. Endothelial progenitor cells biology in diabetes mellitus and peripheral arterial disease and their therapeutic potential. *Stem Cell Rev.* 2019;15(2):157–165.
26. Medina RJ, Barber CL, Sabatier F, et al. Endothelial progenitors: a consensus statement on nomenclature. *Stem Cells Transl Med.* 2017;6:1316–1320.
27. Chan CK, Seo EY, Chen JY, et al. Identification and specification of the mouse skeletal stem cell. *Cell.* 2015;160:285–298.
28. Chan CKF, Gulati GS, Sinha R, et al. Identification of the human skeletal stem cell. *Cell.* 2018;175:43–56.e21.
29. Gonzales KAU, Fuchs E. Skin and its regenerative powers: an alliance between stem cells and their niche. *Dev Cell.* 2017;43:387–401.
30. Stzepourginski I, Nigro G, Jacob JM, et al. CD34+ mesenchymal cells are a major component of the intestinal stem cells niche at homeostasis and after injury. *Proc Natl Acad Sci U S A.* 2017;114:E506–E513.
31. Vicinanza C, Aquila I, Scalise M, et al. Adult cardiac stem cells are multipotent and robustly myogenic: c-kit expression is necessary but not sufficient for their identification. *Cell Death Differ.* 2017;24:2101–2116.
32. Yue F, Bi P, Wang C, et al. Pten is necessary for the quiescence and maintenance of adult muscle stem cells. *Nat Commun.* 2017;8:14328.
33. Paul A, Chaker Z, Doetsch F. Hypothalamic regulation of regionally distinct adult neural stem cells and neurogenesis. *Science.* 2017;356:1383–1386.
34. Batlle E, Clevers H. Cancer stem cells revisited. *Nat Med.* 2017;23:1124–1134.
35. Rando TA, Ambrosio F. Regenerative rehabilitation: applied biophysics meets stem cell therapeutics. *Cell Stem Cell.* 2018;22:306–309.
36. Zhang YS, Yue K, Aleman J, et al. 3D bioprinting for tissue and organ fabrication. *Ann Biomed Eng.* 2017;45:148–163.
37. Lawson JH, Glickman MH, Ilzecki M, et al. Bioengineered human acellular vessels for dialysis access in patients with end-stage renal disease: two phase 2 single-arm trials. *Lancet.* 2016;387:2026–2034.
38. Joseph DB, Borer JG, De Filippo RE, et al. Autologous cell seeded biodegradable scaffold for augmentation cystoplasty: phase II study in children and adolescents with spina bifida. *J Urol.* 2014;191:1389–1395.
39. Kaushik G, Leijten J, Khademhosseini A. Concise review: organ engineering: design, technology, and integration. *Stem Cells.* 2017;35:51–60.
40. Dutta D, Heo I, Clevers H. Disease modeling in stem cell–derived 3D organoid systems. *Trends Mol Med.* 2017;23:393–410.
41. da Cruz L, Fynes K, Georgiadis O, et al. Phase 1 clinical study of an embryonic stem cell–derived retinal pigment epithelium patch in age-related macular degeneration. *Nat Biotechnol.* 2018;36:328–337.
42. Duffy C, Prugue C, Glew R, et al. Feasibility of induced pluripotent stem cell therapies for treatment of type 1 diabetes. *Tissue Eng Part B Rev.* 2018;24:482–492.
43. Mandai M, Watanabe A, Kurimoto Y, et al. Autologous induced stem-cell-derived retinal cells for macular degeneration. *N Engl J Med.* 2017;376:1038–1046.
44. Weissman IL, Shizuru JA. The origins of the identification and isolation of hematopoietic stem cells, and their capability to induce donor-specific transplantation tolerance and treat autoimmune diseases. *Blood.* 2008;112:3543–3553.
45. Bartunek J, Davison B, Sherman W, et al. Congestive Heart Failure Cardiopoietic Regenerative Therapy (CHART-1) trial design. *Eur J Heart Fail.* 2016;18:160–168.
46. Herreros MD, Garcia-Arranz M, Guadalajara H, et al. Autologous expanded adipose-derived stem cells for the treatment of complex cryptoglandular perianal fistulas: a phase III randomized clinical trial (FATT 1: Fistula Advanced Therapy Trial 1) and long-term evaluation. *Dis Colon Rectum.* 2012;55:762–772.
47. Panes J, Garcia-Olmo D, Van Assche G, et al. Expanded allogeneic adipose-derived mesenchymal stem cells (Cx601) for complex perianal fistulas in Crohn's disease: a phase 3 randomised, double-blind controlled trial. *Lancet.* 2016;388:1281–1290.
48. Panes J, Garcia-Olmo D, Van Assche G, et al. Long-term efficacy and safety of stem cell therapy (Cx601) for complex perianal fistulas in patients with Crohn's disease. *Gastroenterology.* 2018;154:1334–1342.e1334.
49. Martin PJ, Uberti JP, Soiffer RJ, et al. Prochymal improves response rates in patients with steroid-refractory acute graft versus host disease (SR-GVHD) involving the liver and gut: results of a randomized, placebo-controlled, multicenter phase III trial in GVHD. *Biol Blood Marrow Transplant.* 2010;16:S169–S170.
50. Bloor A, Patel A, Griffin JE, et al. A phase I trial of iPSC-derived MSCs (CYP-001) in steroid-resistant acute GvHD. *Blood.* 2018;132; 4562–4562.

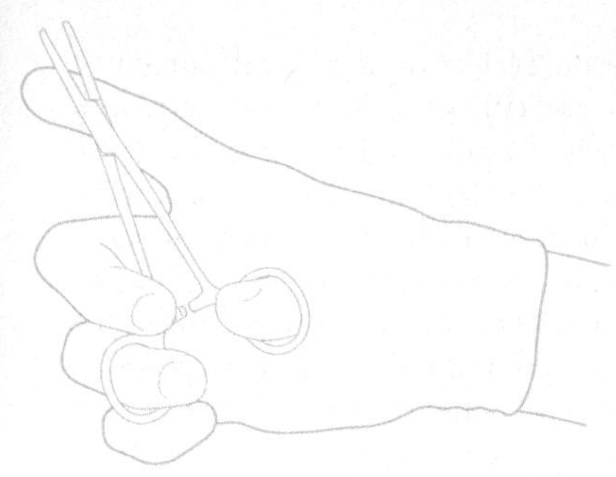

CHAPTER 8

Critical Assessment of Surgical Outcomes and Health Services Research

Benjamin S. Brooke, Samuel R.G. Finlayson

OUTLINE

The practice of surgery has undergone a dramatic evolution over the last century with the availability of new scientific evidence supporting the use of different surgical techniques and management. Central to this mission is the process of critically appraising the surgical evidence base at every opportunity and deciding what can and should be applied to routine clinical practice.

Critical appraisal is defined as the process of carefully and systematically examining research evidence to judge its validity, its value, and its relevance to a particular context.[1] Decisions related to surgical care delivery should be made following a careful assessment of individual patient preferences, clinical experience, and critical appraisal of the evidence in the medical literature. However, given the breadth and complexity of information, surgeons often are challenged to critically evaluate the literature and extrapolate the findings from health services and outcomes studies.

This chapter provides a framework to critically appraise surgical outcomes and health services research. This includes methods to assess the strength of evidence for surgical practices, establish the validity of scientific studies in surgery, and apply evidence-based medicine practices to improve the quality of surgical care. The intent is to provide the reader with conceptual and analytic tools that a modern, evidence-based surgeon needs to navigate the surgical outcomes literature and implement practices that are based on sound science.

EVIDENCE-BASED APPROACH TO SURGERY

Surgeons must be able to understand the evidence-based medicine process in order to identify, access, apply, and integrate new knowledge into their clinical practice and provide high-quality care for their patients. In practice, evidence-based medicine involves the following three fundamental principles.[2] First, the ability to make optimal clinical decisions requires awareness of the best available research evidence. Second, there must be standards by which to judge whether evidence can be trusted. Third, the quality of evidence for benefit must be weighed against the risks, burdens, and costs associated with alternative management strategies, while simultaneously considering individual patients' predicaments, values, and preferences. This evidence-based approach to clinical practice can also be remembered by the five A's—ask, acquire, appraise, apply, and assess (Fig. 8.1).[3] These five steps provide a model for practicing evidence-based medicine that all clinicians are encouraged to use when questions arise during the routine care of patients.

In everyday surgical practice, the evidence-based medicine process often starts when a surgeon learns about a new procedure or technique that could be used to treat a condition managed by their surgical specialty. The next step is to determine whether any research studies provide evidence that support the efficacy and effectiveness of that new procedure. For a study to provide a high level of evidence, it needs to address a significant clinical problem and provide novel results, extend what was previously known, or describe an innovative procedure that represents an improvement over existing technique. The study should include patients who are likely to be offered the intervention in everyday surgical practice. Moreover, it should focus on surgical treatments or strategies that can be replicated in a real-world clinical setting.

Evaluating Research Study Questions

There are several strategies that surgeons can use to review the literature, evaluate research study questions, and determine whether scientific evidence should be applied to their clinical practice. One strategy for evaluating the implications of a research question is outlined by the mnemonic FINER—feasible, interesting, novel, ethical, and relevant.[4] FINER provides a framework that prompts the reader to ask several important questions when considering a research study. Is the study feasible and adequately powered to answer the specific research question? Does the study address a topic that is interesting to the surgical community? Is the research novel or innovative, and does the study meet all ethical standards of research conduct? Finally, do the results from the study change surgical practice or policy, and do they merit further scientific research or evidence.

Another widely accepted approach to developing and accessing a research question is the PICOT framework—population, intervention, comparison, outcome, and time (Table 8.1).[5] PICOT is a structured way to summarize the main components of a research question and can also be used to appraise a study or interpret its

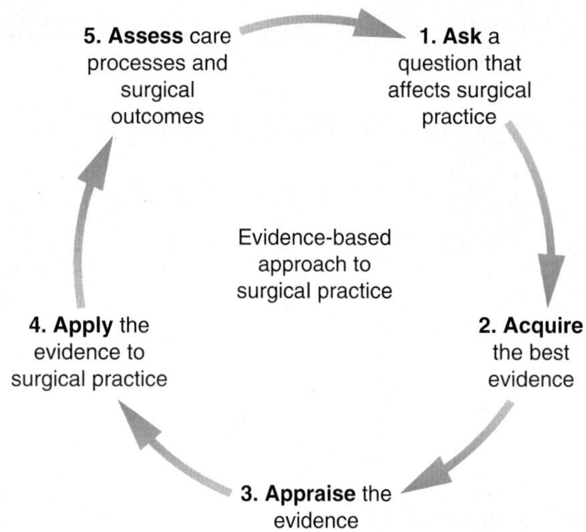

FIG. 8.1 The evidence-based approach to clinical practice.

TABLE 8.1 PICOT framework for evaluating research questions.

ACRONYM	ELEMENT DEFINITION	DESCRIPTION
P	Population or problem	Sample of subjects or problems that will be addressed.
I	Intervention	What is being tested in the study? May apply to therapy, prevention, diagnosis, or exposure groups.
C	Comparator	What is the main intervention being compared to?
O	Outcome	The main results that are being examined and assessed.
T	Time frame	Time for data collection and follow-up assessment.

results.[4] For example, a surgeon evaluating a surgical outcomes study would be prompted to ask: (P) Is the study population or clinical problem comparable with surgical patients or issues that I deal with in routine clinical practice; (I) Is the intervention truly novel, and does it represent an improvement over current standards of care; (C) Are study comparators valid and representative of usual care; (O) Are outcome measures valid and reliable; and (T) Does the duration of treatment and follow-up correspond to the duration important to patients? Using the PICOT framework to ask these questions provides a systematic process for determining whether studies are valid and relevant to clinical practice.

Study Design

There are many study designs used to undertake surgical research, including both experimental and observational designs (Fig. 8.2). The specific study design used to generate evidence is often influenced by practical considerations, such as resource availability and feasibility. Nonetheless, the study design selected to evaluate surgical interventions will largely determine our levels of confidence about cause and effect.

Several criteria have been proposed to establish epidemiological evidence of causal relationships, including the set of nine criteria originally published by Sir Bradford Hill in 1965.[6] Distilled down to the most simplistic terms, causal relationships exist when (1) the cause precedes the effect, (2) the cause was related to the effect, and (3) we can find no other plausible explanation for the effect other than the proposed cause.[7] Experimental studies that are prospective and randomized usually provide the greatest insurance that these criteria are met and are associated with the highest levels of evidence. But even prospective randomized studies can lead to erroneous conclusions if they are not executed or analyzed properly. Evaluating the quality of clinical evidence requires a close look at the strengths and limitations of each type of study design (Table 8.2).

Randomized Controlled Trials

When appropriately designed and conducted, randomized controlled trials (RCTs) are considered the gold standard for evaluating most types of health care interventions. In this study design,

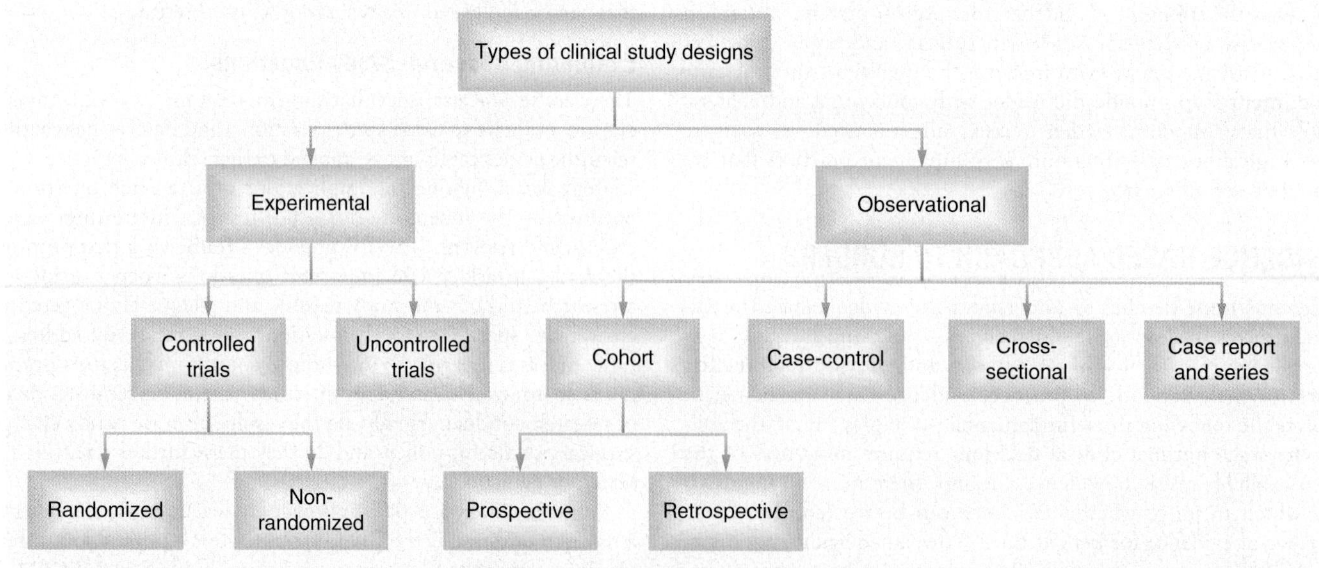

FIG. 8.2 Types of clinical study designs.

TABLE 8.2 **Strengths and weaknesses of common study designs used in clinical research.**

STUDY DESIGN	CHARACTERISTIC	STRENGTHS	WEAKNESSES
Randomized controlled trial	Allocation of subjects to experimental or control group by chance	– Ability to establish causal effects between exposure and outcomes – Can study more than one intervention	– Expensive – Can take a long period – Not suitable for rare events – Often low generalizability due to selection criteria
Cohort study	Cohort of subjects is compared based on different exposure	– High generalizability – Can study rare exposures and multiple outcomes	– Some potential to establish causal effects – Can take a long time (prospective) – Selection bias – Can be expensive
Case control study	Cases are compared with controls with respect to exposure	– Can study rare outcomes and multiple exposures – Relatively inexpensive – Hypothesis generating	– Selection bias – Recall bias – Limited potential to establish causal effects – Can only study one outcome
Cross-sectional study	Exposure and outcomes measures at same point in time	– Use for describing disease prevalence – Fast and inexpensive – Hypothesis generating	– Sample bias – Survival bias – Very limited potential to establish causal effects
Case series and report	Detailed description of one or more subjects (i.e., cases) without a control group	– Very detailed – Inexpensive – Hypothesis generating	– Selection bias – Not generalizable – No ability to establish causal effects

patients are randomly allocated to either a treatment or a control group prior to receiving an intervention using an element of chance to determine the assignments, similar to tossing a coin. After randomization, patients are followed in exactly the same way and the only difference is the treatment group they were allocated to.

The RCT study design has the greatest potential for determining causation between exposure and outcome given that randomization balances both known and unknown prognostic factors (i.e., measured and unmeasured confounders) between comparison groups during the assignment of treatment. As such, the effect of the treatment on outcomes relative to the control group can be determined while other variables are kept constant and selection bias is minimized. Furthermore, randomization can facilitate blinding (also known as masking) of the identity of treatments from investigators, participants, and assessors.

RCTs can be used to compare nearly all types of interventions used in surgical patients. This includes surgical procedures, medications used before or after surgery, screening programs, or diagnostic modalities, to name a few. But while RCTs help us determine the presence and strength of a causal relationship between different surgical interventions and a given outcome, they also have several weaknesses. First, they are very expensive to complete and it can take many years to obtain results when large sample sizes are needed. Second, the results may not be generalizable to patients in everyday practice due to narrow enrollment criteria. Third, many surgical interventions are simply not amenable to randomization. Finally, RCTs can still yield biased results if the study is not well designed or executed properly and lacks methodological rigor.

To assess whether RCT findings are valid, surgeons need complete and transparent information on the methodology and results. This need for adequate RCT reporting fueled the development of the original Consolidated Standards of Reporting Trials (CONSORT) statement in 1996 and its subsequent revision in 2010.[8,9] The most recent CONSORT statement includes a 25-item checklist and flow diagram, which provides guidance for reporting all types of RCTs but focuses on the most common two parallel group design type. This checklist provides an easy way for surgeons to evaluate the quality of evidence derived from these types of studies.

Cross-Sectional Study

A cross-sectional study involves looking at research subjects who differ on one key characteristic at a specific point in time. Exposure and outcome data are collected at the same time point among subjects who are similar in most other characteristics but different in a key factor of interest. For example, this could involve patients undergoing a specific type of surgery who come from different age groups, income levels, or geographic locations.

Cross-sectional studies are commonly used to describe disease prevalence or characteristics that exist in a community or hospital setting. This study design is inexpensive and is often used to make inferences about possible relationships or to gather preliminary data to support further research and experimentation (i.e., hypothesis generating). However, these studies are limited by survival bias and cannot analyze associations over a longitudinal period of time or be used to determine cause-and-effect relationships between exposure and outcome variables. Furthermore, there may be a sampling bias if the timing of the cross-sectional study leads to a sample that is not representative of patients in the general population.

Case-Control Study

The case-control design uses a different sampling strategy in which the investigators identify a group of individuals who exhibit a specific outcome (i.e., the cases) and then compare this group to a set of individuals who do not exhibit the outcome of interest (i.e., the controls). The cases and controls are then compared with respect to the frequency of one or more past exposures. If the cases have substantially higher odds of exposure to a particular factor compared to the control subjects, it suggests an association but does not necessarily provide evidence of causal inference.

There are numerous strengths of case-control studies. This study design allows investigators to examine risk factors associated with outcomes that are uncommon, to examine the association of multiple risk factors with outcomes simultaneously, and to examine outcomes that occur a long period of time after the exposure occurs. They are also relatively inexpensive to complete and can help generate hypotheses. On balance, however, case-control studies are limited by their retrospectively design that allows the potential for recall and selection bias. Moreover, identifying valid control groups to compare to cases can be difficult, estimating the frequency of exposure in the population at-large is often inaccurate, and the design allows evaluation of only one outcome at a time.

Cohort Study

A cohort study is an observational study design in which groups of subjects are identified based on their exposure to a particular risk factor and then compared to a group that have not been exposed to that same factor. This study design can be conducted from either a forward-looking (i.e., prospective) or backward-looking (i.e., retrospective) viewpoint. Prospective cohort studies are planned in advance and carried out over a period of time to assess outcome incidence among exposure groups. In comparison, retrospective cohort studies look at data that already exist and attempt to identify risk factors for outcomes that have already occurred. Retrospective analyses of existing surgical databases, in particular, constitute one of the most common applications of this study design.[10] For both types of cohort studies, a higher incidence of outcomes in the exposed group suggests an association between that factor and the outcome. However, because prospective studies collect information about exposures and outcomes purposefully and systematically, they provide stronger evidence for causation.

There are several strengths and limitations of cohort studies. The advantages of cohort studies are that they are easier and less expensive to conduct than RCTs, the incidence (or rate) of exposure and outcomes can be estimated, and subjects in cohorts can be matched to limit the influence of confounding variables. In addition, enrollment criteria and outcome measures can be standardized, and—unlike case-control studies—multiple simultaneous outcome assessment is possible. However, cohort studies also have several disadvantages. Because there is no randomization, one cannot account for unmeasured imbalances in patient characteristics. Blinding or masking is difficult (or impossible retrospectively), and outcomes of interest can take a long time to occur, requiring many years of information about exposures. For retrospective studies in particular, treatment selection bias and confounding variables may lead to unmeasured differences in exposure groups over time that cannot be controlled for with statistical analysis. Moreover, interpretations can be limited because of missing data that is impossible for researchers go back in time to collect.

In order to assess the evidence quality derived from different types of cohort studies, several simplified checklist methods have been developed. The Strengthening the Reporting of Observational Studies in Epidemiology (STROBE) statement is one of these checklists that provides an organized system for assessing observational study methodology and results that is similar to the CONSORT system used for RCTs.[11] STROBE provides guidance on how to report critical components of research studies from all types of observational study designs, including cohort, case-control, and cross-sectional study designs.

As part of a series of articles on research methods published in a special issue of *JAMA Surgery* in 2018, another checklist was proposed for evaluating the quality of evidence derived from databases commonly used in surgical outcomes research.[10] This checklist consists of 10 items for review that can be used when evaluating the findings of retrospective cohort studies, or considering questions that might be reasonably addressed using these databases. In the same issue of *JAMA Surgery*, in-depth information was provided for 13 of the most popular surgical databases, including the National Inpatient Sample; Surveillance, Epidemiology, and End Results (SEER) Program[12]; Medicare Claims[13]; National Surgical Quality Improvement Program (NSQIP)[14]; Society of Vascular Surgery Vascular Quality Initiative (SVS-VQI)[15]; and the Society of Thoracic Surgeons (STS) National Database.[16]

Case Series and Reports

Historically, the surgical literature has relied upon case series and case reports to describe surgical interventions and patient outcomes. These have been the most highly cited type of study design in the surgical literature until the past couple of decades.[17] Observations are made on a series of individuals, usually all receiving the same surgical intervention, but with no control group. The sampling of a case series is based on either exposure or outcomes, but not both. For example, a series could include all patients who underwent surgery at a single institution over a decade, or a case report might describe patients who experienced some rare adverse event after surgery.

The strength of case series and reports lie in their ability to provide in-depth narrative information on a given topic when other study designs cannot be carried out. This in turn may help to generate new hypotheses. However, the main limitation of this study design is the lack of ability to generalize findings or to establish a cause and effect relationship between exposures and outcomes. Case series and reports cannot be comparative and no absolute risk nor relative effect measures for an outcome can be calculated. As such, studies with these designs are nearly always considered low quality evidence.

Synthetic and Systematic Outcome Studies

Meta Analyses

One of the highest forms of evidence quality comes from a meta-analysis, where the results from multiple studies on the same topic are combined. This includes data generated from either experimental or observational study designs (Fig. 8.2). The basic tenet behind meta analysis is that there is an underlying true association between an exposure and outcome variable assessed within similar studies, but which has been measured with a certain degree of error within each individual study. By combining similar outcomes studies and using statistics to derive a pooled estimate, meta analysis can improve the precision and accuracy of this estimate and have the statistical power to detect the true association. Furthermore, meta analyses allow study results to be generalized to larger populations, permit inconsistency of results between studies to be quantified and analyzed, and identify the presence of publication bias between similar studies.[18]

However, there are several factors that can limit the quality of evidence derived from meta analyses.[19] Often, studies examining a specific topic do not have comparable patient populations, endpoints, or exposure groups. Excess variation or heterogeneity in exposure or outcome variables between individual studies beyond what chance alone would predict indicates that the results of the studies are not compatible and should not be pooled. This is a particular concern when aggregating results from observational studies where selection bias and confounding may have affected the original analysis. Moreover, the evidence derived from a meta-analysis is only as good as the methodology of the studies that are included. Even a well-designed meta analysis cannot correct for poor study design or intrinsic bias that was present when the included studies were originally designed or analyzed.

Cost-Effectiveness Analysis

A cost-effectiveness analysis is an economic evaluation that simultaneously measures the outcomes and costs of alternative interventions. This type of research evidence has become increasingly prevalent in the surgical literature as health policy has increasingly focused on containing surgical costs and defining high-value care. Cost effectiveness refers to analyses that directly compare the costs of one intervention with some other alternative intervention relative to the difference in clinical benefit. This ratio of differential costs to differential benefits is known as an incremental cost-effectiveness ratio (ICER).[20] The ICER is calculated by taking the ratio of the incremental cost (the difference in cost between two strategies) and the incremental effectiveness (the difference in outcomes between two strategies). For example, if intervention A is both more costly and more effective than intervention B, the ICER conveys how much it would cost to produce the incremental increase in effectiveness achieved by choosing intervention A over intervention B.

Effectiveness outcomes in cost-effectiveness studies are often assessed using the quality-adjusted life-years (QALYs) metric, which measures both the quantity and quality of life.[21] The QALY is constructed by weighting the amount of time spent in a health state by the quality of life in that health state. QALYs have been used extensively in surgical outcomes studies to assess different disease states, and health care strategies that cost less than $100,000 per QALY are generally considered to be cost-effective by current accepted standards.[22] For example, in one study, the ICER for coronary artery bypass surgery versus percutaneous coronary intervention for coronary artery disease was calculated to be about $30,000 per QALY gained.[23] As such, coronary artery bypass surgery is deemed by this evidence to be more cost-effective than percutaneous coronary intervention for coronary artery disease. Studies that use a general measure of benefit that considers the qualitative value of health (e.g., QALY) are typically referred to as cost-utility analyses.

Cost-effectiveness and cost-utility studies can help surgeons make clinical decisions by presenting cost and outcome tradeoffs between competing interventions. These tradeoffs can be simulated over time under different conditions using Markov models that incorporate estimates of risk of adverse events and probability of desired outcomes, such as cure, improved function, or longevity. Markov models assume that a patient is always in one of a finite number of discrete health states, each with a specified value and/or cost, and can transition from one health state to another over time based on known or estimated probabilities of events. By modeling the time dependence of probabilities for entering several different health states and outcomes, Markov models allow for many different scenarios to be estimated for any given clinical decision and are thus a valuable and versatile method for modeling the tradeoffs between competing strategies.

Systematic Reviews

Beyond aggregation of data within meta analyses, systematic reviews of outcomes research are another important means used to synthesize and organize bodies of surgical evidence.[18] Systematic reviews start with a question or hypothesis and involve a systematic search of the surgical literature using explicit criteria for selecting studies to answer the research question. This typically begins by developing a comprehensive and detailed search strategy, a priori, that can be used to identify, exclude, evaluate, and synthesize results from all relevant studies on a given topic. Once a search strategy is developed, it can be executed using several online databases including MEDLINE (United States Library of Medicine database), EMBASE (medical and pharmacologic database by Elsevier publishing), CINAHL (cumulative index to nursing and allied health literature), and the Cochrane Collaborative. In comparison to informal or narrative reviews of the literature, the methods used by systematic reviews for evaluating studies and extracting information from them are rigorous and intended to reduce the potential for subjectivity or bias in the findings. Furthermore, systematic reviews are reported in a manner that is conducive to replication of both methodology and findings.

Well-conducted systematic reviews can be an invaluable resource for surgeons given the large volume of published studies each year on any given surgical topic. They can identify high-quality evidence within the literature and help define the exact knowledge base on any given subject. The Cochrane Collaboration Library (https://www.cochranelibrary.com/cdsr/reviews), in particular, provides a large database of systematic reviews on a wide range of topics that impact surgical patients. By critically examining individual research studies, systematic reviews can help identify inconsistencies among different sources of evidence. Finally, these types of studies also help inform whether research findings can be applied to specific subgroups of surgical patients. For example, systematic reviews have been useful for defining the types of high-risk surgical patients who benefit most from perioperative beta blockers and those that have increased risk of adverse side effects from these medications during the postoperative period.[24]

Qualitative Data Analysis

Another important form of surgical research evidence is derived from qualitative data analyses. Qualitative data (also known as descriptive data) is nonnumerical empirical information collected by researchers to describe concepts, opinions, or interpretations of a specific topic. These data are typically captured from interviews, focus groups, document analysis, or notes taken during an observation. Analyzing these forms of qualitative data can reveal consistent patterns or themes among patients, providers, or other research subjects. These analyses may generate hypotheses that can be further tested with quantitative methods or, alternatively, help researchers drill down to better understand the findings from quantitative outcomes studies.

There are several different methodologies commonly used to conduct qualitative data analyses, including phenomenology, content analysis, grounded theory, and ethnography.[25] The goal of phenomenology is to study how individuals derive meaning from their life experiences by understanding how they perceive a specific phenomenon. For example, the long-term quality of life among patients who had undergone primary leg amputation for trauma could be studied this way. Content analysis is another method whereby documents such as interview or focus group transcripts are analyzed to determine frequencies and patterns of words in the textual data. Based on how materials are categorized, researchers are able to make inferences about common messages or themes within the text. In comparison, grounded theory methods are used to collect descriptive data when researchers want to develop new theories about how processes occur. Finally, ethnography is used to understand the norms, values, and social structures of groups, primarily through observation combined with focused interviews of participants.

The need for these types of qualitative research methods in surgery is recognized because they provide a deeper and more detailed understanding of the social and environmental contexts underlying surgical outcomes.[26] The strength of qualitative data analyses rests in their ability to shed light on phenomena that would be nearly impossible to study using quantitative methods alone. For example, grounded theory and ethnography methods have been used to understand operating room workflow or communications among surgical teams practicing in high-volume versus low-volume hospitals and to generate theories surrounding how information is exchanged between surgical and primary care teams during transitions of surgical care.[27] The opinions and experiences of surgeons, nurses, or trainees were solicited using these methods along with the ability to directly observe care processes as well as the technology used during communication. Alternatively, content analysis has been used to explore psychosocial issues related to surgery from patient focus groups, including reasons underlying satisfaction with care or problems that patients perceive as impeding high-quality care during episodes of surgical care.[28]

These different types of qualitative methods can also be combined with quantitative approaches in what is known as *mixed methods research*.[29] Mixed-methods research involves collecting and analyzing both qualitative and quantitative data within the same study. Rather than focus on just one approach, mixed methods allows investigators to define a specific research problem and then use a combination of methodologies in order to elucidate the relevant issues in a broader and more detailed fashion. For example, a recent mixed methods research study looking at provider compliance with surgical safety checklists first analyzed provider usage of a checklist within an institution (i.e., qualitative analysis), and then interviewed providers to explore and contextualize the specific reasons for their checklist use as opposed to noncompliance (i.e., quantitative analysis).[30]

APPRAISING SURGICAL EVIDENCE

The evidence supporting surgical decision-making comes in many diverse forms. At one end of the spectrum, evidence is simply based on the empirical impression that a specific practice makes physiologic sense and seems to work well. Much of what surgeons do in practice falls into this category and has not been formally tested. But at the other end of the spectrum, evidence has accumulated from multiple well-designed and conducted randomized clinical trials with consistent and reproducible results. The task of the evidence-based surgeon is to judge the reliability of scientific evidence and select practices that conform to the best available evidence.

Several different rubrics have been created to evaluate and determine study hierarchies or levels of evidence. These systems provide a method to judge the strength of scientific evidence, ranging from sources that are most reliable to those that are least sure. Although it is understood that not all surgical practices can be subjected to the highest levels of scientific scrutiny, surgeons are advised to base as many of their practices as possible on evidence gleaned from studies at the high end of the evidence hierarchy. This process is aided by several established systems for grading evidence

One established hierarchy is the "levels of evidence" system popularized by the U.S. Preventive Medicine Task Force (USPMTF).[31] The USPMTF assigns evidence certainty at 1 of 3 levels: high, moderate, and low, on the basis of six critical appraisals, and has become part of the vernacular for clinicians across all medical specialties. Well-designed and conducted RCTs are frequently referenced to as "level 1 evidence." When the USPMTF system was originally released, there was debate given that the system simply identified the design of the study from which the evidence was drawn but did not describe important factors that influence the quality of evidence.[32] For example, a randomized double-blind placebo-controlled trial with 20,000 subjects would be awarded the same grade in the USPMTF system as an unblinded randomized trial with 50 subjects. And the latter trial would, in turn, be graded higher than a well-designed, multi-institution, prospective cohort study with 10,000 subjects. In response to these criticisms, changes were subsequently made to the USPMTF grading system in 2012 to take into account factors other than study design, such as quality, consistency, and completeness.[33]

Another system for grading evidence that takes into account study quality and consistency was developed by the Grading, Recommendations, Assessment, Development, and Evaluation (GRADE) Working Group (Table 8.3).[34,35] GRADE has developed a structured scoring process for determining whether evidence should be downgraded or upgraded based on different study characteristics. For example, a multicenter RCT executed with poor allocation concealment and high attrition would be downgraded by the GRADE system from high evidence quality to moderate or even low evidence quality. In comparison, a single-center RCT with a large effect size or a dose-response gradient could be upgraded from moderate to high evidence quality. The updated USPMTF grading system uses similar criteria as GRADE for determining when evidence quality should be increased or

TABLE 8.3 The GRADE system—quality of evidence and strength of recommendation.

QUALITY OF EVIDENCE	DEFINITIONS	STRENGTH OF RECOMMENDATION	EXPLANATION
High	We are very confident that the true effect lies close to that of the estimate of the effect. Further research is very unlikely to change confidence in the estimate of effect.	Strong	Many high-quality trials confirming the effect
Moderate	We are moderately confident in the effect estimate. The true effect is likely to be close to the estimate of the effect, but there is a possibility that it is substantially different. Further research is likely to have an important impact on our confidence in the estimate of effect.	Conditional	Uncertainty about the balance between desirable and undesirable side effects
Low	Our confidence in the effect estimate is limited: The true effect may be substantially different from the estimate of the effect. Further research is very likely to have an important impact on our confidence in the estimate of effect.	Conditional	Uncertainty or variability in values and preferences
Very low	We have very little confidence in the effect estimate. The true effect is likely to be substantially different from the estimate of effect.	Conditional	Uncertainty about whether the intervention represents a wise use of resources

GRADE, Grading, Recommendations, Assessment, Development, and Evaluation.

decreased (Table 8.4). However, it is recognized that no single grading system is perfect, and surgeons are required to judge the quality and applicability of scientific evidence for themselves.

Evaluating Study Quality

Scientific evidence from surgical outcomes and health services research relies on two important inferences. The first inference is that the observed outcome is the result of some specific intervention and cannot be attributed to some alternative explanation. When conclusions are believable and this inference is deemed true, the study is considered to have internal validity. The second inference is that study results are relevant to scenarios outside the study where the surgeon seeks to implement the practice. In other words, do the study results apply to real-world clinical practice? The extent to which this is true is called external validity or generalizability. Whereas internal validity relies on how well the study is conducted and the results analyzed, external validity relies on how well the study plan reflects the clinical question that inspired it and how well the study's conclusions apply to scenarios outside the study. Poor external validity can also refer to the difference between an intervention's efficacy (i.e., how well it works when applied perfectly) and its effectiveness (i.e., whether it has the same effect when applied generally in an uncontrolled environment).

Internal Validity

Assessing the internal validity of a study requires an understanding of the potential influence of bias, confounding, and chance on the study results. Chance refers to the unpredictable randomness of events that might mislead researchers, whereas bias refers to systematic errors in how study subjects were selected or assessed. In comparison, confounding refers to differences in the comparison groups (other than the intended exposure) that lead to differences in outcomes.

Sources of bias. There are multiple sources of bias that might impact a surgical outcomes or health services research study.[36] Bias refers to a systematic problem with a clinical study that results in an inaccurate estimate of the differences in outcomes between comparison groups. While there are several forms of bias that arise in outcomes studies, two general types are most common: selection bias and measurement bias. The former results from errors in the choice of study subjects, whereas the latter results from errors in the way information about exposures or outcomes (or other pertinent data) is obtained.

Selection bias refers to any imperfection in the selection process that results in either the wrong types of subjects (i.e., people who are not typical of the target population) or a sample of subjects that for some reason, unrelated to the intervention, is more likely to have the outcome of interest. For example, paid volunteer subjects may be more motivated to comply with treatment regimens and report favorable results, resulting in an overestimate of the effect of an intervention. This would affect both internal validity (inference about the size of the effect) and external validity (generalizability to other populations). When assessing the validity of scientific evidence, surgeons must carefully consider the characteristics of the subjects selected for study.

Measurement bias refers to problems caused by the way information about outcomes or other pertinent data are obtained. For example, in a study of sexual function after surgery for open abdominal aortic aneurysm, subjects may report symptoms differently during an in-person interview than they would if mailed an anonymous survey. As another example, asking surgeons to assess surgical site infection outcomes in their own patients might result in erroneous reported rates as compared to surgical site infection rates reported by hospital epidemiologists. Retrospective studies, in particular, are prone to a variety of types of measurement bias. For example, "recall bias" may occur because of subjects' selective memory of past events, and "ascertainment bias" may occur if the outcome is likely to influence how hard observers look for information about exposures. Sources of measurement bias may be subtler than selection bias and require careful attention to reported study methods. Efforts to control measurement bias include blinding (not telling the subject or assessor what intervention was performed) and prospective study design.

Confounding. Confounding refers to differences in outcomes that occur because of differences in the baseline risks of the comparison groups. These differences may occur due to selection bias that distributes risk factors known as confounding variables unevenly between comparison groups. Confounding variables influences both the outcome variable and exposure variable causing a spurious association. For example, a comparison of mortality after open versus laparoscopic colectomy might be skewed because of the greater likelihood of open colectomy being performed as an emergency procedure in critically ill patients with perforation. In this example, the severity of the illness is a confounder in the observed association between mortality and surgical approach.

In evaluating the strength of evidence in a published study, readers must assess how well the researchers accounted for the potential effect of confounding. Confounding can be minimized in several ways, in both the design of the study and the analysis of the study's results. In the design of a study, confounding is most effectively addressed with randomization. When subjects are randomized, potentially confounding variables (both recognized and unrecognized) are likely to be evenly distributed across comparison groups. Thus, whereas the baseline rate of outcomes in the entire

TABLE 8.4 Common factors that reduce or increase the quality of evidence using the USPMTF and GRADE evaluation systems.

FACTORS THAT REDUCE EVIDENCE QUALITY	FACTORS THAT INCREASE EVIDENCE QUALITY
Limitations in study design or execution of methods with risk of bias	Large magnitude of effect
Lack of information on important health outcomes	All plausible sources of confounding would reduce the demonstrated effect or increase the effect if no effect was observed
Indirectness of evidence	Dose-response gradient
Imprecision or inconsistency of results across individual studies	Consistency of findings across multiple studies
Publication bias	Randomization employed or other valid methods used to adjust for measured and unmeasured confounding
Findings not generalizable to routine practice	Representative patient populations studied

GRADE, Grading, Recommendations, Assessment, Development, and Evaluation; *USPMTF*, U.S. Preventive Medicine Task Force.

cohort might be influenced by these factors, the differences across comparison groups are less likely to be affected.

When randomization is not practical, restriction or matching can be used to prevent confounding. Restriction refers to the tight control of study entry criteria, for example, only enrolling patients undergoing elective surgery and excluding emergent procedures. However, restrictive entry criteria can sometimes limit generalizability. In comparison, matching refers to using a comparison group of unexposed (control) subjects who are identical to the exposed (case) subjects across a set of characteristics (e.g., age, sex, residence) that have the potential to result in confounding.

In addition to minimizing confounding through good study design, confounding can also be addressed during the analytic phase of a study with statistical risk-adjustment techniques. The most common technique is multivariate regression analysis, including linear and logistic regression models. Logistic regression models are used when the outcome variable is binary, whereas linear regression is used when the outcome is continuous. Both of these approaches involve taking into account differences in the prevalence of recognized confounders across comparison groups. However, statistical risk adjustment has several important limitations. First, only recognized confounders can be addressed in the regression model. Second, every potential confounding variable added to a statistical model decreases the model's statistical power and thereby increases the chance of resulting in a false-negative result (i.e., type II error). Third, regression model estimates are not very reliable when there are very few outcome events. As a rule of thumb, logistic regression must have at least 10 outcome events for every variable adjusted in the model, whereas linear regression requires 10–15 outcomes per variable included in the model to prevent overfitting.[37,38]

Other analytic techniques used to address confounding include stratification (subanalyses in which subjects with similar risk profiles are compared) and propensity score risk adjustment.[39] The latter technique addresses the problem created by unequal chances of receiving treatment caused by differences in health characteristics. In an observational study of the outcomes of a given treatment, a propensity score is a scalar summary of all observed confounders that predict the probability of receiving the treatment. Propensity scores are typically calculated using multivariate regression models and are used as the basis for stratified analysis or for matching cases and controls in observational studies.

Finally, another more complicated technique used to limit the effect of confounding is instrumental variable (IV) analysis. An IV approach involves studying the effect of a given exposure on outcomes by comparing groups with different levels of a third factor (i.e., the IV) that is highly correlated with the exposure but does not independently affect the outcome. For example, a study evaluating the effects of catheterization and revascularization on mortality following acute myocardial infarction would be prone to confounding related to differences in the baseline health characteristics of the populations receiving or not receiving these treatments. To limit this potential source of confounding, researchers studied the effect of receiving catheterization versus no catheterization (the exposure groups) on mortality after myocardial infarction (the outcome) by comparing groups of patients living at different distances from hospitals providing these services (the IV).[40] The researchers assumed that potentially confounding health characteristics would be distributed randomly geographically and that geographic distance would affect mortality only indirectly through its correlation with access to treatment. In this way, they used distance to "pseudo-randomize" their study population to different levels of treatment for acute myocardial infarction.

Hypothesis Testing

In clinical studies that compare outcomes between two or more treatment groups, the underlying assumption that no difference exists between groups is called the null hypothesis. Erroneous conclusions with regard to the null hypothesis can sometimes occur by chance alone. There are two types of chance-related errors: type I and type II. Type I errors (also called "alpha errors") occur when researchers erroneously reject the null hypothesis, that is, infer that there is a difference in outcomes when there is no difference. Type II errors (also called "beta errors") occur when researchers erroneously confirm the null hypothesis. In other words, the study concludes that there is no difference in outcomes between treatment groups when a difference truly exists.

Type I errors. Statistical testing is used to quantify the likelihood of a type I error. A "*P* value" indicates the probability that observed differences between groups might be due to chance alone. In other words, the difference may not be based on the effect of the intervention being tested. The threshold for "statistical significance" is conventionally set at a *P* value of 0.05, signifying that the likelihood of the observed differences being due to chance alone might occur 5 times out of 100 tests. Although a likelihood of 5% falls short of absolute certainty, this level of confidence is generally accepted as scientific proof and used throughout the scientific literature.

Type I errors can occur when the research question and analysis have not been specified a priori or when multiple statistical tests are performed in a study with several subgroups.[41] For example, with a *P* value set at 0.05, 1 out of every 20 comparisons will be expected by chance to be deemed statistically significant and be a false-positive finding. When more than 20 comparisons are necessary in a given study, a Bonferroni correction or Hochberg sequential procedure can be used to protect against a type I error.[42,43]

An alternative expression of statistical likelihood is confidence intervals. A confidence interval is a range of values that one can be certain contains the true mean of the population. Confidence intervals can also be defined as showing the range of the observed difference that would be expected if the same study were repeated an infinite number of times. For example, a 95% confidence interval would include the observed difference 95% of the times that the study was repeated. Factors affecting the width of the confidence interval include the size of the sample, the confidence level, and the variability in the sample. When all other factors are equal, a large sample size will tend to produce a better estimate of the population parameter.

Many statistical tests can be used to calculate *P* values and confidence intervals. The appropriate statistical test must be selected according to several factors. This includes (1) determining the number of observations in the comparison groups, (2) the number of groups being compared, (3) whether two or more groups are being compared with each other or one group is being compared with itself after some interval of time, (4) what kind of numerical data is being analyzed (e.g., continuous or categorical), (5) whether the sample is normally distributed (i.e., bell shaped) or has a skewed distribution, and (6) whether risk adjustment is required. Although most surgeons are unlikely to fully comprehend all of the nuances of more complex statistical analyses, the majority of surgical outcome studies employ simple designs and statistical tests that are within reach of the nonstatistician to interpret.

Type II errors. Type II errors occur in studies where the null hypothesis is falsely accepted. This often arises when the sample size is simply insufficient to detect small but clinically important differences in outcomes. When a study's sample size is too small to detect differences in outcomes between comparison groups, it is said to lack sufficient statistical power. But once a study is complete, no amount of analysis can correct for insufficient statistical power. Before starting a prospective study, researchers should perform a *power calculation*, which involves determining the minimum size of a meaningful difference in outcomes and then calculating the number of observations required to show that difference statistically.[44] Surgeons should be particularly cautious when evaluating studies with null findings, particularly when no power calculation is explicitly reported. Moreover, a post hoc power analysis can also be helpful with interpreting study results from retrospective studies when no statistically significant effects are found.[43] An evidence-based surgeon is wise to remember the adage, "no evidence for effect is not necessarily evidence of no effect."

INTERPRETING AND APPLYING EVIDENCE TO SURGICAL PRACTICE

Once you are convinced that the observed outcome from a clinical study is the result of the exposure or intervention and cannot be attributed to some alternative explanation (i.e., it is internally valid), then the next challenge to the surgeon is judging the study's external validity. In other words, you must determine whether the findings are applicable to the specific clinical scenario you are facing. Interpreting and applying evidence to surgical practice require a careful assessment of each study's external validity.

The assessment of external validity requires attention to core components of a clinical study, including the patient population, the intervention, and the outcomes that were measured. Even evidence derived from a well-designed, prospective RCT may not be valid if the population that was studied is different from the patient groups for which a surgeon is making clinical decisions. For example, consider the well-publicized multicenter randomized clinical trial that was conducted in the Veterans Administration (VA) to compare laparoscopic versus open inguinal hernia repair.[45] This study randomized military veterans who were, on average, older than the nonveteran general population that undergoes hernia repair and concluded that outcomes of open repair are superior to those of laparoscopic repair. But older subjects are more prone to the risks of general anesthesia needed for laparoscopic hernia repair, whereas simple open hernia repair can often be performed using local or minimal alveolar contraction (MAC) anesthesia. In this respect, a surgeon might consider the evidence provided by the RCT applicable to older patients but reserve judgment on the use of laparoscopy to repair hernias in younger, healthier patients.

As noted above, subject selection bias can adversely affect the external validity or generalizability of a study's results. Another example of the potential effect of selection bias on generalizability comes from the Asymptomatic Carotid Artery Stenosis (ACAS) trial.[46] In this large, prospective randomized trial, enrolled subjects were substantially younger and healthier than the average patient who undergoes carotid endarterectomy (CEA). As a result, the observed perioperative mortality rate in the trial was considerably lower than that observed in the general population or even in the very hospitals where the trial was conducted. Although the results of the ACAS trial significantly changed practice, one could argue that the evidence provided by ACAS trial should only be applied to younger patients with asymptomatic carotid stenosis.

The external validity of a clinical study can also be dependent upon the surgeon who intends to apply the evidence, along with their experience and expected outcomes. In the VA hernia trial, surgeons had variable experience with the laparoscopic approach, and the trial reported two fold differences in hernia recurrences between surgeons who had done more than 250 cases and surgeons who had less case experience.[45] Surgeons deciding whether the trial evidence supports the use of laparoscopic repair would need to examine their own experience before determining the generalizability of this study to their practices. Furthermore, the surgeon selection process for the ACAS trial mandated that expected CEA outcomes for any given surgeon must carry a combined stroke plus mortality rate of $\leq 3.0\%$ for asymptomatic patients.[46] As such, surgeons deciding to perform CEA for asymptomatic carotid stenosis based on the trial evidence must also be able to perform this operation with outcomes that are at least as good.

The type of outcome measured can also affect the generalizability of clinical studies. Outcomes chosen for clinical studies may be those that are most convenient or most easily quantified and may not be the outcomes of greatest interest to patients. In the VA hernia trial, several outcomes were studied, including operative complications, hernia recurrence, pain, and length of convalescence. Some of the outcome differences favored open repair, whereas some favored laparoscopic repair. The interpretation of the trial evidence for one type of repair versus the other involves implicit value judgments regarding which outcomes are most important and relevant to patients. This issue was also illustrated by findings from the Carotid Revascularization Endarterectomy Versus Stenting Trial (CREST), where patients with carotid stenosis were randomized to either CEA or carotid artery stenting.[47] While the study composite end-point (stroke, death, or myocardial infarction) did not differ between carotid artery stenting and CEA, there were still significant differences in individual outcome measures. Patients who underwent carotid artery stenting experienced higher rates of stroke than CEA, while patients who underwent CEA were found to have a higher risk of myocardial infarction. As such, surgeons applying evidence from CREST to preoperative decisions about method for carotid revascularization must weigh the relative risk of having a postoperative stroke versus a myocardial infarction outcome for an individual patient.

CONCLUSION

The practice of evidence-based surgery relies upon the judicious and systematic application of research evidence to everyday surgical decision-making. With an ever-expanding body of published surgical outcomes and health services research studies, knowing how to interpret the literature becomes increasingly important. Surgeons must be able to appraise the strength of scientific evidence as well as evaluate the quality of research studies before making decisions whether to apply the evidence to their own clinical practice. Consistently applying evidence-based medicine practices will help maintain high-value surgical care.

SELECTED REFERENCES

Cook DJ, Mulrow CD, Haynes RB. Systematic reviews: synthesis of best evidence for clinical decisions. *Ann Intern Med.* 1997;126:376–380.

Systematic reviews can help surgeons keep abreast of the literature by summarizing large bodies of evidence and helping to explain differences among studies on the same surgical question. This article provides an overview of how systematic reviews are undertaken and can be used by clinical providers.

Finlayson SR, Birkmeyer JD. Cost-effectiveness analysis in surgery. *Surgery*. 1998;123:151–156.

Hanley JA. Appropriate uses of multivariate analysis. *Annu Rev Public Health*. 1983;4:155–180.

Multivariate regression analysis is one of the most common statistical methods used to adjust for known confounders in surgical outcomes research. The article provides a comprehensive overview of different types of multivariate models and how they can be applied for risk adjustment and prediction.

Hlatky MA, Winkelmayer WC, Setoguchi S. Epidemiologic and statistical methods for comparative effectiveness research. *Heart Fail Clin*. 2013;9:29–36.

Observational studies that compare surgical treatments have methodological challenges that threaten the internal validity of their results. This article reviews several approaches to the analysis of observational data that can be used by outcomes and health services researchers to improve internal validity.

Kaji AH, Rademaker AW, Hyslop T. Tips for analyzing large data sets from the *JAMA Surgery* statistical editors. *JAMA Surg*. 2018;153:508–509.

Administrative data sets and patient registries are commonly used for surgical outcomes research but carry risks of bias and measurement error. This article reviews different methodological issues to consider when analyzing large data sets.

Little RJ, Rubin DB. Causal effects in clinical and epidemiological studies via potential outcomes: concepts and analytical approaches. *Annu Rev Public Health*. 2000;21:121–145.

A central focus of experimental and nonexperimental studies is how to make causal inferences about the effect of treatments on patient outcomes. This article reviews analytic approaches to help make causal inferences using different study designs.

Straus SE, Sackett DL. Using research findings in clinical practice. *BMJ*. 1998;317:339–342.

This article provides an overview of evidence-based medicine approaches and how they can be used by providers in routine clinical practice.

Tanner-Smith EE, Grant S. Meta-analysis of complex interventions. *Annu Rev Public Health*. 201;39:135–151.

Meta analysis is a prominent method used to combine the results from multiple studies and estimate the effects of different interventions. This article discusses meta analytic techniques that can be used in research syntheses on the effects of complex interventions such as those used in surgery.

REFERENCES

1. Castle JC, Chalmers I, Atkinson P, et al. Establishing a library of resources to help people understand key concepts in assessing treatment claims—the "Critical thinking and Appraisal Resource Library" (CARL). *PLoS One*. 2017;12:e0178666.
2. Guyatt G, Rennie D, Meade MO, et al. *Users' Guides to the Medical Literature: A Manual for Evidence-Based Clinical Practice*. 3rd ed. New York: McGraw-Hill Education; 2015.
3. Wilton NK, Slim AM. Application of the principles of evidence-based medicine to patient care. *South Med J*. 2012;105:136–143.
4. Farrugia P, Petrisor BA, Farrokhyar F, et al. Practical tips for surgical research: research questions, hypotheses and objectives. *Can J Surg*. 2010;53:278–281.
5. Schardt C, Adams MB, Owens T, et al. Utilization of the PICO framework to improve searching PubMed for clinical questions. *BMC Med Inform Decis Mak*. 2007;7:16.
6. Hill AB. The environment and disease: association or causation? *Proc R Soc Med*. 1965;58:295–300.
7. Shadish WR, Cook TD, Campbell DT. *Experimental and Quasi-experimental Designs for Generalized Causal Inference*. 2nd ed. New York: Houghton Mifflin Company; 2002.
8. Schulz KF, Altman DG, Moher D. CONSORT 2010 statement: updated guidelines for reporting parallel group randomised trials. *BMJ*. 2010;340:c332.
9. Schulz KF, Altman DG, Moher D, et al. CONSORT 2010 changes and testing blindness in RCTs. *Lancet*. 2010;375:1144–1146.
10. Haider AH, Bilimoria KY, Kibbe MR. A checklist to elevate the science of surgical database research. *JAMA Surg*. 2018;153:505–507.
11. von Elm E, Altman DG, Egger M, et al. The Strengthening the Reporting of Observational Studies in Epidemiology (STROBE) statement: guidelines for reporting observational studies. *J Clin Epidemiol*. 2008;61:344–349.
12. Doll KM, Rademaker A, Sosa JA. Practical guide to surgical data sets: Surveillance, Epidemiology, and End Results (SEER) database. *JAMA Surg*. 2018;153:588–589.
13. Ghaferi AA, Dimick JB. Practical guide to surgical data sets: medicare claims data. *JAMA Surg*. 2018;153:677–678.
14. Raval MV, Pawlik TM. Practical guide to surgical data sets: National Surgical Quality Improvement Program (NSQIP) and Pediatric NSQIP. *JAMA Surg*. 2018;153:764–765.
15. Desai SS, Kaji AH, Upchurch Jr G. Practical guide to surgical data sets: Society for Vascular Surgery Vascular Quality Initiative (SVS VQI). *JAMA Surg*. 2018;153:957–958.
16. Farjah F, Kaji AH, Chu D. Practical guide to surgical data sets: Society of Thoracic Surgeons (STS) National Database. *JAMA Surg*. 2018;153:955–956.
17. Brooke BS, Nathan H, Pawlik TM. Trends in the quality of highly cited surgical research over the past 20 years. *Ann Surg*. 2009;249:162–167.
18. Bartolucci AA, Hillegass WB. Overview, strengths, and limitations of systematic reviews and meta-analyses. In: Chiappelli F, Caldeira Brant XM, Neagos N, et al., eds. *Evidence-Based Practice: Toward Optimizing Clinical Outcomes*. Berlin: Springer-Verlag; 2010:17–33.

19. Ioannidis JP, Lau J. Pooling research results: benefits and limitations of meta-analysis. *Jt Comm J Qual Improv.* 1999;25:462–469.
20. Sanders GD, Neumann PJ, Basu A, et al. Recommendations for conduct, methodological practices, and reporting of cost-effectiveness analyses: second panel on cost-effectiveness in health and medicine. *JAMA.* 2016;316:1093–1103.
21. Weinstein MC, Torrance G, McGuire A. QALYs: the basics. *Value Health.* 2009;12(suppl 1):S5–S9.
22. Laupacis A, Feeny D, Detsky AS, et al. How attractive does a new technology have to be to warrant adoption and utilization? Tentative guidelines for using clinical and economic evaluations. *CMAJ.* 1992;146:473–481.
23. Zhang Z, Kolm P, Grau-Sepulveda MV, et al. Cost-effectiveness of revascularization strategies: the ASCERT study. *J Am Coll Cardiol.* 2015;65:1–11.
24. Blessberger H, Kammler J, Domanovits H, et al. Perioperative beta-blockers for preventing surgery-related mortality and morbidity. *Cochrane Database Syst Rev.* 2018;3:CD004476.
25. Denzin NK, Lincoln YS. *The SAGE Handbook of Qualitative Research.* 5th ed. Thousand Oaks, CA: SAGE Publications; 2018.
26. Maragh-Bass AC, Appelson JR, Changoor NR, et al. Prioritizing qualitative research in surgery: a synthesis and analysis of publication trends. *Surgery.* 2016;160:1447–1455.
27. Slager S, Beckstrom J, Weir C, et al. Information exchange between providers during transitions of surgical care: communication, documentation and sometimes both. *Stud Health Technol Inform.* 2017;234:303–308.
28. Brooke BS, Slager SL, Swords DS, et al. Patient and caregiver perspectives on care coordination during transitions of surgical care. *Transl Behav Med.* 2018;8:429–438.
29. Creswell JW, Creswell JD. *Research Design: Qualitative, Quantitative, and Mixed Methods Approaches.* 5th ed. London: SAGE Publications; 2018.
30. Mahmood T, Mylopoulos M, Bagli D, et al. A mixed methods study of challenges in the implementation and use of the surgical safety checklist. *Surgery.* 2019;165:832–837.
31. Harris RP, Helfand M, Woolf SH, et al. Current methods of the US Preventive Services Task Force: a review of the process. *Am J Prev Med.* 2001;20:21–35.
32. Woloshin S. Arguing about grades. *Eff Clin Pract.* 2000;3:94–95.
33. Barton MB, Miller T, Wolff T, et al. How to read the new recommendation statement: methods update from the U.S. Preventive Services Task Force. *Ann Intern Med.* 2007;147:123–127.
34. Atkins D, Eccles M, Flottorp S, et al. Systems for grading the quality of evidence and the strength of recommendations I: critical appraisal of existing approaches. The GRADE Working Group. *BMC Health Serv Res.* 2004;4:38.
35. Guyatt GH, Oxman AD, Vist GE, et al. GRADE: an emerging consensus on rating quality of evidence and strength of recommendations. *BMJ.* 2008;336:924–926.
36. Paradis C. Bias in surgical research. *Ann Surg.* 2008;248:180–188.
37. Peduzzi P, Concato J, Kemper E, et al. A simulation study of the number of events per variable in logistic regression analysis. *J Clin Epidemiol.* 1996;49:1373–1379.
38. Babyak MA. What you see may not be what you get: a brief, nontechnical introduction to overfitting in regression-type models. *Psychosom Med.* 2004;66:411–421.
39. Braitman LE, Rosenbaum PR. Rare outcomes, common treatments: analytic strategies using propensity scores. *Ann Intern Med.* 2002;137:693–695.
40. Stukel TA, Fisher ES, Wennberg DE, et al. Analysis of observational studies in the presence of treatment selection bias: effects of invasive cardiac management on AMI survival using propensity score and instrumental variable methods. *JAMA.* 2007;297:278–285.
41. Assmann SF, Pocock SJ, Enos LE, et al. Subgroup analysis and other (mis)uses of baseline data in clinical trials. *Lancet.* 2000;355:1064–1069.
42. Armstrong RA. When to use the Bonferroni correction. *Ophthalmic Physiol Opt.* 2014;34:502–508.
43. Kaji AH, Rademaker AW, Hyslop T. Tips for Analyzing large data sets from the JAMA Surgery statistical editors. *JAMA Surg.* 2018;153:508–509.
44. Stokes L. Sample size calculation for a hypothesis test. *JAMA.* 2014;312:180–181.
45. Neumayer L, Giobbie-Hurder A, Jonasson O, et al. Open mesh versus laparoscopic mesh repair of inguinal hernia. *N Engl J Med.* 2004;350:1819–1827.
46. Endarterectomy for asymptomatic carotid artery stenosis. Executive Committee for the Asymptomatic Carotid Atherosclerosis Study. *JAMA.* 1995;273:1421–1428.
47. Brott TG, Hobson 2nd RW, Howard G, et al. Stenting versus endarterectomy for treatment of carotid-artery stenosis. *N Engl J Med.* 2010;363:11–23.

9 CHAPTER

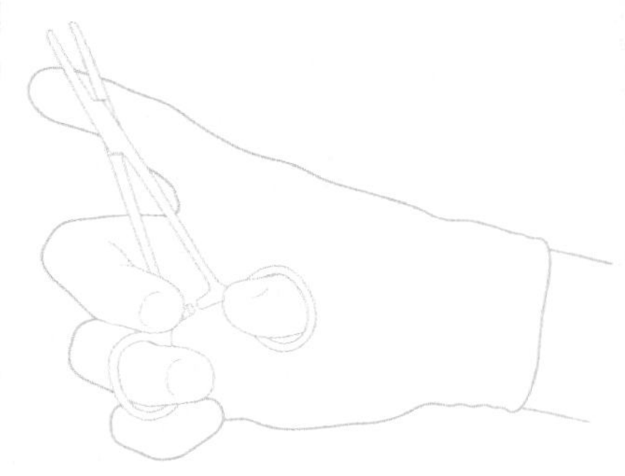

Safety in the Surgical Environment

Warren Sandberg, Roger R. Dmochowski, R. Daniel Beauchamp

OUTLINE

The intent of surgery is to improve health, so it was galvanizing when a series of eye-opening reports published in the 1990s provided clear evidence of high rates of serious adverse events that resulted in serious harm to hospitalized patients. In its landmark report *To Err is Human,* published in 1999, the Institute of Medicine[1] estimated that 1 million people per year were injured and 98,000 per year died as a result of medical errors. When the focus was specifically turned to surgical patients, surgical care accounted for 48% to 66% of adverse events among nonpsychiatric hospital discharges.[2] Adverse events occurred in 3% of operative procedures and deliveries, and surgical adverse events were associated with a 5.6% mortality rate, accounting for 12.2% of hospital deaths. Furthermore, 54% of surgical adverse events were judged to be preventable.

Adverse events in surgical patients encompass adverse events common to all hospitalized patients, such as adverse drug events, falls, missed diagnoses, deep venous thrombosis, pulmonary embolism, aspiration events, respiratory failure, nosocomial pneumonia, myocardial infarction, and cardiac arrhythmias. In addition, adverse events specific to surgery include technique-related complications, wound infections, and postoperative bleeding. In 2000, the Institute of Medicine called for a national effort to reduce medical errors by 50% within 5 years; however, progress fell far short of that goal despite numerous private and public initiatives aimed at finding solutions.[3] Leape and colleagues[3] proposed that these efforts were not adequate because health care organizations had not undertaken the major cultural changes required to accomplish true and lasting improvements in performance. Leape and colleagues[3] proposed that "health care entities must become 'high reliability organizations' that hold themselves accountable to consistently offer safe, effective patient centered care." These authors put forward the following five transforming concepts for adoption by health care organizations seeking such transformative change in culture: (1) Transparency must be a practiced value in everything we do; (2) care must be delivered by multidisciplinary teams working in integrated care platforms; (3) patients must become full partners in all aspects of health care; (4) health care workers need to find joy and meaning in their work; and (5) medical education must be redesigned to prepare new physicians to function in this new environment.

Since the publication of the position paper by Leape and colleagues,[3] significant improvements have occurred, but there still remains much to do. Mortality among patients hospitalized for surgery, while under 1% in most prospective reports, remains higher than what is achievable through more focus on perioperative patient safety. Probably the most reliable prospectively collected data come from large multi-institutional registries such as the National Surgical Quality Improvement Program (NSQIP) database. It should be noted that surgical interventions for traumatic injuries are not included in the NSQIP data and approximately 10% of the cases are emergencies. From NSQIP data obtained from 2012 to 2013, Freundlich and colleagues[4] identified 9255 deaths among 1.2 million patients within 30 days (0.77%) following their index surgical procedures. The most common causes of attributable mortality in this study were bleeding, respiratory failure, septic shock, and renal failure. Furthermore, in the same study, the authors estimated the years of life lost among these patients by using the Centers for Disease Control and Prevention life table and found that unplanned intubation, bleeding, and septic shock were associated with the greatest number of years of life lost (Table 9.1). These data provide important areas of focus in our efforts to prevent avoidable perioperative deaths in North America. In a recent study of perioperative patient outcomes in the African Surgical Outcomes Study published in 2018, reporting on 7-day mortality rates across 247 hospitals in 25 African countries, Biccard and colleagues[5] reported a 2.1% 7-day mortality rate, 94% of deaths occurring after the day of surgery. Importantly, this study included trauma and obstetric patients, and 57% of the entire 11,422 patient cohort had emergency operations and 11% had human immunodeficiency virus (HIV) infection as a comorbidity. Postoperative complications occurred in 18.2%, infection was the most common complication, occurring in 10.2% of all patients, and 9.7% of patients experiencing postoperative infection died. Active, prospective perioperative mortality assessment is possible in resource-constrained environments. For example, perioperative mortality was prospectively measured by a group of Kenyan anesthetists using an open source electronic tool in a rural Kenyan tertiary hospital.[6] The 7-day perioperative mortality was 1.5%, ranging from 0.5% for caesarian delivery to 3.6% for emergency surgery. The electronic tool also captured demographic, health status, and health care process data that highlight the regional differences between health care delivery systems that complicate global comparisons. For example, the Kenyan patients tended to be younger and healthier as a group than North American patients.

TABLE 9.1 Years of life lost associated with each complication, per 1 million patients.

	IN STUDY POPULATION			PER MILLION SURGERIES		
COMPLICATION	WOMEN	MEN	TOTAL	WOMEN	MEN	TOTAL
Bleeding	3474	2378	5852	2895	1981	4876
Unplanned intubation	3110	3367	6477	2592	2806	5397
Septic shock	1357	1284	2641	1131	1070	2202
Superficial infection	1171	816	1987	976	680	1656
Urinary tract infection	1094	613	1707	911	511	1422
Renal failure	679	961	1640	566	801	1367
Myocardial infarction	465	532	997	387	443	830
Stroke	510	441	951	425	368	792
Pneumonia	265	272	537	221	226	447
Renal insufficiency	266	357	623	222	297	519
Failure to wean	192	224	416	160	187	347
Sepsis	255	250	505	212	208	420
Wound infection	314	203	517	261	169	430
Venous thromboembolism	183	124	307	153	103	256
Pulmonary embolus	146	116	262	122	97	219
Wound dehiscence	45	29	74	38	24	62
Organ space infection	0	0	0	0	0	0
Come	0	0	0	0	0	0

From Freundlich RE, Maile MD, Sferra JJ, et al. Complications associated with mortality in the National Surgical Quality Improvement Program Database. *Anesth Analg.* 2018;127:55–62.

Another approach to measure perioperative mortality is to conduct the assessment as a structured sample across a wide range of participating hospitals. In an observational sampling study of 7-day mortality in Europe, there was enormous heterogeneity around a high (mean 3.6%) mortality rate, even in places such as Great Britain.[7] This result provoked numerous reexaminations of perioperative mortality and much lower estimates.[8–13] In a prospective study in a similar patient population by the same research group,[14] the mortality was much lower. Assessing the differences between these works is illustrative: In the prospective work, one of the study assessments was postoperative oxygen saturation determination. The mortality in this prospective study was much lower, only about 1%. Of that mortality, 40% was in the intensive care unit (ICU). One speculation as to the driver of the difference is that in the prospective study, an investigator physically interacts with patients. The investigator recognizes deteriorating patients and sends them to the ICU, where they either die or they are rescued and recover.

Given the apparent simplicity of the perioperative mortality statistic (the number of deaths [within a defined period] divided by the number of operations), it is surprisingly difficult to measure accurately. Prospectively recorded mortality data have the advantage of defined parameters and, in the case of the NSQIP, a robust cross-validation program to ensure that data abstraction is consistent across centers. However, these programs are inherently vulnerable to bias, as the measured endpoints are known to participating organizations and there are strong incentives tied to the mortality statistic. When trying to estimate a rate for perioperative mortality, observational and retrospective studies appear to be the most trustworthy for finding an upper bound on the estimate. These are more "environmentally valid," representing routine practice without unusual oversight or extra observation, but require careful attention to definitions, case finding, and data curation. On the other hand, registries, including those with associated quality improvement efforts, offer the advantage of prospective definitions of perioperative mortality, active data collection, and dedicated data management infrastructure but probably represent optimistic estimates. The picture remains challenging, but the simple solution of "paying more attention"—through leadership commitment to improving the quality of care through education and creating robust multidisciplinary systems of care supported by technology as appropriate—can produce real surgical quality improvements across the arc of perioperative medicine.

Regional differences in patient populations and resource availability hint at why perioperative mortality remains around 1% over time. As techniques and medical management improve, the cohort of operable patients continually becomes older and "sicker," and the persistence of mortality at around 1% reflects expanding access to surgery. Another trend that may drive the persistently high perioperative inpatient mortality is the shift of more and more patients to ambulatory surgery, creating a population of hospitalized patients with the most severe pathophysiology and increased risk of morbidity and mortality. In such a situation, maintaining a stable mortality rate in the face of increased acuity may reflect improvements in care.

Throughout the consideration of system-level efforts to improve safety in the surgical environment, it is important to remember that the individual surgeon's technique still influences outcomes. For example, in a study of 20 bariatric surgeons, there was a strong relationship between summary peer rating of technical skill (derived by expert review of blinded recordings of procedures) and risk-adjusted complication rates after laparoscopic gastric bypass.[15] Each diamond in Fig. 9.1 represents 1 of 20 practicing bariatric surgeons. Technical skill was assigned on a 1-to-5 scale (5 being better) by blinded review performed by at least 10 other surgeons unaware of the identity of the operating surgeon. Complication rates were obtained from a prospective, externally audited clinical outcomes registry after adjustment for patient comorbidities.[15] Surgical skill was predictive of the rate of surgical complications, nonsurgical (medical) complications, reoperations, readmissions, and emergency department visits, indicating that the technical skill of the surgeon is a potential driver of many of the system-level performance domains currently receiving much attention in the area of quality improvement.

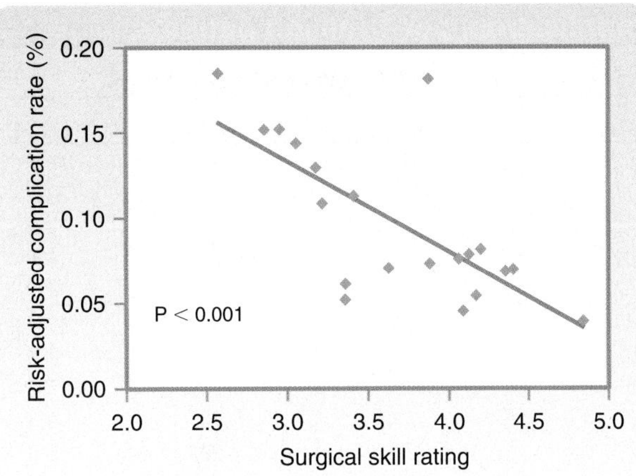

FIG. 9.1 Relationship between summary peer rating of technical skill and risk-adjusted complication rates after laparoscopic gastric bypass. (From Birkmeyer JD, Finks JF, O'Reilly A, et al. Surgical skill and complication rates after bariatric surgery. *N Engl J Med.* 2013;369:1434–1442.)

How then do we create an environment where it is acceptable to acknowledge differences in performance as the first step toward across-the-board performance improvement? Also, how do we collect and report back the data required to assess current performance and monitor progress toward the desired state?

FOSTERING A CULTURE OF SAFETY THROUGH LEADERSHIP

Creating a culture of safety in the perioperative system requires leadership investment from surgeons. In the perioperative system, just as in the operating room (OR) and procedure suite, the surgeon sets the tone, but he or she cannot achieve success alone. Creating a joint governance structure in the perioperative system wherein nursing staff, advance practice nurses, anesthesiologists, and other medical consultants are fully engaged in leadership is vital to capturing the engagement and expertise of these clinicians in the patient safety effort. Health systems are recognizing this fact and trying to cement the multidisciplinary approach by creating service lines wherein all the clinician and nonclinician individuals engaged in the care of selected disease categories or patient populations are grouped into one organizational structure. For example, at Vanderbilt University Medical Center, there are major service lines organized around the care of the surgical patient, and these are jointly led by the chairs of the departments of surgery and anesthesiology and by the nursing leaders of inpatient, outpatient, and perioperative care. The leadership of the perioperative enterprise is tripartite, with the chairs of surgery and anesthesiology and the associate chief nursing officer for perioperative services as coexecutives.

These leadership teams create transparency and fair adjudication of conflicts over scarce resources such as OR time and access to hospital beds, which builds trust and reduces conflict. The tripartite leadership executive models promote behavioral modeling by example. The leaders articulate the expectation of engagement with quality initiatives such as hand hygiene[16] by fully participating themselves and by using executive authority to encourage good performance in subordinates. They also demonstrate commitment to patient safety by investing departmental and institutional resources into the creation and operation of quality and safety organizations within their respective departments and across the service line.

At Vanderbilt University Medical Center, there is a perioperative chief quality officer who works with clinical leadership, nursing, and administration within the patient care areas to identify priorities and to identify necessary resources to support quality improvement and to address safety issues promptly. The Center for Clinical Improvement in the institution provides assistance with resources to support root cause analyses of patient deaths, adverse outcomes, and near misses. Reporting of adverse outcomes and near misses is encouraged in a "blame-free" environment, both in person and via a confidential web-based reporting tool. Within the Perioperative Enterprise, there is a Surgical Site Infection Collaborative and a Perioperative Quality and Safety Committee that collaborate with one another and that receive inputs from the various surgical services, perioperative nursing services, and infection control services. Each surgical service conducts weekly to biweekly morbidity, mortality, and improvement (MMI) conferences. Cases identified in these service-level MMI conferences that exemplify "systems" concerns or issues are referred to a multidisciplinary MMI committee that selects cases for presentation at an institution-wide MMI conference that is held on a quarterly basis. System-level quality projects identified in these various venues are "worked" by quality improvement teams until the quality problems are solved, usually as evidenced by diminution or elimination of the problem for an extended period or a number of cases.

LOCAL ORGANIZATIONAL STRUCTURES TO PROMOTE PERIOPERATIVE SAFETY

When considering the local working environment, procedures, and policies in any health care organization, it is important to remember that almost every step, check, and double-check in the perioperative process, no matter how apparently redundant or pointless, was almost certainly developed as a reaction to a near miss or an event involving patient harm. Nevertheless, it is important to revisit continually and optimize patient care processes in a proactive way to engineer systems deliberately to ensure patient and personnel safety.

Effective health care organizations develop and maintain a multidisciplinary patient safety program that operates in a blame-free culture where deference to expertise is one of the norms of behavior. Input to the program includes proactive scans for opportunities to improve systems but importantly features many routes for reporting nonroutine events, near misses, and critical events for analysis and system redesigns when needed. At Vanderbilt University Medical Center, each of the major role groups has an appointed patient safety officer (PSO) operating in concert with the perioperative chief quality officer. These individuals are chosen for their discretion and effectiveness at taking in and appropriately routing information about safety problems and for their ability to shepherd such investigations and process improvements through to completion. The quality management structure created in the Department of Anesthesiology at Vanderbilt University Medical Center can serve as one illustration of an effective and equitable system (Fig. 9.2). The PSO can receive reports from the confidential web-based reporting system, reports from self-disclosures as part of routine medical documentation, and in-person reports. Institutional Risk Management is also included in report review so as to integrate risk mitigation with improvement activities. The surgical departments have an almost identical quality and safety organizational structure. The surgical and anesthesiology organizational structures are closely associated, and continuous communication links surveillance and intervention activities.

The PSO serves as the primary input point and clearing house for safety considerations and can refer issues to a Quality, Morbidity,

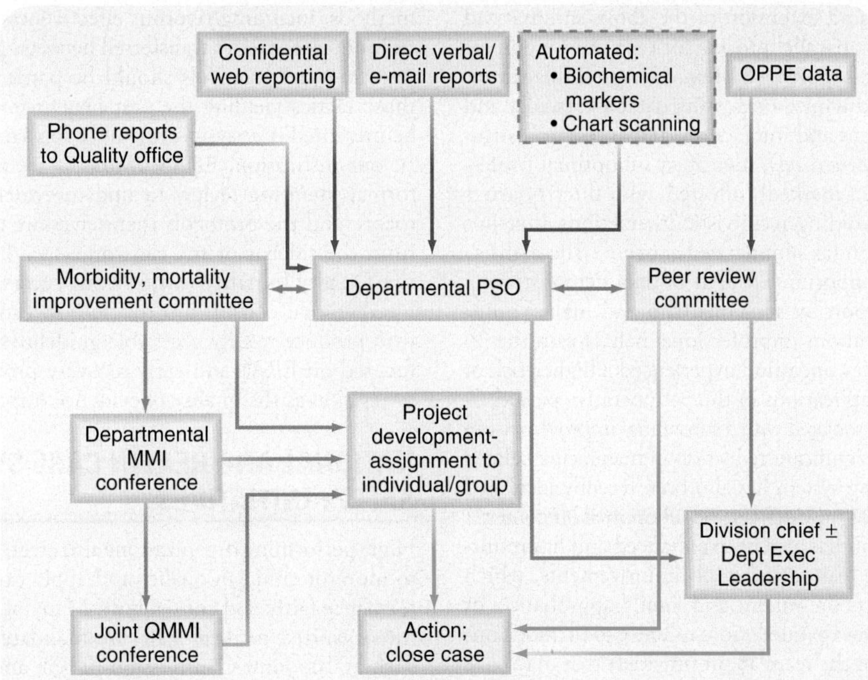

FIG. 9.2 Patient safety officer (PSO) inputs and relationships. The *red arrows* indicate pathways by which information about patient safety events and system quality functions and opportunities for improvements are routed to the PSO. The *blue arrows* indicate communication pathways and potential issue routing between the PSO and the various quality, safety, and performance improvement functions in a procedural department. The *green arrows* indicate information flow and directives to executive and leadership functions for action items developed by the quality and safety functions. The *dashed outline box* indicates a new information input function that is being implemented as of writing. *MMI,* Morbidity, Mortality Improvement; *OPPE,* ongoing professional practice evaluation; *QMMI,* Quality, Morbidity, Mortality Improvement.

Mortality Improvement (QMMI) Committee to deal with system-of-care problems amenable to structural, procedural, and technical solutions or to a Peer Review Committee to deal with events related more to individual performance, knowledge, and decision making, or both. The departmental PSO collaborates with PSOs from other professional departments and from Perioperative Services, all under the umbrella of a multidisciplinary QMMI Committee cochaired by the surgery and anesthesiology PSOs.

Projects referred to the QMMI Committee have included refreshing protocols for cardiac implantable electronic device management, multidisciplinary development of policies and procedures for management of surgical patients receiving dual antiplatelet therapy for maintenance of drug-eluting intracoronary stents, optimization of perioperative assessment and management of the patient with sleep apnea, and adoption of postsurgical structured debriefs. These are public projects. Alternatively, most of the work of the Peer Review Committee is confidential and protected from discovery by legal statute. The Peer Review Committee comprises individual clinicians selected for their clinical acumen, probity, and discretion.

The departmental PSO maintains a confidential database of reports, analyses, projects, and dispositions of QMMI projects as well as Peer Review Committee referrals. Because of the sensitive nature of the work and the need to preserve a safe environment for reporting, the entire safety reporting and peer review process is firewalled from operational leadership (i.e., the people who make decisions about OR access, team assignments, salaries) unless there is a QMMI Committee recommendation or a Peer Review Committee recommendation for executive action. This process is illustrated in Fig. 9.2—the departmental executive leadership charters and supports the quality and safety structures, but they are depicted out of the critical path of function of the structures they sponsor.

Increasing emphasis is now being placed on the experience of the patient and the patient's family and their satisfaction with care, and the importance of optimizing that experience is now a priority for health care delivery systems. Physicians and providers may occasionally have suboptimal interactions with patients and families. Most of these instances represent aberrancies; however, a relatively small number of professionals exhibit patterns of behavior or performance that may affect team performance or the experience of the patient and family.[17,18] At our institution, to promote professionalism, when a single event or pattern of events is observed or reported, timely feedback is provided by trained physician messengers to the individual who is the subject of the report. To facilitate the documentation of events or patient concerns, an electronic record exists to support reporting. This database provides a surveillance tool that can identify events or patterns associated with providers or microenvironments within the institution. Using these data, an intervention algorithm is applied based on the type, frequency, and pattern of events or concerns. Using this accountability model, a nonjudgmental, nondirective conversation occurs between a "concerned professional" and a colleague regardless of hierarchy. When repeated nonprofessional behaviors become manifest, institutional structures exist to provide opportunities to access a variety of resources to support physician and provider wellness, inclusive of counseling support, substance abuse intervention, and psychologic/cognitive evaluation.

The identified importance of team-based interactions centered on collegiality, effective communication, and mutual respect has resulted in an evolution and extension of the above summarized patient-facing system to a parallel process for care team members known as the Co-Worker Reporting System. Using a similar infrastructure (inclusive of anonymized reporting database, faculty and staff leadership engagement and interaction, and access to institutional wellness support structures), identified suboptimal professional behaviors have been markedly affected, with three-quarters of identified providers avoiding recidivistic interactions after initial structured intervention (as summarized above).[19] These observations are particularly important in light of data demonstrating that patients operated upon by surgeons who had higher numbers of coworker reports about unprofessional behavior in the 36 months before the patient's operation experienced a higher risk of surgical and medical complications in the perioperative period.[20]

This system has been associated with a substantial improvement in patient satisfaction and a significant reduction in malpractice-related costs. The patient reporting system has also been recently identified as signaling the potential for provider-centric suboptimal outcomes.[21]

Team-based satisfaction has also been enhanced and has resulted in microenvironment team satisfaction improvements, which have had reciprocal effects on patient and family approbation of care. This system has been expanded more recently to include concerns of other members of the team about providers that may have adverse consequences for health care team interactions and care outcomes. The team-based concerns have identified numerous areas for improvement in provider behaviors and have increased within-team functionality.

Safety in the perioperative environment should also be pursued from the orientation of optimizing surgical and health outcomes, both on the individual patient level and across populations. Accelerating interest in implementing and testing scientifically founded (or at least well-reasoned) approaches to optimize preparation for and recovery from surgery, collectively known as enhanced recovery after surgery (ERAS) techniques, reflects this orientation. To the extent that complications are avoided and recuperation is accelerated and ensured, ERAS approaches improve perioperative safety.

Safety improvements whose benefits include financial ones that drop directly to the bottom line (such as length of stay reductions from effective ERAS programs) are likely to receive interest and support from all stakeholder parties. Thoughtful ERAS implementation can simultaneously reduce length of stay and complications,[22,23] while also favorably impacting topical considerations such as postoperative opioid consumption and postoperative nausea and vomiting.[24] It is important to keep the focus on application of scientifically sound tactics to speed and improve the recuperation from surgery, rather than focus on surrogate endpoints such as cost or length of stay. A well-implemented, patient-centered ERAS program will produce better patient outcomes in which the economic outcomes become incidental, yet are virtually assured.

Despite more than 20 years since the formal description of ERAS pathways, there is much to be discovered and many opportunities for broader implementation. The original ERAS protocol focused on colorectal surgery,[25] and it is unclear whether many of the tactics developed for this patient population are relevant or translatable to other surgical patient populations.[26] The focus on length of stay is an outcome in the ERAS literature along with reflexive transfer of ERAS tactics between surgical domains without reassessment of their benefit/risk profile have led the originator to caution that ERAS interventions should be scientifically based and holistically studied, rather than focused on operational or financial outcomes.[27] Ideally, ERAS protocols should be developed and implemented using formal quality improvement methods, including rigorous effectiveness and risk testing of new techniques or tactics transferred between patient populations. The implemented protocols should be parsimonious, including only those tactics yielding the best benefit-to-ratios, and they should be presented in easy-to-remember formats as shown in Fig. 9.3.[22] At our institution, ERAS protocols are periodically subjected to formal literature review to update evidence and revise the protocols, and the protocols themselves are accessible via direct link from the sidebar of the electronic health record. The Perioperative Quality Initiative (https://.org/, accessed May 19, 2019) is an international consortium focused on early surgical recovery and who produce readily accessible guidelines and evidence syntheses focused on ERAS and early recovery protocols, again, all subject to revision as the quality of evidence improves over time.

NATIONAL AND HEALTH CARE SYSTEM–LEVEL SAFETY INITIATIVES

High-performing organizations also create an efficient bureaucracy to monitor clinician quality and apply expected standards of performance fairly and consistently. Many of these structures, such as the organized medical staff, are mandated by accrediting bodies such as The Joint Commission (TJC), and they serve meaningful purposes in terms of ensuring a consistent level of quality in the medical staff. For example, the requirement for ongoing professional practice evaluation is intended to ensure that all members of the medical staff are frequently evaluated in their specialty practice by methods that are objective and applied more frequently than annually. These evaluations take many forms, ranging from document review to direct observation. Key features of a well-designed ongoing professional practice evaluation process include direct mapping to the clinician's unique medical practice, frequent review, and objective criteria for identifying clinicians whose practice falls outside of normative expectations.

Frequent peer-to-peer assessment via survey is a middle ground between the nonspecific nature of chart reviews and the substantial effort required by direct observations. Box 9.1 demonstrates the series of nine peer-to-peer questions used in the Vanderbilt University Department of Anesthesiology (but transferable to virtually any specialty) to assess specific performance elements that map to the six Accreditation Council for Graduate Medical Education general competencies. There are also summative, general questions. In the Vanderbilt Department of Anesthesiology, these questions are automatically assigned (by a program that runs alongside and is accessible from within the electronic medical record [EMR]) to clinician pairs who have worked together recently. Confidential responses are collected by the same software, and the data are presented to designated individuals (the Peer Review Committee Chair in our case). The Vanderbilt University Medical Center system handles all of the transactions automatically and electronically, but other practices operate such systems using e-mail, for example.

Clinicians who are new members of the medical staff, clinicians who request new or expanded privileges, and clinicians identified as differing from normative expectations all are subject to a focused professional practice evaluation. TJC allows the medical staff organization substantial latitude in the construction of a focused professional practice evaluation; however, in most instances, a focused professional practice evaluation involves some form of direct proctoring in the identified area of medical practice. In addition to a robust and efficient bureaucracy focused on normative expectations of practice, high-performing organizations establish quality and safety improvement teams (see earlier) that operate autonomously but with the support of the departmental or practice hierarchies.

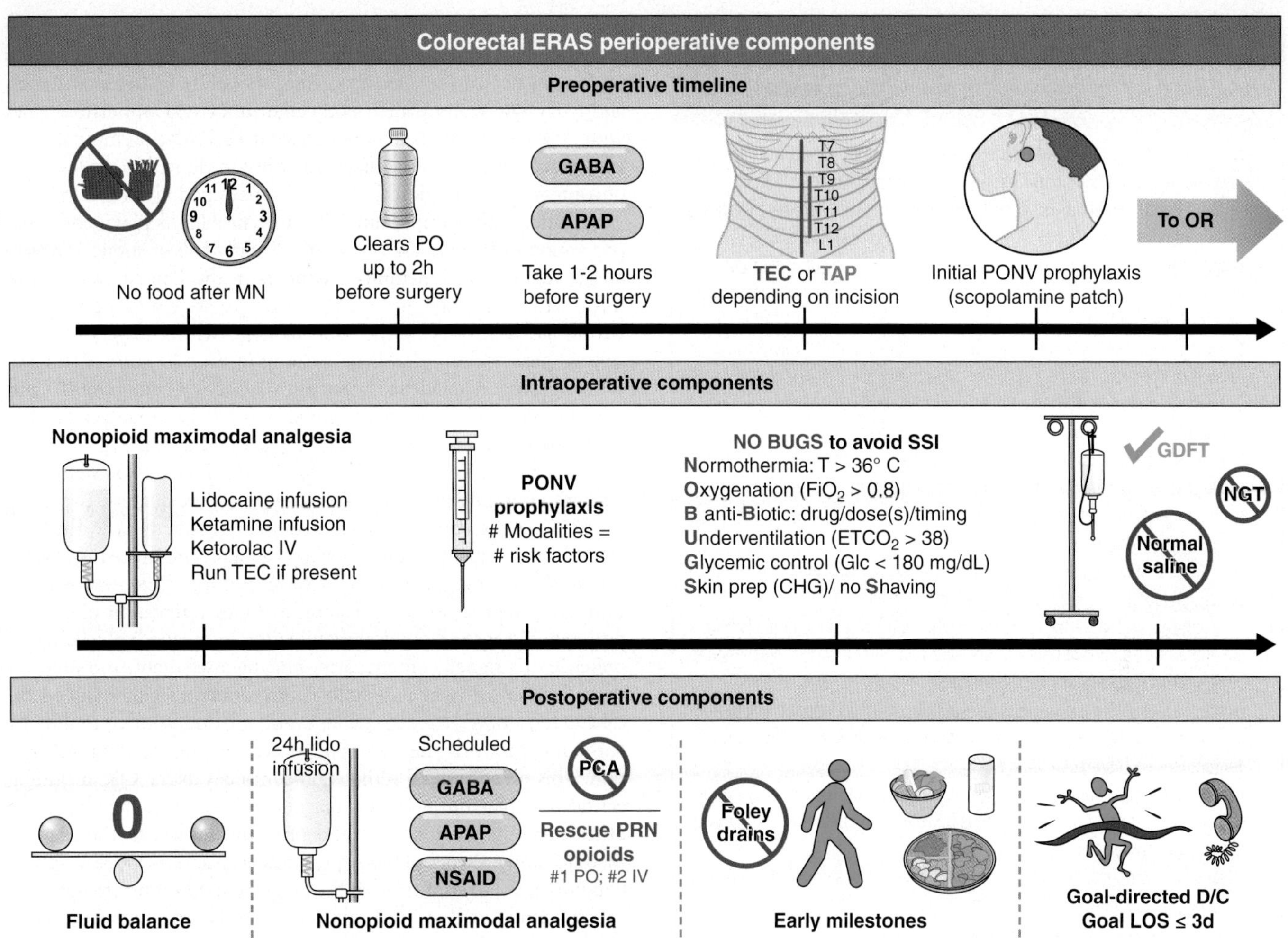

FIG. 9.3 Colorectal enhanced recovery after surgery *(ERAS)* perioperative components. This figure illustrates the principles and goals of the ERAS pathway for colorectal surgical patients at our institution in each phase of care, starting the night before surgery. Of note, the preoperative oral fluid loading on the night before and morning of surgery is currently in the initial implementation phase. (From McEvoy MD, Wanderer JP, King AB, et al. A perioperative consult service results in reduction in cost and length of stay for colorectal surgical patients: evidence from a healthcare redesign project. *Perioper Med (Lond).* 2016;5:3.) *APAP,* Acetaminophen; *CHG,* chlorhexidine gluconate; *D/C,* hospital discharge; *$ETCO_2$,* end tidal carbon dioxide; *FiO_2,* fraction of inspired oxygen; *GABA,* gabapentinoid; *GDFT,* goal-directed fluid therapy; *IV,* intravenous; *lido,* lidocaine; *LOS,* length of stay; *MN,* midnight; *NGT,* XXX; *NSAID,* nonsteroidal antiinflammatory drug; *OR,* operating room; *PCA,* patient-controlled analgesia; *PO,* per os (by mouth); *PONV,* postoperative nausea and vomiting; *PRN,* pro re nata (for which it is needed); *SSI,* surgical site infection; *T,* temperature; *TAP,* transversus abdominus plane block; *TEC,* thoracic epidural catheter.

Major government and third-party payers are becoming increasingly interested in quality and safety in health care, and much attention at the present time focuses on high criticality environments such as perioperative and periprocedural systems. Payers now regularly collect process outcomes (e.g., timely preoperative antibiotic administration) and health outcomes (e.g., surgical site infection) and report them publicly (http://www.medicare.gov/hospitalcompare). Accrediting bodies, specialty boards, and government payers all are applying pressure to clinicians to focus on quality and safety in their practices (Table 9.2).

Perioperative team building has parallels in the aviation industry in that teams intermittently come together for relatively short, defined periods of time to accomplish a complex task requiring the specialized skills of each team member under potentially stressful conditions in which there is inherent danger. Haynes and colleagues[28] demonstrated the impact of implementing a standardized surgical safety checklist on patient outcomes. In a study of more than 3700 surgical patients from eight major hospitals in eight cities worldwide, they found that implementing the checklist reduced complication rates from 11% to 7% and reduced postoperative death rate from 1.5% to 0.8%.

Shortly after the landmark study by Haynes and colleagues,[28] de Vries and coworkers[29] reported that the implementation of a comprehensive, multidisciplinary surgical safety checklist that included medications, marking of the operative site, and postoperative management plans in six hospitals in the Netherlands resulted in a significant decrease in complication rates and in-hospital mortality. These results were compared with data from a control group of five hospitals. When compared with a 3-month baseline period, the rates of total complications in surgical patients were reduced from 27.3 per 100 to 16.7 per 100. The proportion of patients with one or more complications decreased from 15.4% to 10.6%, and the inpatient mortality rate decreased from 1.5% to 0.8% in the surgical population among the study group of hospitals. Control hospitals did not experience a change in these outcomes over the same time intervals.

BOX 9.1 Elements of a survey-based ongoing professional practice evaluation process

Please evaluate the individual in the context of patient care. Rate how you believe the individual demonstrates the following competencies. Choices are: Poor, Fair, Good, Excellent, or Abstain (No basis for knowledge to evaluate this competency).

1. Engages in evidence-based practice. Integrates new evidence to improve his/her own patient care practices (competency in *practice-based learning and improvement*).
2. Demonstrates *medical knowledge* about established and evolving science related to the practice of _________ (specialty).
3. Behaves in a manner that exemplifies *professionalism* (honesty and integrity, work ethic, punctuality, altruism, bringing honor to the profession).
4. Communicates in a manner that demonstrates respect toward coworkers, facilitates interdisciplinary teamwork, and results in effective information exchange and optimal patient care (competency in *interpersonal and communication skills*).
5. Adapts well to changing clinical demands affecting workload and resource allocation (competency in *systems-based practice*).
6. Is organized and well-prepared for his/her clinical assignment. Provides excellent and compassionate patient care and demonstrates excellence in clinical skills (competency in *patient care*).
7. Appropriately seeks and accepts consultation from colleagues (competencies in *practice-based learning and improvement, professionalism,* and *interpersonal and communication skills*).
8. Makes you comfortable handing over care of a patient to, accepting a handover of care from, or sharing responsibility for the care of a patient with him/her (*all* competencies)
9. Makes you comfortable referring a friend or loved one for clinical care by him/her (*all* competencies).

Neily and associates[30] demonstrated that implementation of a medical team training program with intraoperative briefings and debriefings in 74 Department of Veterans Affairs hospitals resulted in 18% improvement in annual risk-adjusted surgical mortality compared with a 7% decrease in mortality among 34 facilities that had not received such training. The mortality rates did not begin to show improvement until the second quarter after such training was completed and improved more through the third quarter. Other improvements reported during structured interviews of participants in the team training included improved communication among OR staff, increased staff awareness, improved overall efficiency, and improved overall teamwork.

In contrast to the aforementioned positive observational studies, Urbach and colleagues[31] reported the results of a group of 101 surgical hospitals in Ontario, Canada, using administrative health data to compare operative mortality, rates of surgical complications, and other 30-day postdischarge outcomes before and after adoption of a surgical safety checklist. In assessment of the 3 months before and after adoption of the surgical safety checklist including more than 100,000 procedures for each time interval, they observed that adjusted risk of death within 30 days of an operation was 0.71% before implementation and 0.65% after implementation of the checklist, a nonstatistically significant difference. Also, there was no significant difference in the adjusted risk of surgical complications in comparing the time periods before and after implementation. On the surface, this study did not support the efficacy of surgical safety checklists, but the study has several important limitations, including the short study intervals of only 3 months, resulting in inadequate levels of adoption of the checklists and inadequate assessment of the compliance and quality of the practice of the checklists. Also, the study included a skewed and likely low-acuity patient population of 60.8% ambulatory cases with 20% of all cases being eye cases and 28.7% being musculoskeletal cases. This low acuity is likely to have contributed to the low rates of complications and deaths observed in both periods in this study.

A different but important focus for checklist deployment is the prevention of rare, devastating events. Nearly half of surgical "never" events resulting in indemnity payments in the United States result from "wrong surgeries"—a concept encompassing a wrong procedure, wrong site, or surgery on the wrong person. Wrong surgery often results in patient death and is devastating to the care team. Estimates of wrong surgery incidence range from 1:112,994[32] to 1:5000[33] and may be increasing. Checklist application[28,34] has reduced the frequency of complications resulting in injury and death. TJC has made the implementation of the Universal Protocol for the prevention of wrong-site, wrong-patient, and wrong-procedure surgery, including the preprocedural time-out, an accreditation requirement.[35] The Universal Protocol includes the following elements: preprocedural verification, site marking, and final verification during the preprocedural time-out. Preprocedural verification includes verification of the appropriate history and physical examination in the medical record, the presence of a signed consent form, nursing assessment, and preanesthesia assessment (when applicable). At Vanderbilt University Medical Center, a nonemergency patient cannot be transported to the OR without completing these components of the preprocedural verification. This preprocedural verification continues in the OR, including verification that the necessary diagnostic laboratory, radiology, and other test results are present and properly displayed. The requirement for and presence of blood products, implants, devices, or special equipment is also confirmed in the preprocedural verification process.

The time-out that occurs immediately before initiation of the procedure provides a final verification of the correct patient, correct site, and correct procedure. The time-out is most effective when it is standardized and conducted consistently in all procedural areas of the hospital; it should be conducted immediately before starting an invasive procedure or making the incision. It is initiated by a designated member of the procedural team and involves the immediate members of the procedure team. During the time-out, other activities are suspended so that team members may focus on active confirmation of the patient, site, and procedure. Any new team members should be introduced. At a minimum, the team members must agree on the correct patient identity, correct procedural site (with the site marking verified when laterality or level is a concern), and correct procedure to be done. Finally, completion of the time-out should be documented for the patient medical record.

This description of the surgical time-out defines the minimal criteria to satisfy TJC requirements; however, if these are the only elements included in the process, the positive impact is limited. The Crew Resource Management training and discipline of the Universal Protocol enables organizations to enhance communication between health care professionals in the perioperative management teams and to incorporate process improvement measures, such as those defined by the Surgical Care Improvement Project, into the checklists. These evidence-based interventions include timely administration of perioperative antibiotics and administration of beta blockers in patients at risk of ischemic heart disease, venous thromboembolism prophylaxis, and intraoperative normothermia. The time-out checklist may also include availability and sterility of instrumentation and implantable devices. The conclusion of the optimal surgical time-out should include an open

TABLE 9.2 Major perioperative and surgical data registries and quality improvement initiatives.

PROJECT NAME	ACRONYM	SPONSOR ORGANIZATIONS	MAJOR INITIATIVES	KEY RESULTS	REFERENCES
Surgical Care Improvement Project	SCIP	CMS, CDC, AHRQ, ACS, AHA, ASA, AORN, VA, IHI, TJC	(1) Reduce incidence and impact of SSIs through timely administration and discontinuation of appropriate antibiotics, appropriate glucose control in selected patient populations, hair removal by clipping, maintenance of normothermia, and appropriate removal of urinary catheters (2) Reduce incidence of perioperative major cardiac events by continuing beta blockade in patients with previous beta blockade (3) Reduce venous thromboembolism and pulmonary embolism by use of thromboprophylaxis when indicated	SCIP process measure compliance is publically reported, sorted by hospital Better compliance with timely antibiotic administration and selection of appropriate antibiotic was associated with a robust reduction in SSI rates* Compliance with the overall process bundle, assessed as an all-or-none score, was associated with an adjusted odds ratio for infection of 0.85 (95% confidence interval, 0.76-0.95), but none of the individual SCIP measures alone were significantly associated with reduced probability of infection†	Fry DE. Surgical site infections and the Surgical Care Improvement Project (SCIP): evolution of national quality measures. *Surg Infect (Larchmt)*. 2008;9:579–584. http://www.jointcommission.org/assets/1/6/Surgical%20Care%20Improvement%20Project.pdf
National Surgical Quality Improvement Program	VA-NSQIP, ACS-NSQIP	VA, ACS	Risk-adjusted outcomes databases comprising up to 135 clinical variables including perioperative risk factors, intraoperative and postoperative events, morbidities, and 30-day mortality, all prospectively abstracted from the medical record by dedicated nursing personnel	Sampling methodology: Hospitals abstract data and send to ACS for analysis. Data are reported back to hospitals along with risk-adjusted comparison to all other hospitals. Hospitals act on data and use subsequent NSQIP performance to monitor (hoped for) performance improvements ACS NSQIP risk calculator (http://riskcalculator.facs.org/) can be used to estimate risks of complications, death, and length of stay	http://site.acsnsqip.org/ For a review of the history, function, and evidence that feedback quality and between-hospital comparisons improve hospital performance and patient outcomes: Maggard-Gibbons M. The use of report cards and outcome measurements to improve the safety of surgical care: The American College of Surgeons National Surgical Quality Improvement Program. *BMJ Qual Saf.* 2014;23:589–599.
Society of Thoracic Surgeons National Database	STS National Database	STS	Prospective, self-reported clinical variables reported to a national database. Three distinct areas of focus are maintained: adult cardiac surgery, general thoracic surgery, and congenital heart surgery. Performance outcomes reports are fed back to participant organizations in risk-adjusted format to allow comparison with local, regional, and national norms	STS public reporting online for CABG, AVR, and AVR + CABG; first public reporting of hospital and surgeon group level performance. Reports are published online and in the consumer journal *Consumer Reports*. Current data are incomplete—not all hospitals and groups have reported data in a form suitable to be listed	http://www.sts.org/national-database
Metabolic and Bariatric Surgery Accreditation and Quality Improvement Program	MBSAQIP	ACS, ASMBS	Accreditation standard setting and monitoring for bariatric surgery programs. All accredited centers report outcomes to MBSAQIP database using a prospective, longitudinal data collection system based on standardized definitions and collected by trained data reviewers, analogous to NSQIP. Provides semiannual, risk-adjusted comparative performance reports to participating centers	In 2011, published comparative morbidity and effectiveness of the major gastric volume reduction procedures were based on data gathered from 109 participating centers‡ Periodically publishes Resources for Optimal Care of the Bariatric Surgery Patient	https://www.facs.org/quality-programs/mbsaqip

Continued

TABLE 9.2 **Major perioperative and surgical data registries and quality improvement initiatives.—cont'd**

PROJECT NAME	ACRONYM	SPONSOR ORGANIZATIONS	MAJOR INITIATIVES	KEY RESULTS	REFERENCES
American College of Surgeons National Trauma Databank	ACS-NTDB	ACS			
Hospital Compare		CMS	Data gathered from multiple mandatory reporting sources or gathered independently by CMS. Includes survey data about experiences as reported by recently discharged patients	Public reporting site that allows individual patients to view and compare hospital performance data within their area as well as regionally and nationally. Ostensibly, patients could use such comparisons to make decisions about where to seek elective care for specific conditions	http://www.medicare.gov/hospitalcompare

ACS, American College of Surgeons; *AHA*, American Heart Association; *AHRQ*, Agency for Healthcare Research and Quality; *AORN*, Association of Perioperative Registered Nurses; *ASA*, American Society of Anesthesiologists; *ASMBS*, American Society for Metabolic and Bariatric Surgery; *AVR*, aortic valve replacement; *CABG*, coronary artery bypass grafting; *CDC*, U.S. Centers for Disease Control and Prevention; *CMS*, Centers for Medicare and Medicaid Services; *IHI*, Institute for Healthcare Improvement; *MBSAQIP*, Metabolic and Bariatric Surgery Accreditation and Quality Improvement Program; *NSQIP*, National Surgical Quality Improvement Program; *NTDB*, National Trauma Databank; *SCIP*, Surgical Care Improvement Project; *SSI*, surgical site infection; *STS*, Society of Thoracic Surgeons; *TJC*, The Joint Commission; *VA*, Department of Veterans Affairs.

*Cataife G, Weinberg DA, Wong HH, et al. The effect of Surgical Care Improvement Project (SCIP) compliance on surgical site infections (SSI). *Med Care*. 2014;52:S66–S73.

†Stulberg JJ, Delaney CP, Neuhauser DV, et al. Adherence to surgical care improvement project measures and the association with postoperative infections. *JAMA*. 2010;303:2479–2485.

‡Hotter MM, Schirmer BD, Jones DB, et al. First report from the American College of Surgeons Bariatric Surgery Center Network: laparoscopic sleeve gastrectomy has morbidity and effectiveness positioned between the band and the bypass. *Ann Surg*. 2011;254:410–420, discussion 420–422.

invitation for any member of the team to speak up at any time during the procedure if they recognize a problem that poses risk to the patient or health care team. Box 9.2 summarizes elements of surgical safety checklists.

Checklists must be performed reliably to be effective, which requires the care team to achieve optimal performance consistently. This is a potential vulnerability. To create a technologic backstop to team performance, Vanderbilt University Medical Center has used automated process monitoring and process control as well as forced function concepts to implement an electronic time-out checklist to reduce the wrong surgery rate. We created an electronic preprocedural briefing and time-out checklist mediated via the intraoperative nursing documentation module of our OR documentation system.[36] Checklist questions are sequentially displayed to the entire care team on a large in-room monitor (Fig. 9.4) interposed as a required documentation step between the "patient-in-OR" and "incision" events. Total development costs were $34,000 and used existing hardware. In a de novo installation, the additional hardware cost would have been $2500 per OR. We were able to recreate the system when changing EMRs, and it operates to the current day.

In our assessment of system effectiveness, all 243,939 main campus OR cases between July 30, 2010, and April 5, 2015, were subject to the electronic time-out procedure, and no wrong surgeries were detected. In the six full years prior to deployment, there were only two wrong surgeries detected (2 in 253,838 cases). We conducted a Bayesian analysis of the probability that the postimplementation rate is lower than the preimplementation rate, using rates reported in the literature. Given the rarity of wrong surgeries in our measured environment, there is substantial statistical uncertainty. The analysis suggests an 84% probability that the wrong surgery rate is lower after implementation, leaving a 16% chance that it is actually higher. Combining sparse published reports of wrong surgery rates suggests an expected rate of about 1 wrong surgery per 23,600 cases, or 4.24×10^{-5} wrong surgeries per case.[36] If our institution performed at this rate, Bayesian analysis indicates we would have expected between 10 and 73 wrong surgeries among the 243,939 cases studied after implementation. Reliable safety depends on continual self-evaluation, process reinforcement, and transparent reporting. Execution of the time-out process, as assessed by "secret shoppers," is highly effective but not always perfect.[37,38] The process was effective in that time-outs led to the discovery and remedy of safety concerns prior to proceeding. Successful completion of a time-out cannot eliminate wrong surgery entirely. Since 2015, two wrong surgeries with unique circumstances unlikely to have been caught by a checklist have been detected and addressed, highlighting the difficulty of completely eliminating error.

Implementation of a surgical continuum of care model and continuum of care for medical/surgical populations within the Geisinger Health Systems hospitals resulted in improvements in mortality rates, reduction in length of stay, and cost savings.[39] These models of care were implemented based on the hypothesis "that a surgical patient with physiological deterioration during the hospital course would have had a variable period of occult deterioration before the 'critical event' that results in activation

BOX 9.2 Elements of the surgical safety checklist

Sign In

Before induction of anesthesia, members of the team (at least the nurse and an anesthesia professional) state that the following have been done:

- The patient has verified his or her identity, surgical site and procedure, and consent.
- The surgical site is marked or site marking is not applicable.
- The pulse oximeter is on the patient and functioning.
- All members of the team are aware of whether the patient has a known allergy.
- The patient's airway and risk of aspiration have been evaluated, and appropriate equipment and assistance are available.
- If there is a risk of blood loss of at least 500 mL (or 7 mL/kg body weight in children), appropriate access and fluids are available.

Time-Out

Before skin incision, the entire team (nurses, surgeons, anesthesia professionals, and any others participating in the care of the patient) or specific members state aloud the following:

- Team confirms that all team members have been introduced by name and role.
- Team confirms the patient's identity, surgical site, and procedure.
- Team reviews the anticipated critical events.
  - Surgeon reviews critical and unexpected steps, operative duration, and anticipated blood loss.
  - Anesthesia professionals review concerns specific to patient.
  - Nurses review confirmation of sterility, equipment availability, and other concerns.
- Team confirms that prophylactic antibiotics have been administered ≤60 minutes before incision is made or that antibiotics are not indicated.
- Team confirms that all essential imaging results for correct patient are displayed in operating room.

Sign-Out

Before the patient leaves the operating room, the following are done:

- Nurse reviews the following aloud with the team:
  - Name of procedure, as recorded
  - That needle, sponge, and instrument counts are complete (or not applicable)
  - That specimen (if any) is correctly labeled, including the patient's name
  - Whether there are any issues with equipment that need to be addressed
- The surgeon, nurse, and anesthesia professional review aloud the key concerns for the recovery and care of the patient.

Adapted from Haynes AB, Weiser TG, Berry WR, et al. A surgical safety checklist to reduce morbidity and mortality in a global population. *N Engl J Med.* 2009;360:491–499.

of code team for cardiopulmonary arrest." The surgical continuum of care and continuum of care models involved redesign of care delivery to include hospitalist comanagement of adult surgical patients in the surgical continuum of care model and the hospital-wide adult population in the continuum of care model. Central elements of the redesigned models of care included multidisciplinary floor-based team building, unit cohort-based placement of patients according to degree of physiologic derangement and anticipated risk of deterioration, the creation of a safety-net unit called the Progressive Care Unit, and intensivist/hospitalist staffing of the Progressive Care Unit. In addition, the care teams organized acuity-stratified rounding on higher risk patients at periodic intervals and implemented a real-time communication

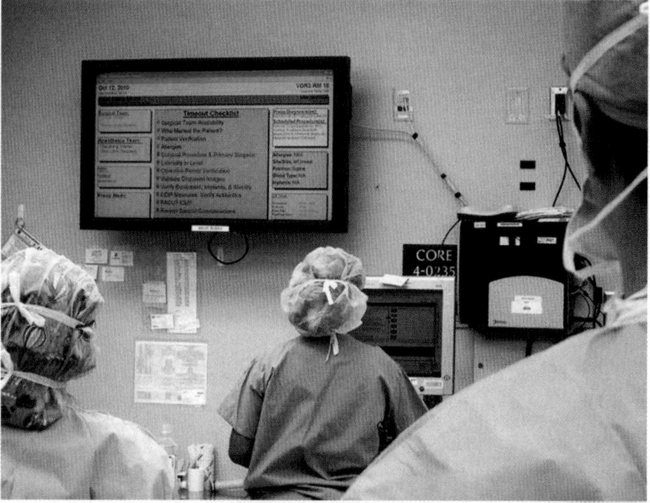

FIG. 9.4 Electronic white-board mediated time-out. Attention of personnel is focused on the display on which the time-out questions are being sequentially addressed. The display serves as a framing system for this important safety step. The view is from the anesthesiologist's position at the head of the bed, with (from left to right) the scrub technician, the circulator nurse, and the surgeon. The circulator's computer (visible to the lower right of the large display) shows the questions on the large display and captures the responses entered by the circulator nurse.

technology system. In a study of more than 100,000 admissions, the above-described interventions resulted in a decrease in the risk-adjusted mortality index from 1.16 before intervention to 0.77 by 6 months after intervention with an unchanged case mix index. The interventions also significantly decreased length of stay and resulted in cost savings in the high-risk and high-acuity populations of patients. Simpler interventions can also improve outcomes. For example, implementation of structured handoffs of care between residents led to a reduction in medical errors and preventable adverse events.[40]

When evaluating the results and impact of quality improvements resulting from mandates or public reporting, it is important to consider the source of the data being reported and the incentives of all of the reporting individuals. Farmer and colleagues[41] drew attention to the precipitous decrease in rates of central line–associated bloodstream infections (CLABSIs) in the course of one quarter after the Centers for Medicare and Medicaid Services (CMS) terminated reimbursement for CLABSI treatment (Fig. 9.5A).[41] These CLABSI rates were derived from a national sample of administrative data used for billing, which heretofore have been assumed to accurately reflect the care provided. However, Lee and associates,[42] using an outcomes data source (outcomes data reported by institutions to a national quality database), saw essentially no immediate change in CLABSI rates around the period when CMS stopped reimbursements.[42] Similarly, Lee and associates[42] saw no change in catheter-associated urinary tract infection or ventilator-associated pneumonia around the time of cessation of reimbursement by CMS for these complications (Fig. 9.5B), whereas Farmer and colleagues[41] detected a precipitous decrease in administrative coding for another surgical complication, retained foreign body, exactly concomitant with the cessation of reimbursement.

Continuous effort to improve surgical outcomes is consistent with the ethos of the surgeon and the right thing to do. However, in the current reimbursement environment, there can be perverse incentives that may limit the impact of quality improvement initiatives. For example, when conducting a complete

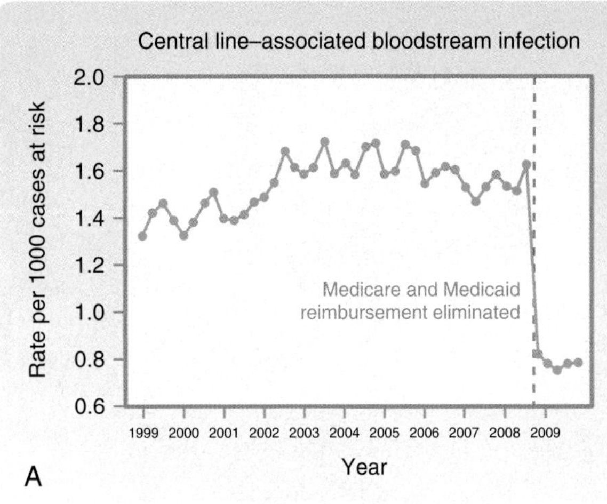

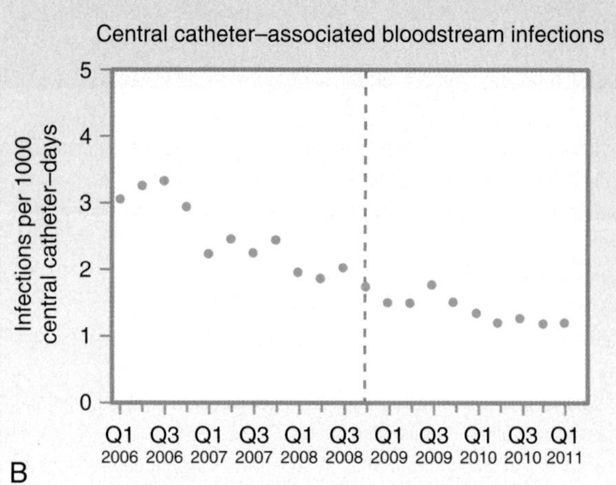

FIG. 9.5 (A) Central line–associated bloodstream infection. (B) Central catheter–associated bloodstream infections. The *red dashed lines* mark the end of reimbursement for patients with central line–associated bloodstream infections. (A, From Farmer SA, Black B, Bonow RO. Tension between quality measurement, public quality reporting, and pay for performance. *JAMA*. 2013;309:349–350. B, From Lee GM, Kleinman K, Soumerai SB, et al. Effect of nonpayment for preventable infections in U.S. hospitals. *N Engl J Med*. 2012;367:1428–1437.)

financial margin analysis of initiatives to reduce complications, a study demonstrated that successful programs may result in a negative cash flow to a hospital unless the hospital's surgical volume is growing sufficiently to fill beds vacated by patients who avoid complications.[43] This finding drives home the importance of sharing the financial benefits of successful quality improvement efforts between the providers and the payers.

SYSTEM-LEVEL INTERVENTIONS IMPROVE SAFETY

The goal of all efforts to improve quality and safety in the perioperative environment is to create systems of care that work efficiently; that rarely, if ever, fail; that alert clinicians of their incipient failure; and that fail into a safe mode. Clinicians working in perioperative systems to improve quality and safety must think of themselves, their plans, their actions, and their quality improvement work as part of an integrated system of care. A useful construct is the notion of perioperative systems design.

Perioperative systems design describes a rational approach to managing the convergent flow of patients having procedures from disparate physical and temporal starting points (frequently home), through the OR, and then to such a place and time (e.g., home or hospital bed) where future events pertaining to the patient have no further impact on OR operations.[44] This process for an individual patient can be envisioned as a set of interdependent activities beginning with the decision to perform an operation and ending when the patient definitively recovers from surgery. The risk of disruption is briefly illustrated in Fig. 9.6,[44] which shows approximately the steps required to bring a patient through an operation and some of the common roadblocks. At each point, physical infrastructure and work processes affect patient progress, quality, safety, and system efficiency. The perioperative process is extremely vulnerable to perturbations, particularly during the critical intraoperative portion. Problems in a single patient's care, regardless of where in the care trajectory they occur, frequently propagate upstream and downstream and ripple across the OR suite or health system as well (e.g., consider the impact of overrunning the booked procedure length for the first case in a room with three cases). Although the perioperative process is commonly conceptualized as a consistent system, workflow analyses reveal that even "defined" workflows have so many exceptions as to be essentially chaotic.[45] Frequently, improvements in one aspect of a perioperative system design highlight fragilities elsewhere. For example, improving OR throughput often unmasks limits to postanesthesia care unit (PACU) capacity.[46] In practice, many steps in the perioperative process are completely dependent on the successful completion of the preceding steps. This tight linkage implies that perioperative systems must be considered globally when making changes to one facet. In particular, upstream and downstream issues must be addressed in an effective perioperative systems design. Any proposed quality, safety, or efficiency improvement effort should be evaluated in terms of its likely and potential positive and negative impacts on the overall perioperative process.

Much hope has been pinned on the propagation of EMRs into the perioperative environment. EMRs allow rapid searches for apparently rare patient safety events within single institutions[47,48] and across multiple facilities.[49] Consortia of major medical facilities (Multicenter Perioperative Outcomes Group [https://www.mpogresearch.org/]) and national professional society efforts (e.g., the Anesthesia Quality Institute of the American Society of Anesthesiologists) now focus on aggregating perioperative EMR data with the aim of estimating incidence and, more importantly, identifying controllable risk factors for poor perioperative outcomes.

The convergence of EMRs and the perioperative system holds out a more proactive possibility for creating a system that performs reliably and fails safely. Specifically, the EMR can serve as the substrate for electronic monitoring of patient progress through the therapeutic encounter and compare this progress with the desired plan. Current technology is insufficient to achieve this ideal in its totality, but there are tractable subtasks that are amenable to electronic process monitoring and process control.[50,51] For example, important perioperative documentation tasks, process steps such as timely administration of perioperative antibiotics, and improvements in intraoperative monitoring have been achieved using systems with computerized ongoing continuous monitoring of the perioperative process and automatic reminders sent directly to the bedside provider when process exceptions are detected.[52–54] At Vanderbilt University Medical Center, electronic systems integrate

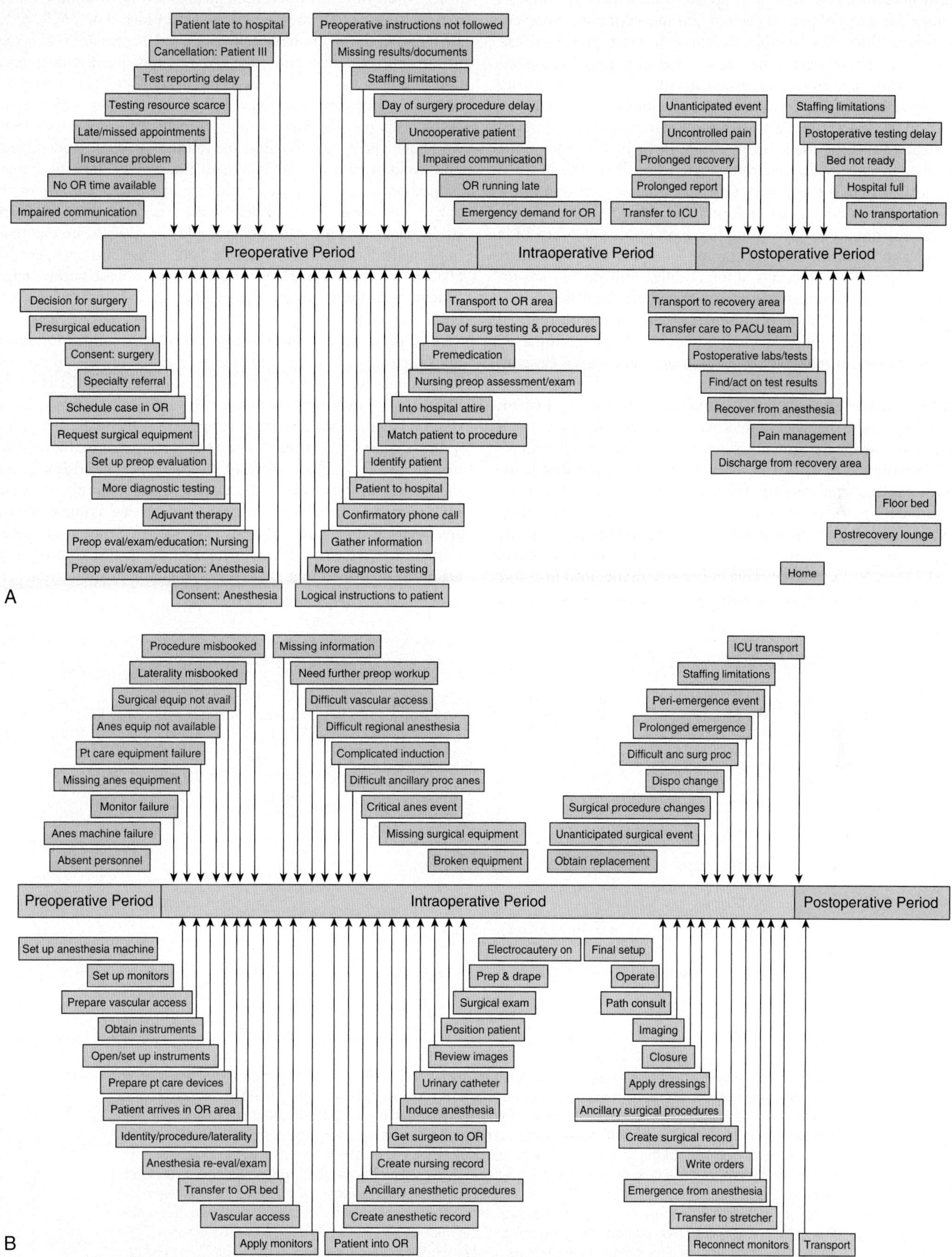

FIG. 9.6 Timeline for intraoperative period. (From Sandberg WS, Ganous TJ, Steiner C. Setting a research agenda for perioperative systems design. *Semin Laparosc Surg.* 2003;10:57–70.). *ICU*, Intensive care unit; *OR*, operating room; *PACU*, postanesthesia care unit.

data from multiple sources and update themselves over time to monitor the status of patients who might meet criteria for preventive interventions. For example, patients who meet certain risk criteria for obstructive sleep apnea (as assessed by required preoperative electronic data collection) automatically trigger a Respiratory Therapy assessment for continuous positive airway pressure in the PACU after surgery. Similarly, electronic systems continually scan for diabetic patients (denoted by diagnosis or oral hypoglycemic agents or insulin in the electronic medication list). The hospital laboratory system is monitored for regular glucose checks for these diabetic patients during the perioperative period. If a diabetic patient is not monitored according to expectations per protocol, a reminder to monitor is sent to the bedside provider. This entire monitoring system functions automatically, with no human intervention required except to receive the notification if action is required. Implementation of this system coincided with reduced deep wound infections for diabetic patients undergoing surgery.[55]

Technology can move electronic decision support even closer to the patient. For example, investigators at Dartmouth were able to reduce the rate of unplanned ICU transfers by the simple expedient of placing a pulse oximeter connected to a system that propagated Spo_2 alarms from the patient's room to the nurse on all patients in the monitored units.[56] The system was so successful that Dartmouth implemented continuous pulse oximetry for all inpatients.

Automatic process monitoring and process control using electronic records and clinical information systems hold substantial promise, but even simple tasks require careful attention to workflow design. Fig. 9.7 provides a simple example from a system intended to ensure that all patients entering the recovery room have a set of postoperative orders by the time handover is complete. In the top workflow, the system is set up to notify the physician to write orders if no PACU orders are found in the computerized physician order entry (CPOE) system by the time the patient enters the PACU. Consequently, the notification, if it fires, technically gives its notification after it is needed and notifies a provider who may have moved on to another task, creating an interruption. The lower workflow in Fig. 9.7 illustrates a better workflow. The system monitors the routine OR clinical documentation workflow and the CPOE system, awaiting the indication that a surgical procedure has moved to the "closing" phase. The system fires only if there are no PACU orders by the time "closing" is documented. In the Dartmouth oximetry example, the design team eventually implemented a system in which the Spo_2 trigger was Spo_2 less than 80% for 30 seconds to achieve an acceptably low false-positive rate.[56] Careful attention to system design was required, and the choice of limits was not intuitively obvious.

Electronic process monitoring and process control for simple tasks such as the electronic time-out described in Fig. 9.4 can help to eliminate wrong surgery related to site, side, and patient identification in environments where it is deployed. Similarly, in our system, when an anesthesiologist opens an OR medical record to create a chart for a surgical operation or procedure, he or she is first greeted by a splash screen of all abnormal and critical laboratory values for that patient, descending chronologically. However, such electronic process monitoring and process control systems are rarely, if ever, part of the feature set of commercial EMRs. Rather, they are either the constructs of the quality improvement teams at the institutions that created them or customizations created for users who insisted on them.

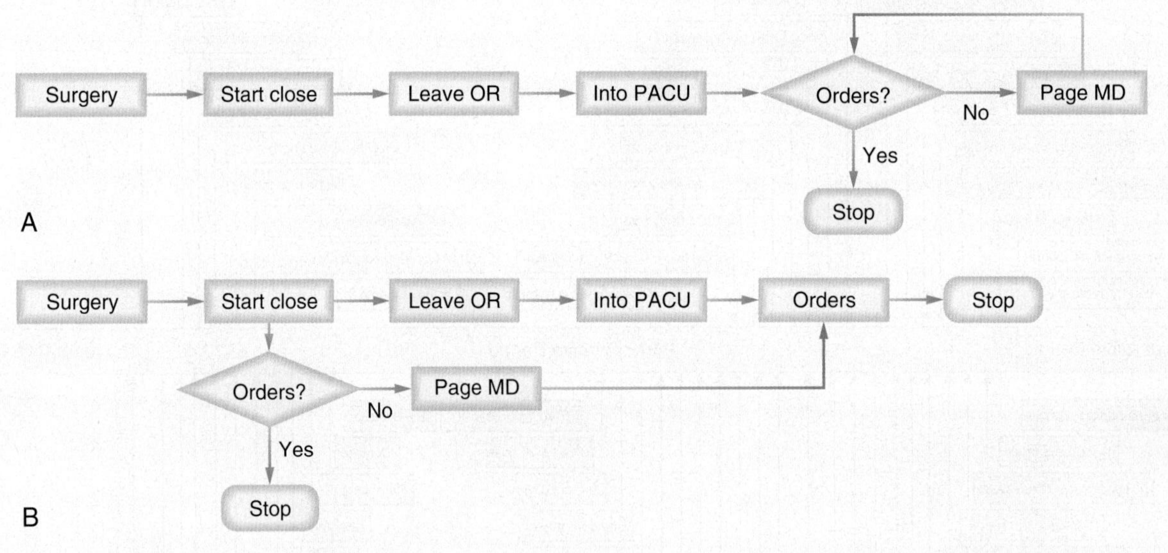

FIG. 9.7 (A) Flowchart of business logic designed to detect and notify a clinician when a process step (in this case, recovery room orders) has been missed. This is the logical flow frequently used in manual process checking and results in many phone calls, pages, and texts related to missing documentation, instructions, and information. It creates at least two interruptions and halts of progress: one for the person detecting the lapse and one for the recipient of the notification. Electronic medical records enable automation of the check for missing process steps, but the flow of work for the physician *(MD)* still creates an interruption as well as a stop in work as the postanesthesia care unit *(PACU)* awaits instructions. (B) Flowchart of business logic wherein the check for complete information needed for the next step is tied to a predicate indicator, in this case, the notion that virtually every case has a detectable "beginning of the end" as the team begins to close the wound. In the specific example, it is reasonable to expect that as the team begins wound closure, most or all of the planned PACU interventions have been specified, and orders can be written by the anesthesiologist for PACU care during the end of the operation and before emergence from anesthesia begins. This avoids both interruptions associated with a traditional workflow. *OR*, Operating room.

What are some of the core feature requirements of an EMR that allow it to facilitate improved perioperative quality and safety? The benefit of a "findable," legible, comprehensive record of all the events that have happened to a patient cannot be overemphasized. Current EMRs may have room for improvement in terms of usability, but they are vastly superior to the paper records they replaced in terms of availability, legibility, and aggregating data. However, these advantages accrue only to the degree that the EMR has access to all of the information about a patient. Most hospital systems still operate their own implementations of commercial EMRs and limit data sharing to comply with patient privacy regulations. Interoperability between commercially available systems is an important goal to achieve greater sharing of currently fragmented data.

CPOE systems are another major component of EMRs. The creation of legible orders by a person with an identifiable signature and contact information is, on its face, a major safety advance, although there have been notable problematic implementations.[57] Order writing is, by its nature, a potential point of risk for patients. A misplaced decimal point is sufficient to cause harm through underdose or overdose. Drug allergies, interactions, and side effects are common. Duplicate orders and orders creating unwanted drug-drug interactions are problematic. However, because CPOE systems are typically self-contained, there is substantial opportunity to mitigate risk through robust decision support. A well-designed and implemented CPOE system should allow writing preoperative orders that can be activated when the patient reports for surgery. Specific orders for the PACU should add to the preoperative orders, but the system should readily suspend (and fence off from the main, active order set) any existing general care orders. Similarly, the PACU orders should automatically expire or "sunset" as the patient moves back to the general care population. Finally, a CPOE system should automatically check for patient-specific drug allergies and drug-drug interactions each time a new entry is made. The system must challenge the clinician to justify orders that violate allergy and drug interaction rules or standard dosing parameters.

CONCLUSION

Perioperative care is in the midst of a transformative renaissance. A major aspect of this change is an evolution in the culture of care. That evolutionary change is being reflected in multiple, somewhat articulated contemporaneous improvement processes being developed or used at the present time. Health care culture must be changed to focus on quality care and patient safety as a societal mandate. As noted earlier, Leape and coworkers[3] have provided the health care system with the critical elements and foundational attributes to promulgate this cultural progression.

Organizational transparency is a key aspect of the progression. Internal and external reporting structures currently exist to accomplish the aim of transparent outcomes and systems reporting (e.g., NSQIP). However, these structures will need to adjust and evolve in consonance with improvements in care and recognition of previously unappreciated or underappreciated factors that disrupt care processes or in other ways affect outcomes. Perioperative provider involvement in the maturation of these reporting structures is of utmost importance. Internal control processes such as standardized adverse event reporting and investigation, coupled with multidisciplinary venues for discussion and education (e.g., MMI meetings) and with linkage of findings to "just in time" improvement processes overseen by entities such as the Perioperative Quality Improvement committee provide real-time institutional process control and improvement.

The importance of team-based care throughout the perioperative episode is vital to integrity of process. Essential to effective team-based care is coherent communication within and among care teams. Checklists and information technology provide components and critical supplements to the process, but other elements are also vital to the care delivery process. All of these processes must be built with the patient's well-being and wishes as the central guiding elements. The process must also seek and respond to feedback from the patient and the patient's family that reflects their experience with the health care environment. Optimized patient literacy, education, and effective communication strategies can substantively improve the overall experience. The recognition that physician and surgeon behaviors can have an impact on the care process has led to the development of methods and tools to identify suboptimal occurrences and initiate specific interventions using structured algorithms. Furthermore, the use of team-based training tools incorporating universal time-out and huddles/debriefs improves caregiver job satisfaction and has been shown to have a positive impact on the culture of safety measures.

The importance of perioperative goals and efforts that harmonize with institutional goals cannot be overemphasized. Leadership commitment to clearly enunciated goals is vital to success. Continuous education links evidence and experience to all members of the care team. Each member of the team contributes to quality care and safety, and this is incorporated into the medical and nursing curriculum.

Just as the last decade has brought tremendous change to the perioperative care arena, it is reasonable to assume that further evolution to our current systems will occur in the near future. The recent concept that any adverse event equates to a "never event" provides a sentinel philosophy for our continued efforts to ensure that perioperative care is of the highest quality and reproducibility.

SELECTED REFERENCES

Birkmeyer JD, Finks JF, O'Reilly A, et al. Surgical skill and complication rates after bariatric surgery. *N Engl J Med.* 2013;369:1434–1442.

Surgeon technique has been an infrequently considered variable in the assessment of surgical outcomes. The authors review the observed technique during surgery of a group of bariatric surgeons with analysis of outcomes related to the procedures.

Cooper WO, Guillamondegui O, Hines OJ, et al. Use of unsolicited patient observations to identify surgeons with increased risk for postoperative complications. *JAMA Surg.* 2017;152:522–529.

Patients whose surgeons received higher numbers of unsolicited patient complaints experience a higher risk of surgical and medical complications.

Cooper WO, Spain DA, Guillamondegui O, et al. Association of coworker reports about unprofessional behavior by surgeons with surgical complications in their patients. *JAMA Surg.* 2019; 154:828–834.

Patients whose surgeons had higher numbers of coworker reports about unprofessional behavior in the 36 months before the patient's operation had an increased risk of surgical and medical complications. Unprofessional behavior by surgeons adversely affects the function of teams in the perioperative setting and puts patients at increased risk of adverse outcomes.

Fry DE. Surgical site infections and the Surgical Care Improvement Project (SCIP): evolution of national quality measures. *Surg Infect (Larchmt)*. 2008;9:579–584.

This is a comprehensive review of the national Surgical Care Improvement Project effort to reduce surgical site infections. The national Surgical Infection Prevention Project was an initiative sponsored jointly by the Centers for Medicare and Medicaid Services and the U.S. Centers for Disease Control and Prevention to decrease the incidence of surgical site infections in major surgical procedures.

Ghaferi AA, Birkmeyer JD, Dimick JB. Variation in hospital mortality associated with inpatient surgery. *N Engl J Med*. 2009;361:1368–1375.

This is a landmark study of 84,730 patients who underwent inpatient general and vascular surgery from 2005 through 2007 that used data from the American College of Surgeons National Surgical Quality Improvement Program.

Haynes AB, Weiser TG, Berry WR, et al. A surgical safety checklist to reduce morbidity and mortality in a global population. *N Engl J Med*. 2009;360:491–499.

Surgery has become an integral part of global health care, with an estimated 234 million operations performed yearly. The article assesses surgical outcomes before and after safety checklist implementation.

Leape L, Berwick D, Clancy C, et al. Transforming healthcare: a safety imperative. *Qual Saf Health Care*. 2009;18:424–428.

Improvement in surgical care and outcomes will require substantial cultural transformation. The elements of the transformative principles are defined and summarized.

Maggard-Gibbons M. The use of report cards and outcome measurements to improve the safety of surgical care: the American College of Surgeons National Surgical Quality Improvement Program. *BMJ Qual Saf*. 2014;23:589–599.

The use of standardized, institution-specific and provider-specific reporting is expanding. Many entities are calculating these reports including governmental and payer groups. Physician involvement is critical to ensure integrity, fairness, and value to these reporting systems.

Webb LE, Dmochowski RR, Moore IN, et al. Using coworker observations to promote accountability for disrespectful and unsafe behaviors by physicians and advanced practice professionals. *Jt Comm J Qual Patient Saf*. 2016;42:149–164.

The use of a coworker observation and reporting system to alert for disrespectful and unsafe behaviors with a timely and graduated feedback system results in improved self-regulation and decreased recidivism of unprofessional behaviors.

REFERENCES

1. Institute of Medicine. *To Err Is Human: Building a Safer Healthcare System*. Washington, DC: National Academy Press; 1999.
2. Gawande AA, Thomas EJ, Zinner MJ, et al. The incidence and nature of surgical adverse events in Colorado and Utah in 1992. *Surgery*. 1999;126:66–75.
3. Leape L, Berwick D, Clancy C, et al. Transforming healthcare: a safety imperative. *Qual Saf Health Care*. 2009;18:424–428.
4. Freundlich RE, Maile MD, Sferra JJ, et al. Complications associated with mortality in the National Surgical Quality Improvement Program Database. *Anesth Analg*. 2018;127:55–62.
5. Biccard BM, Madiba TE, Kluyts HL, et al. Perioperative patient outcomes in the African Surgical Outcomes Study: a 7-day prospective observational cohort study. *Lancet*. 2018;391:1589–1598.
6. Sileshi B, Newton MW, Kiptanui J, et al. Monitoring anesthesia care delivery and perioperative mortality in Kenya utilizing a provider-driven novel data collection tool. *Anesthesiology*. 2017;127:250–271.
7. Pearse RM, Moreno RP, Bauer P, et al. Mortality after surgery in Europe: a 7 day cohort study. *Lancet*. 2012;380:1059–1065.
8. Brodner G, Van Aken H. Mortality after surgery in Europe. *Lancet*. 2013;381:370.
9. van Schalkwyk JM, Campbell D. Mortality after surgery in Europe. *Lancet*. 2013;381:370.
10. Pupelis G, Vanags I. Mortality after surgery in Europe. *Lancet*. 2013;381:369.
11. Mikstacki A. Mortality after surgery in Europe. *Lancet*. 2013;381:369.
12. Franek E, Osinska B, Czech M, et al. Mortality after surgery in Europe. *Lancet*. 2013;381:369–370.
13. Pearse R, Moreno RP, Bauer P, et al. Mortality after surgery in Europe—authors' reply. *Lancet*. 2013;381:370–371.
14. Mazo V, Sabate S, Canet J, et al. Prospective external validation of a predictive score for postoperative pulmonary complications. *Anesthesiology*. 2014;121:219–231.
15. Birkmeyer JD, Finks JF, O'Reilly A, et al. Surgical skill and complication rates after bariatric surgery. *N Engl J Med*. 2013;369:1434–1442.
16. Kenney C. *Transforming Healthcare: Virginia Mason Medical Center's Pursuit of the Perfect Patient Experience*. New York: CRC Press Taylor & Francis Group; 2011.
17. Pichert JW, Hickson G, Moore I. Using patient complaints to promote patient safety. In: Henriksen K, Battles JB, Keyes MA, eds. *Advances in Patient Safety: New Directions and Alternative Approaches (Vol 2: Culture and Redesign)*. Rockville, MD: Agency for Healthcare Research and Quality; 2008:1–10.
18. Sanfey H, Darosa DA, Hickson GB, et al. Pursuing professional accountability: an evidence-based approach to addressing residents with behavioral problems. *Arch Surg*. 2012;147:642–647.
19. Webb LE, Dmochowski RR, Moore IN, et al. Using coworker observations to promote accountability for disrespectful and unsafe behaviors by physicians and advanced practice professionals. *Jt Comm J Qual Patient Saf*. 2016;42:149–164.
20. Cooper WO, Spain DA, Guillamondegui O, et al. Association of coworker reports about unprofessional behavior by surgeons with surgical complications in their patients. *JAMA Surg*. 2019;154:828–834.
21. Cooper WO, Guillamondegui O, Hines OJ, et al. Use of unsolicited patient observations to identify surgeons with increased risk for postoperative complications. *JAMA Surg*. 2017;152:522–529.

22. McEvoy MD, Wanderer JP, King AB, et al. A perioperative consult service results in reduction in cost and length of stay for colorectal surgical patients: evidence from a healthcare redesign project. *Perioper Med (Lond).* 2016;5:3.
23. Hawkins AT, Geiger TM, King AB, et al. An enhanced recovery program in colorectal surgery is associated with decreased organ level rates of complications: a difference-in-differences analysis. *Surg Endosc.* 2019;33:2222–2230.
24. King AB, Spann MD, Jablonski P, et al. An enhanced recovery program for bariatric surgical patients significantly reduces perioperative opioid consumption and postoperative nausea. *Surg Obes Relat Dis.* 2018;14:849–856.
25. Kehlet H. Multimodal approach to control postoperative pathophysiology and rehabilitation. *Br J Anaesth.* 1997;78:606–617.
26. Kehlet H, Joshi GP. Enhanced recovery after surgery: current controversies and concerns. *Anesth Analg.* 2017;125:2154–2155.
27. Memtsoudis SG, Poeran J, Kehlet H. Enhanced recovery after surgery in the United States: from evidence-based practice to uncertain science? *JAMA.* 2019;321:1049–1050.
28. Haynes AB, Weiser TG, Berry WR, et al. A surgical safety checklist to reduce morbidity and mortality in a global population. *N Engl J Med.* 2009;360:491–499.
29. de Vries EN, Prins HA, Crolla RM, et al. Effect of a comprehensive surgical safety system on patient outcomes. *N Engl J Med.* 2010;363:1928–1937.
30. Neily J, Mills PD, Young-Xu Y, et al. Association between implementation of a medical team training program and surgical mortality. *JAMA.* 2010;304:1693–1700.
31. Urbach DR, Govindarajan A, Saskin R, et al. Introduction of surgical safety checklists in Ontario, Canada. *N Engl J Med.* 2014;370:1029–1038.
32. Kwaan MR, Studdert DM, Zinner MJ, et al. Incidence, patterns, and prevention of wrong-site surgery. *Arch Surg.* 2006;141:353–357; discussion 357–358.
33. Rothman G. Wrong-site surgery. *Arch Surg.* 2006;141:1049–1050; author reply 1050.
34. Pronovost P, Needham D, Berenholtz S, et al. An intervention to decrease catheter-related bloodstream infections in the ICU. *N Engl J Med.* 2006;355:2725–2732.
35. The Joint Commission. *2019 National Patient Safety Goals*; 2019. http://www.jointcommission.org/standards_information/npsgs.aspx. Accessed June 10, 2019.
36. Rothman BS, Shotwell MS, Beebe R, et al. Electronically mediated time-out initiative to reduce the incidence of wrong surgery: an Interventional Observational Study. *Anesthesiology.* 2016;125:484–494.
37. Mainthia R, Lockney T, Zotov A, et al. Novel use of electronic whiteboard in the operating room increases surgical team compliance with pre-incision safety practices. *Surgery.* 2012;151:660–666.
38. Freundlich RE, Bulka CM, Wanderer JP, et al. Prospective investigation of the operating room time-out process. *Anesth Analg.* 2020;130:725–729.
39. Ravikumar TS, Sharma C, Marini C, et al. A validated value-based model to improve hospital-wide perioperative outcomes: adaptability to combined medical/surgical inpatient cohorts. *Ann Surg.* 2010;252:486–496; discussion 496–488.
40. Starmer AJ, Spector ND, Srivastava R, et al. Changes in medical errors after implementation of a handoff program. *N Engl J Med.* 2014;371:1803–1812.
41. Farmer SA, Black B, Bonow RO. Tension between quality measurement, public quality reporting, and pay for performance. *JAMA.* 2013;309:349–350.
42. Lee GM, Kleinman K, Soumerai SB, et al. Effect of nonpayment for preventable infections in U.S. hospitals. *N Engl J Med.* 2012;367:1428–1437.
43. Krupka DC, Sandberg WS, Weeks WB. The impact on hospitals of reducing surgical complications suggests many will need shared savings programs with payers. *Health Aff (Millwood).* 2012;31:2571–2578.
44. Sandberg WS, Ganous TJ, Steiner C. Setting a research agenda for perioperative systems design. *Semin Laparosc Surg.* 2003;10:57–70.
45. Meyer MA, Seim AR, Fairbrother P, et al. Automatic time-motion study of a multistep preoperative process. *Anesthesiology.* 2008;108:1109–1116.
46. Schoenmeyr T, Dunn PF, Gamarnik D, et al. A model for understanding the impacts of demand and capacity on waiting time to enter a congested recovery room. *Anesthesiology.* 2009;110:1293–1304.
47. Hobai IA, Gauran C, Chitilian HV, et al. The management and outcome of documented intraoperative heart rate-related electrocardiographic changes. *J Cardiothorac Vasc Anesth.* 2011;25:791–798.
48. Ehrenfeld JM, Agarwal AK, Henneman JP, et al. Estimating the incidence of suspected epidural hematoma and the hidden imaging cost of epidural catheterization: a retrospective review of 43,200 cases. *Reg Anesth Pain Med.* 2013;38:409–414.
49. Bateman BT, Mhyre JM, Ehrenfeld J, et al. The risk and outcomes of epidural hematomas after perioperative and obstetric epidural catheterization: a report from the Multicenter Perioperative Outcomes Group Research Consortium. *Anesth Analg.* 2013;116:1380–1385.
50. Rothman B, Sandberg WS, St Jacques P. Using information technology to improve quality in the OR. *Anesthesiol Clin.* 2011;29:29–55.
51. Wanderer JP, Sandberg WS, Ehrenfeld JM. Real-time alerts and reminders using information systems. *Anesthesiol Clin.* 2011;29:389–396.
52. St Jacques P, Sanders N, Patel N, et al. Improving timely surgical antibiotic prophylaxis redosing administration using computerized record prompts. *Surg Infect (Larchmt).* 2005;6:215–221.
53. Sandberg WS, Sandberg EH, Seim AR, et al. Real-time checking of electronic anesthesia records for documentation errors and automatically text messaging clinicians improves quality of documentation. *Anesth Analg.* 2008;106:192–201, table of contents.
54. Ehrenfeld JM, Epstein RH, Bader S, et al. Automatic notifications mediated by anesthesia information management systems reduce the frequency of prolonged gaps in blood pressure documentation. *Anesth Analg.* 2011;113:356–363.
55. Ehrenfeld JM, Wanderer JP, Terekhov M, et al. A perioperative systems design to improve intraoperative glucose monitoring is associated with a reduction in surgical site infections in a diabetic patient population. *Anesthesiology.* 2017;126:431–440.
56. Taenzer AH, Pyke JB, McGrath SP, et al. Impact of pulse oximetry surveillance on rescue events and intensive care unit transfers: a before-and-after concurrence study. *Anesthesiology.* 2010;112:282–287.
57. Han YY, Carcillo JA, Venkataraman ST, et al. Unexpected increased mortality after implementation of a commercially sold computerized physician order entry system. *Pediatrics.* 2005;116:1506–1512.

SECTION II

Perioperative Management

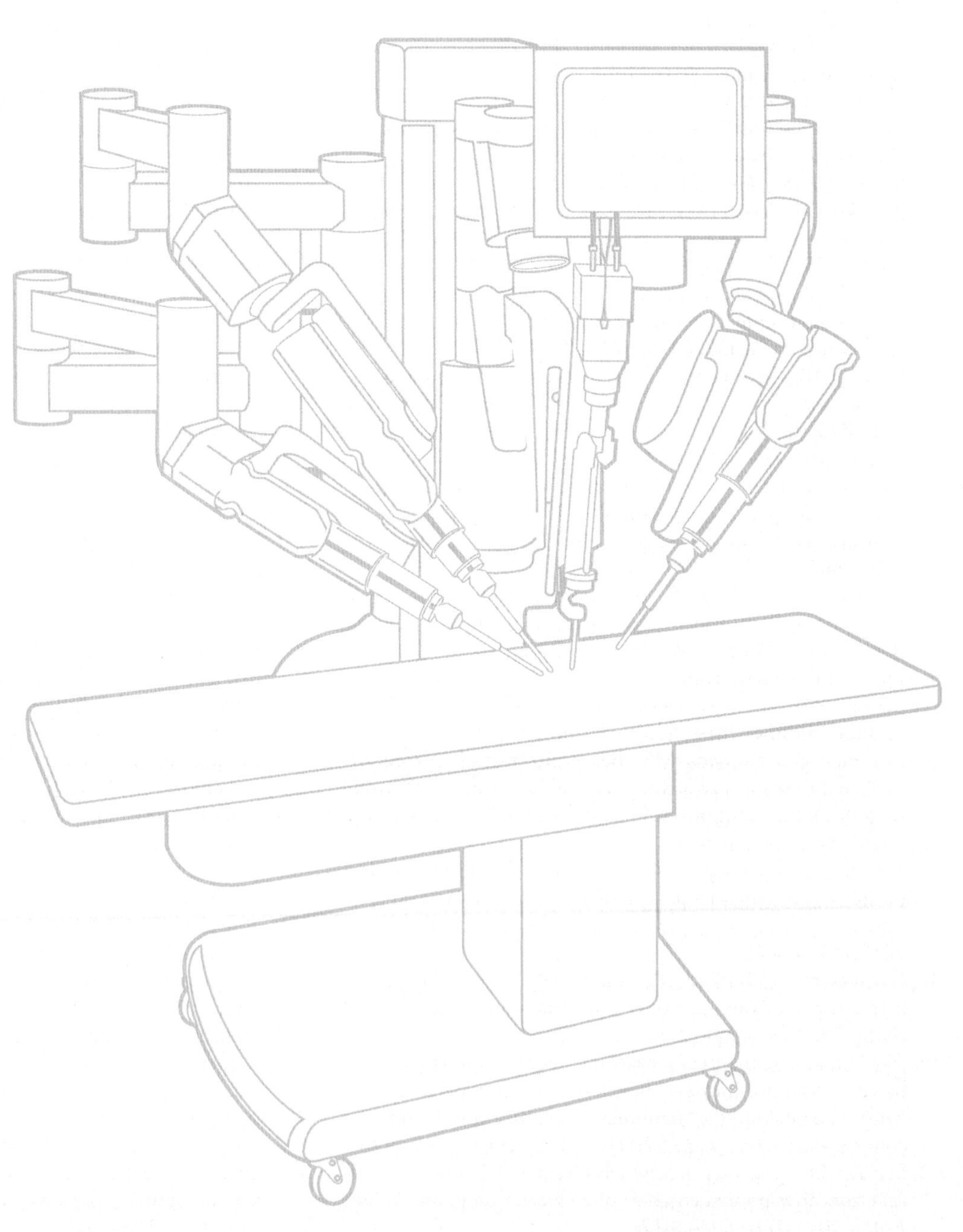

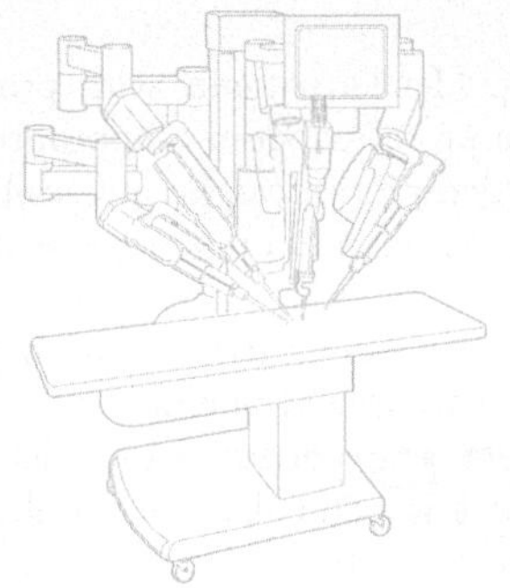

CHAPTER 10

Principles of Preoperative and Operative Surgery

Victor M. Zaydfudim, Yinnin Hu, Reid B. Adams

OUTLINE

PRINCIPLES OF SURGICAL EVALUATION

Patient–Surgeon Relationship

Clear, precise, and unambiguous communication to establish an understanding of mutual expectations and trust is at the pinnacle of the patient–surgeon relationship. A surgeon's initial encounter with a patient most commonly is in the context of a new diagnosis and is initiated by either a professional or self-referral. A history and physical examination, whether in an urgent/emergent or elective setting, initially should focus on confirmation or rebuttal of the suspected diagnosis. Inquiries regarding patients' personal interests, as well as their relationships with their community and society, help create a common bond between the patient and surgeon. In addition to direct communication with the patient, knowledge of their situation is augmented by a thorough review of relevant diagnostic laboratory and imaging results. Through this process, an experienced surgeon effectively recreates the clinical context of a patient's situation during the period preceding evaluation for the illness in question.

Further patient management is directed by the differential diagnosis generated during the initial evaluation. If the differential diagnosis contains items of equipoise that require distinct treatments, further investigations may be necessary to distinguish between these options. In general, the principle of Occam razor or parsimony applies to surgical diagnosis and management; it is important to pursue only those diagnostic studies that have a high likelihood of producing actionable results. Tests with a near-perfect pretest probability, and those unlikely to alter treatment, should be avoided. Once a diagnosis is secured, the objective and urgency of potential surgical therapy are considered.

Surgical Objectives

Achieving a joint understanding of surgical objectives and expectations between patient and surgeon is paramount to improve patient satisfaction and outcomes. There are three broad potential objectives of surgical intervention: disease prevention, disease control, and symptom palliation. Examples of operations aimed at disease prevention include prophylactic mastectomy, colectomy, pancreatectomy or thyroidectomy for heritable cancer syndromes, endarterectomy for asymptomatic carotid stenosis, or appendectomy in the setting of Ladd procedure for intestinal malrotation. These operations are aimed at preempting a disease process. Operations for disease control address a process that is ongoing. Examples include resections for malignancy, cholecystectomy for acute cholecystitis, enterolysis for bowel obstruction, bypass for vascular occlusive disease, or knee replacement for arthritis. With these operations, patients may expect partial or complete resolution of the targeted disease process. Finally, palliative operations are aimed at improving quality of life, rather than curing a disease. Examples include proximal decompression for malignant bowel obstruction or gastrojejunostomy for unresectable pancreatic cancer with gastric outlet obstruction. Inadequate communication of an operation's objectives precludes informed consent and can have dramatic, negative implications for a patient's perioperative decision-making.

Elective, Urgent, and Emergent Indications

Appropriate triage of surgical therapy is important for patient outcomes as well as resource distribution. Accurate categorization of surgical urgency also has implications for quality reporting. The American College of Surgeons (ACS) National Surgical Quality Improvement Program (NSQIP) differentiates between emergency and elective operations and reports different levels of accuracy for patient risk estimates, with emergency cases having both superior predictive accuracy for mortality and significantly higher observed-to-expected ratios.[1] Within ACS NSQIP, emergency surgery is characterized by an ongoing acute process that can result in rapid deterioration in a patient's condition for which unnecessary delay can potentially threaten the clinical outcome. On the other hand, elective operations generally involve a patient who has completed preoperative surgical evaluation during a separate patient–urgeon encounter and is subsequently scheduled for operation. Inpatients, referrals from the emergency department, and direct transfers from clinic are excluded from elective patient categorization. Urgent operations are a relatively ill-defined category and have an acuity level in between those of elective and emergent cases. The World Society of Emergency Surgery created the Timing of Acute Care Surgery classification in 2013, which subdivides urgent cases into those with an ideal time-to-surgery falling between immediate to within 48 hours from diagnosis.[2] Recognition of urgency should be one of the first steps of the preoperative surgical evaluation, as it affects subsequent patient decision-making, counseling, investigatory testing, and perioperative management.

Risk Assessment

Perioperative risk assessment has an impact on all aspects of surgical planning, including the decision to operate, choice of operation, perioperative management, and goals of care discussions. Communication with patients regarding the risks of a proposed operation must be coupled with a thorough review of patient comorbidities and functional status. Hence, patients with prohibitively high operative risk can be protected from inappropriate operations, while those with borderline risk can be medically optimized preoperatively. From the viewpoint of perioperative management, appropriate risk stratification facilitates resource allocation, including intraoperative monitoring, use of intensive care unit (ICU) services after the operation, and potential use of medical consultation. Finally, transparent categorization of patient risk factors improves institutional reporting and allows for multi-institutional comparisons of risk-adjusted patient outcomes.

Risk assessment begins by considering the nature of the disease and patient comorbidities while weighing the risks of possible surgical interventions. For a number of diagnoses, multiple surgical approaches may be available, each with advantages and disadvantages in terms of the morbidity profile, quality outcomes, and durability of the therapy. These must be weighed carefully in the context of each patient's presenting condition and baseline level of health. The American Society of Anesthesiologists (ASA) physical status categorization has frequently served as a simple, initial rubric to summarize baseline patient comorbidity. Patient categorization into ASA 1 to 5 (Table 10.1) helps stratify patients as low risk (1–2), intermediate risk (3), and high risk (4–5). The addition of an "E" designation signifies emergent operation, hence indicating a higher risk. First introduced in 1941, increasing ASA class was shown in a number of landmark studies to be associated with early postoperative mortality. This relationship remains true in the modern era for both emergent and elective operations, with class 5E associated with nearly 20% likelihood of early postoperative mortality.[3]

Next, operations can be categorized into low-, intermediate-, and high-risk groups. This categorization is most commonly approached through expert opinion and consensus guidelines, such as those proposed by the European Society of Cardiology and European Society of Anesthesiology, which stratifies patients based on estimated 30-day risk of cardiac events (Table 10.2). Combination surgical risk models including patient comorbidity and operative risk have been developed using logistic regression with mortality or major complication as the dependent variable.[4] For very low-risk, outpatient procedures, the risk of death is less than 1 in 50,000; conversely, high-risk operations performed for life-threatening conditions in critically ill patients can have expected mortality rates routinely exceeding 20% (Fig. 10.1).

There are a wide variety of tools to help quantify operative risk in the preoperative setting. These tools can predict risks of broad outcomes such as death or length of stay or specific events such as reoperation, intraoperative blood loss, or specific surgical complications. From a methodology standpoint, these tools can be grouped into categorical scales, risk scores, or prediction models. Categorical scales are easy to calculate and are frequently subjective. The most classic example of a categorical scale is the ASA Classification of Physical Status, which is frequently used in preoperative risk estimation. Surgical risk scores combine several predictors, usually chosen using multivariable predictive modeling, to estimate risk of a specific outcome. An example of a risk score is the model for end-stage liver disease (MELD) score used to predict short-term prognoses in patients with end-stage liver disease. More recently, the adoption of advanced statistics to analyze large, multi-institutional datasets has created numerous risk prediction models that account for patient-level risk factors to generate estimated likelihoods of multiple surgical outcomes. The most commonly used and cited example of a surgical risk score is the ACS NSQIP Surgical Risk Calculator (SRC).

TABLE 10.1 American Society of Anesthesiologists physical status (ASA PS) classification.

ASA PS	DEFINITION
I	A normal healthy patient
II	A patient with mild systemic disease
III	A patient with severe systemic disease
IV	A patient with severe systemic disease that is a constant threat to life
V	A moribund patient who is not expected to survive without the operation

Adapted from Cohn SL. Preoperative evaluation for noncardiac surgery. *Ann Intern Med.* 2016;165:ITC81–ITC96.

TABLE 10.2 Surgical risk estimates depending on the type of operation.

LOW RISK: <1%	INTERMEDIATE RISK: 1%–5%	HIGH RISK: >5%
• Superficial surgery • Breast • Dental • Endocrine: thyroid • Eye • Reconstructive • Carotid asymptomatic (CEA or CAS) • Gynecology: minor • Orthopedic: minor (meniscectomy) • Urological: minor (transurethral resection of the prostate)	• Intraperitoneal: splenectomy, hiatal hernia repair, cholecystectomy • Carotid symptomatic (CEA or CAS) • Peripheral arterial angioplasty • Endovascular aneurysm repair • Head and neck surgery • Neurologic or orthopedic: major (hip and spine surgery) • Urologic or gynecologic: major • Renal transplant • Intrathoracic: nonmajor	• Aortic and major vascular surgery • Open lower limb revascularization or amputation or thromboembolectomy • Duodenopancreatic surgery • Liver resection, bile duct surgery • Esophagectomy • Repair of perforated bowel • Adrenal resection • Total cystectomy • Pneumonectomy • Pulmonary or liver transplant

CAS, Carotid artery stenting; *CEA*, carotid endarterectomy.
From Kristensen SD, Knuuti J, Saraste A, et al. 2014 ESC/ESA guidelines on non-cardiac surgery: cardiovascular assessment and management: The Joint Task Force on Non-Cardiac Surgery: cardiovascular assessment and management of the European Society of Cardiology (ESC) and the European Society of Anaesthesiology (ESA). *Eur J Anaesthesiol.* 2014;31:517–573.

The ACS NSQIP universal SRC was developed in 2013 using standardized clinical data from more than 500 NSQIP participant hospitals.[5] This online tool predicts adverse postoperative outcomes based on 20 preoperative patient-level characteristics, including demographics and comorbidities (Table 10.3). Risks associated with procedure type are incorporated using Current Procedural Terminology (CPT) codes. Updated in 2016, the database has been calibrated to predict more accurately outcomes for lowest- and highest-risk patients.[6] It currently contains data from more than 3.8 million cases across 740 hospitals and is publicly accessible at http://riskcalculator.facs.org. Originally designed to predict eight postoperative adverse outcomes, the tool has evolved to currently report likelihoods of 13 specific or composite outcomes within 30 days of surgery (Box 10.1).

Levels of discrimination for these outcomes are generally strong, with c-statistics higher than 0.75 for all predicted outcomes. In particular, discrimination for 30-day postoperative mortality is excellent, with c-statistic exceeding 0.9.[6] Recent investigations have evaluated combining ACS NSQIP SRC models with preoperative biologic markers such as hypoalbuminemia or with organ-specific metrics such as chronic liver disease in patients selected for liver resection. Within the last 5 years, the SRC model has also been adapted for the pediatric population. The Pediatric SRC incorporates nearly 200,000 cases across 67 hospitals and accounts for 382 CPT codes; it has demonstrated excellent predictive accuracy for mortality and morbidity following operations in children. The ACS NSQIP SRC is specifically designed to facilitate patient counseling and consent prior to surgery; as such, it does not take into account intraoperative findings. Despite its excellent calibration within the broad ACS NSQIP dataset, recent studies have identified lapses in predictive accuracy within smaller homogenous patient populations. Therefore, it cannot replace familiarity with institution- and surgeon-specific performance.

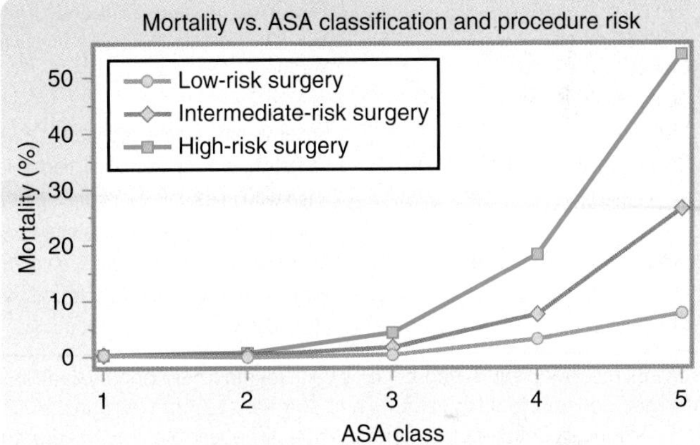

FIG. 10.1 The observed mortality rate as a function of American Society of Anesthesiologists *(ASA)* physical status and surgery-specific risk. (Adapted from Glance LG, Lustik SJ, Hannan EL, et al. The surgical mortality probability model: derivation and validation of a simple risk prediction rule for noncardiac surgery. *Ann Surg.* 2012;255:696–702.)

Informed Consent

Surgeons have an ethical obligation to discuss and pursue informed consent with any patient considering an operation. Comprehensive, transparent, and clear communication of perioperative risks and potential benefits is mandatory. To successfully guide the patient through the consent process, a surgeon must possess a thorough technical understanding of the proposed operation, the most probable perioperative course, and potential pitfalls and complications. A clear and precise communication of risks and expectations is paramount; technical jargon should be avoided. The consent process must take into account all of the preceding facets of surgical objectives, urgency, and patient risk assessment. Systematic reviews indicate that common components of a consent discussion should include (1) the disease diagnosis, (2) the proposed procedure, (3) procedure-related risks, (4) likelihood of success of the procedure, (5) mental capacity of the patient, and (6) alternative treatment options.[7] One of the most challenging impediments to informed consent is the knowledge gap between surgeon and patient. To overcome this, consent processes can be augmented for specific diseases and procedures using decision aids, visual materials, specialized written materials, and previously discussed risk calculators. In general, these supplementary instruments have been shown to improve patient knowledge and satisfaction with decision-making.[8]

TABLE 10.3 ACS NSQIP variables used in the colon-specific and the universal Surgical Risk Calculator.

VARIABLE	CATEGORIES	COLON SPECIFIC	UNIVERSAL
Age group (y)	<65, 65–74, 75–84, ≥85	√	√
Sex	Male, female	√	√
Functional status	Independent, partially dependent, totally dependent	√	√
Emergency case	Yes, no	√	√
ASA class	1 or 2, 3, 4, or 5	√	√
Steroid use for chronic condition	Yes, no	√	√
Ascites within 30 d preoperatively	Yes, no	√	√
System sepsis within 48 h preoperatively	None, SIRS, sepsis, septic shock	√	√
Ventilator dependent	Yes, no	√	√
Disseminated cancer	Yes, no	√	√
Diabetes	No, oral, insulin	√	√
Hypertension requiring medication	Yes, no	√	√
Previous cardiac event	Yes, no	√	√
Congestive heart failure in 30 d preoperatively	Yes, no	√	√
Dyspnea	Yes, no	√	√
Current smoker within 1 y	Yes, no	√	√
History of COPD	Yes, no	√	√
Dialysis	Yes, no	√	√
Acute renal failure	Yes, no	√	√
BMI class	Underweight, normal, overweight, obese 1, obese 2, obese 3	√	√
Colon surgery group (colectomy)	Partial lap with anastomosis, partial lap with ostomy, partial open lap with anastomosis, partial open with ostomy, total lap with ostomy, total open with ostomy	√	
Indication for colon surgery	Diverticulitis, enteritis/colitis, hemorrhage, neoplasm, obstruction/perforation, vascular insufficiency, volvulus, other	√	
CPT-specific linear risk	2805 values		√

From Bilimoria KY, Liu Y, Paruch JL, et al. Development and evaluation of the universal ACS NSQIP Surgical Risk Calculator: a decision aid and informed consent tool for patients and surgeons. *J Am Coll Surg*. 2013;217:833–842, e831–833.

ACS, American College of Surgeons; *ASA*, American Society of Anesthesiologists; *BMI*, body mass index; *COPD*, chronic obstructive pulmonary disease; *CPT*, Current Procedural Terminology; *lap*, laparotomy; *NSQIP*, National Surgical Quality Improvement Program; *SIRS*, systemic inflammatory response syndrome.

ASSESSMENT OF GERIATRIC SURGICAL PATIENTS

The population of the United States continues to age. Currently, 13% of the population is comprised of individuals 65 years or older; by 2030, this proportion will be greater than 20%. Geriatric patients account for greater than 40% of hospital days and one third of all inpatient procedures. The geriatric population presents unique surgical challenges. Tailoring the preoperative work-up to the unique needs of these patients can help surgeons address age-related functional challenges and comorbidities. To ensure that decision-making is appropriately aligned between provider and patient, the patient and their family must clearly understand operative risks, potential effects of surgery-related complications on quality of life, and likely outcomes. Conversely, the surgeon must appreciate, value, and incorporate the patient's personal goals of care in any decision-making process and final assessment.

Comprehensive Geriatric Assessment

Chronologic demarcation of the "geriatric" patient is elusive. A combination of advanced age, comorbidities, and functional and/or cognitive decline contributes to the definition of a geriatric patient. Due to the clinical and social complexities of the geriatric population, an appropriate preoperative evaluation is multifaceted. Collaboration

BOX 10.1 ACS NSQIP universal Surgical Risk Calculator reported outcome measures.

- Serious complication (cardiac arrest, myocardial infarction, pneumonia, etc.)
- Any complication (surgical site infections [SSIs], pulmonary embolus, ventilator >48 hours, etc.)
- Pneumonia
- Cardiac complication
- SSI
- Urinary tract infection
- Venous thromboembolism
- Renal failure
- Readmission
- Return to the operating room
- Death
- Discharge to nursing or rehabilitation facility
- Sepsis

ACS, American College of Surgeons; *NSQIP*, National Surgical Quality Improvement Program.

BOX 10.2 ACS NSQIP/AGS collaborative checklist for preoperative assessment of geriatric surgical patients.

In addition to conducting a complete history and physical examination of the patient, the following assessments are strongly recommended:

- Assess the patient's **cognitive ability** and **capacity** to understand the anticipated surgery.
- Screen the patient for **depression.**
- Identify the patient's risk factors for developing postoperative **delirium.**
- Screen for alcohol and other substance abuse/dependence.
- Perform a preoperative **cardiac** evaluation according to the American College of Cardiology/American Heart Association algorithm for patients undergoing noncardiac surgery.
- Identify the patient's risk factors for postoperative **pulmonary** complications and implement appropriate strategies for prevention.
- Document **functional status** and history of **falls.**
- Determine baseline **frailty** score.
- Assess patient's **nutritional status**, and consider preoperative interventions if the patient is at severe nutritional risk.
- Take an accurate and detailed **medication history**, and consider appropriate perioperative adjustments. Monitor for **polypharmacy.**
- Determine the patient's **treatment goals** and **expectations** in the context of the possible treatment outcomes.
- Determine patient's family and social support system.
- Order appropriate preoperative **diagnostic tests** focused on elderly patients.

ACS, American College of Surgeons; *AGS*, America Geriatrics Society; *NSQIP*, National Surgical Quality Improvement Program.

From Chow WB, Rosenthal RA, Merkow RP, et al. Optimal preoperative assessment of the geriatric surgical patient: a best practices guideline from the American College of Surgeons National Surgical Quality Improvement Program and the American Geriatrics Society. *J Am Coll Surg.* 2012;215:453–466.

BOX 10.3 Cognitive assessment with the Mini-Cog and interpretation of the Mini-Cog.

Cognitive Assessment With the Mini-Cog: Three-Item Recall and Clock Draw[14]

1. GET THE PATIENT'S ATTENTION, THEN SAY:
   "I am going to say three words that I want you to remember now and later. The words are: *banana, sunrise, chair.* Please say them for me now."
   Give the patient three tries to repeat the words. If unable after three tries, go to next item.
2. SAY ALL THE FOLLOWING PHRASES IN THE ORDER INDICATED:
   "Please draw a clock in the space below. Start by drawing a large circle. Put all the numbers in the circle and set the hands to show 11:10 (10 past 11)."
   If the subject has not finished clock drawing in 3 minutes, discontinue and ask for recall items.
3. SAY: "What were the three words I asked you to remember?"

Interpretation of the Mini-Cog[14]

SCORING:
Three-item recall (0 to 3 points): 1 point for each correct word
Clock draw (0 or 2 points): 0 points for abnormal clock
2 points for normal clock
A NORMAL CLOCK HAS ALL OF THE FOLLOWING ELEMENTS:
All numbers 1 to 12, each only once, are present in the correct order and direction (clockwise) inside the circle.
Two hands are present, one pointing to 11 and one pointing to 2.
ANY CLOCK MISSING ANY OF THESE ELEMENTS IS SCORED ABNORMAL. REFUSAL TO DRAW A CLOCK IS SCORED ABNORMAL.
Total score of 0, 1, or 2 suggests possible impairment.
Total score of 3, 4, or 5 suggests no impairment.
Mini-Cog, copyright S. Borson (soon@uw.edu).

Adapted from Borson S, Scanlan J, Brush M, et al. The Mini-Cog: a cognitive 'vital signs' measure for dementia screening in multi-lingual elderly. *Int J Geriatr Psychiatry.* 200;15:1021–1027.

between ACS NSQIP and the American Geriatrics Society (AGS) produced a set of guidelines for multidomain assessment of geriatric patients.[9] This approach was not novel; the concept of comprehensive geriatric assessment (CGA) was first implemented in the 1980s and 1990s in medical inpatient and long-term outpatient settings. Geriatric assessments were shown to improve independent living, physical function, and long-term mortality. Studies reporting the implementation of CGA within surgical populations are rare; a recent systematic review found positive impacts of CGA use on procedural cancellation rate, surgical complications, and length of stay.[10] Importantly, historic data demonstrate that the most effective CGA programs are those that impact direct medical care recommendations. The CGA is comprised of medical, mental health, functional capacity, social, and environmental domains. The ACS NSQIP/AGS collaborative framework (Box 10.2) refocuses the CGA toward themes more relevant to operative and perioperative care. While all aspects of the framework are vital, several are more pertinent within the geriatric population considered for surgery.

Cognitive Impairment and Delirium

Nearly one in five elderly patients has dementia or cognitive impairment. The ACS NSQIP/AGS framework recommends routine neurocognitive assessment for the elderly in the preoperative setting. Specifically, the guidelines recommend cognitive evaluation for any geriatric patient without a preexisting diagnosis of cognitive impairment. Methods include cognitive assessments such as the Mini-Cog (Box 10.3) and/or interviews with the patient's support structure (spouse or family) or affiliated healthcare providers.[11] The Mini-Cog's advantages include the large body of evidence supporting its usefulness, ease of implementation (3 minutes to complete), and focus on attention and executive function. Any findings suggestive of cognitive impairment should prompt referral to a primary care, mental health, or geriatric specialist. Establishing cognitive impairment early in the preoperative setting has direct implications for patient–physician communication, decision-making capacity, and informed consent.

In the postoperative setting, cognitive impairment strongly predicts delirium, which has an incidence of nearly 50% among geriatric patients. Documentation of preexisting cognitive impairment improves interpretation of perioperative mental status and encourages avoidance of medications that may precipitate delirium. In the geriatric population, postoperative delirium has a profound impact on hospital length of stay, long-term postoperative cognition, cost of care, and mortality. Because evidence-based treatments for delirium are few, the majority of studies focus on the identification of risk factors and prevention. The AGS best practice guidelines for delirium recommend preoperative risk factor screening for all geriatric surgical patients (Box 10.4).[12] Identification of these risk factors should raise awareness to avoid second-hit insults (such as high-risk medication administration, sleep cycle disturbance) and to implement simple measures that improve the patient's orientation. Such

BOX 10.4 Risk factors for postoperative delirium.

Age greater than 65 years
Cognitive impairment
Severe illness or comorbidity burden
Hearing or vision impairment
Current hip fracture
Presence of infection
Inadequately controlled pain
Depression
Alcohol use
Sleep deprivation or disturbance
Renal insufficiency
Anemia
Hypoxia or hypercarbia
Poor nutrition
Dehydration
Electrolyte abnormalities (hypernatremia or hyponatremia)
Poor functional status
Immobilization or limited mobility
Polypharmacy and use of psychotropic medications (benzodiazepines, anticholinergics, antihistamines, antipsychotics)
Risk of urinary retention or constipation
Presence of urinary catheter
Aortic procedures

Adapted from Chow WB, Rosenthal RA, Merkow RP, et al. Optimal preoperative assessment of the geriatric surgical patient: a best practices guideline from the American College of Surgeons National Surgical Quality Improvement Program and the American Geriatrics Society. *J Am Coll Surg*. 2012;215:453–466.

measures include holding high-risk medications preoperatively, providing hearing aids, encouraging sleep hygiene with preservation of day/night cycle, and employing the help of the patient's family for reorientation during postoperative in-hospital recovery.

Depression

Increased comorbidity and medical burden, conditions highly prevalent in the geriatric population, can exacerbate depressive symptoms. Additional risk factors include sleep disturbance, low functional status, low education level, and heavy alcohol or polysubstance use. Elderly patients with preoperative depressive symptoms can experience postoperative delirium at a significantly higher rate and longer duration. Depression also may lower the threshold for pain and is a predictor of chronic postoperative pain. In the intensive care setting, depression is associated with increased mortality and reduced quality of life following discharge. Following cardiac surgery, depression and anxiety may increase the likelihood for coronary disease recurrence and mortality. The ACS NSQIP/AGS guidelines recommend the Patient Health Questionnaire-2 as a pragmatic preoperative screening tool for elderly patients; positive findings should be followed by appropriate referral. Optimal management of depression requires a multidisciplinary approach frequently involving both psychiatric medications and cognitive behavioral therapy.

Medication Management

The ACS NSQIP/AGS framework emphasizes the importance of obtaining a comprehensive medication history for all older patients, including over-the-counter medications, eye drops, vitamins, and herbal products. Adverse drug reactions, inappropriate dosing, and polypharmacy can be avoided by considering potential changes in drug metabolism and clearance in the perioperative setting.

The American College of Cardiology (ACC) and American Heart Association (AHA) guidelines for perioperative beta blockade supports continued administration of beta blockers for patients already on this medication. Patients undergoing intermediate-risk surgery with known coronary artery disease or risk factors for ischemic heart disease may be candidates for perioperative beta blockade. If initiation of beta blockers is indicated in the preoperative setting, treatment ideally should start weeks before elective surgery and should be titrated to a target heart rate of 60 to 80 beats/minute. Adverse effects of beta blocker initiation too close to the time of surgery include risk of stroke, hypotension, and death. For patients with limited cardiac risk factors, rapid initiation of beta blockers in the acute preoperative setting is not indicated.

The AGS Beers Criteria for Potentially Inappropriate Medication Use are particularly relevant to elderly patients at risk for polypharmacy. The latest guidelines (updated in 2015) serve as a reference to check for medications with high-risk adverse-effect profiles, common drug-drug interactions, impaired renal and/or hepatic clearance, perioperative sedation, and a predisposition to delirium.[13] Some of the medications, such as benzodiazepines, are categorically contraindicated as they have been demonstrated to increase risk of cognitive impairment, delirium, falls, and other adverse outcomes in older adults.

Functional Status and Frailty

Elderly patients can be impaired in their performance of tasks necessary for independent living. These functional limitations are associated with perioperative complications, discharge to facilities other than home, and postoperative mortality.[14] The association between functional dependence and postoperative mortality is present in patients over 60 but is magnified in patients over 80. A simple way to obtain a broad sense of functional dependence is to inquire about a history of falls. More detailed instruments for scoring functional status include the activities of daily living and instrumental activities of daily living, which describe the ability to perform basic and higher-level functions, respectively (Box 10.5).

The social and family support systems surrounding the patient are intimately interwoven with the functional level of the geriatric patient. The living situation of the patient—independent, with family, in assisted living, or with a neighboring support structure—has far-reaching implications not only for their overall health but also as indicators of postoperative disposition and recovery. Identification and incorporation of the patients' living situation and support system into perioperative decision-making is vital to successful patient-centered recovery processes and management of expectations.

A series reporting on surgical outcomes of octogenarians and nonagenarians have shown that age is often a poor independent marker for surgical risk. A more accurate predictor is frailty. While no single definition of frailty exists, the AGS suggests that frailty is a syndrome comprised of a combination of weakness, fatigue, weight loss, decreased balance, low physical activity, slowed motor processing, social withdrawal, cognitive changes, and vulnerability to stressors. The impact of frailty on postoperative outcomes cannot be overstated. Frailty is associated with major complications and early postoperative mortality for cardiothoracic, orthopedic, otolaryngologic, and elective cancer operations. In a large ACS

BOX 10.5 Functional assessments for activities of daily living.

Activities of Daily Living*
- Bathing
- Dressing
- Toileting
- Transferring
- Continence
- Feeding

Instrumental Activities of Daily Living†
- Telephone ability
- Shopping
- Food preparation
- Housekeeping
- Laundry
- Transportation
- Medication management
- Handling finances

Other
- Muscle strength
- Balance
- Gait
- Walking speed
- Transfer ability

From Knittel JG, Wildes TS. Preoperative assessment of geriatric patients. *Anesthesiol Clin.* 2016;34:171–183.

*Katz S, Ford AB, Moskowitz RW, et al. Studies of illness in the aged. The index of ADL: a standardized measure of biological and psychosocial function. *JAMA.* 1963;185:914–919.

†Lawton MP, Brody EM. Assessment of older people: self-maintaining and instrumental activities of daily living. *Gerontologist.* 1969;9:179–186.

NSQIP study, preoperative frailty index was more strongly associated with postoperative cardiac arrest and death than ASA class or history of myocardial infarction (MI).[15]

Frailty can be measured using exhaustive, multidimensional scales such as the CGA or more pragmatic tests such as the Timed Up and Go (TUG) tool, which measures functional mobility.[16] In a comparison of four frailty scales to predict postoperative outcomes of cardiac surgery, gait speed outperformed several more extensive scales in predicting mortality or major morbidity. As the most pervasive gait speed measure, TUG time is calculated by measuring the time it takes for a patient to rise from a chair, walk 3 m, turn, and return to a sitting position in the same chair (Fig. 10.2). In a multi institutional study of patients undergoing minor and major elective operations for solid malignancies, a TUG time >20 seconds was associated with a 50% risk of major complications among patients older than 70, compared to 14% for patients with a TUG time ≤20 seconds.[17]

Although the physical function domain of frailty may be the easiest and most objective to measure, more comprehensive scales such as CGA may produce more actionable results that can improve optimization in the preoperative setting for elective procedures.

Patient Counseling

Integrated into the process of informed consent is clear communication between physician and patient regarding the patient's individualized

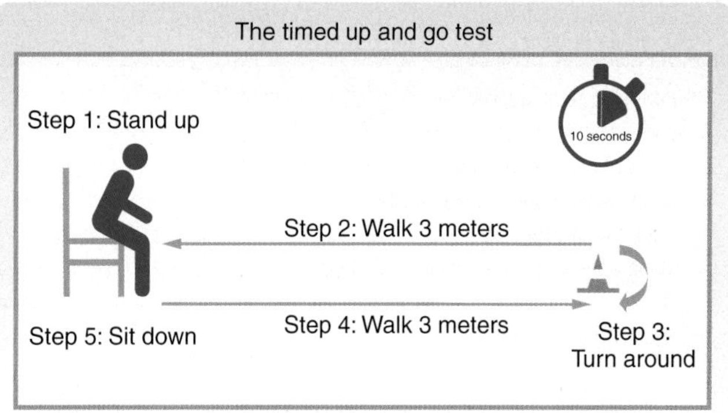

FIG. 10.2 Timed up and go test. (Adapted from www.frailtytoolkit.org.)

goals of treatment. It is critical for the patient to have clear and realistic expectations regarding the likely treatment course and any potential complications. In the case of older patients, conducting this discussion in the presence of the patient's anticipated postoperative support system—including spouse, adult children, or home nurse—can help ensure that both the patient and the support system are informed regarding necessary postoperative care. This is even more vital if the patient has any cognitive impairment. Regardless of baseline cognitive or functional state, it is strongly recommended that older patients anticipating elective surgery should arrange for an advanced directive and designate a health care proxy or surrogate decision maker. These documents should be prominently featured in the medical chart.

SYSTEMS APPROACH TO PREOPERATIVE EVALUATION

Cardiovascular System

As the US population continues to age, patients with heart disease undergoing elective, noncardiac surgery will increase. Perioperative cardiac complications are associated with morbidity, mortality, and cost. However, preoperative cardiac intervention to reduce the risk of noncardiac surgery is rarely needed, except when such an intervention is indicated for management of the patients' baseline condition. In the preoperative setting, the goal of cardiology evaluation (if indicated) is not to provide medical "clearance," but rather to provide information regarding the patient's cardiac risk profile and the management options for this risk. The overarching principle of preoperative cardiovascular evaluation is to obtain supplemental testing only when these tests have a reasonable likelihood of changing management. These changes may involve delaying the operation, preoperative revascularization, medical optimization, modifying perioperative monitoring, or referral to a specialty care center.

The ACC and AHA published collaborative guidelines regarding perioperative cardiac risk in 2007 that included identification of three surgery-specific risk categories.[18] In general, patients undergoing low-risk operations do not require any preoperative cardiac testing.

1. Vascular surgery: Highest risk category. Associated with cardiac morbidity rates greater than 5%. Examples include aortic and peripheral vascular surgery. Endovascular surgery is included in this category.
2. Intermediate-risk surgery: Cardiac morbidity rates range from 1% to 5%. Examples include abdominal and thoracic procedures, carotid endarterectomy, orthopedic surgery, and head and neck surgery.
3. Low-risk surgery: Cardiac morbidity rates are generally less than 1%. Examples include endoscopic, superficial soft tissue, cataract, breast, and ambulatory operations.

BOX 10.6 Revised cardiac risk index.

1. High-risk type of surgery
2. Ischemic heart disease
3. History of congestive heart failure
4. History of cerebrovascular disease
5. Insulin therapy for diabetes
6. Preoperative serum creatinine >2.0 mg/dL

Adapted from Lee TH, Marcantonio ER, Mangione CM, et al. Derivation and prospective validation of a simple index for prediction of cardiac risk of major noncardiac surgery. *Circulation.* 1999;100:1043–1049.

Risk Prediction Scales/Indices

There are numerous published tools that measure patients' risk of perioperative cardiac morbidity. The most pervasive—and the instrument cited by the 2014 ACC/AHA Guideline on Perioperative Cardiovascular Evaluation and Management of Patients Undergoing Noncardiac Surgery—is the Revised Cardiac Risk Index (RCRI). Originally published in 1999 by Lee and colleagues,[19] the RCRI assigns one point to each of six preoperative risk factors (Box 10.6). Patients with 0, 1, 2, or more factors are assigned to classes I, II, III, or IV, respectively. The RCRI has moderate discriminatory power between patients at low versus high risk for cardiac complications; its primary advantage is its ease of implementation and relatively objective criteria. The ACC/AHA guidelines also endorse using the ACS NSQIP risk calculator as an alternative to the RCRI.

Preoperative Testing (Electrocardiogram, Echocardiography, Stress Test, Angiography)

For patients at low risk for perioperative cardiac complications based on surgical and clinical risk factors, no further testing is indicated prior to surgery. For patients with known risk factors for coronary artery disease, the ACC/AHA 2014 guidelines provide a useful stepwise approach to further preoperative testing (Fig. 10.3).[20] First, the surgeon determines the urgency of the operation and identifies patient cardiac risk factors or known coronary artery disease. Any emergent operation should proceed, using patient risk factors to guide perioperative monitoring and management. Second, in cases of urgent or elective surgery, the patient should be assessed for acute coronary syndrome and, if suspected, referred for cardiology evaluation as appropriate. An important component of this assessment is an estimation of patient functional capacity, classically measured in metabolic equivalents of task (METs). An extensive collection of METs for common activities has been compiled by Ainsworth and colleagues.[21] Representative examples are listed in Table 10.4. ACC/ACH guidelines recommend that patients with METs ≥4 without symptoms of cardiac disease proceed with elective or urgent operation. Third, in the absence of acute coronary syndrome, additional testing is pursued on the basis of the combined clinical and surgical risk factors listed above, taking into account baseline functional capacity. Any patient undergoing a low-risk operation—regardless of clinical risk factors even with functional capacity <4 METs—has a low risk for cardiac complication and does not require further testing.

For patients undergoing an operation that is not low risk, a 12-lead electrocardiogram (ECG) is indicated for patients with known coronary disease, arrhythmia, peripheral artery disease, and cerebrovascular disease. Even for asymptomatic patients, ECG may be considered, except for those undergoing a low-risk operation. Assessment of left ventricular function through echocardiography is reasonable for patients with dyspnea of unknown origin or progressive heart failure. For patients with known left ventricular dysfunction, a preoperative echocardiogram should be considered if there has not been an assessment within 1 year preceding surgery or they have a decrement in functional status or change in symptoms. Exercise testing with cardiac imaging may be indicated for patients with elevated risk and poor (<4 METs) or unknown functional capacity if patients have three or more risk factors. Patients fitting these criteria who are unable to complete exercise testing may be referred for pharmacologic stress testing, either through dobutamine stress echocardiography or stress myocardial perfusion imaging.[20] Importantly, all of the aforementioned tests should be pursued only if there is a realistic likelihood that the obtained data could change management.

Surgery After Coronary Revascularization

In general, coronary revascularization for the exclusive purpose of reducing perioperative cardiac risk is not indicated. Revascularization is indicated prior to noncardiac surgery only if it is indicated by baseline clinical practice guidelines. If percutaneous coronary intervention is indicated in the preoperative setting, balloon angioplasty, bare-metal stent implantation, or drug-eluting stent (DES) revascularization may be considered based on preoperative stress imaging and coronary angiographic findings. For patients considering elective noncardiac surgery after recent coronary revascularization, surgery should be delayed a minimum of 14 days after balloon angioplasty and 30 days after bare-metal stent implantation.[20] Ideally, elective surgery should be delayed for 1 year after implantation of DES due to the need for dual antiplatelet therapy. An operation with interruption of dual antiplatelet therapy can be considered after 180 days following DES placement if risk of further surgical delay exceeds the risk of stent thrombosis and ischemia. As with any high-risk patient care situation, direct communication between a surgeon and medical subspecialist, in this instance a cardiologist, is imperative.

Other High-Risk Cardiac Patients

Patients with moderate to severe left-sided heart failure, right-sided heart failure and/or significant pulmonary hypertension (pulmonary artery pressure >25 mm Hg), and severe aortic stenosis (aortic valve area <1 cm^2) are at significantly increased risk of death. Elective or urgent operations in patients with these cardiac comorbidities require a multidisciplinary approach and risk/benefit discussion. While optimization with medical management (e.g., diuretics) or preoperative valve replacement (traditional or transcatheter) might be feasible in some patients, risk of elective operations in patients for whom cardiac function cannot be improved can exceed the potential benefit of the operation, and nonoperative management strategies should be considered.

Perioperative Cardiovascular Medications

Robust evidence supports the use of perioperative beta blockade to reduce cardiac events; however, there is a paucity of data indicating improvement in surgical mortality. Conversely, beta blockers are associated with bradycardia, hypotension, and stroke. As such, the ACC/AHA guidelines recommend that beta blockers should be continued in the perioperative setting for patients for whom it is an established preoperative medication. For patients with intermediate- or high-risk myocardial ischemia and for patients with three or more RCRI risk factors, perioperative beta blockers can

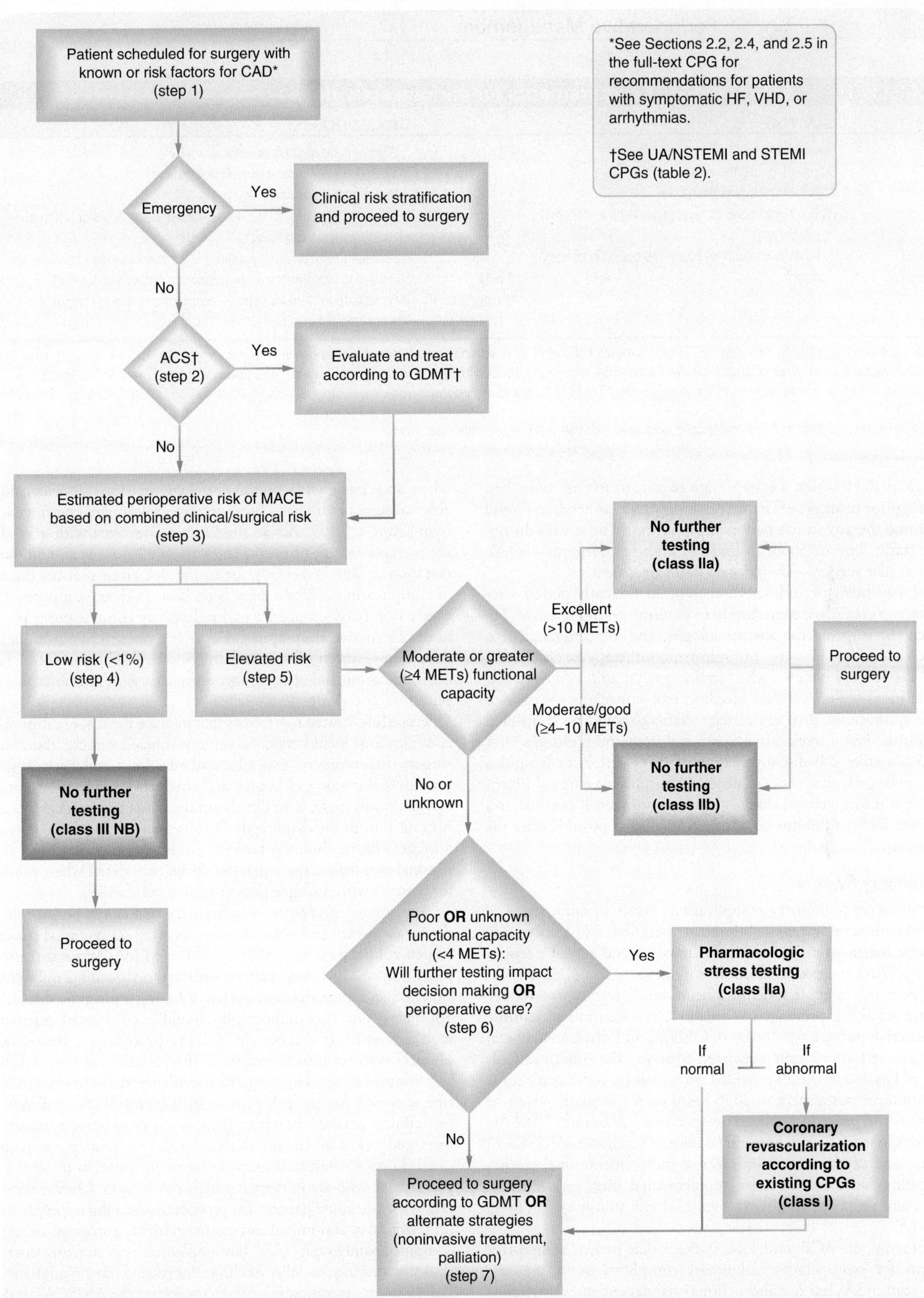

FIG. 10.3 Stepwise approach to perioperative cardiac assessment for coronary artery disease. *ACS*, American College of Surgeons; *CAD*, coronary artery disease; *CPG*, clinical practice guideline; *GDMT*, guideline-directed medical therapy; *HF*, heart failure; *MACE*, major adverse cardiovascular event; MET, metabolic equivalent of the task; *NSTEMI*, non-ST-elevation myocardial infarction; *STEMI*, ST-elevation myocardial infarction; *UA*, unstable angina; *VHD*, valvular heart disease. (Adapted from Fleisher LA, Fleischmann KE, Auerbach AD, et al: 2014 ACC/AHA guideline on perioperative cardiovascular evaluation and management of patients undergoing noncardiac surgery: a report of the American College of Cardiology/American Heart Association Task Force on practice guidelines. *J Am Coll Cardiol*. 2014;64:e77–137.)

TABLE 10.4 Estimated MET requirements for various activities.

	CAN YOU:		CAN YOU:
	Take care of yourself?		Climb a flight of stairs or walk up a hill?
	Eat, dress, or use the toilet?		Walk on level ground at 4 mph (6.4 kph)?
	Walk indoors around the house?		Run a short distance?
	Walk a block or two on level ground at 2 to 3 mph (3.2–4.8 kph)?		Do heavy work around the house like scrubbing floors or lifting or moving heavy furniture?
1 MET 4 METs	Do light work around the house like dusting or washing dishes?	4 METs	Participate in moderate recreational activities like golf, bowling, dancing, doubles tennis, or throwing a baseball or football?
		Greater than 10 METs	Participate in strenuous sports like swimming, singles tennis, football, basketball, or skiing?

Modified from Hlatky MA, Boineau RE, Higginbotham MB, et al. A brief self-administered questionnaire to determine functional capacity (the Duke Activity Status Index). *Am J Cardiol.* 1989;64:651–654, copyright 1989 with permission from Elsevier; and adapted from Fletcher GF, Balady G, Froelicher VF, et al. Exercise standards. A statement for healthcare professionals from the American Heart Association. Writing Group. *Circulation.* 1995;91:580–615.)
kph, Kilometers per hour; *MET,* metabolic equivalent of the task; *mph,* miles per hour.

be initiated. However, it is important to start treatment more than 7 days prior to surgery.[22] Patients taking statins at baseline should continue therapy in the perioperative setting. Those who do not take statins but are about to undergo high-risk surgery—including vascular surgery—should start statin treatment.

Management of antiplatelet therapy in the early period after coronary revascularization should be determined by consensus between the surgeon, the anesthesiologist, and the cardiologist. In general, perioperative use of aspirin monotherapy is safe in the vast majority of patients who require general and cardiovascular operations. Unless surgical bleeding risk outweighs the risk of stent thrombosis, dual antiplatelet therapy should be continued within the first 4 weeks after bare-metal stent and 6 months after DES placement. If discontinuation of $P2Y_{12}$-inhibitor (clopidogrel, prasugrel, ticagrelor) is necessary to prevent surgical bleeding, it is recommended that aspirin be continued if possible and that the $P2Y_{12}$-inhibitor be restarted as soon as possible after the operation.

Pulmonary System

Postoperative pulmonary complications occur in approximately 6% of patients after major abdominal operations and are associated with increased mortality, ICU admission, and a greater length of stay. While the exact definition of pulmonary complication varies, the major categories include pneumonia/infection, respiratory failure requiring prolonged ventilation, exacerbation of chronic obstructive pulmonary disease (COPD), and lobar/parenchymal collapse with or without associated effusion. The American College of Physicians (ACP) provided guidelines for pulmonary complication risk assessment in 2006 based on a systematic review of patient- and procedure-related preoperative risk factors.[23] The Assess Respiratory Risk in Surgical Patients in Catalonia (ARISCAT) study, one of the largest prospective multi-institutional studies on pulmonary complications, supplemented these guidelines in 2010 and proposed an objective scale for risk stratification (Table 10.5).[24]

Broadly, the ACP guidelines indicate that patient-related risk factors for postoperative pulmonary complications include age >50 years, ASA class 2 or above, functional dependence, hypoalbuminemia (<3.5 g/dL), COPD, and heart failure. Although COPD is consistently associated with postoperative morbidity, there is no specific level of preoperative pulmonary impairment that precludes nonthoracic surgery. In fact, congestive heart failure—especially when associated with pulmonary hypertension—is a considerably stronger predictor of postoperative pulmonary complications than severe COPD. Active smoking is associated with a moderate increase in risk of postoperative complications, and smoking cessation at least 4 weeks prior to the operation reduces the risk of complications. While there is no clear evidence supporting an association between obesity and pulmonary complications per se, both obstructive sleep apnea (OSA) and obesity hypoventilation syndrome—which often complement overweight, metabolic syndrome, and morbid obesity—are associated with pulmonary complications and death.

Procedure-related risk factors that increase the risk of pulmonary complications include vascular surgery, thoracic surgery, abdominal surgery, neurosurgery, general anesthesia, head and neck surgery, procedure duration (>3 hours), and emergency surgery. Pulmonary complications increase in likelihood the closer the surgical incision is in relation to the diaphragm. Because general anesthesia conveys a higher risk of clinically relevant pulmonary complications than regional anesthesia, the latter should be considered when possible for patients with multiple patient-related risk factors.

Appropriate preoperative pulmonary evaluation begins with a thorough history and physical exam focusing on potential patient-related risk factors. Spirometry is indicated for physiologic assessment and residual lung volume estimation preceding pulmonary resection and for patients suspected of having undiagnosed COPD. Spirometry and chest radiography should be considered in patients with a preexisting diagnosis of COPD or asthma if history and physical exam cannot determine if the patient is at their optimal baseline physiology. However, these tests should not be used in routine screening for low-risk patients or if results of tests will not affect clinical decision-making. There is no prohibitive spirometric threshold below which nonthoracic surgery is strictly contraindicated. Routine chest radiography may be indicated in patients >50 years of age who are undergoing high-risk surgery. Chest radiography is used in some patients for preoperative staging in preparation for resection of abdominal and gastrointestinal neoplasms, although computed tomography (CT) has supplanted x-ray in many instances as the imaging modality of choice for staging most malignancies. Pulse oxygen saturation is a risk factor within the ARISCAT index, and its low resource utilization allows for routine screening.

There are numerous predictive indices for pulmonary complications; the most frequently cited include the Arozullah index, the ARISCAT index, and the Gupta respiratory failure calculators. The

ARISCAT index is the simplest to use, featuring seven readily available preoperative predictors in a simple score system (Table 10.5).[24] The disadvantage of the ARISCAT index is that it may overestimate postoperative complication rate as its complication definition includes minor morbidities such as small radiographic effusions and bronchospasm/wheezing. The Arozullah index, derived from a veteran population, specifically targets postoperative respiratory failure. More cumbersome for routine implementation, it includes more than 12 risk factors, some of which may not be routinely available. More recently, Gupta and colleagues[25] developed risk calculators using the ACS NSQIP dataset with primary outcomes of postoperative respiratory failure and pneumonia; these calculators are available on the web or as a downloadable mobile app.

OSA and obesity hypoventilation syndrome deserve additional consideration. Older age, obesity, and male sex are associated with a higher prevalence of OSA. A simple STOP-BANG questionnaire has been developed to screen patients for OSA and to stratify patients into risk categories based on presence of symptoms. The eight-question scoring tool includes yes/no responses to (1) snoring, (2) daytime tiredness, (3) observation of stopped breathing or interrupted

TABLE 10.5 ARISCAT risk score system (top) and associated postoperative pulmonary complication rate by intervals (bottom).

	MULTIVARIATE ANALYSIS OR (95% CI) N = 1624*	β COEFFICIENT	RISK SCORE†
Age (y)			
≤50	1		
51–80	1.4 (0.6–3.3)	0.331	3
>80	5.1 (1.9–13.3)	1.619	16
Preoperative SpO_2 (%)			
≥96	1		
91–95	2.2 (1.2–4.2)	0.802	8
≤90	10.7 (4.1–28.1)	2.375	24
Respiratory infection in the last month	5.5 (2.6–11.5)	1.698	17
Preoperative anemia (≤10 g/dL)	3.0 (1.4–6.5)	1.105	11
Surgical incision			
Peripheral	1		
Upper abdominal	4.4 (2.3–8.5)	1.480	15
Intrathoracic	11.4 (4.9–26.0)	2.431	24
Duration of Surgery (h)			
≤2	1		
>2 to 3	4.9 (2.4–10.1)	1.593	16
>3	9.7 (4.7–19.9)	2.268	23
	2.2 (1.0–4.5)	0.768	8
Emergency procedure			

	RISK SCORE INTERVALS*		
	LOW RISK (<26 POINTS)	INTERMEDIATE RISK (26–44 POINTS)	HIGH RISK (≥45 POINTS)
Development subsample, no. (%) of patients†	1238 (76.2)	288 (17.7)	98 (6.0)
Validation subsample, no. (%) of patients	645 (77.1)	135 (16.1)	57 (6.8)
PPC rate, development subsample, % (95% CI)	0.7 (0.2–1.2)	6.3 (3.5–9.1)	44.9 (35.1–54.7)
PPC rate, validation subsample, % (95% CI)	1.6 (0.6–2.6)	13.3 (7.6–19.0)	42.1 (29.3–54.9)

From Canet J, Gallart L, Gomar C, et al. Prediction of postoperative pulmonary complications in a population-based surgical cohort. *Anesthesiology.* 2010;113:1338–1350.

ARISCAT, Assess Respiratory Risk in Surgical Patients in Catalonia; *CI*, confidence interval; *OR*, odds ratio; *PPC*, postoperative pulmonary complications; SpO_2, oxyhemoglobin saturation by pulse oximetry breathing air in supine position.

*Because of a missing value for some variables, three patients were excluded. Logistic regression model constructed with the development subsample, c-index = 0.90; Hosmer-Lemeshow chi-square test = 7.862; $P = 0.447$.

†The simplified risk score was the sum of each β logistic regression coefficient multiplied by 10, after rounding off its value.

CI, Confidence interval; *PPC*, postoperative pulmonary complication.

*Risk intervals were based on division of the development subsample into optimal risk intervals according to the simplified risk score and applying the minimum description length principle.

†Three patients were excluded because of a missing value in some variable.

breathing during sleep, (4) high blood pressure, (5) body mass index (BMI) >35, (6) age >50, (7) neck diameter >40 cm, and (8) male gender.[26] Patients with five or more risk factors are considered at high risk for moderate to severe OSA. If an elective operation is planned, these patients should be considered for a sleep study. If positive, they should have preoperative (continuous positive airway pressure) CPAP machine fitting and optimization. Patients requiring urgent or emergent operations are managed for OSA in the postoperative setting.

Obesity hypoventilation syndrome is defined as a combination of BMI >30 with awake $PaCO_2$ >45 mm Hg indicative of hypercapnia. There are no strict guidelines for arterial gas measurements in obese patients, although the highest risk for hypoventilation are patients with BMI exceeding 50. The problem of hypoventilation can be exacerbated in these patients during the perioperative period by general anesthesia and opioids. Consideration for postoperative capnography and adherence to OSA screening and postoperative CPAP use can decrease the risk of respiratory failure and death.

Renal System

Patients with chronic renal insufficiency—particularly those on hemodialysis—experience substantially greater perioperative morbidity and mortality than the general population. Patients on dialysis have greater pressor requirements, longer periods of mechanical ventilation, and longer ICU and overall hospital stays. The cause of this elevated risk is a high rate of concurrent cardiac disease, perioperative fluid, and electrolyte disturbances and uremia-mediated bleeding diathesis. Preoperative measures to accommodate patients with chronic renal insufficiency primarily focus on a thorough assessment of comorbidities, optimizing fluid and electrolyte status, and securing adequate resources for perioperative care.

Chronic renal disease is a consistent predictor of death and cardiac arrest in the perioperative patient. Assessment of associated cardiac risk begins with a thorough history and physical exam, with attention to predictive indices such as the RCRI (see previous discussion). Because renal insufficiency is a risk factor within the RCRI, preoperative testing for patients with renal insufficiency broadly follow the guidelines put forth by the ACC/AHA. Patients with stage 1 to 2 chronic renal insufficiency and functional capacity >4 METs who are undergoing low- or intermediate-risk surgery do not require additional preoperative studies. Patients who have stage 3 to 5 renal insufficiency or are undergoing high-risk surgery should receive additional cardiac evaluation including ECG, complete blood count, blood chemistry and electrolytes, and urinalysis. Echocardiography should be done in patients with volume overload despite optimal chronic renal disease management to evaluate for concomitant cardiac dysfunction.

For patients on dialysis, preoperative management focuses on fluid and electrolyte optimization and preservation of hemodynamic stability. The ideal timing of preoperative dialysis is the day prior to the operation or the day of surgery. Dialysis goals should include achievement of near-normal electrolyte levels and euvolemia, making the patient close to dry weight. Hyperkalemia is a life-threatening complication of renal disease and must be considered preoperatively in all patients with renal insufficiency and addressed during all perioperative stages. A normal potassium level is a prerequisite for patients with chronic renal disease being considered for an elective or urgent operation because intraoperative medications to counteract hyperkalemia are limited and hyperkalemia can result in intraoperative death. While some experts recommend increasing the amount of peritoneal dialysis for 1 week prior to surgery, objective data do not exist regarding this practice. Patients who have recently initiated dialysis may possess residual renal function. This function is critical for solute clearance and fluid balance during the first year on dialysis and confers a long-term survival benefit for dialysis patients. Thus, its preservation during the perioperative period is critical. Although evidence-based research remains inconclusive, holding diuretics, angiotensin-converting enzyme inhibitors, and angiotensin receptor blockers in the perioperative period should be considered, as these medications can result in variable hemodynamic changes during and after surgery. Once the patient is stable after the operation, these medications should be resumed early in the postoperative period, as they may be associated with long-term preservation of residual glomerular filtration rate.

Chronic renal insufficiency impacts hematologic function as well, and chronic anemia is common in this population. After addressing the various etiologies for chronic anemia, erythropoietin or darbepoietin may be started for preoperative optimization. Although chronic renal insufficiency does not impact platelet count, uremic platelet dysfunction is common. Desmopressin (DDAVP) should be readily available and administered if medical bleeding from platelet dysfunction is encountered. Cryoprecipitate and platelet transfusion can be used if necessary. Intraoperative and postoperative medications must undergo diligent dose adjustment, and nephrotoxic agents—including nonsteroidal anti inflammatory drugs (NSAIDs), aminoglycosides, amphotericin B, and contrast dye—should be avoided if possible in patients with residual renal function.

For all patients with chronic kidney disease, avoidance of secondary renal insults is vital to preservation of any residual renal function. Maintenance of adequate intravascular volume and avoidance of hypotension in the intraoperative and early postoperative periods are particularly important. For patients without residual renal function and on dialysis, use of nephrotoxic medications and agents can be considered.

Hepatobiliary System

Patients with impaired liver function are at elevated risk for surgical and anesthesia-related complications. A thorough preoperative history and physical exam provide cues toward hepatic dysfunction. Acute hepatitis of any etiology (viral, medication-induced, autoimmune, obesity-related, etc.) requires appropriate diagnosis, evaluation, and management. Chronic liver disease, including fibrosis and cirrhosis, can have a significant impact on patients' operative planning and postoperative outcomes. Risk factors for chronic liver disease evident on history can include social behavior factors (e.g., intravenous

TABLE 10.6 Modified Child-Turcotte-Pugh scoring system with historic-associated survival statistics.

	CLASS A	CLASS B	CLASS C
Total points	5–6	7–9	10–15
Historic 1-year survival	100%	80%	45%
Historic 2-year survival	85%	60%	35%

	POINTS		
VARIABLES	**1**	**2**	**3**
Encephalopathy	None	Grade 1–2	Grade 3–4
Ascites	Absent	Slight	Moderate
Serum albumin (g/L)	>3.5	2.8–3.5	<2.8
International normalized ratio	<1.7	1.7–2.3	>2.3
Total bilirubin (mg/dL)or fl.	<2	2–3	>3
I.(mg/dL) in patients with PBC/PSC	<4	4–10	>10

PBC, Primary biliary cirrhosis; *PSC*, primary sclerosing cholangitis.

[IV] drug use, significant alcohol use), long-term obesity, and familial chronic liver disease. Many of the reviews of symptoms findings (pruritus and other manifestations such as jaundice, ascites, gynecomastia) and physical exam features (spider telangiectasias, caput medusae, icterus, splenomegaly, and fluid wave) are usually found in patients with long-standing cirrhosis. For patients without evidence for liver dysfunction on history and physical exam, routine preoperative testing for liver function in the setting of nonhepatobiliary surgery has low predictive value and is not recommended.

Surgical risk in patients with hepatic disease may be stratified by clinical scenarios and objective measures. Contraindications to elective surgery include acute or fulminant hepatitis and alcoholic hepatitis. Acute/fulminant hepatitis can be an indication for liver transplantation. Patients with fibrosis without cirrhosis can usually tolerate elective surgery with low morbidity; however, anesthetic agent modifications might be necessary. Common anesthetics, such as propofol, ketamine, etomidate, benzodiazepines, and opioids undergo hepatic metabolism. Nondepolarizing neuromuscular blockers also pose a pharmacodynamic challenge, as patients with liver disease frequently have greater volume of distribution but a slower drug elimination rate. Cirrhosis is associated with increased mortality across all types of major elective surgery, with odds ratios ranging from 3.4 for cholecystectomy to 8.0 for coronary artery bypass graft.[27]

The three most common objective measures of surgical risk in cirrhotic patients are the Child-Turcotte-Pugh (CTP) score, the MELD score, and residual liver volume. The CTP classification (Table 10.6) of cirrhosis was popularized in the 1980s, given ease of calculation and correlation with perioperative mortality after abdominal surgery. Originally proposed by Child and Turcotte, this score estimated the procedural risk for portosystemic shunting for variceal bleeding. Later, the score was modified by Pugh and colleagues to include prothrombin time (PT) and exclude nutritional status. A CTP score of 5 to 6 is considered class A (well-compensated), 7 to 9 is considered class B (significant compromise), and 10 to 15 is considered class C (decompensated). As surgical technique and perioperative care improved over recent years—particularly with the popularization of laparoscopic surgery—mortality rates for each CTP class have decreased. While outcomes vary by type of procedure, broad estimates of mortality for abdominal operations are 10%, 20%, and 60% for CTP A, B, and C, respectively.[28]

The MELD score is predictive of survival in patients with cirrhosis and was originally developed primarily for transplant selection. In recent years, the MELD score has gradually supplanted CTP classification for both liver-directed operations and nonhepatic surgical risk stratification. Unlike CTP score, which includes subjective components such as encephalopathy and ascites, the MELD score is comprised only of objective measures: total bilirubin (mg/dL), creatinine (mg/dL), and international normalized ratio (INR, %). Thirty-day mortality ranges relatively linearly with MELD score, with MELD <8 associated with 6% mortality, and MELD >20 associated with a greater than 50% mortality.[29]

The relative predictive strengths of CTP and MELD scores have been debated for more than a decade. While some studies suggested that a MELD score of 10 to 14 was a better predictor of death or need for transplantation after abdominal surgery than CTP class C, other analyses demonstrated that CTP score and ASA classification were predictive of mortality among patients selected for nonhepatic abdominal operations and MELD was not. Overall, the predictive utility of both MELD and CTP scores may be greater for urgent than for elective operations; however, appropriate preoperative patient selection and optimization is paramount in patients with cirrhosis selected for an elective surgical procedure. Common general surgical problems encountered in patients with cirrhosis include abdominal wall hernias and biliary tract disease. Significant and poorly controlled ascites predisposes to hernia development through congenital abdominal wall defects. Emergency hernia repair (for repair of a transabdominal defect with leaking ascites) is associated with higher morbidity and mortality. As such, preoperative management and control/reduction of ascites are paramount for successful hernia repair, long-term durability, and perioperative safety. When hernia repair is pursued, abdominal wall closure with suture (without mesh) is both feasible and safe. Numerous studies demonstrated better outcomes after a laparoscopic approach to cholecystectomy when compared to an open approach in patients with cirrhosis. For all patients with cirrhosis, operative risk increases with higher CPT (B–C) and higher MELD (>18–20). Multidisciplinary risk/benefit analysis is paramount in these patients. Patients with decompensated cirrhosis (CPT-C; high MELD) awaiting liver transplantation would benefit from hernia repair after transplantation and/or delaying cholecystectomy to the time of liver transplantation.

When considering hepatic resection, residual liver volume is predictive of postoperative morbidity, particularly posthepatectomy liver failure. Generally defined as PT >50% of normal (INR >1.7) and serum bilirubin >2.9 mg/dL (50 μmol/L) on postoperative day 5—often referred to as the 50-50 criteria—posthepatectomy liver failure is associated with up to 50% mortality rate.[30] For patients without cirrhosis undergoing hepatic resection, a residual liver volume of 20% is generally considered adequate. This minimum is estimated at 40% for patients with compensated cirrhosis. Residual liver volume is most commonly estimated by CT or magnetic resonance imaging volumetry using integrated software, taking into account the proposed liver volume to be resected and patient body surface area.

Patients with chronic liver disease should be medically optimized prior to surgery. Synthetic function should be evaluated through assessment of PT, albumin, and fibrinogen levels. Creatinine and total bilirubin are necessary to complete preoperative MELD risk assessment. However, it is important to note that PT does not directly correlate with bleeding risk in cirrhotic patients. In fact, patients with cirrhosis and elevated PT/INR can have hypercoagulability. By treating ascites with preoperative diuresis or paracentesis, surgeons may reduce the risk for dehiscence or herniation. Renal function is particularly important in cirrhotic patients. Clinicians must be mindful that the impaired synthetic function of cirrhotic patients may artificially lower urea and creatinine synthesis. Finally, malnutrition is very common among patients with cirrhosis and is associated with poor perioperative outcomes. Preoperative nutritional supplementation—including replacement of fat-soluble vitamins as indicated—may be indicated for patients with evidence of recent weight loss or hypoalbuminemia.

Hematologic System

Bleeding and thromboembolism are among the most worrisome, and preventable, operative complications. As such, a thorough hematologic history and physical examination are indicated for every patient considered for an operation. This includes evaluation for symptoms of anemia (fatigue, pallor, hematochezia, dyspnea, palpitations), coagulopathy (petechiae, bleeding diathesis, medications), and hypercoagulability (thrombosis, edema). Physical exam should assess for vital signs, hepatomegaly and splenomegaly, lymphadenopathy, skin tone, extremity edema, and rectal bleeding. A thorough reconciliation of baseline medications is critical, as antithrombotic medications require careful management in the preoperative setting. Information regarding liver and kidney function also impacts risk-assessment for bleeding and perioperative venous thromboembolism prophylaxis.

TABLE 10.7 Approximate risk per unit transfusion of RBCs.

ADVERSE EVENT	APPROXIMATE RISK PER-UNIT TRANSFUSION OF RBCs
Febrile reaction[a]	1:60*
Transfusion-associated circulatory overload[b,c]	1:100†
Allergic reaction[d]	1:250
Transfusion-related acute lung injury[e]	1:12,000
Hepatitis C virus infection[f]	1:1,149,000
Hepatitis B virus infection[g]	1:1,208,000 to 1:843,000‡
Human immunodeficiency virus infection[f]	1:1,467,000
Fatal hemolysis[h]	1:1,972,000

From Carson JL, Guyatt G, Heddle NM, et al. Clinical Practice Guidelines from the AABB: red blood cell transfusion thresholds and storage. *JAMA*. 2016;316:2025–2035.

RBCs, Red blood cells.

*Estimated to be 1:91 with prestorage leukoreduction and 1:46 with poststorage leukoreduction.

†Estimated risk per recipient rather than unit.

‡The estimate is variable depending on the length of the infectious period.

[a]Federowicz I, Barrett BB, Andersen JW, et al. Characterization of reactions after transfusion of cellular blood components that are white cell reduced before storage. *Transfusion*. 1996;36:21–28.

[b]Popovsky MA, Audet AM, Andrzejewski C Jr. Transfusion-associated circulatory overload in orthopedic surgery patients: a multi-institutional study. *Immunohematology*. 1996;12:87–89.

[c]Clifford L, Jia Q, Yadav H, et al. Characterizing the epidemiology of perioperative transfusion-associated circulatory overload. *Anesthesiology*. 2015;122:21–28.

[d]DeBaun MR, Gordon M, McKinstry RC, et al. Controlled trial of transfusions for silent cerebral infarcts in sickle cell anemia. *N Engl J Med*. 2014;371:699–710.

[e]Use of blood products for elective surgery in 43 European hospitals. The Sanguis Study Group. *Transfus Med*. 1994;4:251–268.

[f]Zou S, Dorsey KA, Notari EP, et al. Prevalence, incidence, and residual risk of human immunodeficiency virus and hepatitis C virus infections among United States blood donors since the introduction of nucleic acid testing. *Transfusion*. 2010;50:1495–1504.

[g]Stramer SL, Notari EP, Krysztof DE, et al. Hepatitis B virus testing by minipool nucleic acid testing: does it improve blood safety? *Transfusion*. 2013;53:2449–2458.

[h]US Food and Drug Administration. Transfusion/donation fatalities: notification process for transfusion related fatalities and donation related deaths. Retrieved August 1, 2016.

Anemia

Chronic anemia is one of the most common findings on routine preoperative evaluation. Causes are frequently multimodal including nutritional deficiency, cancer, renal disease, inflammatory disease, infection, and heritable disorders. The vast majority of blood-borne oxygen is delivered via hemoglobin within red blood cells; therefore, anemia can result in significant compromise in tissue oxygenation. However, given the reserve in oxygen delivery compared to tissue utilization, hemoglobin levels considerably below normal ranges are generally well tolerated by healthy patients. Over time, treatment of chronic and perioperative anemia has gravitated from liberal transfusion protocols to restrictive strategies. This is due to a lack of supporting evidence for liberal blood transfusion practice and the measurable risks associated with blood transfusion (Table 10.7).

Triggers for blood transfusion in the setting of anemia should be individualized based on patient and clinical factors; however, general guidelines can be helpful to promote institutional consistency. Based on data from more than 12,000 patients across 31 trials, the AABB (formerly American Association of Blood Banks) provided updated transfusion guidelines in 2016. For most hemodynamically stable, asymptomatic hospitalized patients, transfusion is not indicated until hemoglobin level is ≤7 g/dL. This includes the critically ill patient population. These recommendations are supported by the Transfusion Requirements in Critical Care (TRICC) trial, which demonstrated no difference in 30-day mortality between restrictive and liberal transfusion protocols in critically ill, euvolemic patients with anemia in the intensive care setting. Findings from the TRICC trial were recently corroborated by the Transfusion Requirements in Septic Shock (TRISS) trial in patients with septic shock.[31] Among patients with gastrointestinal bleeding, a restrictive transfusion system is associated with lower 30-day mortality.

Potential exceptions to the 7 g/dL transfusion threshold include patients with cardiovascular disease and those undergoing cardiac surgery, for whom a transfusion threshold of 8 g/dL could be considered. The recent Transfusion Requirements in Cardiac Surgery III (TRICS III) trial found no difference in death, MI, stroke, or renal failure between transfusion thresholds of 7.5 g/dL and 8.5 to 9.5 g/dL in cardiac surgery patients.[32] For asymptomatic patients with baseline cardiovascular disease, the Functional Outcomes in Cardiovascular Patients Undergoing Surgical Hip Fracture (FOCUS) trial suggests that a transfusion threshold of 8 g/dL is not associated with worse postoperative outcomes when compared to a threshold of 10 g/dL.

Anemia in the acutely bleeding patient represents a fundamentally different clinical scenario. In these patients, anemia is more closely associated with hypovolemic shock, and rapid hemodynamic instability often makes laboratory-based transfusion protocols unrealistic. For hemodynamically stable patients, a restrictive transfusion system may be reasonable. However, for patients with ongoing bleeding, hemodynamic instability, or massive trauma, empiric blood transfusion and institutional massive transfusion protocols may be life-saving.

Inherited Coagulopathy

Routine preoperative laboratory screening for bleeding diatheses is discouraged; work-up should be guided by questions that assess bleeding risk. The surgeon should elicit a history of frequent nosebleeds, menorrhagia, intra articular bleeding, and hereditary diseases. Common comorbid conditions that increase bleeding risks include chronic renal or hepatic insufficiency. Prior experiences with invasive procedures and current anticoagulation and antiplatelet medications should be assessed. On physical exam, epistaxis, gingival bleeding, and cutaneous petechiae are suggestive of platelet or collagen disorders. Hemarthrosis, deep hematomas, and large, palpable ecchymoses may indicate factor deficiency. Due to the relatively low incidence of major bleeding in common general surgery operations, studies addressing the value of routine preoperative hemostatic testing are often inadequately powered. If a patient's history and physical exam indicate an increased risk for bleeding, initial laboratory tests should include a complete blood count including platelet count, PT/INR, activated partial thromboplastin time (aPTT), creatinine, and hepatic function panel. Patients with signs of hereditary bleeding disorders should be referred for preoperative hematologic consultation.

When considering the diagnostic approach to hereditary bleeding disorders, the first separation is between disorders of coagulation and those of platelets and vascular integrity. If the work-up includes a normal PT/INR and aPTT, thrombocytopenia or platelet dysfunction should be suspected. Spontaneous bleeding generally does not occur unless the platelet count is below 30,000/μL. Inherited disorders in platelet function or storage include von Willebrand disease (vWD, the most common), Bernard-Soulier, and Glanzmann thrombasthenia. Acquired causes of platelet dysfunction include cirrhosis, myelodysplastic syndromes, uremia, and pharmacologic impacts of aspirin, $P2Y_{12}$ inhibitors, and NSAIDs. A normal PT/INR and aPTT do not rule out coagulopathies outside the measured pathways of these two tests (i.e., factor XIII deficiency) or vascular disorders (inherited and acquired connective tissue disorders, small vessel vasculitis).

Causes of isolated prolongation of aPTT include deficiencies in factors VIII (hemophilia A), IX (hemophilia B), and XI. Hemophilia A and B are by far the most common, and both are X-linked recessive disorders. Isolated prolonged PT, in the absence of pharmacologic contributors or cirrhosis, is indicative of the relatively rare factor VII deficiency. Abnormal results on both PT and aPTT usually indicate a defect in the common coagulation pathway, comprised of factors II (prothrombin), V, X, and fibrinogen. Inherited disorders of the common pathway are rare; an extensive investigation into acquired causes is likely to indicate contributors such as vitamin K deficiency, supratherapeutic warfarin, hepatic insufficiency, or disseminated intravascular coagulation. A broad summary of the screening approach to bleeding disorders is provided in Fig. 10.4.

Institutional protocols for perioperative management in patients with inherited bleeding disorders should be a collaboration between hematologists, anesthesiologists, and surgeons. These protocols vary widely due to differences in available laboratory resources and treatments. However, a few guiding principles are relevant in all scenarios. Elective operations for patients with bleeding disorders should be planned with multidisciplinary input to ensure availability of all laboratory and therapeutic resources in the postoperative period. Multiple avenues of intraoperative venous access should be available for accurate blood sampling away from infusion sites. Perioperative analgesia should not include medications with antiplatelet effects such as aspirin and NSAIDs.

Preoperative treatment for hemophilia A depends on disease severity. Mild phenotypes (fVIII >5%) respond well to DDAVP given the day of surgery, which will raise factor VIII levels up to five fold within 90 minutes. Following administration, factor VIII levels should be measured in the preoperative and postoperative setting, and DDAVP may be redosed on a daily or twice-daily basis as needed. Appropriate attention should be paid to fluid retention, as hyponatremia can be a serious complication of DDAVP, particularly in elderly patients. Because factor IX does not respond

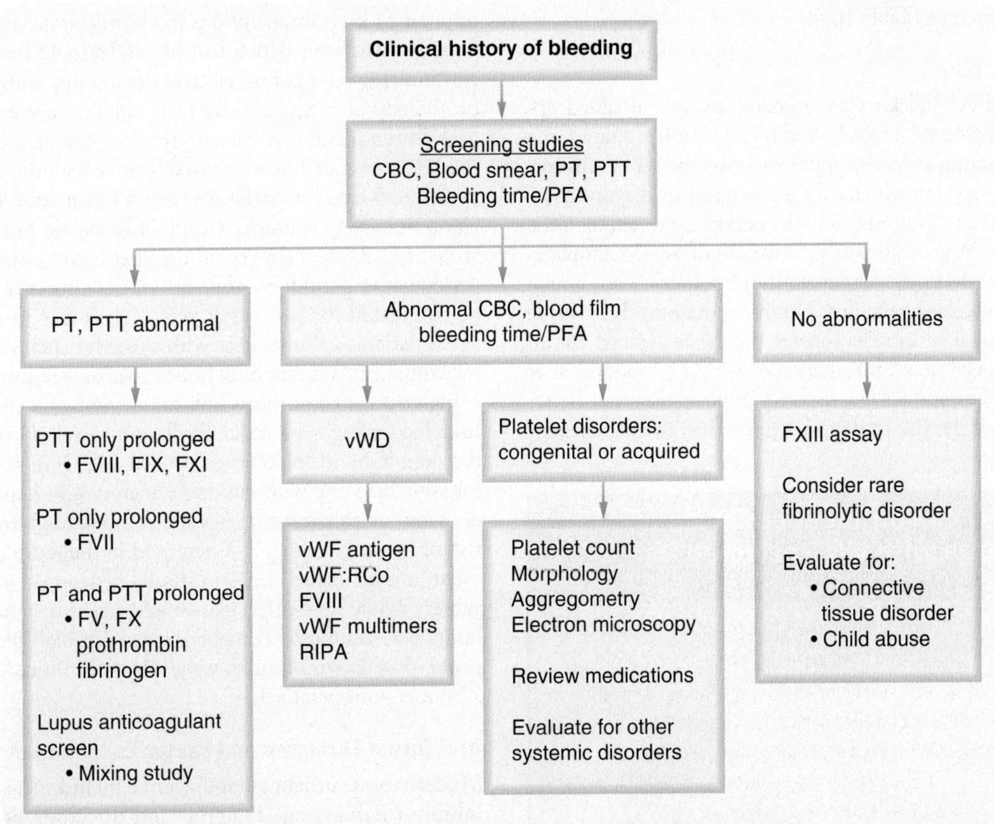

FIG. 10.4 Laboratory evaluation of bleeding disorders. *CBC*, complete blood count; *PFA*, platelet function assay; *PT*, prothrombin time; *PTT*, partial thromboplastin time; *RCo*, Ristocetin Cofactor; *RIPA*, Ristocetin-induced platelet aggregation; *vWD*, von Willebrand disease; *vWF*, von Willebrand factor. (Adapted from Sharathkumar AA, Pipe SW: Bleeding disorders. *Pediatr Rev.* 2008;29:121–129.)

to DDAVP, even mild forms of hemophilia B require factor replacement both before and after major surgery to maintain appropriate levels. For both disorders, severe phenotypes should be treated with administration of factor concentrates in the immediate preoperative setting, within 10 to 20 minutes of incision. Reducing the need for repeat dosing of factor concentrates minimizes the likelihood of inhibitor development. Up to 25% of patients with severe hemophilia A will ultimately develop inhibiting antibodies to factor VIII. Inhibitors reduce the effectiveness of factor replacement therapy. For patients who have had multiple prior treatments with factor replacement, preoperative inhibitor screening should be performed a week before surgery. The presence of inhibitors indicates the need for procoagulant agents that can bypass the intrinsic pathway, such as activated recombinant factor VII or activated prothrombin complex concentrate.

von Willebrand factor (vWF) mediates platelet adhesion to collagen and other platelets. It is the carrier protein for factor VIII. vWD, a disorder of vWF, is subdivided into three broad types. Type 1 is a partial deficiency of vWF. It is the most common version of vWD and responds well to DDAVP administered 1 hour prior to incision. Because vWF is an acute phase reactant, levels generally remain elevated postoperatively. Type 2 vWD comprises a variety of qualitative defects in vWF that can result in decreased binding of factor VIII and disorders in platelet function (2A, 2B, and 2M). While DDAVP may induce a partial response in patients with types 2A and 2M vWD, it is contraindicated in type 2B as it may cause thrombocytopenia. Type 3 vWD is a complete or near-complete deficiency in vWF and universally does not respond to DDAVP. For all patients with type 3 vWD and most patients with type 2 disease, vWF concentrate is the treatment of choice. Preoperative measurement of factor levels should be obtained prior to elective surgery, and minimum target levels should be tailored to surgery type (Table 10.8).

Antiplatelet Therapies

The 2014 ACC/AHA guidelines recommend an individualized approach to weighing risks of surgical bleeding and cardiac risk among patients on chronic antiplatelet therapy.[20] Patients who are on chronic low-dose aspirin therapy but who have not previously undergone coronary stenting should continue aspirin in the perioperative setting if the bleeding risk is low. In general, perioperative use of aspirin antiplatelet monotherapy is safe in the vast majority of patients who require general and cardiovascular operations. Elective operations that require discontinuation of dual antiplatelet therapy should be avoided within 30 days after bare-metal stent implantation or within 12 months after DES implantation. Surgical delay after DES implantation may be reduced to 6 months if the risk of delay is greater than the risk of stent thrombosis. For urgent operations within 4 weeks after bare-metal stent or DES implantation, dual antiplatelet therapy should be continued unless there is significant risk for life-threatening surgical bleeding. If there is a surgical need to discontinue $P2Y_{12}$ inhibitor therapy during this time, aspirin should be continued and the $P2Y_{12}$ inhibitor should be restarted as soon as possible postoperatively. A summarization of the ACC/AHA recommendations for antiplatelet therapy in the setting of recent coronary stenting is shown in Fig. 10.5. Importantly, for patients not previously on aspirin therapy, initiation of aspirin for perioperative cardiac risk reduction is not supported by current evidence. The landmark Perioperative Ischemic Evaluation 2 (POISE-2) trial concluded that administration of aspirin in the perioperative setting has no impact on death or MI and increases the risk of major bleeding.[33]

TABLE 10.8 Recommended levels of vWF in patients with vWD selected for surgery.

Major surgery	100% vWF preoperatively and trough daily levels of 50% until wound healing (5–10 days)
Minor surgery	60% vWF level preoperatively and trough daily levels of 30% until wound healing (2–4 days)
Dental extractions	60% vWF level preoperatively (single dose)
Delivery and puerperium	80%–100% vWF level predelivery and trough levels of 30% (3–4 days)

From Mensah PK, Gooding R. Surgery in patients with inherited bleeding disorders. *Anaesthesia.* 2015;70:112–120, e139–e140. *vWD,* von Willebrand disease; *vWF,* von Willebrand factor.

Anticoagulation

Consideration of perioperative management of anticoagulants balances the risk of bleeding against that of thromboembolic complications. In addition to determining the duration of anticoagulant interruption, clinicians must decide whether a bridging agent is indicated. Patients at exceptionally high risk for thromboembolic complications (i.e., recent ischemic stroke, inadequate anticoagulation in the setting of atrial fibrillation with CHA_2DS_2-VASc >1) should not undergo elective operations until the clotting risk is optimized. Operations with low risk of bleeding—such as many cutaneous operations—can proceed without interruption of chronic anticoagulation. In the case of cardiac interventions for arrhythmia, it may be undesirable to interrupt anticoagulation even in the perioperative setting. The American College of Chest Physicians Evidence-Based Clinical Practice Guidelines (2012) represent the most widely accepted recommendations for perioperative antithrombotic management.[34]

Clinicians should consider the pharmacokinetics of anticoagulants in order to keep interruptions in chronic anticoagulation as short as possible. Warfarin, with a half-life of 36 to 42 hours, should be discontinued 5 days before elective operations, with a PT/INR check on the day of surgery. If the INR remains above 1.5, vitamin K or fresh frozen plasma can be administered preoperatively depending on the extent of coagulopathy and operative planning. Because it usually takes 4 to 5 days for warfarin to attain therapeutic levels of anticoagulation, restarting warfarin within 24 hours after surgery will result in an average of 8 to 9 days of subtherapeutic anticoagulation during the perioperative period. For this reason, bridging anticoagulation should be considered for patients at very high risk of thromboembolism.[34] These patients include those with a recent ischemic stroke, acute arterial embolism, a mechanical heart valve, or venous thromboembolism at high risk for thromboembolism. Previous guidelines recommended bridging for high-risk atrial fibrillation as well. However, results from the double-blind, placebo-controlled BRIDGE trial concluded that forgoing bridging with low-molecular–weight heparin in this setting does not increase risk for arterial thromboembolism and decreases the risk of major bleeding.[35] When used in the setting of bridging treatment, unfractionated heparin should be stopped 4 to 6 hours before surgery, while low–molecular-weight heparin should be stopped 24 hours before surgery. For operations with high bleeding risk, therapeutic-dose low-molecular–weight heparin should be resumed 48 to 72 hours postoperatively.

Oral Direct Thrombin and Factor Xa Inhibitors

Modern oral anticoagulant agents include the direct thrombin inhibitor dabigatran (Pradaxa) and direct factor Xa inhibitors rivaroxaban (Xarelto), apixaban (Eliquis), edoxaban (Savaysa), and betrixaban (Bevyxxa). These agents possess several advantages over the traditional inhibitor of vitamin K–dependent coagulation factors, warfarin. Namely, they offer more rapid onset (less than 4 hours) and shorter half-life, allowing a shorter period of interruption in the perioperative setting. Routine long-term laboratory testing for drug levels is not required. However, perioperative management of these agents requires knowledge of basic pharmacokinetics and options for reversal.[36] A summary of common oral anticoagulants is provided in Table 10.9.

Dabigatran was approved by the US Food and Drug Administration (FDA) for stroke prevention in atrial fibrillation in 2010. Its clearance is renal with a half-life of 12 to17 hours. For patients with normal renal function who are anticipating major surgery, dabigatran should be held for 48 hours prior to surgery and resumed 2 to 3 days after surgery. Dosing adjustments are necessary in the elderly and for those with renal impairment. Dabigatran can be monitored using dilute thrombin time or liquid chromatography-mass spectrometry (LC-MS/MS) drug level. In 2015, the FDA approved idarucizumab (Praxbind) as a specific reversal agent for dabigatran. Rapid reversal is achieved with a single 5-g IV dose.

Rivaroxaban, apixaban, edoxaban, and betrixaban are direct factor Xa inhibitors; they can be monitored using a chromogenic anti-Xa assay or LC-MS/MS. Clearance includes renal excretion in urine and hepatic metabolism via CYP3A4. As such, drug interactions are common

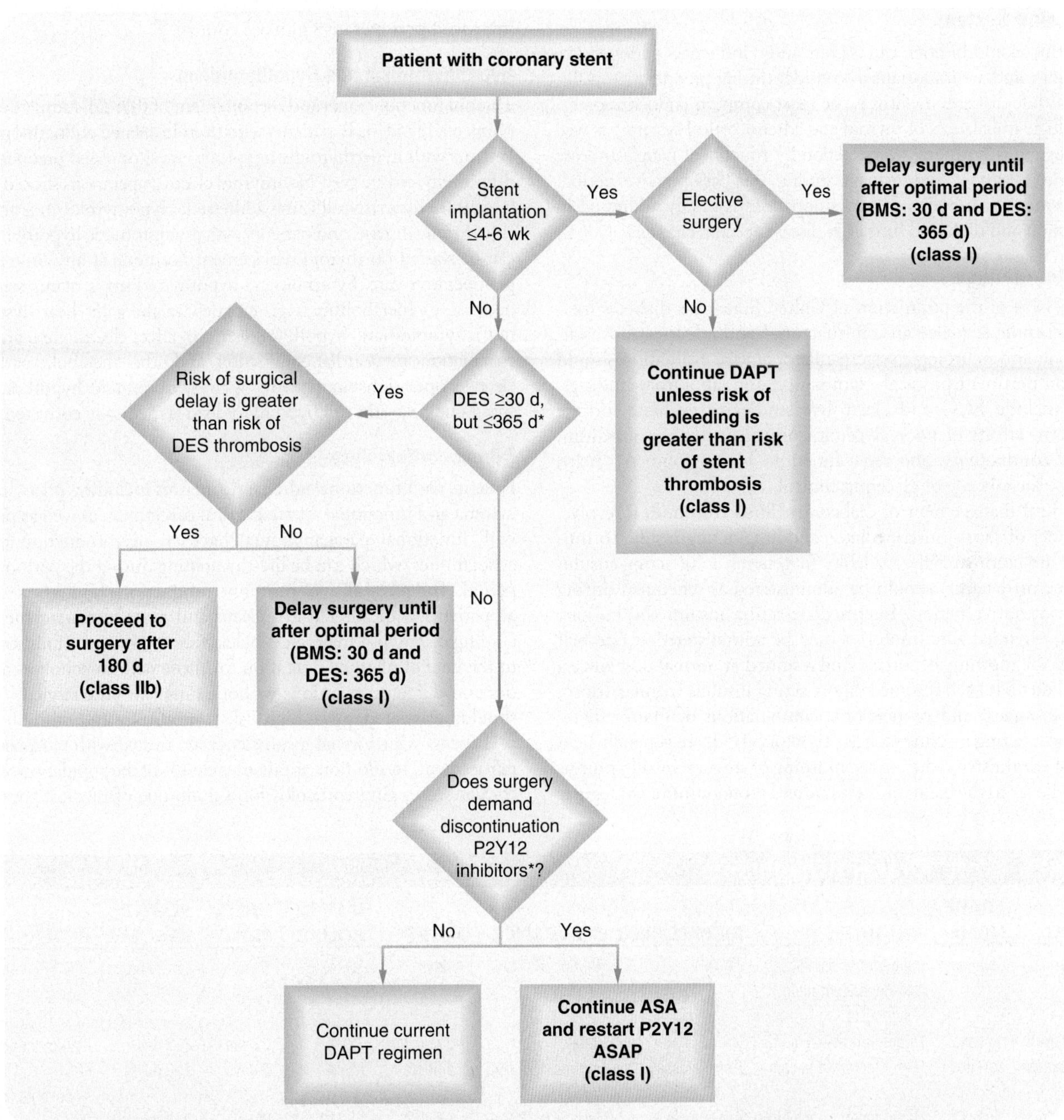

FIG. 10.5 Management of antiplatelet agents in patients with endovascular coronary stent and noncardiac surgery. *Assuming patient is currently on dual antiplatelet therapy (DAPT). *ASA*, Aspirin; *BMS*, bare-metal stent; *DES*, drug-eluting stent; *DAPT*, dual antiplatelet therapy. (Adapted from Fleisher LA, Fleischmann KE, Auerbach AD, et al: 2014 ACC/AHA guideline on perioperative cardiovascular evaluation and management of patients undergoing noncardiac surgery: a report of the American College of Cardiology/American Heart Association Task Force on practice guidelines. *J Am Coll Cardiol.* 2014;64:e77–e137.)

with cytochrome P450 inhibitors (ketoconazole, amiodarone, selective serotonin reuptake inhibitors, cimetidine, etc.) and inducers (carbamazepine, phenytoin, rifampin, etc.). In addition, factor Xa inhibitors are substrates of P-glycoprotein efflux transporters. Therefore, drugs that inhibit both CYP3A4 and P-glycoprotein—the classic example is ketoconazole—can cause profound amplification of anticoagulation effects. Oral Xa inhibitors have rapid onset (2–4 hours) and relatively short half-lives, allowing for short periods of interruption perioperatively. They should be stopped 48 hours prior to surgery and resumed 2 to 3 days postoperatively. In 2018, the FDA approved andexanet alpha (Andexxa) as a targeted reversal agent for oral factor Xa inhibitors. Administration involves an initial bolus of 400 to 800 mg followed by a continuous infusion.

Endocrine System

Endocrine comorbidities can significantly influence perioperative physiology and are important to consider during preoperative evaluation. While diabetes mellitus is the most common endocrinopathy, physiologic imbalances of thyroid and adrenocortical systems, as well as endogenous hormone oversecretion by functional neoplasms, are critical to diagnose and manage during the perioperative period. Management of functional endocrinopathies is briefly addressed in this section and discussed further in disease-specific chapters.

Diabetes Mellitus

Nearly 10% of the population of United States has diabetes mellitus. Chronic sequelae are multifactorial and affect cardiovascular, renal, and neurologic systems. Preoperative evaluation should focus on pertinent physical examination and laboratory findings. These include ECG and electrolyte studies to evaluate for the long-term effects of poor glycemic control on the myocardium, cardiac conductivity, and renal function. Hemoglobin A_{1c} helps evaluate the efficacy of glycemic control.

Medical management of diabetes mellitus continues to evolve. A number of short-, intermediate-, and long-acting insulin formulations are commercially available. In general, long-acting insulin (glargine or detemir) should be administered as scheduled during the perioperative period. Intermediate-acting insulin (NPH, zinc insulin, extended zinc insulin) should be administered at one half dose on the morning of surgery and resumed at normal dose once a normal diet has been resumed. Short-acting insulins (regular, lispro, glulisine, aspart, and proportional combinations of intermediate- with short-acting insulins such as 70/30 or 50/50) are generally held and not administered during the morning of surgery. Insulin pumps should be set to the basal infusion rate and reprogrammed to regular settings once a normal diet has been established. Inpatient endocrinology consultation is frequently helpful in the management of patients with complex insulin regimens or poor glycemic control.

Perioperative management of oral hypoglycemics also has evolved. In general, sulfonylureas (e.g., glyburide, glipizide, glimepiride, and other single-agent or combination sulfonylureas) are withheld the day of surgery. DPP-4 inhibitors (gliptins) typically are administered the morning of surgery. Administration of metformin the morning of surgery is controversial. Historical data suggested an increased risk of lactic acidosis among patients on metformin; thus, liberal withholding parameters were used. More recent data, including a Cochrane systematic review, do not corroborate this increased risk; instead, they note a number of potential benefits of continuing metformin the day of surgery including improved perioperative glucose control.[37]

Hyperthyroidism and Hypothyroidism

Thyroid function panel and measurement of thyroid-stimulating hormone readily identify patients with thyroid-related endocrinopathies. Patients with hyperthyroidism typically are suppressed preoperatively prior to thyroid surgery. Nonthyroid elective operations should be delayed until hyperthyroidism is addressed. Hypothyroidism is an indolent chronic disease, and patients with asymptomatic hypothyroidism can be started on thyroid replacement hormone at any time during perioperative care. Symptomatic hypothyroidism is manifested by a decrease in metabolism (e.g., fatigue, weight gain, heat dysregulation). Symptomatic hypothyroidism can affect electrolyte regulation, coagulation, myocardial conduction, and other metabolic pathways; elective operations in patients with symptomatic hypothyroidism should be delayed until hypothyroidism is medically corrected.

Adrenocortical System

Patients with functional adrenal neoplasms including pheochromocytoma and functional adrenocortical carcinoma, as well as patients with functional paraganglioma, have an overproduction of catecholamines, which can be life-threatening during the perioperative period. The possibility of hormone production should be tested in all patients with adrenal neoplasms and medical management, including α- and β-adrenergic blockade should be accomplished prior to the date of planned operation for those with catecholamine production. Urgent operations without sufficient adrenergic blockade should be avoided, given high risk of morbidity and mortality.

Patients with adrenal insufficiency are treated with glucocorticoid replacement. In addition, approximately 1% of the population of United States uses glucocorticoids for a multitude of medical conditions

TABLE 10.9 Oral anticoagulants.

DRUG	TRADE NAME	MECHANISM	MONITORING	CLEARANCE	ONSET	HALF-LIFE (HOURS)	PREOP HOLD	POSTOP RESUME	REVERSAL
Warfarin	Coumadin	Inhibitor of vitamin K–dependent factor synthesis	PT/INR	Hepatic (CYP1A2, CYP3A4)	>4 days	36–42	5 days	12–24 hours	PCC, FFP, vitamin K
Dabigatran	Pradaxa	Direct thrombin inhibitor	NA	Renal	1–2 hours	12–17	2 days	2–3 days	Idarucizumab
Rivaroxaban	Xarelto	Direct factor Xa inhibitor	Anti-Xa assay	Hepatic (CYP3A4) Renal	2–4 hours	5–9	2 days	2–3 days	PCC Andexanet alpha
Apixaban	Eliquis	Direct factor Xa inhibitor	Anti-Xa assay	Hepatic (CYP3A4) Renal	3–4 hours	8–12	2 days	2–3 days	PCC Andexanet alpha

Adapted from Sunkara T, Ofori E, Zarubin V, et al. Perioperative management of direct oral anticoagulants (DOACs): a systemic review. *Health Serv Insights.* 2016;9:25–36.

FFP, Fresh frozen plasma; *NA*, not applicable; *PCC*, prothrombin complex concentrate; *PT/INR*, prothrombin time/international normalized ratio.

including pulmonary, joint, inflammatory, and other diseases. Traditionally, perioperative high-dose steroid replacement has been used in patients using steroids at baseline. However, recent data suggest that additional (high-dose) steroid administration is not necessary in all patients. Patients with low-dose steroid use (prednisone 5 mg/day or dose equivalent) can continue baseline steroid dosing. Patients with higher daily doses of glucocorticoids can be tested for suppression of hypothalamic-pituitary response to steroid use with low-dose adrenocorticotropic hormone (cosyntropin) stimulation test. Lack of adrenal response to exogenous adrenocorticotropic hormone administration is diagnostic for adrenal insufficiency and administration of physiologic replacement dose of glucocorticoids is indicated. In lieu of stimulation testing for all patients using >5 mg prednisone (or dose equivalent), consensus guidelines recommend glucocorticoid replacement dependent on the extent of the planned operation (Box 10.7).

Neoplastic Endocrinopathies

A number of solid organ neoplasms secrete endogenous hormones. Functional pancreatic neoplasms can secrete excess gastrin, insulin, glucagon, vasoactive intestinal peptide, and other rare peptides. Patients with pancreatic neuroendocrine neoplasms and symptoms concerning for endocrinopathy should complete a preoperative evaluation to establish whether they have a functional tumor. Patients with primary pancreatic, bowel, or lung carcinoid can develop serotonin hypersecretion. In general, clinically significant serotonin production by a primary tumor is rare, and symptoms typically develop in patients with liver metastases.

Carcinoid liver metastases can result in significant hypersecretion of serotonin, histamine, prostaglandins, and other metabolites. Common symptoms of carcinoid syndrome are flushing and diarrhea. Urinary excretion of 5-hydroxyindoleacetic acid can be diagnostic. Patients with symptomatic clinical and/or pathologic diagnosis of carcinoid liver metastases or nonmetastatic but symptomatic (flushing/diarrhea) neuroendocrine neoplasms should be managed with somatostatin-analogue (e.g., octreotide, octreotide LAR, lanreotide) blockade prior to pursuing any operative intervention. Patients with long-standing carcinoid symptoms should be evaluated for valvular heart disease, as they can develop tricuspid regurgitation, pulmonic stenosis, and/or regurgitation. After appropriate somatostatin receptor blockade, clinically significant carcinoid heart disease should be operatively addressed before pursuing tumor-directed surgery. Appropriate perioperative octreotide administration is imperative. This typically takes the form of preoperative admission for octreotide infusion or large-dose octreotide administration prior to anesthetic induction. Intraoperative cardiovascular instability can occur, requiring ongoing high-dose octreotide administration. Intraoperative octreotide infusion is typically weaned in the postoperative period.

Endogenous hypersecretion of antidiuretic hormone causing the syndrome of inappropriate secretion of antidiuretic hormone is a rare manifestation of small cell lung cancer and other lung neoplasms. Syndrome of inappropriate secretion of antidiuretic hormone can also result from neurosurgery (in particular pituitary surgery) or trauma. Management requires maintenance of euvolemia and appropriate correction of serum sodium.

BOX 10.7 Perioperative supplemental glucocorticoid regimens.

No HPAA Suppression

<5 mg of prednisone or equivalent/day for any duration

Alternate-day single morning dose of short-acting glucocorticoid of any dose or duration

Any dose of glucocorticoid for <3 weeks

Treatment: Give usual daily glucocorticoid dose during perioperative period

HPAA Suppression Documented or Presumed

>20 mg of prednisone or equivalent/day for ≥3 weeks

Cushingoid appearance

Biochemical adrenal insufficiency on a low-dose ACTH stimulation test

Minor procedures or local anesthesia

Treatment: Give usual glucocorticoid dose before surgery

No supplementation unless signs or symptoms of adrenal insufficiency, then 25 mg hydrocortisone IV

Moderate surgical stress

Treatment: 50 mg hydrocortisone IV before induction of anesthesia, 25 mg hydrocortisone every 8 hours thereafter for 24–48 hours, then resume usual dose

Major surgical stress

Treatment: 100 mg hydrocortisone IV before induction of anesthesia, 50 mg hydrocortisone every 8 hours thereafter for 48–72 hours, then resume usual dose

HPAA Suppression Uncertain

5–20 mg of prednisone or its equivalent for ≥3 weeks

≥5 mg of prednisone or its equivalent for ≥3 weeks in the year before surgery

Minor procedures or local anesthesia

Treatment: Give usual glucocorticoid dose before surgery

No supplementation

Moderate or major surgical stress

Check low-dose ACTH stimulation test to determine HPAA suppression, *or* give supplemental glucocorticoids as though suppressed.

ACTH, Adrenocorticotropic hormone; *HPAA,* hypothalamic-pituitary-adrenal axis; *IV,* intravenously. Adapted from Schiff RL, Welsh GA. Perioperative evaluation and management of the patient with endocrine dysfunction. *Med Clin North Am.* 2003;87:175–192; and Kohl BA, Schwartz S. Surgery in the patient with endocrine dysfunction. *Med Clin North Am.* 2009;93:1031–1047.

Nutrition and Obesity

Establishing a patient's nutritional status is a vital component of surgical planning. Physiologic stress from surgery or trauma results in a transient catabolic state with rapid consumption of energy and protein. Malnutrition in the perioperative setting can have severe consequences, including impaired wound healing, increased likelihood of infection, electrolyte abnormalities, and organ dysfunction. Optimizing perioperative nutrition counterbalances the effects of systemic stress to minimize these negative effects.

Preoperative Nutrition Assessment

During preoperative evaluation, indicators of malnutrition include history of weight loss and chronic illness. A dietary history should be gathered, including nutritional supplements. On physical exam, relevant findings include BMI, temporal wasting, peripheral edema, muscle mass, skin turgor, and presence of petechiae, ecchymoses, or pressure ulcers. Among the many screening tools for malnutrition, the most used is the Nutritional Risk Screen tool (NRS-2002; Table 10.10). Multiple studies have described associations between greater nutritional risk score as measured by NRS-2002 and postoperative complications, including prolonged hospital length of stay.

Because systemic protein stores are vital for postoperative wound healing, protein status has been a particular focus of preoperative assessment. The most commonly cited serum indicators of protein status are albumin, prealbumin, and transferrin. In a large Veterans Affairs study of noncardiac operations, albumin <3.5 was a strong predictor of early postoperative morbidity and mortality. Given its long half-life (20 days), albumin is generally referenced as an indicator of chronic nutritional status. Prealbumin has a much shorter half-life of 2 days and therefore may reflect more recent nutrition. Importantly, prealbumin and albumin are both negative acute-phase proteins. During acute stress and inflammation, increased production of acute phase proteins results in decreased levels of both albumin and prealbumin, making them less reliable in the perioperative setting. Transferrin has a half-life of 8 to 9 days. In addition to being a negative acute phase protein, transferrin levels also must take into account serum iron levels.

Nutrition Supplementation

Supplementation of nutrition in the perioperative setting is available via enteral or parenteral routes. The enteral route offers several advantages and is preferred in the vast majority of situations. Parenteral nutrition requires special venous access that may be prone to infection. It also confers increased risks of hyperglycemia. Parenteral nutrition frequently lacks immune-bolstering glutamine and omega-3 fatty acids, which support the gastrointestinal tract's important immunologic functions. The intestinal mucosa acts as a physical barrier against infection and produces targeted antibodies including intraluminal immunoglobulin A. During starvation, the mucosa becomes more susceptible to bacterial translocation; enteral feeding helps maintain a healthy intestinal mucosa barrier, decreasing untoward immunologic and translocation effects.

Nutritional prehabilitation before surgery has been the subject of investigation for decades. In 1991, the Veterans Affairs Total Parenteral Nutrition (TPN) Cooperative randomized patients to preoperative TPN or no treatment prior to noncardiac surgery. The TPN group had more infectious complications overall. However, severely malnourished patients receiving TPN experienced fewer noninfectious complications than controls, suggesting that TPN prehabilitation may have a role in select patients. More recent data suggest adopting NRS-2002 as a screening tool and considering parenteral or enteral prehabilitation for patients with severe malnutrition. For patients who are only mildly malnourished, surgery should not be delayed for preoperative nutritional supplementation.

In the postoperative setting, enteral feeding should be initiated early. True contraindications to enteric feeding are few: obstruction, intestinal ischemia, bowel discontinuity, high-output fistulas, and severe malabsorption.[38] Importantly, mechanical ventilation, vasopressor support, and an open abdomen are not strict contraindications to enteral nutrition. Early enteral nutrition (within 24 hours of surgery) is a key component of most enhanced recovery after surgery (ERAS) protocols and may be associated with a reduction in postoperative complications. Awaiting objective signs of bowel function prior to enteral feeding is not necessary. Among patients undergoing upper gastrointestinal tract resection and reconstruction, early enteral feeding is associated with fewer infections and a shorter hospital length of stay. Only when there is an expectation for

TABLE 10.10 Nutritional Risk Screen (NRS-2002) tool.

	IMPAIRED NUTRITIONAL STATUS		SEVERITY OF DISEASE (~INCREASE IN REQUIREMENTS)
Absent **Score 0**	Normal nutritional status	Absent **Score 0**	Normal nutritional requirements
Mild **Score 1**	Weight loss >5% in 3 months or food intake below 50%–75% of normal requirement in preceding week	Mild **Score 1**	Hip fracture* chronic patients, in particular with acute complications: cirrhosis,* COPD.* *Chronic hemodialysis, diabetes, oncology*
Moderate **Score 2**	Weight loss <5% in 2 months or BMI 18.5–20.5 + impaired general condition or food intake 25%–60% of normal requirement in preceding week	Moderate **Score 2**	Major abdominal surgery* Stroke* *Severe pneumonia, hematologic malignancy*
Severe **Score 3**	Weight loss >5% in 1 month (>15% in 3 months) or BMI <18.5 + impaired general condition or food intake 0%–25% of normal requirement in preceding week	Severe **Score 3**	Head injury* Bone marrow transplantation* *Intensive care patients (APACHE >10).*
Score:	+	**Score:**	**= Total score**
Age	if 70 years: add 1 to total score above	**= Age-adjusted total score**	

Score ≥3: the patient is nutritionally at-risk and a nutritional care plan is initiated.
Score <3: weekly rescreening of the patient. If , for example, the patient is scheduled for a major operation, a preventive nutritional care plan is considered to avoid the associated risk status.
NRS-2002 is based on an interpretation of available randomized clinical trials. *Indicates that a trial directly supports the categorization of patients with that diagnosis. Diagnoses shown in *italics* are based on the prototypes given below.
Nutritional risk is defined by the present **nutritional status** and risk of impairment of present status due to **increased requirements** caused by stress metabolism of the clinical condition.
A **nutritional care plan** is indicated in all patients who are:
(1) severely undernourished (score = 3), (2) severely ill (score = 3), (3) moderately undernourished + mildly ill (score 2 + 1), or (4) mildly undernourished + moderately ill (score 1 + 2).
Prototypes for severity of disease. Score = 1: a patient with chronic disease admitted to hospital due to complications. The patient is weak but out of bed regularly. Protein requirement is increased but can be covered by oral diet or supplements in most cases. **Score = 2:** a patient confined to bed due to illness e.g., following major abdominal surgery). Protein requirement is substantially increased but can be covered, although artificial feeding is required in many cases. **Score = 3:** a patient in intensive care with assisted ventilation, etc. Protein requirement is increased and cannot be covered even by artificial feeding. Protein breakdown and nitrogen loss can be significantly attenuated.
From Kondrup J, Allison SP, Elia M, et al. ESPEN guidelines for nutrition screening 2002. *Clin Nutr.* 2003;22:415–421.
APACHE, Acute physiology and chronic health evaluation; *BMI*, body mass index; *COPD*, chronic obstructive pulmonary disease.

greater than 7 days of a nonfunctional gastrointestinal tract should parenteral nutrition be considered in the postoperative setting.

Obesity

Extremes of BMI (>40 or <18.5) are associated with surgical mortality and postoperative morbidity. However, mildly elevated BMI (25–30) may actually be associated with decreased morbidity and mortality, a concept commonly described as the "obesity paradox." Nevertheless, severe obesity is a consistent risk factor for pulmonary, cardiovascular, thromboembolic, and infectious complications. Obese patients experience longer operative times and greater hospital length of stay. Many of these outcomes are attributable to comorbidities associated with obesity, including cardiovascular disease, OSA, obesity hypoventilation syndrome, essential hypertension, and diabetes. Consequently, the AHA recommends a preoperative ECG and chest radiography for all patients with BMI >40 who have a risk factor for heart failure or poor exercise tolerance. The STOP-BANG questionnaire is a sensitive screening test for OSA.[26] Routine implementation of this eight-question survey in the obese population can help direct formal polysomnography testing and anticipate difficult airway problems.

PREOPERATIVE CONSIDERATIONS AND CARE PROTOCOLS

Evaluation of the patient in the preoperative setting on the day of surgery provides the surgeon a final opportunity to assess readiness for the operation. Interval changes in clinical condition since the preceding consultation visit should be queried. A reevaluation of preexisting medications, including the timing of the most recent doses, is performed. Appropriate management of baseline anticoagulant and antiplatelet agents, including timing of the last dose, is confirmed. Informed consent is verified again with the patient to ensure that there is an accurate and appropriate understanding of the procedure's objectives and risks. Orders relevant to the immediate perioperative setting are reviewed with the surgery and anesthesiology teams. Important to every operation is a review of the indications for antibiotic prophylaxis and venous thromboembolism prophylaxis. Perioperative care protocols, such as ERAS protocols and similarly designed pathways, facilitate the standardization of patient care including preoperative expectations, intraoperative management, and postoperative recovery.

Patient Recovery Pathways

A number of patient recovery pathways have been designed and implemented to standardize perioperative care. The ERAS protocols are the best studied and supported by recent literature. Initially introduced in the late 1990s and early 2000s, these pathways were initially implemented in colorectal surgery. Strengths include (1) standardization of care; (2) preoperative patient education, management of expectations, and assessing the need for prehabilitation; (3) intraoperative anesthetic strategies aimed at opioid avoidance and maintenance of intravascular euvolemia; and (4) a postoperative care pathway with standardized early mobilization, multimodality pain management and opioid minimization, avoidance of volume overload, and early resumption of diet.[39]

There has been a proliferation of ERAS-type protocols across abdominal general surgery, thoracic surgery, gynecologic surgery, orthopedics, and other surgical subspecialties. The protocols themselves are very granular, typically enumerating the specific timing of preoperative, intraoperative, and postoperative medications and patient expectations. Patient buy-in and acceptance by multidisciplinary staff including surgeon, anesthesiologist, and nursing staff are vital for success of these patient care pathways. While pathway implementation frequently demonstrates early improvements in postoperative metrics (such as infections, pain scores, length of stay, and others), demonstration of long-term sustained effects have been elusive in some studies. Standardized reporting of compliance and outcomes of such postoperative care protocols has been recommended to understand which elements and/or pathways are best supported by data.

Antibiotic Prophylaxis

Surgical site infections (SSIs) are among the most common causes of nosocomial infection and are associated with increased mortality and postoperative length of stay. SSIs are classified as superficial (involving only the skin or subcutaneous tissue), deep incisional (involving fascia or muscle), and organ space infections. Risk factors for SSIs are numerous, including age, obesity, smoking, malnourishment, diabetes, immunosuppression, radiation, and others. While many risk factors are not modifiable in the immediate perioperative setting, two of the simplest actionable measures that reduce the risk of SSIs are the appropriate selection of perioperative antibiotics and the administration of these antibiotics within 1 hour of incision.

The Centers for Disease Control and Prevention (CDC) categorizes wounds into four classes: clean, clean-contaminated, contaminated, and dirty-infected (Table 10.11). While useful from the standpoint of academic inquiry, recent research has reported limited utility of wound classification, as well as frequent misclassification of surgical incisions as a risk factor for postoperative complications.[40] Antimicrobial prophylaxis may be justified regardless of wound classification for patients at particularly high

TABLE 10.11 Wound classification.

WOUND CLASSIFICATION	DEFINITION
Clean	An uninfected operative wound in which no inflammation is encountered and the respiratory, alimentary, genital, or uninfected urinary tracts are not entered.
Clean-Contaminated	Operative wounds in which the respiratory, alimentary, genital, or urinary tracts are entered under controlled conditions and without unusual contamination. Specifically, operations involving the biliary tract, appendix, vagina, and oropharynx, provided no evidence of infection or major break in technique is encountered.
Contaminated	Open, fresh, accidental wounds. In addition, operations with major breaks in sterile technique or gross spillage from the gastrointestinal tract and incisions in which acute, nonpurulent inflammation is encountered, including necrotic tissue without evidence of purulent drainage.
Dirty-Infected	Old traumatic wounds with retained devitalized tissue and those that involve existing clinical infection or perforated viscera. Organisms causing postoperative infection were present in the operative field before the operation.

Adapted from www.cdc.gov.

risk for SSI due to underlying medical conditions. Nevertheless, unless an indwelling prosthesis is anticipated, antibiotic prophylaxis generally is not required for clean wounds.

The Clinical Practice Guidelines for Antimicrobial Prophylaxis in Surgery, a collaborative rubric developed in 2013, provides surgery-specific recommendations for antibiotic prophylaxis (Table 10.12).[41] Selection of appropriate prophylaxis is guided by a few core principles. First, an antimicrobial agent is chosen to target common surgical site pathogens. Clean procedures encounter primarily skin flora, predominantly *Staphylococcus aureus* and coagulase-negative staphylococcus. Coverage for gram-negative rods and enterococci should be added for clean-contaminated cases involving abdominal viscera, the biliary tract, and the heart. Commonly used FDA-approved agents include cefazolin, cefoxitin, cefotetan, and vancomycin. For most operations, cefazolin is an appropriate choice given its low cost, antimicrobial spectrum, and duration of activity. For patients colonized with methicillin-resistant *Staphylococcus aureus*, vancomycin may be an appropriate alternative.

The second consideration in antimicrobial prophylaxis is timing of the first dose. Historic data from the early 1990s suggested that the lowest rate of surgical wound infection was associated with antibiotic administration within 2 hours prior to incision, compared to earlier or postoperative administration. However, the more recent Trial to Reduce Antimicrobial Prophylaxis Errors, a prospective, multicenter trial comparing antimicrobial timing before a variety of operations, reported the lowest infection risk when antibiotics were administered within 30 minutes of incision or between 31 and 60 minutes before incision.[42] As such, current data support administration of the first dose of prophylactic antibiotics within 60 minutes before surgical incision. For antibiotics that require longer infusion times (vancomycin, fluoroquinolones), administration may begin within 120 minutes before incision. Redosing of antibiotics should be performed to maintain therapeutic serum levels, generally after every two half-lives or if there is blood loss greater than 1500 mL (Table 10.13).

Duration of antimicrobial administration should be limited to the minimal effective length appropriate for each procedure. Most clean and clean-contaminated operations do not require postoperative antimicrobial administration; when indicated, postoperative antimicrobials should be limited to less than 24 hours. The evidence for short-duration or single-dose prophylaxis in cardiothoracic surgery has been inconsistent, and optimal antimicrobial duration following these operations remains contentious. While the Society of Thoracic Surgeons recognizes risks for resistance and superinfection with *Clostridium difficile* with prolonged antibiotic administration, there is evidence that antibiotic duration up to 48 hours reduces the risk of a sternal wound infection. Thus, the Surgical Infection Society and the Society of Thoracic Surgeons both recommend consideration of antimicrobial prophylaxis for up to 48 hours after cardiothoracic surgery.

Review of Medications

Management of home medications on the day of surgery should be tailored to the patient and the operation. The objective is to minimize disruption of baseline homeostasis while limiting risks of surgical bleeding and drug-drug interactions with anesthetic medications. A preoperative review of medications is mandatory, with attention to cardiac, psychiatric, neurologic, and diabetic medications, as well as to anticoagulants and antiplatelet agents. In general, cardiac drugs and inhalers should be continued on the morning of surgery. In the postoperative setting, parenteral substitutes should be administered as indicated to minimize therapeutic lapse and avoid withdrawal symptoms such as rebound hypertension. Drugs that impact perioperative bleeding risk should be discontinued preoperatively based on the drug's half-life. Institutional guidelines regarding timing for withholding antiplatelets and anticoagulants prior to local analgesic procedures such as epidural placement or spinal/regional blockade should be reviewed with the patient during the preoperative clinic visit.

Herbal supplements, vitamins, oral contraceptives, and hormonal therapies are often underreported. Estrogen and tamoxifen should be held for 4 weeks preoperatively due to thromboembolic risk. Many herbal medicines can impact perioperative physiology and should be stopped days to weeks prior to surgery (Table 10.14).

Preoperative Fasting

Bronchopulmonary aspiration can be a life-threatening complication in the perioperative setting. Limiting preoperative oral intake is intended to reduce gastric volume during induction with the objective of minimizing aspiration risk. There is growing evidence, however, that the traditional protocol of fasting prior to surgery is not required for aspiration risk reduction. The ASA provided updated practice guidelines for preoperative fasting in 2017. Broadly, clear liquids—with or without carbohydrate supplementation—are permissible up to 2 hours before elective procedures requiring general anesthesia or procedural sedation. Breast milk may be ingested up to 4 hours before elective procedures. To date, evidence for a specific duration of solid food fasting is lacking. Current guidelines indicate that a light meal may be permissible for up to 6 hours before elective procedures; however, this interval may be lengthened for heavier meals and for patients at higher risk for aspiration (Table 10.15). The ASA does not recommend routine administration of gastrointestinal stimulants, antacids, antiemetics, or anticholinergics for the purpose of reducing aspiration risk or shortening the recommended preoperative fasting period.

OPERATING ROOM

Adequate preparation of the operating room—to ensure the availability and functionality of systems-based resources (e.g., video-endoscopic accessibility, anesthesia team, and blood products) and surgical equipment (e.g., instrument sets, stapler, and/or energy devices)—is as critical to a successful operation as appropriate patient selection and preoperative evaluation.

Systems-based resources include operating room particulars such as temperature control, presurgical cleaning, and availability of anesthesia, pathology, and consultative services. Appropriate preoperative communication with the anesthesia team is imperative, especially when specific perioperative challenges are anticipated. Examples include patients with high-risk cardiac disease, those with significant underlying liver and/or kidney disease, or patients scheduled for high-risk operations where appropriate intraoperative hemodynamic and volume management is imperative. Recent implementation of patient recovery pathways has standardized many aspects of anesthetic care; however, active communication between the surgery and anesthesiology teams remains important to assure the most appropriate intraoperative management. Additional system-based resources include medications and products necessary in the immediate perioperative period such as analgesics, fluids, blood products, antibiotics, anticoagulants, and vasoactive drugs. Also important is the presence of appropriate surgical assistance and back-up. Despite

TABLE 10.12 Recommendations for surgical antimicrobial prophylaxis.

TYPE OF PROCEDURE	RECOMMENDED AGENTS[a,b]	ALTERNATIVE AGENTS IN PATIENTS WITH β-LACTAM ALLERGY	STRENGTH OF EVIDENCE[c]
Cardiac coronary artery bypass	Cefazolin, cefuroxime	Clindamycin,[d] vancomycin[d]	A
Cardiac device insertion procedures (e.g., pacemaker implantation)	Cefazolin, cefuroxime	Clindamycin, vancomycin	A
Ventricular assist devices	Cefazolin, cefuroxime	Clindamycin, vancomycin	C
Thoracic noncardiac procedures, including lobectomy, pneumonectomy, lung resection, and thoracotomy	Cefazolin, ampicillin-sulbactam	Clindamycin,[d] vancomycin[d]	A
Video-assisted thoracoscopic surgery	Cefazolin, ampicillin-sulbactam	Clindamycin,[d] vancomycin[d]	C
Gastroduodenal[e] procedures involving entry into lumen of gastrointestinal tract (bariatric, pancreaticoduodenectomy[f])	Cefazolin	Clindamycin or vancomycin + aminoglycoside[g] or aztreonam or fluoroquinolone[h–j]	A
Procedures without entry into gastrointestinal tract (antireflux, highly selective vagotomy) for high-risk patients	Cefazolin	Clindamycin or vancomycin + aminoglycoside[g] or aztreonam or fluoroquinolone[h–j]	A
Biliary tract open procedure	Cefazolin, cefoxitin, cefotetan, ceftriaxone,[k] ampicillin-sulbactam[h]	Clindamycin or vancomycin + aminoglycoside[g] or aztreonam or fluoroquinolone,[h–j] metronidazole + aminoglycoside[g] or fluoroquinolone[h–j]	A
Laparoscopic procedure			
Elective, low risk[l]	None	None	A
Elective, high risk[l]	Cefazolin, cefoxitin, cefotetan, ceftriaxone,[k] ampicillin-sulbactam[h]	Clindamycin or vancomycin + aminoglycoside[g] or aztreonam or fluoroquinolone,[h–j] metronidazole + aminoglycoside[g] or fluoroquinolone[h–j]	A
Appendectomy for uncomplicated appendicitis	Cefoxitin, cefotetan, cefazolin + metronidazole	Clindamycin + aminoglycoside[g] or aztreonam or fluoroquinolone,[h–j] metronidazole + aminoglycoside[g] or fluoroquinolone[h–j]	A
Small intestine			
Nonobstructed	Cefazolin	Clindamycin + aminoglycoside[g] or aztreonam or fluoroquinolone[h–j]	C
Obstructed	Cefazolin + metronidazole, cefoxitin, cefotetan	Metronidazole + aminoglycoside[g] or fluoroquinolone[h–j]	C
Hernia repair (hernioplasty and herniorrhaphy)	Cefazolin	Clindamycin, vancomycin	A
Colorectal[m]	Cefazolin + metronidazole, cefoxitin, cefotetan, ampicillin-sulbactam,[h] ceftriaxone + metronidazole,[n] ertapenem	Clindamycin + aminoglycoside[g] or aztreonam or fluoroquinolone,[h–j] metronidazole + aminoglycoside[g] or fluoroquinolone[h–j]	A
Head and neck clean	None	None	B
Clean with placement of prosthesis (excludes tympanostomy tubes)	Cefazolin, cefuroxime	Clindamycin[d]	C
Clean-contaminated cancer surgery	Cefazolin + metronidazole, cefuroxime + metronidazole, ampicillin-sulbactam	Clindamycin[d]	A
Other clean-contaminated procedures with the exception of tonsillectomy and functional endoscopic sinus procedures	Cefazolin + metronidazole, cefuroxime + metronidazole, ampicillin-sulbactam	Clindamycin[d]	B
Neurosurgery elective craniotomy and cerebrospinal fluid–shunting procedures	Cefazolin	Clindamycin,[d] vancomycin[d]	A
Implantation of intrathecal pumps	Cefazolin	Clindamycin,[d] vancomycin[d]	C
Cesarean delivery	Cefazolin	Clindamycin + aminoglycoside[g]	A
Hysterectomy (vaginal or abdominal)	Cefazolin, cefotetan, cefoxitin, ampicillin-sulbactam[h]	Clindamycin or vancomycin + aminoglycoside[g] or aztreonam or fluoroquinolone,[h–j] metronidazole + aminoglycoside[g] or fluoroquinolone[h–j]	A
Ophthalmic	Topical neomycin-polymyxin B-gramicidin or fourth-generation topical fluoroquinolones (gatifloxacin or moxifloxacin) given as 1 drop every 5–15 minutes for 5 doses.[o] Addition of cefazolin 100 mg by subconjunctival injection or intracameral cefazolin 1–2.5 mg or cefuroxime 1 mg at the end of procedure is optional.	None	B

Continued

TABLE 10.12 Recommendations for surgical antimicrobial prophylaxis.—cont'd

TYPE OF PROCEDURE	RECOMMENDED AGENTS[a,b]	ALTERNATIVE AGENTS IN PATIENTS WITH β-LACTAM ALLERGY	STRENGTH OF EVIDENCE[c]
Orthopedic clean operations involving hand, knee, or foot and not involving implantation of foreign materials	None	None	C
Spinal procedures with and without instrumentation	Cefazolin	Clindamycin,[d] vancomycin[d]	A
Hip fracture repair	Cefazolin	Clindamycin,[d] vancomycin[d]	A
Implantation of internal fixation devices (e.g., nails, screws, plates, wires)	Cefazolin	Clindamycin,[d] vancomycin[d]	C
Total joint replacement	Cefazolin	Clindamycin,[d] vancomycin[d]	A
Urologic lower tract instrumentation with risk factors for infection (includes transrectal prostate biopsy)	Fluoroquinolone,[h-j] trimethoprim-sulfamethoxazole, cefazolin	Aminoglycoside[g] with or without clindamycin	A
Clean without entry into urinary tract	Cefazolin (addition of a single dose of an aminoglycoside may be recommended for placement of prosthetic material [e.g., penile prosthesis])	Clindamycin,[d] vancomycin[d]	A
Involving implanted prosthesis	Cefazolin ± aminoglycoside, cefazolin ± aztreonam, ampicillin-sulbactam	Clindamycin ± aminoglycoside or aztreonam, vancomycin ± aminoglycoside or aztreonam	A
Clean with entry into urinary tract	Cefazolin (addition of a single dose of an aminoglycoside may be recommended for placement of prosthetic material [e.g., penile prosthesis])	Fluoroquinolone,[h-j] aminoglycoside[g] ± clindamycin	A
Clean-contaminated	Cefazolin + metronidazole, cefoxitin	Fluoroquinolone,[h-j] aminoglycoside[g] + metronidazole or clindamycin	A
Vascular[p]	Cefazolin	Clindamycin,[d] vancomycin[d]	A
Heart, lung, heart-lung transplantation[q]; heart transplantation[r]	Cefazolin	Clindamycin,[d] vancomycin[d]	A (based on cardiac procedures)
Lung and heart-lung transplantation[r,s]	Cefazolin	Clindamycin,[d] vancomycin[d]	A (based on cardiac procedures)
Liver transplantation[q,t]	Piperacillin-tazobactam, cefotaxime + ampicillin	Clindamycin or vancomycin + aminoglycoside[g] or aztreonam or fluoroquinolone[h-j]	B
Pancreas and pancreas-kidney transplantation[r]	Cefazolin, fluconazole (for patients at high risk of fungal infection [e.g., patients with enteric drainage of the pancreas])	Clindamycin or vancomycin + aminoglycoside[g] or aztreonam or fluoroquinolone[h-j]	A
	Cefazolin	Clindamycin or vancomycin + aminoglycoside[g] or aztreonam or fluoroquinolone[h-j]	A
Plastic surgery clean with risk factors or clean-contaminated	Cefazolin, ampicillin-sulbactam	Clindamycin,[d] vancomycin[d]	C

From Bratzler DW, Dellinger EP, Olsen KM, et al. Clinical practice guidelines for antimicrobial prophylaxis in surgery. *Am J Health Syst Pharm.* 2013;70:195–283.

[a]The antimicrobial agent should be started within 60 minutes before surgical incision (120 minutes for vancomycin or fluoroquinolones). Although single-dose prophylaxis is usually sufficient, the duration of prophylaxis for all procedures should be <24 hours. If an agent with a short half-life is used (e.g., cefazolin, cefoxitin), it should be readministered if the procedure duration exceeds the recommended redosing interval (from the time of initiation of the preoperative dose). Readministration may also be warranted if prolonged or excessive bleeding occurs or if there are other factors that may shorten the half-life of the prophylactic agent (e.g., extensive burns). Readministration may not be warranted in patients in whom the half-life of the agent may be prolonged (e.g., patients with renal insufficiency or renal failure).

[b]For patients known to be colonized with methicillin-resistant *Staphylococcus aureus*, it is reasonable to add a single preoperative dose of vancomycin to the recommended agents.

[c]Strength of evidence that supports the use or nonuse of prophylaxis is classified as A (levels I–III), B (levels IV–VI), or C (level VII). Level I evidence is from large, well-conducted, randomized controlled clinical trials. Level II evidence is from small, well-conducted, randomized controlled clinical trials. Level III evidence is from well-conducted cohort studies. Level IV evidence is from well-conducted case-control studies. Level V evidence is from uncontrolled studies that were not well conducted. Level VI evidence is conflicting evidence that tends to favor the recommendation. Level VII evidence is expert opinion.

[d]For procedures in which pathogens other than staphylococci and streptococci are likely, an additional agent with activity against those pathogens could be considered. For example, if there are surveillance data showing that gram-negative organisms are a cause of surgical site infections for the procedure, practitioners may consider combining clindamycin or vancomycin with another agent (cefazolin if the patient is not allergic to β-lactam antibiotics; aztreonam, gentamicin, or single-dose fluoroquinolone if the patient is allergic to β-lactam antibiotics).

[e]Prophylaxis should be considered for patients at highest risk for postoperative gastroduodenal infections, such as patients with increased gastric pH (e.g., patients receiving histamine H_2 receptor antagonists or proton pump inhibitors), gastroduodenal perforation, decreased gastric motility, gastric outlet obstruction, gastric bleeding, morbid obesity, or cancer. Antimicrobial prophylaxis may not be needed when the lumen of the intestinal tract is not entered.

[f]Consider additional antimicrobial coverage with infected biliary tract.

TABLE 10.12 Recommendations for surgical antimicrobial prophylaxis.—cont'd

[g]Gentamicin or tobramycin.
[h]Because of increasing resistance of *Escherichia coli* to fluoroquinolones and ampicillin-sulbactam, local population susceptibility profiles should be reviewed before use.
[i]Ciprofloxacin or levofloxacin.
[j]Fluoroquinolones are associated with an increased risk of tendinitis and tendon rupture in patients of all ages. However, this risk would be expected to be quite small with single-dose antibiotic prophylaxis. Although the use of fluoroquinolones may be necessary for surgical antibiotic prophylaxis in some children, they are not first-choice drugs in pediatric patients because of an increased incidence of adverse events compared with control subjects in some clinical trials.
[k]Ceftriaxone use should be limited to patients requiring antimicrobial treatment for acute cholecystitis or acute biliary tract infections that may not be determined before incision; ceftriaxone should not be used in patients undergoing cholecystectomy for noninfected biliary conditions, including biliary colic or dyskinesia without infection.
[l]Factors that indicate a high risk of infectious complications in laparoscopic cholecystectomy include emergency procedures, diabetes, long procedure duration, intraoperative gallbladder rupture, age >70 years, conversion from laparoscopic to open cholecystectomy, American Society of Anesthesiologists classification of ≥3, episode of colic within 30 days before the procedure, reintervention in <1 month for noninfectious complication, acute cholecystitis, bile spillage, jaundice, pregnancy, nonfunctioning gallbladder, immunosuppression, and insertion of prosthetic device. Because many of these risk factors are impossible to determine before surgical intervention, it may be reasonable to give a single dose of antimicrobial prophylaxis to all patients undergoing laparoscopic cholecystectomy.
[m]For most patients, a mechanical bowel preparation combined with oral neomycin sulfate plus oral erythromycin base or with oral neomycin sulfate plus oral metronidazole should be given in addition to IV prophylaxis.
[n]In cases in which there is increasing resistance to first-generation and second-generation cephalosporins among gram-negative isolates from surgical site infections, a single dose of ceftriaxone plus metronidazole may be preferred over the routine use of carbapenems.
[o]The necessity of continuing topical antimicrobials postoperatively has not been established.
[p]Prophylaxis is not routinely indicated for brachiocephalic procedures. Although there are no data to support it, patients undergoing brachiocephalic procedures involving vascular prostheses or patch implantation (e.g., carotid endarterectomy) may benefit from prophylaxis.
[q]These guidelines reflect recommendations for perioperative antibiotic prophylaxis to prevent surgical site infections and do not provide recommendations for prevention of opportunistic infections in immunosuppressed transplantation patients (e.g., for antifungal or antiviral medications).
[r]Patients who have left ventricular assist devices as a bridge and who experience chronic infection might also benefit from coverage of the infecting microorganism.
[s]The prophylactic regimen may need to be modified to provide coverage against any potential pathogens, including gram-negative (e.g., *Pseudomonas aeruginosa*) or fungal organisms, isolated from the donor lung or the recipient before transplantation. Patients undergoing lung transplantation with negative cultures before transplantation should receive antimicrobial prophylaxis as appropriate for other types of cardiothoracic surgeries. Patients undergoing lung transplantation for cystic fibrosis should receive 7–14 days of treatment with antimicrobials selected according to culture before transplantation and susceptibility results. This treatment may include additional antibacterial or antifungal agents.
[t]The prophylactic regimen may need to be modified to provide coverage against any potential pathogens, including vancomycin-resistant enterococci, isolated from the recipient before transplantation.

diligent preoperative planning, complex operations frequently encounter unforeseen and potentially life-threatening intraoperative challenges. Immediate availability of experienced surgeon partners and consultative services should be verified before every operation.

While the specific assembly of surgical instruments will always depend on the operation at hand, common equipment should be available for any operation. Expected equipment includes appropriate lighting, a properly functioning operating table, surgical instruments, monitors to display preoperative imaging, a suction mechanism, and coagulation instrumentation. For minimally invasive operations, insufflation equipment, trocars, a camera, video monitors, laparoscopic and/or robotic instruments, and resources should be clearly communicated and verified. The patient should be positioned securely while minimizing pressure points to prevent neuromuscular injury. For obese patients and patients in lithotomy position, the risk for extremity compartment syndrome should be acknowledged and minimized, particularly for long operations. Fluid-impermeable drapes and gowns should be used to create a sterile barrier between the operative field and the ambient environment.

The importance of communication between the surgery team, anesthesiology team, and operating room nursing staff cannot be overemphasized. Clear dialogue is necessary to improve focus, eliminate or reduce confusion, and enable anticipation. A preoperative time-out process has been implemented in most institutions (Fig. 10.6); it standardizes immediate preoperative preparation of the "surgical team." Continually updating all parties in the operating room regarding key steps of the operation is vital to minimize risk to the patient and reduce delays due to equipment availability. Finally, best practice uses closed loop communication techniques to ensure communication is heard, understood, and acknowledged by all parties.

Maintenance of Normothermia

Thermoregulation is based on systemic input integrated by the central nervous system, primarily the hypothalamus and spinal cord. Under normal conditions, autonomic control regulates core temperature consistently to between 36°C and 38°C. General anesthesia lowers the cold-response threshold of the body. Volatile and IV anesthetics impair thermoregulation, paralytics prevent the body's shivering response to hypothermia, and compensatory vasoconstriction is downregulated. Neuraxial anesthesia (epidural and spinal) further blunts thermoregulatory control by reducing thermal discomfort and blocking efferent nervous control of vasoconstriction and shivering. The effects of general and neuraxial anesthesia are roughly additive; this factor is particularly relevant due to an increase in usage of neuraxial anesthesia as a component of modern ERAS pathways. An additional factor is large volume cavity exposure (abdominal or thoracic) that significantly contributes to heat loss. Risk of hypothermia

TABLE 10.13 Clinical practice guidelines for antimicrobial prophylaxis in surgery.

	RECOMMENDED DOSE			RECOMMENDED REDOSING INTERVAL (FROM INITIATION OF PREOPERATIVE DOSE)
ANTIMICROBIAL	ADULTS[a]	CHILDREN[b]	HALF-LIFE IN ADULTS WITH NORMAL RENAL FUNCTION (HOURS)[19]	(HOURS)[c]
Ampicillin-sulbactam	3 g (ampicillin 2 g/sulbactam 1 g)	50 mg/kg of ampicillin component	0.8–1.3	2
Ampicillin	2 g	50 mg/kg	1–1.9	2
Aztreonam	2 g	30 mg/kg	1.3–2.4	4
Cefazolin	2 g, 3 g for patients weighing ≥120 kg	30 mg/kg	1.2–2.2	4
Cefuroxime	1.5 g	50 mg/kg	1–2	4
Cefotaxime	1 g[d]	50 mg/kg	0.9–1.7	3
Cefoxitin	2 g	40 mg/kg	0.7–1.1	2
Cefotetan	2 g	40 mg/kg	2.8–4.6	6
Ceftriaxone	2 g[e]	50–75 mg/kg	5.4–10.9	NA
Ciprofloxacin[f]	400 mg	10 mg/kg	3–7	NA
Clindamycin	900 mg	10 mg/kg	2–4	6
Ertapenem	1 g	15 mg/kg	3–5	NA
Fluconazole	400 mg	6 mg/kg	30	NA
Gentamicin[g]	5 mg/kg based on dosing weight (single dose)	2.5 mg/kg based on dosing weight	2–3	NA
Levofloxacin[f]	500 mg	10 mg/kg	6–8	NA
Metronidazole	500 mg	15 mg/kg; neonates weighing <1200 g should receive a single 7.5-mg/kg dose	6–8	NA
Moxifloxacin[f]	400 mg	10 mg/kg	8–15	NA
Piperacillin-tazobactam	3.375 g	Infants 2–9 months: 80 mg/kg of piperacillin component Children >9 months and ≤40 kg: 100 mg/kg of piperacillin component	0.7–1.2	2
Vancomycin	15 mg/kg	15 mg/kg	4–8	NA
Oral Antibiotics for Colorectal Surgery Prophylaxis (Used in Conjunction With Mechanical Bowel Preparation)				
Erythromycin base	1 g	20 mg/kg	0.8–3	NA
Metronidazole	1 g	15 mg/kg	6–10	NA
Neomycin	1 g	15 mg/kg	2–3 (3% absorbed under normal gastrointestinal conditions)	NA

From Bratzler DW, Dellinger EP, Olsen KM, et al. Clinical practice guidelines for antimicrobial prophylaxis in surgery. *Am J Health Syst Pharm.* 2013;70:195–283.

NA, Not applicable.

[a]Adult doses are obtained from different studies.

[b]The maximum pediatric dose should not exceed the usual adult dose.

[c]For antimicrobials with a short half-life (e.g., cefazolin, cefoxitin) used before long procedures, redosing in the operating room is recommended at an interval of approximately two times the half-life of the agent in patients with normal renal function. Recommended redosing intervals marked as *NA* are based on typical case length; for unusually long procedures, redosing may be needed.

[d]Although Food and Drug Administration–approved package insert labeling indicates 1 g, experts recommend 2 g for obese patients.

[e]When used as a single dose in combination with metronidazole for colorectal procedures.

[f]Although fluoroquinolones have been associated with an increased risk of tendinitis or tendon rupture in patients of all ages, use of these agents for single-dose prophylaxis is generally safe.

[g]In general, gentamicin for surgical antibiotic prophylaxis should be limited to a single dose given preoperatively. Dosing is based on the patient's actual body weight. If the patient's actual weight is more than 20% above ideal body weight (IBW), the dosing weight (DW) can be determined as follows: DW = IBW + 0.4 (actual weight – IBW).

is increased in the elderly, in females, and in the malnourished patients during long operations.

The consequences of intraoperative hypothermia are myriad. Platelet aggregation and the coagulation cascade are impaired, resulting in an association between hypothermia and nearly a 20% increased operative blood loss. Due to vasoconstriction and the consequent decreased oxygenation of surgical incisions, hypothermia has been associated with an increased rate of wound infection. Finally, hypothermia alters drug actions/metabolism such that the duration of action of many anesthetics is prolonged and correction of acidosis and electrolyte disarray is impaired. Close monitoring of core body temperature throughout the operation is mandatory. The best and most pragmatic monitoring site is the distal esophagus for intubated patients. Sublingual, axillary,

TABLE 10.14 Perioperative concerns and recommendations for herbal medicines.

COMMON NAME OF HERB	PERIOPERATIVE CONCERNS	RELEVANT PHARMACOLOGIC EFFECT	PREOPERATIVE RECOMMENDATIONS
Echinacea	Allergic reactions; decreased effectiveness of immunosuppressants; potential for immunosuppression with long-term use	Activation of cell-mediated immunity	No data
Ephedra	Risk for myocardial ischemia and stroke from tachycardia and hypertension; ventricular arrhythmias with halothane; long-term use depletes endogenous catecholamines and may cause intraoperative hemodynamic instability; life-threatening interaction with monoamine oxidase inhibitors	Increased heart rate and blood pressure through direct and indirect sympathomimetic effects	Discontinue at least 24 hours before surgery
Garlic	Potential to increase risk for bleeding, especially when combined with other medications that inhibit platelet aggregation	Inhibition of platelet aggregation (may be irreversible); increased fibrinolysis; equivocal hypertensive activity	Discontinue at least 7 days before surgery
Ginkgo	Potential to increase risk for bleeding, especially when combined with other medications that inhibit platelet aggregation	Inhibition of platelet-activating factor	Discontinue at least 36 hours before surgery
Ginseng	Hypoglycemia; potential to increase risk for bleeding; potential to decrease anticoagulative effect of warfarin	Lowers blood glucose; inhibition of platelet aggregation (may be irreversible); increased PT/PTT in animals	Discontinue at least 7 days before surgery
Kava	Potential to increase the sedative effect of anesthetics; potential for addiction, tolerance, and withdrawal after abstinence unstudied	Sedation, anxiolysis	Discontinue at least 24 hours before surgery
St. John's wort	Induction of cytochrome P450 enzymes with effect on cyclosporine, warfarin, steroids, and protease inhibitors and possibly benzodiazepines, calcium channel blockers, and many other drugs; decreased serum digoxin levels	Inhibition of neurotransmitter uptake; monoamine oxidase inhibition is unlikely	Discontinue at least 5 days before surgery
Valerian	Potential to increase the sedative effect of anesthetics; benzodiazepine-like acute withdrawal; potential to increase anesthetic requirements with long-term use	Sedation	No data

From Ang-Lee MK, Moss J, Yuan CS. Herbal medicines and perioperative care. *JAMA*. 2001;286:208–216.
PT/PTT, Prothrombin time/partial thromboplastin time.

TABLE 10.15 Recommended minimum fasting periods between oral intake and general anesthesia for elective operations.

INGESTED MATERIAL	MINIMUM FASTING PERIOD
Clear liquids	2 hours
Breast milk	4 hours
Infant formula	6 hours
Nonhuman milk	6 hours
Light meal	6 hours
Fried foods and meat	8+ hours

Adapted from Practice guidelines for preoperative fasting and the use of pharmacologic agents to reduce the risk of pulmonary aspiration: application to healthy patients undergoing elective procedures: an updated report by the American Society of Anesthesiologists Task Force on Preoperative Fasting and the Use of Pharmacologic Agents to Reduce the Risk of Pulmonary Aspiration. *Anesthesiology*. 2017;126:376–393.

and bladder temperatures also correlate well with core body temperature. Conversely, skin, forehead, external aural canal, and rectal temperatures correlate poorly with core temperature.

Hypothermia is most drastic within the first hour after induction due to the rapid effect of anesthesia-induced vasodilatation. Therefore, it is during this period that rewarming techniques are most critical. Rewarming can take the form of passive or active methods. Passive insulation (blankets, sheets) can reduce cutaneous heat loss by roughly 30%. Increasing ambient room temperature can passively mitigate heat loss but is impractical for raising core body temperature. Active warming with forced air is frequently effective during induction and throughout the operation to compensate for rapid thermal dysregulation. Forced air is the most common approach due to its ease of use, effectiveness, and low cost. Contrary to popular belief, IV fluid warming is relatively ineffective because infused fluid temperatures cannot significantly exceed the body's core temperature. However, patients can be *cooled* by infusion of ambient-temperature fluids, thereby exacerbating anesthesia-induced hypothermia. Therefore, any intraoperative infusion of >1 L/h should be prewarmed.

Preoperative Skin Preparation

SSIs comprise more than 20% of all hospital-acquired infections and are associated with increased length of stay, mortality, and cost. Commensal skin bacteria (*Staphylococci*, *Pseudomonas*, etc.) are responsible for the majority of superficial SSIs. Preoperative antiseptic skin preparation reduces the number of transient and commensal microorganisms. The CDC guidelines recommend the following techniques for application: (1) wide area to include

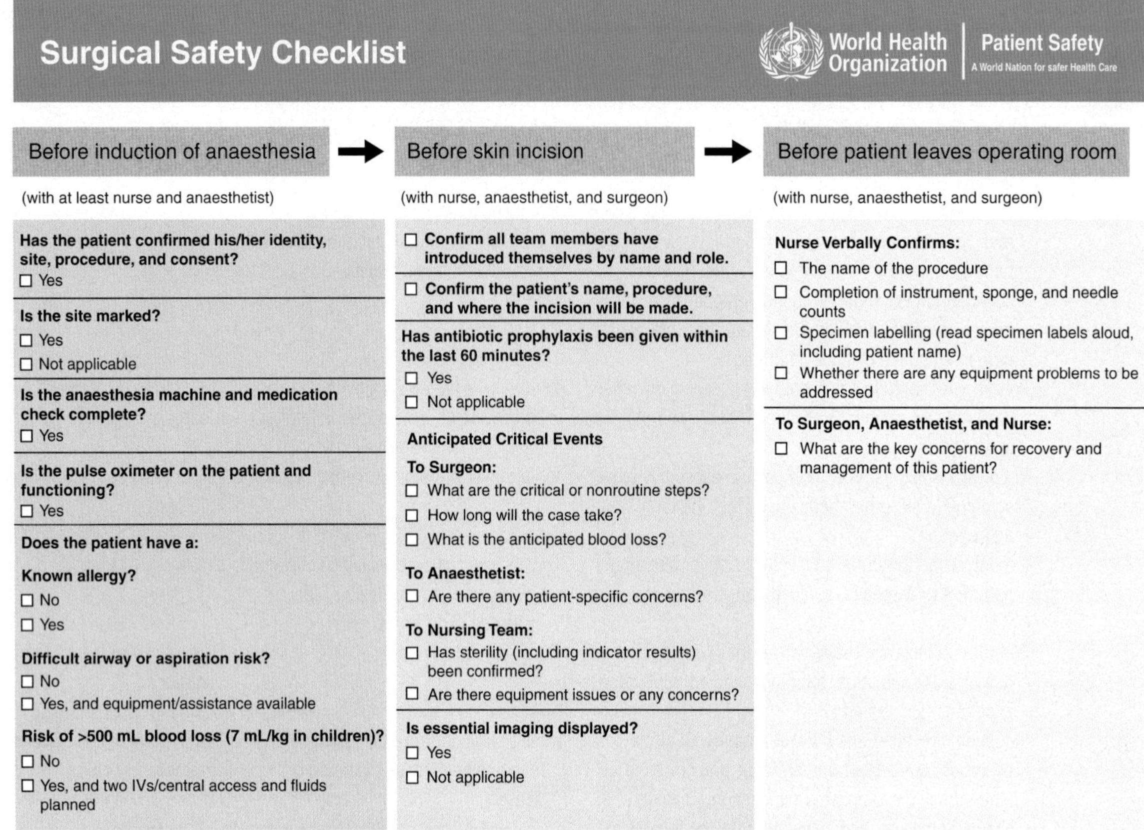
Surgical Safety Checklist

World Health Organization | Patient Safety
A World Alliance for Safer Health Care

Before induction of anaesthesia → Before skin incision → Before patient leaves operating room

Before induction of anaesthesia

(with at least nurse and anaesthetist)

Has the patient confirmed his/her identity, site, procedure, and consent?
☐ Yes

Is the site marked?
☐ Yes
☐ Not applicable

Is the anaesthesia machine and medication check complete?
☐ Yes

Is the pulse oximeter on the patient and functioning?
☐ Yes

Does the patient have a:

Known allergy?
☐ No
☐ Yes

Difficult airway or aspiration risk?
☐ No
☐ Yes, and equipment/assistance available

Risk of >500 mL blood loss (7 mL/kg in children)?
☐ No
☐ Yes, and two IVs/central access and fluids planned

Before skin incision

(with nurse, anaesthetist, and surgeon)

☐ **Confirm all team members have introduced themselves by name and role.**

☐ **Confirm the patient's name, procedure, and where the incision will be made.**

Has antibiotic prophylaxis been given within the last 60 minutes?
☐ Yes
☐ Not applicable

Anticipated Critical Events

To Surgeon:
☐ What are the critical or nonroutine steps?
☐ How long will the case take?
☐ What is the anticipated blood loss?

To Anaesthetist:
☐ Are there any patient-specific concerns?

To Nursing Team:
☐ Has sterility (including indicator results) been confirmed?
☐ Are there equipment issues or any concerns?

Is essential imaging displayed?
☐ Yes
☐ Not applicable

Before patient leaves operating room

(with nurse, anaesthetist, and surgeon)

Nurse Verbally Confirms:
☐ The name of the procedure
☐ Completion of instrument, sponge, and needle counts
☐ Specimen labelling (read specimen labels aloud, including patient name)
☐ Whether there are any equipment problems to be addressed

To Surgeon, Anaesthetist, and Nurse:
☐ What are the key concerns for recovery and management of this patient?

FIG. 10.6 Surgical safety checklist published by the World Health Organization. (From https://www.who.int/patientsafety/safesurgery/checklist/en/.) *IV*, Intravenous;

any potential incision sites, (2) concentric circle motion, (3) use of a dedicated application instrument, and (4) adequate time to allow the solution to dry. Hair removal prior to incision can improve exposure and allow skin marking. However, hair should only be removed with a clipper, as shaving is associated with increased SSI risk.

The benefits of skin preparation depend upon the antiseptic solution used. Common solutions include povidone-iodine scrub and paint (Betadine), chlorhexidine-alcohol scrub (ChloraPrep), and iodine povacrylex with isopropyl alcohol (DuraPrep). Alcohol-containing solutions should be avoided for mucosal surfaces. The optimal choice of antiseptic for intact skin remains controversial. Most randomized trials in the past comparing antiseptic solutions are underpowered. A Cochrane review in 2015 indicated that alcohol-containing products have the greatest probability of being effective but noted the overall low quality of evidence.[43] A multi-institutional randomized comparison of chlorhexidine-alcohol versus povidone-iodine scrub and paint for clean-contaminated surgeries found a lower rate of SSI in the chlorhexidine-alcohol group (9.5% versus 16.1%).[44] Recently, a single-institution randomized trial of colorectal operations failed to conclude non-inferiority of DuraPrep compared to ChloraPrep, with SSI rates of 18.7% vs. 15.9%, respectively. Therefore, based on these data, a skin preparation that contains an alcohol-based agent as part of the preparation appears optimal.

Hemostasis

Meticulous dissection and intimate knowledge of surgical anatomy are mandatory for minimization of intraoperative blood loss. Surgical bleeding obscures the operative field, prolongs operating time, increases hemodynamic stress, induces coagulopathy, and makes postoperative resuscitation more challenging. For certain cancers, perioperative blood transfusion has been consistently associated with an increased risk of recurrence and a decrease in survival.

While capillaries and small veins can be controlled and divided with monopolar electrocautery alone, vessels >1 mm in diameter—including all named vessels—are best controlled with ties, clips, staples, bipolar electrocautery, or ultrasonic devices. To prevent dislodgement of ties or clips, larger vessels may be controlled by suture ligation. Traditionally, vascular structures are ligated with permanent suture material, although use of absorbable suture has not been associated with increased risk of bleeding or reoperation. With the rapid expansion of minimally invasive operations and the associated explosion in manufactured surgical devices, numerous alternatives to the traditional hand-tied ligation have been marketed and popularized. In addition to minimally invasive (robotic or laparoscopic) surgical ties, endoloops are most similar to the hand-tie, with similar vessel burst pressures comparable to hand-ties. On the other end of the spectrum, stapling devices armed with vascular staple loads tolerate lower—but still supraphysiologic—burst pressures (Fig. 10.7).

Wound Closure

In general, incisions for clean and clean-contaminated operations can be closed primarily. Primary fascial closure can utilize permanent or dissolvable suture using running or interrupted techniques. Permanent suture is best suited for malnourished, debilitated patients and for scenarios in which early outpatient follow-up is anticipated. Dissolvable suture, particularly when

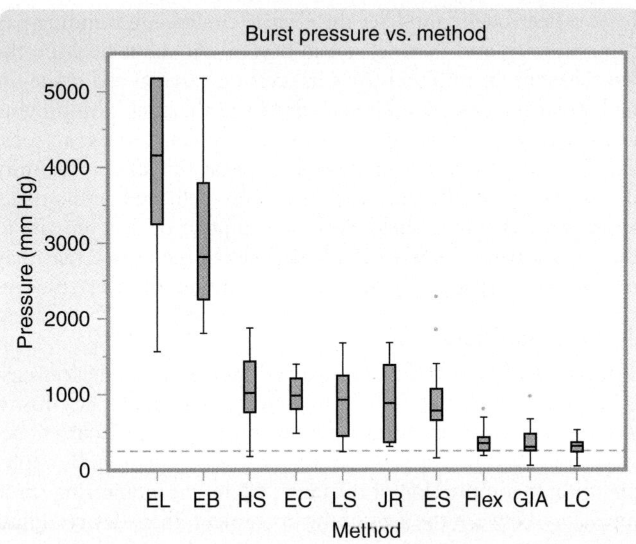

FIG. 10.7 Burst pressure of porcine carotid artery by sealing method. *EB*, ethibond hand-tie; *EC*, endoclip; *EL*, endoloop; *ES*, enseal; *Flex*, endopath stapler; *GIA*, endo GIA stapler; *HS*, harmonic scalpel; *JR*, JustRight; *LC*, proximate linear cutter; *LS*, ligaSure. (Adapted from Tharakan SJ, Hiller D, Shapiro RM, et al. Vessel sealing comparison: OLD school is still hip. *Surg Endosc.* 2016;30:4653–4658.)

used in the subcuticular layer, can often create a cosmetically appealing closure that does not require suture removal. When an incision is anticipated to be under significant tension, vertical mattress sutures distribute tension over two levels of depth at every longitudinal point and approximate the dermal layers effectively. Running suture techniques—especially when used across multiple layers—are more effective at controlling ascites, while interrupted suture allows intermittent wound packing for incisions at high risk for superficial SSI.

Delayed primary closure may be suitable for carefully-selected patients following contaminated operations. Delayed closure is commonly attempted between 2 and 5 days following the index operation. While there is some evidence that delayed primary closure is associated with a reduction in SSI compared to primary closure, there is substantial heterogeneity across existing trials. Heavily contaminated dirty surgical wounds should be left open, allowing for healing by secondary intent with serial packing. Management of open wounds, in particular during the outpatient recovery period, can often be facilitated by applying a negative pressure vacuum device.

Temporary closure of abdominal incisions is useful when a short-interval second-look laparotomy is anticipated, when there is threat of compartment syndrome, and when monitoring of intraabdominal contents is prudent. In almost all cases, temporary closure involves a nonadherent material used as a bridge across an open fascial incision. Traditionally, this was commonly achieved using fenestrated plastic in the form of an IV bag, surgical towel, or cassette covering, covered by foam or surgical towels. An airtight seal is achieved by placing a vacuum drain over the device and covering the bridge with Ioban. The vacuum mechanism reduces intraabdominal fluid accumulation. It also provides a means of monitoring for bleeding, visceral compromise, or infection and has a retention effect that counteracts natural abdominal wall retraction. However, care should be taken to monitor fluid and electrolyte balance in these patients, as massive fluid shifts can occur rapidly. More recently, dedicated vacuum-assisted closure devices such as the V.A.C. Abdominal Dressing System and the ABThera System have gained popularity due to ease of application. Delayed primary fascial closure should be achieved when possible within 7 to 10 days.[45] If this is not possible, serial closure should be initiated using devices such as a Wittman patch, which may be serially tightened every 24 to 48 hours. Once the fascia is less than a few centimeters apart, definitive fascial closure can be attempted. The downside to this technique is that application of a Wittman patch requires suturing the patch to native fascia, which can compromise fascial integrity. For malnourished patients and those who cannot tolerate the abdominal pressure associated with serial closure, an absorbable mesh bridge can allow visceral coverage during the acute phase of illness. However, loss of domain and a large complex hernia will result. More recently, bioprosthetic dermal matrices have gained favor as an alternative material for fascial bridging. Derived from cadaveric dermis (porcine, human, or bovine), acellular dermal matrix is devoid of all cellular components while retaining the extracellular matrix and basement membrane. This structure promotes fibroblast incorporation and collagen deposition and remodeling. Early revascularization results in greater resistance to infection than permanent mesh, while collagen deposition and retained extracellular matrix lend acellular dermal matrix a more durable tensile strength and flexibility than absorbable mesh. However, there is a paucity of large published series capturing experience with acellular dermal matrix, and recurrent hernia and abdominal laxity may develop with longer follow-up.

Use of barrier agents for adhesion prevention has gained popularity over recent years, particularly for patients for whom multiple operations are anticipated. Agents include oxidized regenerated cellulose, polytetrafluoroethylene, and hyaluronic acid-carboxymethylcellulose. These materials are applied to the raw surfaces of abdominal viscera and degenerate into gelatin shortly after surgery. A metaanalysis within the gynecologic literature noted low-quality evidence of efficacy for all three materials over no treatment; however, the relative efficacy between agents remains unclear.[46]

Surgical Adhesives

Tissue adhesives for skin closure were first introduced in the early 1960s. Over the last 25 years, improved tensile strength was brought about by plastic and stabilizer composites. The most common adhesives are Dermabond (octylcyanoacrylate) and Histoacryl (butylcyanoacrylate). Inherent benefits of tissue adhesives include water impermeability, low infection rate, and improved cosmesis. Adhesives can be used without skin sutures for small incisions and is commonly adopted in this manner in the emergency room setting. For larger incisions, tissue adhesives are more commonly used to provide a watertight barrier following subcuticular or dermal closure with absorbable suture. A recent meta-analysis found no significant difference between tissue adhesives and sutures in terms of dehiscence, infection, and surgeon-rated cosmesis.

Fibrin sealant confers both adhesive and hemostatic functions. Blood bank–derived fibrin sealant functions by combining thrombin and fibrinogen to replicate the final step in the clotting cascade. Because the agent contains all necessary components for this reaction, it forms a clot regardless of a patient's intrinsic pathway status. Some data have suggested that the addition of fibrin sealant can serve as a hemostatic adjunct to manual compression in controlling anastomotic hemorrhage following insertion of polytetrafluoroethylene vascular grafts. Although fibrin sealant also has been approved as an adjunct for gastrointestinal anastomoses, application for this purpose has not gained widespread popularity. Fibrin agents have been adopted for a variety of other clinical applications. For perianal fistulae, fibrin glue avoids an adverse impact on continence; however, it exhibits inferior durability compared to conventional surgical treatment. Fibrin glue has been used to treat bronchopleural fistulae, either as a direct injection of fibrinogen followed by topical thrombin or as a diluted pleurodesis agent. As is true for many manufactured and marketed products, primary study data need to be reviewed critically to estimate potential benefit and to balance this benefit against potential harm, noninferiority of alternatives, and associated cost.

SURGICAL DEVICES, ENERGY SOURCES, AND STAPLERS

Technologic advances in energy devices and tissue stapling have revolutionized the way surgeons approach dissection, division, hemostasis, and reconstruction. Energy devices as a whole direct focused energy to the target tissue with the purpose of dissection and division, coagulation, or ablation and cytotoxicity. Stapling devices are traditionally used for alimentary tract division and anastomosis but can also be used for vascular and tissue transection. This section focuses on some of the common energy and stapling devices encountered in the operating room.

Electrosurgery and Electrocautery

While use of electricity to induce thermal cauterization and tissue division has been reported since the mid-1800s, modern electrosurgery as we know it was introduced between 1914 and 1927 by William T Bovie. Diathermy, first described by Karl Franz in 1909, uses high-frequency electric currents to generate heat and penetrate tissues. Bovie developed a commercially available alternating current cautery device between 1914 and 1927, and Harvey Cushing popularized it with a 1928 report of 500 neurosurgical procedures.

Monopolar Electrosurgery

In strict terms, electrocautery implies thermal conduction via a probe heated by a direct electrical current. In modern surgery, this technology most commonly is seen with portable, pen-type cautery devices that function like a soldering iron. Electrosurgery, on the other hand, indicates conduction of an alternating radiofrequency current through a circuit that is completed by the patient's tissue. However, these two terms are often used interchangeably. Classically, monopolar electrosurgery is performed using a current generator, a handheld electrode that delivers current to the patient, and a second large electrode (the "pad") that returns current to complete the circuit. The application electrode has a small area of contact, resulting in focused thermal conversion, while the returning electrode has a large surface area to dissipate energy. With a continuous waveform ("cut" mode), the monopolar device cuts through tissue with little thermal spread and minimal coagulation. With an intermittent waveform ("coagulation" mode), current is delivered over less than 10% of the time that the device is activated and is interspersed with short periods of inactivity. The result is lower thermal energy and greater thermal spread, resulting in tissue dehydration and vessel thrombosis. Many surgeons adopt a blended waveform setting ("blend" mode), which replaces the pure cutting function with small periods of current inactivity to achieve a partial coagulative effect.

Bipolar Electrosurgery

Bipolar devices place the delivering and returning electrodes in close proximity in a single device. In this way, the tissue in between the two electrodes completes the electric circuit. A grounding pad is unnecessary, and thermal spread beyond the tissue between the two electrodes is minimal. By compressing vascularized tissue using bipolar forceps, blood is excluded from the circuit, improving heat delivery to the compressed tissue. Bipolar devices are most useful when precise coagulation is necessary in close proximity to vital structures. Because current is only delivered across tissue between the two hand-held electrodes, bipolar devices are safe to use when a patient has an implanted electronic device that may otherwise be impacted by the delivery of monopolar current.

LigaSure and Enseal

Adaptations of bipolar electrosurgery are bipolar fusion devices such as LigaSure and Enseal. Similar to conventional bipolar electrosurgery, these tissue dissection and division devices transmit current between two adjacent electrodes, causing tissue coagulation. By applying uniform compression of the target tissue and monitoring tissue impedance between the jaws of the instrument, these devices adjust energy delivery during the activation process to minimize thermal spread and seal larger vessels (up to 7 mm). Denaturation followed by cross-linking of collagen and elastin results in a natural tissue sealant. A blade within the instrument then divides the sealed tissue.

Saline-Cooled Radiofrequency Dissectors

A commonly encountered problem when using radiofrequency electrosurgery within highly vascularized parenchyma is the formation of dense eschar that limits coagulation and may result in delayed hemorrhage. Eschar formation occurs when temperature at the contact surface of the target tissue exceeds what is necessary for protein denaturation and vessel sealing. Saline-cooled radiofrequency dissectors (i.e., TissueLink, Aquamantys) overcome this issue by directing a steady irrigation stream of saline to the tissue contact point, thereby maintaining surface temperature <105°C. These devices are used most commonly during dissection of solid-organ parenchyma such as the liver or kidney. Initial division of the organ capsule is necessary (often by traditional Bovie electrosurgery) in order to prevent steam build-up beneath the capsule. Constant pressure with the saline-linked device is then used to achieve a constant depth of coagulation before sharp transection of the denatured tissue or clipping of larger vessels within the treatment zone.

Ultrasonic Dissectors

A distinction should be made between the use of high-frequency oscillation instruments and true ultrasonic energy technology. The classic example of therapeutic ultrasound is extracorporeal shock wave lithotripsy, through which high-energy acoustic shock waves are directed at pathologic stones to shatter material and facilitate passage. While lithotripsy has historically been applied to symptomatic cholelithiasis, current applications are primarily focused on urologic stones and pancreatic duct stones. Shock wave lithotripsy is effective primarily for smaller stones (<2 cm) with lower radiographic density.

Harmonic Scalpel

The harmonic scalpel transduces high-frequency ultrasonic energy through a metallic jaw to generate mechanical vibration. When in contact with tissue, the vibration of a single blade against a static blade results in vaporization and coagulation. The coagulation effect is increased by compressing the target tissue between the two jaws of the instrument. The energy transduced through the metallic jaw is modifiable; high-energy settings result in rapid cutting, while low-energy settings promote coagulation. Since the mechanism for the scalpel is vibration, the instrument divides tissue without the need for a separate cutting blade.

Cavitron Ultrasound Surgical Aspirator

The cavitron ultrasound surgical aspirator uses ultrasonic frequency vibration to selectively dissect parenchymal tissue. The device directs ultrasonic frequency along a hollow titanium tip that vibrates longitudinally to fragment target tissue. Hepatocytes are particularly susceptible to oscillatory fragmentation due to their high water content, while endothelium and epithelium (blood vessels, bile ducts) are selectively spared due to low water content. The cavitron ultrasound surgical aspirator provides a precise dissection plane through this fragmentation process but does not itself confer any vessel-sealing capability. The cavitron ultrasound surgical aspirator tip can be connected to monopolar electrocautery circuit for tissue ablation and is generally used in conjunction with adjunct methods of hemostasis.

Ablation Technology

Radiofrequency Ablation

Radiofrequency energy delivered via a narrow probe is termed *radiofrequency ablation (RFA).* Applications include esophageal dysplasia, atrial fibrillation, and tumors found within solid organ parenchyma. The RFA probe can be directed toward target tissue via a percutaneous approach or during open or laparoscopic surgery. The electrode at the probe tip transmits high-frequency alternating current to the surrounding tissue, which is converted to kinetic and thermal energy and results in denaturation and coagulation. Because RFA has a similar mechanism as electrosurgery, a grounding pad is necessary, and the presence of implantable electronic devices or metallic surgical clips may be a contraindication. Tissue eschar formation surrounding the electrode has an insulator effect and limits the effective radius of RFA. When performed near a blood vessel, thermal energy is dispersed rapidly from the target tissue, creating a "heat sink" and limiting efficacy. Typically, tumors up to 3 cm can be effectively ablated by RFA; an additional margin of 0.5 cm of healthy parenchyma beyond the target lesion should be ablated to ensure complete ablation of the tumor.

Microwave Ablation

Microwave energy lies between infrared and radio waves in frequency. The impact between microwave energy radiation and polar molecules such as water result in oscillation and frictional heat. Applied to target tissue, the outcome is cell death through coagulative necrosis. Similar to RFA, microwave ablation can be performed percutaneously or during open or minimally invasive surgery and is generally image guided via ultrasound or CT. Advantages over RFA include a larger, more homogeneous zone of ablation, an attenuated heat-sink effect, and less time needed to complete ablation. Because the mechanism of microwave ablation does not involve transmission of electric current, a grounding pad is unnecessary and use in the presence of metallic clips and implants is safe. Given advantages over RFA without proven disadvantages, microwave ablation is rising in popularity as the preferred technology for tumor ablation in solid organs including the liver and kidney.

Other Energy Devices

Argon Beam Coagulator

Argon beam coagulation (ABC) was introduced in 1989. Despite its name, ABC is not a laser device but rather an adaptation of monopolar electrosurgery. A focused beam of argon gas—a strong conductor of electricity—is directed at target tissue. Radiofrequency current is transported from a monopolar electrode to the tissue across this pathway of argon gas. Advantages of ABC over conventional electrosurgery include more rapid activity, shallower penetration, and faster heat dispersion.[47] Moreover, the focused jet of argon gas physically disperses blood from the target tissue, providing a dry environment to promote coagulation and reduce eschar formation. For these reasons, ABC is most suitable for achieving hemostasis over surfaces of solid organ parenchyma, such as the spleen, liver, kidney, lung, and peritoneum. Due to its low depth of penetration, ABC is ineffective for control of larger blood vessels. Moreover, the focused jet of argon gas is insoluble in blood, and direct targeting of central veins can result in cardiac arrest due to air (argon) embolism. To minimize this risk, surgeons should keep the flow rate of argon gas low, use an angled approach toward the tissue, and avoid direct argon gas deployment into large veins in direct communication with right atrium.

Surgical Staplers

The surgical stapling device was invented in 1907 to 1908 in Budapest, Austria-Hungary. After initial modifications to decrease weight and complexity in the 1920s, surgical staplers were further modified and popularized for use in alimentary tract surgery in the Soviet Union between the 1940s and 1950s. In 1958, a Soviet model of the surgical stapler was brought to the United States. These initial staplers were hand-made with noninterchangeable parts and required loading of individual staples by hand. Development and commercialization of surgical staplers occurred in the United States in the 1960s and 1970s. Designs were optimized for mass production, including interchangeable and disposable stapler cartridges of various staple heights.

At present, a multitude of different surgical staplers can facilitate tissue closure, division, and reconstruction during open, laparoscopic, and robotic operations. Linear cutting staplers (gastrointestinal anastomosis) vary in length and staple height to accommodate closure, transection, and reconstruction of variable thickness tissues. Similarly, linear noncutting staplers (thoracoabdominal) allow tissue closure without division. Circular cutting staplers (end-to-end anastomosis) allow luminal anastomosis and transection of hollow viscera of variable diameters. In terms of staple height, smaller staples (open 2 mm; closed 1 mm) are best suited for vascular closure and/or transection, and large staples (open 4.5 mm; closed 2 mm) are well suited for closure and/or transection of thicker tissues such as the stomach or pancreas. A number of in-between staple heights are commercially available for use in intermediate tissue types.

POTENTIAL CAUSES OF INTRAOPERATIVE INSTABILITY

With appropriate patient selection and perioperative preparation, untoward events in the operating room should be rare. Management of rare events, however, requires preparation and anticipation. This section addresses common and potentially deadly causes of intraoperative instability including etiology and management strategies.

Malignant Hyperthermia

Malignant hyperthermia (MH) is an acute episode of hypermetabolism as a response to volatile halogenated anesthetic gases (e.g., sevoflurane, isoflurane, and others) and the depolarizing paralytic succinylcholine. Symptoms of MH can occur at any time during general anesthesia or up to 60 minutes after cessation of anesthesia. Intraoperative and/or postoperative manifestations can include fever/hyperthermia, tachycardia, tachypnea, increase in exhaled carbon dioxide *(CO2)*, rhabdomyolysis, and metabolic disarray including hyperkalemia and acidosis. An increase in end-tidal CO_2 despite an increase in minute ventilation is one of the earliest intraoperative harbingers of MH. The prevalence of MH has been reported to range from 1 in 10,000 to 1 in 250,000 anesthetic cases. However, prevalence among susceptible individuals with "at risk" genetic abnormalities is considerably higher. A number of genetic mutations that predispose patients to MH have been described (most commonly a mutation in the RYR1 gene); the majority of these mutations are autosomal dominant with incomplete penetrance.

When suspected, MH is treated by immediate discontinuation of volatile gases, IV administration of dantrolene in doses of 2.5 mg/kg, and body cooling using any available routes. Dantrolene can be redosed every 10 to 15 minutes for ongoing fever, acidosis, and muscle rigidity. Other supportive measures include therapy for arrhythmias, hyperkalemia, and acidosis. Typically, management and observation in the ICU is warranted. With current advances, mortality with MH has decreased from 60% to 80% a few decades ago to less than 5%.

Gas Embolus: Air and Carbon Dioxide

Air embolus is a potentially fatal complication of vascular operations. Similarly, CO_2 embolus can be a fatal complication of minimally invasive laparoscopic or robotic operations. Both are a result of air or CO_2 entering the systemic, most often venous, circulation. In cases of air embolus, air access to the venous system can occur via a planned venotomy during vascular access cases or during repair of great vessels. In contrast, CO_2 embolus occurs more commonly as an unplanned insufflation of gas into the systemic venous circulation. In both cases, an abrupt decrease in end-tidal CO_2 and cardiovascular collapse are the first manifestations, and rapid recognition of symptoms and institution of resuscitative measures are indicated.

In cases of intraoperative cardiovascular collapse due to air or CO_2 embolus, maneuvers allowing access between gas and the vascular system must be terminated. Additionally, cardiopulmonary resuscitation including pharmacologic agents and mechanical cardiopulmonary resuscitation have the best chance to achieve return of spontaneous circulation. Intraoperative transesophageal echocardiography can help confirm the diagnosis and measure the amount of gas trapped within the right heart. If there is appropriate vascular access in the right heart, air aspiration can be attempted. While the Trendelenburg position may be helpful, placing the patient in left lateral decubitus position should only be used in the absence of cardiovascular collapse as meaningful chest compressions cannot be performed in patients who are not supine. Patients with a patent foramen ovale are at risk for collapse of left ventricular function as well as gas-mediated cerebral embolus. Mortality in patients with gas embolus is approximately 20%.

Myocardial Infarction, Pulmonary Embolus, and Pneumothorax

With appropriate preoperative evaluation, both intraoperative MI and intraoperative PE are rare complications among patients selected for elective general surgery operations. Incidences of both are higher in urgent/emergent operations and operations for traumatic injury. Intraoperative monitoring can demonstrate signs of hemodynamic instability (such as tachycardia and hypotension). ECG changes and dysrhythmias are frequently harbingers of cardiac ischemia and/or infarction. Classic ECG changes (e.g., new profound ST elevation) are diagnostic; serum troponin levels can be used to corroborate the diagnosis in hemodynamically stable patients. In the event of a suspected MI and hemodynamic instability, nonemergent operations should be aborted.

PE is rarely suspected when hemodynamic instability is absent. In most cases, for the diagnosis to be considered, intraoperative symptoms include significant tachycardia, hypotension, hypoxia despite high oxygen fraction, and/or cardiovascular collapse. Transesophageal echocardiography can be rapidly used to evaluate for presence of right ventricular dilatation/failure and "right heart strain." In the absence of right heart strain, a clinically significant PE is less likely; with clinically significant right heart strain, right heart failure resulting from MI, PE, and pneumothorax should be under consideration. Treatment of intraoperative PE (systemic anticoagulation vs. directed pharmacologic or mechanical thrombolysis) depends on the clinical symptoms; however, in the presence of hemodynamic instability, elective operations should be terminated.

The etiology of an intraoperative pneumothorax is multifactorial. Interventions leading to pneumothorax include central venous access resulting in iatrogenic lung injury, high ventilator volume/pressure particularly in patients with main-stem bronchial intubation, diaphragmatic injury, and high insufflation pressures during laparoscopy. For patients with large amounts of intrapleural air, hemodynamic instability may be present when sufficient tension is present that increases mediastinal pressures that impede central venous return. The diagnosis can be made by chest auscultation and/or intraabdominal inspection of the diaphragm. In patients without breath sounds and/or a bulging diaphragm, tube thoracostomy is indicated and should lead to symptomatic improvement. If symptoms have resolved and clinical signs of pneumothorax have been reversed, a surgeon may consider completing the ongoing elective operation.

Hemorrhage

When major vascular injuries occur, rapid blood loss into the operative field can be life-threatening and difficult to control. Exposure is immediately compromised, and the next surgical steps should focus on vascular control. If arterial injury is suspected, direct compression and proximal control are frequently the best first steps. Control frequently can be achieved by compression, proximal vascular isolation and clamping, or a combination of these maneuvers with subsequent vascular repair.

When compression is not possible and/or the major artery cannot be readily dissected, proximal control with supraceliac aortic compression can be achieved quickly by caudal retraction of the stomach, division of the gastrohepatic ligament, and compression of the aorta (located just to the left of the esophagus) against the vertebrae. Hands-free control can then be applied by incising the peritoneum, separating the limbs of the right diaphragmatic crus to expose the thoracic aorta and applying an aortic clamp. These measures facilitate exposure of the vascular injury under a controlled environment and allow anesthesiology colleagues to catch up with resuscitation.

In patients with major venous injury, compression of the venotomy combined with direct suture repair is frequently possible. In cases where significant bleeding precludes sufficient visualization of the venotomy, venous compression proximal and distal to the site of injury will help with visualization. Adequate intraoperative exposure and retraction are paramount in any operation. The best preparation for management of vascular injury is sufficient dissection and exposure to allow for management of a vascular injury prior to hemorrhage and exsanguination.

Under some circumstances, particularly in trauma surgery, multiple sites of bleeding, coagulopathy (from hypothermia, prolonged bleeding, sepsis, acidosis), and hemodynamic instability can create a scenario in which definitive control of all sites of bleeding may be impossible or impractical. Goal-directed resuscitation with blood and blood products have been well established in trauma resuscitation[48] and should be used in nontrauma patients with intraoperative hemorrhage. These patients with intraoperative hemorrhage, clinical instability, and coagulopathy are best served with goal-directed blood product resuscitation and temporary abdominal packing, followed by ongoing resuscitation in an intensive care setting. Delayed definitive hemostasis can then be achieved under more controlled conditions either with a return to the operating room or through angiographic embolization.

OUTPATIENT SURGERY

Over recent decades, the volume of operations performed in the outpatient setting has increased dramatically. Driving forces behind this change include improvements in risk assessment and perioperative management, cost differences between outpatient/ambulatory- and inpatient/hospital-based care, patient satisfaction, and increased utilization of ambulatory surgery centers. Ambulatory surgery centers have expanded access to outpatient surgery for patients with suitable operative criteria without associated increases in postoperative mortality or unanticipated admission. Nevertheless, surgeons should determine indications for surgery independent of the operative setting and resist physician-induced demand.[49] Implemented appropriately, outpatient surgery can reduce time away from work and improve patient perception of the postoperative recovery process. However, surgeons and consulting services must exercise caution when selecting patients and cases for the outpatient setting.

The process of preoperative assessment for outpatient surgery should be tailored to the patient and type of operation. In general, only low-risk and some intermediate-risk operations are appropriate in the outpatient setting. Examples include elective plastic operations in patients who will not require postoperative hospitalization, inguinal herniorrhaphy, elective cholecystectomy, superficial excisions, and a number of head-and-neck and orthopedic operations. Patient risk factors should be assessed preoperatively. For patients with ASA status 1 to 2 undergoing low-risk operations, assessments may take place on the day before surgery or even the morning of surgery. Higher-risk patients should undergo assessment in a dedicated preoperative anesthesia clinic, and sufficient time between assessment and day of surgery should be allocated to allow for additional testing, if necessary.

The goals of preoperative evaluation for outpatient surgery are (1) assessment of appropriateness for the outpatient setting, (2) utilization of direct preoperative testing and risk-stratification, and (3) reduction in cancellations on the day of surgery. Preoperative assessment can be performed by a physician, extended provider (nurse practitioner/physician assistant), nurse, or via standardized questionnaires. While physician assessments are reliable and comprehensive, they are also the costliest. Conversely, questionnaire assessments are inexpensive but rely on the patient's own perception of health. When nurse- or questionnaire-based assessments are used, reassessment on the day of surgery by either a surgeon or anesthesiologist is advisable. Risk factors associated with unplanned admission or early postoperative mortality in patients selected for an outpatient operation include advanced age, prior recent hospitalization, and invasiveness of the operation.[50]

Certain populations require additional considerations when assessing appropriateness for outpatient surgery. In general, patients with significant cardiopulmonary comorbidity in whom system-specific or other comorbid condition(s) has not been optimized are not suitable for outpatient surgery. Obese and morbidly obese patients are at increased risk for bronchospasm, hypoventilation, and obstructive airway but are not strictly prohibited from outpatient operations; however, super-morbid obesity with BMI >60 can be considered an absolute exclusion. Organ system–specific exclusion criteria may include cardiac—unstable angina, at-risk-myocardium, cardiomyopathy, moderate to severe heart failure, severe pulmonary hypertension, or valvular disease; pulmonary—noncompliant OSA, STOP-BANG ≥5 with anticipation for postoperative opioids, severe and poorly controlled asthma, cystic fibrosis, or home oxygen use; hematologic—coagulation disorders requiring postoperative infusion of clotting factors and/or procoagulants; renal—end-stage renal disease and additional organ system dysfunction, too long or too short of an interval between dialysis and operation, or uncertain serum potassium or serum potassium >5.5; pregnancy-specific exclusions—complicated pregnancy, fetus >21 weeks, gestation; and other high-risk patient comorbidities—muscular dystrophy, highly contagious airborne infections (e.g., tuberculosis), high-risk for hemorrhage, and others. Patients with chronic reflux, difficult airway, or poorly controlled diabetes are at heightened risk of anesthesia-related complications and should be considered for outpatient surgery only at centers with capabilities for postoperative admission.

Patients considered for outpatient surgery should have adequate supportive resources following discharge. Following sedation, a patient should not be responsible for transportation home and should have an adult to take them home and be available overnight to provide help if needed. Ideally, emergency care facilities should be readily accessible near the patient's residence should unforeseen complications arise. Absence of these outpatient resources should prompt consideration of elective postoperative hospitalization for observation.

SELECTED REFERENCES

Bilimoria KY, Liu Y, Paruch JL, et al. Development and evaluation of the universal ACS NSQIP surgical risk calculator: a decision aid and informed consent tool for patients and surgeons. *J Am Coll Surg.* 2013;217:833–842; e831–833.

Study summarizing development and implementation of the American College of Surgeons National Surgical Quality Improvement Surgical Risk Calculator. The risk calculator is available online to estimate patient-specific postoperative risk of selected morbidities and mortality.

Chow WB, Rosenthal RA, Merkow RP, et al. Optimal preoperative assessment of the geriatric surgical patient: a best practices guideline from the American College of Surgeons National Surgical Quality Improvement Program and the American Geriatrics Society. *J Am Coll Surg.* 2012;215:453–466.

Summary of the best practice management guidelines for geriatric surgical patient developed in collaboration between the American Geriatrics Society and the American College of Surgeons National Surgical Quality Improvement Program.

Canet J, Gallart L, Gomar C, et al. Prediction of postoperative pulmonary complications in a population-based surgical cohort. *Anesthesiology*. 2010;113:1338–1350.

A large prospective study summarizing risk factors associated with postoperative pulmonary complication.

Devereaux PJ, Mrkobrada M, Sessler DI, et al. Aspirin in patients undergoing noncardiac surgery. *N Engl J Med*. 2014;370:1494–1503.

A randomized control trial demonstrating no significant protective effect of aspirin on 30-day mortality or nonfatal myocardial infarction in perioperative noncardiac surgery patients.

Douketis JD, Spyropoulos AC, Kaatz S, et al. Perioperative bridging anticoagulation in patients with atrial fibrillation. *N Engl J Med*. 2015;373:823–833.

A randomized control trial establishing safety of foregoing bridging anticoagulation for patients with atrial fibrillation requiring temporary interruption of chronic anticoagulation for elective invasive procedure or operation.

Douketis JD, Spyropoulos AC, Spencer FA, et al. Perioperative management of antithrombotic therapy: antithrombotic therapy and prevention of thrombosis, 9th ed: American College of Chest Physicians evidence-based clinical practice guidelines. *Chest*. 2012;141:e326S–e350S.

Summary of the best practice management guidelines for management of antithrombotic medications in prevention of venous thromboembolism.

Fleisher LA, Fleischmann KE, Auerbach AD, et al. 2014 ACC/AHA guideline on perioperative cardiovascular evaluation and management of patients undergoing noncardiac surgery: a report of the American College of Cardiology/American Heart Association Task Force on practice guidelines. *J Am Coll Cardiol*. 2014;64:e77–e137.

Summary of the best practice management guidelines for preoperative cardiovascular evaluation and management developed in collaboration between the American College of Cardiology and The American Heart AssociationTask Force.

Holst LB, Haase N, Wetterslev J, et al. Lower versus higher hemoglobin threshold for transfusion in septic shock. *N Engl J Med*. 2014;371:1381–1391.

A randomized control trial demonstrating safety of lower packed red blood cell transfusion threshold (7 g/dL) among critically ill patients with septic shock.

Lee TH, Marcantonio ER, Mangione CM, et al. Derivation and prospective validation of a simple index for prediction of cardiac risk of major noncardiac surgery. *Circulation*. 1999;100:1043–1049.

Study summarizing development and validation of the Revised Cardiac Risk Index, which has served as a backbone for study and risk stratification of patients considered for elective operation.

Steinberg JP, Braun BI, Hellinger WC, et al. Timing of antimicrobial prophylaxis and the risk of surgical site infections: results from the Trial to Reduce Antimicrobial Prophylaxis Errors. *Ann Surg*. 2009;250:10–16.

Study summarizing association between timing of administration of antimicrobial prophylaxis and postoperative surgical site infection.

REFERENCES

1. Hyder JA, Reznor G, Wakeam E, et al. Risk prediction accuracy differs for emergency versus elective cases in the ACS-NSQIP. *Ann Surg*. 2016;264:959–965.
2. Kluger Y, Ben-Ishay O, Sartelli M, et al. World society of emergency surgery study group initiative on Timing of Acute Care Surgery classification (TACS). *World J Emerg Surg*. 2013;8:17.
3. Hopkins TJ, Raghunathan K, Barbeito A, et al. Associations between ASA physical status and postoperative mortality at 48 h: a contemporary dataset analysis compared to a historical cohort. *Perioper Med (Lond)*. 2016;5:29.
4. Glance LG, Lustik SJ, Hannan EL, et al. The Surgical Mortality Probability Model: derivation and validation of a simple risk prediction rule for noncardiac surgery. *Ann Surg*. 2012;255:696–702.
5. Bilimoria KY, Liu Y, Paruch JL, et al. Development and evaluation of the universal ACS NSQIP surgical risk calculator: a decision aid and informed consent tool for patients and surgeons. *J Am Coll Surg*. 2013;217:833–842; e831–833.
6. Liu Y, Cohen ME, Hall BL, et al. Evaluation and enhancement of calibration in the American College of Surgeons NSQIP Surgical Risk Calculator. *J Am Coll Surg*. 2016;223:231–239.
7. Bagnall NM, Pucher PH, Johnston MJ, et al. Informing the process of consent for surgery: identification of key constructs and quality factors. *J Surg Res*. 2017;209:86–92.
8. Kinnersley P, Phillips K, Savage K, et al. Interventions to promote informed consent for patients undergoing surgical and other invasive healthcare procedures. *Cochrane Database Syst Rev*. 2013:CD009445.
9. Chow WB, Rosenthal RA, Merkow RP, et al. Optimal preoperative assessment of the geriatric surgical patient: a best practices guideline from the American College of Surgeons National Surgical Quality Improvement Program and the American Geriatrics Society. *J Am Coll Surg*. 2012;215:453–466.
10. Partridge JS, Harari D, Martin FC, et al. The impact of preoperative comprehensive geriatric assessment on postoperative outcomes in older patients undergoing scheduled surgery: a systematic review. *Anaesthesia*. 2014;69(suppl 1):8–16.
11. Borson S, Scanlan J, Brush M, et al. The mini-cog: a cognitive "vital signs" measure for dementia screening in multi-lingual elderly. *Int J Geriatr Psychiatry*. 2000;15:1021–1027.
12. Postoperative delirium in older adults: best practice statement from the American Geriatrics Society. *J Am Coll Surg*. 2015;220:136–148 e131.
13. American Geriatrics Society 2015 Updated beers criteria for potentially inappropriate medication use in older Adults. *J Am Geriatr Soc*. 2015;63:2227–2246.
14. Knittel JG, Wildes TS. Preoperative assessment of geriatric patients. *Anesthesiol Clin*. 2016;34:171–183.
15. Larsen KD, Rubinfeld IS. Changing risk of perioperative myocardial infarction. *Perm J*. 2012;16:4–9.

16. Podsiadlo D, Richardson S. The timed "up & go": a test of basic functional mobility for frail elderly persons. *J Am Geriatr Soc*. 1991;39:142–148.
17. Huisman MG, van Leeuwen BL, Ugolini G, et al. "Timed up & go": a screening tool for predicting 30-day morbidity in onco-geriatric surgical patients? A multicenter cohort study. *PLoS One*. 2014;9:e86863.
18. Fleisher LA, Beckman JA, Brown KA, et al. ACC/AHA 2007 guidelines on perioperative cardiovascular evaluation and care for noncardiac surgery: executive summary: a report of the American College of Cardiology/American Heart Association Task Force on Practice Guidelines (Writing Committee to Revise the 2002 Guidelines on Perioperative Cardiovascular Evaluation for Noncardiac Surgery): developed in collaboration with the American Society of Echocardiography, American Society of Nuclear Cardiology, Heart Rhythm Society, Society of Cardiovascular Anesthesiologists, Society for Cardiovascular Angiography and Interventions, Society for Vascular Medicine and Biology, and Society for Vascular Surgery. *Circulation*. 2007;116:1971–1996.
19. Lee TH, Marcantonio ER, Mangione CM, et al. Derivation and prospective validation of a simple index for prediction of cardiac risk of major noncardiac surgery. *Circulation*. 1999;100:1043–1049.
20. Fleisher LA, Fleischmann KE, Auerbach AD, et al. 2014 ACC/AHA guideline on perioperative cardiovascular evaluation and management of patients undergoing noncardiac surgery: a report of the American College of Cardiology/American Heart Association Task Force on practice guidelines. *J Am Coll Cardiol*. 2014;64:e77–137.
21. Ainsworth BE, Haskell WL, Herrmann SD, et al. 2011 Compendium of Physical Activities: a second update of codes and MET values. *Med Sci Sports Exerc*. 2011;43:1575–1581.
22. Wijeysundera DN, Duncan D, Nkonde-Price C, et al. Perioperative beta blockade in noncardiac surgery: a systematic review for the 2014 ACC/AHA guideline on perioperative cardiovascular evaluation and management of patients undergoing noncardiac surgery: a report of the American College of Cardiology/American Heart Association Task Force on Practice Guidelines. *Circulation*. 2014;130:2246–2264.
23. Smetana GW, Lawrence VA, Cornell JE. Preoperative pulmonary risk stratification for noncardiothoracic surgery: systematic review for the American College of Physicians. *Ann Intern Med*. 2006;144:581–595.
24. Canet J, Gallart L, Gomar C, et al. Prediction of postoperative pulmonary complications in a population-based surgical cohort. *Anesthesiology*. 2010;113:1338–1350.
25. Gupta H, Gupta PK, Schuller D, et al. Development and validation of a risk calculator for predicting postoperative pneumonia. *Mayo Clin Proc*. 2013;88:1241–1249.
26. Chung F, Abdullah HR, Liao P. STOP-Bang Questionnaire: a practical approach to screen for obstructive sleep apnea. *Chest*. 2016;149:631–638.
27. de Goede B, Klitsie PJ, Lange JF, et al. Morbidity and mortality related to non-hepatic surgery in patients with liver cirrhosis: a systematic review. *Best Pract Res Clin Gastroenterol*. 2012;26:47–59.
28. Neeff H, Mariaskin D, Spangenberg HC, et al. Perioperative mortality after non-hepatic general surgery in patients with liver cirrhosis: an analysis of 138 operations in the 2000s using Child and MELD scores. *J Gastrointest Surg*. 2011;15:1–11.
29. Teh SH, Nagorney DM, Stevens SR, et al. Risk factors for mortality after surgery in patients with cirrhosis. *Gastroenterology*. 2007;132:1261–1269.
30. Balzan S, Belghiti J, Farges O, et al. The "50-50 criteria" on postoperative day 5: an accurate predictor of liver failure and death after hepatectomy. *Ann Surg*. 2005;242:824–828; discussion 828–829.
31. Holst LB, Haase N, Wetterslev J, et al. Lower versus higher hemoglobin threshold for transfusion in septic shock. *N Engl J Med*. 2014;371:1381–1391.
32. Mazer CD, Whitlock RP, Fergusson DA, et al. Restrictive or liberal red-cell transfusion for cardiac surgery. *N Engl J Med*. 2017;377:2133–2144.
33. Devereaux PJ, Mrkobrada M, Sessler DI, et al. Aspirin in patients undergoing noncardiac surgery. *N Engl J Med*. 2014;370:1494–1503.
34. Douketis JD, Spyropoulos AC, Spencer FA, et al. Perioperative management of antithrombotic therapy: antithrombotic therapy and prevention of thrombosis, 9th ed: American College of Chest Physicians Evidence-Based Clinical Practice Guidelines. *Chest*. 2012;141:e326S–e350S.
35. Douketis JD, Spyropoulos AC, Kaatz S, et al. Perioperative bridging anticoagulation in patients with atrial fibrillation. *N Engl J Med*. 2015;373:823–833.
36. Sun Kara T, Ofori E, Zarubin V, et al. Perioperative management of direct oral anticoagulants (DOACs): a systemic review. *Health Serv Insights*. 2016;9:25–36.
37. Salpeter SR, Greyber E, Pasternak GA, et al. Risk of fatal and nonfatal lactic acidosis with metformin use in type 2 diabetes mellitus. *Cochrane Database Syst Rev*. 2010:CD002967.
38. McClave SA, Kozar R, Martindale RG, et al. Summary points and consensus recommendations from the North American Surgical Nutrition Summit. *JPEN J Parenter Enteral Nutr*. 2013;37:99S–105S.
39. Merchea A, Larson DW. Enhanced recovery after surgery and future directions. *Surg Clin North Am*. 2018;98:1287–1292.
40. Levy SM, Lally KP, Blakely ML, et al. Surgical wound misclassification: a multicenter evaluation. *J Am Coll Surg*. 2015;220:323–329.
41. Bratzler DW, Dellinger EP, Olsen KM, et al. Clinical practice guidelines for antimicrobial prophylaxis in surgery. *Surg Infect (Larchmt)*. 2013;14:73–156.
42. Steinberg JP, Braun BI, Hellinger WC, et al. Timing of antimicrobial prophylaxis and the risk of surgical site infections: results from the Trial to Reduce Antimicrobial Prophylaxis Errors. *Ann Surg*. 2009;250:10–16.
43. Dumville JC, McFarlane E, Edwards P, et al. Preoperative skin antiseptics for preventing surgical wound infections after clean surgery. *Cochrane Database Syst Rev*. 2015:CD003949.
44. Darouiche RO, Wall Jr MJ, Itani KM, et al. Chlorhexidine-alcohol versus povidone-iodine for surgical-site antisepsis. *N Engl J Med*. 2010;362:18–26.
45. Diaz Jr JJ, Dutton WD, Ott MM, et al. Eastern Association for the Surgery of Trauma: a review of the management of the open abdomen, part 2: "Management of the open abdomen". *J Trauma*. 2011;71:502–512.
46. Ahmad G, O'Flynn H, Hindocha A, et al. Barrier agents for adhesion prevention after gynaecological surgery. *Cochrane Database Syst Rev*. 2015:CD000475.
47. Sankaranarayanan G, Resapu RR, Jones DB, et al. Common uses and cited complications of energy in surgery. *Surg Endosc*. 2013;27:3056–3072.

48. Nunez TC, Young PP, Holcomb JB, et al. Creation, implementation, and maturation of a massive transfusion protocol for the exsanguinating trauma patient. *J Trauma*. 2010;68:1498–1505.
49. Hollenbeck BK, Dunn RL, Suskind AM, et al. Ambulatory surgery centers and their intended effects on outpatient surgery. *Health Serv Res*. 2015;50:1491–1507.
50. Fleisher LA, Pasternak LR, Herbert R, et al. Inpatient hospital admission and death after outpatient surgery in elderly patients: importance of patient and system characteristics and location of care. *Arch Surg*. 2004;139:67–72.

CHAPTER 11

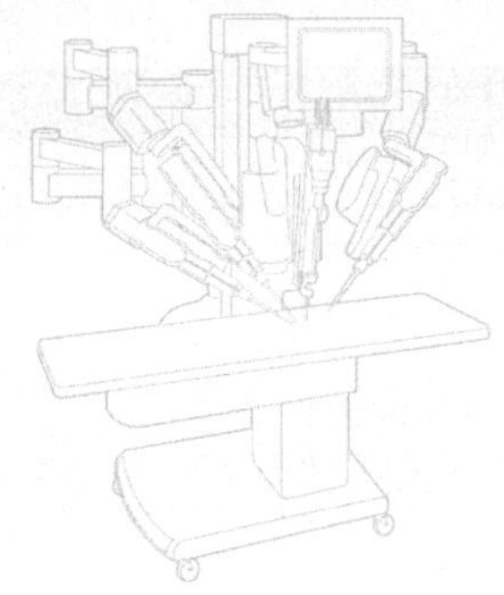

Surgical Infections and Antibiotic Use

Ariel P. Santos, Edwin Onkendi, Sharmila Dissanaike

OUTLINE

Surgical infections encompass a wide-ranging group of diseases, which account for a large burden of mortality and morbidity worldwide. Surgical infections include de novo infectious diseases that require surgery or procedural interventions for cure; common examples include abscesses, intraabdominal infections such as cholangitis and appendicitis, and necrotizing soft tissue infections (NSTIs), all of which are dealt with in detail in this chapter. Another major type of surgical infection is surgical site infections (SSIs)—infections occurring at the site within 30 days of a surgical procedure. SSIs account for 20% of health care–acquired infections and result in significant morbidity and hospital costs.

Surgical infections may lead to sepsis, a life-threatening organ dysfunction due to a dysregulated host response to infection.[1] Sepsis is the leading cause of in-hospital mortality in the United States.[2] Sepsis is estimated to affect 30 million people worldwide each year, although this is likely an underestimate given the paucity of data from low- and middle-income countries.[3] Early and effective source control is important for the successful treatment of sepsis. This requires that the physician recognize when the source of infection is amenable to a surgical cure and effects this without delay in conjunction with other treatments such as fluid resuscitation and antibiotics. The Surviving Sepsis Campaign (SSC) provides expert consensus on guidelines for the treatment of sepsis, which should be familiar to all surgeons treating patients with infection.[4]

SURGICAL SITE INFECTIONS

SSIs are the most common and costly of all hospital-acquired infections, accounting for 20% of all hospital infections. It is associated with increased length of stay and a twofold to eleven fold increase in the risk of mortality.[5] In the United States, there are more than 40 million surgical operations performed and 2% to 5% are complicated by SSIs. There is an estimated annual incidence ranging from 160,000 to 300,000, with an annual cost of SSIs in the United States estimated at $3.5 billion to $10 billion.[6] The increased cost is due to prolonged hospitalization, increase in emergency room visits, readmission, antibiotic costs, and additional procedural costs. About 60% of SSIs are preventable with evidence-based guidelines[6]; as a result, SSI is one of the quality metrics frequently used to assess quality of surgical care, which is then linked to performance ranking, reimbursement, and patient satisfaction.

Classification of Surgical Site Infection

The most commonly used definition of SSI is that of the Centers for Disease Control and Prevention (CDC). The SSI must occur within 30 days after the operative procedure if no implant is left in place, or within 1 year if implant is in place, and the infection appears to be related to the operative procedure.[7] SSIs are classified based on the depth and tissue layers involved as superficial incisional, deep incisional, and organ/space (Table 11.1). Standardization of reporting plays an important role in ensuring accurate data collection for research, quality improvement, and public reporting.

Risk Factors for Surgical Site Infection

The CDC classifies wound into four groups: clean, clean-contaminated, contaminated, and dirty-infected (Table 11.2), with progressively increasing risk of SSIs. In addition, patient, environmental, and treatment factors can increase the risk of subsequent

TABLE 11.1 CDC/NHSN classification of surgical site infection.

CLASSIFICATION	DEFINITION
Superficial incisional SSI (SIS)	Infection occurs within 30 days after the operative procedure and involves only skin and subcutaneous tissue of the incision and had at least one of the following: a. Purulent drainage from the superficial incision. b. Organisms isolated from an aseptically obtained culture of fluid or tissue from the superficial incision. c. At least one of the following signs or symptoms of infection: pain or tenderness, localized swelling, redness, or heat, and superficial incision is deliberately opened by surgeon and is culture positive or not cultured. A culture-negative finding does not meet this criterion. d. Diagnosis of superficial incisional SSI by the surgeon or attending physician.
Deep incisional SSI (DIS)	Infection occurs within 30 days after the operative procedure if no implant is left in place or within 1 year if implant is in place and the infection appears to be related to the operative procedure and involves deep soft tissues (e.g., fascial and muscle layers) of the incision and patient has at least one of the following: a. Purulent drainage from the deep incision but not from organ/space component of the surgical site. b. Deep incision spontaneously dehisces or is deliberately opened by a surgeon and is culture-positive or not cultured when the patient has at least one of the following signs or symptoms: fever (>38°C) or localized pain or tenderness. A culture-negative finding does not meet this criterion. c. An abscess or other evidence of infection involving the deep incision is found on direct examination, during reoperation, or by histopathologic or radiologic examination. d. Diagnosis of a deep incisional SSI by a surgeon or attending physician.Wound that has both superficial and deep incisional infection is classified as DIS.
Organ/space SSI	Infection occurs within 30 days after the operative procedure if no implant is left in place or within 1 year if implant is in place and the infection appears to be related to the operative procedure and infection involves any part of the body, excluding the skin incision, fascia, or muscle layers, that is opened or manipulated during the operative procedure and patient has at least one of the following: a. Purulent drainage from a drain that is placed through a stab wound into the organ/space. b. Organisms isolated from an aseptically obtained culture of fluid or tissue in the organ/space. c. An abscess or other evidence of infection involving the organ/space that is found on direct examination, during reoperation, or by histopathologic or radiologic examination. d. Diagnosis of an organ/space SSI by a surgeon or attending physician.

CDC, Centers for Disease Control and Prevention; *NHSN*, National Healthcare Safety Network; *SSI*, surgical site infection.

development of SSIs (Box 11.1). Of particular interest are risk factors amenable to preoperative optimization such as smoking cessation, protein-calorie malnutrition, and obesity. In general, laparoscopic surgical approaches carry a lower risk of SSIs compared with open techniques for the same procedure.

Surgical Site Infection Prevention

Numerous interventions have been proposed to reduce the risk of SSI. In 2002, the CDC and Center for Medicare and Medicaid Services initiated the Surgical Infection Prevention Project to reduce SSIs, and in 2006, this became the expanded Surgical Care Improvement Program. The U.S. Congress authored the Deficit Reduction Act of 2005, which mandates hospital reporting process and outcome and quality improvement measures to be made available to the public and Center for Medicare and Medicaid Services. The act also allows payment adjustment downward for health care–associated infections that could have been prevented through application of evidence-based strategies.[8] These interventions can be broadly divided into three stages: preoperative, intraoperative, and postoperative strategies.

The CDC provided a new and updated evidence-based recommendation for the prevention of SSIs.[8] Preventive measures for SSI include a full-body bath or shower with soap (antimicrobial or nonantimicrobial) or an antiseptic agent the night before or the morning of the operation, appropriate antimicrobial prophylaxis before incision, and skin preparation with an alcohol-based agent unless contraindicated. In clean and clean-contaminated procedures, additional prophylactic antimicrobial agents should not be administered even in the presence of a drain nor should topical antimicrobials be applied to the surgical incision. Maintenance of normothermia, glycemic control with targets less than 200 mg/dL, and the provision of supplemental oxygen are other adjunct measures proposed to reduce SSI in the perioperative bundle.

In addition to the 2017 CDC guideline for the prevention of SSI, a randomized study showed that prophylactic use of negative pressure dressings for closed laparotomy wounds significantly reduces the incidence of SSI at 30 days postoperatively, concomitantly decreasing length of stay (6.1 vs. 14.7 days; $P = 0.01$).[9]

Treatment of Surgical Site Infection

There are five steps in the treatment of SSI (Box 11.2). Once SSI is diagnosed, it is paramount to obtain a high-quality specimen for Gram stain and culture to identify the causative pathogens. With the increasing prevalence of multidrug resistant organisms associated with wound infection, identification of the causative pathogen and its antimicrobial susceptibility helps guide appropriate antibiotic therapy as well as facilitate rapid de-escalation, which is important in preventing unnecessary antibiotic use that facilitates further development of resistant organisms.

Source control in superficial and deep SSI usually requires opening of the incision site and irrigation, drainage, and debridement of devitalized or infected tissue as needed. Organ space infections often can be controlled by image-guided drainage using computed tomography (CT) scan or ultrasound (US) if localized and well contained. However, where there are multiple sites or widespread infection–interloop abscesses between loops of small

TABLE 11.2 CDC surgical wound classification.

CLASSIFICATION	DESCRIPTION
I—Clean	An uninfected operative wound in which no inflammation is encountered and the respiratory, alimentary, genital, or uninfected urinary tract is not entered. In addition, clean wounds are primarily closed and, if necessary, drained with closed drainage. Operative incisional wounds that follow no penetrating (blunt) trauma should be included in this category if they meet the criteria.
II—Clean-contaminated	An operative wound in which the respiratory, alimentary, genital, or urinary tracts are entered under controlled conditions and without unusual contamination. Specifically, operations involving the biliary tract, appendix, vagina, and oropharynx are included in this category, provided no evidence of infection or major break in technique is encountered.
III—Contaminated	Open, fresh, accidental wounds. In addition, operations with major breaks in sterile technique (e.g., open cardiac massage) or gross spillage from the gastrointestinal tract and incisions in which acute, no purulent inflammation is encountered are included in this category.
IV—Dirty-infected	Old traumatic wounds with retained devitalized tissue and those that involve existing clinical infection or perforated viscera. This definition suggests that the organisms causing postoperative infection were present in the operative field before the operation.

CDC, Centers for Disease Control and Prevention.

intestine, for example, surgical drainage is necessary and can be performed either by laparoscopic or open approach.

NECROTIZING SOFT TISSUE INFECTIONS

NSTIs are rapidly progressing skin and soft tissue infections associated with necrosis of the dermis, subcutaneous tissue, superficial fascia, deep fascia, or muscle. This definition includes a variety of conditions, such as Fournier gangrene affecting the perineum and genitalia, Meleney streptococcal gangrene, and clostridial myonecrosis. While a wide range of organisms might be responsible and different body regions and tissues are affected, these infections are grouped together due to the common characteristics of rapid progression, irreversible tissue necrosis, high rates of sepsis, and mortality rates between 10% and 25%. Patients with NSTIs are often referred to regional burn centers because of the need for intensive care, multiple operations, and resource-intensive complex reconstruction of large tissue and skin defects.

Although uncommon compared with other skin infections such as cellulitis or abscesses, the incidence of NSTI appears to be increasing in the United States. This is often attributed to the increased prevalence of obesity, type 2 diabetes mellitus, and people living with chronic immunosuppression, all of which may predispose an individual to NSTI.[2,5] While these conditions do increase risk, NSTIs may also be diagnosed in previously healthy young adults and even children, although this is rare. NSTIs are rarely "idiopathic"; a minor wound or injury almost always precedes the devastating infection, often by several weeks. NSTI caused by streptococci and clostridia often have a fulminant course with rapid onset of symptoms and worsening over days or even hours and may be rapidly progressing to death if untreated. In contrast, infections caused by mixed flora, staphylococcus, and gram-negative organisms often have an indolent course over days to weeks, which may mislead clinicians into not considering the diagnosis of NSTI.

BOX 11.1 Risk factors for the development of surgical site infection.

Patient Factors

Alcoholism
Ascites
Age
Chronic inflammation
Diabetes
History of skin or soft tissue infection
Hyperbilirubinemia >1 mg/dL
Hypercholesterolemia
Hypoalbuminemia
Hypoxemia
Immunosuppression
Malignancies
Malnutrition
Obesity
Peripheral vascular disease
Postoperative anemia
Preexisting infection
Recent radiotherapy
Smoking
Steroid therapy

Environmental Factors

Contamination
Inadequate antisepsis
Inadequate disinfection
Inadequate ventilation
Increased operating room traffic

Treatment Factors

Blood transfusion
Contamination: poor scrubbing technique, breach in asepsis, poor gloving, etc.
Drains
Emergency surgery
High wound classification
Hypothermia
Hypoxemia
Inadequate or inappropriate antibiotic prophylaxis
Poor glycemic control
Prolonged operation

BOX 11.2 Treatment strategies for surgical site infection.

1. Pathogen identification.
2. Source control by opening the incision in superficial or deep surgical site infections (SSIs) or by image-guided percutaneous drainage, laparoscopic, or open drainage if indicated in organ space SSIs.
3. Immediate empiric antibiotic coverage.
4. Timely antibiotic de-escalation.
5. Local wound care.

TABLE 11.3 Laboratory risk indicator for necrotizing fasciitis (LRINEC) scoring system.

VARIABLE	UNITS	SCORE
C-reactive protein	≥150 mg/L	4 points
White blood cell count	15–25	1 point
(per mm)	>25	2 points
Hemoglobin	11.0–13.5 g/dL	1 point
	<11 g/dL	2 points
Serum sodium	≥135 mmol/L	1 point
	<135 mmol/L	2 points
Serum creatinine	>1.6 mg/dL (or >141 pmol/L)	2 points
Serum glucose	>180 mg/dL (or >10 mmol/L)	1 point
RISK CATEGORY	**LRINEC SCORE, points**	**PROBABILITY OF NSTIS, (%)**
Low	≤5	<50
Intermediate	6–7	50–75
High	≥8	>75

LRINEC, Laboratory risk indicator for necrotizing fasciitis; *NSTIs*, necrotizing soft tissue infections.

Since the progression of NSTI is often fulminant, patient prognosis depends on early recognition and administration of appropriate treatment as soon as possible.

Diagnosis

A major obstacle to the effective treatment of NSTIs and one reason for the high mortality of these conditions is delay in diagnosis. Since these infections affect subcutaneous tissues, muscle, and fascia, visible skin changes on the surface are often underwhelming, misleading clinicians as to the true extent of ongoing necrosis below. The most common clinical features of NSTIs present in 90% of cases are erythema, warmth, and pain—unfortunately, common symptoms and signs that are also present in mild infections such as cellulitis and in almost every case of inflammation from any cause. Crepitus, skin necrosis, and bullae are much more specific to NSTI but unfortunately are present less than 40% of the time, rendering them markedly less useful in diagnosis.[10] Signs of skin and tissue necrosis are pathognomonic and should provoke urgent resuscitation and surgery; however, the lack of obvious necrosis and a superficial appearance similar to cellulitis should not deter the surgeon from further investigation, including local wound exploration, if necessary, based on the patient's systemic signs and symptoms.

Signs and symptoms of systemic illness (i.e., sepsis) are much more likely to be a feature of NSTI than simple skin infections and should prompt serious consideration of the diagnosis. While fever may be present in nearly every infection, hypotension should not be and should serve as a warning sign if present. Similarly, organ failure such as renal failure or hypoxia should not be present with cellulitis or an uncomplicated abscess; these findings on clinical and laboratory examination, in conjunction with pain in a focal body region, should be considered highly suspicious for NSTIs and treated accordingly. The laboratory risk indicator for necrotizing fasciitis scoring system was developed based on laboratory values commonly deranged in NSTIs (Table 11.3); it has been shown to be useful in differentiating NSTI from other infections, although correlation of laboratory risk indicator for necrotizing fasciitis score with outcome in NSTI is less robust, and recent metaanalyses have disputed its value.[11] Nonetheless, whether utilizing a formal scoring system or not, any sign of systemic derangement such as unexpected hyperglycemia, acute renal failure, or hyponatremia will place the burden firmly on the surgical team to disprove the diagnosis of NSTI, requiring further evaluation such as imaging studies or direct surgical exploration.

Imaging

Given the difficulty of diagnosing NSTIs based on physical examination alone, there has been much interest in the use of imaging modalities to differentiate NSTI from other infections. US, magnetic resonance imaging, and CT scans have all been evaluated for their efficacy in NSTI diagnosis; based on ease of access and interpretability of results, CT is the most commonly favored modality for adjuvant imaging. Features suggestive of NSTI on CT include gas in the soft tissues (the easiest finding for nonradiologists to diagnose and the most specific), multiple fluid collections, absence or heterogeneity of tissue enhancement by intravenous (IV) contrast, and significant inflammatory changes under the fascia. Using these criteria, the sensitivity of CT in identifying NSTI was 100%, the specificity 98%, the positive predictive value 76%, and the negative predictive value 100% in one series of 184 patients.[12]

Local Exploration

Given the difficulty in diagnosis and the increase in mortality associated with delays in definitive treatment, surgical exploration of the questionable area is a very reasonable next step when the diagnosis remains in doubt. This requires a full-thickness elliptical excision of all tissues down through fascia and including muscle to rule out necrotizing fasciitis or myositis in addition to subcutaneous infection.

A 2-cm elliptical excision on an extremity will usually suffice and can be performed under local anesthesia at the bedside. In areas of adiposity such as the pannus or groin, this will be easier performed in the operating room. The surgeon should visually inspect for tissue necrosis, dishwater fluid or purulence, greyish discoloration of tissues, or failure of the muscle to react to electrocautery. The tissue at the edges of the incision should be firm and resist pressure—the "push" test. If the surgeon is able to dissect more than a centimeter subcutaneously with blunt finger pressure alone, this is considered a positive finding and wide debridement in the operating room is indicated. Any fluid encountered should be collected and sent for immediate Gram stain and culture in addition to at least 1 cm^3 of skin and subcutaneous tissue and samples from fascia and muscle.

Treatment of Necrotizing Soft Tissue Infections

Surgery

Surgical debridement is the mainstay of NSTI treatment. All affected tissue should be sharply excised with at least 1 cm rim of normal tissue (Fig. 11.1). The "push" test described previously will allow the surgeon to quickly delineate the extent of resection necessary. Bleeding is not an indication of tissue viability, since the presence of active infection will often cause these areas to be hyperemic; significant blood loss is often encountered so the surgical team should be prepared for this eventuality. The use of tourniquets in extremity dissection and attention to hemostasis are necessary to prevent sudden major blood loss from destabilizing an already unstable patient. All questionable tissue should be resected at the initial operation; the need for multiple operations and the spread of infection both increase the risk of mortality.[13]

While skin-sparing procedures have been shown in limited series to improve eventual reconstructive options for both cosmesis and function, it is essential that the skin not be directly involved in these cases and that wide undermining be able to be performed to remove all necrotic tissue, which remains the mainstay of NSTI treatment.

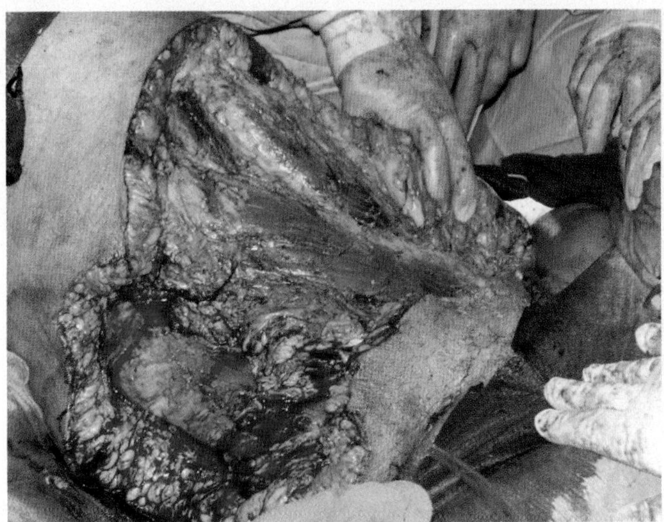

FIG. 11.1 Surgical debridement of necrotizing soft tissue infection.

Antibiotics

Broad-spectrum antibiotics should be initiated as soon as the diagnosis is suspected; once the patient is clinically improving and culture results are available, these may be de-escalated to one or two agents. In general, it is advisable to give one broad-spectrum agent effective against most gram-positive and gram-negative organisms and ensure Methicillin-resistant *S. aureus* coverage and good anaerobic coverage, tailored to local antibiogram. The impact of anaerobes in NSTI outcomes has been underrecognized due to the difficulty of growing anaerobes in conventional culture media; however, recent studies using 16S ribonucleic acid (RNA) sequencing have demonstrated that anaerobes are likely a significant contributor to mortality in NSTIs.[14] Finally, there is evidence that clindamycin has toxin-neutralization properties, especially in streptococcal and clostridial infections; for this reason, we routinely add clindamycin to the initial regimen.

Resuscitation

Patients demonstrating sepsis and septic shock should be managed in an intensive care unit (ICU), using the standard guidelines for sepsis. These include early, goal-directed resuscitation with isotonic fluids, vasopressor support as needed with norepinephrine and vasopressin, and control of hyperglycemia. The use of adjuncts such as IV immunoglobulin and hyperbaric oxygen has been described; however, there is insufficient evidence to recommend routine use. While there is no specific evidence for the use of antioxidants or steroids in NSTIs, recent studies suggest that IV thiamine, vitamin C, and hydrocortisone in combination might improve outcomes in sepsis.[15] Further investigation is warranted as to the utility of this approach in NSTIs.

Wound Care and Reconstruction

The large soft tissue defects that result from appropriate debridement of NSTI will require extensive reconstructive procedures once the patient has recovered from the acute episode. We routinely leave the debrided area completely open to air, sometimes under heat lamps, for the first 48 hours after surgery; a spritz of antibiotic irrigation is used to keep the muscle from drying out excessively, and lubricant is used to cover tendons and other vulnerable areas.[16] This approach allows for continuous evaluation of the wound in the ICU, facilitating the earlier recognition of spreading infection and removing the need for scheduled second-look operations. Removing the need for dressing changes also reduces the pain experienced by the patient, and this approach is surprisingly well tolerated by patients and families alike, after the indications are explained. In body areas such as the groin or under intertriginous folds where it is not possible to leave the tissue exposed to air, we use conventional wet-to-dry gauze dressings changed once or twice a day.

Once the infection is resolved, the wound is placed in a negative pressure vacuum dressing and reconstructive procedures, usually a skin graft, is planned in 2 to 4 weeks. This allows time for the patient to engage in rehabilitation with physical therapy and optimal nutrition in order to optimize the chances of a good long-term outcome. The inclusion of tissue substitutes such as acellular dermal matrix and regeneration templates in reconstruction may improve cosmetic and functional outcomes, although this increases cost significantly.

SPECIFIC INFECTIONS

Intraabdominal Abscess

Intraabdominal infections encompass a wide range of infections that have been classified previously in a variety of ways, including classification based on the nature of the infection (uncomplicated and complicated), the setting of infection (community acquired vs. hospital acquired), and severity of the infection as well as risk of significant morbidity, mortality, and failure of treatment (low, moderate, and high risk).

This chapter focuses on one of these infections (i.e., intra-abdominal abscess) in the surgical patient.

Definition, Etiology, and Classification of Intraabdominal Abscess

Intraabdominal abscess refers to a localized walled-off collection of infected fluid within the confines of the abdomen (peritoneal cavity, retroperitoneum, and pelvic cavity) that occurs as a result of the protective containment of the host's intraabdominal defense mechanisms. Failure of the host intraabdominal defense mechanisms to wall off and localize the infection leads to an uncontained infection with acute diffuse peritonitis and systemic infection associated with a high morbidity and mortality.

An abscess can develop at a later stage of what was previously uncontained intraabdominal "free-floating infection." With the intraabdominal host defense mechanisms against infection in effect, there is, then, the development of a capsular wall around the inflammatory fluid or infected fluid for containment, resulting in a walled-off abscess. A previously uninfected fluid collection that becomes walled off may later become secondarily infected from systemic bacteremia or from external translocation via a drain or instrumentation, for example, secondary infection of a post pancreatitis pseudocyst (Fig. 11.2).

On the other hand, intra-abdominal fluid may already be infected at the onset and then become walled off (e.g. purulent fluid from ruptured acute appendicitis or leaked hollow viscus contaminated fluid like in a colonic anastomotic leak) (Table 11.4).

Intraabdominal abscesses can, therefore, be classified into the following categories based on location, etiology, and severity (Box 11.3).

Diagnostic Evaluation

Patients with intraabdominal abscess usually present with acute abdominal pain associated with signs and symptoms of infection/inflammation (fever, rigors, tachycardia, tachypnea, and

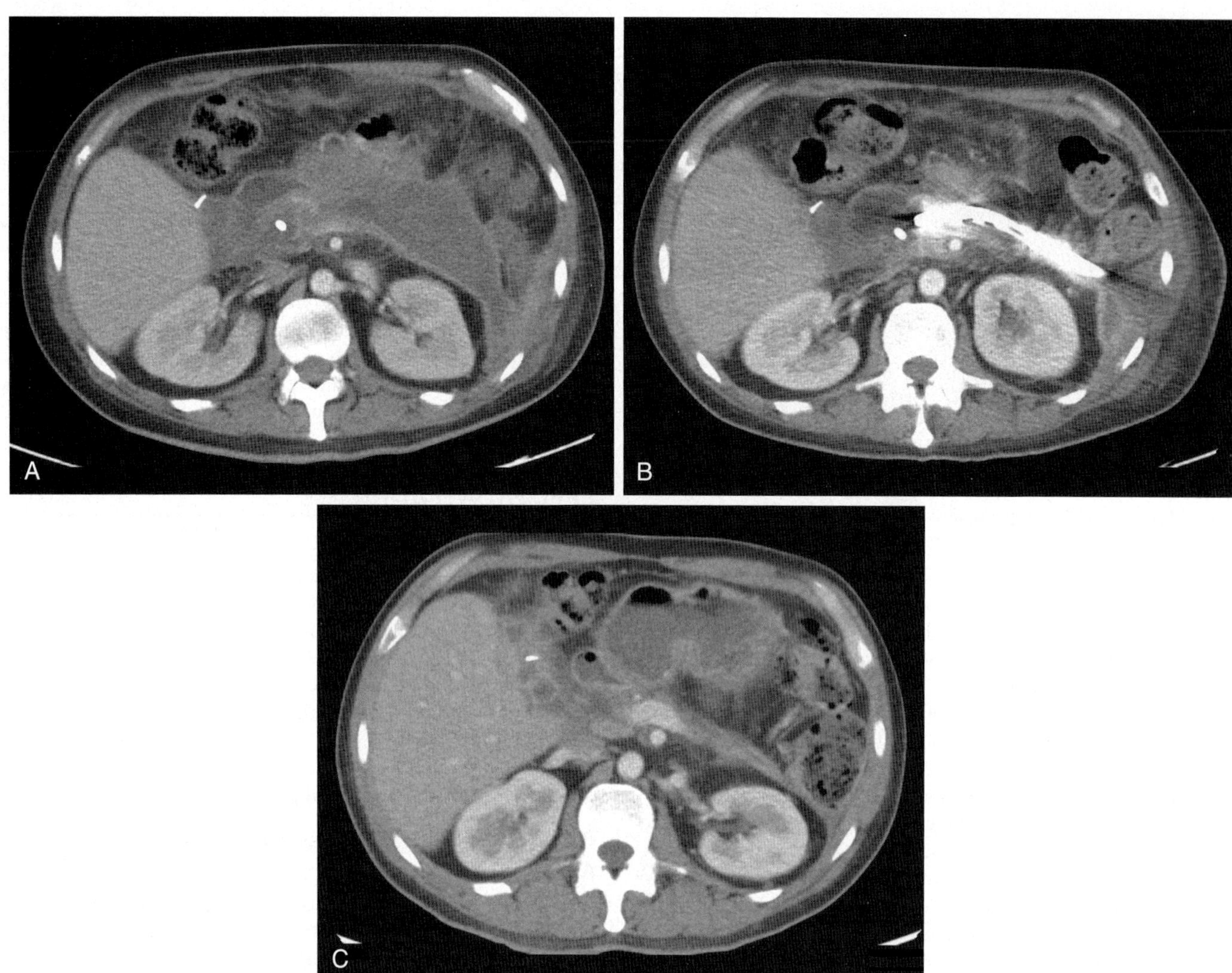

FIG. 11.2 (A) Retroperitoneal abscess that developed in a previously walled-off infected pancreatic necrosis cavity that had been operatively debrided by robotic pancreatic necrosectomy. (B) Percutaneous large bore drainage of the retroperitoneal abscess. (C) Complete resolution of the retroperitoneal abscess 6 weeks after percutaneous drainage.

leukocytosis) as well as gastrointestinal symptoms (nausea, anorexia, emesis, ileus, obstipation, and diarrhea). Initial work-up should include a detailed history and physical examination as well as laboratory tests. These will be suggestive of an underlying infection possibly with abscess in most patients. If the patient's history and physical examination are not available or reliable (e.g., due to patient's altered mental status, intubated patient, or immunocompromised patient), an intraabdominal infection including abscess should be suspected if the patient has features of infection of unknown origin including persistent fever.

Imaging work-up is typically necessary to localize an intraabdominal abscess and determine its characteristics including size, relationship to nearby structures, and presence or absence of multiloculations. CT scan of the abdomen and pelvis with IV contrast is the imaging modality of choice and is the gold standard in high resource countries to assess all these features as well as determine the likely source of the abscess. Whenever possible, CT scan of the abdomen and pelvis should be obtained with IV contrast for better characterization and differentiation of the abscess from surrounding structures. Enteral and per rectal water-soluble contrast may be necessary in patients with suspected gastrointestinal leak.

In areas where there is limited access to CT, US may be helpful in diagnosis. US has become widely available worldwide, with affordable, smaller, portable US machines in widespread use. US in the diagnosis of intraabdominal abscess is especially useful for solid organ abscesses and abscesses not obscured by loops of bowel. It is limited by high user–dependency, limited detail of associated surrounding pathology, and lack of utility for abscesses surrounded by bowel.

Management of Intraabdominal Abscess

Initial resuscitation and management. The treatment approach to intraabdominal abscess should include prompt diagnosis, adequate and early fluid resuscitation, early initiation of IV antibiotic therapy, and early and complete source control by drainage of the abscess and reassessment for clinical improvement/deterioration with as-needed adjustment of therapy.[17] Intraabdominal abscess and associated sepsis and septic shock should be managed as medical emergencies in accordance with the SSC guidelines. Treatment should focus on immediate initial resuscitation followed by frequent hemodynamic reassessments and additional fluid administration as needed. Initial fluid resuscitation and

TABLE 11.4 Types of intraabdominal abscess.

TYPE OF INTRAABDOMINAL ABSCESS	ETIOLOGY/EXAMPLES
Primary intraabdominal abscess (established infections that rupture into peritoneal cavity and become walled-off into abscesses)	Ruptured acute appendicitis abscess, acute diverticulitis with abscess
Delayed primary intraabdominal abscess (microbial-laden hollow viscus fluid leaking into abdomen and transforming into walled-off abscess with time)	Gastrointestinal perforation or postoperative anastomotic leak leading to abscess formation later, subhepatic abscess developing later from infected fluid around after cholecystectomy for acute cholecystitis
Secondary intraabdominal abscess (previously sterile walled-off intra-abdominal fluid collection becomes secondarily infected, transforming into abscess)	Postpancreatitis sterile pseudocyst with secondarily infection from systemic bacteremia or microbial translocation into it via external drain; loculated sterile ascitic/intra-abdominal fluid secondarily infection for external instrumentation or systemic infection.

reassessments should precede diagnostic work-up. Patients with intraabdominal abscess are often volume depleted due to intravascular fluid losses (from tachypnea, fever, vomiting, and diarrhea) and decreased fluid intake (due to nausea, anorexia, emesis, and ileus). If volume depletion is severe, associated acute renal failure may be present. As a result, IV fluid repletion is a necessary part of initial treatment. Even in patients without overt signs of volume depletion, fluid administration may be beneficial as suggested by historical data.

Patients with severe volume depletion associated with septic shock and organ failure should be managed with more aggressive fluid resuscitation according to the SSC guidelines. Key treatment measures according to the "Surviving Sepsis Campaign: International Guidelines for Management of Sepsis and Septic Shock: 2016" include early clinical endpoint-directed fluid therapy (30 mL/kg of crystalloid fluid within the first 3 to 6 hours to restore mean arterial pressure to >65 mm Hg with hemodynamic reassessments and additional fluid therapy guided by serum lactate levels as a marker of tissue perfusion; use of vasopressors in septic shock to maintain mean arterial pressure of 65 mm Hg if not fluid responsive; inotropic support for low cardiac output despite fluid and vasopressor therapy; packed red blood cell transfusion if hemoglobin <7) and early administration of antibiotics and stress-dose steroid therapy if needed.[18] A 2018 update of the SSC guidelines emphasizes immediate initiation of the above measures within the first hour.[4]

Antibiotic therapy with the SSC guideline recommendation of starting antibiotic therapy within 8 hours in patients without septic shock and within 1 hour in those with septic shock should be initiated as soon as an intraabominal abscess is suspected or confirmed.

Source control. Source control is defined as all the measures undertaken to eliminate the source of infection, decrease the bacterial inoculum, and correct or control anatomic derangements to restore normal physiologic function.[19]

BOX 11.3 Intraabdominal abscesses classifications.

Etiology
Primary intraabdominal abscess
Delayed primary intraabdominal abscess
Secondary intraabdominal abscess

Intraabdominal Location
Intraperitoneal abscess
Retroperitoneal abscess
Pelvic abscess
Solid organ intraparenchymal abscess

Risk of Morbidity, Mortality, and Need for Invasive Intervention
Low risk
Moderate risk
High risk

A walled-off abscess creates a low-pH–contained environment that often impairs the host's phagocytic function. In addition, the abscess wall prevents permeation of immune cells and antibiotics into the abscess, therefore decreasing their effectiveness in treatment of the abscess. Due to these factors, an intraabdominal abscess requires some form of drainage (percutaneous or operative) in addition to antibiotic treatment to ensure complete resolution.

Source control can be nonsurgical or surgical. Nonsurgical source control is often performed by percutaneous drainage, which is preferably the first-choice approach to source control for the contained walled-off abscess. Operative drainage should be reserved for failure of percutaneous drainage. For the hemodynamically stable patient, source control via percutaneous drainage should be performed as soon as possible. However, this may be delayed up to 24 hours as long as the patient is covered with appropriate spectrum IV antibiotics and monitored closely. Percutaneous drainage is especially appropriate for single, unilocular abscesses that are accessible via a percutaneous approach and is associated with lower morbidity than operative drainage. Percutaneous drainage requires image guidance. This can be accomplished by US guidance or CT guidance.

Following percutaneous drainage, the patient should be closely monitored for clinical improvement while on antibiotic therapy. Often, a single percutaneous intervention is enough to drain most abscesses and results in resolution of the infection. Small abscesses <5 cm may be adequately managed to full resolution by antibiotics and percutaneous aspiration of the abscess contents alone, without leaving a drain in the abscess cavity. Larger abscesses often need leaving a drain in the abscess cavity for continued drainage until the entire abscess cavity collapses and resolves. This prevents reaccumulation of the abscess contents and allows the collapsed walls of the abscess cavity to adhere to each other and obliterate the cavity space. While the drain is in place, timing of when to remove it can be determined by daily drain output, frequent drain cavity contrast imaging to assess interval changes over time until resolution, and interval cross-sectional imaging.

Percutaneous drainage may be used as an initial immediate treatment approach for an intraabdominal abscess associated with gastrointestinal inflammation or contained perforation with the plan for interval operative intervention at a later stage. With this approach, the significant inflammatory phlegmon associated with acute abscess, which would have required a much more extensive, risky, and complicated resection is avoided in favor of interval resection at a later stage.[20] By this time, often 4 to 6 weeks later, the acute inflammatory phlegmon and periabscess inflammation have resolved resulting in a safer, less extensive resection, which even may be able to be performed in a minimally invasive manner.[21,22] Classic examples include perforated contained acute appendicitis with phlegmon and periappendicular abscess, acute perforated diverticulitis with localized abscess, and acute perforated cholecystitis with intrahepatic abscess.

Surgical source control involves operative drainage of abscess as well as operative measures to manage the underlying etiology of the abscess. These measures include resection of the diseased or perforated viscus (e.g., appendectomy or cholecystectomy), suture repair of perforated viscus (e.g., a perforated peptic ulcer), and debridement of necrotic tissue (e.g., infected necrotizing pancreatitis). Indications for operative drainage include unavailability of percutaneous intervention resources, multiloculated complex abscesses, failure of source control by percutaneous drainage (as indicated by lack of expected clinical improvement or clinical deterioration), poorly localized abscess inaccessible to percutaneous drainage (such as abscess surrounded by small bowel or other critical structures), abscesses associated with diffuse or massive intraperitoneal free air (suspected uncontained hollow viscus perforation), and abscesses associated with diffuse peritonitis. Failure of source control is likely to occur on geriatric patients and patients with malnutrition, immunosuppression, and chronic medical comorbidities. For example, octogenarians and nonagenarians have been shown to have an attenuated inflammatory response and may not present with obvious signs of peritonitis.[23]

Operative drainage may be performed via a minimally invasive approach or via laparotomy. Laparoscopy is ideal in easily accessible abscess including peritoneal cavity, pelvis c, and solid organ abscesses. Complete laparoscopic drainage of retroperitoneal abscesses may be difficult due to the location and the often firm adherence of the surrounding structures to the abscess cavity wall, which limits their mobilization and, therefore, exposure of the abscess for complete drainage. In these cases, it is best to perform open drainage and thorough debridement of the abscess cavity.

Intrathoracic Abscess

Intrathoracic abscess can occur in two main forms:

1. Pleural empyema (abscess)
    - Acute postpneumonic empyema
    - Chronic empyema
    - Postthoracic surgery empyema (postlobectomy, postpneumonectomy, postwedge resection)
    - Posttraumatic empyema
2. Intraparenchymal lung abscess

Both of these are associated with significant morbidity and mortality.

Pleural empyema refers to accumulation of purulent fluid between the parietal and visceral pleura, which may be loculated. Pleural empyema (abscess) often occurs in patients with poor physical and nutritional status and is often associated with prolonged treatment course.

An acute empyema is often a sequelae of pneumonia associated with pleural effusion. Inadequate or delayed drainage of infected acute pleural effusion results in formation of a chronic empyema.

Chronic empyema is an intrapleural abscess that has transformed into a loculated and walled-off abscess. Chronic empyema may develop in a poorly drained postpneumonic infected pleural effusion, postthoracic surgery, often due to a bronchopleural fistula, postthoracic trauma with hemothorax, and rarely from transdiaphragmatic translocation from an intraabdominal infection. Postpneumonectomy empyema is especially feared due to associated high mortality.

Management of Pleural Empyema

Successful treatment of pleural space infection largely depends on the age of the infection. Acute pleural infection that is a few days old consists of thin infected pleural effusion and is therefore amenable to antibiotic therapy and simple tube thoracostomy drainage alone. Conversely, a few-weeks-old pleural space infection usually consists of thick and often loculated fluid with indurated pleural plaque, which makes simple thoracostomy tube drainage not feasible. These require drainage and debridement/decortication to facilitate healing.[24]

Treatment of Acute Empyema

Tube thoracostomy and antibiotic therapy. In the majority of cases, acute empyema can be treated fully with antibiotics and closed tube thoracostomy drainage of the infected pleural effusion. Treatment should be instituted as soon as possible with the goal of complete drainage of the infected pleural space and full reexpansion of the lung to the full space. Sometimes, instillation of fibrinolytic agents may be necessary to facilitate complete drainage by lysing of the fibrinous adhesions that may result in loculations. Repeated reassessment to ensure complete drainage must be done to prevent development of a chronic empyema due to delayed treatment and inadequate drainage. A smaller caliber chest tube may be adequate early on in the course of disease. One chest tube draining the posterior and apical portion of the effusion and an angled chest tube draining the basal and posterior costophrenic recesses may be needed.[25]

Treatment of Chronic Empyema

Closed pleural drainage (tube thoracostomy, thoracoscopy, and thoracotomy). Closed pleural drainage is the approach of choice whenever feasible for management of pleural empyema. This can be accomplished through thoracoscopic drainage and decortication or thoracotomy with drainage and decortication. Rarely, simple thoracostomy tube drainage with instillation of fibrinolytic agents and antimicrobial solutions may be successful in achieving complete drainage and lung reexpansion.[24]

Video-assisted thoracoscopic drainage and decortication and open thoracotomy with drainage and decortication are performed under general anesthesia. Therefore a patient has to be a good operative candidate to undergo these procedures. Simple thoracostomy tube drainage and video-assisted thoracoscopic drainage and decortication are associated with lower morbidity when compared with open thoracotomy with decortication, which may be associated with significant blood loss, persistent air leak, cardiac arrhythmias, and wound complications.[24,26] On the other hand, tube thoracostomy and video-assisted thoracoscopic approaches may not provide adequate and complete decortication and drainage with resolution of the infection. Therefore open drainage may be the only option in some patients.

Open pleural drainage. Open pleural drainage is usually reserved for very sick patients who will not be able to tolerate general anesthesia or are not good operative candidates due to medical comorbidities. A number of approaches have been used, including Eloesser flap, open window thoracostomy with partial resection of two to three ribs, limited thoracic window with dressing changes through this, and closed negative pressure wound system (vacuum therapy).

Eloesser flap thoracostomy window. The Eloesser flap thoracostomy window (EFTW) was described by Leo Eloesser in 1935 as an operative treatment option for tuberculous the pleural space infection associated with bronchopleural fistula to allow passive drainage of the pleural empyema and to act as a one-way valve to drain pleural space fluid without allowing entry of air into the pleural space. As such, the lung is allowed to reexpand and fill up the drained pleural space without collapsing from the pneumothorax.[27] With the advances made in antituberculous and antimicrobial therapy and early treatment of pleural space infection, the EFTW has been of limited use in modern times. However, it may be of use in patients who are poor candidates for operative drainage and decortication due to medical comorbidities and nutritional status. Other indications include failure of the lung to completely reexpand following decortication.

A detailed description of the EFTW is beyond the scope of this chapter. However, the original description of the flap included a 5-cm-wide and two-rib spaces long U-shaped flap of skin and subcutaneous tissue between the posterior axillary line and the caudal portion of the scapula. The base of the flap was two rib spaces over the lowest extent of the empyema cavity. The rib and intercostal muscle deep to the flap are resected, and the flap is placed in the pleural space and sutured to the pleural so that, as the lung reexpands and cavity collapses, the flap acts as a one-way valve.[27]

A modification of the original Eloesser flap was made by Symbas and colleagues in 1971,[28] with the modifications being the use of an inverted-U flap, the base of the flap being directly over the lowest extent of the empyema cavity, and the segment of rib or multiple segments of ribs or multiple ribs being resected depending on the size of the empyema and the patient size.

The Eloesser flap window commits patients to a prolonged time of wound care and dressing changes. Wound care advances have made it easier to manage such a wound, including wound vacuum-assisted closure (VAC). This is described in detail below. Both the EFTW and modified Eloesser flap can be performed under local anesthesia.

Clagett window (open window thoracostomy with partial rib resection). A Clagett open thoracotomy window is a staged procedure performed for the management of chronic empyema and consists of open window thoracostomy, antibiotic irrigation, and subsequent closure of the window. An H-shaped incision is made over the respective intercostal space, and flaps consisting of skin and subcutaneous tissue are raised. The underlying muscles are spared, and a rib or two are isolated and resected. The thickened parietal pleura is bluntly opened, and the empyema is drained, debrided, and decorticated. A pleural washout is performed. The skin flaps are sutured to the pleura with absorbable sutures anchored to the rib stumps, and the skin flaps are sutured to each other at the incision sites. The patient then undergoes daily dressing changes to sterilize the cavity. Eventually, once the lung reexpands and the pleural space has been obliterated, the flaps are released and closed. Alternatively, healing by secondary intention may be allowed.[29,30]

Closed vacuum-assisted closure with open window thoracostomy. This approach has been reported since 2004 and involves open window thoracostomy as described previously combined with wound management using the VAC system. The reported benefits of VAC system therapy include faster sterilization of the pleural space from the added vacuum suction as compared with nonsuction dressing changes, stimulation of granulation tissue formation, quicker obliteration of the pleural space through the vacuum suction force, and potentially enhanced lung reexpansion. All these benefits should lead to faster healing. In addition, VAC therapy may decrease hospital stay through outpatient wound VAC management.[31,32]

Closed vacuum-assisted closure with minimally invasive thoracostomy without rib resection. This minimally invasive approach has been described especially for very ill patients with multiple comorbidities. A mini thoracotomy without rib resection is made, and drainage of empyema and local decortication are performed. The pleural space is packed with continuous VAC sponges, which extend to the exterior and are connected to a vacuum therapy device. Once the infection has been cleared and the lung has reexpanded, the VAC therapy is discontinued and the wound is closed. Wound VAC therapy may also be combined with antimicrobial fluid instillation.[33]

Clostridium difficile Infection

Clostridium difficile infection (CDI) is the most common cause of nosocomial diarrhea in the United States with increasing incidence and severity. It carries significant morbidity and mortality, causing a huge financial burden to the health care system with an annual cost in the United States of $6.3 billion.[34] Common risk factors for CDI include a history of antibiotic use, being immunocompromised, having inflammatory bowel disease, undergoing chemotherapy, prior hospitalization, age over 65, admission to the ICU, and use of proton pump inhibitors. It has been postulated that prior exposure to antimicrobial therapy and widespread use of proton pump inhibitors cause an increase in population of pathologic bacteria in the gastrointestinal tract, causing dysbiosis, leading to an increase in pathogenic flora within the microbiome.

Early diagnosis of CDI is critical. Patients with unexplained and new-onset passage of three or more unformed stools in 24 hours should be tested for CDI. Diagnosis can be made using a stool toxin test as part of a multistep algorithm and colonoscopic or histopathologic findings of pseudomembranous colitis. Repeat testing is discouraged within 7 days unless for epidemiologic studies. Routine testing should not be performed in children younger than 2 years of age, unless other infectious or noninfectious causes have been excluded.

In 2017, the Infectious Diseases Society of America (IDSA) and the Society of Healthcare Epidemiology of America published an evidence-based recommendation for CDI based on severity of disease (see Table 11.5).[35] Oral (PO) vancomycin, 125 mg every 6 hours, or fidaxomicin, 200 mg PO twice daily for 10 days is the recommended treatment for the initial episode of CDI. For fulminant CDI, defined as presence of hypotension, shock, ileus, or toxic megacolon, the recommended treatment is oral vancomycin 500 mg 3 times daily. In the presence of ileus, vancomycin 500 mg in 100 cc normal saline per rectum every 6 hours as a retention enema should be considered. Metronidazole, 500 mg IV every 8 hours, is recommended in addition to rectal vancomycin if ileus is present. Oral metronidazole is an alternative medication if vancomycin or fidaxomicin is limited or unavailable. Fecal microbiota transplantation is associated with symptom resolution and effective for recurrent CDI.[36]

Early surgical consultation is recommended in patients with severe and complicated CDI. The traditional surgical approach for severe CDI is abdominal total colectomy, usually reserved for patients with peritonitis, perforation, ischemia, necrosis, or toxic megacolon. Laparoscopic or open diverting loop colostomy has been described as a less invasive option[37]; this is paired with colonic irrigation using 8 L of warmed polyethylene glycol/electrolyte solution intraoperatively and antegrade colonic enemas with vancomycin (500 mg in 500 mL via ileostomy efferent limb)

TABLE 11.5 **IDSA/SHEA recommendations for the treatment of *Clostridium difficile* infection.**

CLINICAL DEFINITION	CLINICAL SIGNS/ SYMPTOMS	RECOMMENDED TREATMENT	STRENGTH OF RECOMMENDATION/ QUALITY OF EVIDENCE
Initial episode, non-severe	Leukocytosis with WBC ≤15,000 + Creatinine <1.5 mg/dL	Vancomycin 125 mg QID for 10 days, OR Fidaxomicin 200 mg BID for 10 days	Strong/high Strong/high
		Alternate if above agents are unavailable: metronidazole 500 mg TID PO for 10 days	Weak/high
Initial episode (severe)	Leukocytosis with WBC ≥15,000 OR Creatinine ≥1.5 mg/dL	Vancomycin 125 mg QID PO for 10 days, OR Fidaxomicin 200 mg BID for 10 days	Strong/high Strong/high
Initial episode, fulminant	Hypotension or shock, ileus, megacolon	Vancomycin 500 mg PO QID or by NGT.	Strong/moderate
		If ileus, consider adding rectal installation of Vancomycin.	Weak/low
		Metronidazole IV (500 mg every 8 hours) should be administered together with oral or rectal Vancomycin, particularly if ileus is present	Strong/moderate
First recurrence		Vancomycin 125 mg QID for 10 days if metronidazole was used for the initial episode, OR use a prolonged tapered and pulsed Vancomycin regimen if a standard specimen was used for the initial episode (e.g., 125 mg QID for 10–14 days, BID for 1 week, once per day for 1 week, and then every 2 or 3 days for 2–8 weeks), OR	Weak/low Weak/low
		Fidaxomicin 200 mg BID for 10 days if Vancomycin was used for the initial episode.	Weak/moderate
Second or subsequent recurrence		Vancomycin in a tapered and pulsed regimen, OR Vancomycin, 125 mg QID PO for 10 days followed by Rifaximin 400 mg TID for 20 days OR Fidaxomicin 200 mg PO BID for 10 days OR Fecal microbiota transplantation	Weak/low Weak/low Weak/low Strong/moderate

BID, Two times a day; *IDSA*, Infectious Diseases Society of America; *IV*, intravenous; *NGT*, nasogastric tube; *PO*, orally; *QID*, four times a day; *SHEA*, Society for Healthcare Epidemiology of America; *TID*, three times a day; *WBC*, white blood count.
Adapted from McDonald LC, Gerding DN, Johnson S, et al. Clinical practice guidelines for *Clostridium difficile* infection in adults and children: 2017 update by the Infectious Diseases Society of America (IDSA) and Society for Healthcare Epidemiology of America (SHEA). *Clin Infect Dis*. 2018;66:987–994.

postoperatively. One multicenter study showed that diverting loop ileostomy had less mortality than total colectomy and should be considered in the surgical treatment of CDI.[38]

Effective antibiotic stewardship is key to the prevention of CDI. Given the epidemiologic link between proton pump inhibitor and CDI, unnecessary use of proton pump inhibitors should be discontinued. Prevention can be achieved by routine adequate hand washing before and after contact with the patient; importantly, using an alcohol-based hand sanitizer is insufficient to prevent transmission of CDI. Unlike most other nosocomial infections, patients with suspected CDI should be placed on isolation in a private room with a separate toileting area. Gloves and gown should be standard practice for providers and visitors with suspected disease. The recommendation is to continue this practice for at least 48 hours after resolution of the diarrhea.

A recent systematic review with meta regression analysis showed that administering probiotics at the time of first dose of antibiotic reduces the risk of CDI by >50% in hospitalized patients.[39] The optimal dosage, formulation, and species are still under investigation. In 2017, The U.S. Food and Drug Administration approved the use of bezlotoxumab, a human monoclonal antibody to *C. difficile* that can be given as a single IV dose to provide protection against recurrent *C. difficile* infection for up to 2 weeks for patients at high risk for recurrence.[40]

Clostridium septicum and Colorectal Malignancy

In general, gas gangrene, or *Clostridial* myonecrosis, is a rare life-threatening illness resulting from NSTI. More commonly, it is associated with traumatic or surgical wounds, and this type is caused by *Clostridium perfringens*.

However, the much rarer form of gas gangrene is the nontraumatic spontaneous type, which occurs in 16% of cases, and the etiologic organism is the more virulent *Clostridium septicum*. Nontraumatic spontaneous gas gangrene is often associated with underlying malignancy or immunosuppression. Specifically, the association of *C. septicum* infection and colorectal cancer is widely reported in literature. With this strong association, patients with *C. septicum*–positive blood cultures should undergo colonoscopy even if they demonstrate no obvious clinical features of colon cancer. The pathophysiology of this unique association is postulated to be due to malignancy-associated disruption of the colonic mucosa, resulting in a local hypoxic milieu, which in turn facilitates rapid proliferation of *C. septicum* with exotoxin production. Exotoxins lead to increased translocation of the *C. septicum* from the colon to systemic circulation due to exotoxin-induced increase in capillary permeability and subsequent development of infection of nearby tissues.[41] Unlike other *Clostridial* species, *C. septicum* is able to invade and infect healthy tissues. Associated 50% to 60% mortality of *C. septicum* infection is two to three times higher than all other *Clostridial* species' infections.[41] Immediate and early treatment with IV antibiotics and operative debridement is the mainstay of therapy.

HEALTH CARE–ASSOCIATED INFECTIONS

Health care–associated infections are unfortunately common and a major cause of increased morbidity and health care expenditure in the United States. Regulatory bodies and insurers consider these preventable infections and monitor their incidence, with direct impact on hospital reimbursement. Therefore, it is important for multiple reasons that surgeons are familiar with these infections and actively participate in efforts to reduce this preventable harm. Three health care–associated infections that commonly occur in surgical inpatients are briefly discussed.

Catheter-Associated Bloodstream Infections

Central venous lines are commonly used in surgical patients to provide IV access, for advanced monitoring in the ICU and operating room, and for parenteral nutrition and hemodialysis. While catheter-associated bloodstream infections are uncommon, they carry a 25% mortality when they do occur. Efforts to reduce the risk of catheter-associated bloodstream infections include CDC-recommended infection control guidelines and a checklist for all line insertions to ensure attention to sterile technique and removal of the line as soon as possible. Thanks to these efforts, the incidence of catheter-associated bloodstream infections in ICUs was reduced by 58% over the past decade, with a 73% reduction in *Staphylococcus aureus* infections.[42]

Catheter-Associated Urinary Tract Infections

Indwelling urinary catheter use is common in surgical inpatients. They are used to prevent urinary retention as well as monitor urine output on an hourly basis. Despite their utility, each day the indwelling urinary catheter remains increases the risk of the patient acquiring catheter-associated urinary tract infections by 3% to 7%.[43] The definition of catheter-associated urinary tract infection requires that a patient has an indwelling catheter for 2 or more days; clinical symptoms of a urinary infection such as suprapubic tenderness, urgency, frequency or fever; and a urine culture showing $>10^5$ growth of a pathogenic organism. In order to reduce the incidence of catheter-associated urinary tract infections, it is recommended that indwelling catheters be used only when necessary rather than as a routine, be placed using strict aseptic technique, and be removed as soon as feasible. Many institutions have implemented nurse-driven removal protocols to expedite this process.

Ventilator-Associated Pneumonia

Prolonged intubation of the respiratory tract, as happens in many trauma and complex surgical patients, increases the risk of pneumonia. The true incidence of ventilator-associated pneumonia is difficult to discern due to varying definitions and criteria for ventilator-associated events and differing surveillance methodology among institutions. Nonetheless, there is agreement on broad principles for the prevention of ventilator-associated pneumonia, which include attempting noninvasive ventilation where feasible, elevation of the head of the bed above 30 degrees, subglottic suctioning, minimization of interruptions to sterility of the ventilator circuit, and the overall goal of rapid ventilator liberation. Strategies to achieve this goal include reducing sedative use, routine daily sedation vacations with spontaneous breathing trials, and early mobility.[44]

ANTIBIOTIC RESISTANCE

Antimicrobial resistance (AMR) usually occurs naturally as microbes evolve. However, development of resistance has been accelerated by antimicrobial use practices that are inappropriate, unnecessary, and/or suboptimal as defined previously. Widely and rapidly spreading AMR including multidrug and pandrug resistance organisms has complicated treatment of these infections and resulted in increased morbidity, mortality, and cost of health care.

The common mechanisms of AMR include direct antimicrobial inactivation or modification by the microbes; decreased permeability of the antibiotic into the microbial intracellular compartment; active efflux of the antibiotic from the microbial intracellular compartment; antimicrobial target site/receptor alteration or protection, therefore reducing antibiotic-target site binding; and alteration of microbial metabolic pathways usually targeted by the antibiotic. These mechanisms of AMR may occur through intrinsic microbial gene mutations or acquisition of new genes from other strains or species through plasmids, phages, or transposons.

Appropriate Antibiotic Use

Indiscriminate and unnecessary antimicrobial use is associated with significant patient risks, including drug toxicities, *Clostridium difficile* colitis, and multidrug-resistant infections. In a recent study by the CDC, at least 50% of patients receive at least one antibiotic during their hospital stay, and this overall trend had not changed over the preceding decade, but patients are now receiving the more powerful antibiotics more often, including a 37% increased use of carbapenems and a 32% increase in the use of vancomycin. Additionally, antibiotics were often being used without proper microbiologic testing or for too long and when not needed. Such practices are significant contributors to multiple antimicrobial use–associated complications. There is, therefore, a serious need for appropriate antimicrobial use measures and stewardship, as well as monitoring, to eliminate the inappropriate, suboptimal, and unnecessary use and the associated risks and complications.

Up until recently, there was no reference standard regarding appropriate antibiotic use. Now, there are a number of publications that have focused on appropriate antibiotic use and measures to avoid unnecessary, suboptimal, and inappropriate use.

There has been a lack of a standard definition of what **appropriate antimicrobial use** is. However, Spivak and colleagues[45] have recently published proposals for the definition of unnecessary, inappropriate, and suboptimal antimicrobial use applied to days of therapy of specific antimicrobial agents. They emphasized, from an extensive literature review, the difficulty in developing a standard definition of appropriateness of antimicrobial use that is discriminatory yet reproducible and objective. As a result, they proposed that the approach to the ideal definition of appropriate antimicrobial use lies in establishing the correlation between the various definitions and quantitative antimicrobial use data and clinical outcomes. Based on their article, **unnecessary antimicrobial use** was defined as use of antimicrobials for noninfectious syndromes, antibiotics for nonbacterial infections, antimicrobial duration of use beyond the indicated period without clinical indication, and failure to narrow down an empiric antibiotic spectrum after culture and sensitivities reveal that infecting pathogen. **Inappropriate antimicrobial use** was defined as use of antimicrobial agents to which the pathogen is resistant or that are not recommended in the treatment guidelines in the setting of established infection. **Suboptimal antimicrobial use** was defined as the use of an inappropriate antimicrobial drug choice, drug route, or drug dose in the setting of established infection.

On the other hand, van den Bosch and colleagues[46] developed and validated six quality improvement variables defining appropriate antibiotic use. These include prescribing empirical antibiotic therapy according to published guidelines, obtaining at least two sets of blood cultures before starting systemic antibiotic therapy, obtaining specimen for cultures from suspected infection sites before starting systemic therapy, documenting the antibiotic plan in the patient chart at the start of systemic antibiotic therapy, switching IV antibiotic therapy to oral antibiotic therapy within 48 to 72 hours on the basis of clinical condition and when oral treatment is adequate, and switching empirical antibiotic therapy to pathogen-directed therapy once culture sensitivity results become available.[46]

The Global Alliance for Infections in Surgery Working Group, comprising of interdisciplinary task force of 234 experts from 83 countries, has published a global declaration on appropriate use of antimicrobial agents across the surgical pathway. In the declaration, seven detailed principles of appropriate antibiotic prophylaxis and 13 principles for appropriate antibiotic therapy in surgical procedures were published. These are detailed in the article in the 2017 Global Alliance Position Article.

Antibiotic stewardship programs have been shown to optimize treatment of infection while decreasing antibiotic resistance. Antibiotic prescribing needs to be monitored and audited. Audit tools that enable large volume data collection by any member of the medical team (including nurse, microbiologists, physicians, pharmacists, and infection control practitioners) without requiring expert review while allowing for hospital-type comparison are ideal. The CDC has developed objective audit tools that meet these criteria, which can be used to assess appropriate antibiotic use. These tools, when used with the electronic medical records, may facilitate reproducible and large-scale data to assess appropriateness of antibiotic use.

CLINICALLY IMPORTANT PATHOGENS

Carbapenem-Resistant Enterobacteriaceae

Due to their broad-spectrum antimicrobial activity against gram-positive, gram-negative aerobic, and anaerobic pathogens, carbapenems have, up until recently, been used as last-line antibiotics for the treatment of multidrug-resistant Enterobacteriaceae, including the extended-spectrum beta-lactamase–procedure species.[47]

However, there is now a rising spread of carbapenem-resistant Enterobacteriaceae (CRE), which produce enzymes that deactivate beta lactam antibiotics including carbapenems. CRE accounts for 6.6% of approximately 140,000 health care–associated Enterobacteriaceae infections per year in the United States, with carbapenem-resistant *Klebsiella* species accounting for 5.6% and carbapenem-resistant *Escherichia coli* accounting for 1.3%. These two are the most common CREs, resulting in about 10,000 annual infections in the United States.

In Germany, multidrug-resistant gram-negative bacteria *E. coli, Klebsiella pneumoniae*, and *Pseudomonas aeruginosa* account for 6.6% to 9.8% of infections on the regular floor and 11.5% to 13.4% of infections in the ICUs. CREs are resistant to nearly all antibiotics, including the antibiotics of last resort (i.e., carbapenems). Carbapenemases are the enzymes produced by CREs that confer antibiotic resistance by deactivating the beta lactam antibiotics including carbapenems, cephalosporins, penicillins, and monobactam aztreonam. Due to the resultant limited treatment options, CRE infections are associated with a high mortality, with up to 50% of all CRE bloodstream infections leading to death.

Mode of Transmission

The common mode of transmission for CRE is by direct contact from patient to patient, usually through the hands of the health care personnel or indirectly through medical equipment and environmental surfaces.

Reservoirs

Colonized and infected patients are the main reservoirs for CRE organisms, especially because Enterobacteriaceae are part of the normal flora in the gastrointestinal tract. Contaminated colonized surfaces can also act as reservoirs.

Risk Factors for Carbapenem-Resistant Enterobacteriaceae Infections

Factors that increase risk of CRE infection include critical illness, immunosuppression, exposure to the ICU environment, use of broad-spectrum antibiotics, mechanical ventilation, and indwelling urinary and central venous catheters.

Treatment

Despite the increasing incidence of CRE infections worldwide, there is lack of high-quality data regarding the ideal treatment options for CRE infections. There are no randomized controlled trials on this topic, and current available data are limited to retrospective data, case series, and in vitro studies. A number of antimicrobials that may be considered for treatment of CRE infections include carbapenems, tigecycline, polymyxin B, colistin, fosfomycin, and aminoglycosides.[35]

Several case series, retrospective studies, and in vitro studies have shown that monotherapy treatment options against CRE are extremely limited, including pharmacokinetics and susceptibility to a new resistance. As a result, the best treatment strategy includes combined therapy with two or more agents that takes advantage of potential synergistic effects and minimizes the development of resistance. Combined therapy has been shown to be an independent predictor of survival, especially carbapenems with tigecycline or colistin. Tzouvelekis and colleagues[48] and Petrosillo and colleagues[49] showed combined therapy with two or more in vitro active agents to be associated with lower mortality when compared with monotherapy with an in vitro active agent (18.3%–27.4% vs. 38.7%–49.1%).

Vancomycin-Resistant Enterococcus

About one-third of all 66,000 annual Enterococcus infections are cause by drug-resistant bacteria, resulting in significant morbidity and a mortality rate of 6.5%. *E. faecium* accounts for the majority of the vancomycin-resistant Enterococcus (VRE). In the majority of cases, VRE colonization accounts for most cases of VRE positive cultures. However, VRE isolates associated with VRE bacteremia and symptomatic body cavity infection warrant treatment. The treatment options for VRE are few to none.

Mode of Transmission

Transmission is patient to patient by direct contact via temporary carriage on the hands of health care personnel (inadequate or no hand washing) or indirect transfer through patient care equipment or surrounding surfaces including bed rails, sinks, door knobs, testing equipment, etc.

VRE Reservoirs

While VRE can be spread by direct contact or indirectly as indicated previously, most infections are due to the patient's endogenous flora because *Enterococci* comprise part of the normal gastrointestinal and female reproductive tract flora. It is important to account for indirect transmission via environmental and equipment surfaces since VRE can persist for weeks on such surfaces. In addition, residents of long-term care facilities who are VRE-colonized may act as VRE reservoirs to acute care hospitals and vice versa.

Risk Factors for VRE Infection

Patients at high risk for VRE infection include patients who are immunosuppressed, critically ill, on hemodialysis, on broad-spectrum antibiotic therapy, with indwelling urinary or central venous catheters, and postoperative following major abdominal or thoracic procedure.

Treatment

The current treatment for invasive VRE infection primarily involves use of daptomycin or linezolid. Daptomycin is bactericidal against many VRE strains with relatively minimal toxicity. However, selection of nonsusceptible VRE strains is common. Linezolid is bacteriostatic with potential significant toxicity and drug interactions with other drugs. It has excellent oral bioavailability. Resistance to linezolid is very infrequent and may occur with prolonged exposure. Tedizolid has similar mechanism of action to linezolid but is more potent.

Fungal Infections in Surgical Patients

Invasive fungal infections (IFIs) are increasingly becoming prevalent especially due to the increasing use of immunosuppressive therapy in the management of transplantation, autoimmune and connective tissues diseases, malignancy, and inflammatory diseases. Patients admitted to ICUs with severe illness with invasive interventions and catheters are especially vulnerable to IFIs. *Candida* spp. is the leading cause of invasive nosocomial fungal infections and is the third leading cause of bloodstream infections in the ICU and the fourth overall cause of disseminated bloodstream infection. *Candida albicans* accounts for more than half of the *Candida* IFIs. *C. glabrata* and *C. parapsilosis* are the second and third most common, respectively. Other important *Candida* spp. include *C. auris*, *C. lusitaniae*, *C. tropicalis*, and *C. krusei*.

Non-*Candida* IFI often also arises from molds, especially the *Aspergillus* spp. Invasive aspergillosis is now a significant cause of IFIs in critically ill patients in the ICU and in patients with myelosuppression and post–stem cell transplantation.

Less common fungal species–causing infections include *Mucormycosis* spp., *Cryptococcus* spp., and *Fusarium* spp.

Mode of Transmission

Since *Candida* spp. is part of the normal flora in mucosal surfaces, it tends to cause local mucosal infections in the urinary tract and gastrointestinal tract or disseminated infections arising from disruption of the mucosal surfaces where *Candida* is part of the normal flora.

Aspergillus spp. is transmitted via inhalation of conidia as well as contaminated environmental and medical equipment surfaces.

Risk Factors

Patients most vulnerable to IFIs include patients on immunosuppression therapy for organ transplantation, patients with malignancy, burn patients, patients with autoimmune and rheumatologic disorders, critically ill patients in the ICU, and patients with chronic indwelling urinary and central venous catheters. Other risk factors include hematopoietic stem cell transplant, hemodialysis, neutropenia, prolonged mechanical ventilation, total parenteral nutrition, necrotizing pancreatitis, major surgery, and chemotherapy.

Diagnosis

Diagnosis of IFIs can be challenging, and the traditional approaches to diagnosis by clinical signs and symptoms, laboratory evaluation, imaging findings, and culture have significant limitations. To improve on these limitations, rapid diagnostic tests have been developed. These include beta D-glycan text for *Candida* and *Aspergillus* (sensitivity 57%–97%, specificity 56%–93%), nucleic-acid polymerase chain reaction for all fungal species (sensitivity 96%, specificity 97%), Galactomannan test for *Aspergillus* (sensitivity 71% and specificity 89% for serum and 76% to 88% and 87% to 100%, respectively, for bronchoalveolar lavage), and mannan antigen/antimannan antibody test for *Candida* spp. (sensitivity andspecificity for combined antigen and antibody are 83% and 86%, respectively).

Beta D-glycan diagnostic test has been recommended as an adjunct to culture. Mannan is a polysaccharide component of the fungal cell wall specific to *Candida* spp. The mannan antigen and the antimannan antibodies can be evaluated by commercially available tests.

Treatment of Invasive Fungal Infections

The most recent 2016 update by the IDSA guidelines provides the basis for treatment recommendations for IFIs in the surgical patient. The reader is referred to these guidelines for more detailed information on treatment of *Candida* infections[50] and aspergillosis.[51] The following are a few of the recommendations for select fungal infections in the surgical patients.

Candidemia in nonneutropenic patients. Based on the IDSA guidelines, initial therapy should be an echinocandin (caspofungin, micafungin, or anidulafungin). Alternative therapy can be with fluconazole in select patients. If an echinocandin is used as initial therapy, transition to fluconazole within 5 to 7 days is recommended when clinically appropriate and supported by fungal susceptibilities. Amphotericin B may be used in situation of echinocandin intolerance, unavailability, or resistance with transition to fluconazole within 5 to 7 days based on the patient's clinical condition and fungal susceptibilities. Amphotericin B is the recommended treatment in cases of azole- and echinocandin-resistant invasive *Candida* infections. Treatment duration is generally 2 weeks after documented negative blood cultures with clearance of candidemia. Central venous catheters should be removed in the setting of candidemia if suspected to be the source of candidemia.[50]

Candidemia in neutropenic patients. Echinocandins are still recommended as the initial therapy of candidemia in neutropenic patients. Use of amphotericin B, while an effective alternative, is limited by toxicity. In patients who are not critically ill, both fluconazole and voriconazole are appropriate for step-down therapy, following documented clearance of candidemia and with appropriate fungal susceptibilities. A 2-week treatment duration is recommended for candidemia without metastatic complications after documented clearance of candidemia and with appropriate fungal susceptibilities.[50]

Intraabdominal candidiasis. Patients with significant risk of intraabdominal candidiasis include those with recent abdominal surgery, anastomotic leaks, or necrotizing pancreatitis. Treatment includes source control via operative drainage, debridement, and repair or percutaneous drainage, as well as antifungal therapy. Antifungal therapy choices and guidelines are similar to those used for the treatment of candidemia in nonneutropenic patients as detailed previously.

Invasive aspergillosis. The IDSA recommendation for primary treatment is early initiation of voriconazole therapy. Primary treatment with an echinocandin is not recommended. However, an echinocandin may be used with voriconazole as combination antifungal therapy. Strongly recommended duration of therapy is 6 to 12 weeks, depending on the site of infection, response to therapy, and duration of immunosuppression. Surgical intervention should be considered in addition to antifungal therapy in cases of refractory abdominal aspergillosis (including perihepatic biliary obstruction, extrahepatic aspergillosis), *Aspergillus* endocarditis/pericarditis/myocarditis, *Aspergillus* osteomyelitis/septic arthritis, and paranasal aspergillosis.[51]

SELECTED REFERENCES

Fernando SM, Tran A, Cheng W, et al. Necrotizing soft tissue infection: diagnostic accuracy of physical examination, imaging, and LRINEC score: a systematic review and meta-analysis. *Ann Surg.* 2019;269:58–65.

This article showed the poor sensitivity of the laboratory risk indicator for necrotizing fasciitis score, physical examination, and plain radiography in diagnosing necrotizing soft tissue infection; it affirmed that high clinical suspicion warrants immediate surgical consultation.

Marik PE, Khangoora V, Rivera R, et al. Hydrocortisone, vitamin C, and thiamine for the treatment of severe sepsis and septic shock: a retrospective before-after study. *Chest.* 2017;151:1229–1238.

A study demonstrating that early use of vitamin C, steroids, and thiamine may help prevent progressive organ dysfunction and reduce mortality in patients with severe sepsis.

Neal MD, Alverdy JC, Hall DE, et al. Diverting loop ileostomy and colonic lavage: an alternative to total abdominal colectomy for the treatment of severe, complicated *Clostridium difficile* associated disease. *Ann Surg.* 2011;254:423–427; discussion 427–429.

A landmark paper on the alternative surgical management of severe complicated Clostridium difficile *infection.*

Singer M, Deutschman CS, Seymour CW, et al. The third international consensus definitions for Sepsis and Septic Shock (Sepsis-3). *JAMA.* 2016;315:801–810.

Updated international consensus on the definition of sepsis and septic shock for clinical, epidemiologic, and research use.

REFERENCES

1. Singer M, Deutschman CS, Seymour CW, et al. The third international consensus definitions for Sepsis and Septic Shock (Sepsis-3). *JAMA.* 2016;315:801–810.
2. Liu V, Escobar GJ, Greene JD, et al. Hospital deaths in patients with sepsis from 2 independent cohorts. *JAMA.* 2014;312:90–92.
3. Fleischmann C, Scherag A, Adhikari NK, et al. Assessment of global incidence and mortality of hospital-treated sepsis. Current estimates and limitations. *Am J Respir Crit Care Med.* 2016;193:259–272.
4. Levy MM, Evans LE, Rhodes A. The surviving sepsis campaign bundle: 2018 update. *Crit Care Med.* 2018;46:997–1000.
5. Ban KA, Minei JP, Laronga C, et al. American College of Surgeons and Surgical Infection Society: surgical site infection guidelines, 2016 update. *J Am Coll Surg.* 2017;224:59–74.
6. Anderson DJ, Podgorny K, Berrios-Torres SI, et al. Strategies to prevent surgical site infections in acute care hospitals: 2014 update. *Infect Control Hosp Epidemiol.* 2014;35(suppl 2):S66–S88.
7. Horan TC, Andrus M, Dudeck MA. CDC/NHSN surveillance definition of health care–associated infection and criteria for specific types of infections in the acute care setting. *Am J Infect Control.* 20018;36:309–332.
8. Berrios-Torres SI, Umscheid CA, Bratzler DW, et al. Centers for disease control and prevention guideline for the prevention of surgical site infection, 2017. *JAMA Surg.* 2017;152:784–791.
9. O'Leary DP, Peirce C, Anglim B, et al. Prophylactic negative pressure dressing use in closed laparotomy wounds following abdominal operations: a randomized, controlled, open-label trial: the P.I.C.O. Trial. *Ann Surg.* 2017;265:1082–1086.
10. Wong CH, Chang HC, Pasupathy S, et al. Necrotizing fasciitis: clinical presentation, microbiology, and determinants of mortality. *J Bone Joint Surg Am.* 2003;85-A:1454–1460.
11. Fernando SM, Tran A, Cheng W, et al. Necrotizing soft tissue infection: diagnostic accuracy of physical examination, imaging, and LRINEC score: a systematic review and meta-analysis. *Ann Surg.* 2019;269:58–65.
12. Martinez M, Peponis T, Hage A, et al. The role of computed tomography in the diagnosis of necrotizing soft tissue infections. *World J Surg.* 2018;42:82–87.
13. Kobayashi L, Konstantinidis A, Shackelford S, et al. Necrotizing soft tissue infections: delayed surgical treatment is associated with increased number of surgical debridements and morbidity. *J Trauma.* 2011;71:1400–1405.
14. Zhao-Fleming H, Dissanaike S, Rumbaugh K. Are anaerobes a major, underappreciated cause of necrotizing infections? *Anaerobe.* 2017;45:65–70.
15. Marik PE, Khangoora V, Rivera R, et al. Hydrocortisone, vitamin C, and thiamine for the treatment of severe sepsis and septic shock: a retrospective before-after study. *Chest.* 2017;151:1229–1238.
16. Yang D, Davies A, Burge B, et al. Open-to-air is a viable option for initial wound care in necrotizing soft tissue infection that allows early detection of recurrence without need for painful dressing changes or return to operating room. *Surg Infect (Larchmt).* 2018;19:6570.
17. Sartelli M, Chichom-Mefire A, Labricciosa FM, et al. The management of intra-abdominal infections from a global perspective: 2017 WSES guidelines for management of intra-abdominal infections. *World J Emerg Surg.* 2017;12:29.
18. Rhodes A, Evans LE, Alhazzani W, et al. Surviving Sepsis Campaign: international guidelines for management of sepsis and septic shock: 2016. *Crit Care Med.* 2017;45:486–552.
19. Marshall JC. Principles of source control in the early management of sepsis. *Curr Infect Dis Rep.* 2010;12:345–353.
20. Brown CV, Abrishami M, Muller M, et al. Appendiceal abscess: immediate operation or percutaneous drainage? *Am Surg.* 2003;69:829–832.
21. Andersson RE, Petzold MG. Nonsurgical treatment of appendiceal abscess or phlegmon: a systematic review and meta-analysis. *Ann Surg.* 2007;246:741–748.

22. Lai HW, Loong CC, Chiu JH, et al. Interval appendectomy after conservative treatment of an appendiceal mass. *World J Surg*. 2006;30:352–357.
23. Soreide K, Thorsen K, Soreide JA. Clinical patterns of presentation and attenuated inflammatory response in octo- and nonagenarians with perforated gastroduodenal ulcers. *Surgery*. 2016;160:341–349.
24. Taylor MD, Kozower BD. Surgical spectrum in the management of empyemas. *Thorac Surg Clin*. 2012;22:431–440.
25. Ferreiro L, San Jose ME, Valdes L. Management of parapneumonic pleural effusion in adults. *Arch Bronconeumol*. 2015;51:637–646.
26. Tong BC, Hanna J, Toloza EM, et al. Outcomes of video-assisted thoracoscopic decortication. *Ann Thorac Surg*. 2010;89:220–225.
27. Denlinger CE. Eloesser flap thoracostomy window. *Oper Tech Thorac Cardiovasc Surg*. 2010;15:61–69.
28. Symbas PN, Nugent JT, Abbott OA, et al. Nontuberculous pleural empyema in adults. The role of a modified Eloesser procedure in its management. *Ann Thorac Surg*. 1971;12:69–78.
29. Zaheer S, Allen MS, Cassivi SD, et al. Postpneumonectomy empyema: results after the Clagett procedure. *Ann Thorac Surg*. 2006;82:279–286; discussion 286–277.
30. Massera F, Robustellini M, Della Pona C, et al. Open window thoracostomy for pleural empyema complicating partial lung resection. *Ann Thorac Surg*. 2009;87:869–873.
31. Sziklavari Z, Grosser C, Neu R, et al. Complex pleural empyema can be safely treated with vacuum-assisted closure. *J Cardiothorac Surg*. 2011;6:130.
32. Aru GM, Jew NB, Tribble CG, et al. Intrathoracic vacuum-assisted management of persistent and infected pleural spaces. *Ann Thorac Surg*. 2010;90:266–270.
33. Mariani AW, Lisboa JBRM, Rodrigues GD, et al. Mini-thoracostomy with vacuum-assisted closure: a minimally invasive alternative to open-window thoracostomy. *J Brasil Pneumol*. 2018;44:227–230.
34. Zhang S, Palazuelos-Munoz S, Balsells EM, et al. Cost of hospital management of *Clostridium difficile* infection in United States—a meta-analysis and modelling study. *BMC Infect Dis*. 2016;16:447.
35. McDonald LC, Gerding DN, Johnson S, et al. Clinical practice guidelines for *Clostridium difficile* infection in adults and children: 2017 update by the Infectious Diseases Society of America (IDSA) and Society for Healthcare Epidemiology of America (SHEA). *Clin Infect Dis*. 2018;66:987–994.
36. Chapman BC, Moore HB, Overbey DM, et al. Fecal microbiota transplant in patients with *Clostridium difficile* infection: a systematic review. *J Trauma Acute Care Surg*. 2016;81:756–764.
37. Neal MD, Alverdy JC, Hall DE, et al. Diverting loop ileostomy and colonic lavage: an alternative to total abdominal colectomy for the treatment of severe, complicated *Clostridium difficile* associated disease. *Ann Surg*. 2011;254:423–427; discussion 427–429.
38. Ferrada P, Callcut R, Zielinski MD, et al. Loop ileostomy versus total colectomy as surgical treatment for *Clostridium difficile*-associated disease: an Eastern Association for the Surgery of Trauma multicenter trial. *J Trauma Acute Care Surg*. 2017;83:36–40.
39. Shen NT, Leff JA, Schneider Y, et al. Cost-effectiveness analysis of probiotic use to prevent *Clostridium difficile* infection in hospitalized adults receiving antibiotics. *Open Forum Infect Dis*. 2017;4; ofx148.
40. Wilcox MH, Gerding DN, Poxton IR, et al. Bezlotoxumab for prevention of recurrent *Clostridium difficile* infection. *N Engl J Med*. 2017;376:305–317.
41. Cullinane C, Earley H, Tormey S. Deadly combination: *Clostridium septicum* and colorectal malignancy. *BMJ Case Rep*. 2017;2017.
42. Centers for Disease Control and Prevention (CDC). Making health care safer. *CDC Vital Signs Monthly Report*. Atlanta, GA: Centers for Disease Control and Prevention; 2011:1–4.
43. Centers for Disease Control and Prevention (CDC). *Urinary Tract Infection (Catheter-Associated Urinary Tract Infection [CAUTI] and Non-Catheter-Associated Urinary Tract Infection [UTI]) and Other Urinary System Infection [USI]) Events in National Healthcare Safety Network (NHSN) Patient Safety Component Manual, 2019*. Atlanta: 2019:7-1:7–17.
44. Klompas M, Branson R, Eichenwald EC, et al. Strategies to prevent ventilator-associated pneumonia in acute care hospitals: 2014 update. *Infect Control Hosp Epidemiol*. 2014;35:915–936.
45. Spivak ES, Cosgrove SE, Srinivasan A. Measuring appropriate antimicrobial use: attempts at opening the black box. *Clin Infect Dis*. 2016;63:1639–1644.
46. van den Bosch CM, Hulscher ME, Natsch S, et al. Applicability of generic quality indicators for appropriate antibiotic use in daily hospital practice: a cross-sectional point-prevalence multicenter study. *Clin Microbiol Infect*. 2016;22:888.e881–e888, e889.
47. Morrill HJ, Pogue JM, Kaye KS, et al. Treatment options for carbapenem-resistant Enterobacteriaceae infections. *Open Forum Infect Dis*. 2015;2; ofv050.
48. Tzouvelekis LS, Markogiannakis A, Piperaki E, et al. Treating infections caused by carbapenemase-producing Enterobacteriaceae. *Clin Microbiol Infect*. 2014;20:862–872.
49. Petrosillo N, Giannella M, Lewis R, et al. Treatment of carbapenem-resistant *Klebsiella pneumoniae*: the state of the art. *Expert Rev Anti Infect Ther*. 2013;11:159–177.
50. Pappas PG, Kauffman CA, Andes DR, et al. Clinical practice guideline for the management of candidiasis: 2016 update by the Infectious Diseases Society of America. *Clin Infect Dis*. 2016;62:e1–e50.
51. Patterson TF, Thompson 3rd GR, Denning DW, et al. Practice guidelines for the diagnosis and management of aspergillosis: 2016 update by the Infectious Diseases Society of America. *Clin Infect Dis*. 2016;63:e1–e60.

12 CHAPTER

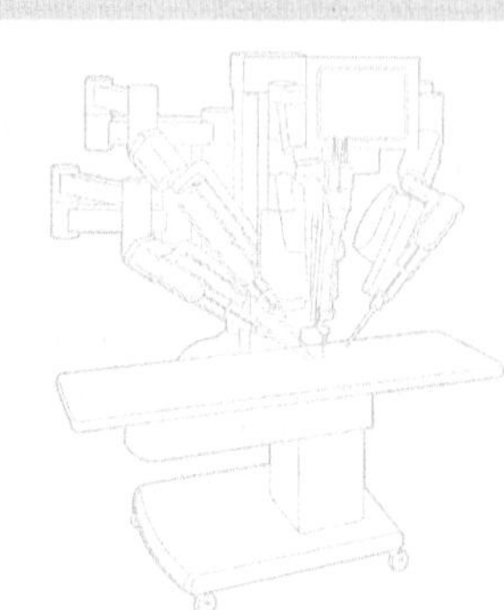

Surgical Complications

Natesh Yepuri, Napat Pruekprasert, Robert N. Cooney

OUTLINE

The current health care environment has increased our focus on the cost and quality of surgical care. As a result, many hospitals and physicians are devoting significant efforts to understand and benchmark the risk of complications in surgical patients. One approach uses risk-adjusted administrative data sets (e.g., Vizient) to generate reports comparing observed to expected complications among different hospitals and departments. Another, the American College of Surgeons National Surgical Quality Improvement Program (NSQIP), collects individual patient data and reports institution-specific, risk-adjusted surgical outcomes.

While most surgeons realize that complications increase the cost of care, the incentives to reduce costs by decreasing complications have been limited in many practice environments. More recently, the Center for Medicare and Medicaid Services has linked professional reimbursement for surgical services with the Merit-Based Incentive Payment System, which links cost and quality outcomes to surgeon payments. As these programs are implemented, there should be a more direct relationship between cost, quality, and surgeon reimbursement.

Although individual surgeon judgment and technique certainly impact the risk of complications, there are many other factors that contribute to surgical outcomes, including specific aspects of the patient population, the perioperative care team, and the environment in which surgical care is provided. Suffice it to say that even the best surgical judgment and technique are only as good as the system in which they practice. Furthermore, the transition to electronic medical records (EMRs) has significantly impacted the perioperative environment. Implementing "evidence-based best practices" to improve quality requires buy-in from multiple individuals, including the patient, the surgery residents, midlevel providers, anesthesiology, nursing, information technology, infectious disease, and others, to bend the cost-quality curve. Clinical care pathways were developed in the 1980s to provide multidisciplinary, evidence-based care for specific patients or surgical procedures. However, with the transition to EMRs, order sets were developed to facilitate the use of standardized patient care. Unfortunately, despite the theoretical potential to extract high-quality data on compliance with order sets and best practices from the EMR, the practical ability to do this has been disappointing at many institutions.

In addition to developing and implementing our own evidence-based surgical practices, we must educate the next generation of surgeons on best practices and quality improvement to reduce complication rates in our patients. With this in mind, the Accreditation Council for Graduate Medical Education developed the Continuous Learning Environment Review program designed to provide teaching hospitals with feedback on their graduate medical education environment as it relates to patient safety, health care quality, care transitions, supervision, duty hours, and fatigue management and professionalism. In addition, the American College of Surgeons developed the Quality in-Training Initiative, which provides a detailed curriculum on quality improvement for surgical residents. These and other initiatives like the Milestones project that require resident involvement and engagement in the Improvement of Care practice domain should help trainees to develop the skills required to improve quality and reduce complications.

Surgical complications is a large topic that has been classified by various methods, including patient risk factors, complication type, severity (e.g., hospital readmission and/or surgical mortality), and organ system. We rely heavily on classification by complication type, severity, and organ system in this chapter.

TABLE 12.1 Recommendations for timing of discontinuation of anticoagulation for elective surgery.

DRUG	TIMING OF DISCONTINUATION		
Warfarin	5 days		
Direct thrombin inhibitors (dabigatran)	CrCl ≥50 mL/min: 1–2 days		
	CrCl <50 mL/min: 3–5 days		
	CrCl (mL/min)	Bleed risk: low	Bleed risk: high (days)
	≥50	2–4 hours	2–3
	30–50	2 days	2–3
	<30	2–4 days	>5
Factor Xa inhibitors			
Rivaroxaban (Xarelto)	≥24 hours		
	ROCKET AF: ≥3 days		
Apixaban (Eliquis)	Low-bleed risk: ≥24 hours		
	High-bleed risk: ≥48 hours		
Antiplatelet agents			
Aspirin	High CV risk/minor: continue		
	Low CV/high-bleed risk: 7–10 days		
Clopidogrel	5 days		

Adapted from McBeth PB, Weinberg JA, Sarani B, et al. A surgeon's guide to anticoagulant and antiplatelet medications part one: warfarin and new direct oral anticoagulant medications. *Trauma Surg Acute Care Open*. 2016;1:e000020.

CrCl, Creatinine clearance; *CV*, cardiovascular.

Stents: bare-mental stents—delay surgery for 6 weeks; drug-eluting stents delay surgery for 6–12 months due to risk of occlusion; otherwise consider continuing agents.

WOUND COMPLICATIONS

Seroma

A seroma is the collection of fluid containing fat, serum, and lymph that develops at surgical wound or dead space from surgery. Seromas are common in surgical procedures, which create dead space or interruption of lymphatic drainage. Examples of this include breast or axillary surgery and hernia surgery. The use of prosthetic mesh in hernia surgery may contribute to poor flap adherence and trigger inflammation which can increase the risk of seroma formation.

Presentation and Management

Seromas frequently present as palpable subcutaneous (SQ) fluid collections under or adjacent to a skin incision. They are more common when there is a significant dead space (e.g., SQ adiposity or large SQ hernia sac) and frequently develop after surgery when the patient is at home. Patients often complain of discomfort at the site of seroma due to pressure from the fluid collection. Some patients may experience swelling, pain, or erythema if infection is present. The diagnosis of seroma can be made clinically based on physical examination or radiologically by ultrasound or computed tomography (CT). Techniques to decrease the risk of seroma include minimization of dead space (e.g., excision of excess skin) and surgical drainage of dead space. Several techniques are used to reduce dead space, including the use of fibrin sealant, quilting sutures, and medical talc with inconsistent results. Many asymptomatic seromas will resolve spontaneously because the fluid can be resorbed by the surrounding tissues. Symptomatic seromas should be aspirated under sterile conditions and have a pressure dressing applied. Care should be taken with repeated seroma aspirations, which may introduce infection. In refractory seromas, a drain can be placed or the surgical site can be opened and packed to heal by secondary intention or treated with negative pressure therapy. Infected seromas should be drained surgically and treated with antibiotics. Prosthetic implants that are exposed should be removed in the setting of severe infection.

Hematoma

A hematoma is collection of blood clot and blood at the surgical site. It includes not only the SQ tissues but may also be found in a deeper tissue space where surgery was performed. Hematomas may be caused by incomplete surgical hemostasis or medical conditions that impair clotting, including coagulation disorders, platelet disorders, or other conditions that impair hemostasis (e.g., uremia, cirrhosis, or sepsis). Medications that alter blood clotting are a major factor in hematoma formation and must be managed properly in the perioperative period to reduce the risks of complications related to bleeding or clotting (Table 12.1). Commonly used antiplatelet agents include aspirin, P2Y12 inhibitors (clopidogrel, prazugrel, ticagrelor), and abciximab. Although warfarin is the most commonly used anticoagulant, the requirement for frequent blood draws to monitor its effects has reduced its popularity. The development of direct-acting oral anticoagulants or novel oral anticoagulants (direct oral anticoagulants) such as rivaroxaban, apixaban, and dabigatran are as effective as coumadin in most conditions requiring anticoagulation and require less frequent testing.

Presentation and Management

Hematomas can occur in various spaces, and clinical presentation differs. Superficial hematomas may present with skin discoloration, SQ swelling, and pain of the affected area due to pressure. Hematomas in other locations may cause pressure effects and irritation depending on the anatomic location. For example, hematomas in the abdominal cavity may present as abdominal compartment syndrome (ACS) or ileus, compartment syndrome in the forearm or leg, and airway compromise from anterior neck hematomas. When clotting disorders are present, the bleeding may persist and patients with large hematomas can present with anemia or hypovolemia. Infected hematomas may cause fever, leukocytosis, or sepsis.

Since coagulopathy is a common cause of hematoma, the perioperative management of surgical patients must include an appropriate evaluation of bleeding disorders and anticoagulant medications. Coagulation tests should be performed selectively since global screening is neither cost effective nor recommended. A patient's history of inappropriate bleeding or bruising, diseases related to hemostasis such as kidney or liver disease, or family history of bleeding disorder should raise the concern of hemostatic abnormality, and a screening test should be performed in these patients before surgery.

Aspirin and clopidogrel are the two most common antiplatelet medications that irreversibly inhibit cyclooxygenase 1 and P2Y12 receptor, respectively. Patients on these medications frequently have a history of coronary artery disease and/or stenting. Current guidelines recommend continuing aspirin and holding anti-P2Y12 agents before surgery, depending on timing after stenting and urgency of surgery. Warfarin is the most common anticoagulant drug used to prevent risk of thromboembolic events in many conditions such as atrial fibrillation, mechanical heart valve implantation, and hypercoagulable disorders. Warfarin use has been shown to be an independent risk factor for bleeding and hematoma in many studies. Therefore, the perioperative management of warfarin and other anticoagulants requires some consideration of the risks of bleeding and benefit of thromboembolic prevention. The risk of thromboembolism varies depending on the medical indication for anticoagulant use. The risk of surgical bleeding can be assessed by using HAS-BLED score (Table 12.2), where a score of 0 to 1 has low risk of bleeding, 2 has intermediate risk, and ≥3 has high risk. Also, surgical procedures can be grouped as high risk of bleeding (2%–4%), such as cardiovascular surgery, orthopedic surgery, surgery of head and neck cancer, urologic surgery, or surgery longer than 45 minutes, or low risk (0%–2%), such as anticipated surgical time <45 minutes, abdominal hernia, or cholecystectomy.[1]

TABLE 12.2 HAS-BLED score evaluating bleeding risk.

HAS-BLED RISK	SCORE
Hypertension, systolic BP >160 mm Hg	1
Abnormal renal or liver function (1 point each)	1 or 2
History of stroke	1
History of bleeding	1
Labile INRs	1
Elderly (>65 years)	1
Drugs or alcohol (1 point each)	1 or 2

BP, Blood pressure; *INR*, international normalized ratio.
Abnormal renal function: chronic dialysis, renal transplant, serum creatinine ≥200 μmol/L; abnormal liver function: chronic hepatic disease such as cirrhosis, bilirubin >2× upper limit normal, aspartate aminotransferase/alanine aminotransferase >3× upper limit normal; history of stroke: sudden focal neurologic deficit from bleeding lasting >24 hours and diagnosed by neurologist; history of bleeding: bleeding that requires hospitalization or causing >2 g/L drop in hematocrit or blood transfusion; labile INRs: therapeutic range <60%; drug and alcohol: antiplatelet, nonsteroidal antiinflammatory drugs, alcohol abuse.

Acute Wound Failure (Dehiscence)

Causes

Despite improvements in surgical techniques, suture materials, and pre- and postoperative care, acute wound failure/or dehiscence remains a dreaded surgical complication. The sequelae of acute wound failure includes fascial dehiscence, evisceration, acute hemorrhage, incisional hernia, anastomotic leaks, and fistulas (discussed later). Abdominal wound dehiscence describes partial or total disruption of the surgical wound, which can be superficial (skin and SQ fat) or deep (fascial), with or without extrusion of abdominal viscera (evisceration). Although the process of wound healing is similar in all tissues, the rate and consequences of failed healing differ by tissue (e.g., failure of bowel healing = anastomotic leak). After an incision, the aponeurosis will never completely regain its original strength and requires relatively longer time to heal.

The physiology of wound healing includes four distinct but overlapping phases (hemostasis, inflammation, proliferation, and remodeling), which are regulated by numerous intercellular interactions (monocytes, lymphocytes, fibroblasts, etc.), the release of local and systemic factors including cytokines, chemokines, growth factors, and inhibitors. Failure of wound healing is usually caused by multiple factors. These include patient-related factors like diabetes, uremia, immunosuppression, jaundice, sepsis, hypoalbuminemia, cancer, obesity, and steroid use. Other factors contributing to wound failure include inadequate closure (technical failure), increased intraabdominal pressure (IAP), and local factors like infection or radiation.

Wound dehiscence occurs in 1% to 3% of all surgical procedures and is more common during the first postoperative week (inflammatory phase of healing) when wound strength is dependent on the suture material and holding capacity of the knot. The fascial layer provides most of the strength and anchor for abdominal incisions. Dehiscence can be caused by technical failure if the suture material breaks, knots become undone, or if the suture material cuts through the suture holding tissues. Over time (during the fibrotic phase), the intrinsic strength of the wound increases, and the integrity of wound is less dependent on the suture and suture technique.

Many factors contribute to failure of wound healing or dehiscence, including advanced age, obesity, malnutrition, cancer, steroid use, intraabdominal sepsis, and local surgical site infection or hematoma. Infection contributes to aponeurotic breakdown and failure in more than half of all cases of wound dehiscence. Infection decreases collagen formation by reducing collagen synthesis and increasing collagen breakdown (via both bacterial and neutrophil collagenase activity). The resulting scar contains dense but fragile collagen fibrils with decreased cellular proliferation, which is prone to disruption. Technical factors can also contribute to wound failure, especially suture placement (too close to the fascial edge, too far apart, or under too much tension). Excessively tight suture lines impair wound perfusion and oxygen delivery needed for adequate wound healing.

Presentation and Management

Wound dehiscence may be an early manifestation of an intraabdominal process (e.g., abscess or anastomotic leak) presenting with serosanguineous fluid drainage from the wound or in some cases sudden evisceration with no warning. Patients with evisceration often note a sudden ripping sensation that occurs with severe coughing or retching. Wound dehiscence is associated with a mortality rate as high as 35% due to associated factors (e.g., malnutrition, sepsis, and cancer).

The optimal suturing technique for fascial closure remains a topic of debate among many surgeons. A suture:wound length ratio of more than 4:1 is recommended for proper fascial closure. The traditional technique of midline laparotomy closure uses continuous monofilament suture with sutures placed 1 cm deep on normal fascia (the bite) followed by 1 cm of progress. Incisional hernia rates of approximately 6% were reported over 5 years with this technique. The small bites versus large bites for closure of abdominal midline incisions (STITCH) trial compared large (1 cm every 1 cm) with small (0.5 cm every 0.5 cm) bite techniques for midline fascial closure.[2] The incidence of incisional hernia was 21% in the large bite group and 13% in the small bite group, suggesting technical superiority of the small bite technique. Wound dehiscence can also occur when the sutures pull through the patient's fascia and many surgeons are hesitant to use the "small bite" technique in obese patients or when they are concerned about tissue quality and sutures "pulling through." General concepts for fascial closure include accurate approximation of anatomic layers, avoiding excessive tension on the suture line, and considering the use of prophylactic mesh or retention sutures in "high-risk" patients.

The management of wound dehiscence depends on the degree of dehiscence (partial or complete), its timing, the presence of evisceration or intraabdominal sepsis, and individual patient factors in many situations. When wound dehiscence presents early after surgery without evisceration, prompt reclosure of the fascia is recommended. However, if the fascial disruption is partial or presents late when the viscera are adherent to the peritoneum, urgent reoperation and fascial reclosure are not always indicated. Local wound care and abdominal binders can be used selectively in some patients if the risk of reoperation and/or bowel injury is felt to be "high." Complete wound dehiscence with evisceration requires immediate reoperation, which is often difficult since many patients are obese or distended with distended and friable bowel due to associated inflammation or infection. The eviscerated bowel should be handled carefully to prevent injury; protection with moist towels during reexploration may help. The peritoneal cavity should be explored when there is concern for an acute intraabdominal process (e.g., anastomotic leak, bowel obstruction, or sepsis). When wound dehiscence occurs due to local soft tissue infection, the fascial edges should be debrided back to healthy tissue and the wound reclosed without tension.

The resultant large open abdominal wound can be treated in several ways. With ongoing abdominal sepsis or massive bowel edema, leaving the abdomen open with a negative pressure dressing may help resolve intraabdominal sepsis or allow for diuresis to decrease bowel edema and facilitate subsequent abdominal closure. In many cases, the use of absorbable (polyglactin or polyglycolic acid) mesh or acellular dermal prosthesis is necessary to close the fascia without undue tension. The use of permanent mesh (polypropylene or polytetrafluoroethylene) is not recommended in most cases due to the presence of associated infection or bowel injury. In some patients, the use of component separation and unilateral or bilateral myofascial advancement flaps can facilitate fascial closure.

In many cases, the skin and SQ tissue will need to be closed over a drain or left open. In general, contaminated or actively infected wounds should be left open. Open wounds can be treated with wet-to-dry dressing changes and delayed primary closure in some cases (usually several days postoperatively). Leaving the wound open, treating with dressing changes, and allowing it to heal by secondary intention are options in cases of severe infection or when the SQ tissues would benefit from local wound care. More recently, the use of negative pressure wound therapy (NPWT) or vacuum-assisted closure (VAC) dressings can be applied. The application of negative pressure to open wounds reduces tissue edema, increases tissue perfusion, and facilitates healing by secondary intention.[3] NPWT also regulates the inflammatory process by recruiting fibroblasts (through mechanical microdeformation) and induces cell migration, directly reducing bacterial populations through impairment of bacterial enzymatic processes. However, NPWT is not recommended in certain situations (e.g., untreated osteomyelitis, necrotic tissue with eschar, and in contact with exposed blood vessels, anastomotic sites, or nerves).

Surgical Site Infection

SSIs are a common complication seen after surgery or invasive procedures. It is one of the most common hospital-associated infections and contributes to increases in morbidity, length of hospital stay, readmission, and cost of care. Estimation of the average additional hospital costs is $5,000–$13,000 per SSI.[4] Approximately half of all SSIs are potentially preventable if evidence-based best practices are followed. For this reason, SSIs are considered to be indicative of the overall quality of surgical care and are routinely monitored by most hospitals. As a result, many institutions have adopted comprehensive programs to reduce the incidence of SSIs. Although the overall incidence of SSIs are trending down, SSIs are reported in 2% to 5% of surgical patients in the United States and up to 11.8% in low-to-medium income countries.[5] These data probably underestimate the true incidence since many infections occur after hospital discharge.

The term SSI refers to infection of the skin incision but also includes infection of the deeper anatomic tissues and organs where surgery was performed. Several standardized definitions of SSI exist, but the most commonly used definition is that of the Centers for Disease Control and Prevention (CDC), which groups SSIs into superficial, deep, and organ/space as outlined in Box 12.1.

Many factors contribute to SSIs, including patient factors and various aspects of surgical management (Table 12.3). SSIs are usually caused by contamination of the surgical site by endogenous bacteria or a break in sterility of the surgical technique and/or instruments. Surgical wounds can be classified as clean, clean contaminated, contaminated, or dirty based on the risk of bacterial contamination by entry of the aerodigestive tract or presence of established infection at the surgical site. As one might expect, each of these categories are associated with specific risks of SSI (Table 12.4). Typical pathogens depend on the procedure performed since surgery breaks the protective barrier of skin or mucosa, and endogenous microorganisms can be introduced into the tissue or organ. Infection after operations involving skin and soft tissue is predominantly gram-positive cocci (*Staphylococcus aureus*, most common). Gram-positive anaerobic cocci frequently cause infections following oral cavity or pharyngeal procedures, and anaerobic bacteria are more likely with

BOX 12.1 Criteria for surgical site infection definition.

Superficial Incisional Surgical Site Infection

Infection occurs within 30 days after the operation *and* infection involves only skin and subcutaneous tissue of the incision *and at last one of the following*:

1. Purulent drainage, with or without laboratory confirmation, from the superficial incision.
2. Organisms isolated from an aseptically obtained culture of fluid or tissue from the superficial incision.
3. At least one of the following signs or symptoms of infection: pain or tenderness, localized swelling, redness, or heat *and* superficial incision is deliberately opened by a surgeon, *unless* incision is culture-negative.
4. Diagnosis of superficial incisional SSI made by a surgeon or attending physician.

Deep Incisional Surgical Site Infection

Infection occurs within 30 days after the operation if no implant is left in place or within 1 year if implant is in place *and* the infection appears to be related to the operation *and* infection involves deep soft tissue (e.g., fascia, muscle) of the incision *and at least one of the following*:

1. Purulent drainage from the deep incision but not from the organ/space component of the surgical site.
2. A deep incision spontaneously dehisced or deliberately opened by a surgeon when the patient has *at least one of the following* signs or symptoms: fever (>38°C) and localized pain or tenderness, unless incision is culture-negative.
3. An abscess or other evidence of infection involving the deep incision found on direct examination, during reoperation, or by histopathologic or radiographic examination.
4. Diagnosis of deep incisional SSI made by a surgeon or attending physician.

Organ/Space Surgical Site Infection

Infection occurs within 30 days after the operation if no implant is left in place or within 1 year if implant is in place *and* the infection appears to be related to the operation *and* infection involves part of the anatomy (e.g., organs and spaces) other than the incision, which was opened or manipulated during an operation *and at least one of the following*.

1. Purulent drainage from a drain that is placed through a stab wound into the organ/space.
2. Organisms isolated from an aseptically obtained culture of fluid or tissue in the organ/space.
3. An abscess or other evidence of infection involving the organ/space that is sound on direct examination, during reoperation, or by histopathologic or radiologic examination.
4. Diagnosis of organ/space SSI made by a surgeon or attending physician.

From Horan TC, Gaynes RP, Martone WJ, et al. CDC definitions of nosocomial surgical site infections, 1992: a modification of CDC definitions of surgical wound infections. *Am J Infect Control.* 1992;20:271–274.

SSI, Surgical site infection.

colonic surgery (Table 12.5). Overall, *S. aureus* is the most common SSI pathogen. Other common pathogens include coagulase negative *Staphylococcus*, *Enterococcus* spp., *Escherichia coli*, *Enterobacter* spp., and *Pseudomonas aeruginosa*.

Methicillin-resistant *S. aureus* (MRSA) is a serious SSI pathogen because it is more virulent, difficult to treat, and associated with longer hospital stay, higher hospital costs, and increased mortality. MRSA infections are increased in patients with nasal

TABLE 12.3 Risk and protective factors of surgical site infections.

PATIENT FACTORS	FACTORS RELATED TO SURGERY AND MANAGEMENT
Advanced age	Duration of surgery
Increased BMI	Implantation of prostheses
High ASA score	Reoperation
High NNIS score	Longer hospital stay before surgery
Diabetic mellitus	Corticosteroid medication
Smoking	Inadequate sterilization, skin antisepsis
Dependence or frailty	Emergency procedure
Malnutrition	Hypothermia
Severe wound class	Intraoperative blood transfusion
Ascites	Perioperative shaving
Coexisting remote infection	Failure to obliterate dead space
Staphylococcal colonization	
Skin disease at surgical site	**PROTECTIVE FACTORS**
Anemia	Laparoscopic procedures
Increased number of comorbidities	Antibiotic prophylaxis

Adapted from Korol E, Johnston K, Waser N, et al. A systematic review of risk factors associated with surgical site infections among surgical patients. *PLoS One.* 2013;8:e83743; *Global Guidelines for the Prevention of Surgical Site Infection.* Geneva: World Health Organization; 2018. https://www.who.int/infection-prevention/publications/ssi-prevention-guidelines/en/; and Berrios-Torres SI, Umscheid CA, Bratzler DW, et al. Centers for Disease Control and Prevention guideline for the prevention of surgical site infection, 2017. *JAMA Surg.* 2017;152:784–791.

ASA, American Association of Anesthesiologists; *BMI*, body mass index; *NNIS*, National Nosocomial Infections Surveillance.

TABLE 12.4 Classification of surgical wounds.

CATEGORY	CRITERIA	INFECTION RATE (%)
Clean	No hollow viscus entered Primary wound closure No inflammation No breaks in aseptic technique Elective procedure	1–3
Clean-contaminated	Hollow viscus entered but controlled No inflammation Primary wound closure Minor break in aseptic technique Mechanical drain used Bowel preparation preoperatively	5–8
Contaminated	Uncontrolled spillage from viscus Inflammation apparent Open, traumatic wound Major break in aseptic technique	20–25
Dirty	Untreated, uncontrolled spillage from viscus Pus in operative wound Open suppurative wound Severe inflammation	30–40

colonization of MRSA, prior MRSA infection, recent hospitalization, and recent antibiotic use.

The majority of SSIs occur within 30 days of surgery and up to 1 year after implantation of a surgical prosthesis. Superficial SSIs present with localized redness, swelling, tenderness, warmth, presence of purulent discharge, or failure of wound healing. Deep SSIs may present with systemic signs and symptoms of infection, including fever, wound dehiscence, and purulent discharge from deep tissues. Organ or deep space infection can present as purulent discharge from surgical drains or with systemic signs of sepsis, including fever, tachycardia, tachypnea, and leukocytosis with associated signs of organ failure (decreased partial arterial oxygen pressure [PaO_2]/fraction of inspired oxygen [FiO_2] ratio, thrombocytopenia, hyperbilirubinemia, hypotension, delirium, or acute kidney injury [AKI]).

Prevention and Management

Patients scheduled for surgery should be managed to minimize the risk of SSI. Before performing surgery, any coexisting infection (skin, urine, and lung) should be treated and resolved. Patients who smoke cigarettes should stop for 1 to 2 months before elective surgery if possible and diabetic patients should have their blood sugar well controlled. Other conditions that may need to be "optimized" include nutritional status, anemia, and obesity. Decolonizing staphylococcal carriers with 2% mupirocin nasal ointment can reduce the risk of postoperative *S. aureus* infection in cardiac and orthopedic surgery. However, there is limited consensus regarding who to screen or for which operations screening should be considered. Preoperative antibiotics should be administered within 60 minutes of the skin incision to reach therapeutic concentration in serum and tissue during the surgical procedure. Vancomycin and fluoroquinolones may need to be started earlier due to their prolonged infusion times and half-lives. Redosing of antibiotics may be required if the duration of surgery exceeds 2 half-lives of the drugs or with massive blood loss. Caution should be used in patients with poor drug clearance (e.g., renal insufficiency or hepatic dysfunction) and the choice of drug should correlate with the common organisms found at the surgical site. In general, prophylactic antibiotics should not be continued after surgery and the duration of antimicrobial prophylaxis should not exceed 24 hours. Table 12.6 summarizes prophylactic antibiotic choice, dosing, and redosing, and Table 12.7 reviews the recommended antibiotic prophylaxis by surgical procedure.

For skin preparation, patients should shower with soap the night before surgery. If hair needs to be removed from the surgical site, a clipper should be used. Skin should be prepared with alcohol-based antiseptic solution (e.g., chlorhexidine) before incision. Perioperative glycemic control has been shown to reduce SSIs with a glucose threshold of <200 mg/dL. Avoiding perioperative hypothermia (core temperature <36°C) has been shown to reduce the risk of SSI and may be achieved with preoperative room warming, warmed intravenous (IV) fluids, etc. Use of increased FiO_2 is recommended during general anesthesia and for 2 to 6 hours postoperatively, especially after colon surgery, to ensure adequate tissue oxygen levels which are associated with reduced risk of SSI. Other considerations include the operating room environment (air handling, etc.), sterile processing of surgical instruments, use of clean instruments to close the abdomen in contaminated cases, etc. In the intraoperative period, using adhesive skin drapes (e.g., Ioban) may help to reduce SSIs in some cases and wound protection devices may help to reduce SSIs in open abdominal surgery by decreasing contamination of the SQ tissues. Antimicrobial coated suture has been developed to reduce bacterial colonization and prevent SSI, but the results remain controversial. Topical NPWT (Provena) is being used by some surgeons to reduce SSI but has not been universally adapted as best practice at this time. However, managing open wounds with NPWT is commonly used to reduce edema, increase blood flow, and decrease bacterial burden. After the operation, the wound should be routinely assessed for infection surveillance.

Infected surgical wounds should be opened to allow the infection to drain, and debridement should be considered if devitalized or infected tissue is present. IV or oral antibiotics should be given when there are signs of systemic infection, including fever >38.5°C, tachycardia >110 beats/min, and leukocytosis >12,000/µL, or when cellulitis (erythema extends >5 cm from wound edge) is present. Patients with risk factors for MRSA infection should be treated with appropriate antibiotics (e.g., vancomycin, daptomycin, linezolid, or ceftaroline). Empiric antibiotics for operations involving axillae, groin, perineum, genital tract, and gastrointestinal (GI) tract should cover gram-negative and anaerobic bacteria. Moreover, patients requiring antibiotics should have drainage or discharge from the wound or site of infection sent for culture to identify the pathogen and its

TABLE 12.5 Common pathogens related to surgical procedures.

TYPE OF SURGERY	LIKELY PATHOGENS
Placement of all grafts, prostheses, or implants	*Staphylococcus aureus*, coagulase-negative staphylococci
Cardiac	*S. aureus*, coagulase-negative staphylococci
Neurosurgery	*S. aureus*, coagulase-negative staphylococci
Breast	*S. aureus*, coagulase-negative staphylococci
Ophthalmic (limited data, however, commonly used in procedures such as anterior segment resection, vitrectomy, and scleral buckles)	*S. aureus*, coagulase-negative staphylococci, streptococci, gram-negative bacilli
Orthopedic (total joint replacement, closed fractured/use of nails, bone plates, other internal fixation device, functional repair without implant/device trauma)	*S. aureus*, coagulase-negative staphylococci, gram-negative bacilli
Noncardiac thoracic (lobectomy, pneumonectomy, wedge resection, other noncardiac mediastinal procedures), closed tube thoracotomy	*S. aureus*, coagulase-negative staphylococci, *Streptococcus pneumoniae*, gram-negative bacilli
Vascular	*S. aureus*, coagulase-negative staphylococci
Appendectomy	Gram-negative bacilli, anaerobes
Biliary tract	Gram-negative bacilli, anaerobes
Colorectal	Gram-negative bacilli, anaerobes
Gastroduodenal	Gram-negative bacilli, streptococci, oropharyngeal anaerobes (e.g., peptostreptococci)
Head and neck (majorly procedures with incision through oropharyngeal mucosa)	*S. aureus*, streptococci, oropharyngeal anaerobes (e.g., peptostreptococci)
Obstetric and gynecologic	Gram-negative bacilli, enterococci, group B streptococci, anaerobes
Urologic	Gram-negative bacilli

From Sganga G, Tascini C, Sozio E, et al. Focus on the prophylaxis, epidemiology and therapy of methicillin-resistant *Staphylococcus aureus* surgical site infections and a position paper on associated risk factors: the perspective of an Italian group of surgeons. *World J Emerg Surg.* 2016;11:26.

antibiotic resistance profile. The wound should be wet dressed with normal saline damped sterile gauze at least daily. Antibiotics should be optimized according to the culture results when available.

THERMAL REGULATION

Hypothermia

Causes

Maintenance of normothermia is important physiologically as even modest deviations in core body temperature contribute to metabolic alterations, resulting in cellular and tissue dysfunction. Hypothermia is a common complication in surgical patients and is defined as core body temperature below 35°C. It can be classified by severity into three categories: mild (32°C–35°C), moderate (28°C–32°C), and severe (<28°C). Vasoconstriction and shivering are the body's major thermoregulatory protective mechanisms, both of which may be impaired in the perioperative period. Risk factors for heat loss and perioperative hypothermia include elderly patients, burn injuries, open surgical procedures, cool operating rooms, prolonged surgeries (>4 hours), infusion of room-temperature fluids, cutaneous vasodilatation from anesthetic agents, and increased evaporative losses from serosal surfaces. Hypothermia can develop during any stage of surgery: preoperatively, intraoperatively, or postoperatively. Preoperatively, the use of muscle relaxants impairs shivering. Intraoperatively, heat loss occurs from large, exposed operative area, anesthetic effects on heat production, cool room temperatures, vasoconstriction, and shivering.

Hypothermia after surgery contributes to organ injury through various mechanisms: ventilation-perfusion (V/Q) mismatch; shift of oxyhemoglobin-dissociation curve to the left causes tissue hypoxia, decreases myocardial contractility and peripheral vasoconstriction, increased blood viscosity; reduced platelet function; and decreased activation of the coagulation cascade. Hypothermia is common after traumatic injury due to shock, alcohol intoxication, environmental exposure, fluid resuscitation, and loss of shivering. Hypothermia is also associated with increased risk of SSI.

TABLE 12.6 Recommendation of prophylactic antibiotic choice, dose, and redosing.

ANTIMICROBIAL	RECOMMENDED DOSE FOR ADULT	REDOSING (HOURS AFTER PREOPERATIVE DOSE)
Ampicillin-sulbactam	3 g	2
Ampicillin	2 g	2
Aztreonam	2 g	4
Cefazolin	2 g, 3 g if body weight >120 kg	4
Cefuroxime	1.5 g	4
Cefotaxime	1 g	3
Cefoxitin	2 g	2
Cefotetan	2 g	6
Ceftriaxone	2 g	NA
Ciprofloxacin	400 mg	NA
Clindamycin	900 mg	6
Ertapenem	1 g	NA
Fluconazole	400 mg	NA
Gentamicin	5 mg/kg*	NA
Levofloxacin	500 mg	NA
Metronidazole	500 mg	NA
Moxifloxacin	400 mg	NA
Piperacillin-tazobactam	3.375 g	2
Vancomycin	15 mg/kg	NA
Neomycin	1 g	NA
Erythromycin-based oral antibiotic (colorectal surgery prophylaxis in conjunction with mechanical bowel preparation)	1 g	NA

Adapted from Bratzler DW, Dellinger EP, Olsen KM, et al. Clinical practice guidelines for antimicrobial prophylaxis in surgery. *Am J Health Syst Pharm.* 2013;70:195–283.

NA, Not applicable.

No redosing needed for typical case duration. For unusually long operations, redosing should be considered.

*Gentamicin is calculated based on actual body weight, if the actual body weight is >20% above ideal body weight (IBW), the dosing weight (DW) can be calculated from DW = IBW + 0.4(Actual body weight - IBW)

Presentation

Intraoperative hypothermia causes significant postoperative discomfort and shivering. Hypothermia significantly impairs cardiovascular function, blood clotting, and wound healing and increases the risk of infection. When the core temperature falls below 32°C, significant reductions in blood pressure and cardiac output occur. Cardiovascular manifestations of hypothermia include cardiac depression, myocardial ischemia, dysrhythmias, peripheral vasoconstriction, impaired tissue oxygen delivery, blunted response to catecholamines, and hypotension. The characteristic electrocardiogram finding of J point elevation, and Osborn wave (notch and deflection at the QST-ST junction), are considered pathognomonic of hypothermia. Adverse myocardial outcomes have been reported in hypothermic patients with preexisting cardiovascular disease (when compared with postoperative normothermic patients). Peripheral vasoconstriction due to shock is the most important impediment to wound oxygenation. Mild core hypothermia results in immune dysfunction by impeding granulocyte chemotaxis and phagocytosis, macrophage function, and antibody production. These changes in immune function, in combination with decreased tissue oxygen tension, abnormal collagen deposition, and poor wound healing, increase susceptibility to infection.

Hypothermia also induces coagulopathy by attenuating hemostatic enzyme function and platelet sequestration, resulting in an increased risk of bleeding. With mild and moderate hypothermia, renal perfusion and glomerular filtration are decreased, resulting in "cold-induced diuresis." Decreased hepatic and renal blood flows, in turn, reduce drug metabolism and excretion, with resultant decreases in plasma clearance and potential prolongations in drug effects, which can lead to delays in emergence from anesthesia and prolonged postoperative anesthesia care unit stays. Also, fluid resuscitation with Ringer's lactate in a patient with existing metabolic acidosis further worsens cardiac function. Severe hypothermia impairs cough reflex and increases the risk of a comatose surgical patient to postoperative pneumonia.

Treatment

Patients at risk for hypothermia should be monitored frequently and every attempt should be made to maintain normal central core temperature. Pulmonary artery, tympanic membrane, urinary bladder, esophagus, trachea, nasopharynx, or rectum have been established as reliable sites for estimation of core temperatures. Continuous temperature monitoring and maintaining normothermia are essential during surgery as anesthesia, cool operating room environment, and significant evaporative cooling occurs during skin preparation making most surgical patients susceptible to hypothermia. Increasing the ambient room temperature, administering warmed IV fluids, covering patients with blankets, and using forced-air warming devices are commonly used techniques to prevent intraoperative hypothermia. Invasive core rewarming techniques can also be used during surgery, including intraperitoneal irrigation with warmed saline and intubation and ventilation with warmed humidified air or gases.[6] Circulating water warmers produce faster rewarming than heat exchanging systems. Inadvertent core hypothermia is commonly seen in the immediate postoperative period. Maintenance of normal body temperature decreases blood loss, fluid requirement, length of intensive care unit (ICU) stay, organ failure, and mortality. Maintenance of intravascular volume and electrolytes is important, particularly in head injuries where mannitol can augment the effects of cold diuresis. However, in the case of major abdominal, cardiothoracic surgery, surgery involving intentional hypothermia (cardiac bypass), or prolonged surgery (>4 hours), forced-air warming, warm IV fluids, and ambient temperature alone are inadequate for maintaining normothermia. When rapid warming is needed, continuous arteriovenous rewarming is more effective. In patients with asystole, defibrillation and drugs have unpredictable efficacy, and cardiopulmonary bypass is essential for rewarming and maintaining perfusion.

Malignant Hyperthermia

Malignant hyperthermia is a life-threatening condition that develops in approximately 1:10,000 to 1:250,000 anesthetic cases, with a higher incidence in younger patients.[7] It is an autosomal dominant pharmacogenetic disorder that presents as hypermetabolic response to inhalation anesthetic agents like halothane, isoflurane, sevoflurane, desflurane, or depolarizing muscle relaxants succinylcholine or suxamethonium.

During muscle contraction, the neuronal signal action potential is transferred to muscle cells, resulting in the release of intracellular calcium from sarcoplasmic reticulum via ryanodine receptors to initiate muscle contraction. The energy used in this process also generates heat and oxygen is consumed with carbon

TABLE 12.7 Recommended antibiotic prophylaxis by surgical procedure.

TYPE OF PROCEDURE	RECOMMENDED AGENTS	ALTERNATIVES FOR PATIENTS WITH β-LACTAM ALLERGY
Gastroduodenal	Cefazolin	Clindamycin or vancomycin + aminoglycoside or aztreonam or fluoroquinolone
Biliary tract	Cefazolin, cefoxitin, cefotetan, ceftriaxone, ampicillin-sulbactam	–Clindamycin or vancomycin + aminoglycoside or aztreonam or fluoroquinolone –Metronidazole + aminoglycoside or fluoroquinolone
Appendectomy for uncomplicated appendicitis	Cefoxitin, cefotetan, cefazolin + metronidazole	–Clindamycin + aminoglycoside or aztreonam or fluoroquinolone –Metronidazole + aminoglycoside or fluoroquinolone
Nonobstructed small bowel	Cefazolin	Clindamycin + aminoglycoside or aztreonam or fluoroquinolone
Obstructed small bowel	Cefazolin + metronidazole, cefoxitin, cefotetan	Metronidazole + aminoglycoside or fluoroquinolone
Hernia repair	Cefazolin	Clindamycin, vancomycin
Colorectal	–Cefazolin + metronidazole, cefoxitin, cefotetan, ampicillin-sul bactam, ceftriaxone + metronidazole, ertapenem	–Clindamycin + aminoglycoside or aztreonam or fluoroquinolone –Metronidazole + aminoglycoside or fluoroquinolone
Head and neck –Clean wound –Clean wound with placement of prosthesis –Clean-contaminated wound	–None –Cefazolin, cefuroxime –Cefazolin + metronidazole, cefuroxime + metronidazole	–None –Clindamycin –Clindamycin
Urologic surgery –Lower urinary tract instrumentation –Clean wound without entry into urinary tract –Involving prosthetic implantation –Clean wound with entry into urinary tract –Clean-contaminated wound	–Fluoroquinolone, trimethoprim-sulfamethoxazole, cefazolin –Cefazolin (addition of aminoglycoside for placement of prosthetic material) –Cefazolin ± aminoglycoside, cefazolin ± aztreonam, ampicillin-sulbactam –Cefazolin (addition of aminoglycoside for placement of prosthetic material) –Cefazolin + metronidazole, cefoxitin	–Aminoglycoside with or without clindamycin –Clindamycin, vancomycin –Clindamycin ± aminoglycoside or aztreonam, vancomycin ± aminoglycoside or aztreonam –Fluoroquinolone, aminoglycoside with or without clindamycin –Fluoroquinolone, aminoglycoside + metronidazole or clindamycin
Vascular	Cefazolin	Clindamycin, vancomycin
Transplant surgery –Liver –Pancreas and pancreas-kidney	–Piperacillin-tazobactam, cefotaxime + ampicillin –Cefazolin, fluconazole (for high risk of fungal infection)	–Clindamycin or vancomycin + aminoglycoside or aztreoman or fluoroquinolone –Clidamycin or vancomycin + aminoglycoside or aztreonam or fluoroquinolone
Plastic surgery	Cefazolin, ampicillin-sul bactam	Clindamycin, vancomycin

From Bratzler DW, Dellinger EP, Olsen KM, et al. Clinical practice guidelines for antimicrobial prophylaxis in surgery. *Am J Health Syst Pharm.* 2013;70:195–283.

dioxide (CO_2) release. Calcium is transported back to storage and muscles are then relaxed. In genetically susceptible patients, most commonly ryanodine receptor mutations, certain triggers can stimulate continuous release of calcium, leading to persistent high levels of intracellular calcium causing constant muscle contraction or rigidity, generation of heat, increased oxygen consumption, and (CO_2) release, which lead to respiratory and metabolic acidosis and eventually, if left untreated, rhabdomyolysis.

Early presentations of malignant hyperthermia include an increase in end-tidal (CO_2) or tachypnea if the patient is not intubated and ventilated, hypoxia, tachycardia, masseter muscle spasm, or trismus. Later presentations of malignant hyperthermia include muscle rigidity, cardiac arrhythmias, respiratory and metabolic acidosis, rhabdomyolysis, and hyperthermia, as the name suggests. Complications from rhabdomyolysis include disseminated intravascular coagulation, AKI, hyperkalemia, and possible cardiac arrest.

Since malignant hyperthermia is an autosomal dominant disorder, patients with a family history of malignant hyperthermia should be carefully evaluated and consider testing before surgery. They should be carefully monitored during anesthesia and trigger-free anesthetic agents should be used. Once malignant hyperthermia develops, the initial management is to discontinue the inciting anesthetic agent and halt the operation if possible. Dantrolene is the medication of choice to treat malignant hyperthermia, and an initial dose of 2.5 mg/kg IV should be given and can be repeated according to the response: end-tidal CO_2, tachycardia, muscle rigidity, and acidosis. Oxygen supplementation should be given with hyperventilation. Blood should be tested for electrolyte and blood gas to assess for acidosis and hyperkalemia, creatine phosphokinase, and renal function and then treated accordingly. The electrocardiogram should be continuously monitored for arrhythmias. Core body temperature should be measured and monitored. Active cooling with ice packs and 4°C normal saline IV should be initiated if the body temperature is more than 39°C but should be stopped when the body temperature decreases to 38.5°C to avoid overcooling and hypothermia. Renal function should be assessed and urine output should be closely monitored. IV hydration should be given with diuresis when rhabdomyolysis is present; hemodialysis may be needed in some cases. Clotting studies and platelet count should be checked for the possibility of disseminated intravascular coagulation. When stable (i.e., end-tidal CO_2 and temperature are decreased, tachycardia or other arrhythmia is improved, and muscle rigidity is resolved), patients should be monitored in the intensive setting for at least 24 hours with dantrolene maintenance. Muscle weakness is a side effect from dantrolene so breathing and oxygenation should be monitored and aspiration should be prevented. Other side effects of dantrolene are hepatitis, phlebitis, and drowsiness. First-degree relatives should be advised of the potential risks and provided with genetic counseling.

Postoperative Fever

Causes

Fever refers to an increase in the body's normal core temperature. Postoperative fevers can be broadly divided into infectious and noninfectious (systemic inflammatory response syndrome [SIRS]) causes (Table 12.8). Fevers are most often transient increases in temperature caused by the systemic inflammatory stimuli as a normal response to injury. However, fever can also be an early sign of potentially life-threatening infection. Pyrogenic cytokines are produced in response to infection and trauma (including surgery) and play an important role in regulating host inflammation and fever. Duration and extent of tissue trauma during surgery cause a release of interleukin-1 (IL-1), a primary activator of the febrile response; IL-1 levels correlate with an increase in core temperature. Also, the timing of fever onset provides an important diagnostic clue; early postoperative fever is characterized by the release of cytokines during surgery. Immediate postoperative fever occurring within the first 48 hours after surgery is most likely due to an inflammatory response to surgery. The proinflammatory mediators (tumor necrosis factor-α [TNF-α], IL-6, and interferon γ), released in response to inflammation, cause a cascade of systemic effects that induce a febrile inflammatory response, also known as SIRS.[8] SIRS is diagnosed when there is presence of two or more of the following criteria: temperature >36°C, heart rate (HR) >90 beats/min, respiratory rate >20/min or $PaCO_2$ <32 mm Hg, white blood cell (WBC) count >12,000/mm^3, or <4000/mm^3 or >10% band forms. A fever that develops 72 hours or more after surgery is more likely to be due to infection. Hence, it can sometimes be clinically challenging to delineate the precise etiology of these fevers since they can result from infectious and/or noninfectious causes.

In the postoperative period, the most common infectious causes are wound infections, urinary tract infections (UTIs), and pneumonia. Prolonged IV access, bladder catheterization, or endotracheal intubation presents ongoing risks of infection that result from disruption of normal host defense mechanisms. Postoperative UTI is more common in patients with preexisting prostrate hypertrophy. Urinary tract instrumentation and indwelling urinary catheters damage the epithelial lining, eliciting an inflammatory response that facilitates bacterial adherence and the risk of UTI increases with duration of bladder catheterization.

Catheter-related bloodstream infection (CRBSI) is the most common cause of nosocomial bacteremia and septicemia. As such, early diagnosis and treatment are vital to reduce the morbidity and mortality involved. The incidence of CRBSI varies

TABLE 12.8 Causes of postoperative fever.

INFECTIOUS	NONINFECTIOUS
Abscess	Acute hepatic necrosis
Acalculous cholecystitis	Adrenal insufficiency
Bacteremia	Allergic reaction
Decubitus ulcers	Atelectasis
Device-related infections	Dehydration
Empyema	Drug reaction
Endocarditis	Head injury
Fungal sepsis	Hepatoma
Hepatitis	Hyperthyroidism
Meningitis	Lymphoma
Osteomyelitis	Myocardial infarction
Pseudomembranous colitis	Pancreatitis
Parotitis	Pheochromocytoma
Perineal infections	Pulmonary embolus
Peritonitis	Retroperitoneal hematoma
Pharyngitis	Solid organ hematoma
Pneumonia	Subarachnoid hemorrhage
Retained foreign body	Systemic inflammatory response syndrome
Sinusitis	Thrombophlebitis
Soft tissue infection	Transfusion reaction
Tracheobronchitis	Withdrawal syndromes
Urinary tract infection	Wound infection

considerably by type of catheter, frequency of catheter manipulation, underlying patient-related factors, and local risk factors such as poor personal hygiene, occlusive transparent dressing, and moisture around the exit site[9]; administration of parenteral nutrition through intravascular catheters choice to treat malignant hyperth risk. The mode of contamination for CRBSI varies with the duration of catheterization (short vs. long). Short-term CRBSIs (<10 days) are extraluminal and are preventable as they result from contamination by normal resident flora of the skin at the insertion site. In contrast, the source of infection is endoluminal that propagates the infection in long-term CRBSI (>10 days) that results in sepsis with multiorgan failure. The organisms most commonly involved in CRBSI are Staphylococci (both *S. aureus* and the coagulase-negative staphylococci), enterococci, aerobic gram-negative bacilli, and fungal species (e.g., *Candida albicans*). The diagnosis of CRBSI requires at least one positive blood culture obtained from a peripheral vein, clinical manifestations of infection (e.g., fever, chills, and/or hypotension), and no apparent source for the blood stream infection (BSI) except the catheter. Antibiotic therapy is often initiated empirically; Vancomycin is recommended for empirical therapy for MRSA. Factors responsible for recurrent bacteremia despite parenteral therapy include antibiotic administration through retained catheter and biofilm formation. Severe sepsis and metastatic infectious complications (e.g., infective endocarditis) prolong the course of CRBSI. Catheters should be removed from patients with CRBSI associated with any local or systemic inflammation or immunocompromised condition.

RESPIRATORY COMPLICATIONS

General Considerations

Surgical interventions (especially thoracic and abdominal) and anesthesia impact pulmonary physiology by decreasing functional residual capacity (FRC). In most patients, this is well tolerated, but patients with underlying pulmonary disease (e.g., chronic obstructive pulmonary disease, emphysema, cigarette smokers, etc.) may be prone to develop pulmonary complications. Identifying "high-risk" patients before surgery can be helpful and preoperative pulmonary function testing, tobacco cessation, or sleep studies may help the surgical team reduce the risk of complications by optimizing the patient's condition before surgery (e.g., preoperative bilevel positive airway pressure ventilation, bronchodilator therapy, etc.). More recently, standard patient care protocols (e.g., iCough) have been developed to decrease the risk of pulmonary complications, which include incentive spirometry, coughing and deep breathing, oral care (brushing teeth and using mouthwash), elevating the head of bed, and getting out of bed three times a day. Multimodal pain control and judicious use of regional analgesia (e.g., thoracic epidurals) may also help to prevent pulmonary complications in surgical patients.

Atelectasis

Atelectasis due to partial or complete collapse of alveoli is the most common respiratory complication in the postoperative patient. Predisposing factors for atelectasis include general anesthesia and upper abdominal or thoracic surgery with stimulation of GI viscera, which can alter diaphragmatic function for several days. The mechanisms include decreased lung compliance (due to reduced FRC), along with accumulated endobronchial secretions, resulting in V/Q mismatch and shunt, which directly correlates with the degree of atelectasis. Anesthesia, cigarettes, morbid obesity, and preexisting pulmonary disease also impair mucociliary clearance and decrease the patient's ability to cough and clear secretions, contributing to an increased risk of atelectasis.

Atelectasis is the most common cause of postoperative fever in the early postoperative period. It may also present with tachypnea, decreased oxygen saturation ± accessory muscle use. On physical examination, breath sounds may be absent or reduced, or "bronchial" in nature. The chest radiograph may reveal loss of the left hemidiaphragm, air bronchograms, or decreased lung volume with tracheal deviation toward the collapsed side in severe cases. Atelectasis can be reversed in the first 24 to 48 hours with early mobilization, deep breathing (five sequential breaths held for 5–6 seconds), incentive spirometry, coughing, chest physiotherapy, bronchodilator therapy, hydration, and tracheal suctioning. Multimodal pain control using acetaminophen, nonsteroidal antiinflammatory agents, and opioids as needed or regional blocks represent the most commonly effective approach for optimal perioperative pain control.

Pneumonia

Nosocomial pneumonia is the second leading cause of nosocomial infection and is more common in surgical patients. The diagnosis of postoperative pneumonia requires the absence of infiltrates prior to admission or before surgery and can be classified as either hospital-acquired pneumonia (developing 48 hours after admission) or ventilator-associated pneumonia (VAP) (pneumonia developing 48–72 hours after endotracheal intubation). Aspiration of oropharyngeal secretions, diminished humoral defense mechanisms, injury to the surface epithelium by instrumentation (endotracheal or nasogastric [NG] tube), azotemia, critical illness, duration of surgery/ventilation, advanced age, preexisting pulmonary conditions (e.g., chronic obstructive pulmonary disease), cigarette smoking within a year prior to surgery, altered sensorium, malnutrition, and prior antibiotic therapy may facilitate colonization. Stress ulcer prophylaxis (histamine 2 [H_2] blockers, antacids) and enteral feeding can increase gastric pH, gastric colonization, and aspiration (gastropulmonary route), which plays an important role in the pathogenesis of VAP.[10]

Postoperative pneumonias are commonly caused by gram-negative, aerobic bacteria, *S. aureus* in neurosurgical patients or fungal organisms in immunocompromised patients. VAP is polymicrobial in nearly half of cases, and the most common organisms include enteric gram-negative bacilli (*Pseudomonas aeruginosa*, *Actinobacter* species, *Enterobacter* species, *Klebsiella* species, *Serratia marcescens*, *Escherichia coli*, *Proteus* species, and *Legionella* species) or gram-positive organisms (*S. aureus*). In surgery, trauma, and critically ill patients, the use of prophylactic antibiotics can alter the microbial flora. In early-onset VAP (<4 days postintubation), the organisms are usually antibiotic (e.g., methicillin) sensitive. In contrast, late-onset VAP (>4 days postintubation) is frequently due to drug-resistant bacteria. Also, risk of VAP is greatest during the first 5 days of mechanical ventilation (3%, with a mean of 3.3 days); thereafter, between 5 and 10 days, the risk declines to 2% per day, further declining to 1% per day after 10 days. Refractory VAP is defined as VAP with failure to improve after 72 hours. Postoperative pneumonia is associated with a high mortality (50%).

Diagnosis

A high index of suspicion is required for the diagnosis of postoperative pneumonia, especially in mechanically ventilated patients. Patients with postoperative pneumonia usually present with fever, leukocytosis, and a new pulmonary infiltrate. In intubated patients, VAP should be suspected when two or more of the following clinical features are present (purulent respiratory secretions, temp >38°C or <36°C, leukocytosis or leukopenia, or hypoxemia). Hypoxemia should be treated supportively by increasing the inspired oxygen level or positive end-expiratory pressure to increase the PaO_2 to 65 mm Hg, and/or the SpO_2 to 92%. If a newer or persistent chest radiographic abnormality is found, tracheobronchial secretions should be cultured (qualitative or quantitative) and empiric therapy should be started.

Treatment

The management of postoperative pneumonia depends on the patient's clinical status, the timing of pneumonia occurrence relative to admission, prior antibiotic exposure, and type of surgery. While intubation and mechanical ventilation may be required, the alternatives to this should be considered (e.g., noninvasive positive-pressure ventilation can be applied to manage hypoxic or hypercarbic failure in some patients) before intubation, which is the main risk factor for VAP. When intubation is considered, the orotracheal route is usually preferred over nasotracheal intubation, which has an increased risk of sinusitis and VAP. In patients intubated for 48 to 72 hours, continuous or intermittent endotracheal and oropharyngeal secretions should be suctioned prior to extubation. Although the use of selective oropharyngeal decontamination is controversial, chlorhexidine may be beneficial in reducing postoperative respiratory infections in cardiac surgery patients. In addition, the risk of VAP can be lowered with preventive care bundles, including hand washing, limiting sedation, elevating the head end of the bed, early mobility, spontaneous breathing trials with early extubation, and low tidal volume ventilation. Prolonged intubation results in biofilm formation and microorganism colonization of the endotracheal tube surface. Coating the endotracheal tube with antibacterial agents (silver, silver sulfadiazine) may help to reduce the risk of VAP in some patients. The use of sucralfate for stress ulcer prophylaxis is associated with a reduced incidence of pneumonia relative to prophylaxis with H_2 receptor antagonists. Patients diagnosed with postoperative pneumonia and VAP should be reevaluated for clinical response (usually marked by improvement of fever, leukocytosis, and infiltrate). Prompt initiation of appropriate antibiotics within 12 hours of diagnosis leads to improved survival, and antibiotic regimen should be modified to specifically cover the pathogens and antibiotic resistance profile of the culture results.

Aspiration Pneumonitis and Aspiration Pneumonia

Causes

Aspiration of gastric contents in the perioperative period is associated with significant pulmonary morbidity and mortality. Aspiration pneumonitis (Mendelson syndrome) refers to an acute inflammatory injury of the lung parenchyma resulting from aspiration of usually sterile acidic gastric contents (critical pH is 2.5). It can also occur due to aspiration of oropharyngeal contents. Aspiration pneumonia is a common infectious complication of enteral nutrition usually resulting either from contamination of the initial aspirate or secondarily from aspiration of colonized oropharyngeal secretions. Although the underlying patient characteristics that predispose to these conditions are similar, the distinction between the two entities is important since aspiration pneumonia requires antibiotic treatment and aspiration pneumonitis is managed supportively. Surgery patients are at increased risk of aspiration pneumonia since tissue injury, hemorrhage, and anesthesia can contribute to impaired host defenses.

The factors that predispose an individual to increase risk of aspiration include emergency surgery, chronic debilitating disease, oropharyngeal or airway instrumentation (e.g., enteral feeding, prolonged intubation, upper GI endoscopy, or tracheostomy), small bowel obstruction, autonomic neuropathy with delaying gastric emptying, and impaired consciousness (e.g., from general anesthesia, epileptic seizure, trauma, alcohol, drug overdose, or cerebrovascular accident). Aspiration risk inversely correlates with the patient's Glasgow Coma score. Older patients are at increased risk of oropharyngeal aspiration secondary due to the combination of pharyngeal dysmotility, gastroesophageal reflux, and poor oral hygiene in this population. The common infectious organisms in aspiration pneumonia are *E. coli*, *Klebsiella*, *Staphylococcus*, *Pseudomonas*, and *Bacteroides* species.

The pathogenesis and outcomes of gastric aspiration depend on the nature of aspirated matter, volume and pH of gastric acid, and immunologic status of the patient. The more acidic (e.g., pH <2.5) and voluminous (>20 mL) the aspirate, the greater the severity of pulmonary damage. However, independent of acidity, aspiration of gastric fluid with particulate matter causes significant and persistent pulmonary damage. The initial parenchymal inflammatory changes (airspace edema, hemorrhage, hyaline membrane) in Mendelson syndrome are similar to acute respiratory distress syndrome (ARDS) and attributed to neutrophil activation and recruitment and inflammatory cytokines (TNF and IL-8) release. Aspiration of particulate matter can result in death from airway obstruction or subsequent granulomatous reaction to the foreign particles.

Some physicians feel the risk of aspiration can be minimized by monitoring of gastric residual volumes in tube-fed patients. However, there is no consensus regarding the safe or unsafe limits of gastric residual volumes in these patients. Bolus feedings possess a higher risk of aspiration than continuous feeding. The use of small-bore NG tubes has been suggested to decrease aspiration pneumonia and reflux. Some centers prefer to use double-lumen feeding tubes that allow simultaneous postpyloric feeding and gastric decompression.

According to the American Society of Anesthesiology, the routine administration of preoperative medications to reduce gastric pH is not routinely recommended for patients with no increased risk of pulmonary aspiration.[11] The risk-benefit ratio for using prophylactic H_2 receptor antagonists or proton pump inhibitors (PPIs) to reduce the gastric acid pH is favorable in high-risk patients. However, none of these drugs are absolutely reliable in preventing the risk of aspiration pneumonitis.

Presentation and Diagnosis

Aspiration of gastric contents in patients undergoing elective surgery rarely results in severe pulmonary manifestations. However, in critically ill patients, aspiration can present with a range of pulmonary sequelae. Gastric aspiration may cause mild, subclinical pneumonitis, or more severe progressive respiratory failure with significant morbidity and mortality. After an aspiration event, the clinical and radiographic changes begin to appear within the next 24 to 36 hours. Common signs and symptoms of gastric aspiration include fever, cough, rales, diminished breath sounds, wheezing, and infiltrates on chest radiograph. Hypoxia is the earliest and most reliable sign. Arterial blood gas analysis should be performed to determine the severity of hypoxemia. The absence of symptoms in the first 2 hours usually correlates with a benign course. The risks of hypercapnia and acidosis are increased in the presence of particulate matter, and tracheobronchial aspirate should be collected for culture and sensitivity tests. In supine patients, infiltrates are seen in the in posterior segments of the upper lobe or superior segments of the lower lobes due to aspiration. However, aspiration pneumonitis differs from other aspiration sequelae, since it frequently has a rapid onset, is self-limiting, and most radiographic changes of simple toxic aspiration usually clear within 48 hours. In contrast, the persistence of symptoms and associated signs of bacterial infection should raise concerns about the possibility of aspiration pneumonia.

Treatment

The risk of aspiration is decreased by reducing the volume of gastric contents, minimizing regurgitation, and protecting the airway. Patients should be NPO (nothing by mouth) for 2 or more hours before elective procedures requiring general or regional anesthesia or deep levels of conscious sedation. In intubated patents with suspected or increased risk of aspiration, extubation can be delayed until the patient is fully awake and has protective airway reflexes. Gastric decompression and rapid sequence induction of anesthesia with cricoid pressure has been advocated as the most effective way to prevent aspiration during intubation in high-risk patents but is not 100% effective.[12] When aspiration occurs, the treatment is usually supportive with supplemental oxygen. The airway should be suctioned, the stomach decompressed, and bronchoscopy should be considered for retrieval of aspirated particulate matter. In more severe cases, the patient requires mechanical ventilation and positive end-expiratory pressure.

Antibiotics are not required in most cases since aspirated gastric content is usually sterile. However, in certain cases (e.g., feculent small bowel contents with intestinal obstruction), antibiotics should be administered. Empiric antibiotics (fluoroquinolones, piperacillin/tazobactam, or ceftriaxone) are recommended in patients with small bowel obstruction or ileus and for pneumonitis that fails to resolve within 48 hours. The administration of corticosteroids to reduce pulmonary inflammation is controversial and not routinely recommended.

Pulmonary Edema and Acute Respiratory Distress Syndrome

Respiratory gas exchange occurs in the alveoli of the lung parenchyma. The alveolar wall is composed of a thin alveolar fluid layer with epithelial cells, a basement membrane, interstitial space, and capillary vessels. Oxygen diffuses through this alveolar wall and is transported primarily by red blood cells (RBCs) in the circulation, while CO_2 is dissolved in the blood and passes from the circulation to the alveolar space in the opposite direction. The pulmonary vessels, their normal endothelial barrier, tissue hydrostatic and oncotic pressures, and the lymphatic drainage system maintain fluid balance in the alveolar and interstitial spaces. When normal fluid balance is disrupted, fluid accumulates in the alveolar wall and spaces, resulting in decreased lung compliance, gas exchange, and hypoxemia. Pulmonary fluid imbalance is multifactorial in etiology and can be caused by increased hydrostatic pressure or capillary leak. Examples of these causes include excess IV fluid administration, congestive heart failure, myocardial infarction, valvular dysfunction, arrhythmias, fluid overload, renal failure, systemic infection or inflammation causing increased capillary permeability, radiation pneumonitis, toxin, gastric fluid aspiration, infection, pancreatitis, trauma, burn, interruption of lymphatic drainage, and lung resection surgery or tumor. A sudden increase in pulmonary blood flow can also raise hydrostatic pressure and cause pulmonary edema. Examples of this include reexpansion pulmonary edema, negative pressure pulmonary edema, and rapid change in inspiratory force with upper airway obstruction such as laryngeal spasm after extubation or facial fracture.

ARDS is a severe form of acute lung injury caused by either direct or indirect insult to the lung parenchyma. Direct lung injury is commonly caused by pneumonia, aspiration, chest trauma, or smoke inhalation. Indirect lung injury is typically caused by severe sepsis and systemic inflammation due to pancreatitis, shock, or ischemia/reperfusion. The pathophysiology of ARDS is characterized by inflammation, increased capillary permeability, alveolar edema, and surfactant deactivation. The resulting injury to alveolar epithelium and endothelial damage results in alveolar edema and collapse with impaired gas exchange and lung compliance. Because the inflammatory pathogenesis of ARDS results in the destruction of epithelial and endothelial cells, the resolution takes longer than pulmonary edema.

Presentation and Diagnosis

Patients with clinical risk factors for ARDS may present with shortness of breath, hypoxia, and coughing. Physical examination may indicate decreased breath sounds with crackles during inspiration, tachypnea, use of accessory respiratory muscle, anxiety, agitation, cold and clammy skin, sweating, cyanosis, and arrhythmias. The differential diagnosis of ARDS includes cardiogenic pulmonary edema, which is more commonly seen in patients with preexisting heart disease as signs or symptoms of congestive heart failure (e.g., lower extremity edema, engorged neck veins, and orthopnea). Chest radiographs show perihilar haziness, Kerley B lines, septal lines, thickening of the fissures, "batwing" distribution of air space opacification, pleural effusions, and possibly cardiomegaly in cardiogenic pulmonary edema. Arterial blood gas may show hypoxia with increased $PaCO_2$ or respiratory acidosis.

Acute lung injury and ARDS are characterized by the acute worsening of respiratory symptoms, usually within 1 week of clinical insult. The chest radiograph in ARDS shows bilateral infiltrates. The normal PaO_2/FiO_2 ratio is approximately 500. The severity of ARDS is categorized as mild, with a PaO_2/FiO_2 ratio ≤ 300; moderate, with a PaO_2/FiO_2 ratio <200; and severe, with a PaO_2/FiO_2 ratio <100.[13] In cases where the etiology of pulmonary edema is unclear, measuring central venous pressure and echocardiography can be used to differentiate between cardiogenic and noncardiogenic pulmonary edema.

Management

Patients with pulmonary edema should be positioned upright, given oxygen and ventilatory support as clinically indicated. Oxygen is given to maintain normoxia (SpO_2 <92%, and <88% in patients with chronic obstructive pulmonary disease). Noninvasive ventilation (e.g., continuous positive airway pressure or bilevel positive airway pressure) can be beneficial in patients with hypoxemia to recruit alveoli and improve oxygenation but should not be used in patients with hypotension or possible pneumothorax. In many cases, intubation and mechanical ventilation are required. Diuretics should be given to patients with objective evidence of volume overload, and urine output as well as total fluid intake and output should be monitored. IV furosemide 40 to 80 mg is commonly used and can be given in higher doses to patients who take diuretics regularly or in patients with renal insufficiency. Associated causes of pulmonary edema should also be treated (e.g., inotropic agents or afterload reducing therapy in patients with congestive heart failure).

In patients with ARDS, treatment is focused on the underlying cause (e.g., smoke inhalation, sepsis, etc.), and the care for lung injury is supportive with mechanical ventilation to optimize oxygenation and allow time for the lungs to recover. Noninvasive ventilation (e.g., continuous positive airway pressure or bilevel positive airway pressure) can be used to support oxygenation in patients with mild ARDS who do not require mechanical ventilation. When mechanical ventilation is necessary in ARDS, care should be taken to prevent additional lung injury by minimizing ventilator-induced lung injury. The patient's ideal or predicted body weight should be calculated and a tidal volume of 6 mL/kg of predicted body weight with plateau pressure of ≤30 mm H_2O should be used initially according to current ARDS net protocols. There is emerging evidence that protective ventilation strategies like airway pressure release ventilation with prolonged inspiratory phase and positive end-expiratory pressure can help to prevent ventilator-induced lung injury. Because the lung injury in ARDS is frequently heterogeneous, prone positioning can be used to decrease V/Q mismatch in some patients. In severe cases, deep sedation and muscle relaxants may be necessary to facilitate patient-ventilator synchrony. Salvage therapy for refractory hypoxemia in severe ARDS includes extracorporeal membrane oxygenation in some cases. While high-frequency oscillatory ventilation has been used in some situations, a recent trial comparing it to standard ARDS net ventilation showed no survival benefit.[14] Importantly, the cause of lung injury must be managed accordingly. Assessment of arterial blood gases can be used to monitor and adjust ventilator settings of intubated patients. Patients should be weaned from the ventilator and endotracheal tube should be removed as soon as possible.

Venous Thromboembolism

Virchow triad (venous stasis, endothelial injury, and hypercoagulability) describes the factors contributing to venous clot formation and deep venous thrombosis (DVT). Venous thromboembolism (VTE) includes DVT and pulmonary embolism (PE). DVT describes a blood clot in the deep venous system of the upper or lower extremities. DVTs often start at venous saccules or valves where blood flow is turbulent. Clot formation slows venous blood flow, which further enhances thrombus propagation and proximal extension of the clot. Newly formed thrombi are not firmly attached to the vessel wall and can detach and embolize through the venous system, ending up in the pulmonary vasculature. These pulmonary emboli are subsequently coated with fibrin and platelets, causing mechanical obstruction of the pulmonary blood flow, pulmonary hypertension, and acute right ventricular strain. VTE is associated with increased postoperative morbidity and mortality in surgery patients but are less significant when they are detected early and properly treated. About 50% of VTE occur in current or recently hospitalized patients, especially if they are admitted for surgery.[15] Conditions related to Virchow triad increase the risk of clot formation and VTE development, including long-distance travel (>4 hours), increased age, obesity, frailty, malignancy, nephrotic syndrome, varicose veins, inflammatory bowel disease, prolonged immobilization, history of VTE, inherited hypercoagulation conditions, pregnancy, use of contraceptive medication, trauma, and indwelling venous catheters.

Presentation and Diagnosis

The clinical symptoms of VTE are variable, and patients can be asymptomatic if the clot is small or nonobstructing. However, many patients with DVT have significant symptoms, including unilateral or bilateral swelling of the extremities, warmth, and localized tenderness. In patients with an acute PE, the most common symptoms are dyspnea or shortness of breath. However, there can be significant variability in PE symptomatology depending on the size of the clot, its location in the pulmonary vasculature, and the patient's underlying cardiac and pulmonary function. Massive PEs can cause obstruction of pulmonary blood flow and acute right heart strain, leading to hemodynamic compromise. Consequently, patients with massive PE can present with life-threatening symptoms of severe hypotension, unconsciousness, and/or cardiac arrest. The majority of PE are not "massive" and do not cause either hemodynamic compromise or right ventricle (RV) dysfunction. Other PE-related symptoms include dyspnea, anxiety, cough, pleuritic or dull chest pain, hemoptysis, and syncope. Physical examination may show tachycardia, low-grade fever, loud P2, or poor perfusion. The arterial blood gas measurement may show hypoxemia with respiratory alkalosis from hyperventilation. Chest radiographs are frequently normal but may show the classic wedge shape opacity (Hampton hump), decreased vascularity, atelectasis, or pleural effusion. Electrocardiography usually demonstrates tachycardia but may also have nonspecific T-wave change, right-axis deviation, right bundle branch block, cor pulmonale, or S1Q3T3. Chest radiography and electrocardiography are not diagnostic, and normal results do not exclude PE. Cardiac biomarkers (troponin T [TnT], TnI, B-type natriuretic peptide [BNP], N-terminal [NT] proBNP) can be elevated due to right ventricular strain and are indicative of higher mortality.[16]

Since clinical findings can be variable, a number of scoring systems have been developed and validated to determine the probability of VTE prior to diagnostic imaging. For example, the Wells criteria categorize patients into likely or unlikely groups and the revised Geneva score categorizes into high-, moderate-, and low-risk group of having VTE. D-dimer is a product of fibrin breakdown, which is increased in VTE but is also elevated in many other conditions and is not useful in patients with recent surgery or trauma. Although these scoring systems and D-dimer level are sensitive screening tools, they are not specific and the diagnosis of VTE should not be made based on these factors alone. In patients where VTE is suspected, imaging studies should be used to confirm or exclude the diagnosis. Moderate-risk and low-risk VTE groups should have D-dimer tested and diagnostic imaging if elevated. However, D-dimer should not be used to screen for VTE in surgery or trauma patients (who have a high incidence of elevated D-dimer) in which diagnostic imaging is preferred. In hemodynamically unstable patients suspected of having massive PE, diagnostic imaging should be done as soon as possible.

Venous duplex ultrasonography is the imaging of choice for DVT showing cross-sectional vein incompressibility, direct thrombus with vein enlargement, abnormal spectral Doppler, and color Doppler flow, which provides useful information regarding clot location and size. For many years, contrast venography was considered the gold standard for DVT diagnosis. However, it is rarely used today because of its invasive nature and its limited availability relative to duplex ultrasonography. Other diagnostic modalities for DVT include CT venography and magnetic resonance (MR) venography. CT pulmonary angiography has become the diagnostic imaging procedure of choice for PE due to the routine availability of the CT scan at most institutions. Conventional pulmonary artery angiography can be useful in select cases but is more invasive and more commonly used when endovascular or surgical intervention is being considered (e.g., pulmonary embolectomy). V/Q scan has high sensitivity in diagnosing V/Q mismatch. Unfortunately V/Q scans can also be abnormal in other pulmonary conditions (e.g., pneumonia, atelectasis, and previous PE). However, V/Q scan is sometimes preferred over CT pulmonary angiography in specific situations like pregnancy, renal insufficiency, and IV contrast allergy. Negative V/Q scans can reliably exclude clinically significant acute PEs. Transthoracic echocardiography (TTE) is commonly used when there are concerns about cardiac function and may show thrombus in the RV strain. A nondiagnostic TTE does not exclude PE, and positive findings provide indirect evidence of PE and should be carefully interpreted. However, TTE is a useful technique for bedside evaluation and follow-up and is especially useful in emergency situations when emergency thrombolytic therapy is used. Transesophageal echocardiography can give better direct visualization of pulmonary thromboembolism than TTE, and transesophageal echocardiography is the preferred over TTE if available.

Management

Many surgery patients are at increased risk of VTE and should be risk stratified for prophylactic therapy. Many validated scoring systems have been developed to quantify the VTE risk, including the Caprini score, the Department of Health VTE risk assessment tool, the Padua score, the IMPROVE score, and the Rogers score. Although pharmacologic DVT prophylaxis is generally considered to be "low risk" for bleeding complications, certain groups are considered "high risk" for bleeding complications. Patients with active GI bleeding, intracranial hemorrhage, liver disease, bleeding disorder, thrombocytopenia, recent head trauma or spinal injury/surgery, or relative contraindication to anticoagulants should be carefully assessed for risk-benefit ratio before initiating pharmacologic VTE prophylaxis.

VTE prophylaxis modalities include pharmacologic prophylaxis with low–molecular-weight heparin (LMWH), unfractionated heparin (UFH), fondaparinux, and mechanical prophylaxis with intermittent pneumatic compression, foot pumps, and graduated compression stockings. Decisions regarding VTE prophylaxis modalities are based on assessment of VTE and bleeding risk in the specific patient or population. In high-risk VTE patients (Caprini score ≥5), pharmacologic prophylaxis is preferred, if not contraindicated. Mechanical prophylaxis is often used in low-risk groups (Rogers score 7–10, Caprini score 1–2) or when patients have high bleeding risk or if anticoagulants are contraindicated. In very low risk (Rogers score <7, Caprini score 0), frequent mobilization and early ambulation are preferred. Vena cava filters are considered on a case-by-case basis in high-risk patients with contraindications to anticoagulation.

Patients diagnosed with acute DVTs are started on therapeutic anticoagulation using LMWH, UFH, or fondaparinux for 5–10 days and usually transitioned to long-term anticoagulant therapy with LMWH, vitamin K antagonist (VKA), or direct oral anticoagulants for at least 3 months. VKA medications are usually given to overlap with parenteral anticoagulant until a target international normalized ratio (INR) of 2 to 3 is reached. Extended treatment with anticoagulants beyond 3 months is considered in specific cases (e.g., inherited hypercoagulable state or chronic medical conditions with high thrombotic risk). Vena cava filters can be considered in patients with contraindications to anticoagulants, bleeding from anticoagulant, or in patients with recurrent VTE despite anticoagulation. However, patients who have recurrent VTE despite anticoagulation and have vena cava filters placed should still be given anticoagulants if possible. In severe cases, such as impending venous gangrene, thrombectomy should be considered.

In suspected PE patients, the management depends on severity and mortality risk assessed by patient conditions: hemodynamic instability, RV failure, cardiac biomarkers, and PE severity index. Patients with hypotension, RV failure by echocardiography or CT, elevated cardiac biomarkers, and PE severity index score of class III or higher are considered high risk for mortality. The first priority is to maintain hemodynamics and ventilation and the patient care team should be prepared for cardiac life support in case of cardiac arrest. Patients may need intubation, mechanical ventilation, and vasopressors to maintain blood pressure and cardiac output. IV fluids should be administered carefully in patients with PE since increased vascular volume can worsen right heart failure. Patients should be cared for in an ICU setting with central venous catheter, arterial line, electrocardiogram monitoring, and bladder catheterization with strict intake and output. Parenteral anticoagulation should be initiated immediately unless strongly contraindicated, and echocardiography should be considered when patients are hemodynamically unstable. Levophed is commonly used as the vasopressor of choice in this situation and interventions to treat obstructing PE causing severe pulmonary hypertension and RV failure should be considered. These include fibrinolytic drugs like streptokinase, urokinase, recombinant tissue plasminogen activator (rTPA) or catheter-directed therapy, and surgical embolectomy. Fibrinolytic therapies are usually preferred over the surgical or catheter-based interventions but have a higher incidence of bleeding complications (e.g., major hemorrhage or intracranial bleeding). Catheter or surgical embolectomy is considered in patients with contraindications to fibrinolytic therapy, patients who do not improve with fibrinolysis, or patients with severe hemodynamic instability. Catheter-directed therapy allows for the administration of fibrinolytic medication at the site of the clot and is associated with fewer systemic bleeding problems. Complications of catheter-directed therapy include pulmonary artery injury, cardiac tamponade, distal embolization, hemoptysis, and groin hematoma.

Extracorporeal membrane oxygenation can both provide hemodynamic support and improve oxygenation and is considered in potentially reversible patients for stabilization prior to embolectomy. Other possible causes of hemodynamic instability should be evaluated, including acute valvular dysfunction, myocardial infarction, cardiac tamponade, and aortic dissection. However, the majority of PE cases are less severe and hemodynamically stable, and the management is similar to DVT with therapeutic anticoagulation and transition to long-term anticoagulants for usually 6 months. The routine use of fibrinolytic medication for PE outweighs the benefits in most patients and should be reserved for hemodynamically unstable patients with clinical deterioration despite anticoagulation and aggressive supportive care.

For management of anticoagulants, SQ LMWH and fondaparinux are preferred over UFH due to lesser risk of major bleeding and lower incidence of heparin-induced thrombocytopenia (HIT). Examples of LMWH are enoxaparin, tinzaparin, dalteparin, and nadroparin. However, they should not be used in patients with renal impairment due to possible accumulation and bleeding complications. IV UFH is preferred in patients whom reperfusion therapy is considered due to its shorter half-life, ease of effect monitoring, availability of rapid discontinuation, and protamine reversal, and UFH should be held during infusion of fibrinolytic medication. An initial bolus of 80 units/kg is administered, and then 18 units/kg/h. The medication effect of UFH is monitored by activated partial thromboplastin time (aPTT), with a target of 1.5 to 2.5 times control value, or plasma heparin antifactor Xa 0.3 to 0.7 IU/mL. Complications include bleeding and HIT. LMWH has better bioavailability and can be given subcutaneously, with a longer half-life. The dose is calculated based on actual body weight: enoxaparin 1 mg/kg 2 times/day or 1.5 mg/kg once daily, tinzaparin 175 U/kg once daily, dalteparin 100 IU/kg 2 times/day, 200 IU/kg once daily, nadroparin 86 IU/kg 2 times/day, 171 IU/kg once daily, and LMWH does not require laboratory monitoring. However, the dose of LMWH must be carefully titrated in patients with renal insufficiency, especially since LMWH is not reversible with protamine. In patients diagnosed with HIT, both UFH and LMWH should be avoided. Direct thrombin inhibitors, hirudin, argatroban, and bivalirudin inhibit conversion of fibrinogen to fibrin and is reserved for patients likely to develop HIT. Hirudin (0.4 mg/kg IV) is given followed by an infusion of 0.15 mg/kg/h; the dose must be adjusted to renal function, and levels are routinely monitored by aPTT to achieve 1.5 to 2.5 times the laboratory normal value. Argatroban is given, 2 μg/kg/min IV, with an aPTT target of 1.5 to 3 times the normal laboratory value. Fondaparinux is given daily at a dose of 5 mg SQ if body weight is less than 50 kg, 7.5 mg SQ if body weight is between 50 and 75 kg, and 10 mg SQ if body weight is more than 100 kg. Fondaparinux is contraindicated in renal insufficiency patients (creatinine clearance <30 mL/min). Oral VKA is started as soon as oral intake is possible until reaching a target INR of 2 to 3 for two consecutive days. Patients are followed up every 4 weeks during VKA treatment for INR testing and dose adjustment if required, or at 6 weeks in stable cases. Patients who have INR >4.5 but <10 are advised to stop taking VKA without giving vitamin K, and patients with life-threatening bleeding are admitted and should receive vitamin K and 4-factor prothrombin complex concentrates or fresh-frozen plasma if not available. Direct oral anticoagulants, dabigatran, rivaroxaban, apixaban, and edoxaban, are recommended as alternative to heparin/VKA treatment. Physicians should be aware of drug interaction in patients receiving anticoagulation.

CARDIAC COMPLICATIONS

Perioperative Myocardial Ischemia and Infarction

Perioperative myocardial ischemia and infarction (PMI) are important and potentially severe complications in noncardiac surgery. They are the most common cardiac complications that increase length of hospital stay and cost of care and worsen prognosis. Normally, acute myocardial infarction is diagnosed by an elevation of cardiac enzyme with either ischemic symptoms, electrocardiographic changes attributable to myocardial ischemia, infarction, or imaging findings. However, 65% of patients with PMI do not experience ischemic symptoms, according to the Perioperative Ischemia Evaluation (POISE) trial,[17] and only 41.8% of patients with myocardial injury after noncardiac surgery met the criteria for myocardial infarction in the Vascular Events in Noncardiac Surgery Patients Cohort Evaluation (VISION) cohort study of 15,065 patients.[18] Elevation of cardiac troponin alone is an independent risk factor of myocardial ischemia and is associated with increased postoperative mortality. In short, if the diagnostic criteria of chest pain with associated signs and symptoms, serum markers, and change in electrocardiogram were used, we would routinely underdiagnose PMI and myocardial injury after noncardiac surgery.

Cause

The cause of PMI is from two main mechanisms. The first is the classic theory of plaque rupture and thrombosis of coronary vessels occluding the blood supply to myocardium. The second is the imbalance between oxygen demand and supply during the perioperative period and postoperative care. Therefore, patients at risk for cardiac complications are those who have underlying coronary artery disease, recent myocardial infarction or stenting, recent stroke, and other risk factors for coronary disease, including peripheral arterial disease, diabetes, hyperlipidemia, smoking, family history, or hypertension. Other risk factors are the types of surgery and perioperative events contributing to alteration of oxygen demand and supply. Major surgeries are more stressful to the patient and can impact normal homeostasis by causing inflammation, hypercoagulability, platelet activation, tachycardia, or high blood pressure, which exert stress on coronary vessels, leading to preexisting plaque rupture. The stress response to surgery activates the sympathetic nervous system, resulting in elevated catecholamines, which can lead to coronary vasoconstriction and increased myocardial oxygen demand. The examples of major surgeries with increased risk of PMI include major vascular surgery, noncardiac transplant surgery, intraperitoneal and thoracic surgery, and emergency surgery. During the perioperative period, alterations in hemodynamics, oxygenation, and ventilation related to surgery can also affect coronary blood flow and cause imbalance of myocardial oxygen demand and supply. Examples include hypoxia, hypothermia, hypotension, hypertension, tachycardia, bleeding, and anemia.

Presentation and Diagnosis

Most patients have perioperative ischemia or infarction within 48 hours after surgery. Symptomatic patients may develop substernal chest pain or pressure radiating to the left shoulder or neck. They may also experience arrhythmia, tachycardia, sweating, dyspnea, or signs of heart failure, hypoxia, acidosis, cardiogenic shock, and cardiac arrest. When these symptoms occur, cardiac biomarkers should be measured and electrocardiography should be performed. Changes in electrocardiography are another indication of cardiac ischemia and range from ST-segment elevation, ST depression, T-wave inversion, or Q waves. However, most patients with perioperative ischemia or infarction are asymptomatic, and there are still no standardized diagnostic criteria for this group. Cardiac biomarkers are associated with perioperative ischemia and infarction and may be the only abnormality detected. Elevations of TnT and TnI are associated with higher mortality since concentrations are normally very low (TnT 0.02 ng/mL, TnI 0.2 ng/mL). Also, preoperative natriuretic peptides (BNP, NTproBNP) are shown to be predictive of ischemia or infarction, and creatine kinase MB fraction is also elevated but has lesser sensitivity and specificity. Screening for PMI by routinely checking troponin levels in surgical patients remains a controversial topic according to recent clinical practice guidelines.[19] The 2014 American College of Cardiology and American Heart Association (ACC/AHA)[20] guidelines recommend troponin screening be considered only in patients with signs and symptoms suggestive of myocardial infarction both before and 48 to 72 hours after surgery. Their rationale is that troponin levels may be elevated in different medical conditions like renal insufficiency, heart failure, PE, and atrial fibrillation. Furthermore, most high-risk patients present with high troponin levels before surgery. There is insufficient evidence that biomarker screening reduces cardiac events; therefore, routine screening is not recommended (2014 AHA guideline).

In contrast, the 2014 European Society of Cardiology and the European Society of Anaesthesiology guidelines[21] recommend screening every high-risk patient both before surgery and 48 to 72 hours after surgery. Consequently, the diagnosis and management of patients with perioperative ischemia who do not fulfill the standard criteria of myocardial infarction should be individualized based on the patient's characteristics, risks, and biomarkers.

Prevention and Management

Identification of patients with increased risk of developing PMI allows their physicians to more carefully evaluate their cardiac risks before surgery. Several methods for cardiac risk stratification are available, and the most commonly used today is the revised cardiac risk index (RCRI). The RCRI assesses the perioperative risk of major cardiac complications, including myocardial infarction, pulmonary edema, ventricular fibrillation, or cardiac arrest, and complete heart block based on six patient characteristics (Box 12.2). Patients with at least two risk factors are at increased risk for cardiac complications. Other common risk-calculating methods are the NSQIP-myocardial infarction or cardiac arrest (www.surgicalriskcalculator.com/miorcardiacarrest) and the NSQIP risk calculator (www.riskcalculator.facs.org) developed by the American College of Surgeons, which are commonly used in the United States. Patients are categorized as low risk (risk <1%) or elevated risk (risk >1%). If categorized by surgical procedure, it can be grouped as low, intermediate, and high risk (Table 12.9).

Before surgery, physicians should obtain and evaluate the patient's functional class since poor functional class is associated with cardiac complications. Electrocardiography should be done within 3 months before surgery, and patients with unknown dyspnea or change in functional class should have left ventricular function examined. Functional class can be assessed by daily activity using metabolic equivalence of the task (MET), where 1 MET is equal to the resting oxygen consumption of a 40-year old, 70-kg man. Simple questions about daily activities can be asked to evaluate the patient's conditions. Examples of activities, which patients with poor functional class (METs <4) are able to do, are walking slowly (3 mph), ballroom dancing, working on a computer, and playing a musical instrument, and activities indicating moderate or great functional class (METs ≥4) include gardening, walking up a hill, biking, and heavy work around the house. Recommendations for perioperative testing by the ACC/AHA are presented in Fig. 12.1 to guide management and reduce risk before surgery. Perioperative beta blockers have been shown to reduce the risk of myocardial infarction and are recommended before surgery; however, beta blockers may also increase the risk of stroke, bradycardia, and mortality in some patients.[22] Therefore, beta blockers should be continued in patients who already take them and initiation of beta blockers should be considered in high-risk patients (≥3 RCRI) several days before surgery. Aspirin and statins are two commonly used medications in patients with coronary disease. Initiating aspirin before surgery is controversial due to the potential risk of bleeding. However, aspirin should be continued in patients taking aspirin with a history of coronary disease or stenting. Statins have also been shown to reduce postoperative cardiovascular events and should be continued or initiated especially in vascular surgery patients.

Patients with coronary disease who have been treated with percutaneous coronary intervention (PCI) ± stents are placed on dual antiplatelet therapy (DAPT) with aspirin and a P2Y12 receptor inhibitor to prevent thrombosis. Thrombotic risk is considered low 4 weeks after balloon angiography), 6 months after bare-metal stents, and 1 year after drug-eluting stents. Elective surgery for PCI patients should be postponed if possible during the high-thrombotic-risk periods described above. Perioperative management of DAPT for noncardiac surgery patients should consider the risk of thrombosis and the risk of hemorrhage. Specific guidelines are available to guide perioperative antiplatelet therapy, but surgeon judgment is required to optimize care for individual patients. Anemia should be corrected to optimize oxygen delivery during operation.

During the operation, surgeons and anesthetists should maintain good blood pressure and oxygenation, minimize bleeding, avoid hypothermia, and provide adequate pain control. However, there is no specific evidence-based intraoperative values or goals of vital signs and measurements. Monitoring these variables should be continued in the postoperative period, and electrocardiography should be obtained if PMI is suspected.

Once myocardial tissue has been damaged, the median time from PMI to death is approximately 12 days.[23] The challenge in management comes in determining the pathophysiology of PMI between plaque rupture/thrombosis (type I) or imbalance of oxygen demand and supply (type II), and there is no standard or international criteria for diagnosis and management. However, ST-elevated myocardial infarction and unstable angina/non-ST-elevated myocardial infarction should be managed according to clinical practice guidelines, but recent major surgery is a relative contraindication of fibrinolytic drugs. Judgment in managing patients

BOX 12.2 Six independent risk predictors for the revised cardiac risk index.

Patients with two or more risk factors are considered elevated risk.

- High-risk type of surgery (intraperitoneal, intrathoracic, suprainguinal vascular surgery)
- History of ischemic heart disease
- History of congestive heart failure
- History of cerebrovascular disease
- Insulin therapy for diabetes
- Preoperative serum creatinine >2 mg/dL

From Lee TH, Marcantonio ER, Mangione CM, et al. Derivation and prospective validation of a simple index for prediction of cardiac risk of major noncardiac surgery. *Circulation.* 1999;100:1043–1049.

TABLE 12.9 Cardiac risk stratification for noncardiac surgical procedures.

LEVEL OF RISK	RISK FACTOR
High (cardiac risk often >5%)	Emergency major operations, particularly in elderly patients Aortic and other major vascular surgery Peripheral vascular surgery Anticipated prolonged surgical procedures associated with large fluid shifts and blood loss
Intermediate (cardiac risk generally <5%)	Carotid endarterectomy Intraperitoneal and intrathoracic surgery Orthopedic surgery Prostate surgery
Low (cardiac risk generally <1%)	Endoscopic procedures Superficial procedures Cataract surgery Breast surgery

From Eagle KA, Berger PB, Calkins H, et al. ACC/AHA guideline update for perioperative cardiovascular evaluation for noncardiac surgery—executive summary. A report of the American College of Cardiology/American Heart Association Task Force on Practice Guidelines (Committee to Update the 1996 Guidelines on Perioperative Cardiovascular Evaluation for Noncardiac Surgery). *Anesth Analg.* 2002;94:1052–1064.

not fulfilling the criteria for ST-elevated myocardial infarction and unstable angina/non-ST-elevated myocardial infarction should be individualized with consideration of a cardiology consult. Patients with suspected type I injury should receive aggressive aspirin therapy, with caution exerted for bleeding risk, and statin therapy with consideration of angiography. Secondary prevention using beta blockers and angiotensin-converting enzyme (ACE) inhibitors should be given when feasible. Patients suspected of type II injury should have optimal hemodynamics and oxygenation therapy with possible angiography during follow-up after surgery. The consequences of severe myocardial infarction can be life-threatening and include cardiogenic shock or cardiac arrest. Life-threatening complications of severe myocardial infarction include free rupture of the cardiac wall or septum, acute mitral valve regurgitation from rupture of chordae tendineae, and complete heart block. Aggressive management is required to prevent death and includes hemodynamic and oxygenation support in case of cardiogenic shock and cardiopulmonary resuscitation in cardiac arrest. However, the mortality in this group is as high as 70%.

Postoperative Hypertension

Causes

Hypertension is a common problem in surgical patients, with an incidence of approximately 30% in patients >20 years and 50% in patients >65 years.[24] Hypertension can increase the perioperative morbidity and mortality in surgical patients due to its long-term effects on coronary disease, impairment of cardiac function, and renal insufficiency. Postoperative hypertension is defined as blood pressure more than 190/100 mm Hg in two consecutive readings after surgery. Many patients with postoperative hypertension were diagnosed with hypertension prior to surgery. Stopping preoperative antihypertensive medications is a common reason for postoperative hypertension in these patients. However, other causes include postoperative pain, anxiety, volume overload, hypercapnia, hypothermia, and volume overload. Other less common conditions, including bladder distension, alcohol or benzodiazepine withdrawal, catecholamine surge in pheochromocytoma, vasoactive tumors, and thyroid storm, should be considered in the differential diagnosis.

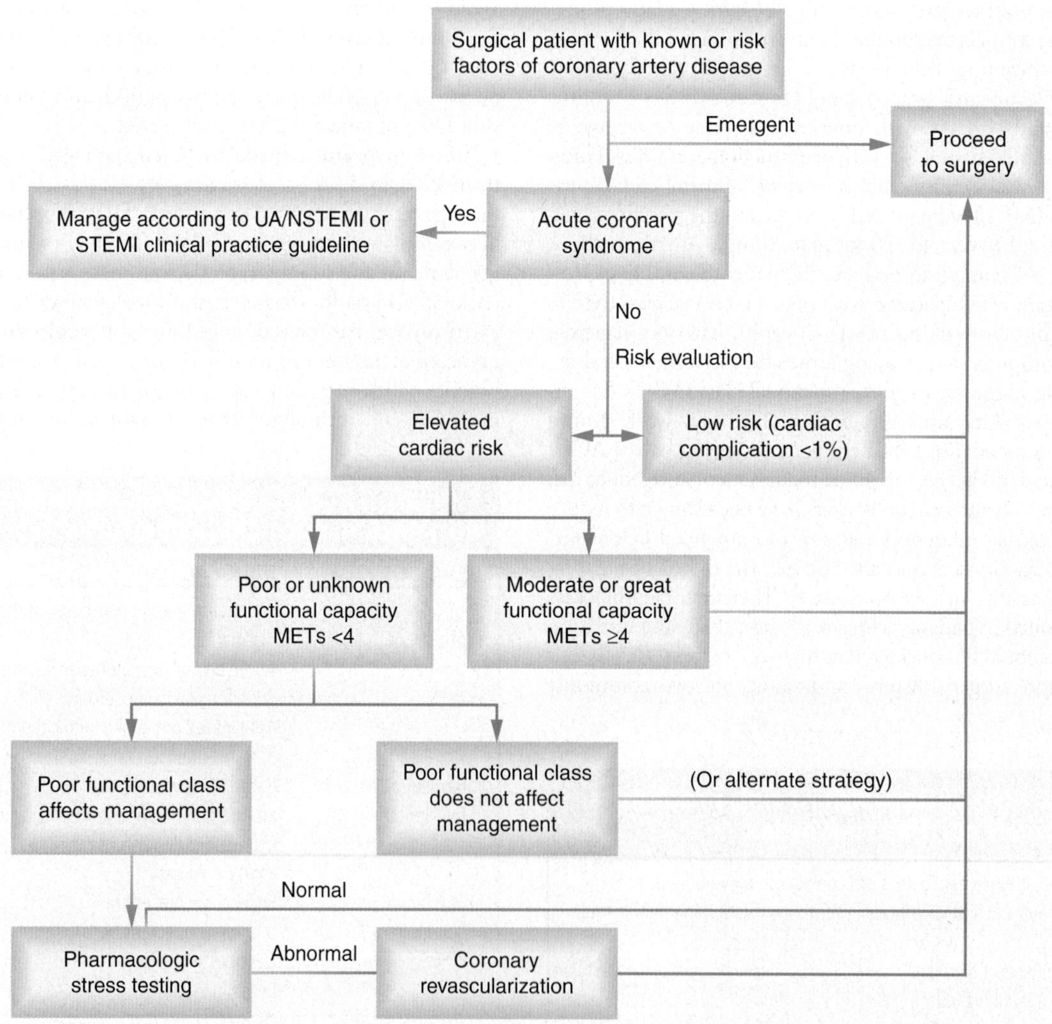

FIG. 12.1 Algorithm for stepwise approach to perioperative cardiac assessment. (*METs*, Metabolic equivalents of the task; *NSTEMI*, non-ST-elevation myocardial infarction; *STEMI*, ST-elevation myocardial infarction; UA, unstable angina. Adapted from Fleisher LA, Fleischmann KE, Auerbach AD, et al. 2014 ACC/AHA guideline on perioperative cardiovascular evaluation and management of patients undergoing noncardiac surgery: a report of the American College of Cardiology/American Heart Association Task Force on Practice Guidelines. *J Am Coll Cardiol.* 2014;64:e77–e137.)

Presentation and Management

Postoperative hypertension commonly begins within 30 minutes after surgery and can last for several hours. Complications include an increased risk of cardiovascular events, cerebrovascular events, and bleeding from surgical sites. When severe hypertension is noted after surgery, postoperative pain and anxiety should be considered and treated as needed. Intraoperative fluid therapy should be reviewed for volume overload, and the patient's respiratory status should be assessed to rule out postanesthesia hypoxia or hypercarbia. Treatment of postoperative hypertension should be carefully titrated to avoid hypotension with associated hypoperfusion. The use of antihypertensives with rapid onset and short half-lives is recommended, with an initial target of lowering blood pressure by 25% and then reevaluating. The most commonly used medications are calcium channel blockers (clevidipine, nicardipine), beta blockers (labetalol, esmolol), vasodilators (nitroglycerin, nitroprusside, hydralazine), and ACE inhibitors (e.g., enalapril).

Preoperative evaluation of patients with preexisting hypertension should focus on organ damage related to hypertension. This includes changes in the electrocardiogram, a change in functional class, history of transient ischemic attacks, stroke, or an increase in serum creatinine. Preoperative echocardiogram or cardiac catheterization should be considered in high-risk surgeries (e.g., major vascular surgery). If target organ damage is present or secondary hypertension is suspected, those issues should be managed preoperatively. Patients with untreated hypertension or poorly controlled blood pressure may have greater hemodynamic instability during anesthesia and surgery. However, mild to moderate elevation of blood pressure alone (<180/110 mm Hg) without evidence of organ damage should not be the reason to postpone surgery. In patients with a diastolic blood pressure of more than 110 mm Hg, there is an increased risk of cardiac complications. Preoperative antihypertensive medications should be continued until the day of surgery, especially sympatholytic drugs such as beta blockers and clonidine, since withdrawal could lead to adverse events. During anesthesia, vascular tone from sympathetic activity is decreased, and blood pressure is maintained by regulation of the renin-angiotensin-aldosterone system (RAAS). Therefore, patients taking ACE inhibitors or angiotensin II receptor blockers (ARBs) should usually stop them the day before surgery. Stopping ACE inhibitors before surgery has been shown to decrease all-cause mortality and vascular events, including myocardial injury and stroke.[25] Antihypertensive medication should be resumed as soon as possible after surgery.

Postoperative Arrhythmias

Arrhythmias are alterations of cardiac electrical impulse including conduction (reentry, delay or blocking) and initiation (premature impulse, change in automaticity). Dysrhythmia-induced changes in HR or rhythm can cause abnormal beating or myocardial contraction of the heart, resulting in increased or decreased HR and possibly cardiac output. Postoperative arrhythmias or dysrhythmias can happen after surgery (especially cardiac surgery) due to direct disturbance of the heart or in patients with underlying structural heart abnormalities like valvular heart disease, ischemia, or scarring. Dysrhythmias may occur after noncardiac surgery due to surgical stress, anesthesia, or complications from surgery. Patients with postoperative arrhythmias tend to have a longer hospital stay and higher mortality. Risk factors include increasing age, male gender, history of arrhythmias, valvular heart disease, hypertension, history of stroke, chronic lung disease, and obesity. In the postoperative period, arrhythmias can be triggered by acid-base and electrolyte abnormalities, inflammatory or surgical stress caused by pain, PMI, heart failure, hypoxia, infections, bacteremia, or sepsis; and medications can also trigger arrhythmias. Withdrawing beta blockers can result in a surge of catecholamines and lead to arrhythmias.

Presentation

Most dysrhythmias after surgery are transient and cause no hemodynamic compromise. Patients may feel nothing or just palpitations. If the dysrhythmias are persistent or severe, they can cause hemodynamic alterations, including signs and symptoms of low cardiac output like chest pain, pulmonary edema, confusion, desaturation, hypotension, low urine output, or even cardiac arrest. Tachydysrhythmias may reduce diastolic time and coronary flow, potentially triggering myocardial ischemia or infarction. Patients with postoperative arrhythmias should be examined with 12-lead electrocardiography and have their hemodynamic status monitored. The two most common arrhythmias after surgery are atrial fibrillation and atrial flutter, which commonly develop within 3 days of surgery.

Management of postoperative atrial fibrillation is similar to new-onset atrial fibrillation. In hemodynamically normal patients, initial treatment involves control of the ventricular rate with beta blockers, calcium channel blockers, or digoxin. Chemical cardioversion may be considered to decrease the risk of thromboembolism when the atrial arrhythmia is less than 48 hours duration. However, if the onset is more than 48 hours or unknown anticoagulation therapy is recommended since the risks of atrial clot formation increase over time. The decision to start anticoagulation for postoperative atrial fibrillation must balance the risks of thromboembolism with the risks of bleeding after surgery. The most commonly used thromboembolic risk stratification tool is the CHA_2DS_2-VASc risk score, which recommends routine anticoagulation if the score is ≥2.[26] Antiarrhythmic drugs commonly used to convert atrial fibrillation are amiodarone, flecainide, dofetilide, propafenone, or ibutilide. In most cases, rate control is indicated prior to initiating chemical conversion. Electrical cardioversion ± anticoagulation should be considered in patients with rapid atrial fibrillation and hemodynamic compromise. In addition, physicians should simultaneously treat and correct potentially precipitating problems, including infection, sepsis, acid-base and electrolyte abnormalities, and anemia. If patients fail to convert to sinus rhythm, long-term anticoagulation should be considered based on the individual patient's risk factors.

Narrow complex supraventricular tachycardia (e.g., from electrical reentry of atrioventricular nodal conduction) can be treated with vagal maneuvers such as carotid sinus massage (in patients with no risk of stroke from carotid artery disease), with IV adenosine, or cardioversion in case of hemodynamic compromise. Ventricular arrhythmias are less common. Premature ventricular contraction, which often is asymptomatic and does not increase the risk of sustained ventricular tachycardia or ventricular fibrillation and may not require perioperative evaluation or management unless it is frequent, multifocal, or symptomatic. Treatment of ventricular dysrhythmias includes correction of electrolyte abnormalities (especially potassium and magnesium) and/or medications. Commonly used medications for ventricular arrhythmias include beta blockers, amiodarone, and lidocaine. In hemodynamically unstable ventricular dysrhythmias, electrical cardioversion or defibrillation should be performed in conjunction with cardiopulmonary resuscitation. Bradyarrhythmias include sinus bradycardia, which is the most common, and different grades of atrioventricular blocks. Medications used to treat symptomatic bradycardias include atropine, aminophylline, or cardiac pacing in patients with sustained symptomatic bradyarrhythmias.

Postoperative Heart Failure

Heart failure is a clinical syndrome indicating poor cardiac function. It can be grouped into two categories according to the pathophysiology: systolic dysfunction caused by reductions in left ventricular ejection fraction (LVEF) and diastolic dysfunction characterized by having a nondilated left ventricle with normal or preserved LVEF. Many medical conditions can contribute to this clinical syndrome, including ischemia or infarction of myocardium, arrhythmias, abnormal heart valve, PE, pericardium abnormality, cardiac tamponade, hypertension, and volume overload. All of these factors ultimately result in an inability to increase stroke volume and cardiac output, leading to congestion of volume. Further, many cardiac risk stratification systems include heart failure as a predictor. Perioperative heart failure is associated with a 63% increased mortality compared to patients with no postoperative heart failure.[27] Patients with diastolic heart failure (preserved LVEF) have lower mortality rate than the ones with systolic heart failure (reduced LVEF), especially LVEF <30%.[27]

Presentation and Management

Most patients with postoperative heart failure have a history of heart failure. Their physicians should look for medical conditions that might lead to poor cardiac function such as previous myocardial infarction, longstanding hypertension, diabetes, or a family history of heart failure. Common symptoms of heart failure include dyspnea on exertion, poor functional status, fatigue, weight gain, orthopnea, and paroxysmal nocturnal dyspnea. Physical examination findings in heart failure include engorgement of neck veins, lower extremity edema, a third heart sound, and rales or wheezing on lung auscultation. Ancillary testing may show pulmonary edema or cardiomegaly on chest x-ray and evidence of previous myocardial infarction, ventricular hypertrophy or arrhythmias on electrocardiogram.

Patients with signs and symptoms of heart failure should be evaluated before surgery using TTE to assess LVEF, diastolic function, and valve function. Patients with a history of cardiac disease should have electrocardiography and chest x-ray in case of suspected pulmonary edema. The natriuretic peptides BNP and NT proBNP are proteins derived from the myocardium and fibroblast responses to cardiac wall stress, which have good sensitivity and specificity in predicting cardiovascular events in noncardiac surgery. Preoperative BNP and NT proBNP in conjunction with RCRI can help assess perioperative cardiac risk. However, the optimal cut point for serum BNP and NT-proBNP levels are not yet defined. In a meta analysis, screening with preoperative BNP, at a cut point of 30 pg/mL, demonstrates a 95% sensitivity and a 44% specificity in predicting MACE at 30 days in vascular surgery patients.[28] BNP levels can be used to detect, monitor, and guide therapy in patients with heart failure. Surgery patients with heart failure should be medically optimized before surgery using beta blockers, ACE inhibitors/ARBs, aldosterone antagonist, digitalis, and/or diuretics in symptomatic patients as clinically indicated. On the day of surgery, discontinuing ACE inhibitors/ARBs to prevent hypotension is reasonable but should be resumed as soon as possible. Patients with LVEF <35% or QRS complex >120 ms should be considered for cardiac resynchronization therapy before surgery. During and after surgery, volume management is very important; patients should be monitored hemodynamically with routine physical examination, biomarker determination, and electrocardiogram to avoid development of heart failure. Patients who develop postoperative heart failure should be treated with diuretics as needed to relieve symptoms. Inotropes, along with invasive hemodynamic monitoring, may be used to increase cardiac contractility, and an aortic balloon pump may be used selectively to decrease workload in critically ill patients. Since heart failure is the result of many conditions, identifying and treating the underlying cause of the heart failure are important too.

RENAL AND URINARY COMPLICATIONS

Acute Kidney Injury

AKI, formerly known as acute renal failure, is a rapid decline in the ability of the kidney to clear waste products. AKI is a common postoperative complication that increases morbidity and mortality especially after major surgical procedures, including complex cardiac, vascular, and major abdominal surgery. The standardized criteria for diagnosing AKI were established by the risk, injury, failure, loss, and end-stage kidney disease (RIFLE) criteria in 2004 and were modified to the Acute Kidney Injury Network (AKIN) criteria in 2007 using the serum creatinine level and urine output as indicators of kidney function. The most recent consensus statement on the diagnosis of AKI are the 2012 Kidney Disease: Improving Global Outcomes (KDIGO) criteria (Table 12.10), which classifies AKI into stages based on severity. The higher stages are associated with worse outcomes, mortality, and need for renal replacement therapy (RRT). Because the serum creatinine may vary with age, muscle mass, and diet, its ability to indicate the origin

TABLE 12.10 The 2012 KDIGO clinical practice guidelines for acute kidney injury.

Definition of Acute Kidney Injury	
Increase in serum creatinine by ≥0.3 mg/dL within 48 hours OR Increase in serum creatinine to ≥1.5 times baseline, which is known or presumed to have occurred within the prior 7 days OR Urine volume <0.5 mL/kg/h for 6 hours.	
Staging of Acute Kidney Injury	
Serum Creatinine	***Urine Output***
Stage 1	
1.5–1.9 times baseline OR ≥0.3 mg/dL increase	<0.5 mL/kg/h for 6–12 hours
Stage 2	
2.0–2.9 times baseline	<0.5 mL/kg/h for ≥12 hours
Stage 3	
3 times baseline OR Increase in serum creatinine to ≥4.0 mg/dL OR Initiation of renal replacement therapy OR In patients <18 years, decrease in eGFR to <35 mL/min/1.73 m^2	<0.3 mL/kg/h for ≥24 hours OR Anuria for ≥12 hours

eGFR, Estimated glomerular filtration rate; *KDIGO*, Kidney Disease: Improving Global Outcomes.

of AKI is limited in certain situations. Therefore, new biomarkers have been identified and are utilized to improve the diagnosis and localization of AKI, including neutrophil gelatinase-associated lipocalin, cystatin C, tissue inhibitor of metalloproteinase-2, and insulin-like growth factor (IGF) binding protein-7. Although many of these biomarkers are used to assess kidney injury in research studies and some are used clinically in several countries, none of them are used routinely at this time.

The pathophysiology of AKI can be characterized as either prerenal, renal, or postrenal. Prerenal AKI or renal hypoperfusion, an important cause of kidney injury in surgical patients, is caused by loss of intravascular volume from bleeding or dehydration, medications that affect regulation of the RAAS or impair the normal regulatory mechanisms of afferent and efferent arterioles, vasodilatation from inflammation, sepsis, or anesthetic agents. Renal etiologies of AKI include medications or chemicals that are directly toxic to the kidney such as nonsteroidal antiinflammatory drugs (NSAIDs), aminoglycosides, and amphotericin B. Trauma patients with crush injuries or impaired blood supply to the extremities may develop rhabdomyolysis. The release of myoglobin from injured muscle in patients with rhabdomyolysis may cause kidney injury by several mechanisms, including renal vasoconstriction, the formation of tubular casts caused by myoglobin precipitation, and most importantly the injury of tubular cell by free oxygen radicals. The use of contrast media in radiographic imaging is one of the most common causes of AKI in surgical patients. The mechanisms of contrast media–induced AKI are complex but involve a combination of medullary vasoconstriction/ischemia and direct injury/cytotoxicity to tubular epithelial cells. Risk factors for developing postoperative AKI include increased age, obesity, diabetes, hypertension, perioperative hypotension, anemia, intraoperative transfusion, preexisting chronic kidney disease, higher ASA grade, poor cardiac function or heart failure, nephrotoxic medications and contrast media, types of surgery especially cardiac surgery, use of cardiopulmonary bypass, and emergency surgery (Table 12.11).

Presentation and Management

It is important to monitor urine output and serum creatinine in patients at risk for AKI. Urine output is easy to measure and can be monitored continuously using indwelling bladder catheters. An acute reduction in urine output (<0.5 mL/kg/h) is an important and useful tool in the diagnosis and prevention of AKI. Despite its utility, reductions in urine output are of limited use in predicting AKI in certain conditions, including hyperglycemia, osmotic diuresis, nonoliguric AKI, and postrenal obstruction.

The signs and symptoms of renal insufficiency present in the later stages as nitrogen waste products accumulate and patients become fluid overloaded. Signs and symptoms of more advanced renal failure can include nausea, vomiting, fatigue, confusion from uremia, asterixis, pericardial rub from uremic pericarditis, and abnormal bleeding. In cases of volume overload, peripheral edema, shortness of breath, and increased pulmonary infiltration on chest x-ray could be noted and are suggestive of congestive heart failure. Laboratory tests that help to discriminate prerenal, renal, and postrenal causes of AKI are summarized in Table 12.12. In prerenal AKI, activation of RAAS and antidiuretic hormone (ADH) retain volume intravascularly by concentrating the urine (urine osmolarity >500 mOsm/L) and reabsorbing sodium (urinary sodium <20 mOsm/L, fractional excretion of sodium <1%), causing increased blood urea nitrogen (plasma urea to creatinine ratio >20). In contrast, the malfunctioning nephron in renal AKI loses the ability to concentrate urine (urine osmolarity close to plasma, urinary sodium >50 mOsm/L, fractional excretion of sodium >3%, plasma urea to creatinine ratio <20). New imaging techniques with promising utility in identifying the risk of AKI have been developed, but there are currently no established indications for clinical use. For example, Doppler ultrasonography measuring renal blood flow, vascular resistance, and compliance can be used to calculate the renal resistive index, which is higher in patients with a higher risk of AKI.

The optimal management strategy for AKI is the identification of high-risk patients and preventively managing their care to minimize the risk of developing AKI. Risk factors for perioperative AKI include age, obesity, high ASA class, preexisting renal disease,

TABLE 12.12 Diagnostic evaluation of acute renal failure.

PARAMETER	PRERENAL	RENAL	POSTRENAL
Urine osmolality	>500 mOsm/L	= Plasma	Variable
Urinary sodium	<20 mOsm/L	>50 mOsm/L	>50 mOsm/L
Fractional excretion of sodium	<1%	>3%	Variable
Urine, plasma creatinine level	>40	<20	<20
Urine, plasma urea level	>8	<3	Variable
Urine, plasma osmolality	<1.5	>1.5	Variable

TABLE 12.11 Risk factors for developing postoperative acute kidney injury.

PRERENAL	RENAL	POSTRENAL	TYPE OF SURGERY	PATIENT FACTORS
Hypovolemia	Nephrotoxic medication –Aminoglycosides –Amphotericin B	Stones	Cardiac surgery	Age
Hemorrhage	Radiocontrast media	Cell debris	Major vascular surgery	Obesity
Third space loss	Rhabdomyolysis	BPH	Emergency surgery	High ASA class
Hypotension		Neurogenic bladder	Laparoscopic surgery	Underlying renal insufficiency
NSAIDs				Impaired cardiac function
RAAS blockers				Diabetes
Intraabdominal pressure				Anemia
Perioperative hypotension				Chronic liver disease
				Hypertension

ASA, American Association of Anesthesiologists; *BPH*, benign prostatic hyperplasia; *NSAIDs*, nonsteroidal antiinflammatory drugs; *RAAS*, renin-angiotensin-aldosterone system.

diabetes, and hypertension. Preventive strategies to reduce perioperative AKI include attention to volume status and hemoglobin levels before surgery, which can reduce the risk of intraoperative renal hypoperfusion and hypoxia. Patients with vomiting, diarrhea, anorexia, preoperative bowel preparation, or bleeding are at increased risk for hypovolemia/prerenal AKI and need to be aggressively resuscitated. Patients with a history of chronic kidney disease or previous episodes of AKI are at risk for postoperative AKI, and the adjustment of nephrotoxic medications should be considered before the operation. During the perioperative period, the goal is to maintain adequate renal perfusion; a mean arterial pressure lower than 60 mm Hg is associated with a higher risk of postoperative AKI. Therefore, during anesthesia, the mean arterial pressure should be maintained above 65 mm Hg or 75 to 80 mm Hg in patients with hypertension. Invasive hemodynamic monitoring (e.g., central venous catheter or arterial line) should be considered in certain cases. Intraoperative urine output should be maintained at ≥0.5 mL/kg/h in the perioperative period if possible.

Once AKI has developed, there is no specific treatment to regain kidney function. The goal is to maintain adequate renal perfusion and to avoid further kidney injury, allowing the return of renal function. Repeated episodes of AKI can lead to permanent deterioration of renal function and chronic renal insufficiency, increasing the risk of long-term RRT. Volume assessment is critical and can be challenging, especially for patients with heart failure or underlying renal insufficiency. Since hypovolemia can cause prerenal AKI and too much of volume can reduce renal blood flow by increasing abdominal pressure and causing renal congestion, the evaluation of volume status and whether the patient is volume responsive is critical and can determine the direction of management. In a complicated situation, using other methods to evaluate intravascular volume such as chest x-ray, echocardiography, variation of hemodynamic parameters (stroke volume, pulse pressure, systolic pressure), diameter of the vena cava, or leg raising test may be considered. The optimal resuscitative fluid for patients with AKI who are thought to be hypovolemic is still controversial. However, many studies recommend avoiding colloid containing hydroxyethyl starches because its use is associated with AKI. Also, normal saline should be used with caution due to the possibility of causing hyperchloremic metabolic acidosis. Resuscitation with a balanced crystalloid solution, which is more similar to human plasma with respect to electrolytes, pH, and buffer capacity, is being studied. Diuretic drugs were initially considered as preventative therapy for AKI by maintaining urine output, blocking ion channels, decreasing energy consumption of renal tubules, reducing oxygen demand, and preventing hypoxia. However, recent studies showed no clinical benefit in the prevention and treatment of AKI; thus, diuretics should be used primarily to prevent volume overload. Managing volume with diuretics should not delay RRT if indicated. Vasopressors should be used to maintain blood pressure in AKI patients as needed. Dopamine was thought to be the vasopressor of choice for AKI due to its ability to increase renal blood flow. However, dopamine does not appear to be more effective than other vasopressors in patients with AKI and vasopressor choice should be individualized based on their underlying medical condition.

Contrast-induced AKI is another important cause of AKI, especially in patients with underlying renal insufficiency. Several strategies have been used to prevent contrast-induced AKI, such as reducing reactive oxygen species by acetylcysteine, vitamin C, or bicarbonate or using diuretic drugs to dilute contrast and reduce exposure time in the renal tubules. Unfortunately, these preventive strategies are still controversial. However, volume expansion appears to be the most beneficial intervention possibly by suppression of vasopressin, inhibition of RAAS, and dilution of contrast. IV fluids of choice include isotonic normal saline or sodium bicarbonate solution and should be started 6 to 12 hours before the procedure and for 4 to 12 hours after the procedure in patients at risk of AKI.

In cases of severe AKI, RRT prevents mortality from volume overload, electrolyte imbalance, and uremia. The indication and timing of RRT is still varied, and there are no standard criteria of RRT initiation. Hemodialysis is continued until renal function is regained, as noted by a reduction of serum creatinine during stable hemodialysis or an increase in creatinine clearance. Patients who fail to regain renal function should have long-term RRT.

Urinary Retention[29]

Postoperative urinary retention has no standardized definition. However, it is a common postoperative complication and refers to the inability to spontaneously empty the urinary bladder after surgery. The urinary bladder has a capacity of approximately 500 mL; overstretching the bladder wall will cause muscular ischemia and reduce sensation and contractility; thus, factors which interfere with the micturition reflex, over distend the bladder, or compromise the outflow of urinary tract can result in urinary retention. Risk factors of urinary retention include increased age, male gender, anesthetic choice, types of surgery, operative time and intraoperative fluid administration, underlying urinary and neurologic conditions, and certain medications (Table 12.13).

Presentation and Management

Patients usually complain of lower abdominal fullness, suprapubic pain, or discomfort. Although uncommon, the massively distended bladder can stimulate the vasovagal reflex causing cardiovascular symptoms, including bradycardia, arrhythmia, hypotension, or asystole. Physical examination may demonstrate a palpable bladder at the lower abdomen. However, some patients show no signs or symptoms of bladder distention and present with overflow incontinence. If left untreated, urinary retention can result in a UTI, which may lengthen hospital stay and increase morbidity. Chronic retention could permanently damage the detrusor muscle and cause long-term complications such as bladder stone, hydronephrosis, incontinence, or renal insufficiency.

Prevention of urinary retention starts with careful evaluation of patient risk factors, minimizing damage during surgery, pain control, fluid administration, and monitoring postoperative urination. Most patients should void within 6 to 8 hours after

TABLE 12.13 Risk factors for urinary retention.

RISK FACTORS	
Age	Degeneration of neurons in micturition reflex and narrowing of urinary passage
Sex	Narrower outflow
Anesthetic choice	Spinal, epidural anesthesia can affect micturition reflex
Intraoperative IV fluid and operation time	Increased total fluid intake and rapid filling of bladder
Medication	Anticholinergic, opioid
Patient comorbidities	BPH, neurologic bladder, DM, neurologic disorders
Types of surgery	Colorectal surgery, spine surgery, hernia

BPH, Benign prostatic hyperplasia; *DM*, diabetes mellitus; *IV*, intravenous.

surgery. When postoperative urinary retention is suspected, ultrasound should be used to estimate the bladder volume. Bladder volumes of 500 mL or more require intervention, most commonly urinary catheterization, and suprapubic tube placement in cases of urethral stricture or trauma.

ENDOCRINE DYSFUNCTION

Adrenal Insufficiency

Causes

Adrenal insufficiency (AI) occurs when the adrenal cortex fails to secrete adrenal hormones, resulting in homeostatic abnormalities. The adrenal cortex is divided into three separate zones secreting mineralocorticoids, glucocorticoids, and androgens. The zona reticularis secretes dehydroepiandrosterone. Aldosterone secretion by the zona glomerulosa is increased in response to hypovolemia or low sodium and results in negative feedback to renin secretion (RAAS). The zona fasciculata secretes glucocorticoids and is regulated by adrenocorticotropic hormone release from the anterior pituitary gland, which is controlled by corticotropin-releasing hormones from the hypothalamus (hypothalamic-pituitary-adrenal [HPA] axis). Cortisol is the prominent corticosteroid from the adrenal cortex, and a stress hormone that signals negative feedback to the anterior pituitary gland and hypothalamus, suppressing the HPA axis. Cortisol is secreted in a pulsatile manner according to the circadian rhythm with highest levels in the morning and lower levels at night.

Primary AI is the inability of the adrenal cortex to produce and secrete hormones. The most common cause of primary AI, or Addison disease, is gradual destruction of the adrenal cortex by the immune system. Less common causes of AI are infectious (e.g., tuberculosis, human immunodeficiency virus, Histoplasma, Cryptococcus), adrenal hemorrhage from meningococcal sepsis, bilateral adrenal metastasis (e.g., lung, breast, colon cancer), drug induced (e.g., ketoconazole, fluconazole, phenobarbital, phenytoin, rifampin, etomidate), or infiltrative disease (e.g., sarcoidosis, amyloidosis, hemochromatosis). Central or secondary AI occurs when the pituitary gland or hypothalamus fails to stimulate the adrenal gland to secrete adrenal hormones. The most common cause is withdrawal of long-term exogenous glucocorticoids, which suppresses the HPA axis and causes atrophy of the zona fasciculata. Other causes of central AI are pituitary or hypothalamic tumors, Sheehan syndrome, neurosurgery of pituitary gland or hypothalamus, trauma, and injury.

Presentation

Primary AI patients lack all hormones from the adrenal cortex (aldosterone, cortisol, and adrenal sex hormones). The symptoms of AI are nonspecific and include weakness, fatigue, anorexia, weight loss, dizziness, depression, diarrhea, and abdominal pain. Decreased adrenal sex hormones may result in decreased potency or libido. Deficiency of mineralocorticoids results in hyponatremia, hyperkalemia, and hypovolemia, and lack of glucocorticoids may present as hypoglycemia. The absence of negative feedback results in high levels of renin-angiotensin, corticotropin, and corticotropin-releasing hormone, and a high corticotropin level causes hyperpigmentation of the skin. In central AI, no hyperpigmentation is observed due to a low corticotropin level, and the mineralocorticoids are not affected. Patients with central AI might have other pituitary hormone deficiencies like hypothyroidism or diabetic insipidus.

The clinical presentation may be variable when there is reduced gland function or when exogenous steroids are held (subclinical AI). Cortisol requirements are higher in times of stress. During severe stress, patients may present in adrenal crisis. Although adrenal crisis has no standardized definition or criteria, it is often described as deterioration in general health with absolute or relative hypotension, which resolves after glucocorticoid administration. The symptoms are nausea, vomiting, abdominal pain, myalgia, joint pain, fatigue, delirium, weakness, loss of consciousness, coma, severe hypotension, and shock refractory to fluids and vasopressors. Adrenal crisis can be a life-threatening complication that requires prompt management. Physicians must have a high index of suspicion especially in patients with history of AI and long-term steroid use. Patients with primary AI have a higher risk of adrenal crisis due to lack of both glucocorticoid and mineralocorticoid functions. Perioperative patients with adrenal crisis may present only with hypotension and shock as other signs and symptoms are suppressed by anesthesia.

Management

Known AI patients usually take exogenous steroids on a regular basis, with dosing based on their individual physiologic response. A careful history and medication review is important to identify underlying AI and to determine if the patient's current steroid dosage has been recently adjusted. The higher the steroid dose and longer duration of steroid use, the greater the risk of HPA suppression and potential to precipitate an adrenal crisis. Patients who have been taking low-dose steroids (e.g., 5–10 mg/day of prednisolone or equivalent) for less than 3 weeks are at low risk of HPA suppression and adrenal crisis. These patients do not require perioperative stress-dose steroids or testing of HPA axis before surgery. Patients taking more than 20 mg/day of prednisone or an equivalent dose for more than 3 weeks or who have a clinical presentation of Cushing syndrome are considered high risk for HPA suppression. These patients should be given stress doses of steroid during surgery. Patients with an unsure history of steroid use can be evaluated with either a corticotropin stimulation test or morning serum cortisol level. If these tests are normal, they do not require stress steroids for surgery. An early morning (8:00 a.m.) cortisol level of <5 mcg/dL is likely to indicate suppression of the HPA axis, whereas morning cortisol levels of more than 15 mcg/dL indicate normal circadian secretion. Cortisol levels >18 mcg/dL 30 minutes after 250 mcg corticotropin stimulation indicates normal HPA response and requires no stress dose before surgery. In patients who are not in a low-risk group and require urgent or emergent surgery, HPA axis evaluation testing should not delay treatment and stress-dose steroids should be given. Although strong evidence-based recommendations of stress-dose steroids are still limited and the recommended dosing is varied depending on type of surgery and patient's condition, the benefit of adrenal crisis prevention often outweighs the risk of side effects from temporary steroid overtreatment.

In patients with adrenal crisis, initial management is to reverse hypotension or shock, correct electrolytes, blood sugar, and pH. Hydrocortisone (100 mg bolus) is given intravenously with 1 L of normal saline over 60 minutes with hemodynamic and electrocardiography monitoring. Other forms of glucocorticoid (e.g., prednisolone) can be given in equivalent dosage if hydrocortisone is not available. If the patient's hemodynamic status does not improve within 1 hour of administering hydrocortisone, other causes of hypotension or shock should be evaluated. After stabilizing the patient's condition, maintenance hydrocortisone 100 to 200 mg/day is given intravenously or in divided doses of 50 mg intramuscularly. Serum electrolytes, pH, and glucose should be monitored and corrected. The precipitating cause and associated comorbidities should be evaluated and treated. Hydrocortisone is tapered and maintenance therapy is continued. Mineralocorticoid supplementation may be needed in primary AI, and androgen supplementation may be needed in women since the adrenal cortex is their main source of androgen. Physicians must be aware of medications that interfere with hepatic enzymes, especially cytochrome P450 3A4, which can interact with glucocorticoid metabolism. All patients must be advised and educated about the disease and importance of lifelong medication and continuous follow-up, physiologic stress recognition, necessity of dose adjustment during illness, the need to inform their physicians of their condition, and carrying medical identification to alert others of their condition.

Hyperthyroid Crisis

Causes

Hyperthyroidism results from sustained overproduction of thyroid hormone by an overactive thyroid gland. Thyrotoxicosis refers to the clinical syndrome of hypermetabolism and hyperactivity caused by excess circulating thyroid hormone levels from either endogenous or exogenous sources. Thyroid hormone levels are regulated by hypothalamic release of thyrotropin-releasing hormone, which stimulates secretion of thyroid-stimulating hormone (TSH) by the pituitary. TSH stimulates the synthesis and release of thyroid hormones by the thyroid, and its release is regulated by a classic negative feedback loop. Thyroid hormones stimulate metabolism in most tissues, but the cardiovascular manifestations are most characteristic.

Hyperthyroid crisis is an urgent medical condition seen in patients with toxic adenoma, goiter, or Grave disease. Hyperthyroid crisis may be precipitated by trauma, emergency surgery conditions, childbirth, diabetic ketoacidosis, or an intercurrent illness such as pneumonia. Although the precise underlying mechanism for this rapid clinical decompensation is unknown, acute illness causes sudden inhibition of the thyroid hormone binding to plasma proteins, results in an increase rise in the already elevated free-hormone pool, and increases the sensitivity of the receptors through increases in target cell adrenergic receptor density or postreceptor modifications in signaling pathways. Cytokine release and acute immunologic disturbances may worsen the thyrotoxic state. Additionally, primary hyperparathyroidism further worsens the thyroid storm through its markedly elevated serum calcium level that augments the action of free thyroxine (T_4) via the role of a secondary messenger. Without treatment, the thyroid storm is associated with a high mortality rate (20%–50%) caused by organ dysfunction, congestive heart failure, respiratory failure, arrhythmia, disseminated intravascular coagulation, GI perforation, hypoxic brain syndrome, and sepsis.

Presentation and Diagnosis

The diagnosis of the thyroid storm is based on clinical signs and symptoms of thyrotoxicosis, including anxiety, palpitations, weight loss, fever (>38°C), tachycardia and tachyarrhythmias (especially atrial fibrillation), congestive heart failure, GI system dysfunction (diarrhea, jaundice), and central nervous system (CNS) symptoms (agitation, delirium, psychosis, coma). As the thyroid storm progresses, coma, hypotension, vascular collapse, and death may ensue unless active therapy is instituted.

Thyroid functions tests do not differentiate between severe thyrotoxicosis and the thyroid storm, although serum-free T_4 levels are significantly higher in patients with the thyroid storm, which may partially explain more severe symptoms. Burch and Wartofsky[30] delineated a scoring system to predict the thyroid storm based on thermoregulatory, cardiovascular, GI, and CNS dysfunction. A score of <25 indicates the thyroid storm is unlikely, whereas a score of 25 to 44 suggests an impending storm, and a score of ≥45 is highly suggestive of the thyroid storm. However, in elderly patients, apathy, severe myopathy, profound weight loss, and congestive heart failure may be the predominant findings. In febrile patients with leukocytosis, an inflammatory or infectious focus should be sought and blood cultures should be obtained. Thyroid scan with technetium-99 helps differentiate between the potential etiologies of thyrotoxicosis. Increased uptake is seen in Grave disease or toxic nodular goiter, whereas low uptake is seen in thyroiditis.

Treatment

Early diagnosis and treatment are critical in the successful management of patients with thyroid storm. Therapy should be initiated rapidly (prior to biochemical confirmation if necessary) as delays in treatment may increase the risk of death. Patients should be monitored continuously in the ICU with supportive care and medications to reduce thyroid hormone synthesis, release, and action. Supportive care includes oxygen, hydration, beta blockers to control HR, acetaminophen for fever, VTE prophylaxis, etc. Thionamides (propylthiouracil, methimazole) block thyroid hormone synthesis, potassium iodide (Lugol solution) blocks the release of T_4 and triiodothyronine (T_3) from the gland, and steroids decrease the extrathyroid conversion of T_4 to T_3 and are also effective in treating any underlying autoimmune cause (e.g., Graves disease) and preventing adrenal crisis (Box 12.3).

BOX 12.3 Management of thyroid crisis.

Identify and Treat Precipitation Factor

Supportive Care

- Oxygen
- Intravenous (IV) fluid therapy with continuous evaluation with central venous catheter monitoring is required.
- Sedation (chlorpromazine) reduces shivering during the rapid induction.
- Prophylaxis against stroke or pulmonary embolism/venous thromboembolism.
- IV hydrocortisone, 300 mg initially followed by 100 mg every 8 hours, to prevent adrenal crisis due to relative adrenal insufficiency.
- Correction of hypoglycemia, hypercalcemia.
- Insulin for diabetic ketoacidosis.

Fever: aggressive treatment with antipyretics and peripheral cooling. Acetaminophen is preferred to salicylates since aspirin elevates free hormone levels by decreasing T_4-binding globin.

Heart failure: digoxin and diuretics

Atrial fibrillation: IV heparin

Beta blockers: oral propranolol (or diltiazem), 60–80 mg every 4 hours, is given to reduce heart rate below 100 beats/min. In acutely ill patients, cardioselective esmolol is given intravenously.

Propylthiouracil or methimazole: The antithyroid drug propylthiouracil blocks new hormone synthesis and decreases extrathyroidal conversion of T_4 to T_3. Methimazole has longer duration of action and lacks extrathyroidal conversion.

Lugol solution, 8 drops every 6 hours, or saturated solution of potassium iodide, 5 drops every 6 hours.

Plasmapheresis and charcoal plasma perfusion or exchange transfusion are reserved for recalcitrant cases if no response in 24–48 hours.

When euthyroidism is achieved, definitive therapy/radioactive ablation must be considered to prevent a second crisis.

T_3, Triiodothyronine; T_4, thyroxine.

To prevent recurrent thyroid storm in patients with Graves disease, definitive therapy with radioactive iodine or thyroidectomy is required as it enables discontinuation of thionamide treatment and its potential side effects (agranulocytosis, hepatotoxicity). The radioactive iodine dose (usual 15–30 mCi) required for complete thyroid ablation depends upon the size of gland and 24-hour radioactive iodine uptake. Over 80% to 90% of patients become euthyroid or hypothyroid after a single dose of radioactive iodine. However, a major side effect is permanent hypothyroidism, and its use is contraindicated in pregnant patients and children. Thyroidectomy for thyroid crisis should be considered only if there is no clinical improvement in 12 to 24 hours with the usual therapy. In patients requiring emergency surgery, stabilization (with hydration, beta blockers, steroids, propylthiouracil, and antipyretics) is required before surgical intervention can be performed. Treatment with propranolol and potassium iodide before surgery can ameliorate cardiovascular symptoms and antithyroid medications must be continued through the morning of surgery.

Hypothyroidism

Causes

Hypothyroidism is caused by inadequate production of thyroid hormone or action of thyroid hormone on target tissues. It can be primary (defect in thyroid hormone synthesis or release, radiation, surgery, drugs) or secondary (hypothalamic-pituitary-thyroid axis defect in either thyrotropin-releasing hormone or TSH signaling). Postoperative hypothyroidism is common after total or near-total thyroidectomy and is correlated with the size of the remnant gland. External beam radiation (head and neck cancer) and radioactive iodine use (Graves disease) also increase the risk of hypothyroidism. Hypothyroidism varies in severity depending on the cause, duration, and severity. Patients with hypothyroidism may be asymptomatic or very ill in cases of severe myxedema coma. Myxedema coma is an extreme manifestation of severe hypothyroidism that results from a combination of failure of adaptive mechanisms to maintain homeostasis and reduced T_3 production. Peripheral conversion of T_4 to T_3 is reduced in many systemic illnesses. Stressors like cold exposure, infection, drugs, trauma, stroke, heart failure, and GI bleeding can precipitate myxedema in patients with previously undiagnosed hypothyroidism.

Presentation and Diagnosis

The symptoms of hypothyroidism are quite variable depending on the degree and duration of thyroid hormone deprivation. Many patients complain of fatigue, cold intolerance, dry skin, constipation, vocal changes, and muscle aches. On physical examination, prolonged ankle-jerk reflex appears to correlate with the degree of hypothyroidism. In primary hypothyroidism, serum total T_4, free T_4, and free T_3 levels are low, whereas the TSH level is elevated. In secondary hypothyroidism, the TSH level, free T_4 index, and free T_3 level are all low. Typical electrocardiogram findings include bradycardia, varying degrees of block, low voltage, flattened or inverted T waves, and prolonged Q-T interval, which can result in torsades de pointes ventricular tachycardia. Myxedema coma is the most severe manifestation of hypothyroidism (mortality rate of 40%–50%) and is characterized by coma, hypothermia (often profound to 80°F), loss of deep tendon reflexes, and cardiopulmonary collapse. With myxedema, T_4 is decreased and TSH is markedly elevated. Patients also demonstrate hypoxemia, hypercapnia, hyponatremia, and increased serum lactate dehydrogenase and creatine kinase levels.

Treatment

Elective surgery should be delayed until the euthyroid state is achieved. When emergency surgery is required in patients with severe hypothyroidism, IV T_4 (200–250 μg L-thyroxine) should be given before surgery to prevent stress-induced myxedema coma. Factors that predispose to postoperative hypothyroidism are not clear. During subtotal thyroidectomy, the smaller thyroid remnant is left in the posterior rim of each lobe to prevent hypothyroidism. However, in most cases, recurrent hyperthyroidism is considered to be a worse complication than hypothyroidism. Supplementation with T_4 is needed to prevent the development of overt hypothyroidism in most patients after thyroidectomy.

Myxedema coma is an emergency condition that requires early diagnosis, rapid administration of thyroid hormone, and aggressive supportive measures (Table 12.14). Treatment with IV hydrocortisone is usually required, too, since pituitary-adrenal function is impaired and cortisol levels are frequently decreased.

Syndrome of Inappropriate Antidiuretic Hormone Secretion

Causes

The syndrome of inappropriate ADH (SIADH) release is caused by unsuppressed vasopressin release from either the pituitary gland or nonpituitary sources (e.g., ADH-producing tumors). Vasopressin or ADH is synthesized in the posterior pituitary and binds to receptors in the collecting ducts of the nephron to promote water absorption. Vasopressin is normally released in response to high serum osmolality but is also released in response to systemic stress (e.g., surgery) and inflammation. SIADH is commonly diagnosed in hospitalized, postoperative patients with hyponatremia (sodium <135 mmol/L) due to the administration of hypotonic fluids, drugs (ACE inhibitors, NSAIDs), and the body's response to stress. Increased arginine secretion in SIADH occurs secondary to underlying disease process (Table 12.15). In general, significant neurologic symptoms occur when serum sodium <125 mEq/L and subsequent coma and respiratory arrest develop at 115 to 120 mEq/L.

Presentation

The clinical syndrome of SIADH consists of hyponatremia, inappropriately elevated urine osmolality, excessive urine sodium, and decreased serum osmolality in a euvolemic patient without edema; there is no diuretic use with normal cardiac, renal, adrenal, hepatic, and thyroid function. Clinical manifestations of SIADH

TABLE 12.14 Management of myxedema coma.

Hypothyroidism	IV T_4 300–500 μg; T_3 in the absence of clinical improvement Or IV 200–300 μg T_4 plus 10–25 μg T_3
Hypocortisolemia	IV hydrocortisone 200–400 mg daily
Hypoventilation	Mechanical ventilation
Hypothermia	Usually resolves with treatment with T_3/T_4
Hyponatremia	Hypertonic saline (50–100 mL 3% NaCl)
Identification and treatment of underlying stressors (e.g., antibiotic for infection)	

IV, Intravenous; *T_3*, triiodothyronine; *T_4*, thyroxine.

depend upon the rapidity of onset and severity of hyponatremia, with symptoms ranging from mild nonspecific (headache and nausea) to more significant disorders (e.g., disorientation, confusion, obtundation, focal neurologic deficits). Idiopathic SIADH in elderly patients over 65 years of age with mild to moderate hyponatremia are at increased risk of fractures due to risk of falls and gait problems.

Treatment

Management of SIADH includes treatment of any underlying disease process and correcting the patient's hyponatremia. Restricting free water intake is the mainstay of treatment in patients with mild to moderate symptoms, while severe symptomatic or resistant hyponatremia may require more aggressive treatment with IV 3% saline. The serum sodium should be monitored frequently during treatment since excessively rapid correction may cause osmotic demyelination syndrome ("locked-in" syndrome), resulting in quadriplegia. Consequently, the rate of correction should not exceed 8 mEq/L per 24 hours or 0.5 to 1 mEq/L per hour. Vasopressin receptor antagonists conivaptan (IV) or tolvaptan (oral) are effective in severe persistent SIADH.

GASTROINTESTINAL COMPLICATIONS

Ileus and Early Postoperative Bowel Obstruction

Causes

Postoperative bowel obstruction can be mechanical or functional. Mechanical bowel obstruction can be classified as either intrinsic or extrinsic, partial or complete, or proximal (pylorus to proximal jejunum), intermediate (mid-jejunum to mid-ileum), or distal (distal ileum to ileocecal valve) in location. With a partial obstruction, luminal contents pass distally despite slow transit time, whereas with complete obstruction, the lumen is totally occluded. Complete obstruction can be described as simple, closed-loop, or strangulated in nature. Early postoperative (mechanical) bowel obstruction is defined as occurring within the first 6 weeks of surgery. Early postoperative bowel obstructions are a distinct clinic entity with a unique pathophysiology that needs to be differentiated from classic mechanical bowel obstruction and postoperative ileus. Adhesions are responsible for the majority of early postoperative bowel obstructions (>90%), with internal herniation, intraabdominal abscess, intramural hematoma, intussusception, and anastomotic edema or leak as less likely causes.

TABLE 12.15 Causes of syndrome of inappropriate antidiuretic hormone release.

Central nervous system disorders	Stroke, hemorrhage, infection, trauma, mental illness, and psychosis
Tumors	Small cell lung cancer (most common), head and neck cancers
Drugs	Carbamazepine, oxcarbazepine, chlorpropamide, cyclophosphamide, and selective serotonin reuptake inhibitors
Surgery	Surgery increases arginine secretion in response mediated by pain afferents
Endocrine disorders	Hypopituitarism and hypothyroidism presents with SIADH and hyponatremia; can be corrected by hormone replacement

SIADH, Syndrome of inappropriate antidiuretic hormone.

Postoperative adhesions may occur after any intraabdominal surgery but are more likely to cause bowel obstructions after pelvic surgery, especially colorectal and gynecologic procedures. Normal peritoneal healing is a complex, but programmed, inflammatory process. Adhesions are bridges of collagen tissue caused by fibrin deposition that forms between visceral and/or parietal peritoneum. During surgery, peritoneal injury triggers an inflammatory response, causing complement and coagulation cascade activation, exudation of fibrinogen rich-fluid that causes apposition of adjacent surfaces resulting in a band (i.e., an adhesion).

After abdominal surgery, there is a normal time course and pattern for return of intestinal motility. The small bowel usually develops contractile activity within several hours, the stomach requires 24 to 48 hours, and the colon recovers 3 to 5 days after surgery. Postoperative ileus is a term to describe a generalized reduction in gut motility with dysfunction after surgery. Postoperative ileus is the most common form of functional bowel obstruction and can be classified as primary or physiologic, secondary, adynamic, or paralytic ileus depending on the etiology, timing, and involvement of the GI tract. The duration of ileus generally correlates with the type of surgery and degree of surgical trauma. Paralytic ileus may be associated with abdominal, pelvic, or retroperitoneal trauma; mesenteric ischemia; electrolyte abnormalities (e.g., hypokalemia, hypomagnesemia); recent abdominal surgery with extensive bowel manipulation; intraabdominal inflammation (e.g., pancreatitis); medications (e.g., opioids); or extra abdominal pathology (pneumonia).

The pathophysiology of postoperative ileus is complex and multifactorial in nature. Neurogenic (enteric nervous system and CNS), inflammatory (histamine, IL-6 and IL-8, monocytes and macrophages), enteric hormones and neuropeptides (motilin, substance P, and vasoactive intestinal peptide [VIP]), perioperative electrolyte disturbances, and opioids are all contributing factors.[31] The combination of these factors results in impaired local neuromuscular function and activation of neurogenic inhibitory pathways, resulting in impaired contractility, motility, relative hypoxemia, and bowel edema. Following intestinal resection and anastomosis, neuromuscular discontinuity can result in impaired downstream intestinal motility due to electromechanical uncoupling with the distal segment. Perioperative electrolyte disturbances, postoperative pain control with opioids, and certain medications (e.g., tricyclic antidepressants) can result in reduced GI motility.

Presentation

The classical presentation of bowel obstruction includes intermittent or colicky abdominal pain, distention, acute obstipation, nausea, and vomiting. Pain and distention usually precede the nausea and vomiting. The presence of severe constant or localized pain may indicate strangulation (especially if subjective pain is disproportional to exam findings). However, the symptoms of early postoperative mechanical obstruction tends to be vague and nonspecific since nausea, vomiting, abdominal distention, and obstipation are relatively common in the early postoperative period. Hence, the differential diagnosis for these symptoms includes early postoperative mechanical bowel obstruction and "paralytic ileus."

Mechanical proximal bowel obstruction typically presents with severe, crampy visceral pain, occurring in short recurrent paroxysms (30 seconds to 2 minutes) in a crescendo/decrescendo pattern. In contrast, with distal mechanical obstruction, the episodes are usually spaced farther apart in time and tend to last longer (minutes rather than seconds). Complete obstruction often presents earlier and with more acute findings than partial obstruction. The more proximal the obstruction, the earlier and more prominent the symptoms of nausea and vomiting (bilious), whereas vomiting with distal bowel obstruction is typically delayed in presentation and feculent in nature. Findings concerning for strangulation include fever, tachycardia, and leukocytosis. Closed-loop obstruction may be caused by incarcerated bowel in a hernia sac or intestinal torsion and is associated with increased risk of vascular compromise and irreversible intestinal ischemia. Closed-loop obstruction presents more rapidly with acute symptoms compared to partial or "open-loop" obstruction.

Bowel sounds are frequently high pitched with metallic "rushes" and "groans" in patients with partial small bowel obstruction. In contrast, bowel sounds are more likely diminished or absent in patients with functional bowel obstruction or ileus. Postoperative ileus is usually characterized by dilated small and large bowel and usually resolves without any serious sequelae. However, substantial volumes of fluid may become sequestered in the dilated bowel, resulting in intravascular volume depletion. The dilated bowels frequently result in abdominal distention, pain, nausea, vomiting, and obstipation.

Diagnosis is suspected clinically depending on the presence of classic signs and symptoms and then confirmed with imaging, such as abdominal radiography or by CT scan. The pattern of bowel gas helps to determine the type and location of the obstruction. Proximal bowel obstruction presents with less intestinal dilatation due to the shorter length of obstructed intestine and decompression proximally into the stomach. In contrast, distal bowel obstruction presents with multiple dilated loops, and proximal decompression is less likely. Postoperatively, imaging studies can be difficult to interpret since early postoperative bowel obstruction and ileus can manifest with similar findings on plain abdominal radiographs. CT imaging can help to identify the presence or absence of a focal site of obstruction. The presence of a dilated proximal small bowel with decompressed distal bowel is concerning, but usually, a clearly defined transition point is seen with mechanical obstruction. CT imaging may also help diagnose the cause of obstruction (hernia, solid mass, inflammatory lesion, or intussusception), the presence of closed-loop obstruction and a mesenteric swirl is frequently seen with internal hernias. The use of IV contrast helps to identify vascular patency, and decreased bowel wall enhancement may indicate ischemic bowel. Barium should not be used in case of suspected perforation, strangulation, or a complete or closed-loop obstruction. The use of enteral contrast with the CT scan is helpful when the diagnosis is uncertain in patients with a nonresolving partial bowel obstruction and to differentiate between partial and complete bowel obstruction. A complete blood cell count, electrolyte panel, urinalysis, arterial blood pH, and serum lactate concentration are useful in evaluation of fluid and electrolyte imbalance, inflammation, and bleeding and to rule out sepsis. Increased serum amylase, serum D-lactate, and intestinal fatty acid binding protein are associated with intestinal ischemia.

Treatment

Ideally, early postoperative bowel obstructions could be prevented with meticulous surgical technique. Minimally invasive surgery typically has fewer adhesions, and presumably, intraoperative peritoneal adhesions can be minimized through meticulous surgical technique. Minimizing tissue trauma by handling tissues gently, constant bathing of the tissues with saline, avoiding ischemia and desiccation, maintaining hemostasis, and avoiding contamination and infection are conceptually associated with fewer adhesions, but their impact is difficult to quantify. Other adjuncts to decrease adhesion formation include the use of antiadhesive agents like polytetrafluoroethylene, hyaluronate, and carboxymethylcellulose.

Early recognition and treatment of early postoperative bowel obstruction prevent irreversible ischemia and transmural necrosis, thereby decreasing morbidity and mortality. Postoperative physiologic ileus is usually self-limiting and can be managed conservatively. In the case of paralytic ileus, treatment of the underlying etiology, such as treatment of electrolyte abnormalities and an associated intraabdominal process (e.g., pancreatitis), will hasten the return of bowel function. Initial management of mechanical obstruction requires appropriate fluid resuscitation, opioid discontinuation, and NG decompression of the obstructed bowel as intraluminal distension results in mucosal ischemia. Patient-controlled epidural analgesia or NSAIDs are alternative choices, instead of opioids, for postoperative pain control.

An initial trial of nonoperative management is appropriate for most cases of partial mechanical obstruction in the early postoperative period in the absence of clinical deterioration and when the patient shows signs of improvement during the first 12 to 24 hours. Nonoperative management begins with aggressive fluid resuscitation and correction of any electrolyte disorders. Contraindications to nonoperative management include suspected ischemia, closed-loop obstruction, strangulated hernia, and perforation. Patients with complete or high-grade partial obstruction and presence of fever, tachycardia, worsening leukocytosis, peritonitis, bowel perforation, or strangulation require immediate surgery. Several centers recommend algorithm-based treatment of small bowel obstruction. NG decompression is followed by water-soluble contrast administration (90 mL gastrografin) down the NG tube with follow-up abdominal plain films to assess contrast in the cecum at 8 and 24 hours. If the contrast reaches the cecum in 8 hours, the NG tube can be removed and liquids started. If the contrast does not reach the cecum in 24 hours, early surgical intervention is recommended. Simple or open-loop obstruction is characterized by no vascular compromise and can be decompressed proximally via emesis or NG tube. If a large segment of bowel appears to be threatened, or if bowel viability cannot be clearly established, the surgeon can leave the abdomen open with plans to return to the operating room in 24 to 48 hours for a repeat assessment.

Abdominal Compartment Syndrome

Cause

ACS describes the physiologic consequences of acute, severe abdominal distention with intraabdominal hypertension (IAH), including hypoxia, hypoventilation, decreased blood pressure, cardiac output, and renal and visceral perfusion. Normally, IAP in a healthy individual is <8 mm Hg. IAH is frequently present in patients with morbid obesity but is not synonymous with ACS. ACS refers to a clinical syndrome caused by an acute increase in IAP with associated organ dysfunction, especially hypotension, oliguria, or respiratory insufficiency. It is defined as sustained increased IAP greater than or equal to 12 mm Hg along with new organ dysfunction or organ failure and improvement after abdominal decompression.

The etiology of ACS can be described as primary or secondary. Primary ACS develops as a result of intraabdominal pathology (blunt or penetrating abdominal trauma, hemorrhage, abdominal aortic aneurysm rupture, intestinal obstruction, retroperitoneal hematoma). In contrast, secondary ACS develops in the absence of abdominal injury and is described in patients with severe burn injury, multiple extremity fractures, and/or septic shock. A common denominator in primary and secondary ACS is the presence of shock and resuscitation. Aggressive resuscitation with large volumes of crystalloid contributes to progressive visceral and soft tissue edema, third spacing of abdominal fluid, decreased abdominal compliance, ileus, and progressive distention with subsequent development of IAH and ACS.[32] Closure of the massively distended abdomen with a noncompliant abdominal wall under tension may further aggravate IAH in critically ill patients with intraabdominal pathology. More recently, the use of damage control surgery and temporary abdominal closure are recommended in "high-risk" patients. Resuscitation of massive hemorrhage with whole blood or a combination of plasma, packed RBCs, and platelets also helps to decrease the edema associated with large volume crystalloid administration.

ACS-mediated organ dysfunction may be caused by direct compressive effects (e.g., IAP-induced pulmonary or renal failure), inadequate end-organ perfusion, or both. Upward displacement of the diaphragm results in decreased diaphragmatic excursion and reduced pulmonary compliance and impairs both oxygenation and ventilation. Increased IAP and intrathoracic pressure negatively impacts cardiac preload, afterload, and contractility. Venous return is decreased despite normal or elevated central venous pressures. The combination of decreased preload, RV function, and increased afterload results in decreased cardiac output, which is largely "volume dependent." Decreased urine output is probably due to the combination of reduced renal arterial perfusion from reduced preload, direct compression of the kidney, decreased venous outflow due to renal vein, and inferior vena cava compression. Increased IAP >15 cm H_2O results in mesenteric and splanchnic hypoperfusion, and persistent elevations above 20 to 25 cm usually require immediate treatment. ACS can also impact cerebral perfusion and worsen traumatic brain injury. The combination of decreased cerebral venous drainage (due to increased intrathoracic pressure) with low cardiac output reduces the effective cerebral perfusion pressure, increases the increased intracranial pressure, and can exacerbate brain injury.

Presentation

The clinical manifestations of ACS are caused by the effects of severe abdominal distention and increased IAP on the pulmonary, cardiovascular, and renal systems. Most patients present with a tense abdominal distention and elevated IAP, difficulty ventilating due to elevated airway pressures, low blood pressure (due to decreased venous return and low cardiac output), decreased urine output, visceral hypoperfusion with progressive acidosis, and an improvement of these findings with abdominal decompression. In trauma patients, a progressive increase in IAP may be due to persistent intraabdominal bleeding, and the degree of initial injury does not always correlate with the subsequent physiologic derangement. Inappropriate response to resuscitation is another sign of ACS.

Diagnosis

ACS is a clinical syndrome that occurs in high-risk patients with severe abdominal distention, elevated IAP, and organ dysfunction, most commonly difficult ventilation, hypoperfusion, and low urine output. IAP can be measured using direct and indirect methods. Most commonly, bladder pressures are commonly monitored either intermittently or continuously (by connecting the transurethral Foley catheter to a pressure transducer) in patients at risk for developing ACS. Elevations in IAP can be classified as Grade 1 (10–15 cm H_2O), Grade II (15–25 cm H_2O), Grade III (25–35 cm H_2O), or Grade IV (>35 cm H_2O). As the IAP increases through Grades II, III and IV, the degree of organ dysfunction progressively worsens. Most patients with Grade III and all patients with Grade IV require abdominal decompression. When the physiologic consequences of increased IAP begin to have cause impaired organ function and decreased perfusion, the diagnosis of ACS can be made, regardless of the absolute IAP.

Treatment

Early recognition and treatment of ACS are important since delays in treatment are associated with increased morbidity and mortality. Recognition of high-risk patients, appropriate monitoring of abdominal pressure, early implementation of preventive measures (e.g., neuromuscular relaxation), and prompt decompressive laparotomy are the keys to successful treatment. Preventive measures include use of neuromuscular relaxants, paracentesis of ascites, and pressure-limiting ventilation strategies to avoid ventilator-induced lung injury. Emergency abdominal decompression can be lifesaving when abdominal distention prohibits adequate oxygenation or ventilation of the patient. Although abdominal decompression is usually very effective in restoring ventilation, it can be accompanied by reperfusion injury in some patients. The sudden release of IAP with visceral reperfusion may cause acidosis and hypotension in some patients. Adequate preload and maintaining appropriate ventilation before decompressive laparotomy helps to avoid this syndrome. Several techniques for temporary abdominal closure have been described, including NPWT and temporary abdominal wound closure with a prosthesis (e.g., Bogota bag, Whitman patch). IAP should still be monitored in "high-risk" patients since recurrent ACS has been reported in up to 50% of patients after damage control laparotomy. Enteral feedings with an open abdomen are safe and could lead to decreased bowel edema and early closure of the abdomen. In general, abdominal reexploration should be performed in 24 to 48 hours and the abdomen should be closed as soon as the patient's physiology and visceral edema allow. The time between the initial decompressive laparotomy and reexploration predicts primary fascial closure.

More recently, considerable efforts have been focused on modifying patient care to reduce the incidence of ACS. The use of damage control laparotomy (hemorrhage and contamination control, abdominal packing, and temporary closure) was popularized on the 1990s in patients with exsanguinating abdominal trauma to prevent the lethal triad of hypothermia, acidosis, and coagulopathy. Following resuscitation in the ICU, these patients returned to surgery for pack removal, restoration of intestinal continuity, enteral access, and abdominal closure. This concept has been extended to include patients with severe peritonitis and abbreviated laparotomy due to physiologic derangements, intestinal ischemia with deferred anastomosis and planned second look, severe bowel edema, retroperitoneal hematoma, etc. Damage control resuscitation with fresh whole blood or balanced transfusion of plasma, platelets, and packed RBCs is more commonly used to resuscitate massive hemorrhage than large volumes of crystalloid. Damage control resuscitation has been shown to reduce the development of ACS in patients with severe intraabdominal bleeding.

Definitive abdominal closure may be difficult in many patients. Recently, the combination of hypertonic saline resuscitation and wound vacuum therapy and early surgery for sequential fascial closure has been suggested.[33] Although this protocol may help decrease visceral edema, in many patients, abdominal wall reconstruction may be necessary to facilitate abdominal closure. Surgical techniques like component separation with bilateral myofascial advancement flaps may be used successfully in many patients. However, in some patients, the combination of primary closure and use of biologic or acellular dermal prosthesis may be required.

Postoperative Gastrointestinal Bleeding

Causes

Postoperative GI bleeding encompasses a large number of clinical scenarios, including primary intestinal disease, stress-related, and/or surgical complications with varying locations and severities. Depending upon the etiology and presentation, GI bleeding is commonly categorized as either upper GI bleeding (UGIB) or lower GI bleeding (LGIB). UGIB is defined as hemorrhage proximal to the ligament of Treitz and is commonly caused by peptic ulcer disease, stress erosions, Mallory-Weiss tear, and gastric varices. LGIB is anatomically located distal to the ligament and is caused by arteriovenous malformations, diverticulosis, or postpolypectomy/colectomy in the colon. LGIB from the small bowel is less common and includes arteriovenous malformations, ulcerated small bowel tumors, and Meckel diverticula in the differential diagnosis. Postoperative GI bleeding is associated with significant morbidity; therefore, it is imperative to recognize risk factors prior to operation, as persistent hemorrhage necessitates reoperation in 2% to 5% of patients. Stress gastritis is more commonly seen in critically ill patients with known risk factors, including mechanical ventilation, coagulopathy (INR >1.5, platelet count <50,000, aPTT >2 times normal), hypoperfusion, significant burn, severe brain or spinal cord injury, multisystem trauma, and sepsis. Prophylaxis with PPIs, H_2 blockers, or sucralfate should be considered in these patients.

Presentation

When evaluating patients with a GI bleed, the patient's medical history provides important diagnostic clues and may help guide management decisions. Despite the increased use of PPIs and understanding of *Helicobacter pylori*, peptic ulcer disease remains the most common cause of nonvariceal UGIB. Mallory Weiss tears are mucosal lacerations at the gastroesophageal junction caused by forceful emesis more commonly seen in alcoholic patients. A history of liver disease, cirrhosis, or the stigmata of portal hypertension on examination suggests variceal etiology of UGIB. The most common sources of LGIB are diverticular and postpolypectomy bleeding. While the former is seen in patients with diverticular disease, the latter manifests as delayed bleeding 1 to 3 weeks after the procedure. In patients with recent intestinal surgery, the anastomotic site should be considered as a potential source of bleeding; however, other potential sources of bleeding should be excluded since the risk for hemorrhage from a colorectal anastomosis is generally less than 1%. In a patient with previous intraabdominal aortic surgery, aortoenteric fistula should be considered. Additionally, coagulopathies due to liver disease, NSAIDs, antiplatelet agents, or anticoagulation therapies increase the risk of bleeding.

Hematemesis, melena, or hematochezia are common manifestations of GI bleeding. UGIB typically presents with hematemesis or melena, but brisk UGIB can also present with hematochezia; however, melena can also manifest as LGIB, especially when there is slow transit time. The redder the blood, the more rapid the bleed. Flexible endoscopy is the standard of care for localization and control of GI bleeding in the stable patient when UGIB suspicion is high. Also, in evaluation of LGIB, upper endoscopy or gastric aspiration should be considered to exclude UGIB sources. Tachycardia, hypoxemia, or hypotension suggest the need for immediate resuscitation.

Diagnosis and Treatment

The basic principles of management of postoperative GI bleeding include the following: fluid resuscitation and restoration of intravascular volume, monitoring clotting parameters and correcting abnormalities, identification and treatment of aggravating factors, transfusion of blood products, and identification and treatment of the source of the bleeding

Stress ulcers are superficial mucosal lesions which are usually confined to the mucosa of the stomach and proximal duodenum. They can cause clinically significant GI bleeding in critically ill patients. However, routine use of ulcer prophylaxis and improvements in critical care have reduced the incidence of major hemorrhage and mortality. Physiologic stresses, including trauma, burns (Curling ulcer), increased intracranial pressure (Cushing ulcer), and sepsis predispose to ulcer formation. Mechanical ventilation and coagulopathy are associated with increased risk. The underlying pathogenic mechanisms causing mucosal injury include mucosal ischemia due to hypoperfusion, vasoconstriction, the loss of cytoprotective substances (prostaglandins), and increased acidity in the gastric lumen secondary to intracranial pressure mediated by the vagus nerve. These lesions typically heal without any sequelae, but, rarely, deep penetration or perforation can cause peritonitis. Intraluminal pH should be maintained above 3.5, and prophylaxis with H_2 blockers, proton pump inhibitors (PPIs), sucralfate, anticholinergics decreases bleeding. However, in patients with uncontrolled bleeding, endoscopic therapy using electrocautery or heater probe hemostasis or angiographic injection of vasopressin or gelfoam may be required. Surgery is occasionally needed and may include gastrostomy with oversewing of focal areas of active bleeding, subtotal gastric resection or total gastrectomy in intractable cases.

Aggressive resuscitation with correction of hemodynamics, hemoglobin, and coagulopathy can reduce mortality in patients with postoperative GI bleeding. Serial blood counts and coagulation studies (prothrombin time, partial thromboplastin time, and bleeding time) should be performed every 6 hours and corrected with appropriate transfusion therapy. Thromboelastography is commonly used to identify coagulation deficits or anticoagulant effects and may facilitate appropriate transfusion therapy. The indications for continuous blood transfusions are unstable vital signs, continued bleeding, symptoms of tissue hypoxia (shortness of breath, dizziness), or persistently low hematocrit values (20% to 25%); hematocrit should be maintained at or above 30% in elderly patients, whereas in younger healthy patients, a hematocrit of 20% to 25% may be satisfactory.

After initial workup, based on the clinical status of the patient (stable or unstable), the localization of the bleeding source to either the upper or lower GI tract aids in determining the appropriate diagnostic and treatment options. The major goals of treatment are to stop active bleeding and prevent recurrent bleeding. Endoscopy is the major diagnostic tool for localization and treatment of UGIB and is indicated for control of active bleeding. Therapeutic interventions include the combination of thermal coagulation, hemoclips, and/or endoscopic band ligation, with or without epinephrine injection. Recurrent bleeding after endoscopic control is seen in 15% to 20% of patients, and the common risk factors include older adults (>65), malignancy, and use of NSAIDs. Repeat endoscopy can control long-term bleeding and has fewer complications when compared with surgery for recurrent bleed. Patients with repeat bleeding after second endoscopic therapy should be considered for angiography with transarterial embolization. Surgical control of the bleeding may be required in patients who failed angiographic therapy.

Localization of LGIB requires a combination of CT angiography, tagged RBC scintigraphy, video capsule endoscopy, and colonoscopy. Upper GI endoscopy should be considered to exclude UGIB sources. Patients who are stable and can tolerate bowel preparation are commonly assessed with colonoscopy. CT angiography is useful in patients with active bleeding, while video capsule endoscopy is commonly used for initial evaluation of suspected small bowel bleeding. The advantage of tagged RBC scintigraphy is that it is highly accurate (75%) in localization even in cases of intermittent and delayed bleeding (>48 hours). Angiography with selective embolization may be used to treat active LGIB and is successful in >90% of cases with a relatively low (<8%) risk of bowel ischemia. Anoscopy or rigid proctoscopy can be used to localize bleeding from a colorectal, coloanal, or ileoanal anastomosis. Bleeding from diverticular and postpolypectomy bleeding can be successfully localized with colonoscopy and treated with epinephrine injection and hemostatic clip placement.

Acute variceal bleeding, especially in patients with decompensated liver cirrhosis (with ascites or hepatic encephalopathy), is associated with a high mortality rate. Correction of hypovolemia, rapid hemostasis, prevention of early rebleeding and complications related to bleeding, and restoration of liver function are most important components in the management. Furthermore, in contrast to patients with nonvariceal bleeding, aggressive fluid administration may result in increased portal venous pressure complicated by pulmonary edema or ascites. Treatment with vasopressors (octreotide and vasopressin) to decrease the portal pressure should be initiated. Hemoglobin level >8 g/dL, systolic blood pressure (>90–100 mm Hg), HR <100/min, and central venous pressure (1–5 mm Hg) are required to achieve hemodynamic stability. In stable patients, endoscopic hemostasis can be achieved either by performing endoscopic variceal ligation or injection of sclerotherapy; transjugular intrahepatic portosystemic shunt (TIPS) can be lifesaving when ligation fails. Use of nonselective beta blockers prevents long-term rebleeding. Also, repeat endoscopic banding is recommended every 10 to 14 days for complete eradication of varices.

Bleeding from Mallory Weiss tears is usually self-limited and does not usually require endoscopic hemostasis. Likewise, bleeding from an intestinal anastomosis during the early postoperative period also resolves spontaneously. However, when bleeding does not spontaneously cease, transfusion with 4 to 6 units of blood and repair of the leak should be done in the operating room either by oversewing or resection of the anastomosis and recreation of an anastomosis or end stoma. Hemorrhage from a low colorectal anastomosis can be managed with transanal suture ligation.

Stomal Complications

Causes

Although the advent of restorative proctocolectomy and stapled low anterior anastomosis has lessened the need for permanent ileostomy and end colostomy, the creation of intestinal stomas for diversion of enteric contents remains an integral component in the surgical management of gastroenterologic disease. Urostomy (bowel for urinary tract reconstruction or diversion) can be either incontinent or continent, indicated for malignancy and underlying neurologic conditions (e.g., spinal cord injury, spina bifida).

Despite extensive surgical experience, complications of intestinal stomas still occur with relative frequency. Early postoperative stomal complications are defined as those occurring less than 1 month postoperatively (Table 12.16), including improper site selection, ischemia, retraction, peristomal skin irritation, peristomal infection/abscess/fistula, acute parastomal herniation, and skin complications.[34] In contrast, delayed stoma complications like stomal stenosis and stricture are usually the result of poor blood supply. The incidence of stomal complications may vary depending on the underlying disease process (e.g., stomas in patients with Crohn disease have more problems with stenosis, peristomal fistulas, and dermatitis compared to stomas created in patients with ulcerative colitis).

Presentation and Diagnosis

Mucocutaneous healing requires adequate blood supply. Ischemia is associated with stenosis and poor stomal healing. Mucocutaneous separation of the stoma from the skin occurs as a result of tension, ischemia, infection, and poor nutrition. Mucocutaneous separations usually heal by secondary intention with appropriate stoma care. A healthy stoma is always pink but turns dark purple or black usually within the first 24 hours when ischemia is present. Stomal congestion can be caused by bowel edema, a tight abdominal wall trephination, or excess tension on the bowel mesentery, resulting in dark, purple discoloration postoperatively. Melanosis coli, a brown-black discoloration of the colonic mucosa caused by anthraquinone laxatives, may also cause a dark or even black stoma postoperatively but requires no treatment.

Ischemia is more common in an end stoma relative to a loop stoma due to its tenuous blood supply. Ischemia may be limited to the part of the stoma above the skin level, or it may extend to the fascial level, the peritoneal level, or the proximal intraabdominal ileum. Vascular integrity of a congested stoma postoperatively can be assessed by transillumination with a flashlight. A viable stoma transilluminates bright red, even in the face of venous congestion; failure to transilluminate indicates ischemia. Additionally, the presence of arterial bleeding with a pinprick test indicates absence of mucosal necrosis.

TABLE 12.16 Stomal complications.

	COMPLICATIONS	
CATEGORY	EARLY	LATE
Stoma	Poor location Retraction* Ischemic necrosis Detachment Abscess formation* Opening wrong end	Prolapse Stenosis Parastomal hernia Fistula formation Gas Odor
Peristomal skin	Excoriation Dermatitis*	Parastomal varices Dermatoses Cancer Skin manifestations of inflammatory bowel disease
Systemic	High output*	Bowel obstruction Nonclosure

*May also develop as a late complication.

Stoma recession or retraction in the immediate postsurgical period is usually a result of tension on the bowel or its mesentery due to inadequate mobilization, a large abdominal defect or inadequate fixation, adhesion between the stoma and the abdominal wall, or poor stomal siting. Patient factors contribute to stoma retraction, including malnutrition, obesity, corticosteroid therapy, intraabdominal sepsis, poor wound healing, and Crohn disease. Stomal recession can be intermittent or fixed. Intermittent recession is posture dependent. In the upright position, the stoma length and protrusion are adequate and above the skin level. However, when the patient lies supine, the stoma is either flush with the skin or recedes below the skin level, resulting in soiling and leakage of contents due to inadequate appliance seal. Stoma stenosis occurs as a consequence of ischemia or infection, relatively small skin or fascia aperture, excessive tension, retraction, or recurrent inflammatory bowel disease, with reported incidence typically less than 10%.

Osteotomy prolapse can occur with any type of abdominal stoma. Transverse loop colostomies constructed for acute large bowel obstruction are associated with increased risk, especially since the hole in the abdominal fascia needs to be large to accommodate the obstructed bowel. Although the exact underlying reason in unclear, a large stomal aperture (particularly when stomas are created in an emergency setting) and a poorly fixed, redundant, distal transverse colon have been implicated. Prolapse can be fixed (present constantly) or sliding (present intermittently). Fixed prolapse is an uncommon condition in which excessive bowel has been everted during stoma construction and rarely requires treatment. Sliding prolapse occurs when a long segment (>50 cm) of ileum or colon protrudes through the stomal orifice intermittently, usually due to increased abdominal pressure and retracts flush with the abdominal wall when the patient lies down, predisposing to leakage.

Parastomal hernias are the most frequent complication of colostomy and can be caused by multiple factors, including poor operative technique, infection, incorrect stoma location, too large a hole (early hernia), high IAP due to obesity, constipation, prostatism, or chronic cough (late hernia). However, early postoperative parastomal hernias are usually caused by creating a fascial defect that is larger than needed to exteriorize the bowel segment. The symptoms of parastomal hernia include nausea and vomiting associated with a painful lump or mass adjacent to the stoma. Patients may also have difficulty maintaining an appliance seal, pain, small bowel obstruction, stoma outlet obstruction, skin excoriation, and difficulty with stoma irrigation. Fever, leukocytosis, and air-fluid levels on upright abdominal radiograph indicate bowel obstruction. Incarceration and/or strangulation occurs in less than 10% of cases. Diligent inspection and palpation of the peristomal skin and abdominal wall will determine the presence or absence of a hernia in most patients.

Peristomal skin irritation may be caused by chemical dermatitis from stoma effluent or traumatic skin desquamation from frequent appliance changes. Appliance leakage and local skin irritation may require more frequent appliance changes, creating a cycle of worsening dermatitis. Peristomal skin irritation is more common with ileostomies than with colostomies due to the more liquid and caustic nature of bilious small intestinal contents. Leakage of ileostomy effluent ranges in presentation from contact dermatitis to full-thickness skin necrosis and ulceration. It is most often caused by stoma neglect, improper stoma placement, or appliance fit. Traumatic dermatitis also presents with painful, peristomal ulceration. Ulceration around the stoma can also be seen with recurrent Crohn disease, whereas ulceration of the stoma itself may be caused by an appliance aperture that is too small, resulting in injury of the stoma causing bleeding and ulceration.

Stomal dermatitis can be caused by either skin irritation or an allergic reaction as a response to skin contact with external agents.[35] Irritant contact dermatitis is the most common type and is caused by mechanical injury to the skin from pouch removal, contact with stomal effluent, or irritation from solvents alone or in combination. Allergic reactions are caused by sensitivity to skin barriers, adhesives, or tape and are fairly common. Leakage of stomal effluent causes proliferation of microorganism under adhesive tape resulting in infectious dermatitis. It can be avoided by proper skin cleaning and application of antimicrobial absorbent silver dressing to reduce the bacterial burden and promote healing. However, *Candida* skin infections are more common in the debilitated host. *Candida* stomal skin infections are characterized by itching and burning bright red primary and satellite papular lesions. Treatment includes topical nystatin powder application during routine pouch changing until the infection has resolved.

Peristomal abscesses in the immediate postoperative period occurs due to preoperative colonization of the peristomal skin and perioperative seeding of the surgical site, infected hematoma, or an infected suture granuloma. Iatrogenic perforation of a colostomy during irrigation is another less common cause of paracolostomy abscesses. A fistula between the emerging bowel and the peristomal skin is uncommon. However, in patients with Crohn disease, a peristomal fistula in conjunction with an ileostomy indicates disease recurrence.

The normal physiologic response to colectomy in most patients manifests as voluminous watery ileostomy output. Diversion colitis is an iatrogenic, inflammatory nutritional complication following the creation of fecal diversion and resolves rapidly once continuity has been reestablished.

The skin conditions associated with stomal leakage include pseudoepithelial hyperplasia, psoriasis, and pyoderma gangrenosum. Pseudoepithelial hyperplasia manifests as painful, wart-like epithelial thickening caused by repeated exposure to highly liquid effluent. Psoriasis can develop on the peristomal skin as sharply demarcated, erythematous, weeping, papular lesions or plaques with scales. Pyoderma gangrenosum is associated with inflammatory bowel disease or malignancy, presents as a painful, large necrotic ulcers, and can be treated with a combination of corticosteroids (topical, systemic, or intralesional) and antibiotics (e.g., dapsone).

Parastomal varices are abnormal portosystemic vascular collaterals that develop between the mesenteric veins of the intestine and the systemic veins of the peristomal skin. They are most commonly seen in patients with portal hypertension caused by sclerosing cholangitis. Parastomal varices can cause intermittent bleeding or life-threatening hemorrhage. Local procedures such as suture ligation or cauterization may be effective for the initial control of bleeding. However, recurrent bleeding is common and reducing portal pressures with TIPS is the most effective way to stop bleeding. Bleeding from stomal varices is usually associated with high mortality due to the patient's underlying liver disease.

Treatment

Improper site selection is one of the most common and preventable complications of stoma surgery (Box 12.4). Poor site selection causes difficulties in self-care and interferes with the maintenance of a secure stoma appliance. The creation of a stoma within the belly of the rectus abdominis muscle reduces the potential late

BOX 12.4 Technical aspects of stoma construction.

Abdominal Wall Aperture
Excision of circular piece of skin (≈2 cm in size)
Preservation of subcutaneous fat to provide support for stoma
Transrectus muscle placement of stoma
Fascial aperture to admit two fingers

Stoma
Selection of normal bowel for stoma
Adequate mobilization of bowel to avoid tension on stoma
Preservation of blood supply to end of bowel (marginal artery of the colon and last vascular arcade of small bowel mesentery must be preserved)
Small bowel serosa must not be denuded of more than 5 cm of mesentery

Maturation
Primary maturation of end stoma or afferent limb of loop ileostomy
Avoidance of traversing skin with sutures during maturation

Other Maneuvers*
Tunneling of bowel through extraperitoneal space of the abdominal wall
Mesenteric-peritoneal closure
Fixation of mesentery or bowel to fascial ring
Use of supportive rod with loop stomas

*May be performed but have not been proved to be effective in preventing postoperative complications.

complications, such as stomal prolapse and parastomal herniation. The ideal stoma site should be centered on a 2-inch flat surface away from scars, skin creases, and bony prominences, with healthy surrounding skin to provide an adequate pouch seal.[36] Ideally, the patient's abdomen should be inspected in several positions when choosing a stoma site preoperatively. This includes prone, sitting, standing, and leaning forward. Selection of the site when the patient is anesthetized on the operating room table does not allow for consideration of abdominal skin folds and their impact on appliance placement. Ideally, the stoma should be sited below the belt line. The SQ tissue between the stoma and skin should be kept clean by the use of stomahesive or absorptive powder until a new junction develops secondarily. Stomal ischemia is primarily due to interruption of segmental arterial supply to the exteriorized segment of bowel. In most instances, it is best to divide and complete preparation of the bowel well in advance of bringing the limb of intestine through the abdominal wall to allow time for demarcation in instances when the vascular supply is in question. When preparing the limb of intestine for an end ileostomy, the mesentery can usually be detached from the bowel for a distance of up to 5 cm without compromising arterial supply due to submucosal collaterals.[37]

In case of stomal ischemia, the first priority is to assess the proximal extent of ischemia. Ischemia limited to mucosa resolves spontaneously and heals by secondary intention. In contrast, vascular compromise below the level of the fascia and peritoneum requires immediate laparotomy and colostomy revision to prevent perforation and peritonitis. Ischemic complications can be minimized by preparing the bowel for stoma formation early in the operation, which provides opportunity to assess for inadequate perfusion at the time of stoma creation. Mild asymptomatic stenosis does not require any treatment. A tight stenosis causing subacute intestinal obstruction can be managed with simple and gentle dilatation in conjunction with a low-fiber diet. In case of recurrent obstructive episodes or pain, the stoma needs to be revised. Skin-level stenosis can be managed by detaching the skin from the mucosa and by excising the stenosed mucocutaneous junction along with a small amount of skin to increase the trephine size, mobilizing the distal intestine and resuturing the fresh, mobilized bowel to the widened skin edge.

In cases of incomplete retraction, local revision with excision of devitalized tissue and resuturing of viable mucosa to the skin using Brooke-type sutures can be done in the presence of viable bowel and absence of undue tension. However, complete stoma retraction with mucocutaneous separation requires immediate laparotomy and revision, as this situation results in subfascial contamination, peritonitis, and sepsis.

Management of acute parastomal herniation and bowel obstruction in the immediate postoperative period requires urgent reoperation, hernia reduction, resection of nonviable bowel if present, and revision of the fascial opening. Management of late prolapse depends upon the frequency and severity of symptoms since mild symptomatic, infrequent prolapse does not require repair and can be managed with appliance modification ± a support belt with the aid of a stoma therapist. However, when the prolapse causes ischemia, obstruction, or difficulty maintaining a functional appliance, surgical intervention is warranted. Strangulation of bowel within a parastomal hernia is an absolute indication for surgery.[38] Several surgical techniques are commonly used for parastomal hernia repair, including local repair, repair with prosthetic material, and stoma relocation. Mesh can be used with all of the three techniques.

Peristomal abscesses requires surgical drainage. A persistent peristomal fistula requires resection of the peristomal disease and construction of a new stoma at a different site to avoid the infection present at the former site. Stoma laceration can be caused by a pouch system that fits too closely against the stoma or by an improperly fitted belt. If recognized early, this problem can be treated by an appropriate size stoma appliance and discontinuing the belt. Ulcers can be treated symptomatically with local enterostomal wound care. Surgical treatment is reserved for ulcerations that extend deep into the ileostomy or extensive, unmanageable peristomal ulcerations. A properly situated stoma has a height of at least 1 cm and can usually be managed with a pouch change every 3 to 7 days.

Local skin irritation is a common problem that is frequently seen in patients with skin-level or retracted stomas. These require more frequent pouch changes, often daily or several times a day. Topical skin management includes providing an adequate appliance seal, controlling wound pain, and infection to enhance skin healing. Definitive treatment requires an appropriate pouching system that protects the parastomal skin from contact with the offending effluent, pouch refitting, and often patient education. Traumatic dermatitis can be prevented with meticulous selection of the stoma site at the time of surgery as well as diligent postoperative attention to appliance fit and replacement at appropriate intervals. Allergic contact dermatitis may be caused by specific stomal products, and patch testing can be used to identify the causative agent and confirm the diagnosis. Stomal or peristomal skin bleeding may be treated with silver nitrate or electrocautery to control bleeding. Additional measures including appliance refitting, direct pressure to the site of bleeding, epinephrine compresses, and/or transfusions can be used as needed.

Clostridioides difficile Colitis

Clostridioides difficile (*C. difficile*), formerly known as *Clostridium difficile*, is a gram-positive, anaerobic, toxin-producing, spore-forming bacillus. The spores are resistant to heat, acid, and antibiotics and can be transmitted through the fecal-oral route. Normally, the indigenous microbiota of the intestine inhibits the growth of *C. difficile* and prevents its proliferation. *C. difficile* infection (CDI) can occur when normal gut flora are disrupted by antibiotic usage or when spores germinate resulting in *C. difficile* overgrowth in the colon. *C. difficile* colitis is caused by the production of enterotoxin A and cytotoxin B, which damage intestinal epithelia, impair cell function, and promote local inflammation. Some strains of *C. difficile* have mutations in the toxin-producing gene, leading to increased toxin secretion and virulence. CDI is the most common cause of nosocomial diarrhea, although not all patients colonized with *C. difficile* will develop symptoms. *C. difficile* spores can survive for months in the environment and asymptomatic carriers can serve as a reservoir for the bacteria. Colonization is more common in hospitalized patients or people who work in health care facilities. Moreover, *C. difficile* can be transferred among hospitalized patients via health care providers. The risk factors of CDI are antibiotic exposure, increased age (>65 years), hospitalization, inflammatory bowel disease, GI surgery, immunosuppressive medication, or an immunologically compromised host. Nearly all antibiotics are associated with CDI, including the ones used to treat the disease (vancomycin, metronidazole). Broad spectrum penicillin and cephalosporins, clindamycin, and fluoroquinolones are the common antibiotics precipitating CDI. The risk of CDI is increased by a prolonged course of antibiotic treatment or the administration of multiple antibiotics. Surgery patients are at risk for CDI since they are usually elderly and hospitalized, have associated comorbidities, and are relatively immunosuppressed. Community-acquired CDI is also increasingly reported.

Clinical Presentation

After *C. difficile* colonization, the incubation time is varied. CDI symptoms range from asymptomatic, mild to moderate diarrhea, or life-threatening fulminant colitis. The distal colon is most commonly affected, but CDI can present as localized colitis in any part of the colon or as diffuse colitis. Most patients develop watery diarrhea during antibiotic therapy or shortly after a course of antibiotics but can also present weeks later. Other symptoms of CDI include abdominal pain, fever, weakness, loss of appetite, nausea, and vomiting. Severe cases of CDI may present with significant dehydration, abdominal distension, ileus, toxic megacolon, bowel ischemia, colonic perforation, peritonitis, renal failure, sepsis, shock, and death. Patients with fulminant CDI present with hypotension, shock, ileus, and toxic megacolon, which is associated with a higher mortality. Rare extracolonic manifestations are reactive arthritis and small intestine infiltration. In recurrent cases of CDI, the infection can be caused by reactivation of the same strain or reinfection with a new strain of *C. difficile*.

Diagnosis

Stool testing for *C. difficile* is commonly performed in patients who have three or more episodes of unexplained loose or watery stools within 24 hours. Laboratory testing can detect either free toxin (toxin A, toxin B) by enzyme immunoassay or the presence of *C. difficile* by detecting common antigen, toxin genes, cells, or spores. The gold standard for detecting the *C. difficile* organism is toxigenic culture, but it is time consuming and requires specialized equipment, which delays the diagnosis. More recently, real-time polymerase chain reaction testing for toxin encoding genes (tcdA, tcdB) is performed and provides a rapid, accurate diagnosis in most cases. The gold standard test for toxin detection is a cell cytotoxicity assay, which takes 1 to 2 days, and enzyme immunoassay of the toxin is the most common test. Fresh stool should be collected and sent to the laboratory as soon as possible. A rectal swab can be done in suspected cases of CDI with associated ileus. Flexible or rigid proctoscopy can be performed at the bedside in critically ill patients when urgent surgical intervention is necessary. Patients with CDI demonstrate white to yellow pseudomembranes about 2 cm in size separated by normal mucosa. Abdominal x-rays may show dilated, edematous colon or toxic megacolon in severe cases. An abdominal CT scan with oral contrast can evaluate toxic megacolon (cecal diameter >12 cm, colon >6 cm) or bowel perforation. Blood tests frequently demonstrate a significant leukocytosis, metabolic acidosis, high lactate, AKI, and hypoalbuminemia in severe cases. Leukocytosis ≤15,000 and serum creatinine <1.5 mg/dL suggest non-severe CDI. Whereas leukocytosis >15,000 and serum Cr >1.5 mg/dL suggest severe CDI. Presence of hypotension, shock, ileus, and toxic megacolon is seen with fulminant CDI.

Prevention and Management

Transmission of *C. difficile* is prevented by contact precaution. Patients with CDI are usually placed in a single room on "isolation precautions" with a separate toilet or on "contact isolation precautions." Patients should be encouraged to wash hands and take regular showers if possible to reduce the risk of spore transmission. All health care providers should wear gowns and gloves and wash hands with soap and water before and after they are in contact with CDI patients since the spores are resistive to alcohol-based solutions. Visitors should also be advised to follow these precautions as well. Sporicidal solutions should be used for cleaning the room to facilitate decontamination after discharge.

Treatment of CDI starts by discontinuing the patient's inciting antibiotics as soon as possible and administering IV fluids to prevent or correct dehydration. Only symptomatic patients with CDI should be treated. The drugs of choice for CDI are vancomycin or fidaxomicin. When the clinical suspicion of CDI is high, laboratory testing should not delay the treatment. For the initial episode of CDI, vancomycin 125 mg is given orally 4 times/day or fidaxomicin 200 mg orally 2 times/day for 10 days.[39] In less severe cases of CDI, metronidazole (500 mg orally 3 times/day for 10 days) is an alternative if vancomycin and fidaxomicin are not available. In fulminant CDI, vancomycin (500 mg orally 4 times/day) is given with additional metronidazole (500 mg IV 3 times/day), and the use of vancomycin enemas (500 mg in 100 mL normal saline enema) is also recommended. Recurrent CDI is treated with the normal vancomycin regimen if metronidazole was used to treat the first episode, but if vancomycin was used in the first episode, vancomycin has to be given for a prolonged period in a tapered and pulse manner (125 mg orally 4 times/day for 10–14 days, followed by 2 times/day for 7 days, and then every 2–3 days for 2–8 weeks). Fidaxomicin (200 mg 2 times/day for 10 days) can be used if vancomycin was used for the first episode of CDI. Subsequent recurrences of CDI can be treated with vancomycin or fidaxomicin as described above, or with vancomycin (125 mg 4 times/day for 10 days) followed by rifaximin (400 mg 3 times/day for 20 days). Fecal microbiota transplantation can be considered in patients with multiple recurrent CDIs. Surgical intervention is considered in patients with peritonitis, colonic perforation, bowel ischemia, ACS, worsening acidosis, sepsis, and shock despite appropriate resuscitation, and worsening clinical presentation of CDI despite adequate medical management. For many years, total abdominal colectomy with ileostomy was viewed as the procedure of choice for life-threatening CDI. More recently, laparoscopic loop ileostomy and colonic lavage with 8 L of polyethylene glycol (PEG 350) and antegrade vancomycin flushes (500 mg in 500 mL Ringer's lactate every 8 hours) and IV metronidazole for 10 days has been adopted at many centers. Colectomy may still be required in refractory cases of CDI but is more commonly used for salvage of nonresponders to the fecal diversion and colonic lavage protocol. Stomal reversal is considered later when the patient is fully recovered, although the reversal rate is low. Repeat testing of *C. difficile* and toxin is generally not recommended in patients with clinical response to treatment since the results might still be positive but the treatment does not need to be continued.

Anastomotic Leak

Intestinal anastomoses are commonly performed in emergency and elective general surgery. Successful intestinal anastomoses require a combination of meticulous surgical technique (correct suture placement or stapling procedure), good blood supply (pink color, peristaltic bowel with pulsatile mesentery), and no tension at the anastomosis (proper mobilization of bowel). Various anastomotic techniques are available including stapled (linear or circumferential), sutured (interrupted, continuous, one or two layer) end-to-end or end-to-side anastomoses. The choice of surgical technique may be influenced by intestinal location, bowel diameter, the presence of bowel edema, patient factors, associated peritoneal infection, cancer, contamination, or surgeon preference. Considerable literature is devoted to the impact of surgical technique on anastomotic leak rates. In general, the anastomotic technique does not appear to be associated with major differences in leak rate, except in specific situations. For example, inflamed, edematous, or thickened bowel (diverticulitis, radiation enteritis, or inflammatory bowel disease) is associated with an increased leak rate with most techniques; some studies show superiority of handsewn and/or two layer anastomoses in these and other special circumstances. If the surgical team is concerned about the anastomosis, anastomotic integrity can be tested intraoperatively by instilling saline, betadine, or air under pressure to distend the bowel at the anastomotic site. If small leaks are noted, they can usually be repaired with a few additional stitches. However, major leaks from failed staple firing may require completely revising the anastomosis. If there are concerns about bowel ischemia or viability, fluorescence vascular angiography can be used to assess bowel perfusion, or damage control surgery with a second look and delayed anastomosis can be performed.

Causes

Numerous factors have been implicated in the failure of anastomotic healing (Table 12.17). These can be broadly categorized as surgeon-related, patient-related, and disease-related factors. While anastomotic integrity depends on the complex interplay of patient factors and underlying disease processes, the surgeon must ensure these factors are considered and the anastomotic technique is appropriate for the clinical situation. Technical factors contributing to early leakage include gaps in the suture line, misplacement of sutures, stapler misfiring, enterotomy, or tear near the suture line. Distal obstruction, ischemia, and underlying disease processes may also contribute to delayed anastomotic leaks. Recent data suggest the intestinal microflora plays an important role in anastomotic leaks. Alterations in intestinal bacteria (e.g., increases in *Enterococcus faecalis*) can increase the risk of anastomotic leak by activating MMP9 and enhancing collagen-degrading activity at the anastomotic site.[40] The tensile strength of an intestinal anastomosis depends on the stapled or sutured collagen fibers in the submucosa, so it makes sense that increased collagenase activity at the anastomosis could contribute to breakdown. Likewise, collagen synthesis is required for proper anastomotic healing. Chemotherapy, radiation, and cofactor deficiencies (e.g., vitamins A, C, and E), which affect the cellular function, proliferation, and tissue repair, can adversely impact the healing process. In uncontrolled diabetes, macrophage number and activity are decreased resulting in impaired angiogenesis, lymphatic vessel formation, and collagen synthesis causing delayed healing. Zinc deficiency can also affect healing by augmenting matrix metalloproteinase activity, altering collagen-type ratio, and reducing cellular proliferation.

Microcirculatory blood flow at the level of the anastomosis is critical to healing, as it provides micronutrients, oxygen, anabolic cells, and growth factors.[41] Conditions like heart failure, mesenteric vascular disease, or hemorrhagic or septic shock may cause hypoperfusion of the anastomotic site and increase the risk of leak or dehiscence. Although hypoxia stimulates angiogenesis, healing is impaired when arterial oxygen tension falls below 35 mm Hg as it affects the formation of mature collagen fibers. Angiogenesis, growth factors, and epithelialization are further impaired when oxygen levels fall below 10 mm Hg. Therefore, it is essential to maintain euvolemia, normoxia, and prevent excessive intraoperative blood loss in order to maintain tissue oxygenation at the anastomosis.

The location of the anastomosis may also contribute to the risk of anastomotic leak. Small bowel anastomoses (enteroenterotomy, ileocolic, and ileorectal anastomoses) are considered "low risk" while esophageal, pancreaticoenteric, and colorectal anastomoses have an increased risk of anastomotic leak. With rectal surgery, the distance from the anal verge is an independent risk factor and colorectal anastomoses have a higher leak rate compared to an ileocolic and colocolic anastomosis. The risk of leak is higher if the anastomosis is below the peritoneal reflection (8%–20%) and for a rectal anastomosis (1%–9%).

Patient-related factors like protein malnutrition (albumin <3.0–3.5 g/dL), weight loss (>10% body weight), diabetes, shock, severe blood loss, immune deficiency, smoking, alcohol

TABLE 12.17 Risk factors associated with anastomotic leak.

DEFINITIVE FACTORS	IMPLICATED FACTORS
Technical aspects	Mechanical bowel preparation
Blood supply	Drains
Tension on suture line	Advanced malignancy
Airtight and watertight anastomosis	Shock and coagulopathy
Location in gastrointestinal tract	Emergency surgery
Pancreaticoenteric	Blood transfusion
Colorectal	Malnutrition
Above peritoneal reflection	Obesity
Below peritoneal reflection	Gender
Local factors	Smoking
Septic environment	Steroid therapy
Fluid collection	Neoadjuvant therapy
Bowel-related factors	Vitamin C, iron, zinc, and cysteine deficiency
Radiotherapy	Stapler-related factors
Compromised distal lumen	Forceful extraction of stapler
Crohn disease	Tears caused by anvil or gun insertion
	Failure of stapler to close

consumption, increased age, and obesity are associated with an increased risk of anastomotic failure in patients undergoing colorectal surgery. Also, underlying disease processes affect healing of a newly formed colorectal anastomosis. Metastatic colorectal cancer is an independent risk for anastomotic leak and both pre- and postoperative use of the chemotherapeutic agent bevacizumab has been reported to increase the risk of anastomotic dehiscence. Therefore, it is recommended that bevacizumab should be administered 6 weeks before an elective colorectal anastomosis and 28 days after surgery.[42] Patients with inflammatory bowel disease (Crohn disease and ulcerative colitis) treated with immunosuppression (e.g., infliximab) or steroids may have an increased risk of anastomotic leak. In general, steroid use impairs healing by lowering transforming growth factor-β, IGF-I, and collagen production.

The risk of anastomotic leak is also influenced by whether the procedure is performed electively or under emergent conditions. Emergency surgery is associated with an increased rate of anastomotic leak for multiple reasons, including the presence of underlying malignancy, immunocompromised state, presence of intra-abdominal contamination or sepsis, hemodynamic instability, etc. Damage control surgery may be used in cases with severe peritoneal contamination and has been shown to improve outcomes when patients have ischemic bowel and are not fully resuscitated or are in septic shock. However, open abdomens with NPWT are associated with higher anastomotic leak rates when compared with those that are primarily closed. It is unclear whether this is due to patient-related factors (e.g., patients that are sicker tend to be left open more often) or factors that are intrinsic to negative pressure therapy. The role of adjuvant measures like pelvic drains, omental wrapping, or tissue reinforcement in modifying the leak rate remains unclear. In the pelvis, the rationale for using drains is that they prevent the accumulation of blood and fluid adjacent to the suture line, which may become infected and contribute to suture line dehiscence. However, studies report mixed results regarding the use of pelvic drains, with some concluding that the use of closed suction pelvic drains results in fewer anastomotic complications and others reporting that the use of pelvic drains is an independent risk factor for anastomotic leak.

When elective intestinal surgery is performed, there are opportunities to optimize patient-related risk factors to decrease the risk of anastomotic leak. These include smoking cessation, nutritional optimization to correct protein malnutrition, and replacement of deficient essential nutrients (e.g., protein, zinc, and copper) and vitamins (e.g., A, C, and E). Patients with significant cardiac or pulmonary disease should be risk stratified and optimized if possible. This could include identifying and treating sleep apnea with continuous positive airway pressure ventilation, preoperative beta blockade or afterload reduction, and/or improving glycemic control in patients with type 2 diabetes mellitus. Another factor to be considered in elective bowel surgery is the role of mechanical and antibiotic bowel preparation. Mechanical bowel preparation has traditionally been considered important in preventing anastomotic dehiscence by reducing the fecal burden at the anastomotic site. However, during the last decade with the advent of effective antibiotic prophylaxis, modern surgical techniques, and improved patient care, many surgeons question the dogma of mechanical bowel preparation. Moreover, several studies have shown that mechanical bowel preparation is not "essential" for successful anastomotic healing.[43] The combination of oral antibiotics, mechanical bowel preparation, and parenteral antibiotics has been shown to reduce the risk of SSI in elective colorectal surgery, and some studies show that oral antibiotics are associated with reduced rates of anastomotic leak. However, in the case of a suspected leak, antibiotics against both aerobes and anaerobes should be started immediately.

Presentation and Diagnosis

The signs and symptoms of anastomotic leak are variable depending on the intestinal location, the size of the leak, the degree and spread of contamination, and the timing of presentation (early vs. late). Fever, tachycardia, increasing abdominal pain, elevated WBC count, decreased urine output, and shortness of breath are commonly seen with intraabdominal leaks. Leaks may present early with severe symptoms, sepsis, and multiple organ failure if intestinal contents are disseminated throughout the peritoneal cavity. Patients may also present in a more delayed and subtle fashion with vague abdominal pain, prolonged ileus, or delayed return of bowel function if they present late or the abscess has been "walled off" by omentum or other viscera. Anastomotic leaks may also present as drainage of intestinal contents from intra-abdominal drains or as SSIs with enterocutaneous fistulas (ECFs) draining from the skin incision. Many symptoms of anastomotic leak are nonspecific and may overlap with other complications or delays in postoperative recovery. The surgical team should have a high index of suspicion and aggressively investigate unexpected symptoms in patients with recent intestinal anastomoses since delays in diagnosis and treatment of anastomotic leaks are associated with worse outcomes.

The timing of presentation may vary with anastomotic location. Gastrojejunal leaks after gastric bypass surgery usually present early (<24 hours) and small bowel or colon leaks more typically present between 5 and 7 days after surgery. When the diagnosis of anastomotic leak is clinically obvious and the patient has peritonitis or severe sepsis, many surgeons will proceed with immediate exploratory laparotomy or diagnostic laparoscopy. Laboratory tests like complete blood test, C-reactive protein, and procalcitonin may be elevated with anastomotic leak but are considered relatively nonspecific. The most common imaging techniques to assess for anastomotic leak are water-soluble contrast studies and CT scans. Fluoroscopic contrast studies are most useful for proximal GI or distal colorectal anastomoses. Abdomen-pelvic CT scans with oral or rectal contrast are used to assess for anastomotic leaks but do not routinely demonstrate contrast leakage from the site of the leak. Signs of local inflammation like stranding and thickened bowel, large amounts of fluid (>300 mL) around the anastomosis ± free air should raise concern for a leak. Interventional radiology sampling or drainage of the fluid may be used to confirm and in some instances treat a small or contained leak.

Depending on the clinical condition of the patient, management of an anastomotic leak ranges from drainage, bowel rest, and antibiotic therapy to exploratory laparotomy with repair, resection, proximal diversion, or ostomies. Asymptomatic, radiographic-discovered leaks may require no treatment. In patients with localized abscesses who are not toxic, successful management may include abscess drainage, broad spectrum antibiotics, and/or bowel rest. A contained leak, along with an abdominal or pelvic abscess and clinical signs of sepsis, requires drainage of the abscess with broad spectrum antibiotic coverage. Surgical intervention is required in the absence of clinical improvement or deterioration, sepsis, or diffuse peritonitis. The surgical treatment of anastomotic leaks is determined by the patient's medical condition and intraoperative findings; small leaks (<1 cm) can be managed with simple repair and drainage when there are healthy tissues and minimal inflammation. When severe peritonitis, bowel edema and inflammation, and systemic sepsis are present, a diverting stoma should be considered. Small leaks with localized inflammation from a low colorectal anastomosis can be managed with pelvic drains and a diverting loop ileostomy. The use of protective stomas are not just limited to rectal surgery but are applicable to all anastomoses. Although a proximal diverting stoma does not prevent an anastomotic leak, it will mitigate the clinical impact of anastomotic failure by diverting the fecal stream away from the newly created anastomosis. Anastomotic breakdown in the pelvis is commonly caused by ischemia and frequently results in peritoneal contamination. In this situation, takedown of the anastomosis is required with complete fecal diversion using a colostomy or ileostomy.

Intestinal Fistulas

Causes

A fistula is defined as an abnormal communication between two epithelialized surfaces. Fistulas in the GI tract originate from the intestinal wall, biliary, or pancreatic ducts and communicate with adjacent organs or intestine (internal fistulas) or externally with the abdominal wall (external fistula). Fistulas can be classified as congenital (e.g., tracheoesophageal fistula) or acquired. Acquired fistulas can be traumatic, spontaneous, or postoperative. Most GI fistulas (75%–85%) are iatrogenic or traumatic and caused by faulty operative technique, injury to the intestine during handling, lysis of adhesions, abdominal fascial closure, or percutaneous drainage. Spontaneous fistulas account for the remaining 15% to 25% and may be caused by previous intestinal irradiation, intraabdominal sepsis, or inflammatory bowel disease, especially Crohn disease. Among the acquired GI fistulas, esophageal fistulas occur as a consequence of instrumentation, head and neck surgery, or trauma (both penetrating and blunt). Gastric fistulas are mostly iatrogenic (85%), resulting from anastomotic leak following peptic ulcer disease, antireflux procedures, and bariatric surgery, while the remainder are due to irradiation, inflammation, ischemia, and malignancy. Duodenal fistulas occur as a complication of gastric resection, duodenal resection, biliary tract procedures, pancreatic resections, trauma, perforated peptic ulcers, and cancer.

Intestinal fistulas are classified as internal, external, or mixed. Mixed fistulas involve two or more hollow viscera with a cutaneous connection and are almost always associated with an abscess. External intestinal fistulas, or ECFs, are the most common type and are usually the result of complications from previous abdominal surgery (e.g., anastomotic leak, bowel injury, iatrogenic injury, or from bowel exposure to large abdominal defects or prosthetic mesh). The ileum is the most common site for an ECF. Proximal ECFs (e.g., small bowel) are usually high output, whereas distal ones (e.g., colon) tend to be low output. Crohn disease is associated with both external fistula and internal fistulas (enteroenteric, enterovesical, or enterocolonic). Colocutaneous fistulas may also be seen with diverticulitis, cancer, inflammatory bowel disease, and appendicitis or radiation therapy. Aortoenteric fistulas occur due to erosion of prosthetic aortic grafts into the surrounding viscera, usually the duodenum.

The fistula output over a 24-hour period is the most important determinant of its physiologic impact (on fluid and electrolyte status) on the patient and guides management. ECFs can be classified as low (<200 mL/day), moderate (200–500 mL/day), or high (>500 mL/day) output. Medical treatment of fistulas commonly include wound management, pharmacologic (e.g., H_2 blockers), nutrition, fluid, and electrolyte management. Fistula closure is considered spontaneous in the absence of radiologic or surgical intervention. Anatomic characteristics associated with nonhealing fistulas include large adjacent abscess, fistula tract <2 cm in length, enteral defects >1 cm, and fistulas arising from certain bowel segments (e.g., stomach, lateral duodenum, ligament of Treitz, and ileum; see Table 12.18). Sepsis is a well-recognized risk factor that negatively impacts spontaneous closure of the fistula. Fistulas associated with concurrent pancreatic fistulas, presence of malnutrition, or adjacent infection have a low rate of spontaneous closure. Low-output fistulas are about three times more likely to close spontaneously than high-output fistulas, and postoperative fistulas are about five times more likely to close than fistulas associated with inflammatory bowel disease or trauma.

Presentation and Diagnosis

Patients with ECFs can present with a wide range of symptoms. They may demonstrate delayed return of bowel function and controlled drainage of enteric contents from an intraabdominal drain with minimal signs of infection. However, sepsis is the most common complication seen in patients with an ECF. With this presentation, patients may demonstrate fever, tachycardia, elevated WBC count, leakage of purulent material, and finally enteric contents draining from their surgical incision. Dehydration, fluid and electrolyte abnormalities, and malnutrition are common in this setting, especially in "high output" fistulas. The diagnosis of ECFs is usually straightforward because the drainage of enteric contents through the skin (enterocutaneous) or vagina (enterovaginal) is clinically obvious. ECFs may also present with severe abdominal wall infections caused by bacterial invasion and chemical erosion that facilitates extension of infectious process through

TABLE 12.18 Factors affecting healing of external intestinal fistulas.

FACTORS	FAVORABLE	UNFAVORABLE
Surgical anatomy of fistula	Long tract, >2 cm	Short tract, <2 cm
	Single tract	Multiple tracts
	No other fistulas	Associated internal fistulas
	Lateral fistula	End fistula
	Nonepithelialized tract	Epithelialized tract
	Origin (jejunum, colon, duodenal stump, and pancreaticobiliary)	Origin (lateral duodenum, stomach, and ileum)
	No adjacent large abscess	Adjacent large abscess
Status of bowel	No intestinal disease	Intrinsic intestinal disease (Crohn disease, radiation enteritis, recurrent or incompletely resected cancer)
	No distal bowel obstruction	Distal bowel obstruction
	Small enteral defect, <1 cm	Large enteral defect, >1 cm
Condition of abdominal wall	Intact	Disrupted (fistula opens into base of disrupted incision)
	Not diseased	Infiltrated with malignancy or intestinal disease
	No foreign body	Foreign body (mesh)
Physiology of patient	No malnutrition	Malnutrition
	No sepsis	Sepsis
Output of fistula	No influence	Influence

fascial planes, SQ tissue, and muscle. In contrast, internal fistulas (e.g., colovesical) may present more subtly and require imaging or endoscopy to diagnose.

CT scans of the abdomen and pelvis are commonly obtained in patients with postoperative sepsis and concerning intraabdominal fluid collections are drained with radiographic guidance to treat infected fluid collections. When oral contrast leaks from the GI tract or enteric contents are drained, the diagnosis is made. Other commonly used methods of diagnosing small bowel fistulas include a fistulogram for external fistulas or upper and lower GI series (internal fistulas). Fistulograms provide information about the length and origin of the fistula, which can help in determining whether the fistula might close spontaneously. However, most ECFs require prolonged hospital stay and are associated with significant morbidity and mortality.

Treatment

Prevention of fistulas is facilitated by the use of healthy bowel for anastomosis, preoperative mechanical bowel preparation, preoperative intraluminal or systemic antibiotics, sound anastomotic techniques (as discussed in anastomotic failure), and preoperative optimization of the nutritional status. Over the last three decades, the reduced mortality (40%–60% to 15%–20%) associated with fistulas has been attributed to advances in fluid, electrolyte, and nutritional management. The overall treatment goals in managing ECFs include control of sepsis, prevent fluid/electrolyte depletion, manage the fistula drainage, prevent skin damage, and enhance healing by optimizing the patient's nutritional status with total parenteral nutrition (TPN) and enteral feeding as tolerated.[44] Restoration of normovolemia, electrolyte replacement, and correcting acid-base balance requires accurate measurement of fistula output and composition. Once sepsis is controlled, initial management includes NPO status, NG decompression, and/or pharmacologic measures (e.g., PPIs or H_2 blockers) to decrease gastric secretions. The use of somatostatin analogues is somewhat controversial, but proponents of using the somatostatin analogue octreotide cite evidence of decreased fistula output, reductions in fistula healing time, and the time required for TPN. Infliximab (monoclonal antibody to TNF-α) may help with fistula closure in patients with Crohn disease.

After the basal fistula output is measured, enteral feeding can be initiated to see how this impacts fistula output. If enteral feeding causes a significant increase in fistula output, the patient should be made NPO and started on TPN with an appropriate volume and electrolyte composition to replace fistula losses.[45] For low-output and colonic fistulas, the use of enteral nutrition facilitates early fistula closure, reduced pneumonia rate, improved intestinal barrier function, and decreased rate of fistula recurrence. However, enteral nutrition usually requires at least 122 cm of bowel. Fistuloclysis (distal enteral feeding) is a technique developed to provide nutrition support in patients with high output, proximal fistulas. Collection and refeeding of fistula drainage, in combination with enteral feeding to the distal bowel, can decrease the need for TPN, help prevent fluid and electrolyte problems, and maintain nutrition in some patients. However, fistuloclysis is unsuccessful in many patients due to the inherent difficulties in wound management, tube dislodgement, and leakage of tube feeds around the tube onto the patient's skin. In many patients with high output fistulas and complex intraabdominal pathology, long-term TPN is necessary to provide nutrition support, maintain normovolemia, and prevent electrolyte disorders.

Wound management is a major consideration in all patients with ECFs, and nurses with experience in wound/ostomy management are critical for this. Spillage of enteral contents causes severe local skin excoriation at the site of an ECF. Fistula output >500 mL/day usually requires a pouch system, whereas output <50 mL/day can be managed with dressing and skin barrier. Various techniques are available to manage these frequently complex wounds, including protective substances (stomahesives, fibrin sealants), wound management systems, and NPWT. In many situations, it becomes a matter of trial and error to see which solution is best for each patient.

Once the sepsis is controlled, the patient's fluid and nutrition status is improving, and the wound is managed, the probability of spontaneous closure and timing of surgical intervention needs to be considered. Medical therapy should be continued as long as the patient is continuing to improve. The majority of fistulas that close spontaneously do so in the first 4 weeks. Therefore, in most cases, patients should be given at least 8 weeks for the fistula to heal spontaneously before surgery is considered. Surgical therapy is inevitable in many cases, especially when unfavorable characteristics are present (Table 12.18). Indications for surgical management of ECFs include persistent drainage, sepsis, or abscess. However, the timing of surgical intervention requires an assessment of the risk-benefit ratio for the individual patient. This requires considering the patient's previous abdominal surgery, the inflammatory status of the abdominal cavity, and the patient's ability to tolerate a major surgical procedure. Surgical intervention for ECFs should be delayed until both the intraabdominal and systemic conditions have been optimized. In many cases, there is a dense peritoneal reaction caused by abdominal sepsis and ECF that peaks around 10 to 21 days and lasts at least 6 to 8 weeks before subsiding. In some cases, delaying surgery even longer (e.g., 3–6 months) may allow peritoneal inflammation to significantly subside and allow the patient to be nutritionally and physiologically optimized before subjecting them to major surgery with its associated complications.

Surgery for ECFs is technically challenging and time consuming. Many patients with ECFs have large abdominal wall defects that need to be repaired in conjunction with the fistula surgery. Entering the abdomen above or below the previous incision may help to access the peritoneal cavity without injuring the underlying viscera. In most cases, the fistulous tract and the surrounding skin will be completely resected, an extensive adhesiolysis is usually required, and the entire bowel is examined to exclude distal pathology or obstruction. The fistula is usually resected, followed by an end-to-end intestinal anastomosis. In some cases (e.g., low rectal fistulas), diverting ostomies may be used to decrease the risk of pelvis sepsis. Many patients require abdominal wall reconstruction procedures with component separation, use of bioabsorbable mesh, and/or acellular dermal prostheses. Meticulous attention to surgical technique is required to prevent recurrent ECFs, which can be seen in up to 10% to 20% of cases. Factors associated with ECF recurrence include inflammatory bowel disease, small bowel fistula location, and anastomotic technique.[45]

Pancreatic Fistulas

Pancreatic fistulas can be internal (e.g., pancreaticopleural fistulas, pancreaticoenteric, pseudocyst) or external (e.g., pancreaticocutaneous) and iatrogenic (e.g., from pancreatic surgery, endoscopic retrograde cholangiopancreatography [ERCP], or trauma) or noniatrogenic (e.g., acute or chronic pancreatitis). Pancreaticopleural fistulas arise subsequent to pseudocyst fluid tracking into the chest cavity, causing pleural ascites; disconnected duct syndrome can occur secondary to acute necrotizing pancreatitis with cellular necrosis, leading to pancreatic fluid leakage into the peritoneal cavity and pancreatic ascites. Pancreaticoenteric fistula, a rare occurrence, develops when a pseudocyst or abscess ruptures into an adjacent hollow viscus (most often into splenic flexure or transverse colon). Pancreaticocutaneous/postoperative pancreatic fistula (POPF) (often seen arising from the pancreatic tail) develops subsequent to pancreatic anastomotic failure, is noted in nearly 33% of high-risk patients, and occurs following pancreatic debridement/resection, pancreaticoduodenectomies (10%–15%), middle and distal pancreatectomies (20%–30%), percutaneous drainage (especially in disconnected duct syndrome), left renal or adrenal surgery, splenic surgery, and splenic flexure mobilization.

Recently, the International Study Group on Pancreatic Fistula redefined clinically significant POPF (CR-POPF) as drain output of any measurable volume with an amylase level more than three times the upper limit of normal and formulated a 10-point scale "Fistula score" based on (1) soft gland texture, (2) small pancreatic duct size, (3) pathology exclusive of pancreatic cancer or pancreatitis, and (4) elevated blood loss, for identifying high-risk anastomoses and to develop universal mitigation strategies for comparison of outcomes across studies.[46] Although their risk is multifactorial, a soft gland parenchyma and small duct size (≤3 mm) are commonly reported risk factors.

A high index of suspicion for fistula formation is required after an inciting event (pancreatitis, operation, or trauma). Most patients with pancreatic ascites, pleural ascites, and external pancreatic fistulas, particularly POPF, respond to conservative management, provided that healing reestablishes ductal continuity, the fistula does not arise from an isolated pancreatic remnant, and in the absence of proximal duct obstruction. Medical management includes NPO, antisecretagogues (octreotide), nasojejunal feeding, fluid drainage with antibiotics to control the inflammation and potential source of infection, correction of fluid and electrolyte imbalances, and skin care. Imaging with CT helps to localize and drain intraabdominal fluid collections. MR cholangiopancreatography (MRCP) is noninvasive and delineates the sites of ductal disruption, especially upstream, that are not visible on ERCP. ERCP additionally facilitates therapeutic interventions including sphincterotomy, stenting, and nasobiliary drainage. However, ERCP is not recommended in the early period as it can exacerbate the inciting condition and also increase the risk of infection. Preoperatively, the prophylactic use of octreotide to facilitate spontaneous fistula closure is controversial; currently available data noted that somatostatin analogues are effective in decreasing external pancreatic fistulas output but do not affect the incidence or time of fistula closure.

POPF occurrence can be minimized with improved anastomotic techniques: pancreaticogastrostomy, pancreaticojejunostomy (most widely applied), duct-to-mucosa technique, invagination, Roux (double) limb creation, or with the use of transanastomotic stents.[47] The use of pancreaticogastrostomy was not effective in lowering CR-POPF rates in cases of a soft gland but was beneficial when a small duct (<3 mm) is present. Duct-to-mucosa anastomosis is not always feasible, especially when the duct is too small (or fragile). Invagination anastomosis is usually created in an end-to-side, duct-to-mucosa anastomosis or invagination of the pancreatic remnant; results from a randomized controlled trial reported significantly lower rates of fistula formation in the invagination group. Anastomotic stents can facilitate the creation of the duct-to-mucosa anastomosis and prevent dehiscence by shunting digestive pancreatic enzymes and reducing the rate of clinically relevant fistulas. Fistulas in the pancreatic head or a small ductal disruption respond to transpapillary stenting.

In patients with a failed conservative or endoscopic procedure, surgery facilitates spontaneous closure through elimination of ductal hypertension and is indicated in patients who are unable to have endoscopic therapies secondary to postsurgical anatomy or failure to cannulate the pancreatic duct due to ductal stricture or the presence of very large defect. Also, operative intervention depends upon the location of the ductal disruption. Injury near the tail of the pancreas is routinely treated with distal pancreatectomy, whereas injury in the neck is best managed with fistula drainage, allowing a fibrous tract to develop, followed by fistula tract-jejunostomy. Persistent fistulas are managed with Roux-en-Y fistula tract-jejunostomy, pancreaticojejunostomy, or pancreatic resection.

HEPATOBILIARY COMPLICATIONS

Bile Duct Injuries

Causes

Bile duct injury (BDI) is the most common severe and problematic complication associated with gallbladder surgery. The likelihood of sustaining a major BDI during cholecystectomy is relatively low (e.g., 3/1000 procedures). However, these potentially preventable injuries can be devastating and are associated with significant morbidity and mortality. In general, BDIs during laparoscopic surgery tend to be more complex than those encountered with open surgery due to the proximal location of BDI and frequent association with vascular injury. Strasberg and colleagues proposed a classification system that encompassed injuries commonly incurred during laparoscopic cholecystectomies.[48] Many factors are associated with the occurrence of BDI, and efforts to understand how they happen may help to decrease their incidence. Risk factors associated with BDI can be characterized as patient factors, local factors, and learning curve effect. Inflammation in the area of the triangle of Calot can result in close approximation of the cystic and common bile ducts (CBDs). A number of other contributing factors have been recognized, such as excessive cephalad retraction on the gallbladder fundus, excessive use of cautery, tenting of the common duct from excessive lateral retraction on the infundibulum resulting in a tear, and aberrant biliary anatomy. Misidentification of the bile duct may also contribute (e.g., misidentification of the CBD or right hepatic duct as the cystic duct).

The CBD is most commonly injured when it is mistaken for the cystic duct. This can be caused by aberrant or distorted anatomy due to inflammation, a short, wide cystic duct, or when the cystic duct runs parallel to the common hepatic duct. The infundibular technique, which is widely used for identification of the cystic duct, is unreliable, especially under conditions of acute inflammation. Consequently, most surgeons prefer the "critical view of safety" technique and often selectively use cholangiography as an adjunct to duct identification. The presence of any of these risk factors should alert the surgeon to the increased possibility of encountering a potentially dangerous situation during laparoscopic cholecystectomy. Additionally, failure to obtain secure closure of the cystic duct (e.g., when the duct is thick, rigid, or wide) can result in biliary leak.

Presentation and Diagnosis

Less than one third of iatrogenic biliary injuries are detected at the time of laparoscopic cholecystectomy. Most biliary injuries are diagnosed in a delayed fashion. Recognition and proper diagnosis of BDIs are advantageous in preventing serious complications. Patients often present with nonspecific symptoms, such as vague abdominal pain, nausea and vomiting, and low-grade fever, usually resulting from uncontrolled bile leakage into the peritoneal cavity. Some patients may present with sepsis from severe bile peritonitis, jaundice, or intraabdominal abscess. Patients who have ligation or early stricture formation may also present with cholangitis and jaundice. Also, excessive use of cautery or laser in the region of the common duct results in biliary strictures that manifest as recurrent cholangitis, obstructive jaundice, or secondary biliary cirrhosis. Cholangiography is considered the gold standard for evaluating BDIs, but the hepatobiliary iminodiacetic acid scan is frequently used to screen for bile leaks. Ultrasound and CT are capable of detecting intraabdominal fluid collections and ductal dilatations.

Treatment

Biliary injuries are best avoided by understanding the circumstances in which biliary injuries are likely to occur and how to avoid injury in these situations. While it may be impossible to completely eliminate BDI, taking care to avoid BDI should be of paramount concern to all surgeons performing laparoscopic cholecystectomy. The surgeon should remember that gallbladder disease is usually a benign condition that is rarely life-threatening. When difficulty is encountered during laparoscopic cholecystectomy, it can be safely converted to open cholecystectomy, cholecystostomy tube placement, or aborted altogether if the operating surgeon feels there is an unacceptable risk in continuing laparoscopically. Failure of progression of the dissection, inability to grasp and retract the gallbladder, anatomic ambiguity, poor visualization of the field due to hemorrhage, and other factors should trigger the surgeon to consider modifying their technique or planned operation (e.g., leaving a portion of the infundibulum).

The management of BDIs can be categorized as early or delayed repairs. The optimal timing and method of repair depend on extent of the injury, the expertise of the operating surgeon and team, the degree of acute inflammation in the area, and the hemodynamic stability of the patient. Immediate detection and repair are associated with an improved outcome. The goals of bile duct repair include the restoration of a durable bile conduit and the prevention of short- and long-term complications such as biliary fistula, intraabdominal abscess, biliary stricture, recurrent cholangitis, and secondary biliary cirrhosis. Some surgeons advocate waiting up to 6 weeks before repair to allow for the inflammation to subside and infection to resolve. The initial management of biliary injuries includes appropriate volume resuscitation and the initiation of antibiotics.

Imaging techniques, such as ultrasound and CT, are extremely valuable during the initial evaluation of a patient with suspected BDI. The presence of obstructed bile within the liver or a subhepatic collection suggests a bile leak that requires prompt drainage. Simple injuries such as cystic duct leak, gallbladder bed leak, and partial duct lacerations can be repaired immediately. Lateral duct injuries that do not result in complete transaction can be repaired primarily over a T-tube in the CBD as long as there is no evidence of significant ischemia or cautery damage at the site of injury. In the case of a bile leak from an aberrant right hepatic duct not in communication with the common duct, reconstruction of the isolated segment can be performed with Roux-n-Y hepaticojejunostomy. Percutaneous transhepatic cholangiography (PTC) is indicated in cases of complete transection to define the proximal anatomy and site of injury. MRCP is becoming the test of choice to diagnose late strictures and define the bile duct anatomy. If complete disruption or occlusion of the proximal bile duct is present, prompt evaluation with PTC is necessary to define the biliary anatomy and decompress the biliary system. The final phase in the management of BDI includes defining biliary anatomy and reestablishing biliary enteric communication.

Vasculobiliary Injury

Vasculobiliary injury is defined as an injury to both a bile duct and a hepatic artery and/or portal vein. The BDI may be caused by operative trauma, may be ischemic in origin or both, and may or may not be accompanied by various degrees of hepatic ischemia. They are classified into two types; one is right hepatic artery, which accounts for about 90% of vasculobiliary injuries, as it lies behind the common hepatic duct at the level of transection in the classical injury as described above. The other variant, extreme vasculobiliary injuries that involve major hepatic arteries and portal veins, is rare but has severe consequences, including infarction of the liver. Extreme vasculobiliary injury can occur when fundus-down cholecystectomy is attempted in the presence of severe inflammation in and around the gallbladder and results in severe hemorrhage due to dissection behind the cystic plate into the right portal pedicle. BDIs that include a vascular injury can result in acute hepatic necrosis, abscess formation, or secondary biliary cirrhosis, and in rare cases, liver transplantation may be required. The most common CT scan finding suggestive of hepatic artery injury is nonenhancement of the right lobe during the arterial phase. Initial symptoms may be nonspecific, typically related to the effects of biliary leak or biliary obstruction rather than due to vascular-related complications. Specific early symptoms related to arterial injury have been reported sporadically and may include bleeding, hemobilia, acute hepatic insufficiency, and sepsis related to right lobe atrophy, necrosis, and abscess formation. Patients with hepatic artery injury are more likely to have ischemic biliary mucosa and a higher risk of stricture formation. Consideration should be given to delaying repair of a biliary injury in patients with occlusion of the right hepatic artery.

The desire to complete a cholecystectomy should be secondary to the aim of completing the operation safely. Contracture of the gallbladder, with puckering of the liver, adhesion of pericholecystic structures, and difficulty in finding the gallbladder can serve as signs to warn the surgeon not to attempt to remove the gallbladder from above, but, instead, to perform a limited safe procedure such as cholecystostomy or subtotal cholecystectomy in which the gallbladder is not taken off the liver bed at all.

Management depends on whether there is evidence of liver injury and the timing of recognition of the hepatic artery injury, which may influence the necessity of performing resection of necrotic liver parenchyma at the time of biliary repair or revisional surgery in case of liver atrophy. The outcome of patients with major BDIs, combined with arterial disruptions, is worse than in patients with an intact blood supply of the bile ducts. The consequences of such injuries are much more extreme. Patients with injuries to the portal vein or proper or common hepatic should be emergently referred to tertiary care centers. Hepatic infarction is common, often with rapid onset and frequently necessitating emergency right hepatectomy or urgent liver transplantation. Death occurred in about 50% of the patients reported.

NEUROLOGIC COMPLICATIONS

Postoperative Delirium

Delirium refers to a state of mental dysfunction that presents with a wide range of neuropsychiatric symptoms. According to the *Diagnostic and Statistical Manual of Mental Disorders,* Fifth Edition, delirium refers to a disturbance of consciousness (reduced clarity and awareness of the environment) and change in cognition (memory deficit, disorientation, language, and perceptual disturbance) that develops in a short period of time, fluctuates during the day, and is not explained by preexisting dementia or neurodegenerative disorders. Delirium is especially common in elderly patients and its causes are multifactorial. The incidence of postoperative delirium (POD) varies from 15% to 53% in elderly surgical patients and represents a significant cause of morbidity. While it remains unclear if POD results in increased mortality, it is associated with increased length of hospital stay, care dependency, and both short- and long-term cognitive dysfunction (postoperative cognitive dysfunction, or POCD). The diagnosis of POCD requires both pre- and postoperative evaluation of cognitive function, and it has no clear diagnostic criteria and reported incidence because of the rarity of cognitive evaluation being routinely done and the variation of cognitive testing tools used.

Cause and Risk Factors

The causes of POD are multifactorial, and there are many hypotheses regarding the pathogenesis of POD, including neuroinflammation from infection or stress of surgery, alterations in blood-brain barrier permeability, poor cerebral perfusion, imbalances in neuroendocrine and neurotransmitter activity (especially cholinergic), cerebral atrophy, and reduction of cognitive reserve in elderly. The risk factors for POD include patient-related risk factors, illness-related factors, and interventions triggering POD. Patient-related factors for POD include advanced age (>65 years), multiple medical comorbidities, malnutrition, polypharmacy, history of cerebral infarction, chronic renal or hepatic disease, depression, and anxiety. POD is common after certain surgical procedures like hip replacement, cardiac surgery, vascular surgery, and emergency surgery. Postoperatively, inadequate pain control or impaired oxygenation can increase the risk of POD. The hospital environment (noise, sleep disturbance due to light/dark cycle and waking patients for vital signs and medication administration, the ICU) and medical/surgical interventions (NG tubes, drains, Foley catheters, endotracheal intubation) are also associated with an increased risk for POD. Patients with lower education level and preexisting cognitive dysfunction are also at increased risk for POCD. Other factors that contribute to developing POD include pain, infection, hypoxia, dehydration, anemia, emotional and physical stress, sleep deprivation, medication such as anticholinergic and benzodiazepines, and physical restraints.

Presentation

POD can present early after surgery in the postanesthetic care unit and, in most cases, presents within 5 days postoperatively. The symptoms of POD are acute, fluctuate over 24 hours, and are often reversible. These include sleep alteration: daytime drowsiness, night time insomnia, and psychomotor alteration with lucid intervals. POD symptoms can be hyperactive, hypoactive, or both. Hyperactive symptoms include agitation, anger, restlessness, verbal and physical aggression, or mood lability. Hypoactive symptoms are more common and present as lethargy, inattention, flat mood, somnolence, and decreased response to stimuli. For this reason, patients with hypoactive POD are less likely to be diagnosed. POCD develops later than POD and may last for weeks to months. The most common cognitive functions affected in POCD are memory and executive functions.

Prevention and Management

Although certain risk factors for POD cannot be changed (e.g., patient age, type of operation, anesthetic choice, etc.), many predisposing POD factors can and should be modified in the perioperative period. Nutritional status, anemia, volume status, and hydration should be corrected before surgery. In addition, anticholinergic and benzodiazepine medications should be avoided unless the patient is "high risk" for alcohol withdrawal or severe anxiety. Prevention of deep sedation by monitoring anesthesia depth during surgery with electroencephalogram (EEG) monitoring or by using dexmedetomidine for light sedation during ICU care reduces the incidence of POD. The Confusion Assessment Method and Richmond Agitation-Sedation Scale scoring systems are commonly used to monitor responsiveness and titrate sedation in ICU patients at risk for POD. In surgical and trauma patients, pain control should be adequate with multimodal analgesia using additional nonopioid medication if possible. Surgical patients should have physical restraints such as Foley catheters, endotracheal tubes, and drains removed and be transferred out of the ICU as soon as possible. Physicians and teams should routinely check for responsiveness and arouse patients during rounds especially in elderly patients to screen for hypoactive symptoms. Sleep disturbance should be avoided if possible and the room environment should be adjusted to enhance patient comfort with access to outside windows for maintenance of circadian rhythms. Family members can be involved in taking care of patients to support daily care and early mobilization is recommended. Many hospitals use geriatric consult services to assess and adjust care to minimize the risks of delirium in "high-risk" elderly patents.

Once delirium is detected, the care-giving team should consider safety of the patients and staff and perform a comprehensive assessment (physical examination, laboratory tests, etc.) to identify possible causes, including myocardial infarction, stroke, seizure, electrolyte imbalance, hypoxia, hypothermia, hypoglycemia, and acidosis. Absent treatable medical causes for POD are nonpharmacologic interventions, including cognitive reorientation, decreasing sleep disturbance, optimizing nutrition, fluid and oxygenation, providing hearing and vision aids, etc., that are preferable. Pharmacologic intervention should be reserved for patients who are not responsive to nonpharmacologic methods or hyperactive patients who are at risk of harming themselves, other patients, or caregivers. Antipsychotics (e.g., haloperidol, olanzapine, and quetiapine) are commonly used to treat hyperactive POD. Gabapentin is used to prevent alcohol withdrawal and benzodiazepines are used to treat alcohol and benzodiazepine withdrawal. In most instances, POD is treated using a small dose of medication, titrating the dose as needed and for the shortest duration possible. POD patients should be closely monitored during treatment and receive follow-up after discharge to assess cognitive function.

Perioperative Seizure

Seizure is a clinical manifestation of abnormal electrical activity in the brain. The cause of seizures in the perioperative period is often due to preexisting epilepsy or intracranial pathology such as tumor, infarction, hemorrhage, cerebrovascular disease, or traumatic brain injury. Other possible causes of perioperative seizure include metabolic disturbances such as electrolyte imbalance, infection or sepsis, hypoglycemia, intoxication, medication side effects, or alcohol withdrawal. Seizures can present as abnormal movements (e.g., convulsion, rhythmic tonic-clonic body movements that are usually self-limited and of short duration). Most seizures are followed by changes in consciousness and frequently amnesia. Seizures can also be prolonged and refractory to treatment with progression to status epilepticus if they continue for more than 30 minutes. Seizures can impact the ability to maintain one's airway and normal ventilation and result in hypoxemia with associated complications. Seizures may also result in the loss of autonomic control with bowel or bladder incontinence and may result in increased intracranial pressure or cerebral edema.

The risk of perioperative seizures can be decreased by careful management of antiepileptic drugs (AEDs) in patients with epilepsy. Patients with recent adjustment of their AED regimen or with long periods of NPO are at increased risk of perioperative seizures. Careful monitoring of circulating AED levels and administering an equivalent dose of parenteral medication can help to prevent seizures in these patients. Initiating preoperative prophylactic AEDs in patients without history of seizure disorder who have never taken AEDs has not been shown to be beneficial.

Management of perioperative seizures includes monitoring vital signs, electrocardiogram, maintaining airway patency and ventilation, preventing aspiration, and obtaining IV access. Blood should be tested for hypoglycemia (and managed promptly), electrolyte imbalance, toxicology, and AED levels. Medications should be given to stop seizure activity and prevent progression to status epilepticus, and imaging (e.g., head CT scan) should be performed if clinically indicated. Benzodiazepines are the first-line medications to stop seizures, especially IV lorazepam or diazepam. Intramuscular midazolam or IV phenobarbital can be used if lorazepam is not available or contraindicated. After seizures are controlled and appropriate airway/IV management, investigation of potentially precipitating causes should be completed and managed accordingly. A neurologic exam should be performed to look for neurologic deficits and evaluate blood test results. Brain imaging such as CT or magnetic resonance imaging (MRI) should be done in patients with new-onset seizure or new neurologic symptoms to look for brain tumor, stroke, or intracranial hemorrhage. Patients with alcohol withdrawal should be given glucose and thiamine. With prolonged seizures or status epilepticus, additional doses of lorazepam or diazepam can be given. If multiple doses of lorazepam are unable to control seizure activity, additional AEDs (e.g., IV fosphenytoin, valproate, levetiracetam, or phenobarbital) should be given. IV anesthetic drugs like propofol or thiopental are given with EEG monitoring in intubated patients in cases of status epilepticus that are difficult to control with standard AEDs. Moreover, drug interaction between AEDs and other medications must be considered. AEDs should be tapered gradually in patients receiving maintenance medication.

Perioperative Stroke

Causes and Presentation

Perioperative stroke is defined as focal or global loss of cerebral function lasting more than 24 hours, which occurs during the perioperative period or within 30 days after surgery. Stroke can result in permanent brain damage with neurologic deficits affecting both quality of life and mortality. The incidence of stroke after noncardiac, nonneurologic surgery is 0.1% to 1.9%. Certain surgical procedures, including head and neck, carotid artery, and cardiac valve surgery and some aortic procedures, have higher incidence due to the risk of emboli. Most perioperative strokes are detected in the hospital and represent a significant portion of all in-hospital strokes.

Perioperative strokes can be either hemorrhagic or ischemic. While ischemic strokes are more common, hemorrhagic strokes account for 1% to 4% of perioperative strokes. Hemorrhagic strokes are caused by bleeding into the intracranial ventricles, brain parenchyma, or subarachnoid space. They are commonly caused by uncontrolled hypertension, vascular malformation, anticoagulants, and antiplatelet medications. Consequently, patients with uncontrolled hypertension, coagulation disorders, or known intracranial vascular malformation are at increased risk for hemorrhagic strokes. Ischemic strokes are caused by poor cerebral perfusion that occurs during or after surgery leading to cerebral ischemia and infarction. Embolism is the most common cause of perioperative ischemic stroke causing cerebrovascular occlusion. Ischemic strokes are also caused by narrowing or occlusion of intracranial vessels, cerebral hypoxia, decreased blood pressure or hypotension, thrombosis, anemia, or hemodilution. Numerous factors are associated with increased risk of perioperative stroke, including atherosclerosis, cardiac emboli, hypercoagulable state, cerebral hypoperfusion, advanced age, family history of stroke, obesity, diabetes, hypertension, smoking, previous stroke or transient ischemic attack, polycythemia, pregnancy, oral contraception, perioperative beta blockers, atrial fibrillation, left atrial enlargement, bacterial endocarditis, ischemic heart disease, heart failure, and carotid stenosis.

Perioperative stroke commonly occurs within 7 days after surgery and presents as an acute neurologic deficit. This could include a decrease or loss of motor function, facial droop, decreased sensation, alteration of speech, or mental status such as delirium, lethargy, or decreased responsiveness, which might be confused with sedation and pain. These acute neurologic deficits may be temporally associated with risk factors like changes in blood pressure, cardiogenic shock, atrial fibrillation, or supratherapeutic anticoagulation.

Treatment

Prevention of ischemic stroke requires optimizing cerebral perfusion and decreasing the risk of embolism. Efforts to reduce the risk of hemorrhagic stroke include controlling hypertension and correction of any coagulation disorders. Stable cerebral perfusion is normally maintained by cerebrovascular autoregulation (i.e., constriction and dilatation of the cerebral vessels). In patients with recent stroke, autoregulation is impaired, hence there is increased risk of perioperative stroke. For these patients, elective surgery should be postponed at least 6 to 12 months. If emergency surgery is required, careful monitoring, control of blood pressure, and intraoperative monitoring of cerebral function with EEG and somatosensory evoked potential monitoring should be considered. Patients with carotid bruits should be evaluated with duplex ultrasonography for possible carotid stenosis and should be treated, if indicated, before surgery. Perioperative beta blockers can increase the risk of stroke but are beneficial in preventing PMI so the risk-benefit ratio should be considered on a case-by-case basis. Statin and aspirin therapy should be continued. Anticoagulants should be held before surgery, and bridge therapy should be considered in patients at high risk for thromboembolic complications. After surgery, sedation should be minimized to decrease the risk of masking the presentation of complications.

Once stroke is suspected, a stroke code or the stroke team should be called immediately and neurologic examination should be performed. Blood glucose level should be tested since hypoglycemia could cause neurologic symptoms, and both hypoglycemia and hyperglycemia worsen stroke outcomes. Baseline electrocardiogram and cardiac troponin should be obtained, and noncontrast CT imaging of the brain should be done as soon as possible to discriminate hemorrhagic versus ischemic stroke. General management is to ensure airway, ventilation, oxygenation, prevention of aspiration in patients with decreased consciousness, and control of blood pressure. In cases of hemorrhagic stroke, all medications affecting coagulation should be held, coagulation abnormalities reversed, blood pressure controlled, and the neurosurgical team consulted. Treatment of an ischemic stroke is challenging because treating with thrombolytic therapy within 3 to 4.5 hours is a relative contraindication in patients after major surgery due to the risk of bleeding. Optimization of blood pressure is essential to restore cerebral perfusion, and mechanical thrombectomy should be considered in select patients. If thrombolytic therapy is initiated, rTPA should be given in the ICU setting or stroke unit. Patients should be routinely monitored for complications of rTPA, including bleeding; angioedema, which is treated by steroid and antihistamine; and intracranial hemorrhagic transformation (i.e., severe headache, nausea, vomiting, sudden hypertension, worsening neurologic examination). If hemorrhagic transformation is suspected, rTPA should be stopped immediately, coagulation corrected, and CT scan performed. Patients should then be followed up with a neurologic examination. Rehabilitation interventions to decrease pressure ulcers, DVT prophylaxis, and depression screening should be included in the routine care of the stroke patient, and speech therapy should evaluate for dysphagia before starting an oral diet. Aspirin should be given for secondary prevention as soon as it is safe to do so. Patients with arrhythmias should be considered for treatment with anticoagulants to prevent secondary embolic events. Patients should be advised to control underlying diseases, such as diabetes and hypertension, quit smoking, and take statins if coronary artery disease is present.

EAR, NOSE, AND THROAT COMPLICATIONS

Epistaxis

Epistaxis results from blood vessel rupture within the nasal mucosa. It can be spontaneous, traumatic, or secondary to other comorbidities or malignancies. Nasal bleeding is often minor and self-limited. However, hypertension and/or coagulation disorders can result in prolonged and severe epistaxis. Epistaxis is commonly divided into anterior and posterior by the site of origin. The major causes of anterior epistaxis are direct nasal trauma by digital manipulation or iatrogenic injury from nasal tubes (e.g., NG or nasal endotracheal). Since the anterior septal area is readily accessible, hemorrhage from this region can be managed with direct pressure by pinching the nose over the cartilaginous septum. If anterior bleeding is not controlled by direct pressure, then packing and otolaryngology consultation should be considered. Appropriate management of severe epistaxis requires careful evaluation and treatment. It is important to protect the airway to prevent aspiration; intubation may be required in patients with facial trauma and/or severe profuse bleeding.

When nasal bleeding continues despite anterior packing, posterior epistaxis should be suspected. The incidence of posterior epistaxis is higher in elderly patients with atherosclerosis due to bleeding from sphenopalatine vessels. The current management of posterior epistaxis includes combined anterior posterior packing, angiographic embolization, arterial ligation, and endoscopic electrocautery. The classic posterior nasal packing consists of using rolled gauze or tonsil packs secured in the posterior choanae by inserting the pack through the oral cavity and then in the nasopharynx via sutures or using a Foley catheter with a 30 mL balloon. However, use of a Foley catheter is associated with higher rates of complications like pressure necrosis, infection, nasal trauma, vagal response, aspiration, infection, airway obstruction, and hypoxia. Failure to control blood loss with less invasive measures requires either surgical exploration or transarterial embolization. If bleeding persists after arterial ligation, endoscopic cauterization and/or medical correction of coagulopathy are required. In the absence of coagulopathy and failed arterial ligation, arterial embolization may be effective in controlling persistent localized bleeding.

After adequate control of bleeding, attention should be redirected to the patient's general state. If the bleeding was significant, the patient volume status and blood count should be checked. IV fluids and blood transfusion should be considered as medically indicated. Similarly, coagulopathy, hypertension, and other aggravating/precipitating factors should be addressed.

Nosocomial Sinusitis

Nosocomial sinusitis (NS) represents a potential cause of occult fever in critically ill patients. Outpatient sinusitis commonly presents with clinically overt symptoms. In contrast, the symptoms of NS are typically masked by more serious illness and the microbiology is more commonly polymicrobial. *Pseudomonas species* and *S. aureus* are commonly isolated pathogens in patients with NS. NS is more commonly seen in ICU patients with nasal instrumentation (e.g., nasotracheal airways or NG tubes), which obstruct the ostial meatal complex, causing inflammation and facilitating fluid accumulation in the sinus cavity. Inflammation and edema of the nasal mucosa decrease sinus ostial patency and impair mucociliary clearance, which favors microbial growth. Other risk factors for NS include Glasgow coma score ≤7, corticosteroid use, drying of mucosal lining due to prolonged oxygen use, anatomic variations, and sepsis-induced inhibition of nitric oxide synthesis in the maxillary sinuses, which can impair mucociliary clearance and epithelium perfusion. Diagnosis of NS is often difficult due to the lack of clinical signs (e.g., facial pain, malaise, fever, purulent nasal discharge) because "at-risk" ICU patients are often unable to communicate. NS should be suspected in patients with a fever of unknown origin and are endotracheally intubated.

CT and MRI imaging are sensitive techniques to evaluate soft tissue changes in the sinuses. The CT findings suggestive of sinusitis are sinus opacification, air-fluid levels, sinus wall displacement, and 4 mm or greater mucosal thickening. Treatment of NS includes antibiotics effective against gram-negative rods and *S. aureus*, topical decongestants, removal of nasal tubes, and head elevation. The majority of patients respond to these measures and become afebrile in 2 to 5 days. Functional endoscopic sinus surgery can be considered for patients who fail medical management as it relieves obstruction, restores drainage, and mucociliary clearance. Early detection and treatment of NS is important since delays in diagnosis can lead to the development of VAP, sepsis, and life-threatening complications such as meningitis, mastoiditis, intracranial abscesses, and cavernous sinus thrombosis.

Acute Hearing Loss

Hearing impairment after surgery is often subclinical and rarely reported. It can either be conductive or sensorineural, unilateral or bilateral, and transient or permanent. In particular, patients with prolonged intubation in an ICU are more likely to develop conductive hearing loss after a surgical procedure due to middle ear effusion, infection, and/or inflammation. Otologic surgery with damage to the ossicular chain causes immediate hearing loss. Restoration of hearing is unlikely if there is no spontaneous recovery within 2 weeks. Cardiopulmonary bypass surgery may also result in irreversible unilateral sensorineural hearing loss due to microembolism of the inner ear causing ischemic damage. Most ototoxic drugs (diuretics, antiinflammatory agents, aminoglycoside antibiotics, and antineoplastic agents) are also nephrotoxic, and impaired renal function further exacerbates functional impairment and/or cellular degeneration of tissues of the inner ear, resulting in bilateral hearing loss. A comprehensive examination with emphasis on identification of underlying cause and subsequent directed therapy may improve the likelihood of hearing recovery. Otoscopic examination may reveal foreign material, inflammation and/or edema, or perforated tympanic membrane. Ototoxicity usually improves when the inciting medication is discontinued; however, hearing should be monitored over the ensuing 2 to 3 days.

Parotitis

Acute suppurative parotitis is most often seen in debilitated and dehydrated postoperative patients with poor oral hygiene. The lack of oral stimulation causes decreased parotid gland secretions, which facilitate retrograde passage of bacteria and ductal obstruction. Parotitis manifests as a sudden painful enlargement of the parotid gland. It is most commonly unilateral and may be associated with painful mastication, erythema of the overlying skin, and purulent discharge from the parotid duct on massage of the gland. Treatment of parotitis includes topical warm compresses, adequate hydration, and administration of parenteral antibiotics. Antimicrobial therapy for parotitis should include coverage for *S. aureus* and hemolytic streptococci. Infection of the parotid gland can extend locally by rupture of the abscess into surrounding tissues, resulting in deep neck space infections. Deep neck space infection is a serious complication that may cause mediastinal empyema, airway compromise, epiglottic/laryngeal edema, and severe sepsis with an associated high mortality rate (20%–40%). In the absence of clinical improvement with 4 to 5 days of medical treatment, surgical drainage should be considered. Since the parotid gland is divided by multiple septa, ultrasound or CT scan is useful to detect abscesses in the absence of localized fluctuation and suppuration. Care should be taken to avoid facial nerve injury when drainage is performed using a preauricular incision.

THE GERIATRIC PATIENT AND FRAILTY

Improvements in health care have led to an increased number of "older adults" (age >65 years), which represents the fastest-growing segment of our society. Although age alone does not translate into increased operative risk or perioperative complications, the geriatric population is prone to increased perioperative complications for multiple reasons, including age-related physiologic changes, associated medical comorbidities, polypharmacy and increased sensitivity to analgesics, poor nutrition, altered balance and mobility, sarcopenia, and frailty. For a comprehensive overview of this subject, the reader is referred to the Optimal Management of the Geriatric Patient NSQIP guidelines by the American College of Surgeons and American Geriatrics Society. Because of the increased risks associated with surgery in elderly patients with frailty, this topic will be discussed in more detail.

Frailty is a state of reduced physiologic reserve affecting multiple organ systems resulting in the catabolism of muscle mass and strength (referred to as sarcopenia).[49] The incidence of frailty is higher in women than men and increases with age, ranging from 4% in patients <65 years old to 26% in patients over 85 years of age. Frailty is commonly defined using the frailty phenotype model as the presence of three or more of the five features of slowness, weakness, exhaustion, weight loss, and low physical activity. Slowness is measured by gait speed, weakness by hand grip, and other features by standard questions. Patients with none of these features are nonfrail, those with one or two are considered "prefrail," and those with three or more are deemed "frail." The key characteristics of the frailty cycle are decreased appetite, chronic malnutrition, and progressive loss of skeletal muscle mass, strength, and power. The Fried criteria are helpful in identifying sarcopenia, which has been linked to increased morbidity and mortality with major surgery. Unfortunately, the phenotype model does not readily identify patients with cognitive impairment, a subcategory of frailty defined by the presence of both physical frailty and cognitive impairment. Although the pathophysiology of frailty is complex, it appears to involve a combination of environmental factors, systemic inflammation, and epigenetic changes caused by increased DNA methylation, which collectively contribute to muscle loss and widespread cellular damage. Suffice it to say that the increased risks of surgery in patients with frailty make it important to properly identify and treat or counsel these patients before surgery.

Frailty state (FS) patients are characterized by a heterogeneous combination of reduced physical ability, nutritional and energy status, cognition, and overall health that can be precipitated by inactivity, poor nutrition, disease, stress, or psychosocial illnesses. Patients with chronic illnesses and disabilities also experience FS; older people presenting with hip fractures are some of the frailest surgical patients. Although no laboratory tests are involved in diagnosing FS, the presence of abnormal results in three or more systems was a significant predictor of frailty; laboratory tests performed to assess for comorbid conditions are helpful. The pathophysiologic effects of FS on different organ systems are listed in Table 12.19.

FS prevalence is higher in surgical preoperative settings, varying from 10% to 46%, depending on the screening instrument selected, the surgical procedure, and patient characteristics. Compared with nonfrail patients, FS patients in ICUs have higher in-hospital mortality rates. In addition, FS patients are five to seven times more common in patients on hemodialysis and cardiac failure is seen in up to 75% of frail patients after major cardiac surgeries. FS has been shown to be a strong tool for evaluating preoperative risk factors for poor postoperative outcomes and a powerful predictive preoperative tool for 30-day postoperative complications. Central muscle mass can predict long-term mortality in elderly patients after major vascular surgery. Abnormal physiologic deterioration measured by FS is an important independent predictor of outcomes after pancreatic surgery. A minor insult may be sufficient to lead to permanent functional decline postsurgery in a very frail patients; these patients would benefit from early recognition and treatment of surgical complications, postoperative infections, monitoring of adequate hydration and nutrition, early mobilization, and rehabilitation to prevent deconditioning. As such, FS has emerged as an essential part of the preoperative assessment and risk stratification of patients prior to surgery, and earlier recognition of complications is likely to reduce the chance of failure to rescue patients and improve outcomes and has been measured by myriads of instruments.

Despite the strong evidence that frailty in surgical patients leads to poorer postoperative outcomes, there is still a lack of a unifying tool to measure frailty that is time-efficient and practical to use. Explaining the higher risk of postoperative complications will preempt potential adverse outcomes and give patients and families realistic expectations after surgery. Those who are extremely frail may accept the high risk of morbidity and mortality while undergoing palliative surgery with the goal of improved quality of life; however, despite being well-recognized, there is no consensus on how FS should be measured.

TABLE 12.19 Pathophysiologic effects of frailty state on different organ systems.

Endocrine system	Low levels of testosterone, insulin-like growth factor, and vitamin D.
Immune system	Impaired immunity results with low levels of lymphocytes and CD8 T-cells.
Coagulation	Procoagulant state with decreased plasminogen activator inhibitor-1.
Renal	Reduced glomerular filtration rate, a reduction in the activity of the cytochrome P450 system.
Cognition	Result from a combination of anticholinergic medications and hypoxic injury of the brain during the perioperative period. This is compounded by the systemic inflammation caused by surgery, releasing proinflammatory cytokines interleukin-1β and tumor necrosis factor-α, activating central nervous system microglia, which further release proinflammatory cytokines, which in turn impair acetylcholine synthesis.
Cardiovascular system	Cardiac autonomic dysfunction results in blood pressure lability and prolonged hypotension in response to the administration of anesthesia.
Drug interactions	Drugs such as benzodiazepines, antihistamines, and tricyclic antidepressants may increase the risk of oversedation, falls, and orthostatic hypotension. The potential benefits of continuing these medications may outweigh the risks.

Treatment

Normal aging-related changes cannot be prevented, but FS can be prevented. Detection of frailty at baseline preoperatively could aid in identification of high-risk patients with potential poor outcomes. The goal of treatment in these patients should be twofold: appropriate management of illnesses that results in FS and prevention of sarcopenia through muscle strengthening exercises and improved nutrition. Exercise decreases inflammatory markers and increases muscle strength. A systematic review of preoperative exercise intervention in cancer patients showed significant improvement in the rate of incontinence, functional walking capacity, and cardiorespiratory fitness.[50] Also, adequate nutrition, proper treatment of chronic illnesses, appropriate vaccination (e.g., for pneumonia, influenza, shingles, and tetanus), prevention of falls through increased home safety, and monitoring the use of medications (e.g., sedatives, diuretics) that can contribute to inactivity and/or exacerbate weakness can prevent FS. Continued medical surveillance is important to quickly identify any physiologic changes that can be reversed. Interventions targeted at underlying reversible conditions (including congestive cardiac failure and chronic renal failure) may be effective in mitigating, or even reversing, frailty. Renal transplantation, for example, can reverse frailty associated with end-stage renal failure.

Recommendations

Recommendations include honest disclosure of prognostic information, emotional support, tailoring suggestions to the individual patient and family, and verifying that the patient and family understand the material presented to them (Box 12.5). Of particular importance is the recognition that prognostic communication should occur as an iterative process. Difficult discussions about aging, frailty, and the approaching end of life require time to reflect and adapt while balancing expectations with realistic forms of hope.

BOX 12.5 Recommendation for the prevention of frailty complications.

- Assess muscle strength, fall risk, and ability to safely ambulate and perform activities of daily living.
- Initiate fall precautions per facility protocol, and maintain patient safety (e.g., airway, circulation, and prevention of injury).
- Promote optimum physiologic status, and reduce the risk of complications.
- Assess vital signs, all physiologic systems, and pain level.
- Administer prescribed medications (e.g., analgesics, medications for comorbid conditions) and immunizations (e.g., influenza, pneumococcal).
- Evaluate weight loss over the past year, and request referral to a nutritionist if weight loss is significant.
- Rehabilitation (good nutrition and physical therapy) after stressful events is important in preventing frailty state.
- Assess recent changes in the patient's mobility, mood, appetite, and ability to perform daily activities independently.
- Assess patient's level of anxiety, stress, and depression.

SELECTED REFERENCES

Afshari A, Ageno W, Ahmed A, et al. European Guidelines on perioperative venous thromboembolism prophylaxis: executive summary. *Eur J Anaesthesiol.* 2018;35:77–83.

This is a comprehensive summary of European guidelines for perioperative venous thromboembolism prophylaxis.

Badrasawi M, Shahar S, Sagap I. Nutritional management in enterocutaneous fistula. What is the evidence? *Malays J Med Sci.* 2015;22:6–16.

Early nutritional support with parenteral nutrition, enteral nutrition, or fistuloclysis plays a significant role in the management of enterocutaneous fistula. This article is a retrospective review of the current evidence on nutritional assessment, protein and calorie requirements, and routes of feeding in enterocutaneous fistula patients.

Fleisher LA, Fleischmann KE, Auerbach AD, et al. 2014 ACC/AHA guideline on perioperative cardiovascular evaluation and management of patients undergoing noncardiac surgery: a report of the American College of Cardiology/American Heart Association Task Force on practice guidelines. *J Am Coll Cardiol.* 2014;64:e77–e137.

This article summarizes the American College of Cardiology and the American Heart Association guidelines for the management of patients with underlying cardiac disease undergoing noncardiac surgery.

Gentilello LM. Advances in the management of hypothermia. *Surg Clin North Am.* 1995;75:243–256.

Postoperative restoration of normal body temperature decreases surgical mortality, blood loss, fluid requirement, organ failure, and length of intensive care unit stay. This important article describes the effect of hypothermia on coagulation and discusses various passive and active rewarming techniques.

Gribovskaja-Rupp I, Melton GB. Enterocutaneous fistula: proven strategies and updates. *Clin Colon Rectal Surg.* 2016;29:130–137.

This article summarizes current classification systems and provides an in-depth review of enterocutaneous fistula management, including fluid and nutrition management, wound care, nonoperative management, timing of surgery, etc.

Harrell BR, Miller S. Abdominal compartment syndrome as a complication of fluid resuscitation. *Nurs Clin North Am.* 2017;52:331–338.

This important article details the pathophysiology of intraabdominal hypertension and abdominal compartment syndrome and provides guidelines for medical and surgical management of patients with these complications.

Harvin JA, Mims MM, Duchesne JC, et al. Chasing 100%: the use of hypertonic saline to improve early, primary fascial closure after damage control laparotomy. *J Trauma Acute Care Surg.* 2013;74:426–430; discussion 431–422.

Early fascial closure after damage control laparotomy is associated with reduced infections, wound, and pulmonary complications. This article is a retrospective review of a single institution experience with hypertonic saline resuscitation that facilitated early fascial closure.

Kann BR. Early stomal complications. *Clin Colon Rectal Surg.* 2008;21:23–30.

Early postoperative stomal complications have significant impact on patient's outcome, both financially and psychologically. This review article is highly relevant because it provided an overview of the early complications and outlines the causative factors, treatment options, and preventative strategies.

Kristensen SD, Knuuti J, Saraste A, et al. 2014 ESC/ESA guidelines on non-cardiac surgery: cardiovascular assessment and management: the Joint Task Force on Non-Cardiac Surgery: cardiovascular assessment and management of the European Society of Cardiology (ESC) and the European Society of Anaesthesiology (ESA). *Eur Heart J.* 2014;35:2383–2431.

This article describes the assessment and perioperative management of cardiac conditions that are potential sources of complications during noncardiac surgery.

Practice guidelines for preoperative fasting and the use of pharmacologic agents to reduce the risk of pulmonary aspiration: application to healthy patients undergoing elective procedures: an updated report by the American Society of Anesthesiologists Committee on Standards and Practice Parameters. *Anesthesiology.* 2011;114:495–511.

American Society of Anesthesiologists Committee on Standards and Practice Parameters offers recommendations for preoperative prevention of aspiration pneumonia.

Singh F, Newton RU, Galvao DA, et al. A systematic review of pre-surgical exercise intervention studies with cancer patients. *Surg Oncol.* 2013;22:92–104.

This systematic review highlights how preoperative conditioning with exercise can reduce frailty complications in cancer patients undergoing surgery.

(2018). Global Guidelines for the Prevention of Surgical Site Infection. Geneva. World Health Organization. Retrieved May 5, 2019, from https://www.who.int/infection-prevention/publications/ssi-prevention-guidelines/en/.

This article summarizes the current multinational evidence and focuses on the prevention of surgical site infection and recommendations for intervention during the pre-, intra-, and postoperative period.

REFERENCES

1. Douketis JD, Johnson JA, Turpie AG. Low-molecular-weight heparin as bridging anticoagulation during interruption of warfarin: assessment of a standardized periprocedural anticoagulation regimen. *Arch Intern Med.* 2004;164:1319–1326.
2. Deerenberg EB, Harlaar JJ, Steyerberg EW, et al. Small bites versus large bites for closure of abdominal midline incisions (STITCH): a double-blind, multicentre, randomised controlled trial. *Lancet.* 2015;386:1254–1260.
3. Heller L, Levin SL, Butler CE. Management of abdominal wound dehiscence using vacuum assisted closure in patients with compromised healing. *Am J Surg.* 2006;191:165–172.
4. Umscheid CA, Mitchell MD, Doshi JA, et al. Estimating the proportion of healthcare-associated infections that are reasonably preventable and the related mortality and costs. *Infect Control Hosp Epidemiol.* 2011;32:101–114.
5. *Global Guidelines for the Prevention of Surgical Site Infection.* Geneva: World Health Organization; 2018. https://www.who.int/infection-prevention/publications/ssi-prevention-guidelines/en/. Accessed May 5, 2019.
6. Gentilello LM. Advances in the management of hypothermia. *Surg Clin North Am.* 1995;75:243–256.
7. Rosenberg H, Pollock N, Schiemann A, et al. Malignant hyperthermia: a review. *Orphanet J Rare Dis.* 2015;10:93.
8. Jaffer U, Wade RG, Gourlay T. Cytokines in the systemic inflammatory response syndrome: a review. *HSR Proc Intensive Care Cardiovasc Anesth.* 2010;2:161–175.
9. Gahlot R, Nigam C, Kumar V, et al. Catheter-related bloodstream infections. *Int J Crit Illn Inj Sci.* 2014;4:162–167.
10. Prescott HC, O'Brien JM. Prevention of ventilator-associated pneumonia in adults. *F1000 Med Rep.* 2010;2.
11. Practice guidelines for preoperative fasting and the use of pharmacologic agents to reduce the risk of pulmonary aspiration: application to healthy patients undergoing elective procedures: an updated report by the American Society of Anesthesiologists Committee on Standards and Practice Parameters. *Anesthesiology.* 2011;114:495–511.
12. Algie CM, Mahar RK, Tan HB, et al. Effectiveness and risks of cricoid pressure during rapid sequence induction for endotracheal intubation. *Cochrane Database Syst Rev.* 2015:CD011656.
13. Ranieri VM, Rubenfeld GD, Thompson BT, et al. Acute respiratory distress syndrome: the Berlin definition. *JAMA.* 2012;307:2526–2533.

14. Young D, Lamb SE, Shah S, et al. High-frequency oscillation for acute respiratory distress syndrome. *N Engl J Med.* 2013;368:806–813.
15. Heit JA, O'Fallon WM, Petterson TM, et al. Relative impact of risk factors for deep vein thrombosis and pulmonary embolism: a population-based study. *Arch Intern Med.* 2002;162:1245–1248.
16. Giannitsis E, Katus HA. Biomarkers for clinical decision-making in the management of pulmonary embolism. *Clin Chem.* 2017;63:91–100.
17. Devereaux PJ, Xavier D, Pogue J, et al. Characteristics and short-term prognosis of perioperative myocardial infarction in patients undergoing noncardiac surgery: a cohort study. *Ann Intern Med.* 2011;154:523–528.
18. Botto F, Alonso-Coello P, Chan MT, et al. Myocardial injury after noncardiac surgery: a large, international, prospective cohort study establishing diagnostic criteria, characteristics, predictors, and 30-day outcomes. *Anesthesiology.* 2014;120:564–578.
19. Royo MB, Fleisher LA. Chasing myocardial outcomes: perioperative myocardial infarction and cardiac troponin. *Can J Anaesth.* 2016;63:227–232.
20. Fleisher LA, Fleischmann KE, Auerbach AD, et al. 2014 ACC/AHA guideline on perioperative cardiovascular evaluation and management of patients undergoing noncardiac surgery: a report of the American College of Cardiology/American Heart Association Task Force on practice guidelines. *J Am Coll Cardiol.* 2014;64:e77–e137.
21. Kristensen SD, Knuuti J, Saraste A, et al. 2014 ESC/ESA guidelines on non-cardiac surgery: cardiovascular assessment and management: the Joint Task Force on Non-Cardiac Surgery: cardiovascular assessment and management of the European Society of Cardiology (ESC) and the European Society of Anaesthesiology (ESA). *Eur Heart J.* 2014;35:2383–2431.
22. Wijeysundera DN, Duncan D, Nkonde-Price C, et al. Perioperative beta blockade in noncardiac surgery: a systematic review for the 2014 ACC/AHA guideline on perioperative cardiovascular evaluation and management of patients undergoing noncardiac surgery: a report of the American College of Cardiology/American Heart Association Task Force on Practice Guidelines. *Circulation.* 2014;130:2246–2264.
23. van Waes JA, Nathoe HM, de Graaff JC, et al. Myocardial injury after noncardiac surgery and its association with short-term mortality. *Circulation.* 2013;127:2264–2271.
24. Fleisher LA. Preoperative evaluation of the patient with hypertension. *JAMA.* 2002;287:2043–2046.
25. Roshanov PS, Rochwerg B, Patel A, et al. Withholding versus continuing angiotensin-converting enzyme inhibitors or angiotensin II receptor blockers before noncardiac surgery: an analysis of the vascular events in noncardiac surgery patients cohort evaluation prospective cohort. *Anesthesiology.* 2017;126:16–27.
26. January CT, Wann LS, Alpert JS, et al. 2014 AHA/ACC/HRS guideline for the management of patients with atrial fibrillation: executive summary: a report of the American College of Cardiology/American Heart Association Task Force on practice guidelines and the Heart Rhythm Society. *Circulation.* 2014;130:2071–2104.
27. Hammill BG, Curtis LH, Bennett-Guerrero E, et al. Impact of heart failure on patients undergoing major noncardiac surgery. *Anesthesiology.* 2008;108:559–567.
28. Rodseth RN, Lurati Buse GA, Bolliger D, et al. The predictive ability of pre-operative B-type natriuretic peptide in vascular patients for major adverse cardiac events: an individual patient data meta-analysis. *J Am Coll Cardiol.* 2011;58:522–529.
29. Afazel MR, Jalali E, Sadat Z, et al. Comparing the effects of hot pack and lukewarm-water-soaked gauze on postoperative urinary retention; a randomized controlled clinical trial. *Nurs Midwifery Stud.* 2014;3:e24606.
30. Burch HB, Wartofsky L. Life-threatening thyrotoxicosis. Thyroid storm. *Endocrinol Metab Clin North Am.* 1993;22:263–277.
31. Vather R, O'Grady G, Bissett IP, et al. Postoperative ileus: mechanisms and future directions for research. *Clin Exp Pharmacol Physiol.* 2014;41:358–370.
32. Harrell BR, Miller S. Abdominal compartment syndrome as a complication of fluid resuscitation. *Nurs Clin North Am.* 2017;52:331–338.
33. Harvin JA, Mims MM, Duchesne JC, et al. Chasing 100%: the use of hypertonic saline to improve early, primary fascial closure after damage control laparotomy. *J Trauma Acute Care Surg.* 2013;74:426–430; discussion 431–422.
34. Kann BR. Early stomal complications. *Clin Colon Rectal Surg.* 2008;21:23–30.
35. Alvey B, Beck DE. Peristomal dermatology. *Clin Colon Rectal Surg.* 2008;21:41–44.
36. Strong SA. The difficult stoma: challenges and strategies. *Clin Colon Rectal Surg.* 2016;29:152–159.
37. Kwiatt M, Kawata M. Avoidance and management of stomal complications. *Clin Colon Rectal Surg.* 2013;26:112–121.
38. Stylinski R, Alzubedi A, Rudzki S. Parastomal hernia—current knowledge and treatment. *Wideochir Inne Tech Maloinwazyjne.* 2018;13:1–8.
39. McDonald LC, Gerding DN, Johnson S, et al. Clinical practice guidelines for *Clostridium difficile* infection in adults and children: 2017 update by the Infectious Diseases Society of America (IDSA) and Society for Healthcare Epidemiology of America (SHEA). *Clin Infect Dis.* 2018;66:987–994.
40. Shogan BD, Belogortseva N, Luong PM, et al. Collagen degradation and MMP9 activation by *Enterococcus faecalis* contribute to intestinal anastomotic leak. *Sci Transl Med.* 2015;7: 286ra268.
41. Thompson SK, Chang EY, Jobe BA. Clinical review: healing in gastrointestinal anastomoses, part I. *Microsurgery.* 2006;26:131–136.
42. Akkouche A, Sideris L, Leblanc G, et al. Complications after colorectal anastomosis in a patient with metastatic rectal cancer treated with systemic chemotherapy and bevacizumab. *Can J Surg.* 2008;51:E52–E53.
43. Gravante G, Caruso R, Andreani SM, et al. Mechanical bowel preparation for colorectal surgery: a meta-analysis on abdominal and systemic complications on almost 5,000 patients. *Int J Colorectal Dis.* 2008;23:1145–1150.
44. Gribovskaja-Rupp I, Melton GB. Enterocutaneous fistula: proven strategies and updates. *Clin Colon Rectal Surg.* 2016;29:130–137.
45. Badrasawi M, Shahar S, Sagap I. Nutritional management in enterocutaneous fistula. What is the evidence? *Malays J Med Sci.* 2015;22:6–16.
46. Bassi C, Marchegiani G, Dervenis C, et al. The 2016 update of the International Study Group (ISGPS) definition and grading of postoperative pancreatic fistula: 11 years after. *Surgery.* 2017;161:584–591.

47. Barreto SG, Shukla PJ. Different types of pancreatico-enteric anastomosis. *Transl Gastroenterol Hepatol.* 2017;2:89.
48. Strasberg SM, Hertl M, Soper NJ. An analysis of the problem of biliary injury during laparoscopic cholecystectomy. *J Am Coll Surg.* 1995;180:101–125.
49. Xue QL. The frailty syndrome: definition and natural history. *Clin Geriatr Med.* 2011;27:1–15.
50. Singh F, Newton RU, Galvao DA, et al. A systematic review of pre-surgical exercise intervention studies with cancer patients. *Surg Oncol.* 2013;22:92–104.

13 CHAPTER

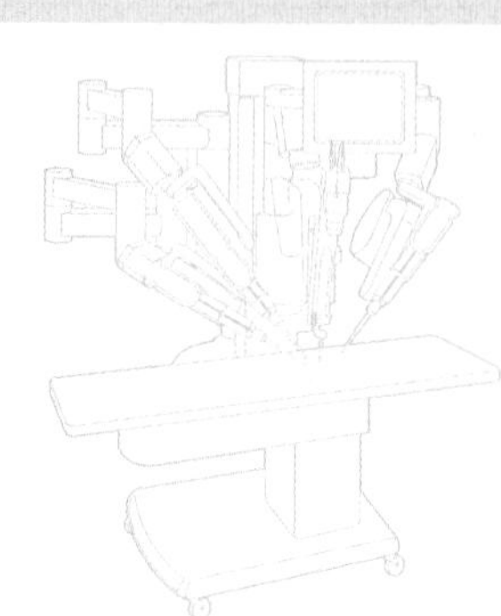

Surgery in the Geriatric Patient

Vanita Ahuja, Ronnie A. Rosenthal

OUTLINE

Life expectancy has increased dramatically in the last several decades. An average 65-year-old woman today can expect to live an additional 20.6 years, nearly twice as long as her counterpart in 1900. An average 80-year-old female can expect to live nearly 9.8 years (Table 13.1).[1] With this increase in life expectancy comes an increase in the number of people living into old age with diseases and chronic conditions that would have caused death in past decades. At present, more than 75% of adults older than age 65 years have at least one chronic condition and 20% of the Medicare population have five or more. Many of these diseases and chronic conditions, such as cancer, degenerative joint disease, coronary artery disease, and visual impairment, have a surgical option as part of the treatment algorithm. Currently, the 15% of the population age 65 years old and older accounts for 40% of the surgical procedures in the United States.

Starting in 2012, nearly 10,000 Americans turn 65 every day. Over the next few decades, as the 78 million people in the Baby Boomer generation (born from 1946 to 1964) begin to reach age 65, there will be a rapid aging of the U.S. population (Fig. 13.1).[2] It is expected that by 2030, one in five people will be older than 65 years old, and by 2050, almost 20 million people will be older than 85 years old. Unlike older persons in prior generations, baby boomer seniors expect to remain active and independent long after retirement. The demand for surgical care is likely to overwhelm the system if new ways to increase supply and improve delivery are not developed.

OUTCOMES OF SURGERY IN OLDER ADULTS

There is no doubt that increasing age appears to have a negative effect on the outcome of surgery. Previous small or single institution studies demonstrated similar outcomes in older and younger patients for even the most complex procedures such as Whipple resection for pancreatic cancer. These studies likely suffered from selection bias with only the fittest of older patients being offered surgery. More recent large database studies indicate that operative mortality of surgery for major gastrointestinal diseases clearly increases with increasing age even after adjustment for comorbid conditions. Mortality from high-risk operations such as esophagectomy or pancreatectomy can be two and three times the mortality for similar procedures in younger adults. Multiple studies, however, now confirm that the age of the patient alone is not the major predictor of poor outcome, but rather how successfully the patient has aged. It is now generally accepted that frailty, rather than chronological age, is the most important predictor of traditional surgical outcomes.

Most studies of surgical outcomes in older and younger adults focus on 30-day mortality and 30-day complications, such as pneumonia and surgical site infections. The American College of Surgeons National Surgical Quality Improvement Program (ACS NSQIP) surgical risk calculator is an extremely useful tool in predicting the likelihood of these outcomes.[3] Preoperatively, individual patient and procedural risk factors can be entered into the NSQIP model and rates of various traditional outcomes for that individual are calculated. This information can be used to help inform shared decision-making. However, other outcomes that are more relevant to older adults, such as cognitive decline, functional decline, and loss of independence, are rarely if ever measured. In one study exploring the treatment preferences of seriously ill adults, patients were much more willing to take a treatment if there was a possibility of death than they were if there was a possibility of cognitive or functional decline (Fig. 13.2).

Unfortunately, because little data are collected on the cognitive or functional outcomes of surgery, it is difficult to advise older adults about the likelihood of these outcomes. In response to the need to provide such data, in 2014, the NSQIP began a new

TABLE 13.1 Life expectancy of older persons at various ages (in years).

	ALL RACES	
AGE (IN YEARS)	MALE	FEMALE
65	17.9	20.6
70	14.4	16.6
75	11.2	12.9
80	8.3	9.8
85	5.9	7.0
90	4.1	4.8
95	2.8	3.3
100	2.0	2.3

From Ortman JM, Velkoff VA, Hogan H. An aging nation: the older population in the United States. *Current Populations Reports*. Washington, DC: U.S. Census Bureau; 2014;P25-1140.

geriatric pilot with 23 volunteer hospitals collecting new risk and outcome variables more relevant to older adults.[4] These variables covered the areas of goals of care, cognition, mobility, and function (Fig. 13.3). Using these data, NSQIP was able to provide participants with benchmarked rates of postoperative delirium and functional decline.[5] These data were also used to create a Geriatric Risk calculator, which can for the first time provide older adults with some information on the likelihood of the outcomes that are more relevant to them.[6]

In addition to the differences in outcomes in older adults, there is great variability in surgical mortality rates in Medicare patients depending on the hospital in which they are treated. Mortality rates can vary as much as threefold between best-preforming hospitals and worst performers. There is also great variability in the rates at which surgical care is provided in older adults. In a study looking at the rates of surgery in patient near the end of life, 31.9% of decedents had surgery in the last year and 18.3% in the last month. What is most remarkable in this study is the variability of these surgical rates across the country, with 34.4% of decedents in Gary, Indiana, having surgery in the last year of life and only 11.2% in Hawaii. Other studies have shown that there is no difference in the end-of-life preferences in Medicare recipients from high- and low-spending areas. It is therefore unlikely that patient preferences explain this difference in surgical rates. It is clear, however, that this variability indicates a lack of standard approach to the surgical care of older adults and those approaching the end of life.

In response to the need to provide more standardization in the surgical care of older adults, the ACS partnered with the John A. Hartford Foundation to form the Coalition for Quality in Geriatric Surgery. The Coalition was comprised of nearly 60 major national and regional organizations representing patients and family advocacy groups, regulators and insurers, surgeons in many specialties, geriatricians and other medical specialists, nurses, social workers, and other health professionals. Together, over a 4-year period, the Coalition developed a set of 30 evidence- and consensus-based standards that form the basis for the ACS Geriatric Surgery Verification program. This ACS Quality program, like those in trauma, bariatrics, cancer, and pediatrics, hopes to improve the outcomes for surgical care in older adults by providing a consistent framework for care that is patient centered, interdisciplinary, and embedded in the function of the hospital at https://www.facs.org/quality-programs/geriatric-surgery.

Improving the outcome of surgery in older adults will require that all those who participate in the care understand the differences inherent in caring for older adults. The following section describes the physiologic changes of aging that leave older adults more vulnerable to poor outcomes when subjected to the stress of surgery and illness; reviews the current recommendations for assessing and addressing these vulnerabilities to be sure the surgical care received is consistent with the individuals healthcare goals; and reviews the current approach to treatment of some of the most common surgical diseases associated with aging.

FRAILTY AND PHYSIOLOGIC DECLINE

With aging, there is a decline in physiologic function in all organ systems, but the magnitude of this decline is variable among organs and individuals. Over the past several decades, an enormous amount of research has been conducted to define the specific changes in organ function that are directly attributable to aging. This task is inherently difficult because aging is also accompanied by increased vulnerability to disease. It is often difficult to determine whether an observed decline in function is secondary to aging per se or to disease associated with aging. The overall effect, however, is still the same—a much smaller margin for error in the care of older patients.

Frailty

Frailty is defined as "a biologic syndrome of decreased reserve and resistance to stressors, resulting from cumulative declines across multiple physiologic systems causing vulnerability to adverse outcomes." The actual mechanism of frailty is complex and beyond the scope of this chapter; however, a conceptual model shows that the frail state is characterized by loss of muscle mass (sarcopenia), chronic undernutrition, weakness, and decreased exercise tolerance (Fig. 13.4). The presence of frailty is associated with many poor health outcomes, such as falls, disability, hospitalization, and death, as well as worse outcomes from any health care intervention, including surgery. The impact of frailty on surgical outcomes has been the subject of many studies over the past decade. These studies are complicated by the many different methods used to define the characteristics of the frail individual; however, the conclusion that frailty is associated with worse outcomes is common to all of them.[7]

The Fried frailty phenotype[8] is the most widely used method to describe frailty. It defines the frail phenotype by five characteristics: weight loss, weak grip strength, self-reported exhaustion, slow walking speed, and low energy expenditure. Using this definition, frail patients undergoing elective surgery were found to have more postoperative complications, longer lengths of stay, and more frequent discharge to a location other than home.

Another method of describing frailty is the multidomain model that includes measures of cognition and mood, function, malnutrition, chronic disease, and geriatric syndromes.[9] Using elements of this model (cognition, activities of daily living [ADLs], low serum albumin, anemia, comorbidity, and falls), frail patients undergoing surgery that required an intensive care unit (ICU) stay were found to have higher rates of mortality at 6 months following surgery.

There are many tools to measure frailty. The Edmonton Frail scale is a questionnaire that covers many of the domains of frailty and can be easily administered by support personnel in the office setting. This tool allows specific deficits in the various domains to be identified preoperatively so interventions designed to address the specific deficits can be planned. There are other simple surrogate measures of frailty that are also easy in the office setting, such as the Timed Up and Go Test, measurement of gait speed, and the

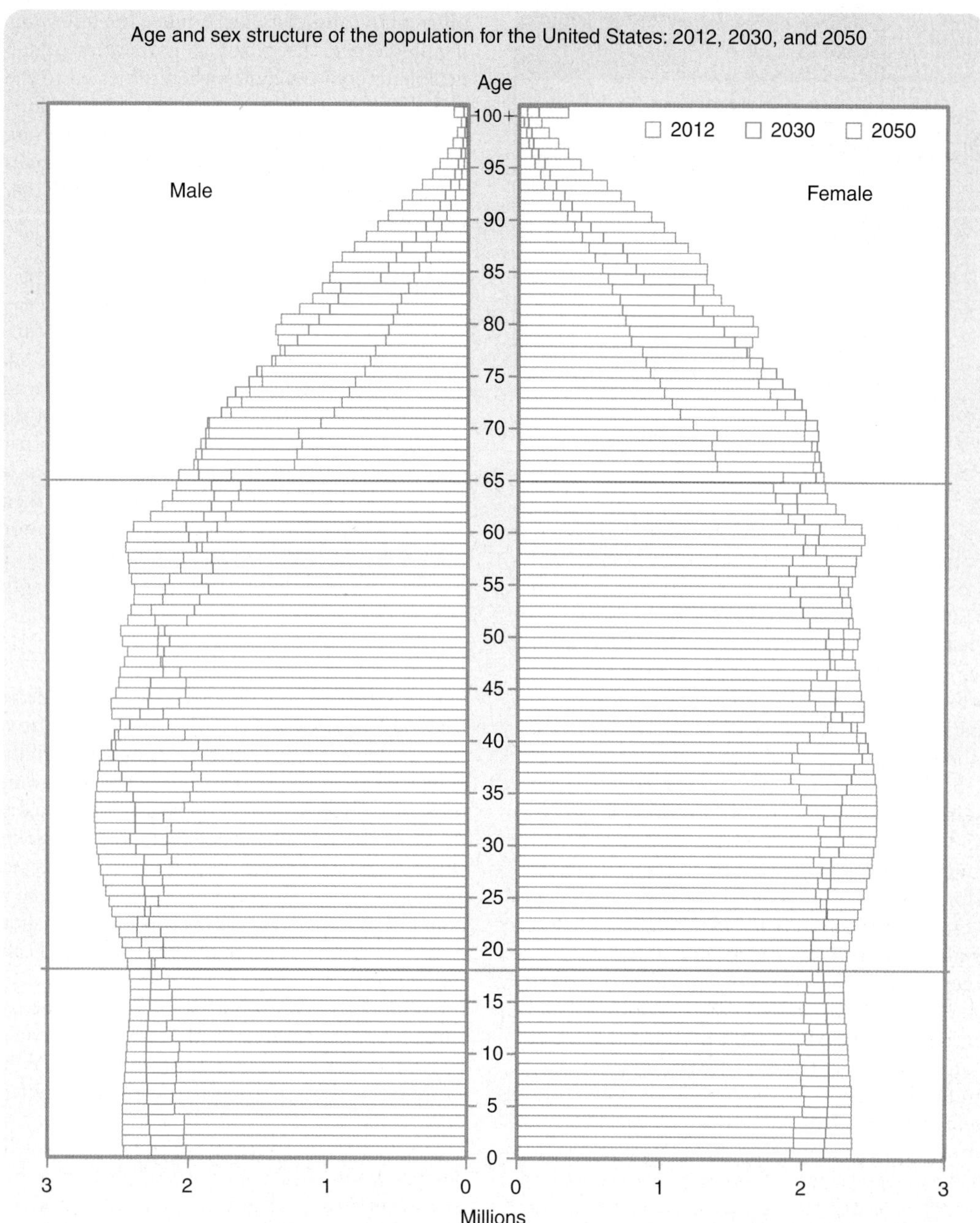

FIG. 13.1 The aging of the Baby Boom generation and their offspring in United States 2013, 2030, and 2050. (From Ortman JM, Velkoff VA, Hogan H. An aging nation: the older population in the United States. *Current Populations Reports*. Washington, DC: U.S. Census Bureau; 2014:P25-1140.)

simplified frailty index, which includes weight loss, low energy level, and the inability to rise from a chair five times in succession without using the arms. Other methods for measuring frailty based on data from large datasets include the Risk Analysis Index and several other administrative claims-based tools.[10]

Regardless of the method used to identify frailty, the presence of this geriatric syndrome is now widely recognized as a significant risk factor for poor surgical outcomes. While frailty cannot be reversed in preparation for surgery, recognition of the increase risk caused by the various components of frailty, such as chronic undernutrition and impaired mobility, can help direct a preoperative preparation program and a postoperative management program that may help mitigate the risk.

Organ-Specific Decline

Cardiovascular System

Cardiovascular disease is the leading cause of death in the United States in men and women. Of these deaths, 83% occur in persons older than 65 years old. Cardiac events account for a significant portion of the complications in older adults in the postoperative period and are attributable to disease and to changes in the structure and function of the heart that accompany aging (Box 13.1). Knowledge of these changes is important in directing the postoperative management of older adults.

Morphologic changes are found in the myocardium, conducting pathways, valves, and vasculature of the heart and great vessels with increasing age. The number of myocytes declines as the collagen and elastin content increases, thereby resulting in fibrotic areas throughout the myocardium and an overall decline in ventricular compliance. Almost 90% of the autonomic tissue in the sinus node is replaced by fat and connective tissue, and fibrosis interferes with conduction in the intranodal tracts and bundle of His. These changes contribute to the high incidence of sick sinus syndrome, atrial arrhythmia, and bundle branch block. Sclerosis and calcification of the aortic valve are common but are usually of no functional significance. Progressive dilatation of all four valvular annuli is probably responsible for the multivalvular regurgitation demonstrated in healthy older persons. Finally, there is a progressive increase in rigidity and decrease in distensibility of the coronary arteries and great vessels. Changes in the peripheral vasculature contribute to increased systolic blood pressure, increased resistance to ventricular emptying, and compensatory loss of myocytes with ventricular hypertrophy.

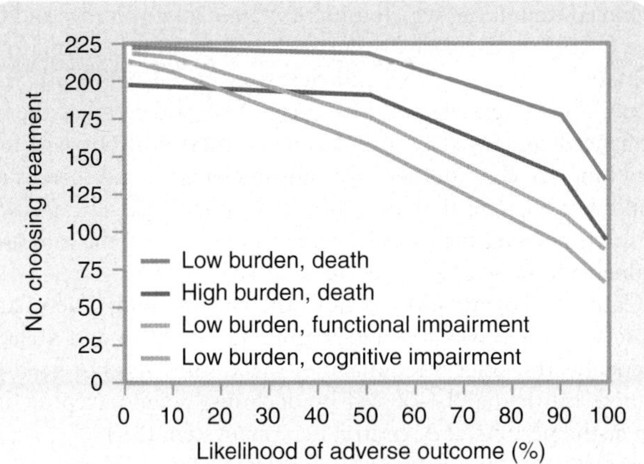

FIG. 13.2 Many patients are willing to undertake high- or low-burden treatments, even if the risk of death is high (up to 50%). However, when there is even a small risk of cognitive or functional decline, the number of patients willing to undergo even a low-burden treatment sharply declines. (From Fried TR, Bradley EH, Towle VR, et al. Understanding the treatment preferences of seriously ill patients. *N Engl J Med.* 2002;346:1061–1066.)

The direct functional implications of these changes are difficult to assess accurately because age-related changes in body composition, metabolic rate, general state of fitness, and underlying disease all influence cardiac performance. It is now generally accepted that systolic function is well preserved with increasing age. Cardiac output and ejection fraction are maintained, despite the increase in afterload imposed by stiffening of the outflow tract. The mechanism whereby cardiac output is maintained during exercise, however, is somewhat different. In younger persons, output is maintained by increasing the heart rate in response to β-adrenergic stimulation. With aging, there is a relative hyposympathetic state in which the heart becomes less responsive to catecholamines, possible secondary to declining receptor function. The aging heart therefore maintains cardiac output not by increasing its rate but by increasing ventricular filling (preload). Because of the dependence on preload, even minor hypovolemia can result in significant compromise in cardiac function.

Diastolic function, however, which depends on relaxation rather than contraction, is affected by aging. Diastolic dysfunction is responsible for up to 50% of cases of heart failure in patients older than 80 years old. Myocardial relaxation is more energy dependent and therefore requires more oxygen than contraction. With aging, there is a progressive decrease in the partial pressure of oxygen. Consequently, even mild hypoxemia can result in prolonged relaxation, higher diastolic pressure, and pulmonary congestion. Because early diastolic filling is impaired, maintenance of preload becomes even more reliant on atrial kick. Loss of the atrial contribution to preload can result in further impairment of cardiac function.

It is also important to remember that the manifestation of cardiac disease in older adults may be nonspecific and atypical. Although chest pain is still the most common symptom of myocardial infarction, atypical symptoms such as shortness of breath, syncope, acute confusion, or stroke will occur in as many as 40% of older patients.

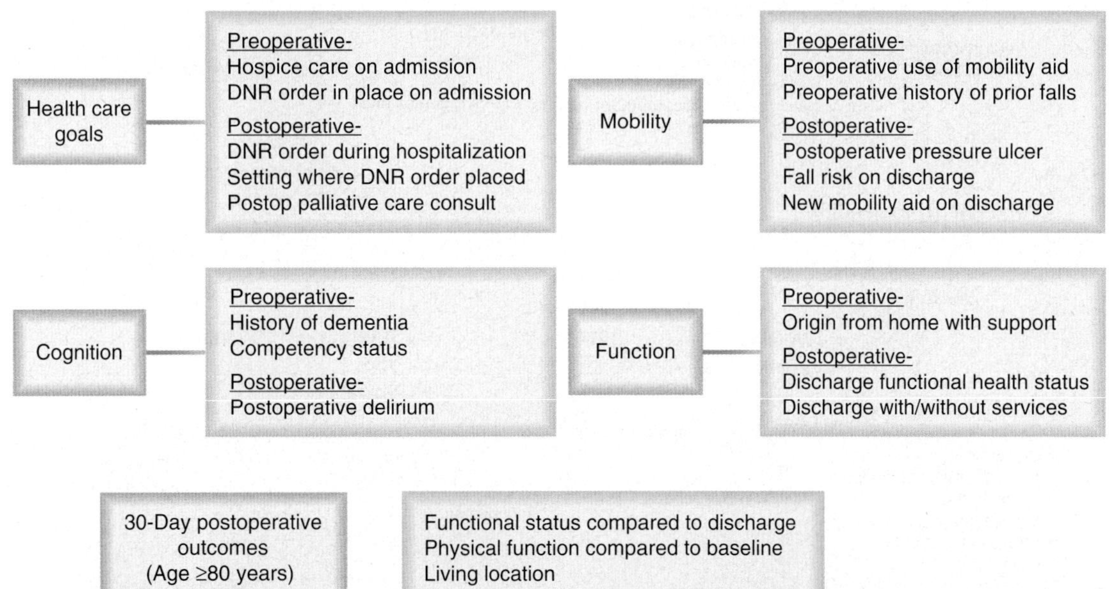

FIG. 13.3 Variables used in the ACS NSQIP Geriatric Pilot Project. (From Robinson TN, Rosenthal RA. The ACS NSQIP Geriatric Surgery Pilot Project: improving care for older surgical patients. *Bull Am Coll Surg.* 2014;99:21e23.) *ACS NSQIP*, American College of Surgeons National Surgical Quality Improvement Program; *DNR*, do not resuscitate.

Aging also impairs blood vessel function and leads to cardiovascular disease. Vascular dysfunction is caused by (1) oxidative stress enhancement, (2) reduction of nitric oxide (NO) bioavailability, by diminished NO synthesis and/or augmented NO scavenging, (3) production of vasoconstrictor/vasodilator factor imbalances, (4) low-grade proinflammatory environment, (5) impaired angiogenesis, and (6) endothelial cell senescence. The aging process in vascular smooth muscle is characterized by (1) altered replicating potential, (2) change in cellular phenotype, (3) changes in responsiveness to contracting and relaxing mediators, and (4) changes in intracellular signaling functions. Systemic arterial hypertension is an age-dependent disorder, and almost half of the elderly human population is hypertensive. Treatment for hypertension is recommended in the elderly. Lifestyle modifications, natural compounds, and hormone therapies are useful for initial stages and as supporting treatment with medication, but evidence from clinical trials in this population is needed. Since all antihypertensive agents can lower blood pressure in the elderly, therapy should be based on its potential side effects and drug interactions.

Respiratory System

Chronic lower respiratory disease is the fourth leading cause of death after heart disease, cancer, and stroke. Respiratory problems are the most common postoperative complications in older patients (Box 13.2). Both disease- and age-related changes in lung structure and function contribute to this vulnerability.[9]

With aging, there is a decline in respiratory function that is attributable to changes in the chest wall and lungs. Chest wall compliance decreases secondary to changes in structure caused by kyphosis and is exaggerated by vertebral collapse. Calcification of the costal cartilage and contractures of the intercostal muscles result in a decline in rib mobility. Maximum inspiratory and expiratory forces decrease by as much as 50% as a result of a progressive decrease in the strength of the respiratory muscles.

In the lung, there is loss of elasticity, which leads to increased alveolar compliance with collapse of the small airways and subsequent uneven alveolar ventilation with air trapping. Uneven alveolar ventilation leads to ventilation-perfusion mismatches, which in turn causes a decline in arterial oxygen tension of approximately 0.3 or 0.4 mm Hg/yr. The partial pressure of carbon dioxide (CO_2) does not change, despite an increase in dead space. This may be caused, in part, by the decline in production of CO_2 that accompanies the falling basal metabolic rates. Air trapping is also responsible for an increase in residual volume, or the volume remaining after maximal expiration.

Loss of support of the small airways also leads to collapse during forced expiration, which limits dynamic lung volumes and flow rates. Forced vital capacity decreases by 14 to 30 mL/yr and forced expiratory volume in 1 second decreases by 23 to 32 mL/yr (in males). The overall effect of loss of elastic inward recoil of the lung is balanced somewhat by the decline in chest wall outward force. Total lung capacity therefore remains unchanged, and there is only a mild increase in resting lung volume, or functional residual capacity. Because total lung capacity remains unchanged, the increase in residual volume results in a decrease in vital capacity.

Control of ventilation is also affected by aging. Ventilatory responses to hypoxia and hypercapnia fall by 50% and 40%, respectively. The exact mechanism of this decline has not been well defined, but it may be caused by declining chemoreceptor function at the peripheral or central nervous system level.

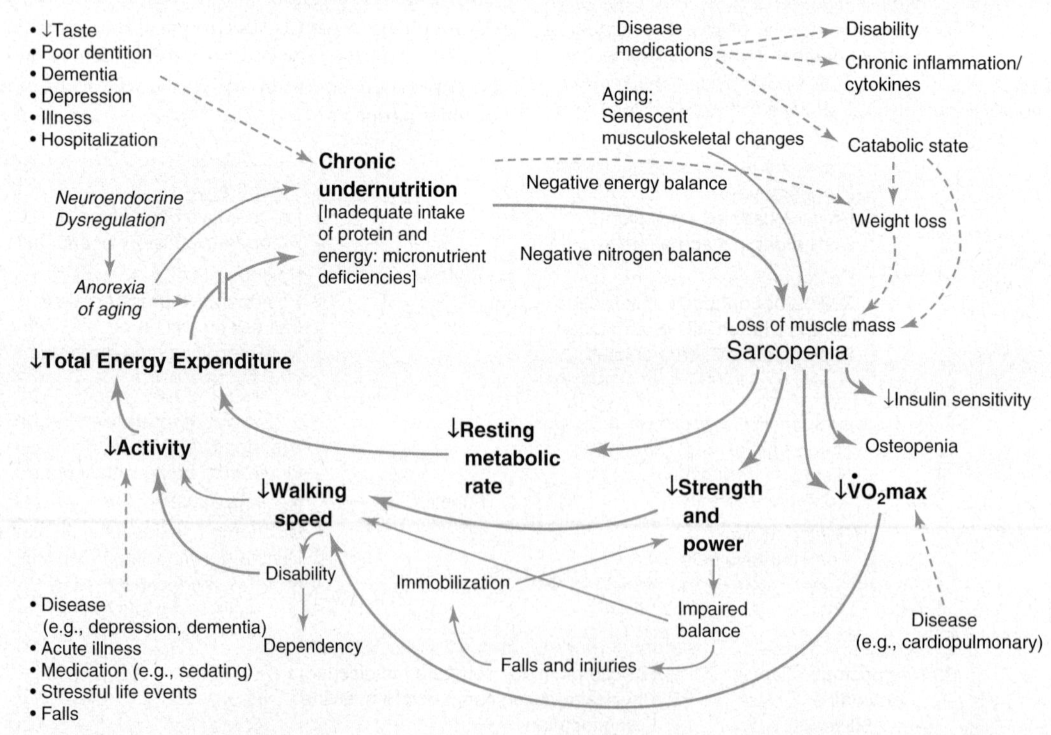

FIG. 13.4 The cycle of frailty is characterized by chronic undernutrition, loss of lean muscle mass (sarcopenia), and decreased exercise tolerance. (From Fried LP, Walston J. Frailty and failure to thrive. In: Hazzard WR, Blass JP, Ettinger WH Jr, Halter JB, Ouslander J, eds. *Principles of Geriatric Medicine and Gerontology*. 4th ed. New York: McGraw Hill; 1998:1387–1402.)

BOX 13.1 Major cardiovascular changes with age.

- Decreased number of myocytes
- Fibrosis of conducting pathways with increased arrhythmias
- Decrease in ventricular and arterial compliance (increased afterload)
- Decreased β-adrenergic responsiveness
- Increased dependence on preload (including atrial kick)
- Increased diastolic dysfunction
- Increased silent ischemia

BOX 13.2 Major respiratory changes with age.

- Decrease in chest wall compliance
- Decline in maximum inspiratory and expiratory force
- Decrease in lung elasticity (small airway collapse)
- Ventilation-perfusion mismatch
- Decrease in PaO_2, no change in $PaCO_2$
- Decreased FVC and FEV_1
- Decline in ventilator responses to hypoxemia and hypercapnia
- Decline in normal airway protective mechanisms (increased risk for aspiration)

FEV_1, Forced expiratory volume in 1 second; *FVC*, forced vital capacity; *$PaCO_2$*, arterial carbon dioxide pressure; *PaO_2*, arterial oxygen pressure.

In addition to these intrinsic changes, pulmonary function is affected by alterations in the ability of the respiratory system to protect against environmental injury and infection. Clearance of particles from the lung through the mucociliary elevator is decreased and associated with ciliary dysfunction. Many complex changes in immunity with aging contribute to increased susceptibility to infections, including a less robust immune response from both the innate and adaptive immune systems.

There is also a decrease in several components of swallowing function. Loss of the cough reflex secondary to neurologic disorders, combined with swallowing dysfunction, may predispose to aspiration. The increased frequency and severity of pneumonia in older persons have been attributed to these factors and to an increased incidence of oropharyngeal colonization with gram-negative organisms. This colonization correlates closely with comorbidity and with the ability of older patients to perform ADLs. This fact lends support to the idea that functional capacity is a crucial factor in assessing the risk for pneumonia in older patients.

Renal System

Approximately 25% of all Americans 70 years old and older have moderately or severely decreased kidney function (Box 13.3). Between the ages of 25 and 85 years, there is a progressive decrease in the renal cortex. Over time, approximately 40% of the nephrons become sclerotic. The remaining functional units hypertrophy in a compensatory manner. Sclerosis of the glomeruli is accompanied by atrophy of the afferent and efferent arterioles and by a decrease in renal tubular cell number. Renal blood flow also falls by approximately 50%. Functionally, there is a decline in the glomerular filtration rate of approximately 45% by age 80 years.

Renal tubular function also declines with advancing age. The ability to conserve sodium and excrete hydrogen ion decreases,

BOX 13.3 Major renal changes with age.

- Decrease in the number of functional nephrons
- Decrease in the number of tubular cells
- Decreased renal blood flow
- Decreased glomerular filtration rate
- Decline in creatinine clearance despite normal serum creatinine level
- Decline in tubular function (loss of concentrating ability)
- Increase susceptibility to dehydration
- Decrease clearance of certain drugs
- Increase in lower urinary track dysfunction and infection

resulting in a diminished capacity to regulate fluid and acid-base balance. Dehydration becomes a particular problem because losses of sodium and water from nonrenal causes are not compensated for by the usual mechanisms. The inability to retain sodium is believed to be caused by a decline in the activity of the renin-angiotensin system. The increasing inability to concentrate the urine is related to a decline in end-organ responsiveness to antidiuretic hormone. The marked decline in the subjective feeling of thirst is also well documented but not well understood. Alterations of osmoreceptor function in the hypothalamus may be responsible for the failure to recognize thirst in spite of significant elevations in serum osmolality.

Circulating levels of erythropoietin (EPO) are higher in the healthy elderly as compared to younger individuals. Increased EPO production in the elderly is interpreted as a counterregulatory mechanism aimed at preserving normal red blood cell mass in response to a higher turnover, as well as to EPO resistance. However, EPO levels are reduced in anemic elderly individuals, suggesting an impaired counterregulatory response to low hemoglobin levels. Elderly people may develop vitamin D deficiency due to the impaired capacity of the aging kidney to convert 25-hydroxyvitamin-D to 1,25 dihydroxyvitamin-D, but extrarenal factors (i.e., 25-OH-vitamin D availability) are at least equally responsible for vitamin D insufficiency in this age group.

Because of the decline in renal function with aging, it is important to measure glomerular filtration rate in older patients as part of preoperative risk assessment and in the hospital to provide accurate medication dosing. In older hospital patients, direct measurement of creatinine clearance (CrCl) is difficult because incontinence and cognitive impairment make 24-hour urine collection unreliable. Serum creatinine level measurement may be an unreliable indicator of renal function status because this value may remain unchanged as a result of a concomitant decrease in lean body mass and, thus, a decrease in creatinine production. A serum creatinine level of 1.0 mg/dL may represent a CrCl of over 100 mL/min in a 30-year-old but less than 60 mL/min in an 85-year old.

To overcome these problems, formulas have been developed to estimate CrCl from plasma creatinine and patient characteristics. The most commonly used formulas are the Cockcroft-Gault equation and the Modification of Diet in Renal Disease equation (Fig. 13.5). In a large study of older hospitalized patients, the Cockcroft-Gault equation has been shown to correlate more closely with directly measured CrCl.

Acute kidney injury (AKI) is defined as a 0.3-mg/dL or 50% or higher change in the serum creatinine level from baseline or a reduction in urine output of less than 0.5 mL/kg/h over a 6-hour interval, within a 48-hour period, and following adequate volume resuscitation. AKI is a frequent occurrence after major surgery. Up

Cockcroft-Gault equation

C_{cr} = [(140 − Age in years) × Weight in kilograms]/(72 × Serum creatinine in mg/dL)

MDRD study equation

GFR = 175 × (Standardized serum creatinine in mg/dL)$^{-1.154}$ × (Age in years)$^{-0.203}$

FIG. 13.5 Equations for calculating creatinine clearance. *MDRD*, Modification of Diet in Renal Disease.

to 7.5% of patients with a normal preoperative serum creatinine level will develop AKI. AKI is associated with increased short-term morbidity and mortality, as well as increased long-term mortality. Age, in addition to emergency surgery, ischemic heart disease, and congestive heart failure, is a risk factor for the development of postoperative AKI. Furthermore, older patients with already compromised renal function are at increased risk of postoperative AKI. The keys to avoiding postoperative AKI is to understand that older patients are at increased risk and to take steps to avoid unnecessary hypovolemia and ensure proper dosing of drugs that are cleared by the kidney and of drugs that are nephrotoxic.

The lower urinary tract also changes with increasing age. In the bladder, increased collagen content leads to limited distensibility and impaired emptying. Overactivity of the detrusor muscle secondary to neurologic disorders or idiopathic causes has also been identified. In women, decreased circulating levels of estrogen and decreased tissue responsiveness to this hormone cause changes in the urethral sphincter that predispose to urinary incontinence. In men, prostatic hypertrophy impairs bladder emptying. Together, these factors lead to urinary incontinence in 10% to 15% of older persons living in the community and 50% of those in nursing homes. There is also an increased prevalence of asymptomatic bacteriuria with age, which varies from 10% to 50% depending on gender, level of activity, underlying disorders, and place of residence. Urinary tract infections alone are responsible for 30% to 50% of all cases of bacteremia in older patients. Alterations in the local environment and declining host defenses are thought to be responsible.

Hepatobiliary System

Overall, hepatic function is well preserved with aging. However, there is an increase in liver disease and in liver disease–related mortality in persons between the ages of 45 and 85 years. Morphologic changes include a reduction in overall liver weight, size, and volume. Hepatocyte size, as well as the number of binucleated cells, increases while the number of mitochondria decreases. Functionally, hepatic blood flow decreases by 35% to 50%.

The synthetic capacity of the liver, as measured by standard tests of liver function, remains unchanged (Box 13.4). However, the metabolism of and sensitivity to certain types of drugs are altered. Drugs requiring microsomal oxidation (phase I reactions) before conjugation (phase II reactions) may be metabolized more slowly, whereas those requiring only conjugation may be cleared at a normal rate. Drugs that act directly on hepatocytes, such as warfarin (Coumadin), may produce the desired therapeutic effects at lower doses in older adults because of an increased sensitivity of cells to these agents. Some recent evidence has also suggested that aging may be associated with a decline in the ability of the liver to protect against the effects of oxidative stress.

The most significant correlate of altered hepatobiliary function in older adults is the increased incidence of gallstones and gallstone-related complications. Gallstone prevalence rises steadily with age, although there is variability in the absolute percentages depending on the population. Stones have been demonstrated in as many as 80% of nursing home residents older than 90 years old. Biliary tract disease is the single most common indication for abdominal surgery in older adults (see later).

BOX 13.4 Major hepatobiliary changes with age.

- Decrease in the number of hepatocytes
- Decrease in hepatic blood flow
- Synthetic capacity remains unchanged
- Increased sensitivity to and decreased clearance of certain drugs
- Increased incidence of gallstones and gallstone-related diseases

Immune Function

Immune competence, like other physiologic parameters, declines with advancing age (Box 13.5). This immunosenescence is characterized by enhanced susceptibility to infections, an increase in autoantibodies and monoclonal immunoglobulins, and an increase in tumorigenesis. In addition, like other physiologic systems, this decline may not be apparent in the unchallenged state. For example, there is no decline in neutrophil count with age, but the ability of the bone marrow to increase neutrophil production in response to infection may be impaired. Older patients with major infections frequently have normal white blood cell (WBC) counts, but the differential count will show a profound shift to the left, with a large proportion of immature forms.

With aging, there is a decline in the hematopoietic stem cell pool in the bone marrow that leads to decreased production of naïve T cells from the thymus and of B cells from the bone marrow. Moreover, involution of the thymus gland, with a decline in thymic hormone levels, further impairs the production and differentiation of naïve T cells and leads to an increased proportion of memory T cells. This change in the population of T cells leaves older adult hosts less able to respond to new antigens.

BOX 13.5 Major changes in immune function with age.

- Involution of the thymus gland
- Decrease production and differentiation of naïve T cells
- Decrease in T cell mitogenic activity
- Increase in inflammatory cytokines
- Increase in autoantibodies

Some B-cell defects have recently been identified, although it is thought that the functional deficits in antibody production are related to altered T-cell regulation rather than intrinsic B-cell changes. In vitro, there is increased helper T-cell activity for nonspecific antibody production, as well as a decreased ability of suppressor T cells from old mice to recognize and suppress specific antigens from self. This is reflected in an increase in the prevalence of autoantibodies to more than 10% by 80 years of age. The mix of immunoglobulins also changes; immunoglobulin M (IgM) levels decrease, whereas IgG and IgA levels increase slightly.

Changes in the immune system with aging are similar to those seen in chronic inflammation and cancer. In addition to the reduced mitogenic responses of T cells, there is an increase in the levels of acute phase proteins. It is hypothesized that persistently elevated levels of inflammatory cytokines may be responsible for the downregulation of interleukin-2 production by chronically stimulated T cells. Markers of inflammation such as interleukin-6 have recently been shown to be increased in older patients. Chronic inflammation has been implicated in the syndrome of frailty, which is characterized by loss of muscle mass (sarcopenia), undernutrition, and impaired mobility. Inflammatory cytokines are also implicated in the normocytic anemia that is common in frail older adults.

The clinical implications of these changes are difficult to determine. When superimposed on the known immunosuppression caused by the physical and psychological stresses of surgery, insufficient immunologic responses are to be expected in older adults. The increased susceptibility to many infectious agents in the postoperative period, however, is more likely the result of a combination of stress and comorbid disease rather than physiologic decline alone.

Glucose Homeostasis

Data from the National Health and Nutrition Examination Survey have shown a clear increase in the prevalence of disorders of glucose homeostasis with age; more than 20% of persons older than 60 years old have type 2 diabetes. An additional 20% have glucose intolerance characterized by normal fasting glucose and a postchallenge glucose level higher than 140 mg/dL but less than 200 mg/dL. This glucose intolerance may be the result of a decrease in insulin secretion, increase in insulin resistance, or both (Fig. 13.6).[11]

There is now general consensus that beta cell function declines with age. This change is manifested by failure of the beta cell to adapt to the hyperglycemic milieu with an appropriate increase in insulin response. The question of insulin resistance is more controversial. Although insulin action has been shown to decrease in older adults, this change is thought to be more a function of changing body composition, with increased adipose tissue and decreased lean body mass, rather than age per se. Others believe that there is an increase in insulin resistance directly attributable to aging, as manifested by a decrease in insulin-mediated glucose uptake in muscle that is normally regulated by the glucose transporter (GLUT)-4. There is also an increase in intracellular lipid accumulation, which interferes with normal insulin signaling. These changes may be associated with the decline in mitochondrial function that also accompanies aging.

These factors, combined with comorbid illness, medications, and genetic predisposition, come together to render older surgical patients at particularly high risk for uncontrolled hyperglycemia when subjected to the usual insulin resistance that accompanies the physiologic stress of surgery. Both the endogenous glucose response to traumatic stress and glycemic response to an exogenous glucose load are exaggerated in injured older patients.

Although most of the data on glucose control and surgical outcomes are in the cardiac surgery literature, recent evidence has confirmed that uncontrolled hyperglycemia in the immediate perioperative period is associated with an increase in infections in almost all types of surgery. The optimum level of glucose control, however, is still controversial. Earlier prospective studies indicated that tight control of blood sugar (80–110 mg/dL) achieved by continuous infusion of insulin improved some outcomes,

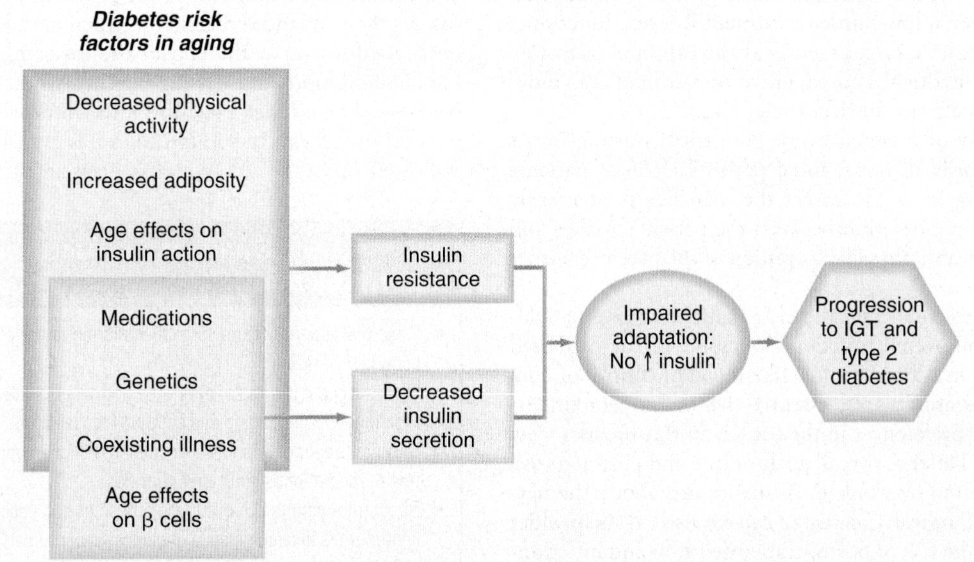

FIG. 13.6 The normal response to hyperglycemia is for the beta cell to adapt and secrete sufficient insulin to restore euglycemia. In aging, there is a decrease in insulin secretion and a probable increase in insulin resistance, which, when combined with comorbid illness, genetic factors, and medications, leads to a failure of this glucoregulatory process. (From Chang AM, Halter JB. Aging and insulin secretion. *Am J Physiol Endocrinol Metab.* 2003;284:E7–E12.) *IGT,* Impaired glucose tolerance.

including mortality in critically ill patients in the surgical ICU, but more recent data have cast some doubt on the benefits of such strict control. In general, maintenance of the blood glucose level below 180 mg/dL in the perioperative period is now widely accepted as an appropriate target, even in older patients.

PREOPERATIVE ASSESSMENT AND DECISION-MAKING

Providing optimal care for the older adult surgical patient depends on the team recognizing the effects aging has had on that individual and carefully designing a perioperative plan to address the individual's specific needs.

Patient Counseling

The first and perhaps the most important consideration in the preoperative assessment is being sure the patient and their family understand the ramifications of the care that is being suggested and that this care is concordant with the patients' goals for that care and for their overall health.

Surgical Decision-Making

Surgeons traditionally measure surgical success in terms of 30-day mortality and morbidity. For older patients, however, the definition of success is more complex. Although we are now able to perform even the most complicated surgery on our oldest patients with traditional surgical success, the quality of the outcome in the patient's view is more likely to depend on whether he or she can continue to function as before surgery. For some older patients, losing functional independence because of a major surgical intervention may be a far worse outcome than living with, or even dying of, the disease for which surgery is offered. In a study of older patients with limited life expectancy because of serious chronic disease, Fried and colleagues examined the impact of treatment burden (low, minor interventions, such as intravenous [IV] antibiotics; high, major interventions, such as surgery) and expected outcome (desirable vs. undesirable) on patient preferences for treatment. Results indicated that more than 70% of older patients would not want even a low-burden treatment if severe functional impairment or cognitive impairment was the expected outcome. The concern for functional and cognitive impairment was more dramatic than the concern for death (Fig. 13.2).

In another study of preferences for permanent nursing home placement in seriously ill hospitalized patients, 56% of patients were very unwilling or would rather die than live permanently in a nursing home. Correlation between the patient's wishes and both the surrogate's and physician's opinion of the patient's wishes was poor.

Therefore, it is essential that the older patient be given a realistic estimate of the overall functional outcome of the proposed surgical treatment, in addition to the likelihood of control or cure of the particular disease. It is also essential that the surgeon understands the patient's preferences in the context of this broader view of surgical success. Patient's overall goals of care and postoperative quality of life are often overlooked. As mentioned above, the new NSQIP Geriatric Surgical Calculator can be used to help older adults understand the risk of postoperative delirium and functional decline and better inform the shared decision-making.

For general and acute care surgeons, the presentation of an abdominal emergency in an older patient with multiple comorbidities presents a particularly difficult problem. When faced with the need to make a decision for surgery in a short time frame, for pathology that is potentially amenable to surgical cure, consideration is often focused entirely on the risk of short-term mortality and morbidity. This "fix it" mentality often leads down a path that neither the patient nor the surgeon intended. Several tools have been developed to help surgeons communicate more effectively with the older patient and his or her family in the acute setting. The "Best Case/Worse Case" model provides a structured way of discussing what the postoperative period will look like for the patient and has been shown to improve the quality of these difficult discussions.[12] Another model provides a structured framework for the discussion that puts the decision-making in the context of the patient's overall health and healthcare goals (Box 13.6).[13]

Advanced Directives

All patients should be encouraged to make a formal advanced directive and identify a surrogate decision maker should the patient become unable to make his or her own decisions.[14] Providers should be sure to discuss the patient's preferences directly with the patient, as discussions of these issues are not always easy and surrogates may not be fully aware of the patient's preferences. Tools, such as "PREPARE" (https://prepareforyourcare.org) and the "Five Wishes" (https://fivewishes.org) are available to help patients and families have these discussions and create advanced care plans. Providers should also be sure when advanced directives do exist that they are clearly documented and easily accessible in the patients' medical record.

Palliative Care

Honoring a patient's preferences for treatment at the end of life is a necessary component of quality health care. Studies have documented that the extent of burden plays a role in patient's decisions to choose aggressive care, and often, if the risk and benefits are appropriately discussed, aging patients may choose less aggressive treatment.

For patients with a poor prognosis, discussions regarding palliative care should happen early in the treatment conversation and do not preclude treatment of the disease or symptoms. Patients and their family members should be encouraged to complete and discuss their advanced directives, which have been shown to make decisions for care at the end of life easier for patients and their families and more in line with patient wishes. Early palliative care has been shown to lead to substantial improvements in quality of life and mood and in some studies has even been shown to have increased survival.[15] As there has been an increased focus on the

BOX 13.6 Goals of a structured communication.

- Place the patient's acute surgical condition in the context of the patient's underlying illness.
- Elicit the patient's goals, priorities, and what is acceptable to the patient regarding life-prolonging and comfort-focused care.
- Describe treatment options—including palliative approaches—in the context of the patient's goals and priorities.
- Direct treatment to achieve these outcomes and encourage the use of time-limited trials in circumstance of clinical uncertainty.
- Affirm continued commitment to the patient's care.

From Cooper Z, Koritsanszky LA, Cauley CE, et al. Recommendations for best communication practices to facilitate goal-concordant care for seriously ill older patients with emergency surgical conditions. *Ann Surg*. 2016;263:1–6.

quality of care, physicians and surgeons have come to understand that treatment is not only about curing disease but also about quality of life and alleviating suffering in patients.

Screening to Identify High-Risk Characteristics

To assure the best surgical decision-making and the best surgical outcome for the individual older patient, the preoperative assessment must be thorough and must address all of the relevant concerns. With this in mind, the American College of Surgeons and the American Geriatric Society worked together to define a set of best practice guidelines for the preoperative assessment of the geriatric patient that can be found at https://www.facs.org/-/media/files/quality-programs/nsqip/acsnsqipagsgeriatric2012guidelines. These guidelines provide a 13-item checklist of cognitive, comorbid, functional, and psychosocial factors that have all been shown to have an impact on the outcome of care for older surgical patients (Fig. 13.7).

Cognitive Assessment

Preoperative cognitive status as a risk factor for negative postoperative outcomes in older patients is often overlooked. Cognitive assessment is rarely a part of the preoperative history and physical examination. However, preoperative cognitive deficits are common; the prevalence of dementia is approximately 1.5% at age 65 years and approximately doubles with every five additional years of life. Over one third of persons older than age 70 years have some cognitive impairment or dementia. Preexisting cognitive dysfunction can impair a patient's capacity to give informed

ACS NSQIP©/AGS BEST PRACTICE GUIDELINES:
Optimal Preoperative Assessment of the Geriatric Surgical Patient

Preoperative Assessment

In addition to conducting a complete and thorough history and physical examination of the patient, the following assessments are strongly recommended:

- ☐ Assess the patient's **cognitive ability** and **capacity** to understand the anticipated surgery (see Section I.A, Section I.B, and Appendix I).
- ☐ Screen the patient for **depression** (see Section I.C).
- ☐ Identify the patient's risk factors for developing postoperative **delirium** (see Section I.D).
- ☐ Screen for **alcohol** and other **substance abuse/dependence** (see Section I.E).
- ☐ Perform a preoperative **cardiac** evaluation according to the American College of Cardiology/American Heart Association (ACC/AHA) algorithm for patients undergoing noncardiac surgery (see Section II and Appendix II).
- ☐ Identify the patient's risk factors for postoperative **pulmonary** complications, and implement appropriate strategies for prevention (see Section III).
- ☐ Document **functional status** and history of **falls** (see Section IV).
- ☐ Determine baseline **frailty** score (see Section V and Appendix III).
- ☐ Assess patient's **nutritional status,** and consider preoperative interventions if the patient is at severe nutritional risk (see Section VI and Appendix IV).
- ☐ Take an accurate and detailed **medication history,** and consider appropriate perioperative adjustments. Monitor for **polypharmacy** (see Section VII, Appendix V, Appendix VI, and Appendix VII).
- ☐ Determine the patient's **treatment goals** and **expectations** in the context of the possible treatment outcomes (see Section VIII).
- ☐ Determine patient's **family** and **social support system** (see Section VIII).
- ☐ Order appropriate preoperative **diagnostic tests** focused on elderly patients (see Section IX).

FIG. 13.7 Best Practice Guidelines checklist. (From Chow WB, Rosenthal RA, Merkow RP, et al. Optimal preoperative assessment of the geriatric surgical patient: a best practices guideline from the American College of Surgeons National Surgical Quality Improvement Program and the American Geriatrics Society. *J Am Coll Surg.* 2012;215:453–466.)

consent and can have significant short- and long-term consequences in the postoperative period. A history of dementia prior to surgery has been associated with increased rates of mortality and serious morbidity. Dementia is also the single greatest risk factor for postoperative delirium.

While there are several methods to assess baseline cognitive status, the Mini-Cog[16] is an accurate test for cognitive impairment that is easy to perform in a busy clinic setting. The Mini-Cog test combines a three-item word learning and recall task (0 to 3 points; each correctly recalled word, 1 point), with a simple clock-drawing task (abnormal clock, 0 points; normal clock, 2 points, used as a distraction before word recall). Total possible Mini-Cog scores range from 0 to 5 points, with 0 to 2 suggesting high and 3 to 5 suggesting a low likelihood of cognitive impairment.

Capacity

In order to give informed consent, a patient must have decision-making capacity. The essentials of decision-making capacity are well described. In essence, the patients must be able to understand the nature of his or her illness, the risks and benefits of the treatment recommended, and the risks and benefits of the treatment alternatives. In order to be considered competent to give consent, the patient must be able to:

1. Clearly indicate a treatment choice
2. Understand the relevant information given
3. Appreciate the medical condition and the consequences of treatments
4. Reason about the treatment options

Delirium Risk

Delirium is defined as an acute disorder of cognition and attention and is among the most common and potentially devastating complications seen in older surgical patients. Delirium occurs in from 5% to over 50% of older surgical patients and is associated with longer hospital stays, increased rates of mortality, morbidity, poor functional recovery, and more discharges to locations other than home. Both cognitive dysfunction and depression are risk factors for delirium; however, other factors must also be assessed. Risk factors for delirium are divided into two groups, the preoperative or predisposing factors and the precipitating factors or those that occur in the postoperative period (Table 13.2). In addition to advanced age and cognitive dysfunction, predisposing factors include functional impairment, malnutrition, comorbid illness, sensory impairment, alcohol/substance abuse, psychotropic medications, severe illness, and type of surgery. Delirium risk can be assessed using a predictive rule that considers the patient's age, comorbidities, and type of surgery. Delirium risk can also be assessed using the ACS NSQIP Geriatric Surgical Risk Calculator described previously.[6]

TABLE 13.2 Risk factors and precipitating factors for delirium.

RISK (PREDISPOSING) FACTORS	PRECIPITATING FACTORS
Advanced age	Infection
Cognitive impairment	Medications
Functional impairment	Hypoxemia
Poor nutrition	Electrolyte abnormalities
Comorbidity	Undertreated/overtreated pain
Alcohol abuse	Neurologic events
Psychotropic medications	Dehydration
Sensory impairment	Sensory deprivation
Type of surgery	Sleep disruption
Severe illness	Use of bladder catheters
	Unfamiliar environment
	Use of physical restraints

Depression

Depression is present in approximately 11% of persons older than age 71 years. Unrecognized depression in the postoperative period may explain poor oral intake, lack of participation in the postoperative treatment plan, and higher requirements for analgesics. Depression also has been associated with higher mortality and longer hospitals stays in patients undergoing cardiac surgery. Screening for depression is easily accomplished using the Patient Health Questionnaire-2, which requires the patient to answer two questions:

1. In the past 12 months, have you ever had a time when you felt sad, blue, depressed, or down for most of the time for at least 2 weeks?
2. In the past 12 months, have you ever had a time, lasting at least 2 weeks, when you did not care about the things that you usually care about or when you did not enjoy the things that you usually enjoy?

Functional Assessment

There are several ways to evaluate function in the preoperative period. Each has value in predicting outcomes of surgery.

Activities of daily living. For older adults, the ability to perform ADLs (e.g., feeding, continence, transferring, toileting, dressing, bathing) and instrumental ADLs (IADLs; e.g., telephone use, transportation, meal preparation, shopping, housework, medication management, managing finances) has been shown to correlate with postoperative mortality and morbidity. In a study of patients over 80 years old, function (defined as independent, partially dependent, or totally dependent in ADLs) was a better predictor of mortality than age. More importantly, evaluating ADLs and IADLs preoperatively is essential for perioperative and discharge planning.

American Society of Anesthesiologists classification. For decades, the physical status classification of the American Society of Anesthesiologists (ASA) has been used successfully to stratify operative risk. This simple classification ranks patients according to the functional limitations imposed by coexisting disease. When curves for mortality versus ASA class are examined with regard to age, there is little difference between younger and older patients, which indicates that mortality is a function of frailty and coexisting disease rather than chronologic age. ASA classification has been shown to predict postoperative mortality accurately, even in patients older than 80 years old.

Exercise tolerance. Of all the methods of assessing overall functional capacity, exercise tolerance is the most sensitive predictor of postoperative cardiac and pulmonary complications in older adults. The metabolic requirements for many routine activities have been determined and are quantitated as metabolic equivalents of the task (METs). One MET, defined as 3.5 mL/kg/min, represents the basal oxygen consumption of a 70-kg, 40-year-old man at rest. Estimated energy requirements for various activities are shown in Fig. 13.8. An inability to function above 4 METs has been associated with increased perioperative cardiac events and long-term risk.[17] By asking appropriate questions about the level of activity, functional capacity can be accurately determined.

ESTIMATED ENERGY REQUIREMENTS FOR VARIOUS ACTIVITIES*

1 MET ↓ 4 METs	Can you take care of yourself? Eat, dress, or use the toilet? Walk indoors around the house? Walk a block or two on level ground at 2–3 mph or 3.2–4.8 km/h? Do light work around the house like dusting or washing dishes?	4 METs ↓ 10 METs	Climb a flight of stairs or walk up hill? Walk on level ground at 4 mph or 6.4 km/h? Run a short distance? Do heavy work around the house like scrubbing floors or lifting or moving heavy furniture? Participate in moderate recreational activities like golf, bowling, dancing, doubles tennis, or throwing a baseball or football? Participate in strenuous sports like swimming, singles tennis, football, basketball, or skiing?

**MET*, Metabolic equivalent of the task (see text).

FIG. 13.8 Estimated energy requirements for various activities. With increasing activity, the number of METs increases. An inability to function above 4 METs has been associated with increased perioperative cardiac events and long-term risk. (From Eagle KA, Berger PB, Calkins H, et al. ACC/AHA guideline update for perioperative cardiovascular evaluation for noncardiac surgery—executive summary: a report of the American College of Cardiology/American Heart Association Task Force on Practice Guidelines [Committee to Update the 1996 Guidelines on Perioperative Cardiovascular Evaluation for Noncardiac Surgery]. *Circulation.* 2002;105:1257–1267.)

Mobility/Fall Risk Assessment

Falls, considered one of the geriatric syndromes, are a leading cause of injury in older adults and are associated with declining overall health. A fall in the hospital is considered a never event. Recent evidence also suggests that a fall in the preoperative period may predict negative postoperative outcomes.[6] Every older patient should be asked about a history of falls and should be assessed for gait and mobility factors that may predispose to a fall. A simple way to assess gait and mobility impairment is the Timed Up and Go Test,[18] which can easily be accomplished in the office setting. The patient is asked to rise from a chair without using the armrests, walk a measured 10 feet, turn and return to the chair, and sit back down. The inability to rise from the chair without the armrests or a test time of more than 15 seconds is considered an indication of a high fall risk. Patients identified as high risk for fall should be considered for preoperative gait and balance training if time allows and should have physical therapy assist with early mobilization in the postoperative period.

Nutritional Status and Swallowing Function

The impact of poor nutrition as a risk factor for perioperative mortality and morbidity such as pneumonia and poor wound healing has long been appreciated. A variety of psychosocial issues and comorbid conditions common to older adults place this population at high risk for nutritional deficits. Malnutrition is estimated to occur in approximately 0% to 15% of community-dwelling older persons, 35% to 65% of older patients in acute care hospitals, and 25% to 60% of institutionalized older adults. Factors that lead to inadequate intake and uptake of nutrients in this population include the ability to obtain food (e.g., financial constraints, availability of food, limited mobility), desire to eat food (e.g., living situation, mental status, chronic illness), ability to eat and absorb food (e.g., poor dentition, chronic gastrointestinal disorders such as gastroesophageal reflux disease [GERD] or diarrhea), and medications that interfere with appetite or nutrient metabolism (Box 13.7).

In the frail older adult, a number of factors contribute to neuroendocrine dysregulation of the signals that control appetite and satiety and lead to what is termed the *anorexia of aging*. Although the anorexia of aging is a complex interaction of many interrelated events and systems, the result is chronic undernutrition and loss of muscle mass (sarcopenia). Malnutrition has also been associated with increased risk of falls and hospital admission.

BOX 13.7 Factors associated with increased risk of malnutrition.

- Recent weight loss
- Limited ability to obtain food
  - Immobility
  - Poverty
- Disinterest in eating
  - Depression
  - Isolation
  - Cognitive impairment
  - Decreased appetite
  - Decreased taste
- Difficulty eating
  - Poor dentition
  - Swallowing disorder
  - GERD
- Increased gastrointestinal losses
  - Diarrhea
  - Malabsorption
- Systemic diseases
  - Chronic lung
  - Liver
  - Cardiac
  - Renal
  - Cancer
- Drugs and medication
  - Alcohol
  - Suppressed appetite
  - Block nutrient metabolism

GERD, Gastroesophageal reflux disease.

Measurement of nutritional status in older adults, however, is difficult. Standard anthropomorphic measures do not take into account the changes in body composition and structure that accompany aging. Immune measures of nutrition are influenced by age-related changes in the immune system in general. Furthermore, criteria for the interpretation of biochemical markers in this age group have not been well established. Complicated markers and indices of malnutrition exist but are not necessary in the routine surgical setting. Subjective assessment by history and physical examination, in which risk factors and physical evidence of malnutrition are evaluated, has been shown to be as effective as objective measures of nutritional status.

Several screening tools may be used, including the Subjective Global Assessment (SGA) and Mini Nutritional Assessment (MNA). The SGA is a relatively simple, reproducible tool for assessing nutritional status from the history and physical examination. SGA ratings are most strongly influenced by loss of subcutaneous tissue, muscle wasting, and weight loss. The SGA has been validated in older and critically ill patients and has been related to the development of postoperative complications.[19] The MNA, which measures 18 factors, including body mass index (BMI), weight history, cognition, mobility, dietary history, and self-assessment, is also a reliable method for assessing nutritional status. Nutritional status, as determined by the SGA and MNA, has been shown to predict outcome in outpatient and hospitalized geriatric medical patients.

Severe nutritional deficits can be identified by measuring the BMI (weight in kilograms/height in meters squared) and serum albumin and inquiring about unintentional weight loss. BMI <18.5 kg/m^2, albumin <3.0 g/dL, and unintentional weight loss $>10\%$ to 15% within 6 months identify patients at high risk for nutritional-related complications. For these patients, a course of preoperative nutritional supplementation may be warranted, even if surgery needs to be delayed for several weeks.

One frequently overlooked part of the nutritional assessment is the evaluations of swallowing function. Swallowing dysfunction is present and often unappreciated in older adults and is associated with aspiration in the postoperative period (see "Aspiration" below). Factors associated with swallowing dysfunction include diseases such as diabetes, GERD, prior stroke, and other neuromuscular diseases and many medications, particularly those that cause dry mouth. It is therefore essential to ask older adults if they have any swallowing difficulties and, if so, to do a formal swallowing assessment so a plan for appropriate postoperative nutrition can be made.

Medication Management

Physiologic changes, such as decreased lean muscle mass and decline in renal function (see Renal Physiology section), affect the distribution and elimination of many drugs. As a result, older patients are at increased risk for adverse events related to inappropriate drugs or inappropriate dosing of drugs. The Beer's list is a comprehensive list of medications that should be avoided or used with caution in the older adult.[20] The most common drugs to be avoided include all benzodiazepines, the analgesic meperidine (Demerol), and the antihistamines diphenhydramine (Benadryl).

Multiple medication use also poses a risk to older patients in the perioperative period. In a random sample of older adults living in the community over 80% were found to take at least one prescription medication, with 68% taking an over-the-counter drug or supplement as well. Over 50% of persons over age 60 take five or more medications and supplements, many of which are unnecessary or inappropriately prescribed. Therefore, a thorough review of all medications should be conducted prior to surgery. All nonessential medications should be stopped, including all supplements as the content of these is frequently unclear.

Other medications, such as those with potential for withdrawal, including beta blockers, should be continued in the perioperative period. For patients with significant cardiac or vascular disease not currently on beta blockers or statin therapy, consideration should be given to starting these medications

BOX 13.8 ACS–geriatric surgery verification requirements for multimodality pain plan.

- Utilize opioid-sparing techniques (nonopioid drugs, regional analgesia).
- Titrate medication for increased sensitivity (start low, go slow).
- Avoid Beer's list of drugs (benzodiazepines, meperidine, skeletal muscle relaxants, etc.).
- Include a prophylactic pharmacologic bowel regimen.
- Consider nonmedication-based strategies for pain control.

From American College of Surgeons optimum resources for geriatric surgery. 2019. https://www.facs.org/quality-programs/geriatric-surgery. Accessed January 16, 2020.
ACS, American College of Surgeons.

INTRAOPERATIVE AND POSTOPERATIVE MANAGEMENT

In order to eliminate the great variability seen in current surgical outcomes in older adults, perioperative processes should be standardized to address the common problems that older adults experience when subjected to the stress of surgery, illness, and hospitalization.

Multimodality Pain Control

Older adults are much more sensitive than are younger adults to the adverse effects of many drugs, including the analgesics, antiemetics, and anxiolytics commonly used in the intra- and postoperative period. Avoidance of opioids is particularly important as they are associated with cognitive impairment, delirium, falls, and constipation. Pain under treatment is also common in older adults and also associated with delirium.

Structured protocols, such as the Enhanced Recovery After Surgery (ERAS) program, formalize the use of multimodality, opioid-sparing pain postoperative treatment regimens. While not designed specifically for older adults, ERAS protocols have been used successfully to improve outcomes in older adults.[21] The new ACS Geriatric Surgery Verification Program has a standard devoted to multimodality postoperative pain management. Components of this standard are found in Box 13.8.[22]

Delirium

Delirium, a disturbance of consciousness and cognition that presents over a short period of time with a fluctuating course is among the most common and potentially devastating postoperative complication seen in older patients. Postoperative delirium is associated with higher rates of morbidity (30 days) and mortality (6 months), longer ICU length of stay, longer hospital length of stay, higher rates of institutionalization after discharge, and higher overall hospital costs.[23] The incidence of postoperative delirium in older patients varies with the type of procedure: less than 5% after cataract surgery, 35% after vascular surgery, and 40% to 60% after hip fracture repair. The incidence in older patients requiring treatment in an ICU is over 50%.

Postoperative delirium is usually the result of an interaction between preexisting conditions (risk factors) and postoperative events or complications (precipitating factors) (Table 13.2). The onset of delirium may be the first indication of a serious postoperative complication. Identifying risk factors preoperatively and minimizing precipitating factors intraoperatively and postoperatively are currently the best strategy to prevent delirium. Recently, the American Geriatric Society has released a formal Guideline for Postoperative Delirium, which can be found at http://geriatricscareonline.org/ProductAbstract/postoperative_delirium/CL018/?param2=search.

Precipitating factors for delirium in the postoperative setting include common postoperative complications (e.g., hypoxia, sepsis, metabolic disturbances), untreated or undertreated pain, medications (e.g., certain antibiotics, analgesics, antihypertensives, beta blockers, benzodiazepines), situational issues (e.g., unfamiliar environment, immobility, loss of sensory assist devices such as glasses and hearing aids), use of bladder catheters and other indwelling devices or restraints, and disruption of the normal sleep-wake cycle (e.g., medications and treatments given during usual sleep hours) (Table 13.2). No association has been found with the route of anesthesia (epidural vs. general) or the occurrence of intraoperative hemodynamic complications. However, intraoperative blood loss, need for blood transfusion, and postoperative hematocrit level lower than 30% are associated with a significantly increased risk for postoperative delirium.

Although delirium is common in older patients following surgery, the diagnosis is frequently not appreciated. Agitation and confusion are usually recognized, but depressed levels of consciousness may also be present. The Confusion Assessment Model (CAM) developed by Wei and colleagues is a simple, well-validated tool to diagnose delirium. A positive CAM requires the following: (1) acute onset with waxing and waning course and (2) inattention, with (3) disordered thinking, or (4) altered level of consciousness.

The best treatment for delirium is prevention. Strategies that focus on maintaining orientation (e.g., family at the bedside, sensory devices available), encouraging mobility, maintaining normal sleep-wake cycles (no medications during sleep hours), and avoiding dehydration and inappropriate medications have been shown to decrease the number and duration of episodes of delirium in hospitalized patients. Pharmacologic prevention trials have not yet shown consistently positive results.

Once delirium is diagnosed, a thorough search for precipitating factors such as infections, hypoxia, metabolic disturbances, inappropriate medications, and undertreated pain should be conducted. Invasive devices and catheters should be removed as soon as possible and restraints should be avoided. A thorough review of the history should also be conducted and the family queried about possible predisposing factors, such as unrecognized alcohol consumption. The use of antipsychotic medications, such as very-low-dose haloperidol, should be reserved only for those patients whose behavior presents a danger to themselves or others.

Aspiration

Aspiration is a common cause of morbidity and mortality in older patients in the postoperative period. The incidence of postoperative aspiration pneumonia increases almost exponentially with increasing age, with patients older than 80 years old having a ninefold to tenfold greater risk than those 18 to 29 years of age.

Swallowing is a complex, coordinated interaction of many neuromuscular events. As many as one third of independent functioning older persons report some difficulty with swallowing. With age, there is a decline in several of the elements of normal swallowing that predispose to aspiration. These include loss of teeth, decrease in the strength of the muscles of mastication, slowing of the swallow time, decreased laryngopharyngeal sensation, and decreased cough strength. Poor oral hygiene and the edentulous state are also associated with an overgrowth of pathologic organisms, which predispose to pneumonia following aspiration.

In general, other risk factors for aspiration in older patients can be categorized as disease-related (e.g., stroke, dementia, neuromuscular disorders such as Parkinson disease, GERD), medication-related (e.g., drugs that cause dry mouth or altered mental status), and iatrogenic factors. The last of these is particularly relevant to surgical patients. The presence of devices crossing the oropharynx (e.g., nasogastric tubes, endotracheal tubes, esophageal thermometers, transesophageal echocardiographic probes) has been shown to disrupt the swallowing mechanism further. The need for prolonged intubation is associated with swallowing dysfunction and aspiration, as is the use of enteral feeding tubes. The routine use of nasogastric tubes in patients undergoing colon resection has been correlated with an increased risk of aspiration pneumonia, as has the use of transesophageal echocardiographic probes in patients undergoing cardiac surgery. The occurrence of postoperative ileus also predisposes to aspiration.

Aspiration risk should be assessed preoperatively in all older patients with risk factors for aspiration and in those with any report of a swallowing abnormality (see earlier, "Preoperative Assessment"). Aspiration precautions should be ordered for any patient thought to be at risk. These include 30- to 45-degree upright positioning, careful evaluation of gastrointestinal function prior to starting feeding and, frequently thereafter, careful monitoring of gastric residuals in patients with feeding tubes, and upright position during meals and for 30 to 45 minutes after meals in those on an oral diet. Prior to feeding patients at risk for aspiration, swallowing function can be assessed by a 3-ounce bedside swallow test. Passing this test is a good indication of the ability to tolerate thin liquids.[24]

Deconditioning

In older patients, the prolonged period of immobility that follows hospitalization for a major surgical procedure often results in functional decline and overall deconditioning. Functional decline has been observed after as little as two days of immobility. Deconditioning is a distinct clinical entity, characterized by specific changes in function of many organ systems (Table 13.3). Deconditioned individuals have ongoing functional limitations, despite improvement

TABLE 13.3 Organ system effects of bed rest.

SYSTEM	EFFECT
Cardiovascular	↓ Stroke volume, ↓ cardiac output, orthostatic hypotension
Respiratory	↓ Respiratory excursion, ↓ oxygen uptake, ↑ potential for atelectasis
Muscles	↓ Muscle strength, ↓ muscle blood flow
Bone	↑ Bone loss, ↓ bone density
Gastrointestinal	Malnutrition, anorexia, constipation
Genitourinary	Incontinence
Skin	Sheering force, potential for skin breakdown
Psychological	Social isolation, anxiety, depression, disorientation

From Kleinpell RM, Fletcher K, Jennings BM. Reducing functional decline in hospitalized elderly. In Hughes RG, ed. *Patient Safety and Quality: An Evidence-Based Handbook for Nurses*. Rockville, MD: Agency for Healthcare Research and Quality; 2008:251–265. AHRQ Publication No. 08-0043.

in the original acute illness. The period for functional recovery may be as much as three times longer than the period of immobility. Prolonged bed rest also leads to other postoperative complications, such as pressure ulcers and falls. Older adult surgical patients who develop functional decline while in the hospital are also at greater risk of readmission, complications, and death within 300 days after discharge.[25]

A major risk factor for deconditioning during hospitalization is a preexisting functional limitation. For example, patients requiring ambulation assist devices such as canes or walkers prior to hospitalization are more likely to suffer significant further functional decline. Other less obvious functional limitations, such as the inability to perform activities such as walking up a flight of steps carrying a bag of groceries (4 METs), are also associated with higher rates of postoperative complications and greater chances of functional decline. Other risk factors include two or more comorbidities, five or more medications, and a hospitalization or emergency room visit in the preceding year. Patients who develop delirium while in the hospital are also at greater risk of developing serious functional decline and of requiring placement in short-term rehabilitation or long-term care facilities.

Assessment of functional capacity is an essential part of the preoperative assessment. In patients identified at risk for functional decline, a plan for early directed methods to promote mobility, including early physical therapy consultation, should be establish prior to surgery. The "out of bed" order may be the most important of all routine postoperative orders for older patients.

Structured models for the in-hospital care of geriatric patients have been developed for patients hospitalized for medical illnesses. Adaptation of these models for surgery patients could promote improvements in functional and cognitive status. Preoperative conditioning to improve function prior to surgery, termed prehabilitation or prehab, has theoretical merit, although evidence to support its usefulness is still lacking.

TRANSITIONS OF CARE

Discharge planning for older adults should begin on the day the decision is made to proceed with surgery. Functional and cognitive deficits present on admission are exacerbated by the stress of surgery and constraints of hospitalization and immobilization, even if the surgery itself is uncomplicated. Not surprisingly, the need for postacute care is higher in older adults, as are the rates of readmission following surgical discharge. Unfortunately, a quarter of these readmissions are to facilities other than the initial treating hospital. New providers lacking knowledge of the events of the surgery and perioperative period are at a great disadvantage when caring complex older adults. Outcomes for these readmissions are much worse than readmissions to the initial treating institution.

Starting early in the perioperative period, it is important to set expectations for both patients and their families regarding length of stay, likelihood of the need for postacute nursing or rehabilitation placement, or the need for special services or equipment in the home. In addition, expectations regarding functional outcomes should be discussed. For patients coming from a nursing home, there may be specific requirements for them to be able to keep their place in the facility. Obviously, in the emergency setting, this is not possible, but as soon as needs are realized, case management should be involved in the care.

Important factors in discharge planning include assessment of family involvement, home readiness (i.e., does the patient have stairs, what will they need to be able to do functionally to return to their home), a physical and occupational therapy evaluation, and an open discussion with the patient about the surgeons' and the physicians' expectations for return of function. Studies have shown that advanced discharge planning, with involved case management, can improve patient outcomes, patient satisfaction, and decrease readmission, even improving cost of care.[26] And, while it may be resource intensive, in these high-risk patients, there is some evidence that a more intensive follow-up by nursing staff aimed at looking for early warning signs (such as dehydration) may promote earlier treatment and decrease rates of readmission.

The importance of a comprehensive discharge discussion and documentation cannot be overstated. Dealing with the aftermath of surgery, with new medications, new functional limitations, and new wounds to care for, is difficult for anyone. Add to that the preexisting functional and cognitive challenges, the effects of immobility and deconditioning, and the long list of prior medications so common in vulnerable older adults, and it is not surprising that serious problems can and do occur. A carefully documented discharge summary that recognizes the individual's vulnerabilities (as identified on the preoperative screens) and gives clear information to the caregivers about how to deal with predictable problems is essential. This, combined with a thorough verbal review of the major concerns described in the summary with the patient and the caregivers, can help avoid some of the more common problems.

Discharge communications should also occur with the postacute care facility when the patient requires nursing home care or postoperative rehabilitation. Clear, frequent, and two-way communication, starting with the thorough discharge summary and a discussion of it (or warm hand off), will help focus the postoperative care on the individual patient vulnerabilities.

SURGERY OF MAJOR ORGAN SYSTEMS

Endocrine Surgery

Thyroid Disease

Thyroid disease, especially hypothyroidism, is common among geriatric patients. This disease occurs in 10% of women and 2% of men older than 60 years old, and hyperthyroidism occurs in 0.5% to 6% of persons older than 55 years old. Hypothyroidism is a disease that can be caused by other factors such as previous radioablation or surgery, and some other causes can be from drugs that interfere with the synthesis of thyroid hormone, such as amiodarone. Another thyroid disease is hyperthyroidism, which is usually caused by toxic multinodular goiter, also known as Graves disease; however, this disease is more common in younger persons compared to geriatric patients. Medical treatment of hypothyroidism in older adults is like that in younger patients. In addition, the surgical treatment of hyperthyroidism may be necessary for large goiters compressing the trachea.

The incidence of thyroid nodules increases throughout life, whether detected by physical examination, ultrasound, or autopsy, although physical examination is less sensitive because of fibrosis of the soft tissues of the neck and the gland. Thyroid nodules are common in the elderly with linear increase with age. By ultrasonography, approximately 50% of patients older than 65 years old have nodules, with some studies showing a higher prevalence. A likely contributor to rising prevalence of thyroid nodules is the increased use of imaging modalities, and with this use is the detection of asymptomatic or incidental nodules. Once the thyroid nodules have been identified, there should be evaluation following American Thyroid Association Guidelines (Fig. 13.9) for examination. The cancer prevalence decreases in clinically relevant thyroid

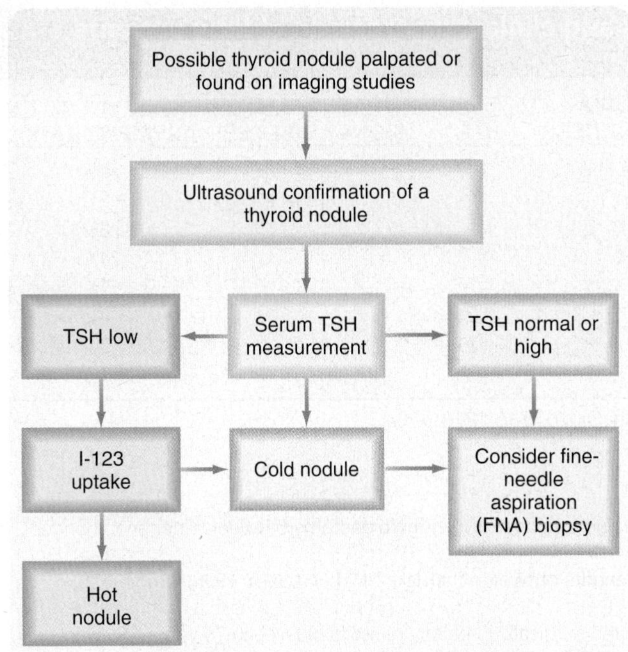

FIG. 13.9 Evaluation of a thyroid nodule. (From Lechner MG, Hershman JM. Thyroid nodules and cancer in the elderly. In Feingold KR, Anawalt B, Boyce A, et al. eds. *Endotext*. South Dartmouth, MA: MD Text com. Inc; 2018.) *TSH*, Thyroid stimulating hormone.

nodules (>1 cm) with increasing age. However, malignant nodules tend to have more aggressive phenotypes in elderly patients, with thyroid cancer–specific mortality being about 8%.

There are two types of well-differentiated thyroid cancers, which is divided into papillary and follicular subtypes. Sporadic papillary thyroid cancer has an almost bell-shaped distribution of age at diagnosis, with a decreasing trend in patients older than 60 years old. Age is a negative prognostic factor for survival and other outcomes. In addition, patients older than 60 years old have an increased risk for local recurrence, and patients younger than 20 years old and older than 60 years old have a higher risk for the development of distant metastasis. Increasing patient age correlates with increased risk for death by approximately twofold over a span of 20 years. Guidelines for the management of thyroid nodules and well-differentiated cancers can be found in the 2009 report of the American Thyroid Association's Guidelines Task Force.

When thyroidectomy is indicated, it can usually be performed safely, even in patients much older than 80 years old. However, older age does confer a higher risk of complications. For example, the patient can have longer hospital stays, higher mean costs, more likely discharges to a location other than home, and higher rates of perioperative mortality. Surgical outcomes in older patients with multiple comorbidities have been shown to be better when the operative volume of the surgeon has more than 30 thyroidectomies per year. Based on the population with complicated comorbidities, there are surgical risks and benefits that must be carefully weighed before operating on the patient.[27]

Parathyroid Disease

The most common reason for the finding of hypercalcemia in an elderly outpatient setting is primarily hyperparathyroidism (HPTH). The incidence of primary HPTH increases with age; it affects approximately 2% of older persons, with a 3:1 female preponderance (1 in 1000 postmenopausal women). The disease is characterized by elevated serum calcium levels. The normal patient usually has 1 mg of serum calcium. However, when compared to HPTH patients, the levels are 1.5 to 2.0 times normal. Most cases in older adults are solitary adenomas.

Elderly patients are less likely to present with kidney stones, but instead, they are more likely to have neuropsychiatric complaints compared to younger patients. With the advent of routine calcium testing, as part of automated chemistry analysis, most cases are now asymptomatic. There is a concern that this may be misclassification as the symptoms may be attributed to "old age." A careful history may reveal the presence of less obvious psychological and emotional symptoms. Other subtle symptoms in older persons include memory loss, personality changes, inability to concentrate, exercise fatigue, and back pain (Table 13.4). Several studies have shown that only 5% to 8% of patients are truly asymptomatic for kidney stones. If surgical treatment had to be done, it would be most cost effective for patients age 50 years or older with an expected life expectancy of 5 years or longer to be surgically treated on.

In response to the controversy regarding treatment of asymptomatic HPTH, the National Institutes of Health consensus conference in 1990 and again in 2002 came together to define parameters for care for patients with HPTH. In 2008, an international workshop on HPTH reviewed the old guidelines and provided updated recommendations as follows. For asymptomatic patients, surgery is recommended if there is elevation in serum calcium by >1 mg/dL above the normal range, increased 24-hour urine calcium excretion (>400 mg), decreased CrCl (<60 cc/min), and reduction in bone density of more than 2.5 standard deviations below peak bone mass (T-score <2.5). Otherwise, follow-up can be difficult because of other comorbidities or if the patient is younger than 50 years old.

Minimally invasive parathyroid surgery should be offered to elderly patients following the same algorithm as younger patients since the rate of multigland disease is not different. The most common complication is transient hypercalcemia, which can result in infection and hoarseness from transient laryngeal nerve injury. There is a significant increase in bone mineral density and a decreased risk of fracture following the surgery. Parathyroid hormone surgery in elderly has shown to improve quality of life and increased fracture-free survival.

Breast Disease

Epidemiology

Increasing age is a major risk factor for developing breast cancer, with an estimated 21% of newly diagnosed cases in patients older than age 70 years. The overall mortality is affected with this diagnosis even when adjusting for comorbidities. This could be due to undertreatment or overtreatment, decreased tolerance to therapy, and possibly decreased patient compliance. However, optimal treatment in elderly remains unknown since they are excluded from trials. Unlike the treatment of younger women with breast cancer, a treatment algorithm requires that a Comprehensive Geriatric Assessment be performed and base the treatment on whether the patient is frail or fit.[28]

Presentation and Screening

The presentation of breast cancer is similar in older and younger populations. The painless mass represents the most common symptom of breast cancer. In older women, a new breast lump is likely to represent a malignancy. Breast pain, skin thickening, breast swelling, or nipple discharge or retraction should be vigorously pursued with biopsy in older women. Breasts become less dense with aging, and this makes the clinical examination easier in older women. This

TABLE 13.4 Most common presenting symptoms and clinical disorders in elderly patients undergoing parathyroid surgery.

STUDY	FATIGUE	MENTAL IMPAIRMENT*	BONE PAIN/ DISEASE	MUSCLE WEAKNESS	HTN	KIDNEY DISEASE†	ASYMPTOMATIC
Bachar et al.[a]	11%		44%	11%	19%	14%	18%
Chen et al.[b]	39%	42%	33%			19%	6%
Chigot et al.[c]	35%	60%	15%				8%
Egan et al.[d]	12%	6%	44%				20%
Irvin and Carneiro[e]	15%	9%	50%	9%		15%	18%
Kebebew et al.[f]			26%		50%		0%
Politz and Norman[g]	62%	57%	44%		62%	15%	3%
Uden et al.[h]	35%		31%	28%	47%		7%

From Morris LF, Zelada J, Wu B, et al. Parathyroid surgery in the elderly. *Oncologist.* 2010;15:1273–1284.
HTN, Hypertension.
*Includes confusion and memory problems.
†Includes nephrolithiasis.
[a]Bachar G, Gilat H, Mizrachi A, et al. Comparison of perioperative management and outcome of parathyroidectomy between older and younger patients. *Head Neck.* 2008;30:1415–1421.
[b]Chen H, Parkerson S, Udelsman R. Parathyroidectomy in the elderly: do the benefits outweigh the risks? *World J Surg.* 1998;22:531–535; discussion 535–536.
[c]Chigot JP, Menegaux F, Achrafi H. Should primary hyperparathyroidism be treated surgically in elderly patients older than 75 years? *Surgery.* 1995;117:397–401.
[d]Egan KR, Adler JT, Olson JE, et al. Parathyroidectomy for primary hyperparathyroidism in octogenarians and nonagenarians: a risk-benefit analysis. *J Surg Res.* 2007;140:194–198.
[e]Irvin GL 3rd, Carneiro DM. "Limited" parathyroidectomy in geriatric patients. *Ann Surg.* 2001;233:612–616.
[f]Kebebew E, Duh QY, Clark OH. Parathyroidectomy for primary hyperparathyroidism in octogenarians and nonagenarians: a plea for early surgical referral. *Arch Surg.* 2003;138:867–871.
[g]Politz D, Norman J. Hyperparathyroidism in patients over 80: clinical characteristics and their ability to undergo outpatient parathyroidectomy. *Thyroid.* 2007;17:333–339.
[h]Uden P, Chan A, Duh QY, et al. Primary hyperparathyroidism in younger and older patients: symptoms and outcome of surgery. *World J Surg.* 1992;16:791–797; discussion 798.

difference also translates into an improved positive predictive value of an abnormal mammogram in women older than 65 years old. There is some controversy in screening guidelines in average-risk patient with age. The American Cancer Society annual mammography begins at age 45 years, with no upper age limit if a woman remains in good health. If a woman's life expectancy is estimated to be less than 3 to 5 years and she has severe functional limitations or has multiple comorbidities that are likely to impair survival, discontinuation of screening is appropriate. There is a general consensus with different groups to perform screening until at least the age of 70 years; the U.S. Preventative Services Task Force (USPSTF) recommends screening up to age 74 years (Table 13.5).[28]

Pathology and Treatment

Overall, breast cancers in older patients tend to be associated with more favorable pathologic prognostic factors. As patients' ages increase, their breast tumors are associated with more favorable tumor biology. This is shown by increased hormone sensitivity, attenuated epidermal growth factor receptor 2 (ERB-b2) overexpression, and lower grades and proliferative indices. However, older patients are more likely to present with larger and more advanced tumors, and recent reports have suggested that the involvement of lymph nodes increases with age. A concerning observation, based off of the data, suggests that older women are less likely to be treated according to the recommended guidelines as follows: less likely to receive definitive surgery, breast-conserving surgery, postlumpectomy radiotherapy, adjuvant hormonal therapy, or adjuvant chemotherapy. Recent studies show that the use of primary endocrine therapy has become a common noninvasive treatment for elderly patients, and it is good for local disease control in the short term (<2 or 3 years). However, this treatment is reserved and or recommended for patients with a shorter life expectancy. The accuracy rates for these models were different, ranging from high accuracy to low accuracy, thus making them range from moderate (69%) to very good (89%). These recent studies show that although there has been significant improvement in recurrence and mortality due to improvements in screening and treatment, this improvement has been smaller among older women.

Surgery. The gold standard for treating localized breast cancer at any age is surgery. Surgical mortality in elderly women in reasonable health is low (<1%). Surgical resection of the primary tumor is recommended for all older patients unless they are poor surgical candidates. Recent studies have indicated that the proportion of older women undergoing breast-conserving therapy is increasing. Omitting surgery exposes patients to a higher risk of local relapse and therefore is considered a suboptimal option, even for unfit older women. Tamoxifen alone had been previously recommended for the treatment of patients unfit for surgery and with short life expectancies, because tamoxifen antagonizes the estrogen receptor.

The role of axillary lymph node dissection (ALND) in the management of women with breast cancer has evolved over the last 10 to 15 years. ALND should be used when there is clinical suspicion of axillary lymph node involvement or a high-risk tumor. In addition, biopsy of sentinel lymph nodes is a safe alternative to ALND in patients with clinically node-negative tumors. Older patients with tumor size smaller than 2 to 3 cm and no clinical evidence of axillary involvement should be offered a sentinel lymph node biopsy.

Radiation therapy. For women 70 years of age or older who have early estrogen-receptor–positive breast cancer, the addition

TABLE 13.5 1 Guideline recommendations about screening mammography in older women

USPSTF GUIDELINES	ACS GUIDELINES	ACR GUIDELINES	AGS GUIDELINES
Offer biennial screening to women aged 50–74 years. Evidence is insufficient to recommend for or against screening in women >74 years of age. "I" Statement*. The Task Force encourages more research on the topic.	Offer screening to women aged ≥45 years and continue as long as a woman is in good health and has life expectancy of ≥10 years.	Offer annual screening to women aged ≥40 years and continue as long as a woman is in good health.	Offer screening to women aged ≤85 years who have life expectancy ≥5 years and for healthy women aged and ≥85 years who have excellent functional status or who feel strongly about the benefits of screening (no screening frequency specified).

From Optimal breast cancer screening strategies for older women: current perspectives. Braithwaite D, Demb J Henderson L. *Clinical Interventions in Aging.* 2016.:11 page 112. Reprinted with the permission of Dove Medical Press.
ACR, American College of Radiology; *ACS*, American Cancer Society: *AGS*, American Geriatrics Society; *USPSTF*, US Preventive Services Task. Force.
*Current evidence is insufficient to address benefits and harms of breast cancer screening in women >74 years of age.

of adjuvant radiation therapy to tamoxifen does not significantly decrease the rate of mastectomy for local recurrence, but there is an increase in the survival rate and an increase in the rate of freedom from distant metastases. Therefore, tamoxifen alone is a reasonable choice for adjuvant treatment in such women. For older women with small, node-negative tumors, the decision to include breast irradiation after lumpectomy should be made on a case-by-case basis. This should be done after careful discussion of the risks of locoregional recurrence and the side effects of radiation therapy. Alternatively, partial-breast irradiation with multicatheter interstitial brachytherapy, balloon catheter brachytherapy, three-dimensional conformal external-beam radiotherapy, and intraoperative radiotherapy can be an option in selected older patients. Older women treated with mastectomy should be offered chest wall irradiation if they have tumors greater than 5 cm or more than four involved axillary lymph nodes.[28]

Chemotherapy. Adjuvant endocrine therapy is generally recommended for older women with estrogen receptor–positive breast cancer. Tamoxifen and aromatase inhibitors, such as anastrozole, improve overall survival, reduce local recurrence, and reduce the risk of contralateral breast cancer for hormone-sensitive tumors in older women. Tamoxifen and anastrozole have side effects that can reduce their tolerance. Tamoxifen is associated with deep vein thrombosis, pulmonary emboli, cerebrovascular events, endometrial carcinoma, vaginal discharge and bleeding, and hot flashes. There are considerably more musculoskeletal complaints, including arthralgias and fractures, with anastrozole. It is important to monitor bone density and treat patients who have bone density loss while on aromatase inhibitors.

Older women who endure adjuvant chemotherapy trials have generally been underrepresented. However, recent data suggest that standard adjuvant chemotherapy has a role in the treatment of fit older women. The added value of chemotherapy in older women who receive endocrine therapy is influenced greatly by comorbidity and life expectancy. Models for estimating the benefits of chemotherapy in hormone receptor–positive older women have been developed. The model demonstrates that a high risk of recurrence is needed to achieve a small survival benefit with adjuvant chemotherapy. For example, to reduce mortality risk at 10 years by 1% with chemotherapy, the risk of breast recurrence at 10 years must be at least 25% for a 75-year-old woman in average health. These data suggest that chemotherapy for older women with hormone receptor–positive breast cancer should be offered only to node-positive patients who are in reasonable health, with a high risk of recurrence and a life expectancy of more than 5 years. Older node-negative patients are unlikely to benefit from chemotherapy unless they have large hormone receptor–positive tumors with adverse pathologic characteristics or hormone receptor–negative tumors larger than 2 cm. An Internet-based tool that incorporates age, health status, and tumor characteristics can help determine the potential benefit of adjuvant chemotherapy for breast cancer patients (available at http://www.adjuvantonline.com).

Gastrointestinal Surgery

Esophagus

Motility disorders. The esophagus undergoes characteristic changes with aging. Dysfunction of the proximal aspects of swallowing is noted during normal aging. Another aspect to take note of is that the resting upper esophageal sphincter pressure and relaxation are decreased in the older normal population compared with a younger control population. The duration of oropharyngeal swallowing and the sensory threshold for initiating a swallow are increased with advancing age. These factors increase the risk of pharyngeal stasis and potential for aspiration. Dysmotility of the cricopharyngeus (upper esophageal sphincter) with increasing age can result in Zenker diverticula. It appears that in normal healthy individuals, the physiologic function of the esophagus itself is preserved until patients reach around 80 years of age. In this group, the amplitude of esophageal contractions is decreased.

Gastroesophageal reflux disease. It has been suggested that there is an association of GERD with the peristaltic dysfunction that occurs with aging. Although the lower esophageal sphincter resting pressure is normal and relaxes appropriately after deglutition, the sphincter fails to contract rapidly back to baseline, resulting in prolonged decreased tone. Due to laxity at the gastroesophageal junction, there is also an increased incidence of sliding hiatal hernia with aging. These conditions, along with delayed gastric emptying in older patients, predispose them to GERD. It is also important to remember that many medications prescribed for older patients increase the relaxation of the lower esophageal sphincter.

The complications of GERD, including erosive esophagitis, Barrett esophagus, and esophageal adenocarcinoma, are seen with an increased frequency in older patients. However, recent studies have demonstrated that symptoms may be attenuated in older adults. Specifically, older patients with severe esophagitis are least likely to have severe heartburn. Instead, they present with more nonspecific symptoms, such as dysphagia, anorexia, anemia, weight loss, and vomiting. The absence of classic symptoms may be the result of an age-related decreased esophageal sensitivity to pain. Therefore, more aggressive diagnosis and/or treatment of GERD may be warranted for older patients, regardless of their presenting symptoms.

The success of laparoscopic Nissen fundoplication for the correction of GERD in older patients provides a viable alternative to lifelong medications, which may also be less effective in older patients. This is seen in 90% of older patients, as they report relief of symptoms, particularly vomiting and aspiration, after a Nissen procedure. In addition, laparoscopic Nissen has been shown to be safe, with comparable outcomes in elderly adults.

Paraesophageal hernias. Paraesophageal hernias also increase with advancing age and can reach enormous size without symptoms. In the past, the fear of gastric volvulus, with subsequent strangulation, has caused us to mandate immediate repair of paraesophageal hernias, even in the absence of symptoms. Recently, watchful waiting is generally recommended, rather than immediate surgery for asymptomatic hernias. It has been demonstrated that asymptomatic hernias to have a low (1.1%) annual probability of requiring an emergency operation. Mortality rates after emergency surgery are about 5.4% to 8% with higher frailty having a tendency to predict higher mortality.

Esophageal cancer. The peak incidence of diagnosis is between 60 and 80 years old with patients 70 years of age or older contributing to 38.9% of all esophageal cancer in the Surveillance Epidemiology and End Results database. Esophageal resection remains the only established curative treatment for cancer of the esophagus and gastric cardia. The elderly patients may have a higher proportion of localized disease, but these elderly patients did not have surgery and/or radiation therapy. However, patients age 70 years or older compared to younger patients with esophageal cancer have worse overall survival. The difference in survival is no longer observed between the elderly and the younger patients if surgical resection is performed. A strategy needs to be developed on a case-by-case basis if surgery can be beneficial in elderly patients with localized disease.

Stomach

A progressive cephalad migration of the antral-fundic junction occurs with age. Studies have shown that between 25% and 80% of older adults have fasting achlorhydria. This is caused by progressive loss of parietal cells and decreased antral and serum concentrations of gastrin. Achlorhydria results in derangements in folate, iron, and vitamin B_{12} absorption.

Peptic ulcer. The incidence of peptic ulcer disease increases with age. Up to 80% of peptic ulcer–related deaths occur in patients older than 65 years old. Other factors that increase the risk of peptic ulcer disease in older adults are the use of nonsteroidal antiinflammatory drugs (NSAIDs) and infection with *Helicobacter pylori.* NSAID use has increased markedly over the past few years, especially in older adults. When compared with younger patients, the use of NSAIDs increases the risk of developing complicated peptic ulcer disease in older patients. The actual NSAID use is also a helpful prognostic indicator, and it has been indicated that the mortality rate from peptic ulcer disease in older patients who take NSAIDs is twice that of those who do not. Similarly, 80% of all ulcer-related deaths are in patients taking NSAIDs. Despite this finding, NSAIDs are frequently prescribed to older patients, even those with previous gastrointestinal problems. *H. pylori* infections are believed to occur at a rate of 1% per year, yielding a substantial percentage of older adults harboring infections.

Older patients typically present for surgical correction of peptic ulcer disease in a delayed fashion and with more advanced disease. This translates to statistically significant increases in operative mortality for older patients undergoing surgery for complicated peptic ulcer disease. However, age alone has not been shown to be an independent predictor of surgical risk. Based on the multivariate analysis, the analysis reveals three risk factors for operative mortality in a perforated ulcer: the presence of concomitant disease, preoperative shock, and more than 48 hours of perforation. In conclusion, the patient's age, amount of peritoneal soilage, and length of history of ulcer disease do not appear to be significant risks.

Gastric cancer. The incidence of gastric cancer rises progressively with age, with most patients between the ages of 50 and 70 years old at presentation. Risks include dietary (e.g., pickled vegetables, salted fish, nitrates, nitrites), occupational (e.g., metal, asbestos, rubber workers), and geographic (Asia vs. Western Hemisphere) factors. Certain medical history can be associated with an increased risk of gastric cancer, for example, chronic atrophic gastritis, previous gastric surgery, and chronic *H. pylori* infection. These results from patient history are more frequently found in older patients and are associated with gastric cancer. Chronic atrophic gastritis and *H. pylori* infection are also risk factors for gastric lymphoma and its precursor, mucosal-associated lymphoid tissue. These patients typically present with this issues in the sixth decade of life.

The presentation of gastric cancer is changing in older persons. This is leading to the need for more aggressive surgery. Older patients who present with a predominance of intestinal-type tumors tend to have the more aggressive diffuse type. There is also a progression of the location of the tumor to more proximal areas of the stomach. As a result, total gastrectomy for cure in this population is now required in 13% to 34% of cases. Between younger and older patients, there is no difference in being able to resect or the rate of positive lymph nodes found at surgery (60%–70%).[29] Early reports of minimally invasive gastrectomy have demonstrated decreased morbidity and cost because of decreased length of stay. Therefore, the long-term outcomes are less clear.

Biliary Tract Disease

In almost all populations including both genders, the prevalence of gallstones increases with increasing age, although the magnitude of this increase varies with the population. Therefore, it is not surprising that biliary tract disease is the single most common cause of acute abdominal complaints in patients older than 65 years old in the United States. In addition, these patients account for approximately one third of all abdominal surgeries in this age group. In 2006, persons older than 65 years old accounted for 50% of the hospital discharges for primary diagnosis cholelithiasis and one third of the over 400,000 inpatient cholecystectomies performed that year.

The indications for treatment of gallstone disease in older persons are the same as in younger patients. Even though complications of the disease are more common in those of advanced age, biliary colic is seen only half as often in older as compared to younger patients. Even in the presence of acute cholecystitis, as many as 25%

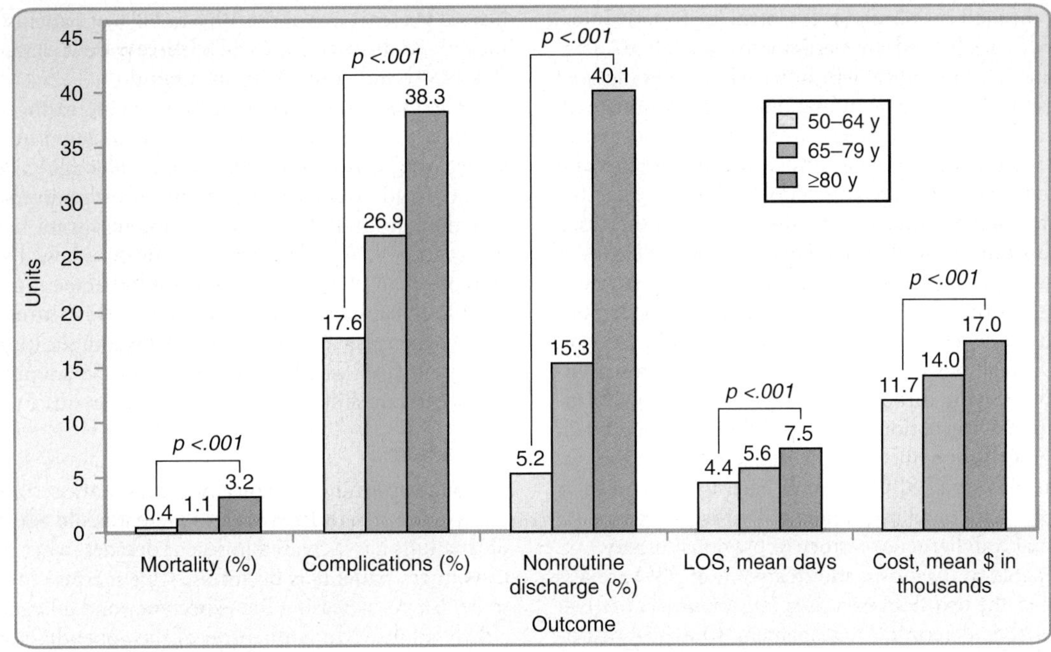

FIG. 13.10 Outcomes of inpatient cholecystectomy with age. (From Kuy S, Sosa JA, Roman SA, et al. Age matters: a study of clinical and economic outcomes following cholecystectomy in elderly Americans. *Am J Surg.* 2011;201:789–796.)

of older patients may have no abdominal tenderness, one third have no elevation in temperature or WBC count, and up to 59% have no peritoneal signs in the right upper quadrant. Older patients admitted to the hospital for cholecystectomy are more likely to have multiple biliary diagnoses, carry a concomitant diagnosis of cholangitis, undergo open operation, and require additional procedures such as endoscopic retrograde cholangiopancreatography (ERCP) or common bile duct (CBD) exploration. When looking at patients who undergo ERCP or cholecystectomy, these patients have a 70% lower risk of biliary disease recurrence within 1 year of operation. Even though ERCP is proven to be safe and effective for the elderly, when used in combination with laparoscopic cholecystectomy, it creates complications such as bile leaks and adhesions. Recurrence of CBD stones after sphincterotomy, even with antecedent or subsequent cholecystectomy, is higher in older than in younger patients (20% vs. 4%). Risk factors for recurrence include a dilated CBD, duodenal diverticulum, angulation of the CBD, and previous cholecystectomy.

Laparoscopic cholecystectomy is more prevalent in the elderly group, but the outcome of biliary tract surgery in vulnerable older patients has not improved much over the past several decades. Older patients still have more complicated disease at the time of surgery. Some complications may be longer lengths of stay, higher rates of in-hospital mortality, and much higher rates of discharge to sites other than home (Fig. 13.10). These complications have been identified, and improving the outcome of biliary tract disease in older adults will be difficult.

Liver

Over the past 20 years, the mortality associated with liver resection in patients older than 65 years old has decreased. Advances in operative technique, anesthetic management, and intensive care have greatly reduced morbidity and mortality. Today, the rates in younger and older patients are comparable. Results are so similar that age alone is not necessarily a contraindication to simultaneous resection of colorectal malignancy and liver metastases. Previous studies on the safety of resection in elderly patients cite mortality and morbidity of around 4% to 5% and 30% to 40%, respectively. Interestingly, postoperative liver function in well-selected elderly patients has proven comparable to their younger counterparts.

Tumors of the liver are 20 times more likely to arise from metastatic disease than from primary cancer. In addition, metastatic tumors from gastrointestinal tract are primarily the most common type when referring to resection. Patients with colon cancer have a 35% risk for recurrence in the liver, but only 10% to 20% of those identified have resectable disease. Patients resected have more than a 30% 5-year survival rate versus 0% if not resected. Resection of colon and rectal liver metastases has been shown to be safe and effective in a select group of elderly patients.

When determining the appropriateness of resection, it is important to consider the prevalence of insulin, resistance, and nonalcoholic fatty liver disease since it is higher in elderly patients. While age itself is not a contraindication, careful consideration of comorbidities must be considered. For patients who are not candidates for surgical intervention, there are other options to treat hepatic cancer, including radiological embolization, cryotherapy, and radiofrequency ablation therapy. The different types of therapies listed above can be performed operatively or transcutaneously in highly comorbid patients.

Small Bowel Obstruction

Small bowel obstruction (SBO) is the most common and surgically relevant disorder of small intestinal function encountered in older persons. Although the exact incidence of SBO in older adults is difficult to assess, the gastrointestinal procedure, lysis of adhesions, is the third most common procedure after cholecystectomy and partial excision of the large bowel. Of the deaths associated with SBO, 50% occur in patients older than 70 years old.

In Western countries, adhesions are responsible for a substantial majority of SBOs, followed by incarcerated hernias, neoplasms, and inflammatory bowel disease. It has been noted that patients with incarcerated hernias are slightly older than patients with adhesive obstruction. In addition, certain types of hernias, such as those that occur through the obturator foramen, are found almost exclusively in older adults and are particularly difficult to diagnose. Luminal obstruction, other than from deliberately ingested objects, accounts for less than 5% of cases. However, most cases of this type of obstruction occur in older adults. The two most common objects obstructing the lumen in adults are phytobezoars and gallstones. Phytobezoars are large concretions of poorly digested fruit and vegetable matter; these concretions form with increased frequency in the stomach of older patients with poor dentition, decreased gastric acid, impaired gastric motility, and previous gastrectomy. In the stomach, these masses can become enormous without any symptoms. However, when a portion breaks free and migrates into the small bowel, obstruction ensues. Gallstones enter the small bowel usually through a fistula between the gallbladder and duodenum. Obstruction of the small bowel lumen by an aberrantly located gallstone, incorrectly termed *gallstone ileus*, accounts for 1% to 3% of all SBOs but has been implicated in as many as 25% of obstructions in patients older than 65 years old with no abdominal wall hernia or history of previous surgery.

The pathophysiology, diagnosis, and treatment of SBO are discussed elsewhere in the text. However, it is important to note two important issues that determine management strategy—distinguishing functional (ileus) from mechanical obstruction and distinguishing simple from strangulated obstruction—both of these issues are even more complex in older patients.

There are many factors associated with ileus, such as systemic infections, intraabdominal infections, metabolic abnormalities, and medications that affect motility and are more common in older persons. In addition, signs and symptoms of underlying infections such as pneumonia, urinary tract infection, or appendicitis may be subtle within geriatric patients. Bowel distention may be erroneously considered the primary problem rather than a secondary event, and vomiting from a variety of nonobstructive causes can rapidly lead to dehydration and subsequent electrolyte abnormalities in older adults. In conclusion, even with the many factors associated with ileus, it is important not to look at the larger problem at hand, not the smaller issues.

In patients of all ages, it is standard that a patient may have adhesive SBO. The suggested initial management is to use nonoperative management with nasogastric decompression and IV hydration. Although rates vary, only approximately 30% of patients with adhesive SBO will require surgery, usually for failure to progress or fear of strangulation. However, an accurate distinction between strangulated and simple mechanical SBO is difficult to make. This is because there are no objective markers that consistently identify which patient will require small bowel resection for ischemia at the time of surgery for SBO. Clinical findings of fever, tachycardia, elevated WBC count, and focal tenderness are notoriously misleading, especially in older adults in whom the risk for strangulation is the highest.

In older patients who have undergone previous abdominal operations for malignant disease, the decision about when to operate is even more difficult. Metastatic obstruction presents several technical and ethical problems. Obstructing lesions are frequently found at a number of points in the bowel and resection may not be possible. Thirty-day operative mortality rates for this form of obstruction in older patients exceed 35%, and most patients die within 6 months. This discouraging outcome has led some to advocate prolonged periods of nonoperative decompression. Unfortunately, this approach produces only transient relief of obstructive symptoms. Furthermore, a previous history of malignancy is not an absolute indication that the obstruction is caused by metastatic disease. As seen, out of the 10% to 38% of patients with suspected malignant obstruction, some of these patients have a benign cause that was found at the time of surgery.

Over the past decade, there has been increasing interest in using minimally invasive techniques to diagnose and treat SBO. At first glance, the laparoscopic approach in older adults has considerable appeal. In addition, early intervention with minimal surgical stress would seem ideal. There are now numerous relatively small series by experienced laparoscopic surgeons that show diagnostic success in more than 90% of cases and total therapeutic success rates of 50% to 90%. However, laparoscopy in this setting can be technically challenging and there are usually complications. It is unclear at present how widely this option will be adopted as more surgeons become skilled in these advanced laparoscopic techniques.[30]

Appendicitis

Although appendicitis typically occurs in the second and third decades of life, 5% to 10% of cases present in old age. Appendicitis in older adults has increased in recent decades, whereas the incidence in younger patients is declining. This increase in part is thought to be due to increasing life expectancy and a larger proportion of elderly adults.[31] Inflammation of the appendix now accounts for 2.5% to 5% of acute abdominal disease in patients older than age 60 to 70 years old. The overall mortality from appendicitis is only 0.8%, but the vast majority of deaths occur in the very young and the very old. In adults, the mortality rate after an appendectomy is strongly related to age, ranging from a minimum of 0.07/1000 appendectomies in patients aged 20 to 29 years old to a maximum of 164/1000 in nonagenarians.

The classic presentation of appendicitis is only present in less than 20% of older patients. Although almost all older patients with acute appendicitis will present with abdominal pain, only 50% to 75% will have pain localized to the right lower quadrant. Almost one-third of patients will have diffuse nonlocalizable abdominal pain. It is common that an older patient may have vague abdominal pain. However, its significance may be overlooked, leading to delays in treatment. Other signs of acute appendicitis are also unreliable in older adults. The WBC count and temperature are normal in 20% to 50% of older patients with appendicitis. Other symptoms like nausea, vomiting, and anorexia are also found less frequently in older patients.

The indolent and nonspecific nature of the initial symptoms of appendicitis in older adults usually leads to delays of 48 to 72 hours before medical attention is sought. These delays are compounded by a delay in diagnosis once the patient reaches the hospital. Delays to operation longer than 24 hours are three times more likely to occur in older than in younger patients. As a result of these delays, over 50% of older patients will have perforated appendicitis identified at operation. Older patients undergoing appendectomy for perforated appendicitis have a higher risk of complications and death than those undergoing simple appendectomy for appendicitis without peritonitis.

The use of computed tomography (CT) scanning in the diagnosis of acute appendicitis has increased dramatically. Prior to urgent appendectomy, fewer than 20% of patients underwent preoperative CT in 1998, which was compared with over 90% of patients in 2007. It is important to note that the negative appendectomy rate in older adults has not changed during this same time period. CT scanning has been advocated because of the atypical presentation of appendicitis, which is a high rate of perforation at the time of presentation, and the expanded differential diagnosis in older adults. If an abscess is found, percutaneous drainage and

IV antibiotics are often preferable to exploration. In older adults, recurrent appendicitis after resolution of the abscess is uncommon and interval appendectomy is therefore not necessary in all cases. However, patients with complicated appendicitis in this age group mandate a thorough evaluation of the colon when the acute process is controlled. When an older patient presents with signs and symptoms of acute appendicitis, but with a longer duration of symptoms and a lower hematocrit than expected, these signs should raise the concern for colon or appendiceal cancer.

The use of laparoscopic surgery for the treatment of acute appendicitis has increased dramatically over the past decade. During laparoscopy, a significantly higher incidence of complicated appendicitis and other pathology is observed in older adults. These factors lead to a higher conversion rate to open surgery in older patients. There is no difference in infectious-related morbidity between younger and older patients undergoing laparoscopic appendectomy. However, older patients do experience a higher rate of cardiopulmonary complications. Importantly, laparoscopic appendectomy is associated with a higher likelihood of discharge to their home compared with discharge to a skilled or unskilled nursing facility. Despite improvements in diagnosis and management of appendicitis in elderly patients, morbidity and mortality for this group remain high, ranging between 28% to 60% and 10%, respectively, and much of this may be caused due to the delay in diagnosis, so clinical suspicion should remain high.

Carcinoma of the Colon and Rectum

Colorectal cancer is predominantly a disease of aging and is a major cause of morbidity and mortality in the older population. Colorectal cancer incidences are directly associated with increasing age, with most cases affecting older adults; 71% of new cases occur in patients 65 years and older, and 42% occur in those 75 years old and older. The annual incidence of colon cancer is almost 40 times higher for patients older than 85 years old compared with individuals who are 40 to 44 years of age.

Increasing age is a poor prognostic factor in colorectal cancer. Patients older than 75 years old have a significantly decreased 5-year, disease-free survival compared with younger patients. Although there are differences in the survival of colorectal cancer, it could be attributed to the cancer's biology and physiologic function, which is specific to older adults.[32] The presenting signs and symptoms of colorectal cancer depend on the location of the tumor and do not vary substantially with age. However, because fatigue, falls, constipation, and bowel dysfunction are accepted as common sequelae of aging, these symptoms are frequently ignored by the patient and the physician. Therefore, the diagnosis is often not made until a complication occurs.

Older patients, regardless of the number of comorbidities they have, are less likely to receive screening for colorectal cancer. As a result, older adults are more likely to present with more advanced disease than younger patients. In addition, the proportion of unstaged cancers increases with advancing age. The USPSTF recommends screening for colorectal cancer in adults beginning at age 50 and continuing until age 75 for average risk individuals. Recommendations for screening include annual fecal occult blood testing and flexible sigmoidoscopy every 5 years, with a full colonoscopy for positive occult blood or an adenomatous polyps on flexible sigmoidoscopy, or a colonoscopy every 5 to 10 years. Since older patients have an increased incidence of right-sided cancers, more than 50% of patients with right-sided cancers have no lesions within reach of the flexible sigmoidoscope. Therefore, it would be more effective to use the colonoscopy screening tool in older patients. Colorectal cancer screening for older adults is not advised for individuals unlikely to live 5 years or for those who have significant comorbid medical conditions precluding treatment. Screening trials indicate that a difference in colorectal cancer mortality between screened and unscreened persons does not become noticeable until at least 5 years after screening.

Surgical resection is the only curative treatment for resectable colorectal cancer, regardless of the patient's age. Regarding tumors of the abdominal colon, the use of anesthetic should be prohibitive due to the risk of secondary to severe comorbidity. This should especially be emphasized in the presence of advanced metastatic disease. These are the only factors that negatively influence the decision for surgery. There has been some concern about the ability of older patients to tolerate resection procedures for low rectal cancers. This includes abdominoperineal resection, low anterior resection, and sphincter-saving coloanal anastomosis. Although the procedure coloanal anastomosis is technically more demanding than the traditional abdominoperineal resection, coloanal anastomosis provides a sphincter-saving alternative that is well tolerated by older adults in terms of operative mortality and postoperative complications. Several studies have shown that in highly selected patients, the long-term results for coloanal anastomosis and abdominoperineal resection are comparable. Coloanal reconstruction can achieve continence in almost 80% of older individuals. Assessment of anal function is extremely important when selecting patients for low rectal anastomosis, since many of these patients will have poor functional results after sphincter-preserving surgery. Fecal incontinence may result in a worse quality of life than a well-controlled end-sigmoid colostomy, and it is important for physicians to talk about these risks with their patients.

Several randomized studies comparing laparoscopic colectomy to open colectomy have been completed; however, older patients are underrepresented. Available series data suggest that, in elderly patients, there was no significant difference between laparoscopic colectomy and open colectomy in the perioperative mortality rates, no need for blood transfusion, or no incidence of reoperation. As seen, elderly patients may actually benefit more from the minimally invasive approach than younger patients. Cardiopulmonary morbidity appears to be lower in older patients undergoing minimally invasive approach to resection of colorectal cancer. After laparoscopic colectomy, there has been a quicker gastrointestinal and respiratory recovery. In addition, patients have reported less pain, required less narcotic analgesia, experienced a shorter hospital stay, and are more likely to return to independent status. Finally, when comparing laparoscopic colectomy and open colectomy, the oncologic clearance is equivalent in both treatment groups.

For patients with significant comorbidities, local excision of low-lying rectal cancers may be an option for patients with early-stage cancers. Although the local recurrence rate is significantly higher for local excision, the overall 5-year survival is similar when being compared. For the frail older or high-risk patient, lesser procedures, including transanal excision and fulguration, can provide local control of the tumor without disrupting continence. Local control of rectal tumors with chemoradiation is also possible to control pain and bleeding in poor-risk patients with metastatic disease and a short life expectancy. The use of colonic stents to palliate poor surgical candidates with impending obstruction should be considered when technically feasible.

In patients with little or no comorbidity, operative mortality is similar, regardless of age. Even in patients older than 80 years old, elective operative mortality rates are only approximately 2%. Unfortunately, because of the issues described, older patients are

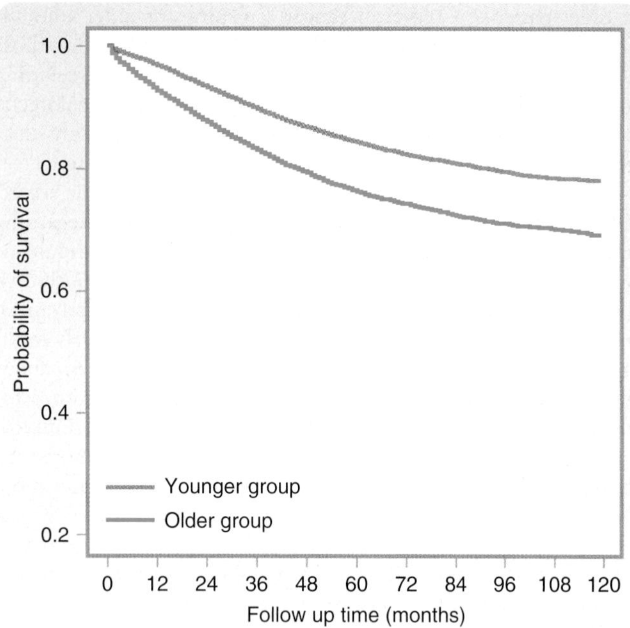

FIG. 13.11 A Kaplan-Meier survival curve for colon specific survival by age. (Frin Fu J, Ruan H, Zheng H, et al. Impact of old age on resectable colorectal cancer outcomes. *PeerJ*. 2019;7:e6350.)

more likely to require emergency surgery compared to younger patients. In addition, colorectal cancer patients 85 years of age are twice as likely to need emergency surgery as those 65 years of age. With advancing age, a decreasing proportion of patients undergo curative resection at the time of surgery. When surgery is performed as an emergency, mortality increases threefold to fourfold over elective mortality for similar procedures with an increase in the length of hospital stays and hospital costs. The survivors of emergent operations are only half as likely to return to independent living as are those elective emergency surgeries.

Long-term survival after a diagnosis of colorectal cancer in older adults is disproportionately poor compared with that in younger patients (Fig. 13.11). Methodology taking into account competing causes of death has established that older patients die more frequently from colorectal cancer, which is above the expected age-related rates of death. In older patients with both colon and rectal cancers, the 5-year mortality following surgical resection is 1.5 to 2.5 times greater than for younger patients. The poorer survival seen in older patients with colorectal cancer may be a result of the reduced use of adjuvant therapy in this group. Despite the fact that most patients with colorectal cancer are older than 70 years old, only 20% of patients in randomized trials are older than 70 years old. The efficacy and tolerance of adjuvant chemotherapy for colon cancer and neoadjuvant chemoradiotherapy for rectal cancer in older patients have been demonstrated; however, less than 30% of patients older than age 75 years will receive adjuvant therapy. Moreover, of those who do receive adjuvant therapy, more than 50% will not receive the appropriate therapy for the recommended duration.

Surgical therapy directed to the treatment of colorectal liver metastasis is being used with increasing frequency. The resection of metastatic lesions is associated with improved survival and operative morbidity, and mortality rates have been declining. However, older patients are poorly represented in studies evaluating liver resection for colorectal cancer liver metastasis due to the inaccurate provider perceptions of high postoperative mortality and the lack of oncologic concerns. Although there are some physiologic changes in liver function with increasing age, these changes are not usually sufficient enough to influence the outcome of liver resection. Mortality rates after liver resection in older adults are less than 5%. Older adults do derive a significant benefit from a surgical approach to colorectal liver metastases and have reasonable morbidity and mortality. Five-year survival after resection has been reported to be 32% compared with 10.5% in those not undergoing hepatectomy.[33]

Abdominal Wall Hernias

Repair of an abdominal wall hernias represent the most common surgical procedure in the United States. The lifetime risk for inguinal hernia is 27% for men and 3% for women, with about 27% performed in adults younger than 65 years old. More than 750,000 inguinal hernias are repaired every year in the United States with a bimodal distribution. Most develop for the first time in patients younger than 1 year old and in those aged 55 to 85 years. The estimated incidence of abdominal wall hernia in persons older than 65 years old is 13/1000, with a fourfold to eightfold higher incidence in men than in women. In patients older than 70 years old, 65% of all hernias are inguinal, 20% are femoral, 10% are ventral, 3% are umbilical, and 1% are esophageal hiatal. Whereas the overwhelming majority of all groin hernias occur in men, 80% of femoral hernias occur in women. Older adults are also at risk for the more occult types of hernias, such as paraesophageal hernias and obturator hernias that do not become apparent until a complication has occurred.

In the older adult, hernias pose some additional challenges. For example, they are often long-standing, and many have been present for less than 10 years. As a result of the chronic nature of these hernias, often, the normal anatomy is distorted and there is loss of tissue planes. In addition, loss of tissue strength may make an anatomic repair more difficult. Even with these challenges, it is clear that symptomatic groin and umbilical hernias in older adults should preferentially be repaired electively. Open, tension-free mesh repair of inguinal, femoral, and umbilical hernias can be performed as an outpatient procedure under epidural or local anesthesia with IV sedation. Mortality rates are low, even in patients with concomitant medical disease, and many reports have demonstrated mortality rates of 0%. Laparoscopic repair requires a general anesthetic in most cases, takes more operative time to complete, and incurs greater hospital costs. In older adults, the decreased economic benefit to society of an earlier return to normal activities and work seems to obviate the overall cost-benefit of the laparoscopic operation. The trend in most centers is for laparoscopic repair to be restricted to bilateral and recurrent inguinal hernias, for which the results are excellent.

The issue of watchful waiting instead of immediate repair of asymptomatic and mildly symptomatic hernia in older adults remains controversial. Although some randomized studies have favored watchful waiting, others have suggested that repair may improve general health and decrease possible serious morbidity. Most studies agree that the risk of incarceration of asymptomatic hernias is small. One consideration that is most important in the decision to choose watchful waiting over repair is how the presence of the hernia might limit the activities of the aging individual. An important predictor of long-term survival and quality of life in older persons is maintenance of function and mobility. A recent trial showed that watchful waiting was safe. Family members were surveyed about the ability of the hernia patient to perform four activities—normal activities around the home, normal work, social activities, and recreational activities. Based off the family members who were surveyed, 25% to 30% reported some level of concern about the patient's ability to perform these activities. It was suggested these results favor repair.

Approximately 15% to 30% of hernia repairs for older adults are performed on an emergent basis. Incarceration, if it does occur, can be catastrophic, particularly for the frail older person. This is mainly the result of the high incidence of strangulation found at the time of surgery. Intestinal resection is required in up to 12% to 20% of incarcerated inguinal hernias and in as many as 40% of incarcerated femoral hernias. The decision to operate for asymptomatic or mildly symptomatic hernias is made on an individual basis by balancing the possible consequences of watchful waiting with the risks of the surgery. Care should be taken to determine whether the patient has limited his or her activities to avoid mild discomfort by seeking input from the family. Decreased activity presents more of a risk to the overall health of older persons than the operative risk associated with inguinal hernia repair.

Incisional hernias in older adults are common and may be challenging to repair. Unlike laparoscopic inguinal hernia repair, there is a clear benefit to utilizing this technique as long as preexisting comorbidities and technical difficulty do not preclude the use of laparoscopic techniques. Recent studies have shown decreased wound complication and length of stay in the laparoscopic groups.

Vascular Diseases

The most frequent peripheral vascular diseases seen in older patients are abdominal aortic aneurysms (AAAs), carotid artery disease, and peripheral arterial occlusive disease. Under elective conditions and in patients with well-managed concomitant disease, vascular surgery remains safe and effective. In addition, in many cases, endovascular technology is changing patterns of intervention.

Abdominal Aortic Aneurysm

Despite the high incidence of comorbidities in this age group, mortality from elective AAA repair is generally considered to be less than 5% in patients 65 years old and older. However, recent evidence has called into question the effects of age on the outcome of AAA repair. It has now been shown that there is a strong effect of age on mortality. This has been shown in a recent study that looked at perioperative mortality rate in younger and older males and females. The results shows that males 85 years old and older have almost five times the perioperative mortality rate of younger men, and females 85 years old and older have over 10 times the mortality rate of younger women. Similarly, 5-year mortality after AAA repair in older male and female patients is approximately 80% to 90% compared with 25% to 30% in younger patients. Octogenarians are more difficult to treat by endovascular aneurysm repair (EVAR) than younger patients due to poorer anatomic suitability and a higher incidence of complications. Recovery of quality of life in octogenarians takes longer (>12 months) than expected. As EVAR has become more prevalent, experience with open AAA repair is diminishing, with concomitant increased mortality and morbidity associated with open surgery. In older patients, complications occur in approximately one third of open AAA repairs with infrarenal clamping and in over 50% of those with suprarenal clamping. Also, suprarenal clamping continues to be associated with increases in 30-day mortality, renal insufficiency, intraoperative blood loss, hospital length of stay, and rate of discharge to a nursing home. These results suggest that open AAA repair is becoming even less appropriate for most older patients, especially as the mean age of "older" patients increases.

This is supported by recent data from the Veterans Affairs Cooperative Study Group in a prospective randomized trial comparing EVAR to open repair in 881 patients with asymptomatic AAA. The previously reported reduction in perioperative mortality with endovascular repair was sustained at 2 years and at 3 years, but not thereafter. There were 10 aneurysm-related deaths in the endovascular-repair group (2.3%) versus 16 in the open-repair group (3.7%, $P = 0.22$). Six aneurysm ruptures were confirmed in the endovascular-repair group versus none in the open-repair group ($P = 0.03$). A significant interaction was observed between age and type of treatment ($P = 0.006$); survival was increased among patients younger than 70 years of age in the endovascular-repair group, but these patients tended to be better among the patients who were 70 years of age or older in the open-repair group (Fig. 13.12).[34] The true usefulness of EVAR may be with the repair of ruptured AAA. Emergency open repair for rupture is still associated with an operative mortality rate higher than 50% and an extremely high morbidity rate in those who do survive. However, based off of the reports of EVAR, ruptured aneurysms are encouraging, which means there is reduced mortality rate. A recent collective review of worldwide experience with more than 1700 patients with ruptured aneurysms has shown a 30-day mortality rate of 19.7% in patients treated with EVAR compared with 36.3% in patients treated with open repair. In addition, the outcome of ruptured AAA might be improved by wider use of local anesthesia for EVAR.[34] It is probable that the durability of stent grafts will increase over time. This suggests that EVAR is likely to be appropriate for older patients with suitable anatomy for repair. In conclusion, future directions involve fenestrated grafts for juxtarenal and pararenal aneurysms. This will extend the seal zone to include the superior mesenteric and celiac arteries.

Carotid Artery Disease

Treatment of carotid disease for the prevention of stroke remains a common issue for older patients. In patients older than 65 to 80 years old, the stroke rate from surgery is approximately 2.8% and the mortality rate is 2.4%. Survival of patients older than 80 years old after carotid endarterectomy is similar to that in the general population. The incidence of neurologic symptoms after endarterectomy is lower than in an unoperated patient (13% vs. 33%), and the incidence of late stroke is much lower as well (2% vs. 17%). Based off of the data, there is confirmation on the efficacy of endarterectomy in older patients. Suitable indications in octogenarians are similar to those in younger patients and include high-grade carotid lesions and hemispheric symptoms, with well-controlled concomitant disease. The development of carotid artery angioplasty and stenting was originally thought to be a breakthrough, as the procedure is a minimally invasive treatment for carotid disease, with wide applicability. Among elderly patients with symptomatic or asymptomatic carotid stenosis, there is a risk of the composite primary outcome of stroke, myocardial infarction, or death, and these outcomes did not differ significantly when comparing the groups undergoing carotid artery stenting and the groups undergoing carotid endarterectomy (Fig. 13.13). During the periprocedural period, there was a higher risk of stroke with stenting and a higher risk of myocardial infarction with endarterectomy. Patients older than 75 years old have increased arch calcium deposits and increased arch tortuosity compared with younger patients. This suggests that increased stroke risk is inherent to standard femoral approaches generally used for carotid artery angioplasty and stenting, so age should be considered when planning a carotid intervention. Carotid stenting has an increased risk of adverse cerebrovascular events in elderly patients,

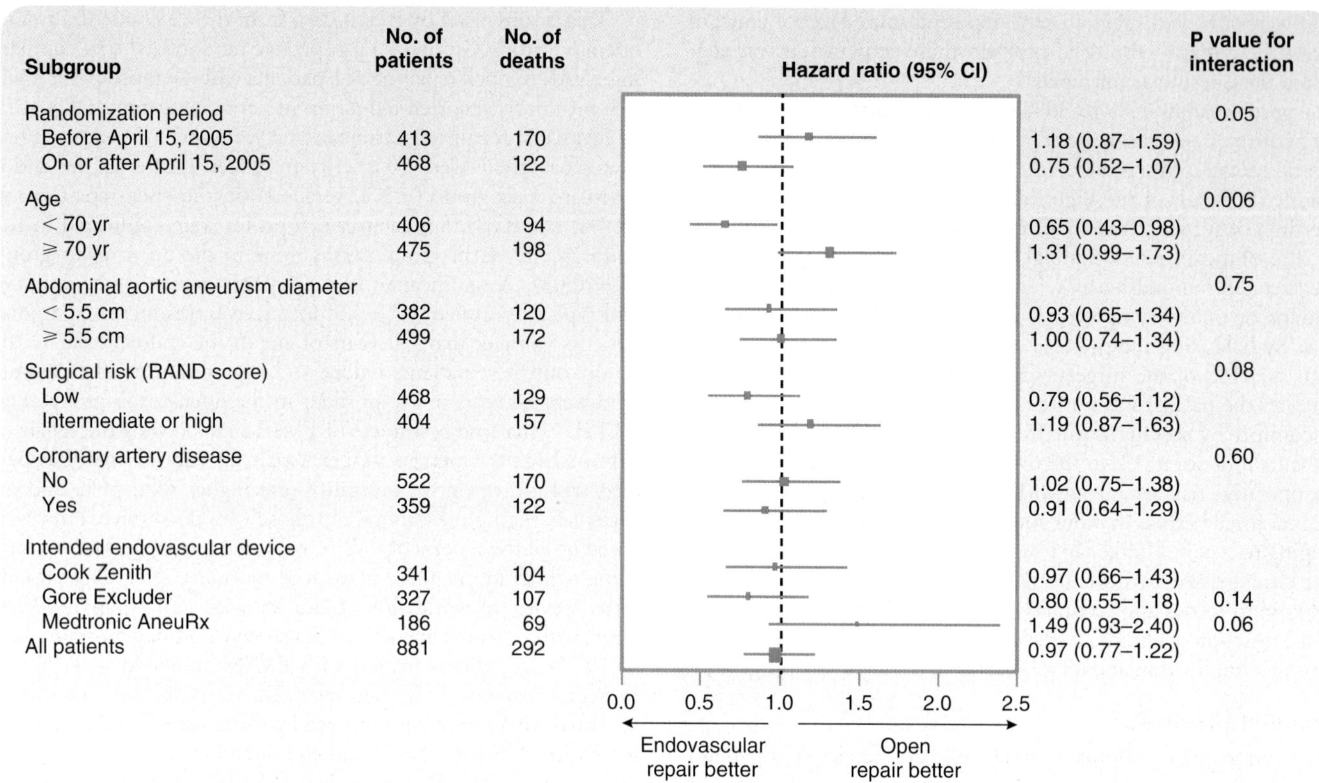

FIG. 13.12 Factors predictive of death in endovascular and open repair. (From Lederle FA, Freischlag JA, Kyriakides TC et al. Long-term comparison of endovascular and open repair of abdominal aortic aneurysm. *N Engl J Med.* 2012;367:1988–1997.)

but mortality is equivalent to younger patients. At the expense of increased mortality, carotid endarterectomy is associated with similar neurologic outcomes in elderly and young patients.[35]

Peripheral Vascular Disease

Peripheral vascular surgery for limb salvage is indicated for ischemic pain at rest, nonhealing ulcers, or frank gangrene. Although reports continue to show that age older than 80 years is a relative risk factor for increased perioperative mortality, surgery can generally be safely performed in older patients, especially when performed electively. In patients older than 80 years old, the mortality rate associated with surgery is less than 5%, and limb salvage rates over a period of 3 to 5 years are 50% to almost 90%. Five-year graft patency rates have been reported to be better in older than in younger patients with both prosthetic and autologous graft materials. However, there are only a small number of patients who have been studied, so this suggests that larger series are still needed to validate these single-center reports. Nevertheless, it is clear that older patients certainly do no worse than younger patients after infrageniculate bypass surgery. Treatment of graft infections in older patients is morbid, but aggressive wound care and muscle flap coverage are an option with good results (>50% graft salvage and 90% limb salvage). Endovascular approaches can also be used in the periphery in older patients, with reasonable durability in those with limited life expectancy. Angioplasty of the superficial femoral artery has a 5-year cumulative primary patency rate higher than 50% and a secondary patency rate of up to 70% in older patients. It is unclear whether these results will lead to increased treatment of older claudicant patients, as it has in younger patients. In a recent study of mostly elderly patients, at 5 years, endovascular-first and open-first revascularization strategies had equivalent limb salvage rates and amputation-free survival in patients with critical limb ischemia when properly selected.[36]

After the procedure has been performed, the quality of life and preservation or restoration of functional independence are the most important considerations in older patients. Amputation can be performed safely in older patients, with rates of perioperative mortality less than 10%. However, long-term survival after amputation is poor, with 1-year survival rates of approximately 50%. In addition, there are independent risk factors for mortality which include high-level amputation, congestive heart failure, and the inability to ambulate in the community. These functionally poor results of amputation lead many surgeons to continue to offer an aggressive approach to limb salvage in older patients.

Cardiothoracic Diseases

Cardiovascular disease has been the leading cause of death in the United States for almost 100 years. In the new millennium, cardiovascular disease is still present in approximately 64 million Americans, or 23% of the population. Most deaths attributable to cardiovascular disease occur in older patients.

Cardiac surgery is usually a dramatic event for patients and, accordingly, is one of the most frequently studied surgical procedures. Older patients have excellent results after cardiac surgery; as minimally invasive treatment of cardiac atherosclerosis changes patterns of referral to cardiac surgeons, patients are becoming older, with more frequent and severe comorbid conditions. Mortality in nonagenarians is approximately 14% but 5-year survival is approximately 59%. Factors associated with excellent outcome in older patients include technically flawless surgery, meticulous

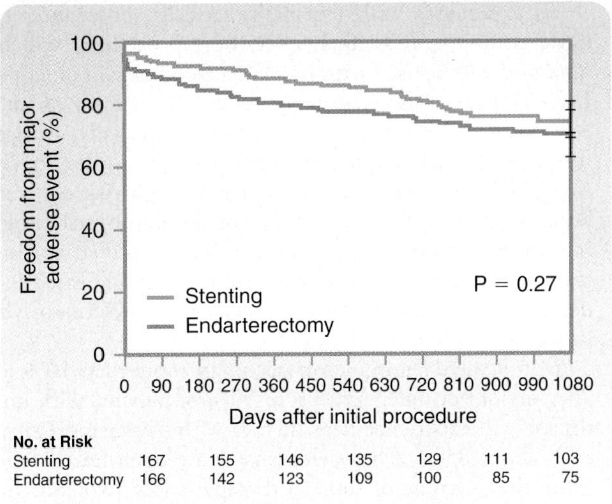

A

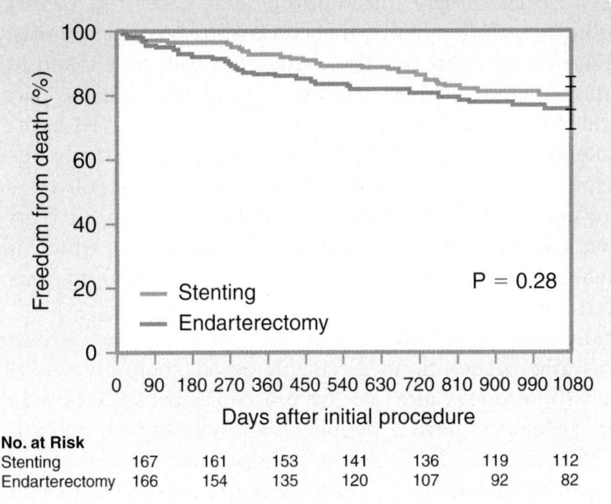

B

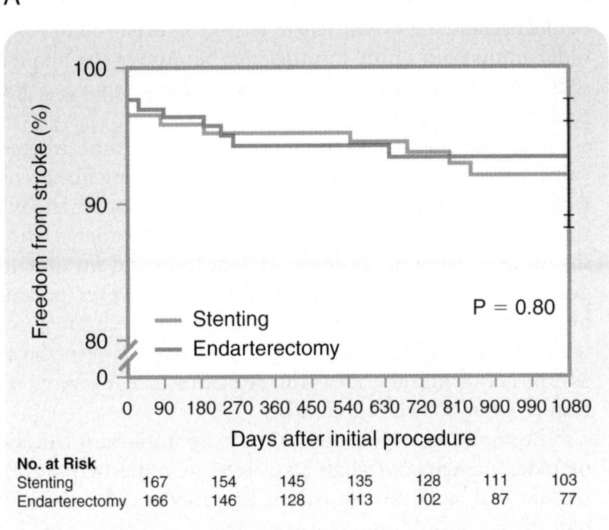

C

FIG. 13.13 Kaplan-Mier curves depicting outcomes of major adverse events, stroke, and death in patients undergoing carotid endarterectomy and carotid stenting. (From Gurm HS, Yadav JS, Fayad P, et al. Long-term results of carotid stenting versus endarterectomy in high-risk patients. *N Engl J Med.* 2008;358:1572–1579.)

hemostasis, excellent myocardial protection, and perfect anesthesia management. Frailty has been shown to be a predictor of mortality and morbidity after cardiac surgery and has been recommended to be added to the cardiac surgery risk score.

Coronary Artery Disease

The number of coronary artery bypass grafting (CABG) procedures performed on patients older than 65 years old rose from 2.6 operations/1000 in 1980 to 13.0 operations/1000 in 1993. However, with the increasing use and success of percutaneous coronary artery interventions, the rate of CABG cases in persons older than 65 years old has fallen to 8.9/1000. This pattern is reflective of the performance of CABG cases in the general population, increasing from 7.2/1000 discharges in 1988 to 12.2/1000 in 1997, decreasing to 9.1/1000 in 2003; nevertheless, overall mortality after CABG decreased from 5.4% in 1988 to approximately 3.3% in 2003.

Patients who are now referred for bypass usually have more complex disease or have failed alternative procedures. More than 50% of CABG procedures are now performed on patients older than 65 years old. As the mortality and morbidity associated with cardiac surgical procedures have decreased, there has been a growing willingness to offer surgical therapy to older patients with reconstructible coronary artery disease. Unfortunately, older patients referred for cardiac surgery have a higher incidence of advanced disease (e.g., triple-vessel disease, left main or main equivalent disease, poor left ventricular function) and more symptomatic disease (90% of octogenarians are preoperatively classified as New York Heart Association [NYHA] functional class III or IV) and require emergency or urgent procedures more often.

Comorbid disease must be considered in older patients and may be extensive in some. Several preoperative risk factors for mortality after coronary bypass surgery have been identified, including an emergency procedure, severe left ventricular dysfunction, mitral insufficiency requiring a combined procedure, NYHA functional class IV, elevated preoperative creatinine level, chronic pulmonary disease, anemia (hematocrit <34%), and previous vascular surgery. In addition, some other risk factors for morbidity include obesity, diabetes mellitus, aortic stenosis, and cerebrovascular disease. These risk factors must be taken in the context of global patient comorbidity and considered as part of informed decision-making for an individual patient. Risks attributable to patients age 70 to 79 years are not significantly different from risks attributable to patients younger than 60 years old. However, when compared to patients older than 80 years old, these patients have increased age-associated risk, which is equivalent to the presence of shock or acute (<6 hours) myocardial infarction.

In individuals older than 80 years old, coronary artery bypass surgery is associated with an acceptable overall mortality of 7% to 12%, with mortality after elective procedures being lower than 3%. Nonagenarians have a perioperative mortality of approximately 15% to 20%, but a 5-year postoperative survival of approximately 50%, and this represents a significant survival benefit associated with surgery. In addition, early elective surgery is clearly preferable to emergency surgery, which is associated with 2 to 10 times higher mortality.

In elderly patients undergoing percutaneous coronary intervention, major adverse coronary event rates are relatively high, but successful revascularization is associated with a reduction in these outcomes at 5-year follow-up. When examining the outcomes of elderly patients treated with drug-eluting stents, the rates of 1-year all-cause death were nearly four times higher in octogenarians than in nonoctogenarians.

Morbidity after coronary surgery in older adults is high in many series. Pulmonary failure can be due to requiring prolonged intubation, neurologic events such as cerebrovascular accidents and delirium, and sternal wound infections, which increase with age, and all of these factors are associated with postoperative mortality. Other complications include reoperation for bleeding, the need for pacemaker insertion, perioperative myocardial infarction, and superficial wound infections. These complications occur with equal frequency in both younger and older patients even though some studies have noted a slightly higher incidence of sternal wound infection in older patients. Older patients with end-stage heart failure have traditionally been excluded from the option of cardiac transplantation because of the scarcity of donor hearts and an inability to tolerate pharmacologic immunosuppression easily. Recent reports of partial left ventriculostomy are encouraging especially since the mortality and functional outcome in patients older than 65 years old are similar to that in younger patients.

Valvular Disease

Since 1975, there have not been enough data accumulated that support the safety and efficacy of aortic valve replacement in older adults. Operative mortality is 3% to 10%, and the long-term survival rate is approximately 75% to 80%. Although mortality in older patients is slightly higher than that in younger patients, most differences were not statistically significant. The vast majority of older patients receiving new aortic valves have great improvement in their quality of life. As many as 90% of older patients who were classified as NYHA functional class III or IV preoperatively and survive are reclassified postoperatively as class I or II. Since the average life expectancy for a healthy 70-year-old is approximately 13 years and for an 80-year-old is approximately 8 years, safe aortic valve replacement surgery is preferable to the approximately 80%, 4-year mortality associated with untreated symptomatic aortic stenosis.

As experience with minimally invasive procedures become more common, it is likely that these procedures will become safer and will be used with increased frequency in older patients. Early clinical trials confirm the safety and efficacy of transcatheter aortic valve replacement (TAVR), especially in high- and intermediate-risk surgical patients. Recent studies are showing that TAVR may be a safe approach in high-risk octogenarians because there is lower likelihood of developing AKI, bleeding, requiring blood transfusion, or transfer to a skilled nursing facility. The number of TAVR have progressively increased in young octogenarians with >95% of octogenarians in Germany with this procedure with aortic disease.

Mitral valve regurgitation occurs in more than 10% of those 75 years old or older, and up to 50% of patients with untreated disease will experience heart failure with 5-year mortality. However, about 85% of octogenarians refuse open-heart surgery because the outcome of surgical therapy is less favorable, having a slightly higher operative mortality after mitral valve replacement compared with the mortality rate after aortic valve replacement in octogenarians. Left ventricular reserve is often compromised in older adults with mitral insufficiency because of the frequently associated ischemic disease. Also, low cardiac output is a particular problem after mitral valve replacement.

Transcatheter mitral valve replacement and transcatheter mitral valve repair are emerging as an alternative therapy for severe mitral regurgitation in high-risk surgical patients. Repair is considered the gold standard especially in acceptable risk patients with extensive bi-leaflet or anterior leaflet calcification and myxomatous degermation without extensive calcification. However, patients with high prohibitive risks may benefit from interventional approach with MitraClip. This device allows a bridge between the anterior and posterior mitral leaflet. The rate of recurrent severe regurgitation is about 55% at 12 months.

The choice of valve material is also an important consideration in older patients. Mechanical valves are extremely durable but require lifelong anticoagulation. In patients older than 75 years old, the mortality from long-term anticoagulation alone is almost 10%/yr. Bioprosthetic valves do not require anticoagulation and are somewhat less durable, but bioprosthetic valves may suffice for patients with a life expectancy of less than 10 years.[37]

Lung Cancer

Lung cancer, usually adenocarcinoma or squamous cell carcinoma, remains a leading cause of death in industrialized countries. More than 150,000 deaths are still caused by lung cancer in the United States annually. Also, smoking remains the most important risk factor for lung cancer, and smoking cessation is an appropriate preventive measure for all patients. Appropriate therapy is critically dependent on accurate staging from a CT scan, and ^{18}F-fluorodeoxyglucose positron emission tomography is currently playing increasing diagnostic roles.

The incidence of non–small-cell lung cancer (NSCLC) increases with age. As seen, the recommendations of the American Association of Thoracic Surgery Task Force for Lung Cancer Screening and Surveillance differed from other professional society's recommendations in two particular areas: an increase in the age of the screened population to age 79 years and an annual scan schedule that extends beyond a 3-year start.[38] There is still bias that older patients with early-stage (I–III) NSCLC do poorly with surgical resection, and, thus, these patients are often referred for limited resection or radiation therapy. Aggressive chemotherapy, particularly platinum-based adjuvant therapy, is often poorly tolerated by older patients. Recent studies including elderly patients and mainly stage IB to IIIA NSCLC patients show that preoperative chemotherapy significantly improves overall survival, time to distant recurrence, and recurrence-free survival in resectable NSCLC. These findings suggest that a valid treatment option for most of these patients is the use of preoperative chemotherapy. Toxic effects could not be assessed in the study, however.[38] As such, many older patients have less than a full staging workup, incomplete histologic diagnoses, or undocumented performance status. Stage IV disease is initially diagnosed in most patients with NSCLC, and they may be treated with combined chemotherapy and radiation therapy. However, older patients are not often considered candidates for this therapy. The use of single agent (oral etoposide) is not recommended in this population based on inferior survival compared with multidrug IV treatment. Likewise, dose attenuation of standard cisplatin/etoposide regimen was associated with poorer outcome. There is a significant interaction in poor performance status with age, favoring cisplatin-based treatment in younger patients (<70 years old) and carboplatin-based treatment in older patients. Neoadjuvant therapy is generally prescribed in older patients who are borderline candidates for surgery, would benefit from tumor downstaging, or would best be treated definitively by radiation therapy.

Evidence has suggested improved outcomes in older patients after surgical treatment of lung cancer.[38] Surgical resection for lung cancer is associated with an operative mortality rate of approximately 6%, although approximately 50% of patients still suffer some postoperative morbidity, such as atrial fibrillation, pneumonia, or retained secretions requiring bronchoscopy. Five-year survival in older patients after pulmonary resection for cancer is approximately 35%, with up to 40% survival in patients undergoing just lobectomy. Video-assisted thoracic surgery (VATS) is finding increased application, with some surgeons performing VATS for lung cancer resection. The potential for less operating time and blood loss, as well as short hospital length of stay and improved recovery time, holds great promise for all patients, especially older adults. In addition, the perioperative mortality rate for octogenarians treated with VATS is as low as 2%. VATS is associated with a similar 5-year survival rate compared with conventional open surgery, and the increased age remains associated with more complications but only marginally worse survival. Results such as these suggest that VATS may increase the number of older patients who will be candidates for surgical therapy. In a recently published review of retrospective series, lobectomy emerged as the surgical treatment of choice for carefully selected, operable octogenarians with early stage lung cancer. The reported 5-year survival for stage I NSCLC was 56% and reached 62% for stage Ia.

It is likely that future reports will define combinations of adjuvant and neoadjuvant therapy and the analysis of oncologic genomic signatures. Therefore, there will be an increase in the number of older patients who will be surgical candidates and achieve disease-free survival. However, the outlook for older patients with preexisting pulmonary disease or other severe comorbid conditions remains poor.

Trauma

Trauma is currently the fifth leading cause of death in older adults. Persons older than 65 years old account for up to one third of trauma cases and 30% to 40% of trauma deaths, with more recent rates being the highest. Older patients have increased mortality, longer hospital stays, increased morbidity, and worse functional outcomes than younger patients. Motor vehicle accidents are the most common form of fatal injury in patients younger than 80 years old, and falls are the most frequent fatal injury after the age of 80 years. Interestingly, the incidence of death from motor vehicle accidents in older adults is the same whether they are passengers or pedestrians.

Older persons are at an increased risk for blunt trauma and its complications. Age-associated central nervous system changes decrease coordination and mobility and therefore lead to an increase of risk for accidents. Cerebral atrophy and decreased viscoelastic properties within the cranial vault make the brain more susceptible to blunt injury. Increased bone fragility results in an increased tendency for fracture. Decreased cardiac reserve and inability to increase cardiac output prevent avoidance of accidents. Concomitant use of drugs such as anticoagulants and antiplatelet agents increases the morbidity associated with traumatic events in older patients.

Significant injury can result from even simple falls from a level surface to the ground. The incidence of fracture or serious injury from such a fall is as high as 40% in an older person. After a fall with injury, there is significant morbidity. Of those hospitalized after a fall, up to 50% of patients need to be discharged from the hospital to a nursing facility, and only 50% are alive 1 year later. Elevator injuries in older patients are most commonly a slip, trip, or fall but are associated with 15% hospital admission; 40% of these admissions are for a fractured hip.

Older patients have increased morbidity and mortality after head trauma, particularly when taking anticoagulant medications. Older people have increased rates of traumatic brain injury after head trauma and have longer disability. They take much longer time to recover from head trauma than younger people and require more intensive rehabilitation. Blunt head trauma in an older person carries a particularly high mortality. Mortality in older patients with a Glasgow Coma Scale score of 5 is more than twice that of patients aged 20 to 40 years, and only 2% of older patients have a favorable recovery as compared with 38% of younger patients.

Injury from burns accounts for 8% of trauma in older patients. Older adults are at particular risk for burns because of impaired vision, decreased reaction time, depressed alertness, and decreased sensation of pain. In most older burn victims, injuries occur as a result of actions during ADLs—scalding, cooking accidents with flame, and electrical burns. In all patients, survival from burns is directly related to the total body surface area (TBSA) affected, but this association is more pronounced in older adults. In general, burns involving more than 40% of the TBSA in older persons have a poor prognosis. Reasons for the increased mortality are concomitant medical disease, burn wound sepsis, and multisystem failure, including pneumonia. For survivors of serious burns for patients who are 59 years old or older, fewer than 50% are discharged to independent living, one third to assisted living at home, and 20% to nursing facilities.

Older patients, whether they live with relatives or are institutionalized, are at risk for trauma as a result of elder abuse. It is estimated that 5% of older adults living in the community are subject to this type of maltreatment. It has also been shown that only 1 in 13 or 14 cases of elder abuse is reported. Maltreatment of older people can take one or more of six basic forms: physical abuse, sexual abuse, neglect, psychological abuse, financial exploitation, and violation of rights. As the older adult population increases, surgeons treating older trauma victims must learn to detect and report signs of physical and sexual abuse in addition to providing physical care of the patient's injuries, much as they have been mandated to do with children.[39]

Transplantation

In 1946, the first successful renal transplantation was performed. Early results with cadaveric renal transplants in patients older than 45 years old were poor. The introduction of cyclosporine in the 1980s led to dramatic improvements, particularly in high-risk patients. As experience at transplantation centers has grown and the population of those older than 60 years old has increased, the number of older patients who could potentially benefit from transplantation has also increased. Over the past two decades, the rate of persons older than 65 years old requiring renal replacement therapy in the United States has doubled, and the rate in those older than 75 years old has tripled.

There is proven benefit of renal transplantation for the elderly; however, this may be compromised due to difficulties in access to a transplant. In one study of renal transplantation, patients older than 60 years old had more delayed graft function and a longer initial hospital stay, but the incidence of acute rejection episodes was lower. Patient survival, graft survival, and death-censored graft survival did not differ between older and younger patients, although follow-up of older patients was shorter (4.1 vs. 6.7 years). The main cause of organ loss in older patients was death with a functioning kidney. Other studies have shown that 10-year allograft survival is higher in older patients than in patients younger than 60 years old. However, the survival rate at 10 years in those older than 60 years old is 44% versus 81% for younger patients. Given the shortage of organ donors, the ethics of transplantation in older individuals with a higher likelihood of dying with a functioning allograft is questioned, although many believe that the evidence does not justify denying transplantation on the basis of age alone. Consideration of factors such as physical and cognitive function and frailty in addition to comorbidity may enhance the process of evaluation for transplant in the geriatric population. Kidneys with high Kidney Donor Profile Index scores and living donor organs may become the most realistic transplant options for seniors in light of amended allocation policy.

The number of older persons requiring liver transplantation has also increased. The percentage of liver recipients older than 65 years old has increased from 4.9% in 1991 to 6.8% in 2002. Although age has been identified as a risk factor for a poorer outcome after liver transplantation, when patients are in better health (e.g., living at home at the time of transplantation), age is not a factor. Many studies have supported liver transplantation in low-risk, properly evaluated older adults.[40] As the number of older transplant patients has increased, one important factor has emerged. The rate of acute and chronic rejection is clearly lower in older patients. This has been attributed to the overall decline in immunocompetence with age. However, this decline also renders older patients more susceptible to infection and malignancy. The high incidence of lymphoproliferative disorders in older transplant patients in general and the high rate of recurrent hepatitis C in older liver transplant patients in particular may be the result of excessive immunosuppression in this already compromised population. Decreasing immunosuppression in older patients may, in fact, improve both long- and short-term survival.

SELECTED REFERENCES

Chow W, Rosenthal RA, Merkow RP, et al. Optimal preoperative assessment of the geriatric surgery patient: a best practice guideline from the american college of surgeons national surgery quality improvement program and the american geriatrics society. *J Am Coll Surg*. 2012;215:453–466.

With the support of the John A. Hartford Foundation, the American College of Surgeons National Surgical Quality Improvement Program and the American Geriatrics Society assembled a 21-member expert panel to create best practice guidelines for the optimal preoperative assessment of the geriatric patient. These guidelines are based on evidence where available and on consensus expert opinion where evidence is not available. It provides a comprehensive checklist and supporting tools to help clinicians perform a thorough evaluation of factors that impact the surgical outcomes of older adults.

Finlayson E, Wang L, Landefeld CS, et al. Major abdominal surgery in nursing home residents: a national study. *Ann Surg*. 2011;254:921–926.

Using national Medicare claims data and the nursing home Minimum Data Set, nursing home patients were compared to nonnursing home patients. Results show that nursing home residents experience substantially higher rates of mortality and invasive interventions after surgery than other Medicare beneficiaries. These findings should be used to council patients and for physicians to consider in their discussion.

Fried TR, Bradley EH, Towle VR, et al. Understanding the treatment preferences of seriously ill patients. *N Engl J Med*. 2002;346:1061–1066.

Elderly patients were asked about their preferences for treatment based on the likelihood of an adverse outcome. The authors found that the burden of treatment, its outcomes, and the likelihood of outcomes all influence patient treatment preferences. Most patients chose low burden therapy. If patients felt they had a risk of severe cognitive impairment, most would not want to receive the therapy. This work supports the importance of talking with patients about treatment options and outcomes.

Garg K, Kaszubski PA, Moridzadeh R, et al. Endovascular-first approach is not associated with worse amputation-free survival in appropriately selected patients with critical limb ischemia. *J Vasc Surg*. 2014;59:392–399.

This was a retrospective analysis of patients with critical limb ischemia that were initially revascularized with either an endovascular or open approach. The endo-first was performed in 187 (62%), open-first in 105 (35%), and 10 (3%) had hybrid procedures. The authors showed that at 5 years, the endo-first and open-first revascularization strategies had equivalent limb salvage rates and amputation-free survival rates in patients with critical limb ischemia when properly selected. A patient-centered approach with close surveillance improves long-term outcomes for both open and endo approaches.

Rostagno C. Heart valve disease in elderly. *World J Cardiol.* 2019;11:71–83.

There is an increased prevalence of degenerative disease in the elderly with heart valve abnormalities leading to high morbidity and mortality. Heart valve disease represents in about 5% of older patients aged ≥75 years old for both mitral and aortic disease. The author reviews the epidemiology and pathophysiology in aortic and mitral valve disease in older adults. The article evaluates the recent surgical options and reviews current developments in interventional procedures for intermediate and high-risk patients.

REFERENCES

1. Arias E, Xu J. United States life tables, 2017. *Natl Vital Stat Rep.* 2017;68:1–66.
2. Ortman JM, Velkoff VA, Hogan H. *An Aging Nation: The Older Population in the United States. Current Population Reports.* Washington, DC: U.S. Census Bureau; 2014:P25–1140.
3. Liu Y, Cohen ME, Hall BL, et al. Evaluation and enhancement of calibration in the american college of surgeons NSQIP surgical risk calculator. *J Am Coll Surg.* 2016;223:231–239.
4. Robinson TN, Rosenthal RA. The ACS NSQIP geriatric surgery pilot project: improving care for older surgical patients. *Bull Am Coll Surg.* 2014;99:21–23.
5. Berian JR, Zhou L, Hornor MA, et al. Optimizing surgical quality datasets to care for older adults: lessons from the american college of surgeons NSQIP geriatric surgery pilot. *J Am Coll Surg.* 2017;225:702–712 e701.
6. Hornor MA, Ma M, Zhou L, et al. Enhancing the american college of surgeons NSQIP surgical risk calculator to predict geriatric outcomes. *J Am Coll Surg.* 2020;230:88–100 e101.
7. Fried LP, Walston J. Frailty and failure to thrive. In: Hazzard WR, Blass JP, Ettinger Jr WH, Halter JB, Ouslander J, eds. *Principles of Geriatric Medicine and Gerontology.* 4th ed. New York: McGraw Hill; 1998:1387–1402.
8. Fried LP, Tangen CM, Walston J, et al. Frailty in older adults: evidence for a phenotype. *J Gerontol A Biol Sci Med Sci.* 2001;56:M146–M156.
9. Rockwood K, Mitnitski A. Frailty defined by deficit accumulation and geriatric medicine defined by frailty. *Clin Geriatr Med.* 2011;27:17–26.
10. Kim DH, Patorno E, Pawar A, et al. Measuring frailty in administrative claims data: comparative performance of four claims-based frailty measures in the United States Medicare data [published online ahead of print September 30, 2019]. *J Gerontol Biol Sci Med Sci.*
11. Chang AM, Halter JB. Aging and insulin secretion. *Am J Physiol Endocrinol Metab.* 2003;284:E7–E12.
12. Kruser JM, Nabozny MJ, Steffens NM, et al. "Best case/worst case": qualitative evaluation of a novel communication tool for difficult in-the-moment surgical decisions. *J Am Geriatr Soc.* 2015;63:1805–1811.
13. Cooper Z, Koritsanszky LA, Cauley CE, et al. Recommendations for best communication practices to facilitate goal-concordant care for seriously ill older patients with emergency surgical conditions. *Ann Surg.* 2016;263:1–6.
14. Sharp T, Moran E, Kuhn I, et al. Do the elderly have a voice? Advance care planning discussions with frail and older individuals: a systematic literature review and narrative synthesis. *Br J Gen Pract.* 2013;63:e657–e668.
15. Ernst KF, Hall DE, Schmid KK, et al. Surgical palliative care consultations over time in relationship to systemwide frailty screening. *JAMA Surg.* 2014;149:1121–1126.
16. Marcantonio ER, Goldman L, Mangione CM, et al. A clinical prediction rule for delirium after elective noncardiac surgery. *JAMA.* 1994;271:134–139.
17. Eagle KA, Berger PB, Calkins H, et al. ACC/AHA guideline update for perioperative cardiovascular evaluation for noncardiac surgery—executive summary a report of the american college of cardiology/american heart association task force on practice guidelines (committee to update the 1996 guidelines on perioperative cardiovascular evaluation for noncardiac surgery). *Circulation.* 2002;105:1257–1267.
18. Podsiadlo D, Richardson S. The timed "up & go": a test of basic functional mobility for frail elderly persons. *J Am Geriatr Soc.* 1991;39:142–148.
19. D'Alegria B, Cohen C, Medeiros F, et al. Nutritional diagnosis obtained by subjective global assessment in surgical patients and occurrence of post operative complications. *Nutr Hosp.* 2008;23:621.
20. American geriatrics society updated beers criteria for potentially inappropriate medication use in older adults. *J Am Geriatr Soc.* 2012;60:616–631.
21. Slieker J, Frauche P, Jurt J, et al. Enhanced recovery ERAS for elderly: a safe and beneficial pathway in colorectal surgery. *Int J Colorectal Dis.* 2017;32:215–221.
22. American College of Surgeons Optimum Resources for Geriatric Surgery. 2019. https://www.facs.org/quality-programs/geriatric-surgery. Accessed January 16, 2020.
23. Berian JR, Zhou L, Russell MM, et al. Postoperative delirium as a target for surgical quality improvement. *Ann Surg.* 2018;268:93–99.
24. Suiter DM, Leder SB. Clinical utility of the 3-ounce water swallow test. *Dysphagia.* 2008;23:244–250.
25. Berian JR, Mohanty S, Ko CY, et al. Association of loss of independence with readmission and death after discharge in older patients after surgical procedures. *JAMA Surg.* 2016;151:e161689.
26. Naylor MD, Brooten D, Campbell R, et al. Comprehensive discharge planning and home follow-up of hospitalized elders: a randomized clinical trial. *JAMA.* 1999;281:613–620.
27. Lechner MG, Hershman JM. Thyroid nodules and cancer in the elderly. In: Feingold KR, Anawalt B, Boyce A, et al., eds. *Endotext.* South Dartmouth, MA: MD Text com. Inc; 2018:1–40.
28. Tesarova P. Specific aspects of breast cancer therapy of elderly women. *Biomed Res Int.* 2016;2016:1381695.
29. Liguigli W, Tomasello G, Toppo L, et al. Safety and efficacy of dose-dense chemotherapy with TCF regimen in elderly patients with locally advanced or metastatic gastric cancer. *Tumori.* 2017;103:93–100.
30. Bower KL, Lollar DI, Williams SL, et al. Small bowel obstruction. *Surg Clin North Am.* 2018;98:945–971.
31. Buckius MT, McGrath B, Monk J, et al. Changing epidemiology of acute appendicitis in the United States: study period 1993–2008. *J Surg Res.* 2012;175:185–190.
32. Li Z, Coleman J, D'Adamo CR, et al. Operative mortality prediction for primary rectal cancer: age matters. *J Am Coll Surg.* 2019;228:627–633.
33. Booth CM, Nanji S, Wei X, et al. Management and outcome of colorectal cancer liver metastases in elderly patients: a population-based study. *JAMA Oncol.* 2015;1:1111–1119.

34. Patel R, Sweeting MJ, Powell JT, et al. Endovascular versus open repair of abdominal aortic aneurysm in 15-years' follow-up of the UK endovascular aneurysm repair trial 1 (EVAR trial 1): a randomised controlled trial. *Lancet*. 2016;388:2366–2374.
35. Perkins WJ, Lanzino G, Brott TG. Carotid stenting vs endarterectomy: new results in perspective. *Mayo Clin Proc.* 2010;85:1101–1108.
36. Garg K, Kaszubski PA, Moridzadeh R, et al. Endovascular-first approach is not associated with worse amputation-free survival in appropriately selected patients with critical limb ischemia. *J Vasc Surg*. 2014;59:392–399.
37. Rostagno C. Heart valve disease in elderly. *World J Cardiol.* 2019;11:71–83.
38. Detillon D, Veen EJ. Postoperative outcome after pulmonary surgery for non-small cell lung cancer in elderly patients. *Ann Thorac Surg*. 2018;105:287–293.
39. Kwan E, Straus SE. Assessment and management of falls in older people. *CMAJ*. 2014;186:E610–E621.
40. Chen HP, Tsai YF, Lin JR, et al. Recipient age and mortality risk after liver transplantation: a population-based cohort study. *PLoS One*. 2016;11:e0152324.

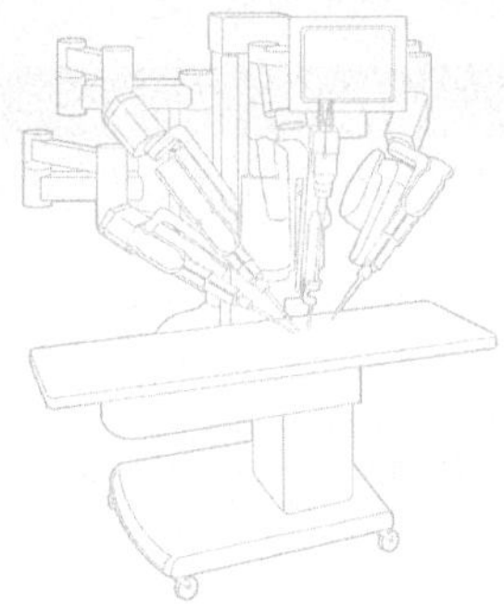

CHAPTER 14

Anesthesiology Principles, Pain Management, and Conscious Sedation

Antonio Hernandez, Edward R. Sherwood

OUTLINE

The history of anesthesiology began only a little more than 150 years ago with the administration of the first ether anesthetic. Throughout much of the subsequent history, the risk of anesthesia-related mortality and morbidity was unacceptably high as a consequence of primitive equipment, complication-prone drugs, and lack of adequate monitors. However, during the past four decades, rapid technological and pharmacologic progress has resulted in the ability to provide anesthesia safely for complex surgical procedures, even in patients with severe underlying disease.

The most notable advances in anesthesia equipment have been the development of anesthetic machines that reduce the possibility of providing hypoxic gas mixtures, vaporizers that provide accurate doses of potent inhalational agents, advanced airway devices that facilitate ventilation in difficult airway scenarios, and intraoperative anesthesia ventilators that provide more precise and sophisticated respiratory support. Pharmacologic advances have generally consisted of shorter-acting drugs with fewer important side effects. However, the greatest advances have been in monitoring devices. These include in-circuit oxygen analyzers, capnometers to assess the presence of exhaled carbon dioxide (CO_2), pulse oximeters, and anesthetic vapor–specific analyzers. Although these monitors do not guarantee a successful outcome, they markedly increase its probability. Advances in ultrasound have facilitated safe and effective execution of peripheral nerve blocks, central venous access, and hemodynamic monitoring. This chapter sets the stage for discussing anesthetic management by reviewing the unique aspects of the anesthetic environment: the drugs, equipment, and monitors that are the basis for safe practice. Subsequent sections address preanesthetic assessment and preparation for anesthesia, selection of anesthetic techniques and drugs, airway management, conscious sedation, postanesthetic care, and management of acute postoperative pain.

PHARMACOLOGIC PRINCIPLES

The initial practice of anesthesiology used single drugs such as ether or chloroform to abolish consciousness, prevent movement during surgery, ensure amnesia, and provide analgesia. In contrast, current anesthesia practice combines multiple agents, often including

TABLE 14.1 Important characteristics of inhalational agents.

ANESTHETIC	POTENCY	SPEED OF INDUCTION AND EMERGENCE	SUITABILITY FOR INHALATIONAL INDUCTION	SENSITIZATION TO CATECHOLAMINES	METABOLIZED (%)
Nitrous oxide	Weak	Fast	Insufficient alone	None	Minimal
Diethyl ether	Potent	Very slow	Suitable	None	10
Halothane	Potent	Medium	Suitable	High	20+
Enflurane	Potent	Medium	Not suitable	Medium	<10
Isoflurane	Potent	Medium	Not suitable	Minimal	<2
Sevoflurane	Potent	Rapid	Suitable	Minimal	<5
Desflurane	Potent	Rapid	Not suitable	Minimal	0.02

regional techniques, to achieve specific end points. Although inhalational agents remain at the core of modern anesthetic combinations, intravenous (IV) anesthetics, especially propofol, are gaining prominence. Most anesthesiologists initiate anesthesia with IV induction agents and then maintain anesthesia with inhalational or IV agents supplemented by adjuncts such as opioids, ketamine, lidocaine, and muscle relaxants. Benzodiazepines are often added to induce anxiolysis and amnesia. In many cases, total IV anesthesia is desirable and is executed through administration of anesthetics such as propofol in combination with opioids and other adjuncts.

Inhalational Agents

The original inhalational anesthetics—ether, nitrous oxide, and chloroform—had important limitations. Ether was characterized by notoriously slow induction and equally delayed emergence but could produce unconsciousness, amnesia, analgesia, and lack of movement without the addition of other agents. In contrast, both induction and emergence were rapid with nitrous oxide, but the agent lacked sufficient potency to be used alone. Nevertheless, nitrous oxide is still used in combination with other agents in modern practice. Chloroform was associated with hepatic toxicity and, occasionally, fatal cardiac arrhythmias.

Subsequent drug development emphasized inhalational agents that facilitate rapid induction and emergence and are nontoxic. Such drugs include isoflurane, sevoflurane, and desflurane. Although halothane and enflurane were also commonly used in the past, the use of both agents has decreased dramatically during the last 5 to 10 years. The important aspects of each volatile anesthetic can be summarized in terms of key clinical attributes (Table 14.1). Two of the most important characteristics of inhalational anesthetics are the blood/gas solubility coefficient and the minimum alveolar concentration (MAC). The blood/gas solubility coefficient is a measure of the uptake of an agent by blood. In general, less soluble agents (lower blood/gas solubility coefficients), such as nitrous oxide and desflurane, are associated with more rapid induction of and emergence from anesthesia, whereas induction and emergence are slower with agents having high solubility in blood, such as halothane. Isoflurane and sevoflurane have intermediate rates of induction and emergence. MAC is the concentration of volatile agent required to prevent movement in response to a skin incision in 50% of patients and is a way of describing the potency of a volatile anesthetic. A higher MAC represents a less potent volatile anesthetic. Among modern volatile agents, halothane is the most potent, with a MAC of 0.75%, while desflurane has a MAC of 6% and is the least potent of the hydrocarbon-based volatile agents. Nitrous oxide has a MAC of 104% at sea level, meaning that nitrous oxide alone is generally not suitable for maintenance of general anesthesia. The pungency of anesthetic agents also has practical implications. Agents with low pungency, such as halothane and sevoflurane, do not cause significant airway irritation when delivered at commonly used concentrations and are useful for inhalation induction of anesthesia. Desflurane is highly irritating to the airways and is not useful for inhalation induction under most conditions.

Nitrous Oxide

Nitrous oxide provides only partial anesthesia at atmospheric pressure because its MAC is 104% of inspired gas at sea level. Nitrous oxide minimally influences respiration and hemodynamics. In addition, it has low solubility in blood. Therefore, it is often combined with one of the potent volatile agents to permit a lower dose of the potent volatile agent, thus limiting side effects, reducing cost, and facilitating rapid induction and emergence. The most important clinical problem with nitrous oxide is that it is 30 times more soluble than nitrogen and diffuses into closed gas spaces faster than nitrogen diffuses out, thus increasing gas volume and pressure within the closed space. Because of this characteristic, nitrous oxide is contraindicated in the presence of closed gas spaces such as pneumothorax, small bowel obstruction, or middle ear surgery, as well as in retinal surgery in which an intraocular gas bubble is created. Because nitrous oxide gradually accumulates in the pneumoperitoneum, some clinicians prefer to avoid its use during laparoscopic procedures. However, periodic venting can prevent gas accumulation.[1]

The Evaluation of Nitrous Oxide in the Gas Mixture for Anaesthesia (ENIGMA) Trial, reported in 2007, indicated that patients having major surgical procedures lasting more than 2 hours had a higher incidence of postoperative complications and severe postoperative nausea and vomiting (PONV) if they received 70% nitrous oxide as part of their anesthetic regimen compared to patients randomized to not receive nitrous oxide.[2] However, the more recent ENIGMA II Trial, published in 2014, reported that use of nitrous oxide was not associated with an increased incidence of death, cardiovascular complications, or wound infection in high-risk surgical patients. Although the incidence of severe PONV was higher (15% vs. 11%) in patients receiving nitrous oxide compared to controls, the occurrence of PONV in the nitrous oxide group was effectively controlled by antiemetic prophylaxis.[3] A one-year follow-up of ENIGMA II patients did not show an increase in long-term morbidity and mortality with nitrous oxide administration.[4]

Isoflurane

Approved by the U.S. Food and Drug Administration (FDA) in 1979, isoflurane rapidly replaced halothane as the most commonly used potent inhalational agent. Despite the recent release of sevoflurane and desflurane, isoflurane remains commonly used in modern operating rooms, in part because the cost of the now-generic compound is well below that of the newer agents. Isoflurane has several advantages over halothane, including less reduction in cardiac output, less sensitization to the arrhythmogenic effects of catecholamines, and minimal metabolism (Tables 14.1 and 14.2). However, isoflurane-induced

TABLE 14.2 **Cardiopulmonary effects of inhalational anesthetics.**

INHALATIONAL AGENT	BLOOD PRESSURE	HEART RATE	CARDIAC OUTPUT	SENSITIZATION TO CATECHOLAMINES	VENTILATORY DEPRESSION	BRONCHO DILATATION
Nitrous oxide	Little effect	Little effect	Little effect	No	Minimal	No
Halothane	Marked dose-dependent decrease	Moderate decrease	Marked dose-dependent decrease	Marked	Moderate dose-dependent effect	Moderate
Enflurane	Marked dose-dependent decrease	Moderate decrease	Moderate dose-dependent decrease	Moderate	Marked dose-dependent effect	Minimal
Isoflurane	Moderate dose-dependent decrease	Variable increase	Minimal decrease	Minimal	Marked dose-dependent effect	Moderate
Sevoflurane	Moderate dose-dependent decrease	Little effect	Moderate dose-dependent decrease	Minimal	Moderate dose-dependent effect	Moderate
Desflurane	Minimal decrease	Variable; marked increase with rapid increase in concentration	Minimal decrease	Minimal	Marked dose-dependent effect	Moderate

tachycardia, a variable response, can increase myocardial oxygen consumption. Careful observation and management of the heart rate are necessary when it is used in patients with coronary artery disease. In concentrations of 1.0 MAC or less, isoflurane causes little increase in cerebral blood flow and intracranial pressure (ICP) and depresses cerebral metabolic activity more than halothane or enflurane does. Its pungent odor virtually precludes use for inhalational induction.

Sevoflurane

Sevoflurane's relatively low blood solubility facilitates rapid induction and relatively rapid emergence. Sevoflurane is associated with faster emergence than isoflurane is, especially in longer cases, although its slightly faster emergence does not result in earlier discharge after outpatient surgery. Sevoflurane is associated with a lower incidence of postoperative somnolence and nausea in the postanesthesia care unit (PACU) and in the first 24 hours after discharge than isoflurane is. Unlike isoflurane, sevoflurane is pleasant to inhale, thus making it suitable for inhalational induction in children. However, the clinical differences between halothane and sevoflurane are subtle. In premedicated pediatric patients undergoing bilateral myringotomy and tube placement and randomized to receive sevoflurane or halothane, anesthesiologists correctly identified the agent (to which they were blinded) in only 56.6% of cases.

Sevoflurane is clinically suitable for outpatient surgery, mask induction of patients with potentially difficult airways, and maintenance of patients with bronchospastic disease. When sevoflurane, halothane, and isoflurane were compared, all three of the potent agents decreased respiratory resistance in endotracheally intubated nonasthmatics; sevoflurane reduced airway resistance more than halothane or isoflurane did. Another advantage of sevoflurane is that its cardiovascular side effects are minimal.

Considerable metabolic transformation of sevoflurane takes place and results in increases in the serum fluoride ion concentration and, in the presence of soda lime or Baralyme, production of compound A, a metabolite that is nephrotoxic in experimental animals. However, β-lyase, the enzyme responsible for the formation of compound A, has 8 to 30 times greater activity in rat kidney tissue than in human kidney tissue. Therefore, the toxicity of compound A in humans appears to be theoretical and not clinically important.

Desflurane

Desflurane is rapidly taken up and eliminated. After anesthesia lasting more than 3 hours, desflurane was associated with more rapid recovery than isoflurane was. The most volatile and least potent of the volatile anesthetics, desflurane must be administered through specialized electrically heated vaporizers. Its pungent odor precludes inhalational induction. In addition, desflurane is associated with tachycardia and hypertension if the inspired concentration is increased too rapidly.

When exposed to dry CO_2 absorbent, desflurane, isoflurane, and enflurane are partially converted to carbon monoxide. Desflurane, enflurane, and isoflurane produce more carbon monoxide than halothane or sevoflurane does. Carbon monoxide production is greater with dry CO_2 absorbent, with Baralyme than with soda lime, at higher temperatures, and at higher anesthetic concentrations. Because continued gas flow in an unused machine will desiccate the CO_2 absorbent, turning gas flow off in anesthesia machines when they are not in use can reduce carbon monoxide production.

Intravenous Agents

Since the introduction of thiopental, IV agents have become an indispensable component of modern anesthetic practice. IV agents are used primarily for induction of anesthesia and as part of a multidrug combination to produce total IV anesthesia.

Induction Agents

For most adult patients and many older children, IV induction is preferable to inhalational induction. IV induction is rapid, pleasant, and safe for the vast majority of patients; however, there are situations in which IV induction introduces hazards. Although several agents can be used for IV induction of anesthesia, propofol is the most widely used agent in the United States. Other agents include sodium thiopental, ketamine, methohexital, etomidate, and midazolam (Table 14.3).

Propofol is a short-acting induction agent that is associated with smooth, nausea-free emergence. Small doses are also useful for short-term sedation during brief procedures such as retrobulbar or peribulbar eye blocks, and propofol is commonly used as a continuous infusion during total IV anesthesia and for sedation during less invasive procedures such as gastrointestinal endoscopy. The primary

TABLE 14.3 Clinical characteristics of intravenous induction agents.

INTRAVENOUS INDUCTION AGENT	DOSE mg/kg	COMMENTS	SIDE EFFECTS	SITUATIONS REQUIRING CAUTION	RELATIVE INDICATIONS
Thiopental	2–5	Inexpensive; slow emergence after high doses	Hypotension	Hypovolemia; compromised cardiac function	Suitable for induction in many patients
Ketamine	1–2	Psychotropic side effects controllable with benzodiazepines; good bronchodilator; potent analgesic at subinduction doses	Hypertension; tachycardia	Coronary disease; severe hypovolemia	Rapid-sequence induction of asthmatics; patients in shock (reduced doses)
Propofol	1–2	Burns on injection; good bronchodilator; associated with low incidence of postoperative nausea and vomiting	Hypotension	Coronary artery disease; hypovolemia	Induction of outpatients; induction of asthmatics
Etomidate	0.1–0.3	Cardiovascularly stable; burns on injection; spontaneous movement during induction	Adrenal suppression (with continuous infusion)	Hypovolemia	Induction of patients with cardiac contractile dysfunction; induction of patients in shock (reduced doses)
Midazolam	0.15–0.3	Relatively stable hemodynamics; potent amnesia	Synergistic ventilatory depression with opioids	Hypovolemia	Induction of patients with cardiac contractile dysfunction (usually in combination with opioids)

limitations of propofol are pain on injection and blood pressure reduction. Thus propofol should be used with caution in patients who may be hypovolemic or who may tolerate hypotension poorly, such as those with severe coronary artery disease.

Propofol produces excellent bronchodilatation. In asthmatic patients, 0% of those who received propofol wheezed at 2 or 5 minutes after intubation versus 45% of those who received a thiobarbiturate and 26% of those who received an oxybarbiturate. In nonasthmatic patients, three quarters of whom smoked, airway resistance was less after induction with propofol than after induction with thiopental or etomidate. Evidence indicates that the bronchodilatory effects of propofol and ketamine are mediated through blockade of vagus nerve–mediated cholinergic bronchoconstriction.

Ketamine, which produces a dissociative state of anesthesia, is the only IV induction agent that increases blood pressure and heart rate and decreases bronchomotor tone. Usually associated with increased sympathetic tone, ketamine causes direct cardiac depression that may become evident if given to patients with high preanesthetic sympathetic tone, as in patients in hemorrhagic shock. In markedly reduced doses (15%–20% of the usual induction dose), ketamine is an appropriate choice for IV induction of severely hypovolemic patients in whom it causes the least fall in blood pressure of any of the induction agents. Ketamine is an appropriate agent for IV induction of asthmatic patients because it reduces the increase in bronchomotor tone associated with endotracheal intubation. Among the IV induction agents, ketamine also causes the least amount of ventilatory depression and loss of airway reflexes. However, because of the induction of copious oropharyngeal secretions, a drying agent such as glycopyrrolate is generally administered with ketamine.

Ketamine can be used as the sole anesthetic for brief, superficial procedures because it produces profound amnesia and somatic analgesia. It is less useful, however, for abdominal cases or delicate surgery because it produces no muscular relaxation, does not control visceral pain, and may not completely control patient movement. The potent pain-relieving effects of ketamine have been exploited for preemptive analgesia. In patients in whom ketamine was infused continuously before incision and continued through wound closure, postoperative morphine consumption was significantly lower on postoperative days 1 and 2 than in patients who did not receive ketamine.

In patients with coronary artery disease, ketamine is usually avoided because tachycardia and increased blood pressure may cause myocardial ischemia. In patients with increased ICP (e.g., after traumatic brain injury), ketamine may further increase ICP because it is the only IV agent that increases cerebral blood flow. Another clinically important side effect of ketamine is emergence delirium. In adults and older children, supplemental benzodiazepines or volatile agents are generally effective in preventing emergence delirium.

Etomidate is an imidazole compound that produces minimal hemodynamic changes. Because it preserves blood pressure in most patients, etomidate is often chosen as an alternative for induction of patients with cardiovascular disease or severe hypovolemia. Major drawbacks include burning pain on injection, abnormal muscular movements (myoclonus), and adrenal suppression when given as a prolonged infusion for sedation of critically ill patients.

Induction with thiopental, the oldest IV induction agent, is rapid and pleasant. Although the drug is remarkably well tolerated by a wide variety of patients, it is not commonly used in modern anesthetic practice and several clinical situations necessitate caution (Table 14.3). In hypovolemic patients and those with congestive heart failure, thiopental-induced vasodilatation and cardiac depression can lead to severe hypotension unless doses are markedly reduced. In such patients, etomidate or ketamine is an alternative agent. Although thiopental does not directly precipitate bronchospasm, bronchospasm may develop in patients with reactive airway disease in response to the intense airway stimulation produced by endotracheal intubation. Consequently, propofol or ketamine is often chosen as an alternative for induction in patients with reactive airway disease. In the usual doses used for induction of anesthesia, thiopental is associated with rapid emergence because of redistribution of the agent from the brain to peripheral tissues, particularly fat. In higher doses, circulating blood levels increase and the action of thiopental must be terminated by hepatic metabolism, which eliminates only about 10% per hour.

Midazolam is sometimes used for induction because it usually causes minimal cardiovascular side effects and has a much shorter duration of action than diazepam does. Its onset of action is acceptably rapid and, even in smaller doses, induces profound amnesia for painful or anxiety-producing events. Midazolam is frequently selected for induction of patients for cardiovascular surgery. Because midazolam combines powerful anxiolytic and amnesic effects, smaller doses also are commonly used to premedicate anxious patients and as a component of a multidrug anesthetic.

Opioids

Opioids are used in the majority of patients undergoing general anesthesia and are given systemically to a large proportion of patients receiving regional or local anesthesia. As a component of a multifaceted anesthetic, opioids produce profound analgesia and minimal cardiac depression. Their disadvantages include ventilatory depression and inconsistent hypnosis and amnesia, which must usually be provided by other agents.

Several reasons explain the popularity of opioids in anesthetic management. First, they reduce the MAC of potent inhalational agents. For example, fentanyl (3 ng/mL plasma concentration) decreased the MAC of sevoflurane by 59% and reduced MAC_{awake} (the alveolar concentration at which an emerging patient responds to commands) by 24%. Second, they blunt the hypertension and tachycardia associated with manipulations such as endotracheal intubation and surgical incision. Third, they provide analgesia that extends through the early postemergence interval and facilitates smoother awakening from anesthesia. Fourth, in doses 10 to 20 times the analgesic dose, opioids act as complete anesthetics in a high proportion of patients by providing not only analgesia but also hypnosis and amnesia. This characteristic has prompted their use in cardiac surgery patients, sometimes as sole anesthetic agents and more often as a major component of a multimodal anesthetic. Finally, they are now often added to local anesthetic solutions in epidural and intrathecal blocks to improve the quality of analgesia.

Morphine, hydromorphone, and meperidine are inexpensive, intermediate-acting agents that are less commonly used for maintenance of anesthesia than for postoperative analgesia. Fentanyl, a synthetic opioid that is 100 to 150 times more potent than morphine, is commonly used for maintenance of anesthesia because of its shorter duration of action and rapid onset. Newer synthetic, short-acting opioids, including sufentanil and alfentanil, are also used during anesthesia because they are quickly metabolized and excreted. Remifentanil, an opioid metabolized by serum esterases, is particularly short acting. Remifentanil does not accumulate during prolonged infusions and is therefore often used as part of IV anesthetics. Methadone is a long-acting opioid that is not only a potent μ-opioid receptor agonist but also interacts with *N*-methyl-D-aspartate (NMDA) receptors and alters the reuptake of serotonin and norepinephrine in the brain. A recent study comparing intraoperative methadone to hydromorphone in patients undergoing posterior spinal fusion showed that methadone administration decreased postoperative opioid requirements, decreased pain scores, and improved patient satisfaction with pain management.[5]

Neuromuscular Blockers

Fifty years ago, anesthesia was typically conducted with single potent inhalational agents that produced all the components of general anesthesia, including the degree of muscle relaxation that was necessary for the conduct of surgery. Among the drawbacks of this approach was the fact that the depth of anesthesia necessary to produce profound muscle relaxation was much deeper than that necessary to provide hypnosis and amnesia. The addition of muscle relaxants afforded the opportunity to deliver only enough of the inhalational and IV agents to achieve hypnosis, amnesia, and analgesia while still providing satisfactory operating conditions.

The two categories of neuromuscular blockers in clinical use are depolarizing (noncompetitive) and nondepolarizing (competitive) agents. The depolarizing agents exert agonistic effects at the cholinergic receptors of the neuromuscular junction, initially causing contractions evident as fasciculations followed by an interval of profound relaxation. The nondepolarizing neuromuscular blockers compete for receptor sites with acetylcholine in the neuromuscular junction, with the magnitude of block dependent on the availability of acetylcholine, the concentration of neuromuscular blocker in the neuromuscular junction, and the affinity of the agent for the receptor.

Succinylcholine, the only depolarizing agent still in clinical use, remains popular for endotracheal intubation because of its rapid onset and short duration of action. However, it is associated with serious hazards, including hyperkalemia and malignant hyperthermia, in a small proportion of patients. The drug can be administered in a relatively high dose for intubation because it is rapidly metabolized by plasma pseudocholinesterase, except in a small fraction of patients with atypical or absent pseudocholinesterase. At high doses, onset of muscle relaxation is rapid (60–90 seconds), which facilitates rapid intubation in patients at risk for aspiration. Because its duration of action is only 5 minutes, a patient who cannot be successfully intubated can be ventilated by mask for a short time until spontaneous respiration resumes. However, a patient who cannot be ventilated by mask after succinylcholine administration will likely not resume spontaneous breathing before the onset of life-threatening hypoxemia.

The side effects of succinylcholine include bradycardia, especially in children, and severe, life-threatening hyperkalemia in patients with burns, paraplegia, quadriplegia, and massive trauma. Succinylcholine, alone or when combined with a volatile agent, is also implicated in triggering malignant hyperthermia in susceptible individuals. Therefore, it is best avoided in patients at risk for malignant hyperthermia, including those with muscular dystrophy or a family history of malignant hyperthermia. Some anesthesiologists avoid succinylcholine in children because masseter spasm is a common occurrence that may presage malignant hyperthermia, but it is usually a benign effect. Because succinylcholine is a depolarizing agent that causes visible muscle fasciculations, it has been implicated in causing postoperative muscle pain, which can be reduced by pretreatment with a small, precurarizing dose of a nondepolarizing agent. As a result of the multiple sporadic problems associated with the use of succinylcholine, some anesthesiologists now reserve its use only for situations in which an airway must be rapidly secured (i.e., rapid-sequence induction). In other situations, nondepolarizing agents, chosen largely on the basis of their mode of excretion and duration of action, are preferable. For instance, cisatracurium is largely metabolized in serum by Hoffman degradation

TABLE 14.4 Dose-response relationships of nondepolarizing neuromuscular blocking drugs in humans.

DRUG	DURATION	ED_{50} (mg/kg)	ED_{95} (mg/kg)	INTUBATING DOSE (mg/kg)
d-Tubocurarine	Long	0.23 (0.16–0.26)	0.48 (0.34–0.56)	0.5–0.6
Pancuronium	Long	0.036 (0.022–0.042)	0.067 (0.059–0.080)	0.08–0.12
Vecuronium	Intermediate	0.027 (0.015–0.031)	0.043 (0.037–0.059)	0.1–0.2
Cisatracurium	Intermediate	0.026 (0.15–0.31)	0.04 (0.32–0.55)	0.15–0.2
Rocuronium	Intermediate	0.147 (0.069–0.220)	0.305 (0.257–0.521)	0.6–1.0

ED_{50}, Dose effective for surgical relaxation in 50% of patients; ED_{95}, dose effective for surgical relaxation in 95% of patients.
Data are mean (95% confidence limits). Somewhat larger doses are required to facilitate endotracheal intubation.
Modified from Naguib M, Lien CA. Pharmacology of muscle relaxants and their antagonists. In: Miller RD, Fleisher LA, Johns RA, et al, eds. *Miller's Anesthesia.* 6th ed. Philadelphia, PA; Churchill Livingstone; 2005:481–572.

and is suitable for patients with reduced renal function in whom pancuronium and vecuronium would be unsuitable because they are partially eliminated by the kidneys.

Nondepolarizing relaxants are used when succinylcholine is contraindicated as an alternative to succinylcholine for patients in whom easy endotracheal intubation is anticipated and when intraoperative relaxation is required to facilitate surgical exposure. Knowledge of the side effects of individual agents (often related to vagolysis or release of histamine) and routes of metabolism plays a major role in the selection of specific agents for individual cases. Doses required to provide satisfactory operating conditions are summarized in Table 14.4. Dosing of nondepolarizing agents requires knowledge of several important characteristics. First, the use of neuromuscular blockers prevents movement in response to noxious stimuli. Therefore, chemical paralysis can mask the signs of inadequate anesthesia (or sedation or analgesia in postoperative patients). Medicolegal claims of intraoperative awareness during general anesthesia were more than twice as frequent in patients receiving intraoperative muscle relaxants. Second, higher doses are required to provide satisfactory conditions for intubation than for surgical relaxation. Therefore, if a nondepolarizer is used only after intubation, smaller doses are required. Third, other anesthetic drugs potentiate the actions of nondepolarizing agents. Succinylcholine used for intubation decreases subsequent requirements for nondepolarizers. Potent inhalational agents dose-dependently potentiate the effects of competitive neuromuscular blockers. The newer inhalational agent desflurane potentiates the effects of vecuronium approximately 20% more than isoflurane does. Fourth, individual responses to muscle relaxants vary widely, with patients demonstrating both markedly increased and markedly decreased neuromuscular blockade in comparison to expected levels.

Fifth, and most important, subtle blockade can be difficult to detect and can be associated with postoperative complications. The importance of subtle residual paralysis has recently been quantified by using the train-of-four (TOF) fade ratio, a semiquantitative monitoring technique used to assess the adequacy of neuromuscular blockade and the adequacy of pharmacologic reversal. At the conclusion of anesthesia, a TOF ratio greater than 0.90 has been considered adequate return of neuromuscular function. This ratio means that the fourth of four muscle twitches in response to supramaximal stimuli delivered at 0.5-second intervals to the ulnar nerve is at least 90% of the magnitude of the first twitch. In a 2003 study, at TOF ratios less than 0.90, subjects had diplopia and difficulty tracking objects in all directions. The ability to strongly oppose the incisors did not return until the TOF ratio was higher than 0.90. The authors concluded that satisfactory return of neuromuscular function requires return of the TOF ratio to greater than 0.90 and ideally to 1.0.[6] In patients who received the intermediate-acting neuromuscular blockers atracurium, vecuronium, or rocuronium only for endotracheal intubation, the TOF ratio was lower than 0.9 in 37% of patients 2 hours after receiving the muscle relaxant. More recent studies show that patients with TOF ratios lower than 0.9 have an increased incidence of postoperative respiratory complications and delayed PACU discharge.[7] Thus, it is important to optimize return of neuromuscular function at the end of surgery through judicious use of muscle relaxants and reversal agents.

The use of neuromuscular blocking agents in general and nondepolarizing agents in particular necessitates a strategy to ensure adequate muscular function at the conclusion of anesthesia. Many of the complications associated with neuromuscular blockers relate to inadequate reversal at the conclusion of cases or inadequate assessment of reversal. Historically, nondepolarizing relaxants are generally pharmacologically reversed with an anticholinesterase (neostigmine or edrophonium) accompanied by atropine or glycopyrrolate to counteract the muscarinic effects of the anticholinesterase. However, recovery depends both on the intensity of neuromuscular blockade at the time that reversal is attempted and on the effects of the reversal agent. At the end of anesthesia, profound neuromuscular blockade may preclude reliable antagonism by an anticholinesterase within 5 to 10 minutes. With the longer-acting muscle relaxants, residual blockade can potentially complicate postoperative recovery. In a clinical trial of reversal of muscle relaxation, 691 patients undergoing abdominal, gynecologic, or orthopedic surgery under general anesthesia were randomized to receive pancuronium, vecuronium, or atracurium. After reversal with neostigmine, a higher proportion (26%) of patients who had received pancuronium had residual neuromuscular blockade (TOF <0.70) than did patients who had received vecuronium or atracurium (5.3% combined). Patients who received pancuronium and had a TOF ratio less than 0.70 had a higher incidence of atelectasis or pneumonia on postoperative chest radiographs (16.9% of 59 patients in that category). There was no association between postoperative pulmonary complications and residual blockade with the other two muscle relaxants. However, the development of sugammadex has overcome many of the problems associated with using anticholinesterases to reverse neuromuscular blockade. Sugammadex is a cyclodextrin that directly binds nondepolarizing steroidal neuromuscular blocking agents such as rocuronium and vecuronium. Sugammadex rapidly reverses neuromuscular blockade and avoids the muscarinic side effects associated with use of anticholinesterases. Dosing of sugammadex is based on the depth of neuromuscular blockade. Therefore, monitoring of blockade depth with a twitch monitor is required

BOX 14.1 Routine and specialized electronic monitors used in anesthetic practice and their indications.

Routine Monitors

Pulse oximetry
- Blood oxygen saturation
- Heart rate
- Tissue perfusion (via plethysmography)

Automated blood pressure cuff
- Blood pressure

ECG
- Heart rhythm
- Heart rate
- Monitor of myocardial ischemia

Capnography
- Adequacy of ventilation
- Intratracheal placement of endotracheal tube
- Pulmonary perfusion

Oxygen analyzer
- Monitoring of delivered oxygen concentration

Ventilator pressure monitor
- Ventilator disconnection during general anesthesia
- Monitoring of airway pressure

Temperature monitoring

Specialized Monitors

Monitoring of urine output (Foley catheter)
- Gross indicator of intravascular volume status and renal perfusion

Arterial catheter
- Continuous measurement of arterial blood pressure
- Sampling of arterial blood

Central venous catheter
- Continuous measurement of central venous pressure
- Delivery of centrally acting drugs
- Rapid administration of fluids and blood

Pulmonary artery catheter
- Measurement of pulmonary artery pressure
- Measurement of left ventricular pressure
- Measurement of cardiac output
- Measurement of mixed venous oxygenation

Precordial Doppler
- Detection of air embolism

Transesophageal echocardiography
- Evaluation of myocardial performance
- Assessment of heart valve function
- Assessment of intravascular volume
- Detection of air embolism

Esophageal Doppler
- Assessment of descending aortic blood flow
- Assessment of cardiac preload

Transpulmonary indicator dilution
- Measurement of cardiac output
- Measurement of preload

Esophageal and precordial stethoscope
- Auscultation of breathing and heart sounds

EEG/BIS
- Depth of anesthesia

BIS, Bispectral index; *ECG*, electrocardiography; *EEG*, electroencephalography.

for optimal reversal of neuromuscular blockade with sugammadex. Nevertheless, comparison of sugammadex to neostigmine for reversal of neuromuscular blockade in patients undergoing abdominal surgery showed that sugammadex administration eliminated residual neuromuscular blockade in the PACU and shortened the time of readiness for discharge from the operating room.[8]

One key factor determining recovery from neuromuscular blockade is the ability to metabolize and excrete the drugs. In patients with renal disease, the half-lives of D-tubocurarine, rocuronium, vecuronium, and pancuronium are prolonged. In such patients, alternative drugs such as cisatracurium, which is metabolized by Hoffman degradation and thus does not have a prolonged half-life in patients with renal dysfunction, should be considered. The sugammadex-neuromuscular blocking agent complex is excreted in the kidney. Therefore, complexes will persist longer in the circulation of patients with renal insufficiency. However, sugammadex binds neuromuscular binding agents irreversibly, so return of neuromuscular blockade is not a concern.

ANESTHESIA EQUIPMENT

Anesthesia equipment has undergone rapid development over the past few decades. The central piece of equipment for delivery of anesthesia is the modern anesthesia machine. The anesthesia machine functions primarily to deliver oxygen and volatile anesthetics to the patient. In addition, modern anesthetic machines have sophisticated ventilators that allow for effective respiratory support and have integrated monitors that accurately measure oxygen delivery, inspired and end-tidal gas concentrations, airway pressures, minute ventilation, and fresh gas flows. Despite many years of improving design, hazards of gas delivery systems must still be considered. The primary concern is inadvertent delivery of a hypoxic gas mixture. Adverse anesthetic outcomes were associated with gas delivery equipment in 72 of 3791 cases in the American Society of Anesthesiologists (ASA) closed claims database. Misuse of equipment occurred in 75% of incidents, and 78% could have been detected with monitoring of pulse oximetry or capnography. The essential elements of an anesthesia machine are gas sources (oxygen, nitrous oxide, and air), flowmeters, and a flow-proportioning device. In most cases, gases are delivered to the anesthesia machine from a bank of large H cylinders housed in a central area within the hospital. A backup system of E cylinders is attached directly to the anesthesia machine and provides a source of gases, particularly oxygen, if the central gas source becomes unavailable. The flowmeters allow independent administration of individual gases. So-called fail-safe valves that require pressurization of the oxygen line before nitrous oxide can be delivered and flow-proportioning devices that automatically reduce the flow of nitrous oxide if the flow of oxygen is reduced below a safe concentration are present to minimize the chance of delivering a hypoxic gas mixture. The measurement of inspired oxygen concentration provides a further safeguard against delivering hypoxic gas mixtures.

In addition to the anesthesia machine, the other major components of anesthesia equipment are monitors. The use of monitors to assess changes in respiratory and cardiovascular function during anesthesia and surgery has been instrumental in improving overall safety (Box 14.1).

PATIENT MONITORING DURING AND AFTER ANESTHESIA

Effective monitoring is a critical aspect of anesthesia care. The essential components of monitoring include observation and vigilance, instrumentation, data analysis, and institution of corrective measures, if indicated. The goal of patient monitoring is to provide optimal anesthetic management and detect abnormalities early in their course so that corrective measures can be instituted before serious or irreversible injury occurs. Although it is difficult to directly relate improved patient outcomes with specific monitors, the reduction in anesthesia-related morbidity and mortality has paralleled the institution of current monitoring practices.

The indications as well as risks and benefits associated with the use of noninvasive and invasive electronic monitors must be assessed for each individual patient (Box 14.1). These decisions are guided by the patient's medical condition, the type of surgery, and the potential complications associated with invasive monitoring. However, the proliferation of electronic monitoring devices does not circumvent the need for clinical skills such as observation, inspection, auscultation, and palpation. The ASA has established standards for basic anesthetic monitoring that were most recently updated in 2015 (https://www.asahq.org/standards-and-guidelines/standards-for-basic-anesthetic-monitoring). These standards are designed to integrate clinical skills and electronic monitoring with the goal of enhancing patient safety.

Standard I asserts that a qualified anesthesia care provider must be continuously present in the operating room during the administration of anesthesia. The practitioner must continuously monitor the status of the patient and alter anesthesia care based on the patient's response to the dynamic changes associated with anesthesia and surgery.

Standard II mandates continuous assessment of ventilation, oxygenation, circulation, and temperature during all anesthetics. Specific requirements include the following:

1. The use of an oxygen analyzer with a low–oxygen–concentration alarm during general anesthesia.
2. Quantitative assessment of blood oxygenation such as by pulse oximetry.
3. The adequacy of ventilation must be continuously ensured by clinical evaluation. Quantitative monitoring of the CO_2 content in expired gas and the volume of expired gas is strongly recommended.
4. Clinical assessment and monitors to determine the presence of CO_2 in expired gases to ensure correct endotracheal tube placement after intubation. A device capable of detecting disconnection of breathing system components during mechanical ventilation must be in continuous use. This device must give an audible signal when its alarm threshold is exceeded. During moderate or deep sedation, adequacy of ventilation shall be evaluated by assessment of clinical signs and monitoring of the presence of exhaled CO_2 unless precluded or invalidated by the clinical situation.
5. The electrocardiogram (ECG) must be continuously monitored during anesthesia, and blood pressure and the heart rate must be evaluated at least every 5 minutes. In patients undergoing general anesthesia, adequacy of circulatory function must be continuously monitored by electronic means, palpation, or auscultation.
6. A means of temperature evaluation must be readily available in the operating room and is used during periods of intended or expected changes in body temperature.

Blood Pressure Monitoring

Blood pressure monitoring is required during all anesthetics. Noninvasive blood pressure monitoring is appropriate for the majority of surgical cases, and most modern operating rooms are equipped with automated oscillometric blood pressure analyzers. Indications for invasive blood pressure monitoring include intraoperative use of deliberate hypotension, continuous blood pressure assessment in patients with significant end-organ damage or during high-risk surgical procedures, anticipation of wide perioperative blood pressure swings, need for multiple blood gas analyses, and inadequacy of noninvasive blood pressure measurements, such as in morbidly obese patients. Several sites for arterial cannulation are available, each with inherent advantages and potential for complications. The radial artery is most commonly cannulated because of its superficial location, relative ease of cannulation, and in most patients, adequate collateral flow from the ulnar artery. Other potential sites for percutaneous arterial cannulation include the femoral, brachial, axillary, ulnar, dorsalis pedis, and posterior tibial arteries. Possible complications of intraarterial monitoring include hematoma, neurologic injury, arterial embolization, limb ischemia, infection, and inadvertent intraarterial injection of drugs. Intraarterial catheters are not placed in extremities with potential vascular insufficiency. However, with proper patient selection, the complication rate associated with intraarterial cannulation is low and its benefits can be important.

Electrocardiography

ECG monitoring is a standard of care during the administration of anesthesia. Information regarding dysrhythmias and cardiac ischemia can be readily obtained from ECG data. Analysis of ECG tracings is the cornerstone of cardiopulmonary resuscitation protocols.

Ventilation Monitoring

Sedation and opioid administration and the induction of general or regional anesthesia can depress or abolish spontaneous ventilation and thus necessitate intraoperative ventilator support. Several means are available to assess the adequacy of ventilation, among which are physical assessment of chest expansion, auscultation of breath sounds, and evaluation for evidence of upper airway obstruction and stridor. Precordial and esophageal stethoscopes provide continuous input regarding air movement and the development of wheezing. During mechanical ventilation, monitors of airway pressure and minute ventilation alert the anesthesiologist to conditions that can impair ventilation, such as disconnection of the ventilatory circuit, dislodgement of the endotracheal tube, obstruction of the gas delivery system, and changes in airway resistance or compliance, or both.

The advent of end-tidal CO_2 ($ETCO_2$) monitoring has greatly enhanced the monitoring of ventilation and detection of esophageal intubation. In normal individuals, the difference between $ETCO_2$ and $PaCO_2$ is 2 to 5 mm Hg. The gradient between end-tidal and arterial CO_2 reflects dead space ventilation, which is increased in cases of decreased pulmonary blood flow, such as pulmonary air embolism or thromboembolism and decreased cardiac output. Therefore, $ETCO_2$ monitoring can also provide important information regarding systemic perfusion. Specifically,

$ETCO_2$ will decrease during periods of decreased cardiac output and pulmonary perfusion.

Oxygenation Monitoring

Monitoring the fractional concentration of oxygen in inspired gas (FiO_2) and hemoglobin oxygen saturation is a standard of care during all general anesthetics. Modern anesthesia machines are equipped with oxygen analyzers that detect the delivered oxygen concentration (FiO_2). This monitor, in combination with fail-safe devices, low–oxygen delivery alarms, and oxygen ratio monitors, greatly decreases the chance of delivering a hypoxic gas mixture during anesthesia.

Temperature Monitoring

Temperature is monitored in all patients undergoing general anesthesia. The site of measurement is dependent on the surgical procedure and the physical characteristics of the patient. Esophageal temperature is most commonly measured during general anesthesia. Other sites of temperature monitoring include rectal, cutaneous, tympanic membrane, bladder, nasopharynx, and, in patients with pulmonary artery catheters, the pulmonary artery. Because of the potential morbidity associated with hypothermia and hyperthermia, it is important to monitor body temperature and institute measures to maintain temperature as close to normal as possible.

Neuromuscular Blockade Monitoring

Because of variability in sensitivity to and metabolism of neuromuscular blockers among patients, it is essential to monitor neuromuscular function in patients receiving intermediate- and long-acting muscle relaxants. The most common sites of monitoring are at the ulnar or orbicularis oculi muscles. The basis of neuromuscular monitoring is assessment of muscle activity after proximal nerve stimulation (Box 14.2). This evaluation gives an indication of acetylcholine receptor blockade at the neuromuscular junction. The degree of neuromuscular blockade is indicated by a decreased evoked response to twitch stimulation. As noted earlier in this chapter, it is essential to monitor neuromuscular blockade and to assure resolution of blockade at the end of anesthesia to minimize the incidence of postoperative complications related to residual neuromuscular blockade.

Central Nervous System Monitoring

Awareness during anesthesia is an uncommon, but a disturbing, complication. Many years of experience with intraoperative electroencephalogram signal processing has resulted in the development of the bispectral index (BIS) array, which is believed to monitor awareness during anesthesia. The monitor is essentially a modified electroencephalogram that assesses brain wave activity and reports numbers from 0 to 100, which correlate with the level of awareness. A value of 100 represents complete awareness and 0 represents complete suppression of brain wave activity. Data suggest that BIS is an accurate indicator of the depth of anesthesia.[9] Monitoring the depth of anesthesia may allow for more precise titration of volatile and IV anesthetics and may improve time to awakening and discharge in the outpatient setting. Furthermore, some reports indicate that BIS values of less than 40 for more than 5 minutes during general anesthesia may be associated with increased perioperative morbidity, including myocardial infarction and stroke in high-risk patients.[10] A recent metaanalysis concluded that BIS monitoring can reduce intraoperative awareness in high-risk patients, but it is unclear if the use of BIS monitoring provides advantages in that regard over monitoring end-tidal anesthetic gas concentration in most patients.[11] In addition to intraoperative use, BIS monitors are gaining acceptance as a means of assessing awareness in locations such as emergency departments and intensive care units (ICUs).

BOX 14.2 Techniques for assessing neuromuscular blockade.

Train-of-Four: Four Successive 200-μsec Stimuli Over a 2-Second Period

Twitch height progressively fades with increasing blockade

- Loss of the fourth twitch indicates 75% receptor blockade
- Loss of the third twitch indicates 80% blockade
- Loss of the second twitch indicates 90% blockade
- Loss of the first twitch indicates 100% blockade
- Clinical relaxation requires 75% to 95% blockade

Presence of four twitches without fade suggests adequate reversal of neuromuscular blockade

Double-Burst Stimulation: Two Successive Sets of 50-Hz Bursts (Three Stimuli/Burst) Separated by 750 msec (Appears as Two Twitches)

Easier to detect fade visually with this technique than with train-of-four

Loss of the second twitch indicates 80% receptor blockade

Presence of two twitches without fade suggests adequate reversal of neuromuscular blockade

Tetany: Sustained 50- or 100-Hz Burst

Duration of sustained contraction fades with increasing blockade

Sustained contraction for 5 seconds suggests adequate reversal of neuromuscular blockade

Accelerometry

Provides a quantitative comparison of the first and fourth twitches of the train-of-four and generates a train-of-four ratio (ratio of the fourth twitch over the first twitch)

A train-of-four ratio of less than 0.9 signifies clinically significant residual neuromuscular blockade

Hemodynamic Monitoring (Transesophageal Echocardiography/Right Heart Catheter)

Hemodynamic monitoring techniques have become less invasive with greater yield to include devices that provide continuous oximetry information via a central venous catheter, arterial pulse-contour continuous cardiac output monitoring, and even transcutaneous bioimpedance monitoring. The use of pulmonary artery catheters has subsided due to insufficient data to support their use and emergence of evidence that suggested an increase in morbidity and mortality. This also applies to the cardiac surgery population where there also appears to be an association with increased morbidity and mortality.[12] However, with a rise in heart failure and pulmonary arterial hypertension in patients undergoing surgery, there has been a resurgence in the use of pulmonary artery catheters. Even in these patient populations, there are insufficient data to support their use. As for intraoperative monitoring, the use of ultrasound has had a significant impact on monitoring for surgery. The use of transesophageal echocardiography (TEE) has also played a significant role in cardiac and noncardiac surgery for identification of occult pathology and as an aid in the rescue and guidance of management for patients in shock.[13] The impact of TEE in the hands of an anesthesiologist has evolved from rescue, to qualitative assessment, to quantitative analysis, and, in the recent past, onto critical procedural guidance and monitoring.[14]

Point-of-Care Ultrasound

Emergency medicine physicians and trauma surgeons have been early adopters of point-of-care ultrasound with the implementation of the Focused Assessment with Sonography in Trauma protocol. Anesthesiologists also adopted ultrasound with the use of TEE. More recently, the use of ultrasound in the preoperative clinic and just prior to surgery led to a significant impact to avoid delays for further work-up and, in remote cases, identification of occult pathology that changed the trajectory of management for these patients.[15] The use of ultrasound in the operating room has found a niche for multiple facets in the care of surgical patients to include confirmation of the airway, assessment of the cardiac and pulmonary systems, and identification of gastric contents prior to surgery.[16] Furthermore, the use of ultrasound in postoperative care has also had impact in the assessment of patients and for the management of patients on extracorporeal membrane oxygenation.[17] In some cases, the use of ultrasound has also had an impact on survival for those in septic shock.[18]

PREOPERATIVE EVALUATION

The ASA has established basic standards for preanesthetic care in which an anesthesiologist is required to evaluate the medical status of the patient, derive a plan for anesthetic care, and discuss the plan with the patient (https://www.asahq.org/standards-and-guidelines/standards-for-basic-anesthetic-monitoring). The Joint Commission for Accreditation of Healthcare Organizations requires that all patients receiving anesthesia undergo a preanesthetic evaluation. Because a decreasing percentage of patients are admitted to the hospital on the day before surgery, preoperative testing clinics have been developed to facilitate preoperative evaluation. The advent of preoperative clinics has facilitated efficient use of operating room resources. Ferschl and colleagues[19] reported that the development of an anesthesia preoperative evaluation clinic in a teaching hospital reduced day-of-surgery cancellations and delays. Optimally, preoperative clinics need to be efficient, predictable, and thorough. In modern practice, many patients without complicated medical problems who are scheduled for elective, low-risk procedures are interviewed by telephone prior to surgery and given preoperative instructions.

The anesthesia preoperative evaluation serves multiple purposes. First, the patient has the opportunity to speak to an anesthesiologist and discuss the expected impact of anesthesia, including the patient's fears and concerns regarding anesthesia and postoperative pain management. Second, the preanesthetic interview focuses on the type of surgery, the underlying conditions necessitating surgery, any history of previous anesthetics, and the presence of coexisting diseases. The preoperative interview allows evaluation of the patient's medical status to determine whether additional medical evaluation or treatment is needed before surgery. This process requires a focused history, physical examination, and, if indicated, laboratory evaluation. Current medications must be reviewed to anticipate potential drug interactions and manage medical problems during the perioperative period. Instructions regarding oral intake, changes in medication use, and other important issues that need to be addressed prior to surgery are communicated to the patient during the preoperative interview.

A well-focused history will allow the practitioner to perform targeted physical and laboratory examinations. Laboratory tests performed within 6 months of surgery generally do not need to be repeated unless a significant change in the patient's medical status has occurred. Healthy patients undergoing elective procedures may not need any preoperative laboratory testing. In the current climate of cost containment, preoperative testing must be minimized but effective. The use of routine preoperative testing is associated with significant costs, both in dollars and potential harm. False-positive tests can cause needless delays in surgery and could require follow-up, which will increase costs and could lead to harm or injury associated with further tests and procedures. Studies have shown that routine testing adds to costs but has little impact on patient care. However, targeted testing based on results of the history and physical exam can significantly improve overall patient care. Investigation of conditions associated with increased perioperative morbidity is important for reducing the risks related to anesthesia and surgery. Coexisting conditions that must be carefully evaluated include intravascular volume status, airway abnormalities, cardiovascular disease, pulmonary disease, neurologic disease, renal and hepatic disease, and disorders of nutrition, endocrinology, and metabolism. Preoperative pregnancy testing is controversial. The rationale for performing preoperative pregnancy testing is the potential for spontaneous abortion and birth anomalies associated with surgery and anesthesia. There is no clear evidence to demonstrate an association of anesthetic drugs with the development of fetal anomalies in humans, but animal studies have shown that some anesthetics, such as nitrous oxide, may cause developmental abnormalities. A clear sexual history and documentation of the last menstrual cycle are obtained in women of childbearing age. In ambiguous situations, a preoperative pregnancy test is indicated.

Airway Examination

Assessing the airway is a crucial step in developing an anesthetic plan. Even if regional anesthesia is planned, general anesthesia and the need to maintain a patent airway could be necessary in the advent of failed block, surgical needs, or complications. The goal of the airway examination is to identify characteristics that could hinder assisted mask ventilation or tracheal intubation. A history of diseases or conditions that are associated with airway closure or difficult laryngoscopy will alert the practitioner to potential airway difficulties. Review of previous anesthetic records can provide invaluable information regarding previous airway management. The airway examination is completed by systematic inspection of the mouth opening, thyromental distance, neck mobility, and the size of the tongue in relation to the oral cavity (Box 14.3). The patient is observed in both frontal and profile views because many airway abnormalities, such as a receding mandible, will not be evident from a frontal view. The size of the tongue in relation to the oral cavity can be graded by using the Mallampati classification (Fig. 14.1). The Mallampati examination is performed with the patient sitting and the head in a neutral position, the mouth opened as wide as possible, and the tongue protruded maximally. The observer views the oral and pharyngeal structures that are evident. In general, a patient in whom the uvula, tonsillar pillars, and soft palate are visible (class I) will be easy to mask ventilate and intubate. Patients in whom only the hard palate is visible, a class IV airway, have a higher likelihood of being difficult to mask ventilate and intubate. However, the Mallampati classification is only one component of the airway examination and must be used in conjunction with other aspects of the airway examination and the

BOX 14.3 Important factors in performing an airway examination.

Patient History
Previous anesthetic history
Medical history (e.g., history of oropharyngeal mass, pharyngeal disease)
Review of the chart to assess prior airway management during previous anesthetics

Physical Examination
Mouth opening (should be 6–8 cm [three to four fingerbreadths])
Cervical spine mobility
Mallampati classification
Thyromental distance (should be 6–8 cm [three to four fingerbreadths])
Frontal and profile view
Neck circumference
Assessment for disease-associated airway abnormalities
Presence of facial hair

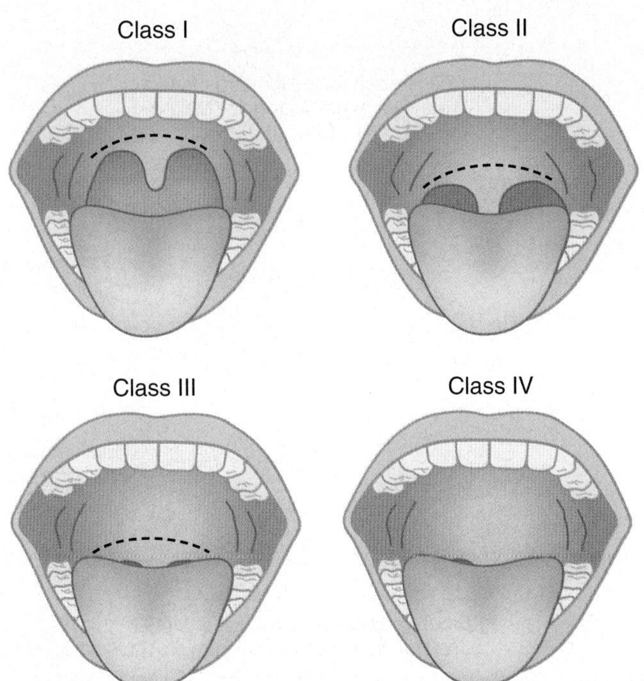

FIG. 14.1 The Mallampati classification relates tongue size to pharyngeal size. This test is performed with the patient in the sitting position, the head held in a neutral position, the mouth wide open, and the tongue protruding to the maximum. The subsequent classification is assigned according to the pharyngeal structures that are visible: class I, visualization of the soft palate, fauces, uvula, and anterior and posterior pillars; class II, visualization of the soft palate, fauces, and uvula; class III, visualization of the soft palate and the base of the uvula; and class IV, soft palate not visible at all. (From Mallampati SR, Gatt SP, Gugino LD, et al. A clinical sign to predict difficult tracheal intubation: a prospective study. *Can Anaesth Soc J.* 1985;32:429–434.)

patient's history to provide a complete airway assessment. Other physical factors that are associated with uncomplicated airway management are adequate mouth opening, neck extension, and thyromental distance. In a metaanalysis examining more than 50,000 patients, Shiga and coauthors[20] reported that individual physical characteristics, by themselves, have poor predictive value for identifying airway difficulties. However, the combined presence of two or more physical endpoints that predict difficult airway management increasingly improves sensitivity and specificity.

Cardiovascular Disease

The risk for perioperative myocardial ischemia and infarction and the risk for cardiac death have become important issues as progressively more complex surgery has been offered to patients with increasingly severe systemic disease. The apparent incidence of perioperative myocardial ischemia depends on the perspective of the study (prospective or retrospective), the sensitivity of the markers used, and the type of surgical procedure. Based on review of the available literature, the American College of Cardiology (ACC) and American Heart Association (AHA) have published guidelines for perioperative cardiovascular evaluation and management of patients undergoing noncardiac surgery.[21] The guidelines focus on the patient's history of cardiovascular disease, exercise tolerance, and the type of surgery proposed. A detailed history and physical are required to assess the presence of underlying cardiovascular disease. Assessment of functional status and the ability to perform common daily tasks is a critical part of the assessment. Patients with active major cardiovascular conditions require evaluation and treatment before undergoing elective noncardiac surgery.

In the 2014 revision of the ACC/AHA guidelines, the committee developed a revised, algorithm-based approach for assessment of cardiovascular risk and determination of the need for perioperative cardiovascular testing.

Functional status is a reliable predictor of perioperative and long-term cardiovascular risk. Patients with poor functional status are at increased risk of cardiovascular events, whereas patients with good exercise tolerance are at lower risk. In the absence of recent exercise testing, a patient's functional status can be assessed based on determination of ability to perform common activities. Functional capacity is commonly expressed in terms of metabolic equivalents of the task (METs), where 1 MET is the resting or basal oxygen consumption of a 40-year-old, 70-kg man. In the perioperative literature, functional capacity is classified as excellent (>10 METs), good (7–10 METs), moderate (4–6 METs), poor (<4 METs), or unknown. Perioperative cardiac and long-term risks are increased in patients unable to perform 4 METs of work during daily activities. Examples of activities requiring <4 METs are slow ballroom dancing, golfing with a cart, playing a musical instrument, and walking at approximately 2 to 3. Examples of activities requiring >4 METs are climbing a flight of stairs or walking up a hill, walking on level ground at 4 mph, and performing heavy work around the house. Assessment tools such as the Duke Activity Status Index and the Specific Activity Scale allow for more detailed assessment of functional status. Fig. 14.2 provides a framework for determining which patients are candidates for preoperative cardiac testing. The clinician must consider the urgency of surgery, the patient's functional capacity, and type of surgery and give them appropriate weight. Since publication of the perioperative cardiovascular evaluation guidelines in 2002 and the revision in 2007, several new randomized trials and cohort studies have led to modification of the original algorithm. For a detailed overview of the current ACC/AHA guidelines, clinicians should refer to the most recently published update. The following stepwise approach is recommended.[21]

Step 1: In patients scheduled for surgery with risk factors for or known coronary artery disease, heart failure, valvular heart disease, or arrhythmias, determine the urgency of surgery. If an emergency, then determine the clinical risk factors that may

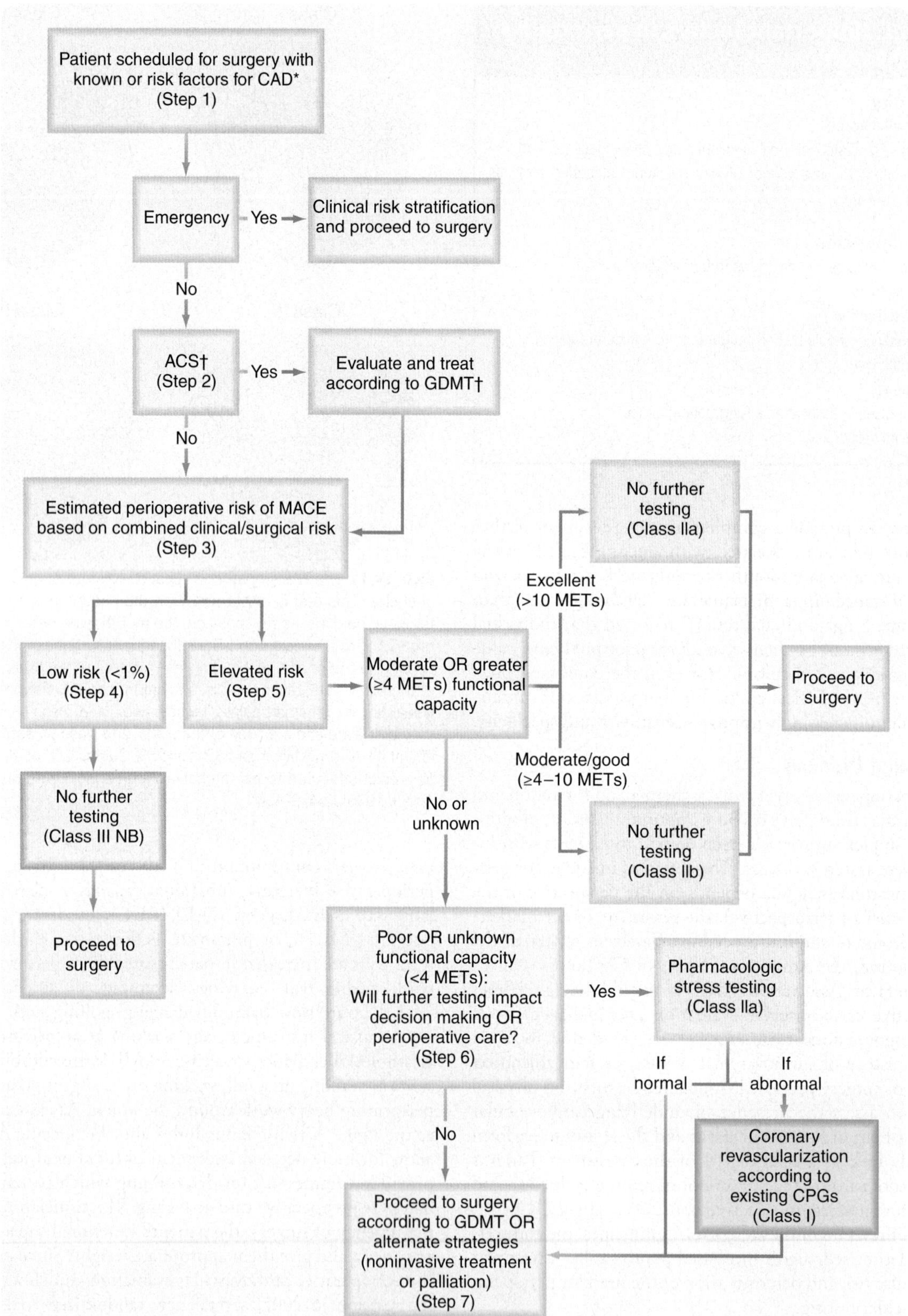

FIG. 14.2 Stepwise approach to perioperative cardiovascular assessment for patients undergoing noncardiac surgery. The need for preoperative testing is based on the patient's functional status, type of surgery, and urgency of surgery. (From Fleisher LA, Fleischmann KE, Auerbach AD, et al. 2014 ACC/AHA guideline on perioperative cardiovascular evaluation and management of patients undergoing noncardiac surgery: a report of the American College of Cardiology/American Heart Association Task Force on practice guidelines. *J Am Coll Cardiol.* 2014;64:e77–137.) *ACS,* Acute coronary syndrome; *CAD,* coronary artery disease; *CPG,* clinical practice guideline; *GDMT,* goal-directed medical therapy; *MACE,* major adverse cardiac event; *METs,* metabolic equivalents of the task.

influence perioperative management and proceed to surgery with appropriate monitoring and management strategies based on the clinical assessment.

Step 2: If the surgery is urgent or elective, determine if the patient has an active coronary syndrome. If yes, then refer patient for cardiology evaluation and management according to guideline-directed medical therapy.

Step 3: If the patient has risk factors for stable coronary artery disease, then estimate the perioperative risk of a major adverse cardiac event (MACE) on the basis of the combined clinical/surgical risk. This estimate can be determined based on use of the American College of Surgeons National Surgical Quality Improvement Program risk calculator (http://www.surgicalriskcalculator.com) or by incorporating the revised cardiac risk index with an estimation of surgical risk. For example, a patient undergoing very-low–risk surgery (e.g., ophthalmologic surgery), even with multiple risk factors, would have a low risk of MACE, whereas a patient undergoing major vascular surgery with few risk factors would have an elevated risk of MACE.

Step 4: If the patient has a low risk of MACE (<1%), then no further testing is needed, and the patient may proceed to surgery.

Step 5: If the patient is at elevated risk of MACE, then determine functional capacity with an objective measure or scale such as the Duke Activity Status Index. If the patient has moderate, good, or excellent functional capacity (≥4 METs), then proceed to surgery without further evaluation.

Step 6: If the patient has poor (<4 METs) or unknown functional capacity, then the clinician should consult with the patient and perioperative team to determine whether further testing will impact patient decision-making (e.g., decision to perform original surgery or willingness to undergo coronary artery bypass grafting or percutaneous coronary intervention, depending on the results of the test) or perioperative care. If yes, then pharmacologic stress testing is appropriate. In those patients with unknown functional capacity, exercise stress testing may be reasonable to perform. If the stress test is abnormal, consider coronary angiography and revascularization depending on the extent of the abnormal test. The patient can then proceed to surgery with guideline-directed medical therapy or consider alternative strategies, such as noninvasive treatment of the indication for surgery (e.g., radiation therapy for cancer) or palliation. If the test is normal, proceed to surgery according to guideline-directed medical therapy.

Step 7: If testing will not impact decision-making or care, then proceed to surgery according to guideline-directed medical therapy or consider alternative strategies, such as noninvasive treatment of the indication for surgery (e.g., radiation therapy for cancer) or palliation.

The need for specific testing is dependent on the patient's exercise tolerance, comorbidities, and the type of surgery proposed. Box 14.4 defines current recommendations on specific perioperative testing including preoperative electrocardiography, echocardiography, stress testing, radionuclide perfusion scans, and coronary angiography. It is recommended that practitioners refer to the most recent ACC/AHA guidelines for detailed recommendations and level of evidence to support the guidelines.[21]

Perioperative medical management is guided by the patient's cardiovascular status, current drug regimen, and the type of surgery proposed. The need for preoperative coronary revascularization is limited to patients who are candidates for emergency or urgent revascularization under any circumstances. Such patients include those with unstable angina, active myocardial infarction, or arrhythmias caused by active ischemia. Elective coronary revascularization to decrease perioperative cardiovascular complications in most patients undergoing noncardiac surgery is not supported by current evidence. For patients who have undergone angioplasty, it is recommended that surgery be delayed a minimum of 14 days and for 30 days for patients

BOX 14.4 Summary of recommendations for supplemental preoperative evaluation.

The 12-Lead ECG

Preoperative resting 12-lead ECG is reasonable for patients with known coronary heart disease or other significant structural heart disease, except for low-risk surgery.

Preoperative resting 12-lead ECG may be considered for asymptomatic patients, except for low-risk surgery.

Routine preoperative resting 12-lead ECG is not useful for asymptomatic patients undergoing low-risk surgical procedures.

Assessment of LV Function

It is reasonable for patients with dyspnea of unknown origin to undergo preoperative evaluation of LV function.

It is reasonable for patients with heart failure with worsening dyspnea or other change in clinical status to undergo preoperative evaluation of LV function.

Reassessment of LV function in clinically stable patients may be considered.

Routine preoperative evaluation of LV function is not recommended.

Exercise stress testing for myocardial ischemia and functional capacity.

For patients with elevated risk and excellent functional capacity, it is reasonable to forgo further exercise testing and proceed to surgery.

For patients with elevated risk and unknown functional capacity, it may be reasonable to perform exercise testing to assess for functional capacity if it will change management.

For patients with elevated risk and moderate to good functional capacity, it may be reasonable to forgo further exercise testing and proceed to surgery.

For patients with elevated risk and poor or unknown functional capacity, it may be reasonable to perform exercise testing with cardiac imaging to assess for myocardial ischemia.

Routine screening with noninvasive stress testing is not useful for low-risk noncardiac surgery.

Cardiopulmonary Exercise Testing

Cardiopulmonary exercise testing may be considered for patients undergoing elevated risk procedures.

Noninvasive Pharmacologic Stress Testing Before Noncardiac Surgery

It is reasonable for patients at elevated risk for noncardiac surgery with poor functional capacity to undergo either DSE or MPI if it will change management.

Routine screening with noninvasive stress testing is not useful for low-risk noncardiac surgery.

Preoperative Coronary Angiography

Routine preoperative coronary angiography is not recommended.

Adapted from Fleisher LA, Fleischmann KE, Auerbach AD, et al. 2014 ACC/AHA guideline on perioperative cardiovascular evaluation and management of patients undergoing noncardiac surgery: a report of the American College of Cardiology/American Heart Association Task Force on practice guidelines. *J Am Coll Cardiol*. 2014;64:e77–e137. *DSE*, Dobutamine stress echocardiogram; *ECG*, electrocardiogram; *LV*, left ventricular; *MPI*, myocardial perfusion imaging.

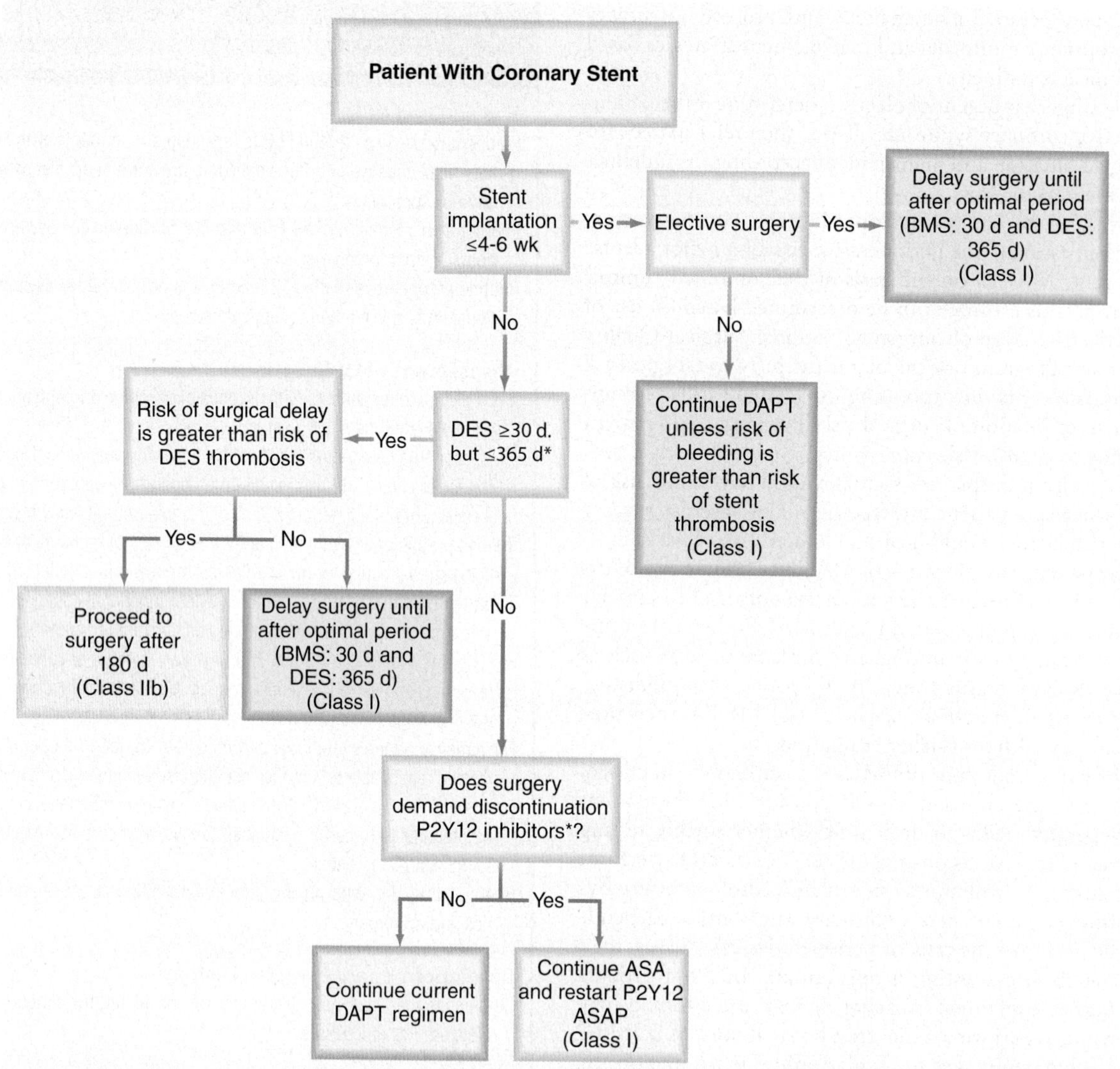

FIG. 14.3 Stepwise approach to patients who have received recent coronary stenting and present for surgery. (From Fleisher LA, Fleischmann KE, Auerbach AD, et al: 2014 ACC/AHA guideline on perioperative cardiovascular evaluation and management of patients undergoing noncardiac surgery: A report of the American College of Cardiology/American Heart Association Task Force on practice guidelines. *J Am Coll Cardiol.* 2014;64:e77–137.) *ASA,* Acetylsalicylic acid; *ASAP,* as soon as possible; *BMS,* bare metal stent; *DAPT,* dual antiplatelet therapy; *DES,* drug-eluting stent.

receiving bare metal stents (BMSs). In patients receiving drug-eluting stents (DESs), current evidence indicates that the risk of stent thrombosis is stabilized at 6 months after DES placement. Although the risk of restenosis is higher with BMS compared to DES, thrombosis is generally not life-threatening in patients receiving BMS and can be treated with repeat angioplasty. Thus, in cases in which the need for noncardiac surgery is time sensitive, consideration should be given to insertion of BMS. If noncardiac surgery is urgent or an emergency and the risk of bleeding is high, then the risks and benefits of coronary revascularization should be weighed and coronary artery bypass grafting should be considered as a revascularization strategy. Recommendations for management of patients who have undergone recent coronary revascularization are presented in Fig. 14.3.

Numerous investigators have assessed the efficacy and safety of beta blockers in the management of cardiovascular disease during the perioperative period. Current studies suggest that beta blockers reduce perioperative myocardial ischemia and may reduce the risk of myocardial infarction and cardiovascular death in high-risk patients. Currently, the ACC/AHA recommends continuation of beta blocker therapy in those patients who are on chronic beta blocker therapy.[21] The use of beta blockers should be considered based on risk stratification and titrated based on clinical circumstances. In beta blocker–naïve patients, perioperative beta blocker therapy should be initiated with caution and based on clinical judgment. Similarly, the perioperative use of calcium channel blockers should be based on patient comorbidities and clinical judgment. Statins should be continued in patients on chronic statin therapy. Perioperative initiation of statin therapy should be considered in patients undergoing vascular surgery and patients at risk for cardiovascular disease who are undergoing high risk procedures. It is reasonable to continue treatment with angiotensin converting enzyme inhibitors and angiotensin receptor antagonists during the perioperative period and to reinitiate those agents postoperatively in patients in whom the drugs were withheld preoperatively. The use of α2-agonists for prevention of cardiac events is not recommended, based on the current literature. An overview of recommendations for perioperative medical management is provided in Box 14.5.[21]

BOX 14.5 Summary of recommendations for perioperative medical management.

Coronary Revascularization Before Noncardiac Surgery

Revascularization before noncardiac surgery is recommended when indicated by existing clinical practice guidelines.

Coronary revascularization is not recommended before noncardiac surgery exclusively to reduce perioperative cardiac events.

Timing of Elective Noncardiac Surgery in Patients With Previous PCI

Noncardiac surgery should be delayed after PCI 14 days after balloon angioplasty and 30 days after BMS implantation.

Noncardiac surgery should be delayed 365 days after DES implantation.

A consensus decision as to the relative risks of discontinuation or continuation of antiplatelet therapy can be useful.

Elective noncardiac surgery after DES implantation may be considered after 180 days.

Elective noncardiac surgery should not be performed in patients in whom DAPT will need to be discontinued perioperatively within 30 days after BMS implantation or within 12 months after DES implantation.

Elective noncardiac surgery should not be performed within 14 days of balloon angioplasty in patients in whom aspirin will need to be discontinued perioperatively.

Perioperative Beta Blocker Therapy

Continue beta blockers in patients who are on beta blockers chronically.

Guide management of beta blockers after surgery by clinical circumstances.

In patients with intermediate- or high-risk preoperative tests, it may be reasonable to begin beta blockers.

In patients with ≥3 RCRI factors, it may be reasonable to begin beta blockers before surgery.

Initiating beta blockers in the perioperative setting as an approach to reduce perioperative risk is of uncertain benefit in those with a long-term indication but not in those with other RCRI risk factors.

In patients with a long-term indication but no other RCRI risk factors. , it may be reasonable to begin beta blockers.

It may be reasonable to begin perioperative beta blockers long enough in advance to assess safety and tolerability, preferably >1 day before surgery.

Beta-blocker therapy should not be started on the day of surgery.

Perioperative Statin Therapy

Continue statins in patients currently taking statins.

Perioperative initiation of statin use is reasonable in patients undergoing vascular surgery.

Perioperative initiation of statins may be considered in patients procedures.

α2-Agonists

α2-Agonists are not recommended for prevention of cardiac events.

ACE Inhibitors

Continuation of ACE inhibitors or ARBs is reasonable perioperatively.

If ACE inhibitors or ARBs are held before surgery, it is reasonable to restart as soon as clinically feasible postoperatively.

Antiplatelet Agents

Continue DAPT in patients undergoing urgent noncardiac surgery during the first 4 to 6 weeks after BMS or DES implantation, unless the risk of bleeding outweighs the benefit of stent thrombosis prevention.

In patients with stents undergoing surgery that requires discontinuation P2Y12 inhibitors, continue aspirin and restart the P2Y12 platelet receptor–inhibitor as soon as possible after surgery.

Management of perioperative antiplatelet therapy should be determined by consensus of treating clinicians and the patient.

In patients undergoing nonemergency/nonurgent noncardiac surgery without prior coronary stenting, it may be reasonable to continue aspirin when the risk of increased cardiac events outweighs the risk of increased bleeding.

Initiation or continuation of aspirin is not beneficial in patients undergoing elective noncardiac noncarotid surgery who have not had previous coronary stenting.

Perioperative Management of Patients With CIEDs

Patients with ICDs should be on a cardiac monitor continuously during the entire period of inactivation, and external defibrillation equipment should be available. Ensure that ICDs are reprogrammed to active therapy.

Adapted from Fleisher LA, Fleischmann KE, Auerbach AD, et al. 2014 ACC/AHA guideline on perioperative cardiovascular evaluation and management of patients undergoing noncardiac surgery: a report of the American College of Cardiology/American Heart Association Task Force on practice guidelines. *J Am Coll Cardiol.* 2014;64:e77–e137.

ACE, Angiotensin-converting enzyme; *ARB,* angiotensin receptor blocker; *BMS,* bare metal stent; *CIED,* cardiac implantable electronic device; *DAPT,* dual antiplatelet therapy; *DES,* drug-eluting stent; *ICD,* implantable cardioverter-defibrillator; *PCI,* percutaneous coronary intervention; *RCRI,* Revised Cardiac Risk Index.

Endocarditis Prophylaxis

Some patients with congenital or valvular heart disease are at increased risk for the development of infective endocarditis (IE). The AHA previously proposed long-standing guidelines that recommended antibiotic prophylaxis for patients at risk for the development of IE who underwent dental, urinary, gastrointestinal, or respiratory surgical procedures. However, the AHA guidelines for endocarditis prophylaxis were changed significantly in 2007.[22] The revised recommendations are based on research that indicates that the chance of developing IE is much more likely to

TABLE 14.5 Regimens for dental procedures.

SITUATION	AGENT	REGIMEN: SINGLE DOSE 30 TO 60 MIN BEFORE PROCEDURE ADULTS	CHILDREN
Oral	Amoxicillin	2 g	50 mg/kg
Unable to take oral medication	Ampicillin or cefazolin or ceftriaxone	2 g IM or IV	50 mg/kg IM or IV
		1 g IM or IV	50 mg/kg IM or IV
Allergic to penicillins or ampicillin—oral	Cephalexin*,† or clindamycin or azithromycin or clarithromycin	2 g	50 mg/kg
		600 mg	20 mg/kg
		500 mg	15 mg/kg
		1 g IM or IV	50 mg/kg IM or IV
Allergic to penicillins or ampicillin and unable to take oral medication	Cefazolin or ceftriaxone† or clindamycin	600 mg IM or IV	20 mg/kg IM or IV

IM, Intramuscular; *IV*, intravenous.
*Or other first- or second-generation oral cephalosporin in equivalent adult or pediatric dosage.
†Cephalosporins should not be used in an individual with a history of anaphylaxis, angioedema, or urticaria with penicillins or ampicillin.

result from random bacteremias caused by daily activities such as chewing and tooth brushing rather than as a result of bacteremia generated by dental and surgical procedures. Therefore, antibiotic prophylaxis is not recommended based solely on an increased lifetime risk of developing IE and should be reserved for patients at highest risk (Table 14.5). The AHA panel recommends that antibiotic prophylaxis is reasonable for dental procedures that involve manipulation of gingival tissues, periapical region of teeth, or perforation of oral mucosa as well as respiratory tract procedures or procedures that manipulate infected skin or musculoskeletal structures in patients at highest risk. Antibiotic prophylaxis solely to prevent IE is not recommended for genitourinary or gastrointestinal tract procedures. For recommended procedures and indications, oral amoxicillin is the drug of choice. Alternative drugs and routes are recommended for patients who are unable to take oral medications or those with penicillin allergy (Box 14.6).

BOX 14.6 Cardiac conditions associated with the highest risk of adverse outcome from endocarditis for which prophylaxis with dental procedures is reasonable.

Prosthetic cardiac valve or prosthetic material used for cardiac valve repair
Previous infective endocarditis
CHD*

- Unrepaired cyanotic CHD, including palliative shunts and conduits
- Completely repaired congenital heart defect with prosthetic material or device, whether placed by surgery or by catheter intervention, during the first 6 months after the procedure†
- Repaired CHD with residual defects at the site or adjacent to the site of a prosthetic patch or prosthetic device (which inhibit endothelialization)

Cardiac transplantation recipients who develop cardiac valvulopathy

CHD, Congenital heart disease.
*Except for the conditions listed above, antibiotic prophylaxis is no longer recommended for any other form of CHD.
†Prophylaxis is reasonable because endothelialization of prosthetic material occurs within 6 months after the procedure.

Pulmonary Disease

Surgical patients often have obstructive or restrictive pulmonary disease. The preoperative history focuses on functional status, exercise tolerance, severity of the disease, and current medications. Recent worsening of symptoms needs to be closely evaluated. A thorough chest physical examination must be performed. Findings on the history and physical examination, as well as an understanding of the planned surgical procedure, suggest appropriate preoperative testing, which may include chest radiography, arterial blood gas analysis, and pulmonary function testing. The goal of preoperative evaluation is to detect and treat reversible pulmonary pathology, optimize medical management, and allow planning for postoperative ventilatory support, if indicated.

The perioperative risk associated with preexisting pulmonary disease has been extensively studied. Qaseem and coworkers,[23] reviewing the topic of preoperative pulmonary evaluation, identified patient-related risk factors, factors related to the surgical site, and other factors related to surgery, such as the duration of surgery, the choice of general anesthesia, and intraoperative use of pancuronium (Table 14.6). Major patient-associated risk factors are ASA class greater than II, age older than 60 years, functional dependence, and the presence of chronic obstructive pulmonary disease or congestive heart failure. A serum albumin concentration of less than 3.5 g/dL was also a strong predictor of pulmonary complications. Current smoking was a minor predictor of pulmonary complications. The presence of obesity or mild to moderate asthma was not significantly associated with perioperative pulmonary complications.

Obstructive sleep apnea (OSA) is an increasingly common condition in surgical patients that requires preoperative evaluation and optimization. Patients with OSA present significant challenges regarding perioperative decision-making. OSA is characterized by periodic upper airway obstruction during sleep resulting in repetitive arousal from sleep to restore airway patency. The condition can result in daytime somnolence, episodic hypoxia, and hypercarbia as well as cardiovascular dysfunction. Perioperative complications include exaggerated respiratory depression from anesthetics and analgesics, postoperative pulmonary complications, cardiac dysrhythmias, and prolonged hospital stays.[24] The ASA has developed Practice Guidelines for the Perioperative Management of Patients with OSA.[25] The guidelines emphasize the importance of preoperative evaluation and development of protocols to optimize the perioperative care of patients with OSA.

Patients with asthma or chronic obstructive pulmonary disease should be evaluated preoperatively and optimized prior to surgery. Assessment should include physical examination and history to assess bronchodilator and steroid use, number and severity of recent respiratory exacerbations, history of previous intubation, and precipitating factors.[26] The approach to preoperative optimization is

TABLE 14.6 Risk factors associated with postoperative pulmonary complications.

PATIENT-ASSOCIATED RISK FACTORS	RELATIVE RISK ASSOCIATED WITH FACTOR	PROCEDURE-ASSOCIATED RISK FACTORS	RELATIVE RISK ASSOCIATED WITH FACTOR
Age >60 years	2.1–3.0	Surgery >3 hours	2.1
Functional dependence	2.5	General anesthesia	1.8
ASA class >II	4.9	Emergency surgery	2.2
Congestive heart failure	2.9		
Smoking	1.3		
Obesity	1.3		
COPD	1.8		

Modified from Qaseem A, Snow V, Fitterman N, et al. Risk assessment for and strategies to reduce perioperative pulmonary complications for patients undergoing noncardiothoracic surgery: a guideline from the American College of Physicians. *Ann Intern Med.* 2006;144:575–580.
ASA, American Society of Anesthesiologists; *COPD*, chronic obstructive pulmonary disease.

dependent on the patient's history and current disease severity and includes use of inhaled β2- agonists, anticholinergics, and steroids, as well as treatment of other existing comorbidities. The choice of anesthetic agents and technique is dependent on patient condition and type of surgery. In patients with active disease, elective surgery should be postponed until the patient is adequately treated.

The other major factors predicting perioperative pulmonary complications are related to surgical and anesthetic interventions and include surgery lasting longer than 3 hours, emergency surgery, and the use of general anesthesia. Procedures with an increased risk for pulmonary complications include abdominal surgery, thoracic surgery, neurosurgery, head and neck surgery, and vascular surgery.

Pulmonary function testing remains controversial, in part, because of changing expectations regarding the ability of patients with chronic pulmonary disease to tolerate extensive surgery. Pulmonary function testing has variable predictive value, cannot define a threshold above which the risk associated with surgery is prohibitive, and identifies no group at high risk but without clinical evidence of pulmonary disease. Arterial blood gas analysis also does not identify a group for whom the risk of surgery is prohibitive. Spirometry may be helpful in a patient who has unexplained cough, dyspnea, or exercise intolerance or if there is a question regarding optimal improvement of airflow obstruction. Warner and associates[27] compared 135 patients who had undergone spirometry, were undergoing abdominal surgery, and met objective criteria for obstructive pulmonary disease (mean forced expiratory volume in 1 second, 0.9 ± 0.2 L) to 135 patients matched for gender, surgical site, smoking history, and age. Although there was a significantly greater incidence of bronchospasm, the incidence of prolonged endotracheal intubation, prolonged ICU admission, or readmission was no different. These results are reiterated in the metaanalysis performed by Qaseem and colleagues.[23]

Renal and Hepatic Disease

Renal and hepatic dysfunctions alter the metabolism and disposition of many anesthetic agents, as well as impair many systemic functions. Patients with acute renal or hepatic insufficiency do no undergo elective surgery until these conditions can be adequately stabilized. Chronic renal insufficiency (CRI) provides many perioperative management challenges, including acid-base abnormalities, electrolyte disturbances, and coagulation disorders. A thorough history must include the cause of CRI, the presence of systemic complications related to CRI, and other systemic diseases. Current daily urinary output, the type and frequency of dialysis, and dialysis-related complications must also be evaluated. The physical examination focuses on identifying systemic complications of CRI, including evidence of altered volume status, coagulopathy, anemia, pericardial effusion, and encephalopathy. Laboratory evaluation includes assessment of anemia, electrolyte abnormalities, coagulopathy, and cardiovascular disease. Dialysis is performed 18 to 24 hours before surgery to avoid the fluid and electrolyte shifts that occur immediately after dialysis.

A patient with chronic liver disease poses many perioperative challenges. The presence of liver disease alters anesthetic drug metabolism, and hypoalbuminemia increases the free fraction of many drugs, thus making these patients sensitive to both the acute and long-term effects of many anesthetics. The perioperative risks associated with anesthesia and surgery are dependent on the severity of hepatic dysfunction. The preoperative evaluation focuses on hepatic synthetic and metabolic function and the presence of coagulopathy, encephalopathy, and ascites, as well as the nutritional status of the patient.

Nutrition, Endocrinology, and Metabolism

Diabetes mellitus warrants discussion because of its high prevalence and potential for comorbidity. Preanesthetic evaluation focuses on the duration and type of diabetes, as well as the current medical regimen. Review of end-organ function with emphasis on autonomic dysfunction, cardiovascular disease, renal insufficiency, retinopathy, and neurologic complications is mandatory. Patients with diabetes are considered to have delayed gastric emptying and to be at risk for gastroesophageal reflux. Perioperative plasma glucose levels need to be well controlled, yet hypoglycemia must be prevented. Appropriate control of perioperative blood sugar in diabetics is difficult to define. Over the long-term, there is compelling evidence of a correlation between hyperglycemia and long-term diabetic and perioperative complications.[28] It is much less clear whether blood sugar must be tightly controlled during the acute stress of surgery. However, there is a strong correlation between mortality and tight control of glucose in critically ill patients, including surgical patients. Furthermore, given the heterogeneity of the diabetic population, it is unlikely that a single standard approach is appropriate for all patients.

In diabetic patients undergoing surgery, several principles of management are generally accepted.

1. Insulin pumps should be continued at sleep basal rates.
2. Provide a reduced dose of intermediate-acting or long-acting insulin and hold short-acting insulin on the morning of surgery.
3. Once a diabetic who is receiving nothing by mouth is given insulin, provide glucose in IV fluids or closely monitor plasma glucose concentrations.

4. Plasma glucose concentrations should be checked before surgery and before discharge as a minimum.
5. In patients with type 2 diabetes, most authors suggest holding oral antidiabetic medications and noninsulin injectables on the day of surgery.
6. Metformin is usually stopped because of a slight risk for perioperative drug-induced lactic acidosis. Perioperative insulin requirements vary depending on body weight, liver disease, steroid therapy, infection, and the use of cardiopulmonary bypass.

Patients who have received systemic glucocorticoids prior to surgery may not be able to respond adequately to surgical stress. Because of the remote risk for adrenal insufficiency during anesthesia, patients who receive chronic glucocorticoids generally receive perioperative glucocorticoid coverage. Recommendations regarding identification of patients at risk and appropriate dosing are based on anecdote. Newer recommendations are based on the preoperative dosage of glucocorticoid, the duration of therapy, and the type of surgery. For minor surgical stress, the equivalent of 25 mg of hydrocortisone on the operative day is recommended; for moderate surgical stress, 50 to 75 mg equivalent for 1 to 2 days; and for major surgical stress, 100 to 150 mg/day for 2 to 3 days.

Fasting Before Surgery

Pulmonary aspiration of gastric contents during anesthesia is an uncommon, but serious, complication. To prevent aspiration, *nil per os* (NPO; nothing by mouth) guidelines have been developed for patients scheduled for anesthesia and surgery. Traditionally, orders for "NPO after midnight" forbade any intake of liquids and solids. However, applying the same guidelines for clear liquids (gastric emptying time, 1–2 hours) and solids (gastric emptying time, 6 hours) has been questioned. The ASA adopted guidelines in 1998 that recommended a minimum fasting period of 2 hours after the ingestion of clear liquids and 6 hours for solids and nonclear liquids such as milk or orange juice (Table 14.7). *Clear liquids* are defined as liquids that you can see through and do not contain solids or particulates. The routine use of gastrointestinal stimulants, gastric acid secretion blockers, antacids, and antiemetics is not recommended. However, many patients have medical conditions that cause decreased gastric emptying. In these patients, the use of agents to improve gastric emptying and neutralize gastric acid may be warranted. In addition, precautions are instituted to decrease the risk for aspiration during anesthesia in patients undergoing emergency procedures.

The reported incidence of aspiration during anesthesia in various studies has varied from 1.4 to 11 per 10,000 anesthetics. A higher incidence has been noted during emergency surgery and in patients with underlying disease processes that cause decreased gastric emptying. Interestingly, some reports suggest that aspiration is at least as common during emergence from anesthesia as during the induction phase. Of patients in whom aspiration is suspected, less than half exhibit evidence of pulmonary injury. In one study, approximately one-third of patients with suspected aspiration during anesthesia required postoperative intubation and ventilation. Most of these patients were extubated within 6 hours of surgery. About 10% of patients required intubation and ventilation for 24 hours or longer. Approximately half the patients requiring ventilation for longer than 24 hours after aspiration of gastric contents died of pulmonary complications.

TABLE 14.7 Summary of preoperative fasting recommendations to reduce the risk of pulmonary aspiration.*

INGESTED MATERIAL	MINIMUM FASTING PERIOD
Clear liquids[†]	2 hours
Breast milk	4 hours
Infant formula	6 hours
Nonhuman milk	6 hours
Solid food	6 hours

Adapted from Practice guidelines for preoperative fasting and the use of pharmacologic agents to reduce the risk of pulmonary aspiration: application to healthy patients undergoing elective procedures: a report by the American Society of Anesthesiologist Task Force on Preoperative Fasting. *Anesthesiology*. 1999;90:896–905.
*Applies to healthy patients undergoing elective procedures.
[†]Examples of clear liquids are water, fruit juices without pulp, black coffee, clear tea, carbonated beverages.

Assessment of Physical Status

The ASA has developed a graded, descriptive scale as a means of categorizing preoperative comorbidity. The classification is independent of operative procedure and serves as a standardized method of communicating patient physical status to anesthesiologists and other health care providers. Patients are categorized as follows:

ASA I—No organic, physiologic, biochemical, or psychiatric disturbance.
ASA II—A patient with mild systemic disease that results in no functional limitation. Examples are well-controlled hypertension and uncomplicated diabetes mellitus.
ASA III—A patient with severe systemic disease that results in functional impairment. Examples are diabetes mellitus with vascular complications, previous myocardial infarction, and uncontrolled hypertension.
ASA IV—A patient with severe systemic disease that is a constant threat to life. Examples are congestive heart failure and unstable angina pectoris.
ASA V—A moribund patient who is not expected to survive with or without the surgery. Examples are ruptured aortic aneurysm and intracranial hemorrhage with elevated ICP.
ASA VI—A declared brain-dead patient whose organs are being harvested for transplantation.
E—Emergency surgery is required. For example, *ASA IE* represents an otherwise healthy patient undergoing emergency appendectomy.

SELECTION OF ANESTHETIC TECHNIQUES AND DRUGS

Selection of anesthetic techniques and drugs begins with the preoperative anesthetic evaluation. Recognition of important preexisting conditions and chronic medication use may suggest that certain approaches are preferable. Then the requirements of the surgical procedure and surgeon are considered. What is the operative site? How will the patient be positioned? What is the expected duration of surgery? Is the patient expected to return home after an ambulatory procedure or is hospital admission anticipated? Finally, in this era of cost constraints, are the costs of newer drugs and approaches justified by probable clinical benefit? Evidence of the increasing safety of anesthesia is the fact that multiple options can often be used safely and effectively for the same procedure and the same patient.

After completing the preanesthetic evaluation, the anesthesiologist discusses various options regarding anesthetic care with the patient. Together, sometimes with input from the patient's surgeon, the anesthesiologist and patient choose an anesthetic technique. Continued progress in the pharmacology of anesthetic drugs, improvements in the accuracy and applicability of monitoring devices, and parallel improvements in the management of chronic disease processes have resulted in the ability to extensively customize the anesthetic management of individual patients.

Risk of Anesthesia

Patients often desire information regarding the risk of death or major complications associated with anesthesia. However, because perioperative death and major complications have become so uncommon, the risk associated with anesthesia is difficult to quantify. An estimated 234 million surgical cases occur worldwide each year. In developed nations, surgical mortality is estimated to be 0.4% to 0.8%, with morbidity rates of 3% to 17%.[29] The risk for cardiac arrest attributable to anesthesia appears to be less than 1 in 10,000 cases.[30] Schwilk and colleagues[31] prospectively studied preoperative risk factors as predictors of perioperative adverse events in 26,907 patients undergoing noncardiac surgery. Fourteen variables proved to be independent risk factors, including gender, age, ASA status, functional status, nutritional state, coronary disease, airway and lung pathology, Mallampati classification, fluid and electrolyte balance, metabolic state, grade of urgency, operative site, duration of surgery, and anesthetic technique (lower risk with regional than with general anesthesia). With the use of a point system, patients could be reliably separated into low- and high-risk groups.

Because so many surgical procedures are now performed without admission to the hospital, the risk associated with ambulatory anesthesia is particularly important. To assess this risk, 38,598 patients who had undergone 45,090 consecutive ambulatory surgical procedures were contacted within 72 hours and 30 days of surgery (99.94% and 95.9% of patients, respectively). No patient died of a medical complication within 1 week of surgery. The total death rate was 1 in 11,273 (4 deaths), and the total complication rate was 1 in 1366. A more recent study by Fleisher and colleagues[32] reported similar findings with mortality rates of 0.025% to 0.05% for patients undergoing outpatient surgery in physician offices, ambulatory surgery centers, and outpatient hospital facilities. Patient and procedure selection are important factors in determining the safety of outpatient anesthesia and surgical procedures. The associated risk is a summation of surgery and anesthesia. The individual contributions of each component are difficult to determine.

Selection of a Specific Technique

The first step in selecting a specific anesthetic technique for an individual patient is to consider whether the procedure can be appropriately performed with monitored anesthesia care (also sometimes abbreviated as MAC, to be distinguished from the identical abbreviation for minimum alveolar concentration), regional anesthesia (including regional upper and lower extremity blocks, subarachnoid blocks, and epidural anesthesia), or general anesthesia. Monitored anesthesia care supplements local anesthesia performed by surgeons. Anesthesiologists usually participate because an individual patient or procedure requires higher doses of potent sedatives or opioids or because an acutely or chronically ill patient requires close monitoring and hemodynamic or respiratory support. Regional anesthesia (discussed in detail in a later section) is useful for operations on the upper and lower extremities, pelvis, and lower part of the abdomen. Certain other procedures, such as carotid endarterectomy and awake craniotomy, can also be successfully performed under a regional or field block. Patients receiving regional anesthesia can generally remain awake and, if needed, can receive IV sedation or analgesics. Although regional anesthesia avoids general anesthesia and intuitively appears to be safer, hazards specific to regional anesthesia must be considered. Such hazards include, among others, postdural puncture headache, local anesthetic toxicity, high neuraxial block, and peripheral nerve injury. In addition, an inadequate regional anesthetic may require rapid transition to heavy sedation or general anesthesia.

Regardless of the suitability of a particular technique for a specific surgical procedure, other factors, including the patient's preferences, must be considered. For instance, regional anesthesia might not be chosen if a patient were extremely anxious or could not communicate effectively because of a language barrier. Monitored anesthesia care might be inappropriate if a patient were unlikely to lie quietly during delicate or prolonged surgery. Any procedure planned under regional anesthesia or monitored anesthesia care can require conversion to general anesthesia if the original choice proves unsatisfactory.

AIRWAY MANAGEMENT

Airway management is perhaps the most critical skill in anesthesiology. As discussed earlier, the preoperative evaluation focuses on recognition of patients who may be difficult to mask ventilate or intubate. Knowledge of and skill with various techniques for establishment of a patent airway constitute the central group of skills that are critical for the safe practice of anesthesiology. Fortunately, the incidence of difficult intubations is low. Difficult direct laryngoscopy occurs in 1.5% to 8.5% of general anesthetics, and failed intubation occurs in 0.13% to 0.3% of general anesthetics. The laryngeal mask airway, the lighted stylet, and an array of videolaryngoscopes are recent developments that make ventilation and intubation possible in many patients who have failed intubation with a conventional laryngoscope. The fiberoptic bronchoscope is an additional tool for the management of a difficult airway.

Because of the importance of a prompt, effective response to difficult intubation, the ASA has developed guidelines for managing difficult airways (Fig. 14.4). A key factor is the initial airway examination and recognition of the patient with a potentially difficult airway. If the practitioner suspects that mask ventilation and tracheal intubation will be difficult, it is recommended that spontaneous ventilation be preserved. Approaches to these patients include awake intubation or the use of anesthetic techniques that preserve spontaneous ventilation. In some cases, establishment of a surgical airway in an awake patient under local anesthesia may be indicated. However, some patients are found to have a difficult airway only after anesthesia and muscle relaxation have been induced. This is an emergency situation that must be rectified quickly to avoid hypoxemia, brain injury, or death. A variety of airway adjuncts are available to preserve ventilation and facilitate tracheal intubation under emergency conditions. The practitioner always must call for assistance in these situations to optimize patient care and consider reestablishment of spontaneous ventilation. It is essential to have alternate means for securing the airway available for all patients in the event of an unanticipated difficult airway.

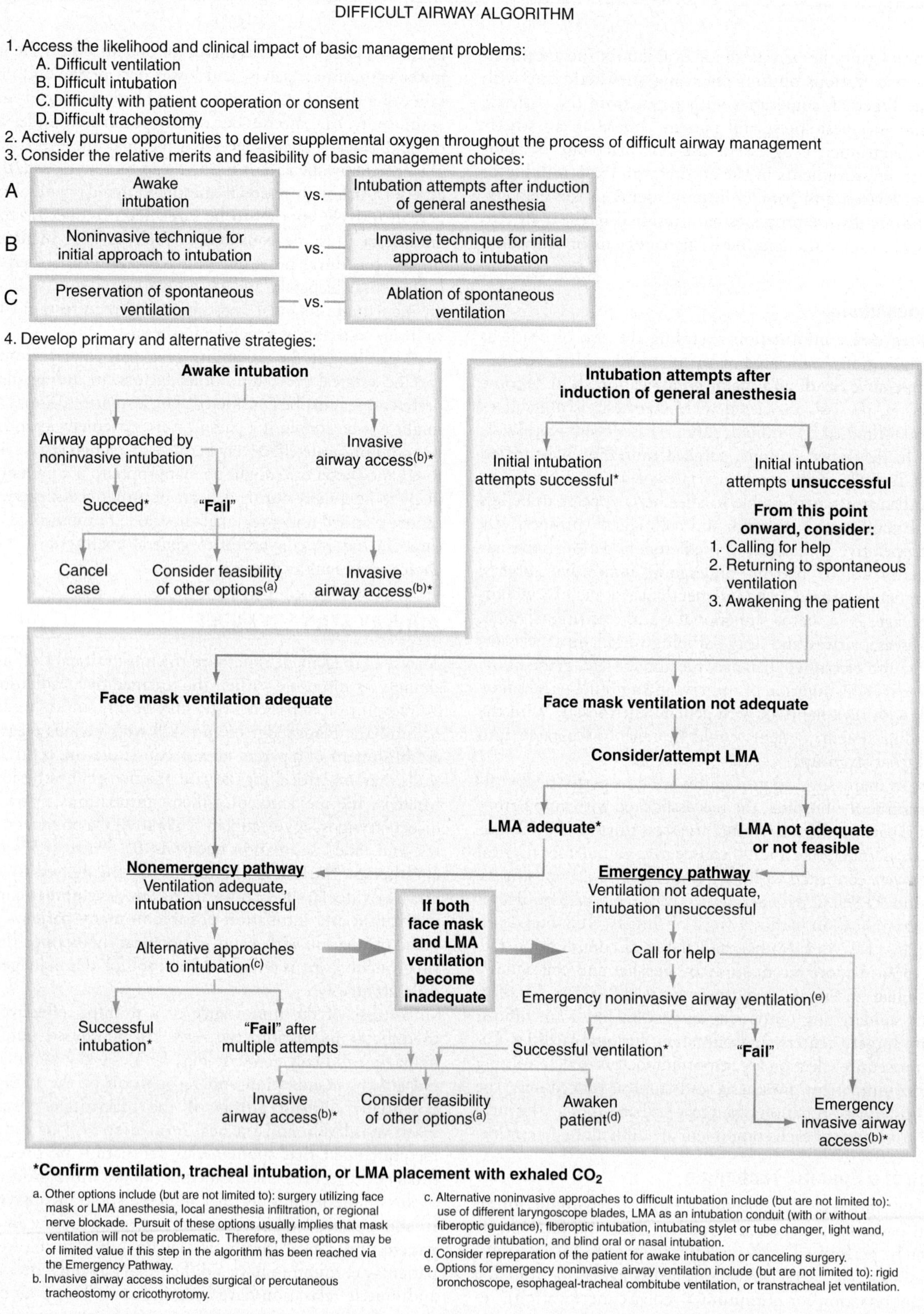

DIFFICULT AIRWAY ALGORITHM

1. Access the likelihood and clinical impact of basic management problems:
   A. Difficult ventilation
   B. Difficult intubation
   C. Difficulty with patient cooperation or consent
   D. Difficult tracheostomy
2. Actively pursue opportunities to deliver supplemental oxygen throughout the process of difficult airway management
3. Consider the relative merits and feasibility of basic management choices:

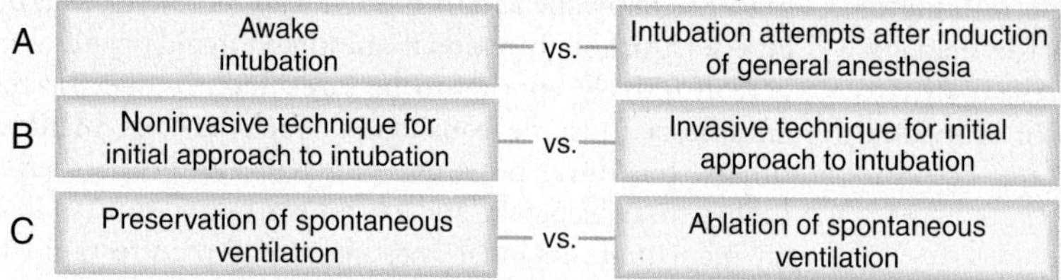

4. Develop primary and alternative strategies:

Awake intubation

Airway approached by noninvasive intubation

Invasive airway access(b)*

Succeed*

"Fail"

Cancel case

Consider feasibility of other options(a)

Invasive airway access(b)*

Intubation attempts after induction of general anesthesia

Initial intubation attempts successful*

Initial intubation attempts **unsuccessful**

From this point onward, consider:
1. Calling for help
2. Returning to spontaneous ventilation
3. Awakening the patient

Face mask ventilation adequate

Face mask ventilation not adequate

Consider/attempt LMA

LMA adequate*

LMA not adequate or not feasible

Nonemergency pathway
Ventilation adequate, intubation unsuccessful

Alternative approaches to intubation(c)

If both face mask and LMA ventilation become inadequate

Emergency pathway
Ventilation not adequate, intubation unsuccessful

Call for help

Emergency noninvasive airway ventilation(e)

Successful intubation*

"Fail" after multiple attempts

Successful ventilation*

"Fail"

Invasive airway access(b)*

Consider feasibility of other options(a)

Awaken patient(d)

Emergency invasive airway access(b)*

***Confirm ventilation, tracheal intubation, or LMA placement with exhaled CO_2**

a. Other options include (but are not limited to): surgery utilizing face mask or LMA anesthesia, local anesthesia infiltration, or regional nerve blockade. Pursuit of these options usually implies that mask ventilation will not be problematic. Therefore, these options may be of limited value if this step in the algorithm has been reached via the Emergency Pathway.

b. Invasive airway access includes surgical or percutaneous tracheostomy or cricothyrotomy.

c. Alternative noninvasive approaches to difficult intubation include (but are not limited to): use of different laryngoscope blades, LMA as an intubation conduit (with or without fiberoptic guidance), fiberoptic intubation, intubating stylet or tube changer, light wand, retrograde intubation, and blind oral or nasal intubation.

d. Consider repreparation of the patient for awake intubation or canceling surgery.

e. Options for emergency noninvasive airway ventilation include (but are not limited to): rigid bronchoscope, esophageal-tracheal combitube ventilation, or transtracheal jet ventilation.

FIG. 14.4 American Society of Anesthesiologists difficult airway algorithm. The likelihood and clinical impact of basic management problems such as difficult intubation, difficult mask ventilation, and difficulty with patient cooperation or consent should be assessed in all patients in whom airway management is being contemplated. The clinician should consider the relative merits and feasibility of basic management choices, including the use of awake intubation techniques, preservation of spontaneous ventilation, and the use of surgical approaches to establish a secure airway. Primary and alternative strategies should be considered: (a) other options include, but are not limited to, surgery under mask anesthesia, surgery under local infiltration or nerve block, and intubation attempts after induction of general anesthesia; (b) alternative approaches include the use of different laryngoscope blades, awake intubation, blind oral or nasal intubation, fiberoptic intubation, an intubating stylet or tube changer, light wand, retrograde intubation, and surgical airway access; (c) see awake intubation; (d) options for an emergency nonsurgical airway include transtracheal jet ventilation, laryngeal mask airway, and Combitube. (From Practice guidelines for management of the difficult airway. A report by the American Society of Anesthesiologists Task Force on Management of the Difficult Airway. *Anesthesiology*. 1993;78:597–602.)

GENERAL ANESTHESIA

General anesthesia is a reversible state of unconsciousness. Although the mechanism of general anesthetics remains speculative and controversial, the four components of general anesthesia (amnesia, analgesia, inhibition of noxious reflexes, and skeletal muscle relaxation) are usually achieved in modern anesthesia by a combination of IV anesthetics and analgesics, inhalational anesthetics, and, frequently, muscle relaxants. Because the drugs that produce these components cause both desirable and undesirable physiologic changes, the pharmacologic effects of the agents must be matched to the pathophysiology of the patient's comorbidities. The major adverse changes associated with anesthetic drugs are respiratory depression, cardiovascular depression, and loss of airway maintenance and protection. Important complications of general anesthesia include hypoxemia (with possible central nervous system [CNS] damage), hypotension, cardiac arrest, and aspiration of acidic gastric contents (which can lead to severe pulmonary damage). Dental damage is more frequent but not life-threatening. General anesthesia can be maintained by inhalation of volatile agents or by infusion of IV agents. Both techniques can have advantages under certain conditions, and individual patient factors should be considered. General anesthesia is required for major intraabdominal and thoracic procedures, most neurosurgical operations, and any procedure in which airway protection and mechanical ventilation are required.

REGIONAL ANESTHESIA

Regional anesthesia is an attractive anesthetic option for many types of operative procedures and can provide excellent postoperative pain management in selected patients. However, like any anesthetic technique, the risks and benefits associated with regional anesthesia must be assessed for each individual. Several regional techniques are in common use, including spinal, epidural, and peripheral nerve blocks. Each technique has specific benefits and risks, which depend in part on the choice of local anesthetic drugs.

Local Anesthetic Drugs

Local anesthetics have played a critical role in intraoperative anesthesia almost since they were first described. The two classes of local anesthetic drugs in common use are aminoesters and aminoamides (often described as *esters* and *amides*). The mechanism of action of local anesthetics is dose-dependent blockade of sodium currents in nerve fibers. Local anesthetic drugs differ in terms of their physicochemical characteristics. Of these characteristics, the most important are pK_a, protein binding, and the degree of hydrophobicity. pK_a refers to the pH at which half the drug exists in the basic uncharged form and half exists in the cationic form. In general, agents with a lower pK_a have a faster onset than do agents with a higher pK_a, although some agents, such as chloroprocaine, can be given at much higher concentrations, thereby offsetting the effects of a high pK_a. Because all commonly used local anesthetics have relatively high pK_a values, they are largely ineffective in acidotic (inflamed) environments in which local anesthetics exist primarily in the ionized form, which does not penetrate nerves. In general, greater hydrophobicity is associated with greater potency, and increased protein binding correlates with a longer duration of action. The development of liposomal bupivacaine has the potential to prolong analgesia after local administration. Liposomal bupivacaine is composed of bupivacaine encapsulated in multivescicular liposomes and can provide up to 72 hours of analgesia after local infiltration. Liposomal bupivacaine was approved by the FDA for local wound infiltration and for interscalene block. The superiority of liposomal bupivacaine compared to other modes of analgesia is currently unclear and a topic of current research. However, local infiltration of liposomal bupivacaine to provide postoperative analgesia has been widely accepted for some procedures. The speed of onset, duration of action, and typical doses of agents commonly used for regional anesthesia or local anesthesia are summarized in Table 14.8.

In using local anesthetics clinically, the priority is to prevent local anesthetic toxicity. When used for regional anesthesia, the toxicity of local anesthetics is dependent on the site of injection and the speed of absorption. Inadvertent intravascular injection of local anesthetics produces toxicity with much smaller doses. The main symptoms of local anesthetic toxicity involve the CNS and cardiovascular system. The earliest signs of an overdose or inadvertent intravascular injection are numbness or tingling of the tongue or lips, a metallic taste, light-headedness, tinnitus, or visual disturbances. Signs of toxicity can progress to slurred speech, disorientation, and seizures. With higher doses of local anesthetics, cardiovascular collapse will ensue.

The best defenses against local anesthetic toxicity are aspiration to detect unplanned vascular entry before injecting large doses of local anesthetics and knowledge of the maximal safe dose of the drug being injected. Adding epinephrine, which slows absorption, also decreases the likelihood of a toxic response secondary to rapid absorption. The primary treatments of local anesthetic toxicity are oxygen and airway support. If a seizure does not terminate spontaneously, a benzodiazepine (e.g., midazolam) or thiopental is given. Cardiovascular support may be needed.

Cardiovascular toxicity from bupivacaine may be particularly difficult to treat. One approach intended to reduce the cardiovascular toxicity of bupivacaine (a racemic mixture of the *levo* and *dextro* isomers) has been to produce a solution consisting of only the *levo* isomer. In healthy male volunteers, slow IV infusion of levobupivacaine reduced the mean stroke index, acceleration index,

TABLE 14.8 Important characteristics of local anesthetics for major nerve blocks.

LOCAL ANESTHETIC	AMINOAMIDE OR AMINOESTER	SPEED OF ONSET (MIN)	DURATION OF ACTION (MIN)	MAXIMAL DOSE* (AXILLARY BLOCK)
Lidocaine	Aminoamide	10–20	60–180	5 mg/kg
Mepivacaine	Aminoamide	10–20	60–180	5 mg/kg
Bupivacaine	Aminoamide	15–30	180–360	3 mg/kg
Ropivacaine	Aminoamide	15–30	180–360	3 mg/kg

*Maximal dose without epinephrine; doses of lidocaine and mepivacaine can be increased to 7 to 8 mg/kg if epinephrine is added. Lower doses may be toxic if infiltrated subcutaneously, as for intercostal nerve blocks; larger doses of lidocaine and mepivacaine may be tolerated if given by epidural injection.

and ejection fraction less than racemic bupivacaine did. Ropivacaine, a newer potent amide local anesthetic, was compared to bupivacaine and lidocaine in volunteers receiving a slow IV infusion until CNS symptoms first occurred. Echocardiography and electrocardiography were used to quantify systolic, diastolic, and electrophysiologic effects. Bupivacaine increased QRS width during sinus rhythm as compared to the other two treatments and reduced both systolic and diastolic function, whereas ropivacaine reduced only systolic function. The anesthetic properties of ropivacaine are similar to bupivacaine, and, based on its decreased toxicity profile, it is commonly used as an alternative to bupivacaine by many practitioners. Many case reports and experimental studies have reported the efficacy of lipid emulsion infusion as a means of rescuing subjects from severe local anesthetic toxicity. Although the mechanisms of action of lipid emulsion therapy are not completely understood, the use of lipid emulsion therapy in cases of systemic local anesthetic toxicity has been adopted by the American Society of Regional Anesthesia and Pain Medicine, who recommend bolus injection of 1.5 mL/kg (lean body mass) of 20% lipid emulsion over 1 minute followed by an infusion of 0.25 mL/kg/min. In cases of refractory toxicity, the bolus may be repeated and the infusion rate doubled.[33]

An area of intense research interest has been the use of α_2-adrenergic agents to potentiate or substitute for local anesthetics. Regional anesthesia was first produced with cocaine (also a local anesthetic) for subarachnoid block in the late 1800s, although the specific receptors involved were not established until much later. The α_2-adrenergic drug clonidine was first used epidurally in 1984 after extensive characterization in animals. Despite side effects such as hypotension, bradycardia, and sedation, experience in thousands of patients has demonstrated considerable safety when used alone or with local anesthetics or opioids for epidural anesthesia and analgesia, subarachnoid block, or peripheral nerve block. In general, clonidine prolongs or intensifies the effects of local anesthetics or opioids and produces pain relief when used alone.

Spinal Anesthesia

Spinal anesthesia or subarachnoid block has many applications for urologic, lower abdominal, perineal, and lower extremity surgery. Spinal anesthesia is induced by the injection of local anesthetic, with or without opiates, into the subarachnoid space. A well-performed subarachnoid block provides excellent sensory and motor blockade below the level of the block. The block generally has a relatively rapid and predictable onset. Several factors determine the level, speed of onset, and duration of spinal blockade.

1. Local anesthetic agent. Local anesthetics have varying potencies, durations of action, and speeds of onset after subarachnoid administration. Typical doses and durations of action are shown in Table 14.9. Bupivacaine and tetracaine have significantly longer durations of action than lidocaine does. These properties are determined by the lipid solubility, protein binding, and pK_a of each agent.
2. Volume and dose of the local anesthetic. Increasing the dose will generally increase the extent of cephalad spread and duration of subarachnoid blockade. Rapidly injecting local anesthetic solutions leads to turbulent flow and unpredictable spread.
3. Patient position and local anesthetic baricity. Local anesthetic solutions can be prepared as hypobaric, isobaric, and hyperbaric solutions. Cerebrospinal fluid (CSF) has low specific gravity (i.e., only slightly greater than that of water). Local anesthetic solutions prepared in water have slightly lower specific gravity than CSF does and will therefore ascend within CSF. Plain local anesthetic solutions are isobaric, and local anesthetics mixed in 5% dextrose are hyperbaric relative to CSF. The baricity of the local anesthetic solution and the position of the patient at the time of injection and until the local anesthetic firmly binds to nervous tissue will determine the level of block. For example, administration of hyperbaric bupivacaine at the low lumbar level to a patient in the sitting position will result in intense lumbosacral blockade. The longer the patient remains in the sitting position, the less the cephalad spread of the block.
4. Vasoconstrictors. The addition of epinephrine or phenylephrine, particularly to short-acting local anesthetics, will increase the duration of action.
5. Addition of opioids. The addition of small doses of fentanyl (e.g., 20 μg) or morphine (e.g., 0.25 mg) will prolong the duration of analgesia and increase the duration of analgesia and tolerance for tourniquet pain.
6. Anatomic and physiologic factors. A higher-than-expected level of spinal anesthesia can result from anatomic factors that decrease the relative volume of the subarachnoid space, such as obesity, pregnancy, increased intraabdominal pressure, previous spine surgery, and abnormal spinal curvature. Elderly patients tend to be more sensitive to intrathecally injected local anesthetics.

Spinal anesthesia provides the advantage of avoiding manipulation of the airway and the potential complication of tracheal intubation, as well as the potential side effects of general anesthetics such as nausea, vomiting, and prolonged emergence or drowsiness. Spinal anesthesia also provides advantages for several types of surgery, including endoscopic urologic procedures, particularly transurethral resection of the prostate in which an awake patient provides a valuable monitor for assessment of hyponatremia or bladder perforation. Less confusion and postoperative delirium have been reported in elderly patients after repair of hip fractures under spinal anesthesia. Intrathecal opiate administration can provide high-quality

TABLE 14.9 Local anesthetics used for subarachnoid block.

DRUG	USUAL CONCENTRATION (%)	USUAL VOLUME (mL)	TOTAL DOSE (mg)	BARICITY	GLUCOSE CONCENTRATION (%)	USUAL DURATION (MIN)
Lidocaine	1.5, 5.0	1–2	30–100	Hyperbaric	7.5	30–60
Tetracaine	0.25–1.0	1–4	5–20	Hyperbaric	5.0	75–200
	0.25	2–6	5–20	Hypobaric	0	75–200
	1.0	1–2	5–20	Isobaric	0	75–200
Bupivacaine	0.5	2–4	10–20	Isobaric	0	75–200
	0.75	1–3	7.5–22.5	Hyperbaric	8.25	75–200

From Berde CB, Strichartz GR. Local anesthetics. In: Miller RD, ed. *Anesthesia.* 5th ed. Philadelphia: Churchill Livingstone; 2000:491–522.

postoperative analgesia for patients undergoing abdominal, lower extremity, urologic, and gynecologic procedures.

In most cases, spinal anesthesia is administered as a single bolus injection. Therefore, the block is of limited duration and is not suitable for prolonged procedures. The practice of continuous spinal anesthesia with the use of small-bore catheters has largely been abandoned because of neurologic complications associated with local anesthetic toxicity. However, continuous spinal anesthesia with relatively large-bore epidural catheters can provide the advantages of incremental titration and the ability to administer additional doses in selected elderly patients. Unfortunately, this technique has a high likelihood of inducing a postdural puncture headache in young patients.

Complications of subarachnoid block include hypotension (sometimes refractory), bradycardia, postdural puncture headache, transient radicular neuropathy, backache, urinary retention, infection, epidural hematoma, and excessive cephalad spread resulting in cardiorespiratory compromise. Frank neurologic injury, although recently described with continuous techniques using small-bore catheters, is quite rare. Hypotension, which occurs as a consequence of sympathectomy, usually responds readily to fluids and small doses of pressors such as ephedrine. The efficacy of fluid preloading in providing prophylaxis against hypotension is controversial.

Postdural puncture headache occurs after a small proportion of subarachnoid blocks. Factors that increase its incidence include female gender, younger age, and larger needles. Epidural analgesia would appear to avoid the complication but, if the dura is inadvertently punctured, it leaves a much larger dural rent. When compared to epidural anesthesia, spinal anesthesia has a quicker onset, is more predictably satisfactory for surgery, and is less frequently associated with backache. Transient radicular neuropathy, a painful but usually self-limited condition, recently became evident in association with an increase in enthusiasm for the use of lidocaine for subarachnoid block.

When cardiac arrest results from excessive cephalad spread of subarachnoid block or protracted hypotension, cardiopulmonary resuscitation is notoriously difficult. Patients who suffer cardiac arrest during subarachnoid block have poor survival, possibly because the profound sympathectomy causes difficulty in generating adequate coronary perfusion pressure. Relatively large doses of epinephrine may be necessary to achieve adequate perfusion pressure during cardiopulmonary resuscitation after spinal anesthesia. Absolute contraindications to spinal anesthesia include sepsis, bacteremia, infection at the site of injection, severe hypovolemia, coagulopathy, therapeutic anticoagulation, increased ICP, and patient refusal.

Epidural Anesthesia

Epidural block, another form of neuraxial regional block, has application in a wide variety of abdominal, thoracic, and lower extremity procedures. Induction of epidural anesthesia or analgesia results from injection of local anesthetics, with or without opiates, into the lumbar or thoracic epidural space. Generally, a catheter is inserted after the epidural space has been located with a needle. The presence of the catheter provides several advantages. First, local anesthetic can be added in a controlled fashion so that the time to onset of the block can be well controlled. Second, the catheter can be used for repeated dosing so that anesthesia can be provided for the duration of lengthy procedures. Third, local anesthetics or opiates can be administered for several days to provide postoperative analgesia.

Epidural anesthesia has specific advantages for thoracic surgery, peripheral vascular surgery, and gastrointestinal surgery. Epidural anesthesia has also been shown to decrease blood loss and deep venous thrombosis during total joint arthroplasty. Postoperative epidural analgesia for thoracic surgery provides superior pain control, less sedation, and better pulmonary function than parenteral opiates do.

In a recent Cochrane Database analysis, it was determined that the use epidural anesthesia was associated with a significant decrease in 0- to 30-day mortality and a decrease incidence of pneumonia compared to the use of general anesthesia in a broad group of surgical procedures. The incidence of perioperative myocardial infarction was not different among groups. Similarly, the use of epidural analgesia after general anesthesia decreased the incidence of postoperative pneumonia compared to the use of general anesthesia alone but did not change 0- to 30-day mortality or incidence of myocardial infarction.[34]

The use of low concentrations of local anesthetics in conjunction with epidural opiates has been associated with earlier ambulation and less postoperative ileus after abdominal surgery. Thoracic epidural anesthesia, but not lumbar epidural anesthesia, appears to be associated with more rapid recovery of gastrointestinal function after major abdominal surgery. However, IV lidocaine also resulted in more rapid return of bowel function (flatus and bowel movement). Thus, circulating systemic lidocaine may account for at least some of the effects of epidural anesthesia on postoperative bowel function. A study by Swenson and colleagues[35] did not show a significant difference in return to bowel function, hospital length of stay, or postoperative pain control when comparing epidural analgesia with continuous lidocaine infusion in patients undergoing colon resection. A continuing controversy relates to whether epidural or subarachnoid analgesia reduces subsequent analgesic requirements after the block has resolved (so-called preemptive analgesia).

The complications and contraindications associated with epidural anesthesia are similar to those for spinal anesthesia. However, a special cautionary note is indicated regarding epidural anesthesia and anticoagulation. Because of the risk of spinal hematoma, placement and removal of epidural catheters in patients receiving oral or parenteral anticoagulation are performed in conjunction with an anesthesiologist. The recent advent of low–molecular-weight heparin (LMWH) for prophylaxis of deep venous thrombosis has resulted in an increase in the incidence of epidural hematomas associated with the removal or placement of epidural catheters. Although LMWH is effective as prophylaxis against venous thromboembolism, spinal hematomas have occurred in association with perioperative use of LMWH in patients given neuraxial analgesia. The timing of catheter placement and removal in the setting of LMWH use is critical to avoiding this rare but catastrophic complication. Although many of the guidelines are based on evidence provided by small clinical studies and case reports, a general consensus exists regarding the placement and removal of epidural catheters in patients receiving LMWH.[36] In general, an epidural catheter should not be placed earlier than 24 hours after treatment with LMWH, and LMWH should not be started before 6 hours after epidural catheter placement. An epidural catheter should not be removed earlier than 12 hours after the last dose of LMWH, and LMWH should not be restarted earlier than 2 hours after catheter removal. A high index of suspicion of epidural hematoma must be maintained in patients undergoing neuraxial blockade who have received or will receive LMWH. All persons involved in the care of patients receiving continuous epidural analgesia need to be aware of the signs of epidural hematoma, including back pain, lower extremity sensory and motor dysfunction, and bladder and bowel abnormalities. To reduce the risk, needle placement is not done less than 10 to 12 hours after the last dose, and subsequent dosing is delayed at least 2 hours. Epidural catheters are withdrawn at least 10 to 12 hours after the last dose of LMWH.

A final rare complication, epidural abscess, is considered in patients in whom back pain develops after epidural injection; magnetic resonance imaging is an effective diagnostic tool in such patients.

Peripheral Nerve Blocks

Blockade of the brachial plexus, lumbar plexus, and specific peripheral nerves is an effective means of providing surgical anesthesia and postoperative analgesia for many surgical procedures involving the upper and lower extremities. The advantage of peripheral nerve blocks is reduced physiologic stress in comparison to spinal or epidural anesthesia, avoidance of airway manipulation and the potential complications associated with endotracheal intubation, and avoidance of the potential side effects associated with general anesthesia. However, successful nerve block anesthesia requires a cooperative patient, an anesthesiologist skilled in peripheral nerve blocks, and a surgeon who is accustomed to operating on awake patients. All patients undergoing peripheral nerve block receive full preoperative evaluation under the assumption that general anesthesia could be used if the block is inadequate.

Improvements in nerve block equipment and methodology, as well as the availability of a wide range of local anesthetics, have greatly improved the effectiveness and safety of peripheral nerve blocks. In addition to providing surgical anesthesia, peripheral nerve blocks and the placement of indwelling catheters for a prolonged nerve block provide excellent analgesia for many types of upper extremity surgery and trauma. An additional application of indwelling catheters is enhancement of blood flow after reattachment of amputated limbs and in patients with peripheral vascular disease. Each particular block has specific associated risks and benefits. However, general complications of peripheral nerve blocks include local anesthetic toxicity, neurologic injury, inadvertent neuraxial block, and intravascular injection of local anesthetics.

Abdominal Wall Blocks

The use of anterior abdominal wall blocks has increased over the last decade due to the adoption of minimally invasive and laparoscopic surgical procedures. Transversus abdominis plane and rectus sheath blocks are relatively easy to place under ultrasound guidance and are generally safe and effective when applied in the proper clinical context. Other abdominal wall blocks include ilioinguinal-iliohypogastric and quadratus lumborum blocks. Prospective clinical trials and metaanalyses have generally shown that abdominal wall blocks confer analgesic benefit in adult and pediatric patients undergoing minimally invasive or laparoscopic intraabdominal procedures.[37] Abdominal wall blocks also have the potential to provide analgesic benefit in patients undergoing open intraabdominal surgery who have contraindications to epidural analgesia.

Enhanced Recovery After Surgery Pathways

Enhanced recovery pathways have been increasingly applied to standardize perioperative management of surgical patients with the goal of optimizing patient outcomes and improving healthcare efficiency. This approach emphasizes a multidisciplinary, multimodal application of care beginning with preoperative optimization and education, intraoperative use of minimally invasive surgical approaches, and standardized nonopioid multimodal anesthesia and analgesia followed by early postoperative ambulation and oral intake.[38]

CONSCIOUS SEDATION

When anesthesiologists participate in the sedation of patients undergoing surgical procedures, the procedure is termed *monitored anesthesia care.* Monitored anesthesia care encompasses a wide range of depths of sedation ranging from minimal sedation to brief intervals of complete unconsciousness (for instance, during placement of a retrobulbar block by an ophthalmologist). When nonanesthesia personnel administer sedation for surgical procedures, the process is generally termed *conscious sedation*, although the term *moderate sedation* is preferable. Moderate sedation implies that the patient can respond purposefully to verbal or tactile stimulation, has a patent airway requiring no intervention, demonstrates adequate spontaneous ventilation, and has maintained cardiovascular function. There is a narrow margin between minimal sedation, which may be inadequate for surgery to continue, and deep sedation, which may result in airway compromise and cardiovascular and respiratory depression. Although relatively rare in this setting, a closed claim analysis showed that hypoventilation and hypoxemia were the most common major complications.[39] Because of the risks associated with moderate sedation, the Joint Commission for Accreditation of Healthcare Organizations requires that patients be managed with precautions similar to what they would receive if an anesthesiologist were managing the sedation. Important factors include the necessity for preprocedure evaluation, continuous presence of a trained monitoring assistant who has no other responsibilities throughout the procedure, immediate availability of airway and resuscitation equipment, monitoring after the procedure until the effects of sedation have resolved, and specific written postoperative instructions. Physicians who perform procedures under conscious sedation are granted privileges in line with their training and experience in the appropriate resuscitative procedures.

Drugs used for moderate sedation usually consist of opioids such as fentanyl or morphine, often combined with an anxiolytic such as midazolam. Titration of these agents requires careful assessment of a patient's level of pain or anxiety and the requirements for the surgical procedure. Induction agents such as propofol are becoming increasingly popular for induction of moderate sedation outside of the operating room. While generally safe when used under the proper conditions, those agents introduce an added element of risk and increase the need for caution due to potentially rapid progression to deep sedation or even general anesthesia. Most hospitals now have specific policies and procedures governing moderate sedation. Those who use moderate sedation outside hospitals (e.g., in office-based surgical practices) need to follow the same precautions as practiced in the hospital environment.

POSTANESTHESIA CARE

The PACU is the area designated for the care of patients recovering from the immediate physiologic and pharmacologic consequences associated with anesthesia and surgery. The PACU ideally is located close to the operating rooms. Monitors for the assessment of ventilation, oxygenation, and circulation must be available for all recovering patients. Care also includes periodic assessment of neuromuscular function, mental status, temperature, pain, fluid status, urine output, nausea and vomiting, and bleeding and drainage. The extent of monitoring depends on the condition of the patient. The ASA has established standards of postanesthesia care.[40] Recovery from anesthesia is usually uneventful and routine. Most patients stay in the PACU for 30 to 60 minutes until they are fully reactive and can move to a second-stage recovery area (for ambulatory patients who are returning home that day) or to a bed on a surgical floor. However, several criteria need to be met before the patient can be safely discharged from the PACU. All patients must be awake and oriented and have stable vital signs. Patients must be breathing without difficulty, able to protect their airways, and oxygenating appropriately. Pain, shivering, nausea, and vomiting must be adequately controlled. Patients receiving regional anesthesia must be observed for resolution of the block. There can be no evidence of surgical complications such as postoperative bleeding.

Several types of anesthesia-related complications can be encountered in the PACU and must be promptly recognized and treated to prevent serious injury.

Postoperative Agitation, Delirium, and Cognitive Decline

Pain and anxiety are often manifested as postoperative agitation. However, agitation may also signal serious physiologic disturbances such as hypoxemia, hypercapnia, acidosis, hypotension, hypoglycemia, surgical complications, and adverse drug reactions. Serious underlying conditions must be excluded as the cause of agitation before empirically treating patients with pain medications, sedatives, or physical restraints.

Postoperative delirium is a common complication of surgery and anesthesia that occurs in up to 70% of patients over the age of 60 who undergo major procedures requiring inpatient care. Development of postoperative delirium in the elderly is associated with increased mortality, persistent cognitive decline, and prolongation of in-hospital care. Factors contributing to postoperative delirium are multifactorial and include preoperative cognitive function, extent of surgery, and the need for postoperative intensive care. Approaches to minimize postoperative delirium are under investigation, but no definitive recommendations can be given at this time.

Respiratory Complications

Respiratory problems are the most frequently occurring major complications in the PACU. Airway obstruction is most commonly due to obstruction of the oropharynx by the tongue or oropharyngeal soft tissues as a result of the residual effects of general anesthetics, pain medications, or muscle relaxants. Other causes of airway obstruction include laryngospasm; blood, vomitus, or debris in the airway; glottic edema; vocal cord paralysis; and external compression of the airway by a hematoma, dressing, or cervical collar. Oxygen must be administered to a patient with airway obstruction as measures are taken to relieve the obstruction. The characteristic physical signs of airway obstruction are sonorous respiratory sounds and paradoxical chest movement.

Many obstructions can be relieved by applying a head-tilt and jaw-thrust maneuver with or without placement of an oral or nasopharyngeal airway. Suctioning the airway may also be beneficial, and the patient needs to be examined for evidence of external airway compression. In cases of laryngospasm, continuous positive airway pressure is applied, followed by the administration of 10 to 20 mg of succinylcholine if continuous positive airway pressure is ineffective. Patients may require mask ventilation and endotracheal intubation if the laryngospasm does not resolve promptly. In children, glottic edema or postextubation croup can result in airway obstruction. Mild cases are treated with humidified oxygen. Refractory obstruction may require the administration of systemic steroids and racemic epinephrine by nebulization. Reintubation may also be required.

Hypoxemia is a surprisingly common problem, and administration of supplemental oxygen during transportation to the PACU and during immediate postoperative period decreases the incidence and severity of hypoxemia. The incidence of mild hypoxemia (Spo_2 = 86%–90%) and severe hypoxemia (Spo_2 ≤85%) was 7% and 0.7%, respectively, in the PACU for patients undergoing superficial elective plastic surgery; 38% and 3%, respectively, for patients undergoing upper abdominal surgery; and 52% and 20%, respectively, for patients undergoing thoracoabdominal surgery. Hypoxemia can result from hypoventilation, ventilation-perfusion mismatching, or right-to-left intrapulmonary shunting. Reluctance to inspire deeply after abdominal or thoracic surgery may also result in hypoxemia. Clinically, hypoxemia must be suspected as an underlying problem in patients exhibiting restlessness, tachycardia, or cardiac irritability. Bradycardia, hypotension, and cardiac arrest are late signs. Hypoxemia in the PACU may be secondary to atelectasis, which may respond to incentive spirometry or vigorous encouragement to inspire deeply and cough. Treatment of hypoxemia requires the administration of oxygen, assurance of adequate ventilation, and treatment of the underlying causes.

Hypoventilation (synonymous with hypercapnia) can result from airway obstruction, central respiratory depression caused by the residual effects of anesthetic agents, hypothermia, CNS injury, or restriction of ventilation secondary to muscle relaxants, abdominal distention, and electrolyte abnormalities. Signs can include prolonged somnolence, a slow (or rapid) respiratory rate, airway obstruction, shallow breathing, tachycardia, and arrhythmias. Severe hypoventilation can result in hypoxemia, although augmented inspired oxygen will limit the severity of hypoventilation-induced hypoxemia. Treatment is aimed at identification and treatment of the underlying problem. In all cases, ventilation must be supported until corrective measures are instituted. Obtundation, circulatory depression, and severe respiratory acidosis are indications for endotracheal intubation and ventilatory support.

Postoperative Nausea and Vomiting

Perhaps one of the most annoying problems for both patients and personnel in the PACU is PONV. A wide variety of agents have varying degrees of effectiveness for the prevention or treatment of PONV (Table 14.10). No single technique has yet proved to be both uniformly therapeutic and cost-effective. The use of propofol for induction of anesthesia has also been shown to be effective in decreasing the incidence of PONV. One important complication related to the IV coadministration of ondansetron and metoclopramide has been the production of bradyarrhythmias, including a slow junctional escape rhythm and ventricular bigeminy. More recently, the FDA has placed a so-called black box warning on the use of droperidol in which additional ECG monitoring is required before and after administration of the drug because of an alleged increase in serious cardiac arrhythmias caused by QT prolongation. The FDA warning has been controversial because of the good safety profile of droperidol during the past 30 years and relative lack of scientific evidence to support the recommendation.[41] A study comparing droperidol and saline did not show a

TABLE 14.10 Commonly used antiemetic agents.

DRUG CLASS	COMMON SIDE EFFECTS
Dopamine Receptor Antagonists (DA-2)	
Phenothiazines	
Fluphenazine	
Chlorpromazine	
Prochlorperazine	Sedation
Butyrophenones	Dissociation
Droperidol	Extrapyramidal effects
Haloperidol	
Substituted benzamide	
Metoclopramide	
Antihistamines (H_1)	
Diphenhydramine	Sedation
Promethazine	Dry mouth
Anticholinergics	
Scopolamine	Sedation
Serotonin Receptor Antagonists	
Ondansetron	Headache
Dolasetron	
Corticosteroids	
Dexamethasone	Glucose intolerance
Methylprednisolone	Altered wound healing
Hydrocortisone	Immunosuppression
	Renal effects

significant effect of either intervention on the QT interval during or after anesthesia.[42] Nevertheless, the FDA recommendation has caused a significant reduction in the use of droperidol for the treatment of PONV.

The approach to the prophylaxis and treatment of PONV is guided by an understanding of the mechanisms causing nausea and vomiting. Areas in the brainstem that control nausea and vomiting reflexes, such as the chemoreceptor trigger zone, contain receptors for dopamine, acetylcholine, histamine, and serotonin. Binding of all of these receptors may precipitate nausea, vomiting, or both. Effective pharmacologic approaches to the treatment of PONV include the use of anticholinergics, serotonin receptor antagonists, antidopaminergics, corticosteroids, and antihistamines (Table 14.10). The use of any particular agent is based on efficacy, potential side effects, and cost. In patients at high risk of PONV or in those with a history of PONV, it is often effective to employ a multimodal approach.

Hypothermia

Hypothermia has been extensively studied as a perioperative complication. The most important issues related to perioperative hypothermia include the risk of increased oxygen consumption postoperatively due to shivering, alterations in drug metabolism, effects on blood coagulation, and the possibility that hypothermia could increase the rate of surgical infections. Increased oxygen consumption could be a particular problem in patients with coronary artery disease in whom shivering could trigger myocardial ischemia. However, the risk associated with mild hypothermia has not been well defined in otherwise healthy patients. Nevertheless, the Centers for Medicare and Medicaid Services has designated perioperative normothermia as a Pay for Performance issue. This means that hospitals and medical centers that report on and achieve perioperative normothermia (36°C within 30 minutes of arrival in the PACU for procedures lasting for more than 1 hour) receive financial incentives.

General anesthesia has profound effects on thermoregulatory mechanisms, and active intraoperative warming is required to maintain normothermia under most conditions. Forced air and circulating water warmers are the most effective techniques for providing active intraoperative warming, each having advantages under different conditions. IV fluid warmers and airway warming devices can also be useful for minimizing heat loss but do not allow for active warming. Because of the effects of anesthesia on heat redistribution to the skin and peripheral tissues, preoperative warming is required to minimize core hypothermia in patients undergoing procedures lasting less than an hour. Studies indicate that prophylactic warming will decrease the incidence of postoperative hypothermia and need for intervention in the outpatient surgical setting. However, time to PACU discharge and patient satisfaction were not affected. The use of prophylactic warming is associated with a significant increase in cost. Therefore, guidelines for temperature management during short, outpatient surgical procedures remain to be fully implemented.

Circulatory Complications

Hypotension in the PACU is most commonly due to hypovolemia, left ventricular dysfunction, or arrhythmias. Other causes include anaphylaxis, transfusion reactions, cardiac tamponade, pulmonary emboli, adverse drug reactions, adrenal insufficiency, and hypoxemia. Treatment involves support of the circulation with fluids, administration of inotropic agents, use of the Trendelenburg position, and delivery of oxygen until the underlying cause is diagnosed and treated.

Hypertension is a common finding in the PACU. Common causes include pain, anxiety, and inadequately managed essential hypertension. Hypoxemia and hypercapnia always need to be ruled out. Other less common causes include hypoglycemia; drug reactions; diseases such as hyperthyroidism, pheochromocytoma, or malignant hyperthermia; and bladder distention. The fundamental goal in control of postoperative hypertension is to identify and correct the underlying cause.

Postoperative Visual Loss

Postoperative visual loss is a rare but devastating complication that occurs most commonly in patients undergoing prolonged surgery in the prone position (spine surgery) or cardiac surgery. The overall incidence is reported as 0.02%. Causes include retinal artery occlusion, cortical blindness, and ischemic optic neuropathy. Risk factors for the development of postoperative visual loss are not completely understood, but recent studies have identified obesity, prolonged length of surgery, high intraoperative blood loss, and lack of use of colloids for resuscitation as possible risk factors. Because of the seriousness of the complication, the ASA has released practice advisory on postoperative visual loss.[43]

ACUTE PAIN MANAGEMENT

Pain, one of the most common symptoms experienced by surgical patients, has historically been poorly evaluated and frequently undertreated. There have been important changes in medical care with respect to pain management, with inclusion of pain management in medical school curricula, establishment of institutional protocols and procedures for pain management, development of the subspecialty of pain medicine, creation of organizations focused on pain, and increased interest on the part of governmental and third-party payers. These changes will continue into the future, and medical personnel must continue to increase their knowledge of pain control and their commitment to provide optimal analgesia as a key component of patient care. Surveys demonstrate that continued improvement is necessary to further reduce the high incidence of moderate to severe acute postoperative pain.

Acute pain occurs frequently in the setting of surgery and trauma. The pain experience may be part of the symptom complex that prompts the patient to seek medical care, or it may be caused by tissue injury sustained as a result of surgery or trauma. The term *acute pain* refers to pain that is expected to be of relatively short duration and that should resolve with tissue healing or withdrawal of the noxious stimulus. Acute pain generally resolves within minutes, hours, or days. *Chronic pain*, which can persist for years, is defined as pain that persists for at least 1 month beyond the usual course of an acute disease or beyond a reasonable time in which an injury would be expected to heal. The acute stress response associated with acute pain serves a useful function, although undertreatment may result in harmful pathophysiologic changes. Chronic pain serves no useful function and is now recognized not only as a part of certain disease processes such as cancer but also often as a disease itself.

Mechanisms of Acute Pain

The International Association for the Study of Pain defines *pain* as "an unpleasant sensory and emotional experience associated with actual or potential tissue damage or described in terms of such damage." This definition emphasizes not only the sensory experience but also the affective component of pain. The tissue injury that leads to the complaint of pain results in a process called *nociception*, which has four steps: transduction, transmission, modulation, and perception. With transduction, the noxious stimulus is converted into an electrical signal at free nerve endings, which are also known as nociceptors. Nociceptors are widely distributed throughout the body in both somatic and visceral tissues.

With transmission, the electrical signal is sent via nerve pathways toward the CNS. Nerve pathways include primary sensory afferents (primarily Aδ and C fibers) that project to the spinal cord, ascending tracts (including the spinothalamic tract) to the brainstem and thalamus, and thalamocortical pathways to the cortex. Modulation, the process that either enhances or suppresses the pain signal, occurs primarily in the dorsal horn of the spinal cord, in particular, the substantia gelatinosa. Perception, the final step in the nociceptive process, occurs when the pain signal reaches the cerebral cortex. The first three steps in nociception are important for the sensory and discriminative aspects of pain. The fourth step, perception, is integral to the subjective and emotional experience.

Methods of Analgesia

Multiple agents, routes of administration, and modalities are available for effective management of acute pain (Fig. 14.5). Analgesic agents include opioids, nonsteroidal antiinflammatory drugs (NSAIDs), acetaminophen, and local anesthetics. Less traditional agents that may be used more frequently in the future include clonidine, dexmedetomidine, guanfacine, dextromethorphan, and gabapentin. Routes of administration include the oral, parenteral, epidural, and intrathecal routes. The oral route is the preferred route for analgesic delivery. Patients experiencing mild to moderate acute pain and who can receive agents orally can obtain effective analgesia. Parenteral administration is preferred for patients experiencing moderate to severe pain, patients who require rapid control of pain, and those who cannot receive agents through the gastrointestinal tract. The IV route is preferred over intramuscular and subcutaneous injections when the parenteral route is indicated. Intramuscular injections are painful, result in erratic absorption, and lead to variable blood levels of the administered agent.

Opioids

Opioids are potent analgesic agents that are effective but frequently underused. By binding to opioid receptors in the CNS and probably also in peripheral tissues, opioids modulate the nociceptive process. The best-characterized opioid receptors are μ1, μ2, δ, κ, ε, and σ receptors. The μ1 receptors are involved in supraspinal analgesia. The δ and κ receptors are involved in spinal analgesia. Opioids can be administered by multiple routes, including oral, parenteral, neuraxial, rectal, and transdermal.

Opioids have varying degrees of potency. Strong opioids are ideal for moderate to severe pain and for pain that is constant in frequency. Weak opioid agents are suitable for mild to moderate pain that is intermittent in frequency. Morphine, the prototype strong opioid, can be delivered by a variety of routes and techniques. Other strong opioids include hydromorphone, fentanyl, and meperidine. Morphine is metabolized to morphine-3-glucoronide and morphine-6-glucoronide, which can accumulate in patients who have renal impairment. For moderate to severe pain in patients with renal dysfunction, fentanyl and hydromorphone are more suitable agents. Historically, meperidine has frequently been the preferred strong opioid. This practice has declined because meperidine is metabolized to normeperidine, a unique toxic metabolite that can accumulate and cause seizure-like activity. Patients who are particularly vulnerable to this side effect include the elderly, patients who are dehydrated, and those with renal impairment. Fentanyl is available in a transdermal preparation, but this route is not recommended for acute pain management.

Weak opioid agents, such as hydrocodone and codeine, are commonly combined with aspirin or acetaminophen. Tramadol is an analgesic that is a nonopioid but has some opioid-like effects. It is a centrally acting agent that is administered orally and can be used for mild to moderate pain. Common opioid-related side effects include nausea, pruritus, sedation, mental clouding, decreased gastric motility, urinary retention, and respiratory depression. Appropriate selection of agents, monitoring, and treatment can prevent or ameliorate these side effects.

One major barrier to the effective use of opioid agents by patients, physicians, and other health care providers is the fear of addiction, which can be manifested as underdosing, use of excessively wide dosing intervals, administration of weak opioids for moderate to severe pain, and underreporting of pain. In the setting of acute postoperative pain, the use of opioids has not been shown to be a risk factor for the development of an addiction disorder. Key terms to understand include *tolerance*, *addiction* (psychological dependence), and *physical dependence*. Tolerance occurs when a previously effective opioid dose fails to provide adequate analgesia. It is a normal physiologic effect and should not be confused with addiction. Tolerance develops not only to the analgesic effect of opioids but also to most opioid-related side effects. The duration of opioid exposure also plays a role in the development of tolerance. In patients manifesting tolerance, an increased dose is

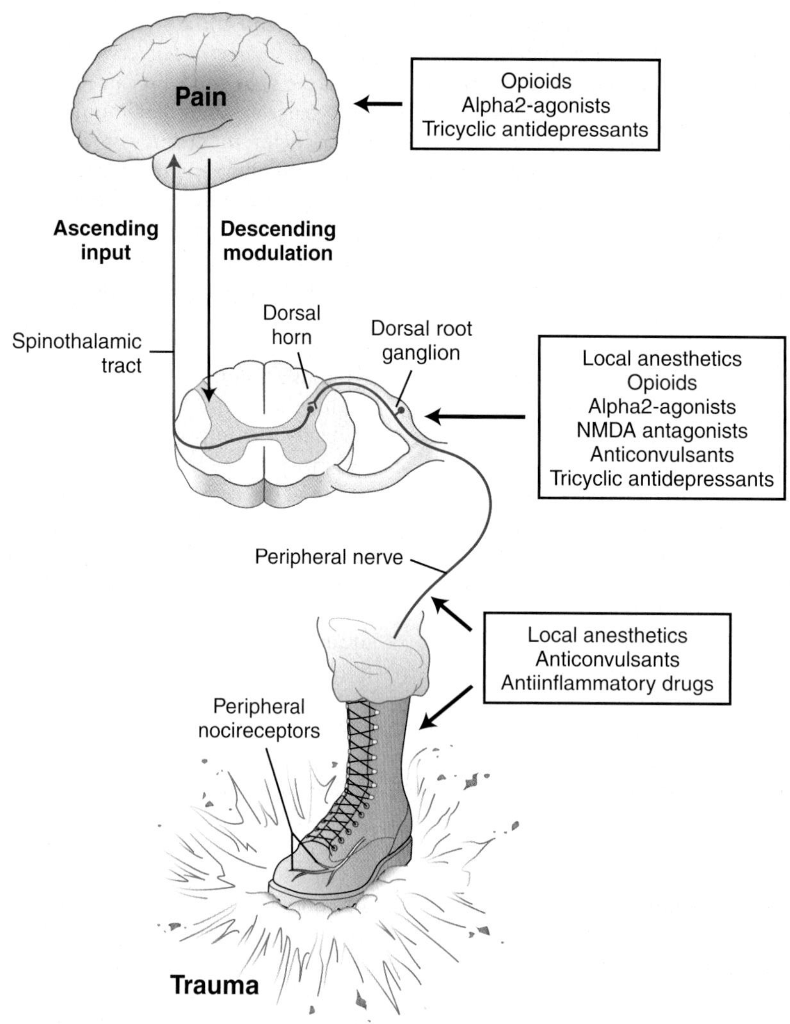

FIG. 14.5 Schematic diagram outlining the nociceptive pathway for transmission of painful stimuli. Interventions that prevent nociceptive transmission are shown at the points in the pathway that are thought to be their sites of action. (From Buckenmaier CC III, Bleckner LL, eds. *Military Advanced Regional Anesthesia and Analgesia.* Washington, DC: Borden Institute, Walter Reed Army Medical Center; 2008.) NMDA, *N*-methyl-D-aspartate.

required to achieve effective analgesia. Addiction or psychological dependence is a compulsive disorder manifested by preoccupation with obtaining and inappropriate use of a substance, continued use despite harm, decreased quality of life, and denial. Psychological dependence should not be confused with physical dependence, which is a normal physiologic process. Physical dependence is manifested by the occurrence of a withdrawal syndrome when use of a drug is stopped suddenly or when an antagonist is given. The duration of opioid treatment is a factor in the development of physical dependence. The short-term use of opioids in the perioperative period rarely results in physical dependence. Slow tapering of opioids generally prevents withdrawal symptoms.

Nonsteroidal Anti-inflammatory Drugs

NSAIDs are an important component of perioperative analgesia that, when used as a part of a multimodal analgesic approach, reduce pain and can decrease opioid consumption. Their mechanism of action is achieved through inhibition of cyclooxygenase (COX) enzyme activity, which results in decreased production of prostaglandins. Prostaglandins are potent mediators of pain that act directly at nociceptors and also increase nociceptor sensitivity. Inhibition of prostaglandin production results in analgesia but can also lead to side effects such as gastric ulceration, bleeding, and renal injury. These side effects have limited the use of NSAIDs in the perioperative period. Contrary to previous evidence that NSAIDs act mainly in peripheral tissues, there is now evidence that NSAIDs also work in the CNS.

There is a wide range of compounds in this analgesic class with differing chemical structures. Most of these agents are intended for oral administration, which limits their use perioperatively. Ketorolac is available for parenteral administration and has been shown to be effective for analgesia and safe with appropriate patient selection. Ketorolac is avoided in patients with a history of gastropathy, platelet dysfunction, or thrombocytopenia; in those with a history of allergy to the agent; and in patients with renal impairment or hypovolemia. It is used with caution in elderly patients. A loading dose of 30 mg IV followed by 15 mg IV every 6 hours for a short course can provide effective analgesia for mild to moderate pain or can be a useful adjunct for moderate to severe pain when combined with opioids or other analgesic techniques. Moodie and colleagues[44] conducted a double-blinded placebo-controlled trial in patients undergoing abdominal and orthopedic surgery. Subjects received intranasal 30 mg or 10 mg of ketorolac or placebo spray upon recovering from anesthesia. Patient-controlled analgesia

(PCA) morphine pump dose over 40 hours was lowest in the 30-mg ketorolac group (37.8 mg) versus ketorolac 10 mg (54.3 mg) versus placebo (56.5 mg). Ketorolac 30 mg was associated with lower pain at 6 hours but was not significant beyond this time point nor was the incidence of nausea or pruritus.[44]

The most recent advance in this analgesic category involves the introduction of agents that are selective in their inhibition of subtypes of the COX enzyme. There are at least two subtypes of this enzyme: COX-1 (constitutive) and COX-2 (inducible). Traditional NSAIDs are nonselective inhibitors of COX. The newer agents (celecoxib, rofecoxib, valdecoxib) are selective COX-2 inhibitors. COX-2 inhibitors appear to offer similar analgesia with a somewhat reduced risk of causing gastrointestinal bleeding, bleeding diathesis, and renal compromise. They have mostly been studied and used clinically in the management of arthritis-related pain but are becoming more frequently used in the perioperative period. Currently available COX-2 inhibitors are for oral administration. In a study by Huang and colleagues,[45] the COX-2 selective inhibitor celecoxib was administered to patients undergoing total knee arthroplasty under subarachnoid blockade. Celecoxib 200 mg was administered 1 hour before surgery and every 12 hours thereafter for 5 days. PCA morphine use was lower in the celecoxib group (15.1 mg) versus placebo (19.7 mg). Celecoxib use was associated with a lower pain score during the first postoperative 48 hours, and increased knee range of motion during the first three postoperative days. Morphine-related adverse effects (nausea and vomiting) did not differ between groups.[45] Parecoxib is being studied for parenteral use. There are indications that COX-2 inhibitors are associated with a lower incidence of gastropathy. Concerns about the use of these selective NSAIDs include the risk for cardiovascular events and their effects on bone healing. Some of these agents (rofecoxib, valdecoxib) have been removed from the market because of the risk for cardiovascular complications. Valdecoxib was removed from commercial distribution because of the risk for severe skin reaction and cardiovascular complications.

NMDA antagonists. Ketamine has long been recognized as a powerful induction agent with strong analgesic properties, albeit at the expense of psychotropic adverse effects to include dysphoria and, at higher doses of the drug, psychosis. Discovery of NMDA antagonists and its role in sensitizing the CNS has led to a reemergence of this class of agents for the use in management of acute pain in perioperative medicine. A prospective randomized, double-blinded placebo controlled study by Zakine and colleagues[46] compared two ketamine regimens against placebo. They used intraoperative ketamine (500 μg/kg load followed by 2 μg/kg/min) or intraoperative and postoperative ketamine (2 μg/kg/min) against placebo in patients undergoing major abdominal surgery under general anesthesia. The authors noted lower morphine PCA use in the perioperative (intra- and postoperative) ketamine group (27 mg) versus intraoperative ketamine (48 mg) versus placebo (50 mg). Of note, pain scores were lower in both ketamine groups as compared to placebo, and the incidence of nausea and vomiting was highest in the placebo group.[46] Similar results were noted in a study of total knee replacement surgery patients. Furthermore, a study by Remerand and colleagues[47] demonstrated perioperative ketamine to be associated with 6-month reduction in chronic pain, 8% in the ketamine group as compared to 21% in the placebo. If, however, ketamine is not administered via continuous infusion (i.e., PCA or intraoperative alone), it seems to be ineffective as noted in a gynecologic surgery study and pediatric scoliosis surgery study, respectively. Lastly, in the NMDA group, magnesium has also been recognized to possess NMDA antagonist properties. However, it seems to be ineffective as an analgesic unless administered in high doses.

Alpha2-Adrenergic agonists. It has been recognized that there is a high density of α2-adrenergic receptors in the substantia gelatinosa of the dorsal horn in humans, where it is believed that α2-adrenergic agonists impair the transmission of pain signals. Clonidine, due to its potent antihypertensive properties is of limited use in perioperative medicine. However, dexmedetomidine has been demonstrated to be effective in perioperative medicine with only transient effects on hemodynamics in exchange for improved analgesia and lower opiate use and lower related opiate side effects. In a study by Tufanogullari and colleagues[48] that involved patients undergoing laparoscopic bariatric surgery under general anesthesia, patients were randomized into one of four groups. The groups included IV dexmedetomidine 0.2, 0.4, or 0.8 μg/kg/hr or placebo infusion therapy during the operation alone. The authors noted less PCA morphine use up to 48 hours in the dexmedetomidine groups. Incidence of nausea and vomiting was lower in the dexmedetomidine groups, as was the PACU stay. However, pain scores were no different between groups, which the authors suggest may have been a result of not continuing the infusion in the postoperative period.[48] Aside from analgesic benefits, dexmedetomidine seems to have other preoperative advantages. Ji and colleagues,[49] in a recent study, evaluated the association of dexmedetomidine in cardiac surgery patients beginning the infusion upon weaning from cardiopulmonary bypass and continuing into the ICU for less than 24 hours. In their study, they noted reduction in hospital, 30-day, and 1-year mortality as well as reduction of complications to include delirium. Pain scores were not described by the authors, and therefore we cannot conclude if pain was lower with the administration of dexmedetomidine.[49] Guanfacine is another α2-adrenergic agonist that is receiving attention as an agent to decrease postoperative delirium and serve as an adjunct for pain management. Guanfacine is delivered orally and has minimal cardiovascular side effects. Further study is needed to determine the efficacy of guanfacine as a perioperative adjunct.

Local Anesthetics for the Management of Acute Pain

Local anesthetics work by blocking conduction in nerve fibers, the second step in the process of nociception. These agents are used to provide regional anesthesia for surgery, but their effects last into the postoperative period and contribute to preemptive analgesia. Local anesthetics used in doses lower than that required for anesthesia can also provide analgesia by a variety of application techniques, including local infiltration, topical application, epidural infusion, and peripheral nerve infusion. It was previously considered that local anesthetic infiltration was beneficial to aid with postoperative analgesia, but emerging evidence suggests that this therapy may lead to inconsistent results. In a study by Hariharan and colleagues,[50] patients undergoing abdominal hysterectomy were randomized into one of four groups to include local anesthetic (1% lidocaine with 0.25% bupivacaine, with 2 μg/mL epinephrine). Patients either received local anesthetic infiltration under the skin preoperatively and postoperatively, preoperatively alone, postoperatively alone, or placebo. PCA morphine and pain scores were not different among all four groups, suggesting that these techniques are ineffective for perioperative analgesia in this patient population.[50] Topical application of local anesthetic includes the use of agents such as eutectic mixture of local anesthetics (EMLA cream), which contains prilocaine and lidocaine. This agent can be used for superficial procedures and can be placed before the surgical incision. Placement of peripheral nerve catheters for local anesthetic infusion is becoming a frequently used technique for postoperative pain management. The development of disposable and lightweight infusion pumps is leading to the increasing use of peripheral nerve infusion in the ambulatory setting. Peripheral nerve infusion analgesia has been shown to provide improved postoperative pain control when compared to opioid administration.

Combination Analgesic Therapy

By combining agents from different analgesic classes, synergy may be obtained. Synergy results in potentiation of effect and reduced dosage of each individual agent with fewer and less severe side effects from each agent. Common combinations include opioids and NSAIDs in an analgesic regimen or epidural administration of a local anesthetic with an opioid. The choice of agent and technique depends on factors such as the patient's medical history, the patient's preference, the extent of surgery, the expected degree of postoperative pain, the experience of the staff providing care for the patient, and the postoperative setting in which the patient will recover. Gabapentin, an anticonvulsant used for the management of chronic neuropathic pain, has shown efficacy for analgesia in the acute postoperative period, including improved pain control and reduced opioid-related side effects. However, it should be noted that studies demonstrating benefit from gabapentin used doses of 900 or 1200 mg to demonstrate an analgesic benefit. In a study by Khan and colleagues,[51] involving lumbar laminectomy patients, patients received either 900 or 1200 mg of gabapentin in the preoperative or postoperative period. The authors found reduced morphine use in the first 24 hours postoperatively as well as pain score with lower side effects, regardless of the timing of (preoperative or postoperative) gabapentin administration.[51] Aside from acute pain benefits, gabapentin may play a role in chronic pain as well. Although not new, the role of pregabalin in acute pain remains to be determined. There are a few negative trials, but emerging evidence may demonstrate an optimal strategy that will likely involve therapy beyond the hospitalization period.[52] In the study by Buvanendran and colleagues,[52] patients underwent a total knee arthroplasty under combined epidural-intrathecal anesthesia for postoperative epidural analgesia. Epidural analgesia was used up until 32 to 42 hours postoperatively. Pregabalin 300 mg or placebo was administered preoperatively and tapered over 14 days. Epidural use was lower in the pregabalin group at the expense of increased sedation and confusion on postoperative day 0. However, there was an associated reduction in neuropathic pain at 3 and 6 months in the pregabalin group. Other studies are ongoing, and we look forward to their results.

The concept of preemptive analgesia continues to be actively explored and used in the perioperative period. Induced by a variety of agents and techniques, the goal of preemptive analgesia is to influence the analgesic process before initiation of the noxious stimulus (e.g., surgical incision). This minimizes sensitization of the nervous system and moderates the process of nociception described previously. Effective preemptive analgesia results in decreased postoperative pain, reduced postoperative analgesic requirement, decreased side effects from analgesics, increased compliance with postoperative rehabilitation, and decreased incidence of chronic postsurgical pain syndromes.

Neuraxial Analgesia

Neuraxial routes of administration include the epidural and intrathecal (subarachnoid) routes. These modes of administration require consultation from acute pain specialists, usually anesthesiologists who receive specialized training in use of the neuraxial route for the administration of anesthesia and analgesia. Neuraxial agents are delivered by a single injection into the epidural or subarachnoid space, by intermittent injections through an indwelling epidural catheter, by continuous infusion through an indwelling epidural catheter, or by patient-controlled epidural analgesia through an indwelling catheter. Indwelling subarachnoid catheters are rarely used for acute pain. An important consideration in selecting patients for neuraxial analgesia is the presence of abnormal coagulation, including concurrent use of antiplatelet and anticoagulant agents. Knowledge of such coagulation issues is important to minimize the risk for intraspinal bleeding and spinal hematoma formation, which can lead to severe neurologic injury. The neuraxial route requires education of the medical and nursing staff and the use of protocols and guidelines. In general, patients can be managed on surgical floors with these analgesic techniques. However, monitoring procedures need to be in place to minimize the development of side effects and enhance patient safety.

Agents such as opioids and local anesthetics are given via the neuraxial route to achieve analgesia. Other agents that have been used neuraxially include clonidine, neostigmine, and acetaminophen. Opioids, when delivered by the neuraxial route, provide analgesia by their action at opioid receptors located in the dorsal horn of the spinal cord. An important determinant of opioid action when delivered by the neuraxial route is the drug's degree of lipid solubility. Morphine is hydrophilic, which accounts for its slow onset of analgesia, long duration of action, ability to provide analgesia over a wide dermatomal distribution, and the risk for late respiratory depression. Fentanyl is lipophilic, which accounts for its fast onset and short duration of action, ability to provide segmental analgesia, and limited risk for late respiratory depression. A hydrophilic opioid such as morphine, when delivered into the epidural or subarachnoid space, remains in the CSF longer than a lipophilic opioid does. The drug can travel rostrally to the brain and influence the respiratory centers hours after initial delivery.

Local anesthetics, when used for neuraxial analgesia, provide analgesia by blocking nerve conduction. To achieve neuraxial analgesia, local anesthetics are delivered in smaller doses and weaker concentrations than those required to achieve surgical anesthesia. This resulting sensory blockade is sufficient to provide analgesia but not sufficiently profound to interfere with motor function and mask complications. Analgesic concentrations of local anesthetics also cause less impairment of sympathetic tone. Bupivacaine and ropivacaine are the most commonly used local anesthetics for epidural analgesia and peripheral nerve infusion analgesia. They affect sensory fibers more than motor fibers (differential blockade) and have a lower incidence of tachyphylaxis (tolerance to local anesthetic action). Neuraxial analgesia for acute pain commonly combines opioids and local anesthetics. Each agent has a different mechanism of action; combining these agents produces synergistic analgesia and thereby results in reduced doses of each agent and a decreased incidence and severity of side effects. A recent metaanalysis of the efficacy of postoperative epidural analgesia concluded that epidural analgesia, regardless of agent, location of catheter placement, and type of pain assessment, provided analgesia superior to that of parenteral opioids.[53]

Intravenous Patient-Controlled Analgesia

An increasingly popular and effective modality using the parenteral route of administration is IV PCA. This modality minimizes the steps involved in the delivery of analgesia and increases patient autonomy and control. Opioids are the agent of choice for

IV PCA. In comparing IV PCA with conventional intermittent nurse-administered opioid delivery, patients obtain prompt analgesia, receive smaller doses of opioids at more frequent intervals, can maintain blood concentration of drug in the analgesic range, and have a lower incidence of drug-related side effects. Candidates for IV PCA are patients who can understand the basic steps involved in use of the device, who are willing to assume control of their analgesia, and who are physically capable of activating the device. Such patients include children as young as 4 years of age and most adults, including geriatric patients.

The preferred agents for IV PCA are opioids, with morphine sulfate most commonly chosen. Other opioids used for IV PCA include hydromorphone, fentanyl, and meperidine. Methadone IV PCA has been described. Physicians' orders for IV PCA must specify the drug, drug concentration, loading dose, bolus dose, continuous infusion rate (basal rate), lockout interval, and dose limits. Selection of these parameters is based on the patient's age, medical status, and level of pain. The routine use of a continuous basal infusion rate with IV PCA remains controversial. With a continuous infusion, drug is delivered to the patient regardless of demand, thus resulting in the potential for a higher incidence of drug-related side effects, including respiratory depression. It is safest to restrict the use of basal infusions to patients in special categories, including those with severe pain from extensive surgery or trauma and patients who are tolerant because of chronic opioid use.

The use of structured protocols and guidelines is encouraged for facilities using IV PCA. The medical and nursing staff need to receive training in the care of patients using this modality. There is an increased risk for complications if staff members are not trained to understand the concept of IV PCA; to perform appropriate patient selection, education, and assessment; to use appropriate drug and dose selection; and to establish appropriate monitoring requirements and protocols for management of side effects.

Selection of Methods of Postoperative Analgesia

The choice of postoperative pain management strategies is a function of patient factors, surgeon preferences, the anesthesiologist's skills, and the availability of resources for postoperative care and monitoring.

Chronic Pain

In a subset of patients, pain persists after the expected healing time despite the lack of sufficient pathology to account for the pain. Pain that persists for 1 month beyond the expected time for recovery or initial onset is considered evidence of a chronic pain syndrome. Such patients with persistent pain frequently use words such as *burning*, *shooting*, and *shock-like* to describe their pain, which is generally associated with a neuropathic pain syndrome. Neuropathic pain syndromes occur when there has been injury to the nervous system (central, peripheral, or both). Central sensitization is believed to underlie the development of neuropathic pain. Examples include patients with persistent pain after head and neck surgery, thoracotomy, mastectomy, hernia repair, and amputation. Certain factors that may increase the risk for chronic pain include infection at the surgical site, intraoperative trauma to nerves, diabetes mellitus, and nerve entrapment by cancer. There is some evidence that preemptive analgesia may help minimize the occurrence of these syndromes.

Because chronic pain syndromes can be difficult to diagnose in the early postoperative period, it is important for physicians to perform appropriate pain assessment during postoperative follow-up. For instance, after amputation, patients might consider it strange to continue to feel sensation and pain in the location of an amputated limb and might be reluctant to volunteer information that they believe could suggest psychological instability. In such circumstances, appropriate questioning may elicit the complaint and result in patient reassurance and appropriate treatment. Referral to a pain medicine consultant is appropriate when the diagnosis of a chronic postoperative pain syndrome is made. Treatment modalities include the use of adjuvant medications such as antidepressants and anticonvulsants, nerve blocks, physical therapy, and psychological techniques.

Specific Types of Acute Pain Patients

Patients With a History of Chronic Pain

Patients who have a history of chronic pain may experience acute pain as a result of surgery or trauma differently from patients who have no history of chronic pain. Their experience of pain is affected by their experience with chronic pain. Some of these patients may be receiving chronic opioid therapy as a part of their chronic pain management. It is likely that these patients will manifest tolerance to opioid therapy and have a decreased pain threshold, which may result in the patient reporting higher levels of pain and the physician increasing the opioid dose. Obtaining a pain history preoperatively, choosing anesthetic and surgical techniques to minimize tissue trauma and the response to trauma, and appropriate planning for postoperative analgesia can assist in achieving effective analgesia.

Patients With a History of Substance Abuse

Patients with a history of substance abuse are frequently undertreated for acute pain complaints. The stigma associated with drug abuse, misunderstanding on the part of health care providers, and inappropriate pain behavior contribute to undertreatment in this patient population. Effective analgesia can be obtained with strict guidelines, patient education, and appropriate use of consultants and modalities such as regional analgesia.

Pediatric Patients

Pediatric patients experience similar severity of acute postoperative and posttraumatic pain as adults. A major historical myth that has been refuted is the belief that neonates, infants, and children do not perceive pain as adults do. Effective analgesia for a pediatric patient experiencing acute pain can be achieved with pain assessment tools that are tailored for this population and the use of modalities and agents similar to those used for adults. Dosage selection in a pediatric patient must be guided by calculations based on patient weight. With neonates, nurse-controlled analgesia is standard. Older children can effectively use PCA. Regional anesthesia is increasingly being used for pediatric surgery, with the benefits of analgesia extending into the postoperative period and reduced opioid requirements. Epidural analgesia, usually via a caudally placed catheter or a single injection into the caudal canal, can provide effective analgesia. Placement of a peripheral catheter for infusion of local anesthetics can also be used. Topical anesthesia with local anesthetics such as the application of EMLA cream can likewise minimize pain from IV catheter placement and superficial procedures.

Elderly Patients

As the proportion of elderly in the general population increases, a growing percentage of geriatric patients are undergoing surgery or being treated for trauma. These patients will require pain assessment and evaluation tailored to their mental status and cognitive abilities. The modalities and agents used to manage acute pain in this population must take into consideration underlying disease states and decreased organ function.

CONCLUSION

Modern anesthesia is safe and effective for the vast majority of patients, in large part because of important advances in anesthesia equipment, monitors, and drugs. With a wide variety of specific techniques to choose from, selection of anesthetic and postoperative pain regimens for each patient can be based on the requirements of the surgical procedure, the patient's preferences, and the experience and expertise of the anesthesiologist. Over time, patients with more significant comorbidities are receiving surgical care. Anesthesia practice is evolving to provide adequate risk assessment and risk adjustment and to optimize the care of the perioperative patient.

SELECTED REFERENCES

Abbott TEF, Fowler AJ, Pelosi P, et al. A systematic review and consensus definitions for standardised end-points in perioperative medicine: pulmonary complications. *Br J Anaesth.* 2018;120:1066–1079.

Report of a consensus conference that reviewed the topic of postoperative pulmonary outcomes. This group reviewed current definitions of perioperative pulmonary complications and developed practical definitions to guide pulmonary care and improve postoperative pulmonary outcomes.

Benumof JL, Dagg R, Benumof R. Critical hemoglobin desaturation will occur before return to an unparalyzed state following 1 mg/kg intravenous succinylcholine. *Anesthesiology.* 1997;87:979–982.

Using a combination of pharmacologic and physiologic information from the literature, the authors provide a detailed discussion of factors that influence the rate at which clinically important hypoxemia occurs in relation to the expected duration of succinylcholine. This contributes an important counter to the common misconception that succinylcholine will be metabolized before hypoxemia-induced harm occurs.

Fleisher LA, Fleischmann KE, Auerbach AD, et al. 2014 ACC/AHA guideline on perioperative cardiovascular evaluation and management of patients undergoing noncardiac surgery: a report of the American college of cardiology/American heart association task force on practice guidelines. *J Am Coll Cardiol.* 2014;64:e77–137.

In this extensive review, a joint task force of the American College of Cardiology and the American Heart Association reports guidelines for evaluation of patients with cardiovascular disease who are scheduled for noncardiac surgery. They thoroughly examine the importance of the history, physical findings, functional status, and the influence of various types of surgery as well as current recommendations on the perioperative use of beta blockers, statins, and other medications. The value of preoperative testing is also evaluated. This is a valuable update of a consensus approach to this topic.

Grosse-Sundrup M, Henneman JP, Sandberg WS, et al. Intermediate acting non-depolarizing neuromuscular blocking agents and risk of postoperative respiratory complications: prospective propensity score matched cohort study. *BMJ.* 2012;345:e6329.

In a study of 18,579 surgical patients, the authors determined that the use of intermediate-acting neuromuscular blocking agents is associated with a higher incidence of respiratory complications during the postoperative period. The importance of assuring adequate reversal of neuromuscular blockade at the end of surgery is emphasized.

Myles PS, Leslie K, Chan MT, et al. The safety of addition of nitrous oxide to general anaesthesia in at-risk patients having major non-cardiac surgery (ENIGMA-II): a randomised, single-blind trial. *Lancet.* 2014;384:1446–1454.

In contrast to previous trials, the Evaluation of Nitrous Oxide in the Gas Mixture for Anaesthesia (ENIGMA) II Trial reported that use of nitrous oxide was not associated with an increased incidence of death, cardiovascular complications, or wound infection in high-risk surgical patients. Although the incidence of severe postoperative nausea and vomiting (PONV) was higher (15% vs. 11%) in patients receiving nitrous oxide compared to controls, the occurrence of PONV in the nitrous oxide group was effectively controlled by antiemetic prophylaxis.

Practice guidelines for the perioperative management of patients with obstructive sleep apnea: an updated report by the American society of anesthesiologists task force on perioperative management of patients with obstructive sleep apnea. *Anesthesiology.* 2014;120:268–286.

Guidelines for the preoperative assessment, perioperative management, and postoperative disposition of patients with obstructive sleep apnea.

Punjasawadwong Y, Phongchiewboon A, Bunchungmongkol N. Bispectral index for improving anaesthetic delivery and postoperative recovery. *Cochrane Database Syst Rev.* 2014:CD003843.

The metaanalysis concluded that bispectral index (BIS) monitoring can reduce intraoperative awareness in high-risk patients, but it is unclear if the use of BIS monitoring provides advantages in that regard over monitoring end-tidal anesthetic gas concentration in most patients.

Sprung J, Warner ME, Contreras MG, et al. Predictors of survival following cardiac arrest in patients undergoing noncardiac surgery: a study of 518,294 patients at a tertiary referral center. *Anesthesiology.* 2003;99:259–269.

Cardiac arrest occurred in 223 of 518,294 patients (4.3 per 10,000) undergoing noncardiac surgery between January 1, 1990, and December 31, 2000. The frequency of arrest in patients receiving general anesthesia decreased over time (7.8 per 10,000 during 1990–1992; 3.2 per 10,000 during 1998–2000). The immediate survival rate after arrest was 46.6%, and the hospital survival rate was 34.5%. Twenty-four patients (0.5 per 10,000) had cardiac arrest related primarily to anesthesia.

REFERENCES

1. Diemunsch PA, Van Dorsselaer T, Torp KD, et al. Calibrated pneumoperitoneal venting to prevent N_2O accumulation in the CO_2 pneumoperitoneum during laparoscopy with inhaled anesthesia: an experimental study in pigs. *Anesth Analg.* 2002;94:1014–1018.
2. Myles PS, Leslie K, Chan MT, et al. Avoidance of nitrous oxide for patients undergoing major surgery: a randomized controlled trial. *Anesthesiology.* 2007;107:221–231.
3. Myles PS, Leslie K, Chan MT, et al. The safety of addition of nitrous oxide to general anaesthesia in at-risk patients having major non-cardiac surgery (ENIGMA-II): a randomised, single-blind trial. *Lancet.* 2014;384:1446–1454.
4. Leslie K, Myles PS, Kasza J, et al. Nitrous oxide and serious long-term morbidity and mortality in the evaluation of nitrous oxide in the gas mixture for anaesthesia (ENIGMA)-II trial. *Anesthesiology.* 2015;123:1267–1280.
5. Murphy GS, Szokol JW, Avram MJ, et al. Clinical effectiveness and safety of intraoperative methadone in patients undergoing posterior spinal fusion surgery: a randomized, double-blinded, controlled trial. *Anesthesiology.* 2017;126:822–833.
6. Debaene B, Plaud B, Dilly MP, et al. Residual paralysis in the PACU after a single intubating dose of nondepolarizing muscle relaxant with an intermediate duration of action. *Anesthesiology.* 2003;98:1042–1048.
7. Grosse-Sundrup M, Henneman JP, Sandberg WS, et al. Intermediate acting non-depolarizing neuromuscular blocking agents and risk of postoperative respiratory complications: prospective propensity score matched cohort study. *BMJ.* 2012;345:e6329.
8. Brueckmann B, Sasaki N, Grobara P, et al. Effects of sugammadex on incidence of postoperative residual neuromuscular blockade: a randomized, controlled study. *Br J Anaesth.* 2015;115:743–751.
9. Kreuer S, Bruhn J, Larsen R, et al. A-line, bispectral index, and estimated effect-site concentrations: a prediction of clinical end-points of anesthesia. *Anesth Analg.* 2006;102:1141–1146.
10. Leslie K, Myles PS, Forbes A, et al. The effect of bispectral index monitoring on long-term survival in the B-aware trial. *Anesth Analg.* 2010;110:816–822.
11. Punjasawadwong Y, Phongchiewboon A, Bunchungmongkol N. Bispectral index for improving anaesthetic delivery and postoperative recovery. *Cochrane Database Syst Rev.* 2014:CD003843.
12. Chiang Y, Hosseinian L, Rhee A, et al. Questionable benefit of the pulmonary artery catheter after cardiac surgery in high-risk patients. *J Cardiothorac Vasc Anesth.* 2015;29:76–81.
13. Schulmeyer C, Farias J, Rajdl E, et al. Utility of transesophageal echocardiography during severe hypotension in non-cardiac surgery. *Rev Bras Anestesiol.* 2010;60:513–521.
14. Cronin B, Khoche S, Maus TM. The year in perioperative echocardiography: selected highlights from 2017. *J Cardiothorac Vasc Anesth.* 2018;32:1537–1545.
15. Canty DJ, Royse CF, Kilpatrick D, et al. The impact of pre-operative focused transthoracic echocardiography in emergency non-cardiac surgery patients with known or risk of cardiac disease. *Anaesthesia.* 2012;67:714–720.
16. Diaz-Gomez JL, Renew JR, Ratzlaff RA, et al. Can lung ultrasound be the first-line tool for evaluation of intraoperative hypoxemia? *Anesth Analg.* 2018;126:1769–1773.
17. Diaz-Gomez JL, Via G, Ramakrishna H. Focused cardiac and lung ultrasonography: implications and applicability in the perioperative period. *Rom J Anaesth Intensive Care.* 2016;23:41–54.
18. Kanji HD, McCallum J, Sirounis D, et al. Limited echocardiography-guided therapy in subacute shock is associated with change in management and improved outcomes. *J Crit Care.* 2014;29:700–705.
19. Ferschl MB, Tung A, Sweitzer B, et al. Preoperative clinic visits reduce operating room cancellations and delays. *Anesthesiology.* 2005;103:855–859.
20. Shiga T, Wajima Z, Inoue T, et al. Predicting difficult intubation in apparently normal patients: a meta-analysis of bedside screening test performance. *Anesthesiology.* 2005;103:429–437.
21. Fleisher LA, Fleischmann KE, Auerbach AD, et al. 2014 ACC/AHA guideline on perioperative cardiovascular evaluation and management of patients undergoing noncardiac surgery: a report of the American college of cardiology/American heart association task force on practice guidelines. *J Am Coll Cardiol.* 2014;64:e77–e137.
22. Wilson W, Taubert KA, Gewitz M, et al. Prevention of infective endocarditis: guidelines from the American heart association: a guideline from the American heart association rheumatic fever, endocarditis and kawasaki disease committee, council on cardiovascular disease in the young, and the council on clinical cardiology, council on cardiovascular surgery and anesthesia, and the quality of care and outcomes research interdisciplinary working group. *J Am Dent Assoc.* 2007;138(739–745):747–760.
23. Qaseem A, Snow V, Fitterman N, et al. Risk assessment for and strategies to reduce perioperative pulmonary complications for patients undergoing noncardiothoracic surgery: a guideline from the American college of physicians. *Ann Intern Med.* 2006;144:575–580.
24. Park JG, Ramar K, Olson EJ. Updates on definition, consequences, and management of obstructive sleep apnea. *Mayo Clin Proc.* 2011;86:549–554; quiz 554–545.
25. Practice guidelines for the perioperative management of patients with obstructive sleep apnea: an updated report by the American society of anesthesiologists task force on perioperative management of patients with obstructive sleep apnea. *Anesthesiology.* 2014;120:268–286.
26. Yamakage M, Iwasaki S, Namiki A. Guideline-oriented perioperative management of patients with bronchial asthma and chronic obstructive pulmonary disease. *J Anesth.* 2008;22:412–428.

27. Warner DO, Warner MA, Barnes RD, et al. Perioperative respiratory complications in patients with asthma. *Anesthesiology.* 1996;85:460–467.
28. Sebranek JJ, Lugli AK, Coursin DB. Glycaemic control in the perioperative period. *Br J Anaesth.* 2013;111(suppl 1):i18–i34.
29. Moonesinghe SR, Mythen MG, Grocott MP. High-risk surgery: epidemiology and outcomes. *Anesth Analg.* 2011;112:891–901.
30. Sprung J, Warner ME, Contreras MG, et al. Predictors of survival following cardiac arrest in patients undergoing noncardiac surgery: a study of 518,294 patients at a tertiary referral center. *Anesthesiology.* 2003;99:259–269.
31. Schwilk B, Muche R, Treiber H, et al. A cross-validated multifactorial index of perioperative risks in adults undergoing anaesthesia for non-cardiac surgery. analysis of perioperative events in 26907 anaesthetic procedures. *J Clin Monit Comput.* 1998;14:283–294.
32. Fleisher LA, Pasternak LR, Herbert R, et al. Inpatient hospital admission and death after outpatient surgery in elderly patients: importance of patient and system characteristics and location of care. *Arch Surg.* 2004;139:67–72.
33. Neal JM, Mulroy MF, Weinberg GL. American society of regional anesthesia and pain medicine checklist for managing local anesthetic systemic toxicity: 2012 version. *Reg Anesth Pain Med.* 2012;37:16–18.
34. Guay J, Choi P, Suresh S, et al. Neuraxial blockade for the prevention of postoperative mortality and major morbidity: an overview of cochrane systematic reviews. *Cochrane Database Syst Rev.* 2014:CD010108.
35. Swenson BR, Gottschalk A, Wells LT, et al. Intravenous lidocaine is as effective as epidural bupivacaine in reducing ileus duration, hospital stay, and pain after open colon resection: a randomized clinical trial. *Reg Anesth Pain Med.* 2010;35:370–376.
36. Horlocker TT, Wedel DJ, Benzon H, et al. Regional anesthesia in the anticoagulated patient: defining the risks (the second ASRA consensus conference on neuraxial anesthesia and anticoagulation). *Reg Anesth Pain Med.* 2003;28:172–197.
37. Chin KJ, McDonnell JG, Carvalho B, et al. Essentials of our current understanding: abdominal wall blocks. *Reg Anesth Pain Med.* 2017;42:133–183.
38. Cummings JJ, Ehrenfeld JM, McEvoy MD. A guide to implementing enhanced recovery after surgery protocols: creating, scaling, and managing a perioperative consult service. *Int Anesthesiol Clin.* 2017;55:101–115.
39. Metzner J, Domino KB. Risks of anesthesia or sedation outside the operating room: the role of the anesthesia care provider. *Curr Opin Anaesthesiol.* 2010;23:523–531.
40. Apfelbaum JL, Silverstein JH, Chung FF, et al. Practice guidelines for postanesthetic care: an updated report by the American society of anesthesiologists task force on postanesthetic care. *Anesthesiology.* 2013;118:291–307.
41. White PF. Droperidol. a cost-effective antiemetic for over thirty years. *Anesth Analg.* 2002;95:789–790.
42. White PF, Song D, Abrao J, et al. Effect of low-dose droperidol on the QT interval during and after general anesthesia: a placebo-controlled study. *Anesthesiology.* 2005;102:1101–1105.
43. Practice advisory for perioperative visual loss associated with spine surgery: an updated report by the American society of anesthesiologists task force on perioperative visual loss. *Anesthesiology.* 2012;116:274–285.
44. Moodie JE, Brown CR, Bisley EJ, et al. The safety and analgesic efficacy of intranasal ketorolac in patients with postoperative pain. *Anesth Analg.* 2008;107:2025–2031.
45. Huang YM, Wang CM, Wang CT, et al. Perioperative celecoxib administration for pain management after total knee arthroplasty—a randomized, controlled study. *BMC Musculoskelet Disord.* 2008;9:77.
46. Zakine J, Samarcq D, Lorne E, et al. Postoperative ketamine administration decreases morphine consumption in major abdominal surgery: a prospective, randomized, double-blind, controlled study. *Anesth Analg.* 2008;106:1856–1861.
47. Remerand F, Le Tendre C, Baud A, et al. The early and delayed analgesic effects of ketamine after total hip arthroplasty: a prospective, randomized, controlled, double-blind study. *Anesth Analg.* 2009;109:1963–1971.
48. Tufanogullari B, White PF, Peixoto MP, et al. Dexmedetomidine infusion during laparoscopic bariatric surgery: the effect on recovery outcome variables. *Anesth Analg.* 2008;106:1741–1748.
49. Ji F, Li Z, Nguyen H, et al. Perioperative dexmedetomidine improves outcomes of cardiac surgery. *Circulation.* 2013;127:1576–1584.
50. Hariharan S, Moseley H, Kumar A, et al. The effect of preemptive analgesia in postoperative pain relief—a prospective double-blind randomized study. *Pain Med.* 2009;10:49–53.
51. Khan ZH, Rahimi M, Makarem J, et al. Optimal dose of pre-incision/post-incision gabapentin for pain relief following lumbar laminectomy: a randomized study. *Acta Anaesthesiol Scand.* 2011;55:306–312.
52. Buvanendran A, Kroin JS, Della Valle CJ, et al. Perioperative oral pregabalin reduces chronic pain after total knee arthroplasty: a prospective, randomized, controlled trial. *Anesth Analg.* 2010;110:199–207.
53. Block BM, Liu SS, Rowlingson AJ, et al. Efficacy of postoperative epidural analgesia: a meta-analysis. *JAMA.* 2003;290:2455–2463.

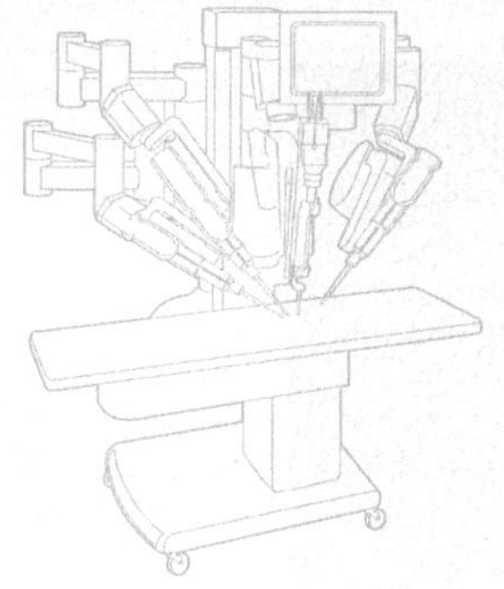

CHAPTER 15

Emerging Technology in Surgery: Informatics, Electronics

Amin Madani, Carmen L. Mueller, Gerald M. Fried

OUTLINE

Please access Elsevier eBooks for Practicing Clinicians to view the videos for this chapter https://expertconsult.inkling.com/.

There has been a dramatic change in surgical care over the past 30 years with the introduction of digitization, miniaturization, improved optics, advanced diagnostic and therapeutic tools, and computerized information systems in the operating room (OR). Whereas surgery has traditionally required large incisions sufficient to allow the surgeon to introduce his/her hands into the body and to allow sufficient light to see the structures being operated upon, innovations have stimulated a radical change in the way surgical procedures are performed. For many surgical procedures, image-guided techniques have now become the standard of care, and the technology continues to evolve, rendering it safer and more seamless for optimizing patient outcomes. These can be done by manipulating instruments from outside the patient, while directing them by looking at displays of direct images of the target tissues (e.g., endoscopic or laparoscopic surgery) or at indirect images of the region of interest (e.g., endovascular catheter-based treatments, image-guided energy ablation of specific targets). Image-guided surgery has enabled the use of significantly smaller incisions to introduce surgical instruments into specific compartments and perform a procedure that would otherwise not be possible without a traditional incision (Fig. 15.1). In other cases, the surgical instruments can access the target tissues through anatomic conduits (e.g., arteries or veins) or natural orifices (e.g., mouth, anus, vagina, or urethra) without the need for any visible incision. These digital platforms have also opened the door to an entire world of opportunities to provide surgeons with real-time data and guidance to improve performance and patient safety, including the use of augmented reality, telementoring by an expert outside the operating theater, and the emerging field of artificial intelligence (AI) to provide computer-augmentation of intraoperative performance. Furthermore, newer technologies have created an explosion of available diagnostic and therapeutic tools that can potentially be used to improve patient outcomes after surgery.

Although patients may benefit substantially from new technologies that minimize the invasiveness of surgical therapies and improve the safety of surgery altogether, employment of novel techniques often requires an entirely new set of skills for the surgeon and his/her team. While the concept of the procedure itself may be familiar to the operating team, the aptitudes required to perform the procedure using a new approach and using new tools are different (e.g., developing a mental model of the anatomic landmarks from a different vantage point or developing the psychomotor skills necessary to effectively maneuver a new tool). Learning and practice have become fundamental aspects of introducing new technologies in the OR in order to avoid the risk of complications during this transition phase. In addition, "new" does not always equate to "better," and critical assessment of the utility, safety, and cost-effectiveness of new technology remains a cornerstone of the process of adopting innovations in surgery.

This chapter describes recent groundbreaking surgical innovations, highlights emerging technologies that are poised to change the OR significantly in the near future, discusses important elements and hurdles for introducing technologies in the OR, and addresses approaches to training and establishing proficiency as new technologies emerge.

RECENT SIGNIFICANT ADVANCES IN SURGICAL TECHNOLOGY

Continuing Evolution of Minimal-Access Surgery

Accessing internal body cavities, such as the chest, abdomen, and pelvis, requires making an incision, the size of which is determined by the surgeon's need to visualize, feel, and manipulate the target tissues, and knowing the dimensions of any tissues that need to be extracted. Minimal-access surgery (such as laparoscopic surgery) provides the means to diminish the trauma of access using image-guided systems to perform the operation without compromising its overall goal. The "cost" to the patient of the access incision is multifactorial. Generally, larger incisions are associated with more postoperative pain, longer recovery periods, a period of physical disability, greater morbidity in cases of wound infection, more risk of incisional hernias, a higher rate of symptomatic adhesive bowel obstruction in the future, and poorer

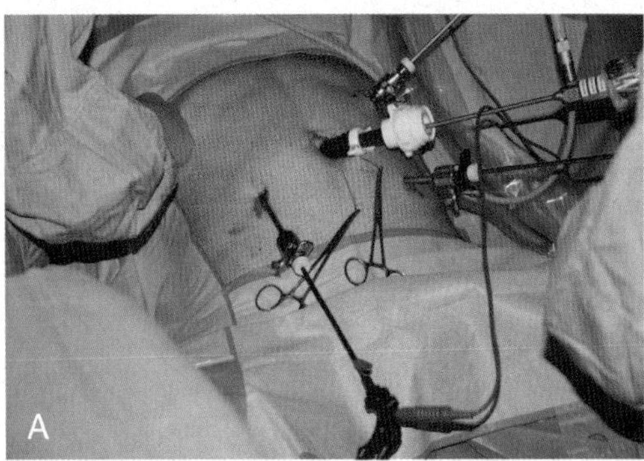

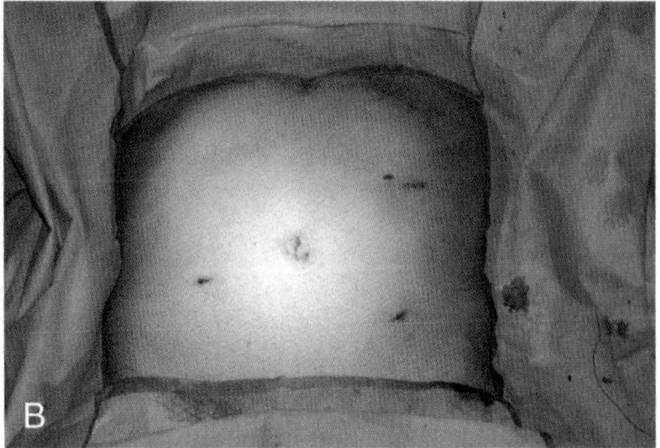

FIG. 15.1 Surgical field for laparoscopic colectomy. (A) Instruments are passed through trocars in the abdominal wall. (B) The small incisions at the completion of the surgery. The largest incision at the umbilicus is used to extract the specimen.

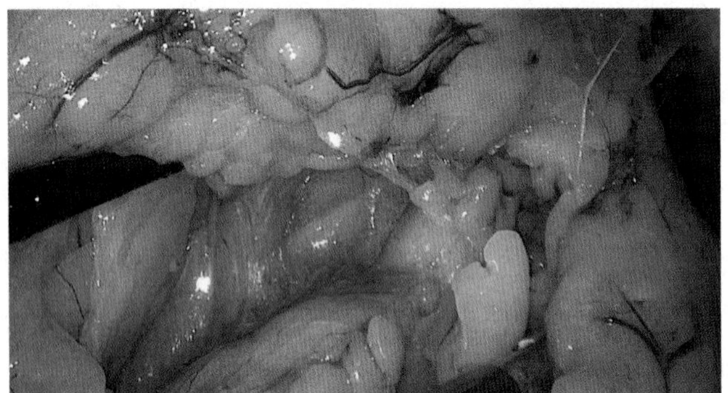

FIG. 15.2 During a left retroperitoneoscopic adrenalectomy, images are provided with a magnified, high-definition view of the operating field.

cosmetic results. While minimally invasive surgery has already been widely adopted as the standard of care for many surgical procedures for over two decades, it nevertheless continues to evolve, with more advanced optical systems, integrated digital platforms, and incorporation of more sophisticated therapeutic and diagnostic tools. As surgeons have become more skilled in laparoscopy, these systems are increasingly being adopted for procedures that have traditionally been either too complex or difficult to accomplish without an open approach, bolstered by evidence of effectiveness and safety. Relative contraindications have continued to diminish, and, currently, most elective and many emergency abdominal surgical procedures are frequently done laparoscopically. Despite their advantages, the smaller incisions present some specific challenges to the operating surgeon, and conversion to an open operation should always be considered a possibility.

One of the advantages of minimally invasive image-guided surgery is the illumination of target tissues, which conveys a bright, magnified, high-definition image to the surgeon through an attached or incorporated camera system (i.e., endoscope). This view, particularly when using newer platforms with high-definition (4K or 8K) cameras, is startling in its clarity (Fig. 15.2). It eliminates shadows and affords all members of the operating team an identical view of the surgery. An important limitation of endoscopic imaging is that it is generally monocular (compared to the binocular view of open surgery), since traditional scopes have a single lens system. With a monocular scope, the surgeon obtains a two-dimensional view of the body displayed on a video monitor. Other sensory cues must be used as part of the surgeon's mental model to appreciate the relative positions of the instruments and tissues in a three-dimensional (3D) space. This depth perception is a learned skill, and most surgeons are able to adjust to laparoscopic imaging with adequate training. Newer platforms have recently emerged to provide minimally invasive surgeons with binocular perception to provide a better sense of stereopsis. Evidence suggests 3D camera technology shortens the learning curve during the acquisition of laparoscopic skills for novices and may enhance proficiency in complex tasks such as fine dissection and suturing for even experienced surgeons.[1,2] Limitations involve increased cost, the need for the surgeon to wear 3D glasses in order to properly see the image, and reduced visualization when using energy devices due to the snow-like appearance of surgical smoke that can obstruct visualization of the field.

Another drawback of endoscopic surgery is the limited field of view, requiring the scope to be moved dynamically to maintain an ideal image. The closer the scope is to the target, the better the illumination, magnification, and image detail but the more limited the field of view. Constant communication between the surgeon performing the operation and the assistant managing the telescope is essential for safe surgery. New automated navigation systems for both endoscopic and robotic surgery have begun to be developed and could potentially be integrated into the operating theater of the future.

Whereas in open surgery the surgeon can palpate and compress tissues to evaluate tissue and assess pathology, including that which lies beneath the surface, laparoscopic images give the surgeon a view of the surface of tissues without the ability for direct manual assessment. Interposing the laparoscopic instrument between the surgeon's hands and the target tissue significantly dampens tactile feedback. This significantly limits the acquisition of tactile feedback from the environment that helps surgeons fine-tune their understanding of relevant anatomy and pathology (i.e., their mental model). In order to augment one's mental model intraoperatively, various methods have been introduced, including the use of augmented reality platforms that can superimpose anatomic reconstructions onto the display monitor (see section below), intraoperative imaging modalities (e.g., laparoscopic ultrasound), or other innovations such as near-infrared fluorescent imaging (e.g., real-time indocyanine green cholangiography). Novel instruments for minimally invasive surgery that incorporate tactile feedback have also recently been developed and have shown to improve kinesthetic perception.[3]

Perhaps some of the greatest advances in minimal-access surgery are in cardiovascular surgery using catheter-based therapies. Vascular surgery has traditionally involved replacing or bypassing occluded or aneurysmal vessels. For several decades, endovascular procedures have revolutionized vascular surgery in much the same way that laparoscopy has impacted abdominal and thoracic surgery. Imaging is provided by fluoroscopy, and contrast solution is injected to outline the vascular anatomy. By accessing the vascular system through puncture or cut-down, instruments can be threaded inside the vessel, stenotic vessels can be dilated with balloons, and intraluminal stents can be threaded into position, guided by real-time fluoroscopic imaging. Large incisions required for access in patients with serious comorbidity can be avoided entirely. Short-term results of endovascular procedures are excellent, recovery is hastened, and the requirements for prolonged hospitalization and intensive care unit care are reduced.[4,5] Newer and more sophisticated tools, such as drug-eluting stents, drug-coated balloons, and fenestrated and branched endografts for thoracoabdominal aortic aneurysms, are being used with increasing technical success and long-term patency to treat complex pathologies. In cardiac surgery, similar transcatheter endovascular approaches have been used to treat coronary artery disease, close septal defects, dilate stenotic valves, and even replace cardiac valves. The idea of avoiding the stress and morbidity of a major incision is particularly appealing in these patients with serious underlying disease. Despite this, the effectiveness and durability of these less invasive therapies must be compared to traditional surgical approaches, and selection of appropriate candidates for these operations is paramount.

One of the limitations to image-guided surgery is the constraint in range of motion afforded to the operator to perform very delicate and complex tasks in a confined and restricted space (e.g., hand-sewn anastomosis). Unlike in open surgery, whereby the surgeon has the flexibility to utilize many degrees of freedom via the shoulder, elbow, wrist, and joints of the hand, laparoscopic instruments have a long shaft whose translational motions within an internal cavity are largely limited to a single axis via a trocar through the abdominal wall and to rotational motions along three axes of the instrument about a fulcrum. This has stimulated the development of novel laparoscopic instruments that offer additional degrees of freedom with articulating components within the instrument in order to overcome this limitation. However, similar to other technologies, the psychomotor skills required to operate these instruments effectively are not inherent to a laparoscopic surgeon and require training prior to their utilization in the OR.

Advances in Endoscopy as a Surgical Platform

Having realized the tremendous benefit of laparoscopy, there has been a consistent desire to further reduce the overall stress of surgery and improve recovery after surgery by diminishing the trauma of access to internal body cavities. This has promoted a trend to using flexible endoscopy and other transluminal approaches to accomplish increasingly complex procedures. Natural orifice transluminal endoscopic surgery (NOTES) is a method whereby access to a body cavity is achieved without any incision in the body wall. This is truly scarless surgery, conducted by accessing the target organ through a natural orifice (such as the mouth, rectum, or vagina). After placing a flexible or rigid endoscope through a natural orifice, an organ (esophagus, stomach, colon, or vagina) is intentionally perforated and the scope is advanced directly to the target tissue. One way this is accomplished is by passing a flexible endoscope through the mouth into the stomach, then through the stomach wall into the abdominal cavity. Other surgical instruments are then advanced through or around the gastroscope, out this opening, and into the abdominal cavity. After the procedure is completed, the resected tissue is retrieved through the mouth and the organ perforation is closed with clips or sutures.

This concept has similarly been adopted for nongastrointestinal operations, such as in transoral endoscopic thyroidectomy vestibular approach, whereby the thyroid gland is excised endoscopically by obtaining access through the mouth. In this technique, standard laparoscopic equipment is used to develop a working space in the neck and perform the dissection. Preliminary case series have demonstrated feasibility and safety with this approach, but, while its cosmetic advantages seem promising compared to a traditional cervical incision, its role currently remains unknown.[6] In colorectal surgery, transanal total mesorectal excision has gained significant popularity to address tumors in the lower third of the rectum, which tend to pose significant technical challenges due to the anatomic constraints of the bony pelvis and thin mesorectum at that level.[7] In this approach, the total mesorectal excision (one of the core surgical principles to optimizing long-term oncologic outcomes for rectal cancer) proceeds transanally ("bottom-up"), enhancing the surgeon's view of the total mesorectal excision planes compared to conventional transabdominal total mesorectal excision (Fig. 15.3). Despite this, the procedure is technically challenging and is fraught with potential complications (e.g., urethral injury) during the initial learning curve if performed with inadequate training.[8]

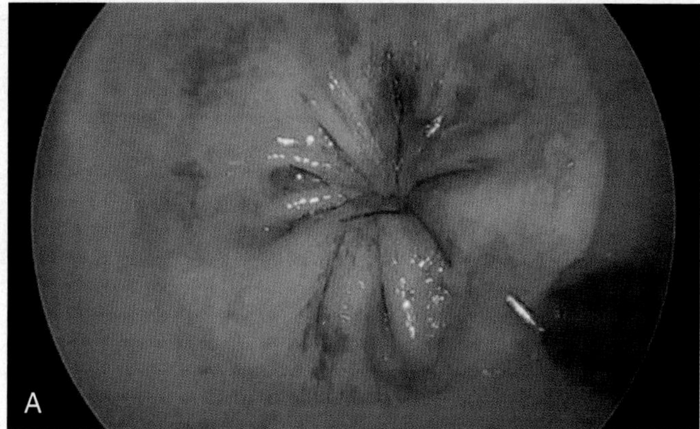

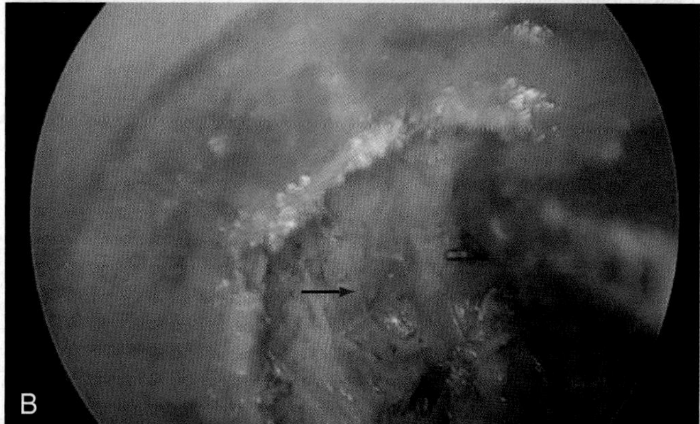

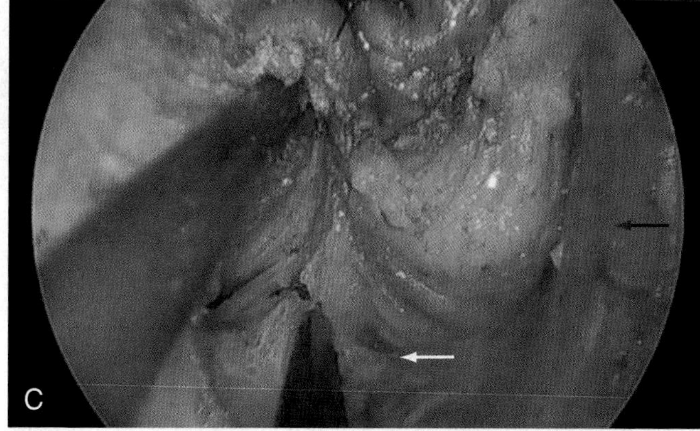

FIG. 15.3 Transanal total mesorectal excision (TaTME): TME dissection from the perineal approach using an advanced endoscopic operating platform. (A) Rectal purse-string closure from transanal view. (B) Dissection of the anterior plane. The *black arrow* points to the TME plane between the prostate and mesorectum. (C) Dissection of the posterior plane. The *white arrow* points to the TME plane between the mesorectum and pelvic floor. The *hatched arrow* demonstrates the levator ani. (Images courtesy of Dr. Lawrence Lee.)

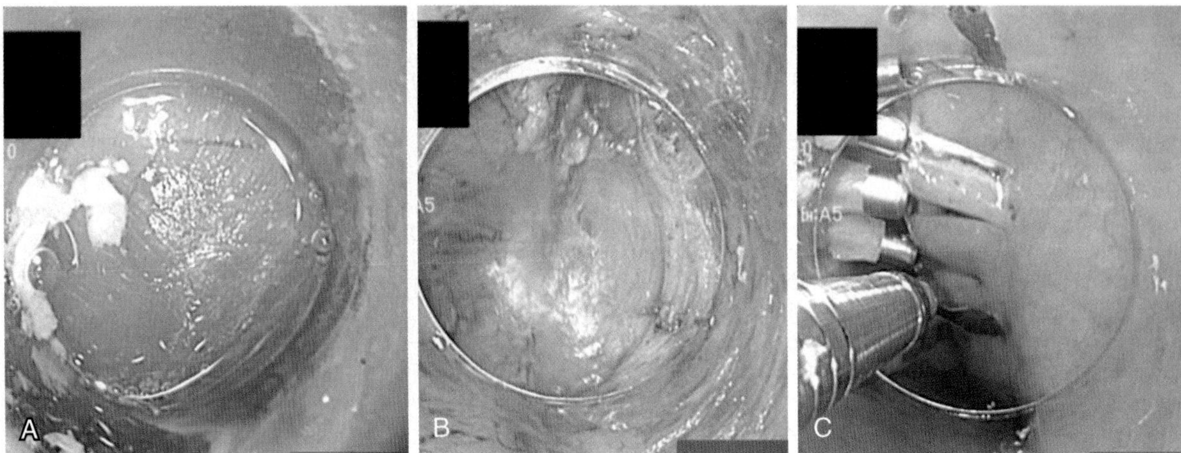

FIG. 15.4 Peroral endoscopic myotomy. (A) View of the endoscopic submucosal tunnel after an incision is made in the mucosa. (B) Almost complete myotomy with only a few circular muscle fibers remaining to be divided. (C) Closure of mucosal incision with clips. (Images courtesy of Dr. Melina Vassiliou and Dr. Daniel Von Renteln.)

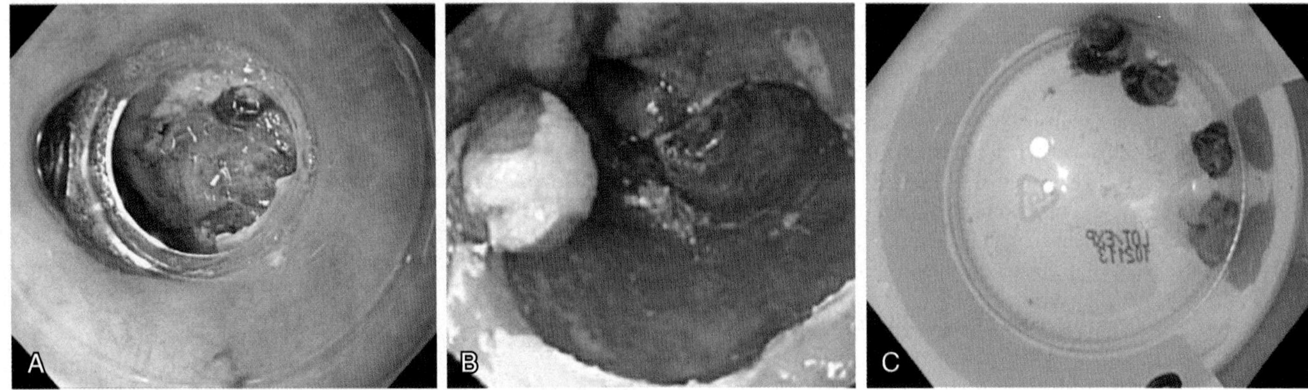

FIG. 15.5 Endoscopic mucosal resection. (A) View of the target lesion through the endoscopic cap. (B) Target lesion is raised off the underlying tissues by submucosal injection and banded to create a pseudopolyp, which is removed by a technique similar to snare polypectomy. (C) Large lesions must be removed piecemeal using this technique. (Images courtesy of Dr. Lorenzo Ferri.)

As might be imagined, natural orifice surgery is challenging, including the need for very long instruments, which are difficult to maneuver without also moving the field of view from the visualization platform (endoscope). In addition, NOTES requires an iatrogenic perforation to obtain access. Any failure of healing can result in serious consequences, such as peritonitis or dyspareunia.

Novel platforms are increasingly pushing the boundaries of what can be treated endoscopically through the upper and lower gastrointestinal (GI) tract. This can be an attractive option, especially if the procedure can be performed with only topical anaesthesia or intravenous sedation. Endoscopes can now be equipped with more advanced functions to perform more complex tasks, such as endoscopic suturing, balloon dilatation, and placement of more intricate stents.[9,10] These devices have paved the way for surgeons to perform procedures endoscopically that were traditionally performed using an open or laparoscopic approach. For instance, peroral endoscopic myotomy (POEM procedure; Fig. 15.4) has gained popularity over the last decade for the treatment of achalasia. This is a natural orifice technique that involves creation of a long esophageal myotomy using a flexible GI endoscope. After incising the esophageal mucosa, a tunnel is created in the esophageal wall, the circular muscle is divided to a point distal to the lower esophageal sphincter, and the esophageal mucosal opening is closed with clips. While long-term data are still lacking, preliminary data in skilled hands have shown short-term effectiveness with POEM, equivalent to the gold-standard laparoscopic Heller myotomy to control dysphagia, with low morbidity and rapid recovery. However, the procedure does appear to be associated with a higher rate of gastroesophageal reflux compared to a Heller myotomy combined with an antireflux procedure.[11,12]

As the scope and breadth of advanced endoscopic procedures continue to gain momentum, this technology has also been used to resect tumors in the esophagus, stomach, colon, and rectum, thereby sparing the patient an anatomic organ resection for early stage cancers in which lymphadenectomy is not required or would not be tolerated due to poor performance status. Techniques currently employed include endoscopic mucosal resection (Fig. 15.5) and endoscopic submucosal dissection (Fig. 15.6). While these techniques are not necessarily new, there is a constant evolution of highly specialized equipment required to perform them, including endoscopes with enhanced range of motion at the tip and additional working and water irrigation channels, as well as specialized endoscopic dissection and hemostasis tools.

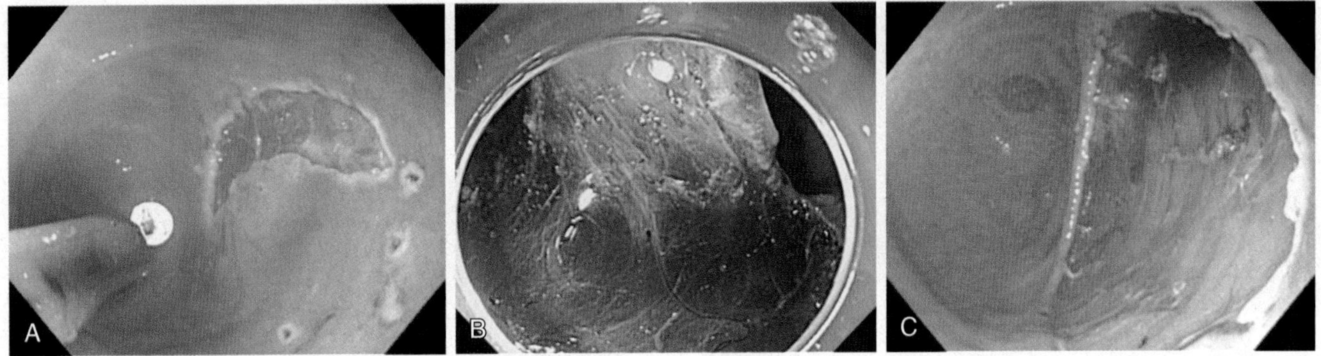

FIG. 15.6 Endoscopic submucosal dissection. (A) The target lesion is mapped out with radiofrequency energy and raised off the underlying tissues through submucosal injection. The mucosa is then circumferentially cut around the target lesion. (B) The mucosal lesion is dissected from the submucosa. (C) The resulting mucosal defect after en bloc removal of the target lesion. (Images courtesy of Dr. Lorenzo Ferri.)

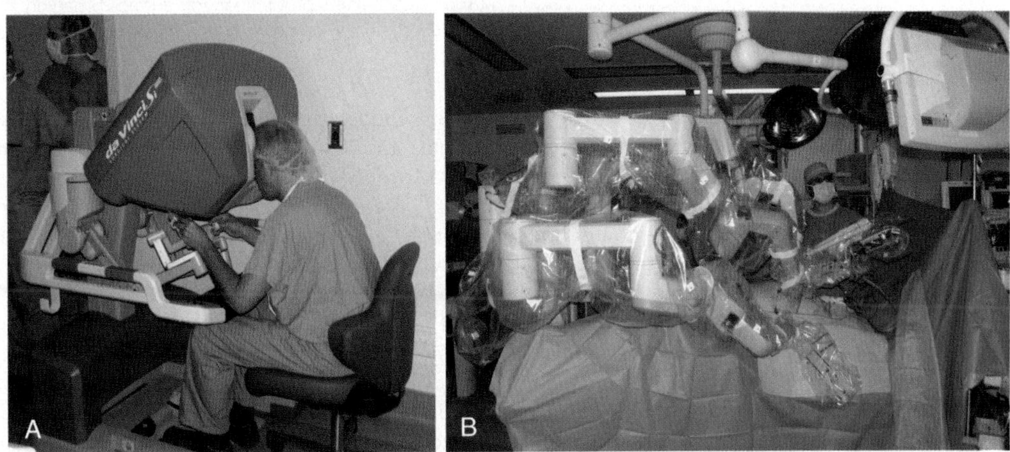

FIG. 15.7 Robotic surgery. (A) The surgeon at the console uses his hands and feet to control the robot arms. (B) Robotic setup at the patient.

Recent advances have also combined the outstanding imaging capability of the flexible endoscope with an ultrasound transducer at the distal end. Applications in the GI tract (endoscopic ultrasound [EUS]) and bronchial tree (endobronchial ultrasound) extend the capability of the endoscope to visualize the complete thickness of the wall of the organ (for staging of tumors), adjacent lymph nodes that can be biopsied, and adjacent structures (e.g., evaluation of the common bile duct or pancreas through the duodenum or stomach during EUS). Surgical procedures can now be performed using EUS guidance, such as drainage of pancreatic pseudocysts, debridement of walled-off pancreatic necrosis into the stomach, and gastrojejunal stenting to palliate obstructing pancreatic tumors. While technically challenging, the endoscopic approach in these cases is associated with significantly lower morbidity and mortality compared to an open approach.[13]

Evolution of Minimally Invasive Robotic Surgery

Robotic surgical systems were designed to overcome some of the limitations of endoscopic surgery by using enabling characteristics of robots to improve the capabilities of the surgeon compared to working freehand.[14,15] Unlike the use of robotics in industry, surgical robots rarely work autonomously but rather act as an interface between the operating surgeon and the patient. In this master-slave relationship, the master (surgeon) sits at a console in an ergonomically sound position and uses movements of both hands and feet to control movements of the laparoscope and wristed instruments inside the patient attached to the robot arms (slave) (Fig. 15.7). The most widely used robotic system in North America uses a proprietary laparoscope with two optical systems providing binocular (3D) vision and additional depth perception. The surgical instruments have additional articulating components near their distal tips (i.e., "wristed") so that the movements of the surgeon's hands can be reproduced by the instruments without the usual limitations of the fulcrum effect seen with traditional laparoscopic instruments. This enables surgeons to perform finer motor movements within a small, confined, and deep space. For a demonstration of robotic-assisted dissection, see Video 1.

Since there is no direct contact between the surgeon at the console and the instruments, the surgeon can also work from a remote location or even long distances, paving the way for telesurgery. Robotic surgical platforms are especially appealing for providing care to patients in hostile environments, such as those in the military, on outer space missions, on deep-sea explorations, and on polar expeditions. Despite the theoretical advantages of providing surgical care to remote regions, the costs and resources required to deploy such a system have limited its practicality and implementation. For instance, trained personnel would still be required on site to prepare the patient, insert the ports, dock the robot, change instruments, and intervene to treat complications or unexpected findings that cannot be controlled robotically. Also, issues relating

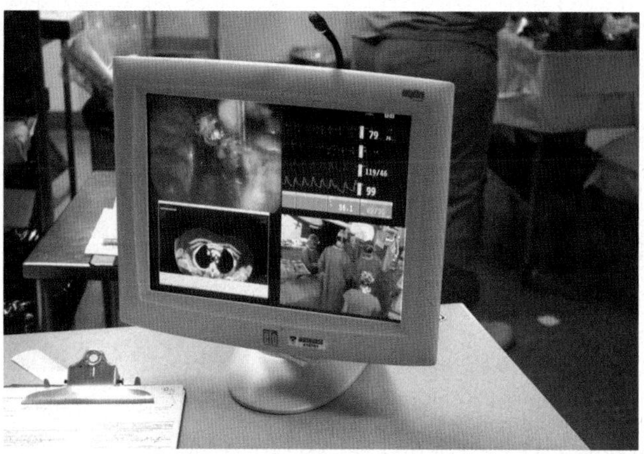

FIG. 15.8 In this quad-screen display, the surgeon can select up to four images to be displayed simultaneously on a monitor. This display at the nursing station shows the endoscopic image, preoperative image, preoperative computerized tomography images, vital signs, and room view.

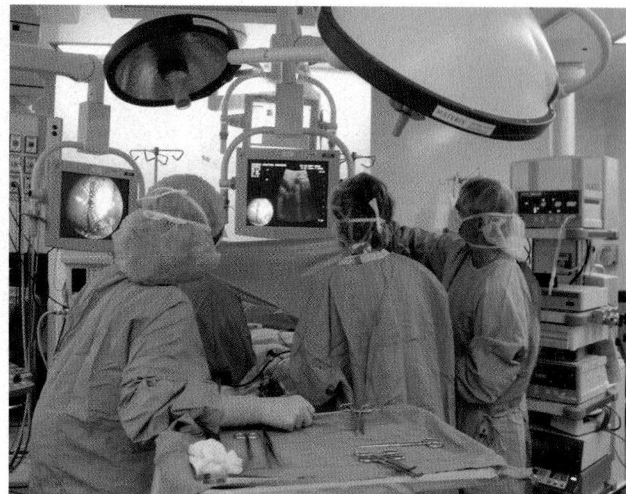

FIG. 15.9 The combination of surface imaging by laparoscopy and cross-sectional imaging with laparoscopic ultrasound are complimentary.

to licensing and liability have yet to be addressed, and latent delays between motions performed by the surgeon and the movement of the instrument on site must be resolved. The longer the distance that the data needs to be transmitted from the console to the patient, the greater the latent delay, as even 250 millisecond can have significant impact on the quality of the operation.[16] It is important to highlight that a negative feature of this interface is that the surgeon has no tactile sense of the tissues and, as a result, must adapt by using only visual data. However, integrated tactile feedback into the next generation of minimally invasive robotic systems has thus far shown to improve tissue handling and will undoubtedly help address some of the platform's limitations in the future.[17]

Robotic surgery provides other exciting opportunities to enhance surgical performance. Since there is an interface between the surgeon and the effector instruments, it is possible to modulate the relationship between the surgeon's movement and that of the instrument using complex computer algorithms. The platform can adjust the gain or the scale of movement. In this way, the surgeon may make larger movements to affect very fine movements of the instrument tip. This can be very helpful for procedures that require precise movements, such as microvascular anastomosis. Algorithms can also be incorporated to dampen tremor using embedded filters. Over the last few years, robotic surgery has been carried out in conjunction with robotic-assisted anesthesia. This is an automated platform in which anesthesia agents are controlled using computer-assisted devices that calculate moment-to-moment anesthesia doses in a closed-loop system to provide optimal dosing—as either a completely automated or a semiautomated system.

Currently, minimally invasive robotic systems are widely used in urologic surgery and gynecology and to a lesser extent in cardiac surgery, general surgery, and endocrine surgery.[15,18,19] The main drawbacks are costs, bulkiness, and set-up time for the equipment and absence of compelling data to show superiority of robotic operations over those done by well-trained laparoscopic surgeons. Nevertheless, several new robotic surgery platforms have recently entered the market and will undoubtedly stimulate competition and innovation to overcome these limitations and expand the role of robotics in surgical care.[14] Indeed, one of the greatest influences of robotics may be in flexible endoscopic procedures. The single-operator nature of contemporary endoscopes strongly limits the ability to expose tissues and perform advanced motor movements (e.g., traction/countertraction, dissection, suturing). As a result, robotic endoscopes have been equipped with advanced navigation systems and instruments that can be maneuvered and articulated with more flexibility, making it possible to execute complex tasks.[20] Various platforms have recently become commercially available, and preliminary data demonstrating their effectiveness, safety, and feasibility will begin to surface in the near future.

Digitization and Augmentation of Surgery

Today's integrated ORs have been completely redesigned so that all devices, lighting, and image routing can be controlled from the surgical field or a control station (Fig. 15.8). By controlling the interface, any digital image or combination of images can be routed to any monitor, depending on the needs of the operating team. Any image can be recorded to document the surgical findings. The images or video clips can be annotated by verbal recordings or by textual description. This provides very valuable documentation of the operative findings for the medical record. Another major opportunity presented by image-guided surgery is that the display monitor can provide multiple pieces of information simultaneously to augment the mental model of the surgeon in real-time. Most data required by the surgical team (e.g., hemodynamic parameters or preoperative or intraoperative imaging) are available digitally and can be routed to any display device. This can be extremely useful in a situation when this information can affect intraoperative decision-making, such as when operating on an unstable patient and deciding whether to proceed with a damage-control tactic based on the physiology of the patient. Another example is when performing a complicated dissection near important anatomic structures that are at risk of injury and deciding where are the safe planes and dangerous planes. Display of preoperatively acquired images or images generated intraoperatively by ultrasound, flexible endoscopy, or fluoroscopy can be very helpful to guide the surgeon and add safety and efficiency to the operation (Fig. 15.9). Further, the use of touchscreens has been adapted to provide telestration capabilities by making annotations on a monitor in order to communicate specific anatomic and pathologic findings from the operating field (Fig. 15.10). Digitization of image-guided surgery and the ability to equip the operating theater with a system of cameras make videoconferencing a reality, bringing consultant surgical specialists and other members of the patient care team directly into the previously closed surgical arena. The ubiquitous use

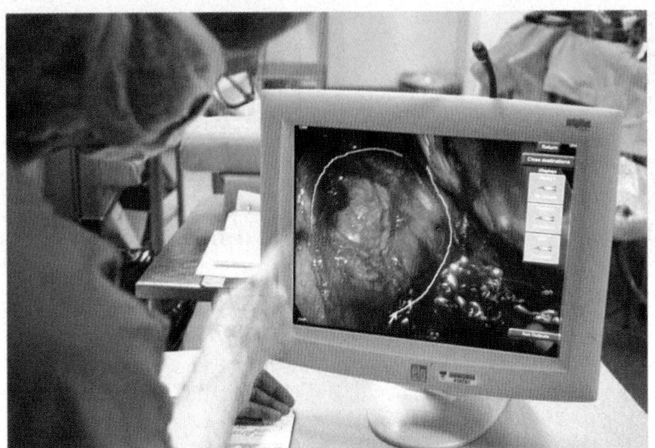

FIG. 15.10 Telestration allows the surgeon to use the touchscreen interface to make annotations on the image for documentation and teaching purposes.

of head-mounted cameras in extreme sports and other activities has now also been adapted in the OR, allowing members of the operating team to record open operations with high-definition. In digitally augmented surgery, the surgeon can have access to a whole dashboard of information and select the relevant data for heads-up display during the procedure. The routing of digital information to display(s) can be carried out using voice controls or touchscreens in the surgical field. This means that with the appropriate cybersecurity and privileges, access can be obtained remotely in real-time, making videoconferencing technology a useful tool for remote training and mentoring through the processes of telementoring and teleproctoring—both in the OR and in surgical simulation.[21] Video feeds of live surgical procedures can include audio commentating and allow large groups of surgeons to simultaneously learn from a single expert, a trend that has become quite popular at many professional conferences and courses.

One of the most exciting areas in surgery is the adoption of augmented-reality–assisted surgery to provide intraoperative guidance and navigation. Computer-generated 3D image reconstructions can be acquired and superimposed onto the field of view, providing a digital overlay using image-guided surgery or, more recently, using augmented-reality platforms. Using proprietary software that utilizes preoperative digital imaging (e.g., computerized tomography, magnetic resonance imaging, ultrasonography), complex anatomic and pathologic models can be created to assist with the operation. This is especially useful in endoscopic and robotic surgery in which there is loss of tactile feedback to establish one's mental model of the surgical field (as is done in open procedures). For instance, additional data displaying the location of a tumor and critical structures (e.g., major vascular structures, ureters, major bile ducts) can assist a surgical oncologist to assess their relative location and help potentially avoid inadvertent injuries during a difficult dissection. In breast surgery, augmented reality systems have been developed to provide guidance on tumor location and to minimize the rate of positive margins with lumpectomies.[22] Another method to provide this information is the use of fluorescence markers (such as indocyanine green). While this technology has been used for decades by ophthalmologists, it has only recently become popular for visualizing biliary anatomy to avoid major bile duct injuries and for assessing the vascular supply to bowel during a GI anastomosis.[23,24] Preliminary data regarding the usefulness of these tools are promising, and surgical centers are increasingly using this technology to augment decision-making during surgery.

EVOLVING TECHNOLOGIES IN SURGERY

3D Printing and Bioprinting

3D printing technology emerged in the mid-1980s and was originally known as additive manufacturing. The process involves the deposition of materials other than ink from printer-like nozzles onto a moving platform according to computerized algorithms to create 3D objects. Originally used in the manufacture of simple objects, such as those containing glass, plastic, and metal, 3D printing technology could conceivably be applied to create objects involving food, electronics, and even human tissue. The potential uses in medicine are vast, and this technology has only just begun to be explored for medical and surgical applications. In 2019, only approximately 2% of a $700-million industry is being directed toward medical applications, but this is projected to expand to a US$1.9-billion industry for medical applications alone within the next few years.

At present in medicine, 3D printing applications are being investigated for remote "printing" of prescription drugs, custom-fit prosthesis modeling, and preoperative fracture modeling for surgical planning and simulation training, among other applications. Indeed, one of the greatest potentials for this form of technology is in the domain of transplantation and reconstructive surgery, where advances in tissue engineering and stem cell research are starting to be used to recreate cells, tissues, and organs de novo. 3D bioprinting has also been projected to recreate native tissues, which can reproduce clinically relevant physiologic functions that are dysfunctional or lacking in disease states, a feat that has thus far only been feasible using transplantation.[25] While this technology has not been widely adopted and clinical trials demonstrating safety, feasibility, and clinical effectiveness have yet to be done prior to its translation into clinical practice, several groups have shown the ability to bioprint various tissues, including bone, skin, cartilage, nerves, blood vessels, and adipose tissue for breast reconstruction. Bioprinting 3D models can also provide surgeons the means to rehearse an operation using patient-specific anatomic data as opposed to relying purely on preoperative imaging.

Artificial Intelligence

Perhaps one of the most exciting new areas of surgical innovation is the cross-pollination between surgery and advances in computer science, data science ("big data"), and AI algorithms. Indeed, potential benefits of AI have attracted massive venture capital investments, including as much as $5 billion in 2016. There are several ways in which AI can potentially impact surgical care in the future. For instance, using machine learning, a program can be used to learn and to make predictions regarding a specific outcome or to identify subtle patterns within a very large data set that would otherwise be unperceivable to human analysis. This can be useful to clinicians when attempting to predict clinical outcomes (e.g., complications or long-term oncologic outcomes) based on a multitude of patient-related, pathology-related, system-related, perioperative, and intraoperative variables. Such nonlinear algorithms have so far been shown to potentially outperform conventional statistical methodologies performed manually, especially when using artificial neural networks—a framework of different machine learning algorithms designed to process and compute large quantities of data in a manner similar to biologic nervous systems.[26] Similarly, the concept of "computer vision" has emerged in AI, whereby images and videos can be used for identification and pattern recognition of particular scenes and objects (Fig. 15.11). Computer-aided diagnostic programs have already been developed and shown to have strong

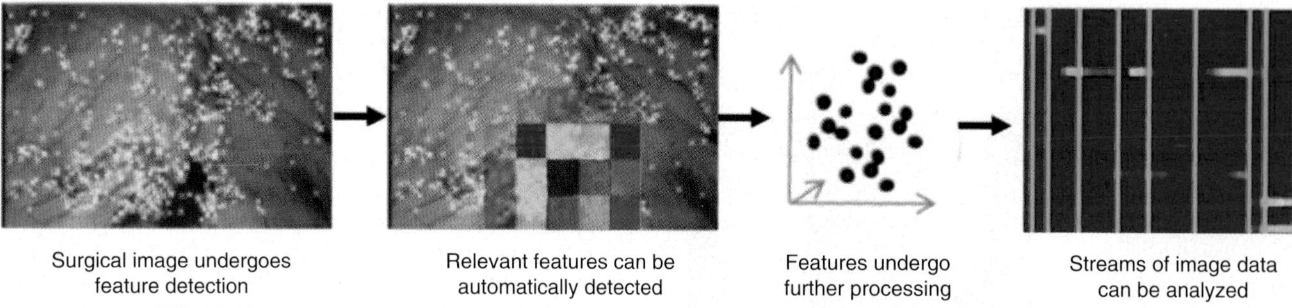

FIG. 15.11 Computer vision utilizes complex mathematical algorithms to analyze images or video streams using quantifiable factors such as color, texture, and position. These data are subsequently used within a large dataset to identify statistically meaningful events. (Adapted from Hashimoto DA, Rosman G, Rus D, et al. Artificial intelligence in surgery: promises and perils. *Ann Surg.* 2018;268:70–76.)

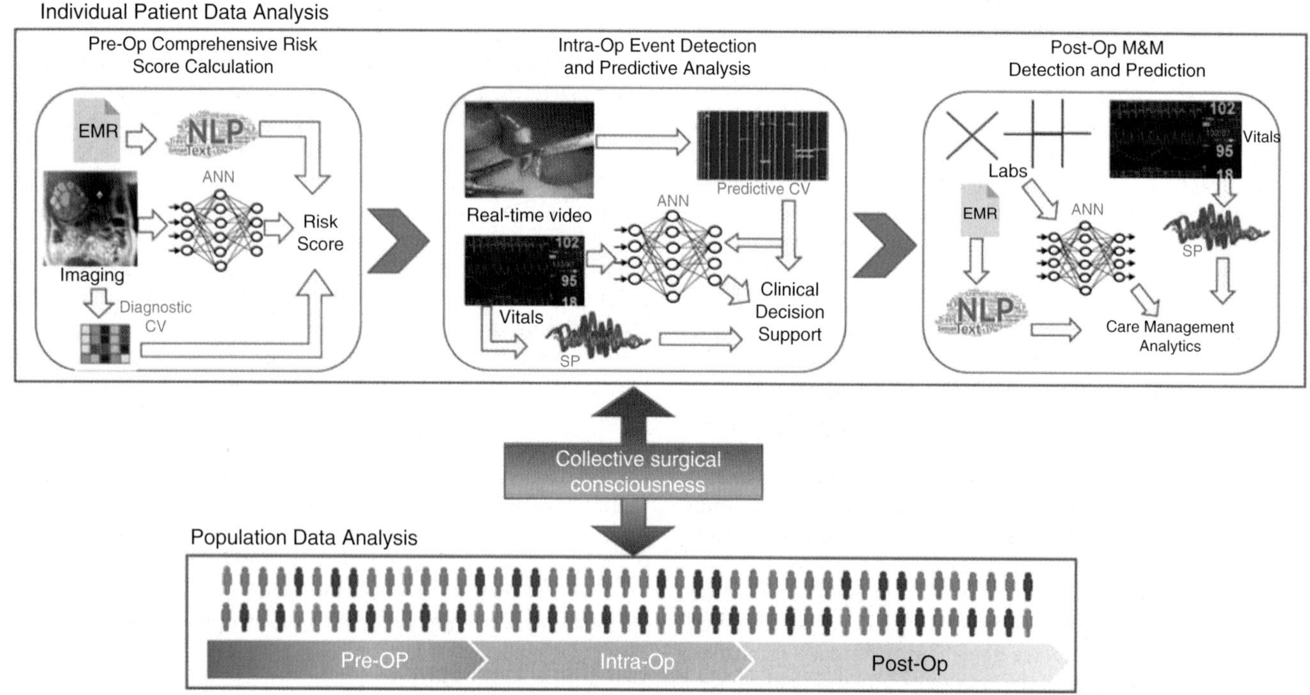

FIG. 15.12 Integration of multimodal data using artificial intelligence could be leveraged to augment surgical decision-making across all phases of care, the so-called "collective surgical consciousness." These data can potentially impact care on an individual or population level. (Adapted from Hashimoto DA, Rosman G, Rus D, et al. Artificial intelligence in surgery: promises and perils. *Ann Surg.* 2018;268:70–76.) *ANN,* Artificial neural network; *CV,* computer vision; *NLP,* natural language processing; *SP,* signal processing. *EMR,* electronic medical record; *M&M, XXX;*

potential in improving patient care.[27] It is also conceivable that, with the development of complex algorithms using large datasets of intraoperative videos and perioperative outcomes, specific behaviors can be coded, identified, and correlated with adverse events and clinical outcomes. While this concept has yet to be demonstrated at a more practical level, it is certainly on the horizon. AI algorithms that can process intraoperative data and provide real-time feedback to surgeons during a procedure are being developed with an aim to improve judgment and performance. Ultimately, analyzing data obtained from all phases of patient care may one day be used to augment surgical decision-making—a concept referred to as "collective surgical consciousness" (Fig. 15.12).[26]

Intraoperative Diagnostic Tools for Targeted Surgery

Another trend in surgical innovation has been to improve the precision of an operation (e.g., excision of a mass or ablation of tissues), minimizing the extent of surgery and subsequent physiologic toll of an operation, with the goal of improving outcomes. To address this need, various intraoperative diagnostic tools have been developed to provide surgeons with real-time on-the-spot data regarding the biologic nature of target tissues. For instance, mass spectrometry, an analytic technique used to ionize chemicals and detect their charge-to-mass ratio, has recently been embedded into surgical devices to detect the specific molecular profiles of target tissues and correlate it with a specific phenotype (e.g., cancer vs. benign).[28,29] The concept of in vivo real-time detection of tumor cells can be potentially useful in scenarios where it is not possible to tell if microscopic disease remains at the surgical margins and whether additional resection would have significant impact on the course of the operation. This can also be useful when surgeons encounter thick fibrotic benign tissue that is indiscernible from cancer (e.g., prior radiation therapy, adhesions from prior operation, or locoregional inflammatory tissue effects). Several imaging techniques have also been used to provide real-time diagnostic data on the phenotype of target tissues in order to detect disease that may otherwise not be detectable, such as during the treatment of cancerous and precancerous conditions (e.g., endoscopic radiofrequency ablation or resection of dysplastic Barrett esophagus). These include confocal laser endomicrosurgery (microscopic imaging of tissues), chromoendoscopy (using various dyes such as indigo carmine to accentuate dysplastic tissue), virtual chromoendoscopy (e.g., narrow band imaging), and optical coherence tomography (cross-sectional tissue imaging using backscattering of light) to name a few.[30–32] Finally, development of biomarkers in concert with advances in optics in the OR has been used in various applications for improving the quality of resected specimens, such as in neurosurgery.[33] In a manner similar to indocyanine green injection to illuminate target tissues during hepatobiliary and GI surgery, these diagnostic tools ultimately serve the same purpose: to augment the mental model of the operating team in order to improve performance, patient safety, and outcomes.

PROCESS OF INNOVATION IN SURGERY

As exemplified in the previous sections, innovation in surgery has provided the means to revolutionize the management of surgical patients and has opened the door to possibilities that were once considered improbable. Innovations can include anything from incremental modifications of an existing device (e.g., new generation of laparoscopic instruments with articulating components) to disruptive devices and technologies that revolutionize surgical care (e.g., cardiopulmonary bypass, image-guided surgery). Despite the enthusiasm to introduce novel technologies into the OR, it is important to emphasize that the translation of ideas into tangible products that can subsequently be applied into practice and improve patient care is a long, expensive, and high-risk endeavor with very high rates of long-term failure and poor rates of adoption by end-users.[34,35] This innovation pathway requires a thorough needs assessment, a process of ideation, many rounds of prototyping and experimentation, adequate commitment of capital and resources, and a team of individuals with diverse backgrounds to tackle issues related to intellectual property, regulatory approval, commercialization, and corporate and product development (Fig. 15.13).[36] Any of these elements can potentially derail an idea from conception to implementation. Indeed, bringing an idea into market can often take more than a decade, with a failure rate estimated at greater than 90% after 10 years.[35] It is also important for innovators and clinicians to take into consideration the various consequences that can result from introducing medical technologies into the clinical environment. Specifically, patients need to be protected from harm as new technologies can often lead to unexpected adverse events, such an alarmingly higher rate of bile duct injuries arising during the early days of laparoscopic cholecystectomy compared to the open approach.[37] Prior to using a new product on patients, end-users (including surgeons and other members of the operating team) need to undertake the appropriate level of training, with adequate supervision and proctorship, to ensure a smooth transition. This can often be challenging when attempting to convince surgeons to retrain themselves to incorporate a new technology into their practice. However, with adequate support and resources, including dedicated simulation-based training and objective metrics to ensure proficiency has been met, this can be achieved. Furthermore, hospital administrators, insurance companies, and various other stakeholders are becoming increasingly more cost-conscious in today's health care climate. In order for an innovation to be successfully implemented, it needs to be cost-effective and provide significant value (in terms of improving patient outcomes) relative to its costs to the institution, patients, and health care system. Ultimately, surgery provides a very fertile ground for creativity and novel ideas for introducing tools and devices in the OR, and as technology continues to evolve, surgeons play a central role in conceptualizing, developing, introducing, and evaluating the impact of new technologies on patient care.

INNOVATIONS IN SIMULATION: SURGICAL TRAINING AND OPERATIVE PLANNING

Use of new technology in surgery, whether performed by laparoscopy, robotics, flexible endoscopy, transcatheter methods, or by other techniques, generally requires a set of specific technical, cognitive, and interpersonal skills distinct from those required for traditional open surgical procedures. Ensuring adequate training of surgeons remains a critical step in the transition of a new technology from inception to a widely accepted practice norm. Each technique makes specific demands on the surgeon, requiring specific training programs. It cannot be assumed that a surgeon who is proficient at performing pancreaticoduodenectomy by laparotomy can smoothly adopt the robotic or laparoscopic approach for this operation without further training. Moreover, many of these new techniques require a different level of interactivity and teamwork with various members of the OR in order to achieve optimal performance.

There is a concept of the learning curve during which the surgical team acquires proficiency with a technique in the course of applying the technique in surgical practice. As a result, the evaluation of a new technology or techniques can be biased by evaluating the outcome of the procedure in the hands of a surgeon during the learning curve phase, and it may not be clear when the learning curve is completed. In this regard, outcomes measured at the introduction of a new technology may be more reflective of the surgeon's experience or proficiency with the technique than the merits of the procedure itself, leading to negative opinions within the surgical community and lay press and consequently limiting the adoption of the innovation.

To overcome this obstacle, learning a surgical technique in a simulation environment can present many practical advantages. Specific learning objectives can be defined and modeled for learning, allowing the surgeon to repeatedly and deliberately practice the specific skills that are required to make the transition to using a new technique. Practice in a simulated environment focuses the experience on the learner and not on the patient, without risking any inadvertent injuries to the latter. The learner can be allowed to progress at his/her own pace and eventually progress beyond his or her comfort level and experiment with different techniques or approaches. Learners can be allowed to make errors and develop the ability to correct them. Performance can be measured in a standardized and objective way and compared to accepted performance standards (proficiency level).[38–40] Simulation allows for the acquisition of skills through learner-centered, deliberate practice in a safe environment, analogous to practicing a sport. Coaching can be performed by designing drills that emphasize specific and difficult aspects and/or areas of weakness and by providing learners with focused feedback and ample opportunities for repetition.[41] For example, instead of learning how to dissect the gallbladder from the liver bed during laparoscopic cholecystectomy

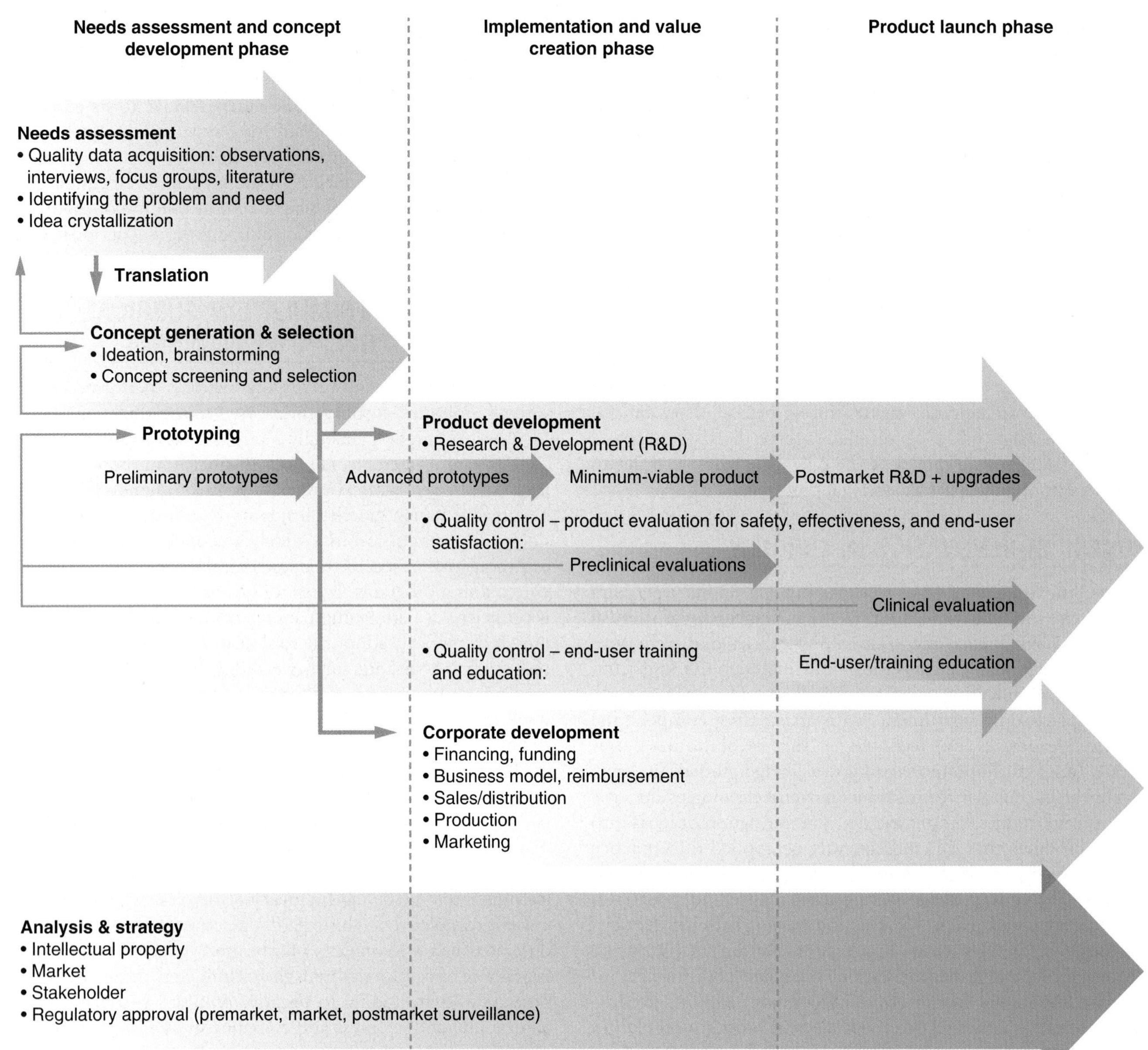

FIG. 15.13 A conceptual framework from the Simnovate collaborative defining and characterizing the product development pathway for health care innovation. (Adapted from Madani A, Gallix B, Pugh CM, et al. Evaluating the role of simulation in healthcare innovation: recommendations of the Simnovate Medical Technologies Domain Group. *BMJ Simul Technol Enhanced Learn.* 2017;3:S8–S14.)

in the OR, trainees acquire the fundamental psychomotor skills in a simulation center, allowing them to focus on operative strategy, anatomy, and judgment with their clinical proctor in the OR. As such, simulation is best seen as a potentially important adjunct to clinical experience, especially during early training for a particular skill or procedure and ideally within a developed curriculum. Simulations can occur using a number of different platforms, including live animals, human cadavers, inanimate objects (e.g., box trainers in laparoscopy), or computer-based models such as virtual reality (VR) trainers. Simulations can be designed to teach and assess fundamental skills (part-task trainers) or entire procedures, teamwork, and interprofessional skills. Innovations such as the integration of trainers with actors to create human-simulator hybrids may enhance effectiveness. Unfortunately, simulation often can be very costly in terms of its development, as well as the material and human resources required to run training sessions. As a result, choosing the form of simulation depends on the educational objectives that one aims to achieve. For instance, advanced VR simulators can be designed to incorporate a very high degree of fidelity and haptic feedback to accurately mimic real tissues. In some circumstances, this is an important feature of the simulator's design and useful for the specific skills that are targeted in the curriculum. In other cases, however, developing a very advanced simulator may not always improve learning and performance compared to cheaper alternatives, and it is critical for educators to choose the most cost-effective and practical method for designing a simulation model. Just as importantly, simulation centers may not always be optimally located for ease of access, and these issues can act as significant obstacles for integrating simulation into a pedagogical model for busy clinicians.

Objective assessment of performance is an important aspect of simulation-based training to set practice goals, guide remediation, and judge the effectiveness of these new educational interventions. The best incentive to improve particular skills is to measure them. Having a measure of performance allows the establishment of norms, proficiency target goals for training, comparison to peers, and an objective standard for certification. This is only possible when performance can be assessed using metrics that have passed the standards of validity evidence required to use these measures in a high-stakes environment (i.e., "how well do these metrics reflect the underlying skill that is being assessed?"). The parameters measured must reflect and predict clinical performance, must be practical to apply, must be meaningful to the learner, and must be generalizable to different learning environments. The attraction of measuring performance in a simulated environment is that the context for testing can be standardized, unaffected by patient differences in body habitus, anatomy, and pathology. The level of difficulty can be altered systematically and in a reproducible and standardized fashion. By providing a consistent test environment, the metrics can be evaluated scientifically and improvement and learning curves can be tracked. For example, in the Fundamentals of Laparoscopic Surgery curriculum, a low-fidelity part-task training program developed for surgeons to practice basic psychomotor skills required to perform image-guided laparoscopic surgery,[42] efficiency, and accuracy are measured using a combination of time and errors to score a trainee. However, developing these metrics can be difficult and much of what we know about surgical errors, intraoperative performance, and patient safety over the past three decades is centered around skillsets that go well beyond psychomotor skills, relating to advanced mental processes such as decision-making, judgment, and various interpersonal skills such as communication and teamwork.[43–46] Developing objective and reproducible metrics to accurately measure these cognitive behaviors is one of the biggest challenges in surgical education.[47] Traditionally, checklists or performance assessments using Likert rating scales have been used with some success. However, more recently, the incorporation of technology-enhanced learning environments has allowed novel methods to be used to measure advanced cognitive skills in a more meaningful manner to provide learners with focused feedback and opportunities to deliberately practice these highly important skills. For instance, the visual concordance test is a method where a learner is provided with a scenario in the form of an intraoperative video and is asked to make annotations on the surgical field in relation to a critical and specific aspect of the case (e.g., "identify the plane" or "where do you want to dissect"). These annotations are given accuracy scores according to prior response from experts, and this data is provided to the learner in the form of a heat map to provide the learner with on-the-spot expert feedback regarding their decisions for that given scenario.[48]

One of the exciting and innovative areas in surgical education is in the use of augmented and VR platforms using commercially available headsets that have become very popular in the video game industry. This technology provides the means to fully immerse a learner into an environment such as the OR and practice a variety of different tasks. Newer and more advanced handset controllers have been developed to simulate the handling of surgical instruments and allow the participant to manipulate or interact with objects and tissues in a virtual world. One potential application is toward the concept of preoperative surgical rehearsal based on patient-specific anatomy and pathology. Since sophisticated imaging techniques provide anatomic and functional information in a digital format, 3D computer models can be constructed preoperatively that simulate the operative environment. Patient-specific imaging data could even be modeled into a VR simulator with realistic haptic properties and with tissue deformation that mimics the viscoelastic properties of actual human tissues. The surgeon could then explore different approaches to performing a complex or high-risk surgical procedure before actually undertaking the operation in the real patient, having previously been able to interact with the patient's unique anatomy and pathology in the safety of a VR environment. Such modeling systems have been developed in neurosurgery, allowing surgeons to determine the optimal operative approach to challenging surgical problems, such as arteriovenous malformations.[49] The application for neurosurgery is particularly attractive, since the skull forms a rigid framework to the brain, allowing accurate stereotactic representation. Ongoing work in this area is also resulting in the application of such technology to abdominal procedures, such as liver resection.[50] Preoperative imaging modalities such as computerized tomography and magnetic resonance imaging can be used to render 3D composite images that can be manipulated by the surgeon in VR preoperatively and intraoperatively. Information from these models could be used to guide the operative approach, predict the anatomy to be encountered at each operative step, and even customize port placement to optimize operative ergonomics based on each patient's unique anatomy. Theoretically, an operation could be orchestrated in advance, similar to developing a movie, practicing and refining parts of the procedure until optimization is reached, recording all the movements and playing back the perfect operation in the OR as guidance. Limitations in animation and graphic design have so far limited the capabilities of VR for simulating subtle differences in tissue effects necessary to truly recapitulate the intricacies of complex operations. However, this industry has grown exponentially in the past five years and will only continue to become increasingly relevant for surgical training.

CONCLUSION

Surgery is going through a rapid growth spurt as advancements in technology continue to be adapted to the OR. This is a stimulating time. The rate of innovation holds great promise for the rapid advancement in diverse areas such as image-guided surgery, robotics, diagnostics, and advanced computer systems to augment surgical performance and patient care. As previously distinct technologies such as surgery, endoscopy, and radiology continue to overlap in the ORs of tomorrow, surgeons will be progressively challenged to embrace and master new techniques throughout their careers. In this landscape, simulation is predicted to feature prominently as a key training tool for surgeons of all disciplines.

SELECTED REFERENCES

Hashimoto DA, Rosman G, Rus D, et al. Artificial intelligence in surgery: promises and perils. *Ann Surg*. 2018;268:70–76.

This review article provides an excellent description and overview of the potential applications of artificial intelligence in surgery, including machine learning, natural language processing, artificial neural networks, and computer vision.

Madani A, Gallix B, Pugh CM, et al. Evaluating the role of simulation in healthcare innovation: recommendations of the Simnovate Medical Technologies Domain Group. *BMJ Simul Technol Enhanced Learn*. 2017;3; S8–S14.

This article describes the various challenges required to introduce a medical technology in the operating room, as well as the role of simulation technologies for accelerating and facilitating this process.

Marcus HJ, Payne CJ, Hughes-Hallett A, et al. Making the leap: the translation of innovative surgical devices from the laboratory to the operating room. *Ann Surg*. 2016;263:1077–1078.

This original article describes the very long process required to translate a great and innovative idea into a device that is used in the clinical environment.

Peters BS, Armijo PR, Krause C, et al. Review of emerging surgical robotic technology. *Surg Endosc*. 2018;32:1636–1655.

This review article describes the current and future landscape in minimally invasive robotic surgery, as well as the various platforms that are poised to change the operating room in the next 5 to 10 years.

Seol YJ, Kang HW, Lee SJ, et al. Bioprinting technology and its applications. *Eur J Cardiothorac Surg*. 2014;46:342–348.

The principles of three-dimensional printing technology and the current and soon-to-emerge applications of bioprinting in medicine are summarized.

Valdes PA, Roberts DW, Lu FK, et al. Optical technologies for intraoperative neurosurgical guidance. *Neurosurg Focus*. 2016;40:E8.

This review article summarizes novel innovations in biomedical optics and their diagnostic and therapeutic value in neurosurgery to provide the means for more targeted resections.

REFERENCES

1. Sakata S, Watson MO, Grove PM, et al. The conflicting evidence of three-dimensional displays in laparoscopy: a review of systems old and new. *Ann Surg*. 2016;263:234–239.
2. Smith R, Schwab K, Day A, et al. Effect of passive polarizing three-dimensional displays on surgical performance for experienced laparoscopic surgeons. *Br J Surg*. 2014;101:1453–1459.
3. Alleblas CCJ, Vleugels MPH, Coppus S, et al. The effects of laparoscopic graspers with enhanced haptic feedback on applied forces: a randomized comparison with conventional graspers. *Surg Endosc*. 2017;31:5411–5417.
4. van Beek SC, Conijn AP, Koelemay MJ, et al. Editor's choice—endovascular aneurysm repair versus open repair for patients with a ruptured abdominal aortic aneurysm: a systematic review and meta-analysis of short-term survival. *Eur J Vasc Endovasc Surg*. 2014;47:593–602.
5. Patel R, Sweeting MJ, Powell JT, et al. Endovascular versus open repair of abdominal aortic aneurysm in 15-years' follow-up of the UK endovascular aneurysm repair trial 1 (EVAR trial 1): a randomised controlled trial. *Lancet*. 2016;388:2366–2374.
6. Anuwong A, Ketwong K, Jitpratoom P, et al. Safety and outcomes of the transoral endoscopic thyroidectomy vestibular approach. *JAMA Surg*. 2018;153:21–27.
7. Ma B, Gao P, Song Y, et al. Transanal total mesorectal excision (taTME) for rectal cancer: a systematic review and meta-analysis of oncological and perioperative outcomes compared with laparoscopic total mesorectal excision. *BMC Cancer*. 2016;16:380.
8. Francis N, Penna M, Mackenzie H, et al. Consensus on structured training curriculum for transanal total mesorectal excision (TaTME). *Surg Endosc*. 2017;31:2711–2719.
9. Kumbhari V, Tieu AH, Khashab MA. Common indications for transoral flexible endoscopic suturing. *Gastrointest Endosc*. 2015;81:1000.
10. Stavropoulos SN, Modayil R, Friedel D. Current applications of endoscopic suturing. *World J Gastrointest Endosc*. 2015;7:777–789.
11. Bhayani NH, Kurian AA, Dunst CM, et al. A comparative study on comprehensive, objective outcomes of laparoscopic Heller myotomy with per-oral endoscopic myotomy (POEM) for achalasia. *Ann Surg*. 2014;259:1098–1103.
12. Pescarus R, Shlomovitz E, Swanstrom LL. Per-oral endoscopic myotomy (POEM) for esophageal achalasia. *Curr Gastroenterol Rep*. 2014;16:369.
13. van Brunschot S, Hollemans RA, Bakker OJ, et al. Minimally invasive and endoscopic versus open necrosectomy for necrotising pancreatitis: a pooled analysis of individual data for 1980 patients. *Gut*. 2018;67:697–706.
14. Peters BS, Armijo PR, Krause C, et al. Review of emerging surgical robotic technology. *Surg Endosc*. 2018;32:1636–1655.
15. Steffens D, Thanigasalam R, Leslie S, et al. Robotic surgery in uro-oncology: a systematic review and meta-analysis of randomized controlled trials. *Urology*. 2017;106:9–17.
16. Lum MJ, Rosen J, King H, et al. Teleoperation in surgical robotics—network latency effects on surgical performance. *Conf Proc IEEE Eng Med Biol Soc*. 2009;2009:6860–6863.
17. Wottawa CR, Genovese B, Nowroozi BN, et al. Evaluating tactile feedback in robotic surgery for potential clinical application using an animal model. *Surg Endosc*. 2016;30:3198–3209.
18. Prete FP, Pezzolla A, Prete F, et al. Robotic versus laparoscopic minimally invasive surgery for rectal cancer: a systematic review and meta-analysis of randomized controlled trials. *Ann Surg*. 2018;267:1034–1046.
19. Pettinari M, Navarra E, Noirhomme P, et al. The state of robotic cardiac surgery in Europe. *Ann Cardiothorac Surg*. 2017;6:1–8.
20. Yeung BP, Chiu PW. Application of robotics in gastrointestinal endoscopy: a review. *World J Gastroenterol*. 2016;22:1811–1825.
21. Bilgic E, Turkdogan S, Watanabe Y, et al. Effectiveness of telementoring in surgery compared with on-site mentoring: a systematic review. *Surg Innov*. 2017;24:379–385.
22. Lan L, Xia Y, Li R, et al. A fiber optoacoustic guide with augmented reality for precision breast-conserving surgery. *Light Sci Appl*. 2018;7:2.
23. Shen R, Zhang Y, Wang T. Indocyanine green fluorescence angiography and the incidence of anastomotic leak after colorectal resection for colorectal cancer: a meta-analysis. *Dis Colon Rectum*. 2018;61:1228–1234.
24. Vlek SL, van Dam DA, Rubinstein SM, et al. Biliary tract visualization using near-infrared imaging with indocyanine green during laparoscopic cholecystectomy: results of a systematic review. *Surg Endosc*. 2017;31:2731–2742.

25. Seol YJ, Kang HW, Lee SJ, et al. Bioprinting technology and its applications. *Eur J Cardiothorac Surg*. 2014;46:342–348.
26. Hashimoto DA, Rosman G, Rus D, et al. Artificial intelligence in surgery: promises and perils. *Ann Surg*. 2018;268:70–76.
27. Garcia-Martinez A, Vicente-Samper JM, Sabater-Navarro JM. Automatic detection of surgical haemorrhage using computer vision. *Artif Intell Med*. 2017;78:55–60.
28. Fatou B, Saudemont P, Leblanc E, et al. In vivo real-time mass spectrometry for guided surgery application. *Sci Rep*. 2016;6:25919.
29. Phelps DL, Balog J, Gildea LF, et al. The surgical intelligent knife distinguishes normal, borderline and malignant gynaecological tissues using rapid evaporative ionisation mass spectrometry (REIMS). *Br J Cancer*. 2018;118:1349–1358.
30. Canto MI, Anandasabapathy S, Brugge W, et al. In vivo endomicroscopy improves detection of Barrett's esophagus-related neoplasia: a multicenter international randomized controlled trial (with video). *Gastrointest Endosc*. 2014;79:211–221.
31. Carns J, Keahey P, Quang T, et al. Optical molecular imaging in the gastrointestinal tract. *Gastrointest Endosc Clin N Am*. 2013;23:707–723.
32. di Pietro M, Boerwinkel DF, Shariff MK, et al. The combination of autofluorescence endoscopy and molecular biomarkers is a novel diagnostic tool for dysplasia in Barrett's oesophagus. *Gut*. 2015;64:49–56.
33. Valdes PA, Roberts DW, Lu FK, et al. Optical technologies for intraoperative neurosurgical guidance. *Neurosurg Focus*. 2016;40:E8.
34. Gani F, Ford DE, Pawlik TM. Potential barriers to the diffusion of surgical innovation. *JAMA Surg*. 2016;151:403–404.
35. Marcus HJ, Payne CJ, Hughes-Hallett A, et al. Making the leap: the translation of innovative surgical devices from the laboratory to the operating room. *Ann Surg*. 2016;263:1077–1078.
36. Madani A, Gallix B, Pugh CM, et al. Evaluating the role of simulation in healthcare innovation: recommendations of the Simnovate Medical Technologies Domain Group. *BMJ Simul Technol Enhanc Learn*. 2017;3; S8–S14.
37. A prospective analysis of 1518 laparoscopic cholecystectomies. The Southern Surgeons Club. *N Engl J Med*. 1991;324:1073–1078.
38. Dawe SR, Windsor JA, Broeders JA, et al. A systematic review of surgical skills transfer after simulation-based training: laparoscopic cholecystectomy and endoscopy. *Ann Surg*. 2014;259:236–248.
39. Faulkner H, Regehr G, Martin J, et al. Validation of an objective structured assessment of technical skill for surgical residents. *Acad Med*. 1996;71:1363–1365.
40. Reedy GB, Lavelle M, Simpson T, et al. Development of the human factors skills for healthcare instrument: a valid and reliable tool for assessing interprofessional learning across healthcare practice settings. *BMJ Simul Technol Enhanc Learn*. 2017;3:135–141.
41. Ericsson KA, Krampe RT, Teschromer C. The role of deliberate practice in the acquisition of expert performance. *Psychol Rev*. 1993;100:363–406.
42. Fried GM, Feldman LS, Vassiliou MC, et al. Proving the value of simulation in laparoscopic surgery. *Ann Surg*. 2004;240:518–525; discussion 525–518.
43. Forster AJ, Asmis TR, Clark HD, et al. Ottawa Hospital Patient Safety Study: incidence and timing of adverse events in patients admitted to a Canadian teaching hospital. *CMAJ*. 2004;170:1235–1240.
44. Gawande AA, Zinner MJ, Studdert DM, et al. Analysis of errors reported by surgeons at three teaching hospitals. *Surgery*. 2003;133:614–621.
45. Rogers Jr SO, Gawande AA, Kwaan M, et al. Analysis of surgical errors in closed malpractice claims at 4 liability insurers. *Surgery*. 2006;140:25–33.
46. Way LW, Stewart L, Gantert W, et al. Causes and prevention of laparoscopic bile duct injuries: analysis of 252 cases from a human factors and cognitive psychology perspective. *Ann Surg*. 2003;237:460–469.
47. Madani A, Vassiliou MC, Watanabe Y, et al. What are the principles that guide behaviors in the operating room?: creating a framework to define and measure performance. *Ann Surg*. 2017;265:255–267.
48. Madani A, Watanabe Y, Bilgic E, et al. Measuring intra-operative decision-making during laparoscopic cholecystectomy: validity evidence for a novel interactive Web-based assessment tool. *Surg Endosc*. 2017;31:1203–1212.
49. Ferroli P, Tringali G, Acerbi F, et al. Brain surgery in a stereoscopic virtual reality environment: a single institution's experience with 100 cases. *Neurosurgery*. 2010;67:79–84.
50. Mutter D, Dallemagne B, Bailey C, et al. 3D virtual reality and selective vascular control for laparoscopic left hepatic lobectomy. *Surg Endosc*. 2009;23:432–435.

16 CHAPTER

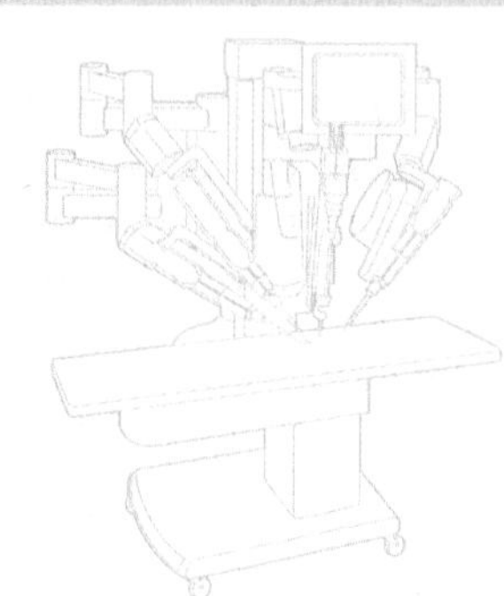

Robotic Surgery

Yanghee Woo, Yuman Fong

OUTLINE

PREFACE

Robotic surgery is arguably the most disruptive and perhaps the most enabling twenty-first century surgical innovation. Born of military technology, developed by industry, and championed by surgeon pioneers, robotic surgery is increasingly adopted as an alternative to laparoscopy to perform a wide breadth of surgical procedures for both benign and malignant diseases (Box 16.1). Since the U.S. Food and Drug Administration (FDA) approval in 2000 of the da Vinci Surgical System (Intuitive Surgical Inc., Sunnyvale, CA), the most utilized commercially available surgical robot, surgeons have performed over 5 million robotic surgical procedures worldwide with more than 10,000 peer-reviewed publications reporting its safety, feasibility, and efficacy compared to open and laparoscopic procedures (Fig. 16.1).

The field of robotic surgery has challenged our traditional concepts of laparoscopic surgery with novel perceptions of the surgical view, methods of operative exposure, tissue manipulation, and instrument use. Robotic surgery capitalizes on the "master-slave" concept to offer surgeons control over a system that provides enhanced visualization, augmented dexterity and precision, sophisticated articulating instruments, and improved ergonomics. This alternative minimally invasive surgical (MIS) approach offers the potential to overcome the limitations of laparoscopy and increase MIS benefits to a diverse surgical patient population.

As an evolution from traditional laparoscopic surgery, numerous studies have demonstrated that robotic assisted laparoscopic techniques are safe and feasible and provide MIS benefits of improved patient outcomes with smaller incisions, less pain, less blood loss, shorter length of hospital stay, quicker return of bowel function, and more rapid overall recovery when compared to open procedures. Moreover, studies evaluating intraoperative oncologic parameters support the reliable use of robotic surgery in the treatment of malignant diseases including gastric, colorectal, pancreatic, and liver cancers. The oncologic parameters evaluated include negative margin status, adequate number of nodes, and proper extent of lymph node dissection in cancer operations. On the other hand, the consistently longer operative time and higher cost of robotic surgery continue to challenge the field of robotic surgery. Comparative results of these studies for rectal resections, pancreaticoduodenectomies, distal pancreatectomies, and liver resections are summarized and presented in Tables 16.1 to 16.4.

Not surprisingly, the perceived technical advantages of the robotic system experienced by the surgeon have yet to be fully documented by data. It is clear that the robotic approach for many operations produce equivalent results to laparoscopic procedures perfected over decades of surgical development. However, clear superiority for a robotic approach over laparoscopic techniques has been difficult to demonstrate by traditional parameters. In coming years, it is likely that the ease of adaption, the shorter learning curve, and the ergonomic superiority will emerge as the inducements for entering the robotic surgery field. It is also expected that cost of robotic surgery and laparoscopic surgery will become similar. This will result from both an increased cost of laparoscopic procedures as technologies are developed in advanced MIS and robotic surgery becomes adopted and a decrease in robotic surgery cost accompanying additional robotic entries into the surgical market. As the field of robotic surgery matures with optimization of surgeon integration of robotic technology into clinical practice and with evolution of the technology that continues to enhance the surgeon's operative performance and the cost of robotic surgery decreases, the benefits of robotic surgery may be redefined.

In this textbook's first robotic surgery chapter, we present an overview of robotic surgery by covering the history of robotics in surgery, familiarizing the reader with results of the studies describing the advantages and disadvantages of the robotic approach, offering insight into safe and effective methods of adopting robotic surgery in clinical practice. Who will adopt robotic surgery into their practice and how its adoption will impact the field of surgical robotics and transform MIS depend on how surgeons address these challenges and embrace the opportunities robotics offers to improve outcomes for surgical patients, including the elderly and the frail.[1,2]

HISTORY

The concept of robotic surgery is based on teleoperated robots and emerged from its foundations in robotics research funded by the National Aeronautics and Space Administration (NASA) and the Defense Advanced Research Project Administration starting in the 1970s.[3] The initial goal of surgical robotics was to develop a system that would enable remotely controlled surgical procedures and replace patient-side surgeons in dangerous or difficult-to-reach places, such as in the battlefield and in space aircrafts. Its commercial development over the last half century has integrated the advances in robotic engineering, computer programming, and concepts of MIS. Most notable developments in surgical robotics are chronologically represented in Fig. 16.2.

Notably, in 1992, Computer Motion Inc. (Goleta, CA), with a NASA-JPL grant, developed Automated Endoscopic System for Optimal Positioning (AESOP), the first FDA-approved commercial robot that enabled surgeons to command and manipulate a laparoscopic camera during surgical procedures. With the addition of three arms capable of being remotely controlled by the surgeon, the AESOP system was soon developed into the Zeus Robotic Surgical System.[4] Using this new robotic system, a landmark telerobotic surgery was performed in 2002 by Dr. Jacques Marescaux and his team.[4] They successfully performed the first robot-assisted transatlantic cholecystectomy with the surgeon seated at the robotic manipulator located in New York City with the "patient-side" robot-system in Strasburg, France.[4]

The da Vinci Surgical Systems (Intuitive Surgical, Sunnyvale, CA) came to dominate the field in robotic-assisted laparoscopic abdominal operations when Zeus Robotic Surgical System was discontinued after a merger between Computer Motion and Intuitive Surgical in 2003. Since the FDA approved Intuitive Surgical's da Vinci Standard System in the year 2000, three newer generations of da Vinci Surgical Systems, each with increasingly more sophisticated features, were developed: the S System (2003), the Si System (2009), and the Xi System (2014). Over 4500 da Vinci Robotic Surgical Systems have been installed as of March 2018 with more than 50% of the robotic operations being performed in the United States.[5]

The initial system was intended for cardiac bypass surgery, but it failed to gain acceptance by cardiac surgeons. Urologists popularized the surgical application of the robotic system with robotic

BOX 16.1 Selected list of the most commonly performed robotic abdominal operations

Foregut/Upper Abdominal Operations
- Heller myotomy
- Antireflux surgery
- Bariatric surgery (Roux-en-Y gastric bypass, sleeves)
- Esophagogastrectomy with gastric pull-up
- Radical gastrectomy for gastric cancer (subtotal distal, total, D1+ and D2 lymphadenectomies)
- Splenectomy

Hepatopancreaticobiliary Operations
- Liver resection (left lateral segmentectomy, right lobectomy, right posterior segmentectomy)
- Pancreatic resections (pancreaticoduodenectomy, central and distal pancreatectomies)
- Cholecystectomy (simple, radical)

Colorectal Operations
- Right colectomy
- Left colectomy
- Low anterior resection with total mesorectal excision
- Abdominoperineal resection

Other General Surgical Procedures
- Hernias (inguinal, ventral incisional, hiatal)
- Thyroidectomy (transaxillary, retroauricular)

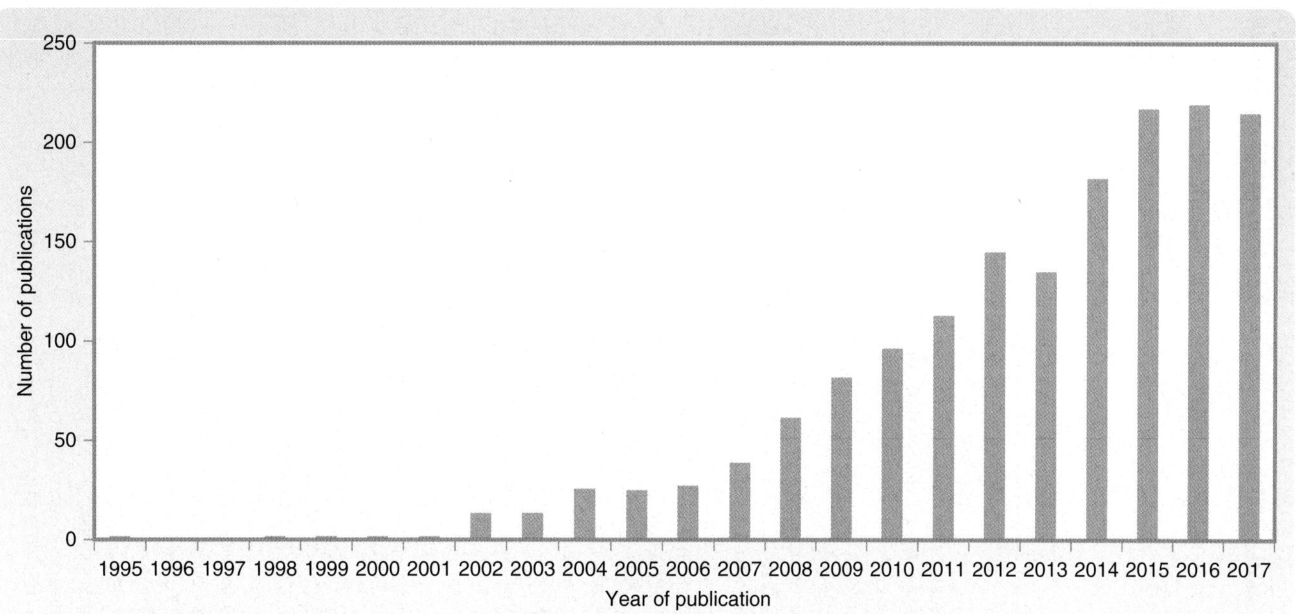

FIG. 16.1 Increase in peer-reviewed publications in robotic surgery (PubMed search for "robotic surgery, robot-assisted surgery").

TABLE 16.1 **Summary of recently comparative studies, randomized control trials, and meta analyses focusing on the key outcomes of laparoscopic versus robotic total mesorectal excision.***

	STUDY CHARACTERISTICS	OUTCOMES										
		NUMBER OF PATIENTS		OPERATION TIME (MINUTES)			LENGTH OF STAY (DAYS)			MAJOR COMPLICATION RATE (%) CD III–V		
STUDY	STUDY DESIGN	laTME	rTME	laTME	rTME	*P* VALUE	laTME	rTME	*P* VALUE	laTME	rTME	*P* VALUE
Baik SH, Ko YT, Kang CM, et al. Robotic tumor-specific mesorectal excision of rectal cancer: short-term outcome of a pilot randomized trial. *Surg Endosc.* 2008;22:1601–1608.	RT	18	18	204	217	NS	8.7 ± 1.3	6.9 ± 1.3	<0.001	0.0%	0.0%	
Patriti A, Ceccarelli G, Bartoli A, et al. Short- and medium-term outcome of robot-assisted and traditional laparoscopic rectal resection. *JSLS.* 2009;13:176–183.	CCS	37	29	208	202	NS	9.6 ± 6.9	11.9 ± 7.5	NS	NR	NR	
Park JS, Choi GS, Lim KH, et al. Robotic-assisted versus laparoscopic surgery for low rectal cancer: case-matched analysis of short-term outcomes. *Ann Surg Oncol.* 2010;17:3195–3202.	MCC	82	41	169	232	<0.001	9.4 ± 2.9	9.9 ± 4.2	NS	7.3%	9.8%	0.641
Bianchi PP, Ceriani C, Locatelli A, et al. Robotic versus laparoscopic total mesorectal excision for rectal cancer: a comparative analysis of oncological safety and short-term outcomes. *Surg Endosc.* 2010;24:2888–2894.	CCS	25	25	237	240	NS	6 (4–20)	6.5 (4–15)	NS	0.12	0.8%	
Baek JH, Pastor C, Pigazzi A. Robotic and laparoscopic total mesorectal excision for rectal cancer: a case-matched study. *Surg Endosc.* 2011;25:521–525.	MCC	41	41	315	296	NS	6.6 (3–20)	6.5 (2–33)	NS	NR	NR	
Kwak JM, Kim SH, Kim J, et al. Robotic vs laparoscopic resection of rectal cancer: short-term outcomes of a case-control study. *Dis Colon Rectum.* 2011;54:151–156.	MCC	59	59	228	270	<0.001	NR	NR		NR	NR	
Park JS, Choi GS, Lim KH, et al. S052: a comparison of robot-assisted, laparoscopic, and open surgery in the treatment of rectal cancer. *Surg Endosc.* 2011;25:240–248.	CCS	123	52	–	–	–				4.9%	7.7%	0.331
Kim JY, Kim NK, Lee KY, et al. A comparative study of voiding and sexual function after total mesorectal excision with autonomic nerve preservation for rectal cancer: laparoscopic versus robotic surgery. *Ann Surg Oncol.* 2012;19:2485–2493.	CCS	39	30	–	–	–	NR	NR		NR	NR	

Kang J, Yoon KJ, Min BS, et al. The impact of robotic surgery for mid and low rectal cancer: a case-matched analysis of a 3-arm comparison—open, laparoscopic, and robotic surgery. *Ann Surg.* 2013;257:95–101.	MCC	165	165	277	309	<0.001	13.5 ± 9.2	10.8 ± 5.5	<0.001	NR	NR	
Park SY, Choi GS, Park JS, et al. Short-term clinical outcome of robot-assisted intersphincteric resection for low rectal cancer: a retrospective comparison with conventional laparoscopy. *Surg Endosc.* 2013;27:48–55.	CCS	40	40	185	236	0.001	11.3 ± 3.6	10.6 ± 4.2	NS	2.5%	5.0%	1.0
D'Annibale A, Pernazza G, Monsellato I, et al. Total mesorectal excision: a comparison of oncological and functional outcomes between robotic and laparoscopic surgery for rectal cancer. *Surg Endosc.* 2013;27:1887–1895.	CCS	50	50	280	270	<0.001	10 (8–14)	8 (7.11)	0.034	NR	NR	
Barnajian M, Pettet D, 3rd, Kazi E, et al. Quality of total mesorectal excision and depth of circumferential resection margin in rectal cancer: a matched comparison of the first 20 robotic cases. *Colorectal Dis.* 2014;16:603–609.	MCC	20	20	180	240	0.066	7 (5–36)	6 (4–31)	NS	NR	NR	
Tam MS, Abbass M, Abbas MA. Robotic-laparoscopic rectal cancer excision versus traditional laparoscopy. *JSLS.* 2014;18:e2014.00020.	CCS	21	21	240	260	0.04	5 (3–14)	6 (4–23)	0.05	NR	NR	
Cho MS, Baek SJ, Hur H, et al. Short and long-term outcomes of robotic versus laparoscopic total mesorectal excision for rectal cancer: a case-matched retrospective study. *Medicine (Baltimore).* 2015;94:e522.	MCC	278	278	272	362	<0.001	10.7 ± 6.6	10.4 ± 5.6	NS	12.2%	12.2%	1.0
Melich G, Hong YK, Kim J, et al. Simultaneous development of laparoscopy and robotics provides acceptable perioperative outcomes and shows robotics to have a faster learning curve and to be overall faster in rectal cancer surgery: analysis of novice MIS surgeon learning curves. *Surg Endosc.* 2015;29:558–568.	CCS	106	92	262	285		9.9 (8.5–11.3)	9.6 (8.3–11.0)		4.7%	6.5%	
Serin KR, Gultekin FA, Batman B, et al. Robotic versus laparoscopic surgery for mid or low rectal cancer in male patients after neoadjuvant chemoradiation therapy: comparison of short-term outcomes. *J Robot Surg.* 2015;9:187–194.	CCS	65	14	140	182		5 (4–10)	6 (2–32)	NS	NR	NR	

Continued

TABLE 16.1 Summary of recently comparative studies, randomized control trials, and meta analyses focusing on the key outcomes of laparoscopic versus robotic total mesorectal excision.*—cont'd

	STUDY CHARACTERISTICS	OUTCOMES										
		NUMBER OF PATIENTS		OPERATION TIME (MINUTES)			LENGTH OF STAY (DAYS)			MAJOR COMPLICATION RATE (%) CD III–V		
STUDY	STUDY DESIGN	laTME	rTME	laTME	rTME	*P* VALUE	laTME	rTME	*P* VALUE	laTME	rTME	*P* VALUE
Allemann P, Duvoisin C, Di Mare L, et al. Robotic-assisted surgery improves the quality of total mesorectal excision for rectal cancer compared to laparoscopy: results of a case-controlled analysis. *World J Surg.* 2016;40:1010–1016.	MCC	40	20	313	291	<0.001	NR	NR		22.5%	20.0%	0.38
Kim YS, Kim MJ, Park SC, et al. Robotic versus laparoscopic surgery for rectal cancer after preoperative chemoradiotherapy: case-matched study of short-term outcomes. *Cancer Res Treat.* 2016;48:225–231.	MCC	66	33	277	441		13.1 ± 12.8	10.9 ± 6.2	NS	NR	NR	
Kim JC, Yu CS, Lim SB, et al. Comparative analysis focusing on surgical and early oncological outcomes of open, laparoscopy-assisted, and robot-assisted approaches in rectal cancer patients. *Int J Colorectal Dis.* 2016;31:1179–1187.	CCS	486	553	205	441	<0.001	10.9 ± 6.2	13.1 ± 12.8		3.0%	3.0%	
Feroci F, Vannucchi A, Bianchi PP, et al. Total mesorectal excision for mid and low rectal cancer: laparoscopic vs robotic surgery. *World J Gastroenterol.* 2016;22:3602–3610.	CCS	58	53	192	342	<0.001	8 (5–53)	6 (3–17)	<0.001	17.2%	7.5%	0.297
Ramji KM, Cleghorn MC, Josse JM, et al. Comparison of clinical and economic outcomes between robotic, laparoscopic, and open rectal cancer surgery: early experience at a tertiary care center. *Surg Endosc.* 2016;30:1337–1343.	CCS	27	26	240	407	NS	11.3 ± 13.7	7 ± 3.4	NS	0.0%	12.0%	0.11
Shiomi A, Kinugasa Y, Yamaguchi T, et al. Robot-assisted versus laparoscopic surgery for lower rectal cancer: the impact of visceral obesity on surgical outcomes. *Int J Colorectal Dis.* 2016;31:1701–1710.	CCS	109	127	237	236		8.0 (6–44)	7.0 (6–29)	<0.001	6.4%	3.1%	0.19

Yamaguchi T, Kinugasa Y, Shiomi A, et al. Robotic-assisted vs. conventional laparoscopic surgery for rectal cancer: short-term outcomes at a single center. *Surg Today*. 2016;46:957–962.	CCS	239	203	227	233	NS	9.3 ± 6.7	7.3 ± 2.3	<0.001	NR	NR	
Colombo PE, Bertrand MM, Alline M, et al. Robotic versus laparoscopic total mesorectal excision (TME) for sphincter-saving surgery: is there any difference in the transanal TME rectal approach?: a single-center series of 120 consecutive patients. *Ann Surg Oncol.* 2016;23:1594–1600.	CCS	60	60	228	274	0.005	11 (6–60)	12 (6–27)	NS	20.0%	28.3%	0.246
Bedirli A, Salman B, Yuksel O. Robotic versus laparoscopic resection for mid and low rectal cancers. *JSLS*. 2016;20.	CCS	28	35	208	252	0.027	5.1 ± 3.7	4.6 ± 2.8	>0.05	NR	NR	
Silva-Velazco J, Dietz DW, Stocchi L, et al. Considering value in rectal cancer surgery: an analysis of costs and outcomes based on the open, laparoscopic, and robotic approach for proctectomy. *Ann Surg*. 2017;265:960–968.	CCS	118	66	239	288	<0.001	6 (3–33)	5 (2–28)		NR	NR	
Lim DR, Bae SU, Hur H, et al. Long-term oncological outcomes of robotic versus laparoscopic total mesorectal excision of mid-low rectal cancer following neoadjuvant chemoradiation therapy. *Surg Endosc*. 2017;31:1728–1737.	CCS	64	74	312	364	0.033	NR	NR		NR	NR	
Kim J, Baek SJ, Kang DW, et al. Robotic resection is a good prognostic factor in rectal cancer compared with laparoscopic resection: long-term survival analysis using propensity score matching. *Dis Colon Rectum*. 2017;60:266–273.	CCS MCC	460 224	272 224	234 250	288 285	<0.001 <0.002	14.4 ± 19.2 13.8 ± 10.9	13.2 ± 13.5 13.5 ± 14.1	NS NS	NR NR	NR NR	
Law WL, Foo DCC. Comparison of short-term and oncologic outcomes of robotic and laparoscopic resection for mid- and distal rectal cancer. *Surg Endosc* 2017;31: 2798–2807.	CCS	171	220	225	260	<0.003	6 (2–83)	6 (2–64)	NS	NR	NR	
Kim MJ, Park SC, Park JW, et al. Robot-assisted versus laparoscopic surgery for rectal cancer: a phase II open label prospective randomized controlled trial. *Ann Surg*. 2018;267:243–251.	RCT	82	83	228	339	<0.001	10.8 (7.4)	10.3 (3.4)	NS	5.4%	9.4%	0.227

Continued

TABLE 16.1 Summary of recently comparative studies, randomized control trials, and meta analyses focusing on the key outcomes of laparoscopic versus robotic total mesorectal excision.*—cont'd

	STUDY CHARACTERISTICS	OUTCOMES										
		NUMBER OF PATIENTS		OPERATION TIME (MINUTES)			LENGTH OF STAY (DAYS)			MAJOR COMPLICATION RATE (%) CD III–V		
STUDY	STUDY DESIGN	laTME	rTME	laTME	rTME	*P* VALUE	laTME	rTME	*P* VALUE	laTME	rTME	*P* VALUE
Valverde A, Goasguen N, Oberlin O, et al. Robotic versus laparoscopic rectal resection for sphincter-saving surgery: pathological and short-term outcomes in a single-center analysis of 130 consecutive patients. *Surg Endosc.* 2017;31:4085–4091.	CCS	65	65	226	215	NS	12 ± 10	11 ± 8	NS	15.0%	23.0%	0.26
Harslof S, Stouge A, Thomassen N, et al. Outcome one year after robot-assisted rectal cancer surgery: a consecutive cohort study. *Int J Colorectal Dis.* 2017;32:1749–1758.	CCS	141	208	NR	NR			7 (2–61)			NR	
Jayne D, Pigazzi A, Marshall H, et al. Effect of robotic-assisted vs conventional laparoscopic surgery on risk of conversion to open laparotomy among patients undergoing resection for rectal cancer: the ROLARR Randomized Clinical Trial. *JAMA.* 2017;318:1569–1580.	RCT	234	237	261	298		8.2 ± 6.0	8.0 ± 5.9			NR	NR

	OUTCOMES (CONT.)											
	CONVERSION RATE (%)			COMPLETENESS OF TME (%)			POSITIVE CIRCUMFERENTIAL MARGIN (%)			HARVESTED LYMPH NODES		
STUDY	laTME	rTME	*P* VALUE	laTME	rTME	*P* VALUE	laTME	rTME	*P* VALUE	laTME	rTME	*P* VALUE
Baik SH, Ko YT, Kang CM, et al. Robotic tumor-specific mesorectal excision of rectal cancer: short-term outcome of a pilot randomized trial. *Surg Endosc.* 2008;22:1601–1608.	11.1%	0.0%	NS	72.2%	94.4%	NS	NR	NR		18 (6–49)	22 (9–42)	NS
Patriti A, Ceccarelli G, Bartoli A, et al. Short- and medium-term outcome of robot-assisted and traditional laparoscopic rectal resection. *JSLS.* 2009;13:176–183.	18.9%	0.0%	NS	NR	NR		0.0%	0.0%		10.3 ± 4	11.2 ± 5	>0.05
Park JS, Choi GS, Lim KH, et al. Robotic-assisted versus laparoscopic surgery for low rectal cancer: case-matched analysis of short-term outcomes. *Ann Surg Oncol.* 2010;17:3195–3202.	0.0%	0.0%	NS	94.4%	76.5%	NS	NR	NR		20.0 ± 9.1	17.4 ± 10.6	NS

Bianchi PP, Ceriani C, Locatelli A, et al. Robotic versus laparoscopic total mesorectal excision for rectal cancer: a comparative analysis of oncological safety and short-term outcomes. *Surg Endosc.* 2010;24:2888–2894.	4.0%	0.0%		NR	NR		4.0%	0.0%	NS	18	17	NS
Baek JH, Pastor C, Pigazzi A. Robotic and laparoscopic total mesorectal excision for rectal cancer: a case-matched study. *Surg Endosc.* 2011;25:521–525.	22.0%	7.3%	NS	NR	NR		4.9%	2.4%	NS	13.1 (3–33)	16.2 (5–39)	NS
Kwak JM, Kim SH, Kim J, et al. Robotic vs laparoscopic resection of rectal cancer: short-term outcomes of a case-control study. *Dis Colon Rectum.* 2011;54:151–156.	3.4%	0.0%	NS	NR	NR		0.0%	1.7%	NS	20 (12–27)	21 (14–28)	NS
Park JS, Choi GS, Lim KH, et al. S052: a comparison of robot-assisted, laparoscopic, and open surgery in the treatment of rectal cancer. *Surg Endosc.* 2011;25:240–248.	0.0%	0.0%		NR	NR		2.4%	1.9%	NS	19.4 ± 10.2	15.9 ± 10.1	NS
Kim JY, Kim NK, Lee KY, et al. A comparative study of voiding and sexual function after total mesorectal excision with autonomic nerve preservation for rectal cancer: laparoscopic versus robotic surgery. *Ann Surg Oncol.* 2012;19:2485–2493.	NR	NR		94.9%	96.5%	NS	2.5%	6.0%	NS		–	
Kang J, Yoon KJ, Min BS, et al. The impact of robotic surgery for mid and low rectal cancer: a case-matched analysis of a 3-arm comparison—open, laparoscopic, and robotic surgery. *Ann Surg.* 2013;257:95–101.	1.8%	0.6%	NS	NR	NR		6.7%	4.2%	NS	15.0 ± 9.4	15.6 ± 9.1	NS
Park SY, Choi GS, Park JS, et al. Short-term clinical outcome of robot-assisted intersphincteric resection for low rectal cancer: a retrospective comparison with conventional laparoscopy. *Surg Endosc.* 2013;27:48–55.	0.0%	0.0%	NS	NR	NR		5.0%	7.5%	NS	12.9 ± 7.5	13.3 ± 8.6	NS
D'Annibale A, Pernazza G, Monsellato I, et al. Total mesorectal excision: a comparison of oncological and functional outcomes between robotic and laparoscopic surgery for rectal cancer. *Surg Endosc.* 2013;27:1887–1895.	12.0%	0.0%	0.011	NR	NR		12.0%	0.0%	0.022	16.5 ± 7.1	13.8 ± 6.7	NS
Barnajian M, Pettet D, 3rd, Kazi E, et al. Quality of total mesorectal excision and depth of circumferential resection margin in rectal cancer: a matched comparison of the first 20 robotic cases. *Colorectal Dis.* 2014;16:603–609.	10.0%	0.0%	NS	95.0%	80.0%	NS	NR	NR		14 (3–22)	11 (4–18)	NS
Tam MS, Abbass M, Abbas MA. Robotic-laparoscopic rectal cancer excision versus traditional laparoscopy. *JSLS.* 2014;18:e2014.00020.	0.0%	5.0%	NS	NR	NR		5.0%	0.0%	NS	17 (8–40)	15 (8–21)	0.03

Continued

TABLE 16.1 Summary of recently comparative studies, randomized control trials, and meta analyses focusing on the key outcomes of laparoscopic versus robotic total mesorectal excision.*—cont'd

	STUDY CHARACTERISTICS	OUTCOMES										
		NUMBER OF PATIENTS		OPERATION TIME (MINUTES)			LENGTH OF STAY (DAYS)			MAJOR COMPLICATION RATE (%) CD III–V		
STUDY	STUDY DESIGN	laTME	rTME	laTME	rTME	*P* VALUE	laTME	rTME	*P* VALUE	laTME	rTME	*P* VALUE
Cho MS, Baek SJ, Hur H, et al. Short and long-term outcomes of robotic versus laparoscopic total mesorectal excision for rectal cancer: a case-matched retrospective study. *Medicine (Baltimore)*. 2015;94:e522.	0.7%	0.4%	NS	NR	NR		4.7%	5,0%	NS	15 ± 8	16± 8	NS
Melich G, Hong YK, Kim J, et al. Simultaneous development of laparoscopy and robotics provides acceptable perioperative outcomes and shows robotics to have a faster learning curve and to be overall faster in rectal cancer surgery: analysis of novice MIS surgeon learning curves. *Surg Endosc*. 2015;29:558–568.	3.8%	1.1%		NR	NR		2.8%	3.3%		17 (15–20)	16 (14–18)	
Serin KR, Gultekin FA, Batman B, et al. Robotic versus laparoscopic surgery for mid or low rectal cancer in male patients after neoadjuvant chemoradiation therapy: comparison of short-term outcomes. *J Robot Surg*. 2015;9:187–194.	3.0%	0.0%		80.0%	100.0%	NS	NR	NR		32 (17–56)	23 (4–67)	0.008
Allemann P, Duvoisin C, Di Mare L, et al. Robotic-assisted surgery improves the quality of total mesorectal excision for rectal cancer compared to laparoscopy: results of a case-controlled analysis. *World J Surg*. 2016;40:1010–1016.	20.0%	5.0%	NS	55.0%	95.0%	0.0003	25.0%	10.0%	NS	24 ± 14	20 ± 7	NS
Kim YS, Kim MJ, Park SC, et al. Robotic versus laparoscopic surgery for rectal cancer after preoperative chemoradiotherapy: case-matched study of short-term outcomes. *Cancer Res Treat*. 2016;48:225–231.	0.0%	6.1%	NS	91.0%	97.0%	NS	6.7%	16.1%	NS	22.3 ± 11.7	21.6 ± 11.0	NS
Kim JC, Yu CS, Lim SB, et al. Comparative analysis focusing on surgical and early oncological outcomes of open, laparoscopy-assisted, and robot-assisted approaches in rectal cancer patients. *Int J Colorectal Dis*. 2016;31:1179–1187.	0.0%	6.1%		NR	NR		1.1%	1.5%	NS	23.2 ± 10	20.9 ± 8.5	<0.001

Feroci F, Vannucchi A, Bianchi PP, et al. Total mesorectal excision for mid and low rectal cancer: laparoscopic vs robotic surgery. *World J Gastroenterol.* 2016;22:3602–3610.	1.7%	3.8%	NS	NR	NR		1.7%	1.9%	NS	18 (4–49)	11 (3–27)	<0.001
Ramji KM, Cleghorn MC, Josse JM, et al. Comparison of clinical and economic outcomes between robotic, laparoscopic, and open rectal cancer surgery: early experience at a tertiary care center. *Surg Endosc.* 2016;30:1337–1343.	37.0%	12.0%	NS	44.0%	60.0%	NS	0.0%	0.0%		16.7 ± 6.8	16.8 ± 7.7	NS
Shiomi A, Kinugasa Y, Yamaguchi T, et al. Robot-assisted versus laparoscopic surgery for lower rectal cancer: the impact of visceral obesity on surgical outcomes. *Int J Colorectal Dis.* 2016;31:1701–1710.	0.9%	0.0%	NS	NR	NR		0.9%	0.0%	NS	26.0 (11–60)	26.0 (7–63)	NS
Yamaguchi T, Kinugasa Y, Shiomi A, et al. Robotic-assisted vs. conventional laparoscopic surgery for rectal cancer: short-term outcomes at a single center. *Surg Today.* 2016;46:957–962.	3.3%	0.0%	0.009	NR	NR		NR	NR		30.0 ± 10.3	29.3 ± 11.8	NS
Colombo PE, Bertrand MM, Alline M, et al. Robotic versus laparoscopic total mesorectal excision (TME) for sphincter-saving surgery: is there any difference in the transanal TME rectal approach?: a single-center series of 120 consecutive patients. *Ann Surg Oncol.* 2016;23:1594–1600.	4.8%	3.2%	NS	90.0%	93.3%	NS	90.0%	93.3%	NS	15 (6–71)	19 (6–68)	NS
Bedirli A, Salman B, Yuksel O. Robotic versus laparoscopic resection for mid and low rectal cancers. *JSLS.* 2016;20.	NR	NR		NR	NR		3.6%	2.9%	>0.05	27 ± 11	23 ± 8	NS
Silva-Velazco J, Dietz DW, Stocchi L, et al. Considering value in rectal cancer surgery: an analysis of costs and outcomes based on the open, laparoscopic, and robotic approach for proctectomy. *Ann Surg.* 2017;265:960–968.	15.4%	9.1%	NS	90.4%	89.4%	NS	3.4%	7.6%	NS	22 (7–106)	24 (3–129)	NS
Lim DR, Bae SU, Hur H, et al. Long-term oncological outcomes of robotic versus laparoscopic total mesorectal excision of mid-low rectal cancer following neoadjuvant chemoradiation therapy. *Surg Endosc.* 2017;31:1728–1737.	6.4%	1.4%	NS	98.4%	95.9%	NS	1.6%	4.0%	NS	11.6 ± 6.9	14.7 ± 6.5	NS
Kim J, Baek SJ, Kang DW, et al. Robotic resection is a good prognostic factor in rectal cancer compared with laparoscopic resection: long-term survival analysis using propensity score matching. *Dis Colon Rectum.* 2017;60:266–273.	0.9% 0.9%	0.0% 0.0%	NS	NR NR	NR NR		3.5% 4.9%	5.5% 4.0%	NS NS	19.7 ± 12.3 20.2 ± 12.1	21.7 ± 14.3 21.0 ± 14.4	0.049 NS

Continued

TABLE 16.1 **Summary of recently comparative studies, randomized control trials, and meta analyses focusing on the key outcomes of laparoscopic versus robotic total mesorectal excision.*—cont'd**

	STUDY CHARACTERIS-TICS	OUTCOMES										
		NUMBER OF PATIENTS		OPERATION TIME (MINUTES)			LENGTH OF STAY (DAYS)			MAJOR COMPLICATION RATE (%) CD III–V		
STUDY	STUDY DESIGN	laTME	rTME	laTME	rTME	*P* VALUE	laTME	rTME	*P* VALUE	laTME	rTME	*P* VALUE
Law WL, Foo DCC. Comparison of short-term and oncologic outcomes of robotic and laparoscopic resection for mid- and distal rectal cancer. *Surg Endosc.* 2017;31:2798–2807.	3.5%	0.8%	NS	NR	NR		8.2%	4.1%	NS	12	14	0.002
Kim MJ, Park SC, Park JW, et al. Robot-assisted versus laparoscopic surgery for rectal cancer: a phase II Open Label prospective randomized controlled trial. *Ann Surg.* 2018;267:243–251.	0.0%	1.5%	NS	78.1%	80.3%	NS	5.5%	6.1%	NS	18 (7–59)	15 (4–40)	
Valverde A, Goasguen N, Oberlin O, et al. Robotic versus laparoscopic rectal resection for sphincter-saving surgery: pathological and short-term outcomes in a single-center analysis of 130 consecutive patients. *Surg Endosc.* 2017;31:4085–4091.	17.0%	5.0%	0.044	82.0%	88.0%	NS	89.0%	6.0%	NS	17 ± 9	19 ± 10	
Harslof S, Stouge A, Thomassen N, et al. Outcome one year after robot-assisted rectal cancer surgery: a consecutive cohort study. *Int J Colorectal Dis.* 2017;32:1749–1758.	21.0%	31.0%	0.06	NR	NR			7.0%			20 (6–47)	
Jayne D, Pigazzi A, Marshall H, et al. Effect of robotic-assisted vs conventional laparoscopic surgery on risk of conversion to open laparotomy among patients undergoing resection for rectal cancer: the ROLARR Randomized Clinical Trial. *JAMA.* 2017;318:1569–1580.	12.2%	8.1%	NS	77.6%	76.4%	NS	6.3%	5.1%	NS	24.1 ± 12.9	23.2 ± 12.0	

CCS, Case control study; *CD III–V*, Clavien-Dindo III–V class surgical complications; *laTME*, laparoscopic total mesorectal excision; *MCC*, matched case control; *NR*, not reported; *NS*, nonsignificant; *RCT*, randomized controlled trial; *RT*, retrospective trial; *rTME*, robotic total mesorectal excision.

*No significant difference was observed between laTME and rTME regarding gender and body mass index.

TABLE 16.2 Selected results from studies comparing robotic versus open pancreaticoduodenectomy.

STUDY	STUDY DESIGN	APPROACH	NUMBER OF CASES	OPERATION TIME (MIN)	ESTIMATED BLOOD LOSS (mL)	LENGTH-OF-STAY (DAYS)	COMPLICATIONS (MAJOR)	MORTALITY
Baker EH, Ross SW, Seshadri R, et al. Robotic pancreaticoduodenectomy: comparison of complications and cost to the open approach. *Int J Med Robot.* 2016;12:554–560.	Retrospective Cohort	RPD OPD	22 49	454 (294–529) 364 (213–948) $P = 0.035$	425 (50–2200) 650 (150–6100) $P = 0.42$	7 (4–25) 9 (5–48) NS	40.7% (13.6%) 67.4% (20.4%) $P = 0.036$* NS	0 4.1% NS
Zureikat AH, Postlewait LM, Liu Y, et al. A multi-institutional comparison of perioperative outcomes of robotic and open pancreaticoduodenectomy. *Ann Surg.* 2016;264:640–649.	Retrospective Comparative	RPD OPD	211 817	402 (257–685) 300 (107–840) $P < 0.001$	200 (30–4500) 300 (20–7350) $P < 0.001$	8 (4–58) 8 (4–148) NS	NA (23.7%)[†] NA (23.9%) NS	1.9% 2.82% NS
Boggi U, Napoli N, Costa F, et al. Robotic-assisted pancreatic resections. *World J Surg.* 2016;40:2497–2506.	Retrospective	RPD OPD	83 36	527 ± 166 425.3 ± 93 $P < 0.0001$	NA NA	17 (14–26) 14 (13–28) $P = 0.06$	74% (18.1%) 78% (11.2%) NS	1.2% 0 NS
Chen S, Chen JZ, Zhan Q, et al. Robot-assisted laparoscopic versus open pancreaticoduodenectomy: a prospective, matched, mid-term follow-up study. *Surg Endosc.* 2015;29:3698–3711.	NR Prospective	2010–2012 RPD OPD 2013 RPD OPD	 40 80 20 40	 445 ± 88 322 ± 73 $P < 0.001$ 340 ± 98 324 ± 92 NS	 500 (310–738) 500 (400–800) NS 200 (100–450) 500 (300–700) $P = 0.002$	All RPD 20 ± 7.4 All OPD 25 ± 11.2 $P = 0.002$	All RPD 35% (11.7%) All OPD 40% (13.3%) NS	All RPD 1.7% All OPD 2.5% NS
Bao PQ, Mazirka PO, Watkins KT. Retrospective comparison of robot-assisted minimally invasive versus open pancreaticoduodenectomy for periampullary neoplasms. *J Gastrointest Surg.* 2014;18:682–689.	Retrospective	RPD OPD	28 28	431 (340–628) 410 (190–621) $P = 0.038$	100 (50–300) 300 (100–800) $P = 0.0001$	7.4 (5.5–17.1) 8.1 (6.5–15.3) NS	NS Grade B/C PF SSI	7% 7% NS
Lai EC, Yang GP, Tang CN. Robot-assisted laparoscopic pancreaticoduodenectomy versus open pancreaticoduodenectomy—a comparative study. *Int J Surg.* 2012;10:475–479.	Retrospective	RPD OPD	20 67	719 ± 186 265 ± 64 $P = 0.01$	247 (50–889) 774 (50–8000) $P = 0.03$	13.7 ± 6.1 25.8 ± 23 $P = 0.02$	50% 49% NS	0 3% NS
Chalikonda S, Aguilar-Saavedra JR, Walsh RM. Laparoscopic robotic-assisted pancreaticoduodenectomy: a case-matched comparison with open resection. *Surg Endosc.* 2012;26:2397–2402.	Prospective	RPD OPD	30 30	476 366 $P = 0.0005$	485 775 NS	9.8 13.3 $P = 0.043$	30% 43% NS	4% 0 NS
Zhou NX, Chen JZ, Liu Q, et al. Outcomes of pancreatoduodenectomy with robotic surgery versus open surgery. *Int J Med Robot.* 2011;7:131–137.	Retrospective Case-matched	RPD OPD	8 8	719 ± 187 420 ± 127 $P = 0.011$	154 ± 43 210 ± 53 $P = 0.045$	16.4 ± 4.1 24 ± 7 $P = 0.04$	25% 75% $P = 0.05$	0 12.5% $P = 0.05$
Buchs NC, Addeo P, Bianco FM, et al. Robotic versus open pancreaticoduodenectomy: a comparative study at a single institution. *World J Surg.* 2011;35:2739–2746.	Retrospective Comparative	RPD OPD	44 39	444 ± 93.5 559 ± 135 $P = 0.0001$	387 ± 334 827 ± 439 $P = 0.0001$	13 ± 17.5 14.6 ± 9.5 NS	36.4% 48.7% NS	4.5% 2.6% NS

NA, Not available; *NR*, not reported; *NS*, nonsignificant; *OPD*, open pancreaticoduodenectomy; *PF*, pancreatic fistula; *RPD*, robotic pancreaticoduodenectomy; *SSI*, surgical site infection.
*No difference in delayed gastric emptying, marginal ulcers, pancreatic fistula, anastomotic leak, urinary tract infection, deep vein thrombosis, pulmonary emboli, pneumonia, sepsis; difference seen mostly due to surgical site infections: 26.5% versus 0 ($P = 0.007$). Study found statistical increase in Grade B/C pancreatic fistula rates in RPD: 13.7% versus 9.1% ($P = 0.04$).

TABLE 16.3 Results of comparative studies on robotic versus laparoscopic and open distal pancreatectomy.

STUDY	STUDY DESIGN	NUMBER OF PATIENTS	BODY MASS INDEX	INDICATIONS % PDAC/PNET/ IPMN/MC	OPERATION TIME (MIN)	ESTIMATED BLOOD LOSS (mL)	SPLEEN PRESERVATION	CONVERSION RATE	LENGTH-OF-STAY (DAYS)	FISTULA (GRADE B–C)	MAJOR MORBIDITY AND MORTALITY
Waters JA, Canal DF, Wiebke EA, et al.	Retro	17	NA	0/29/35/18	298	279	65	12*	4	NA	18/0
Robotic distal pancreatectomy: cost	Robot	18		11/28/11/17	224	667	28	11	6		33/0
effective? *Surgery.* 2010;148:814–823.	Lap	22		50/18/18/9	234	681	14	–	8		18/0
	Open				*P* = 0.01	*P* = 0.17	*P* = 0.04	NS	*P* = 0.0.4		*P* = 0.4
Kang CM, Choi SH, Hwang HK, et al.	Retro	20	24.2	0/15/10/25	349	372	95	NA	7.1	NA	18/0
Minimally invasive (laparoscopic and		25	23.4	0/12/40/8	258	420	64		7.3		16/0
robot-assisted) approach for solid pseudo-papillary tumor of the distal pancreas: a single-center experience. *J Hepatobiliary Pancreat Sci.* 2011;18:87–93.					*P* = 0.024	NS	*P* = 0.27		NS		NS
Daouadi M, Zureikat AH, Zenati MS,	Retro	30	27.9	43/27/17/13	293	150		0	6	26	20
et al. Robot-assisted minimally invasive		94	29.0	15/22/12/31	372	150		16	7	17	14
distal pancreatectomy is superior to the laparoscopic technique. *Ann Surg.* 2013;257:128–132.					*P* = 0.01	NS		*P* < 0.05		NS	NS
Duran H, Ielpo B, Caruso R, et al. Does	Retro	16	NA	56/25/12/0	315	NA	13	13	8	0	0
robotic distal pancreatectomy surgery	Robot	18		44/27/0/0	250		12	27	19.1	11	44
offer similar results as laparoscopic	Lap	13		46/30/15/0	366			–	20.4	15	8
and open approach? A comparative study from a single medical center. *Int J Med Robot.* 2014;10:280–285.	Open				NS		NS	NS	*P* = 0.035	NS	*P* = 0.014
Butturini G, Damoli I, Crepaz L, et al. A	PNRCT	22	25.3	14/4/0/3	265	NA	27	4.5	7	3	
prospective non-randomised single-		21	24.2	10/4/0/3	195		19	4.9	7	4	
center study comparing laparoscopic and robotic distal pancreatectomy. *Surg Endosc.* 2015;29:3163–3170.							*P* = 0.78	*P* = 0.84	*P* = 0.84	*P* = 0.61	
Lee SY, Allen PJ, Sadot E, et al. Distal	Retro	37	28.7	11/21/11/16	213	193	8	38	5	8	43/0
pancreatectomy: a single institution's		131	28.2	15/31/14/12	193	262	22	31	5	8	33/0
experience in open, laparoscopic, and		637	28.4	39/23/6/4	185	596	14	–	7	12	35/0.6
robotic approaches. *J Am Coll Surg.* 2015;220:18–27.				*P* < 0.05	*P* < 0.05	*P* < 0.05	*P* = 0.02		*P* = 0.16	*P* = 0.45	*P* = 0.26
Chen S, Zhan Q, Chen JZ, et al. Robotic	PNRCT	69	24.6	23 (Malignant)	200	100	45/47	0	14.7	32	10/0
approach improves spleen-preserving rate		50	24.6	23 (Malignant)	150	290	13/33	6	12.9	24.6	9/0
and shortens postoperative hospital stay of laparoscopic distal pancreatectomy: a matched cohort study. *Surg Endosc.* 2015;29:3507–3518.					*P* < 0.001	*P* < 0.001	*P* < 0.001	*P* = 0.072	*P* = 0.023	*P* = 0.376	*P* = 0.808
Lai EC, Tang CN. Robotic distal	Retro	17	23.5	65	221.4	100.3	52.9	NA	14	35	39/0
pancreatectomy versus conventional		18	11.1	78	173.6	268.3	38.9		11	28	47/0
laparoscopic distal pancreatectomy: a comparative study for short-term outcomes. *Front Med.* 2015;9:356–360.					*P* = 0.026	*P* = 0.290	*P* = 0.505		*P* = 0.46	*P* = 0.73	*P* = 73

IPMN, Intraductal papillary mucinous neoplasm; *Lap*, laparoscopy; *MCN*, mucinous cystic neoplasm; *NA*, not available; *NS*, nonsignificant; *PDAC*, pancreas ductal adenocarcinoma; *PNET*, pancreatic neuro endocrine tumor; *PNRCT*, prospective nonrandomized clinical trial; *Retro*, retrospective.

TABLE 16.4 Results of the comparative studies evaluating robotic versus laparoscopic liver resections.

STUDY	STUDY TYPE	APPROACH	RESECTION TYPE	NUMBER OF CASES	TUMOR SIZE (cm)	MALIGNANT/ BENIGN	OPERATION TIME (MIN)	ESTIMATED BLOOD LOSS (mL)	LENGTH-OF-STAY (DAYS)	COMPLICATIONS (MAJOR)	CONVERSION
Berber E, Akyildiz HY, Aucejo F, et al. Robotic versus laparoscopic resection of liver tumours. *HPB (Oxford).* 2010;12:583–586.	Retro Comp	RLR LLR	Minor	9 23	3.2 ± 1.3 2.9 ± 1.3	9/0 23/0	259 ± 28 234 ± 16	136 ± 61 155 ± 54	NA NA	1 (NA) 4 (NA)	1 0
Ji WB, Wang HG, Zhao ZM, et al. Robotic-assisted laparoscopic anatomic hepatectomy in China: initial experience. *Ann Surg.* 2011;253:342–348.	Retro CC	RLR LLR	Major & minor	13 20	6.4 (1.8–12) NA	8/5 NA	338 ± 167 130 ± 43	NA NA	NA	1 (0) 2 (0)	0 2
Wu YM, Hu RH, Lai HS, et al. Robotic-assisted minimally invasive liver resection. *Asian J Surg.* 2014;37:53–57.	Retro Comp	RLR LLR	Major & minor	38 41	6.3 ± 1.7 2.5 ± 1.6	38/0 41/0	380 ± 166 227 ± 80	325 ± 480 173 ± 165	7.9 ± 4.7 7.2 ± 4.4	3 (NA) 4 (NA)	2 5
Yu YD, Kim KH, Jung DH, et al. Robotic versus laparoscopic liver resection: a comparative study from a single center. *Langenbecks Arch Surg.* 2014;399:1039–1045.	Retro Comp	RLR LLR	Major & minor	13 17	3.1 ± 1.6 3.5 ± 1.8	10/3 5/12	241 ± 69 292 ± 85	389 ± 65 343 ± 85	7.8 ± 2.3 9.5 ± 3.0	0 (NA) 2 (NA)	0 0
Tsung A, Geller DA, Sukato DC, et al. Robotic versus laparoscopic hepatectomy: a matched comparison. *Ann Surg.* 2014;259:549–555.	Retro CC	RLR LLR	Major & minor	57 114	3.2 (2.1–5.0) 3.5 (2.0–6.0)	26/10 54/18	253 ± 44 199 ± 21	200 ± 77 100 ± 50	4.1 ± 0.6 4.0 ± 0.3	11 (1) 29 (1)	4 10
Tranchart H, Ceribelli C, Ferretti S, et al. Traditional versus robot-assisted full laparoscopic liver resection: a matched-pair comparative study. *World J Surg.* 2014;38:2904–2909.	Retro Comp	RLR LLR	Minor	28 28	3.5 (0.6–11.5) 4.0 (0.6–13.0)	13/15 11/17	236 ± 109 197 ± 98	562 ± 589 331 ± 323	7.0 ± 3.5 15.5 ± 12.3	5 (3) 6 (3)	4 2
Spampinato MG, Coratti A, Bianco L, et al. Perioperative outcomes of laparoscopic and robot-assisted major hepatectomies: an Italian multi-institutional comparative study. *Surg Endosc* 28:2973–2979.	Retro Comp	RLR LLR	Major	25 25	NA NA	NA NA	456 ± 121 375 ± 105	625 ± 450 513 ± 288	10.5 ± 4.5 10.2 ± 4.3	4 (1) 9 (3)	1 1
Montalti R, Scuderi V, Patriti A, et al. Robotic versus laparoscopic resections of posterosuperior segments of the liver: a propensity score-matched comparison. *Surg Endosc.* 2016;30:1004–1013.	Retro CC	RLR LLR	Minor	36 72	4.4 ± 3.1 5.0 ± 3.5	NA NA	306 ± 182 295 ± 107	415 ± 414 437 ± 523	6.0 ± 2.9 4.9 ± 3.0	13 (4) 16 (5)	6 7

Continued

TABLE 16.4 **Results of the comparative studies evaluating robotic versus laparoscopic liver resections.—cont'd**

STUDY	STUDY TYPE	APPROACH	RESECTION TYPE	NUMBER OF CASES	TUMOR SIZE (cm)	MALIGNANT/ BENIGN	OPERATION TIME (MIN)	ESTIMATED BLOOD LOSS (mL)	LENGTH-OF-STAY (DAYS)	COMPLICATIONS (MAJOR)	CONVERSION
Lee KF, Cheung YS, Chong CC, et al. Laparoscopic and robotic hepatectomy: experience from a single centre. *ANZ J Surg.* 2016;86:122–126.	Retro Comp	RLR LLR	Major & minor	70 66	2.5 (0.6–9.0) 2.5 (1.0–12.0)	56/16 57/9	305 ± 131 260 ± 78	675 ± 625 453 ± 401	8.5 ± 5.0 6.8 ± 3.3	8 (NA) 3 (NA)	4 8
Kim JK, Park JS, Han DH, et al. Robotic versus laparoscopic left lateral sectionectomy of liver. *Surg Endosc.* 2016;30:4756–4764.	Retro Comp	RLR LLR	Minor	12 31	2.3 (2.0–3.6) 2.4 (1.7–3.0)	7/5 24/7	404 ± 139 246 ± 101	225 ± 43 150 ± 94	7.3 ± 1.1 6.8 ± 0.8	3 (2) 6 (3)	NA NA
Lai EC, Tang CN. Long-term survival analysis of robotic versus conventional laparoscopic hepatectomy for hepatocellular carcinoma: a comparative study. *Surg Laparosc Endosc Percutan Tech.* 2016;26:162–166.	Retro Comp	RLR LLR	Major & minor	100 35	3.3 ± 1.9 2.7 ± 1.3	100/0 35/0	207 ± 77 134 ± 42	335 ± 583 335 ± 583	7.3 ± 5.3 7.1 ± 2.6	14 (NA) 7 (NA)	4 2
Croner RS, Perrakis A, Hohenberger W, et al. Robotic liver surgery for minor hepatic resections: a comparison with laparoscopic and open standard procedures. *Langenbecks Arch Surg.* 2016;401:707–714.	Retro CC	RLR LLR	Minor	10 19	4.8 (2.9–10.5) 4.1 (1.8–8.5)	10/0 15/4	321 ± 93 242 ± 93	NA NA	NA NA	5 (0) 6 (0)	NA NA
Magistri P, Tarantino G, Guidetti C, et al. Laparoscopic versus robotic surgery for hepatocellular carcinoma: the first 46 consecutive cases. *J Surg Res.* 2017;217:92–99.	Retro Comp	RLR LLR	Major & minor	22 24	3.4 ± 1.4 2.7 ± 1.1	22/0 24/0	318 ± 114 211 ± 78	588 ± 432 464 ± 293	5.1 ± 2.4 6.2 ± 2.6	15 (2) 24 (3)	0 4
Fruscione M, Pickens R, Baker EH, et al. Robotic-assisted versus laparoscopic major liver resection: analysis of outcomes from a single center. *HPB (Oxford).* 2019;21:906–911.	Retro Comp	RLR LLR	Major	57 116	NA NA	37/22 54/62	194 (152–255) 204 (149–280) *P* = 0.189	250 (125–255) 400 (150–750) *P* = 0.129	4 (3–5) 5 (3–6) *P* = 0.136	16 (4) 41 (11) *P* = 0.339	NA NA

CC, Case control; *LLR*, laparoscopic liver resection; *NA*, not available; *Retro Comp*, retrospective comparative; *RLR*, robotic liver resection.
Variables presented with standard deviations are mean numbers; variables presented with ranges are median numbers.

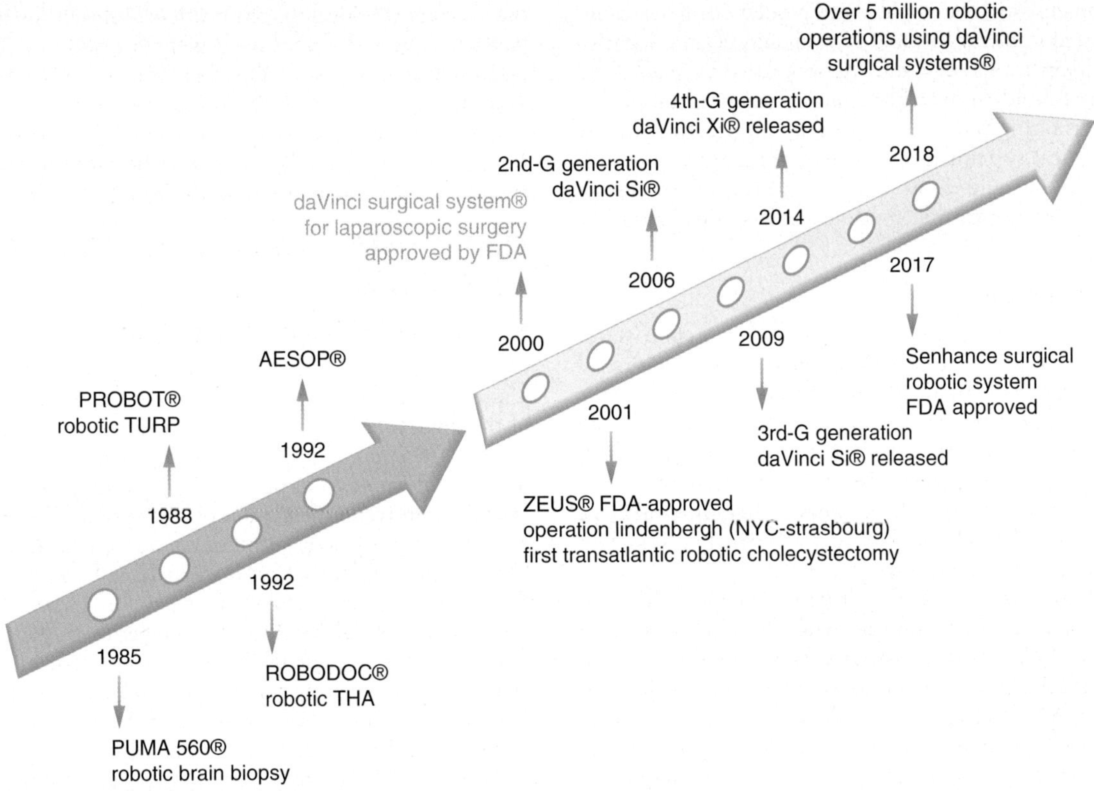

FIG. 16.2 Important dates in robotic surgery development.

prostatectomies that eventually took over 90% of market share of prostatectomies. In urology and gynecology, use of robotics has become standard practice and part of routine practice and training. Recently, robotic surgery adoption in complex abdominal operations is moving at an increased rate with the Xi System, outpacing the rate of laparoscopic application.

The remainder of the chapter covers the understanding and mastery of the robotic surgical platform, namely da Vinci Si and Xi Robotic Systems. We review the clinical outcomes, indications for robotic surgery, selection of patients, and the procedural steps for the following selected robotic operations: robotic radical distal gastrectomy with D2 lymphadenectomy, robotic hepatic posterior segmentectomies, robotic low anterior resection with total mesorectal excision (TME), robotic distal pancreatectomy, and robotic ventral hernia repairs.

PREPARING FOR ROBOTIC SURGERY

Preparation and training are key to adopting robotic surgery into clinical practice and becoming a successful robotic surgeon. Before starting any robotic operation, the surgeon should (1) understand the robotic surgical system, its features and function, and optimal instrument selection and their use; (2) establish a safe and efficient robotic operating room; (3) study the necessary steps of the procedure and the specific steps of the robotic approach; and (4) be knowledgeable about the available literature on robotic surgery.

Understanding da Vinci Si and Xi Surgical Systems

The da Vinci Si and Xi Surgical Systems are composed of the surgeon console, the patient-side cart with robotic arms, and the vision cart. A comprehensive web-based educational module to familiarize users with the da Vinci Surgical System is available through the Intuitive website (www.intuitive.com). Unlike open and laparoscopic operations, the primary surgeon is not scrubbed during the procedure; instead, the surgeon sits at the console a short distance away from the patient's bedside. The surgeons have complete control of robotic function and instrument movements using a master console. Seamless maneuvering of the four arms and attached instruments requires the surgeon's constant hand-eye-foot coordination throughout the operation.

The robotic surgery platform offers the surgeon several technological advantages over laparoscopy: (1) enhanced operative view, (2) ability to control four arms, (3) increased precision of instrument movements, and (4) more sophisticated articulating dissecting, cutting, ligating, suturing, and stapling instruments. ***Enhanced operative view*** is offered by a high-definition three-dimensional camera with up to 10× magnification of surgical anatomy, steady control of camera movements, ready on and off capability of near-infrared, and multiview capabilities by Firefly and Tilepro, respectively. Firefly provides intraoperative fluorescence-guided identification of surgical anatomy including liver perfusion, vascular perfusion, lymph nodes, and lymphatic drainage. The Tilepro program is a multidisplay imaging capability that allows the surgeon to simultaneously view other images, such as intraoperative ultrasound, endoscopy, and radiologic pictures, on the console in real-time during an operation.

The ***precision of instrumentation*** is provided by scaling of motion with a tremor filter and 7 degrees of the Endowristed function. Several ***advanced surgical instruments*** can be employed during robotic operation, including Endowristed needle drivers, with or without suture-cutting capabilities; Endowristed energy devices (vessel sealers with bipolar energy and cutting capabilities);

cutting instruments with monopolar and bipolar energy capabilities; Endowristed staplers (30-mm, 45-mm, and 60-mm lengths) with SmartClamp technology and intraoperative feedback; and Harmonic Ultrasound Shears without articulating capabilities.

Lastly, for training purposes, simulators to practice the use of robotic surgical systems in task-oriented modules are available for both the Si and Xi Systems, as well as an increasing number of procedure-specific modules now available for the Xi System.

Operating Room Setup

Proper operating room setup is essential for safe and effective robotic procedures and requires coordination and consideration of the five elements: the patient, the anesthesiologist, the primary surgeon, the bedside assistant, the robotic patient-side cart, and the surgeon's console. While many operating room setups exist, general concepts can be applied to all robotic operations of the abdomen and pelvis. In general, the anesthesiologist should be positioned to either the right or left side of the patient's head with ready access to the patient's airway.

With the Si System, there is very little flexibility on the positioning of the robotic patient-side cart, which needs to be brought over the patient in line with the trocars for proper docking. For upper gastrointestinal (GI) operations, there are two positions for the patient's cart: (1) brought in straight over the patient's head and docked or (2) brought in off to the left side of the patient's head in a slight angle. In lower GI operations, specifically in left-sided resections, the Si Robotic System must be brought to the left lower side of the patient.

The surgeon's console is usually positioned somewhere in a corner of the operating room facing the patient with ready view of the entire room. If stapling is to be performed by the bedside assistant, it is recommended that the bedside assistant be positioned on the patient's right side and the assistant's video monitor placed on the opposite side, facing the assistant. However, if the robotic stapling device is used, then the placement of the robotic trocar for the stapler should be considered, and which side the bedside assistant stands is not as important.

In the case of the Xi Surgical System, the docking of the robotic patient-side cart is easier, with the cart's ability to rotate 180 degrees to reach its proper position. Therefore, the robot cart can be positioned on either the patient's right or left side, avoiding over-the-head docking all together.

Choosing Robotic Instruments

Selection of instruments for the operation should be done prior to the start of the operation. The instruments to be selected include instruments for retraction, dissection, and ligation and hemostasis. Vessel sealer extension, which is available only on the Xi System, is probably the most versatile of the da Vinci energy devices developed to provide slimmer profile and allow for grasping ability, as well as sealing and cutting. An alternative to the vessel sealer is a Harmonic scalpel (Ethicon, Somerville, NJ) used just as in laparoscopy. It is the only nonarticulating instrument besides the camera that can be controlled by the robotic arm. A Maryland forceps is ideal for dissection and isolation of vessels with its narrow tip and bipolar energy capabilities to achieve hemostasis around soft tissues. At times, a cautery hook monopolar device is useful and can be used just like a Bovie. Monopolar sheers provide sharp dissection and cause less collateral thermal injury; however, they cannot substitute as a grasper. The most often used grasper during GI operations is the Cadiere forceps. It is the least traumatic of the graspers and ideal for retraction of stomach, small bowel, and pancreas, but it does not have energy capabilities. Care must be taken not to grasp the small bowel for a prolonged period of time as delayed perforation from pressure necrosis can occur. Alternative graspers, ProGrasp/fenestrated bipolar graspers are also options for graspers but with more force between the jaws, therefore, should be used with caution on the bowel.

CURRENT STATUS OF SELECTED ROBOTIC OPERATIONS

Robotic Ventral Hernia Repair With Mesh

More than 350,000 ventral hernias are repaired annually in the United States.[6] Expert consensus reached after a systematic review of the highest level of evidence recommends mesh reinforcement in hernias ≥2 cm and against elective repairs in patients ≥50 kg/m^2, current smokers, or patients whose hemoglobin A1C is ≥8%. However, no recommendation on the approach of the repair was made. Numerous open techniques and now laparoscopic ventral hernia repairs (LVHRs) with mesh have been described. With the recent adoption of robotic surgery for ventral hernia repairs, the transabdominal retromuscular preperitoneal hernia repair has found favor among general surgeons as it capitalizes on the advantages of the articulating robotic instruments for improved ability to close the fascial defect, for suturing the mesh in place, and for closing the peritoneal defect over the mesh.[7]

Since LVHR was first reported in the early 1990s, several comparative studies have been conducted and reported to date. Two systematic reviews of laparoscopic versus open abdominal wall and incisional hernia repairs were identified. One study by Al Chalabi and colleagues (2015)[8] included results of five randomized controlled trials (RCTs) (306 patients in the laparoscopic group and 305 patients in the open group), and the other systemic review by Sauerland and colleagues (2011)[9] included 10 non-RCTs with a total number of 880 patients. The study by Al Chalabi and colleagues (2015)[8] revealed no difference between the laparoscopic and the open group in recurrences with 2 to 35 months of follow-up (P = 0.30), a clear decrease in wound infections in the laparoscopic group (P < 0.001), and a trend toward longer operative time in the laparoscopic group (P = 0.5). The latter study was a meta analysis performed for the Cochrane Review, which demonstrated no difference in recurrence rates between the two groups with less than 2 years of follow-up in all 10 studies and a significant decrease in wound infections for the laparoscopic approach (relative risk, 0.26; 95% confidence interval [CI], 0.15–0.45). While numerous LVHR techniques have been reported, several limitations were found in its wide adoption due to technically demanding maneuvers hampered by the lack of instrument articulation and difficulty in closing the abdominal wall defects.

Robotic ventral herniorrhaphy addresses the limitations of laparoscopy demonstrating improved clinical outcomes compared to the open approach. While still in the early phase of adoption, robotic techniques in ventral hernia repair have been reported and found to be particularly beneficial in intracorporeal closure of the hernia defect and suturing of the mesh to the fascia. Comparative studies demonstrate significant decrease in length of hospital stay for the robotic approach compared to LVHRs.[10,11] In a 2:1 propensity match multi-institutional study conducted by the American Hernia Society Quality Collaborative, which included data from patients operated on between 2013 and 2016, the length of stay for the robotic retromuscular ventral hernia repair (RRVHR) group (n = 111) was shorter than the laparoscopic group (n =

222), 2 days and 3 days, respectively. They showed no difference in 30-day readmission rates and surgical site infections.

In a retrospective comparative study of all LVHRs (n = 103) and RRVHRs (n = 53) performed at one institution between June 2013 and May 2015, the patients were older in the robotic group (60.2 vs. 52.9 years, P = 0.001), but other demographics and hernia width (6.9 vs. 6.5 cm, P = 0.508) were similar between groups.[7] A significant difference in achieving fascial closure favored the RRVHR (96.2% vs. 50.5%, P < 0.001). Operative time was longer in the RRVHR (245 vs. 122 minutes, P < 0.001). Seroma at the repair site was more common after RRVHR (47.2% vs. 16.5%, P < 0.001), but surgical site infection was similar (3.8% vs. 1%, P = 0.592). Median length of stay was shorter after RRVHR (1 day vs. 2 days, P = 0.004).

A retrospective review of 215 patients undergoing ventral hernia repair (142 robotic and 73 laparoscopic) at two large academic centers was reported by Walker and colleagues (2018)[11] evaluating recurrence, primary fascial closure, and surgical site occurrences. This study demonstrated that robotic repair was associated with a decreased incidence of recurrence (2.1% vs. 4.2%, P<0.001), surgical site occurrence (4.2% vs. 18.8%, P<0.001), and increased rates of primary fascial closure (77.1% vs. 66.7%, P<0.01).[11] This study, however, has a limitation with a lower body mass index (BMI) (28.1 ± 3.6 vs. 34.2 ± 6.4, P<0.001) and fewer comorbidities in the robotic group, indicating selection bias favoring the robotic group.[11]

The adoption of robotic ventral hernia repair is increasing despite the absence of randomized prospective clinical trials. Studies designed to investigate the efficacy, safety, and cost effectiveness of robotic techniques for ventral hernia repair are needed to support its continued use as higher cost of technology continues to require justification for integration of surgical innovation into our clinical practice.

Robotic Total Mesorectal Excision for Rectal Cancer

TME is the gold standard and surgical technique of choice for locally advanced rectal cancer.[12] We have selected robotic lower anterior resection (rLAR) with TME as one of the procedures to present in this chapter for the potential of robot assistance to facilitate a successful MIS approach to rectal cancer.

In the past 25 years since the results of landmark clinical trials demonstrated laparoscopic noninferiority in oncologic outcomes and benefits of MIS such as less blood loss, faster recovery of bowel function, and shorter length of hospital stay for colorectal cancer surgery, the laparoscopic approach has become well accepted for colorectal operations.[13–16] However, the initial conversion rates of up to 34%, high positive circumferential margins (12%), and increased complication and recurrence rates with decreased disease-free survival attest to the difficulty of laparoscopic TME (laTME) and limit the broad adoption of MIS techniques for these patients.[17] Colorectal surgeons report laTME to be feasible but technically difficult with steep learning curves of between 50 and 150 cases.[18,19]

Robotic surgical systems were gradually adopted to various colorectal surgical procedures starting in the early phase of clinical adoption.[18,19] The first robotic TME (rTME) was described in 2006,[20] and the results of rTME with attention to nerve preservation was reported in 2007.[21] Early adopters of robotic rectal surgery emphasize the technical advantages gained from the enhanced robotic features for fine dissection in difficult-to-reach pelvic anatomy during a TME. There is particular interest in capitalizing on the robotic advantages in overcoming major challenges posed by low-lying bulky tumors in obese patients with narrow male pelvises, which were all independent risk factors for longer operations and open conversions. Especially considering the relatively short learning curve for rTME, reported to be less than 20 cases, robotics promised greater MIS penetration in rectal surgery.[22,23]

Consistent with the robotics approach for other procedures, the benefits of rLAR with TME have paralleled that of laparoscopy when rLAR is compared to open operations. However, the comparative outcomes of rLAR with TME versus laparoscopic LAR with TME remain controversial. The initially reported advantages of lower conversion rates, less positive circumference margins, and shorter length of stay did withstand the rigors of two RCTs. In clinical practice, however, the initial positive results of rLAR with TME studies cannot be dismissed as they provide insight into the ability of robotic technique to offer the patients equivalent outcomes to laparoscopic operations even in the early phase of robotic adoption as most surgeons participating in the studies had more laparoscopic experience than robotic experience in rectal operations. A summary of the results of recently published comparative studies, RCTs, and meta analyses focusing on the key intraoperative, postoperative, pathologic, and long-term oncologic and functional outcomes is presented in Table 16.1.

Two RCTs showed comparable outcomes for both robotic and laparoscopic approaches for rectal cancer, with the exception of two disadvantages of the robotic group that included longer operative time and higher cost.[24,25] A Phase II RCT of 165 rectal cancer patients undergoing robotic low anterior resection (rLAR) with TME or laparoscopic LAR with TME demonstrated several differences. There was longer operative time with rTME (rTME 339.2 vs. laTME 227.8 minutes, P < 0.001). There was improved sexual function after rTME after 12 months of follow-up as reported on the quality of life questionnaire for colorectal cancer (QLQ-CR) 38 scores (mean, 35.2; 95% CI, 26.9–43.5 vs. 23.0 and 15.7–30.2, P = 0.32). There was no difference in length of stay (rTME 10.3 days vs. laTME 10.8 days, NS) and no significant difference in major complications (rTME 9.4% vs. laTME 5.4%, P = 0.227). There were no differences in minor complications (rTME 25.8% vs. laTME 17.8%, P = 0.227), conversion rate (rTME 1.2% vs. laTME 0.0%, P = 0.475), or positive circumference margins (5.5% vs. 6.1%, P = 0.999).[25]

The most recent international multi-institutional RCT comparing rLAR with TME to laparoscopic LAR with TME, the ROLARR RCT of 471 patients with rectal adenocarcinoma revealed no difference between the robotic and laparoscopic approaches in conversion to open laparotomy (8.1% vs. 12.2%, P = 0.16), operative time (298.5 vs. 261.0 minutes, NS), positive circumference margins (5.1% vs. 8.1%, P = 0.56), 30-day mortality (0.8% vs. 0.9%, NA), length of stay (8.0 vs. 8.2 days, NS), or postoperative 30-day complication rate (14.4% vs. 16.5%, P = 0.84).[26] This study also conducted a health care cost analysis in the subgroup of patients enrolled from the United States and UK and determined that robotic approach was more expensive than laparoscopy due to longer operation usage and instrument cost. Informatively, obesity did not have any impact on the operative times, open conversion, estimated blood loss during surgery, and length of hospital stay in rLAR with TME; however, significant differences were demonstrated for these outcomes between obese and nonobese patients in the laparoscopic group.

A totally rLAR with TME is not often reported nor practiced. Most experienced laparoscopic colorectal surgeons comfortably mobilize the left colon and take down the splenic flexure laparoscopically. A stepwise adoption with hybrid techniques combining laparoscopic mobilizations and rTME has been suggested.

Especially since robotic rectal resection with TME are multiquadrant operations requiring redocking of the robotic arms and repositioning of the robotic cart, surgeons have been less inclined to perform the entire procedure as a totally robotic operation. However, with the Xi System with its boom rotation capabilities, interchangeability of the camera position among all the robotic trocars and the ability to synchronize the robot to the operating room table for intraoperative repositioning, a totally rLAR with TME has become more appealing to the surgeon, during which the portion of the operation to employ the robotic system remains the surgeon's choice.

Robotic Pancreatic Surgery

Pancreatic operations, including pancreaticoduodenectomy (PD) and distal pancreatectomy, are considered the most complicated and technically challenging abdominal procedures performed by general surgeons. This is no different when an MIS approach is applied. Minimally invasive pancreatic surgery began with the first report of laparoscopic PD (LPD) by Michal Gagner in 1994,[27] who later attested to the difficulty of laparoscopic technique in pancreatic surgery when he reported a series of 23 patients who had undergone a planned LPD (n = 10), laparoscopic distal pancreatectomy (n = 9), and laparoscopic enucleation (n = 4) with a conversion rate of 40%, operative time of 8.5 hours, and length of hospitalization of 22.3 days.

Despite the initially discouraging results, minimally invasive pancreatic resections have persisted, and its adoption continues to grow worldwide in the hand of expert surgeons working to bring MIS benefits to patients undergoing pancreatic resection. The technical feasibility and the safety of the laparoscopic approaches to pancreatic resections have been demonstrated in numerous studies pending randomized clinical trial results of ongoing trials in laparoscopic versus open distal pancreatectomy (the Dutch LEOPARD-1 multicenter RCT [minimally invasive vs. open distal pancreatectomy] and the Swedish LAPOP single-center RCT [laproscopic vs. open distal pancreatectomy]), but none are pending PDs.[28,29]

The caution and systematic development of robotic pancreatic procedures parallel that of laparoscopic approach, which began a decade later in 2003 with Giulianotti and colleagues[30] reporting a series of robotic operations including robotic pancreatic resections and Melvin and colleagues[31] describing robotic distal pancreatectomy. Thus far, the evidence on robotic pancreatic surgery is based on nonrandomized comparative studies, most of which come from single-institutional experience. These results are summarized in Tables 16.2 and 16.3.

Robotic Pancreaticoduodenectomy

Robotic PD (RPD) is feasible and can safely be performed by expert surgeons at high-volume centers who are supported by an experienced robotic surgical team. In the field of pancreatic surgery, RPD is being developed in parallel to LPD (Table 16.2). Two major review articles on RPD were published in 2017 (systematic review) and 2018 (meta analysis comparing RPD vs. open PD), including 13 and 11 non-RCTs, respectively.[32,33] Additionally, RPDs and LPDs were compared in a recent study using the 2014–2015 pancreas-targeted American College of Surgeons National Surgical Quality Improvement Program (NSQIP) database of 428 patients who underwent minimally invasive pancreaticoduodenectomies.[34] The results of the systematic review demonstrated RPD to have lower conversion rates (11.4% vs. 26.0%, P = 0.004), lower odds of conversions (odds ratio [OR], 0.46; 95% CI, 0.26–0.81), overall morbidity rates between 25% and 73%, mortality rates ranging from 1% to 12.5%, and no difference in operative time, length of hospital stay, readmission rates, 30-day mortality rates, and major complication rates when compared to LPD.

Eleven non-RCTs comparing RPD versus open PD were included in the systematic review and meta analysis recently published by Zhao and colleagues.[35] The results of the pooled analysis demonstrated that RPD had significantly longer operative times with a mean weighted difference (MWD) of 88.7 minutes (95% CI, 38.38–138.99 minutes, P = 0.0005) but had less blood loss with a MWD of −197.0 mL (95% CI, −313.42 to −80.61 mL, P = 0.0009), and RPD was associated with a lower positive margin rate (MWD, 0.29; 95% CI, 0.15–0.56; P = 0.0003), lower overall complications (OR, 0.67; 95% CI, 0.47–0.95; P = 0.02), and a faster time to postoperative out of bed (MWD, −2.24; 95% CI, −3.51 to −0.96; P = 0.0006). No significant difference was seen in the number of lymph nodes or in the rate of other perioperative parameters such as pancreatic fistula, delayed gastric emptying, return to operating room, length of hospital stay, and mortality between the two groups.

An NSQIP study aimed to compare the rate of postoperative 30-day overall complications between laparoscopic (n = 235) and robotic (n = 193) pancreaticoduodenectomies. The study determined that there was no association of complications with the type of MIS approach, whether laparoscopic or robotic. However, overall complications as well as 30-day overall complications were associated with higher BMI (OR, 1.05; 95% CI, 1.02–1.09), vascular resection (OR, 2.10; 95% CI, 1.23–3.58), and longer operative time (OR, 1.002; 95% CI, 1.001–1.004).[34]

Examination of the learning curve of robotic pancreatic resections is instructional. A study by Boone et al. (2015)[36] examined the number of cases required to achieve optimization of perioperative outcomes in RPD. The study included a retrospective review of 200 consecutive patients who underwent RPD in a large academic center over a 6.5-year period and evaluated important perioperative quality metrics (morbidity, mortality, estimated blood loss, open conversion, incidence of pancreatic fistula, operative time, length of stay, and readmission rate) in groups of 20 cases. The results showed that there was no statistically significant change in mortality rates or major morbidity during the evaluated time period. However, after 20 cases, improvements in estimated blood loss (600 vs. 250 mL, P=0.002) and in open conversion rates (35.0% vs. 3.3%, P<0.001) were observed. Moreover, a decreased incidence of pancreatic fistula after 40 cases (27.5% vs. 14.4%, P = 0.04) and decreased operative time after 80 cases (581 vs. 417 minutes, P<0.001) were reported.

Interestingly, the study concluded that the optimized metrics beyond the learning curve included a mean operative time of 417 minutes, a median estimated blood loss rate of 250 mL, a conversion rate of 3.3%, a 90-day mortality of 3.3%, a clinically significant (Grade B/C) pancreatic fistula rate of 6.9%, and a median length of stay of 9 days. This study further confirms the challenging nature of pancreatic surgery and RPD, suggesting that at least 80 RPDs are required to overcome the learning curve and provide optimized outcomes.

Robotic Distal Pancreatectomy

Pancreatic resections are complex abdominal surgeries requiring a high level of technical skill and a high volume of experience to provide optimum outcome.[37,38] Understandably, they are considered one of the most challenging fields of MIS. Twenty-four years after the first report of laparoscopic distal pancreatectomy in 1994 by Cuschieri,[39] laparoscopic distal pancreatectomies have become the preferred approach by some experts over the traditional open approach, attesting to its safety, feasibility, and association with improved patient outcomes such as less blood loss, decreased pain, and shorter length of hospital stay. However, less than 15% of all pancreatic operations in the United States are laparoscopically performed, with persistent and significant barriers to its widespread clinical adoption mainly due to the difficulty of vascular control and high open conversion rates. Additionally, concerns over the ability to perform the proper extent of oncologic resection persist, and debate over the implementation of minimally invasive pancreatic cancer surgery remain.

Early adopters of robotic technology have implemented robotic pancreatic resections in their practice with the first report of robotic distal pancreatectomy in a 46-year-old woman with a pancreatic neuroendocrine tumor in the tail of the pancreas by Melvin and colleagues in 2003.[31] The potential for robotic surgery to facilitate distal pancreatic resections has been evaluated and compared to laparoscopic approach. While no randomized control trials are available, several retrospective and prospective comparative studies offer insight into the possible benefits and disadvantages among the robotic, laparoscopic, and open techniques for distal pancreatectomy and are summarized in Table 16.3.

Theoretically, the enhanced operative visualization provided by 3D camera, Tile Pro and Firefly; the articulating instruments; and the increased precision of the steady tremor filtered movements of the robotic arms should offer the surgeon and the patient improved surgical outcomes when compared to laparoscopic techniques for distal pancreatectomy. The recent meta analysis including 10 studies comparing robotic (n = 267 patients) and laparoscopic (n = 546 patients) distal pancreatectomies concluded that there were no differences in pancreatic fistula rates (30.3% vs. 33.5%, respectively; OR, 0.93; P = 0.75), operative time (262.8 vs. 233.2 minutes, P = 0.17), and major complications (16% vs. 17%; OR, 1.19; P = 0.52). There were differences in open conversion rates that were lower in the robotic distal pancreatectomy group (8.2% vs. 21.6%; OR, 0.33; 95% CI, 0.12–0.92; P = 0.03). Robotic distal pancreatectomy also had a higher rate of spleen preservation (48.9% vs. 27%; OR, 2.89; 95% CI, 1.78–4.71; $P < 0.0001$) and a shorter length of hospital stay (7.18 vs. 9.08 days, P = 0.01) but a higher cost of the operation (P = 0.00001). The surgeon should consider these findings when adopting robotic surgery for distal pancreatic resections.

The indications for robotic distal pancreatectomy are the same as those for the laparoscopic approach and include the following diseases involving the distal pancreas: pancreatic adenocarcinoma, pancreatic neuroendocrine tumors, intraductal papillary neoplasm, mucinous cystic neoplasm, serous cystadenoma, pseudopapillary solid tumors, and pancreatic stricture.

Careful selection of patients should be considered based on the patient's health, the experience of the surgeon, and the nature (benign, premalignant, or malignant), size, and location of lesions. Patients who are younger, with lower BMIs, with limited comorbid conditions, and who are otherwise in good health are ideal initial candidates. Lesions that are more distally located away from the major vessels (superior mesenteric and portal vein) can be considered for first cases based on surgeon comfort and experience. These characteristics may affect the ability to successfully complete the operations robotically and decrease the risk of open conversion. Moreover, the surgeon and the operating room team should be prepared with an emergency open conversion plan as intraoperative hemorrhage during a robotic operation, especially during spleen preservation (due to loss of exposure, insufficient visualization of vascular anatomy, inability to gain rapid control of the bleeding, and the surgeons' comfort level), is one of the major reasons for open conversion.

In brief, robotic surgery has been shown to have MIS benefits equivalent to the laparoscopic procedure, allows for increased rates of successful splenic preservation when desired, suggests a shorter learning curve in some reports, and consistently costs more per operation. Most of the benefits of the robotic approach remain subjective, and adoption of the approach over laparoscopy or open depends on the surgeon perception and expertise.

Robotic Liver Resections

Since the first laparoscopic liver resection was reported in 1991 by Reich and colleagues[40] for benign liver disease, numerous methods of minimally invasive techniques in liver surgery have been described. Studies have demonstrated the benefits of minimally invasive liver surgery to be safe and feasible and to improve perioperative patient outcomes for totally laparoscopic, hand-assisted laparoscopic, and robotic wedge resections to trisegmentectomies for both benign and malignant indications.[41] Minimally invasive liver resections are now the standard approach for peripheral hepatic lesions as recommended by the international position on laparoscopic liver surgery: the Louisville statement in 2008.[42]

Laparoscopic liver resections, however, are technically challenging minimally invasive procedures with high learning curves and notable open conversion rates.[43] The difficulties have been attributed to the lack of depth perception, the constraints of straight instruments with only 4 degrees of freedom and fixed maneuverability, and surgeon fatigue in long procedures. These are especially true for laparoscopic major hepatectomies for lesions located in difficult-to-reach places such as the posterior segments of the liver.

With the advent of new robotic technology, the opportunities for increased adoption of MIS have been appealing with promising initial studies demonstrating perioperative benefits over open procedures and lower open conversion rates than the laparoscopic approach. However, systematic evaluations of robotic versus laparoscopic liver resections do not provide satisfying results, and the robotic benefits are still being explored. One leading philosophy that may yield superior outcomes is to better define the patient selection criteria for robotic hepatectomy (RH). For example, robotic liver surgery may be most beneficial to patients with incision-dominant procedures in patients with poorly placed tumors such as those located in the posterosuperior segments where laparoscopic approach is difficult if not prohibitive due to tumor location and least beneficial for patients undergoing major hepatectomies such as right trisegmentectomy in which recovery and outcomes are determined by liver physiology and not by incision size. A summary of the robotic versus laparoscopic studies is provided in Table 16.4.

Robotic Versus Laparoscopic Liver Resections

No RCTs exist to compare robotic versus laparoscopic liver resection. However, several metaanalyses of high-quality non-RCTs have systematically analyzed the available evidence in this field. The most recent meta analysis performed by Guan and colleagues[44] systematically reviewed and selected 13 nonrandomized control studies that included patients diagnosed with focal liver lesions (hepatocellular carcinoma, cholangiocarcinoma, focal nodular hyperplasia, hemangioma, hepatic adenoma, and metastatic lesions) and reported at least one perioperative outcome of interest (operation time, intraoperative blood loss, blood transfusion rate, complications, conversion rate, R1 resection rate, and the hospital stays).[44] The studies involved 938 patients (RH = 435; laparoscopic hepatectomy = 503), where the robotic group was found to have longer operative times of an average of 65.5 minutes (95% CI, 42.0–89.0; $P < 0.00001$), decreased intraoperative blood loss on average of 69.9 mL (95% CI, 27.1–112.7; $P < 0.001$), and a higher cost (4.24; 95% CI, 3.08–5.39; $P < 0.00001$). There were no significant differences for the two groups in the transfusion rate, complication rate, conversion rate, R1 resection rate, and hospital stay.

Difference in Lesion Location

Indications for the robotic approach are the same as for laparoscopy and include primary tumors (e.g., hepatocellular carcinoma and intrahepatic cholangiocarcinoma), metastatic lesions from colorectal and breast cancers, benign tumors (e.g., enlarging hemangiomas, adenomas, focal nodular hyperplasia), and symptomatic lesions (e.g., cysts and abscesses). In case-by-case selection of patients who would most benefit from a robotic approach, however, one should consider patients with posterosuperior segments (a1, 4A, 7, 8) when the tumor is poorly located; open surgery would require a large incision when tumors are difficult to reach by conventional laparoscopic methods.[45,46]

In a recent retrospective study evaluating 97 patients who underwent robotic liver sections including major resections (n = 13) and minor resections (segments 2, 4B, 5, and 6 [n = 51] or segmentectomies 1, 2, 4A, 7, and 8 [n = 33]), Melstrom and colleagues[45] offered insight into the benefits of robotic surgery for "incision-dominant" operations. The study found that two-thirds of the patients were discharged within 3 days of the robotic procedure, including three patients who had undergone hemihepatectomies. Risk for length of hospital stay >3 days included extent of resection ($P = 0.003$), occurrence of complications ($P = 0.009$), and operative time greater than 210 minutes ($P = 0.001$).

A multinational retrospective study evaluated 51 robotic and 145 open minor liver resections performed between 2009 and 2016 by high-volume liver surgeons.[46] The final 1:1 propensity-matched analysis of 31 robotic and 31 open posterosuperior segments demonstrated the safety, feasibility, and shorter length of hospital stay in the robotic group (median 4 vs. 8 days, $P <$ 0.001). No differences were found in median operative time, estimated blood loss, major complications rates, readmission rates, and mortality (0% for both groups). Again, this study highlights the importance of case selection in harnessing the strengths of robotic techniques. It utilizes the advantages of the robotic system's enhanced 3D visualization, simultaneous multiview on the console (during intraoperative ultrasound-guided tumor location), near-infrared imaging capability (localizing the margin of tumor), the articulating instruments such as dissectors, energy devices, and staplers to help to reach the most difficult-to-approach liver lesions in the right posterior sections and overcome the limitations of laparoscopic approach to provide minimally invasive liver surgery benefits to patients.

As for the adoption of any new technology, patient safety is the primary consideration when initiating robotic liver surgery in clinical practice. Several useful practices to ensure safe and successful integration of robotic liver surgery into one's surgical armamentarium include partnering with another experienced liver surgeon, establishing predetermined time limits and thresholds for open conversion, and being prepared for intraoperative emergencies such as hemorrhage or uncertainty of surgical anatomy.

CONCLUSION

Surgical practice is changing. The concepts underlying open surgical techniques rooted in century-old traditions have been challenged by MIS with improved outcomes for patients. Robotic surgery has emerged as an alternative approach to laparoscopy, offering surgeons more sophisticated surgical instruments to overcome the limitations of laparoscopy that hinder widespread adoption of MIS. Unlike other fields of medicine, in which evaluation of new drugs has a well-defined testing pathway prior to reaching standard of care use, the adoption of surgical innovation is charting a new course toward widespread adoption and implementation.[47–49] Testing a new technology requires additional training and experience, development of new procedures, and expertise and continues to challenge not only the field of surgery but also the individual surgeon.[50,51] In the absence of RCT demonstrating the superiority of robotic surgery over laparoscopy for many of the commonly performed general surgical procedures, the decision whether or not to adopt and offer a robotic operation is a surgeon's choice based on the surgeon's access to the robotic system and his or her knowledge, training, and experience.

SELECTED REFERENCES

Carbonell AM, Warren JA, Prabhu AS, et al. Reducing length of stay using a robotic-assisted approach for retromuscular ventral hernia repair: a comparative analysis from the americas hernia society quality collaborative. *Ann Surg*. 2018;267:210–217.

A propensity-matched study of patients undergoing retromuscular ventral hernia repair (open 222: robotic 111) from the Americas Hernia Society Quality Collaboration between 2013 and 2016. This study showed reduced length of stay but increased seroma production.

George EI, Brand TC, LaPorta A, et al. Origins of robotic surgery: from skepticism to standard of care. *JSLS*. 2018;22.

A comprehensive review of the history of robotic surgery.

Jayne D, Pigazzi A, Marshall H, et al. Effect of robotic-assisted vs conventional laparoscopic surgery on risk of conversion to open laparotomy among patients undergoing resection for rectal cancer: the ROLARR Randomized Clinical Trial. *JAMA*. 2017;318:1569–1580.

A multinational randomized control trial comparing robotic-assisted (n = 237) versus conventional laparoscopic (n = 234) rectal resection including 40 surgeons. No difference in conversion rates were found between robotic and laparoscopic approaches for the treatment of rectal cancer.

Nota CL, Woo Y, Raoof M, et al. Robotic versus open minor liver resections of the posterosuperior segments: a multinational, propensity score-matched study. *Ann Surg Oncol*. 2019;26:583–590.

A multinational propensity-matched retrospective study comparing 31 robotic and 31 open posterosuperior segments (1, 4A, 7, 8). This study demonstrated the safety, feasibility, and shorter length of hospital stay in the robotic group.

Zhao W, Liu C, Li S, et al. Safety and efficacy for robot-assisted versus open pancreaticoduodenectomy and distal pancreatectomy: a systematic review and meta-analysis. *Surg Oncol.* 2018;27:468–478.

A meta analysis of nonrandomized control trials (11 robot-assisted pancreaticoduodenectomy vs. open pancreaticoduodenectomy and 4 robot-assisted distal pancreatectomy vs. open distal pancreatectomy) including 3690 patients. Robot-assisted pancreaticoduodenectomy improves outcome compared to open but has longer operative times.

REFERENCES

1. Konstantinidis IT, Lewis A, Lee B, et al. Minimally invasive distal pancreatectomy: greatest benefit for the frail. *Surg Endosc.* 2017;31:5234–5240.
2. Ceccarelli G, Andolfi E, Biancafarina A, et al. Robot-assisted surgery in elderly and very elderly population: our experience in oncologic and general surgery with literature review. *Aging Clin Exp Res.* 2017;29:55–63.
3. George EI, Brand TC, LaPorta A, et al. Origins of robotic surgery: from skepticism to standard of care. *JSLS.* 2018;22.
4. Marescaux J, Leroy J, Gagner M, et al. Transatlantic robot-assisted telesurgery. *Nature.* 2001;413:379–380.
5. Gosrisirikul C, Don Chang K, Raheem AA, et al. New era of robotic surgical systems. *Asian J Endosc Surg.* 2018;11:291–299.
6. Kennedy M, Barrera K, Akelik A, et al. Robotic TAPP ventral hernia repair: early lessons learned at an inner city safety net hospital. *JSLS.* 2018;22.
7. Warren JA, Cobb WS, Ewing JA, et al. Standard laparoscopic versus robotic retromuscular ventral hernia repair. *Surg Endosc.* 2017;31:324–332.
8. Al Chalabi H, Larkin J, Mehigan B, et al. A systematic review of laparoscopic versus open abdominal incisional hernia repair, with meta-analysis of randomized controlled trials. *Int J Surg.* 2015;20:65–74.
9. Sauerland S, Walgenbach M, Habermalz B, et al. Laparoscopic versus open surgical techniques for ventral or incisional hernia repair. *Cochrane Database Syst Rev.* 2011; CD007781.
10. Carbonell AM, Warren JA, Prabhu AS, et al. Reducing length of stay using a robotic-assisted approach for retromuscular ventral hernia repair: a comparative analysis from the Americas Hernia Society Quality Collaborative. *Ann Surg.* 2018;267:210–217.
11. Walker PA, May AC, Mo J, et al. Multicenter review of robotic versus laparoscopic ventral hernia repair: is there a role for robotics? *Surg Endosc.* 2018;32:1901–1905.
12. Mortenson MM, Khatri VP, Bennett JJ, et al. Total mesorectal excision and pelvic node dissection for rectal cancer: an appraisal. *Surg Oncol Clin N Am.* 2007;16:177–197.
13. Nelson H, Sargent DJ, Wieand HS, et al. A comparison of laparoscopically assisted and open colectomy for colon cancer. *N Engl J Med.* 2004;350:2050–2059.
14. Jayne DG, Thorpe HC, Copeland J, et al. Five-year follow-up of the Medical Research Council CLASICC trial of laparoscopically assisted versus open surgery for colorectal cancer. *Br J Surg.* 2010;97:1638–1645.
15. Jeong SY, Park JW, Nam BH, et al. Open versus laparoscopic surgery for mid-rectal or low-rectal cancer after neoadjuvant chemoradiotherapy (COREAN trial): survival outcomes of an open-label, non-inferiority, randomised controlled trial. *Lancet Oncol.* 2014;15:767–774.
16. Buunen M, Veldkamp R, Hop WC, et al. Survival after laparoscopic surgery versus open surgery for colon cancer: long-term outcome of a randomised clinical trial. *Lancet Oncol.* 2009;10:44–52.
17. Jayne DG, Guillou PJ, Thorpe H, et al. Randomized trial of laparoscopic-assisted resection of colorectal carcinoma: 3-year results of the UK MRC CLASICC Trial Group. *J Clin Oncol.* 2007;25:3061–3068.
18. Luglio G, De Palma GD, Tarquini R, et al. Laparoscopic colorectal surgery in learning curve: role of implementation of a standardized technique and recovery protocol. A cohort study. *Ann Med Surg (Lond).* 2015;4:89–94.
19. Miskovic D, Ni M, Wyles SM, et al. Learning curve and case selection in laparoscopic colorectal surgery: systematic review and international multicenter analysis of 4852 cases. *Dis Colon Rectum.* 2012;55:1300–1310.
20. Pigazzi A, Ellenhorn JD, Ballantyne GH, et al. Robotic-assisted laparoscopic low anterior resection with total mesorectal excision for rectal cancer. *Surg Endosc.* 2006;20:1521–1525.
21. Baik SH, Kim NK, Lee YC, et al. Prognostic significance of circumferential resection margin following total mesorectal excision and adjuvant chemoradiotherapy in patients with rectal cancer. *Ann Surg Oncol.* 2007;14:462–469.
22. Akmal Y, Baek JH, McKenzie S, et al. Robot-assisted total mesorectal excision: is there a learning curve? *Surg Endosc.* 2012;26:2471–2476.
23. Ng SS, Lee JF, Yiu RY, et al. Laparoscopic-assisted versus open total mesorectal excision with anal sphincter preservation for mid and low rectal cancer: a prospective, randomized trial. *Surg Endosc.* 2014;28:297–306.
24. Colombo PE, Bertrand MM, Alline M, et al. Robotic versus laparoscopic total mesorectal excision (TME) for sphincter-saving surgery: is there any difference in the transanal TME rectal approach?: a single-center series of 120 consecutive patients. *Ann Surg Oncol.* 2016;23:1594–1600.
25. Kim MJ, Park SC, Park JW, et al. Robot-assisted versus laparoscopic surgery for rectal cancer: a phase II open label prospective randomized controlled trial. *Ann Surg.* 2018;267:243–251.
26. Jayne D, Pigazzi A, Marshall H, et al. Effect of robotic-assisted vs conventional laparoscopic surgery on risk of conversion to open laparotomy among patients undergoing resection for rectal cancer: the ROLARR randomized clinical trial. *JAMA.* 2017;318:1569–1580.
27. Gagner M, Pomp A. Laparoscopic pylorus-preserving pancreatoduodenectomy. *Surg Endosc.* 1994;8:408–410.
28. de Rooij T, van Hilst J, Vogel JA, et al. Minimally invasive versus open distal pancreatectomy (LEOPARD): study protocol for a randomized controlled trial. *Trials.* 2017;18:166.
29. Björnsson B. *Prospective, Randomized Comparison of Laparoscopic Vs. Open Distal Pancreatectomy, Multicentre, Ongoing Trial.* Springer Nature; 2014. http://www.isrctn.com/ISRCTN26912858. Accessed March 19, 2019.
30. Giulianotti PC, Coratti A, Angelini M, et al. Robotics in general surgery: personal experience in a large community hospital. *Arch Surg.* 2003;138:777–784.
31. Melvin WS, Needleman BJ, Krause KR, et al. Robotic resection of pancreatic neuroendocrine tumor. *J Laparoendosc Adv Surg Tech A.* 2003;13:33–36.

32. Kornaropoulos M, Moris D, Beal EW, et al. Total robotic pancreaticoduodenectomy: a systematic review of the literature. *Surg Endosc*. 2017;31:4382–4392.
33. Zhao W, Liu C, Li S, et al. Safety and efficacy for robot-assisted versus open pancreaticoduodenectomy and distal pancreatectomy: a systematic review and meta-analysis. *Surg Oncol*. 2018;27:468–478.
34. Nassour I, Wang SC, Porembka MR, et al. Robotic versus laparoscopic pancreaticoduodenectomy: a NSQIP analysis. *J Gastrointest Surg*. 2017;21:1784–1792.
35. Zhao Z, Yin Z, Hang Z, et al. A systemic review and an updated meta-analysis: minimally invasive vs open pancreaticoduodenectomy. *Sci Rep*. 2017;7:2220.
36. Boone BA, Zenati M, Hogg ME, et al. Assessment of quality outcomes for robotic pancreaticoduodenectomy: identification of the learning curve. *JAMA Surg*. 2015;150:416–422.
37. Fong Y, Gonen M, Rubin D, et al. Long-term survival is superior after resection for cancer in high-volume centers. *Ann Surg*. 2005;242:540–544; discussion 544–547.
38. Birkmeyer JD, Siewers AE, Finlayson EV, et al. Hospital volume and surgical mortality in the United States. *N Engl J Med*. 2002;346:1128–1137.
39. Cuschieri A. Laparoscopic surgery of the pancreas. *J R Coll Surg Edinb*. 1994;39:178–184.
40. Reich H, McGlynn F, DeCaprio J, et al. Laparoscopic excision of benign liver lesions. *Obstet Gynecol*. 1991;78:956–958.
41. White M, Fong Y, Melstrom L. Minimally invasive surgery of the liver. *Cancer Treat Res*. 2016;168:221–231.
42. Buell JF, Cherqui D, Geller DA, et al. The international position on laparoscopic liver surgery: the Louisville Statement, 2008. *Ann Surg*. 2009;250:825–830.
43. Lee SY, Goh BKP, Sepideh G, et al. Laparoscopic liver resection difficulty score—a validation study. *J Gastrointest Surg*. 2019;23:545–555.
44. Guan R, Chen Y, Yang K, et al. Clinical efficacy of robot-assisted versus laparoscopic liver resection: a meta analysis. *Asian J Surg*. 2019;42:19–31.
45. Melstrom LG, Warner SG, Woo Y, et al. Selecting incision-dominant cases for robotic liver resection: towards outpatient hepatectomy with rapid recovery. *Hepatobiliary Surg Nutr*. 2018;7:77–84.
46. Nota CL, Woo Y, Raoof M, et al. Robotic versus open minor liver resections of the posterosuperior segments: a multinational, propensity score-matched study. *Ann Surg Oncol*. 2019;26:583–590.
47. Lewis TL, Furness HN, Miller GW, et al. Adoption of a novel surgical innovation into clinical practice: protocol for a qualitative systematic review examining surgeon views. *BMJ Open*. 2018;8:e020486.
48. Vyas D, Cronin S. Peer review and surgical innovation: robotic surgery and its hurdles. *Am J Robot Surg*. 2015;2:39–44.
49. Garas G, Cingolani I, Panzarasa P, et al. Network analysis of surgical innovation: measuring value and the virality of diffusion in robotic surgery. *PLoS One*. 2017;12:e0183332.
50. Krummel TM, Gertner M, Makower J, et al. Inventing our future: training the next generation of surgeon innovators. *Semin Pediatr Surg*. 2006;15:309–318.
51. Tom CM, Maciel JD, Korn A, et al. A survey of robotic surgery training curricula in general surgery residency programs: how close are we to a standardized curriculum? *Am J Surg*. 2019;217:256–260.

SECTION III

Trauma and Critical Care

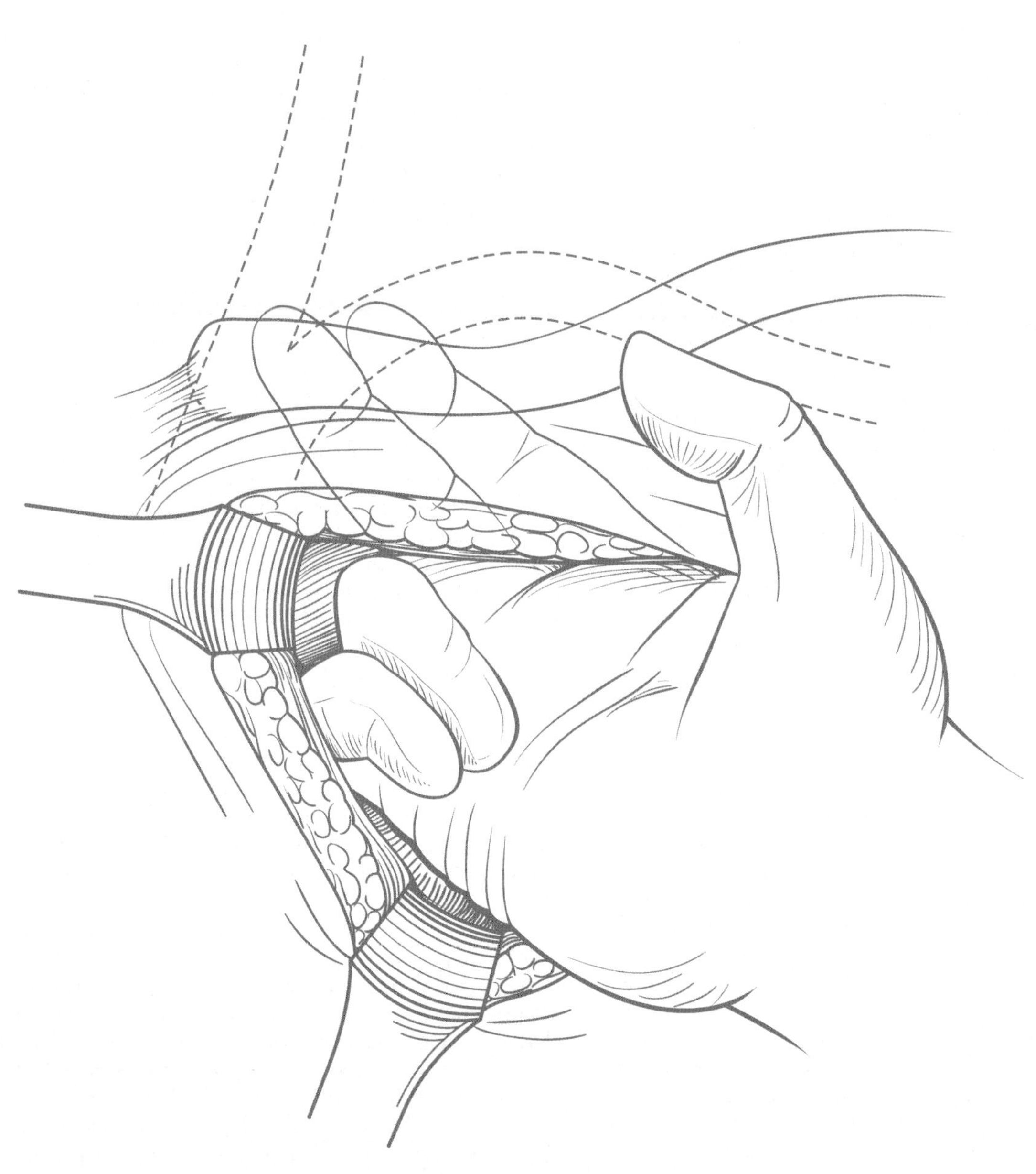

17

Management of Acute Trauma

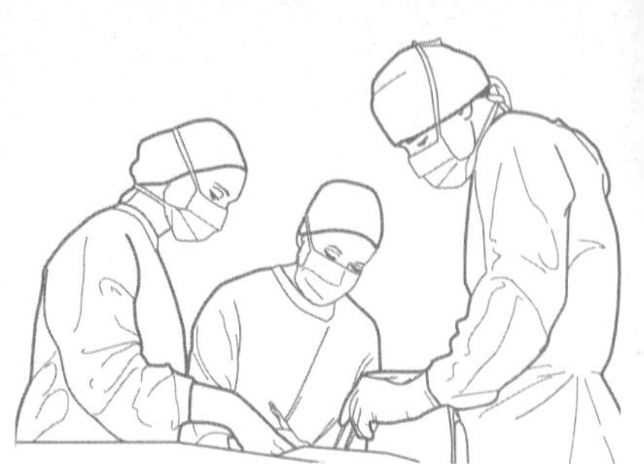

Samuel P. Carmichael II, Nathan T. Mowery, R. Shayn Martin, J. Wayne Meredith

OUTLINE

OVERVIEW AND HISTORY

Injury management has been an important assignment of the practicing surgeon. Throughout the history of medical care, the treatment of trauma necessitates a mastery of diverse skills spanning all areas of anatomy and physiology. Because of the great disease burden due to injury sustained in conflict, care for the trauma patient has been advanced most profoundly during wartime. Box 17.1 lists some major contributions to trauma care that were developed during major U.S. wars. Common themes that have evolved over time include improvements in wound management, resuscitation, and systems of care. Military-based programming and funding continue to formalize this research in the development of care provided in austere and civilian environments. Likewise, advancements in civilian care have had a reciprocal effect within the military. Civilian training of military providers and clinical research on hemostasis and damage control techniques have saved the lives of countless service personnel across the globe.

Traumatology has matured into a distinct surgical field with a unique infrastructure over the last century. After the formation of the American College of Surgeons in 1913, the leadership of the organization appointed a committee to report on the management of fractures. Created in 1922 and chaired by Charles L. Scudder, the Committee on Fractures evolved in 1949 to become the Committee on Trauma (COT), as the need for formal oversight became evident. Beginning with the publication of *Early Care of the Injured*, the COT has been instrumental in advancing trauma care throughout the world via initiatives such as the Advanced Trauma Life Support (ATLS) course, verification of trauma centers, and the development of trauma systems to improve access to care. One of the ways in which the COT has been highly effective is through creation of state-level divisions. Activities of the state committees frequently include (1) trauma system development with the creation of triage documents, maximizing the use of local prehospital and hospital resources, (2) injury prevention initiatives, (3) maintenance of statewide trauma registries, and (4) advancement of performance improvement efforts. To standardize the way in which trauma centers define appropriate structure, process, and outcome, the COT first created in 1976 the *Resources for the Optimal Care of the Injured Patient* reference manual, now freely and electronically accessible in its sixth edition on the American College of Surgeons' website with an associated update for 2019.[1] The COT has also developed the National Trauma Data Bank (NTDB), which is the largest database of trauma ever assembled, currently including more than 7 million patients from 747 trauma centers.[2] Data from the NTDB are included throughout this chapter to provide the reader with up-to-date information on specific injuries.

Beyond the COT, several other professional organizations have been developed with the primary goal of promoting the improvement of trauma care. The American Association for the Surgery of Trauma (AAST) originated in 1938 and is the oldest and largest of all trauma professional organizations. The AAST conducts an annual scientific conference in September that recently has become the Annual Meeting of the AAST and Clinical Congress of Acute Care Surgery. The maturation of this meeting reflects the inclusion of emergency general surgery as a component of acute care surgery into the scientific proceedings. The AAST has also been the lead organization in the development of the acute care surgery training paradigm, which now includes advanced education in trauma, emergency general surgery, and surgical critical care.

BOX 17.1 Advances and discoveries in trauma care during war.

French and Indian War (1754–1763)
Wound contraction during healing
Primary and secondary healing
Description of granulation tissue and epithelialization

American Revolutionary War (1775–1783)
Exhaustive therapy (bleeding, diarrhea, vomiting, salivation, sweating)
Centralization of medical care
Establishment of first medical school

American Civil War (1861–1865)
Primary amputation (vs. secondary)
Use of topical antiseptic agents
Whole blood transfusion
Development of specialty hospitals (eye/ear, orthopedics, hernia)
Extremity traction splinting

World War I (1914–1918)
Laparotomy for penetrating abdominal trauma
Wound debridement and delayed closure
Early use of plasma and crystalloid
First blood bank

World War II (1939–1945)
Guillotine amputation and delayed primary closure
Exteriorization of colon injuries
Mobile surgical teams
Organ dysfunction after injury described

Korean War (1950–1953)
Vascular surgery for limb salvage
Hypovolemic shock recognition
Mobile Army Surgical Hospital (MASH) units

Vietnam War (1955–1964)
Aeromedical transfer (helicopter)
Sulfamylon for burn care
Recognition of acute respiratory distress syndrome (Da Nang lung)

Operation Enduring Freedom (Iraq, 2003 to Present)
Damage control resuscitation
Highly efficient trauma systems
Re-emergence of tourniquet use

Since program inception in 2008, there are currently 21 centers providing training in acute care surgery in accordance with a standardized curriculum. In addition to the AAST, the Eastern Association for the Surgery of Trauma (EAST) and the Western Trauma Association (WTA) comprise partnering academic organizations that promote the exchange of scientific knowledge in trauma care. Both groups contain active multi-institutional trial committees and have focused on the development of practice management guidelines, available electronically on their respective websites. Furthermore, the American Trauma Society, founded in 1968, has been an instrumental part of injury prevention and trauma systems development by advocating for the injured patient and promoting trauma-related legislation. Finally, the Orthopedic Trauma Association, American Association of Neurological Surgeons, and Society of Trauma Nurses represent three organizations whose members are part of the multidisciplinary team dedicated to improving the care of the injured patient.

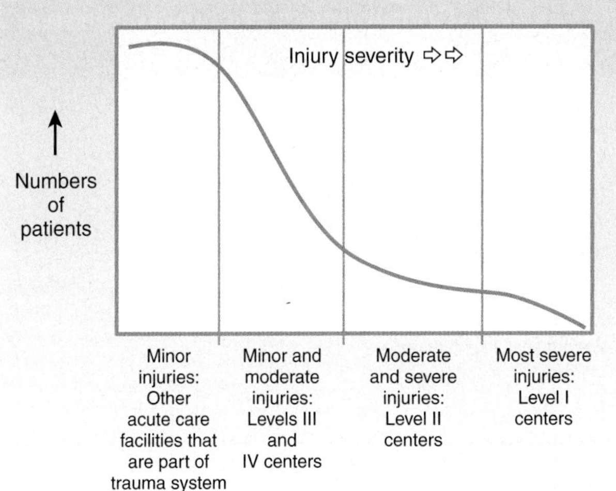

FIG. 17.1 The inclusive trauma system including the relationship between number of patients and severity of injury with respect to trauma facilities. The system is designed to optimally match the level of injury with the capabilities of the medical center. (From American College of Surgeons Committee on Trauma. *Resources for the Optimal Care of the Injured Patient 2014.* 6th ed. Chicago: American College of Surgeons; 2014.)

TRAUMA SYSTEMS

At the most basic level, the primary goal of a trauma system is to get *the right patient to the right place at the right time.* Outcomes in trauma are highly dependent on the geography of injury, and regions that respond best have developed an organized approach to providing all the key elements to maximize meaningful recovery, called a *trauma system.* The ideal trauma system includes the entire care continuum, beginning with prevention and encompassing prehospital care, acute hospital services, postinjury rehabilitation, and research.[1]

As the American healthcare system developed, trauma care was initially centered on the large, academic hospital. All patients were transported to the major trauma center, regardless of the degree of injury. Although this "exclusive" trauma system was beneficial to the severely injured, it resulted in the movement of a significant number of minimally injured patients and failed to capitalize on local resources. Data emerged, revealing similar outcomes and improved measures of efficiency in minimally injured patients managed outside of Level 1 trauma centers.

The solution was the development of a trauma system that includes all hospitals to address the needs of injured patients, regardless of designation (Fig. 17.1). Inclusive trauma systems identify roles for facilities as a continuum, from critical access hospitals to the large Level I and Level II trauma centers. Guided by triage protocols, injured patients are transported to facilities that are appropriate to the severity of the injuries. Although this may require transfer of patients from smaller hospitals to trauma centers, most can receive appropriate treatment within the local network. Box 17.2 lists the common components of an inclusive trauma system that must be coordinated to maximize the effectiveness of care. The benefits of this approach include a reduction in wastefulness of medical resources and allowance of appropriate care within the community.

BOX 17.2 Components of comprehensive inclusive trauma system.

- Injury prevention efforts
- Prehospital care
- Triage
- Communication
- Transportation
- Acute care facilities
- Trauma center designation and verification
- Postacute care and rehabilitation
- Performance improvement
- Education and outreach
- Legislation

The genesis of trauma systems in the United States followed the publication of "Accidental Death and Disability: The Neglected Disease of Modern Society," a landmark report by the National Academy of Sciences in 1966. Congressional legislation (National Highway Safety Act of 1966) was subsequently passed to allocate funding for care of the injured following motor vehicle accidents. Maryland, Illinois, and Florida capitalized on this initiative, first implementing state trauma infrastructures approximately 40 years ago with demonstrable reductions in mortality. A follow-up report, "Injury in America: A Continuing Public Health Problem," was published in 1985 and revealed trauma to be an ongoing issue at the national level. The National Center for Injury Prevention and Control was subsequently installed into the Centers for Disease Control and Prevention (CDC), and Congress legislated the Trauma Care Systems Planning and Development Act of 1990, which formally addressed the need and funding of new or revised state trauma systems. Further advancement occurred in 1992 when the Health Resources and Services Administration released the "Model Trauma Care System Plan," intending to provide each state with a template for systems development. Revised in 2006 and renamed the "Model Trauma System Planning and Evaluation," this work applied a public health disease-based approach to trauma and identified three critical functions: (1) epidemiological assessment, (2) policy implementation for public protection, and (3) high-quality well-regulated care provision.[3]

Evidence for the mortality benefit of trauma system care is provided by two seminal publications. In 2006, the National Study on Costs and Outcomes of Trauma (NSCOT) was performed to evaluate variations in the care provided between trauma centers and nontrauma center hospitals. Supported by the National Center for Injury Prevention and Control of the CDC, NSCOT represents one of the largest epidemiological studies ever to evaluate the care of the injured patient. Including more than 5000 patients from 69 hospitals, NSCOT established that patient outcomes are improved when care is provided at a trauma center versus a nontrauma center. After correction for injury severity, care at a trauma center was associated with a 20% in-hospital mortality reduction and a 25% reduction in 1-year mortality.[4] At the system level, Nathens and colleagues[5] demonstrated the value of a coordinated response to injury after studying 400,000 patients during a 17-year period. The study spanned a length of time (1979–1995) during which trauma systems were established and optimized. After accounting for all possible contributors to improved outcomes, the development of a trauma system resulted in an 8% reduction in mortality during a 15-year period.[5]

TABLE 17.1 Abbreviated Injury Scale (AIS) body regions.

AIS FIRST DIGIT	BODY REGION
1	Head
2	Face
3	Neck
4	Thorax
5	Abdomen
6	Spine
7	Upper extremity
8	Lower extremity
9	Unspecified

Despite the clear progress that has been made in national trauma care over prior decades, there is no "one size fits all" approach and systems implementation must be tailored to locations ranging from rural to urban geographies. In 2015, the COT developed the Needs-Based Assessment of Trauma Systems (NBATS) tool to assist with designation or creation of new trauma centers within a region. Criteria for the tool include point values assigned to six categories within a trauma service area: (1) population, (2) median transport time, (3) community support for a trauma center, (4) number of severely injured patients (Injury Severity Score [ISS] >15) discharged from nontrauma acute care facilities, (5) number of Level 1 trauma centers, and (6) number of severely injured patients evaluated at trauma centers already in the trauma service area.[3] Given overestimations of trauma centers required in rural areas and underestimations of centers already existent in urban areas, a second version (NBATS-2) was created in 2018 to incorporate predictive geospatial modeling. Benefits of this update include assessment of how established center volumes and payer mixes would be affected by the addition of a new trauma center. As the current understanding of trauma systems continues to evolve, tools like these will provide valuable insight into structure and organization unique to each region of the country.

INJURY SCORING

Concurrent with the development of trauma systems has been the need for a reliable method of injury comparison. Scoring systems are typically based on either injury anatomy or the physiology demonstrated after one or more injuries are sustained. The Abbreviated Injury Scale (AIS) has been the most used anatomic system of injury classification since it was first described in 1971. Injuries are characterized by a six-digit taxonomy that includes the body region, type of anatomic structure, and specific anatomic detail of the injury. Table 17.1 demonstrates the body regions and the associated first digit code within the AIS lexicon that allow users of this system to know clearly the location of the injury. Perhaps of even more widespread use is the AIS severity code (frequently described as the post-dot code). This seventh digit describes the severity and potential risk of death for each injury in the AIS system. Post-dot codes range from 1 (minimal severity) to 6 (presumably fatal) and are frequently used to cohort injuries and to compare outcomes. The Association for the Advancement of Automotive Medicine frequently embarks on the rigorous process of refining the AIS to be sure that is stays current in its ability to accurately characterize injury.

The AIS represents the foundation for other scoring systems that are better able to account for the severity of multiple

TABLE 17.2 **Glasgow Coma Scale.**

Eye opening	Spontaneous	4
	To voice	3
	To pain	2
	None	1
Verbal response	Oriented	5
	Confused	4
	Inappropriate	3
	Incomprehensible	2
	None	1
Motor response	Obeys commands	6
	Localizes pain	5
	Withdraws to pain	4
	Flexion	3
	Extension	2
	None	1
Total Glasgow Coma Scale score		3–15

TABLE 17.3 **Revised trauma score.**

Glasgow Coma Scale score	13–15	4
	9–12	3
	6–8	2
	4–5	1
	3	0
Systolic blood pressure (mm Hg)	>89	4
	76–89	3
	50–75	2
	1–49	1
	0	0
Respiratory rate (breaths/min)	10–29	4
	>29	3
	6–9	2
	1–5	1
	0	0
Total revised trauma score		0–12

combined injuries. In 1974, Baker and colleagues presented the ISS, calculated by summing the squares of the AIS severity codes for the three most severely injured body regions. The ISS ranges from 1 to 75, with severity groupings being defined as minor injury (ISS less than 9), moderate injury (ISS between 9 and 16), serious injury (ISS between 16 and 25), and severe injury (ISS more than 25). The ISS has been commonly used throughout the literature to quantify the overall burden of injury sustained by a patient. As a further development in anatomic injury scoring, the Organ Injury Scale (OIS) released by the AAST has been incorporated into the more recent versions of the AIS. By introducing the concept of injury grades, the OIS has added greater anatomic detail for specific organs and incorporated the ability to better delineate organ injury severity. This OIS severity has been validated with the NTDB to optimize the associated risk of morbidity and mortality.

In addition to anatomic scoring systems, other scales have been developed that include the physiologic insult from injury. These physiologic scoring systems are more capable of identifying the overall condition and can also better guide real-time decision-making. One commonly used scale of this type is the Glasgow Coma Scale (GCS), which reflects level of consciousness. With scores ranging from 3 to 15, the GCS is composed of a measure of eye opening, verbal response, and motor function. The GCS, specifically the motor score alone, has been found to be reflective of outcomes after traumatic brain injury (TBI).[6] The Revised Trauma Score is another well-studied physiologic scoring system that characterizes the condition of the injured patient by incorporating the GCS, systolic blood pressure, and respiratory rate. These scores have been of value for research purposes and have been successfully used to make triage decisions. To better demonstrate the way in which the GCS and Revised Trauma Score are designed, Tables 17.2 and 17.3 reflect how these scores are calculated.

PREHOSPITAL TRAUMA CARE

Immediately after a patient is injured, the trauma system engages the prehospital phase of care. The goal of the prehospital system is to move a patient to a location capable of providing definitive injury management as quickly as possible. The prehospital team plays an integral role in the management of the trauma patient because of the time-dependent nature of injury. The initial approach to the injured patient in the prehospital setting includes four key priorities:

1. Evaluate the scene.
2. Perform an initial assessment.
3. Make triage-transport decision.
4. Initiate critical interventions and transport the patient.

After-scene safety is ensured to protect our prehospital providers. The initial assessment should be rapidly completed. The initial assessment consists of a systematic approach to immediately identify life-threatening conditions that require urgent intervention. The ABC mnemonic guides the initial assessment, during which **a**irway, **b**reathing, and **c**irculation are sequentially evaluated and addressed. While the spine is protected, the airway is secured and assisted ventilation is provided as necessary. External hemorrhage is identified and immediately controlled while resuscitation is initiated.

Emergent interventions in the field can be immediately lifesaving, but optimal outcomes ultimately depend on quickly making an effective triage and transport decision. Using the "load and go" approach, all essential prehospital interventions can be provided while the patient is being transported. A recent NTDB review by Chen and colleagues[7] demonstrated that trauma patients with prehospital hypotension (<90 mm Hg), GCS of ≤8, and nonextremity firearm injury have higher mortality with increasing prehospital time.

All prehospital teams know that immediate departure from the scene is paramount, but identifying where to go and how to get there can be more challenging. Well-defined protocols should guide the field triage process so that teams know immediately where to transport a patient. Fig. 17.2 demonstrates the Field Triage Decision Scheme, which was developed by the CDC and included in recent editions of the COT reference, *Resources for the Optimal Care of the Injured Patient*, and the *Advanced Trauma Life Support (ATLS)*, 10th edition 2018 update.[8] Using physiologic status, mechanism of injury, and other indicators of a high-risk patient, this tool assists in determining which patients might benefit from care at a trauma center. Most prehospital agencies attempt to assess a patient rapidly and initiate the transport process while minimizing the scene time to less than 15 minutes.

The initial clinical concern that the prehospital team must assess is the airway. The "gold standard" for airway maintenance

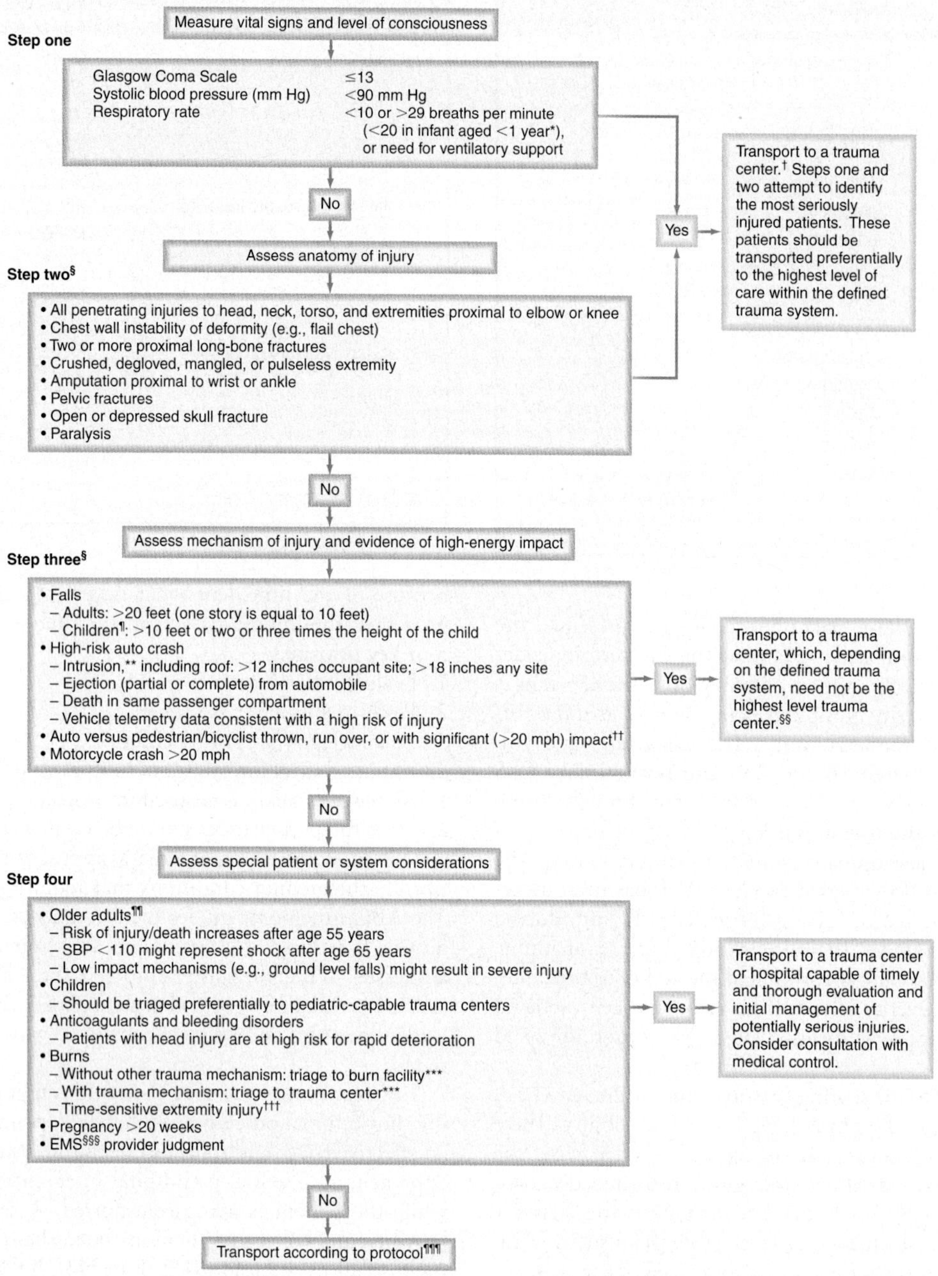

FIG. 17.2 Guidelines for field triage of injured patients, which were created to guide the development of state and local EMS systems triage protocols. The guidelines use four decision steps (physiologic, anatomic, mechanism of injury, and special considerations) to direct triage decisions within the local trauma system. (From Sasser SM, Hunt RC, Faul M, et al. Centers for Disease Control and Prevention: Guidelines for field triage of injured patients: recommendations of the National Expert Panel on Field Triage, 2011. *MMWR Recomm Rep.* 2012;61:1–20.). *EMS*, Emergency medical services; *SBP*, systolic blood pressure. Source: Adapted from American College of Surgeons. *Resources for the Optimal Care of the Injured Patient.* Chicago, IL: American College of Surgeons; 2006. Footnotes have been added to enhance understanding of field triage by persons outside the acute injury care field. *The upper limit of respiratory rate in infants is >29 breaths per minute to maintain a higher level of overtriage for infants. †Trauma centers are designated Level I–IV, with Level I representing the highest level of trauma care available. §Any injury noted in steps two and three triggers a "yes" response. ¶Age <15 years. **Intrusion refers to interior compartment intrusion, as opposed to deformation, which refers to exterior damage. ††Includes pedestrians or bicyclists thrown or run over by a motor vehicle or those with estimated impact >20 mph with a motor vehicle. §§Local or regional protocols should be used to determine the most appropriate level of trauma center; appropriate center need not be Level I. ¶¶Age >55 years. ***Patients with both burns and concomitant trauma for whom the burn injury poses the greatest risk for morbidity and mortality should be transferred to a burn center. If the nonburn trauma presents a greater immediate risk, the patient may be stabilized in a trauma center and then transferred to a burn center. †††Injuries such as an open fracture or fracture with neurovascular compromise. §§§Emergency medical services. ¶¶¶Patients who do not meet any of the triage criteria in steps 1 through 4 should be transported to the most appropriate medical facility as outlined in local EMS protocols.)

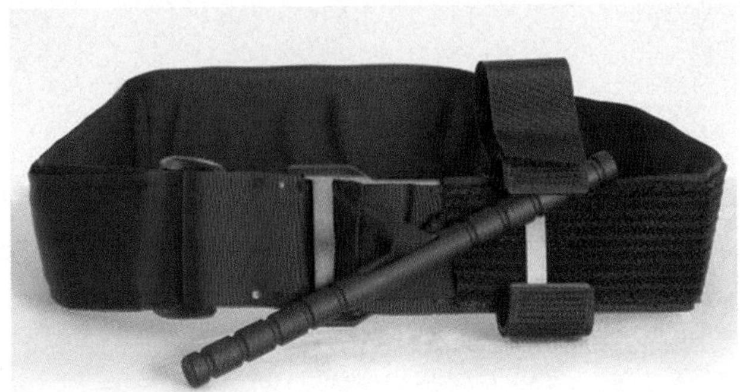

FIG. 17.3 Example of a tourniquet. Tourniquets are commonly being used to prevent extremity exsanguination in military and civilian prehospital environments.

in the severely injured patient remains endotracheal intubation, typically using a rapid-sequence intubation (RSI) or drug-assisted intubation (DAI) technique. One must always assume that the patient has a spine injury and appropriately maintain spinal precautions. The utility of advanced airway management in the field has been questioned, with no high-quality prospective evidence in the literature. Previous studies have reported that airway management with endotracheal intubation is associated with increased mortality when compared to noninvasive techniques. Conversely, other investigators have suggested the benefit of advanced prehospital airway support in a select group of patients (i.e., neurologic outcome in severe TBI).[9] In reality, the decision to establish a prehospital advanced airway is a complex decision, weighing the technical and physiologic consequences of RSI (i.e., cardiovascular collapse in hemorrhagic shock) against the possible benefits of airway protection and oxygen delivery. As an alternative, blind insertion supraglottic airway devices have become common and add great value in providing a bridge to a more definitive solution. Regardless of the approach implemented by the prehospital agency, personnel need to have the ability to manage all levels of airway compromise while transporting the patient to definitive care.

External hemorrhage control and initiation of resuscitation are critical needs during the prehospital phase of care. Direct pressure remains the mainstay of hemorrhage control, although tourniquet use has become more common in the management of exsanguinating extremity trauma. For some time, tourniquets were infrequently used because of concern about causing unnecessary muscle and nerve injury. Driven by military experience and advances in device development, tourniquets have demonstrated benefit in select situations. Recent publications now report a mortality benefit related to the use of prehospital tourniquets in the civilian sector. In response, the American College of Surgeons has developed the Stop the Bleed campaign, whereby laypeople are instructed in proper application of extremity tourniquets. Prehospital agencies now commonly include tourniquets on their standard equipment lists so that they may be used when a patient with uncontrolled extremity bleeding is encountered. Many commercial devices are available, and Fig. 17.3 illustrates an example of a tourniquet that can be used in the prehospital setting.

As hemorrhage is the primary cause of preventable trauma mortality, patients in shock require initiation of prehospital resuscitation concurrent with efforts toward temporary hemorrhage control. Prior studies have demonstrated that large-volume crystalloid-based resuscitation is detrimental, suggesting that blood products may be the superior resuscitative fluid. In a recent pragmatic, multicenter, cluster randomized trial of helicopter transported patients in hemorrhagic shock, packed red blood cells (PRBCs) administered with plasma conferred the greatest survival benefit, followed by plasma alone and PRBC alone. Among patients who would have qualified to receive blood products, administration of crystalloid increased mortality incrementally by dose.[10] These data are in contrast to a second randomized controlled trial in which ground ambulance teams administered either 2 units of plasma or crystalloid alone to hypotensive patients en route to the hospital. No associated survival benefit was noted in the group receiving plasma-based resuscitation.[11] Ultimately, prehospital plasma may be of greatest benefit to a select group of patients with moderate transfusion requirements, as the mortality-reducing effect was not seen in patients who went on to receive ongoing massive transfusion (>10 units PRBC in initial 24 hours).[12] Although the ideal resuscitative scheme has yet to be identified, many of the challenges limiting prehospital transfusion are logistical in nature (i.e., supply, storage, cost). As a result, many prehospital agencies provide mixed crystalloid and product-based resuscitation practices, based on local resources.

INITIAL ASSESSMENT AND MANAGEMENT

The mainstay of the initial approach to the injured patient is the ATLS course. Since its development in 1980, ATLS has instructed more than 1 million students of trauma in 86 countries. The course has provided a structured, standardized approach to the injured patient that is based on the concept of rapidly identifying and addressing life-threatening conditions during the initial assessment of the patient.[8] More specifically, ATLS conveys three important concepts that greatly enhance the ability to manage injured patients, regardless of where care is provided:

1. Treat the greatest threat to life first.
2. The lack of a definitive diagnosis should not delay the application of an indicated urgent treatment.
3. An initial, detailed history is not essential to begin the evaluation of a patient with acute injuries.

Following a defined order of assessment, life-threatening conditions are immediately addressed at the time of identification. This initial assessment, also termed the *primary survey*, follows the mnemonic ABCDE (Fig. 17.4):

Airway and cervical spine protection
Breathing
Circulation
Disability or neurologic condition
Exposure and environmental control

In addition, the primary survey can be repeated any time there is a change in condition. Despite being simple in design, the primary survey offers a tool that the surgeon can trust to identify what life-threatening condition exists and where to direct clinical effort. The following outlines describe the performance of the primary survey.

Airway

Upon arrival of the patient to the trauma bay, the status of the airway should be immediately assessed. Simply eliciting a verbal response provides the most meaningful information, as the ability to speak usually indicates adequate airway protection. Patients who cannot speak have either mental status depression or some obstruction to air flow, both of which are indications for airway management. Further indicators of airway compromise include

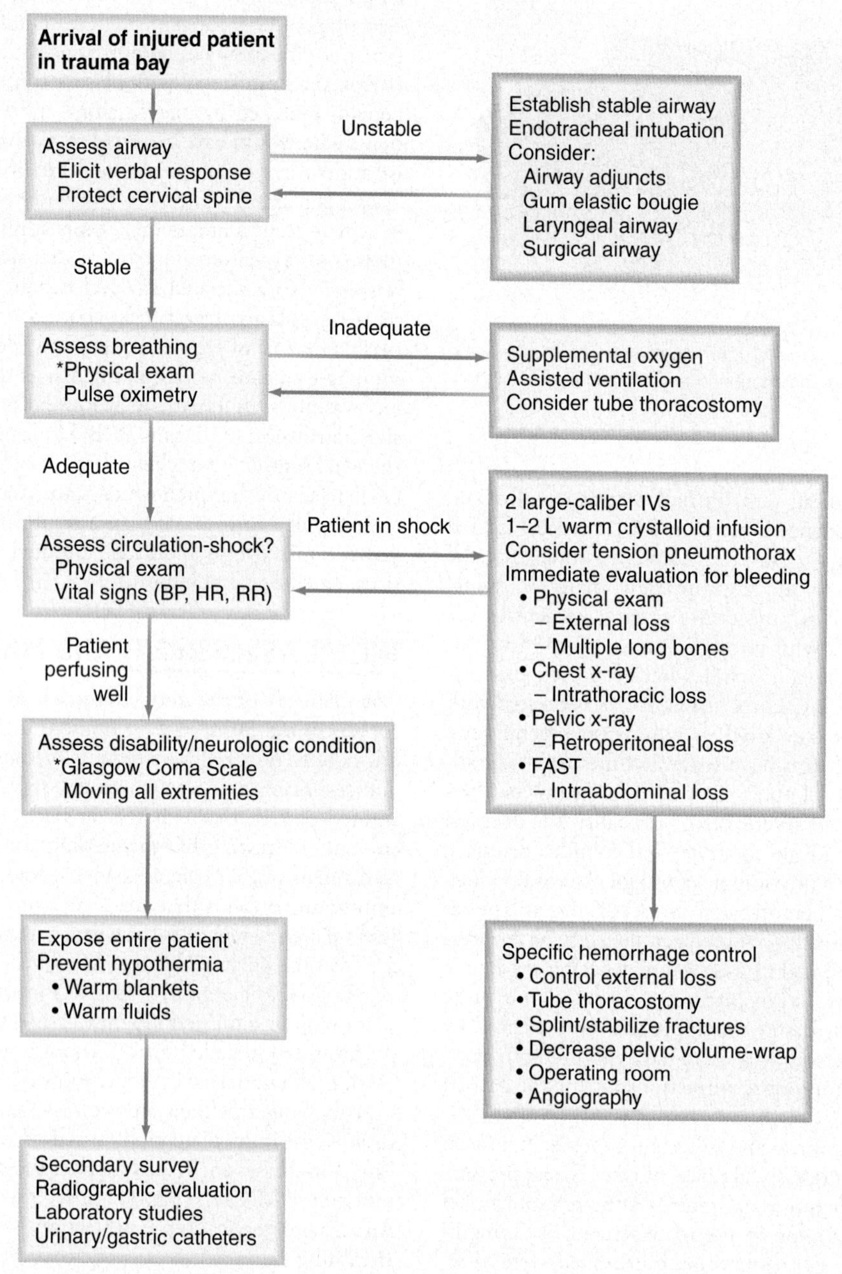

FIG. 17.4 Algorithm for the initial assessment of the injured patient. *BP*, Blood pressure; *FAST*, focused abdominal sonography in trauma; *HR*, heart rate; *RR*, respiratory rate.

noisy breathing, severe facial trauma (specifically with oropharyngeal blood or foreign body), and patient agitation. A determination of the adequacy of the airway, as well as the decision to obtain improved airway control, should be completed within seconds of arrival. After the initial assessment, frequent reassessment for deterioration and the development of airway compromise is paramount.

Until it is ruled out with an appropriate evaluation, all injured patients should be assumed to have an injury to the vertebral column and have the appropriate precautions maintained. This is of significant importance during the manipulation of the head and neck while the airway is being managed. Cervical spine protection includes the use of a hard cervical collar and the maintenance of the log roll technique for all movement of the patient. During airway assessment and management, the anterior portion of the cervical collar can be removed to optimize exposure, but manual stabilization from an assistant should be provided when the collar is not securely in place. Rigid long spine boards may be of value during transport of the patient but should be removed as soon as possible to avoid pressure-related wounds that can occur within a short time.

When the airway is deemed inadequate, a definitive airway must be established. The definitive airway of choice for most injured patients remains oral endotracheal intubation provided by RSI or DAI (*ATLS* 10th edition) technique. While the patient is being prepared for intubation, adjuncts such as oropharyngeal

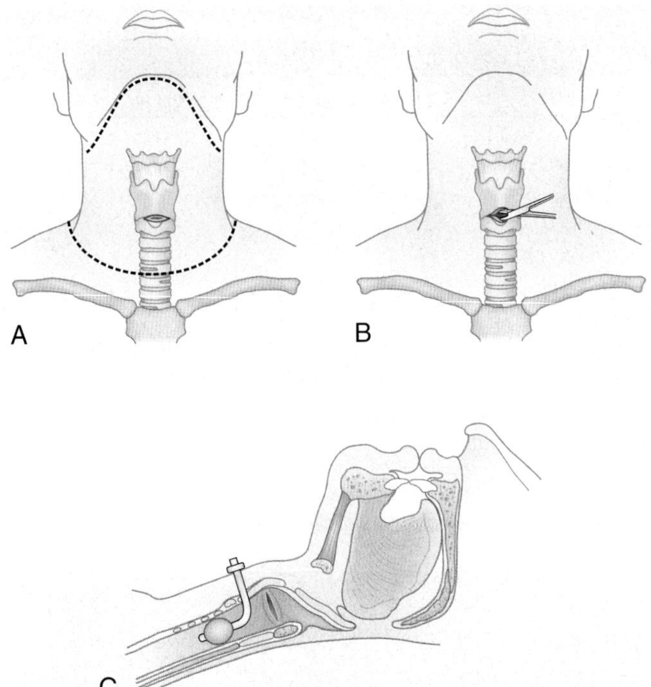

FIG. 17.5 Technique of cricothyroidotomy. The cricothyroid membrane is identified by palpation, and a longitudinal incision is first made along the trachea (A). The incision and dissection are continued through the cricothyroid membrane in transverse fashion, and the cricothyroidotomy is spread (B), allowing the passage of a tracheal tube (C).

and nasopharyngeal airways may assist in maintaining airway patency during preoxygenation. The patient is provided a sedative and fast-acting neuromuscular blocker, such as succinylcholine or rocuronium, to enhance glottic visualization maximally. Direct laryngoscopy and endotracheal intubation are performed, with care taken to avoid cervical spine motion. The appropriate position of the tube in the trachea is confirmed by chest auscultation, end-tidal carbon dioxide measurement, and a chest radiograph. The presence of experienced airway personnel is critical and, particularly in trauma centers, is often an important component of the trauma alert system.

Common adjuncts in the difficult airway scenario include the gum elastic bougie, video-assisted laryngoscopy, and blind insertion airway device. When the normal view of the glottis is obscured, the bougie may be placed with a limited view of the vocal cords, assisting with appropriate placement the endotracheal tube. Although prior studies have suggested improvement in success rates of intubation with bougie, a recent systematic review and metaanalysis concluded that equivalent rates of first-attempt intubation, intubation duration, and esophageal intubation were observed with techniques incorporating either bougie or stylet. The authors further note that available studies comprising the analysis include small sample sizes and heterogeneous types of providers performing the procedure.[13]

Several devices are now available that provide the clinician a view of the upper airway anatomy that is displayed on a video monitor. Despite this mitigation of challenges related to the angle of the airway, recent data have yielded conflicting results as to any improvement in successful first-pass orotracheal intubation.[14] In parallel to the utility of the bougie, a device is only as functional as the provider employing it. Whichever adjunct, or combination thereof, is selected in the setting of a difficult airway, familiarity with benefits, risks, and limitations of the tool is upon the person performing the procedure.

The blind insertion airway device offers an additional instrument to be applied when attempts at orotracheal intubation are unsuccessful. Devices such as the laryngeal mask airway, multilumen esophageal airway (Combitube), and laryngeal tube airway (King LT-D) are placed blindly and function by occluding the esophagus and the posterior pharynx, allowing assisted ventilation to pass selectively down the trachea.

As airway specialists are transitioning to advanced techniques, preparation for a surgical airway should begin. Before physiologic deterioration, a cricothyroidotomy should be performed when other approaches have failed. The inability to maintain oxygenation with a bag valve mask between intubation attempts is a reasonable indication for establishment of a surgical airway. A cricothyroidotomy (Fig. 17.5) is performed in a three-step maneuver:

1. Spreading retraction with the nondominant hand of the tissues overlying the cricothyroid space (typically performed from patient's right side).
2. Keeping lateral tension on the tissues, vertically incise in the tracheal midline, beginning at the thyroid cartilage and extending inferior to the cricoid cartilage.
3. Transversely incising the cricothyroid membrane, which can be palpated between the thyroid cartilage and cricoid ring, followed by insertion of a 6-0 endotracheal tube or tracheostomy appliance.

It is critical that the surgeon frequently palpate the underlying structures to guide the dissection and avoid injury to more lateral structures of the neck. Care must be taken also to avoid advancing an endotracheal tube past the carina, which is common in these situations. Tube position is immediately confirmed with lung auscultation and end-tidal carbon dioxide determination. Finally, patients suspected of having a laryngeal injury may have abnormal anatomy in the vicinity of the cricothyroid membrane and therefore require a tracheostomy rather than a cricothyroidotomy.

Breathing

Following the management of the airway, breathing is evaluated by visualizing chest movement, auscultating breath sounds, and measuring oxygen saturation. Limited respiratory effort or dyspnea requires support of ventilation and further assessment of the chest. Ventilatory problems may be secondary to tension pneumothorax, massive hemothorax, or flail chest with pulmonary contusion. Tension pneumothorax may cause respiratory deterioration but may also be in the form of unstable hemodynamics or cardiovascular collapse. It is a clinical diagnosis that should be recognized on the primary survey without need for radiographic confirmation before treatment. Deviation of the trachea in the sternal notch with unilaterally absent or diminished breath sounds and cardiopulmonary compromise should immediately suggest tension pneumothorax. Thoracic decompression should be rapidly performed with a large-bore needle or tube thoracostomy, depending on the availability of equipment and supplies. Massive hemothorax also requires tube thoracostomy with evacuation of blood and reexpansion of the lung. Severe pulmonary contusion commonly requires aggressive mechanical ventilation, often with elevated levels of positive end-expiratory pressure. To avoid loss of positive end-expiratory pressure, one should resist repeated disconnection from the ventilator to suction or manually ventilate the patient, as oxygenation will only improve with an uninterrupted circuit.

BOX 17.3 Indicators of shock in the injured patient.

- Agitation or confusion
- Tachycardia
- Tachypnea
- Diaphoresis
- Cool, mottled extremities
- Weak distal pulses
- Decreased pulse pressure
- Decreased urine output
- Hypotension

Circulation

The primary goal of a cardiovascular assessment is determining the presence or absence of shock. ATLS defines shock clinically as evidence of end-organ hypoperfusion present on physical exam. Clinical signs of shock are demonstrated in Box 17.3. Although hypotension is a clear indicator of cardiovascular decompensation, patients may be in shock well before the onset of hypotension, given physiologic compensatory mechanisms. By far, the most common cause of shock in the injured patient is hemorrhage, and acute blood loss must be ruled out before other causes are considered. Table 17.4 indicates the different classes of hemorrhagic shock.

Upon recognizing the presence of shock, ATLS recommends intravenous (IV) access with two large-bore, short, peripheral IV catheters, an intraosseous needle, or a central venous catheter and initial resuscitation with 1 L of warmed crystalloid solution. Patients who fail to respond appropriately to initial crystalloid resuscitation should undergo product-based resuscitation, recognizing that crystalloid resuscitation beyond 1.5 L increases risk of death.[8]

The patient must next undergo a rapid screen to identify the cause of life-threatening blood loss. There are essentially five major locations through which exsanguination may occur: chest, abdomen, retroperitoneum, pelvis, and/or long bone fractures. The initial physical examination identifies sources of external blood loss and long bone fractures. These are managed immediately with direct pressure and fracture splinting, respectively. Adjunctive imaging to the primary survey includes x-ray examinations (i.e., chest and pelvis) and ultrasound. A chest film quickly evaluates for hemothorax and a pelvic film will identify pelvic fracture. The focused abdominal sonography in trauma (FAST) scan is a rapidly obtainable ultrasound examination that assesses for intraperitoneal fluid. Specifically, the FAST scan assesses the hepatorenal, splenorenal, and pelvic spaces for fluid, which is presumed to be blood in the setting of trauma. The value of the FAST scan is that it can be performed quickly in the trauma bay and rapidly repeated, if necessary. As an example, blood in the hepatorenal space on FAST scan is demonstrated by Fig. 17.6.

After the initial administration of IV fluid, patients are assessed for ongoing signs of shock. Those who respond by demonstrating a normalizing physiologic state then undergo a comprehensive evaluation to identify all injuries. A common pitfall during this time is to continue administering IV fluids at a high rate that may mask ongoing blood loss. As mentioned previously, failure to respond to the initial crystalloid bolus likely indicates continued bleeding, necessitating immediate intervention. Ongoing intrathoracic bleeding after chest tube placement may require thoracotomy. Intraabdominal bleeding in the hemodynamically unstable patient warrants emergent laparotomy. Pelvic fractures require immediate management of any increased pelvic volume with a binder or sheet, followed by operative or angiographic treatment with embolization for arterial hemorrhage.

TABLE 17.4 Types of shock in the injured patient.

	CLASS I	CLASS II	CLASS III	CLASS IV
Blood volume loss (%)	<15	15–30	30–40	>40
Heart rate	—	—/↑	↑	↑↑
Blood pressure	—	—	—/↓	↓
Pulse pressure	—	↓	↓	↓
Respiratory rate	—	—	—/↑	↑
Urine output	—	—	↓	↓↓
GCS	—	—	↓	↓
Base deficit (mEq/L)	0 to −2	−2 to −6	−6 to −10	−10 or <
Need for transfusion	Monitor	Possible	Yes	MTP

Modified from American College of Surgeons: Committee on Trauma. *Advanced Trauma Life Support*. 10th ed. Chicago: American College of Surgeons; 2018.

GCS, Glasgow Coma Scale; *MTP*, massive transfusion protocol.

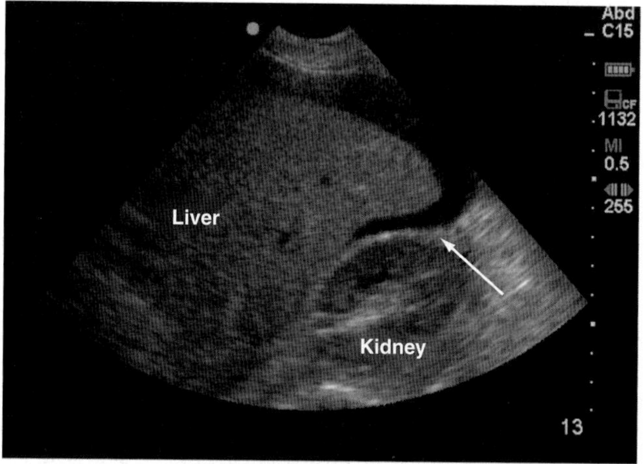

FIG. 17.6 Focused abdominal sonography in trauma scan demonstrating fluid in the hepatorenal space (Morison pouch). The *arrow* identifies fluid (blood) between the liver and the right kidney.

Disability and Exposure

During the primary survey, it is valuable to make a rapid determination of neurologic function. Of particular importance is globally characterizing neurologic function to assess for traumatic brain and spinal cord injuries (SCIs). The GCS score should be determined to identify deficits in eye opening, verbal ability, and motor responses to potentially reflect the degree of neurologic injury. When sedating medications are required, noting the baseline level of neurologic function before administration can be beneficial. The spinal cord is grossly assessed by visualizing movement of the extremities. While neurogenic shock should always be considered in the setting of hypotension with lack of extremity movement, the provider must be careful in attributing shock to an SCI due to the frequency of hemorrhage in the trauma patient. It is important to recognize that classic teaching requires a cervical or high thoracic spine injury to produce neurogenic shock. If a patient is able to move their upper extremities, the likelihood of neurogenic shock is greatly diminished.

All clothing is removed at this time to allow for an adequate examination, core body temperature measurement, and any required intervention. As hypothermia is one of the components in the "terrible triad of death" in trauma (coagulopathy, acidosis, hypothermia), efforts to restore physiologic body temperature with blankets, heating elements (i.e., Bair Hugger), elevated room/operating room (OR) temperature, and warmed resuscitative fluids are of critical importance.

Resuscitative Thoracotomy and Endovascular Aortic Occlusion

After critical injury, select patients who experience cardiac arrest may benefit from resuscitative thoracotomy (RT) in the emergency department. First formally described by Cooley and Debakey over 50 years ago for penetrating cardiovascular trauma, RT provides opportunity for four therapeutic maneuvers: release of cardiac tamponade, temporary repair of cardiac injury, cross-clamping the distal thoracic aorta, and management of intrathoracic bleeding. Given risks to health care providers performing the procedure and overall low rates of salvage, multiple studies have attempted to define what groups of patients should be candidates for the procedure on the basis of injury mechanism and physiology at the time of presentation. Patients with the best outcomes after RT are those with penetrating thoracic injuries and signs of life (reactive pupils, spontaneous ventilation, carotid pulse, measurable or palpable blood pressure, extremity movement, or cardiac electrical activity) upon reaching the emergency department. Seamon and colleagues reviewed 72 studies with 10,238 patients, concluding that patients presenting after penetrating chest mechanism, with and without signs of life, survived at 21.3% and 8.3%, respectively. By converse, blunt trauma patients presenting with and without signs of life reveals 4.6% and 0.7% survival from RT, respectively.[15] Moreover, an NTDB review of 11,380 patients undergoing RT revealed a 100% mortality in both blunt and penetrating mechanisms for patients above the age of 57.[16] In these circumstances, bilateral thoracostomy tubes with conservative transfusion measures are likely more appropriate. RT should only be performed in locations with readily available surgical support for definitive repair of thoracic injuries if return of spontaneous circulation is achieved.

Resuscitative endovascular balloon occlusion of the aorta (REBOA) has emerged over the past decade as a promising method of obtaining temporary hemorrhage control in the decompensating trauma patient. Although traditionally employed in the setting of abdominal aortic aneurysm repair, application for combat casualty care in noncompressible truncal hemorrhage was first described during the Korean War. With the evolution of this technology for rapid deployment in both military and civilian sectors, REBOA is now being used in approximately 51 domestic trauma centers (median 6 cases per center per year) in the setting of advanced shock and imminent cardiac arrest. Depending on the zone of trauma, REBOA is introduced through the common femoral artery, advanced proximal to level of injury, and inflated, effectively shunting blood to the heart and brain while also decreasing hemorrhage. Currently, there is no high-grade evidence to support indications or the superiority of REBOA beyond standard care, and a comparison of technique to RT introduces both survival and indication biases. Deployment of this technology should only take place within a trauma system capable of managing definitive surgical hemostasis and the multiple possible complications of placement (i.e., vascular injury, extremity ischemia, spinal cord ischemia). At present, protocols for utility are developed by multidisciplinary committee and may vary by institution.[17]

Secondary Survey

ATLS defines the secondary survey as a thorough head-to-toe examination and patient history. This is often performed immediately after the primary survey in patients who are stable and not requiring emergent intervention. Findings identified during the secondary survey often prompt further evaluation with imaging or other diagnostic modalities. A more detailed neurologic evaluation can be completed at this time and abnormalities of the face and neck are identified. Posterior surfaces that are more difficult to visualize because of the cervical collar are now better examined. The torso is evaluated to identify evidence of pulmonary dysfunction, and findings consistent with peritonitis must be recognized. Seat belt marks or other superficial injury to the neck and abdomen may prompt further evaluation. The pelvis is assessed for tenderness and instability, with care taken to avoid excessive compression. A rectal examination with a nonbloody glove to assess the position of the prostate and the presence of gross gastrointestinal (GI) blood should be included. The extremities are manipulated to identify open or closed deformities and distal perfusion must be carefully assessed. Formal evaluation consisting of distal blood pressure measurements with comparison to uninjured extremities (i.e., ankle-brachial indices) is valuable to obviate further imaging for major vascular injuries. The patient is rolled to evaluate the spine for deformity or tenderness and the long spine board should be removed. In the setting of penetrating trauma, all possible areas of skin must be visualized, including those within body folds, scalp, posterior neck, mouth, axilla, perineum, and back. Marking of penetrating injuries with radiopaque markers can be extremely helpful if subsequent imaging studies are obtained.

MANAGEMENT OF SPECIFIC INJURIES

Damage Control Principles

The concept of damage control arose in contrast to the traditional approach of definitive injury repair at index operation. It was noted that a portion of patients in the latter group would develop progressive intraoperative physiologic derangement with exacerbation of hypothermia, coagulopathy, and metabolic acidosis. Therefore, damage control emerged as a method of halting this rapid deterioration by expeditious hemostasis, including application of packs, management of GI contamination with repair or resection, and temporary abdominal closure. The patient was then transported to the intensive care unit, and definitive reconstruction could be delayed until resuscitation had been completed. Rotondo and associates first coined the term "damage control" to describe this approach to management in a series of 46 patients operated for penetrating abdominal injury. While actual survival rates were similar between damage control and definitive laparotomy groups (55% vs. 58%, respectively), a significant improvement in survival was noted in a subset of patients with major vascular injury and two or more visceral injuries (77% vs. 11%, $P < 0.02$).[18] Although damage control began as a method to manage severe abdominal injuries, it is now universally used in the chest, pelvis, and extremities.

Functioning in tandem with damage control surgery, massive transfusion protocols (MTPs) have emerged from the military experience to reveal improved survival with transfusion of equivalent blood component ratios (1:1:1—plasma, platelets, PRBC) in

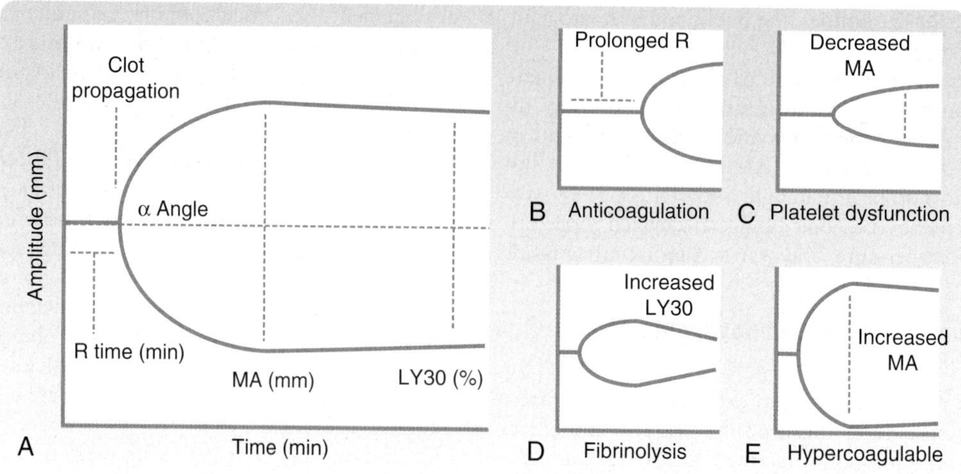

FIG. 17.7 Thromboelastogram (TEG) with standard parameters and pathologies. (A) Normal TEG. (B) Delayed clot formation with prolonged R time, treated with plasma transfusion. (C) Decreased maximum amplitude with low platelet function, treated with platelet transfusion. (D) Elevated LY30 representing fibrinolysis, treated with tranexamic acid. (E) Decreased R time and elevated MA representing hypercoagulable state. *α Angle*, Clot formation/polymerization; *LY30*, percent amplitude decrease at 30 minutes, index of clot breakdown (lysis); *MA*, maximum amplitude, clot strength; *R time*, time to clot formation.

order to approximate whole blood. This approach to the severely injured patient was termed damage control resuscitation and defined by permissive hypotension, facilitation of rapid hemostasis with early balanced transfusion, treatment of coagulopathy, and minimization of crystalloid.[19] To inform initiation of MTP, the Assessment of Blood Consumption score provides a 4-point metric (penetrating mechanism, positive FAST, arrival systolic blood pressure 90 mm Hg, and arrival pulse >120 bpm) whereby clinicians may request product coolers based on prehospital (if available) or initial vital signs. A score of at least 2 was predictive of MTP need (75% sensitivity, 86% specificity) and a delay in initiation is associated with a 5% increase in mortality per minute.[20] Many trauma centers have adopted this strategy and now have well-defined MTPs.

In certain locations, thromboelastography (TEG) provides adjunctive guidance to ongoing MTP and is rapidly obtainable as a point-of-care metric. Originally developed approximately 70 years ago for assessment of inherited bleeding disorders, TEG has historically been employed in liver transplant and cardiac surgery. In traditional analyzers, clot formation is assessed based on resistance transduced from a pin in a small quantity (360 μL) of whole blood. As the blood oscillates, a real-time graphic is produced, providing a dynamic representation of clot generation. Component deficiencies are illustrated as morphologic changes to the clot cylinder (Fig. 17.7). Potential advantages to utilization of TEG-based resuscitation include rapid results for individualized component transfusion, overall conservation of blood products, and a survival benefit with fewer deaths due to hemorrhagic shock in the first 6 hours after injury.[21]

Lastly, an additional treatment adjunct to MTP in damage control resuscitation is tranexamic acid (TXA). TXA is a synthetic derivative of lysine with high affinity for lysine binding sites on plasminogen, thus inhibiting fibrinolysis via antagonism of plasmin binding to fibrin surfaces. It has been shown previously to reduce the need for blood transfusion in elective surgery by one third. The Clinical Randomization of an Antifibrinolytic in Significant Hemorrhage (CRASH)-2 trial randomized 20,211 injured patients to either early administration of TXA (within 8 hours) versus placebo. Patients who received TXA demonstrated a decrease in all-cause mortality compared with placebo (14.5% vs. 16%, P = 0.0035) and a reduction in risk of death due to bleeding (4.9% vs. 5.7%, P = 0.0077). Notably, there was no observed difference in rates of vascular occlusive events between the treatment and placebo groups (1.7% vs. 2.0%, respectively). While the study had limitations due to the inclusion of large numbers that did not require transfusion, it has led to TXA becoming a standard part of the initial resuscitation within many prehospital systems and trauma centers.[22]

Injuries to the Brain

Even in the setting of optimal care, TBIs result in substantial morbidity and account for approximately one-third of all trauma-related mortality, resulting in an annual cost of $75 billion to the U.S. economy. Those who survive often experience permanent disability that ranges from mild deficits to conditions requiring permanent total care. Outcomes faced by patients who sustain polytrauma are often dictated predominantly by the TBI. As injury epidemiology has evolved, falls are now the most common cause of brain injuries, with those at the extremes of age being most vulnerable. Although further high-quality evidence for TBI is needed, comprehensive guidelines for management are described by the Brain Trauma Foundation, American College of Surgeons, EAST, and WTA.[23]

At the tissue level, brain injuries are the result of either direct transmission of energy, the accumulation of blood within the cranium, or a combination of the two. Energy transmitted to the cranium and the underlying brain tissue can cause direct injury both at the location of contact and on the contralateral side (coup contrecoup). Further, the shearing of blood vessels at the time of injury can result in the accumulation of blood within the cranium. As is the case with most tissue, injured brain develops inflammation and edema after trauma that can be worsened by ongoing ischemia. According to the Monro-Kellie doctrine, any increase in the volume of intracranial contents (from extravascular blood or edema) results in an elevation of intracranial pressure (ICP) with an associated decrease in the volume of other tissues (i.e., brain parenchyma, intravascular blood, and cerebrospinal fluid [CSF]).

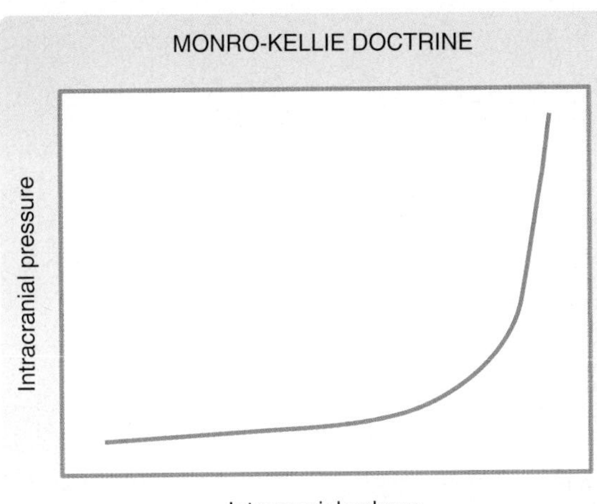

FIG. 17.8 Monro-Kellie doctrine, which describes the increase in intracranial pressure as intracranial volume increases from hemorrhage or edema. This relationship of pressure to volume is a result of the rigid cranial vault that exhibits a fixed volume.

As seen in Fig. 17.8, an increase in intracranial volume ultimately results in an exponential increase in ICP, thereby worsening cerebral perfusion pressure (CPP), oxygenation, and increasing the risk of herniation.

In terms of specific TBI, epidural hematomas (Fig. 17.9) typically result from a lateral fracture of the cranium, causing bleeding from the middle meningeal artery or a nearby vessel. Classically, the clinical course consists of an initial loss of consciousness followed by a lucid interval, during which time the hematoma expands. Upon reaching a significant size, the epidural hematoma causes profound neurologic deterioration. Recognition of this clinical course early may result in treatment with decompression, leading to a favorable outcome. Fortunately, the underlying brain tissue is often not severely injured in the setting of an epidural hematoma. This is in distinction to subdural hematomas, which commonly are associated with severe underlying brain tissue injury (see Fig. 17.9). Subdural hematomas are commonly caused by tearing of the bridging veins deep to the dura mater and superficial to the arachnoid mater. Although the hematoma itself can be compressive, it is usually the underlying contusion and axonal injury that predict the outcome after these injuries. Bleeding within the subarachnoid space is indicative of diffuse bleeding from brain tissue and in itself is not deleterious. Despite this, subarachnoid hemorrhages are not benign, and surveillance is mandated to identify deterioration. Parenchymal contusions of brain tissue result from the direct transmission of energy to the cranium and underlying brain as well as from movement of the brain within the rigid cranial vault, resulting in contrecoup injury. Finally, diffuse axonal injury describes the phenomenon of axonal disruption of from the neuronal body secondary to severe rotational forces. Imaging often underestimates the severity of diffuse axonal injury, revealing only punctate hemorrhages and loss of gray and white matter differentiation. Commonly, diffuse axonal injury becomes evident when patients demonstrate poor neurologic status in the setting of underwhelming imaging studies, although ultimate functional prognosis remains difficult to predict based on this finding.[24]

Immediate Management

Prevention of secondary brain injury, or treatment of recoverable cells (penumbra) around the traumatic focus, is the primary goal of TBI management. As the primary brain injury process cannot be reversed or corrected, outcomes after TBI are dictated by how well secondary injury is prevented. Thus, the mainstay of preventing secondary brain injury consists of standardized ATLS-based resuscitative efforts to facilitate normative brain physiology as quickly as possible. Airway control and ventilatory support are therefore critical immediately after TBI, as transient episodes of hypoxia may increase mortality up to fourfold. Although permissive hypotension is attendant to damage control resuscitation, its role in the setting of TBI is less clear and may worsen outcomes by exacerbating the ischemic insult. In the hypotensive polytrauma patient with severe TBI, military guidelines recommend 3% saline 250 mL bolus followed by 50 to 100 mL infusion for hemodynamic resuscitation and ICP reduction, possibly conferring survival benefit.[23] Anticoagulant medications can worsen intracranial bleeding and urgent reversal is indicated, based upon institutional protocols. Currently, the same paradigm cannot be applied to antiplatelet agents, as limited evidence of benefit exists to support platelet transfusion or treatment with desmopressin (DDAVP) to mitigate intracranial hemorrhage progression. Results of the recent international CRASH-3 trial suggest a mortality benefit in mild-moderate but not severe TBI patients receiving TXA within 3 hours of injury and may be included in future protocols.[25] Patients who are considered candidates for operative decompression should be immediately transferred to a facility capable of neurosurgical procedures.

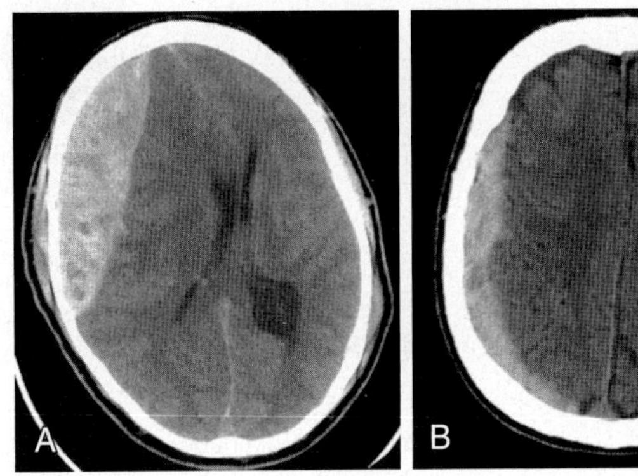

FIG. 17.9 Cranial computed tomography demonstrating (A) an epidural hematoma and (B) a subdural hematoma. Blood appears as high-density fluid *(white)* identified on the right side of both images. The epidural hematoma is associated with a significant midline shift. Note how the subdural hematoma follows the contour of the underlying brain.

Evaluation

A brief neurologic assessment is first performed during the primary survey when the GCS score is determined. The motor function component of the GCS is the most predictive of future neurologic outcome, with the ability to localize stimulation or follow commands being most favorable. An assessment of pupillary size and reactivity is also included, as this can be indicative of intracranial hypertension with impingement on the third cranial (oculomotor) nerve. When possible, a neurologic examination should be performed before the administration of any sedating or paralyzing agents so as not to obscure pertinent findings.

Following the management of airway, breathing, and circulation, patients with TBI benefit from immediate cranial imaging to expedite decompression when needed. Computed tomography (CT) without the administration of IV contrast is the most important diagnostic study during the initial evaluation of TBI because it is highly sensitive for detecting intracranial hemorrhage.

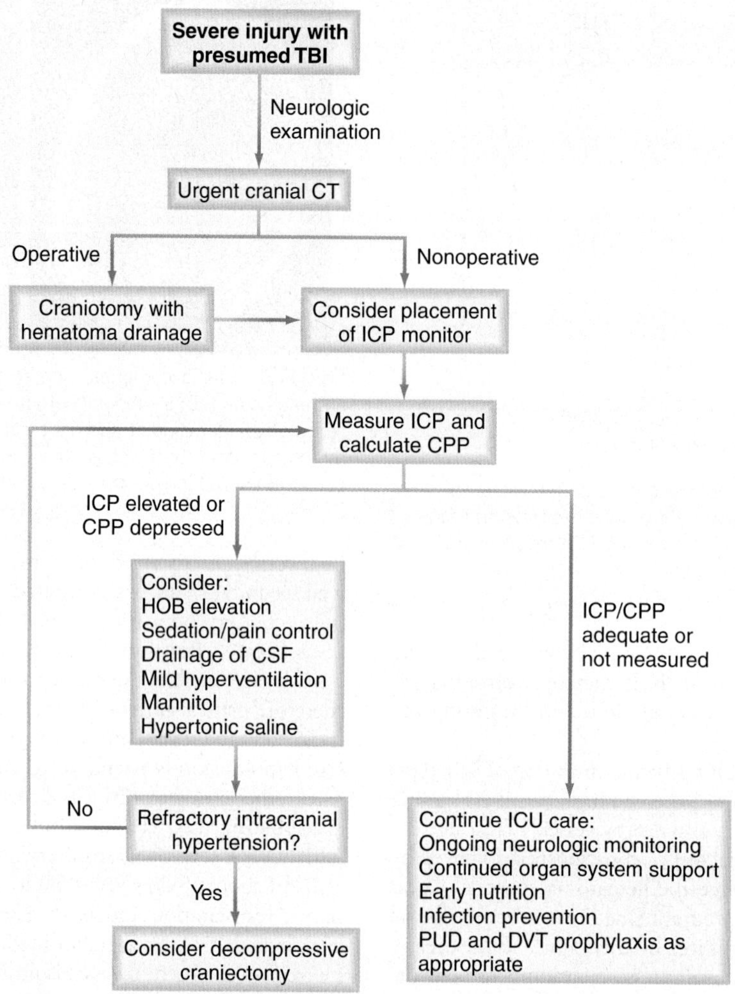

FIG. 17.10 Algorithm for the management of traumatic brain injury *(TBI)*. *CPP*, Cerebral perfusion pressure; *CSF*, cerebrospinal fluid; *CT*, computed tomography; *DVT*, deep venous thrombosis; *HOB*, head of bed; *ICP*, intracranial pressure; *ICU*, intensive care unit; *PUD*, peptic ulcer disease.

Acute blood appears as high-density fluid in various locations and mass effect with lateral shifting of parenchyma is a key finding. Contusions within the brain with associated local or global edema can also be visualized. In general terms, indications for primary decompressive craniectomy include space occupying intracranial hemorrhage with mass effect, recently and temporally associated with a decline in exam. Magnetic resonance imaging (MRI) may be able to provide better anatomic detail, but it has no role in the initial evaluation of the brain-injured patient.

Management

Most commonly, epidural and subdural hematomas with mass effect benefit from immediate decompression in the OR, although craniectomy for severe TBI is rarely needed (1.6%).[23] Depressed skull fractures may also require early surgical intervention to manage hemorrhage and to elevate the displaced bone. After surgery, management includes ongoing surveillance of neurologic function and avoidance of intracranial hypertension. In the setting of medically recalcitrant severe intracranial hypertension, patients may be considered for decompressive craniectomy, although operative salvage has recently been shown only to improve mortality but not functional outcomes.

Patients with severe TBI, whether managed operatively or medically, frequently require close neurologic monitoring in the intensive care unit. ICP is often measured directly to guide treatment (goal <22 mm Hg), although the necessity of invasive monitoring has been called into question by the Benchmark Evidence from South American Trials - Treatment of Intracranial Pressure (BEST-TRIP) trial data, suggesting noninferiority with serial imaging and clinical exam. In general terms, indications for ICP monitor placement include GCS <8 with evidence of intracranial lesion on CT. Although external ventricular drains have the added ability beyond parenchymal monitors to drain CSF and treat elevated pressures, no single device has demonstrated superiority over another. CPP, the difference between the mean arterial pressure (MAP) and ICP, is also commonly used to guide severe TBI management with goal 60 to 70 mm Hg. Although MAP, and consequently CPP, may be synthetically augmented by the addition of vasopressor, this does not obviate the need for maintenance of ICP within an acceptable range. While ICP and CPP are both frequently used to guide the management of patients with severe TBI, neither has been found to be superior. A suggested approach to the management of severe TBI is presented in Fig. 17.10.

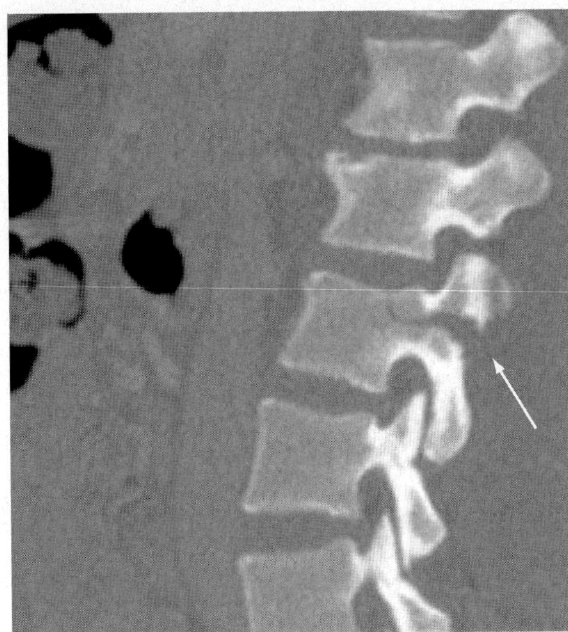

FIG. 17.11 Chance fracture on lumbar spine computed tomography scan in sagittal view. Note the fracture involvement of all posterior elements as identified by the *arrow*.

Persistent intracranial hypertension often requires a tiered approach to management. Head-of-bed elevation (or reverse Trendelenburg), midline facial positioning, and appropriately fitted cervical collars are simple techniques that can provide gravity drainage reductions in ICP. Tier 1 approaches include adequate anesthesia and analgesia, often initially in the form of short-acting continuous infusions that are paused intermittently for evaluation of clinical exam. A ventriculostomy may be placed to drain CSF. Tier 2 includes hyperosmolar therapy with hypertonic saline or mannitol, creating a gradient to reduce edema in regions of the brain with intact blood-brain barrier. Neuromuscular paralysis may be added at this time, with consideration of repeat CT imaging. Tier 3 (rescue/salvage) therapies include interventions to decrease brain metabolism with barbiturate class medications and mild hypothermia, neither of which have demonstrated outcome benefit. Although the use of significant hyperventilation has been found to be deleterious, increased ventilation resulting in a Pco_2 between 30 and 35 mm Hg results in an optimal therapeutic vasoconstriction but should only be used as a bridge to initiation of additional treatment. All available evidence continues to demonstrate that corticosteroid administration has no role in the management of TBI. As ICP tends to peak at 48 to 72 hours, patients who respond to management will experience a subsequent slow decrease in ICP with reductions in tissue edema and improvement in neurologic function.

Injuries to the Spinal Cord and the Vertebral Column

With an annual incidence of approximately 12,000 cases, SCIs are not a common cause of early mortality, although they result in severe long-term effects and years of disability.[26] Except for high cervical spine injuries, mortality directly related to SCIs is low, although the associated morbidity is substantial and currently irreversible. For young patients with SCI, the years of disability and lost productivity can be significant. In blunt trauma patients, vertebral column fracture alone is over 10 times more frequent than SCIs. Although more frequent, mortality associated with to blunt vertebral spine injuries is approximately 8%.[2]

Blunt and penetrating mechanisms result in different causes of SCI. Blunt trauma to the spine can cause cord injury through direct impingement by bony aspects or secondarily by accumulation of blood or edema. In the cervical spine, where mobility is maximal, incidence of SCI is highest (55%).[8] Injuries at this level are due to axial loading (Jefferson fracture), flexion, extension (Hangman's fracture), rotation (C1 rotary subluxation), lateral force (odontoid), and distraction. The 5th to 6th cervical vertebrae are within the zone of greatest mobility and hence most susceptible to injury. The thoracic and lumbar spines are more limited in mobility and mechanisms of injury to this region include axial loading (anterior wedge compression, burst injury) and flexion-extension (Chance fracture, fracture-dislocations). Chance fractures occur most commonly with motor vehicle accidents and have a high association with retroperitoneal or abdominal visceral injury (Fig. 17.11). Penetrating mechanisms either directly lacerate the spinal cord or cause indirect injury through ischemia or vertebral fracture. Lastly, patients present on occasion with a neurologic deficit that is not explained by any vertebral column abnormality. This SCI without radiographic abnormality can be challenging to diagnose and treat, given the lack of bone irregularity.

Immediate Management

Spinal immobilization with a rigid cervical collar and a long spine board is an immediate priority for prehospital personnel as a scene is approached. All blunt trauma patients are assumed to have an injury to the spine until a proper evaluation can exclude the diagnosis. High cervical SCI (C3–C5) may have immediate respiratory suppression requiring airway management and ventilatory support due to paresis of the phrenic nerves. Injuries to descending sympathetic pathways (T6 and above, intermediolateral column) may affect vasomotor tone, resulting in unopposed parasympathetic vagal outflow and neurogenic shock. Such patients may require intravascular volume expansion and vasopressor support. The classic presentation of *neurogenic shock* is hypotension in the setting of warm, well-perfused extremities in the paralyzed patient. Bradycardia may also be present, requiring atropine or inotropic support. This should be distinguished from *spinal shock*, which refers to the loss of reflexes and muscle tone that occurs after SCI.

Evaluation

A gross assessment of spinal cord function occurs during the primary survey by observing extremity movement. A more thorough evaluation of neurologic function occurs during the secondary survey when deficits are better characterized by dermatome (sensory level) or myotome (motor level). The *ATLS* 10th edition has produced a MyATLS companion app (myatls.com) that provides supplemental guides for dermatomes, myotomes, and muscle strength assessment. This information can assist in identifying the location of the injury and tracking progression of symptoms, which may affect therapeutic decisions. SCIs are characterized as *complete* or *incomplete*, depending on whether all neurologic function is absent below the level of injury or a portion is retained. To assist with standardization of SCI assessment, the International Standards for Neurological Classification of Spinal Cord Injury worksheet, produced by the American Spinal Injury Association, generates and impairment scale as follows: A (complete injury), B (sensory incomplete), C/D (motor incomplete), E (normal). Finally, tenderness over the injured vertebrae or the presence of a deformity consistent with disruption of the vertebral column is often indicative of associated acute fracture. Most importantly, reassessment is key whenever there is concern for new deficit. The

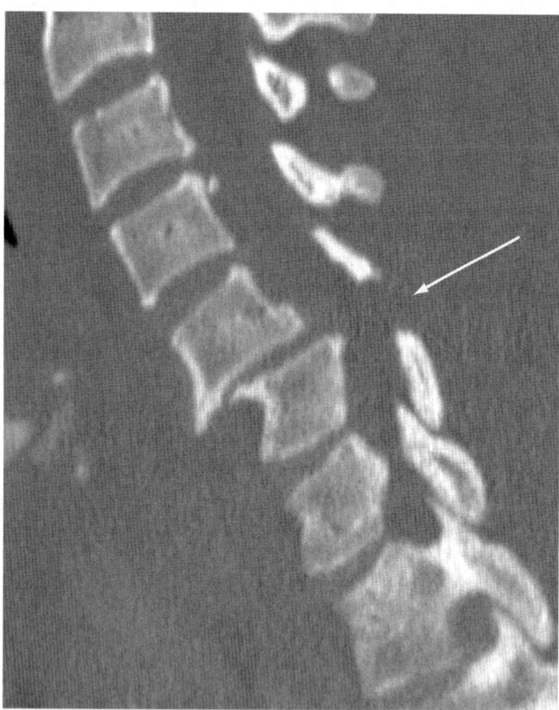

FIG. 17.12 Cervical spine fracture with severe anterior subluxation and compromise of the spinal canal. The *arrow* identifies the severe narrowing of the spinal canal.

involvement of a spine surgeon upon identification of an injury may guide further evaluation and expedite operative intervention when it is needed. Prehospital screening tools, such as the Canadian C-spine Rule or the National Emergency X-Radiography Utilization Study (NEXUS), provide a means by which patients who have no findings on examination, demonstrate no decreased level of consciousness, and have no distracting injuries can undergo clearance of the spine by clinical means alone. Interestingly, a recent AAST multi-institutional trial revealed a negative predictive value of approximately 99% with negative physical exam with and without attendant distracting injury. Patients older than 65 years old were included in the analysis and did not demonstrate increased rates of missed injury.[27]

Imaging of the cervical, thoracic, and lumbar portions of the spine is commonly required to evaluate further for vertebral column injury. Although plain radiographs of the spine (anteroposterior, lateral, odontoid) are acceptable, the high-quality images, superior sensitivity, and rapid availability associated with CT have made this the modality of choice in most emergency departments.[8] Because of the challenges of visualizing the cervicothoracic junction on plain radiography, a dedicated cervical spine CT scan is now often obtained during the initial imaging of the patient and may be considered sufficient to remove a cervical collar in the intoxicated patient with negative findings.[28] Sagittal and coronal reconstruction of CT imaging of the spine provides better anatomic visualization. CT imaging offers excellent evaluation of bone injuries, but SCIs are poorly delineated because of limited soft tissue detail. Nevertheless, spinal canal compromise and soft tissue edema on CT are highly suggestive of injury to the spinal cord. MRI is often needed to better characterize soft tissue injury, particularly in the setting of neck pain and normal radiography, if performed within the first 72 hours of trauma, and may provide valuable information to guide early operative intervention. Fig. 17.12 demonstrates a severe cervical spine fracture with subluxation and anterior displacement of the vertebral body. Obtaining these images, especially in the acute setting, must be carefully considered with respect to overall level of stability.

Management

As a general rule, the spine should be protected from further injury by maintaining strict immobilization until injuries can be ruled out. An important exception is in the setting of penetrating trauma, where there has been no demonstrable neurologic benefit, inclusive of patients with direct neck injury, and is associated with increased mortality.[29] Raising the head of the bed in these patients facilitates their participation with airway management until the appropriate setting for intubation (i.e., OR) may be provided. Notwithstanding, early removal of the long spine board to avoid the development of pressure wounds is extremely important. On recognition of an SCI in the resuscitation bay, consultation with a spine surgeon should be obtained promptly. Immediate arrangements should be made for transfer when spine surgery services are not available. To avoid delays, subsequent imaging should be avoided unless the results will have an immediate impact on the care provided.

Cervical SCIs with neurogenic shock require resuscitation with volume expansion and often vasopressor/inotropic therapy. No agent or combination thereof has demonstrated superiority in this setting. Brief periods of hypotension (<90 mm Hg), not unlike TBI, have been shown previously to be detrimental to long-term outcomes in SCI; thus, shock should be treated aggressively. Such resuscitations can be challenging in the setting of shock combinations (i.e., hemorrhagic and neurogenic). Following shock resolution, questions remain as to the benefit of MAP augmentation in SCI. Although society guidelines include recommendations for MAP goals 85 to 90 mm Hg for 7 days following injury, data are associative in nature.[26] Future studies are needed to elucidate the impact of sustained pressure elevation beyond normotension upon SCI outcomes.

Corticosteroid therapy for SCI has been well studied but remains controversial. Several large randomized trials (National Acute Spinal Cord Injury Study series) have demonstrated motor improvement at 6 weeks and 6 months following methylprednisolone administration if initiated within 8 hours of injury. Functional recovery is similar whether methylprednisolone is administered as bolus-infusion for a duration of 24 or 48 hours in patients receiving treatment within 3 hours or 3 to 8 hours after injury, respectively. Patients treated for 48 hours demonstrated higher rates of severe sepsis and severe pneumonia, although mortality was not different. Taken together, short-duration steroids remain a potentially therapeutic option following SCI, although they should be considered in consultation between trauma and neurosurgical services.[26]

Surgical management of spine injuries varies greatly, depending on the injury pattern and the associated vertebral column stability. In appropriate candidates, spinal cord decompression has been shown in trial data to improve functional outcomes if performed within 24 hours of injury.[26] Cervical fracture-dislocation injuries may benefit from the application of traction in the emergency department to restore vertebral column alignment. Vertebral column injuries with instability often require operative fixation as soon as emergent issues are managed and the patient can safely undergo spine surgery. Fractures without instability may require only immobilization with a hard collar or brace and follow-up upright x-rays until bone healing can occur. Table 17.5

TABLE 17.5 **Fractures of the vertebral column.**

FRACTURE	DESCRIPTION	TYPICAL MANAGEMENT
C1 Jefferson fracture	Disruption of C1 ring in multiple locations; blow-out of ring	Stable transverse ligament: hard collar Unstable transverse ligament: traction or surgery
Odontoid fractures	Type I: tip of odontoid Type II: through base Type III: involves C2 body	Type I: hard collar Type II: halo vest or surgery Type III: halo vest
C2 hangman fracture	Bilateral C2 pedicles with spondylolisthesis	Halo vest or surgery if displacement is severe
Cervical vertebral body fractures	Compression or burst of vertebral body with or without retropulsion into canal	Mild loss of height: hard collar Involvement of multiple columns or presence of retropulsion into canal: surgical stabilization
Thoracic vertebral body fractures	Compression or burst of vertebral body with or without retropulsion into canal	Anterior column only: TLSO Anterior and posterior columns: surgical stabilization
Lumbar vertebral body fractures	Compression or burst of vertebral body with or without retropulsion into canal	Anterior column only: TLSO Anterior and posterior columns: surgical stabilization
Chance fracture	Avulsion of posterior elements of lumbar vertebrae seen with high seat belt use	Surgical stabilization

TLSO, Thoracolumbosacral orthosis.

lists the previously described and commonly encountered vertebral column fractures with the associated management options. After stabilization of the bony spine, early involvement of physical therapy is the next best influence over functional outcomes in SCI. Although there are currently no regenerative options for SCI with deficits, promise has been shown in animal models with stem cell treatment.[26]

Injury to the Maxillofacial Region

The face is commonly injured in the setting of blunt and penetrating trauma, although these injuries are rarely life-threatening. Of foremost concern is tissue damage that compromises the airway and/or obstructs access to oral endotracheal intubation. Bleeding from facial vasculature can be significant and contribute to the need for urgent airway management. Facial bone fractures are routinely identified in this setting. One specific injury pattern includes the Le Fort class of facial fractures, consisting of three variations of midface disruption from the surrounding facial bones. Significant morbidity can result from injuries to the face, particularly when there is associated sensory disruption from trauma to the eyes, ears, nose, or mouth. Nonetheless, poor functional outcomes after facial trauma are often due to a concomitant TBI rather than the injuries themselves.

Immediate Management

Injury to the face requires prompt assessment and management of the airway, particularly when lower face soft tissue and bone involvement is present. Because edema can worsen rapidly, early intubation can be lifesaving if there is concern about airway stability. Blood or debris in the oropharynx can greatly complicate intubation, and the application of backup airway options, including a surgical approach, should be anticipated and may be necessary. Given the vascularity of the face, bleeding can be an immediate concern and should be managed with direct pressure, suture ligature, and the initiation of resuscitation. Rapid closure of wounds may be required, although facial bleeding is sometime challenging to identify. Bleeding from deep vessels or fractured bone may require angioembolization for definitive control to be obtained. Frequently, bleeding from the face is exacerbated by hypothermia and coagulopathy, which should be aggressively prevented or treated.

Evaluation

Facial injuries are first identified on physical examination, during which the extent of soft tissue involvement is determined. The eyes are grossly examined for diplopia and subjective changes in visual acuity. The condition of the globe and the surrounding orbit requires careful evaluation for rupture or extraocular muscle entrapment, which requires urgent treatment. The external ear is examined, and drainage from the ear canal is identified when present. Midface and mandibular stability, proper occlusion, and quality of the dentition are assessed. Forehead and midface deformities are indicative of underlying frontal and maxillary bone fractures, respectively. When fractures or soft tissue injuries are identified, the motor function of the face should be assessed to evaluate facial nerve function.

Injuries to the face often benefit from three-dimensional imaging with thin-cut CT to adequately visualize the facial bones. Sagittal and coronal as well as three-dimensional reconstructions can aid in thorough structural assessment and evaluation of deep soft tissue. CT is indicated when severe external injury is identified on secondary survey or when facial abnormality is identified on cranial CT. Imaging of the face should be performed only after life-threatening injuries have been addressed, as management of facial trauma is not time sensitive in the majority of cases.

Management

Facial fractures and severe soft tissue injuries often benefit from the involvement of a maxillofacial surgical consultation to assist in management. As previously described, airway management and bleeding are the most immediate priorities. Direct pressure and wound closure are often effective in managing facial bleeding. In severe cases, angiography with embolization may be necessary. Before wound closure, jagged or nonviable skin edges should be debrided, followed by irrigation of the wound with sterile fluid. Lacerations can frequently be closed with local anesthesia using deep absorbable sutures followed by closure of the skin with 5-0 or 6-0 interrupted or running sutures. Lacerations to the lip, nose, ear, and orbit are more complex in nature, and closure requires special consideration to facilitate optimal wound healing.

The management of facial fractures is infrequently required in the acute setting and can be deferred until after other injuries are addressed. Severely depressed facial bone fractures are the exception because these may involve the underlying brain and require urgent reduction. Most facial fractures are repaired after time allows for reduction in the associated soft tissue edema. Large open wounds and fractures involving sinuses or the aerodigestive tract may require antibiotics shortly after admission, but over-extending this course should be avoided. When repair is appropriate, fractures often benefit from open reduction and internal fixation, typically with screws and plates. Reconstructive efforts are aimed at optimizing functional and cosmetic outcomes. This includes the preservation of normal extraocular motor function by addressing orbital fractures with rectus muscle involvement. Mandibular fractures can be treated with maxillary-mandibular fixation, although significant fracture displacement may require internal fixation with plating.

Injuries to the Neck

The neck contains multiple vital structures in close proximity, complicating diagnosis, exposure, and treatment in the setting of injury. Nevertheless, as with other areas of the body, managing neck injuries can be made reasonable by implementing an organized approach. Trauma to the neck is relatively uncommon but results in the highest mortality of all body regions (17% mortality for AIS ≥3 injuries in the NTDB).[2] Penetrating injuries from gunshot and stab wounds are the most common mechanisms. Penetrating injuries can directly lacerate vascular and aerodigestive structures, resulting in substantial bleeding or contamination, respectively. Although uncommon, blunt mechanisms can cause sudden compression, with subsequent fracture of the larynx or trachea. Blunt pharyngeal or esophageal injuries are even less common but can result in tissue devitalization, leakage into the surrounding soft tissues with consequent abscess, or mediastinitis. Blunt force to the neck may also cause injury to the carotid or vertebral arteries. These blunt cerebrovascular injuries (BCVIs) result from seat belt compression or severe flexion-extension mechanisms. BCVI severity ranges from intimal tears (Grade I), with or without thrombosis, to full-thickness injury with pseudoaneurysm formation (Grade III) and transection (Grade V). The morbidity associated with BCVI is predominantly due to ischemic stroke from acute thromboembolic phenomenon.

Immediate Management

Neck injuries often require rapid intervention due to the vulnerability of the contained vital structures. In keeping with ATLS, highest priority concern is the establishment of a secure airway. Deterioration can occur rapidly, necessitating timely recognition and definitive care. Direct injury to the larynx or trachea is the most common cause of airway compromise and presents one of the most challenging circumstances to airway management. Expanding neck hematomas quickly compress the upper airway, leading to inadequate ventilation. Immediate intubation should occur in the setting of an expanding neck hematoma or if there is concern for impending airway compromise. Importantly, patients who are maintaining their own airway should have a planned approach to airway management that may include intubation or awake tracheostomy in the OR. Attempted intubation could worsen a tenuous situation and should not be performed without a well-developed backup plan. A loss of airway requires emergent intervention, including performance of a cricothyroidotomy or tracheotomy. The surgical airway of choice for an upper airway injury is a tracheotomy because injury to the larynx may make cricothyroidotomy ineffective.

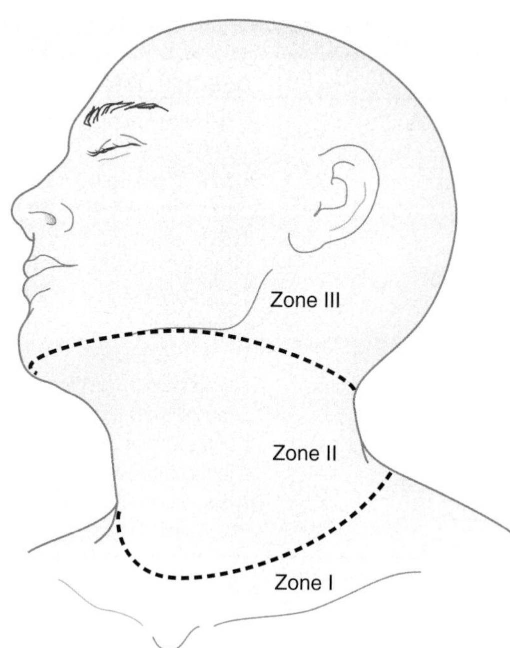

FIG. 17.13 Zones of the neck. *Zone 1* extends from the thoracic inlet to the cricoid cartilage. *Zone 2* is between the cricoid cartilage and the angle of the mandible. *Zone 3* extends from the angle of the mandible to the skull base.

In the immediate setting, hemorrhage is the other major concern after neck trauma. Injury to the carotid sheath vasculature will often require surgical control and MTP-based resuscitation should be rapidly and concurrently initiated when needed. Direct pressure with either finger or Foley balloon effectively manages most bleeding from the neck during transport to the OR. Similar to patients with significant aerodigestive injury, patients requiring surgical intervention for bleeding in the neck are best served by airway management in the OR immediately prior to treatment of hemorrhage.

Evaluation

Patients with hemodynamic instability and/or hard signs of vascular or aerodigestive injury (i.e., airway compromise, massive subcutaneous emphysema, air bubbles necessitating through wound, expanding or pulsatile hematoma, active bleeding, neurologic deficit, hematemesis) should be taken immediately to the OR for surgical exploration.[30] Stable patients may undergo further evaluation for neck injury with thin-slice multidetector CT angiography (MDCTA) imaging.

Penetrating injuries are classically characterized by anatomic location and surgical accessibility (Fig. 17.13). Zone I extends from the thoracic inlet to the cricoid cartilage and contains large vascular structures as well as the trachea and esophagus. Stretching from the cricoid cartilage to the angle of the mandible, zone II is the most accessible surgically and contains the carotid and vertebral arteries, jugular veins, and structures of the aerodigestive tract. Zone III includes the neck between the angle of the mandible and the base of the skull. Structures within zone III include blood vessels that are difficult to expose surgically. Although zone II injuries with physical exam are indicators for depth of injury (i.e., violation of platysma) traditionally mandated operative exploration, it has since been recognized that only those patients with hard signs of vascular or aerodigestive injury require immediate operation while the remainder may undergo radiographic assessment (so-called "no-zone" approach).

BOX 17.4 Indicators of high risk for blunt cerebrovascular injury.

Signs and Symptoms

Expanding neck hematoma
Arterial hemorrhage from neck, nose, or mouth
Focal neurologic deficit
Cervical bruit (patient <50 years old)
Stroke on CT or MRI
Neurologic deficit unexplained by CT findings

Risk Factors

Severe midface fracture, Le Fort II or III
Basilar skull fracture involving the carotid canal
Diffuse axonal injury and GCS score ≤6
Significant cervical spine fracture or ligamentous injury
Significant soft tissue injury to anterior neck (i.e., seat belt mark)
Near-hanging with anoxia

CT, Computed tomography; *GCS*, Glasgow Coma Scale; *MRI*, magnetic resonance imaging.

CT angiographic evaluation of the neck, performed in the emergency department, has become readily available and decreased the rate of negative neck explorations for penetrating injury. A prospective multicenter study (n = 453) revealed that, on 40 or 64 multislice CT scanners, the sensitivity and specificity for penetrating vascular or aerodigestive injuries were 100% and 97.5%, respectively. Specificity was depreciated by two patients with falsely positive vascular imaging, resulting in a negative exploration and catheter angiography, and three patients with air tracking concerning for aerodigestive injury subsequently ruled out endoscopically. Versus evaluation of the neck by anatomic zones, MDCTA in appropriate patients allows for evaluation of the neck as a unit and obviates the need for additional invasive testing (i.e., bronchoscopy, rigid/flexible endoscopy, esophagram, digital subtraction angiography [DSA]) in many cases. Only those patients with equivocal MDCTA, as may occur with retained ballistic, require additional selective diagnostics. Standard DSA does not suffer from scatter limitation and may provide added information in this setting.[31]

Blunt trauma to the neck often manifests in the form of BCVI. The improved technology of MDCTA has cast light upon this entity, which is now recognized as a major source of morbidity. Initially considered uncommon, the emergence of high-risk screening criteria and improved detection have led to a significant increase in the diagnosis of BCVI. DSA subsequently confirmed BCVI in 30% of this high-risk cohort. Commonly referred to as the Denver criteria, these risk factors were used to screen patients and to prompt further evaluation (Box 17.4). The emergence and evolution of MDCTA have since replaced DSA as the study of choice for diagnosis of BCVI and recent studies report incidence as approximately 2% to 3% of all blunt trauma patients. Contemporary screening criteria liberally prompts the evaluator toward MDCTA in the setting of (1) any injury above the clavicle, regardless of mechanism, (2) neurologic exam not explained by brain imaging, and (3) Horner syndrome.[32] As blunt aerodigestive injury is exceedingly rare, diagnostics will likely favor a tailored approach with MDCTA, esophagoscopy, esophagography, and/or bronchoscopy if there is concern.

Management

As previously mentioned, hard signs of vascular or aerodigestive injury require immediate neck exploration, as outlined in the WTA 2013 guidelines (Fig. 17.14). Most commonly, structures of the neck are exposed by an incision along the anterior border of the sternocleidomastoid on the side of the injury. A collar incision may be more versatile, especially if a bilateral neck exploration is required. The platysma is divided to expose the anterior border of the sternocleidomastoid, which is dissected from the underlying tissue to expose the carotid sheath (common carotid artery, vagus nerve, internal jugular vein). An injured internal jugular vein may require direct repair with Prolene suture or ligation, if closure is not possible. The facial vein is identified entering the anterior surface of the internal jugular vein. Ligation and division of the facial vein allow the deep structures of the vascular compartment to be exposed. With the internal jugular vein retracted laterally, the carotid artery and vagus nerves are exposed. If necessary, the carotid artery may be controlled proximally and distally. Care should be taken to avoid injury to either the vagus or hypoglossal nerves, which lie adjacent to and superiorly crossing the carotid artery, respectively. Short-segment carotid artery injuries should be repaired with either simple closure or end-to-end anastomosis. More extensive injuries require reconstruction with a synthetic graft or autologous vein. In damage control situations, the carotid artery can be shunted or ligated in extreme circumstances, although cerebral blood flow may be compromised.

Exploration of the trachea and esophagus is achieved via lateral retraction of the carotid artery. Dissection is continued medially and the esophagus is identified immediately anterior to the cervical vertebral bodies, detection of which may be aided by nasogastric tube placement. Injuries to the esophagus should be debrided to expose the entirety of the mucosal perforation. Closure of the esophageal wall can be in one or preferably two layers (mucosal/muscular) and wide drainage is important. Covering the esophageal repair with vascularized muscle pedicle, commonly sternocleidomastoid, may be highly beneficial, particularly in the setting of adjacent tracheal or vascular repair. Massive tissue loss or delayed presentation poses a significant challenge and may require esophageal diversion with esophagostomy followed by delayed reconstruction. Tracheal lacerations can be primarily closed with absorbable suture if the injury is small and will approximate in a tension-free fashion. Large tracheal defects may require resection and anastomosis, although some anterior tracheal injuries can be managed by creating a tracheostomy through the injury. After the tracheostomy tract matures, the tube can be removed, and closure usually occurs spontaneously.

As the evaluation of BCVI has evolved, treatment has also become more advanced. To decrease the risk of thromboembolic stroke (37%–4.8%), anticoagulation or antiplatelet therapy is initiated, although neither has demonstrated superiority. Endovascular stenting may be considered in select circumstances involving pseudoaneurysm and dissection with 70% flow limitation. Given the potential for ischemic complications, employment of this therapy is roughly 10% overall.[32] Bleeding risk from associated injuries often limits the ability to begin immediate anticoagulation or antiplatelet therapy, but treatment should be initiated as soon as safely possible. Although the majority of strokes occur in the first few days after injury, a significant percentage occur in the following days to weeks and therefore still benefit from delayed initiation of therapy. Fig. 17.15 presents a graded approach to the diagnosis and management of BCVI. Anticoagulation with heparin should be started with the goal of achieving a partial thromboplastin time

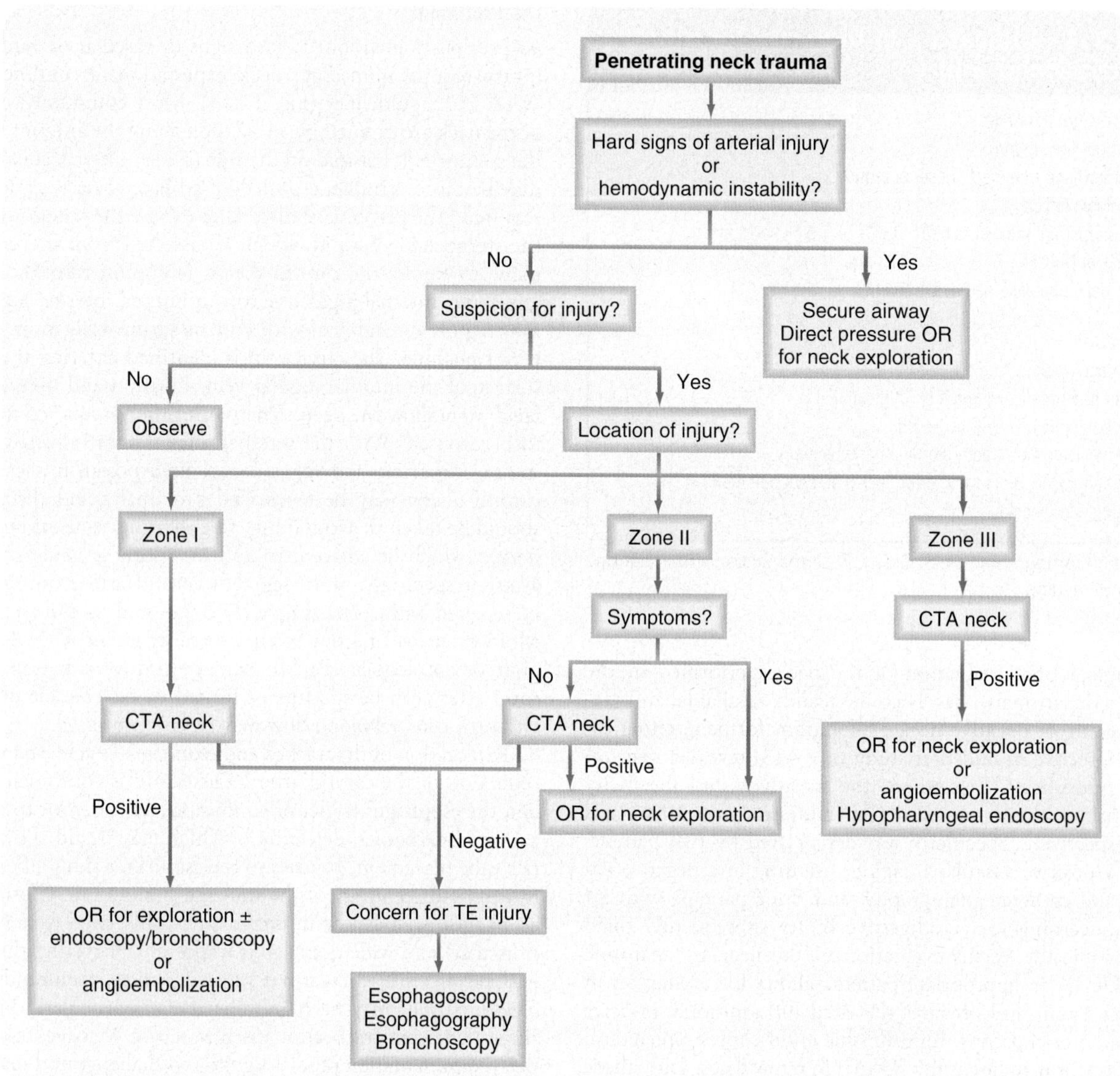

FIG. 17.14 Algorithm for the management of penetrating neck injuries. Hard signs of vascular or aerodigestive injury include airway compromise, massive subcutaneous emphysema, air bubbles necessitating through wound, expanding or pulsatile hematoma, active bleeding, neurologic deficit, and hematemesis. (Modified from Sperry JL, Moore EE, Coimbra R, et al. Western Trauma Association critical decisions in trauma: penetrating neck trauma. *J Trauma Acute Care Surg.* 2013;75:936–940.). *CTA,* Computed tomography angiography; *OR,* operating room; *TE,* tracheoesophageal.

between 40 and 50 seconds, although daily 325 mg aspirin (ASA) presents an equivalent therapeutic option. MDCTA may be repeated in 24 to 48 hours if findings are indeterminate on initial scan. All confirmed injuries should undergo repeat imaging at 7 to 10 days to evaluate for progression or resolution and subsequent discontinuation of therapy. Persistent injury requires treatment for 3 months, followed by outpatient follow-up MDCTA.

Injuries to the Chest

Injuries to the thorax are common, occurring in 22% of trauma patients annually with an associated 9.5% mortality in the NTDB.[2] These injuries can be life-threatening, as the chest contains vital cardiopulmonary structures. Falls and motor vehicle crashes comprise the majority of blunt chest injuries via transmission of energy to the chest wall and direct compression or deceleration forces to underlying structures. The relative prominence of the chest makes it vulnerable to penetrating mechanisms, such as gunshot and stab wounds. Penetrating mechanisms result in direct laceration of pulmonary and mediastinal structures. High energy blunt and penetrating trauma can also cause significant lung contusion to tissue, local to the site of focal impact, or diffusely in the setting of blast injury. Despite the serious nature of these injuries, less than 10% of blunt and between 15% and 30% of penetrating trauma to the chest require surgical management.[8]

Immediate Management

Thoracic injuries often require intervention during the primary survey because of the impact upon cardiopulmonary function. Chest trauma with pulmonary compromise requires immediate management of the airway and ventilatory assistance. Decreased breath sounds and poor pulmonary compliance in the setting of shock is consistent with possible tension pneumothorax and may require

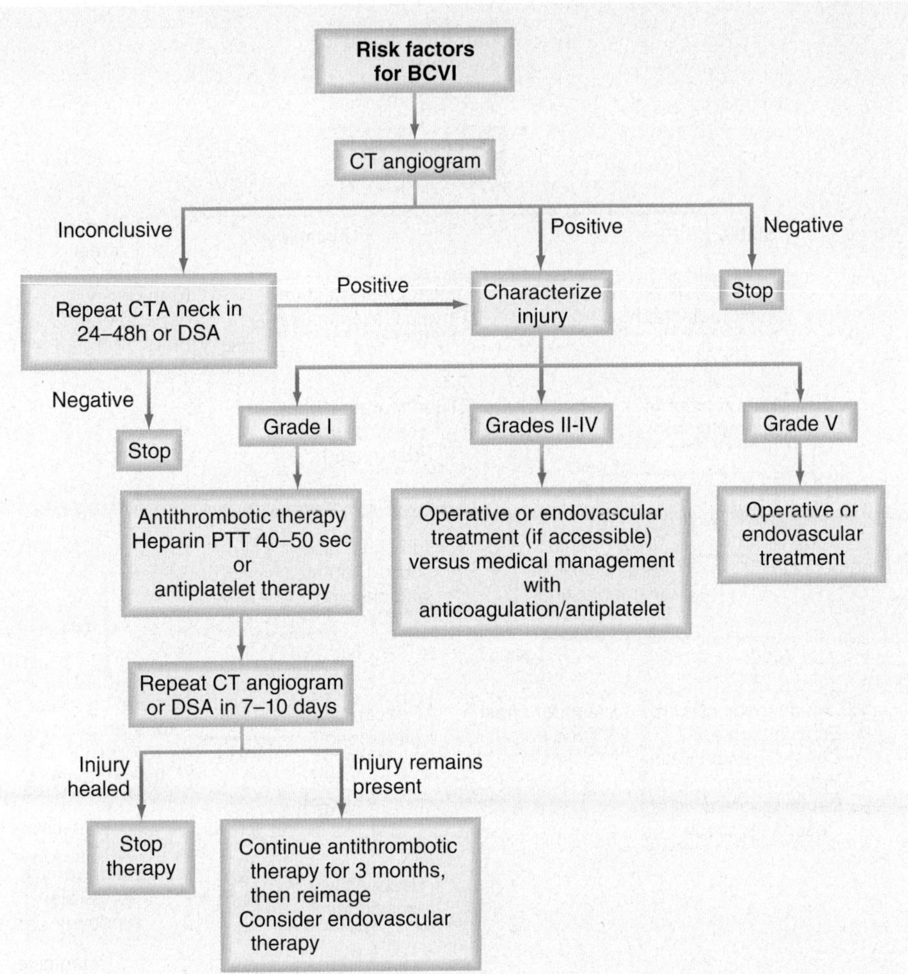

FIG. 17.15 Algorithm for the management of blunt cerebrovascular injury *(BCVI)*. (Modified from Biffl WL, Cothren CC, Moore EE, et al. Western Trauma Association critical decisions in trauma: screening for and treatment of blunt cerebrovascular injuries. *J Trauma*. 2009;67:1150–1153.). *CT*, Computed tomography; *CTA*, computed tomography angiography; *DSA*, digital subtraction angiography; *PTT*, partial thromboplastin time.

urgent decompression with tube thoracostomy. External bleeding should be controlled with direct pressure while resuscitation is initiated. Although hemodynamic instability most commonly indicates hemorrhage until proven otherwise, cardiac dysfunction secondary to pericardial tamponade, cardiac contusion, or coronary air embolism may represent other possible sources in this setting. Following an assessment for sources of blood loss, a search for pericardial fluid with ultrasound or pericardial window may be required, especially following penetrating trauma. Patients with persistent shock despite resuscitation and ongoing blood loss from the chest often require operative intervention. Cardiac arrest, particularly in the setting of penetrating mechanisms, may benefit from RT (see earlier section). Fig. 17.16 demonstrates an approach to the initial evaluation and management of penetrating chest injuries.

Evaluation

The majority of chest injuries can be diagnosed with physical examination and plain chest radiography. External injuries, such as chest wall defects and penetrating wounds, will be identified on physical examination. Chest wall tenderness and paradoxical movement can be identified to reflect segmental injuries to the ribs (flail) and sternum. Deviation of the trachea at the sternal notch may reveal intrathoracic tension on the side opposite the trachea.

Chest radiography is almost universally performed during the initial assessment on patients at risk for thoracic injuries. In blunt trauma, the chest is evaluated for the presence of a large-volume pneumothorax or hemothorax that would require immediate tube thoracostomy. Whereas the chest radiograph may contain findings suggestive of blunt aortic injury (i.e., widened mediastinum, obliteration of the aortopulmonary window, apical capping), this modality lacks sufficient detail for screening. Thoracic MDCTA has become the standard approach to evaluation of the chest and provides superior visualization of the chest wall, vasculature, pleural spaces, and lung parenchyma. It is, however, unreliable for evaluation of pericardium, given cardiac motion degradation. Importantly, CT angiography has become accepted as sufficient to guide operative intervention without the need for standard angiography of the chest.

Penetrating trauma to the chest should be identified rapidly on physical exam and marked with adhesive radio-opaque markers for x-ray. Injuries that are believed to involve or cross the mediastinum require further evaluation. Wounds within the area defined by the sternal notch superiorly, the costal margin inferiorly, and the nipples laterally ("the cardiac box") constitute these high-risk injuries. Immediate ultrasound is performed to evaluate the pericardium for effusion, although decompression into a hemothorax

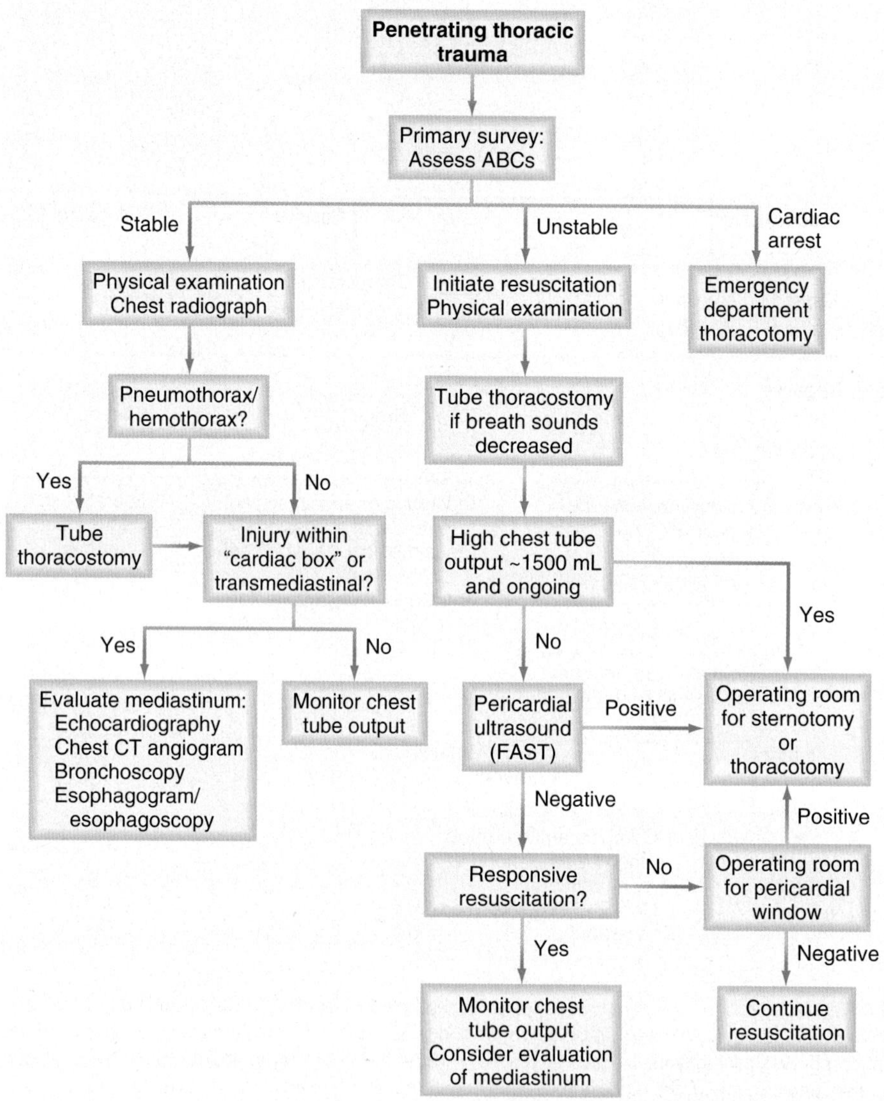

FIG. 17.16 Algorithm for the management of penetrating thoracic injuries. *ABCs*, Airway, breathing, and circulation; *CT*, computed tomography; *FAST*, focused abdominal sonography in trauma.

through traumatic pericardiotomy may yield false-negative results.[33] As with blunt trauma, the great vessels are evaluated for injury with MDCTA, although this can be impeded by the presence of retained missile fragments, necessitating standard catheter-based angiography if there is concern. Depending on the trajectory of the penetrating object, the trachea and proximal airways may require evaluation with bronchoscopy and a combination of esophagoscopy with contrast esophagography are diagnostic for esophageal injuries. As described in the neck injury section, these studies have an approximate 20% false-negative rate in isolation, although their combined sensitivity approaches 100%.

Management

Thoracic injuries are often straightforward to manage, with up to 85% successfully treated with tube thoracostomy alone. Although chest tubes are often urgently required, placement may still be performed in a controlled manner to include strict sterile preparation and excellent surgical technique. To avoid the development of an empyema (3% overall incidence in chest trauma), the chest should be prepared appropriately by wide preparation with chlorhexidine as well as wide draping to maintain the sterility of the field. External landmarks for reliable placement should include the level of the nipple or inframammary fold inferiorly, midaxillary line posteriorly, and the hypotenuse of the two sides ("triangle of safety"). After infusion of local analgesia, a skin incision roughly equivalent to the circumference of the chest tube should be made within the triangle at or just above the level of the nipple (5th–6th intercostal spaces). This location successfully avoids intraabdominal placement or injury to the diaphragm. A subcutaneous tunnel is created in a superior direction and the chest is entered bluntly at an interspace above the skin incision. Accomplishing the tunnel naturally directs the chest tube into an apical position. The lung is palpated to confirm chest entry and to evaluate for intrathoracic adhesions. Chest tube sizing for trauma has typically ranged from 32 to 36 Fr, although accumulating evidence suggests equivalent success in drainage of hemothorax irrespective of luminal diameter. To confirm that the tube is not kinked, it is helpful to be sure that the tube freely spins before completion of the procedure. The tube is then connected to an underwater drainage device providing 20 cm H_2O suction.

The traditional indications for immediate thoracotomy include (1) more than 1500 mL of blood drained on chest tube insertion, (2) 150 to 200 mL/hr of drainage for two to four consecutive hours, or (3) persistent hemodynamic instability in the setting of ongoing transfusion requirement.[34] Nonetheless, it is paramount to remember that these indications are based upon Vietnam war–era data from patients who died due to chest injury rather than contemporary trials examining predictors of survivorship; there are no absolute values that mandate operation. Arguably more important questions to be asking are: Does the chest tube output represent ongoing bleeding or accumulated blood (i.e., "is bleeding" vs. "has bled")? Is the bleeding surgical in nature? Is it impacting physiology? For example, chest tubes that initially drain 1500 mL then have little ongoing output in the setting of hemodynamic stability may not require thoracotomy. Like other zones of injury, the patient physiology and response to resuscitation should guide operative planning. Other indications for thoracotomy include a massive air leak with associated pneumothorax and drainage of esophageal or gastric contents from the chest tube.

When thoracotomy is required, the choice of surgical approach depends on the suspected injury. Access to the lungs, pulmonary vasculature, and hemidiaphragm is achieved through a posterolateral thoracotomy that is best performed through the fifth interspace, with possible removal of the fifth rib. On the right, this incision also exposes the proximal and mid esophagus as well as the trachea and bilateral mainstem bronchi. The distal esophagus, left lung, left ventricle, descending aorta, and left subclavian artery are best approached through a left thoracotomy. A median sternotomy can be a highly versatile approach, providing exposure to the right side of the heart, ascending aorta, aortic arch with right-sided arch vessels, and pulmonary vasculature.

Chest Wall and Pleural Space Injuries. With more than 65% of blunt trauma patients sustaining one or more rib fractures, chest wall injuries are the most common thoracic injury. Similarly, rib fractures occur in more than one out of four cases of penetrating chest trauma in the NTDB. The mortality rate associated with chest wall injuries after blunt trauma is approximately 7%, whereas it exceeds 19% for penetrating injuries. Rib fractures typically occur secondary to compression of the thoracic cage in an anteroposterior or lateral direction, which often dictates the location of the cortical disruption along the rib. During motor vehicle crashes, the steering wheel and seat belt are commonly the cause of chest wall deformation. Large amounts of energy transferred to the chest wall can result in a flail segment, which includes two or more adjacent ribs fractured in two or more locations. Clinically, a flail segment results in a portion of the chest wall that moves independently and paradoxically in relation to the remainder of the chest. Although abnormal chest wall mechanics occur in this setting, the associated pulmonary contusion causes the greatest physiologic insult and may ultimately require the most supportive energies. Some volume of air (pneumothorax) or blood (hemothorax) is commonly associated with chest injury, owing to compressive forces upon the lung or penetrating mechanisms.

The evaluation of the chest wall begins during the primary and secondary surveys, during which chest wall tenderness, wall motion abnormalities, and changes in pulmonary mechanics are suggestive of trauma. Injuries involving the chest wall or pleural space can frequently be identified on chest radiographs, in which a pneumothorax appears as a lucency peripheral to the standard lung markings (Fig. 17.17) and hemothorax is revealed as dependent opacification. Chest CT is often a valuable part of the evaluation and identifies chest wall trauma as well as pleural air and blood with a great degree of sensitivity. An occult pneumothorax is defined by identification on chest CT without evidence on plain radiography. Finally, CT easily recognizes significant chest wall deformities, such as flail segment, displaced ribs, and sternal fractures, and may be used to guide considerations of chest wall reconstruction.

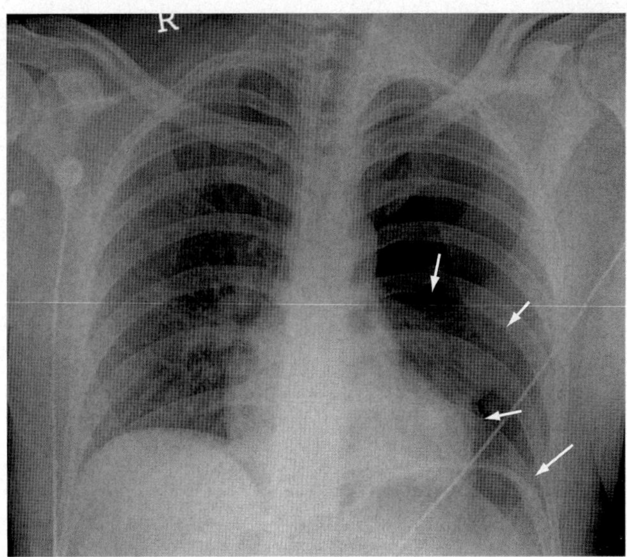

FIG. 17.17 Large left-sided pneumothorax on plain chest radiograph. The *arrows* identify the lateral border of the collapsed lung.

All pneumo- or hemothoraces visible on a chest radiograph should be considered for tube thoracostomy, yet routine utility remains a controversial topic. Although large-volume pneumothoraces are typically detected on x-ray, up to half are subsequently discovered on CT chest. In the absence of hemodynamic instability and respiratory compromise, recent data suggest that observation for pneumothoraces with CT radial diameter of up to 35 mm may be safe for both blunt and penetrating trauma.[35] Occult pneumothoraces not accompanied by respiratory compromise can be managed with observation and a repeated chest radiograph 12 to 24 hours later to demonstrate stability. Hemothoraces visible on upright chest x-ray represent an approximate volume of 400–500 mL and should be evacuated with thoracostomy. Residual hemothorax that does not resolve after insertion of a chest tube should be considered for video-assisted thoracosopic (VATS) drainage. This approach results in shorter duration of chest tube drainage, shorter hospital length of stay, lower hospital costs, and prevention of a surgical procedure later in the hospital course when compared to the placement of a second chest tube. Moreover, retained hemothorax following chest tube placement has been associated with a 33% risk of empyema. Timing of VATS intervention is best undertaken in days 3 to 7 of hospitalization to reduce the risk of conversion to thoracotomy.[34] Chest tubes may be safely removed following demonstrated pleural space evacuation, on underwater seal, with <300 mL output over prior 24 hours.

The impact of rib fractures upon patient physiology may vary greatly, depending on the morphology of injury and patient characteristics. Of greatest concern is the associated inability to perform pulmonary toilet due to pain with subsequent development of respiratory compromise. To this end, institutional protocols involve multimodal narcotic-sparing pain regimens, often with the assistance of an acute pain service and consideration of epidural catheterization. Adequate analgesia allows for optimal pulmonary toilet and avoidance of pneumonia. Technological

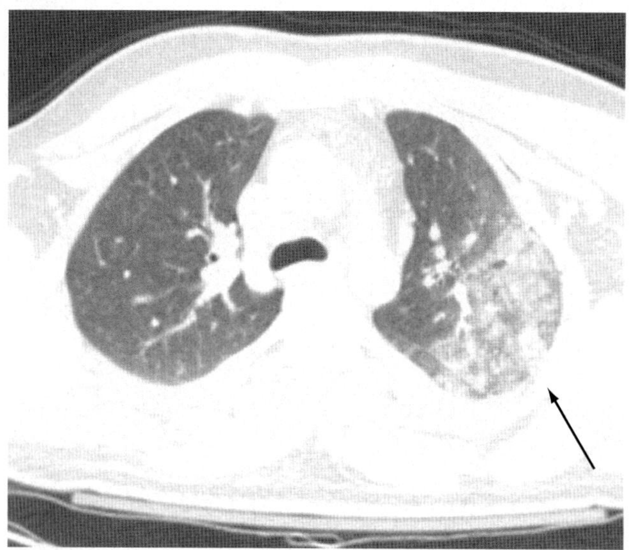

FIG. 17.18 Left pulmonary contusion on thoracic computed tomography scan. The *arrow* identifies contused lung, which appears as higher density tissue because of air space hemorrhage and associated edema.

advances and data demonstrating benefit in flail segment repair have prompted renewed interest in the surgical stabilization of rib fractures. In nonsegmental fractures, recent trial data show decreased numeric pain scores and improved quality-of-life metrics at 2 weeks following surgical stabilization of rib fractures.[36] Sternal fractures are most often managed similarly to nonoperative rib fractures, although certain patterns may benefit from reconstruction. Taken together, as questions persist regarding the role for surgical stabilization of rib fractures in chest wall injury management, operative planning is best undertaken on a case-by-case basis and couched in risk/benefit conversations with the patient and surgical partnership.

Pulmonary Injuries. Approximately one in three patients in the NTDB sustains a pulmonary contusion after chest trauma. Mortality after pulmonary contusion is predominately a result of respiratory failure from acute respiratory distress syndrome (ARDS) or pneumonia. Trauma to the lung is caused by energy transfer through the chest wall to the pulmonary parenchyma, resulting in tissue damage as well as hemorrhage into the alveolar and interstitial spaces. This tissue damage is manifested as a physiologic shunt with hypoxemia. The majority of morbidity is secondary to a profound inflammatory response that can progress to multiple organ dysfunction or failure. Frequently, pulmonary contusion occurs with a flail segment and is often more clinically important than the bony trauma. Lung injury can also be caused by penetrating mechanisms, with gunshot wounds (GSWs) being the most common. Typically, the missile directly lacerates the parenchyma and then can cause significant contusion of the surrounding tissue.

Beyond clinical suspicion, chest radiographs obtained in the trauma bay shortly after arrival may be the first suggestion of underlying pulmonary injury. Lung contusions are occasionally present on the initial chest radiograph, but typically require time (24–48 hours) to become visualized. Pulmonary contusions that are identified early on chest film are frequently severe and often rapidly progress to respiratory failure. Thoracic CT is valuable for the identification of pulmonary contusion, although it can be challenging at times to differentiate contusion from atelectasis. A valuable rule of thumb is that atelectasis does not cross pulmonary fissures, whereas contusions are not limited by ventilatory segments. Furthermore, injured pulmonary tissue in the vicinity of chest wall trauma, especially in nondependent segments, is highly suggestive of pulmonary contusion. Injured lung tissue on CT appears as a higher density, as depicted in Fig. 17.18.

Pulmonary contusion is typically managed with supportive care (aggressive pulmonary toilet, adequate pain control). Patients should be monitored for hypoxemia, increased work of breathing, and agitation, the sum of which indicates respiratory decompensation. Although the majority of pulmonary contusions resolve with time, some may progress to mechanical ventilation and extracorporeal membrane oxygenation (ECMO). A recent large retrospective review of trauma patients managed with primarily venovenous ECMO demonstrated at 70% survival from cannulation and 60% to hospital discharge. ARDS was the most common indication following chest trauma and the median duration of cannulation was 8 to 9 days.[37]

Nonoperative measures and thoracostomy manage the majority of thoracic trauma. Although there are classic guidelines for operative chest exploration as defined by chest tube output, the decision to operate should be based on the likelihood of *ongoing* bleeding. For this reason, persistent drainage of blood from the chest tube in the physiologically compromised patient is more important than the amount of initial output upon insertion. In most cases, tube thoracostomy alone with lung expansion adequately manages low-pressure lung bleeding and small air leaks. Ongoing bloody effluent indicates a more central, high-pressure source, which should prompt intervention for control of bleeding. While endovascular management for injuries to the thorax is best described for aortic and thoracic outlet injury, embolization of bleeding vessels within the pulmonary circulation may be an alternative to surgery at institutions with interventional radiology support.

Blunt trauma results in severe diffuse lung injury and is more difficult to treat surgically with worse outcomes compared to penetrating injury. Where stapled incision of a missile tract (tractotomy) and stapled wedge resection (20%–40%) are more common in penetrating mechanisms, anatomic lobectomy and pneumonectomy are more commonly performed if resection is required in association with blunt trauma (15%–20%). Hilar control with either clamp or "hilar twist" should be the initial maneuver performed if significant bleeding is encountered upon entry into the chest. Bleeding from the pulmonary parenchyma is controlled through suture (3-0 polypropylene) ligation of bleeding vessels. Stapled tractotomy exposes injured vessels and bronchi for individual ligation. Trauma pneumonectomy is extremely morbid with high mortality (>50%) and should only be performed for the patient *in extremis*, having quickly exhausted other attempts at hemostasis. Damage control principles may also be applied to the chest with laparotomy sponges and temporary closure over chest tubes. As opposed to abdominal packing, packs in the chest should occupy minimal space and be constructed to allow maximal lung expansion.

Cardiac Injuries. Despite being uncommon, cardiac injuries are some of the most severe injuries sustained by patients after penetrating and blunt trauma. Penetrating injury to the heart occurred in 1% to 2% of patients with penetrating trauma in the NTDB and in less than 10% of the subset with penetrating chest trauma alone. These statistics likely underestimate the true incidence of penetrating cardiac injuries, as up to 94% are immediately lethal and never present to a hospital. Mortality among patients arriving to a trauma center with a penetrating cardiac injury ranges from 17% to 58%.[38]

The location of penetrating injury on initial examination will often be suggestive of cardiac injury ("the cardiac box," described previously). Patients may present in extremis with pericardial tamponade or bleeding into one of the pleural spaces. Those who require immediate RT in the emergency department may have a cardiac injury identified at that time. In others, indicators of pericardial tamponade may be present (Beck triad—hypotension, distended neck veins, and muffled heart sounds) although inconsistently. Ultrasound is a valuable tool for quickly assessing the pericardium for fluid and should be performed in all patients with hemodynamic instability. When the results of ultrasound are inconclusive or potentially falsely negative, as in the setting of left or right hemothorax, a subxiphoid pericardial window is required to evaluate for the presence of blood in the pericardium. On making a small opening in the pericardium, the pericardial space can be directly visualized. The pericardial window may then be extended to perform a median sternotomy in the setting of visualized blood. Recent evidence suggests a safe alternative approach to sternotomy following positive subxiphoid window with pericardial drain placement in those patients for whom bloody effluent is self-limiting and remain hemodynamically stable.[38]

For cardiac injuries that cause cardiovascular collapse, a left anterolateral thoracotomy is performed in the emergency department as previously described and may be extended to a contralateral ("clamshell") incision if need be. When time permits, most cardiac injuries are best approached through a median sternotomy. Injuries to the atria can be grasped in a side-biting fashion with a Satinsky clamp and then closed with running permanent monofilament sutures on a long taper needle (i.e., 3-0 prolene). Ventricular injuries can be more challenging and usually are associated with significant bleeding. The laceration can be held together manually while the defect is closed with horizontal mattress sutures, avoiding ligation of adjacent coronary vessels, and reinforced with pledgets. To gain temporary control and allow transport to the OR, skin staples may provide short-term closure of the cardiac laceration. Another option is the passage of a Foley catheter through the wound, followed by inflation of the balloon and maintenance of outward tension. This technique must be performed carefully as it runs the risk of dilating the cardiotomy with excessive tension.

Blunt injury to the heart occurs less commonly, being seen in only 2.2% of blunt chest trauma cases. Most of these cases represent a contusion of the myocardium that results in arrhythmias and is frequently self-limited. In rare cases, blunt cardiac injury results in heart failure with cardiogenic shock. The diagnosis of cardiac contusion has been well studied but remains controversial. Patients suspected of having a blunt cardiac injury should undergo electrocardiography and troponin I evaluation at the time of initial workup. These studies in tandem rule out blunt cardiac injury if both are negative.[39] A new abnormality on the electrocardiogram (ECG), most commonly tachyarrhythmia, should result in admission for continuous ECG monitoring. Clinical findings of cardiac contusion that are absent on admission are unlikely to develop and, in their continued absence, require no further evaluation. The presence of hemodynamic instability with evidence of heart failure should prompt echocardiography to assess cardiac wall and septal motion as well as valvular function. Cardiogenic shock may require treatment with inotropic support and right ventricular afterload reduction, given the frequent involvement of the right side of the heart. Patients who demonstrate structural abnormalities, such as valvular incompetence, may require urgent operation for repair.

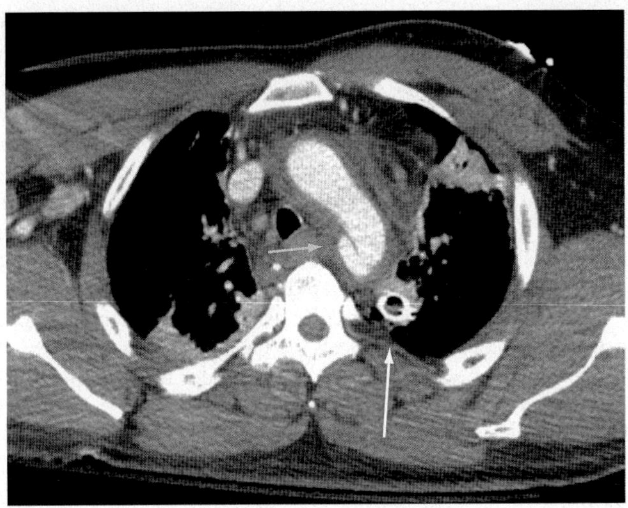

FIG. 17.19 Aortic transection with pseudoaneurysm and associated hematoma on thoracic computed tomography. This injury occurred at the typical location, just distal to the left subclavian artery at the aortic isthmus. The *yellow arrow* identifies a pseudoaneurysm; the *white arrow* identifies a left-sided tube thoracostomy.

Thoracic Aortic Injuries. Thoracic aortic injuries are fortunately uncommon but are associated with poor outcomes. Approximately 80% of trauma patients with blunt traumatic aortic injury (BTAI) die before they reach a hospital and 50% of those surviving to the hospital die within 24 hours.[40] As with other severe injuries, the described incidence of these injuries underestimates the actual frequency, given an unknown denominator. BTAI are believed to be a result of rapid deceleration, which tears the aortic wall in the vicinity of the ligamentum arteriosum. Other theories suggest that lateral mechanisms also contribute, during which the aortic arch acts as a lever and causes torque to develop at the aortic isthmus. The result of these mechanisms can range from a tear in the aortic intima to full-thickness transection of the vessel wall. With full-thickness injuries, only those who experience containment of the rupture by the surrounding adventitial and mediastinal tissues survive to hospital presentation. Penetrating aortic injury is also uncommon, being present in approximately 3% of penetrating chest trauma, with the associated mortality approaching 90%.

In the setting of BTAI, a chest radiograph may demonstrate findings such as a widened mediastinum, apical capping, loss of the aortic knob, or deviation of the left mainstem bronchus. Because of a high rate of missed injuries with use of chest radiography as a screening study, most patients involved in high-energy injury mechanisms undergo helical CT angiography of the chest to evaluate for aortic injury. On this modality, an aortic injury ranges from a disruption in the intima (Grade I), intramural hematoma (Grade II), pseudoaneurysm (Grade III) to rupture (Grade IV). As technology has evolved, chest CT alone is usually sufficient to plan operative repair and standard angiography is rarely necessary. Fig. 17.19 reveals a chest CT image that demonstrates a contained pseudoaneurysm from an aortic transection. Similarly, aortic injury from penetrating trauma may be identified on CT imaging or at the time of exploration, often in the setting of a patient in extremis.

BTAI with pseudoaneurysm will require operative repair, as the natural history of these injuries is slow expansion to free aortic rupture. Despite this, the progression is usually slow and allows for other more urgent issues, such as acute hemorrhage and resuscitation, to be addressed in the first 24 hours of admission. It is essential that aortic wall stress be controlled until repair is performed. This is usually adequately achieved with beta-receptor antagonist medications (i.e., labetalol or esmolol infusions). The majority of these injuries are now addressed via thoracic endovascular aortic repair. This change in treatment has evolved during the last 10 years, now demonstrating equivalent mortality and in-hospital morbidity to open repair. Thus the appeal of the minimally invasive approach with the rapid progression of catheter-based technology has made endovascular repair the treatment of choice at most trauma centers.[40] Access to the thoracic aorta is through the groin, and the stent graft is placed under fluoroscopic guidance. On occasion, the graft will cover the ostia of the left subclavian artery, at which time a carotid-to-subclavian bypass may also be required if symptoms develop. When open surgical repair is required, the aorta is exposed through a left thoracotomy. Large penetrating injuries and blunt transection require replacement of a segment of the aorta with a prosthetic graft. This is most commonly performed with the assistance of cardiopulmonary bypass, including full bypass through a femoral-femoral approach or with a centrifugal pump and left-sided heart bypass. The use of cardiopulmonary bypass has been associated with a decreased incidence of paraplegia, which can result from cessation of aortic blood flow if a clamp and sew technique is used.

As the ability to visualize small intimal defects on CT has evolved, there are aortic injuries that may not require operative repair. Some patients with only a small intimal tear may be candidates for nonoperative management, as many of these injuries will heal without intervention. Patients should be treated with beta-blocker therapy and undergo follow-up imaging to ensure the absence of expansion and ultimately the resolution of the injury.

Tracheobronchial Injuries. Tracheobronchial tree injuries are uncommon but associated with significant morbidity and mortality. Penetrating mechanisms are the most common cause, although these injuries historically represent only rare occurrences (<1%). Blunt injury to the tracheobronchial tree can occur but is similarly uncommon, resulting from the application of a large amount of energy to the anterior chest. These forces pull the lungs laterally and avulse the bronchi from the fixed carina. Furthermore, a tracheal rupture may occur when lungs and airways are rapidly compressed against a closed glottis, perforating the trachea along the membranous portion. Penetrating tracheobronchial injuries are predominantly a result of GSWs that cause direct laceration of the tracheobronchial tree.

The location of the airway disruption will dictate the clinical presentation and the method of injury identification. Injuries that involve the thoracic trachea and proximal bronchi may result in large amounts of pneumomediastinum identified by chest radiography or CT imaging. More distal airway injuries will typically cause a pneumothorax requiring insertion of a tube thoracostomy. A continuous air leak with persistent pneumothorax is highly suggestive of an injury to a bronchus or large bronchiole. Significant subcutaneous air may also be present on physical examination. Diagnosis is made with either rigid or flexible bronchoscopy, depending on the location of the injury and the ability to manipulate the neck. Bronchoscopy allows the identification of the injury and a detailed characterization, such as the location and severity of the disruption.

The management of tracheobronchial injuries begins with careful assessment and control of the airway. With the placement of any airway, avoidance of further disruption is vital, and it may benefit from bronchoscopic guidance under direct visualization. Bronchial injuries that occupy less than one third of the luminal circumference may be considered for nonoperative management if lung expansion with a chest tube results in resolution of the pneumothorax and associated air leak. Management includes humidified oxygen, careful suctioning, and close observation to monitor for infectious sequelae that may develop. Operative management of the trachea, right-sided airways, and proximal left mainstem bronchus is best approached through a right posterolateral thoracotomy. Distal left-sided injuries are repaired through a left thoracotomy. A vascularized intercostal muscle flap should be mobilized and preserved during creation of the thoracotomy, as placement of a retractor will prevent harvest of this valuable tissue coverage. Devitalized tissue should be debrided and injures closed with absorbable monofilament suture. Large injuries may require segmental resection with anastomosis. Coverage of the repair with a tissue pedicle, such as the previously created intercostal muscle flap, may improve healing. If possible, patients who require ongoing mechanical ventilation should have the endotracheal tube advanced so that the end of the tube is distal to the repair and protected from positive pressure. Other options include dual-lung ventilation and extracorporeal life support during the immediate postoperative period.

Esophageal Injuries. Similar to the tracheobronchial tree, the thoracic esophagus is uncommonly injured by either blunt or penetrating mechanisms. Penetrating injury is slightly more common; however, historically, less than 1% of chest injuries in the NTDB had involvement of the esophagus by blunt or penetrating mechanism. Most penetrating injuries are caused by GSWs, followed by stab wounds. The mortality associated with penetrating esophageal injuries is substantial (35%), as a result of mediastinal sepsis and injury to the adjacent vital structures. Although these injuries are rare, the mortality is significant because of challenges with timely diagnosis and treatment. Whereas penetrating injury causes direct tissue laceration, blunt esophageal injury is likely to be caused by a rapid elevation in intraluminal pressure during compression of the chest or abdomen. An impact to the upper abdomen can compress the distended stomach, leading to transmission of air and fluid up the esophagus and resulting in a perforation of the wall, usually in the distal segment.

The location of penetrating injuries and the presumed trajectory are often suggestive of esophageal injury. Penetrating injuries in the vicinity of the mediastinum require consideration of possible esophageal injury. The esophagus is best evaluated through a combination of contrast esophagography (water-soluble first, followed by thin barium) and esophagoscopy. Together, these two modalities result in a sensitivity of almost 100% for esophageal injury. Diagnostic studies may reveal leak of contrast material from the esophageal lumen or a disruption of the mucosa visualized during endoscopy. Helical CT esophagography may be a reasonable alternative to a fluoroscopic esophagram, obviating the need for patient participation (i.e., intubated patients) and radiologist administration of the study. In the absence of contrast, chest CT reveals air adjacent to the esophagus but outside the lumen with surrounding soft tissue inflammation. High-resolution CT imaging may even demonstrate an esophageal wall defect. The location of the injury should be determined to assist in operative planning.

Esophageal injuries with associated mediastinal contamination require immediate identification and repair, as delays are associated with worse outcomes. Esophageal injuries require operative repair to close the esophageal defect, ideally in two layers (mucosal/muscular), with provision of adequate drainage. Management of injuries to the cervical esophagus is described previously in "Injuries to the Neck." The upper and midthoracic esophagus is best approached through a right posterolateral thoracotomy through the fourth or fifth interspace, whereas the lower esophagus is exposed from the left through the sixth or seventh interspace. As with tracheobronchial injuries, creation of a vascularized intercostal muscle flap on entry into the chest will allow excellent coverage of the repair. Alternatives to the intercostal muscle include pleura, pericardium, or diaphragm.

When the location of the injury is at the gastroesophageal junction, it may best be approached through a laparotomy. The injury is entirely exposed, which usually requires opening of the muscle layer superiorly and inferiorly to reveal the extent of the mucosal defect, which is commonly larger than the muscle disruption. The esophageal injury is then closed in one or two layers, frequently with an absorbable mucosal suture followed by interrupted muscle sutures of a permanent material. Coverage of the repair with a muscle flap or adjacent tissue may help reduce the high rate of leak. Esophageal repairs at the gastroesophageal junction can be covered with a fundoplication of gastric tissue. Wide drainage of the mediastinum and chest is extremely important to control any leak that may develop. Decompression of the stomach and distal feeding access are necessary, whether through nasoenteral tube placement or surgical gastrostomy and feeding jejunostomy. Following repair, an esophagram may be performed at day 5 to confirm healing and liberalization of oral intake.

Inflammation within the mediastinum develops quickly, and primary repair of injuries that are identified late may not be possible. Salvage techniques to be considered in these circumstances include repair of the defect over a T-tube for creation of a controlled fistula, esophageal diversion through a cervical incision, or esophageal stenting. Esophagectomy, although rare in the setting of trauma, may be the only option to allow recovery followed by planned elective reconstruction.

Diaphragmatic Injuries. Traumatic diaphragmatic injuries were analyzed in a large series by the NTDB in 2012, including >800,000 patients. Results revealed an overall incidence of 0.46%. Penetrating trauma was more common than blunt (67% vs. 33%, respectively). GSWs outnumbered stab wounds and motor vehicle collisions were among the commonest mechanisms. Higher mortality was identified among blunt over penetrating trauma (19.8% vs. 8.8%).[41] Almost all of these deaths are a result of injury to adjacent vital organs because diaphragmatic injuries themselves are usually of limited threat to life. As opposed to direct laceration of the tissue by missile, blunt diaphragmatic injuries are believed to be a result of a rapid increase in intraabdominal pressure during an anterior impact, causing a blow-out of the diaphragmatic tissue. The left side of the diaphragm is the injured location in approximately 75% of the cases because of the coverage of the right side with the liver. The morbidity related to diaphragmatic injuries is occasionally identified months to years later when the perforation was not initially repaired. The natural history of these injuries includes progressive enlargement with herniation of abdominal viscera into the chest.

Injuries to the diaphragm can be a diagnostic challenge and require a high index of suspicion, even with the most subtle indicators. The chest radiograph may demonstrate the presence of abdominal viscera, most commonly the stomach, within the chest (Fig. 17.20). Passage of a nasogastric tube can be of assistance if the tube is identified in the lower left hemithorax. The injection of gastric contrast material may add to the detection with this modality. CT scans may demonstrate the presence of abdominal viscera in the chest or an abnormality of the diaphragm itself, such as thickening, elevation, or defect. Penetrating diaphragmatic injuries are usually discovered on operative exploration of the chest or abdomen. During exploration, following the trajectory of the injury will usually allow identification of the diaphragmatic defect. In the hemodynamically stable patient without peritonitis, laparoscopy is recommended over CT scanning alone to decrease the incidence of missed traumatic diaphragmatic injuries. Given the rare incidence of right-sided delayed diaphragmatic hernia, penetrating thoracoabdominal trauma to the right hemibody may be considered for nonoperative management.[41] In the absence of radiographic stigmata, blunt injuries can be more elusive and laparoscopic evaluation may be required when imaging is suggestive. The application of VATS has been reported as an alternative means of visualizing the diaphragm, although no demonstrable superiority exists compared to laparoscopy.

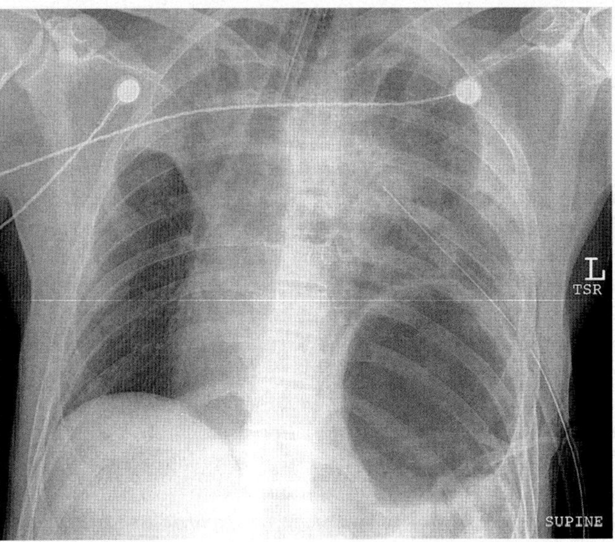

FIG. 17.20 Left-sided diaphragmatic injury on plain chest radiograph. The gas-filled stomach can be visualized on the left side of the chest because of herniation through a large diaphragmatic laceration.

Diaphragmatic injuries are typically repaired by debriding nonviable tissue and then closing the defect. The diaphragm exhibits enough redundancy for all, but the largest defects to be closed primarily. Closure is performed with a single layer of nonabsorbable suture incorporating large full-thickness bites of healthy diaphragmatic tissue. It is important to obtain hemostasis because diaphragmatic injuries can bleed significantly from branches of the phrenic artery that can be exposed at the edges of the tear. Large areas of tissue loss are rare in traumatic rupture, but when present may require reconstruction with a prosthetic. Nonabsorbable synthetic materials can be used to reconstruct the diaphragm in clean surgical fields but should be avoided in the setting of contamination. A peripheral detachment of the diaphragm from the wall of the torso can be repaired by reinserting the injured tissue one or two interspaces superior.

Injuries to the Abdomen

The abdomen is a commonly injured body region and frequently requires the care of a surgeon for definitive management. Within the 2016 NTDB, 11.7% of all patients sustained abdominal injuries with an associated case fatality rate of 12.9%.[2] The vital nature of the organs contained within the abdomen makes evaluation and management a priority. The predominant sources of morbidity and mortality are bleeding and visceral perforation with associated sepsis. In the setting of blunt trauma, solid organs often sustain contusion or laceration, causing bleeding that may require surgical management. Furthermore, blunt forces can cause rupture of hollow viscera due to rapid compression of a segment of intestine containing fluid and air. Penetrating mechanisms directly lacerate solid and hollow viscera, resulting in bleeding and intraabdominal contamination that often require operative repair.

As described for other cavities, the initial evaluation of the abdominally injured patient varies on the basis of blunt versus penetrating mechanisms, although a common priority is rapidly determining the presence or absence of ongoing hemorrhage. Although metric definitions of this are nonstandard, patients who respond to resuscitation and maintain appropriate hemodynamics are termed *responders*. This population is considered likely to "have bled" rather than suffering persistent bleeding. On the contrary, patients who do not respond to resuscitation with persistent physiologic instability are considered *nonresponders* and likely require immediate intervention. *Transient responders* are those in whom an improvement in metrics is initially noted with resuscitation but return to instability within a short time period. In the trauma bay, ATLS surveys are designed for expeditious identification of cavitary hemorrhage, following assessment of airway and breathing.

Blunt Abdominal Trauma Evaluation

Ultrasound has become a nearly ubiquitous technology in emergency departments internationally and has found routine application in the assessment of intraabdominal hemorrhage following blunt trauma. It is considered an adjunct to the primary survey in ATLS and has the advantage of being rapidly performed at the bedside (*ATLS* 10th edition, FAST video on MyATLS mobile app).[8] Ultrasound for trauma evaluates the pericardium, hepatorenal fossa, splenorenal fossa, and retrovesicular space (pouch of Douglas). Resuscitationists may choose to obtain a FAST in the presence or absence of hemodynamic instability, as this exam may be repeated should physiologic decline develop at a later point. Abdominal exploration is classically indicated in blunt trauma patients who are nonresponders in the presence of intraabdominal fluid on FAST. If FAST examination capabilities are unavailable, ATLS recommends performance of diagnostic peritoneal lavage. Peritoneal aspiration revealing GI contents, bile, or more than 10 mL of gross blood suggests operative intraabdominal trauma. Notably, neither technique of rapid assessment is flawless. FAST is limited by operator familiarity, body habitus, and subcutaneous emphysema/bowel gas. Diagnostic peritoneal lavage is very rarely performed, associated with iatrogenic injury, relatively contraindicated in obesity, and suffers from low specificity. Both techniques are unable to evaluate the retroperitoneum, which may represent a considerable source of hemorrhage.

Technological advancements and increased availability of CT over the past two decades have made it the primary method for comprehensive workup of the blunt trauma patient. This evolution has supported the development of nonoperative management strategies for many solid abdominal organ injuries. Abdominal CT for trauma is typically performed with IV administration of a contrast agent additionally timed to capture the portal venous phase, which best demonstrates the perfusion of the solid abdominal organs. This technique provides the necessary visualization of the solid organs to allow the determination of injury severity, including the presence of active bleeding. Imaging findings prompt management decisions, such as the need for operative, nonoperative, or angiographic therapy. Historically, blood within the abdomen mandated laparotomy, although commonly, the bleeding from solid organs was self-limited by the time of exploration. Subsequently, surgeons recognized that the physiologic state was likely more indicative of the need for laparotomy than the presence of injury alone. Thus, consideration of nonoperative management in the presence of hemoperitoneum with stable vital signs became an accepted pathway. As practice continues to evolve with the proximity and speed of CT scanning in the emergency department, damage control resuscitation under trauma team management is able to continue throughout the ever shortening diagnostic window. The unclear sources of shock often germane to the blunt trauma patient have led some contemporary practices to advocate whole-body CT scanning in the presence of hypotension (systolic <90). The resultant information from rapidly obtained CT scanning may lead the surgeon down vastly different treatment algorithms (i.e., operative, endovascular, supportive).

Despite being sensitive for solid organ injury, CT is less capable of detecting injuries to the hollow viscera. This ability has improved as CT technology evolves, although there are still significant limitations. Injury to the GI tract is suggested by bowel wall thickening, inflammation in the surrounding adipose tissue (stranding), or the presence of free intraperitoneal fluid. Oral contrast material is uncommonly provided as it adds little to the value of the study. Unexplained free fluid must be carefully considered, given a high risk for associated bowel injury. In a significant percentage of cases, unexplained free fluid represents blood from a mesenteric tear that is no longer bleeding. Clinical findings such as the presence of an abdominal seat belt mark or tenderness on examination raise concern in the setting of a suggestive CT. Serial examinations of the abdomen to monitor for worsening tenderness and peritoneal irritation are important and required for those patients who are not taken directly for exploration. Alternatively, laparoscopy may be a safe and feasible alternative to open exploration in patients without shock or other indications for surgery. A representative flow diagram of blunt abdominal trauma evaluation is depicted in Fig. 17.21.

Penetrating Abdominal Trauma Evaluation

The evaluation of penetrating abdominal trauma requires an approach unique from that for blunt mechanisms. Per typical ATLS approach, airway and breathing should be assessed first, followed by identification of all penetrating trauma. In the setting of GSWs, injuries should be identified with radiopaque markers and plain radiographs obtained to establish possible trajectory and pneumoperitoneum. The role of FAST in abdominal GSWs is of controversial utility. When positive, it may support the need for abdominal exploration but is insufficient to rule out major hemorrhage or other operative trauma. The number of missiles and skin wounds should add up to an even number or a more intense search for retained ballistics is required. Patients in extremis, although protecting their airway, should go directly to the OR with intubation immediately prior to incision. In the presence of normal physiology, abdominal GSW patients may proceed to CT scan for further delineation of their injuries. GSWs involving the thoracoabdomen may also require evaluation of the chest for mediastinal, pleural, or pulmonary injuries.[42]

Similar to patients with GSWs, abdominal stab wound patients with hemodynamic instability, peritonitis, or evisceration require immediate laparotomy. In patients who are not examinable, evaluation for peritoneal violation may be conducted via local wound exploration, ultrasound, CT, or diagnostic laparoscopy. All others can be managed by one of several pathways depending upon location of the wound. For stab wounds to the flank or back, contrasted CT imaging (+/- rectal contrast) should be undertaken to identify signs of operative injury. If solid organ

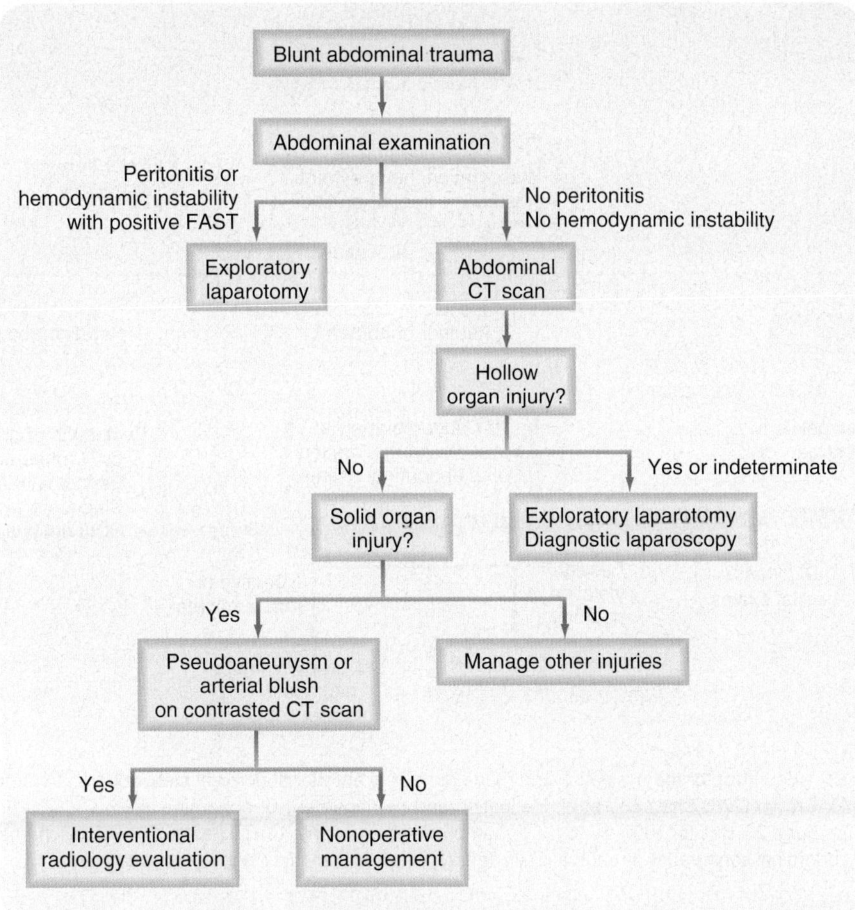

FIG. 17.21 Algorithm for the evaluation and management of blunt abdominal trauma. *CT,* Computed tomography; *FAST,* focused abdominal sonography in trauma.

injury is identified with active extravasation, angioembolization should be considered. Anterior stab wounds allow for discretion of the attending surgeon. Local wound exploration to determine fascial violation, serial clinical exams, or diagnostic imaging for the hemodynamically appropriate patient represent equivalent pathways to safe management. Patients without any fascial penetration can be considered for discharge. If the local wound exploration reveals any evidence of possible fascial penetration, patients should be monitored with serial abdominal examinations, undergo CT imaging or be considered for diagnostic laparoscopy. Diagnostic laparoscopy is highly accurate for the identification of peritoneal violation but remains controversial for identification of intraabdominal injury and is highly user-dependent.

The development of peritonitis, hemodynamic instability, significant decreases in hemoglobin level, or leukocytosis should prompt further evaluation, usually with laparotomy. Patients without clinical change after 24 hours can have a diet instituted and be considered for discharge. Of note, this approach does require the presence of an infrastructure that allows close surveillance of these patients, which may not be available in all facilities. Lastly, thoracoabdominal stab wounds should employ a chest x-ray for evaluation of pneumothorax and pericardial ultrasound for effusion. Stab wounds to the left upper quadrant will likely require laparoscopy for diaphragmatic assessment, although this may be optional in the right upper quadrant due to liver presence.[43] A suggested abdominal stab wound algorithm is demonstrated in Fig. 17.22.

Management

A laparotomy is performed to explore the abdomen and repair injuries that are identified. It is important that the exploration of the abdomen be performed systematically to avoid missing injuries that may be subtle. As described in the setting of damage control, this approach may require abbreviation in the setting of a deteriorating physiologic condition. As a standard technique, the abdomen is opened from the xiphoid process to the pubic symphysis to provide adequate exposure. The falciform ligament can be divided, separating the liver from the abdominal wall to improve retraction and to facilitate perihepatic packing. With use of a handheld retractor, blood is quickly evacuated from all four quadrants of the abdomen and laparotomy sponges are placed to provide temporary hemostasis. A fixed retractor can be placed to facilitate optimal exposure. Sponges placed in the four quadrants are removed to address bleeding but can be replaced as needed in the setting of damage control. The entire GI tract is carefully evaluated, from the gastroesophageal junction to the proximal rectum at the peritoneal reflection. The lesser sac is also entered to visualize the posterior stomach and the pancreas. When injuries are identified, they are repaired, as detailed in subsequent sections. The development of physiologic compromise prompts the need to abbreviate the operation and proceed with damage control methods, including temporary abdominal closure. This recognition benefits greatly from effective two-way communication between the surgical and anesthesia teams. If the operation can be completed without conversion to damage

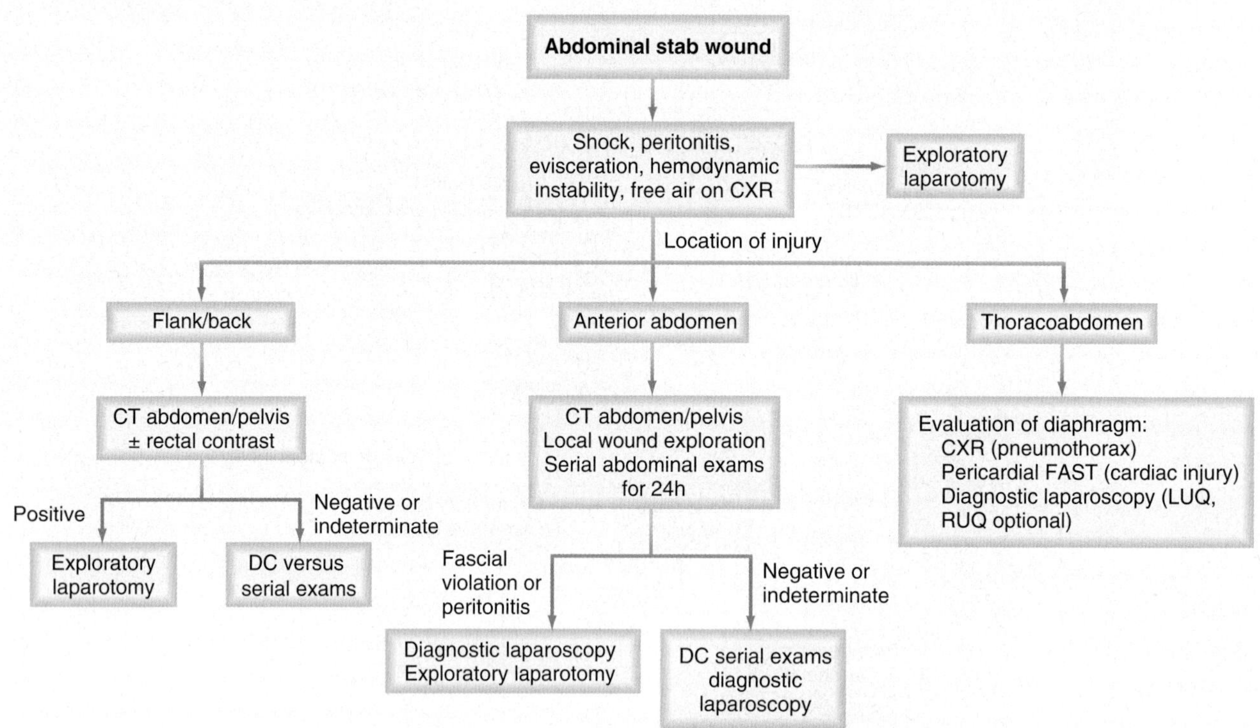

FIG. 17.22 Algorithm for the evaluation and management of anterior abdominal stab wounds. (Adapted from Martin MJ, Brown CVR, Shatz DV, et al. Evaluation and management of abdominal stab wounds. *J Trauma Acute Care Surg.* 2018;85(5):1007–1015.). *CT*, Computed tomography; *CXR*, chest x-ray; *DC*, discharge; *FAST*, focused abdominal sonography in trauma; *LUQ*, left upper quadrant; *RUQ*, right upper quadrant.

control, the abdominal fascia is closed and the subcutaneous wound addressed as dictated by the level of intraabdominal contamination.

Splenic Injuries. The spleen, in alternation with the liver, is the first or second most commonly injured abdominal organ, and isolated splenic injury comprises approximately 42% of abdominal trauma.[44] The frequency of these injuries requires the surgeon to possess a sound understanding of management strategies in splenic injury. In reality, splenic trauma represents a spectrum of diseases, ranging from self-limitation and observation to immediate splenectomy in the setting of hemodynamic instability.

In blunt trauma, direct compression of the spleen with parenchymal fracture is a common pathophysiologic mechanism at the tissue level. Additionally, injury can be secondary to rapid deceleration that tears the splenic capsule and/or parenchyma where it is fixed to the retroperitoneum. This mechanism can create a subcapsular hematoma, which is demonstrated in Fig. 17.23. Penetrating splenic trauma is less common but is still present in 8.5% of all penetrating abdominal injuries in the 2012 NTDB. Hemorrhage from a splenic injury can be ongoing with instability at the time of presentation or, more commonly, will have resolved spontaneously. As with other abdominal injuries, patients who are nonresponders to resuscitation with intraabdominal fluid on FAST require exploration. Patients who respond to resuscitation with normalized physiology can often be managed nonoperatively, although this group is at risk for delayed reinitiation of hemorrhage (majority <72 hours). Over the past several decades, rates of nonoperative management in splenic trauma has increased from roughly 40% to 70% with coincident decreases in mortality among the higher grades of injury.[44]

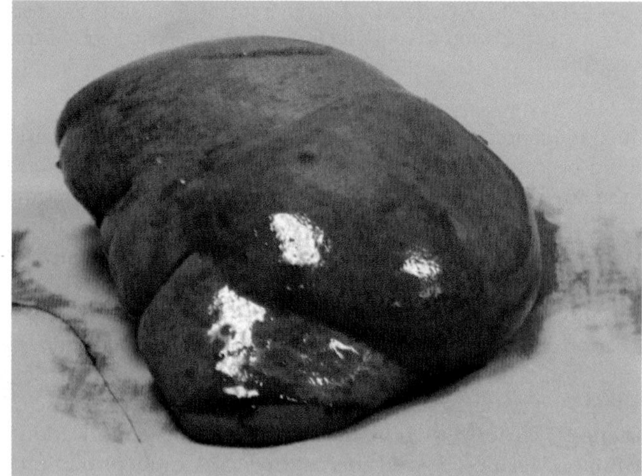

FIG. 17.23 Splenic injury with subcapsular hematoma. Despite only a 1-cm capsular tear, this injury demonstrated ongoing hemorrhage.

Unstable patients with abdominal trauma who are taken emergently to the OR may have a splenic injury identified at the time of laparotomy (10% of blunt splenic injury). In all other patients, abdominal CT with IV administration of a contrast agent is the most valuable study for identifying and characterizing splenic injuries (sensitivity/specificity 96%–100%). Splenic injuries appear as disruptions in the normal splenic parenchyma, frequently with surrounding hematoma and free intraabdominal blood. Active bleeding can be identified by visualizing extravasation of contrast material (i.e., high-density blush or accumulation of contrast-laden blood). At times, this extravasation will be free into the peritoneal space or contained within an intraparenchymal pseudoaneurysm. A splenic injury with active extravasation into a pseudoaneurysm is demonstrated in Fig. 17.24. Other types of splenic injury can include a hematoma confined to the subcapsular space and even complete devascularization of the organ caused by injury of the hilar vessels. Spleen injuries are characterized by the AAST Injury Scoring Scale, which grades injuries on the basis of parenchymal or subcapsular abnormality and the presence of vascular involvement (Table 17.6).

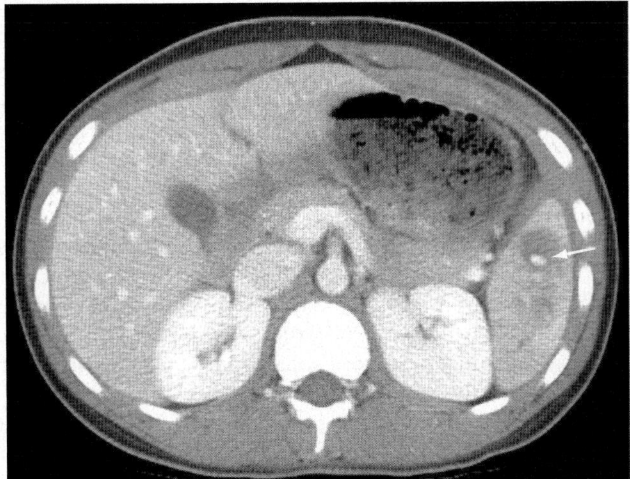

FIG. 17.24 Grade III splenic laceration on abdominal computed tomography. Note the focus of active extravasation of contrast material within the injured splenic parenchyma as identified by the *arrow*.

The overall success rate for nonoperative management is approximately 90% in blunt splenic trauma for high-volume centers. Advantages to this approach include reductions in hospital costs, intraabdominal complications, blood transfusions, nontherapeutic laparotomies, and mortality. Due to the increasing use of splenic angiography and embolization over the past decade, nonoperative management failure rates of 5% are achievable in AAST Grades III to V.[44] To protocolize this approach, our institution has developed a practice guideline whereby stable patients who demonstrate imaging concerning for active extravasation or pseudoaneurysm are evaluated by interventional radiology or angiography and embolization. Furthermore, patients without these findings but high-grade injuries (III–V) are also evaluated by interventional radiology and proceed to angiography and embolization within 24 hours. Despite a great deal of prior investigation, there is no constellation of risk factors (i.e., age, AAST grade, volume of hemoperitoneum, etc.) for failure of nonoperative management that, when present, identifies patients who would benefit from prophylactic operative management in the setting of hemodynamic stability. Moreover, previous studies have demonstrated a lack of increase in complications and mortality with delayed operative intervention.[44] Nonetheless, patients with high-grade injures should undergo intensive care monitoring on admission, maintaining a low threshold for surgical management in the setting of decline.

Operative management of splenic injuries may be required in the setting of instability at the time of admission or after failed nonoperative management. Regardless, the best approach is through a

TABLE 17.6 AAST Spleen Injury Scale (2018 revision).

GRADE	AIS SEVERITY	IMAGING CRITERIA (CT FINDINGS)	OPERATIVE CRITERIA	PATHOLOGIC CRITERIA
I	2	Subcapsular hematoma <10% surface area	Subcapsular hematoma <10% surface area	Subcapsular hematoma <10% surface area
		Parenchymal laceration <1 cm depth	Parenchymal laceration <1 cm depth	Parenchymal laceration <1 cm depth
		Capsular tear	Capsular tear	Capsular tear
II	2	Subcapsular hematoma 10%–50% surface area	Subcapsular hematoma 10%–50% surface area	Subcapsular hematoma 10%–50% surface area
		Intraparenchymal hematoma <5 cm	Intraparenchymal hematoma <5 cm	Intraparenchymal hematoma <5 cm
		Parenchymal laceration 1–3 cm	Parenchymal laceration 1–3 cm	Parenchymal laceration 1–3 cm
III	3	Subcapsular hematoma >50% surface area	Subcapsular hematoma >50% surface area or expanding	Subcapsular hematoma >50% surface area
		Ruptured subcapsular or intraparenchymal hematoma ≥5 cm	Ruptured subcapsular or intraparenchymal hematoma ≥5 cm	Ruptured subcapsular or intraparenchymal hematoma ≥5 cm
		Parenchymal laceration >3 cm depth	Parenchymal laceration >3 cm depth	Parenchymal laceration >3 cm depth
IV	4	Any injury in the presence of a splenic vascular injury or active bleeding confined within the splenic capsule	Parenchymal laceration involving segmental or hilar vessels producing >25% devascularization	Parenchymal laceration involving segmental or hilar vessels producing >25% devascularization
		Parenchymal laceration involving segmental or hilar vessels producing >25% devascularization		
V	5	Any injury in the presence of a splenic vascular injury with active bleeding extending beyond the spleen into the peritoneum	Hilar vascular injury, which devascularizes the spleen	Hilar vascular injury which devascularizes the spleen
		Shattered spleen	Shattered spleen	Shattered spleen

AAST, American Association for the Surgery of Trauma; *AIS*, Abbreviated Injury Scale; *CT*, computed tomography.

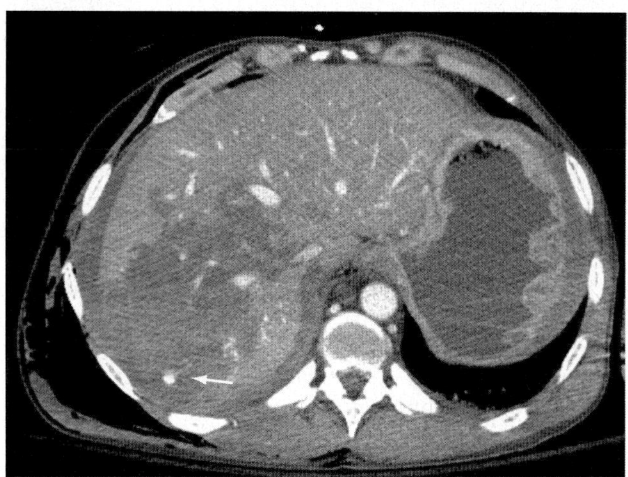

FIG. 17.25 Grade IV liver laceration involving the right hepatic lobe on abdominal computed tomography. Note the focus of active extravasation of contrast material within the injured liver parenchyma at the periphery of the injury as identified by the *arrow*.

midline incision, followed by packing of all four quadrants. A fixed retractor can improve exposure, and the packs are removed to expose the injured spleen. To mobilize the spleen, the peritoneum is divided laterally by retracting the spleen posteromedially to expose the retroperitoneal attachments. This division of the peritoneum begins at the white line of Toldt (splenocolic ligament) and then continues superiorly until the short gastric vessels are encountered. After the peritoneum is opened laterally, a blunt plane is created posterior to the spleen in a medial direction, extending behind the tail of the pancreas. This maneuver mobilizes the entire spleen and distal pancreas, allowing the spleen to be delivered up into the wound. While avoiding the greater curve of the stomach, the short gastric vessels are ligated and divided. Finally, the spleen is removed after the hilar vessels are clamped and ligated, taking care not to injure the tail of the pancreas or greater curve of the stomach. A drain should be placed only if there is concern that the tail of the pancreas was injured. Postsplenectomy vaccines must be provided to ensure protection from encapsulated bacteria (*Streptococcus pneumoniae*, *Neisseria meningitidis*, and *Haemophilus influenzae*) and prevention of overwhelming postsplenectomy sepsis (incidence 0.5%–2%, mortality 30%–70%). Whereas splenic salvage techniques are well described, their utility is limited in the era of highly effective nonoperative management and endovascular approaches to splenic trauma.

Hepatic Injuries. Liver injuries are extremely common after blunt trauma at a rate of 22.2% within the 2012 NTDB. Similarly, the liver is the most commonly injured abdominal organ after penetrating trauma, present in 26.1% of cases. Mechanisms of blunt hepatic trauma include compression with direct parenchymal damage and shearing forces, which tear hepatic tissue and disrupt vascular and ligamentous attachments. The liver is partially protected by the thoracic cage, although the ribs provide little support during high-energy mechanisms. Penetrating mechanisms directly lacerate the hepatic parenchyma while also causing adjacent tissue contusion. Mortality from liver injury, not unlike the management of other abdominal solid organs, has decreased over time as practices have evolved from primarily operative to nonoperative management with endovascular and endoscopic treatments. Associated morbidity from liver injury includes bleeding, biliary, fistula (i.e., hemobilia, biliary fistula), infection, and hepatic necrosis.

Similar to other abdominal organs, liver injuries are often first diagnosed on entering the abdomen in the unstable patient explored for free fluid on FAST examination. Those who do not require immediate operation should be imaged with abdominal CT enhanced with IV administration of a contrast agent. CT is capable of providing excellent anatomic detail that allows highly accurate characterization of injuries. Timing of contrast for delineation of hepatic injury occurs in three phases (noncontrast, arterial, portal venous), giving insight into the hemorrhage type. Common findings on CT indicative of liver injury include disruption of the hepatic parenchyma with perihepatic blood or hematoma and hemoperitoneum. Bleeding from the liver can be seen on CT as extravasation of contrast material either within the liver parenchyma or into the peritoneal space, as seen in Fig. 17.25. The characteristics of the liver injury on CT can be used to categorize the injury with the AAST OIS, which accounts for parenchymal involvement and the presence of vascular injury (Table 17.7).

Treatment of liver trauma has progressed over prior decades from aggressive operative to largely nonoperative care, coinciding with decreased in-hospital mortality. As described by Peitzman and Richardson, the period of 1960 to 1975 presented multiple series of patients who underwent resectional management, hepatic artery ligation, and T-tube choledochostomy for liver injury. At that time, morbidity and mortality, ranging from 27% to 65%, were suspected to arise from biliary/septic complications rather than hemorrhage. In 1976, Lucas and Ledgerwood shifted the focus of care to prioritize bleeding management in hepatic trauma with subsequent decrease in mortality to 22%. Furthermore, the partners described the use of temporary abdominal packing for control of liver bleeding. This approach was later promoted by Feliciano, Mattox, and Jordan for critically ill patients in whom surgical solutions for bleeding had failed. Following these practice changing reports, the AAST OIS for liver, spleen, and kidney was first described in 1989 and remains a consistent scheme for defining solid abdominal organ injury. As data began to accumulate for a nonoperative management option in blunt liver trauma, a review of the literature by Pachter and Hofstetter concluded that nonoperative management should be the approach of choice for the hemodynamically stable patient, regardless of AAST grade. The continued development of CT technology in tandem with endovascular/endoscopic support has resulted in the majority of patients with Grades I to III injuries being successfully managed nonoperatively, while two-thirds of Grades IV and V residually require surgical care. Polanco and colleagues, in review of resectional management for complex blunt and penetrating liver trauma, report a mortality from liver injury of 9%. They attribute the improved mortality within their series to early decision for major operation, intraoperative resuscitation technique, and senior surgical/subspecialty assistance.[45]

Patients who are hemodynamically stable in the setting of blunt and penetrating liver trauma should be considered primarily for nonoperative management. Parenchymal bleeding or pseudoaneurysm on contrasted imaging should prompt consultation to interventional radiology for evaluation. The natural history of hepatic pseudoaneurysms is not entirely elucidated, but it is believed that they may be associated with an increased risk of delayed bleeding, especially when associated with hepatic arterial branches. After successful embolization, patients need intensive care surveillance for all hepatic injuries managed nonoperatively, although there is no standardized laboratory monitoring interval. In appropriately selected patients, the use of angioembolization has improved the rate of successful nonoperative management with a reduction in conversion to surgical treatment.

TABLE 17.7 **AAST liver injury scale (2018 revision).**

GRADE	AIS SEVERITY	IMAGING CRITERIA (CT FINDINGS)	OPERATIVE CRITERIA	PATHOLOGIC CRITERIA
I	2	Subcapsular hematoma <10% surface area	Subcapsular hematoma <10% surface area	Subcapsular hematoma <10% surface area
		Parenchymal laceration <1 cm depth	Parenchymal laceration <1 cm depth	Parenchymal laceration <1 cm depth
		Capsular tear	Capsular tear	Capsular tear
II	2	Subcapsular hematoma 10%–50% surface area	Subcapsular hematoma 10%–50% surface area	Subcapsular hematoma 10%–50% surface area
		Intraparenchymal hematoma <10 cm in diameter	Intraparenchymal hematoma <10 cm in diameter	Intraparenchymal hematoma <10 cm in diameter
		Laceration 1–3 cm in depth and ≤10 cm length	Laceration 1–3 cm in depth and ≤10 cm length	Laceration 1–3 cm in depth and ≤10 cm length
III	3	Subcapsular hematoma >50% surface area	Subcapsular hematoma >50% surface area	Subcapsular hematoma >50% surface area
		Ruptured subcapsular or parenchymal hematoma	Ruptured subcapsular or parenchymal hematoma	Ruptured subcapsular or parenchymal hematoma
		Intraparenchymal laceration >10 cm, laceration >3 m depth	Intraparenchymal laceration >10 cm, laceration >3 m depth	Intraparenchymal laceration >10 cm, laceration >3 m depth
		Any injury in the presence of a liver vascular injury or active bleeding contained within liver parenchyma		
IV	4	Parenchymal disruption involving 25%–75% of a hepatic lobe	Parenchymal disruption involving 25%–75% of a hepatic lobe	Parenchymal disruption involving 25%–75% of a hepatic lobe
		Active bleeding extending beyond the liver parenchyma into the peritoneum		
V	5	Parenchymal disruption >75% of a hepatic lobe	Parenchymal disruption >75% of a hepatic lobe	Parenchymal disruption >75% of a hepatic lobe
		Juxtahepatic venous injury to include retrohepatic vena cava and central major hepatic veins	Juxtahepatic venous injury to include retrohepatic vena cava and central major hepatic veins	Juxtahepatic venous injury to include retrohepatic vena cava and central major hepatic veins

AAST, American Association for the Surgery of Trauma; *AIS*, Abbreviated Injury Scale; *CT*, computed tomography.

Even successful nonoperative management may require the treatment of complications (12%–14%), such as bile leaks with biloma formation, hemobilia, and development of liver abscesses.[45] Frequently, these are suggested by the development of abdominal symptoms with, at times, the addition of systemic infection or inflammation. CT or ultrasound imaging can be valuable in evaluating for abscess and biloma; these can usually be managed with percutaneous drainage guided by CT or ultrasound. Endoscopic retrograde cholangiopancreatography (ERCP) with stent placement is occasionally required to decompress the biliary tree and to promote healing of a bile leak. Biliary ascites not amenable to percutaneous drainage may require laparoscopy or laparotomy for adequate drainage to be obtained. Hemobilia is managed with angiography, which includes embolization of the hepatic vessel that is communicating with the biliary tree.

Although there have been great advances in the nonoperative management of liver injuries, it should not be overlooked that unstable patients require operative management of bleeding. In blunt trauma, a recent systematic review reported a pooled nonoperative management failure rate of 9.5%, predictive factors including signs of shock and peritoneal signs on presentation, high ISS, and associated intraabdominal trauma.[45] Similarly, analysis from LA county demonstrates failure of selective nonoperative management in approximately 5% of patients suffering GSWs to the liver.[46] Polanco and colleagues, in a review of resectional management for complex blunt and penetrating liver trauma, report a mortality from liver injury of 9%. The surgical approach to hepatic injuries as developed by the WTA is presented in Fig. 17.26. When operative management is required, a midline laparotomy is the most versatile approach for managing any liver injury that might be encountered. The falciform ligament is divided, and perihepatic sponges are placed to temporarily manage bleeding from the liver. A fixed retractor can be placed to improve exposure of the right upper quadrant structures. When needed, perihepatic packing and manual compression can temporize bleeding to provide the opportunity to catch up with the resuscitation. Once the patient is reasonably stable, the packs are removed and the injuries to the liver are evaluated. Mild injuries with minimal ongoing bleeding may be managed with further compression, topical hemostatic agents, or suture hepatorrhaphy. Management of liver injuries may be facilitated by dividing the triangular ligaments to mobilize the right or left hepatic lobes. This will allow injuries to be better exposed for repair but may also allow more effective packing by optimizing anterior to posterior compression. Any mobilization of the liver must be carefully considered if there is any chance that the attachments of the liver are providing lifesaving tamponade of retrohepatic bleeding. Most liver injuries will require only superficial techniques for hemostasis to be obtained.

When more severe bleeding from the liver is present, a Pringle maneuver is a valuable adjunct to slow blood flow enough to visualize the injury. The hepatoduodenal ligament is encircled with a vessel loop or vascular clamp to occlude hepatic blood flow from the hepatic artery and portal vein. This maneuver helps distinguish hepatic arterial and portal venous bleeding from hepatic

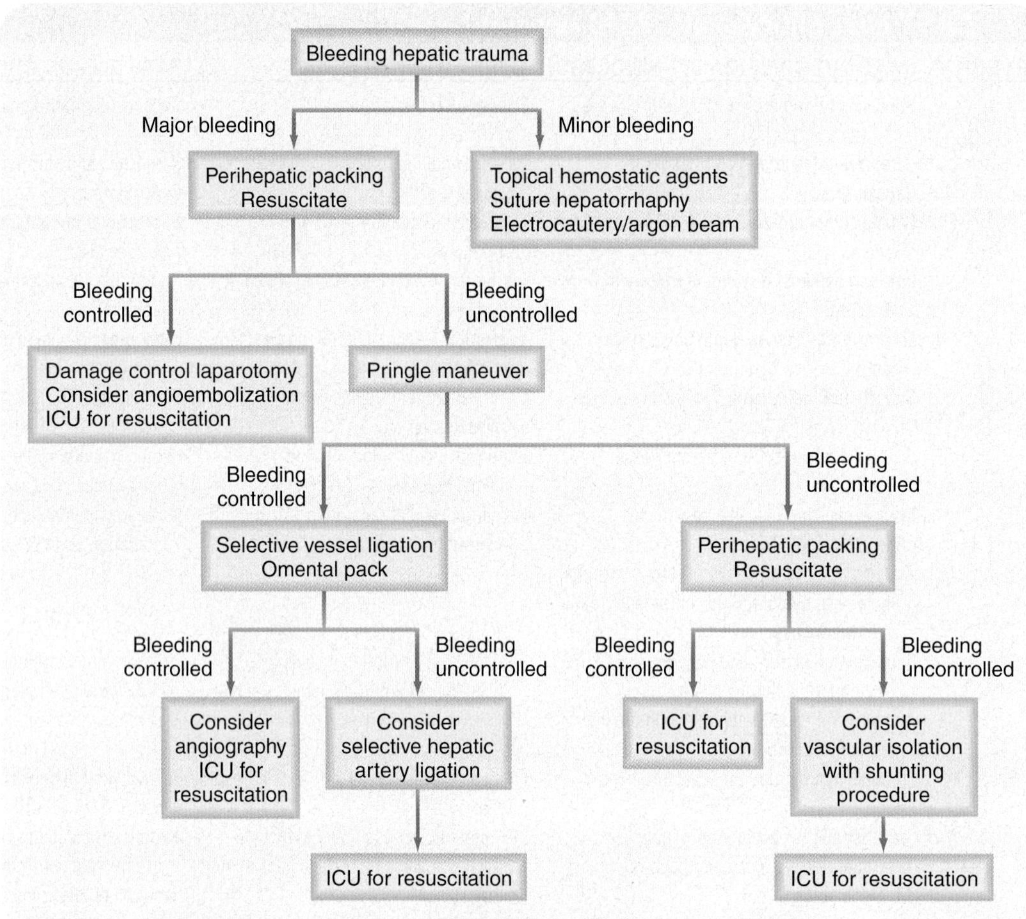

FIG. 17.26 Algorithm for the operative management of hepatic injuries. (Modified from Kozar RA, Feliciano DV, Moore EE, et al. Western Trauma Association/critical decisions in trauma: Operative management of adult blunt hepatic trauma. *J Trauma.* 2011;71:1–5.). *ICU,* Intensive care unit.

vein bleeding, which will persist with the hepatoduodenal ligament clamped. In many cases, the liver laceration can then be explored and any actively bleeding vessels controlled with suture ligation. Hepatic parenchyma that appears to be devitalized should be debrided and drains placed when injuries appear to be at risk for a bile leak. A vascularized pedicle of omentum may reduce parenchymal bleeding and promote healing of the laceration when it is packed within the liver injury.

Liver injuries in the vicinity of the retrohepatic vena cava that are not actively bleeding should be packed and not explored. There are many heroic techniques described in the literature that outline the repair of retrohepatic vena cava injuries, but the approach with the greatest likelihood of success is preserving the natural tamponade of this low-pressure region when feasible. An atriocaval (Shrock) shunt is one method that includes isolation of the retrohepatic vena cava by placing an intravascular shunt between the right atrium and infrahepatic vena cava. Isolation of the liver with an atriocaval shunt with the addition of a Pringle maneuver theoretically allows repair of the vena cava or hepatic veins with less ongoing blood loss.

Damage control techniques are often required because many patients who require operative intervention for liver injuries have already deteriorated physiologically. Control of surgical bleeding is obtained and the liver is packed, followed by temporary abdominal closure. It is inappropriate to leave surgical bleeding in the hope that packing alone will provide adequate control. Conversely, diffuse liver bleeding due to coagulopathy will not respond to repeated attempts at placement of suture. Instead, this should be treated with reversal of physiologic derangements. Patients are then resuscitated in the intensive care unit until hypothermia, coagulopathy, and acidosis resolve, at which time the abdomen can be reexplored and packs removed. After damage control, angiography with embolization may provide additional assistance with management of ongoing bleeding from hepatic artery branches. Nonetheless, the mortality in this cohort of patients remains high.

Gastric Injuries. Injuries to the stomach by penetrating mechanism (11%–18%) far outweigh the incidence due to blunt modalities (<1%).[47] However, the mortality associated with blunt gastric trauma is significant, reaching 28.2% in an EAST multi-institutional trial. A closer evaluation of these patients reveals a significantly higher ISS compared to other groups, suggesting that mortality associated with blunt perforation of the stomach is consequential to high energy mechanisms. Rupture is caused by an acute increase in intraluminal pressure from external forces that result in bursting of the gastric wall. Because of the high-energy nature of this mechanism, associated injury to the liver, spleen, pancreas, and small bowel is common, and mortality is frequently attributed to these associated injuries. In contrast, death from penetrating injury to the stomach is relatively low at 2.2%.[47]

Penetrating gastric injuries often cause full-thickness perforations with spillage of gastric contents into the abdomen.

Like other hollow visceral injuries, gastric injuries may be identified on physical examination by the presence of peritonitis. The onset of this finding may be faster compared to small bowel perforation, given the lower pH of gastric contents.[47] Furthermore, the location of penetrating wounds may be suggestive of gastric injury. Although, historically, injuries to the hollow viscus were identified on exploration for solid organ trauma, CT is now a commonly employed modality in the stable trauma patient prior to operation. The overall sensitivity and specificity for hollow visceral injury on CT are limited (sensitivity 55%–95%, specificity 48%–92%) and depends upon the presence of secondary signs: bowel wall thickening, irregular wall enhancement, mesenteric defects, and abdominal free fluid in the absence of solid organ trauma. The latter finding of free fluid is an unreliable single metric for operation, in the setting of which therapeutic laparotomy ranges from 27% to 54%. Similarly, isolated pneumoperitoneum in blunt trauma may also be an untrustworthy indicator for hollow viscus injury.[47] As described previously, the algorithmic evaluation of blunt or penetrating abdominal trauma may include a period of observation, whereby injury to the hollow viscus becomes clinically apparent. Importantly, if suspicion is high based upon multiple metrics, the decision to explore should be expeditiously made, as mortality increases proportional to surgical delay.

A full evaluation of the stomach includes visualization of the anterior and posterior walls, requiring entry into the lesser sac. Failure to accomplish this may lead to missed injuries with subsequent morbidity. The approach to repair is based on the amount of tissue loss and the injury location. Hematomas within the gastric wall should be evacuated to ensure the absence of perforation. This is followed by control of bleeding and closure of the seromusculature with nonabsorbable suture. Injuries that are full thickness should have all nonviable tissue debrided; the gastric wall is then closed in one or two layers. A common approach is to close the perforation with absorbable suture and then to invert the suture line with nonabsorbable seromuscular stitches. A stapler can also be used to close a perforation due to the redundancy of gastric tissue and the unlikelihood of overly decreasing the volume of the stomach lumen. Injuries involving the gastroesophageal junction, lesser curve, fundus, and posterior wall may be more challenging to approach and require better exposure of the upper abdomen. Rarely, highly destructive injuries that cause the loss of large portions of the stomach will require partial or even total gastrectomy. Reconstruction could require Billroth I or II gastroenterostomy or creation of a Roux-en-Y esophagojejunostomy, depending on the extent of the resection.

Duodenal Injuries. Duodenal injuries are uncommon after blunt and penetrating mechanisms, comprising under 2% of abdominal trauma. Because of the retroperitoneal location of the duodenum, most injuries are due to penetrating modalities, owing to GSWs in approximately 80% of cases. In a recent multi-institutional series, nearly 70% had associated abdominal injuries and the associated mortality was 24%. On univariate analysis, mortality was related to arrival hemodynamics, transfusion requirement, ISS, renal failure, and associated pancreatic injury.[48] Blunt injuries are caused by a blow to the epigastrium with a narrow object, resulting in contusion of the wall or a rupture secondary to acute elevation of intraluminal pressure. The classic description includes abdominal impact by a steering wheel or, in children, a bicycle handlebar. Morbidity in duodenal injury is most commonly related to septic complications, particularly in the setting of repair failure. As such, surgical treatment for duodenal injury has produced multiple and complex treatment options.

Duodenal trauma can often pose a diagnostic and therapeutic challenge. Penetrating duodenal injuries are commonly first diagnosed at laparotomy, initiated on the basis of penetrating wound location. Blunt duodenal injuries can be more challenging to identify and therefore require a high index of suspicion to avoid missed injuries. Physical examination findings can be lacking due to the retroperitoneal location of the duodenum. Even full-thickness duodenal perforations may not demonstrate peritoneal signs unless the perforation involves an intraperitoneal segment. The most valuable tool for diagnosis is abdominal CT with a low threshold for operative exploration. Imaging may demonstrate a thickened duodenal wall with periduodenal air and fluid. Low-grade injuries, such as a duodenal hematoma, may also be identified by CT. If initial emergent imaging in hemodynamically stable patients is suggestive of duodenal trauma, repeat imaging in the form of oral contrast-enhanced CT, timed for duodenal transit, or upper GI fluoroscopy should be performed. Any evidence of duodenal perforation on imaging requires immediate operative intervention. Findings may be subtle, but a low threshold for exploration must be maintained because of the potential for false-negative abdominal CT results.

The approach to management of duodenal injuries depends on the location of the injury and the amount of tissue destruction. Hematomas of the duodenal wall will often resolve without intervention and are an issue only if they cause a gastric outlet obstruction. Treatment of obstructing hematomas consists of gastric decompression, initiation of total parenteral nutrition, and reevaluation of gastric emptying with a contrast study after 5 to 7 days. If the duodenal obstruction persists after approximately 14 days, operative exploration is warranted to evacuate hematoma, evaluate for perforation, stricture, or associated pancreatic injury. Hematomas will frequently decompress spontaneously during mobilization of the duodenum and the intestinal wall should then be evaluated for injury. Duodenal hematomas identified incidentally during laparotomy should not be intentionally opened unless there is a concern for full-thickness injury.

A retrospective study from the Panamerican Trauma Society found that 98% of patients with operative duodenal injury were amenable to primary repair, inclusive of all AAST grades.[48] Duodenal wall perforations can be repaired by a single- or double-layer approach after debridement of devitalized tissue. Complete mobilization of the duodenum with a wide Kocher maneuver is required to provide necessary exposure and to ensure a tension-free repair. Larger amounts of tissue loss or duodenal transection can be managed with resection and primary anastomosis as long as the ampulla is not involved and the injured segment is short. Longer segments of duodenal injury or areas adjacent to the ampulla may require enteric bypass with a Roux-en-Y reconstruction. If possible, a healthy piece of omentum should be placed over any repair for reinforcement. Additional maneuvers for protection of suture lines from enteric contents (i.e., duodenal diverticulization, pyloric exclusion with gastrojejunostomy, tube duodenostomy) has been questioned in previous reviews and should be individualized to select cases. Similarly, drain placement following definitive repair is not mandatory, although a potential benefit may be controlled fistula creation if leak occurs. In the damage control setting, the use of resection with wide drainage and temporary discontinuity is highly effective for controlling contamination.

Pancreatic Injuries. Pancreatic injuries commonly occur in association with injury to the duodenum because of their proximity.

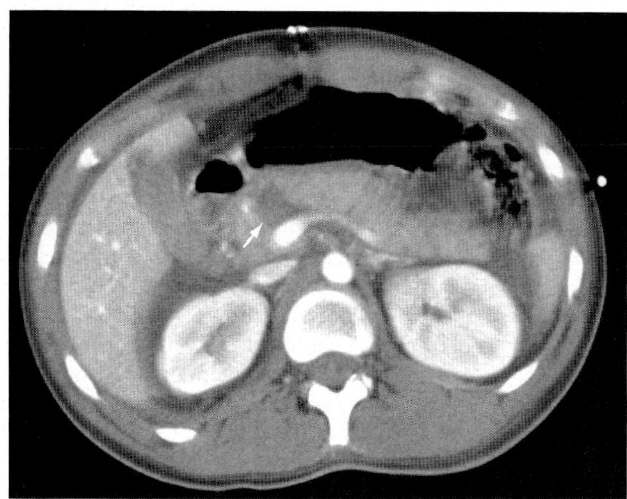

FIG. 17.27 Pancreatic injury on abdominal computed tomography. The injury involves the pancreatic neck and appears as a 2-cm segment of nonperfused pancreas tissue with surrounding edema as identified by the *arrow*.

However, the overall incidence in abdominal trauma is relatively low (0.2%–12%).[49] A penetrating mechanism is more commonly the cause, with 4.4% of patients with penetrating abdominal trauma sustaining a pancreatic injury. True pancreatic trauma-related mortality is difficult to identify, as deaths are often attributable to associated pathology. Nonetheless, morbidity and mortality are noted to increase with AAST grade (up to 40% in Grade V injury) along with delays in diagnosis and management.[49] Pancreatic enzymes are caustic; thus ductal injury with leak (≥Grade III) is the most significant contributor to organ-specific morbidity and mortality. Pancreas tissue injury can result from direct laceration of the organ or through the transmission of blunt force energy to the retroperitoneum. A common mechanism of blunt pancreatic injury involves crushing of the body of the pancreas between a rigid structure, such as a steering wheel or seat belt, and the vertebral column. The impact to the pancreas causes injury that ranges from mild contusion to complete transection with ductal disruption.

The identification of pancreas injuries can be challenging, particularly because available imaging modalities are not highly effective. As with the duodenum, the retroperitoneal location of the pancreas makes physical examination findings less helpful for diagnosis. Three-dimensional imaging with IV contrast–enhanced abdominal CT provides the best view of the pancreas and associated injury. Despite this, sensitivity/specificity for the detection of parenchymal injury (sensitivity 47%–79%) and the presence of ductal involvement (sensitivity 52%–54%, specificity 90%–95%) remain inconsistently reported in the literature, potentially reflecting variations in radiologic interpretation between centers.[49] CT alone may not be satisfactory to rule out a clinically significant pancreatic injury, and a high index of suspicion must be maintained. On abdominal CT, findings suggestive of pancreatic injuries include malperfusion of the pancreatic parenchyma, surrounding fluid, or hematoma and stranding in the adjacent soft tissue. An injury involving the neck of the pancreas on CT is demonstrated in Fig. 17.27.

The identification of clinically significant pancreatic injuries may require the use of other diagnostic studies. Reported incidence of missed pancreatic trauma on CT approximates 15%.[49] Repeated CT imaging may suggest a pancreatic injury that required time to develop inflammation in the patient who remains persistently unwell. When obtained more than 3 hours after injury occurrence, an elevated serum amylase level may reflect pancreatic trauma. Used in this way, serum amylase levels are reasonably sensitive but lacking in specificity and are of limited value. Imaging of the pancreatic ducts with ERCP or magnetic resonance cholangiopancreatography may increase diagnostic yield, especially for those patients who have a suggestion of pancreatic injury. These additional modalities continue to be studied and may occasionally be valuable in planning therapy and the operative approach.

Pancreatic injuries of any significance require surgical management. Exposure of the entire pancreas is required to evaluate for injury and to develop an effective surgical plan. This exposure includes mobilization of the hepatic flexure and division of the gastrocolic ligament, allowing retraction of the transverse and mesocolon inferiorly. A Kocher maneuver will mobilize the pancreatic head and facilitate visualization. Assessment of the pancreas includes determining the amount of parenchymal involvement, location of the injury, and presence of ductal trauma. Pancreatic ductal injuries to the left of the superior mesenteric vessels are managed with a distal pancreatectomy. The proximal pancreatic stump can be managed by individually ligating the duct, then oversewing the parenchyma or using a stapling device. Healing of the retained pancreas may be enhanced by coverage with a piece of healthy omentum. A closed suction drain should be placed to manage any pancreatic enzyme leak.

Treating injuries of the ductal system within the head of the pancreas can be more challenging. When tissue destruction is limited, managing these injuries with drainage alone often diverts the leakage of pancreatic fluid externally, creating a controlled fistula that frequently will close spontaneously. The closure of a fistula may be facilitated by biliary decompression through the placement of stents by ERCP. Massive destruction of the pancreatic head with devitalized parenchyma (Grade V) or combined pancreatic and duodenal injuries may require a pancreaticoduodenectomy (Whipple procedure). This presents the patient with a large surgical burden and is associated with a high postoperative complication rate. Only patients with normalized physiology should be considered candidates for pancreaticoduodenectomy; others undergo an abbreviated operation with later reconstruction. Damage control for pancreatic injury includes hemorrhage control, external drainage, and temporary abdominal closure with plans for reexploration.

Effective external drainage is an important component in the management of pancreatic injuries, the value of which cannot be overstated. Pancreatic enzyme diversion is required to prevent retroperitoneal exposure to caustic enzymes, which will provoke a massive inflammatory response and progressive organ dysfunction. Less severe pancreatic injuries that do not involve the pancreatic duct (Grades I and II), including hematomas, parenchymal contusions, and lacerations of the capsule or superficial parenchyma, should be managed with external drainage. Closed suction systems are associated with a reduced rate of abscess development compared with open-style drains.[49] Distal feeding access may be valuable to provide early enteral nutrition, depending on the overall clinical picture. Fig. 17.28 demonstrates an approach to the operative management of pancreatic injuries.

Small Bowel Injuries. Although the small intestine is one of the more frequently injured organs after penetrating abdominal trauma, it is a rarely injured entity by blunt mechanism (0.3%). Mortality rates range from 15% to 20%, with most caused by associated vascular injuries.[47] At the tissue level, injury can be secondary to crushing, rupture, and shearing mechanisms. Penetrating injuries

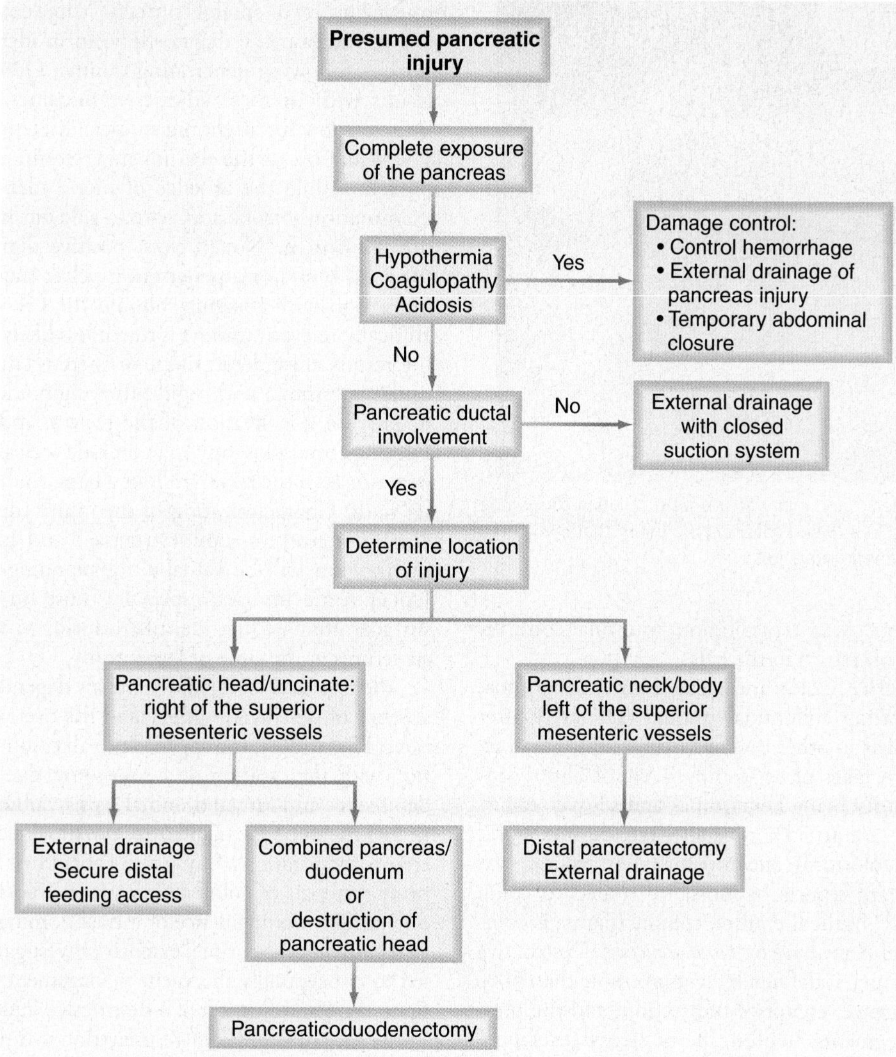

FIG. 17.28 Algorithm for the operative management of pancreatic injury.

can range from tiny perforations to large destructive injuries that devitalize circumferential segments of small bowel. Direct blunt tissue injury can occur when the small bowel is crushed between the steering wheel or seat belt and a rigid structure, such as the vertebral column. Small bowel rupture occurs when the intraluminal pressure rapidly increases, causing a blow-out along the antimesenteric border. Deceleration mechanisms can result in a shearing of the serosa or muscularis throughout a segment of small bowel. Finally, injuries to the small bowel mesentery can result in devascularization and subsequent intestinal necrosis without direct tissue injury.

In the setting of penetrating mechanisms, small bowel injuries are often identified at the time of abdominal exploration. Patients may have peritonitis on presenting examination or their abdominal findings may worsen in the hours after arrival. As with other hollow abdominal viscera, the evaluation can be challenging and is similar to the evaluation of the stomach and duodenum as described earlier. Abdominal CT imaging has significant limitations, and a high index of suspicion must exist to avoid a missed injury.

The repair of small bowel injuries depends on the amount of intestinal wall destruction in relation to the overall luminal circumference. Injuries to the intestinal serosa can be reinforced with interrupted nonabsorbable suture, which imbricates the injury. Small perforations can be repaired primarily with one or two layers after debridement of devitalized tissue. Care must be taken to avoid overly compromising the size of the intestinal lumen. In the setting of multiple perforations, primary repair can still be safely performed as long as the injuries are not so close as to result in narrowing of the bowel lumen when closed. Despite this, many surgeons choose to perform a resection with anastomosis when multiple perforations are present within a segment of bowel. When injuries involve more than 50% of the intestinal wall circumference, bowel resection with anastomosis should be performed. There has been no difference in leak rates demonstrated between stapled and hand-sewn anastomoses following resection. Selection of the anastomosis technique should be based on the preference of the surgeon and the amount of experience with the chosen technique. Hand-sewn anastomoses are frequently constructed in two layers, but single-layer methods are equally efficacious. Damage control for small bowel injuries includes rapid closure of perforations to control contamination with resection when large injuries are present. Patients in shock may benefit from resection without immediate anastomosis because of a higher risk of anastomotic dehiscence and the need for an abbreviated operation. The abdomen is temporarily closed and the patient is resuscitated to correct

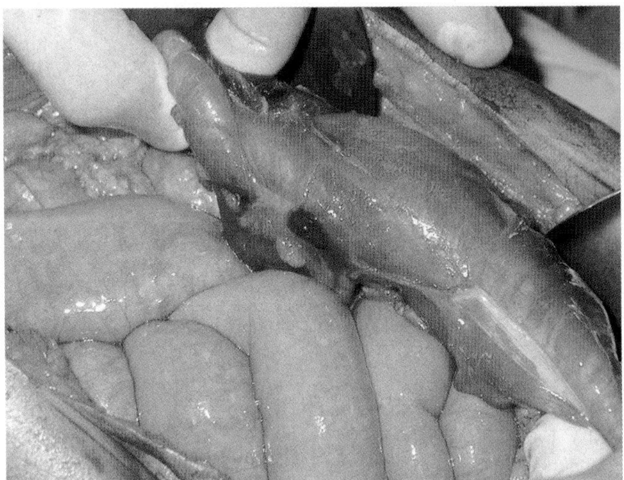

FIG. 17.29 Blunt left-sided colon injury at the time of laparotomy. The injury mechanism resulted in a deserosalizing-type injury that involved a segment of colon several centimeters long.

physiologic derangements. After resuscitation, intestinal continuity can be reestablished on return to the OR.

Colon and Rectal Injuries. Colon and rectal injuries occur most commonly after penetrating abdominal trauma and rarely after blunt mechanisms. Similar to other hollow visceral injury, trauma to the colon and rectum takes place in only 0.3% of bluntly injured patients, the majority being hematomas and serosal tears.[47] Historical data reveal a 22% to 35% mortality rate during World War II, at which time colostomy creation for colon trauma was mandatory. Contemporary reports of mortality related to colon injury are as low as 1%.[50] In the literature, colonic trauma is commonly classified as either *destructive* or *nondestructive*. Destructive injury in penetrating trauma is defined by wounds more than 50% of the colonic circumference, complete transection, and the presence of devascularized segments. In blunt injury, serosal tears more than 50% colon circumference, full-thickness perforation, and mesenteric devascularization are considered destructive. These pathologies in blunt trauma are produced by direct crush or rupture when the rate of compression results in a rapid elevation in intraluminal pressure. Importantly, depending upon the involved colonic segment, colon injury with perforation can occur into the retroperitoneum. Most commonly seen in the retroperitoneal portions, shearing forces can cause a separation of the serosa or muscularis from the underlying mucosa over a long segment. The results of this injury mechanism are evident in Fig. 17.29. Finally, in addition to GSWs, injury to the rectum may also occur when severe pelvic fractures with sharp bone fragments cause a laceration.

From an examination standpoint, patients may present with a wide range of physiology. Peritonitis may be present on exam in the setting of free perforation, yet the retroperitoneal location of the right and left colon may obscure this finding. Furthermore, colonic injuries may first be identified at the time of laparotomy prompted by hemodynamic instability or a suggestive penetrating mechanism. For the physiologically stable patient, the evaluation of the colon is similar to that of previously described hollow viscus injury. Abdominal CT is limited in capability, although it may demonstrate colonic wall thickening with surrounding stranding or fluid. Imaging may identify the track of a penetrating mechanism, allowing the surgeon to assess proximity to the colon. Finally, care must be taken to adequately assess the segments of the colon that are retroperitoneal in location. This has led some authors to advocate for routine utility of enteral contrast ("triple contrast": oral, rectal, and IV) to increase CT diagnostic yield in identification of operative injuries following penetrating trauma. Others contend equivalent results without these adjunctive measures, leading recent guidelines to allow for attending surgical discretion.[42]

Evaluation of the rectum may require a slightly different approach. While the absence of blood identified on digital rectal examination may be adequate to rule out injury, its presence does not confirm it. Nonetheless, positive digital rectal examination for gross blood or a penetrating pelvic trajectory requires further evaluation with imaging. Should the CT be negative for injury, clinically relevant trauma is much less likely. However, if the imaging results are indeterminate or there is clinical concern, an exam under anesthesia with rigid proctosigmoidoscopy can be valuable to provide visualization of the rectum and distal sigmoid colon. Findings on endoscopy may include a clear injury to the rectum, hematoma in the rectal wall, or a large amount of blood in the rectal vault. Characterization of the injury (destructive rectal [>25% circumference] vs. nondestructive) and location relative to the peritoneum will be valuable for planning surgical management. Upper rectal injuries, especially those on the anterior or lateral surfaces, may be first identified during visualization of the pelvic structures at the time of laparotomy.

The approach to operative repair depends upon the presence or absence of destructive injury and the overall physiology of the patient. Historically, the approach to all colon injuries included resection with the creation of a colostomy, due to fear of anastomotic dehiscence and intraabdominal sepsis. Subsequent experience questioned the need for mandatory proximal fecal diversion to manage colonic perforations. Stone and Fabian first prospectively described primary repair of colon injury versus colostomy creation in 1979, observing lower incidence of intraabdominal infection with primary repair. Since that time, extensive investigation from Memphis has led to conceptually divergent management of colon injuries based upon the identification of a destructive injury. Destructive wounds in the face of significant resuscitation (>6 units PRBC) and medical comorbidity were noted to experience anastomotic leak at 42% versus 3% in otherwise healthy, minimally transfused patients following resection. Thus was developed surgical stratification for optimal outcomes in operative colon injury, recommending primary repair (one or two layers) in all nondestructive injuries, resection, and anastomosis for destructive injury in the healthy patient without extremis and diversion for destructive injury in the comorbid patient requiring resuscitation.[50] This schema holds true for both penetrating and blunt injury and are not impacted by the degree of intraabdominal contamination. Distal injuries require segmental resection with colocolonic anastomosis.

Destructive colon injuries that are encountered during damage control laparotomy in the unstable patient should be resected, but immediate anastomosis should be avoided because of an unacceptably high leak rate. Depending on the need to abbreviate the operation, colostomy can be created or the GI tract left in discontinuity until after the patient has been adequately resuscitated. Delayed primary anastomosis or creation of a colostomy can be performed on return to the OR. Discerning between these approaches has led to a spectrum of conclusions, from equivalency in outcomes to mandatory colostomy for patients requiring open abdomen as part of their management.[50] Regardless, the most recent WTA guidelines suggest bias toward ostomy creation in patients with ongoing shock, concomitant abdominal injuries, chronic illness, immunosuppression, or inability to close fascia. A question that remains unanswered is whether a diverting loop ileostomy following colonic anastomosis would serve the same function in this population as it has in other inflammatory states.

Rectal injuries that result in perforation can cause significant contamination leading to pelvic sepsis. For this reason, operative management is often required. Destructive rectal injuries (>25% circumference) are predominantly managed with fecal diversion (loop ileostomy or colostomy) and consideration of presacral drainage until healing has occurred. A rectal contrasted enema will serve to define wound resolution with subsequent ostomy reversal. Evidence for routine proximal diversion and presacral drainage of all injuries, irrespective of tissue destruction, is based on limited data in small trials. More recent evidence suggests that extraperitoneal rectal injuries may be managed without drainage and diversion alone.[50] Of note, if an extraperitoneal rectal injury is found at laparotomy, management should convert to treatment of intraperitoneal colon trauma.

Abdominal Great Vessel Injuries. The major blood vessels of the abdomen are predominantly located within the retroperitoneum, with some larger vessels also in the intestinal mesenteries. Because of massive associated blood loss, visualization of the vessels can be compromised, making management of these injuries challenging. Most commonly, major abdominal vascular injuries are secondary to penetrating mechanisms. In the setting of blunt trauma, hematomas within the retroperitoneum are often secondary to pelvic fractures with bleeding from pelvic blood vessels that dissect superiorly. Abdominal vascular injuries are addressed elsewhere in this text (Chapter 64); thus only those concepts related to initial assessment and management are presented here.

Abdominal vascular injuries are often first recognized at the time of laparotomy being performed for penetrating abdominal trauma. These injuries are frequently associated with significant ongoing blood loss and hemodynamic instability. The specific vascular injury is better delineated after exploration and exposure of the retroperitoneal structures. Penetrating injuries to the back frequently benefit from three-dimensional imaging, given that most do not enter the peritoneal cavity. CT is often used to identify the path of the injury and therefore to suggest possible involvement of adjacent structures. Similarly, evaluation of the abdominal vasculature after blunt trauma is best achieved with contrast-enhanced CT. On occasion, retroperitoneal vascular injury is identified during urgently performed laparotomy, although further identification of specific injuries depends on the location of the hematoma.

Penetrating injuries to the retroperitoneum identified during laparotomy require exploration and repair. Although the details of these repairs are discussed elsewhere, knowledge of the basic exposure of these structures is important. Hematomas of the infrarenal vasculature or the right renal hilum are exposed with a right medial visceral mobilization, also known as the Cattell-Braasch maneuver. A wide Kocher maneuver is performed, and the peritoneal dissection is continued inferiorly to mobilize the right colon. The dissection continues around the cecum and superiorly up the mesenteric root. Retraction of the abdominal viscera superior and to the left will expose the lower midline vascular structures (right colon should eviscerate to lay upon the chest). Basic tenets of vascular repair including proximal and distal control of the injured vessel are achieved when possible. Injuries to the suprarenal great vessels or the left renal hilum are exposed by performing a left medial visceral mobilization (the Mattox maneuver). This is achieved by dividing the peritoneum along the entire left side of the abdomen, from above the spleen down to the distal left colon. The plane posterior to the colonic mesentery and the pancreas is

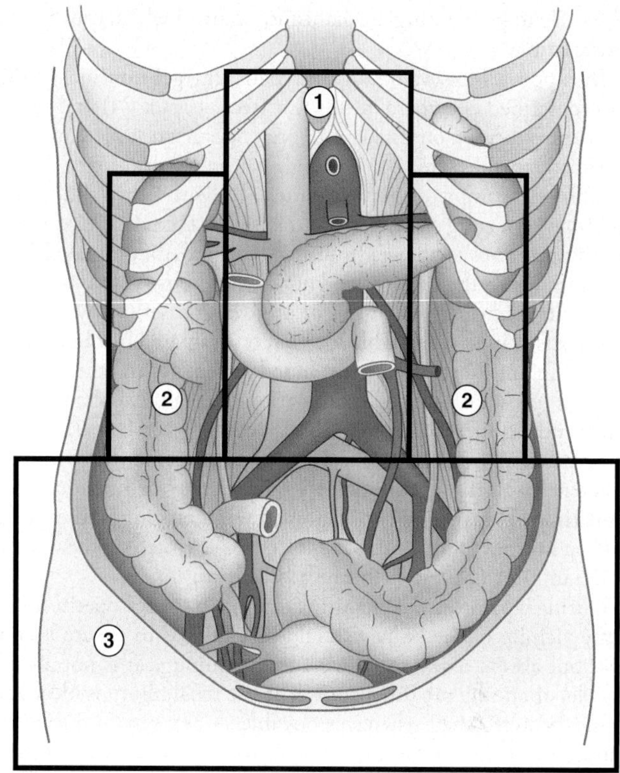

FIG. 17.30 Zones of the retroperitoneum visualized at the time of laparotomy. *Zone 1* includes the central vascular structures, such as the aorta and vena cava. *Zone 2* includes the kidneys and adjacent adrenal glands. *Zone 3* describes the retroperitoneum associated with the pelvic vasculature.

developed, and the abdominal viscera are retracted to the right to expose the superior retroperitoneal vasculature.

Blunt abdominal vascular injuries that are not actively bleeding may require operative repair or may be considered for endovascular therapy, depending on the nature of the vascular disease. During laparotomy, the location of retroperitoneal hematoma guides surgical decision-making. As seen in Fig. 17.30, the retroperitoneum can conceptually be divided into three zones. Zone 1 hematomas require exploration because these frequently involve the aorta, proximal visceral vessels, or inferior vena cava, although an exception may be the dark hematoma behind the liver, which suggests a retrohepatic vena cava injury. Injuries to the retrohepatic vena cava are best served by not exposing the contained, low-pressure injury and by gently packing the surrounding area. A hematoma in the region of zone 2, which predominantly contains the kidneys, should be explored only if it appears that the hematoma is expanding and continuing to lose blood. Finally, a hematoma in zone 3 is usually secondary to pelvic fracture bleeding and should not be explored unless exsanguinating hemorrhage is obvious.

Genitourinary Injuries. The genitourinary organs include the kidneys, ureters, bladder, and urethra, all of which are contained within the retroperitoneum. Bleeding and extravasation of urine are the major concern with injuries to these structures. Blunt mechanisms can result in renal laceration or bladder rupture, which can occur into the peritoneal space or the soft tissue of the pelvis. The typical mechanism for bladder injuries is the transmission of significant energy to the urine-filled bladder, resulting in wall rupture. This is almost universally associated with some amount of pelvic fracture. All genitourinary structures are vulnerable to penetrating mechanisms, many of which cause urine extravasation.

The approach to evaluating and managing genitourinary injuries is described elsewhere in this text (see Chapter 74) and therefore is only briefly outlined. The presence of gross hematuria is the most valuable screen for injuries to the genitourinary organs and should prompt further evaluation. As with other abdominal structures, imaging with IV contrast–enhanced CT frequently identifies injuries to the genitourinary organs. Abdominal CT reveals injuries to the kidneys and adjacent adrenal glands and can demonstrate findings suggestive of urine extravasation. When suspicion exists, injury to the bladder can be evaluated by obtaining a CT cystogram. In male patients, blood at the urethral meatus or a displaced prostate on rectal examination is suggestive of a urethral injury and requires evaluation. This is best achieved by performing retrograde urethrography, especially before placement of a urinary catheter. Penetrating genitourinary injuries may be first identified at the time of laparotomy or diagnosed with imaging studies. Penetrating injuries to the back benefit from CT, which can characterize the injury track and delineate adjacent organs.

During laparotomy, penetrating trauma to the retroperitoneum in the vicinity of the kidney should be explored to ensure hemostasis but also to assess for a urine leak. Although it is not always feasible, obtaining proximal control at the renal hilum is ideal and should be performed whenever possible. Many renal injuries are hemostatic at the time of exploration, whereas many will respond favorably to simple techniques. Conversely, devastating renal injuries, especially in the setting of shock with ongoing bleeding, may require nephrectomy. Assessment of the contralateral side for a kidney is valuable, but the potential for renal salvage should be dictated by the physiologic condition of the patient. The repair of ureteral injuries can be achieved in several different ways ranging from primary repair to nephrectomy. Intraperitoneal bladder injuries can be repaired in two layers of absorbable suture and the bladder drained with a Foley catheter or suprapubic cystostomy tube. Extraperitoneal bladder ruptures require only decompression with a urinary catheter, followed by cystography to confirm healing after a period of recovery.

Blunt injury to genitourinary structures is commonly identified on imaging and can be managed nonoperatively in most cases. Bleeding from the kidneys and adrenal glands is often self-limited and requires no specific intervention. Injuries that demonstrate no evidence of ongoing bleeding are candidates for nonoperative management. Physiologic deterioration requires laparotomy with management of uncontrolled bleeding. Patients with hemodynamic stability but pseudoaneurysm from a renal injury on imaging may benefit from angioembolization. As described before, a renal hematoma after blunt trauma identified at laparotomy should be explored only if it appears that the hematoma is expanding.

Injuries to the Pelvis and Extremities

The majority of injuries sustained by trauma patients involve the musculoskeletal system. Orthopedic injuries to the pelvis and extremities are extremely common and described in depth elsewhere in this text (Chapter 19). A basic approach to management as it relates to the general or trauma surgeon is presented here. Orthopedic injuries constituted the greatest number of cases in the 2016 NTDB report, with 31.66% of patients having upper extremity and 40.09% having lower extremity trauma. Although the mortality is low for each group (approximately 4%–5%), the long-term morbidity and functional implications can be significant.[2] A variety of physical mechanisms are responsible for orthopedic injuries, with falls and motor vehicle crashes being the most common causes.

Evaluation for musculoskeletal injuries begins with a thorough physical examination, which easily identifies fractures that are open or demonstrate severe deformity. Plain radiography remains highly effective for diagnosis, although some fractures, such as complex pelvic fractures, benefit from CT. Pelvic fractures are typically identified on initial pelvic radiography and then better characterized on abdominal CT. In addition to evaluating the bone structures, CT can identify associated hematomas and the presence or absence of active extravasation of contrast medium, which appears as high-density material within the hematoma. Extremity examination must include a thorough vascular assessment and evaluation for compartment syndrome. Clinical evidence of vascular injury may require angiography to localize and to characterize the abnormality. CT angiography has evolved and now constitutes a major contributor to the evaluation of peripheral vascular trauma.

Bleeding from complex pelvic fractures presents a unique challenge and requires a coordinated approach. As depicted in Fig. 17.31, unstable patients should have a pelvic radiograph quickly obtained and interpreted for pelvic fracture. An important point is that although some pelvic fracture patterns are higher risk, any fracture is capable of bleeding and should be addressed in the unstable patient. Pelvic fractures that demonstrate an increase in pelvic volume should be compressed with a pelvic binder or sheet wrapped around the hips to reduce the space available for hematoma formation. Pelvic compression will frequently address venous bleeding, but ongoing instability suggests an arterial source, which should be addressed with angiography and embolization. Some recent work has suggested that packing of the pelvis may be an alternative to embolization, especially when endovascular therapy is not immediately available. Stabilization of the pelvic ring with external fixation or definitive repair is then performed to maintain reduction of the pelvic volume and to limit ongoing venous bleeding.

REHABILITATION

Although the acute management of injuries plays the greatest role in the reduction of mortality, it is the process of rehabilitation that limits the long-term morbidity of injury. The rehabilitation process can be substantially longer than the hospital phase of care and is indispensable in restoring functionality and allowing patients to return to productive lives after injury. Despite a great deal of emphasis being placed on trauma-related fatalities, there were approximately 31 million nonfatal injuries in 2013, many of which required rehabilitative services.

The rehabilitation process begins immediately after the acute needs of the injured patient have been met. Early mobilization is extremely important to circumvent deconditioning. Physical and

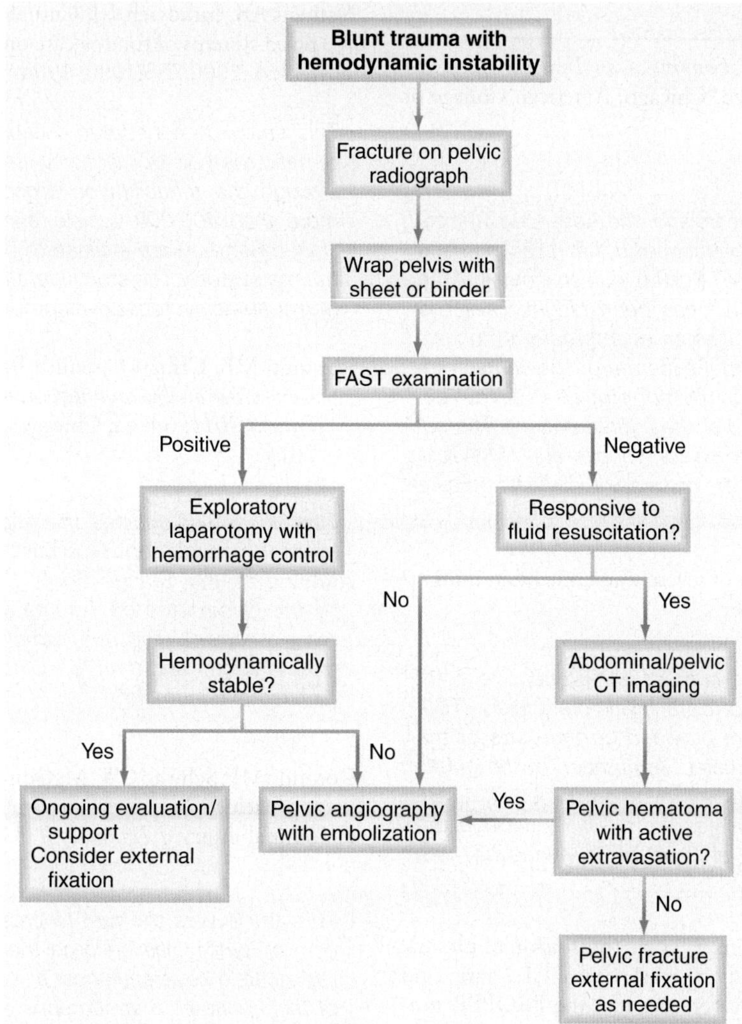

FIG. 17.31 Algorithm for the evaluation and management of pelvic fractures with associated hemorrhage. *CT*, Computed tomography; *FAST*, focused abdominal sonography in trauma.

occupational therapists frequently begin the process by initiating therapy and determining what resources may be required when the patient leaves the hospital. With these recommendations available, case managers and social workers can begin the process of identifying the inpatient or outpatient resources required to address the unique rehabilitation needs of the patient. Early engagement by the rehabilitation team can expedite referrals and transfer to appropriate facilities. Select populations of patients may benefit from rehabilitation centers that focus on the recovery from specific conditions, such as TBIs and SCIs. These two patient cohorts have specific needs that are best addressed at centers with specialized expertise. Health systems committed to trauma care must place a high priority on supporting the rehabilitation process, given that this is one of the most important aspects of a patient's long-term recovery.

SELECTED REFERENCES

American College of Surgeons. *Committee on Trauma. Advanced Trauma Life Support*. 10th ed. Chicago: American College of Surgeons; 2018.

First released more than 35 years ago, the Advanced Trauma Life Support (ATLS) course revolutionized the initial approach to the injured patient. The ATLS 10th edition contains the same systematic approach that has been taught since the initiation of the course as well as an even greater emphasis on the underlying support from the literature. The course provides a framework to successfully perform an initial evaluation, stabilization, and transfer of the injured patient. The addition of online tools and companion mobile app (MyATLS) further support the trainee in the process of internalizing care for the injured.

Guidelines for the management of severe traumatic brain injury. *J Neurotrauma*. 2007;24:S1–S106.

These guidelines represent the most comprehensive compilation of all literature related to traumatic brain injury (TBI). Evidence-based guidelines are provided on the basis of the strength of the associated studies. Application of the guidelines has been associated with improved outcomes after TBI. Current editions of the guidelines are available through the Foundation website, as they are updated continuously as a living document.

Holcomb JB, Tilley BC, Baraniuk S, et al. Transfusion of plasma, platelets, and red blood cells in a 1:1:1 vs a 1:1:2 ratio and mortality in patients with severe trauma: the PROPPR randomized clinical trial. *JAMA*. 2015;313:471–482.

This trial solidified the concepts of damage control resuscitation with transfusion of reapproximated whole blood to the injured trauma patient. It was the first randomized multicenter trial of its kind to demonstrate optimal resuscitative practices within the civilian population. Data revealed that a 1:1:1 transfusion strategy (plasma, platelets, RBC) resulted in more patients achieving hemostasis with decreased death due to exsanguination at 24 hours versus 1:1:2.

MacKenzie EJ, Rivara FP, Jurkovich GJ, et al. A national evaluation of the effect of trauma-center care on mortality. *N Engl J Med*. 2006;354:366–378.

The National Study on Costs and Outcomes of Trauma is a large multicenter project supported by the Centers for Disease Control and Prevention that was initiated to define variations in injury care and outcomes between trauma centers and nontrauma centers. The project included more than 5000 patients from 69 hospitals spanning 12 states. This study demonstrated the benefit of care provided at a trauma center versus a nontrauma center. After correction for injury severity, trauma center care was associated with a reduction of in-hospital mortality (7.6% vs. 9.5%; relative risk, 0.80; 95% confidence interval, 0.66 to 0.98) as well as 1-year mortality (10.4% vs. 13.8%; relative risk, 0.75; 95% confidence interval, 0.60–0.95).

Nathens AB, Jurkovich GJ, Cummings P, et al. The effect of organized systems of trauma care on motor vehicle crash mortality. *JAMA*. 2000;283:1990–1994.

This study demonstrated the benefit of establishing a systematic method of managing trauma from the time of injury through the rehabilitation process. During a 17-year span, more than 400,000 vehicle-related fatalities throughout the United States were evaluated for the effect of establishing a trauma system. The study identified a mortality benefit of 8% from trauma system development.

Rotondo MF, Cribari C, Smith RS. *American College of Surgeons Committee on Trauma: Resources for Optimal Care of the Injured Patient 2014*. 6th ed. Chicago: American College of Surgeons; 2014.

This document outlines the necessary components for the optimal management of injured patients in a trauma center. Known as the Orange Book, this resource was developed by the Committee on Trauma and is frequently updated to remain current. The requirements to become verified as a trauma center and then to maintain verification are contained within this document.

Rotondo MF, Schwab CW, McGonigal MD, et al. 'Damage control': an approach for improved survival in exsanguinating penetrating abdominal injury. *J Trauma*. 1993;35:375–382.

This article was the first to present the concept of damage control, which has become the standard of care in managing multiple severe injuries. It was not until the development of this approach that surgeons employed the abbreviation of abdominal surgery to prevent the deadly cycle of worsening hypothermia, coagulopathy, and acidosis. Based on the success of this methodology, other areas of trauma management, such as orthopedics and resuscitation, have developed similar approaches.

REFERENCES

1. Rotondo MF, Cribari C, Smith RS. *American College of Surgeons Committee on Trauma: Resources for Optimal Care of the Injured Patient 2014*. 6th ed. Chicago: American College of Surgeons; 2014.
2. Committee on Trauma American College of Surgeons. *National Trauma Data Bank Annual Report 2016*. Chicago: American College of Surgeons; 2016.
3. Pigneri DA, Beldowicz B, Jurkovich GJ. Trauma systems: origins, evolution, and current challenges. *Surg Clin North Am*. 2017;97:947–959.
4. MacKenzie EJ, Rivara FP, Jurkovich GJ, et al. A national evaluation of the effect of trauma-center care on mortality. *N Engl J Med*. 2006;354:366–378.
5. Nathens AB, Jurkovich GJ, Cummings P, et al. The effect of organized systems of trauma care on motor vehicle crash mortality. *JAMA*. 2000;283:1990–1994.
6. Healey C, Osler TM, Rogers FB, et al. Improving the Glasgow Coma Scale score: motor score alone is a better predictor. *J Trauma*. 2003;54:671–678; discussion 678–680.

7. Chen X, Guyette FX, Peitzman AB, et al. Identifying patients with time-sensitive injuries: association of mortality with increasing prehospital time. *J Trauma Acute Care Surg*. 2019;86:1015–1022.
8. American College of Surgeons. *Committee on Trauma. Advanced Trauma Life Support*. 10th ed. Chicago: American College of Surgeons; 2018.
9. Hudson AJ, Strandenes G, Bjerkvig CK, et al. Airway and ventilation management strategies for hemorrhagic shock. To tube, or not to tube, that is the question!. *J Trauma Acute Care Surg*. 2018;84:S77–S82.
10. Guyette FX, Sperry JL, Peitzman AB, et al. Prehospital blood product and crystalloid resuscitation in the severely injured patient: a secondary analysis of the prehospital air medical plasma trial. *Ann Surg*. 2019.
11. Moore HB, Moore EE, Chapman MP, et al. Plasma-first resuscitation to treat haemorrhagic shock during emergency ground transportation in an urban area: a randomised trial. *Lancet*. 2018;392:283–291.
12. Anto VP, Guyette FX, Brown J, et al. Severity of hemorrhage and the survival benefit associated with plasma: results from a randomized prehospital plasma trial. *J Trauma Acute Care Surg*. 2020;88:141–147.
13. Sheu YJ, Yu SW, Huang TW, et al. Comparison of the efficacy of a bougie and stylet in patients with endotracheal intubation: a meta-analysis of randomized controlled trials. *J Trauma Acute Care Surg*. 2019;86:902–908.
14. Lascarrou JB, Boisrame-Helms J, Bailly A, et al. Video laryngoscopy vs direct laryngoscopy on successful first-pass orotracheal intubation among ICU patients: a randomized clinical trial. *JAMA*. 2017;317:483–493.
15. Seamon MJ, Haut ER, Van Arendonk K, et al. An evidence-based approach to patient selection for emergency department thoracotomy: a practice management guideline from the Eastern Association for the Surgery of Trauma. *J Trauma Acute Care Surg*. 2015;79:159–173.
16. Gil LA, Anstadt MJ, Kothari AN, et al. The National Trauma Data Bank story for emergency department thoracotomy: how old is too old? *Surgery*. 2018;163:515–521.
17. Bulger EM, Perina DG, Qasim Z, et al. Clinical use of resuscitative endovascular balloon occlusion of the aorta (REBOA) in civilian trauma systems in the USA, 2019: a joint statement from the American College of Surgeons Committee on Trauma, the American College of Emergency Physicians, the National Association of Emergency Medical Services Physicians and the National Association of Emergency Medical Technicians. *Trauma Surg Acute Care Open*. 2019;4:e000376.
18. Rotondo MF, Schwab CW, McGonigal MD, et al. 'Damage control': an approach for improved survival in exsanguinating penetrating abdominal injury. *J Trauma*. 1993;35:375–382; discussion 382–373.
19. Holcomb JB, Tilley BC, Baraniuk S, et al. Transfusion of plasma, platelets, and red blood cells in a 1:1:1 vs a 1:1:2 ratio and mortality in patients with severe trauma: the PROPPR randomized clinical trial. *JAMA*. 2015;313:471–482.
20. Meyer DE, Vincent LE, Fox EE, et al. Every minute counts: time to delivery of initial massive transfusion cooler and its impact on mortality. *J Trauma Acute Care Surg*. 2017;83:19–24.
21. Subramanian M, Kaplan LJ, Cannon JW. Thromboelastography-guided resuscitation of the trauma patient. *JAMA Surg*. 2019;154:1152–1153.
22. Shakur H, Roberts I, Bautista R, et al. Effects of tranexamic acid on death, vascular occlusive events, and blood transfusion in trauma patients with significant haemorrhage (CRASH-2): a randomised, placebo-controlled trial. *Lancet*. 2010;376:23–32.
23. Alam HB, Vercruysse G, Martin M, et al. Western Trauma Association critical decisions in trauma: management of intracranial hypertension in patients with severe traumatic brain injuries. *J Trauma Acute Care Surg*. 2020;88:345–351.
24. Humble SS, Wilson LD, Wang L, et al. Prognosis of diffuse axonal injury with traumatic brain injury. *J Trauma Acute Care Surg*. 2018;85:155–159.
25. Effects of tranexamic acid on death, disability, vascular occlusive events and other morbidities in patients with acute traumatic brain injury (CRASH-3): a randomised, placebo-controlled trial. *Lancet*. 2019;394:1713–1723.
26. Hachem LD, Ahuja CS, Fehlings MG. Assessment and management of acute spinal cord injury: from point of injury to rehabilitation. *J Spinal Cord Med*. 2017;40:665–675.
27. Khan AD, Liebscher SC, Reiser HC, et al. Clearing the cervical spine in patients with distracting injuries: an AAST multi-institutional trial. *J Trauma Acute Care Surg*. 2019;86:28–35.
28. Martin MJ, Bush LD, Inaba K, et al. Cervical spine evaluation and clearance in the intoxicated patient: a prospective Western Trauma Association Multi-Institutional Trial and Survey. *J Trauma Acute Care Surg*. 2017;83:1032–1040.
29. Velopulos CG, Shihab HM, Lottenberg L, et al. Prehospital spine immobilization/spinal motion restriction in penetrating trauma: a practice management guideline from the Eastern Association for the Surgery of Trauma (EAST). *J Trauma Acute Care Surg*. 2018;84:736–744.
30. Sperry JL, Moore EE, Coimbra R, et al. Western Trauma Association critical decisions in trauma: penetrating neck trauma. *J Trauma Acute Care Surg*. 2013;75:936–940.
31. Inaba K, Branco BC, Menaker J, et al. Evaluation of multidetector computed tomography for penetrating neck injury: a prospective multicenter study. *J Trauma Acute Care Surg*. 2012;72:576–583; discussion 583–574.
32. Shahan CP, Croce MA, Fabian TC, et al. Impact of continuous evaluation of technology and therapy: 30 years of research reduces stroke and mortality from blunt cerebrovascular injury. *J Am Coll Surg*. 2017;224:595–599.
33. Ball CG, Williams BH, Wyrzykowski AD, et al. A caveat to the performance of pericardial ultrasound in patients with penetrating cardiac wounds. *J Trauma*. 2009;67:1123–1124.
34. Mowery NT, Gunter OL, Collier BR, et al. Practice management guidelines for management of hemothorax and occult pneumothorax. *J Trauma*. 2011;70:510–518.
35. Bou Zein Eddine S, Boyle KA, Dodgion CM, et al. Observing pneumothoraces: the 35-millimeter rule is safe for both blunt and penetrating chest trauma. *J Trauma Acute Care Surg*. 2019;86:557–564.
36. Pieracci FM, Leasia K, Bauman Z, et al. A multicenter, prospective, controlled clinical trial of surgical stabilization of rib fractures in patients with severe, nonflail fracture patterns (Chest Wall Injury Society NONFLAIL). *J Trauma Acute Care Surg*. 2020;88:249–257.
37. Swol J, Brodie D, Napolitano L, et al. Indications and outcomes of extracorporeal life support in trauma patients. *J Trauma Acute Care Surg*. 2018;84:831–837.
38. Chestovich PJ, McNicoll CF, Fraser DR, et al. Selective use of pericardial window and drainage as sole treatment for hemopericardium from penetrating chest trauma. *Trauma Surg Acute Care Open*. 2018;3:e000187.
39. Clancy K, Velopulos C, Bilaniuk JW, et al. Screening for blunt cardiac injury: an Eastern Association for the Surgery of

Trauma practice management guideline. *J Trauma Acute Care Surg*. 2012;73:S301–306.
40. Shackford SR, Dunne CE, Karmy-Jones R, et al. The evolution of care improves outcome in blunt thoracic aortic injury: a Western Trauma Association multicenter study. *J Trauma Acute Care Surg*. 2017;83:1006–1013.
41. McDonald AA, Robinson BRH, Alarcon L, et al. Evaluation and management of traumatic diaphragmatic injuries: a practice management guideline from the Eastern Association for the Surgery of Trauma. *J Trauma Acute Care Surg*. 2018;85:198–207.
42. Martin MJ, Brown CVR, Shatz DV, et al. Evaluation and management of abdominal gunshot wounds: a Western Trauma Association critical decisions algorithm. *J Trauma Acute Care Surg*. 2019;87:1220–1227.
43. Martin MJ, Brown CVR, Shatz DV, et al. Evaluation and management of abdominal stab wounds: a Western Trauma Association critical decisions algorithm. *J Trauma Acute Care Surg*. 2018;85:1007–1015.
44. Coccolini F, Montori G, Catena F, et al. Splenic trauma: WSES classification and guidelines for adult and pediatric patients. *World J Emerg Surg*. 2017;12:40.
45. Coccolini F, Catena F, Moore EE, et al. WSES classification and guidelines for liver trauma. *World J Emerg Surg*. 2016;11:50.
46. Schellenberg M, Benjamin E, Piccinini A, et al. Gunshot wounds to the liver: no longer a mandatory operation. *J Trauma Acute Care Surg*. 2019;87:350–355.
47. Coleman JJ, Zarzaur BL. Surgical management of abdominal trauma: hollow viscus injury. *Surg Clin North Am*. 2017;97:1107–1117.
48. Ferrada P, Wolfe L, Duchesne J, et al. Management of duodenal trauma: a retrospective review from the Panamerican Trauma Society. *J Trauma Acute Care Surg*. 2019;86:392–396.
49. Ho VP, Patel NJ, Bokhari F, et al. Management of adult pancreatic injuries: a practice management guideline from the Eastern Association for the Surgery of Trauma. *J Trauma Acute Care Surg*. 2017;82:185–199.
50. Biffl WL, Moore EE, Feliciano DV, et al. Management of colorectal injuries: a Western Trauma Association critical decisions algorithm. *J Trauma Acute Care Surg*. 2018;85:1016–1020.

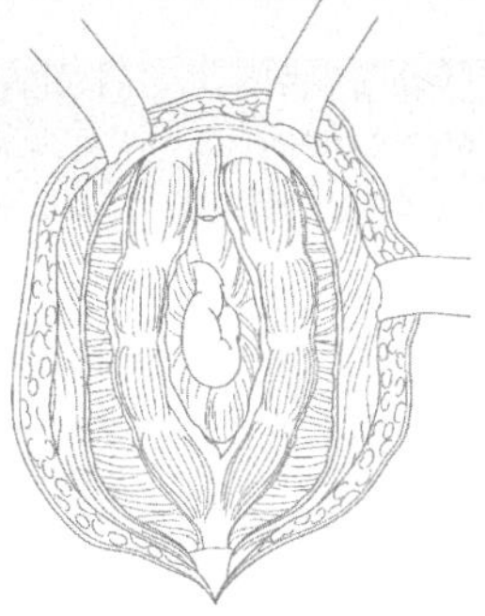

CHAPTER 18

The Difficult Abdominal Wall

Michael C. Smith, Oliver L. Gunter, Richard S. Miller

OUTLINE

Please access Elsevier eBooks for Practicing Clinicians to view the videos for this chapter https://expertconsult.inkling.com/.

Although the midline laparotomy is a common incision used in abdominal surgery, there is little evidence to guide surgeons regarding the optimal closure of the abdominal wall. The goal of this chapter is to illustrate techniques of both temporary and permanent closure of the abdominal wall. We pay particular attention to difficult and high-risk abdominal closures.

SUTURE MATERIAL

Abdominal wall closure has changed over time in large part due to improvements in suture materials and characteristics. The ideal suture material for abdominal wall closure is one that resists infection, provides adequate tensile strength to prevent abdominal wall disruption, minimizes tissue damage, and is absorbable. In current practice, a significant percentage of abdominal wall incisions are closed with slow-absorbing monofilament sutures such as polydioxanone (PDS, Ethicon, Johnson & Johnson). Polydioxanone has an advantage over polyglactin with longer strength retention profile and absorption time, as well as being a monofilament that may resist infection to a greater degree than the braided suture. Use of nonabsorbable sutures for abdominal closure (e.g., polypropylene) has been associated with increased patient pain and sinus tract formation, and their use has shown no significant difference in the incidence of incisional hernia formation, wound dehiscence, or surgical site infection (SSI) as compared to that of absorbable suture.[1,2]

Barbed sutures are increasingly being used for fascial closure. This suture has tiny barbs in a helical arrangement that allow an even distribution of tension across the incision rather than just at the knots. In a porcine model, barbed and smooth sutures had a similar burst strength. Barbed sutures have also been shown to have a similar hernia recurrence rate in fascial plication for rectus diastasis. They are secured without knots, thus allowing for faster placement, and eliminate the knot as a nidus for infection.[3,4]

CLOSURE TECHNIQUE

The principles of wound closure applied for the closure of the abdominal wall are essentially the same for closure of any surgical incision. Minimization of tissue damage is imperative, and this may be done by limiting the incorporation of the abdominal wall musculature in the closure. A 4:1 ratio of suture to wound length has been advocated. Recent evidence suggests that a strategy of taking smaller (5 mm) bites with smaller (5 mm) space between them is associated with a lower rate of incisional hernia.[5,6] This strategy achieves a ratio of suture to wound length even greater than 4:1. Layered closure of the abdominal wall to include separate layered closure of the peritoneum and subcutaneous tissues in addition to the skin and fascia is discouraged, and mass closure is preferred. A continuous suture of slowly absorbable suture material is the recommended method of closure in elective abdominal surgery, although there is little evidence to guide closure in the emergency setting.[1]

Although retention sutures are frequently employed, there is little evidence to suggest benefit to their use.[7] While they are intended to prevent evisceration, there is no consensus on the ideal adjunct to standard techniques of abdominal wall closure. Retention sutures have been associated with increased pain, increased wound inflammation, wound complications and skin breakdown, and problems with ostomy appliance placement. Thus, routine use of retention sutures, while theoretically advantageous, is not without potential complications. Patients at high risk of acute fascial dehiscence may benefit from some method of evisceration prophylaxis, and some have promoted the use of synthetic mesh in high-risk abdominal wall closures.[8] Identification of the patient who is at higher risk of abdominal wall dehiscence may alter surgical technique of abdominal wall closure and should be considered in any abdominal operation.

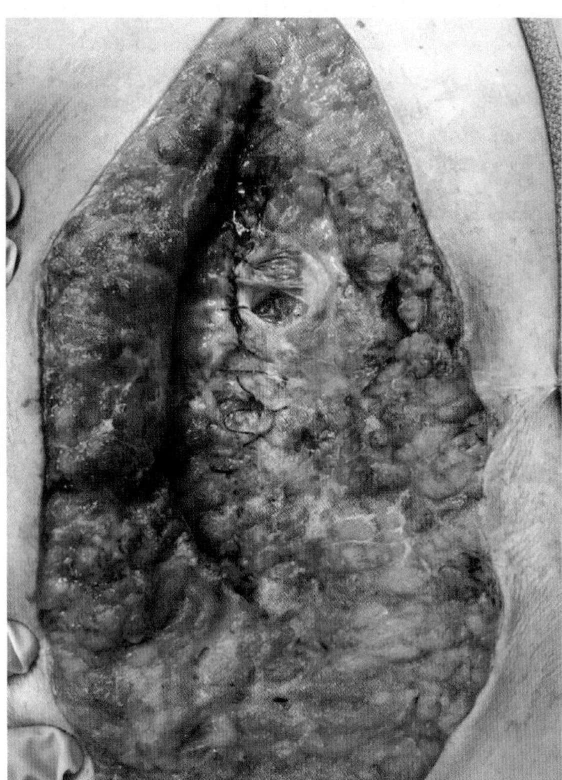

FIG. 18.1 Fascial dehiscence.

PROPHYLACTIC MESH

With incisional hernia rates after midline laparotomy in high-risk groups of 30% or more in some series, placement of prophylactic mesh at the index laparotomy for high-risk patients has drawn a large interest. Both the onlay and sublay positions have been utilized for this purpose. In multiple studies, there is a decrease in incisional hernia rates when a mesh is utilized, with no increase in surgical site occurrence (SSO) rates. Postoperative seroma rates are increased in the population that undergoes mesh placement, particularly in the onlay position. Additionally, prophylactic mesh placement has been shown to be cost effective.[9–12]

ABDOMINAL FASCIAL DEHISCENCE

The incidence of fascial dehiscence has been reported in the literature to be between 3% and 3.5% after major abdominal surgery and is associated with significant morbidity and mortality.[13] Acute fascial dehiscence may be heralded by increased serosanguinous drainage from the laparotomy wound and often can be confirmed on physical exam (Fig. 18.1). Patient risk factors and disease/surgical risk factors for abdominal wall suture complications are illustrated in Boxes 18.1 and 18.2. Several different multifactor scoring systems predictive of abdominal wall suture complications have been described in the literature, including the Veterans Affairs Medical Center (VAMC) score and the Rotterdam score.[14]

Surgical management of acute dehiscence is based on the underlying cause, with SSI and intraabdominal abscess being the most common. The technical causes of acute fascial dehiscence are knot failure and fascial damage related to tension, ischemia, or suture material failure. Although the risk of fascial dehiscence may persist beyond 3 weeks postoperatively, the usual time frame is within the first 7 days after primary closure.

BOX 18.1 Patient risk factors for abdominal wall suture complications.

- Age >70
- Obesity
- Cigarette use/chronic obstructive pulmonary disease
- Steroid use
- Diabetes mellitus
- Malnutrition
- Ascites
- Previous laparotomies

BOX 18.2 Disease: surgical risk factors for abdominal wall suture complications.

- Abdominal trauma
- Ruptured abdominal aortic aneurysm
- Retroperitoneal hematoma
- Pancreatitis
- Peritonitis/sepsis
- Bowel occlusion surgery with resection or suture
- Wound infection
- Wound Class III (contaminated) or Class IV (dirty)
- Presence of enterocutaneous fistula
- Synthetic mesh infection
- Necrotizing fasciitis
- Abdominal wall defect >10 cm width

There is no consensus management strategy for fascial wound dehiscence. The decision to proceed with immediate or delayed primary fascial closure is based on the infectious source (if one is present) and the appearance of the wound. If a superficial wound infection is the source, drainage and local wound management with dressing changes are often used. Once the infectious source is dissipated, placement of a negative pressure wound therapy (NPWT) can be effective in promoting granulation tissue and closure at the expense of developing an incisional hernia that would require delayed repair. Alternatively, operative debridement and delayed primary fascial repair, if feasible, can lead to faster healing and decreased incidence of ventral hernia.

Depending on the degree of any intraperitoneal inflammation, the abdomen may be inaccessible for repeated laparotomy at the time of dehiscence. This should then be managed as a planned ventral incisional hernia, with reconstruction in a delayed fashion, once the acute physiologic process has dissipated. The use of a biologic mesh to bridge the fascial defect in this circumstance is discussed later in the chapter.

TEMPORARY ABDOMINAL CLOSURE

Damage control laparotomy is now a well-established method to control hemorrhage and contamination at the index operation, replete physiologic reserve, and then restore abdominal continuity thereafter. In civilian trauma, between 8.8% and 36.3% of patients undergoing a trauma laparotomy require a damage control procedure during the preliminary procedure and thus a method of temporary abdominal closure (TAC).[15] Techniques in damage control have become standard adjuncts in trauma, general surgery, and subspecialty surgical procedures. Indications for TAC are shown in Box 18.3, and current options for TACs are illustrated in Table 18.1.

The goal of all TAC techniques is to minimize damage to the abdominal contents and minimize adherence of abdominal contents to the anterior abdominal wall while retaining the ability to close the fascia primarily at a subsequent operation. Current options for TAC include a tension-free, atraumatic abdominal visceral coverage using the vacuum-pack technique popularized by Barker, commercially available vacuum systems (VAC or ABThera, KCI International, San Antonio, TX), or the use of dynamic techniques in which the fascial edges are closed with serial plication. This includes serial suture closure starting at the upper and lower edges of the incision, use of absorbable or nonabsorbable synthetic mesh, an artificial Velcro/burr technique (Wittmann Patch, Star Surgical, Burlington, WI) with or without a dynamic retention suture, or silicone elastomer techniques (TAWT, Star Surgical, or ABRA System, Canica Design, Inc., Almonte, Ontario, Canada).

A recent systematic review of publications on TAC management reported that the Wittmann patch, dynamic retention sutures, and VAC methods all have similar pooled delayed primary fascial closure rates of 78% (8 series), 71% (3 series), and 61% (38 series) respectively.[16] However, this was a heterogeneous patient population with a lack of technique uniformity and outcome definitions.[17]

NPWT has gained wide acceptance for the use in a variety of complex abdominal wall circumstances (Fig. 18.2). In a contaminated environment, NPWT techniques have the ability to remove peritoneal fluids rich in inflammatory mediators, reducing the concentration of intraperitoneal cytokines. Several studies have shown that in an inflamed setting, this method achieves the highest delayed primary closure rate, lowest mortality, and lowest incidence of enterocutaneous fistula formation.[18] The artificial burr and dynamic retention suture techniques prevent lateral fascial retraction and can be sequentially tightened to allow eventual fascial closure without undue tension. A significant disadvantage of any these techniques is their requirement to be sutured to the abdominal wall musculature and fascia, which may complicate future reconstructive procedures. Incorporating dynamic serial fascial closure in conjunction with commercial NPWT has demonstrated 90% delayed primary fascial closure rates. This technique extends beyond the 8-day benchmark, with low complications rates in several series.[18–22]

Our five-stage management algorithm has helped minimize variability in patients with an open abdomen, with the goal to successfully close the abdominal fascia during Stage 3 of this

BOX 18.3 Indications for temporary abdominal closure.

- Damage control
  - Severe hemorrhage
  - Hypothermia, acidosis, coagulopathy
  - Delayed definitive operation secondary to patient's physiologic state
- Intraabdominal hypertension or compartment syndrome
- Major abdominal and/or retroperitoneal tissue edema
- Questionable visceral viability
- Planned acute reoperation
- Severe intraabdominal sepsis
- Triage

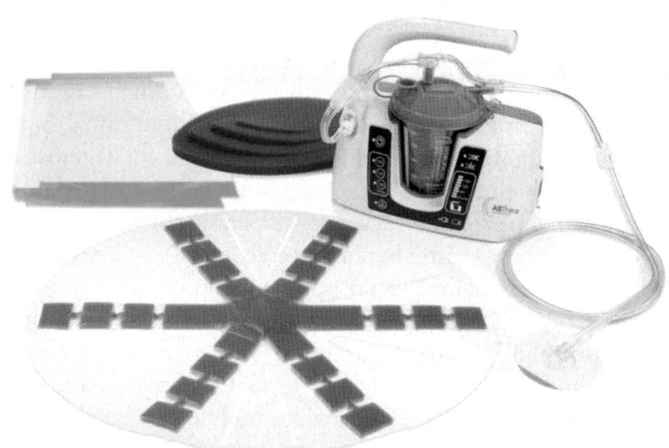

FIG. 18.2 ABThera wound management system.

TABLE 18.1 Current techniques for temporary abdominal closure.

TECHNIQUE (EXAMPLE)	DESCRIPTION	MECHANISM
Vacuum pack technique (Barker Vacuum Pack)	Perforated polyethylene sheet placed under fascia, covering abdominal viscera. Sterile surgical towels and two surgical drains placed in the wound, covered with adhesive plastic drape with drains placed to continuous suction.	Negative pressure keeps constant tension on facial edges, collects abdominal fluid
Vacuum-assisted closure (KCI VAC)	Perforated plastic sheet placed under fascia, covering abdominal viscera, and sponge placed between the facial edges. Adhesive plastic drape, pierced by suction drain connected to suction pump.	Negative pressure supplied by pump keeps constant tension on fascial edges, collects abdominal fluid, potentially helps resolve edema.
Negative pressure wound therapy (ABTHERA VAC)	Unique capsulated foam extension system incorporated into polyethylene sheet placed over abdominal viscera.	Extension runs deep into paracolic gutters to allow more efficient suctioning of ascites fluid, potentially decreasing bowel edema.
Artificial burr (Wittmann Patch)	Two opposing Velcro sheets with hooks and loops sutured to facial edges. Velcro sheets connected in the midline.	Stepwise reapproximation of fascial edges by pulling sheets tighter together over time. Helps reduce lateral retraction of rectus muscle complex.
Dynamic retention systems (A, TAWT—horizontal sutures B, ABRA—silicone elastomers)	Sutures of elastomers placed transabdominally, just lateral to rectus fascia bilaterally.	Keeps tension on fascia and progressive tightening over time to aid in reapproximating fascial edges.

algorithm in the majority of patients (Fig. 18.3).[23] Staging of abdominal reconstruction serves several vital functions: intensive care unit resuscitation, reduction of contamination and control of intraabdominal sepsis, debridement of devitalized or contaminated tissue, and allowance for decisions on subsequent reconstruction.

The goal of delayed primary fascial closure is to have the fascia closed as soon as possible, ideally within the first 8 days, to minimize complications related to the open abdomen management.[23] However, the risk for development of intraabdominal hypertension and abdominal compartment syndrome from an ongoing inflammatory response, visceral edema, retraction of abdominal wall musculature (loss of domain), lack of source control, intraabdominal abscess, or enterocutaneous fistula may all be reasons to delay primary closure. In this setting, the surgeon may have to accept a planned delayed abdominal wall reconstruction and use alternative means of visceral coverage (Stages 4 and 5).

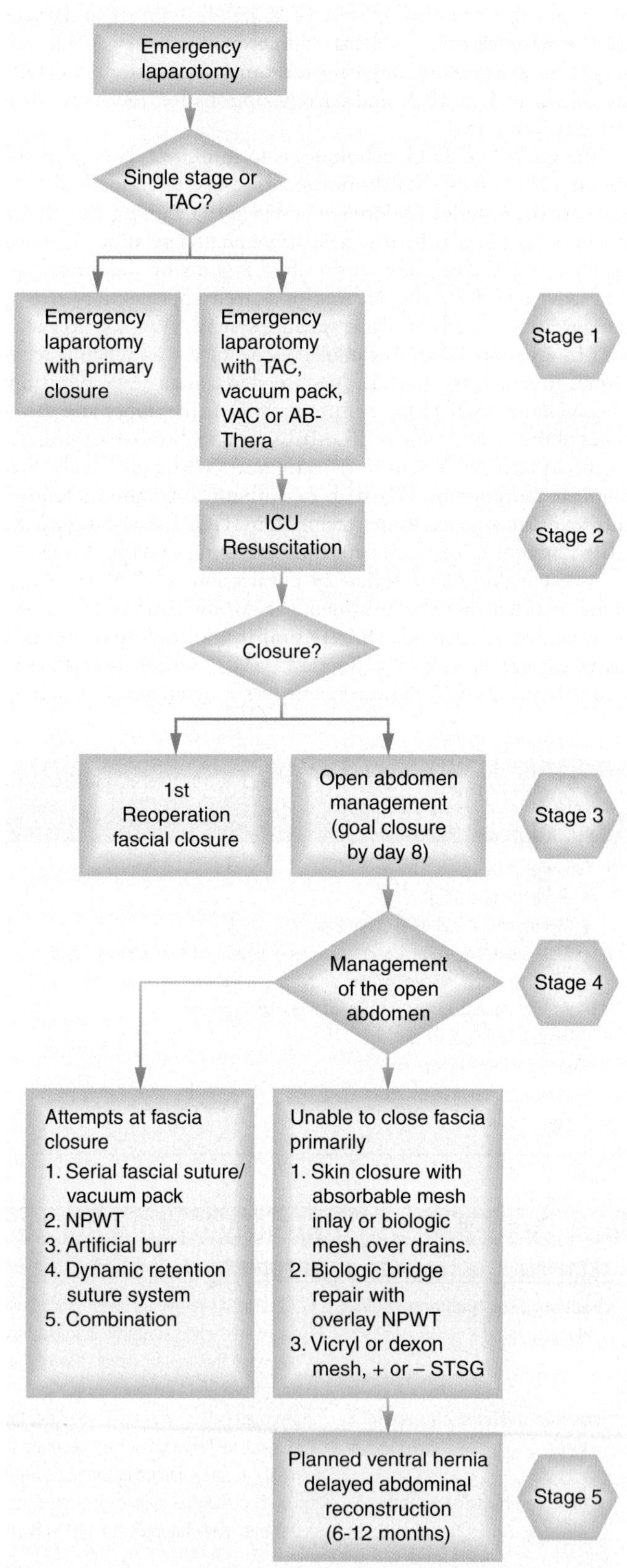

FIG. 18.3 Five-stage proposed algorithm for management of the open abdomen. *ICU*, Intensive care unit; *NPWT*, negative pressure wound therapy; *STSG*, split-thickness skin graft; *TAC*, temporary abdominal closure; *VAC*, vacuum-assisted closure.

MANAGEMENT OF THE OPEN ABDOMEN AND ASSESSING READINESS FOR ABDOMINAL CLOSURE

After hemorrhage and/or contamination control, intraoperatively, the primary goal in the initial resuscitation of the patient with an open abdomen is correction of hypothermia, coagulopathy, and acidosis. For the trauma patient, this can usually be accomplished within 24 to 36 hours. Massive transfusion protocols and minimizing crystalloid infusions during this period have shown to expedite and improve successful first reoperative fascial closure.[24–26] Injured or devitalized tissues are resected, and the gastrointestinal injuries can be anastomosed safely, minimizing the need for enterostomy. However, for high-risk patients (e.g., those with sepsis related to gastrointestinal perforation, severe postoperative bleeding, multiple injuries, and intraoperative hypotension requiring vasopressors), enterostomy often remains the most prudent approach.[27]

Timing of initial reexploration can usually be achieved within 24 to 72 hours. Fluids should be restricted with attempts at diuresis, if indicated, and infections strictly controlled. Definitive closure should only be attempted when the underlying condition is resolving.

During Stage 3 or 4, it is important to assess the ability to close the fascia without undue tension due to tissue edema or loss of domain. This can be assessed by measuring intraabdominal pressure and/or changes in peak inspiratory pressure during closure. Sustained intraabdominal hypertension (>20–25 mm Hg) and a rise of peak inspiratory pressure of 10 cm H_2O during attempts at fascial closure are warning signs of high fascial tension with the potential for compromise to the abdominal wall, underlying viscera, renal function, and ventilation. Delayed closure of the fascia or a planned ventral hernia may be prudent for this subgroup of critically ill patients with an open abdomen.[22,28]

Additionally, early enteral nutrition in the patient with an open abdomen should be strongly considered in all patients with a viable gastrointestinal tract. Multiple studies have shown the benefits of enteral nutrition use in decreasing the time to abdominal fascial closure, decreased complication rates, and decreased mortality.[29,30]

PHARMACOLOGIC ADJUNCTS TO CLOSURE

In patients with open abdomens, the fascia often retracts laterally, making a tension-free closure difficult. Continuous neuromuscular blockade was thought to mitigate this, but in a retrospective cohort of trauma patients, this did not reduce time to abdominal closure.[31] However, use of botulinum toxin type A (BTA) injection in the abdominal wall musculature has been shown to decrease the thickness and increase the length of the abdominal wall muscles in a rat model. This method has been shown to be useful in both the elective setting for interval hernia repair after management with an open abdomen and in the index hospitalization. In the elective setting, 250 units total of BTA was injected at five points bilaterally between the internal and external oblique muscles under ultrasound guidance. This resulted in a decreased thickness and increased length of muscles for better approximation at the midline. In patients with an open abdomen, 300 units total of BTA was injected in a similar fashion under ultrasound guidance with an 83% primary fascial closure rate.[32,33]

SYNTHETIC MESH FAILURE

The use of synthetic prosthetic mesh is well established as the surgical treatment of choice for repair of ventral incisional hernias and, in the majority of cases, can provide a long-lasting repair with low recurrence rates. The development of synthetic mesh material was a major advancement in hernia surgery, and its advantages include decreased recurrence rates, ease of use, and a low cost compared to biologic mesh.[34] This has resulted in synthetic mesh being the most commonly used prosthetic for reinforcement for initial incisional and recurrent hernia repairs.

Although the application of synthetic mesh has resulted in a significant improvement in failure and recurrence rates, the use of these mesh materials may result in specific complications that range from minor to potentially life-threatening. Synthetic mesh may variably become infected dependent on the degree of contamination of the wound and the nature of the prosthetic material utilized.

Infections should be eradicated before considering any major repair, and measures should be taken to heal open wounds, as the bacterial colonization may be significant even in the absence of a frank infection. In the case of mesh infection, this often requires removal of the infected mesh material or anchoring sutures, drainage of any abscesses, and debridement of the wound. Lighter-weight, macroporous meshes carry a lower risk of infection compared to the heavier microporous meshes such as extended polytetrafluoroethylene (ePTFE).[35] Any mesh that is not incorporated should be excised completely from the edge of the wound to healthy tissues. If the wound has a large amount of contamination, it requires major debridement, a bowel resection, or enterocutaneous fistula takedown, etc.; a multistage approach may be required to achieve a clean wound before definitive abdominal wall reconstruction is entertained. Challenges to hernia repair in an infected field are multiple.

When there is insufficient autologous tissue for layered closure, often the case after emergent surgery in the setting of peritonitis, the surgeon is then faced with several challenges that must be addressed in a prioritized fashion. After the infection is eradicated, bowel resection performed, and necrotic tissue debrided, the visceral sac must then be contained. In this scenario, it is generally not advisable to create large skin flaps or perform myofascial component separations during this acute phase of management. After source control and treatment of infections, preparation of the wound for definitive repair should not interfere with possible reconstruction options in the future. Tissue repair during this time period is an anabolic process, and malnourished or actively catabolic patients have impaired healing. Additionally, the open abdomen creates an environment that is conducive to the development

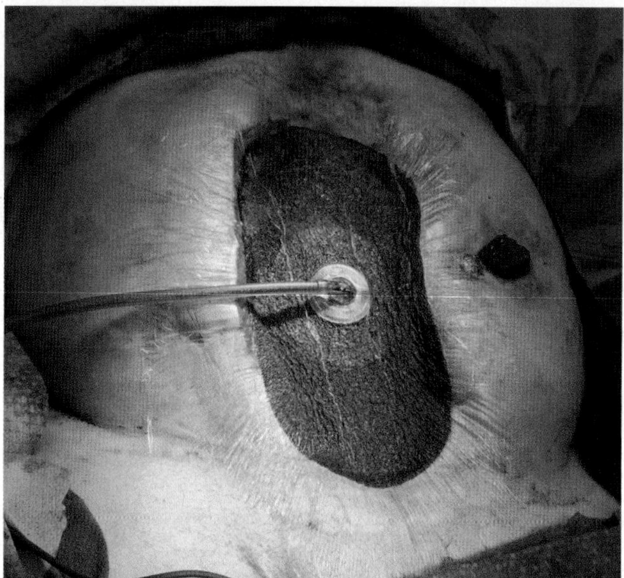

FIG. 18.4 Negative pressure wound therapy over a bridged repair.

of enterocutaneous fistulas and can represent a significant source of protein calorie malnutrition.

Although less than ideal, it may be necessary to rely on TAC and fascial bridge techniques to first reduce the biologic mesh burden and then develop a clean wound for later definitive repair. Determining the proper way to deal with this residual defect is still the source of controversy. Negative pressure devices have been used to help in this situation, first to eradicate all infection and then to cover a biologic mesh bridged repair (Fig. 18.4).

CHALLENGES IN THE CONTAMINATED FIELD

There are many challenges to hernia repair in an infected field. After an infection is eradicated, bowel resection performed, and necrotic tissue debrided, the visceral sac must then be contained. In this scenario, we advise against creating large skin flaps or performing myofascial component separation during the acute phase of management. After source control and treatment of infections, preparation of the wound for definitive repair should not interfere with possible reconstruction options in the future. Tissue repair during this time is an anabolic process, and malnourished or actively catabolic patients may have significantly impaired wound healing. In addition, the open abdomen probably contributes to the systemic inflammatory response and catabolic state.

Although less than ideal, it may be necessary to rely on TAC and fascial bridge techniques first to reduce the bacterial burden and then to develop a clean wound for later definitive repair. The most efficacious management strategy of a ventral hernia in a contaminated wound continues to be debated and includes methods of staging the repair with the use of negative pressure devices, primary fascial closure alone, the use of permanent or absorbable synthetic mesh, or biologic mesh.

Biologic mesh was developed and promoted primarily for use in contaminated fields in which synthetic mesh use was contraindicated. A variety of biologic mesh material currently used includes sources from human, porcine, and bovine species with variable amounts of elastin and collagen and may or may not be cross-linked. The donor sites include dermis, intestinal mucosa, and pericardium. The processing of these materials removes all cellular elements, microbes, and epitopes responsible for rejection,

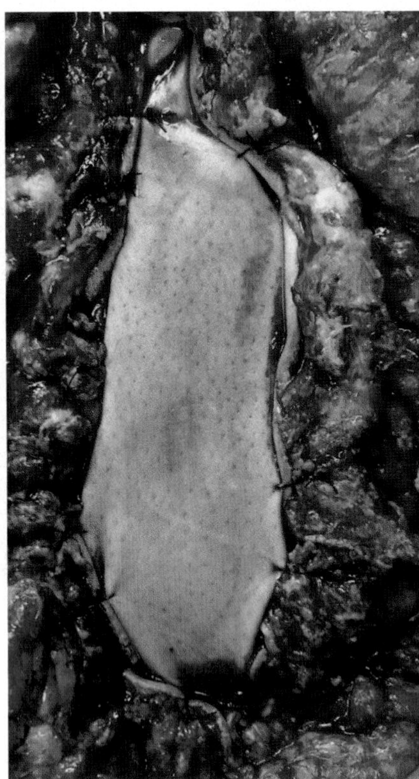

FIG. 18.5 Bridged repair with biologic mesh.

leaving only the extracellular matrix and vascular channels intact. The theoretical benefits of biologic mesh over synthetic mesh include revascularization and incorporation into the host tissues, thus causing less of an inflammatory reaction, less adhesion formation, and improvement of bacterial clearance in a contaminated wound.[36] There still are many unanswered questions as to the ideal source material, processing methods, and most appropriate placement techniques.[37,38]

In the case of sepsis and/or a prolonged inflammatory process with a large abdominal wound defect or major fascial dehiscence, our current practice involves the use of a non–cross-linked biologic mesh as an inlay bridge repair to cover the fascial gap (Fig. 18.5). This method can help protect the abdominal viscera from desiccation and fistula formation. Coverage of the biologic mesh with an NPWT technique and skin coverage over drains are accepted bailout maneuvers in this circumstance. Wound management systems that use topical antimicrobials and moist sponge materials can minimize desiccation and limit the bacterial burden to the biologic mesh while it incorporates into native tissue. Delayed ventral hernia repair can then be performed once the patient has recovered and their protein calorie malnutrition has been repleted.

This biologic bridge technique is useful for patients with significant comorbidities, for the acutely ill, and in cases in which definitive reconstruction is a prohibitive risk. There is clear evidence that if the biologic mesh is used as a bridge repair, the result is a high recurrence rate because of stretching of the biologic mesh over time, causing laxity and bulging, or an actual recurrence within a year. Thus, the bridge repair should be thought of not as a definitive reconstruction alternative, but more as a biologic mesh covering of the peritoneal cavity that prevents desiccation and enterocutaneous fistula formation. Complications related to biologic mesh use include seroma and hematoma formation, SSO, graft degradation, and desiccation. Ensuring ongoing hydration of the biologic mesh with the use of hydrating gels, enzymatic debriding agents, and overlying skin or VAC therapy can reduce these complications.[39]

Since the introduction of these bioprosthetic materials, there has been an ever-expanding market of both new biologic, biosynthetic, and lightweight macroporous synthetic materials that claim superiority in the contaminated field. Few of these materials have been subject to critical evaluation of their outcomes in humans for complex abdominal wall reconstruction.

The Ventral Hernia Working Group and a recent systematic review and metaanalysis recommend consideration of biologic mesh in contaminated or dirty wounds (Grades 3 and 4).[40] The primary benefits when biologic mesh is used in contaminated cases are less need for removal as compared to synthetic grafts and their 30-day SSI is not increased based on the degree of wound contamination in contrast to synthetic mesh.

A multicenter prospective study utilizing a porcine biologic mesh for repair of infected or contaminated ventral hernias demonstrated an SSO rate of 66% and an SSI rate of 30%.[41] A 5-year follow-up of this patient population found a 50% recurrence rate at 3 years with a two times higher recurrence when the biologic mesh was placed intraperitoneal versus retrorectus. The mean fascial defect size was 236 cm^2 with 80% ability of complete fascial closure over the biologic mesh.

A large multicenter, longitudinal study for contaminated ventral hernia repair (Complex Open Bioabsorbable Reconstruction of the Abdominal Wall [COBRA] trial) using biosynthetic mesh (biologic with absorbable synthetic mesh) found at 24 months an SSO rate of 28%, an SSI rate of 18%, and a recurrence rate of 17%.[42] This is less than the Repair of Infected or Contaminated Ventral Incisional Hernias (RICH) study, but critical reviews comparing the two studies state that they were different patient populations and mean hernia size in the COBRA study was significantly less (137 cm^2) with a compete fascial closure rate of 100%. Multiple studies now clearly demonstrate that a bridged repair is a significant predictor of hernia recurrence.[43,44]

Recent literature now suggests that lightweight permanent synthetic mesh may be an option to biologic mesh in the contaminated environment with comparable risk of SSO and need for mesh removal. Carbonell and colleagues[45] challenged the fact that permanent mesh is contraindicated in contaminated fields, reviewing 100 patients with clean-contaminated or contaminated ventral hernia repairs using lightweight polypropylene mesh. SSO was 26.2% in clean-contaminated wounds and 34% in contaminated wounds. The recurrence rate was 7% with a mean follow-up of 10.8 months.[45]

SEROMA AND SKIN NECROSIS

Seroma and skin necrosis are frequent complications related to major abdominal wall reconstruction (Fig. 18.6). Seromas occur especially in cases with wide subcutaneous dissection or with premature drain dislodgement or clogging. Release of fascial planes or creation of large tissue flaps creates a potential space that can fill with exudate that exceeds the capacity to be reabsorbed. To reduce seroma formation, closed suction drains should be placed in the subcutaneous and/or retrorectus space. These drains should be stripped regularly during the early postoperative period and are typically removed when less than 25 to 30 mL in a 24-hour period has been recorded. In addition, external compression with abdominal binders may aid in the abdominal wall and skin flap adherence and may hinder fluid collection formation.

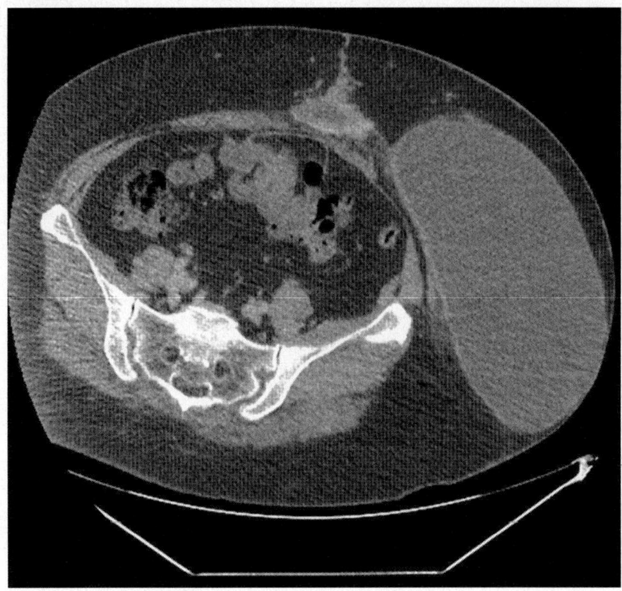

FIG. 18.6 Seroma after skin flap creation.

Methods that have been described in the literature to decrease seroma formation include quilting stiches, talc application, or, most recently, surgical tissue adhesive application under skin flaps or over mesh application in the retrorectus space. However, there are no large studies to definitively show the benefit of these methods, and they should be considered on a case-by-case basis. If the seroma is asymptomatic and small, it will often resorb without any invasive intervention. Aspiration or reoperative drainage may be required if the seroma enlarges or shows signs of infection.[46]

The blood supply to the skin is primarily distributed through the subcutaneous fat and perforators originating from the deep inferior epigastric artery. Intraoperative methods for optimizing and preserving the circulation to the skin and preventing postoperative skin necrosis are essential. In creating any skin flap, dissection should be in the plane between the subcutaneous layer and the underlying fascia. Techniques to preserve the perforators are well described in the literature. The perforators' density is highest around the periumbilical area, and thus it is important to spare a circular distance of about 3 cm around the umbilicus area during dissection.

Impending skin necrosis can be manifested as duskiness, blistering, and blanching redness that can progress to definitive necrotic tissue. Management varies by the depth and the total area of necrosis. Superficial skin necrosis can be treated locally with hydrating gels or enzymatic debriding agents. These products reduce the bacterial and necrotic tissue burden and maintain a moist environment for healing. Full-thickness wounds require skin and subcutaneous sharp debridement. Negative pressure wound management systems can aid in sterile wound coverage for this complication.

PREPARATION FOR ABDOMINAL WALL RECONSTRUCTION

The goal of definitive reconstruction is first to optimize the patient's condition and then to restore the structure and functional continuity of the musculofascial system in order to provide stable and durable wound coverage to minimize additional complications. Once the decision has been made to operate, preoperative risk factors must be carefully evaluated and optimized before an elective complex abdominal wall reconstruction is performed. Understanding of preoperative risk factors during the process of patient and procedure selection is essential to minimize adverse postoperative occurrences.

Every effort should be made to control diabetes and obtain a hemoglobin A1C less than 8 and optimize protein-calorie repletion and cardiopulmonary status. Mandatory cigarette smoking cessation is required for at least 4 to 6 weeks before repair. In patients with a previous methicillin-resistant *Staphylococcus aureus* infection, consideration should be given to decolonizing the patient or suppressing methicillin-resistant *S. aureus* carriers preoperatively and using vancomycin prophylaxis perioperatively.

DEFINITIVE REPAIR—CREATING A DYNAMIC ABDOMINAL WALL

Even with a great deal of preoperative planning, there is still no single approach that will solve all the needs for the reconstruction of a complex abdominal wall defect. It is essential that the surgeon review all prior operative reports and have a clear understanding of what remains in the wound and in what location. A preoperative computed tomography scan of the abdominal wall is essential prior to any consideration of major reconstruction.

In cases of previous contamination or infection, the surgeon is often faced with the difficult task of having to decide when to utilize mesh for reinforcement, the type of mesh to use, and where to place it. There is still little supportive evidence and it will require a prospective randomized trial to definitively determine the type of mesh to be used in each category of the previously described grading system. The only large multi-institutional single arm study for ventral hernias in contaminated fields utilized a porcine acellular dermal matrix for repair. The incidence of wound complications was 33.8% at 6 months, and none of the patients required mesh removal. To date, there is no comparative trial to evaluate different biologic repair materials. There is currently an ongoing comparison between biologic mesh and lightweight macroporous synthetic mesh in contaminated ventral hernia cases.

There is now widespread belief that a tension-free, fascia-to-fascia closure utilizing component separation techniques combined with underlay reinforcement with mesh is the ideal method for abdominal wall reconstruction. Expert opinion in the literature states that the most important factor in preventing postoperative complications is placement of the mesh in the retrorectus space utilizing a sublay technique. In general, the retrorectus repair and the sublay placement of mesh have resulted in the lowest complication rate, including less infection, seroma formation, and hernia recurrence, as compared to the onlay or inlay techniques.

Various techniques for mobilization of the fascia medially with the component separation provide a tension-free repair of the rectus fascia and subsequent protection from infection from the overlying subcutaneous fat and skin. The classically described Ramirez technique for component separation requires large subcutaneous flaps to gain access to the lateral abdominal wall and release the external oblique fascia. This technique has high wound morbidity and is, in general, not recommended for high-risk patients. Recently developed endoscopic methods to perform component separation release of the external oblique aponeurosis by using an endoscopic camera and avoiding division of the perforators have now been described.[47]

The appreciation of abdominal wall function to create a dynamic abdominal wall unit has popularized two ideal reconstruction techniques: the Rives-Stoppa-Wantz repair and the transversus abdominis release. Both utilize a retromuscular sublay of mesh

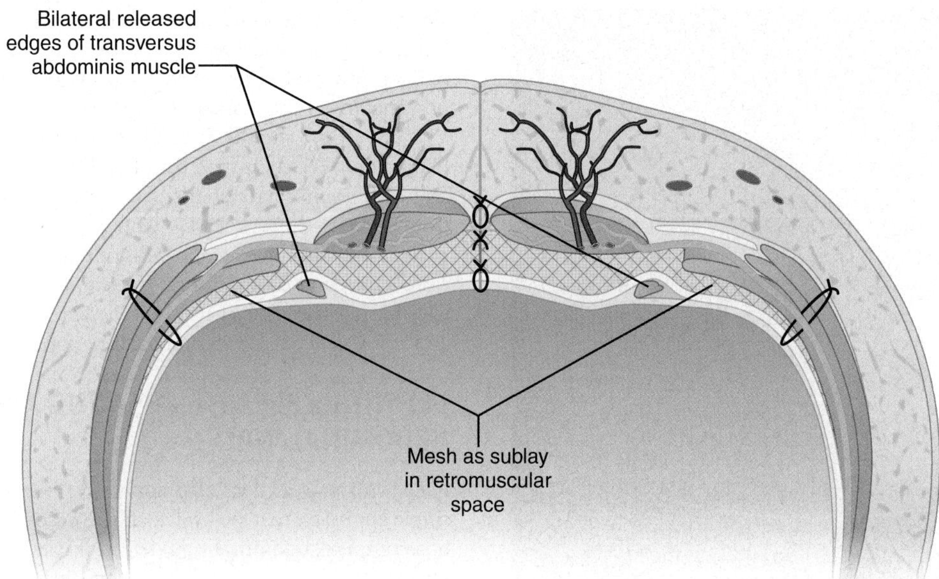

FIG. 18.7 Retrorectus positioning of mesh after Rives-Stoppa-Wantz repair.

and have become the gold standard repair by the American Hernia Society. The retromuscular space has a rich vascularization, and these two techniques preserve the abdominal wall neurovascular bundle with favorable outcomes. Both techniques utilize a posterior component separation and the placement of lightweight macroporous synthetic mesh in the retrorectus space and outside of the peritoneal cavity. These techniques serve as optimal protection of the bowel from the mesh provided by the posterior rectus sheath, peritoneum, and omentum.

RIVES-STOPPA-WANTZ AND TRANSVERSUS ABDOMINIS RELEASE TECHNIQUES

In this technique, the posterior rectus sheath is incised approximately one half of a centimeter from the fascial edge of the defect. The retrorectus plane is then developed to the lateral extent of the dissection: the linea semilunaris. If this dissection is insufficient to close the posterior rectus fascia, an extension of this technique includes the transversus abdominis release. In this technique, the transversus abdominis muscle is divided, which then allows entrance into the space between the transversalis fascia and the lateral edge of this divided transversus abdominis muscle. This allows the creation of a wide lateral dissection plane with substantial posterior and anterior fascial advancement. Both procedures avoid a major subcutaneous dissection and preserve the neurovascular bundle (Figs. 18.7 and 18.8).

PERIOPERATIVE CONSIDERATIONS

Reconstruction of large abdominal defects can markedly change the physiology of respiration and alter the function of the diaphragm and respiratory musculature. Many surgeons have advocated the use of the plateau pressure as an intraoperative method for gauging the effects of hernia repair on pulmonary function. Postoperative respiratory complications have been found to be significantly increased when the plateau pressure was raised above 6 mm Hg, and patients were nine times more likely to have complications with this finding.[48] Additionally, intraoperative and postoperative monitoring of abdominal pressures indirectly using bladder pressure measurements is routinely recommended when the abdominal wall defect is more than 600 cm^2.[48]

Pain management is essential in this patient population, and the use of epidural catheters and transversus abdominis plane blocks substantially improves pain relief. These reduce narcotic use within the postoperative phase and decrease costs and postoperative morbidity.[49] Both techniques increase early mobilization, thus reducing additional complications related to this extensive surgery. Long-acting injectable bupivacaine medication can provide prolonged relief of pain and reduce the use of narcotics. Abdominal binders can also improve patient ambulation, pain control, and comfort.

Finally, a thorough understanding of the determinants of outcomes may be the most important factor in reducing complications and even death in this patient population. Nonoperative close observation strategies for asymptomatic large incisional hernias may be prudent in certain patient populations. Currently, there is no study evaluating patients with known incisional hernias who are managed nonoperatively.

Most recently, the American Hernia Society has developed a quality collaborative (AHSQC) to improve the value of hernia care delivered to patients. It was formed in 2013 by hernia surgeons both in private practice and in academic centers. The goal of the AHSQC is to utilize concepts of continuous quality improvement, improve outcomes, and optimize costs. Ongoing data collection, performance feedback, and collaborative learning will no doubt improve patient outcomes by providing optimal timing and operation selection for this challenging patient population.

SUMMARY

In most damage control laparotomies for trauma, vascular surgery, and/or emergency general surgery, primary fascial closure can be achieved in 60% to 90% of the cases. Patients for whom the abdomen cannot be closed make up the category of those with a difficult abdominal wall. This can then give rise to the complex ventral hernia. The causes of the difficult abdominal wall share features in common—loss of abdominal domain, risk of the development of intraabdominal hypertension and/or abdominal compartment

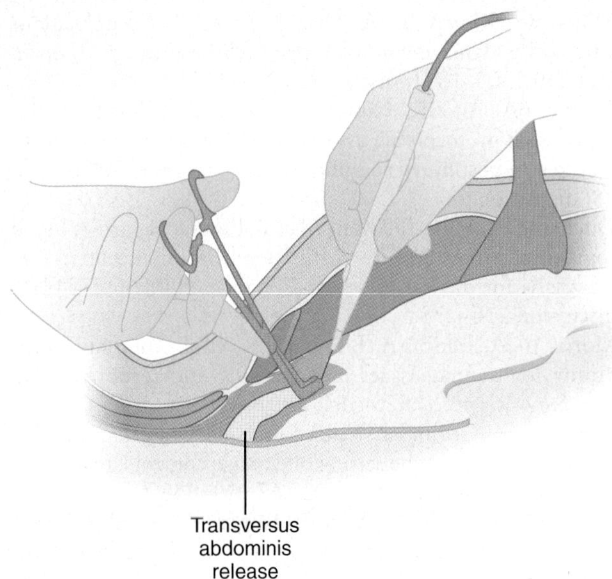

FIG. 18.8 Transversus abdominis release.

syndrome, development of intraabdominal abscess or fistula, systemic inflammatory response syndrome, and a higher than 50% risk of hernia formation. When temporary coverage of the abdomen is necessary, the technique should be easy to apply, tension-free, atraumatic, and inexpensive and allow ultimately for delayed primary fascial closure.

Following normalization of physiology, reexploration and a staged repair may be performed. It is not advisable to attempt delayed primary fascial closure if there is undue tension on the fascia or if the peak inspiratory pressure rises more than 10 cm H_2O. However, the inability to close the open abdomen by 8 days is associated with a significant increase in complications, including enteroatmospheric fistulas. For this reason, some surgeons have bridged an abdominal wall defect with biologic mesh to protect the abdominal viscera. However, this repair should be considered as a temporizing measure because most bridging repairs will develop bulging and/or laxity within 1 year of closure. Delayed ventral hernia repair using component separation reinforced with biologic mesh has produced excellent results and is recommended for the closure of the complicated abdominal wall.

SELECTED REFERENCES

Boele van Hensbroek P, Wind J, Dijkgraaf MG, et al. Temporary closure of the open abdomen: a systematic review on delayed primary fascial closure in patients with an open abdomen. *World J Surg*. 2009;33:199–207.

This is a systematic review of studies involving management of the open abdomen, comparing the relative closure rates of the various techniques.

Carbonell AM, Criss CN, Cobb WS, et al. Outcomes of synthetic mesh in contaminated ventral hernia repairs. *J Am Coll Surg*. 2013;217:991–998.

Contamination of the surgical field has long been thought to be an absolute contraindication to the use of prosthetic mesh for hernia repair. There is growing evidence that synthetic materials may be safely used despite the presence of contamination, potentially resulting in improved long-term outcomes of hernia repair.

Diener MK, Voss S, Jensen K, et al. Elective midline laparotomy closure: the INLINE systematic review and meta-analysis. *Ann Surg*. 2010;251:843–856.

This is a systematic review of the literature regarding closure of midline laparotomy. It evaluates the various techniques and suture materials. It does caution that there is no evidence to guide closure of emergency laparotomies.

Miller RS, Morris Jr JA, Diaz Jr JJ, et al. Complications after 344 damage-control open celiotomies. *J Trauma*. 2005;59:1365–1371.

This study evaluated a large number of damage control abdomens. Morbidity is associated with the timing and method of wound closure and transfusion volume but is independent of injury severity. Best outcomes occurred with delayed primary fascial closure before 8 days.

Novitsky YW, Elliott HL, Orenstein SB, et al. Transversus abdominis muscle release: a novel approach to posterior component separation during complex abdominal wall reconstruction. *Am J Surg*. 2012;204:709–716.

This is a landmark surgical anatomy description that expounds on the knowledge of the retrorectus space by describing a closed internal component separation method. The anatomic details of the transversus abdominis space are described that set the basis for the transversus abdominis release hernia repair.

REFERENCES

1. Diener MK, Voss S, Jensen K, et al. Elective midline laparotomy closure: the INLINE systematic review and meta-analysis. *Ann Surg*. 2010;251:843–856.
2. Fortelny RH. Abdominal wall closure in elective midline laparotomy: the current recommendations. *Front Surg*. 2018;5:34.
3. Oni G, Brown SA, Kenkel JM. A comparison between barbed and nonbarbed absorbable suture for fascial closure in a porcine model. *Plast Reconstr Surg*. 2012;130:535e–540e.
4. Rosen A, Hartman T. Repair of the midline fascial defect in abdominoplasty with long-acting barbed and smooth absorbable sutures. *Aesthet Surg J*. 2011;31:668–673.
5. Seiler CM, Bruckner T, Diener MK, et al. Interrupted or continuous slowly absorbable sutures for closure of primary elective midline abdominal incisions: a multicenter randomized trial (INSECT: ISRCTN24023541). *Ann Surg*. 2009;249:576–582.
6. Deerenberg EB, Harlaar JJ, Steyerberg EW, et al. Small bites versus large bites for closure of abdominal midline incisions

(STITCH): a double-blind, multicentre, randomised controlled trial. *Lancet.* 2015;386:1254–1260.

7. Khorgami Z, Shoar S, Laghaie B, et al. Prophylactic retention sutures in midline laparotomy in high-risk patients for wound dehiscence: a randomized controlled trial. *J Surg Res.* 2013;180:238–243.
8. Caro-Tarrago A, Olona Casas C, Jimenez Salido A, et al. Prevention of incisional hernia in midline laparotomy with an onlay mesh: a randomized clinical trial. *World J Surg.* 2014;38:2223–2230.
9. Borab ZM, Shakir S, Lanni MA, et al. Does prophylactic mesh placement in elective, midline laparotomy reduce the incidence of incisional hernia? A systematic review and meta-analysis. *Surgery.* 2017;161:1149–1163.
10. El-Khadrawy OH, Moussa G, Mansour O, et al. Prophylactic prosthetic reinforcement of midline abdominal incisions in high-risk patients. *Hernia.* 2009;13:267–274.
11. Fischer JP, Basta MN, Wink JD, et al. Cost-utility analysis of the use of prophylactic mesh augmentation compared with primary fascial suture repair in patients at high risk for incisional hernia. *Surgery.* 2015;158:700–711.
12. Jairam AP, Timmermans L, Eker HH, et al. Prevention of incisional hernia with prophylactic onlay and sublay mesh reinforcement versus primary suture only in midline laparotomies (PRIMA): 2-year follow-up of a multicentre, double-blind, randomised controlled trial. *Lancet.* 2017;390:567–576.
13. Shanmugam VK, Fernandez SJ, Evans KK, et al. Postoperative wound dehiscence: predictors and associations. *Wound Repair Regen.* 2015;23:184–190.
14. van Ramshorst GH, Nieuwenhuizen J, Hop WC, et al. Abdominal wound dehiscence in adults: development and validation of a risk model. *World J Surg.* 2010;34:20–27.
15. Higa G, Friese R, O'Keeffe T, et al. Damage control laparotomy: a vital tool once overused. *J Trauma.* 2010;69:53–59.
16. Quyn AJ, Johnston C, Hall D, et al. The open abdomen and temporary abdominal closure systems—historical evolution and systematic review. *Colorectal Dis.* 2012;14:e429–e438.
17. Sharrock AE, Barker T, Yuen HM, et al. Management and closure of the open abdomen after damage control laparotomy for trauma. A systematic review and meta-analysis. *Injury.* 2016;47:296–306.
18. Mukhi AN, Minor S. Management of the open abdomen using combination therapy with ABRA and ABThera systems. *Can J Surg.* 2014;57:314–319.
19. Atema JJ, Gans SL, Boermeester MA. Systematic review and meta-analysis of the open abdomen and temporary abdominal closure techniques in non-trauma patients. *World J Surg.* 2015;39:912–925.
20. Haddock C, Konkin DE, Blair NP. Management of the open abdomen with the abdominal reapproximation anchor dynamic fascial closure system. *Am J Surg.* 2013;205:528–533; discussion 533.
21. Salamone G, Licari L, Guercio G, et al. Vacuum-assisted wound closure with mesh-mediated fascial traction achieves better outcomes than vacuum-assisted wound closure alone: a comparative study. *World J Surg.* 2018;42:1679–1686.
22. Boele van Hensbroek P, Wind J, Dijkgraaf MG, et al. Temporary closure of the open abdomen: a systematic review on delayed primary fascial closure in patients with an open abdomen. *World J Surg.* 2009;33:199–207.
23. Miller RS, Morris Jr JA, Diaz Jr JJ, et al. Complications after 344 damage-control open celiotomies. *J Trauma.* 2005;59:1365–1371; discussion 1371–1364.
24. Cotton BA, Au BK, Nunez TC, et al. Predefined massive transfusion protocols are associated with a reduction in organ failure and postinjury complications. *J Trauma.* 2009;66:41–48; discussion 48–49.
25. Duchesne JC, Hunt JP, Wahl G, et al. Review of current blood transfusions strategies in a mature level I trauma center: were we wrong for the last 60 years? *J Trauma.* 2008;65:272–276; discussion 276–278.
26. Morris Jr JA, Eddy VA, Blinman TA, et al. The staged celiotomy for trauma. Issues in unpacking and reconstruction. *Ann Surg.* 1993;217:576–584; discussion 584–576.
27. Weinberg JA, Griffin RL, Vandromme MJ, et al. Management of colon wounds in the setting of damage control laparotomy: a cautionary tale. *J Trauma.* 2009;67:929–935.
28. Turza KC, Campbell CA, Rosenberger LH, et al. Options for closure of the infected abdomen. *Surg Infect (Larchmt).* 2012;13:343–351.
29. Burlew CC, Moore EE, Cuschieri J, et al. Who should we feed? Western trauma association multi-institutional study of enteral nutrition in the open abdomen after injury. *J Trauma Acute Care Surg.* 2012;73:1380–1387; discussion 1387–1388.
30. Collier B, Guillamondegui O, Cotton B, et al. Feeding the open abdomen. *JPEN J Parenter Enteral Nutr.* 2007;31:410–415.
31. Smith SE, Hamblin SE, Guillamondegui OD, et al. Effectiveness and safety of continuous neuromuscular blockade in trauma patients with an open abdomen: a follow-up study. *Am J Surg.* 2018;216:414–419.
32. Ibarra-Hurtado TR, Nuno-Guzman CM, Miranda-Diaz AG, et al. Effect of botulinum toxin type a in lateral abdominal wall muscles thickness and length of patients with midline incisional hernia secondary to open abdomen management. *Hernia.* 2014;18:647–652.
33. Zielinski MD, Goussous N, Schiller HJ, et al. Chemical components separation with botulinum toxin a: a novel technique to improve primary fascial closure rates of the open abdomen. *Hernia.* 2013;17:101–107.
34. Fischer JP, Basta MN, Mirzabeigi MN, et al. A comparison of outcomes and cost in VHWG grade II hernias between Rives-Stoppa synthetic mesh hernia repair versus underlay biologic mesh repair. *Hernia.* 2014;18:781–789.
35. Diaz-Godoy A, Garcia-Urena MA, Lopez-Monclus J, et al. Searching for the best polypropylene mesh to be used in bowel contamination. *Hernia.* 2011;15:173–179.
36. Harth KC, Broome AM, Jacobs MR, et al. Bacterial clearance of biologic grafts used in hernia repair: an experimental study. *Surg Endosc.* 2011;25:2224–2229.
37. Harris HW. Clinical outcomes of biologic mesh: where do we stand? *Surg Clin North Am.* 2013;93:1217–1225.
38. Rosen MJ, Denoto G, Itani KM, et al. Evaluation of surgical outcomes of retro-rectus versus intraperitoneal reinforcement with bio-prosthetic mesh in the repair of contaminated ventral hernias. *Hernia.* 2013;17:31–35.
39. Piccoli M, Agresta F, Attina GM, et al. "Complex abdominal wall" management: evidence-based guidelines of the Italian Consensus Conference. *Updates Surg.* 2018.
40. Breuing K, Butler CE, Ferzoco S, et al. Incisional ventral hernias: review of the literature and recommendations regarding the grading and technique of repair. *Surgery.* 2010;148:544–558.

41. Itani KM, Rosen M, Vargo D, et al. Prospective study of single-stage repair of contaminated hernias using a biologic porcine tissue matrix: the RICH Study. *Surgery.* 2012;152:498–505.
42. Rosen MJ, Bauer JJ, Harmaty M, et al. Multicenter, prospective, longitudinal study of the recurrence, surgical site infection, and quality of life after contaminated ventral hernia repair using biosynthetic absorbable mesh: the COBRA Study. *Ann Surg.* 2017;265:205–211.
43. Booth JH, Garvey PB, Baumann DP, et al. Primary fascial closure with mesh reinforcement is superior to bridged mesh repair for abdominal wall reconstruction. *J Am Coll Surg.* 2013;217:999–1009.
44. Garvey PB, Giordano SA, Baumann DP, et al. Long-term outcomes after abdominal wall reconstruction with acellular dermal matrix. *J Am Coll Surg.* 2017;224:341–350.
45. Carbonell AM, Criss CN, Cobb WS, et al. Outcomes of synthetic mesh in contaminated ventral hernia repairs. *J Am Coll Surg.* 2013;217:991–998.
46. Kohler G, Koch OO, Antoniou SA, et al. Prevention of subcutaneous seroma formation in open ventral hernia repair using a new low-thrombin fibrin sealant. *World J Surg.* 2014;38:2797–2803.
47. Dauser B, Ghaffari S, Ng C, et al. Endoscopic anterior component separation: a novel technical approach. *Hernia.* 2017;21:951–955.
48. Blatnik JA, Krpata DM, Pesa NL, et al. Predicting severe postoperative respiratory complications following abdominal wall reconstruction. *Plast Reconstr Surg.* 2012;130:836–841.
49. Fischer JP, Nelson JA, Wes AM, et al. The use of epidurals in abdominal wall reconstruction: an analysis of outcomes and cost. *Plast Reconstr Surg.* 2014;133:687–699.

19 CHAPTER

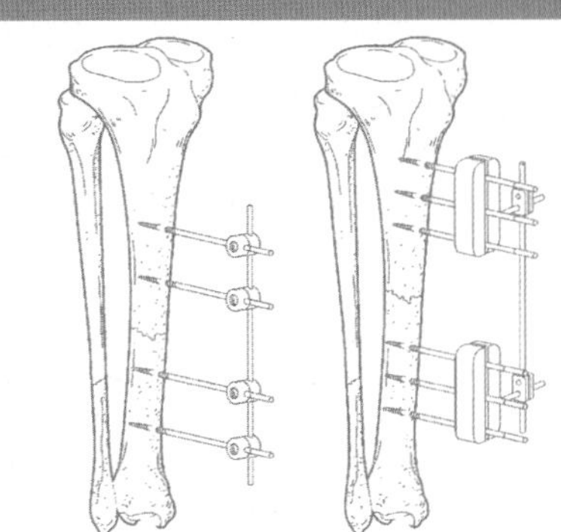

Emergency Care of Musculoskeletal Injuries

Jack Dawson, Omar Atassi, Daniel Sun, Mihir Sheth

OUTLINE

EPIDEMIOLOGY OF ORTHOPEDIC INJURIES

Fractures occur when the applied load to the bone exceeds its load-bearing capacity. Fracture patterns relate to bone strength and the forces that cause the injury. The patient's age and the mechanism of injury are both strong determinants of the fracture pattern and the soft tissue injury that occurs concurrent with the fracture, both of which will drive the treatment strategy. In general, basic physics is implied: kinetic energy equals ½(mass)(velocity).[1,2] Thus, the greater the velocity is, an exponentially higher amount of energy is stored within a system. Upon impact, that energy is absorbed by the body and the musculoskeletal system. This energy is realized as comminution (multifragmentary fractures) and local damage to soft tissue. In practice, we see these differences quite clearly. Young, active individuals have strong bone, and elderly, osteoporotic individuals have diffusely weak bone. A femur fracture in a young individual is more likely to have resulted from a high energy mechanism and will often have other bodily injuries, whereas a femur fracture in an elderly patient is most often from a ground-level fall and is usually isolated.

Tumors, infection, and dysplasia can cause focal bone defects that may weaken a bone so significantly that it fails under a load that the bone should normally withstand: a young patient who sustains a hip fracture after a ground-level fall, for example. A clinical history that does not "match" the fracture pattern should prompt the provider to dig a little deeper with that patient.

Accidents continue to be a leading cause of death and disability throughout the world. In general, the amount of energy absorbed by a multiply injured patient corresponds to the extent of the musculoskeletal injuries. Because high energy is frequently involved, fractures and soft tissue injuries are common. It has been estimated that 46% of patients sustaining a traumatic injury in the United States have an orthopedic injury, and between 13% and 25% of these patients require an orthopedic traumatologist.[2] Given that trauma is one of the leading causes of disability in younger generations of patients, the financial burden to both the individual patients as well as society in general is tremendous.[1,3] Trauma in the United States accounts for billions of dollars in lost productivity, medical costs, and property damage each year, and orthopedic trauma remains one of the most cost-effective forms of medicine.

Fractures may result from both low- and high-energy forces and may occur in either isolation or as multiple injuries. The mechanism of injury defines the specific individual fracture pattern and is important for dictating both temporizing as well as definitive fixation. Typical fracture mechanisms include blunt versus penetrating trauma, low-energy versus high-energy forces, and twisting, bending, or crushing forces. Extremity injuries compromise functional outcome and can lead to long-term pain, abnormal gait, degenerative joint disease, chronic infection, and limb loss.

At the national and global levels, substantial improvements in transportation safety and delivery of medical care have helped address this growing pandemic. Seat belt and helmet laws, enforcement of drunk driving laws, mandates for improved safety features in automobiles, rapid deployment of emergency medical teams, and establishment of trauma centers have decreased the number of accident scene fatalities. These changes have led to an increased number of patients who survive high-energy crashes and who consequently sustain higher severity lower extremity injuries. Shock Trauma in Baltimore noted a decrease in the mortality associated with bilateral femur fractures from 26% to 7% over a 15-year period. There was an associated drop in Injury Severity Score (ISS) that suggests that a contribution to this decrease in mortality is directly related to changes in motor vehicle design.[4]

With more victims now likely to survive accidents that might have been fatal in the past, caregivers will be challenged with managing more complex fractures and soft tissue wounds. These realities demand that trauma teams be aware of the frequency and consequences of musculoskeletal injuries in every trauma patient. In particular, the immediate assessment and determination of severity are of the utmost importance as it facilitates the correct triage of patients. An appreciation for the unique features of skeletal injury in patients who may also have severe head, thoracic, or intraabdominal trauma is essential. In this way, a cohesive, integrated approach to the diagnosis and treatment of musculoskeletal injuries may be used in the care of the multiply injured patient.

TABLE 19.1 Important fracture descriptors.

TERM	MEANING
General Terms	
Skeletal maturity	Open versus closed growth plate (physis)
Pathologic	Failure of bone through an area of preexisting disease
Insufficiency, fragility	Osteoporotic bone
Open	Communication of the fracture with the skin
Closed	No communication of the fracture with the skin
Children	
–Greenstick	Incomplete cortical disruption
–Physeal	Partial or complete involvement of the growth plate (physis)
–Buckle, torus	Axial crush with small buckling of cortex
Location	
–Diaphyseal	The shaft
–Metaphyseal	The flare between the shaft and the joint surface
–Epiphyseal	The joint surface
–Supracondylar	Proximal to the epicondyles (humerus and femur)
–Intracondylar	Between the articular condyles (humerus and femur)
–Intraarticular	Extending into the joint surface
Pattern	
–Transverse	Perpendicular to the long axis of the bone
–Oblique	Angular to the long axis of the bone
–Spiral	Torsional failure
–Butterfly	Separate fragment at the fracture
–Comminuted	Multiple pieces
Displacement	
–Translation	Percent displacement of the distal fragment relative to the proximal
–Angulation	Apex volar or dorsal, apex valgus or varus
–Length	Shortened or distracted
–Rotation	Relative to the proximal fragment

TERMINOLOGY

Communication among collaborating specialists is central to patient care. Trauma and emergency department (ED) findings need to be relayed precisely to consulting specialists. This task is particularly challenging in view of the variety of anatomic locations, fracture patterns, and associated soft tissue injuries encountered in orthopedics. Although many injuries are identified by eponyms within the orthopedic community, the most practical and universally understood characterizations of injuries are those that adhere to basic anatomic and mechanical principles. The common fracture descriptors are summarized in Table 19.1 but will be reviewed in the following section as well.

Fracture Types

A fracture is a disruption of the normal architecture of bone. Fractures can be acute, subacute, or chronic. Subacute and chronic fractures, while frequently needing treatment, can often be managed on an ambulatory basis and do not require emergent care. Radiographically, acute fractures can be differentiated from older fractures by the identification of sharp, well-defined edges of the fragments. Older fractures will have evidence of callus formation and a blunting of the fracture edges. Chronic fractures can be radiographically dramatic because of bony hypertrophy and/or adjacent structure destruction. A simple history from the patient usually determines that these do not require emergent management (Fig. 19.1).

Because of increased plasticity, a more substantial periosteum, and the presence of growth plates, children's bones are at risk for a different set of fractures (Fig. 19.2). Plastic deformity of a long bone in a pediatric patient is deformation of the bone without actual disruption of the bone cortex. Radiography of the contralateral extremity can aid in diagnosis. Diagnosis of the deformity often necessitates radiography of the contralateral extremity to confirm asymmetry. Axial loads of long bones in children can lead to buckling of the cortex without a visible fracture line, appropriately termed a *buckle fracture.* Incomplete disruptions of the cortex are termed *greenstick fractures* in children or *infractions* in adults. A greenstick fracture consists of a cortical disruption on one side of the bone, with a buckle fracture or plastic deformation on the opposite side. The dense periosteal layer in children can contribute stability to many of these fractures if the layer remains intact. In some cases, radiographs will be normal, yet the child will not use

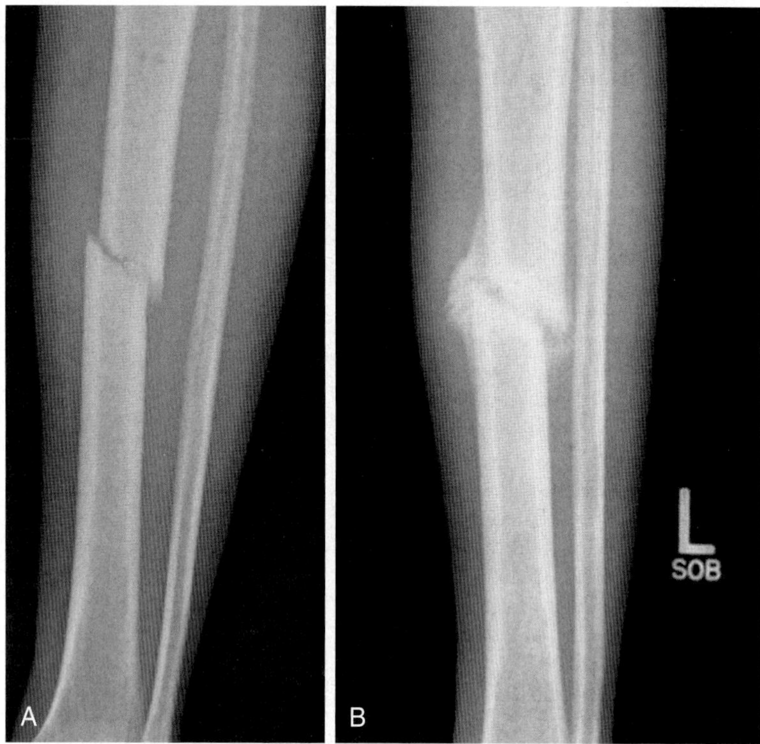

FIG. 19.1 (A) Acute fracture. Note the sharp, well-defined edges. (B) Nonunion. 6 months later, the fracture line is still clearly visible, the edges of this fracture are blunted, and the bone ends are sclerotic with callus formation. There was still motion at the fracture site on clinical examination. The patient had significant chronic pain.

the extremity. Care must be taken to ensure that there is no missed partial or complete fracture through the cartilaginous growth plate (physis). Physeal fractures are described by the Salter-Harris classification (Fig. 19.3A). These centers of bony growth around the ends of each bone ossify at different points in a child's life. Disruption of one of these "ossification centers" can alter the future growth of the affected bone, leading to length discrepancies or angular deformities. A high level of clinical suspicion is necessary to diagnose these injuries.

When a bone fails through an area weakened by preexisting disease, it is termed a *pathologic fracture.* Causes may include weakness from primary bone tumors, metastatic lesions, infection, metabolic disease, and injury to an old fracture site. Although they are not commonly referred to in this way, fractures in osteoporotic bone are technically pathologic. However, the term *insufficiency* or *fragility fracture* is most frequently used to describe these injuries. In contradistinction to acute fractures in healthy bone, fragility fractures normally result from accidents with much lower energy, such as a fall from standing height. Hip fractures, compression fractures of the vertebral bodies, and distal radius fractures in older adults are common examples.

A fracture is considered *open* when an overlying wound produces communication between the fracture site and the outside environment. This is a very important determination that has ramifications for the immediate treatment, the definitive treatment, and the long-term outcomes. Open fractures can range from small poke-holes to severe soft tissue degloving. The Gustilo classification is typically used to grade the degree of soft tissue; but in practice, the authors have found that this can be simplified to *high energy* and *low energy*, leading to a more consistent determination of treatment. High-energy fracture patterns indicate that the soft tissues as well as the bones have absorbed large forces. Although the skin laceration is the most obvious component, the energy of the fracture, degree of contamination, and soft tissue injury must all be taken into account in grading the severity of the injury. Final grading of open fractures occurs in the operating room, after thorough debridement and evaluation of the soft tissue envelope. Contamination of bone can lead to the development of osteomyelitis and all its catastrophic consequences and thus necessitates emergency treatment.

A fracture that extends into a joint is termed *intraarticular.* These injuries are normally caused by an axial load across the joint. The joint surface must be perfectly smooth in order to function correctly, so displaced intraarticular fractures require anatomic reduction and rigid fixation to minimize the risk of posttraumatic arthritis. This is distinctly different from a fracture of the diaphysis (shaft) of a long bone. A shaft fracture must only be held in good alignment and at the appropriate length. If the bone heals imperfectly in appearance but is mechanically sound, then the end goal is achieved. Articular fractures must not only be in sound mechanical alignment but also must be perfectly reduced in order to achieve the best possible long-term outcome. In some instances, there is enough cartilage damage from the injury itself that posttraumatic arthritis is unavoidable.

Long bone fractures are characterized by the anatomic location of the fracture (Fig. 19.3B). The epiphysis includes the area between the physis, or physeal scar, and articular surface. The metaphysis is located between the epiphysis and shaft and includes the growth plate. The diaphysis encompasses the shaft of the bone between the proximal and distal metaphysis. The diaphysis is made up of mostly dense cortical bone, which has less vascularity than the soft cancellous bone of the metaphysis. This difference in vascularity affects the rate at which the bone heals. Fractures can be described according to location within these three sections

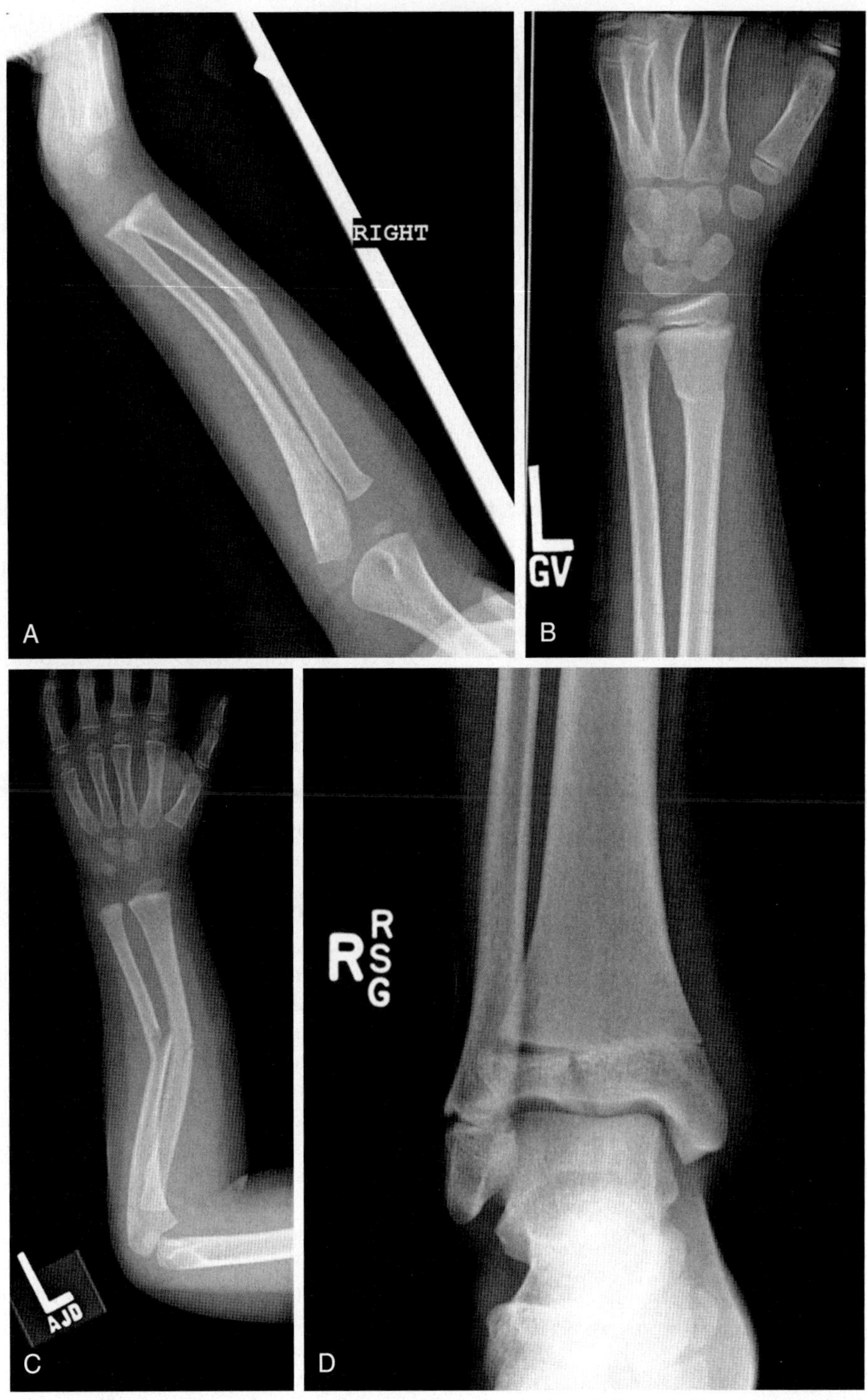

FIG. 19.2 (A) Plastic deformity. Note the bowing of the ulna. (B) Buckle fracture. The cortex of the distal radius is deformed but intact. (C) Greenstick fracture. Disruption of radial cortices, without disruption of the ulnar cortices, in this forearm fracture in both bones. (D) Physeal fracture. Note the gapping of the lateral tibial physis.

or according to the location in the bone—proximal, middle, and distal. Often, these fractures occur around muscular attachments to the bone, thus affecting how the fracture is displaced and how the reduction of the fracture will be achieved.

Metaphyseal fractures of the distal humerus and femur are referred to as *supracondylar* or *intracondylar* in reference to the adjacent epicondyles, the medial and lateral bony prominences to which the stabilizing ligaments and muscles of the elbow and knee are attached. The articular surfaces distal to the epicondyles are known as condyles. Intracondylar fractures are intraarticular and may extend proximally. Such distinctions are important because they can drive the decision for type of definitive treatment as well as the intraoperative surgical plan.

After describing the location of a fracture, the actual fracture pattern should be described (Fig. 19.4). The orientation of the primary fracture line may be transverse, oblique, or spiral. Bones are weakest in torsion, and spiral fractures result from torsional forces. Transverse and oblique fractures result from directly applied forces where the bone is "bent" over an object or fails under off-axis loading. Often, there is a combination of these various forces. Local

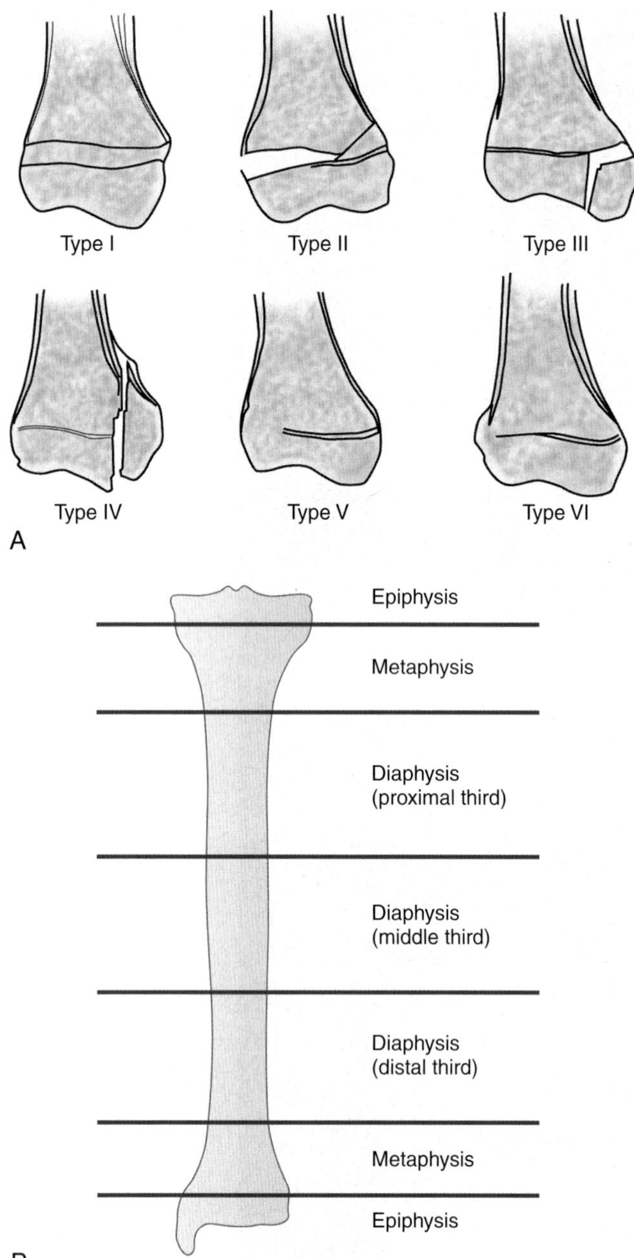

FIG. 19.3 (A) Salter-Harris classification of growth plate injuries. (B) Anatomic regions of the tibia. (A, From Janicki JA. Salter-Harris fractures. In: Miller M, Hart JF, MacNight JM, eds. *Essential Orthopaedics*. Philadelphia: Saunders Elsevier; 2010;939–943.)

comminution can occur in the form of wedge or "butterfly" fragment. When a bending moment is applied to a bone, there is a resultant compressive force on the bone on the concave side of the bend and a reciprocal tension on the convex side. Bone initially fails on tension side, and as the fracture propagates toward the concave side, the fracture will move around the compressed bone both proximal and distal to it, creating a wedge-shaped fragment, or butterfly. Comminution refers to the presence of multiple fragments within an individual fracture site and usually indicates a higher energy injury or weakened bone in an older patient. Segmental fractures occur at multiple levels in the same bone.

Displacement, if present, is described from a combination of principles. These deformities may occur in any plane. When viewed on plain radiographs, all injuries will be resolved into pure coronal or sagittal displacement. However, the true displacement usually occurs in a plane that is somewhere in between. Translation, angulation, rotation, and shortening are all components of fracture displacement. Translation is the relationship of the proximal fracture fragment to the distal one. It is described in terms of percentage of overlap. A fracture with 100% translation in any plane is completely displaced. Angulation is simply the angle created by the displaced fracture fragments. It is conventionally described in two ways. The first is by the direction of displacement of the distal fragment, and the second is by the direction of the apex of the fracture. For example, the fracture shown in Fig. 19.5 may be described as dorsally angulated or apex volar angulated. The final component is rotation. To describe rotation exactly, a full-length film of the limb segment involved, including the joints above and below, must be examined. Alternatively, rotational deformity may be assessed clinically by comparing the injured limb with the contralateral side.

Once a fracture has been identified, it must be described in a consistent, systematic manner. All descriptions begin with whether the fracture is open or closed. The amount of soft tissue involvement is described. A closed fracture is assumed if, after careful evaluation, there is no observed communication between the fracture and outside world. The presence of an intraarticular fracture is then communicated. The side of the body and injured bone are stated next. A description of the pattern, followed by its location in the bone, is indicated. The displacement of the fracture fragments is related. Finally, it is important to indicate any associated, nonorthopedic injuries that may alter the timing and type of initial orthopedic management. Adherence to this scheme allows complete understanding of the fracture.

Other Injuries

Ligamentous injuries are commonly encountered in association with traumatic injuries to bones and joints. When a ligament is damaged but is still in continuity, it is termed a *sprain.* Sprains can range in severity from minor injuries to significant instability about a joint. Grade I ligamentous injuries are caused by stretching of a ligament or ligament complex. They do not normally result in instability. A simple ankle sprain is a typical example of this type of injury. Partial ruptures of ligaments can result in minor instability and are considered Grade II injuries. Complete ruptures, or Grade III injuries, lead to significant instability at the associated joint. Avulsion fractures at the insertion of ligamentous structures also fall into this category. Ligamentous injuries cannot be overlooked because they can produce significant joint instability and endanger the surrounding soft tissue and neurovascular structures. This detail is critical in evaluating musculoskeletal injuries. A full neurovascular examination should be performed whenever there is suspicion of joint instability. Although most ligamentous injuries do not require urgent orthopedic management, stabilization or immobilization of the joint with a splint or brace is usually advisable.

A strain is an injury to a muscle or tendon. These injuries are most commonly of an overuse nature. Further loading of the already weakened structure can compound these injuries and lead to muscle or tendon rupture. Rest, ice, compression, and elevation are the mainstays of treatment for a strain; however, more urgent orthopedic management is necessary for a rupture. Although many tendon ruptures can be treated nonoperatively, proper positioning of the joint is important to ensure that the tendon scars down in a functional position. If operative management is pursued, it should occur fairly urgently. Scarring of the tendon tract and contracture of the muscle significantly complicate the operative procedure.

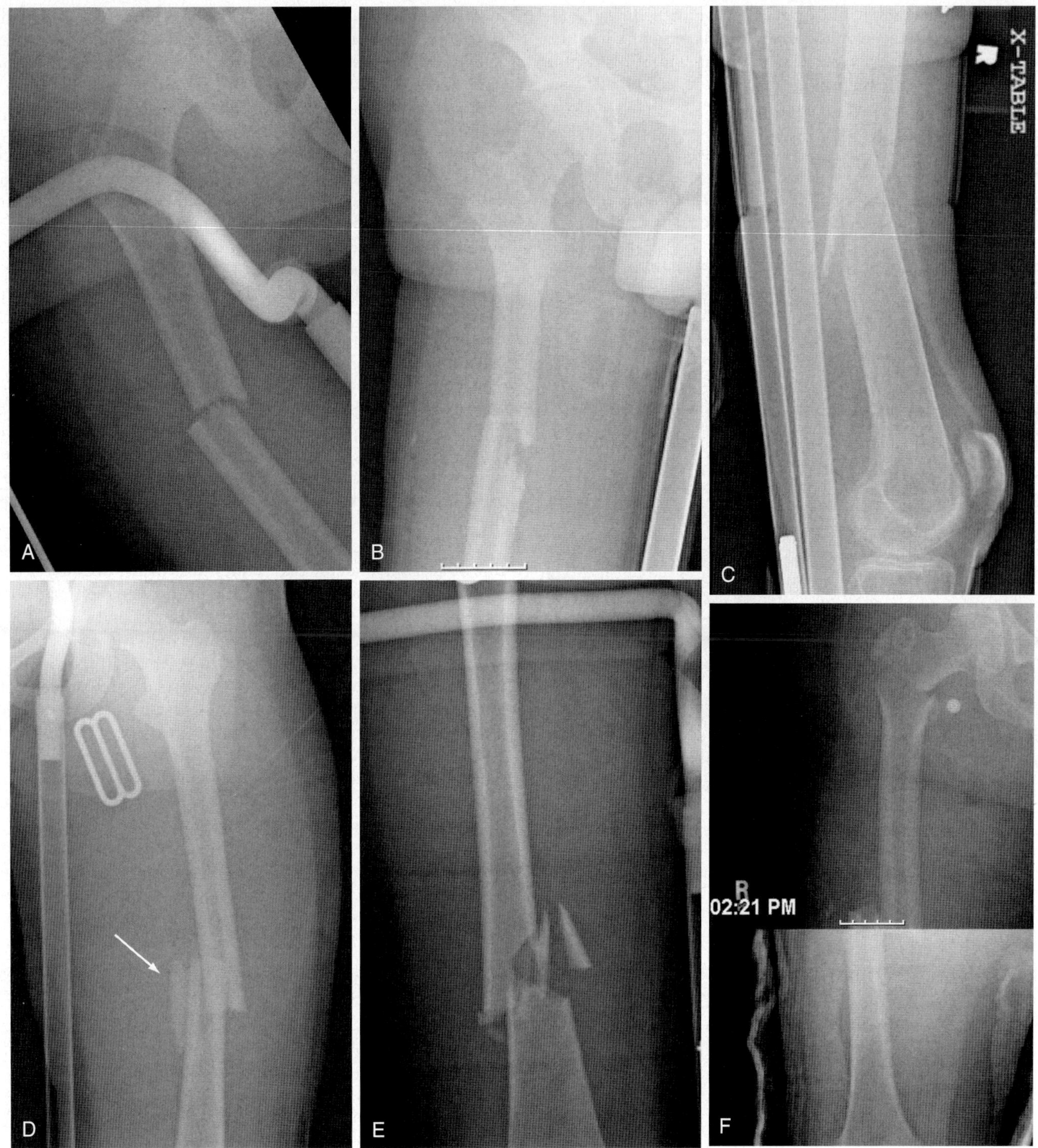

FIG. 19.4 Femur fracture patterns. (A) Transverse. (B) Oblique. (C) Spiral. (D) Butterfly fragment *(arrow)*. (E) Comminuted. (F) Segmental.

Joint injury without fracture is common in axial load injuries. Articular contusions, or bone bruises, usually heal with a period of rest and restricted weight bearing but can lead to late degenerative changes in the joint. A more significant osteochondral defect occurs when a piece of articular cartilage, along with its underlying subchondral bone, is separated from the surrounding joint surface. Small osteochondral defects can be asymptomatic; however, many of these lesions can lead to chronic pain and joint degeneration. In some cases, the osteochondral fragment is large enough to be seen on plain radiographs. In these cases, it is important to immobilize the joint to minimize joint damage from the free-floating bone fragment. Other commonly injured joints are the intervertebral discs in the spine. These discs are made up of a viscoelastic nucleus pulposus surrounded by a dense, fibrous anulus fibrosus. With a great enough axial load, the nucleus pulposus can herniate through the anulus, resulting in a disc herniation. This disc bulge can impinge on nerve roots, causing back and radicular pain. Disc herniations rarely need surgical intervention and often resolve with a course of physical therapy. Very rarely, severe disc bulge in the lumbar spine can cause significant impingement on the cauda equina, resulting in cauda equina syndrome. This is a surgical emergency and is discussed in more detail later in the chapter.

FIXATION PRINCIPLES

There are multiple ways to stabilize the injured extremity, varying in how stable they hold the bone. Table 19.2 summarizes the types of fixation and some of their common indications. Each type of fixation has certain clinical situations in which it is particularly warranted. The fixation types are arranged in order of increasing stability of the bone. The defining characteristics between fixation types fall into several categories.

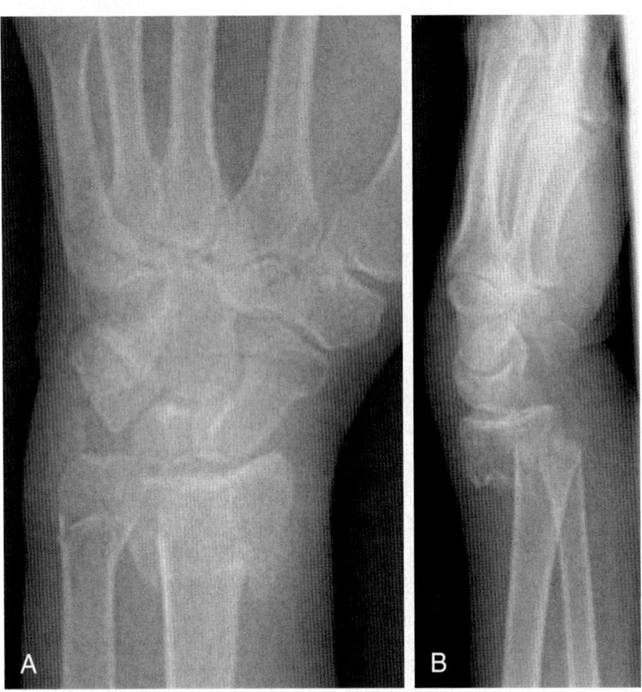

FIG. 19.5 Posteroanterior (A) and lateral (B) left wrist radiographs of a 75-year-old woman who fell and sustained a dorsally translated, apex volar angulated, distal radius fracture and a comminuted displaced distal ulna fracture. (From Foster B, Bindra R. Intrafocal pin plate fixation of distal ulna fractures associated with distal radius fractures. *J Hand Surg.* 2012;137:356–350.)

First, is the bone directly or indirectly controlled? Splinting, which is the easiest and most common form of limb stabilization, is the only form of fixation that does not directly attach to the bone. Attaching directly to the bone improves the control of that segment of the limb, but it also carries with it the inherent risk of infection. Other than the placement of skeletal traction, most other forms of fixation generally require regional or general anesthesia. The closer the fixation is to the bone, the better it is controlled. Thus, a plate resting on the surface of the bone or a nail on the inside of the bone will control it much better than a frame that is built several centimeters above the level of the skin.

Second, does the fixation traverse both the skin and the bone? Skeletal traction, percutaneous pins, and all forms of external fixation all create a pathway between the outside world and the bone. This is an infection risk, and pin-site infections are common. There is an advantage, however: in the event of an infection, removal of the pin/wire usually facilitates eradication of the infection.

Finally, does the surgeon have direct visualization of the fracture or not? Any fracture that is not intraarticular does not necessarily require anatomic fixation. The primary goal of long bone fracture fixation is reestablishment of the mechanical axis. While some fracture patterns are amenable to anatomic fixation (a transverse radial shaft fracture), other fractures are not (a comminuted femoral shaft fracture). In contrast, intraarticular fractures almost always require direct visualization of the fracture for fixation. The downside of direct visualization is that it necessarily involves removing the soft tissue from around the bone. Not only does this decrease the vascularity of the injured bone but there is also more soft tissue damage from the surgical approach. There is also an increased risk of an infection.

Every fixation strategy has pros and cons. Often there is more than one way to accomplish the end goal of getting the bone to heal. Choosing the correct mode of fixation depends on the clinical situation, the resources available, and the surgeon's capabilities.

TABLE 19.2 Methods of skeletal stabilization.

FIXATION TYPE	DETAILS	COMMON INDICATIONS	PROS	CONS
Splinting	Plaster or fiberglass	Temporary stabilization of acute extremity injuries	Accommodates soft tissue swelling	Indirect control of the bone, not length stable
Skeletal traction	Transosseous pin with traction weight	Temporary stabilization of femur and pelvis fractures	Helps control pain and bleeding, maintains length	Indirect control of the bone, does not allow for patient mobilization
External fixation (pins/bars)	Multiple transosseous pins with attached external bars	Temporary stabilization of acute extremity	Improved control of the bones and thus improved soft tissue control Length stable	Allows too much motion for most fractures to heal
Closed reduction and percutaneous pins (CRPP)	Transosseous pins across a fracture site	Small bone fixation; pediatric fixation	Limited soft tissue disruption; removed once fracture healed	Risk of pin-site infection; indirect reduction of fracture
External fixation (pins/wires, rings)	Multiple transosseous pins/wires with attached external rings	Definitive fixation with the ability to manipulate the bones	Can be used for complex deformities	Risk of pin-site infection; indirect reduction of fracture
Intramedullary nailing (IMN)	Intraosseous nail	Long bone fracture treatment	Limited soft tissue disruption; excellent mechanical stability	Indirect reduction of fracture: limited utility in articular injuries
Open reduction and internal fixation (ORIF)	Plates and screws	Articular fractures; upper extremity long bone fractures	Direct reduction and absolute stability feasible	Larger soft tissue disruption; mechanical less stable than nails

PATIENT EVALUATION

History

Obtaining a detailed history of a skeletally injured patient is essential for accurate diagnosis and treatment. This can be challenging with multiply injured and older patients in the trauma setting; however, it is important to gather as much information as possible about the mechanism of injury. Often, trauma patients are unable to give accurate histories because of unconsciousness, intoxication, dementia, or delirium. In these cases, an account of the mechanism of injury and patient history should be obtained from family members, emergency medical response crew members, or other witnesses to the accident. Descriptions from the injury scene can be helpful because common patterns of injury follow from specific mechanisms (Table 19.3).

A general history that includes demographic information, past medical history, past surgical history, and social history is obtained. Knowledge of allergies, current medications, and time since last oral intake is useful in guiding treatment. One should adhere to the normal ED protocol of not allowing food or drink while under assessment. Information about the position of the limb before and after the injury as well as the direction of the deforming force can help predict the resulting injuries. Ambulatory status before the injury helps determine realistic goals for functional recovery, and it can also drive treatment decisions, in particular, knowing if a patient ambulates in the community or primarily only within his/her household. Any transient neurologic symptoms, such as loss of consciousness, numbness, dysesthesias, and spasm, must be documented. Loss of bowel or bladder control in patients with back or neck pain must also be noted. The time elapsed since injury becomes critical information in a patient with a vascular injury, open wound, or dislocation.

TABLE 19.3 Common patterns and associated injuries.

INJURY PATTERN OR MECHANISM	ASSOCIATED INJURIES
Fall from a height	• Calcaneus fracture • Tibial plateau fracture • Fractures around the hip (proximal femur, acetabulum) • Vertebral burst fracture

Fall on outstretched hand	• Distal radius fracture
	• Posterior elbow dislocation
	• Pediatric
	  • Both-bones forearm fracture
	  • Supracondylar humerus fracture

Ejection from a vehicle	• Closed head injury • Spinal fractures
T-bone motor vehicle accident	• Lateral compression–type pelvic fracture • Closed head injury • Thoracic injury

Head-on motor vehicle accident	• Abdominal visceral injury
	• Open-book pelvic fracture
	• Retroperitoneal bleeding
	• Injuries caused by floor board intrusion
	  • Calcaneal fracture
	  • Tibial plateau fracture
	  • Posterior hip dislocation

Posterior knee dislocation	• Popliteal artery injury
Supracondylar humerus fracture	• Brachial artery injury • Nerve injury (median or radial)
Anterior shoulder dislocation	• Axillary nerve injury
Posterior hip dislocation	• Sciatic (peroneal division) nerve injury

Trauma Room Evaluation

Examination of a multiply injured patient must first follow advanced trauma life support (ATLS) protocols in a systematic fashion and must be accompanied by appropriate treatment. The concept of life before limb demands that the ABCs (*a*irway, *b*reathing, and *c*irculation) be addressed before evaluating for any orthopedic injuries. Hemodynamically unstable patients are assumed to be in hemorrhagic shock until proven otherwise. A search for the source of hemorrhage is undertaken and may include examination of the pleural cavities, abdomen, extremities, retroperitoneum, and pelvis. A plain chest radiograph may quickly reveal a hemothorax. Chest tubes are placed if necessary.

Pelvic instability and the need for rapid external pelvic fixation are addressed. A single examination of the pelvis for instability, performed by an experienced examiner, can be undertaken. There is debate about whether the anteroposterior (AP) pelvic film, which has traditionally been considered part of the standard trauma radiographic series, is justified with the advent of newer, ultrafast computed tomography (CT) scanners. Paydar and associates found that in hemodynamically stable blunt trauma patients with normal findings on physical examination, 99.7% of pelvic radiographs were negative.[5] Should a pelvic fracture be suspected, plain radiography initially can be done not just for injury characterization but also as a baseline for follow-up examinations. Intraperitoneal hemorrhage can be evaluated by a focused assessment with sonography in trauma (FAST) examination, diagnostic peritoneal lavage, or CT scan. Pelvic fracture patients require special consideration in the use of these tests. FAST scanning has been shown to lack sensitivity in detecting intraperitoneal bleeding in patients with a pelvic fracture.[6] Diagnostic peritoneal lavage has increased sensitivity; however, false-positives in patients with pelvic fractures can occur. The current recommendation for hemodynamically stable patients with a pelvic fracture is to undergo CT of the abdomen and pelvis with intravenous (IV) administration of a contrast agent to evaluate for intraperitoneal bleeding, regardless of FAST results.[7]

The patient's neurologic status is noted on admission, and the Glasgow Coma Scale score is calculated. Patients with suspected head injury need to be evaluated as soon as possible by CT. Peripheral vascular injuries and musculoskeletal injuries are next in priority, followed by maxillofacial injuries.

In the initial care of musculoskeletal injuries, open fractures or those with vascular injury or compromise, such as compartment syndrome, take precedence. Although the previous dictum of addressing open fractures in the operating room within 6 hours of injury may no longer hold true, open fractures still require relatively urgent operative care. More important, emergent trauma room management, including administration of appropriate antibiotics, tetanus prophylaxis, gross debridement, copious irrigation, splinting, and wound coverage, is imperative for preventing future infection. Sterile dressings placed in the trauma room need to be left in place until the patient reaches the operating room. This practice has led to decreased infection rates compared with routine redressing of wounds in the trauma area.

Unstable pelvic fractures are addressed in the primary survey because of the possibility of exsanguination. Traumatic spine injuries with associated neurologic compromise also deserve immediate attention. These exceptions aside, examination and management of the extremities are deferred to the secondary survey after the airway has been controlled and hemodynamic stability has been obtained. In a team approach, these examinations and treatments take place simultaneously. One caveat to this protocol is the conscious patient who is able to follow commands but will need intubation to protect the airway. In this case, a cursory neurologic examination of the extremities should be performed before sedation or intubation. Documentation of motor and sensory function in the upper and lower extremities is valuable information and takes only seconds to carry out. Throughout the resuscitation phase and during the remainder of the hospital course, reexamination in the form of the tertiary survey will ensure that no injury goes unrecognized.

Evidence of pelvic fractures is assessed early in the resuscitative effort. Massive flank or buttock contusions and swelling are indicative of significant bleeding. The Morel-Lavallée lesion is an ecchymotic lesion over the greater trochanter that represents a subcutaneous degloving injury. This lesion is frequently associated with acetabular fractures. Blood at the urethral meatus, signifying injury to the genitourinary tract, may be a sign of an underlying pelvic fracture. Palpation of the symphysis pubis and the sacroiliac joints can help determine the presence of disruption of these joints. Gentle rocking and lateral compression (LC) through the anterior iliac crests can provide helpful clues to the stability of the pelvic ring. Any opening or looseness signifies instability and may represent a source of hemorrhage. Rectal and vaginal examinations are performed, noting the presence of gross blood, lacerations, bone fragments, hematomas, or masses. Wounds and palpable bone fragments found on either of these examinations are diagnostic of an open pelvic fracture, which carries a poor prognosis. Rectal examination can also reveal a high-riding prostate gland, another indication of injury to the genitourinary tract.

The trauma team must always take steps to protect the patient from self-inflicted or iatrogenic spinal cord injury. Therefore, full spine precautions must be observed until it is confirmed that the patient's vertebral column is intact, either by physical examination and clinical findings or by radiologic confirmation, when warranted. Fitting the patient with a hard, cervical collar stabilizes the cervical spine. Maintaining the patient in a supine flat position at all times protects the thoracic, lumbar, and sacral segments of the spine. If the patient is to be moved, a strict log roll technique is used. At times, a patient may have to be physically restrained to prevent potential self-inflicted injury by head or lower extremity movements that could impart rotational, translational, or bending moments to the vertebral column. Special care must be taken with combative patients or those with altered mental status who may have lost the ability to protect themselves from further injury. On examination of the back, the examiner notes the presence of deformity, edema, or ecchymosis. Tenderness elicited on palpation of the spine is recorded for each level at which the patient complains of pain. Distinction is made regarding whether the pain is midline or paraspinal. Perianal sensation and rectal sphincter tone should be evaluated to test sacral nerve root function. Deep tendon reflexes and pathologic reflexes, such as the bulbocavernosus and Babinski reflexes, are tested.

Plain radiographs of the cervical spine, including AP, lateral, and open-mouth odontoid views, were previously considered part of the standard trauma series of radiographs. Recently, however, Mathen and associates[8] have shown that the standard plain films fail to identify 55.5% of clinically relevant fractures identified by multislice CT and add no clinically relevant data. Similarly, CT of the thoracic, lumbar, and sacral spine is faster and more accurate than radiography at identifying traumatic injury. With most trauma patients undergoing CT of the chest, abdomen, and pelvis, reformatting of the data into spinal reconstructions adds neither time nor radiation exposure. With these data, plain films are no longer indicated.

Examination of the extremities in either a patient with isolated injuries or a polytrauma patient follows a simple, systematic, and reproducible pattern. Even when an isolated extremity injury is the primary reason for evaluation, the entire skeleton must be examined. The examiner must not be distracted from the task by obvious or severe injuries. Deformity, edema, ecchymosis, crepitus, tenderness, and pain with motion are the cardinal signs of an acute fracture. Each limb segment needs to be examined for lacerations and the signs of trauma described earlier. All joints are put through passive range of motion, at a minimum. Active range of motion is tested whenever possible. Joint effusions are evidence of intraarticular disease (e.g., ligament or cartilage damage or an intraarticular fracture). The joints are then manually stressed to assess the integrity of the ligamentous structures. A neurovascular examination is performed and documented. Pulses are recorded and compared with the opposite uninvolved extremity when possible. Doppler signals are obtained when palpable pulses are not present or are weak. Measuring the ankle-brachial index (ABI) is important when vascular injury is suspected. Motor function and sensation must be documented for the extremity dermatomes as well as for the trunk in a patient with thoracic spine pain. To avoid the complications of a missed compartment syndrome, palpation of the involved compartments is performed. Any firm or tense compartments are checked for increased pressure if time and the patient's condition allow. Fasciotomies are performed urgently if pressures are elevated. Gross alignment and interim immobilization of long bone fractures are achieved before transportation of the patient from the trauma room. This helps prevent further damage to underlying soft tissues, reduces the patient's discomfort, facilitates transportation, and may help prevent further embolization of intramedullary (IM) contents. Traction splints or skeletal traction is applied when indicated.

Diagnostic Imaging

Radiographic examination is used to supplement and to enhance the information gathered during the primary survey, history, and physical examination. In a multiply injured patient, the ATLS protocol calls for a lateral cervical spine film and AP views of the pelvis and chest. However, as noted earlier for a stable, conscious patient with no physical examination findings of pelvic trauma, the pelvic film may be deferred for the pelvic CT scan. Cervical spine radiographs should be deferred for a CT scan of the cervical spine (if available). The secondary survey then dictates which extremity radiographs are necessary.

In filming long bone injuries, it is important to verify the integrity of adjacent limb segments because of the relatively high incidence of concurrent articular injuries. Therefore, the joints above and below the level of injury are always included in the films. They are filmed separately if the cassette is not large enough to accommodate the entire view. Similarly, when pathologic change is suspected in a joint, the long bones above and below are also imaged. This practice helps identify commonly associated injuries to the adjacent limb segments that might otherwise be missed.

Because bone is a three-dimensional object, a single two-dimensional radiograph cannot describe a fracture. To understand the position and direction of the fracture fragments, orthogonal

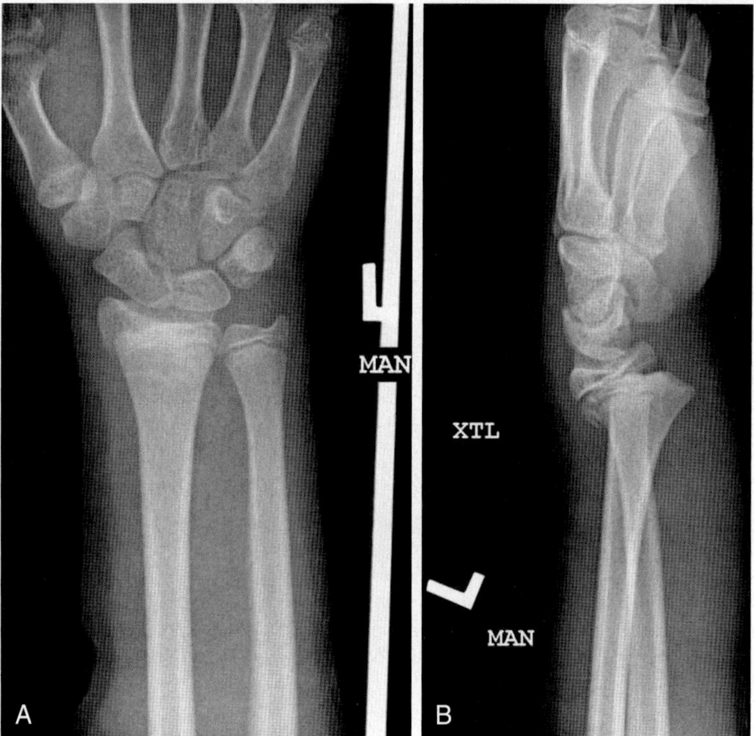

FIG. 19.6 (A) Anteroposterior radiograph of the wrist showing disruption of the distal radial physis but adequate alignment. (B) Lateral view showing complete physeal separation with 50% dorsal displacement and significant angulation.

views (images taken at 90 degrees to one another) must be obtained. A bone may appear minimally displaced in one plane but in another view may be significantly displaced (Fig. 19.6). All extremities with deformity need to be rotated to the anatomic position before radiographs are taken to help decrease confusion in describing the fracture.

If at any point a reduction of a fracture or dislocated joint is performed, imaging should be obtained after the reduction to verify improvement in position or alignment or congruency of the joint reduction.

Some patients will have anatomic variants. If there is a question regarding the presence of an injury, imaging of the contralateral, uninjured side can be very useful in determining what is normal for that individual patient. When finer detail is necessary—such as in the assessment of an intraarticular injury or to confirm the findings of an equivocal radiograph—a CT scan should be ordered.

Magnetic resonance imaging (MRI) has become a particularly useful imaging modality. It is used to evaluate soft tissue, acute fractures, stress fractures, spinal cord injuries, and intraarticular disease. Its role in the trauma setting has expanded as well, and it is particularly helpful in the setting of spinal cord injury. More frequently, MRI is used in the outpatient setting to evaluate soft tissue injuries and pathologic lesions. MRI is now commonly used for the diagnosis of acute fractures when plain films are negative.

Shoulder

Frequently, an AP and lateral view of the shoulder is obtained with just rotation of the humerus and no movement of the x-ray tube. This is not an adequate assessment of the shoulder. True AP and lateral views of the shoulder must be taken in relation to the scapula because of the orientation of the joint (Fig. 19.7). The most useful lateral view is an axillary radiograph (Fig. 19.8). The tube is angled cephalad, with the plate on the superior aspect of the abducted shoulder. This view is often difficult to obtain because of pain or instability at the proximal end of the humerus. The Velpeau view is a modified axillary view that provides orthogonally equivalent images. While wearing a sling, the patient leans backward 30 degrees over the cassette on the table. The x-ray tube is placed above the shoulder, and the beam is projected vertically down through the shoulder onto the cassette (Fig. 19.9). This allows the radiograph to be taken with the shoulder adducted and in a sling, allowing acquisition of the axillary images without the pain of shoulder abduction. A third option is the scapula "Y" view that obtains an image of the scapula down its long axis (Fig. 19.10).

Elbow

AP and lateral views of the elbow provide visualization of most of the bone anatomy. Internal and external oblique views are included in a complete elbow series and allow better visualization of the medial and lateral epicondyles. On the lateral view, look for the fat pad sign or the sail sign for evidence of an occult fracture. The sail sign can be noted when hemarthrosis from an intraarticular fracture forces the anterior and posterior fat pads out of the coronoid and olecranon fossae, respectively. On radiography, the visualized fat pads resemble a sail (Fig. 19.11). Although the anterior fat pad can be visualized in a normal elbow, the presence of a posterior fat pad sign is strongly suggestive of occult fracture and, if clinically appropriate, warrants a CT scan. A CT scan is sometimes ordered if there is a question of intraarticular extension, as this changes the operative plan.

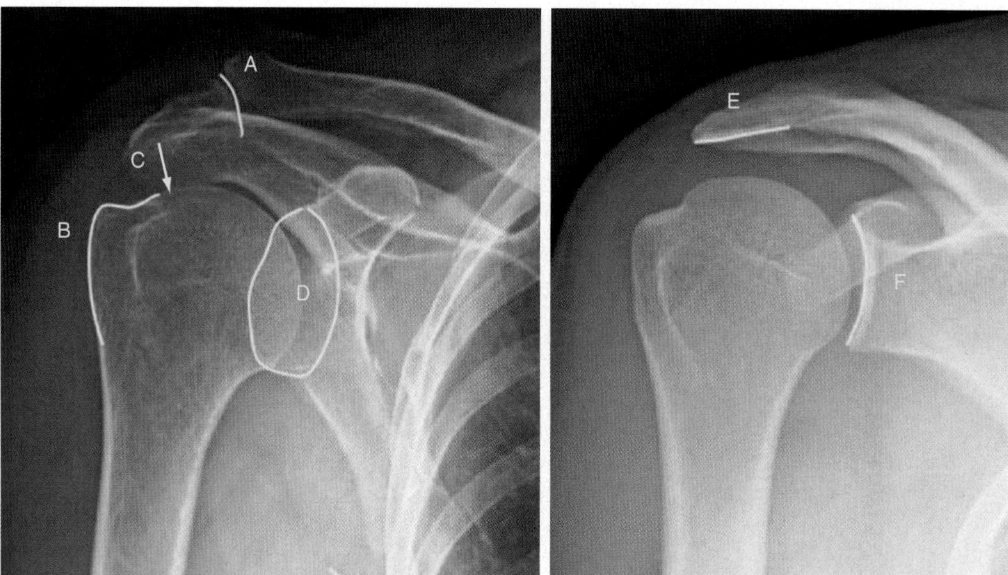

FIG. 19.7 Anteroposterior view of the shoulder showing the acromioclavicular joint *(A)*, greater tuberosity *(B)*, acromiohumeral distance of 7 mm on average *(C)*, and glenoid fossa viewed at an angle to its face *(D)*. Grashey view of the shoulder showing the acromion down its longitudinal axis *(E)* and the glenoid fossa down its longitudinal axis *(F)*.

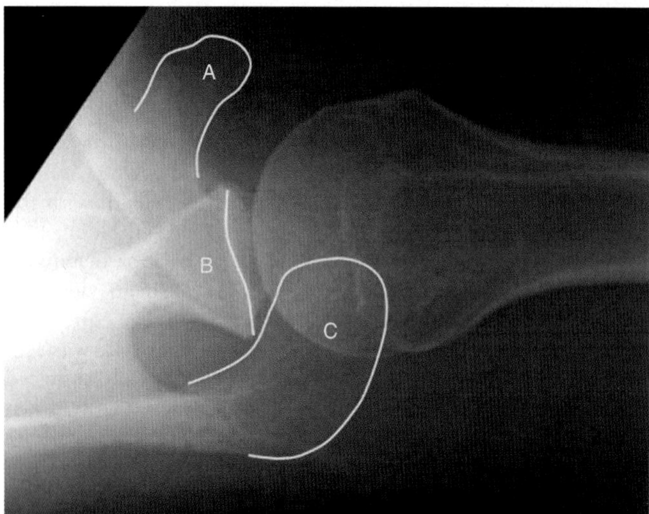

FIG. 19.8 Axillary lateral view of the shoulder showing the coracoid process *(A)*, glenoid fossa *(B)*, and acromion process *(C)*. This view allows for the assessment of anterior to posterior translation of the humeral head relative to either the glenoid fossa (dislocations) or the humeral shaft (fractures).

Another option is a traction view of the elbow, which can even be obtained prior to surgical prep.

Forearm and Wrist

The forearm should be imaged entirely on a single x-ray cassette in both the AP and lateral planes. The elbow and wrist should always be included. The radius and ulna have a close relationship and move relative to each other. An injury to one may necessarily involve the other, and injuries at the wrist can sometimes affect the elbow joint.

The wrist should be imaged in the AP, oblique, and lateral views. Any wrist fracture that undergoes a closed reduction should have postreduction imaging as well.

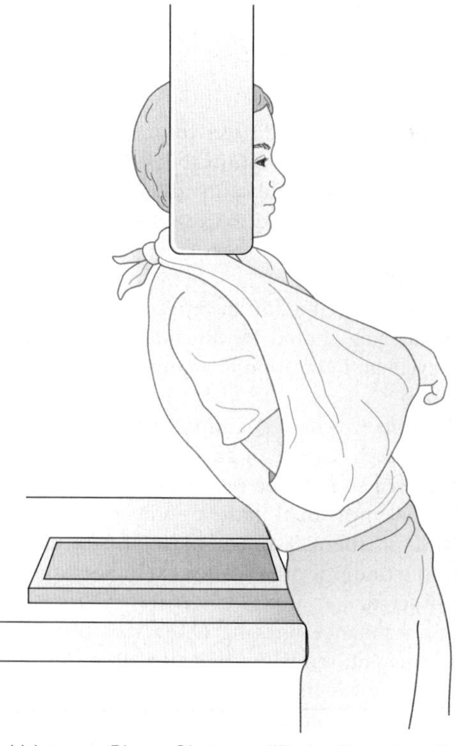

FIG. 19.9 Velpeau or Bloom-Obata modified axillary view. (From Green A, Norris TR. Proximal humeral fractures and glenohumeral dislocations. In Browner BD, Levine AM, Jupiter JB, et al, eds. *Skeletal Trauma: Basic Science, Management, and Reconstruction*. 4th ed. Philadelphia: WB Saunders; 2008.)

Pelvis and Acetabulum

The pelvis is large in all planes and has a very unique anatomy. Because of that, radiographs remain an important tool of pelvic assessment despite the ubiquity of CT scans. Radiographs allow for the visualization of the entire pelvis at one time, which allows

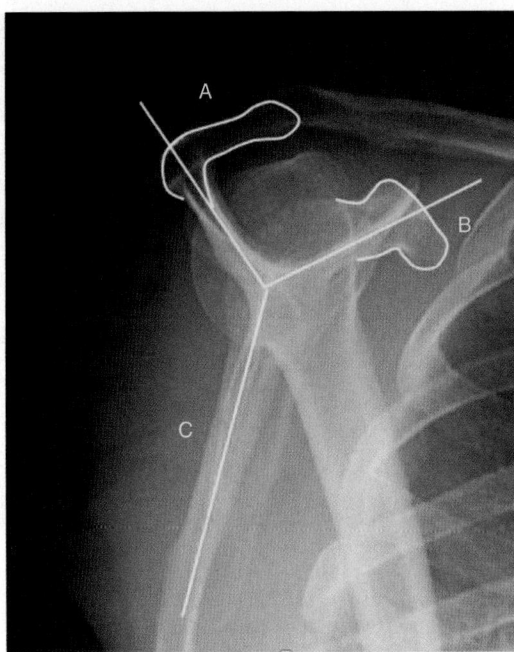

FIG. 19.10 Scapula "Y" view showing the acromion process *(A)*, coracoid process *(B)*, and scapula body *(C)*. This view allows for the assessment of anterior to posterior translation of the humeral head relative to either the glenoid fossa (dislocations) or the humeral shaft (fractures).

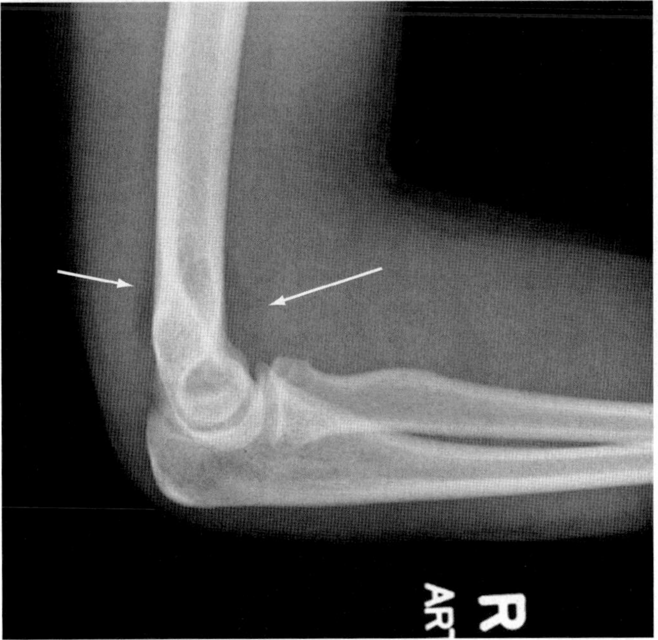

FIG. 19.11 Positive fat pad or sail sign in a patient with a nondisplaced radial neck fracture. Note the anterior and posterior areas of radiolucency *(arrows)* representing the extruded fat pads.

for the bony relationships to be assessed. The standard AP radiograph of the pelvis provides an overview to the structural integrity of the hips and pelvic ring. If pelvic disease is noted on this film or suspected from physical examination, further views are necessary. Judet views, or 45-degree oblique views of the pelvis, are used to evaluate the acetabula (Fig. 19.12).

Similarly, inlet and outlet views of the pelvis allow closer examination of the sacroiliac joints and the sacrum itself, as well as identifying AP disruption in the pelvic ring. The inlet view is taken with the beam angled 60 degrees caudad, thus making the beam perpendicular to the pelvic brim. The sacral ala, displacement of the sacroiliac joints, and displacement of the pubic symphysis in the AP plane are easily seen. The outlet view is a 30-degree oblique view, with the tube angled cephalad. The sacrum is pictured en face, and the neural foramina are easily evaluated.

If it has not already been obtained as part of the trauma workup, pelvic CT should be ordered to evaluate fractures of the acetabula and sacrum. This allows detailed evaluation of the amount of articular involvement or displacement and of the presence of bone fragments within the joint. It also provides information about sacral displacement or neural foraminal involvement. Finally, it allows evaluation for intrapelvic hematoma. MRI has little role in acute, traumatic pelvic ring injury; however, it is the imaging modality of choice for suspected osteomyelitis or pelvic abscess.

Hip

A hip series consists of AP and cross-table lateral radiographs. An AP pelvis radiograph is also included in the hip assessment to allow for comparison to the contralateral side. In an adult patient with acute groin pain and inability to bear weight, an occult hip fracture should be ruled out with an MRI. Failure to identify this early can lead to this developing into an outright hip fracture, which is drastically more morbid than an operation to reinforce the femur before it breaks.

In patients with femoral shaft fractures, the incidence of ipsilateral femoral neck fracture is as high as 9%. A protocol of intraoperative live fluoroscopic rotation views can prevent this injury from being missed, as recent data have shown that preoperative radiographs and CT scans have poor sensitivity for diagnosis of these occult injuries.[9]

Knee

AP, lateral, and internal or external oblique plain films allow visualization of most traumatic osseous abnormalities of the knee. If possible, standing films are useful for evaluating knee alignment and joint space narrowing. Imaging both knees on a single weight-bearing AP allows for easy comparison to the contralateral side. The lateral film can show an effusion, patellar fracture, posterior tibial plateau fracture, or tibial tubercle injury. If there is any doubt as to the degree of articular involvement, displacement, or depression, a CT scan should be ordered (Fig. 19.13). Although MRI can be helpful in the acute setting, evaluation of ligamentous derangement is not urgent and can be deferred to the outpatient setting. In the setting of a knee dislocation, vascular injury should be assumed until proven otherwise. Serial measurements of the ABI are useful to monitor for vascular compromise, but vascular imaging in the form of CT angiography or MR angiography should be strongly considered in the setting of an acute knee dislocation.

Ankle

Most ankle injuries are rotational in nature, and a variety of injuries can be cause be the same rotational forces, depending on where the body fails. Like the forearm, the relationship between the tibia and fibula can be considered as a single joint that runs the length of the leg. Rotational injuries at the ankle can affect the proximal leg: energy that enters the medial ankle or leg when the body moves above a planted foot must exit at some point. That exit may be through the distal fibula at the level of the joint, or it may be at the top of the fibula. The distal tibia shaft may break instead of the ankle. Imaging must

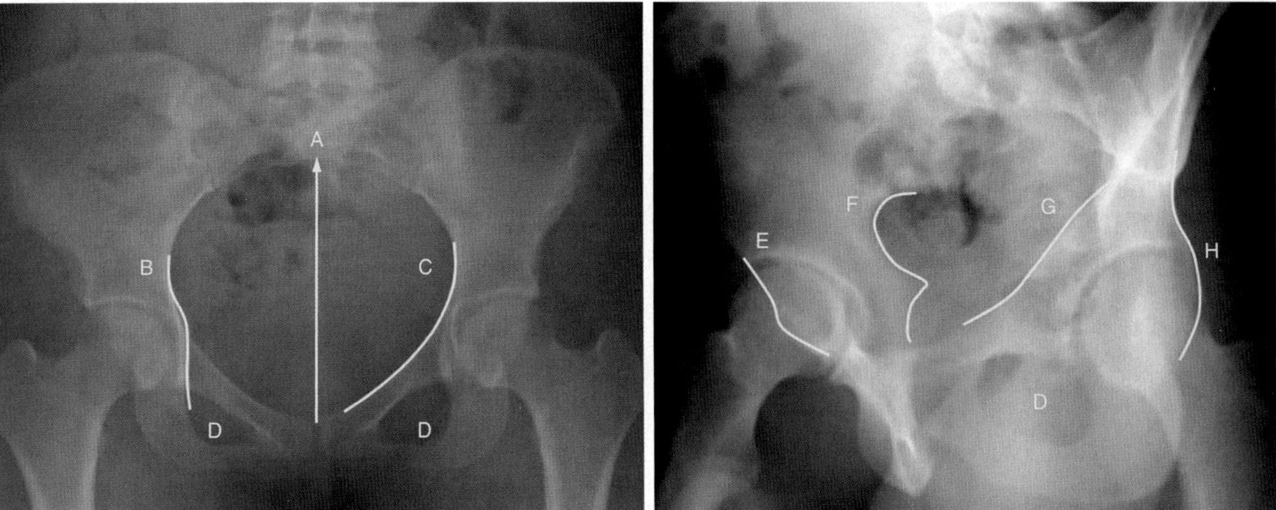

FIG. 19.12 Anteroposterior and Judet pelvic radiographs. *A*, The pubic symphysis should line up with the center of sacrum to ensure no rotation. *B*, The ilioischial line. *C*, The iliopectineal line. *D*, The obturator foramen are even in size and shape, ensuring no rotation. The obturator oblique is so named because the obturator foramen is visualized en face. The obturator oblique of one acetabulum is the iliac oblique of the contralateral hip in which the *(E)* anterior wall and *(F)* the posterior column are visualized. The *(G)* anterior column and *(H)* posterior wall are visualized on the obturator oblique.

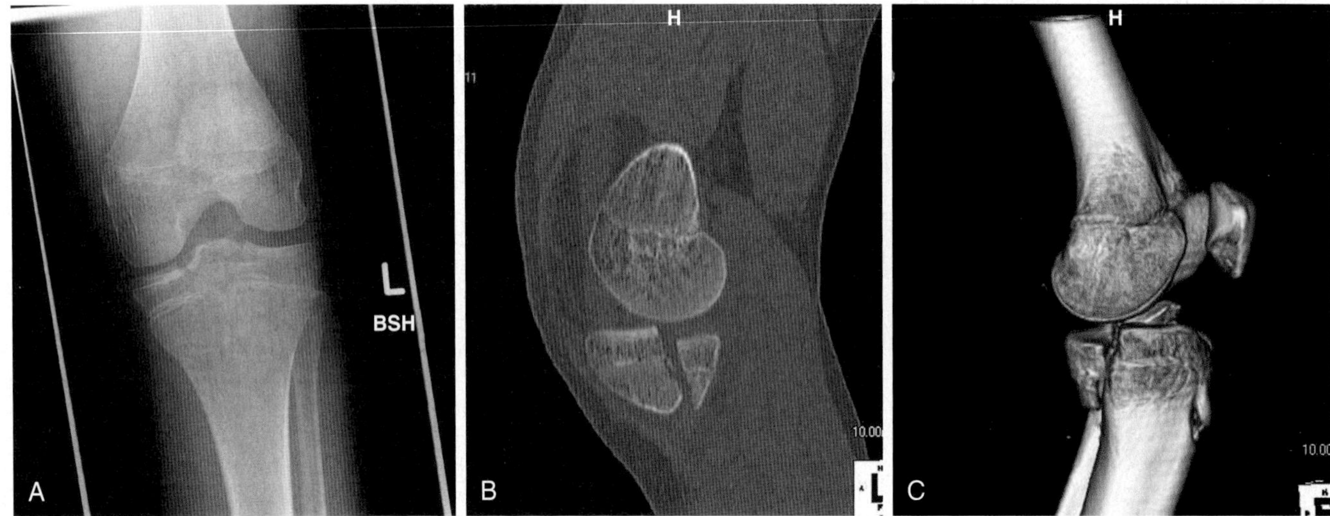

FIG. 19.13 (A) Minimally displaced fracture of the tibial eminence. (B) Computed tomography scan of the knee shows a significant step-off of the posterior medial tibial plateau. (C) Three-dimensional reconstruction.

be ordered with sustained vigilance that the entire leg may be affected.

In the ankle, it is important to confirm congruency of the mortise. The stability of the mortise depends on bone and ligamentous support. With AP, mortise, and lateral radiographs, disruptions in the bone anatomy can be visualized directly. Although the ligamentous structures cannot be visualized directly, assumptions about their continuity can be made by evaluating the spaces between the bones. Three main parameters commonly used are the tibia-fibula overlap, tibia-fibula clear space, and medial clear space (Fig. 19.14). When internally rotating the ankle from the AP to the mortise view, the medial clear space and tibia-fibula overlap will change. The tibia-fibula clear space should stay relatively the same.

While bimalleolar and trimalleolar ankle fractures are operative, isolated distal fibula fractures can potentially be treated conservatively with a splint or fracture boot. A radiographic stress exam should be performed when evaluating any distal fibula fracture. The ankle is stressed on the mortise x-ray. This can either be done manually or by using gravity. The latter is performed by laying the patient on the ipsilateral side with a stack of sheets under the lateral leg. This allows the affected ankle to hand freely to the lateral side. In a positive stress exam, either or both the medial clear space and the tibia-fibula clear space will widen. A positive stress x-ray is demonstrative of an unstable ankle joint that requires operative fixation.

As noted in other sections, articular injuries of the tibial plafond (pilon fractures) necessarily require a CT scan. One difference, however, is that pilon fractures almost always must be placed in an ex-fix for 7–14 days to allow for soft tissue recovery prior to definitive treatment. The CT scan should be deferred until after the ankle joint and the fracture fragments are distracted in an ex-fix.

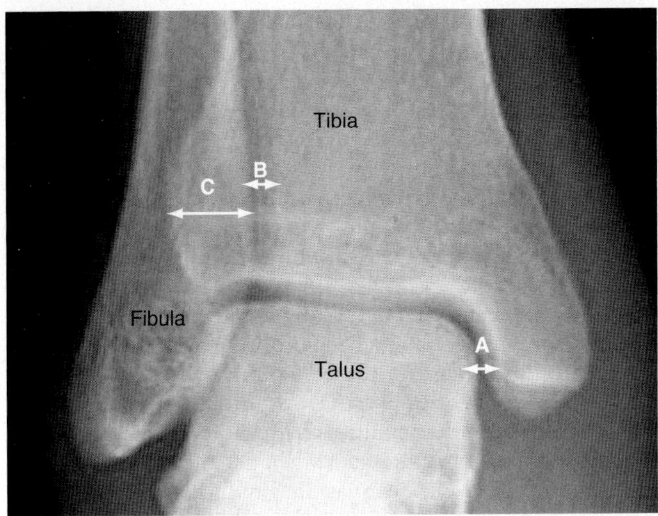

FIG. 19.14 Anteroposterior radiograph of the ankle showing medial clear space *(A)*, tibia-fibula clear space *(B)*, and tibia-fibula overlap *(C)*.

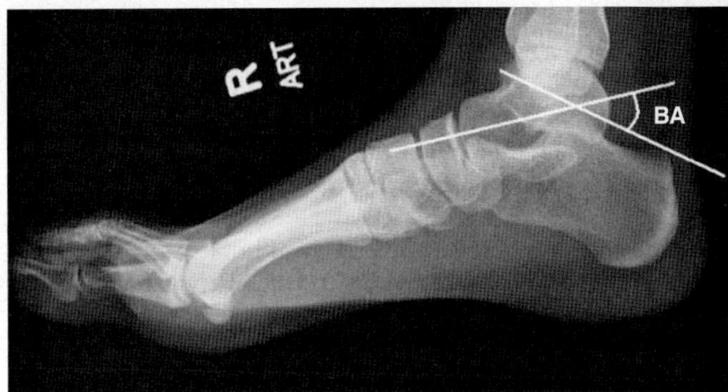

FIG. 19.15 Lateral radiograph of the foot showing Bohler angle *(BA)*.

Foot

When an injury of the foot is suspected, the workup should start with a standard series of AP, lateral, and oblique radiographs. However, because of the complex three-dimensional structure of the foot, this standard series of films may not be adequate to visualize certain bones. In the case of a calcaneus fracture, a Harris axial view should be added to evaluate the varus-valgus alignment of the tuberosity as well as any sagittal splits in the bone. Bohler angle—an angle formed by the bisection of a line drawn from the superior aspect of the calcaneal tuberosity to the superior aspect of the posterior facet and a line drawn from the tip of the anterior process to the superior aspect of the posterior facet—should be evaluated in the lateral view (Fig. 19.15). A normal Bohler angle is between 20 and 40 degrees. A decrease in this angle usually indicates fracture, with depression of the posterior facet. When in doubt, films of the uninjured foot should be taken for comparison.

For fractures of the talus, the AP and lateral films should be evaluated for articular congruence at the tibiotalar, subtalar, and talonavicular joints. There are specialized views of the bone (e.g., Canale view for the talar neck and Broden view for evaluation of the subtalar joint); however, these views are radiology technician dependent. In many cases, if a fracture is seen on the AP or lateral view, a CT scan is a faster and more cost-effective way to evaluate the displacement pattern. If radiographs are negative or equivocal and the patient has evidence of fracture—ecchymosis, pain out of proportion to plain film findings, significant soft tissue swelling—a CT scan should be ordered. All but the most minimally displaced intraarticular fractures of the talus and calcaneus warrant a CT scan to define the fracture pattern and extent of articular displacement better. Except in the case of suspected osteomyelitis, MRI of the foot is of little use in the emergency setting.

Spine

In patients with acute back pain, AP and lateral radiographs of the spine can be useful to look for fractures, spondylolisthesis, malalignment, or congenital anomalies. In most cases of traumatic injury presenting with a complaint of back pain, suggestive findings on plain films, back pain out of proportion to radiographic findings, or neurologic deficit, further imaging is needed. CT is useful for defining bone anatomy. If ligamentous injury or neurologic compromise is suspected, MRI should be performed. In patients for whom MRI is contraindicated, a bone scan can be considered if occult fracture is suspected, and CT myelography can be used to look for compromise of the spinal canal or intervertebral foramina.

Vascular Injuries

Angiography is another important modality used for the evaluation of extremity and pelvic injuries. It is indicated whenever signs of distal ischemia are noted in an extremity. In addition, it should be considered for a patient with pelvic fractures who is hemodynamically unstable. Knee dislocations are concerning because of the high incidence of associated vascular injury. There is a reported 18% to 30% rate of vascular injury after traumatic knee dislocation.[10] Current recommendations for evaluation of the leg after a knee injury include serial vascular examinations, using both manual palpation of pulses and the ABI, followed by selective arteriography of patients with abnormal examination findings.[11]

Initial Management

Care of musculoskeletal injuries begins in the prehospital phase of care. The extent of fracture and wound management differs with the level of training and experience of the first responders—laypeople, police, and emergency medical personnel. Therefore, it is essential that the initial treating physician perform a thorough assessment and begin initial management, including splinting and wound care.

Wound Management

After a thorough physical examination, treatment is begun immediately. All wound dressings and nontraction splints placed in the field should be removed by a single examiner to evaluate the degree of deformity and soft tissue injury. If an open fracture is suspected, tetanus prophylaxis and appropriate antibiotic prophylaxis should be given immediately.[12,13] Superficial contamination by dirt, gravel, or grass may be removed. Using sterile technique, wounds should be irrigated with sterile saline and mechanically debrided in the ED; however, this is expected to be cursory given the setting. A more thorough debridement will necessarily occur later in the controlled environment of the operating room. External bleeding in the extremities is controlled by direct manual pressure. Sterile saline solution or povidone-iodine–soaked dressings are then applied. After sterile dressings are placed over the wounds in the ED, they should remain in place until the time of operative irrigation and debridement. Immobilization is then undertaken in the same manner as for a closed injury.

Reduction and Immobilization

All displaced fractures and dislocations are gently reduced to reestablish limb alignment provisionally. If the patient's condition allows, precise reductions are performed, and the extremities are splinted formally to maintain the fracture reduction. With time, the difficulty of reduction increases because of edema and muscle spasm. Therefore, reduction needs to be attempted as soon as possible and with the patient as relaxed as possible. Often, narcotic analgesics and sedatives are necessary, particularly with large joint dislocations. Muscle spasm can obstruct atraumatic reduction of these injuries. If a joint is still dislocated after adequate sedation and relaxation, general anesthesia may be necessary.[14]

Reduction maneuvers follow the same principles for all fracture and dislocation types. First, in-line traction is applied to the limb. If the soft tissue envelope surrounding the fracture fragments is intact, in-line traction alone may produce satisfactory alignment through ligamentotaxis. In most cases, the deformity must be recreated and exaggerated to unhook the fractured ends. While still pulling traction, the mechanism of injury is reversed, and the fracture reduced. Neurovascular status is documented before and after any reduction maneuver or splint application. Once satisfactory reduction or alignment is achieved, it must be maintained by immobilization through casting, splinting, or continuous traction. The joints above and below the fracture must be included to prevent displacement. Postreduction radiographs are required to confirm alignment and rotation. Nondisplaced fractures are treated like displaced fractures, without reduction. Most nondisplaced fractures do not require surgical treatment. Splints are placed initially and then changed to circumferential casts after the swelling subsides.

Ligamentous injuries may also require immobilization. The joint is fully evaluated as described earlier, and a thorough neurovascular examination is performed on the limb. Frequently, pain, effusions, or hemarthroses occur; these represent intraarticular injury. Therapeutic aspiration of a traumatic hemarthrosis is not recommended because this can lead to iatrogenic infection. In addition, release of the pressure of the effusion can precipitate more bleeding. The limb is then immobilized and reevaluated after the acute pain and swelling decrease.

The rationale for immobilization is threefold. First, splinting, particularly with traction or compression devices, reduces bleeding by reducing the volume of the muscle compartments. Second, additional soft tissue injury may be averted, and the chance of converting a closed to an open fracture by sharp bone fragments is reduced. Third, immobilization of the fracture reduces the patient's discomfort and facilitates transportation and radiographic evaluation of the patient. All fractures and dislocations are splinted or immobilized in the ED. Splints are usually fashioned from padded plaster or fiberglass. Different splinting techniques are used to immobilize each type of fracture. A volar or ulnar gutter splint is used for fractures of the hand. A sugar tong splint (Fig. 19.16A–D) is used for wrist or forearm fractures. This splint prevents flexion and extension at the wrist and elbow as well as pronation and supination of the forearm. Fractures about the elbow are placed in a posterior long arm splint. For humeral shaft fractures, a coaptation or posterior splint is used. When there is minimal swelling present with a humeral shaft fracture, a functional fracture brace may be applied in the ED.[15] A short leg splint consisting of a posterior slab and a U or stirrup component (Fig. 19.16E–H) is used for disease of the foot and ankle. With the addition of side slabs crossing the knee, this splint can be extended into a long leg splint for tibial fractures or knee dislocations (Fig. 19.16I and J). Splints can be secured with a bias-cut stockinette, elastic wraps, or gauze bandage, provided they are wrapped in a nonconstrictive fashion.

For fractures that require reduction, it is important to mold the initial splint or cast to maintain the reduction. The natural tendency of many fractures is to displace back into their injured position. Three-point molding of the splint is required to maintain the reduction in the proper position. Common examples of molding include a slight valgus mold for humeral shaft fractures and a volarly directed mold for dorsally displaced distal radius fractures (Fig. 19.17).

The role of circumferential casting in the acute setting is questionable. Because swelling of the injured extremity increases for 48 to 72 hours, a circular cast can be too constrictive and may lead to pressure necrosis or compartment syndrome. In select cases, in which a cast will be the definitive treatment (pediatric fractures or select nondisplaced fractures in adults), the initial circumferential cast can be applied and then cut longitudinally on two sides to allow swelling without splitting of the padding. This technique is called bi-valving the cast; it maintains a reduction more effectively than an open splint while still allowing soft tissue swelling.

Traction

Traction is used to immobilize fractures or dislocations displaced by muscle forces that cannot be adequately controlled with simple splints. The most common indications are vertical shear injuries of the pelvis, unstable hip dislocations, acetabular fractures, and fractures of the proximal femur or femoral shaft.[16,17] Traction may be applied through the skin using a Buck traction boot or through the bone using a skeletal traction pin placed through the bone distal to the fracture (Fig. 19.18). Traction of more than 8 pounds through the skin for any extended period causes skin damage. Therefore, skin traction is practical only for geriatric hip fractures and pediatric injuries requiring limited distraction force. The Hare traction splint applies a distraction force through an ankle stirrup and can provide effective immobilization for femoral shaft fractures (Fig. 19.19). It can be applied in the field and helps facilitate transport and mobilization, but it should be used only temporarily because of the risk of skin breakdown from the stirrup.

Skeletal traction may be maintained for longer periods with more weight than that possible with skin traction. It is applied using Steinmann pins or Kirschner wires. Up to 10% of body weight may be applied to a lower extremity skeletal traction pin. Radiographs of the anticipated pin site should be obtained before placement. Neurovascular structures must be avoided during placement of the pins. As a rule of thumb, pins should be placed from the side of the extremity containing the known structure at risk. This allows control over where the pin enters in relation to these structures. In the distal femur, the pin should be passed from medial to lateral to avoid the adductor hiatus containing the femoral artery and nerve. The pin should be placed parallel to the knee joint slightly proximal to the superior pole of the patella and in the midpoint of the bone on the lateral radiograph. In the proximal tibia, the pin should be passed from lateral to medial to avoid the common peroneal nerve passing around the fibular head. The ideal pin placement is parallel to the joint, approximately 2 cm distal and 2 cm posterior to the top of the tibial tubercle. In the calcaneus, the pin should be passed medial to lateral to avoid the neurovascular bundle passing around the medial malleolus. The pin should be placed in the tuberosity, parallel to the ankle joint, as far posterior and inferior as possible while still passing through good bone. Once the pins are placed, the skin is checked for tension, which is relieved with incisions if necessary. The wounds are

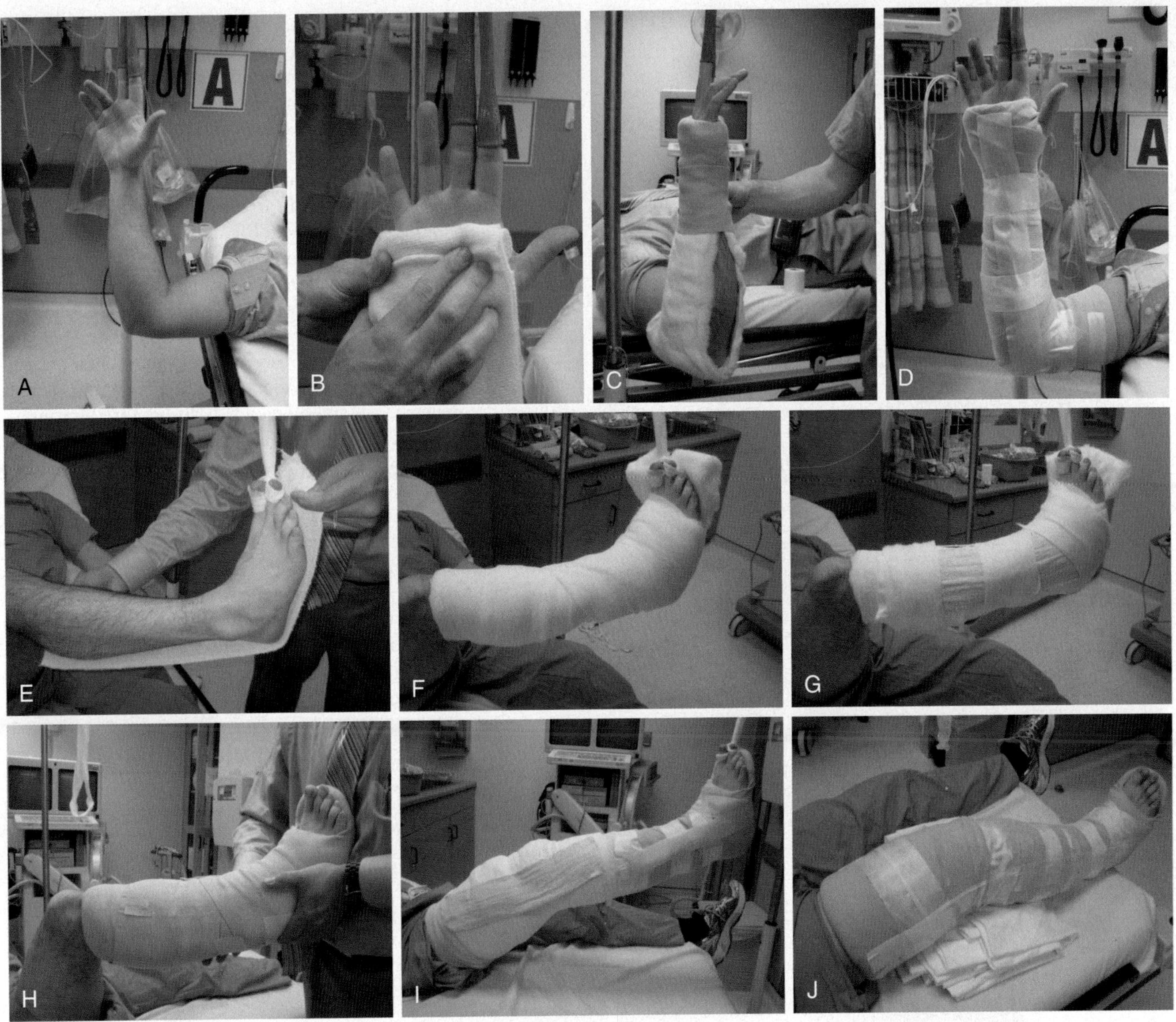

FIG. 19.16 Application of sugar tong (A–D), short leg (E–H), and long leg (I and J) splints. (A) Finger traps are used to apply gravity traction. (B and C) A well-padded splint (plaster or fiberglass) is measured and applied to the limb. The splint should extend from the distal palmar crease volarly (B) to the metacarpophalangeal joints dorsally. This allows motion of the metacarpophalangeal joints. (D) The compressive wrap (bias bandage or elastic wrap) is applied and secured with tape. (E) Gravity traction is applied by hanging the limb by the toes in a figure-4 position across the bed. This serves two functions. First, flexion at the knee relaxes the pull of the gastrocnemius muscle across the ankle; second, the inversion produced by this position helps maintain fibular length and the reduction of the medial malleolus. Both a posterior slab and a U or stirrup component (plaster or fiberglass) are measured. (F) The limb is protected with a soft dressing (circumferential Robert Jones cotton). (G) The posterior followed by the stirrup splints are applied to the injured extremity and held in place with cast padding. (H) The compressive wrap (bias bandage or elastic wrap) is applied and secured with tape. When possible, the knee is flexed and the ankle is placed in neutral position to prevent equinus contracture. (I) The short leg splint may be extended into a long leg splint by protecting the remainder of the limb with a soft dressing and then applying medial and lateral side slabs overlapping the short leg splint and extending to the proximal thigh. (J) Again, the compressive wrap (bias bandage or elastic wrap) is applied and secured with tape.

then dressed with petrolatum gauze and sterile sponges. While pin track infections are a rare complication, they can lead to osteomyelitis or septic arthritis in the worst cases.[18,19] Pin site care should be performed twice daily with a half-strength hydrogen peroxide solution and sterile dressings.

The availability of an operating room and expected time to surgery should be considered before applying skeletal traction. A study by Even and colleagues prospectively evaluated 65 patients with diaphyseal femur fractures randomized to cutaneous (Buck's) versus skeletal traction.[20] All patients underwent fixation within 24 hours of hospitalization. There was no difference in preoperative pain control or intraoperative time to reduction between groups. For patients predicted to undergo operative fixation within 24 hours, application of cutaneous traction can avoid any unnecessary risks of ED traction pin placement. Polytrauma patients or those likely not to be taken in a timely manner to the operating room should have skeletal traction placed.

Prioritization of Surgical Care

After the secondary survey is completed and necessary diagnostic studies are obtained, a multiply injured patient may be moved to the operating room. Because operative decisions are made on a continuous basis as the patient's condition evolves, the trauma surgeon serves as the coordinator of care and prioritizes all surgical procedures after consulting with the anesthesiologist, neurosurgeon, and orthopedic surgeon. Critical procedures are carried out first, and each additional intervention is reviewed as the patient's status evolves. Intraabdominal, intrapelvic, thoracic, retroperitoneal, and intracranial hemorrhages are immediate surgical priorities. These injuries include acute visceral hemorrhage, aortic or caval injuries, injuries to the heart and pulmonary vessels, intracranial mass lesions, depressed skull fractures, and pelvic fractures with associated instability. In addition to hemorrhage, immediate surgery is indicated for the prevention of local and systemic infections from open or devitalized wounds and for limb salvage.

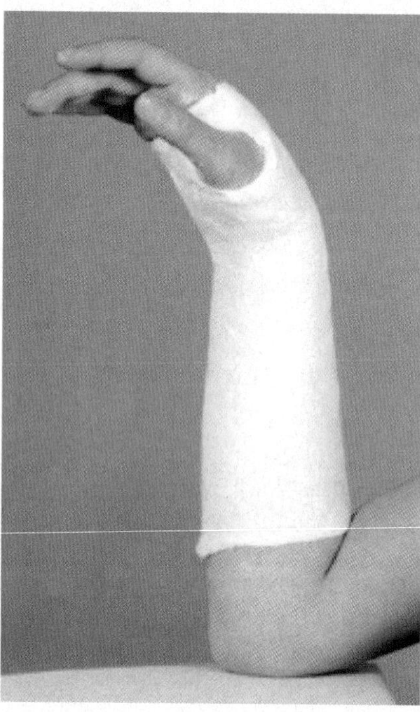

FIG. 19.17 Distal radius mold. (© The Royal Children's Hospital, Melbourne, Australia. <http://www.rch.org.au/fracture-education/management_principles/Management_Principles/>.)

Stabilization of severe open fractures or long bone fractures may be performed simultaneously with or after hemodynamic stabilization of the surgical patient. Limb-threatening vascular injuries are managed on an emergency basis because limiting the warm ischemia time to 6 hours is essential for optimal recovery.[21] Decisions about limb viability, compartment syndrome, and the need for amputation of a mangled extremity are made in concert with all services involved. Consideration must also be given to unreduced joint dislocations and time-sensitive fractures, such as fractures of the spine, pelvic ring, acetabulum, or proximal and diaphyseal femur.[22,23] Definitive care of other fractures is undertaken if the patient's condition permits. Development of a hospital protocol to standardize resuscitation and treatment of the multiply injured patient has been shown to reduce complications and length of hospital stay.[23–25]

TIME-DEPENDENT ORTHOPEDIC INJURIES

Open Fractures

Open fractures are complex injuries resulting from high-energy trauma. A fracture is considered open when there is a break in the skin that allows the fracture site to communicate with the outside

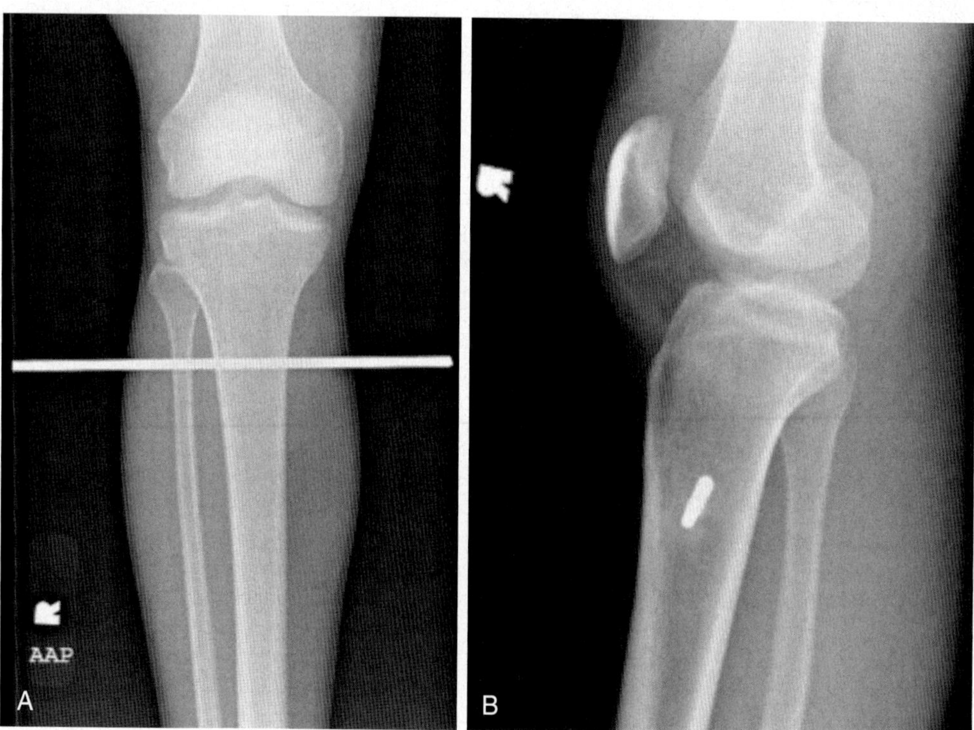

FIG. 19.18 (A and B) Proximal tibial traction pin.

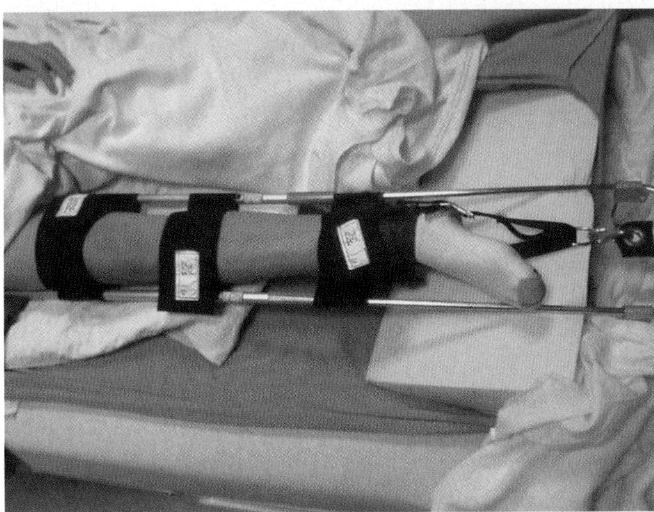

FIG. 19.19 Hare traction splint placed at the scene of the accident to stabilize a femoral shaft fracture.

environment. The communication poses an infection risk, and historically, these injuries were treated with early amputation due to high rates of sepsis and gangrene.[26] The high-energy mechanisms causing these injuries frequently involve multiple surgical disciplines, and thus, nonorthopedic trauma providers should be familiar with the fundamentals of management.

Classification

The most widely used classification scheme for open fractures is the Gustilo-Andersen classification. The classification is based on the size of the skin break, with larger skin breaks representing a more severe soft tissue injury (Table. 19.4).

Both the authors of the scheme and numerous other centers have demonstrated its prognostic value, with each successive grade having a higher risk for developing infection. Various studies have reported infection rates of 0% to 2% for Grade I fractures, from 2% to 10% for Grade II fractures, and from 10% to 50% for Grade III fractures, with Grade IIIC fractures exhibiting the highest rates of infection.[27–30]

The limitations of the scheme include 53% to 60% interobserver reliability, which most orthopedic surgeons feel is related to the inaccuracy of assessing the extent of deep soft tissue injury based on the skin changes alone.[31,32] For example, in Fig. 19.20A, a lateral ankle is seen with a two small lacerations, each less than 1 cm. However, in Fig. 19.20B, the radiograph for that ankle is shown. Per the Gustilo-Anderson grading scheme, this would be labeled a "Grade I open distal tibia fracture." However, upon closer examination, there is considerable evidence that this is a high-energy injury. First, there is comminution at the fracture site. Second, there is air in the soft tissue on the radiograph suggesting considerable soft tissue injury. Third, the skin itself appears contused and mottled, suggesting a higher severity injury. Finally, the patient was in a high-speed motor vehicle accident and also has lumbar spine and pelvis fractures. For all of these reasons, a more appropriate preoperative description of this fracture would be a "Grade IIIA open distal tibia fracture."

That said, the true Gustilo-Anderson classification should be made in the operating room. If, in the operating room, a lot of necrotic tissue and periosteal stripping is noted, then the label of "Grade IIIA" will be confirmed. If, however, the lateral skin is noted to be too damaged to survive and must be debrided, then the fracture will become a "Grade IIIB."

TABLE 19.4 Gustilo-Anderson classification of open fractures.

FRACTURE TYPE	DESCRIPTION	ANTIBIOTICS
I	Skin opening <1 cm, clean; most likely inside-to-outside lesion; minimal muscle contusion; simple transverse or oblique fracture	First-generation cephalosporin
II	Laceration >1 cm with extensive soft tissue damage, flaps, or avulsion; minimal to moderate crushing; simple transverse or short oblique fracture with minimal comminution	First-generation cephalosporin ± aminoglycoside
III	Extensive soft tissue damage including muscle, skin, and neurovascular structures; often a high-velocity injury with a severe crushing component (barnyard injuries)	First-generation cephalosporin + aminoglycoside + penicillin G
IIIA	Extensive laceration, adequate bone coverage; segmental fracture; gunshot injuries	
IIIB	Extensive soft tissue damage with periosteal stripping and bone exposure necessitating formal soft tissue coverage; usually associated with massive contamination	
IIIC	Any open fracture with a vascular injury requiring repair	

From Gustilo R, Mendoza R, Williams DN. Problems in the management of type III (severe) open fractures. *J Trauma.* 1984;24:742–746.

The authors have found that, particularly in an academic trauma center, it is much more reliable to divide injuries into either *high-* or *low*-energy injuries. Even somebody relatively unfamiliar with trauma can—when given an x-ray, a picture of the soft tissue injury, and the mechanism of injury—determine the energy that created an injury. Low-energy injuries will be equivalent to Gustilo Grades I and II, and high-energy injuries will be equivalent to Grades IIIA, B, and C.

Initial Management

The initial management of open fractures is the same as all other high-energy traumatic injuries: a thorough understanding of the injury mechanism and appropriate treatment for other injuries based on the ATLS protocol. Table 19.5 is an example of the open fracture protocol used at the authors' institution. Every institution should have a document similar to this that defines this treatment algorithm.

The most important aspect of the treatment of open fractures is the early administration of antibiotics.[33–35] The general expectation is that antibiotics should be administered within 60 minutes of a patient arriving to the ED. There is evidence to suggest that that 60-minute clock really starts at the time of injury, and thus, some centers have begun prehospital antibiotic administration for severe open fractures.[13,36]

While there is general agreement that early administration of antibiotics is a priority when treating open fractures, the standard practice for the remainder of care varies some from center to center. The antibiotic used generally relies upon the clinical grading of

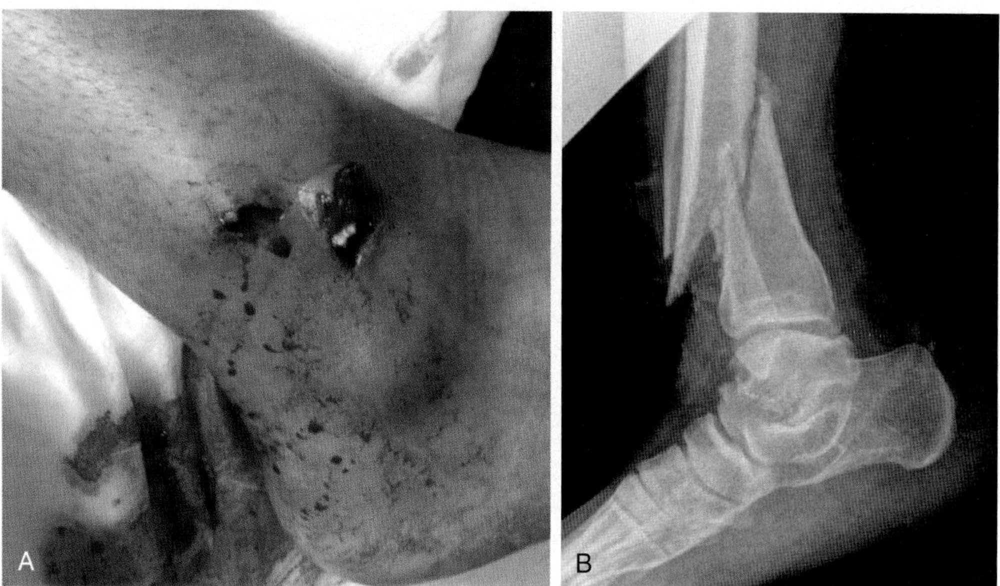

FIG. 19.20 Two small lateral ankle lacerations (A) above a comminuted distal tibia fracture with intraarticular extension (B).

the fracture as described above. All grades of open fracture should receive gram-positive coverage, usually in the form of Cefazolin. Its use has been historically supported by numerous Level 1 and 2 studies.[37] For patients with Grades II and III open fractures, it is standard practice to add an aminoglycoside for gram-negative coverage. This is based on historical data showing late infections from gram-negative organisms that significantly increase morbidity, number of operations, duration of hospital stay, and duration of antibiotics.[29] There have been recent efforts to demonstrate the efficacy of alternative antibiotics due to aminoglycoside nephrotoxicity. A recent prospective study showed piperacillin-tazobactam to be as effective as aminoglycosides in preventing deep infection.[38] Despite this, a survey of Orthopedic Trauma Association surgeons showed that 25% to 75% still use aminoglycosides.[39]

It is the authors' opinion that institutional protocol should be defined based on the bacteria endemic to the geographic region of the institution. For example, the authors' institution is in the Southern United States and local epidemiological studies have found a community rate of *Methicillin Resistant S. aureus* that approaches 40%. For this reason, vancomycin is used to treat Grade III open fractures. As mentioned in the last section, the authors also distill the grading system down to *high-* and *low-*energy injuries (see Table 19.5).

The duration of antibiotics after wound closure is controversial. The common practice is continuation for 24 hours after primary closure or for 48 hours between operative debridements. Two major guidelines agree that antibiotics should be delivered for 24 hours after closure in Grade I and 48 to 72 hours for Grade III fractures; however, they differ in their recommendations for Grade II, with one recommending 24 hours and the other 48 hours.[40,41] Despite this, numerous orthopedic trauma providers continue antibiotics for longer than 72 hours in Grade IIIA fractures, which is concerning given our knowledge of increasing antibiotic resistance.[39]

While not supported by evidence, it is common practice to remove superficial debris (i.e., leaves, stones), gently irrigate the wound with saline solution, reduce the fracture, apply moist dressings (i.e., wet-to-dry with saline), and place the limb in a well-padded splint. It is also useful to take pictures of the wound prior to the applying the splint; if possible, this should be done using the electronic medical record.

There is currently no evidence for an optimal time to debridement. However, numerous studies have demonstrated that the historical time limit of 6 hours to debridement does not have a lower deep infection rate than after 6 hours.[42–44] Given these data as well as the benefits associated with waiting for a more experienced daytime operating room team, open fractures are generally treated as an urgency rather than emergency.

Surgical debridement should be meticulous and systematic. All foreign and devascularized tissue should be removed, including any bone without soft tissue attachments. The wound should be debrided every 24 to 48 hours until a viable tissue bed is obtained. Muscle viability is assessed by the "4 C's" of color, contractility, consistency, and capacity to bleed; however, a recent histopathologic study suggests that these criteria may lead to debridement of viable muscle.[45]

No studies have defined the optimal volume, but expert consensus is to use 3 L of normal saline for Grade I fractures, 6 L for Grade II fractures, and 9 L for Grade III fractures. Irrigation is typically performed using gravity and regular surgical tubing: animal studies have demonstrated that low-pressure lavage has shown to produce lower rebound bacterial levels at 48 hours than high-pressure lavage. It is thought that high-pressure irrigation may push contamination deeper into the wound bed.[46]

Antibiotic delivery devices, such as tobramycin- or vancomycin-based beads, are commonly used between debridements due to the higher local bioavailability and decreased systemic toxicity.[39] Numerous studies assessing the value of antibiotic or detergent additives have demonstrated no benefit compared to normal saline.[47–49]

In cases when the wound cannot be closed primarily, negative pressure wound therapy should be used. This has been shown to reduce infection rates compared to normal dressing techniques combined with antibiotics between debridements.[50] Planning for wound coverage begins with the initial debridement. Early plastic surgery consultation may be helpful. If skin grafting or muscle flap coverage is necessary, it should be performed within the first 72 hours before secondary colonization and wound fibrosis develop.

TABLE 19.5 **Open fracture guidelines.**

Treatment Goals

- Antibiotic therapy initiated within 1 hour of arrival
- Operative debridement within 6–24 hours
- When necessary, soft tissue coverage within 7 days of injury

Prophylactic Antibiotics

Low grade (I/II)	Ancef	48 hours from presentation 24 hours after subsequent intervention
High grade (IIIA/B/C)	Vancomycin/cefepime	48 hours from presentation 24 hours after subsequent intervention
Soil contamination	Penicillin	Single dose
Marine contamination	Levaquin	Single dose
Gunshot injury with fracture	Vancomycin/cefepime	48 hours from presentation, 24 hours after subsequent intervention
Transcolonic gunshot injury to the spine or pelvis	Vancomycin/cefepime/flagyl	7 days from presentation, 24 hours after subsequent intervention

Emergency Room Management

- Prophylactic antibiotics (see above)
- Radiographs, irrigation and removal of gross contamination from wound, reduce fracture and loosely approximate skin, splint
- NPO, obtain acute care surgery clearance

Operative Management

- Prewash with chlorohexidine scrub/alcohol; prep with chlorohexidine
- Sharp excisional debridement of nonviable tissue and foreign material
- Irrigation with plain normal saline and GU tubing
  - Low grade (I–II) 3–6 L; high grade (III) = 9 L
- Vancomycin/tobramycin—1 g/1.3 g per 20 g cement (1 vial of each and a half bag of cement) beads when staged treatment planned and soft tissue allows
- Grade IIIB—call plastic surgery preoperatively and intraoperatively for assessment of the wound
- Apply external fixation versus definitive fixation dependent upon type of injury, location, and grade

Specific Fractures

- Upper extremities—often treated definitively at initial debridement
- Pelvic ring—almost always treated without internal fixation in the front
- Femur shaft and supracondylar femur—often treated definitively at initial debridement
- Periarticular fractures in the leg—staged treatment with ex-fix followed by definitive treatment
- Low-grade (I–II) tibia shaft—definitive treatment at initial debridement with reamed intramedullary nailing
- High-grade (III) tibia fractures—ex-fix followed by unreamed nail or Ilizarov
- IIIB fractures
  - Repeat debridements/antibiotic bead placement by orthopedic service
  - Plastic surgery presence in the operating room at initial and final debridement prior to coverage
- Ankle fractures—definitive treatment at initial debridement when soft tissues permit
- Calcaneus fractures—often treated with debridement alone
- Spine fractures
  - Nontranscolonic injuries will be treated the same as a Grade III fracture 2/2 GSW
  - Transcolonic injuries will require 7 days of vancomycin/cefepime/flagyl

GSW, Gunshot wound; *GU*, genitourinary; *NPO*, nothing by mouth.

The desire to avoid nosocomial infection has promoted a trend toward immediate coverage of open fracture wounds.

Fixation and soft tissue reconstruction strategies for every open fracture are beyond the scope of this text. External fixation has the benefit of stabilizing the fracture while allowing the soft tissues to recover prior to definitive fixation. Internal fixation, such as IM fixation or plate-screw constructs, can be considered when the soft tissues are ready. The usage of external fixation and the timing of definitive fixation is very institution dependent; however, the authors do advise defining institutional guidelines in order to achieve some level of standardization.

Limb Salvage Versus Primary Amputation

The choice between primary amputation and salvage of a severely injured extremity is a difficult one. Successful salvage depends on a number of factors, including vascular status, extent of soft tissue injury, degree of comminution, bone loss, and neurologic function. In addition to these local factors, ultimate success depends on systemic and psychological elements. Patients with poor nutrition, multisystem injuries, or psychoses and those unable to cooperate with a lengthy reconstructive process may not be candidates for limb salvage. Several scoring systems have been devised to help assess the need for primary amputation objectively. These systems were developed retrospectively in reference to injuries involving the lower part of the leg. Severely injured upper extremities have a far greater impact on the overall functioning status of the patient, and thus, indications for upper extremity amputation are significantly more limited.

The Mangled Extremity Severity Score (MESS) is the most widely validated classification systems. It is the product of a retrospective review of 25 charts of patients with severe open fractures of the lower extremity.[21] Investigators found that limb salvage was related to vascular status, age of the patient, duration of ischemia, and absorbed energy. A score of 7 or higher consistently predicted the need for amputation, whereas all limbs with initial scores of 6 or less remained viable in the long term. This system has been validated prospectively, and subsequent studies have almost uniformly supported the specificity of MESS in evaluating a severely injured lower leg. Subsequent studies have confirmed the high specificity (i.e., a low score reliability predicts limb salvage); however, these studies have also shown the sensitivity of the MESS to be low (i.e., a high score does not necessarily predict the need for amputation).[51] Other scoring systems have been shown to be equally poor predictors of the need for amputation.

The combined experiences of the U.S. military dealing with combat-related blast injuries and the Lower Extremity Assessment Project (LEAP) have shaped the current trends in dealing with the mangled extremity. The LEAP study was a prospective, multicenter trial conducted to study patients with severe lower extremity injuries.[52] This study represents the highest evidence available on the management of the mangled lower extremity, and several key findings were noted in this group's 7-year follow-up. The first finding was that functional outcomes were similar in patients 2 and 7 years after limb salvage or amputation. Similar rates of pain, return to work, and disability were also found. The lifetime cost to the patient was noted to be higher in the amputation group, mostly because of the cost of prosthetics. The study also raised questions about a previously held absolute indication for amputation, which was lack of plantar foot sensation on arrival indicating disruption of the tibial nerve. A subgroup study showed that many patients with this finding managed with limb salvage had sensation return within 2 years from the index injury, and outcomes for these patients were no different from those of patients with intact sensation on presentation.[53] The MESS, the Limb Salvage Index, and many other scoring systems were found in this study to have poor utility in predicting which limbs required amputation.

The military conflicts of the last decade resulted in an increased experience with combat-related blast injuries. Lower extremity amputations versus limb salvage in this population were studied in the Military Extremity Trauma Amputation/Limb Salvage (METALS) study.[54] This was a retrospective cohort of 324 patients who underwent limb salvage versus amputation after a wartime injury. The study found similar rates of depression and return to any activity (work and school) as in the LEAP study; however, functional outcomes were notably higher in the amputation group. It is thought that the lower average age as well as the ability immediately to begin structured rehabilitation in the military may have contributed to this finding.

These studies have influenced our current management of the mangled extremity. Absolute indications for amputation are few and include a severe crush injury, a mangled stump or distal tissue not amenable to repair, and a missing extremity. An extremity with warm ischemia time of more than 6 hours should be strongly considered for amputation as well. Finally, if possible, a discussion with the patient should be undertaken to determine the patient's wishes. This may take place after an initial limb salvage procedure if the patient is obtunded on presentation. Visits with the prosthetic team during the patient's hospitalization can help the patient reach a decision. Should primary amputation be indicated, thorough documentation must take place. It is important to document all pertinent local and systemic factors accurately. A MESS should be calculated for each patient but should be used with caution as a guideline to supplement the clinical findings. Whenever possible, pictures should be taken and added to the permanent medical record. When the indications are not absolute, it is essential that several surgeons evaluate the patient independently and document their opinions in the medical record.

After amputation, multidisciplinary management is critical. Patients should be screened for symptoms of depression and posttraumatic stress disorder and referred appropriately. Physical therapy and orthotics providers should be involved with the patient as soon as the condition permits. Future expectations, including possible repeated surgeries for infection, neuroma, heterotopic ossification, and stump revision, should be discussed with the patient early in the course of treatment.

Fractures Secondary to Firearm Injury

Firearm injuries are common in the United States and frequently can involve injury to the musculoskeletal system. Fractures secondary to firearm injury are typically classified according to whether a high-energy (>2000 ft/s projectile velocity) or low-energy (<2000 ft/s) weapon was involved. Most handguns have low muzzle velocity, whereas most hunting and military rifles have a high muzzle velocity. The velocity of the weapon translates into the energy imparted and, thus, the damage caused to the soft tissues of the body.

Fractures caused by low-velocity weapons are typically treated as sterile, closed fractures. Irrigation and debridement in the ED, tetanus prophylaxis, and a short course of antibiotics are the typical treatment for these fractures. Fracture stabilization is dictated by the fracture pattern, as if it was a closed injury. Entrance and exit wounds are usually left open to allow drainage and healing by secondary intention.

Fractures caused by high-velocity weapons are treated per an open fracture protocol. Aggressive debridement, tetanus prophylaxis, and IV antibiotics are the standard of care for these injuries. Temporary stabilization with external fixation is employed to allow soft tissue management until definitive fixation can occur. Most fractures caused by close-range shotguns, despite that they are lower energy weapons, are typically treated in this manner, given the concomitant soft tissue injury. Gunshot wounds at the metaphysis may have nondisplaced intraarticular extension and thus may warrant further imaging with CT.[55]

Intraarticular gunshot injuries deserve special attention. Bullets or fragments that remain lodged in a joint can lead to plumbism or systemic lead toxicity. They can also lead to a breakdown of articular cartilage and the development of early osteoarthritis from third-body wear. These risks warrant urgent exploration and removal of intraarticular bullets. This can be performed with formal open arthrotomy or with arthroscopic assistance. Bullets that traverse the joint without retention of the bullet are not associated with increased infection rates and thus do not necessitate formal irrigation and debridement.[56]

Bullets traversing the intraabdominal cavity are associated with fractures of the hip, pelvis, and spine. A review has noted that even in injuries that involve a hollow viscus perforation, retained bullet fragments in nonoperative fractures to the pelvis or spine may be managed with a simple course of IV antibiotics for the prevention of osteomyelitis.[57] Broad-spectrum coverage for gram-positive and gram-negative organisms is required. For periarticular gunshots, a CT scan can be a useful adjunct to determine if any fragments remain in the joint. Retained fragments with an incomplete or evolving spinal cord injury or evolving neurologic exam warrant consideration for removal.

Skeletal Stabilization

Skeletal stabilization has been shown to be crucial for soft tissue healing, especially in the setting of an open fracture. Compared with cast and splints, internal or external fixation permits greater access for wound care and is more effective in controlling pain during mobilization. At the cellular level, the inflammatory response is shortened, and the spread of bacteria is diminished. The decision to use one mode of fixation over another is dependent on the fracture pattern, the degree of contamination, and the surgeon's preference.

One of the most widely accepted methods of fixation has been external fixation. In unstable patients or grossly contaminated wounds, standard or ringed external fixation can be used for temporary stabilization or for definitive fixation. External fixation minimizes dissection and avoids the insertion of large metallic implants. It is easily removed, replaced, and adjusted and can be combined with other means of fixation. However, external fixators are not without their problems. Although pin track osteomyelitis has become rare with changes in design and the technique of pin insertion, superficial infection with drainage occurs with relative frequency. Because of their size and location, further debridement and coverage can be cumbersome. In the tibia, for example, pin insertion through the subcutaneous anteromedial border reduces pin track infection but often results in obstructed access for plastic and reconstructive surgery. In other cases, more extensive fracture patterns may require more complex frame constructs that further limit access. Although effective in providing skeletal stabilization during soft tissue reconstruction, external fixation is not ideal for achieving fracture union. Additional surgery, including bone grafting or conversion to internal fixation, is often necessary.

For these above reasons, IM nailing appears to be an attractive option. Definitive fracture care usually can be accomplished in a single operation. Without bulky exposed hardware, mobilization and daily wound care are facilitated. Concerns about infection have been raised since these methods have been in use, particularly with reamed IM nails. Originally, the increased infection rate was believed to be caused by destruction of cortical blood flow by reaming. The injury itself causes periosteal stripping and significant soft tissue loss. The loss of the medullary blood supply potentially further weakens the bone's healing potential and resistance to infection. However, studies in animals have shown that the endosteal blood supply is reconstituted during a relatively short time. Reaming the IM canal before insertion of the nail allows placement of a larger diameter nail and forces bone marrow in between the fractured bone ends, which facilitates healing. However, studies have shown a higher risk of reoperation when reamed IM nails are used, with higher energy mechanisms of injury, and when a fracture gap is left over the nail.[58] Previous metaanalyses, however, have shown no difference specifically in infection rate between reamed and unreamed nails. Although there is still controversy about reamed versus unreamed nailing, the general consensus is that, in a stable patient, IM nailing is the fixation of choice for open tibial fractures. High rates of infection have been shown when delayed conversion from external fixation to IM nailing is performed; however, the infection rate is significantly reduced when the conversion happens within 2 weeks. Open periarticular fractures and fractures of the upper extremity should be treated with plate fixation if the patient's condition warrants. Many fractures that in isolation are treated conservatively (clavicle fractures, humeral shaft fractures) are operatively stabilized in the polytrauma patient to allow earlier weight bearing in those limbs for physical therapy.

ACUTE COMPARTMENT SYNDROME

Compartment syndrome occurs when there is increased pressure within a confined myofascial space that causes permanent and irreversible damage. Increased compartment pressure can result from either increased volume within the compartment or a limitation on compartment expansion secondary to an external source, such as a tight dressing or cast. While hemorrhage can increase the volume within a compartment, the most common cause of increased volume is edema secondary to muscle injury. Muscle injury frequently results from direct trauma but may also develop during postischemic reperfusion and in the setting of burns.

Rapid diagnosis and management of compartment syndrome are paramount to achieve a successful clinical outcome. The most important attribute of treating this very morbid condition is maintaining vigilance: there have been case reports of compartment syndrome all over the body and resulting from a wide variety of causes. This section addresses the pathogenesis, diagnosis, and management of acute compartment syndrome, specifically in the forearm and lower part of the leg.

Early recognition and treatment of compartment syndrome are critical in a trauma patient to avoid limb dysfunction, limb amputation, and even death. Volkmann was the first to describe the sequelae of postischemic contracture more than a century ago. He attributed permanent muscle contracture to trauma, swelling, and tight bandaging. As the late complications of compartment syndrome of the upper and lower extremities have been elucidated, the importance of early recognition and fasciotomy has become apparent. Failure to diagnose and to treat this complication has resulted in numerous cases of preventable morbidity, rare cases of mortality, and litigation. Missed or delayed diagnosis of compartment syndrome is one of the most common causes of malpractice litigation for orthopedic surgeons. Increasing time from the onset of symptoms to the actual fasciotomy is linearly associated with an increase in indemnity payments.[59]

Pathogenesis

Compartment syndrome occurs secondary to increased pressure in the enclosed fascial space. The most common cause of compartment syndrome in an orthopedic patient is muscle edema from direct trauma to the extremity or reperfusion after vascular injury. This edema causes an increase in compartment pressure, which prevents venous outflow from the affected extremity. The backflow congestion furthers the cycle of increasing pressure and muscle ischemia. As muscle is deprived of oxygen, there is an inflammatory release and capillary permeability is increased, both of which lead to localized swelling, which further increases the compartment pressure. As such, this cyclic process is difficult to reverse once it has begun.

Diagnosis

The diagnosis of acute compartment syndrome requires a high degree of clinical suspicion, a full understanding of the mechanism of injury, and careful serial physical examinations. It is highly recommended that an institution establishes a protocol involving nursing and the medical staff that delineates the various treatment algorithms. The authors' institutional protocol was developed as a collaboration between Acute Care Surgery, Orthopedic Surgery, and Vascular Surgery and is illustrated in Fig. 19.21. The diagnosis of compartment syndrome relies on an understanding of high-risk injury patterns, the subjective complaints of the patients, and an appreciation of early and late physical and clinical findings. Common clinical situations that are prone to see the development of compartment syndrome include crush injuries, severely comminuted or segmental fractures, widely displaced joint or fracture pieces, and high-energy injuries with impaired sensorium.

Repeated clinical exams with consistent documentation remain the crux of diagnosing compartment syndrome reliably. While pulses may be present, patients will often have worsening pain that is out of proportion to the injury as well as with passive extension of the involved muscle compartment. Dysesthesias will be noted in the digits as the nerves are asphyxiated proximally.

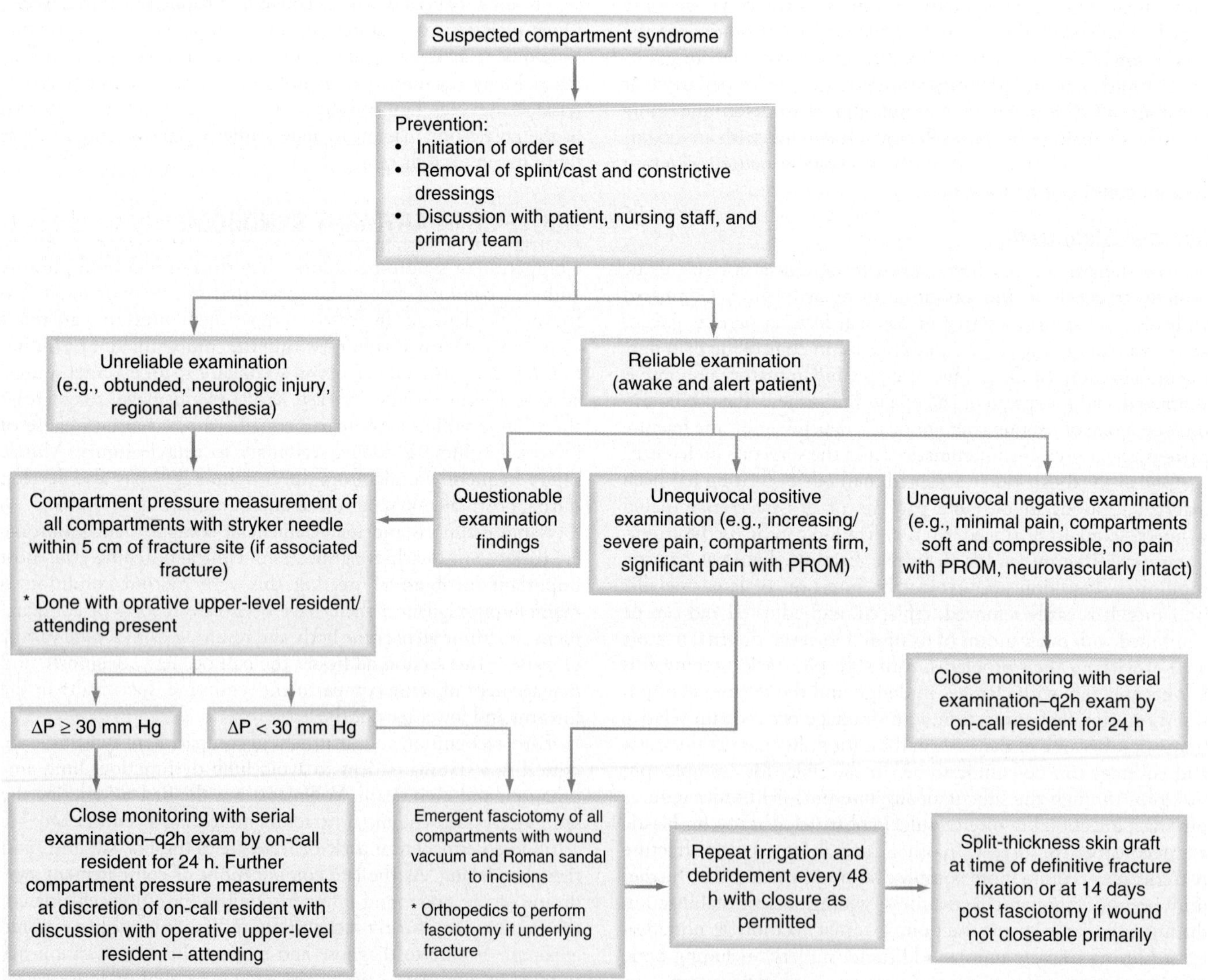

FIG. 19.21 Algorithm for the management of a patient with suspected compartment syndrome. *PROM,* passive range of motion.

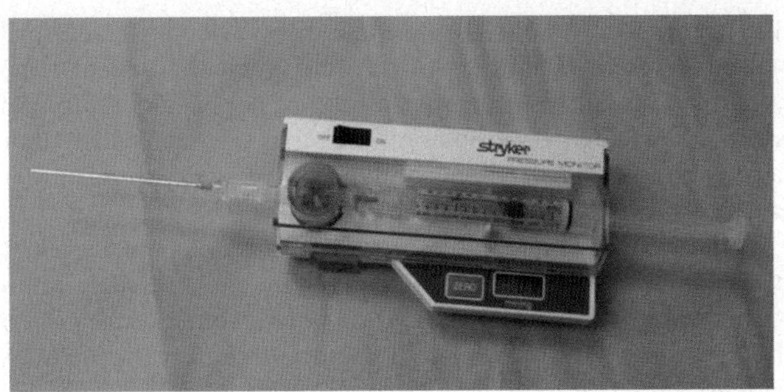

FIG. 19.22 Stryker Intra-Compartmental Pressure Monitor System (STIC) catheter.

An individual provider's clinical exam is not always reliable: 386 tibia shaft fractures were evaluated at a Level 1 hospital and the rate of fasciotomy between attending surgeons ranged from 2% to 24%.[60] This illustrates the need for a system to be in place that involves multiple providers on multiple levels.

Compartment pressure monitoring is an important adjunct to serial clinical exams. In patients with altered mental status or who are unreliable upon exam, measuring the compartment pressures is an important objective finding (and sometimes the only objective finding), and it can be used to drive treatment decisions. That said, compartment pressure measurements are far from perfect and there are numerous potential pitfalls in their utilization.

First, pressure measurements should be taken using a side-port needle and a pressure measurement system. The most common method of measurement is the Stryker Intra-Compartmental Pressure Monitor System (STIC; Stryker, Mahwah, NJ), which uses the side port needle technique (Fig. 19.22). Alternative measurement systems include a wick or slit catheter or an arterial line setup. Slit catheters can be used in continuous monitoring systems. Arterial line setups are widely available, but they have a tendency to artificially elevate the measure pressure. There are some noninvasive methods of monitoring pressures, but these are not yet widely used.

Second, pressure measurement should be done correctly, or it will yield inaccurate measurements. All compartments of the limb should be measured: four in the leg and two in the forearm. If a fracture is present, measure should occur within 5 cm of the fracture.[61] The measurement system needs be even with the area being measured, and care must be taken to avoid iatrogenically elevating compartment pressures by inserting too much fluid while zeroing the device. The measured pressure is compared to the diastolic blood pressure of the patient, and ΔP less than 30 mm Hg is the generally accepted threshold. Previously, absolute values have been used, but these have been shown to have a high false-positive rate of diagnosis.[62]

Third, single time-point compartment pressure measurement has a notable false-positive rate. Compartment pressures are a moving target, and if they are only measured one time, there is a possibility that one will have a high false-positive rate of diagnosis of compartment syndrome. In 48 patients with a tibia shaft fracture that had no clinical suspicion of compartment syndrome, elevated pressures a ΔP less than 30 mm Hg were noted in 35% of the patients.[60] Continuous monitoring of patients has confirmed that elevated pressures can be transient.[63]

Ideally, continuous pressure can be used in all patients in whom compartment syndrome is suspected. This is expensive, however, and not available to most centers. A robust system of clinical escalation has been shown to be as sensitive at correctly diagnosing compartment syndrome as a continuous pressure monitoring system.[64] Such a system relies primarily on a reliable clinical exam in an awake and cooperative patient. Unequivocal negative physical exam findings that persist across serial exams are treated without the addition of pressure monitoring. If the patient has positive physical exam findings, the next step is emergent fasciotomies. If the patient is obtunded or intubated and compartment syndrome is suspected, then pressure monitoring, either one-time or continuous, is utilized and fasciotomies performed for a persistent ΔP less than 30 mm Hg.

Surgical Treatment

The treatment for compartment syndrome is either a single or a double incision fasciotomy. This is not a benign procedure. While the complications of compartment syndrome are catastrophic for a limb, fasciotomies should not be thrown around lightly as a panacea to the risk of missing a compartment syndrome. In the setting of a fracture, the fasciotomy incisions effectively turn the fracture into an open fracture, increasing the risk of infection. This significantly increases the length of time to union as well as the risk of nonunion.[65] In addition, there is scarring, muscle weakness, and prolonged pain. There are necessarily multiple operations, and the patient's length of stay as well as the total cost incurred more than double.[66]

The two-incision approach to fasciotomy (Fig. 19.23) of the lower part of the leg is a reliable and straightforward procedure, given that the anatomy is well understood. This approach involves making an anterolateral incision over the anterior and lateral compartments and a medial incision just posterior to the medial aspect of the tibia. The anterolateral incision is centered halfway between the fibular shaft and tibia. Once the fascia is identified, a small transverse incision is made to identify the anterior and lateral compartments as well as the superficial peroneal nerve traveling in the lateral compartment. It is important to release the entire compartment, including the most proximal and distal aspects. The posteromedial incision is used to decompress the superficial and deep posterior compartments. The incision is made approximately 2 cm posterior to the tibial shaft. Care must be taken to preserve the saphenous nerve and vein. Once the fascia is identified, a transverse incision is made to delineate the superficial and deep compartments. The superficial posterior compartment is released first, proximal and distal to the medial malleolus. In similar fashion, the deep posterior compartment is released. To decompress the deep compartment completely, the soleus muscle must be taken down off the medial side of the tibia.

Although it is different at every institution, it is the authors' preference that the orthopedic surgery service performs the fasciotomies in the setting of a fracture with compartment syndrome. There are some instances where the incisions for the definitive fixation of the fracture either should be avoided or be included in the fasciotomy incisions.

The skin incisions should not be closed primarily after fasciotomy (although closing one incision may be appropriate if a tension-free closure is possible). Even though the fascia has been released, closing the skin can lead to a dangerous increase in intramuscular pressures. Secondary closure may be attempted when limb swelling has been reduced (3–5 days). Wound management before closure consists of wet to dry dressing changes or placement of a negative pressure dressing. Negative pressure dressings help reduce swelling and may help bring the skin edges together without undue tension. Skin closure of the fasciotomy can also be facilitated with vessel loops laced through staples placed along the skin edges. The vessel loops can be tightened daily at the bedside

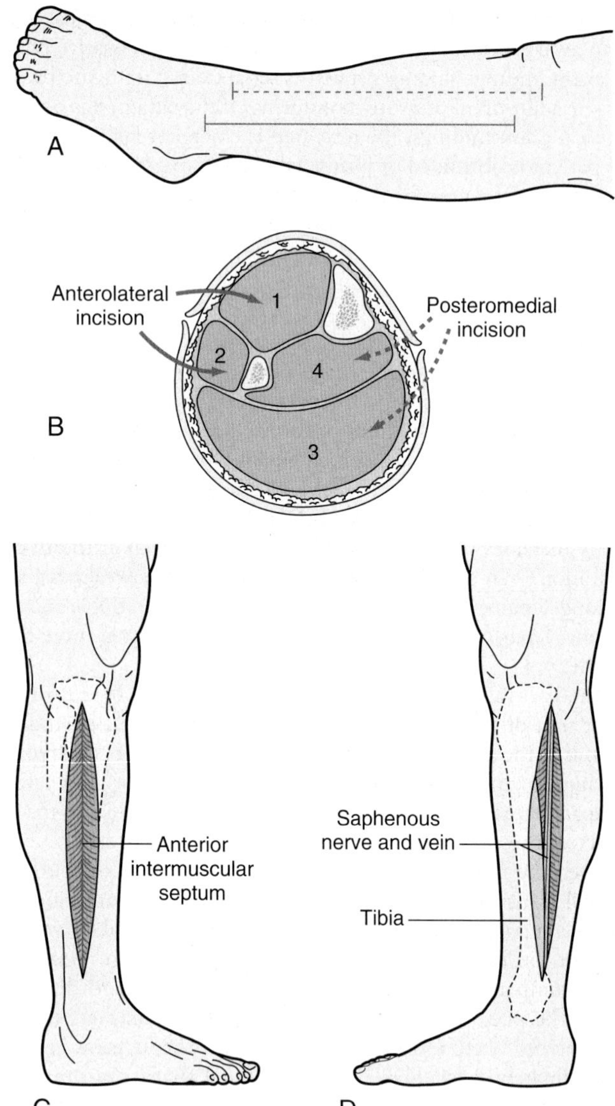

FIG. 19.23 (A) Double-incision technique for performing fasciotomies of all four compartments of the lower extremity. (B) Cross-section of the lower extremity showing positions of anterolateral and posteromedial incisions that allow access to the anterior and lateral compartments *(1* and *2)* and the superficial and deep posterior compartments *(3* and *4).* (C) The anterior intramuscular septum should be identified in the lateral incision as it marks the division of the anterior and lateral leg compartments. (D) The saphenous nerve and vein are identified in the medial incision and should be protected during compartment release.

as the soft tissue swelling diminishes, which may eliminate the need for skin grafting. If a tension-free closure is not possible, the exposed muscle can be covered with a split-thickness skin graft.

PELVIC RING DISRUPTION

Pelvic ring disruption is a major cause of morbidity and mortality in multiply injured patients with a high rate of associated injuries. Because of the high force necessary to disrupt the pelvic ring in young patients, it is not surprising that up to 80% of these patients also have additional musculoskeletal injuries. Mortality rates vary from 15% to 25%, resulting from uncontrolled hemorrhage or other associated injuries.[67] Higher ISS scores, shock on arrival, greater transfusion requirements, and patient age are risk factors to mortality in patients with pelvic ring fractures.[68] Mortality increases almost thirteen fold when the patient is hypotensive. In combination with a head or abdominal injury that requires surgical intervention or if the pelvis fracture is open, mortality increases to 50%. When both procedures are necessary, mortality approaches 90%.[7]

Long-term disability, such as low back or pelvic pain, leg length discrepancies, dyspareunia, difficulty with childbearing, impotence, and incontinence is caused by nonanatomic restoration of the pelvic ring. Even with successful restoration of the anatomy, patients can have long-term disability from the associated genitourinary and neurologic injuries effecting the lower extremity.[69]

Classification

Pelvic ring disruption can be broadly classified into two major groups, stable and unstable. A stable pelvis is defined as one that can withstand normal physiologic forces without being displaced. This stability depends on the integrity of the osseous and ligamentous structures (Fig. 19.24). Instability can be divided into rotational and vertical components (Fig. 19.25). Historically, stable injuries have been defined by less than 2.5 cm of translation of the anterior structures, either through the symphysis or through rami fractures. Instability in the vertical plane is translation of more than 1 cm through either a sacral fracture or the sacroiliac joint. This amount of injury requires injury of the posterior sacroiliac ligaments. Transverse process fractures of the L5 vertebrae should raise suspicion for pelvic instability secondary to disruption of the iliolumbar ligament. Because the pelvis is a true ring structure, significant anterior displacement must be accompanied by posterior disruption. Disruptions in the pelvic ring are usually a combination of osseous and ligamentous injury.

Early recognition of an unstable pelvic ring is essential because pelvic instability is associated with potentially fatal hemorrhage. In addition, these injuries require intervention to reestablish the pelvic ring anatomy and to minimize late disability. Determination of the stability of the injured hemipelvis must be established through a combination of physical examination and review of the imaging studies. An anterior defect can sometimes be detected by palpation at the symphysis pubis. Rotational instability can be appreciated with LC of the pelvis through the anterior iliac spines. Because repeated manipulation can cause iatrogenic injury, such handling needs to be done only once. Vertical instability may be appreciated with push-pull radiographs. These are obtained by taking two separate AP pelvic radiographs, one view with lower extremity traction and one with an axial load applied to the leg on the affected side. In the vast majority of cases, the physical examination and AP pelvic radiograph are sufficient to assess stability and to guide initial treatment. Anterior injuries are easily identified on this projection, and most unstable posterior injuries can also be appreciated.

More recently, we have come to appreciate pelvic injuries as dynamic. Our historical definitions of stability are defined on static radiographic imaging, and while helpful, they sometimes do not correctly predict the need for fixation. First, frequently, the actual severity of the injury is not fully appreciated on initial imaging. There is some recoil of the pelvis immediately following the original impact force. In reality, the static images obtained in the ED only catch a "snap-shot" into a truly dynamic injury process. Patients often enter CT scanners with pelvic binders on that, while vital to the resuscitation process, can mask the severity of the pelvic ring.[70] Failure to obtain initial pelvic radiographs prior to binder placement limits key information needed in order

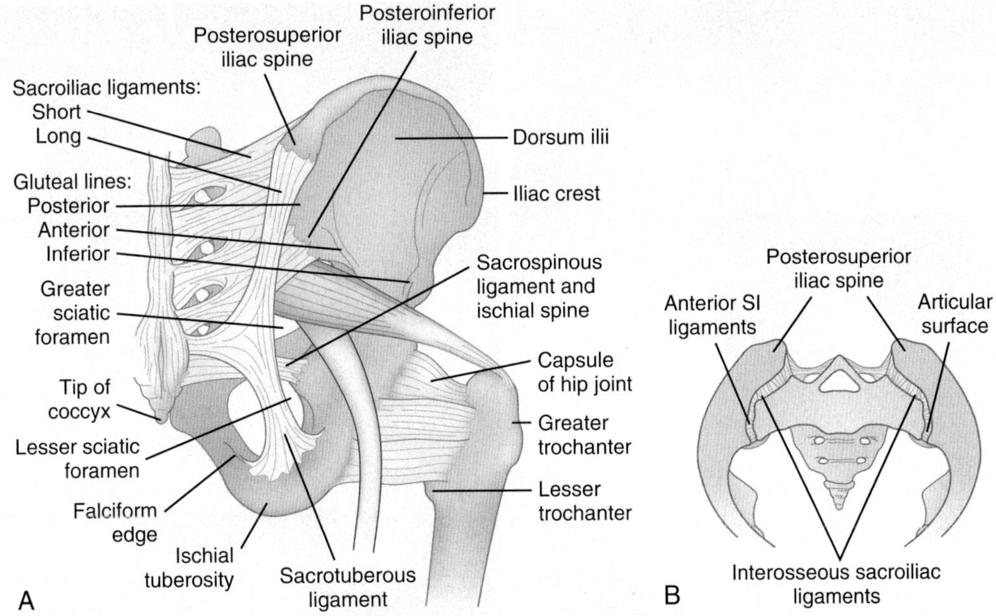

FIG. 19.24 Ligamentous complexes of the pelvis. (A) Posteriorly, the major ligaments noted in the region of the sacroiliac *(SI)* joint are the posterior SI ligaments, both long and short. The long ligaments blend with the sacrospinous and sacrotuberous ligaments. (B) In cross-section, the orientation of the very thick posterior interosseous SI ligaments is noted. (From Stover MD, Mayo KA, Kellam JF. Pelvic ring disruptions. In: Browner BD, Levine AM, Jupiter JB, et al, eds. *Skeletal Trauma: Basic Science, Management, and Reconstruction.* 4th ed. Philadelphia: WB Saunders; 2008.)

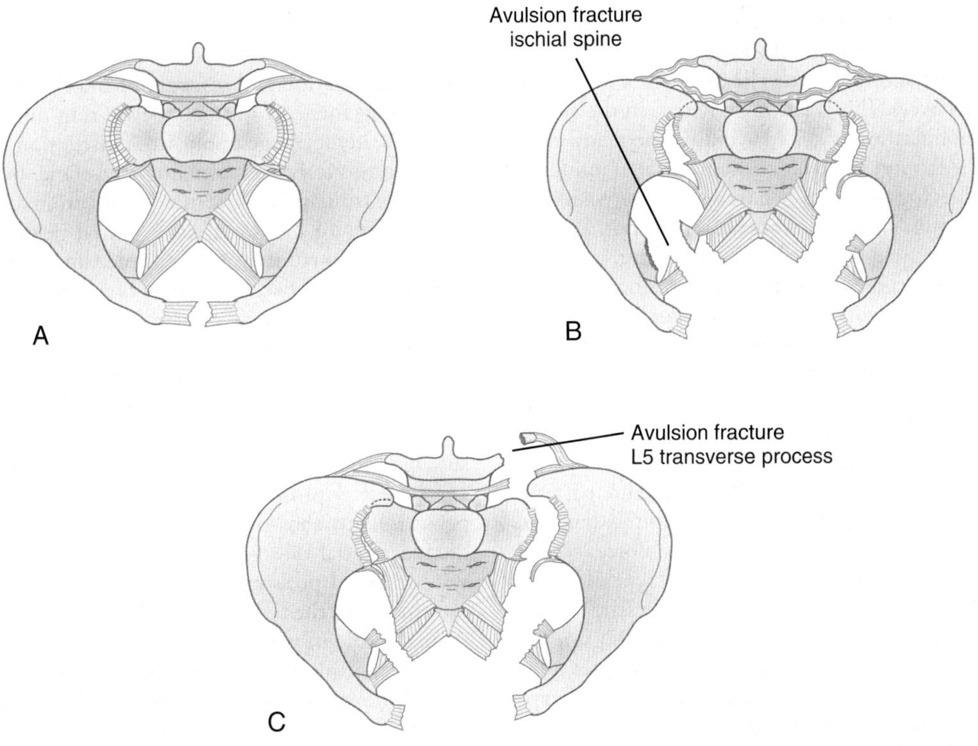

FIG. 19.25 (A) Division of the symphysis pubis allows the pelvis to open to approximately 2.5 cm with no damage to any posterior ligamentous structures. (B) Division of the anterior sacroiliac and sacrospinous ligaments, either by direct division of their fibers (*right*) or by avulsion of the tip of the ischial spine (*left*), allows the pelvis to rotate externally until the posterior superior iliac spines abut the sacrum. Note, however, that the posterior ligamentous structures (e.g., the posterior sacroiliac and iliolumbar ligaments) remain intact. Therefore, no displacement in the vertical plane is possible. (C) Division of the posterior band ligaments, that is, the posterior sacroiliac as well as the iliolumbar, causes complete instability of the hemipelvis. Note that global displacement is now possible. (From Stover MD, Mayo KA, Kellam JF. Pelvic ring disruptions. In: Browner BD, Levine AM, Jupiter JB, et al, eds. *Skeletal Trauma: Basic Science, Management, and Reconstruction.* 4th ed. Philadelphia: WB Saunders; 2008.)

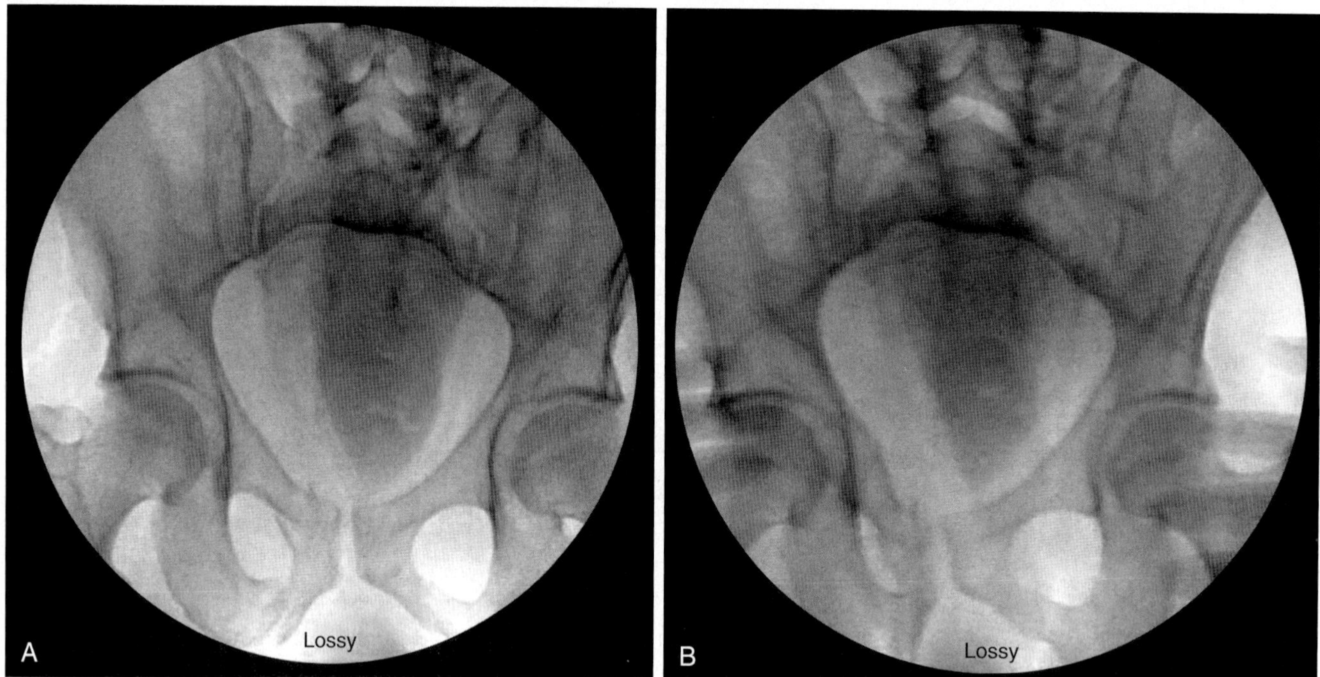

FIG. 19.26 (A) The intraoperative anteroposterior fluoroscopic shot of a complex pelvis injury as the patient lies on the bed. (B) The same shot with an internal rotation manual stress placed. The complexity of the injury is illustrated by this dynamic exam.

for the orthopedic team to make immediate decisions. At times, even with proper acute imaging, the final definitive fixation may not be fully determined until intraoperative stress radiographs are obtained with the patient fully anesthetized (Fig. 19.26).[71]

Second, some stable fractures prove to be too painful for the patient to mobilize effectively. This is particularly true in the elderly population where mobilization is key to avoiding the many complications of being bedbound when old. Often, a trial of mobilization with physical therapy over 2 to 3 days will prove whether a patient can be successfully treated nonoperatively or not. Patients generally will either progress well each day with therapy or they will not get out of bed because of the pain. Often, the pelvis can be stabilized relatively easily with percutaneous screw fixation, and the patient usually progresses quickly from that point forward.

Detailed classification systems have been developed on the basis of the direction of force, stability of the pelvis, location of the fracture, and whether it is an open or closed injury. The Young and Burgess classification characterizes pelvic ring fractures on the basis of the mechanism of injury (Fig. 19.27).[72] Fracture patterns are divided into three types (A, B, C), depending on the direction of the deforming force. Type A results from an LC force, type B results from an AP compression (APC) force, and type C results from a vertical shear force. Type A and type B fractures are further subdivided into types I, II, and III patterns, depending on the amount of ligamentous or osseous disruption. In both cases, type I fractures are stable, type II are rotationally unstable, and type III are rotationally and vertically unstable. APC injuries have the greatest risk for retroperitoneal hemorrhage. The APC III, also known as an open-book pelvis, significantly increases the volume of the pelvis, allowing massive blood loss in a short time (Fig. 19.28). Intrapelvic visceral injuries are also more common with the AP patterns. Mortality in APC injuries is related to a combination of retroperitoneal bleeding and visceral injuries. LC and vertical shear fractures are associated with intraabdominal and head injuries. Whereas intrapelvic hemorrhage occurs in LC fractures, the most common cause of death in a patient with this injury pattern is associated closed head trauma.[7]

Management

Pelvic stabilization and control of hemorrhage are the goals of initial management of unstable pelvic ring injuries. In most pelvic fractures, hemorrhage results from disruption of the pelvic venous plexus posteriorly and bleeding cancellous bone. Most bleeding resulting from pelvic fracture comes from the presacral venous plexus (Fig. 19.29). As a result, initial treatment of hemorrhage must focus on control of venous bleeding by reduction and stabilization of the pelvic ring. Reduction leads to a decrease in pelvic volume and tamponade of the bleeding vessels through compression of the viscera and pelvic hematoma. Stabilization maintains the reduction and avoids movement of the hemipelvis, thereby reducing pain and limiting disruption of any organizing thrombus. In patients who remain hemodynamically unstable after initial resuscitation and stabilization, a source of arterial bleeding must be considered. A prospective study of 143 patients with high-energy pelvic fracture showed that 10% had arterial injury.[73] Factors predicting arterial bleeding included a base deficit of 6 mmol/L, a systolic blood pressure less than 104 mm Hg, and the need for transfusion in the ED.[73] CT angiography is another useful tool to evaluate patients who may benefit from angiographic or open control of pelvic bleeding. The significance of a "pelvic blush" finding on CT, however, remains controversial. A study by Verbeek and coworkers demonstrated that, of 42% of patients with pelvic ring injuries who had a pelvic blush on CT, only 47% required pelvic hemorrhage control. The negative predictive value of CT angiography is much higher, typically greater than 90%.[6]

Stabilization of pelvic ring injuries accomplishes more than simply control of hemorrhage. Patients with a stabilized pelvis may more easily be transferred in bed, be repositioned, and have the head of the bed elevated. This facilitates the care of these usually multiply injured patients in the intensive care unit (ICU).

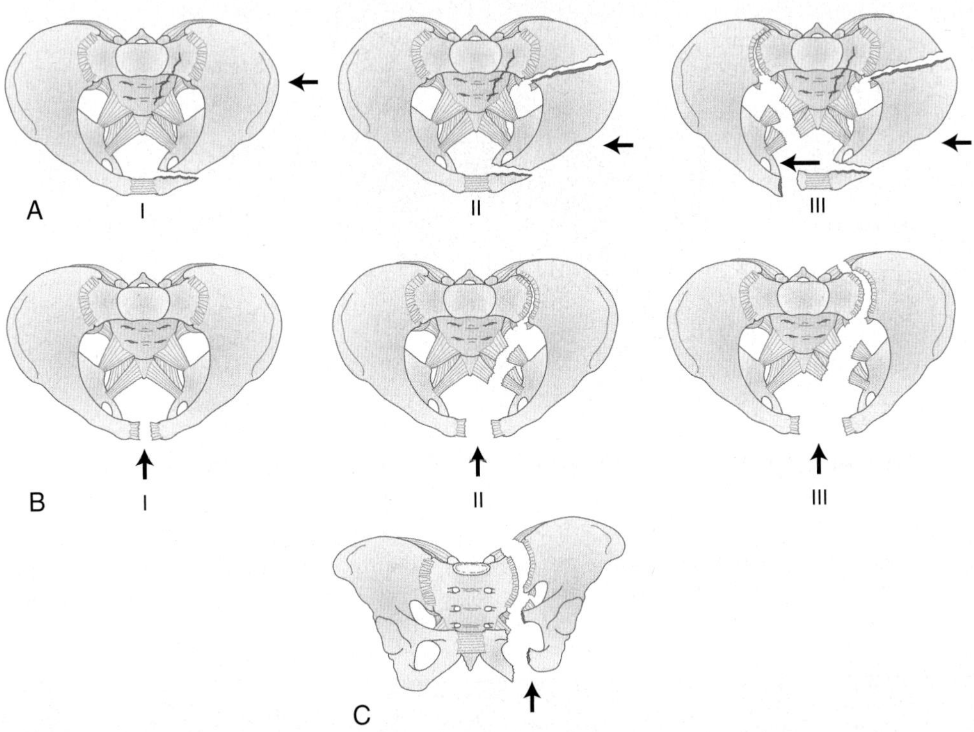

FIG. 19.27 Young and Burgess classification. (A) Lateral compression force. *Type I,* a posteriorly directed force causing a sacral crushing injury and horizontal pubic ramus fractures ipsilaterally. This injury is stable. *Type II,* a more anteriorly directed force causing horizontal pubic ramus fractures with an anterior sacral crushing injury and either disruption of the posterior sacroiliac joints or fractures through the iliac wing. This injury is ipsilateral. *Type III,* an anteriorly directed force that is continued and leads to a type I or type II ipsilateral fracture with an external rotation component to the contralateral side; the sacroiliac joint is opened posteriorly, and the sacrotuberous and spinous ligaments are disrupted. (B) Anteroposterior compression fractures. *Type I,* an anteroposterior-directed force opening the pelvis but with the posterior ligamentous structures intact. This injury is stable. *Type II,* continuation of a type I fracture with disruption of the sacrospinous and potentially the sacrotuberous ligaments and an anterior sacroiliac joint opening. This fracture is rotationally unstable. *Type III,* a completely unstable or vertical instability pattern with complete disruption of all ligamentous supporting structures. (C) A vertically directed force at right angles to the supporting structures of the pelvis leading to vertical fractures in the rami and disruption of all the ligamentous structures. This injury is equivalent to an anteroposterior type III or a completely unstable and rotationally unstable fracture. (Adapted from Young JWR, Burgess AR. *Radiologic Management of Pelvic Ring Fractures.* Baltimore: Urban and Schwarzenberg; 1987.)

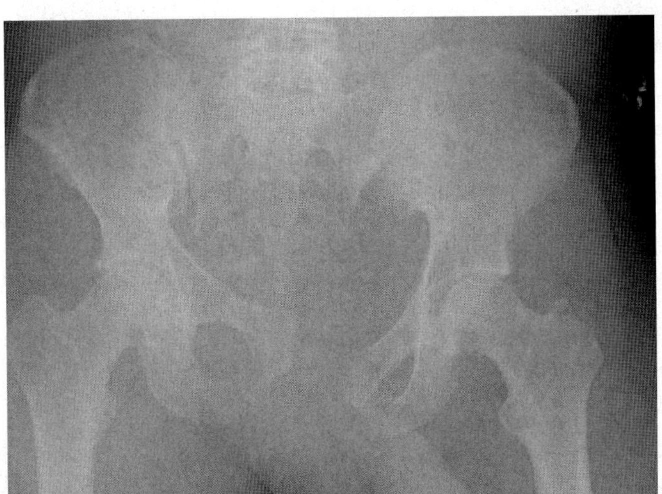

FIG. 19.28 Anteroposterior pelvic radiograph showing the so-called open-book pelvis. Complete disruption of the anterior and posterior ligamentous structures leaves this pelvis rotationally and vertically unstable.

Pain management and the decrease in the inflammatory cascade associated with an unstable, mobile fracture site are also benefits.

Initial Stabilization

The initial stabilization of a patient with a pelvic ring injury occurs in the prehospital setting. When field personnel detect unstable pelvic ring disruptions on physical examination, they can begin treatment by binding the pelvis with a rolled sheet, pelvic binder, or applying pneumatic antishock garments (PASGs). Like air splints applied to the extremities, the garment functions by compressing the pelvis. If they are applied in the field, PASGs should not be deflated until the patient is being resuscitated in the trauma room. A PASG has the advantage of ease of use, application in the field, and reusability. However, it blocks access to the patient and restricts excursion of the diaphragm, and there have been reports of gluteal and thigh compartment syndromes developing after extended use of PASGs in hypotensive patients. Because of these disadvantages, the use of the pelvic binder has become more common. These devices have been shown through biomechanical studies and clinical experience to effectively reduce

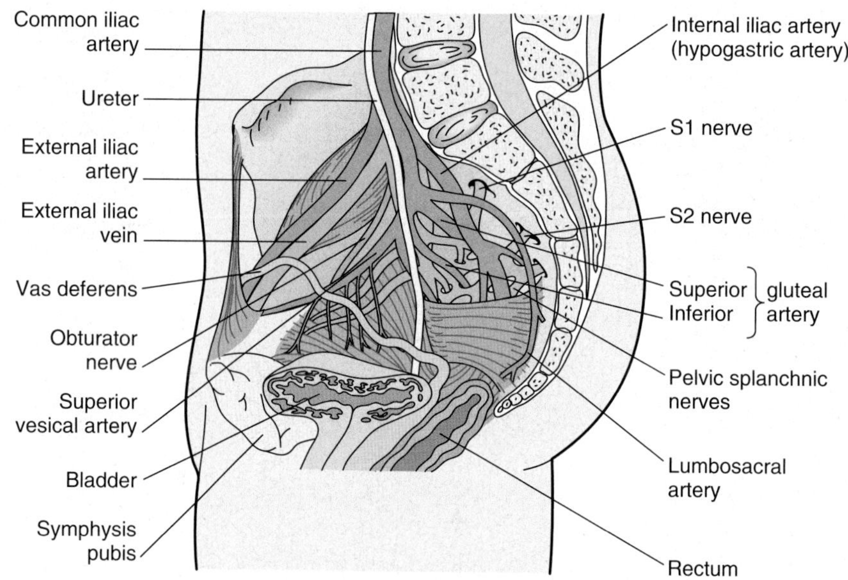

FIG. 19.29 Internal aspect of the pelvis showing the great vessels and lumbosacral plexus as well as the pelvic floor, bladder, and rectum. (From Stover MD, Mayo KA, Kellam JF. Pelvic ring disruptions. In: Browner BD, Levine AM, Jupiter JB, et al, eds. *Skeletal Trauma: Basic Science, Management, and Reconstruction.* 4th ed. Philadelphia: WB Saunders; 2008.)

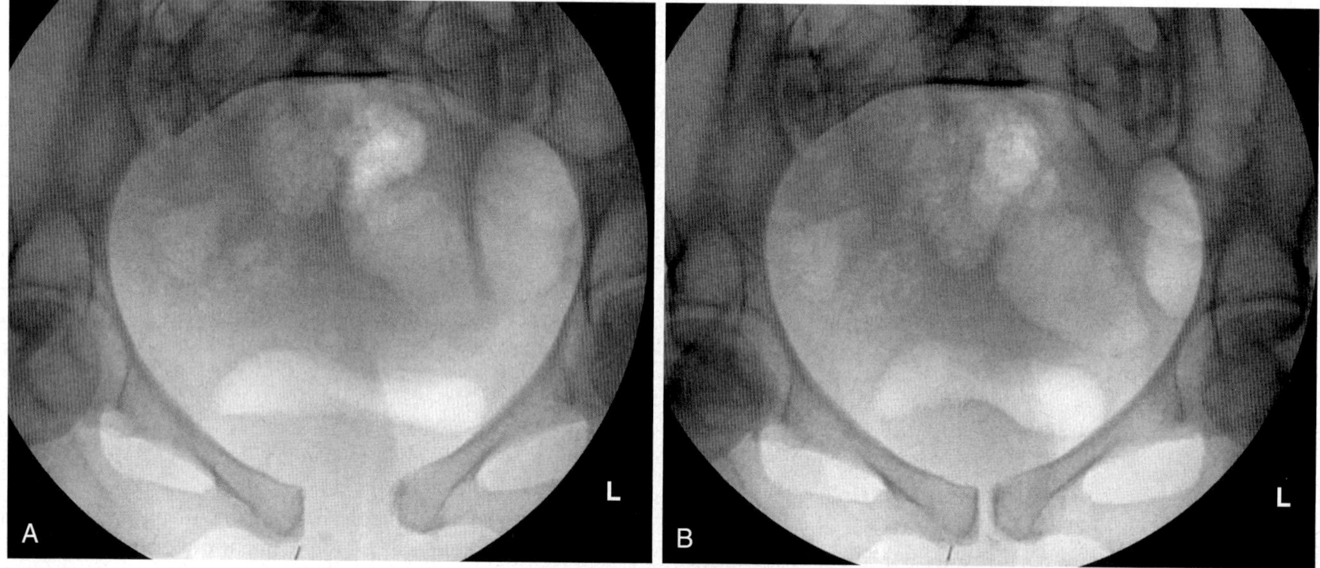

FIG. 19.30 (A) Pelvic ring with bilateral anteroposterior compression 2 injuries demonstrating widening of the pubic symphysis and bilateral anterior sacroiliac joints. (B) Internal rotation of the legs with compression on the greater trochanters bilaterally anatomically reduces the pelvic ring

pelvic volume.[74] Binders or sheets are properly applied by centering them over the greater trochanters and applying pressure. The more proximal part of the construct may be cut away to allow access to the lower abdomen if necessary. Internally rotating both legs and holding this position with tape across the ankles or knees also assist in pelvic reduction (Fig. 19.30). These devices should be removed from the patient as soon as possible as skin breakdown can begin to occur quickly. In LC-type pelvic injuries, the binder may theoretically over-reduce the fracture and injure intrapelvic structures. Overall, the use of binders and sheets should be limited to APC injuries with associated hemodynamic instability. Patients who do not respond to binder or sheet placement may necessitate other interventions including pelvic artery embolization (PAE) or pelvic packing.

PAE can be performed in either the internal iliac artery (nonselective) or distal to the internal iliac artery (selective). Although the benefits of PAE in the pelvic fracture patients with refractory hypotension are well documented, there are complication rates of 11%, including muscle necrosis, surgical wound breakdown, infection, and impotence. Complication rates are particularly high when associated with bilateral or nonselective PAE: a recent retrospective review by Lindvall and colleagues showed a 20% complication rate associated with nonselective PAE.[75]

Pelvic packing is another option that can be used to control venous and/or bony bleeding. Pelvic packing can be considered in the patient who does not respond to resuscitation efforts in the ED/ICU. Additionally, if the patient has a pelvic hematoma and remains unstable after abdominal exploration and intervention, pelvic packing may be considered. An external fixator is recommended to be placed prior to pelvic packing in order to provide fracture stabilization and prevent inadvertent expansion of the pelvic volume during packing. Six to nine laps are placed, starting posteriorly at the sacrum and moving anteriorly to the pubis. Packing should be removed after resuscitation in 24 to 48 hours. Delays in removal of the packing or repeat packing have been associated with increased infection rates.[76] Ultimately, the decision of when to perform PAE or pelvic packing requires a multidisciplinary treatment approach with the trauma surgeon, interventional radiologist, and orthopedic surgeon in order to improve outcomes and decrease complications.

Definitive Management

Long-term definitive care of pelvic ring disruption is dependent on the pattern of injury and its severity as well as the associated injuries. The exact timing of definitive fixation of the pelvis is in debate with institutional variations, but it should generally be performed within the first week. The overall goal is to perform definitive fracture management once the patient has been adequately resuscitated.[77]

Stable fracture patterns usually require no more than protected weight bearing. External fixator is typically used as an initial temporizing stabilization before definitive open reduction internal fixation. However, there are circumstances in which a well-fixed external fixator can be used definitively. Complex anterior fracture patterns or patient anatomy may preclude fixation of the anterior pelvis with plates and or screws. Patients with a large panniculus, associated open perineal wounds, or complex urinary injuries may pose increased infection risks in the setting of internal instrumentation.[78] In women of child-bearing age, temporary external fixation may be considered in order to prevent difficulties with vaginal delivery seen with internal fixation of the pelvis.[79] In cases in which the fixator may be obstructing access to the abdomen or an interim binder has been applied, open reduction with internal fixation or closed reduction and percutaneous fixation may be indicated. When rotational or vertical instability is present, the anterior and posterior pelvis must be stabilized. Anteriorly, the symphysis is often secured with open plating or percutaneous screws. The sacroiliac joint or sacral fractures can be secured with plates, bars, or percutaneously inserted cannulated screws (Fig. 19.31). The fixation strategies are constantly evolving, particularly with the popularization and better understanding of percutaneous methods. In the end, the definitive fixation is determined by a multitude of factors, including fracture pattern, associated injuries, and surgeon preference (Fig. 19.32).

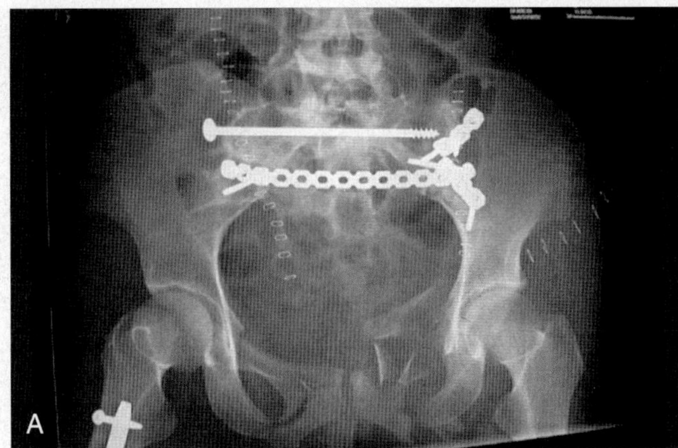

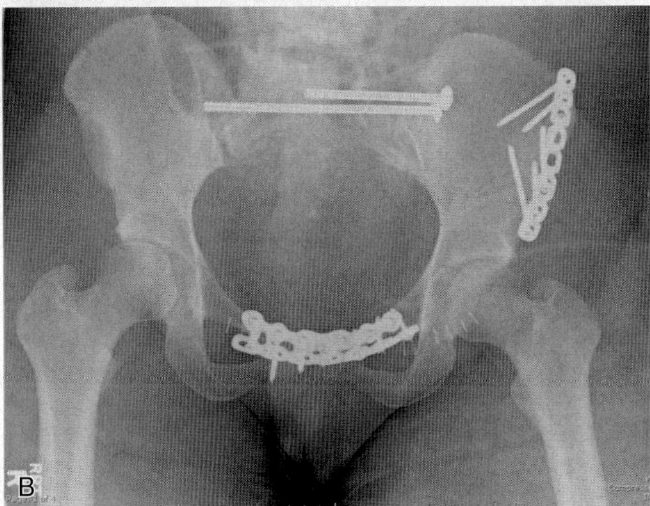

FIG. 19.31 Fixation of unstable pelvic fractures. (A) One transiliac screw, one transiliac plate, and two left sacroiliac plates were used to stabilize the posterior elements in this fracture. (B) One transiliac screw and one sacroiliac screw were used to stabilize the posterior elements of this fracture. Plates were used to stabilize the pubic symphysis. An iliac crest plate was used to fix the left iliac wing fracture.

SPINAL INJURIES

Evaluation

The initial evaluation of the trauma patient for spinal injuries follows the ATLS protocol as described earlier in this chapter. All trauma patients are typically placed in a cervical collar in the prehospital or ED phase of care, especially if neck pain is present or the patient has a distracting injury. Level 1 evidence suggests that the awake, sober, neurologically intact patient without distracting injury should have the collar removed as soon as possible if certain criteria are met.[80] To have the collar removed, these patients must have no tenderness to palpation in the cervical spine and must have full pain-free active range of motion. If midline neck pain or tenderness is present, CT evaluation is indicated. Likewise, the intoxicated patient or those with multiple distracting injuries should also have a CT evaluation and the collar maintained. MRI may be used to identify injury to the posterior ligamentous structures.

Acute compression of the spinal cord can lead to spinal shock, which is detectable by physical examination. For diagnosis of spinal shock, the bulbocavernosus reflex is tested by tugging on the Foley catheter or squeezing the glans penis and looking for an anal wink. An absent reflex indicates spinal shock. As spinal shock resolves, usually within 48 hours, this reflex returns. Examination at this point will provide a more accurate indication of neurologic deficits. The presence of sacral sparing (intact perianal sensation, rectal tone, or great toe flexion) represents at least partial continuity of the white matter long tracts. After a full neuromotor examination, an American Spinal Injury Association (ASIA) classification may be assigned to the spine-injured patient (Fig. 19.33).

Management

The spinal cord is divided into three columns (Fig. 19.34). The anterior column consists of the anterior two-thirds of the vertebral body as well as the anterior longitudinal ligament. The middle column includes the posterior third of the vertebral body and the posterior longitudinal ligament. The posterior column includes all bone and ligamentous structures posterior to the posterior longitudinal ligament. In general, injury to one column results in a stable injury. Injury to two or three columns results in an unstable spinal

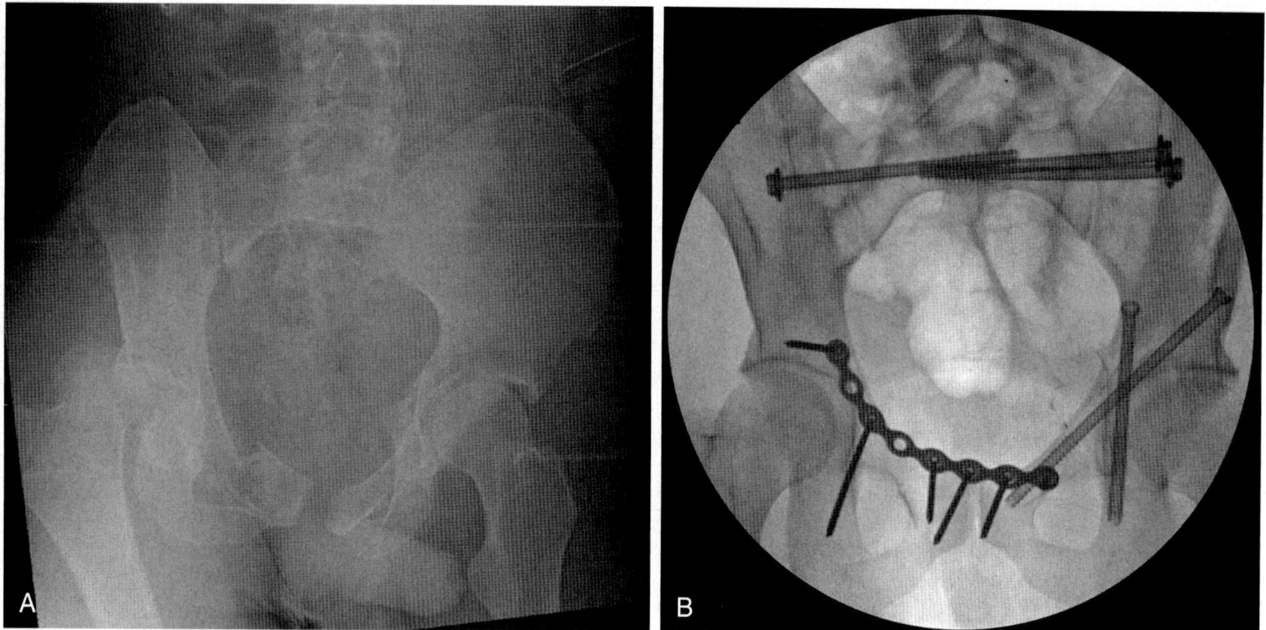

FIG. 19.32 (A) Anteroposterior pelvis radiograph demonstrating a combined mechanism injury with bilateral sacroiliac injuries, a left acetabulum fracture, right rami fractures, and a disruption of the pubic symphysis. (B) Postoperative fluoroscopic anteroposterior with percutaneous posterior pelvic fixation, percutaneous fixation of the left acetabulum, and open reduction and internal fixation of the pubic symphysis and right superior ramus.

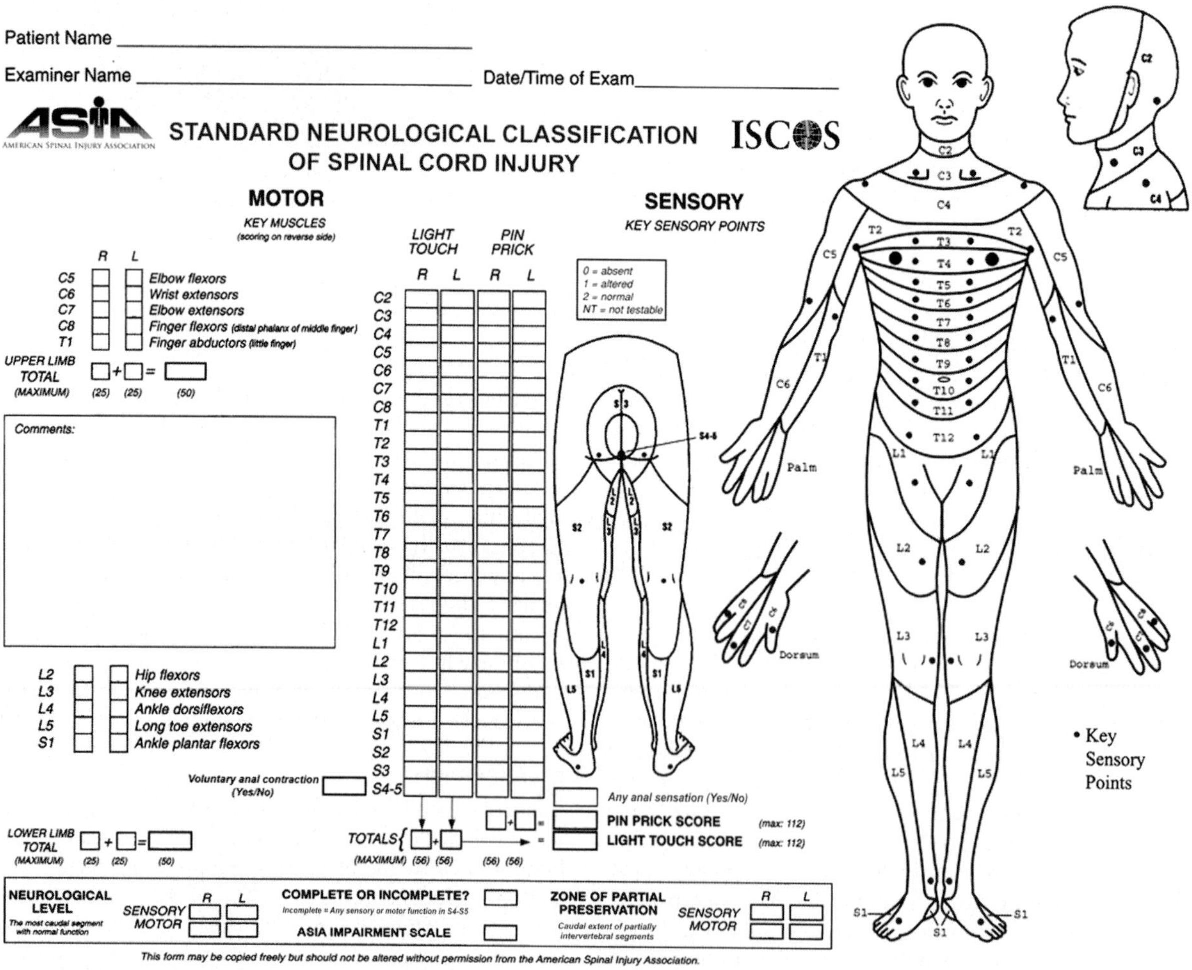

Patient Name ______________________

Examiner Name ______________________ Date/Time of Exam______________

ASIA AMERICAN SPINAL INJURY ASSOCIATION **STANDARD NEUROLOGICAL CLASSIFICATION OF SPINAL CORD INJURY** ISCoS

MOTOR

KEY MUSCLES *(scoring on reverse side)*

	R	L	
C5			Elbow flexors
C6			Wrist extensors
C7			Elbow extensors
C8			Finger flexors (distal phalanx of middle finger)
T1			Finger abductors (little finger)
UPPER LIMB TOTAL (MAXIMUM)	(25)	(25)	= (50)

Comments:

	R	L	
L2			Hip flexors
L3			Knee extensors
L4			Ankle dorsiflexors
L5			Long toe extensors
S1			Ankle plantar flexors

Voluntary anal contraction (Yes/No)

LOWER LIMB TOTAL (MAXIMUM) (25) + (25) = (50)

SENSORY

KEY SENSORY POINTS

	LIGHT TOUCH R	LIGHT TOUCH L	PIN PRICK R	PIN PRICK L
C2				
C3				
C4				
C5				
C6				
C7				
C8				
T1				
T2				
T3				
T4				
T5				
T6				
T7				
T8				
T9				
T10				
T11				
T12				
L1				
L2				
L3				
L4				
L5				
S1				
S2				
S3				
S4-5				
TOTALS (MAXIMUM)	(56)	(56)	(56)	(56)

0 = absent
1 = altered
2 = normal
NT = not testable

Any anal sensation (Yes/No)

PIN PRICK SCORE (max: 112)

LIGHT TOUCH SCORE (max: 112)

NEUROLOGICAL LEVEL The most caudal segment with normal function		R	L
	SENSORY		
	MOTOR		

COMPLETE OR INCOMPLETE? Incomplete = Any sensory or motor function in S4-S5

ASIA IMPAIRMENT SCALE

ZONE OF PARTIAL PRESERVATION Caudal extent of partially intervertebral segments		R	L
	SENSORY		
	MOTOR		

This form may be copied freely but should not be altered without permission from the American Spinal Injury Association.

FIG. 19.33 ASIA classification. (©American Spinal Injury Association. <http://www.asia-spinalinjury.org/elearning/ISNCSCI.php>.)

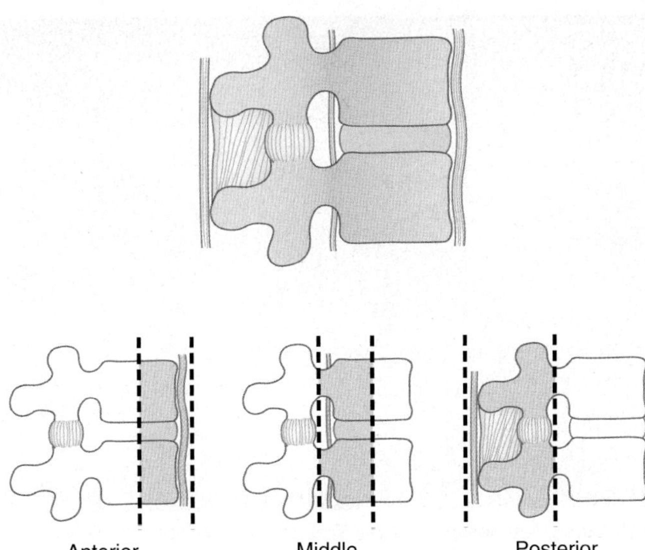

FIG. 19.34 Denis' three-column model of the spine. The anterior column consists of the anterior two-thirds of the vertebral body and anterior longitudinal ligament. The middle column includes the posterior third of the vertebral body and posterior longitudinal ligament. The posterior column includes all bone and ligamentous structures posterior to the posterior longitudinal ligament. (From Lee Y, Templin C, Eismont F, et al. Thoracic and upper lumbar spine injuries. In: Browner BD, Levine AM, Jupiter JB, et al, eds. *Skeletal Trauma: Basic Science, Management, and Reconstruction.* 4th ed. Philadelphia: WB Saunders; 2008.)

segment. Instability in the spinal column puts the spinal cord at risk. Burst fractures, by definition, involve injury to the anterior and middle columns. These fractures are to be differentiated from compression fractures, which involve the anterior column only and are rarely associated with spinal cord injury. Burst fractures commonly occur after a fall from a height in which an axial load is transmitted to the upper axial skeleton when the feet strike the ground first.[81] This mechanism results in a common pattern of fractures, including calcaneus, tibial plateau, and proximal femur fractures (see Table 19.3). Depending on the fracture pattern, treatment of spine injuries may range from observation with bracing to surgical fixation or external halo fixation. However, treatment of all injuries begins with strict immobilization and spine precautions.

Cervical spine injuries can occur by several mechanisms, which can be divided into three main categories. The first involves direct trauma to the neck itself. The second mechanism involves motion of the head relative to the axial skeleton. This injury can occur by direct trauma to the head or continued movement of the head relative to the fixed body (whiplash), as often occurs in blunt trauma such as motor vehicle accidents, when the body is restrained. In attempting to tether the head against motion, the cervical spine endures a large bending or twisting moment that results in flexion-extension injuries or rotational injuries, respectively. A third mechanism of cervical spine injury involves a direct axial load imparted on the cranium that causes axial compression forces across the cervical vertebrae. This may result in a burst fracture and potential spinal cord injury. This pattern of injury is more commonly seen in the lumbar spine. An algorithm for diagnosis of cervical spine injuries is presented in Fig. 19.35.

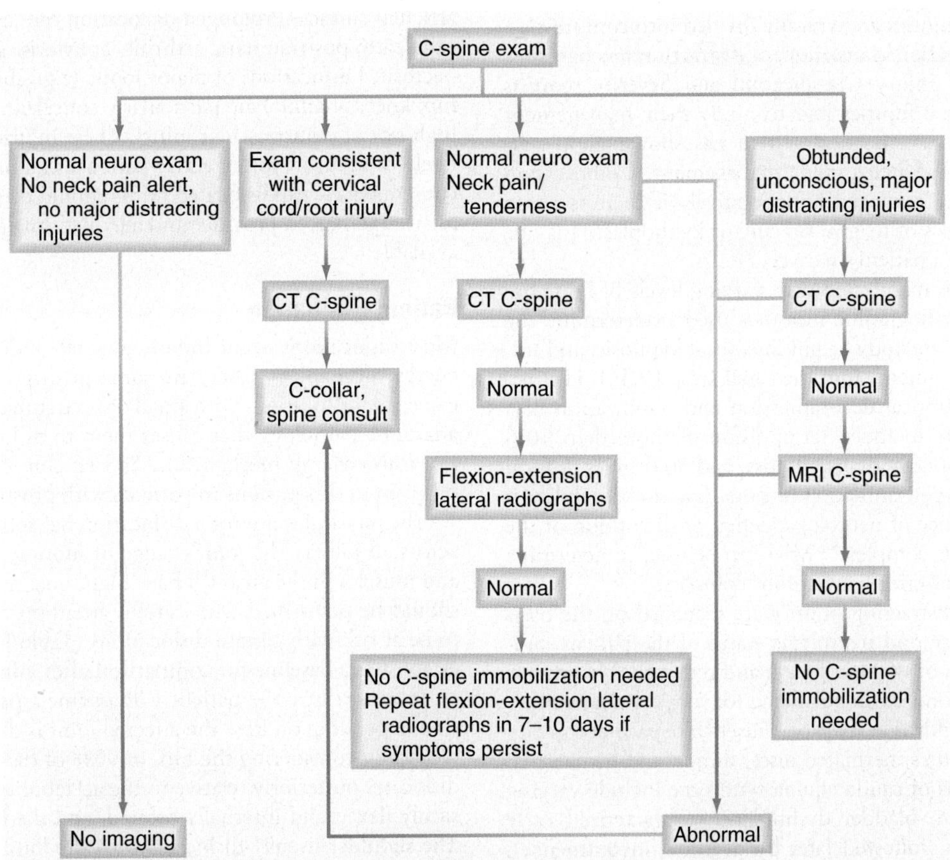

FIG. 19.35 Algorithm for imaging diagnosis of cervical spine (C-spine) injury. (Adapted from Lee Y, Templin C, Eismont F, et al. Thoracic and upper lumbar spine injuries. In: Browner BD, Levine AM, Jupiter JB, et al, eds. *Skeletal Trauma: Basic Science, Management, and Reconstruction.* 4th ed. Philadelphia: WB Saunders; 2008.) *CT,* Computed tomography; *MRI,* magnetic resonance imaging; *neuro,* neurologic.

TABLE 19.6 Point system for the Thoracolumbar Injury Classification and Severity score.

	POINTS
Type	
Compression	1
Burst	2
Translational/rotational	3
Distraction	4
Integrity of Posterior Ligamentous Complex	
Intact	0
Suspected/indeterminate	2
Injured	3
Neurologic Status	
Intact	0
Nerve root	2
Cord, conus medullaris, complete	2
Cord, conus medullaris, incomplete	3
Cauda equina	3

From Patel AA, Vaccaro AR. Thoracolumbar spine trauma classification. *J Am Acad Orthop Surg*. 2010;18:63–71.

Clinical qualifiers: extreme kyphosis, marked collapse, lateral angulation, open fractures, soft tissue compromise, adjacent rib fractures, inability to brace, multisystem trauma, severe head injury, sternum fracture.

Thoracolumbar injuries are typically divided into compression (simple or burst), rotation/translation, or distraction mechanisms. The Thoracolumbar Injury Classification and Severity score is used to describe these injuries and to guide their management (Table 19.6).[82] The classification system has shown good reliability and validity and helps guide management. Compression fractures are typically managed nonoperatively if there is not a significant (>25%) loss of height. Bracing or kyphoplasty may be offered if pain limits a patient's recovery.[83]

Burst fractures are manifested with varying levels of bone deformity. The three radiographic measures used to determine the severity of the injury are body height loss, focal kyphosis, and retropulsion of bone fragments into the canal (Fig. 19.36). Historical indications for surgical decompression and stabilization of a lumbar burst fracture included retropulsion of more than 50% of the spinal canal, 50% body height loss, and 30 degrees of focal kyphosis. Currently, determination of burst fracture instability is defined by the presence of neurologic deficit or disruption of the posterior ligamentous complex.[84] MRI can be used to determine the stability of the posterior ligamentous complex.

Translational or distracting injuries are managed on the basis of the fracture pattern and neurologic status of the patient. Spinal stabilization with or without fusion and removal of fragments causing canal compromise can be offered for surgical treatment.

Cauda equina syndrome may be caused by space-occupying lesions, such as fractures, herniated discs, tumor, and hematoma. The classic symptoms of cauda equina syndrome include varying degrees of back pain, bladder dysfunction (characterized early by urinary retention, followed later by overflow incontinence), saddle anesthesia, lower extremity numbness, and weakness and reduced rectal tone (a late finding). If cauda equina syndrome is suspected, MRI should be ordered immediately to look for canal

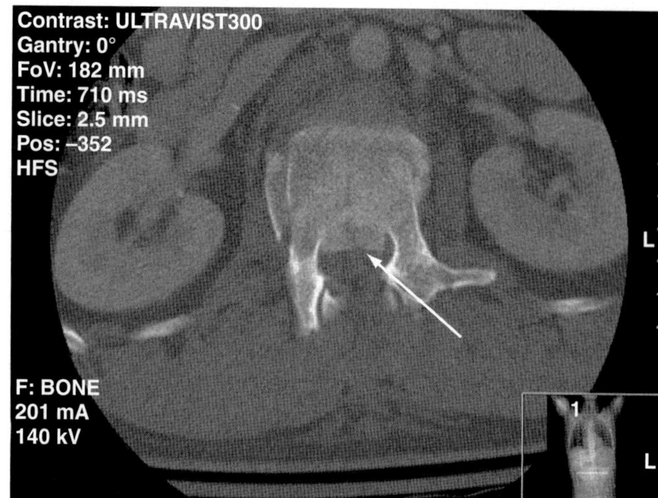

FIG. 19.36 Lumbar-level burst fracture showing 50% retropulsion of bone fragments into the canal. *CT, Computed tomography; MRI, magnetic resonance imaging.*

compromise. If MRI is not available or the patient cannot undergo MRI, CT myelography can be performed. When a diagnosis of cauda equina syndrome is confirmed, surgical exploration and decompression should be performed immediately.

DISLOCATIONS

A dislocated joint is considered an orthopedic emergency because of the possibility of neurovascular injury and damage to the articular surface. Prolonged dislocation can lead to cartilage cell death, posttraumatic arthritis, ankylosis, and avascular necrosis. Dislocations of major joints (e.g., shoulder, elbow, hip, knee, or ankle) are particularly concerning because of the high risk of neurovascular injury. These injuries, which are more likely to occur in young active patients, can have devastating consequences. All dislocated joints should be reduced as soon as an experienced provider and adequate analgesia or sedation is available.

Patient Evaluation

Most dislocations occur in young, active individuals from a high energy mechanism. There are some predisposing conditions that can cause dislocations with small or no trauma: shoulders can have anatomic pathology that causes them to dislocate frequently and from low energy mechanisms. Special consideration should also be given to dislocations in patients with prosthetic joints.

The physical exam for a dislocation has some common features across all joints. The joint's range of motion will be very limited and muscles in the area will have high tone. A neurovascular exam should be performed with careful attention to structures known to be at risk with certain dislocations (Table 19.7). The exam also establishes a baseline for comparison after joint reduction.

In most cases, the patient will assume a pathognomonic position depending on how the affected joint is dislocated. For example, when considering the hip, in 90% of cases, the femoral head dislocates posteriorly relative to the acetabulum. The thigh is classically flexed and internally rotated, and the limb is shortened.[85] The shoulder usually dislocates with the humerus anterior to the glenoid. The arm is held in an externally rotated and adducted position. In thin patients, the normally rounded contour of the deltoid will be obviously disrupted.[85]

TABLE 19.7 Dislocated joints and associated injuries.

JOINT	STRUCTURE AT-RISK	ASSOCIATED INJURIES OR LONG-TERM CONSEQUENCES
Hip	• Sciatic nerve (ankle and toe function; e.g., foot drop) • Femoral artery	• Avascular necrosis of the femoral head • Degenerative joint disease
Knee	• Popliteal artery • Common peroneal nerve (ankle eversion, foot drop)	• Peroneal nerve palsy • Multiligamentous knee injury
Shoulder	• Axillary nerve (shoulder abduction, sensation over deltoid) • Axillary artery	• In patients <40 years old, labral tear • In patients >40 years old, rotator cuff tear
Elbow	• Brachial artery • Radial, ulnar, and median nerves (wrist extension, crossing fingers, flexion of index DIP and thumb IP joints, respectively)	• Rotatory instability • Stiffness

DIP, Distal interphalangeal; *IP*, interphalangeal.

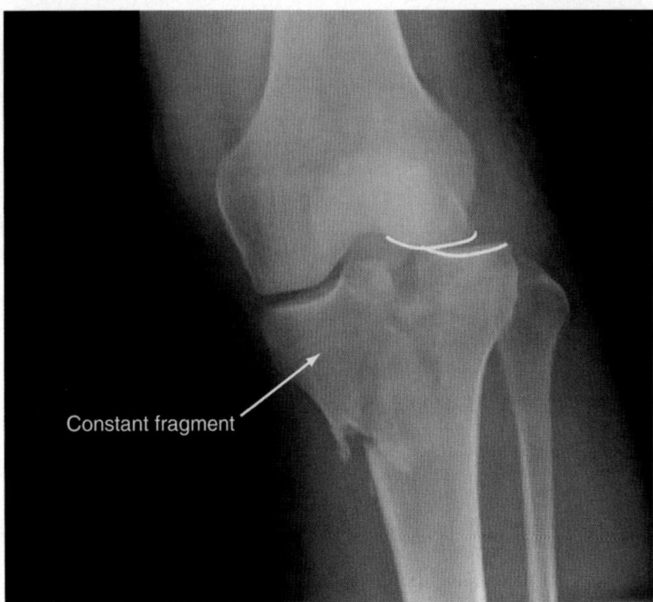

FIG. 19.37 Medial tibial plateau fracture with a concomitant dislocation of the knee joint. While it appears that the medial "constant fragment" is fractured off of the tibia shaft, this fractured fragment is maintaining its attachments to the distal femur. The tibia shaft is actually fractured off of the "constant fragment" and dislocated laterally. The incongruence of the latèral tibial plateau is noted.

Radiographs should be ordered to establish the diagnosis and identify associated fractures. Seventy percent of hip dislocations have associated acetabular fractures, and many shoulder dislocations will have impaction injuries to the humeral head or fractures of the glenoid rim.[86] Standard orthogonal views are usually enough to establish the direction of dislocation; however, as mentioned in the section on radiography, these must be true orthogonal images of the shoulder and not just internal and external rotation views of the proximal humerus.

Special Considerations for the Trauma Setting

Hip and knee dislocations require special discussion because of the extreme consequences of failure to recognize and address them in timely fashion.

Delay in the reduction of a dislocated hip can lead to sciatic nerve injury, cartilage cell death, and avascular necrosis. Avascular necrosis and the subsequent femoral head collapse are devastating sequela that lead to significant dysfunction and, in many cases, total hip arthroplasty. A recent metaanalysis showed that reduction after 12 hours has an odds ratio of 5.6 for development of avascular necrosis.[86]

Knee dislocations should be evaluated for popliteal artery injury. A recent systematic review found the rate of popliteal artery injury after knee dislocation to be 18%, of which 80% underwent vascular repair.[10] The popliteal artery is tethered proximal to the knee joint at the adductor hiatus and distal to the joint by the soleus. Up to 50% of knee dislocations will reduce spontaneously, but if the knee presents dislocated, it should be reduced promptly.[87] Some knee dislocations can masquerade as fractures (Fig. 19.37), and vigilance should be maintained when considering all distal femur and proximal tibia fractures.

The workup for arterial injury is historically controversial, with some authors arguing for universal arteriography. Current evidence supports the use of selective arteriography, reserved for patients with abnormal exams. A common protocol uses sequentially timed vascular exams at presentation, 4 to 6 hours later, and then 24 to 48 hours later. The exam includes symmetry of distal pulses, gross evaluation of color and temperature, and the ABI. Two prospective studies and eight retrospective studies using this type of protocol, totaling 545 patients, reported zero patients who had a normal vascular exam with a clinically significant arterial injury.[88–91] When the vascular exam is abnormal, CT angiography has been shown to be an effective and efficient next step in diagnosing the injury.

Treatment

While descriptions for reduction maneuvers of each dislocated joint are easy to find, the approach and principles to each one are the same.

IV sedation is very helpful in reducing muscle tone that can resist reduction but is not always necessary if the patient has adequate analgesia. A neurovascular exam should be performed before reduction to provide a baseline for comparison after reduction. This is useful because there is a risk of iatrogenic entrapment of neurovascular structures.

The general reduction technique is to recreate the deforming force, apply traction, and then reverse the deforming force. For example, in a posterior hip dislocation, the position of the hip at the time of dislocation was most likely flexed and internally rotated. When the hip dislocates, the femoral head usually hinges on the posterior wall of the acetabulum, which inhibits reduction. To reduce the joint, it should first be flexed and internally rotated, unhinging it from the posterior wall. Next, traction clears the head anterior to the posterior wall. Finally, external rotation and will ensure that the joint remains reduced.

Knee dislocations usually occur with the tibia posterior to the femur. These can be reduced by a posterior translating force to the tibia, followed by gentle traction, and then guiding the tibia forward into a reduced position. Skin furrowing at the anteromedial aspect of the femur, also known as the "dimple sign," suggests femoral condyle protrusion through the soft tissue; these can be irreducible and multiple attempts should not be made due to the risk of skin necrosis.

Shoulder dislocations can be reduced in several ways. One technique, called the "FARES" (Fast, Reliable, Safe) technique involves gentle traction applied at the wrist, oscillation of the arm while abducting and simultaneously moving it from anterior to posterior, and then externally rotating the arm once 90 degrees of abduction is reached.[92]

If a joint is irreducible in the ED, the patient should be brought to the operating room for an attempt at closed reduction under general anesthesia. Staff and instruments for open reduction should be available if this fails.

Most reduced dislocations are immobilized using well-padded splints (i.e., elbow, wrist, ankle) or joint-specific immobilizers (i.e., shoulder sling, knee immobilizer). All dislocations require either in-hospital or outpatient evaluation by an orthopedic surgeon.

VASCULAR INJURIES

Incidence and Recognition

The rate of vascular injuries associated with blunt and penetrating extremity trauma is estimated to be 1.6% for adults, but the morbidity associated with these injuries is significant.[93]

There are five basic types of vascular injury: (1) intimal injury (flaps, disruptions, or subintimal and intramural hematomas), (2) complete wall defects with pseudoaneurysms or hemorrhage, (3) complete transections with hemorrhage or occlusion, (4) arteriovenous fistulas, and (5) spasm.[94] Blunt trauma generally causes intimal injury with possible subsequent true aneurysm development. Penetrating trauma can cause the latter four types of vascular injury.[95]

Recognizing these injuries can be difficult. Normal pulses are present in 5% to 15% of patients with a vascular injury, and overt hemorrhage causing obvious blood pressure changes is rare in orthopedic trauma.[96] However, certain findings on clinical exam, especially when compared to the unaffected limb, have a sensitivity of greater than 90%.[97] These include pulselessness, pallor, paresthesia, paralysis, rapidly expanding hematomas, relative loss of Doppler signals, obvious massive bleeding, and a palpable thrill or audible bruit.[95] For lower extremity trauma, an ABI of less than 0.9 warrants further workup for vascular injury.[90] CT angiography has supplanted conventional angiography as the definitive test to identify vascular injury. Note that patients with prolonged or severe ischemia are better served by expeditious surgical exploration; therefore, a complete diagnostic workup may be deferred.

Certain orthopedic injuries are known to have frequent clinically significant vascular injuries. These include knee dislocations, supracondylar humerus fractures, elbow dislocations, and unstable pelvic fractures. While these injuries are classically known to have vascular injuries, it is better to correlate clinical or radiographic deformity to basic vascular anatomy.

The prognosis of vascular injuries is complex, but generally related to the injured vessel's level within the extremity (i.e., proximal vs. distal) and the adequacy of collateral circulation. To illustrate the latter point, consider vascular injuries to the popliteal versus the superficial femoral artery. There is poor collateral circulation past the popliteal artery into the leg; therefore, injuries affecting the patency of the popliteal artery (i.e., knee dislocations) may lead to end-vessel thrombosis in situ secondary to low flow and subsequent need for amputation. By contrast, injury to the superficial femoral artery rarely results in amputation because of the rich collateral circulation with the profunda femoris artery.

Management

A comprehensive description of surgical techniques for vascular injuries is beyond the scope of this chapter. Typically, vascular repair involves shunt or graft placement to provide a bypass over the injured area. Damaged segments of the proximal and distal vessels are resected. An arteriogram is routinely obtained at the end of the procedure to evaluate for arterial patency, which has implications on limb salvage. All major vein injuries are repaired to increase the patency rate of the arterial repair and to prevent the sequelae of chronic venous congestion.

More relevant to this chapter, there are considerations specific to patients with concomitant orthopedic injuries that require skeletal stabilization.

The sequence of skeletal stabilization and vascular repair is controversial. Proponents of beginning with skeletal stabilization argue that traction placed during fracture stabilization could damage a repaired vessel. The counterargument is that delaying vascular repair prolongs ischemia and tissue injury. In addition, at times, the external fixation that is placed precludes adequate exposure of the injured vascular structure.

The sequence should be individualized to each patient through discussion between both surgical teams. Generally, it is recommended that the orthopedic procedure be performed first if (1) the patient does not have cold ischemia or prolonged warm ischemia or (2) the fracture pattern is so unstable (i.e., comminution, shortened) that its stability would benefit vascular repair. The vascular procedure should be performed first if (1) there is cold ischemia or (2) the patient has or is currently experiencing a prolong period of warm ischemia.[95]

Temporary versus definitive fracture fixation at the time of vascular repair is also controversial. Generally, most studies have shown benefit to temporary external fixation at the index procedure.[95,98] The external fixator should be placed away from the zone of vascular injury with the goals of maintaining the length and stability of the fracture site to protect the vascular repair.

Prophylactic fasciotomies should be considered in all patients who have restored blood flow after a vascular procedure. This practice has been associated with four times less risk for amputation and other complications after limb revascularization and supersedes any concerns about wound management.[99]

COMMON LONG BONE FRACTURES

Femur Fractures

Epidemiology and Significance

A closed femoral shaft fracture is considered a major injury in calculating the ISS. Therefore, another major injury in any other organ system qualifies the patient as multiply injured. With the exception of pathologic or insufficiency fractures in older patients, these fractures are the result of a high-energy injury. Frequently, these injuries lead to significant bleeding. Because of the geometry of the thigh, several units of blood can be lost into the tissues, with little external evidence of bleeding. Transfusion with packed red blood cells is often necessary. In addition to concerns about bleeding, the treating team should have a high suspicion of concomitant femoral neck fractures for all patients with femoral shaft fractures. As noted, there is almost a 10% incidence of these associated injuries.

Initial Management

All femur fractures must be immobilized before the patient is transported from the scene of the accident. Without immobilization, displaced femoral shaft fractures can cause increased edema, bleeding, and further damage to the surrounding soft tissues. Continued motion at the fracture site also results in increased fat embolization and contributes to the development of adult respiratory distress syndrome (ARDS). Proper immobilization begins with in-line traction in the field (see Fig. 19.19), which decreases the diameter of the thigh compartment, reducing its volume. The soft tissues are then under tension and can tamponade bleeding at the fracture site. For patients in extremis, a posterior splint alone will suffice until formal traction or immobilization can be achieved. As previously discussed, a traction pin can be placed through the proximal tibia to provide skeletal traction and to allow access to the distal femur (see Fig. 19.18). Up to 10% of a patient's body weight can be applied to a properly placed skeletal traction.

Definitive Stabilization

The recommended timing of definitive fixation of femoral shaft fractures has followed a parabolic course over the last few decades. In the 1970s, femoral shaft patients were often thought of as being "too sick to operate on." In the 1980s, this changed to become that they were "too sick *not* to operate on."[100] During this period, there was a big push to operate on femoral shaft fractures within 24 hours after admission. This treatment algorithm was dubbed early total care (ETC). In the 1990s, the pendulum started to swing the other way. Pulmonary complications were shown to be more prevalent in patients who had both chest injuries as well as early femoral fracture fixation.[101] The reasoning behind these observations was that the systemic inflammatory system was primed after the initial injury, and the pulmonary load and subsequent inflammatory response of a femoral nail being placed into the femoral canal caused a second hit to the lungs that pushed them over the threshold into ARDS. This was the birth of damage control orthopedics (DCO).

DCO primarily consists of the placement of an external fixator on the femur to hold the fracture fragments in good alignment and out to length. The goals of DCO include provisional fracture fixation that allows mobilization of the patient, hemorrhage control, soft tissue management, and the important avoidance of a major surgery (second hit).

Since the 1990s, the debate of DCO versus ETC has been lively. For the patient in extremis, DCO is definitely the best option. Similarly, the evidence has consistently held the standard of care for a stable femoral shaft patient to be ETC within 24 hours. The main points of controversy concern those patients who fall into the "borderline" category. These are multiply injured patients with both soft organ and musculoskeletal injuries. Since the 1990s, there have been multiple studies that have disputed the idea that DCO is the best first-line treatment for borderline patients. When considering the incidence of ARDS, mortality, and length of stay, these studies have found either no difference between DCO and ETC or, if there was a difference in those endpoints, it was almost always in favor of ETC.[72,102–105]

Another salient point is that, over these last few decades, we have improved how we resuscitate patients. The "borderline" patient is a moving target, and that patient frequently becomes a "stable" patient within 24 hours of admission. Assuming prompt resuscitation, the overwhelming majority of patients should have definitive fixation of a femoral shaft fracture within 24 to 48 hours. DCO is indicated if the patient is going to the operating room and there is persistent hypotension, metabolic acidosis, or a severe head injury. If DCO is performed, it is best to wait for longer than 5 days before performing definitive fixation to avoid any second hit. If the patient is not going to the operating room, the skeletal traction can be used until the patient is resuscitated.

Tibial Shaft Fractures

Epidemiology and Significance

Fractures of the diaphysis of the tibia occur by direct and indirect mechanisms. Common mechanisms are bumper injuries, gunshot wounds, and bending or torsional injuries with a firmly planted foot. Due to the anatomy of the blood supply in the tibia and the high energy involved in these injuries, treatment of tibial shaft fractures can present many difficulties. Further complicating matters, because of the minimal soft tissue coverage—especially over the medial tibia—tibia shaft fractures are often open injuries.

Blood Supply

Tibial shaft fractures tend to be slow healing as a result of their tenuous blood supply and limited soft tissue envelope. A single nutrient artery that branches from the posterior tibial artery serves the entire diaphysis. It enters the medullary canal and travels proximally and distally to anastomose with metaphyseal endosteal vessels. Although there is some contribution from the penetrating branches of the periosteal arteries that supply the outer third of the cortex, a diaphyseal fracture can easily compromise the nutrient arterial blood supply. Concomitant soft tissue stripping may leave an entire segment of tibia devascularized. This fragile environment predisposes tibial shaft fractures to impaired healing and, with open fractures, to osteomyelitis.

Associated Soft Tissue Injuries

Aside from injuries to the overlying skin and muscle, tibial shaft fractures often have other associated soft tissue injuries. Ligamentous injuries causing knee instability are common and are often identified later as a source of continued morbidity. The incidence of compartment syndrome in tibial shaft fractures is as high as 10%, so close monitoring of the patient's symptoms and, if necessary, compartment pressures is important.[106] Neurovascular injury should always be suspected and a careful examination must always be performed. The dorsalis pedis and posterior tibial arterial pulses should be palpated, and capillary refill assessed. If injury is suspected, a Doppler probe can be used to assess arterial blood flow further. ABIs should also be calculated.

Neurologic examination includes assessment of all five major nerves that travel distally in the leg. The deep peroneal nerve, traveling in the anterior compartment, can be evaluated by testing first dorsal web space sensation and foot and toe dorsiflexion. Testing of sensation along the dorsum of the foot and eversion strength can assess the superficial peroneal nerve, which travels in the lateral compartment. The tibial nerve travels in the deep posterior compartment and provides sensation to the sole of the foot and motor function to the foot and toe plantar flexors. The sural and saphenous nerves travel superficially to the muscle compartments and are both pure sensory nerves. The sural nerve supplies sensation to the lateral aspect of the heel, and the saphenous nerve supplies sensation to the medial malleolus.

In particular, vigilance should be maintained when treating proximal tibia fractures as both vascular and nerve injuries can occur. The popliteal artery and peroneal nerves are both tethered as they pass the knee and prone to being stretched. Some tibial plateau fractures are actually knee dislocations and should be treated as such.

Management and Treatment

Management and treatment of tibial shaft fractures have evolved over the years. A closed fracture with minimal displacement can be treated by cast immobilization and functional bracing. However, most fractures are now treated surgically to allow early weight bearing and rehabilitation. Reamed IM nailing is the technique of choice, when appropriate.

Plate fixation has fallen out of favor for diaphyseal fractures because of the high risk for wound healing complications. However, it remains a valuable treatment option for diaphyseal fractures that extend proximally or distally into the metaphysis, which are less amenable to IM stabilization. Minimally invasive percutaneous plating techniques have improved the results of plate fixation by limiting surgical dissection in the zone of injury. External fixation is an option for a patient who is unstable or when soft tissue injury precludes definitive fixation. Although it is generally reserved for temporary stabilization, with a good reduction, an external fixator can be used as definitive fixation. For complex fractures, a ringed external fixator is a powerful tool for correcting significant deformity or bone defects.

Humerus Shaft Fractures

Epidemiology, Acceptable Alignment, and Associated Injuries

Historically, studies have shown a nearly 95% rate of union and 85% return to full shoulder and elbow function following nonoperative treatment with a functional (Sarmiento) brace.[107] More recent data suggest that the nonunion rate may be closer to 20% and that operative management with compression plating has a significantly lower rate of malunion and nonunion.[108] Despite this, nonoperative management is the mainstay of treatment for fractures that maintain acceptable alignment. These parameters are less than 20 degrees of sagittal plane deformity, 30 degrees of coronal plane deformity, and 3 cm of shortening.[109]

Radial nerve injuries occur in up to 6% to 18% of these fractures, especially mid-shaft fractures with significant displacement.[110] This is due to the close association of the radial nerve with the posterior humeral shaft as it travels from medial to lateral in the spiral groove. The nerve enters the shaft at an average of 11 cm and exits at an average of 16 cm from the acromion; this roughly corresponds to the middle of the humeral shaft (Fig. 19.38).[111] In the trauma setting, right-sided humeral shaft fractures can be predictive of concomitant injury to the liver and other intraabdominal organs.[112]

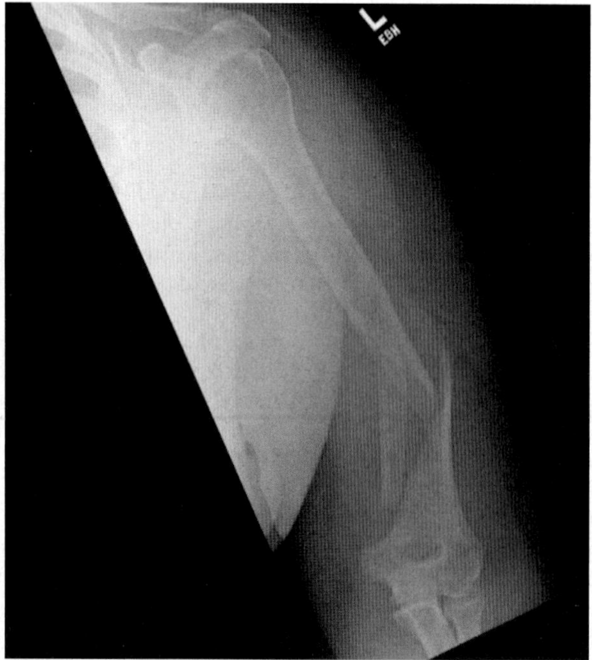

FIG. 19.38 Holstein-Lewis fracture of the humeral shaft. This patient had no radial nerve function at presentation. At the time of surgery, the nerve was found to be intact but interposed between two fracture fragments. Full radial nerve function returned by 6 months.

Treatment

There are multiple nonoperative treatment methods: coaptation splints, hanging arm casts, "sling and swathe," and functional bracing. While there are studies showing minor benefits to each method, the most common treatment is an initial coaptation splint followed by transition to functional brace (Sarmiento brace) at clinic follow-up (usually 3–7 days later). Functional bracing is not initiated in the acute setting because it relies on the compression of soft tissues to exert a hydraulic, stabilizing force on the fracture; that pressure in the face of an acute injury is painful to the patient compared to a coaptation splint. During the functional brace stage, patients are allowed free elbow flexion-extension and arm abduction to 60 degrees because motion generates hydraulic compression as the muscles change shape with motion, helping maintain alignment as well as compressing the fracture ends together.

If a patient fails closed reduction, has an unstable fracture pattern (i.e., comminution, segmental), has an ipsilateral forearm or elbow fracture, or is a polytrauma patient who could benefit from earlier mobility to rehabilitate from other injuries, operative management should be considered. Morbid obesity is also a relative indication because the thicker soft tissues limit the stabilizing force of a functional brace.[113] The mainstay of surgical management is compression plating with four bicortical screws on each side of the fracture. Other less common techniques include IM nailing and external fixation. An algorithm for treatment of this problem is presented in Fig. 19.39. There is a recent trend toward minimally invasive approaches where the plate is slid underneath muscle without full exposure; this has shown equivalent results, but its practice is not widespread at this time.[114]

When a radial nerve injury is encountered, it is likely a neuropraxia and will recover spontaneously within 3 to 4 months in 90% of patients.[110] The patient should be placed in a removable forearm splint during that time to support the wrist and fingers. If the nerve function does not return by then, an electromyography can be ordered to determine if exploration is indicated. If a coaptation splint is placed and the patient develops a radial nerve palsy afterward, then the splint should be promptly reduced. If the nerve function does not return, the nerve should be explored as it is likely in the fracture site.

CHALLENGES AND COMPLICATIONS

Missed Injuries

Missed musculoskeletal injuries account for a large proportion of delays in diagnosis within the first few days of care of a critically injured patient. Severely injured patients, especially those with a high ISS and a Glasgow Coma Scale score below 8, are more likely to have missed injuries.[115] Clinical reassessment of trauma patients within 24 hours has reduced the incidence of missed injuries by almost 40%.[115] Patients should be reexamined as they regain consciousness and resume activity. Repeated assessments should be routinely performed in all patients, especially unstable and neurologically impaired patients. The tertiary trauma survey includes a comprehensive examination and review of laboratory results and radiographs within 24 hours of initial evaluation. Specific injury patterns should be reviewed closely, especially in patients with multiple injuries and severe disability. External soft tissue trauma may be indicative of a more severe underlying injury. Formal radiology rounds can facilitate increased recognition of occult injuries.

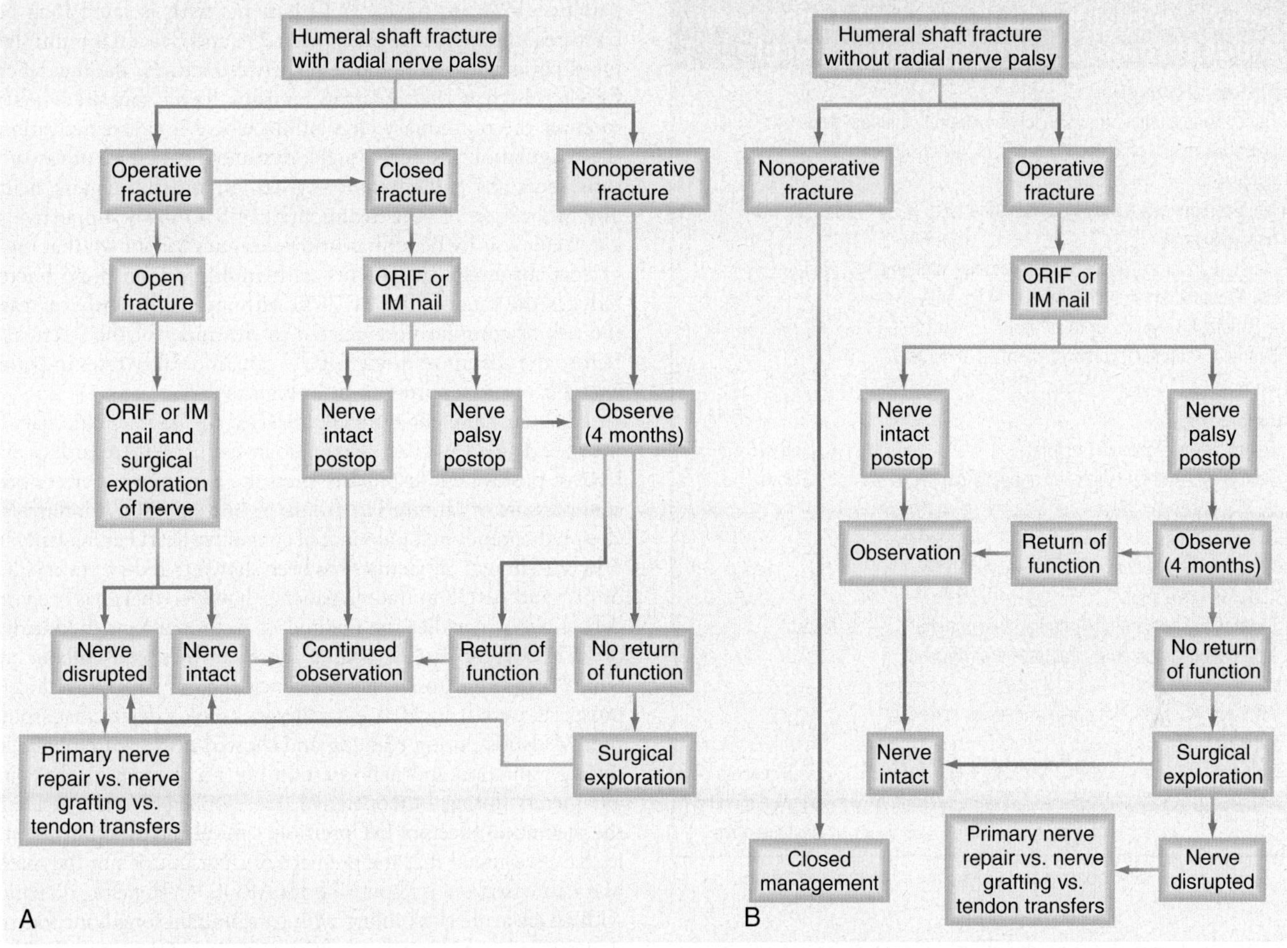

FIG. 19.39 Algorithms for management of a patient presenting with a humeral shaft fracture with (A) and without (B) radial nerve palsy. *IM,* Intramedullary; *ORIF,* open reduction internal fixation.

Drug and Alcohol Use

The incidence of drug and alcohol use in patients with musculoskeletal injuries has been reported to be as high as 50%. Prescription opiate use and abuse have also become more common in recent years and is a well-documented societal problem. Orthopedic trauma patients have a higher preinjury use of opioids than the general population. In addition, lower-income and unemployed patients are more likely to feel that their surgeon is not prescribing them enough pain medicine. Unemployed patients are also more likely to self-medicate on top of the prescribed amount of opioids.[116]

ISS have been correlated with higher inpatient opioid use. This, in turn, correlates with higher postdischarge opioid use.[117] Many institutions have instituted multimodal pain management guidelines with good success at abating opioid overuse, and this is recommended. There are ongoing multicenter trials looking at specific protocol, some of which contains nonsteroidal antiinflammatory drugs, commonly avoided by orthopedic surgeons postoperatively because of the supposed risk of nonunion.[118]

Alcohol and drug use result in more severe orthopedic injuries and more frequent injuries requiring longer hospitalization. Associated complications include those from cocaine use, such as fever, hypertension, acute myocardial ischemia, arrhythmias, and stroke. Cocaine can also facilitate cardiac arrhythmias when it is combined with halothane, nitrous oxide, or ketamine. Furthermore, the use of alcohol or drugs can adversely affect the administration of premedicating drugs. Prophylaxis for delirium tremens in postoperative patients should be performed when indicated. Inpatient detoxification consultation should be obtained before discharge.

Thromboembolic Complications

Orthopedic and trauma patients are at significantly higher rate of developing deep venous thrombosis (DVT) and pulmonary embolism (PE), each of which is associated with significantly morbidity and even mortality. Inpatient chemoprophylaxis has been shown to significantly decrease the rate of DVT and PE after both orthopedic and polytrauma admission; however, the duration to continue anticoagulation as an outpatient and in which patients remains controversial. DVT risk factors include trauma, lower extremity fractures, immobilization, hospitalization, and recent surgery.[119] Within orthopedic patients, studies have shown that fractures of the pelvis and femur are at highest risk of DVT; however, there still remains increased risk for DVT and PE after any fracture of the lower extremity.[120–122] Despite the clinical incidence of both symptomatic DVT and PE, there remains no agreed-upon protocol for routine chemoprophylaxis following orthopedic surgery and wide variation in protocols used by surgeons across the country.[123] See Table 19.8 for the authors' institutional protocol. This protocol is designed for a patient population that is almost entirely unfunded.

TABLE 19.8 Inpatient and outpatient deep venous thrombosis prophylaxis protocol.

Inpatient (Nonspine)	
• Direct trauma admission with lower extremity injuries	Lovenox 30 BID
• Lower extremity ambulatory surgery/delayed surgical admission	
• Isolated upper extremity trauma patients, nonambulatory	
• Isolated upper extremity trauma patients, ambulatory	None
*Pelvis/acetabulum fractures preoperative: hold lovenox beginning the *night prior to surgery*	
*All others, continue lovenox on morning of surgery	
Outpatient	
• Femur/hip/acetabulum fracture:	Aspirin 325 daily × 35 days
• Any lower extremity with any of below risk factors	
○ Obesity (BMI >29)	
○ Admitted to ICU	
○ Associated abdominal OR thoracic trauma	
○ Motorcycle injury	
• Isolated lower extremity trauma, tibia or distal	None
• Isolated upper extremity fractures with/without above risk factors	
• Ambulatory/outpatient upper and lower extremity surgeries	
• Spine	Case-by-case basis pending mobility postoperative

BID, Twice daily; *BMI*, body mass index; *ICU*, intensive care unit.

Multiple studies have shown high efficacy for routine chemoprophylaxis following surgery for acetabulum, hip, and femur fractures.[123–125] It is estimated that patients remain at increased risk for a DVT or PE for up to 35 days following major orthopedic surgery about the hip.[124] Additionally, there is significant literature within the joint arthroplasty field showing the benefit of routine outpatient anticoagulation following joint arthroplasty.[125,126] Studies have shown that there is no clinical benefit to routine chemoprophylaxis after hospitalization in lower extremity fractures of the tibia and distal.[120,127]

While it is relatively agreed upon that, following lower extremity fracture repair, patients remain on routine mechanical and chemoprophylaxis, the type and duration of outpatient anticoagulation patients take upon discharge vary greatly.[123] The American Academy of Chest Surgeons has a strong recommendation for chemoprophylaxis for 35 days following total hip arthroplasty, total knee arthroplasty, or hip fracture surgery.[124,128] Multiple options are available for outpatient anticoagulation, including low–molecular-weight heparin, enoxaparin, and direct clotting cascade inhibitors, all of which have been shown to decrease the incidence of both DVT and PE with similar side effect profiles.[126,129]

Pulmonary Failure: Fat Emboli Syndrome and ARDS

Fat emboli syndrome (FES) is a condition characterized by respiratory distress, altered mental status, and skin petechiae. First described in humans in 1862, it occurs in multiply injured patients, especially those with orthopedic injuries. Clinical signs are evident hours to days after an injury involving long bone or pelvic fractures. Recent literature has suggested a higher rate of fat embolism found at autopsy in trauma patients compared with nontrauma patients (82% vs. 63%).[130] In patients with isolated long bone fractures, the incidence is between 2% and 5%. In a multiply injured patient with long bone or pelvic fractures, the incidence of FES is as high as 19%. Marrow fat from the fracture site is believed to enter the pulmonary circulation, where it causes activation of the coagulation cascade, platelet dysfunction, release of vasoactive substances and inflammatory cytokines, and subsequent neutrophil infiltration.[131] The treatment of FES is mostly supportive, but a metaanalysis by Bederman and colleagues has shown that the use of corticosteroids in patients with multiple long bone fractures reduces the rate of FES by 78% without significantly increasing the risk of complications related to treatment of the fractures.[132] Before the advent of modern ICU care, mortality rates in patients with FES were reported to be as high as 20%.

FES may represent a subset of ARDS. ARDS is a pulmonary failure state defined as a Pao_2/Fio_2 ratio lower than 200 regardless of the level of positive end-expiratory pressure, a pulmonary artery occlusion pressure of 18 mm Hg or less, or bilateral diffuse infiltrates on chest radiographs in the absence of congestive heart failure. Early fixation (<24 hours) of fractures has been shown to reduce the incidence of FES and ARDS in trauma patients; however, there has been some debate about whether the method of fixation affects the incidence of FES.[77] In theory, IM nailing causes an increased embolic load, which could lead to an increased incidence of FES. A multicenter prospective study by Hall and colleagues took a device that aspirates the IM debris during reaming and showed decreased embolic load during aspiration and nail insertion but no changes in physiologic parameters during intraoperative transesophageal echo.[133] Despite the theoretical effects of IM insertion, clinical and experimental studies have suggested that the presence of chest injury, not the method of fracture fixation, is responsible for ARDS.[134] Therefore, in patients with severe acute chest injury with concomitant long bone fractures, it may be advisable to delay definitive fixation of the fracture with IM devices until the patient's pulmonary status has stabilized. Temporary stabilization with external fixation may be warranted, which not only helps with resuscitation and pain control but also decreases the embolization of fat seen with moving fracture ends.

POSTOPERATIVE MOBILIZATION

The benefits of early fixation and mobilization of multiply injured patients have been discussed. However, a distinction between mobilization and weight bearing is essential. Mobilization is transfer of the patient from the supine position, either under the patient's own power or with the help of nurses or therapists. This includes turning the patient every shift by the nurse, sitting the patient up in bed, or transferring the patient to a chair. All patients should be mobilized by the first or second postoperative day if their general condition permits. Mobilization helps prevent the development of pulmonary and septic complications.

Weight bearing, in contrast, is transmission of a load through an extremity. For a patient to be allowed to bear weight on an injured extremity, the following three conditions must be met:

1. There must be bone-to-bone contact at the fracture site as demonstrated intraoperatively or on postreduction radiographs. Without contact of the fracture ends, the fixation devices will be subjected to all the stresses applied to the extremity. While the implants are robust, if the bone does not heal, eventually, the metal will fatigue and fail.
2. Stable fixation of the fracture must be achieved. By definition, stable fixation is not disrupted when it is subjected to normal physiologic loads. Stable fixation is dependent on a number

of factors. Fixation may be less than ideal in patients with osteopenic bone or severely comminuted fractures. When excessive loads are anticipated, such as with heavy or obese patients, the typical fixation may not be adequate.

3. The patient must be able to comply with the weight-bearing status. Frequently, reliability of the patient is a significant consideration in the determination of weight-bearing status. Social, psychological, or emotional circumstances can affect a patient's ability to comply with weight-bearing restrictions.

Unless all three criteria are met, the fixation will need to be protected with restricted weight-bearing status. Touch-down weight bearing allows the patient to place the foot of the affected extremity flat on the floor, without bearing any of the patient's body weight. Touch-down weight bearing is often permitted in patients with injuries around the hip and allows extension of the hip and knee and dorsiflexion at the ankle. This natural position relaxes the hip musculature and minimizes joint reactive forces. Crutch walking with the foot off the floor (non–weight bearing) leads to a significant increase in force across the hip joint because of contraction of the muscles around the hip. Toe-touch weight bearing, a phrase often used synonymously with touch-down weight bearing, is an unfortunate use of terminology. Most patients attempt to walk while touching only the toe of the injured extremity to the ground. In this position, the hip and knee are flexed, and the ankle is held in equinus. When this status is maintained for any significant amount of time, contractures at the hip, knee, and ankle are common. For this reason, use of this terminology is discouraged.

Partial weight bearing is defined in terms of the percentage of body weight applied to an injured extremity. It is gradually increased as the fracture gains stability through healing. With the use of a scale, the patient can learn what different amounts of body weight feel like. When a fracture and the patient are stable enough to withstand normal loads, weight bearing as tolerated is instituted. It is believed that reliable patients limit their own weight bearing according to their pain.

Even when weight bearing is not allowed, mobilization of affected and adjacent joints is typically performed within a few days. After surgical treatment, joints are typically immobilized briefly and then allowed passive or active range of motion in bed if weight bearing is not prudent. Early joint mobilization decreases the likelihood of fibrosis and therefore increases early mobility. Furthermore, joint motion is necessary for the good health of articular cartilage. Cartilage is nourished from synovial fluid most efficiently when the joint is moving. Early joint mobilization has become a basic tenet of orthopedic care and has led to a decrease in the morbidity associated with musculoskeletal injuries.

SUMMARY

In the setting of acute trauma, preservation of a patient's life takes precedence over preservation of a limb. However, injuries to the extremities and axial skeleton may be life-threatening in rare circumstances (e.g., hemorrhage secondary to vascular injury from pelvic or long bone fractures). These must be recognized early and managed appropriately. Once the critical period has passed, musculoskeletal injuries are a major cause of posttraumatic morbidity, as demonstrated by increased healthcare costs, lost work days, physical disability, emotional distress, and diminished quality of life. Accordingly, it is essential that a detailed and complete extremity and axial musculoskeletal survey be performed on every patient, that injuries be identified early, and that the consulting orthopedic surgical team be notified of the specifics of these injuries in a timely fashion. It is essential that the trauma team have a high index of suspicion for the orthopedic emergencies discussed for any patient who has experienced high-energy trauma. Moreover, the patient should not be transported from the trauma room, unless necessary for lifesaving interventions, until the orthopedic team has evaluated and stabilized the involved extremity to protect it against further injury and morbidity. Finally, appropriate treatment of musculoskeletal injuries is a multidisciplinary undertaking. With cooperation and collaboration of all treating teams—general surgery, vascular surgery, neurosurgery, plastic surgery, internal medicine, and physical therapy—we will be able to ensure the best possible outcome for our patients.

SELECTED REFERENCES

Bosse MJ, McCarthy ML, Jones AL, et al. The insensate foot following severe lower extremity trauma: An indication for amputation? *J Bone Joint Surg Am.* 2005;87:2601–2608.

One of the many seminal articles to come out of the Lower Extremity Assessment Project, this article is representative of that collective set of publications in its longitudinal effect on the practice of orthopedic trauma.

Egol KA, Koval KJ, Zuckerman JD. *Handbook of Fractures.* 2nd ed. Philadelphia: Wolters Kluwer; 2014.

This conveniently sized handbook is the ideal reference for physicians managing musculoskeletal injuries in the emergency setting. Comprehensive but concise, this guide discusses epidemiology, anatomy, mechanism of injury, clinical evaluation, radiologic evaluation, classification, treatment, and management of complications of most acute musculoskeletal injuries.

Petrisor B, Sun X, Bhandari M, et al. Fluid lavage of open wounds (FLOW): a multicenter, blinded, factorial pilot trial comparing alternative irrigating solutions and pressures in patients with open fractures. *J Trauma.* 2011;71:596–606.

This multicenter trial illustrated that what is most simple is sometimes best: low-flow normal saline was the cheapest, best option for irrigating open fractures.

Vallier HA, Moore TA, Como JJ, et al. Teamwork in trauma: system adjustment to a protocol for the management of multiply injured patients. *J Orthop Trauma.* 2015;29:e446–e450.

This recent article is representative of the recent push back toward early total care (ETC). Dr. Vallier and associates have published extensively on this topic, and they have several well-done studies published supporting aggressive resuscitation and ETC.

REFERENCES

1. Court-Brown CM, Caesar B. Epidemiology of adult fractures: a review. *Injury*. 2006;37:691–697.
2. Clement RC, Carr BG, Kallan MJ, et al. Who needs an orthopedic trauma surgeon? An analysis of US national injury patterns. *J Trauma Acute Care Surg*. 2013;75:687–692.
3. MacKenzie EJ, Bosse MJ, Kellam JF, et al. Early predictors of long-term work disability after major limb trauma. *J Trauma*. 2006;61:688–694.
4. O'Toole RV, Lindbloom BJ, Hui E, et al. Are bilateral femoral fractures no longer a marker for death?. *J Orthop Trauma*. 2014;28:77–81; discussion 81–72.
5. Paydar S, Ghaffarpasand F, Foroughi M, et al. Role of routine pelvic radiography in initial evaluation of stable, high-energy, blunt trauma patients. *Emerg Med J*. 201330:724-727 .
6. Verbeek DO, Ponsen KJ, van Delden OM, et al. The need for pelvic angiographic embolisation in stable pelvic fracture patients with a "blush" on computed tomography. *Injury*. 2014;45:2111.
7. Deunk J, Brink M, Dekker HM, et al. Predictors for the selection of patients for abdominal CT after blunt trauma: a proposal for a diagnostic algorithm. *Ann Surg*. 2010;251:512–520.
8. Mathen R, Inaba K, Munera F, et al. Prospective evaluation of multislice computed tomography versus plain radiographic cervical spine clearance in trauma patients. *J Trauma*. 2007;62:1427–1431.
9. O'Toole RV, Dancy L, Dietz AR, et al. Diagnosis of femoral neck fracture associated with femoral shaft fracture: blinded comparison of computed tomography and plain radiography. *J Orthop Trauma*. 2013;27:325–330.
10. Medina O, Arom GA, Yeranosian MG, et al. Vascular and nerve injury after knee dislocation: a systematic review. *Clin Orthop Relat Res*. 2014;472:2621–2629.
11. Levy BA, Fanelli GC, Whelan DB, et al. Controversies in the treatment of knee dislocations and multiligament reconstruction. *J Am Acad Orthop Surg*. 2009;17:197–206.
12. Saveli CC, Morgan SJ, Belknap RW, et al. Prophylactic antibiotics in open fractures: a pilot randomized clinical safety study. *J Orthop Trauma*. 2013;27:552–557.
13. Lack WD, Karunakar MA, Angerame MR, et al. Type III open tibia fractures: immediate antibiotic prophylaxis minimizes infection. *J Orthop Trauma*. 2015;29:1–6.
14. Bommiasamy AK, Opel D, McCallum R, et al. Conscious sedation versus rapid sequence intubation for the reduction of native traumatic hip dislocation. *Am J Surg*. 2018;216:869–873.
15. Updegrove GF, Mourad W, Abboud JA. Humeral shaft fractures. *J Shoulder Elbow Surg*. 2018;27:e87–e97.
16. Gosling T, Giannoudis PV. Femoral shaft fractures. In: Browner BD, Jupiter JB, Krettek C, et al., eds. *Skeletal Trauma: Basic Science, Management, and Reconstruction*. 5th ed. Philadelphia: Elsevier Saunders; 2015:1787–1821.
17. Routt Jr MLC, Gary J. Surgical treatment of acetabular fractures. In: Browner BD, Jupiter JB, Krettek C, et al., eds. *Skeletal Trauma: Basic Science, Management, and Reconstruction*. 5th ed. Philadelphia: Elsevier Saunders; 2015:1107–1161.
18. Bumpass DB, Ricci WM, McAndrew CM, et al. A prospective study of pain reduction and knee dysfunction comparing femoral skeletal traction and splinting in adult trauma patients. *J Orthop Trauma*. 2015;29:112–118.
19. Austin DC, Donegan D, Mehta S. Low complication rates associated with the application of lower extremity traction pins. *J Orthop Trauma*. 2015;29:e259–e265.
20. Even JL, Richards JE, Crosby CG, et al. Preoperative skeletal versus cutaneous traction for femoral shaft fractures treated within 24 hours. *J Orthop Trauma*. 2012;26:e177–182.
21. Johansen K, Daines M, Howey T, et al. Objective criteria accurately predict amputation following lower extremity trauma. *J Trauma*. 1990;30:568–572; discussion 572–563.
22. Lewis PM, Waddell JP. When is the ideal time to operate on a patient with a fracture of the hip?: a review of the available literature. *Bone Joint J*. 2016;98-B:1573–1581.
23. Vallier HA, Dolenc AJ, Moore TA. Early appropriate care: a protocol to standardize resuscitation assessment and to expedite fracture care reduces hospital stay and enhances revenue. *J Orthop Trauma*. 2016;30:306–311.
24. Vallier HA, Moore TA, Como JJ, et al. Teamwork in trauma: system adjustment to a protocol for the management of multiply injured patients. *J Orthop Trauma*. 2015;29:e446–e450.
25. Vallier HA, Wang X, Moore TA, et al. Timing of orthopaedic surgery in multiple trauma patients: development of a protocol for early appropriate care. *J Orthop Trauma*. 2013;27:543–551.
26. Buckwalter JA. Advancing the science and art of orthopaedics. Lessons from history. *J Bone Joint Surg Am*. 2000;82-A:1782–1803.
27. Chang Y, Kennedy SA, Bhandari M, et al. Effects of antibiotic prophylaxis in patients with open fracture of the extremities: a systematic review of randomized controlled trials. *JBJS Rev*. 2015;3.
28. Gustilo RB, Gruninger RP, Davis T. Classification of type III (severe) open fractures relative to treatment and results. *Orthopedics*. 1987;10:1781–1788.
29. Gustilo RB, Merkow RL, Templeman D. The management of open fractures. *J Bone Joint Surg Am*. 1990;72:299–304.
30. Papakostidis C, Kanakaris NK, Pretel J, et al. Prevalence of complications of open tibial shaft fractures stratified as per the Gustilo-Anderson classification. *Injury*. 2011;42:1408–1415.
31. Brumback RJ, Jones AL. Interobserver agreement in the classification of open fractures of the tibia. The results of a survey of two hundred and forty-five orthopaedic surgeons. *J Bone Joint Surg Am*. 1994;76:1162–1166.
32. Horn BD, Rettig ME. Interobserver reliability in the Gustilo and Anderson classification of open fractures. *J Orthop Trauma*. 1993;7:357–360.
33. Merritt K. Factors increasing the risk of infection in patients with open fractures. *J Trauma*. 1988;28:823–827.
34. Patzakis MJ, Wilkins J. Factors influencing infection rate in open fracture wounds. *Clin Orthop Relat Res*. 1989:36–40.
35. Zalavras CG. Prevention of infection in open fractures. *Infect Dis Clin North Am*. 2017;31:339–352.

36. Lack W, Seymour R, Bickers A, et al. Prehospital antibiotic prophylaxis for open fractures: practicality and safety. *Prehosp Emerg Care.* 2019;23:385–388.
37. Gosselin RA, Roberts I, Gillespie WJ. Antibiotics for preventing infection in open limb fractures. *Cochrane Database Syst Rev.* 2004:CD003764.
38. Redfern J, Wasilko SM, Groth ME, et al. Surgical site infections in patients with type 3 open fractures: comparing antibiotic prophylaxis with cefazolin plus gentamicin versus piperacillin/tazobactam. *J Orthop Trauma.* 2016;30:415–419.
39. Obremskey W, Molina C, Collinge C, et al. Current practice in the management of open fractures among orthopaedic trauma surgeons. Part A: initial management. A survey of orthopaedic trauma surgeons. *J Orthop Trauma.* 2014;28:e198–202.
40. Hauser CJ, Adams Jr CA, Eachempati SR, et al. Surgical Infection Society guideline: prophylactic antibiotic use in open fractures: an evidence-based guideline. *Surg Infect (Larchmt).* 2006;7:379–405.
41. Hoff WS, Bonadies JA, Cachecho R, et al. East Practice Management Guidelines Work Group: update to practice management guidelines for prophylactic antibiotic use in open fractures. *J Trauma.* 2011;70:751–754.
42. Spencer J, Smith A, Woods D. The effect of time delay on infection in open long-bone fractures: a 5-year prospective audit from a district general hospital. *Ann R Coll Surg Engl.* 2004;86:108–112.
43. Schenker ML, Yannascoli S, Baldwin KD, et al. Does timing to operative debridement affect infectious complications in open long-bone fractures? A systematic review. *J Bone Joint Surg Am.* 2012;94:1057–1064.
44. Skaggs DL, Friend L, Alman B, et al. The effect of surgical delay on acute infection following 554 open fractures in children. *J Bone Joint Surg Am.* 2005;87:8–12.
45. Sassoon A, Riehl J, Rich A, et al. Muscle viability revisited: are we removing normal muscle? A critical evaluation of dogmatic debridement. *J Orthop Trauma.* 2016;30:17–21.
46. Svoboda SJ, Bice TG, Gooden HA, et al. Comparison of bulb syringe and pulsed lavage irrigation with use of a bioluminescent musculoskeletal wound model. *J Bone Joint Surg Am.* 2006;88:2167–2174.
47. Anglen JO. Comparison of soap and antibiotic solutions for irrigation of lower-limb open fracture wounds. A prospective, randomized study. *J Bone Joint Surg Am.* 2005;87:1415–1422.
48. Crowley DJ, Kanakaris NK, Giannoudis PV. Irrigation of the wounds in open fractures. *J Bone Joint Surg Br.* 2007;89:580–585.
49. Petrisor B, Sun X, Bhandari M, et al. Fluid lavage of open wounds (FLOW): a multicenter, blinded, factorial pilot trial comparing alternative irrigating solutions and pressures in patients with open fractures. *J Trauma.* 2011;71:596–606.
50. Webb LX. New techniques in wound management: vacuum-assisted wound closure. *J Am Acad Orthop Surg.* 2002;10:303–311.
51. Ly TV, Travison TG, Castillo RC, et al. Ability of lower-extremity injury severity scores to predict functional outcome after limb salvage. *J Bone Joint Surg Am.* 2008;90:1738–1743.
52. Higgins TF, Klatt JB, Beals TC. Lower Extremity Assessment Project (LEAP)—the best available evidence on limb-threatening lower extremity trauma. *Orthop Clin North Am.* 2010;41:233–239.
53. Bosse MJ, McCarthy ML, Jones AL, et al. The insensate foot following severe lower extremity trauma: an indication for amputation? *J Bone Joint Surg Am.* 2005;87:2601–2608.
54. Doukas WC, Hayda RA, Frisch HM, et al. The Military Extremity Trauma Amputation/Limb Salvage (METALS) study: outcomes of amputation versus limb salvage following major lower-extremity trauma. *J Bone Joint Surg Am.* 2013;95:138–145.
55. Hwang JS, Koury KL, Gorgy G, et al. Evaluation of intra-articular fracture extension after gunshot wounds to the lower extremity: plain radiographs versus computer tomography. *J Orthop Trauma.* 2017;31:334–338.
56. Nguyen MP, Reich MS, O'Donnell JA, et al. Infection and complications after low-velocity intra-articular gunshot injuries. *J Orthop Trauma.* 2017;31:330–333.
57. Miller AN, Carroll EA, Pilson HT. Transabdominal gunshot wounds of the hip and pelvis. *J Am Acad Orthop Surg.* 2013;21:286–292.
58. Schemitsch EH, Bhandari M, Guyatt G, et al. Prognostic factors for predicting outcomes after intramedullary nailing of the tibia. *J Bone Joint Surg Am.* 2012;94:1786–1793.
59. Bhattacharyya T, Vrahas MS. The medical-legal aspects of compartment syndrome. *J Bone Joint Surg Am.* 2004;86-A:864–868.
60. Whitney A, O'Toole RV, Hui E, et al. Do one-time intracompartmental pressure measurements have a high false-positive rate in diagnosing compartment syndrome? *J Trauma Acute Care Surg.* 2014;76:479–483.
61. Heckman MM, Whitesides Jr TE, Grewe SR, et al. Compartment pressure in association with closed tibial fractures. The relationship between tissue pressure, compartment, and the distance from the site of the fracture. *J Bone Joint Surg Am.* 1994;76:1285–1292.
62. Prayson MJ, Chen JL, Hampers D, et al. Baseline compartment pressure measurements in isolated lower extremity fractures without clinical compartment syndrome. *J Trauma.* 2006;60:1037–1040.
63. McQueen MM, Court-Brown CM. Compartment monitoring in tibial fractures. The pressure threshold for decompression. *J Bone Joint Surg Br.* 1996;78:99–104.
64. Al-Dadah OQ, Darrah C, Cooper A, et al. Continuous compartment pressure monitoring vs. clinical monitoring in tibial diaphyseal fractures. *Injury.* 2008;39:1204–1209.
65. Reverte MM, Dimitriou R, Kanakaris NK, et al. What is the effect of compartment syndrome and fasciotomies on fracture healing in tibial fractures? *Injury.* 2011;42:1402–1407.
66. Crespo AM, Manoli 3rd A, Konda SR, et al. Development of compartment syndrome negatively impacts length of stay and cost after tibia fracture. *J Orthop Trauma.* 2015;29:312–315.
67. Smith W, Williams A, Agudelo J, et al. Early predictors of mortality in hemodynamically unstable pelvis fractures. *J Orthop Trauma.* 2007;21:31–37.
68. Starr AJ, Griffin DR, Reinert CM, et al. Pelvic ring disruptions: prediction of associated injuries, transfusion requirement, pelvic arteriography, complications, and mortality. *J Orthop Trauma.* 2002;16:553–561.
69. Lybrand K, Bell A, Rodericks D, et al. APC injuries with symphyseal fixation: what affects outcome? *J Orthop Trauma.* 2017;31:27–30.

70. Gibson PD, Adams MR, Koury KL, et al. Inadvertent reduction of symphyseal diastasis during computed tomography. *J Orthop Trauma*. 2016;30:474–478.
71. Avilucea FR, Archdeacon MT, Collinge CA, et al. Fixation strategy using sequential intraoperative examination under anesthesia for unstable lateral compression pelvic ring injuries reliably predicts union with minimal displacement. *J Bone Joint Surg Am*. 2018;100:1503–1508.
72. Morshed S, Miclau 3rd T, Bembom O, et al. Delayed internal fixation of femoral shaft fracture reduces mortality among patients with multisystem trauma. *J Bone Joint Surg Am*. 2009;91:3–13.
73. Toth L, King KL, McGrath B, et al. Factors associated with pelvic fracture-related arterial bleeding during trauma resuscitation: a prospective clinical study. *J Orthop Trauma*. 2014;28:489–495.
74. Knops SP, Schep NW, Spoor CW, et al. Comparison of three different pelvic circumferential compression devices: a biomechanical cadaver study. *J Bone Joint Surg Am*. 2011;93:230–240.
75. Lindvall E, Davis J, Martirosian A, et al. Bilateral internal iliac artery embolization results in an unacceptably high rate of complications in patients requiring pelvic/acetabular surgery. *J Orthop Trauma*. 2018;32:445–451.
76. Burlew CC, Moore EE, Stahel PF, et al. Preperitoneal pelvic packing reduces mortality in patients with life-threatening hemorrhage due to unstable pelvic fractures. *J Trauma Acute Care Surg*. 2017;82:233–242.
77. Vallier HA, Super DM, Moore TA, et al. Do patients with multiple system injury benefit from early fixation of unstable axial fractures? The effects of timing of surgery on initial hospital course. *J Orthop Trauma*. 2013;27:405–412.
78. Lee C, Sciadini M. The use of external fixation for the management of the unstable anterior pelvic ring. *J Orthop Trauma*. 2018;32(suppl 6):S14–S17.
79. Vallier HA, Cureton BA, Schubeck D. Pregnancy outcomes after pelvic ring injury. *J Orthop Trauma*. 2012;26:302–307.
80. Anderson PA, Gugala Z, Lindsey RW, et al. Clearing the cervical spine in the blunt trauma patient. *J Am Acad Orthop Surg*. 2010;18:149–159.
81. Vaccaro AR, Lehman Jr RA, Hurlbert RJ, et al. A new classification of thoracolumbar injuries: the importance of injury morphology, the integrity of the posterior ligamentous complex, and neurologic status. *Spine (Phila Pa 1976)*. 2005;30:2325–2333.
82. Patel AA, Vaccaro AR. Thoracolumbar spine trauma classification. *J Am Acad Orthop Surg*. 2010;18:63–71.
83. Robinson Y, Heyde CE, Forsth P, et al. Kyphoplasty in osteoporotic vertebral compression fractures—guidelines and technical considerations. *J Orthop Surg Res*. 2011;6:43.
84. Gjolaj JP, Williams SK. Thoracic and lumber spinal injuries. In: Garfin S, Eismont F, Bell G, et al., eds. *Rothman-Simeone and Herkowitz's the Spine*. 7th ed. Philadelphia: Elsevier Saunders; 2018:1333–1363.
85. Adams MR, Reilly MC. Hip dislocations and associated fractures of the femoral head. In: Stannard JP, Schmidt AH, eds. *Surgical Treatment of Orthopaedic Trauma*. 2nd ed. New York: Thieme; 2016:2591–2643.
86. Kellam P, Ostrum RF. Systematic review and meta-analysis of avascular necrosis and posttraumatic arthritis after traumatic hip dislocation. *J Orthop Trauma*. 2016;30:10–16.
87. Stannard JP, Fanelli GC. Knee dislocations and ligamentous injuries. In: Stannard JP, Schmidt AH, eds. *Surgical Treatment of Orthopaedic Trauma*. 2nd ed. New York: Thieme; 2016:3378–3492.
88. Stannard JP, Sheils TM, Lopez-Ben RR, et al. Vascular injuries in knee dislocations: The role of physical examination in determining the need for arteriography. *J Bone Joint Surg Am*. 2004;86:910–915.
89. Miranda FE, Dennis JW, Veldenz HC, et al. Confirmation of the safety and accuracy of physical examination in the evaluation of knee dislocation for injury of the popliteal artery: a prospective study. *J Trauma*. 2002;52:247–251; discussion 251–242.
90. Long B, April MD. What is the utility of physical examination, ankle-brachial index, and ultrasonography for the diagnosis of arterial injury in patients with penetrating extremity trauma? *Ann Emerg Med*. 2018;71:525–528.
91. Martinez D, Sweatman K, Thompson EC. Popliteal artery injury associated with knee dislocations. *Am Surg*. 2001;67:165–167.
92. Maity A, Roy DS, Mondal BC. A prospective randomised clinical trial comparing FARES method with the Eachempati external rotation method for reduction of acute anterior dislocation of shoulder. *Injury*. 2012;43:1066–1070.
93. Barmparas G, Inaba K, Talving P, et al. Pediatric vs adult vascular trauma: a National Trauma Databank review. *J Pediatr Surg*. 2010;45:1404–1412.
94. Feliciano DV, Moore FA, Moore EE, et al. Evaluation and management of peripheral vascular injury. Part 1. Western Trauma Association/critical decisions in trauma. *J Trauma*. 2011;70:1551–1556.
95. Mavrogenis AF, Panagopoulos GN, Kokkalis ZT, et al. Vascular injury in orthopedic trauma. *Orthopedics*. 2016;39:249–259.
96. Barnes CJ, Pietrobon R, Higgins LD. Does the pulse examination in patients with traumatic knee dislocation predict a surgical arterial injury? A meta-analysis. *J Trauma*. 2002;53:1109–1114.
97. Inaba K, Branco BC, Reddy S, et al. Prospective evaluation of multidetector computed tomography for extremity vascular trauma. *J Trauma*. 2011;70:808–815.
98. Howard PW, Makin GS. Lower limb fractures with associated vascular injury. *J Bone Joint Surg Br*. 1990;72:116–120.
99. Farber A, Tan TW, Hamburg NM, et al. Early fasciotomy in patients with extremity vascular injury is associated with decreased risk of adverse limb outcomes: a review of the National Trauma Data Bank. *Injury*. 2012;43:1486–1491.
100. Bone LB, Johnson KD, Weigelt J, et al. Early versus delayed stabilization of femoral fractures. A prospective randomized study. *J Bone Joint Surg Am*. 1989;71:336–340.
101. Pape HC, Regel G, Dwenger A, et al. Influence of thoracic trauma and primary femoral intramedullary nailing on the incidence of ARDS in multiple trauma patients. *Injury*. 1993;24(suppl 3):S82–103.
102. Nahm NJ, Como JJ, Wilber JH, et al. Early appropriate care: definitive stabilization of femoral fractures within 24 hours of injury is safe in most patients with multiple injuries. *J Trauma*. 2011;71:175–185.
103. Tuttle MS, Smith WR, Williams AE, et al. Safety and efficacy of damage control external fixation versus early definitive stabilization for femoral shaft fractures in the multiple-injured patient. *J Trauma*. 2009;67:602–605.

104. Nicholas B, Toth L, van Wessem K, et al. Borderline femur fracture patients: early total care or damage control orthopaedics? *ANZ J Surg*. 2011;81:148–153.
105. Nahm NJ, Vallier HA. Timing of definitive treatment of femoral shaft fractures in patients with multiple injuries: a systematic review of randomized and nonrandomized trials. *J Trauma Acute Care Surg*. 2012;73:1046–1063.
106. Park S, Ahn J, Gee AO, et al. Compartment syndrome in tibial fractures. *J Orthop Trauma*. 2009;23:514–518.
107. Papasoulis E, Drosos GI, Ververidis AN, et al. Functional bracing of humeral shaft fractures. A review of clinical studies. *Injury*. 2010;41:e21–e27.
108. Denard Jr A, Richards JE, Obremskey WT, et al. Outcome of nonoperative vs operative treatment of humeral shaft fractures: a retrospective study of 213 patients. *Orthopedics*. 2010;33.
109. Klenerman L. Fractures of the shaft of the humerus. *J Bone Joint Surg Br*. 1966;48:105–111.
110. Shao YC, Harwood P, Grotz MR, et al. Radial nerve palsy associated with fractures of the shaft of the humerus: a systematic review. *J Bone Joint Surg Br*. 2005;87:1647–1652.
111. Guse TR, Ostrum RF. The surgical anatomy of the radial nerve around the humerus. *Clin Orthop Relat Res*. 1995:149–153.
112. Adili A, Bhandari M, Sprague S, et al. Humeral shaft fractures as predictors of intra-abdominal injury in motor vehicle collision victims. *Arch Orthop Trauma Surg*. 2002;122:5–9.
113. Jensen AT, Rasmussen S. Being overweight and multiple fractures are indications for operative treatment of humeral shaft fractures. *Injury*. 1995;26:263–264.
114. Kim JW, Oh CW, Byun YS, et al. A prospective randomized study of operative treatment for noncomminuted humeral shaft fractures: conventional open plating versus minimal invasive plate osteosynthesis. *J Orthop Trauma*. 2015;29:189–194.
115. Pfeifer R, Pape HC. Missed injuries in trauma patients: a literature review. *Patient Saf Surg*. 2008;2:20.
116. Gangavalli A, Malige A, Terres G, et al. Misuse of opioids in orthopaedic postoperative patients. *J Orthop Trauma*. 2017;31:e103–e109.
117. Flanagan CD, Wysong EF, Ramey JS, et al. Understanding the opioid epidemic: factors predictive of inpatient and post-discharge prescription opioid use after orthopaedic trauma. *J Orthop Trauma*. 2018;32:e408–e414.
118. Castillo RC, Raja SN, Frey KP, et al. Improving pain management and long-term outcomes following high-energy orthopaedic trauma (Pain Study). *J Orthop Trauma*. 2017;31(suppl 1):S71–S77.
119. Cushman M. Epidemiology and risk factors for venous thrombosis. *Semin Hematol*. 2007;44:62–69.
120. Patterson JT, Morshed S. Chemoprophylaxis for venous thromboembolism in operative treatment of fractures of the tibia and distal bones: a systematic review and meta-analysis. *J Orthop Trauma*. 2017;31:453–460.
121. Whiting PS, Jahangir AA. Thromboembolic disease after orthopedic trauma. *Orthop Clin North Am*. 2016;47:335–344.
122. Decker S, Weaver MJ. Deep venous thrombosis following different isolated lower extremity fractures: what is known about prevalences, locations, risk factors and prophylaxis? *Eur J Trauma Emerg Surg*. 2013;39:591–598.
123. Sagi HC, Ahn J, Ciesla D, et al. Venous thromboembolism prophylaxis in orthopaedic trauma patients: a survey of OTA Member Practice Patterns and OTA Expert Panel recommendations. *J Orthop Trauma*. 2015;29:e355–e362.
124. Francis CW. Prevention of VTE in patients having major orthopedic surgery. *J Thromb Thrombolysis*. 2013;35:359–367.
125. Forster R, Stewart M. Anticoagulants (extended duration) for prevention of venous thromboembolism following total hip or knee replacement or hip fracture repair. *Cochrane Database Syst Rev*. 2016;3:CD004179.
126. Bala A, Huddleston 3rd JI, Goodman SB, et al. Venous thromboembolism prophylaxis after TKA: aspirin, warfarin, enoxaparin, or factor Xa inhibitors? *Clin Orthop Relat Res*. 2017;475:2205–2213.
127. Selby R, Geerts WH, Kreder HJ, et al. A double-blind, randomized controlled trial of the prevention of clinically important venous thromboembolism after isolated lower leg fractures. *J Orthop Trauma*. 2015;29:224–230.
128. Falck-Ytter Y, Francis CW, Johanson NA, et al. Prevention of VTE in orthopedic surgery patients: antithrombotic therapy and prevention of thrombosis, 9th ed: American College of Chest Physicians evidence-based clinical practice guidelines. *Chest*. 2012;141:e278S–e325S.
129. Douketis JD, Eikelboom JW, Quinlan DJ, et al. Short-duration prophylaxis against venous thromboembolism after total hip or knee replacement: a meta-analysis of prospective studies investigating symptomatic outcomes. *Arch Intern Med*. 2002;162:1465–1471.
130. Eriksson EA, Rickey J, Leon SM, et al. Fat embolism in pediatric patients: an autopsy evaluation of incidence and etiology. *J Crit Care*. 2015;30:221; e221–e225.
131. Blankstein M, Byrick RJ, Nakane M, et al. Amplified inflammatory response to sequential hemorrhage, resuscitation, and pulmonary fat embolism: an animal study. *J Bone Joint Surg Am*. 2010;92:149–161.
132. Bederman SS, Bhandari M, McKee MD, et al. Do corticosteroids reduce the risk of fat embolism syndrome in patients with long-bone fractures? A meta-analysis. *Can J Surg*. 2009;52:386–393.
133. Hall JA, McKee MD, Vicente MR, et al. Prospective randomized clinical trial investigating the effect of the reamer-irrigator-aspirator on the volume of embolic load and respiratory function during intramedullary nailing of femoral shaft fractures. *J Orthop Trauma*. 2017;31:200–204.
134. Morley JR, Smith RM, Pape HC, et al. Stimulation of the local femoral inflammatory response to fracture and intramedullary reaming: a preliminary study of the source of the second hit phenomenon. *J Bone Joint Surg Br*. 2008;90:393–399.

20 CHAPTER

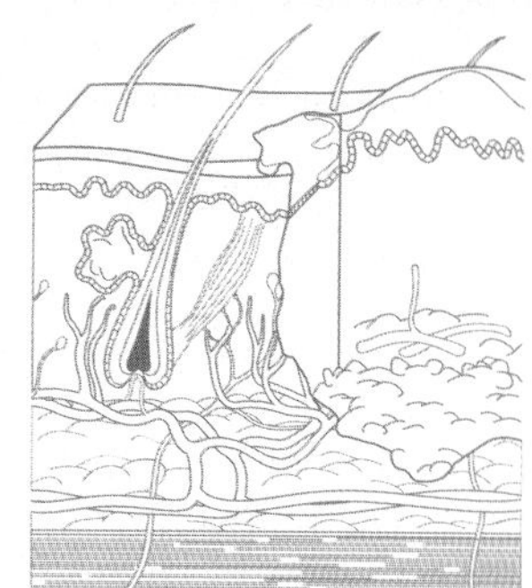

Burns

Steven E. Wolf

OUTLINE

GENERAL CONSIDERATIONS

In 2017, approximately 400,000 people were burned in the United States, of whom 3400 died. The epidemiological trends from 2001 to 2017 demonstrate that the U.S. population has increased from 285,000,000 to 326,000,000 people, a nominal 14% increase. Correspondingly, the incidence of burns decreased from 520,000 to 403,000, a 23% decrease. Fatal burns also decreased from 3800 deaths in 2001 to 3400 deaths in 2017 (10% decrease).[1] From these data, we conclude that the number of burns has decreased per capita over this time period at an appreciable rate; however, burns remains a real public health threat, as these changes seem to be leveling off at about 125 recorded burns per 100,000 people (Fig. 20.1). If the population continues to increase, we expect that burns will continue to be commonly encountered. When separated into children (0–18 years), adults (19–65 years), and the elderly (>65 years), these trends remain for some, decreasing mostly in children and moderate decreases in adults. However, the number of burns in the elderly has actually increased, likely in association with the growing percentage of the population (Fig. 20.2). Therefore, this is the best group for new targeted prevention strategies.

Fortunately, most burn cases are mild to moderate and are commonly treated in the outpatient setting. However, approximately 40,000 burns per year in the United States are severe enough to receive inpatient hospitalization for treatment.[2] It is estimated by the Centers for Disease Control and Prevention that the annual direct healthcare cost for burns is $1.5 billion.[1] For context, in 2014, about 10% of the United States population sustained some form of injury receiving recorded treatment, but very few sustained fatal injuries (0.6 per 1000); for comparison, the mortality rate for those with burns is about 1 per 1000, a 67% increase in injury-related mortality. For deaths from injury, those with burns represented 1.6% of all injury fatalities but only 1.3% of recorded injuries. Thus, it can be surmised that burns have a higher severity in terms of outcomes than other forms of injury.

Burn deaths generally occur in a bimodal distribution, either immediately after the injury or weeks later as a result of multiple organ failure, a pattern similar to all trauma-related deaths and in keeping with the maxim espoused by Basil Pruitt, "burns is the universal trauma model."[3] Therefore, burns remain a major morbid problem in the United States as a representative of high-income countries. However, it is likely even worse in low- and middle-income countries.

Approximately 41% of burns in the United States are due to fire and flame, 33% from scalding with hot liquid or grease burns, 9% from contact burns, 3% from chemical burns, and 3% from electrical burns.[4] Two-thirds of all burns occur at home and commonly involve children less than 10 years of age, adult males, and increasingly the elderly. In a 10-year average from 2005 to 2014 in the United States, 15% of burns occurred in the 0 to 4-year-old age group and another 15% in the 5- to 18-year-old age group, for a 30% total for burns sustained in children. Approximately 45% of burns occurred in the 19- to 45-year-old adult age group and another 19% in those from 46 to 65 years old, for a total of 64% sustained in young and middle-aged adults. Finally, the remaining 6% were in the elderly over 65 years old. In terms of gender, 67% of burns in the United States occur in males, and, by ethnicity, 58%

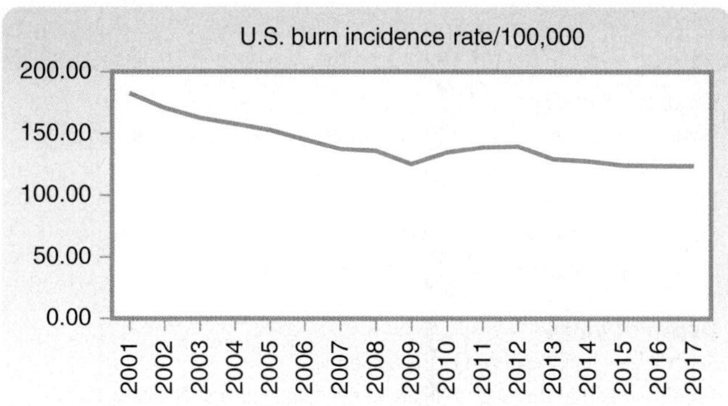

FIG. 20.1 U.S. burn incidence rate per 100,000 people.

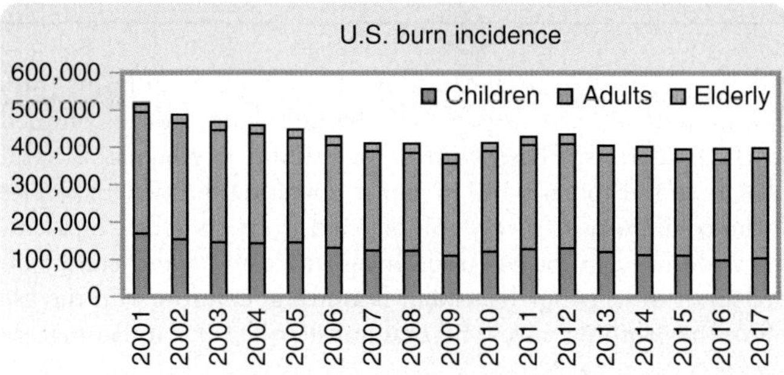

FIG. 20.2 U.S. burn incidence.

occur in persons of European descent, 21% in those of African descent, 13% occur in those of Hispanic descent, 5% occur in persons of other ethnicities, and 3% occur in those of Asian descent.

Seventy-five percent of all burn-related deaths occur in house fires commonly associated with food preparation or heating equipment. Interestingly, the cause of fire with the highest mortality is from cigarette smoking, which leads to 22% of house-fire–related deaths. Young adults are frequently burned with flammable liquids, whereas toddlers are often scalded by hot liquids at a proportion of 60%. A significant percentage of burns in children are due to child abuse. Other risk factors include low socioeconomic class and unsafe environments.[5] These generalizations emphasize that most of these injuries are preventable and therefore amenable to prevention strategies.

A recent probit analysis on the overall mortality from burns regardless of age in the United States showed an LD50 at a 55% total body surface area (TBSA) burn; therefore, in current times, a 55% TBSA burn has a 50% probability of death. When a similar analysis was done with Baux score (age + TBSA burned) accounting for improved survival probability in younger age groups, the LD50 was 105 and LD90 at 130.[5]

Prevention strategies have decreased the number and severity of injuries. Successful approaches included legislation for fire-safe cigarettes, changes in the National Electrical Code, elevation of hot water heaters from the ground, and increased smoke alarm use, which decreased fire death rates by 50%. In addition, mortality rate from all causes of burns has improved for patients sustaining severe injuries. In 1949, Bull and Fisher from the Birmingham Burns Centre in the United Kingdom first reported an LD50 for children 14 years old and younger with burns of 49% TBSA; LD50 for those 15 to 44 years old was 46% TBSA, those aged 45 to 64 years was 27% TBSA, and those 65 years and older with burns was 10% TBSA. These dismal statistics have improved, with the latest studies from the same institution with an LD50 of 85% TBSA for ages 0 to 14, 66% TBSA for ages 15 to 44, 46% TBSA for ages 45 to 64, and 23% TBSA for those over 65 years of age.[6] Therefore, a healthy young patient with even massive burns is expected to survive using modern treatment techniques.[7] Advances in treatment are based on improved understanding and implementation of resuscitation, rapid wound coverage, and improved critical care techniques. Further improvements can be made in these areas, and investigators are active in all these fields to discover means to further improve survival and outcomes.

BURN UNITS

Improvements in burn care originated principally in specialized units dedicated to the care of burned patients, first developed in the United Kingdom during WWII by Gilles and MacIndoe. These consist of experienced personnel with dedicated resources to maximize outcome from these devastating injuries (Box 20.1). The American Burn Association and the American College of Surgeons Committee on Trauma currently provide a program to verify whether burn units meet a series of qualifications for personnel, space, equipment, supplies, and processes to ensure best outcomes. They also recommend that patients with the following criteria should be referred to a designated burn center[8]:

1. Partial-thickness burns greater than 10% TBSA.
2. Burns involving the face, hands, feet, genitalia, perineum, or major joints.
3. Any full-thickness burn.
4. Electrical burns, including lightning injury.
5. Chemical burns.
6. Inhalation injury.
7. Burns in patients with preexisting medical disorders that could complicate management, prolong recovery, or affect outcome.
8. Any patient with burns and concomitant trauma (such as fractures) in which the burn injury poses the greater immediate risk of morbidity and mortality. In such cases, if the trauma poses the greater immediate risk, the patient may be initially stabilized in a trauma center before being transferred to a burn unit. Physician judgment is necessary in such situations and should be in concert with the regional medical control plan and triage protocols.
9. Burned children in hospitals without qualified personnel or equipment to care for children.
10. Burns in patients who will benefit from special social, emotional, or long-term rehabilitative intervention.

PATHOPHYSIOLOGY OF BURNS

Local Changes

Thermal burns, in particular, cause damage to the skin and occasionally underlying structures through abrupt temperature change that exceed biologic tolerance. This leads to membrane disruption, protein denaturation, and necrosis. The injury extends from the skin surface to deeper structures in a first-order logarithmic distribution depending on the temperature of the burning agent and duration of exposure.[9] Severe burns to the skin reaching over 280°F induce a Maillard-type reaction with changes in consistency and color common with flame full-thickness burns. Burns that induce necrosis of the surface with temperatures below 280°F, such as scald burns from hot water, have a different appearance and texture and are commonly mistaken for partial-thickness burns.

BOX 20.1 Burn unit organization and personnel.

- Experienced burn surgeons (burn unit director and qualified surgeons)
- Dedicated nursing personnel
- Physical and occupational therapists
- Social workers
- Dietitians
- Pharmacists
- Respiratory therapists
- Psychiatrists and clinical psychologists
- Prosthetists

The thermal conductivity of the causative agent for scald and contact burns also affects the depth, which is typically by conduction rather than convection or radiation common with flame burns, particularly those sustained during explosions. Thermal conductivity is the ability to transfer heat; for water, it is 0.61 W/m/°C, and for hot cooking oil, it is 4.2 joule/g °C, while that for grease is 1.8 joule/g °C; therefore, with cooling being the opposite of heating, more energy is transferred more rapidly.

Burns are classified into five different causal categories and depths of injury (Box 20.2). The causes include injury from flame, hot liquids (scald), contact with hot or cold objects (contact), conduction of electricity, and chemical exposure. The first three induce cellular damage primarily by the transfer of energy, inducing coagulative necrosis (except for cold injuries, which do not engender protein denaturation). Electricity and chemicals cause direct injury to cellular membranes in addition to the transfer of heat.

The skin provides a robust barrier to transfer of energy to deeper tissues; therefore, much of the injury is confined to this layer. Further, transfer of energy generally follows a first-order distribution; thus, distance from the source induces logarithmic decreases in damage. Time is also a key component, with direct correlation to the severity and depth of the injury. This is important to note, since people often attempt to quickly remove themselves from environments where burns occur, with enthusiasm, thus limiting the severity of injury.

After the inciting focus is removed, however, the response of local tissues can lead to injury in the deeper layers. The area of cutaneous injury has been divided into three zones: zone of coagulation, zone of stasis, and zone of hyperemia.[10] The necrotic area of burn where cells were directly disrupted is termed the *zone of coagulation*. This tissue is irreversibly damaged at the time of injury. The area immediately surrounding the necrotic zone has a moderate degree of insult with decreased tissue perfusion. This is termed the *zone of stasis* and, depending on the wound environment, can either survive or go on to coagulative necrosis. The zone of stasis is associated with vascular damage and vessel leakage. The last area is termed the *zone of hyperemia*, which is characterized by vasodilatation from inflammation surrounding the burn wound. This region contains the clearly viable tissue from which the healing process begins and is generally not at risk for further necrosis. This concept, termed "Jackson levels," has been questioned recently with the development of new molecular and imaging techniques for measurement of the process, although it remains as the basis for the physiologic description of burn wound progression and results.[11]

Burn Depth

Burn depth depends on the initial tissue damage, classified by penetrance from the surface to the epidermis, dermis, subcutaneous fat, and underlying structures (Fig. 20.3). Superficial burns (previously termed "first-degree") are, by definition, injury confined to the epidermis. These injuries are painful, erythematous, and blanch to the touch with an intact epidermal barrier. Examples include sunburn or a very minor scald from a kitchen incident. These do not disrupt any underlying structures, and therefore do not result in scarring. Treatment is aimed at comfort with the use of topical soothing salves and oral nonsteroidal anti inflammatory agents.

BOX 20.2 Burn classifications.

Causes of Injury

Flame—damage from superheated oxidized air by convection and radiation
Scald—damage from contact with hot liquids
Contact—damage from contact with hot or cold solids
Chemical—contact with noxious chemicals
Electrical—conduction of electrical current through tissues

Depth of Injury

Superficial—injury confined to the epidermis
Superficial partial-thickness—injury to the epidermis and papillary dermis
Deep partial-thickness—injury to the epidermis and reticular dermis
Full-thickness—injury extending through the epidermis and dermis into subcutaneous fat

Partial-thickness burns (formerly called "second-degree") are divided into two types, superficial and deep. All partial-thickness burns have some degree of dermal damage, and the division is based on the depth of injury into this structure. Superficial partial-thickness burns are limited to the papillary dermis and are erythematous, painful, blanch to touch, and often blister. Hair follicles remain viable and intact; thus, a finding on physical exam is retention of hairs to gentle pulling. Examples include scald injuries sustained in kitchen incidents and flash flame burns. These wounds spontaneously reepithelialize from retained epidermal structures in rete ridges and hair follicles in the follicular dermis in 7 to 14 days. After healing, these burns may have some slight skin discoloration and textural differences without other significant scarring. Deep partial-thickness burns within the reticular dermis appear more pale and mottled, do not blanch to touch, but remain painful to pinprick. These burns heal in 15 to 21 days by reepithelialization from deep hair follicles and sweat gland keratinocytes, often with severe scarring as a result of loss of dermal integrity.

Full-thickness burns (formerly termed as "third-degree") extend through the epidermis and dermis into the underlying fat and are characterized by a hard leathery eschar that is painless and black, white, or cherry red in color depending on the temperature of the source. No epidermal or dermal keratinocytes remain; thus, these wounds must heal by reepithelialization from the wound edges. Deep dermal and full-thickness burns benefit from excision of the eschar with autologous skin grafting in order to heal in a timely fashion and minimize contraction. Full-thickness burns can extend below the superficial fat to involve other structures, such as muscle and bone.

Currently, burn depth is most accurately assessed by judgment of experienced practitioners, although modern imaging technologies, such as laser Doppler flowmetry, laser speckle imaging, and optical coherence with or without artificial intelligence techniques hold the promise of improving the assessment and guiding better treatment and outcomes.[12–14] Accurate assessment of depth is critical to determine optimal treatment for each affected area

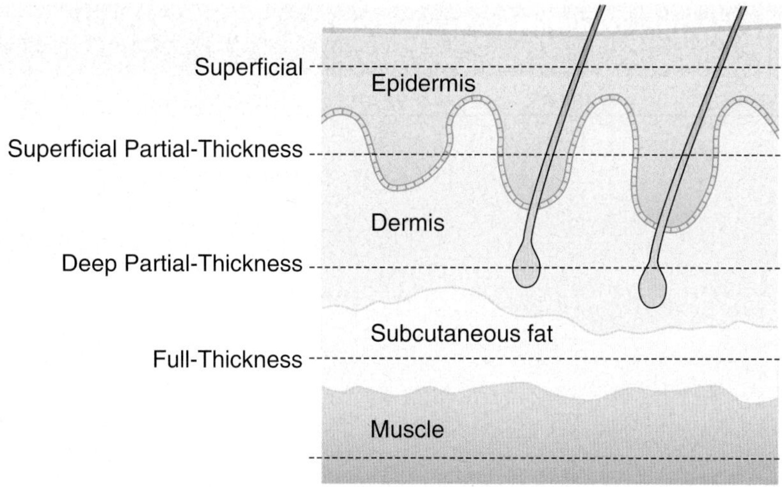

FIG. 20.3 Depths of a burn. Superficial burns are confined to the epidermis. Superficial partial-thickness burns are limited to the epidermis and papillary dermis. Deep partial-thickness burns extend through the epidermis and reticular dermis. Full-thickness burns extend through the epidermis and dermis into subcutaneous fat and can involve injury to underlying tissue structures, such as muscle, tendons, and bone.

and ensure best outcomes in terms of scarring and distress during treatment. Examination of the entire wound by the surgeons ultimately responsible and accountable for management then is the "gold standard" to guide treatment decisions. Imaging techniques and decision-support algorithms, some of which can be used sequentially, hold the promise to make such improvements.

Burn Size

Determination of burn size estimates the extent of injury. Burn size is traditionally assessed manually by the "rule of nines." In adults, each upper extremity and the head and neck are 9% of the TBSA, the lower extremities and the anterior and posterior trunk are 18% each, and the perineum and genitalia are assumed to be 1% of the TBSA. Another method of estimating smaller burns is to equate the area of the open hand (including the palm and the extended fingers) of the patient as approximately 1% TBSA, and then to transpose that measurement visually onto the wound for a determination of its size. This method is helpful when evaluating splash burns and other burns of disparate distribution.

Children have a relatively larger portion of the body surface area in the head and neck, which is compensated by a relatively smaller surface area in the lower extremities. Infants have 21% of the TBSA in the head and neck and 13% in each leg, which incrementally approaches the adult proportions with increasing age. The Berkow formula is used to accurately determine burn size in children (Table 20.1).

Systemic Changes

Inflammation and Edema

Burns induce a massive increase in inflammation in response to the injury, in the wound first that is then generalized to all other tissues. The Glue Grant Investigators demonstrated that over 80% of the genes in circulating immune cells are radically changed following severe injury, including burns.[15] The changes involve most, if not all, cellular functions and pathways and was termed a "genomic storm." This breadth and degree of change was not anticipated by the investigators, identifying that circulating leukocytes are radically activated in the response to severe injury with dramatically increased expression of genes in the inflammatory, innate immunity, and antiinflammatory spheres. They also noted a significant downregulation of genes associated with adaptive immunity. Perhaps most interestingly, they found that later complications such as infection and organ failure were not related genomic changes during the course of recovery, differing only in the magnitude and duration of the initial changes. Persons with many types of injury were included in the study, but many of them had severe burns. They further found no differences in the response by injury type, and therefore, these findings are clearly applicable to burned patients. In particular, it is prudent to recognize that severe burns induce massive physiologic and immune changes that are prolonged. Further, tracking genomic and inflammatory mediator changes along the course of treatment is not likely to be fruitful to predict complications and infections, as these are already established with the injury.[16]

Mediators that are produced locally induce vasoconstriction and vasodilatation, increased capillary permeability, and edema. The whole-body response then ensues based on the extent of injury, with changes in permeability and activity of mediators to cause generalized edema through Starling forces in both burned and unburned skin.[17] Initially, the interstitial hydrostatic pressures in the burned skin decrease dramatically with an associated slight increase in nonburned skin interstitial pressures. As plasma oncotic pressures decrease and interstitial oncotic pressures increase, edema forms in the burned and nonburned tissues. The edema is greater in the burned tissues because of lower interstitial pressures.

Many mediators have been proposed to account for the changes in permeability after burn, including histamine, bradykinin, vasoactive amines, prostaglandins, leukotrienes, activated complement, and catecholamines, among others. Recently, investigators showed that shedding glycocalyx from plasma membranes are also instrumental in the process.[18] Mast cells in the burned skin release histamine in large quantities immediately after injury, which elicits a characteristic response in venules by increasing intercellular junction space formation. The use of antihistamines in the treatment of burn edema, however, has had limited success. In addition, aggregated platelets release serotonin to play a major role in edema formation. This agent acts directly to increase pulmonary vascular

TABLE 20.1 **Berkow formula to estimate burn size (%) based on area of burn in an isolated body part.***

BODY PART	0–1 YEAR	1–4 YEARS	5–9 YEARS	10–14 YEARS	15–18 YEARS	ADULT
Head	19	17	13	11	9	7
Neck	2	2	2	2	2	2
Anterior trunk	13	13	13	13	13	13
Posterior trunk	13	13	13	13	13	13
Right buttock	2.5	2.5	2.5	2.5	2.5	2.5
Left buttock	2.5	2.5	2.5	2.5	2.5	2.5
Genitalia	1	1	1	1	1	1
Right upper arm	4	4	4	4	4	4
Left upper arm	4	4	4	4	4	4
Right lower arm	3	3	3	3	3	3
Left lower arm	3	3	3	3	3	3
Right hand	2.5	2.5	2.5	2.5	2.5	2.5
Left hand	2.5	2.5	2.5	2.5	2.5	2.5
Right thigh	5.5	6.5	8	8.5	9	9.5
Left thigh	5.5	6.5	8	8.5	9	9.5
Right leg	5	5	5.5	6	6.5	7
Left leg	5	5	5.5	6	6.5	7
Right foot	3.5	3.5	3.5	3.5	3.5	3.5
Left foot	3.5	3.5	3.5	3.5	3.5	3.5

*Estimates are made, recorded, and then summed to gain an accurate estimate of the body.

resistance, and it indirectly aggravates the vasoconstrictive effects of various vasoactive amines. Serotonin also plays a key local role, and when the antiserotonin agent methysergide was given to animals after scald injury, wound edema formation decreased as a result of local effects.[19] In addition, decreases in resuscitation fluid is seen with high-dose vitamin C therapy immediately after burn, presumably because of its antiinflammatory effects,[20] although this has been questioned recently as the doses given are likely to have an independent osmotic diuretic effect.[21]

Microvascular changes induce cardiopulmonary alterations characterized by loss of plasma volume, increased peripheral vascular resistance, and subsequent decreased cardiac output immediately after injury. Studies in efforts to sustain intravascular volume by increasing oncotic pressure with colloid solutions, such as albumin, are currently underway. Cardiac output remains depressed from decreased blood volume and increased blood viscosity, as well as decreased cardiac contractility. Ventricular dysfunction in this period is attributed to a circulating myocardial depressant factor present in lymphatic fluid, although the specific factor has never been isolated.[22] Cardiac output is almost completely restored with resuscitation.[23]

Effects on the Renal System

Diminished blood volume and cardiac output result in decreased renal blood flow and glomerular filtration rate; this is mitigated somewhat by intravenous volume resuscitation. Other stress-induced hormones and mediators such as angiotensin, aldosterone, vasopressin, and thromboxane B_2 further reduce renal blood flow immediately after the injury. These effects result in oliguria, which, if left untreated, will cause acute tubular necrosis and renal failure. Before 1984, acute renal failure in burn injuries was almost always fatal; after 1984, however, techniques in intermittent dialysis became widely used to support the kidneys during recovery.[24] Since that time, developments in continuous renal replacement therapies have radically changed outcomes related to renal failure in the severely burned. It was shown that 28-day mortality and in-hospital mortality in the severely burned with renal failure decreased by 50% and 25%, respectively, with the use of continuous venovenous hemofiltration compared to intermittent hemodialysis controls.[25] This is a massive improvement that has received significant attention, and has been corroborated by several other studies.[26]

Effects on the Immune System

Burns cause a global depression in immune function, which is demonstrated most prominently by prolonged allograft skin survival on burn wounds. As stated previously, after severe injury, adaptive immunity is downregulated in favor of innate immune mechanisms. Burned patients are then at great risk for a number of infectious complications, including bacterial wound infection, pneumonia, and fungal and viral infections. These susceptibilities and conditions are based on depressed cellular function in all parts of the immune system, including activation and activity of neutrophils, macrophages, T lymphocytes, and B lymphocytes. With burns of more than 20% TBSA, impairment of these immune functions is proportional to burn size.

Macrophage production after burn is relatively diminished, which is related to spontaneous elaboration of negative regulators of myeloid growth. This effect is enhanced by the presence of endotoxin and can be partially reversed with granulocyte colony-stimulating factor treatment or inhibition of prostaglandin E2.[27] Total neutrophil counts are initially increased after burn by demargination and decreased cell death by apoptosis. However, neutrophils that are present are dysfunctional in terms of diapedesis, chemotaxis, and phagocytosis, this related to abnormalities in granulopoiesis and lifespan, cell trafficking, and antimicrobial effector functions.[28] After 48 to 72 hours, neutrophil counts decrease somewhat like macrophages with similar causes.

T-cell function is depressed after a severe burn. Until recently, T helper cells were categorized as Th1 and Th2 phenotypes, but this has been dramatically expanded to other phenotypes such as Th9,

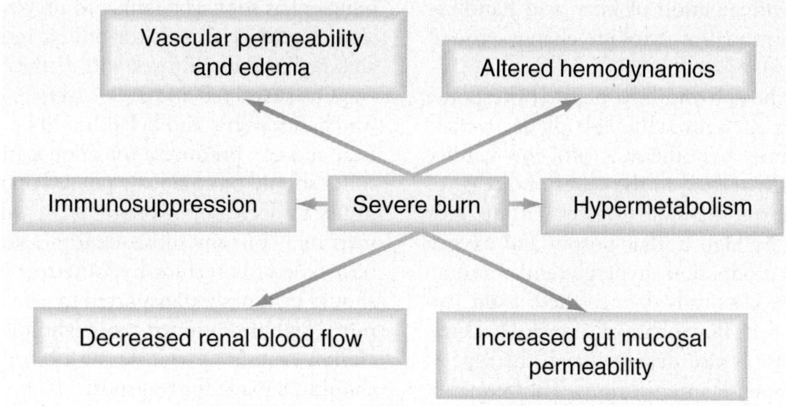

FIG. 20.4 Systemic effects of a severe burn.

Th17, Th22, and T-regs; work on this categorization and relevant functions is ongoing. In particular, the Th17 phenotype is likely to play a significant role in the burn wound given its association with adaptive immunity on mucosal surfaces and the skin.[29] This field continues to evolve as we examine the roles of each phenotype in response to antigens. Each is associated with typical cytokines, such as interleukin-2 (IL-2) for Th1 responses, IL-4 and IL-10 for Th2, and IL-17 and 22 for Th17. Burns also impairs cytotoxic T-lymphocyte activity as a function of burn size, thus increasing the risk of infection, particularly from fungi and viruses. Early burn wound excision improves cytotoxic T-cell activity.[30]

Hypermetabolism

After severe burn and resuscitation, typically 3 to 4 days after injury, the condition of *hypermetabolism* develops, characterized by tachycardia, increased cardiac output, elevated energy expenditure, increased oxygen consumption, and massive proteolysis and lipolysis (Fig. 20.4). This response is seen in all major injuries but is present in its most dramatic form in severe burns. The condition is likely related to the massive inflammatory response already mentioned, but delivery of nutrition to support recovery from the wound and bed rest and immobility associated with treatment is also likely to play a major role. Hypermetabolism may be sustained for months, leading to massive weight loss and decreased strength, particularly when muscle strength is needed to recover from the injury. These changes in metabolic activity are due in part to the release of catabolic hormones, such as catecholamines, glucocorticoids, and insulin/glucagon among others. Catecholamines act directly and indirectly to increase glucose availability through hepatic gluconeogenesis and glycogenolysis, and fatty acid availability through peripheral lipolysis. Effects are direct through alpha- and beta-adrenergic receptors on myocytes, lipocytes, and hepatocytes. The indirect effects are mediated through stimulation of adrenergic receptors in endocrine tissue within the pancreas, which causes a relative increase in glucagon release compared with insulin. Normally, glucagon increases hepatic glucose production and peripheral lipolysis, whereas insulin has the opposite effects. Catecholamine stimulation of beta-adrenergic receptors within the pancreas increases the release of both glucagon and insulin, but concurrent stimulation of alpha-receptors has a greater inhibitory effect on insulin than on glucagon, resulting in a greater net release of glucagon compared with insulin. The effects of catecholamine-stimulated glucagon release then outweigh the effects of insulin on glucose and fatty acid production and release. Glucocorticoid hormones, released by way of the hypothalamic-pituitary-adrenal axis, are mediated through neural stimulation. Cortisol has similar actions on energy substrates and it induces insulin resistance, which is an additive to the hyperglycemia because of the release of liver glucose. Catecholamines, when combined with glucagon and cortisol, augment glucose release, which initially could be beneficial because glucose is the principal fuel of inflammatory cells as well as neural tissue.

Substrate supply for hepatic gluconeogenesis is produced through feeding, proteolysis of existing muscle tissue, and to some extent by peripheral lipolysis. Structural and constitutive proteins degraded to amino acids enter into (1) the tricarboxylic acid cycle for energy production, (2) the liver to be used as substrate for gluconeogenesis, or (3) the synthesis of acute-phase proteins. Lactate and alanine are important intermediates that are released in proportion to the extent of injury. Glutamine is also released in massive quantities, depleting muscle tissue stores to 50% of normal concentrations. After conversion to pyruvate or oxaloacetate, these amino acids form glucose with a net loss of adenosine triphosphate (ATP). Eighteen of the 20 amino acids are gluconeogenic. Increased acute-phase protein synthesis in the liver includes representative factors such as C-reactive protein, fibrinogen, $alpha_2$-macroglobulin, and complement. These are often used as proxies for the degree of hypermetabolism that is present, but, as discussed, the inflammatory response is so massive that most treatments will have little effect; perhaps the best strategy is to address the inflammatory condition of the wound through wound closure rather than untoward attention to the effects.

Peripheral lipolysis, mediated through the catabolic hormones, is another principal component of the metabolic response to severe burn. Elevation of catecholamines, glucagon, and cortisol levels stimulates the same or similar intracellular hormone-sensitive lipases in the adipocyte to release free fatty acids. These are circulated to the liver, where they are oxidized for energy, reesterified to triglyceride, and deposited in the liver or further packaged for transport to other tissues by way of very low-density lipoproteins. Glycerol from fat breakdown enters the gluconeogenic pathway at the glyceraldehyde 3-phosphate level after phosphorylation. In severely burned patients, the rates of lipolysis are dramatic, and the processing of lipid by the liver can be compromised from the increasing amounts of circulating fat. Fatty liver often develops akin to nonalcoholic fatty liver disease and is thought to be secondary to the overload of normal processing enzymes or perhaps to a downregulation of fatty acid handling mechanisms as a result of hormonal or cytokine changes associated with the injury (Fig. 20.5).[31]

The classic description of the ebb and flow phases of response to illness and trauma deserve mention. The ebb phase is characterized by low metabolic rate, hypothermia, and low cardiac output. This is often temporally related to the onset of disease or time of injury. After resuscitation, this state gives way to the flow phase, which is characterized by high cardiac output and oxygen consumption, increased heat production, hyperglycemia, and an elevated metabolic rate. Moore classically defined these as the *catabolic* and *anabolic* portions of the flow phase of recovery.[32] Duration of the catabolic flow phase is also dependent on the type of injury and the efficacy of therapeutic interventions. The frequency and severity of complications also have a bearing on the length of time of this phase of recovery, which in critically ill patients can last for weeks or months. The anabolic flow phase is characterized by a slow reaccumulation of protein and fat that extends for even years after the injury.[33]

INITIAL TREATMENT OF BURNS

Prehospital

During and immediately after injury, burned patients must be removed from the source and the burning process stopped. In the prehospital setting, this should be achieved first, but care must be taken so that the rescuer does not become another victim. Universal precautions include wearing gloves and protective eyewear during retrieval. Burning clothing should be extinguished and removed as soon as possible to prevent further injury. Next attention should be directed at initial resuscitation, starting with the airway. For those burned with flames, inhalation injury should always be suspected and 100% oxygen given by facemask. All rings, watches, jewelry, and belts should be removed because they retain heat and can produce a tourniquet-like effect. Room temperature water should be copiously poured on the wound within 3 hours of injury to decrease the depth of the wound to improve healing and scarring,[34] but any subsequent measures to cool the wound should be avoided to preclude hypothermia during resuscitation. Patients should be rapidly transported to a local emergency department for initial stabilization; for those who meet the American Burn Association criteria for transfer to a burn center, timely arrangements should be made for transport.

Initial Assessment

As with any injured patient, the initial assessment of a burn patient is divided into the primary and secondary survey. First, immediate life-threatening conditions are quickly identified and treated; in the secondary survey, a more thorough head-to-toe evaluation of the patient is undertaken.

Exposure to heated gases and smoke often results in damage to the upper respiratory tract. Direct injury to the upper airway results in localized edema, which, in combination with generalized whole-body edema associated with severe burn, may obstruct the airway over the course of hours (not minutes). Airway injury must be suspected with facial burns, singed nasal hairs, carbonaceous sputum, and tachypnea, and respiratory status must be continually monitored to assess for airway intervention and ventilatory

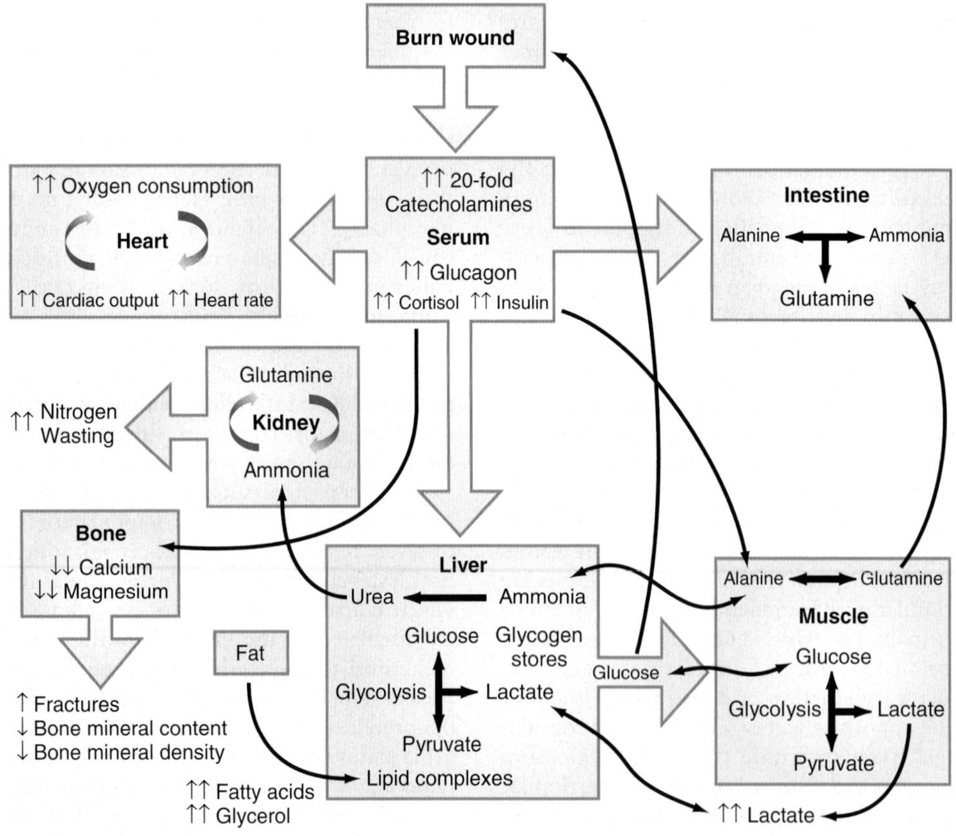

FIG. 20.5 Effects of metabolic dysfunction after burn injury. (From Williams FN, Jeschke MG, Chinkes DL, et al. Modulation of the hypermetabolic response to trauma: temperature, nutrition, and drugs. *J Am Coll Surg.* 2009;208:489–502.)

support. Progressive hoarseness is a sign of impending airway obstruction, and endotracheal intubation should be instituted early before edema irretrievably distorts the upper airway anatomy. This is especially important in patients with massive burns, who may appear to breathe without problems early in the resuscitation period until several liters of volume are given to maintain homeostasis, resulting in significant airway edema. In general, those with over 40% TBSA burns should be prophylactically intubated for this reason.

The chest should be exposed to assess breathing; airway patency alone does not ensure adequate ventilation. Chest expansion and equal breath sounds with CO_2 return from the endotracheal tube ensure adequate air exchange.

Blood pressure may be difficult to obtain in burned patients with edematous or charred extremities. Pulse rate can be used as an indirect measure of circulation; however, most burn patients remain tachycardic even with adequate resuscitation. For the primary survey of burned patients, the presence of pulses or Doppler signals in the distal extremities may be adequate to determine adequate circulation of blood until better monitors, such as arterial pressure measurements and urine output, can be established.

In those who have been in an explosion or deceleration incident, a possibility exists for spinal cord injury and other fractures. Appropriate cervical spine stabilization must be accomplished by whatever means necessary, including using cervical collars to keep the head immobilized until the condition can be evaluated and excluded.

Wound Care

Prehospital care of the burn wound is basic and simple, as only protection from the environment with application of a clean dry dressing or sheet to cover the involved part; damp dressings should not be used. Irrigation to cool the wound in the first 3 hours after injury might be considered in controlled conditions, but this should be done actively and not passively with dressings. Further, the patient should be wrapped in a blanket to minimize heat loss and for temperature control during transport. The first step in diminishing pain is to cover the wounds to prevent contact to exposed nerve endings. Intramuscular or subcutaneous narcotic injections for pain should never be used because drug absorption is decreased as a result of the peripheral vasoconstriction, resulting in later and unexpected release with respiratory complications. Small doses of intravenous morphine may be given after complete assessment of the patient and after it is determined to be safe by an experienced practitioner.

Although prehospital management is simple, it is often difficult to accomplish appropriately, particularly in at-risk populations. Studies showed that initial burns first-aid treatment was inadequate in many patients.[35] These authors also showed that inadequate first-aid care was clearly associated with poorer outcomes. They suggested that defined education programs targeted upon at-risk populations might improve these outcomes.

Transport

Rapid, uncontrolled transport of the burn victim is not a priority, except when other life-threatening conditions coexist. In most incidents involving major burns, ground transportation of victims to the receiving hospital is appropriate, with air transport of greatest use when the distance between the accident and the hospital is 30 to 150 miles. For distances greater than 150 miles, transport by fixed-wing aircraft is most appropriate. Whatever the mode of transport, it should be of appropriate size and have emergency equipment available with trained personnel on board, such as a nurse, physician, paramedics, or respiratory therapists who are familiar with multiply injured trauma patients.

Resuscitation

Adequate resuscitation of the burned patient involves establishing and maintaining reliable intravenous access. Increased times to beginning resuscitation of burned patients result in poorer outcomes, and delays should be minimized. Venous access is best attained through short peripheral catheters in unburned skin; however, veins in burned skin can be used and are preferable to no intravenous access. Superficial veins are often thrombosed in full-thickness injuries and, therefore, are not suitable for cannulation. Saphenous vein cut-downs are useful in cases of difficult access and are used in preference to central vein cannulation because of lower complication rates. In children younger than 6 years of age, experienced practitioners can use intramedullary access in the proximal tibia until intravenous access is accomplished. Lactated Ringer's solution without dextrose is the fluid of choice except in children younger than 2 years, who should receive 5% dextrose Ringer's lactate. The initial rate can be rapidly estimated by multiplying the TBSA burned by 10 in adults.[36] Thus, the rate of infusion for a man with a 40% TBSA burn would be 400 mL/hr; this rate should be continued until a formal calculation of resuscitation needs is performed.

$$80 \text{ kg} \times 40\% \text{ TBSA}/8 = 400 \text{ mL/hr}$$

Formulas are used to estimate fluid volumes for resuscitation of a burned patient, all originating from classical experimental studies on the pathophysiology of burn shock (Table 20.2). Baxter and Shires established the basis for modern fluid resuscitation protocols.[37] They showed that edema fluid in burn wounds is isotonic and contains the same amount of protein as plasma and that the greatest loss of fluid is into the interstitium. They used various volumes of intravascular fluid to determine the optimal amount in terms of cardiac output and extracellular volume in a canine burn model, and this was applied to the clinical realm with the Parkland formula. Plasma volume changes were not related to the type of resuscitation fluid in the first 24 hours, but thereafter, colloid solutions increased plasma volume by the amount infused. From these findings, they concluded that colloid solutions should not be used in the first 24 hours until capillary permeability returned closer to normal. Others have argued that normal capillary permeability is restored somewhat earlier after burn (6 to 8 hours), and therefore, colloids could be used earlier.[38]

Concurrently, Moncrief and Pruitt showed the hemodynamic effects of fluid resuscitation in burns, which culminated in the Brooke formula. They found that fluid resuscitation caused an obligatory 20% decrease in both extracellular fluid and plasma volume that concluded after 24 hours. In the second 24 hours, plasma volume returned to normal with the administration of colloid. Cardiac output was low in the first day despite resuscitation, but it subsequently increased to supernormal levels as the flow phase of hypermetabolism was established.[39] Since these studies, investigators found that much of the fluid needs are due to "leaky" capillaries that permit passage of large molecules into the interstitial space to increase extravascular colloid osmotic pressure. Intravascular volume follows the gradient to tissues, both into the burn wound and the nonburned tissues. Approximately 50% of fluid resuscitation needs are sequestered in nonburned tissues in 50% TBSA burns.[40]

TABLE 20.2 Resuscitation formulas.

FORMULA	CRYSTALLOID VOLUME
Parkland	4 cc/kg/% TBSA burned
Brooke	2 cc/kg/% TBSA burned
Galveston (pediatric)	5000 cc/m^2 burned + 1500 cc/m^2 total surface area

TBSA, Total body surface area.

Hypertonic saline solutions have theoretical advantages in burn resuscitation. These solutions are purported to decrease net fluid intake, decrease edema, and increase lymph flow, probably by the transfer of volume from the intracellular space to the interstitium. When using these solutions, hypernatremia must be avoided, and it is recommended that serum sodium concentrations should not exceed 160 mEq/dL. However, it must be noted that patients with more than 20% TBSA burns who were randomized to either hypertonic saline or lactated Ringer's solution resuscitation did not have significant differences in volume requirements or changes in percent weight gain.[41] Other investigators have found an increase in renal failure with hypertonic solutions that has tempered further efforts in this area of investigation.[42] Many of these studies are quite dated, but the use of hypertonic saline does not appear to have entered the marketplace with any enthusiasm. Currently, we cannot recommend its widespread use unless new data emerge in its favor.

Most burn units use something akin to either the Parkland or Brooke formula, which call for administering varying amounts of crystalloid and colloid for the first 24 hours. In general, these volumes should be given as a continuous infusion; bolus administration is not recommended. The fluids are generally changed in the second 24 hours with an increase in colloid use. These are guidelines to direct resuscitation of the amount of fluid necessary to maintain adequate perfusion. Of note, the use of Parkland formula for the initial estimates of fluid delivery demonstrated that much more was actually given, at 5.2 cc/kg/% TBSA.[43]

The use of decision-support technology in medicine is on the rise, including in burn resuscitation. Investigators showed that the use of one such system conclusively lowered volumes given during resuscitation, using initial weight and burn size to give an initial estimate for volume infusion. It then tracked urine output across time to give hourly recommendations for fluid volume. The use of this system significantly decreased resuscitation volumes compared to historical controls with improvements in goal urine outputs.[44] Such systems have a significant promise to improve outcomes in burned patients for not only burn resuscitation but many other areas as well. These allow for continuous monitoring and recommendations for treatment during the period of resuscitation, using data from the patient to guide therapy. Other methods are of course available through manual monitoring volume of urine output with adjustments to meet a goal of 0.5 mL/hr in adults and 1.0 mL/kg/hr in children. Changes in intravenous fluid infusion rates should be made on an hourly basis determined by the response of the patient to the particular fluid volume administered.

For burned children, formulas are commonly used that account for changes in surface area to mass ratios and baseline insensible losses. The Galveston formula recommends 5000 mL/m^2 per TBSA burn in m^2 + 1500 mL/m^2 TBSA for maintenance in the first 24 hours to account for resuscitation volumes and maintenance needs. All the formulas listed in Table 20.2 calculate recommendations for the amount of volume given in the first 24 hours after injury (not arrival to the hospital), one half of which is to be given in the first 8 hours after injury. Ongoing monitoring and adjustment are indicated.

To combat any complications of aspiration, a nasogastric tube should be inserted in all patients with major burns. This is especially important for all patients being transported in aircraft at high altitudes. Additionally, all patients should be restricted from taking anything by mouth until the transfer has been completed. Decompression of the stomach is usually indicated since the apprehensive patient will swallow considerable amounts of air and distend the stomach.

Recommendations for tetanus prophylaxis are based on the condition of the wound and the patient's immunization history. All patients with burns of greater than 10% TBSA should receive 0.5 mL tetanus toxoid. If prior immunization is absent or unclear, or the last booster dose was more than 10 years ago, 250 units of tetanus immunoglobulin is also given.

Escharotomies

When deep partial-thickness or full-thickness burns encompass the circumference of an extremity, peripheral circulation to the limb can be compromised. Development of generalized edema beneath a nonyielding eschar impedes venous outflow and eventually affects arterial inflow to the distal beds. This is recognized by numbness and tingling in the limb and increased pain in the digits. Arterial flow can be assessed by determination of Doppler signals in the digital arteries and the palmar and plantar arches in affected extremities; capillary refill and compartment pressures can also be assessed. Extremities at risk are identified either on clinical examination or on measurement of tissue pressures greater than 30 mm Hg. These extremities should undergo escharotomy, which are releases of the burn eschar only. This procedure is generally performed at the bedside by incising the lateral and medial aspects of the extremity with a scalpel or electrocautery unit. The entire constricting eschar must be incised longitudinally to completely relieve impediment to venous blood flow. For the upper extremities, incisions are carried down onto the thenar and hypothenar eminences and potentially the fingers to completely open the hand if it is involved (Fig. 20.6). If it is clear that the wound will undergo excision and grafting because of its depth, escharotomies are safest to restore perfusion to the underlying nonburned tissues until formal excision. If vascular compromise has been prolonged, reperfusion after an escharotomy may cause reactive hyperemia and further edema formation in the muscle, making continued surveillance of the distal extremities necessary. Increased muscle compartment pressures after escharotomiesmay indicate fasciotomies. The most common complications associated with these procedures are blood loss and the release of anaerobic metabolites, causing transient hypotension. If distal perfusion does not improve with these measures, central hypotension from hypovolemia should be suspected and treated.

A constricting truncaleschar can cause a similar phenomenon, except the effect is to decrease ventilation by limiting chest excursion. Any acute decrease in ventilation of a burn patient should produce inspection of the chest with appropriate escharotomies to relieve the constriction and allow adequate tidal volumes. This becomes evident for patients whose peak airway pressures increase.

INHALATION INJURY

One major factor contributing to death in severe burns is the presence of inhalation injury. Smoke damage adds another inflammatory focus and impedes normal airway function for

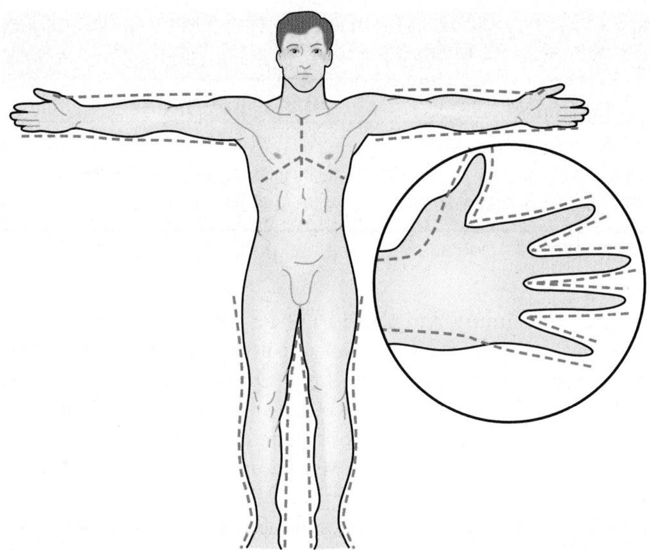

FIG. 20.6 Recommended escharotomies. In limbs requiring escharotomies, the incisions are made on the medial and lateral sides of the extremity through the eschar. In the case of the hand, incisions are made on the medial and lateral digits and on the dorsum of the hand.

critically injured patients. Inhalation injury increases the amount of time spent on mechanical ventilation, a strong predictor of mortality.[45] Early diagnosis and prevention of complications are of interest to decrease morbidity and mortality rates related to this condition.

With inhalation injury, damage is primarily from chemical burns associated with inhaled toxins. Heat is dispersed in the upper airways, whereas the cooled particles of smoke and toxins are carried distally into the major airways principally, and occasionally to the lower airways and the alveoli depending on the type of smoke and duration of exposure. Direct thermal damage to the lung is rarely seen because of dispersal of the heat in the pharynx. The exception is high-pressure steam inhalation, which has 4000 times the heat-carrying capacity of dry air.

The response of the airways to smoke inhalation is an immediate dramatic increase in blood flow from the bronchial arteries with edema formation and increased lung lymph flow. The lung lymph in this situation is similar to serum, indicating that permeability at the capillary level is markedly increased. The edema that results is associated with an increase in lung neutrophils, and it is postulated that these cells may be the primary mediators of pulmonary damage with this injury.[46] Neutrophils release proteases and oxygen free radicals to produce conjugated dienes by lipid peroxidation. High concentrations are present in the lung lymph and pulmonary tissues after inhalation injury, suggesting that the increased concentration of neutrophils is active in producing cytotoxic materials. When neutrophils are depleted before injury by nitrogen mustard, increases in lung lymph flow and conjugated diene levels are markedly reduced.[47]

Another hallmark of inhalation injury is separation of the ciliated epithelial cells from the basement membrane followed by exudate formation within the airways. The exudate consists of proteins found in the lung lymph, and, eventually, it coalesces to form fibrin casts. Clinically, these fibrin casts can be difficult to clear with standard airway suction techniques. These casts also add distal barotrauma to localized areas of lung by forming a ball valve that is open with inspiration/airway dilatation and closes during expiration; the additional volume of air adds pressure that is associated with numerous complications, including pneumothorax and decreased lung compliance.

Smoke inhalation is commonly associated with a clinical history of closed-space smoke exposure, hoarseness, wheezing, and carbonaceous sputum. It may also be associated with facial burns and singed nasal hairs. Each of these findings individually has poor sensitivity and specificity; therefore, the definitive diagnosis should be further clarified by the use of bronchoscopy. Bronchoscopy reveals early inflammatory changes such as erythema, ulceration, and prominent vasculature in addition to infraglottic soot. The findings of airway erythema and ulceration alone are also nonspecific, and these findings must be placed with the entire clinical presentation to verify significant inhalation injury. Initial treatment for severe inhalation injury is institution of mechanical ventilation for airway management and lung support to maintain gas exchange. Repeated bronchoscopy often reveals continued ulceration of the airways with granulation tissue formation, exudate formation, inspissation of secretions, and focal edema. Eventually, the airway heals by replacement of the sloughed cuboidal ciliated epithelium with squamous cells and scar.

Combustion products of organic and inorganic materials found in smoke cause direct damage to the airway cells, but also have significant systemic effects. Most notably, carbon monoxide (CO) and hydrogen cyanide (HCN) can cause physiologic derangements that can lead to death if not recognized and treated appropriately.

CO exposure should be presumed in all cases of suspected inhalation injury. CO is impossible to detect without special equipment due to its properties of being colorless, odorless, tasteless, and nonirritating. Once inhaled, CO rapidly crosses the pulmonary capillary membrane and binds to hemoglobin with approximately 200 times the affinity of oxygen, forming carboxyhemoglobin. CO also causes a conformational change to hemoglobin that diminishes oxygen off-loading ability in peripheral tissues (left-shift in the hemoglobin dissociation curve). Oxygen delivery is further impaired by hypoxia-induced cardiac dysfunction. Intracellularly, CO also has been shown to bind cytochrome c oxidase, disrupting the electron transport chain in mitochondria, resulting in a functional shift from aerobic to anaerobic metabolism and worsening oxidative stress. The impact of CO is most apparent in organ systems with high metabolic output such as the brain and heart; CO poisoning therefore most commonly manifests as neurologic changes such as dizziness or altered mental status and cardiovascular findings such as arrhythmias and even infarction.

Widespread use of synthetic materials in construction and home furnishings has led to production of increased levels of HCN gas during house fires. Cyanide is a potent and rapidly acting poison, which, under normal conditions, is converted into thiocyanide that is excreted through the urine. This system is easily overwhelmed in the setting of inhalation injury, leading to accumulation of circulating cyanide ions. The cyanide ion interferes with cellular energy production, leading to rapid depletion of ATP stores and the subsequent development of lactic acidosis. These events aside, debate exists as to whether HCN is truly a significant contributor to inhalation injury, in large part due to the fact that HCN has a low flash point and will therefore be rapidly consumed by the fire, thus limiting exposure. Unfortunately, the unpredictable nature of the gaseous compounds iteratively generated and consumed during a fire limits our ability to study their subsequent effects both systemically and as a direct pulmonary irritant.

CO poisoning is measured by carboxyhemoglobin levels, with elevations above 5% considered to have toxicity ramifications.

Headaches are generally present with levels above 10%, dizziness and impaired judgment at 20%, dyspnea above 30%, and syncope, seizures, and obtundation over 40%. Initial treatment is 100% oxygen to decrease the half-life of carboxyhemoglobin from 4 hours on room air to 1 hour. For extreme conditions, hyperbaric oxygen might be considered. For cyanide toxicity, removal from the source is indicated as well as hydroxocobalamin might be given intravenously; this will result in orange coloration of the urine.

The clinical course of patients with inhalation injury is divided into three stages. The first is acute pulmonary insufficiency. Patients with severe lung injuries may begin to show signs of pulmonary failure from the time of injury with asphyxia, CO poisoning, bronchospasm, and upper airway obstruction. Clinical signs of parenchymal damage with hypoxia are not common during this phase. The second stage occurs from 72 to 96 hours after injury and is associated with increased extravascular lung water, hypoxia, and development of diffuse lobar infiltrates. This condition is similar clinically to adult respiratory distress syndrome (ARDS), which occurs in nonburned injured and critically ill patients. In the third stage, clinical bronchopneumonia dominates and appears in up to 60% of these patients. These infections generally occur 3 to 10 days after burn injury and are associated with the expectoration of large mucous casts formed in the tracheobronchial tree. The differentiation of pneumonia from tracheobronchitis is difficult at this stage, and bronchoscopy with lavage may be of assistance. Early pneumonias are usually caused by penicillin-resistant *Staphylococcus* species, whereas after 5 to 7 days, the changing flora of the burn wound is reflected in the appearance in the lung of gram-negative species, especially *Pseudomonas* and *Klebsiella*. Ball-valve effects and ventilator-associated barotrauma are also hallmarks of this period.

Management of inhalation injury is directed at maintaining open airways and maximizing gas exchange while the lung heals. A coughing patient with a patent airway can clear secretions much more effectively than any suctioning technique (including bronchoscopy), and efforts should be made to manage patients without mechanical ventilation if at all possible. If respiratory failure is imminent, intubation should be instituted with frequent chest physiotherapy and suctioning performed to maintain pulmonary toilet (Table 20.3). Frequent bronchoscopy may be indicated to clear inspissated secretions. Mechanical ventilation should be used to provide gas exchange with as little barotrauma as possible using permissive hypercapnia and ARDS net ventilation protocols. Arterial oxygen tensions of greater than 60 (or an oxygen saturation of 92%) are also tolerated to minimize oxygen toxicity to the lungs. When the clinical condition improves to the point of weaning from ventilatory support, oxygen concentration, positive end-expiratory pressure, and ventilator volumes and rate should be decreased in a graduated manner until the patient can be extubated. This may take several weeks.

Inhalation treatments have been effective in improving the clearance of tracheobronchial secretions and decreasing bronchospasm (Table 20.3). Intravenous heparin has been shown to reduce tracheobronchial cast formation, minute ventilation, and peak inspiratory pressures after smoke inhalation.[48] When heparin was administered directly to the lungs in a nebulized form, it had similar effects on casts without causing systemic coagulopathy. When n-acetylcysteine treatments are added to nebulized heparin in burned children with inhalation injury, reintubation rates and mortality rates are decreased.[49] In addition to the measures already discussed, adequate humidification and treatment of bronchospasm with beta-agonists are indicated. Steroids are not of benefit in inhalation injury and should not be given unless the patient is steroid dependent before injury or if the patient has bronchospasm resistant to standard therapy. Other potential treatments are hypertonic saline to induce coughing and racemic epinephrine to reduce mucosal edema for those who are extubated.

TABLE 20.3 Inhalation treatments of smoke inhalation injury.

TREATMENT	TIME AND DOSE
Bronchodilators (e.g., albuterol)	q2h
Nebulized heparin	5000 units in 3 cc normal saline q4h
Nebulized acetylcysteine	20%, 3 cc q4h

q2,4h, Every 2,4 hours.

In addition to conventional ventilator methods, novel ventilator therapies have been devised to minimize barotrauma, including high-frequency percussive ventilation. This method combines standard tidal volumes and respirations (ventilator rates 6–20/minute) with smaller high-frequency respirations (200–500/minute) and permits adequate ventilation and oxygenation in patients who failed conventional ventilation. One reason for the greater utility of this method is that it recruits alveoli at lower airway pressures. This ventilator method may also have a percussive effect that loosens inspissated secretions and improves the pulmonary toilet, although the percussive effects can lead to additional airway injury.[50]

Several clinical studies have shown that pulmonary edema is not prevented by fluid restriction. Indeed, fluid resuscitation appropriate for the patient's other needs results in a decrease in lung water, has no adverse effect on pulmonary histology, and improves survival rate. Although overhydration could increase pulmonary edema, inadequate hydration increases the severity of pulmonary injury by sequestration of neutrophils, leading to increased risk of death. In both animal and clinical studies, resuscitation was adequate if normal cardiac index or urine output was maintained.

Prophylactic antibiotics for inhalation injury are not indicated but are clearly to be used for diagnosed lung infections. Empirical choices for treatment of pneumonia before culture results are returned should include coverage of methicillin-resistant *Staphylococcus aureus* and gram-negative organisms (especially *Pseudomonas*).

As patients recover from lung injury, extubation should ensue as soon as possible. Patients are able to clear their own airways through coughing more effectively than suction through an endotracheal tube. This is preferably done as soon as upper airway edema has resolved (injury day 1–2) in those who were intubated to control the airway or for burn excision. It is our experience that patients who are extubated with the same degree of inhalation injury do better than those who are intubated. Standard extubation criteria can be used, although many patients who do not meet these criteria may also do well without mechanical ventilation. If the airway is easily accessible by airway experts, a trial of extubation might be of benefit in patients with borderline weaning parameters.

WOUND CARE

After the airway is assessed and resuscitation is underway, attention must be turned to the burn wound. Treatment depends on the characteristics and size of the wound, and all treatments are aimed at rapid and less painful healing. Current therapy directed specifically toward burn wounds can be divided into three stages: assessment, management, and rehabilitation. Once the extent and depth of the wounds have been assessed and the wounds have been thoroughly cleaned and debrided, the management phase begins. Each wound should be dressed with an appropriate covering that serves several functions. First, it should protect the damaged epithelium, minimize bacterial and fungal colonization, and provide splinting action to maintain the desired position of function. Second, the dressing should be occlusive to reduce evaporative heat loss and minimize cold stress. Third, the dressing should provide comfort over the painful wound.

The choice of dressing is based on the characteristics of the treated wound. Superficial epidermal wounds are minor, with minimal loss of barrier function; thus, no dressing is indicated with treatment by topical salves to keep the skin moist. Systemic nonsteroidal antiinflammatory agents given by mouth assist in pain control. Partial-thickness wounds are treated with daily dressing changes with topical antibiotics, cotton gauze, and elastic wraps or with one of the longer-lasting dressings containing silver as an antimicrobial. Alternatively, the wounds can be treated with a temporary biologic or synthetic covering to close the wound that may or may not be applied in the operating room (Table 20.4). Deep partial-thickness or full-thickness wounds benefit from excision and grafting for sizable burns, and the choice of initial dressing should be aimed at holding bacterial proliferation in check and providing occlusion until the operation is performed.

Antimicrobials

The timely and effective use of antimicrobials has revolutionized burn care by decreasing invasive wound infections. The untreated burn wound rapidly becomes colonized with bacteria and fungi because of the loss of innate skin barrier mechanisms. As the organisms proliferate to high wound counts (>10^5 organisms per gram of tissue), they may penetrate into viable tissue. Organisms then invade blood vessels, causing a systemic infection that often leads to the death of the patient. This scenario has become uncommon in most burn units because of the effective use of antibiotics and wound care techniques. The antimicrobials that are used can be divided into those given topically and those given systemically.

Available topical antibiotics can be divided into three classes: salves, soaks, and antimicrobial dressings. Salves are generally applied directly to the wound with cotton dressings placed over them (Table 20.5), soaks are solutions poured into cotton dressings on the wound, and antimicrobial dressings contain active agents to inhibit microbial growth, generally some form of silver ion or other antibiotic. Each of these classes of antimicrobials has advantages and disadvantages. Salves may be applied daily but may lose their effectiveness between dressing changes. Frequent dressing changes can result in shearing with loss of grafts or underlying healing cells as well as procedural pain. Soaks remain effective because antibiotic solution can be added without removing the dressing; however, the underlying skin can become macerated. Longer-term antimicrobial dressings have the advantage of less frequent painful changes, decreasing both pain and provider effort, but some of these must remain moist and thus must be monitored.

Topical antibiotic salves include 11% mafenide acetate (Sulfamylon), 1% silver sulfadiazine (Silvadene), polymyxin B, neomycin, bacitracin, mupirocin, and the antifungal agent nystatin among others. No single agent is completely effective, and each has advantages and disadvantages. Silver sulfadiazine was very commonly used before the development of antimicrobial dressings. It has a broad spectrum of activity because its silver and sulfa moieties are effective against gram-positive, most gram-negative, and some fungal forms. Some *Pseudomonas* species possess plasmid-mediated resistance. Silver sulfadiazine is relatively painless upon application, has a high patient acceptance, and is easy to use. However, it must be changed daily, which induces significant repeated painful episodes. Occasionally, patients complain of a burning sensation after it is applied, and, in a few patients, a transient leukopenia develops 3 to 5 days following its continued use. This leukopenia is generally harmless and resolves with or without treatment cessation. Of some concern is the recent finding of wound healing inhibition by the agent.[51]

TABLE 20.4 Biologic coverings.

Xenograft	Occlusive closure of the wound, some immunologic benefits
Allograft	Occlusive closure of the wound, provides normal functions of skin, dermal elements can engraft and worsen scarring

Mafenide acetate is another topical agent with a broad spectrum of activity owing to its sulfa moiety. It is particularly useful against resistant *Pseudomonas* and *Enterococcus* species. It also can penetrate eschar, which silver sulfadiazine cannot. Disadvantages include painful application on skin, such as in second-degree wounds. It also can cause an allergic skin rash, and it has carbonic anhydrase inhibitory characteristics that can result in a metabolic acidosis when applied over large surfaces. For these reasons, mafenide sulfate is typically reserved for small full-thickness injuries.

Petroleum-based antimicrobial ointments with polymyxin B, neomycin, and bacitracin are clear on application, painless, and allow for easy wound observation. These agents are commonly used for treatment of facial burns, graft sites, healing donor sites, and small partial-thickness burns. Mupirocin is a petroleum-based ointment that has improved activity against gram-positive bacteria, particularly methicillin-resistant *S. aureus* and selected gram-negative bacteria. Nystatin, either in a salve or powder form, can be applied to wounds to control fungal growth. Nystatin-containing ointments can be combined with other topical agents to decrease colonization of both bacteria and fungus. The exception is the combination of nystatin and mafenide acetate; each inactivates the other.

Available agents for application as a soak include 0.5% silver nitrate solution, 0.05% Dakin (sodium hypochlorite with buffers), 0.25% Domboro (acetic acid with buffers), and mafenide acetate as a 5% solution. Silver nitrate has the advantage of being painless on application and having complete antimicrobial effectiveness. The disadvantages include its staining of surfaces to a dull gray or black when the solution dries. This can become problematic in deciphering wound depth during burn excisions and in keeping the patient and his or her surroundings clean of the black staining. The solution is hypotonic as well, and continuous use can cause electrolyte leaching, with rare methemoglobinemia as another complication. Dakin's solution, which is a dilute solution of sodium hypochlorite with added buffering agents, has effectiveness against most microbes; however, it also has cytotoxic effects on the healing cells of patients' wounds. Low concentrations of sodium hypochlorite have less cytotoxic effects while maintaining most of the antimicrobial effects. Hypochlorite ion is inactivated by contact with protein, so the solution must be continually changed. The same is true for acetic acid solutions, which may be more effective against *Pseudomonas*. Mafenide acetate soaks have the same characteristics of the mafenide acetate salve, except in liquid form.

TABLE 20.5 Burn wound dressings.

DRESSING	ADVANTAGES AND DISADVANTAGES
Salves	
Silver sulfadiazine	Broad-spectrum, painful daily dressing changes, does not penetrate eschar, inhibition of epithelialization
Mafenide acetate 11%	Broad-spectrum, penetrates eschar, painful application to partial-thickness burns, painful daily dressing changes, potential for metabolic acidosis, inhibition of epithelialization
Bacitracin	Gram-positive coverage, painful daily dressing changes
Neomycin	Gram-positive coverage, painful daily dressing changes
Bactroban	Gram-positive coverage, painful daily dressing changes
Polymyxin B	Gram-negative coverage, painful daily dressing changes
Nystatin	Fungal coverage, cannot be used in combination with mafenide acetate
Solutions	
Silver nitrate 0.5%	Effective against all microbes, stains contacted areas, associated with methemoglobinemia
5% Mafenide acetate	Broad-spectrum, penetrates eschar, painful application to partial-thickness burns, painful daily dressing changes, potential for metabolic acidosis, inhibition of epithelialization
Dakin's solution	0.5% sodium hypochlorite with buffers, effective against all microbes, inhibits epithelialization
Domboro's solution	0.25% acetic acid with buffers, effective against most microbes particularly *Pseudomonas*, inhibits biofilm formation
Antimicrobial Dressings	
Silver containing dressings	Broad-spectrum, long-term use minimizing painful wound care, does not penetrate eschar, difficult to assess the wound

Many new antimicrobial dressings containing silver ions have reached the marketplace and provide the advantages listed above. Most wound care companies offer a dressing with these characteristics, and therefore, the choice among them is principally based on these characteristics rather than the antimicrobial properties. The advantage is that these can be applied and left in place for several days, providing for prolonged occlusive treatment for 3 to 7 days typically, and antimicrobial activity. Monitoring of the patient and wound is still indicated since these dressings typically do not allow direct observation of the wound.

The use of perioperative systemic antimicrobials also has a role in decreasing burn wound sepsis until the burn wound is closed. Common organisms that must be considered when choosing a perioperative regimen include *S. aureus*, *Pseudomonas* species, and *Klebsiella*, which are prevalent in burn wounds.

Synthetic and Biologic Dressings

Synthetic and biologic dressings are an alternative to antimicrobial dressings. These types of dressings provide for stable coverage without painful dressing changes, provide a barrier to evaporative losses, and decrease pain in the wounds. They do not inhibit epithelialization, which is a feature of all topical antimicrobials. These coverings include allograft (cadaver skin), xenograft (pig skin), Biobrane, Suprathel, and dermal equivalent-like products. These should generally be applied within 72 hours of the injury, before high bacterial colonization of the wound occurs. Most often, synthetic and biologic dressings are used to cover second-degree wounds while the underlying epithelium heals or it is used to cover full-thickness wounds for which autograft is not yet available. Each type of dressing has its advantages and disadvantages.

Biologic dressings include xenografts from swine and allografts from cadaver donors. These human skin equivalents are applied to the wounds in the manner of skin grafts, where they engraft and perform the immunologic and barrier functions of normal skin. Thus, these biologic dressings are the optimal wound coverage in the absence of normal skin. Some of these are live tissue, such as fresh or frozen human allograft, while other formulations are treated with glycerol to lyse any live cells, leaving the extracellular matrix and proteins intact. Eventually, these biologic dressings will be rejected by usual immune mechanisms, causing the grafts to slough. They can then be replaced, or the open wound can be covered with autograft skin from the patient. Generally, severely burned patients are immunosuppressed, and biologic dressings that have adhered will not reject for several weeks. Biologic dressings can be used to cover any wound as a temporary dressing. They are particularly well suited to massive partial-thickness injuries (>50% TBSA) to close the wound and allow for healing to take place underneath the dressing. Disadvantages include the possible transmission of viral diseases with allograft and the possibility that a residual mesh pattern will be left from engrafted cadaver dermis if meshed allograft is used.

Biobrane consists of collagen-coated silicone manufactured into a sheet. Suprathel is another like formulation. These are placed on the wound and becomes adherent in 24 to 48 hours with dried wound transudate. This sheet then provides a barrier to moisture loss, and it provides a relatively painless wound bed without dressing changes. When the epithelium is complete under the sheet, it is easily peeled off the wound. Caution must be exercised when using this product to ensure that copious exudate does not form under the sheet, which provides an optimum environment for bacterial proliferation and eventual invasive wound infection. Biobrane has no antimicrobial activities, while Suprathel has some effects. These agents should be used primarily in superficial second-degree burns and split-thickness skin graft donor sites.

Dermal equivalents such as Integra combine a collagen matrix (dermal substitute) with a silicone sheet outside layer (epidermal substitute). The collagen matrix engrafts into the wound, and after 2 weeks, the silicone layer is removed and replaced with available autograft. The advantages of this product are that it can be used in full-thickness burns to close the wound. It also provides a dermal equivalent that has the theoretical advantage of inhibiting future scarring of the burn wound, although this has not been clinically confirmed to date. The disadvantages are similar to those of all synthetic products, in that it has no antimicrobial properties; thus, its use can be complicated by invasive wound infections. Additionally, it takes two operations for wound coverage, as the silicone layer simulating the epidermis must be replaced 2 to 3 weeks after application with autograft.

Excision and Grafting

Deep partial-thickness and full-thickness burns do not heal in a timely fashion without autografting. In fact, the practice of leaving these dead tissues only serves as a nidus for inflammation and infection that could lead to the patient's death. It leads to the maxim, "there is no advantage to unexcised eschar." Early excision and grafting of these wounds, first used by Janzekovich in the 1970s, are followed by most burn surgeons since reports show benefit over serial debridement and dressing changes in terms of survival, blood loss, incidence of sepsis, and length of hospitalization.[52] The technique of early excision and grafting has made conservative treatment of full-thickness wounds a practice to be used only in those with very high operative risks. Attempts are made to excise tangentially to optimize cosmetic outcome. Rarely, excision to the level of fascia is necessary to remove all nonviable tissue, or it may become necessary at subsequent operations for infectious complications. These excisions can be performed with tourniquet control or with application of topical epinephrine and thrombin to minimize blood loss.

After a burn wound has been excised, the wound must be covered. This covering is ideally the patient's own skin. Wounds covering 20% to 30% TBSA can usually be closed at one operation with autograft split-thickness skin taken from the patient's available donor sites. In these operations, the skin grafts are not meshed, or they are meshed with a narrow ratio (2:1 or less), to maximize cosmetic outcome. In major burns, autograft skin may be limited to the extent that the wound cannot be completely closed. The availability of cadaver allograft skin has changed the course of modern burn treatment for these massive wounds. A typical method of treatment is to use widely expanded autografts (4:1 or greater) covered with cadaver allograft to completely close the wounds for which autograft is available. The 4:1 skin heals underneath the cadaver skin in approximately 21 days, and the cadaver skin falls off (Fig. 20.7). The portions of the wound that cannot be covered with even widely meshed autograft are covered with allograft skin in preparation for autografting when donor sites are healed. Ideally, areas with less cosmetic importance are covered with the widely meshed skin to close most of the wound before using nonmeshed grafts at later operations for the cosmetically important areas, such as the hands and face.

Most surgeons excise the burn wound in the first week, sometimes in serial operations by removing 20% of the burn wound per operation on subsequent days. Others remove the whole of the burn wound in one operative procedure; however, this can be limited by the development of hypothermia or continuing massive blood loss. It is our practice to perform the excision immediately after stabilization of the patient after injury because blood loss diminishes if the operation can be done early. This may be due to the relative predominance of vasoconstrictive substances, such as thromboxane and catecholamines, and the natural edema planes that develop immediately after the injury. When the wound becomes hyperemic after 2 days, blood loss can be a considerable problem. The use of hemostatic agents such as epinephrine, thrombin, and tourniquets sometimes aid in this approach.

Occasionally, split-thickness skin grafts do not adhere Loss of skin grafts is due to one or more of the following reasons: fluid collection under the graft, shearing forces that disrupt the adhered graft, presence of infection causing graft lysis, or an inadequate excision of the wound bed with remaining necrotic tissue. Of these, inadequate excision is by far the most common, followed by shearing forces and then fluid accumulation under the graft. With the use of topical antimicrobial agents, infection is the least common. Technical attention to the depth of excision by excising to punctate bleeding, meticulous hemostasis, appropriate meshing of grafts, or "rolling" of sheet grafts or bolsters over appropriate areas minimizes fluid collections. Shearing is decreased by immobilization of the grafted area. Infection is controlled by the appropriate use of perioperative antibiotics and covering the grafts with topical antimicrobials at the time of surgery.

One alternative to split-thickness autografts typically used for skin grafting is cultured keratinocytes from the patient's own skin. Keratinocytes can be cultured in sheets from full-thickness skin biopsies, which are used as autografts. This technology has been used to greatly expand the capacity of a donor site, such that most of the body can be covered with grafts from a single small full-thickness biopsy sample. Cultured epithelial autografts are of use

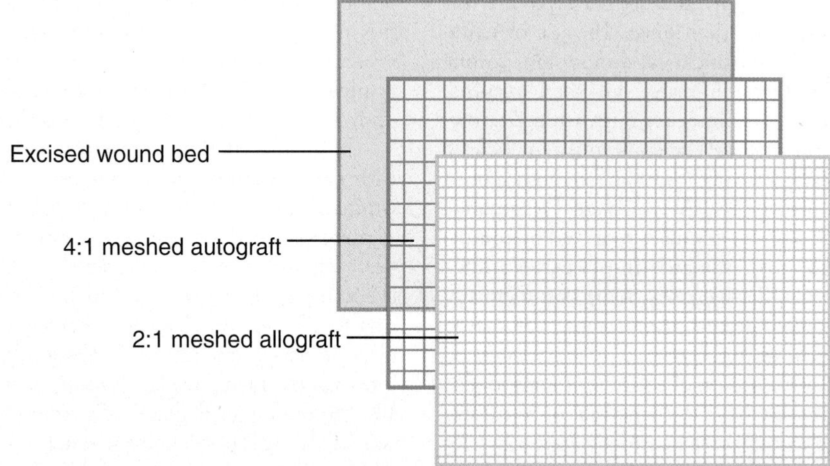

FIG. 20.7 Diagram of skin closure using widely meshed autografts. A widely meshed autograft is placed on a freshly excised viable wound bed. The remaining open wound between the interstices of the autograft is closed with an overlying layer of allograft, which can also be meshed to allow transudate, exudate, and hematoma to escape.

in truly massive burns (>80% TBSA) because of their limited donor sites. The disadvantages of cultured epithelial autografts are the length of time required to grow the autografts (2–3 weeks), a 50% to 75% take rate of the grafts after initial application, the low resistance to mechanical trauma over the long-term, a proposed increase in scarring potential associated with the lack of dermis, and the potential for squamous cell cancer. These grafts are also very expensive to produce. When a group of patients with greater than 80% TBSA burns who received cultured epithelial autografts were compared with a group who received conventional treatment, the acute hospitalization length of stay and the number of subsequent reconstructive operations were lower in the conventional group. These results demonstrate that more research and experience are needed to further optimize this technique. Technologies like cultured epithelial autografts hold the promise to radically limit donor sites, and it may be the optimal closure in combination with a dermal equivalent in the future. In this vein, recent technological advancements in cell separation and expansion by spraying on the operating table have been tested. Potential benefits are the potential for 100:1 expansion ratios and inclusion of keratinocyte stem cells in the grafts, which are not present in cultured cell preparation. This technology is now on the market, and it is expected that innovations will take place with its use in association with other standard techniques.

In all burned patients, every effort should be made to maximize the long-term appearance of the wound, because almost all patients will survive to bear the scars of their injury. Burn wound scarring causes both functional and cosmetic deficits associated with wound contracture. Experience has shown that full-thickness skin grafts that include the entire dermal and epidermal layer provide the best scarring outcomes, with diminished contracture and superior skin appearance compared with split-thickness skin grafts. Split-thickness and full-thickness grafts have a complete epidermal layer; therefore, the superior function and appearance of full-thickness grafts must lie in the uninterrupted complete dermal layer. The challenge to burn surgeons in terms of minimizing scarring, then, is to provide complete dermis during wound coverage. This might be addressed through using thicker split-thickness skin grafts, but our experience suggests that thicker split-thickness grafts do not result in better scarring. Therefore, it is reasonable to conclude that standard-thickness skin grafts are appropriate for acute coverage of burn wounds.

Full-thickness skin grafts to supply the dermal layer are not plentiful and cannot be used more than once. The use of tissue expanders to increase available full-thickness donor skin is conceivable, but impractical for most injuries. For these reasons, these grafts are not commonly used in acute burn wound coverage. Engrafted cadaver dermis that has the epidermis removed by dermabrasion 1 to 2 weeks after placing it on the wound has been used with some success to provide the dermal layer. Presumably, the sparse cellular component of the dermis is removed by immunologic processes, leaving the dermal matrix in place as scaffolding for the ingrowth of normal dermal cells. Some commercially available decellularized preserved dermis products are available to provide a dermal equivalent in wound coverage. As discussed earlier, the product Integra also has a dermal equivalent component to form a neodermis. All of these have the potential to minimize scarring contractures and to maximize the cosmetic appearance of burn scars. The long-term results with the use of these techniques are not yet known.

Recently, the use of vacuum-assisted closure of wounds has been reported. These vacuum-assisted devices have been used successfully for closure of complicated decubitus ulcers, among other uses, and are now in common use in burn wounds for treatment and to secure skin grafts and improve take rates.

MINIMIZING COMPLICATIONS

Early aggressive resuscitation regimens have improved survival rates dramatically. With the advent of vigorous fluid resuscitation, irreversible burn shock has been replaced by sepsis and subsequent multiple organ failure as the leading cause of death associated with burns. What is required is an inflammatory focus, which in severe burns is the massive skin injury with associated inflammation that is required to heal.

Etiology and Pathophysiology

The progression to multiple organ failure after severe burn is not well explained, although some of the responsible mechanisms are recognized. As shown in the Glue Grant data, massive changes in the inflammatory genome are already present in those who are severely burned; development of infectious sources is not uncommon, mostly associated with the burn wound but also from other sources such as the lungs. As organisms proliferate out of control, mediators are liberated, from both microbes as well as endogenous sources such as mitochondria. Their release is associated with a cascade of inflammatory mediators that can result, if unchecked, in further damage and progression toward organ failure.

Inflammation from the presence of necrotic tissue and open wounds can incite a similar inflammatory mediator response.[53] It is known that a cascade of systemic events is set in motion either by invasive organisms or from open wounds that initiates massive inflammation, which may progress to multiple organ failure. Evidence from animal studies and clinical trials suggests that these events converge to a common pathway. Those circulating mediators can, if secreted in excessive amounts, damage organs distal from their site of origin. Among these mediators are endotoxin, the arachidonic acid metabolites, mitochondrial fragments, cytokines, neutrophils and their adherence molecules, nitric oxide, complement components, and oxygen free radicals.

Prevention

Because different cascade systems are involved in the pathogenesis of burn-induced multiple organ failure, it is so far impossible to pinpoint a single mediator that initiates the event. Thus, because the mechanisms of progression are not well known, prevention is currently the best solution. The current recommendations are to prevent the development of organ dysfunction and to provide optimal support to avoid conditions that promote the onset.

The great reduction of mortality rate from large burns was seen with early excision and an aggressive surgical approach to deep wounds; thus, the best solution is likely early wound closure.

Removal of devitalized tissue prevents wound infections and decreases inflammation associated with the wound. In addition, it eliminates small-colonized foci, which are a frequent source of transient bacteremia. Transient bacteremia during surgical manipulations may prime immune cells to react in an exaggerated fashion to subsequent insults, leading to whole body inflammation and remote organ damage. We recommend complete early excision of clearly full-thickness wounds within 48 hours of the injury with rapid closure of the wound by autologous skin grafting.

Oxidative damage from reperfusion after low-flow states makes early aggressive fluid resuscitation imperative. This is particularly important during the initial phases of treatment and operative excision with its attendant blood losses. Furthermore, the volume of fluid may not be as important as the timeliness with which it is given. In the study of children with greater than 80% TBSA burns, it was found that one of the most important contributors to survival was the time to starting intravenous resuscitation, regardless of the initial volume given.[45]

Topical and systemic antimicrobial therapy has significantly diminished the incidence of invasive burn wound sepsis. Perioperative antibiotics clearly benefit patients with injuries greater than 30% TBSA burns. Vigilant and scheduled replacement of intravascular devices minimizes the incidence of catheter-related sepsis. Where possible, peripheral veins should be used for cannulation, even through burned tissue. The saphenous vein, however, should be avoided because of the high risk of thrombophlebitis.

Pneumonia, which contributes significantly to death in burned patients, should be vigilantly anticipated and aggressively treated. Every attempt should be made to wean patients as early as possible from the ventilator to reduce the risk of ventilator-associated nosocomial pneumonia. Furthermore, early ambulation is an effective means of preventing respiratory complications. With sufficient analgesics, even patients on continuous ventilatory support can be out of bed and in a chair.

The most common sources of sepsis are the wounds and/or the tracheobronchial trees; efforts to identify causative agents should be concentrated there. Another potential source, however, is the gastrointestinal tract, which is a natural reservoir for bacteria. Starvation and hypovolemia shunt blood from the splanchnic bed and promote mucosal atrophy and failure of the gut barrier. Early enteral feeding reduces septic morbidity and prevents failure of the gut barrier. At our institution, patients are fed immediately through a nasogastric tube. Early enteral feedings are tolerated in burn patients and preserve the mucosal integrity and may reduce the magnitude of the hypermetabolic response to injury. Support of the gut goes along with carefully monitored hemodynamics. One other infection to consider, usually late in the course, is endocarditis with microbes associated with the cardiac valves usually late in the course of treatment. This can be detected with echocardiography and should be considered in the face of infection for which no other source is identified.

Organ Failure

Even with the best efforts at prevention, the presence of the systemic inflammatory syndrome that is ubiquitous in burn patients may progress to organ failure. It was found that approximately 28% of patients with greater than 20% TBSA burns develop severe multiple organ dysfunction, of which 14% will also develop severe sepsis and septic shock.[54] Others found that 40% of deaths after severe burn were related to organ failure, which universally involved the renal system with on average at least three other systems.[55] The general development begins in the renal or pulmonary systems and can progress through the liver, gut, hematologic system, and central nervous system. The development of multiple organ failure does not predict mortality, however, and efforts to support the organs until they heal are justified.

Renal Failure

With the advent of early aggressive resuscitation, the incidence of renal failure coincident with the initial phases of recovery has diminished significantly in severely burned patients. However, a second period of risk for the development of renal failure 2 to 14 days after resuscitation is still present. Renal failure is hallmarked by decreasing urine output, hypervolemia, electrolyte abnormalities including metabolic acidosis and hyperkalemia, the development of azotemia, and increased serum creatinine. Treatment is aimed at averting complications associated with these conditions.

Urine output of more than 1 mL/kg/hr in children and 30 cc/hr in adults is an adequate measure of renal perfusion in the absence of underlying renal disease. Decreasing the volume of fluid given can alleviate volume overload in burned patients. These patients have increased insensible losses from the wounds, which can be roughly calculated at 1500 mL/m^2 TBSA +3750 mL/m^2 TBSA burned. Decreasing the infused volume of intravenous fluids and enteral feedings to less than the expected insensate losses alleviates hypervolemia problems. Almost invariably, severely burned patients receive exogenous potassium because of the heightened aldosterone response that results in potassium wasting; therefore, hyperkalemia is rare even with some renal insufficiency.

If the problems listed earlier overwhelm the conservative measures, some form of dialysis may be indicated. The indications for dialysis are hypervolemia unresponsive to diuretics or electrolyte abnormalities not amenable to other treatments. Kidney Disease: Improving Global Outcomes (KDIGO) criteria may be used to determine utility of dialysis, and level 3 or severe acute renal failure indicates use. Hemodialysis and hemofiltration are the most common modalities, either intermittent or continuous. With the advent of relatively simple continuous renal replacement technologies, these treatments can often be managed by critical care specialists with consultation from experienced nephrologists in difficult cases. After beginning dialysis, renal function is expected to return associated with the abundant regeneration properties of the kidney. Therefore, patients undergoing such treatment rarely undergo lifelong dialysis.

Pulmonary Failure

Many burn patients undergo mechanical ventilation to protect the airway in the initial phases of their injury. We recommend that these patients be extubated as soon as possible after the risk is diminished. A trial of extubation is often warranted in the first few days after injury, and reintubation in this setting is not a failure. Performing this technique safely, however, requires the involvement of experts in obtaining an airway. The goal is extubation as soon as possible to allow the patients to clear their own airways, because they can perform their own pulmonary toilet better than through an endotracheal tube or tracheostomy. The first sign of impending pulmonary failure is a decline in oxygenation. This is best monitored with continuous oximetry, and a decrease in saturation to less than 92% is indicative of failure. Increasing concentrations of inspired oxygen are necessary, and when ventilation begins to fail, denoted by increasing respiratory rate and hypercarbia, intubation is indicated.

Some have stated that early tracheostomy (within the first week) might be indicated in those with significant burn who are likely to require long-term ventilation. A randomized study comparing those severely burned patients who underwent early tracheostomy with those who did not found some improvements in oxygenation; however, no significant differences could be found in outcome measures such as ventilator days, length of stay, incidence of pneumonia, or survival. In fact, 26% of those not undergoing tracheostomy were successfully extubated within 2 weeks of admission, implying that they would not have benefited from tracheostomy at all.[56] It seems that although tracheostomy may benefit some severely burned patients on ventilatory support, the advantages of early tracheostomy do not outweigh the disadvantages.

Hepatic Failure

The development of hepatic failure in burned patients is a challenging problem without many solutions. The liver synthesizes circulating proteins, detoxifies the plasma, produces bile, and provides immunologic support. When the liver begins to fail, protein concentrations of the coagulation cascade decrease to critical levels and the patient becomes coagulopathic. Toxins are not cleared from the bloodstream, and concentrations of bilirubin increase. Complete hepatic failure is not compatible with life, but a gradation of liver failure with some decline of the functions is common. Efforts to prevent hepatic failure are the only effective methods of treatment.

With the development of coagulopathies, treatment should be directed at replacement of factors II, VII, IX, and X until the liver recovers. Albumin replacement may also be required. Attention to obstructive causes of hyperbilirubinemia, such as acalculouscholecystitis, should be considered as well. Initial treatment of this condition should be gallbladder drainage, which can be done percutaneously.

Hematologic Failure

Burn patients may become coagulopathic through two mechanisms: (1) depletion and impaired synthesis of coagulation factors or (2) thrombocytopenia. Factors associated with factor depletion are through disseminated intravascular coagulation associated with sepsis. This process is also common with coincident head injury. With breakdown of the blood-brain barrier, brain lipids are exposed to the plasma, which activates the coagulation cascade. Varying penetrance of this problem results in differing degrees of coagulopathy. Treatment of disseminated intravascular coagulation should include infusion of fresh frozen plasma and cryoprecipitate to maintain plasma levels of coagulation factors. For disseminated intravascular coagulation–induced by brain injury, following the concentration of fibrinogen and repleting levels with cryoprecipitate are the most specific indicators. Impaired synthesis of factors from liver failure is treated, as alluded to earlier.

Thrombocytopenia is common in severe burns from depletion during burn wound excision and is one of the best signs of the development of sepsis.[57] Platelet counts of less than 50,000 are common and do not require treatment. Only when the bleeding is diffuse and is noted from the intravenous sites should consideration for exogenous platelets be given.

Paradoxically, it was found that severely burned patients are also at risk for thrombotic and embolic complications likely related to immobilization. Complications of deep venous thrombosis was associated with increasing age, weight, and TBSA burned.

NUTRITION

The response to injury known as hypermetabolism is dramatically exhibited after severe burn. Increases in oxygen consumption, metabolic rate, urinary nitrogen excretion, and lipolysis are directly proportional to the size of the burn. This response can be as high as 200% of the normal metabolic rate and continues unabated for 9 to 12 months after injury. Because the metabolic rate is so high, energy utilization is immense. Endogenously, these are met by mobilization of available carbohydrate, fat, and protein stores. Because the demands are prolonged, these energy stores are quickly depleted, leading to loss of active muscle tissue and malnutrition. Immobilization for treatment further worsens the condition, leading to malnutrition. This is associated with functional impairment of many organs, delayed and abnormal wound healing, and decreased immunocompetence. Malnutrition in burns can be subverted to some extent by delivery of adequate exogenous nutritional support, but the goals of this treatment is principally to prevent nutritional complications.

Several formulas are used to calculate caloric requirements in burn patients. One multiplies the basal energy expenditure determined by the Harris-Benedict formula by 2 in burns greater than 40% TBSA, assuming a 100% increase in total energy expenditure. When total energy expenditure was measured by the doubly labeled water method, actual expenditures were found to be 1.3 times the predicted basal energy expenditure for pediatric patients with burns greater than 40% TBSA.[58] When measured during convalescence after initial hospitalization, it remained elevated at 1.1 times predicted energy expenditure.[59] These studies indicate that the calculation of 2 times the predicted basal energy expenditure might be too high.

Another common used calculation is the Curreri formula, which calls for 25 kcal/kg/day plus 40 kcal per percent TBSA burned per day. This formula provides for maintenance needs plus the additional caloric needs related to the burn wounds. This formula was devised as a regression from nitrogen balance data in severely burned adults. In children, formulas based on body surface area are more appropriate because of the greater body surface area per kilogram of weight. We recommend the following formulas depending on the child's age (Table 20.6). These formulas were determined to maintain body weight in severely burned children. The formulas change with age based on the body surface area alterations that occur with growth.

The composition of the nutritional supplement is also important. The optimal dietary composition contains 1 to 2 g/kg/day of protein, which provides a calorie-to-nitrogen ratio at around 100:1 with the earlier suggested caloric intakes. This amount of protein provides for the synthetic needs of the patient, thus sparing to some extent the proteolysis occurring in the active muscle tissue. Nonprotein calories can be given either as carbohydrate or as fat. Carbohydrates have the advantage of stimulating endogenous insulin production, which may have the beneficial effects on muscle and the burn wounds as an anabolic hormone.[60] In addition, it was shown that almost all of the fat transported in very-low-density lipoprotein after severe burn is derived from peripheral lipolysis and not from de novo synthesis of fatty acids in the liver from dietary carbohydrates.[61] Additional fat to deliver noncarbohydrate calories then has little support.

The diet may be delivered in two forms, either enterally through enteric tubes or parenterally through intravenous catheters. Parenteral nutrition may be given in isotonic solutions through peripheral catheters or with hypertonic solutions in central catheters; however, the caloric demands of burn patients prohibit the use of peripheral parenteral nutrition. Total parenteral nutrition delivered centrally in burned patients has been associated with increased complications and mortality rate compared with enteral feedings.[62] Total parenteral nutrition is reserved only for those patients who cannot tolerate enteral feedings. Enteral feeding has been associated with some complications, however, which can be disastrous. These include mechanical complications, enteral feeding intolerance, and diarrhea.

Nutritional adjunctive treatment with anabolic agents has received attention as a means to decrease lean mass losses after severe injury. Agents used include growth hormone, insulin-like growth factor, insulin, oxandrolone, testosterone, and propranolol. Studies supporting the use of each are now over 10 years old, and the market test suggested that oxandrolone and propranolol are now the most commonly used. Each of these agents has different

TABLE 20.6 **Formulas to predict calorie needs in severely burned children.**

AGE GROUP	MAINTENANCE NEEDS	BURN WOUND NEEDS
Infants (0–12 months)	2100 kcal/% TBSA burned/24 hours	1000 kcal/% TBSA burned/24 hours
Children (1–12 years)	1800 kcal/% TBSA burned/24 hours	1300 kcal/% TBSA burned/24 hours
Adolescents (12–18 years)	1500 kcal/% TBSA burned/24 hours	1500 kcal/% TBSA burned/24 hours

TBSA, Total body surface area.

actions to stimulate protein synthesis through an increase in protein synthetic efficiency. Put simply, the free amino acids available in the cytoplasm from protein breakdown with severe injury or illness are preferentially shunted toward protein synthesis rather than export out of the cell.

ELECTRICAL BURNS

Initial Treatment

Of all admitted burned patients, 3% to 5% are injured from electrical contact. Electrical injury is unlike other burns in that the visible areas of tissue necrosis represent only a small portion of the injured tissue. Electrical current enters a part of the body, such as the fingers or hand, and proceeds through tissues with the lowest resistance to current, generally the nerves, blood vessels, and muscles. The skin has a relatively high resistance to electrical current and is therefore mostly spared. The current then leaves the body at a "grounded" area on some other part of the body. Heat generated by the transfer of electrical current and passage of the current itself then injures the tissues. During this exchange, the muscle is the major tissue through which the current flows and thus sustains the most damage. Most muscle is in close proximity to bones; therefore, that is where the most injury is evident. The bone itself does not sustain any increase in temperature or injury. Blood vessels transmitting much of the electricity initially remain patent, but they may proceed to progressive thrombosis as the cells either die or repair themselves, thus resulting in further tissue loss from ischemia that might be evident days later.

Injuries are divided into high- and low-voltage injuries. Low-voltage injury is similar to thermal burns without transmission to the deeper tissues; zones of injury from the surface extend into the tissue. Most household currents (110–220 volts) produce this type of injury, which causes only local damage. The worst of these injuries are those involving the edge of the mouth (oral commissure) sustained when children gnaw on household electrical cords with alternating current. Most households are on direct current, and therefore, these types of injuries are now rare.

The syndrome of high-voltage injury consists of varying degrees of cutaneous burn at the entry and exit sites, combined with hidden destruction of deep tissue. Often, these patients also have cutaneous burns associated with ignition of clothing from the discharge of electrical current. Of note, the burns on the skin are mostly thermal, and not electrical. Initial evaluation consists of cardiopulmonary resuscitation if ventricular fibrillation is induced. Thereafter, if the initial electrocardiogram findings are abnormal or there is a history of cardiac arrest associated with the injury, continued cardiac monitoring is indicated along with pharmacologic treatment for any dysrhythmias. The most serious derangements occur in the first 24 hours after injury. If patients with electrical injuries have no cardiac dysrhythmias on initial electrocardiogram or recent history of cardiac arrest, no further monitoring is necessary.

Patients with electrical injuries are at risk for other injuries, such as being thrown from the electrical jolt or falling from heights after disengaging from the electrical current. In addition, the violent tetanic muscular contractions that result from alternating current sources may cause a variety of fractures and dislocations. These patients should be assessed as any other patient with blunt traumatic injuries.

The key to managing patients with an electrical injury lies in the treatment of the wound. The most significant injury is within the deep tissue, and subsequent edema formation can cause vascular compromise to any area distal to the injury. Assessment should include circulation to distal vascular beds, because immediate escharotomy and fasciotomy may be indicated. If the muscle compartment is extensively injured and necrotic, such that the prospects for eventual function are dismal, early amputation may be necessary. We advocate early exploration of affected muscle beds and debridement of devitalized tissues, with attention given to the deeper periosteous planes, because this is the area with the most muscle. Fasciotomies should be complete and may include nerve decompressions, such as carpal tunnel and Guyon canal releases. Tissue that has questionable viability should be left in place, with planned reexploration. Many such reexplorations may be required until the wound is completely debrided. Electrical damage to vessels may be delayed, and the extent of necrosis may extend after the initial debridements.

After the devitalized tissues are removed, closure of the wound becomes paramount. Although skin grafts suffice as closure for most wounds, flaps may offer a better alternative, particularly with exposed bones and tendons. Even exposed and superficially infected bones and tendons can be salvaged with coverage by vascularized tissue. Early involvement by reconstructive surgeons versed in the various methods of wound closure is optimal.

Muscle damage results in release of hemochromogens (myoglobin), which are filtered in the glomeruli and may result in obstructive nephropathy. Therefore, vigorous hydration and infusion of intravenous sodium bicarbonate (5% continuous infusion) and mannitol (25 g every 6 hours for adults) are indicated to solubilize the hemochromogens and maintain urine output if significant amounts are found in the serum. These patients also benefit from additional intravenous volumes over predicted amounts for the wound area because most of the wound is deep and cannot be assessed by physical examination.

Delayed Effects

Neurologic deficits may occur that may seem somewhat random. Serial neurologic evaluations should be performed as part of routine examination in order to detect any early or late neuropathology. Central nervous system effects such as cortical encephalopathy, hemiplegia, aphasia, and brainstem dysfunction injury have been reported up to 9 months after injury; others report delayed peripheral nerve lesions characterized by demyelination with vacuolization and reactive gliosis. Another devastating long-term effect is the development of cataracts, which can be delayed for several years. These complications may occur in up to 30% of patients with significant high-voltage injury, and patients should be made aware of their possibility even with the best treatment.

CHEMICAL BURNS

Most chemical burns are incidental from mishandling of household cleaners, although some of the most dramatic presentations involve industrial exposures. Thermal burns are, in general, short-term exposures to heat, but chemical injuries may be of longer duration, even for hours in the absence of appropriate treatment. The degree of tissue damage, as well as the level of toxicity, is determined by the chemical nature of the agent, concentration of the agent, and the duration of skin contact. Chemicals cause their injury by protein destruction, with denaturation, oxidation, formation of protein esters, or desiccation of the tissue. In the United States, the composition of most household and industrial chemicals can be obtained from the Poison Control Center in the area, which can give suggestions for treatment.

Speed is essential in the management of chemical burns. For all chemicals, lavage with copious quantities of clean water should be done immediately after removing all clothing. Dry powders should be brushed from the affected areas before irrigation. Early irrigation dilutes the chemical, which is already in contact with the skin, and timeliness increases effectiveness of irrigation; several liters of irrigant may be used. For example, 10 mL of 98% sulfuric acid dissolved in 12 L of water decreases the pH to 5.0, a range that can still cause injury. If the chemical composition is known (acid or base), monitoring of the spent lavage solution pH gives a good indication of lavage effectiveness and completion. A reasonable rule of thumb is to lavage with 15 to 20 L of tap water or more for significant chemical injuries. The lavage site should be kept drained in order to remove the earlier, more concentrated effluent. Care should be taken to drain away from uninjured areas to avoid further exposure (Fig. 20.8).

All patients must be monitored according to the severity of their injuries. They may have metabolic disturbances, usually from pH abnormalities, because of exposure to strong acids or caustics. If respiratory difficulty is apparent, oxygen therapy and mechanical ventilation must be instituted. Resuscitation should be guided by the body surface area involved (burn formulas); however, the total fluids given may be dramatically different from the calculated volumes. Some of these injuries may be more superficial than they appear, particularly in the case of acids because of coagulative necrosis, and therefore have less resuscitation volume. Injuries from bases, however, may penetrate beyond that which is apparent on examination (liquefactive necrosis), and therefore, more volume might be indicated. For this reason, patients with chemical injuries should be observed closely for signs of adequate perfusion, such as urine output. All patients with significant chemical injuries should be monitored with indwelling bladder catheters to accurately measure outputs.

Operative excision if indicated by clinical assessment of wound depth should take place as soon as the patient is stable and resuscitated. Following adequate lavage and excision, burn wounds are covered with antimicrobial agents or skin substitutes. Once the wounds have stabilized with the indicated treatment, they are taken care of as with any loss of soft tissue. Skin grafting or flap coverage is performed as needed.

Alkali

Alkalis, such as lime, potassium hydroxide, bleach, and sodium hydroxide, are among the most common agents involved in chemical injury. Incidental injury frequently occurs in infants and toddlers exploring cleaning cabinets. Three factors are involved in the mechanism of alkali burns: (1) saponification of fat causes the loss of insulation of heat formed in the chemical reaction with tissue, (2) massive extraction of water from cells causes damage because of the hygroscopic nature of alkali, and (3) alkalis dissolve and unite with the proteins of the tissues to form alkaline proteinates, which are soluble and contain hydroxide ions. These ions induce further chemical reactions, penetrating deeper into the tissue. Treatment involves immediate removal of the causative agent with lavage of large volumes of fluid, usually water. Attempts to neutralize alkali agents with weak acids are not recommended because the heat released by neutralization reactions induces further injury through the thermoplastic reaction. Particularly strong bases should be treated with lavage and consideration for the addition of wound debridement in the operating room. Tangential removal of affected areas is performed until the tissues removed are at a normal pH.

Cement (calcium oxide) burns are alkali in nature, occur commonly, and are usually work-related injuries. The critical substance responsible for the skin damage is the hydroxyl ion. Often, the agent has been in contact with the skin for prolonged periods, such as underneath the boots of a cement worker who seeks treatment hours after the exposure, or after the cement penetrates clothing and, when combined with perspiration, induces an exothermic reaction. Treatment consists of removing all clothing and irrigating the affected area with water and soap until all the cement is removed and the effluent has a pH of less than 8. Injuries tend to be deep because of exposure times, and surgical excision and grafting of the resultant eschar may be indicated.

Acids

Acid injuries are treated initially like any other chemical injury, with removal of all chemicals by disrobing the affected area and copious irrigation. Acids induce protein breakdown by hydrolysis and coagulative necrosis, which results in a hard eschar that does not penetrate as deeply as the alkalis. These agents also induce thermal injury by heat generation with contact of the skin, further causing soft tissue damage.

Formic acid injuries are relatively rare, usually involving an organic acid for industrial descaling and as a hay preservative. Electrolyte abnormalities are of great concern for patients who have sustained extensive formic acid injuries, with metabolic acidosis, renal failure, intravascular hemolysis, and pulmonary complications being common. Acidemia detected by a metabolic acidosis on arterial blood gas analysis should be corrected with intravenous sodium bicarbonate. Hemodialysis may be indicated when extensive absorption of formic acid has occurred. A formic acid wound typically has a greenish appearance and is deeper than what it initially appears to be; it is best treated by surgical excision.

Hydrofluoric acid is a toxic substance used widely in both industrial and domestic settings and is the strongest inorganic acid known. Management of these burns differs from other acid burns in general. Hydrofluoric acid produces dehydration and corrosion of tissue with free hydrogen ions. In addition, the fluoride ion complexes with bivalent cations such as calcium and magnesium to form insoluble salts. Systemic absorption of the fluoride ion then can induce intravascular calcium chelation and hypocalcemia, which causes life-threatening arrhythmias. Beyond initial copious irrigation with clean water, the burned area should be treated immediately with copious 2.5% calcium gluconate gel. These wounds in general are very painful because of the calcium chelation and associated potassium release; this finding can be used to determine the effectiveness of treatment. The gel should be changed at 15-minute intervals until the pain subsides, an indication of removal of the active fluoride ion. If pain relief is incomplete after several applications or symptoms recur, intradermal injections of 10% calcium gluconate (0.5 mL/cm^2 affected),

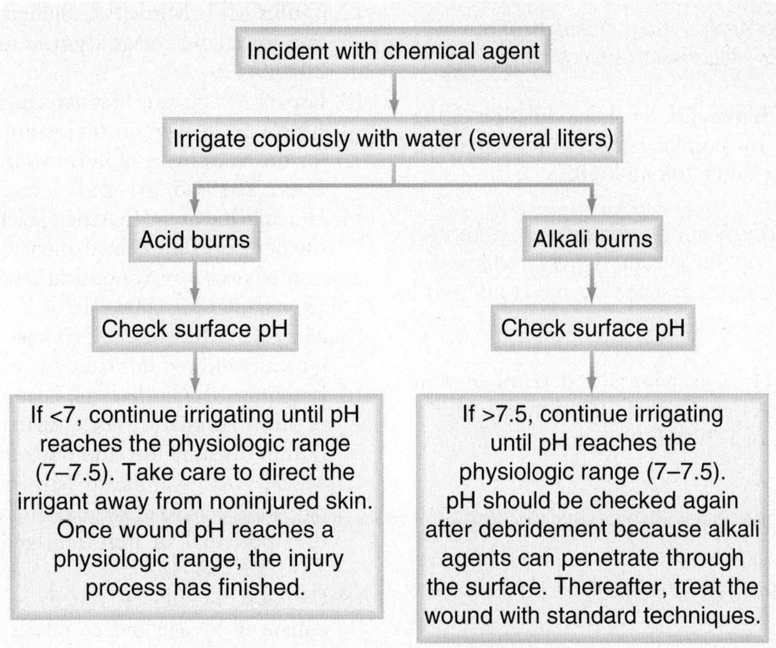

FIG. 20.8 Treatment of acid and alkali burns.

intra-arterial calcium gluconate into the affected extremity, or both may be required to alleviate symptoms. If the burn is not treated in such a fashion, decalcification of the bone underlying the injury and extension of the soft tissue injury may occur.

All patients with hydrofluoric acid burns should be admitted for cardiac monitoring, with particular attention paid to prolongation of the QT interval. A total of 20 mL of 10% calcium gluconate solution should be added to the first liter of resuscitation fluid, and serum electrolytes must be closely monitored. Any electrocardiographic changes should institute a rapid response by the treatment team with intravenous calcium chloride to maintain heart function. Several grams of calcium may be needed in the end until the chemical response has run its course. Serum magnesium and potassium also should be closely monitored and replaced. Speed is the key to effective treatment.

Hydrocarbons

The organic solvent properties of hydrocarbons promote cell membrane dissolution and skin necrosis. Symptoms include erythema and blistering, and the burns are typically superficial and heal spontaneously. If absorbed systemically, toxicity can produce respiratory depression and eventual hepatic injury thought to be associated with benzenes. Ignition of the hydrocarbons on the skin induces a deep full-thickness injury.

SUMMARY

The treatment of burns is complex. Minor injuries can be treated in the community by knowledgeable physicians. Moderate and severe injuries, however, benefit from treatment in dedicated facilities with resources to maximize the outcomes from these often-devastating events. Care of patients has markedly improved such that most patients even with massive injuries survive. Challenges for the future will be in the areas of scar minimization and control and acceleration of the healing time to result in functional and visually appealing outcomes.

SELECTED REFERENCES

Baxter CR. Fluid volume and electrolyte changes of the early postburn period. *Clin Plast Surg*. 1974;1:693–703.

This article defined the development and use of the Parkland formula for the resuscitation of burned patients.

Bull JP, Squire JR. A study of mortality in a burns unit: standards for the evaluation of alternative methods of treatment. *Ann Surg*. 1949;130:160–173.

This landmark article was one of the first to describe the incidence of burn mortality.

Herndon DN, Hart DW, Wolf SE, et al. Reversal of catabolism by beta-blockade after severe burns. *N Engl J Med*. 2001;345:1223–1229.

This landmark clinical trial showed that propranolol, a nonselective beta receptor antagonist, attenuates the profound hypermetabolic response and the muscle-protein catabolism after severe burn injury.

Herndon DN, Tompkins RG. Support of the metabolic response to burn injury. *Lancet*. 2004;363:1895–1902.

This review was one of the premier articles to highlight the many methods to attenuate the hypermetabolic response and to thoroughly describe the physiologic and metabolic derangements postburn.

Jeschke MG, Chinkes DL, Finnerty CC, et al. Pathophysiologic response to severe burn injury. *Ann Surg*. 2008;248:387–401.

This landmark clinical trial delineated the complexity of the hypermetabolic, hypercatabolic response to severe burn injury.

Williams FN, Jeschke MG, Chinkes DL, et al. Modulation of the hypermetabolic response to trauma: temperature, nutrition, and drugs. *J Am Coll Surg.* 2009;208:489–502.

This review highlights the significant pharmacologic and nonpharmacologic modulators of the postburn hypermetabolic response that have been shown to improve morbidity and mortality.

Wolf SE, Rose JK, Desai MH, et al. Mortality determinants in massive pediatric burns. An analysis of 103 children with > or = 80% TBSA burns (> or = 70% full-thickness). *Ann Surg.* 1997;225:554–565.

The treatment of severely burned pediatric patients and the major determinants of mortality are described in this article. A formula was also devised to predict those who will survive or succumb to their injuries.

REFERENCES

1. Centers for Disease Control and Prevention. *Injury Prevention & Control: Data & Statistics (WISQARS)*; 2016. https://www.cdc.gov/injury/wisqars/index.html. Accessed June 19, 2019.
2. American Burn Association. *Burn Incidence Fact Sheet*; 2016. Available at https://ameriburn.org/who-we-are/media/burn-incidence-fact-sheet/. Accessed June 19, 2019.
3. Pruitt Jr BA. The universal trauma model. *Bull Am Coll Surg.* 1985;70:2.
4. America Burn Association. *National Burn Repository 2019 Update: Report of Data from 2009–2018*; 2019. http://ameriburn.org/wp-content/uploads/2019/04/2019_aba_annual_report_website-content.pdf. Accessed June 19, 2019.
5. Wolf SE, Cancio LC, Pruitt Jr BA. Epidemiological, demographic, and outcome characteristics of burns. In: Herndon DN, ed. *Total Burn Care.* 5th ed. Edinburgh: Elsevier; 2018:14–27.
6. Jackson PC, Hardwicke J, Bamford A, et al. Revised estimates of mortality from the Birmingham Burn Centre, 2001–2010: a continuing analysis over 65 years. *Ann Surg.* 2014;259:979–984.
7. Spies M, Herndon DN, Rosenblatt JI, et al. Prediction of mortality from catastrophic burns in children. *Lancet.* 2003;361:989–994.
8. American Burn Association. *Burn Center Transfer Criteria*; 2017. ameriburn.org/wp-content/uploads/2017/05/burncenterreferralcriteria.pdf. Accessed June 20, 2019.
9. Abraham JP, Stark J, Gorman J, et al. Tissue burns due to contact between a skin surface and highly conducting metallic media in the presence of inter-tissue boiling. *Burns.* 2019;45:369–378.
10. Jackson DM. The diagnosis of the depth of burning. *Br J Surg.* 1953;40:588–596.
11. Shupp JW, Nasabzadeh TJ, Rosenthal DS, et al. A review of the local pathophysiologic bases of burn wound progression. *J Burn Care Res.* 2010;31:849–873.
12. Cirillo MD, Mirdell R, Sjoberg F, et al. tensor decomposition for colour image segmentation of burn wounds. *Sci Rep.* 2019;9:3291.
13. Jaspers MEH, van Haasterecht L, van Zuijlen PPM, et al. A systematic review on the quality of measurement techniques for the assessment of burn wound depth or healing potential. *Burns.* 2019;45:261–281.
14. Heredia-Juesas J, Thatcher JE, Lu Y, et al. Burn-injured tissue detection for debridement surgery through the combination of non-invasive optical imaging techniques. *Biomed Opt Express.* 2018;9:1809–1826.
15. Xiao W, Mindrinos MN, Seok J, et al. A genomic storm in critically injured humans. *J Exp Med.* 2011;208:2581–2590.
16. Bergquist M, Hastbacka J, Glaumann C, et al. The time-course of the inflammatory response to major burn injury and its relation to organ failure and outcome. *Burns.* 2019;45:354–363.
17. McGee MP, Morykwas MJ, Argenta LC. The local pathology of interstitial edema: surface tension increases hydration potential in heat-damaged skin. *Wound Repair Regen.* 2011;19:358–367.
18. Osuka A, Kusuki H, Yoneda K, et al. Glycocalyx shedding is enhanced by age and correlates with increased fluid requirement in patients with major burns. *Shock.* 2018;50:60–65.
19. Zhang XJ, Irtun O, Zheng Y, et al. Methysergide reduces nonnutritive blood flow in normal and scalded skin. *Am J Physiol Endocrinol Metab.* 2000;278:E452–E461.
20. Matsuda T, Tanaka H, Reyes HM, et al. Antioxidant therapy using high dose vitamin C: reduction of postburn resuscitation fluid volume requirements. *World J Surg.* 1995;19:287–291.
21. Lin J, Falwell S, Greenhalgh D, et al. High-dose ascorbic acid for burn shock resuscitation may not improve outcomes. *J Burn Care Res.* 2018;39:708–712.
22. Ferrara JJ, Franklin EW, Kukuy EL, et al. Lymph isolated from a regional scald injury produces a negative inotropic effect in dogs. *J Burn Care Rehabil.* 1998;19:296–304.
23. Cioffi WG, DeMeules JE, Gamelli RL. The effects of burn injury and fluid resuscitation on cardiac function in vitro. *J Trauma.* 1986;26:638–642.
24. Chrysopoulo MT, Jeschke MG, Dziewulski P, et al. Acute renal dysfunction in severely burned adults. *J Trauma.* 1999;46:141–144.
25. Chung KK, Lundy JB, Matson JR, et al. Continuous venovenous hemofiltration in severely burned patients with acute kidney injury: a cohort study. *Crit Care.* 2009;13:R62.
26. Clark AT, Li X, Kulangara R, et al. Acute kidney injury after burn: a cohort study from the parkland burn intensive care unit. *J Burn Care Res.* 2019;40:72–78.
27. Gamelli RL, He LK, Liu H, et al. Burn wound infection-induced myeloid suppression: the role of prostaglandin E2, elevated adenylate cyclase, and cyclic adenosine monophosphate. *J Trauma.* 1998;44:469–474.
28. McDonald B. Neutrophils in critical illness. *Cell Tissue Res.* 2018;371:607–615.
29. Rendon JL, Choudhry MA. Th17 cells: critical mediators of host responses to burn injury and sepsis. *J Leukoc Biol.* 2012;92:529–538.
30. Hultman CS, Yamamoto H, deSerres S, et al. Early but not late burn wound excision partially restores viral-specific T lymphocyte cytotoxicity. *J Trauma.* 1997;43:441–447.
31. Martini WZ, Irtun O, Chinkes DL, et al. Alteration of hepatic fatty acid metabolism after burn injury in pigs. *JPEN J Parenter Enteral Nutr.* 2001;25:310–316.

32. Moore FD. Bodily changes in surgical convalescence. I. The normal sequence observations and interpretations. *Ann Surg.* 1953;137:289–315.
33. Hart DW, Wolf SE, Mlcak R, et al. Persistence of muscle catabolism after severe burn. *Surgery.* 2000;128:312–319.
34. Harish V, Tiwari N, Fisher OM, et al. First aid improves clinical outcomes in burn injuries: evidence from a cohort study of 4918 patients. *Burns.* 2019;45:433–439.
35. Frear CC, Griffin B, Watt K, et al. Barriers to adequate first aid for paediatric burns at the scene of the injury. *Health Promot J Austr.* 2018;29:160–166.
36. Chung KK, Salinas J, Renz EM, et al. Simple derivation of the initial fluid rate for the resuscitation of severely burned adult combat casualties: in silico validation of the rule of 10. *J Trauma.* 2010;69(suppl 1):S49–S54.
37. Baxter CR. Fluid volume and electrolyte changes of the early postburn period. *Clin Plast Surg.* 1974;1:693–703.
38. Navickis RJ, Greenhalgh DG, Wilkes MM. Albumin in burn shock resuscitation: a meta-analysis of controlled clinical studies. *J Burn Care Res.* 2016;37:e268–e278.
39. Pruitt Jr BA, Mason Jr AD, Moncrief JA. Hemodynamic changes in the early postburn patient: the influence of fluid administration and of a vasodilator (hydralazine). *J Trauma.* 1971;11:36–46.
40. Demling RH, Mazess RB, Witt RM, et al. The study of burn wound edema using dichromatic absorptiometry. *J Trauma.* 1978;18:124–128.
41. Gunn ML, Hansbrough JF, Davis JW, et al. Prospective, randomized trial of hypertonic sodium lactate versus lactated Ringer's solution for burn shock resuscitation. *J Trauma.* 1989;29:1261–1267.
42. Huang PP, Stucky FS, Dimick AR, et al. Hypertonic sodium resuscitation is associated with renal failure and death. *Ann Surg.* 1995;221:543–554; discussion 554–547.
43. Klein MB, Hayden D, Elson C, et al. The association between fluid administration and outcome following major burn: a multicenter study. *Ann Surg.* 2007;245:622–628.
44. Salinas J, Chung KK, Mann EA, et al. Computerized decision support system improves fluid resuscitation following severe burns: an original study. *Crit Care Med.* 2011;39:2031–2038.
45. Wolf SE, Rose JK, Desai MH, et al. Mortality determinants in massive pediatric burns. An analysis of 103 children with > or = 80% TBSA burns (> or = 70% full-thickness). *Ann Surg.* 1997;225:554–565; discussion 565–559.
46. Rehberg S, Yamamoto Y, Sousse LE, et al. Antithrombin attenuates vascular leakage via inhibiting neutrophil activation in acute lung injury. *Crit Care Med.* 2013;41:e439–e446.
47. Basadre JO, Sugi K, Traber DL, et al. The effect of leukocyte depletion on smoke inhalation injury in sheep. *Surgery.* 1988;104:208–215.
48. Deutsch CJ, Tan A, Smailes S, et al. The diagnosis and management of inhalation injury: an evidence based approach. *Burns.* 2018;44:1040–1051.
49. Desai MH, Mlcak R, Richardson J, et al. Reduction in mortality in pediatric patients with inhalation injury with aerosolized heparin/*N*-acetylcystine [correction of acetylcystine] therapy. *J Burn Care Rehabil.* 1998;19:210–212.
50. Chung KK, Wolf SE, Renz EM, et al. High-frequency percussive ventilation and low tidal volume ventilation in burns: a randomized controlled trial. *Crit Care Med.* 2010;38:1970–1977.
51. Nimia HH, Carvalho VF, Isaac C, et al. Comparative study of Silver Sulfadiazine with other materials for healing and infection prevention in burns: a systematic review and meta-analysis. *Burns.* 2019;45:282–292.
52. Ong YS, Samuel M, Song C. Meta-analysis of early excision of burns. *Burns.* 2006;32:145–150.
53. Zhang Q, Raoof M, Chen Y, et al. Circulating mitochondrial DAMPs cause inflammatory responses to injury. *Nature.* 2010;464:104–107.
54. Cumming J, Purdue GF, Hunt JL, et al. Objective estimates of the incidence and consequences of multiple organ dysfunction and sepsis after burn trauma. *J Trauma.* 2001;50:510–515.
55. Kallinen O, Maisniemi K, Bohling T, et al. Multiple organ failure as a cause of death in patients with severe burns. *J Burn Care Res.* 2012;33:206–211.
56. Saffle JR, Morris SE, Edelman L. Early tracheostomy does not improve outcome in burn patients. *J Burn Care Rehabil.* 2002;23:431–438.
57. Wolf SE, Jeschke MG, Rose JK, et al. Enteral feeding intolerance: an indicator of sepsis-associated mortality in burned children. *Arch Surg.* 1997;132:1310–1313; discussion 1313–1314.
58. Goran MI, Peters EJ, Herndon DN, et al. Total energy expenditure in burned children using the doubly labeled water technique. *Am J Physiol.* 1990;259:E576–E585.
59. Prelack K, Yu YM, Dylewski M, et al. Measures of total energy expenditure and its components using the doubly labeled water method in rehabilitating burn children. *JPEN J Parenter Enteral Nutr.* 2017;41:470–480.
60. Hart DW, Wolf SE, Zhang XJ, et al. Efficacy of a high-carbohydrate diet in catabolic illness. *Crit Care Med.* 2001;29:1318–1324.
61. Aarsland A, Chinkes D, Wolfe RR, et al. Beta-blockade lowers peripheral lipolysis in burn patients receiving growth hormone. Rate of hepatic very low density lipoprotein triglyceride secretion remains unchanged. *Ann Surg.* 1996;223:777–787; discussion 787–779.
62. Herndon DN, Barrow RE, Stein M, et al. Increased mortality with intravenous supplemental feeding in severely burned patients. *J Burn Care Rehabil.* 1989;10:309–313.

21 CHAPTER

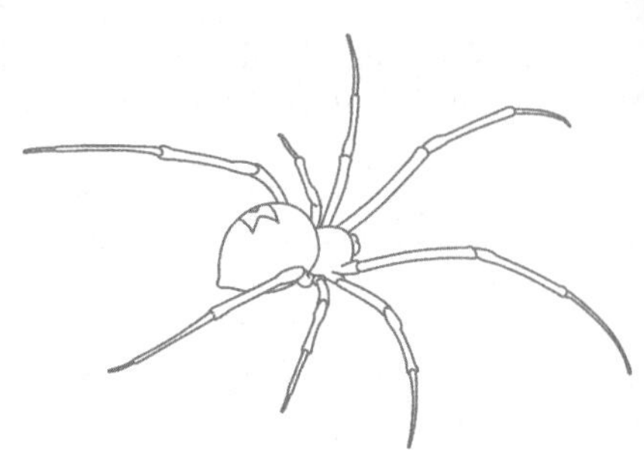

Bites and Stings

Lillian Liao, Robert L. Norris, Elaine E. Nelson, Ronald M. Stewart

OUTLINE

SNAKEBITES

Epidemiology

Snakebites are a public health problem primarily in warm areas across the globe. The burden of injury is greatest in the tropical and subtropical regions of the world, primarily affecting Southeast Asia, India, Australia, South America, and parts of Africa. The World Health Organization reports approximately 5.4 million snakebites worldwide, with 2.7 million snakebite envenomations each year resulting in 81,000 to 138,000 deaths with an estimated threefold number of amputations or permanent disabilities.[1] The actual number of bites may be underreported. In the United States, approximately 5000 venomous bites occur annually, with approximately five deaths reported annually.[2] It is estimated that more deaths would occur if injured individuals did not seek medical care. Long-term morbidity from snakebites is unknown because extended long-term follow-up of these patients is not usually conducted.

Venomous Species Indigenous to United States

Clinically important venomous snakes that inhabit the United States can be divided into two broad classes, Crotalinae and Elapidae. Crotalinae are a subfamily of Viperidae, more commonly known as pit vipers, named for their infrared sensing facial pit. Crotalinae species are numerous and occupy a broad range of habitats, present throughout all of the contiguous United States, with the exception of Maine. Crotalinae include rattlesnakes (Fig. 21.1), copperheads (Fig. 21.2), and cottonmouths/water moccasins. Several characteristics distinguish Crotalinae from nonvenomous snakes. Crotalinae tend to have relatively triangular heads, elliptical pupils, heat-sensing facial pits, and large, retractable anterior fangs (Figs. 21.3 and 21.4). All but one species of rattlesnakes have a terminal rattle as a typical distinguishing feature (see Fig. 21.1). Non-Crotalinae, which with the exception of coral snakes are nonvenomous, have more rounded heads, circular pupils, and no fangs. The only indigenous Elapidae of the United States is the coral snake (Fig. 21.5), which encompasses three distinct species: the eastern coral snake (*Micrurus fulvius*), Texas coral snake (*Micrurus tener*), and Sonoran coral snake (*Micruroides euryxanthus*). North American coral snakes have distinctly colored stripes arranged in a typical pattern on their skin, perhaps remembered best through folk rhymes as "red on yellow, kill a fellow; red on black, venom lack."

Lower extremity bites are more common when the victim is not intentionally handling the snake. Upper extremity bites predominate in victims intentionally handling venomous snakes. Most patients with Crotalinae envenomations present with swelling and pain to the site of injury.[3–5] Coral snake envenomations may have minimal or no local findings.

Pathophysiology

Clinical findings of envenomation from the two subfamilies of snakes differ. Snakes in the Crotalinae family cause 95% of venomous snakebites in the United States. Crotalinae envenomation is typically deposited into the subcutaneous tissue by the fangs of the viper. Less commonly, it is deposited into intramuscular compartments or intravenously and causes major local effects of tissue necrosis and sometimes severe systemic effects with hematologic

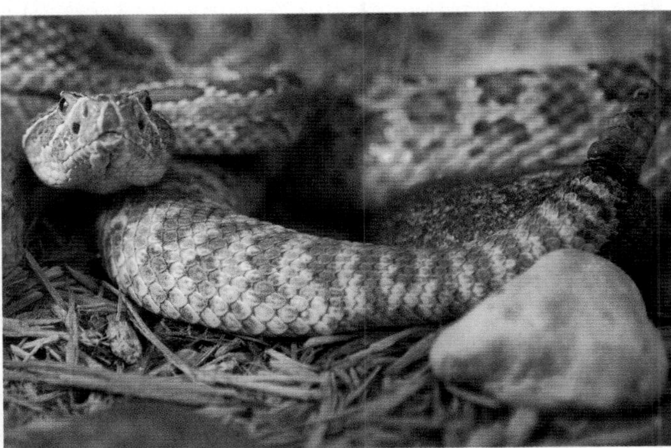

FIG. 21.1 A typical rattlesnake of the Crotalinae subfamily. There are 32 different species in North America, and all but one species have the terminal rattle. (Courtesy Ronald M. Stewart.)

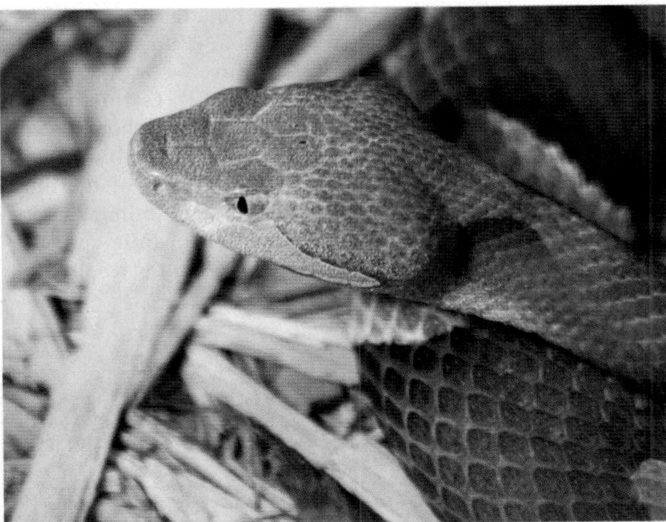

FIG. 21.2 Typical features of a North American copperhead. Many, if not most, copperhead and water moccasin envenomations are less severe than the related rattlesnake species. (Courtesy Ronald M. Stewart.)

abnormalities as a result of its hemotoxic affects.[4,5] Envenomation, which leads to diffuse capillary leakage, can result in pulmonary edema, hypotension, and shock. In addition to primary hemotoxins, a consumptive coagulopathy may follow the severe tissue injury.[6,7] Envenomation can result in diffuse bleeding within 1 hour of envenomation. Although intravenous (IV) envenomation is exceedingly rare, it produces profound shock and organ dysfunction, with onset of these symptoms within minutes.

Crotalinae venom contains a wide array of complex components, including peptides and various enzymes. The venom typically contains zinc-dependent metalloproteinases. These enzymes cause damage at the basement membrane level, disrupting the endothelial cell connections, causing hemorrhage and fluid extravasation.[5] Bite severity in each case is related to the volume deposited and the concentrations of toxin produced by the species of Crotalinae. Rattlesnake envenomations are typically more severe and more likely to require antivenin therapy.

Elapidae venom contains alpha neurotoxin, which results in a direct neurotoxic effect. Toxins affect presynaptic and postsynaptic receptors. The venom can result in respiratory depression with progression to neurogenic shock. Patients with these symptoms have a high risk of mortality, and immediate medical attention is required.[8]

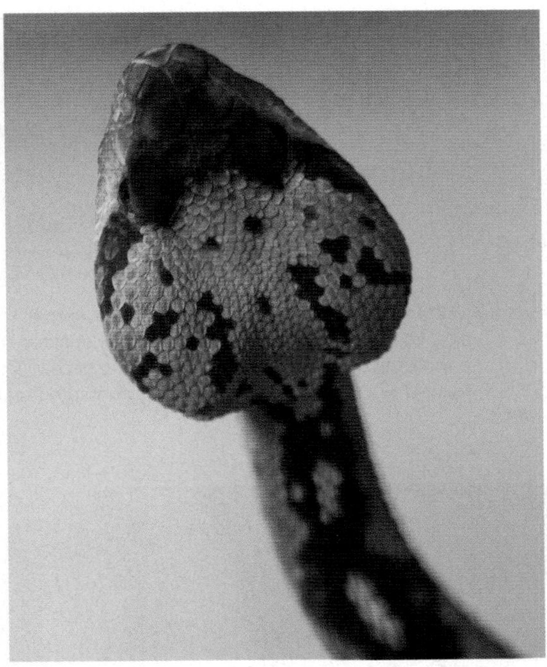

FIG. 21.3 This rattlesnake displays the typical broad, triangular head characteristic of Crotalinae species. (Courtesy Ronald M. Stewart.)

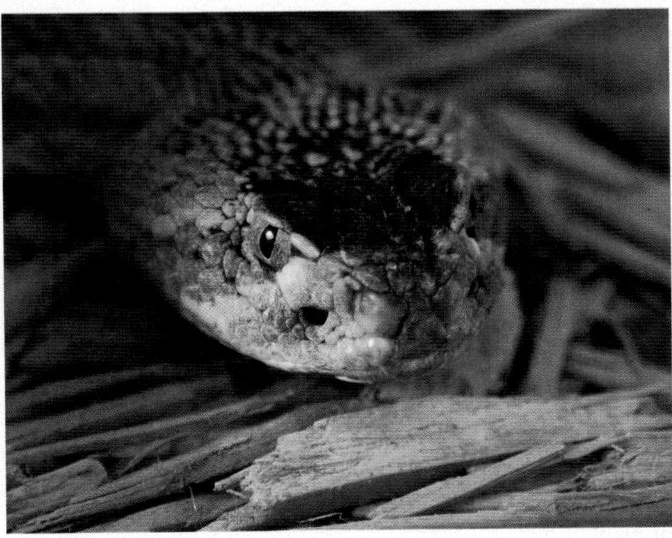

FIG. 21.4 Crotaline species have characteristic facial pits that are extremely sensitive to infrared radiation and elliptical pupils. (Courtesy Ronald M. Stewart.)

Clinical Manifestations

Local signs and symptoms of Crotalinae snakebites include swelling, pain, and ecchymosis. Swelling may progress to bullae formation and typically progresses along the path of the lymphatic drainage of the region bitten (Fig. 21.6). Pain is reported as a burning that starts within minutes of envenomation. Swelling, if progressive, can develop into compartment syndrome of the

Coral snake species, Micrurus sp., remembered through folk rhymes as "red on yellow, kill a fellow; red on black, venom lack."

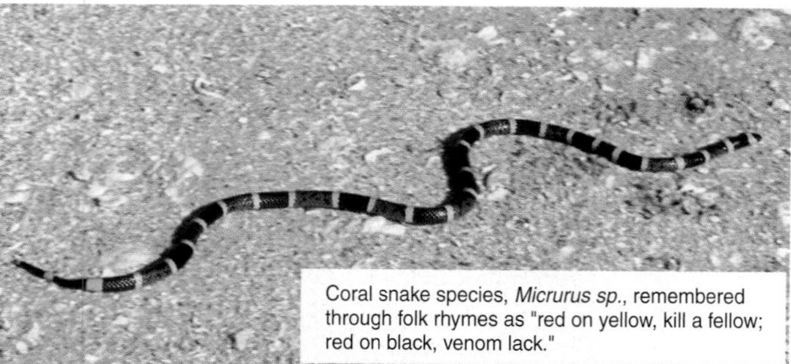

FIG. 21.5 Typical markings of North American coral snakes. It is uncommon to see the furtive coral snake in broad open spaces. (Courtesy Luther C. Goldman, U.S. Fish and Wildlife Service, annotated by Ronald M. Stewart.)

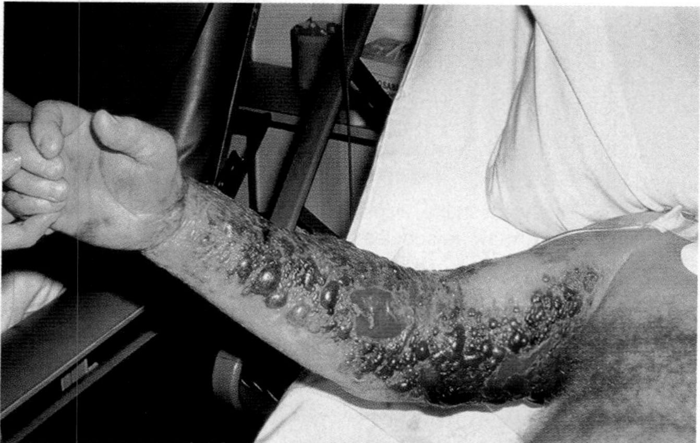

FIG. 21.6 Signs of a severe envenomation (grade 3) with extensive bullae formation after a rattlesnake bite to the hand. This appearance is now uncommon in patients treated early with antivenin.

extremity. Tissue necrosis can also occur, with delays in treatment resulting in loss of function from Crotalinae bites. Systemic signs are due to diffuse circulatory collapse as a result of envenomation. Patients report initial nausea, perioral paresthesias, metallic taste, and muscle twitching. Laboratory derangements include increased partial thromboplastin time, prothrombin time, fibrin split products, elevated creatinine, creatine phosphokinase, proteinuria, hematuria, and anemia.[9]

In contrast, patients with coral snake envenomation, which primarily causes neurotoxicity, may present with respiratory failure or neurologic symptoms with minimal local findings. Systemic signs of coral snakebites, including cranial nerve dysfunction and loss of deep tendon reflexes, may progress to respiratory depression and paralysis over several hours. Differences in therapy make it important to distinguish between coral snake and pit viper bites.[7–9]

Management

Initial management of a snakebite victim is to remove the victim from the area of danger. The wound should be cleaned locally, the affected area should be elevated to the level of the heart if possible, and the patient should be transported to a nearby hospital for determination of need for antivenin administration. Historical recommendations of x-cut aspiration, freshly killed bird, cryotherapy, suction, tourniquets, and electrical shock therapy are harmful and should not be used for first aid or treatment (Table 21.1).

Initial hospital evaluation should follow the protocols and guidelines according to the Advanced Trauma Life Support Course.[10] A detailed history should be obtained from the patient or field health care provider regarding the timing of injury, type of snake involved, and prior history of envenomation. Patients or their family members often bring in the snake (alive or dead); however, these animals should not be handled because bite reflex can occur for up to 1 hour after the snake has been dead. The area of the bite should be marked, and the affected area should be assessed every 15 minutes for progression until the progression has stabilized.[7–9]

Complete laboratory evaluation is needed for patients with Crotalinae bites. Patients with Elapidae bites also need respiratory monitoring. A chest radiograph and electrocardiogram is needed for older patients or patients with systemic symptoms. All patients with signs of envenomation should be observed for at least 24 hours in the hospital. Patients with Crotalinae bites without signs of envenomation or laboratory abnormalities can be discharged after 6 to 8 hours of observation. Potential coral snake envenomations should be observed for a longer time, typically 24 hours.

A grading scale has been used for estimating the severity of Crotalinae bites.[11] The grading tool helps to evaluate progression of injury and determine the need for antivenin administration. This is an important tool because CroFab (BTG International Inc., West Conshohocken, PA) is expensive, and, although generally safe, it can have adverse side effects. The snakebite severity grading scale (Table 21.2) should be used as part of the initial assessment for use of antivenin. Patients with minimal severity without progression would likely not benefit from antivenin. Conversely, patients with moderate to severe bites would likely benefit from antivenin administration (Fig. 21.7).[8–12]

TABLE 21.1 Outdated or disproven treatment modalities for snakebites.

X-CUT ASPIRATION	CONSTRICTOR BAND
Freshly killed bird dressing	Partial or radical excision of wounds
Electrical stimulation	Steroids
Ice—ligature cryotherapy	Heat
Fasciotomy (prophylactic)	Tourniquet

TABLE 21.2 Snakebite severity grading scale.

0	Fang mark; local swelling, ecchymosis <2.5 cm; minimal pain and tenderness; no systemic symptoms
1	Fang mark; history of immediate pain with bite; swelling and erythema 5–15 cm; no systemic symptoms
2	Fang mark; history of immediate severe pain; swelling and erythema 15–40 cm; mild systemic symptoms or abnormal laboratory findings or both
3	Fang mark; history of immediate severe pain; swelling and erythema >40 cm; petechiae and bullae; moderate systemic symptoms; bleeding or disseminated intravascular coagulopathy or both; abnormal laboratory values
4	Fang mark; signs of multiple envenomation sites; history of immediate severe pain; severe systemic signs—coma, shock, bleeding, disseminated intravascular coagulation, and paralysis

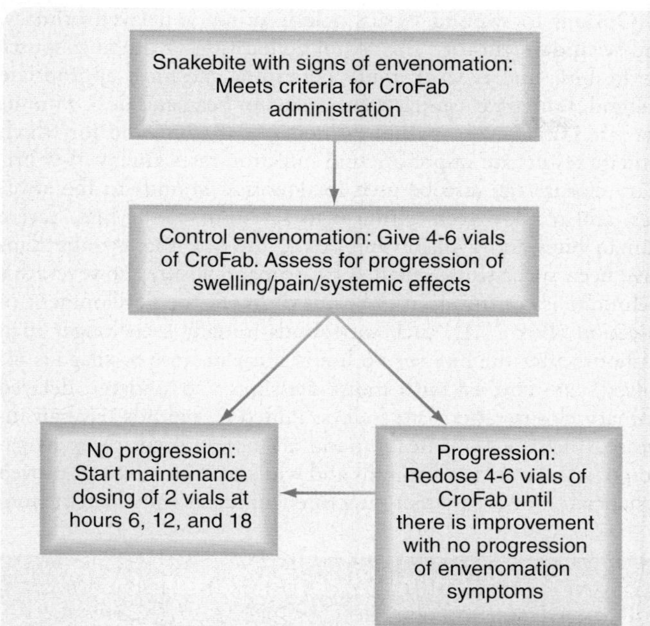

FIG. 21.7 Straightforward algorithm for management of patients with significant envenomation. Dosing is based on an estimate of the degree of envenomation, not on weight.

Antivenin Therapy

Antivenin therapy is the mainstay of treatment for significant envenomations from Crotalinae and Elapidae species.[13] A decision to use antivenin therapy requires clinical judgment, and consultation with experienced clinicians is recommended. Administration of antivenin is time-sensitive in both categories of envenomation: The earlier antivenin is administered, the more effective the therapy. CroFab is a commercially available polyvalent antivenin effective against a wide range of Crotalinae species in the United States. The antibodies used for this product are derived from sheep, and clinical experience has demonstrated the product to be significantly safer than the polyvalent antivenom used before 2000. Antivenin therapy is mediated by antibody to antigen binding. CroFab, as its name implies, consists of fragment antigen-binding segments of the antibodies (Fab). Because there must be enough antibodies to neutralize a given amount of antigen, antivenin dosing is determined by the amount of venom injected by the snake rather than the mass or size of the patient. The initial standard dosing is four to six vials in pediatric and adult patients. The bolus is repeated until the signs and symptoms are stabilized, after which two vials of CroFab are given every 6 hours for three additional doses. Pregnancy is not a contraindication to CroFab.[11–13]

Coral snake (*Micrurus fulvius*) antivenin was produced by Pfizer (New York, NY) and is available in limited quantities for coral snakebites. The antivenin is not currently being produced, and the expiration dates of available antivenin supply have been extended since 2011. The U.S. Food and Drug Administration, in partnership with Pfizer, has been trying to secure more coral snake antivenin. However, at the present time, the supply is highly uncertain, and contacting hospital pharmacies and the regional poison control center is mandatory to assess treatment options. Antivenin treatment should be started early for patients who definitively sustained coral snakebites, as signs and symptoms initially can be minimal. The antivenin carries a risk of anaphylaxis, so administration in a facility where treatment for anaphylaxis is ready available (epinephrine, steroids, antihistamine, and airway control) is mandatory. For envenomations from nonindigenous species in the United States, poison control centers and zoos can provide important information regarding the procurement of antivenin and management. The American Association of Poison Control Centers (800-222-1222) is a useful source of information for physicians needing help in managing venomous snakebites. Given the shortage of some antivenin products, the poison control center contacts are particularly important.[12]

Coagulopathy of Envenomation

Crotalinae envenomation can result in a cascade of systemic coagulopathy.[14] Blood product is required only if the coagulation defect is not reversed by antivenin, or if there is active, significant hemorrhage. Serious bleeding requires the administration of appropriate blood product components based on laboratory values. However, antivenin should begin before replacement of any blood products because treating the primary cause of bleeding is of utmost importance. Coagulopathy can last 2 weeks after injury, and elective surgery must be avoided during this time.[5,9,12]

Fasciotomy

Based on probability, most venom is injected into the subcutaneous space, so fasciotomy is very rarely required; however, venom occasionally is injected into muscle compartments (Fig. 21.8). Children and patients with bites to the hands or fingers are most likely to sustain intramuscular injection of venom. In cases of intramuscular injection, compartment syndrome may develop, and evaluation must be done serially. There is no role for prophylactic fasciotomy.[15] Animal data demonstrate that fasciotomy may increase the severity of local myonecrosis, and antivenin is effective in reducing compartment syndrome[16]; however, if adequate antivenin has been administered and a compartment syndrome is highly likely or demonstrated by increased compartmental pressures, fasciotomy may be required. One must refrain from debridement of injured muscle groups because the usual evaluation of muscle viability (contraction, coloration, general appearance)

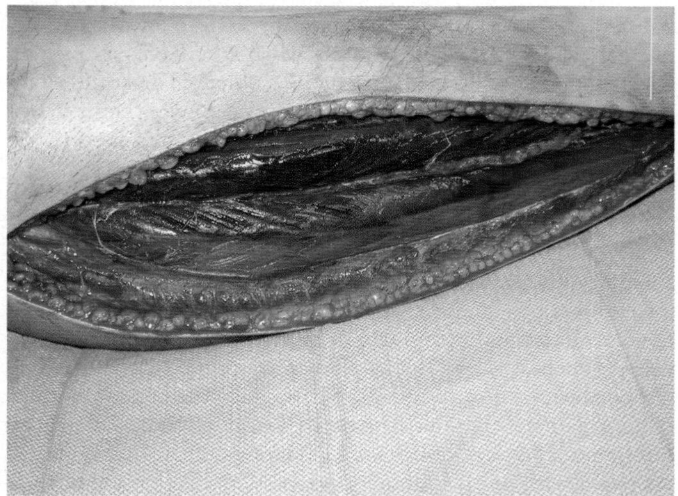

FIG. 21.8 Fasciotomy of the lower extremity in a victim of a severe rattlesnake bite on the lower leg. Intracompartmental pressures were documented to be exceedingly elevated in this patient, despite limb elevation and large doses of antivenom. (Courtesy Ronald M. Stewart.)

is unreliable in the setting of intramuscular envenomation, as this may be a sign of venom injury rather than muscle necrosis. Premature debridement can result in unnecessary morbidity.[15] Antivenin administration is the primary treatment for these patients. Additionally, negative pressure wound therapy is appropriate for coverage of fasciotomy sites.

MAMMALIAN BITES

Epidemiology

The incidence of mammalian bite injuries is unknown because most patients with minor wounds never seek medical care. The majority of human deaths by nonhuman mammals in the United States result from injuries from horses or cattle, not bites.[17] Death from mammalian bites is uncommon in the United States, but thousands of people are killed around the world each year, primarily by large animals such as lions and tigers. Dogs are responsible for 80% to 90% of mammalian bites in the United States, followed by cats and humans; an estimated 4.7 million dog bites occur annually in the United States and account for 1% of emergency department visits.[18] Most of these bites are from a family pet or a neighborhood dog. Pit bulls and Rottweilers account for most fatal dog bites in the United States.[18] Animal bites occur most frequently on the extremities of adults and on the head, face, and neck of children, which increases the risk for death and serious morbidity in children. More than 60% of reported bites occur in children, especially boys 5 to 9 years old. Demographically, the greatest risk of death from dog bites in the United States are in children ages 0 to 4 years old (75 deaths per year) and those greater than 65 years of age (74 deaths per year).[17]

Treatment

Evaluation

Humans attacked by animals are at risk for blunt and penetrating trauma. Animals produce blunt injuries by striking with their extremities, biting with their powerful jaws, and crushing with their body weight. Teeth and claws can puncture body cavities, including the cranium, and amputate extremities. Patients with serious injuries are managed in a similar fashion as other potentially seriously injured victims, with special attention given to wound management. Useful laboratory tests are the same as in other causes of trauma and also include cultures when an infection is present. Radiographs are obtained to diagnose potential fractures, joint penetration, severe infections, and retained foreign bodies, such as teeth. The patient's tetanus immunization status needs to be updated as necessary.

Wound Care

Local wound management reduces the risk for infection and maximizes functional and esthetic outcomes. Early wound cleaning is the most important therapy for preventing infection and zoonotic diseases such as rabies. Intact skin surrounding dirty wounds is scrubbed with a sponge and 1% povidone-iodine or 2% chlorhexidine gluconate solution. Alternatively, a dilute povidone-iodine solution can be used for irrigation, as long as the wound is flushed afterward with normal saline or water. Wounds that are dirty or contain devitalized tissue are cleaned lightly with gauze or a porous sponge and sharply debrided. Optimal wound management may require treatment in the operating room under general or regional anesthesia.

Options for wound repair include primary, delayed primary, and secondary closure. The anatomic location of the bite, source of the bite, and type of injury determine the most appropriate method. Primary closure is appropriate for head and neck wounds that are initially seen within 24 hours of the bite and for which esthetic results are important and infection rates are low.[19,20] Primary closure can also be used for low-risk wounds to the arms, legs, and trunk if seen within 6 to 12 hours of the bite. Severe human bites and avulsion injuries of the face that require flaps have been successfully repaired by primary closure; however, this technique is controversial. Wounds prone to the development of infection (Box 21.1), such as wounds initially seen longer than 24 hours after the bite (or >6 hours if ear or nose cartilage is involved), are covered with moist dressings and undergo delayed primary closure after 3 to 5 days. Puncture wounds have an increased incidence of infection and are not sutured. Deep irrigation of small puncture wounds and wide excision have not proved beneficial. However, larger puncture wounds usually benefit from

BOX 21.1 Animal bite risk factors for infection.

High Risk

Location

Hand, wrist, or foot
Scalp or face in infants (high risk of cranial perforation)
Over a major joint (possible perforation)
Through-and-through bite of a cheek

Type of Wound

Puncture (difficult to irrigate)
Tissue crushing that cannot be debrided
Carnivore bite over a vital structure (artery, nerve, joint)

Patient

>50 years old
Asplenic
Chronic alcoholism
Altered immune status
Diabetes
Peripheral vascular insufficiency
Long-term corticosteroid therapy
Prosthetic or diseased heart valve or joint

Species

Domestic cat
Large cat (deep punctures)
Human (hand bites)
Primates
Pigs

Low Risk

Location

Face, scalp, or mouth

Type of Wound

Large, clean lacerations that can be thoroughly irrigated

Adapted from Keogh S, Callaham ML. Bites and injuries inflicted by domestic animals. In Auerbach PS, ed. *Wilderness Medicine: Management of Wilderness and Environmental Emergencies.* 4th ed. St Louis: Mosby; 2001:961–978.

irrigation and debridement. Healing by secondary intention generally produces unacceptable scars in cosmetically sensitive areas. The clinician should be alert to the fact that significant dog bites may have extensive undermined areas created by the large canine teeth. These wounds require operative intervention under general or regional anesthesia.

Bites involving the hands or feet have a much greater chance of becoming infected and are left open.[20] The primary goal in repairing bite wounds on the hand is to maximize functional outcome. Even with adequate therapy, approximately one-third of dog bites on the hand become infected.[20] Healing by secondary intention is recommended for most hand lacerations. After thorough exploration, irrigation, and debridement, the hand is immobilized, wrapped in a bulky dressing, and elevated. Although high-quality data are limited, preventive, empirical antibiotics in these settings may be warranted.[21]

A common human bite wound associated with high morbidity is a clenched fist injury (fight bite) resulting from striking the tooth of another person's mouth. Regardless of the history obtained, injuries over the dorsum of the metacarpophalangeal joints are treated as clenched fist injuries. Although these wounds appear minor, they often result in serious injury to the extensor tendon or joint capsule and have significant oral bacterial contamination. The extensor tendon retracts when the hand is opened, so evaluation needs to be carried out with the hand in the open and clenched positions. Minor injuries are irrigated, debrided, and left open. Potentially deeper injuries and infected bites require exploration and debridement in the operating room and administration of IV antibiotics.[22] All bite injuries are reevaluated in 1 or 2 days to rule out secondary infection.

Microbiology

Given the large variety and concentration of bacteria in mouths, it is not surprising that wound infection is the main complication of bites, with 3% to 18% of dog bite wounds and approximately 50% of cat bite wounds becoming infected. Infected wounds contain aerobic and anaerobic bacteria and yield an average of five isolates/culture (Box 21.2). Although many wounds are infected by *Staphylococcus* and *Streptococcus* spp. and anaerobes, *Pasteurella* spp. are the most common bacterial pathogen, found in 50% of dog bites and 75% of cat bites. Human bite wounds, as in other bite wounds, are related to the oral flora of the biting offender. These wounds are typically contaminated with *Eikenella corrodens* in addition to the microorganisms found after dog and cat bites.[22,23]

Systemic diseases such as rabies, cat-scratch disease, cowpox, tularemia, leptospirosis, and brucellosis can be acquired through animal bites. Human bites can transmit hepatitis B and C, tuberculosis, syphilis, and human immunodeficiency virus (HIV).[24] Although HIV transmission from human bites is rare, seroconversion is possible when a person with an open wound, either from a bite or a preexisting injury, is exposed to saliva containing HIV-positive blood.[24] In this scenario, baseline and 6-month postexposure HIV testing is performed, and prophylactic treatment with anti-HIV drugs is considered.

BOX 21.2 Common bacteria found in mouths of animals.

- *Acinetobacter* spp.
- *Actinobacillus* spp.
- Aeromonas hydrophila
- *Bacillus* spp.
- *Bacteroides* spp.
- *Bordetella* spp.
- Brucella canis
- Capnocytophaga canimorsus
- Clostridium perfringens
- *Corynebacterium* spp.
- Eikenella corrodens
- *Enterobacter* spp.
- Escherichia coli
- *Eubacterium* spp.
- *Fusobacterium* spp.
- Haemophilus aphrophilus
- Haemophilus haemolyticus
- *Klebsiella* spp.
- Leptotrichia buccalis
- *Micrococcus* spp.
- *Moraxella* spp.
- *Neisseria* spp.
- Pasteurella aerogenes
- Pasteurella canis
- Pasteurella dagmatis
- Pasteurella multocida
- *Peptococcus* spp.
- *Peptostreptococcus* spp.
- *Propionibacterium* spp.
- Proteus mirabilis
- *Pseudomonas* spp.
- Serratia marcescens
- Staphylococcus aureus
- Staphylococcus epidermidis
- *Streptococcus* spp.
- Veillonella parvula

Adapted from Keogh S, Callaham ML. Bites and injuries inflicted by domestic animals. In: Auerbach PS, ed. *Wilderness Medicine: Management of Wilderness and Environmental Emergencies.* 4th ed. St Louis: Mosby; 2001:961–978.

Antibiotics

Although data are limited, preventive antibiotics are recommended for patients with high-risk bites.[21] The initial antibiotic choice and route are based on the type of animal and severity and location of the bite. Cat bites often cause puncture wounds that require antibiotics. Patients with low-risk dog and human bites do not benefit from prophylactic antibiotics unless the hand or foot is involved.[23] Patients seen 24 hours after a bite without signs of infection do not usually need prophylactic antibiotics. Routine cultures of uninfected wounds have not proved useful and are reserved for infected wounds.

Initial antibiotic selection needs to cover *Staphylococcus* and *Streptococcus* spp., anaerobes, *Pasteurella* spp. for dog and cat bites, and *E. corrodens* for human bites. Amoxicillin-clavulanate is an acceptable first-line antibiotic for most bites. Alternatives include second-generation cephalosporins, such as cefoxitin, or a combination of penicillin and a first-generation cephalosporin. Patients who are allergic to penicillin can receive clindamycin combined with trimethoprim-sulfamethoxazole.[18] Infections developing within 24 hours of the bite are generally caused by *Pasteurella* spp. and are treated by antibiotics with appropriate coverage. Patients with serious infections require hospital admission and parenteral antibiotics such as piperacillin-tazobactam, ampicillin-sulbactam, and ticarcillin-clavulanate. For penicillin-allergic patients, options include clindamycin combined with either fluoroquinolone or trimethoprim-sulfamethoxazole and/or doxycycline.

Rabies

Annually, thousands of people die of rabies worldwide, with dog bites or scratches being the major source.[25] In the United States, rabies is primarily found in wildlife, with raccoons being the primary source, followed by skunks, bats, and foxes.[26] Cats and dogs account for less than 5% of cases since the establishment of rabies control programs. Although the number of infected animals in the United States continues to increase, with the total approaching 8000/year, human infection rates remain constant at one to three cases annually. Bats have been the main source of human rabies reported in the United States during the past 20 years, although a history of bat contact is absent in most victims.

Rabies is caused by a rhabdovirus found in the saliva of animals and is transmitted through bites or scratches. Acute encephalitis develops, and patients almost invariably die. The disease usually begins with a prodromal phase of nonspecific complaints and paresthesias, with itching or burning at the bite site spreading to the entire bitten extremity. The disease progresses to an acute neurologic phase. This phase generally takes one of two forms. The more common encephalitic or furious form is typified by fever and hyperactivity that can be stimulated by internal or external factors such as thirst, fear, light, or noise, followed by fluctuating levels of consciousness, aerophobia or hydrophobia, inspiratory spasm, and abnormalities of the autonomic nervous system. The paralytic form of rabies is manifested by fever, progressive weakness, loss of deep tendon reflexes, and urinary incontinence. Both forms progress to paralysis, coma, circulatory collapse, and death.

Adequate wound care and postexposure prophylaxis can prevent the development of rabies.[27] Wounds are washed with soap and water and irrigated with a virucidal agent such as povidone-iodine solution. If rabies exposure is strongly suspected, consider leaving the wound open. The decision to administer rabies prophylaxis after an animal bite or scratch depends on the offending species and nature of the event. Guidelines for administering rabies prophylaxis can be obtained from local public health agencies or from the Advisory Committee on Immunization Practices and the U.S. Centers for Disease Control and Prevention.[27] Research indicates that rabies prophylaxis is not being administered according to guidelines, which results in costly overtreatment or potentially life-threatening undertreatment.

Worldwide, almost 1 million people receive rabies prophylaxis each year; this includes 40,000 people from the United States.[25] Unprovoked attacks are more likely to occur by rabid animals. All wild carnivores must be considered rabid, but birds and reptiles do not contract or transmit rabies. In cases of bites by domestic animals, rodents, or lagomorphs, the local health department needs to be consulted before beginning rabies prophylaxis. A bite from a healthy-appearing domestic animal does not require prophylaxis if the animal can be observed for 10 days (see Boxes 21.1 and 21.2).

Rabies prophylaxis involves passive (with rabies immune globulin) and active (with rabies vaccine) immunization. Passive immunization consists of administering 20 IU/kg body weight of rabies immune globulin. As much of the dose as possible is infiltrated into and around the wound. The rest is given intramuscularly at a site remote from where the vaccine was administered. If the human rabies immune globulin is not given immediately, it can still be administered for up to 7 days. Active immunization for healthy patients consists of administering 1 mL of human diploid cell vaccine or 1 mL of purified chick embryo cell vaccine intramuscularly into the deltoid of adults and into the anterolateral aspect of the thigh in children on days 0, 3, 7, and 14. For immunocompromised patients, a five-dose schedule is recommended on days 0, 3, 7, 14, and 28.[27] Patients with preexposure immunization do not require passive immunization and need active immunization only on days 0 and 3.[27]

ARTHROPOD BITES AND STINGS

Although mammalian and reptilian bites inflict more serious injuries and are generally more dramatic in their presentations, many more people in the United States die from insect bites and stings, most often caused by anaphylaxis. Also, even more people contract vector-related infectious diseases from the bites of insects.

Black Widow Spiders

Widow spiders (genus *Latrodectus*) are found throughout the world. At least one of five species inhabits all areas of the United States except Alaska. The best-known widow spider is the black widow (*Latrodectus mactans*). The female has a leg span of 1 to 4 cm and a shiny black body with a distinctive red ventral marking (often hourglass-shaped) (Fig. 21.9). Variations in color occur among other species, with some appearing brown or red and some without the ventral marking. The nonaggressive female widow spider bites in defense. Males are too small to bite through human skin.

Toxicology

Widow spiders produce neurotoxic venom with minimal local effects. The major component is alpha-latrotoxin, which acts at presynaptic terminals by enhancing the release of neurotransmitters.

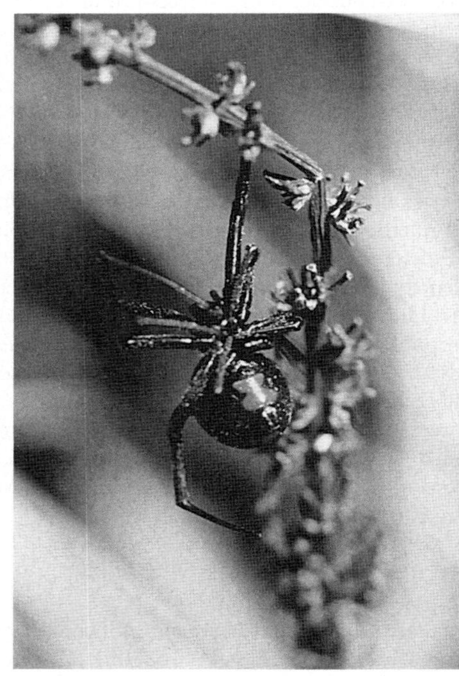

FIG. 21.9 Female black widow spider (*Latrodectus mactans*) with the characteristic hourglass marking. (Courtesy Paul Auerbach.)

The ensuing clinical picture results from excess stimulation of neuromuscular junctions as well as the sympathetic and parasympathetic nervous systems.

Clinical Manifestations

The bite itself may be painless or felt as a pinprick. Local findings are minimal. The patient may have systemic complaints and no history of a spider bite, making the diagnosis challenging. Neuromuscular symptoms may occur 30 minutes after the bite and include severe pain and spasms of large muscle groups. Abdominal cramps and rigidity could mimic a surgical abdomen, but rebound is absent. Dyspnea can result from chest wall muscle tightness. Autonomic stimulation produces hypertension, diaphoresis, and tachycardia. Other symptoms include muscle twitching, nausea and vomiting, headache, and paresthesias.

Treatment

Mild bites are managed with local wound care—cleansing, intermittent application of ice, and tetanus prophylaxis as needed. The possibility of delayed severe symptoms makes an observation period of several hours prudent. The optimal therapy for severe envenomation is controversial. IV calcium gluconate, previously recommended as a first-line drug to relieve muscle spasms after widow spider bites, has no significant efficacy. Narcotics and benzodiazepines are more effective agents to relieve muscular pain. Antivenin has been shown to reduce or eliminate symptoms of latrodectism.[28]

In the United States, antivenom derived from horse serum is available (Black Widow Spider Antivenin; Merck, West Point, PA). Because this antivenom can cause anaphylactoid reactions or serum sickness, it must be reserved for serious cases. Antivenom is currently recommended for pregnant women, children younger than 16 years, adults older than 60 years, and patients with severe envenomation and uncontrolled hypertension or respiratory distress. Skin testing for possible allergy to the U.S. antivenom is recommended by the manufacturer and is outlined in the package insert, although the reliability of such testing is low. Patients about to receive antivenom may be pretreated with antihistamines to reduce the likelihood or severity of a systemic reaction to the serum. The initial recommended dose is one vial intravenously or intramuscularly, repeated as necessary, although it is exceedingly rare for more than two vials to be required. Studies have demonstrated that antivenom can decrease a patient's hospital stay, with discharge several hours after administration.[28] A high-quality antivenom is also available in Australia for *Latrodectus* bites, and a new purified Fab fragment *Latrodectus mactans* antivenom (Analatro) is currently undergoing clinical trials (ClinicalTrials.gov Identifier: NCT00657540) (manufacturer: Instituto Bioclon S.A. de C.V., Mexico City, Mexico).

Brown Recluse Spiders

Envenomation by brown spiders of the genus *Loxosceles* is termed *necrotic arachnidism* or *loxoscelism*. These arthropods primarily inhabit North and South America, Africa, and Europe. Several species of *Loxosceles* are found throughout the United States, with the greatest concentration in the Midwest. Most significant bites in the United States are by *Loxosceles reclusa*, the brown recluse. The brown spiders are varying shades of brownish gray, with a characteristic dark brown, violin-shaped marking over the cephalothorax—hence, the name *violin spider* (Fig. 21.10). Although most spiders have four pairs of eyes, brown spiders have only three pairs. Male and female spiders can bite and may do so when threatened.

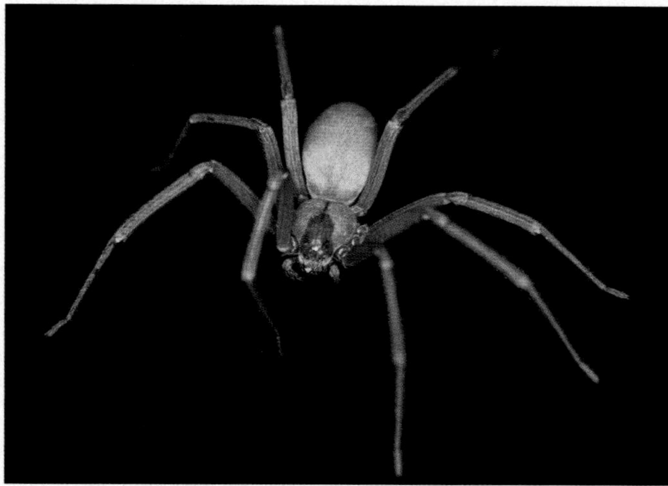

FIG. 21.10 Brown recluse spider (*Loxosceles reclusa*) with a typical violin-shaped marking on the cephalothorax. (Courtesy Rose Pineda, www.rosapineda.com.)

Toxicology

Although several enzymes have been isolated from the venom, the major deleterious factor is sphingomyelinase D, which causes dermonecrosis and hemolysis. It is a phospholipase that interacts with the cell membranes of erythrocytes, platelets, and endothelial cells and causes hemolysis, coagulation, and platelet aggregation. Host responses have some significance in determining the severity of envenomation because functioning polymorphonuclear leukocytes and complement are necessary for the venom to have maximal effect.

Clinical Manifestations

Local findings at the bite site range from mild irritation to severe necrosis with ulceration.[29] The patient is often completely unaware of the bite or may have felt a slight stinging. It is unusual for the victim to see or capture the spider. This can make the diagnosis very challenging because similar skin lesions can represent bites by other arthropods, skin infections (including methicillin-resistant *Staphylococcus aureus*), herpes zoster, dermatologic manifestation of a systemic illness, or other causes of dermatitis and vasculitis.[30] Within several hours of a *Loxosceles* bite, local tissue ischemia develops in some patients, with resulting pain, itching, swelling, and erythema. A blister may form at the site. In more severe bites, the central area turns purple as a result of microvascular thrombosis. Peripheral vasoconstriction can also create a pale border surrounding the central region of necrosis. Over the next several days, an eschar develops over the widening necrotic area. The eschar separates and leaves an ulcer that usually heals over a period of many weeks to months, but occasionally skin grafting is required. Necrosis is most severe in fatty areas such as the abdomen and thigh.

Systemic features include headache, nausea and vomiting, fever, malaise, arthralgia, and maculopapular rash. Additional findings may include thrombocytopenia, disseminated intravascular coagulation, hemolytic anemia, coma, and possibly death. Renal failure can result from intravascular hemolysis.

In patients with lesions consistent with brown spider bites, a search for evidence of systemic involvement (viscerocutaneous or systemic loxoscelism) is initiated, particularly if the victim has any systemic complaints. Appropriate laboratory tests include a complete blood count with platelet count and a bedside urine test for blood. If the results of any of these tests are abnormal, electrolyte, liver function, and coagulation studies are in order, but no truly diagnostic studies are available. Systemic loxoscelism is more common in children and can occur with minimal local findings.

Treatment

All recommended management is controversial, and recommendations should be viewed with a measure of healthy skepticism, especially when the etiology is uncertain. The bite site is splinted, elevated, and treated with cold compresses. Cold therapy inhibits venom activity and has been reported to reduce inflammation and necrosis. Heat application, in contrast, enhances tissue damage and ulcer development. Although controversial, a lipophilic prophylactic antibiotic such as erythromycin or cephalexin can be administered in standard doses for a few days. Tetanus status is updated as needed. Brown spider bites in which necrosis does not develop within 72 hours generally heal well and require no additional therapy. No commercial antivenom is available in the United States.

Some research has suggested that more severe lesions may benefit from dapsone if administered within the first few days after the bite, even though the drug is not approved for this indication.[31] Dapsone may reduce local inflammation and necrosis by inhibiting neutrophil function. The suggested adult dosage is 100 mg/day. Dapsone can cause methemoglobinemia and is contraindicated in patients with glucose-6-phosphate dehydrogenase deficiency. Levels of this enzyme are checked as therapy begins, and dapsone is discontinued if the enzyme level is found to be deficient. Dapsone is not approved for use in children. Given the conflicting data on efficacy, the often uncertain etiology of the lesion, and the side-effect profile of dapsone, the risks of dapsone use likely outweighs any potential benefits. Diphenhydramine has been suggested to be of benefit and is associated with a much more favorable risk profile.[32]

Early surgical intervention, other than simple conservative debridement of obviously necrotic tissue, is avoided. It is difficult or impossible to predict with any certainty the extent of eventual necrosis, and early surgery is apt to be overaggressive and needlessly disfiguring. Pyoderma gangrenosum, manifested as nonhealing ulcers and failure of skin grafts, occurs more often in patients undergoing early excision and debridement, possibly as a result of the rapid spread of venom.[28] After 1 to 2 weeks, when eschar margins are defined, debridement can be performed as necessary. In severe cases, wide excision and split-thickness skin grafting are necessary while dapsone therapy is continued.

Patients with rapidly expanding necrotic lesions or a clinical picture suggesting systemic loxoscelism are admitted for close observation and management. Primary staphylococcal soft tissue infections are much more prevalent than brown recluse spider bites and are often attributed to "spider bites"; alternative diagnoses that may cause rapid expanding tissue necrosis should also be strongly considered in this situation, including serious soft tissue infection. Patients with less serious lesions can be monitored on an outpatient basis with frequent wound checks. Visits during the first 72 hours include reassessment for any evidence of systemic involvement based on symptoms and signs and possibly a bedside urine test for blood.

Scorpions

Significant scorpion envenomation occurs worldwide by species belonging to the family Buthidae. In this group, the bark scorpion (*Centruroides sculpturatus*) is the only potentially dangerous species in the United States. It is found throughout northern Mexico, Arizona, and southern California. Numerous other *Centruroides* species exist throughout the southern United States extending as far north as Nebraska. The bark scorpion is a yellow-to-brown crablike arthropod up to 5 cm in length. Approximately 15,000 scorpion stings were reported during 2004 in the United States, and this is almost certainly a significant underestimate of the total number of stings that occurred. Scorpions tend to be nocturnal and sting when threatened.

Toxicology

Neurotoxic scorpion venoms, such as that produced by the bark scorpion, contain multiple low-molecular-weight basic proteins but possess very little enzymatic activity. The neurotoxins target excitable tissues and work primarily on ion channels, particularly sodium and potassium channels. They cause massive release of multiple neurotransmitters throughout the autonomic nervous system and the adrenal medulla.[33] Almost any organ system can be adversely affected, either by direct toxin effects or by the flood of autonomic neurotransmitters. Because of the speed of their systemic absorption, these neurotoxic scorpion venoms can cause rapid systemic toxicity and potentially death.

Clinical Manifestations

Most scorpion stings in the United States cause short-lived, searing pain and mild, local irritation with slight swelling. Stings by the bark scorpion typically produce local paresthesias and burning pain. Systemic manifestations may include cranial nerve and neuromuscular hyperactivity and respiratory distress.[33] Signs of adrenergic stimulation, accompanied by nausea and vomiting, may also develop. Young children are at greatest risk for severe stings from the bark scorpion. Death can occur from bark scorpion stings, but this is very rare in the United States. As with spider bites, the clinician is advised to consider other common conditions when the etiology is uncertain, as methamphetamine overdose has been misdiagnosed as scorpion envenomation.

Treatment

All patients receive tetanus prophylaxis if indicated, application of cold compresses to the sting site, and analgesics for pain. Victims of bark scorpion stings with signs of systemic envenomation require supportive care, with close monitoring of cardiovascular and respiratory status in an intensive care setting. If systemic signs are present, an equine-derived Fab antivenin approved by the Food and Drug Administration is available for use; Centruroides Immune F(ab′)2 (Anascorp) is manufactured by Rare Disease Therapeutics Inc. (Franklin, TN). This antivenin was studied in a very small randomized clinical trial and found to be effective in reducing systemic symptoms.[34]

Ticks

Several potentially serious diseases occur from tick bites, including Rocky Mountain spotted fever, ehrlichiosis, tularemia, babesiosis, Colorado tick fever, relapsing fever, and Lyme disease. Timely and adequate removal of the tick is important to prevent disease. Common lay recommendations for tick removal, such as the application of local heat, gasoline, methylated spirits, and fingernail polish, are ineffective. Proper removal involves grasping the tick by the body as close to the skin surface as possible with an instrument and applying gradual, gentle axial traction, without twisting. Commercial tick removal devices are superior to standard tweezers for this purpose.[35] An alternative removal method involves looping a length of suture material in a simple overhand knot around the body of the tick. The loop is slipped down as close to the patient's skin surface as possible. The knot is tightened, and the tick is pulled backward and out, over its head in a somersault action. Crushing the tick is avoided because potentially infectious secretions may be squeezed into the wound. After extraction, the wound is cleansed with alcohol or povidone-iodine. Any retained mouthparts of the tick are removed with the tip of a needle. If the tick was embedded for less than 24 hours, the risk of transmitting infection is very low. Tetanus immunization needs to be current. Occasionally, a granulomatous lesion requiring steroid injection or surgical excision may develop at the tick bite site a few weeks after the incident.[36] Patients in whom a local rash or systemic symptoms develop within 4 weeks of exposure to tick-infested areas, even in the absence of a known bite, need to be evaluated for infectious complications such as Lyme disease, the most common vector-borne disease in the United States.

Lyme disease is caused by the spirochete *Borrelia burgdorferi* and may initially be seen in any of three stages—early localized (stage 1), early disseminated (stage 2), or late-persistent (stage 3). Stage 1 findings of limited infection include a rash in at least 80% of patients that develops after an incubation period of approximately 3 to 30 days.[37,38] The rash, termed *erythema migrans*, is typically a round or oval erythematous lesion that begins at the bite site and expands at a relatively rapid rate, up to 1 cm/day, to a median size of 15 cm in diameter.[39] As the rash expands, there may be evidence of central clearing and, less commonly, a central vesicle or necrotic eschar. Fatigue, myalgia, headache, fever, nausea, vomiting, regional lymphadenopathy, sore throat, photophobia, anorexia, and arthralgia may accompany the rash. Without treatment, the rash fades in approximately 4 weeks. If untreated, the infection may disseminate, and multiple erythema migrans lesions (generally smaller than the primary lesion) and neurologic, cardiac, or joint abnormalities may develop 30 to 120 days later. Neuroborreliosis occurs in approximately 15% of untreated patients and is characterized by central or peripheral findings such as lymphocytic meningitis, subtle encephalitis, cranial neuritis (especially facial nerve palsy, which may be unilateral or bilateral), cerebellar ataxia, and motor neuropathies.[40] Cardiac findings occur in approximately 5% of untreated patients and are usually manifested as atrioventricular nodal block or myocarditis. Oligoarticular arthritis is a common finding in early disseminated Lyme disease and occurs in approximately 60% of untreated victims. There is a particular propensity for larger joints such as the knee, which becomes recurrently and intermittently swollen and painful. Findings of early disseminated Lyme disease eventually disappear with or without treatment. Over time, up to 1 year after the initial tick bite, Lyme disease can progress to its chronic form, manifested by chronic arthritis, chronic synovitis, neurocognitive disorders, chronic fatigue, or any combination of these findings.

The diagnosis of Lyme disease is based largely on the presence of classic erythema migrans in a patient with a history of possible tick exposure in an endemic area or the presence of one or more findings of disseminated infection (e.g., nervous system, cardiovascular system, or joint involvement) and positive serology. Serologic testing is done in two stages. The first test is an enzyme-linked immunosorbent assay for immunoglobulin M (IgM) and IgG antibodies to *B. burgdorferi*. If this test is reactive or indeterminate, it needs to be confirmed with a second test, a Western blot. If the patient has been ill for longer than 1 month, only IgG is assayed because an isolated positive IgM antibody level is probably a false-positive finding at this stage. Patients from highly endemic areas with the classic findings of stage 1 disease, including erythema migrans, can be treated without serologic confirmation because testing may be falsely negative at this early stage.[41]

First-line treatment of early or disseminated Lyme disease, in the absence of neurologic involvement, is oral doxycycline for 14 to 21 days. The second-line agent for use in children 8 years of age or younger and pregnant women is amoxicillin. An equally effective third choice is cefuroxime axetil. Each of these oral agents provides a cure in more than 90% of patients.[38] In more complex management situations, including the possibility of neuroborreliosis or patients with cardiac manifestations, treatment consists of daily IV ceftriaxone for 14 to 28 days with consultation with appropriate infectious disease physicians.[39,42] Treatment of persistent arthritis after antibiotic therapy consists of anti-inflammatory agents or arthroscopic synovectomy.

Decisions to treat a victim of a tick bite prophylactically to prevent Lyme disease are controversial. Some authors condemn such an approach given the low (approximately 1.4%) risk for transmission after a tick bite, even in an endemic area.[39] However, research has shown that a single dose of doxycycline 200 mg orally given within 72 hours of a tick bite can further reduce the already low risk of disease transmission.[38,43] A vaccine against Lyme disease has been withdrawn from the market. The best prevention for tick-borne diseases such as Lyme disease is the use of insect repellent and frequent body checks for ticks when traveling through their habitat.

Hymenoptera

Most arthropod envenomation occurs by species belonging to the order Hymenoptera, which includes bees, wasps, yellow jackets, hornets, and stinging ants. In the United States, Hymenoptera account for most human fatalities, more than snake and mammalian bites combined. The winged Hymenoptera are located throughout the United States, whereas so-called fire ants are currently limited to the southeastern and southwestern regions. The Africanized honeybee, which characteristically attacks in massive numbers, has migrated into the southwestern United States.

Toxicology

Hymenoptera sting humans defensively, especially if their nests are disturbed. The stingers of most Hymenoptera are attached to venom sacs located on the abdomen and can be used repeatedly. However, some bees have barb-shaped stingers that prevent detachment from the victim and render the bees capable of only a single sting. Hymenoptera venom contains vasoactive compounds such as histamine and serotonin, which are responsible for the local reaction and pain. The venom also contains peptides, such as melittin, and enzymes, primarily phospholipases and hyaluronidases, which are highly allergenic and elicit an IgE-mediated response in some victims.[44] Fire ant venom consists primarily of nonallergenic alkaloids that release histamine and cause a mild local necrosis. Allergenic proteins constitute only 0.1% of fire ant venom.

Clinical Reactions

A Hymenoptera sting in a nonallergic individual produces immediate pain followed by a wheal and flare reaction. Stings from fire ants characteristically produce multiple pustules from repetitive stings at the same site. Multiple Hymenoptera stings can produce a toxic reaction characterized by vomiting, diarrhea, generalized edema, cardiovascular collapse, and hemolysis, which can be difficult to distinguish from an acute anaphylactic reaction.

Large exaggerated local reactions develop in approximately 17% of envenomed subjects.[44] These reactions are manifested as erythematous, edematous, painful, and pruritic areas larger than 10 cm in diameter and may last 2 to 5 days. The precise pathophysiology of such reactions is unclear, although they may be partly IgE mediated.[45] Patients in whom large local reactions develop are at risk for similar episodes with future stings but do not appear to be at increased risk for systemic allergic reactions.

Bee sting anaphylaxis develops in 0.3% to 3% of the general population and is responsible for approximately 40 reported deaths annually in the United States.[44] Fatalities occur most often in adults, usually within 1 hour of the sting. Symptoms generally occur within minutes and range from mild urticaria and angioedema to respiratory arrest secondary to airway edema and bronchospasm and finally cardiovascular collapse. A positive IgE-mediated skin test to Hymenoptera extract helps predict an allergic sting reaction. Unusual reactions to Hymenoptera stings include late-onset allergic reactions (>5 hours after the sting), serum sickness, renal disease, neurologic disorders such as Guillain-Barré syndrome, and vasculitis. The cause of these reactions is thought to be immune-mediated.

Treatment

If an offending bee has left behind a stinger, it is removed as quickly as possible to prevent continued injection of venom.[46] The sting site is cleaned and locally cooled. Topical or injected lidocaine can help decrease pain from the sting. Antihistamines administered orally or topically can decrease pruritus. Blisters and pustules (typically sterile) from fire ant stings are left intact. Tetanus status is updated as needed.

Treatment of an exaggerated, local envenomation includes the aforementioned therapy in addition to elevation of the extremity and analgesics. A 5-day course of oral prednisone (1 mg/kg/day) is also recommended.[44] Isolated local reactions, typical or exaggerated, do not require epinephrine or referral for immunotherapy.

Mild anaphylaxis can be treated with 0.01 mg/kg (up to 0.5 mg) of 1:1000 (1 mg/mL, or 0.1%) intramuscular (mid-anterolateral thigh) epinephrine and an oral or parenteral antihistamine. More severe cases are also treated with steroids and may require oxygen, endotracheal intubation, IV epinephrine infusion, bronchodilators, IV fluids, or vasopressors. These patients are observed for approximately 24 hours in a monitored environment for any recurrence of severe symptoms.

Venom immunotherapy effectively prevents recurrent anaphylaxis from subsequent stings in patients with positive skin tests.[47] Patients with previous severe, systemic allergic reactions to Hymenoptera stings or in whom serum sickness develops are referred to an allergist for possible immunotherapy. Referral is also recommended for adults with purely generalized dermal reactions, such as diffuse hives. Children with skin manifestations alone appear to be at relatively low risk for more serious anaphylaxis after subsequent stings and do not need referral. Patients with a history of systemic reactions resulting from Hymenoptera stings need to carry injectable epinephrine with them at all times; they also need to wear an identification medallion identifying their medical condition.[47]

MARINE BITES AND STINGS

Of all living creatures, 80% reside underwater. Humans primarily in temperate or tropical seas encounter hazardous marine animals. Exposure to marine life through recreation, research, and industry leads to frequent encounters with aquatic organisms. Injuries generally occur through bites, stings, or punctures and infrequently through electrical shock from creatures such as the torpedo ray.

Initial Assessment

Injuries from marine organisms can range from mild local irritant skin reactions to systemic collapse from major trauma or severe envenomation. Several environmental aspects unique to marine trauma may make treatment of these patients challenging. Immersion in cold water predisposes patients to hypothermia and near-drowning. Rapid ascent after an encounter with a marine organism can cause air embolism or decompression illness in a scuba diver. Anaphylactic reaction to venom may further complicate an envenomation. Late complications include unique infections caused by a wide variety of aquatic microorganisms and immune-mediated phenomena.

Microbiology of Marine-Related Soft Tissue Infections

There are a range of potential marine-related microbial pathogens that can cause serious soft tissue infections with even minor skin breaks or abrasions.[48] In the Gulf of Mexico, *Vibrio* spp. are of primary concern, particularly in immunocompromised hosts and patients with cirrhosis. In fresh water, the related vibrio-like organisms *Aeromonas* spp. can be particularly aggressive pathogens. *Staphylococcus* and *Streptococcus* spp. are also frequently cultured from infections. Other marine specific pathogens that should be considered include *Chromobacterium violaceum*, *Edwardsiella tarda*, *Erysipelothrix rhusiopathiae*, *Mycobacterium fortuitum*, *Mycobacterium marinum*, *Shewanella putrefaciens*, *Streptococcus iniae*, and *Vibrio vulnificus*. The laboratory is notified that cultures are being requested for aquatic-acquired infections to alert them of the need for appropriate culture media and conditions.

General Management

Initial management is focused on the airway, breathing, and circulation. Anaphylaxis needs to be anticipated and the victim treated accordingly. Patients with extensive blunt and penetrating injuries are managed as major trauma victims. Patients who have been envenomed receive specific intervention directed against a toxin (discussed separately, according to the marine animal), in addition to general supportive care. Contact of the regional poison control center is highly advised. Antivenom can be administered, if available, and should be directed by experienced clinicians or the poison control center. Antitetanus immunization is updated after a bite, cut, or sting. Radiographs are obtained to locate foreign bodies and fractures. Magnetic resonance imaging is more useful than ultrasound or computed tomography to identify small spine fragments.

Selection of antibiotics is tailored to marine bacteriology. Third- and fourth-generation cephalosporins provide adequate coverage for gram-positive and gram-negative microorganisms found in ocean water, including *Vibrio* spp.[48] Ciprofloxacin, cefoperazone, gentamicin, carbapenems, and trimethoprim-sulfamethoxazole are acceptable antibiotics. For significant soft tissue infections, these agents should be used in combination directed toward the most likely pathogens in the region. Regional patterns of common pathogens include *V. vulnificus* in the Gulf of Mexico, *C. violaceum* in the Western Pacific, and *Shewanella* infections in the Mediterranean and Western Pacific. Initial antibiotic therapy in cases of unknown bacterial etiologies should be based on the initial clinical manifestations of impetigo, erysipelas, cellulitis, pyodermas, or necrotizing soft tissue infections. Most marine infections and all gram-negative and mycobacterial marine infections will require therapy with combination antibiotic regimens.[48] Outpatient regimens include ciprofloxacin, trimethoprim-sulfamethoxazole, or doxycycline. Patients with large abrasions, lacerations, puncture wounds, or hand injuries and immunocompromised patients should receive prophylactic antibiotics. Infected wounds are cultured.

Wound Care

Meticulous wound care is necessary to reduce the risk for infection and optimize the esthetic and functional outcomes.[49] Wounds are irrigated with normal saline. Debridement of devitalized tissue can decrease infection and promote healing. Large or complex wounds require exploration and management in the operating room. As noted with other bite wounds, the decision to close a wound primarily must balance the cosmetic result against the risk for infection.[50] Given the risk of serious infection, marine-related wounds should generally be managed with healing by secondary intention or delayed primary closure following aggressive irrigation and debridement of any nonviable tissue. For large shark wounds, postoperative management may be prolonged, and common complications and sequelae of shock, massive blood transfusion, myoglobinuria, and respiratory failure may occur.

Antivenom

Antivenom is available for several types of envenomation, including from the box jellyfish, sea snake, and stonefish.[50] Patients demonstrating severe reactions to such envenomation benefit from antivenom. Skin testing to determine which patients might benefit from pretreatment with diphenhydramine or epinephrine can be performed before antivenom is administered, but it is not an absolute predictor of severe reactions. Ovine-derived antivenom (Commonwealth Serum Laboratories, King of Prussia, PA) to treat severe *Chironex fleckeri* (box jellyfish) envenomation has been administered intramuscularly by field rescuers for many years without reports of a serious adverse reaction. Serum sickness is a complication of antivenom therapy and can be treated with corticosteroids. In the case of managing one of these envenomations in the United States, the regional poison control center is contacted, or major marine aquariums or zoos may be helpful.

Injuries From Nonvenomous Aquatic Animals

Sharks

Approximately 50 to 100 shark attacks are reported annually. However, these attacks cause fewer than 10 deaths/year.[49] Tiger, great white, gray reef, and bull sharks are responsible for most attacks. Most incidents occur at the surface of shallow water within 100 feet of the shore.[40] Sharks locate prey by detecting motion, electrical fields, and sounds and by sensing body fluids through smell and taste. Most sharks bite the victim once and then leave. Most injuries occur to the lower extremities.

Powerful jaws and sharp teeth produce crushing, tearing injuries. Hypovolemic shock and near-drowning are life-threatening consequences of an attack.[49] Other complications include soft tissue and neurovascular damage, bone fractures, and infection. Most wounds require exploration and repair in the operating room (see Chapter 6). Radiographs may reveal one or more shark teeth in the wound. Occasionally, bumping by sharks can produce abrasions, which are treated as second-degree burns.

Moray Eels

Morays are bottom dwellers that reside in holes or crevices. Eels bite defensively and produce multiple small puncture wounds and, rarely, gaping lacerations. The hand is most frequently bitten. Occasionally, the eel remains attached to the victim, with decapitation of the animal required for release. Puncture wounds and bites on the hand from all animals, including eels, are at high risk for infection and must not be closed primarily if the capability exists for delayed primary closure.

Alligators and Crocodiles

Crocodiles can attain a length of more than 20 feet and travel at speeds of 20 mph in water and on land. Similar to sharks, alligators and crocodiles attack primarily in shallow water. These animals can produce severe injuries by grasping victims with their powerful jaws and dragging them underwater, where they roll while crushing their prey. Injuries from alligator and crocodile attacks are treated similarly to shark bites.

Miscellaneous

Other nonvenomous animals capable of attacking include the barracuda, giant grouper, sea lion, mantis shrimp, triggerfish, needlefish, and freshwater piranha. Except for the needlefish, which spears a human victim with its elongated snout, these animals bite. Barracuda are attracted to shiny objects and have bitten fingers, wrists, scalps, or dangling legs adorned with reflective jewelry.

Envenomation by Invertebrates

Coelenterates

The phylum Cnidaria (formerly Coelenterata) consists of hydrozoans, which include fire coral, hydroids, and Portuguese man-of-war; scyphozoans, which include jellyfish and sea nettles; and anthozoans, which include sea anemones. Coelenterates carry specialized living stinging cells called cnidocytes that encapsulate intracytoplasmic stinging organelles called cnidae, which include nematocysts.[49,50]

Mild envenomation, typically inflicted by fire coral, hydroids, and anemones, produces skin irritation. The victim notices immediate stinging followed by pruritus, paresthesias, and throbbing pain with proximal radiation. Edema and erythema develop in the involved area, followed by blisters and petechiae. This can progress to local infection and ulceration.

Severe envenomation is caused by anemones, sea nettles, and jellyfish.[49,50] Patients have systemic symptoms in addition to the local manifestations. An anaphylactic reaction to the venom may contribute to the pathophysiology of envenomation. Fever, nausea, vomiting, and malaise can develop. Any organ system can be involved, and death is attributed to shock and cardiorespiratory arrest. One of the most venomous creatures on earth, found primarily off the coast of northern Australia, is the box jellyfish *Chironex fleckeri* (sea wasp). In the United States, *Physalia physalis*, *Chiropsalmus quadrigatus*, and *Cyanea capillata* are substantial stingers.

Therapy consists of detoxification of nematocysts and systemic support. Dilute (5%) acetic acid (vinegar) can inactivate most coelenterate toxins and is applied for 30 minutes or until the pain is relieved.[49,50] This treatment is critical with the box jellyfish. If a detoxicant is unavailable, the wound may be rinsed in seawater and gently dried.[49,50] Fresh water and vigorous rubbing can cause nematocysts to discharge. For a sting from the box jellyfish, Australian authorities previously recommended the pressure immobilization technique, but this is no longer recommended. Instead, the envenomed limb is kept as motionless as possible, and the victim is promptly taken to a setting in which antivenom and advanced life support are available.

To decontaminate other jellyfish stings, isopropyl alcohol is used only if vinegar is ineffective. Baking soda may be more effective than acetic acid for inactivating the toxin of U.S. eastern coastal

Chesapeake Bay sea nettles. Baking soda must not be applied after vinegar without a brisk saline or water rinse in between application of the two substances to avoid an exothermic reaction. Powdered or solubilized papain (meat tenderizer) may be more effective than other remedies for sea bather's eruption (often misnamed sea lice) caused by thimble jellyfishes or larval forms of certain sea anemones. Fresh lime or lemon juice, household ammonia, olive oil, or sugar may be effective, depending on the species of stinging creature.

After the skin surface has been treated, any remaining nematocysts must be removed. One method is to apply shaving cream or a flour paste and shave the area with a razor. The affected area again is irrigated, dressed, and elevated. Medical care providers need to wear gloves for self-protection. Cryotherapy, local anesthetics, antihistamines, and steroids can relieve pain after the toxin is inactivated. Prophylactic antibiotics are not usually necessary. Safe Sea jellyfish-safe sun block (Nidaria Technology, Jordan Valley, Israel) has been shown to reduce the risk of being stung and may be recommended as a preventive measure before entering the water.

Sponges

Two syndromes occur after contact with sponges.[50] The first is an allergic plant–like contact dermatitis characterized by itching and burning within hours of contact. This dermatitis can progress to soft tissue edema, vesicle development, and joint swelling. Large areas of involvement can cause systemic toxicity with fever, nausea, and muscle cramps. The second syndrome is an irritant dermatitis after penetration of the skin with small spicules. Sponge diver's disease is caused by anemones that colonize the sponges rather than by the sponges themselves.

Treatment consists of gently washing and drying the affected area. Dilute (5%) acetic acid (vinegar) is applied for 30 minutes three times daily.[50] Any remaining spicules can be removed with adhesive tape. A steroid cream can be applied to the skin after decontamination. Occasionally, a systemic glucocorticoid and an antihistamine are required.

Echinodermata

Starfish, sea urchins, and sea cucumbers are members of the phylum Echinodermata. Starfish and sea cucumbers produce venom that can cause contact dermatitis.[49,50] Sea cucumbers occasionally feed on coelenterates and secrete nematocysts, so local therapy for coelenterates also needs to be considered. Sea urchins are covered with venomous spines capable of causing local and systemic reactions similar to those from coelenterates. First aid consists of soaking the wound in warm, but tolerable, water. Residual spines can be located with soft tissue radiographs or magnetic resonance imaging. Purple skin discoloration at the site of entrance wounds may be indicative of dye leached from the surface of an extracted urchin spine. This temporary tattoo disappears in 48 hours, which often confirms the absence of a retained foreign body. A spine is removed only if it is easily accessible or closely aligned to a joint or critical neurovascular structure. Reactive fusiform digit swelling attributed to a spine near a metacarpal bone or flexor tendon sheath may be alleviated by a high-dose glucocorticoid administered in an oral 14-day tapering schedule. Retained spines may cause the formation of granulomas that are amenable to excision or intralesional injection with triamcinolone hexacetonide, 5 mg/mL.

Mollusks

Octopuses and cone snails are the primary envenoming species in the phylum Mollusca. Most harmful cone snails are found in Indo-Pacific waters. Envenomation occurs from a detachable harpoon-like dart injected via an extensible proboscis into the victim.[49,50] Blue-ringed octopuses can bite and inject tetrodotoxin, a paralytic agent. Both species can produce local symptoms such as burning and paresthesias. Systemic manifestations are primarily neurologic and include bulbar dysfunction and systemic muscular paralysis. Management of the bite site is best achieved by pressure and immobilization to contain the venom. Immediate transport to a medical facility is mandatory to assess the bandage and for supportive care.

Annelid Worms (Bristleworms)

Annelid worms (bristleworms) carry rows of soft, easily detached fiberglass-like spines capable of inflicting painful stings and irritant dermatitis. Inflammation may persist for 1 week. Visible bristles are removed with forceps and adhesive tape or a commercial facial peel. Alternatively, a thin layer of rubber cement may be used to trap the spines and then peel them away. Household vinegar, rubbing alcohol, or dilute household ammonia may provide additional relief. Local inflammation is treated with a topical or systemic glucocorticoid.

Envenomation by Vertebrates

Stingrays

Rays are bottom dwellers ranging from a few inches to 12 feet long (tip to tail). Venom is stored in whiplike caudal appendages. Stingrays react defensively by thrusting their spines into a victim, causing puncture wounds and lacerations. The most common site of injury is the lower part of the leg and top of the foot. Local damage can be severe, with occasional penetration of body cavities; this is worsened by the vasoconstrictive properties of the venom, which produce cyanotic-appearing wounds. The venom is often myonecrotic. Systemic complaints include weakness, nausea, diarrhea, headache, and muscle cramps. The venom can cause vasoconstriction, cardiac dysrhythmias, respiratory arrest, and seizures.

If an experienced medical provider is present, the wound is irrigated and soaked in nonscalding hot water (up to 45°C [113°F]) for 1 hour. Caution with hot water is warranted. Debridement, exploration, and removal of spines are carried out during or after hot water soaking. Immersion cryotherapy is thought to be detrimental. The wound is not closed primarily. Lacerations heal by secondary intention or are repaired by delayed closure. The wound is dressed and elevated. Pain is relieved locally or systemically. Radiography is performed to locate any remaining spines. Acute infection with aggressive pathogens is anticipated and prophylactic therapy based on the most likely pathogens should be employed.[48] In the event of a nonhealing draining wound, retention of a foreign body is suspected.

Miscellaneous Fish

Other fish with spines that can produce injuries similar to those of stingrays include lionfish, scorpionfish, stonefish, catfish, and weeverfish. Each can cause envenomation, puncture wounds, and lacerations, with spines transmitting venom. Clinical manifestations and therapy are similar to those pertaining to stingrays. In the case of lionfish, vesiculations are sometimes noted. An equine-derived antivenom (Commonwealth Serum Laboratories) is available for administration in case of significant stonefish envenomation.

Sea Snakes

Sea snakes of the family Hydrophiidae appear similar to land snakes. They inhabit the Pacific and Indian Oceans. The venom produces neurologic signs and symptoms, with possible death from paralysis and respiratory arrest. Local manifestations can be minimal or absent. Therapy is similar to that for coral snake (Elapidae) bites. The pressure immobilization technique is recommended in the field. Polyvalent sea snake antivenom is administered if any signs of envenomation develop. The initial dose is one ampule, repeated as needed. Consultation with an experienced clinician, toxicologist, or poison control center is mandatory.

SELECTED REFERENCES

Auerbach PS, Cushing TA, Harris NS. *Wilderness Medicine*. 7th ed. Boston: Elsevier; 2017.

This textbook is an authoritative, in-depth review of wilderness medicine. Bites and stings by many organisms are discussed in detail by experts from each field. Many pertinent studies are reviewed.

Casale TB, Burks AW. Clinical practice. Hymenoptera-sting hypersensitivity. *N Engl J Med*. 2014;370:1432–1439.

The reactions to Hymenoptera stings are well organized in this practical monograph. The natural history of stinging insect allergy is reviewed, and therapeutic considerations regarding acute management, immunotherapy to prevent recurrent anaphylaxis, and who should receive immunotherapy are discussed.

Gold BS, Dart RC, Barish RA. Bites of venomous snakes. *N Engl J Med*. 2002;347:347–356.

This article is a concise, practical review of snake venom poisoning in the United States. Proper use of North American antivenom is well summarized.

Isbister GK, Bawaskar HS. Scorpion envenomation. *N Engl J Med*. 2014;371:457–463.

This article provides an excellent review of the use of antivenom in spider bites around the world.

Mebs D. *Venomous and Poisonous Animals*. Boca Raton, FL: CRC Press; 2002.

This book is a superbly illustrated collection of fascinating, detailed information about venoms and poisons in the animal kingdom, including marine and terrestrial animals.

Shapiro ED. Clinical practice. Lyme disease. *N Engl J Med*. 2014;370:1724–1731.

This article provides a thorough review of the current understanding of Lyme borreliosis and outlines diagnosis and treatment.

Williamson JA, Fenner PJ, Burnett JW, eds. *Venomous and Poisonous Marine Animals*. Sydney, Australia: University of New South Wales Press; 1996.

This book discusses all common and uncommon toxic marine animals.

REFERENCES

1. *Snakebite Envenoming. World Health Organization Fact Sheet.*; 2019. https://www.who.int/news-room/fact-sheets/detail/snakebite-envenoming. Accessed November 20, 2019.
2. Chippaux JP. Incidence and mortality due to snakebite in the Americas. *PLoS Negl Trop Dis*. 2017;11:e0005662.
3. Spano S, Macias F, Snowden B, et al. Snakebite survivors club: retrospective review of rattlesnake bites in central california. *Toxicon*. 2013;69:38–41.
4. Corneille MG, Larson S, Stewart RM, et al. A large single-center experience with treatment of patients with crotalid envenomations: outcomes with and evolution of antivenin therapy. *Am J Surg*. 2006;192:848–852.
5. Moss ST, Bogdan G, Dart RC, et al. Association of rattlesnake bite location with severity of clinical manifestations. *Ann Emerg Med*. 1997;30:58–61.
6. Hall EL. Role of surgical intervention in the management of crotaline snake envenomation. *Ann Emerg Med*. 2001;37:175–180.
7. Correa JA, Fallon SC, Cruz AT, et al. Management of pediatric snake bites: are we doing too much? *J Pediatr Surg*. 2014;49:1009–1015.
8. Balde MC, Chippaux JP, Boiro MY, et al. Use of antivenoms for the treatment of envenomation by elapidae snakes in guinea, sub-saharan africa. *J Venom Anim Toxins Incl Trop Dis*. 2013;19:6.
9. Walker JP, Morrison RL. Current management of copperhead snakebite. *J Am Coll Surg*. 2011;212:470–474; discussion 474–475.
10. *Advanced Trauma Life Support Course (ATLS)*. 10th ed. Chicago: American College of Surgeons; 2018.
11. Dart RC, Hurlbut KM, Garcia R, et al. Validation of a severity score for the assessment of crotalid snakebite. *Ann Emerg Med*. 1996;27:321–326.
12. Cribari C. *Management of Poisonous Snakebites*. Chicago; 2004. https://www.facs.org/-/media/files/quality-programs/trauma/publications/snakebite.ashx. Accessed December 3, 2019.
13. Chippaux JP, Lang J, Eddine SA, et al. Clinical safety of a polyvalent f(ab')2 equine antivenom in 223 african snake envenomations: a field trial in cameroon. VAO (Venin Afrique de l'Ouest) investigators. *Trans R Soc Trop Med Hyg*. 1998;92:657–662.
14. Budzynski AZ, Pandya BV, Rubin RN, et al. Fibrinogenolytic afibrinogenemia after envenomation by western diamondback rattlesnake (*Crotalus atrox*). *Blood*. 1984;63:1–14.
15. Stewart RM, Page CP, Schwesinger WH, et al. Antivenin and fasciotomy/debridement in the treatment of the severe rattlesnake bite. *Am J Surg*. 1989;158:543–547.
16. Tanen DA, Danish DC, Clark RF. Crotalidae polyvalent immune fab antivenom limits the decrease in perfusion pressure of the anterior leg compartment in a porcine crotaline envenomation model. *Ann Emerg Med*. 2003;41:384–390.
17. Forrester JA, Weiser TG, Forrester JD. An update on fatalities due to venomous and nonvenomous animals in the United States (2008–2015). *Wilderness Environ Med*. 2018;29:36–44.
18. Nonfatal dog bite-related injuries treated in hospital emergency departments—United States, 2001. *MMWR Morb Mortal Wkly Rep*. 2003;52:605–610.
19. Paschos NK, Makris EA, Gantsos A, et al. Primary closure versus non-closure of dog bite wounds. A randomised controlled trial. *Injury*. 2014;45:237–240.

20. Maimaris C, Quinton DN. Dog-bite lacerations: a controlled trial of primary wound closure. *Arch Emerg Med.* 1988;5:156–161.
21. Callaham M. Prophylactic antibiotics in common dog bite wounds: a controlled study. *Ann Emerg Med.* 1980;9:410–414.
22. Perron AD, Miller MD, Brady WJ. Orthopedic pitfalls in the ED: fight bite. *Am J Emerg Med.* 2002;20:114–117.
23. Broder J, Jerrard D, Olshaker J, et al. Low risk of infection in selected human bites treated without antibiotics. *Am J Emerg Med.* 2004;22:10–13.
24. Vidmar L, Poljak M, Tomazic J, et al. Transmission of HIV-1 by human bite. *Lancet.* 1996;347:1762.
25. *Rabies Surveillance and Control: The World Survey Of Rabies. No. 35 for the year 1999.* World Health Organization; 1999. http://www.who.int/rabies/resources/wsr1999/en. Accessed December 3, 2019.
26. Krebs JW, Wheeling JT, Childs JE. Rabies surveillance in the United States during 2002. *J Am Vet Med Assoc.* 2003;223:1736–1748.
27. Use of a reduced (4-dose) vaccine schedule for postexposure prophylaxis to prevent human rabies: recommendations of the Advisory Committee on Immunization Practices. *MMWR Morb Mortal Wkly Rep.* 2010;59:RR-2. http://www.cdc.gov/mmwr/pdf/rr/rr5902.pdf.
28. Offerman SR, Daubert GP, Clark RF. The treatment of black widow spider envenomation with antivenin latrodectus mactans: a case series. *Perm J.* 2011;15:76–81.
29. Sams HH, Dunnick CA, Smith ML, et al. Necrotic arachnidism. *J Am Acad Dermatol.* 2001;44:561–573.
30. Swanson DL, Vetter RS. Bites of brown recluse spiders and suspected necrotic arachnidism. *N Engl J Med.* 2005;352:700–707.
31. King Jr LE, Rees RS. Dapsone treatment of a brown recluse bite. *JAMA.* 1983;250:648.
32. Carlton PK. Brown recluse spider bite? Consider this uniquely conservative treatment. *J Fam Pract.* 2009;58:E1–E6.
33. LoVecchio F, McBride C. Scorpion envenomations in young children in central arizona. *J Toxicol Clin Toxicol.* 2003;41:937–940.
34. Boyer LV, Theodorou AA, Berg RA, et al. Antivenom for critically ill children with neurotoxicity from scorpion stings. *N Engl J Med.* 2009;360:2090–2098.
35. Stewart RL, Burgdorfer W, Needham GR. Evaluation of three commercial tick removal tools. *Wilderness Environ Med.* 1998;9:137–142.
36. Metry DW, Hebert AA. Insect and arachnid stings, bites, infestations, and repellents. *Pediatr Ann.* 2000;29:39–48.
37. Montiel NJ, Baumgarten JM, Sinha AA. Lyme disease—part II: clinical features and treatment. *Cutis.* 2002;69:443–448.
38. Shapiro ED. Clinical practice. Lyme disease. *N Engl J Med.* 2014;370:1724–1731.
39. Shapiro ED, Gerber MA. Lyme disease. *Clin Infect Dis.* 2000;31:533–542.
40. Steere AC. A 58-year-old man with a diagnosis of chronic lyme disease. *JAMA.* 2002;288:1002–1010.
41. DePietropaolo DL, Powers JH, Gill JM, et al. Diagnosis of lyme disease. *Am Fam Physician.* 2005;72:297–304.
42. Dinser R, Jendro MC, Schnarr S, et al. Antibiotic treatment of lyme borreliosis: what is the evidence? *Ann Rheum Dis.* 2005;64:519–523.
43. Nadelman RB, Nowakowski J, Fish D, et al. Prophylaxis with single-dose doxycycline for the prevention of Lyme disease after an *Ixodes scapularis* tick bite. *N Engl J Med.* 2001;345:79–84.
44. Wright DN, Lockey RF. Local reactions to stinging insects (Hymenoptera). *Allergy Proc.* 1990;11:23–28.
45. Reisman RE. Insect stings. *N Engl J Med.* 1994;331:523–527.
46. Visscher PK, Vetter RS, Camazine S. Removing bee stings. *Lancet.* 1996;348:301–302.
47. Casale TB, Burks AW. Clinical practice. Hymenoptera-sting hypersensitivity. *N Engl J Med.* 2014;370:1432–1439.
48. Diaz JH, Lopez FA. Skin, soft tissue and systemic bacterial infections following aquatic injuries and exposures. *Am J Med Sci.* 2015;349:269–275.
49. McGoldrick J, Marx JA. Marine envenomations. Part 2: invertebrates. *J Emerg Med.* 1992;10:71–77.
50. McGoldrick J, Marx JA. Marine envenomations; part 1: vertebrates. *J Emerg Med.* 1991;9:497–502.

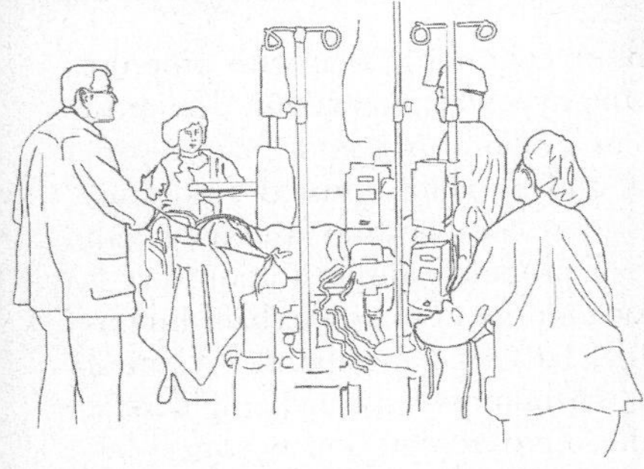

CHAPTER 22

Surgical Critical Care

John P. Saydi, Vamsi Aribindi, S. Rob Todd

OUTLINE

Intensive care units (ICUs) represent a triumph of medicine: the ability to support and replace a large number of bodily functions. And yet, these actions are not cost free. Nearly every intervention has side effects and risks, all of which must be mitigated. While rapid decision-making is often possible and desired in the management of emergency center or ward patients, this approach can be prone to errors in the ICU environment and must be used in the appropriate clinical situations. In much of academic medicine, there are two overarching approaches to patients, those being a "problem-based" approach and a "systems-based" approach. In the ICU, the "systems-based" approach is preferred because of the need to thoroughly consider the patient's needs and status from every angle. And this too is the layout of this chapter, covering each organ system and their common dysfunctions and treatments.

In the United States, critical care medicine has numerous educational pathways to include surgery, anesthesia, and internal medicine fellowships. Similarly, many larger hospitals have separate ICUs focused on patient subsets: cardiothoracic ICUs, medical ICUs, neuroscience ICUs, surgical ICUs, transplant ICUs, etc. Other smaller hospitals dispense of any such distinction. Each specialty brings a unique perspective and advantage to the field of critical care medicine. Surgical intensivists possess a strong grasp of the expected course of surgical diseases as well as comfort with many commonly needed procedures such as bronchoscopy, esophagogastroduodenoscopy, percutaneous tracheostomy, etc.

Finally, it must be emphasized that providing quality ICU care is not solely dependent on the intensivist, but also on the entire multidisciplinary ICU team. To the greatest extent possible, joint guidelines and standardization of care in conjunction with nursing, pharmacy, physical therapy, respiratory therapy, and other members of the healthcare team should be developed. It is well documented that this standardization of care improves outcomes. Although exceptions may exist to every guideline, having standard processes with the ability to adjust improves the quality of care. These guidelines are often unique to an institution based on best evidence and local expertise, capabilities, etc.

NEUROLOGIC SYSTEM

Pain and Agitation

Pain is a ubiquitous but often underrecognized and inadequately treated symptom for the critically ill patient. In the ICU setting, sources of pain include traumatic injuries, burns, surgical wounds, underlying illness, and/or noxious stimuli (e.g., tracheal intubation, mechanical ventilation, invasive lines, etc.). Pain is a source of fear and anxiety that, if not properly addressed, contributes to physiologic alterations that can negatively impact patient outcomes and delay recovery. Although the sensation of pain is subjective, there are several measuring tools and scales to quantify pain as an objective data point that can be treated and easily reassessed for improvement. In patients who are able to communicate, the visual analog scale and numeric rating scale are used and provide reliable means for assessment and treatment; however, noncommunicative, altered, or comatose patients must rely upon the observant and attentive physician or nurse to identify the visual cues and physiologic alterations (e.g., tachycardia, hypertension, tachypnea, diaphoresis, etc.) that coincide with uncontrolled pain. If objective data are unavailable, one is better off to presume the presence of pain and provide appropriate treatment.

Opioids have traditionally been the first-line therapy for pain as they are centrally acting, highly effective for nonneuropathic pain, have a rapid onset, and can be administered via multiple routes (enteral, intravenous [IV], transdermal, etc.). Unfortunately, opioids are often overprescribed, leading to untoward side effects, patient abuse, and addiction. Deleterious side effects including nausea, vomiting, pruritis, sedation, respiratory depression, and bowel dysfunction result in unnecessary complications, prolonged hospital length of stay, and increased morbidity. Prolonged use can also result in physiologic dependence, tolerance, and opioid-induced hyperalgesia. Enhanced recovery after surgery protocols and the practice of utilizing multimodal therapies that work synergistically to alleviate pain and provide sedation are paramount in combating the opioid epidemic that currently plagues the United States. Combining the ability to perform regional anesthetic blocks along with nonopioid adjuncts with varying mechanisms of action such as acetaminophen, nonsteroidal anti inflammatory agents, gabapentinoids, tramadol, and muscle relaxants results in more effective analgesia and lower overall opioid requirements.[1] The use of multimodal pain medications has become the standard of care to reduce opioid reliance and should be implemented widely.

In the same manner that pain is assessed and treated, agitation is quantified using various scoring systems to include the Richmond Agitation-Sedation Scale. When a patient is agitated, it is important that a thorough assessment of any underlying treatable etiologies is completed prior to initiating a pharmacologic intervention. Clinical guidelines have been recently updated and published by the Society of Critical Care Medicine as to the management of the agitated ICU patient. The most commonly used sedatives in the ICU include propofol, benzodiazepines, and dexmedetomidine. When deciding on which agent to use, considerations must include the expected duration and depth of sedation required, comorbidities, which may affect pharmacokinetics or metabolic clearance, and potential drug interactions with other medications the patient may already be receiving.

Propofol is a highly protein-bound, lipophilic molecule that is frequently utilized in the ICU. The exact mechanism of action is not fully elucidated, but it is thought to potentiate γ-aminobutyric acid (GABA) receptors resulting in amnesia but without analgesia. Because propofol is highly lipophilic, it readily traverses the blood-brain barrier and results in rapid onset of action in less than 1 minute as well as a short duration of action as it is quickly distributed into peripheral tissues and readily metabolized by the liver. Rapid clearance of propofol makes it the ideal drug for daily sedation weans to assess a patient's neurologic status. Hypotension and cardiovascular depression are commonly seen with propofol administration, especially in the hypovolemic patient. The most serious potential side effects of propofol infusion include pancreatitis, hypertriglyceridemia, and propofol infusion syndrome. Propofol infusion syndrome is a rare complication associated with prolonged and/or high doses of propofol administration that is thought to be caused by mitochondrial respiratory chain inhibition or impaired mitochondrial fatty-acid metabolism. Clinical features include bradycardia, rhabdomyolysis, hyperlipidemia, hepatomegaly, and renal failure. Early recognition is critical because it has a high mortality rate and treatment is fairly limited to supportive care and discontinuing propofol administration.

Benzodiazepines are GABA receptor agonists that produce anxiolysis at low doses and sedation, amnesia, and cardiorespiratory depression at higher doses. The most common benzodiazepines used in the ICU setting are midazolam, lorazepam, and diazepam. Both midazolam and lorazepam can be administered as continuous infusions, whereas all three can be administered intermittently and have rapid onsets of action. The duration of action for each of these drugs is relatively short on initial administration as they are lipophilic and readily distributed to peripheral tissues. However, repeated administration or prolonged infusions result in saturation of adipose tissues and prolonged sedation even after discontinuation. Age, obesity, and altered hepatic or renal function all can alter benzodiazepine clearance and must be considered when deciding on the appropriate medication. The side effects of benzodiazepine administration include cardiovascular and respiratory depression, delirium especially in the elderly, as well as propylene glycol toxicity. Propylene glycol is used as the solvent for IV lorazepam and diazepam, and toxicity is rare. It is characterized as an anion gap metabolic acidosis, renal failure, and eventual multisystem organ failure. Treatment is limited to dialysis and discontinuing the offending agent.

Dexmedetomidine is a centrally acting α2- adrenoreceptor agonist that binds to receptors within the locus ceruleus to provide sedation and anxiolysis and receptors in the spinal cord to provide for analgesia.[2] It has a relatively quick onset of action between 5 and 15 minutes and a duration of action between 60 and 120 minutes. Dexmedetomidine is hepatically metabolized by glucuronidation and the cytochrome P450 system, and, as such, alterations in dosing may be required when other cytochrome P450 altering medications are being given. One of the main advantages of dexmedetomidine is that it has no effect on respiratory drive, so patients can be sedated without the need for mechanical ventilation. Studies have also demonstrated that dexmedetomidine usage results in extubation almost 2 days sooner compared to midazolam use.[2] The adverse effects of dexmedetomidine use include bradycardia, hypotension, atrial fibrillation, and reflex hypertension with abrupt cessation of administration. Currently, the US. Food and Drug Administration (FDA) states the use of dexmedetomidine for initial sedation should be limited to 24 hours with the idea that prolonged use can exacerbate reflex hypertension when stopped.

It is not uncommon for ICU patients to receive continuous infusions of sedatives as it increases patient comfort and provides a reliable and consistent level of sedation. That being said, randomized trials have demonstrated that protocol-driven daily sedation interruption decreases the duration of mechanical ventilation and length of stay in the ICU and improves the ability to perform daily neurologic assessments.[3] Sedation holidays are also cost-effective as they decrease amounts of medication administration and reduce unnecessary diagnostic testing obtained to evaluate a patient's neurologic status.[3]

Altered Mental Status and Delirium

Assessing and accurately diagnosing alterations in a patient's mental status is an often overlooked and underestimated aspect of critical care. Alterations in mental status among the critically ill can be hard to recognize and include a spectrum of disorders including delirium, encephalopathy, and coma. Patients who are elderly and those with preexisting mental illness or cognitive impairment are at increased risk for developing alterations in mental status when critically ill. When a patient has an acute change in mental status, it is important to rule out any organic or potentially reversible causes because the diagnosis of delirium of critical illness is otherwise a diagnosis of exclusion. Some examples of organic causes that can lead to an acute change in mental status include hypoxia, hypercapnia, hypoglycemia, medication side effects or withdrawal, infection, metabolic derangements, cerebrovascular accidents, seizures, and changes in intracranial pressure.

When a patient becomes confused, they lose their sense of orientation and are no longer able to identify who they are or where they are and/or will lack a general perception of time. Delirium is defined as confusion along with a disturbance in focus, attention, or awareness that occurs over a short period of time. The delirious patient will also develop cognitive deficits such as memory loss and difficulty with language or visuospatial abilities. Identifying and trying to reverse the effects of delirium are important because those who develop ICU delirium have an increased mortality, residual functional disabilities, and higher rates of dementia after discharge.[4] In general, hyperactive delirium is easier and more quickly detected as these patients are agitated and restless. However, the opposite is true for patients who develop hypoactive delirium, as they are quiet, inattentive, and lethargic, which can be easily overlooked and ignored. The elderly and patients with prior mental illness or decreased cognition are at higher risk for developing hypoactive delirium and should be evaluated carefully.

Assessment for delirium has been standardized by utilizing either the Confusion Assessment Method for the ICU or the Intensive Care Delirium Screening Checklist. Both assessment tools have been validated in the ICU setting and can also be utilized for the mechanically ventilated patient. Utilizing either one of these assessment tools on a regular and scheduled basis allows for an objective assessment of a patient's mental status and increases the chances for early detection of delirium.

When a diagnosis of delirium has been established, prompt intervention is important in order to begin the process of reorienting the patient and identifying any precipitating factors. The basis of treatment includes identifying and reversing any potential organic causes and providing supportive measures that bring the patient's behavioral alterations back to baseline. Supportive measures serve to limit abnormalities around a patient's environment that would not necessarily be present and to provide a calm, secure, and safe environment. Modifiable behavioral and environmental factors include limiting circadian rhythm abnormalities and maintaining normal sleep-wake cycles by opening blinds or shades during the day and turning off lights at night, reducing ancillary and unnecessary noises or noxious stimuli, avoiding the use of restraints when safe, mobilizing the patient, providing the patient with their eyeglasses or hearing aids if needed, and having family or friends help to reorient and reassure the patient. New-onset delirium has been documented to result in a statistically significant increase in the 90-day mortality rate, which increased in a graded manner when these patients were exposed to noxious stimuli, placed in restraining devices, or developed hospital-acquired conditions such as falls or pressure ulcers. Altering a patient's environment and normalizing their daily lives can be readily done and drastically affects mortality and outcomes.

If patient behavior interferes with their care or they are disoriented to the point of potentially harming themselves or others, low-dose antipsychotic medications such as haloperidol can be safely utilized. Benzodiazepine use should be limited to cases of sedative or alcohol withdrawal as they can precipitate delirium, especially in the elderly population. When sedative infusions are necessary, dexmedetomidine has been found to decrease the rate of delirium by more than 20% when compared to using midazolam, although no one agent is ideal and the proper choice of sedative needs to be made on a case-by-case basis. The medical workup of delirium should include a thorough review and cessation of any unnecessary medications, physical and neurologic examination with possible computed tomography (CT) imaging of the brain, and evaluation for potential infectious etiologies with sampling of cerebrospinal fluid with lumbar puncture when clinically indicated. If no obvious etiology is found, one must consider magnetic resonance imaging (MRI) of the brain, electroencephalogram, measuring drug or toxin levels, or prophylactic supplementation with vitamin B_{12} or folate if there is concern for alcoholism.

Often confused with delirium, which describes the mental manifestations of the disease, encephalopathy is a term to describe an altered mental state per the underlying pathophysiologic process. Encephalopathy develops as a syndrome of overall brain dysfunction and can occur from many organic and inorganic causes that directly induce brain injury or remotely affect the brain from other systemic causes. Encephalopathy can be described as acute or chronic based on the timing and potential reversibility of the syndrome. Chronic encephalopathy is slow to progress and results in structural changes in the brain that are usually irreversible. Acute encephalopathy can potentially be reversed with a return to baseline functional status if the inciting insult is removed or treated in a timely fashion. Examples of causes of encephalopathy include chronic traumatic encephalopathy, Wernicke-Korsakoff syndrome, heavy metal poisoning, electrolyte abnormalities, liver failure, medications, and sepsis.

At the furthest end of the spectrum of altered mental status is coma. A comatose patient is unarousable and unaware of their environment. Most cases of coma that present to the emergency department are due to trauma, cerebrovascular accidents, metabolic derangements, medications, seizures, and infections. The Glasgow Coma Scale (GCS) is a neurologic assessment tool that provides a reliable and objective measurement of a patient's conscious state. It is composed of three elements (eye, verbal, and motor responses) and scaled from 3 to 15. The lowest possible score is 3 when a patient has no response to stimuli, and the highest possible score is 15 when a patient is fully awake and interactive. When comatose patients have a GCS score of 8 or lower, their brain injury or dysfunction is deemed severe and they should be intubated as they cannot reliably protect their airway. As is the case with most causes of altered mentation, treatment for a comatose patient is based on identifying and treating any reversible organic causes and providing supportive care.

Traumatic Brain Injury

One of the leading causes of disability in the United States, traumatic brain injury (TBI) is a devastating and life-altering event that often leads to heavy familial and socioeconomic burden. It is the most common cause of death and disability in people between the ages of 15 and 30, and the most severe cases result in prolonged periods of coma and unresponsiveness. The severity of TBI is classified using GCS scoring, as it is simple, reproducible, and a prognosticator for outcomes. Neuroimaging is utilized to identify pathologic injuries such as skull fractures, cerebral contusions, hemorrhage or hematoma, and diffuse axonal injury. Primary and secondary brain injuries are the two phases during which neuronal injury occurs. Primary brain injury occurs during the initial insult, whereas the focus of critical care management of TBI is to limit secondary brain injury. Secondary brain injury is a consequence of pathologic and physiologic alterations that manifest after the initial injury usually due to concomitant multiorgan injury. Examples of causes of secondary brain injury resulting in further neuronal injury and death include ischemia, hypoxia, hypotension, cerebral edema, acidosis, and elevated intracranial pressure.

Management and treatments are focused on optimizing intracranial pressure and blood pressure in order to maintain adequate cerebral perfusion, avoiding hypoxia, and maintaining normothermia and normoglycemia. Often, antiseizure medications are prescribed as antiseizure prophylaxis, although the ideal medication, dosage, and duration of treatment are not clearly established.[5] Recovery after TBI can be a prolonged and lengthy process. Approximately 10% to 15% of patients with severe TBI (GCS <8) are discharged in a vegetative state, with approximately 50% regaining consciousness by 1 year. Medication adjuncts to accelerate and maintain long-term recovery are sparse. A randomized control trial investigating the use of amantadine has shown that, over a 4-week treatment period, patients showed accelerated recovery; however, over the long-term, there was no difference between the treatment and placebo groups. Long-term prognosis and recovery are variable and difficult to predict and are highly dependent on the severity of TBI, patient comorbidities, and postinjury complications.

CARDIOVASCULAR SYSTEM

Cardiovascular issues commonly encountered in the ICU can be separated broadly into three categories: cardiac arrhythmias, shock, and myocardial ischemia. All of these areas are affected in the setting of primary cardiac dysfunction such as heart failure or a myocardial infarction (MI) and may be affected by extracardiac disease processes (e.g., pulmonary embolism [PE] can lead to right heart failure, hyperthyroidism can lead to arrhythmias, and increased metabolic demand can lead to cardiac ischemia). This section begins by briefly covering normal physiology, continues on to disorders encountered in these three areas and their treatments, and concludes with invasive and noninvasive methods of monitoring the heart and fluid status.

Cardiac Physiology

The heart is a two-pump circuit in sequence. All blood that goes out of the right ventricle to the pulmonary circulation must then be pumped out of the left ventricle to the system circulation, with important exceptions that arise in the setting of congenital cardiac anomalies and a minor exception from bronchial arteries and veins. There is a vast difference in resistance between the pulmonary vascular bed faced by the right heart and the systemic vascular bed faced by the left heart, with the pulmonary pressures and resistance being significantly lower. The heart's ultimate function is to supply oxygenated blood to the tissues of the human body. This ability is captured by the oxygen delivery (Do_2) equation:

$$\text{Oxygen Delivery} = (\text{Cardiac Output [CO]})(\text{Hemoglobin} * 1.3 * \text{Oxygen Saturation} + 0.003 \text{ Partial Pressure of Dissolved Oxygen})$$

CO is defined as the blood flow put out by the heart per unit time, typically expressed in liters/min. An average, CO is 4 to 6 L/min. Overall, one observation is evident: the primacy of the hemoglobin and oxygen saturation in determining the carrying capacity of oxygen by the blood and the relatively trivial contribution of dissolved oxygen.

Vascular resistance is the collective resistance of all vessels including arteries and veins against the flow of blood, and there are two such resistances: the systemic vascular resistance (SVR) faced by the left ventricle and the pulmonary vascular resistance (PVR) faced by the right. The relationship between flow, pressure, and resistance is defined by Ohm's law:

$$\text{Mean Arterial Pressure} - \text{Right Atrial Pressure} = (\text{SVR})(\text{CO})$$

$$\text{Mean Pulmonary Arterial Pressure} - \text{Left Atrial Pressure} = (\text{PVR})(\text{CO})$$

These relationships guide decisions about fluid and vasopressor therapy, which are elucidated later. The lower PVR consequently requires a smaller right heart muscle volume (lower pulmonary artery pressure) to supply the lungs with the same CO as the rest of the body. This means that the right heart is unable to maintain its CO in the face of large, acute rises in PVR, and this lack of reserve has significant consequences both in trauma surgery when a trauma pneumonectomy is performed and in thromboembolic disease in the lung. In both these situations, a sudden rise in PVR, particularly in the context of a low preload, can lead to cardiovascular collapse.

The heart muscle is supplied primarily by the coronary arteries. During systole, the subendocardial vessels experience retrograde flow, and thus the heart is primarily supplied during diastole. This has important implications for cardiopulmonary resuscitation, as failure to allow for full recoil of the chest may reduce blood supply to the subendocardium during resuscitation.

The heart's rhythm is controlled by pacemaker cells. The primary node is the sinoatrial node, which is influenced by sympathetic stimulation from the sympathetic trunk mainly arising from the T1–T4 spinal levels, which stimulate positive chronotropy. Parasympathetic stimulation results in negative chronotropy and is mediated via the vagus nerve. The heart has a series of escape pacemakers, which are, in order, the atria, the atrioventricular node, and the ventricles themselves. As long as the sinoatrial node paces above the intrinsic rate of these escape pacemakers and as long as those impulses are transmitted through the atrioventricular node and to the ventricles, impulses from the sinoatrial node control the heart rate.

Cardiac Arrhythmias

Supraventricular Tachycardias

Atrial fibrillation. Postoperative atrial fibrillation is common, occurring in 8% of major surgeries and 45% of cardiac ones. Recent work has noted that the risk of thromboembolism after the development of atrial fibrillation after noncardiac surgery is similar to that of patients with nonvalvular atrial fibrillation.[6] However, while the 2016 European Society of Cardiology guidelines now recommend anticoagulation for postoperative atrial fibrillation following cardiac surgery, they do not address other major surgical procedures.

For atrial fibrillation with rapid ventricular response, the acute management is dependent on the hemodynamic stability of the patient. If the patient is acutely unstable, immediate electrocardioversion is mandated as it is for any tachyarrhythmia causing acute instability. In the context hemodynamic stability, pharmacologic methods should be employed, including amiodarone, beta blockers, and calcium channel blockers. Amiodarone is favored in the context of heart failure, as it does not depress cardiac function as is done by beta blockers and calcium channel blockers. That being said, a recent retrospective review documented that metoprolol had the greatest success in the treatment of acute atrial fibrillation, defined by rate control without the need for a second agent.[7] Other studies have noted more rapid control of atrial fibrillation with diltiazem in both the emergency department and the ICU but also noted an increased rate of hypotension with its use relative to amiodarone. More recent data from the emergency medicine literature suggests that procainamide may be an efficacious option for cardioversion of atrial fibrillation (Ottawa Aggressive Protocol). Acutely, digoxin alone is not recommended owing to its slow onset and comparative lack of success in controlling atrial fibrillation.

Two points of caution should be noted. Traditionally, it was held that cardioversion of an atrial rhythm into sinus could safely occur up to 48 hours after initiation of the rhythm. Thereafter, either a transesophageal echocardiogram to verify lack of clot formation in the left atrium or 4 weeks of anticoagulation were recommended prior to cardioversion, except in cases of acute hemodynamic compromise. However, recent work suggests that the safe period of cardioversion may be much shorter, as little as 12 hours.[7] While all drugs used to treat atrial fibrillation may induce cardioversion into sinus rhythm, amiodarone is especially prone to do so. Thus, it should be used with caution in patients with longer time periods of atrial fibrillation due to its higher tendency to result in a return to sinus rhythm. Second, in patients with an accessory pathway, such as Wolf-Parkinson-White syndrome, atrial fibrillation with preexcitation may develop. The use of calcium channel blockers, beta blockers, amiodarone, and digoxin is contraindicated in such instances due to the risk that following suppression of the atrioventricular node, the accessory pathway will result in an exacerbated tachycardia. In this scenario, ibutilide or procainamide is recommended by the most recent guidelines.

Multifocal atrial tachycardia. Multifocal atrial tachycardia is most commonly associated with hypomagnesemia. Pulmonary insufficiency, hypokalemia, and coronary artery disease are other known precipitating factors. If correcting hypomagnesemia and hypokalemia (in that order) are not effective, then beta blockers and calcium channel blockers should be tried. Interestingly enough, data show that an empiric push of 6 mg of IV magnesium sulfate terminated multifocal atrial tachycardia 88% of the time, regardless of serum magnesium levels, a result possibly explained by a systemic deficiency of magnesium with normal blood levels.

Atrial flutter. Atrial flutter is commonly caused by the same disorders that give rise to atrial fibrillation. It is also not infrequent following the treatment of atrial fibrillation with amiodarone. It is an unstable rhythm and has the potential to spontaneously degenerate into atrial fibrillation or to revert to normal sinus rhythm, particularly if the underlying factors have been addressed. The management of atrial flutter is similar to that of atrial fibrillation, with rate and rhythm control options, but electrocardioversion is the preferred therapy. Antiarrhythmic drug therapy is also an option and may be selected for stable patients who are too high risk to undergo the sedation that would typically be required prior to electrocardioversion. Additionally, ibutilide is FDA approved for the conversion of atrial flutter to normal sinus rhythm and has shown superiority to amiodarone and procainamide in this setting. It should be remembered that all antiarrhythmic drugs have proarrhythmic tendencies and ibutilide is no exception with a significant risk of torsades de pointes. It must be used with caution in patients at high risk for torsades de pointes, and patients should be in a monitored setting following its use. IV magnesium given alongside ibutilide both enhance its ability to break atrial flutter and prevent torsades de pointes.

Paroxysmal supraventricular tachycardia. There are numerous other subtypes of supraventricular tachycardias, of which the most common is atrioventricular nodal reentrant tachycardia. The pathophysiology is a reentrant circuit. While sometimes difficult to distinguish from sinus tachycardia and ventricular tachycardia, blocking the atrioventricular node by using vagal maneuvers can reveal the underlying rhythm. Agents acting at the atrioventricular node (adenosine, beta blockers, and calcium channel blockers) are all options to terminate these rhythms. It is important to distinguish a paroxysmal supraventricular tachycardia with a block from a ventricular tachycardia, as both may present with a widened QRS. A history of heart disease or operation portends a ventricular tachycardia. Furthermore, adenosine will aid in distinguishing the rhythms, as it will stop a supraventricular tachycardia but not a ventricular tachycardia. Additionally, ventricular tachycardia will not respond to beta or calcium channel blockers.

Ventricular Tachycardia

Monomorphic ventricular tachycardia. Ventricular arrhythmias are rare in young patients and those without a history of heart disease. Options for treatment in stable patients include lidocaine, amiodarone, and procainamide; these are also adjuncts to consider if initial defibrillation for stable or unstable patients fails to convert a ventricular tachycardia into a sinus rhythm. Additionally, a recent study demonstrated the superiority of procainamide to amiodarone in the conversion of stable ventricular tachycardia. Seeing as procainamide is a therapeutic option for atrial fibrillation with rapid ventricular response, supraventricular tachycardias, and ventricular tachycardias, it may be considered a go to option if one is uncertain of the rhythm. While some patients with ventricular tachycardia may appear stable, they are at high risk for sudden deterioration and must be monitored closely and treated expeditiously.

Polymorphic ventricular tachycardia. Fundamentally, a monomorphic ventricular tachycardia indicates that ectopic beats are arising from one often ischemic focus in the ventricles, typically secondary to coronary artery disease. Polymorphic ventricular tachycardia indicates either multiple foci of ectopic beats or a more commonly global dysfunction. The latter is a rhythm classically known as torsades de pointes, a feared rhythm for which a predisposing factor is a prolonged QT interval. This can be caused by a variety of drugs and by an inherited condition. Ironically, many antiarrhythmics, including procainamide, lidocaine, and ibutilide, prolong the QT interval, as do commonly used antipsychotic drugs such as haloperidol. The treatment is focused on unsynchronized cardioversion if unstable and aggressive administration of magnesium.

Bradycardia

While the treatment of tachycardia involves extensive pharmacologic options backed up with electrical cardioversion, the treatment of bradycardia focuses more on electrical pacing, either transcutaneous or transjugular, as well as reversing the underlying cause. Such causes of bradycardia include acute spinal cord injury, MI, hypoxia, and various toxicologic states, as well as global dysfunction from severe sepsis. Bradycardia is most prevalent in general ICU populations, as it is a sign of profound cardiac dysfunction and sometimes a periarrest rhythm. The acute management includes atropine, epinephrine, and pacing; however, these are temporary supports (apart from spinal cord injury), and the priority must be reversal of the underlying cause.

Sinus bradycardia. Sinus bradycardia may be a normal resting rhythm for many fit, young individuals, and no treatment is required. It may also be seen in profound shock states, as a periarrest rhythm. Sinus bradycardia secondary to a spinal cord injury can occur in high (cervical) spinal cord injuries and should be treated with atropine and concomitant vasopressor therapy to treat neurogenic shock as required. Similarly, sinus bradycardia associated with MI, commonly seen in inferior wall infarctions due to involvement of the sinoatrial node, can be treated with atropine as well. Sinus bradycardia secondary to the use of dexmedetomidine requires a different mindset. If this occurs, treatment of the resultant hypotension with vasopressors is required until the drug wears off, and/or pacing may be required if the hypotension is significant and unresponsive to moderate vasopressor use. Atropine and epinephrine will be ineffective with this etiology due to the α1-antagonist effect of dexmedetomidine.

Junctional or ventricular bradycardia. Junctional or ventricular bradycardia is due to profound atrioventricular node dysfunction. There is no atrial activity apparent. Treatment with temporary pacing may be required if the CO falls. Atropine is not effective in this scenario because it acts upon the dysfunctional atrioventricular node.

Shock

The most severe hemodynamic alteration is shock, which is a condition of circulatory failure resulting in end organ dysfunction secondary to reduced perfusion. A shock state itself is indicated by signs of end-organ dysfunction such as rising lactate, altered mental status, falling urine output, and liver enzyme elevation. Each form of shock demands different responses, and when different forms of shock are combined, the appropriate management can be challenging. There are numerous forms of shock, classified broadly into four categories: distributive, hypovolemic, cardiogenic, and obstructive.

Distributive Shock

Neurogenic shock. Neurogenic shock occurs secondary to the loss of sympathetic tone after a spinal cord injury. The overall etiology is decreased vascular resistance; however, there are two variants based on the location of the spinal cord injury. In lower spinal cord injuries, below C5, the hypotension causes an appropriate reflex tachycardia. In higher spinal cord injuries, C5 and above, the patient is often bradycardic, in that the heart does not respond appropriately to the increased vagal tone due to the lack of sympathetic innervation to the heart. This results in a "warm" shock. Treatment consists of vasopressor support to maintain blood pressure. While norepinephrine is considered the first-line therapy, no agent has been proven to be superior.

Of note, neurogenic shock does not equate to spinal shock. Spinal shock is not a hemodynamic phenomenon and results in the temporary loss of reflexes following a spinal cord injury, most commonly the bulbocavernosus and cremasteric reflexes. It is temporary in nature.

Septic shock. Septic shock arises from inflammatory mediators released by the body in response to bacterial or fungal pathogens and is considered a dysregulated immune response. Traditionally, sepsis was defined as a systemic inflammatory response syndrome (SIRS) accompanied by a suspected source of infection, with SIRS being defined as derangements in two or more of four parameters: white blood cell count, temperature, heart rate, and respiratory rate. Septic shock was then sepsis unresponsive to fluid resuscitation requiring vasopressor support to maintain the blood pressure. While still commonly used, these definitions have been superseded by new guidelines that base the definition of sepsis and septic shock on sequential organ failure assessment (SOFA) scores.[8] Specifically, organ dysfunction represented by an increase in SOFA score of 2 or more represents sepsis, while sepsis with hypotension despite fluid resuscitation and/or a serum lactate greater than 2 despite a lack of hypovolemia represents septic shock.

Previous sepsis management guidelines included immediate lactate measurement (and other laboratory values), an empiric 2-L fluid bolus, empiric antibiotic administration following cultures being drawn, appropriate measurement and titration of fluid resuscitation to central venous pressure and central venous oxygen saturation, and potentially a Swan-Ganz catheter to accurately capture hemodynamic variables. This was known as an early goal-directed therapy. Subsequent randomized controlled trials suggest that this bundle has no benefit; however, proponents maintain that these studies are flawed in that much of early goal-directed therapy has become standard of care.[9] This issue is even more complicated as many aspects of early goal directed therapy have been indoctrinated as quality metrics, meaning failure to comply results in the hospital or clinician being penalized. What is widely accepted is that early recognition and administration of antibiotics lead to increased survival, although this must be balanced against the risk of increasing antibiotic resistance and the harms associated with administering antibiotics to patients who do not require them. Early source control of the infection is also positively associated with outcomes.

While it may seem logical that vasopressors are the first choice for septic shock, given that the derangement is systemic vasodilatation, this is counterbalanced by the fact that a critical portion of the pathophysiology of septic shock is leakage of fluid into the interstitial spaces due to an increase in vascular permeability. Consequently, increasing vasoconstriction alone will not by itself reverse the shock state. Traditionally fluid resuscitation followed by vasopressor therapy only when fluids no longer produced an increase in blood pressure (fluid responsiveness) has been standard. This is currently being studied in a major randomized controlled trial.

The most recent updated guidelines for the overall management of sepsis were released by the Surviving Sepsis Campaign in 2017.[10] It controversially continued to recommend an empiric crystalloid bolus of fluid to all patients. Less controversially, it is recommended continued close monitoring, a target mean arterial pressure of 65 mm Hg, and using lactate as a measure of tissue hypoperfusion and as a guide to resuscitation. The use of central venous pressure to guide fluid resuscitation has been largely discredited, owing to its inability to reliably predict fluid responsiveness. In its place, the guidelines recommend the use of so-called dynamic parameters, including passive leg raise, fluid challenges, pulse pressure variation in response to mechanical ventilation, and other techniques. Many devices and techniques exist to predict fluid responsiveness, but ultimately, clinical judgment must still be used to guide fluid resuscitation and vasopressor therapy in septic shock states.

Currently, when crystalloid fluid resuscitation is not effective at raising blood pressure, the vasopressor of choice is norepinephrine, which has been shown to be superior to the other vasopressors.

Epinephrine can be substituted if norepinephrine is inadequate; however, it may lead to falsely elevated lactate concentrations and difficulty in using this as an endpoint for resuscitation. Phenylephrine has been associated with higher in-hospital mortality in septic shock.

When norepinephrine requirements increase significantly (past a value of approximately 5 mcg/min), low-dose vasopressin should be added. This is based upon research suggesting a relative vasopressin deficiency in inflammatory vasodilatory shock. The dosing is 0.04 units/min, a relatively low dose thought to correct this relative deficiency, and may decrease norepinephrine requirements to maintain the blood pressure. High-dose vasopressin is not recommended. When high doses of norepinephrine and added vasopressin are insufficient, epinephrine may then be added, with no data suggesting a clear benefit. Dobutamine may also be used to augment tissue perfusion if the CO is low.

The use of corticosteroids in septic shock has been controversial for over two decades. The current recommendation by the Surviving Sepsis Campaign is for low-dose steroids in vasopressor-dependent, volume-replete septic shock. Additional therapies being investigated include a bundle of vitamin C, thiamine, and hydrocortisone, the "Marik" protocol, which showed dramatic results in a single-center before and after trial.[11] Similarly, foundational concepts such as initial fluid resuscitation versus vasopressor use and even the meaning of lactate as a resuscitation endpoint remain in dispute and are being investigated. The critical care physician is advised to remain abreast of the literature in this rapidly changing arena.

Other etiologies of distributive shock. Other etiologies of distributive shock include anaphylactic and endocrine shock. The former occurs in response to an allergic stimulus, with the first-line treatment being epinephrine. Optionally, adjuncts such as Benadryl and steroids may be used. While the former does not manage airway symptoms and may cause hypotension, the latter takes several hours to be effective and has never proven to be of benefit.

Endocrine shock results from severe myxedema coma from thyroid deficiency and Addisonian crisis from acquired or iatrogenic hypothalamic-pituitary-adrenal axis suppression. The diagnosis depends on an accurate history and physical examination in both cases. Often, until laboratory tests rule out coexisting Addison disease, the treatment for myxedema coma includes empiric steroids alongside levothyroxine and liothyronine.

Hypovolemic Shock

Hypovolemic shock is characterized by increased SVR and decreased CO, with the latter being secondary to decreased preload. This is a so-called "cold shock," meaning the skin is cold and clammy from the vasoconstriction. For hypovolemic shock from dehydration or fluid losses, such as from prolonged physical activity in warm temperatures or excessive gastrointestinal (GI) losses and lack of oral intake, the treatment is relatively straightforward to include fluid resuscitation with crystalloid.

Hemorrhagic Shock

In hemorrhagic shock, blood products are the resuscitative fluid of choice. In these situations, crystalloid administration leads to increased coagulopathy and can increase the blood pressure, resulting in more bleeding, which is exacerbated by the aforementioned coagulopathy. Two resuscitation strategies are possible: empiric resuscitation with packed red blood cells (PRBCs), fresh frozen plasma (FFP), and platelets in a ratio designed to roughly approximate whole blood; or resuscitation based upon analysis of clotting via thromboelastography (TEG) or rotational thromboelastometry, which are tests that purport to accurately measure derangements in coagulation and guide resuscitation strategy. The first strategy, administration of blood products in an empiric ratio, is commonly employed in many centers as part of a massive transfusion protocol to be administered until control of bleeding can be obtained and/or resuscitation endpoints have been met. Alongside this are adjuncts such as the administration of tranexamic acid, which too is highly controversial. It should be noted that a strict 1:1:1 ratio was shown to be no better than a 1:1:2 ratio of FFP to platelets to PRBCs in patients with severe trauma.[12]

Cardiogenic Shock

Cardiogenic shock is a "cold" shock in that it is characterized by decreased CO due to intrinsic failure of the heart as a pump, with compensatory vasoconstriction. Numerous causes for heart failure resulting in cardiogenic shock exist, but the most commonly seen is the acute or long-term sequelae of coronary artery disease. This shock state has multiple variants to include diastolic versus systolic failure and left heart versus right heart failure. Valvular obstruction may also be a cause of dysfunction. Heart failure progresses through three stages. Initially, the filling pressure of the ventricle increases, but contractility is preserved at the expense of increased pressure and congestion in the lungs. Next, the stroke volume begins to fall, but an increase in heart rate preserves CO. Finally, CO begins to fall.

Right heart failure. The mainstay of right heart failure therapy is straightforward. This includes fluid boluses until the central venous pressure (or wedge pressure if available) is above 15 mm Hg, followed by inodilator therapy with dobutamine or milrinone. This being said, fluid therapy must be used judiciously, as dilatation of the right ventricle may cause the septum to bow out into the left ventricle, resulting in decreased left ventricular function, a phenomenon called interventricular interdependence. Inodilators both dilate the vasculature, reducing blood pressure, and promote CO by increasing contractility. They are ideal choices when the CO is low and the SVR high, but often are not options if systemic blood pressure is low. For this reason, inodilators in conjunction with vasopressors such as norepinephrine are a commonly pursued strategy, with the inodilator titrated to the CO and the vasopressor titrated to an appropriate systemic blood pressure.

Left heart failure. The two questions in left heart failure are: what is the patient's blood pressure and is the patient fluid overloaded? While diuretics historically have been given to almost all patients in left heart failure on the theory that such patients are past the inflection point on the Starling curve, in reality, patients who are in cardiogenic shock may be fluid overloaded, underloaded, or euvolemic. Alternative measures should be used to determine volume status, including weight, pedal edema, inferior vena cava ultrasound, and other newer noninvasive tools.

The other decision point is blood pressure. If the patient is hypertensive, then nitroglycerin, nitroprusside, or nicardipine may be used. All three will decrease the afterload, allow for forward flow of blood to peripheral tissues, reduce the myocardial oxygen demand, and protect the heart from ischemic damage. Nitroprusside has the risks of worsening coronary ischemia and of causing cyanide toxicity and so is less preferred compared to the other agents. If the blood pressure is normal in a state of cardiogenic shock, inodilators may be used. Vasodilators can also be used with caution as long as the blood pressure is maintained. Finally, if both the blood pressure and CO are low, epinephrine or dopamine infusions may be tried; however, due to their peripheral vasoconstriction, they can further increase the afterload and worsen the patient's condition. This state has an extremely high mortality, and, often times, mechanical circulatory support is one of the few options left. These options include intra aortic balloon pumps, left ventricular assist devices, and extracorporeal membrane oxygenation (ECMO). If a facility does not have these resources in-house, the patient should be considered for transfer to a center with these capabilities, possibly by having a mobile unit from the accepting facility arrive at bedside and placing the patient on mechanical circulatory support prior to transfer.

Obstructive Shock

The etiologies of obstructive shock include tension pneumothorax, cardiac tamponade, constrictive pericarditis, and massive PE. In all cases, the treatment is interventional in that they require removal of the cause of the obstructive shock. Options include a needle decompression or thoracostomy tube in the case of pneumothorax; pericardiocentesis or thoracotomy in the case tamponade; and heparinization and systemic or catheter-directed thrombolysis in the case of PE. A high index of suspicion is required in making these diagnoses.

Myocardial Infarction

Both myocardial ischemia and MI are feared entities in the perioperative period, both of them portending significant morbidity and mortality. The lack of ischemic symptoms or electrocardiogram (EKG) changes associated with a rise in troponins is not a sign of safety, as mortality remains high. Two fundamental types of MI exist.[13] Type I MI is based upon atherosclerotic plaque rupture, and consequent ischemia and infarction of muscle that was being supplied by that blood vessel. In contrast, type 2 MI is based upon a mismatch of the supply of blood and the heart's demand for it and is also commonly referred to as demand ischemia. The treatments for each type of MI flow naturally from their causes: revascularization for type I MI and reduction of cardiac oxygen demand for type 2 MI.

Type 1 MIs can be broken down into ST elevation MI (STEMI) and non-STEMI (NSTEMI). As its name indicates, a STEMI classically involves symptoms and elevations in cardiac enzymes as well as evidence of ST elevations on EKG, while an NSTEMI is similar but without EKG evidence of infarction. Unstable angina is a symptom of ischemia, but without cardiac biomarker elevation indicating injury. These critical distinctions drive differences in the immediate management, and it should be noted that unstable angina and NSTEMI are indistinguishable in the first 6 hours as that is how long it takes troponins to become positive after cardiac injury. All three together form part of the spectrum of acute coronary syndrome.

The treatment of a type I MI in the postoperative period focuses on a percutaneous coronary intervention with thrombolysis as an option if timely percutaneous coronary intervention is unavailable.[14] In NSTEMI, intervention can be delayed in some cases up to 72 hours. However, the overall intervention decision is complicated by the added burden of deciding on the risks and benefits of full-dose systemic anticoagulation in postoperative patients. In certain populations, such as those who recently underwent neurosurgical procedures, the risks of stroke or death from hemorrhage make percutaneous coronary intervention with its attendant anticoagulation unacceptable, while in other patients, the risks can be accepted.

In addition to the primary intervention, the complications of an acute MI must be managed. Cardiogenic shock should be managed as previously discussed. Nitroglycerin, either sublingual or IV, can be given for hypertension and for chest pain. The distinction between a right- and left-sided MI is critical, as giving nitroglycerin to reduce the afterload and myocardial oxygen demand in the setting of presumed left-sided MI may reduce the preload, resulting in right-sided heart failure if in fact the patient is suffering a right-sided MI. This could have catastrophic consequences. Pain control with any IV opiate such as morphine can be used to control chest pain symptoms if not relieved by nitroglycerin. The patient should be given aspirin and additional anticoagulant medications as specified by local protocol and depending upon the course of therapy chosen. Beta blockers should be initiated if there are no signs of cardiogenic shock, as these are cardioprotective. However, if the patient is hypotensive or has a decreased ejection fraction or bradycardia, avoid these. Above all else, have the defibrillator close by, pads preferably on the patient, ready to shock any life-threatening arrhythmias or pace the patient if they go into bradycardia secondary to heart block.

RESPIRATORY SYSTEM

ICUs in many ways were defined by the mechanical ventilator. The first ICU was arguably established by Dr. Bjørn Aage Ibsen in 1953 in response to a polio outbreak in Denmark. The use of positive pressure ventilation, initially supplied by medical students working in shifts, in combination with intubation, prevented secretions from causing aspiration pneumonitis and pneumonia, saving hundreds of lives. This basic combination of intubation and mechanical ventilation continues to represent a common function of critical care units of all types, and familiarization with both airway management and mechanical ventilation is fundamental to the practice of critical care medicine.

Respiratory Physiology

Respiratory physiology is characterized by two linked processes, oxygenation and ventilation. Oxygenation refers to the addition of oxygen (O_2) to the blood stream from the air, which is typically at a concentration of 21%, also known as the fraction of inspired oxygen (FiO_2). Ventilation is the clearance of carbon dioxide (CO_2) from the blood stream, after the latter has been generated by cellular respiration. It can help to think of these two processes as entirely separate, although in reality, this abstraction breaks down at extremely low minute ventilations.

Both processes rely upon air coming down the oral cavity, into the trachea, through the bronchi and into the lung parenchyma, where blood brought from the pulmonary artery goes through the pulmonary capillaries. This alveolar-capillary interface is where gas exchange occurs. If too much blood flow relative to oxygenation capacity is present, it is referred to as shunt physiology. Air exchange in areas that do not have sufficient blood supply is known as dead space physiology. Some amount of both of these is normal: less than 10% of total CO does not participate in gas exchange and 20% to 30% of total ventilation does not equilibrate with blood. Increases in shunt fraction occur secondary to asthma, to distention of alveoli from pulmonary edema or pneumonia, to atelectasis, or to PE, where excessive CO flows through nonembolized regions. Dead space ventilation takes place when the alveolar-capillary interface is destroyed by emphysema, when the CO is low, or when air overdistends the alveoli during positive pressure ventilation. Oxygen delivery was previously discussed in the "Cardiovascular System" section and is not further discussed here.

In respiratory physiology, compliance is the increase in volume of a lung in response to a given pressure applied to it. Diseased, fibrotic lungs in interstitial lung disease or acute respiratory distress syndrome (ARDS) have low compliance. Critically, in the era of mechanical ventilation, low compliance can be a viscous cycle. An initial insult from pneumonia, pulmonary contusion, severe systemic disease like pancreatitis, or other cause can result in a decrease in compliance. Using mechanical ventilation, air is forced into the lungs to deliver a set amount of ventilation. This results in barotrauma, or trauma to the lungs from increased pressure. This barotrauma further decreases compliance. Thus, preventing barotrauma is a key goal of the ARDSNet protocol, which is discussed later.

Oxygen Therapy

It is difficult to find a patient in the ICU or floor who does not have a nasal cannula in place, delivering a few liters per minute of oxygen. Nonetheless, it must be emphasized that oxygen itself is a drug, with risks and benefits. 100% FiO_2 can be lethal to SCUBA divers, and supplemental oxygen given to heart attack patients who did not have hypoxia (O_2 saturation >94%) caused increased infarct size at 6 months and no mortality benefit. It should be used only when indicated. In intubated and mechanically ventilated patients, a target FiO_2 should be less than 50% if tolerated, as this setting appears to be safe and without risks of pulmonary toxicities. While theoretically the FiO_2 should be dropped to 21% if tolerated, this is not commonly done.

Noninvasive Ventilation

Some patients in impending respiratory failure may avoid intubation with noninvasive ventilatory support via continuous or bilevel positive airway pressure (CPAP or BIPAP). Both are often worn at night by many patients with sleep apnea at home and should be provided to such patients in the hospital if indicated. BIPAP in particular has been shown to significantly benefit patients with pulmonary edema from a congestive heart failure exacerbation. They provide the equivalent of positive end-expiratory pressure (PEEP), helping to keep the alveoli open at the end of expiration. In BIPAP, there are two settings: expiratory positive airway pressure and inspiratory positive airway pressure. The inspiratory positive airway pressure is provided with each inspiratory breath, while expiratory positive airway pressure is the constant support, analogous to what CPAP would provide. These machines are thus well suited to providing support over CPAP in cases of hypercarbic ventilatory insufficiency.

It is important to remember the contraindications to such devices to include altered mental status and consequent inability to protect the airway being a near absolute one. Both machines involve a mask worn over the face, and any large volume emesis event can rapidly turn into a large volume aspiration and cardiac arrest event in a tenuous patient. Furthermore, the use of these modalities in patients with fresh esophageal, gastric, or duodenal anastomoses is relatively contraindicated, as the positive pressure can increase upper GI insufflation. Although the normal resting pressure of the lower esophageal sphincter is greater than 10 mm Hg, and normal BIPAP settings would be an inspiratory positive airway pressure of 10 mm Hg and an expiratory positive airway pressure of 5 mm Hg, many conditions and patient characteristics can reduce this protective mechanism and make the use of BIPAP a riskier proposition. BIPAP can also be used as a bridge from extubation. A recent small-randomized trial suggested that extubating a patient directly onto BIPAP reduced reintubation rates.

Intubation and Mechanical Ventilation

Intubation and mechanical ventilation are most commonly required to protect the airway from aspiration due to neurologic deficits or loss of patency or to assist with inadequate oxygenation and/or ventilation. The first indication, protection of the airway, is well known by the saying "GCS less than 8, intubate." While this is treated practically as a commandment in critical care, it should be remembered that significant risks exist during intubations and that there are exceptions to every rule. Impending loss of patency can be caused by airway edema secondary to hereditary angioedema, to airway trauma, to severe allergic reactions, and to airway burns. The latter is often a delayed phenomenon, so assessment of a burn patient for signs of airway injury is essential. The second indication represents a failure of the lungs to accomplish their two tasks without assistance. Rising respiratory acidosis and hypoxia are both reasons to intubate, which can arise from many causes including pneumonia, pulmonary contusion, severe illness, flash pulmonary edema, congestive heart failure exacerbation, and exhaustion from increased work of breathing secondary to metabolic acidosis. High spinal cord injury patients, above C5, may have a delayed presentation of ventilatory failure as their diaphragm weakens, while it was initially compensated for by the use of accessory muscles.

Recent work in a multi-institutional study found that 3% of patients who are intubated in the ICU arrest during the procedure, of which 29% could not be resuscitated.[15] Previous work established hypotension and hemodynamic instability as the most predictive factors in peri-intubation arrests, but the causes for these arrests are multifactorial, including hemodynamic shifts induced by induction agents, temporary hypoxia during the procedure itself, and the influence of positive pressure ventilation on venous return to the heart. It is essential to resuscitate patients adequately prior to intubation and to use adjuncts such as vasopressors prior to and during intubation if indicated. Ultimately, while laboratory tests such as arterial blood gas measurements and measurement of tidal volumes using noninvasive ventilators can assist in determining whether or not a patient needs to be intubated, nothing can replace clinical judgment in determining whether a patient requires intubation.

Standard Modes of Mechanical Ventilation

Volume Assist Control

Assist control is one of the most commonly utilized modes of mechanical ventilation, specifically volume assist control. The four basic settings in this mode (and most all standard modes) include respiratory rate, tidal volume, PEEP, and FiO_2. Tidal volume is the amount of air delivered to the lungs, while PEEP represents backpressure that keeps the alveoli open and distended at the end of expiration. Respiratory rate and FiO_2 have previously been described. Volume assist control delivers a set tidal volume at a set minimum respiratory rate. If the patient is not breathing spontaneously, that rate is exactly what the patient will receive. If the patient is awake and breathing spontaneously, they will receive that minimum number of breaths unless they are overbreathing the mechanical ventilator, during which time every breath the patient takes, whether spontaneous or ventilator directed, will be driven to the minimum set tidal volume. These two parameters multiplied (respiratory rate and tidal volume) equal the minute ventilation. It is adjustment in minute ventilation that affects clearance of CO_2 from the bloodstream. In contrast, adjustments in FiO_2 and PEEP affect the oxygen saturation. An alternative to this is pressure assist control, which delivers a set pressure of air at a set respiratory rate, but with varying tidal volumes based on the lung's compliance.

With both modes of mechanical ventilation, the free variable (airway pressure in volume assist control and tidal volume in pressure assist control) must be carefully monitored. Peak airway pressures greater than 35 mm Hg are potentially deleterious. The equation for airway pressure is:

Airway Pressure = (Air Flow)(Airway Resistance) + Alveolar Pressure

Thus, the measured airway pressure itself is not necessarily harmful, but the alveolar pressure is and can lead to barotrauma. When faced with elevated peak airway pressures, a first step is to rule out causes of increased airway resistance such as a kinked tube, auto-PEEP from breath stacking, and other causes such as tension pneumothorax or asthma. Ways to diagnose this include measuring the pressure during an inspiratory breath pause, also known as the plateau pressure. This is a direct reflection of the alveolar pressure. A high plateau pressure in conjunction with a high peak airway pressure indicates that the problem is poor pulmonary compliance. But a low plateau pressure indicates the problem is more proximal.

Synchronized Intermittent Mandatory Ventilation

Synchronized intermittent mandatory ventilation (SIMV) is another commonly used mode. The primary difference between assist control and SIMV involves the spontaneous breaths. In assist control, every patient-initiated breath receives full support up to the set tidal volume. In SIMV, a fifth parameter is set, pressure support. This value is analogous to the inspiratory positive airway pressure setting on BIPAP and provides a set level of pressure support for all spontaneous breaths. Thus, in SIMV, all spontaneous breaths generate whatever the patient is capable of doing with the applied pressure support. Whether assist control or SIMV forms the "default" mode of mechanical ventilation in an ICU is typically practitioner and unit specific.

Pressure Support Ventilation

Another fundamental mode of mechanical ventilation is pressure support ventilation. It is directly analogous to a BIPAP machine. Every breath the patient takes is supported by a set pressure support with additional PEEP that is constant throughout the respiratory cycle. This mode is an excellent tool to wean the patient from mechanical ventilation and is discussed further under extubation.

Advanced Modes of Mechanical Ventilation

High-Frequency Oscillatory Ventilation

High-frequency oscillatory ventilation is an infrequently utilized mode involving extremely low tidal volumes at a high rate. It is often used as a salvage mode and/or a bridge to ECMO in severe ARDS. Two high-quality randomized controlled trials showed no mortality benefit, and possible increased mortality from use of this mode.[16] However, in the neonatal population, which is beyond the scope of this chapter, there are data documenting benefit.

Airway Pressure Release Ventilation and Biphasic Positive Airway Pressure Ventilation

Both airway pressure release ventilation and BIPAP ventilation provide two levels of CPAP that allow a mixture of spontaneous and ventilator mandated breaths. They minimize the pressures seen by the alveoli and are thus most commonly used in patients with significantly reduced lung compliance, such as ARDS. Specifically, airway pressure release ventilation consists of a high CPAP (P_H) for a greater period of time (T_H), which then falls to a lower pressure (P_L) for a shorter period of time (T_L). Bilevel is similar, but with a prolonged T_L. The specifics of these modes settings are beyond the scope of this text, but in brief, the P_H is set at a level to ensure oxygenation, while P_L and T_L are set to ensure adequate ventilation. While the data on these modes support improved oxygenation, they have not been shown decreased mortality. Opponents of these modes maintain that they can achieve similar results by adjusting the inspiratory and expiratory times in assist control with resultant inverse ratio ventilation.

Pressure Regulated Volume Control and Adaptive Support Ventilation

These are patented modes of mechanical ventilation and are only available with certain manufacturers. Pressure regulated volume control adjusts the driving pressure from breath to breath to achieve a set tidal volume, with set limits on maximum inspiratory pressure. In doing so, one is able to reap the benefits of a pressure mode (primarily a decreased risk of barotrauma) with the ease of use of a set volume control mode. There has been no mortality benefit documented with this mode, although it does decrease the plateau pressure. Adaptive support ventilation seeks to minimize the patient's work of breathing in achieving a target minute ventilation. It too has no mortality benefit; however, secondary outcomes such as ventilator days were reduced.

Extracorporeal Membrane Oxygenation

ECMO is an option in those patients with refractory hypoxemia to all other interventions. It is not without risks, as the anticoagulation required can cause devastating bleeds and cerebrovascular accidents, and limb ischemia may also occur. In considering ECMO, ethical issues may arise. In the setting of irreversible pulmonary pathology, ECMO may not be an option. It is too high risk and resource-intensive as a destination therapy, unless the patient qualifies as a lung transplant candidate. Cannulation for ECMO may be performed bedside and can be venovenous or venoarterial, with the latter mode providing circulatory support as well as oxygenation and ventilation.

Extubation or Tracheostomy

Unless significant hemodynamic instability or other considerations prevent, one should always be weaning the patient from the mechanical ventilator. So much so that even an open abdomen is not a contraindication to liberation from the mechanical ventilator. There are a plethora of weaning techniques, and none have truly been documented superior. The decision to extubate a patient is based on the following broad concepts:

1. Is the patient's airway patent (and can they protect it)?
2. Can the patient support themselves with sufficient oxygenation and ventilation?

Various parameters are in play for each decision. In assessing airway patency, a leak test is performed. Following deflation the endotracheal tube cuff, a loss of 10% to 20% of the ventilated volume should be observed. If this is not the case, one may still proceed with extubation; however, it is advisable to extubate over a bougie and to have equipment bedside for possible reintubation. Alternately, IV steroids and reassessment in 24 hours are a more conservative approach. The patient must also be able to protect their airway, which is evaluated by the patient's GCS and/or one's ability to follow commands. Lack of ability to follow commands is not an absolute contraindication to extubation, particularly in neurosurgical patients; however, such decisions should be made by experienced clinicians.

There are numerous means of assessing the oxygenation and ventilation capabilities of the intubated patient. The successful tolerance of a spontaneous breathing trial is the best predictor of successful extubation. A spontaneous breathing trial is performed by placing the patient on pressure support ventilation 5/5 at 40% FiO_2. These settings (5/5) essentially provide compensation for the endotracheal tube. Tolerance for 30 minutes equates with "passing the spontaneous breathing trial." The rapid shallow breathing index is another commonly employed measure. While the patient is on pressure support, it is calculated by dividing the respiratory rate by the tidal volume (L). While a rapid shallow breathing index less than 105 is predictive (yet not a guarantee) of a successful extubation, a value >105 is essentially a guarantee of extubation failure. Other respiratory mechanics to include respiratory rate <25, negative inspiratory force more negative than −20, tidal volume >5 cc/kg, minute ventilation <10 L/min, and vital capacity >10 cc/kg are all indicative of successful extubation.

If a patient is likely to remain intubated for an extended period of time, conversion to a tracheostomy should be considered. While the data on when to perform a tracheostomy are debatable, a commonly used date for evaluation is on mechanical ventilator day 7. Advocates for early tracheostomy cite decreased sedation needs, decreased airway risks, and more expedient liberation from the mechanical ventilator as benefits.

Pulmonary Pathology

Pulmonary Embolism

While labeled "pulmonary," this is a disorder of the clotting system more than a primary insult to the lung parenchyma, and its primary pathophysiology is to increase PVR and, ultimately, right heart failure. Nonetheless, it is important to recognize that PEs can cause significant dead space physiology with resultant hypoxia. Prevention is the best weapon to include early ambulation, intermittent pneumatic compression devices, and prophylactic anticoagulation in at risk populations. The treatment is systemic anticoagulation (heparin drip or weight-based low-molecular weight heparin), to prevent clot propagation, and acute thrombolytics or catheter directed therapies or surgery in rare cases. ECMO may also serve as a bridging therapy in extreme cases.

Pneumonia

Pneumonia is diagnosed by a new infiltrate on chest radiograph together with fever, leukocytosis, and/or purulent secretions. That being said, almost every patient in an ICU will have alternate reasons for some or all of those findings, and thus the diagnosis can be difficult.

Community-acquired pneumonia. For patients presenting to the emergency center with community acquired pneumonia, the Infectious Diseases Society of America and the American Thoracic Society offer extensive guidelines.[14] For those patients presenting with three of the following factors: tachypnea, PaO_2/FiO_2 ratio <250, multilobar infiltrates, confusion, uremia, leukopenia, thrombocytopenia, hypothermia, or hypotension requiring fluid boluses, the recommendation is for direct ICU admission. In those patients originally admitted to the ward and then who required transfer to the ICU, there was noted to be increased mortality.[14] Of course, those patients in septic shock and/or requiring intubation and mechanical ventilation mandate ICU admission.

The mainstay of the treatment of community-acquired pneumonia is either a respiratory fluoroquinolone or a beta-lactam together with a macrolide. Recent evidence about the risk of aortic aneurysm and dissection with the use of fluoroquinolones and the increased mortality with macrolides suggests caution with the use of either regimen. A mortality benefit has been noted with macrolides.

Healthcare—associated pneumonia and ventilator-associated pneumonia. The diagnoses of healthcare-associated pneumonias (HAPs) and ventilator-associated pneumonias (VAPs) are loosely defined as pneumonia diagnosed within 48 hours of hospital admission and within 48 hours of intubation, respectively. That being said, the diagnoses of these two entities are controversial, not least because they are tracked as hospital quality measures. This has inevitably led to significant efforts by hospitals to adopt practices to reduce (and in some instances artificially reduce) the rates of these two entities.

Prior to initiating therapy in both HAP and VAP, it is critical to send cultures (bronchoalveolar lavage or by endotracheal aspirate). If the patient has risk factors for multidrug resistant pathogens, defined as prior antibiotics within 90 days, HAP should be treated with a regimen of vancomycin, cefepime, and levaquin.[15] Patients with VAP are at higher risk for multidrug resistant organisms, and any with septic shock, ARDS, 5 or more hospitalization days, and/or renal replacement therapy should be covered with the same antibiotics, until cultures allow targeting of therapy, for a total of 8 days. Patients without these risk factors should be treated with cefepime alone. However, it should be noted that local practices, formularies, and antibiotic resistance patterns vary widely throughout the United States and the world. Development of guidelines in conjunction with an ICU pharmacist will lead to improved quality of care and outcomes.

A key in managing HAPs and VAPs is prevention. All patients should have the head of their bed elevated to 30 degrees, a measure that can prevent HAPs, along with incentive spirometry and early mobilization. Additionally, patients on the mechanical ventilator should have daily chlorhexidine rinses and interruptions of sedation. But the ultimate prevention measure for VAP is liberation from the mechanical ventilator as early as safely possible.

Acute Respiratory Distress Syndrome

ARDS is a response of the lung to multiple inciting factors to include blood product transfusions, sepsis (pneumonia etc.), severe pancreatitis, pulmonary contusion from trauma, and bleeding and/or hypotension. It is characterized by decreasing ability to oxygenate and decreased compliance of the lung. The formal definition (known as the Berlin definition [or criteria]) was adopted by a joint effort of several societies. It requires bilateral infiltrates on chest radiograph or CT scan, a PaO_2/FiO_2 ratio <300 (<300 is mild, <200 is moderate, and <100 is severe), an inciting factor within 7 days prior to the diagnosis, and a rule-out of hydrostatic edema as a cause of the bilateral infiltrates. It should be noted that patients can have hydrostatic edema from heart failure and ARDS simultaneously.

The management of ARDS revolves around mechanical ventilator settings, as previously discussed in this chapter. In a landmark trial (ARDSNet), the mainstay of treatment was labeled lung protective ventilation.[17] It consists of several goals:

- 4 to 6 cc/kg tidal volumes
- Pa_{O_2} 55 to 80 mm Hg or Sp_{O_2} 88% to 95%
- Requires higher PEEP settings
- Plateau pressure ≤30 cm H_2O
- pH 7.30 to 7.45

These are often met via a comprehensive guideline/algorithm (Fig. 22.1). As shown here, there are many adjuncts to assist in meeting oxygenation requirements, etc. Fluid diuresis and optimization of fluid status to reduce any extrapulmonary edema are a sensible first step. Additionally, deep sedation and/or neuromuscular blockade with paralytics can then be employed to ensure lack of any ventilator asynchrony, although some authorities maintain this step is unnecessary if sedation is sufficiently deep. Finally, prone positioning is one of the few options that have been shown

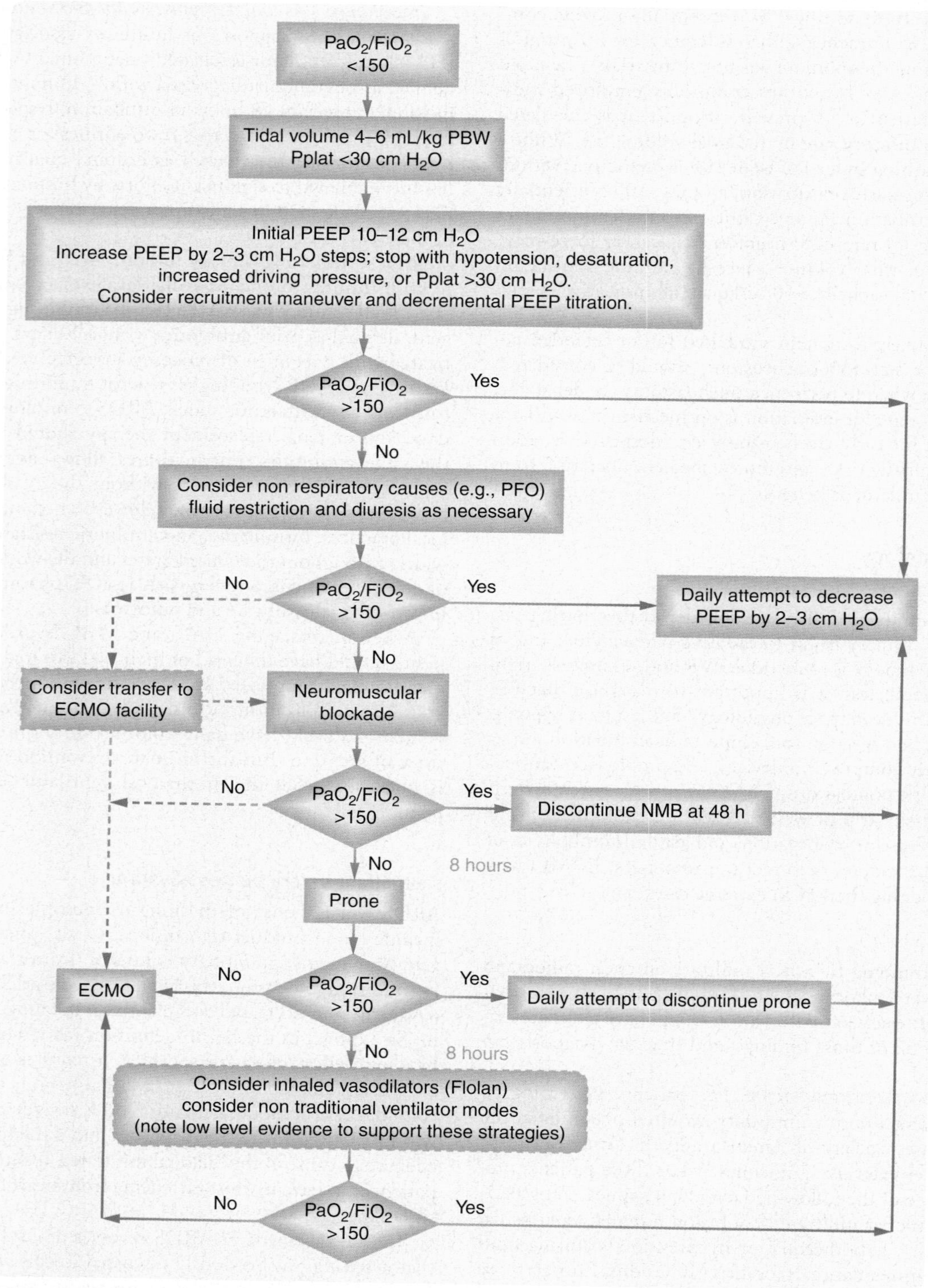

FIG. 22.1 Ben Taub Hospital refractory hypoxemia guideline (September, 2017). *ECMO*, Extracorporeal membrane oxygenation; *FiO_2*, Fraction of inspired oxygen; *NMB*, neuromuscular blockade; *PBW*, predicted body weight; *Pa_{O_2}*, XXXX; PEEP, positive end-expiratory pressure; *PFO*, XXX; *Pplat*, XXX.

to reduce mortality in a randomized controlled trial. However, this intervention should be used with caution and in a unit with experienced personnel in this technique. Placing a patient prone significantly reduces access, and turning a patient who has many lines and other attachments is not a risk-free endeavor. Close coordination with nursing staff and all ancillary staff is required. If utilized, it should be used early in the course of ARDS.

ECMO serves as a final option for refractory ARDS. The CESAR trial documented reduced mortality for patients with ARDS referred to ECMO centers. That being said, approximately 25% of the group of patients transferred for possible ECMO did not actually receive ECMO. The more recent EOLIA trail concluded that there was no significant benefit for ECMO and was terminated early for futility.[18] However, at the time of termination, there was an absolute 10% mortality benefit in the ECMO arm. Ultimately, it seems the availability of ECMO may be a correlate for an institution that is skilled in treating ARDS and sees a high volume of such patients. As such, adoption of standard guidelines and algorithms is likely to improve quality of care and mortality.

Steroids, inhaled nitric oxide, inhaled epoprostenol, and high-frequency oscillatory ventilation techniques have all been shown to have no mortality benefit and are not commonly used, although they do improve hypoxia. Similarly, the alternative modes of mechanical ventilation previously discussed, as well as inverse ratio ventilation, do not have a proven mortality benefit.

GASTROINTESTINAL SYSTEM

Nutritional Requirements of the Critically Ill Patient

The energy requirements of the critically ill patient are higher than the baseline caloric demands of the average patient due to the hypermetabolic state that is induced by acute stressors. Major trauma, surgery, burns, or critical illness such as sepsis, congestive heart failure, or respiratory failure induce a catabolic state with an increase in inflammation, cytokines, and subsequent loss of weight and lean body mass. Combined with underlying comorbidities, bed rest and inactivity, and poor oral feeding, it becomes easy for the overall metabolic demands of a patient to exceed nutritional intake and result in malnutrition, poor healing, and an increase in complications.

The metabolic demands of critical illness require the mobilization of macronutrients to adequately supply the immediate high-energy demands of acute illness. The stress response is characterized by an increase in tissue catabolism, high oxygen consumption, and a net negative nitrogen balance due to proteolysis and amino acid oxidation.[19] Catabolic hormones including glucagon, cortisol, and catecholamines induce glycogenolysis, gluconeogenesis, and mobilization of free fatty acids and cause skeletal muscle breakdown.[19] The resultant stress hyperglycemia and accompanying insulin resistance ensure that an adequate supply of energy is immediately available in an attempt to satisfy the increased metabolic strain.

The nutritional needs of the patient will vary as they shift from an acute catabolic phase to an anabolic recovery phase. There are several contradictory studies demonstrating that underfeeding or overfeeding both have their advantages and disadvantages when it comes to managing critically ill patients. However, it should be stressed that each patient's nutritional requirements are unique and the etiology of illness, comorbidities, and barriers to nutrition should always be taken into consideration. The components of a patient's overall energy expenditure include the resting energy expenditure (60%–70%), physical activity and exercise (20%–30%), and thermic effect of food (10%–15%). Indirect calorimetry remains the gold standard for calculating a patient's overall energy expenditure. It is based on the fact that nutrients (carbohydrates, fats, and proteins) are converted into CO_2, water (H_2O), and heat in the presence of O_2 to produce adenosine triphosphate.[20] Thus, a patient's overall energy expenditure can be calculated by measuring the amount of O_2 consumed ($\dot{V}O_2$) and CO_2 produced ($\dot{V}CO_2$) by the body.[2] These values can then be applied to the modified Weir calculation in order to calculate a patient's overall energy expenditure:

$$\text{Energy Expenditure (kcal/day)} = ([\dot{V}O_2 \times 3.941] + [\dot{V}CO_2 \times 1.11]) \times 1440$$

Despite its accuracy and usefulness, there are several limitations that preclude the universal application of indirect calorimetry for all critically ill patients. The high cost of the machines and necessary training make widespread use fiscally impossible. Prerequisites to testing include the patient being in a quiet and relaxed environment, fasting for at least 5 hours, without exercise for at least 4 hours, and having had no stimulatory medications or supplements such as nicotine or caffeine.[20] Additional variables that can affect the accuracy of indirect calorimetry measurements include supplemental oxygen administration, significant ventilatory support, presence of air leaks or chest tubes, recent anesthetic use, and continuous renal replacement therapy.[21] There are several predictive equations available that can be used to measure a patient's overall energy expenditure; however, their accuracy is poor when compared to indirect calorimetry. Many of them include variables that are constantly changing and affect a patient's overall energy expenditure, such as weight, medications, and body temperature.[21]

According to guidelines published in 2016 by Society of Critical Care Medicine and the American Society of Parenteral and Enteral Nutrition, optimal nutrition requirements for the critically ill patient are roughly 25 to 30 kcal/kg/day.[21] Of this, protein is the most important macronutrient, and weight-based equations can be used to estimate daily protein requirements (1.2–2 g/kg/day).[21] Compared to carbohydrates and fats, protein requirements are proportionally higher and vital for wound healing, maintaining, and preventing loss of lean body mass, and supporting immune function.

Initial identification of patients at risk for malnutrition is pivotal for early intervention and avoidance of potential complications. Upon admission to the ICU, every patient should have a nutritional assessment, calculation of their energy and protein requirements, and a tentative plan for initiation of enteral or parenteral feeding. Traditional serum protein markers can be obtained to establish a general idea of a patient's nutritional status, but each has its limitations. Serum albumin, transferrin, and prealbumin are all created in the liver and their levels can be reflective of a patient's overall protein status. Serum albumin has a longer half-life of approximately 18 to 20 days, which can help to establish what a patient's most recent nutritional status has been prior to hospitalization. However, hepatic disease and renal disease can decrease serum albumin levels, and neither acute starvation nor nutritional supplementation will result in a measurable change in the acute ICU setting. Serum transferrin has a half-life of approximately 8 to 9 days, but levels can be altered based on a patient's serum iron levels and systemic inflammation. Transferrin should only be considered as a marker of protein status when serum iron levels are normal. Lastly, prealbumin has a half-life of 2 to 3 days and levels rapidly fluctuate as a representation of catabolism, inflammation, or transition to an anabolic state. Unfortunately, these serum markers are negative acute phase reactants, and in the setting of significant stress or trauma, their levels will decrease due to increases in vascular permeability and reallocation of hepatic protein synthesis. Their values should be interpreted in conjunction with a patient's hospital course and clinical status. C-reactive protein may serve as an overall marker of inflammation and stress with which to take into account.

Tissue imaging techniques are now recognized as accurate and validated means of analyzing a patient's body composition and estimating lean body mass. CT imaging allows for cross-sectional measurements and quantification of skeletal muscle that can be easily compared to prior or subsequent studies. Cross-sectional imaging at the third lumbar vertebra provides precise estimates of total body composition of adipose tissue, total body muscle volume, and lean muscle volume. Investigations into alterations of psoas muscle quality and density correlate with changes in a patient's nutritional status and length of hospital stay.[22] Despite these benefits, CT imaging is quite limited by cost and potentially unnecessary exposure to ionizing radiation. Bedside use of ultrasound has developed as an easily reproducible and harmless means to measure a patient's muscle mass that can be repeated for comparison. Although ultrasound lacks the negative effects of CT scan, its use has not yet been validated for patients in the ICU. Without a single modality to reliably and accurately measure a patient's overall nutritional status, one must continue to assess the patient with a complete physical exam, use clinical judgment, and gather additional data from ancillary studies to develop an individualized and comprehensive plan for nutritional support.

Enteral and Parenteral Nutrition

Along with timing and proportion of nutrients, the route of administration of nutrition is an important decision that is based on the patient's clinical status and risk for complications. Enteral nutrition refers to the administration of feeds and fluids via the intestinal route, be it orally or via a feeding tube, and should be the first choice for nutrition administration when possible. In addition to being the physiologic manner in which we nourish ourselves on a daily basis, there are several additional benefits. Enteral nutrition aids in preserving gut integrity by maintaining tight junctions between intraepithelial cells, induces blood flow to the intestine, promotes intestinal microbial diversity and intestine-mediated immunity, and stimulates the release of endogenous hormones and digestive enzymes.[21,23]

Patients who are intubated, altered, sedated, at risk for aspiration, or require additional caloric support can be initiated on enteral nutrition via a nasogastric tube or Dobhoff tube. When placed, these tubes should have their positions confirmed radiographically before they are used. Nasogastric tubes have the advantage of being able to be used for feeds, medications, and gastric decompression and are less likely to clog. Dobhoff tubes are softer, more flexible, can be positioned post–ligament of Treitz, and are better tolerated when needed for longer periods of time but are unable to be used for decompression and have a tendency to clog due to their smaller diameter. Post–ligament of Treitz feeding has been shown to decrease infectious morbidity and ICU length of stay compared to intragastric feeding. Post–ligament of Treitz positioning is most beneficial for patients who are at high risk of aspiration, have delayed gastric emptying, or have proven intolerant to gastric feeding. Proper tube positioning can be difficult and if timely placement is not possible, then it is best to avoid delay and initiate early gastric feeding while awaiting small bowel positioning.

Barriers to enteral nutrition often result in patients not meeting their daily caloric requirements. Tube feeds are frequently interrupted for patient care, bedside procedures, diagnostic imaging, and prior to operative intervention among other things. Absolute contraindications to the administration of enteral nutrition include ileus, bowel discontinuity, bowel obstruction, active intestinal hemorrhage, and hemodynamic instability. If a patient is hypotensive or has new onset and/or increasing vasopressor requirements, enteral feeds should be held until the patient is stabilized. Administration of enteral feeds in the setting of hypotension has the potential to worsen bowel ischemia leading to necrosis and bacterial overgrowth. Conversely, patients who have minimal and stable vasopressor requirements do better with early enteral nutrition administration. While there are no set guidelines regarding enteral nutrition in the setting of vasopressor support, it is important to recognize any potential signs of bowel ischemia including feeding intolerance, abdominal distention, new-onset ileus, and worsening metabolic acidosis.[21]

Parental nutrition provides nutrients and fluids through an IV and is typically reserved for patients with contraindications to enteral nutrition. It is a much more reliable means of providing calories as there are less interruptions to administration and the caloric needs of the patient are met more rapidly. Parenteral nutrition is also customizable to meet each patient's individual needs by altering the total amount of fluids, dextrose, amino acids, lipids, electrolytes, vitamins, and trace elements. When a patient is receiving parenteral nutrition, they should have a daily set of chemistries, a triglyceride level prior to initiation of lipid emulsion, and a weekly set of liver enzymes. Parenteral nutrition can be given in two forms: as total parenteral nutrition via central venous access or as partial parenteral nutrition via peripheral IV access when a patient is able to tolerate minimal oral feedings but needs supplementation or is awaiting central venous access.

Although IV nutrition seems ideal, studies have shown that early parenteral nutrition within 48 hours of critical illness does not convey any mortality benefit and may be associated with increased infectious morbidity. In well-nourished patients, it is typical to wait up to 7 days before starting parenteral nutrition in the hopes that the patient will be able to feed enterally. Complications associated with parenteral nutrition include central line–associated bloodstream infection (CLABSI), vascular thrombosis, hypertriglyceridemia, hyperglycemia, hepatic steatosis, and cholestasis. Patients receiving parenteral nutrition are at higher risk for CLABSI compared to patients with a central line not receiving nutrition. The most common organism is staphylococci, and parenteral nutrition is the strongest risk factor for nosocomial candidemia. Metabolic complications include refeeding syndrome and overfeeding. Refeeding syndrome occurs secondary to full caloric administration after a period of starvation resulting in hypokalemia, hypophosphatemia, and hypomagnesemia and can be avoided by slowly introducing calories and increasing to full caloric requirements over time. Overfeeding results in electrolyte imbalances, hyperglycemia, and hypertriglyceridemia and complicates weaning from mechanical ventilation. Disuse of the GI tract results in intestinal mucosal atrophy and loss of microvilli, bile stasis, cholelithiasis, and hepatic steatosis. Long-term parenteral nutrition places patients at risk for developing acute cholecystitis, cirrhosis, and liver failure and is a major cause of mortality related to patients with short bowel syndrome.

Comparisons between enteral and parenteral nutrition administration have found no impact on mortality in critically ill patients.[23] However, patients receiving enteral nutrition have less infectious complications and decreased ICU length of stay.[23] In the general population, patients receiving enteral over parenteral nutrition have lower rates of pneumonia and CLABSI, and trauma patients have lower rates of abdominal abscess formation.[21] There are also cost differences as outlined by the CALORIES trial indicating that overall patient care costs were higher with parenteral administration.[24] Overall, when faced with the choice of initiating enteral or parenteral nutrition in the absence of absolute contraindications, there are clear benefits for the patient and overall cost savings with the use of enteral nutrition.

Stress Ulcer Prophylaxis

The GI mucosa is highly sensitive to the hemodynamic alterations often experienced by the critically ill patient. Splanchnic hypoperfusion, mucosal ischemia, reperfusion injury, and decreased mucosal protection all can result in the formation of ulcerations that have the potential to bleed or cause viscus perforation. Mechanical ventilation influences a patient's hemodynamics, especially in cases that utilize high PEEP and/or higher than normal tidal volumes. Increased intrathoracic pressures decrease venous return and right heart filling, thus decreasing CO. Gastric ulcerations can be found in up to 90% of patients after severe trauma or hypotension, but their consequence is not clear as only a small percentage of these patients go on to have clinically relevant GI bleeding.[25]

Classically, patients requiring mechanical ventilation for greater than 48 hours and the development of coagulopathy have been identified as the two main risk factors associated with the formation of GI ulcerations and GI bleeding. These patients are often administered gastric acid suppressants such as proton pump inhibitors (PPIs), histamine-2 receptor antagonists, or gastric mucosa protective agents either as prophylaxis or treatment.[8] A recent inception cohort study looking at 1034 patients with overt GI bleeding in the ICU secondary to gastric ulceration identified the following risk factors: three or more comorbidities, liver disease, renal replacement therapy, acute coagulopathy, and a high SOFA score on ICU day 1.[25] Additional clinical considerations for which prophylaxis may be given include patients with elevated intracranial pressures (Cushing ulcer), burns (Curling ulcer), septic shock, cardiogenic shock, high-dose corticosteroid use, chronic or high-dose nonsteroidal anti inflammatory drug use, kidney or liver failure, and prior history of gastric ulceration or GI bleed.[26] With such a broad range of risk factors, it is reported that >80% of critically ill patients are routinely administered either a PPI or histamine-2 receptor antagonist as stress ulcer prophylaxis.[25]

Gastric acid suppression with histamine-2 receptor antagonists has been shown superior to gastric mucosal protection with sucralfate in preventing GI bleeding, making PPIs and histamine-2 receptor antagonists the main choice for prophylaxis and treatment.[26] When comparing PPIs to histamine-2 receptor antagonists, PPI administration is associated with decreased GI bleeding rates, but no difference in mortality.[8] However, gastric acid suppression has been shown to result in increased morbidity secondary to nosocomial pneumonia, infection with *Clostridioides* (previously *Clostridium) difficile*, and less commonly, thrombocytopenia, MI, and drug interactions.[26] Gastric acid is a natural barrier against pathogens, and suppression can lead to gastric and duodenal bacterial overgrowth and increased survival rates of *C. difficile*. For these reasons, histamine-2 receptor antagonists are preferred for stress ulcer prophylaxis.

Despite prior evidence demonstrating the efficacy of GI prophylaxis in decreasing the incidence of significant GI bleeding, these data are now in question. There is controversy regarding the necessity of GI prophylaxis in light of significantly improved ICU care, better hemodynamic monitoring, early goal-directed resuscitation, and the practice of early enteral feeding for GI mucosal maintenance and protection. For now, until better data from a high-quality randomized placebo-controlled trial can be conducted, stress ulcer prophylaxis remains the standard of care.

HEPATIC SYSTEM

Perioperative Management of the Cirrhotic Patient

Cirrhosis in the critically ill patient is a difficult and complex medical condition to manage because of its effects on almost all other organ systems. The prevalence of cirrhosis has and will continue to increase as the obesity epidemic in the United States worsens. Many patients with subclinical cirrhosis are unaware of their disease, and any patient who is admitted to the ICU with risk factors for the development of cirrhosis should be adequately screened. Risk factors for liver disease include chronic alcohol or substance use, sexual promiscuity, blood transfusions, tattoos, a history of jaundice, and family history of liver disease.[27] A thorough review of a patient's medications and specific questions regarding the use of herbal medications are important as some herbal medications can be hepatotoxic. Clinical features that should raise suspicion for underlying liver disease include fatigue, pruritis, jaundice, obesity, temporal wasting, palmar erythema, spider telangiectasias, gynecomastia, ascites, splenomegaly, caput medusae, and testicular atrophy.[27]

Laboratory evaluation for suspected cirrhosis includes a complete blood count looking for anemia and thrombocytopenia, a basic metabolic panel to evaluate renal function, a coagulation panel to assess the liver's intrinsic ability to generate clotting factors, and a hepatic function panel. Radiologic examination should start with a right upper quadrant ultrasound with duplex as it is safe for the patient, relatively inexpensive, can be done at the bedside, is easily repeatable, and is highly sensitive for vascular abnormalities such as thrombus. Evaluation with elastography also allows for a quantitative measurement of liver stiffness that occurs with cirrhosis. Ultrasound is, however, limited by the patient's body habitus and the variability in quality of images obtained that can occur as it is technician dependent. Alternatively, contrast-enhanced cross-sectional imaging using CT or MRI allows for very detailed visualization of the entire liver, spleen, and portal system; is reliably reproducible with little variation; and is not limited by patient habitus other than the patient being able to physically fit in the scanner. In comparison to ultrasound testing, cross-sectional imaging is more expensive, often requires transportation that can be dangerous in unstable patients, and can result in nephrotoxicity with iodine or gadolinium contrast administration; CT imaging requires exposure to ionizing radiation, and MRI cannot be obtained if the patient has a metal device or implant.

The systemic alterations caused by cirrhosis lead to a number of complications that occur when the body is no longer able to compensate for the diseased state. The clinical manifestations of decompensated cirrhosis include ascites, esophageal variceal bleeding, hemorrhoid formation and bleeding, bacterial peritonitis, hepatic encephalopathy, hepatopulmonary syndrome, and hepatorenal syndrome.[27] The mortality rate at 1 year with decompensated cirrhosis is 20%, which increases to 57% when esophageal bleeding occurs, and the overall median survival is less than 2 years.[27] Patients with decompensated cirrhosis have limited physiologic compensatory reserve to be able to tolerate a significant insult such as trauma or emergency general surgery. Severe complications include acute liver failure, coagulopathy, portal vein thrombosis, acute renal failure, significant fluid and electrolyte imbalances, and sepsis.[27]

Preoperative risk stratification is an important piece of data that can help guide therapy for cirrhotic patients when surgical intervention is nonurgent. Considerations must include not only the severity of liver disease but also the urgency of intervention in addition to comorbid conditions. The stage of cirrhosis can be estimated using the Child-Pugh-Turcot Score to categorize a patient as compensated (class A), mildly decompensated (class B), or severely decompensated (class C; Table 22.1).[28] The Child-Pugh-Turcot Score was originally developed to predict operative mortality in patients presenting with cirrhosis and esophageal bleeding and is now used to estimate a patient's overall prognosis. It is calculated utilizing a patient's prothrombin time (PT) (standardized and calculated as an international normalized ratio [INR]), serum total bilirubin, serum albumin, and grading of ascites and hepatic encephalopathy.

Child-Pugh-Turcot class A corresponds with a 10% perioperative mortality for abdominal surgery, 30% for class B, and 80% for class C. While the Child-Pugh-Turcot Score was created as a means of surgical risk stratification, it does not take into consideration renal function and is limited by subjective assessment of ascites and hepatic encephalopathy. An alternative risk stratification tool is the model for end-stage liver disease (MELD) scoring system (Table 22.2). The MELD score was developed as a means of predicting the 3-month mortality rate after a transjugular intrahepatic portosystemic shunt procedure used to treat cirrhosis induced portal hypertension and has since been found useful for assessing long-term prognosis with cirrhosis and prioritizing candidates for liver transplantation.[27] A patient's MELD score is reproducibly calculated using objective data: serum sodium, serum creatinine, serum total bilirubin, and INR level.[28]

There are many caveats that alter a patient's MELD score, such as the presence of hepatocellular carcinoma or hepatopulmonary syndrome, but those are more applicable for liver allocation and will not be discussed here. Calculated MELD scores ≤11 have a 3-month mortality between 5% and 10%; scores between 12 and 25, between 25% and 54% mortality; and scores ≥26, 55% to 80% mortality.[28] Because neither of these calculators were developed with the intention to be used as predictors for general operative mortality for cirrhotic patients, the Mayo Clinic has since developed a risk stratification tool assessing postoperative mortality for abdominal, orthopedic, and cardiac surgery in cirrhotic patients.[28] Regardless of which assessment tool is utilized, it should not be used to decide clinical decisions but should be treated as additional data to help guide the clinician to better manage such a complex disease.

TABLE 22.1 Child-Pugh-Turcot classification for severity of cirrhosis.

	POINTS		
CLINICAL AND LAB CRITERIA	**1**	**2**	**3**
Encephalopathy	None	Grade 1 or 2	Grade 3 or 4
Ascites	None	Mild to moderate (diuretic responsive)	Severe (diuretic refractory)
Bilirubin (mg/dL)	<2	2–3	>3
Albumin (g/dL)	>3.5	2.8–3.5	<2.8
Prothrombin time	<4	4–6	>6
Seconds prolonged	<1.7	1.7–2.3	>2.3
International normalized ratio			

CLASS	DESCRIPTION	POINTS
A	Mild: well-compensated disease	5–6
B	Moderate: significant functional compromise	7–9
C	Severe: decompensated disease	10–15

TABLE 22.2 Model for end-stage liver disease (MELD) scoring system.

MELD = $3.78 \times \log_e$ serum bilirubin (mg/dL) +
$11.2 \times \log_e$ INR +
$9.57 \times \log_e$ serum creatinine (mg/dL) +
6.43 (constant for liver disease etiology)
If the patient received dialysis twice within the past 7 days, the value for serum creatinine used should be 4.0
MELD-Na = MELD + $1.59 \times (135 - Na^+$ [mEq/L])

MELD SCORE	3-MONTH MORTALITY RATE
≤9	1.9%
10–19	6.0%
20–29	19.6%
30–39	52.6%
≥40	71.3%

INR, International normalized ratio; *Na*, sodium.

Surgery is generally considered safe in patients that are Child-Pugh-Turcot class A or have a MELD score <10; however, preoperative optimization can be difficult especially in advanced stages of disease.[29] Coagulopathy is a major concern in the pre- and postoperative period as these patients often have decreased production of coagulation factors, thrombocytopenia, and dysfunctional platelets secondary to malnutrition, sequestration, myelosuppression, and renal failure.[29] Platelet count goals prior to surgery are institutional and surgeon dependent, but counts <50,000/μL for moderate-risk and <100,000/μL for high-risk procedures should be corrected.[29] Correction of coagulopathy with vitamin K and cryoprecipitate is preferred over FFP in order to minimize fluid overload and should be guided by TEG, which assesses not only coagulation but also platelet function, clot strength, and fibrinolysis.[29] Patients with cirrhosis are often malnourished, which is associated increased perioperative complications as previously discussed. Nutritional optimization is important to support the immune system and promote wound healing and recovery. Complications of ascites, fluid overload, and electrolyte abnormalities can lead to respiratory failure and hemodynamic collapse. Portal hypertension results in splanchnic vasodilatation, reduces preload, and causes compensatory retention of water and sodium to increase the circulatory volume, resulting in hyponatremia and fluid overload.[29]

Management of Liver Injuries

The liver is the most commonly injured abdominal organ in blunt trauma and the second most common in penetrating injuries. Liver injuries are graded according to the American Association for the Surgery of Trauma (AAST) fr om I to VI based on hematoma, laceration, size, and vascular involvement. The decision for operative or nonoperative management of liver injuries should be based not solely on AAST guidelines, but more so on the hemodynamic status of the patient and associated injuries. Although higher-grade injuries more often require operative intervention, it is the anatomic injury and its physiologic effects that should dictate management.

Patients with blunt liver injuries and either hemodynamic instability or peritonitis should be taken to the operating room emergently for exploratory laparotomy. If the patient is hemodynamically stable and without peritonitis and does not have associated injuries requiring emergent operative intervention, then a CT scan with IV contrast should be obtained to properly grade the injury and assess for active extravasation of contrast (blush). Any arterial extravasation or pseudoaneurysm on CT scan should be further assessed/managed with angiography for selective embolization. Proximal hepatic, right hepatic, or left hepatic artery embolization should be avoided. Injury grade alone is not an indication for embolization in the absence of active extravasation. Patients with blunt liver injuries should be admitted to a monitored setting for continuous vital sign monitoring, assessment of urine output, and frequent laboratory draws.

Management of penetrating abdominal injuries has been an evolving practice as more institutions become comfortable with nonoperative and expectant management. As with blunt injuries, any patient with hemodynamic instability or peritonitis should be taken for emergent exploration. Patients undergoing CT imaging with findings of hollow organ injury should undergo laparotomy, and those with thoracoabdominal injuries concerning for diaphragm involvement should undergo either laparotomy or laparoscopy for further evaluation and repair.[30] Nonoperative management can be successful, proving that selective cases of penetrating injuries can be successfully managed in the appropriate trauma center environment with adequate resources.[30]

Complications of nonoperative management of liver injuries include delayed hemorrhage, bile leak and biloma, hemobilia, necrosis, and abscess formation. Delayed hemorrhage with hemodynamic instability should be managed with surgical intervention but otherwise evaluated by triple phase CT imaging with subsequent angiography and embolization if stable. Hemobilia, often presenting as upper GI bleeding, should be initially managed with angiography and embolization but may require surgical intervention if uncontrolled. Bile leak and biloma formation may be managed by percutaneous drainage, with endoscopic retrograde cholangiopancreatography with stenting strongly encouraged. Preferred management of delayed bile peritonitis or rupture of subcapsular hematoma is with laparoscopy with early endoscopic retrograde cholangiopancreatography for suspected bile leak. For most hepatic abscesses, image-guided percutaneous drainage is the preferred management with surgical intervention on a case-by-case basis as initial therapy or following failure of percutaneous drainage. Patients who develop hepatic necrosis may be managed by observation only, although in cases where surgical management is required, formal resection of involved segments is preferred to serial debridement.

RENAL SYSTEM

Physiology

Renal dysfunction results in significant morbidity and mortality in the critically ill patient, and some element is seen in up to 15% of ICU patients. Not only does is affect the key functions of the kidney, electrolyte, acid-base, and volume homeostasis, it also affects drug disposition and other critically stressed organ systems.

Anatomically, the kidneys are supplied by the right and left renal arteries and drained by the right and left renal veins. At the glomerular level, blood is supplied by the afferent arteriole, traverses the glomeruli, and exits via the efferent arteriole. Relative vasoconstriction of the afferent and efferent arterioles dictates the filtration levels of the kidney. Additional concentration and dilution of urine in the collecting system occur in response to stimuli such as antidiuretic hormone (ADH), atrial natriuretic peptide, and aldosterone. Overall, the kidneys respond to different states to maintain homeostasis in volume, acid-base, and electrolyte status.

Acid Base Disturbances

Acid base disorders are common in the ICU and require a thoughtful approach to determining their etiology such that appropriate therapy can be instituted to avoid potentially fatal complications. Be mindful that a primary derangement in one area often results in a compensatory derangement in the other (i.e., metabolic acidosis will result in a compensatory respiratory alkalosis).

Metabolic Acidosis

There are many causes of a metabolic acidosis, with all being categorized as either a high or normal anion gap acidosis. High anion gap acidosis occurs when there is excessive ingestion, production, or retention of a strong acid. Etiologies include lactate, ketones, sulfates, or metabolites of ethylene glycol, methanol, or salicylate among others. Normal or nonanion gap acidosis exists when chloride is reabsorbed in place of bicarbonate resulting in a hyperchloremic metabolic acidosis. This is most commonly associated with diarrhea and renal tubular acidosis.

High anion gap acidosis may be differentiated by assessing lactate, ketones, creatinine, and osmolality while the urine anion gap may aid in differentiating normal anion gap acidosis. The treatment of metabolic acidosis is reversal of the underlying insult, with bicarbonate therapy being reserved for normal anion gap acidosis. Dialysis is rarely required.

Metabolic Alkalosis

Metabolic alkalosis occurs with acid loss or bicarbonate gain. It is most commonly seen with upper GI losses (vomiting) or overdiuresis. In assessing metabolic alkalosis, urinary chloride is helpful and aids in determining if it is a saline (chloride) responsive or nonresponsive alkalosis. Management includes normal saline resuscitation in saline responsive cases. Nonsaline responsive alkalosis requires correcting mineralocorticoid excess and primary hyperaldosteronism.

Respiratory Acidosis

Respiratory acidosis is secondary to inadequate ventilation with resultant excess CO_2. The causes are multiple to include sleep apnea, overmedication, and increased respiratory workload from metabolic acidosis with exhaustion, to name a few. The management is supportive (pharmacologic therapies, O_2 supplementation, and noninvasive mechanical ventilation) yet may require mechanical ventilation if not already in place.

Respiratory Alkalosis

Respiratory alkalosis is an acid-base disturbance secondary to alveolar hyperventilation with resultant hypocapnia. Etiologies include a physiologic response to hypoxia, pain, and anxiety, to name a few. Management is directed at the underlying disorder.

Electrolyte Abnormalities

Although a comprehensive overview of electrolyte abnormalities is beyond the scope of this chapter, a brief overview is provided here.

Hyponatremia

Hyponatremia is the most common electrolyte disorder seen in the hospitalized population, including the ICU. It occurs secondary to H_2O gain or salt loss. The most common cause in the hospital and ICU is the use of hypotonic maintenance solutions. This practice has been rebuked via compelling evidence in the both the surgical and nonsurgical populations.[31] Additionally, ADH is released in response to stress and contributes in many patients, a form of syndrome of inappropriate ADH. Diuretics also give rise to hyponatremia. Other etiologies include diarrhea, heart failure, liver disease, and renal disease. Serum and urine electrolytes and osmolality, along with the assessment of volume status, are utilized in diagnosing hyponatremia causes.

Management strategies include fluid restriction alone or with a diuretic (in hypervolemic states), normal saline (in hypovolemic states), and treatment of the underlying etiology (in euvolemic states). Correction of chronic severe (serum sodium <121 mEq/L) hyponatremia too quickly may result in osmotic demyelination syndrome, previously known as central pontine myelinolysis. For this reason, the goal is to correct the hyponatremia no quicker than 0.5 mEq/hr. Acute hyponatremia can be corrected more quickly, along with symptomatic hyponatremia resulting in seizures, which should be corrected more quickly until the seizures cease, followed by a slower correction rate.

Hypernatremia

Hypernatremia is caused by either a H_2O deficit or salt gain. Water losses may occur with invasive mechanical ventilation, open abdomens following damage control surgery, central or nephrogenic diabetes insipidus from loss of ADH, and insensible losses. A major symptom is thirst. Treatment is correction of the free water deficit, which is calculated via the following formula:

$$\text{Free } H_2O \text{ Deficit} = (\text{Total Body } H_2O)[(\text{Serum Na}/140)-1]$$

Acute hypernatremia (occurring within the last 24 hours) should be corrected over 24 hours, and chronic or unknown hypernatremia should be corrected over 48 hours with a correction rate of no more than 0.5 mOsm/L/hr to avoid cerebral edema.

Other Electrolyte Abnormalities

Hypocalcemia, hypokalemia, hypomagnesemia, and hypophosphatemia. All commonly occur in the ICU secondary to nutritional deficits and anabolic demands of the critically ill patient, among other etiologies. Hypocalcemia often does not require replacement unless clinically symptomatic. All others should be replaced per institutional practices.

Hypercalcemia, hyperkalemia, hypermagnesemia, and hyperphosphatemia. Hyperkalemia and hyperphosphatemia will be covered later under acute kidney injury (AKI). Hypermagnesemia is rare in the ICU setting, with the most common cause being an excessive magnesium load in the face of renal impairment. Hypercalcemia too is rarely seen in the ICU, with the most common causes being primary hyperparathyroidism and malignancy overall. Mild cases do not require treatment; however, severe cases with altered mental status do. Management includes volume resuscitation with balanced crystalloid solutions, along with calcitonin and bisphosphonates. Dialysis remains an option for severe cases in the setting of renal failure.

Acute Kidney Injury

AKI is a common complication in the ICU. Most typically, the etiology is multifactorial to include hypotension, drugs, and infection. There have been numerous consensus definitions of AKI. The RIFLE criteria were initially proposed by the Acute Dialysis Quality Initiative and subsequently revised by the Acute Kidney Injury Network (AKIN). Most recently, the Kidney Disease: Improving Global Outcomes criteria were adopted as a revision of AKIN.[32] These criteria include:

- Increase in serum creatinine by ≥0.3 mg/dL (≥26.5 μmol/L) within 48 hours; or
- Increase in serum creatinine to ≥1.5 times baseline, which is known or presumed to have occurred within the prior 7 days; or
- Urine volume <0.5 mL/kg/hr for 6 hours.

Once identified, one must determine if the AKI is prerenal, intrarenal, or postrenal. Prerenal causes account for the majority of hospital-acquired AKI and include hypovolemia, congestive heart failure, and decompensated liver disease. Fortunately, prerenal AKI typically does not result in permanent kidney damage. Prerenal AKI may be confirmed by a fractional excretion of sodium <1%. Intrarenal AKI is most commonly caused by acute tubular necrosis. Etiologies of acute tubular necrosis include medications, contrast media,[33] and sepsis to name a few. Intrarenal AKI may be confirmed by a fractional excretion of sodium >1%. Postrenal AKI is uncommon in the ICU setting. It is the result of obstruction to urinary flow. Evaluation includes assessment of the postrenal system and a renal ultrasound.

Once diagnosed, the initial management of AKI is supportive in nature and includes managing the inciting cause and the sequelae of AKI. These sequelae include hyperkalemia, volume overload, metabolic acidosis, and, often paired, hyperphosphatemia and hypocalcemia. If this is unsuccessful, dialysis may be required. Similarly, dialysis may be required to manage life-threatening sequelae.

Hyperkalemia

Hyperkalemia is the result of impaired potassium excretion (AKI) or transcellular potassium shifts. Its most critical effect is a reduction in the myocardial resting membrane potential with conduction system abnormalities. EKG findings include peaked T waves (most common finding), widening QRS complexes, loss of P waves, sine wave, ventricular arrhythmias, and ultimately asystole.

In managing hyperkalemia, it is most critical to prevent life-threatening arrhythmias. Measures include counteracting potassium's effect at the cellular level, shifting potassium to the intracellular space, and removing potassium from the body. Calcium chloride (1 g) is used to antagonize hyperkalemia-induced arrhythmias, while insulin (10 units) increases the cellular uptake of potassium. It is the most successful agent at shifting potassium to the intracellular space. Insulin must be followed by dextrose to avoid the resultant hypoglycemia. Additional agents that shift potassium to the intracellular space are nebulized albuterol and sodium bicarbonate. All of these maneuvers are temporizing, so measures to remove potassium from the body must be employed likewise.

Sodium polystyrene sulfonate (kayexalate) exchanges sodium for potassium in the colon and effectively removes potassium from the body. That being said, it requires 24 hours to do so (1 g of kayexalate removes 1 mEq of potassium) and has been associated with intestinal necrosis and bowel perforation.[34] Newer agents (patiromer and sodium zirconium cyclosilicate) are on the horizon; however, they are not fully vetted as of yet. Dialysis remains the gold standard for potassium removal from the body. It should be used liberally when indicated.

Volume Overload

AKI and volume overload are intimately related. As such, the pulmonary status of patients in AKI must be closely watched, and endotracheal intubation may be required. The management of such overload includes diuretics if the patient is still producing urine or, more commonly, dialysis.

Metabolic Acidosis

The kidney's function in excreting acid and generating bicarbonate may be impaired leading to significant acidosis, in addition to the effect of the underlying insult that caused the AKI. While bicarbonate therapy serves as a temporizing maneuver, dialysis should be considered definitive therapy. Generally, treatment is deferred unless the pH drops below 7.1, at which point there is risk for serious metabolic effects such as left ventricular depression and hemodynamic instability.

Hypocalcemia and Hyperphosphatemia

The kidney's ability to excrete phosphorous is impaired in AKI, leading to hyperphosphatemia and resultant hypocalcemia. The hypocalcemia should be repleted only if the patient is symptomatic; however, if the patient's hypocalcemia is secondary to hyperphosphatemia, calcium administration may cause metastatic calcification, a devastating complication. Typically, dialysis is the treatment of choice, with IV calcium reserved for instances of severe symptomatic hypocalcemia.

HEMATOLOGIC SYSTEM

Thromboelastography

TEG was devised in the 1950s to assess the clotting capability of whole blood. Despite its potential applications, its widespread use was limited by a lack of accessibility and complexity in testing, and so the more common and conventional coagulation tests such as PT/INR, partial thromboplastin time (PTT), platelet count, and fibrinogen level were preferred. It was not until the 1980s when testing became more practical, quicker, and reproducible that TEG was used to guide resuscitation during transplant and cardiac surgeries and was found to decrease the total administration of blood products and mortality.[35]

Treating patients with various hematologic abnormalities ranging from acute hemorrhage to thromboembolic disease requires an intimate knowledge of the clotting cascade and objective data to be able to assess where deficiencies or abnormalities exist in order to maintain the delicate balance between coagulation and fibrinolysis. While the basic tests of coagulation provide information regarding the quantity of coagulation factors, they do not assess the quality and functionality of those factors. Thromboelastogram provides a functional assay of clotting and clot lysis that can be used to guide resuscitation and treatment efforts.

There are three phases of coagulation that are measured with TEG: clot initiation, clot strength, and clot stability (Fig. 22.2). The test begins by exposing an aliquot of whole blood to an activator, which induces the clotting cascade. The time required for the first evidence of clot formation is measured as the "R-time." Fibrin cross-linking propagates clot enlargement and the time required to form 20 mm of clot is defined as the "K-time." The rate of clot enlargement is the "α-angle," measured as the tangent to the curve of the TEG tracing as the K-time is reached. Platelet aggregation continues and the widest part of the TEG tracing represents the point of maximal clot strength, termed the "maximum amplitude." The assay continues for an additional 30 minutes and the degree of fibrinolysis is measured as a percentage of clot lysed (LY-30). Alterations in the R-time, K time, α-angle, maximum amplitude, and LY30 result in varying TEG tracings that correspond to coagulation abnormalities that can be treated with transfusions of either FFP, platelets, or cryoprecipitate.

It is insufficient to rely upon the basic hematologic assays of PT, INR, and PTT when assessing a patient's overall coagulation status as these tests do not provide information on the quality of coagulation factors nor what factors in the clotting cascade are deficient or altered.[36] Thromboelastogram provides a reliable functional assay of coagulation that identifies the specific phases of coagulation that are altered and can be improved. It also accurately predicts the need for transfusion for the first 24 hours after a penetrating injury as demonstrated by Plotkin and colleagues.[36] Beyond the ability to guide resuscitation, additional consideration must be placed into the time necessary to obtain a test result. A standard PT, INR, PTT, and platelet count require roughly 45 to 60 minutes due to logistic restraints of a hospital laboratory, while the initial results from a TEG require only 10 to 15 minutes and can often be examined real time.[36] Because a TEG study provides real-time data for various phases of coagulation, preliminary results can be obtained early while awaiting the full testing results.

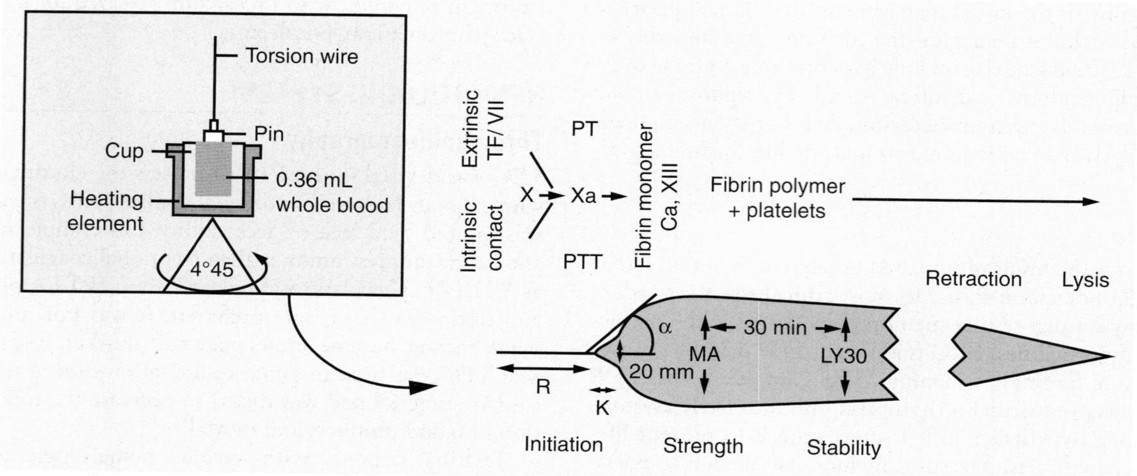

FIG. 22.2 Diagram of thromboelastography, thromboelastogram tracing, and its relation to the clotting cascade. (Adapted from Hackner SG, Rousseau A. Bleeding disorders. In: Silverstein DC, Hopper K, eds. *Small Animal Critical Care Medicine*. 2nd ed. St. Louis: Elsevier Saunders; 2015:554–566.). *MA*, Maximum amplitude; *PT*, prothrombin time; *PTT*, partial thromboplastin time; *TF*, tissue factor.

Heparin-Induced Thrombocytopenia

Heparin-induced thrombocytopenia (HIT) is a life-threatening complication that occurs in a small percentage of patients exposed to any of the forms of heparin. There are two types of HIT that are distinguishable based on timing and degree of thrombocytopenia and can be confirmed with laboratory testing. Type 1 HIT is a mild, transient thrombocytopenia that affects approximately 10% of patients within 2 days of heparin exposure. Thrombocytopenia occurs due to a nonimmune-mediated direct effect of heparin on platelets, causing aggregation. Platelet counts typically nadir at approximately 100,000/μL and recover to normal levels without intervention. Type 1 HIT generally has no clinical significance, does not cause thrombosis, and is managed expectantly.

Alternatively, type 2 HIT is a serious and life-threatening immune mediated thrombocytopenia that affects 1% to 5% of patients exposed to heparin. Heparin will bind to circulating platelet factor 4 molecules and form immunogenic complexes that can be bound by immunoglobulin G antibodies. These immune complexes release additional prothrombotic molecules, thus propagating platelet consumption. The reticuloendothelial system eliminates these circulating immune complexes, leading to thrombocytopenia. Studies demonstrate that 20% to 68% of patients who develop type 2 HIT will also have arterial and venous thromboembolic events.[37] The degree of thrombocytopenia seen with type 2 HIT is more pronounced, with a roughly 50% decrease in platelet count and nadir approaching 50,000/μL. The development of type 2 HIT usually occurs approximately 5 to 7 days after heparin administration or sooner if there is prior heparin exposure.

There are many potential etiologies for thrombocytopenia in an ICU patient, but when there is clinical suspicion for HIT, further investigation is warranted. The "4 Ts score" is a quantifiable clinical assessment tool providing a pretest probability for the presence of HIT. Factors assessed include the degree of thrombocytopenia and platelet nadir, timing of thrombocytopenia after heparin exposure, presence of thrombosis, and the possibility of alternative etiologies for thrombocytopenia. Laboratory assessment for HIT generally begins with an enzyme-linked immunosorbent assay (ELISA), which is sensitive but not specific for HIT, and a confirmatory assay such as the serotonin release assay. Although serotonin release assay is considered the "gold standard," it is not as readily available and requires testing in a reference laboratory. Patients at moderate risk for HIT based on the 4 Ts score should have all sources of heparin discontinued, start on an IV direct thrombin inhibitor unless there are relative contraindications, and have an ELISA assay obtained. If the ELISA is negative, then the direct thrombin inhibitor is discontinued unless the probability of HIT has increased since the ELISA assay was sent. Patients at high risk for HIT are also started on a direct thrombin inhibitor, but even if an ELISA is negative, they are presumed to have HIT until a confirmatory serotonin release assay is obtained.

Over 40% of patients in the ICU develop thrombocytopenia, but HIT is rarely the cause, with an overall incidence of only 0.02% to 0.45%.[37] Despite its rarity, even with treatment mortality rates associated with HIT can be as high as 14.5% to 25%.[37] In any patient with clinical suspicion for HIT, it is prudent to avoid all heparin exposure until a definitive diagnosis is obtained.

Venous Thromboembolism

Critically ill patients are at high risk for developing venous thromboembolism (VTE) as they have all the components of Virchow triad to some degree: endothelial injury, venous stasis, and hypercoagulability. VTE is a preventable cause of death that is common but often undiagnosed and clinically silent. All patients admitted to the ICU should be assessed for and treated against the development of VTE as recommended by the American College of Chest Physicians Evidence-Based Clinical Practice Guidelines, and yet approximately 40% of patients at risk of VTE remain untreated.[38] Most cases where thromboprophylaxis is held is due to physician perception that the risk of bleeding outweighs the risk of VTE. However, delays over 24 hours in initiating pharmacologic VTE prophylaxis after ICU admission are associated with a threefold increase in VTE formation after major trauma.[38] Omission of thromboprophylaxis after 24 hours conveys an attributable mortality of approximately 3.9% to 15.4% in patients with major trauma, sepsis, cardiac arrest, or heavy cancer burden. Data and statistics from the Centers for Disease Control and Prevention convey the significant morbidity and mortality of VTE: approximately 10% to 30% of patients with VTE die within 1 month of diagnosis, sudden death is the first symptom in 25% of PEs, and 50% of patients with deep vein thrombosis (DVT) will have long-term complications of swelling, pain, and discoloration of the affected limb.

Absolute contraindications to chemical thromboprophylaxis include active bleeding or intracranial hemorrhage, coagulopathy, and severe thrombocytopenia. However, in patients with relative contraindications such as recent GI bleeding, recent surgery, and moderate thrombocytopenia, the decision to initiate chemical thromboprophylaxis must be made on a case-by-case basis. At a minimum, mechanical thromboprophylaxis should be provided by means of intermittent pneumatic compression devices. Mechanical compression is used to promote venous blood flow and is thought to activate tissue plasminogen and local fibrinolysis. When no absolute contraindications are present, chemical thromboprophylaxis should be administered as it is proven superior to mechanical compression for the prevention of DVTs and PEs. Low–molecular-weight heparin is shown to be more effective than unfractionated heparin for the prevention of DVTs but is renally excreted and should not be used in the setting of AKI or renal failure. Despite adherence to chemical thromboprophylaxis administration, obesity and proinflammatory states such as sepsis convey higher rates of VTE prophylaxis failure. In these cases, goal-directed therapy and titration of low-molecular-weight heparin dosing based on anti-Xa levels have been proven effective. In patients in whom chemical thromboprophylaxis is contraindicated for an extended period of time, one must consider placement of an inferior vena cava filter to prevent large DVT embolization and clinically significant PEs.

Hemoglobin Transfusion Strategies

Along the same lines as antibiotic stewardship, the good faith practice is required when deciding to transfuse a patient. Although guidelines exist, they are not intended to replace clinical judgment and do not apply universally to all patients. Along with hemoglobin level, other factors to consider regarding the need for a transfusion include the rate of hemoglobin decline, overall volume status, tachycardia or hypotension not responsive to fluid administration, and subjective findings of shortness of breath, light-headedness, and chest pain.[39] Currently, the American Association of Blood Banks (AABB) strongly recommends a restrictive transfusion threshold of a hemoglobin level of 7 g/dL for all hemodynamically stable patients including the critically ill.[39] A slightly more liberal transfusion threshold of hemoglobin level of 8 g/dL is recommended by the AABB for patients undergoing orthopedic or cardiac surgery.[6] A recently released multicenter trial examining 5243 adults undergoing cardiac surgery showed that a restrictive transfusion threshold of hemoglobin level of 7.5 g/dL was noninferior to a more liberal threshold of 9.5 g/dL.[40] When transfusing PRBCs, standard practice is to transfuse 1 unit of PRBC with a recheck of hemoglobin prior to transfusing further. It is also important to note that transfusion-related complications are not infrequent to include allergic or anaphylactic reactions, fluid overload, iron overload, transmission of blood-borne infections, transfusion-related acute lung injury, immunosuppression, hypersensitivity reactions, and life-threatening hemolysis from ABO incompatibility.

ENDOCRINE SYSTEM

Glucose Control

Hyperglycemia in severely ill patients was originally thought of as an adaptive response to critical illness but has since proven to be associated with poor outcomes. As mentioned earlier in the GI section, stress hyperglycemia in the acute setting is secondary to many factors, including glucose production and release in response to catabolic hormones and accompanying insulin resistance. Hyperglycemia is an independent risk factor for adverse outcomes after trauma, sepsis, and TBI, as it is associated with increase rates of infections, a state of immunosuppression, and resultant organ dysfunction. Conversely, tight glycemic control in the ICU setting can be difficult to maintain, especially in patients with variable caloric intake, and can easily lead to severe hypoglycemic episodes resulting in stupor, coma, seizures, and neurologic injury.

While the optimal glucose target range is still up for debate, there are numerous studies proving that tight glycemic control is associated with worse outcomes. As was demonstrated by the NICE-SUGAR trial, patients managed with tight glycemic control between 81 to 109 mg/dL as compared to a more conventional glucose target goal of <180 mg/dL were found to have a statistically significant increased 90-day mortality rate.[41] Rates of severe hypoglycemia (glucose level <40 mg/dL) occurred in 6.5% of patients within the tight glycemic control group as opposed to 0.5% of patients with conventional glucose management.[41] Subsequent studies have since confirmed the dangerous effects of tight glycemic control in the ICU, and a more liberal and attainable glucose target of between 140 and 180 mg/dL is now the standard of care.

Adrenal Insufficiency

Critical illness–related corticosteroid insufficiency occurs when a patient is unable to generate sufficient corticosteroids to compensate for the severe stress and shock state they are experiencing. Severe trauma, sepsis, and the significant metabolic demands of critical illness lead to upregulation of the hypothalamic-pituitary-adrenal axis in an attempt to increase corticosteroid release. However, when these demands are not met, the patient will remain hypotensive and unresponsive to fluid or vasopressor administration. The most severe cases of critical illness–related corticosteroid insufficiency can be seen secondary to adrenal hemorrhage in the setting of trauma, burns, thromboembolic disease, coagulopathy or sepsis, and secondary to pituitary apoplexy from sudden necrosis of pituitary tumors.

The use of steroids for treatment of refractory shock began as an anecdotal finding with minimal corroboration. However, the CORTICUS trial demonstrated that corticosteroid administration had no effect on survival or reversal of shock in the setting of sepsis but did quicken shock reversal in patients who recovered.[42] While the quality of evidence is variable, current recommendations are for corticosteroid administration in the form of hydrocortisone when a patient is unresponsive to vasopressors when they are volume replete. For patients with chronic, long-term steroid use, equivalent IV dosages should utilized until the patient is able to resume oral intake. As these patients have no intrinsic corticosteroid production, exogenous administration is necessary to prevent an Addisonian crisis.

Thyroid Dysfunction

Dysregulation of the thyroid gland and thyroid hormone production in the setting of critical illness can have systemic consequences that can be fatal if not promptly recognized and treated. Thyrotoxicosis due to Graves disease, a toxic nodular goiter, or toxic adenoma can precipitate into a thyroid storm in the setting of acute trauma, critical illness, infection, iodine contrast administration, and medication reactions. Thyroid storm is a very rare and life-threatening condition with a mortality rate of approximately 10% to 30% that can occur when normal autoregulatory and biofeedback mechanisms become altered and ineffective.[43] Clinical manifestations include altered mental status, anxiety, high fevers commonly up to 105°F, tachycardia, tremors, and GI dysfunction including nausea, vomiting, and diarrhea. Severe forms can result in seizures, coma, atrial fibrillation, heart failure, and hepatic dysfunction.

The diagnosis of thyroid storm is based on clinical evidence and laboratory evaluation demonstrating suppression of thyroid stimulating hormone and elevation of free thyroxine and/or triiodothyronine. Grading scales to predict the presence of thyroid storm do exist, but the clinical manifestations can be very nonspecific with innumerable etiologies. As such, a high index of suspicion is required to diagnose thyroid storm to include patients with very high fevers. Of note, establishing an underlying diagnosis for the cause of thyroid storm should not delay treatment. When thyroid storm is suspected, treatment should be started immediately and is focused on minimizing the clinical manifestations and decreasing thyroid hormone production. Beta blockers such as propranolol or esmolol control the tachycardia and hypertension and reduce anxiety. Thionamides such as methimazole or propylthiouracil inhibit new thyroid hormone synthesis, and when not contraindicated, propylthiouracil is preferred as it also decreases peripheral conversion of thyroxine to the more active triiodothyronine. Iodine is then given as potassium iodine or Lugol solution to inhibit thyroid hormone release but must be delayed 1 to 2 hours after thionamide administration to prevent the iodine substrate from being used for new thyroid hormone synthesis. Glucocorticoids can also be given to decrease peripheral conversion of thyroxine to triiodothyronine and may help treat an underlying Graves disease as the cause of thyroid storm. Patients who fail medical management or have contraindications to thionamides should undergo therapeutic plasma exchange or surgery for definitive treatment.[43]

INFECTIOUS DISEASES

General Principles

One of the greatest challenges to diagnosing and treating infections in the ICU is that findings classically associated with infection (or not) are quite nonspecific in the ICU setting. For example, an elevated white blood cell count or fever may simply be secondary to a postoperative or postinjury inflammatory response. Conversely, a normal body temperature may not be reassuring, as patients undergoing continuous renal replacement therapy, those on ECMO, or those with large surface area burns may not manifest a fever. Additionally, other nonspecific findings may portend an untreated infection, such as a new-onset ileus representing an intra abdominal source of infection. Ultimately, clinical judgment is key. As for the optimal processes for evaluating a possible infectious etiology, there are no widely agreed upon guidelines regarding the optimal indications and timing for cultures. Much of this has to do with the lack of meaning of blanket (or pan) cultures, with the majority of blood cultures obtained being negative.[44]

With regard to the evaluation and management of sepsis, most institutions have enacted sepsis protocols. Such systems, along with astute clinicians, are critical seeing as the early suspicion and diagnosis of sepsis and the prompt administration of antibiotics convey a significant mortality benefit.[45] Additionally critical is adequate source control. In all cases, broad-spectrum antibiotics should be administered while awaiting source control with de-escalation once culture sensitivities have returned. As for the broad antibiotic approach, this should be driven by the suspected source and the local/institutional antibiogram.

Central Line–Associated Bloodstream Infections

CLABSIs are a source of significant morbidity and mortality in hospitals and are the most expensive of all healthcare-associated infections, accounting for approximately $46,000 per case. By definition, a CLABSI is a laboratory confirmed bloodstream infection in a patient with a central line, where the cultured organism is unaffiliated with an infection from a different site. As most critically ill patients with central lines have many other possible infectious sources, one must be keenly aware of the central access that a patient has and its possibility of infection. In situations of concern, one may simply observe the patient, obtain appropriate blood cultures, or remove the central line, among other options. If the line is to be removed, catheter tip cultures are not to be obtained, as they are often misleading.

Once diagnosed, the mainstay treatment for a CLABSI is line removal and antibiotic therapy. That being said, the specifics are poorly established. Attempts at catheter salvage with antibiotics alone are not recommended in the critically ill population. Empiric antibiotic therapy should be initiated upon suspicion and continued until cultures return negative or deescalated based on antimicrobial susceptibility. The duration of treatment varies by organism and ranges from 7 days to 6 weeks.

That said, the best treatment for CLABSIs is prevention. Most effective is strict aseptic technique to include proper hand hygiene before and after insertion, full-barrier precautions during insertion, and 2% alcoholic chlorhexidine use for skin preparation. Avoidance of the femoral vein site and the prompt removal of unwarranted lines are also critical.[46]

Catheter-Associated Urinary Tract Infections

Urinary tract infections (UTIs) are the most commonly reported healthcare-associated infection. Approximately 75% of these are catheter-associated UTIs (CAUTIs). Technically, a CAUTI is a UTI in which the positive urinary culture is from an indwelling urinary catheter that has been in place for more than two calendar days. Similar to CLABSIs, CAUTIs in the ICU often present with vague symptoms and can be challenging to diagnose. Many symptoms/signs suggestive of a UTI, such as penile pain, pyuria, and bacterial growth, may be found normally with colonized Foley catheters. However, the absence of pyuria and bacterial growth strongly suggests against the diagnosis of CAUTI. The diagnosis of a CAUTI is per urinalysis and urine culture with 10^5 colony-forming units.

The management of a CAUTI includes initial empiric antibiotics, replacement of the catheter, and supportive measures. Subsequently, antibiotics are deescalated based on culture and sensitivity testing. Optimal duration of treatment is not firmly established, yet 7 to 14 days is widely accepted based on the organism.

As with CLABSI, the best treatment of CAUTI is prevention. This includes the use of sterile technique on insertion of a urinary catheter and aggressive attempts to remove the catheter as soon as possible. Intermittent straight catheterization is another option to consider in place of Foley catheters in certain patient populations.

Diarrhea and *Clostridioides difficile*

Diarrhea in the ICU setting is not terribly uncommon, often secondary to enteric feeds or iatrogenic secondary to motility agents.

Most concerning of these is that caused by *C. difficile*. The occurrence of hospital acquired *C. difficile* infections have been increasing over the years. Many factors such as antibiotic exposure, older age, and recent hospitalizations increase the risk for patients to develop *C. difficile* diarrhea. In screening for *C. difficile* infection, a thoughtful approach is key. Indications to sample include three or more watery stools in 24 hours, or significantly increased ostomy quantity and output; no laxatives or bowel regimen for the prior 48 hours; and not having tested for *C. difficile* (or a positive test) within the past 7 days.

The management of *C. difficile* is comprised of discontinuing any antibiotics if possible, avoiding antimotility agents, and an appropriate antibiotic regimen based on if this is an initial bout or a recurrence and disease severity. Initial bouts of mild disease are managed with oral vancomycin over oral metronidazole.[47] Initial severe bouts may require surgery, while fulminant bouts do require surgery in addition to oral vancomycin and IV metronidazole. Recurrent bouts require an oral vancomycin taper.

In severe cases, *C. difficile* can progress to toxic megacolon with high morbidity and mortality In toxic megacolon, diarrhea ceases and is replaced by a paralytic ileus. The severe metabolic derangements and end-organ failure that occur with toxic megacolon often mandate a total colectomy and end-ileostomy.

While *C. difficile* is an important cause of diarrhea, it is not the only infectious cause in the ICU setting. Patients should be assessed for a history of travel or food consumption, and persistent and/or bloody diarrhea without evidence of *C. difficile* should be investigated for etiologies such as *Salmonella*, *Escherichia coli*, *Shigella*, *Campylobacter jejuni*, and *Giardia*. In immunocompromised patients, cryptosporidium and cytomegalovirus are other etiologies to consider.

Other Common Infectious Issues in the ICU

Intra abdominal Infections

In surgical ICUs, a common infectious etiology is an intra abdominal infection secondary to a multitude of sources. If a generic patient has persistent fevers and leukocytosis, but no obvious source of infection, a CT of the abdomen and pelvis should be considered to assess for an intra abdominal source. Similar to aforementioned, the mainstays of therapy are source control and antibiotics, with the antibiotic therapy being dependent on the exact source, the risk level of the patient, and the possibility of the infection being hospital acquired. Recent (extrapolated) data suggest that antibiotics for intra abdominal infections can be discontinued 4 days after source control has been achieved, as there is no benefit to a longer duration.[48]

Thrombophlebitis

Superficial venous thrombus and infection are not infrequent in the ICU, most commonly being related to IV catheterization. Treatment is removal of the IV, elevation of the extremity, warm compresses, and possibly a nonsteroidal anti inflammatory agent. Antibiotics are not routinely indicated. In severe cases, excision of the vein for source control may be required.

SPECIAL ISSUES

The Open Abdomen

The open abdomen is not commonly found in the ICU. It results from several situations, most commonly damage control surgery and abdominal compartment syndrome. Damage control surgery is a technique whereby patients who are critically ill but require urgent surgery to control traumatic hemorrhage, abdominal sepsis, etc., are taken to the operating room.[49] There, the surgeon performs life-saving maneuvers (i.e., control of hemorrhage, control of hollow viscus injuries, shunting of critical vascular injuries, etc.), and brings the patient to the ICU with a temporary abdominal closure. In the ICU, the goal is to return the patient to normal physiologic status to include correction of coagulopathy, hypothermia, and acidosis. Once stabilized, the patient returns to the operating room, where definitive repairs are performed. Abdominal compartment syndrome is a potentially lethal condition caused by an inciting event that yields intra abdominal hypertension and resultant organ dysfunction (i.e., decreased lung compliance, decreased urinary output, decreased venous return to the heart, etc.), the definitive treatment being a decompressive laparotomy, the abdomen left open, and a temporary closure.

Patients in the ICU with an open abdomen require special attention. Volume management is per routine; however, one must be cognizant as to potential fluid losses from the open abdomen and assure appropriate replacement. Contrary to popular belief, patients with an open abdomen do not need to remain intubated and on the mechanical ventilator, provided they are otherwise physiologically stable. Most commonly, patients with an open abdomen are managed with vacuum-assisted closure therapy. This provides a temporarily closed environment where negative-pressure is applied to the wound. Such systems are changed at 48-hour intervals until the abdomen is closed. Failure of the vacuum-assisted closure therapy system often requires replacement either at the bedside or in the operating room.

A concept gaining traction for severe abdominal trauma and its resultant inflammation is direct peritoneal resuscitation. This modality involves continuously bathing an open abdomen with what is essentially peritoneal dialysis fluid. In several studies, this technique has been documented to decrease the inflammation and abdominal complications but has not shown any survival benefit.

Palliative Care

As the population ages and medical technologies improve especially the life-sustaining efforts of the ICU, the management of end-of-life issues, it is a crucial skill set for the surgical intensivist. Palliative care is the multidisciplinary approach to those patients with life-threatening illnesses. This includes pain and symptom management, psychosocial support, planning beyond the immediate hospitalization, etc. As such, its integration into the ICU is critical. That being said, such integration is often easier said than done. Transitioning from a curative to a palliative mode is challenging and requires excellent communication with the patient, the patient's family, and the care team.

Multisystem Organ Failure and Futility

Multisystem organ failure, also known as multiple organ dysfunction, involves altered organ function in the critically ill patient, and carries extremely high morbidity and mortality. The management includes that for the failing systems: inotropes, intra aortic balloon pumps, left ventricular assist devices for heart failure; mechanical ventilation for acute respiratory failure; continuous renal replacement therapy or dialysis for AKI; etc. While there is no widely available liver replacement therapy, in certain pediatric populations, molecular adsorbent recirculating systems are being used. It is imperative to realize that as the number of organ systems failing increases, so does the mortality. The SOFA score is one of several options for assessing mortality rates in multisystem organ failure.[50]

As multisystem organ failure develops and progresses, it is critical to have candid conversations with the patient's family. Although these discussions are difficult and nuanced, if performed well, the patient's family and care team can often come to a resolution that has the patient's best interest in mind. In instances where the patient's management is without benefit and potentially inflicting pain and prolonged suffering, it is even more critical to engage in such conversations. Such conversations of futility are the most challenging of all. Medical futility refers to interventions that are unlikely to yield any sort of benefit to the patient. Such determination is ethically challenging and, as such, controversial. Engaging local experts to include palliative care specialists and the hospital's ethics committees can be quite beneficial and is recommended. Critical care physicians need to be intimately involved in such processes and also in setting institutional and governmental policies in this arena.

SELECTED REFERENCES

Ho KM, Chavan S, Pilcher D. Omission of early thromboprophylaxis and mortality in critically ill patients: a multicenter registry study. *Chest*. 2011;140:1436–1446.

This large study of 175,665 patients showed a significant association between omission of early thromboprophylaxis (within the first 24 hours) and increased intensive care and hospital mortality.

Holcomb JB, Tilley BC, Baraniuk S, et al. Transfusion of plasma, platelets, and red blood cells in a 1:1:1 vs a 1:1:2 ratio and mortality in patients with severe trauma: the proppr randomized clinical trial. *JAMA*. 2015;313:471–482.

This multicenter randomized controlled trial among patients with severe trauma and major bleeding showed no significant differences in mortality at 24 hours or 30 days between transfusion protocols of plasma, platelets, and red blood cells in a 1:1:1 versus 1:1:2 ratio.

Kress JP, Pohlman AS, O'Connor MF, et al. Daily interruption of sedative infusions in critically ill patients undergoing mechanical ventilation. *N Engl J Med*. 2000;342:1471–1477.

This randomized controlled trial was a landmark study of mechanically ventilated adults demonstrating that scheduled daily interruption of sedative infusions decreases the duration of mechanical ventilation and intensive care unit length of stay.

Marik PE, Khangoora V, Rivera R, et al. Hydrocortisone, vitamin c, and thiamine for the treatment of severe sepsis and septic shock: a retrospective before-after study. *Chest*. 2017;151:1229–1238.

This retrospective before-after clinical study of septic patients showed that early treatment with intravenous vitamin C together with hydrocortisone and thiamine are effective in preventing progressive organ dysfunction and reduced mortality in patients with severe sepsis and septic shock.

Sawyer RG, Claridge JA, Nathens AB, et al. Trial of short-course antimicrobial therapy for intraabdominal infection. *N Engl J Med*. 2015;372:1996–2005.

This randomized controlled trial demonstrated that, in patients with intra abdominal infections who had undergone a source-control procedure, a shorter, fixed duration of antibiotic treatment (4 days) resulted in similar outcomes compared to longer antibiotic courses and significantly decreased antibiotic exposure.

REFERENCES

1. Wick EC, Grant MC, Wu CL. Postoperative multimodal analgesia pain management with nonopioid analgesics and techniques: a review. *JAMA Surg*. 2017;152:691–697.
2. Riker RR, Shehabi Y, Bokesch PM, et al. Dexmedetomidine vs midazolam for sedation of critically ill patients: a randomized trial. *JAMA*. 2009;301:489–499.
3. Kress JP, Pohlman AS, O'Connor MF, et al. Daily interruption of sedative infusions in critically ill patients undergoing mechanical ventilation. *N Engl J Med*. 2000;342:1471–1477.
4. Salluh JI, Wang H, Schneider EB, et al. Outcome of delirium in critically ill patients: systematic review and meta-analysis. *BMJ*. 2015;350:h2538.
5. Hazama A, Ziechmann R, Arul M, et al. The effect of keppra prophylaxis on the incidence of early onset, post-traumatic brain injury seizures. *Cureus*. 2018;10:e2674.
6. Butt JH, Olesen JB, Havers-Borgersen E, et al. Risk of thromboembolism associated with atrial fibrillation following noncardiac surgery. *J Am Coll Cardiol*. 2018;72:2027–2036.
7. Moskowitz A, Chen KP, Cooper AZ, et al. Management of atrial fibrillation with rapid ventricular response in the intensive care unit: a secondary analysis of electronic health record data. *Shock*. 2017;48:436–440.
8. Singer M, Deutschman CS, Seymour CW, et al. The third international consensus definitions for sepsis and septic shock (sepsis-3). *JAMA*. 2016;315:801–810.
9. Yealy DM, Kellum JA, Huang DT, et al. A randomized trial of protocol-based care for early septic shock. *N Engl J Med*. 2014;370:1683–1693.
10. Rhodes A, Evans LE, Alhazzani W, et al. Surviving sepsis campaign: international guidelines for management of sepsis and septic shock: 2016. *Intensive Care Med*. 2017;43:304–377.
11. Marik PE, Khangoora V, Rivera R, et al. Hydrocortisone, vitamin C, and thiamine for the treatment of severe sepsis and septic shock: a retrospective before-after study. *Chest*. 2017;151:1229–1238.
12. Holcomb JB, Tilley BC, Baraniuk S, et al. Transfusion of plasma, platelets, and red blood cells in a 1:1:1 vs a 1:1:2 ratio and mortality in patients with severe trauma: the proppr randomized clinical trial. *JAMA*. 2015;313:471–482.
13. Thygesen K, Alpert JS, Jaffe AS, et al. Fourth universal definition of myocardial infarction (2018). *Eur Heart J*. 2019;40:237–269.
14. Patel MR, Calhoon JH, Dehmer GJ, et al. ACC/AATS/AHA/ASE/ASNC/SCAI/SCCT/STS 2016 appropriate use criteria for coronary revascularization in patients with acute coronary syndromes: a report of the American College of Cardiology Appropriate Use Criteria Task Force, American Association For Thoracic Surgery, American Heart Association, American Society of Echocardiography, American Society of Nuclear Cardiology, Society For Cardiovascular Angiography

and Interventions, Society of Cardiovascular Computed Tomography, and the Society of Thoracic Surgeons. *J Am Coll Cardiol*. 2017;69:570–591.
15. Kalil AC, Metersky ML, Klompas M, et al. Management of adults with hospital-acquired and ventilator-associated pneumonia: 2016 clinical practice guidelines by the Infectious Diseases Society of America and the American Thoracic Society. *Clin Infect Dis*. 2016;63:e61–e111.
16. Ranieri VM, Rubenfeld GD, Thompson BT, et al. Acute respiratory distress syndrome: the berlin definition. *JAMA*. 2012;307:2526–2533.
17. Brower RG, Matthay MA, Morris A, et al. Ventilation with lower tidal volumes as compared with traditional tidal volumes for acute lung injury and the acute respiratory distress syndrome. *N Engl J Med*. 2000;342:1301–1308.
18. Combes A, Hajage D, Capellier G, et al. Extracorporeal membrane oxygenation for severe acute respiratory distress syndrome. *N Engl J Med*. 2018;378:1965–1975.
19. Ndahimana D, Kim EK. Energy requirements in critically ill patients. *Clin Nutr Res*. 2018;7:81–90.
20. Gupta RD, Ramachandran R, Venkatesan P, et al. Indirect calorimetry: from bench to bedside. *Indian J Endocrinol Metab*. 2017;21:594–599.
21. McClave SA, Taylor BE, Martindale RG, et al. Guidelines for the provision and assessment of nutrition support therapy in the adult critically ill patient: Society of Critical Care Medicine (SCCM) and American Society for Parenteral and Enteral Nutrition (A.S.P.E.N.). *JPEN J Parenter Enteral Nutr*. 2016;40:159–211.
22. Yeh DD, Ortiz-Reyes LA, Quraishi SA, et al. Early nutritional inadequacy is associated with psoas muscle deterioration and worse clinical outcomes in critically ill surgical patients. *J Crit Care*. 2018;45:7–13.
23. Elke G, van Zanten AR, Lemieux M, et al. Enteral versus parenteral nutrition in critically ill patients: an updated systematic review and meta-analysis of randomized controlled trials. *Crit Care*. 2016;20:117.
24. Harvey SE, Parrott F, Harrison DA, et al. A multicentre, randomised controlled trial comparing the clinical effectiveness and cost-effectiveness of early nutritional support via the parenteral versus the enteral route in critically ill patients (CALORIES). *Health Technol Assess*. 2016;20:1–144.
25. Krag M, Perner A, Wetterslev J, et al. Prevalence and outcome of gastrointestinal bleeding and use of acid suppressants in acutely ill adult intensive care patients. *Intensive Care Med*. 2015;41:833–845.
26. Buendgens L, Koch A, Tacke F. Prevention of stress-related ulcer bleeding at the intensive care unit: risks and benefits of stress ulcer prophylaxis. *World J Crit Care Med*. 2016;5:57–64.
27. Abbas N, Makker J, Abbas H, et al. Perioperative care of patients with liver cirrhosis: a review. *Health Serv Insights*. 2017;10; 1178632917691270.
28. Hackl C, Schlitt HJ, Renner P, et al. Liver surgery in cirrhosis and portal hypertension. *World J Gastroenterol*. 2016;22:2725–2735.
29. Lopez-Delgado JC, Ballus J, Esteve F, et al. Outcomes of abdominal surgery in patients with liver cirrhosis. *World J Gastroenterol*. 2016;22:2657–2667.
30. Demetriades D, Hadjizacharia P, Constantinou C, et al. Selective nonoperative management of penetrating abdominal solid organ injuries. *Ann Surg*. 2006;244:620–628.
31. Wang J, Xu E, Xiao Y. Isotonic versus hypotonic maintenance IV fluids in hospitalized children: a meta-analysis. *Pediatrics*. 2014;133:105–113.
32. Kellum JA, Lameire N. Diagnosis, evaluation, and management of acute kidney injury: a KDIGO summary (part 1). *Crit Care*. 2013;17:204.
33. Luk L, Steinman J, Newhouse JH. Intravenous contrast-induced nephropathy-the rise and fall of a threatening idea. *Adv Chronic Kidney Dis*. 2017;24:169–175.
34. Abuelo JG. Treatment of severe hyperkalemia: confronting 4 fallacies. *Kidney Int Rep*. 2018;3:47–55.
35. Park MS, Martini WZ, Dubick MA, et al. Thromboelastography as a better indicator of hypercoagulable state after injury than prothrombin time or activated partial thromboplastin time. *J Trauma*. 2009;67:266–275; discussion 275–266.
36. Plotkin AJ, Wade CE, Jenkins DH, et al. A reduction in clot formation rate and strength assessed by thrombelastography is indicative of transfusion requirements in patients with penetrating injuries. *J Trauma*. 2008;64:S64–S68.
37. East JM, Cserti-Gazdewich CM, Granton JT. Heparin-induced thrombocytopenia in the critically ill patient. *Chest*. 2018;154:678–690.
38. Ho KM, Chavan S, Pilcher D. Omission of early thromboprophylaxis and mortality in critically ill patients: a multicenter registry study. *Chest*. 2011;140:1436–1446.
39. Carson JL, Guyatt G, Heddle NM, et al. Clinical practice guidelines from the AABB: red blood cell transfusion thresholds and storage. *JAMA*. 2016;316:2025–2035.
40. Mazer CD, Whitlock RP, Fergusson DA, et al. Restrictive or liberal red-cell transfusion for cardiac surgery. *N Engl J Med*. 2017;377:2133–2144.
41. Finfer S, Chittock DR, Su SY, et al. Intensive versus conventional glucose control in critically ill patients. *N Engl J Med*. 2009;360:1283–1297.
42. Sprung CL, Annane D, Keh D, et al. Hydrocortisone therapy for patients with septic shock. *N Engl J Med*. 2008;358:111–124.
43. Wang HI, Yiang GT, Hsu CW, et al. thyroid Storm in a patient with trauma—a challenging diagnosis for the emergency physician: case report and literature review. *J Emerg Med*. 2017;52:292–298.
44. Linsenmeyer K, Gupta K, Strymish JM, et al. Culture if spikes? indications and yield of blood cultures in hospitalized medical patients. *J Hosp Med*. 2016;11:336–340.
45. Levy MM, Evans LE, Rhodes A. The surviving sepsis campaign bundle: 2018 update. *Crit Care Med*. 2018;46:997–1000.
46. Parienti JJ, Mongardon N, Megarbane B, et al. Intravascular complications of central venous catheterization by insertion site. *N Engl J Med*. 2015;373:1220–1229.
47. McDonald LC, Gerding DN, Johnson S, et al. Clinical practice guidelines for *Clostridium difficile* infection in adults and children: 2017 update by the Infectious Diseases Society of America (IDSA) and Society for Healthcare Epidemiology of America (SHEA). *Clin Infect Dis*. 2018;66:e1–e48.
48. Sawyer RG, Claridge JA, Nathens AB, et al. Trial of short-course antimicrobial therapy for intraabdominal infection. *N Engl J Med*. 2015;372:1996–2005.
49. Bogert JN, Harvin JA, Cotton BA. Damage control resuscitation. *J Intensive Care Med*. 2016;31:177–186.
50. Falcao ALE, Barros AGA, Bezerra AAM, et al. The prognostic accuracy evaluation of SAPS 3, SOFA and APACHE II scores for mortality prediction in the surgical ICU: an external validation study and decision-making analysis. *Ann Intensive Care*. 2019;9:18.

23 CHAPTER

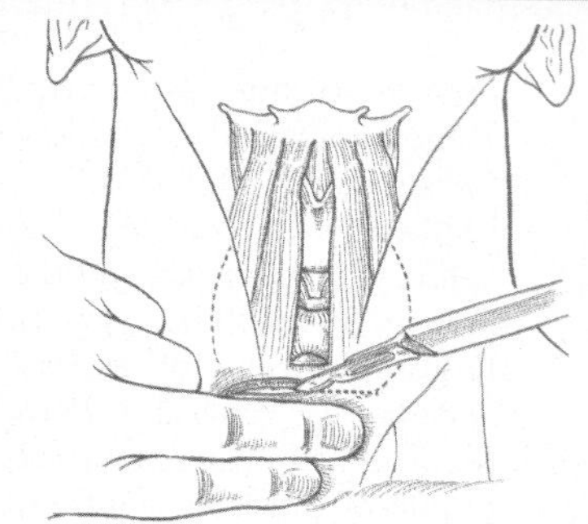

Bedside Surgical Procedures

Bradley M. Dennis, Oliver L. Gunter, Jose J. Diaz

OUTLINE

Bedside surgical procedures have become a standard in many intensive care units (ICUs), replacing the operating room (OR) as the preferred location for select procedures in critically ill patients.[1] Performing appropriately selected procedures within the ICU limits the risk of transporting critically ill patients, facilitates flexibility in timing and scheduling, and reduces cost.[2–9] The ability to perform some operations at the bedside may be lifesaving in critically ill patients too unstable to transport safely to the OR. Advancements in monitoring and sedation, in endoscopic and percutaneous techniques, and in bedside imaging have enabled the transition of several procedures traditionally performed in the OR and endoscopy and interventional radiology suites to the ICU. Some procedures now regularly performed in the ICU include bedside laparotomy, tracheostomy, percutaneous endoscopic feeding access, percutaneous drainage procedures, and the placement of inferior vena cava filters. For example, between 2006 and 2014, more than 2800 percutaneous tracheostomies, 900 percutaneous endoscopic gastrostomy (PEG) or percutaneous endoscopic gastrojejunostomy (PEGJ) tube placements, 450 exploration and irrigation of open abdomens, and 50 exploratory laparotomies were performed at the bedside in the ICUs at Vanderbilt University Medical Center. In the unstable patient, other procedures may be performed at the bedside including irrigation and debridement of wounds, orthopedic stabilization with external fixation, fasciotomies, amputations, and diagnostic laparoscopy.

Although bedside operative procedures can be performed safely, with complication rates equal to those in the OR, doing so mandates that cases are appropriately selected and that appropriate safety practices are consistently implemented. The ICU represents a complex environment in which to perform complex processes and procedures. Recognition of the numerous potentials for error and adverse events in such settings is important. Based on the experience of industry and other high-reliability organizations, prevention of error and adverse events requires standardization of processes and elimination of variability.[10] Protocols and safety practices specifically for bedside operative procedures should be in place to ensure the ability to perform these procedures safely, with low infection rates, and with the assurance of comfort and amnesia. In this chapter, we discuss the following topics:

1. The rationale for bedside surgical procedures.
2. Process of bringing the OR to the bedside.
3. Systematic safety methodologies and practices to ensure safe performance of bedside procedures.
4. Selection of patients for bedside surgical procedures.
5. Specific considerations for common bedside procedures:
   a. Bedside laparotomy
   b. Percutaneous tracheostomy
   c. Percutaneous endoscopic feeding tubes
   d. Bronchoscopy.

RATIONALE FOR BEDSIDE SURGICAL PROCEDURES

For good reasons, most surgical procedures are performed in the OR. The centralization of resources, including anesthesia personnel and equipment, surgical equipment, radiology, specialized nursing and procedural support staff, and safety policies and principles, makes the modern surgical suite an ideal venue for most operations (Fig. 23.1). However, OR demand may exceed available resources, complicating timely access to the OR and scheduling of unplanned, urgent, or emergent cases. Competition for OR space may delay or prevent timely operative procedures for critically ill patients. Additionally, performance of procedures in the OR mandate transportation of critically ill patients from the ICU and back and requires substantial resource utilization and costs. As the complexity and severity of illness of critical care patients have increased, so too has the risk related to their transport. The transport of critically ill patients frequently requires multiple personnel, including nursing staff, transport staff, respiratory care, and anesthesia staff. Furthermore, the change of venue and personnel caring for the patient necessitates detailed communication for handoff and represents a potential source of medical error. The transport of a patient from the ICU to the OR is a resource sink, adds cost, and increases risk. Consideration of transport to the OR should be evaluated in the same manner as other treatments by assessing risk versus benefit for the individual patient.[11] Each hospital should have guidelines for the inter- and intrahospital

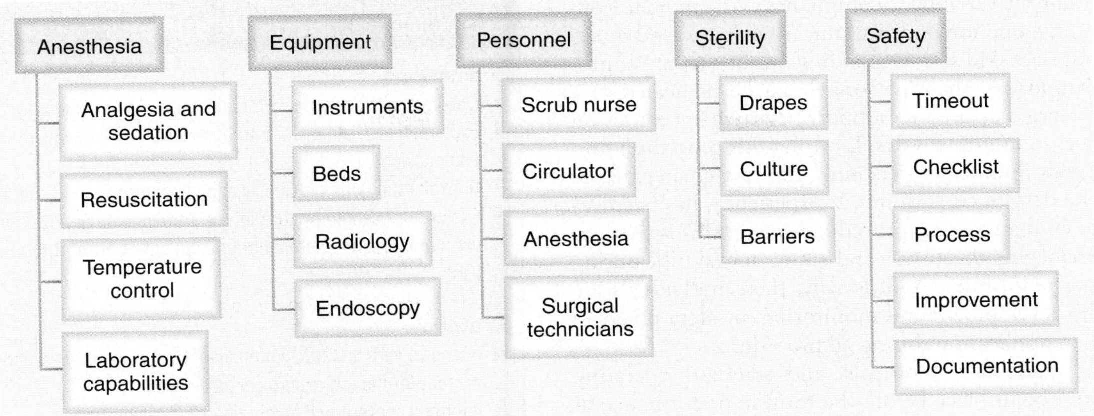

FIG. 23.1 Resources available in the operating room.

transport of critically ill patients to various parts of the hospital for various imaging, tests, or procedures and to the OR to decrease inherent risk.[12]

TAKING THE OPERATING ROOM TO THE BEDSIDE

While the vast majority of surgical procedures should be performed in the OR, the ICU is a logical alternative location for some surgical procedures. The two locations are similar in many ways. Both locations have monitoring equipment capable of real-time monitoring of cardiovascular, respiratory, and neurologic monitoring. The ICU and OR both have mechanical ventilation capability. In fact, many ICUs have ventilators with more advanced functionalities than their corresponding ORs. Although lacking inhalational anesthetic administration capabilities, intravenous sedation and analgesia can be administered in the ICU to allow for the performance of bedside procedures. Lastly, and most importantly, there are analogous staff in ICU. In the ICU, the roles of circulating OR nurse and anesthesia providers can be filled by the teamwork of a critical care nurse, respiratory therapist, and intensivist. The one crucial OR role not easily translated to the ICU setting is the scrub nurse/technician. Dedicated procedure support personnel have been described in the ICU setting to bridge this gap.[3] In this role, the procedure support nurse is responsible for many of the same functions as the scrub nurse. Dedicated procedure support personnel not only decrease the variability in how an individual procedure is performed, but also they play important roles in compliance to guidelines, both of which are significant factors in reducing error.

Multiple factors are required to create and maintain a successful system for performing bedside procedures (Fig. 23.2). Management guidelines may include standard operating procedures, preprocedure checklists including time-out procedures, and sedation protocols. Appropriate access to supplies may require temporary storage of core equipment in an individual ICU with standardized restocking mechanisms, streamlining the supply chain. Finally, a facilitative mindset among staff is vital to the success of such a system.

SAFETY PRACTICES FOR BEDSIDE SURGICAL PROCEDURES

To ensure the safety of operative procedures performed at the bedside in the ICU, systematic measures should be in place for appropriate patient selection; adequate expertise of supporting personnel; limited procedural variability; adequate monitoring and anesthesia; and facilitation of concise, accurate, and specific

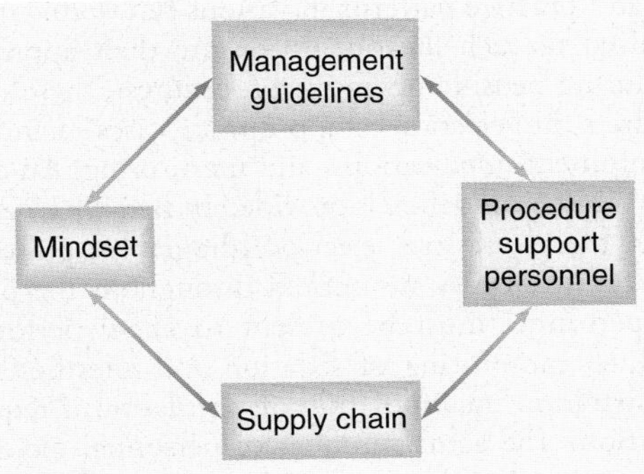

FIG. 23.2 Fundamentals vital to the success of bedside surgical procedures.

intrateam communication. Measures shown to increase safety in the OR are also appropriate for procedures performed at bedside in the ICU. Implementation of the Safe Surgery Saves Lives program developed by the World Health Organization (WHO) has been associated with a significant global reduction in perioperative morbidity and mortality.[13] The 10 safety objectives outlined in the WHO Guidelines for Safe Surgery 2009 are as follows[14]:

1. The team will operate on the correct patient at the correct site.
2. The team will use methods known to prevent harm from administration of anesthetics while protecting the patient from pain.
3. The team will recognize and effectively prepare for life-threatening loss of airway or respiratory function.
4. The team will recognize and effectively prepare for risk of high blood loss.
5. The team will avoid inducing an allergic or adverse drug reaction for which the patient is known to be at significant risk.
6. The team will consistently use methods known to minimize the risk for surgical site infection.
7. The team will prevent inadvertent retention of instruments and sponges in surgical wounds.
8. The team will secure and accurately identify all surgical specimens.
9. The team will effectively communicate and exchange critical information for the safe conduct of the operation.
10. Hospitals and public health systems will establish routine surveillance of surgical capacity, volume, and results.

The use of specifically trained procedure support personnel to support bedside operative procedures within the ICU greatly facilitates reduction in variability, compliance with standard operative procedures, reduction of communication errors, and maintenance of appropriate skill sets. Depending on the volume of procedures to be supported, these personnel can be dedicated to a specific unit or service or used to support bedside procedures on numerous services in multiple ICUs. Limiting this procedure support role to a small number of personnel allows a greater degree of expertise to be developed and, in our experience, has been extremely valuable in maintaining procedural safety; this is particularly true with managing the airway and endotracheal tube during percutaneous tracheostomies. Additionally, these individuals are charged with the development and monitoring of safety practices and ensuring their application during all procedures.

Management guidelines, protocols, and standard operating procedures should be in place before the routine performance of bedside operative procedures. They should be in line with procedures developed for the OR and be easily accessible, and compliance should be monitored. Because of variations in specific personnel and practice patterns in various ICUs, documents may be customized to each location to ensure their appropriate application during bedside operative procedures. These documents should address the selection of appropriate cases, mandatory personnel, equipment, medications, and monitoring. An example of a bedside operative guideline is provided in Box 23.1.[5] All patients should have blood pressure, electrocardiography, pulse oximetry, and ventilation routinely monitored throughout the procedures. Adequate personnel must be present to allow performance of the procedure, monitoring of sedation and anesthesia, medication administration, manipulation of ventilation if required, and documentation. The actual number of personnel required varies depending on the procedure and expertise of particular personnel. Analgesia and sedation must be ensured with appropriate medications under the direction of the adequately credentialed personnel. Additionally, guidelines and protocols should include standards for adequate preparation, equipment, and instrument accounting.

The use of preprocedure time-out and procedural checklists aids in ensuring appropriate safety practices. Use of these tools helps limit communication errors, facilitates compliance with standard operating procedures, and can be used to aid in documentation and compliance monitoring. These tools should be consistent with practices employed in the OR to reduce variability where appropriate. Fig. 23.3 provides an example of such a procedural checklist. Ideally, these tools can be combined with forms required for documentation, and information can be captured for quality and performance analysis.

Ensuring a high degree of safety of bedside operative procedures and providing documentation of such when required mandate that mechanisms for tracking procedure performance, compliance monitoring, and adverse event review and reporting are developed. These mechanisms must be applicable locally to facilitate consistent, nonvariable performance and interface with global hospital safety mechanisms and initiatives. Development of process mapping flow charts and diagrams facilitates the integration of unit-specific, departmental, and hospital-wide processes and helps delineate lines of communication and authority.

SELECTION OF PATIENTS FOR BEDSIDE SURGICAL PROCEDURES

As noted previously, if selected appropriately, bedside operative procedures can be performed with similar risk of complications as when performed in the OR, at lower cost, and without transportation risks.[4–7,9] However, there are no randomized studies and few retrospective reviews that evaluate the safety of bedside operative procedures or help delineate what the appropriate patient populations and operative procedures are. The safety and efficacy of bedside procedures vary depending on the local experience and application of safety practices. As experience is gained, indications may broaden, and frequency may increase. The decision to perform an operative procedure at the bedside requires a careful risk-benefit analysis. This decision considers the difficulty and risk of transport; the complexity of the operation; the ability to achieve timely OR space; and the safety, ease, and cost savings of performing the procedure at the bedside. Most major operative procedures should be performed in the OR. In general, the indications for bedside operative procedures fall into two categories: (1) the patient requires a lifesaving intervention but is too unstable

BOX 23.1 Bedside surgery protocol.

Indications

- Decompressive celiotomy for abdominal compartment syndrome
- Exploratory celiotomy for intraabdominal hemorrhage after damage control and packing
- Reexploration of a previously open abdomen for washout or closure
- Exploratory celiotomy to rule out intraabdominal sepsis in a patient with ventilatory requirements that prohibit safe transport to the operating room (OR)

Protocol

a) Intensive care unit (ICU) attending physician and operating surgeon will be present for the entire surgical procedure.
b) Informed consent will be obtained (if possible).
c) Preprocedure checklist will be reviewed by the bedside nurse.
d) Bedside nurse and a respiratory therapist will monitor patient and record procedure (conscious sedation sheet).

Indications to proceed to OR (level 1):

- Surgical bleeding
- Dead bowel
- Need to open another body cavity
- Surgeon preference

For laparotomies:

- A sterile perimeter will be set up in the patient's room. All individuals must wear a surgical head covering and mask.
- The ICU attending physician will oversee anesthetic management of the patient.
- General anesthesia will include narcotics, benzodiazepines, propofol, paralytics, and ventilator management.
- A sterile hand wash will be performed by the operating team.
- Preoperative antibiotics are indicated only if a new surgical wound is to be made (e.g., cefazolin [Ancef], 1–2 g intravenously).
- A povidone-iodine (Betadine)–chlorhexidine abdominal preparation will be used.
- A standard Bovie will be set up (when indicated).
- Wall suction canisters will be set up.
- A 4-L warm irrigation with normal saline will be used.
- A standard bedside celiotomy tray will be set up with suture on a sterile field.

Adapted from Vanderbilt University Medical Center, Division of Trauma and Surgical Critical Care. Emergency general surgery protocols: bedside surgery protocol, 2005. http://www.vumc.org/trauma-and-scc/sites/vumc.org.trauma-and-scc/files/public_files/Manual/BedsideSurgeryProtocolRev2005.pdf.

SICU Procedure "TIME-OUT" Check List		
Complete this form (a) just prior to beginning the procedure and (b) at the location where the procedure is to be performed.		
Patient's Name: ______________ Medical record number: ______________		
Procedure Type: ☐ Planned nonemergent ☐ Not planned nonemergent ☐ Emergent		
VERIFICATION		
1. Invasive procedure to be performed:	Circle one	
2. H&P completed if patient admitted within past 24 hours	Yes	No
3. Informed consent obtained? (Verified by Bedside RN and Procedure RN)	Yes	No
4. Correct patient identity? ☐ Arm Band ☐ MRN ☐ Consent If procedure is emergent, Bedside RN, Procedure RN, and Physician performing procedure need to verify patient ID and initial this form.	Yes	No
5. Agreement on procedure (Agreement b/w Physician performing procedure and Procedure RN)	Yes	No
6. Correct side/site verified and marked? ☐ NA ☐ Right ☐ Left ☐ Site: (Verified and marked by Physician performing procedure and Procedure RN)	Yes	No
7. Correct equipment available? (Verified by Physician performing procedure and Procedure RN)	Yes	No
8. Required resources available? (Verified by Physician performing procedure and Procedure RN)	Yes	No
9. Ready to set up procedure? (Verified by Procedure RN)	Yes	No
9. Ready to proceed with procedure? (Verified by Procedure RN)	Yes	No
TIME-OUT: All individuals performing and assisting with the procedure are to review the checklist and sign below.		
Physician performing procedure:		
Procedure RN name:		
Bedside RN name:		
Other:	Other:	Other:
Staff calling "TIME-OUT": (Title and signature)		

FIG. 23.3 Surgical intensive care unit procedure time-out checklist.

for transport to the OR and (2) low complexity procedures in which the risk of transport, difficulties of OR scheduling, and cost and resource utilization of the OR favor a bedside procedure. Factors that generally favor performance of procedures in the OR include complex procedures, complex or extensive equipment needs, risk of encountering significant bleeding, need for insertion of prosthetic materials, significant lighting requirements, and lengthy procedures. Commonly performed bedside procedures include percutaneous and open tracheostomy, PEG or PEGJ tube placement, bronchoscopy, soft tissue debridement, decompressive laparotomy for abdominal hypertension, washout and packing removal after a damage control laparotomy, placement of inferior vena cava filters, and damage control orthopedic procedures (e.g., placement of external fixator). Occasionally, the condition of extremely critically ill patients can be temporized at the bedside by the performance of a bedside operative procedure with subsequent performance of the definitive operation in the OR.

BEDSIDE LAPAROTOMY

Bedside laparotomy was initially a procedure of last resort in patients too sick to proceed to the OR—a heroic attempt to identify reversible intraabdominal pathology as the patient was near death.[5] However, the recognition of abdominal compartment syndrome (ACS) as a frequent complication of resuscitation of acutely ill patients and the acceptance of the "damage control" approach to the management of acutely ill patients with intraabdominal pathology has resulted in a dramatic increase in the application of bedside laparotomy in more controlled settings.[4,5,15] Damage control and management of ACS use an open abdomen approach in which the fascia remains open and necessitates the use of various temporary abdominal closure techniques. Indications for bedside laparotomy can be classified as emergent or semielective. Common emergent indications include (1) decompressive laparotomy for ACS, (2) control and packing for recurrent bleeding after a previous damage control laparotomy, and (3) suspicion of intraabdominal infection in patients too critically ill to be transported to the OR. Common semielective indications include (1) pack removal after damage control laparotomy, (2) irrigation and debridement of the open abdomen, (3) source control for sepsis resulting from intraabdominal pathology, and (4) management of traumatic abdominal defects.

Historically, the most common emergent indication for bedside laparotomy was for decompression of abdominal hypertension. Recognition and understanding of the pathophysiology of increased intraabdominal pressure leading to organ system dysfunction—ACS—have increased significantly since first described the measurement of intraabdominal pressure as an indication for abdominal reexploration.[16–18] ACS can be classified as primary, resulting from intraabdominal processes, or secondary, resulting from bowel edema and intraabdominal fluid secondary to the treatment and resuscitation of extraabdominal pathology. Increasing intraabdominal pressure leads to alterations in abdominal perfusion pressure, restricted venous return, and reduction of pulmonary compliance. These alterations can lead to cardiac failure, pulmonary decompensation, and oliguria. Severe elevations in abdominal pressure can lead to organ hypoperfusion and ischemia, although the pressure at which this occurs may vary depending on mean arterial pressure. Grading systems for the degree of abdominal hypertension have been proposed with Grades III (21–25 mm Hg) and IV (>25 mm Hg) considered to be significantly elevated, defining ACS.[19] Management of ACS may involve only measures to ensure adequate abdominal perfusion pressures at lower pressures, but as intraabdominal pressure increases, abdominal decompression by laparotomy is indicated. Appropriate treatment requires recognition of development of this syndrome. Routine monitoring of bladder pressures of patients requiring significant resuscitation after abdominal procedures and patients being resuscitated from a significant shock (base deficit >10) who receive 6 L or more of crystalloid or 6 units or more of packed red blood cells in a 6-hour period is indicated. With changes in resuscitation strategies in critically unstable patients, the incidence of ACS may be declining.

The acceptance of damage control, an abbreviated laparotomy to salvage trauma patients with exsanguination, has led to an increased application of bedside laparotomy for control of recurrent bleeding within the abdomen before correction of the patient's systemic physiology and for removal of abdominal packs, irrigation, and debridement.[20] Bedside laparotomy is common in most level I trauma centers where damage control and temporary abdominal closure for patients in extremis are frequently used. Numerous methods of temporary abdominal closure have been described and continue to evolve. We prefer to use negative pressure systems, and a facility with the applications of these systems is required for patient management.

The open abdominal approach is also applied to the general surgery population, most commonly for the management of necrotizing pancreatitis, necrotizing soft tissue infection of the abdominal wall, diffuse peritonitis in patients at high risk of failure of source control, and mesenteric ischemia.[5] Damage control techniques with staged gastrointestinal reconstruction, serial abdominal washouts for source control, and delayed abdominal wall closure can be used in the management of these very complex patients. Controlled trials of these techniques are limited, and the indications and settings in which the open abdominal approach is most appropriate are not fully determined.

Surgical rescue of the critical ill patient has become an increasing area of awareness. In select critically ill patients, with severe cardiopulmonary instability precluding transport to the OR, a resuscitative bedside laparotomy may be indicated.[21] Patients who require an emergent bedside laparotomy have an extremely high rate of death, with over 50% mortality. This information may be useful in the setting of preintervention counseling with patient's families.[22]

TRACHEOSTOMY

Tracheostomy is the most common surgical procedure in critically ill patients requiring prolonged mechanical ventilation.[23] Table 23.1 shows some of the common indications and contraindications for tracheostomy. Nearly all contraindications are relative ones, and most are temporary. Indications for tracheostomy in critically ill patients fall broadly into three categories:

- Upper airway obstruction
- Prolonged mechanical ventilation
- Neurologic condition preventing safe extubation

The ease and convenience of bedside tracheostomy in critically ill patients have made performance at the bedside the standard in many institutions. Open and percutaneous dilatational tracheostomy (PDT) can be performed safely at the bedside in the ICU.[3,6,24,25] Evidence-based guidelines do not recommend one specific technique over another with respect to reducing complications or mortality.[26] PDT has become widely used for elective tracheostomy in critically ill adult patients. Ciaglia and colleagues[27] first described elective PDT in 1985, and since that time, numerous modifications to the technique have been made. When comparing PDT with standard surgical tracheostomy performed in the OR, PDT demonstrated decreased wound infection and clinically relevant bleeding.[24] Percutaneous tracheostomy has also been demonstrated to be more cost-effective in critically ill ICU patients.[2,6,25,28] Perioperative mortality related to PDT in randomized studies appears to be less than 0.2%.[2,3,6,24] The safety of bedside PDT was confirmed in a retrospective analysis of more than 3000 consecutive procedures.[3] This analysis revealed a periprocedural major complication rate of 0.15% and a periprocedural mortality rate of less than 0.1% within this population of

TABLE 23.1 Indications and contraindications for tracheostomy.

INDICATIONS	CONTRAINDICATIONS
Upper airway obstruction	Recent anterior neck surgery (<7 days)
Difficult airway	High ventilator settings
Significant maxillofacial trauma	Fraction of inspired oxygen >70%
Angioedema	Positive end expiratory pressure >10 cm H_2O
Upper airway tumors	Advanced ventilator modes
Neurologic condition preventing safe extubation	Elevated intracranial pressure
Brain injury—acute or progressive	Hemodynamic instability
Spinal cord injury (including halo fixation)	Significant bleeding risk
Severe agitation or delirium	Local infection or malignancy at proposed site
Prolonged altered mental status	Predicted early mortality
Prolonged mechanical ventilation	

critically ill patients. Additionally, this review demonstrated the safety of bedside PDT in obese and superobese patients. These data are useful for decisions regarding the indications for tracheostomy in critically ill patients; patients in whom the risks of failure of extubation or airway loss are estimated to result in fatal outcome are greater than 1 in 1000 should be considered for tracheostomy. Timing of tracheostomy is controversial in patients with predicted prolonged mechanical ventilation. Most studies have shown no difference in relevant clinical outcomes such as mortality, pneumonia rates, and hospital length of stay.[29–32] Studies have supported early tracheostomy (up to 7 days) versus delayed tracheostomy (after 7 days) with shorter ICU stays and less mechanical ventilation but with no difference in mortality in trauma and nontrauma populations.[29,33] However, a randomized study of medical ICU patients demonstrated a significant reduction in mortality (32% vs. 62%), pneumonia (5% vs. 25%), and accidental extubation (0 vs. 6) when early tracheostomy (48 hours) was compared with delayed tracheostomy (14–6 days) for patients predicted to require 14 days of mechanical ventilation.[34] The early group also had significantly decreased ICU length of stay and ventilator days.

Long-term complications have not been adequately studied in randomized trials to draw conclusions. Reported perioperative complications of percutaneous tracheostomy include the following:

- Peristomal bleeding from injury to the anterior jugular veins or thyroid isthmus
- Injury of the posterior trachea and/or esophagus by laceration through the back wall of the trachea
- Extraluminal placement by creating a false tract during placement of the tracheostomy tube
- Loss of airway.

Major perioperative complications can be minimized by employing safety measures outlined in the previous sections. We find that specifically trained support personnel managing the airway is particularly helpful in limiting airway mishaps. Dedicated multidisciplinary tracheostomy teams have been shown to reduce time to decannulation, length of stay, and adverse events.[35] Additionally, one of two techniques should be used to ensure proper positioning of the tracheostomy tube and to minimize risk of loss of airway by inadvertent extubation during the procedure: bronchoscopic guidance or semiopen technique with blunt dissection to the anterior trachea.[36] However, bronchoscopic guidance does not eliminate severe tracheal injuries, and involvement of experienced personnel is important to prevent these complications Recently, the use of preprocedure ultrasound to identify the neck anatomy is helpful in decreasing potential risk of bleeding from crossing veins, identifying enlarge thyroid lobes, and decreasing the number of sticks.[37,38] This has been especially helpful in the morbidly obese patient. Long-term, the incidence of serious tracheal stenosis after percutaneous tracheostomy is low with reports of 6%,[39] and tracheal stenosis usually occurs early in the subglottic position. Subclinical tracheal stenosis is found in 40% of patients.[40] Follow-up of patients discharged from the ICU with tracheostomies is important to minimize and identify complications.

PERCUTANEOUS ENDOSCOPIC GASTROSTOMY

Gauderer and coworkers[41] first described PEG in 1980 for access into the stomach for enteral feedings using a "pull" technique. Various other techniques have since been described. The principle of a sutureless approximation of the stomach to the anterior abdominal wall has allowed the pull technique to become the most popular method used. The other two most commonly used techniques are the "push" and introducer techniques, both of which require the use of stay sutures to approximate the stomach to the anterior abdominal wall. Newer PEGJ tubes combine gastric and jejunal ports to allow distal feeding and proximal decompression.

Accepted primary indications for a PEG or PEGJ include inability to swallow, high risk of aspiration, severe facial trauma, and indications for mechanical ventilation for longer than 4 weeks.[42] Other indications include nutritional access for debilitated patients and patients with dementia with severe malnutrition. PEG tubes have been associated with reducing overall hospital cost.

Numerous gastrostomy and gastrojejunostomy tubes are commercially available. Most allow simple gastrostomy assessment with or without a valve. Some are flush with the skin and require a tube to be attached only during feeding. For critically ill patients with increased risk of aspiration, multilumen percutaneous endoscopic transgastric jejunostomy tubes are available. These tubes allow drainage of the stomach while feeding the proximal jejunum. A third lumen connects to a balloon that maintains apposition of the gastric and abdominal walls. Although feeding can be started on the same day as the PEG is placed, most critically ill patients are not started on feedings for 24 hours.[43] This allows for a period of time for no unseen complication to manifest itself prior to starting enteral feeds. Contraindications for PEG placement include the following:

- No endoscopic access
- Significant ascites
- Severe coagulopathy
- Gastric outlet obstruction or previous gastric resection
- Gastric bypass surgery
- Survival less than 4 weeks
- Inability to bring the gastric wall in approximation to the abdominal wall
- Severe immunosuppression (white blood cell count <1).

There are a few relative contraindications, such as an inability to transilluminate through the anterior abdominal wall, gastric varices, and diffuse gastric cancer. The super morbidly obese patient may make placing a PEG nearly impossible due to the thickness of the abdominal wall. Anterior wall inflammation or infection should be treated before the procedure. If there are no other options, ascites may be drained before the procedure to facilitate PEG tube placement.[44] PEG tubes may be placed in the presence of a ventriculoperitoneal shunt or a dialysis catheter. However, placement should be separated by 1 to 2 weeks or more to minimize the risk of catheter infection.[45] History of a previous or recent laparotomy is not a contraindication for PEG. However, one may consider a preprocedure CT scan to confirm there is a clear window for PEG placement. A discrete indentation of the stomach when palpating the anterior abdominal wall and adequate transillumination should be ensured.[46]

PEG is thought to be a safe procedure whether it is performed in the gastrointestinal laboratory, the OR, or at bedside in the ICU. However, because PEG tube placement is frequently performed in debilitated or critically ill patients, complications are associated with a higher mortality than would be expected for most elective procedures.[47] Free intraperitoneal air after PEG is common and can persist for 4 weeks.[48] Abdominal wall infection can occur as an early complication of PEG placement; an ample skin incision that prevents creation of a closed space around the feeding tube and administration of antibiotics before the procedure have been demonstrated to decrease PEG site infections.[49] Dislodgment of the PEG from the stomach can occur and may be life-threatening. Dislodgment may occur acutely through the application of traction on the gastrostomy tube, pulling it partially or completely through the abdominal wall. Alternatively, the tube may necrose through the stomach wall if the PEG flange or balloon applies too much pressure on the gastric wall. If this complication occurs before development of a fibrous tract during the initial 10 to 14 days, it should be considered a surgical emergency because gastric contents would spill into the abdominal cavity. Operative closure of the gastrostomy is required. To minimize the risk of this complication, methods that prevent inadvertent movement of the gastrostomy tube should be used and meticulously followed. These methods include ensuring adequate fixation of the tube to the external abdominal wall, recording of the position of the gastrostomy tube at the skin surface immediately after the procedure with routine verification, and application of binders or other devices that limit the inadvertent application of traction of the tube.

BRONCHOSCOPY

Fiberoptic bronchoscopy of surgical critical care patients is indicated for diagnostic and therapeutic indications. Therapeutic indications include insertion of an endotracheal tube, removal of foreign bodies inadvertently aspirated, removal of mucous plugs, reversal of atelectasis in mechanically ventilated patients, suctioning of thick tenacious secretions, and diagnosis of obstructive pneumonia.[50]

Diagnostic bronchoscopy is most commonly used for obtaining pulmonary specimens for diagnosis and management of pneumonia.[51] Quantitative cultures obtained via fiberoptic bronchoscopy have been shown to eliminate the diagnosis of pneumonia in nearly 50% of patients with clinical signs of pneumonia, to decrease inappropriate antibiotic use, and to improve mortality compared with nonquantitative techniques. Standardization of culture techniques should be undertaken.

The risk associated with diagnostic bronchoscopy is related more to the need for conscious sedation and the required medications if performed in a nonintubated patient. Medication use could possibly result in depressed mental status progressing to hypoventilation, airway vulnerability, and the risk of aspiration. The risks of the procedure itself are pneumothorax, hypoxia, airway hyperreactivity, pulmonary hemorrhage, loss of pulmonary reserve in patients on high ventilator settings, and systemic hypotension or hypertension.

SELECTED REFERENCES

Delaney A, Bagshaw SM, Nalos M. Percutaneous dilatational tracheostomy versus surgical tracheostomy in critically ill patients: a systematic review and meta-analysis. *Crit Care.* 2006;10:R55.

This metaanalysis of percutaneous dilatational tracheostomy (PDT) versus standard open surgical tracheostomy supports the benefits of PDT.

Dennis BM, Eckert MJ, Gunter OL, et al. Safety of bedside percutaneous tracheostomy in the critically ill: evaluation of more than 3,000 procedures. *J Am Coll Surg.* 2013;216:858–865.

This article, which is the largest review of the safety of bedside percutaneous dilatational tracheostomy, documents safety across body mass index distribution.

Diaz Jr JJ, Mejia V, Subhawong AP, et al. Protocol for bedside laparotomy in trauma and emergency general surgery: a low return to the operating room. *Am Surg.* 2005;71:986–991.

This primary article examines outcomes of bedside laparotomy with a protocol for indications and support.

Fagon JY. Diagnosis and treatment of ventilator-associated pneumonia: fiberoptic bronchoscopy with bronchoalveolar lavage is essential. *Semin Respir Crit Care Med.* 2006;27:34–44.

The indications, benefits, and performance of bronchoscopy for the diagnosis of pneumonia are reviewed.

Moore AF, Hargest R, Martin M, et al. Intra-abdominal hypertension and the abdominal compartment syndrome. *Br J Surg.* 2004;91:1102–1110.

This article provides a review of the pathophysiology and treatment of abdominal compartment syndrome.

Raimondi N, Vial MR, Calleja J, et al. Evidence-based guidelines for the use of tracheostomy in critically ill patients. *J Crit Care.* 2017;38:304–318.

This article provides a systematic review and evidence-based recommendations for the use of tracheostomy in critically ill patients including technique, timing, cost, and special populations.

Rumbak MJ, Newton M, Truncale T, et al. A prospective, randomized study comparing early percutaneous dilational tracheotomy to prolonged translaryngeal intubation (delayed tracheotomy) in critically ill medical patients. *Crit Care Med.* 2004;32:1689–1694.

This primary article examining the benefit of tracheostomy at 48 hours versus 14 days demonstrated a significant reduction in complications and mortality when tracheostomy is performed early.

Shapiro MB, Jenkins DH, Schwab CW, et al. Damage control: collective review. *J Trauma*. 2000;49:969–978.

This article is a collective review of the history, indications, and performance of damage control laparotomy.

Van Natta TL, Morris Jr JA, Eddy VA, et al. Elective bedside surgery in critically injured patients is safe and cost-effective. *Ann Surg*. 1998;227:618–624.

This article is the first report of the safety and effectiveness of bedside surgical procedures.

REFERENCES

1. Barba CA. The intensive care unit as an operating room. *Surg Clin North Am*. 2000;80:957–973, xi.
2. Bowen CP, Whitney LR, Truwit JD, et al. Comparison of safety and cost of percutaneous versus surgical tracheostomy. *Am Surg*. 2001;67:54–60.
3. Dennis BM, Eckert MJ, Gunter OL, et al. Safety of bedside percutaneous tracheostomy in the critically ill: evaluation of more than 3,000 procedures. *J Am Coll Surg*. 2013;216:858–865; discussion 865–857.
4. Diaz Jr JJ, Mauer A, May AK, et al. Bedside laparotomy for trauma: are there risks? *Surg Infect (Larchmt)*. 2004;5:15–20.
5. Diaz Jr JJ, Mejia V, Subhawong AP, et al. Protocol for bedside laparotomy in trauma and emergency general surgery: a low return to the operating room. *Am Surg*. 2005;71:986–991.
6. Freeman BD, Isabella K, Cobb JP, et al. A prospective, randomized study comparing percutaneous with surgical tracheostomy in critically ill patients. *Crit Care Med*. 2001;29:926–930.
7. Porter JM, Ivatury RR, Kavarana M, et al. The surgical intensive care unit as a cost-efficient substitute for an operating room at a level I trauma center. *Am Surg*. 1999;65:328–330.
8. Porter JM, Ivatury RR. Preferred route of tracheostomy—percutaneous versus open at the bedside: a randomized, prospective study in the surgical intensive care unit. *Am Surg*. 1999;65:142–146.
9. Van Natta TL, Morris Jr JA, Eddy VA, et al. Elective bedside surgery in critically injured patients is safe and cost-effective. *Ann Surg*. 1998;227:618–624; discussion 624–616.
10. Pronovost PJ, Thompson DA. Reducing defects in the use of interventions. *Intensive Care Med*. 2004;30:1505–1507.
11. Szem JW, Hydo LJ, Fischer E, et al. High-risk intrahospital transport of critically ill patients: safety and outcome of the necessary "road trip". *Crit Care Med*. 1995;23:1660–1666.
12. Warren J, Fromm Jr RE, Orr RA, et al. Guidelines for the inter- and intrahospital transport of critically ill patients. *Crit Care Med*. 2004;32:256–262.
13. Haynes AB, Weiser TG, Berry WR, et al. A surgical safety checklist to reduce morbidity and mortality in a global population. *N Engl J Med*. 2009;360:491–499.
14. Haugen AS, Softeland E, Almeland SK, et al. Effect of the World Health Organization checklist on patient outcomes: a stepped wedge cluster randomized controlled trial. *Ann Surg*. 2015;261:821–828.
15. Miller RS, Morris Jr JA, Diaz Jr JJ, et al. Complications after 344 damage-control open celiotomies. *J Trauma*. 2005;59:1365–1371; discussion 1371–1364.
16. Kirkpatrick AW, Balogh Z, Ball CG, et al. The secondary abdominal compartment syndrome: iatrogenic or unavoidable? *J Am Coll Surg*. 2006;202:668–679.
17. Leppaniemi A, Kemppainen E. Recent advances in the surgical management of necrotizing pancreatitis. *Curr Opin Crit Care*. 2005;11:349–352.
18. Moore AF, Hargest R, Martin M, et al. Intra-abdominal hypertension and the abdominal compartment syndrome. *Br J Surg*. 2004;91:1102–1110.
19. Sugrue M. Abdominal compartment syndrome. *Curr Opin Crit Care*. 2005;11:333–338.
20. Shapiro MB, Jenkins DH, Schwab CW, et al. Damage control: collective review. *J Trauma*. 2000;49:969–978.
21. Schreiber J, Nierhaus A, Vettorazzi E, et al. Rescue bedside laparotomy in the intensive care unit in patients too unstable for transport to the operating room. *Crit Care*. 2014;18:R123.
22. Martin ND, Patel SP, Chreiman K, et al. Emergency laparotomy in the critically ill: futility at the bedside. *Crit Care Res Pract*. 2018;2018:6398917.
23. Cools-Lartigue J, Aboalsaud A, Gill H, et al. Evolution of percutaneous dilatational tracheostomy—a review of current techniques and their pitfalls. *World J Surg*. 2013;37:1633–1646.
24. Delaney A, Bagshaw SM, Nalos M. Percutaneous dilatational tracheostomy versus surgical tracheostomy in critically ill patients: a systematic review and meta-analysis. *Crit Care*. 2006;10:R55.
25. Heikkinen M, Aarnio P, Hannukainen J. Percutaneous dilational tracheostomy or conventional surgical tracheostomy? *Crit Care Med*. 2000;28:1399–1402.
26. Raimondi N, Vial MR, Calleja J, et al. Evidence-based guidelines for the use of tracheostomy in critically ill patients. *J Crit Care*. 2017;38:304–318.
27. Ciaglia P, Firsching R, Syniec C. Elective percutaneous dilatational tracheostomy. A new simple bedside procedure; preliminary report. *Chest*. 1985;87:715–719.
28. Bacchetta MD, Girardi LN, Southard EJ, et al. Comparison of open versus bedside percutaneous dilatational tracheostomy in the cardiothoracic surgical patient: outcomes and financial analysis. *Ann Thorac Surg*. 2005;79:1879–1885.
29. Terragni PP, Antonelli M, Fumagalli R, et al. Early vs late tracheotomy for prevention of pneumonia in mechanically ventilated adult ICU patients: a randomized controlled trial. *JAMA*. 2010;303:1483–1489.
30. Young D, Harrison DA, Cuthbertson BH, et al. Effect of early vs late tracheostomy placement on survival in patients receiving mechanical ventilation: the TracMan randomized trial. *JAMA*. 2013;309:2121–2129.
31. Trouillet JL, Luyt CE, Guiguet M, et al. Early percutaneous tracheotomy versus prolonged intubation of mechanically ventilated patients after cardiac surgery: a randomized trial. *Ann Intern Med*. 2011;154:373–383.
32. Diaz-Prieto A, Mateu A, Gorriz M, et al. A randomized clinical trial for the timing of tracheotomy in critically ill patients: factors precluding inclusion in a single center study. *Crit Care*. 2014;18:585.

33. Arabi Y, Haddad S, Shirawi N, et al. Early tracheostomy in intensive care trauma patients improves resource utilization: a cohort study and literature review. *Crit Care.* 2004;8:R347–352.
34. Rumbak MJ, Newton M, Truncale T, et al. A prospective, randomized, study comparing early percutaneous dilational tracheotomy to prolonged translaryngeal intubation (delayed tracheotomy) in critically ill medical patients. *Crit Care Med.* 2004;32:1689–1694.
35. Garrubba M, Turner T, Grieveson C. Multidisciplinary care for tracheostomy patients: a systematic review. *Crit Care.* 2009;13:R177.
36. Paran H, Butnaru G, Hass I, et al. Evaluation of a modified percutaneous tracheostomy technique without bronchoscopic guidance. *Chest.* 2004;126:868–871.
37. Saritas A, Kurnaz MM. Comparison of bronchoscopy-guided and real-time ultrasound-guided percutaneous dilatational tracheostomy: safety, complications, and effectiveness in critically ill patients. *J Intensive Care Med.* 2017; 885066617705641.
38. Song JQ, Xuan LZ, Wu W, et al. Comparison of percutaneous dilatational tracheostomy guided by ultrasound and bronchoscopy in critically ill obese patients. *J Ultrasound Med.* 2018;37:1061–1069.
39. Norwood S, Vallina VL, Short K, et al. Incidence of tracheal stenosis and other late complications after percutaneous tracheostomy. *Ann Surg.* 2000;232:233–241.
40. Walz MK, Peitgen K, Thurauf N, et al. Percutaneous dilatational tracheostomy—early results and long-term outcome of 326 critically ill patients. *Intensive Care Med.* 1998;24:685–690.
41. Gauderer MW, Ponsky JL, Izant Jr RJ. Gastrostomy without laparotomy: a percutaneous endoscopic technique. *J Pediatr Surg.* 1980;15:872–875.
42. Adams GF, Guest DP, Ciraulo DL, et al. Maximizing tolerance of enteral nutrition in severely injured trauma patients: a comparison of enteral feedings by means of percutaneous endoscopic gastrostomy versus percutaneous endoscopic gastrojejunostomy. *J Trauma.* 2000;48:459–464; discussion 464–455.
43. Stein J, Schulte-Bockholt A, Sabin M, et al. A randomized prospective trial of immediate vs. next-day feeding after percutaneous endoscopic gastrostomy in intensive care patients. *Intensive Care Med.* 2002;28:1656–1660.
44. Wejda BU, Deppe H, Huchzermeyer H, et al. PEG placement in patients with ascites: a new approach. *Gastrointest Endosc.* 2005;61:178–180.
45. Schulman AS, Sawyer RG. The safety of percutaneous endoscopic gastrostomy tube placement in patients with existing ventriculoperitoneal shunts. *JPEN J Parenter Enteral Nutr.* 2005;29:442–444.
46. Eleftheriadis E, Kotzampassi K. Percutaneous endoscopic gastrostomy after abdominal surgery. *Surg Endosc.* 2001;15:213–216.
47. Lockett MA, Templeton ML, Byrne TK, et al. Percutaneous endoscopic gastrostomy complications in a tertiary-care center. *Am Surg.* 2002;68:117–120.
48. Dulabon GR, Abrams JE, Rutherford EJ. The incidence and significance of free air after percutaneous endoscopic gastrostomy. *Am Surg.* 2002;68:590–593.
49. Sharma VK, Howden CW. Meta-analysis of randomized, controlled trials of antibiotic prophylaxis before percutaneous endoscopic gastrostomy. *Am J Gastroenterol.* 2000;95:3133–3136.
50. Labbe A, Meyer F, Albertini M. Bronchoscopy in intensive care units. *Paediatr Respir Rev.* 2004;(5 suppl A):S1–S19.
51. Fagon JY. Diagnosis and treatment of ventilator-associated pneumonia: fiberoptic bronchoscopy with bronchoalveolar lavage is essential. *Semin Respir Crit Care Med.* 2006;27:34–44.

CHAPTER 24

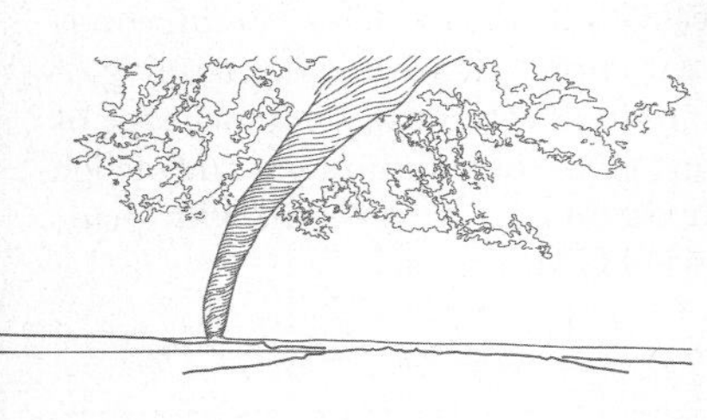

The Surgeon's Role in Mass Casualty Incidents

Jennifer M. Gurney, Matthew J. Martin

OUTLINE

"Those who are dangerously wounded should receive the first attention, without regard to rank or distinction. They who are injured in a less degree may wait until their brethren in arms, who are badly mutilated, have been operated on and dressed, otherwise the latter would not survive many hours; rarely, until the succeeding day."

Dr. Baron Larrey, Memoirs of Military Surgery, 1812

Mass casualty (MASCAL) incidents or events are characterized by a large number of people becoming injured or ill in a specific event or series of related events. These events can include intentional or terrorist-type attacks (mass shooting, bombing), nonintentional events (industrial accident, building fire), and natural disasters (hurricane, earthquake). MASCAL events are relatively uncommon outside of the military or battlefield setting but are an ever-present risk that every medical provider and medical system must be prepared for. There has been a particular focus on education and preparation for these events over the past decade, likely due to the increased numbers of events related to terrorist groups, civilian bombings such as the 2013 Boston Marathon event, and the continuing series of mass shootings at schools and other public venues.[1,2]

One of the hallmarks of almost all MASCAL events is the presence of major traumatic injuries that require rapid triage, evaluation, and surgical or other procedural interventions. In this respect, the surgeon has a critical and obvious role in nearly every aspect of MASCAL management, from preparation and training to the execution and recovery phases. Although the role of the surgeon in providing clinical care and emergent/urgent surgery during a MASCAL event is obvious, it is critical that surgeons be actively involved in all of the key nonclinical aspects of MASCAL care, particularly in the local and regional MASCAL planning and preparation activities. In many systems these tasks have been assigned to nonsurgeons and even to nonclinicians, with a common result being an unrealistic MASCAL plan and a resultant suboptimal clinical response to the actual event.

Another frequently underappreciated and misunderstood concept in MASCAL care is the critical role and importance of triage. Among the earliest changes in the way that patients are managed during a MASCAL event is the "sifting and sorting" into categories and their priorities for receiving emergent/urgent care.[3] Although the injury severity and urgency of injured patients will vary somewhat between events, the majority of patients presenting for care will not have major or life-threatening injuries (Fig. 24.1). In addition, these minimally injured patients will tend to arrive before the more severely injured cohorts, rather than the most severely injured arriving first. We believe that appropriate high-quality triage is the most critical physician-driven aspect of MASCAL management and that all surgeons should be familiar with the principles and practices of triage in these scenarios. Appropriate and effective triage will set the stage for the success or failure of any MASCAL response by optimizing the match between the injuries and injury severity of the presenting patients and the available critical resources of the facility or system that will be providing care.[4,5]

HISTORY

The term "triage" was coined by Napoleon's surgeon, Dr. Baron Larrey. Dr. Larrey poignantly describes the importance of addressing the most seriously injured patients first. The military's earliest documented systems of triage date back to the eighteenth century, and triage is a principal component of battlefield care. MASCAL events are becoming increasingly common, and there are many lessons that can be learned from both the military and civilian

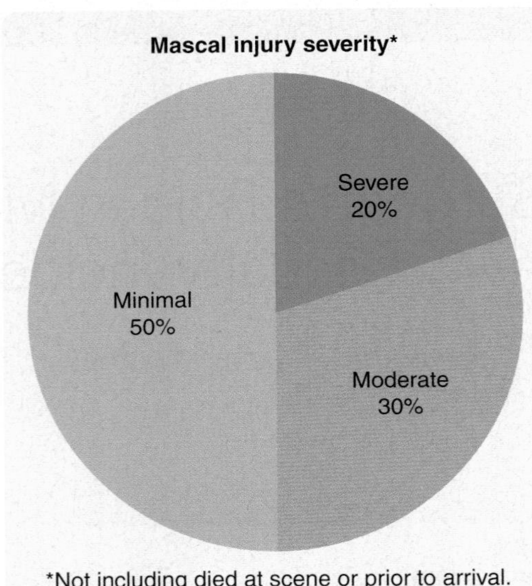

FIG. 24.1 Typical injury severity breakdown for an average mass casualty event. Note that only 20% of patients will have severe or immediately life-threatening injuries, and 50% or more will have minor or minimal injuries.

systems in terms of triage and trauma systems in order to optimize care and outcomes for as many casualties as possible.

Triage is a term with its roots in military trauma, and the practice of triage arose from the demands of large amounts of battlefield casualties during war; the original triage concepts were primarily focused on MASCAL situations during battlefield trauma. Dr. Larrey was known for his surgical leadership and skill and is credited with the development of the concept of "sorting" patients to salvage the greatest number of casualties in a resource scarce battlefield environment. Dr. Larrey's principals of sorting also included evacuating patients according to the severity of wounding and prioritizing their care based on both the severity of the injury and the likelihood of survival.

With each subsequent war since Napoleon's time, the U.S. military and civilian medical communities have continued to advance the concepts of triage and MASCAL management. Simultaneously, developments in order to provide lifesaving care and procedures closer to the point of injury have evolved. Triage occurs along a continuum of tiered care in the military system with higher echelons of care having increasing capabilities. On the battlefield, appropriate triage of patients directs the patients to an appropriate level of care and helps manage a chaotic situation where large numbers of casualties receive appropriate and effective care. The tiered triage system used by the military has evolved and is still used in current wars with tiered levels of care from point of injury to advance care and rehabilitation in the United States. Other principals of current military triage, point of injury care, en route care, and the movement of advanced capabilities closer to the place and time of wounding have saved the lives of military patients and have the potential to do the same in civilian MASCAL situations.[3,6]

As the world becomes increasingly tumultuous with the higher frequency of MASCAL events, shootings, and natural disasters, the potential for surgeons to be involved in MASCAL situations is increasing. Surgeon leadership, hospital planning, and community preparation are the first steps to the successful management of these dreadful events. Surgeon involvement in every tier of MASCAL management is ideal. While the modern-day surgeon is rarely a prehospital provider, the comprehensive understanding of the system of trauma care, combined with intricate knowledge of the physiologic effects of injury, gives surgeons unique knowledge for oversight, leadership, and training to be involved with planning, leadership training for MASCAL events.[7]

KEY DEFINITIONS

In the normal, nonmass casualty trauma system functions, triage most frequently applies to the sorting of trauma or critically ill patients in order to direct them to the medical treatment facility with the appropriate level of capability. Accurate triage results in distributing patients to appropriate hospitals that can expertly manage their condition, whether it is traumatic injury, myocardial infarction, stroke, or sepsis. In terms of trauma, the standard civilian use of trauma triage refers to the day-to-day function of sending patients to the appropriate hospital/trauma center in order to avoid over- and undertriage. Basic triage (outside of MASCAL incidents) optimizes care delivery and resource allocation, and it is not the focus of this chapter. The chapter focuses on the surgeons' role in MASCAL incidents, the trauma system, and triage. Optimizing triage in the face of multiple casualties and potentially limited resources requires leadership, planning, and an established trauma system.[8,9] Surgeon leadership in triage process and the trauma system helps establish a well-organized response to MASCAL incidents; surgeon involvement in the triage planning and process should occur at every level in a healthcare system: individual, local, regional, and national.

Triage is the process of sorting patients to provide the greatest amount of good for the highest number of patients. Triage is an essential component of any trauma system and is pivotal for optimizing survival in multiple casualty incidents (MCIs). Triage can occur in the absence of a MASCAL—but MASCALs always require triage. Success or failure is measured in lives saved or lives lost and resources wasted or appropriately utilized; success or failure depends on accurate and effective triage.[4]

- **Field triage**

  Done at or near the scene of the event. The process by which emergency medical service (EMS) providers decide which hospital to send patients injured by a disaster or traumatic event.
- **Undertriage**

  Occurs when seriously injured patients are transported to nontrauma centers or centers that do not have the expertise or capability to manage the severity of the injury.
- **Overtriage**

  Occurs when patients with minor or nonurgent injuries are transported to major trauma centers or triaged to an immediate care bed. In a MASCAL situation, this bogs down the system, results in significant bottlenecking, and can result in increased rates of adverse outcomes (Fig. 24.2).

- The goal of field triage is to efficiently concentrate injured patients to major trauma centers without overwhelming these centers with patients who have minor injuries.
- The national benchmarks for field trauma triage are set by the American College of Surgeons Committee on Trauma and are based on system level rates of undertriage and overtriage.

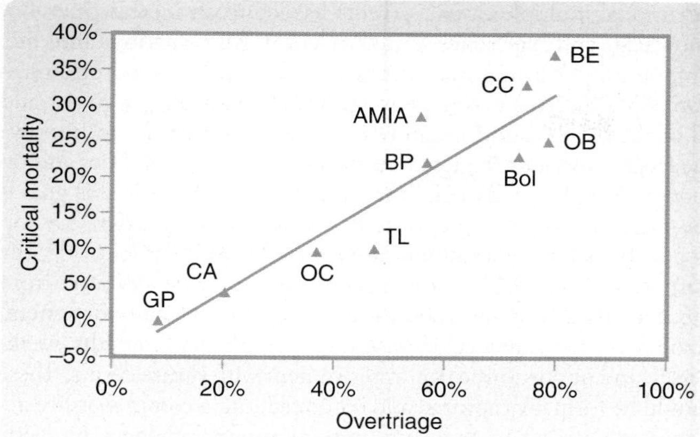

FIG. 24.2 Graphic relation of overtriage rate to critical mortality rate, in ten terrorist bombing incidents from 1969 to 1995, demonstrating linear increase in mortality with higher overtriage rates. Linear correlation coefficient (*r*) 0.92. (From Frykberg ER. Medical management of disasters and mass casualties from terrorist bombings: how can we cope? *J Trauma*. 2002;53:201–212.) *AMIA*, Buenos Aires; *BE*, Beirut; *Bol*, Bologna; *BP*, Birmingham pubs; *CA*, Craigavon; *CC*, Cu Chi; *GP*, Guildford pubs; *OB*, Od Bailey; *OC*, Oklahoma City; *TL*, Tower of London.

- **Hospital triage**

  Sorting patients into predefined categories in order to determine their relative priority of treatment. Patients are separated into groups based on the local triage system that is used. Patients are sorted into categories: those not expected to survive even with treatment; those who will recover with minimal treatment; and the highest priority group, those who will not survive without treatment.
- **Standard trauma incident**

  Typically involves one or several patients and there are an excess of available resources and expertise to manage these patients. These are the most common trauma incidents that occur in rural and urban trauma centers.
- **MCI**

  Multiple injured patients present simultaneously, but adequate resources are present and the system is not significantly stressed. An MCI for a large trauma center could be routine, but an MCI may result in a MASCAL scenario for a small hospital.
- **MASCAL incident**

  When the number of injured patients or the resources required to care for the patients exceed what is available and put a significant stress on the trauma system, hospital, and providers.
- **Disaster incident**

  Large-scale natural or manmade MASCAL event that often results in overwhelming numbers of patients injured or ill, as well as frequent destruction or degradation of local infrastructure, which may include the healthcare facilities.

There is a critical distinction between an MCI and a true MASCAL event that must be understood and appreciated by the surgeon.[10] While an MCI requires little to no change to the usual practices and the standard of care, a true MASCAL requires major alterations from the usual patient care protocols at that facility and a focus on optimizing group outcomes versus individual patient outcomes. The primary factor that distinguishes these two categories is the relationship between the presenting injuries and the available resources and expertise to care for them, and not purely the number of patients. This is commonly referred to as the surge capacity for a given facility or system. As shown in

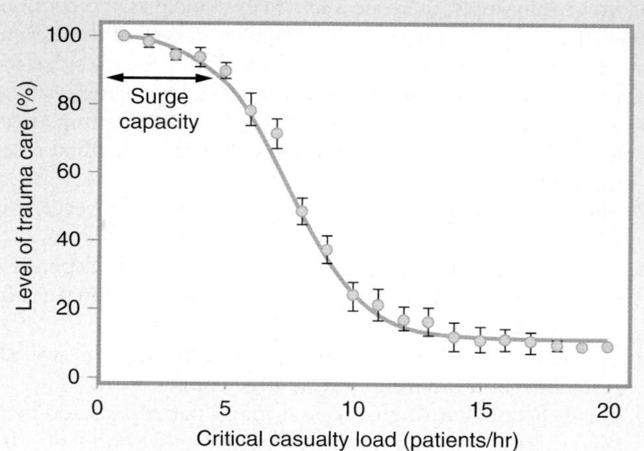

FIG. 24.3 Graphic depiction of the results of a computer simulation of the flow of casualties of an urban bombing through the trauma service line of an urban trauma center and the impact on the global level of care. The level of care for a single patient on a normal working day is defined as 100%. The *upper flat portion* of the curve corresponds to an MCI, the *steep portion* represents a mass casualty situation, and the *lower flat portion* represents a major medical disaster. The surge capacity of the hospital trauma service line is the maximal critical casualty load that can be managed without a precipitous drop in the level of care. (From Hirshberg A, Scott BG, Granchi T, et al. How does casualty load affect trauma care in urban bombing incidents? A quantitative analysis. *J Trauma*. 2005;58:686–693.)

Fig. 24.3, the standard level of care can be maintained for a finite number of patients, but once this number is exceeded, there is a precipitous decline in the level of care and associated outcomes. A well-resourced Level 1 trauma center may be easily able to handle 20 severely injured patients from one incident, whereas a smaller rural nontrauma center may be overwhelmed with more than two to three severely injured patients.

We have found that many of the events described as MASCALs are actually MCIs and should be labeled accordingly. A true MASCAL event rapidly exceeds the facility surge capacity and has the potential to quickly overwhelm an individual facility or the entire local/regional trauma system and evacuation processes. MASCAL events due to a local manmade or natural disaster (earthquake, flood, etc.) have the potential to result in the greatest number of injured and/or ill patients that can quickly overwhelm the local/regional facilities.[11] In addition, these events can be particularly devastating when they are coupled with severe damage or destruction of critical local infrastructure, utilities, or even major damage to the healthcare facility itself.[12,13] Surgeon involvement in every level of training, education, and system refinement will help ensure a successful system when it is stressed with multiple casualties. The triage process is pivotal to the successful execution of any MASCAL plan, and surgeons must have both expertise in triage and be involved in system, regional, and hospital triage planning.

MASCAL KEY PRINCIPLES

Multiple casualty and MASCAL events can occur via a wide variety of mechanisms or causes and will be highly heterogeneous in terms of the number and severity of presenting patients, the need for resources and specialty care, and the ultimate impact on the local healthcare facilities and system. Although it is impossible to develop a single inclusive protocol or set of detailed guidelines that will universally apply, there are a set of key principles and commonalities that have been observed across a wide variety of these events. The following is a list of the "top 10" MASCAL principles that have been reported across a broad range of events and experiences:

1. Triage is a dynamic process and should be happening at each level of care from the point of injury/scene to the final receiving hospital or other facility.
2. The MASCAL goal: do the best for the most, not everything for everyone.
3. Success of failure during an MCI or MASCAL depends on accurate and effective triage. The success of regional trauma systems depends on good Field Triage.
4. Triage starts with understanding and assessing the available system capabilities, resources, and personnel.
5. For in-hospital or single hospital triage, patients should be triaged through one entry point and with one-way only flow into the facility.
6. There must be redundancy of capability, not duplication of action, to avoid inefficiencies in an already stressed system.
7. Prearranged electronic or paper MASCAL chart and patient admission packets should be prepared and ready at the facility triage intake point.
8. There are multiple well-validated triage systems. Select and train with the optimal one for your system, and ensure all personnel know the system (DIME, START, SALT, etc.).
9. The triage officer should be one of the most experienced and organized personnel and should ideally have a deputy to facilitate communications and recording.
10. Scene security and safety is necessary for safe and effective care. Ensure scene safety prior to rushing into an unsecure scene; do not become a victim and put more stress on the system.

As emphasized in the list above, MASCAL preparation and effective triage are among the most important aspects associated with success and optimization of both patient and system outcomes. Although the first step of triage is often assumed to be the sorting of arriving patients into categories or a prioritized order for evaluation and interventions, this requires a clear understanding of the capabilities, capacity, and available resources before effective triage can be started. Thus, the first step of any experienced triage officer is to perform what we have termed the "zero survey."[3] This entails rapidly, assessing the current status and availability of critical resources at that facility and simultaneously activating the local MASCAL plan and the notification system for all hospital personnel. Although the natural focus in these scenarios tends to be on the emergency room (ER) bed status, it is important to also assess and optimize the availability of beds and staff in the operating room (OR), intensive care units (ICUs), and hospital wards. Key ancillary services including the blood bank, pharmacy, radiology, and laboratory must be notified to cease any nonurgent activities and prepare for the expected large influx of patients requiring their services. Two particularly critical nonclinical areas that also must be activated and in place prior to patient arrival (when possible) are patient administration (PAD) and security. Getting the incoming patients identified, registered, and entered into the hospital's medical records system is a frequently overlooked issue that can create chaos and danger due to misidentification and medication or blood administration errors.[2,14]

CRITICAL MASCAL LESSONS LEARNED

The past decade-plus of sustained combat operations by the U.S. military and the increased frequency of civilian terrorist and other intentional multiple casualty events has led to an increased level of knowledge and experience related to MASCAL operations and care. Among the most important principles for readiness and optimization of MASCAL outcomes is to optimize the learning from any and all of these events and to apply these "lessons learned" to improve the facility and local/regional healthcare system's capabilities and response. A widely accepted "best practice" for achieving this goal is the performance of in-depth after-action reviews (AARs) as soon as possible after any multiple casualty or MASCAL event.[15,16] The purpose of these AARs, which should be held at every level from the individual hospital section/unit to the entire facility or system, is to review the sequence of events and identify key strengths, weaknesses, and opportunities for improvement with future events. These should be formally captured and compiled into a comprehensive action plan with adequate follow-up to ensure that changes are made and that the MASCAL plan is continually adjusted based on this feedback. Similar to the key principles listed previously, there have been a number of key common MASCAL "lessons learned" that have been reported across a wide variety of disparate events. Among the most important and widely applicable of these are the following:

1. No one is safe! MASCAL events can occur anywhere at any time and are likely to increase in frequency…be prepared.
2. Know your assets and capabilities at every level of care: prehospital, evacuation/transport, individual hospitals, and the system of care when there are multiple roles of care in the affected area.
3. Leadership and a chain of command are important especially when allocating trauma system and evacuation resources; reread #2.
4. Appropriate scene triage and point-of-injury care can turn a potential MASCAL into a more orderly MCI.
5. The most important job is that of the senior triage officer, who should be an experienced and trusted provider who is able to work well with others.
6. Scene control and scene safety are crucial. An organized security plan must be part of any MASCAL plan in order to prevent additional casualties, protect personnel, and limit entry points. MASCAL events create vulnerable situations, and secondary injury must be avoided. Hospitals are easy targets during MCIs or MASCALs. A good security plan is imperative.
7. Execution of a good MASCAL plan requires good patient flow and throughput with minimal congestion at the bottlenecks (ED, radiology). Establishment of one-way flow through the ED facilitates patients' evaluation and disposition expeditiously to avoid congestion in the ED.
8. In true MASCAL events that exceed the capacity of the ED, establish a separate area for the minimally injured and the "walking wounded" that is outside of the ED and triage area. In hospitals, outpatient clinics are ideal for this and they should be staffed by providers who can examine and retriage patients if necessary.
9. Hemorrhage control, airway, and breathing issues are the initial priority for most MASCAL situations. Hemorrhage control can and should occur along the continuum of care.
10. Blood products are often a scarce resource in the initial phases of a MASCAL event. Have a plan to never run out of blood. Blood should be pushed far forward to triage sites if there is the potential for long transport times or extrications.

The initial triage and patient management/disposition schemes will set the precedent and the tone for the subsequent phases of any MASCAL event, starting with the prehospital/scene phase and continuing to the in-hospital phase. Triage at the scene is typically managed by the scene commander or their designated triage officer and should focus on the initial sorting into triage categories, performing needed immediate lifesaving interventions and then prioritizing and directing transport to the appropriate hospital facility. Tight control of this process at the scene and then appropriate and balanced distribution of patients from the scene to the available local facilities can convert what is a MASCAL event at the point of injury into multiple MCI events at the hospital level. The 2013 Boston Marathon bombing provides a ready example in which excellent scene care and triage were able to evenly distribute the seriously injured patients to multiple local hospitals rather than overwhelming the single closest center.[17,18]

Triage at the hospital level is arguably the most important of the key clinical leadership roles during the initial phases of any true MASCAL event. Historically, the importance of the role of the senior triage officer has been underappreciated and often assigned to the "least clinically useful" person on the medical team.[19] This approach has now been widely recognized to be inappropriate and potentially disastrous, and the triage officer should be someone who is selected carefully for their advanced expertise in trauma management, leadership skills, and ability to communicate effectively. In our experience, this is usually best performed by an experienced trauma surgeon or emergency medicine provider. In scenarios in which there is a need to establish both an external (primary) and internal (secondary) triage area for the facility, then the senior triage office and assistant or secondary triage officer must work in a highly coordinated and consistent fashion.

MASCAL MANAGEMENT AND THE SURGEON'S ROLE IN TRIAGE

Although there are numerous methods and reported systems for MASCAL management, no one approach has proven clearly superior or universally applicable. What has been clearly demonstrated is that complex and confusing systems that are not understood and well rehearsed by the frontline clinicians are doomed to failure. Arguably more important than which particular system is selected are the principles of simplicity, familiarity, and effective and realistic rehearsal drills as part of a comprehensive MASCAL/Disaster preparation program.[3,10] We propose the use of the mnemonic TRIAGE (Box 24.1) as a memory aid and guide to the core principles of MASCAL management and the role of the surgeon in the preparation for and execution of these events.

Training

"Training is everything…"

Mark Twain

Training for MASCAL events requires surgeon involvement at the local and regional levels. Effective leadership and training are foundational for a successful response to an MCI or MASCAL event; while surgeons are not involved with point-of-injury care or rarely with field triage, surgeon involvement with the planning and training is extremely important. Any trauma system, even the most established, can be burdened by large volumes of patients. Successful triage requires significant training and sorting and prioritizing of casualties according to their injuries while considering for the tactical situation and resources available; it is a skill that, in addition to training, requires education and leadership.

For both field and in-hospital triage, the choice of the triage officer should be determined as part of a MASCAL plan and the triage officer should be one of the most experienced and organized personnel; for in-hospital triage, the triage officer is frequently an experienced surgeon; and for field triage, either an ED physician or an experienced prehospital provider. It is essential that the triage officer be able to quickly recognize life-threatening injuries. The experience and expertise of the triage officer are crucial; the triage officer must be able to rapidly identify life-threatening injuries and injury patterns and place the patients in the correct triage category. The decision for who is going to be the triage officer should not be made at the time of the MASCAL event. Each hospital and field triage system should have redundancy in the personnel who can serve as the triage officer.

The triage officer must also have been informed and understand the tactical situation in order to appropriately manage resources and meet the goal of doing the best for the most, not everything for everyone. Awareness of the event, the situation, estimated number of casualties, risk for secondary event, effectiveness of field triage, etc., is important information to give the hospital triage officer perspective to facilitate optimization of resources. The triage officer should be one of the most experienced and organized personnel and should ideally have a deputy to facilitate communications and recording. While most triage officers are surgeons, experienced providers in emergency medicine can be excellent triage officers. MASCAL plans in the hospital should be trained and rehearsed. More than one potential triage officer should be identified and train for that role to provide redundancy in the available expertise and also to prepare for scenarios in which the primary triage officer is injured/ill, otherwise engaged, or in which multiple triage points need to be established.

The location for the triage point(s) should be predetermined and clearly spelled out in the written MASCAL plan and any rehearsal drills. One of the most common errors that we have observed in hospital MASCAL planning is the development of only one triage plan and location, which fails to appreciate the highly variable nature of these events.[7,20] We recommend the development of at least two flexible triage schemas that allow for the different triage requirements that will be seen in smaller-scale MASCAL events versus larger-scale or disaster-type events. In general, smaller-scale MASCAL events (relative to the available ED and hospital bed space) where all patients can be immediately brought inside the facility require only one primary triage point that is usually optimal to locate near the ED entrance. Larger-scale events that exceed the available bed space or providers necessitate the establishment of an external primary triage site where patients are categorized, prioritized, and held until they can be moved into the facility (Fig. 24.4).[21,22] Secondary triage would then occur as patients are filtered into the facility and then directed to the appropriate location based on their needed level of care. The external triage location should have climate control, be well lit, and have prestocked supplies for immediate patient needs including hemorrhage control and airway/breathing interventions. All patients who arrive at the facility must be triaged and ideally enter the

BOX 24.1 Simple mnemonic for TRIAGE.

T Training (in-hospital response/local)
R Readiness (regional/field triage readiness)
I Integration of Systems
A Adaptable
G Grow (remember system lessons learned)
E Exsanguination Control (along the continuum)

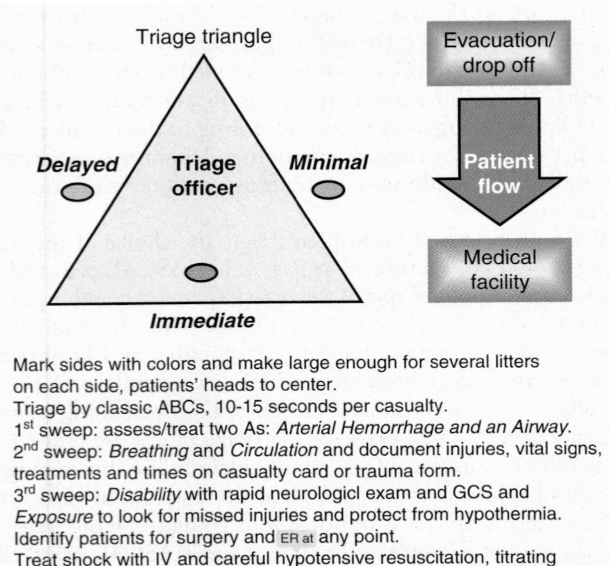

FIG. 24.4 The "Triage Triangle" arrangement for setting up an external triage point during a large mass casualty event. This allows the triage officer or team to be centrally located and to categorize and group patients as immediate, delayed, or minimal. (From Martin MJ, Beekley A, Eckert MJ. *Front Line Surgery: A Practical Approach*. 2nd ed. New York: Springer Science+Business Media; 2017.)

hospital through one tightly controlled entry point, with all other facility entrances protected by assigned security personnel.

Accompanying the triage officer during hospital triage should be a PAD officer, a nurse coordinator who acts as a "bed manager," and a nurse or medic equipped with basic bleeding control supplies. The triage team organized in this fashion can sort, communicate, track, and treat casualties. As patients get sorted/prioritized by the triage officer, the PAD officer can tag the patient, keep accountability, and communicate the disposition to the centralized PAD center. The nurse coordinator is essential to help relay the plan for disposition of the patient and communicate this plan to the patient care areas in the hospital. If patients need to go straight to the OR for emergent surgery or into the ED for an urgent airway, the nurse coordinator can help communicate and facilitate the triage officer's plans. Lastly, having a clinically experienced nurse, medic, or EMT on the triage team allows for immediate treatment of hemorrhage with tourniquet placement, wound packing, or the use of hemostatic adjuncts.[23–25] Bringing a hemorrhage control capability to the triage team also helps patients move into lower-acuity triage categories; e.g., an immediate patient with a traumatic amputation can get triaged to a delayed category with tourniquet hemorrhage control. If advanced warning is received, these personnel and resources should be prepositioned in accordance with the (well-rehearsed) MASCAL plan. Triage starts with understanding the system capabilities, resources, and personnel; resource utilization and appropriation are the keys to effective triage. The plan, patient flow, and ancillary services (blood bank, pharmacy, PAD, incident command system, patient movement) all must be included in the training.

While there are many triage categorization schemes, each hospital and trauma system should choose one, keep it simple, and train with it regularly.[8,20,26] Training requires a significant time, energy, and resource investment; perfunctory training without stressing the weak areas in the process or involving the entire system will only lead to potential failures should the system be stressed with a MASCAL event. Surgeon leadership is necessary for MASCAL training; there is a tendency for triage and MASCAL training to involve prehospital providers and the initial hospital response, but the training does not get brought into the hospital beyond the ED phase of care. Not involving the ORs and the ICUs in the MASCAL training makes it less realistic and can portend a false sense of success when patients get rapidly moved out of the ED to go to the ORs without planning and training the times that it takes for multiple operations to occur.[7,27] While the details and nuances may be second nature to the triage officer, weak areas in the system will be amplified in the event of a MASCAL event. Realistic and typically resource-intensive training with surgeon involvement at all levels will improve the triage and initial response to a MASCAL situation.

Triage Systems

There are a number of useful and well-validated triage systems that are currently utilized for guiding the initial evaluation and then categorization of patients during a MASCAL event. However, many of these are primarily used and validated for initial evaluation and triage sorting at the point of injury or the scene triage point and may be less useful for performing triage at the hospital level. These typically combine a rapid assessment of clinical factors (mental status, ambulating, vital signs) and obvious injuries followed by categorization that prioritizes that patient for immediate interventions and for rapid transport to a trauma center. Several of the more commonly utilized include the following: Sort, assess, lifesaving interventions, and treatment/transport (SALT), Simple Treatment and Rapid Transport (START), JumpSTART (pediatric version of START), Care Flight Triage, the Sacco Triage Method, and Secondary Assessment of Victim Endpoint (SAVE).[9,20,26] Fig. 24.5 shows an example of the SALT triage system, which has been endorsed by the American College of Surgeons (ACS) and other professional organizations.[26] Although there are strengths and weaknesses with each system, they can all be highly effective when used properly by a trained triage officer.

At the hospital level, similar rapid triage and categorization are again performed either as the patient is entering the facility or at an established external triage point. The above-mentioned prehospital triage systems are generally less useful at this level, where the primary focus now is to identify patients who require immediate intervention or surgery, those who require additional detailed workup, and those with negligible injuries who do not require urgent care or evaluation.[28] In lower-volume MASCAL events at robust centers, the arriving patients can generally be triaged into only two categories: (1) the highest-acuity ED beds for patients with major or urgent injuries and (2) lower-acuity areas of the ED for less urgent or minimal injuries. However, in higher-volume events or at less robust facilities where the patient volume clearly outweighs the available ED staff and bed space, more traditional triage into multiple categories or priorities should be performed. In these instances, we recommend use of the North Atlantic Treaty Organization (NATO) triage categorization system based on the mnemonic DIME (also used by the SALT system shown in Fig. 24.5).[29] This groups patients into categories of delayed, immediate, minimal, and expectant, as shown in Fig. 24.6.[30] In addition to these categories, it is also important to have a clear plan and identified location for those patients who are

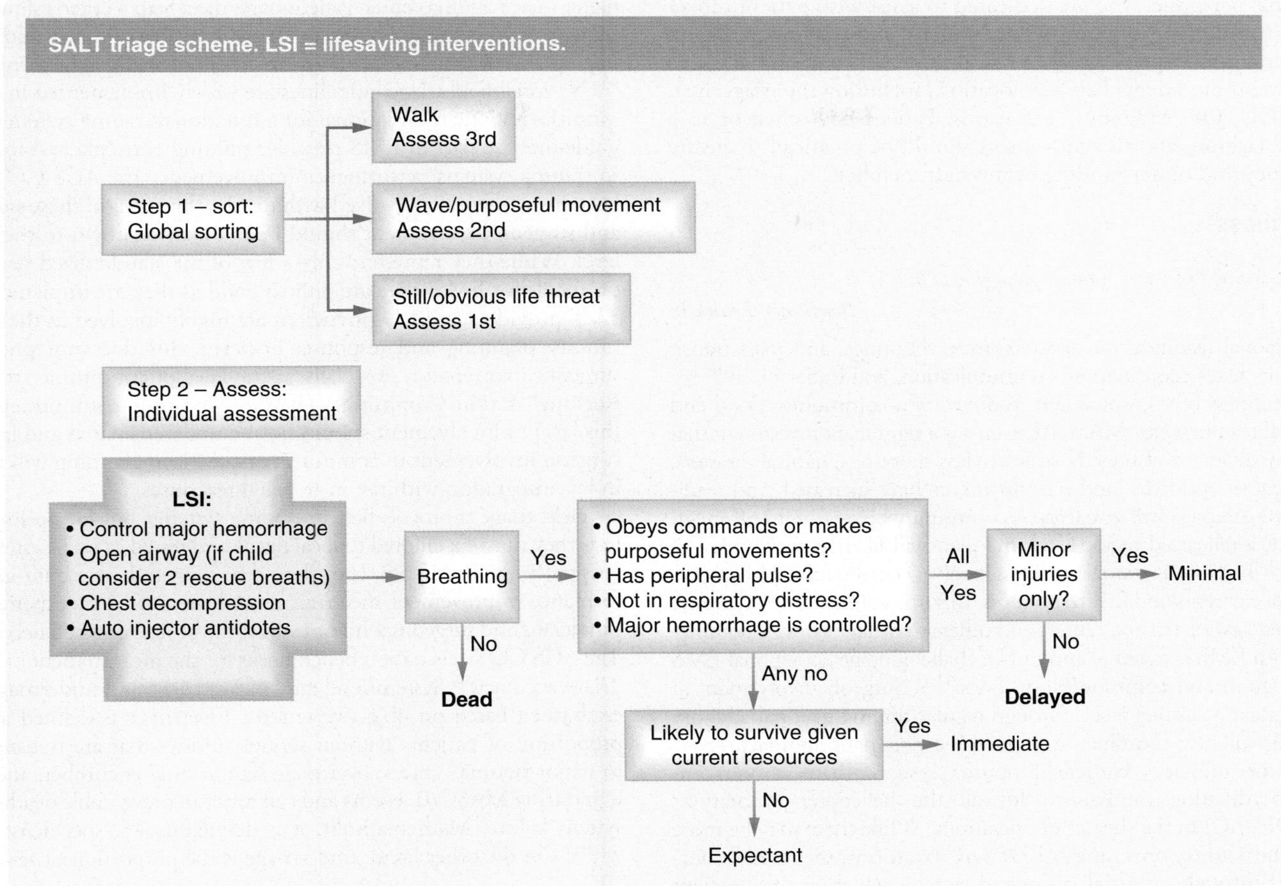

FIG. 24.5 Algorithm for the sort, assess, life interventions, treatment/transport (SALT) triage scheme, which is composed of a first step of global sorting by patient mobility and responsiveness and then individual prioritized assessment into the triage categories of dead, delayed, immediate, minimal, or expectant. (From SALT mass casualty triage: concept endorsed by the American College of Emergency Physicians, American College of Surgeons Committee on Trauma, American Trauma Society, National Association of EMS Physicians, National Disaster Life Support Education Consortium, and State and Territorial Injury Prevention Directors Association. *Disaster Med Public Health Prep.* 2008;2:245–246.)

Triage and evacuation categories

- Standard NATO nomenclature is recommended, often called "DIME"
- – **Delayed** (yellow tag) – may be life-threatening, but intervention may be delayed for several hours with frequent reassessment – (fractures, tourniquet-controlled bleeding, head or maxillofacial injuries, burns)
- – **Immediate** (red tag) – immediate attention required to prevent death – usually "AABC" issue – airway, arterial bleed, ventilation, circulatory
- – **Minimal** (green tag) – ambulatory, minor injuries such as lacerations, minor burns or musculoskeletal injuries – can wait for definitive attention
- – **Expectant** (black tag) – survival unlikely, such as extensive burns, severe head injuries

FIG. 24.6 The NATO DIME triage categorization system and color codes that also are utilized by multiple civilian triage schemes. Patients are categorized as delayed (requires treatment but not emergent), immediate (requires emergent/urgent evaluation and intervention), minimal (minor injuries, also referred to as "walking wounded"), and expectant (fatal injuries or injuries that are untreatable and have a low probability of survival within the existing mass casualty scenario limitations).

dead on arrival or who die shortly after presentation to the facility. Some key bullet points related to hospital level triage are listed below:

➢ Retriage is a crucial component of the triage process. Triage is a fluid process at all levels; a change in the situation or resource availability may result in a change in the patient triage category at any time.

➢ As the situation changes and resources become more or less available, retriage of delayed and expectant patients should occur.

➢ Patients in the minimal category can undergo a secondary and tertiary survey and usually be discharged. Occasionally, they will have missed injuries discovered during the retriage process and should be immediately reassigned into the delayed or immediate category.

Patient inflow and movement into and out of the triage area are crucial to prevent bottlenecking and chaos. Not having a well-planned map of patient movement and patient triage category areas will lead to significant confusion and potentially have a negative impact on patient care. This attention to patient flow and throughput should be made clear to all personnel and should also be rehearsed regularly. In addition, there should be a diagrammatic map that is well displayed and accessible. Another frequently overlooked aspect of MASCAL execution is the need for a group of available personnel who are dedicated to assist with patient movement, running for supplies and equipment, and relaying messages. This "manpower pool" will be critical to the efficient and effective movement of patients between locations including the triage area, ED, ICU, OR, radiology, and wards. Patient flow must be in a logical fashion, and this movement should be practiced to ensure efficiency and understanding of the staff members.

Readiness

"By failing to prepare, you are preparing to fail."

Benjamin Franklin

Regional readiness for disasters, mass shootings, and mass transit accidents takes coordination, communication, and leadership.[7,10,21,31] The readiness of a hospital and readiness of a community (local and regional readiness) for MASCAL events is a significant investment that will pay dividends if tragedy strikes. Mass shootings, natural disasters, mass transit accidents, and terrorist events have increased, and readiness/preparedness will save lives. A community being caught off-guard without a rehearsed regional trauma plan will likely pay the price in terms of lives lost. Regional readiness involves coordination with all prehospital elements and first responders. In some communities, there are multiple Level 1 trauma centers and others may have none. Coordination with EMS is essential and can be challenging given regional EMS organization and communication lines.[32,33] Surgeon involvement at the regional planning levels through regular trauma regional advisory councils will help coordinate and provide a systematic approach.

In the military's battlefield trauma system, there is one central coordinating mechanism for all the helicopter evacuations (MEDEVAC) in the theater of operations. While there may be more than one country operating MEDEVAC platforms, they are all coordinated through a central command system, which enables patient movement coordination across the theater of operations.[6,23] Having a centralized regional command enables a lead agent for the entire area of operations and gives situational oversight regarding capabilities available and remaining capacity at the different treatment facilities. This unified regional command is more of a challenge in the civilian setting given multiple ambulance companies, many of them privatized as well as hospitals that do not share a similar leadership paradigm; however, in the case of MASCAL events in which patients will be delivered to multiple hospitals, having regional coordination is essential for success.

Community MASCAL readiness involves a well-rehearsed field triage plan and situational awareness of this plan among all medical elements in a community. Field triage is integral in a regional trauma response because it guides EMS personnel in identifying and transporting high-risk patients to major trauma centers.[34] The process of field triage is guided by national triage guidelines, which have been widely implemented in the U.S. regional trauma systems and are supported by the ACS Committee on Trauma (COT).[35] The most recent Field Triage Guidelines were updated in 2011 and can be found at: https://www.cdc.gov/mmwr/preview/mmwrhtml/rr6101a1.htm.

The national field triage guidelines have four steps:

1. Assessing physiologic criteria.
2. Assessing anatomic criteria.
3. Assessing mechanism-of-injury criteria.
4. Special considerations (elderly, child, burn, pregnancy).

Steps 1 and 2 attempt to identify the most seriously injured patients. The patients should be transported preferentially to the highest level of care within the defined trauma system. For Step 3, patients meeting these criteria should be transported to a trauma center, which, depending on the defined trauma system, need not necessarily be the highest-level trauma center. Patients who meet Step 4 criteria should be transported to a trauma center or hospital capable of timely and thorough evaluation and initial management of potentially serious injuries.

National field triage guidelines are widely implemented in communities and are foundational for a functional trauma system—the guidelines are part of EMS provider training curricula and integral to trauma systems performance improvement. The ACS COT has been instrumentally involved with the development of these systems and surgeon involvement should be maintained down to the local level. While they represent only a few of the standardized national protocols for EMS, they are only as good as they are implemented. EMS providers and ED physicians are highly involved in the community planning and response; however, this does not preclude surgeon involvement, especially at the level of community trauma Regional Action Committees (RACs). The time commitment for this level of involvement should not be underestimated and lack of surgeon involvement in community field triage planning will result in less integration with the in-hospital responses.

Field triage protocols benefit trauma systems, but for optimal effect, they must be tailored to local needs and tested in each system for sensitivity and specificity. They should be trained, have a built-in performance improvement mechanism, and monitored by experienced physicians and surgeons who can adjust the protocols when necessary. The ACS COT sets nation benchmarks for the measurement of Field Triage accuracy.[36] System-level rates of overtriage and undertriage are established based on objective criteria. Overtriage is defined as the proportion of patients without serious injuries that are transported to major trauma centers; overtriage significantly encumbers the system during MASCAL events and can result in preventable deaths and system failure. Mathematically, it is defined as 1 – specificity (Fig. 24.7). On the other hand, undertriage is the proportion of seriously

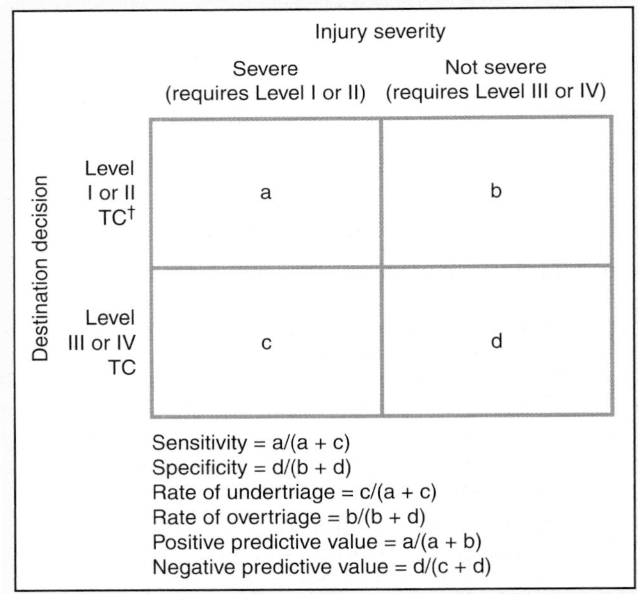

FIG. 24.7 Four-by-four box graph plotting the injury severity versus the destination decision. The performance of the triage system and the under and overtriage rates can be easily calculated as shown. (From Sasser SM, Hunt RC, Sullivent EE, et al. Guidelines for field triage of injured patients. Recommendations of the National Expert Panel on Field Triage. *MMWR Recomm Rep*. 2009;58:1–35.)

injured patients transported to nontrauma centers or triaged to an inappropriate category at the hospital and is mathematically defined as 1 – sensitivity (Fig. 24.7). In usual trauma practice, there is a focus on avoiding undertriage at all costs, while accepting the resultant high levels of overtriage. In MASCAL events, this relationship changes to one in which there must be equal or greater focus on avoiding overtriage as there is on minimizing undertriage in order to optimize outcomes and preserve scarce or critical resources (Fig. 24.2).

Casualty identification and tracking can be a serious challenge in any MASCAL event.[14] A large number of different triage cards are widely used and can be beneficial if their use is standardized and trained within a given system. The most common triage cards used are standardized Field Triage Cards.[37,38] As shown in the example in Fig. 24.8, these cards can rapidly display critical information, including vital signs, major injuries, and then easily identify what category or priority has been assigned to that patient. Although these cards have the advantage of simplicity and ease of use, there are downsides and logistic challenges such as getting lost or not staying with the patient as they move through the system. Writing can also be obscured by blood or be illegible. Like everything else in a MASCAL situation, they must be practiced with and the utilization must be rehearsed.

While there should be a redundancy of capability, there should not be a redundancy of action; inefficiency must be avoided. As patients are being triaged to different hospitals in the system, both the capability and capacity must be considered, and this should part of the triage training. Capabilities would refer to the current clinical services that would be immediately available at the hospital (neurosurgery, vascular, interventional radiology). Capacity, on the other hand, would refer to bed status, hospital status, blood available at the hospital, and

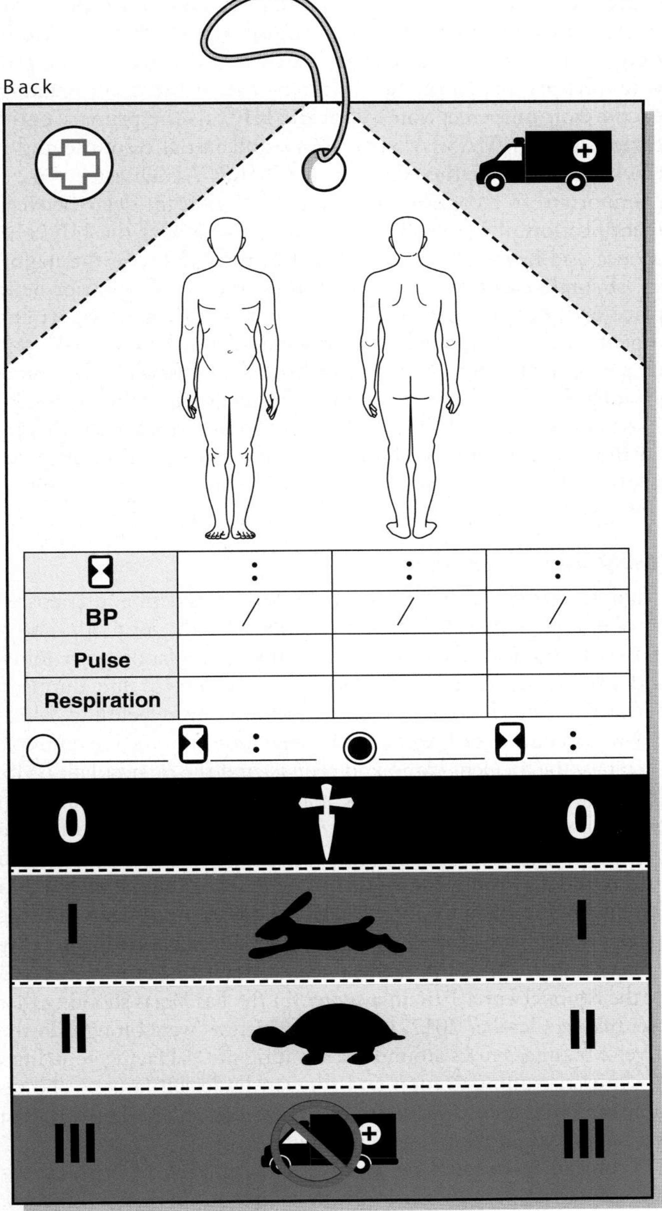

FIG. 24.8 Example of a triage card and patient tag that allows for documentation of the initial evaluation and vital signs as well as identification of the color-coded triage category that has been assigned to that individual patient.

OR availability. In a large MASCAL event, this information is necessary for appropriate field triage. Variations in both capability and capacity status should be rehearsed in regional MASCAL training. Coordination with hospital and regional incident command centers is necessary for this to occur successfully. Newer web-based tools are now widely available that can greatly aid this process by monitoring and continually updating the status and capabilities of all available hospitals in a given health system or region.[21,39]

Understanding the Hospital Incident Command System

The currently utilized organizational plan and structure in the US for sustained responses to large-scale emergency events is the Incident Command System, and at the hospital, this is known as the Hospital Incident Command System (HICS). This provides a generalized and flexible crisis leadership infrastructure that can be implemented across all types of events (the "all hazards" approach), including MASCAL events.[40,41] The HICS system broadly consists of an incident commander and four subordinate sections of Operations, Finance, Logistics, and Planning. Additional key personnel serve under each of these sections or provide advisory or liaison functions for the incident commander. A common misperception is that the HICS is the primary entity responsible for MASCAL operations and initial response and is the key element at the center of any MASCAL/Disaster plan. It is important to recognize that there is a significant delay between identification of the crisis event with activation of the HICS response and having an operational system in place. In the majority of single-event MASCAL responses, the HICS will not be in place or functional before all of the initial patient transport and urgent care is completed and thus should not be counted upon to perform or assist in the early MASCAL response. For more prolonged events, typically natural disasters such as the Hurricane Katrina events, the HICS will have a more critical role in supporting key functions including resupply, coordination of rescue efforts, maintenance and repair of critical equipment or facilities, and coordination with local and federal agencies.[11,41]

Integration of Systems

Multiple systems come into play when considering a prepared community response for a MASCAL. Both local (in-hospital) and regional (field) triage coordination, planning, training, and process leadership will help minimize loss of life during a MASCAL. The chaos of multiple casualties is overwhelming, which is why systems coordination and integration among the multiple hospitals, the incident command centers, and the prehospital, EMS, and in-hospital elements are essential. Trauma system coordination occurs through the function of the ACS COT among Level 1 trauma centers; however, as more regional Level 2 trauma centers enter into communities, it is imperative that surgeon leadership be involved in the integration of not only the regional triage process but also the incident command centers. These lower-level facilities frequently play a major role in MASCAL events that can even exceed the role played by the regional Level 1 trauma center. In the Las Vegas shooting that occurred in October 2017, most of the victims were brought to the Level 2 trauma centers around the shooting site.[42] Having good lines of clinician communication and surgeon leadership among the regional trauma centers will continue to integrate and build the system to function well during large casualty events.

From an in-hospital perspective, the function of hospital departments such as the blood bank, patient transport, radiology, PAD, ORs, etc., relies on integration and coordination within the hospital in order for there to be good patient flow and no bottlenecks. Without reliable integration of the hospital functional areas of the hospital, there is more likely to be increased disorganization chaos and delays in patient care. Good system integration does not come without a significant training investment. Surgeon leaders, trauma director, the ED leadership, and nursing leadership must all participate in system integration with the incident command center and the hospital department; these plans cannot just be on paper, they have to be invested in with rehearsals and mock events that stress the system in order to determine the weak areas of system integration. Events that create large numbers of patients are naturally chaotic and stressful, and a systems integration plan (including back-up mechanisms for communication between hospital departments) helps mitigate the chaos inherent to MASCAL situations from permeating into the clinical care arena and improves hospital function.

Security

The triage area at a hospital as well as in the field must be secure. Security is often overlooked given that first responders and providers are more concerned with saving lives. Scene safety prior to medical providers rushing into a potentially dangerous environment is paramount. An unsecured scene has the potential to result in increased casualties and induce more stress on the system. Scene security and safety are necessary for effective triage. In MASCAL planning, surgeons must remember that security is one of the most important yet frequently overlooked components. Security personnel should always be involved in MASCAL planning in both local and regional MASCAL drills. In today's world, safety and security in a disaster or MASCAL event are essential. Effective triage cannot occur in an unsafe and unsecure area. Examples of this are the Boston Marathon with the second bomb, active shooter events, building collapses, and other MASCAL incidents. As part of trauma system planning, coordination with security forces and local law enforcement ensure good communication regarding scene security for field triage.

For local (in-hospital) triage, the most important protection that the security team provides is not from enemies, but rather from media, frenzied families, and onlookers.[3] *Crowd control is essential*; large crowds of well-intentioned bystanders in a hospital ED or triage area hinder optimal care. Security personnel should be trained to allow only mission-critical staff into the hospital during a MASCAL. Points of entry into the triage area and into the hospital should be identified and secured. Additionally, disasters and MASCALs generate psychiatric casualties and combative patients. Once again, as with any other aspect, this must be rehearsed and trained. Surgeon leadership advocating for hospital security staff to be part of the training exercises is important. At Level 1 trauma centers, the trauma surgeons and ED physicians are familiar with security personnel from working in the trauma bay; however, at other hospitals, this may not be the case. Having surgeon leadership know the security leadership and awareness of the security staff and including the security team in the MASCAL training exercises will help keep the patients and staff safe during a MASCAL event. MASCAL situations also may create psychiatric casualties. Security personnel and designated medical staff should manage psychiatric casualties, combative patients, and individuals who are disruptive and create danger to themselves and other patients.

Communications

Multiple communication systems are essential for effective management in MASCAL events. Communication must occur regionally from the site of the situation and also occur effectively within the hospital. Like everything else, communication channels must be rehearsed, and during training for these events, they must participate on a full scale. From a regional standpoint, essential prehospital communications—from EMS notification, EMS coordination, to first responders—and the determination of which facility to transport the patient to happen every day on a routine basis. When large-scale events occur, this communication can get chaotic. Training for MASCAL events should include EMS coordination (many times there are multiple different private companies covering a regional area) with the centralized dispatch hub as well as with the regional hospitals. This should be rehearsed with different scenarios.

Regional

- ✔ EMS notifications.
- ✔ EMS coordination with first responders.
- ✔ Setting up known triage area at site (with security).
- ✔ Ground coordination of ambulance movement to and from triage area.
- ✔ Communication with security.
- ✔ Ground commander (triage site incident commander) should have communication with regional hospitals to get **capability** and **capacity** updates (see above).
- ✔ Triage site command should establish communications with regional hospitals to help ensure the "immediate" patients (using the DIME system) get sent to the right hospital.
- ✔ Must have contingency plans for communication between triage sites and hospitals. For example, if cell service is disabled, use of radios or land-lines are alternates that can be used for communication if planned and rehearsed. Without a reliable communication system, EMS cannot communicate with hospitals to inform them of incoming casualties and get bed status updates.

Local Integration

At the hospital level, as the Incident Command Center organizes and sets up their area, the staff should be being notified through a predetermined alert roster. Given the extent of social media and ease of communication, there is a good chance the hospital staff will be aware of the event and many of them will be headed to the hospital prior to receiving the official notification.[43] As part of the MASCAL plan, each staff member should report to a predetermined area and receive direction from the leadership. The MASCAL notification system must include all hospital departments, clinical and nonclinical.

In large MASCAL events, standard forms of communication will likely be nonfunctional. Cell towers will be overwhelmed and potentially even nonfunctional for security reasons. Backup communications such as pagers and even alerts through social media should be considered as contingency plans.[43] Hospital Public Affairs Office should be prepared to deal with the media and keep the media well informed but not interfering with MASCAL operations or the delivery of care. Interviews and statements to the media should all be handled through one office or approving authority, and official statements or announcements should be handled by one of the clinical or administrative leaders with the knowledge and experience to convey critical information and respond effectively to media questions and concerns.

Documentation and Patient Tracking

Patients can be easily misidentified or even lost during a MASCAL or disaster response. Record keeping is a challenge and usual forms of electronic documentation are unlikely to be successful.[14,44] Record keeping during a MASCAL has to balance expediency with standards. It is imperative to efficiently and accurately track patients as well as their course of care, both in the prehospital setting and during the hospital stay. Patients may move to multiple areas and can easily be "misplaced" or misidentified. Simple and low-tech solutions for initial triage and MASCAL tracking should be understood and rehearsed. This includes switching to paper-based charting and ordering systems for the initial phases of care, particularly if the local electronic medical record is unable to perform adequately with a large acute influx of patients. Documenting critical information by writing directly on the patient and/or dressings is a highly effective method of communicating important information, particularly when the patient is being moved from one location to another (Fig. 24.9). Hospitals should have preprepared MASCAL packets with simplified charting and ordering mechanism in place in case the

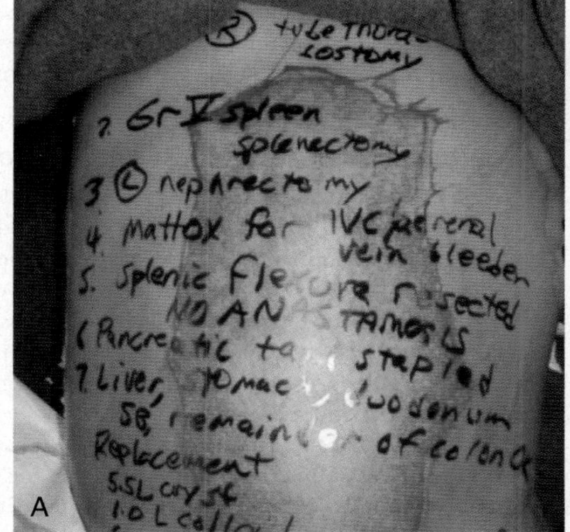

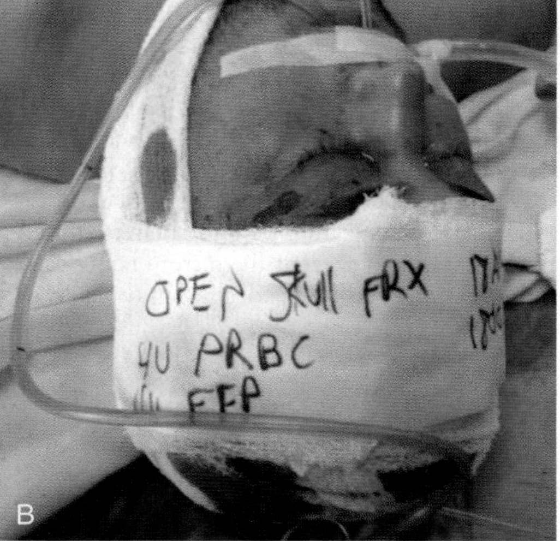

FIG. 24.9 Examples of improvised documentation to facilitate communication of critical information during mass casualty events when patients are being transferred between provider teams or between facilities. (A) documentation on a temporary abdominal closure dressing conveying critical information about the initial damage controls, surgical procedures, and resuscitation and (B) clearly marked dressing conveying the underlying injuries and the time/date of the most recent dressing change.

electronic medical record fails, is damaged by the inciting event, or is unable to adequately perform patient care functions.

Community Elements and Other Considerations

For disasters or MASCAL events that affect an entire community/region, certain provisions should be considered, and, of course, these should be incorporated into the regional and hospital MASCAL plan. Social media and news broadcasting will certainly report on the event; it is important that accurate messages are relayed. Additionally, social media can be leveraged, but effective and accurate messaging is imperative. For example, if blood or platelet donors are needed, the request could be disseminated through social medial sites. Blood Donor Centers could also communicate shortages of certain blood types through official social media sites. Social media can be also leveraged for notifications regarding road closures and traffic issues around hospitals and the MASCAL site.

A potential challenge for MASCAL events is if a large number of patients arrive who do not speak English. In the military, it is not uncommon to have MCI or MASCAL events that involved host nation patients who do not speak English. Linguists are essential to communicate with the casualties and are necessary to provide effective and compassionate care. In the Asiana Airline crash that occurred at San Francisco Airport in July 2013, 187 patients were sent to hospitals in the San Francisco Bay Area—the majority of the patients were from Korea and China and were non–English speaking. Hospitals will unlikely have enough linguists for these types of international events. While not ideal, social media can be used to request additional medical linguist support. Certainly, any individuals who arrive at the hospital to help with linguist support would have to be screened expeditiously by security to ensure there were no overt safety issues with their presence. Ideally, there would be contracts with medical linguist companies that could help provide support; however, there are practical and logistic challenges to be able to have contingency plans for multiple languages.

Large casualty-producing events can create dilemmas for patient disposition. Whether homes are destroyed from natural disasters or patients injured are not from the area of the event (Boston Marathon, Las Vegas concert), there may not be a safe place for them to go if they are treated for minor injuries and discharged from the hospital. Taxi companies and transportation services should have prearranged plans with the hospitals to help with the transport of patients discharged. This needs to be predetermined and included in the MASCAL plan. Additionally, in order to avoid hospitals from becoming shelters, not only should a transportation plan exist, but also predetermined places in the community such as churches, schools, and regional hospitals should assist with patient disposition. In the case of displaced persons (infrastructure collapse, fire), churches and shelters should help decompress the hospitals and prevent them from being used as shelters. Psychological support should ideally be available to these patients as well.

Adaptable

"Do what you can, with what you have, where you are."

Theodore Roosevelt

The success or failure of a MASCAL response pivots on many different factors. The best plans may not be able to be implemented secondary to unforeseen events. MASCAL plans cannot predict every possible contingency or event. While leadership, effective triage, and training are all crucial components to succeed managing MCI or MASCAL events, the plan must be able to adapt to unforeseen circumstances. No disaster, MCI event, or MASCAL event will be the same; however, triage principals and patient management concepts remain the same, but they must be able to adapt to the situation.

Military triage and Tactical Combat Casualty Care is no different: the principals remain the same, but being able to adapt to the tactical situation is where the art of effective triage and early MASCAL management saves the most lives. Resource availability at the regional and hospital level will dictate various triage decisions, and situational awareness is imperative.

When plans need to be quickly adapted because of the situation, leadership is crucial. If leaders are unable to adapt, the system will be unable to adapt. Triage, regional and in-hospital, and overall MASCAL management are dynamic processes that unfold as the casualty-producing event progresses. Management of triage patients as they move through the system must be performed within the constraints of the scenario and environment with the considerations of the tactical situation.

Understanding the hospital, prehospital, en route, and regional resources is crucial. Being able to adapt the situation depending on information from law enforcement is also important because the tactical situation can change. Natural disasters, floods, and fires have the potential to take out communications and leave some facilities nonfunctional, and expertise in the regional hospital capabilities would be necessary for adequate field triage. Setting up off-site treatment areas and mobilizing treatment teams can be life-saving if hospitals are overburdened with patients or if there are infrastructure problems. The military has been pushing capabilities closer to the point of injury, and while this may not always be feasible in an urban MASCAL, if there are teams trained for this contingency, the capability could be utilized.[1,20]

Being adaptable is most necessary and critical for the senior triage officer. During MCI and MASCAL events, patients do not arrive in any order of precedence, and frequently, some of the sickest casualties arrived after many casualties with minor injuries have been brought inside the EDs. The triage officer must have good situational awareness and ensure that casualties get treated in a timely and appropriate manner utilizing resources appropriately to maintain capability for the additional influx of casualties. Coordination and communications are key factors in being able to adapt; there must be redundancy and fail safes in the communication systems so that, as the system adapts to overcome situations not accounted for in MASCAL planning, all elements of the local and regional teams are kept aware.

Grow (Elements of a Learning Health System)

Among the most important and frequently overlooked aspects of improving MASCAL care at every level is the need to capture, process, and then act on the feedback and lessons learned from past events. While success or failure during an MCI or MASCAL depends on accurate and effective triage, the success or failure of the next event depends upon a structured AAR of each event in order to improve individuals, groups, and systems. Although there are many different formats and techniques for performing an effective AAR, they all have several characteristics in common that should be highlighted. The AAR should be done as soon after the event as possible, in order to capture events while they are fresh in people's minds and to ensure maximal participation. They should be done at every level, from an individual department or area (ED, OR, ICU) up to the facility and even the system level. The AAR should focus on gathering input in two categories: things that went well or worked and things that did not work or need to be improved. In particular, any obvious areas that resulted in suboptimal outcomes, patient/provider harm, or near-misses should be identified. This should be done in an entirely nonjudgmental and nonpunitive manner, and input from all levels should be encouraged. A formal write up of the AAR should be created and submitted up the chain of command to be integrated into the hospital or system-level AAR. Finally, and most importantly, an action plan based on the AAR feedback and review should be created that identifies and prioritizes changes to be implemented in order to better prepare for future MASCAL events. Institutionalization of processes like this, with the aim of continual improvement of the delivery of care and focused with the patient at the center, characterize the "Learning Health System." This was emphasized and codified in a recent National Academies of Science, Engineering, and Medicine (NASEM) report on "Zero Preventable Deaths," calling for an overhaul of the national trauma systems in the United States.[31,45]

Exsanguination Control Along the Spectrum

"The fate of the wounded lays with those who apply the first dressing."

Colonel Nicholas Senn

Dr. Larrey, the father of triage and a surgeon in Napoleon's army, did rapid and effective amputations on the forward line of battle, markedly improving survival from major bleeding extremity injuries. Basic hemorrhage control and airway management should be part of the triage process from the most forward point of care and not relegated to only the in-hospital phase. The triage team and any primary or secondary triage points should have personnel trained in hemorrhage control and airway interventions and should be adequately supplied with tourniquets, and hemostatic dressings. Multiple military and civilian studies have now demonstrated that most potentially preventable trauma deaths occur prior to the patient reaching surgical care and are secondary to hemorrhage.[16,46–48] In many MASCAL events, and particularly events such as explosive blasts or mass shootings, exsanguinating hemorrhage will be an even more common issue than in usual trauma settings.

Triage is part of a large organizational structure or system of care. The success of managing MASCALs or MCI resulting from disasters, shootings, or terrorist events pivots on an effective, efficient, rehearsed and well-trained personnel and "ready" systems of care. However, ensuring adequate preparation and training for these events can be challenging and can meet with significant resistance due to the time and financial commitments that are required. It is therefore imperative to optimize the already available resources and expertise within any system and to be as efficient as possible in selecting and then delivering high-yield and high-quality training. Universal training in basic hemorrhage control and the use of widely available adjuncts such as tourniquets and hemostatic dressings is one area that should be considered the highest priority and can be done efficiently and cost-effectively. As part of the ACS "Stop the Bleed" campaign, the newly developed and promulgated Basic Control of Hemorrhage (BCON) Course can provide familiarization with these techniques to both medical providers and lay people with minimal time and supply investment.[25,49] We recommend that all personnel who may be involved in MASCAL care at every step along the continuum of care be BCON certified (or some equivalent training) and have access to modern hemorrhage control devices and adjuncts.[24]

CONCLUSIONS

MASCAL and disaster events are among the most challenging and high-stress settings that can be encountered in the delivery of health care and are a "perfect storm" of factors that can lead to errors, lapses in care, and suboptimal outcomes. As medical providers who are highly trained in the delivery of emergency trauma care and lifesaving interventions, surgeons are uniquely positioned to be critical elements of any MASCAL response. In addition to expertise in emergency operative management, the experienced surgeon is ideally positioned to function in key MASCAL leadership roles such as senior triage officer or local incident commander. In order to optimize the medical care and population outcomes from large-scale trauma events, all surgeons should be familiar with the key principles of effective MASCAL management and triage. Triage in these situations is a tactical art, embodying skills such as leadership, communication, flexibility, and adaptability. There are three core components that are required for successful preparation for MASCAL responses and optimal execution during these events: leadership, expertise, and training (Box 24.2). If any of these three components have not been optimized, then there will be deficiencies in the delivery of care and unnecessary (and preventable) morbidity and mortality. Creating a truly ready and integrated system for MASCAL care requires training at all levels, regional readiness, integration of multiple systems along the care continuum, and refining the system through the capture and promulgation of lessons learned. Among the most important and highest volumes of these lessons have been accrued by the military over the past decade-plus of sustained combat operations. As stated in the NASEM Zero Preventable Deaths report, full integration of the military and civilian trauma systems is critical to the future of trauma care in the United States and particularly for integrating the large volume of military experience with MASCAL care.[1,31,45] Such a comprehensive integration would leverage the relative strengths of each component to standardize and optimize MASCAL readiness and systems of care nationwide (Fig. 24.10).

What can be learned from the military system of care?

- ➢ The military applies damage control principals across the continuum of care.
  - ○ When patients are unable to rapidly get to definitive care, they get triaged along the continuum of care to undergo damage control surgery or resuscitation in order to bridge the time and space gap from wounding to definitive care.
- ➢ Centralized leadership and C2 (command and control).
  - ○ Imposes strict order on the regional (battlefield) trauma ecosystem.

BOX 24.2 Simple mnemonic for some of the core and critical concepts to successful mass casualty (MASCAL) planning and execution.

M Minimize chaos—remain calm and confident
A Assess—perform accurate, ongoing triage; assess weather, supply status, personnel, etc.
S Safety—do not create additional patients; take care of self and staff
C Communication—can never be enough; make it clear and concise
A Alert—be ready for more casualties; reconstitute and resupply
L Lost—do not lose patients or staff; use tracking system for patients; maintain accountability of the team.

Courtesy of Colonel Jorge Klajnbart, Chief of Surgery Evans Army Community Hospital.

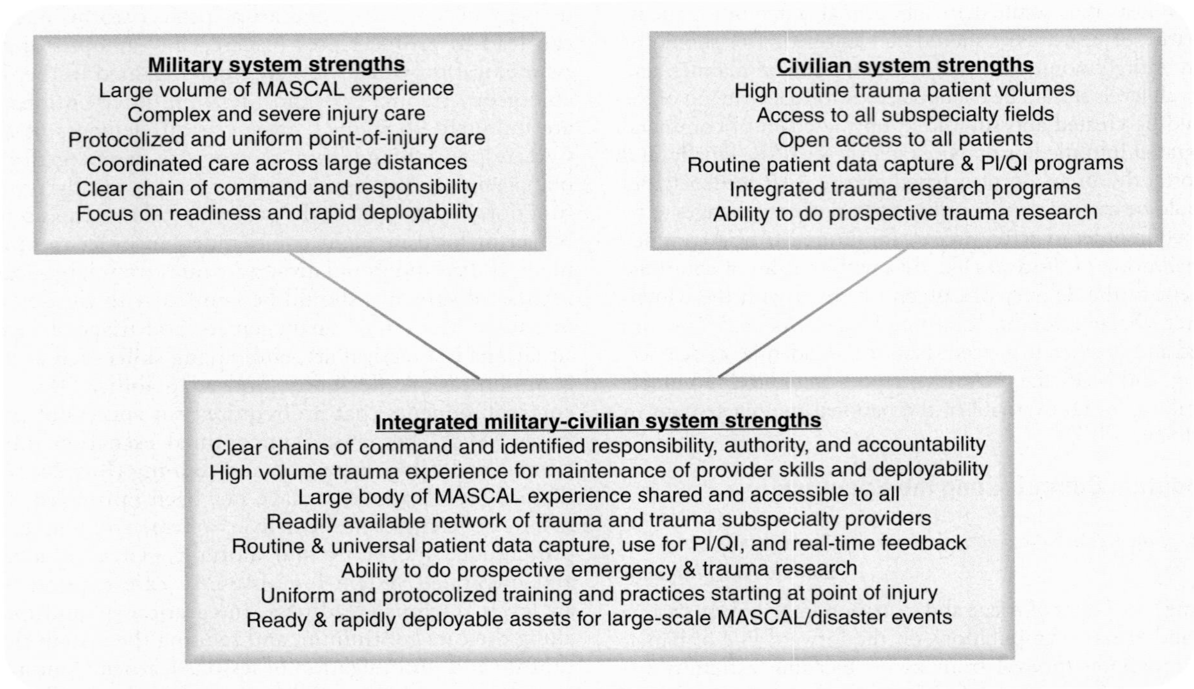

FIG. 24.10 Graph listing the individual strengths and weaknesses of the military versus civilian trauma systems related to MASCAL care, and the potential benefits of a fully integrated national military-civilian trauma system. *MASCAL*, Mass casualty; *PI/QI*, performance improvement/quality improvement. (From Martin MJ, Rasmussen TE, Knudson M, et al. Heeding the call: Military-civilian partnerships as a foundation for enhanced mass casualty care in the United States. *J Trauma Acute Care Surg*. 2018;85:1123–1126.)

- Intentional positioning of surgical capabilities on the battlefield.
  - Gets major trauma and complex injuries to the correct capability.
  - While this is not always possible in civilian communities, in areas with long transport times, contingencies can be put in place at smaller hospitals to facilitate hemorrhage control until patients can reach definitive care.
  - Military triage principals can be applied to many civilian scenarios.
- Lessons learned from tourniquet use, pain control, airway management (TCCC) can be trained to the level of the first responders—but this level of training requires significant commitment, funding, community, and trauma center leadership.
- The tactical setting, leadership, and imposing system order on chaos are crucial components to regional/field triage.
- Flexibility and adaptability are essential especially in disaster scenarios that threaten infrastructure and communication networks.
- Redundancy in systems helps mitigate these factors.
- Bring the capability (hemorrhage control, transfusion) as far forward as possible.
  - The overarching goal in military, regional (field), or local (hospital) triage is to prioritize, stabilize, sort, and move the injured to definitive care.
  - Going for the acceptable, not always the optimal…but optimal is always the goal.

SELECTED REFERENCES

Berwick DM, Downey AS, Cornett EA. National academies of sciences, engineering, and medicine; health and medicine division; board on health sciences policy; board on the health of select populations; committee on military trauma care's learning health system and its translation to the civilian sector. *A National Trauma Care System: Integrating Military and Civilian Trauma Systems to Achieve Zero Preventable Deaths After Injury*. Washington, DC: The National Academies Press; 2016.

A landmark National Academies report analyzing the existing military and civilian trauma systems, identifying critical areas of excellence and opportunities for improvement, and then setting forward a set of clear recommendations for national integration and improvement in mass casualty (MASCAL) and routine trauma care.

Carli P, Pons F, Levraut J, et al. The french emergency medical services after the paris and nice terrorist attacks: what have we learnt? *Lancet*. 2017;390:2735–2738.

Excellent summary of the medical response to multisite terrorist attacks in Paris in 2015 and Nice in 2016 and the efforts of the French medical system to prepare for future events by incorporating best practices from the civilian and military sectors. This viewpoint also identifies key areas of "shortfalls" in the response to the events, including communication/coordination challenges and difficulty in identifying victims.

Frykberg ER. Medical management of disasters and mass casualties from terrorist bombings: how can we cope? *J Trauma*. 2002;53:201–212.

This is the first overview of the medical response to urban terrorism that emphasizes the role of effective triage and looks at the medical response in quantitative terms. Of particular importance in this work is the emphasis of the adverse effects of overtriage during mass casualty (MASCAL) events. Dr. Frykberg was a pioneer in bringing the importance of disaster preparedness to the attention of surgeons.

Gates JD, Arabian S, Biddinger P, et al. The initial response to the Boston marathon bombing: lessons learned to prepare for the next disaster. *Ann Surg*. 2014;260:960–966.

Detailed analysis of the mass casualty (MASCAL) event and medical response following the multiple explosive detonations at the 2013 Boston Marathon. This work highlights the critical importance of scene triage and smart distribution of casualties to local hospitals, transitioning from routine to MASCAL care at the hospital level, and expected injury patterns after a blast event. Importantly, key areas for improvement, such as the lack of tourniquets and hemostatic dressings, communication challenges, and difficulties with the electronic medical record, are highlighted.

Hirshberg A, Scott BG, Granchi T, et al. How does casualty load affect trauma care in urban bombing incidents? A quantitative analysis. *J Trauma*. 2005;58:686–693; discussion 694–685.

A computer model was used to simulate the response of a major U.S. trauma center to an urban bombing using casualty profiles from an Israeli hospital. The model predicts the now classic sigmoid-shaped relationship between the level of trauma care and increasing casualty load and defines the surge capacity of the hospital trauma service line.

Kuckelman J, Derickson M, Long WB, et al. Management from Baghdad to Boston: top ten lessons learned from modern military and civilian MASCAL events. *Curr Trauma Rep*. 2018;4:138–148.

A summary and "top 10" list of key lessons learned from over a decade of military and civilian mass casualty (MASCAL) events. These include the importance of high-quality triage, initial management and evaluation prioritization and rationing, facility security and patient flow, and centralized command and communication practices.

REFERENCES

1. Martin MJ, Rasmussen TE, Margaret Knudson M, et al. Heeding the call: military-civilian partnerships as a foundation for enhanced mass casualty care in the United States. *J Trauma Acute Care Surg*. 2018;85:1123–1126.
2. Wild J, Maher J, Frazee RC, et al. The fort hood massacre: lessons learned from a high profile mass casualty. *J Trauma Acute Care Surg*. 2012;72:1709–1713.
3. Kuckelman J, Derickson M, Long WB, et al. Management from Baghdad to Boston: top ten lessons learned from modern military and civilian MASCAL events. *Curr Trauma Rep*. 2018;4:138–148.
4. Frykberg ER. Medical management of disasters and mass casualties from terrorist bombings: how can we cope? *J Trauma*. 2002;53:201–212.
5. Hirshberg A, Scott BG, Granchi T, et al. How does casualty load affect trauma care in urban bombing incidents? A quantitative analysis. *J Trauma*. 2005;58:686–693; discussion 694–685.
6. Elster EA, Butler FK, Rasmussen TE. Implications of combat casualty care for mass casualty events. *J Am Med Assoc*. 2013;310:475–476.
7. Callaway DW. A review of the landscape: challenges and gaps in trauma response to civilian high threat mass casualty incidents. *J Trauma Acute Care Surg*. 2018;84:S21–S27.
8. Khajehaminian MR, Ardalan A, Keshtkar A, et al. A systematic literature review of criteria and models for casualty distribution in trauma related mass casualty incidents. *Injury*. 2018;49:1959–1968.
9. Briggs S. Triage in mass casualty incidents: challenges and controversies. *Am J Disaster Med*. 2007;2:57.
10. Spruce L. Back to basics: mass casualty incidents. *AORN J*. 2019;109:95–103.
11. Yarmohammadian MH, Atighechian G, Shams L, et al. Are hospitals ready to response to disasters? Challenges, opportunities and strategies of Hospital Emergency Incident Command System (HEICS). *J Res Med Sci*. 2011;16:1070–1077.
12. Huber-Wagner S, Lefering R, Kay MV, et al. Duration and predictors of emergency surgical operations—basis for medical management of mass casualty incidents. *Eur J Med Res*. 2009;14:532–540.
13. Brevard SB, Weintraub SL, Aiken JB, et al. Analysis of disaster response plans and the aftermath of Hurricane Katrina: lessons learned from a level I trauma center. *J Trauma*. 2008;65:1126–1132.
14. Landman A, Teich JM, Pruitt P, et al. The Boston Marathon bombings mass casualty incident: one emergency department's information systems challenges and opportunities. *Ann Emerg Med*. 2015;66:51–59.
15. Tami G, Bruria A, Fabiana E, et al. An after-action review tool for EDs: learning from mass casualty incidents. *Am J Emerg Med*. 2013;31:798–802.
16. Brunner J, Rocha TC, Chudgar AA, et al. The Boston Marathon bombing: after-action review of the Brigham and Women's Hospital emergency radiology response. *Radiology*. 2014;273:78–87.
17. Gates JD, Arabian S, Biddinger P, et al. The initial response to the Boston marathon bombing: lessons learned to prepare for the next disaster. *Ann Surg*. 2014;260:960–966.
18. Hupp JR. Important take-aways from the Boston marathon bombing. *J Oral Maxillofac Surg*. 2013;71:1637–1638.
19. Janousek JT, Jackson DE, De Lorenzo RA, et al. Mass casualty triage knowledge of military medical personnel. *Mil Med*. 1999;164:332–335.
20. Romero Pareja R, Castro Delgado R, Turegano Fuentes F, et al. Prehospital triage for mass casualty incidents using the META method for early surgical assessment: retrospective validation of a hospital trauma registry. *Eur J Trauma Emerg Surg*. 2020;46:425–433.

21. Shartar SE, Moore BL, Wood LM. Developing a mass casualty surge capacity protocol for emergency medical services to use for patient distribution. *South Med J*. 2017;110:792–795.
22. Moran CG, Webb C, Brohi K, et al. Lessons in planning from mass casualty events in UK. *BMJ*. 2017;359:j4765.
23. Schauer SG, April MD, Simon E, et al. Prehospital interventions during mass-casualty events in Afghanistan: a case analysis. *Prehosp Disaster Med*. 2017;32:465–468.
24. Robaina JA, Crawford SB, Huerta D, et al. Mass casualty incidents and B-Con training. *J Emerg Manag*. 2018;16:397–404.
25. Butler FK. Stop the bleed. Strategies to enhance survival in active shooter and intentional mass casualty events. The Hartford consensus. A major step forward in translating battlefield trauma care advances to the civilian sector. *J Spec Oper Med*. 2015;15:133–135.
26. SALT mass casualty triage: concept endorsed by the American College of Emergency Physicians, American College of Surgeons Committee on Trauma, American Trauma Society, National Association of Ems Physicians, National Disaster Life Support Education Consortium, and State and Territorial Injury Prevention Directors Association. *Disaster Med Public Health Prep*. 2008;2:245–246.
27. Massalou D. The French surgical services after the paris and nice terrorist attacks: what have we learnt? *Lancet*. 2017;390:1581.
28. Khajehaminian MR, Ardalan A, Hosseini Boroujeni SM, et al. Criteria and models for the distribution of casualties in trauma-related mass casualty incidents: a systematic literature review protocol. *Syst Rev*. 2017;6:141.
29. Fink BN, Rega PP, Sexton ME, et al. START versus SALT triage: which is preferred by the 21st century health care student? *Prehosp Disaster Med*. 2018;33:381–386.
30. Martin MJ, Beekley A, Eckert MJ. *Front Line Surgery: A Practical Approach*. 2nd ed. New York: Springer Science+Business Media; 2017.
31. Berwick DM, Downey AS, Cornett EA. A national trauma care system to achieve zero preventable deaths after injury: recommendations from a National Academies of Sciences, Engineering, and Medicine Report. *J Am Med Assoc*. 2016;316:927–928.
32. Kearns RD, Marcozzi DE, Barry N, et al. Disaster preparedness and response for the burn mass casualty incident in the twenty-first century. *Clin Plast Surg*. 2017;44:441–449.
33. Jenkins DH, Cioffi WG, Cocanour CS, et al. Position statement of the coalition for national trauma research on the National Academies of Sciences, Engineering and Medicine report, A National Trauma Care System: integrating military and civilian trauma systems to achieve zero preventable deaths after injury. *J Trauma Acute Care Surg*. 2016;81:816–818.
34. Carli P, Pons F, Levraut J, et al. The French emergency medical services after the Paris and nice terrorist attacks: what have we learnt? *Lancet*. 2017;390:2735–2738.
35. Newgard CD, Fu R, Zive D, et al. Prospective validation of the National Field Triage guidelines for identifying seriously injured persons. *J Am Coll Surg*. 2016;222:146–158.e142.
36. Committee on Trauma. *Resources for Optimal Care of the Injured Patient, 6*. Chicago: American College of Surgeons; 2014.
37. Radestad M, Lennquist Montan K, Ruter A, et al. Attitudes towards and experience of the use of triage tags in major incidents: a mixed method study. *Prehosp Disaster Med*. 2016;31:376–385.
38. Field K, Norton I. Australian triage tags: a prospective, randomised cross-over trial and evaluation of user preference. *Emerg Med Australas*. 2012;24:321–328.
39. Hall TN, McDonald A, Peleg K. Identifying factors that may influence decision-making related to the distribution of patients during a mass casualty incident. *Disaster Med Public Health Prep*. 2018;12:101–108.
40. Sauer LM, Romig M, Andonian J, et al. Application of the incident command system to the hospital biocontainment unit setting. *Health Secur*. 2019;17:27–34.
41. Shooshtari S, Tofighi S, Abbasi S. Benefits, barriers, and limitations on the use of hospital incident command system. *J Res Med Sci*. 2017;22:36.
42. Lozada MJ, Cai S, Li M, et al. The las vegas mass shooting: an analysis of blood component administration and blood bank donations. *J Trauma Acute Care Surg*. 2019;86:128–133.
43. Callcut RA, Moore S, Wakam G, et al. Finding the signal in the noise: could social media be utilized for early hospital notification of multiple casualty events? *PloS One*. 2017;12:e0186118.
44. Bergeron K. Lessons in disaster: the Boston marathon bombing. *Radiol Manage*. 2014;36:46–48.
45. Berwick DM, Downey AS, Cornett EA. National academies of sciences, engineering, and medicine; health and medicine division; board on health sciences policy; board on the health of select populations; committee on military trauma care's learning health system and its translation to the civilian sector. *A National Trauma Care System: Integrating Military and Civilian Trauma Systems To Achieve Zero Preventable Deaths After Injury*. Washington, DC: The National Academies Press; 2016.
46. Beekley AC, Martin MJ, Spinella PC, et al. Predicting resource needs for multiple and mass casualty events in combat: lessons learned from combat support hospital experience in operation iraqi freedom. *J Trauma*. 2009;66:S129–S137.
47. Frykberg ER, Tepas 3rd JJ. Terrorist bombings. Lessons learned from Belfast to Beirut. *Ann Surg*. 1988;208:569–576.
48. Martin M, Oh J, Currier H, et al. An analysis of in-hospital deaths at a modern combat support hospital. *J Trauma*. 2009;66:S51–S60; discussion S60–S51.
49. Goolsby C, Jacobs L, Hunt RC, et al. Stop the bleed education consortium: education program content and delivery recommendations. *J Trauma Acute Care Surg*. 2018;84:205–210.

SECTION IV

Transplantation and Immunology

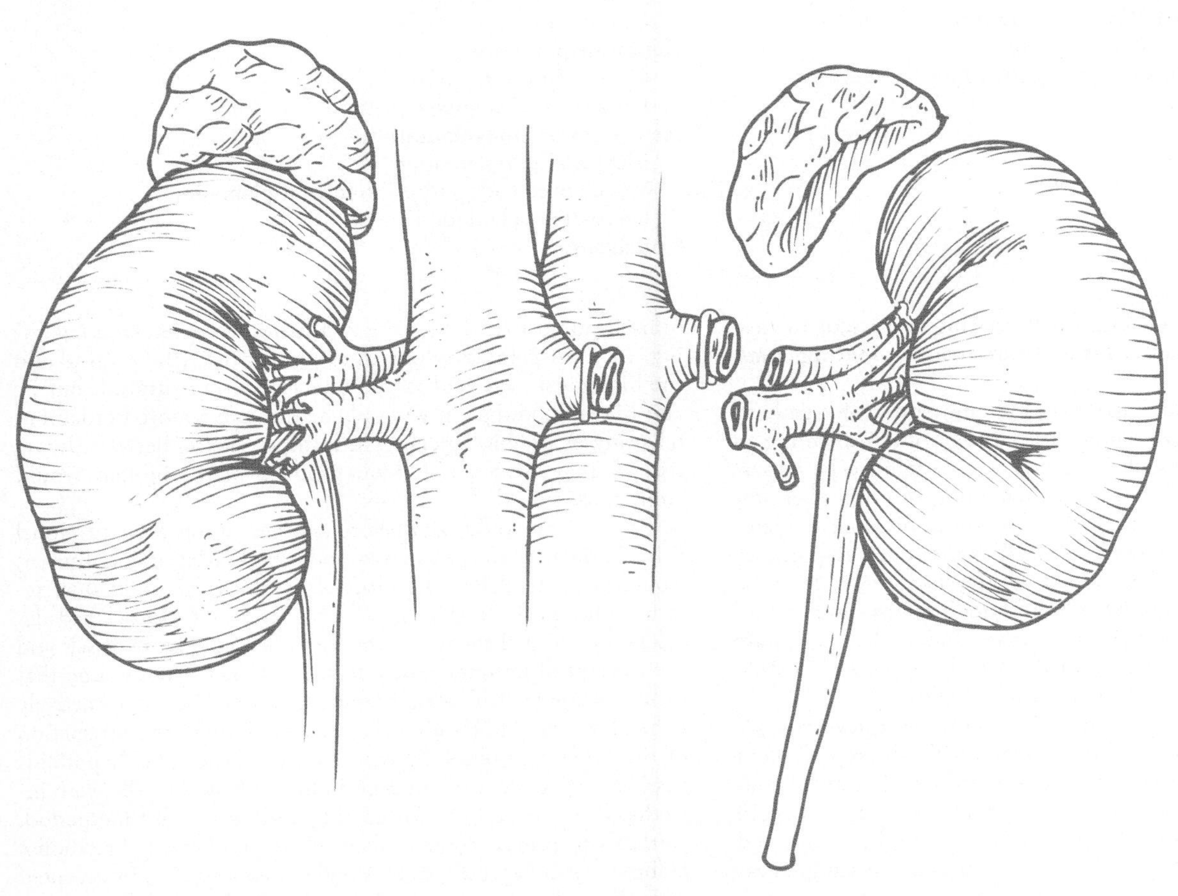

25 CHAPTER

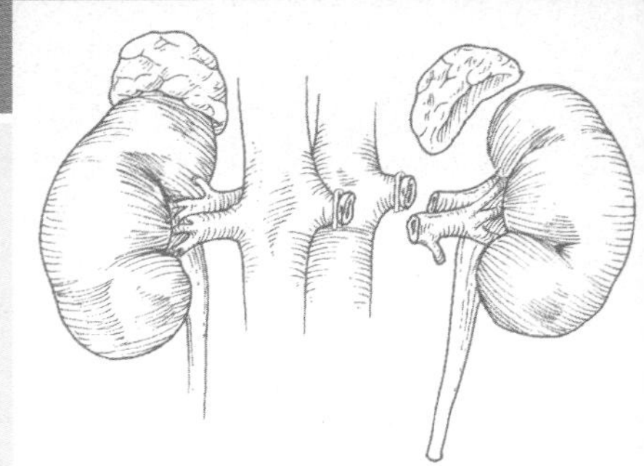

Transplantation Immunobiology and Immunosuppression

I. Raul Badell, Andrew B. Adams, Christian P. Larsen

OUTLINE

Please access Elsevier eBooks for Practicing Clinicians to view the videos for this chapter https://expertconsult.inkling.com/.

Only a few short decades ago, there were no options for patients dying of end-stage organ failure. The concept of transplanting an organ from one individual to another was thought to be impossible. The evolution of clinical transplantation and transplant immunology is one of the bright success stories of modern medicine. It was through understanding of the immune response to the transplanted tissue that pioneers in the field were able to develop therapies to manipulate the immune response and to prevent rejection of the transplanted organ. Today, there are more than 25,000 transplants performed annually, and over 100,000 patients are currently listed and awaiting an organ.

The concept of transplantation is certainly not new. History is replete with legends and myths recounting the replacement of limbs and organs. An oft-repeated myth of early transplantation is derived from the miracle of Saints Cosmas and Damian (brothers and subsequently patron saints of physicians and surgeons) in which they successfully replaced the gangrenous leg of the Roman deacon Justinian with a leg from a recently deceased Ethiopian (Fig. 25.1). It was not, however, until the French surgeon Alexis Carrel developed a method for joining blood vessels in the late nineteenth century that the transplantation of organs became technically feasible and verifiable accounts of transplantation began (Fig. 25.2). He was awarded the Nobel Prize (Medicine) in 1912 "in recognition of his work on vascular suture and the transplantation of blood vessels and organs." Having established the technical component, Carrel himself noted that there were two issues to be resolved regarding "the transplantation of tissues and organs…the surgical and the biological." He had solved one aspect, the surgical, but he also understood that "it will only be through a more fundamental study of the biological relationships existing between living tissues" that the more difficult problem of the biology would come to be solved.

Forty years would pass before another set of eventual Nobel Prize winners, Peter Medawar and Frank Macfarlane Burnet, would begin to define the process by which one individual rejects another's tissue (Fig. 25.3).[1] Medawar and Burnet had developed an overall theory on the immunologic nature of self and the concept of immunologic tolerance. Burnet hypothesized that the definition of "self" was not preprogrammed but rather actively defined during embryonic development through the interaction of the host's immune cells with its own tissue. This hypothesis implied that tolerance could be induced if donor cells were introduced to the embryo within this developmental time period. Burnet was proven correct when Medawar showed that mouse embryos receiving cells from a different mouse strain accepted grafts from the strain later in life while rejecting grafts from other strains. These seminal studies were the first reports to demonstrate that it was possible to manipulate the immune system to accept allografts.[1]

Shortly thereafter, Joseph Murray, Nobel Laureate 1990, performed the first successful renal transplant between identical twins in 1954.[2] At the same time, Gertrude Elion, who worked as an assistant to George Hitchings at Wellcome Research Laboratories, developed several new immunosuppressive compounds including

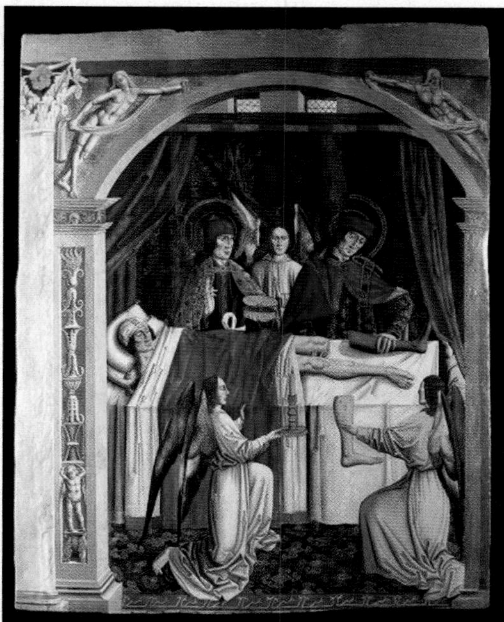

FIG. 25.1 A fifteenth century painting of Cosmas and Damian, patron saints of physicians and surgeons. The legend of the Miracle of the Black Leg depicts the removal of the diseased leg of Roman Justinian and replacement with the leg of a recently deceased Ethiopian man.

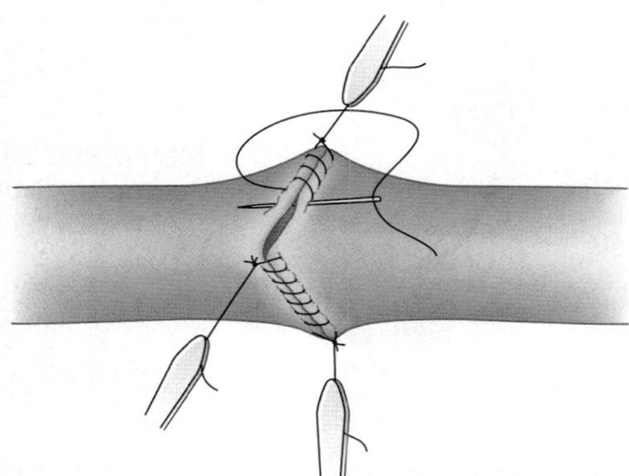

FIG. 25.2 Triangulation technique of vascular anastomosis by Alexis Carrel. (Reprinted from Edwards WS, Edwards PD. *Alexis Carrel: Visionary Surgeon*. Springfield, IL: Charles C Thomas; 1974.)

6-mercaptopurine and azathioprine. Roy Calne, a budding surgeon-scientist who came from the United Kingdom to study with Murray, subsequently tested these reagents in animals and then introduced them into clinical practice, permitting nonidentical transplantation to be successful. Elion and Hitchings later shared the Nobel Prize in 1988 for their work on "the important principles of drug development." Subsequent discovery of increasingly effective agents to suppress the rejection response has led to the success in allograft survival that we enjoy today. It is this collaboration between scientists and surgeons that has driven our understanding of the immune system as it relates to transplantation. In this chapter, we provide an overview of the immune response with specific attention to transplant immunity and the rejection process, review the specific immunosuppressive agents that are employed to prevent rejection, and provide a glimpse into the future of the field.

THE IMMUNE RESPONSE

The immune system, of course, did not evolve to prevent the transplantation of another individual's tissue or organs; rejection, rather, is a consequence of a system that has developed over thousands of years to protect against invasion by pathogens and to prevent subsequent disease. To understand the rejection process and in particular to appreciate the consequences of pharmacologic suppression of rejection, a general understanding of immune response as it functions in a physiologic setting is required.

The immune system has evolved to include two complementary divisions to respond to disease: the innate and acquired immune systems. Broadly speaking, the innate immune system recognizes general characteristics that have, through selective pressure, come to represent universal pathologic challenges to our species (ischemia, necrosis, trauma, and certain nonhuman cell surfaces). The acquired arm, on the other hand, recognizes specific structural aspects of foreign substances, usually peptide or carbohydrate moieties, recognized by receptors generated randomly and selected to avoid self-recognition. Although the two systems differ in their specific responsibilities, they act in concert to influence each other to achieve an optimal overall response.

Innate Immunity

The innate immune system is thought to be a holdover from an evolutionarily distant response to foreign pathogens. In contrast to the acquired immune system, which employs an innumerable host of specificities to identify any possible antigen, the innate system uses a select number of protein receptors to identify specific motifs consistent with foreign or altered and damaged tissues. These receptors can exist on cells, such as macrophages, neutrophils, and natural killer (NK) cells, or free in the circulation, as is the case for complement. Whereas they fail to exhibit the specificity of the T-cell receptor (TCR) or antibody, they are broadly reactive against common components of pathogenic organisms, for example, lipopolysaccharides on gram-negative organisms or other glycoconjugates. Thus, the receptors of innate immunity are the same from one individual to another within a species and, in general, do not play a role in the direct recognition of a transplanted organ. They do, however, exert their effects indirectly through the identification of "injured tissue" (e.g., as is the case when an ischemic, damaged organ is moved from one individual to another).

Once activated, the innate system performs two vital functions. It initiates cytolytic pathways for the destruction of the offending organism, primarily through the complement cascade (Fig. 25.4). In addition, the innate system can convey the encounter to the acquired immune system for a more specific response through byproducts of complement activation by activation of antigen-presenting cells (APCs). Macrophages and dendritic cells not only engulf foreign organisms that have been bound by complement, but they can also distinguish pathogens as they can be identified through receptors for foreign carbohydrates (e.g., mannose receptors). Recently, a highly evolutionarily conserved family of proteins known as Toll-like receptors (TLRs) has been described to play an important role as activation molecules for innate APCs. They bind to pathogen-associated molecular patterns, motifs common to pathogenic organisms. Some examples of TLR ligands include lipopolysaccharide, flagellin (from bacterial flagella), double-stranded viral RNA, unmethylated CpG islands of bacterial and viral DNA, zymosan (β-glucan found in fungi), and numerous heat shock proteins. In contrast to pathogen-associated molecular patterns, which

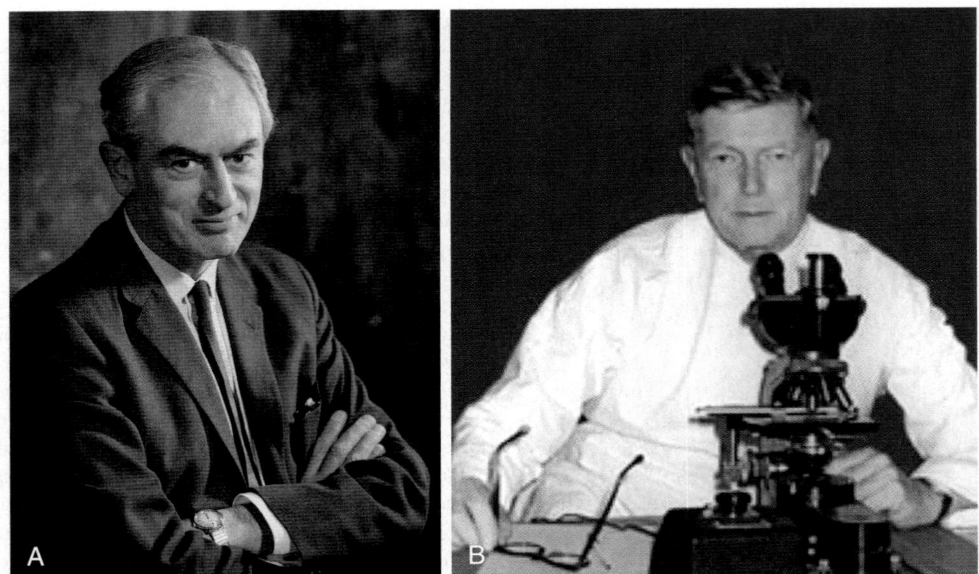

FIG. 25.3 (A) Sir Peter Medawar. (Courtesy Bern Schwartz Collection, National Portrait Gallery, London.) (B) Sir Frank Macfarlane Burnet. (Courtesy Walter and Eliza Hall Institute of Medical Research.)

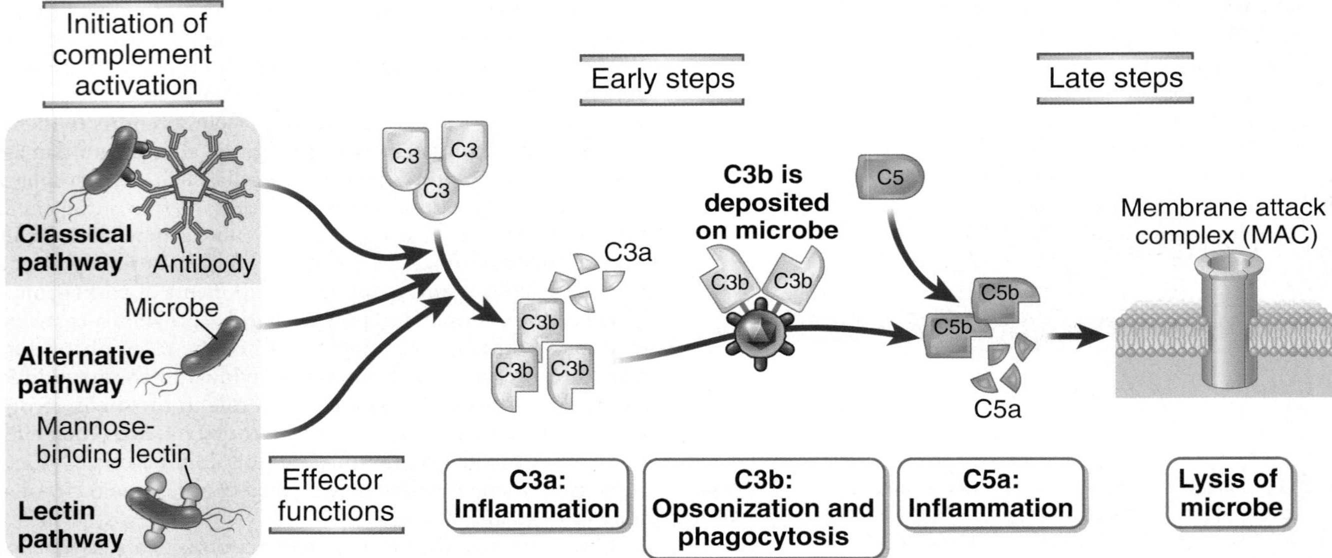

FIG. 25.4 Complement activation. There are three distinct pathways that lead to complement activation. All three pathways lead to production of *C3b*, which initiates the late steps of complement activation. *C3b* binds to the microbe and promotes opsonization and phagocytosis. *C5a* stimulates the local inflammatory response and catalyzes formation of the membrane attack complex, which results in microbial cell membrane disruption and death by lysis. (Adapted from Abbas AK, Lichtman AH, Pillai S. *Cellular and Molecular Immunology*. 9th ed. Philadelphia: Saunders Elsevier; 2018.)

initiate a response to an infectious challenge, danger-associated molecular pattern molecules (DAMPs), also called alarmins, trigger the innate inflammatory response to noninfectious cell death and injury. Many DAMPs are nuclear or cytosolic proteins or even DNA that is released or exposed in the setting of cell injury. These signals alert the innate immune system that injury has occurred and a response is required. DAMP receptors include some of the TLRs, including TLR2 and TLR4, but also a variety of other proteins, such as receptor for advanced glycosylation end-products (RAGE) and triggering receptor expressed on myeloid cells 1 (TREM-1). In the setting of a transplant surgery where an organ is cut out of one individual with a period of obligatory ischemia, cooled to near freezing, and then replaced in another individual, DAMPs play an active role in stimulating the innate inflammatory response. Once an injury or infectious insult has been identified, the cellular components of the innate system begin to initiate a response.

Monocytes

Mononuclear phagocytes are bone marrow–derived cells that initially emerge as monocytes within peripheral blood. In the setting of certain inflammatory signals, they are home to sites of injury or inflammation, where they mature and become macrophages. Their function is to acquire, process, and present antigen as well as to serve as effector cells in certain situations. Once activated, they elaborate various cytokines that regulate the local immune response. They play a significant role in facilitating the acquired T-cell response through antigen presentation, and their cytokines induce substantial tissue dysfunction in sites of inflammation. Thus, their recruitment to sites of injury and cell death can subsequently provoke T-cell activation and rejection.

Dendritic Cells

Dendritic cells are specialized macrophages that are regarded as professional APCs. They are the most potent cells that present antigen and are distributed throughout the lymphoid and nonlymphoid tissues of the body. Immature dendritic cells can be found along the gut mucosa, within the skin, and in other sites of antigen entry. Once they have encountered antigen in sites of injury, they undergo a process of maturation, including the upregulation of both major histocompatibility complex (MHC) molecules, class I and class II, as well as various costimulatory molecules. They also begin to migrate toward peripheral lymphoid tissue (i.e., lymph nodes), where they can interact with antigen-specific T cells and potentiate their activation. The dendritic cell is involved in the licensing of CD8+ T cells for cytotoxic function, stimulates T-cell clonal expansion, and provides signals for helper T cell (Th) differentiation. There are also subsets of dendritic cells that serve distinct functions in inducing and regulating the cellular response. For example, myeloid dendritic cells are more immunogenic, whereas plasmacytoid dendritic cells are more tolerogenic and may work to suppress the immune response.

Natural Killer Cells

NK cells are large granular lymphocytes with potent cytolytic function that constitute a critical component of innate immunity. They were initially discovered during studies focused on tumor immunology. There was a small subset of lymphocytes that exhibited the ability to lyse tumor cells in the absence of prior sensitization, described as "naturally" reactive. These "natural killer" cells exhibited rapid cytolytic activity and existed in a relatively mature state (i.e., morphology characteristic of activated cytotoxic lymphocytes—large size, high protein synthesis activity with abundant endoplasmic reticulum, and rapid killing activity). Further studies have indicated that NK cells lyse cell targets that lack expression of self class I MHC, termed the missing self hypothesis, a situation that could arise as a result of viral infection with suppression of self class I molecules or in tumors under strong selection pressure of killer T cells. Since those initial studies, NK cells have been found to express cell surface inhibitory receptors, which include killer inhibitory receptors. These molecules function to deliver inhibitory signals when they bind class I MHC molecules, thus preventing NK-mediated cytolysis on otherwise healthy host cells. NK cells produce various cytokines, including interferon-γ (IFN-γ), which may function to activate macrophages, which can in turn eliminate host cells infected by intracellular microbes. Similar to macrophages, NK cells express cell surface Fc receptors, which bind antibody and participate in antibody-dependent cellular cytotoxicity. NK cells also play an important role in the immune response after bone marrow transplantation and xenotransplantation. Their role in solid organ transplantation is less well defined.

Acquired Immunity

The distinguishing feature of the acquired immune system is specific recognition and disposition of foreign elements as well as the ability to recall prior challenges and to respond appropriately. Highly specific receptors, discussed later, have evolved to distinguish foreign from normal tissue through antigen binding. The term *antigen* is used to describe a molecule that can be recognized by the acquired immune system. An epitope is the portion of the antigen, generally a carbohydrate or peptide moiety, that actually serves as the binding site for the immune system receptor and is the base unit of antigen recognition. Thus, there may be one or many epitopes on any given antigen. The acquired response is divided into two distinct arms: cellular and humoral. The predominant effector cell in each arm is the T cell and B cell, respectively. Accordingly, the two main types of receptors that the immune system employs to recognize any given epitope are the TCR and B-cell receptor or antibody. In general, individual T or B lymphocytes express identical receptors, each of which binds only to a single epitope. This mechanism establishes the specificity of the acquired immune response. The antigenic encounter alters the immune system such that future challenges with the same antigen provoke a more rapid and vigorous response, a phenomenon known as immunologic memory. There are vast differences in the way each division of the acquired immune response identifies an antigen. The B-cell receptor or antibody can identify its epitope directly without preparation of the antigen, either on an invading pathogen itself or as a free-floating molecule in the extracellular fluid. T cells, however, recognize only their specific epitope after it has been processed and bound to a set of proteins, unique to the individual, which are responsible for presentation of the antigen. This set of proteins, crucial to antigen presentation, are termed histocompatibility proteins and, as their name suggests, were defined through studies examining tissue transplantation. The case of the immune response in tissue transplantation is unique and is discussed in its own section.

Major Histocompatibility Locus: Transplant Antigens

The MHC refers to a cluster of highly conserved polymorphic genes on the sixth human chromosome. Much of what we know about the details of the immune response grew from initial studies defining the immunogenetics of the MHC. Studies began in mice in which the MHC gene complex, termed *H-2*, was described by Gorer and Snell as a genetic locus that segregated with transplanted tumor survival. Subsequent serologic studies identified a similar genetic locus in humans called the human leukocyte antigen (HLA) locus. The products of these genes are expressed on a wide variety of cell types and play a pivotal role in the immune response. They are also the antigens primarily responsible for human transplant rejection, and their clinical implications are discussed later.

MHC molecules play a role in both the innate and acquired immune systems. Their predominant role, however, lies in antigen presentation within the acquired response. As mentioned earlier, the TCR does not recognize its specific antigen directly; rather, it binds to the processed antigen that is bound to cell surface proteins. It is the MHC molecule that binds the peptide antigen and interacts with the TCR, a process called antigen presentation. Thus, all T cells are restricted to an MHC for their response. There are two classes of MHC molecules, class I and class II. In general, CD8+ T cells bind to antigen within class I MHC, and CD4+ T cells bind to antigen within class II MHC.

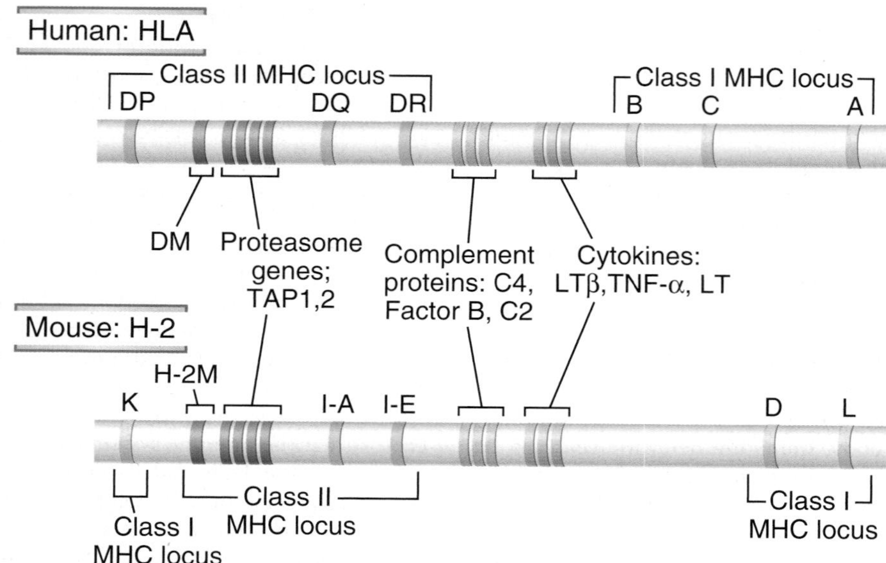

FIG. 25.5 Location and organization of the HLA complex on human chromosome 6 and H-2 complex on murine chromosome 17. The complex is conventionally divided into regions I and II. (Adapted from Abbas AK, Lichtman AH, Pillai S. *Cellular and Molecular Immunology*. 9th ed. Philadelphia: Saunders Elsevier; 2018.) *TAP*, Transporter associated with antigen processing; *TNF-α*, tumor necrosis factor-α.

Human Histocompatibility Complex

The antigens primarily responsible for human allograft rejection are those encoded by the HLA region of chromosome 6 (Fig. 25.5). The polymorphic proteins encoded by this locus include class I molecules (HLA-A, B, and C) and class II molecules (HLA-DP, DQ, and DR). There are additional class I genes with limited polymorphism (E, F, G, H, and J), but they are not currently used in tissue typing for transplantation and are not considered here. There are class III genes as well, but they are not cell surface proteins involved in antigen presentation directly but rather include molecules that are pertinent to the immune response by various mechanisms: tumor necrosis factor-α (TNF-α), lymphotoxin β, components of the complement cascade, nuclear transcription factor-β, and heat shock protein 70. Other conserved genes within the HLA include genes necessary for class I and class II presentation of peptides, such as the peptide transporter proteins TAP1 and TAP2 and proteasome proteases LMP2 and LMP7.[3] Although other polymorphic genes, referred to as minor histocompatibility antigens, exist in the genome outside of the HLA locus, they play a less significant role in transplant rejection and are not covered here. It is, however, important to point out that even HLA-identical individuals are subject to rejection on the basis of these minor differences. The blood group antigens of the ABO system must also be considered transplant antigens, and their biology is critical to humoral rejection.

Although initially identified as transplant antigens, class I and class II MHC molecules actually play vital roles in all immune responses, not just those to transplanted tissue. HLA class I molecules are present on all nucleated cells. In contrast, class II molecules are found almost exclusively on cells associated with the immune system (macrophages, dendritic cells, B cells, and activated T cells) but can be upregulated and appear on other parenchymal cells in the setting of cytokine release due to an immune response or injury.

The importance to transplantation of MHC gene products stems from their polymorphism. Unlike most genes, which are identical within a given species, polymorphic gene products differ in detail while still conforming to the same basic structure. Thus, polymorphic MHC proteins from one individual are foreign alloantigens to another individual. Recombination within the HLA locus is uncommon, occurring in approximately 1% of molecules. Consequently, the HLA type of the offspring is predictable. The unit of inheritance is the haplotype, which consists of one chromosome 6 and therefore one copy of each class I and class II locus (HLA-A, B, C, DP, DQ, and DR). Thus, donor-recipient pairings that are matched at these HLA loci are referred to as HLA-identical allografts, and those matched at half of the HLA loci are termed *haploidentical.* Note that HLA-identical allografts still differ genetically at other genetic loci and are distinct from isografts. Isografts are organs transplanted between identical twins and are immunologically indistinguishable and thus are not naturally rejected. The genetics of HLA is particularly important in understanding clinical living related donor transplantation. Each child inherits one haplotype from each parent; therefore, the chance of siblings being HLA identical is 25%. Haploidentical siblings occur 50% of the time, and completely nonidentical or HLA-distinct siblings occur 25% of the time. Biologic parents are haploidentical with their children unless there has been a rare recombination event. The degree of HLA match can also improve if the parents are homozygous for a given allele, thus giving the same allele to all children. Likewise, if the parents share the same allele, the likelihood of that allele being inherited improves to 50%. This is even more important in the field of bone marrow transplantation in which the risks of donor-mediated cytotoxicity and resultant graft-versus-host disease become a more relevant issue.

Each class I molecule is encoded by a single polymorphic gene that is combined with the nonpolymorphic protein β2-microglobulin (chromosome 15) for expression. The polymorphism of each class I molecule is extreme, with 30 to 50 alleles per locus. Class II molecules are made up of two chains, α and β, and individuals differ not only in the alleles represented at each locus but also in the number of loci present in the HLA class II region. The polymorphism of class II is thus increased by combinations of α and β chains as well as by hybrid assembly of chains from one class II locus to another. As the HLA sequence varies, the ability of various peptides to bind to the molecule and to be presented for T-cell recognition changes. Teleologically, this extreme diversity is thought to improve the likelihood that a given pathogenic peptide will fit into the binding site of these antigen-presenting molecules, thus preventing a single viral agent from evading detection by T cells of an entire population.[4]

Class I Major Histocompatibility Complex

The three-dimensional structure of class I molecules (HLA-A, B, and C) was first elucidated in 1987.[5] The class I molecule is composed of a 44-kDa transmembrane glycoprotein (α chain) in a noncovalent complex with a nonpolymorphic 12-kDa polypeptide called β_2-microglobulin. The α chain has three domains, α_1, α_2, and α_3. The critical structural feature of class I molecules is the presence of a groove formed by two α helices mounted on a β pleated sheet in the α_1 and α_2 domains (Fig. 25.6). Within this groove, a 9–amino acid peptide, formed from fragments of proteins being synthesized in the cell's endoplasmic reticulum, is mounted for presentation to T cells. Almost all the significant sequence polymorphism of class I is located in the region of the peptide-binding groove and in areas of direct T-cell contact (Fig. 25.7). The assembly of class I is dependent on association of the α chain with β2-microglobulin and native peptide within the groove. Incomplete molecules are not expressed. In general, all peptides made by a cell are candidates for presentation, although sequence alterations in this region favor certain sequences over others. The α_3 immunoglobulin (Ig)-like domain, which is the domain closest to the membrane and interacts with the CD8 molecule on the T cell, demonstrates limited polymorphism and is conserved to preserve interactions with CD8+ T cells.

Human class I presentation occurs on all nucleated cells, and expression can be increased by certain cytokines, thus allowing the immune system to inspect and to approve of ongoing protein synthesis. IFNs (IFN-α, IFN-β, and IFN-γ) induce an increase in the expression of class I molecules on a given cell by increasing levels of gene expression. T-cell activation occurs when a given T cell encounters a class I MHC molecule carrying a peptide from a nonself protein presented in the proper context (e.g., viral protein is processed in an infected cell and the peptide fragments are presented on class I molecules for T-cell recognition). So-called cross-presentation may also occur in which certain APCs, namely, a subset of dendritic cells, have the ability to take up and process exogenous antigen and present it on class I molecules to CD8+ T cells.[6] In the case of transplantation, this activation is not only possible when foreign peptide is identified after the donor MHC has been processed and presented on recipient APCs but is thought to more commonly occur when a T cell interacts directly with the donor nonself class I MHC, the so-called direct alloresponse.

Class II Major Histocompatibility Complex

The class II molecules are products of the HLA-DP, HLA-DQ, and HLA-DR genes. The structural features of class II molecules are strikingly similar to those of class I molecules. The three-dimensional structure of class II molecules was inferred by sequence homology to class I in 1988 and eventually proven by x-ray crystallography in 1993 (Fig. 25.8).[7] The class II molecules contain two polymorphic chains, one approximately 32 kDa and the other approximately 30 kDa. The peptide-binding region is composed

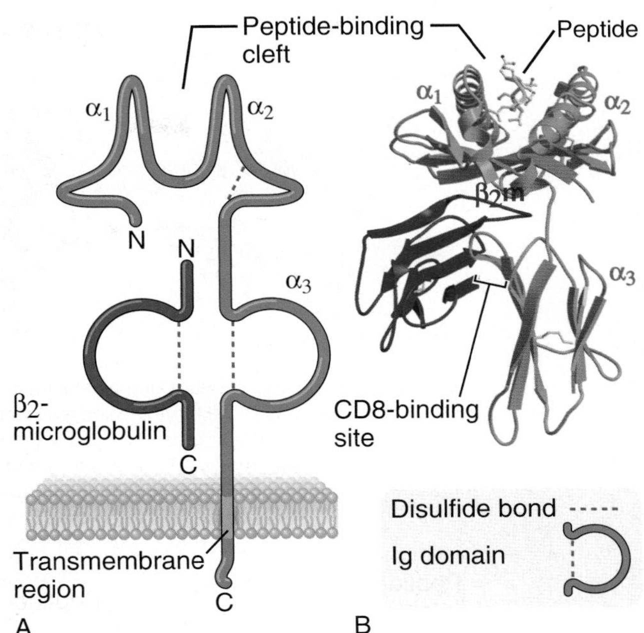

FIG. 25.6 Structure of the major histocompatibility complex class I molecule. Class I molecules are composed of polymorphic α chain noncovalently attached to the nonpolymorphic β_2-microglobulin (β_2m). (A) Schematic diagram. (B) The ribbon diagram shows the extracellular structure of a class I molecule with a bound peptide. (Adapted from Abbas AK, Lichtman AH, Pillai S. *Cellular and Molecular Immunology*. 9th ed. Philadelphia: Saunders Elsevier; 2018.)

of the α1 and β1 domains. As with the class I molecule, significant polymorphic residues of class II are located in the peptide-binding clefts and in the alpha helices around these clefts (Fig. 25.7). The Ig-like domain is composed of the α2 and β2 segments. Similar to the class I Ig-like α3 domain, there is limited polymorphism in these segments, and the β2 domain, in particular, is involved in the binding of the CD4 molecule, helping to restrict class II interactions to CD4+ T cells. Class II molecule assembly requires association of both the α chain and β chain in combination with a temporary protein called the invariant chain.[8] This third protein covers the peptide-binding groove until the class II molecule is out of the endoplasmic reticulum and is sequestered in an endosome. Proteins that are engulfed by a phagocytic cell are degraded at the same time as the invariant chain is removed, allowing peptides of external sources to be associated with and presented by class II. In this way, the acquired immune system can inspect and approve of proteins that are present in circulation or that have been liberated from foreign cells or pathogens through the phagocytic process. Accordingly, class II molecules, in contrast to class I molecules, are confined to cells related to the immune response, particularly APCs (macrophages, dendritic cells, B cells, and monocytes). Class II expression can also be induced on other cells, including endothelial cells, under the appropriate conditions. After binding class II molecules, CD4+ T cells participate in APC-mediated activation of CD8+ T cells and antibody-producing B cells. In the case of transplanted organs, ischemic injury at the time of transplantation accentuates the potential for T-cell activation by upregulation of both class I and class II molecules locally on the recipient. The trauma of surgery and ischemia also upregulate class II on all cells of the allograft, making nonself MHC more abundant. Host CD4+ T cells may then recognize donor MHC directly (direct alloresponse) or after antigen processing on the

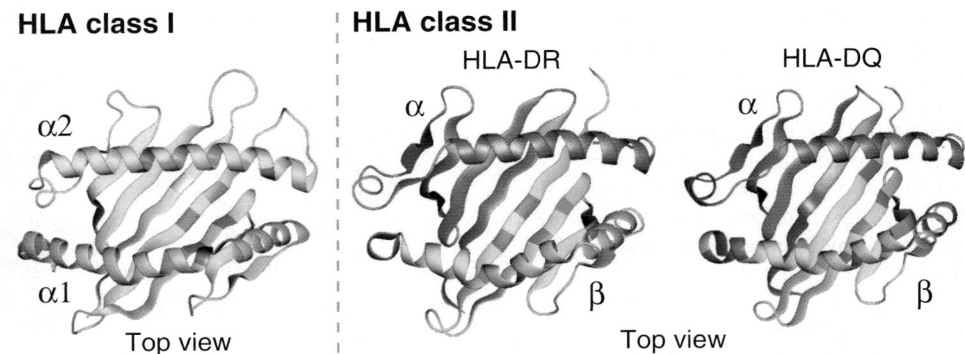

FIG. 25.7 Polymorphic residues of major histocompatibility complex (MHC) molecules. The polymorphic residues of class I and class II MHC molecules are located in the peptide-binding grooves and the α helices around the grooves. The regions of greatest variability among different human leukocyte antigen *(HLA)* alleles are indicated in *red*, of intermediate variability in *green*, and of the lowest variability in *blue*. (Adapted from Abbas AK, Lichtman AH, Pillai S. *Cellular and Molecular Immunology*. 9th ed. Philadelphia: Saunders Elsevier; 2018.)

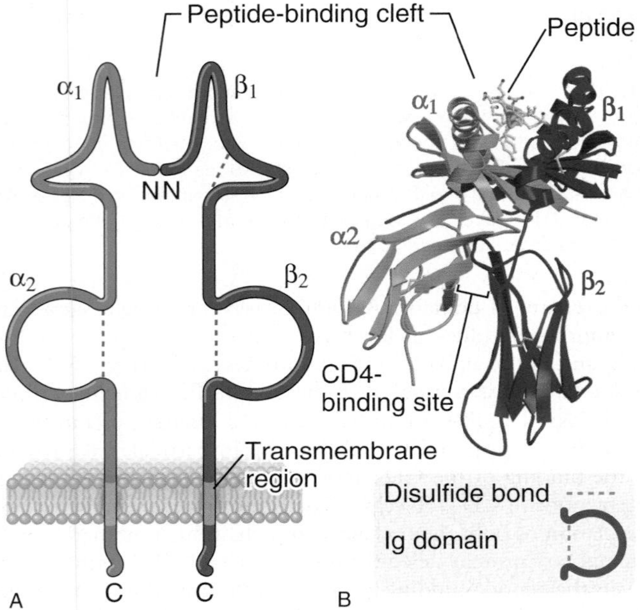

FIG. 25.8 Structure of the major histocompatibility complex class II molecule. Class II molecules are composed of a polymorphic α chain noncovalently attached to a polymorphic β chain. (A) Schematic diagram. (B) The ribbon diagram shows the extracellular structure of a class II molecule with a bound peptide. (Adapted from Abbas AK, Lichtman AH, Pillai S. *Cellular and Molecular Immunology*. 9th ed. Philadelphia: Saunders Elsevier; 2018.)

recipient's own MHC (indirect alloresponse) and then proceed to participate in rejection.

Human Leukocyte Antigen Typing: Implications for Transplantation

For the reasons already discussed, closely matched or less mismatched transplants are less likely to be recognized and rejected than are similar grafts differing by multiple alleles at the MHC. HLA matching has clear influence on the prolongation of graft survival. Humans potentially have two different HLA-A, B, and DR alleles (one from each parent, six in total). Although clearly biologically important, the HLA-C, DP, and DQ loci have historically been administratively dismissed in general organ allocation. However, reporting requirements on the genetic typing of donors have recently been expanded to include HLA-C, DP, and DQ so that these HLA molecules can also be considered for the purpose of organ allocation. Whereas current immunosuppressive regimens negate much of the impact of matching, several studies have demonstrated better renal allograft survival when the six primary alleles (A, B, and DR) are matched between donor and recipient, a so-called six-antigen match or zero-antigen mismatch (Fig. 25.9). Historically, MHC compatibility had been defined using two cellular assays: the lymphocytotoxicity assay and the mixed lymphocyte reaction. Both assays identify MHC epitopes but do not comprehensively define the entire antigen or the exact HLA genetic disparity involved. More precise molecular techniques now exist for genotyping that distinguish the nucleotide sequence of an individual's MHC.

The mixed lymphocyte reaction is performed by incubating recipient T cells with irradiated donor cells in the presence of ^{3}H-thymidine (the irradiation treatment ensures that the assay measures only proliferation of recipient T cells). If the cells differ at the class II MHC locus, recipient CD4+ T cells produce interleukin-2 (IL-2), which stimulates proliferation. Proliferating cells incorporate the labeled nucleotide into their newly manufactured DNA, which can be detected and quantified. Whereas class II polymorphism is detected by this assay, it takes several days to complete one assay. Thus, use of the mixed lymphocyte reaction as a prospective typing assay is limited to living related donors. The specific MHC alleles are not identified with this assay; instead, they are inferred from a series of reactions. Although this assay has been extremely valuable historically, it has now been largely supplanted by more modern molecular techniques. The lymphocytotoxicity assay involves taking serum from individuals with anti-MHC antibodies of known specificity and mixing it with lymphocytes from the individual in question. Exogenous complement is added, as is a vital dye, which is not taken up by intact cells. If the antibody binds to MHC, it activates the complement and leads to cell membrane disruption, and the cell takes up the vital stain. Microscopic examination of the cells can then determine if the MHC antigen was present on the cells. This, too, has been supplanted by more modern methods of MHC-specific antibody detection.

The sequencing of the HLA class I and class II loci has allowed several genetic-based techniques to be used for histocompatibility testing. These methods include restriction fragment length

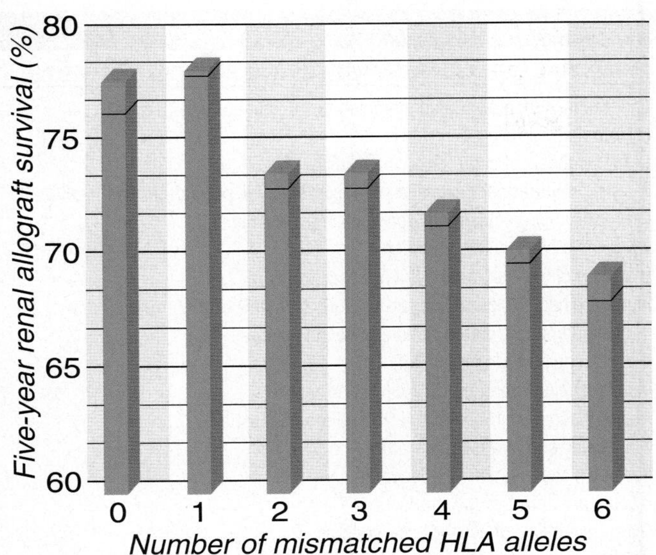

FIG. 25.9 Influence of human leukocyte antigen *(HLA)* matching on renal allograft survival. Matching of HLA alleles between donor and recipient significantly improves renal allograft survival. The data are shown for deceased donor renal allografts stratified by number of matched HLA alleles. (Adapted from Abbas AK, Lichtman AH, Pillai S. *Cellular and Molecular Immunology.* 9th ed. Philadelphia: Saunders Elsevier; 2018.)

polymorphism, oligonucleotide hybridization, and polymorphism-specific amplification using the polymerase chain reaction and sequence-specific primers. Of these methods, the polymerase chain reaction with sequence-specific primers technique is most commonly employed for class II typing. Serologic techniques are still the predominant method for class I typing because of the complexity of class I sequence polymorphism. Sequence polymorphisms that do not alter the TCR-MHC interface are unlikely to affect allograft survival; thus, the enhanced precision of molecular typing may provide more information than is actually clinically relevant.

Cellular Components of the Acquired Immune System

The key cellular components of the immune system, T cells, B cells, and APCs, are hematopoietically derived and arise from a common progenitor stem cell. The development of the lymphoid system begins with pluripotent stem cells in the liver and bone marrow of the fetus. As the fetus matures, the bone marrow becomes the primary site of lymphopoiesis. B cells were named after the primary lymphoid organ that produces B cells in birds, the bursa of Fabricius. In humans and most other mammals, precursor B cells remain within the bone marrow as they mature and fully develop. Although precursor T cells also originate in the bone marrow, they soon migrate to the thymus, the primary site of T-cell maturation, where they become "educated" to self and acquire their specific cell surface receptors and the ability to generate effector function. Mature lymphocytes are then released from the primary lymphoid organs, the bone marrow and thymus, to populate the secondary lymphoid organs including lymph nodes, spleen, and gut, as well as peripheral tissues. Each of these cells has a unique role in establishing the immune response. The highly coordinated network is regulated in part through the use of cytokines (Table 25.1).

Both B and T cells are integral components of a highly specific response that must be prepared to recognize a seemingly endless array of pathogens. This is accomplished through a unique method that allows random generation of almost unlimited receptor specificity yet controls the ultimate product by eliminating or suppressing those that might react against self and perpetuate an autoimmune response. There are fundamental differences in the manner in which T and B cells recognize antigen. B cells are structured to respond to whole antigen and in response synthesize and secrete antibody that can interact with antigen at distant sites. T cells, on the other hand, are responsible for cell-mediated immunity and of necessity must interact with cells in the periphery to neutralize and to eliminate foreign antigens. From the peripheral blood, T cells enter the lymph nodes or spleen through highly specialized regions in the postcapillary venules. Within the secondary lymphoid organ, T cells interact with specific APCs, where they receive the appropriate signals that in effect license them for effector function. They then exit the lymphoid tissues through the efferent lymph, eventually percolating through the thoracic duct and returning to the bloodstream. From there, they can return to the site of the immune response, where they encounter their specific antigen and carry out their predefined functions.

T-Cell Receptor

Considerable progress has been made in defining the mechanisms of T-cell maturation and the development of a functional TCR. The formation of the TCR is fundamental to the understanding of its function.[9] When precursor T cells migrate from the fetal liver and bone marrow to the thymus, they have yet to obtain their specialized TCR or accessory molecules. On arrival to the thymus, T cells undergo a remarkable rearrangement of the DNA that encodes the various chains of the TCR (α, β, γ, and δ) (Fig. 25.10). The order of genetic rearrangement recapitulates the evolution of the TCR. T cells first attempt to recombine the γ and δ TCR genes and then, if recombination fails to yield a properly formed receptor, resort to the more diverse α and β TCR genes. The $\gamma\delta$ configuration is typically not successful, and thus, most T cells are $\alpha\beta$ T cells. T cells expressing the $\gamma\delta$ TCR have more primitive functions, including recognition of heat shock proteins and activity similar to NK cells as well as MHC recognition, whereas $\alpha\beta$ T cells are more typically limited to recognition of MHC complexed with processed peptide.

Regardless of the genes used, individual cells recombine to express a TCR with only a single specificity. These rearrangements occur randomly and can theoretically produce 10^{15} different TCRs; however, 10^{15} T cells would weigh 500 kg and cannot all be contained in the human body. Based on computational models of homeostasis of multiclonal populations of T cells, it is estimated that approximately 10^9 naïve T-cell clonotypes (i.e., T cells with the same TCR specificity) are present at any point in time.[10] As a result, the frequency of naïve T cells available to respond to any given pathogen is relatively small, estimated to be between 1 in 200,000 and 1 in 500,000. These developing T cells also express both CD4 and CD8, accessory molecules that strengthen TCR binding to MHC. These accessory molecules further increase the binding repertoire of the population to include either class I or class II MHC molecules. If the process of T-cell maturation ended at this stage, there would be a host of T cells that could recognize self MHC–peptide complexes, resulting in an uncontrolled, global autoimmune response. To avoid the release of autoreactive T cells, developing cells undergo a process following recombination known as thymic selection (Fig. 25.11).[11] Cells initially interact with the MHC-expressing cortical thymic epithelium, which produces hormones (thymopoietin and thymosin) as well as cytokines

TABLE 25.1 **Summary of cytokines.**

CYTOKINE	SOURCE	PRINCIPAL CELLULAR TARGETS AND BIOLOGIC EFFECTS
Interleukin-1	Macrophages, endothelial cells, some epithelial cells	Endothelial cell: activation (inflammation, coagulation) Hypothalamus: fever Liver: synthesis of acute-phase proteins
Interleukin-2	T cells	T cells: proliferation, ↑ cytokine synthesis, survival, potentiates Fas-mediated apoptosis, promotes regulatory T-cell development NK cells: proliferation, activation B cells: proliferation, antibody synthesis (in vitro)
Interleukin-3	T cells	Immature hematopoietic progenitor cells: stimulates differentiation into myeloid lineage, proliferation of myeloid lineage cells
Interleukin-4	CD4+ T cells (Th2), mast cells	B cells: isotype switching to IgE T cells: Th2 differentiation, proliferation Macrophages: inhibition of IFN-γ–mediated activation Mast cells: stimulates proliferation
Interleukin-5	CD4+ T cells (Th2)	Eosinophils: activation, ↑ production B cells: proliferation, IgA production
Interleukin-6	Macrophages, endothelial cells, T cells	Liver: ↑ synthesis of acute-phase proteins B cells: proliferation of antibody-producing cells
Interleukin-7	Fibroblasts, bone marrow stromal cells	Immature hematopoietic progenitor cells: stimulates differentiation into lymphoid lineage T and B cells: important for survival during development as well as for T-cell memory
Tumor necrosis factor	Macrophages, T cells	Endothelial cells: activation (inflammation, coagulation) Neutrophils: activation Hypothalamus: fever Liver: ↑ synthesis of acute-phase proteins Muscle, fat: catabolism (cachexia) Many cell types: apoptosis
Interferon-γ	T cells (Th1, CD8+ T cells), NK cells	Macrophages: activation (increased microbicidal functions) B cells: isotype switching to IgG subclasses that facilitate complement fixation and opsonization T cells: Th1 differentiation Various cells: ↑ expression of class I and class II MHC, ↑ antigen processing and presentation to T cells
Type I interferons (IFN-α, IFN-β)	Macrophages: IFN-α Fibroblasts: IFN-β	All cells: stimulates antiviral activity including ↑ class I MHC expression NK cells: activation
Transforming growth factor-β	T cells, macrophages, other cell types	T cells: inhibition of proliferation and effector functions B cells: inhibition of proliferation, ↑ IgA production Macrophages: inhibits activation, stimulates angiogenic factors Fibroblasts: increased collagen synthesis
Lymphotoxin	T cells	Lymphoid organogenesis Neutrophils: increased recruitment and activation
BAFF (CD257)	Follicular dendritic cells, monocytes, B cells	B cells: survival and proliferation
APRIL (CD256)	T cells, follicular dendritic cells, monocytes	B cells: survival and proliferation
Interleukin-8	Lymphocytes, monocytes	Stimulates granulocyte activity Chemotactic activity
Interleukin-9	Activated Th2 lymphocytes	Enhances proliferation of T cells, mast cells
Interleukin-10	Macrophages, T cells (mainly regulatory T cells)	Macrophages and dendritic cells: inhibition of IL-12 production, stimulates expression of costimulatory molecules and class II MHC
Interleukin-11	Bone marrow stromal cells	Megakaryocytes: thrombopoiesis Liver: induces acute-phase proteins B cells: stimulates T-dependent antibody production
Interleukin-12	Macrophages, dendritic cells	T cells: Th1 differentiation NK and T cells: IFN-γ synthesis, increased cytotoxic activity
Interleukin-13	CD4+ T cells (Th2), NKT cells, mast cells	B cells: isotype switching to IgE Epithelial cells: increased mucus production Fibroblasts and macrophages: increased collagen synthesis
Interleukin-14	T cells, some B-cell tumors	B cells: enhances proliferation of activated B cells, stimulates Ig production

Continued

TABLE 25.1 Summary of cytokines.—cont'd

CYTOKINE	SOURCE	PRINCIPAL CELLULAR TARGETS AND BIOLOGIC EFFECTS
Interleukin-15	Macrophages, others	NK cells: proliferation T cells: proliferation (memory CD8+ T cells)
Interleukin-17	T cells	Endothelial cells: increased chemokine production Macrophages: increased chemokine/cytokine production Epithelial cells: GM-CSF and G-CSF production
Interleukin-18	Macrophages	NK and T cells: IFN-γ synthesis
Interleukin-21	Th2, Th17, Tfh	Drives development of Th17 and Tfh B cells: activation, proliferation, differentiation NK cells: functional maturation
Interleukin-22	Th17	Epithelial cells: production of defensins, increased barrier functions Promotes hepatocyte survival
Interleukin-23	Macrophages, dendritic cells	T cells: maintenance of IL-17–producing T cells
Interleukin-27	Macrophages, dendritic cells	T cells: inhibits production of IL-17/Th17 cells, promotes Th1 differentiation NK cells: IFN-γ synthesis
Interleukin-33	Endothelial cells, smooth muscle cells, keratinocytes, fibroblasts	Th2 development and cytokine production

Adapted from Abbas AK, Lichtman AH, Pillai S. *Cellular and Molecular Immunology*. 9th ed. Philadelphia: Saunders Elsevier; 2018.
APRIL, A proliferation-inducing ligand; *BAFF*, B cell–activating factor; *G-CSF*, granulocyte-colony stimulating factor; *GM-CSF*, granulocyte-macrophage colony-stimulating factor; *IFN*, interferon; *Ig*, immunoglobulin; *MHC*, major histocompatibility complex; *NK*, natural killer; *NKT*, natural killer T cell; *Tfh*, T follicular helper.

(e.g., IL-7) that are critical to T-cell development. If binding does not occur to self MHC, those cells are useless to the individual (e.g., they cannot bind self cells to assess for infection), and they are permitted to die by neglect through apoptosis, a process called positive selection. Thus, positive selection ensures that T cells are restricted to self MHC. Cells surviving positive selection then move to the thymic medulla and normally eventually lose either CD4 or CD8. If binding to self MHC in the medulla occurs with an unacceptably high affinity, there is an active process whereby death-promoting signals are delivered and programmed cell death is initiated, a process termed negative selection. Negative selection stands in contrast to the death that occurs by neglect when immature lymphocytes are not positively selected. Another possible, although less common, outcome of a high-affinity interaction with self peptide–MHC is the development of a regulatory T-cell (Treg) phenotype. The precise nature of this affinity threshold remains a matter of intense investigation and involves interaction with hematopoietic cells that reside in the thymus as well as medullary thymic epithelial cells. These thymically derived "natural" Tregs emerge from the thymus and are involved in the suppression of autoreactive T cells in the periphery, which is discussed later.

The only cells released into the periphery are those that can both bind self MHC and avoid activation. Whereas T cells are restricted to bind self MHC–peptide complexes without activation, the selection process does not consider foreign MHC. Thus, by random chance, some cells with appropriate affinity for self MHC survive and have inappropriately high affinity for the MHC molecules of other individuals. In the setting of transplantation, these recipient T cells are able to recognize donor MHC–peptide complexes because there are sufficient conserved motifs shared between donor and self MHC molecules. However, because donor MHC was not present during the thymic education process, the binding of donor MHC by an "alloreactive" T cell leads to activation, and rejection ensues. The precursor frequency or the number of alloreactive T cells is much higher than the 1 in 200,000 or 1 in 500,000 T cells available to react toward any given antigen. Because T cells are selected to bind self MHC, the frequency specific for a similar, nonself MHC (i.e., alloreactive) is estimated to be between 1% and 10% of all T cells.[12]

In addition to thymic selection, it is now clear that mechanisms exist for peripheral modification of the T-cell repertoire. Many of these mechanisms are in place for removal of T cells after an immune response and downregulation of activated clones. CD95, a molecule known as Fas, is a member of the tumor necrosis factor (TNF) receptor superfamily and is expressed on activated T cells. Under appropriate conditions, binding of this molecule to its ligand, CD178, promotes programmed cell death of a cohort of activated T cells. This method is dependent on TCR binding and the activation state of the T cell. Complementing this deletional method to TCR repertoire control are nondeletional mechanisms that selectively anergize (make unreactive) specific T-cell clones. In addition to signaling through the TCR complex, T cells require additional costimulatory signals (described in detail later). TCR binding leads to T-cell activation only if the costimulatory signals are present, generally delivered by APCs. In the absence of costimulation, the cell remains unable to proceed toward activation and in some circumstances becomes refractory to activation even with the appropriate signals. Thus, TCR binding that occurs to self in the absence of appropriate antigen presentation or active inflammation results in an aborted activation and prevents self-reactivity.

T-Cell Activation

T-cell activation is a sophisticated series of events that has only recently been more fully described. The TCR, unlike antibody, recognizes its ligand only in the context of MHC. By requiring that T cells respond only to antigen encountered when it is physically embedded on self cells, the system avoids constant activation by soluble molecules.

T cells can then specifically recognize and destroy cells that make peptide products of mutation or viral infection. Because the number of potential antigens is high and the likelihood is that self-antigens vary minimally from foreign antigens, the nature of the TCR-binding event has evolved such that a single interaction with an MHC molecule is not sufficient to cause activation. In fact, a T

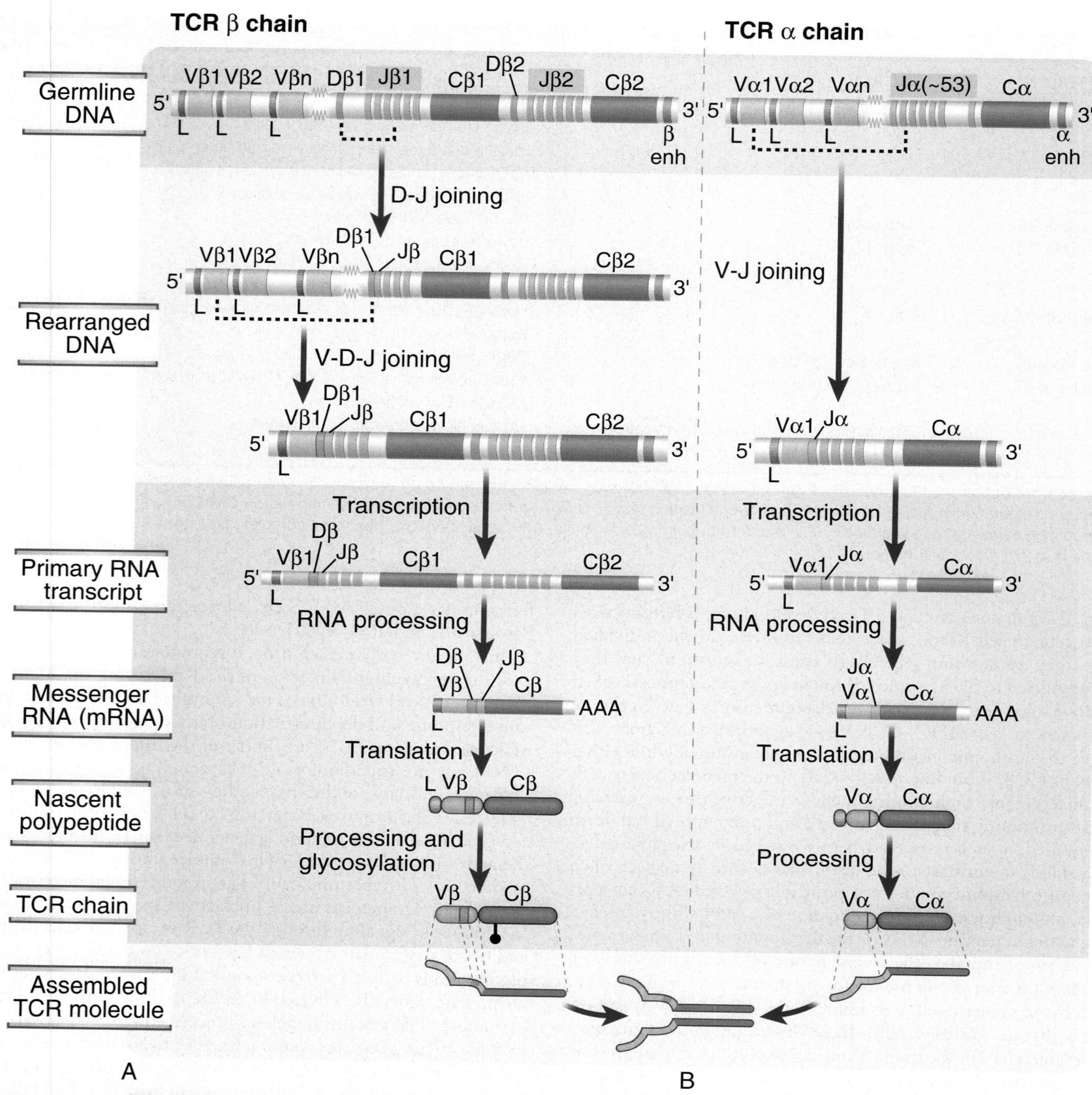

FIG. 25.10 T-cell receptor *(TCR)* recombination and expression (α and β loci shown here). There is an elaborate genetic rearrangement that leads to the formation of a diverse repertoire of TCRs. Genomic DNA is spliced under the direction of specific enzymes active during T-cell development within the thymus. Random segments from regions termed variable *(V)*, joining *(J)*, diversity *(D)*, and constant *(C)* are brought together to form a unique gene responsible for a unique TCR chain. The γ and δ loci recombine first, and if successful, a γδ TCR is formed. If unsuccessful, then α and β regions recombine to form an αβ TCR. Approximately 95% of T cells progress to express an αβ TCR. (Adapted from Abbas AK, Lichtman AH, Pillai S. *Cellular and Molecular Immunology*. 9th ed. Philadelphia: Saunders Elsevier; 2018.)

cell must register a signal from approximately 8000 TCR-ligand interactions with the same antigen before a threshold of activation is reached. Each event results in the internalization of the TCR. Because resting T cells have low TCR density, sequential binding and internalization during several hours are required. Transient encounters are not sufficient. This threshold is reduced considerably by appropriate costimulation signals (detailed later).

Most TCRs are heterodimers composed of two transmembrane polypeptide chains, α and β. The αβ-TCR is noncovalently associated with several other transmembrane signaling proteins, including CD3 (composed of three separate chains, γ, δ, and ε) and ζ chain molecules, as well as the appropriate accessory molecule from the T cell, either CD4 or CD8, which associates with its respective MHC molecule. Together, these proteins are known as

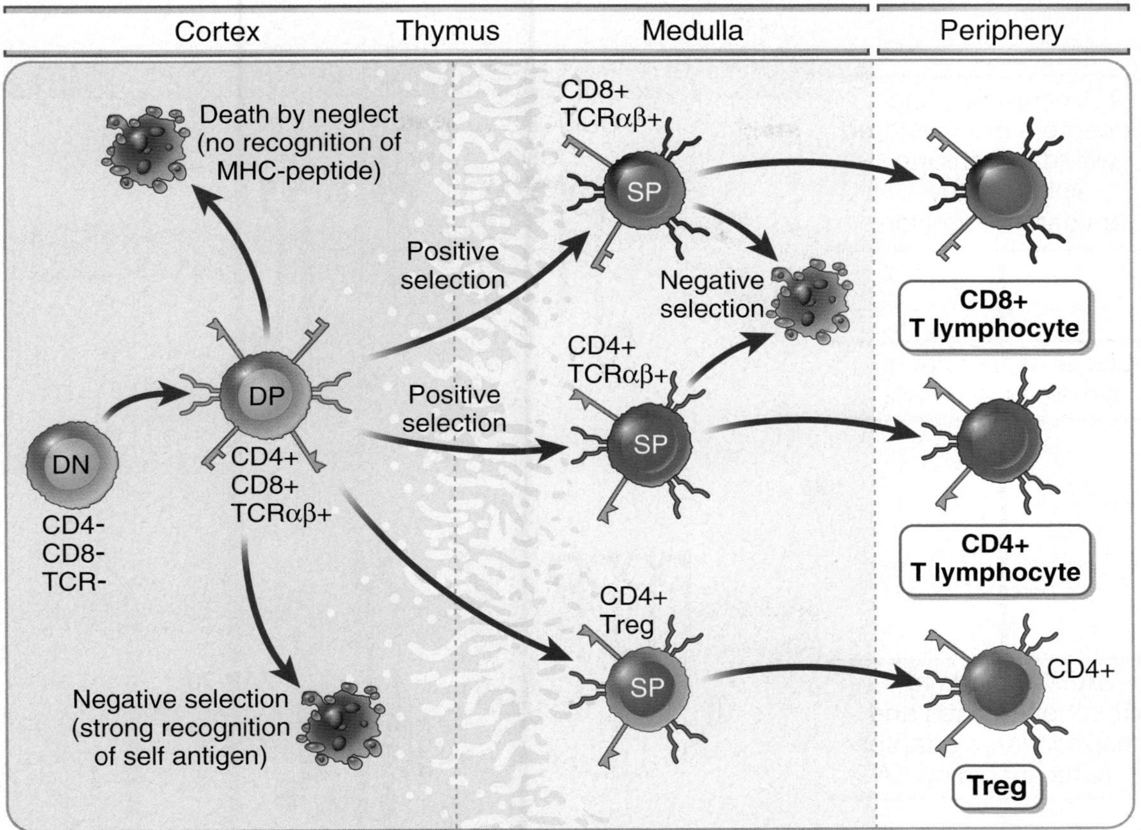

FIG. 25.11 T-cell maturation. Initially, bone marrow-derived T-cell precursors arrive in the thymic cortex lacking CD4, CD8, or a T-cell receptor *(TCR)* and are referred to as double negative. The genes responsible for expression of the TCR chains subsequently undergo a series of recombination events resulting in expression of either a γδ TCR or, more commonly (>90%), an αβ TCR on the cell surface. The γδ T cells proceed through a distinct selection process that is independent of major histocompatibility complex *(MHC)* restriction. The αβ T cells acquire expression of both CD4 and CD8 and are then referred to as double positive. They then proceed to undergo the process of positive and negative selection and ultimately express only CD4 or CD8, depending on which class of MHC they restrict to. (Adapted from Abbas AK, Lichtman AH, Pillai S. *Cellular and Molecular Immunology*. 9th ed. Philadelphia: Saunders Elsevier; 2018.)

the TCR complex. When the TCR is bound to an MHC molecule and the proper configuration of accessory molecules stabilizes its binding, a signal is initiated by intracytoplasmic protein tyrosine kinases (Fig. 25.12). These protein tyrosine kinases include p56lck (on CD4 or CD8), p59Fyn, and ZAP-70, the last two of which are associated with CD3. Repetitive binding signals combined with the appropriate secondary costimulation eventually activate phospholipase-γ1, which in turn hydrolyzes the membrane lipid phosphatidylinositol bisphosphate, thereby releasing inositol trisphosphate and diacylglycerol. Inositol trisphosphate binds to the endoplasmic reticulum, causing a release of calcium that induces calmodulin to bind to and activate calcineurin. Calcineurin dephosphorylates the critical cytokine transcription factor nuclear factor of activated T cells (NFAT), prompting it, with the transcription factor nuclear factor κB (NF-κB), to initiate transcription of cytokines including IL-2 and its receptor. Resting T cells express only low levels of the IL-2 receptor (CD25), but with activation, IL-2R expression is increased. As the activated T cell begins to produce IL-2 secondary to events initiated by TCR activation, the cytokine begins to work in both autocrine and paracrine fashions, potentiating diacylglycerol activation of protein kinase C. Protein kinase C is important in activating many gene regulatory steps critical for cell division. This effect, however, is restricted only to T cells that have undergone activation after encountering their specific antigen leading to IL-2R expression. Thus, the process limits proliferation and expansion to only those clones specific for the offending antigen. As the antigenic stimulus is removed, IL-2R density decreases and the TCR complex is reexpressed on the cell surface. There is a negative feedback system between the TCR and the IL-2R, resulting in a highly regulated and efficient system that is reactive only in the presence of antigen and ceases to function once antigen is removed. Not surprisingly, many of these steps in T-cell activation have been targeted in the development of immunosuppressive agents. These are discussed in detail in a subsequent section of this chapter.

Costimulation

Recognition of the antigenic peptide–MHC complex through TCR binding is usually not sufficient alone to generate a response in a naïve T cell. Additional signals through so-called costimulatory pathways are required for optimal T-cell activation.[13,14] In fact, receipt of TCR complex signaling, often referred to as signal 1, in the absence of costimulation or signal 2 not only fails to achieve activation but also can lead to a state of inaction or anergy (Fig. 25.13).

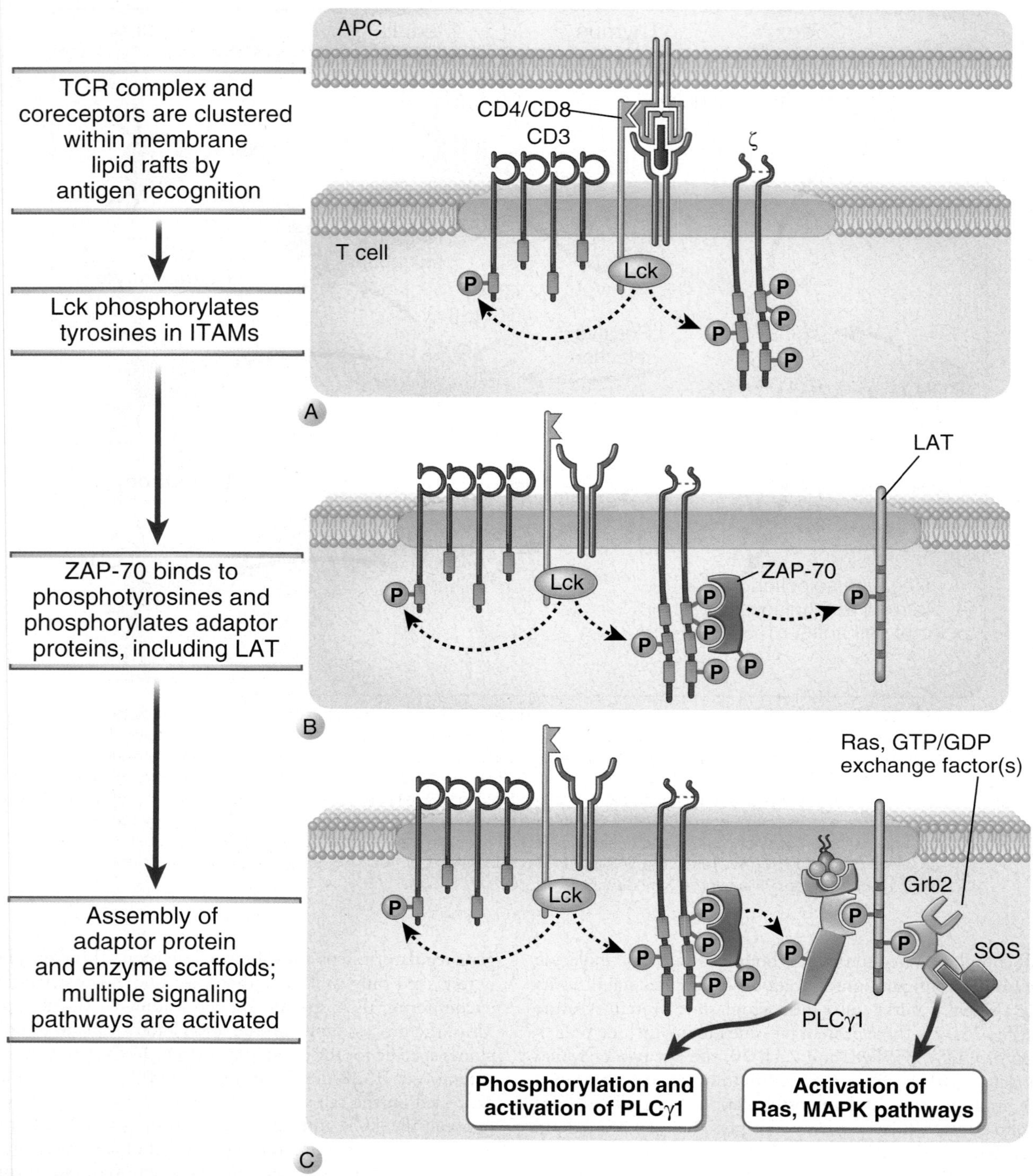

FIG. 25.12 T-cell activation. On antigen recognition, there is a clustering of T-cell receptor *(TCR)* complexes and coreceptors that initiates a cascade of signaling events within the T cell. Tyrosine kinases associated with the coreceptors (e.g., Lck) phosphorylate CD3 and the ζ chain (A). The ζ chain association protein kinase (ZAP-70) subsequently associates with these regions and becomes activated. ZAP-70 phosphorylates various adaptor molecules, such as LAT (B). These adaptors become docking sites for other enzymes such as PLCγ1 that ultimately lead to the activation of upstream cellular enzymes (e.g., Ras and MAPK pathways) (C). These enzymes then activate transcription factors that promote expression of various genes involved in proliferation and T-cell responses. (Adapted from Abbas AK, Lichtman AH, Pillai S. *Cellular and Molecular Immunology*. 9th ed. Philadelphia: Saunders Elsevier; 2018.)

An anergic T cell is rendered unable to respond even if given both of the appropriate stimuli.[15] This characteristic of the immune system is thought to be one of the major mechanisms in tolerance to self-antigens in the periphery, crucial in the prevention of autoimmunity. Researchers have exploited this discovery using antibodies or receptor fusion proteins designed to block interactions between key costimulatory molecules at the time of antigen exposure. Much of the research to date has focused on the interactions of two costimulatory pathways, the CD28/B7 pathway (Ig-like superfamily members) and CD40/CD154 pathway (TNF/TNFR superfamily

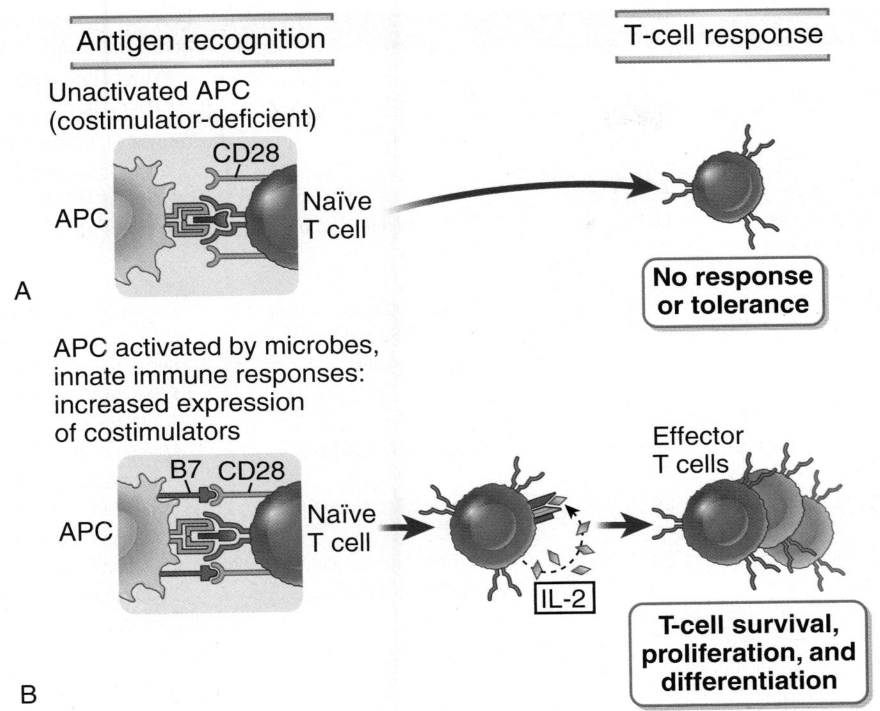

FIG. 25.13 T-cell costimulation. Naïve T cells require multiple signals for efficient activation. (A) Signal 1 occurs when the T-cell receptor (TCR) recognizes its putative major histocompatibility complex–peptide combination. In the absence of any additional signals, there is an aborted response or anergy, a state in which the cell is no longer available for stimulation. (B) TCR signaling in conjunction with signals received through costimulatory molecules (e.g., B7 molecules), signal 2, promotes effective T-cell activation and function. (Adapted from Abbas AK, Lichtman AH, Pillai S. *Cellular and Molecular Immunology*. 9th ed. Philadelphia: Saunders Elsevier; 2018.) *APC*, Antigen-presenting cell; *IL-2*, interleukin-2.

members). There have been, however, many additional pairings within these same families and others that have been found to have distinct roles in costimulatory function (Table 25.2).

CD28, present on T cells, and the B7 molecules CD80 and CD86 on APCs were among the first costimulatory molecules to be described. Ligation of CD28 is necessary for optimal IL-2 production and can lead to the production of additional cytokines, such as IL-4 and IL-8, and chemokines, such as Regulated upon Activation, Normal T Cell Expressed and Presumably Secreted (RANTES), as well as protect T cells from activation-induced apoptosis through the upregulation of antiapoptotic factors such as Bcl-X_L and Bcl-2. CD28 is expressed constitutively on most T cells, whereas the expression of CD80 and CD86 is largely restricted to professional APCs, such as dendritic cells, monocytes, and macrophages. The kinetics of CD80/CD86 expression is complex, but they are typically increased with the induction of the immune response. Another ligand for CD80 and CD86 is CTLA-4 (CD152). This molecule is upregulated and expressed on the surface of T cells after activation, and it binds CD80/CD86 with 10 to 20 times greater affinity than CD28. CTLA-4 has been shown to have a negative regulatory effect on T-cell activation and proliferation, an observation supported by the fact that CTLA-4–deficient mice develop a lethal lymphoproliferative disorder. The negative regulatory effect of CTLA-4 is mediated through both cell intrinsic activation of intracellular phosphatases and cell extrinsic mechanism in which CTLA-4 binding actually removes CD80/CD86 from the surface of the APC, thereby limiting the availability of ligands for CD28 costimulation. The therapeutic potential of costimulation blockade was first made apparent through the development of CTLA-4–Ig, an engineered fusion protein composed of the extracellular portion of the CTLA-4 molecule and a portion of the human Ig molecule. This compound binds CD80 and CD86 and prevents costimulation through CD28. Several clinical trials in autoimmunity have demonstrated the efficacy of CTLA-4–Ig (abatacept). More recently, a higher-affinity, second-generation version, belatacept, has been tested with success as a replacement for calcineurin inhibitors and was approved in 2011 for kidney transplant recipients.[16,17]

Closely related to the CD28/B7 pathway is the CD40/CD154 (CD40L) pathway. Evidence for the crucial role of the CD40/CD154 pathway in the immune response came to light after the observation that hyper-IgM syndrome results from a mutational defect in the gene encoding CD154. In addition to defects in the generation of T cell–dependent antibody responses, patients with hyper-IgM syndrome also have defects in T cell–mediated immune responses. CD40 is a cell surface molecule expressed on endothelium, B cells, dendritic cells, and other APCs. Its ligand, CD154, is primarily found on activated T cells. Upregulation of CD154 after TCR signaling allows signals to be sent to the APC through CD40; in particular, it is a critical signal for B-cell activation and proliferation. CD40 binding is required for APCs to stimulate a cytotoxic T-cell response. It leads to the release of activating cytokines, particularly IL-12, and the upregulation of B7 molecules. It also initiates innate functions of APCs, including nitric oxide synthesis and phagocytosis. Interestingly, CD154 is also released in soluble form by activated platelets. Thus, sites of trauma that attract activated platelets simultaneously recruit the ligand required to activate tissue-based APCs, providing a link

TABLE 25.2 Costimulatory molecules.

RECEPTOR	DISTRIBUTION	LIGAND	DISTRIBUTION	PRINCIPAL EFFECTS AND FUNCTIONS
CD28	T cells	CD80/CD86	Activated APCs	Lowers the threshold for T-cell activation Promotes survival, ↑ antiapoptotic factors Promotes Th1 phenotype
CD40	Dendritic cells, B cells, macrophages, endothelial cells	CD154	T cells, soluble platelets	Induces CD80/CD86 expression on APCs
CD27	T cells, NK cells, B cells	CD70	Thymic epithelium, activated T cells, activated B cells, mature dendritic cells	Enhances T-cell proliferation and survival Acts after CD28 to sustain effector T-cell survival Influences secondary responses more than primary Promotes B-cell differentiation and memory formation
CD30	Activated T cells, activated B cells	CD153	B cells, activated T cells	Maintains survival of primed and memory T cells Promotes Th2 > Th1
CD95 (Fas)	T cells, B cells, APCs, stromal cells	CD178 (FasL)	T cells, APCs, stromal cells	Involved in peripheral T-cell homeostasis through "fratricide," may deliver costimulatory signal
CD134 (OX40)	Activated T cells CD4+ > CD8+	CD252 (OX40L)	Activated T cells, mature dendritic cells, activated B cells	Important for CD4+ T-cell expansion and survival ↑ Antiapoptotic factors Functions after CD28 to sustain CD4+ T-cell survival Enhances cytokine production Augments effector and memory CD4+ T-cell function Promotes Th2 > Th1
CD137 (4-1BB)	Activated T cells CD8+ > CD4+ Monocytes, follicular dendritic cells, NK cells	4-1BBL	Mature dendritic cells, activated B cells, activated macro phages	Sustains rather than initiates CD8+ T-cell responses Functions after CD28 to sustain T-cell survival Important in antiviral immunity Promotes CD8+ effector function and cell survival
CD152 (CTLA-4)	Activated T cells	CD80/CD86	Activated APCs	Higher affinity for CD80/CD86 than CD28, inhibits T-cell response
HVEM	T cells, monocytes, immature dendritic cells	CD258 (LIGHT)	Activated lymphocytes, immature dendritic cells, NK cells	Augments T-cell responses, CD8+ > CD4+ Promotes dendritic cell maturation
		CD272 (BTLA)	Activated T cells, B cells, dendritic cells	Negative costimulator, inhibits IL-2 production BTLA remains expressed on Th1 but not Th2
		CD160	NK cells, cytolytic CD8+ T cells, γδ T cells	Negative regulator of CD4+ T-cell activation Inhibits proliferation and cytokine production
CD265 (RANK)	Dendritic cells	CD254 (TRANCE)	Activated T cells CD4+ > CD8+	Enhances dendritic cell survival, upregulates Bcl-xl, possibly enhances IFN-γ production
CD279 (PD-1)	T cells	CD274 (PD-L1)	T cells, B cells, APCs, some parenchymal cells	Inhibits activation, proliferation, and acquisition of effector cell function Th1 > Th2
		CD273 (PD-L2)	Dendritic cells, macrophages	Inhibits activation, proliferation, and acquisition of effector cell function Th2 > Th1
CD278 (ICOS)	Activated T cells, memory T cells	CD275 (ICOSL)	Dendritic cells, B cells, macrophages	Promotes survival and expansion of effector T cells, possibly promotes Th2 responses
GITR	Tregs, CD8+ T cells, B cells, macrophages	GITRL	B cells, dendritic cells, macrophages, endothelial cells	Marker for Tregs, allows proliferation of Tregs Promotes T-cell proliferation and cytokine production Negative regulator for NK function

APC, Antigen-presenting cell; *BTLA*, B and T lymphocyte–associated; *CTLA*, cytotoxic T lymphocyte–associated; *GITR*, glucocorticoid-induced tumor necrosis factor receptor; *GITRL*, glucocorticoid-inducted tumor necrosis factor receptor ligand; *HVEM*, herpes virus entry mediator; *ICOS*, inducible costimulator; *ICOSL*, inducible costimulator ligand; *NK*, natural killer; *PD*, programmed death; *RANK*, receptor activator of NFκB; *Treg*, regulatory T cell.

between innate and acquired immunity. Antibody preparations against CD154 have shown great promise in experimental models, but initial clinical trials were halted because of concern for unexpected thrombotic complications. There continues to be hope that anti-CD154 antibodies that bind distinct epitopes, Fc-silent domain antibodies devoid of cross-linking abilities, or antibodies directed toward CD40 may circumvent this issue (See "Immunosuppression" section).

Since earlier investigations, multiple other pairings of molecules have been characterized and shown to demonstrate costimulatory or coinhibitory activity. It is the sum of these positive costimulatory and negative coinhibitory signals that shapes the character and magnitude of the T-cell response.[18] CD278 (inducible costimulator, or ICOS) is a CD28 superfamily expressed on activated T cells, and its ligand, CD275 (ICOSL or B7-H2), is expressed on APCs. Unlike CD28, ICOS is not present on naïve T cells, but instead expression is upregulated after T-cell activation and persists on memory T cells. ICOS can function to boost activation of effector T cells in general but in particular plays a critical role in the function of T follicular helper (Tfh) cells, a specialized CD4+ T-cell subset involved in the germinal center reaction and generation of class-switched antibody. Another member of the CD28 superfamily, programmed death (PD-1) (CD279), and its ligands PD-L1 (CD274) and PD-L2 (CD273), both B7 family members, have been shown to be involved in negative regulation of cellular immunity. More recently, coinhibitory molecules PD-1H (also known as VISTA for V domain Ig suppressor of T cell activation) and B and T lymphocyte–associated (BTLA) have joined this list. Several members of the TNF/TNFR superfamily have been shown to play important roles in T-cell costimulation. These include CD134/CD252 (OX40/OX40L), CD137/CD137L (4-1BB/4-1BBL), CD27/CD70, CD95/CD178 (Fas/FasL), CD30/CD153, receptor activator of NFκB/TNF-related activation-induced cytokines (RANK/TRANCE), and others. Furthermore, members of the CD2 family function in both costimulatory (i.e., CD2) and coinhibitory (i.e., 2B4) roles during the execution of an alloimmune response. Finally, the T cell–Ig mucin-like family of molecules has been shown to play important coinhibitory roles during alloimmunity, both on effector cells and on Tregs.

In addition to the multitude of costimulatory molecules, many other adhesion molecules expressed on the cell surface (intercellular adhesion molecule, selectins, integrins) control the movement of immune cells through the body, regulate their trafficking to specific areas of inflammation, and nonspecifically strengthen the TCR-MHC binding interaction. They differ from costimulation molecules in that they enhance the interaction of the T cell with other cell types and antigen without directly influencing the quality of the TCR response. There are two main families of cellular adhesion molecules within the immune system: the selectins and the integrins. The selectin family of adhesion molecules is responsible for "rolling," the initial attachment of leukocytes to vascular endothelial cells at sites of tissue injury and inflammation before their firm adhesion (mediated by integrin binding). The selectin family of proteins is composed of three closely related molecules, each having differential expression on immune cells: L-selectin is expressed on leukocytes, P-selectin is expressed on platelets, and E-selectin is expressed on endothelium. Structurally, all selectins share an amino-terminal lectin domain that interacts with a carbohydrate ligand, an epidermal growth factor–like domain, and two to nine short repeating units that share homology with sequences found in some complement-binding proteins. In contrast to most other adhesion molecules that also possess some signaling or costimulatory functionality, selectins function solely to facilitate leukocyte binding to vascular endothelium. This selectin-mediated loose binding is converted into tight adhesion after activation of leukocyte integrins. Integrins are transmembrane receptors that serve as bridges for cell-cell as well as for cell–extracellular matrix interactions. Many are expressed constitutively on cells of the immune system (i.e., leukocyte function antigen 1) but on sensing inflammatory cytokine or chemokine signals, such as IL-8, are induced to change conformation that results in higher avidity interaction with integrin ligands, resulting in leukocyte extravasation into inflamed tissue. Both selectins and integrins are potential therapeutic targets to inhibit access of donor-reactive T cells into the allograft and weaken proimmune interactions.

T-Cell Effector Functions

During thymic education, most T cells initially express both CD4 and CD8 molecules, but subsequently, T cells become either CD4+ or CD8+, depending on which MHC class they restrict to. Thus, these accessory molecules govern which type of MHC and by extension which types of cells a given T cell can interact with and evaluate. Because there is nearly ubiquitous expression of class I MHC, all cell types are surveyed. These class I molecules display peptides that are generated within the cell (e.g., peptides from normal cellular processes or from internal viral replication). T cells responsible for inspecting all cells express the accessory molecule CD8, which in turn binds to class I and specifically stabilizes a TCR interaction with a class I–presented antigen. Thus, CD8+ T cells evaluate most cell types and mediate destruction of altered cells. Appropriately, they have been termed cytotoxic T cells.

APCs are the predominant cell type that expresses class II MHC molecules in addition to class I. Class II molecules display peptides that have been sampled from surrounding extracellular spaces through phagocytosis and thus usually represent the presentation of newly acquired antigen. Cells initiating an immune response need to have access to this newly processed antigen. CD4 binds class II MHC and stabilizes the interaction of the TCR with the class II–peptide complex. Thus, under physiologic conditions, CD4+ T cells are first alerted to an invasion of the body by hematopoietically derived APCs that present their newly acquired antigen in the form of processed peptide in a class II molecule. As a consequence of their MHC restriction, these subpopulations of T cells have several different functions. CD4+ T cells typically contribute to the response in a helper or regulatory role, whereas CD8+ T cells are much more likely to play a part in cell elimination through cytotoxic functions.

After activation, CD4+ T cells initially play a critical role in the expansion of the immune response. After encountering an APC that expresses the specific antigenic peptide–MHC class II pairing, the CD4+ T cell can then signal back to the APC to promote factors that allow CD8+ T-cell activation. This process is accomplished by expression of specific costimulatory molecules and the release of certain cytokines. This licensing of CD8+ T cells for cytotoxic function is a key step within the immune response. This describes in part how CD4+ T cells become helper cells. More recently, there has been further elucidation of their cellular differentiation into several well-defined Th subsets, including Th1, Th2, Th17, and Tfh cells, which are largely defined on the basis of the distinct transcription factors they express and the cytokines they elaborate (Fig. 25.14). The main cytokine driving the differentiation of Th1 cells is IL-12, and mature Th1 cells mediate effector function through the release of IFN-γ and TNF. The predominant role of IFN-γ is to enhance macrophage function and activity as well as

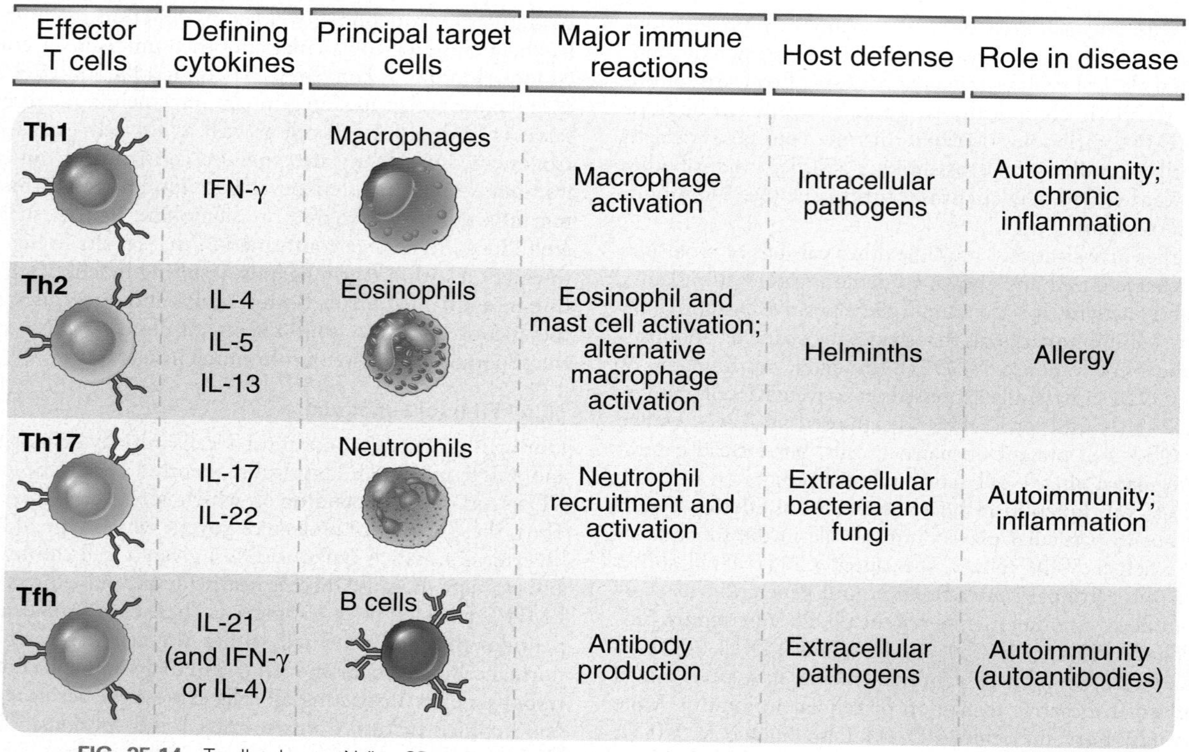

Effector T cells	Defining cytokines	Principal target cells	Major immune reactions	Host defense	Role in disease
Th1	IFN-γ	Macrophages	Macrophage activation	Intracellular pathogens	Autoimmunity; chronic inflammation
Th2	IL-4 IL-5 IL-13	Eosinophils	Eosinophil and mast cell activation; alternative macrophage activation	Helminths	Allergy
Th17	IL-17 IL-22	Neutrophils	Neutrophil recruitment and activation	Extracellular bacteria and fungi	Autoimmunity; inflammation
Tfh	IL-21 (and IFN-γ or IL-4)	B cells	Antibody production	Extracellular pathogens	Autoimmunity (autoantibodies)

FIG. 25.14 T-cell subsets. Naïve CD4+ T cells may differentiate into distinct subsets of effector cells in response to antigen, costimulatory, or coinhibitory signals and cytokines. Th1 cells produce interferon-γ *(IFN-γ)*, which activates macrophages to kill intracellular microbes. Th2 cells produce cytokines (interleukin *[IL]*-4, IL-5, and others) that stimulate immunoglobulin E production and activate eosinophils in response to parasitic infection. Th17 cells secrete IL-17 and IL-22; they play an important role in responses to fungi and contribute to several autoimmune inflammatory diseases. Tfh cells produce IL-21 and provide help to B cells for antibody production. (Adapted from Abbas AK, Lichtman AH, Pillai S. *Cellular and Molecular Immunology*. 9th ed. Philadelphia: Saunders Elsevier; 2018.)

to promote cell-mediated immunity. Activated macrophages then proceed to ingest and to kill invading microbes, and at the same time, the acquired immune system is directed to produce antibodies that promote opsonization, thereby enhancing the overall process. Th2 cell differentiation, in contrast, is driven by the presence of IL-4 and results in release of IL-4, IL-5, IL-10, and IL-13, which ultimately inhibit macrophage activation and promote IgE production and eosinophil activation. Th17 cells are an inflammatory CD4+ subset that plays a major role in the protective immune response against fungal pathogens and extracellular bacteria. Th17 cells are generated in the presence of transforming growth factor-β (TGF-β) and IL-6 and are potent secretors of the inflammatory cytokines IL-17 and IL-23. Interestingly, in addition to their role in protective immunity, Th17 cells have been associated with several autoimmune diseases, including multiple sclerosis, rheumatoid arthritis, and psoriasis, and several immunomodulatory therapies are being developed to impair their activity in these patients. Finally, Tfh cells are ICOS+ PD-1+ cells that home to lymphoid germinal centers by virtue of their expression of the chemokine receptor CXCR5, where they provide help for the generation of class-switched, high-affinity IgG responses. Tfh cells provide this help in the form of CD154 expression and the secretion of IL-21.

An important feature of these CD4+ Th cells is the ability of one subset to regulate the activity of the other. For example, IL-10 produced by Th2 cells and Tregs negatively regulates transcription of IFN-γ mRNA. Thus, the initial steps in differentiation depend greatly on the surrounding immunologic milieu, which ultimately influences the character of the immune response. Furthermore, more recent fate mapping studies have revealed a high degree of plasticity between Th subsets, demonstrating that cells of one Th subset can under certain conditions transdifferentiate into another Th subset.

Another subset of CD4+ T cells that has been described to play a critical role in the ability of the immune system to temper its response is the Treg population. Tregs suppress immune responses either through direct cell-cell contact with effector cells or indirectly through their interaction with APCs. These cells not only have the ability to suppress cytokines, adhesion molecules, and costimulatory signals but are also able to focus this response by expression of integrins, which allow Tregs to home to the location of immune engagement. The most extensively studied population of Tregs are those CD4+ T cells that express CD25 (the high-affinity α chain of the IL-2 receptor).[19] CD4+CD25+ cells express the transcription factor Foxp3, a protein that has been shown to be both necessary and sufficient for the differentiation of CD4+ T cells into Tregs. Indeed, both mice and humans that lack functional Foxp3 molecule develop severe systemic autoimmunity. Thus, CD4+CD25+ Foxp3+ T cells have been the target of numerous attempts to alter immune function and are being tested in clinical trials of cellular immunotherapy to control graft rejection after transplantation and to mitigate autoimmunity. Foxp3+ Tregs develop during T-cell thymic development after recognition of self-antigen in the thymus (with signal strength that is not sufficient to induce negative selection). These so-called natural Tregs (also termed thymic Tregs) express a TCR repertoire distinct from that of conventional T cells and are important for maintaining immune homeostasis and preventing autoimmunity. However, Foxp3+ Tregs can also develop extrathymically during the course of an immune response, and studies have shown that these cells are elicited by stimulation with low-dose antigen or under conditions of limited CD154 costimulation. These so-called induced Tregs (also termed peripheral Tregs) are highly specific for the antigen by which they were elicited and thus may be more potent suppressors of autoimmunity and transplant rejection when used as cellular immunotherapy.

Unlike CD4+ T cells, CD8+ T cells function primarily to eliminate infected or defective cells. As mentioned before, licensing occurs through APC interactions, and subsequent cell killing occurs by either a calcium-dependent secretory mechanism or a calcium-independent mechanism that requires direct cell contact. In the calcium-dependent mechanism, the rise in intracellular calcium after activation triggers exocytosis of cytolytic granules. These granules contain a lytic protein called perforin and serine proteases called granzymes. Perforin polymerization creates defects in the target cell's membrane, allowing granzyme activity to lyse the cell. In the absence of calcium, T cells can induce apoptosis of a target cell through a Fas-dependent mechanism. It occurs when surface CD95 (Fas) is bound by its ligand CD178 (FasL). Cytotoxic T cells upregulate CD178 on activation. This, in turn, binds CD95 on target cells, resulting in programmed cell death.

Cytokines

Cell surface receptors provide an interface through which adjacent cells can transfer signals vital to the immune response. Whereas this cell-to-cell contact is a critical component of cellular communication, soluble mediators are also used extensively to accomplish similar tasks. These polypeptides, termed cytokines, are critical to the development and function of both the innate and acquired immune processes. The action of cytokines, also known as interleukins (see Table 25.1), may be autocrine (on the same cell) or paracrine (on adjacent cells), but it is usually not endocrine. They are released by multiple cell types and may function to activate, to suppress, or even to amplify the response of adjacent cells. The prototypical cytokine of T-cell activation is IL-2. Once a given T cell encounters its specific antigen in the setting of appropriate costimulation, it will subsequently produce and release IL-2 as well as other cytokines that will influence any cell within its vicinity. As mentioned before, Th cellular subsets are differentiated on the basis of the pattern of cytokine expression. Th1 cells, which mediate cytotoxic responses such as delayed-type hypersensitivity, express IL-2, IL-12, IL-15, and IFN-γ. Th2 cells support the development of humoral or eosinophilic responses and consequently express IL-4, IL-5, IL-10, and IL-13. Th17 cells, a more recently described subset, are distinguished by their production of IL-17, IL-21, and IL-22.

Cytokine receptors are now known to function through Janus kinase (JAK) signal transduction proteins. They convey signals to signal transducers and activators of transcriptions (STATs), DNA-binding proteins that translocate to the nucleus to influence gene transcription. As is the case with most of the immune response, this pathway is tightly regulated. For example, suppressors of cytokine signaling proteins act in a negative feedback loop to inhibit STAT phosphorylation by binding and inhibiting JAKs or competing with STATs for phosphotyrosine-binding sites on cytokine receptors. There is evidence emerging for the involvement of suppressors of cytokine signaling proteins in human disease, which raises the possibility that therapeutic strategies based on the manipulation of suppressors of cytokine signaling activity might be of clinical benefit.

One particular subset of cytokines is termed chemokines for their ability to influence the movement of leukocytes and to regulate their migration to and from secondary lymphoid organs, blood, and tissues. Chemokines, or chemotactic cytokine chemokines, are a unique set of cytokines that are structurally homologous, 8- to 10-kDa polypeptides that have a varying number of cysteine residues in conserved locations that are key to forming their three-dimensional shape. The two major families are CC chemokines (also called β), in which the two defining cysteine residues are adjacent, and the CXC (or α) chemokine family, in which these residues are separated by one amino acid. There are numerous CC (1–28) and CXC (1–16) chemokines with various targets and functions. The CC and CXC chemokines are produced not only by leukocytes but also by several other cell types, such as endothelial and epithelial cells as well as fibroblasts. In many circumstances, these cell types are stimulated to produce and to release the chemokines after recognition of microbes or other tissue injury signals detected by the various cellular receptors of the innate immune system discussed earlier. Although there are exceptions, recruitment of neutrophils is mainly mediated by CXC chemokines, monocyte recruitment is more dependent on CC chemokines, and lymphocyte homing is modulated by both CXC and CC chemokines. Chemokine receptors are G protein–coupled receptors containing seven transmembrane domains. These receptors initiate intracellular responses that stimulate cytoskeletal changes and polymerization of actin and myosin filaments, resulting in increased cell motility. These signals may also change the conformation of cell surface integrins, increasing their affinity for their ligands, thus affecting migration, rolling, and diapedesis. Thus, chemokines work in concert with adhesion molecules, such as integrins and selectins, and their ligands to regulate the migration of leukocytes into tissues. Distinct combinations of chemokine receptors are expressed on various types of leukocytes, resulting in the differential patterns of migrations of those leukocytes. Chemokines or their receptors have been exploited by viruses such as human immunodeficiency virus (HIV) (CCR5 and CXCR4 expressed on CD4 T cells are used as entry coreceptors) or used as therapeutic targets, such as CCR7 (FTY720 or fingolimod, an S1PR1 modulator, promotes sequestration of T cells in the lymph node through a CCR7-dependent mechanism; see later). In addition to cytokines, there are a host of other soluble, small-molecule mediators that are released during an immune response or with other types of inflammation. These function to increase blood flow to the area and to improve the exposure of the area to lymphocytes and the innate immune system.

B Cells and Antibody Production

The primary lymphoid organ responsible for B-cell differentiation is the bone marrow. Similar to all other cells in the immune system, B cells are derived from pluripotent bone marrow stem cells. IL-7, produced by bone marrow stromal cells, is a growth factor for pre-B cells. IL-4, IL-5, and IL-6 are cytokines that stimulate the maturation and proliferation of mature primed B cells. The principal function of B cells is to produce antibodies against foreign antigens (i.e., the humoral immune response) as well as to be involved in antigen presentation. B-cell development occurs through several stages, each stage representing a change in the genomic content at the antibody loci. During the differentiation

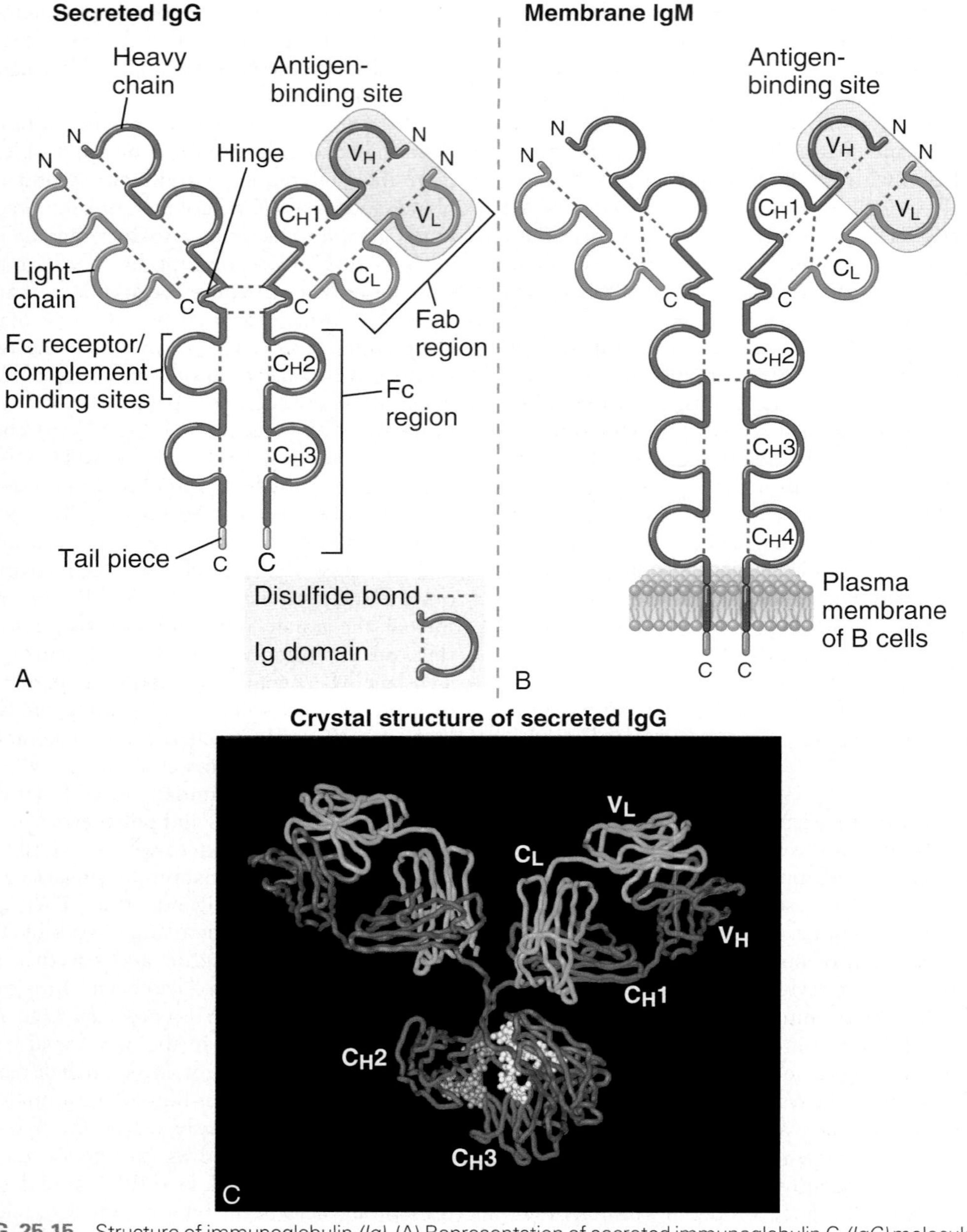

FIG. 25.15 Structure of immunoglobulin *(Ig)*. (A) Representation of secreted immunoglobulin G *(IgG)* molecule. The antigen-binding regions are formed by the variable regions of both light *(V_L)* and heavy *(V_H)* chains. The constant region of the heavy chain *(C_H)* is responsible for the Fc receptor and complement-binding sites. (B) Schematic diagram of membrane-bound immunoglobulin G *(IgM)*. The membrane form of the antibody has C-terminal transmembrane and cytoplasmic portions that anchor the molecule in the plasma membrane. (C) X-ray crystallography representation of IgG molecule. Heavy chains are colored *blue* and *red*, light chains are colored *green*, and carbohydrates are shown in *gray*. (Adapted from Abbas AK, Lichtman AH, Pillai S. *Cellular and Molecular Immunology*. 9th ed. Philadelphia: Saunders Elsevier; 2018.)

process, there is an elegant series of nucleotide rearrangements that results in a nearly unlimited array of specificities, allowing for a diverse recognition repertoire.

Similar to the T cell and its receptor, each B cell has a unique membrane-bound receptor through which it recognizes specific antigen. In the case of the B cell, this Ig molecule may also be produced in a secreted form that can interact with the extracellular environment far from its cellular origin. Each mature B cell produces antibody of a single specificity.

Each antibody is composed of two heavy chains and two light chains. Five different heavy chain loci (μ, γ, α, ε, and δ) are found on chromosome 14 and two light chain loci (κ and λ) are located on chromosome 2. Each chain is composed of V, D, J, and C regions, which are brought together randomly by the RAG1 and RAG2 complex to form a functional antigen receptor. Ig has a basic structure of four chains, two of which are identical heavy chains and two of which are identical light chains (Fig. 25.15). Both heavy and light chains have a constant region as well as a

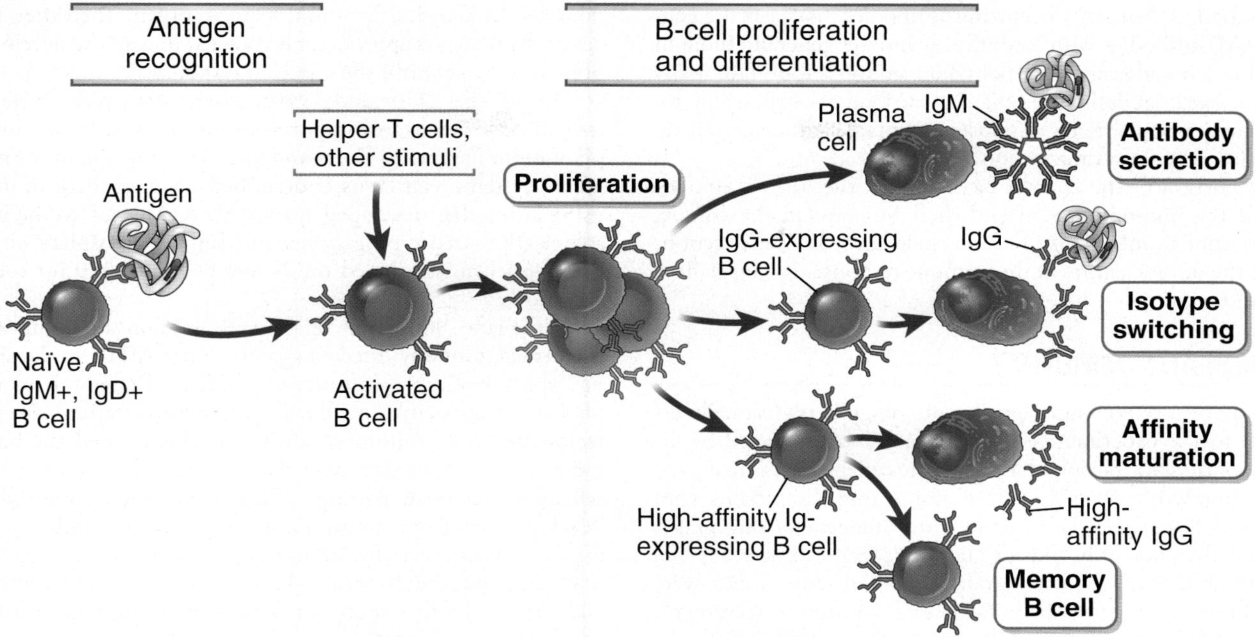

FIG. 25.16 B-cell differentiation. Naïve B cells recognize their specific antigen as it binds to surface-bound antibody. Under the influence of helper T cells, costimulatory signals, and other stimuli, B cells become activated and clonally expand, producing many B cells of the same specificity. They also differentiate into antibody-secreting cells, plasma cells. Some of the activated B cells undergo heavy chain class switching and affinity maturation. Ultimately, a small subset become long-lived memory cells, primed for future responses. (Adapted from Abbas AK, Lichtman AH, Pillai S. *Cellular and Molecular Immunology*. 9th ed. Philadelphia: Saunders Elsevier; 2018.) *Ig*, Immunoglobulin; *IgD*, immunoglobulin D; *IgG*, immunoglobulin G; *IgM*, immunoglobulin M.

variable, antigen-binding region. The antigen-binding site is composed of both the heavy and light chain variable regions. The ability of antibody to neutralize microbes is entirely a function of this antigen-binding region.

In humans, there are nine different Ig subclasses or isotypes: IgM, IgD, IgG1, IgG2, IgG3, IgG4, IgA1, IgA2, and IgE. Heavy chain use defines the subtype of any given antibody. Whereas the variable regions are involved in antigen binding, the constant regions have functionality as well. The fragment crystallizable region or Fc region is in the tail portion composed of the two heavy chain constant regions. It interacts with Fc receptors on phagocytic cells of the innate immune system to facilitate opsonization and subsequent destruction of the antigen to which the antibody is bound, as well as facilitating antigenic peptide processing. The Fc portion of IgM and some classes of IgG also serves to activate complement. Distinct immune effector functions are assigned to each isotype. IgM and IgG antibodies provide a pivotal role in the endogenous or intravascular immune response. IgA is primarily responsible for mucosal immunity and is largely confined to the gastrointestinal and respiratory tracts. Resting B cells that have not yet been exposed to antigen express IgD and IgM on their cell surface. After interaction with antigen, the first isotype produced is IgM, which is efficient at binding complement to facilitate phagocytosis or cell lysis. Further activation and differentiation of the B cell occur after interactions with CD4+ Tfh cells. B cells undergo isotype switching, which results in a decrease in IgM titer with a concomitant rise in IgG titer. Unlike the TCR, the Ig loci undergo continued alteration after B-cell stimulation to improve the affinity and functionality of the secreted antibody. A primed B cell may undergo further mutation within the variable regions that leads to increased affinity of antibody, termed somatic hypermutation. Such B cells are retained to provide the ability to generate a more vigorous response if the antigen happens to be re-encountered (Fig. 25.16).

B-cell activation occurs when antigen is bound by two surface antibodies (or a multimeric form of antibody) and the antibodies are brought together on the cell surface in a process known as cross-linking. This event stimulates B-cell activation, proliferation, and differentiation into various B-cell subsets and antibody-secreting plasma cells. As for T cell, the threshold for B-cell activation is high. This can be lowered 100-fold by costimulatory signals received by the transmembrane complex CD19-CD21. B cells can also internalize antigens bound to surface antibodies and process them for presentation to T cells, thus participating in antigen presentation. As discussed earlier, B cells may provide and receive certain costimulatory signals. For example, B cells express CD40, and when bound by CD154 expressed on activated T cells, the result is upregulation of B7 molecules on the B cell and delivery of important costimulatory signals to T cells as well.

Plasma cells reside in the bone marrow and are distinguished histologically by their hypertrophied Golgi apparatus resulting from their high degree of protein synthesis. They secrete large amounts of monoclonal (single specificity) antibody and exhibit phenotypic and functional characteristics distinct from other B cells that are the focus of therapeutic strategies to target plasma cells either for oncologic purposes or for the control of alloantibodies in transplantation.

In addition to being secreted in an adaptive manner after exposure to antigen, antibody can also exist as part of the innate or natural immune repertoire in the circulation for initial response to common pathogens. Antigen exposure generally leads to B-cell affinity maturation and isotype switching and produces high-affinity

IgG antibodies. Naturally occurring antibodies, however, are generally IgM antibodies with low affinity and are generally thought to bind to a broad array of carbohydrate epitopes found on many common bacterial pathogens. Natural antibody is responsible for ABO blood group antigen responses and discordant xenograft rejection (see "Xenotransplantation").

This portion of the chapter has reviewed the various components of the immune system and their function in the context of conventional, infectious immune challenges. The next sections address the unique nature of the immune response to transplanted tissue and organs.

TRANSPLANT IMMUNITY

The study of modern transplant immunology is traditionally attributed to the experiments of Sir Peter Medawar fueled by attempts to use skin transplantation as a treatment for burned aviators during World War II. While monitoring the victims with autologous (syngeneic) and homologous (allogeneic) skin grafts, he noted that not only did all allogeneic grafts universally fail promptly, but also secondary grafts from the same donor were rejected even more vigorously, suggesting immune involvement. He pursued this hypothesis with extensive experiments in rabbits, wherein he confirmed his previous observation and noted the presence of a heavy lymphocyte infiltrate in the rejecting graft. It was N.A. Mitchison, working in the early 1950s, who definitively identified a role for lymphocytes in the rejection of foreign tissue. Subsequent studies in tumor immunology as well as work by Snell using strains of genetically identical mice identified the genetic basis for graft rejection as the MHC, known in humans as HLA and in mice as the H-2 locus. These series of experiments during a short period of several years demonstrated that rejection of transplanted tissue was an immunologic process, implicated lymphocytes as the principal effector cells, and identified the MHC as the primary source of antigen in the rejection response. These pivotal studies laid the groundwork for the transition of transplantation from the experimental to the clinical realm.

Whereas the technical skill for the transplantation of skin and other organs had been available for some time, the vigorous rejection of allografts had prevented its widespread use for many years. It was not until 1954, after Medawar's critical studies had been published, that the first successful organ transplantation was performed. Despite Medawar's claim that the "biological force" responsible for rejection would "forever inhibit transplantation from one individual to another," Joseph Murray, a surgeon-scientist, persevered in his pursuit of making clinical transplantation a reality. At the time, there was evidence to suggest that the overall immunologic barrier was lacking between identical twins, and coincidentally, Murray was busily perfecting a surgical technique for kidney transplantation in dogs. In 1954, the opportunity presented itself to test the hypothesis. Richard Herrick, who had incurable kidney damage, was the first candidate, and his identical sibling, Ronald, was willing to donate a kidney for transplantation to his brother. Murray confirmed the lack of immunologic reactivity between the two brothers by first placing skin grafts from each twin onto the other. Once he confirmed the lack of a response, he used the technique that he had perfected in the canine model, performing the first successful kidney transplant between identical twins in December 1954.[2] The operation proceeded without complication, and the kidney functioned well without the need for immunosuppression. Despite this landmark advance in transplantation, the majority of individuals in need of a transplant did not have an identical twin to donate an organ. Thereafter, the focus of the field was appropriately directed toward the development of methods to control the rejection response.

During the 1950s and 1960s, several discoveries were made that were of the utmost importance for future successes in transplantation. Following Gorer and Snell's description of the murine MHC system, Jean Dausset described the equivalent in humans using antibodies developed against HLA. This led to the first serologically based typing system for human transplant antigens. Snell and Dausset shared the Nobel Prize in 1980 for their observations.

In the late 1960s, Paul Terasaki reported on the significance of preformed antibody directed against donor MHC molecules and its impact on kidney graft survival.[20] He developed the microlymphocyte cytotoxicity test, allowing pretransplantation detection of recipient-derived antidonor antibody. This formed the basis for the physical crossmatch assay that is used today to screen potential donor-recipient pairings. These techniques, along with the development of new immunosuppressive compounds, including 6-mercaptopurine and azathioprine, led to the first successful kidney transplantation between relatives who were not identical twins and also to the first successful transplant using a kidney from a deceased donor.

Although early attempts at immunosuppression permitted extended allograft survival in selected patients, both the reproducibility and durability of results were far from adequate. In the 1970s, investigators sought novel treatments to improve the success rate for transplantation; these modalities included thoracic duct drainage and the use of antilymphocyte serum. Despite these efforts, the results for kidney transplantation remained poor, with the best centers achieving 1-year survival rates of 70% for living related kidney grafts and 50% for deceased donor kidney transplants. Then a chance discovery of a promising agent from a fungal isolate dramatically changed the outlook for kidney and other types of transplantation. Jean-François Borel identified an active metabolite, cyclosporine A (CsA), that showed selective in vitro inhibition of lymphocyte cultures but no significant myelotoxic effects. Promising results in dogs eventually led to clinical trials in humans, and the modern era of transplantation had begun.

The introduction of CsA ushered in the most dramatic improvement in the field of transplantation. Liver and heart transplant survival rates doubled, and the improved immunosuppression encouraged transplant teams around the world to begin broader investigational use, transplanting lung, small bowel, and pancreas. Now, with the use of CsA and newer agents such as tacrolimus, 1-year graft survival has exceeded 90% for virtually all organs except the small intestine. Despite the discovery and clinical introduction of ever increasingly potent immunosuppressants, the field of transplantation has many areas in need of improvement. Drug-related side effects and the intractable problem of chronic rejection still plague practitioners. One area of focus of current research is the development of a clinically applicable strategy to promote "transplantation tolerance," thereby eliminating the pitfalls and shortcomings of current immunosuppressive therapy.

Rejection

There are three classic histopathologic definitions of allograft rejection that are based on not only the predominant mediator but also the timing of the process (Fig. 25.17).

1. Hyperacute rejection occurs within minutes to days after transplantation and is primarily mediated by preformed antibody.

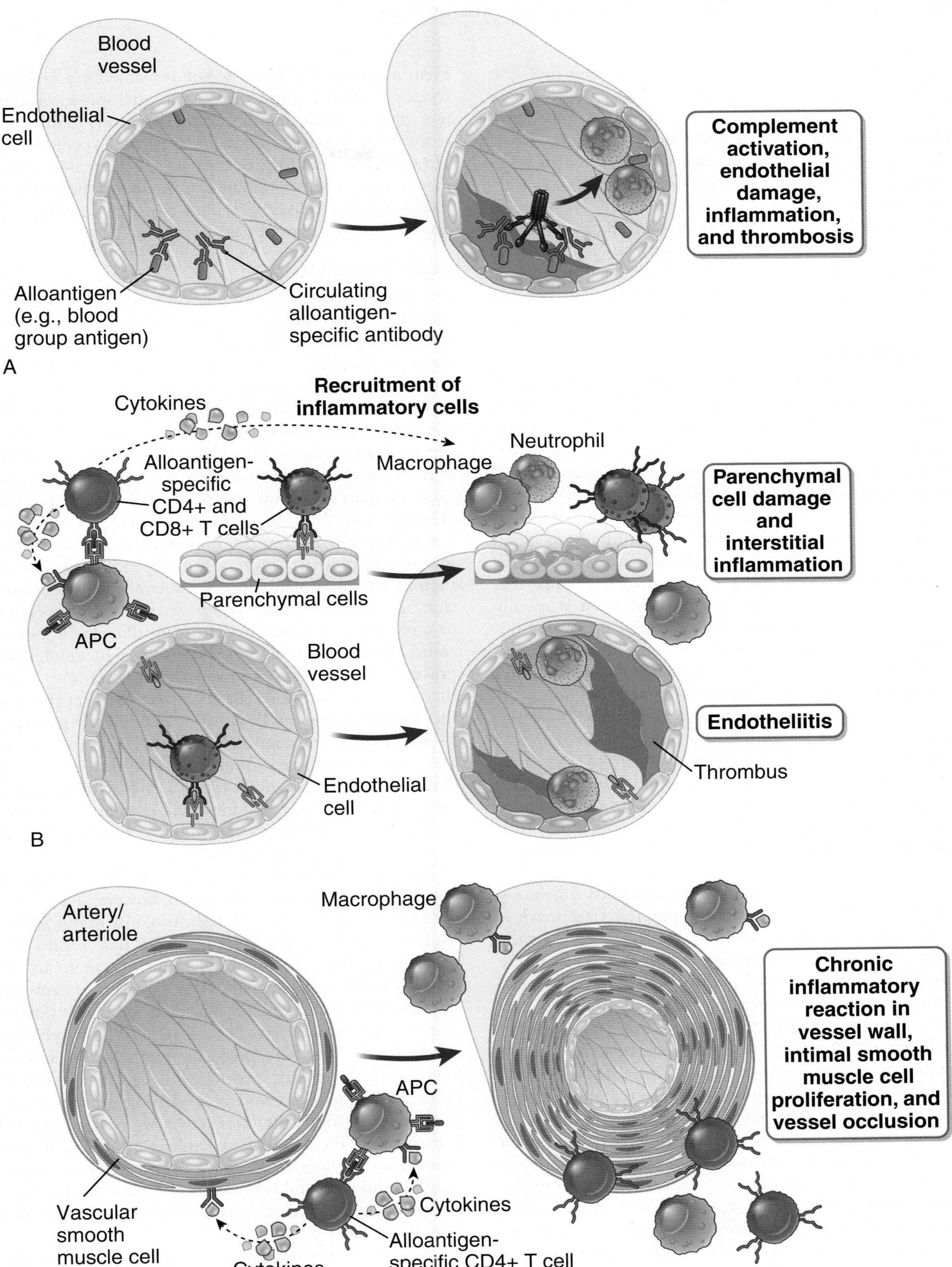

FIG. 25.17 Mechanisms of rejection. (A) Hyperacute rejection occurs when preformed antibodies react with donor antigens on the vascular endothelium of the graft. Subsequent complement activation triggers rapid intravascular thrombosis and graft necrosis. (B) Acute cellular rejection is predominantly mediated by a cellular infiltrate of alloreactive T cells that attack donor cells both in the endothelium and in the parenchyma. Alloreactive antibodies can also develop after engraftment and lead to antibody-mediated rejection that contributes to parenchymal and vascular injury. (C) Chronic rejection is characterized by graft arteriosclerosis and fibrosis. Immune- and non–immune-mediated mechanisms are responsible for abnormal proliferation of cells within the intima and media of the vessels of the graft, eventually leading to luminal occlusion. (Adapted from Abbas AK, Lichtman AH, Pillai S. *Cellular and Molecular Immunology*. 9th ed. Philadelphia: Saunders Elsevier; 2018.) *APC*, Antigen-presenting cell.

2. Acute rejection is a process mediated most commonly by T cells but is often accompanied by an acquired antibody response and generally occurs within the first few weeks to months of transplantation but can occur at any time.
3. Chronic rejection is a common contributing cause of long-term allograft loss and is an indolent fibrotic process that occurs over months to years. It is thought to be secondary to chronic immunologic injury from both T and B cell–mediated processes (including antidonor antibodies) but is difficult to completely separate from nonimmune mechanisms of chronic organ damage (e.g., drug toxicity and cardiovascular comorbid diseases).

Hyperacute Rejection

Although essentially untreatable, hyperacute rejection is nearly universally avoidable with the proper use of the lymphocytotoxic crossmatch or other means of detecting antidonor antibodies before transplantation. This form of rejection occurs when preformed antibodies against the donor, commonly referred to as donor-specific antibodies, are present in the recipient's system before transplantation. These antibodies may be the result of "natural processes," such as the formation of antibody to blood group antigens, or the product of prior exposure to antigens with similar enough specificities as those expressed by the donor that cross-reactivity can occur. In the latter, sensitization is usually the result of prior transplantation, transfusion, or pregnancy but may also result from prior environmental antigen exposure. As expected, hyperacute rejection can occur within the first minutes to hours after graft reperfusion. Antibodies bind to the donor tissue or endothelium and initiate complement-mediated lysis and endothelial cell activation, resulting in a procoagulant state and immediate graft thrombosis. On histologic evaluation, there may be platelet and fibrin thrombi, early neutrophil infiltration, and positive staining for the complement product C4d on the endothelial lining of small blood vessels (Fig. 25.18). Thankfully, this type of rejection is avoidable with pretransplantation testing by current crossmatch assays.

Similar to the lymphocytotoxicity assay described previously that is used for MHC class I typing, the physical crossmatch is performed by mixing cells from the donor with serum from the recipient and the addition of complement if needed. Lysis of the donor cells indicates that antibodies directed against the donor are present in the recipient's serum; this is called a positive crossmatch. Thus, a negative crossmatch assay coupled with proper ABO matching will effectively prevent hyperacute rejection in 99.5% of transplants. Newer crossmatch techniques have become increasingly sophisticated, including those directed at both class I and class II antibodies, flow cytometric techniques, and bead-based screening assays to exclude non-HLA antibodies. As a given patient's sensitivity status may change over time, a more common technique for screening a patient's sensitization status is to screen a potential recipient's serum against a panel of random donor cells representing the anticipated regional donor pool. Known as the panel reactive antibody (PRA) assay, the results are expressed as a percentage of the panel within the randomly selected cell set that lyses when recipient serum is added. Thus, a nonsensitized patient would be given a score of 0%, and a highly sensitized patient might have a PRA score up to 100%. These screens can now be performed without the need for cells by using polystyrene beads coated with HLA antigens. In this situation, the laboratory detects all anti-HLA antibodies and calculates a PRA score on the basis of the expected frequency of the HLA types in the donor pool. In the event a compatible donor is not available for a highly sensitized recipient, clinical protocols exist to attempt desensitization that uses plasmapheresis or intravenous immune globulin (IVIG) to reduce circulating antibody and prevent hyperacute rejection.[21] However, the need for desensitization is decreasing with advancements in deceased donor allocation algorithms and living donor paired donor exchange programs aimed at avoiding crossmatch-positive donor-recipient pairs.

Acute Rejection

Of the three types of rejection, only acute rejection can be successfully reversed once it is established. T cells constitute the core element responsible for acute rejection, often termed *T cell–mediated rejection*. There is also a form of acute rejection that is particularly aggressive and involves vascular invasion by T cells known as acute vascular rejection. Finally, a more recently recognized form of acute rejection mediated by the humoral immune system, known as antibody-mediated rejection (AMR), is discussed briefly later. With the advent of increasingly effective immunosuppression, allograft loss from acute cellular rejection has become increasingly rare. Acute rejection can occur at any time after the first few postoperative days, the time needed to mount an acquired immune response; it most commonly occurs within the first 6 months after transplantation. Without adequate immunosuppression, the cellular response will progress during the course of days to a few weeks, ultimately destroying the allograft. As described earlier, there are two main pathways through which rejection can proceed, the direct and indirect alloresponses (Fig. 25.19). In either case, alloreactive T cells encounter their specific antigen (either processed donor MHC peptides indirectly presented on self MHC or directly recognized donor MHC), undergo activation, and promote similar rejection responses. The precursor frequency of T cells specific for either direct allorecognition or indirect allorecognition differs.[12] Indirect allorecognition is theoretically similar to that of any given pathogen. Donor MHC protein is processed into peptides and presented on self MHC. The number of T cells specific for this antigen is approximately 1 in 200,000 to 1 in 500,000. Direct allorecognition, however, has a much higher precursor frequency. These T cells recognize donor MHC directly without processing (Fig. 25.20). Given that T cells are selected to recognize self MHC molecules and that there are similarities between donor and recipient MHC, it is no surprise that a substantial number of T cells are alloreactive. Some estimates suggest that somewhere between 1% and 10% of all T cells are directly alloreactive.[12] This high precursor frequency likely overwhelms many of the regulatory processes in place to control the much lower cell frequencies involved in physiologic immune responses. These alloreactive T cells, once activated, move to attack the graft. Subsequently, there is massive infiltration of T cells and monocytes into the allograft, resulting in organ injury through direct cytolysis and a general inflammatory milieu that leads to generalized parenchymal dysfunction and endothelial injury resulting in thrombosis (see Fig. 25.18).

The bulk of current immunosuppressive agents are directed toward the T cells themselves or interruption of pathways essential to their activation or effector functions. In an effort to prevent acute cellular rejection, induction therapy is generally used during the initial stages after transplantation. These agents are discussed in the subsequent section but are most often antibody therapies that serve to globally deplete or inactivate T cells during the immediate postoperative period of engraftment when ischemia-reperfusion injury is most likely to promote immune recognition.

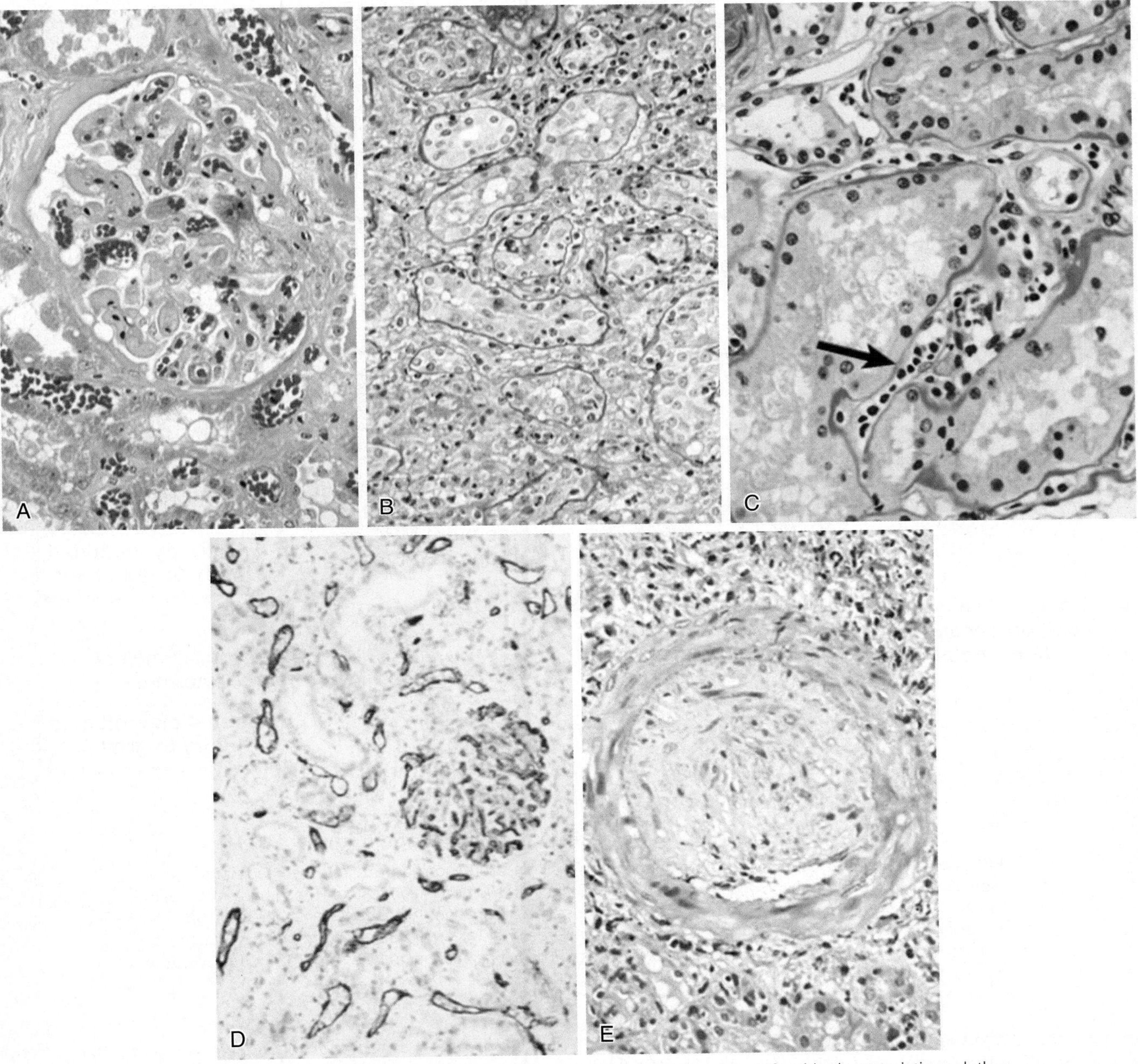

FIG. 25.18 Histology of rejection. (A) Hyperacute rejection of a kidney allograft with characteristic endothelial damage, thrombus, and early neutrophil infiltrates. (B) Acute cellular rejection of kidney with inflammatory cells within the connective tissue around the tubules and between tubular epithelial cells. (C) Acute antibody-mediated rejection of kidney allograft with inflammatory reaction within a graft vessel resulting in endothelial disruption *(arrow)*. (D) C4d deposition in the small vessels of the transplanted kidney. (E) Chronic rejection in a transplanted kidney with graft arteriosclerosis. The vascular lumen has been replaced with smooth muscle cells and fibrotic response. (Adapted from Abbas AK, Lichtman AH, Pillai S. *Cellular and Molecular Immunology*. 8th ed. Philadelphia: Saunders Elsevier; 2015.)

Immunosuppressive regimens are frequently designed to favor more intensive initial immunosuppression in the immediate postoperative period and are then tapered to lower, less toxic levels over time.

T cell–specific treatments lead to the prevention of acute rejection in approximately 70% of transplants, and when it does occur, it can be reversed in most cases. Similar to hyperacute rejection resulting from preformed antibody responses, T-cell presensitization will result in an accelerated form of cellular rejection mediated by memory T cells. It generally occurs within the first 2 or 3 days after transplantation and can be accompanied by a significant humoral response.

The humoral equivalent to acute cellular rejection is AMR. This occurs when offending antibodies specific for alloantigen exist in the circulation at levels undetectable by crossmatch assays or, alternatively, B-cell clones capable of producing donor-specific antibody are activated and stimulated to produce de novo alloantibodies. These antibodies are thought to bind HLA antigens

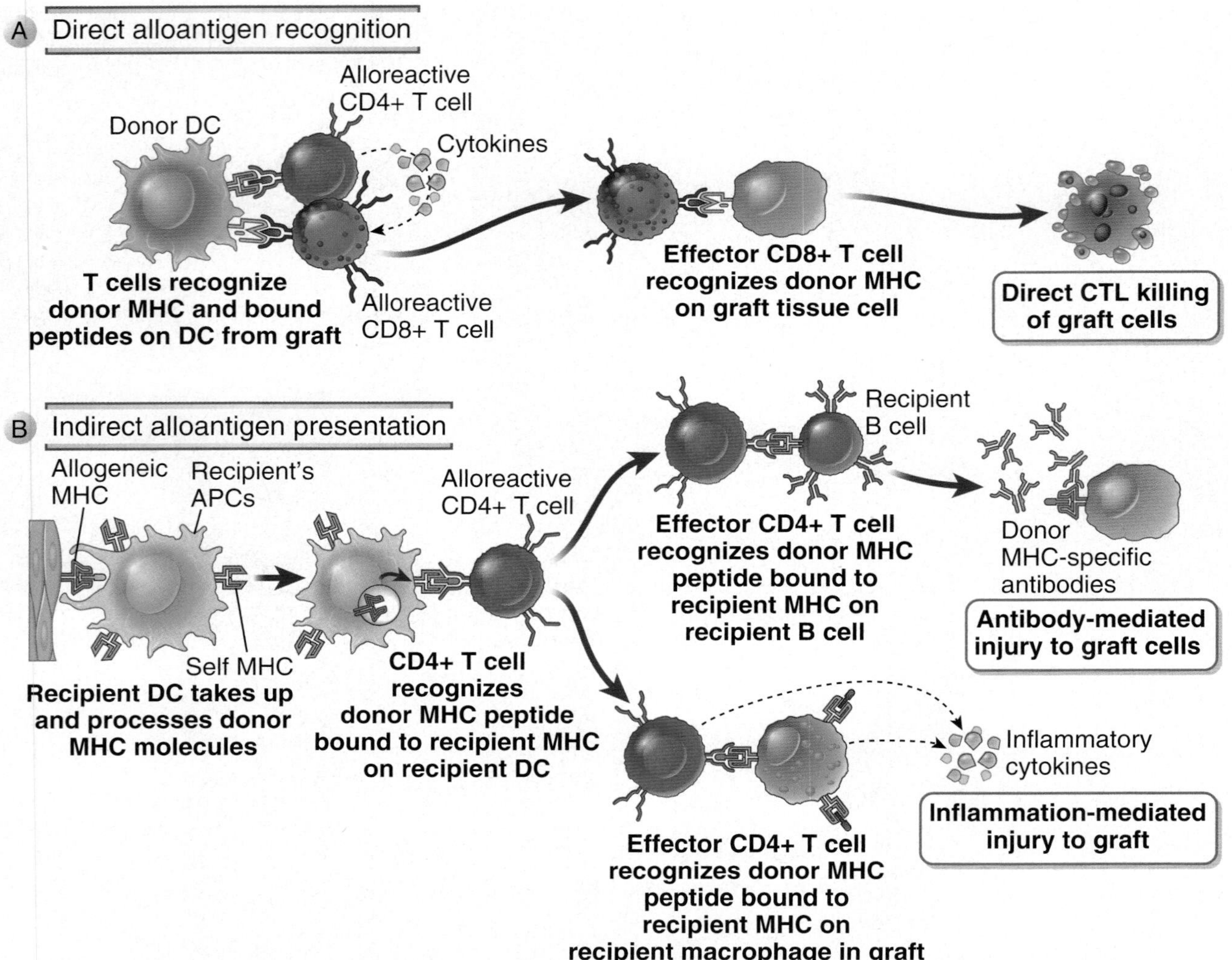

FIG. 25.19 Direct versus indirect allorecognition. (A) Direct allorecognition occurs when recipient T cells bind directly to donor MHC molecules on graft cells. (B) Indirect allorecognition results when recipient antigen-presenting cells *(APCs)* take up donor MHC and process the alloantigen. Allopeptides are then presented on recipient (self) MHC molecules in standard fashion to alloreactive T cells. (Adapted from Abbas AK, Lichtman AH, Pillai S. *Cellular and Molecular Immunology.* 9th ed. Philadelphia: Saunders Elsevier; 2018.) *CTL,* Cytotoxic lymphocyte; *DC,* dendritic cell; *MHC,* major histocompatibility complex.

within the graft, recruit innate and adaptive immune mechanisms, and acutely injure the transplanted organ (Fig. 25.18). The former scenario is often seen in patients with a high PRA score that has decreased over time. Transplantation presumably leads to restimulation of memory B cells responsible for the donor-specific antibodies. The result is initial graft function, followed by rapid deterioration within the first few postoperative days. Implementation of a more aggressive immunosuppressive regimen, including higher doses of steroids combined with nonspecific antibody reduction by plasmapheresis or IVIG (nonspecific Ig), is occasionally successful in acutely reversing AMR.

Prompt recognition of acute rejection is essential to ensure optimal graft survival. Untreated rejection leads to expansion of the immune response to involve multiple pathways, some of which are less sensitive to T cell–specific therapies. In addition, damage to the allograft, particularly for kidney, pancreas, and heart, is generally accompanied by a permanent loss of function that is proportional to the magnitude of involvement. Most acute rejection episodes are initially asymptomatic until the secondary effects of organ dysfunction occur. By this point, the rejection process has proceeded to a point that it is often more difficult to reverse. Accordingly, monitoring for acute rejection is usually intense initially, particularly during the first year after transplantation. In general, any unexplained graft dysfunction should prompt biopsy and evaluation for the lymphocytic infiltration, antibody deposition, and parenchymal necrosis characteristic of acute rejection.

Chronic Rejection

Whereas the mechanisms of acute and hyperacute rejection have been better described, chronic rejection remains less understood. True chronic rejection is an immune-based process derived from repeated or indolent T cell–mediated rejection or AMR, but the clinical phenotype of chronic graft fibrosis and deterioration is often secondary to a combination of both immune and nonimmune effects. Appropriately, the term *chronic rejection* has been substituted with more descriptive terms: interstitial fibrosis and tubular atrophy (previously chronic allograft nephropathy) for kidneys,

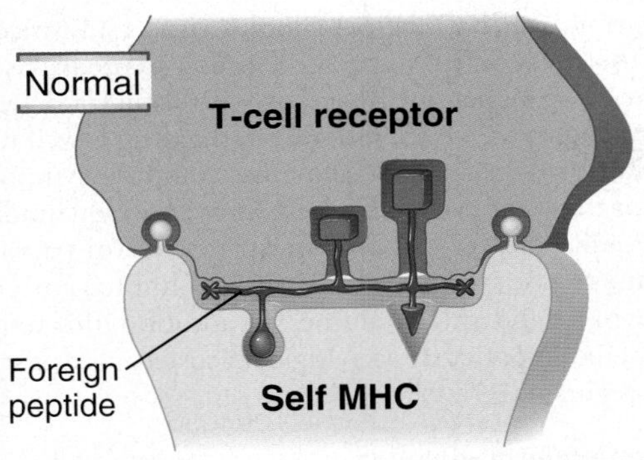

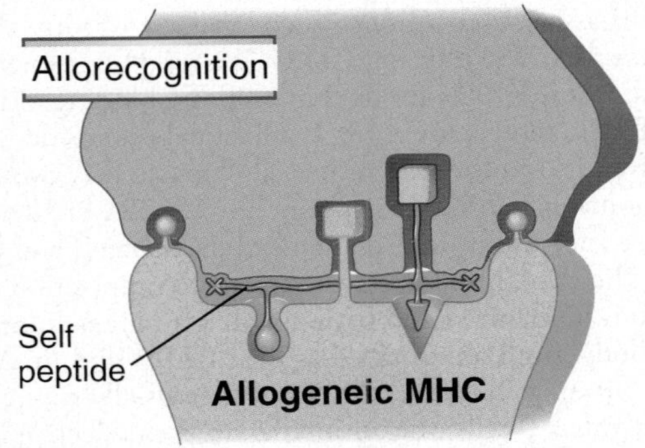

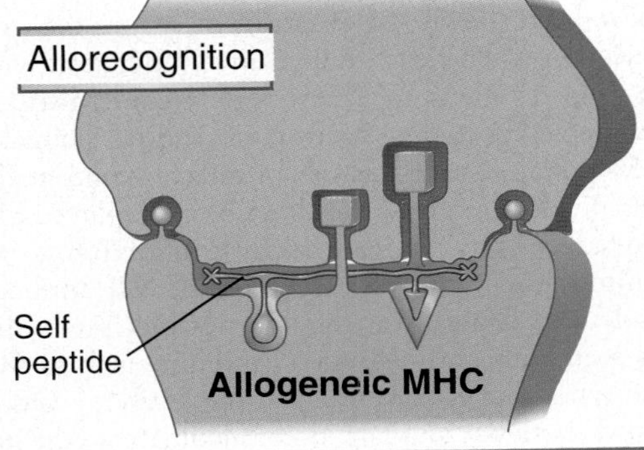

FIG. 25.20 Molecular basis for direct allorecognition. Recipient T cells may recognize donor major histocompatibility complex *(MHC)* molecules directly because of the similarities between MHC alleles but become activated because only T cells strongly reactive to self MHC were deleted in the thymus through negative selection. (A) Normally, T cells encounter self MHC complexed with foreign peptide and become activated in the appropriate context. (B) T cells may encounter allogeneic MHC complexed with endogenous peptide that together resemble self MHC bound with foreign peptide. (C) Alternatively, allogeneic MHC alone may contribute to allorecognition and T-cell activation independent of self peptide. (Adapted from Abbas AK, Lichtman AH, Pillai S. *Cellular and Molecular Immunology*. 9th ed. Philadelphia: Saunders Elsevier; 2018.)

chronic coronary vasculopathy for hearts, vanishing bile duct syndrome for livers, and bronchiolitis obliterans for lungs.[22] The process is insidious, usually occurring during a period of years, but it can be accelerated and occur within the first year. Regardless of the organ involved, it is characterized by parenchymal replacement by fibrous tissue with a relatively sparse lymphocytic infiltrate but may contain macrophages or dendritic cells (see Fig. 25.18). Organs with epithelium show a disappearance of the epithelial cells as well as endothelial destruction. The events that ultimately trigger this response are certainly related to the transplantation, including but not limited to the response to alloantigen as well as the ischemia-reperfusion injury associated with the actual transfer of the organ itself. These events set the stage for expression of various soluble factors, including TGF-β, leading to a remodeling of the parenchyma and ensuing fibrous replacement. Chronic inflammatory insults can also evoke a process of epithelial to mesenchymal dedifferentiation, leading to epithelial cells that regress into fibrocytes. Although to date these processes remain essentially untreatable once identified, several factors have been identified that predispose toward the development of chronic rejection. The most important of these is prior acute rejection episodes. Another important factor is the presence of donor-specific antibody, which often portends premature allograft loss. Thus, the more effectively immune control is exerted to limit acute rejection episodes and the development of donor-specific antibodies in the early stages after transplantation, the less likely chronic rejection related to immune injury is to occur.

IMMUNOSUPPRESSION

Current immunosuppressive therapies in transplantation achieve excellent results, especially in terms of relatively short-term patient and allograft survival rates. Despite tremendous progress during the past 60 years, all agents designed to prevent rejection remain nonspecific to the alloimmune response. Given the redundancy of the immune system, recipients almost always need multiple agents to adequately control the normal immune response. In addition, none of these therapies specifically inhibit the response to the allograft; instead, most immunosuppressants target the immune response globally. In other words, all drugs that prevent rejection do so at the cost of suppressing the normal host response to bacterial and viral pathogens as well as tumor surveillance. Whereas some of the newer therapies are more precise in their mechanisms and selective for immune cells, many target not only the mediators of the immune response but also any cells undergoing maturation or division. Consequently, there are many nonimmune side effects associated with immunosuppressive therapy that can directly or indirectly contribute to graft dysfunction and loss. In addition, the societal costs are not trivial, considering that transplant recipients may take dozens of pills a day at an annual cost of $10,000 to $15,000.

The most critical time for immune protection is the first few days to months after transplantation. The graft is fresh, and there is a heightened state of inflammation secondary to inevitable graft injury from ischemia-reperfusion as well as the physical transfer of the organ itself. In addition, this is the time of initial antigen exposure, which plays a large role in determining the long-term status of immune responsiveness. For this reason, immunosuppression is extremely intense in the early postoperative period and normally tapered thereafter. This initial conditioning of the recipient's immune system is known as induction immunosuppression. It most commonly involves depletion or at least aggressive reduction of T cells and consequently is tolerated only for a short time without lethal consequences. After this initial period, the agents used to prevent acute rejection for the remainder of the life of the transplanted organ are called maintenance immunosuppressants. These medications still carry with them a host of immune and nonimmune side effects that may also ultimately contribute to long-term graft failure. Immunosuppressants used to reverse an acute rejection episode are called rescue agents. They are generally the same as those agents used for induction therapy. The mechanisms of the various immunosuppressants are described here and detailed in Table 25.3.

Induction Therapy

Most of the current induction regimens involve the use of some depleting antilymphocyte antibody preparation. Their mechanism of action is probably not fully understood but involves some combination of either selective or nonselective depletion and inactivation. They cause profound immunosuppression, placing the recipient at increased risk for opportunistic infections or malignancies such as lymphoma, and are consequently generally limited to short-term use on the order of days to weeks.

Antithymocyte Globulin

Antithymocyte globulin preparations are produced by immunizing another species with an inoculum of human thymocytes consisting primarily of lymphocytes, followed by collection of the sera and purification of the gamma globulin fraction. The result is a polyclonal antibody preparation that contains antibodies directed against a multitude of antigens on lymphocytes. The two most commonly used preparations are rabbit antithymocyte globulin (RATG) and horse antithymocyte globulin (ATGAM). RATG seems to be more effective than ATGAM at reducing the incidence of acute rejection episodes and consequently is the preferred preparation at most U.S. transplantation centers.[23] The polyclonal preparation consists of hundreds of polyclonal antibodies that coat dozens of epitopes over the surface of the T cell. The result is T-cell clearance through complement-mediated lysis and opsonization. In addition to simple depletion mechanisms, the antisera also interfere with effective TCR signaling and can promote inappropriate cross linking of key cell surface molecules, including adhesion and costimulatory receptors, resulting in unresponsiveness or anergy.

These preparations are used as induction agents as well as rescue treatment for acute rejection episodes. Most commonly, RATG is used as part of a multidrug induction protocol that includes a calcineurin inhibitor, an antiproliferative agent such as mycophenolate mofetil (MMF), and prednisone. One strategy in renal transplantation is the sequential use of RATG followed by a calcineurin inhibitor to avoid the nephrotoxic effects of the calcineurin inhibitor in the early posttransplantation period as well as to maximize the effects of RATG by depleting or inactivating the majority of T cells at the critical time of graft introduction. More recently, RATG has been used as a key component of newer steroid-minimization or calcineurin inhibitor–free regimens.[24,25]

Many of the side effects associated with RATG administration are related to its polyclonal composition. Surprisingly, only a small fraction of the known specificities are actually directed at defined T-cell epitopes. One major side effect is profound thrombocytopenia secondary to platelet-specific antibodies within the polyclonal preparation. In addition to T-cell depletion, leukopenia and anemia may also result. Overimmunosuppression is also a concern; given that these preparations are extremely effective at T-cell depletion, there is an increase in viral reactivation and primary viral infections, including cytomegalovirus (CMV), Epstein-Barr virus (EBV), herpes simplex virus, and varicella-zoster virus. The effect on EBV-specific T cells also predisposes treated patients to a higher incidence of EBV-associated lymphoid malignant neoplasms. Overall, however, the drug is well tolerated by most transplant recipients. The most common symptoms are the result of transient cytokine release after antibody binding and cell lysis. Chills and fevers occur in up to 20% of patients, but this cytokine release syndrome is usually self-limited and treatable with antipyretics and antihistamines. In addition, this response is often tempered in patients receiving corticosteroids as part of the induction regimen.

Anti–IL-2 Receptor Antibodies

The cytokine IL-2 plays a critical role in T-cell activation and function. After antigen recognition and signal transduction through the TCR complex, expression of IL-2 and its receptor is markedly upregulated. The receptor consists of three chains: α (CD25), β (CD122), and the common cytokine receptor γ chain (CD132). These chains associate in a noncovalent manner to form the IL-2 receptor complex. The α chain, CD25, is a type I transmembrane protein that is responsible for the high-affinity binding of IL-2 on activated T cells and is critical for T-cell clonal expansion (see Fig. 25.21). Given its importance in the cellular response, two nondepleting monoclonal antibodies specific for CD25 were developed and approved for use in transplantation: daclizumab and basiliximab.[26,27] The two antibodies differ in their composition in that daclizumab is humanized and basiliximab is a mouse-human chimeric antibody. Both are directed against CD25 and function to block IL-2 binding. Because CD25 is preferentially expressed on recently activated T cells, the antibodies are semiselective in their effects, presumably affecting only T cells specific for the allograft that have been activated at the time of graft implantation. Once the T-cell response is well under way, effector T cells are much less dependent on CD25 expression, and these antibodies are much less effective. For this reason, both anti-CD25 antibodies are used during the induction phase only. Much like antithymocyte globulin, they have been shown to prevent or to reduce the frequency of acute rejection when they are used in combination with standard three-drug regimens.[26,27] However, in contradistinction to lymphocyte depleting agents, daclizumab and basiliximab, while generally less potent, confer less risk of infection and malignancy posttransplant. More recently, they have been employed as part of regimens to reduce or to eliminate calcineurin inhibitors or within steroid-minimization protocols. These anti-IL-2R antibodies are very well-tolerated clinically as they do not precipitate the same side effects seen with antithymocyte globulin, such as the cytokine release syndrome. Unlike the murine antibody OKT3 (see OKT3 below), both daclizumab and basiliximab are the products of genetic engineering, with the some or all of the structural components of the mouse antibody having been replaced with human IgG, and thus, they are much less likely to invoke neutralizing antibody responses themselves. Daclizumab has since been discontinued as a result of diminished demand, leaving basiliximab as the sole anti-IL-2 receptor option.

OKT3

Muromonab-CD3 (OKT3), a murine monoclonal antibody directed against the human CD3 ε chain (a component of the TCR signaling complex), was approved by the U.S. Food and Drug Administration (FDA) for use in patients in 1986 and is now of pure historical interest. It was the first commercially available monoclonal antibody preparation for use in organ transplantation

TABLE 25.3 **Summary of immunosuppressive drugs.**

DRUG	DESCRIPTION	MECHANISM	NONIMMUNE TOXICITY AND COMMENTS
Prednisone	Corticosteroid	Binds nuclear receptor and enhances transcription of IκB, which inhibits NF-κB and T-cell activation	Diabetes, weight gain, psychological disturbances, osteoporosis, ulcers, wound healing, adrenal suppression
CsA	11–Amino acid cyclic peptide from *Tolypocladium inflatum*	Binds to cyclophilin; complex inhibits calcineurin phosphatase and T-cell activation	Nephrotoxicity, hemolytic uremic syndrome, hypertension, neurotoxicity, gingival hyperplasia, skin changes, hirsutism, posttransplantation diabetes, hyperlipidemia
Tacrolimus (Prograf)	Macrolide antibiotic from *Streptomyces tsukubaensis*	Binds to FK-BP12; complex inhibits calcineurin phosphatase and T-cell activation	Effects similar to CsA but with lower incidence of hypertension, hyperlipidemia, skin changes, hirsutism, and gingival hyperplasia but higher incidence of posttransplantation diabetes and neurotoxicity
Sirolimus (Rapamycin)	Triene macrolide antibiotic from *Streptomyces hygroscopicus* from Easter Island (Rapa Nui)	Binds to FK-BP12; complex inhibits target of rapamycin and IL-2–dependent T-cell proliferation	Hyperlipidemia, increased toxicity of calcineurin inhibitors, thrombocytopenia, delayed wound healing, delayed graft function, mouth ulcers, pneumonitis, interstitial lung disease
Everolimus (Zortress)	Derivative of sirolimus, similar mechanism and toxicities		
Mycophenolate mofetil (CellCept)	Mycophenolic acid from *Penicillium stoloniferum*	Inhibits synthesis of guanosine monophosphate nucleotides; blocks purine synthesis, preventing proliferation of T and B cells	Gastrointestinal symptoms (mainly diarrhea), neutropenia, mild anemia
Azathioprine (Imuran)	Prodrug that undergoes hepatic metabolism to form 6-mercaptopurine	Converts 6-mercaptopurine to 6-thioinosine-5′-monophosphate, which is converted to thioguanine nucleotides that interfere with DNA and purine synthesis	Leukopenia, bone marrow depression, liver toxicity (uncommon)
Antithymocyte globulin	Polyclonal IgG from rabbits or horses immunized with human thymocytes	Blocks T-cell membrane proteins (CD2, CD3, CD45), causing altered function, lysis, and prolonged T-cell depletion	Cytokine release syndrome, thrombocytopenia, leukopenia, serum sickness
OKT3 (muromonab-CD3)	Anti-CD3 murine monoclonal antibody	Binds CD3 associated with the TCR, leading to initial activation and cytokine release, followed by blockade of function, lysis, and T-cell depletion	Severe cytokine release syndrome, pulmonary edema, acute renal failure, central nervous system changes
Basiliximab	Anti-CD25 chimeric monoclonal antibody	Binds to high-affinity chain of IL-2R (CD25) on activated T cells, causing depletion and preventing IL-2–mediated activation	Hypersensitivity reaction, uncommon
Daclizumab	Anti-CD25 humanized monoclonal antibody	Similar to that of basiliximab	Hypersensitivity reaction, uncommon
Rituximab	Anti-CD20 chimeric monoclonal antibody	Binds to CD20 on B cells and causes depletion	Infusion and hypersensitivity reactions, uncommon
Alemtuzumab	Anti-CD52 humanized monoclonal antibody	Binds to CD52 expressed on most T and B cells, monocytes, macrophages, and NK cells, causing lysis and prolonged depletion	Mild cytokine release syndrome, neutropenia, anemia, autoimmune thrombocytopenia, thyroid disease
FTY720	Sphingosine-like derivative of myricin from the fungus *Isaria sinclairii*	Functions as an antagonist for sphingosine-1-phosphate receptors on lymphocytes, enhancing homing to lymphoid tissues and preventing egress, causing lymphopenia	Reversible first-dose bradycardia, potentiated by general anesthetics and beta blockers, nausea, vomiting, diarrhea, increased liver enzyme levels
Belatacept (LEA29Y)	High-affinity homologue of CTLA-4–Ig	Binds to CD80/CD86 and prevents costimulation through CD28	In clinical trials, results show improved glomerular filtration rate and improved outcomes to CsA

Adapted from Halloran PF. Immunosuppressive drugs for kidney transplantation. *N Engl J Med.* 2004;351:2715–2729.
CsA, Cyclosporine A; *CTLA*, cytotoxic T lymphocyte–associated; *IgG*, immunoglobulin G; *IL*, interleukin; *NF-κB*, nuclear factor κB; *NK*, natural killer; *TCR*, T-cell receptor.

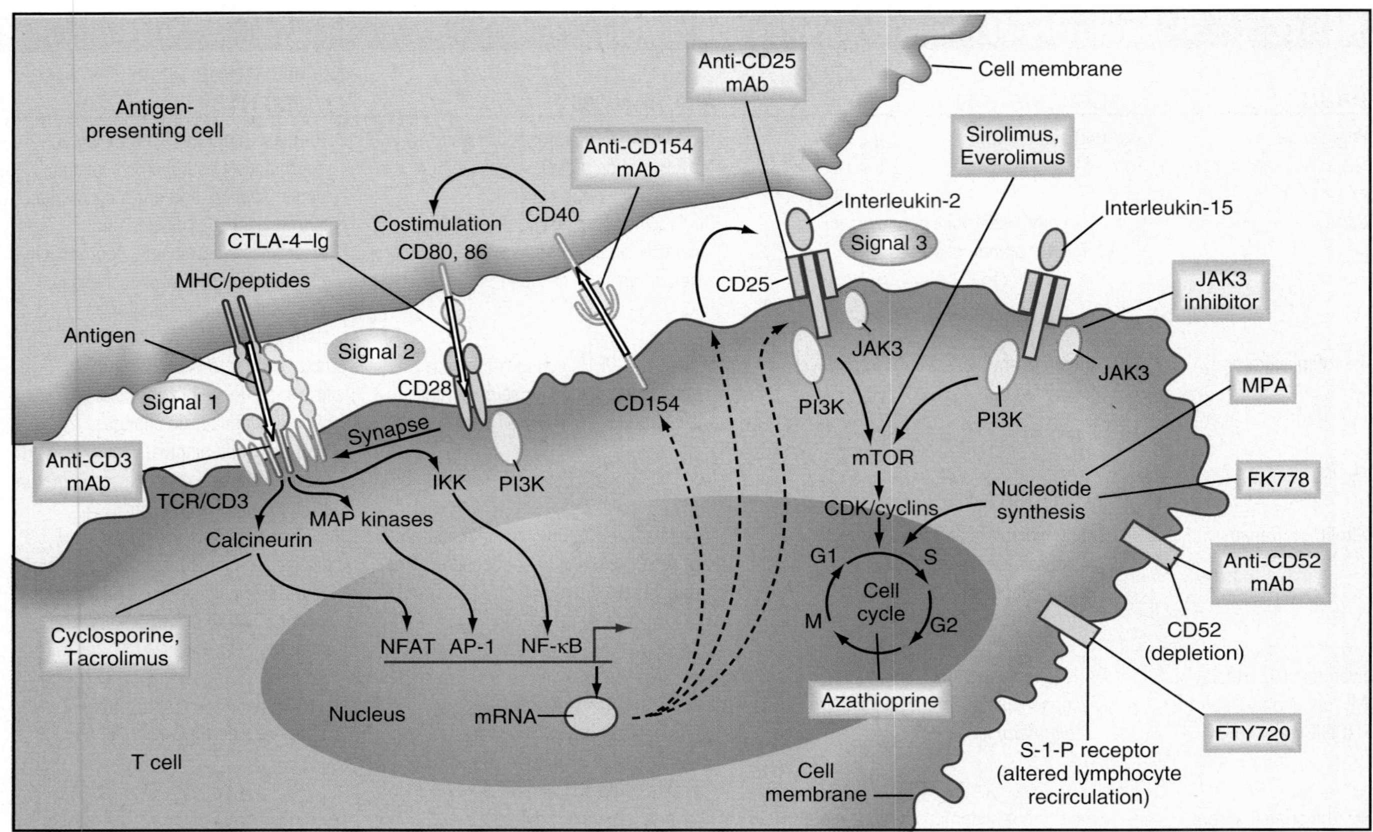

FIG. 25.21 Molecular mechanisms of immunosuppression. Immunosuppressants may be small molecules, antibodies, or fusion proteins that block various pathways critical for T-cell activation. TCR binding facilitates kinase activity by CD3 and the coreceptors (CD4 or CD8). The costimulatory molecules CD28, CD154, and others determine the relative potency of these signals. TCR signal transduction proceeds through a calcineurin-dependent pathway, resulting in dephosphorylation of NFAT, which subsequently enters the nucleus and acts in concert with nuclear factor κB *(NF-κB)* to facilitate cytokine gene expression. IL-2 functions in an autocrine fashion, binding to the IL-2R once the high-affinity chain (CD25) is expressed, to promote cell division. Cyclosporine and tacrolimus block TCR signal transduction by inhibiting calcineurin. Sirolimus and everolimus target mTOR to effectively block IL-2R signaling. Azathioprine and MMF/MPA interrupt the cell cycle by interfering with nucleic acid metabolism. Monoclonal antibodies (OKT3, anti–IL-2 receptor, alemtuzumab, anti-CD154, and others) or fusion proteins (CTLA-4–Ig, belatacept) function to deplete T cells or to interrupt key surface interactions required for T-cell function. (From Halloran PF. Immunosuppressive drugs for kidney transplantation. *N Engl J Med.* 2004;351:2715–2729.) *CTLA,* Cytotoxic T lymphocyte–associated; *Ig,* immunoglobulin; *IKK,* IkB kinase; *IL,* interleukin; *mAb,* monoclonal antibody; *MMF,* mycophenolate mofetil; *MPA,* mycophenolic acid; *mTOR,* mammalian target of rapamycin; *NFAT,* nuclear factor of activated T cell; *TCR,* T-cell receptor.

with T-cell specificity devoid of the unintended bystander effects observed with polyclonal preparations. Similar to the polyclonal preparations, there are several proposed mechanisms of action for OKT3. On binding to CD3, OKT3 triggers internalization of the TCR complex, preventing antigen recognition and subsequent signal transduction. In addition, it also labels cells for elimination through opsonization and phagocytosis. OKT3 was shown to be superior to conventional steroid therapy in reversing rejection and consequently improved allograft survival.[28] Because OKT3 is a mouse antibody, it can elicit an immune response to itself, and the recipient will generate antimurine antibodies directed against the structural regions of the antibody or the actual binding site, thereby limiting its therapeutic effect. In addition, the cytokine release syndrome associated with OKT3 administration can be vigorous, resulting in hypotension, pulmonary edema, and myocardial depression. In fact, a high dose of intravenous steroid is often given as premedication before the first few administrations of OKT3 in an attempt to minimize the adverse reactions. Because of this vigorous response, its immunogenicity and the availability of alternative therapeutic options, OKT3 has been withdrawn from production. There are newer monoclonal antibodies, either chimeric or humanized, with a similar mechanism of action and specificity as OKT3; these include otelixizumab, teplizumab, and visilizumab. They have been tested for the treatment of autoimmune conditions like Crohn disease, ulcerative colitis, and type 1 diabetes.

Alemtuzumab

Alemtuzumab was originally developed in the oncology field for the treatment of lymphoma. It is a humanized antibody against human CD52, a cell surface protein expressed on most mature lymphocytes and monocytes but not on their stem cell precursors. It has been used not only in patients with lymphoma but also in autoimmune processes, such as multiple sclerosis and rheumatoid arthritis. Administration of alemtuzumab is extremely effective at reducing the number of T cells both in the peripheral blood and in secondary lymphoid organs. In addition, it depletes, to a lesser extent, both B cells and monocytes. Unlike other strategies, this depletion may last for weeks to months after dosing. Investigational studies in transplantation employing alemtuzumab as an induction agent have allowed minimization of immunosuppression, particularly when it is combined with a calcineurin inhibitor.[29,30] Its optimal use in transplantation remains to be established.

Maintenance Immunosuppression

Following the immediate posttransplant period of induction, transplant recipients continue on long-term maintenance immunosuppression. Practice has evolved to maintain patients on standard multidrug regimens that have facilitated lower doses of individual agents to minimize toxicity and enhanced the quality of net immunosuppression through the use of various mechanisms of action. With outstanding short-term transplant outcomes, chronic use of maintenance agents and their attendant off-target toxicities has driven dose-reduction protocols over time and efforts to develop more selective and less toxic novel therapies.

Corticosteroids

Steroids, in particular glucocorticoids, remain one of the most commonly employed medications to prevent rejection. They are almost exclusively used in combination with other agents with which they seem to act synergistically to improve graft survival. They may also be used in higher doses as induction or rescue therapy for acute rejection episodes. Although steroids possess potent immunosuppressive properties, they can contribute significantly to the morbidity of transplantation by their effects on wound healing and propensity to cause diabetes, hypertension, and osteoporosis. With the advent of more effective and alternative immunosuppressive options over time, there has been an emphasis on developing steroid-minimization or steroid-sparing protocols to avoid these well-known side effects. Nonetheless, low-dose steroids remain a common component of current standard immunosuppressive regimens.

Although the Nobel Prize was awarded more than 50 years ago for work on the hormones of the adrenal cortex, the mechanism of the immunosuppressive effect of glucocorticoids was only recently better understood.[31] Similar to other steroid hormones, glucocorticoids bind to an intracellular receptor after passing into the cytoplasm through nonspecific mechanisms. The receptor-steroid complex then enters the nucleus, where it acts as a transcription factor. One of the most important genes upregulated is the gene encoding IκB. This protein binds to and inhibits the function of NF-κB, a key activator of proinflammatory cytokines and an important transcription factor involved in T-cell activation. Through this mechanism, steroids also act to diminish transcription of IL-1 and TNF-α by APCs as well as to prevent upregulation of MHC expression. Phospholipase A2, and consequently the entire arachidonic acid cascade, is also inhibited. They decrease the leukocyte response to various chemokines and chemotactins and by inhibiting vasodilators, such as histamine and prostacyclin, thus dampen the inflammatory response globally. This broad antiinflammatory response quickly mollifies the intragraft environment and thus substantially improves graft function long before the offending cells have actually left the graft. The most commonly used oral glucocorticoid formulation is prednisone; its intravenous equivalent is methylprednisolone.

Antiproliferative Agents

Azathioprine. The purine analogue azathioprine was first described in the 1960s and remained a mainstay of immunosuppression for the next 30 years.[32] It is still used today in organ transplantation and in the treatment of some autoimmune diseases, such as autoimmune hepatitis. Similar to other antiproliferative agents, it is a nucleotide analogue that targets cells undergoing rapid division; in the case of an immune response, its goal is to limit the clonal expansion of T and B cells. Azathioprine undergoes hepatic conversion to several active metabolites, including 6-mercaptopurine and 6-thioinosine monophosphate. These derivatives inhibit DNA synthesis by alkylating DNA precursors and interfering with DNA repair mechanisms. In addition, they inhibit the enzymatic conversion of thioinosine monophosphate to adenosine monophosphate and guanosine monophosphate, effectively depleting the cell of adenosine. The effects of azathioprine are relatively nonspecific, and like other antiproliferative agents, it acts on all rapidly dividing cells requiring nucleotide synthesis. Consequently, its predominant toxicities are seen in the bone marrow, gut mucosa, and liver. Azathioprine has been used as a maintenance agent in combination with other medications, such as a corticosteroid and calcineurin inhibitor. Although it has largely been replaced by MMF as the first-line antiproliferative agent, azathioprine remains the agent of choice during pregnancy.

Mycophenolate mofetil. MMF is an immunosuppressive agent with a similar mechanism of action to azathioprine. It is derived from the fungus *Penicillium stoloniferum*. Once ingested, it is metabolized in the liver to the active moiety mycophenolic acid. The active compound inhibits inosine monophosphate dehydrogenase, the enzyme that controls the rate of synthesis of guanosine monophosphate in the de novo pathway of purine synthesis, a critical step in RNA and DNA synthesis. Importantly, however, is the presence of a "salvage pathway" for guanosine monophosphate production in most cells except lymphocytes (hypoxanthine-guanine phosphoribosyltransferase–catalyzed guanosine monophosphate production directly from guanosine). Thus, MMF exploits a critical difference between lymphocytes and other body tissues, resulting in relatively lymphocyte-specific immunosuppressive effects. MMF blocks the proliferative response of both T and B cells, inhibits antibody formation, and prevents the clonal expansion of cytotoxic T cells.

There have been numerous clinical trials to evaluate MMF. Specifically, MMF has been shown to decrease the rate of biopsy-proven rejection and the need for rescue therapy compared with azathioprine.[33] Accordingly, MMF has replaced azathioprine in most standard three-drug immunosuppressive regimens, although recent evidence suggests that its therapeutic difference is less pronounced when it is used with more modern immunosuppressive therapies. It has also been used in combination with either a calcineurin inhibitor or sirolimus by many centers in steroid-sparing protocols. MMF is not, however, effective enough to be used alone without either steroids or calcineurin inhibitors. The major clinical side effects include leukopenia and diarrhea.

Calcineurin Inhibitors

Cyclosporine A. Jean-François Borel is credited with the discovery of CsA in 1972 while working as a microbiologist for Sandoz Laboratories (now Novartis). He apparently was vacationing in Norway and while there had collected soil samples for analysis in search of new antibiotics. Although the samples failed to show any significant antimicrobial activity, they did show potent immunosuppressive characteristics. Further studies demonstrated that the active component is a cyclic, nonribosomal peptide of 11 amino acids produced by the fungus *Tolypocladium inflatum*.[34] The mechanism of action of CsA is mediated primarily through its ability to bind the cytoplasmic protein cyclophilin. The CsA-cyclophilin complex binds to the calcineurin-calmodulin complex within the cytoplasm and blocks calcium-dependent phosphorylation and activation of NFAT, a critical transcription factor involved in T-cell activation including upregulation of the IL-2 transcript (Fig. 25.21). The result is blockade of IL-2 production. Thus, CsA is used as a maintenance agent, blocking the initiation of an immune response, but it is ineffective as a rescue agent once IL-2 has already been produced. In addition, CsA acts to increase transcription of TGF-β, a cytokine involved in the normal processes that limit the immune response by inhibiting T-cell activation, reducing regional blood flow, and stimulating tissue remodeling and wound repair. As discussed later, the toxicity and side effects of CsA may be in large part related to the effects of TGF-β.

CsA has poor water solubility and consequently must be given in a suspension or emulsion. This becomes a particular concern in liver transplantation because the oral absorption of CsA is dependent on bile flow; fortunately, this was addressed through the development of a microemulsion form that is less bile dependent. CsA is metabolized by the hepatic cytochrome P450 enzymes, and blood levels are therefore influenced by agents that affect the P450 system. P450 inhibitors, which include ketoconazole, erythromycin, calcium channel blockers, and grapefruit juice, result in higher CsA levels; inducers of P450, including rifampin, phenobarbital, and phenytoin, result in lower CsA levels.

The discovery of CsA and its subsequent development as an immunosuppressant contributed enormously to the advancement of organ transplantation. It was first approved for clinical use in 1983 and led to substantial improvement in the outcome of deceased donor renal transplantation and permitted the widespread practice of heart and liver transplantation.[35] Whereas its potent immunosuppressive activity was welcomed, its attendant toxicities were less than ideal. CsA induces the expression of TGF-β, and much of CsA toxicity can be linked to increased TGF-β activity. One of the most important side effects of CsA is renal toxicity. CsA has a significant vasoconstrictor effect on proximal renal arterioles, resulting in a 30% decrease in renal blood flow. This action is most likely mediated through increased TGF-β levels that act to increase the transcription of endothelin, a potent vasoconstrictor, resulting in activation of the renin-angiotensin pathway and resultant hypertension. The remodeling effects of TGF-β also induce fibrin deposition, which is thought to play a role in the fibrosis typically seen during chronic allograft nephropathy. CsA frequently causes neurologic side effects consisting of tremors, paresthesias, headache, depression, confusion, somnolence, and, rarely, seizures. Hypertrichosis (increased hair growth) is another frequent side effect, predominantly occurring on the face, arms, and back in up to 50% of patients. Gingival hyperplasia may also occur. The use of CsA in combination with other immunosuppressive agents permitted lower doses of CsA to limit toxicity, but current mainstay immunosuppression now favors the calcineurin inhibitor tacrolimus.

Tacrolimus. Tacrolimus was isolated from Japanese soil samples in 1984 as part of an effort to discover novel immunosuppressants. A macrolide produced by the fungus *Streptomyces tsukubaensis*, tacrolimus was found to possess potent immunosuppressive properties.[36] Similar to CsA, it blocks the effects of NFAT, prevents cytokine transcription, and arrests T-cell activation. The intracellular target is an immunophilin protein distinct from cyclophilin known as FK-binding protein (FK-BP). In vitro, tacrolimus was found to be 100 times more potent in blocking IL-2 and IFN-γ production than CsA and is clinically more effective at preventing acute rejection.[37] Tacrolimus, like CsA, also increases TGF-β transcription, leading to both the beneficial and toxic effects of this cytokine. The side effect profile for tacrolimus is similar to that of CsA with regard to renal toxicity, but the cosmetic side effects, such as abnormal hair growth and gingival hyperplasia, are substantially reduced. Neurotoxicity, including tremors and mental status changes, is more pronounced with tacrolimus, as is its diabetogenic effect. Tacrolimus has been shown to be extremely effective for solid organ transplantation and has become the cornerstone drug of choice for most centers.

Mammalian Target of Rapamycin Inhibitors

Sirolimus and everolimus. Sirolimus (rapamycin) was isolated from a soil sample taken from Easter Island, a Polynesian island in the southeastern Pacific Ocean also known as Rapa Nui, hence the name rapamycin. It is a macrolide derived from the bacterium *Streptomyces hygroscopicus* with potent immunosuppressive properties. Everolimus is a derivative of rapamycin that possesses similar properties. Both are similar in structure to tacrolimus and bind to the same intracellular target, FK-BP, but neither agent affects calcineurin activity and consequently does not inhibit expression of NFAT or IL-2 expression. Instead, the sirolimus–FK-BP complex inhibits the mammalian target of rapamycin (mTOR), specifically the mTOR complex 1 (see Fig. 25.21). mTOR is also called FRAP (FK-BP–rapamycin-associated protein) or RAFT (rapamycin and FK-BP target). RAFT-1 is a critical kinase involved in the IL-2 receptor signaling pathway. The result is inhibition of p70 S6 kinase activity, an enzyme essential for ribosomal phosphorylation, and arrest of cell cycle progression. Other receptors are also affected, including those for IL-4, IL-6, and platelet-derived growth factor.

Both sirolimus and everolimus are potent inhibitors of rejection in experimental models. Sirolimus and tacrolimus can act synergistically to impair rejection, but the combination can result in intolerable clinical toxicity. More often, sirolimus is used as an alternative to calcineurin inhibitors in a multidrug regimen or combined with other agents, allowing a reduction in the dose and minimization of side effects, including calcineurin inhibitor–related nephrotoxicity or steroid-specific side effects. In addition to immunosuppressive properties, mTOR inhibitors have been shown to have promising antitumor effects as well. For example, sirolimus has been shown to promote programmed cell death in B-cell lymphomas, and everolimus has demonstrated activity against EBV. Thus, both agents may play an important role in the prevention of posttransplantation lymphoproliferative disorder (PTLD). Sirolimus and everolimus have also been used in the development of drug-eluting coronary stents to limit the rate of in-stent restenosis because of their antiproliferative properties. There is an increased incidence of hypercholesterolemia and hypertriglyceridemia with both agents that often requires treatment with cholesterol-lowering agents or discontinuation of the drug. Oral ulcers, wound healing complications (in particular an increased incidence of lymphoceles), elevated levels of proteinuria, and thrombocytopenia remain frequent problems and limit universal application.

Costimulation Blockade

Belatacept. Costimulation is a critical component of naïve T-cell activation and has been extensively studied as a potential target for immune modulation in organ transplantation. One of the

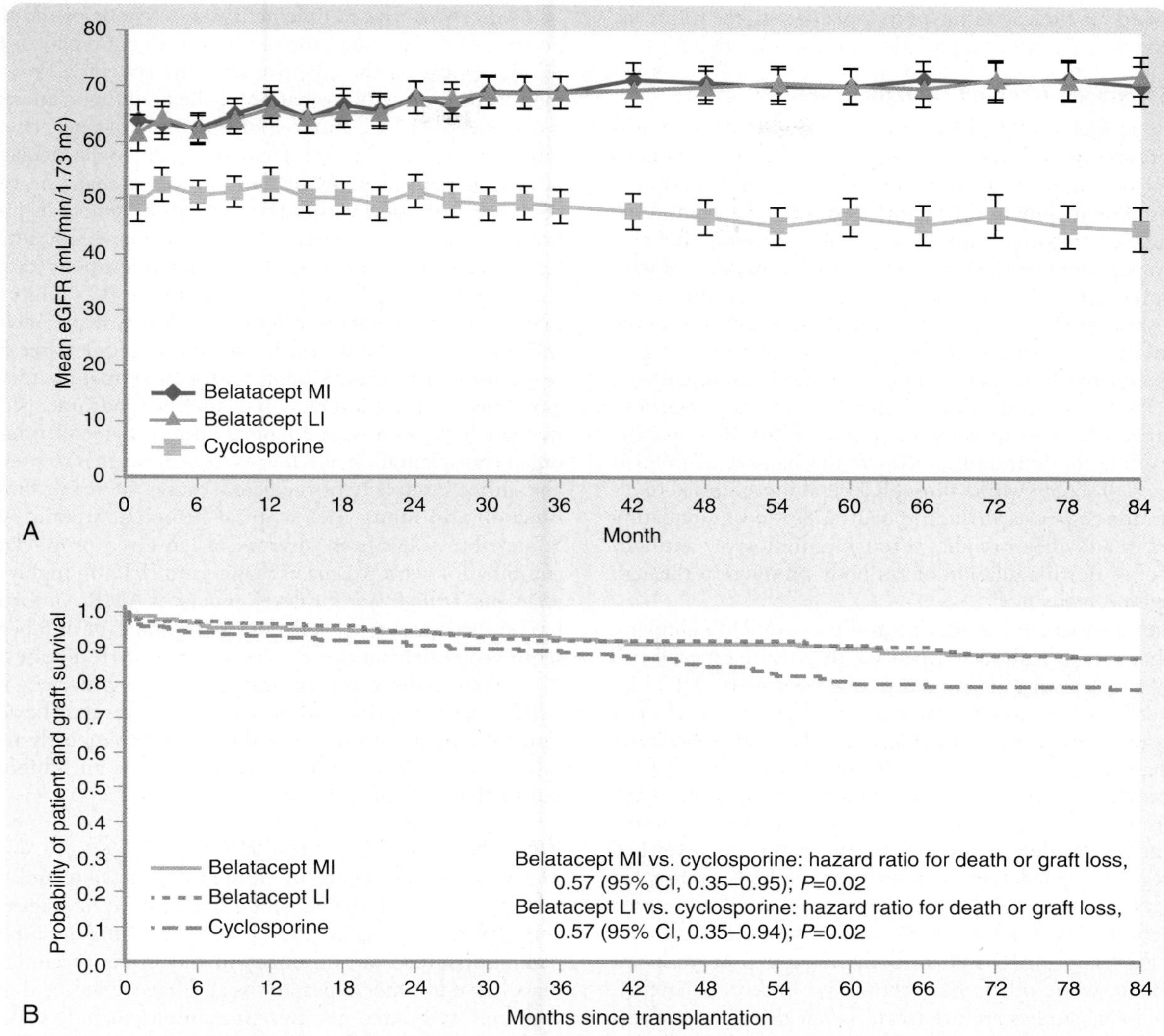

FIG. 25.22 Long-term outcomes with belatacept. Seven-year outcomes of the phase 3 BENEFIT study demonstrated significantly higher renal function as measured by mean estimated glomerular filtration rate (eGFR) over time (A) and improved patient and graft survival (B) with more intense (MI) and less intense (LI) belatacept as compared to the calcineurin inhibitor cyclosporine. (From Vincenti F, Rostaing L, Grinyo J, et al. Belatacept and long-term outcomes in kidney transplantation. *N Engl J Med.* 2016;374:333–343.)

most important costimulation pathways is the interaction between CD28 and CD80/CD86. Signaling through CD28 allows effective IL-2 production and promotes cell survival through upregulation of antiapoptotic molecules. CD152 (CTLA-4) is another cell surface molecule expressed on activated T cells that is more effective in binding CD80 and CD86 than CD28. Once activated, T cells begin to express CD152, which interacts with CD80 and CD86 with a higher affinity and effectively interferes with CD28 binding and may deliver inhibitory signals to the T cell as part of a downregulatory mechanism for the immune response. CTLA-4–Ig is a fusion protein consisting of the extracellular component of CTLA-4 and the heavy chain of human IgG1 that was developed to block CD28-CD80/CD86 interactions and consequently to impair costimulation and T-cell activation (see Fig. 25.21). CTLA-4–Ig (abatacept) is used clinically for several autoimmune indications, including rheumatoid arthritis and psoriasis. However, the observed immunosuppressive strength of abatacept in preclinical transplant studies was suboptimal; thus, efforts to improve the efficacy of CTLA-4–Ig resulted in a novel mutant form, LEA29Y (belatacept). LEA29Y is a second-generation CTLA-4–Ig molecule that differs by two amino acid residues within the ligand binding domain, resulting in increased affinity for CD80 and CD86. The resultant improvement in binding affinity led to more potent immunosuppressive properties in vitro and in vivo.[17] Belatacept has since been tested in both preclinical nonhuman primate studies and phase 3 clinical trials in human renal transplantation and was FDA approved for use in kidney transplantation in 2011. Seven-year clinical trial data demonstrated improved long-term outcomes with better renal function and a significant reduction in the risk of patient death and allograft loss with belatacept in a calcineurin inhibitor–free regimen compared to CsA-based immunosuppression (Fig. 25.22).[16] Higher-than-expected acute rejection rates and logistic challenges related to intravenous infusion administration requirements have slowed large-scale uptake of belatacept. However, with proven improvement in long-term transplant outcomes and a favorable toxicity profile, along with new generation blockers and alternative delivery methods poised for clinical testing in transplantation, the future for costimulation-based immunosuppression strategies is bright.

B-Cell and Antibody-Directed Therapies

Intravenous immune globulin. IVIG is composed of pooled plasma fractions from thousands of donors and essentially contains a representative sample of all antibodies found within that population. It is used frequently in the treatment of several autoimmune diseases, such as idiopathic thrombocytopenic purpura, Guillain-Barré syndrome, and myasthenia gravis, as well as in patients with severe immune deficiencies featuring low or absent antibody levels. IVIG is also used in organ transplantation, specifically in the treatment of humoral rejection or before transplantation in highly sensitized recipients as a desensitization method in an attempt to reduce the PRA score and risk for hyperacute or early rejection. More recently, it has also been used as part of ABO-incompatible protocols. While the immunosuppressive mechanism of IVIG is not known, it probably works through several mechanisms to alter the immune response, including neutralization of circulating autoantibodies and alloantibodies through antiidiotypic antibodies and selective downregulation of antibody production through Fc-mediated mechanisms.[38]

Rituximab. Rituximab is a murine antihuman CD20 chimeric antibody that was initially developed for the treatment of B-cell lymphoma and has since been used in the treatment of PTLD. CD20 is a cell surface protein expressed on all mature B cells but not on plasma cells. Rituximab binds to CD20 and facilitates antibody-dependent cellular cytotoxicity and complement-dependent cytotoxicity of B cells as well as promoting programmed cell death. More recently, rituximab has been used in a wide variety of autoimmune disorders and as a component in some investigational strategies designed as induction therapy in highly sensitized transplant recipients undergoing kidney transplantation or even in ABO-incompatible pairings. Some studies have indicated a reduction in the risk of AMR and antibody rebound posttransplant with rituximab, while others have shown no benefit. Therefore, additional clinical studies are needed to better define its optimal role in solid organ transplantation. Interestingly, the fact that CD20 is not expressed on antibody-producing plasma cells may explain the mixed clinical results with rituximab, and its beneficial effects may relate to the role of B cells in antigen presentation and memory B cells in antibody recall responses.

Antiplasma Cell Therapies

In an effort to specifically target antibody-secreting plasma cells, the anti-CD38 mAb daratumumab and two proteasome inhibitors have emerged. In contrast to CD20, CD38 is expressed on the surface of short- and long-lived plasma cells and may be a better target for the control of AMR resulting from plasma cell-derived alloantibodies. However, daratumumab mediates potent depletion of not only plasma cells but also potentially beneficial immunoregulatory T- and B-cell subsets. Therefore, the net effect of this anti-CD38 mAb remains to be carefully investigated in human transplantation. The proteasome inhibitors bortezomib and carfilzomib also selectively target antibody-producing plasma cells due to their high rate of Ig synthesis and reliance on their proteasomes to breakdown damaged proteins. The use of these agents to treat AMR in transplantation has also led to mixed results, and while proteasome inhibition may be effective at controlling acute antibody production, combination with other agents may be needed to achieve sustained control of alloantibodies and improve long-term outcomes in transplantation.

Eculizumab. The complement system is one of the main components of the innate immune response but also plays a significant role in regulating the adaptive immune system as well. Complement activation with formation of the membrane attack complex is the end point of a number of inflammatory processes that can cause damage to the transplanted organ. In particular, the role of complement in AMR or other processes that lead to immune complex deposition within the allograft or xenograft has recently been recognized as a potential target of therapeutic intervention. Eculizumab is a humanized monoclonal antibody targeting the complement component C5. Its binding to C5 inhibits the formation of complement components downstream, including the split product C5a and membrane attack complex (see Fig. 25.4). It is approved to treat patients with paroxysmal nocturnal hemoglobinuria and atypical hemolytic uremic syndrome. More recently, there have been several reports employing eculizumab in solid organ transplantation as a means to treat or even to prevent AMR and other complement-mediated causes of renal allograft dysfunction and injury (i.e., atypical hemolytic uremic syndrome). Some efficacy has been observed when given prophylactically in combination with plasma exchange and IVIG in highly sensitized recipients at high risk for development of AMR. Unfortunately, it has not been universally effective as a significant number of highly sensitized patients proceed to experience AMR despite treatment. This likely reflects the complexity of the processes leading to AMR, suggesting that additional mechanisms may be at play. Additional ongoing studies have shown promising early results with other complement-specific reagents, such as an inhibitor of C1, but further trials are needed.

Novel Immunosuppressive Agents

The vast improvements in immunosuppression and transplant outcomes have led to a very high standard for new agents to overcome. While agents in the clinical development pipeline have had rational mechanisms of action and strong preclinical efficacy, many have not met expectations and have failed to show efficacy and improved outcomes. Recent examples include a sphingosine-1-phosphate receptor modulator (fingolimod) and JAK3 inhibitor (tofacitinib).

Fingolimod. Fingolimod has a unique mechanism of action that results in sequestration of lymphocytes within lymph nodes, thereby preventing them from participating in allograft rejection. Fingolimod requires phosphorylation by sphingosine kinase 2 to become active, after which it binds to a sphingosine-1-phosphate receptor (specifically S1PR1) (see Fig. 25.21) and results in aberrant internalization of the receptor deprives lymphocytes of the signals necessary for egress from secondary lymphoid organs, and functionally traps them within lymph nodes. Unfortunately, despite promising experimental data, fingolimod failed to show an improvement in efficacy in the prevention of renal allograft rejection in two large phase 3 studies. Without improved efficacy and new, unexpected side effects in these studies, clinical trials were halted in renal transplantation.

Tofacitinib. There has been an intense effort to develop other therapeutic targets by exploiting the other pathways that are critical for T-cell activation and effector function. As was covered earlier in this chapter, cytokines are critical signals and growth factors that influence T-cell proliferation and differentiation. Cytokine receptors found on the T-cell surface transduce their signal through the use of the JAK/STAT pathways; thus, several JAK inhibitors have been developed. One in particular, the JAK3 inhibitor tofacitinib, has been tested in kidney transplantation. JAK3, unlike other subtypes, is restricted in its expression to primarily hematopoietic cells and associates with the common γ chain, a shared component of the receptor for IL-2 and numerous other cytokines. JAK3 inhibition has been an effective treatment for autoimmune disorders, and in a phase 2b clinical trial, tofacitinib was found to be equally effective at preventing rejection as CsA in renal transplant recipients and led to better renal function, less chronic damage on kidney biopsy, and lower rates of posttransplantation diabetes. Unfortunately, treatment with tofacitinib was associated with more anemia and neutropenia and a trend toward more infections, including BK virus and CMV infections, and cases of PTLD, resulting in reduced interest for development in transplantation. Tofacitinib is, however, approved for rheumatoid arthritis and other autoimmune conditions.

CD40/CD154 pathway blockade. Beyond the CD28/B7 pathway, blockade of the CD40/CD154 costimulation pathway remains of significant interest in transplantation. Although the clinical development of CD154-specific therapies has been circuitous and challenged by an association with thromboembolic events in preclinical and clinical studies, experimentally targeting this pathway continues to show profound effects on alloimmunity. The recognition that anti-CD154 mAbs may cause thromboembolism by binding and cross-linking CD154 on platelets has left open the possibility that therapeutic targeting of CD40 or alternative methods of blocking CD154 may achieve the immunosuppressive effects of inhibiting this pathway without disrupting hemostatic mechanisms. Successful targeting of CD40 as an alternative to CD154 has been achieved in preclinical nonhuman primate studies, as well as blockade of CD154 with a novel Fc silent domain antibody devoid of cross-linking ability. The anti-CD40 monoclonal antibody ASKP1240 has recently been tested in early phase clinical trials, but under the regimens tested, higher rates of acute rejection and infectious complications were observed, rendering the optimal immunosuppressive regimen to utilize blockers of the CD40/CD154 pathway and the clinical future of this agent uncertain. More recently, CFZ533, an Fc-silent anti-CD40 antibody, is being tested in humans after demonstrated efficacy and safety in preclinical primate studies. Because targeting CD154 has generally been observed to be more potent than its receptor CD40, efforts to test novel CD154 blockers in human transplant recipients are ongoing in the hopes of one day introducing this promising immunosuppressive strategy into the clinic.

Complications of Immunosuppression

The development of immunosuppressive agents was the key step in the advancement of the field of transplantation. Unfortunately, these same agents are responsible for much of the morbidity associated with organ transplantation as well. All current immunosuppressants function to a greater or lesser degree in a nonspecific fashion (i.e., global immunosuppression instead of donor-specific or allospecific immunosuppression). The consequence is occasional overzealous suppression of the immune system, resulting in infectious complications, primarily viral infections, as well as an increased risk of malignant disease. In addition, many of these agents modify the function of proteins and pathways required for normal cell function, and consequently, their inhibition results in undesired, nonimmune side effects, including direct organ injury.

Risk of Infection

There is a fine balance between sufficient immunosuppression to prevent rejection and preservation of the host response to nontransplant antigens and pathogens. Introduction of tissue from one individual to another always introduces the potential for transfer of new organisms. Currently, an extensive battery of testing is performed on both the donor and recipient before transplantation. These examinations have greatly decreased the potential exposure to the recipient, but no test is perfect, and testing can be limited by available technology and the time interval between procurement and implantation. Some infections may still be transferred unknowingly for various reasons, including early infection and lack of seropositivity. Infections may be donor derived, such as a CMV+ organ placed into a CMV− recipient, or may arise from less commonly transferred viruses, resulting in primary infections of HIV, hepatitis C virus, hepatitis B virus, tuberculosis, *Trypanosoma cruzi*, West Nile virus, lymphocytic choriomeningitis virus, or rabies.[39]

The threat comes not only from new pathogens but, more importantly, from those to which the recipient has likely already been exposed and harbors in a state of dormancy or latency. Normally, these pathogens are controlled after the initial infection and remain quiescent. After the immune system is rendered impotent by pharmacologic suppression, these pathogens can spring to life and quickly become uncontrollable. Recipient-derived infections are much more common after transplantation than donor-derived infections. One common example is CMV reactivation. The majority of the population has been exposed to CMV at some point in their lives. In the setting of induction and maintenance immunosuppressive therapy in transplantation, CMV reactivation can occur, resulting in pneumonitis, hepatitis, pancreatitis, or colitis. CMV has also been implicated in the lesions of heart transplant recipients with chronic rejection, highlighting the interplay between the immune response and chronic viral infections or the inflammation they may induce. Other recipient-derived infections include tuberculosis, certain parasites (*Strongyloides stercoralis*, *Trypanosoma cruzi*), viruses (e.g., CMV, EBV, herpes simplex, varicella-zoster, hepatitis B, hepatitis C, and HIV), and endemic fungi (e.g., *Pneumocystis jiroveci*, *Histoplasma capsulatum*, *Coccidioides immitis*, and *Paracoccidioides brasiliensis*).

Fortunately, patterns of opportunistic infections after transplantation have been altered by the use of routine antimicrobial prophylaxis. The risk for reactivation is highest approximately 6 to 12 weeks after transplantation and again after periods of increased immunosuppression for acute rejection episodes. Transplant programs use various prophylactic regimens, depending on the organs transplanted. Many regimens include pneumococcal vaccine, hepatitis B vaccine, and trimethoprim-sulfamethoxazole for *Pneumocystis* pneumonia and urinary tract infections; ganciclovir or valganciclovir for CMV infections; and clotrimazole troche or nystatin for oral and esophageal fungal infections. As immunosuppressive strategies have evolved, resulting in increases in both allograft and patient survival, the specific pathogens as well as the pattern of infection have also evolved. For example, the polyomaviruses BK and JC have been recognized to play a more important role in transplantation than previously understood. Infection with the polyomavirus BK has been found in association with a progressive nephropathy and ureteral obstruction, and the JC virus has been associated with progressive multifocal leukoencephalopathy. Detection of BK viral DNA in blood and urine has been useful for monitoring response to therapy, which includes minimizing immunosuppression and treatment with antiviral therapies.

Risk for Malignant Disease

The immune system not only plays a critical role in defending the host against attack from pathogens, it also plays an important role in the surveillance and detection of cancer, particularly those cancers driven by viral infection. The consequence is a nearly ten fold increase in rates of malignant disease. Skin cancers, particularly squamous cell cancers, are the most common malignant conditions in transplant recipients and account for substantial morbidity and mortality.[40] As expected, virally mediated tumors tend to occur much more frequently in transplant recipients. For example, human papillomavirus is associated with cancer of the cervix, hepatitis B and C viruses with hepatocellular carcinoma, and human herpesvirus 8 with Kaposi sarcoma. EBV, in particular, can be associated with the development of PTLD, a broad term used to describe EBV-associated lymphomas that occur in transplant recipients. PTLD varies from asymptomatic to life-threatening, and, accordingly, treatment varies from simple reduction or withdrawal of immunosuppression to vigorous chemotherapeutic regimens. More recently, patients have been treated with antiviral agents targeting EBV or even chemotherapy including antibody therapy against the tumor cells, such as rituximab.

Nonimmune Side Effects

Although current immunosuppressants have become increasingly more specific, in general, they are still directed at pathways that play an important role in multiple systems other than immunity. Thus, inhibition of a pathway for the sake of immunosuppression can also lead to unintended consequences if the target is critical to other processes. For example, calcineurin inhibitors are potent suppressors of T-cell activation, but their activity not only decreases IL-2 transcription, it also increases TGF-β expression. Elevated levels of TGF-β result in an increase in endothelin expression and eventually lead to hypertension. In addition, TGF-β is thought to play a critical role in the development of chronic allograft nephropathy, previously thought to be immune mediated but now likely to be, at least partly, secondary to nonimmune side effects secondary to calcineurin inhibitor use.

Histologic evidence of calcineurin inhibitor–associated nephrotoxicity is essentially universal in renal transplants by 10 years. Furthermore, these deleterious effects are not limited to only renal transplant recipients. The incidence of chronic renal failure in nonrenal transplant recipients is an astonishing 16.5%.[41] New-onset diabetes after transplantation is also an important problem, particularly in individuals receiving tacrolimus or steroids. The incidence of new-onset immunosuppressive-related diabetes mellitus approaches 30% in the first 2 years after renal transplantation, conferring a significantly higher risk of death. In addition to renal failure, hypertension, and diabetes, immunosuppressive therapy can also lead to hyperlipidemia, anemia, and accelerated cardiovascular disease, which is a leading cause of death in long-term transplant survivors. Thus, it appears that the very reagents that ushered in a new era of short-term success in organ transplantation have proven to be major contributors in the demise of the transplanted organ or recipient over the long-term. Clearly, there is a pressing clinical need to develop novel immunosuppressive agents that are effective and more specific yet less toxic, or to devise strategies to induce immune tolerance so that long-term immunosuppression may eventually be eliminated altogether.

TOLERANCE

Immunologic tolerance, or the maintenance of allograft function without immune suppression, has been fittingly thought of as the "holy grail" of transplantation biology, as it has been the subject of noble scientific pursuit that remains a mystery and has yet to be discovered. Self-tolerance as discussed before involves regulation of the immune response to prevent undesired effects toward host tissues or proteins. This is established and maintained through both central (i.e., thymic selection and deletion) and peripheral mechanisms. The ability to selectively inactivate the host response toward only the transplanted donor antigens while maintaining immunocompetence would be highly desirable. This would avoid the need for lifelong immunosuppression with its associated toxicities as well as eliminate chronic rejection, a major cause of late graft failure.

It has been more than 50 years since the first reports of acquired tolerance. The discovery of neonatal transplantation tolerance has been credited to Ray Owen, a geneticist who studied the inheritance of red blood cell antigens in cattle. He reported in 1945 that dizygotic twins had mixtures of their own cells and their twin partner's cells. Earlier observations had demonstrated that bovine dizygotic twins develop a fusion of their placentas during embryonic life. This results in a common intrauterine circulation and the unabated passage of sex hormones, explaining the phenomenon of freemartin cattle. Owen also recognized that this common circulation allows the exchange of hematopoietic cells during embryonic life and the establishment of a chimeric state. Interestingly, these calves did not develop isoantibodies to their twin, suggesting a state of immunologic tolerance.

Peter Medawar acknowledged the importance of Owen's observation and predicted that an exchange of skin grafts between dizygotic calves could verify the tolerance hypothesis, and together with his postdoctoral fellow, Rupert Billingham, he performed a series of grafting experiments that provided direct support for the concept of neonatally acquired transplantation tolerance. Subsequent experiments by Billingham, Leslie Brent, and Medawar demonstrated that neonatally acquired transplantation tolerance could be achieved in mice by inoculation of embryos or intravenous injection of newborn mice with allogeneic cells. Medawar shared the Nobel Prize in 1960 for the discovery of acquired immunologic tolerance.

Just as there are multiple methods to provide for self-tolerance in any given individual, there have been many proposed strategies to induce transplantation tolerance exploiting these pathways. Some of these include clonal deletion or elimination of donor-reactive cells, clonal anergy or functional inactivation of donor-reactive cells, and regulation or suppression of donor-reactive cells. There are rare reports of patients who have discontinued immunosuppression for various reasons and have not experienced rejection. Ongoing studies within this small population of operationally tolerant patients seek to determine what mechanisms are responsible for graft maintenance in the absence of immunosuppression. One such study suggests that those kidney transplant patients who discontinue their immunosuppressive treatments for whatever reason and continue to enjoy stable allograft function also have elevated numbers of naïve and transitional B cells in their peripheral blood compared with those patients who remain on immunosuppression, suggesting a role for this cell population in the tolerant state.[42]

There are numerous reports of intentionally induced tolerance in experimental models, but most of these are not effective when translated to higher animal models such as nonhuman primates. Although there are several exciting avenues of research and even clinical trials in humans, currently there is no proven regimen to reliably induce transplantation tolerance that would be widely applicable. Here are a few strategies of particular interest that are currently under investigation.

Lymphocyte Depletion

Most currently employed immunosuppressive regimens involve the use of induction therapy. Many rely on some form of antilymphocyte preparation, most commonly RATG, to eliminate or to inactivate recipient cells at the time of transplantation. They are used in the very early posttransplantation period, which corresponds to the time when ischemia and reperfusion of the graft accompanied by the surgical trauma significantly increase immune recognition. These preparations successfully remove T cells from the circulation for several days, and those that are present remain anergic for some period. Use of these agents has significantly reduced the rate of acute rejection and allowed minimization of immunosuppression in several different protocols. A number of groups have undertaken clinical trials using early recipient T-cell depletion in combination with various other immunosuppressive strategies in an attempt to induce tolerance. The prevailing concept is one of T-cell clone reduction in an effort to allow existing tolerance mechanisms to be effective. Several studies have used alemtuzumab to induce profound T-cell depletion for this purpose. Despite achieving depletion that was similar to promising preclinical studies with respect to kinetics, magnitude, and effectiveness within the secondary lymphoid tissues, treatment with alemtuzumab alone or in combination with deoxyspergualin was not sufficient to induce tolerance in adult humans.[30] Newer studies have combined alemtuzumab with belatacept and rapamycin with promising results, although tolerance was not achieved.[43] The failure of these T cell–centric approaches suggests that other components of the immune system, such as B cells, NK cells, or monocytes, may also need to be specifically targeted to achieve tolerance. Whereas depletion alone has not been able to establish tolerance, it has allowed minimization of immunosuppression to a single agent in some cases and likely facilitates other protolerant approaches.

Costimulation Blockade

T-cell activation requires not only interaction between the TCR complex and MHC-bound peptide but also sufficient costimulatory signals to promote a successful response. TCR ligation in the absence of appropriate costimulation results in T-cell inactivation or anergy. This mechanism is used presumably as a mechanism of peripheral tolerance to control any aberrant, self-reactive T cell that may have escaped the thymic selection process. Researchers have tried to exploit this through the development of antibodies or fusion proteins designed to block these costimulatory interactions. Interruption of costimulatory pathways at the time of transplantation should thus selectively inactivate or anergize only those cells specific for donor antigen, leaving nonreactive cells unaffected. Preexisting immunity and innate responses should be unaffected by this approach. There are multiple animal models of transplantation in which this has proven to be the case, particularly with simultaneous blockade of the CD28 and CD40 pathways.[44] This approach in both rodents and primates has resulted in prolonged survival of cardiac and renal allografts without the need for any subsequent immunosuppression and without significant infectious or malignant side effects. However, the extrapolation of these results to clinical practice has been thus far disappointing. In the only human tolerance trial of costimulation blockade, hu5C8, a humanized anti-CD154 monoclonal antibody, demonstrated limited efficacy and was associated with potential thromboembolic toxicity. Newly developed agents that block the CD28 pathway are now being tested as maintenance agents, which may pave the way for their use in future tolerance trials. In addition, there are numerous other therapeutic reagents that have been or are in development (such as antibodies to CD40, CD134 [OX40L], ICOS, and many other costimulatory pathways). It remains to be seen which of these will make it through the gauntlet of drug development, but there are exciting possibilities for future tolerance regimens.

Chimerism

Hematopoietic chimerism is associated with a particularly robust form of donor-specific tolerance. This approach involves both central and peripheral mechanisms for induction and maintenance of tolerance. Complete chimerism classically occurs in bone marrow transplantation where all bone marrow–derived cells in a recipient are eliminated and replaced by donor cells. However, the morbidity associated with the myeloablative conditioning required to achieve complete chimerism precludes it as a viable method of tolerance induction in solid organ transplantation. Hence, mixed chimerism refers to a recipient who possesses both self- and donor-derived hematopoietic cells after bone marrow transplantation and requires less morbid and milder forms of preconditioning to achieve. In chimeric states, similar to the normal physiologic process, donor marrow elements migrate to the thymus and participate in thymic selection, resulting in central deletion of potentially donor-reactive T cells. Presumably similar events occur within the bone marrow for B-cell selection. The peripheral compartment can be pharmacologically deleted in a nonspecific fashion at the time of transplantation, or alternatively, donor antigen delivered at the time of bone marrow infusion engages donor-reactive cells in the absence of appropriate costimulation as a result of concomitantly administered immunosuppression, causing peripheral deletion, anergy, or regulation and resulting in donor-specific nonresponsiveness.

In humans, successful bone marrow transplantation and complete chimerism allow the acceptance of subsequent organ allografts from the same donor in the absence of immunosuppression. Conventional bone marrow transplantation regimens, however, are typically myeloablative in nature, and the associated toxicities are too great for them to be employed as part of a solid organ tolerance trial. Newer advances in nonmyeloablative techniques with less toxicity have since paved the way for the clinical application and testing of mixed chimerism–based strategies. An initial trial to test the efficacy of a mixed chimerism strategy to induce tolerance was performed in highly selected patients suffering from both end-stage renal failure and multiple myeloma. These patients simultaneously received bone marrow and a kidney from an HLA-identical sibling. The regimen led to chimerism in all six patients; four had transient chimerism, and the remaining two progressed into full chimeras. Three patients remain operationally tolerant without any immunosuppression after a reported follow-up of up to 7 years. The same group of investigators reported on a similar protocol in haploidentical living related donor-recipient pairs that resulted in the successful induction of transient chimerism and tolerance. None of these patients possessed concomitant indications for bone marrow transplantation, such as multiple myeloma, as was the case in the first trial. One allograft was lost to irreversible humoral rejection, but remarkably, the other four recipients have sustained stable renal allograft function for up to 5 years after complete withdrawal of immunosuppressive drugs.[45] The conditioning regimen required resulted in profound T, B, and NK cell depletion and substantial myelosuppression, leading to severe leukopenia and capillary leak syndrome. Interestingly, the biologic phenomenon that inspired the protocol, mixed chimerism, was not achieved in any patient, suggesting that the predominant effect is one of intensive induction.

Newer approaches have involved nonmyeloablative techniques combined with cell-based therapies to facilitate chimerism and tolerance induction. Cell-based therapies have consisted of a variety of different cell types, including modified hematopoietic stem cell preparations, Tregs, tolerogenic dendritic cells, and regulatory macrophages, among others. One notable phase 2 trial combined reduced intensity conditioning with facilitator cell enriched hematopoietic stem cell transplantation in HLA-mismatched living donor kidney transplant recipients. Of 31 subjects with more than 12 months of follow-up, 22 patients achieved stable donor chimerism and were weaned off immunosuppression. However, not all subjects achieved chimerism and discontinuation of immunosuppression, and several experienced recurrent autoimmunity and infectious complications resulting in graft loss.[46] Two patients developed graft-versus-host disease, resulting in one death. Therefore, while these approaches show promise for immunosuppression withdrawal in a portion of transplant recipients, the incidence and durability of tolerance, the rate and severity of graft-versus-host disease, and the long-term effects of intensive conditioning remain to be determined before these regimens find a role in clinical practice.

XENOTRANSPLANTATION

The most pressing problem in clinical transplantation is the shortage of available organs. More than 100,000 individuals are currently listed and awaiting organ transplantation. Many more individuals could benefit from transplantation but, given the shortage of organs, are not currently considered. Those who are placed on the list for transplantation must often wait a significant amount of time before an organ becomes available, during which time their clinical status can deteriorate, diminishing their ability to survive and to recover from surgery. An alternative source of organs could potentially come from another species, namely, xenotransplantation. In addition to increasing the supply of available organs, xenotransplantation could also offer some of the same benefits realized with living donors, such as decreased ischemic time and injury as well as optimization of the recipient's health status prior to transplantation. There are potential novel disadvantages with xenotransplantation, such as ethical considerations and zoonotic viral transmission. Xenografts may be concordant and discordant, depending on the proximity in evolution of the given species to humans. This proximity markedly influences the immune response, and the implications are discussed here.

Concordant Xenografts

Concordant xenografts refer to transplants between closely related species; for humans, these include Old World monkeys and apes. The critical element defining an animal as concordant is the assembly of carbohydrate antigens on the cell surface. Similar to humans, concordant species lack galactosyltransferase, and as a result, their carbohydrates are the typical blood group antigens and they lack the N-linked disaccharide galactose-α(1-3)-galactose (α-Gal). Thus, the natural antibodies present in the circulation of potential human recipients can be predicted by straightforward blood group typing, thereby avoiding the problem of hyperacute rejection. Even though hyperacute rejection is not a threat, the typical mechanisms of graft rejection remain, including acute cellular rejection, acute vascular rejection, and, presumably, chronic rejection. Surprisingly, most of the critical molecular elements responsible for antigen presentation and T cell–mediated rejection are evolutionarily conserved in mammals. That is to say, MHC molecules, adhesion proteins, and costimulatory molecules are similar across species and are adequate for immune function. Consequently, concordant xenografts undergo cellular and humoral rejection in a similar fashion as would a totally MHC-mismatched allograft in the absence of immunosuppression.

Several experimental models of concordant xenograft transplantation, as well as occasional ventures into the clinical arena, have clearly demonstrated that concordant xenotransplantation is feasible. The most famous case occurred almost 25 years ago when clinicians at Loma Linda transplanted a baboon heart into an infant born with hypoplastic heart syndrome. The child survived for 20 days after the transplantation before eventually succumbing to primarily humoral-mediated rejection.[47] This foray into the realm of clinical xenotransplantation highlighted the ethical issues associated with primate to human transplantation. Widespread application of concordant xenografts would quickly deplete the supply of nonhuman primates, particularly when a loss rate extrapolated from poorly matched allografts is taken into consideration. In addition, there is significant concern that zoonotic transfer of disease, in particular retroviral transmission, will put the patient and the public at undue risk. Given these factors, it is unlikely that concordant xenotransplantation will ever gain widespread application.

Discordant Xenografts

Transplant concordance among species is predominantly determined on the basis of the expression of the enzyme galactosyltransferase. This enzyme is responsible for differential expression of carbohydrate moieties on the cell surface of discordant species, primarily α-Gal expression. In considering human recipients, discordant xenograft donors would include New World monkeys and other mammals, but for physiologic concerns (e.g., organ size, availability), pigs would be the preferred animal donor. When organs from discordant species are transplanted into humans, they rapidly undergo hyperacute rejection. The primary mechanism relies on the presence of preformed IgM antibodies against cell surface carbohydrate moieties, particularly α-Gal. These so-called natural antibodies are similar to those antibodies that define the blood group antigens. In transplantation, they bind to the endothelial cells on the donor organ and in concert with complement precipitate an irreversible reaction of cell damage, thrombosis, and immediate graft failure. As with concordant xenografts, the remainder of the acquired and innate immune responses may also play an important role in the rejection process.

Despite the aggressive immune response elicited by discordant xenograft transplantation, enthusiasm and research continue toward establishing a xenogeneic source of donor organs. Several groups have now developed transgenic pigs that express various human complement regulator proteins, such as CD59, CD55 (decay-accelerating factor), and membrane cofactor protein. Other groups have developed α(1-3)-galactosyltransferase knockout animals, eliminating the expression of α-Gal and removing the major target of natural antibodies and complement activation (Fig. 25.23). Baboons transplanted with hearts from decay-accelerating factor transgenic pigs enjoy prolonged survival compared with control pig donors. More recently, there have been exciting reports of prolonged xenograft survival (in some cases >1 year) in preclinical nonhuman primate models of heart, islet, and kidney

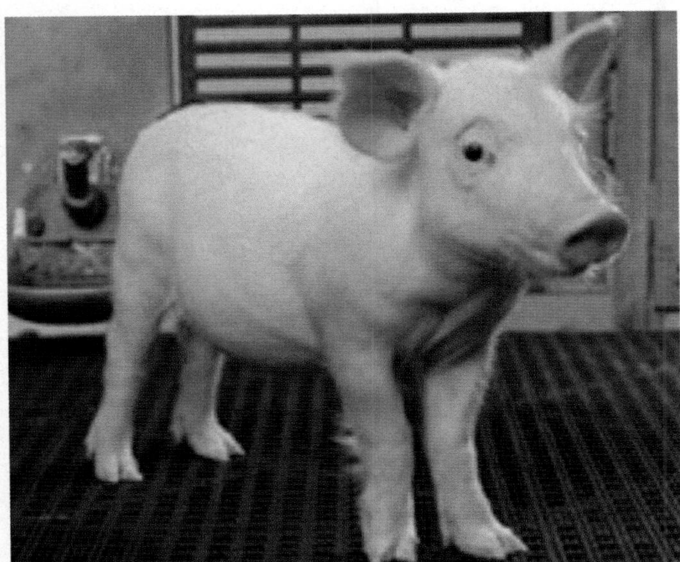

FIG. 25.23 Xenotransplantation using genetically engineered porcine donors. Example of an α-galactosyltransferase knockout, human decay-accelerating factor transgenic donor pig. (Courtesy National Swine Resource and Research Center [NSRRC]; http://www.nsrrc.missouri.edu/NSRRC0009info.asp.)

transplantation.[48] Whereas there are significant barriers before clinical application, genetic engineering may conceivably allow an endless supply of made-to-order organs.

NEW AREAS OF TRANSPLANTATION

Islet Cell Transplantation

The concept of islet cell transplantation to treat diabetes is not novel, but reliable reversal of diabetes after islet transplantation is a relatively recent accomplishment. Techniques for islet isolation have undergone refinement for most of the latter half of the last century. Clinical application of this technique, however, was largely hampered by both the lack of efficient isolation techniques and the lack of effective immunosuppressive regimens, many of which included diabetogenic drugs such as steroids, which promoted diabetes themselves, resulting in poor outcomes (~10% of recipients became insulin independent after transplantation). In 2000, a group from Edmonton, Alberta, demonstrated successful, consistent insulin independence after islet transplantation. The principal change was the development of a steroid-free immunosuppressive protocol composed of low-dose tacrolimus, sirolimus, and daclizumab. The initial report ignited incredible enthusiasm within the diabetes community, but the optimism has since been tempered by less promising long-term results. In a subsequent multicenter trial, less than half of the 36 patients achieved insulin independence 1 year after transplantation, and those who initially did achieve independence lost it over time. In addition to the questions of long-term efficacy, islet transplantation is associated with substantial costs, and there are questions about its safety and ultimate utility. Given these more recent results, the number of clinical islet transplantations performed worldwide has dramatically decreased in the last few years. Despite these setbacks, there is promise for the field of islet transplantation, including research focusing on ex vivo islet expansion and the use of stem cells, newer more effective yet less toxic immunosuppressive protocols, tolerance regimens, and xenotransplantation.

Vascularized Composite Tissue Transplantation

Vascularized composite tissue transplantation involves the transfer of multiple tissue types, including skin, fat, muscle, nerves, blood vessels, tendon, and bone, within one functional unit, such as a hand or face. Annually, there are millions of patients with lost limbs or extensive soft tissue injuries who could potentially benefit from reconstruction with composite tissue transfer. Several of these cases have been highlighted within the media in the last few years, and the ethical debate over non-lifesaving transplantation has generated extensive discussion. The first successful hand transplantation was performed in Lyon, France, in 1998, and since that time, over 70 patients have undergone single- or double-hand transplants. Many have recovered remarkable levels of function, including tying shoes, dialing a cell phone, turning door knobs, and throwing a ball, as well as sensitivity to hot and cold. Unfortunately, some patients have required amputation of the transplanted hand after uncontrolled rejection, most of which has been attributed to noncompliance. Shortly after the early reports of hand transplantation, there have been numerous descriptions of other successful composite tissue allografts, including larynx, trachea, and face.[49]

The first successful face composite allograft was reported by a group of surgeons from France in 2005. Not long after, the first near-total human face transplantation in the United States was performed in 2008 on a patient with severe midface trauma after a gunshot wound. Many patients regain the ability to perform many normal daily activities, such as breathing through the nose, recovering a sense of smell and taste, speaking intelligibly, and using the mouth to eat solid foods and to drink from a cup (Fig. 25.24).[49] Unlike traditional solid organ transplantation, many of the cases of composite tissue transplantation provoke ethical, economic, and clinical dilemmas. Some may argue that subjecting recipients to the risks of surgery and lifelong immunosuppression for a non–life-sustaining transplant may not be appropriate. Nevertheless, these transplants can totally transform the life of a severely disabled or disfigured patient, improving both form and function. With the advent of increasingly less toxic immunosuppressants and possible tolerance strategies, composite tissue transplantation could become an ever-increasing part of standard clinical treatment.

Uterus Transplantation

The advent of nonvital tissue or organ transplantation as with composite tissue transplantation introduced the concept of utilizing transplantation to address medical problems that significantly limit quality of life. As such, uterus transplantation research began shortly after the first reported human hand transplant in 1998 and has culminated with numerous successful uterus transplants in humans throughout the world. It is estimated that 3% to 5% of females suffer from absolute uterine factor infertility resulting either from congenital agenesis or malformation, or acquired conditions related to surgical removal or uterine malfunction (e.g., fibroids). For many women desiring pregnancy with absolute uterine factor infertility, gestational surrogacy is not a viable option due to legal, ethical, or religious concerns and uterus transplantation offers these women with infertility a novel and alternative option for gestation. The first technically successful uterus transplant was performed in 2011, and the first functionally successful transplanted uterus to lead to a healthy live birth occurred in 2014

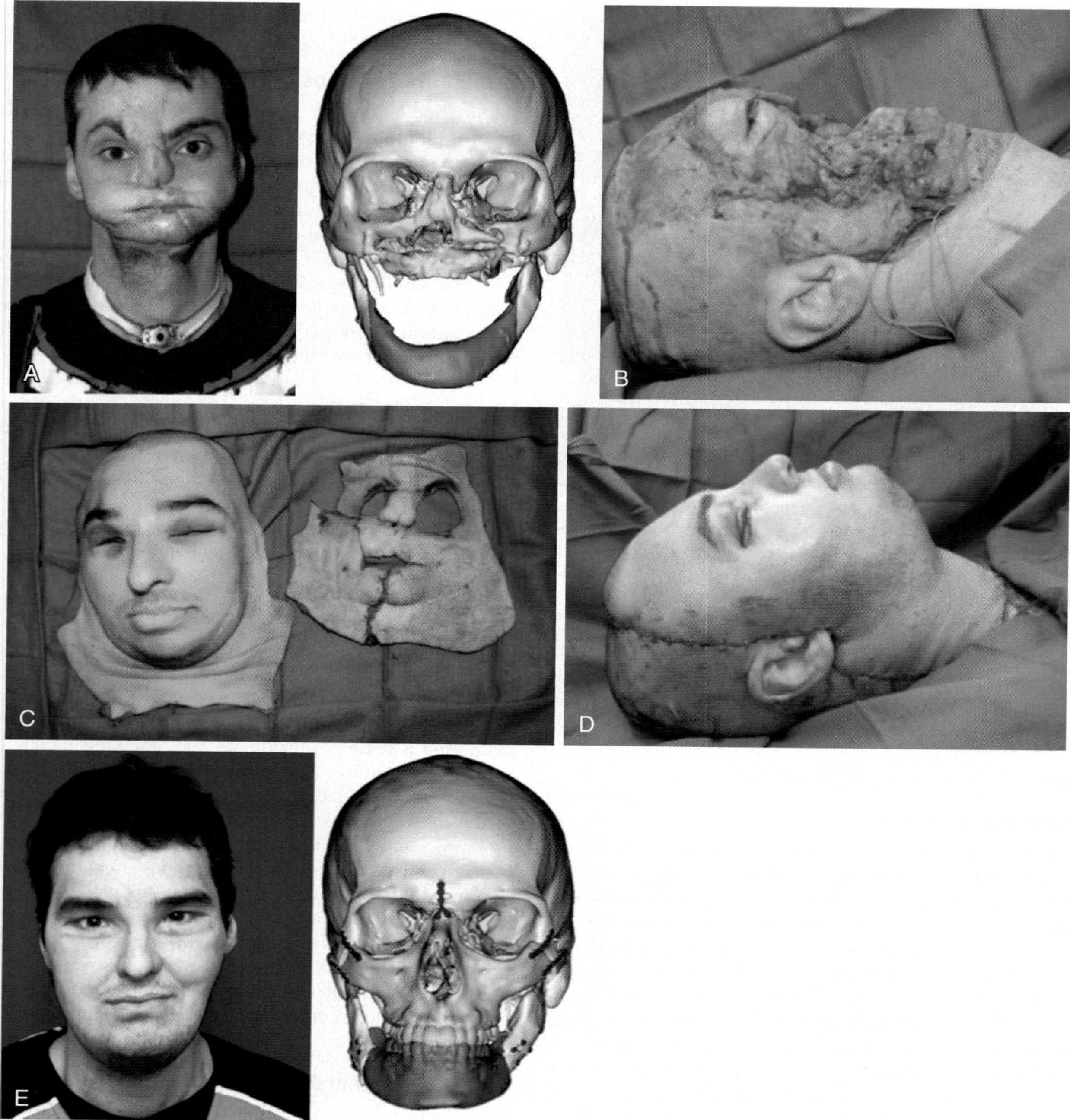

FIG. 25.24 (A) Frontal view and computed tomography scan reconstruction of patient before transplantation. (B) Intraoperative photograph after removal of disfigured tissue, hardware, and bone. (C) Side-by-side comparison of the donor face attached to its underlying skeletal architecture on the left and the recipient's face on the right. (D) Intraoperative photograph of final facial reconstruction. (E) Frontal view and computed tomography scan reconstruction 16 months after transplantation. (From Dorafshar A, Branko, B, Christy, M, et al. Total face, double jaw, and tongue transplantation: an evolutionary concept. *Plast Reconstr Surg*. 2013;131:241–251; Khalifian A, Brazio P, Mohan R, et al. Facial transplantation: the first 9 years. *Lancet*. 2014;384:2153–2163. Courtesy Eduardo D. Rodriguez, MD, DDS.)

in Sweden (Fig. 25.25).[50] While this form of solid organ transplantation remains largely experimental, several programs have been initiated throughout the world and more than 30 uterus transplants have been performed from both deceased and living donors. Given the global clinical interest, seemingly large demand from women with absolute uterine factor infertility, and ongoing advances in transplantation, the field expects continued growth of this largely experimental treatment in the form of increasing research and clinical trials. Uterus transplantation introduces the unique considerations of cyclical physiologic function and undulating periods of immunological activity and potential for hosting a fetus. Protocols with limited immunosuppressive courses may be indicated once desired pregnancies have occurred and the transplanted uterus is no longer functionally needed, minimizing or

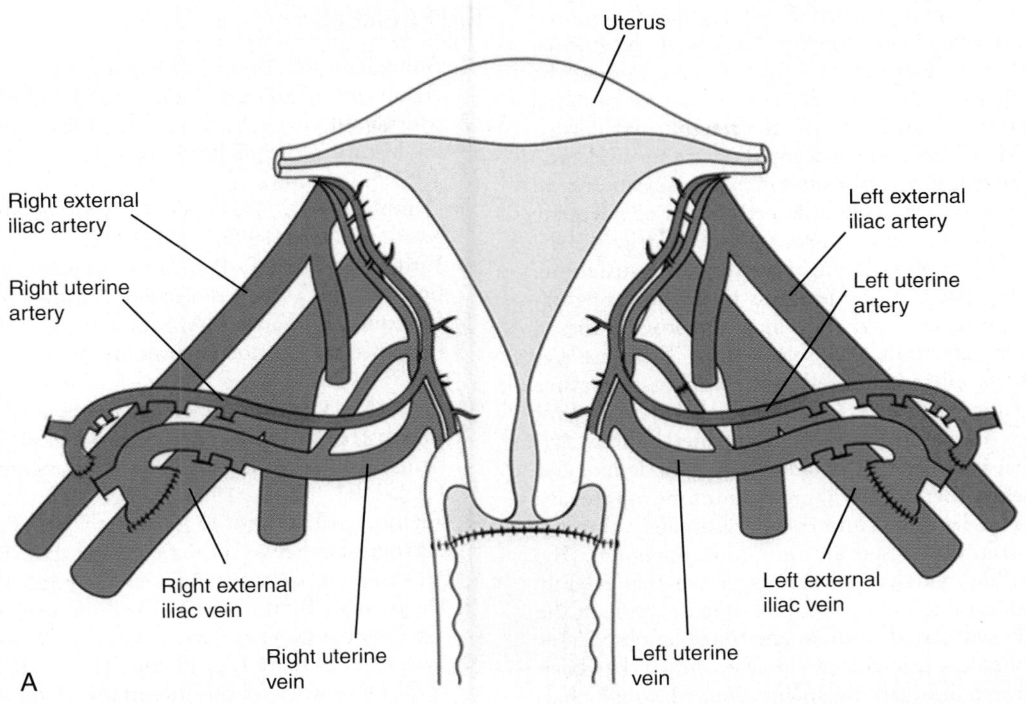

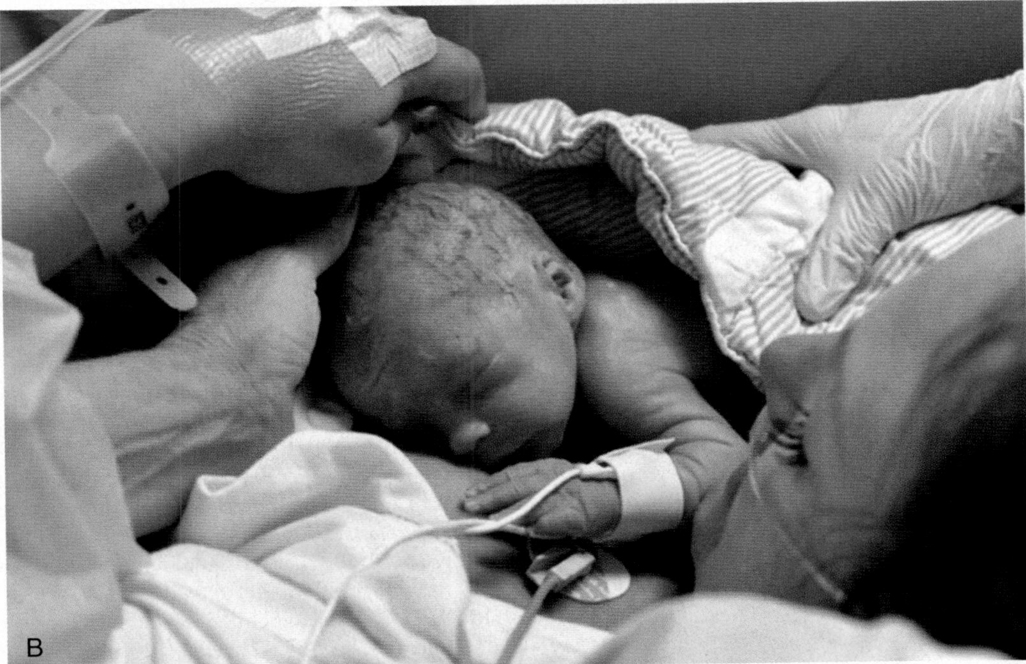

FIG. 25.25 Uterus transplantation. (A) Schematic of the vascular anastomoses performed in a uterus transplant. The uterine veins and arteries are connected end-to-side to the external iliac veins and arteries, respectively. (B) First newborn baby to result from a transplanted uterus shortly after birth. (From Brannstrom M, Johannesson L, Bokstrom H, et al. Livebirth after uterus transplantation. *Lancet*. 2015;385:607–616.)

avoiding the long-term side effects and risks of infection and malignancy observed with standard immunosuppression.

CONCLUSION

More than a half-century has passed since the first successful solid organ transplantation. Today, thousands of patients with end-stage diseases undergo lifesaving transplantation each year. That which was once considered impossible is now an everyday occurrence, and most transplant recipients are leading healthy, productive lives with an organ from another individual functioning inside of them. The idea of replacing a diseased organ with a healthy one is simple in concept, yet the details of managing the rejection response is very complex. The immune system typically generates a highly organized yet regulated response when challenged. Many of the principal details of the normal immune response were described by researchers examining the mechanisms of allograft rejection. In fact, surgeons garnered multiple Noble Prizes in Medicine for their significant contributions to the field. Whereas short-term allograft survival rates have steadily improved, long-term outcomes remain an area in need of significant improvement. The availability of adequate donor organs remains the most pressing issue restricting the majority of potential recipients from receiving a life-sustaining transplant. There continues to be progress in xenotransplantation and tissue engineering, and they may yet provide for an unlimited supply of safe, transplantable organs. There are significant drawbacks to current nonselective immunosuppressive therapies, such as increased risks of infections and malignant disease, economic constraints, and long-term metabolic toxicities, including renal insufficiency, diabetes, hyperlipidemia, and cardiovascular disease. Increasingly targeted immunosuppressive agents continue to be developed and tested. Ultimately, the goal is to achieve low-risk, donor-specific immunosuppression. The development of a safe, widely applicable regimen that reliably produces transplantation tolerance would eliminate many of the problems currently associated with organ transplantation. Indeed, one of the medical miracles of the last century has been the success and growth of organ transplantation. Although challenges remain, transplant surgeons and scientists will undoubtedly continue to be at the forefront of discovery and innovation as the field marches forward.

SELECTED REFERENCES

Abbas AK, Lichtman AH, Pillai S. *Cellular and Molecular Immunology*. 9th ed. Philadelphia: Saunders Elsevier; 2018.

Concise and well-established textbook of immunology that comprehensively surveys fundamental immunology.

Brent L. *A History of Transplantation Immunology*. San Diego: Academic Press; 1997.

Interesting historical perspective on the development and evolution of transplantation immunology.

Chong AS, Alegre ML. The impact of infection and tissue damage in solid-organ transplantation. *Nat Rev Immunol*. 2012;12:459–471.

Excellent review on the importance of the innate immune response in the rejection process.

Halloran PF. Immunosuppressive drugs for kidney transplantation. *N Engl J Med*. 2004;351:2715–2729.

Excellent overview of immunosuppression in the context of clinical transplantation.

Vincenti F, Rostaing L, Grinyo J, et al. Belatacept and long-term outcomes in kidney transplantation. *N Engl J Med*. 2016;374:333–343.

Seminal report of clinical trial demonstrating improved long-term outcomes in kidney transplantation with the biologic co-stimulation blocker belatacept.

REFERENCES

1. Billingham RE, Brent L, Medawar PB. Actively acquired tolerance of foreign cells. *Nature*. 1953;172:603–606.
2. Murray JE, Lang S, Miller BF. Observations on the natural history of renal homotransplants in dogs. *Surg Forum*. 1955;5:241–244.
3. Campbell RD, Trowsdale J. Map of the human MHC. *Immunol Today*. 1993;14:349–352.
4. Parham P, Ohta T. Population biology of antigen presentation by MHC class I molecules. *Science*. 1996;272:67–74.
5. Bjorkman PJ, Saper MA, Samraoui B, et al. Structure of the human class I histocompatibility antigen, HLA-A2. *Nature*. 1987;329:506–512.
6. Bevan MJ. Cross-priming. *Nat Immunol*. 2006;7:363–365.
7. Brown JH, Jardetzky TS, Gorga JC, et al. Three-dimensional structure of the human class II histocompatibility antigen HLA-DR1. *Nature*. 1993;364:33–39.
8. Teyton L, O'Sullivan D, Dickson PW, et al. Invariant chain distinguishes between the exogenous and endogenous antigen presentation pathways. *Nature*. 1990;348:39–44.
9. Davis MM, Bjorkman PJ. T-cell antigen receptor genes and T-cell recognition. *Nature*. 1988;334:395–402.
10. Lythe G, Callard RE, Hoare RL, et al. How many TCR clonotypes does a body maintain? *J Theor Biol*. 2016;389:214–224.
11. Kappler JW, Roehm N, Marrack P. T cell tolerance by clonal elimination in the thymus. *Cell*. 1987;49:273–280.
12. Suchin EJ, Langmuir PB, Palmer E, et al. Quantifying the frequency of alloreactive T cells in vivo: new answers to an old question. *J Immunol*. 2001;166:973–981.
13. Chambers CA, Allison JP. Co-stimulation in T cell responses. *Curr Opin Immunol*. 1997;9:396–404.
14. Larsen CP, Pearson TC. The CD40 pathway in allograft rejection, acceptance, and tolerance. *Curr Opin Immunol*. 1997;9:641–647.
15. Schwartz RH. A cell culture model for T lymphocyte clonal anergy. *Science*. 1990;248:1349–1356.
16. Vincenti F, Rostaing L, Grinyo J, et al. Belatacept and long-term outcomes in kidney transplantation. *N Engl J Med*. 2016;374:333–343.
17. Larsen CP, Pearson TC, Adams AB, et al. Rational development of LEA29Y (belatacept), a high-affinity variant of CTLA4-Ig with potent immunosuppressive properties. *Am J Transplant*. 2005;5:443–453.
18. Ford ML. T cell cosignaling molecules in transplantation. *Immunity*. 2016;44:1020–1033.
19. Wood KJ, Sakaguchi S. Regulatory T cells in transplantation tolerance. *Nat Rev Immunol*. 2003;3:199–210.
20. Patel R, Terasaki PI. Significance of the positive crossmatch test in kidney transplantation. *N Engl J Med*. 1969;280:735–739.
21. Gloor JM, DeGoey SR, Pineda AA, et al. Overcoming a positive crossmatch in living-donor kidney transplantation. *Am J Transplant*. 2003;3:1017–1023.
22. Gourishankar S, Halloran PF. Late deterioration of organ transplants: a problem in injury and homeostasis. *Curr Opin Immunol*. 2002;14:576–583.
23. Hardinger KL, Rhee S, Buchanan P, et al. A prospective, randomized, double-blinded comparison of thymoglobulin versus Atgam for induction immunosuppressive therapy: 10-year results. *Transplantation*. 2008;86:947–952.

24. Swanson SJ, Hale DA, Mannon RB, et al. Kidney transplantation with rabbit antithymocyte globulin induction and sirolimus monotherapy. *Lancet*. 2002;360:1662–1664.
25. Matas AJ, Kandaswamy R, Gillingham KJ, et al. Prednisone-free maintenance immunosuppression—a 5-year experience. *Am J Transplant*. 2005;5:2473–2478.
26. Vincenti F, Kirkman R, Light S, et al. Interleukin-2-receptor blockade with daclizumab to prevent acute rejection in renal transplantation. Daclizumab Triple Therapy Study Group. *N Engl J Med*. 1998;338:161–165.
27. Nashan B, Moore R, Amlot P, et al. Randomised trial of basiliximab versus placebo for control of acute cellular rejection in renal allograft recipients. CHIB 201 International Study Group. *Lancet*. 1997;350:1193–1198.
28. A randomized clinical trial of OKT3 monoclonal antibody for acute rejection of cadaveric renal transplants. *N Engl J Med*. 1985;313:337–342.
29. Calne R, Friend P, Moffatt S, et al. Prope tolerance, perioperative campath 1H, and low-dose cyclosporin monotherapy in renal allograft recipients. *Lancet*. 1998;351:1701–1702.
30. Kirk AD, Hale DA, Mannon RB, et al. Results from a human renal allograft tolerance trial evaluating the humanized CD52-specific monoclonal antibody alemtuzumab (CAMPATH-1H). *Transplantation*. 2003;76:120–129.
31. Rhen T, Cidlowski JA. Antiinflammatory action of glucocorticoids—new mechanisms for old drugs. *N Engl J Med*. 2005;353:1711–1723.
32. Calne RY, Murray JE. Inhibition of the rejection of renal homografts in dogs by Burroughs Wellcome 57-322. *Surg Forum*. 1961;12:118–120.
33. Sollinger HW. Mycophenolate mofetil for the prevention of acute rejection in primary cadaveric renal allograft recipients. U.S. Renal Transplant Mycophenolate Mofetil Study Group. *Transplantation*. 1995;60:225–232.
34. Borel JF, Feurer C, Gubler HU, et al. Biological effects of cyclosporin A: a new antilymphocytic agent. *Agents Actions*. 1976;6:468–475.
35. Merion RM, White DJ, Thiru S, et al. Cyclosporine: five years' experience in cadaveric renal transplantation. *N Engl J Med*. 1984;310:148–154.
36. Kino T, Hatanaka H, Miyata S, et al. FK-506, a novel immunosuppressant isolated from a Streptomyces. II. Immunosuppressive effect of FK-506 in vitro. *J Antibiot (Tokyo)*. 1987;40:1256–1265.
37. Pirsch JD, Miller J, Deierhoi MH, et al. A comparison of tacrolimus (FK506) and cyclosporine for immunosuppression after cadaveric renal transplantation. FK506 Kidney Transplant Study Group. *Transplantation*. 1997;63:977–983.
38. Samuelsson A, Towers TL, Ravetch JV. Anti-inflammatory activity of IVIG mediated through the inhibitory Fc receptor. *Science*. 2001;291:484–486.
39. Fishman JA. Infection in solid-organ transplant recipients. *N Engl J Med*. 2007;357:2601–2614.
40. Euvrard S, Kanitakis J, Claudy A. Skin cancers after organ transplantation. *N Engl J Med*. 2003;348:1681–1691.
41. Ojo AO, Held PJ, Port FK, et al. Chronic renal failure after transplantation of a nonrenal organ. *N Engl J Med*. 2003;349:931–940.
42. Newell KA, Turka LA. Tolerance signatures in transplant recipients. *Curr Opin Organ Transplant*. 2015;20:400–405.
43. Kirk AD, Guasch A, Xu H, et al. Renal transplantation using belatacept without maintenance steroids or calcineurin inhibitors. *Am J Transplant*. 2014;14:1142–1151.
44. Larsen CP, Elwood ET, Alexander DZ, et al. Long-term acceptance of skin and cardiac allografts after blocking CD40 and CD28 pathways. *Nature*. 1996;381:434–438.
45. Kawai T, Sachs DH, Sprangers B, et al. Long-term results in recipients of combined HLA-mismatched kidney and bone marrow transplantation without maintenance immunosuppression. *Am J Transplant*. 2014;14:1599–1611.
46. Leventhal JR, Ildstad ST. Tolerance induction in HLA disparate living donor kidney transplantation by facilitating cell-enriched donor stem cell infusion: the importance of durable chimerism. *Hum Immunol*. 2018;79:272–276.
47. Bailey LL, Nehlsen-Cannarella SL, Concepcion W, et al. Baboon-to-human cardiac xenotransplantation in a neonate. *JAMA*. 1985;254:3321–3329.
48. Higginbotham L, Mathews D, Breeden CA, et al. Pre-transplant antibody screening and anti-CD154 costimulation blockade promote long-term xenograft survival in a pig-to-primate kidney transplant model. *Xenotransplantation*. 2015;22:221–230.
49. Siemionow M, Papay F, Alam D, et al. Near-total human face transplantation for a severely disfigured patient in the USA. *Lancet*. 2009;374:203–209.
50. Brannstrom M, Johannesson L, Bokstrom H, et al. Livebirth after uterus transplantation. *Lancet*. 2015;385:607–616.

26 CHAPTER

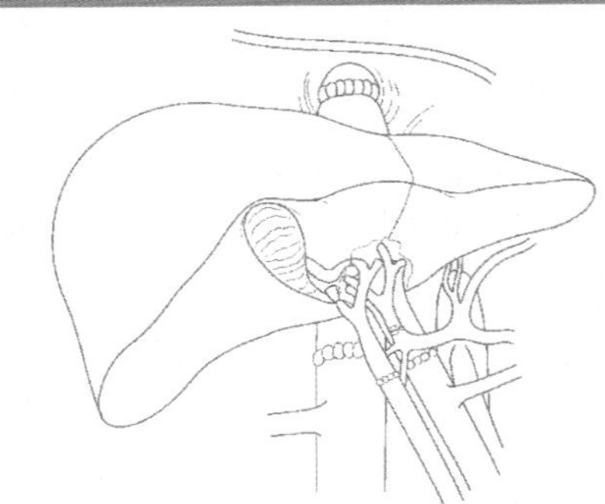

Liver Transplantation

Seth J. Karp, Sophoclis Alexopoulos

OUTLINE

HISTORY

More than 90% of patients receiving a liver transplant in the United States will be alive 1 year after the surgery, and almost 85% will be alive after 3 years.[1] This extraordinary achievement arose as the result of the syntheses of a myriad of discoveries in disparate fields. Liver transplantation represents a triumph of scientific achievement, collaboration, and teamwork.

Seminal discoveries instrumental in developing transplantation trace back more than 100 years. These include the technical achievements of Alexis Carrel in creating vascular anastomoses in the first decade of the 20th century. While performing research on skin grafting for soldiers in World War II in the early 1940s, Sir Peter Medawar discovered graft loss was due to immunological factors, specifically cell-mediated immunity.[2] His subsequent studies established the efficacy of steroids to protect against graft injury.[3] In 1952, the chemists Gertrude Eillion and George Hitchings at Burroughs-Wellcome synthesized azathioprine and 6-mercaptopurine, which would become cornerstones of early immunosuppressive therapy. In 1954, Joseph Murray proved transplantation could be successful by performing a renal transplant using an identical twin as a donor.[4] In 1959, Dr. Murray went on to demonstrate the feasibility of transplantation across immunological barriers using total body irradiation to suppress the immune system.[5] All of these investigators earned a Nobel Prize in recognition of their accomplishments.

Despite these advancements allowing limited success for kidney transplantation, early attempts at human liver transplantation were marked by failure (expertly chronicled in the book *The Puzzle People* by Thomas Starzl).[6] Technical complexities of the operation, coagulopathy, metabolic derangements, and poor understanding of the immunological basis of graft loss conspired to produce poor outcomes. The first attempt at human liver transplantation in 1963 by Dr Starzl failed, as did subsequent attempts in Berlin, Boston, and Paris. Things looked so grim that Starzl himself placed a 3-year moratorium on liver transplantation, returning exclusively to the lab to determine how to best move forward.[6]

With advances in technique and immunosuppression, limited success was achieved. In the 1970s, Starzl reported 1-year survival rates around 30%.[7] Nearly two decades after the first liver transplant was attempted, Jean Borel discovered that cyclosporine, initially investigated as an antifungal agent, had immunosuppressive properties.[8] This discovery ushered in the modern era of liver transplantation as cyclosporine became the mainstay of antirejection therapy.

As outcomes improved, attention turned toward maximizing the number of available donors. In 1989, Mies and colleagues[9] in Brazil described two cases of liver transplantation from live adult donors into children, although neither achieved long-term survival. The first generally accepted successful living donor liver transplantation (LDLT) in a pediatric recipient was performed by Strong and colleagues.[10] A Japanese group led by Koichi Tanaka produced excellent outcomes using these techniques and established the reliability of this approach.[11] Approximately 10 years later, the first adult-to-adult LDLT using the left lobe was performed by Hashikura and colleagues.[12]

Other efforts to expand the donor pool include the use of grafts produced after circulatory determination of death and grafts with significant fibrosis or fat content for selected recipients. There is increasing interest in the use of machine perfusion to allow transplantation of grafts that might otherwise be discarded.

INDICATIONS

Indications for adult liver transplantation fall into two main categories: (1) symptomatic liver failure or (2) hepatocellular cancer if tumor location or accompanying liver disease prevents resection. Disease states causing liver failure that may be successfully treated with transplant include noncholestatic and cholestatic

BOX 26.1 Disease states causing liver failure that may be successfully treated with transplant.

Noncholestatic Cirrhosis
Alcoholic
Nonalcoholic fatty liver disease
Hepatitis C
Cryptogenic cirrhosis
Autoimmune cirrhosis
Hepatitis B
Drug or exposure induced

Cholestatic Cirrhosis
Primary biliary cirrhosis (PBC)
Primary sclerosing cholangitis (PSC)
Caroli disease
Choledochol cyst

cirrhosis (Box 26.1), cancer, fulminant hepatic failure, metabolic diseases, biliary atresia, and relatively rare mix of other causes including Budd-Chiari syndrome, hyperalimentation-induced liver disease, large adenomas, and polycystic liver disease. With the advent of effective antiviral therapy for hepatitis C, the most common reason for listing for liver transplantation has become alcoholic liver disease, followed by nonalcoholic steatohepatitis (NASH), which has risen dramatically in the late 2010s, followed by hepatitis C.

Noncholestatic Cirrhosis

The common theme in these diseases is hepatocyte injury. Although the liver has a unique potential to regenerate, over time, chronic hepatocyte injury results in stellate cell activation leading to widespread collagen deposition. This process disrupts the unique liver microstructure that allows low-pressure portal blood flow, nutrient exchange, and bile secretion. This in turn leads to portal hypertension and associated varices and ascites. As hepatocyte synthetic and excretory function fails, coagulopathy, jaundice, hypoalbuminemia, fatigue, pruritus, and encephalopathy may occur. Additional complications, the development of which is poorly understood, include hepatorenal syndrome, hepatopulmonary syndrome, and portopulmonary hypertension. The term "noncholestatic" reflects that the primary injury is to the hepatocytes and not the bile ducts, despite the fact that patients can and often do present with jaundice.

Alcoholic

Alcoholic liver disease encompasses steatohepatitis, alcoholic cirrhosis, and alcoholic hepatitis.[13] Chronic alcohol ingestion is the most common indication for liver transplantation, responsible for approximately 25% of all listings. The absolute number of patients listed with this diagnosis is growing. Ingestion of 30 g of alcohol per day seems to be a relevant threshold and will cause chronic liver damage in approximately 6% of people; risk increases with increasing use.[14]

Toxicity of ethanol is incompletely understood but likely depends on conversion to acetaldehyde via alcohol dehydrogenase, catalase, or cytochrome P450. Over time, pericentral fibrosis progresses to panlobar fibrosis with associated manifestations of cirrhosis. Aspartate aminotransferase (AST)/alanine aminotransferase (ALT) ratio is typically greater than 2, and transaminase elevation tends to be relatively mild (<500).

Alcoholic hepatitis is a subset of alcohol-associated liver disease that occurs in patients with a long history of alcohol use who present with an acute inflammatory syndrome with a bilirubin of greater than 3.0. Episodes can be self-limited or lead to complete liver failure. This diagnosis is increasingly common as an indication for liver transplantation.

Historically, decisions regarding whether to list a patient with alcoholic liver disease for transplantation depended on a period of sobriety prior to transplant, typically 6 months, due to concern for recidivism and injury to the transplanted liver. Although policies vary by center, in general, over time, these guidelines have been relaxed as it has been difficult to demonstrate differences in outcomes among those with less than 18 months of sobriety.[15] Unfortunately, this extended time period is unlikely to be survived by many patients who present with advanced liver disease. Current expert review practice guidelines from the American Gastroenterological Association for acute alcoholic hepatitis recommend referral for transplant if the model for end-stage liver disease (MELD) is greater than 26 given high short-term mortality.[16]

Nonalcoholic Fatty Liver Disease

Nonalcoholic fatty liver disease consists of nonalcoholic fatty liver and NASH and is the most common liver disorder in Western nations. In America, approximately 19% of adults have nonalcoholic fatty liver disease by ultrasound imaging.[17] Risk factors include diabetes, central obesity, dyslipidemia, and metabolic syndrome.

First recognized by Caldwell in 1999 as a cause of end-stage liver disease, NASH is now the second most common indication for liver transplantation in the United States. Biopsy in NASH demonstrates hepatocyte steatosis, ballooning degeneration, and lobular inflammation most commonly in zone 3. Over time, this can progress to fibrosis, cirrhosis, and liver failure, leading to the need for liver transplantation.

Hepatitis C

In 2016, Bartenschlager, Rice, and Sofia were awarded the Lasker-DeBakey Clinical Medical Research Award for efforts instrumental in developing effective therapies for hepatitis C.[18] Their work and that of many others revolutionized the care and treatment of patients with advanced liver disease in two fundamental ways. First, it greatly reduced the burden of hepatitis C and the number of patients being listed with this diagnosis, and second, it allowed the use of organs from donors with hepatitis C, significantly increasing the organ supply. As a result, hepatitis C has gone from the most common to the third most common indication for liver transplantation in the United States.

Patients who present with advanced cirrhosis should be considered for liver transplantation consistent with usual clinical indications. Patients with mild disease should be treated in the hope of delaying or arresting disease progression. In some cases, fibrosis will even improve. In patients with advanced disease, the decision to treat is individualized to the patient. Even patients who achieve a sustained virologic response to therapy remain at a 3% per year risk of the development of hepatocellular cancer or disease progression and therefore must be followed carefully with liver transplant based on clinical and radiologic criteria.[19]

Cryptogenic

As a diagnosis of exclusion, what was previously classified as "cryptogenic cirrhosis" is generally now thought to be advanced NASH cirrhosis. Indeed, there is debate in the literature about whether cryptogenic cirrhosis should be considered its own pathological entity.[20,21] The diagnosis, treatment, and decision-making are similar to patients with NASH.

Autoimmune

Autoimmune hepatitis is an inflammatory disease of the liver that occurs mostly in women (4:1 for type I). The course can be self-limited or recurrent leading to chronic liver disease and cirrhosis requiring transplantation. The etiology is poorly understood. Diagnosis is typically one of exclusion. Characteristic findings on laboratory evaluation include high elevations in AST and ALT with lesser elevations in alkaline phosphatase, and elevated gamma globulins. Antinuclear and antismooth muscles are often elevated. Histologic findings include a mononuclear cell infiltrate primarily in the portal regions, and piecemeal necrosis may be present at the periportal region. Most patients will have ductal injury, and plasma cell infiltrates are common. In the initial stages of the disease, fibrosis may be absent. As the disease progresses, fibrosis occurs and may develop into cirrhosis. Transplantation should be considered for patients who develop cirrhosis.

Hepatitis B

Approximately 2 billion people worldwide have been exposed to hepatitis B, and nearly 250 million are chronic carriers,[22] making hepatitis B a major public health problem. Acute infection with hepatitis B is subclinical in 70% of patients. Approximately 30% will develop jaundice. Less than 1% will develop fulminant hepatic failure. These patients should be considered for emergent liver transplantation. In patients who develop chronic infection, progression to cirrhosis is influenced by the age of onset. For perinatal acquired infection, 90% will progress to chronic infection, with rates decreasing as the age of transmission increases.[23]

Up through the late 1990s, transplantation for patients with hepatitis B produced poor outcomes due to disease recurrence. This changed with the discovery of lamivudine and, in combination with hepatitis B immunoglobulin, allowed successful transplantation of these patients.[24] In current practice, patients with hepatitis B routinely receive liver transplants, and donors with hepatitis B can be used with appropriate antiviral therapy.

Cholestatic Liver Disease

The common thread in this group of diseases is chronic biliary damage. As ducts become injured, bile stasis occurs, leading to infection and a vicious cycle of damage, inflammation, and recurrent infection. Pruritis can be debilitating. Recurrent cholangitis may produce the classic Charcot triad of jaundice, fever, and right upper quadrant pain. Ongoing biliary damage predisposes the patient to the development of cholangiocarcinoma, especially in patients with primary sclerosing cholangitis (PSC).

Primary Biliary Cholangitis

Primary biliary cholangitis is an autoimmune disease in which inflammatory injury to the bile ducts results in cholestatic liver disease. Granulomatous destruction of the intralobar ducts causes obstruction and jaundice. Patients often suffer from jaundice and pruritis. Laboratory evaluation typically reveals elevated alkaline phosphatase, and positive antimitochondrial antibodies are often present. History often reveals fatigue and pruritis, with physical exam showing jaundice and xanthomata. Osteoporosis commonly develops. Positive antimitochondrial antibodies are the hallmark of the disease.

Primary Sclerosing Cholangitis

Patients with PSC develop fibrosis of the intrahepatic and/or extrahepatic biliary tree leading to inflammation. The disease is more common in men. Diffuse structuring leads to jaundice, pruritis, fibrosis, recurrent biliary sepsis, and liver failure. Many patients with PSC also have a history of inflammatory bowel disease. These patients are at high risk for cholangiocarcinoma and require careful screening. Laboratory evaluation most commonly shows elevated alkaline phosphatase. In addition, gammaglobulin, serum immunoglobulin M levels, atypical perinuclear antineutrophil cytoplasmic antibodies, and human leukocyte antigen DRw52a, antinuclear, antismooth muscle, anticardiolipin, thyroperoxidase, and rheumatoid factor may be elevated and can provide clues to the diagnosis. Antimitochondrial antibodies are generally negative in contrast to primary biliary cholangitis.

Patients with PSC carry significant risk of cholangiocarcinoma of 13%. With the onset of cholangiocarcinoma, CA19-9 levels typically rise and should be followed serially.

Caroli Disease

Caroli disease is a poorly understood congenital disorder of the large intrahepatic bile ducts. Most commonly, the disease is transmitted as an autosomal recessive fashion associated with polycystic renal disease. When associated with congenital hepatic fibrosis, the term "Caroli syndrome" is used. Similar to PSC, stasis, recurrent infection, and ongoing fibrosis lead to liver failure in some patients, although the severity of disease is variable. Patients are at risk for the development of cholangiocarcinoma.

Acute Liver Failure

Acute liver failure is a clinical syndrome of hepatic encephalopathy and elevated prothrombin time (PT)/international normalized ratio (INR) due to injury to the liver in patients without preexisting liver disease. Terminology can be confusing. In general, fulminant liver failure, acute hepatic necrosis, fulminant hepatic necrosis, or fulminant hepatitis can refer to the same clinical entity. Importantly, the presence of encephalopathy is required for the diagnosis and for listing in the most urgent category for liver transplant, a status 1A designation.

Acute liver failure can be further divided based on the duration between onset of symptoms and encephalopathy. Hyperacute liver failure occurs within 7 days of symptom onset; acute, from 7 to 21 days; and subacute, between 21 days and 26 weeks. The shorter the duration of symptoms, the more common it is for patients to develop cerebral edema. In contrast, patients with disease of longer duration more commonly present with portal hypertension.

The most common causes of acute liver failure are given in Box 26.2, with acetaminophen overdose being the most common cause.

Patients presenting with acute liver failure present with challenging management decisions, centered around determining who needs a transplant and who will improve with supportive management. Although successful transplantation is associated with excellent survival, it is inferior to the survival of patients who spontaneously recover. On the other hand, failure to list and perform a transplant in a patient who needs one will result in death. Further complicating matters are the need for an expeditious workup and transplantation. This is especially challenging in patients with

BOX 26.2 Common causes of acute liver failure

- Acetaminophen overdose
- Drug ingestion
- Indeterminate
- Hepatitis B
- Hepatitis A
- Autoimmune
- Ischemia
- Wilson disease

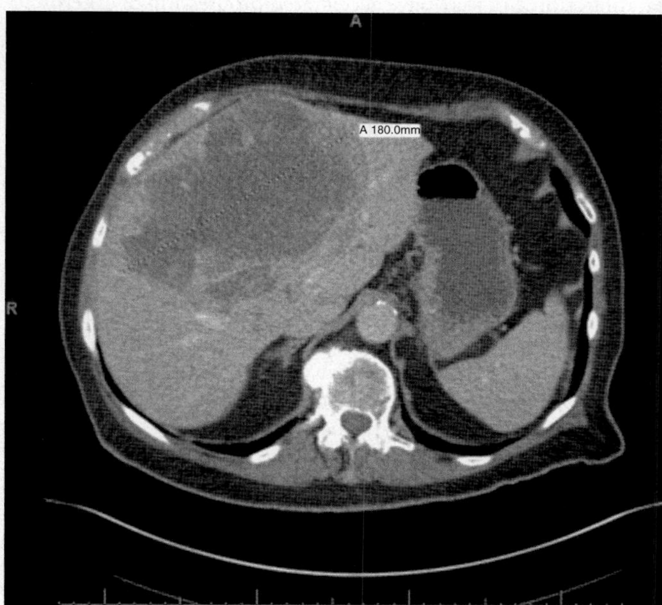

FIG. 26.1 Unresectable hepatocellular cancer.

acetaminophen overdose who tend to be young but may have a history of multiple suicide attempts or poor social support.

Progression of hepatic encephalopathy to stage II can be used as a guideline to move forward with transplant, although this differs among transplant centers. More precise determination uses King's College criteria.[25] In a patient with acetaminophen overdose, arterial pH less than 7.3 after resuscitation, or high PT, creatinine, and grade III or IV encephalopathy suggest need for transplant. Use of serial computed tomography (CT) scans or an intracranial pressure monitor (bolt) can help guide therapy and, importantly, the decision to proceed with transplantation.

Malignant Neoplasms

Hepatocellular Cancer

According to the Scientific Registry of Transplant Recipients, approximately 16% of transplants performed in the United States carry malignancy as the primary indication (Fig. 26.1).[26]

Initial efforts performing liver transplantation for hepatocellular cancer produced dismal results with very high recurrence rates. Over time, it became apparent that early-stage lesions did quite well, as demonstrated by a series of patients reported in Milan, which subsequently defined the Milan Criteria.[27] These early-stage lesions have equivalent survival to nonmalignant indications for transplantation. In order to prioritize these patients for transplant to receive a graft prior to the development of metastatic disease, exception points are granted for patients with up to three lesions, each between 1 and 3 cm in diameter, or one lesion 2 to 5 cm in diameter. In addition, many centers employ locoregional therapies, including transarterial chemoembolization, radiofrequency ablation, and radioembolization using Y90 to "downstage" patients into Milan Criteria. These patients are then eligible for exception points. Recent modifications recognize the poor prognosis carried by high alphafetoprotein levels and require special exception point applications for these patients.

Nearly all patients with hepatocellular cancer have significant fibrosis or cirrhosis. The primary treatment modality for hepatocellular cancer is surgical resection. The determination must be made as to whether the underlying liver disease will allow successful resection. In general, 30% of the liver must be preserved to ensure adequate synthetic function; however, in the setting of significant liver disease, this proportion may be higher. Severe portal hypertension with varices, significant ascites, debilitation, malnutrition, and encephalopathy are all contraindications to resection. In addition, the location of the lesion may also make resection impossible. Lesions adjacent to the confluence of major vascular or biliary structures may not allow surgical options. In this case, transplantation is the preferred treatment.

While on the transplant waiting list, minimally invasive ablative therapies may be employed to prevent the progression of disease. These show great usefulness in preventing progression.

Cholangiocarcinoma

Cholangiocarcinoma is a highly lethal lesion with poor long-term survival. Early reports demonstrated that chemoradiation protocols followed by liver transplantation provided good long-term survival for patients with early-stage hilar lesions.[28] This remains a controversial indication for transplant, with some reports suggesting that selected patients benefit from liver transplantation.[29] Others feel these patients have been carefully selected and show equivalent survival to patients that undergo liver resection. A key principle is the need to obtain a negative margin either with transplantation or resection.

Other

Budd-Chiari Syndrome

Budd-Chiari syndrome is a rare condition that occurs when hepatic venous outflow is occluded, typically due to thrombosis of the hepatic veins or vena cava at the level of the hepatic veins. It can also occur due to extrinsic compression. Presentation is variable and can be divided into acute, subacute, and chronic. Approximately 5% of patients will present with acute liver failure. In these patients, ascites and pain are more common, whereas patients with chronic obstruction more frequently present with portal hypertension. An underlying hypercoagulable or other reason is identified in over 80% of patients[30] and should be actively sought with a hypercoagulable workup and imaging to look for masses (Fig. 26.2).

In early stages, side-to-side portacaval shunt decompresses the liver and can provide excellent long-term survival.[31] In patients with established fibrosis or cirrhosis, liver transplantation should be considered. Operative planning must consider suitable outflow options, particularly side-to-side cavocavostomy.

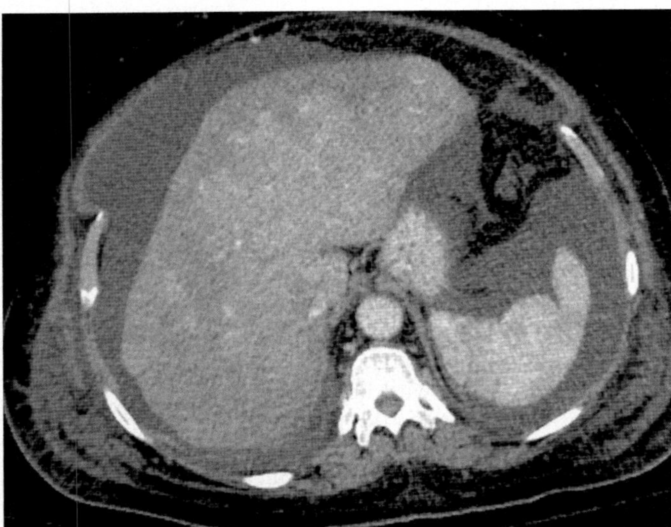

FIG. 26.2 Budd-Chiari syndrome.

Very Rare Causes of Liver Failure That Can Be Addressed With Liver Transplantation

Total Parenteral Nutrition/Hyperalimentation-Induced Liver Disease

In patients with short bowel syndrome or intestinal failure, liver failure can follow for reasons that are not well understood. In these patients, combined liver/intestinal transplant can be lifesaving.

Polycystic Liver Disease

In rare cases, patients with polycystic liver disease can present with debilitating pain, intestinal obstruction, malnutrition, hemorrhage, or liver failure. For these patients, liver transplantation may be indicated.

Hepatic Adenoma

Patients with large, unresectable hepatic adenomas may present with pain or bleeding and carry increased risk of malignancy.

Metastatic Cancer

Certain types of metastatic disease can be treated with transplantation, including neuroendocrine tumors. In general, this is a controversial indication that should be considered on a case-by-case basis.

Hemangioendothelioma

This is a slow-growing and rare malignancy. In the case of unresectable disease, transplant can provide excellent outcomes.

Wilson Disease

Occurring at a frequency of 1 in 30,000, Wilson disease an autosomal recessive disease of copper transport. Over time, copper accumulation leads to cirrhosis. A small subgroup of patients will present with liver failure, which is generally an acute presentation on the background of undiagnosed cirrhosis. These patients benefit from transplant with good long-term survival.

CONTRAINDICATIONS

As techniques and technologies for liver transplantation improved, the number of patients who could benefit increased at a rate that outpaced organ availability. To be good stewards of the limited resource, the decision-making around listing patients for liver transplant is more complex than in other areas of surgery. Contraindications are based on whether the patient can survive the operation and whether they can achieve a long-term survival, including whether they can properly care for the organ.

Patients with advanced cardiac disease are usually excluded from consideration of transplant. Severe valvular disease can make intraoperative management prohibitively difficult. Hypotension may occur due to rapidly shifting intravascular volume with significant hemorrhage or clamping of major vasculature. This can also lead to life-threatening arrhythmias. A particularly difficult problem is pulmonary hypertension, which may result in unrecoverable right heart failure on reperfusion of the new liver. Patients with coronary heart disease are at risk for intraoperative myocardial infarction and may have accelerated progression of atherosclerosis due to immunosuppression after transplant.

Similarly, patients with severe respiratory conditions are generally not candidates for liver transplantation. Intraoperative hypoxia may be uncorrectable, and long-term outcomes are poor. Portopulmonary hypertension uncorrectable to less than 50 mm Hg is generally considered a contraindication, as is hepatopulmonary syndrome if the PaO_2 cannot be corrected on 100% oxygen.

Other contraindications include irreversible neurological impairment. In the setting of encephalopathy, this can be difficult to determine. A careful history is needed to exclude chronic, progressive causes. Infection must be carefully considered but in many cases is not an absolute contraindication. For example, in patients with PSC and liver abscesses, liver excision may be the only way to eradicate the infection. Uncontrolled sepsis or other infection that will not be cured by the transplant is a relative contraindication. In most cases, extrahepatic cancer is a contraindication for transplant. Recent cancer may require a waiting period. The Israel Penn International Transplant Tumor Registry maintains a database that can provide guidance around waiting times needed for different types of cancer. Patients with human immunodeficiency virus (HIV), previously thought to be an absolute contraindication to transplant, can undergo successful transplantation.[32]

The transplant community generally feels that the ability to take care of the graft depends on adequate social and financial support and resources, so that lack of this resource is an absolute contraindication to transplantation, although recent work suggests this may be a disadvantage to certain groups of patients.[33]

Active alcohol use is considered a contraindication for transplant, although selected centers will perform transplants in these patients, and in fact the number of these transplants is increasing rapidly.[26] Liver transplant programs generally include specialists in social, psychiatric, and finance to help sort out relevant issues.

Advances in surgical technique have made exclusion of patients for anatomic reasons very rare in experienced centers. Methods for dealing with difficult anatomy are discussed in the section on surgical considerations.

MELD AND ALLOCATION

Originally developed to predict 3-month mortality in patients after transjugular portosystemic shunt placement, the MELD was found also to predict mortality in patients waitlisted for transplant.[34] Currently, the MELD score determines priority for liver transplantation. A great success of the system was in creating objective criteria (laboratory results) that were not subject to interpretation by individual centers. In its original formulation, it was based on serum creatinine, INR, and bilirubin. Serum sodium has

BOX 26.3 Current calculation for the model for end-stange liver disease (MELD) score.

MELD = 3.8*loge(serum bilirubin [mg/dL]) + 11.2*loge(INR) + 9.6*loge(serum creatinine [mg/dL]) + 6.4 + 1.32 * (137-Na) – [0.033*MELD* (137-Na)]

subsequently been added to improve the predictive value of the score. The current calculation is included in Box 26.3, although the calculation changes from time to time. When a donor liver becomes available, a list of patients eligible to receive the transplant is generated, ranked by MELD score. The liver is offered sequentially to each person on the list until it is accepted.

Status 1 patients suffer from fulminant liver failure with expected death on the order of days. These patients are prioritized above patients with MELD scores.

Although MELD is recognized as good predictor of mortality, there are certain conditions thought to carry higher mortality than the MELD score would suggest. In particular, patients with hepatocellular cancer can be cured with liver transplantation but typically have low MELD scores and would likely not come to transplant prior to disease progression. For these patients, additional points are given, termed "exception points," to reflect the desire of the community to prioritize these patients. Prioritization algorithms are reviewed and adjusted from time to time. Additional diagnoses generally accepted for additional points are listed in Boxes 26.4 and 26.5. If patients do not fit into these categories, a review board exists to consider particular cases.

How organs are distributed across the country is a distinct question from which patients in a group receive priority for the transplant offer. This complex question perennially is one of the most hotly debated in the transplant community. Within this decision resides the intersection of ethical principles of justice, utility, and fairness, as well as public preferences, resource utilization, and disparities in access and outcomes of care due to socioeconomic factors.[35] Finally, whether and how to incorporate performance of local organ procurement organizations remain contentious.

There is general agreement that most patients with low MELD scores (less than 15) do not benefit from transplantation, and this has been reflected in national allocation policies.[36]

DONOR SELECTION

The ideal liver donor is young, healthy, and thin with normal liver function tests and no history of liver disease or risk factors for infectious disease. The patient is pronounced brain dead and with normal hemodynamics is taken semielectively for the donation procedure. This "perfect" scenario is quite rare, however, and each deviation from these characteristics carries quantifiable risks. It is critical to consider that the risk of accepting any individual donor must be balanced with the risk of the potential recipient declining the liver and dying prior to receiving the next offer. From a public health standpoint, use of livers with high risk is, in general, preferable to not using the liver given the number of waiting list deaths.

Older donors carry additional risk of short- and long-term graft loss, and older age is an independent risk factor for mortality. On the other hand, in general, outcomes with older donors are very good.[37]

Donors with significant health problems need to be considered on a case-by-case basis. In general, disease in other organs should not be a contraindication to use the liver. A notable exception is

BOX 26.4 Common indications for exception points for liver transplant.

- Hepatocellular carcinoma
- Hepatopulmonary syndrome
- Portopulmonary hypertension (provided the mean arterial pressure can be maintained at <35 mm Hg with treatment)
- Familial amyloid polyneuropathy
- Primary hyperoxaluria
- Cystic fibrosis
- Hilar cholangiocarcinoma
- Hepatic artery thrombosis (occurring within 14 days of liver transplantation but not meeting criteria for status 1A)

BOX 26.5 Diagnoses that may be appropriate for exception points.

- Recurrent cholangitis in patients with primary sclerosing cholangitis who are on antibiotic suppressive therapy or require repeated biliary interventions
- Refractory ascites
- Refractory hepatic encephalopathy
- Refractory variceal hemorrhage
- Portal hypertensive gastropathy leading to chronic blood loss
- Intractable pruritus in a patient with primary biliary cirrhosis

cancer, but again this must be considered on a case-by-case basis. Severe atherosclerosis can affect the hepatic artery, and this must be assessed at the time of donation.

Livers from patients who are obese may have nonalcoholic fatty liver disease or steatohepatitis. In general, livers more than 60% steatosis or with significant fibrosis for any reason should be used with caution.

Interestingly, ongoing infection in the donor is not an absolute contraindication for use of the organ. Suspicion of viral etiology for the donor death, however, in general, is an absolute contraindication for the use of any organs. Spread of the virus to immunosuppressed recipients can cause multiple deaths. Patients with risk factors for infection such as intravenous drug abuse carry a small risk of transmission of disease even though nucleic acid testing is routinely performed and is very sensitive for hepatitis C and HIV. The use of hepatitis C infected donors is becoming routine given the success of specific antiviral therapy.

A class of organs is procured from the donors declared dead body based on circulatory criteria. These are termed *donation after circulatory determination of death (DCDD) organs*. In this case, after determination that the patient experienced a devastating, nonsurvivable injury and that the patient wishes to donate, support measures are withdrawn and the patient is allowed to progress to death. Once the patient is declared dead, a rapid perfusion technique with organ removal is performed. DCDD organs are a significant source of organs for transplant, with excellent outcomes in selected hands.[38] Ischemic cholangiopathy, a diffuse structuring disease, can occur in these cases, which may require retransplantation.

PREOPERATIVE EVALUATION

Evaluation of a patient for liver transplantation is complex and seeks to determine whether a candidate would benefit from a

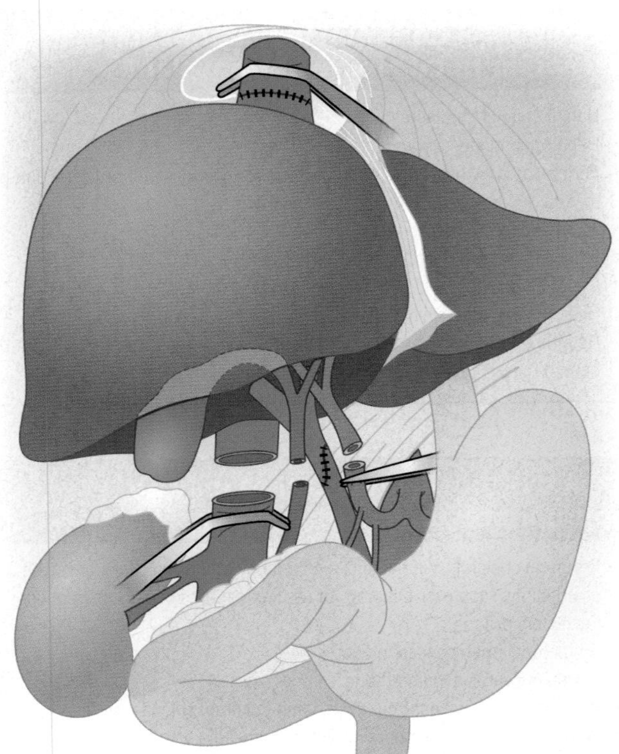

FIG. 26.3 Steps of the liver transplant operation.

transplant, whether there are alternative therapies available, and whether the predicted outcome is good enough to justify use of this scarce resource in this individual.

Work-up therefore includes a detailed history and physical exam. Full laboratory evaluation is appropriate for patients considering the magnitude of the operation. Cardiac and pulmonary workup is similarly essential including stress testing and pulmonary function tests in patients with appropriate risk factors. All screening testing should be up-to-date, including mammography, colonoscopy, prostate cancer screening, etc.

Liver transplantation requires long-term follow-up and medications to prevent rejection and other complications. For this reason, adequate financial and social support must be available to the recipient. Patients in the United States meet with financial coordinators as well as social workers to ensure that they can adequately care for the organ postoperatively. This also assesses risk of recidivism in patients with a history of alcohol or other substance abuse.

SURGICAL CONSIDERATIONS

The major steps of the liver transplant operation are pictured in Fig. 26.3. Many techniques are used: here, we will outline a relatively common general approach. Access to the abdomen is generally obtained using a right subcostal incision and either a midline extension or a left subcostal extension, and sometimes both. Often, portal hypertension is severe, occurring in combination with severe coagulopathy. Care must be taken to prevent exsanguinating hemorrhage. Portal dissection involves ligating the right and left branches of the hepatic artery and transecting the bile duct high in the hilum. Ligation of lymphatics leaves only the intact portal vein for later transection prior to excision of the liver. The triangular and coronary ligaments are lysed. In an orthotopic placement, the inferior vena cava is encircled above the renal veins and the suprahepatic cava above the hepatic veins in preparation to remove the entire cava. The recipient liver is removed with the retrohepatic cava and the donor liver is then placed with the donor cava anastamosed to the recipient cava both above the renal veins and below the diaphragm. In the piggyback technique, the caudate is dissected off of the retrohepatic cava, leaving the recipient cava intact. The donor cava is anastamosed to the cloaca fashioned using the confluence of the three hepatic veins. Once this is done, the liver is perfused with saline to remove the potassium contained in the preservation solution. The portal vein anastomosis is performed, followed by the hepatic artery and then bile duct, usually in a duct to duct fashion (Fig. 26.3).

Major hemodynamic shifts occur during the operation. Patients with cirrhosis typically have very low systemic vascular resistance and can quickly become hypotensive with blood loss. Either total caval occlusion using the orthotopic technique or hepatic vein occlusion using the piggyback technique diminishes blood flow to the heart, causing hypotension and increased renal vein pressure leading to kidney injury. After the liver is implanted, reperfusion leads to a massive bolus of volume to the right heart on opening the cava, which can lead to right heart strain or even failure, which can be life-threatening.

In recipients with portal vein thrombosis, first attempts should be to open the vein with thrombectomy catheters and thromboendovenectomy if needed. If this fails, inflow can be obtained from the superior mesenteric vein, nearby varices, and even the left renal vein in patients in whom there is significant splenorenal shunting. For arterial inflow, much of the splanchnic circulation can be used, as can grafts from the suprarenal or infrarenal aorta. Difficult biliary anastomoses can be managed with a Roux-en-Y technique or even direct choledochoduodenostomy. A particularly difficult problem is trying to place a large liver into a small recipient. If the right lobe is very large, it can be difficult to perform the portal anastomosis. Similarly, if the liver is too large in the dorsal ventral direction, the donor portal vein can lay on top of the recipient portal vein in a fashion where it cannot be cut back far enough to permit anastomosis. In this case alternative inflow must be sought.

POSTOPERATIVE MANAGEMENT

After a complex surgery with significant hemodynamic derangements, good postoperative management is essential to ensure optimal outcomes. Liver transplantation creates particular challenges.

Given the hemodynamic changes, patients often come out of the operating room after receiving a significant amount of fluid and blood products. It is critical to have a good sense of the patient's total body volume and intravascular volume. The vast majority of patients will be total volume overloaded but intravascular volume can be low, normal, or high. The best way to determine total body volume status is an accurate patient weight taking into account preoperative ascites. If the patient is massively volume overloaded but hypotensive, a vasopressor may mitigate the need for massive ongoing fluid resuscitation. Pulmonary artery catheters or noninvasive echocardiographic assessment may help determine intravascular volume to guide decision-making around fluids. Once the blood pressure is normalized, restoring whole-body normovolemia is an important goal to prevent soft tissue and pulmonary edema. Volume management is complicated by potential ongoing bleeding and acute renal injury, which is common. Very careful attention must be paid to these possibilities.

Respiratory management consists of extubation as soon as feasible with the understanding that many patients will be severely debilitated and may not be able to perform the work of breathing. In these cases, early tracheostomy is indicated.

Feeding should begin as early as is safe, and there should be a low threshold for placing a feeding tube should the patient demonstrate an inability to consume adequate calories after normal gastrointestinal (GI) function returns. Early ambulation and incentive spirometry are critical, and early discharge should be a goal to prevent nosocomial infection.

Most programs will use drains for additional fluid and to diagnose bile leaks. These should be inspected multiple times a day for output and color.

COMPLICATIONS AND THEIR TREATMENT

Early complications: Careful attention to the patient in the immediate postoperative setting is essential to ensure optimal outcomes. Frequent assessment of graft function is essential and quick action must be taken when indicated. Postoperative hypotension can be caused by many factors, but bleeding must always be considered. Abdominal drains will usually, but not always, help establish this diagnosis. Drains can become clotted or sequestered from areas of massive hemorrhage. Frequent hematocrit checks should be obtained. Ongoing hemorrhage requiring continuous blood replacement is generally an indication to return to the operating room. The exception may be a patient with severe coagulopathy and or hypothermia who may benefit from a longer observation period with factor replacement and warming to determine if the bleeding is surgical in nature. A good practice is to set a threshold transfusion limit after which abdominal exploration is considered. In addition, patients who develop a compartment syndrome must return to the operating room.

Primary nonfunction is a serious complication requiring retransplantation. The most common causes are an unrecognized procurement error, use of certain types of higher-risk grafts (fatty, fibrotic, DCDD), or arterial complication after the transplant. Typically, the patient will not wake up, the lactate will remain very high, bilirubin will continue to rise, and the AST and ALT will rise into the 5000 to 10,000 range. In these cases, an ultrasound should be obtained to interrogate the artery. In this situation, plans should be made for urgent retransplantation.

Arterial complications not producing primary nonfunction occur in approximately 2% to 4% of patients.[39] This usually manifests as increased AST and ALT, high bilirubin, and poor synthetic function with elevated INR. Arterial stenosis or thrombosis can be diagnosed on ultrasound or contrast CT and must be addressed as soon as possible if discovered. Early arterial thrombosis, even if not associated with primary nonfunction, should lead to relisting for transplantation (Fig. 26.4).

Portal vein stenosis or thrombosis may present with normal liver function tests and synthetic function. Over time, however, these patients develop signs and symptoms of portal hypertension and require intervention. Portal stents are often successful in these situations.

Biliary issues are the most common complication in the postoperative period and occur in approximately 20% of patients. This can present as bile in the drain in the case of a leak or in a patient who returns with a biloma. Stricture leads to increased bilirubin and alkaline phosphatase. Modern management of bile duct issues employs endoscopic management for stent placement and dilations. Early major biliary issues should prompt an ultrasound to ensure vessel patency and reoperation to check for bile duct ischemia and to consider reanastomosis, possibly as a Roux-en-Y reconstruction.

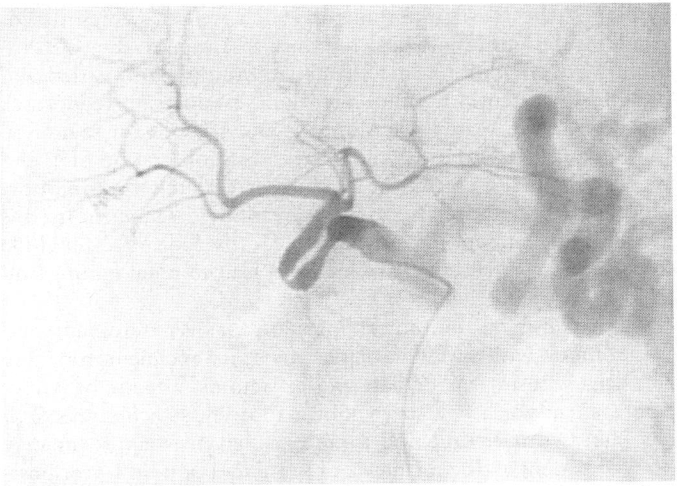

FIG. 26.4 Hepatic artery stenosis demonstrated by arteriogram.

Rejection typically presents with elevated liver function tests and is diagnosed on biopsy characterized by portal inflammatory infiltrate, bile duct injury, and endotheliitis. In many cases, mild rejection can be treated by raising the immunosuppression level and bolus steroids. More severe rejection may require antibody therapy.

Recurrent hepatitis C is becoming much less common with the advent of highly active viral therapy.

Late complications include arterial or portal venous structuring, bile duct strictures, and opportunistic infections. Chronic rejection is poorly understood and often leads to the need for retransplantation. Chronic immunosuppression often leads to renal dysfunction and increased risk of certain types of cancer, especially skin cancer associated with sun exposure.

IMMUNOSUPPRESSION

Liver grafts are recognized by the recipient as foreign based on major histocompatibility complex antigens. Hepatocytes express low levels of class I antigen and no class II antigen. During ongoing immune surveillance, T cells recognize the graft as foreign and initiate an immune response. Distinct from renal transplantation, liver transplantation does not require matching between donor and recipient human leukocyte antigen, although there is some concern that the effect of human leukocyte antigen mismatch may be greater than previously appreciated.

Modern immunosuppression chooses from a variety of classes of agents. Induction agents, if used, are administered at implantation. Choices include antithymocyte globulin, an anti-T-cell antibody, which binds to and depletes T cells, delivering potent and relatively nonspecific immunosuppression. These are very potent agents that can increase the rate of infection. Basiliximab is an antibody to the interleukin-2 (IL-2) receptor, which blocks IL-2 signaling and is not as immunosuppressive as antithymocyte globulin.

Maintenance immunosuppression generally involves agents of three different classes. Steroids inhibit transcription of cytokines, the most important of which is IL-2, which downregulates the immunological response to antigen. They also inhibit T-cell migration. Side effects are multiple and varied and include hypertension, fluid retention, cataracts, osteoporosis, diabetes, and increased risk of infection. Mycophenolate mofetil inhibits purine synthase, which decreases proliferation of T and B cells. The major side effect is GI upset. Calcineurin inhibitors block signal 2 required for T-cell activation. Calcineurin itself is a calcium-dependent phosphatase in T cells. Side effects include hypertension, renal toxicity which can lead to renal failure, and lipid abnormalities.

The mainstay of immunosuppression for liver transplantation is tacrolimus, with over 90% of liver transplant recipients receiving this drug with mycophenolate and/or steroids. The use of induction agents, which have been shown to decrease acute rejection, has increased over time and is currently given to approximately 35% of patients.[1] The incidence of acute rejection by 1-year post-transplant is approximately 10%.

LIVING DONOR LIVER TRANSPLANTATION INCLUDING DONOR SELECTION

LDLT arose from the intersection of an improved understanding of segmental liver anatomy, technical advances in hepatic parenchymal transection, and an inadequate supply of deceased donor liver allografts. LDLT draws on the ability of the liver to regenerate. A portion of liver with sufficient quality and mass, when provided with adequate arterial and venous inflow, as well as venous drainage, will recreate adequate mass to meet the metabolic demands of both donor and recipient. The first LDLT consisted of an adult segment II/III graft including the left hepatic vein, left hepatic artery, left portal vein, and left hepatic duct that was transplanted into a small child. The field quickly developed to allow for adult-to-adult liver transplantation with right lobe grafts consisting of segments V/VI/VII/VIII along with the right hepatic veins, right hepatic arteries, right portal veins, and right hepatic ducts and left lobe grafts consisting of segments II/III/IV along with the left hepatic vein, left hepatic arteries, left portal vein, and left hepatic ducts. The rapid increase in the number of LDLTs has led to a better understanding of both recipient selection and donor risk with significant improvements in patient and graft survival.

Donor

The safety of the donor is of paramount importance. Increased experience with LDLT in several high-volume centers helped define general criteria to maximize donor safety. Specifically, the donor should be left with an adequate amount of hepatic mass to ensure full recovery postoperatively. Donors with acute or chronic liver diseases or extrahepatic disease that may subsequently impair regeneration are excluded from becoming living liver donors. Donors should undergo a thorough medical and psychosocial evaluation to ensure that they are able to donate and recover from surgery safely. A donor should be left with a residual liver volume of no less than 30%.[40] This may be increased if the donor is older or has hepatic steatosis. While laparoscopic live liver donation has been reported, most centers perform an open hepatectomy.[41] Donation is associated with a mortality rate of 1 in 400 to 1 in 500.[1] Forty percent of donors will experience at least one complication within the first-year postdonation. The most frequent complications include infection (13%–15%), bile leak/biloma (7%–9%), reoperation (2%–3%), and hernia (11%–16%).[1,42] Despite both short- and long-term complications, most donors would choose to donate again.[43]

Recipient

Successful living donor transplantation requires a liver allograft of adequate parenchymal mass to support the recipient's metabolic needs as determined by the donor graft-recipient weight ratio (GRWR). Although successful liver transplantation has been performed with living donor grafts resulting in GRWR as low as 0.5%, the risk of morbidity and mortality due to small-for-size syndrome significantly increases with decreasing GRWR. Small-for-size syndrome develops when the amount of functioning transplanted liver parenchyma is inadequate to support the recipient and manifests with jaundice, coagulopathy, ascites, encephalopathy, and renal impairment that may progress to death. Retransplantation with a larger allograft may be necessary.

A GRWR of 0.8% to 1% is generally accepted as safe; however, donor liver quality and recipient degree of illness both affect the minimum safe GRWR. Donor steatosis, donor age older than 50 years old, and high recipient MELD score frequently necessitate higher GRWR up to or in excess of 1.[40] Ensuring adequate hepatic arterial and portal venous inflow to the live donor allograft is of critical importance for immediate graft function and subsequent graft hypertrophy. Hepatic parenchymal mass is regulated based on portal vein flow, and inadequate portal flow due to portosystemic shunting can be deleterious to allograft regeneration and perpetuate graft failure. Alternatively, exposure of a healthy liver allograft to sudden and persistent portal hypertension can lead to centrilobular injury and small-for-size syndrome.

LDLT is technically challenging due to the microvascular and biliary reconstructions necessary between the donor graft and recipient. The biliary reconstructions are particularly complication prone with biliary structuring occurring in nearly 30% of recipients.[44] Despite the challenges, LDLT is currently associated with 1-year patient survival of 90% and is an important and life-saving option.[1]

PEDIATRIC LIVER TRANSPLANTATION

The indications for pediatric liver transplantation are generally grouped into diseases leading to cirrhosis, inborn errors of metabolism, primary hepatic malignancies, and acute liver failure. Biliary atresia is the most common cause of end-stage liver disease in children and accounts for one third of all pediatric liver transplants. It is a congenital disease of unknown etiology leading to progressive fibroinflammatory obliteration of the biliary tree and the rapid development of cirrhosis. A diagnosis of biliary atresia should be suspected in all infants with persistent neonatal jaundice. Early intervention within the first several months of life is associated with superior outcome.[45] Reestablishing adequate biliary-enteric drainage prior to the development of end-stage liver disease is critical. This is typically accomplished by surgical anastomosis of the intestine to the biliary tree at the hepatic hilum. Pioneered by Kasai in the 1950s, the procedure is known as a hepatic portoenterostomy and has long-term success when the disease process is limited to the extrahepatic biliary tree.[46] Unfortunately, most children with biliary atresia have disease involvement of the intrahepatic biliary tree with progression of cirrhosis and death without liver transplantation.[47] Failure to normalize bilirubin at 3 months posthepatic portoenterostomy is predictive of the need of salvage liver transplantation, as are growth failure and recurrent bouts of cholangitis.[48] Nearly half of children with biliary atresia treated with portoenterostomy will need a liver transplant by 2 years of life. Other diseases such as autoimmune hepatitis and PSC can also lead to cirrhosis requiring liver transplantation in children.

Unlike adult liver transplantation, pediatric liver transplantation is frequently performed for indications beyond the treatment of end-stage liver disease. The liver is the major site of nitrogen metabolism in the body, and inherited genetic abnormalities involved in any aspect of the urea cycle or amino acid catabolism can lead to the accumulation of toxic metabolites and neurologic injury. Significant enzymatic dysfunction within the urea cycle of either N-acetylglutamate, carbamoyl phosphate synthase I, ornithine transcarbamylase, or argininosuccinate lyase deficiency impairs the body's ability to dispose of nitrogenous waste through the conversion of ammonia to urea. The neurotoxic hyperammonemia that ensues, particularly in the interval shortly after birth, causes the rapid development of lethargy, cerebral edema, seizures, and death. Other enzyme deficiencies within the urea cycle, including those of argininosuccinate synthase or citrin with resultant citrullinemia, arginase with resultant hyperargininemia, and ornithine translocase deficiency with resultant hyperornithinemia and homocitrullinuria, result in more insidious hyperammonemia and progressive neurologic injury. Similarly, enzymatic dysfunction in amino acid catabolism as seen in Maple Syrup Urine disease, methylmalonic acidemia, propionic acidemia, and tyrosinemia results in the accumulation of certain amino acids and their metabolites with resultant cellular toxicity and neurologic injury. Children with inborn errors of nitrogen metabolism are particularly vulnerable to neurologic injury resulting from the metabolic stress associated with growth, injury, or infections. Routine viral infections of childhood including common colds or influenza can be life-threatening events. The synthetic function of the liver in patients with inborn errors of metabolism is normal and liver transplantation is performed to provide normal enzymatic function and minimize or arrest further neurological injury. Early liver transplantation minimizes or arrests neurologic injury.[49]

Liver transplantation treats primary malignancies of the liver including hepatoblastoma and hepatocellular carcinoma. Hepatoblastoma arises from fetal or embryonal hepatocyte progenitor cells and is the most common primary pediatric liver malignancy. It is often diagnosed in children less than 3 years of age when they present with abdominal distension, feeding intolerance, or abdominal pain. The goal of treatment of hepatoblastoma is complete surgical resection. The PRETEXT (pretreatment extent of disease) classification is used to stage the extent of hepatic involvement and the likelihood of successful treatment with partial hepatectomy.[50] Although most hepatoblastomas can be successfully treated with partial hepatic resection, approximately 10% are surgically unresectable and benefit from liver transplantation, which provides for a 3-year survival of 75% with most mortality secondary to disease recurrence.[51] Hepatocellular carcinoma is very rare in the pediatric population and has a different pathology than that in adults. Excellent long-term survival approaching 80% at 5 years is reported with liver transplantation for hepatocellular carcinoma even when exceeding Milan Criteria.[52]

Most pediatric recipients who undergo orthotopic liver transplantation are younger than 5 years of age, and many receive a deceased donor whole liver allograft. However, the number of children needing a liver transplant greatly exceeds the number of pediatric whole liver deceased donors. This imbalance between the supply of size-appropriate pediatric deceased donors and demand of pediatric recipients necessitated the development of techniques for liver transplantation utilizing reduced size adult allografts. The introduction of deceased donor split liver allografts in 1998 allowed the transplantation of infants and small children utilizing the left lateral section of an adult liver based on the vasculobiliary anatomy of the left lobe.[53] LDLT further increased liver allograft availability for all pediatric patients with end-stage liver disease.[10] The transplantation of left lateral segment and live donor grafts necessitates the utilization of a cava-preserving technique. The vascular anastomoses in infants and small children have an increased complication rate, and microvascular techniques as well as anticoagulation are routinely used to minimize thrombotic events. Long-term results for pediatric liver transplantation are excellent, with a 5-year graft survival of 85% for biliary atresia followed by a 5-year graft survival slightly above 75% for hepatoblastoma and acute liver failure (Fig. 26.5).[1]

NEW TECHNOLOGIES INCLUDING MACHINE PERFUSION

A major advance in liver transplantation was the development of cold storage solutions in the 1980s. Pioneered by Belzer and colleagues at the University of Wisconsin, this technology quickly became standard of care.

Recent work suggests that machine perfusion may be a superior alternative to cold storage.[54] Although there are a number of different protocols and configurations, these devices maintain perfusion of the organs after procurement from the donor. This can be beneficial in a number of different ways: (1) Perfusion can allow for assessment of the quality of the graft. For liver considered marginal or when there is concern for their quality, examination of the perfusate can differentiate good livers, which could then be used with confidence from damaged livers unlikely to work.[55] (2) Perfusion can be used either to rehabilitate grafts from ongoing oxygenation or to administer drugs to enhance function.[56] (3) Perfusion can be used to extend the viability of the organ to improve logistics and allow safer transportation (Fig. 26.6).[57]

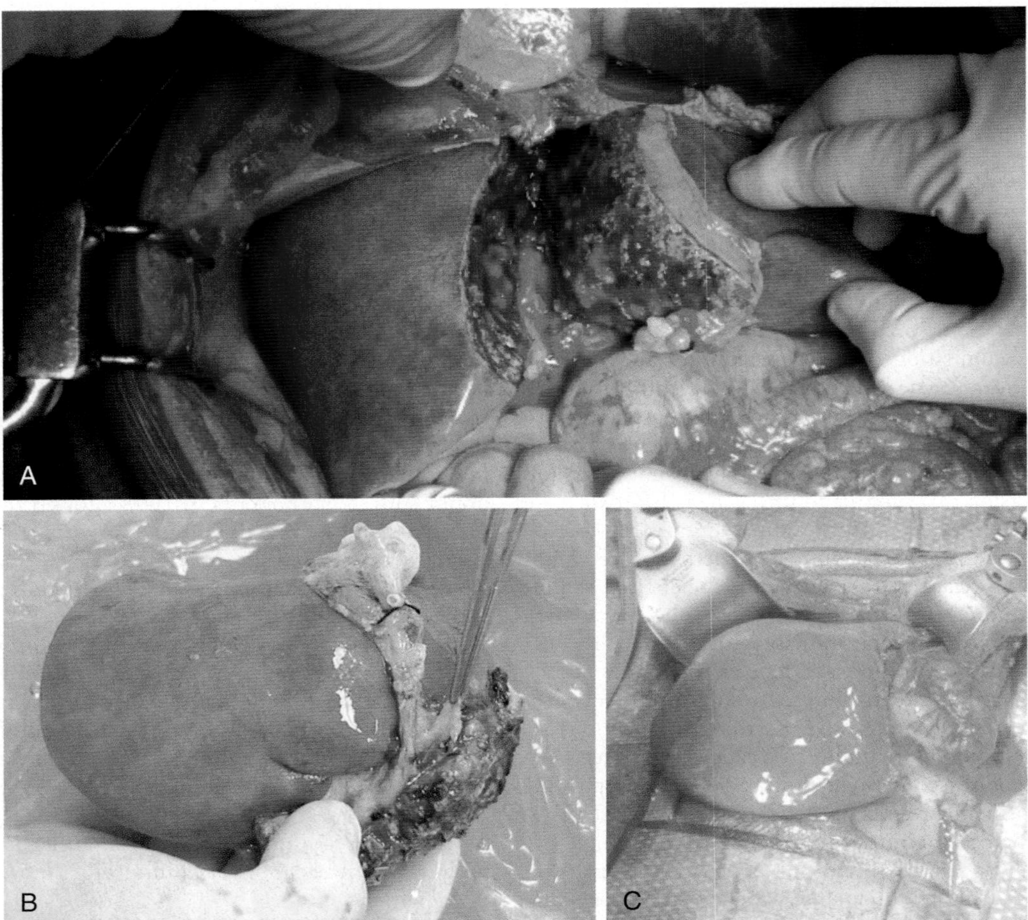

FIG. 26.5 Split liver transplant for a child. (A) In situ resection of live donor graft. (B) Segment prepared for transplant. (C) Graft reperfused in recipient.

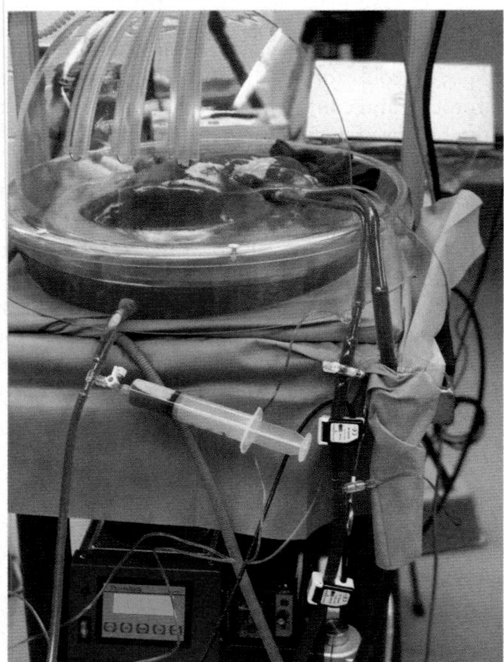

FIG. 26.6 Machine perfusion of a liver.

SELECTED REFERENCES

Kim WR, Lake JR, Smith JM, et al. OPTN/SRTR 2017 annual data report: liver. *Am J Transplant*. 2019;19(suppl 2):184–283.

Current liver transplantation by the numbers.

Mazzaferro V, Regalia E, Doci R, et al. Liver transplantation for the treatment of small hepatocellular carcinomas in patients with cirrhosis. *N Engl J Med*. 1996;334:693–699.

This work forms the basis for modern treatment of unresectable hepatocellular cancer.

Starzl TE. *The Puzzle People. Memoirs of a Transplant Surgeon*. Pittsburgh: University of Pittsburgh Press; 1992.

An engaging history of liver transplantation by its pioneer.

Wiesner R, Edwards E, Freeman R, et al. Model for end-stage liver disease (MELD) and allocation of donor livers. *Gastroenterology*. 2003;124:91–96.

Early results after institution of model for end-stage liver disease scoring for organ allocation.

REFERENCES

1. Kim WR, Lake JR, Smith JM, et al. OPTN/SRTR 2017 annual data report: liver. *Am J Transplant.* 2019;19(suppl 2):184–283.
2. Medawar PB. Relationship between the antigens of blood and skin. *Nature.* 1946;157:161.
3. Medawar PB, Sparrow EM. The effects of adrenocortical hormones, adrenocorticotrophic hormone and pregnancy on skin transplantation immunity in mice. *J Endocrinol.* 1956;14:240–256.
4. Guild WR, Harrison JH, Merrill JP, et al. Successful homotransplantation of the kidney in an identical twin. *Trans Am Clin Climatol Assoc.* 1955;67:167–173.
5. Dealy Jr JB, Dammin GJ, Murray JE, et al. Total body irradiation in man: tissue patterns observed in attempts to increase the receptivity of renal homografts. *Ann N Y Acad Sci.* 1960;87:572–585.
6. Starzl TE. *The Puzzle People. Memoirs of a Transplant Surgeon.* Pittsburgh: University of Pittsburgh Press; 1992.
7. Starzl TE, Porter KA, Putnam CW, et al. Orthotopic liver transplantation in ninety-three patients. *Surg Gynecol Obstet.* 1976;142:487–505.
8. Borel JF. Immunosuppressive properties of cyclosporin A (CY-A). *Transplant Proc.* 1980;12:233.
9. Mies S, Baia CE, Almeida MD, et al. Twenty years of liver transplantation in Brazil. *Transplant Proc.* 2006;38:1909–1910.
10. Strong RW, Lynch SV, Ong TH, et al. Successful liver transplantation from a living donor to her son. *N Engl J Med.* 1990;322:1505–1507.
11. Yamaoka Y, Tanaka K, Ozawa K. Liver transplantation from living-related donors. *Clin Transpl.* 1993:179–183.
12. Hashikura Y, Makuuchi M, Kawasaki S, et al. Successful living-related partial liver transplantation to an adult patient. *Lancet.* 1994;343:1233–1234.
13. Godfrey EL, Stribling R, Rana A. Liver transplantation for alcoholic liver disease: an update. *Clin Liver Dis.* 2019;23:127–139.
14. Bellentani S, Saccoccio G, Costa G, et al. Drinking habits as cofactors of risk for alcohol induced liver damage. The Dionysos Study Group. *Gut.* 1997;41:845–850.
15. Egawa H, Nishimura K, Teramukai S, et al. Risk factors for alcohol relapse after liver transplantation for alcoholic cirrhosis in Japan. *Liver Transpl.* 2014;20:298–310.
16. Mitchell MC, Friedman LS, McClain CJ. Medical management of severe alcoholic hepatitis: expert review from the Clinical Practice Updates Committee of the AGA Institute. *Clin Gastroenterol Hepatol.* 2017;15:5–12.
17. Lazo M, Hernaez R, Eberhardt MS, et al. Prevalence of nonalcoholic fatty liver disease in the United States: the Third National Health and Nutrition Examination Survey, 1988–1994. *Am J Epidemiol.* 2013;178:38–45.
18. Bartenschlager RF, Rice CM, Sofia MJ. Hepatitis C virus-from discovery to cure: the 2016 Lasker-DeBakey Clinical Medical Research Award. *JAMA.* 2016;316:1254–1255.
19. van der Meer AJ, Feld JJ, Hofer H, et al. Risk of cirrhosis-related complications in patients with advanced fibrosis following hepatitis C virus eradication. *J Hepatol.* 2017;66:485–493.
20. Thuluvath PJ, Kantsevoy S, Thuluvath AJ, et al. Is cryptogenic cirrhosis different from NASH cirrhosis? *J Hepatol.* 2018;68:519–525.
21. Giannini EG, Bodini G, Furnari M, et al. NASH-related and cryptogenic cirrhosis similarities extend beyond cirrhosis. *J Hepatol.* 2018;69:972–973.
22. Schweitzer A, Horn J, Mikolajczyk RT, et al. Estimations of worldwide prevalence of chronic hepatitis B virus infection: a systematic review of data published between 1965 and 2013. *Lancet.* 2015;386:1546–1555.
23. Stevens CE, Beasley RP, Tsui J, et al. Vertical transmission of hepatitis B antigen in Taiwan. *N Engl J Med.* 1975;292:771–774.
24. Yao FY, Osorio RW, Roberts JP, et al. Intramuscular hepatitis B immune globulin combined with lamivudine for prophylaxis against hepatitis B recurrence after liver transplantation. *Liver Transpl Surg.* 1999;5:491–496.
25. O'Grady JG, Alexander GJ, Hayllar KM, et al. Early indicators of prognosis in fulminant hepatic failure. *Gastroenterology.* 1989;97:439–445.
26. *Scientific Registry of Transplant Recipients*; 2019. https://www.srtr.org/. Accessed July 23, 2019.
27. Mazzaferro V, Regalia E, Doci R, et al. Liver transplantation for the treatment of small hepatocellular carcinomas in patients with cirrhosis. *N Engl J Med.* 1996;334:693–699.
28. Rea DJ, Heimbach JK, Rosen CB, et al. Liver transplantation with neoadjuvant chemoradiation is more effective than resection for hilar cholangiocarcinoma. *Ann Surg.* 2005;242:451–458; discussion 458–461.
29. Lunsford KE, Javle M, Heyne K, et al. Liver transplantation for locally advanced intrahepatic cholangiocarcinoma treated with neoadjuvant therapy: a prospective case-series. *Lancet Gastroenterol Hepatol.* 2018;3:337–348.
30. Darwish Murad S, Plessier A, Hernandez-Guerra M, et al. Etiology, management, and outcome of the Budd-Chiari syndrome. *Ann Intern Med.* 2009;151:167–175.
31. Orloff MJ, Daily PO, Orloff SL, et al. A 27-year experience with surgical treatment of Budd-Chiari syndrome. *Ann Surg.* 2000;232:340–352.
32. Roland ME, Barin B, Huprikar S, et al. Survival in HIV-positive transplant recipients compared with transplant candidates and with HIV-negative controls. *AIDS.* 2016;30:435–444.
33. Ladin K, Emerson J, Berry K, et al. Excluding patients from transplant due to social support: results from a national survey of transplant providers. *Am J Transplant.* 2019;19:193–203.
34. Wiesner R, Edwards E, Freeman R, et al. Model for end-stage liver disease (MELD) and allocation of donor livers. *Gastroenterology.* 2003;124:91–96.
35. Ladin K, Zhang G, Hanto DW. Geographic disparities in liver availability: accidents of geography, or consequences of poor social policy? *Am J Transplant.* 2017;17:2277–2284.
36. Merion RM, Schaubel DE, Dykstra DM, et al. The survival benefit of liver transplantation. *Am J Transplant.* 2005;5:307–313.
37. Gao Q, Mulvihill MS, Scheuermann U, et al. Improvement in liver transplant outcomes from older donors: a US National Analysis. *Ann Surg.* 2019;270:333–339.
38. Goldberg DS, Karp SJ, McCauley ME, et al. Interpreting outcomes in DCDD liver transplantation: first report of the Multicenter IDOL Consortium. *Transplantation.* 2017;101:1067–1073.
39. Maynard E. Liver transplantation: patient selection, perioperative surgical issues, and expected outcomes. *Surg Clin North Am.* 2019;99:65–72.

40. Lee SG. A complete treatment of adult living donor liver transplantation: a review of surgical technique and current challenges to expand indication of patients. *Am J Transplant*. 2015;15:17–38.
41. Samstein B, Griesemer A, Halazun K, et al. Pure laparoscopic donor hepatectomies: ready for widespread adoption? *Ann Surg*. 2018;268:602–609.
42. Abecassis MM, Fisher RA, Olthoff KM, et al. Complications of living donor hepatic lobectomy--a comprehensive report. *Am J Transplant*. 2012;12:1208–1217.
43. Sotiropoulos GC, Radtke A, Molmenti EP, et al. Long-term follow-up after right hepatectomy for adult living donation and attitudes toward the procedure. *Ann Surg*. 2011;254:694–700; discussion 700–691.
44. Baker TB, Zimmerman MA, Goodrich NP, et al. Biliary reconstructive techniques and associated anatomic variants in adult living donor liver transplantations: the Adult-to-Adult Living Donor Liver Transplantation Cohort Study experience. *Liver Transpl*. 2017;23:1519–1530.
45. Serinet MO, Wildhaber BE, Broue P, et al. Impact of age at Kasai operation on its results in late childhood and adolescence: a rational basis for biliary atresia screening. *Pediatrics*. 2009;123:1280–1286.
46. Hartley JL, Davenport M, Kelly DA. Biliary atresia. *Lancet*. 2009;374:1704–1713.
47. Superina R, Magee JC, Brandt ML, et al. The anatomic pattern of biliary atresia identified at time of Kasai hepatoportoenterostomy and early postoperative clearance of jaundice are significant predictors of transplant-free survival. *Ann Surg*. 2011;254:577–585.
48. Shneider BL, Brown MB, Haber B, et al. A multicenter study of the outcome of biliary atresia in the United States, 1997 to 2000. *J Pediatr*. 2006;148:467–474.
49. Kido J, Matsumoto S, Momosaki K, et al. Liver transplantation may prevent neurodevelopmental deterioration in high-risk patients with urea cycle disorders. *Pediatr Transplant*. 2017;21.
50. Hafberg E, Borinstein SC, Alexopoulos SP. Contemporary management of hepatoblastoma. *Curr Opin Organ Transplant*. 2019;24:113–117.
51. Cruz Jr RJ, Ranganathan S, Mazariegos G, et al. Analysis of national and single-center incidence and survival after liver transplantation for hepatoblastoma: new trends and future opportunities. *Surgery*. 2013;153:150–159.
52. Pham TA, Gallo AM, Concepcion W, et al. Effect of liver transplant on long-term disease-free survival in children with hepatoblastoma and hepatocellular cancer. *JAMA Surg*. 2015;150:1150–1158.
53. Pichlmayr R, Ringe B, Gubernatis G, et al. Transplantation of a donor liver to 2 recipients (splitting transplantation)—a new method in the further development of segmental liver transplantation. *Langenbecks Arch Chir*. 1988;373:127–130.
54. Ceresa CDL, Nasralla D, Coussios CC, et al. The case for normothermic machine perfusion in liver transplantation. *Liver Transpl*. 2018;24:269–275.
55. Mergental H, Perera MT, Laing RW, et al. Transplantation of declined liver allografts following normothermic ex-situ evaluation. *Am J Transplant*. 2016;16:3235–3245.
56. Goldaracena N, Echeverri J, Spetzler VN, et al. Anti-inflammatory signaling during ex vivo liver perfusion improves the preservation of pig liver grafts before transplantation. *Liver Transpl*. 2016;22:1573–1583.
57. Liu Q, Nassar A, Buccini L, et al. Ex situ 86-hour liver perfusion: pushing the boundary of organ preservation. *Liver Transpl*. 2018;24:557–561.

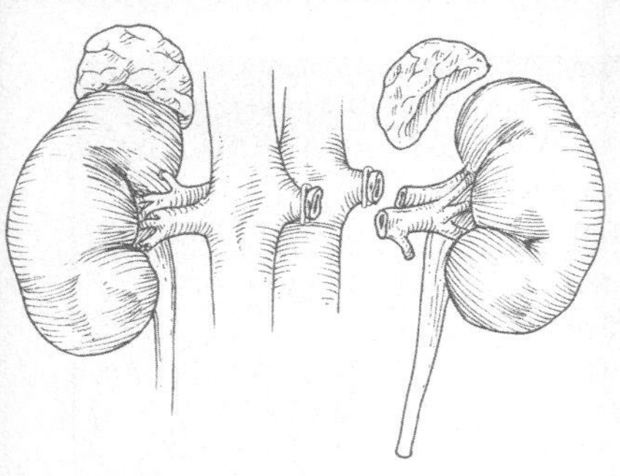

CHAPTER 27

Kidney and Pancreas Transplantation

Yolanda Becker

OUTLINE

HISTORICAL PERSPECTIVE

The field of organ transplant has contributed to the development of surgical technique as well as to the advancement of immunology. Attempts at transplant to cure organ failure date back several centuries. Alexis Carrel developed techniques of triangulation of vascular anastomoses by performing various organ transplants in animals and received the Nobel Prize in 1912. Organ function was minimal, and further attempts at organ transplantation were abandoned. However, in the early 1950s, Medawar and colleagues described the prevention of rejection in mice, and human organ transplantation was again attempted. Joseph Murray performed the first successful renal transplantation in 1954 between identical twins. He received the Nobel Prize in 1990 for his groundbreaking work. Other major milestones in transplantation have included the discovery of cyclosporine and other effective immunosuppressive medications, the description of the histocompatibility antigens, and the perfecting of preservation solutions (Box 27.1). Current efforts target improving graft survival so that a recipient needs only one transplant for life.

Pancreas transplantation has developed as a durable way to provide constant insulin to the type 1 diabetic. Hedon performed the first pancreas transplantation in an animal in 1913. He attempted placement of a pancreas allograft in the neck of pancreatectomized dogs. William Kelly and Richard Lillehei at the University of Minnesota performed the first successful human pancreas transplantation. They transplanted a duct-ligated segmental pancreas graft simultaneously with a kidney graft from the same deceased donor. The pancreas failed because of thrombosis and was removed on the seventh postoperative day. Management of the exocrine pancreas secretions has remained a problem with many surgical revisions developed over the years. The first attempts included duct ablation by injection, but this was mired in complications from leakage of digestive enzymes. Subsequent efforts include the duodenal button technique, bladder drainage, and finally enteric drainage. There has been renewed interest in islet transplantation since it is a cellular therapy with much promise. Debate has arisen about the efficacy of pancreas or islet transplant in comparison to newer insulin delivery systems. While islet transplantation has been recognized as an approved alternative to whole organ pancreas transplantation in Canada, Australia, and much of Europe, this therapy is considered experimental in the United States and is currently performed under research protocols.

KIDNEY TRANSPLANTATION

Indications

Kidney transplantation offers patients a chance to be free from dialysis. Patients state that their quality of life is improved and transplant is the preferred modality of renal replacement rather than remaining on dialysis. The largest study to date showed that kidney transplant is clearly lifesaving, and over 25 years, 1,373,272 life years have been saved (4.4 life-years per recipient).[1] The kidney waiting list continues to grow, and, currently, over 95,000 patients are awaiting kidney transplants (https://optn.transplant.hrsa.gov/data/view-data-reports, accessed January 2, 2019). There continues to be a trend of patients who are removed from the waitlist due to deteriorating health status.[2] The waitlist is increasingly comprised of patients in an older demographic (222,681 patients older than 65 years old waiting), and ethnicity has remained stable. With the implementation of a new allocation system in 2014 that used years on dialysis as a metric for waiting time points, the number of patients listed in an inactive status has decreased.

The most common causes of renal disease in patients on the transplant waiting list continue to be hypertension and diabetes. Overall, the percentage of patients with diabetes has increased to

BOX 27.1 Major milestones in the history of transplantation.

1954	Joseph Murray performs the first successful kidney transplantation between identical twins
1966	Kelly and Lillehei perform the first pancreas transplantation
1967	First simultaneous kidney and pancreas transplantation
1970s	Borel, Stahelin, Calne, and White initiate trials of use of cyclosporine in transplantation
1980s	Belzer and Southard develop University of Wisconsin Solution (ViaSpan)
1990	Murray receives the Nobel Prize in Medicine
1990	Scharp and Lacy report the first successful human clinical islet transplantation
2015	HOPE Act passes allowing HIV+ donors to be considered for HIV+ recipients

HIV, Human immunodeficiency virus.

36% from 28%. An increasing percentage of the waitlisted patients have had end-stage renal disease (ESRD) requiring dialysis for more than 10 years.[3] Older patients with longer times on dialysis are a surgical challenge. Given that more than 600,000 patients in the United States have kidney disease and 468,000 are on dialysis (https://www.niddk.nih.gov/health-information/health-statistics/kidney-disease), transplant remains a sought-after therapy for renal replacement.

Patient Selection

The evaluation of patients as appropriate candidates for transplantation is an arduous process for both the patient and the transplant center professionals. Patients with ESRD have significant comorbidities, and these must be taken into account in evaluating for transplantation. Guidelines for evaluation of these patients have been established. Emphasis should be placed on obtaining the original cause of renal disease so the patient can be given reasonable expectations for dialysis-free survival. Recurrence of native kidney disease can occur in up to 20% of patients and may be the cause of graft failure. Depending on the cause for recurrence, changes in immunosuppression may be warranted.[4] Table 27.1 shows common diseases that recur after transplant and the percentage of loss if disease recurs. Mortality rates are above 20% per year with dialysis. Long-term follow-up of kidney transplant recipients has shown a clear survival advantage over remaining on dialysis. The most important consideration in addressing patients who seek transplant is the improvements gained in quality of life and participation measures.[5]

Recipients must be carefully evaluated for surgical technical risk as well as for their ability to tolerate long-term immunosuppression. The absolute and relative contraindications for transplant candidacy are shown in Box 27.2. Patients do not need to be on dialysis to be listed for kidney transplant, and those patients whose glomerular filtration rate (GFR) falls below 20 mL/min/1.72 m^2 should be evaluated for possible transplant if they do not have an absolute contraindication.

TABLE 27.1 Primary renal diseases and recurrence rates.

DISEASE	RECURRENCE RATE (%)	GRAFT LOSS (%)
FSGS	30–60 first transplant; 80 second	40–50
MPGN type 1	25–65	30
MPGN type 2	90	10–20
IgA nephropathy	30–60	10–30
Membranous nephropathy	40	Up to 50
Hemolytic uremic syndrome	25–50	40–60
Systemic lupus	≤10	Rare

From Morozumi K, Takeda A, Otsuka Y, et al. Recurrent glomerular disease after kidney transplantation: an update of selected areas and the impact of protocol biopsy. *Nephrology (Carlton)*. 2014;19(suppl 3):6–10.
FSGS, Focal segmental glomerulonephritis; *IgA*, immunoglobulin A; *MPGN*, membranoproliferative glomerulonephritis.

BOX 27.2 Contraindications to renal transplantation.

Absolute
Active malignant disease
Active infection
Unreconstructable peripheral vascular disease
Severe cardiac or pulmonary disease
Active intravenous drug abuse
Significant psychosocial barriers that interfere with the patient's ability to comply with a complex medical regimen

Relative
Limited life expectancy
History of nonadherence to medication regimen
History of noncompliance with dialysis
Financial barriers
Psychiatric issues
Renal disease with high recurrence rate
Morbid obesity (BMI is center dependent)
Frailty

BMI, Body mass index.

Human immunodeficiency virus (HIV) infection was once a contraindication to transplantation; however, select patients with appropriate cell counts (CD4+ above 400 cells/mm^3) and an undetectable viral load have good results with transplantation as a treatment modality for HIV-associated nephropathy. There has been an increase in transplantation as a treatment modality for HIV-associated nephropathy and currently 300 patients on the waiting list have HIV-associated nephropathy (https://optn.transplant.hrsa.gov/data/view-data-reports, accessed 1/2/2019). The HIV Organ Policy Equity (HOPE) Act passed by Congress in 2015 has allowed organs from HIV-positive donors to be transplanted to HIV-positive recipients.

Screening of potential recipients should begin with a detailed history and careful physical exam. The length of time on dialysis has been noted to be an independent risk factor for poorer outcomes; however, the death rate is highest in the first year after transplant and survival benefit is gained by 2 years after transplant.[3] In addition to queries about chronic illnesses and the etiology of kidney failure, it is important to gather information about exposures to infectious diseases (especially tuberculosis, cytomegalovirus [CMV], Epstein-Barr virus, hepatitis), recent travel history, and any history of malignancy. Cardiac risk factors should be evaluated. Family history of renal disease or other systemic illnesses should be documented. Routine age-appropriate screening examinations, such as Papanicolaou smears, mammograms, colonoscopy, prostate specific antigen, dental prophylaxis, and bone density, should be obtained as recommended by clinical practice guidelines. In addition, the patient should be questioned about thrombotic events, such as miscarriages, multiple dialysis access thrombectomies, deep venous thrombosis, and pulmonary embolism, so a hypercoagulable profile can be obtained. The ability of the patient to tolerate immunosuppression should be evaluated. This involves consideration not only of the medical conditions but also of the ability to comply with a complex medical regimen and the financial ability to obtain lifelong immunosuppression.

Patients with chronic kidney disease (CKD) are 10 to 20 times more likely to have significant cardiovascular disease compared to the general population.[6] Hence, a careful preoperative cardiac screening must be completed. There is little consensus as to the optimal screening algorithm; however, dobutamine stress echocardiography has been shown to have superiority in accuracy and predictability for perioperative cardiac events.[7] Patients should have a baseline electrocardiogram, recognizing that nearly 75% will have evidence of left ventricular hypertrophy. The patient's risk profile should be assessed to determine whether any risk factors can be modified (diet, weight management). Low-risk patients include those who have good functional capacity and no cardiac disease previously identified. These are typically patients with isolated renal disease, such as immunoglobulin A nephropathy or polycystic kidney disease, and have little comorbidity. Moderate-risk patients should undergo stress testing. It is important to ensure that the stress test is diagnostic and a reasonable heart rate was achieved. Moderate-risk patients include those without cardiac symptoms but who have diabetes, a prior history of heart disease, or two or more other risk factors for coronary disease (smoking, strong family history, hyperlipidemia, hypercholesterolemia). High-risk patients include those with a positive result on noninvasive testing, long-standing diabetes, or history of severe congestive heart failure. These patients require cardiac catheterization before being accepted for the transplant list. Cardiac revascularization should occur before transplantation. Fig. 27.1 shows our current algorithm for cardiac evaluation. Patients who are awaiting deceased donor transplant may be listed for many years and will undergo reevaluation. At any reevaluation, the cardiac status should be routinely reviewed and updated.

Renal failure patients are at increased risk for cerebrovascular events, and the stroke risk is 10 times higher than that of the general population. If carotid bruits are discovered, patients should be screened for significant carotid stenosis. Atrial fibrillation can also be discovered on physical examination. The femoral, dorsalis pedis, and posterior tibial arteries should be palpated and any bruits documented. If the pulses are abnormal or the patient has undergone previous amputation for vascular disease, further diagnostic vascular evaluation should be obtained to assess the level of peripheral vascular disease. It may be that iliac inflow is significantly compromised, which would prevent the patient from having a successful outcome. If inflow is compromised, one can consider whether a revascularization with conduits is warranted before or at the time of transplantation.[8]

Kidney organs can be obtained from living or deceased donors. The demand for kidney transplant and appropriate organs has continually increased, given the increase in the burden of ESRD. The number of living donor transplant has remained flat for several years. A worrisome trend is the increase in discard rate in donors over age 65 or donors with diabetes. In 2014, a new allocation system was adopted in which donor kidneys receive a kidney donor profile index (KDPI) score. This score is derived using 10 clinical parameters shown in Table 27.2. A KDPI score of greater than 85% is associated with decreased graft survival and increases in delayed graft function.[9] This may lead to surgeons hesitating to accept these high-score kidneys for transplant.

Deceased donation occurs after the patient has been declared brain dead or the family has given permission for donation after circulatory (cardiac) death (DCD). In DCD, the care team has determined that the patient is unlikely to make a reasonable recovery and the patient is being maintained on mechanical ventilation but has not met the criteria for brain death (Box 27.3). If the family consents for DCD, the ventilator is disconnected in either the operating room or intensive care unit. If the heart stops within a designated time frame (usually 60–90 minutes), the team waits several minutes to ensure cardiac standstill. The patient is then declared dead by the care team (not a member of the organ recovery team), and the organs are procured en bloc.

Living Donor Selection

The first successful living kidney donation was performed in 1954. Since that time, data continue to show that living kidney donation provides the best graft and patient survival results in recipients. Donors may or may not be genetically related to their intended recipient. In some cases, living donors are anonymous. There are several reports of extended altruistic donor chains. In these cases, an initial donor-recipient pair cannot go forward with transplantation, usually because of ABO incompatibility or sensitization of the recipient. A reciprocal exchange with another incompatible pair allows a "domino transplant" with multiple exchanges, with centers across the country participating. There has been no difference in outcomes of kidneys requiring shipping in paired donation versus traditional living kidney donation.[10] The 5-year survival of an unrelated kidney transplant is the same as that of a kidney transplant from a related donor. The underlying premise of living donation is that the donor will not suffer any medical consequences from the donation and has minimal surgical risk.

Currently accepted eligibility criteria include the following: age, 18 to 70 years; body mass index (BMI) below 35; no cancer or active infection; and adequate renal function. ABO compatibility is also a consideration. However, recipients can undergo desensitization protocols, and transplantation can be performed across ABO barriers. The donor should be informed in these circumstances of an increased risk of rejection of the kidney by the recipient. There is some individual variation among transplant centers concerning acceptable GFR or BMI. Relative contraindications include renal stones, impaired glucose tolerance with a family history of type 2 diabetes, GFR of 70 to 80 mL/min/1.72 m^2, hypertension, and BMI above 35. Absolute contraindications are listed in Box 27.4. For screening, all donors should have a thorough history and physical examination completed. Potential donors should be asked about nonsteroidal use in addition to questions about any medical illnesses. Potential donors should be made aware of the need to be away from work for a time, and their willingness to donate free of

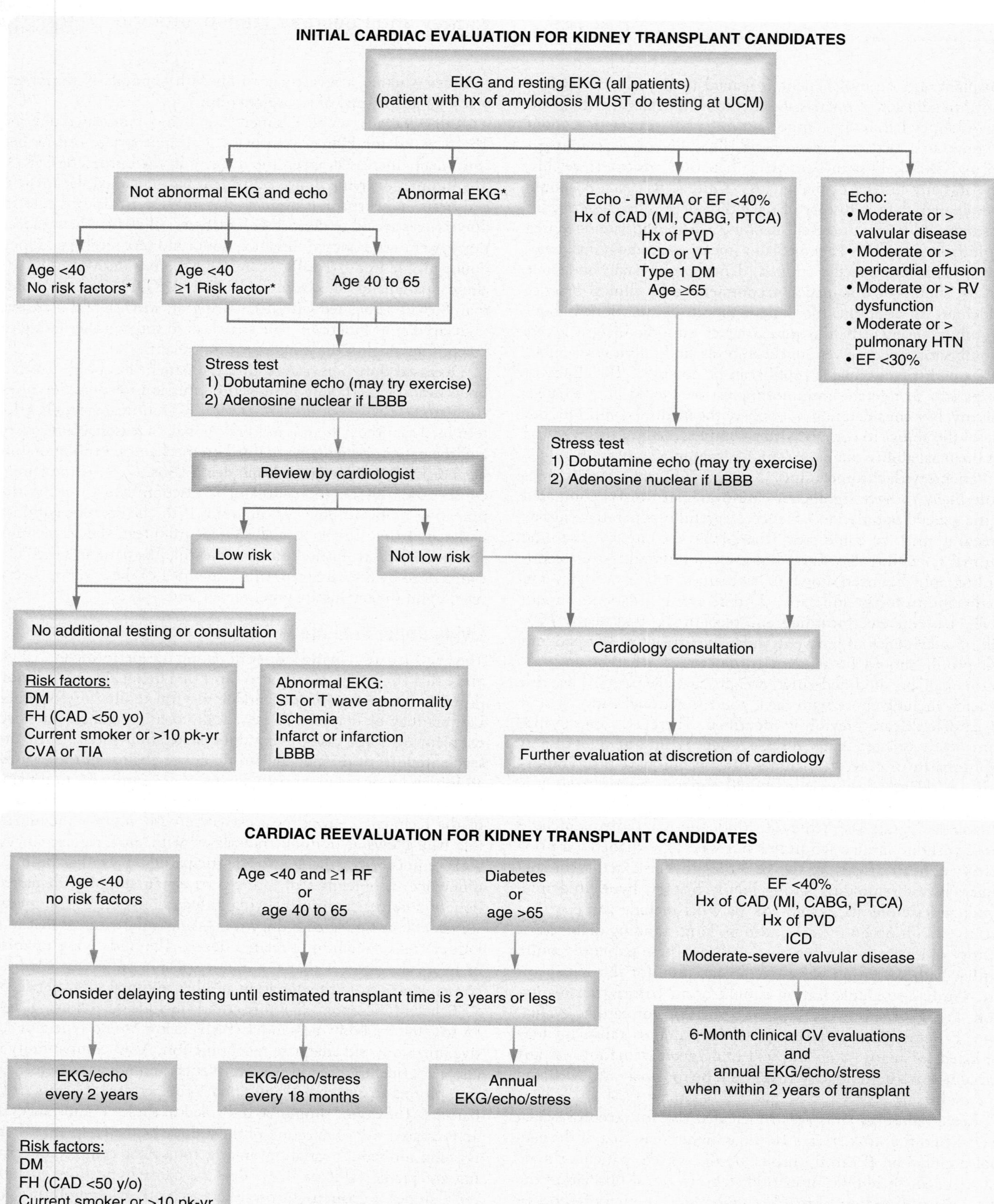

FIG. 27.1 Algorithm for the evaluation of cardiac disease in potential transplant candidates. *CABG*, Coronary artery bypass graft; *CAD*, coronary artery disease; *CV*, cardiovascular; *CVA*, cardiovasclar accident; *DM*, diabetes mellitus; *echo*, echocardiogram; *EF*, ejection fraction; *EKG*, electrocardiogram; *FH*, family history; *HTN*, hypertension; *Hx*, history; *ICD*, implantable cardioverter-defibrillator; *LBBB*, left bundle branch block; *MI*, myocardial infarction; *PTCA*, percutaneous transluminal coronary angioplasty; *PVD*, peripheral vascular disease; *RF*, risk factor; *RV*, right ventricular; *RWMA*, right wall motion abnormality; *TIA*, transient ischemic attack; *UCM*, University of Chicago Medicine; *VT*, ventricular tachycardia.

TABLE 27.2 Kidney donor profile index score components.

Age	Height
Weight	Ethnicity
Brain death or circulatory death	Creatinine level
Stroke	Hypertension
Diabetes	Hepatitis C

BOX 27.3 Confirmatory testing for a determination of brain death.

Cerebral Angiography

The contrast medium should be injected under high pressure in both anterior and posterior circulation.

No intracerebral filling should be detected at the level of entry of the carotid or vertebral artery to the skull.

The external carotid circulation should be patent.

The filling of the superior longitudinal sinus may be delayed.

Electroencephalography

A minimum of eight scalp electrodes should be used.

Interelectrode impedance should be between 100 and 10,000 Ω.

The integrity of the entire recording system should be tested.

The distance between electrodes should be at least 10 cm.

The sensitivity should be increased to at least 2 μV for 30 minutes with inclusion of appropriate calibrations.

The high-frequency filter setting should not be set below 30 Hz, and the low-frequency setting should not be above 1 Hz.

Electroencephalography should demonstrate a lack of reactivity to intense somatosensory or audiovisual stimuli.

Transcranial Doppler Ultrasonography

There should be bilateral insonation. The probe should be placed at the temporal bone above the zygomatic arch or the vertebrobasilar arteries through the suboccipital transcranial window.

The abnormalities should include a lack of diastolic or reverberating flow and documentation of small systolic peaks in early systole. A finding of a complete absence of flow may not be reliable because of inadequate transtemporal windows for insonation.

Cerebral Scintigraphy (Technetium-99m Hexametazime)

The isotope should be injected within 30 minutes after its reconstitution.

A static image of 500,000 counts should be obtained at several time points: immediately, between 30 and 60 minutes later, and at 2 hours.

A correct intravenous injection may be confirmed with additional images of the liver, demonstrating uptake (optional).

From Wijdicks EF. The diagnosis of brain death. *N Engl J Med.* 2001;344:1215–1221.

coercion should be ascertained. An electrocardiogram and chest radiograph should be obtained. Routine laboratory work should include urinalysis, complete blood count, liver function testing, creatinine concentration (with estimated GFR), chemistries, lipid profile, microalbumin level, and oral glucose tolerance test. All age-appropriate screening examinations should be complete prior to donation. Radiographic evaluation of the anatomy of the renal arteries, veins, and collecting system should be performed and can be done by computed tomography (CT) angiography, magnetic resonance imaging, or arteriography on the basis of local expertise. In addition, all donors must be evaluated by an independent donor advocate. The independent donor advocate is not influenced by a relationship with the intended recipient or the transplant center. The donor and recipient pair must also adhere to the National Organ Transplant Act of 1984, which states, "It is unlawful for any person to knowingly acquire, receive, or otherwise transfer any human organ for valuable consideration for use in human transplantation." Many transplant centers ask potential donors to undergo a psychological or psychiatric evaluation.

BOX 27.4 Contraindications to living kidney donation.

- BMI >40
- Diabetes
- Active malignant disease
- GFR <70 mL/min/1.72 m^2 (center dependent)
- Significant albuminuria
- Hypertension requiring multiple medications
- Pelvic or horseshoe kidney
- Significant psychiatric impairment
- Nephrolithiasis with a high chance of recurrence (cystine, struvite)

BMI, Body mass index; *GFR*, glomerular filtration rate.

Potential donors should be informed that the risk of perioperative mortality regardless of surgical technique is approximately 0.03%. Lentine and colleagues[11] combined data obtained from the Organ Procurement and Transplant Network (OPTN) and hospital administrative records. They reported that, overall, 16.8% reported a perioperative complication, with the most common being gastrointestinal (4.4%) and bleeding (3%). Risk factors for complications include being male, being African American, or having preexisting conditions (genitourinary, hematologic, or psychiatric disorders).

Donor nephrectomy may be performed by open or laparoscopic techniques. The open technique is performed through a flank incision. There are variations in the technique of laparoscopic donor nephrectomy. Some centers use a hand-assisted approach; others perform the procedure entirely laparoscopically and make a Pfannenstiel incision to retrieve the kidney, and still, others perform the procedure robotically. Some centers perform a single-incision donor nephrectomy and dissect the renal hilum using instruments placed through a GelPort system, which is ultimately the site of kidney retrieval. There is no difference in outcome based on technique so the exact placement of ports and the retrieval incision is best left to the operative surgeon. If unexpected anatomy or bleeding is encountered, it is important to promptly convert to open techniques to prevent any donor complications or prolonged surgery.

Laparoscopic Surgical Technique

Either the right or left kidney can be procured laparoscopically. The left renal anatomy is generally preferred as the renal vein is longer. Many studies have shown that the right kidney can be procured safely.[12] A left kidney dissection is described here as it is far more common. A 5-mm entry site is placed in the left lower quadrant, and a Veress needle is used to insufflate the abdomen to a pressure of 10 to 15 mm Hg. A 12-mm port is placed at the umbilicus. Two additional 5-mm ports are placed, one at the left costal margin and the last in the midaxillary line to retract the kidney.

The left colon and splenic flexure are taken down at the line of Toldt with the harmonic scalpel. The ureter and gonadal vein complex are identified at the pelvic brim and isolated from surrounding tissue. The renal vein is identified by following the gonadal vein to its entry point. The artery is identified, and lymphatic tissue overlying the artery and vein is divided with the harmonic scalpel.

The adrenal gland is visualized at the upper pole of the kidney and divided from the upper pole of the kidney. The adrenal vein is dissected free from surrounding tissue and transected. The kidney is retracted medially, and the posterior and lateral attachments outside of Gerota fascia are divided with the harmonic scalpel. A Pfannenstiel incision is made approximately three fingerbreadths above the pubis. The rectus abdominis muscles are split at the midline, and a purse-string suture with 0 Vicryl suture is made in the peritoneum. Electrocautery is used to enter the peritoneum, and an Endo Catch bag is introduced for retrieval of the kidney. The ureter and gonadal vein are transected with the linear Endo gastrointestinal anastomosis (GIA) white load stapler at the pelvic brim. The artery is isolated and divided with an Endo GIA white load linear cutting stapler. The vein is also divided with the Endo GIA stapler. The kidney is placed in the Endo Catch bag and brought out through the Pfannenstiel incision and given to the recipient surgeon for flushing.

Open Surgical Technique

The patient is placed in the lateral decubitus position. A subcostal incision is made from the tip of the 12th rib anteriorly extending approximately 10 to 12 cm. The latissimus dorsi and posterior serratus are divided. The external and internal oblique muscles are divided starting at the posterior border. The retroperitoneal space is exposed, and Gerota fascia is identified and incised. The 12th rib may need to be resected to allow better exposure. The ureter is identified and dissected down to the iliac vessels, at which point it is clipped and divided, preserving an appropriate length for subsequent transplantation. Tissue overlying the renal artery and vein is identified and divided. At this point, the kidney is isolated on its vascular pedicle. When the recipient team is ready, a right-angle clamp is placed on the renal artery and the artery is divided. A Satinsky clamp is placed around the inferior vena cava for a right nephrectomy or on the renal vein for a left nephrectomy. The renal vein is divided, and the kidney is given to the recipient team. The renal artery stump is then suture ligated. The renal vein stump is oversewn with a 5-0 Prolene suture in a running fashion.

Postoperative Care and Follow-up of Living Donors

Postoperatively, the patient should be kept well hydrated and careful attention paid to urine output. The diet can be advanced quickly in either open or laparoscopic cases. The most common complications are urinary retention and ileus. Other less common complications are bleeding, deep venous thrombosis or pulmonary embolism, rhabdomyolysis, injury to the bowel or bladder, and injury to the spleen. Patients who undergo laparoscopic donor nephrectomy tend to have shorter hospital stays (2–4 days) compared with patients who undergo open nephrectomy (3–7 days). The group at Duke implemented a protocol for enhanced recovery after surgery that safely allows the patient to be discharged on postoperative day 1 (see Table 27.3). Patients report great satisfaction with pain control and early discharge.[13] The OPTN requires that data be submitted for all living kidney donors at 6 months and 1 and 2 years after surgery. Survival and the development of ESRD do not appear to be affected by living donation. In a study of 3698 kidney donors from 1963 to 2007 at a single center, it was shown that ESRD developed in 180 cases per million persons per year in donors compared with 268 cases per million persons per year in the general population.[14] Scores of physical and mental health in the living kidney donor population were significantly better than those of the general US population.

The long-term consequences of kidney donation have been of concern to the transplant community for many years. However, a long-term donor registry is still not a reality. The long-term consequences of decreased GFR seen in living kidney donors and the risk of subsequent renal failure were studied by the group at Johns Hopkins.[15] At issue has been whether original control groups

TABLE 27.3 Duke enhanced recovery after donor nephrectomy protocol.

	PREOPERATIVE HOLDING	INTRAOPERATIVE	POSTOPERATIVE
DIET	CHO drink 2 hours, preoperative	NPO	Resume early diet
MULTIMODAL ANALGESIA	a. Acetaminophen 975 mg PO b. Gabapentin 600 mg	a. Fentanyl boluses b. Subfascial Exparel (bupivacaine liposome suspension) injected by surgeon c. Acetaminophen 1 g IV toward end of case d. Ketorolac 15 mg IV toward end of case	a. Acetaminophen PO b. Ketorolac IV (first 24 hours) c. Gabapentin PO d. PRN Tramadol PO
ANTIEMETICS	a. Scopolamine patch Emend for high risk PONV patients (failed scopolamine patch in the past)	a. Dexamethasone 4 mg IV at start of case b. Zofran 4 mg IV when closing	a. Scopolamine patch b. Zofran c. Phenergan (if needed)
VTE PROPHYLAXIS	Heparin 5000 units SC	SCDs	SCDs early ambulation
ANTIBIOTIC PROPHYLAXIS	Cefazolin 1–2 g IV or Clindamycin 600 mg IV (if allergic to Cefazolin)	Repeat if procedure >4 hours	None

Duke ERAS pathway. This table highlights the various details of pre-, intra-, and postoperative aspects of the ERAS protocol implemented at Duke for laparoscopic living done nephrectomy.

From Rege A, Leraas H, Vikraman D, et al. Could the use of an enhanced recovery protocol in laparoscopic donor nephrectomy be an incentive for live kidney donation? *Cureus*. 2016;8:e889.

CHO, Carbohydrate; *IV*, intravenous; *NPO*, nothing by mouth; *PONV*, postoperative nausea and vomiting; *PO*, by mouth; *PRN*, as needed; *SC*, subcutaneous; *SCDs*, sequential compressive devices; *VTE*, venous thromboembolism.

were appropriate in comparing living donors with an unscreened population. In the current study, the authors compared donors to the third National Health and Nutrition Examination Survey (NHANES III). They found that kidney donors had a higher risk for development of ESRD throughout their life (90 per 10,000) compared with a healthy population (14 per 10,000), but the risk was still much lower than in the general population (326 per 10,000). There was increased risk noted in African American, older, and related donors. However, a recent metaanalysis of 53 recent studies revealed that the relative risk of development of ESRD is quite small, with an incidence of 0.5 events per 1000 patient years.[16] Previous living donors who develop ESRD are granted 4 points in the kidney allocation system, thus they have a shorter waiting time.

Deceased Donor Surgical Technique

The criteria for establishing brain death were published in the *New England Journal of Medicine* in 2001. A complete neurologic examination must first be completed when the patient has a core temperature above 32°C and there is no evidence of drug intoxication, poisoning, or neuromuscular blocking agents. There can be no other medical conditions that can confound the clinical assessment, such as severe electrolyte, acid-base, or endocrine disturbances or hypotension. A complete clinical neurologic examination includes documentation of coma, the absence of brainstem reflexes, and apnea. Confirmatory testing is also completed as outlined in Box 27.3.

A careful medical and social history is obtained from the medical record and the family. Potential donors are excluded if there is active infection or malignant disease. Renal function and urine output are assessed. If a donor has increased risk behavior as defined by the Centers for Disease Control and Prevention (CDC) for transmission of HIV infection or hepatitis C, the intended recipient must be informed that the donor is high risk, and a written consent for transplantation with an increased-risk CDC donor must be obtained (Box 27.5). In managing a donor, it is important to monitor urine output carefully. Vasopressin may need to be given if diabetes insipidus develops. Many organ procurement specialists administer hormonal therapy to stabilize the donor after the catecholamine release that is common in acute brain death.[15] This catecholamine release can result in significant decreases in thyroid hormone, cortisol, and insulin levels.

Usually, kidney procurement takes place after the thoracic and liver procurements are complete. The retroperitoneum is fully exposed. The ureters are identified and divided as close to the bladder as possible. In procuring the right kidney, it is important to preserve the vena cava cuff so that the renal vein can be lengthened if needed to facilitate the recipient operation.

On the back table, Gerota fascia is removed. The renal artery and vein are identified. The ureter is identified, and the periureteric tissue as well as the tissue along the lower pole of the kidney is preserved to prevent ureter ischemia. If any lower pole renal arteries are identified, these must be reconstructed to ensure adequate blood supply to the ureter.

Preservation and Storage

Once the kidneys are procured, they must be transported to the respective transplant centers by the organ procurement organization. During this time, the kidneys experience changes from cold ischemia. The goal of preservation is to extend the period of organ viability. Delayed graft function significantly increases at 24 hours. Various preservation solutions have been developed over the years. The predominant storage solutions currently used in the United States are ViaSpan (Dupont, University of Wisconsin Solution) and Custodial (histidine-tryptophan-ketoglutarate). Kidneys may be stored in static cold solution. However, there is increasing evidence supporting the use of pulsatile machine perfusion in the preservation of kidneys. With use of this technology, flow is maintained throughout the kidney and vasoconstriction can be minimized. A landmark study by Ploeg and colleagues[17] showed that machine perfusion significantly decreased the risk of delayed graft function, and recipient creatinine concentration was significantly lower for the first 2 weeks after transplantation. If delayed graft function developed, the duration was 3 days shorter in machine-perfused kidneys (10 vs. 13 days; $P = 0.04$). These findings have been confirmed in several follow-up studies.

Recipient Operation

The kidney is usually placed in a retroperitoneal position in the recipient. The donor renal vein is anastomosed to the common or external iliac vein, and the donor artery or Carrell patch is anastomosed to the recipient common or external iliac artery. It should be noted if the recipient has significant upstream iliac atherosclerotic disease as this may affect transplant outcomes. The ureter is then spatulated, and an end-to-side anastomosis is completed to the bladder mucosa. A ureteral stent is placed that is then removed 4 to 6 weeks postoperatively.

BOX 27.5 Increased risk CDC donor.

Donors meeting one or more of the following 11 criteria should be identified as being at increased risk for recent human immunodeficiency virus (HIV), hepatitis B virus (HBV), and hepatitis C virus (HCV) infection:

1. Men who have had sex with another man (MSM) in the preceding 12 months
2. Women who have had sex with a man with a history of MSM behavior in the preceding 12 months
3. People who have had sex with a person who has injected drugs by intravenous, intramuscular, or subcutaneous route for nonmedical reasons in the preceding 12 months
4. People who have injected drugs by intravenous, intramuscular, or subcutaneous route for nonmedical reasons in the preceding 12 months
5. People who have engaged in sex in exchange for money or drugs in the preceding 12 months
6. Persons who have had sex in the preceding 12 months with a person known or suspected to have HIV, HBV, or HCV infection
7. Persons who have had sex with a person who has had sex in exchange for money or drugs in the preceding 12 months
8. People who have been in lockup, jail, prison, or a juvenile correctional facility for more than 72 hours in the preceding 12 months
9. A child who is ≤18 months of age and born to a mother known to be infected with or at increased risk for HIV, HBV, or HCV infection
10. A child who has been breastfed within the preceding 12 months and the mother is known to be infected with or at increased risk for HIV infection
11. People who have been newly diagnosed with or have been treated for syphilis, gonorrhea, chlamydia, or genital ulcers in the preceding 12 months

CDC, Centers for Disease Control and Prevention.

Patients with abnormal bladders due to neurogenic causes (diabetes, spina bifida) or obstruction (posterior urethral valves, primary reflux) may require bladder reconstruction prior to transplant.[18]

Kidney Allocation

Significant concerns were raised that the kidney allocation system that had been in place for nearly three decades before 2013 was outdated and created unintended consequences such as racial disparity. In June 2013, the Organ Procurement and Transplantation Network Board of Directors approved sweeping changes to the current kidney allocation system. In the new system, recipients will receive an Estimated Post Transplant Survival score, which is calculated on the basis of four variables: recipient age, diabetic status, time on dialysis, and number of prior solid organ transplants.

Prior to allocation, all deceased donor kidneys receive a KDPI score, which is based on 10 variables (see Table 27.2). Kidneys with the top 20% KDPI are preferentially allocated to the top 20% Estimated Post Transplant Survival score candidates. Those kidneys with a KDPI greater than 85% will be an "opt in" system that will require recipients to sign prior consent for these kidneys. Kidneys with a KDPI greater than 85% will be allocated on the basis of waiting time and local or regional area (https://optn.transplant.hrsa.gov/media/1200/optn_policies.pdf#nameddest=Policy_08, accessed January 1, 2019).

Recent data analysis has shown that the new kidney allocation system accomplished the goals of decreasing racial disparity and making donor kidneys more available to highly sensitized patients.[2]

Postoperative Surgical Complications

The overall rate of technical complications in kidney transplantation is low (5%–10%). Most complications are manifested as a sudden drop in urine output. However, some recipients experience delayed graft function, so urine output is not a reliable marker of a surgical complication. Daily monitoring of serum creatinine and hemoglobin levels is crucial in the first days after kidney transplantation. Other parameters, such as β_2-microglobulin, can also be helpful to differentiate early rejection from a surgical complication. The most common surgical complications are outlined here.

Hemorrhage

If the kidney transplant was placed in the retroperitoneal space and no window was created to the peritoneal cavity, bleeding will be limited. Patients will commonly present with the acute onset of flank pain, and there may be a palpable mass at the incision site. An acute decrease in hematocrit or hemoglobin may also be seen. Because of compression of the kidney parenchyma, patients will sometimes present with hypertension rather than with the expected hypotension. Many patients are receiving beta blockers, so tachycardia is also not a reliable sign. The patient must be examined, and a high clinical suspicion should be maintained. Risk factors include increased midabdominal circumference,[19] antiplatelet agents, and anticoagulation.[20] An ultrasound examination can be helpful if time permits. Often, the bleeding site cannot be identified, and evacuation of a large hematoma is completed. Biopsy of the kidney should be performed as hyperacute rejection can lead to kidney swelling and disruption of the parenchyma as the cause of the bleed (Fig. 27.2).

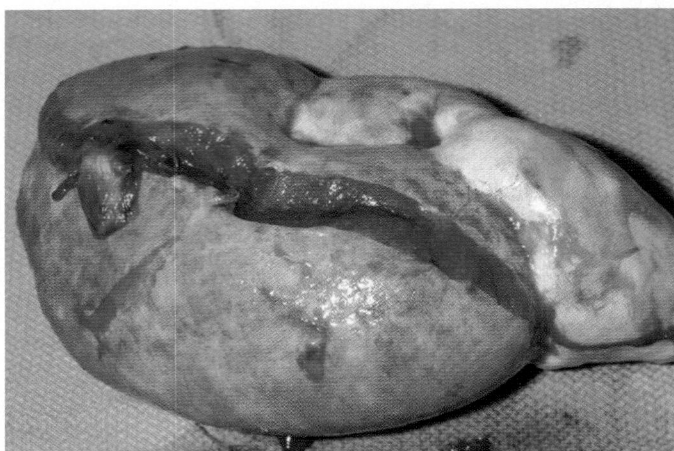

FIG. 27.2 Acute rejection causing kidney parenchymal disruption and hemorrhage.

Venous Thrombosis

Venous thrombosis is rare and occurs in less than 3% of cases and usually is manifested within the first week postoperatively.[21] The patient may develop sudden hematuria or a decrease in urine output. Ultrasound examination may still reveal dampened arterial flow but there will be high resistance and venous flow is absent. The transplanted renal vein might be kinked at the time of the original transplantation because of compression in the retroperitoneal position or possibly external compression for a lymphocele or hematoma. Dialysis patients also have a high incidence of hypercoagulable states. A preoperative hypercoagulable workup should be completed if the patient reports multiple dialysis access thrombosis events (especially of native fistulas), a history of deep venous thrombosis or pulmonary embolism, or a high incidence of miscarriages. The graft is usually unable to be salvaged after renal vein thrombosis. There are case reports of salvage if the patient is able to be taken to the operating room within the hour after the diagnosis.[22] However, this is rare, and a transplant nephrectomy is usually required.

Arterial Thrombosis

Arterial thrombosis occurs in less than 1% of cases. The patient may have sudden cessation of urine output, or the failure of the β_2-microglobulin levels to fall after transplantation may herald the problem. Ultrasound is diagnostic. If there is normal anatomy and a single renal artery, the chance of salvage is minimal. The kidney will not tolerate warm ischemia, and a transplant nephrectomy is warranted. In rare cases, if a segmental artery or upper pole branch is affected, the remaining renal mass may be able to sustain the patient for a time. However, if a lower pole artery is thrombosed, the ureter becomes ischemic, and a urine leak may develop from ureteral necrosis.

Arterial Stenosis

Stenosis of the renal artery is a late complication. The incidence varies from 1% to 23%. Patients usually present with an asymptomatic rise in creatinine concentration. The etiology of stenosis is varied and may be due to a clamp injury of the native iliac artery, preexisting atherosclerotic disease in the donor or recipient, or the development of later fibrosis from ongoing rejection. Patients often present with bilateral lower extremity edema and worsening

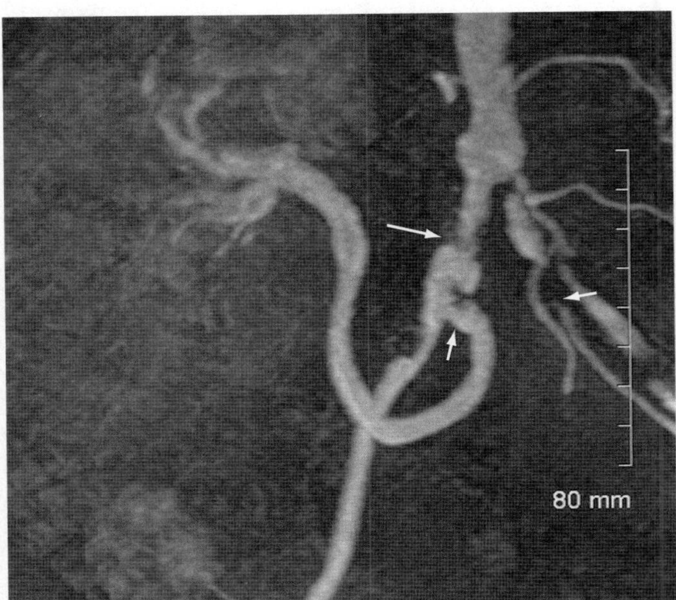

FIG. 27.3 Angiogram demonstrating native iliac disease limiting arterial inflow to the transplant kidney.

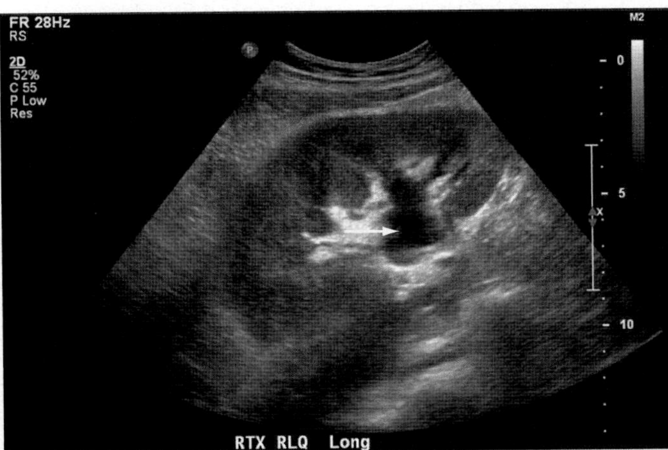

FIG. 27.4 Ultrasound image demonstrating hydronephrosis.

hypertension. Magnetic resonance imaging, CT angiography, or ultrasound can be performed to confirm the diagnosis. The ultrasound is diagnostic if the renal artery velocity is ≥300 cm/sec, spectral broadening is seen (indicating turbulence), and tardus parvus waveforms are present.[23] Patients may have upstream iliac disease, which will mimic transplant renal artery stenosis as the transplant is still ischemic. Many modalities can be used to treat the stenosis. If the native iliac artery is diseased, balloon angioplasty has been successful. Fig. 27.3 demonstrates native iliac artery atherosclerotic disease. In this case, the renal artery was anastomosed to the recipient's hypogastric artery at the initial operation because of native atherosclerotic disease. Balloon angioplasty of transplant renal artery stenosis has success rates varying between 20% and 80%.

Urologic Complications

Urologic complications are rare. The blood supply to the ureter comes from multiple sources including the gonadal artery, superior and inferior vesicular arteries, and common iliac and hypogastric arteries. During procurement of the donor kidney, it is important to avoid injury to the periureteric tissue in the "golden triangle," an anatomic area defined by the renal artery, the lower pole of the kidney, and the ureter. Approximately 15% to 20% of donors have a lower pole renal artery that is a major source of arterial inflow to the ureter. Complications of the ureter include leak, obstruction, and stenosis. Use of a stent at the time of implantation has been associated with fewer mechanical urologic complications.[24] However, there is an increased incidence of urinary tract infections when stents are used. Stenosis may occur early or late in up to 5% of recipients.[24] Early in the course of transplantation, stenosis may be caused by extrinsic compression from a lymphocele or acute ischemia. Polyomavirus (BK) is a cause of late multiple strictures. In obstruction or stenosis, an ultrasound examination will demonstrate hydronephrosis (Fig. 27.4) and may also show a lymphocele obstructing the ureter. The acute obstruction can be relieved by placing a percutaneous nephrostomy tube. A more definitive study can then be performed to demonstrate the exact location of the obstruction. A short, very distal obstruction or stenosis can be repaired by reimplanting the ureter. A long stricture or very proximal stricture will need to be repaired by performing a ureteropyelostomy and using the native ureter. It is important to determine that the patient has a normal native ureter before this reconstruction.

Urine leak can also develop. This occurs in 1% of cases overall but accounts for 25% of all urologic complications.[24] Patients present with pelvic pain as well as swelling at the transplant site, usually within the first week after transplantation. The creatinine concentration is also elevated. The diagnosis can be made by aspirating the perinephric fluid and checking the creatinine level. A nuclear medicine scan can also be performed. Delayed images will reveal the urine leak when the contrast material is seen outside of the bladder. Placement of a double-J stent at the time of transplantation may decrease the risk of this complication. Graft loss is rare with urologic complications.

Lymphocele

During the routine recipient operation, the lymphatics overlying the iliac vessels are divided. Since the transplant is located in the retroperitoneal space, a lymphocele will develop if the lymphatics leak. Drain placement at the time of the transplant does not prevent this complication.[25] Careful ligation or sealing of lymphatics with energy devices such as the LigaSure at the time of transplantation can help decrease the incidence of this complication, but it does not completely eliminate the risk. Many lymphoceles are asymptomatic. However, some patients may present with a swollen leg and increased creatinine concentration because of compression on the iliac vein or transplanted ureter. Ultrasound is diagnostic (Fig. 27.5). The treatment of symptomatic lymphoceles is surgical, with a peritoneal communication being established either by open techniques or laparoscopically. Percutaneous aspiration has poor results with a high rate of recurrence and carries the risk of infecting the fluid collection. Laparoscopic techniques are successful and are associated with less postoperative pain and a slight decrease in hospital stay. Care must be taken not to injure the transplanted ureter when creating a window. The lymphocele fluid should be sent for creatinine levels at the time of surgery to ensure that there is no occult urine leak.

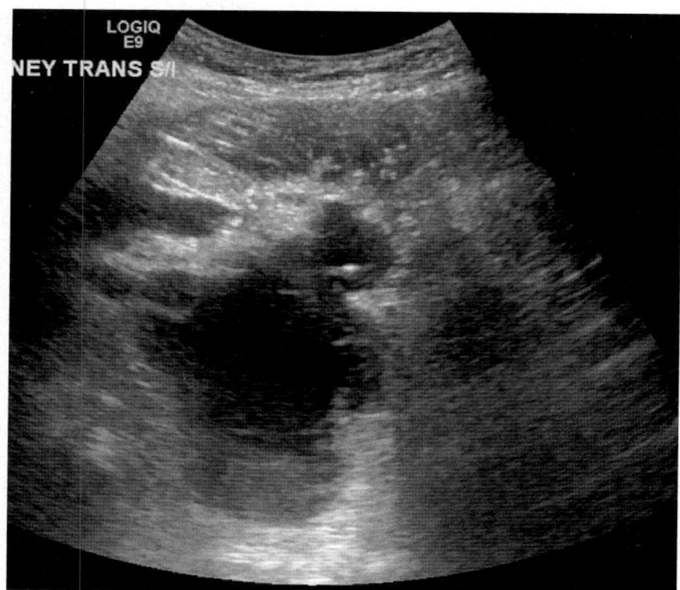

FIG. 27.5 Ultrasound image demonstrating a lymphocele.

Infections

Infectious complications are common after transplantation in large part because of the use of immunosuppression. Up to 80% of recipients experience a urinary tract infection.[18] There is a 1% to 10% chance of wound infections immediately after surgery. As expected, diabetes, obesity, and the use of steroids increase the risk. Viral infections are also common in the first 3 months after transplantation as this is the time that the patient is receiving the highest levels of maintenance immunosuppression and the effects of induction therapy are the most pronounced. Common viral infections include CMV, Epstein-Barr virus, and polyomavirus (BK-type). For this reason, many transplant centers will treat patients in the early posttransplantation phase with antivirals including ganciclovir, acyclovir, and valganciclovir. Another common opportunistic infection is *Pneumocystis jiroveci*, and trimethoprim-sulfamethoxazole (Bactrim) or pentamidine is used as prophylaxis.

Outcomes

Transplantation offers patients a better quality of life compared with dialysis. It is also a cost-effective form of kidney replacement therapy associated with improved survival, especially if the patient can be transplanted before initiation of dialysis. Patient and graft survival remain excellent. Over 80% of living donor kidneys transplanted in 2006 were still functioning in 2016 and death censored 10-year graft failure improved from 33.7% to 26.2%. As expected, KDPI scores correlated with graft survival, and declared brain dead vs. DCD grafts showed no difference in survival. In a large single center study, KDPI was shown to be an accurate predictor of graft half-life and the contribution of donor factors to transplant outcomes (Table 27.4).[9]

Long-surviving grafts still have immunity and the diagnosis of chronic T cell–mediated or antibody mediated rejection and the choice of therapy remains challenging. The Banff process for revising diagnostic criteria for the pathologic diagnosis and differentiation of types of rejection continues to be robust. Interstitial fibrosis and tubular atrophy in the renal cortex has been shown to precede T cell–mediated rejection and may drive treatment

TABLE 27.4 **Adult kidney graft half-life (years) by KDPI and donor type.**

	DECLARED BRAIN DEAD	DONATION AFTER CIRCULATORY (CARDIAC) DEATH
KDPI 0–60	12.5	13.0
KDPI 61–84	8.5	8.25
KDPI >85	7.25	100

From Zens TJ, Danobeitia JS, Leverson G, et al. The impact of kidney donor profile index on delayed graft function and transplant outcomes: a single-center analysis. *Clin Transplant*. 2018;32:e13190.
KDPI, Kidney donor profile index.

decisions. While no specific recommendations are given regarding which transcripts to test, the Banff group recommends obtaining biopsy tissue to analyze and enhance our understanding of antibody and T-cell mediated rejection.[26]

PANCREAS TRANSPLANTATION

Diabetes is a major health concern in the United States and is the leading cause of ESRD. In 1999, the American Diabetes Association clinical guidelines advocated whole organ pancreas transplantation as a viable treatment option for type 1 diabetes. The guidelines state "Pancreas transplantation should be considered an acceptable therapeutic alternative to continued insulin therapy in diabetic patients with imminent or established end-stage renal disease who have had or plan to have a kidney transplant, because the successful addition of a pancreas does not jeopardize patient survival, may improve kidney survival, and will restore normal glycemia" (www.guideline.gov). To date, over 42,000 pancreas transplants have been performed worldwide with over 27,000 in the United States alone.[27] Successful pancreas transplantation can improve the quality of life of patients with type 1 diabetes by eliminating the need for frequent glucose monitoring and decreasing the need for strict dietary monitoring. In addition, patients and their families no longer need to monitor for hypoglycemic events that are life-threatening.

Diabetes is also a leading cause of blindness worldwide. In strictly controlled diabetic patients, the risk of progression of diabetic retinopathy is much lower. Early after transplant, retinopathy may worsen in young patients with the abrupt onset of euglycemia. However, in long-term follow up, progression of retinopathy was reduced and there was less need for panretinal photocoagulation.[28]

Many options exist for pancreas transplantation. Patients with kidney failure may undergo simultaneous pancreas and kidney transplant (SPK) or pancreas after kidney transplant (living or deceased donor). Patients with significant hypoglycemic unawareness are appropriate candidates for pancreas transplant alone (PTA). The history of pancreas transplantation has been marked by the limitations of surgical complications and rejection. In the early era of pancreas transplantation, 25% of grafts were lost because of technical issues. Given that patients with type 1 diabetes have a mortality rate of 33% in the first 5 years after starting dialysis and that glycemic control minimizes the microvascular complications of diabetes, pancreas transplant should be considered a reasonable therapeutic modality.

Patient Selection

Patients requiring pancreas transplantation are usually type 1 diabetics with a clear C-peptide deficiency. There have been a select group of patients with type 2 diabetes that have undergone pancreas transplant.[27] Barbas and colleagues[29] have recently reported pancreas transplantation in patients with pancreatic insufficiency due to extensive native resection for chronic pancreatitis. Patients who are accepted as transplant recipients must balance the effects of lifelong immunosuppression and potential surgical risk with the opportunity to improve their quality of life and perhaps decrease the progression of microvascular complications. Controversy exists concerning recommending the use of closed loop systems or transplant to patients seeking euglycemia.[30] For patients who choose PTA, there should be clear documentation of significant hypoglycemic events, severe metabolic complications such as ketoacidosis, or consistent failure of exogenous insulin. The candidates for PTA should have evidence of stable renal function. Because the patients will require calcineurin inhibitor therapy after PTA, a GFR of more than 70 to 80 mL/min/1.72 m^2 and proteinuria of less than 1 g are required in our program. In pancreas after kidney transplant candidates, a GFR of more than 50 mL/min/1.72 m^2 is required to maintain renal function with a temporary increase in immunosuppression. Patients with minimal secondary complications are the best candidates for pancreas transplantation. Reversal and slowed progression of renal disease can be seen after pancreatic transplant. An analysis of SPK patients showed normalization of circulating micro-RNA profiles association with nephropathy and microvascular damage.[31]

Diabetes is a major risk factor for cardiac disease, and careful pretransplant screening is necessary. Cardiovascular disease is the leading cause of death among type 1 diabetics.[32] There is no universally accepted algorithm for the evaluation of cardiac reserve in the type 1 diabetics. Although concerns about preserving renal function are important, correction of cardiac lesions before transplantation is paramount to a successful outcome, and dye studies are warranted. Posttransplant cardiac events are markedly increased in patients with valvular disease and pulmonary circulation abnormalities.[32] Given the burden of disease in this population, cardiac catheterization is recommended for evaluation. A careful physical examination, with particular attention paid to the peripheral dorsalis pedis and posterior tibial pulses as well as the presence of carotid bruits, can help determine if further screening studies are required.

SPK has recently been offered to a growing number of patients with type 2 diabetes. The overall rate increased from 2% in 1995 to 7% in 2010. According to the same database, approximately 8% of SPK, 5% of pancreas after kidney transplant, and 1% of PTA transplantations were performed in patients with type 2 diabetes in 2010. However, current results from all single-center and database studies do not provide a clear message about the pros and cons of SPK in type 2 diabetes with CKD, and many physicians remain skeptical about its definite role as it carries significant surgical challenges, and it is not an immediately lifesaving procedure.[33]

Pancreas Donor

To assess factors that affect graft survival, a pancreas donor risk index (PDRI) has been developed. The PDRI uses 10 donor factors (Table 27.5) and one transplant factor to calculate the risk of graft failure at 1 year compared to a reference donor with a PDRI of 1.0. Alhamad and colleagues[34] have shown that pancreata obtained from mildly obese donors (BMI 30–35) was not associated with an increased risk of early graft failure. Nevertheless, clinical judgment must be made at the time of procurement to determine the quality of a pancreas.[34] The ideal pancreas is neither fatty nor edematous (Fig. 27.6). Pancreas organs can be safely procured from DCD with outcomes similar to donation after brain death.[35] In DCD, we recommend warm ischemia times of less than 45 minutes. The ideal age range is 10 to 45 years. Pediatric donors can be safely used. In a registry review of all pediatric pancreas donors from 2000 to 2015, there were 4015 pancreas donors younger than 18 years. The average pediatric donor weight was 65 kg (range 10.8–159.0). The lower limit of weight in this review was 10.8 kg and the subanalysis of extra small donors (less than 20 kg) showed comparable results to adult donors.[36]

TABLE 27.5 Pancreas donor risk index donor components.

Age	Cause of death
Sex	Preservation time
Race	DCD
BMI	Terminal creatinine
Height	Cold ischemia time

BMI, Body mass index; *DCD*, donation after circulatory (cardiac) death.

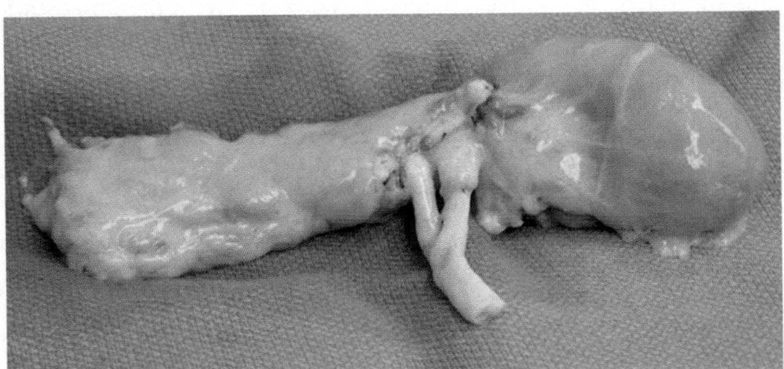

FIG. 27.6 Photograph of the "ideal pancreas."

Pancreas Procurement, Preparation, and Transplantation

During the procurement, minimal handling of the pancreas is optimal. A generous midline incision is made and a median sternotomy is accomplished. It is most common to procure the liver and pancreas en bloc and then to separate the organs in ice to minimize warm ischemia time. The right and left colon is mobilized, and a Kocher maneuver is accomplished to free the duodenum and head of the pancreas. The gastrohepatic ligament is carefully inspected to identify a replaced left hepatic artery. The gastrohepatic ligament is divided as well as the omentum along the greater curvature of the stomach. The pancreas is visualized and inspected for fibrosis or masses. The splenic attachments are freed, and the tail of the pancreas is mobilized from its attachments, with care taken to stay away from the pancreatic parenchyma. The left gastric artery is ligated and divided. The pancreas is mobilized to the level of the vena cava. The bowel mesentery is ligated and divided. The mesenteric vessels may be ligated with ties before flushing, or a vascular stapling device may be used after flushing. If a stapling device is used, the mesentery should be carefully oversewn as the pancreas is prepared for transplantation to prevent any mesenteric vessels from retracting and causing a significant hematoma at the head of the pancreas after organ reperfusion. The stomach is divided at the level of the pylorus with a TA stapler, and the small bowel is divided with a GIA 55 or 75 stapler just distal to the ligament of Treitz. The superior mesenteric artery (SMA) root is identified. The aorta is cross-clamped, and 2 L of University of Wisconsin solution (ViaSpan) is flushed through the organs. University of Wisconsin solution remains the preferred solution as histidine-tryptophan-ketoglutarate preservation solution has been associated with increased risk of thrombosis. This may be due to the increased viscosity of ViaSpan with lower flow rates through the pancreas and decreases in peak amylase and lipase after transplant.[37] The pancreas and liver are removed en bloc and separated on the back table. If there are two different teams procuring liver and pancreas, then the separation is performed in situ with particular attention paid to the division of the portal vein.

On the back table, the SMA is identified, and care is taken to preserve a replaced right hepatic artery if it is present. The splenic artery is identified, and a small 6-0 Prolene suture is used to mark the splenic artery as it enters the pancreatic body. The splenic artery is then divided. Division of the portal vein must be done carefully to ensure adequate length for both the liver and pancreas transplant recipients. At least 1 cm of portal vein should be preserved for the pancreas anastomosis. Extension of the portal vein for pancreas transplantation results in an unacceptable risk of transplant thrombosis.

Once the pancreas and liver are separated, the pancreas is bathed in University of Wisconsin solution and further back table preparation ensues. The spleen is removed from the tail of the pancreas. A probe is placed in the splenic artery and SMA to check patency. The duodenal segment is then prepared. The segment is stapled with a GIA 55 stapler just distal to the pylorus, with care taken to preserve the pancreatic duct drainage. The excess distal small bowel is also shortened with a GIA stapler. Both staple lines are oversewn with 3-0 silk in a Lembert fashion. The portal vein is then dissected. There is usually one small peripancreatic venous branch that can be safely ligated and divided, thereby lengthening the portal vein. The splenic artery and SMA are clearly identified. The excess celiac plexus tissue between the arteries is carefully ligated and divided. Extreme care must be taken to prevent injury to the pancreas at this point. Several figure-of-eight silk sutures are placed in this area to prevent bleeding after reperfusion.

The vascular reconstruction is then completed. The iliac artery is used as a Y-graft, and an end-to-end anastomosis of the external and internal iliac arteries to the pancreas splenic artery and SMA, respectively, is completed with 6-0 Prolene sutures in a running fashion.

The recipient is then prepared. A midline incision is made, and the iliac arteries are exposed for systemic drainage. The pancreas transplant is usually placed on the right side to prevent undue stretching of the venous anastomosis. For systemic venous drainage, the portal vein is anastomosed to the distal vena cava in an end-to-side fashion. The iliac artery graft is sutured to the common iliac artery of the recipient. For portal drainage, the donor portal vein is anastomosed to the recipient proximal superior mesenteric vein (SMV). A path is created in the small bowel mesentery so that the arterial Y-graft can be anastomosed to the iliac artery (usually the right). The vascular clamps are then removed. Slow, sequential removal of the clamps is essential to prevent hematoma formation. The venous clamp is slowly removed, and venous bleeding is controlled. The distal arterial clamp is removed, and hemorrhage is controlled. The proximal arterial clamp is then removed. For enteric drainage of exocrine secretions, there are many technical options. We prefer a side-to-side hand-sewn double-layer duodenojejunostomy. A Roux-en-Y anastomosis may be created, which has the advantage of taking the transplant out of the fecal stream and possible decreasing tension on the transplant to recipient anastomosis. Both techniques have similar outcomes.[38] Direct duodenal anastomosis and gastric drainage are other options.

The exocrine secretions may also be drained to the bladder. A 4- to 5-cm cystostomy is made on the anterior dome of the bladder. A two-layer anastomosis is completed; the outer layer is created with nonabsorbable 3-0 or 4-0 suture and the inner layer with absorbable 4-0 or 5-0 suture.

After completion of the exocrine drainage anastomosis, another careful inspection of the graft should be accomplished to identify any delayed bleeding that may have developed after warming of the transplant.

Drainage Techniques

Exocrine Drainage

Enteric drainage or bladder drainage. Managing the exocrine secretions of the pancreas transplant remains a challenge. A multitude of techniques have been used over the years, including duct exclusion by injection, duct ligation, and even open drainage to the peritoneal cavity. In the past, the duodenal stump was thought to be a cause for rejection and the size was minimized by a "button technique" or the stump was eliminated altogether and a direct duct anastomosis was completed. However, all these techniques were complicated by significant leak rates. The duodenal stump is now left intact and anastomosed to either the bladder or bowel as described in the previous section.

Bladder drainage offers the advantages of decreasing the risk of enteric content contamination from the native enterotomy and allowing monitoring of urinary amylase level as an early diagnostic tool for dysfunction or rejection of the transplant. However, significant metabolic acidosis as well as urinary tract complications may develop. There is a high incidence of urinary tract infections, dysuria, urethritis, and even urethral disruption. Leaks can occur in the early postoperative course, and patients may present with abdominal discomfort or there may be an asymptomatic rise in amylase or lipase. Urinary anastomotic leaks can be diagnosed with a bladder contrast-enhanced CT scan with delayed images. A leak from the bladder anastomosis can be managed nonoperatively by placement of a Foley catheter and rarely leads to graft loss.[39] A normal amylase level with normoglycemia represents clinical resolution of the leak, and no further imaging studies are required. However, if a large amount of fluid is seen, the surgeon should be concerned that there could be compromise of the duodenal stump.

Enteric drainage is clearly more physiologic. Many patients who were bladder drained required conversion to enteric drainage due to complications. Given the good outcomes in patients who underwent conversion of bladder to enteric drainage, interest was renewed in enteric drainage beginning in early 2000. Currently, more than 80% of patients are enterically drained.[39] Follow-up studies have shown that enteric drainage is not associated with significant increases in infection, and by use of this technique, the complications of bladder drainage can be avoided.

Endocrine Drainage

Systemic drainage versus portal drainage. Hyperinsulinemia has been noted in pancreas transplant recipients who have systemic drainage. To allow for the "first-pass" effect through the liver, several groups advocate portal venous drainage through the superior mesenteric vein (SMV). In long-term studies comparing systemic drainage and portal drainage, there has been no clear advantage seen in portal drainage. While theoretical concern exists about atherosclerosis, no clear metabolic advantages of portal drainage have been proved. At this point, the choice of systemic drainage or portal drainage lies with the surgeon.[38]

Surgical Complications

Leak

Leak from the enteric anastomosis was the Achilles heel of early attempts at pancreas transplantation. The incidence varies from 2% to 10%. Enteric leak presents with signs and symptoms similar to intestinal perforation, including abdominal pain, nausea and vomiting, fever, and tachycardia. Patients may have an elevated white blood cell count, but this is often nonspecific as patients are receiving steroids. The amylase levels are not always affected. However, serum creatinine levels are often elevated and can signal ongoing infection. As a consequence of immunosuppression, transplant patients may not display overt signs of infection or leak, and a high index of suspicion is critical to timely diagnosis and treatment. Clinical suspicion may be sufficient to mandate reoperation, but radiographic imaging can often provide confirmatory evidence in equivocal cases. The most useful imaging test in this setting is CT, with oral administration of a contrast agent. CT is especially useful for identifying the duodenal stump and recipient small bowel because ultrasound may be hampered by overlying bowel.[40] Findings include free or loculated intraperitoneal fluid, extraluminal air, and extravasation of contrast material.

Enteric leak almost always requires reoperation. Early leaks are most often anastomotic, and treatment depends on the size of the leak and the condition of the donor duodenum. Simple oversewing may be sufficient for small leaks. If part of the duodenum is compromised, that portion may be resected and the remaining duodenum shortened. If the original anastomosis was performed in a side-to-side fashion, a Roux-en-Y limb may be created to divert the intestinal stream away from the graft. In the case of significant leak with sepsis or advanced peritonitis or in the setting of devitalized tissue, graft pancreatectomy is the procedure of choice.

Most leaks occur in the first several weeks after transplantation. However, there is a subset of patients who experience leaks late in their transplant course. When leaks from the bladder anastomosis occur after 10 years, the duodenal stump can be thin walled, and conversion is associated with a higher rate of anastomotic leak from the newly created enteric anastomosis. For this reason, we recommend that enteric conversion in a transplant after 10 years be created with a Roux-en-Y anastomosis to divert the intestinal stream. We also place perianastomotic drains at the time of the conversion.

Vascular Complications

Bleeding. Immediate posttransplantation bleeding can occur from the pancreatic parenchyma, particularly near the SMA or splenic arteries. The patient presents with hypotension, tachycardia, and abdominal distention. It is our practice to place several figure-of-eight superficial silk sutures in the peripancreatic tissue lying between the SMA and splenic arteries to prevent bleeding in this difficult to approach area.

Delayed gastrointestinal bleeding can also occur from the enteric anastomosis. This usually is manifested from postoperative days 6 to 10 and is self-limited. Patients present with a sudden drop in hemoglobin and are usually hemodynamically stable. It is important to correct any coagulopathy that may be preexisting. Single doses of vasopressin at 0.3 μg/kg as well as initiation of an octreotide infusion at 25 μg/hr are also helpful in limiting blood loss. Endoscopy or radiographic studies are usually not diagnostic in this instance. However, if the patient becomes hemodynamically unstable, another diagnosis, such as duodenal ulcer, should be considered.

Late gastrointestinal bleeding can ensue as a result of CMV infection, duodenal ulcers of the duodenal stump from ischemia, or rejection or development of pseudoaneurysms.[41] Most cases of late bleeding are associated with graft loss. An aortoenteric fistula must be taken into consideration as a source of the hemorrhage in the differential diagnosis as this can be life-threatening.[41] In such cases, the source of bleeding is not identified on upper and lower endoscopy. Findings on angiography of the celiac trunk and superior and inferior mesenteric arteries may be normal as the source of the fistula is the iliac vessel. The proper approach requires immediate diagnostic iliac artery angiography and therapeutic placement of a covered stent if aortoenteric fistula or pseudoaneurysm is identified and there has been a gradual evolution to endovascular techniques. Both aortoenteric fistulas and pseudoaneurysms are prone to develop in cases of chronic rejection, infection, or in proximity to already failed organs.

Thrombosis. Graft thrombosis represents the most common nonimmunologic cause of pancreas transplant failure. This usually presents early in the postoperative course with an acute risk in glucose as well as the onset of severe abdominal pain. The risk factors for graft thrombosis are multifactorial and include donor factors such as injury during procurement and reperfusion injury. Recipient factors such as decreased fibrinolysis found in diabetic patients or obesity can contribute to loss.[42] Use of a venous interposition graft to extend the portal vein may also increase the risk for thrombosis. Recipient factors likely also play a part in graft thrombosis. Coagulopathy related to uremia may confer protection from thrombosis in recipients of SPK transplants, whereas the diabetic state is known to be associated with hypercoagulability. There is a need to balance the risk of bleeding with thrombosis. Results from a study of 152 patients indicate that low-dose heparin (200–400 units/hr or 5 units/kg/hr) for 48 hours postoperatively may provide a protective benefit in prevention of early graft loss resulting from thrombosis without an increased risk of bleeding.[43]

The majority of graft thromboses occur early after transplantation and are suspected in the setting of graft tenderness, hyperglycemia, elevation in serum amylase and lipase, or decrease in urinary amylase for bladder-drained pancreas transplants. Patients with arterial thrombosis may have an acute rise in glucose concentration without pain as the graft is not swollen after arterial thrombosis. Graft thrombosis leads to a rapid decline in the patient's clinical status, with hypotension and tachycardia developing soon after the rise in glucose. Emergent exploratory laparotomy with transplant pancreatectomy is often necessary. In the case of partial arterial thrombosis, the graft may occasionally be rescued with a combination of mechanical or pharmacologic thrombolysis and resection. The appearance of the graft on reexploration is critical. It is usually obvious whether there is sufficient viable pancreas to save.

Pancreas transplant ultrasound is the initial diagnostic test of choice. Doppler flow imaging can provide an overall view of parenchymal vascularity, and flow signals should be identified in both the arterial and venous systems. Limitations of ultrasonography include operator dependence and interference from surrounding structures and overlying bowel.

Other considerations. Infections, bowel obstruction, and pancreatitis can also occur after transplantation. Most often, these do not require open surgical therapy but must be considered in the differential diagnosis of transplant dysfunction.

Infection. After pancreas transplantation, infection may develop in the superficial or deep wound spaces. The appropriate use of perioperative antibiotics can limit this complication. Pancreas transplant recipients should be treated with 48 hours of gram-positive, gram-negative, and fungal coverage.

Surgical site infection, most commonly from gram-positive organisms, may occur in up to 50% of patients. Superficial wound infections are generally treated with local wound care and additional antibiotics. Deep space or intraabdominal infections are less common but carry a significantly greater morbidity. Signs and symptoms of intraabdominal infection are similar to those for enteric leak. Ultrasound and CT are the mainstays of diagnosis.

The stable patient with a localized abscess can generally be treated with percutaneous abscess drainage. Patients with widespread infection or hemodynamic instability should be reexplored. Culture specimens should be obtained to focus antimicrobial therapy. Intraabdominal infection, especially when it is close to the vascular anastomosis, may predispose to pseudoaneurysm formation. Unexplained intraabdominal bleeding in a patient with a history of abdominal abscess should raise the possibility of anastomotic pseudoaneurysm as described before.

Pancreatitis. Graft pancreatitis is common after transplantation, occurring in as many as 35% of patients. Early pancreatitis is likely to be related to reperfusion injury to the graft. The diagnosis is made in the setting of abdominal pain and hyperamylasemia. It is important to rule out the possibility of acute rejection, although abdominal pain is less likely with rejection. CT imaging of the graft reveals a swollen, hypervascular organ, often with a significant amount of surrounding fluid. Our treatment of graft pancreatitis includes aggressive fluid resuscitation, withholding of enteral nutrition with institution of total parenteral nutrition as required, treatment of superimposed or concurrent infection, and supportive management. Most cases of pancreatitis are self-limited.

Bowel obstruction. Significant intraabdominal dissection is required in pancreas transplantation. In contrast to the retroperitoneal kidney transplantation alone, the intraperitoneal nature of the pancreas operation increases the risk of bowel complications. Small bowel obstruction may be caused by postsurgical adhesions or by internal hernia formation.

Patients typically present with nausea, vomiting, obstipation, and abdominal pain. Plain radiographs demonstrate air-fluid levels, and CT confirms the diagnosis. In the stable patient, resuscitation and nasogastric tube decompression may be sufficient. Unstable patients or those with peritonitis should be explored in the operating room.

Outcomes

Pancreas transplantation is a safe and reliable treatment for type 1 diabetes. There is a significant survival benefit, with a waitlist mortality of 30% compared with 9% after transplantation.[44] Normoglycemia is restored, and patients demonstrate normal hemoglobin A1c levels. Importantly, patients do not suffer from hypoglycemic unawareness. Early efforts at pancreas transplantation were hindered by surgical complications and difficulty with the diagnosis and treatment of rejection. However, with improvements in surgical technique, immunosuppression, and tissue typing, outcomes have significantly improved in the current decade. Graft survival is excellent for all forms of solid organ pancreas transplants, with a 1-year patient survival at 97% to 98% and survival at 3 years above 90%.[45] Acute rejection rates have fallen to below 10% in the current era of immunosuppression with prednisone, mycophenolate mofetil, and tacrolimus. A major consideration for pancreas transplantation is the potential for prevention of the secondary complications of diabetes. However, there are no randomized clinical trials comparing the efficacy of pancreas transplantation to tight glycemic control with insulin therapy. It has become increasingly apparent that benefits may not be seen until 5 to 10 years after transplantation. Peripheral neuropathy is improved with improvements seen in motor and sensory nerve conduction.[46] There has been debate about the effect of consistent normoglycemia on diabetic retinopathy. The grade of disease before transplantation may affect the response. Those with severe disease before transplantation may still progress to blindness. However, in long-term follow-up, retinopathy stabilizes and there is less need for photocoagulation in patients with successful transplantation.[28]

Successful pancreas transplantation normalizing glucose control for at least 1 year significantly improves kidney graft survival not only when the pancreas is implanted simultaneously, but also, to a lesser extent, when pancreas transplantation follows deceased or living donor kidney transplantation.

The major cause of death in pancreas transplant recipients is cardiovascular disease. A careful preoperative screening is necessary in these patients to treat any silent cardiac disease before transplantation. In addition to normalization of hemoglobin A1c levels and nearly normal fasting glucose levels, patients enjoy freedom from hypoglycemic events, which significantly improves the quality of life for both the patients and their families.

ISLET TRANSPLANTATION

Because the main goal of pancreas transplantation is to replace beta cell function, endocrine tissue only (islet) transplantation has the potential to provide the same therapeutic effect without the need for major surgery. Islet transplantation is a minimally invasive procedure, thereby avoiding complex intraabdominal surgery and related surgical complications as well as those related to exocrine secretions of the pancreas. Interest in this cellular therapy was rejuvenated after Shapiro and colleagues[47] reported the outcomes of seven patients who were insulin free 1 year after islet transplantation on a steroid-free protocol of immunosuppression. This was a pivotal change in the field. In patients with severe peripheral vascular disease, islet injection may offer the only chance for improved glucose control and an insulin-free life without fear of hypoglycemic unawareness. Unique indications for islet transplant have developed. Nijhoff and colleagues[48] reported a case of islet isolation and rescue transplant infusion in a pancreas allograft that had been removed for bleeding. Either autotransplant or allotransplant may be indicated in patients with extensive pancreatectomy. Also, patients with a failed solid organ transplant may be candidates for islets alone.[49] Transplanting only the islets also obviates the need to manage the complications secondary to the exocrine secretions of the pancreas. The patient and physician must consider the balance between the secondary complications of diabetes and the side effects of immunosuppression.

Isolation and Infusion Techniques

For islet transplantation, the pancreas is procured and preserved from a deceased donor in the same fashion as for whole organ transplantation, with special attention paid to proper cooling of the organ during the entire procedure and not injuring the capsule of the organ. Because blood vessels are not used during islet isolation, in the case of a replaced right hepatic artery in the donor, the SMA might be easily dissected and sent with the liver and the pancreas used for islet transplantation. In most countries, the best-quality donor pancreata are first allocated for whole organ transplantation; if rejected, they are then offered for islets. However, fatty organs from donors with a BMI above 32 might go directly to islet centers with high isolation yields.

Choosing donors carefully allows centers to save time and money by minimizing the risk of a low yield or failed isolation. Islet cell processing takes place in clinical-grade facilities meeting Good Manufacture Practice requirements. First, the pancreas is dissociated during enzymatic digestion with collagenase, and then the islets are separated from acinar tissue during gradient purification. Next, islets can be cultured for up to 72 hours, allowing an elective procedure and preparation of the patient. Islets are infused into the portal vein by an interventional radiologist. The entire procedure can be performed under local anesthesia with minimal sedation. Intraabdominal bleeding occurs in 3% to 15% of cases and is the main risk related to the procedure. However, less than 1% of patients who have a bleeding episode require surgery. The initial cohorts reported a small chance of portal vein thrombosis. In the current era, use of heparin and modern purification techniques that result in low pellet volume minimizes this risk.

Outcomes

During the last 14 years, new islet isolation and transplantation techniques have been optimized. New immunosuppressive protocols have been tested. The 10th report of Collaborative Islet Transplant Registry shows that more than 1000 patients have undergone islet transplantation worldwide from 1999 to 2015 (https://citregistry.org/system/files/10th_AR.pdf, accessed December 20, 2018). Use of T-cell depleting agents in combination with tumor necrosis factor-α blocker, mammalian target of rapamycin inhibition, and/or calcineurin inhibitors leads to improved clinical outcomes. Freedom from insulin outcomes is comparable to that of PTA.[50] Of note, this group showed that patients who resumed insulin after islet transplant remained free from hypoglycemic events. Subsequent sequential islet infusions may safely extend the insulin-free period and patients report a durable reduction in the fear and anxiety associated with hypoglycemia.[51] It should be highlighted that 90% of patients maintained islet function more than 5 years after the procedure, expressing normal levels of C-peptide in the bloodstream. Nephrotoxicity of the immunosuppressive agents has been one of the major concerns of islet transplantation compared with remaining on insulin. Results from a crossover study indicated that the progression of kidney disease is faster in "brittle" type 1 diabetics remaining on the waiting list on optimal insulin therapy compared with patients who received islet transplants and maintained a therapeutic dose of tacrolimus.[51]

For highly selected patients with the brittle form of type 1 diabetes and hypoglycemic unawareness, islet transplantation offers a vital minimally invasive therapeutic option with durable long-term results. Because of the high cost and limited funding, further progress in the field in the United States requires approval and reimbursement of the procedure by the insurance payers.

SELECTED REFERENCES

Hart A, Smith JM, Skeans MA, et al. OPTN/SRTR 2016 annual data report: kidney. *Am J Transplant.* 2018;18(suppl 1):18–113.

Kandaswamy R, Stock PG, Gustafson SK, et al. OPTN/SRTR 2016 annual data report: pancreas. *Am J Transplant.* 2018;18(suppl 1):114–171.

These yearly summaries of outcomes and trends are important to review when deciding the best therapy for treatment of organ failure.

Muzaale AD, Massie AB, Wang MC, et al. Risk of end-stage renal disease following live kidney donation. *JAMA.* 2014;311:579–586.

This paper sparked a careful review of outcomes after kidney donation, prompted a change in information provided to potential donors, and pushed forward a requirement for longer follow-up in living kidney donors.

Shapiro AM, Lakey JR, Ryan EA, et al. Islet transplantation in seven patients with type 1 diabetes mellitus using a glucocorticoid-free immunosuppressive regimen. *N Engl J Med.* 2000;343:230–238.

This classic article reinvigorated the clinical interest in pancreas islet transplantation.

REFERENCES

1. Rana A, Gruessner A, Agopian VG, et al. Survival benefit of solid-organ transplant in the United States. *JAMA Surg.* 2015;150:252–259.
2. Hart A, Smith JM, Skeans MA, et al. OPTN/SRTR 2016 annual data report: kidney. *Am J Transplant.* 2018;18(suppl 1):18–113.
3. Rose C, Gill J, Gill JS. Association of kidney transplantation with survival in patients with long dialysis exposure. *Clin J Am Soc Nephrol.* 2017;12:2024–2031.
4. Morozumi K, Takeda A, Otsuka Y, et al. Recurrent glomerular disease after kidney transplantation: an update of selected areas and the impact of protocol biopsy. *Nephrology.* 2014;19(suppl):3:6–10.
5. Purnell TS, Auguste P, Crews DC, et al. Comparison of life participation activities among adults treated by hemodialysis, peritoneal dialysis, and kidney transplantation: a systematic review. *Am J Kidney Dis.* 2013;62:953–973.
6. Ortiz A, Covic A, Fliser D, et al. Epidemiology, contributors to, and clinical trials of mortality risk in chronic kidney failure. *Lancet.* 2014;383:1831–1843.
7. Wang LW, Fahim MA, Hayen A, et al. Cardiac testing for coronary artery disease in potential kidney transplant recipients: a systematic review of test accuracy studies. *Am J Kidney Dis.* 2011;57:476–487.
8. Coleman S, Kerr H, Goldfarb D, et al. Utilization of vascular conduits to facilitate renal transplantation in patients with significant aortoiliac calcification. *Urology.* 2014;84:967–970.
9. Zens TJ, Danobeitia JS, Leverson G, et al. The impact of kidney donor profile index on delayed graft function and transplant outcomes: a single-center analysis. *Clin Transplant.* 2018;32:e13190.
10. Treat EG, Miller ET, Kwan L, et al. Outcomes of shipped live donor kidney transplants compared with traditional living donor kidney transplants. *Transpl Int.* 2014;27:1175–1182.

11. Lentine KL, Lam NN, Axelrod D, et al. Perioperative complications after living kidney donation: a national study. *Am J Transplant*. 2016;16:1848–1857.
12. Kumar S, Witt RG, Tullius SG, et al. Hand-assisted laparoscopic retroperitoneal donor nephrectomy: a single-institution experience of over 500 cases—operative technique and clinical outcomes. *Clin Transplant*. 2018;32:e13261.
13. Rege A, Leraas H, Vikraman D, et al. Could the use of an enhanced recovery protocol in laparoscopic donor nephrectomy be an incentive for live kidney donation? *Cureus*. 2016;8:e889.
14. Ibrahim HN, Foley R, Tan L, et al. Long-term consequences of kidney donation. *N Engl J Med*. 2009;360:459–469.
15. Muzaale AD, Massie AB, Wang MC, et al. Risk of end-stage renal disease following live kidney donation. *J Am Med Assoc*. 2014;311:579–586.
16. O'Keeffe LM, Ramond A, Oliver-Williams C, et al. Mid- and long-term health risks in living kidney donors: a systematic review and meta-analysis. *Ann Intern Med*. 2018;168:276–284.
17. Moers C, Smits JM, Maathuis MH, et al. Machine perfusion or cold storage in deceased-donor kidney transplantation. *N Engl J Med*. 2009;360:7–19.
18. Salman BM, Hassan AI, Sultan SM, et al. Renal transplant in patients with abnormal bladder: impact of causes on graft function and survival. *Exp Clin Transplant*. 2017;15:609–614.
19. Taha M, Davis NF, Power R, et al. Increased mid-abdominal circumference is a predictor for surgical wound complications in kidney transplant recipients: a prospective cohort study. *Clin Transplant*. 2017;31:e12960.
20. Koch M, Kantas A, Ramcke K, et al. Surgical complications after kidney transplantation: different impacts of immunosuppression, graft function, patient variables, and surgical performance. *Clin Transplant*. 2015;29:252–260.
21. de Freitas RAP, de Lima ML, Mazzali M. Early vascular thrombosis after kidney transplantation: can we predict patients at risk? *Transplant Proc*. 2017;49:817–820.
22. Harraz AM, Shokeir AA, Soliman SA, et al. Salvage of grafts with vascular thrombosis during live donor renal allotransplantation: a critical analysis of successful outcome. *Int J Urol*. 2014;21:999–1004.
23. Fananapazir G, Troppmann C. Vascular complications in kidney transplant recipients. *Abdom Radiol (NY)*. 2018;43:2546–2554.
24. Abrol N, Dean PG, Prieto M, et al. Routine stenting of extravesical ureteroneocystostomy in kidney transplantation: a systematic review and meta-analysis. *Transplant Proc*. 2018;50:3397–3404.
25. Heer MK, Clark D, Trevillian PR, et al. Functional significance and risk factors for lymphocele formation after renal transplantation. *ANZ J Surg*. 2018;88:597–602.
26. Haas M, Loupy A, Lefaucheur C, et al. The Banff 2017 Kidney Meeting Report: revised diagnostic criteria for chronic active T cell–mediated rejection, antibody-mediated rejection, and prospects for integrative endpoints for next-generation clinical trials. *Am J Transplant*. 2018;18:293–307.
27. Kandaswamy R, Stock PG, Gustafson SK, et al. OPTN/SRTR 2016 annual data report: pancreas. *Am J Transplant*. 2018;18(suppl 1):114–171.
28. Kim YJ, Shin S, Han DJ, et al. Long-term effects of pancreas transplantation on diabetic retinopathy and incidence and predictive risk factors for early worsening. *Transplantation*. 2018;102:e30–e38.
29. Barbas AS, Al-Adra DP, Goldaracena N, et al. Pancreas transplantation with portal-enteric drainage for patients with endocrine and exocrine insufficiency from extensive pancreatic resection. *Transplant Direct*. 2017;3:e203.
30. Thabit H, Hovorka R. Coming of age: the artificial pancreas for type 1 diabetes. *Diabetologia*. 2016;59:1795–1805.
31. Dean PG, Kukla A, Stegall MD, et al. Pancreas transplantation. *BMJ*. 2017;357:j1321.
32. Kim J, Schulman-Marcus J, Watkins AC, et al. In-hospital cardiovascular complications after pancreas transplantation in the United States from 2003 to 2012. *Am J Cardiol*. 2017;120:682–687.
33. Fourtounas C. Transplant options for patients with type 2 diabetes and chronic kidney disease. *World J Transplant*. 2014;4:102–110.
34. Alhamad T, Malone AF, Lentine KL, et al. Selected mildly obese donors can be used safely in simultaneous pancreas and kidney transplantation. *Transplantation*. 2017;101:1159–1166.
35. Siskind E, Akerman M, Maloney C, et al. Pancreas transplantation from donors after cardiac death: an update of the UNOS database. *Pancreas*. 2014;43:544–547.
36. Spaggiari M, Bissing M, Campara M, et al. Pancreas transplantation from pediatric donors: a united network for organ sharing registry analysis. *Transplantation*. 2017;101:2484–2491.
37. Hameed AM, Wong G, Laurence JM, et al. A systematic review and meta-analysis of cold in situ perfusion and preservation for pancreas transplantation. *HPB*. 2017;19:933–943.
38. Laftavi MR, Gruessner A, Gruessner R. Surgery of pancreas transplantation. *Curr Opin Organ Transplant*. 2017;22:389–397.
39. Siskind EJ, Amodu LI, Pinto S, et al. Bladder versus enteric drainage of exocrine secretions in pancreas transplantation: a retrospective analysis of the united network for organ sharing database. *Pancreas*. 2018;47:625–630.
40. Tirkes T, Sandrasegaran K. Pancreas transplantation. In: Fananapazir G, Lamda R, eds. *Transplantation Imaging*. New York: Springer; 2018:105–122.
41. Yadav K, Young S, Finger EB, et al. Significant arterial complications after pancreas transplantation—a single-center experience and review of literature. *Clin Transplant*. 2017;31:e13070.
42. Aboalsamh G, Anderson P, Al-Abbassi A, et al. Heparin infusion in simultaneous pancreas and kidney transplantation reduces graft thrombosis and improves graft survival. *Clin Transplant*. 2016;30:1002–1009.
43. Scheffert JL, Taber DJ, Pilch NA, et al. Clinical outcomes associated with the early postoperative use of heparin in pancreas transplantation. *Transplantation*. 2014;97:681–685.
44. van Dellen D, Worthington J, Mitu-Pretorian OM, et al. Mortality in diabetes: pancreas transplantation is associated with significant survival benefit. *Nephrol Dial Transplant*. 2013;28:1315–1322.
45. Gruessner AC, Gruessner RWG. The current state of pancreas transplantation in the United States: a registry report. *Curr Transplant Rep*. 2018;5:304–314.
46. Samoylova ML, Borle D, Ravindra KV. Pancreas transplantation: indications, techniques, and outcomes. *Surg Clin North Am*. 2019;99:87–101.
47. Shapiro AM, Lakey JR, Ryan EA, et al. Islet transplantation in seven patients with type 1 diabetes mellitus using a glucocorticoid-free immunosuppressive regimen. *N Engl J Med*. 2000;343:230–238.

48. Nijhoff MF, Dubbeld J, van Erkel AR, et al. Islet alloauto-transplantation: allogeneic pancreas transplantation followed by transplant pancreatectomy and islet transplantation. *Am J Transplant.* 2018;18:1016–1019.
49. Gerber PA, Hochuli M, Benediktsdottir BD, et al. Islet transplantation as safe and efficacious method to restore glycemic control and to avoid severe hypoglycemia after donor organ failure in pancreas transplantation. *Clin Transplant.* 2018;32:e13153.
50. Moassesfar S, Masharani U, Frassetto LA, et al. A comparative analysis of the safety, efficacy, and cost of islet versus pancreas transplantation in nonuremic patients with type 1 diabetes. *Am J Transplant.* 2016;16:518–526.
51. Rickels MR, Robertson RP. Pancreatic islet transplantation in humans: recent progress and future directions. *Endocr Rev.* 2019;40:631–668.

28 CHAPTER

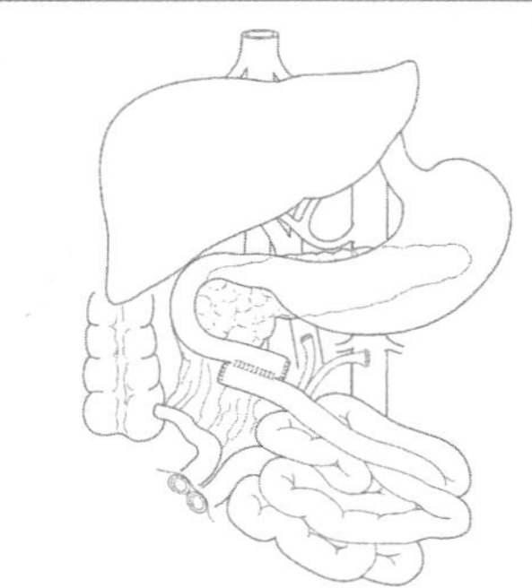

Small Bowel Transplantation

Samuel J. Kesseli, Debra L. Sudan

OUTLINE

HISTORY

Intestine transplantation has become a lifesaving treatment option for patients with intestinal failure. The term *intestinal failure* encompasses multiple disorders of inadequate intestinal length or function that prevent adequate nutrient absorption. In contrast, *enteral autonomy* is a term describing the ability of an individual to absorb all nutrient needs from the gastrointestinal tract. For the subset of patients who have intestinal failure because of loss of bowel length, the terms *short gut syndrome* and *short bowel syndrome* are used interchangeably. The causes of short bowel syndrome include congenital malformations, traumatic injury, infection, and ischemia. The absolute length of remnant bowel required to sustain nutrient absorption varies among individuals and on the basis of age. As a rule of thumb, however, short bowel syndrome and lack of enteral autonomy are expected after resection of more than 75% of the native intestine.

Intestinal failure may also describe a subset of patients with normal or nearly normal intestinal length but with abnormal function as a result of Crohn disease, motility disorders (such as intestinal pseudo-obstruction and long-segment Hirschsprung disease), or diseases of the enterocytes (such as intestinal epithelial dysplasia). Disorders of intestinal function are less common than short bowel syndrome but share the same devastating consequences, leaving patients unable to absorb nutrients from the gut. In fact, before the 1960s, any cause of intestinal failure was nearly always fatal. Today, however, numerous treatment strategies have been developed, and the management of intestinal failure continues to vary greatly by treatment center. To better understand the natural history and clinical outcomes in these patients, the British Association for Parental and Enteral Nutrition recently established first national intestinal failure registry, which will include surgical outcomes and help define the role for intestinal transplantation as a life-saving therapy in select patients.

The first investigation of intestine transplantation as therapy for intestinal failure is attributed to Alexis Carrel in 1905.[1] Given the lack of understanding of transplant immunology at that time, it was not surprising that these early efforts were unsuccessful. Approximately 50 years later, in 1959 (after the first reports of successful kidney transplantation), Lillehei and colleagues[2] at the University of Minnesota published their successful experimental work transplanting intestines in a canine model. In 1962, Starzl (also working in a dog model) described transplantation of multiple abdominal organs, including the liver and entire gastrointestinal tract (from stomach through colon), termed homotransplantation of multiple visceral organs.[3] Human intestinal transplantation was subsequently attempted by Lillehei and coworkers in 1967.[4] Like Carrel's work, this effort and several additional attempts during the next two decades were unsuccessful in achieving complete enteral autonomy, although several intestine recipients survived for several months after transplantation.[5] The primary reasons for failure were early technical complications and the inability to control rejection, leading to development of overwhelming infections or posttransplantation lymphoma.

The clinical course of intestinal failure was dramatically altered when Dudrick and associates[6] described hyperalimentation, which is arguably one of the most significant medical breakthroughs of the century. Their work demonstrated that puppies could achieve nearly normal growth patterns while exclusively sustained by hyperalimentation, more commonly referred to currently as total parenteral nutrition (TPN). The clinical introduction of long-term TPN led to increased survival in individuals with intestinal failure, and contemporary studies have now reported overall survival in parenteral nutrition–dependent patients at 84% and 73% in pediatric populations[7] and 88% and 64% in adults[8] at 1 and 5 years, respectively. Given the success of parenteral nutritional support in the early 1970s and the abysmal results after early attempts at intestine transplantation, there was diminished enthusiasm for further clinical trials of intestine transplantation during this era.

Over time, potentially fatal complications associated with TPN administration were identified. These included severe catheter-associated bloodstream infections; technical difficulties in

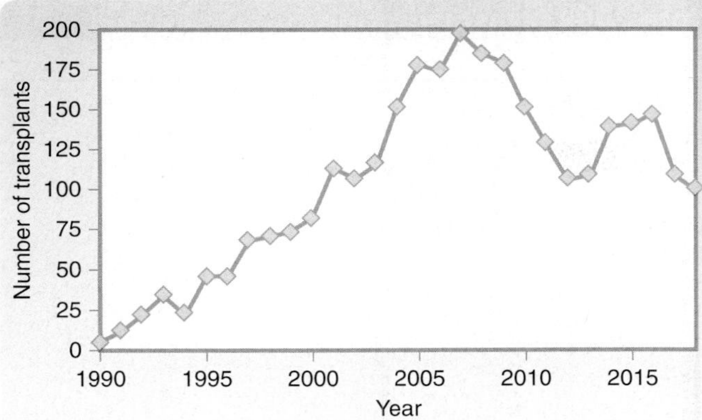

FIG. 28.1 Number of intestinal transplants performed annually in the United States 1990–2018. (Number of intestinal transplants performed annually in the United States 1990–2018. U.S. Department of Health & Human Services. https://optn.transplant.hrsa.gov/data/view-data-reports/national-data/#. Accessed January 22, 2019.)

maintaining venous access because of catheter-associated venous thrombosis; and cholestasis leading to liver failure, also referred to as parenteral nutrition–associated liver disease (PNALD) or intestinal failure–associated liver disease (IFALD). Although a formal consensus definition for IFALD is lacking, it is often biochemically characterized as a conjugated bilirubin level greater than 2 mg/dL in patients who have been on TPN for greater than 2 weeks. IFALD develops in approximately 50% of pediatric patients and is closely related to the duration of TPN (>3 months).[9] Risk of IFALD-induced steatosis in adults receiving home parenteral nutrition is lower, with reported rates of 15% to 40%. Once IFALD develops, however, it is associated with a 43% 5-year mortality in patients with remnant jejunum and ileum length of less than 50 cm.[7]

Concurrent with reports of severe TPN-associated complications, cyclosporine immunosuppression was introduced, resulting in marked improvements in kidney and liver allograft survival. With advances in immunosuppression, there was renewed interest in the field of intestine transplantation. The first successful human isolated intestine allograft (with the achievement of enteral autonomy) was reportedly performed by Deltz and colleagues[10] in 1988 with a living donor allograft procured from the sister of the 42-year-old recipient. Although rejection episodes recurred, these episodes were controlled with the use of cyclosporine, bolus steroids, and antilymphocyte treatments, eventually achieving enteral autonomy. A few months later, Grant and coworkers[11] performed the first cadaveric combined liver-intestine transplant to achieve complete enteral autonomy and more than 1-year patient and graft survival using cyclosporine. Despite these individual successes, 1-year expected patient survival after intestine transplantation using cyclosporine immunosuppression was approximately 25%, and failure to achieve enteral autonomy and risk for early death persisted.[5] In the early 1990s, the introduction of tacrolimus immunosuppression improved control of intestine allograft rejection, resulting in improved patient and graft survival after intestine transplantation.[12] While this led to a mild increase in volume, the overall volume and experience with intestine transplantation have been dramatically less than with transplantation of other solid organ allografts. In the United States, the United Network for Organ Sharing (UNOS) has reported that only 3000 intestine transplants have been performed as of December 2018, with 100 performed in the year 2018 (Fig. 28.1).

INDICATIONS FOR INTESTINE TRANSPLANTATION

Dependence on parenteral nutrition alone is not considered an indication for intestine transplantation in light of the excellent survival of most patients receiving parenteral nutrition. Indications for transplantation of the intestine were proposed by experts in the field at the Sixth International Small Bowel Transplant Symposium in 2001 and have not changed appreciably since. These include irreversible intestinal failure *and* one or more of the following[13]: (1) overt or impending liver failure caused by PNALD; (2) multiple thromboses of central veins limiting central venous access; (3) more than two episodes of catheter-related infection requiring hospitalization in any year; (4) single episode of fungal line infection; and (5) frequent and severe episodes of dehydration, despite intravenous (IV) fluid supplementation and TPN. Additional indications for intestine transplantation have subsequently been added, including intestinal failure that typically results in early death despite TPN (e.g., unreconstructible gastrointestinal tract) and diseases for which no alternative therapy is available (such as complete splanchnic venous thrombosis and unresectable benign or slow-growing mesenteric tumors).[14,15] Other potential indications include patients with high morbidity, poor quality of life, and severe fluid or electrolyte abnormalities that require frequent hospitalization, although these are not uniformly accepted.

The international Intestinal Transplant Registry (ITR) has collected demographic and outcome data on nearly all intestine transplants worldwide since the first successful cases in the late 1980s. The most common primary underlying disease states prompting intestinal transplantation reported by the ITR are shown in Table 28.1. In both pediatric and adult patients, short gut syndrome accounts for about two thirds of patients, although secondary to different underlying pathologies; in pediatric patients, these include gastroschisis (22%), volvulus (16%), and necrotizing enterocolitis (14%), while in adults, ischemia (24%), Crohn disease (11%), volvulus (8%), and trauma (7%) are more common.[16]

EVALUATION

Recipient Evaluation

Timely referral to an intestine transplantation center (before or soon after the development of complications of parenteral nutrition administration) is the first step for the potential intestine transplant candidate. Evaluation for transplantation includes determination of residual intestine length, anatomy and function, extent of complications of intestinal failure, and presence and extent of comorbid conditions. Although each center develops its own protocols, diagnostic studies frequently performed during the evaluation are listed in Table 28.2. After the evaluation, a multidisciplinary team (including transplant surgery, gastroenterology, anesthesia, social work, finance, nutrition, pharmacy, finance, and medical psychology) determines if a patient is an appropriate candidate on the basis of center-specific inclusion and exclusion criteria. If the patient is deemed a candidate, the center places the patient on the waiting list within the donor service area of UNOS. UNOS has developed allocation strategies for available cadaveric donor organs, which are publicly available (http://www.unos.org).

Donor Evaluation

An appropriate cadaveric donor is selected on the basis of compatible blood type and size of the donor compared with the recipient. Size is a significant consideration for the intestine donor because substantial loss of abdominal domain is common in the recipients who have typically

TABLE 28.1 Underlying conditions necessitating intestinal transplantation.

PEDIATRIC	INCIDENCE (%)	ADULT	INCIDENCE (%)
Short bowel syndrome	63	Short bowel syndrome	64
–Gastroschisis	22	–Ischemia	24
–Volvulus	16	–Crohn disease	11
–Necrotizing enterocolitis	14	–Other	10
–Atresia	4	–Volvulus	8
–Ischemia	1	–Trauma	7
–Trauma	1		
–Unspecified	3		
Motility disorders	18	Tumor	13
Malabsorption syndromes	8	Motility disorders	11
Retransplantation	8	Other	9
Other	5	Retransplantation	7

Adapted from Grant D, Abu-Elmagd K, Mazariegos G, et al. Intestinal Transplant Registry report: global activity and trends. *Am J Transplant.* 2015;15:210–219.

TABLE 28.2 Diagnostic studies for evaluation of the intestine transplant candidate.

DIAGNOSTIC STUDIES	TESTS AND PROCEDURES
Laboratory evaluation	Serum chemistries, liver function tests, complete blood count, prothrombin time–international normalized ratio, partial thromboplastin time, platelet count, albumin
Immunologic evaluation	HLA typing, HLA antibody, panel reactive antibody (PRA)
Serologic tests for infectious diseases	CMV immunoglobulin G/immunoglobulin M, EBV antibodies, hepatitis B virus, hepatitis C virus, HIV
Endoscopy	Upper gastrointestinal endoscopy, colonoscopy with biopsy
Pathology	Percutaneous liver biopsy
Radiographic evaluation	Upper gastrointestinal series with small bowel follow-through, barium enema
	Computed tomography of abdomen and pelvis, liver ultrasound
	Doppler ultrasonography of jugular and subclavian veins (or magnetic resonance venography) to assess patency
	Gastric emptying study, motility testing
	Two-dimensional echocardiography
Other	Nutrition, psychosocial, cardiopulmonary, and anesthesia assessment

CMV, Cytomegalovirus; *EBV*, Epstein-Barr virus; *HIV*, human immunodeficiency virus; *HLA*, human leukocyte antigen.

undergone extensive resection. To address the problem of loss of domain, some centers have advocated that an ideal donor should have a body weight 50% to 75% that of the recipient.[17] Additionally, an extensive abdominal surgical history in the donor may preclude procurement.

Another important aspect of donor selection is cold ischemia time. Compared to other abdominal organs, intestinal allografts are particularly sensitive to cold ischemia owing to the highly vascularized and metabolically active mucosa. Prolonged cold storage of the graft may lead to loss of mucosal integrity, and thus, bacterial translocation or intestinal perforation early after implantation; therefore, many protocols advise a maximum cold ischemia time of 6 to 8 hours. As a result, optimal small bowel donors are hemodynamically stable, require minimal vasopressor support, and are geographically close to the recipient transplant center.[18]

Lastly, viral serologic testing of the cadaveric donor for Epstein-Barr virus (EBV) and cytomegalovirus (CMV) is important due to the associated risk for primary viral transmission, leading to post-transplantation lymphoproliferative disorder (PTLD) and severe enteritis, respectively.[19,20]

Donor and Recipient Surgical and Technical Considerations

Isolated Intestine Transplantation

Isolated intestine (or small bowel) allografts typically include the entire jejunum and ileum with the associated vasculature, that is, the superior mesenteric artery (SMA) and vein (SMV) (Fig. 28.2). The most common variable in this type of allograft is the site of vascular transection (above or below the pancreas), which primarily depends on whether the pancreas from the intestine donor is allocated independent of the intestine allograft. In the neonatal donor or in any donor for whom the isolated pancreas has not been allocated separately for transplantation, the SMA is divided at the level of the aorta and the portal vein is divided at the superior border of the pancreas to provide maximum lengths of vessels to the intestine allograft. The donor jejunum is divided with a surgical stapler just distal to the ligament of Treitz, and the ileum is transected proximal to the ileocecal valve. In contrast, in adult and older pediatric donors without significant aberrations in anatomy, isolated intestine can be safely procured while still allowing use of the liver and pancreas from the same donor for other recipients. In these circumstances, the donor operation requires additional careful dissection of the mesentery from the retroperitoneal organs, and the SMA and SMV are divided at the mesenteric root at the inferior border of the pancreas. Carotid or iliac arteries and iliac or jugular veins are also procured from the cadaveric donor to allow vascular reconstruction in the recipient.

During the recipient operation, arterial inflow is established by direct anastomosis of the donor SMA to the recipient infrarenal aorta or by interposition of a donor arterial conduit. Venous outflow from the allograft is provided by anastomosis of the donor SMV to the recipient portal vein or inferior vena cava, with or

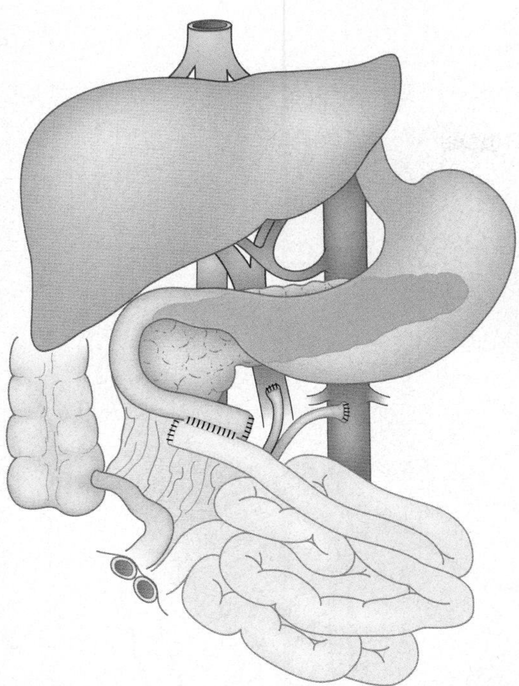

FIG. 28.2 Isolated intestine transplant. Arterial inflow is established through anastomosis of the donor superior mesenteric artery with the recipient infrarenal aorta. Venous drainage is achieved by anastomosis of the donor superior mesenteric vein to the native portal vein or inferior vena cava. Bowel continuity is established through anastomosis of the proximal graft jejunum to the recipient duodenum, and the distal ileum is brought out as an ileostomy.

without an interposition of donor venous conduit. The continuity of the bowel is established proximally and distally by standard techniques for enteric anastomoses. Finally, a distal ileostomy is created to allow routine monitoring of the graft (Fig. 28.2).

Intestine Allograft in Combination with Other Abdominal Organs

The nomenclature of grafts that include additional abdominal organs along with the intestine is less consistent than the isolated intestine graft and has varied over time and among various centers. A liver–small bowel graft as described by Grant and colleagues[11] refers to the individual liver and intestine grafts procured from the same cadaveric donor, but each implanted separately. The technical aspects of donor procurement for grafts planned to be implanted separately are the same as those described for isolated intestine transplantation and in standard liver procurement. This composite graft requires a loop of defunctionalized (Roux-en-Y) allograft small bowel for biliary drainage. In this situation, the pancreas allograft could potentially be allocated to a different recipient. The second variant of the liver and intestine allograft is the en bloc version, in which the liver and intestine, along with the duodenum and pancreas (or head of the pancreas), are procured and transplanted in continuity, thus preserving the extrahepatic biliary system (Fig. 28.3).[21] However, when the liver–small bowel graft is planned to be implanted en bloc, after complete mobilization of the abdominal organs along the avascular planes, the cadaveric donor procurement differs from that described before in that (1) no hilar dissection is performed (leaving the hepatic hilum, donor duodenum, and donor pancreas undisturbed), (2) the donor thoracic aorta is excised in continuity with the abdominal aorta (including the orifices of both the celiac axis and SMA), and (3) the donor spleen is typically removed from the tail of the pancreas on the back table. The sites for division of the bowel (just distal to the pylorus and proximal to the ileocecal valve) and division of the inferior vena cava (above and below the liver) are the same as in isolated liver or isolated intestine transplantation.

During the recipient operation, the native liver is excised along with most (or all) of the remnant small bowel to make room for the intestine allograft. The extent of native visceral resection may include the distal native stomach, native duodenum, pancreas, and spleen. Conditions that may affect the extent of native visceral resection include the extent or location of hilar or mesenteric root tumors, presence of enterocutaneous fistulas or anatomic abnormalities in any of these structures, and loss of abdominal domain that precludes placement of the graft because of size discrepancy. The suprahepatic inferior vena cava anastomosis is performed first as in a liver-only transplantation procedure. Reconstruction of the vena cava can be performed in either caval replacement or piggyback fashion (largely dependent on the presence or absence of size discrepancy between the donor and recipient or preference of the center or surgeon). The caval anastomosis allows venous drainage of the composite organs because the donor portal system remains intact. Next, the arterial inflow is reestablished. Fig. 28.3A demonstrates use of the donor thoracic aorta as a conduit for arterial inflow to the donor celiac trunk and SMA. This donor aortic conduit may be anastomosed to the recipient's infrarenal aorta or supraceliac aorta as shown in Fig. 28.3B. Once the graft is revascularized, bowel continuity is restored proximally and distally; however, the site of anastomosis depends on the recipient's anatomy and the extent to which native viscera have been removed. In Fig. 28.3A, the proximal bowel reconstruction is shown at the level of the native duodenum and allograft proximal jejunum, and the distal reconstruction is at the level of the allograft distal ileum and remnant native transverse colon.

When the recipient foregut is retained, a portacaval (or splenorenal) shunt must be performed to allow venous drainage of the native foregut (stomach, pancreas, spleen, and duodenum) to prevent formation of esophagogastric varices or refractory ascites from venous outflow obstruction. In this instance, the proximal bowel reconstruction is performed between the proximal native remnant jejunum and the donor allograft proximal jejunum.

The strategic advantage of individual implantation is the potential to explant a failed intestine allograft without disrupting the liver allograft if discordant injury occurs after transplantation, which was clearly a concern in the early experience in light of the high incidence and recurrent nature of intestine allograft rejection. The advantages of the en bloc strategy are the simplified recipient operation and the decreased potential for technical complications, given that reconstruction of the biliary drainage and portal vein is not necessary. In addition, the en bloc strategy requires a single vascular anastomosis to either a cuff or conduit of donor aorta, in contrast to individual reconstruction of the celiac artery and SMA, in which the grafts are implanted separately.[21] The major criticism for the nomenclature liver–small bowel for both of these techniques is that it does not distinguish when the donor duodenum and pancreas are included as part of the graft, nor does it distinguish what native viscera are retained or removed.

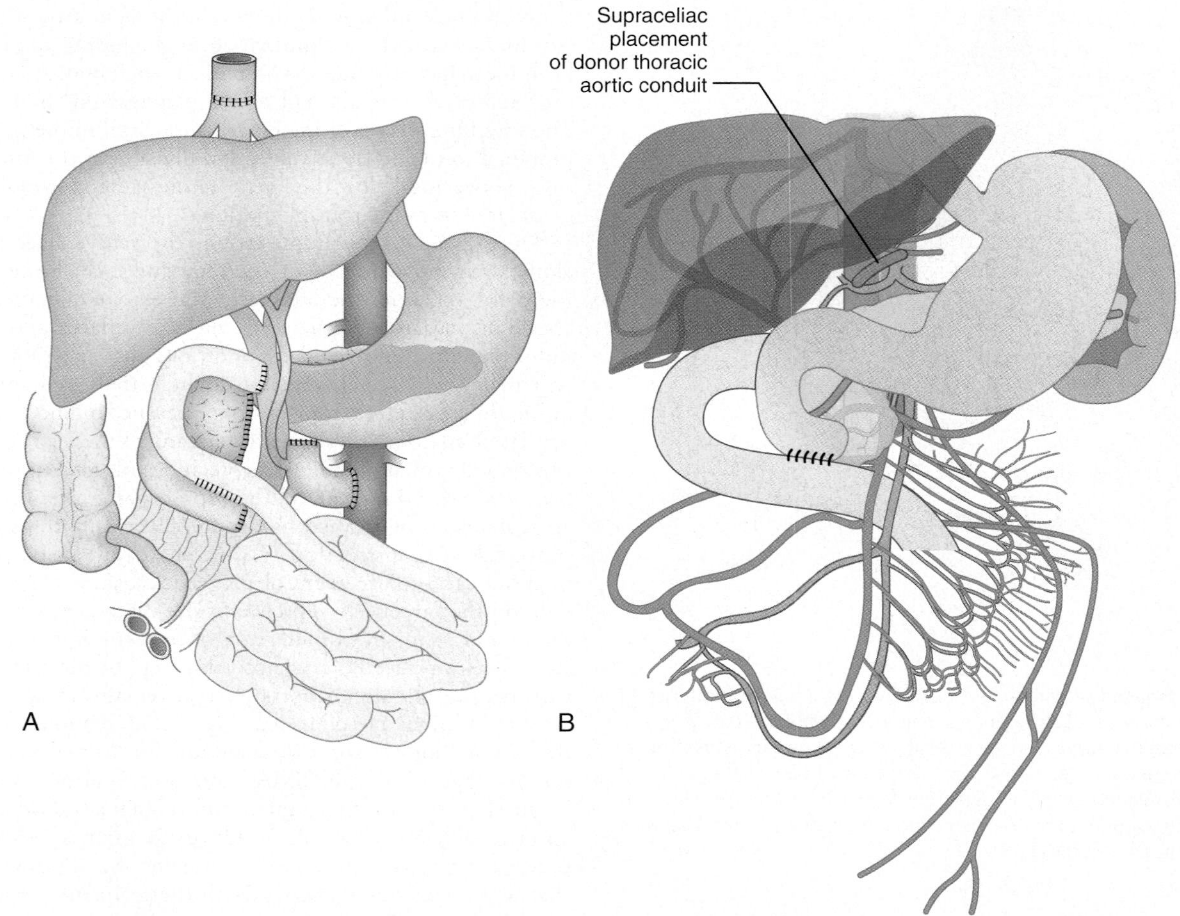

FIG. 28.3 Liver-intestine-pancreas transplant. (A) The donor celiac axis and superior mesenteric arteries are left on an aortic conduit, which is anastomosed to the recipient aorta infrarenally. Venous outflow is through the anastomosis between the donor hepatic veins and the recipient suprahepatic inferior vena cava. The donor duodenum and the head of the pancreas (shown) or the entire donor pancreas are left intact to preserve the donor common bile duct. The donor jejunum is anastomosed to the native stomach, duodenum (shown), or proximal jejunum, depending on the native remnant anatomy. (B) Supraceliac placement of donor thoracic aortic conduit.

Other Technical Variations

Technical variations in the donor and recipient operations are common for multiorgan intestine-containing allografts; however, the nuances of these variations are difficult to assess in terms of contribution to patient outcomes because of the nonspecific nature of the nomenclature used to describe these techniques and inconsistency in use of the various terms. In addition to the liver–small bowel allograft described earlier, three additional terms are presently (or have been previously) used in reference to multiorgan intestine-containing allografts: cluster, multivisceral, and modified multivisceral grafts. In the initial papers using the term *multivisceral* in the description of multiorgan intestine-containing allografts in dogs, the graft included the entire gastrointestinal tract from proximal stomach to transverse colon along with the liver.[3] As more commonly used today, *multivisceral* has been reserved for a multiorgan intestine-containing allograft that specifically contains donor stomach as part of the allograft, whether or not the colon is included as part of the graft.[22] Historically, the right and transverse colon, which receive their arterial supply based on the SMA, were included as part of the intestine transplant. The colon was placed orthotopically and anastomosed to the recipient colon or brought out as an end colostomy. An early series from Pittsburgh[23] described increased risk of graft loss with inclusion of the colon, and inclusion of the colon in multivisceral grafts was largely abandoned for many years thereafter. More recent reports have refuted this perceived negative impact, and centers are increasingly including the colon (and thus ileocecal valve) with intestine allografts, which has been shown to augment stool formation and therefore improve quality of life and continence.[24,25] The ITR report presented in 2013 showed that the rate of colon inclusion has increased from 4% in 2000 to 30% in 2012.[16] In addition to these variations, the term *multivisceral* has also been used by some to refer to the multiorgan en bloc liver–small bowel–duodenum–pancreas allograft (as described earlier) or more extensive explantation of native upper abdominal viscera in the recipient (i.e., complete upper abdominal exenteration). The term *modified multivisceral* has been used to describe a multiorgan intestine-containing graft that includes donor stomach when the donor liver is excluded (with or without inclusion of donor colon). The term *cluster* overlaps a bit with multivisceral but emphasizes the anatomic structure of various organs with vascular supply from a common pedicle (i.e., the donor aorta), and the particular organs included or excluded could be altered on the basis of the needs for the particular recipient. As originally described, the cluster graft

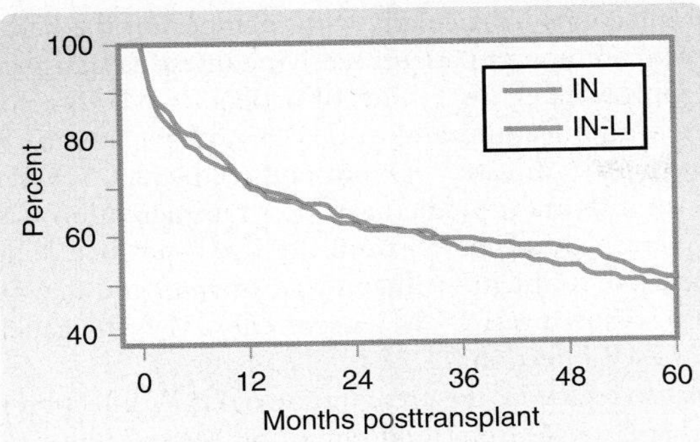

FIG. 28.4 Graft survival within the first 60 months after transplantation among adult deceased donor intestine transplant recipients. (From Smith JM, Weaver T, Skeans MA, et al. OPTN/SRTR 2016 annual data report: intestine. *Am J Transplant.* 2018;18(suppl 1):254–290.) *IN*, Intestine; *IN-LI*, intestine-liver.

was used primarily for the transplantations performed for tumor, and the organs included were selected on the basis of the extent of native organ involvement.[26]

For a number of years, there has been suspicion that the liver was protective immunologically for the intestine allograft[27]; however, data from the 2016 Organ Procurement and Transplantation Network/Scientific Registry of Transplant Recipients (OPTN/SRTR) has demonstrated equivalent graft survival between isolated intestinal and combined intestine-liver grafts (Fig. 28.4).[28] The more detailed anatomic data collection in the most recent ITR report compared with the UNOS data set has allowed preliminary analysis of factors that may affect outcome, including the various organ combinations. Further studies are required to identify the advantages and disadvantages of the various techniques of donor organ implantation and the contribution to outcome based on the extent of recipient native organ removal.

IMMUNOSUPPRESSION

The increased immunogenicity of the intestine requires more potent immunosuppression regimens than are typically used with other solid organs. It has been hypothesized this is related to mucosal associated lymphoid tissue and bacterial colonization present in the graft.[29] The introduction of cyclosporine was the key to the successful introduction of intestine transplantation. However, it was not until the introduction of tacrolimus (FK-506, Prograf), which formed the basis for most maintenance immunotherapy regimens today, that successful intestine transplantation reached acceptable rates. Steroids are also widely used, although the use of a steroid avoidance protocol has been reported with apparent success.[30] Belatacept (Nulojix) has also been successfully employed as maintenance therapy in intestinal transplant recipients who did not tolerate tacrolimus due to nephrotoxic side effects.[31] Most centers use induction immunosuppression intraoperatively with a monoclonal antibody (e.g., alemtuzumab [Campath] or basiliximab [Simulect]) or polyclonal antibody (e.g., antithymocyte globulin [Thymoglobulin]) preparation. Induction therapy has been associated with a substantial decrease in the incidence of early rejection, and the most recent review by the ITR suggests a survival advantage for depletional induction therapy.[16] Use of other immunosuppressive agents (including mycophenolate mofetil [CellCept] and sirolimus [Rapamune]) has been reported at various centers either routinely or when side effects of the standard immunosuppressive regimens are encountered.[22] Similar to the anatomic considerations in surgical techniques and choice of induction agent, no specific maintenance regimen has proved to be superior to another, and centers continue to use regimens based on preference of the physician, experience, and needs of the individual patient.

COMPLICATIONS

Surgical and Perioperative Complications

Despite the advances in intestine transplantation, it remains a surgical procedure with high morbidity, and reported complication rates approach 50%. The most common types of technical complications are bowel anastomotic leaks, intestine perforations, and wound complications. These can be catastrophic and require a high index of suspicion because of the extensive immunosuppression and at times lack of typical signs and symptoms. The management of these surgical complications in the intestine allograft recipient uses standard surgical principles to provide coverage to the bowel loops, to drain or to debride infectious material or tissue, and to close enteric defects. Vascular complications are rare but include both bleeding and thrombosis. Postoperative hemorrhage may result from recipient coagulopathy (especially in the case of native or allograft hepatic dysfunction) and be amplified by the extensive dissection usually required as a result of multiple adhesions from previous surgeries. Thrombosis of arterial inflow or venous outflow conduits is typically associated with devastating sudden graft necrosis and results in patient or graft loss. Biliary complications can be largely avoided in liver-intestine transplantations by including the duodenum and pancreas, thus avoiding any hilar dissection as noted before. Rare instances of intrahepatic biliary strictures due to preservation injury, prolonged cold ischemia, or late immunologic injury have been observed.

Monitoring and Rejection

Historically, rejection was frequent and often severe in intestine transplant recipients, with incidence as high as 70% to 80%.[11] More recently, with the evolution of various immunosuppressive strategies, a decrease in the incidence of rejection has been observed that correlates with improved patient survival.[30] Acute cellular rejection usually occurs within the first year after transplantation but can occur at any time. The most frequent clinical signs and symptoms of rejection may mimic those of viral gastroenteritis, including unexplained fever, abdominal pain or cramping, and increased stoma or stool output. Because of the insidious onset, lack of distinctive features, and absence of specific biomarkers, diagnosis may potentially be delayed. For this reason, rejection remains closely associated with rates of graft failure and mortality.

Unlike in hepatic or renal transplantation, no convenient serochemical marker exists to monitor intestinal function. Stool calprotectin and serum citrulline levels have been examined as potential markers, but due to limited access and prolonged testing time, neither of these tests is widely used at this time.[32,33] Although a serologic biomarker is lacking, perhaps one advantage unique to intestinal transplants is that tissue for biopsy can be readily obtained endoscopically. Ileoscopy through the ostomy provides a method of visualizing the mucosa and directly obtaining tissue for pathologic examination. Routine ileoscopy and biopsy typically begin between postoperative days 5 and 7, and most centers will obtain biopsy specimens once or twice weekly for the first 1 to 3 months and as needed for symptoms thereafter.

Recent investigation has also highlighted the role of donor-specific antibodies (DSAs) in accelerating both acute and chronic rejection.[29] These antibodies bind donor human leukocyte antigen (HLA) and are present in 11% to 31% of patients before transplant and develop de novo in up to 18% to 25% of patients posttransplant; their presence indicates up to 30% risk of graft loss within 2 years.[29,34] Monitoring DSA is accomplished via enzyme-linked immunosorbent assay or HLA bound microbead assay (Luminex); however, currently there is no consensus protocol in using these assays or for the treatment of DSA. In clinical investigation, however, DSA has been measured at 1-, 3-, 6-, and 12-month intervals following transplant (in addition to anytime rejection is clinically suspected) and is treated on a case-by-case basis.[34]

Acute cellular rejection is characterized histologically in mild forms by an inflammatory response that is localized to the lamina propria and the crypts, with increased numbers of apoptotic bodies seen in the crypts but with maintenance of an intact mucosal lining and normal or nearly normal villous height. Moderate acute cellular rejection is defined by markedly increased inflammation within the lamina propria, increased apoptotic bodies within the crypts, and blunting or distortion of the villous architecture. In severe acute cellular rejection, the damage to crypts is so marked that the intestinal architecture may be lost and severe mucosal ulceration or exfoliation is identified.[35] Although the mechanism is presently unclear, some centers have reported a higher incidence or severity of acute cellular rejection in isolated intestine transplants compared with intestine transplants in combination with the liver; however, this protective effect is lost in patients with persistent circulating DSA following transplant.[29]

Once rejection has been established, treatment usually consists of large steroid doses and an increase in the target levels of maintenance immunosuppression. Resistant cases may be treated with more potent immunosuppression, such as rabbit antithymocyte globulin with or without additional immunosuppressive medications (e.g., sirolimus, mycophenolate mofetil) or rarely infliximab (a murine monoclonal antibody to tumor necrosis factor-α; Remicade).[36] During treatment for rejection, the combination of increased immunosuppression and potential compromise of the gut mucosal barrier can lead to secondary infections, requiring close follow-up and a high index of suspicion for infections.

Infection

Following intestinal transplantation, infection is a leading cause of morbidity and mortality and is the most common cause of graft loss.[16] Bacterial infections are prevalent, with incidence as high as 70% to 90% after intestine transplantation.[37] A number of preoperative and intraoperative factors contribute to a high rate of bacterial infection, including prolonged operative time, multiple blood transfusions, potential contamination from enteric spillage, preexisting liver disease, preexisting infections, and frequent need for prolonged central venous access. Ischemia-reperfusion injury may also lead to loss of the gut mucosal barrier and bacterial translocation or intestinal anastomotic leak in the immediate postoperative period. Rejection leads to a similar impairment of the gut mucosal barrier, but later in the postoperative course. Bacterial infections can be manifested as intra abdominal infection, catheter-related infections, pneumonia, or wound infections, with central line infections being the most common. Organisms include typical gut flora such as *Escherichia coli*, *Klebsiella*, *Enterobacter*, and enterococci. Special consideration is also given to fungal infections (most commonly invasive candidiasis),[38] and most centers now incorporate antifungal prophylaxis as part of their perioperative regimen.

Viral infections (particularly with members of the herpesvirus family) are common in patients receiving intestine transplants, affecting approximately two thirds of patients. CMV is a common pathogen with infection rates from 18% to 25%, and a 7% incidence of invasive disease.[39] Donor and recipient CMV serologic status is an important predictor of posttransplantation CMV infection. Transplanting bowel from the CMV-positive donor to a CMV-negative recipient facilitates transmission and may increase the risk for tissue-invasive CMV, recurrent CMV, and ganciclovir-resistant CMV infection.[40]

Similar to rejection, the presentation of CMV infection may be insidious and ranges from mild symptoms (fever, increased stoma or stool output, cramping, and abdominal pain) to severe symptoms (intestinal ulceration, bleeding, perforation, or frank ischemia). The potential severity of primary CMV infections has led some to propose the restriction of transplantation from a CMV-positive donor intestine into a CMV-negative recipient. Because the symptoms of CMV infection may mimic those of intestine allograft rejection, biopsy of the allograft may be needed to differentiate the two causes of graft injury. The presence of CMV inclusion bodies on hematoxylin and eosin stain or identification of CMV by immunohistochemistry or stool electron microscopy confirms the diagnosis of CMV enteritis. Fortunately, with appropriate antimicrobial treatment, typically IV ganciclovir (Cytovene) alone or in combination with CMV immune globulin (CytoGam), and reduction in immunosuppression, graft loss can be avoided in most cases.[41]

EBV, another member of the herpesvirus family, presents a unique challenge to intestine transplant recipients because of the association with development of PTLD. In intestine transplant recipients, the reported incidence of PTLD is 10% to 20%, which is considerably higher compared with kidney recipients (1%–2%), liver recipients (2%–5%), and lung-heart recipients (5% to 10%).[42] In addition, EBV-associated PTLD is more common after primary infection and therefore more common in children than in adults. According to the 2003 ITR report, the incidence of PTLD in pediatric recipients was 11% (intestine), 10% (liver-intestine), and 19% (multivisceral) compared with 3.4%, 2.9%, and 6% in adult recipients, respectively.[23] The 2015 ITR report also detailed the declining incidence of PTLD with transplant era, with an overall incidence of 19.2% in patients transplanted in 1985 to 1995, 10% for patients transplanted in 1995 to 2001, and 6.2% for those transplanted in 2001 to 2011.[16]

PTLD usually is manifested within the first year after intestine transplantation and has a variable presentation, ranging from mild to moderate symptoms of infection (fever, malaise, lymphadenopathy) to life-threatening malignant disease (solid masses at extranodal sites, such as the transplanted intestine, lung, liver, or central nervous system). Routine screening for seroconversion by a serum quantitative EBV polymerase chain reaction assay is common to try to identify primary infections before severe symptoms occur. Other risk factors for the development of PTLD include transplantation of organs from an EBV-positive donor to an EBV-negative recipient, use of more potent immunosuppression, history of rejection, and history of retransplantation.[43] Reduction of immunotherapy (with or without antiviral medication) is the first line of treatment with more severe cases (patients who develop Burkitt or T-cell lymphoma) requiring chemotherapy. Anti-CD20 monoclonal antibodies (e.g., rituximab) may also be useful in the treatment of PTLD when the EBV infection appears to be leading to B-cell tumors or proliferation. Surgical excision of localized disease, if possible (e.g., tonsillectomy, splenectomy, lobectomy,

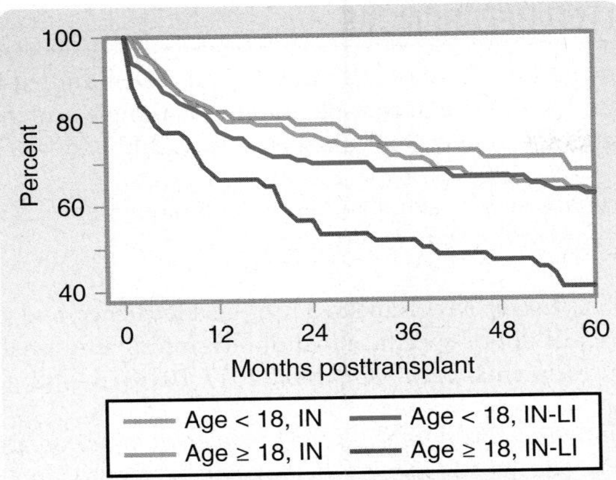

FIG. 28.5 Patient survival among intestinal transplant recipients, 2009–2011. (From Smith JM, Weaver T, Skeans MA, et al: OPTN/SRTR 2016 annual data report: intestine. *Am J Transplant.* 2018;18(suppl 1):254–290.) *IN*, Intestine; *IN-LI*, intestine-liver.

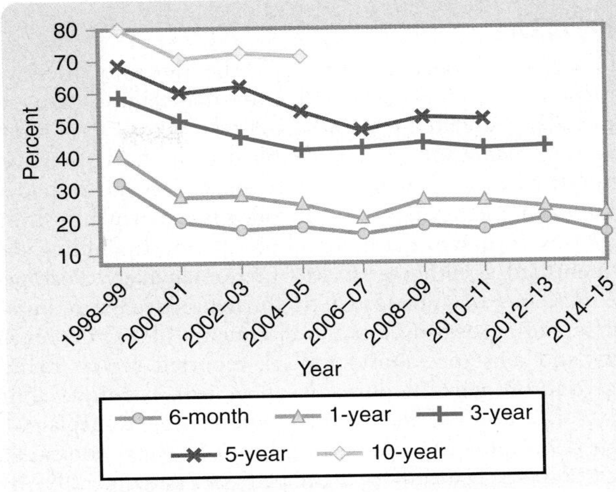

FIG. 28.6 Graft failure rates among intestinal transplant recipients without liver. (From Smith JM, Weaver T, Skeans MA, et al. OPTN/SRTR 2016 annual data report: intestine. *Am J Transplant.* 2018;18(suppl 1):254–290.)

or enterectomy), is also highly effective. Despite these treatments, EBV-associated PTLD has a mortality rate exceeding 25%.[43]

Graft-versus-host disease occurs when donor lymphoid cells begin to target recipient tissues, most notably the epithelial cells in the skin and intestine. Because of the large amount of lymphoid tissue present in the intestine, it was predicted that an intestine recipient might be at higher risk for graft-versus-host disease, but surprisingly, it has been relatively uncommon. The reported incidence is approximately 9%.[44] Increasing immunosuppression, mainly through the increase or addition of steroids or antithymocyte globulin, has been the mainstay of treatment, but the outcome varies according to severity, with a high rate of mortality in the most severe cases.

OUTCOMES

Patient and Graft Survival

Patient and graft survival rates have improved with time. The 2015 ITR report analyzed 2699 patients from 82 transplant centers, finding overall patient survival of 77%, 58%, and 47% at 1, 5, and 10 years, respectively, for patients transplanted after year 2000.[16] Data from the most recent OPTN/SRTR annual report has also shown that patient survival is influenced by patient age and the type of transplant (isolated intestinal vs. multivisceral); survival is best in isolated intestine recipients under age 18 (82.3% and 67.% at 1 and 5 years, respectively) and lowest in adult patients who received combined liver-intestinal grafts (66.1% and 40.3% at 1 and 5 years, respectively; Fig. 28.5).[28]

Rates of graft failure have remained relatively stable in the last decade (Figs. 28.6 and 28.7).[28] The ITR report demonstrated overall graft survival rates of 71%, 58%, and 47% at 1, 5, and 10 years, respectively.[16] Sepsis is the leading cause of graft loss (50%), followed by rejection (13%), cardiovascular events (8%), PTLD (6.8%–9.9%), and technical complications (6.1%).[16] Age appears to influence the cause of graft loss, as children younger than 18 years are more likely than adults to lose grafts as a result of rejection (62.4% vs. 47.8%) and lymphoma (2.2% vs. 0%).[16] In general, graft function after transplantation is good in survivors; at 6 months posttransplant, 67% are free from TPN. In patients receiving a colon segment with their intestine graft, there is a 5% higher rate of freedom from parenteral nutrition or IV fluid support.

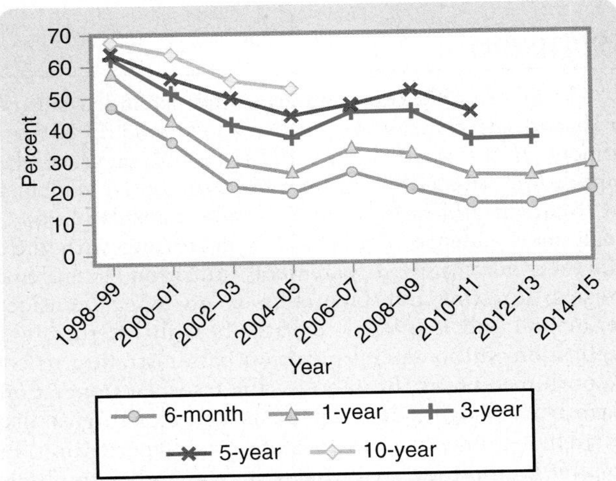

FIG. 28.7 Graft failure rates among intestinal transplant recipients with liver (includes multiorgan transplants). (From Smith JM, Weaver T, Skeans MA, et al. OPTN/SRTR 2016 Annual Data Report: Intestine. *Am J Transplant.* 2018;18(suppl 1):254–290.)

Cost

Given the substantial cost to manage intestinal failure, many patients rely on government payers (state Medicaid or Medicare) prior to transplantation. As a result of these financial constraints, access to experienced centers can be a challenge as there are only 28 U.S. centers performing intestinal transplant, which has led to differential access to multidisciplinary intestinal failure programs. Estimates of the annual cost for home TPN range from $100,000 to $250,000, including costs of supplies and infusion solutions (ranging from $75,000–$122,000) and costs of hospitalizations for parenteral nutrition–related complications (ranging from $10,000–$196,000).[45] Comparatively, the cost of intestinal transplantation has been estimated between $130,000 and $250,000.[46] Despite the high cost of the initial transplant procedure, immunosuppressive medications, and subsequent hospitalizations, transplantation typically becomes cost effective within 1 to 3 years.[46]

Quality of Life

While intestinal transplantation may be the only life-saving treatment for select patients with intestinal failure, many will suffer challenges related to health care–related quality of life following transplantation. A series published by the University of Pittsburgh Medical Center evaluated quality of life in patients who survived greater than 5 years following transplant, finding that 75% were able to maintain an occupation (including those who identified as either a student or homemaker). Postoperatively, 24% met diagnostic criteria for neuropsychiatric impairment (including hearing loss, developmental delay, depression, anxiety, and substance abuse) and self-reported surveys demonstrated improvement in domains of anxiety, cognitive ability, sleep, social support, and recreation following transplant (although depression and financial obligations were worsened).[47] In studies that specifically evaluate pediatric patients, 29% have developmental delay (often recognized prior to transplant) and 60% require specialized educational programming.[48] Parents of intestine recipients tend to perceive a slightly worse quality of life; however, pediatric patients rate their quality of life similar to that of normal age-matched children.[49]

CONCLUSION

The field of intestine transplantation has expanded slowly in part due to successful widespread use of home TPN for the treatment of intestinal failure. PNALD and catheter-related complications (infections or venous thrombosis) remain the most frequent indications for intestine transplantation, although the incidence of PNALD is decreasing with the introduction of improved parenteral nutrition management strategies. Intestine transplantation is no longer considered experimental and is offered to patients with life-threatening complications of parenteral nutrition administration or complete portomesenteric thrombosis. The transplant operation is frequently challenging due to patients' complex surgical history, altered anatomy, and presence of portal hypertension. Furthermore, the postoperative course is frequently complicated. Readmission to the hospital is often required for treatment of diarrhea, dehydration, infection, or rejection; however, after initial recovery, independence from TPN is achieved in most patients. Patient survival has been increasing, similar to survival on long-term TPN. These improvements in morbidity and mortality have led to acceptance of intestine transplantation as a standard treatment for intestinal failure in appropriately selected patients.

Future directions in the field of intestinal transplantation include conducting multi-institutional studies to aide in standardizing immunosuppression protocols, development of universal postoperative monitoring guidelines (including use of ileoscopy, biomarkers, and DSA testing), and elucidating the mechanisms underlying DSA-mediated rejection.

SELECTED REFERENCES

Abu-Elmagd KM, Costa G, Bond GJ, et al. Five hundred intestinal and multivisceral transplantations at a single center: major advances with new challenges. *Ann Surg*. 2009;250:567–581.

A landmark single-center series, which highlights outcomes between different transplant eras.

Cheng EY, Everly MJ, Kaneku H, et al. Prevalence and clinical impact of donor-specific alloantibody among intestinal transplant recipients. *Transplantation*. 2017;101:873–882.

A recent study characterizing the prevalence of donor-specific antibody and its association with accelerated intestinal graft rejection.

Deltz E, Schroeder P, Gebhardt H, et al. Successful clinical small bowel transplantation—report of a case. *Clin Transplant*. 1988;3:89–91.

A case report of what is considered the first successful living donor small intestine transplant.

Dudrick SJ, Vars HM, Rhoads JE. Growth of puppies receiving all nutritional requirements by vein. *Fortschr Parenteral Ernahrung*. 1967;2:16–18.

This is the landmark paper in which prolonged survival was demonstrated to be feasible in puppies using only hyperalimentation (intravenous nutrition, more commonly referred to today as parenteral nutrition).

.Fryer JP. Intestinal transplantation: current status. *Gastroenterol Clin North Am*. 2007;36:145–159; vii.

A review of intestinal transplantation and its current practices.

Grant D, Abu-Elmagd K, Mazariegos G, et al. Intestinal Transplant Registry report: global activity and trends. *Am J Transplant*. 2015;15:210–219.

This is a summary of data from the Intestinal Transplant Registry database that includes statistics compiled from intestinal transplant recipients at transplant centers from 21 countries.

Smith JM, Weaver T, Skeans MA, et al. OPTN/SRTR 2016 annual data report: intestine. *Am J Transplant*. 2018;18(suppl 1):254–290.

The most recent report from the Organ Procurement and Transplantation Network, which summarizes trends in intestinal transplantation over the last decade.

REFERENCES

1. Carrel A. Landmark article, Nov 14, 1908: results of the transplantation of blood vessels, organs and limbs. By Alexis Carrel. *JAMA*. 1983;250:944–953.
2. Lillehei RC, Goott B, Miller FA. The physiological response of the small bowel of the dog to ischemia including prolonged in vitro preservation of the bowel with successful replacement and survival. *Ann Surg*. 1959;150:543–560.
3. Starzl TE, Kaupp Jr HA, Brock DR, et al. Homotransplantation of multiple visceral organs. *Am J Surg*. 1962;103:219–229.
4. Lillehei RC, Idezuki Y, Feemster JA, et al. Transplantation of stomach, intestine, and pancreas: experimental and clinical observations. *Surgery*. 1967;62:721–741.
5. Starzl TE, Rowe MI, Todo S, et al. Transplantation of multiple abdominal viscera. *JAMA*. 1989;261:1449–1457.
6. Dudrick SJ, Vars HM, Rhoads EJ. Growth of puppies receiving all nutritional requirements by vein. *Fortschr Parenteral Ernahrung*. 1967;2:16–18.
7. Messing B, Crenn P, Beau P, et al. Long-term survival and parenteral nutrition dependence in adult patients with the short bowel syndrome. *Gastroenterology*. 1999;117:1043–1050.
8. Joly F, Baxter J, Staun M, et al. Five-year survival and causes of death in patients on home parenteral nutrition for severe chronic and benign intestinal failure. *Clin Nutr*. 2018;37:1415–1422.
9. Lauriti G, Zani A, Aufieri R, et al. Incidence, prevention, and treatment of parenteral nutrition-associated cholestasis and intestinal failure-associated liver disease in infants and children: a systematic review. *JPEN J Parenter Enteral Nutr*. 2014;38:70–85.
10. Deltz E, Schroeder P, Gebhardt H, et al. Successful clinical small bowel transplantation— report of a case. *Clin Transplant*. 1988;3:89–91.
11. Grant D, Wall W, Mimeault R, et al. Successful small-bowel/liver transplantation. *Lancet*. 1990;335:181–184.
12. Abu-Elmagd KM, Reyes J, Fung JJ, et al. Evolution of clinical intestinal transplantation: improved outcome and cost effectiveness. *Transplant Proc*. 1999;31:582–584.
13. Kaufman SS, Atkinson JB, Bianchi A, et al. Indications for pediatric intestinal transplantation: a position paper of the American Society of Transplantation. *Pediatr Transplant*. 2001;5:80–87.
14. Sudan D. The current state of intestine transplantation: indications, techniques, outcomes and challenges. *Am J Transplant*. 2014;14:1976–1984.
15. Fishbein TM, Matsumoto CS. Intestinal replacement therapy: timing and indications for referral of patients to an intestinal rehabilitation and transplant program. *Gastroenterology*. 2006;130:S147–S151.
16. Grant D, Abu-Elmagd K, Mazariegos G, et al. Intestinal Transplant Registry report: global activity and trends. *Am J Transplant*. 2015;15:210–219.
17. Fryer JP. Intestinal transplantation: current status. *Gastroenterol Clin North Am*. 2007;36:145–159, vii.
18. Matsumoto CS, Kaufman SS, Girlanda R, et al. Utilization of donors who have suffered cardiopulmonary arrest and resuscitation in intestinal transplantation. *Transplantation*. 2008;86:941–946.
19. Ming YC. Post transplant lymphoproliferative disorders and intestinal transplant in children—single center experience. *Transplantation*. 2017;101: S36–S36.
20. Nagai S, Mangus RS, Anderson E, et al. Cytomegalovirus infection after intestinal/multivisceral transplantation: a single-center experience with 210 cases. *Transplantation*. 2016;100:451–460.
21. Sudan DL, Iyer KR, Deroover A, et al. A new technique for combined liver/small intestinal transplantation. *Transplantation*. 2001;72:1846–1848.
22. Reyes J, Mazariegos GV, Abu-Elmagd K, et al. Intestinal transplantation under tacrolimus monotherapy after perioperative lymphoid depletion with rabbit anti-thymocyte globulin (thymoglobulin). *Am J Transplant*. 2005;5:1430–1436.
23. Grant D, Abu-Elmagd K, Reyes J, et al. 2003 report of the intestine transplant registry: a new era has dawned. *Ann Surg*. 2005;241:607–613.
24. Matsumoto CS, Kaufman SS, Fishbein TM. Inclusion of the colon in intestinal transplantation. *Curr Open Organ Transplant*. 2011;16:312–315.
25. Kato T, Selvaggi G, Gaynor JJ, et al. Inclusion of donor colon and ileocecal valve in intestinal transplantation. *Transplantation*. 2008;86:293–297.
26. Starzl TE, Todo S, Tzakis A, et al. Abdominal organ cluster transplantation for the treatment of upper abdominal malignancies. *Ann Surg*. 1989;210:374–385; discussion 385–376.
27. Abu-Elmagd KM, Costa G, Bond GJ, et al. Five hundred intestinal and multivisceral transplantations at a single center: major advances with new challenges. *Ann Surg*. 2009;250:567–581.
28. Smith JM, Weaver T, Skeans MA, et al. OPTN/SRTR 2016 annual data report: intestine. *Am J Transplant*. 2018;18(suppl 1):254–290.
29. Abu-Elmagd KM, Wu G, Costa G, et al. Preformed and de novo donor specific antibodies in visceral transplantation: long-term outcome with special reference to the liver. *Am J Transplant*. 2012;12:3047–3060.
30. Abu-Elmagd KM, Costa G, Bond GJ, et al. Evolution of the immunosuppressive strategies for the intestinal and multivisceral recipients with special reference to allograft immunity and achievement of partial tolerance. *Transpl Int*. 2009;22:96–109.
31. Vrakas G, Weissenbacher A, Chen M, et al. Belatacept and basiliximab in intestinal transplantation: a single centre experience. *Transplantation*. 2017;101: S7–S7.
32. Hibi T, Nishida S, Garcia J, et al. Citrulline level is a potent indicator of acute rejection in the long term following pediatric intestinal/multivisceral transplantation. *Am J Transplant*. 2012;12(suppl 4):S27–S32.
33. Sudan D, Vargas L, Sun Y, et al. Calprotectin: a novel noninvasive marker for intestinal allograft monitoring. *Ann Surg*. 2007;246:311–315.
34. Cheng EY, Everly MJ, Kaneku H, et al. Prevalence and clinical impact of donor-specific alloantibody among intestinal transplant recipients. *Transplantation*. 2017;101:873–882.
35. Remotti H, Subramanian S, Martinez M, et al. Small-bowel allograft biopsies in the management of small-intestinal and multivisceral transplant recipients: histopathologic review and clinical correlations. *Arch Pathol Lab Med*. 2012;136:761–771.
36. Berger M, Zeevi A, Farmer DG, et al. Immunologic challenges in small bowel transplantation. *Am J Transplant*. 2012;12(suppl 4):S2–S8.
37. Guaraldi G, Cocchi S, Codeluppi M, et al. Outcome, incidence, and timing of infectious complications in small

bowel and multivisceral organ transplantation patients. *Transplantation*. 2005;80:1742–1748.
38. Florescu DF, Sandkovsky U. Fungal infections in intestinal and multivisceral transplant recipients. *Curr Opin Organ Transplant*. 2015;20:295–302.
39. Florescu DF, Langnas AN, Grant W, et al. Incidence, risk factors, and outcomes associated with cytomegalovirus disease in small bowel transplant recipients. *Pediatr Transplant*. 2012;16:294–301.
40. Kotton CN, Kumar D, Caliendo AM, et al. The third international consensus guidelines on the management of cytomegalovirus in solid-organ transplantation. *Transplantation*. 2018;102:900–931.
41. Florescu DF, Abu-Elmagd K, Mercer DF, et al. An international survey of cytomegalovirus prevention and treatment practices in intestinal transplantation. *Transplantation*. 2014;97:78–82.
42. Allen UD, Preiksaitis JK. Epstein-Barr virus and posttransplant lymphoproliferative disorder in solid organ transplantation. *Am J Transplant*. 2013;13(suppl 4):107–120.
43. Wozniak LJ, Mauer TL, Venick RS, et al. Clinical characteristics and outcomes of PTLD following intestinal transplantation. *Clin Transplant*. 2018;32:e13313.
44. Wu G, Selvaggi G, Nishida S, et al. Graft-versus-host disease after intestinal and multivisceral transplantation. *Transplantation*. 2011;91:219–224.
45. Hofstetter S, Stern L, Willet J. Key issues in addressing the clinical and humanistic burden of short bowel syndrome in the US. *Curr Med Res Opin*. 2013;29:495–504.
46. Sudan D. Cost and quality of life after intestinal transplantation. *Gastroenterology*. 2006;130:S158–S162.
47. Abu-Elmagd KM, Kosmach-Park B, Costa G, et al. Long-term survival, nutritional autonomy, and quality of life after intestinal and multivisceral transplantation. *Ann Surg*. 2012;256:494–508.
48. Karabala A, Yazigi NA, Khan KM, et al. Features of life quality in long-term survivors of intestinal transplantation in childhood. *Transplantation*. 2017;101: S145–S145.
49. Ngo KD, Farmer DG, McDiarmid SV, et al. Pediatric health-related quality of life after intestinal transplantation. *Pediatr Transplant*. 2011;15:849–854.

SECTION V

Surgical Oncology

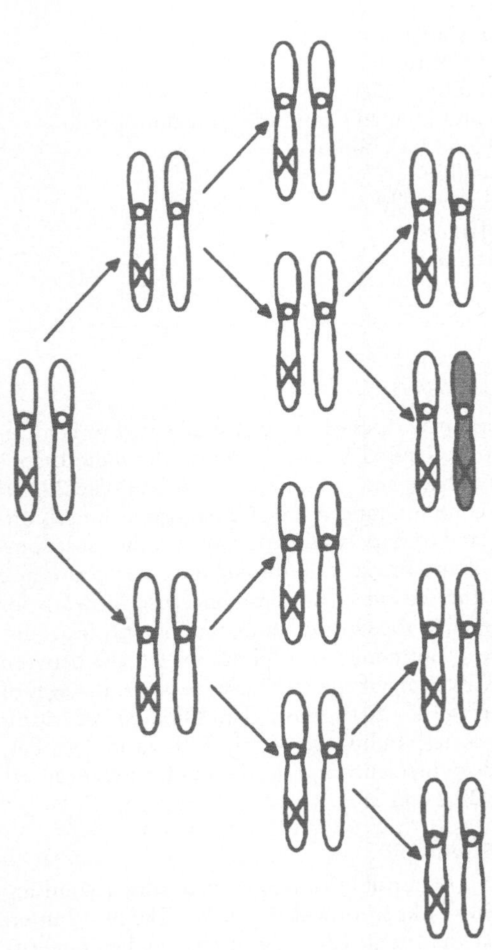

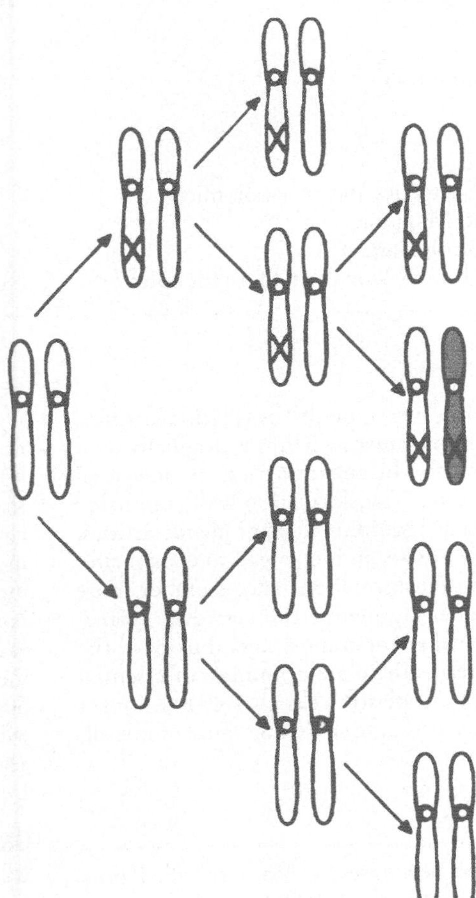

29 CHAPTER

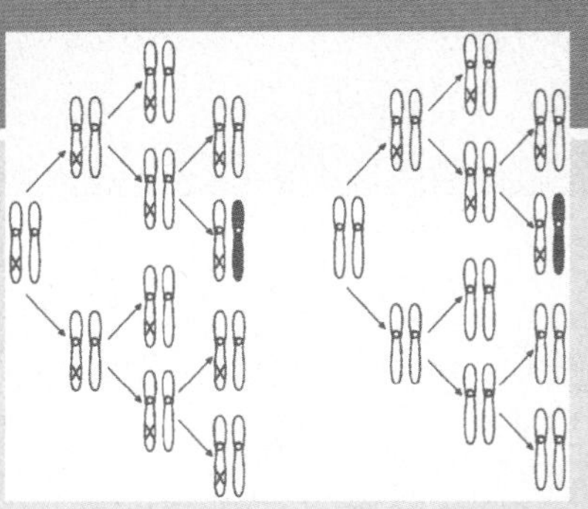

Tumor Biology and Tumor Markers

Bradley A. Krasnick, S. Peter Goedegebuure, Ryan Fields

OUTLINE

Neoplasia (literally meaning "new growth") is the uncontrolled proliferation of cells. The term *tumor*, which was originally used to describe the swelling caused by inflammation, is now used interchangeably with neoplasm. Transformation is the multistep process in which normal cells acquire malignant characteristics, such as the ability to invade tissues and to spread to distant sites (metastasize). Each step-in transformation reflects one or more genetic alterations that confer a growth advantage over normal cells. Cancers are simply malignant tumors and thus have the capacity for metastatic spread. There are a number of essential characteristics expressed by neoplastic cells that enable cancer progression.[1] These characteristics are shared by most, if not all, human cancers.

EPIDEMIOLOGY

Incidence is the number of new cases within a specified time frame, usually expressed as cases per 100,000 people per year. Prevalence is the number of patients with a disease in the population at a given point in time. A person's risk of developing or dying of cancer is usually expressed in terms of lifetime risk (risk during the course of a lifetime) or, in describing the relationship of specific risk factors with a particular cancer, the relative risk (comparing those with a certain exposure or trait with those who do not have it).

Over 1.7 million new cases of cancer are expected to be diagnosed in 2018 in the United States, excluding the more than 1 million new cases of basal and squamous cell cancers (Fig. 29.1).[2] In men, the most common cancers are of the prostate, lung/bronchus, colorectum, and urinary bladder. In women, the most common cancers are of the breast, lung/bronchus, colorectum, and uterus. Cancer is the second most common cause of death for both men and women in the United States, trailing only heart disease, and is the most common cause of death for females between the ages of 40 and 79 years of age and males between the ages of 60 and 79 years of age. In 2018, more than 600,000 Americans will die of cancer, corresponding to roughly 1700 deaths per day. The national trends in incidence and death rates for select cancers are shown in Figs. 29.2 and 29.3.

Global Burden of Cancer

Worldwide, cancer is responsible for one in six deaths, accounting for 9.6 million total deaths worldwide in 2018.[3] The distribution and types of cancer that occur continue to change, being affected primarily by the growth and aging of populations, as well as changing prevalence of multiple risk factors associated with cancer development—many which are associated with increasing socioeconomic development. Although overall cancer incidence rate is two-to threefold higher in the developed, as compared to the developing, world, differences in overall cancer mortality are small

Estimated New Cases*

Males			Females		
Prostate	233,000	27%	Breast	232,670	29%
Lung & bronchus	116,000	14%	Lung & bronchus	108,210	13%
Colorectum	71,830	8%	Colorectum	65,000	8%
Urinary bladder	56.390	7%	Uterine corpus	52,630	6%
Melanoma of the skin	43,890	5%	Thyroid	47,790	6%
Kidney & renal pelvis	39,140	5%	Non-Hodgkin lymphoma	32,530	4%
Non-Hodgkin lymphoma	38,270	4%	Melanoma of the skin	32,210	4%
Oral cavity & pharynx	30,220	4%	Kidney & renal pelvis	24,780	3%
Leukemia	30,100	4%	Pancreas	22,890	3%
Liver & intrahepatic bile duct	24,600	3%	Leukemia	22,280	3%
All Sites	**855,220**	**100%**	**All Sites**	**810,320**	**100%**

Estimated Deaths

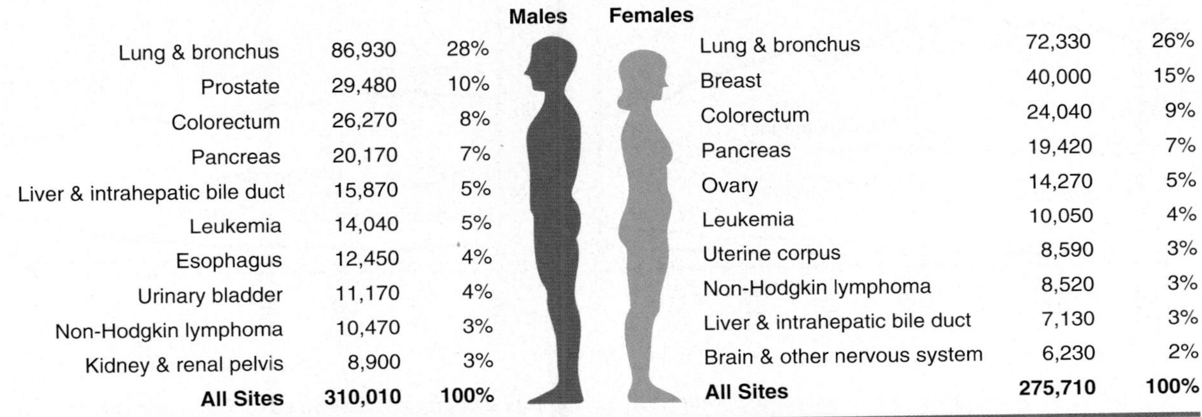

Males			Females		
Lung & bronchus	86,930	28%	Lung & bronchus	72,330	26%
Prostate	29,480	10%	Breast	40,000	15%
Colorectum	26,270	8%	Colorectum	24,040	9%
Pancreas	20,170	7%	Pancreas	19,420	7%
Liver & intrahepatic bile duct	15,870	5%	Ovary	14,270	5%
Leukemia	14,040	5%	Leukemia	10,050	4%
Esophagus	12,450	4%	Uterine corpus	8,590	3%
Urinary bladder	11,170	4%	Non-Hodgkin lymphoma	8,520	3%
Non-Hodgkin lymphoma	10,470	3%	Liver & intrahepatic bile duct	7,130	3%
Kidney & renal pelvis	8,900	3%	Brain & other nervous system	6,230	2%
All Sites	**310,010**	**100%**	**All Sites**	**275,710**	**100%**

FIG. 29.1 Top 10 cancer types for estimated new cancer cases and deaths by sex in 2018 for the United States. *Estimates are rounded to the nearest 10 and exclude basal cell and squamous cell skin cancers and in situ carcinoma except urinary bladder. (From Siegel RL, Miller KD, Jemal A. Cancer statistics, 2018. *CA Cancer J Clin.* 2018;68:7–30.)

due to higher case fatality rates for most cancers in developing countries. Europe and the Americas account for 23.4% and 21%, respectively, of the global incidence of cancer but only 20.3% and 14.4%, respectively, of the global burden of cancer mortality. Meanwhile global cancer incidence in Asia and Africa (48.4% and 5.8%, respectively) is substantially less than their contributions to global mortality, which stands at 57.3% and 7.3%, respectively.

Overall, lung cancer is the most commonly diagnosed cancer worldwide and the leader in cancer death. For males, lung, prostate, and colorectal cancer are the leading cancer by incidence globally, while lung, liver, and stomach cancer are the leading cancers by mortality. For females, breast, colorectal, and lung cancer are the leading cancers by global incidence, while breast, lung, and colorectal cancer are the leading cancers by mortality. However, the leading cancer by incidence and mortality for males and females differs significantly by country. In the United States, Canada, the United Kingdom, and Australia, lung cancer remains the most common cause of cancer mortality for males and females. When looking at developing countries such as Thailand and Mongolia, liver cancer is the leading cause of cancer mortality irrespective of sex. Finally, throughout much of Africa, Mexico, and parts of South America, prostate and breast cancer are the leading cause of cancer death in males and females, respectively. This all translates to significant global economic burden, with total costs for cancer care in the United States alone projected at a staggering $174 billion by 2020.

Aging and Cancer

The incidence of cancer increases with age; thus, cancer disproportionately affects people aged 65 years and older (SEER.gov). In the United States, the incidence of cancer in people 65 years old and older is nearly nine times that of people younger than 65 years of age. In people older than 70 years old, the incidence of invasive cancer is one in three for males and one in four for females.[2] Worldwide, approximately 80% of cancers are diagnosed in people 50 years of age or older. The median age of cancer diagnosis in the United States is 66 years of age.

The proportion of the U.S. population aged 65 years old and older is growing rapidly. From 2010 to 2050, this segment of the U.S. population is expected to more than double in size, which is a recognized trend throughout the developed world. With an expanding older population, the incidence of cancer will increase,

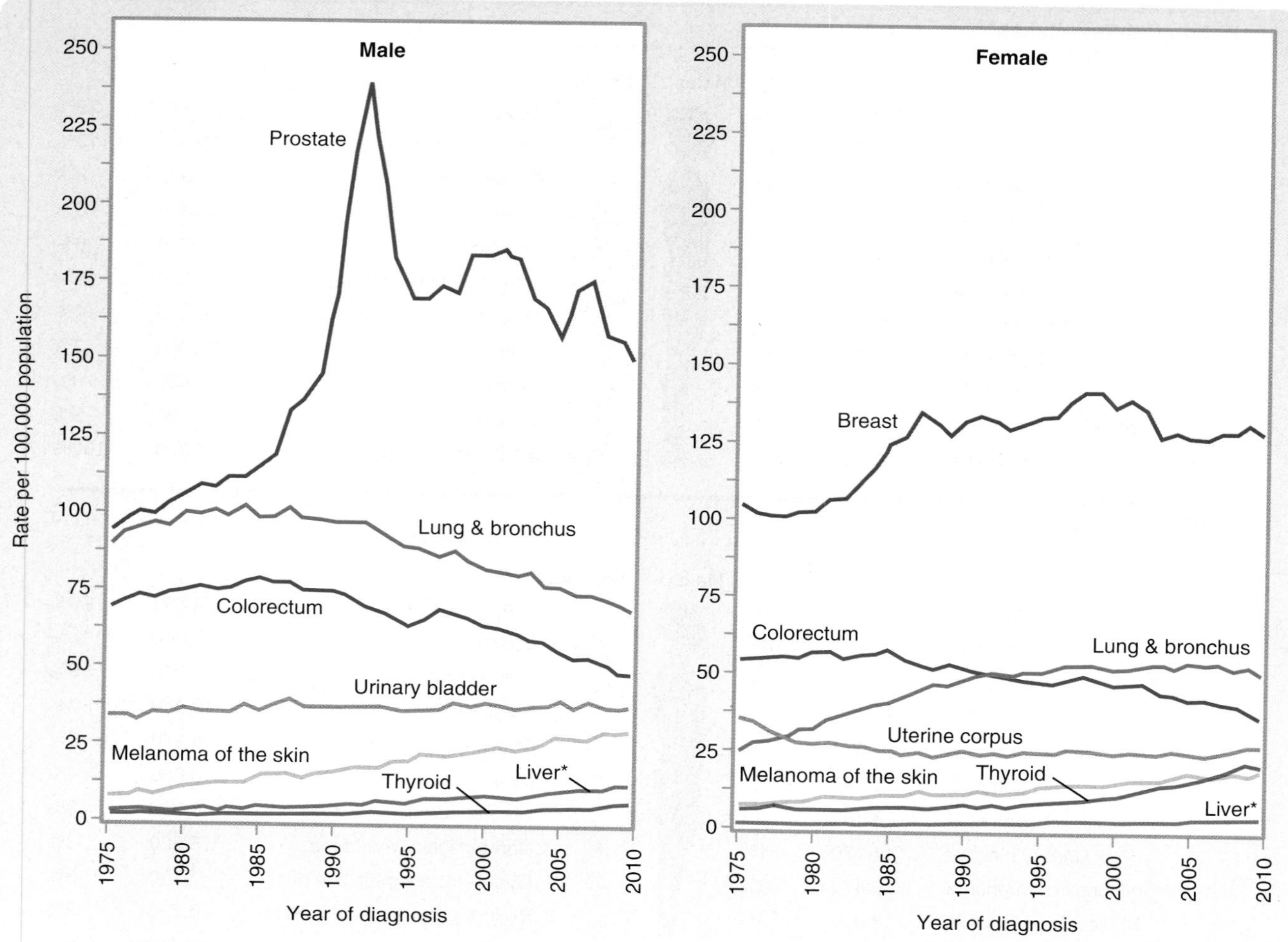

FIG. 29.2 Annual age-adjusted cancer incidence rates for males and females for selected cancers in the United States, 1975–2014. *Includes intrahepatic bile duct. (From Siegel RL, Miller KD, Jemal A. Cancer statistics, 2018. *CA Cancer J Clin.* 2018;68:7–30.)

thereby raising the overall cancer burden on society. In addition, cancer care will also be of increasingly greater complexity in this population; reasons for this include more comorbidities of greater severity in the setting of declining physiologic reserve, difficulties with access to care, and lack of social support.

Cancer treatment in the elderly is less well studied, and it has been shown that the elderly population is underrepresented in clinical trials. Clearly, surgeons must more carefully weigh individuals' operative risk in the context of the morbidity of the procedure with greater consideration for quality of life and functional status. A number of reports have demonstrated underuse of adjuvant therapy in the aging population, despite evidence that adjuvant therapies can be beneficial for this group of patients.[4] Thus, age alone should not be the sole reason for withholding systemic therapy in these patients.

The major mechanism driving increased cancer with aging relies on the accumulation of mutations over time that confer a growth advantage to the cell. Many of these mutations occur due to chance, and thus the more cell divisions a given cell goes through (as one ages), the more chances it has for a mistake to occur. It was beautifully demonstrated that there is a striking linear relationship (Spearman rho=0.81) between the total stem cell divisions over the lifetime of a given tissue and the risk of invasive cancer in the corresponding tissue.[5]

Obesity, Physical Activity, and Cancer

The prevalence of overweight (body mass index [BMI] of 25–29.9 kg/m^2) and obesity (BMI ≥30 kg/m^2) in most developed countries (and in urban areas of many less developed countries) has increased markedly during the past two decades. In the United States, more than one-third of the population is now classified as obese, and 5% of men and 10% of women have a BMI greater than 40 kg/m2. Although obesity has long been recognized as an important cause of diabetes and cardiovascular disease, the relationship between obesity and cancer has historically received less attention. Epidemiological studies indicate that obesity is a risk factor for cancers at multiple sites, including esophageal cancer, colorectal cancer, gallbladder cancer, pancreatic cancer, liver cancer, gastric cancer, postmenopausal breast cancer, uterine cancer, ovarian cancer, renal cell carcinoma, meningioma, multiple myeloma, and thyroid cancer.[6] Globally, increased BMI is third, only behind infection and smoking, as a risk factor for cancer and contributes to up to 20% of cancer-related deaths. Encouragingly, bariatric surgery has been demonstrated to have the potential to offset some of the cancer risk in this population, with a recent study demonstrating a 33% reduction in cancer risk for obese patients undergoing bariatric surgery as compared to weight matched controls.[7]

In concert with the obesity epidemic, decreased physical activity has been shown to be associated with an increased incidence of

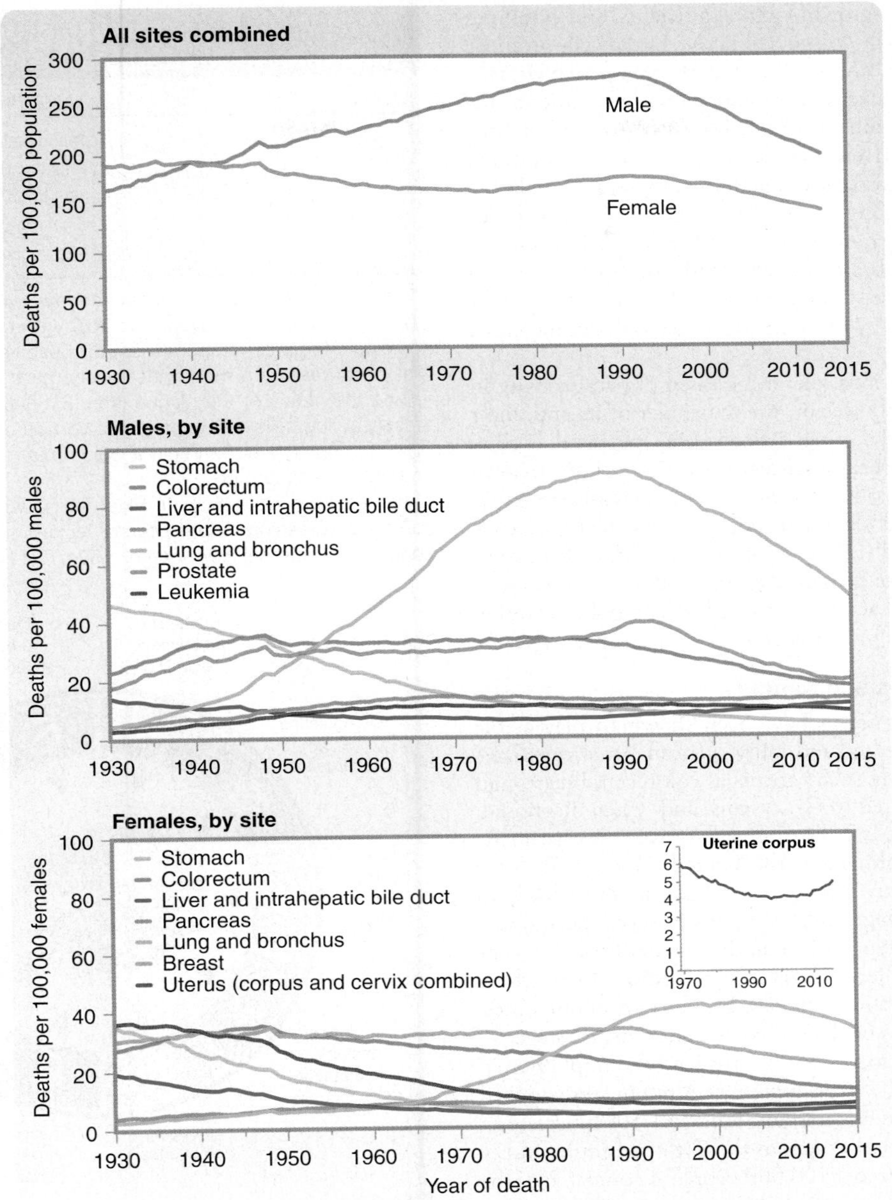

FIG. 29.3 Trends in cancer death rates by sex overall and for selected cancers, United States, 1930 to 2015. (From Siegel RL, Miller KD, Jemal A. Cancer statistics, 2018. *CA Cancer J Clin.* 2018;68:7–30.)

many different cancers. In a recent metaanalysis, the cancers where increased exercise is most protective are esophageal adenocarcinoma, gallbladder, and liver cancer, with hazard ratios (HRs) of 0.58, 0.72, and 0.73, respectively.[8] Of 26 cancer subtypes looked at, 13 were associated with decreased rates in people participating in moderate to vigorous physical activity, most of which remained significant predictors even after adjusting for BMI. Interestingly, physical activity was associated with increased risk of melanoma (HR 1.27) and prostate cancer (HR 1.05). For some cancer types, such as colorectal adenocarcinoma, increased physical activity has been tied to decreased cancer risk in a dose-dependent manner. In addition to increased overall cancer incidence seen with increased sedentary behavior, cancer outcomes have been shown to be inferior in sedentary individuals, with cancer mortality being increased by ~20% for individuals in the least active quartile of the population.

Mechanistically, immune, metabolic, endocrine, and inflammatory properties of excess adipose tissue appear to lead to the increased incidence of malignancy in overweight/obese individuals.[6] For example, greater amounts of adipose tissue lead to increased circulating levels of free fatty acids. This in turn causes liver, muscle, and other tissues to increase their use of fats for energy production, thereby reducing their need for uptake and metabolism of glucose and eventually leading to hyperglycemia. This functional insulin resistance forces an increase in pancreatic insulin secretion. Epidemiological and experimental evidence suggests that chronic hyperinsulinemia increases the risk of cancers of the colon and endometrium and probably other tumors (e.g., those of the pancreas and kidney). Obesity can also lead to increased adipocyte-derived stem cell and adipose tissue deposition in the tumor microenvironment, leading to extracellular matrix (ECM) deposition, altered immune profiles as compared to nonobese subjects, as well as a rich supply of growth factors, nutrients, and cytokines beneficial to tumor growth. Adipocyte-derived stem cells promote fibrosis and can become cancer associated fibroblasts, which have been tied to more aggressive cancer biology. In obese patients, increased adiposity in the omentum has been tied to a proinflammatory state that can drive cancer at multiple sites via immune cell activation and inflammatory signaling pathways. Circulating levels of estrogens are strongly related to adiposity. For cancers of the breast (in postmenopausal women) and endometrium, the effects of overweight and obesity on cancer risk are largely mediated by increased estrogen levels. For patients with breast cancer, adiposity has been associated with both worse survival and increased likelihood of recurrence.

In addition to the obvious role of increased physical activity in helping maintain a healthy weight, the remainder of its anticancer properties are still actively being defined. One potential mechanism for estrogen-driven breast cancers is the association between increased physical activity and decreased blood estradiol concentrations. Physical activity has also been shown to upregulate cell cycle and deoxyribonucleic acid (DNA) repair pathways in male patients undergoing surveillance for prostate cancer. In addition to potential positive effects of physical activity, increased sedentary behavior has been tied to increased insulin resistance and C-reactive protein levels.

Healthcare Disparities and Cancer

Race and socioeconomic status have been shown to play a role in both cancer incidence and mortality. African Americans have a higher risk of developing such cancers as colorectal, breast, and prostate cancer as compared to Caucasians, and, when diagnosed, the cancer phenotype tends to be more aggressive.[9] Five-year survival for all cancers combined in the United States is 68% for whites and 61% for blacks.[2] African Americans are more likely to be diagnosed at a later stage and have a lower stage-specific survival for most cancer subtypes. Overall, the risk of death after cancer diagnosis is 33% higher in blacks than whites. Other ethnic minorities have also been shown to have inferior cancer outcomes, with Hispanics tending to be diagnosed at a later disease stage.

In addition to race, socioeconomic status has been implicated in the incidence of cancer, as well as outcomes. A recent study looked at all counties in the United States and found a ~50% increase in the number of cancer-related deaths in the 90th percentile county for number of cancer deaths per 100,000 people as compared to the 10th percentile county.[10] Differences in socioeconomic status, geographic risk factors, and access to quality healthcare explain a significant portion of these differences. One major factor entwined with these disparities is health insurance status. In one analysis of patients aged 18 to 64 years old in the United States, those without insurance or covered by Medicaid (as compared to nonMedicaid insurance) were more likely to present with later stage disease and were less likely to undergo cancer-directed therapy (e.g., surgery or radiation therapy). In addition, cancer-related mortality was increased for these patients (HR 1.44 Medicaid and 1.47 for uninsured).

TUMOR BIOLOGY

Solid tumors are composed of neoplastic cells and stroma. It has become clear that these two compartments are interdependent and function as a unit to promote tumor growth, therapeutic resistance, invasion, and metastasis. Much has been learned about the multistep process of tumorigenesis. For example, the transformation of melanocytes into malignant melanoma can be divided histopathologically and clinically into five major identifiable steps (Table 29.1). Successive genetic changes confer a physiologic growth advantage leading to progressive conversion of normal cells into cancer cells. Genetic changes that lead to cancer classically occur in proto-oncogenes or tumor suppressor genes, whereby an activating mutation of a proto-oncogene (e.g., *KRAS;* when activated referred to as an oncogene) leads to tumor survival/growth ("pressing on the accelerator"), and an inactivating mutation of a tumor suppressor gene (e.g., *p53)* leads to decreased suppression of protumor survival/growth signaling ("taking your foot off of the brake").[11] In addition to changes in tumor cells, the cells of the nearby stroma undergo phenotypic changes that further perpetuate tumor progression. A number of distinct physiologic changes are essential to tumorigenesis (discussed later), many of which are therapeutic targets (Fig. 29.4).

TABLE 29.1 Stepwise progression from melanocyte to metastatic melanoma.

STEP*	CHARACTERISTICS
1	Common melanocytic nevus
2	Dysplastic nevus
3	Radial growth phase of melanoma
4	Vertical growth phase of melanoma
5	Metastatic melanoma

*Common acquired and congenital nevi without cytologic atypia (step 1) may progress into dysplastic nevi with clear atypical histologic and cytologic features (step 2). Most of these lesions are stable, but a few may progress to a malignant melanoma that tends to grow outward along the radius of the plaque (step 3). Within the plaque, a nodule of fast-growing cells that expand in a vertical direction develops, invading the dermis and elevating the epidermis (step 4). Finally, the tumor metastasizes (step 5).

Adapted from Clark WH, Jr, Elder DE, Guerry D 4th, et al. A study of tumor progression: The precursor lesions of superficial spreading and nodular melanoma. *Hum Pathol.* 1984;15:1147–1165.

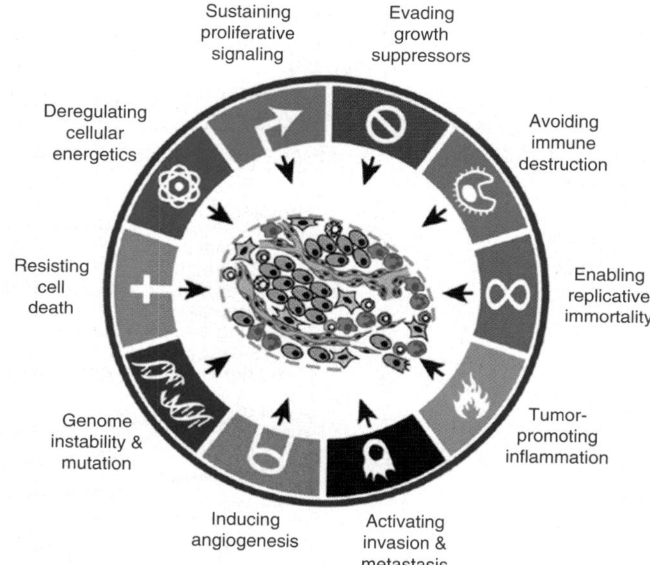

FIG. 29.4 Key physiologic changes associated with progressive conversion of normal cells into malignant tumor cells. The indicated traits are common to the majority of human cancers, together conferring cell survival or tumor expansion. (Adapted from Hanahan D, Weinberg RA. Hallmarks of cancer: The next generation. *Cell.* 2011;144:646–674.)

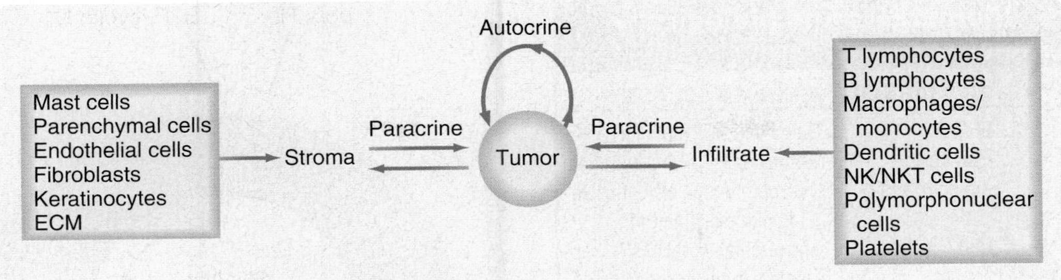

FIG. 29.5 Paracrine and autocrine growth mechanisms. Both stromal cells and infiltrating cells secrete paracrine factors that affect tumor development. In addition, tumor cells secrete autocrine as well as paracrine factors that in turn act on stromal cells and infiltrating cells. *ECM,* Extracellular matrix; *NK,* natural killer; *NKT, XXX.*

Sustained Proliferative Signaling

Cells within normal tissues are largely instructed to grow by neighboring cells (paracrine signals) or through systemic (endocrine) signals. Likewise, cell-to-cell growth signaling occurs in the majority of tumors as well. The immediate tumor cell environment (the stroma) contains residing nonmalignant cells, such as parenchymal cells, epithelial cells, fibroblasts, and endothelial cells. In addition, most tumors are characterized by infiltrating immune cells, such as lymphocytes, polymorphonuclear cells, mast cells, and macrophages. Altered differentiation of cell subsets, and/or selective recruitment and integration of nonmalignant cells results in coevolution with the tumor cells to sustain the growth of the tumor cells. Finally, basement membranes form the ECM that provides a scaffold for proliferation of fibroblast and endothelial cells. Together, tumor cells and stroma produce factors (autocrine and paracrine factors) that, in cell-bound, matrix-bound, or soluble form, directly or indirectly influence tumor development. Autocrine factors secreted by tumor cells promote growth of tumor cells but may also stimulate neighboring tumor cells. In addition, tumor cells secrete paracrine factors that act on host cells or ECMs, generating a supportive microenvironment. For example, transforming growth factor-β (TGF-β) may induce angiogenesis, production of ECM molecules, and production of other cytokines by fibroblasts and endothelial cells. Simplified, tumor growth is dependent on the response of tumor cells to paracrine and autocrine factors (Fig. 29.5). These factors include angiogenesis factors, growth factors, chemokines (polypeptide signaling molecules originally characterized by their ability to induce chemotaxis), cytokines, hormones, enzymes, and cytolytic factors that may promote or reduce tumor growth (Table 29.2). A classic example of hormone signaling in cancer is breast cancer, whereby in many tumors, overexpression of the nuclear estrogen receptor, leads to estrogen-dependent tumor cell proliferation. Taking away the supply of estrogen from the tumor (e.g., letrozole) or blocking the receptor (e.g., trastuzumab) leads to decreased tumor cell proliferation and cell death.

During the evolution of a tumor, its responsiveness to growth signals changes. Paracrine growth mechanisms are dominant during the early development of tumor. Tumors become resistant to paracrine growth inhibitors and gain responsiveness to paracrine growth promoters. However, autocrine growth mechanisms become more prominent as tumors further develop. The observation that metastatic tumor cells tend to spread more randomly through the body in late-stage tumors suggests that autocrine growth mechanisms may be more dominant than paracrine growth mechanisms. It is even possible for a tumor to grow completely autonomously (acrine state) and to be independent of growth factors and inhibitors.

TABLE 29.2 Cells and soluble factors affecting tumor development.*

CELLS	SOLUBLE FACTORS
Stroma	
Parenchymal cells Endothelial cells Fibroblasts Mast cells Extracellular matrix Keratinocytes	Growth factors, growth inhibitors, nutritional factors, hormones, degradative enzymes, cytokines, angiogenesis factors
Infiltrate	
T lymphocytes B lymphocytes Natural killer cells Natural killer T cells Macrophages-monocytes Dendritic cells Polymorphonuclear cells Platelets	Cytokines, chemokines, cytolytic factors, angiogenesis factors, growth (inhibitory) factors, degradative enzymes, cytostatic factors, antibodies
Tumor	
Tumor cells	Chemokines, cytokines, angiogenesis factors, degradative enzymes, growth (inhibitory) factors

*The list of cells and soluble factors is not meant to be complete but to illustrate the complexity of factors affecting tumor development.

To achieve growth self-sufficiency, growth signaling pathways are altered. This involves alteration of extracellular growth signals, of transmembrane transducers of those signals, or of intracellular signaling pathways that translate those signals into action. Growth factor receptors are overexpressed in many cancers. Receptor overexpression may enable the cancer cell to respond to low levels of growth factor that normally would not trigger proliferation. For example, the epidermal growth factor receptor family (ErbB) is a family of receptor tyrosine kinases that includes both epidermal growth factor receptor (EGFR) and HER2/neu receptor, which are overexpressed in several cancer types. *EGFR* mutations leading to EGFR pathway overexpression in non–small cell lung cancer may be sensitive to small molecular tyrosine kinase inhibitors, such as gefitinib (Table 29.3). *HER2* mutation and overexpression seen in some breast and gastric cancers (and others) leads to sensitivity to HER2 inhibition with trastuzumab (Table 29.3). Another clinically relevant example is the growth factor receptor

TABLE 29.3 Biomarkers and biologically targeted therapies.

CANCER	BIOMARKER	THERAPY (CLASS)*
Breast	BRCA	Olaparib (PARP inhibitor)
Breast	Estrogen/ progesterone receptor	Tamoxifen (selective estrogen receptor modifier)/Letrozole (aromatase inhibitor)
Breast	HER2/neu	Trastuzumab (antiHER2)
Chronic myelogenous leukemia	bcr-abl	Imatinib (tyrosine kinase inhibitor)
Colorectal cancer	KRAS	Cetuximab (antiEGFR)
Colorectal cancer (tumor agnostic)	MSI	Pembrolizumab (antiPD1)
Gastrointestinal stromal tumor	c-kit	Imatinib (tyrosine kinase inhibitor)
Lymphoma	CD20	Rituximab (antiCD20)
Melanoma	BRAF	Dabrafenib (antiBRAF) + Trametinib (antiMEK)
Non–small cell lung cancer	ALK or ROS1	Crizotinib (tyrosine kinase inhibitor)
Non–small cell lung cancer	EGFR	Gefitinib (tyrosine kinase inhibitor)
Non–small cell lung cancer	PD-L1	Pembrolizumab (antiPD1)

Biomarker expression is being increasingly used, often independent of formal staging criteria, to decide which patients receive biologically targeted therapies. Key examples of biomarker directed therapeutics shown, but not meant to be exhaustive list.
ALK, Anaplastic lymphoma kinase; *BRCA*, breast cancer gene; *BRAF*, v-Raf murine sarcoma viral oncogene homolog B; CD20, cluster of differentiation 20; *EGFR*, epithelial growth factor receptor; *HER2*, human epithelial growth factor receptor; *MEK*, mitogen-activated protein kinase; *MSI*, Musashi gene; *PARP*, polymerase 1 gene; *PD-1*, programmed cell death protein 1; *PD-L1*, programmed death ligand 1.
*Example of therapeutic in class, often several options available.

tyrosine kinase c-kit, whereby activating mutations (95% of gastrointestinal stromal tumors) leads to activation of multiple protumor signaling cascades. In the majority of *c-kit* mutations, therapy with the tyrosine kinase inhibitor imatinib leads to therapeutic response (Table 29.3). In some cases growth factor receptors can signal independent of ligand binding. This can be achieved through structural alteration of receptors, such as truncated versions of EGFR that lack much of its cytoplasmic domain and are constitutively activated—seen in gliomas and head and neck squamous cell carcinoma.

Cancer cells can also modulate their stromal environment, including the ECM, through secretion of factors such as basic fibroblast growth factor (FGF), platelet-derived growth factor (PDGF), TGF-β, and others. ECM components, such as collagens, fibronectins, laminins, and vitronectins, may bind to two or more receptors and may also bind other ECM molecules. The matrix molecule–receptor interaction induces signals that influence cell behavior, including entrance into the active cell cycle. Cancer cells can switch the types of ECM receptors (integrins and heparan sulfate proteoglycans) they express, favoring ones that transmit progrowth signals. Similarly, fibroblasts and immune cell subsets such as macrophages undergo differentiation into cancer-associated fibroblasts and tumor-associated macrophages, respectively, that promote tumor growth and spread.

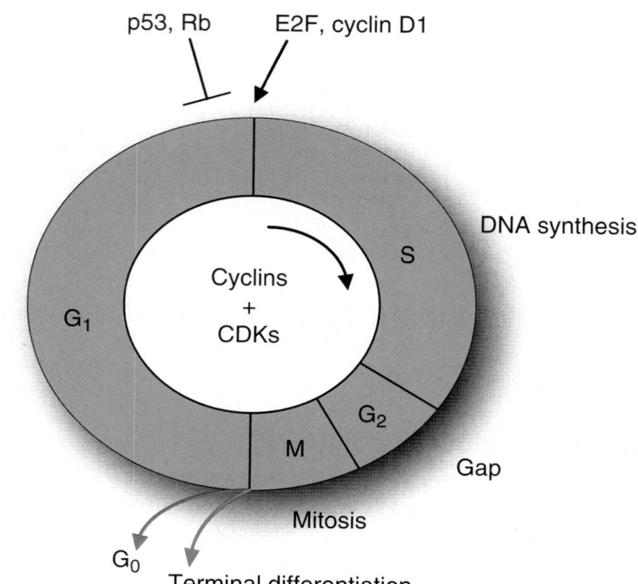

FIG. 29.6 Schematic overview of the cell cycle. Cell division is governed by cyclin proteins and cyclin-dependent kinases *(CDKs)*. After mitosis, a cell can terminally differentiate, enter a quiescent state, or re-enter the cell cycle. A critical point in the cell cycle control is the transition from G_1 to S. After passing this checkpoint, the cell is committed to division. Tumor suppressor genes such as the retinoblastoma *(Rb)* gene and *p53* block G_1 to S transition, whereas oncogenes such as cyclin D1 and E2F promote transition.

A more complex mechanism for acquisition of self-sufficiency in growth signals stems from changes in intracellular signaling pathways, some of which actively engage in crosstalk. Many of the oncogenes mimic normal growth signaling and induce mitogenic signals without stimulation from upstream regulators. For instance, *KRAS* mutations are seen across a wide variety of cancers, with activating mutations leading to receptor independent signaling. This constitutive activation of the KRAS signaling cascade leads to multiple protumor events (e.g., sustained proliferation, immune evasion, resistance to apoptosis, cell migration, and metastasis).[11] KRAS targeting has been the subject of extensive, ongoing research. Another clinically relevant mutated oncogene is *BRAF*, for which activating mutations (e.g., V600E) lead to constitutive activation (seen in such cancers as melanoma, colorectal cancer, and thyroid cancer), upregulation of MEK and ERK signaling, and increased transcription of protumor survival and proliferation factors. BRAF signaling pathway activation can be clinically targeted with BRAF and MEK inhibition (Table 29.3). Finally, negative-feedback mechanisms that help regulate normal signaling pathways can be disrupted and thereby enhance proliferative signaling.

Evading Growth Suppressors

Cell division is an ordered, tightly regulated process involving both stimulatory and inhibitory signals. Thus, in addition to acquiring stimulatory growth signals, tumor cells need to overcome or to neutralize growth-inhibitory signals. These signals include both soluble growth inhibitors and immobilized inhibitors embedded in the ECM and on the surfaces of neighboring cells. Similar to many of the stimulatory signals, the growth-inhibitory signals are transduced by transmembrane receptors coupled to intracellular signaling pathways that target genes regulating the cell cycle. The cell cycle can be divided into an interphase and a mitotic (M) phase (Fig. 29.6). The interphase is further subdivided into two gap phases (G_1 and G_2), separated by a phase of DNA synthesis (S phase). The two gap phases involve crucial regulatory events that prepare the cell for DNA replication and mitosis. Central to cell cycle progression are the cyclin-dependent kinases that bind to the cyclin proteins. These proteins are regulated by numerous other proteins including tumor suppressors and oncogenes that induce stimulatory or inhibitory signals. Antigrowth signals can block cell division by two distinct mechanisms. Cells may be forced to exit the cell cycle into a quiescent (G_0) state (Fig. 29.6).

Alternatively, cells may be induced to enter a postmitotic state, usually associated with terminal differentiation. Many of the signaling pathways that enable normal cells to respond to antigrowth signals are associated with the cell cycle block, specifically with the components governing the restriction point in the G_1 phase of the cell cycle. The restriction point marks the point between early and late G_1 phase passage that represents an irreversible commitment to undergo one cell division. Cells monitor their external environment during this period and, on the basis of sensed signals, decide whether to proliferate, to be quiescent, or to enter into a postmitotic state. At the molecular level, many antiproliferative signals involve the retinoblastoma protein (pRb) and its two family members, p107 and p130. pRb is a key negative regulator at the restriction point. In quiescent cells, pRb is hypophosphorylated and blocks cell division by binding E2F transcription factors that control the expression of many genes essential for progression from G_1 into S phase (Fig. 29.6). In contrast, growth-stimulatory signals induce phosphorylation of pRb that does not bind E2F factors and is considered functionally inactive. Likewise, disruption of the pRb pathway liberates E2Fs and thus allows cell proliferation, rendering cells insensitive to antigrowth factors that normally operate along this pathway to block advance through the G_1 phase of the cell cycle. For example, TGF-β prevents the phosphorylation of pRb, which inactivates pRb and thereby blocks advance through G_1. In some tumors, such as breast, colon, liver, and pancreatic cancers, TGF-β responsiveness is lost through downregulation of TGF-β receptors or through expression of mutant, dysfunctional receptors. In others, such as colon, lung, and liver cancers, the cytoplasmic SMAD4 protein, which transduces signals from ligand-activated TGF-β receptors to downstream targets, may be eliminated through mutation of its encoding gene. Alternatively, in cervical carcinomas induced by human papillomavirus, the viral oncoprotein E7 binds pRb and thereby induces dissociation of E2F and subsequent transcription of genes necessary for cell cycle progression. In addition, cancer cells can also turn off expression of integrins and other cell adhesion molecules (CAMs) that send antigrowth signals. In summary, the antigrowth signaling pathways converging onto Rb and the cell cycle are disrupted in a majority of human cancers. Cyclin–cyclin-dependent kinase complexes, essential for cell cycle progression, are regulated by two families of cyclin–cyclin-dependent kinase inhibitors in normal cells. However, in tumor cells, these regulatory proteins, such as the p16 member of the INK4 family, are frequently deleted, allowing tumor cells to bypass cell cycle arrest.

In addition to avoiding antigrowth signals, tumor cells may also avoid terminal differentiation, for example, through overexpression of the oncogene c-*myc*, which encodes a transcription factor regulating expression of cyclins and cyclin-dependent kinases or through upregulation of Id (short for inhibitor of DNA-binding/differentiation) family members. Likewise, during human colon carcinogenesis, mutations of adenomatous polyposis coli (APC), a negative regulator of β-catenin, lead to the constitutive activation of Wnt/β-catenin signaling, which serves to block the terminal differentiation of enterocytes in colonic crypts.

Resisting Cell Death

The growth of tumors is determined by the ability of tumor cells to proliferate, offset by cell death. Most if not all types of tumors are characterized by defects in cell death signaling pathways and are resistant to cell death. Cell death in tumors is caused primarily by programmed cell death, or apoptosis, which is the most common and well-defined form of cell death. Apoptosis is a physiologic cell suicide program essential for embryonic development, functioning of the immune system, and maintenance of tissue homeostasis. Apoptosis is characterized by disruption of membranes and chromosomal degradation in a matter of hours. The general apoptosis signaling pathway involves the release of cytochrome *c* from mitochondria that activates various caspases (a family of proteases) in sequence (Fig. 29.7).

Activation of caspase cascades leads to DNA fragmentation and apoptosis. Induction of apoptosis is either death receptor dependent (extrinsic pathway) or independent (intrinsic pathway). The two best described receptor pathways are the Fas receptor and death receptor 5 that bind the extracellular Fas ligand and TRAIL, respectively. Binding of the ligands triggers activation of caspase 8 and promotes the cascade of procaspase activation, leading to release of cytochrome *c* from mitochondria and eventually apoptosis. The intrinsic pathway is triggered by various extracellular and intracellular stresses, such as growth factor withdrawal, hypoxia, DNA damage, and oncogene induction. Receptor-independent pathways involve translocation of proapoptotic molecules from the cytoplasm to the mitochondria, causing mitochondrial damage and release of cytochrome *c*. Cytochrome *c* is directly involved in the activation of caspase 9, which activates caspase 3, which then leads to apoptosis.

The idea that apoptosis forms a constraint to cancer was first raised in 1972 when massive apoptosis was observed in the cells populating rapidly growing, hormone-dependent tumors after hormone withdrawal. The discovery of *bcl-2* oncogene as having antiapoptotic activity opened up the investigation of apoptosis in cancer at the molecular level. Bcl-2 promotes formation of B cell lymphomas through a chromosomal translocation linking the *bcl-2* gene to an immunoglobulin locus, which results in constitutive activation of *bcl-2*, driving lymphocyte survival. Further research has demonstrated that altering components of the apoptotic machinery allows a cell to resist death signals, providing it with a selective growth advantage. For example, functional inactivation of the tumor suppressor p53 is observed in more than 50% of human cancers in many series. p53 is a key regulator of apoptosis by sensing DNA damage that cannot be repaired and subsequent activation of the apoptotic pathway. Other abnormalities, such as hypoxia and oncogene overexpression, are also channeled in part through p53 to the apoptotic machinery and fail to elicit apoptosis when p53 function is lost. In addition, alterations in cell survival pathways can suppress or alter apoptosis. For example, the phosphatidylinositol 3-kinase/AKT pathway, which transmits antiapoptotic survival signals, is likely involved in inhibiting apoptosis in many human tumors. This signaling pathway can be activated by extracellular factors such as insulin-like growth factors I and II or interleukin-3 (IL-3), by intracellular signals from Ras, or by loss of the PTEN tumor suppressor that negatively regulates the phosphatidylinositol 3-kinase/AKT pathway. A final example is the discovery of nonsignaling decoy receptors such as

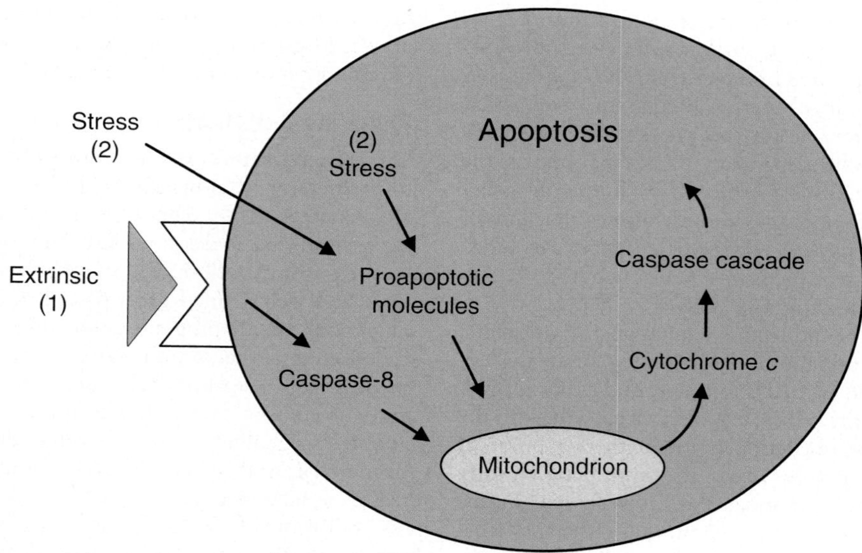

FIG. 29.7 Apoptotic pathways. Extracellular and intracellular stresses can induce apoptosis in tumor cells. Extracellular triggering can occur through a receptor-dependent (1) or receptor-independent (2) pathway. Both pathways induce release of cytochrome *c* from mitochondria, which triggers activation of various caspases in sequence, ultimately leading to apoptosis.

the membrane-bound decoy receptors DcR1 and DcR2 in acute promyelocytic leukemia and prostate cancer. Alternatively, soluble death receptors osteoprotegerin and DcR3 neutralize death-inducing ligands such as TRAIL and FAS ligand in breast cancer, and a high fraction of lung and colon cancers, respectively. Expression of these decoy receptors dilutes the death signal mediated through death receptors.

Nonapoptotic types of cell death that can promote tumor growth include necrosis, autophagy, ferroptosis, and mitotic catastrophe. Necrosis is normally induced by pathophysiologic conditions such as infection, inflammation, and ischemia. Necrosis is characterized by unregulated cell destruction associated with the release of proinflammatory signals. Inflammatory cells, in particular those of myeloid origin that are recruited to the tumor environment, actively promote tumor growth through induction of angiogenesis, immune suppression, tumor invasiveness, and metastasis formation. Autophagy is triggered by growth factor withdrawal, hypoxia, DNA damage, and differentiation and developmental triggers. Degraded intracellular organelles give rise to metabolites that allow survival of tumor cells in stressed, nutrient-limited environments. Autophagy is particularly important for growth of RAS-mutated cancers such as pancreatic, lung, and colon cancers. Ferroptosis is a recently discovered form of cell death that results from iron-dependent lipid peroxide accumulation. When iron-involving oxidative phosphorylation in mitochondria produces reactive oxygen species (ROS), along with ATP, that exceeds the cell's antioxidation capacity, the oxidative stress response damages lipids and proteins, causing cell death.[12] Finally, aberrant mitosis caused by failure of the G_2 checkpoint to block mitosis when DNA is damaged can lead to cell death, known as mitotic catastrophe. Defects in nonapoptotic cell death pathways have been linked to cancer. For example, deletion of the autophagy-regulating gene *beclin-1* is seen in high percentages of ovarian, breast, and prostate cancers. In addition to cell death, cells can undergo permanent growth arrest, called senescence, when repair of damaged DNA fails. Senescent cells lose their clonogenicity, but defects in the senescent program contribute to tumor development.

Enabling Replicative Immortality

Acquired disruption of cell-to-cell signaling by itself does not ensure expansive tumor growth on its own. This is due to the intrinsic programmed decline in replication potential that limits multiplication of normal somatic cells. This program must be disrupted for a clone of cells to develop into a macroscopic tumor. Normal cells have a finite replicative potential. Once a cell population has progressed through a certain number of doublings, they stop growing but remain viable, a process termed *senescence*.

With the exception of stem cells, activated lymphocytes, and germline cells, normal cells have a limited replicative potential. Stem cells give rise to progenitor cells that can progress through a certain number of doublings with an increasing degree of differentiation. Fully differentiated cells do not have replicative potential. The number of doublings is controlled by telomeres, the ends of chromosomes that are composed of several thousand repeats of a short 6–base pair sequence element. Telomeres prevent end-to-end chromosomal fusion. However, each DNA replication is associated with a loss of 50 to 100 base pairs of telomeric DNA from the ends of every chromosome. The progressive shortening of telomeres through successive cycles of replication eventually causes them to lose their ability to protect the ends of chromosomal DNA. When the critical length is bridged, the unprotected chromosomal ends participate in end-to-end chromosomal fusions, yielding a karyotype disarray that almost inevitably results in the death of the affected cell. Telomeric attrition is negated by the enzyme telomerase that elongates telomeric DNA. Telomerase activity is high during embryonic development and in certain cell populations, such as stem cells in adults. However, many tumors are characterized by elevated telomerase activity. Alternatively, telomeres are maintained through recombination-based interchromosomal exchanges of sequence information. Thus, by maintaining a telomere length above a critical threshold, the tumor cells have unlimited proliferative potential and are considered immortal.

Evidence has recently been obtained for the existence of cancer stem cells (CSCs), or cancer-initiating cells, that give rise to tissue-specific progenitor cells and phenotypically diverse cancer cells with limited replicative potential. The definition of CSCs is still a subject of some debate, but a CSC subclass has now been described in most types of cancer. Characteristic of CSCs is the exponentially enhanced ability to seed new tumors, relative to the nonCSC population, in immunodeficient mice. These cells are extraordinarily rare within the tumor and usually make up less than 10%, and often less than 5%, of neoplastic cells. CSCs may generate tumors through self-renewal as well as through differentiation into multiple cell types. Various cell surface markers have been used to define CSCs, such as CD44, CD133, and CXCR4. A recent study identified Lgr5 as a key marker of intestinal colorectal CSCs in mice and showed that CSCs are critical for metastasis formation. In this study, targeting of the CSC population led to the $Lgr5^-$ nonCSC population transitioning into $Lgr5^+$ stem cells, and thus the CSC population can be repopulated even after eradication.[13] Interestingly, CSCs possess similar transcriptional profiles with normal tissue stem cells, further supporting their designation as stem-like. Furthermore, evidence suggests that CSCs are more resistant to traditional therapeutic modalities, such as chemotherapy and radiation.

Inducing Angiogenesis

Based on the observation that many individuals who died of non-cancer-related causes had in situ tumors at the time of autopsy, physicians and scientists concluded that these microscopic tumors are in a dormant state. The reason for tumor dormancy is that the body blocks the tumor from recruiting its own blood supply to provide tumor cells with the required oxygen and nutrients. The growth of new blood vessels, angiogenesis, is a highly regulated process to ensure supply to all cells within an organ. Surprisingly, the microscopic tumors lack the ability to induce angiogenesis, and only an estimated 1 in 600 acquire angiogenic activity. Research pioneered by pediatric surgeon Judah Folkman has demonstrated that naturally occurring endogenous angiogenesis inhibitors prevent tumors from expanding. The angiogenesis inhibitors keep the tumors in check by counterbalancing the angiogenic signals. These signals are mediated by soluble factors and their receptors on endothelial cells as well as by integrins and adhesion molecules mediating cell-matrix and cell-cell interactions. Angiogenic activity is induced by growth factors such as vascular endothelial growth factor (VEGF), basic and acidic FGF, and PDGF. Each binds to transmembrane tyrosine kinase receptors displayed primarily by endothelial cells that are connected to intracellular signaling pathways. Angiogenesis inhibitors are associated with specific tissues or circulate in the blood. The first inhibitor, IFN-α, was reported in 1980, and additional endogenous inhibitors have been identified since then. These include thrombospondin, tumstatin, canstatin, endostatin, and angiostatin. Evidence for the importance of inducing and sustaining angiogenesis in tumors is overwhelming. For example, the switch of dormant human tumors into fast-growing tumors in immune-compromised mice is associated with an angiogenesis gene signature. Most telling are the results of clinical studies with the antiVEGF antibody bevacizumab (Avastin), the first angiogenesis inhibitor approved by the Food and Drug Administration for treatment of colon cancer. Bevacizumab significantly prolongs the survival of some patients with advanced cancer. It should be noted, however, that a minority of tumors are nonangiogenic, while others may contain a mixture of both angiogenic and nonangiogenic areas.[14] Both primary and metastatic tumors may be nonangiogenic, and are most commonly observed in lung, liver, and brain lesions.

The ability to induce and to sustain angiogenesis seems to be acquired in a discrete step (or steps) during tumor development through a switch to the angiogenic phenotype. Tumors appear to activate the angiogenic switch by changing the balance between the total angiogenic stimulation and the total angiogenic inhibition. This occurs in most cases when the angiogenesis stimulators overwhelm the angiogenesis inhibitors. In some tumors, these changes may be linked. It is likely that such disruption in the angiogenic balance is under control of the genetic makeup of the individual tumor cell and its microenvironment. Angiogenesis inducers and inhibitors may be genetically controlled by tumor suppressor genes such as *p53*, whereas oncogenes (e.g., *RAS*) may downregulate transcription of endogenous inhibitors or activate inducers. For example, *Bcl-2* activation leads to significantly increased expression of VEGF and angiogenesis. Another dimension of regulation is through proteases, which can control the bioavailability of angiogenic activators and inhibitors. Thus, a variety of proteases can release basic FGF stored in the ECM, whereas plasmin, a proangiogenic component of the clotting system, can cleave itself into an angiogenesis inhibitor form called angiostatin. Another angiogenesis inhibitor, endostatin, is an internal fragment of the basement membrane collagen XVIII. Finally, hypoxia and other metabolic stressors, mechanical stress from proliferating cells, or inflammatory immune responses can trigger angiogenesis. The coordinated expression of proangiogenic and antiangiogenic signaling molecules and their modulation by proteolysis appear to reflect the complex homeostatic regulation of normal tissue angiogenesis and of vascular integrity. Different types of tumors use distinct molecular strategies to activate the angiogenic switch.

Endothelial cells are key in the formation of new blood vessels through production or expression of angiogenesis-promoting factors. These factors include proinflammatory cytokines such as IL-6, VEGF, and hematopoietic growth factors such as colony-stimulating factors that recruit and activate bone marrow–derived progenitor cells. Among the progenitor cells are myeloid precursors that further promote the proinflammatory responses at the tumor and actively contribute to angiogenesis by producing matrix metalloprotease-9, a critical regulator of tumor angiogenesis through the induced release of VEGF. Bone marrow–derived endothelial precursors foster tumor blood vessel assembly.

Activating Invasion and Metastasis

Progressing tumors give rise to distant metastases that are the cause of 90% of human cancer deaths. For tumors to successfully metastasize, primary tumor cells have to break off from the primary tumor; enter the vasculature (intravasation), extravasate at distant sites, and colonize destination organ sites. Invasion and metastatic growth of tumor cells do not appear to be random processes. Paget observed in 1889 that breast carcinoma often metastasized to the liver, lungs, bone, adrenals, or brain. He hypothesized that tumor cells (the "seed") would grow only in selective environments (the "soil"), where conditions supported tumor growth, hence the so-called seed-and-soil hypothesis. Since then, additional studies have confirmed this hypothesis. For example, malignant melanoma metastasizes to the brain, but ocular malignant melanoma frequently metastasizes to the liver. Prostate cancer metastasizes to the bone and colon carcinoma to the liver.

Whereas metastatic spread is in part determined by circulation patterns, the retention of disseminated tumor cells in distant organs and successful development suggest the existence of specific molecular interactions.[15] Molecular analysis has provided several theories to explain preferential outgrowth of tumor cells.

One theory, the growth factor theory, proposes that tumor cells in the blood or lymphatics invade organs at similar frequency, but only those that find favorable growth factors multiply. Transferrins, for example, are iron-transferring ferroproteins required for cell growth that have additional mitogenic properties beyond their iron-transporting function. Increased concentrations of transferrin are found in lung, bone, and the brain and are associated with elevated levels of transferrin receptors on metastasizing tumor cells. Another theory, the adhesion theory, proposes that endothelial cells lining the blood vessels in certain organs express adhesion molecules that bind tumor cells and permit extravasation. A third theory is that chemokines secreted by the target organ can enter the circulation and selectively attract tumor cells that express receptors for the chemokines. Examples include the chemokine receptor-ligand axis between elevated levels of CXCR4 on breast cancer cells and CXCL12 secreting bone marrow, liver, lymph nodes, and lung, which explains why these organs are preferred sites for breast cancer metastasis. A similar phenomenon was observed for melanoma cells that were found to express elevated levels of the receptors CXCR4, CCR7, and CCR10 compared with normal melanocytes. Lymph nodes, lung, liver, bone marrow, and skin express the highest levels of the ligands for these receptors and are the preferred sites for metastatic spread of melanomas. Because chemokines are now known to affect angiogenesis and expression of cytokines, adhesion molecules, and proteases in addition to inducing migration, it appears that chemokines and their receptors play an essential role in the successful outgrowth of tumors at preferential sites. While the exact mechanism for the so-called organotropism is still unclear, recent discoveries have shown that primary tumors induce the formation of microenvironments in distant organs that permit the homing and outgrowth of tumor cells before their arrival. These premetastatic niches are initiated by tumor-secreted factors and tumor-derived extracellular vesicles that in concert trigger a cascade of events involving increased vascular permeability in microvessels in organs, and recruitment of various bone marrow-derived cell subsets that aid in local tissue remodeling and recruitment of cancer cells.[15]

Detailed analysis of primary tumors indicates that gene functions mediating metastatic activities are present early in the disease. These functions result from genetic or epigenetic alterations. The genes can be grouped into classes, such as metastasis-initiating genes that control invasion, angiogenesis, circulation, and bone marrow mobilization. Similarly, metastasis progression genes control extravasation, survival, and reinitiation, whereas metastasis virulence genes regulate organ-specific colonization. These intrinsic properties of the tumor together with its cellular origin determine the organ specificity and temporal course of metastasis formation.

The epithelial-to-mesenchymal transition (EMT) program plays an essential role in progression from primary to metastatic cancer. The EMT program is a cell-biologic program, orchestrated by certain transcription factors, in which epithelial cells convert into more mesenchymal cell states. The extent of EMT depends on both extracellular signals and intracellular gene circuitry. The EMT program is not only essential at multiple stages during embryonic morphogenesis, but also in wound healing, tissue fibrosis, and cancer progression. Recent work suggests that cells in EMT acquire similar stem-like properties to CSCs, and thus EMT could give rise to CSCs. Cancer cells use EMT to become invasive and to metastasize. During EMT, cancer cells downregulate the expression of cellular adhesion molecules, such as epithelial (E)–cadherin, and become spindle shaped, thus allowing them to invade surrounding tissues, to intravasate into the bloodstream, and to metastasize. Once cells in EMT arrive at distant sites of metastasis, they extravasate and undergo a process of mesenchymal-epithelial transition, whereby these cells revert back to their original epithelial phenotype for clonal expansion and establishment of metastasis.

Both intravasation and extravasation are characterized by changes in ECMs and their interactions with tumor cells. The cell-cell and cell-matrix interactions are mediated through CAMs, primarily by members of the immunoglobulin and calcium-dependent cadherin families, the hyaluronan receptor CD44, selectins, and integrins, which link cells to ECM substrates. Studies have shown that the molecules mediating adhesion are also capable of signal transduction. As such, changes in expression of adhesion molecules will alter signaling pathways, and conversely, signaling molecules can directly affect the function of adhesion molecules in tumor cells.

E–cadherin is the prototype cadherin responsible for cell polarity and organization of epithelium. In normal cells, extracellular domains of E-cadherin on opposing cells couple and form cell-cell junctions. The cytoplasmic cell adhesion complex is linked to the actin cytoskeleton through catenins (α, β, and γ). E-cadherin function is lost in most epithelial tumors during progression to tumor malignancy and may in fact be a prerequisite for tumor cell invasion and metastasis formation. Mechanisms that include mutational inactivation of the E-cadherin or β-catenin genes, transcriptional repression, or proteases of the extracellular cadherin domain induce loss of E-cadherin function. This prevents catenins from binding and leads to their accumulation in the cytoplasm. Inactivation of nonsequestered β- and γ-catenin is dependent on the presence of the tumor suppressor gene *APC* and an inactive Wnt signaling pathway. However, when *APC* function is lost, as is the case in many colon cancers or in the case of Wnt activation, β-catenin is not degraded but instead translocates to the nucleus, where transcription of genes involved in cell proliferation and tumor progression is activated, such as c-*myc*, cyclin D1, CD44, and others.

Changes in expression of CAMs in the immunoglobulin superfamily also appear to play critical roles in the processes of invasion and metastasis. Neuronal-CAM, for example, undergoes a switch in expression from a highly adhesive isoform to poorly adhesive (or even repulsive) forms in Wilms tumor, neuroblastoma, and small cell lung cancer. In invasive pancreatic cancer and colorectal cancers, the overall expression of neuronal-CAM is reduced.

Selectins are a family of transmembrane molecules consisting of endothelial, leukocyte, and platelet selectins that normally mediate blood cell–endothelial cell interactions. However, alterations in the expression level of selectins or their ligands, such as the endothelial- and leukocyte-selectin ligand CD44, have been associated with increased invasiveness and poor survival in several malignant neoplasms, such as breast cancer and colorectal cancer.

Changes in integrin expression are also evident in invasive and metastatic cells. For invading and metastasizing cells to be successful, they need to adapt to changing tissue microenvironments. This is accomplished through shifts in the spectrum of integrin α and β subunits displayed on the cell surface by the migrating cells. The large extracellular domain of integrins can bind to ECM molecules (such as collagens, laminin, and fibronectin), to ligands associated with vascular and coagulation physiology (such as thrombospondin and factor X), or with other CAMs. In addition, integrins may exhibit different specificities when expressed on different cell types. Thus, carcinoma cells facilitate invasion by shifting their expression of integrins from those that favor ECM present in normal epithelium to other integrins that preferentially bind the degraded stromal components produced by extracellular proteases.

The second general parameter of the invasive and metastatic capability involves extracellular proteases that regulate ECM turnover. It has become clear that tumor progression may involve an increased expression of proteases, decreased expression of protease inhibitors, and inactive zymogen forms of proteases that are converted into active enzymes. Expression of the protease tenascin, which neutralizes adhesion to fibronectin, is increased ten fold in invasive breast carcinoma compared with normal breast tissue. Matrix metalloproteases are overexpressed in melanoma, invasive breast carcinoma, and invasive squamous cell carcinoma. Matrix-degrading proteases are characteristically associated with the cell surface by synthesis with a transmembrane domain, binding to specific protease receptors, or association with integrins. One imagines that docking of active proteases on the cell surface can facilitate invasion by cancer cells into nearby stroma, across blood vessel walls, and through normal epithelium cell layers. That notion notwithstanding, it is difficult to unambiguously ascribe the functions of particular proteases solely to this capability, given their evident roles in other hallmark capabilities, including angiogenesis and growth signaling, which in turn contribute directly or indirectly to the invasive and metastatic capability. A further complexity derives from the multiple cell types involved in protease expression and display, including stromal and inflammatory cells such as neutrophils and macrophages.

The activation of extracellular proteases and the altered binding specificities of cadherins, CAMs, selectins, and integrins are clearly central to the acquisition of invasiveness and metastatic potential. The clonal and genetic diversity of tumors permits adhesion and detachment from the same matrix. Some tumor cells within a primary tumor may have the correct genotype and phenotype to permit both detachment from the surrounding tissue and entry into blood vessels or lymphatic vessels. Likewise, extravasation may be mediated by a few tumor cells that express the required receptors for certain ECM molecules. In general, those mutations that confer escape from homeostatic control mechanisms in the host or that give the tumor cell a growth advantage over others are favorably selected. Thus, tumor clones that best complement the environment with expression of particular ECM receptors may thrive because this provides an advantage over other clones. However, the regulatory pathways and molecular mechanisms that govern these changes are incompletely understood and appear to differ from one tissue environment to another.

Avoiding Immune Destruction

In the early 1900s, it was proposed by Paul Ehrlich that the frequency of cancerous transformations would be very high if it were not for the defense system of the host. This concept was later substantiated in the 1950s and 1960s. Burnet hypothesized that the development of T lymphocyte–mediated immunity during evolution was specific for elimination of transformed cells. He further proposed that there is a continuous surveillance of the body for transformed cells, hence the term *immunosurveillance*. It was not until the early 2000s that immune-mediated elimination of tumor cells was conclusively demonstrated in animal models. Extensive studies on immune infiltrate in primary human cancers have established that memory T cells, particularly of the T helper (CD4+) type 1 subtype, and cytotoxic (CD8+) T cells are prognostic factors for disease-free and overall survival at all stages of clinical disease. Alternatively, tumors infiltrated with abundant myeloid cells, particularly macrophages, correlate with worse prognosis in many types of cancers, such as pancreas and breast. Data from mouse and human studies combined suggest that immune surveillance of cancer does exist, mediated through immune cells and soluble factors. Whereas the immune system may eliminate most transformed cells, some cells manage to escape and may develop into tumors.

The continuous pressure of the immune system in an immunocompetent host determines to a great degree if and how tumors evolve, a process called *immunoediting* (Fig. 29.8).[16] In this process, the immune system plays a dual role in the interactions between tumor and the host. On one hand, the immune system effectively eliminates highly immunogenic tumor cells. At the same time, however, the immune system fails to eliminate tumor cells with reduced immunogenicity, thereby selecting for tumor variants that have acquired immune evasion mechanisms. Over time, this selection leads to outgrowth of tumor cells that fail to induce an effective immune response. As such, the interactions between an intact immune system and tumor cells evolve through three phases, referred to as the elimination phase, the equilibrium phase, and the escape phase. The recognition and elimination of transformed cells is a concerted effort between innate and adaptive immunity, representing the two arms of the immune system. Local disruption of tissue that occurs as a result of expansion of transformed cells is associated with release of chemokines and proinflammatory cytokines such as interferons, IL-1, IL-6, and tumor necrosis factor-α that trigger innate immunity.

The innate immune system represents the first line of defense against transformed cells (and microorganisms). The most important outcome of these initial events is the production of IFN-γ by activated innate immune cells. IFN-γ has direct antitumor effects and further boosts tumor cell lysis by innate immune cells. The resulting availability of tumor antigen triggers an adaptive immune response. Key in this process is the uptake of tumor antigen by antigen-presenting cells, primarily dendritic cells. The dendritic cells migrate to tumor-draining lymph nodes and stimulate T and B lymphocytes. The development of adaptive immunity represents the second line of defense against tumors and, together with innate immunity, could completely eliminate the tumor. However, this does not always occur and may lead to what is referred to as the *equilibrium phase*. This phase is characterized by a balance between tumor growth and tumor elimination, as the name suggests. Antitumor immunity leads to destruction of immunogenic tumor cells, whereas tumor cells with reduced immunity go unnoticed.

Over time, genetic instability and heterogeneity of the tumor cells may give rise to tumor variants better able to withstand the immunologic pressure. Contributing to the failure of the immune system are tumor-induced immune suppressor mechanisms. Once this point has been reached, referred to as the escape phase, the immune system can no longer contain the tumor, and the tumor grows progressively. During the last decade, multiple mechanisms have been identified through which tumors escape from elimination by the immune system. These mechanisms include host-related factors, tumor-related factors, and a combination of both. Among host-related factors are treatment-related immunosuppression, acquired or inherited immunodeficiency, and aging. The list of tumor-related escape mechanisms includes loss of major histocompatibility complex alleles, reduced antigen processing or presentation, decreased expression of costimulatory molecules

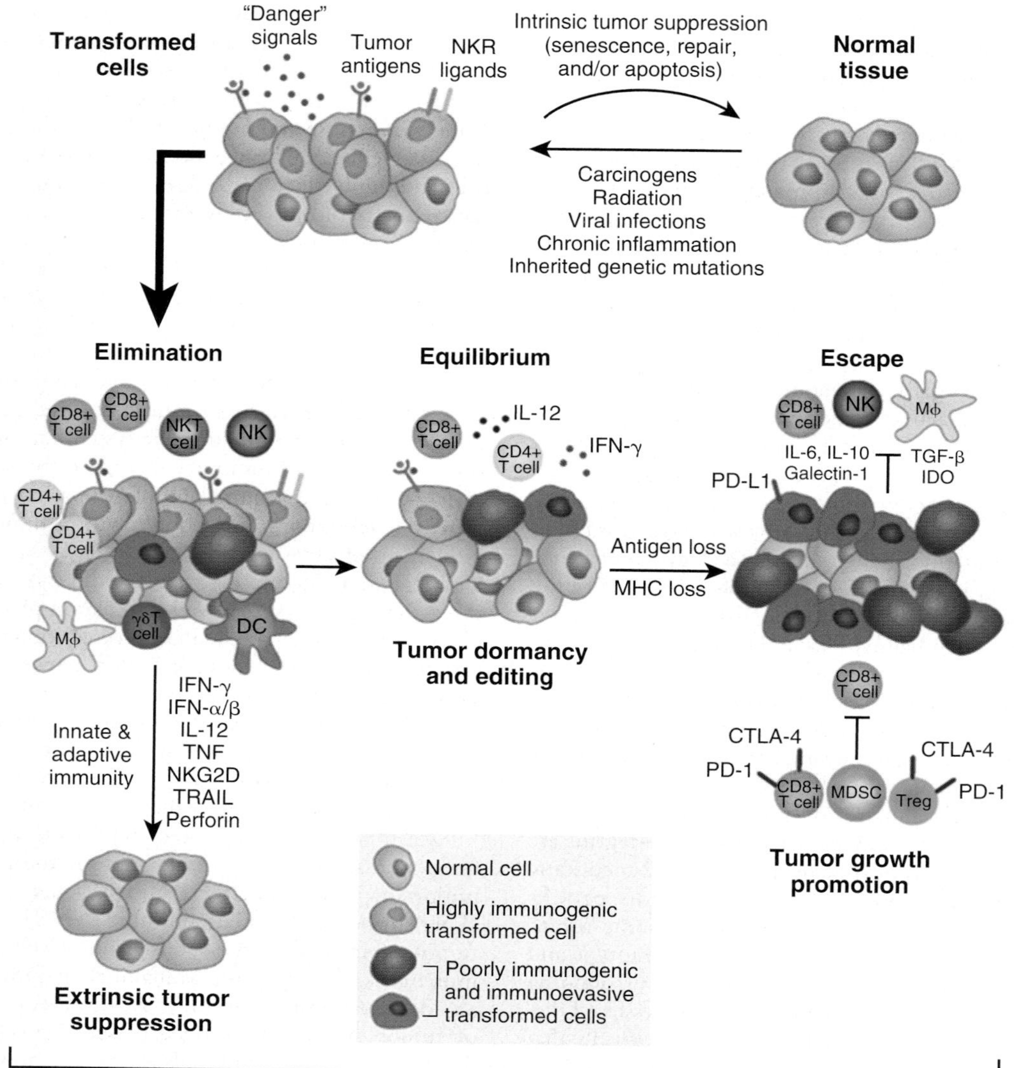

FIG. 29.8 Schematic overview of immunoediting. When developing tumors disrupt local tissue structures, proinflammatory cytokines are released and, together with secreted chemokines, attract innate immune cells, such as macrophages, natural killer *(NK)* cells, NKT cells, and γ/δ cells. Innate immune cells can directly recognize and lyse tumor cells but also induce an adaptive immune response mediated by CD8+ and CD4+ lymphocytes. Whereas most tumor cells are eliminated (elimination phase), tumor cell variants may survive and expand. However, the activated immune system keeps the tumor in check by eliminating those tumor cells that are sufficiently immunogenic (equilibrium phase). The immunologic pressure may cause selection toward tumor cell variants with reduced immunogenicity that are capable of escaping from immune recognition (escape phase). These variants can expand in an immunologically intact environment. (From Schreiber RD, Old LJ, Smyth MJ. Cancer immunoediting: integrating immunity's roles in cancer suppression and promotion. *Science*. 2011;331:1565–1570.)

required for T cell recognition, secretion of immunosuppressive factors (TGF-β, IL-10), stimulation of suppressor cells, and mechanisms that actively induce tolerance or apoptosis in activated immune cells. In addition, when looking across a large number of tumors over 33 cancer types, six unique immune profiles can be identified: TGF-β dominant, immunologically quiet, lymphocyte depleted, inflammatory, IFN-γ dominant, and wound healing.[17] These different classes reflect different cancer outcomes, and differing tumor evolutions in the presence of the host. A thorough discussion of tumor immunology and immunotherapy is found in Chapter 30 of this edition.

Deregulating Cellular Energetics and Metabolomics

Generally, reprogrammed and/or rewired cellular metabolism provides for the energy needs of growing tumors. Otto Warburg first described the anomalous predilection of cancer cells to limit their energy metabolism to glycolysis, even in the presence of oxygen (aerobic glycolysis), an observation termed the *Warburg effect*. Because glycolysis has a roughly eighteen fold lower energy yield compared with aerobic metabolism through mitochondrial oxidative phosphorylation, cancer cells must dramatically upregulate the rate of glycolysis (up to 200-fold higher than normal cells) to keep up with the rapid metabolism of rapidly dividing neoplastic cells. One mechanism used by tumor cells to increase the rate of glycolysis is to upregulate the expression of glucose transporters, such as GLUT1. Clinically, the Warburg effect is used to diagnose or to stage cancers, such as visualizing glucose uptake by positron emission tomography with ^{18}F-fluorodeoxyglucose.

Different classes of metabolic reprogramming activities have been identified: (1) transforming activities, (2) enabling activities and (3) neutral activities.[18] Transforming activities are directly tied to cell transformation, with the most studied examples being mutations of *isocitrate dehydrogenases 1 and 2* (*IDH1, IDH2*), *succinate dehydrogenase,* and *fumarate hydratase. IDH1* and *IDH 2* mutations lead to a now mutated IDH enzyme not able to properly do its normal job in the citric acid cycle, and instead it converts alpha ketoglutarate to the oncometabolite 2-hydroxyglutarate. *Succinate dehydrogenase* and *fumarate hydratase* catalyze reactions in the citric acid cycle, and mutations lead to oncometabolite succinate or fumarate buildup. Succinate, fumarate, and 2-hydroxyglutarate all interfere with dioxygenase function, which leads to multiple downstream effects, including impaired DNA and histone demethylation (see Cancer Epigenetics). This mechanism cooperates with other drivers to help promote cancer growth.

Enabling activities refers to activities that are altered in cancer cells but are not involved in transformations as previously described. For instance, mutant *KRAS* leads to increased nutrient acquisition and macromolecule synthesis, all of which are crucial for continued tumor growth and viability. Indeed, suppressing of these pathways inhibits KRAS-driven tumorigenesis. Finally, neutral activities involve metabolic programs in the cancer cell that are not necessarily needed for continued cancer growth and survival.

All this has led to excitement in trying to determine if aspects of the cancer metabolic cycle can be targeted to suppress tumor growth and in the emergence of the cancer field of metabolomics. Examples include drugs targeting IDH1 and IDH2, now in clinical trials. In addition, drugs targeting amino acids crucial for cancer progression, such as arginine in hepatocellular carcinoma (HCC), are under investigation. It is likely that we have only scratched the surface on this exciting, and evolving area of research.

Genomic Instability and Mutation

Genomic alteration is emerging as a key enabling characteristic to many of the traits outlined before. Under normal physiologic conditions, the genome is maintained under extraordinary fidelity by important caretaker genes. Alterations of this important cellular machinery can result in loss of the ability to detect DNA damage, loss of the ability to directly repair damaged DNA, and inability to inactivate or to intercept mutagenic molecules before DNA damage can occur. Mutant copies of some caretaker genes can predictably result in an increased incidence of certain types of cancer. *TP53* is an important tumor suppressor gene, and it plays a key role in orchestrating the detection and resolution of mutations; hence, it is often referred to as the guardian of the genome. However, *TP53* is the most commonly mutated tumor suppressor gene in cancer. Once proper maintenance of the genome is lost, cells are free to accumulate multiple genetic alterations, any of which can convey the key characteristics for tumor progression discussed previously. Two recently described classes of tumor genomic rearrangements include chromothrypsis and chromopexy. In chromothrypsis, a massive chromosomal rearrangement event occurs in a localized genomic region, while in chromopexy there is coordinated rearrangement across multiple chromosomes. This can lead to tumor beneficial gene mutations and subsequent tumor progression.

Tumor-Promoting Inflammation

Tumor-promoting inflammation is also emerging as a key enabling characteristic of many types of cancer. As previously described, immune cells may play an important role in antitumor defense. However, paradoxically, these same immune cells can also enhance tumor progression. It has long been recognized that many tumors are densely infiltrated by various immune cells. Similar to a chronic wound, leukocytes in the tumor produce various growth factors, which can promote tumor growth, angiogenesis, and therapeutic resistance. Often, inflammation is an early event in tumorigenesis and can incite the conversion of a premalignant lesion into a full-blown cancer. For example, leukocytes can elaborate various ROS that can cause damage to the DNA of nearby cells, thus fostering the progression to malignancy.

As discussed more later in this chapter (Chronic Inflammation), inflammatory changes can lead to upregulation of transcription factors NF-κB, STAT3, and/or hypoxia-inducible factor-1α (HIF1α), which work to mediate cytokine and chemokine expression (e.g., IL6), as well as inflammatory enzymes such as COX-2, leads to inflammatory changes in the tumor microenvironment. Leukocytes, macrophages, mast cells, T cells, and dendritic cells are recruited and further mediate the immune response.[19] Tumors can alter the functionality of infiltrating immune cells, causing functional leukocytes to become anergic or even immunosuppressive. For example, macrophages isolated from tumors, such as pancreatic cancer, are potently immunosuppressive and prevent antitumor immune responses by T cells; however, monocytes from the blood of these same cancer patients are capable of promoting immune responses, suggesting that the tumor environment can alter the functionality of infiltrating leukocytes to escape immune-mediated elimination.

Timing and Pattern of Tumor Growth and Distant Spread

As discussed previously, depending on cancer type and location, metastatic risk and specific site of likely distant organ spread differs. Different cancers undergo progression from normal cell to clinically evident mass in different time horizons. For instance, in an elegant analysis of pancreatic cancer specimens, it was conservatively estimated to take nearly 12 years from initiation of tumorigenesis to formation of the parental pancreatic adenocarcinoma clone. It was estimated that another 7 years would pass prior to the index lesion clinically presenting in the patient and 2 to 3 more years until distant metastatic spread (a total of >20 years from initial founding mutation until distant metastatic spread).[20] Estimates for colorectal carcinoma place the time between initial index mutation and growth into a clinically detectable lesion at ~18 years. This number likely varies significantly between tumor types and within tumor types, but, overall, the time it takes for a clinically detectable tumor to form is on the order of many years, if not decades, in some cases.

When it comes to pattern of distant metastasis, four different metastatic patterns have been described (Fig. 29.9).[21] One, simple linear evolution model, whereby clones arise sequentially from the primary tumor with metastases occurring late from the most recent subclone. Second, early dissemination with parallel evolution model, whereby tumor cells disseminate early and evolve in parallel with the primary lesion. Third, late dissemination from a single primary tumor subclone, whereby a late arising subclone is able to seed multiple metastases. And finally, late dissemination from multiple subclones, whereby multiple subclones from the primary are able to undergo metastatic spread and do so relatively later on during the tumor evolution time course. Overall, the late

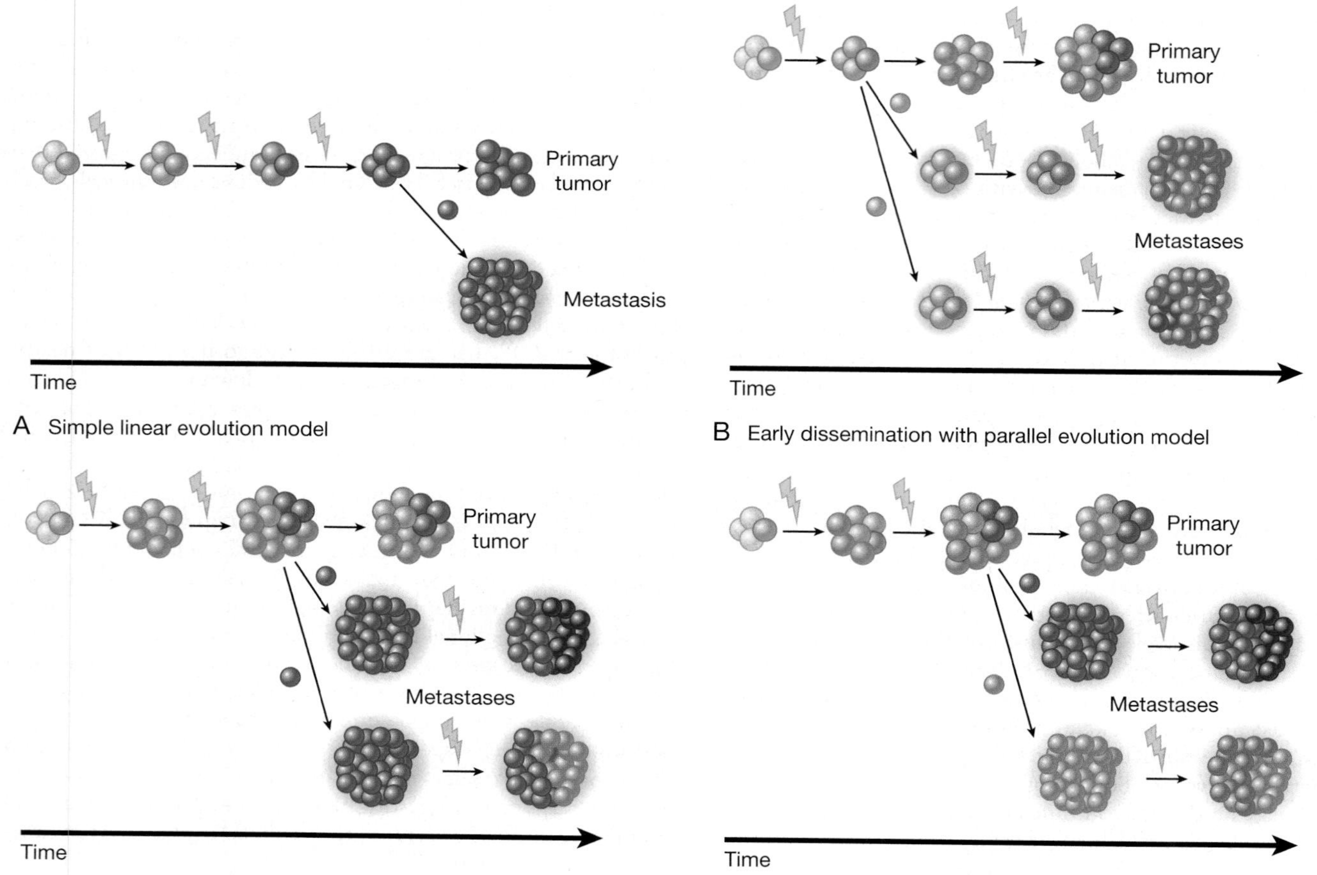

FIG. 29.9 Models of solid tumor metastasis. (A) Linear evolution model with late metastasis. (B) Early dissemination with early distant metastasis and parallel evolution. (C) Late dissemination from a late-arising subclone that has the propensity to see multiple metastases. (D) Late distant metastasis from multiple late-occurring subclones in the primary tumor. (From Hunter KW, Amin R, Deasy S, et al. Genetic insights into the morass of metastatic heterogeneity. *Nat Rev Cancer*. 2018;18:211–223.)

dissemination model is favored by the literature. A recent study of colorectal cancer evolution found that distant lesions were most similar to each other, while still retaining similarity to the primary tumor, thereby favoring the late dissemination model. An analysis of matched primary and metastatic breast cancer samples demonstrated that on average the metastases disseminated at 87% of the molecular age of the primary lesion, again favoring late dissemination. Despite this, some studies do support early (or both early and late) dissemination, and it is likely that across all cancers these two theories are not mutually exclusive.

Another subject of much debate has been regarding dissemination from a single or multiple subclones. In a recent study of colorectal cancer, in two thirds of cases, the distant organ metastasis was more similar to the primary tumor clone than the metastatic lymph node clone, thus supporting dissemination from multiple subclones theory in the majority of cases. This type of spread directly contradicts the classic tumor node metastasis (TNM) paradigm that is taught beginning in medical school, and may be partly to explain why there has been a lack of therapeutic success for recent trials of extended lymph node dissection in breast cancer and melanoma.[22] Finally, there is potential that lymph node metastases could in theory seed distant organ metastases outside of the classic lymphatic to thoracic duct to subclavian vein pathway. In fact, recent work in murine models has demonstrated the ability for lymph node metastases to leave lymph nodes by way of local blood vessels, and then lead to distant metastatic spread.[23]

CARCINOGENESIS

Cancer Genetics

Malignant transformation is the process by which a clonal population of cells acquires alterations that confer a growth advantage over normal cells. Many of these alterations occur at the genetic level, involving the gain of function by oncogenes or the loss of function by tumor suppressor genes (either of which may be referred to as a cancer driver gene). A classic multistep model for colorectal tumorigenesis has been described (Fig. 29.10). Designation as an oncogene or tumor suppressor gene relates to the directionality of effect, without implications about molecular detail. Indeed, the original name for what came to be known as tumor suppressor genes was in fact antioncogenes. A recent analysis looking at over 9000 tumors across 33 cancer subtypes identified 299 distinct mutated cancer driver genes.[11] Many driver mutations of oncogenes (e.g., *KRAS* and *HER2*) as well as loss of function mutation of tumor suppressor genes (e.g., *TP53)* were discussed

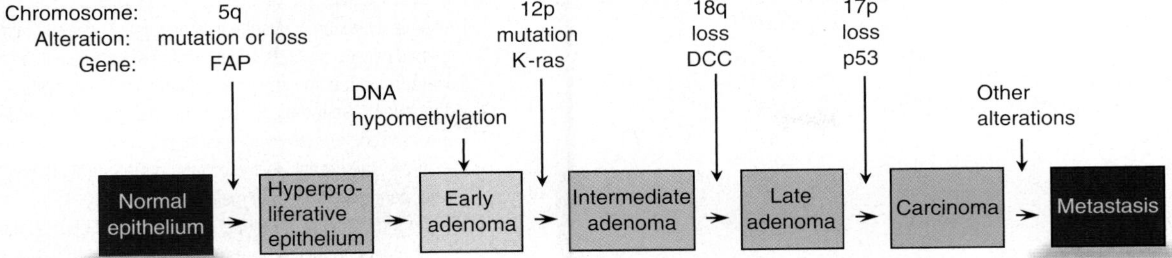

FIG. 29.10 A generic model for colorectal tumorigenesis. Tumorigenesis proceeds through a series of genetic alterations involving oncogenes *(ras)* and tumor suppressor genes (particularly those on chromosomes 5q, 12p, 17p, and 18q). The three stages of adenomas in general represent tumors of increasing size, dysplasia, and villous content. In patients with familial adenomatous polyposis *(FAP)*, a mutation on chromosome 5q (*APC* gene) is inherited. This alteration may be responsible for the hyperproliferative epithelium present in these patients. Hypomethylation is present in very small adenomas in patients with or without polyposis, and this alteration may lead to aneuploidy, resulting in the loss of suppressor gene alleles. The *ras* gene mutation appears to occur in one cell of a preexisting small adenoma and, through clonal expansion, produces a larger and more dysplastic tumor. Allelic deletions of chromosome 17p and 18q usually occur at a later stage of tumorigenesis than do deletions of chromosome 5q or *ras* gene mutations. The order of these changes is not invariant, however, and accumulation of these changes, rather than their order with respect to one another, seems most important. Tumors continue to progress once carcinomas have formed, and the accumulated loss of suppressor genes on additional chromosomes correlates with the ability of the carcinomas to metastasize and cause death. (From Fearon ER, Vogelstein B. A genetic model for colorectal tumorigenesis. *Cell.* 1990;61:759–767.)

previously in this chapter (Tumor Biology, Sustaining Proliferative Signaling and Resisting Cell Death subsections).

Genetic mutations that are inherited from one's parents and are present in all cells of the body are called *germline* (or constitutional) mutations; in contrast, *somatic* mutations are acquired during an individual's lifetime and cannot be passed on to one's children. Somatic mutations, which account for most mutations in cancer, may be caused by exposure to carcinogens in the form of radiation, chemicals, or chronic inflammation (see below in this chapter for more detailed discussion of carcinogens).

A tumor that arises in an individual may be classified as either hereditary or sporadic. In hereditary cases, a germline mutation is responsible for the predisposition to neoplasia. The index case or *proband* is the individual who is first diagnosed as having the syndrome, even if earlier generations are later recognized as also having had the syndrome. If the patient with a tumor does not have an inherited predisposition and the tumor's genetic mutations are all somatic, the tumor is classified as sporadic. In some hereditary cancer syndromes, the germline mutation causes a tendency for the cell to accumulate somatic mutations.

Although hereditary cancer syndromes are rare, their study has provided powerful insights into more common forms of cancer (Table 29.4). Key germline mutations in hereditary cancers are often the same as somatic mutations present in sporadic cancers. *TP53* gene mutations, if inherited, cause Li-Fraumeni syndrome. Familial adenomatous polyposis (FAP) is caused by a germline mutation in the *APC* gene. More than 80% of sporadic colorectal cancers also have a somatic mutation of this same gene. Similarly, mutation in the *RET* proto-oncogene is responsible for the predisposition to development of the familial form of medullary thyroid cancer (MTC). Somatic mutations of *RET* are found in about 50% of sporadic MTCs.

Predisposition in familial cancer syndromes is generally inherited in an autosomal dominant fashion (Table 29.4). Notable exceptions include ataxia-telangiectasia and xeroderma pigmentosum, which are transmitted in an autosomal recessive manner. Not all inherited genetic mutations have complete penetrance. There is almost complete penetrance of colorectal cancer in FAP and of MTC in multiple endocrine neoplasia type 2 (MEN2). In contrast, penetrance is less than 50% for pheochromocytoma in neurofibromatosis. Penetrance can also vary considerably for different characteristics of the same syndrome. The exact factors determining penetrance for a given mutation remain largely unknown, but factors felt to be commonly implicated include interplay between genes and the environment, sex, and age.

There are a number of features of hereditary cancers that distinguish them phenotypically from their sporadic counterparts. The former tend to cause the development of multifocal, bilateral cancer at an early age, whereas in the latter, cancer occurs later and is usually unilateral. Hereditary cancers will display clustering of the same cancer type in relatives and may be associated with other conditions, such as mental retardation and pathognomonic skin lesions.

Selected Familial Cancer Syndromes

Retinoblastoma

Retinoblastoma is a pediatric retinal tumor that holds an important place in the history of cancer genetics because the causative gene, *RB1*, was the first tumor suppressor gene to be cloned. Most cases are detected by the age of 5 years (95%, with 66% detected by 2 years), but bilateral disease is manifested earlier, usually within the first year of life. It is associated with extraocular malignant neoplasms including sarcomas, melanomas, and tumors of the central nervous system. Distinct sporadic and hereditary forms of retinoblastoma have long been recognized, with predisposition conferred by a germline mutation in approximately 40% of cases. Knudson reasoned that the germline mutation is necessary, but not by itself sufficient, for tumorigenesis because some children with an affected parent do not develop a tumor but later produce an affected child, indicating that they are carriers of the germline mutation. Most affected children with an affected parent develop tumors bilaterally. He further hypothesized that hereditary retinoblastoma requires two mutations, one of which is germline and the other somatic. In children with unilateral disease and no family history, both mutations are somatic. The hereditary and nonhereditary forms of the tumor require the same number of

TABLE 29.4 Familial cancer syndromes.

SYNDROME	GENES	LOCATIONS	MODE OF INHERITANCE	CANCER SITES AND ASSOCIATED TRAITS
Ataxia-telangiectasia	*ATM*	11q22	AR	Leukemia, lymphoma, ovarian cancer, gastric cancer, brain tumors, thyroid cancer, parotid cancer, pancreatic cancer, colorectal cancer
Birt-Hogg-Dubé syndrome	*FLCN*	17p11	AD	Renal tumors, benign subcutaneous tumors, lung cysts
Beckwith-Wiedemann syndrome	*CDKN1C, NSD1*	11p15	AD	Wilms tumor, hepatoblastoma, adrenal carcinoma, gonadoblastoma
Breast/ovarian syndrome	*BRCA1*	17q21	AD	Cancers of the breast, ovary, colon, prostate
	BRCA2, PALB2	13q12.3	AD	Cancers of the breast, ovary, colon, prostate, gallbladder and biliary tree, pancreas, stomach; melanoma
Carney complex	*PRKAR1A*	17q22-24	AD	Myxoid tumors (subcutaneous, atrial), adrenal cortical nodular hyperplasia, testicular tumors, pituitary adenoma, mammary fibroadenoma, thyroid cancer, schwannoma
Cowden disease	*PTEN*	10q23	AD	Cancer of the breast, endometrium, and thyroid
Familial adenomatous polyposis	*APC*	5q21	AD	Colorectal carcinoma, duodenal and gastric neoplasms, desmoid tumors, thyroid cancer, osteomas
Familial gastrointestinal stromal tumor	*c-KIT; PDGFRA*	4q12	AD	Gastrointestinal stromal tumors
Melanoma cancer syndrome	*CDKN2A/p16; CDK4*	9p21; 12q14	AD	Melanoma, pancreatic cancer, dysplastic nevi, atypical moles
Gorlin syndrome	*PTCH*	9q22.3	AD	Basal cell cancer, medulloblastoma, ovarian cancer
Hereditary diffuse gastric cancer	*CDH1*	16q22	AD	Gastric cancer
Hereditary nonpolyposis colorectal cancer (Lynch syndrome)	*MLH1; MSH2 (including EPCAM); MSH6; PMS1; PMS2*	3p21; 2p22-21; 2p16; 2q31; 7p22	AD	Colorectal cancer; endometrial cancer; transitional cell carcinoma of the ureter and renal pelvis; and carcinomas of the stomach, small bowel, pancreas, ovary
Hereditary papillary renal cell carcinoma	*MET*	7q31	AD	Renal cell cancer
Hereditary paraganglioma and pheochromocytoma	*SDHB; SDHC; SDHD*	1p36.1-p35; 1q21; 11q23	AD	Paraganglioma, pheochromocytoma
Juvenile polyposis coli	*BMPRIA; SMAD4/DPC4*	10q21-q22; 18q21	AD	Juvenile polyps of the gastrointestinal tract, gastrointestinal malignant neoplasms, pancreatic cancer
Leiomyosarcoma renal cell cancer syndrome	*FH*	1q43	AD	Papillary renal cell cancer, leiomyosarcoma
Li-Fraumeni	*p53; hCHK2*	17p13; 22q12	AD	Breast cancer, soft tissue sarcoma, osteosarcoma, brain tumors, adrenocortical carcinoma, Wilms tumor, phyllodes tumor (breast), pancreatic cancer, leukemia, neuroblastoma
Multiple endocrine neoplasia type 1	*MEN1*	11q13	AD	Pancreatic islet cell tumors, parathyroid hyperplasia, pituitary adenomas
Multiple endocrine neoplasia type 2	*RET*	10q11.2	AD	Medullary thyroid cancer, pheochromocytoma, parathyroid hyperplasia
MYH-associated adenomatous polyposis	*MYH*	1p34.3-p32.1	AR	Cancer of the colon, rectum, breast, stomach
Neurofibromatosis type 1	*NF1*	17q11	AD	Neurofibromas, neurofibrosarcoma, acute myelogenous leukemia, brain tumors
Neurofibromatosis type 2	*NF2*	22q12	AD	Acoustic neuromas, meningiomas, gliomas, ependymomas
Peutz-Jeghers syndrome	*STK11*	19p13.3	AD	Gastrointestinal carcinomas, breast cancer, testicular cancer, pancreatic cancer, benign pigmentation of the skin and mucosa
Retinoblastoma	*RB*	13q14	AD	Retinoblastoma, sarcomas, melanoma, malignant neoplasms of the brain and meninges
Tuberous sclerosis	*TSC1; TSC2*	9q34; 16p13	AD	Multiple hamartomas, renal cell carcinoma, astrocytoma
von Hippel–Lindau syndrome	*VHL*	3p25	AD	Renal cell carcinoma, hemangioblastomas of the retina and central nervous system, pheochromocytoma
WAGR	*WT*	11p13	AD	Wilms tumor, aniridia, genitourinary abnormalities, mental retardation
Werner syndrome	*WRN*	8p12	AR	Sarcoma/osteosarcoma, meningioma
Xeroderma pigmentosum	*XPA; ERCC4; ERCC2; POLH; XPC; ERCC3; DDB2; ERCC5*	9q22; 16p13; 19q13; 6p21; 3p25; 2q14; 11p11; 13q33	AR	Melanoma, leukemia, skin cancer

Adapted from Marsh D, Zori R. Genetic insights into familial cancers—update and recent discoveries. *Cancer Lett*. 2002;181:125–164.
AD, Autosomal dominant; *ADP*, adenomatous polyposis coli ;*AR*, autosomal recessive; *ATM*, ataxia-telangiectasia mutated serine/threonine kinase; *BMPR1A*, bone morphogenic protein receptor type 1A; *BRCA*, breast cancer gene; *CDH1*, cadherin 1; *CDK*, cyclin-dependent kinase; *CDKN*, cyclin-dependent kinase inhibitor; *DDB*, damage-specific DNA-binding protein; *EPCAM*, epithelial cell adhesion molecule; *ERCC*, excision repair cross-complementation; *FH*, Fumarate hydratase; *FLCN*, folliculin; *hCHK*, human checkpoint kinase; *MEN*, multiple endocrine neoplasia; *MET*, met proto-oncogene receptor tyrosine kinase; *MLH*, mutL homolog; *MSH*, propiomelanocortin; *MYH*, mutYDNA glycosylase; *NF*, neurofibromin; *PALB2*, partner and localizer of BRCA2; *PDGFRA*, platelet-derived growth factor receptor type A; *PMS1*, PMS1 homolog 1; *POLH*, DNA polymerase eta; *PRKAR1A*, protein kinase cAMP-dependent type 1 regulatory subunit alpha; *PTCH*, patched; *PTEN*, phosphatase and tensin homolog; *RB*, retinoblastoma; *RET*, ret proto-oncogene; *SDH*, succinate dehydrogenase complex; *SMAD*, smad family member; *STK11*, serine/threonine kinase; *TSC*, solute carrier family 12 member 3; *VHL*, von Hippel-Lindau tumor suppressor; *WRN*, Werner syndrome RecQ like helicase; *WT*, Wilms tumor; *XPA*, xpa DNA damage recognition and repair factor; *XPC*, xpc complex subunit, DNA damage recognition and repair factor.

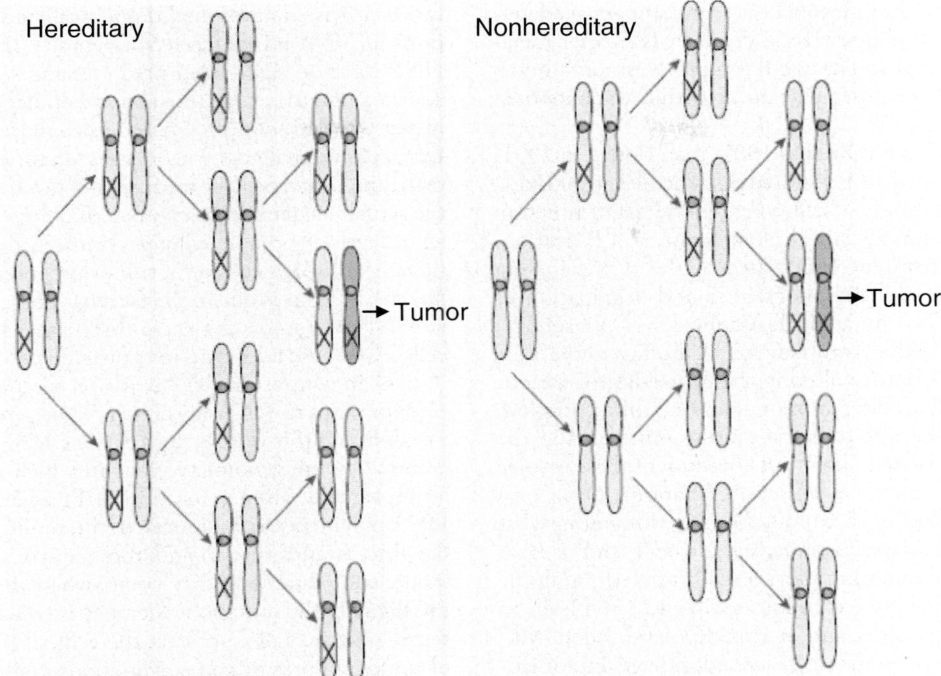

FIG. 29.11 Two genetic hits to cancer. In hereditary retinoblastoma, all retinoblasts are heterozygous for the mutant allele (indicated by X); they all have already sustained "one hit." In contrast, the preneoplastic clone in nonhereditary retinoblastoma must acquire this mutation before sustaining the "second hit" to complete malignant transformation. (Modified from Knudson AG. Two genetic hits (more or less) to cancer. *Nat Rev Cancer.* 2001;1:157–162.)

events—the "two-hit" hypothesis (Fig. 29.11). The *RB1* protein product is a key regulator of the cell cycle, and its loss results in failure of retinoblasts to differentiate properly.

Li-Fraumeni Syndrome

In 1969, Li and Fraumeni reported a new familial syndrome involving sarcomas (of both soft tissue and bone), breast cancers (the most common malignant neoplasm in this syndrome), brain tumors, leukemias, adrenocortical carcinomas, and a variety of other cancers. The syndrome now bears their name, and so called Chompret criteria have been identified to describe four clinical scenarios where there should be high suspicion for Li-Fraumeni syndrome and genetic counseling and testing should be offered: (1) a proband diagnosed with a Li-Fraumeni spectrum tumor prior to the age of 46 years, and at least one first or second degree relative with a Li-Fraumeni syndrome spectrum tumor; (2) proband with multiple malignancies (except two breast cancers), of which at least two are considered Li-Fraumeni syndrome associated, before 46 years of age; (3) patients with adrenocortical carcinoma, choroid plexus carcinoma or embryonal anaplastic subtype rhabdomyoscarcoma (independent of family history); and (4) breast cancer before the age of 31 years old.[24] Approximately 70% of Li-Fraumeni kindreds have mutations in *TP53* gene, which produces the protein p53. Inheritance is in an autosomal dominant fashion. Penetrance is 50% by the age of 31 years among females and 50% by the age of 46 among males, and nearly 100% by the age of 70 years. Patients exhibit increased sensitivity to radiation; the irradiated field is susceptible to the development of new malignant neoplasms. For those kindreds who lack germline *TP53* mutations, a number of candidate genes have been proposed, including the cell cycle checkpoint kinases *CHK1* and *CHK2*, which directly phosphorylate p53. It is likely that other causative mutations involve p53 gene telomere length, aberrant gene methylation, and variant micro ribonucleic acids (RNAs) that modify p53 cell regulation, as well as accumulation of copy number variants.

Familial Adenomatous Polyposis and Related Polyposis Syndromes

FAP accounts for ~1% of the total colorectal cancer burden. It is an autosomal dominant condition caused by mutation in the *APC* gene, located on chromosome 5q21. Penetrance is extremely high, with colorectal cancer incidence approaching 100% by age 50.[25] It is characterized clinically by the development of several hundred to more than a thousand adenomatous polyps that carpet the colon. The first clear FAP kindreds were described in 1925 by the surgeon Lockhart-Mummery. The phenotype usually emerges during the second and third decades of life. The polyps are indistinguishable (macroscopically and microscopically) from sporadic adenomatous polyps, and each individual polyp does not have a greater propensity to undergo malignant degeneration than sporadic polyps. Rather, it is the sheer number of polyps that makes the collective risk of malignancy so high. Untreated individuals typically present with colorectal cancer at 35 to 40 years of age, around 30 years earlier than the median age for sporadic colorectal cancer. Extracolonic manifestations of FAP include upper gastrointestinal polyps (nearly 100% for duodenal adenomas, 10% for gastric adenomas, and 20%–84% fundic gland polyps), desmoid tumors (15%), thyroid cancer (2%–3%, usually papillary), congenital hypertrophy of the retinal pigment epithelium (70%–80%), fibromas (25%–50%), epidermoid cysts (50%), osteomas (50%–90%), and dental abnormalities. Polyps of the duodenum most commonly occur in the periampullary region. Surveillance is necessary of the upper gastrointestinal tract, and duodenal adenocarcinoma is the third leading cause of death in FAP, after metastatic colorectal carcinoma and desmoid tumors. Desmoid tumors are locally invasive fibromatoses that occur within the abdomen or abdominal wall.

The *APC* gene was first localized in 1987, then cloned in 1991, after mutation analyses of FAP kindreds. It encodes a 300-kDa protein, expressed in a variety of cell types, whose major function is as a scaffolding protein, affecting cell adhesion and migration. It is part of a protein complex, modulated by the Wnt signaling pathway, that regulates the phosphorylation and degradation of β-catenin. When *APC* is mutated, β-catenin is not phosphorylated and accumulates in the cytoplasm, where it binds to the TCF family of transcription factors, altering the expression of various genes involved in cell proliferation, migration, differentiation, and apoptosis. More than 700 disease-causing mutations in the *APC* gene have been reported. The most common of these involve a frameshift mutation (68%), a nonsense mutation (30%), or a large deletion (2%). Most of these mutations are located in what is referred to as the *mutation cluster region*, at the 5′ end of exon 15. The location of the mutation plays a role in determining the phenotype.[26] Mutations between codons 1250 and 1464 leads to profuse FAP, with earlier onset and increased polyp burden. Mutations between codon 157 and 1595 are considered intermediate FAP, and is associated with the classic phenotype. Congenital hypertrophy of the retinal pigment epithelium is associated with mutations between codons 311 and 1465. Gardner syndrome is variant of FAP associated osteomas of the mandible or skull, epidermal cysts, and multiple skin and soft tissue tumors, especially desmoids and thyroid tumors. Attenuated FAP is a phenotypically distinct variant of FAP in which (1) affected individuals have fewer than 100 adenomas, (2) the polyps are more proximally distributed in the colon, and (3) the onset of colorectal cancer is about 15 years later than in patients with FAP. Mutations responsible for this variant occur in the extreme upstream or downstream portions of the *APC* gene.

MYH-associated polyposis (MAP) is a syndrome caused by mutations in the human *MutY homologue (MYH)* gene. It accounts for about 20% of patients who have attenuated polyposis but who test negative for *APC* mutations. Unlike FAP, MAP is inherited in an autosomal *recessive* manner, although heterozygote carriers have a threefold increased risk for colorectal cancer (vs. fifty fold for biallelic carriers).[25] Phenotypically, MAP-associated colorectal cancer typically presents with an attenuated polyposis phenotype, often with less than 100 polyps, with a mean age of diagnosis of 50. The polyps are distributed throughout the colon. Extracolonic manifestations are common and, in some cases, indistinguishable from true FAP. Penetrance is estimated at 50% by age 60. The *MYH* gene encodes a DNA glycosylase involved in the base excision repair pathway, important in preventing mutations due to oxidative damage. The mutations Y179C on exon 7 and G396D on exon 13 account for ~80% of all cases. Mutation leads to chromosomal instability in which there is an accelerated rate of chromosomal misaggregation during cell division. This leads to aneuploidy, which has been recognized as an early genetic change in the stepwise carcinogenesis of both FAP and MAP tumors. Polyps bearing *MYH* mutations have twice the overall incidence of aneuploidy compared with those in patients with FAP.

Hereditary Nonpolyposis Colorectal Cancer

Also known as Lynch syndrome, hereditary nonpolyposis colorectal cancer (HNPCC) accounts for 2% to 3% of all colorectal cancers. It is an autosomal dominant condition caused by mutations in DNA mismatch repair genes.[25] The broad phenotype of HNPCC is of right-sided predominance of colonic cancers that appear at an earlier age (median age of diagnosis is 45 years), with increased likelihood of synchronous and metachronous cancers. Extracolonic malignant neoplasms occur, especially of the endometrium, ovary, urinary tract, small bowel, and stomach. Whereas the actual incidence of adenomatous polyps is the same as for those who develop sporadic colorectal cancer, once a tumor develops, there is an increased rate of tumor progression (accelerated carcinogenesis). This is due to the fact that the rate of genetic mutation in HNPCC tumors is two to three times higher than in normal cells. A colonic adenoma may progress to carcinoma within 2 to 3 years, in contrast to the 8 to 10 years typical of sporadic cases.

Mutations in DNA mismatch repair genes cause microsatellite instability (MSI, often referred to as MSI-high or MSI-H). Mi crosatellites are genomic regions in which short DNA sequences are repeated. During replication of these sequences, slippage of the DNA polymerase complex can occur, resulting in the formation of daughter strands that contain too many or too few copies of these sequences. Mutations may occur when these microsatellites are misaligned. The mutations then persist when the DNA mismatch repair proteins fail to correct the errors. This causes inactivation of tumor suppressor genes. Mutations in a number of DNA mismatch repair genes have been identified in patients with HNPCC, including *MSH2, PMS2, PMS1, MLH1, MSH6,* as well as *MSH2* promoter hypermethylation secondary to a germline epithelial cell adhesion molecule (EPCAM) mutation. Lifetime risk of colorectal cancer is nearly 70% in males and just over 50% in females. Gene mutation effects phenotype, with *MLH1, PMS1,* and *MSH2* leading to a higher lifetime risk of colorectal cancer. It should be noted that 15% of sporadic colorectal cancers have MSI, but it occurs through methylation silencing of the *MLH1* gene rather than through mutation as in HNPCC.

Currently, it is recommended that all newly diagnosed colorectal and endometrial cancers undergo testing for MSI. MSI-H tumors, regardless of primary tumor location, have been shown to respond remarkably well to antiprogrammed death receptor-1 immunotherapy, likely due to their characteristic high mutational burden.[27] In 2017, this led to the first ever tumor type agnostic cancer therapeutic approval for the programmed death receptor 1 drug pembrolizumab, for the treatment of metastatic MSI-H tumors.

BRCA1 and BRCA2

About 5% to 10% of all breast cancers are hereditary and attributable to mutations in high-penetrance susceptibility genes. These mutations are predominately linked to *BRCA1* and *BRCA2* and are found more often in people of Ashkenazi Jewish descent. In families with a history of hereditary breast and ovarian cancer, it is estimated that 90% are attributable to *BRCA1* or *BRCA2* mutations. The cumulative breast cancer risk at age 80 for a female *BRCA1* carrier is 72%, and 69% for a *BRCA2* carrier.[28]

Carriers are at risk for other cancers, especially of the ovary. Cumulative risk through age 80 for ovarian cancer in a female who is a carrier for *BRCA1* or *BRCA2* is 44% and 17%, respectively. Male carriers of *BRCA1* and *BRCA2* are at greater risk for prostate cancer, while breast cancer in males is most commonly attributed to *BRCA2*. *BRCA2* mutation is also associated with increased risk of melanoma and cancers of the pancreas, stomach, gallbladder, and biliary system. In a recent analysis, *BRCA2* mutation conferred a 6.2 times increased risk of pancreatic cancer, which was a similar risk to that seen in both Ataxia-Telangiectasia and Li-Fraumeni syndrome.[29]

The *BRCA1* gene is located on the long arm of chromosome 17. It is a large gene of some 100,000 nucleic acids, with many different mutations reported. The *BRCA2* gene, on chromosome 13, is even larger than *BRCA1*. As for *BRCA1*, the majority of alterations are frameshift or nonsense mutations, which produce a truncated protein. Both *BRCA1* and *BRCA2* are tumor suppressor genes; they are nonfunctional in malignant cells as a result of combined germline mutation followed by inactivation of the second allele in the tumor (the Knudson two-hit hypothesis). These genes have key roles in DNA damage repair, regulation of gene expression, and cell cycle control. Recent analysis has tied particular mutation location on *BRCA1* and *BRCA2* to distinct phenotypes. For instance, for *BRCA1* the c.68_69delAG mutation, the most frequent mutation among Ashkenazi Jews, confers an 84% risk of breast cancer by age 70, while for those with the c.2282 to c.4071 mutations, cumulative breast cancer risk at 70 was only 56%.[28]

Multiple Endocrine Neoplasia Type 1

MEN1 is an autosomal dominant condition characterized phenotypically by tumors of the parathyroid gland (leading to hyperparathyroidism), pancreatic islet cells, and the pituitary gland. Affected individuals can also develop lipomas, adenomas of the adrenal and thyroid glands, cutaneous angiofibromas, and carcinoid tumors.

Mutations in the tumor suppressor gene called *MEN1*, located on chromosome 11q13, are responsible for this syndrome; 80% of mutations identified result in the loss of function of the gene product, called *menin*. Menin is a 67-kDa protein predominantly found in the nucleus. It binds with a variety of proteins with roles in the regulation of transcription, DNA repair, and organization of the cytoskeleton. None of these menin pathways has yet been found to be critical in *MEN1* tumorigenesis.

Multiple Endocrine Neoplasia Type 2

All affected individuals with MEN2 develop MTC. It is subclassified into type A and type B. MEN2A is characterized by pheochromocytoma (50%) and hyperparathyroidism (25%). In addition to MTC and pheochromocytoma, MEN2B is characterized by mucosal neuromas on the tongue and lips and subconjunctival areas, intestinal ganglioneuromatosis, and a marfanoid body habitus. The majority of cases of MEN2B are the result of spontaneous new *RET* mutations.

Both types are caused by germline mutations in the *RET* (rearranged during transfection) proto-oncogene, located on chromosome 10q11. It encodes a transmembrane tyrosine kinase receptor, which is expressed on a wide variety of neuroendocrine and neural cells, including thyroid C cells, adrenal medullary cells, and autonomic ganglion cells. Once mutated, the receptor constitutively activates various signaling pathways, including p38/MAPK and JNK pathways.

von Hippel–Lindau Syndrome

von Hippel–Lindau (VHL) is a rare, autosomal dominant syndrome characterized by the development of highly vascularized tumors in multiple organs. VHL affects approximately 1 in 35,000 live births. Tumors associated with VHL include hemangioblastomas of the retina and central nervous system, renal cysts that develop into clear cell renal cell cancer, pheochromocytomas, endolymphatic sac tumors of the middle ear, and epididymal or round ligament cysts. It is caused by mutations in the *VHL* gene. Penetrance is 90% by the age of 65 years, with the mean age at diagnosis being 26 years. Since the discovery of the role of the *VHL* gene in this syndrome, mutations of this same gene have been found in the majority of sporadic clear cell renal cell carcinomas. That loss of *VHL* function is a critical event during renal cell carcinogenesis is supported by experiments in which introduction of wild-type *VHL* into *VHL*-deficient renal cancer cell lines resulted in suppression of tumor growth.

The protein product of the *VHL* gene is a 213 amino acid protein, pVHL. pVHL functions as a tumor suppressor and is part of the cell's response mechanism to hypoxia. Under conditions of low cellular oxygen tension, HIF1α and HIF2α regulate genes involved in metabolism, angiogenesis, erythropoiesis, and cell proliferation. pVHL targets the α subunit of HIF for oxygen-dependent proteolysis. Therefore, lack of pVHL results in persistence of the HIF complex with increased HIF transcriptional activity and upregulation of HIF target genes, including *VEGF*, *GLUT1*, and *erythropoietin*, independent of cellular oxygen levels. pVHL also has roles in regulating ECM turnover and microtubule stability.

Cancer Epigenetics

Epigenetic inheritance is defined as cellular information, other than the nucleotide sequence, that is heritable during cell division. There are three main interrelated forms: DNA methylation, genomic imprinting, and histone modification. These epigenetic templates control gene expression and can be transmitted to daughter cells independently of the DNA sequence.

DNA methylation and cancer has been the subject of much recent research. One of the best studied types of epigenetic change involving increased methylation is cytosine methylation at CpG dinucleotides. CpG islands are approximately 1-kilobase stretches of DNA containing clusters of CpG dinucleotides that are usually unmethylated in normal cells and are often located near the 5′ ends of genes. In normal cells, the cytosines of CpG islands are predominately unmethylated, while in cancer this pattern is often altered and referred to as CpG island methylator phenotype.[30] CpG island methylator phenotype can lead to silencing of the tumor suppressor *p16* and of DNA mismatch repair genes (e.g., *MLH1*). Another example of hypermethylation is seen in tumors with gain of function *IDH* mutations, which is common to gliomas, leukemias, as well as other tumors. Mutant IDH generates an oncometabolite that inhibits hydroxylases, and specifically TET enzymes, which function normally to catalyze demethylation. Therefore, DNA is hypermethylated and subsequently prevents binding of the DNA binding protein CTCF, which typically serves to protect genes from overactivation. This leads to increased gene activation and tumor growth. Finally, promoter methylation can lead to silencing of a given gene that has been implicated in cancer. For instance, *MGMT* encodes a DNA repair factor, and in some colorectal tumors hypermethylation of *MGMT* has been implicated. In this situation, *MGMT* promoter hypermethylation leads to gene silencing and thus increased ability of a cell to propagate errors in the DNA code. This epigenetic change is typically part of a field defect whereby multiple colorectal tumors arise within a given area of tissue—thus likely implicating environmental factors as the underlying inciting event.

Conversely, genes that are hypomethylated, leading to increased transcription, have been identified in tumors. A recent analysis identified a subset of testicular germ cell tumors with genome wide DNA hypomethylation.[31] Loss of methylation is particularly severe in pericentromeric satellite sequences, and cancers of the ovary and breast frequently contain unbalanced chromosomal translocations with breakpoints in the pericentromeric regions of chromosomes 1 and 16. The demethylation of these satellite sequences may predispose to their breakage and recombination.

Genomic imprinting refers to the conditioning of the maternal and paternal genomes during gametogenesis, such that a specific parental allele is more abundantly (or exclusively) expressed in the offspring. In Wilms tumors, loss of imprinting has been demonstrated to lead to pathologic biallelic expression of *IGF2*. This appears to occur in combination with hypermethylation of regions of the reciprocally imprinted *H19* gene. These two phenomena are the earliest detectable genetic changes in this cancer, strongly suggesting a gatekeeper role for epigenetic alterations in cancer.

The modification of histones (e.g., by acetylation, methylation, or phosphorylation) is important in the compaction of chromatin structure and is also crucial in cancer pathogenesis. For instance, histone lysine demethylases (KDMs) have been shown to play a role in cancer progression. It has been shown *in vitro* H3K4 demethylases (KDM5 family) enable lung cancer and melanoma cell lines to transition to a slow cycling state and thus evade anti proliferative therapy.[30] Overall, epigenetic changes in cancer are a crucial and exciting area of active research, with therapies targeting these changes being the subject of several ongoing trials.

Cancer Microbiome

Up until recently, the role of the microbiome in cancer pathogenesis and treatment response had been largely ignored. It is now believed that microbial pathogens drive tumorigenesis in 15% to 20% of cancers, with an altered microbiome being present in an even greater percentage of patients. Some of the tumor drivers associated with the microbiome, such as *Helicobacter pylori*, is touched on later in this chapter (see Carcinogenesis, Carcinogens subsection).

Dysbiosis of the gastrointestinal tract involves shifts in the abundance of commensal bacteria. It has been shown that colorectal cancers often have decreased abundance of *Bacteroidetes* and *Firmicutes* species, with overrepresentation of *Fusobacterium*.[32] In addition, the gut microbiome plays a crucial role in immunity, including tumor immunity. Multiple mechanisms have been implicated, for instance, via byproducts that activate components of the immune system (e.g., microbial-derived butyrate can induce naïve T cells to become regulatory T cells) and by in some cases disrupting gut barrier function and leading to altered mucosal immunity. More recently, intratumoral *Gammaproteobacteria*, found in pancreatic cancer specimens, was shown to metabolize gemcitabine and convert it to an inactive form.[33] There is also emerging evidence that an altered microbiota can be detrimental when treating cancer patients with immunotherapeutics.

Carcinogens

Any agent that can contribute to tumor formation is referred to as a carcinogen, which can be chemical, physical, or biologic. The International Agency for Research on Cancer (IARC) maintains a registry of human carcinogens that is available on the Internet (www.iarc.fr). The compounds are categorized into five groups based on epidemiological studies, animal models, and short-term mutagenesis tests. Group 1 contains what are considered to be proven human carcinogens (120 agents). Group 2A agents are probable human carcinogens for which there is limited evidence of carcinogenicity in humans but sufficient evidence to prove carcinogenicity in experimental animals (82 agents). The group 2B category includes agents that are possibly carcinogenic to humans for which there is limited evidence of carcinogenicity in humans and less than sufficient evidence of carcinogenicity in experimental animals (311 agents). There is inadequate evidence for carcinogenicity in humans or experimental animals for agents included in group 3 (499 agents). Group 4 agents are probably not carcinogenic to humans (1 agent).

Chemical Carcinogens

Chemicals that initiate carcinogenesis are extremely diverse in structure and function and include both natural and synthetic products (Tables 29.5 and 29.6). They fall into one of two categories: direct-acting compounds, which do not require chemical transformation for their carcinogenicity; and indirect-acting compounds, or procarcinogens, which require metabolic conversion in vivo for their carcinogenic effects. All these compounds, or their active metabolites in the latter category, share the essential property of being highly reactive electrophiles (have electron-deficient atoms) that can react with nucleophilic (electron-rich) sites in the cell. These reactions are nonenzymatic and result in the formation of covalent adducts between the chemical carcinogens and (almost always) DNA.

The majority of chemical carcinogens require metabolic activation for their carcinogenic effects. The metabolic pathway that produces the active metabolite may be just one of a number of metabolic pathways required for the degradation of the parent compound. Thus, the carcinogenic potency of the carcinogen is determined not just by the reactivity of the electrophilic derivatives but also by the balance between the metabolic activation and inactivation reactions. Most of the known carcinogens are metabolized by cytochrome P450–dependent mono-oxygenases. Because these enzymes are essential for the activation of procarcinogens, individual susceptibility to carcinogenesis is regulated in part by polymorphisms in the genes that encode these enzymes. For example, the product of the P450 gene *CYP1A1* metabolizes polycyclic aromatic hydrocarbons such as benzo(a)pyrene. About 10% of the white population has a highly inducible form of this enzyme that is associated with an increased risk of lung cancer in smokers. Light smokers with the susceptible genotype of *CYP1A1* have a sevenfold higher risk for development of lung cancer compared with smokers without the permissive genotype. Age, sex, and nutritional status also have an effect on the metabolism of carcinogens and thus their probability of inducing malignancy.

DNA is the primary target of chemical carcinogens. The ability of these compounds to induce mutations is termed mutagenic potential. The Ames test is the most common method for evaluating mutagenic potential and measures the ability of a chemical to induce mutations in the bacterium *Salmonella typhimurium*. The majority of known chemical carcinogens score positive on the Ames test, so it is useful for screening. However, not all compounds with mutagenic potential in vitro also have in vivo effects. Whereas there is no one mutation unique to all chemical carcinogens, individual compounds have been found to induce characteristic changes in DNA. For example, aflatoxin B1 induces a G:C→T:A transconversion in codon 249 of the *TP53* gene (249^{ser} *p53* mutation). Individuals from areas where there is a high level of exposure to aflatoxin B1 develop HCC with this characteristic mutation. This mutation is an otherwise uncommon occurrence in HCC caused by other agents, such as the hepatitis B virus (HBV).

The carcinogenicity of some chemicals is augmented by subsequent administration of other agents, called *promoters,* which are by themselves nontumorigenic. Such chemicals include phorbol esters, hormones, and phenols. Their fundamental characteristic is their ability to induce cell proliferation. Promotion may involve multiple compounds acting as promoters acting on different

TABLE 29.5 Selected IARC Group 1 chemical carcinogens.

CHEMICAL CARCINOGEN	MEANS OF EXPOSURE	PREDOMINANT TUMOR TYPE
Aflatoxins	Ingestion of contaminated maize and peanuts grown in hot, humid climates	Hepatocellular carcinoma
Alcohol	Ingestion	Squamous cell carcinoma of the oropharynx and esophagus, breast cancer, colorectal cancer, hepatocellular carcinoma, and intrahepatic cholangiocarcinoma
Arsenic	Ingestion; also inhalation by smelter workers	Skin cancer, lung cancer, hepatic angiosarcoma
Asbestos	Inhalation, historically shipbuilding and exhaust/ventilation system installation	Mesothelioma, lung cancer
Benzene	Inhalation, especially in gasoline-related industries or in the production of other chemicals from benzene	Leukemia
Benzidine	Inhalation by workers in the dye industry	Cancer of the urinary bladder
Beryllium	Inhalation by workers in the refining of the metal and production of beryllium-containing products; also those in the aircraft, aerospace, electronics, and nuclear industries	Lung cancer
Cadmium	Inhalation by workers in cadmium production and refining, nickel-cadmium battery manufacturing, and other cadmium-related industries	Lung cancer
Coal tars	Inhalation, transcutaneous absorption in a variety of industrial settings	Skin cancer, scrotal cancer
Chromium compounds	Inhalation during chromium plating, chromate production, welding	Lung cancer
Diethylstilbestrol	In-utero exposure (1938–1971)	Clear cell adenocarcinoma of the vagina and cervix
Ethylene oxide	Inhalation during production of various industrial chemicals (e.g., ethylene glycol)	Leukemia, lymphoma
Naphthylamine	Dye industry	Cancer of urinary bladder
Nickel	Inhalation, ingestion, or skin contact in nickel or nickel alloy production plants, welding, or electroplating operations	Lung cancer, nasal cancer
Radon	Inhalation in underground mines, basements	Lung cancer
Silica	Quarry and granite workers, ceramics, refractory brick	Lung cancer
Thorium-232/Thorotrast	Medical use as contrast agent until 1950s, well water use near factory using thorium (e.g., aerospace)	Hepatic angiosarcoma, lung cancer, pancreatic cancer, gallbladder, bile duct cancer
Tobacco smoke	Inhalation	Lung cancer, oropharyngeal cancer, laryngeal cancer, esophageal cancer, pancreatic cancer
Vinyl chloride	Inhalation during production of polyvinyl chloride (e.g., PVC pipes)	Hepatic angiosarcoma, hepatocellular carcinoma, brain tumors, lung cancer, hematopoietic malignant neoplasms

Based on information from IARC Monographs on the Evaluation of Carcinogenic Risks to Humans: International Agency for Research on Cancer (IARC), 2018. (https://monographs.iarc.fr/wp-content/uploads/2018/07/Table4.pdf). *IARC*, International Association for Research on Cancer.

TABLE 29.6 Selected IARC Group 1 pharmaceutical carcinogens.

PHARMACEUTICAL CARCINOGEN	PREDOMINANT TUMOR TYPE
Azathioprine	Non-Hodgkin lymphoma, squamous cell cancer of the skin, hepatocellular carcinoma, cholangiocarcinoma
Cyclophosphamide	Cancer of the urinary bladder, leukemia
Chlorambucil	Leukemia
Cyclosporine	Leukemia, lymphoma, nonmelanoma skin cancer
Tamoxifen	Endometrial cancer
Estrogens (OCP, HRT)	Cancer of the breast and endometrium

Based on information from IARC Monographs on the Evaluation of Carcinogenic Risks to Humans: International Agency for Research on Cancer (IARC), 2018 (https://monographs.iarc.fr/wp content/uploads/2018/07/Table4.pdf). *HRT,* Hormone replacement therapy; *IARC,* International Agency for Research on Cancer;*OCP,* oral contraceptive pill.

regulatory pathways. The end result is the clonal expansion of initiated cells.

Radiation Carcinogenesis

The two most important forms of radiation causing malignant change in humans are ultraviolet (UV) radiation and ionizing radiation (IR). Whereas IR has been found to cause a variety of cancers, UV radiation is principally implicated in the causation of skin cancers. There is typically a long latency period between radiation exposure and clinical development of cancer.

UV radiation is a known risk factor for squamous cell carcinoma, basal cell carcinoma, and possibly malignant melanoma (the latter of which is tied more so to severe sunburn events, while the former two cancers are tied to cumulative UV radiation). The degree of risk depends on the type of UV rays, the intensity of exposure, and the quantity of melanin present in the individual's skin. The UV portion of the electromagnetic spectrum can be divided into three wavelength ranges: UVA (320–400 nm), UVB (280–320 nm), and UVC (200–280 nm). Of these, UVB is the most important. UVC, also a potent mutagen, is filtered out by the planetary ozone layer. The carcinogenicity of UVB is due to its formation of pyrimidine dimers in DNA. This damage may be repaired by the nucleotide excision repair pathway. This is a multistep process involving recognition of the damaged DNA strands, their incision and removal, and synthesis of a patch containing the correct nucleotide sequence, which is then annealed to the DNA structure. With excessive sun exposure, it is postulated that the capacity of this pathway is overwhelmed, and some DNA damage remains unrepaired. Xeroderma pigmentosum, characterized by extreme photosensitivity and a 2000-fold increased risk of skin cancer, is caused by mutations in the genes involved in nucleotide excision repair.

IR includes both electromagnetic (x-rays, gamma rays) and particulate (alpha particles, beta particles, protons, neutrons) forms. IR can act both a carcinogen and a therapeutic agent. IR is composed of electrically charged particles that pass through tissue and deposit energy, with the goal being that they will lead to death of rapidly dividing cancer cells. IR works via directly causing single and double stranded DNA breaks, as well as indirectly by causing radiolysis of water inside cells, leading to ROS generation. The predominant ROS formed are hydroxyl free radicals, which go on to cause further DNA damage. IR also works indirectly by inducing the cytosolic Rac1/NADPH oxidase system, which further leads to ROS formation and resultant DNA damage. ROS are key to cellular damage, and cancer cells that are surviving under hypoxic conditions are three times as resistant to radiation induced damage, as compared to aerobic cells. In addition to effects on tumor cells, it has been shown that modern day targeted radiotherapy often leads to upregulation of antitumor immune markers, and there may be a synergistic role when combining radiotherapy with immune-based therapy.

The goal of IR is to kill tumor cells while sparing as much of the normal cell mass as possible. Normal cells are often able to upregulate DNA damage repair enzymes, such as PARP1, which recognizes single cell DNA breaks and recruits enzymes to repair the damage. Double-stranded breaks are recognized by ATM, together with MRE-RAD50 and NBS1, and repaired. It thus makes sense that *ATM* biallelic mutation, as seen in patients with ataxia-telangiectasia, is considered an absolute contraindication to radiation therapy. Radiation therapy has typically been employed in diseases such as breast cancer and rectal cancer to improve locoregional control. This has largely been shown, but, due to the described potential off-target effects, there is a small but real risk of secondary malignancy. In a recent study of nearly 400,000 women with predominantly early stage breast cancer who underwent adjuvant radiotherapy, 13% of patients had a secondary malignancy at a median follow up of ~9 years, of which 3.4% were tied to radiation therapy treatment.[34]

Survivors of the atomic bombs dropped on Hiroshima and Nagasaki were exposed to a large burden of IR, and many developed leukemias at an average latency period of seven years. Survivors have also suffered an increased incidence of solid organ tumors (e.g., breast, colon, thyroid, and lung). Irradiation of the head and neck in childhood has been associated with a high incidence of thyroid cancer in adulthood.

There is a defined vulnerability of different tissues to radiation-induced carcinogenesis. Most vulnerable is the hematopoietic cell line, causing leukemias (except chronic lymphocytic leukemia), followed by the thyroid gland. In the intermediate category are breast, lung, and salivary glands. The skin, bone, and gastrointestinal tract are relatively radioresistant.

TABLE 29.7 Selected IARC Group 1 infectious carcinogens.

INFECTIOUS CARCINOGENS	PREDOMINANT TUMOR TYPE
DNA Viruses	
Epstein-Barr virus	Burkitt lymphoma, Hodgkin disease, immunosuppression-related lymphoma, nasopharyngeal carcinoma
Hepatitis B	Hepatocellular carcinoma
Human papillomavirus types 16, 18	Cervical cancer, anal cancer
Kaposi sarcoma-associated herpesvirus (HHV-8)	Kaposi sarcoma
RNA Viruses	
Hepatitis C	Hepatocellular carcinoma
Human immunodeficiency virus type 1/AIDS	*AIDS Defining:* Kaposi sarcoma, cervical cancer, non-Hodgkin lymphoma *Non-AIDS Defining:* Lung cancer, anal cancer, Hodgkin lymphoma, oropharyngeal cancer, hepatocellular carcinoma, vulvar, penile cancer
Human T-cell lymphotropic virus type 1	Adult T-cell leukemia/lymphoma
Bacteria	
Helicobacter pylori	Gastric adenocarcinoma, gastric MALT lymphoma, gastric diffuse large B cell lymphoma
Parasites	
Clonorchis sinensis, Opisthorchis viverrini	Cholangiocarcinoma, hepatocellular carcinoma
Schistosoma haematobium	Cancer of the urinary bladder

Based on information from IARC Monographs on the Evaluation of Carcinogenic Risks to Humans: International Agency for Research on Cancer (IARC), 2018 (https://monographs.iarc.fr/wp-content/uploads/2018/07/Table4.pdf). *AIDS*, Acquired immunodeficiency syndrome; *DNA*, deoxyribonucleic acid; *HHV-8*, human herpesvirus type 8; *IARC*, International Agency for Research on Cancer; *MALT*, mucosa-associated lymphoid tissue; *RNA*, ribonucleic acid.

Infectious Carcinogens

One of the first observations that cancer may be caused by transmissible agents was by Peyton Rous in 1911, when he demonstrated that cell-free extracts from sarcomas in chickens could transmit sarcomas to other animals injected with these extracts. This was subsequently discovered to represent viral transmission of cancer by the Rous sarcoma virus. Infectious agents (Table 29.7) may cause or increase the risk of malignancy by a number of mechanisms, including direct transformation, expression of oncogenes that interfere with cell cycle checkpoints or DNA repair, expression of cytokines or other growth factors, and alteration of the immune system.

Viral Carcinogenesis. Approximately 12% of all human tumors worldwide are caused by viruses, with over 80% of these cases occurring in the developing world.[35] This number reflects predominantly two malignant neoplasms: cervical cancer caused by human papillomavirus and hepatocellular cancer caused by HBV and hepatitis C virus (HCV).

BOX 29.1 Principles and strategies of viral carcinogenesis.

Common Traits of Viral Oncogenesis

- Oncoviruses are necessary but not sufficient for viral carcinogenesis.
- Viral-related cancers occur in the context of persistent infection and only many years after initial infection.
- The immune system can play a provirus or an antivirus role.

Human Oncovirus Replication and Persistence Strategies

- Find/create conditions for replication.
  - Induce cell cycle; metabolic reprogramming; inducing angiogenesis
- Ensure correct replication.
  - Recruit or inhibit DDR*
- Maximize virus production.
  - Prevent apoptosis until virion matures; immune evasion
- Multiply latent episomes or provirus.
  - Cell survival; cell immortalization; cell proliferation

Adapted from Mesri EA, Feitelson MA, Munger K. Human viral oncogenesis: A cancer hallmarks analysis. *Cell Host Microbe.* 2014;15:266–282.

DDR, DNA damage response.

*If viruses contain a DNA genome, viral DNA is sensed by host DDR, which can lead to viral growth inhibition. But, when the virus evades DDR mechanisms and survives, the upregulated DDR pathway leads to increased cell mutation acquisition, some of which may lead to oncogenesis.

Tenets of Viral Carcinogenesis. Oncoviruses and their human hosts have both evolved in parallel, which the goal of each being to survive. Humans have developed immune defenses to eradicate viruses, and viruses have evolved mechanisms to evade host defenses. Oncoviruses work to establish long-term infection while evading the immune system. These oncoviruses employ several strategies to survive and proliferate (Box 29.1).

DNA Oncoviruses. DNA tumor viruses are often dependent on the host cell machinery to replicate the viral genome, with several viruses in this class harboring oncogenic potential. For example, Epstein-Barr virus (EBV) is associated with several types of lymphoma and nasopharyngeal carcinoma. EBV can remain latent in host B cells and, in certain instances, is able to lead to cancer formation. Through a series of well-defined events, EBV is able to drive B cells to become resting memory B cells, where only EBV RNA is expressed and not EBV protein products. In dividing memory B cells, EBV is able to switch to one of three discrete cellular programs (so called Latency I, II, and III) that leads to cancer formation (Latency I: Burkitt lymphoma, Latency II: Hodgkin disease and nasopharyngeal carcinoma, and Latency III: immunosuppression-related lymphoma).

Human papillomavirus, which accounts for 5% of cancer worldwide, is a DNA virus with 150 subtypes. Of these subtypes, types 16 and 18 are considered highest risk for oncogenic potential. These high-risk subtypes encode E6 and E7 proteins. E6 binds to the tumor suppressor p53 and targets it for ubiquitin-mediated degradation, while E7 targets the tumor suppressor Rb, leading to Rb proteosomal degradation. These tumorigenic events lead to cervical and anal cancer. A vaccine is now available that prevents these high-risk subtypes of human papillomavirus.[36]

Another DNA oncovirus is Merkel cell polyomavirus, which is associated with up to 80% of cases of Merkel cell carcinoma. Viral positivity seen in Merkel cell carcinoma leads to the presentation of highly immunogenic viral antigens to lymphocytes, which enabled a remarkable response rate to antiPD1 immunotherapy (objective response rate [ORR] 56% in advanced Merkel cell carcinoma).[37] Other DNA oncoviruses include Kaposi sarcoma–associated herpesvirus, and HBV (see Table 29-7).

RNA Oncoviruses. The genetic machinery of RNA viruses consists of RNA, as opposed to DNA. Some RNA oncoviruses termed retroviruses, are comprised of a single-stranded RNA viral genome that is transcribed into a double-stranded DNA copy, which is then integrated into the chromosomal DNA of the cell. Two oncogenic viruses under this family are human T-cell leukemia and lymphoma virus 1, which leads to adult T-cell leukemia/lymphoma and human immunodeficiency virus-1. Human T-cell leukemia and lymphoma virus 1 infects mature CD4+ T cells, and drives oncogenesis via two distinct and well-defined stages. First, the viral oncoprotein Tax is upregulated, and leads to cell survival and proliferation. Later, human T-cell leukemia and lymphoma virus 1 bZIP (HBZ) protein is upregulated. HBZ serves to promote cell survival and replication (e.g., by increasing transcription of the E2F promoter) and also by evading immune destruction. These two stages of oncogenic process lead to the development of adult T-cell leukemia and lymphoma. Human immunodeficiency virus-1 is associated with several different cancers. The mechanism of cancer formation includes chronic inflammation, Ag stimulation, altered cytokine release, and increased oncovirus infection rate. In addition, CD4+ T-cell counts under 200 (thus being termed AIDS) lead to potential AIDS-defining malignancies (e.g., Kaposi sarcoma, non-Hodgkin lymphoma, and cervical cancer).

Hepatitis B and C Viruses. HBV is a small enveloped DNA virus, while HCV is a small RNA virus. Both are spread primarily via blood transmission (HBV and HCV) or bodily fluids (HBV). Chronic infection with HBV or HCV can lead to liver inflammation, hepatocyte destruction, and fibrosis, which can lead to cirrhosis and HCV. HCC is a major cause of cancer related mortality, and currently stands as the third leading cause of cancer death globally. HBV and HCV undergo endocytosis by hepatocytes, whereby HBV DNA, but not HCV RNA, is integrated into the genome of hepatocytes. There are eight well described HBV genotypes, with type C being predominant in the United States. This genotype has a propensity to lead to advanced liver fibrosis and higher rates of HCC. The rate of development of chronic infection in acutely infected individuals is 5% to 10% (90% in infants). For those with chronic infection, without treatment, 40% will develop cirrhosis. HCV has 6 major genotypes, with type 1 being the most common and the most difficult to treat. Unlike with HBV, the majority of those infected with HCV (~75%) will go on to develop chronic disease.

One major player in chronic HBV-mediated HCC carcinogenesis is HBV-encoded X Ag (HBx). HBx stimulates cell division and growth by activating both cyclins and cyclin-dependent kinases and also by directly suppressing p53 (via direct binding) and Rb (by phosphorylation).[35] Hbx also stimulates pathways such as RAS and JAK/STAT, and nuclear HBx leads to increased activation of transcription factors such as SMAD4 and ATF-3. HBx further prevents apoptosis by blocking caspases-8 and -3 and by activating NF-κB. HBx also leads to increased inflammatory cytokine production. Furthermore, HBx increases formation of ROS while promoting cell survival via upregulation of HIF1α, which activates angiogenesis. All of these factors, and others not mentioned, help lead to liver damage and HCC formation. HBx can also promote HCC invasion and distant metastasis by increasing expression of matrix metalloproteinases. HCV encodes the proteins NS3 and NS5A, both of which act via β-catenin to increase hepatocyte proliferation. In addition, HCV-encoded core protein leads to cyclin E and CDK2 expression and thus increased cell cycle progression and cell growth. Furthermore, HCV core and NS3 protein block multiple tumor suppressors, and core protein inhibits caspase-8, thus inhibiting cellular apoptosis. miR-181 has been shown to promote stem markers in HCC and is upregulated in both HBV and HCV. VEGF, which promotes angiogenesis, has also been shown to be upregulated in both HBV and HCV. Luckily, there are now active drugs available to fight chronic HBV and HCV infection, and there has been an effective vaccine available to prevent HBV since the 1980s.[36]

Bacterial Carcinogenesis. *H. pylori* infection is the only bacterial infection listed as a level I carcinogen by the IARC. It was the first bacterium ever directly linked to human cancer. Infection with strains of *H. pylori* that carry the cytotoxin-associated antigen A *(cagA)* gene is associated with gastric carcinoma. The *cagA* gene product, CagA, is delivered into gastric epithelial cells by the bacterial type IV secretion system—in essence, a molecular syringe.[38] Once it is intracellular, CagA is tyrosine phosphorylated by SRC family kinases and then is able to specifically bind and activate the oncogenic phosphatase SHP2. Activated SHP2 has been implicated in several cancers. In addition, in gastric epithelial cells, CagA can lead to p53 degradation. Finally, the Type 4 secretion mechanism described interacts with integrin-β1, which then recruits NF-κB and leads to transcription of prosurvival NF-κB genes. *H. pylori* also leads to a chronic inflammatory state and β-catenin pathway activation.

In addition to *H. pylori,* several other bacteria are felt to contribute to cancer formation, although no other bacteria are listed as level 1 carcinogens. One example is *Chlamydia trachomatis* of which infection targets the lower urogenital tract. Infection leads to epigenetic changes and induces host DNA damage. In addition, p53 degradation is promoted. It is felt to contribute to cervical carcinoma risk.

Parasite Carcinogenesis

Parasites have also been demonstrated to drive tumor formation. The liver flukes *Clonorchis sinensis* and *Opisthorchis viverrini*, endemic in several countries in the eastern hemisphere, are both level 1 carcinogens and have been implicated as causative factors in some cases of cholangiocarcinoma and are also associated with (although to a lesser degree) HCC. Both *C. sinensis* and *O. viverrini* feed on the biliary epithelial cells.[39] Damage to these cells, along with excretory products released from the flukes, leads to biliary tree damage and ulceration. Chronic, longstanding infection is thought to progress to metaplasia, followed by dysplasia and then cancer. The blood fluke *Schistosoma haematobium* is also considered to be a level 1 carcinogen and has been implicated in cancers of the urinary bladder. *S. haematobium* is predominately present in Africa and the Middle East and infects the urogenital tract. It leads to chronic inflammation, which proceeds to dysplasia and cancer. First-line treatment for infection with all flukes discussed is praziquantel.

Chronic Inflammation

Chronic inflammation in the absence of infection has long been linked with the development of cancer. Examples include the development of squamous cell carcinoma of the skin in areas of chronic ulceration (Marjolin ulcer), the high risk for colorectal cancer in patients with ulcerative colitis, and the recently discussed cholangiocarcinoma risk seen in people with longstanding *C. sinensis* infection. One mechanism of cancer development involves inflammation leading to expression of proinflammatory transcription factors such as NF-κB, HIF1α, and/or STAT3.[19] These transcription factors lead to upregulation of different enzymes (e.g., COX2), as well as cytokines and chemokines (e.g., IL-6 and TNFα). This leads to the recruitment of multiple different immune cells, which drive tumorigenesis. There is also some data that antiinflammatory drugs can prevent and/or help treat cancer in some patient subsets, thus further suggesting a role of inflammation driving a portion of tumorigenesis.

TUMOR MARKERS

Tumor markers are indicators of cellular, biochemical, molecular, or genetic alterations by which neoplasia can be recognized. They are surrogate measures of the biology of the cancer, providing insight into the clinical behavior of the tumor. This is particularly useful when the cancer is not clinically detectable. The information provided may help to distinguish benign from malignant disease; it may correlate with the amount of tumor present ("tumor burden"); it may allow subtype classification to more accurately stage patients; it may be prognostic, either by the presence or absence of the marker or by its concentration; and it may guide choice of therapy and predict response to therapy.

The ideal tumor marker has three defining characteristics. First, the marker should be expressed exclusively by the particular tumor. Second, collection of the specimen for the tumor marker assay should be easy. Third, the assay itself should be reproducible, rapid, and inexpensive. Currently, there is no one marker that fulfils all these criteria for any cancer, nor is there any specific cancer for which there are biomarkers that completely describe its behavior.

Tumor markers fall into four broad categories: whole cells, proteins, RNA, and DNA (Box 29.2). Tumor markers found in body fluids, particularly blood and urine, have the greatest potential for clinical application because of the ease of access to these fluids for analysis and because repeated sampling allows in vivo monitoring

BOX 29.2 Tumor biomarkers.

Whole Cells
Whole tumor cells

Proteins
Tumor-associated proteins

RNA-Based Markers
Tumor RNA
- mRNA, miRNA, lncRNA

DNA-Based Markers
Tumor DNA
- Single-nucleotide polymorphisms
- Gene fusions
- Changes in DNA copy number

Epigenetic changes
- Differential methylation

Overview of potential tumor biomarkers. Whole cells: at tumor site or in circulation; Proteins/DNA/RNA: in context of biopsy from tumor or secreted/shed from tumor.
lncRNA, Long noncoding RNA; *mRNA,* messenger RNA: *miRNA,* micro RNA.

of the malignant disease for such things as progression or recurrence, metastasis, and response to therapy.

Rather than provide an exhaustive review of all tumor markers, this section outlines the major categories of tumor markers and focuses on the evidence for the tumor markers currently in clinical use. Of note, protein biomarkers and DNA mutational analysis are part of FDA- and CLIA-approved laboratory testing that are routinely used for clinical evaluation of patients with various solid tumors. Analysis of RNA, proteomics, circulating tumor DNA (ctDNA), circulating tumor cells (CTCs), and epigenetics are currently not approved for clinical use but will likely have approval based on a wealth of preclinical data that is emerging, supporting their use as predictive and prognostic diagnostics.

Protein Tumor Markers

Proteins were the first type of tumor marker identified and hence are considered the "classic" tumor markers. However, despite decades of research, relatively few are in clinical use. Those routinely used generally fall short when it comes to both sensitivity and specificity. Their concentrations in serum or plasma generally correlate with tumor burden as they are shed from the expanding neoplasm.

Carcinoembryonic Antigen

Carcinoembryonic antigen (CEA) is probably the most studied cancer tumor marker and is predominantly used clinically in patients with colorectal cancers. It is an oncofetal protein that is normally present during fetal life but can be present in low concentrations in healthy adults.[40] Structurally, it is a glycoprotein with a molecular mass of 200 kDa and is a component of the glycocalyx, located on the luminal side of the cell membrane of normal epithelial intestinal cells. CEA is a member of a large family of proteins that are related to the immunoglobulin gene superfamily. The molecule itself is secreted into the circulation and is also found in the mucous secretions of the stomach, small intestine, and biliary tree. CEA has been shown to be involved in cell adhesion and is able to inhibit apoptosis induced by loss of anchorage to the ECM.

Testing. Immunoassay kits allow determination of serum CEA levels accurately, reproducibly, and relatively inexpensively. Serum levels of less than 2.5 ng/mL are normal; 2.5 to 5.0 ng/mL, borderline; and greater than 5.0 ng/mL, elevated. Borderline levels may occur with benign disorders such as inflammatory bowel disease, pancreatitis, cirrhosis, and chronic obstructive pulmonary disease. Smoking can also increase CEA; the upper limit of normal in smokers should be 5 ng/mL.

Screening. CEA is not useful as a screening test because of its low sensitivity in early-stage disease. Elevated CEA levels occur in only 5% to 40% of patients with localized disease.

Prognosis. Elevated CEA levels reflect the burden of tumor present. The degree of CEA elevation correlates with increasing stage of disease, and therefore CEA levels have prognostic value. Preoperative serum CEA is an independent predictor of survival; the higher the preoperative serum level, the poorer the prognosis. This effect persists even after patients are stratified for resectability and extent of local tumor invasion.

Monitoring. The most common application of CEA is in monitoring of patients for recurrent disease. A CEA level of greater than 5 ng/mL in any patient who has undergone treatment for colorectal adenocarcinoma should be considered tumor recurrence unless proven otherwise.[40] A 5-ng/mL cutoff for recurrence has a sensitivity of 71% and specificity of 88%, while using a 10- ng/mL cutoff has a sensitivity for of 68% and specificity of 97%. A recent Cochrane review therefore recommends using a 10-mg/mL cutoff during monitoring.[41]

CEA is also useful in monitoring response to chemotherapy in patients with metastatic colorectal cancer. An elevated CEA level is an independent factor associated with poor survival and progression on 5-fluorouracil–based chemotherapy in patients with metastatic colorectal cancer. Moreover, patients with advanced cancer whose CEA levels fall during chemotherapy survive significantly longer than those patients whose CEA levels do not change or increase.

α-Fetoprotein

α-Fetoprotein (AFP) is used in the detection and management of HCC. It is an oncofetal antigen consisting of a single-chain polypeptide with molecular mass of 700 kDa. Levels are elevated in the fetus, fall to low levels after birth, and are elevated during pregnancy. It is synthesized by hepatocytes and endodermally-derived gastrointestinal tissues.

Testing. AFP is measured with immunoassay kits. The upper limit of normal for a healthy, nonpregnant adult is less than 10 ng/mL. Unfortunately, AFP is far from a perfect tumor marker, and in one study using a cutoff as 20 ng/mL as elevated, sensitivity for positivity in patients with known HCC was only 54%. Levels of AFP are also raised in nonseminomatous testicular cancer, for which it is a valuable tumor marker (see Tumor Markers, Alpha Fetoprotein and Human Chorionic Gonadotropin in Testicular Germ Cell Tumors subsection). AFP can also be elevated with intrahepatic cholangiocarcinoma, some colorectal cancer metastases, or in patients with liver disease and no underlying HCC.

Screening. For screening purposes in high-risk populations, AFP is used in addition to ultrasound imaging. A cutoff of 100 ng/mL is typically used, although this varies significantly. In a recent metaanalysis of HCC screening for cirrhotic patients, ultrasound and AFP had a sensitivity of 97% picking up HCC (78% ultrasound alone),[42] although sensitivity for early stage disease for combined ultrasound for AFP screening is predictably lower (sensitivity 63%). Of note, AFP elevation cutoffs for these studies ranged from 15 to 200 ng/mL. AFP on its own is a poor screening tool, with a sensitivity of only 31%.

Prognosis. AFP concentration reflects tumor size, with levels above 400 ng/mL associated with larger tumors. As a result, it has been shown that AFP correlates with stage and prognosis. The rate of increase, expressed as AFP doubling time, has also been associated with poorer prognosis. In addition, AFP response to therapy has been correlated with both recurrence-free and overall survival.

Monitoring. AFP has been shown to decline after resection or ablation, and levels after complete resection should be less than10 ng/mL. In addition, AFP levels usually decline in response to effective chemotherapy. Monitoring of AFP therefore avoids prolonged use of ineffective chemotherapy. AFP is part of the standard surveillance regimen for HCC patients on the transplant list.

Carbohydrate Antigen 19-9

Carbohydrate antigen 19-9 (CA 19-9) is widely used as a serum marker of pancreatic ductal adenocarcinoma, but its use is limited to monitoring responses to therapy, not as a diagnostic marker. It is a mucin-type glycoprotein expressed on the surface of pancreatic cancer cells and was initially detected by monoclonal antibodies raised against colon cancer cell lines in a mouse model. The CA 19-9 epitope is normally present within the biliary tree. Biliary tract disease, both acute and chronic, can elevate serum CA 19-9 levels.

Testing. CA 19-9 is detected by an immunoassay, with the upper limit of normal for a healthy adult being 37 U/mL. The utility of CA 19-9 as a diagnostic marker is limited in a number of ways. First, patients with negative Lewis[a] blood group antigen (10% of population) cannot synthesize CA 19-9, and therefore it should not be used as a serologic marker in these individuals. Second, patients with benign biliary tract disease can have elevated levels. Third, besides pancreas cancer, CA 19-9 levels are also elevated in patients with other cancers, including those of the biliary tree (95%), stomach (5%), colon (15%), liver (HCC, 7%), and lung (13%).

Screening. Serum CA 19-9 greater than 37 U/mL in the diagnosis of pancreatic ductal adenocarcinoma has a sensitivity of 79% to 80% and aspecificity of 82% to 90% in clinically symptomatic patients. Unfortunately, positive predictive value for pancreatic cancer when used as a screening modality in the general population is a mere 0.9%. Thus, CA 19-9 is not considered to be useful as a screening tool. In symptomatic patients, increasing levels of CA 19-9 make the diagnosis of pancreatic cancer more accurate. In this population, when a cutoff level of 100 U/mL is used, the specificity is a near perfect 98%.

Prognosis. In those patients with pancreatic cancer who have CA 19-9 detectable in their serum, the level has been shown to correlate with tumor burden. For example, higher CA 19-9 levels typically correlate with higher tumor stage. Of patients who undergo curative resection, those whose CA 19-9 levels returned to normal survive longer than those whose levels do not.

Monitoring. Serial measurement of CA 19-9 is used to monitor response to therapy. In addition, a rise in CA 19-9 level after curative resection has been shown to precede clinical or imaging evidence of recurrence. In patients with unresectable or metastatic disease, failure of CA 19-9 levels to fall with chemotherapy reflects poor tumor response. However, in both settings, the lack of alternative effective therapies limits the utility of serial monitoring of CA 19-9.

Prostate-Specific Antigen

Prostate-specific antigen (PSA) is a serine protease that is formed in the prostatic epithelium and is secreted into the prostatic ducts. Its function is to digest the gel that is formed in seminal fluid after ejaculation. Under normal circumstances, only small amounts of PSA leak into the circulation. With enlargement of the gland (e.g., in patients with benign prostatic hyperplasia) or distortion of its architecture, serum PSA levels increase. Thus, PSA is considered a tissue-specific rather than a prostate cancer–specific marker; patients who have undergone curative radical prostatectomy as well as women have no detectable PSA.

Testing

PSA is detected with an immunoassay. Besides benign prostatic hyperplasia, other instances in which serum PSA levels may be elevated include prostatitis, prostatic massage, prostatic biopsy, and digital rectal examination—although elevation after digital rectal examination is minimal and testing for PSA level can be done even after a digital rectal examination in the same clinic visit. Initial studies set the upper limit of normal for PSA at 4 ng/mL, with levels greater than 10 ng/mL suggestive of malignancy and levels of 4 to 10 ng/mL being indeterminate. Since then, it has been found that the upper limit of the normal range of PSA increases with age. The typical limit is 2.5 ng/mL for those aged 40 to 49 years, 3.5 ng/mL for those 50 to 59 years, 4.5 ng/mL for those 60 to 69 years, and 6.5 ng/mL for those 70 years and older. The rate of increase of PSA in a normal 60-year-old is 0.04 ng/mL /year, and a change of 0.75 ng/mL/year or greater is generally considered abnormal. The ratio of free to total PSA has also been found to improve the specificity of prostate cancer diagnosis in the PSA range of 4 to 10 ng/mL, with a free to total PSA ratio of less than 10% being considered abnormal.

Screening

PSA is widely used as a screening tool for prostate cancer, enabling early detection and diagnosis of this disease. However, its use has been called into question. The European Randomized Study of Screening for Prostate Cancer (ERSPC) randomized 162,387 men to either screening with PSA or no screening. At a 13-year follow-up, there was a statistically significant, but small, decrease in prostate cancer specific mortality in those assigned to screening. There was a mere 1.1 increase in prostate cancer deaths per 10,000 person-years improvement in those assigned to PSA screening versus those not screened (4.3 vs. 5.4 prostate cancer-specific deaths per 10,000 person-years, respectively). In the Prostate, Lung, Colorectal and Ovary Cancer (PLCO) trial, 76,693 U.S. men were randomized, and with a median 14.8 years of follow-up, there was no significant difference in prostate cancer mortality (4.8 vs. 4.6 prostate cancer-specific deaths per 10,000 person-years for control and screening groups, respectively). This has led the United States Preventative Service Task Force (USPSTF) to provide an evidence grade of C (offer service on a selected basis) to screening men between 55 and 69 years of age, and a grade of D (discourage use) for screening in men 70 years of age or older.

Prognosis and Monitoring Response to Therapy

After operative resection, the PSA level is expected to normalize after 2 to 3 weeks. Patients whose PSA level remained elevated 6 months after radical prostatectomy typically develop recurrent disease. In contrast, it takes 3 to 5 months for the PSA level to normalize after radiotherapy. However, failure of the PSA level to normalize after radiotherapy also predicts relapse. Rise in serum PSA level is usually the first sign of either local recurrence or metastatic progression. In patients with advanced disease, PSA levels are also used to monitor response to systemic therapy.

Carbohydrate Antigen 125

Carbohydrate antigen 125 (CA 125, also known as MUC16) is a carbohydrate epitope on a glycoprotein carcinoma antigen. It is present in the fetus and in derivatives of the coelomic epithelium, including peritoneum, pleura, pericardium, and amnion. In healthy adults, CA 125 has been detected by immunohistochemistry in the epithelium of the fallopian tubes, endometrium, and endocervix. However, ovarian epithelium does not normally express any CA 125.

Testing

CA 125 levels are measured by an immunoassay, with the upper limit of normal set at 35 U/mL. Elevated levels are detected in 50% of patients with early stage and 80% of patients with later stage ovarian cancer. In patients with ovarian masses, an elevated CA 125 level has a sensitivity of 83% to 90% and a specificity of 87% to 97% for ovarian cancer prediction in pre- and postmenopausal women, respectively.[43] It is also detectable in a high percentage of patients with cancer of fallopian tube, endometrium, and cervix as well as in some nongynecologic malignant neoplasms of the pancreas, colon, lung, and liver. Benign conditions in which

CA 125 is elevated include endometriosis, adenomyosis, uterine fibroids, pelvic inflammatory disease, cirrhosis, and ascites.

Screening

By itself, CA 125 is not useful as a screening tool for ovarian cancer because of its poor specificity. In the recently published results from United Kingdom Collaborative Trial of Ovarian Cancer Screening, over 200,000 postmenopausal women aged 50 to 74 were randomized to no screening, annual multimodal screening with CA 125 in the context of a risk calculator (MMS), or transvaginal ultrasound.[44] At a median follow up of 11.1 years, they found a mortality reduction of 15% in the MMS screening group and 11% in the ultrasound group, as compared to the usual care group—although these differences were nonsignificant. A similar large randomized trial in the United States of ultrasound combined with CA 125 showed neither a significant reduction in ovarian cancer mortality with screening nor a trend hinting at a potential benefit. The USPSTF continues to recommend against routine screening for ovarian cancer with CA 125 (grade D).

Prognosis

Patients with elevated CA 125 levels at the time of diagnosis have a worse prognosis compared with those patients with normal levels. Absolute levels of CA 125 do not clearly correlate with tumor stage, although with increasing stage, greater percentages of patients have elevated CA 125 levels: 50% of stage I patients, 70% of stage II patients, 90% of stage III patients, and 98% of stage IV patients.

Monitoring Response to Therapy

CA 125 is of value in monitoring disease course. Partial or complete response to therapy is associated with a decrease in the CA 125 level in more than 95% of patients. Increasing levels of CA 125 correlate with disease recurrence and precede clinical or imaging evidence of recurrence by a median time of three months. When rising CA 125 levels are used as an indication for second-look laparotomies, recurrent disease is found approximately 90% of the time.

α-Fetoprotein and Human Chorionic Gonadotropin in Testicular Germ Cell Tumors

Nonseminomatous testicular cancers comprise several different histologic types, including embryonal carcinoma, syncytiotrophoblasts (choriocarcinoma), yolk sac tumors, and teratomas. Marker expression can be predicted on the basis of the predominant histologic type. Human chorionic gonadotropin is detected in more than 90% of choriocarcinomas, whereas AFP is expressed by 90% to 95% of yolk sac tumors, 20% of teratomas, and 10% of embryonal carcinomas.

Proteomic Profiling

In contrast to single circulating protein tumor biomarkers as discussed previously, proteomics is the study of all the proteins expressed by the genome. In cancer, this can amount to more than 1.5 million proteins.[45] Ultimately, genetic mutations are manifested at the protein level, involving derangements of protein function and communication within diseased cells and with their microenvironment. Execution of the disease process occurs through altered protein function. Clinically, proteomics offers the potential to allow for enhanced cancer diagnosis and treatment decision making. The field relies on the remarkable technological advances that allow investigators to elucidate the vast array of proteins in a given group of cells and then apply systems biology to make meaning of the data.

Protein tumor biomarkers are thought to be low abundance proteins shed from tumor cells or from the tumor-host interface into the circulation. Detection and measurement of these proteins provide information about the clinical behavior of the cancer. Proteomic profiling uses mass spectrometry technologies to generate complex fingerprints of ion peaks corresponding to protein concentrations that can be correlated with disease states. Numerous studies, using samples from blood (plasma or serum), urine, and pancreatic juice, have demonstrated the feasibility of this technology for biomarker discovery and for potential early detection of ovarian, breast, prostate, and pancreas cancer. Identification of reproducible protein signatures of specific diseases has the potential to achieve much higher diagnostic sensitivity and specificity than of currently available biomarkers.

Circulating Tumor Cells

As their name suggests, CTCs are tumor cells that have been shed from the primary (or metastatic) tumor deposit and are found circulating in the blood stream. CTCs were initially described in the 1800s, but only recently have investigators begun to bridge the gap to make them clinically useful biomarkers. In a patient with metastatic cancer, CTCs are estimated to comprise one of every billion cells.[46] Isolation has relied on unique properties of the CTCs, such as via size and other biophysical characteristics or via surface markers (e.g., EPCAM in epithelial cancer). These isolation techniques have to be combined with other techniques to distinguish true malignant cells as opposed to nontumor cells (e.g., normal epithelial cells expressing EPCAM). Investigators have isolated CTCs from patients and shown ability in some cases to create mouse models or cell lines and demonstrated a similar therapeutic response to treatment as the patient being treated. CTCs are an extremely active area of current research.

RNA-Based Markers

Circulating RNA

In 1996, circulating messenger RNA was found in the blood of a patient with melanoma. Since then, much tumor-derived RNA has been identified circulating, the majority of which is micro RNA. Micro RNAs are often carried in exosomes, tumor-educated platelets, apoptotic bodies, or proteins. The NETest was developed based on isolated messenger RNA from a whole blood sample, with 51 genes analyzed.[47] It reports a score that makes the diagnosis of a neuroendocrine tumor more or less likely (score 0–8, with 3 or more consistent with a neuroendocrine tumor), and supplies a second score of risk of disease progression (low, medium, or high). Positive predictive value for a score of three or greater for gastropancreatic neuroendocrine tumor diagnosis is 95%. Initial data suggests it can be used to predict who needs further therapy, as well as who to monitor for treatment response.

Tissue-Derived RNA

RNA-based markers have been identified in the context of global messenger RNA expression using high-throughput technologies. These microarrays ("gene chips") provide a means to measure the expression of multiple human genes in a single experiment. Statistical modeling then allows selection of groups of genes, "fingerprints," that best distinguish disease states.

In 2004, Paik and colleagues[48] described an algorithm to predict likelihood of distant recurrence in patients with node-negative, tamoxifen-treated breast cancer based on the expression of 21 genes in tumor tissue. It is able to extract RNA from formalin-fixed, paraffin-embedded tissue blocks and to use this RNA for the subsequent assay. This assay is known as Oncotype DX and includes 16 tumor-associated genes and 5 reference genes, with the result expressed as a recurrence score. Higher expression levels of "favorable" genes result in a lower recurrence score, whereas higher expression of "unfavorable" genes results in a higher score. Scores of less than 11 are considered favorable (6.8% distant recurrence at 10 years), from 11 to 25 intermediate (14.3% distant recurrence at 10 years), and over 25 consistent with more aggressive disease (30.5% distant recurrence at 10 years). It has been validated for use in decision making for adjuvant chemotherapy (in addition to standard endocrine therapy), with chemotherapy being omitted in low-risk patients and given in high-risk patients. A recent study demonstrated that for most patients with intermediate scores, chemotherapy could be safely omitted as well.[49] The Oncotype Dx score was incorporated as part of the most recent AJCC 8th edition breast cancer staging systems. Other breast cancer multigene assays such as MammaPrint and PAM 50 are also clinically available. Several multigene panels have been developed to predict recurrence and survival in other cancers, such as Oncotype DX for colon cancer, ColoPrint for colorectal cancer, and Decision-Dx-UM for uveal melanoma. Many more panels are currently under development.

DNA-Based Markers

Specific mutations in oncogenes, tumor suppressor genes, and mismatch repair genes can serve as biomarkers for cancer. In addition, tumor cells can shed DNA, which has the potential to diagnose cancer prior to its clinical appearance, as well as track treatment response. In addition, epigenetic changes are often dysregulated and altered in malignancy (see Carcinogenesis, Cancer Epigenetics subsection) and can also serve as tumor markers.

Gene Mutations

Tumor-associated mutations include the *RET* proto-oncogene of MEN2 and the *APC* gene of FAP or *p53* mutations in a wide variety of tumors. Chromosomal abnormalities such as the 9:22 translocation that creates the *bcr-abl* oncogene are also useful biomarkers. Specific single-nucleotide polymorphisms have been identified that are associated with increased risk for specific cancers, and haplotype assessment has been shown to predict susceptibility to several cancers, including prostate, breast, lung, and colon. *HER2* mutation in breast cancer (see Tumor Biology, Sustained Proliferative Signaling subsection) leads to increased copies of the *HER2* gene and resultant increased expression of the protein product. Status of *HER2* routinely guides treatment for patients with breast cancer. This mutation can be identified via fluorescence in-situ hybridization, whereby a probe can identify the increased gene copies. The protein product of *HER2* can also be probed for using immunohistochemistry. It is recommended that all patients with metastatic colorectal carcinoma who are candidates for antiEGFR antibody therapy should have their tumor tested for *KRAS* mutation. If *KRAS* mutation in codon 12 or 13 is detected, these patients should not receive antiEGFR antibody therapy as part of their treatment. This testing is done by isolating DNA from the tumor and looking to see if a mutation is present.

Circulating Tumor DNA

Cell-free DNA (cfDNA) from tumors was first identified by Mandel and Metais in 1948. In 1977 investigators observed that there was more cfDNA in cancer patients than in patients without cancer. Within this cfDNA, it was noted that many of neoplastic changes associated with cancer were present, thus the term *ctDNA* is often used. It is felt that ctDNA is shed secondary to several factors: (1) necrosis leading to DNA release, (2) macrophage phagocytosis of necrotic cancer cells, followed by tumor DNA release, and (3) apoptotic degradation of cellular DNA. Due to low amounts of ctDNA present, sensitive detection methodologies such as droplet PCR or next-generation sequencing with molecular barcodes are commonly used. As a whole, using cfDNA, many different tumor-specific alterations can be identified: gene mutations, copy number alterations, gene fusions, and DNA methylation events.[50]

Early diagnosis of cancer has been an attractive potential application of ctDNA. In one recent study, a 61-amplicon panel was used on patient blood samples, followed by multiplex-PCR, with the goal of identifying potential cancer-driver mutations in the cfDNA.[51] This was combined with 39 secreted oncoprotein biomarkers. The assay, termed *CancerSEEK,* was validated in 1005 nonmetastatic clinically detected known cancer patients and was found to have a sensitivity of 69% to 98% for five of the cancer types looked at and a specificity of over 99%. Overall, eight tumor types were looked at, with sensitivity of 98% for ovarian cancer (highest) and 33% for breast cancer (lowest). Once the presence of cancer cells was identified, correct site of origin was able to be determined in 83% of cases. Other investigators have used alternative strategies for cancer screening with cfDNA. In a recent Chinese study, ctDNA was isolated from plasma and analyzed for EBV DNA as a screen for nasopharyngeal carcinoma in this at-risk population. Sensitivity and specificity in this study were both over 97%. In addition to blood-based testing, urine, stool, ascites fluid, pleural fluid, saliva, and cerebrospinal fluid can all be probed for ctDNA.[50] For instance, the FDA-approved Cologuard uses a combination of stool DNA and fecal immunochemical testing to identify colorectal cancers (92% sensitivity) and advanced adenomas (42% sensitivity).

In addition to diagnosis, ctDNA can be used to guide treatment, treatment response, or relapse. The cobase EGFR Mutation test uses cfDNA to identify the T790M gatekeeper mutation that can be seen in patients with progressive disease after treatment with EGFR inhibitors. Patients with this mutation can be treated successfully with third-generation EGFR inhibitors. In addition to guiding therapeutics, the short half-life of ctDNA allows one to quickly monitor treatment response, with ctDNA dropping precipitously in 1 to 2 weeks in patients who have therapeutic responses to systemic therapy. In addition, it was shown that, for patients with colorectal cancer, cfDNA drawn several weeks after curative surgery could identify patients with residual disease and predict future relapse.

Epigenetic Changes

Testing for epigenetic changes is another exciting emerging modality to apply as a cancer biomarker. Advantages include the fact that (1) DNA assays for aberrant methylation are easier and more sensitive than those for point mutations, (2) cancer-specific DNA methylation patterns can be detected in ctDNA in the bloodstream and in epithelial tumor cells shed into the lumen, and (3) DNA methylation profiles are more chemically and biologically stable than RNA or most proteins.

Methylation biomarker studies have been performed in a variety of cancers, including breast, esophageal, lung, gastric, colorectal, ovarian, and prostate. Hypomethylated CpG islands have been associated with the activation of nearby genes. For example, hypomethylation of the promoter for the cancer/testis antigen CAGE correlates with the gene's increased expression and is found in premalignant lesions of the stomach. Similar instances of demethylated promoters activating their downstream genes have been found in numerous other cancers, including those of the colon, pancreas, liver, uterus, lung, and cervix. In a study of ovarian carcinogenesis, hypomethylation of centromeric and juxtacentromeric satellite DNA was found to be increased in tumors of advanced stage or high grade, and this strong hypomethylation was an independent marker of poor prognosis.

The role of biomarkers in cancer is expanding rapidly. Clearly, the future holds great promise for the use of biomarkers in the clinical management of patients with cancer (Table 29.3). It is likely that biomarkers will play an increasingly important role in cancer prognosis and therapeutic selection as well as, perhaps, in early detection.

SELECTED REFERENCES

Corcoran RB, Chabner BA. Application of cell-free DNA analysis to cancer treatment. *N Engl J Med*. 2018;379:1754–1765.

A concise recent review that lays out the fundamentals of cell-free deoxyribonucleic acid, and its current role in cancer diagnosis, treatment, and monitoring.

Hanahan D, Weinberg RA. Hallmarks of cancer: The next generation. *Cell*. 2011;144:646–674.

In this landmark paper, the authors beautifully take the reader through the current understanding of common physiologic and molecular characteristics of cancer.

Hunter KW, Amin R, Deasy S, et al. Genetic insights into the morass of metastatic heterogeneity. *Nat Rev Cancer*. 2018;18:211–223.

A review of the mechanisms by which a tumor may spread from its primary site of origin to distant locations.

Mesri EA, Feitelson MA, Munger K. Human viral oncogenesis: A cancer hallmarks analysis. *Cell Host Microbe*. 2014;15:266–282.

A great overview of the mechanisms oncoviruses employ in the human host that lead to cancer formation.

Peinado H, Zhang H, Matei IR, et al. Pre-metastatic niches: Organ-specific homes for metastases. *Nat Rev Cancer*. 2017;17:302–317.

A detailed description of the premetastatic niche and the cross-talk between tumors and sites of future distant spread that eventually culminate in clinical metastatic progression.

Schreiber RD, Old LJ, Smyth MJ. Cancer immunoediting: integrating immunity's roles in cancer suppression and promotion. *Science*. 2011;331:1565–1570.

This paper reviews the evidence and theory behind immunoediting in cancer and the dual role the immune system plays in malignancy.

Siegel RL, Miller KD, Jemal A. Cancer statistics, 2018. *CA Cancer J Clin*. 2018;68:7–30.

The 2018 report from the American Cancer Society laying out cancer incidence and mortality in the United States, with further breakdown by sex, ethnicity, and cancer type.

Sparano JA, Gray RJ, Makower DF, et al. Adjuvant chemotherapy guided by a 21-gene expression assay in breast cancer. *N Engl J Med*. 2018;379:111–121.

A recent report on the Oncotype DX assay in patients with node-negative, HER2-negative, hormone receptor–positive breast cancer that demonstrates the ability of a low (<11) or intermediate (<26) Oncotype DX score to enable most patients to forgo cytotoxic chemotherapy.

Yachida S, Jones S, Bozic I, et al. Distant metastasis occurs late during the genetic evolution of pancreatic cancer. *Nature*. 2010;467:1114–1117.

An elegant analysis of pancreatic adenocarcinoma in which they lay out the clonal evolution of this disease and use mathematical modeling to demonstrate an ~15-year time frame between founder mutation and the development of a cancer with metastatic capability.

REFERENCES

1. Hanahan D, Weinberg RA. Hallmarks of cancer: the next generation. *Cell*. 2011;144:646–674.
2. Siegel RL, Miller KD, Jemal A. Cancer statistics, 2018. *CA Cancer J Clin*. 2018;68:7–30.
3. Bray F, Ferlay J, Soerjomataram I, et al. Global cancer statistics 2018: GLOBOCAN estimates of incidence and mortality worldwide for 36 cancers in 185 countries. *CA Cancer J Clin*. 2018;68:394–424.
4. Ko JJ, Kennecke HF, Lim HJ, et al. Reasons for underuse of adjuvant chemotherapy in elderly patients with stage III colon cancer. *Clin Colorectal Cancer*. 2016;15:179–185.
5. Tomasetti C, Vogelstein B. Cancer etiology. Variation in cancer risk among tissues can be explained by the number of stem cell divisions. *Science*. 2015;347:78–81.
6. O'Sullivan J, Lysaght J, Donohoe CL, et al. Obesity and gastrointestinal cancer: The interrelationship of adipose and tumour microenvironments. *Nat Rev Gastroenterol Hepatol*. 2018;15:699–714.
7. Schauer DP, Feigelson HS, Koebnick C, et al. Bariatric surgery and the risk of cancer in a large multisite cohort. *Ann Surg*. 2019;269:95–101.
8. Moore SC, Lee IM, Weiderpass E, et al. Association of leisure-time physical activity with risk of 26 types of cancer in 1.44 million adults. *JAMA Intern Med*. 2016;176:816–825.
9. Akinyemiju T, Wiener H, Pisu M. Cancer-related risk factors and incidence of major cancers by race, gender and region;

analysis of the NIH-AARP diet and health study. *BMC Cancer*. 2017;17:597.
10. Mokdad AH, Dwyer-Lindgren L, Fitzmaurice C, et al. Trends and patterns of disparities in cancer mortality among US counties, 1980–2014. *JAMA*. 2017;317:388–406.
11. Bailey MH, Tokheim C, Porta-Pardo E, et al. Comprehensive characterization of cancer driver genes and mutations. *Cell*. 2018;173:371–385 e318.
12. Stockwell BR, Friedmann Angeli JP, Bayir H, et al. Ferroptosis: A regulated cell death nexus linking metabolism, redox biology, and disease. *Cell*. 2017;171:273–285.
13. de Sousa e Melo F, Kurtova AV, Harnoss JM, et al. A distinct role for Lgr5(+) stem cells in primary and metastatic colon cancer. *Nature*. 2017;543:676–680.
14. Donnem T, Reynolds AR, Kuczynski EA, et al. Non-angiogenic tumours and their influence on cancer biology. *Nat Rev Cancer*. 2018;18:323–336.
15. Peinado H, Zhang H, Matei IR, et al. Pre-metastatic niches: Organ-specific homes for metastases. *Nat Rev Cancer*. 2017;17:302–317.
16. Schreiber RD, Old LJ, Smyth MJ. Cancer immunoediting: Integrating immunity's roles in cancer suppression and promotion. *Science*. 2011;331:1565–1570.
17. Thorsson V, Gibbs DL, Brown SD, et al. The immune landscape of cancer. *Immunity*. 2018;48:812–830 e814.
18. Vander Heiden MG, DeBerardinis RJ. Understanding the intersections between metabolism and cancer biology. *Cell*. 2017;168:657–669.
19. Crusz SM, Balkwill FR. Inflammation and cancer: advances and new agents. *Nat Rev Clin Oncol*. 2015;12:584–596.
20. Yachida S, Jones S, Bozic I, et al. Distant metastasis occurs late during the genetic evolution of pancreatic cancer. *Nature*. 2010;467:1114–1117.
21. Hunter KW, Amin R, Deasy S, et al. Genetic insights into the morass of metastatic heterogeneity. *Nat Rev Cancer*. 2018;18:211–223.
22. Faries MB, Thompson JF, Cochran AJ, et al. Completion dissection or observation for sentinel-node metastasis in melanoma. *N Engl J Med*. 2017;376:2211–2222.
23. Pereira ER, Kedrin D, Seano G, et al. Lymph node metastases can invade local blood vessels, exit the node, and colonize distant organs in mice. *Science*. 2018;359:1403–1407.
24. Kratz CP, Achatz MI, Brugieres L, et al. Cancer screening recommendations for individuals with Li-Fraumeni syndrome. *Clin Cancer Res*. 2017;23:e38–e45.
25. Wells K, Wise PE. Hereditary colorectal cancer syndromes. *Surg Clin North Am*. 2017;97:605–625.
26. Leoz ML, Carballal S, Moreira L, et al. The genetic basis of familial adenomatous polyposis and its implications for clinical practice and risk management. *Appl Clin Genet*. 2015;8:95–107.
27. Le DT, Uram JN, Wang H, et al. PD-1 Blockade in tumors with mismatch-repair deficiency. *N Engl J Med*. 2015;372:2509–2520.
28. Kuchenbaecker KB, Hopper JL, Barnes DR, et al. Risks of breast, ovarian, and contralateral breast cancer for BRCA1 and BRCA2 mutation carriers. *JAMA*. 2017;317:2402–2416.
29. Hu C, Hart SN, Polley EC, et al. Association between inherited germline mutations in cancer predisposition genes and risk of pancreatic cancer. *JAMA*. 2018;319:2401–2409.
30. Flavahan WA, Gaskell E, Bernstein BE. Epigenetic plasticity and the hallmarks of cancer. *Science*. 2017;357; eaal2380.
31. Corces MR, Granja JM, Shams S, et al. The chromatin accessibility landscape of primary human cancers. *Science*. 2018;362.
32. Bhatt AP, Redinbo MR, Bultman SJ. The role of the microbiome in cancer development and therapy. *CA Cancer J Clin*. 2017;67:326–344.
33. Geller LT, Barzily-Rokni M, Danino T, et al. Potential role of intratumor bacteria in mediating tumor resistance to the chemotherapeutic drug gemcitabine. *Science*. 2017;357:1156–1160.
34. Burt LM, Ying J, Poppe MM, et al. Risk of secondary malignancies after radiation therapy for breast cancer: Comprehensive results. *Breast*. 2017;35:122–129.
35. Mesri EA, Feitelson MA, Munger K. Human viral oncogenesis: A cancer hallmarks analysis. *Cell Host Microbe*. 2014;15:266–282.
36. Cuzick J. Preventive therapy for cancer. *Lancet Oncol*. 2017;18:e472–e482.
37. Nghiem PT, Bhatia S, Lipson EJ, et al. PD-1 Blockade with pembrolizumab in advanced Merkel-cell carcinoma. *N Engl J Med*. 2016;374:2542–2552.
38. Gagnaire A, Nadel B, Raoult D, et al. Collateral damage: Insights into bacterial mechanisms that predispose host cells to cancer. *Nat Rev Microbiol*. 2017;15:109–128.
39. Harrington D, Lamberton PHL, McGregor A. Human liver flukes. *Lancet Gastroenterol Hepatol*. 2017;2:680–689.
40. Kim SS, Donahue TR, Girgis MD. Carcinoembryonic antigen for diagnosis of colorectal cancer recurrence. *JAMA*. 2018;320:298–299.
41. Nicholson BD, Shinkins B, Pathiraja I, et al. Blood CEA levels for detecting recurrent colorectal cancer. *Cochrane Database Syst Rev*. 2015:CD011134.
42. Tzartzeva K, Obi J, Rich NE, et al. Surveillance imaging and alpha fetoprotein for early detection of hepatocellular carcinoma in patients with Cirrhosis: A meta-analysis. *Gastroenterology*. 2018;154; 1706–1718 e1701.
43. Romagnolo C, Leon AE, Fabricio ASC, et al. HE4, CA125 and risk of ovarian malignancy algorithm (ROMA) as diagnostic tools for ovarian cancer in patients with a pelvic mass: An Italian multicenter study. *Gynecol Oncol*. 2016;141:303–311.
44. Jacobs IJ, Menon U, Ryan A, et al. Ovarian cancer screening and mortality in the UK Collaborative Trial of Ovarian Cancer Screening (UKCTOCS): A randomised controlled trial. *Lancet*. 2016;387:945–956.
45. Panis C, Pizzatti L, Souza GF, et al. Clinical proteomics in cancer: Where we are. *Cancer Lett*. 2016;382:231–239.
46. Siravegna G, Marsoni S, Siena S, et al. Integrating liquid biopsies into the management of cancer. *Nat Rev Clin Oncol*. 2017;14:531–548.
47. Modlin IM, Kidd M, Malczewska A, et al. The NETest: The clinical utility of multigene blood analysis in the diagnosis and management of neuroendocrine tumors. *Endocrinol Metab Clin North Am*. 2018;47:485–504.
48. Paik S, Shak S, Tang G, et al. A multigene assay to predict recurrence of tamoxifen-treated, node-negative breast cancer. *N Engl J Med*. 2004;351:2817–2826.
49. Sparano JA, Gray RJ, Makower DF, et al. Adjuvant chemotherapy guided by a 21-gene expression assay in breast cancer. *N Engl J Med*. 2018;379:111–121.
50. Corcoran RB, Chabner BA. Application of cell-free DNA analysis to cancer treatment. *N Engl J Med*. 2018;379:1754–1765.
51. Cohen JD, Li L, Wang Y, et al. Detection and localization of surgically resectable cancers with a multi-analyte blood test. *Science*. 2018;359:926–930.

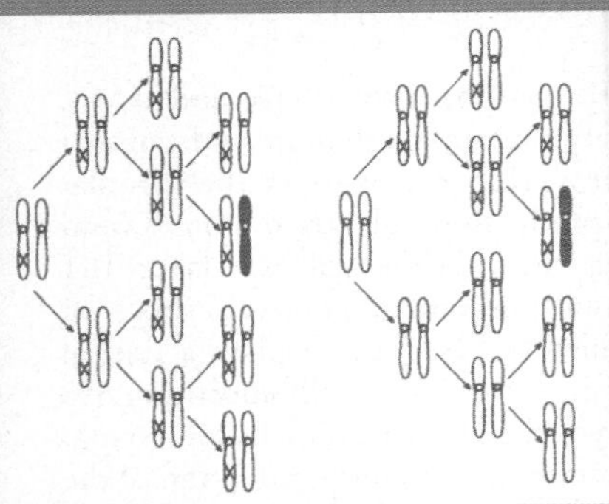

CHAPTER 30

Tumor Immunology and Immunotherapy

James S. Economou, James C. Yang, James S. Tomlinson

OUTLINE

Cancer immunotherapy has had a long and generally disappointing clinical history, until recently. There were clues from early landmark clinical trials using high-dose interleukin-2 (IL-2), which effected dramatic and durable complete responses in small subsets of patients with metastatic melanoma and renal cell cancer; these regressions that were mediated by the infiltration of these tumors with cytotoxic lymphocytes. Another major advance was the demonstration that T cells found within the tumor microenvironment (tumor-infiltrating lymphocytes [TIL]) of some solid cancers could be isolated, expanded ex vivo, and then adoptively transferred back to the patient, producing even higher response rates. These ex vivo activated and expanded TILs could recognize autologous tumor cells in a major histocompatibility complex (MHC) restricted manner, which indicated that these metastatic tumor deposits were enriched with tumor-specific T cells. The ability of melanoma TIL in particular to also recognize other MHC-matched melanoma cell lines led to the early identification of several melanocyte-lineage proteins, thus demonstrating that a least a portion of the antitumor response in melanoma was in fact anti-"self" (autoimmune).

These important discoveries introduced an era of immune-based therapies directed toward lineage-specific targets. These included various vaccine formulations that incorporated these lineage antigens (as whole protein, peptides, DNA, or RNA), which were delivered to the immune system (in adjuvant, by profession antigen-presenting cells, or encoded in viral vectors), all with disappointingly low or absent clinical activity and largely restricted to melanoma. T-cell receptors (TCRs) that recognized these lineage-specific antigens were cloned, placed in viral vectors, and used to engineer large numbers (in the tens of billions) of lineage-specific and highly activated T cells that were then readministered to the patients. This adoptive cell therapy, viewed as a gene therapy version of TIL therapy, has not recapitulated the TIL experience and in fact produced far fewer durable complete responses despite increasing the precursor frequency of these tumor-reactive T cells by orders of magnitude. For some lineage-specific antigens, these therapies were accompanied by off-tumor toxicities directed against the normal lineage cell type. These somewhat surprising results indicated that the composition of the whole TIL cell product must have antitumor effectors with specificities not yet identified.

An important advance in T cell–based immunotherapy was the development of chimeric antigen receptors (CARs; a single chain composed of extracellular immunoglobulin–derived heavy and light chains to confer specificity, linked to intracellular T-cell–activating domains), which could recognize a cell surface "antigen" in a non–MHC-restricted manner. CAR T-cell adoptive therapy directed against CD19—confined to B lymphocytes and many B-cell malignancies—produces dramatic and durable regressions in patients with refractory and recurrent disease; this therapy also causes transient B-cell aplasia. Other CAR targets are undergoing clinical study.

However, arguably the most important breakthrough in human cancer immunotherapy followed seminal studies in the basic biology of immune regulation. T lymphocytes have both stimulatory and inhibitory receptors, and an important balance exists that maintains tolerance to "self." It was discovered that blocking the inhibitory signaling of cytotoxic T lymphocyte–associated antigen 4 (CTLA-4) with its ligands B7.1 and B7.2, subsequently the programmed cell death receptor 1 (PD-1) with its ligands PD-L1 and PD-L2, led to enhancement of the endogenous T-cell response to tumors. These resulted in the development of therapeutic monoclonal antibodies that antagonize the T-cell "checkpoints" that are now in routine clinical use. The simple blockade of inhibitory signaling unleashes remarkably beneficial adaptive immune response against a broad range of common human malignancies—melanoma, genitourinary cancer, lung cancer, and subsets of colorectal cancer. The availability of biospecimens from responding patients, next-generation high-throughput sequencing, and single-cell TCR cloning led to the remarkable realization that the vast majority of these antitumor T cells recognized nonsynonymous cancer-specific mutations (point mutations, insertion-deletion, frameshift

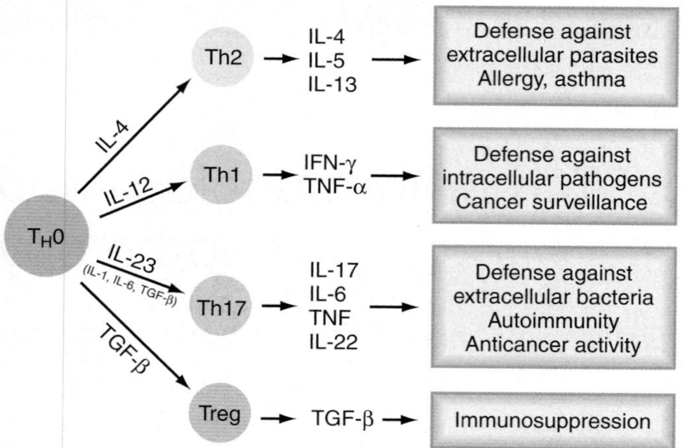

FIG. 30.1 CD4 T-cell subsets and their properties. A T_H0 cell is a naïve T cell that has differentiated successfully and undergone positive and negative selection in the thymus. Naïve helper T cells (CD4+) can differentiate into several subsets whose general properties and predominant cytokine production are shown. *IFN,* Interferon; *IL,* interleukin; *TGF-β,* transforming growth factor-β; *TNF,* tumor necrosis factor.

mutations)—so-called "neoantigens (neoAg)," uniquely expressed by each tumor. Cancers, which accumulate large neoAg mutational burdens, have a higher probability of having several neoAg mutant peptides processed and presented on the tumor cell surface in the context of MHC. This essentially results in a set of xenoantigens—foreign to the patient's immune system and unique for each patient's cancer—being presented to the host immune system whose TCR repertoire can recognize these as foreign. These revolutionary findings have ushered in a new era in cancer immunotherapy for human cancer histologies never before viewed as controllable by the immune system. It also appears that, for some patients, immunotherapy can achieve complete and durable regressions of widely metastatic solid cancers, something difficult to achieve with the majority of other systemic therapies.

The field of human cancer is now legitimately the fourth cancer treatment modality. Future advances may include combinations of strategies (cell based, small molecule, vaccines) that will broaden its effectiveness in common epithelial cancers.

OVERVIEW OF TUMOR IMMUNOLOGY

T Lymphocytes and Natural Killer Cells

Bone marrow–derived progenitor cells enter the thymus from which T cells eventually emerge. In the thymus, an enormous repertoire of TCRs is randomly generated by recombinations and mutations in their α and β chains. Progenitors with TCRs of high affinity for self-antigens undergo deletion (negative selection). Some of those with low affinity for self-antigens survive and are positively selected so that a significant percentage of self-reactive T cells emerge from the thymus. Only a very small percentage of the cells entering and proliferating within the thymus survive this education process. Several types of T cells emerge into the periphery. CD8+ T cells recognize antigen in the context of MHC class I molecules, express αβ TCRs, are commonly referred to as cytotoxic T cells, and produce a number of cytokines. CD4+ T cells recognize antigen in the context of MHC class II molecules. There are several subsets of CD4+ T cells (Fig. 30.1). Among the better recognized are Th1 cells (helper type 1 T cells) that secrete IL-2, tumor necrosis factor-α (TNF-α), and interferon-γ (IFN-γ) and Th2 cells that produce IL-4, IL-5, IL-6, IL-10, and IL-13. Th1 cells promote cytotoxicity and inflammation and combat intracellular pathogens, whereas Th2 cells assist in the stimulation of B cells for antibody production, allergic responses, and addressing extracellular pathogens. T helper cells will favor Th1 (cell-mediated) or Th2 (humoral) immune responses. A subset of CD4 regulatory cells (T regulatory [Treg] cells) plays a critical role in dampening autoimmunity. These Treg cells constitute 5% to 10% of CD4+ cells, express the transcription factor Foxp3, and dominantly suppress autoimmune responses; mutation of the Foxp3 gene in humans and mice leads to multiorgan autoimmune disease. Another T-cell subtype is the so-called Th17 cell, which preferentially produces IL-17, IL-21, and IL-22 and is important in the pathogenesis of autoimmune diseases.

CD4+ T cells also play an important role in the initiation and maintenance of CD8+ T-cell responses.[1] They may do this through a variety of mechanisms. Activated CD4+ T cells can interact with dendritic cells (DCs), which are professional antigen-presenting cells, through an interaction between the CD40 receptor and its ligand CD40L. This activation or "licensing" of DCs allows these antigen-presenting cells to promote the differentiation of CD8+ T cells and to establish a durable memory T-cell response. CD4+ T cells also produce IL-2 and IFN-γ, which could potentially support CD8 function. Thus, CD4+ T cells are important in shaping a productive antitumor response.

Another T-cell subset (γδ) represents a minor population (1%–10%) of CD3+ T cells that is even more enriched in mucosal epithelium and expresses TCRs that recognize bacterial and viral antigens. Natural killer T (NKT) cells express phenotypic markers of T and NK cells and express a specific family of TCRs that recognize glycolipid antigens presented by CD1d molecules. These NKT cells are thought to help initiate T-cell responses through the production of large amounts of the cytokines IFN-γ and IL-4.

Mature T cells have a broad repertoire of αβ TCRs with diverse antigen specificity. This diversity is generated during T-cell differentiation by a process of gene rearrangement of variable (V), joining (J), and diversity (D) gene segments. TCRs are composed of α and β chains; it is estimated that recombination events could potentially yield a repertoire exceeding 10^{12} unique TCRs. These TCRs recognize antigen in the context of MHC proteins found on the surface of cells for MHC class I, proteins within the cell cytoplasm are digested in the proteasome complex into short peptide fragments (8–12 amino acid residues), which are transported to the cell surface bound in the groove of MHC class I molecules; the specific peptide sequence presented is determined by the MHC (in humans, also called human leukocyte antigen [HLA]) allele. These class I–presented peptides are usually recognized by CD8+ T cells. MHC class II extracellular antigens are internalized by antigen-presenting cells into endosomes, where they are degraded into small peptides and mounted on MHC class II molecules for display on the cell surface and typically recognized by CD4 cells. These two pathways provide the immune system with continuous surveillance for intracellular pathogens, such as viruses, and foreign cells as well as noxious proteins and pathogens in extracellular milieu. The activation of resting T cells requires engagement of the correct MHC-peptide complex by the TCR (so-called signal 1) and additional costimulatory signals (signal 2). Professional antigen-presenting cells (DCs) provide either CD80 or CD86 (B7 family genes), which engages the CD28 receptor on the T cell, a requirement for T-cell activation. T cells then upregulate another receptor, CTLA-4, which also binds B7 but with

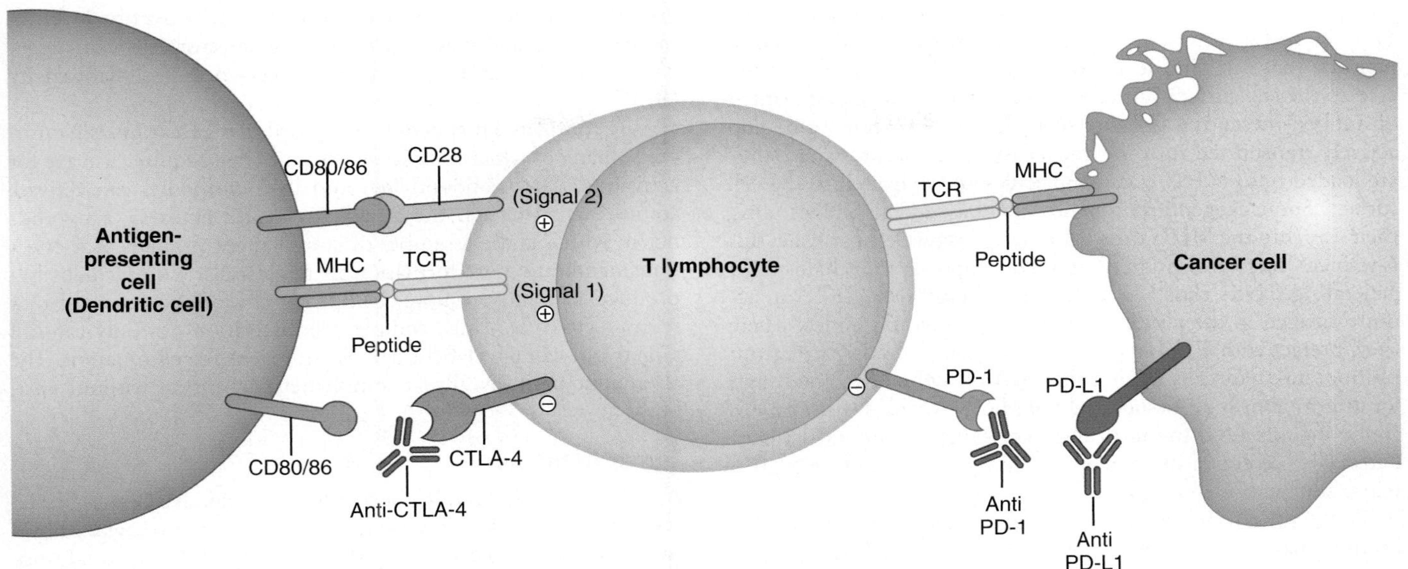

FIG. 30.2 Important activation and inhibitory signaling in T lymphocytes and modern therapeutic interventions. Activation of T cells requires TCR engagement of antigen in the context of MHC and a second costimulatory signal, CD80/86 and CD28. Inhibitory signaling by CTLA-4 or PD-1/PD-L1 can be blocked with monoclonal antibodies. *CTLA-4*, Cytotoxic T lymphocyte–associated antigen 4; *MHC*, major histocompatibility complex; MHLC abbreviation is not in figure. *PD-1*, programmed cell death receptor 1; *PD-L1*, programmed cell death receptor 1 ligand; *TCR*, T-cell receptor.

a higher affinity than CD28. Engagement of CTLA-4 induces an inhibitory signal that downregulates T-cell activation.[2] This is a natural immunomodulatory mechanism for dampening immune responses. Monoclonal antibodies that bind to CTLA-4 can block this interaction and inhibit the negative regulatory signaling (Fig. 30.2). Studies in human subjects have demonstrated that CTLA-4 blockade can break peripheral tolerance to self-antigens and induce both antitumor and anti-"self" (autoimmune) responses.

Another important pathway is the PD-1/PD-L1 axis in which the inhibitory ligand (PD-L1), commonly expressed in many cancers, can engage T-cell PD-1, thereby abrogating lymphocyte activation (Fig. 30.2).[3] Interruption of this negative signaling benefits a significant proportion of patients with several solid tumors.

Although much emphasis in antitumor immunity has been focused on adaptive responses (T lymphocytes and antibodies), effector cells of the innate immune system, specifically NK cells, can act alone or in concert with adaptive immunity.[4,5] NK cells can recognize and kill target cells without prior sensitization. These cells express activating and inhibitory cell surface receptors and, when their activating receptors are engaged without concomitant ligation of their inhibitory receptors, can kill targets directly. NK cells have been traditionally viewed as providing a first line of defense against virally infected cells. NK cells can also interact with the adaptive immune system. They can modulate the function of professional antigen-presenting cells (e.g., DCs), promote the generation of Th1 responses, and potentially dampen autoimmune immunopathologic changes. Because their inhibitory receptors engage MHC molecules, NK cells specifically recognize cells that have lost MHC class I molecules, which can occur during viral infections or malignant transformation. NK cells are strongly activated by exogenous cytokines such as IL-2 and have been termed "lymphokine-activated killer (LAK) cells." LAK cells have greatly enhanced cytotoxicity for a much broader range of target cells.

The cytotoxic T cell (CTL) response is initiated by engagement of their TCR with professional antigen-presenting cells (e.g., DCs) that have processed and presented cognate antigen in the context of MHC class I. This activation event enables resting CD8 T cells to proliferate and differentiate into effector CTL with significant alterations in migratory behavior and function. These CTLs traffic to tumor sites, and their TCR engage antigen peptide presented on the surface of tumor cells and are able to deliver death signals. CTLs are able to kill multiple tumor cells, termed "serial killing": The mechanisms of killing include ligation of so-called "death receptors" (FasL/CDaSL, Apo2L/TRAIL) or cytolytic granule (perforin, granulysin) exocytosis.[6,7] They also elaborate proinflammatory cytokines, which may, through various mechanisms, promote antitumor activity through recruitment of the other cytotoxic effectors such as NK cells.

Antigen-Presenting Cells

DCs are professional antigen-presenting cells whose role is to take up, process, and present antigen to the immune system[8]; they are essential during the initial activation of resting T cells. There are different subtypes of DCs with specialized functions that depend on their anatomic location. DCs are found in lymphoid tissues, in the skin, and on the mucosal surfaces of many organs. DCs in the gastrointestinal tract can sample bacteria in the intestinal lumen and initiate secretory immunoglobulin A (IgA) responses. In the lung, DCs help maintain tolerance to inhaled allergens. In the peripheral blood, DC precursors can migrate to sites of inflammation and initiate immune responses. DC function is powerfully modulated by a variety of receptors including Toll-like receptors (TLRs) and surface C-type lectin receptors. DCs at different stages of differentiation vary in their ability to migrate, to take up antigen by phagocytosis, and to effectively stimulate T cells. Immature DCs patrol their environment, sampling by pinocytosis and receptor-mediated endocytosis. Extracellular antigens are taken up into endosomes, which fuse with protease-containing lysosomes, and within these compartments antigens are cleaved into peptides that can bind to MHC class II molecules and be delivered to the cell surface. Proteins in the cytoplasmic compartment of antigen-presenting cells are degraded by the proteosome and actively transported into the endoplasmic reticulum, where they are loaded onto MHC class I molecules and delivered to the cell surface. Some exogenous or environmental antigens can also find their way into the MHC class I antigen-presentation pathway; this is termed "cross-presentation" and is an important mechanism for generating CD8+ class I–restricted T-cell responses. DCs can acquire antigen in the periphery and travel to lymph nodes, where they interact with T cells and present antigen. DCs originate from pluripotent stem cells from bone marrow, enter the blood, and localize to almost all tissues and lymphoid organs. Myeloid DCs (these include DCs found in deep epithelial tissues and Langerhans cells present in the epidermis) and plasmacytoid DCs are a major source of type I IFN.

DCs have cell surface receptors termed "pattern recognition receptors" that screen the environment for pathogens. The TLR family is the best characterized; these can recognize bacterial products (e.g., lipopolysaccharide, flagellin), viral products such as double-stranded RNA, and specific cytosine-guanine (CpG)–rich DNA motifs, more common in microbial genomes. These signals, along with various proinflammatory cytokines, can deliver a danger signal to DCs that establishes the context within which they see and present antigens. TLR signaling drives immature DCs into a more mature phenotype with much higher expression of MHC, costimulatory molecules, and DC-derived cytokines (such as IL-12). Immature DCs are migratory and highly efficient in antigen capture, whereas mature DCs are less mobile but more efficient in processing and presenting antigen in an immunostimulatory context.

Distinct sets of molecules govern migration of DCs to and from the periphery and to lymph nodes. Prominent among these signals are a variety of chemokines and their receptors (e.g., CCR7, CCL19, CCL21). Signals that induce maturation of immature DCs include CD40 ligand delivered by T cells as well as signals by NK cells, a variety of proinflammatory cytokines (e.g., IL-1, TNF, IL-6), and engagement of TLR and C-type lectins. The context of antigen presentation and the maturational phenotype of DCs will determine and shape the type of T-cell response. Immature DCs have the potential to be tolerogenic, perhaps because they present antigen without an appropriate costimulatory second signal. Activated mature DCs have greater potency in activating and expanding antigen-reactive T cells. This is an oversimplified overview of the complex central role of various DC subsets that orchestrate adaptive and innate antitumor responses.

Antibody

Cell surface and circulating antigens can be recognized by immunoglobulins (antibody molecules). Immunoglobulins serve as membrane-associated receptors on the surface of B cells, which can then be secreted as soluble molecules as these cells differentiate into plasma cells. There are five distinct classes of immunoglobulin molecules: IgG, IgA, IgM, IgD, and IgE. There are several isotypes of IgG and IgA. The basic structure of antibody molecules includes two identical light and two identical heavy polypeptide chains linked by interchain disulfide bridges. Variable regions within the heavy and light chains create a so-called hypervariable region responsible for antigen binding. Antibody binding to antigen is reversible and of variable avidity. The C-terminal portion of certain antibody classes can bind to Fc receptors, which are expressed among a range of mononuclear cells. Antibody binding to antigen and engagement of these effector cells can trigger phagocytosis or antibody-dependent cell-mediated cytotoxicity (ADCC).

The complement system is composed of a series of plasma proteins, many of which exist as proenzymes that require cleavage for activation. Surface-bound IgG and IgM antibodies can activate complement through the so-called classical pathway, a byproduct of which is the assembly of complement proteins that effect transmembrane pore formation in target cells. Complement byproducts can also promote chemotaxis of mononuclear cells that release cytokines. Thus, complement activation not only can kill targets but can also label them as pathogens for elimination. The alternative pathway allows complement activation without antibody.

Tumor Antigens

A molecular understanding of tumor recognition has been achieved only recently. The first molecularly defined antigen recognized by a tumor-reactive T cell was only discovered in 1991.[9] This advance first required elucidation of the biology of antigen processing and presentation and its interaction with MHC molecules, which occurred in the late 1980s. These discoveries demonstrated that any intracytoplasmic protein was a candidate to be degraded by the proteasome complex, bound to MHC class I molecules, and displayed on the cell surface for T-cell recognition, which was crucial to our early understanding of tumor antigens. Mature T cells express the CD8 or CD4 coreceptor, which binds to invariant portions on all class I or class II MHC molecules, respectively. This additional ligation increases the affinity of the T-cell interaction with the antigen-presenting cell. Therefore, T cells expressing CD4 typically recognize antigens presented by MHC class II molecules, and CD8+ T cells usually recognize class I–presented antigens.

Cancer cells can overexpress or abnormally express a variety of normal cellular proteins. Because the human T-cell repertoire can sometimes recognize self-proteins, some of these self-proteins could potentially serve as targets for immune-based therapies. As discussed in detail later, gene products resulting from tumor-specific mutations are much better T-cell targets precisely because they are "nonself" xenoantigens never before experienced during thymic selection. One characteristic of an ideal cancer antigen is its immunogenicity, or its ability to elicit a T cell or antibody response. A gene product associated with the neoplastic process (e.g., a growth factor receptor) with a high degree of specific expression by malignant cells may prove to be an excellent target because it cannot be deleted or downregulated by the tumor cells under selective immune pressure (so-called antigen-loss variants). General classifications of known tumor-associated antigens include:

- Lineage-specific tumor antigens associated with tissue differentiation or function, such as the melanocyte-melanoma lineage antigens MART-1/Melan-A (MART-1), gp100 protein, mda-7 protein, tyrosinase and tyrosinase-related protein (TRP-1 and TRP-2), the prostate antigens (prostate-specific membrane antigen and prostate-specific antigen), and carcinoembryonic antigen
- A class of proteins expressed during ontogeny and in adult germline tissues and tumors (cancer-testis or cancer-germline antigens)
- Epitopes derived from genes specifically mutated in tumor cells (so called neoantigens)
- Epitopes derived from oncoviral processes, such as human papillomavirus oncoproteins E6 and E7 or Epstein-Barr virus–derived proteins; and

BOX 30.1 Cancer cell defense mechanisms.

T regulatory (Treg) cells: CD4+-CD25+ T-cell population, which inhibits T-cell function and proliferation
- In mice, deletion of these cells can induce autoimmunity
- In mice, adversely affects antitumor immunity
- Circumstantial evidence for a role in humans

Cytotoxic T lymphocyte–associated antigen 4 (CTLA-4) (CD152): Inhibitory receptor induced by T-cell activation that binds to CD80 and CD86 ligands
- Blockade can induce tumor regression in some patients

Programmed cell death receptor 1 (PD-1) (CD279; programmed death 1): Another inhibitory receptor on T cells, prevalent on lymphocytes in the tumor microenvironment
- Binds to ligand PD-L1 (CD274); also present on some human tumors

Suppressors of cytokine signaling (SOCS): Family of proteins that bind and inhibit kinases in the JAK/STAT pathway through which a number of cytokines signal

Myeloid suppressor cells: Cells of myeloid lineage that inhibit T cells
- Inhibited by a variety of putative mechanisms, including effects on dendritic cells and modulation of arginine and nitric oxide metabolism
- Accumulate in tumor-bearing state

Transforming growth factor-β (TGF-β): Multifunctional and complex cytokine with many effects on the immune response, some of which are inhibitory

- Nonmutated proteins with tumor-selective expression contributing to the malignant phenotype, including HER2/neu and hTERT.

A cytotoxic response to any nonmutated self-protein has a risk of causing autoimmune toxicity. Directing immune responses to tumor-specific mutated antigens avoids this risk, but the patient-specific nature of such mutations hampers the generation of reagents for use in multiple patients.

Immunosuppressive Tumor Microenvironment

There is abundant evidence that cancer cells have acquired an array of defense mechanisms to thwart their destruction by the immune system.[10] These are summarized in Box 30.1. Most human cancers present peptide epitopes in the context of MHC molecules that can be recognized by antigen-reactive T cells, but tumor cells themselves do not present antigen in an immunostimulatory context. Human T cells require additional signaling through costimulatory molecules, such as CD80/86 (B7 family), for optimal T-cell activation and expansion. Without these other signals, T cells can become anergic. Tumor cells can also downregulate antigen expression by a variety of mechanisms, such as epigenetic silencing, loss of MHC expression, and loss of function of the intracellular machinery that processes and transports peptides to the cell surface.

The immune system also has complex and generally fine-tuned down regulatory signaling to modulate responses.[11] Contraction of an acute immune response after 1 to 2 weeks may be appropriate for a viral infection but will be counterproductive to rejecting a large mass of malignant tissue. Autoimmune and allograft immune responses represent the types of chronic ongoing processes that would favor antitumor immune responses and underscore the need for a better understanding of the basic biology of immune regulation.

In addition to CTLA-4 signaling (see earlier), negative signaling can also be transduced through PD-1. DCs express the programmed death receptor ligand PD-L1 (or B7-H1); its expression by DCs can skew T cells toward an unresponsive phenotype.[2,12] DCs found within the tumor microenvironment have been shown to express high levels of PD-L1, which contribute to decreased local T-cell function. Some tumor cells themselves can present this inhibitory ligand, and expression of PD-L1, as with renal cancer, is associated with a poorer clinical outcome. Blockade of this PD-L1/PD-1 interaction using decoy receptors or antibodies is effective in improving immune therapies in animal models and when translated into human cancer immunotherapy trials has yielded impressive antitumor responses (see later).

Approximately 80% of human cancers do not respond to currently available modern immunotherapies.[13] Since there is a positive correlation between tumor mutational burden and immune checkpoint agents, cancers with few mutations may not present an adequate density of neoAg to the immune system. Impairment of antigen processing or antigen-presenting machinery (e.g., mutation in β_2 microglobulin) may also reduce neoAg display. Immunoediting and antigen loss, the progressive loss of more immunogenic cancer cell clones under the selective pressure of an evolving adaptive immune response, may yield more poorly immunogenic subclones that escape immune control.

Other immunity-avoidance mechanisms may be operative in the tumor microenvironment for cancers with an otherwise adequate threshold of neoAg density. The presence of immune suppressor cell populations within the tumor microenvironment Treg, myeloid-derived suppressor cells and M2-polarized tumor associates macrophages may dominantly suppress otherwise functional neoAg-reactive T cells.

Treg comprise a small subpopulation of CD4+ T cells (5% to 10%) that constitutively express the α chain of the IL-2 receptor CD25; most of these cells also express transcription factor Foxp3 (a forkhead-winged helix family member) and GITR (glucocorticoid-induced TNF receptor), as well as CTLA-4. These cells, Treg cells, produce immunosuppressive cytokines such as IL-10 and transforming growth factor-β (TGF-β) and can also inhibit through cell contact–dependent mechanisms. Mice or humans with a genetic mutation in Foxp3 lack Treg cells and develop a fulminant and lethal autoimmune disorder. Animal studies have clearly shown that Treg cells are responsible for suppressing the self-reactive T-cell repertoire, and the clinical manifestations from genetic loss of Foxp3 suggest that this may also be true in humans. Human Treg cells are enriched in tumor specimens and in draining lymph nodes of many solid tumors, and there is emerging evidence supporting a dominant role in suppressing self-reactive antitumor immune responses. Moderating Treg cell function could potentially favor antitumor immune responses. The use of lymphodepleting strategies before adoptive cell therapy (described later), which clearly enhances the antitumor biology of adoptively transferred T cells, may in part act through depletion of host resident Treg cells.

Myeloid-derived suppressor cells, which include granulocyte and immature myelomonocytic precursors, are expanded in settings of inflammation and cancer and elaborate immunosuppressive factors that include TGF-β, arginase 1, and inducible nitric oxide syntheses. Some strategies under current investigation seek to pharmacologically reduce their infiltration into and function within the tumor microenvironment.

Tumors themselves, and at times tumor stroma, can produce immunosuppressive substances; a prominent factor is TGF-β. TGF-β directly inhibits CTL activation, cytokine production, helper T-cell responses, and activation of DC and can promote the differentiation of Treg cells. Inhibition of TGF-β can have a salutary effect on antitumor immunity. T cells rendered insensitive to TGF-β signaling using a dominant-negative receptor have enhanced function in vivo. Neutralizing antibodies, small molecule inhibitors, and engineered T cells are currently under study in clinical trials. Vascular endothelial growth factor (VEGF) is important in angiogenesis but can also inhibit the function of DC. Thus, anti-VEGF therapy could also function through an immune mechanism. An isoform of the enzyme cyclooxygenase 2 is overexpressed in many tumors and catalyzes the synthesis of prostaglandin E2. Prostaglandin E2 has a generally adverse impact on the immune system, particularly on DC and T-cell function.

The enzymes indoleamine 2, 3-dioxgenase and arginase metabolize the essential amino acids *L*-trytophan and arginine, respectively. Their depletion impairs T-cell and DC function. Specific small molecule inhibitors of these enzymes are being studied preclinically and clinically.

IMMUNOTHERAPY

Cytokine Therapy

The cellular immune system often communicates among its component cells and exerts its effector functions using secreted proteins that bind to specific receptors. These secreted proteins are referred to as cytokines, and most often, they act in a paracrine fashion, exerting their actions on cells in their local environment. The family of interleukins (which currently includes more than 35 members) has a protean scope of interactions. In clinical use, several cytokines have been demonstrated to be of value, typically administered in supraphysiologic doses as systemic agents.

Although the IFNs (type I IFNs, consisting of the many species of IFN-α and IFN-β; and type II IFN, which consists only of IFN-γ) have important and diverse roles in immunity, they have limited clinical utility. Systemically administered IFN-α has some activity against renal cancer, hairy cell leukemia, chronic myeloid leukemia, and HIV-associated Kaposi sarcoma, but IFN-based immunotherapies have largely been superseded by other more effective biologicals.

IL-2 was the first cytokine to demonstrate reproducibly curative outcomes in patients with several types of widely metastatic cancer. Multiorgan toxicity is observed with high-dose IL-2 administration, including hypotension, capillary leak, transient hepatic and renal insufficiency, and mental status changes, which are in many ways reminiscent of events in sepsis. Toxicity is managed by judicious limitations on IL-2 dosing, fluid management, and supportive care because these toxicities are almost always self-limited and fully reversible. In an experienced clinical environment, the treatment-related mortality of high-dose IL-2 should be no more than 1%, with some centers reporting more than 800 consecutive courses administered without treatment-related mortality.[14] Initial studies of IL-2 included patients with tumors of many histologic types, but it soon became apparent that the two most consistently responsive cancers are melanoma and renal cell cancer. For patients with metastatic disease, the objective response rates (partial and complete) for melanoma and renal cell cancer were approximately 15% and 20%, respectively.[15,16] Some of these patients (4%–7%) achieved complete regression of widespread disease, responses that have proved durable more than 30 years (Fig. 30.3).[17,18] The ability to cure widely metastatic solid tumors with any systemic treatment is rare. However, for patients with renal cell cancer and melanoma, those achieving a complete response rarely relapsed. Considerable efforts have failed to provide predictors of which patients will respond to IL-2.

For patients with metastatic clear cell renal cancer, two randomized studies have suggested that high-dose IL-2 regimens produce higher response rates (22% partial and complete responses with high-dose treatments vs. 12% with lower dose regimens) as well as more durable responses than with low-dose regimens, but they were underpowered to evaluate differences in overall survival.[19]

There have been numerous clinical efforts to combine cytokines with other agents, particularly chemotherapy, to improve efficacy. Biochemotherapy using combinations of cisplatin, vinblastine, and dacarbazine (DTIC) with IL-2 and IFN-α, in general, has failed to show any survival benefit and had increased toxicity. Combinations of IL-2 and IFN-α had a similar clinical trials history: no improvement in response but increased toxicity. Use of biologic therapies in the adjuvant setting after complete resection of high-risk local regional melanoma remains controversial. The U.S. Food and Drug Administration (FDA) has approved the use of high-dose IFN-α (1 month of maximal-dose intravenous therapy followed by 11 months of lower dose subcutaneous treatment) after resection of node-positive melanoma on the basis of a randomized prospective study showing a delay in time to progression and borderline improved overall survival. Use of this toxic regimen has declined as other better tolerated and more effective agents have become available.

Several other cytokines have been studied in patients with cancer. IL-15 is a T cell and NK cell growth factor that also inhibits antigen-induced T-cell death in contrast to IL-2. IL-7 is another T-cell growth factor with a role in homeostatic T-cell expansion in response to lymphopenia; it causes dramatic increases in total body CD4+ and CD8+ T cells when it is administered to human subjects. IL-21 is another T-cell growth factor that has been reported to cause tumor regressions in one early clinical study. Yet the systemic use of these agents as monotherapy for the treatment of cancer has not progressed beyond these early studies. Ultimately, their role may be in combination with other more potent immunotherapeutic agents.

Vaccines

Successful presentation of a peptide epitope on an MHC molecule does not automatically result in a brisk T-cell response (see Fig. 30.2). To initiate a good T-cell response, an antigen must be presented to the immune system along with appropriate costimulatory molecules (signal 2, where the peptide MHC complex is signal 1), or it may be rendered anergic instead of reactive. The CD28 receptor usually serves this coreceptor function, although other mechanisms exist. Another important principle is that even well-presented normal self-proteins are general weak immunogens; the most avid self-reactive T-cell clones have been deleted in the thymus.

Early cancer vaccine strategies used autologous or allogeneic tumor cell–based vaccines. These efforts were based on half-century-old studies with carcinogen-induced murine tumor models. Whole cell vaccines contain multiple antigens that could be cross-presented by host antigen-presenting cells (DCs) and whose function could be further enhanced with an adjuvant. Initial crude adjuvants such as alum and the tuberculosis vaccine bacille Calmette-Guérin (BCG) have been replaced by molecules such as imiquimod or unmethylated CpG dinucleotides, which stimulate antigen-presenting cells through TLRs. The results of vaccine trials have been disappointing. Several large randomized trials using allogenic tumor vaccine or recombinant poxviruses failed to show benefit. We now understand why at least allogeneic vaccines failed—except for lineage-specific proteins, the neoAg expressed

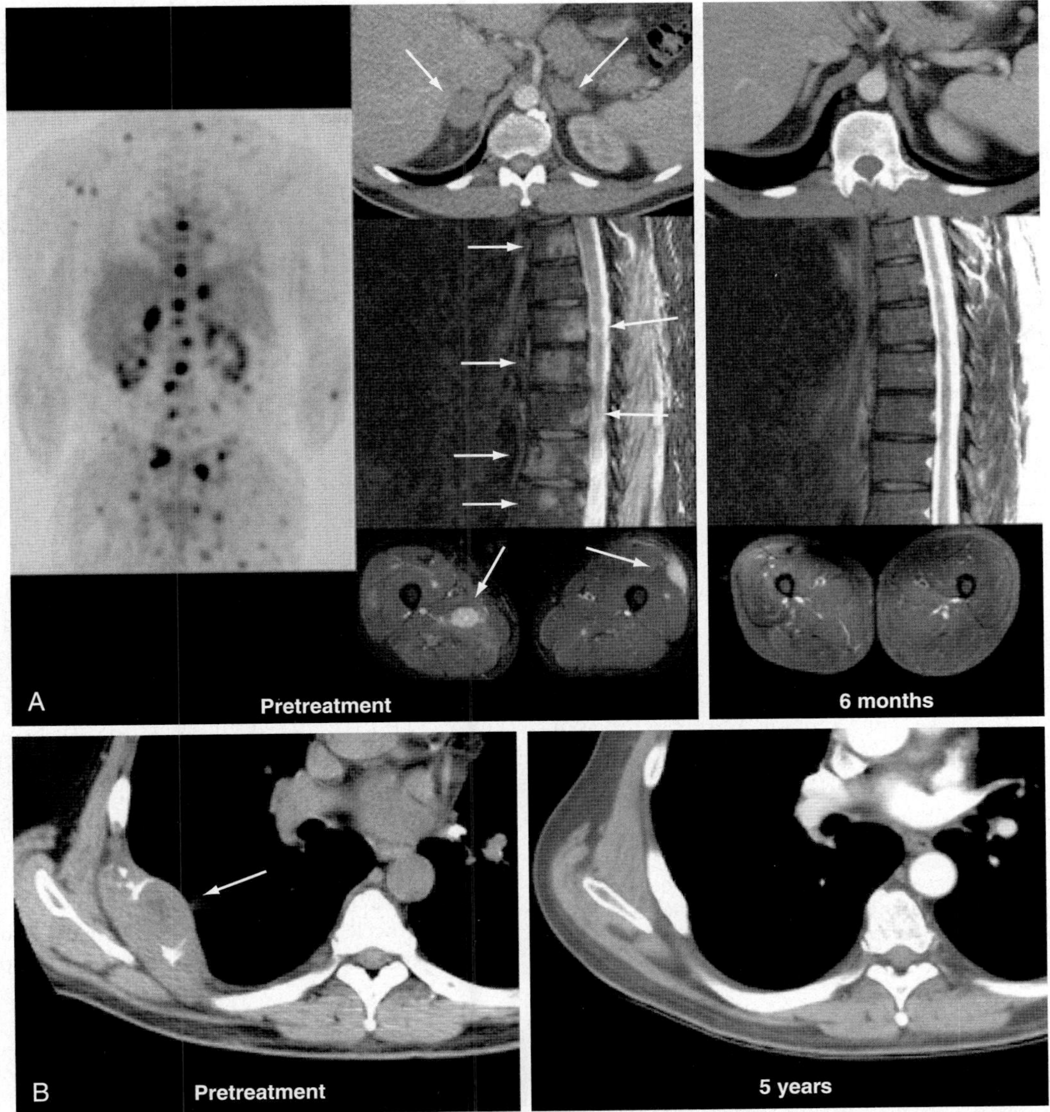

FIG. 30.3 Complete responses to high-dose interleukin-2 (IL-2). (A) Patient with diffuse metastatic melanoma by computed tomography and positron emission tomography scanning who received high-dose IL-2 therapy and had complete regression of all measurable disease, which is still ongoing 2 years later. (B) Patient with multiple bone metastases from renal cell cancer with a complete response sustained 5 years later.

by the allogeneic cancer cells were unique and unrelated to those expressed by the cancers in the vaccinated patient.

The identification of shared tumor rejection antigens and their specific epitopes has allowed new molecularly driven approaches to tumor vaccines. These include the use of synthetic peptides instead of whole cells or proteins (thus bypassing inefficient antigen-processing pathways) and incorporation of genes encoding these antigens into recombinant viral vectors to allow specific antigens to be more effectively targeted. Cell-based vaccines have employed in vitro–generated DCs. These DC-based vaccines have incorporated a variety of strategies—pulsing DCs with immunogenic peptide, genetically engineering with defined tumor antigens using recombinant viral vectors—and result in clinically meaningful tumor responses in a very small percentage of patients with melanoma and perhaps a few other cancers (Fig. 30.4). The application of multiple vaccination approaches against cancer-associated antigens has not led to consistent success in causing cancer regression. Dozens of vaccine approaches against dozens of target antigens in hundreds of clinical trials have largely been unsuccessful against measurable metastatic disease. Many trials have reported infrequent anecdotal responses, primarily in patients with melanoma confined to the skin and nodal sites, which appear to be somewhat more amenable to immunotherapy. A review of more than 1200 patients vaccinated for cancer reported an overall objective response rate of 3.6%.[20] Analyses of these trials have shown that there is little evidence for the generation of significant numbers of new tumor-reactive T cells by most vaccines. Whereas there is clear evidence that some vaccine formulations can activate and expand tumor antigen–reactive T cells, they are still clinically inadequate as stand-alone treatments.

Cancer mutation-derived neoAg serve as excellent targets for antitumor immune responses unleashed by checkpoint blockade. Combined immunotherapy (α-CTLA-4, α-PD-1/PD-L1) has renewed interest in creating individualized neoAg vaccine formulations. High-throughput sequencing of cancer and normal exomes is now cost-effective, and predictive algorithms are iteratively improving the selection of putative cancer neoAg for each patient's tumor. Peptide, RNA, or DNA-based neoAg vaccines are currently under study, alone and in combination with checkpoint blockade, with the goal of increasing the precursor frequency of neoAg-reactive T cells. Yet, the potential for vaccines as systemic therapy in the oncology armamentarium has not yet been realized.

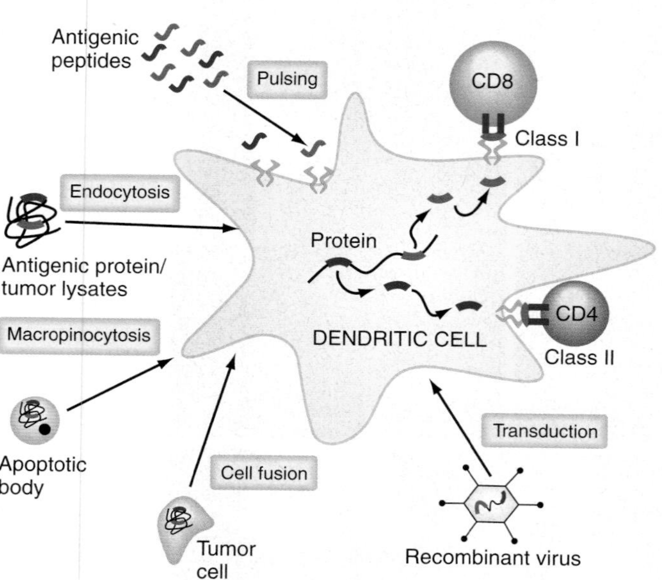

FIG. 30.4 Tumor antigen acquisition by dendritic cells. These professional antigen-presenting cells can acquire and process antigen through endocytosis or pinocytosis or be manipulated ex vivo with peptide loading or genetic engineering to produce a cell-based vaccine.

Targeting Immunomodulatory Pathways

Although the two-signal model (TCR engagement plus costimulatory signal) has been largely validated, the adaptive immune response is modulated by additional costimulatory and coinhibitory signals as it orchestrates an appropriate antigen-reactive response. With respect to antitumor immunity, preclinical animal studies that have been translated into human cancer trials have shown, in particular, that the blockade of coinhibitory molecules such as CTLA-4 and PD-1/PD-L1[21, 22] can yield dramatic and durable tumor regressions in several types of solid tumors (Fig. 30.5). CTLA-4, through engagement with its ligands CD80 and CD86, attenuates activation and expansion of antigen-reactive T cells; it can be thought of as one of the "braking" mechanisms of the immune system. Monoclonal antibodies that block CTLA-4 in humans have been developed: ipilimumab, now FDA approved (a fully human IgG1k monoclonal antibody), and tremelimumab (a fully human IgG2 monoclonal antibody). CTLA-4 blockade has demonstrated a significant survival advantage and long-term benefit in a minority of melanoma patients (approximately 10%).[23]

A second coinhibitory receptor expressed on T cells is PD-1, which is engaged by its ligands PD-L1 and PD-L2. PD-L1 and to a lesser extent PD-L2 are expressed by a broad range of human malignant neoplasms—melanoma, non–small cell lung cancer, colon, breast, urothelial, ovarian, and pancreatic as well as hematologic cancers (Fig. 30.6). Engagement of PD-1 by these tumor-expressed ligands now appears to be an important mechanism by which some human cancers evade an otherwise effective antitumor immune response. Monoclonal antibodies directed against PD-1 or PD-L1, with the goal of interrupting this inhibitory signaling, have now been shown to be even superior to CTLA-4 blockade in a broad range of human cancers.[24] The FDA approved PD-1/PD-L1 inhibitors for non–small cell lung cancer, head and neck squamous cancer, Hodgkin lymphoma, Merkel cell carcinoma, urothelial carcinoma, gastroesophageal cancer,

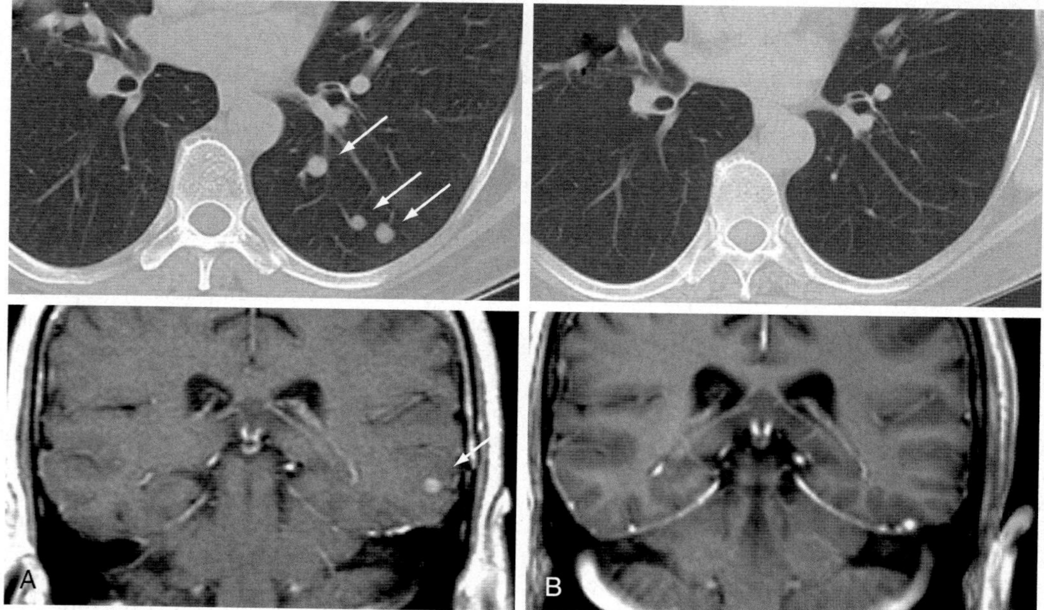

FIG. 30.5 Regression of lung and brain metastases from melanoma in a patient treated with ipilimumab (anti–CTLA-4 antibody). (A) Patient with lung, subcutaneous, and brain metastases received ipilimumab. (B) He then developed immune-mediated hypopituitarism but achieved a complete regression of all disease, which is ongoing 7 years later.

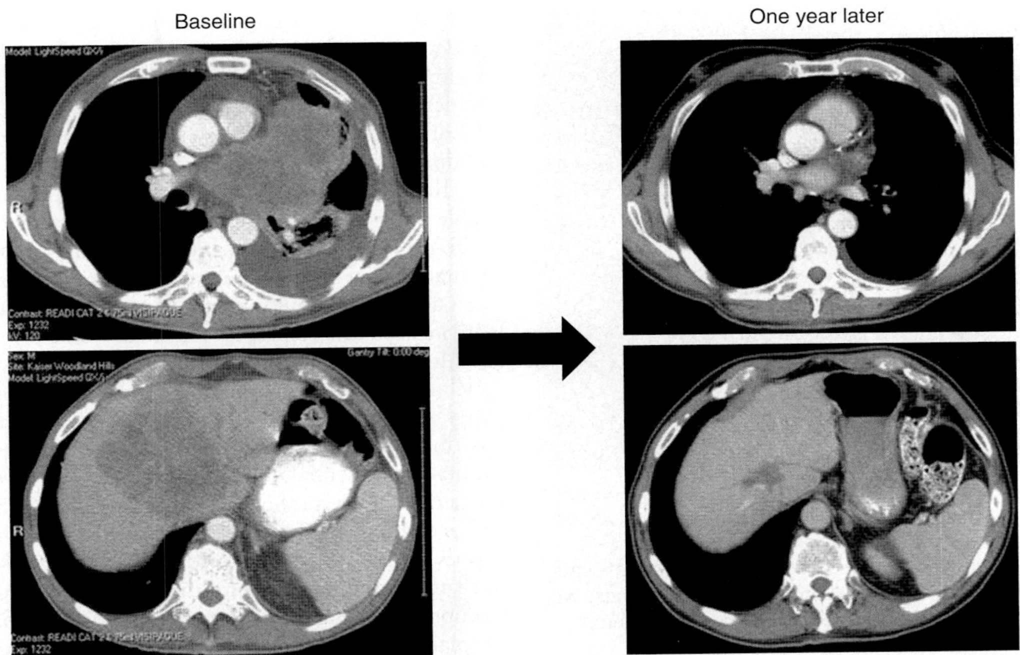

FIG. 30.6 Response of bulky metastatic melanoma to PD-1–blocking antibody. A dramatic response during a period of a year in a patient who failed to respond to biochemotherapy, high-dose interleukin-2 and cytotoxic T lymphocyte–associated antigen 4–blocking antibody.

renal cell cancer, colorectal cancer (microsatellite instability—high or mismatch repair deficient), and hepatocellular carcinoma.[25] Combined PD-1/CTLA-4 therapy was also approved for metastatic melanoma, demonstrating superior response rates to either monotherapy. These immune therapies had overall response rates from between 10% and 70% depending on the cancer type, with improvement in relapse-free and overall survival. For some histologies, complete durable responses have been recorded. Predicting tumor responses has been challenging. Cancers with high mutational burdens have higher response rates to checkpoint blockade. High densities of CD8 T cells along the tumor periphery, or their infiltration into tumor metastases after even a single dose of PD-1, seem to correlate with response. While PD-L1 expression is associated with a higher likelihood of response to PD-1/PD-L1 blockade, its absence does not preclude a response.[26] Other factors, such as genetic polymorphism and gut microbiome, are currently being studied. Mechanisms of resistance and relapse likewise are being intensely studied.[27] The use of checkpoint inhibitors has also been approved for use in an adjuvant setting in resected high-risk melanoma.

The majority of patients receiving CTLA-4, PD-1 checkpoint inhibitors, or the two in combination experience autoimmune-related adverse events.[28] These autoimmune toxicities span almost all organ systems: skin (rash, dermatitis), gastrointestinal (diarrhea, colitis), hepatic (autoimmune, hepatitis), endocrine (thyroiditis, hypophysitis, rarely diabetes), pulmonary (pneumonitis), renal (acute interstitial nephritis), musculoskeletal (arthralgias, myalgias), hematologic (rare), ocular (rare), cardiac (rare but can be life threatening), pancreas (rare), and neurologic (also rare). As expected, higher incidence and severity of adverse events are observed with combination therapy, and with CTLA-4 monotherapy greater than PD-1. Close follow-up therapy, treatment cessation, and use of glucocorticoids have reduced treatment-related mortality to less than 1%.

Our improved understanding of human tumor immune biology afforded by these clinically active checkpoint inhibitors provides many opportunities for their use in combination, with modern cancer vaccines and with T cell–based therapies (see later).

The objective response criteria for immune therapies cannot be accommodated by the response criteria in use for many decades with cytotoxic chemotherapies. For these immunomodulatory therapies, the kinetics of response may be very slow and the achievement of a complete response may evolve over 1 to 2 years, making overall survival the most significant objective response criterion. These observations underscore the need for better biomarkers to predict and confirm responses.

Immune modulation can also be positively driven by stimulation of coreceptors, which enhances immunity. A receptor-like protein expressed on CD4+ and CD8+ T cells after activation is 4-1BB (CD137); cross-linking of 4-1BB with a ligand or antibody delivers a costimulatory signal to the T cell. Preclinical animal studies have demonstrated enhanced tumor rejection in established tumor models. This strategy for immunomodulation using an agonist anti-CD137 human monoclonal antibody is undergoing trials in human subjects. Agonist antibody to CD40, an activating receptor on DCs, likewise is being studied clinically. Combining such activating strategies with blocking of inhibitory receptors and perhaps vaccines may be needed to achieve more impressive and consistent clinical responses.

T-Cell Adoptive Therapy

With the recognition that T lymphocytes are the effectors of tumor rejection and immunologic memory in animal models, early human studies focused on tumor-reactive lymphocytes isolated from patients with IL-2-responsive cancers, largely in melanoma.[29] The basic approach was to isolate, expand, and readminister tumor-reactive T cells as a means to overcome the weak expansion of such cells in vivo by vaccination. In patients with melanoma,

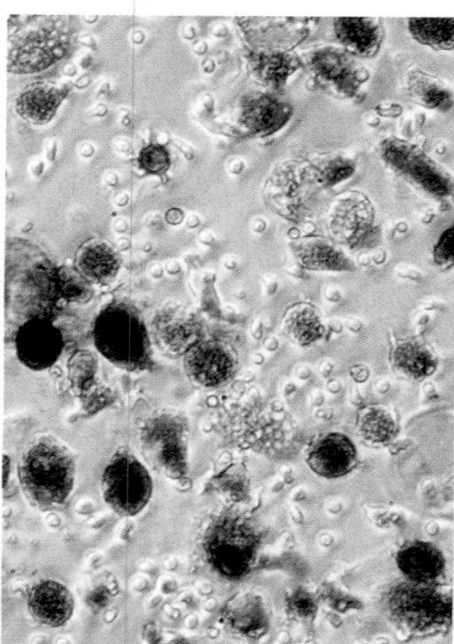
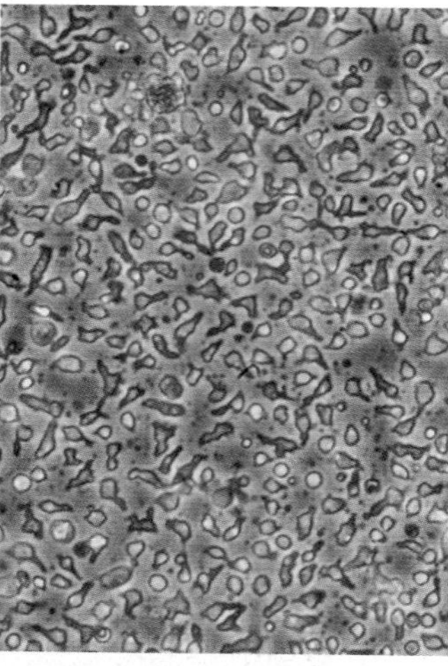

FIG. 30.7 Expansion of tumor-infiltrating lymphocytes from resected metastatic melanoma in culture with interleukin-2 (IL-2). Photomicrograph of fresh melanoma after enzymatic dispersal *(left)* shows tumor cells and small numbers of infiltrating lymphocytes. After several weeks of culture in IL-2, there is T-cell outgrowth and lysis of all tumor cells *(right)*, with most cultures then demonstrating immunologic recognition of tumor.

more than 80% of metastatic lesions were enriched with such resident tumor-reactive T cells, which could be activated and expanded in vitro simply by adding IL-2 to cell culture. These TIL cultures yielded large numbers of oligoclonal populations of MHC-restricted, melanoma-reactive effector cells (Fig. 30.7). This rich source of polyclonal tumor-reactive T cells not only served as a discovery tool for numerous shared antigens in human melanoma but also was critical in demonstrating that the transfer of ex vivo expanded autologous tumor-reactive T cells could cause complete and durable regressions of metastatic cancer. The initial attempt at such an approach used huge numbers of cells grown in vitro (a median of 2×10^{11} cells were administered to patients), supported with high-dose systemic IL-2 to enhance TIL survival and in vivo function.[30] An overall objective response rate of 33% was seen and was not influenced by prior IL-2 failure. However, the major shortcoming of this study was that most responses were of short duration (median, 7 months).

The first protocol to administer genetically modified cells to humans was used to track TILs after administration using a marker gene and showed that almost all infused TILs had disappeared from the circulation within days.[31,32] A chemotherapy-induced lymphodepletion regimen before adoptive transfer was found to enhance lymphocyte survival and to improve T-cell persistence and efficacy. Murine models suggest that the mechanisms were (1) removal of suppressive Treg cells; (2) stimulation of T-cell growth factors in the host in response to lymphodepletion (homeostatic proliferation); (3) reduction in competition for these homeostatic cytokines from endogenous T cells or NK cells; and (4) increased immunostimulatory microbial factors, such as lipopolysaccharide. In clinical protocols, several immunosuppressive regimens have been used to deplete host lymphocytes. The basic regimen consisted of high-dose cyclophosphamide and fludarabine, with some patients also receiving total body irradiation. When peripheral leukocyte counts are essentially zero, a median of 5×10^{10} cultured TILs are given, again followed by systemic IL-2 support (Fig. 30.8).[33] Overall, in 93 patients with metastatic melanoma, of whom 86% had visceral tumor involvement and 84% had prior IL-2, the objective response rate was 56% and the 5-year survival was 30%. Nearly identical results were seen in an additional 101 patients treated more recently with a variety of lymphodepleting regimens. Most strikingly, in these two experiences, was that 44 achieved complete regressions with only two relapses; years later, 19 of the 20 patients achieving complete regressions remain free of disease 5 to 10 years later.

There is emerging evidence that the TILs mediating these durable regressions may in fact be directed not toward shared lineage-specific melanocytic antigens but rather to tumor-associated mutations (neoAg) unique to each patient's tumor. Human cancers accumulate multiple mutations in their gene products, some driving the cancer process and many other "bystander" proteins resulting from carcinogens and genetic instability. Theoretically, such mutated proteins would be the ideal tumor rejection targets; they are limited to the tumor, may be seen by the immune system as "foreign" rather than "self," and in some cases may be "driver" mutations essential to the malignancy. These observations have generated the hypothesis that human cancers with larger numbers of accumulated mutations may present more mutated "neoepitopes," which in turn provides for a more robust antitumor T-cell repertoire, a repertoire that can be exploited clinically with adoptive cell transfer or release of inhibitory signaling.[34] This may explain the responsiveness of cutaneous melanoma to immunotherapy as ultraviolet exposure results in this cancer having the highest frequency of mutations among common human cancers. This is further supported by the fact that microsatellite unstable cancers and lung cancer in smokers (vs. nonsmokers) are also more responsive to checkpoint inhibition.

In the field of adoptive T-cell therapy, the advent of efficient gene engineering methods for human T cells has enabled novel approaches to generate tumor-reactive T cells. Recombinant gamma retroviruses and lentiviruses can introduce new genes into mature human peripheral blood T cells with high efficiency. These techniques have been applied to introduce genes encoding a variety of receptors that can recognize targets on tumors and trigger a T-cell response. There are several types of such receptors in clinical trials. The traditional two-chain TCR consists of α and β chains that engage the peptide-MHC complex of a tumor antigen and transduce a signal by noncovalent association with the CD3 complex in the T cell. Another receptor, termed CAR, uses an antigen-binding extracellular domain (often a single-chain version of the Fab fragment of a monoclonal antibody) covalently linked in tandem to a transmembrane domain and the CD3 ζ molecule for signal transduction (Fig. 30.9). Several generations of CAR receptors also incorporate additional intracellular signaling moieties, such as CD28 or CD137 (4-1BB).[35] These antibody-based CARs bind to a target molecule expressed on the external surface of the cell membrane and therefore have the advantage of not being MHC restricted without apparent normal tissue toxicity.

The most successful CAR effort to date has been in targeting the CD19 molecule on B-cell malignant neoplasms (Fig. 30.10). Several versions of an anti-CD19 CAR have now been FDA approved, having shown dramatic durable complete responses against chemotherapy-refractory chronic lymphocytic leukemia, diffuse large B-cell lymphoma, and acute lymphocytic leukemia.[36] Patients undergoing CD19 CAR treatment also generally develop B-cell aplasia because CD19 is expressed by normal B cells; this can be successfully managed with immunoglobulin infusion and infection control and is considered an acceptable toxicity. Other CAR targets expressed by hematopoietic and solid malignancies are undergoing clinical

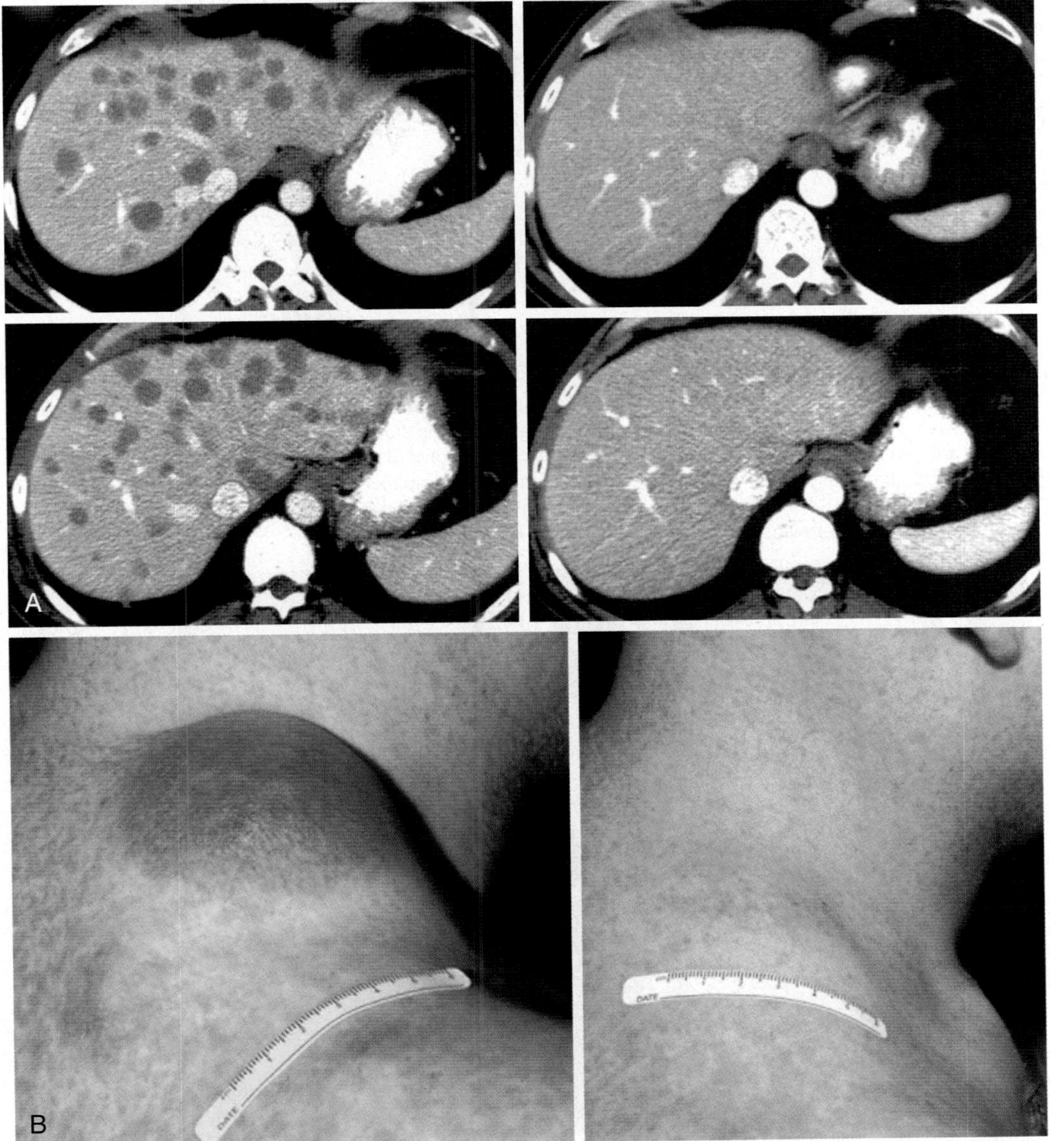

FIG. 30.8 Clinical response in a patient with metastatic melanoma to adoptive transfer of in vitro expanded tumor-infiltrating lymphocytes with systemic interleukin-2 (IL-2), following preparative lymphodepletion. Responses can be durable and rapid. (A) Patient with extensive liver disease remains free of disease more than 5 years after one T-cell transfer. (B) Another patient showed rapid regression of bulky subcutaneous disease only 12 days after cell transfer, achieving a complete response, durable at 4 years.

study, with encouraging early results reported from targeting B-cell maturation antigen expressed on the surface of multiple myeloma.[37]

Ultimately, it may be traditional alpha-beta T-cells (natural or receptor-engineered) that will be most effective against the common solid cancers of epithelial origin. As outlined above, antigens encoded by tumor-specific mutations seem to drive the safest and most effective immune attack against cancer. Antigens recognized by T cells do require specific MHC presentation, but unlike CAR targets, every protein made in the cytoplasm or released into the extracellular milieu is a potential target for a classical CD8 or CD4 T cell. New ways to display a tumor's mutations have been developed to facilitate the identification of tumor antigen-reactive T cells from common epithelial cancers, where autologous tumor lines are rarely available.[38] In preliminary trials, cells identified using these methods have been able to cause regression of widespread metastatic cancers of breast, colon, cervix, and bile duct origin (Fig. 30.11).[39] Overall, these various T-cell adoptive therapy trials have demonstrated that the infusion of tumor-reactive T cells can be a potent new therapeutic modality but will require target antigens of the highest specificity to be administered safely.

Bispecific Antibodies

Bispecific antibodies (BsAbs) are engineered to have two Fab variable sites—one binding to a tumor target cell surface molecule and the other to an effector T cell—with the objective of bringing the two cells in close proximity.[40,41] The BsAb also retains an Fc domain. The goal of this chimeric antibody is to effect T-cell cytotoxicity and Fc-mediated cytotoxicity. A BsAb (Blinatunomab), bispecific for CD3a and CD19, is FDA approved for certain B-cell malignancies.

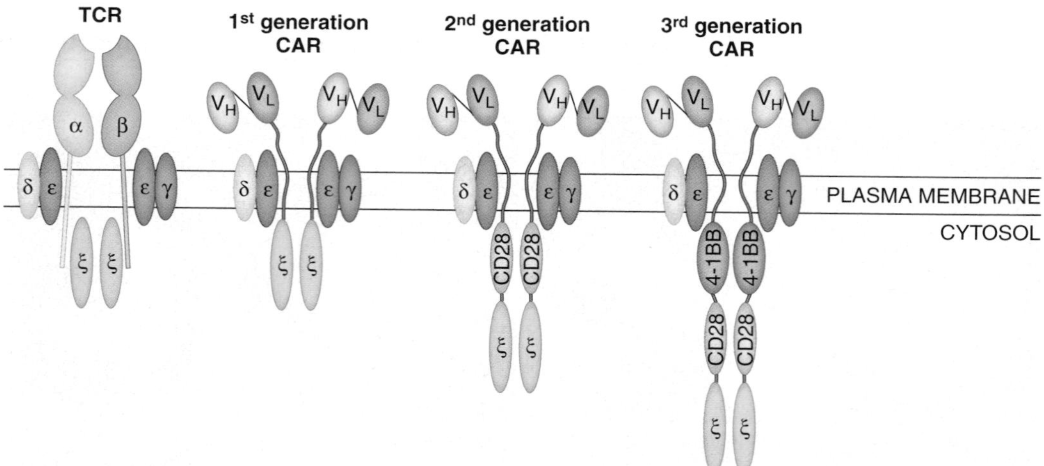

FIG. 30.9 Illustration of a native T-cell receptor *(TCR)* and various chimeric antigen receptors *(CARs)*. The native TCR α and β chains noncovalently associate with the CD3 complex consisting of two ζ chains, two ε chains, one γ chain, and one δ chain to transduce a T-cell activation signal. First-generation CARs covalently attach an antigen-binding domain from a single-chain variable fragment of a monoclonal antibody to the ζ chain of CD3, which then associates with the remainder of the CD3 complex to signal. Second- and third-generation CARs add one or two interposed costimulation domains (respectively) from a variety of T-cell costimulators to enhance activation (here illustrated with CD28 and 4-1BB).

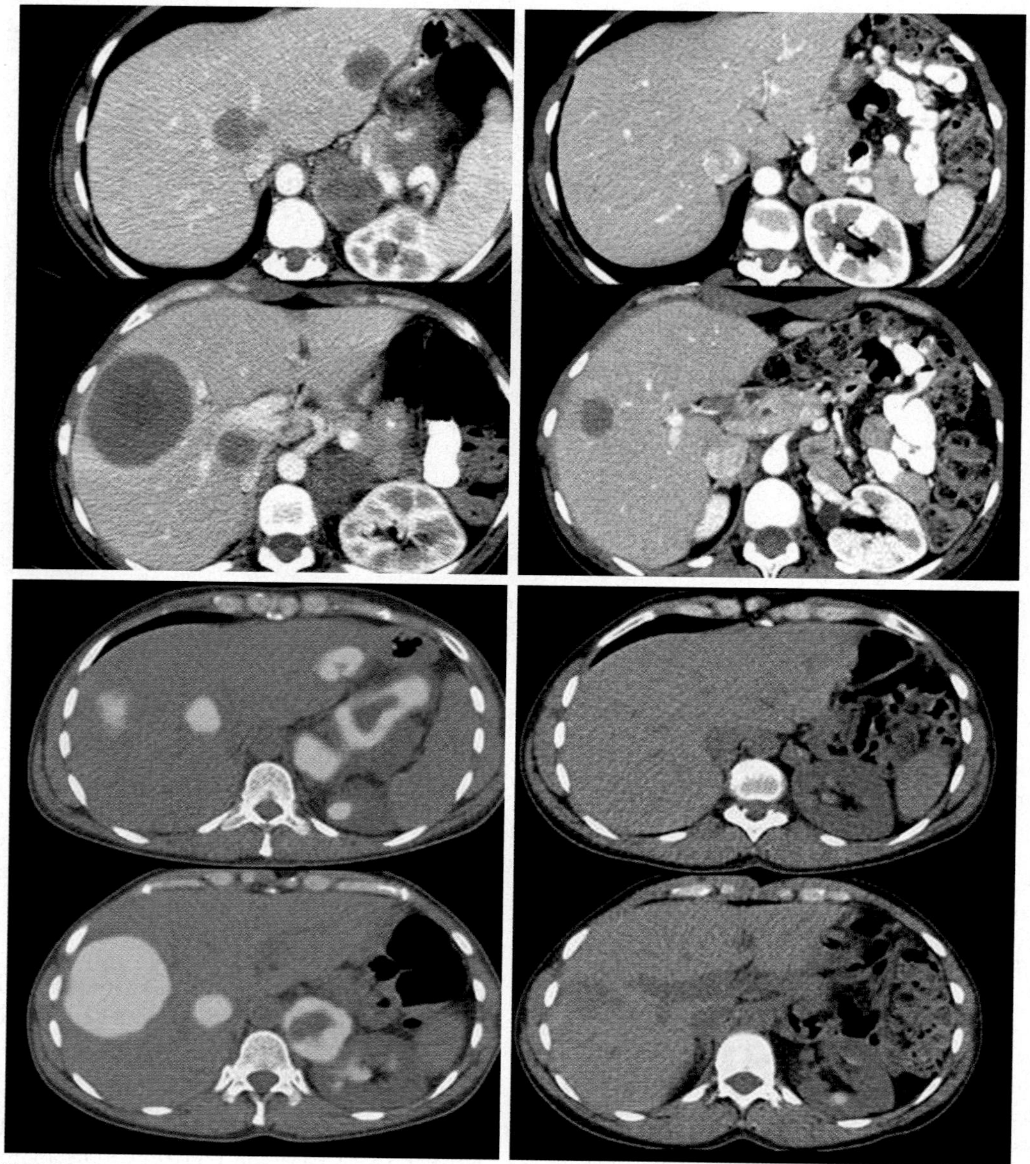

FIG. 30.10 Positron emission tomography/computed tomography scan of a patient with chemotherapy-resistant diffuse large B-cell lymphoma. Pretreatment scan on the *left* demonstrates liver, gastric, and retroperitoneal lymph node involvement. The patient received CD19 chimeric antigen receptor adoptive cell therapy and achieved complete response. Scan on *right* taken at 13 months of follow-up (liver residual metabolically inactive).

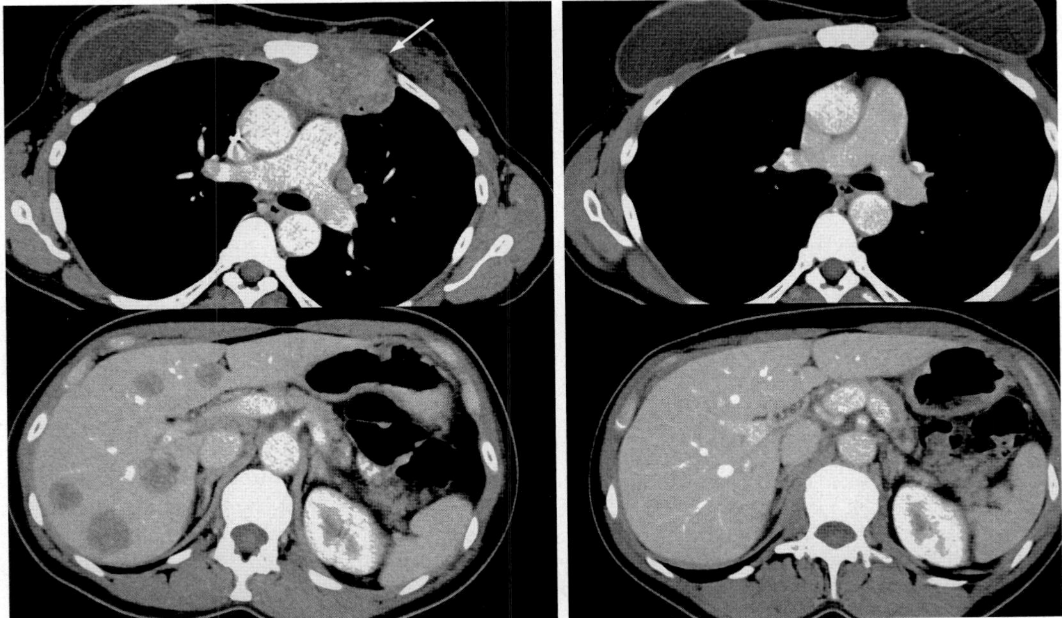

FIG. 30.11 Computed tomography scans of a patient with metastatic breast cancer before *(left)* and 28 months after *(right)* receiving an adoptive transfer of tumor infiltrating lymphocytes selected for recognition of two tumor-specific mutated neoantigens. Complete resolution of mediastinal disease *(arrow)* and large hepatic metastases is seen. (From Zacharakis N, Chinnasamy H, Black M, et al. Immune recognition of somatic mutations leading to complete durable regression in metastatic breast cancer. *Nat Med.* 2018;24:724–730.)

Monoclonal Antibody Therapy

The concept of a patient's immune system providing targeted therapy in the treatment of disease has its origins in experiments performed in 1890 by von Behring and Kitasato. They determined that immunity to infectious diseases could be transferred from one rat to the next through a serum transfusion; they coined the term *passive serotherapy.* The first application of passive serotherapy in the treatment of cancer was performed in 1895 by Hericourt and Richet, when they immunized dogs with human sarcoma and transferred the serum to patients in an attempt to provide cancer immunity. After almost 100 years since the first cancer immunotherapy trial, the FDA approved the first monoclonal antibody to be used in the treatment of cancer. Today, therapeutic monoclonal antibodies are considered to be the fastest growing class of new therapeutic agents.[42,43] Although many had predicted the therapeutic potential of monoclonal antibodies during the past century, it was not until mouse hybridoma technology was developed by Kohler and Milstein in 1975 that the ability to produce monoclonal antibodies directed against a specific target antigen became a reality.[44,45]

Unfortunately, monoclonal antibodies created from mouse hybridoma technology were specific but limited in their therapeutic potential secondary to xenogeneic reasons. First, they are recognized by the immune system as foreign and stimulate the production of human antimouse antibodies, commonly referred to as the HAMA response. This immunogenic response usually limits murine monoclonal antibodies to a single dose. Second, murine monoclonal antibodies are unable to activate other effector functions (e.g., complement, NK cells, phagocytes) of the human immune system. Finally, murine monoclonal antibodies suffer from a much reduced serum half-life compared with human antibodies, resulting in decreased time of exposure to the target antigen. To overcome many of these limitations, molecular engineering techniques were developed to generate antibodies in which the murine sequences were partially or fully replaced by human protein sequences. A "chimeric" monoclonal antibody refers to a murine antibody in which the variable regions responsible for the antigen specificity remain murine and the constant region (Fc) is replaced by human sequences. A "humanized" monoclonal antibody refers to a monoclonal antibody created by engrafting murine complementarity-determining regions onto a human monoclonal antibody variable region. Most recently, fully human antibodies have been produced through human hybridomas and transgenic mice expressing human immunoglobulin genes.[46] Also, engineered monoclonal antibody fragments have been developed and characterized that have unique pharmacokinetic and therapeutic properties (Fig. 30.12).[47,48]

It is estimated that monoclonal antibodies account for approximately 30% of new biotech drugs in development. To date, the FDA has approved more than 76 monoclonal antibody/antibody-based therapeutics to treat various diseases, such as cancer, autoimmune diseases, and transplant rejection, with many more currently in clinical trials. Currently, there are more than 2700 active clinical trials evaluating antibodies in the treatment of cancer in the United States alone. Given the rapid introduction and development of monoclonal antibody therapeutics, the U.S. Adopted Names Council, in collaboration with the World Health Organization International Nonproprietary Names Committee, has established guidelines for the naming of new monoclonal antibodies. Each name is composed of four syllables, with each syllable providing information. The first syllable is a unique prefix. The second syllable describes the indication; for example, all monoclonal antibodies intended to treat tumors will have the second syllable of *-tu* for tumor. The third syllable identifies the source of the antibody (murine, *-o*; chimeric, *-xi*; human, *-u*). The last syllable is always *-mab*, identifying the therapeutic agent as a monoclonal antibody.

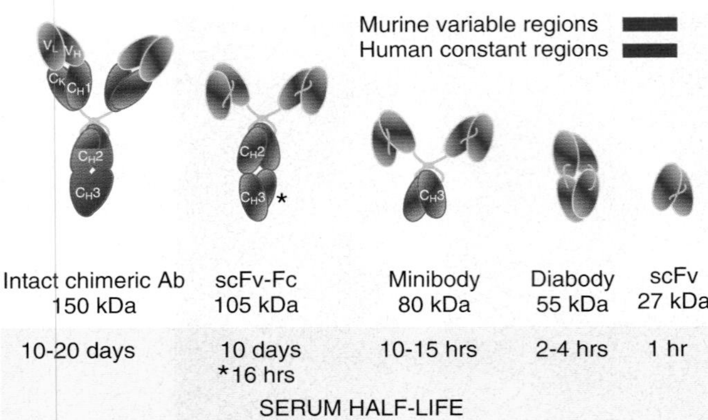

FIG. 30.12 Chimeric monoclonal antibody (Ab) and engineered antibody fragments. A chimeric intact monoclonal antibody is depicted, showing the retained murine domains *(green)* and human domains *(red)*. Engineered antibody fragments are depicted to the right of the intact chimeric antibody. These fragments are listed in decreasing size from right to left, with their corresponding serum half-life. Note that the 105-kDa fragment *(scFv-Fc)* normally has a half-life of 10 days. However, when a point mutation is introduced *(star)*, the fragment has a half-life of 16 hours, comparable to the much smaller 80-kDa minibody fragment. This is the result of a point mutation introduced into the FcRn-binding region in the C_H3 domain, which decreases the fragment's affinity for the FcRn, resulting in a much decreased serum half-life.

To highlight the clinical potential of and challenges to monoclonal antibody therapeutics, the remaining portion of this section describes monoclonal antibody therapy as it pertains to cancer.[49,50] The mechanism of action used by monoclonal antibodies in the fight against cancer can be divided into two types. The first results from the physical binding of the monoclonal antibody to the specific tumor antigen. Many antigenic targets are cell surface receptors connected to signaling pathways, which are important in cancer progression. The best example of this is trastuzumab (Herceptin), which blocks signaling through an overexpressed growth factor receptor (HER2/neu) in a subset of breast cancers. Second, and perhaps more important, a monoclonal antibody directed against a tumor antigen can activate the patient's own immune system to attack the tumor tissue. This mechanism is mediated through interactions of the Fc region of the antibody and effector cells of the immune system bearing the Fcγ receptor, such as NK cells, phagocytes, and neutrophils. Activation of these professional phagocytes leads to tumor cell destruction and is referred to as ADCC.[51] Also, the Fc domain of the antibody can activate the complement system through interactions with complement-activating protein (C1q), resulting in the formation of the membrane attack complex, which causes cell lysis. This is referred to as complement-dependent cytotoxicity. Furthermore, there is mounting evidence that monoclonal antibodies are likely to enhance tumor antigen presentation by professional antigen-presenting cells such as DCs, which may ultimately lead to the induction of tumor antigen–specific CTL responses and result in lasting immunity. Amplification of the immune response to other tumor antigens may also occur because it is likely after ADCC or complement-dependent cytotoxicity that many tumor peptides have the opportunity to undergo professional antigen presentation, with the potential of also inciting a CTL response.[52,53]

Factors Governing the Therapeutic Potential of Monoclonal Antibodies

Endogenous IgG has a half-life of approximately 3 weeks. This relatively long serum persistence is a result of its interaction with the FcRn (neonatal or Brambell receptor) on endothelial cells. Most serum proteins undergo pinocytosis followed by progressive acidification of the endosome, which eventually fuses with a lysosome and results in the destruction of entrapped proteins. IgG, however, binds the FcRn of the endosomal membrane under acidic conditions and is thus protected from lysosomal degradation; it is shuttled back to the serum and released from FcRn under a physiologic pH (7.4). Site-specific mutagenesis has identified the specific amino acid residues responsible for the Fc-FcRn interaction that leads to the long serum half-life of IgG antibodies. Thus, by introducing specific amino acid changes into the Fc region of an engineered antibody, one can tailor the pharmacokinetic properties to fit the clinical or therapeutic indication.[54] For example, by substitution of one amino acid (H310A), the serum half-life of an engineered chimeric monoclonal antibody fragment was reduced by 90%, from 10 days to 16 hours. One can imagine therapeutic applications in which a shorter serum half-life would be beneficial, such as a conjugated monoclonal antibody with toxin or radionuclide in which rapid clearance would serve to decrease the exposure of the normal tissues of the body to the toxin.

Monoclonal antibodies of the IgG subtype are large (150-kDa) proteins. Their relatively large size may limit their ability to penetrate tissues to bind the targeted tumor antigen. It is estimated that the average intervessel distance in tumors is approximately 40 to 100 μM. Obviously, in hypoxic areas of a tumor, this distance is probably increased. Therefore, a smaller molecule will be able to diffuse or to penetrate farther and more quickly. Also, small molecules have different clearance mechanisms. It is generally accepted that molecules smaller than 80 kDa are below the renal threshold and are able to be cleared solely through the kidney. To this end, protein engineers have been able to create very small antibody fragments that retain the antigen-binding specificity but no longer retain the ability to bind the FcRn. The smallest of these entities is the single-chain Fv, with a molecular mass of 27 kDa. Many of these fragments, with ultrashort half-lives, are being tested in mouse models for the ability to target tumors for imaging, diagnostics, and potential transport of larger toxic molecules and chemotherapeutic agents to the tumor.

Compared with traditional chemotherapy, the side-effect profile of nonconjugated monoclonal antibody immunotherapy is rather mild. Most of the toxicity is related to hypersensitivity reactions caused by the protein sequences of mouse origin present in chimeric and humanized monoclonal antibodies. Although fatal infusion reactions are rare, they have been reported. These reactions usually occur during or just after the first dose of the monoclonal antibody. Other side effects may occur as a result of the binding of the monoclonal antibody to its cognate antigen. For example, cetuximab, a chimeric monoclonal antibody that binds the epidermal growth factor receptor (EGFR), is associated with skin eruptions secondary to the blockade of EGFR signaling. Also, bevacizumab (Avastin), a humanized monoclonal antibody that binds VEGF, is associated with hemorrhagic and thrombotic events associated with the decreased signaling through the VEGF receptor (VEGFR).

Unconjugated Antibodies

As noted, the treatment of disease with unconjugated monoclonal antibodies became popular in the 1980s, after murine monoclonal antibodies became available secondary to hybridoma technology. These early therapeutic monoclonal antibodies suffered from poor clinical efficacy and immunogenicity secondary to the HAMA response, leading to the termination of most clinical monoclonal antibody studies. It was not until the development of chimeric, humanized, and fully human therapeutic monoclonal antibodies that clinical efficacy was routinely witnessed in monoclonal antibody studies. Although many therapeutic monoclonal antibodies start as murine monoclonal antibodies, much of the murine antibody is replaced by human IgG protein sequences. For example, a chimeric IgG molecule is approximately 75% human and 25% murine. A humanized murine monoclonal antibody is approximately 95% human, with only the complementarity-determining regions of the variable region remaining murine.

Rituximab is an excellent example of the development of a monoclonal antibody clinically effective against a cancer after transitioning to the chimeric form of the antibody from the parent murine monoclonal antibody. Rituximab, but not its parent murine monoclonal antibody, has demonstrated cytotoxicity in experimental systems. Rituximab is a chimeric monoclonal antibody directed against a cell surface antigen found on mature B cells of non-Hodgkin lymphoma and was the first monoclonal antibody to be approved by the FDA, in 1997, for use in the treatment of a human malignant neoplasm. Initially, rituximab was used as single-agent therapy for recurrent or refractory low-grade B-cell lymphomas and demonstrated an overall response rate of 48% and a complete response rate of 10%.[55] The cytotoxic activity of rituximab is thought to be a combination of complement-dependent cytotoxicity and ADCC; this clarifies the inactivity of the parent murine monoclonal antibody, which lacks the human Fc region to interact with the serum complement protein (C1q) and the Fcγ receptor of the professional phagocytes to elicit ADCC. Evidence in support of ADCC as the mechanism of action was the finding that Fcγ receptor polymorphisms predict response rates in patients with follicular lymphoma treated with rituximab. With high response rates and limited toxicity in the setting of recurrent or refractory non-Hodgkin lymphoma, studies were undertaken to investigate rituximab as a first-line therapy. Initially, rituximab was shown to increase the sensitivity of chemotherapy-resistant cell lines, which spawned a trial of rituximab added to a first-line chemotherapy regimen of cyclophosphamide, doxorubicin, vincristine, and prednisolone (CHOP). The addition of rituximab to CHOP, commonly referred to as R-CHOP, resulted in a 95% overall response rate, including a 55% complete response rate. Long-term follow-up revealed a statistically improved survival without significant differences in toxicity.

Trastuzumab is a humanized antibody derived from a murine monoclonal antibody directed against HER2/neu. This receptor tyrosine kinase is a member of the EGFR family, which was noted to be overexpressed because of gene amplification in approximately 25% of breast cancers. Therefore, the strategy was undertaken to target this overexpressed cell surface receptor that was associated with a more aggressive biology in an attempt to disrupt the cancer-promoting mitogenic signaling through antibody blockade of this receptor. Initial phase 2 trials, conducted in the setting of metastatic HER2/neu-positive breast cancers, demonstrated modest objective response rates of 12% to 16%. Given the evidence for single-agent activity, further trials were conducted with trastuzumab in combination with standard chemotherapy regimens that demonstrated a doubling of the response rates (25% to 57%) compared with chemotherapy alone. In addition, trastuzumab utilized in the adjuvant setting has been associated with a 50% reduction in 1-year recurrence rates in phase 3 trials.[56,57] The mechanism of action responsible for the response rates of trastuzumab in the treatment of breast cancer has not been fully elucidated. Although some studies have provided evidence that the interruption of intracellular signaling by HER2/neu plays a major role in its antitumor activity, others consider ADCC to be a major component of the antitumor activity of trastuzumab. Cardiomyopathy is the major side effect of trastuzumab therapy, especially when it is combined with taxanes and anthracyclines.

Cetuximab (Erbitux) also targets a receptor tyrosine kinase, EGFR. This chimeric monoclonal antibody binds to the receptor in a nonactivating manner with a much higher affinity than the natural ligands. This causes receptor blockade and eventual internalization of the receptor, leading to an overall decrease in receptor signaling. Cetuximab was approved for use in the treatment of colorectal cancer in 2004 on the basis of a trial that compared cetuximab with cetuximab plus irinotecan in patients with metastatic disease. The addition of cetuximab to irinotecan demonstrated superior activity. Interestingly, cetuximab demonstrated moderate response rates in previously chemoresistant patients and appeared to be synergistic when combined with chemotherapy.[58] Recently, cetuximab has been approved for use in squamous cell head and neck cancers in combination with radiotherapy.[59] The addition of cetuximab to radiotherapy has decreased local regional recurrence by 32% and significantly improved overall survival. Toxicity associated with cetuximab therapy is an acneiform rash. There is some evidence that the severity of the rash is associated with improved antitumor activity. Moreover, some medical oncologists are proposing that dosing should be escalated until a rash forms.

Bevacizumab (Avastin) is a humanized monoclonal antibody that targets VEGF, the soluble ligand of the VEGFR expressed on endothelial cells. Signaling through VEGFR is thought to play a major role in the development of new vessels or angiogenesis. Many tumors are known to be associated with increased production of VEGF, leading to increased tumor angiogenesis, which is thought to play an important role in cancer progression and metastases. Bevacizumab has been approved for use in the treatment of metastatic colorectal cancer.[60] Currently, it is combined with fluorouracil and oxaliplatin or irinotecan as first-line therapy for metastatic colorectal cancer. A proposed mechanism of action is actually to normalize tumor vasculature, which helps in the delivery of cytotoxic chemotherapy. Also, bevacizumab has received FDA approval for use in some patients with other cancers, such as renal cell cancer (combined with IFN-α), non–small cell lung cancer, breast cancer, and glioblastoma. Associated toxicities reported are delayed wound healing and hemorrhagic events. It is customary to delay elective surgical procedures until 6 weeks after the last dose of bevacizumab.

Immunoconjugates

Antibodies conjugated to radionuclides were among the first immunoconjugates. External beam radiation delivers focused high-dose radiation during several weeks to treat local areas of cancer. Targeted radioimmunotherapy such as that provided by an immunoconjugate could be delivered intravenously as a systemic therapy to treat tumor deposits throughout the body. Another important difference with external beam radiation is that the radiation source is delivered to the site of the tumor; thus, the tumor is continually exposed to the radiation. Radionuclides can be categorized with respect to the characteristics of the energy emitted on nuclear decay. Some radionuclides are considered high-energy beta emitters (yttrium-90 and rhenium-188), and the path length of cytotoxic radiation can penetrate a tumor up to a distance of 1 cm. This relatively long path length of cytotoxic radiation could overcome some of the limitations of radioimmunoconjugates, such as poor tumor penetration and heterogeneous antigen expression, by achieving a large bystander effect. Radionuclides such as lutetium-177 and iodine-131 are considered medium-energy beta emitters whose energy can traverse approximately 1 mm. If one considers the diameter of a cell to be approximately 20 μm, the bystander effect should encompass approximately 50 cells in all directions. One could imagine that radioimmunoconjugates transporting medium-energy beta emitters could be used in the treatment of micrometastatic disease. Using these radionuclides may limit the radiation dose to the normal tissue surrounding the small tumor deposits.

Two anti-CD20 IgG radioimmunoconjugates are currently FDA approved for the treatment of non-Hodgkin lymphoma. Ibritumomab (Zevalin) is conjugated to yttrium-90, and tositumomab (Bexxar) is conjugated to iodine-131. Interestingly, both are murine monoclonal antibodies, yet the feared HAMA response rarely occurs. The lack of this immunogenic response is thought to be related to the destruction of the CD20-positive B-cell population, the very cells responsible for the HAMA response. Both of these radioimmunoconjugates are associated with high response rates. Patients treated with tositumomab had an overall response rate of 67%, and patients with bulky disease also demonstrated a significant clinical response. Also, in a head-to-head comparison of tositumomab conjugated to 131-I versus the unconjugated antibody, the addition of the radionuclide improved overall response rates, and, importantly, complete response rates were tripled.[61] Moreover, these complete responses proved to be durable compared with responses achieved by rituximab, an unconjugated anti-CD20 monoclonal antibody. The primary toxicity associated with radioimmunotherapy is the exposure of the highly sensitive bone marrow to radioactivity, resulting in dose-limiting myelosuppression.

CONCLUSION

Future work in human tumor immunotherapy will need to define and then address the underlying mechanisms that limit a productive antitumor response. These include strategies to optimize the delivery of defined tumor antigens to professional antigen-presenting cells, such as DCs, and in an immunostimulatory context to initiate a robust CD8+ and CD4+ T-cell response. Provision of adequate precursors, through genetic engineering of T cells or hematopoietic stem cells, may also be needed. T-cell activation and expansion can be promoted in vivo through a variety of strategies that include blocking of negative regulatory signaling and provision of cytokines. As antigen-reactive effector T cells enter a tumor, they encounter a hostile immunosuppressive microenvironment. Tumor cell targets have also frequently acquired constitutively active survival pathways. However, there are promising strategies being developed to address each of these limiting steps, as evidenced by the progressive improvement in clinical tumor immunotherapy occasioned by our better understanding of the underlying basic science.

Financial disclosure: JSE is a scientific advisor and investor in Allogene Therapuetics, Neogene Therapeutics and IconVir Therapeutics for all cancer immunotherapy companies.

SELECTED REFERENCES

Cheever MA. Twelve immunotherapy drugs that could cure cancers. *Immunol Rev.* 2008;222:357–368.

An overview of the most promising strategies to enhance antitumor immunity.

Dudley ME, Wunderlich JR, Yang JC, et al. Adoptive cell transfer therapy following nonmyeloablative but lymphodepleting chemotherapy for the treatment of patients with refractory metastatic melanoma. *J Clin Oncol.* 2005;23:2346–2357.

A phase II study showing the effectiveness of adoptively transferring cultured melanoma-reactive T cells to a patient after preparative lymphodepletion. The response rate of 51% and the achievement of durable complete responses in some patients illustrate the potential of this approach to immunotherapy.

Jakobovits A, Amado RG, Yang X, et al. From XenoMouse technology to panitumumab, the first fully human antibody product from transgenic mice. *Nat Biotechnol.* 2007;25:1134–1143.

One of the major drawbacks to therapeutic monoclonal antibody development and efficacy is the immunogenicity of murine protein sequences. This review summarizes the powerful development of a transgenic mouse (XenoMouse) in which the mouse antibody production genes were replaced by human immunoglobulin heavy- and light-chain loci. Panitumumab was the first fully human monoclonal antibody developed by immunizing the XenoMouse against a cancer cell line that overexpresses epidermal growth factor receptor.

Rosenberg SA, Lotze MT, Yang JC, et al. Experience with the use of high-dose interleukin-2 in the treatment of 652 cancer patients. *Ann Surg.* 1989;210:474–484.

A broad experience in the use of interleukin-2 to treat melanoma and renal cancer, documenting its ability to cause regressions and some apparent cures of metastatic disease.

van der Bruggen P, Traversari C, Chomez P, et al. A gene encoding an antigen recognized by cytolytic T lymphocytes on a human melanoma. *Science.* 1991;254:1643–1647.

A groundbreaking description of the first molecular characterization of a tumor-associated antigen recognized by a T cell. This was an impressive accomplishment, following so quickly after the first understanding of how antigens are processed, presented by major histocompatibility complex, and recognized by T cells. It proved to be the MAGE-1 antigen on a melanoma, presented by human leukocyte antigen A1.

REFERENCES

1. Zhang S, Zhang H, Zhao J. The role of CD4 T cell help for CD8 CTL activation. *Biochem Biophys Res Commun.* 2009;384:405–408.
2. Yao S, Zhu Y, Chen L. Advances in targeting cell surface signalling molecules for immune modulation. *Nat Rev Drug Discov.* 2013;12:130–146.
3. Ribas A. Tumor immunotherapy directed at PD-1. *N Engl J Med.* 2012;366:2517–2519.
4. Cheever MA. Twelve immunotherapy drugs that could cure cancers. *Immunol Rev.* 2008;222:357–368.
5. Topham NJ, Hewitt EW. Natural killer cell cytotoxicity: how do they pull the trigger? *Immunology.* 2009;128:7–15.
6. Halle S, Halle O, Forster R. Mechanisms and dynamics of t cell-mediated cytotoxicity in vivo. *Trends Immunol.* 2017;38:432–443.
7. Martinez-Lostao L, de Miguel D, Al-Wasaby S, et al. Death ligands and granulysin: mechanisms of tumor cell death induction and therapeutic opportunities. *Immunotherapy.* 2015;7:883–882.
8. Ferrantini M, Capone I, Belardelli F. Dendritic cells and cytokines in immune rejection of cancer. *Cytokine Growth Factor Rev.* 2008;19:93–107.
9. van der Bruggen P, Traversari C, Chomez P, et al. A gene encoding an antigen recognized by cytolytic T lymphocytes on a human melanoma. *Science.* 1991;254:1643–1647.
10. Pittet MJ. Behavior of immune players in the tumor microenvironment. *Curr Opin Oncol.* 2009;21:53–59.
11. Peggs KS, Quezada SA, Allison JP. Cancer immunotherapy: co-stimulatory agonists and co-inhibitory antagonists. *Clin Exp Immunol.* 2009;157:9–19.
12. Merelli B, Massi D, Cattaneo L, et al. Targeting the PD1/PD-L1 axis in melanoma: biological rationale, clinical challenges and opportunities. *Crit Rev Oncol Hematol.* 2014;89:140–165.
13. Ott PA, Hodi FS, Kaufman HL, et al. Combination immunotherapy: a road map. *J Immunother Cancer.* 2017;5:16.
14. Kammula US, White DE, Rosenberg SA. Trends in the safety of high dose bolus interleukin-2 administration in patients with metastatic cancer. *Cancer.* 1998;83:797–805.
15. Smith FO, Downey SG, Klapper JA, et al. Treatment of metastatic melanoma using interleukin-2 alone or in conjunction with vaccines. *Clin Cancer Res.* 2008;14:5610–5618.
16. Klapper JA, Downey SG, Smith FO, et al. High-dose interleukin-2 for the treatment of metastatic renal cell carcinoma: a retrospective analysis of response and survival in patients treated in the surgery branch at the National Cancer Institute between 1986 and 2006. *Cancer.* 2008;113:293–301.
17. Rosenberg SA, Yang JC, White DE, et al. Durability of complete responses in patients with metastatic cancer treated with high-dose interleukin-2: identification of the antigens mediating response. *Ann Surg.* 1998;228:307–319.
18. Rosenberg SA, Lotze MT, Yang JC, et al. Experience with the use of high-dose interleukin-2 in the treatment of 652 cancer patients. *Ann Surg.* 1989;210:474–484; discussion 484–475.
19. Yang JC, Sherry RM, Steinberg SM, et al. Randomized study of high-dose and low-dose interleukin-2 in patients with metastatic renal cancer. *J Clin Oncol.* 2003;21:3127–3132.
20. Rosenberg SA, Yang JC, Restifo NP. Cancer immunotherapy: moving beyond current vaccines. *Nat Med.* 2004;10:909–915.
21. Gong J, Chehrazi-Raffle A, Reddi S, et al. Development of PD-1 and PD-L1 inhibitors as a form of cancer immunotherapy: a comprehensive review of registration trials and future considerations. *J Immunother Cancer.* 2018;6:8.
22. Popovic A, Jaffee EM, Zaidi N. Emerging strategies for combination checkpoint modulators in cancer immunotherapy. *J Clin Invest.* 2018;128:3209–3218.
23. Pardoll DM. The blockade of immune checkpoints in cancer immunotherapy. *Nat Rev Cancer.* 2012;12:252–264.
24. Topalian SL, Hodi FS, Brahmer JR, et al. Safety, activity, and immune correlates of anti-PD-1 antibody in cancer. *N Engl J Med.* 2012;366:2443–2454.
25. Hargadon KM, Johnson CE, Williams CJ. Immune checkpoint blockade therapy for cancer: an overview of FDA-approved immune checkpoint inhibitors. *Int Immunopharmacol.* 2018;62:29–39.
26. Gibney GT, Weiner LM, Atkins MB. Predictive biomarkers for checkpoint inhibitor-based immunotherapy. *Lancet Oncol.* 2016;17:e542–e551.
27. Draghi A, Chamberlain CA, Furness A, et al. Acquired resistance to cancer immunotherapy. *Semin Immunopathol.* 2019; 41:31–40.
28. Hassel JC, Heinzerling L, Aberle J, et al. Combined immune checkpoint blockade (anti-PD-1/anti-CTLA-4): evaluation and management of adverse drug reactions. *Cancer Treat Rev.* 2017;57:36–49.
29. Yang JC, Rosenberg SA. Adoptive T-cell therapy for cancer. *Adv Immunol.* 2016;130:279–294.
30. Rosenberg SA, Yannelli JR, Yang JC, et al. Treatment of patients with metastatic melanoma with autologous tumor-infiltrating lymphocytes and interleukin 2. *J Natl Cancer Inst.* 1994;86:1159–1166.
31. Rosenberg SA, Aebersold P, Cornetta K, et al. Gene transfer into humans—immunotherapy of patients with advanced melanoma, using tumor-infiltrating lymphocytes modified by retroviral gene transduction. *N Engl J Med.* 1990;323:570–578.
32. Dubinett SM, Patrone L, Huang M, et al. Interleukin-2-responsive wound-infiltrating lymphocytes in surgical adjuvant cancer immunotherapy. *Immunol Invest.* 1993;22:13–23.
33. Dudley ME, Yang JC, Sherry R, et al. Adoptive cell therapy for patients with metastatic melanoma: evaluation of intensive myeloablative chemoradiation preparative regimens. *J Clin Oncol.* 2008;26:5233–5239.
34. Tran E, Turcotte S, Gros A, et al. Cancer immunotherapy based on mutation-specific CD4+ T cells in a patient with epithelial cancer. *Science.* 2014;344:641–645.
35. June CH, Sadelain M. Chimeric antigen receptor therapy. *N Engl J Med.* 2018;379:64–73.
36. Kochenderfer JN, Dudley ME, Kassim SH, et al. Chemotherapy-refractory diffuse large B-cell lymphoma and indolent B-cell malignancies can be effectively treated with autologous T cells expressing an anti-CD19 chimeric antigen receptor. *J Clin Oncol.* 2015;33:540–549.
37. Liegel J, Avigan D, Rosenblatt J. Cellular immunotherapy as a therapeutic approach in multiple myeloma. *Expert Rev Hematol.* 2018;11:525–536.
38. Tran E, Ahmadzadeh M, Lu YC, et al. Immunogenicity of somatic mutations in human gastrointestinal cancers. *Science.* 2015;350:1387–1390.
39. Zacharakis N, Chinnasamy H, Black M, et al. Immune recognition of somatic mutations leading to complete durable regression in metastatic breast cancer. *Nat Med.* 2018;24:724–730.
40. Kobold S, Pantelyushin S, Rataj F, et al. Rationale for combining bispecific T cell activating antibodies with checkpoint blockade for cancer therapy. *Front Oncol.* 2018;8:285.
41. Krishnamurthy A, Jimeno A. Bispecific antibodies for cancer therapy: a review. *Pharmacol Ther.* 2018;185:122–134.

42. Elgundi Z, Reslan M, Cruz E, et al. The state-of-play and future of antibody therapeutics. *Adv Drug Deliv Rev.* 2017;122:2–19.
43. Lee A, Sun S, Sandler A, et al. Recent progress in therapeutic antibodies for cancer immunotherapy. *Curr Opin Chem Biol.* 2018;44:56–65.
44. Kohler G, Milstein C. Continuous cultures of fused cells secreting antibody of predefined specificity. *Nature.* 1975;256:495–497.
45. Jakobovits A, Amado RG, Yang X, et al. From XenoMouse technology to panitumumab, the first fully human antibody product from transgenic mice. *Nat Biotechnol.* 2007;25:1134–1143.
46. Lonberg N. Human antibodies from transgenic animals. *Nat Biotechnol.* 2005;23:1117–1125.
47. Beckman RA, Weiner LM, Davis HM. Antibody constructs in cancer therapy: protein engineering strategies to improve exposure in solid tumors. *Cancer.* 2007;109:170–179.
48. Wu AM, Senter PD. Arming antibodies: prospects and challenges for immunoconjugates. *Nat Biotechnol.* 2005;23:1137–1146.
49. Griggs J, Zinkewich-Peotti K. The state of the art: immune-mediated mechanisms of monoclonal antibodies in cancer therapy. *Br J Cancer.* 2009;101:1807–1812.
50. Campoli M, Ferris R, Ferrone S, et al. Immunotherapy of malignant disease with tumor antigen-specific monoclonal antibodies. *Clin Cancer Res.* 2010;16:11–20.
51. Steplewski Z, Lubeck MD, Koprowski H. Human macrophages armed with murine immunoglobulin G2a antibodies to tumors destroy human cancer cells. *Science.* 1983;221:865–867.
52. Weiner LM, Dhodapkar MV, Ferrone S. Monoclonal antibodies for cancer immunotherapy. *Lancet.* 2009;373:1033–1040.
53. Selenko N, Majdic O, Jager U, et al. Cross-priming of cytotoxic T cells promoted by apoptosis-inducing tumor cell reactive antibodies? *J Clin Immunol.* 2002;22:124–130.
54. Olafsen T, Kenanova VA, Wu AM. Tunable pharmacokinetics: modifying the in vivo half-life of antibodies by directed mutagenesis of the Fc fragment. *Nat Protoc.* 2006;1:2048–2060.
55. McLaughlin P, Grillo-Lopez AJ, Link BK, et al. Rituximab chimeric anti-CD20 monoclonal antibody therapy for relapsed indolent lymphoma: half of patients respond to a four-dose treatment program. *J Clin Oncol.* 1998;16:2825–2833.
56. Piccart-Gebhart MJ, Procter M, Leyland-Jones B, et al. Trastuzumab after adjuvant chemotherapy in HER2-positive breast cancer. *N Engl J Med.* 2005;353:1659–1672.
57. Romond EH, Perez EA, Bryant J, et al. Trastuzumab plus adjuvant chemotherapy for operable HER2-positive breast cancer. *N Engl J Med.* 2005;353:1673–1684.
58. Jonker DJ, O'Callaghan CJ, Karapetis CS, et al. Cetuximab for the treatment of colorectal cancer. *N Engl J Med.* 2007;357:2040–2048.
59. Bonner JA, Harari PM, Giralt J, et al. Radiotherapy plus cetuximab for squamous-cell carcinoma of the head and neck. *N Engl J Med.* 2006;354:567–578.
60. Hurwitz H, Fehrenbacher L, Novotny W, et al. Bevacizumab plus irinotecan, fluorouracil, and leucovorin for metastatic colorectal cancer. *N Engl J Med.* 2004;350:2335–2342.
61. Davis TA, Kaminski MS, Leonard JP, et al. The radioisotope contributes significantly to the activity of radioimmunotherapy. *Clin Cancer Res.* 2004;10:7792–7798.

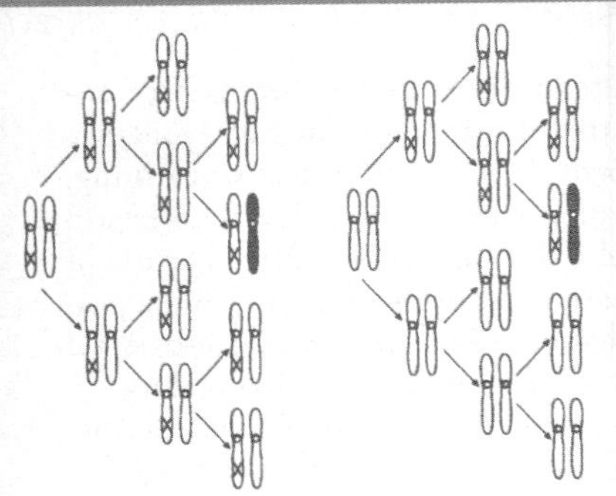

CHAPTER 31

Melanoma and Cutaneous Malignancies

Kelly M. McMasters, Douglas S. Tyler, Michael E. Egger

OUTLINE

Skin cancer is the most common form of cancer, accounting for at least half of all malignant neoplasms. Almost one in five Americans will be diagnosed with skin cancer in their lifetime. The high incidence of skin cancer is largely attributable to environmental exposures, particularly sunlight. Squamous cell carcinoma (SCC) and basal cell carcinoma (BCC) comprise the majority of all skin cancer diagnoses, while melanoma represents the most common cause of skin cancer–related deaths. This chapter focuses primarily on these three malignant neoplasms while mentioning a few less common cutaneous neoplasms that are encountered by surgeons.

MELANOMA

Historical descriptions of what was likely melanoma can be found in the writings of Hippocrates. John Hunter provided the first modern published account of the surgical treatment of melanoma in 1787. René Laennec, who identified metastatic melanoma deposits in distant viscera, described it as "cancer noire" and subsequently named the disease *melanosis*. Our understanding of melanoma and its clinical behavior, molecular mechanisms, and targetable pathways has steadily improved over decades of research.

Epidemiology

Even though melanoma accounts for less than 2% of skin cancer cases, it is currently the fifth most common cancer in men and the sixth most common cancer among women in the United States. Melanoma also causes the majority of skin cancer–related deaths. The American Cancer Society estimated that there would be 91,270 new cases of melanoma diagnosed in the United States in 2018, with 9320 deaths. The incidence of melanoma has steadily increased in the United States and worldwide over the last four decades (Fig. 31.1). Worldwide, the highest incidence rates of melanoma are in Australia, New Zealand, North America, and northern Europe. The steady rise in incidence has been attributed to lifestyle changes leading to increased sun exposure as well as to improved surveillance and detection of early lesions.

The degree of pigmentation in the skin is a relative protective factor against cutaneous melanoma; those with lighter skin tones are at increased risk. As a result, cutaneous melanoma is predominantly a disease of whites. In particular, patients with a fair complexion, blonde or red hair, and blue eyes are at increased risk, as are those who sunburn easily, have a tendency to develop freckles, or have an inability to tan. In the United States, the average annual age-adjusted melanoma incidence per 100,000 persons is 32.2 for non-Hispanic white men and 19.4 for non-Hispanic white women, compared with 4.8 for Hispanic men and 4.6 for Hispanic women, 4.2 for Native American men (including Alaska Natives) and 4.6 for Native American women, 1.6 for Asian/Pacific Islander men and 1.1 for Asian/Pacific Islander women, and 1.1 for Black men and 1.0 for Black women.[1] As one can see from these numbers, melanoma is slightly more common in men across most races/ethnicities.

Melanoma is predominantly seen in middle-age adults, although it occurs across all ages (Fig. 31.2). Importantly, approximately one in six new cases of melanoma occurs in patients younger than 45 years old; accordingly, melanoma-related deaths can result in a high number of potential years of life lost. Genetic risk factors for melanoma include high-risk skin types (Fitzpatrick types I and II), family history of melanoma, and xeroderma pigmentosum. Patients with a prior history of melanoma or other skin cancers, as well as those with a large number of melanocytic nevi, dysplastic nevi, or giant congenital nevi, are also at increased risk. Environmental risk factors include episodes of intense intermittent sun exposure associated with severe blistering sunburns, immunosuppression, and upper socioeconomic status.

There is a clear association between ultraviolet (UV) radiation exposure and the development of melanoma. Intermittent, intense UV radiation exposure appears to be a strong causative factor for melanoma, as opposed to chronic sun exposure and the associated

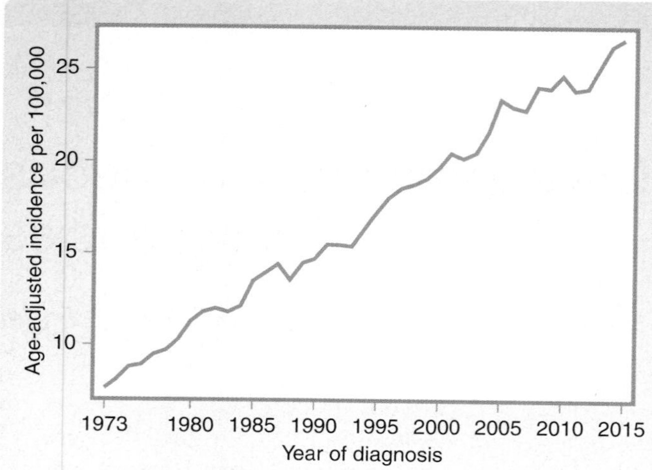

FIG. 31.1 Age-adjusted incidence of cutaneous melanoma in the United States, 1973–2015, SEER. (From SEER Fact Sheets: Melanoma of the skin. http://seer.cancer.gov/statfacts/html/melan.html.)

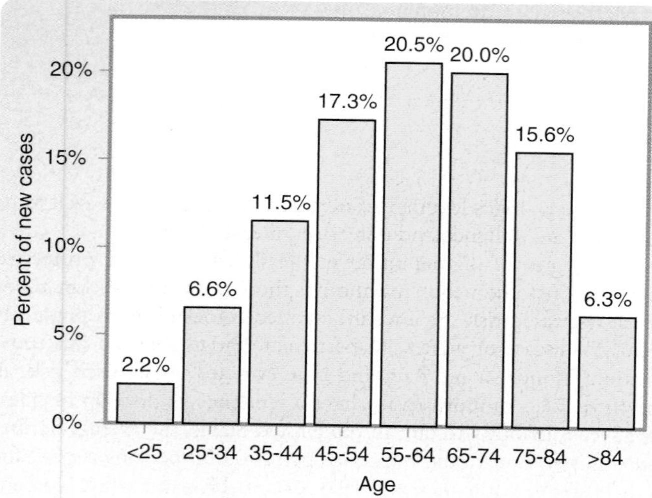

FIG. 31.2 New cases by age group of cutaneous melanoma in the United States, 1973–2015, SEER. (From SEER Fact Sheets: Melanoma of the skin. http://seer.cancer.gov/statfacts/html/melan.html.)

risk of nonmelanoma skin cancers (NMSCs). UV light can be classified as either UVA or UVB; UVA has a longer wavelength and penetrates more deeply into the skin than UVB. Although UVA radiation has long been known to play a major role in skin aging and wrinkling, growing evidence has implicated UVA radiation as a cause of melanoma skin cancer and NMSC alike. UVA is the predominant wavelength in tanning beds. Emerging evidence has demonstrated an epidemiological link between tanning bed use (even without sunburn) and melanoma. [2] Another major risk factor for melanoma is UVB exposure from natural sunlight, especially among those with fair skin. UVB damages the skin's more superficial epidermal layers and is the chief cause of sunburns. A direct link between UVB exposure and specific melanoma oncogenes has been demonstrated.[3] A UV signature consistent with mutations caused by UV damage was found in over 90% of three of the four melanoma subtypes identified in The Cancer Genome Atlas project.[4]

From a public health perspective, melanoma is a cancer for which there are clear primary prevention strategies that can prevent its development and reduce preventable deaths. Recommendations for reducing the risk of melanoma include avoidance of sunbathing and tanning beds, use of sun-protective clothing, and use of sunscreens. Population-based case-control studies and some randomized clinical trials have suggested that regular use of sunscreen can reduce the development of melanoma. From a policy standpoint, one strategy that has been used on a state-by-state basis in the United States is the ban of indoor tanning bed use by minors (age <18 years). Some countries, including Brazil and Australia, have banned commercial indoor tanning salons outright.

Precursor Lesions

Melanomas frequently arise de novo in otherwise normal skin; however, up to 40% may arise within preexisting lesions, including dysplastic nevi, congenital nevi, and Spitz nevi. Upward of 5% to 10% of melanoma patients will have a family history of the disease. Variously termed *dysplastic nevus syndrome, familial atypical multiple mole–melanoma syndrome,* and *B-K mole syndrome,* these syndromes include patients with melanoma in one or more first- or second-degree relatives and large numbers of melanocytic nevi (often >100). These nevi will often be classified as atypical or dysplastic on close clinical and histologic examination. Other cancers may also be present in the family history, particularly pancreatic cancer. These patients require detailed dermatologic evaluation several times annually, with periodic biopsies of the most suspicious lesions.

In general, a dysplastic nevus is a 6- to 15-mm macular (flat) pigmented skin lesion with indistinct margins and variable color. The clinical distinction between a nevus with dysplasia and a nevus without dysplasia is often difficult; therefore, these lesions require careful monitoring over time to evaluate for progression. Most nevi are benign, but some may reflect early atypia associated with increased intracellular growth signaling and can progress to invasive disease with the accumulation of additional mutations. Although most dysplastic nevi do not progress to melanoma, suspicious lesions require biopsy. Dysplastic nevi are typically described as having mild, moderate, or severe dysplasia on histologic examination. Nevi with mild dysplasia usually do not require excision with negative margins but should be closely observed over time. It has been common practice to excise moderately or severely dysplastic nevi with negative margins, although wide local excision (WLE) is unnecessary. However, there is controversy about whether moderately dysplastic nevi require negative-margin excision.[5] The risk of melanoma in those patients with congenital nevi is proportional to the size and number of nevi. Small- or medium-sized congenital nevi represent a low risk and therefore are not observed unless they change in appearance. Giant congenital nevi (>20 cm in diameter) are rare and are estimated to occur in anywhere from 1 in 20,000 to 1 in 500,000 newborns, but they carry an increased lifetime risk for the development of melanoma (Fig. 31.3). These patients are also at increased risk for other tumors, particularly sarcomas. Complete excision should be considered when possible. At a minimum, these patients should undergo regular dermatologic evaluation.

Spitzoid melanocytic lesions constitute a wide range of histopathology from the typical benign Spitz nevus to spitzoid melanoma. A Spitz nevus is a rapidly growing, pink or brown, benign skin lesion with little or no risk for further progression to melanoma. Whereas benign Spitz nevi are most common in children, lesions in adults are more likely to have atypical features or to represent melanoma with spitzoid features. Atypical features include size larger than 10 mm, asymmetry, ulceration, and poor

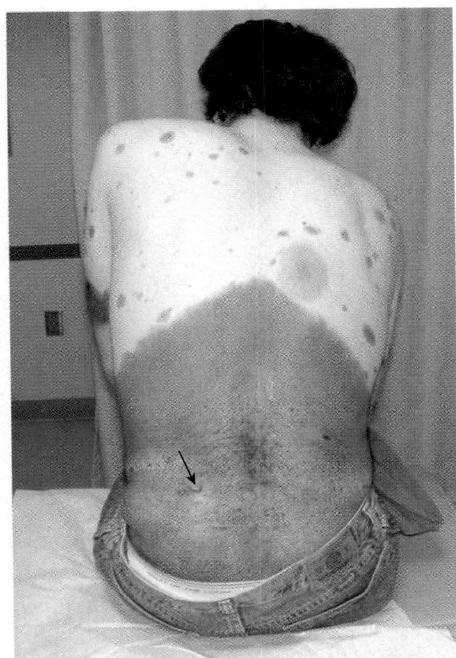

FIG. 31.3 Giant congenital nevus of the trunk with an associated melanoma *(arrow)*.

circumscription; these lesions can be difficult to distinguish histologically from melanoma. Consultation with an expert dermatopathologist is recommended; however, even the most experienced dermatopathologists may have difficulty in determining the malignant potential of spitzoid tumors. Although complete excision with negative margins is adequate for an unequivocal Spitz nevus, the diagnosis is often unclear. If there is any concern that the lesion may be melanoma, WLE with margins appropriate for melanoma is performed. Sentinel lymph node (SLN) biopsy is appropriate for invasive spitzoid melanomas and can be used as a prognostic measure in indeterminate cases. The routine use of SLN biopsy for atypical Spitz tumors is controversial because atypical cells are often seen in SLNs that may not have any prognostic significance.

Pathogenesis

In general, melanoma has the highest mutational burden of any malignancy that has been studied in humans.[6] Our understanding of the molecular mechanisms that underlie melanoma progression has increased greatly over the last decade through collaborative efforts such as The Cancer Genome Atlas Network. In a landmark study in 2015, the collaborative published a study in which 331 cutaneous melanoma tumors underwent an integrative genomic analysis.[4] Using DNA, RNA, and protein-based analyses, the group identified four distinct subtypes of cutaneous melanoma based on the most prevalent significantly altered genes: mutant *BRAF*, mutant *RAS*, mutant *NF1*, and triple-wild-type.

The *BRAF* subtype is the most common genomic subtype in cutaneous melanoma, comprising of approximately one-half of all cutaneous melanoma. The most common mutation is the V600E, followed by the V600K mutation. *BRAF* subtype patients are relatively younger compared to the other subtypes. The second most common subtype was the *RAS* subtype, which described about 30% of cutaneous melanoma. The third most frequent subtype was the *NF1* subtype, found in approximately 15% of samples; these patients were typically older than the other subtypes. Finally, the triple-wild-type was a heterogeneous subtype lacking any of the three major mutations previously mentioned. This subtype had the lowest rate of UV signature changes (30%). The prognostic and therapeutic implications of these genomic subtypes are the subject of intense ongoing research as we attempt to further target our therapies for melanoma in the age of personalized medicine.

The canonical pathway through which nearly all of the genomic subtypes exert melanogenic effect is the mitogen-activated protein kinase (MAPK) signaling pathway (Fig. 31.4). Normally, signals generated by extracellular receptors initiate a signaling cascade that passes down the MAPK pathway to modulate gene expression in the nucleus. Gain-of-function mutations affecting any of the constituent steps along this cascade (*BRAF* and *RAS* subtypes) or loss of inhibitory steps (*NF1*) can result in unchecked cellular growth.

Gain-of-function mutations alone are likely not enough to generate melanoma; *BRAF* mutations are observed at a similar frequency in some benign nevi and malignant disease. Additional loss of key tumor suppressor genes is necessary for further neoplastic development. For instance, an inactivating mutation in the gene *CDKN2A* occurs in 25% to 40% of familial melanomas. A well-characterized gene with key roles in cell cycle control, *CDKN2A* codes for two separate tumor suppressor proteins, INK4A ($p16^{INK4A}$) and ARF ($p14^{ARF}$). In the event of DNA damage or activated oncogenes, INK4A prevents the cyclin-dependent kinase 4 from stimulating the cell to progress through the cell cycle. Through the regulation of p53 levels, ARF also acts as a tumor suppressor in the face of DNA damage or amplified growth signals. ARF prevents degradation of p53, allowing this key regulatory protein to accumulate and either to arrest the cell cycle or to initiate apoptosis. Loss of either ARF or INK4A therefore removes a checkpoint in the cell cycle, increasing the risk of uncontrolled replication.

The second major canonical pathway in melanoma pathogenesis is the PI3/AKT pathway (Fig. 31.4). The PI3/AKT pathway is potentially altered in all four genomic subtypes. Phosphatidylinositol 3,4,5-trisphosphate (PI3) stimulates AKT to increase cellular proliferation through the mammalian target of rapamycin signaling molecule. Phosphatase and tensin homologue (PTEN), whose gene is located on chromosome 10, inhibits PI3/AKT signaling. Loss of PTEN occurs in approximately 25% to 50% of nonfamilial melanomas and is a common culprit pathway for the development of resistance to therapies targeting BRAF/MEK inhibition.

Initial Evaluation

Melanoma commonly presents as an irregular pigmented skin lesion that has grown or changed over time. The ABCDE criteria are used to guide diagnosis and the decision to perform a biopsy of suspicious cutaneous lesions (Box 31.1). The first and most important step in the evaluation of a patient diagnosed with melanoma is a thorough history and physical examination. The history should elicit factors related to the primary melanoma, including duration, change over time, and symptoms such as itching and bleeding. Other risk factors, such as sun exposure, tanning bed use, immunosuppression, prior history of cancer, and family history should be sought. A detailed physical examination should specifically include a complete skin examination with inspection and palpation of the skin to detect any other suspicious skin lesions, including in-transit disease. Palpation of the cervical, axillary, and inguinal lymph nodes should always be performed with palpation of the epitrochlear or popliteal nodes as appropriate for distal upper or lower extremity melanomas. Although it is widely recognized that

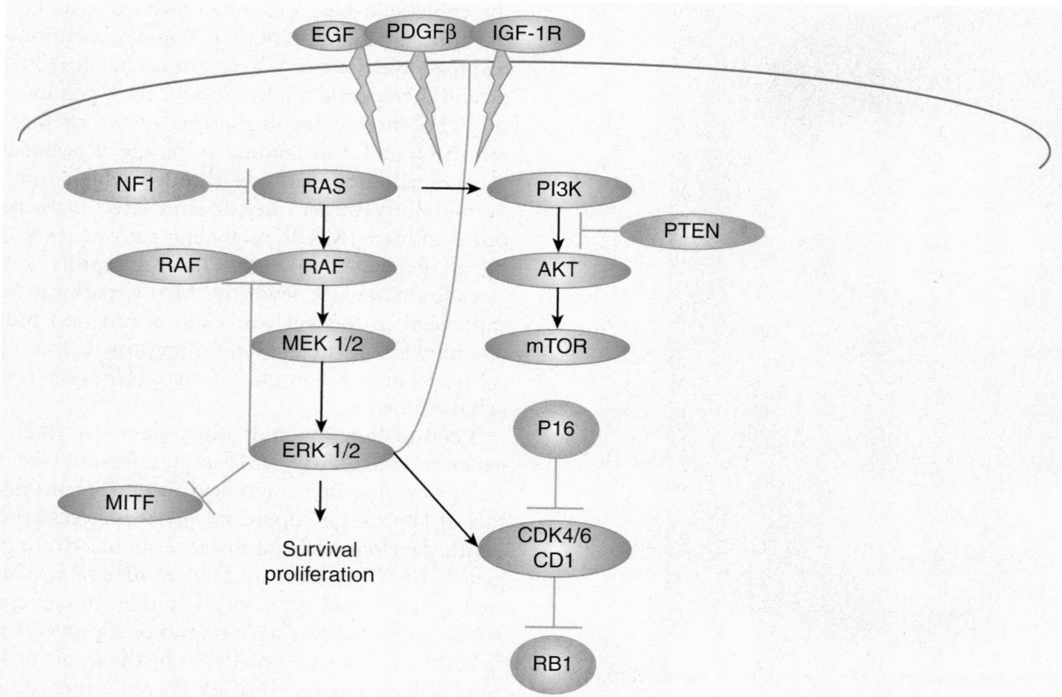

FIG. 31.4 The mitogen-activated protein kinase (RAS-RAF-MEK-ERK) and PI3/AKT pathways; two canonical pathways in melanoma pathogenesis. (From Amaral T, Sinnberg T, Meier F, et al. The mitogen-activated protein kinase pathway in melanoma part I—activation and primary resistance mechanisms to BRAF inhibition. *Eur J Cancer.* 2017;73:85–92.)

BOX 31.1 ABCDE criteria of suspicious skin lesions.

A. **A**symmetry
B. Irregular **B**orders
C. **C**olor variegation
D. **D**iameter >6 mm
E. **E**volution or changes over time

a skin examination should be part of the routine physical examination by primary care physicians and others, it is rarely adequately performed. A full skin examination requires only that the patient undress, and it may take only 1 minute to perform a complete survey. Many lives have been saved by early detection of melanomas by physicians who took the time to evaluate the skin.

Most melanomas occur de novo but some can arise within a congenital or acquired nevus. Even for experienced clinicians, distinguishing between a benign nevus and an early melanoma can be difficult. Benign pigmented lesions are so prevalent that it is challenging to detect an early melanoma among many benign lesions. The most common benign pigmented skin lesions are seborrheic keratoses (Fig. 31.5). Known for their propensity to accumulate over time in elderly patients, typically these are scaly, waxy, raised lesions with a stuck-on look that makes them appear as if they could easily be scraped off with a fingernail. The characteristic appearance usually is completely diagnostic and these lesions do not need to be removed. However, even the most experienced dermatologists have been fooled by what appeared to be an irritated seborrheic keratosis that turned out to be melanoma.

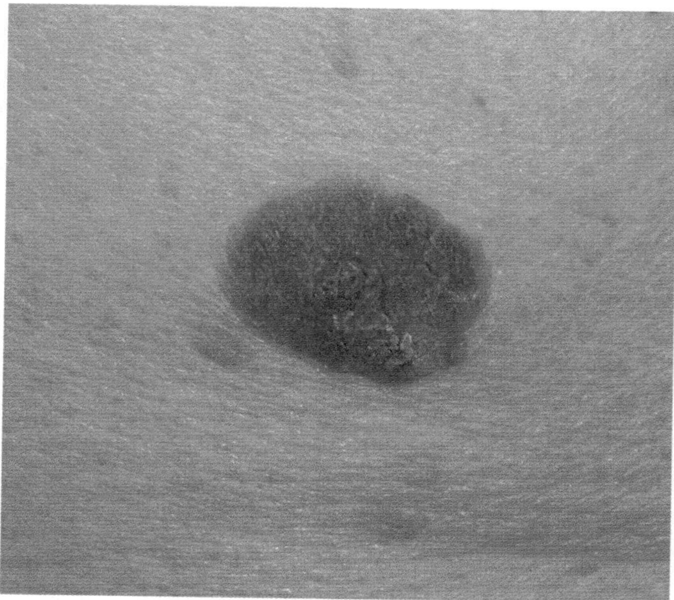

FIG. 31.5 Seborrheic keratosis.

Additional atypical presentations include amelanotic melanoma; these lesions are not pigmented and present as a raised pink or flesh-colored skin lesion. A high index of clinical suspicion is needed, and particular attention should be paid to any history of change in a lesion. If a patient presents with a skin lesion that has changed in size, color, or shape and/or is itching or bleeding, there should be a low threshold for biopsy. Telling a patient that "we should keep an eye on it" usually means that it will be ignored.

Given the increased awareness of this disease, it is uncommon for patients to have advanced regional or distant metastatic disease at the time of initial melanoma diagnosis. Nonetheless, roughly 10% of patients will present with regional disease, while up to 5% may present with metastases. Regional disease refers to the lymphatic spread of tumor to the regional nodal basin, which are the lymph nodes that receive the first drainage from the site of the primary tumor. In-transit melanoma is a form of regional lymphatic metastasis in which the tumor spreads within the draining lymphatic channels and becomes evident as cutaneous or subcutaneous nodules between the site of the primary tumor and regional lymph nodes. Distant metastasis refers to the hematogenous spread of melanoma to distant organs. Although uncommon at the time of initial diagnosis, it is important to elicit symptoms of metastatic disease, such as any masses, neurologic symptoms or headaches, anorexia, weight loss, bone pain, or respiratory symptoms.

Biopsy

Primary care physicians, in addition to dermatologists and surgeons, should be trained to perform a skin biopsy. There are three basic types of skin biopsy—excisional, incisional (including punch biopsy), and shave biopsy. An excisional biopsy completely removes a pigmented skin lesion and is particularly well suited to diagnosis and completely remove small lesions. Using local anesthesia, a narrow margin excision is performed with the subsequent defect closed by sutures. The depth of excision should extend to the subcutaneous fat to ensure a full-thickness biopsy. Attention should be paid to the orientation, as a fusiform excision should be oriented in such a way to easily allow subsequent wide excision if that becomes necessary. In particular, a longitudinal orientation on the extremities is best. In other areas, consideration should be given to an orientation that would allow closure with the least tension and best cosmetic outcome in the event wider excision is needed.

For larger lesions, it may be appropriate to get a tissue diagnosis with a full-thickness incisional biopsy prior to performing complete excision. The simplest way to perform an incisional biopsy is through a punch biopsy. In a punch biopsy, a sharp disposable instrument is twisted into the anesthetized skin to remove a 2-mm to 8-mm cylinder of skin and subcutaneous tissue, generally followed by closure of the defect with one or two simple sutures. Punch biopsies of at least 4 mm should be performed, since smaller tissue samples often do not provide adequate tissue for pathologic evaluation. The punch biopsy should be performed through the thickest or most suspicious-looking area of the lesion, and multiple punch biopsies can be performed to sample larger lesions.

Although traditionally discouraged because of the potential to confound accurate assessment of Breslow thickness, shave biopsy is frequently performed by dermatologists and is the most common technique by which melanomas are biopsied and diagnosed. Shave biopsy is performed by elevating the skin lesion with forceps or inserting a small needle beneath the lesion, followed by shaving the lesion with a razor blade or scalpel. Hemostasis is achieved using topical agents or by electrocautery. The patient then treats the area with topical ointment and the wound heals by secondary intention. Since a shave biopsy is easy to perform and does not require sutures, it is a popular method of biopsy. However, a potential drawback to the use of a shave biopsy to diagnose melanoma is that the lesion may be transected, compromising the ability to accurately assess tumor thickness. To circumvent this problem, dermatologists often perform deep shave or saucerization biopsies, which completely remove the lesion down to subcutaneous fat. In the hands of experienced clinicians, this can be an effective biopsy technique. In reviewing the pathology report of a newly diagnosed melanoma, surgeons should take care to note whether the deep margin is free of tumor.

All pigmented lesions should be sent for pathologic evaluation using fixation and permanent section. Ablation of pigmented skin lesions using cryotherapy, cautery, or lasers should be specifically discouraged; there are many examples of prolonged delays in diagnosis as a result of these practices.

Pathology

The biopsy report is the most important piece of information needed by the surgeon to evaluate a new skin lesion and to develop a treatment plan. Given the consequences of a missed diagnosis of melanoma, pathologists often have a low threshold to classify equivocal lesions as melanoma. It is now common for a pathology report to contain a long description essentially stating that the lesion may be anything from a severely dysplastic nevus to melanoma in situ to early invasive melanoma. In such cases, the prudent decision is to treat such lesions as an early invasive melanoma with a 1-cm margin WLE. Although melanoma in situ does not invade beyond the basement membrane into blood vessels and lymphatics, it may be considered a premalignant lesion given that there remains a significant likelihood of progression to invasive melanoma. For this reason, at least 5-mm margins are recommended for these lesions (see "Wide Local Excision").

Histology. Histologically, invasive cutaneous melanoma is divided into four major types based on growth pattern and location. These include lentigo maligna melanoma, superficial spreading melanoma, acral lentiginous melanoma, and nodular melanoma. All melanomas initially proliferate in the basal layer of the skin. As they multiply, these cells expand radially in the epidermis and superficial dermal layer, termed the radial growth phase. With time, growth begins in a vertical direction and the skin lesion may become palpable, known as the vertical growth phase. The vertical growth phase allows invasion into the deeper layers of the skin, where the tumor may ultimately achieve metastatic potential by invasion of blood vessels and lymphatic channels. While the histologic subtype is not a major factor in prognosis, some histologic subtypes progress to the vertical growth phase earlier in tumor development and are therefore more likely to present at an advanced stage.

The most common histologic type is superficial spreading melanoma (Fig. 31.6). It is not necessarily associated with sun-exposed skin and most commonly appears on the trunk and proximal extremities. As the name suggests, superficial spreading melanoma initially appears as a flat-pigmented lesion growing radially. These lesions are often asymmetric with irregular borders and can display a wide variety of pigments. Untreated, these melanomas will subsequently develop a vertical growth phase, invade more deeply into the skin, and possibly ulcerate.

Lentigo maligna melanoma occurs most commonly on the sun-exposed areas of older individuals and presents as a flat, dark, variably pigmented lesion, with irregular borders and a history of slow development (Fig. 31.7). Lentigo maligna melanomas may become relatively large prior to diagnosis, as the slow progression can escape the patient's notice. The prognosis of lentigo maligna melanoma is better than for the other subtypes given the superficial nature of these tumors. Nonetheless,

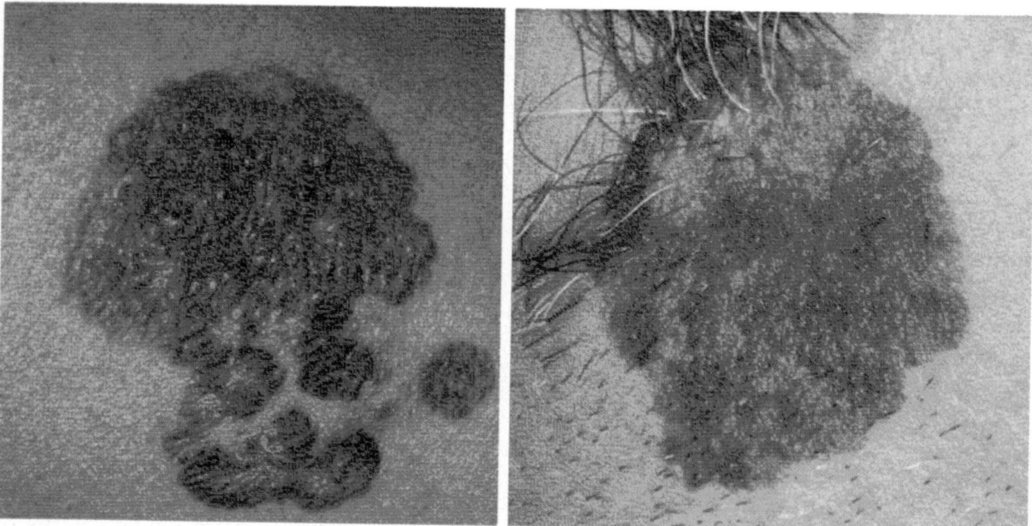

FIG. 31.6 Superficial spreading melanoma.

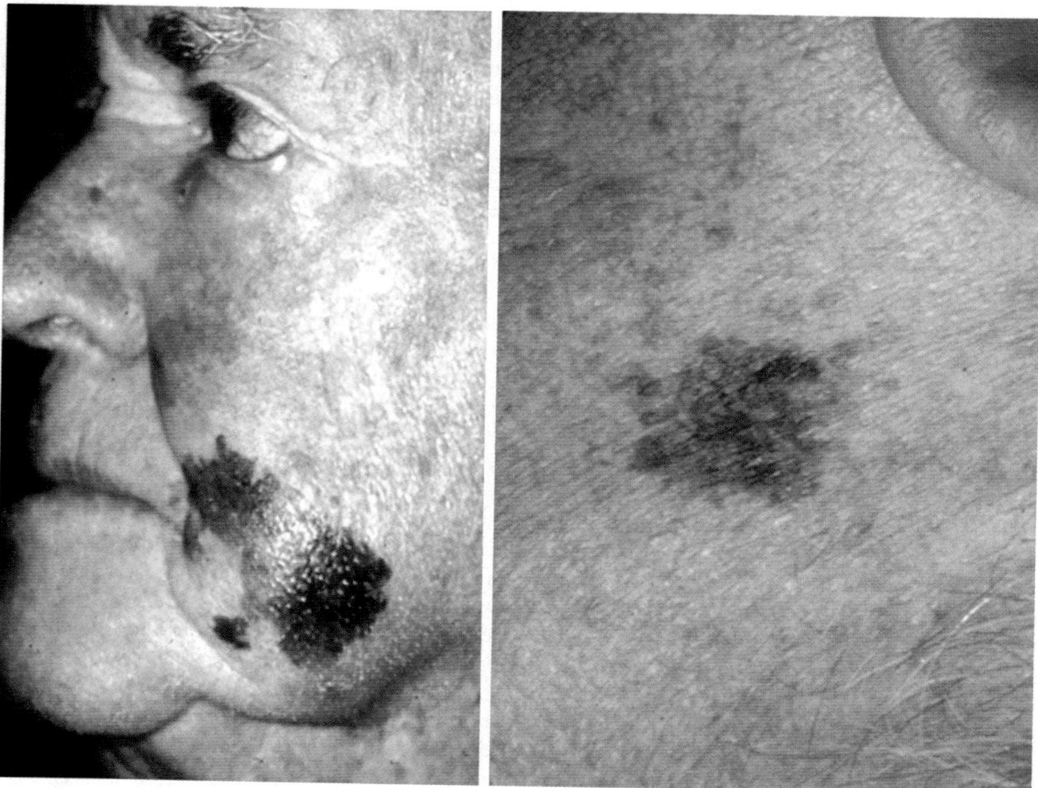

FIG. 31.7 Lentigo maligna melanoma.

these lesions can pose challenging management problems because of their propensity to develop in cosmetically challenging areas such as the face. The histologic extent of the lesion may extend well beyond the clinically apparent borders of the pigmented lesion, hampering efforts to achieve negative margins. Before proceeding with complex tissue flaps for closure, it is prudent to ensure negative margins. This may necessitate delaying the closure until the final pathology report indicates negative margins of excision.

Acral lentiginous melanoma is classified by its anatomic site of origin. These tumors develop in the subungual areas beneath fingernails and toenails and on the palms of the hands and soles of the feet (Fig. 31.8). This is the most common type of melanoma in nonwhite patients. The histologic appearance of acral lentiginous melanomas is similar to melanomas arising on the mucous membranes. The diagnosis is often made at an advanced stage, which accounts for the general poor prognosis of these tumors. Subungual acral lentiginous melanomas are often mistaken for subungual hematomas, leading to a delay in diagnosis. The distinguishing feature of subungual melanomas is that they do not change in position underneath the nail, while a hematoma should migrate distally with growth of the nail. Biopsy of subungual melanomas

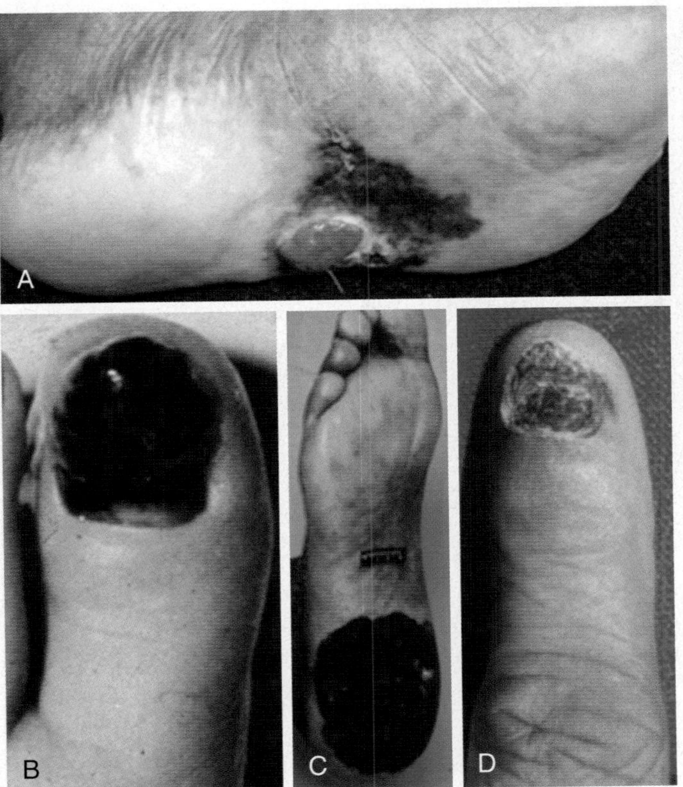

FIG. 31.8 Acral lentiginous melanoma. (A) Arch of the sole of the foot. (B) Subungual. (C) Heel. (D) Subungual.

can be accomplished by performing a digital block with local anesthesia and removing the nail or by performing a punch biopsy through the nail itself.

Nodular melanomas are raised papular lesions that can occur anywhere on the body and tend to develop a vertical growth pattern early in their course (Fig. 31.9). These melanomas can have atypical presentations that do not always conform to ABCDE criteria, including a higher rate of amelanotic lesions compared to the other subtypes. Nodular melanomas often have a poor prognosis because of greater average tumor thickness and frequent ulceration at initial presentation.

A fifth type of melanoma that has a distinct histologic character is desmoplastic melanoma. These lesions are characterized by a combination of melanoma cells with a prominent stromal fibrosis. The diagnosis can be challenging and the presentation delayed because these lesions are often amelanotic. Desmoplastic melanomas are classified as either pure or mixed depending upon the degree of desmoplasia present. Desmoplastic melanomas have a greater propensity for local recurrence and often exhibit neurotropism. Pure desmoplastic melanomas have a low risk of lymph node metastases and some have advocated forgoing a SLN biopsy in these lesions. Mixed desmoplastic melanomas have lymph node metastatic rates that are similar to other histologic subtypes; therefore, SLN biopsy should be considered for the usual indications in these lesions.[7]

Depth Assessment. Dr. Wallace Clark first described a classification system for melanoma that correlated with survival in 1969. Known as Clark level of invasion, this scheme was based on the extent of invasion into the anatomic layers of the skin. Shortly after Clark introduced his levels of invasion, Dr. Alexander Breslow described a simpler system based on a

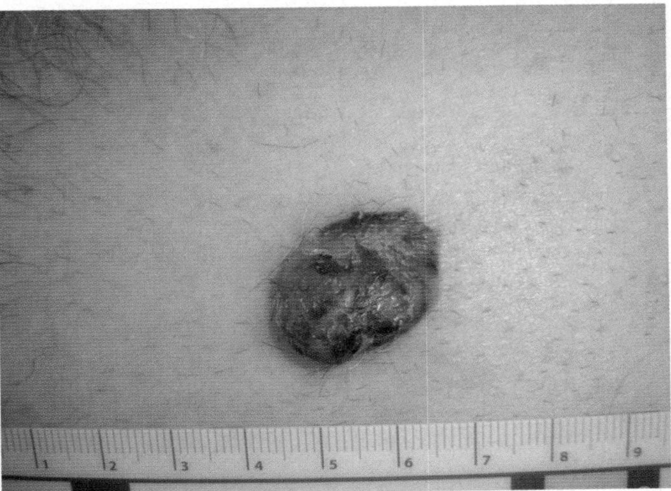

FIG. 31.9 Nodular melanoma.

measurement of the vertical thickness of the melanoma. Now known as Breslow thickness, this is the distance from the top of the granular layer down to the lowest tumor cell. Over time, Breslow thickness has largely supplanted Clark level, as it has been shown to be a more accurate method of predicting prognosis. Melanomas are commonly referred to as thin (<1 mm Breslow thickness), intermediate thickness (1–4 mm), and thick (>4 mm). As the thickness of the melanoma increases, the prognosis worsens.

Staging

AJCC Staging

The American Joint Committee on Cancer (AJCC) Melanoma Staging Committee uses a tumor-node-metastasis (TNM) classification for cutaneous melanoma based on an analysis of data gathered from centers across North America, Europe, and Australia (Table 31.1). Important prognostic factors in the staging system include Breslow thickness, ulceration, nodal status, and other manifestations of lymphatic spread (e.g., satellite lesions, in-transit disease), as well as the presence of distant metastatic disease. Taking all these factors into consideration, the system provides good discrimination of survival among different patient groups. There are two types of staging classifications provided by the AJCC: clinical staging is what can be determined by biopsy of the primary lesion and physical exam, while pathologic staging is only complete once a full assessment of the regional lymph nodes, when indicated, is performed—usually by SLN biopsy.

T Stage. The eight edition of the AJCC staging guidelines designates T classification based on Breslow thickness measured to the nearest one-tenth of a millimeter, while further subclassifying T1–4 based on ulceration. The cut-points for designating T1–4 melanoma are 1.0, 2.0, and 4.0 mm. Ulceration is a critically important prognostic factor. It is defined histologically by the absence of an intact epithelium over the melanoma. Across all T classifications, ulceration portends worse prognosis. The eighth of the AJCC staging system made an important change to the subclassification of T1 melanomas. T1b melanomas are now defined as the presence of either (1) ulceration at any thickness or (2) thickness of 0.8 to 1.0 mm without ulceration. Mitotic rate, which was adopted in the AJCC seventh edition, is no longer used to designate T1b melanomas.

TABLE 31.1 Tumor-node-metastasis–based eighth edition AJCC staging system for cutaneous melanoma.

T Category	Thickness	Ulceration Status
TX: primary tumor thickness cannot be assess (e.g., diagnosis by curettage)	Not applicable	Not applicable
T0: no evidence of primary tumor (e.g., unknown primary or completely regressed melanoma)	Not applicable	Not applicable
Tis (melanoma in situ)	Not applicable	Not applicable
T1	≤1.0 mm	Unknown or unspecified
T1a	<0.8 mm	Without ulceration
T1b	<0.8 mm 0.8–1.0 mm	With ulceration With or without ulceration
T2	>1.0–2.0 mm	Unknown or unspecified
T2a	>1.0–2.0 mm	Without ulceration
T2b	>1.0–2.0 mm	With ulceration
T3	>2.0–4.0 mm	Unknown or unspecified
T3a	>2.0–4.0 mm	Without ulceration
T3b	>2.0–4.0 mm	With ulceration
T4	>4.0 mm	Unknown or unspecified
T4a	>4.0 mm	Without ulceration
T4b	>4.0 mm	With ulceration
N Category	**Number of Tumor-Involved Regional Lymph Nodes**	**Presence of in-Transit, Satellite, and/or Microsatellite Metastases**
NX	Regional nodes not assessed (e.g., SLN biopsy not performed, regional nodes previously removed for another reason) **Exception:** pathologic N category is not required for T1 melanomas, use cN.	No
N0	No regional metastases detected	No
N1	One tumor-involved node or in-transit, satellite, and/or microsatellite metastases with no tumor-involved nodes	
N1a	One clinically occult (i.e., detected by SLN biopsy)	No
N1b	One clinically detected	No
N1c	No regional lymph node disease	Yes
N2	Two or three tumor-involved nodes or in-transit, satellite, and/or microsatellite metastases with one tumor-involved node	
N2a	Two or three clinically occult (i.e., detected by SLN biopsy)	No
N2b	Two or three, at least one of which was detected clinically	No
N2c	One clinically occult or clinically detected	Yes
N3	Four or more tumor-involved nodes or in-transit, satellite, and/or microsatellite metastases with two or more tumor-involved nodes, or any number of matted nodes without or with in-transit, satellite, and/or microsatellite metastases	
N3a	Four or more clinically occult (i.e., detected by SLN biopsy)	No
N3b	Four or more, at least one of which was clinically detected, or presence of any number of matted nodes	No
N3c	Two or more clinically occult or clinically detected and/or presence of any number of matted nodes	Yes
M Category	**Anatomic Site**	**LDH Level**
M0	No evidence of distant metastases	Not applicable
M1	Evidence of distant metastasis	See below
M1a	Distant metastasis to skin, soft tissue including muscle, and/or nonregional lymph node	Not recorded or unspecified
M1a(0)		Not elevated
M1a(1)		Elevated
M1b	Distant metastasis to lung with or without M1a sites of disease	Not recorded or unspecified
M1b(0)		Not elevated
M1b(1)		Elevated
M1c	Distant metastasis to non-CNS visceral sites with or without M1a or M1b sites of disease	Not recorded or unspecified
M1c(0)		Not elevated
M1c(1)		Elevated

TABLE 31.1 **Tumor-node-metastasis–based eighth edition AJCC staging system for cutaneous melanoma.—cont'd**

M1d M1d(0) M1d(1)	Distant metastasis to CNS with or without M1a, M1b, or M1c sites of disease	Not recorded or unspecified Normal Elevated

Amin MB, Edge SB, Greene FL, et al. *AJCC Cancer Staging Manual*, 8th ed. New York: Springer; 2017.
AJCC, American Joint Committee on Cancer; *CNS*, central nervous system; *LDH*, lactate dehydrogenase; *SLN*, sentinel lymph node.
Suffixes for M category: (0) LDH not elevated, (1) LDH elevated. No suffix is used if LDH is not recorded or is unspecified.

N Stage. For patients with regional lymph node disease, independent prognostic factors include the number of involved nodes and nodal tumor burden at the time of staging, in addition to the thickness and ulceration status of the primary tumor. Tumor burden is characterized as either clinically occult disease detected by SLN biopsy or as clinically apparent disease that is subsequently confirmed on pathology. Clinically apparent nodal disease includes palpable, enlarged lymph nodes or those lymph nodes identified on imaging as abnormal and confirmed by needle biopsy to contain metastatic melanoma. In a change from the seventh edition, the current eighth edition of the AJCC staging guidelines stratify nonnodal regional disease, which includes in-transit cutaneous and/or subcutaneous metastases, microsatellite, or satellite metastases, by N category according to the number of regional lymph nodes (N1c, N2c, or N3c).

M Stage. The new eighth edition of the AJCC staging guidelines stratify M categories by both anatomic site of distant disease and serum lactate dehydrogenase (LDH) levels. Four subgroups (instead of three) are defined by distant skin, soft tissue, and nonregional lymph nodes (M1a), lung (M1b), noncentral nervous system viscera (M1c), and central nervous system (M1d). Elevated serum LDH levels further subclassify M1a-d groups with a (0) or (1) designation. An elevated serum LDH levels indicates worse prognosis across all types of metastatic disease.

Additional Factors. Several factors that have consistently been shown to impact survival are not incorporated into the current AJCC staging system. Older patients have a greater risk of melanoma mortality than younger patients, despite the fact that younger patients are more likely to have nodal metastasis. Patients with axial (trunk, head, and neck) melanomas have a worse prognosis than those with extremity tumors. Women have a better prognosis than men, for reasons that are unclear.

Surgeons involved in the care of melanoma patients should also be familiar with several additional features that are commonly mentioned in pathology reports. Tumor infiltrating lymphocytes (TILs) can indicate the presence of a host immune response and are associated with a more favorable prognosis. TILs are classified as brisk, nonbrisk, or absent. Brisk indicates that TILs infiltrate diffusely throughout the lesion or along the base, while nonbrisk indicates only a focal presence of lymphocytes. Regression, defined as partial or complete loss of tumor cells, has not clearly been shown to be an important factor affecting metastasis or survival. There is no compelling evidence that the presence of regression should be used as an indication for SLN biopsy. Although nodular melanoma and acral lentiginous melanoma often present at a more advanced stage, once controlling for tumor thickness and other factors, there is no survival difference based upon histologic subtype.

Even though mitotic rate is no longer used to subclassify T1 melanoma, the AJCC does suggest that it continue to be reported in pathology reports and in prospective research datasets. The number of mitoses per square millimeters is an important predictor of survival across all thickness categories, and the presence of mitoses in thin (<1.0 mm) melanoma may still be used to select patients for SLN biopsy (especially in the 0.76- to 0.99-mm thickness category or in the 0.8- to 1.0-mm thickness category in the eighth edition AJCC staging system).

Beyond the AJCC TNM Staging

Staging systems must perform dual functions that are at odds with one another. On one hand, a staging system should try to identify as many groups as possible that have distinct survival differences. On the other hand, a good staging system should not be overly complex. Thus, the AJCC staging system provides a parsimonious classification of patients into relatively large categories within which there still remains a fair amount of heterogeneity with regard to prognosis. For these reasons, clinical prediction tools are becoming more popular to provide precise, patient-specific assessments of risks using multiple clinical and pathologic risk factors. Two examples of these predictions tools include the AJCC electronic prediction tool (www.melanomaprognosis.org) and the Melanoma Calculator (www.melanomacalculator.com), which is based on data from the Sunbelt Melanoma Trial. Ultimately, tools like these will allow for more accurate risk assessments that can be used to formulate patient-specific treatment and surveillance plans. Molecular signatures that inform prognosis, such as those outlined in The Cancer Genome Atlas project, will likely be incorporated into these models as our understanding of the interaction between clinical, pathologic, and genomic factors matures.

Additional Workup and Imaging

Most melanoma patients who seek surgical consultation will have already been diagnosed with melanoma. Patients clinically staged with localized stage I or II disease do not require any further tests unless symptoms prompt further evaluation. Liver function tests or serum LDH levels were commonly ordered in the past; however, there is no evidence that blood tests are helpful for detecting metastatic disease in patients with localized melanoma. Similarly, additional imaging studies are unnecessary for most patients with localized disease, although patients with thick primary tumors (stage IIC) can be considered for imaging to detect metastatic disease. In patients with stage III disease detected by SLN biopsy, additional imaging workup is controversial. The probability of detecting actual disease in patients with microscopic nodal metastasis using radiographic studies such as positron emission tomography (PET) and computed tomography (CT) scanning is low.[8] Patients with advanced stage III disease who have clinically detectable nodal metastasis or patients in earlier disease stages who present with symptoms suggestive of metastasis should undergo further imaging studies. The distinction between stage III and IV melanoma is important in deciding the appropriate treatment options, and imaging can determine the extent and resectability of any metastatic lesions in stage IV disease. For these advanced presentations, PET/CT or CT scans of the chest, abdomen, and pelvis and magnetic resonance imaging (MRI) of the brain are generally recommended. The National Comprehensive Cancer Network (NCCN) routinely updates guidelines including the appropriate work-up, surgical treatment, and adjuvant therapy for patients with melanoma. These are available for reference online at http://www.nccn.org.

Treatment

Wide Local Excision

Historically, aggressive surgical resection was recommended for cutaneous melanoma. Excision margins of 5 cm were surgical dogma for much of the previous century. Beginning in the 1970s, studies began to report no adverse outcomes in patients who underwent excision with narrower margins. Since that time, multiple randomized controlled trials evaluating excision margins have established current guidelines, summarized in Table 31.2. The principal determinant for appropriate excision margins is the thickness of the primary tumor.

Based largely upon clinical experience and consensus guidelines, 5-mm excision margins are generally recommended for melanoma in situ. There are two potential issues with 5-mm margins for melanoma in situ. One is that negative margins may not be routinely achieved with gross 5-mm margins; a near 100% margin negative rate can be achieved with gross margins closer to 10 mm versus 5 mm. The second issue is that there may be some diagnostic uncertainty with melanoma in situ. In those situations in which an invasive component is found once the entire tumor is excised (as opposed to the biopsy specimen), a 5-mm gross margin would be inadequate and reexcision would be needed for an oncologically sound operation. With this in mind, it may be prudent to attempt 1-cm margins for some melanoma in situ lesions in anatomic areas that will allow for easy primary closure.

In general, the randomized trials that have focused on margins of excision have focused on intermediate thickness melanoma. The general consensus and practice for thin (<1.0 mm) melanomas is that 1-cm margins are sufficient. Several randomized controlled trials have evaluated the margins needed for intermediate thickness melanoma. As in most solid organ malignancies, no benefit in overall survival has been shown with wider excision margins for melanoma, although locoregional recurrence may be influenced by the margin of excision.

TABLE 31.2 Recommended margins of wide local excision (WLE).

THICKNESS	WLE MARGIN*
In situ	0.5 cm
<1 mm	1 cm
1–2 mm	1–2 cm†
>2–4 mm	2 cm
>4 mm	2 cm‡

*Lesser margins may be justified in specific cases in order to achieve better functional or cosmetic outcome.

†A 1-cm margin may be associated with a slightly greater risk of local recurrence in this Breslow thickness category.

‡There is no evidence that margins >2 cm are beneficial; however, greater margins may be considered for advanced melanomas when local recurrence risk is high.

The British Collaborative Trial randomized 900 patients with melanomas at least 2 mm in thickness to a 1-cm versus 3-cm margin excision. Locoregional recurrences (defined as recurrence within 2 cm of excision or in-transit recurrence) were higher in the 1-cm margin group compared to the 3-cm margin group (hazard ratio [HR], 1.26; $P = 0.05$), with no difference in overall survival.[9] Based on this study, 1-cm margins are generally considered inadequate for intermediate or thick melanomas. The Swedish Melanoma Study group trial randomized 936 patients in nine European centers with cutaneous melanoma at least 2 mm in thickness to 2-cm versus 4-cm margins of excision. No statistically significant difference in overall survival was found, and the local recurrence rates were not statistically different.[10] Based on these trials and others, the general consensus is that 2-cm margins should be attempted for all melanoma at least 2.0 mm in thickness. For 1 to 2-mm thick lesions, 2-cm margins are recommended, although narrower (1-cm) margins are acceptable in areas in which wider margins are not anatomically feasible. These narrower margins come with the understanding that local recurrence may be higher with 1-cm margins.

Technique. WLE can be performed under local anesthesia in most cases, although general anesthesia is preferred for patients who will also undergo SLN biopsy or lymphadenectomy. The appropriate margins of excision are measured from the edge of the lesion or previous biopsy scar. This usually is achieved with a fusiform incision that encompasses the margins of excision to allow primary closure (Fig. 31.10). The incision is carried down to the muscular fascia so all of the skin and underlying subcutaneous tissue are in the margin of excision. Excision of the fascia is not necessary in most cases but may be performed for patients with thick primary tumors and limited subcutaneous tissue in whom the deep margin is of concern. The specimen is submitted for permanent section pathology; frozen section analysis of margins is not performed. In most cases, the incision is closed by mobilizing the skin without the need for complex tissue rearrangement or skin grafting. Rotational tissue flaps or skin grafts are rarely necessary, except for melanomas of

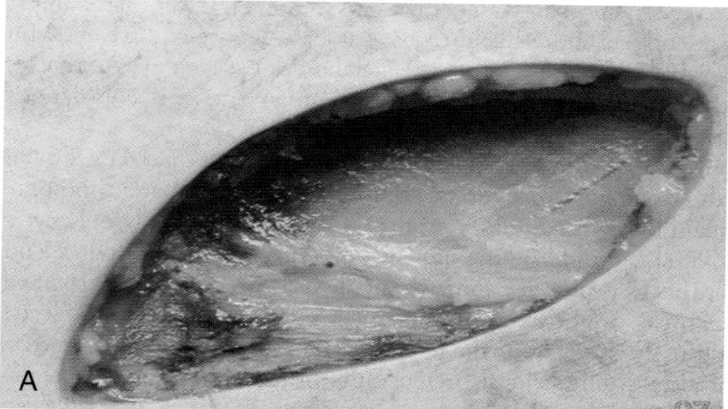

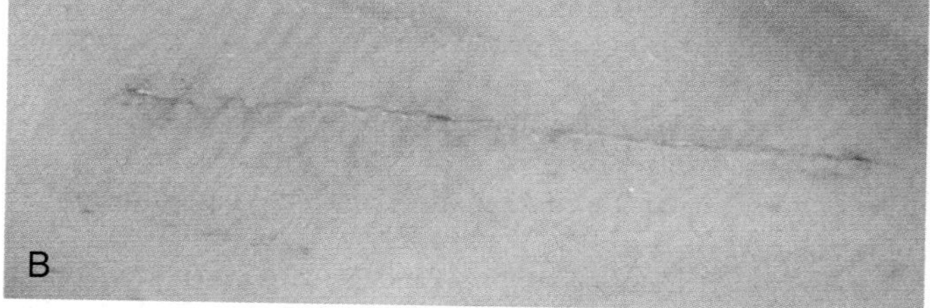

FIG. 31.10 Fusiform incision (A) allowing primary closure (B) for wide local excision of a melanoma.

the head and neck and distal extremities. In these anatomic areas, grafting or tissue rearrangements are useful techniques to achieve skin closure. Tumors arising in proximity to structures such as the nose, eye, and ear may require a compromise of conventionally oncologically sound margins to avoid deformities or disabilities. Subungual melanomas are treated with amputation of the distal digit. For fingers, ray amputations are unnecessary because the melanoma commonly involves only the distal phalanx, and amputation at the distal interphalangeal joint is sufficient. In all cases, resection should achieve histologically negative margins. It should be noted that the recommended margins of excision are the grossly measured margins; it is unnecessary to reexcise the melanoma if the final pathology report indicates that the measured distance from the melanoma to the edge of the excised skin is less than the recommended margin, unless the margin is involved or almost involved by tumor.

Mohs micrographic surgery (MMS) involves the sequential tangential excision of skin cancers with immediate pathologic margin assessment. It is used most often for NMSCs such as SCCs and BCCs with good results. In melanoma, Mohs surgery is used primarily for in situ lesions, although some centers have begun to use MMS for invasive melanoma. MMS is preferred for cosmetically sensitive areas such as the face, where it may minimize the skin defect while still achieving negative margins of excision. Success can be highly operator dependent and requires full pathologic examination of the excised margins. Although there have been several single-institution reports indicating that MMS results in low local recurrence rates for melanoma, it remains controversial. In general, MMS is not considered oncologically acceptable for melanoma, except in the hands of experienced centers in highly selected cases.

Evaluation and Management of Regional Lymph Nodes

The evaluation and management of regional lymph nodes in melanoma have changed rapidly in the last three decades. Elective lymph node dissection to stage clinically node negative patients is a relic of the past. SLN biopsy has been widely adopted and is the foundation of the assessment of intermediate and thick cutaneous melanoma. Indications have changed for a completion lymph node dissection (CLND) following a tumor-positive SLN biopsy based on two landmark studies. All together, the evaluation and management of the regional lymph nodes in melanoma have evolved over time based on clinical research and the willingness of surgical investigators to question the status quo.

Sentinel Lymph Node Biopsy. Since it was introduced by Dr. Donald Morton in 1992, the SLN biopsy has become an indispensable tool in staging patients with cutaneous melanoma. The accuracy of the technique has been well validated and it is now a required part of staging for melanoma greater than 1.0 mm in thickness according to the AJCC. The status of the SLNs is the single most important prognostic factor in melanoma patients without clinical evidence of nodal metastases. The results from the SLN biopsy directly impact treatment and surveillance decisions. A thorough understanding of the indications for SLN across the spectrum of melanoma thickness and the technical execution of the operation is critical for any surgeon who treats melanoma.

Indications. SLN biopsy is relatively simple and straightforward to perform; however, it is not without morbidity and costs. Like other staging tests, it should not be overused in patients at low risk for lymph node metastases or with comorbidities that make general anesthesia prohibitively risky. The NCCN guidelines recommend consideration of SLN biopsy in all patients with T2 or greater (>1.0 mm) melanomas and in those with thinner lesions with a 5% or greater risk of a positive SLN. Some controversy exists regarding the circumstances under which SLN biopsy should be offered to patients with thin (T1) melanomas and if patients with thick (T4, >4.0 mm) benefit from SLN biopsy.

In the United States, approximately 70% of melanomas present as thin melanomas (defined as ≤1.0 mm in thickness). While the overall risk of nodal metastasis in these patients is estimated at 5% or less, certain subsets of this population have rates of nodal disease that approach those seen with thicker lesions. While routine use of SLN biopsy is not recommended for thin melanomas, if these lesions have any features that are associated with an increased risk for nodal spread, then SLN biopsy may be indicated. Features of the primary lesion that have been linked to an increased risk of nodal metastasis include ulceration and mitotic rate (≥1 mitosis/mm^2).

The recent changes to the AJCC staging classification of T1 melanomas have complicated the assessment and risk stratification of thin melanomas for SLN biopsy. Previously, a T1b melanoma was defined by the presence of either ulceration and/or at least 1 mitosis/mm^2. Since these two factors are the strongest risk factors for SLN metastases in thin melanoma, it made for a fairly straightforward recommendation that SLN biopsy be considered for T1b melanomas. However, T1b is now defined by either ulceration or thickness of 0.8 to 1.0 mm, with no consideration for mitotic rate. This was done because of a slight difference in survival based on thickness alone in thin melanomas.[11] T1b is now a group defined by a slightly worse survival than T1a, but not necessarily a group with higher risk of SLN metastases. Mitotic rate, while not formally considered in the AJCC staging criteria, should still be used to identify thin melanomas with an increased risk of SLN metastases. Other factors that can be used to identify higher than average risk thin melanomas include age and thickness ranging from 0.8 to 1.0 mm.[12] Younger-age patients with thin melanomas have an increased risk of SLN metastases. Our general practice is to offer SLN biopsies to any patient with acceptable risk of general anesthesia who has a T1 melanoma with ulceration or those between 0.76 and 0.99 mm thick with a mitotic rate of at least 1 mitosis/mm^2. We selectively offer SLN biopsy to younger patients without these adverse features, especially with thickness approaching 1.0 mm. Any patient with a mitotic rate of at least 1 mitosis/mm^2, thickness of 1.0 mm, and age older than 56 years or mitotic rate of at least 1 mitosis/mm^2 and age 56 years or younger have a greater than 5% risk of SLN metastases and SLN biopsy should be considered.[13]

Because thick (>4 mm) primary melanomas have an increased risk for distant metastatic disease, prior thinking held that the status of the SLN did not add much additional prognostic information. However, a number of studies have shown that thick melanoma patients with tumor-negative SLN have a better prognosis than those with tumor-positive SLN. Because there is a continuum of risk that does not abruptly end at 4-mm thickness, SLN biopsy for thick melanomas provides important risk stratification in these patients, especially for the consideration of adjuvant therapy. SLN biopsy can also be considered for patients with nonnodal regional disease (i.e., in-transit disease) with clinically negative nodes, because the number of positive nodes is prognostically important in this group.

Technical Details. The technical details of a proper SLN biopsy are worthy of attention. All patients should undergo preoperative lymphoscintigraphy, typically performed on the same day

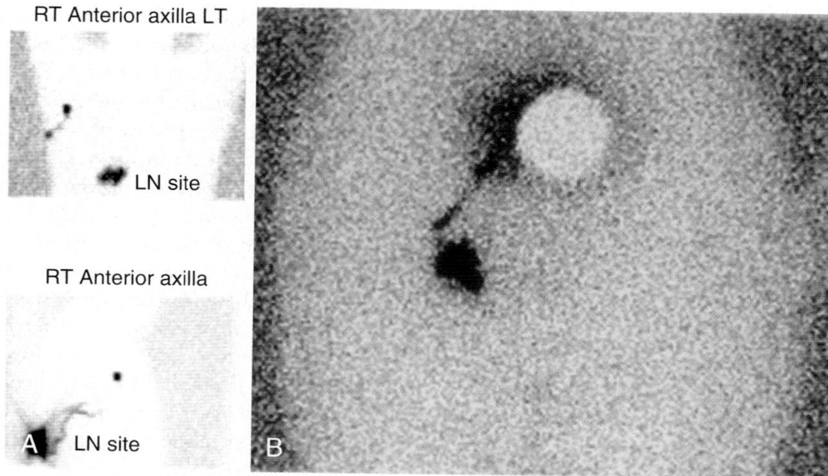

FIG. 31.11 Preoperative lymphoscintigraphy can aid in identification of sentinel lymph nodes. (A) Melanoma of the back with drainage to the axilla. (B) Periumbilical melanoma with drainage to the left inguinal lymph nodes. *LN,* Lymph node; *LT,* left; *RT,* right.

as the operation to perform SLN biopsy and WLE (Fig. 31.11). Technetium-99 sulfur colloid (0.5 mCi) should be injected into the dermis, raising a wheal in four aliquots around the melanoma or biopsy site. It is important to inject the tracer into the normal skin approximately 0.5 cm away from the melanoma or scar from the biopsy and not into the melanoma itself or biopsy scar. A common mistake is to inject the radioactive tracer too deeply into the subcutaneous tissue, which will result in failure to detect a sentinel node. If no sentinel nodes are identified after the initial injection, repeat injection should be performed with the proper technique by an experienced clinician. In almost all cases, this will result in identification of sentinel nodes. Imaging is performed with a gamma camera, with dynamic and static images that allow identification of lymphatic channels and sentinel nodes. Although patterns of lymphatic drainage can be predictable at times, lymphoscintigraphy often identifies lymph nodes in locations that are not anticipated. This is especially true for melanomas in ambiguous lymphatic drainage areas, such as the trunk, head, or neck, where anatomic predictions of nodal spread are unreliable. In such cases, lymphoscintigraphy may identify sentinel nodes in more than one nodal basin. Furthermore, it is not uncommon to identify sentinel nodes outside the traditional cervical, axillary, and inguinal nodal basins. So-called interval, intercalated, or in-transit nodes may be found in subcutaneous locations or between muscle groups. For distal upper or lower extremity melanomas, it is important to assess the presence of epitrochlear or popliteal sentinel nodes, respectively. These interval nodes have the same risk of harboring melanoma cells as sentinel nodes in traditional nodal basins; therefore, it is recommended that they be removed at the time of sentinel node biopsy. In addition, 85% of the time, the interval lymph node is the only positive node, even for those patients with other SLNs identified in traditional basins. Therefore, all sentinel nodes identified by preoperative lymphoscintigraphy should be removed (Fig. 31.12).

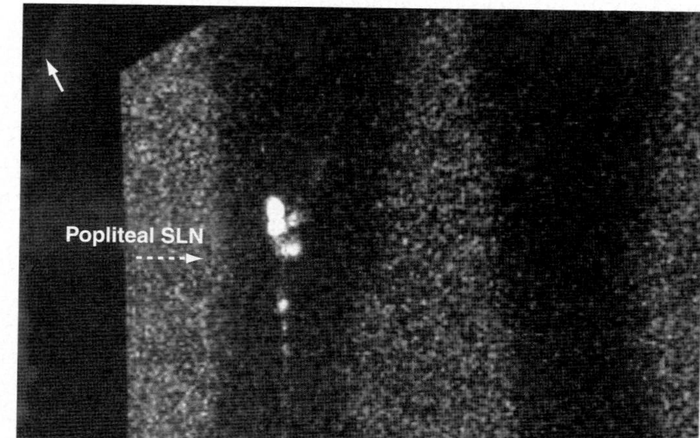

FIG. 31.12 Popliteal sentinel lymph node *(SLN)* on lymphoscintigraphy.

At operation, which is generally performed under general anesthesia, a vital blue dye (e.g., isosulfan blue) is injected into the dermis around the melanoma site in a manner similar to that for injection of the radioactive tracer (Fig. 31.13). This combined lymphatic mapping technique allows for the identification of the sentinel nodes in 99% of patients. Because the blue dye will not

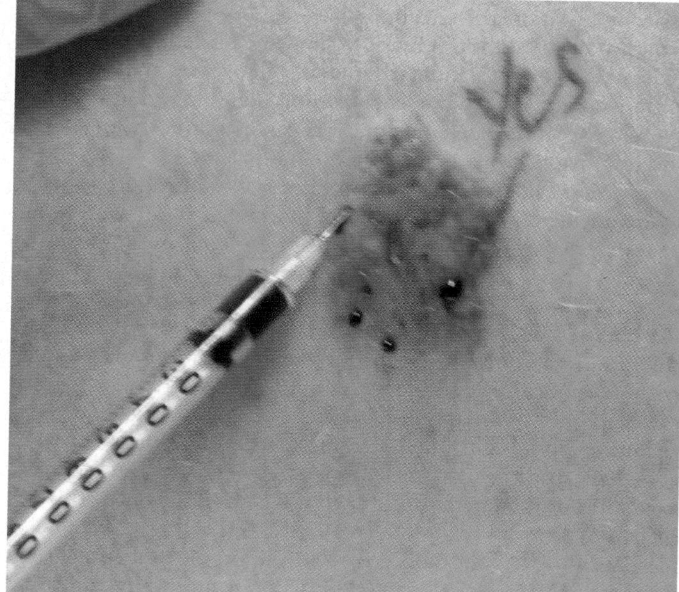

FIG. 31.13 Intradermal injection of isosulfan blue dye for intraoperative lymphatic mapping and sentinel lymph node biopsy.

persist in the sentinel nodes for prolonged periods, it is injected just before the operation; 1 to 5 mL is used, depending on the size of the melanoma. Because blue dye will persist in the skin for many months after injection; it is best to inject it within the margins of the planned WLE. A handheld gamma probe is used to identify the location of the sentinel node(s), and dissection is performed to identify blue lymphatic channels entering into any blue lymph nodes (Fig. 31.14). A sentinel node is defined as any lymph node that is the most radioactive node in the nodal basin, any node that is blue, any node that has a radioactive count of 10% or higher of the most radioactive node in that basin, or any node that is palpably abnormal and suspicious for tumor. All such nodes require resection. By following these guidelines, the risk of a false-negative SLN biopsy is minimized. Although multiple radioactive lymph nodes may be evident within a nodal basin on lymphoscintigraphy, many of these represent mildly radioactive second-echelon nodes and not true sentinel nodes. There is often a poor correlation between the number of nodes visualized on the lymphoscintigram and the number of SLNs identified. In general, the average number of sentinel nodes identified is two per nodal basin. Sentinel nodes should be sent for permanent section histopathology with immunohistochemical stains for melanoma markers (e.g., S-100, HMB-45, and Melan-1). Immediate frozen section histology should be avoided because even expert pathologists have difficulty diagnosing micrometastatic melanoma in the SLN on frozen sections.

SLN biopsy is more challenging in the head and neck than for other regions because of the rich lymphatic drainage network in this location. Correspondingly, the false-negative rate for SLN biopsy is generally higher for melanomas in these locations. Cross-sectional imaging, such as with a single-photon emission CT, can allow the surgeon to identify the exact anatomic location of the SLNs more accurately than with the planar lymphoscintograms. Precise knowledge of the anatomy in this region is essential to avoid inadvertent neurologic injury. Parotid SLNs can be identified and removed, usually without the need for superficial parotidectomy. However, if there is any concern for facial nerve injury, superficial parotidectomy may be a safer option. A common site for cervical SLN is directly adjacent to the spinal accessory nerve, which should be visualized and preserved.

Multicenter Selective Lymphadenectomy Trial. The only randomized control trial to compare outcomes between SLN biopsy and nodal observation is the first Multicenter Selective Lymphadenectomy Trial (MSLT-I).[14] The trial randomized 1347 patients with intermediate-thickness melanoma (1.2–3.5 mm thick) and 314 patients with thick melanoma (>3.5 mm thick) to either SLN biopsy or observation. Patients with disease identified by SLN biopsy underwent immediate completion lymphadenectomy. The frequency of nodal metastasis across all groups was 20.8% and was similar within each treatment arm. No difference in 10-year melanoma-specific survival was found between SLN biopsy and observation group in either the intermediate thickness (81.4% vs. 78.3%; $P = 0.18$) or thick melanoma groups (58.9% vs. 64.4%; $P = 0.56$). However, improved 10-year disease-free was observed with SLN biopsy in both intermediate and thick melanomas. The status of the sentinel node was the strongest predictor of recurrence or death from melanoma: in patients with intermediate thickness melanoma, 10-year survival was 85.1% with a negative SLN biopsy, compared to 62.1% for positive nodes (HR, 3.09; $P < 0.001$). Interestingly, on subgroup analysis limited only to patients with nodal metastasis (disease identified either on SLN biopsy or that developed while under observation), improved melanoma-specific survival, disease-free survival, and distant disease-free survival was observed in the SLN biopsy arm among patients with intermediate thickness lesions.

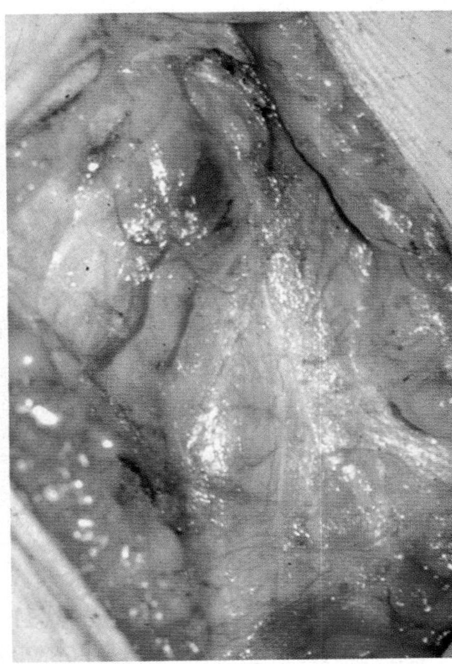

FIG. 31.14 Blue lymphatic channels leading to a blue sentinel lymph node.

Lymph Node Dissection

Historical. Lymph node dissection, historically, was an important component of the surgical treatment of melanoma, but with the development of the SLN biopsy technique and an improved understanding of the biology of melanoma, it has become less important. Prior to the use of SLN biopsy, an elective lymph node dissection of the draining regional nodal basin was often performed for high-risk melanomas in order to identify early, clinically occult lymph node metastases and provide accurate staging. The SLN technique accomplishes the same objectives with decreased morbidity; therefore, elective lymph node dissection is of historical interest only. Lymph node dissection does still play an important role in the treatment of melanoma; therefore, the surgeon treating melanoma should be familiar with the technical details of the operation and its indications.

Completion Lymphadenectomy. Completion lymphadenectomy or CLND is used to remove the remaining lymph nodes in a regional nodal basin that is found to have metastatic melanoma by SLN biopsy. A wide range of prognosis exists in stage III, SLN-positive melanoma. CLND allows one to identify nonsentinel node metastases. This is an important prognostic factor, as multiple studies have demonstrated that metastases to the nonsentinel nodes represent an additional echelon of metastatic disease with more aggressive biology and worse prognosis compared to disease limited to the SLNs. CLND may have a potential therapeutic benefit by removing additional lymph nodes with micrometastatic disease, improving disease-free survival as seen in MSLT-I. CLND

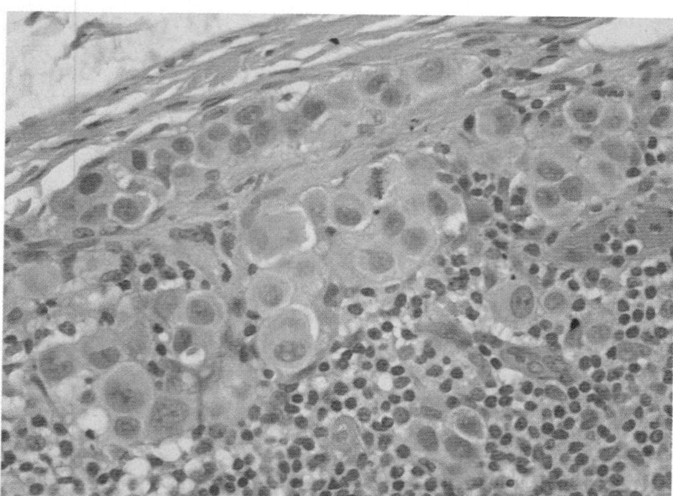

FIG. 31.15 Subcapsular micrometastatic melanoma deposits within the lymph node.

does, however, greatly increase the short- and long-term morbidity to the patients. Complications include wound complications, paresthesias, and permanent lymphedema. Only 15% to 20% of patients with SLN-positive micrometastatic lymph node disease have additional micrometastatic nonsentinel nodes after CLND; thus, 5 out of 6 patients undergoing CLND for SLN-positive disease derive no therapeutic benefit from the procedure and experience all the morbidity associated with the CLND.

Efforts to predict nonsentinel node metastases have focused on clinical and pathologic factors that identify high- and low-risk patients in whom a CLND could either be selectively omitted (in patients at low risk for non-SLN disease) or in whom a CLND would be particularly beneficial. Multiple different scoring systems evaluating the burden of micrometastatic disease within the lymph node have been developed, with criteria including location of tumor deposits, tumor cross-sectional area, tumor diameter (either summed across all foci or only within the largest focus), or depth of invasion into the lymph node (Fig. 31.15). In general, the maximum diameter of the largest tumor deposit is the most prognostically significant tumor burden measure that can predict survival and non-SLN metastases.[15,16] Ongoing research that harmonizes these clinical and pathologic factors with novel genetic markers of increased risk, either in the primary tumor or SLN biopsy, will allow development of comprehensive risk models that can give a patient-specific assessment of the risk of non-SLN metastases. The ability to predict non-SLN metastases may be used in the future to select patients for adjuvant therapy, rather than a CLND, based on two landmark studies discussed below.

Multicenter Selective Lymphadenectomy Trial II and German Dermatologic Cooperative Group Trial (DeCOG-SLT). Two studies were conducted to answer the question concerning whether CLND after a tumor-positive SLN biopsy improved survival compared to observation alone. The rationale for the observation approach is that, as discussed above, upward of 85% of patients do not have any additional micrometastatic disease after a positive SLN biopsy; therefore, no survival benefit is achieved from routine CLND.

The DeCOG-SLT study was a multicenter, randomized clinical trial conducted in Germany, the results of which were published in 2016.[17] In the study, 483 patients with a positive SLN biopsy were randomized to either a CLND of the positive lymph node basin or observation. The trial was closed early due to difficulties in accrual and low event rates; the planned enrollment was 550. With a median follow-up of 35 months, there were no differences in the primary endpoint or distant metastasis-free survival between the two groups (77% vs. 75%). There were no differences in recurrence-free or overall survival. Subgroup analysis of the primary endpoint based on micrometastatic tumor burden (≤1 mm or >1 mm) showed no differences in distant metastasis-free survival. The study has been criticized as being underpowered and failing to meet accrual, but it is an important study that establishes the safety of an observation strategy with SLN-positive melanoma.

The MSLT-II was a larger, multicenter randomized clinical trial that confirmed the findings of the DeCOG study. In MSLT-II, 1939 patients with a tumor-positive SLN biopsy were randomized to a CLND or observation, which consisted of ultrasound-based surveillance of the involved nodal basin.[18] There was no difference in the primary endpoint, melanoma-specific survival, between the two groups. The 3-year melanoma-specific survival rate was 86% in both groups, while the 3-year disease-free survival rate was numerically (but not statistically) greater in the CLND group compared to the observation group (68% vs. 63%; $P = 0.05$). There was an increase in the cumulative incidence of non-SLN metastases in the observation group versus the CLND group (26% vs. 20% at 5 years; $P = 0.005$).

Taken together, the findings of DeCOG-SLT and MSLT-II have been practice-changing. Only in very selective circumstances, in which there is a high degree of concern for non-SLN metastases and failure of regional nodal control, or inability to follow the observation surveillance strategy, is CLND considered after a positive SLN. Although not universally accepted at all centers, the DeCOG and MSLT-II studies firmly establish that it is safe and reasonable to avoid CLND for the vast majority of patients with positive SLN. The issues of this approach and the selection of patients for adjuvant therapy will be discussed below.

Therapeutic Lymph Node Dissection. A therapeutic lymph node dissection, which is a lymphadenectomy of a regional nodal basin with clinically apparent nodal metastases, remains an important part of the armamentarium of the surgeon treating melanoma. It is an excellent procedure for achieving locoregional disease control, and given the findings of MSLT-II and DeCOG-SLT, it will likely be the most common reason for performing a lymphadenectomy in the future. Suspected nodal metastases based on palpable lymph nodes or radiographic abnormalities should be confirmed by fine needle aspiration. On occasion, benign lymphadenopathy may be found, but in a patient with cutaneous melanoma, palpable lymph nodes should be concerning for metastatic disease until proven otherwise. Palliative resection of bulky, painful regional lymphadenopathy can be considered, recognizing that there will be a high risk of regional and distant metastatic recurrence in the absence of effective adjuvant therapy (Fig. 31.16).

A therapeutic lymph node dissection should remove all the fibrofatty and lymphatic tissue in the involved regional nodal basin according to standard anatomic boundaries. For the axilla, a thorough level I, II, and III axillary dissection is performed. This includes complete removal of all fibrofatty tissue around the axillary vein, thoracodorsal and medial pectoral neurovascular bundles, and long thoracic nerve. The pectoralis minor muscle may need to be divided near its insertion on the coracoid process in order to clear bulky level II and III nodes. On rare occasions, the pectoralis

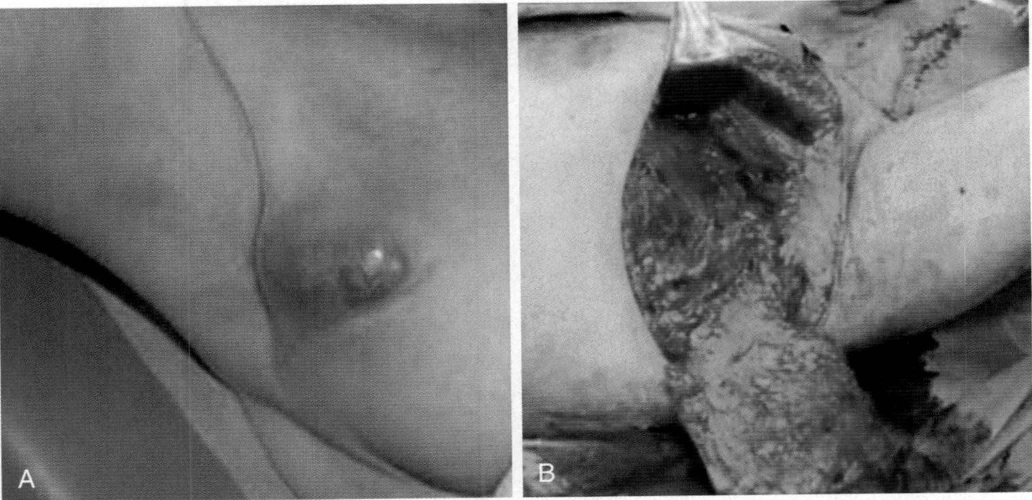

FIG. 31.16 (A) Advanced axillary lymph node metastases. (B) Levels I, II, and III axillary lymph node dissection.

major muscle may need to be divided as well. The axillary vein may be ligated and divided if it becomes involved with tumor, often with less consequence in terms of edema than one might anticipate.

Inguinal lymph node dissection includes the superficial inguinal (femoral) lymph nodes, and may also include dissection of deep or pelvic (internal iliac, external iliac, and obturator) nodes. There is no consensus as to when pelvic nodal dissection should be performed for patients with macroscopic disease confined to the superficial inguinal nodal basin. For patients with palpable nodal disease or with imaging suggestive of involved pelvic lymph nodes, the deep nodes should be dissected in most cases. Metastasis to Cloquet node, which links the femoral and iliac nodal chains underneath the inguinal ligament, has traditionally been a common indication for pelvic nodal dissection. Similarly, gross involvement of multiple femoral nodes is another traditional indication for pelvic dissection.

For cervical lymphadenectomy, a functional neck dissection with sparing of the internal jugular vein and spinal accessory nerve is usually sufficient. The need for superficial parotidectomy may be guided by the lymphoscintigraphy and SLN results. Epitrochlear or popliteal lymphadenectomy is frequently unnecessary but requires careful attention to the particular anatomy in these regions (Fig. 31.17).

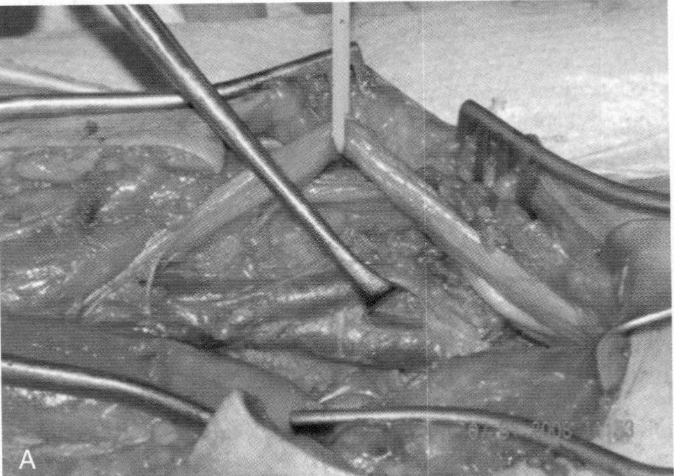

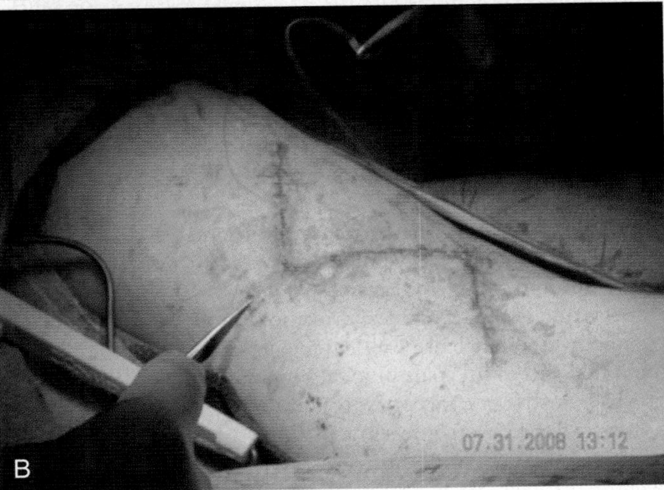

FIG. 31.17 Popliteal lymph node dissection with (A) exposed popliteal artery and vein and (B) closure.

Adjuvant Therapy

As with most solid organ malignancies, the dismal prognosis historically associated with advanced melanoma was the result of lack of effective systemic therapies. Melanoma biology has historically trumped the locoregional disease control strategies of the surgeon. With the exception of some increase in the sophistication of our understanding of the evaluation and management of the regional lymph nodes, vis-á-vis SLN biopsy and indication for completion lymphadenectomy, the operative treatment of melanoma has not changed much in the last few decades. The same cannot be said for systemic treatment options. It is an exciting time to be treating melanoma, as advances in targeted therapy and immunotherapy have been occurring at breakneck speed. We now have multiple adjuvant therapy options that are safe and effective, which offer melanoma patients the hope for durable disease remission after operative therapy (Table 31.3).

Historical. Prior to 2015, the only adjuvant systemic therapy approved for melanoma by the U.S. Food and Drug Administration (FDA) was high-dose interferon alfa-2b. This drug was quite

TABLE 31.3 Summary of adjuvant therapy trials for BRAF-MEK inhibition and immunotherapy in cutaneous melanoma.

TRIAL NAME	STUDY POPULATION	INTERVENTION TREATMENT	CONTROL TREATMENT	PRIMARY OUTCOME	NOTES
EORTC 18071 (Eggermont et al)[21]	IIIA (with >1 mm micrometastasis), IIIB, IIIC (with no in-transit metastases)	Ipilimumab 10 mg/kg every 3 weeks × 4, then every 3 months × 3 years	Placebo	Improved recurrence-free survival (HR, 0.76; 95% CI, 0.64–0.89)	Improved overall survival at 5 years (65.4% vs. 54.4%; HR, 0.72; 95% CI, 0.58–0.88)
COMBI-AD (Long et al)[19]	IIIA (with >1 mm micrometastasis), IIIB, IIIC *BRAF* V600 mutation	Daily dabrafenib/ trametinib x 12 months	Placebo	Improved relapse-free survival (3 year RFS 58% vs. 39%; HR, 0.47; 95% CI, 0.39–0.58)	Improved 3-year overall survival (86% vs. 77%; HR, 0.57; 95%, CI 0.42–0.79)
CheckMate 238 (Weber et al)[22]	Completely resected IIIB, IIIC, or IV	Nivolumab every 2 weeks × 12 months	Ipilimumab 10 mg/kg every 3 weeks × 4, then every 12 weeks × 12 months	Improved 12-month recurrence-free survival with nivolumab (70.5% vs. 60.8%; HR, 0.65; 97.5% CI, 0.51–0.83)	Better safety profile with nivolumab (grade 3 or 4 adverse events, 14.4% vs. 45.9%)
EORTC 1325 (Eggermont, et al)[23]	IIIA (with >1 mm micrometastasis), IIIB, IIIC (with no in-transit metastases)	Pembrolizumab every 3 weeks x 12 months	Placebo	Improved recurrence-free survival (HR, 0.57; 98.4% CI, 0.43–0.74)	Improved RFS in both PD-L1-positive and PD-L1-negative tumors

CI, Confidence interval; *HR*, hazard ratio; *PD-L1*, programmed death ligand 1; *RFS*, recurrence-free survival.

toxic, with a prolonged treatment course and numerous serious adverse events. Therapy was typically delivered for 1 month via intravenous therapy, followed by 11 months of thrice-weekly subcutaneous injections. Common side effects included influenza-like symptoms, fatigue, malaise, anorexia, neuropsychiatric side effects, and hepatic toxicity.

The therapy was marginally effective at best and quite toxic at worst. The FDA approval was based largely on the Eastern Cooperative Oncology Group E1684 trial, in which high-risk patients with palpable nodal disease experienced short-term disease-free and overall survival benefit with adjuvant interferon; longer follow-up demonstrated a modest difference in disease-free survival only. Alternative dosing strategies, including intermittent dosing and use of pegylated interferon alfa-2b, were tried. The Sunbelt Melanoma Trial demonstrated that in lower-risk patients with a single positive SLN, there was no benefit to adjuvant interferon in terms of disease-free or overall survival. The summary assessment of adjuvant interferon for melanoma is that it reproducibly improved disease-free survival, with minimal effect on overall survival at the cost of serious toxicity. Better adjuvant therapy options were needed; these options came in the form of targeted therapy and immunotherapy.

Targeted Therapy. The first successful targeted therapy developed for melanoma was vemurafenib, a small molecule tyrosine kinase inhibitor targeted against the *BRAF* V600E mutation. *BRAF* is one of the recognized driver mutations in melanoma that is present in about half of all cutaneous melanoma. Building on the initial successful trials in metastatic melanoma, BRAF inhibition as a treatment concept evolved into dual BRAF-MEK inhibition in order to overcome some of the resistance issues seen with single-agent BRAF inhibition (Fig. 31.18). The promising experience with BRAF-MEK inhibition in metastatic melanoma led to the development of an adjuvant trial for patients with resected stage III BRAF-mutant melanoma.

The landmark COMBI-AD trial was published by Long and colleagues in 2017.[19] In this multicenter, international study, 870 patients with completely resected stage III melanoma with either the *BRAF* V600E or V600K mutation were randomly assigned to dual BRAF (dabrafenib) and MEK (trametinib) inhibition therapy or placebo for 12 months after resection. The initial findings were simply remarkable: 3-year relapse-free survival was improved from 39% to 58% in the treatment group (HR, 0.47) and 3-year overall survival was improved from 77% to 86% (HR, 0.57). Subgroup analyses showed that the benefit of dual BRAF-MEK inhibition was consistent across multiple cohorts, including age, disease stage (IIIA, IIIB, and IIIC), micrometastatic versus macrometastatic disease, ulceration, and number of nodal metastases. The therapy was well tolerated, with a reasonable adverse event profile. Importantly, the trial enrolled patients with stage III disease who had undergone a completion lymphadenectomy for SLN-positive disease. High-risk micrometastatic disease was selected by only enrolling patients with a lymph node metastasis of more than 1 mm.

This trial has established the potential role of adjuvant targeted BRAF-MEK inhibition for stage III melanoma in patients with BRAF-mutant melanoma; however, there are some issues with how we incorporate this strategy in light of some of the other adjuvant therapy options. There is some concern about the long-term durability of this strategy, as we know that patients who initially respond to targeted therapy often eventually develop resistance. Long-term follow-up of this study will shed some light on this issue. Adjuvant immunotherapy is also very promising (discussed below). Thus, it is not clear what the optimal adjuvant treatment strategy is for BRAF-mutant melanoma patients who are also candidates for adjuvant immunotherapy. Finally, one must reconcile the findings of this trial with the current paradigm for managing SLN-positive melanoma. All patients in this study underwent completion lymphadenectomy for SLN-positive disease; however, the current treatment strategy for SLN-positive disease in light of the MSLT-II and DeCOG studies is to forgo completion lymphadenectomy in favor of nodal surveillance.

Immunotherapy. Adjuvant immunotherapy developed in a similar manner to BRAF-targeted therapy, in which early experience with treatment of metastatic disease developed into an adjuvant therapy concept. The first immunotherapy agent to gain approval for adjuvant therapy was the monoclonal anti-CTLA-4 antibody

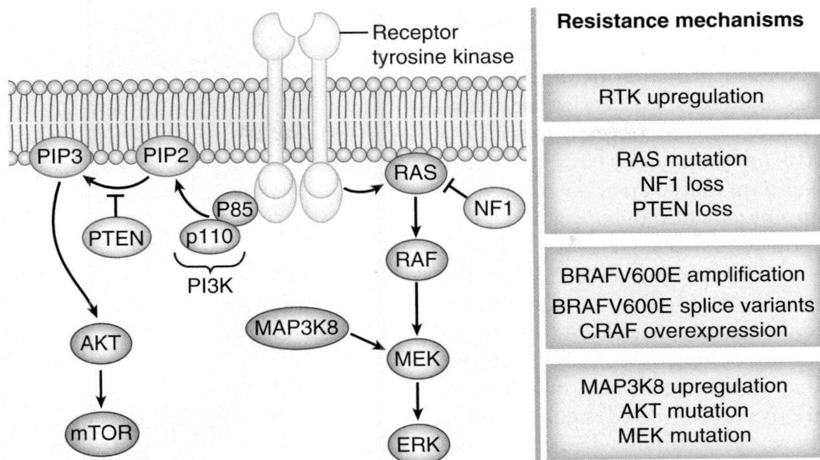

FIG. 31.18 BRAF-MEK signaling pathway and potential mechanisms of resistance. (From Welsh SJ, Rizos H, Scolyer RA, et al. Resistance to combination BRAF and MEK inhibition in metastatic melanoma: where to next? *Eur J Cancer.* 2016;62:76–85.)

ipilimumab in 2015. The FDA approved ipilimumab based on the initial findings of the EORTC 18071 study published in 2015.[20] In this trial, 951 patients with resected stage III melanoma were randomized to treatment with ipilimumab at a dose of 10 mg/kg for up to 3 years or placebo. All patients with SLN-positive disease underwent a completion lymphadenectomy and patients with micrometastatic lymph node disease of 1 mm or less were excluded. Median recurrence-free survival was improved from 17.1 months to 26.1 months in the ipilimumab group (HR, 0.75). With longer follow-up (median follow-up, 5.3 years), the recurrence-free survival benefit was maintained and an overall survival benefits was demonstrated.[21] Five-year recurrence-free survival was 40.8% in the ipilimumab group compared to 30.3% (HR, 0.76) and the 5-year overall survival rate was improved from 54.4% to 65.4% (HR, 0.72). The rate of distant metastasis-free survival was also improved. These benefits did not come without increased risk of serious adverse events and even death from adjuvant ipilimumab. Serious adverse events occurred in 54% of the patients treated with ipilimumab compared to 26% of the placebo group. Five patients (1.1%) died due to complications from adjuvant ipilimumab. The promising results from this trial led to the first new drug approved by the FDA for adjuvant therapy of melanoma in nearly 20 years. However, the side effects and risk of death were of significant concern.

The newer programmed death 1 (PD-1) inhibitors nivolumab and pembrolizumab offered the promise of safer, better-tolerated immunotherapy with just as effective and durable a response as ipilimumab. The Checkmate 238 trial demonstrated that adjuvant nivolumab was more effective than ipilimumab at preventing recurrence in resected stage III and stage IV melanoma.[22] In this trial, 906 patients with complete resection of stage IIIB, IIIC, or IV (as defined by AJCC seventh edition) melanoma were randomly assigned to 1 year of adjuvant nivolumab or ipilimumab. At a minimum follow-up of 18 months, the 12-month recurrence-free survival was 70.5% in the nivolumab group and 60.8% in the ipilimumab group (HR, 0.65). Serious (grade 3 or 4) adverse events were lower in the nivolumab group (14%) compared to the ipilimumab group (46%). The relative benefit of nivolumab compared to ipilimumab was consistent across multiple subgroups, including age, gender, stage (IIIB, IIIC, and IV), ulceration, and micro- versus macrometastatic lymph node disease. Adjuvant pembrolizumab has also been reported to improve recurrence-free survival in resected stage III melanoma. In the EORTC 1325 (KEYNOTE-054) trial, 1019 patents with resected stage III melanoma (by seventh edition AJCC) were randomized to 1 year of adjuvant pembrolizumab or placebo.[23] With a median follow-up of 15 months, adjuvant pembrolizumab was associated with improved 1-year recurrence-free survival compared to placebo (75.4% vs. 61.0%; HR, 0.57). The low rate of serious adverse events reported in the pembrolizumab group (14.7%) was similar to that of nivolumab in the Checkmate 238 trial. Like nivolumab, pembrolizumab was effective across multiple subgroups, including PD-1 ligand (PD-L1) expression, gender, stage (IIIA, IIIB, IIIC), number of positive lymph node, micro- versus macrometastatic lymph node disease, ulceration, and BRAF mutation status.

Based on these landmark trials, the PD-1 inhibitors nivolumab and pembrolizumab have become the preferred adjuvant immunotherapy option for patients with resected stage III and IV melanoma. Ipilimumab has fallen out of favor because of its toxicity profile compared to the PD-1 inhibitors, but it may still play a role in salvage therapy or in combination with PD-1 inhibitors (discussed in more detail below). Preference for nivolumab or pembrolizumab is usually institution specific, as there are no data to suggest one is more effective than the other. The issue that surgeons and medical oncologists face, as alluded to in the Targeted Therapy section previously, is the reconciliation of the adjuvant trial study populations, in which all SLN-positive patients underwent CLND, with the current treatment paradigm of omission of CLND in most SLN-positive patients. Checkmate 238 excluded stage IIIA patients, and EORTC 1325/KEYNOTE-054 allowed IIIA patients, but only if the micrometastatic lymph node burden was larger than 1 mm in diameter (using the seventh edition AJCC staging criteria). The majority of patients with nodal metastases detected by SLN biopsy have a single microscopically positive lymph node. We are thus facing a population of stage III patients that are mostly IIIA, with an adjuvant treatment strategy that we know is effective in IIIB and IIIC patients. The risk stratification of these single positive SLN patients into groups that will and will not benefit from adjuvant immunotherapy will be the focus of a great deal of research in the future as we try to tailor our adjuvant treatment strategy to maximize effectiveness and minimize excess utilization.

Radiation Therapy. Although melanoma has been historically believed to be relatively resistant to radiation, several newer studies suggest that there may be roles for radiation treatment in the adjuvant and palliative settings as well as a potential adjunct to systemic immunotherapy. Adjuvant radiation therapy may have a role in select patients at high risk for lymph node basin recurrence after lymphadenectomy. In long-term follow-up of the ANZMTG 01.02/TROG 02.01 trial, adjuvant radiation therapy after regional lymphadenectomy reduced the cumulative incidence of lymph node field relapse from 36% to 21% (adjusted HR, 0.52).[24] The trial randomized 250 patients considered to be at high risk for nodal recurrence to either adjuvant radiotherapy (48 Gy in 20 fractions) or observation following lymphadenectomy. High risk was defined as one or more involved parotid nodes, two or more cervical or axillary nodes, three or more involved inguinal nodes, presence of extranodal extension, or maximum diameter of the largest lymph node greater than 4 cm (3 cm for cervical nodes). After long-term follow-up, there remained no difference in overall survival or relapse-free survival. Adjuvant radiation therapy does appear to offer some improvement in control of regional lymph node disease in high-risk patients after lymphadenectomy; however, the importance of this regional control with disease that is clearly high risk for systemic metastases is not clear. It is likely that patients with high-risk regional nodal disease would derive more benefit from better adjuvant systemic therapy (immunotherapy) to reduce the risk of metastatic recurrence rather than adjuvant radiation therapy to improve nodal basin disease control.

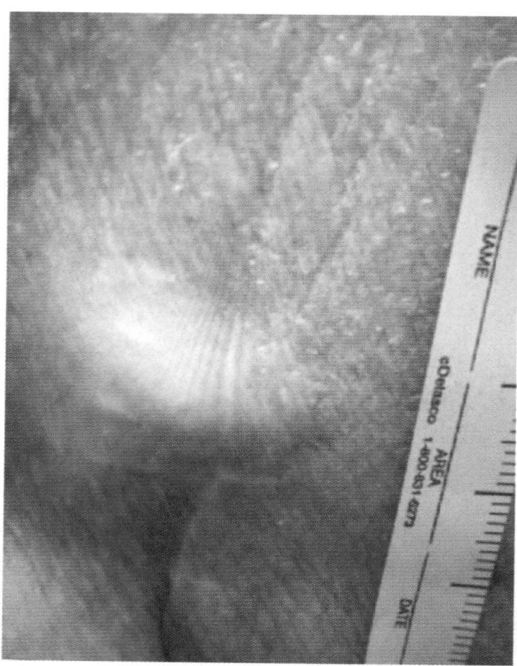

FIG. 31.19 Local recurrence of melanoma within the scar of the primary melanoma excision.

Surveillance

There are no definitive guidelines on appropriate follow-up for patients with resected melanoma who are disease free, although the NCCN does offer some suggested surveillance approaches. The general principle that should be considered is that the intensity of the surveillance strategy and incorporation of imaging studies should be individualized according to the patient's risk and likely site of recurrence. Most recurrences are detected within the first 5 years after treatment, although melanoma is notorious for delayed recurrences, sometimes decades after treatment, in seemingly low-risk lesions.

Patients with early stage, localized disease (0–II) are at low risk of recurrence and should be observed by history and physical examination at least every 6 months for the first 3 years and at least annually thereafter. A careful history is necessary to elicit symptoms such as new skin lesions, nodal masses, pain, headaches, neurologic changes, weight loss, and gastrointestinal and pulmonary symptoms. Patients should be educated about common symptoms and signs of recurrence so that they can report any important changes that arise between scheduled visits. Physical examination should include a complete skin inspection, including palpation to detect regional nodal or in-transit recurrence. Most recurrences in these patients will be reported by the patients themselves.[25]

For stage III melanoma and those with high-risk stage II disease (thick and/or ulcerated primaries), a reasonable follow-up schedule is a history and physical examination every 3 or 4 months for the first 3 years, every 6 months for the next 2 years, and annually thereafter. The use of laboratory tests and imaging tests such as CT, MRI, or PET/CT is controversial but not unreasonable for these patients. Even though there has never been any proven benefit to early detection of recurrent melanoma with radiographic or laboratory studies, it stands to reason that in this age of effective immunotherapy for metastatic melanoma, there may be some utility in early detection of low-volume disease. Patients with stage IV melanoma will have regular clinical, laboratory, and radiologic evaluations to monitor the response to treatment.

The survivorship team, which will likely include the surgeon, dermatologist, and potentially the medical oncologist, should consider both recurrence of the primary melanoma and development of a second primary melanoma. Survivors of melanoma continue to exhibit high-risk UV exposure and suboptimal risk reduction behavior.[26] Melanoma survivors have a ten fold increased risk of a subsequent melanoma compared to the general population and a cumulative risk of the development of a second primary melanoma of approximately 5%.[27] Melanoma survivors should have regular skin exams for the rest of their lives.

Treatment of Locoregional Recurrent Disease

Local recurrence. Recurrences within 5 cm of the WLE scar or skin graft are considered local recurrences and represent aggressive tumor biology associated with a poor overall survival (Fig. 31.19). Recurrence risk increases with tumor thickness and has been estimated as 0.2%, 2%, 6%, and 13% for melanomas less than 0.75 mm, 0.75 to 1.5 mm, 1.5 to 4 mm, and larger than 4 mm, respectively. Treatment for local recurrence is operative resection to histologically negative margins. Although WLE guidelines for primary tumors do not apply, at least a 1-cm margin should be attempted with complete resection of the prior WLE scar. SLN biopsy of local recurrences is technically feasible, and the results may have some prognostic value. The rate of a positive SLN biopsy when performed for recurrence may be as high as 40%, and this may offer valuable risk stratification to select patients for additional surgery or adjuvant therapy.[28]

In-transit disease. In-transit tumors, either at presentation or as a recurrence after initial local therapy, are subcutaneous or cutaneous tumor nodules between the primary tumor site and draining nodal basin formed by tumor deposits within the lymphatic channels (Fig. 31.20). They are often subtle in appearance, lack pigmentation, and may only be appreciated as a palpable

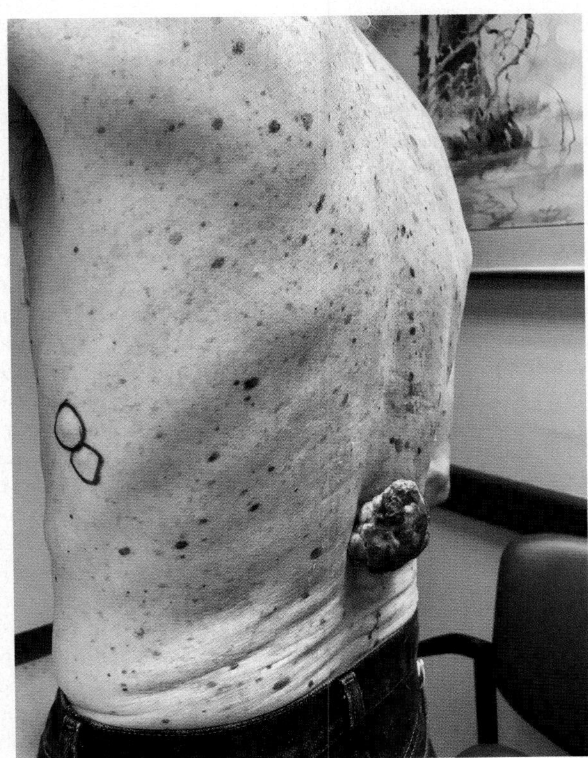

FIG. 31.20 In-transit metastases *(circled on left flank)* between the large primary tumor of the mid lower back and the draining nodal basin.

nodule. Fine needle aspiration or core biopsy can confirm the diagnosis. Once diagnosed, whole body imaging should be performed, as there is a high risk of distant metastatic disease. Limited in-transit disease may be adequately treated with simple excision to negative margins, but a high suspicion for a more aggressive disease biology that will require additional treatment must be in the mind of the surgeon. In approximately 20% of patients, local excision alone may be sufficient treatment, but they may require repeat excision in the future. SLN biopsy in the setting of in-transit disease should be considered, as the results carry prognostic significance.[28]

Historically, extensive or recurrent in-transit disease confined to the extremity was treated with regional chemotherapy. Methods of delivering high-dose chemotherapy into the limb that was otherwise isolated from the rest of the body included hyperthermic isolated limb perfusion or isolated limb infusion. Melphalan was the most common chemotherapy agent delivered into the circuit. Isolated limb infusion was developed as a less invasive, less resource-intensive technique with comparable oncologic outcomes and less limb toxicity. These treatments are used less often now, as intralesional and systemic immunotherapies are now preferred as an effective way to achieve locoregional disease control of in-transit disease with less morbidity for patients.

Unresectable stage III disease, including in-transit disease, was included in many of the early immunotherapy trials that evaluated CTLA-4 or PD-1 inhibition. Both agents showed good response rates and improved progression-free survival, used alone or in combination. Talimogene laherparepvec (T-VEC) is a herpes simplex virus type 1–derived oncolytic immunotherapy that is serially injected into palpable target lesions to induce both a direct local effect and potentially a systemic response. In the OPTiM trial, 436 patients with unresected stage IIIB to IV melanoma by the seventh edition AJCC staging were randomized to either serial intralesional T-VEC injection or granulocyte macrophage colony-stimulating factor as a control.[29] A durable response rate of 16% was seen in the T-VEC group compared to 2% in the control group (odds ratio, 8.9). The overall response rate was also greater in the T-VEC group (26% vs. 6%) and median overall survival was marginally improved (23 months vs. 19 months). The best responses were seen in IIIB, IIIC, and M1a disease. There were systemic, off-target responses as well. Investigators observed a 34% response rate in uninjected nonvisceral lesions and 15% response rate in uninjected visceral lesions, defined by a size reduction of at least 50%. Based on this trial, T-VEC received FDA approval for intralesional therapy of stage III or IV cutaneous melanoma. The addition of T-VEC to systemic immunotherapy appears to improve the response rate to immunotherapy in unresectable stage III/IV disease; this combination strategy will continue to be investigated.[30–32]

Given the successes seen with intralesional and systemic immunotherapies, these have become the first-line treatment for patients with extensive in-transit disease that is not amenable to simple resection. Regional infusion of chemotherapy continues to have a role, mostly in salvage situations in which immunotherapy has been ineffective and the disease remains isolated to an extremity. These situations are increasingly uncommon, as our experience with intralesional and systemic immunotherapy continues to grow.

Regional nodal recurrence. Therapeutic lymph node dissection for isolated regional nodal recurrences was historically the preferred treatment in patients who had not previously had a lymph node dissection. Strictly following the protocols used in the adjuvant immunotherapy trials discussed above, this strategy is still acceptable. After confirming the absence of metastatic disease, a therapeutic lymph node dissection of the involved nodal basin can be performed to achieve reasonable disease control, followed by adjuvant immunotherapy. If nodal recurrence occurs after adjuvant immunotherapy, an alternative adjuvant therapy strategy can be considered after regional lymphadenectomy.

An alternative strategy can be considered, which takes lessons from the treatment of other solid organ malignancies in which a neoadjuvant treatment strategy is used. The approach recognizes that patients with regional nodal recurrences in fact have a form of systemic metastatic disease. Most of these patients will eventually develop systemic recurrences. Recognizing that the concern in these patients should be first and foremost systemic disease control, a neoadjuvant treatment strategy can be used in which disease biology and treatment response can be assessed prior to surgery. The first group to show the potential effectiveness of this strategy is the group from the MD Anderson Cancer Center, using targeted BRAF-MEK inhibition in high-risk, resectable stage III and oligometastatic stage IV melanoma. In this study, 21 patients with BRAF-mutant melanoma with resectable stage III or oligometastatic stage IV melanoma were randomized to upfront surgical resection and adjuvant dabrafenib/trametinib or neoadjuvant dabrafenib/trametinib, followed by surgical resection and adjuvant BRAF-MEK inhibition.[33] The trial was stopped early because of the remarkable benefit seen in the neoadjuvant group, who enjoyed a median event-free survival of 19.7 months versus 2.9 months in the surgery first group (HR, 0.016). With a median follow-up of 18 months, 71% of the neoadjuvant treatment group were alive without disease progression compared to none in the upfront resection group.

The next logical extension of this experience is to apply a neoadjuvant immunotherapy treatment strategy that can be used regardless of BRAF mutation status in patients with regional nodal recurrences. Several clinical trials are underway, evaluating the safety and efficacy of neoadjuvant immunotherapy in patients with stage III or oligometastatic stage IV melanoma followed by resection. These studies will give us some insight into the pathologic response rate that can be expected with this approach and the potential markers that can be identified to predict a favorable response with this treatment strategy. Operative resection of these patients for persistent or recurrent regional lymph node recurrence still plays a role; however, we predict that these operations will become less common in the future as our immunotherapy treatments improve. However, the surgeon must still be able to offer a safe, effective operation that often will improve a patient's quality of life with bulky nodal disease. This may often be in a palliative situation in which short-term relief from pain may be enjoyed by the patient, even though recurrence is almost certain.

Treatment of Metastatic Disease

Treatment options for metastatic melanoma have expanded greatly in the last decade (Table 31.4). Metastatic melanoma, which once carried a dismal prognosis measured in months, can now be treated effectively with multiple agents that prolong survival and improve quality of life. It is indeed an exciting time to be treating melanoma as our therapies expand and our ability to treat patients with metastatic disease continues to improve.

Historical. Historically, the only two agents approved for metastatic melanoma were dacarbazine and high-dose interleukin-2. These agents were found to induce moderate response rates without any benefit in overall survival. Biochemotherapy, which was a highly toxic combination of cytotoxic chemotherapy with interleukin-2 and interferon, would sometimes result in limited successes. This approach was never able to demonstrate a consistent improvement in overall survival. Some individuals would respond well and achieve a durable response; however, these events were too infrequent to demonstrate a benefit to a large population of patients. These therapies were associated with significant toxicity and potential fatal complications. Better therapies for metastatic melanoma were desperately needed.

Immunotherapy. Melanoma was always considered a cancer that was susceptible to immunotherapy treatment strategies. Prior to the development of immune checkpoint blockade, interleukin-2, interferon, granulocyte-macrophage colony-stimulating factor, and multiple vaccines were tried in an attempt to boost the inherent immune response to melanoma. Through a better understanding of the regulation of the immune response, newer strategies focusing on blocking the negative feedback systems that suppress T-cell activity were developed, specifically the CTLA-4 and PD-1 pathways (Fig. 31.21).

Ipilimumab is a monoclonal anti–CTLA-4 antibody that was the first systemic agent to demonstrate improved overall survival in patients with metastatic melanoma. In activated T cells, the CTLA-4 receptor traffics to the extracellular membrane, where it inhibits costimulatory ligands on antigen-presenting cells and thereby prevents continued antigen-presenting cell stimulation of the T cell. By blocking CTLA-4, ipilimumab effectively prolongs the T-cell response. In one of the early-randomized trials to show that ipilimumab could improve survival, 502 patients with metastatic melanoma were randomized to standard of care dacarbazine or dacarbazine plus ipilimumab.[34] The group treated with ipilimumab had improved overall survival at 1 and 3 years (HR, 0.72). Based on this study and other subsequent studies, ipilimumab was approved by the FDA for metastatic melanoma. Significant autoimmune toxicities, including potentially fatal bowel perforations, prompted additional studies to find less toxic but equally effective immunotherapy options.

The PD-1 inhibitors represent a newer family of immune checkpoint regulators that work to suppress the natural inhibitory system of the T-cell immune response. The interaction of PD-1 receptor with its ligands PD-L1 and PD-L2 promote T-cell anergy and apoptosis. Some tumors express PD-L1 as a mechanism to promote T-cell tolerance and evade the immune system. Multiple randomized clinical trials have demonstrated that PD-1 inhibitors can improve survival in patients with metastatic melanoma. Patients treated with pembrolizumab alone or nivolumab alone have improved overall survival compared to those treated with ipilimumab alone.[35,36] The PD-1 inhibitors have an improved safety profile compared to ipilimumab and are more effective; thus, they have become the preferred first line agents for metastatic melanoma. Combining PD-1 inhibitors (nivolumab) with CTLA-4 inhibition has been attempted to improve response rates. There does appear to be marginally improved response rates and survival when nivolumab is combined with ipilimumab, but at the cost of increased risk of serious adverse events. When nivolumab or ipilimumab alone is used, the rates of serious adverse treatment-related events were 21% and 28%, while when used in combination, the rates of serious adverse treatment-related events doubled to 59%.[36]

The next generation of immunotherapy for melanoma will likely include the use of TIL or chimeric antigen receptor T-cell therapy. The TIL technique involves the isolation and expansion of tumor-specific T cells collected from the peritumor stroma. With this technique, these melanoma-specific TIL cells are clonally expanded, then reinfused into the patient after lymphodepletion. The TIL cells then enhance the patient's own adoptive immunity in order to evoke a heightened immune response to the tumors. Current studies are underway evaluating the safety and efficacy of this technique. Chimeric antigen receptor T-cell therapy involves genetically engineering an extracellular antigen-binding domain that targets melanoma or other target malignant cells with the intracellular signaling portion of the T cell receptor. Initial experience with chimeric antigen receptor T-cell therapy in hematologic malignancies is promising, but more work needs to be done to understand its potential role for treating metastatic melanoma.

Targeted therapy. The first agent used to target metastatic melanoma with the *BRAF* V600E mutation was vemurafenib. For BRAF-mutant patients, vemurafenib demonstrated significant improvement in overall and progression-free survival and was approved by the FDA for treatment of BRAF-mutant metastatic melanoma. The major issue with single-agent BRAF inhibition, including vemurafenib and dabrafenib, is the development of treatment resistance. This is not the result of a change in the target *BRAF* gene, rather it is felt to be the result of upregulation of alternative signaling pathways, including the MAPK pathway. Dual BRAF-MEK inhibition with trametinib and dabrafenib has been shown to improve overall response rates and survival compared to single agent trametinib or dabrafenib in BRAF-mutant metastatic melanoma.[37,38] Long-term follow-up for these studies is ongoing, as there remain concerns regarding the durability of the response to targeted therapy inhibition.

Dual BRAF-MEK inhibition is a good treatment option for patients with BRAF-mutant metastatic melanoma who cannot

TABLE 31.4 Summary of important targeted therapy and immunotherapy trials for metastatic melanoma.

TRIAL NAME	STUDY POPULATION	INTERVENTION TREATMENT	CONTROL TREATMENT	PRIMARY OUTCOME	NOTES
Hodi et al[51]	Unresectable stage III or IV	Ipilimumab 3 mg/kg with or without gp100	gp100	Improved overall survival with ipilimumab plus gp100 vs. gp100 alone (median OS, 10 vs. 6.4 months; HR, 0.68)	Ipilimumab alone as effective as ipilimumab + gp100
Robert et al[34]	Previously untreated, unresectable IIIB or IV	Ipilimumab 10 mg/kg + dacarbazine	Dacarbazine	Improved overall survival with ipilimumab + dacarbazine (median OS, 11.2 vs. 9.1 months; HR, 0.72)	
COMBI-d (Long et al)[37]	Unresectable stage III or IV melanoma with *BRAF* V600E or V600K mutations	Dabrafenib + trametinib	Dabrafenib + placebo	Improved progression-free survival (HR, 0.75; 95% CI, 0.57–0.99)	Improved response rate (67% vs. 51%) and 6-month OS (93% vs. 85%; HR, 0.63)
COMBI-v (Robert et al)[38]	Unresectable stage III or IV melanoma with *BRAF* V600E or V600K mutations	Dabrafenib + trametinib	Vemurafenib	Improved overall survival at 12 months (72% vs. 65%; HR, 0.69; 95% CI, 0.53–0.89)	Stopped early for efficacy, improved objective response rate (64% vs. 51%)
CheckMate 066 (Robert et al)[52]	Previously untreated, unresectable stage III or IV melanoma without *BRAF* mutations	Nivolumab	Dacarbazine	Improved overall survival (HR, 0.42; 99.79% CI, 0.25–0.73)	Improved progression-free survival and improved objective response rate
CheckMate 069 (Postow et al)[53]	Previously untreated, unresectable stage III or IV melanoma	Nivolumab + ipilimumab	Ipilimumab	Improved objective response rate in *BRAF* wild type (61% vs. 11%, *P* <0.001)	Increased serious adverse events with nivolumab + ipilimumab (54% vs. 24%)
CheckMate 067 (Wolchok et al)[36]	Previously untreated, unresectable stage III or IV	Nivolumab + ipilimumab Nivolumab alone	Ipilimumab	Improved overall survival in nivolumab/ipilimumab (HR, 0.55) and nivolumab alone (HR, 0.65) vs. ipilimumab alone	Similar 3-year OS in nivolumab alone (52%) compared to nivolumab/ipilimumab (58%), both better than ipilimumab alone (34%)
KEYNOTE-006 (Schachter et al)[35]	Unresectable stage III or IV melanoma?	Pembrolizumab every 2 or 3 weeks	Ipilimumab	Overall survival better in both pembrolizumab groups compared to ipilimumab (HR, 0.68 compared to ipilimumab for both treatment regimens)	No differences in every 2 week or every 3 week pembrolizumab

CI, Confidence interval; *gp100*, glycoprotein 100; *HR*, hazard ratio; *OS*, overall survival.

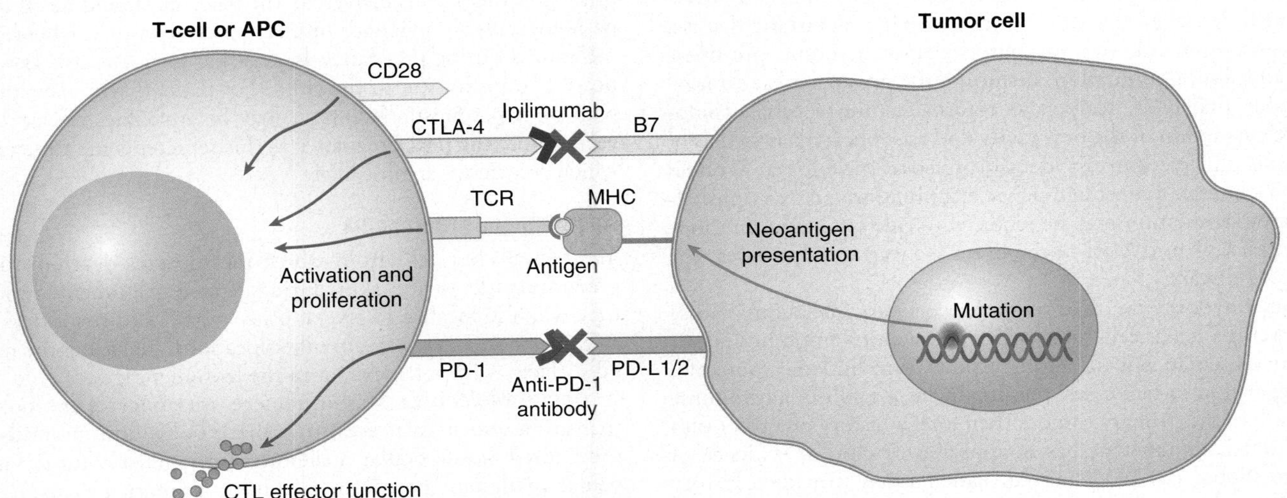

FIG. 31.21 The CTLA-4 and PD-1 pathways that are integral to immunotherapy for melanoma. *APC*, Antigen-presenting cell; *CTL*, cytologic T lymphocyte; *CTLA*, cytotoxic T lymphocyte antigen; *MHC*, major histocompatibility complex; *PD-1*, programmed death 1; *TCR*, T cell receptor. (From Herzberg B, Fisher DE. Metastatic melanoma and immunotherapy. *Clin Immunol.* 2016;172:105–110.)

tolerate immunotherapy, usually because of existing autoimmune comorbidities. Immunotherapy is probably the preferred treatment strategy for those patients who are BRAF-mutant but also eligible for immunotherapy in most centers. Patients not eligible for immunotherapy with BRAF-wild type melanoma continue to have limited effective treatment options.

Metastasectomy. Although most patients with stage IV melanoma will present with disseminated lesions that are not amenable to resection, patients with limited metastatic disease should be considered for resection if the disease is stable or responds to systemic therapy. Operative resection may not only offer symptom palliation, but also in some highly selected patients, it may provide a survival advantage similar to that seen after lymphadenectomy for advanced stage III patients. Resection of oligometastatic disease in well-selected patients can lead to 5-year survival rates ranging from 15% to 40%. Even patients with brain metastases may benefit from complete resection, further emphasizing that complete extirpation of all disease may be the best treatment, even for advanced disease. Careful selection of patients is paramount. Important things to consider in evaluating a patient for resection of metastatic disease include the patient's underlying functional status and comorbidities, the location and number of metastatic lesions, and the features reflective of the underlying tumor behavior, such as the disease-free interval from the time of primary resection. Failure to respond to systemic immunotherapy is usually a poor prognostic sign that signifies aggressive disease biology. However, medical and surgical oncologists are more often encountering the phenomenon of mixed response to immunotherapy. Oftentimes, in patients with multiple sites of metastatic disease, there will be a good radiologic response to immunotherapy in most, but not all, of the distant metastases. In these situations, if these nonresponding sites are amenable to resection, it makes sense to perform metastasectomy to remove the nonresponding lesions.

Special Situations and Noncutaneous Melanoma

Unknown Primary Melanoma

In rare cases, patients will present with stage III or stage IV melanoma and no preceding diagnosis of a primary cutaneous melanoma. This occurs in less than 2% of melanoma cases overall and in less than 5% of all cases involving metastatic disease. A diagnosis of unknown primary melanoma should prompt a thorough skin examination, including the perianal area, external genitalia, nail beds, scalp, and external auditory canal. Endoscopic evaluation of the oral cavity and nasopharynx as well as of the anus and rectum can identify mucosal melanoma. Women should undergo a thorough pelvic examination, and an ophthalmology examination may be required to rule out ocular melanomas. PET/CT and MRI of the brain are warranted to assess the extent of disease.

Some hypothesize that unknown primary melanomas arise from benign nevus cells already trapped within lymph nodes. Alternatively, cutaneous melanoma is known to undergo spontaneous regression in rare cases, presumably as a result of an immune response to the primary tumor. Therefore, a history of a prior pigmented skin lesion that has disappeared or clinical evidence of vitiligo should not be dismissed. Patients may provide a history of pigmented skin lesions that have been excised, cauterized, or treated with lasers. Pathology review of any previously excised skin lesions should be performed.

In the setting of lymph node metastasis without a primary lesion, the patient should be treated as a patient with stage III melanoma, as discussed above. Interestingly, patients with unknown primary melanomas who present with lymph node involvement have equivalent or possibly better overall survival compared with patients with a known primary lesion. This may suggest a stronger immune response in these patients that resulted in regression of the primary melanoma.

Melanoma and Pregnancy

As many as one third of women diagnosed with melanoma are of childbearing age; treatment of melanoma in pregnant women involves some difficult decision-making. Whether there is a link between pregnancy and the overall risk for development of melanoma is not well understood. Early studies suggested that hormonal changes during pregnancy led to increasing pigmentation and an environment conducive to melanoma development; however, current evidence does not support this theory. Any nevus or pigmented lesion with suspicious changes during pregnancy should not be attributed to hormones or the expected physiology of pregnancy; appropriate workup is required. Some evidence has suggested worse outcomes for melanoma in pregnancy; however, after controlling for other relevant risk factors, it appears that the prognosis of patients with melanoma treated during pregnancy is no different from that of nonpregnant patients.[39]

The evaluation and treatment of a pregnant patient with melanoma should follow guidelines similar to those for the nonpregnant patient. There is no therapeutic benefit to early termination of the pregnancy. WLE can be safely performed under local anesthesia. Based on experience with pregnant patients with breast cancer, SLN biopsy may be performed if indicated by the pathologic factors of the primary tumor, although vital blue dye should not be used. Not only is there an unknown risk to the fetus, but also there is an estimated 1 in 10,000 risk of an anaphylactic reaction if isosulfan blue dye is used. Lymphoscintigraphy is considered safe since the dose used is well below the teratogenic threshold. Nevertheless, some physicians and patients are uncomfortable with the use of radioactive materials during pregnancy. In such situations, WLE under local anesthesia with a 1-cm margin can be performed, with wider margin excision and SLN biopsy reserved until after the baby is delivered. The placenta should be examined pathologically for evidence of melanoma in women who develop melanoma during pregnancy as a marker for metastasis as well as possible transmission to the child. For patients who have tumors with poor prognostic factors, it may be advisable to wait 2 to 3 years before the next pregnancy as this represents the time during which recurrence is most likely.

Noncutaneous Melanoma

The neural crest cells from which melanocytes develop migrate predominantly to the skin during fetal development; however, they will also localize to several other organs and tissues. As a result, melanoma may arise in other locations, including the mucosal surfaces, within the eye, or in the leptomeninges.

Ocular Melanoma. Within the eye, melanocytes are found in the retina and uveal tract (iris, ciliary body, and choroids). In the United States, ocular melanoma is the most common intraocular malignant neoplasm in adults. Primary treatment consists of enucleation or iodine-125 brachytherapy, although other options include photocoagulation and partial resection. Unlike cutaneous melanoma, given the lack of lymphatic vessels in the uveal tract, metastatic spread of ocular melanoma occurs hematogenously. Metastases develop almost exclusively in the liver. Resection is rarely possible because the pattern of metastases is often a diffuse, miliary one. Dedicated liver imaging is needed to detect these lesions. Ocular melanoma is less responsive to immunotherapy compared to cutaneous melanoma. One hypothesis is that ocular melanoma carries less of a mutational burden compared to cutaneous melanoma, thus rendering immunotherapy less effective.

Mucosal Melanoma. The most common sites for mucosal melanoma are the head and neck (oral cavity, oropharynx, nasopharynx, and paranasal sinuses), anal canal, rectum, and female genitalia. Because of the occult location of many of these lesions, patients tend to present with more advanced disease and have a poor prognosis. These tumors should be excised to negative margins when possible. Given the high risk of metastatic disease, extensive local resections, such as abdominoperineal resection or pelvic exenteration, do not improve overall survival. These procedures may still be necessary for local disease control. Radiation therapy may be used to improve locoregional disease control. In general, the role for SLN biopsy has not been well established. We perform SLN biopsy routinely for anal and other mucosal melanomas when feasible. For anal melanoma, a negative SLN biopsy in the superficial inguinal region would omit that region from the radiation fields. Unlike ocular melanoma, it appears that the response rate to immunotherapy for mucosal melanoma is similar to that of cutaneous melanoma, thus some have recommended that these agents be considered for use in the adjuvant setting or for treatment of metastatic disease.

NONMELANOMA SKIN CANCERS

NMSC represents the most common type of malignant neoplasm in the world. In the United States, it is estimated that almost one in five Americans will develop NMSC during their lifetime. Approximately 80% are BCCs, with SCC representing nearly 20%. Much rarer types of NMSC make up the remainder of cases. Sun exposure is the predominant risk factor. Similar to cutaneous melanoma, the overall incidence of NMSC is increasing. Accurate estimates of NMSC incidence are difficult to ascertain as many are treated without obtaining a histologic diagnosis, and most cases are not reported in cancer registries. The American Cancer Society estimated that there are more than 5 million cases of BCC and SCC diagnosed in over 3 million people per year in the United States. Patients diagnosed with a BCC or SCC have an increased risk of additional cancers, including a second NMSC, melanoma, and nonskin cancers. For this reason, patients with a prior diagnosis of skin cancer require long-term surveillance.

Squamous Cell Carcinoma

Presentation and Risk Factors

Risk factors for the development of SCC include exposure to sunlight, susceptible skin types, compromised immunity, environmental exposures, and underlying genetic disorders. Most SCCs occur on sun-exposed surfaces, particularly the head and neck. In susceptible individuals (those with fair skin, blond hair, and blue eyes), prolonged sun exposure correlates directly to an increased risk for SCC. In contrast to melanoma or BCC, the cumulative effect of chronic UV radiation likely plays a larger role in SCC than intermittent, intense exposures. As with melanoma, individuals with dark complexions have a lower risk of SCC, even with prolonged sun exposure. The risk for SCC increases with occupational or recreational sun exposure, advancing age, and proximity to the equator. The amount of sun exposure is also proportional to the incidence of known precursor lesions for SCC, including actinic keratosis.

UV radiation, and UVB in particular, increases the risk of SCC through several mechanisms. There is the direct carcinogenic effect of UV light on the frequently dividing keratinocytes within the basal layer of the epidermis. Unrepaired mutations from UV light damage can drive tumor proliferation and growth. UVB-induced silencing of the *p53* tumor suppressor gene occurs in more than 90% of SCCs. With loss of p53, keratinocytes are unable to arrest the cell cycle or to initiate apoptosis in the face of cellular damage from UV radiation. With subsequent mutations, cells can then progress from dysplasia to in situ or invasive disease.

Occupational and environmental carcinogens, including arsenic, organic hydrocarbons, ionizing radiation, and cigarette smoke are associated with an increased risk for SCC. Genetic disorders, including xeroderma pigmentosum and albinism, are associated with increased risk for many types of skin cancer, including SCC. A history of chronic inflammation from burn scars (Marjolin ulcer), draining sinuses, infections (including osteomyelitis), and nonhealing ulcers can precede the development of SCCs. In the setting of chronic nonhealing wounds, or even with previously healed wounds that subsequently break down, biopsy may be prudent to rule out SCC.

Immunosuppression is a well-established risk factor for SCCs of the skin, particularly with the suppression of cell-mediated immunity after solid organ transplantation. Skin cancer is the most frequent malignant neoplasm in organ transplant recipients, with SCC and BCC representing 95% of these cancers. Whereas the risk of BCC increases ten fold after transplantation, the incidence of SCC in posttransplant patients is 65 times that of the normal population (Fig. 31.22). SCC that develops in immunosuppressed patients are more aggressive and have an increased risk of systemic metastases. The intensity of immunosuppression and the duration of therapy both correlate with the risk of malignancy. Whereas malignant neoplasms develop in 10% to 27% of patients after 10 years of immunosuppression, this number increases to 40% to 60% after 20 years. Other conditions associated with impairments of cell-mediated immunity (lymphoma, leukemia, autoimmune disease, etc.) are associated with an increased risk of SCC. Human papillomavirus, an infection associated with immunosuppression, is a proposed risk factor for the development of SCCs. BRAF inhibition used to treat melanoma is also associated with the development of SCC.

Most SCCs begin with a proliferation of keratin cells in the basal layer of the epidermis that appear as red or pink areas, clinically termed actinic keratoses (solar keratoses). Local symptoms may wax and wane for a period of many months. Lesions are scaling, with an uneven surface and an erythematous base (Fig. 31.23). Individual lesions are usually smaller than 1 cm in diameter and appear in chronically sun-damaged skin. The diagnosis is both clinical and histologic as actinic keratoses share many microscopic features with SCC in situ. The risk of malignant transformation of actinic keratosis to SCC is approximately 0.01%–0.6% over 1 year and up to 2.5% over 4 years. Bowen disease, which appears histologically as SCC in situ, initially manifests as a reddened area that progresses to thickened plaques of variable size. When it is confined to the glans penis or vulva, Bowen disease is sometimes referred to as erythroplasia of Queyrat.

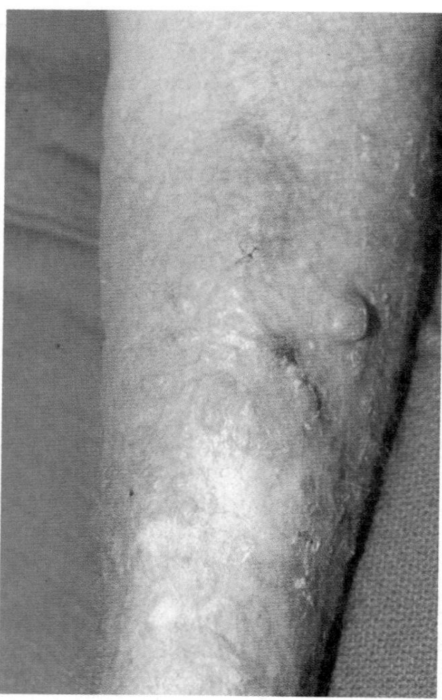

FIG. 31.22 Multiple squamous cell carcinomas on the forearm of a patient on immunosuppression after kidney transplant.

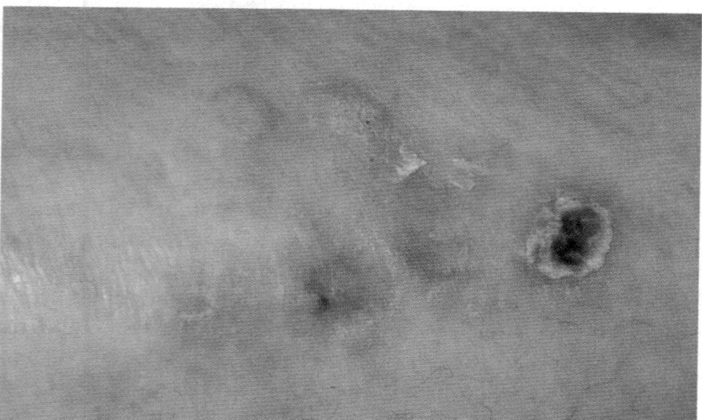

FIG. 31.23 Squamous cell carcinoma with red, scaling skin.

Invasive SCCs are palpable scaling lesions that become ulcerated centrally and have elevated, firm edges. In addition to spreading horizontally, these lesions may grow vertically and become fixed to underlying tissue. They may be confused with keratoacanthoma, a benign lesion that can also thicken and ulcerate. Biopsy may be required to differentiate between these two conditions.

Treatment

Unlike melanoma, SCC T category is based on the diameter of the lesion. Other high-risk features for SCC of the skin have been defined by the NCCN (Table 31.5). These high-risk features include assessment of size, location, histology, and individual patient factors. Most SCCs can be treated with local excision with excellent results. The typical margin of excision is a gross 5-mm resection, although MMS can be used when a cosmetically sensitive area demands skin conservation. MMS may also be preferred for recurrent or high-risk tumors. For higher-risk lesions, 10 mm margins are recommended.

Field therapies, which treat a generalized area but do not define the status of the margin, can also be used. Examples of field therapies include radiation therapy, cryosurgery, photodynamic therapy, electrodessication and curettage, and topical agents like imiquimod. Cryotherapy is best suited for small superficial lesions and can be expected to achieve local control rates greater than 90%. Treated areas are allowed to heal slowly by secondary intention, often resulting in pale scars. Curettage may be used for patients with superficial lesions less than 2 cm. In precursor lesions of SCC, such as actinic keratosis, cryotherapy is a commonly performed therapy. Alternative treatments include topical 5-fluorouracil, electrodessication and curettage, carbon dioxide laser, dermabrasion, and chemical peel. Tissue biopsy is indicated when the actinic keratosis is raised or recurrent after topical therapy.

SLN biopsy may have a role in high-risk lesions, as clinically occult lymph node metastases may be identified in 7% to 20% of patients. The indications for SLN biopsy and subsequent nodal management strategy (completion lymphadenectomy with or without radiation therapy) are not as well defined as they are for cutaneous melanoma. Adjuvant radiation to the primary tumor is recommended by the NCCN for any SCC with extensive perineural or large nerve involvement.[40]

Locally advanced or metastatic SCC of the skin is fortunately rare; advanced disease is difficult to treat. Systemic cytotoxic chemotherapies are usually platinum based with variable response rates. Targeted epidermal growth factor receptor agents have been used with moderate success as primary and salvage systemic therapy for metastatic SCC.[41–43] A new PD-1 inhibitor, cemiplimab, was recently approved by the FDA based on a phase 1 study using PD-1 inhibition in refractory advanced cutaneous SCC in which a response rate of 50% was observed, with the duration of response exceeding 6 months in over half of the responders.[44]

Basal Cell Carcinoma

Presentation and Risk Factors

BCC is the most common NMSC, and lesions are most commonly found on the sun-exposed areas of the head and neck. Risk factors for the development of BCC are similar to those for SCC, although basal cell lesions are more often associated with intense, intermittent exposure to UV radiation. The hedgehog-signaling pathway is a key signaling pathway in embryonic development but is largely inactive in mature adult tissue. The pathway is mutated in up to 90% of BCCs. In the presence of hedgehog signaling peptides, the Patched receptor releases the transmembrane Smoothened (SMO) protein, allowing SMO to initiate a signaling cascade that activates the expression of several target genes. Normally, Patched will inhibit SMO in the absence of hedgehog signals. Both activating mutations in SMO and inactivating mutations in Patched have been linked to BCC, ultimately leading to unrestricted growth signaling.

In contrast to SCCs and actinic keratoses, there is no precursor skin lesion for BCCs. These lesions may have an appearance that varies from nodules in the skin to a large nonhealing sore with drainage and crusting. In comparison to SCCs, they have a slow growth rate, often leading to a delay in diagnosis. BCCs commonly infiltrate locally but rarely metastasize. Metastases are associated with advanced age and large, neglected lesions. The primary site will often undergo resection multiple times before metastases appear. Once metastatic disease develops, the median survival decreases to less than 1 year.

BCCs grow in multiple distinctive patterns, and although there is not a universally accepted classification system, there are several common subtypes. The nodular growth pattern is characterized

TABLE 31.5 Risk factors for local recurrence or metastases in squamous cell carcinoma of the skin.

	LOW RISK	HIGH RISK
Location/size	Area L <20 mm Area M <10 mm	Area L ≥20 mm Area M ≥10 mm Area H
Borders	Well defined	Poorly defined
Primary vs. recurrent	Primary	Recurrent
Immunosuppression	No	Yes
Site of prior radiation therapy or chronic inflammatory process	No	Yes
Rapidly growing tumor	No	Yes
Neurologic symptoms	No	Yes
Degree of differentiation	Well or moderately differentiated	Poorly differentiated
Acantholytic (adenoid), adenosquamous (showing mucin production), desmoplastic, or metaplastic (carcinosarcomatous) subtypes	No	Yes
Depth, thickness, or Clark level	<2 mm, or I, II, III	≥2 mm, or IV, V
Perineural, lymphatic, or vascular involvement	No	Yes

Area H: "mask areas" of face (central face, eyelids, eyebrows, periorbital nose, lips [cutaneous and vermillion], chin, mandible, preauricular and postauricular skin/sulci, temple, ear), genitalia, hands, and feet. Area M: cheeks, forehead, scalp, neck, and pretibial. Area L: trunk and extremities (excluding pretibial, hands, feet, nail units, and ankles).

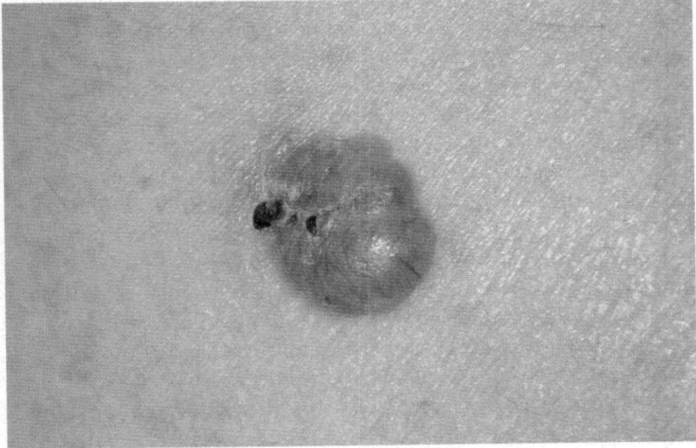

FIG. 31.24 Nodular basal cell carcinoma.

by a well-defined, elevated lesion with a waxy appearance (Fig. 31.24). As the lesion grows, pearly opalescent nodules develop along the margins. A central depression with umbilication or ulceration and rolled edges is a classic sign. Distinct blood vessels (telangiectasia) may be seen across the surface or along the edges of the lesion. Although most BCCs are pink or skin-colored, they may also have shades of brown or black pigmentation, thereby mimicking a benign mole or melanoma. Cystic BCCs are less common but have a distinctive translucent appearance. Their blue or gray appearance may lead to misdiagnosis as a blue nevus. Superficial BCCs have a more macular growth patterns and may extend over the surface of the skin in a multicentric pattern. The center can ulcerate, and the margins are often irregular and ill-defined. These lesions may appear similar to those of psoriasis, tinea, or eczema. In micronodular lesions, there may be several mildly elevated pink or red lesions that pepper the skin. Associated with a more aggressive growth pattern, these lesions often have extension well beyond visible changes in the skin surface. The white scarring varieties of this growth pattern are termed morpheaform BCC; these lesions are among the most locally invasive subtypes and can penetrate deep into the underlying subdermis (Fig. 31.25).

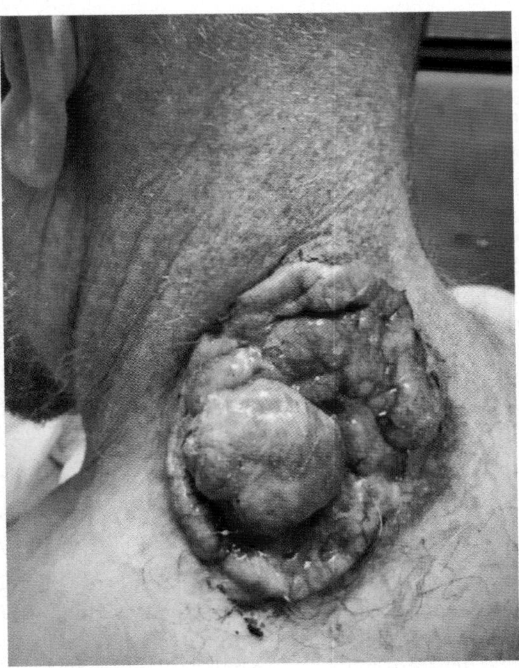

FIG. 31.25 Locally advanced basal cell carcinoma.

Treatment

Since the vast majority of BCCs are locally confined, treatment is directed at a margin negative resection. Similar to SCC, a gross 5-mm margin is usually adequate for local disease control. For higher-risk lesions, wider margins may help reduce local recurrence, but the exact width of the margins has not been defined. MMS can be used for the same indications as SCC. High-risk features of BCC have been defined by the NCCN (Table 31.6).

Similar to local SCCs, field therapies can be used for BCC, including radiation therapy, cryosurgery, photodynamic therapy, electrodessication and curettage, and topical agents like imiquimod. Adjuvant radiation therapy for high-risk lesions can reduce

TABLE 31.6 Risk factors for recurrence in basal cell carcinoma of the skin.

	LOW RISK	HIGH RISK
Location/size	Area L <20 mm Area M <10 mm	Area L ≥20 mm Area M ≥10 mm Area H
Borders	Well defined	Poorly defined
Primary vs. recurrent	Primary	Recurrent
Immunosuppression	No	Yes
Site of prior radiation therapy	No	Yes
Pathologic subtype	Nodular, superficial	Aggressive growth pattern
Perineural invasion	No	Yes

Area H: "mask areas" of face (central face, eyelids, eyebrows, periorbital nose, lips [cutaneous and vermillion], chin, mandible, preauricular and postauricular skin/sulci, temple, ear), genitalia, hands, and feet. Area M: cheeks, forehead, scalp, neck, and pretibial. Area L: trunk and extremities (excluding pretibial, hands, feet, nail units, and ankles). Aggressive growth pattern: having (mixed) infiltrative, micronodular, morpheaform, basosquamous, sclerosing, or carcinosarcomatous differentiation features in any portion of the tumor.

the risk of local recurrence. Evaluation of the lymph nodes by SLN biopsy is not necessary for BCC, as lymph node metastases are exceedingly rare.

In the very rare circumstances in which locally advanced or metastatic BCC develops and cannot be resected, there have been major advances in systemic therapy based on the hedgehog signaling pathway. The small molecule inhibitor of the hedgehog pathway vismodegib demonstrated a 30% response rate in locally advanced BCC and a 43% response rate in metastatic BCC; the complete response rate was 21%.[45] Long-term follow-up confirmed the durability of response in both the metastatic and locally advanced patients, with a median duration of response of nearly 15 months in the metastatic patients and 26 months in the locally advanced patients.[46] A second hedgehog pathway inhibitor, sonidegib, has shown similar efficacy, with objective response rates on the order of 30% to 40% in metastatic or locally advanced BCC.[47]

Merkel Cell Carcinoma

Merkel cell carcinoma (MCC) is a rare but aggressive malignant neoplasm of the skin. It is locally aggressive with high local recurrence rates and has the potential for regional and distant metastases. There is debate as to whether Merkel cells arise from epidermal or neural crest progenitors, but on histologic evaluation, MCC may be indistinguishable from small cell carcinoma and other small round blue cell tumors. There is emerging evidence to suggest that a novel virus, the Merkel cell polyomavirus, is associated with the development of MCC.[48] The incidence of MCC appears to be rising at a faster rate than cutaneous melanoma; the reasons for this are unclear.

MCC usually appears as a painless, raised nodule, often red or purplish, but it can be of the same color as the surrounding skin (Fig. 31.26). It is more commonly found in sun-exposed areas. Workup is similar to melanoma in that a tangential shave biopsy or punch biopsy makes the diagnosis. An experienced dermatopathologist may be needed to confirm the diagnosis. A careful clinical exam of the draining lymph node basis is required, as MCC will often present with clinically apparent lymph nodes. Clinically

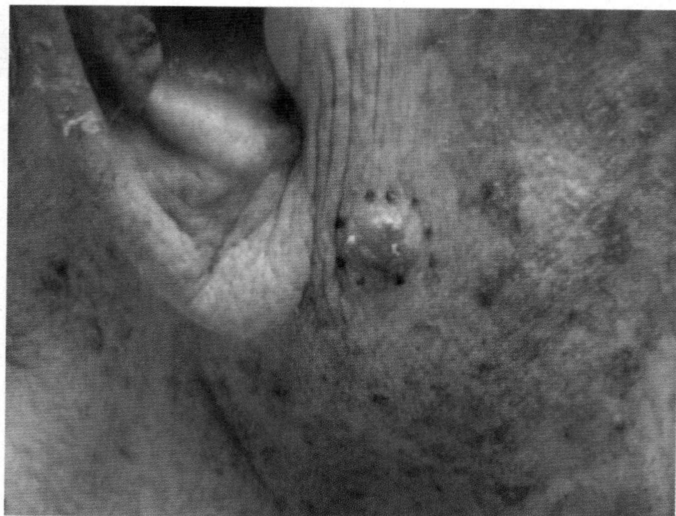

FIG. 31.26 Merkel cell carcinoma.

staging with radiographic imaging, such as cross-sectional CT scan, is reasonable.

The AJCC has a separate staging system for MCC, based on maximum tumor diameter, rather than depth of invasion. The primary treatment is WLE (1- to 2-cm margins), although MMS has been used for some lesions where tissue conservation is necessary. SLN biopsy is generally recommended for all T stages of MCC to identify patients with occult regional lymphatic metastases, which may occur in up to one third of cases. Nodal status affects prognosis, and patients with nodal disease have a significantly decreased overall survival. MCC is a relatively radiosensitive tumor, and adjuvant radiation has been shown to reduce the local recurrence rate at the primary tumor site. If the SLN is positive, adjuvant radiation to the nodal basin after CLND may decrease the rate of regional recurrence and improve overall survival. Although metastases may be responsive to chemotherapy, there is currently little evidence to support adjuvant systemic therapy. Chemotherapy is usually platinum-based, with or without etoposide. As with melanoma and most other solid organ malignancies, immunotherapy has been tried for advanced MCC. An approximately 50% response rate has been reported with the PD-1 inhibitor pembrolizumab; these responses, like those with melanoma, appear durable.[49] The PD-L1 inhibitor avelumab has also shown good responses in advanced MCC.[50] Based on these studies, both of these immunotherapy agents have been approved for use in MCC. Future systemic therapies for MCC will likely include immunotherapies in addition to traditional cytotoxic chemotherapies.

Other Cutaneous Malignancies

Cutaneous Angiosarcoma

Cutaneous angiosarcoma is a rare, aggressive, soft tissue sarcoma derived from blood or lymphatic vessel endothelium. Cutaneous angiosarcoma predominantly occurs in elderly whites and most commonly arises on the head and neck. In addition, angiosarcoma has been observed in the setting of chronic lymphedema after axillary dissection for breast cancer (Stewart-Treves syndrome) and may arise in irradiated tissues after prolonged intervals. The typical finding is a smooth, firm, or spongy subcutaneous growth that develops a violaceous erythema similar to a bruise (Fig. 31.27). Advanced tumors may grow in excess of 10 cm in size and become ulcerated. On histologic evaluation, angiosarcomas are high grade

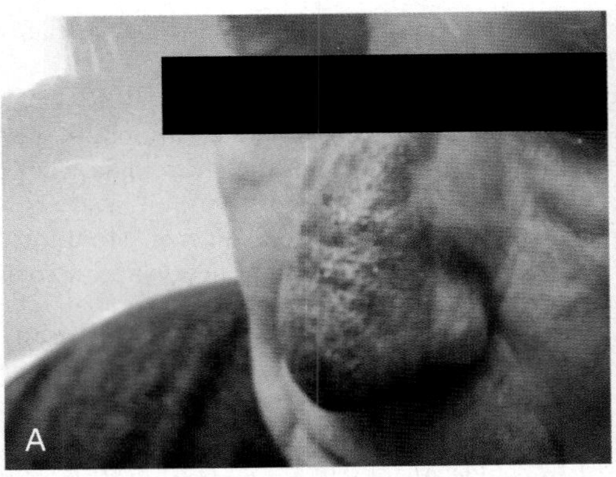

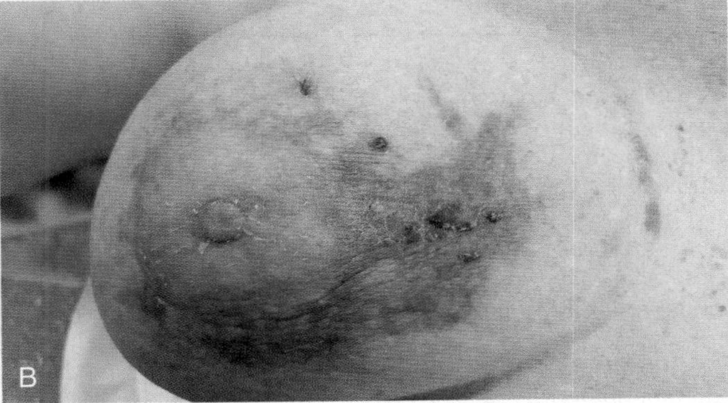

FIG. 31.27 Primary cutaneous angiosarcoma of the nose (A) and secondary cutaneous angioscarcoma of the breast in the setting of radiation therapy for breast cancer (B).

and often multifocal, with skip areas of normal-appearing skin. Abnormal, pleomorphic, malignant-appearing endothelial cells are pathognomonic. Like most sarcomas, the principal route of metastatic spread is hematogenous, although it falls into the small category of sarcomas that has an increased propensity for lymph node metastases. Treatment consists of complete resection with histologically negative margins and radiotherapy of the involved field. Like most sarcomas, a gross margin of approximately 2 cm is attempted at the time of operation to achieve the desired negative pathologic margin. SLN biopsy is not usually performed. Lymph node dissection is indicated for regional lymph node metastases in the absence of metastatic disease. There is no consensus about the role of adjuvant chemotherapy.

Dermatofibrosarcoma Protuberans

Dermatofibrosarcoma protuberans (DFSP) is a low-grade sarcoma arising from dermal fibroblasts. Lesions appear as smooth, flesh-colored nodules in or immediately beneath the skin and generally occur in relatively young patients between 20 and 50 years of age. Most appear on the trunk (50%), with the remainder on the proximal extremities (20%–35%) or in the head/neck region (10%–15%). DFSP grows slowly, so the lesions are usually not grossly very large at the time of diagnosis unless they have been neglected for a long period of time. Their external appearance belies their true character as tumor cells will frequently invade the underlying soft tissues and contribute to incomplete excision and local recurrence. A margin positive resection is an all too common occurrence when managing DFSP. Treatment consists of WLE with a gross 2- to 4-cm margin. Specimen orientation and pathologic analysis of margins are required. Because the margins are often microscopically positive and the wide margin of excision often requires flap reconstruction, a temporary wound coverage strategy, like with a negative pressure dressing, may be employed to confirm histologically negative margins prior to flap reconstruction. Another strategy is to "map out" the planned margin of excision with punch biopsies in the office to confirm that the planned excision will be adequate prior to surgery. Distant metastases are uncommon and are often preceded by multiple local recurrences. A variant of DFSP is associated with fibrosarcomatous change on pathologic examination; these lesions have a more aggressive character with a higher risk for distant metastases. Adjuvant radiation therapy may be considered for margin-positive resection or for recurrences. Imatinib has been used with reasonable results in patients with locally advanced or metastatic disease and sometimes as neoadjuvant therapy in an attempt to improve the odds of negative-margin resection for advanced tumors or in anatomically-constrained areas.

Kaposi Sarcoma

Kaposi sarcoma is a low-grade soft tissue, malignant neoplasm that arises from lymphatic vascular endothelial cells in the skin. The incidence of Kaposi sarcoma has been increasing over the last several decades because it is most often seen in patients with acquired immunodeficiency syndrome (AIDS) and other immunosuppressed states. Human herpesvirus 8 has been identified as the causative agent of Kaposi sarcoma in patients infected with human immunodeficiency virus. There is also a classic variant not associated with an immunosuppressed state seen on the lower extremities of older men of eastern European and Mediterranean descent. The clinical picture is variable; asymptomatic purple to brown bruises develop and progress to spots, plaques, or nodules on both lower extremities. In AIDS patients, the most effective treatment is aggressive antiretroviral therapy. Symptomatic skin lesions can be treated with radiation therapy, intralesional injection of chemotherapeutic agents, cryotherapy, or excision.

Extramammary Paget Disease

Extramammary Paget disease (EMPD) is a rare form of adenocarcinoma that arises from apocrine glands of the skin, most commonly in the perianal area, vulva, and scrotum. The clinical appearance is that of an erythematous plaque, but white or depigmented areas with crusts and scaling may also be present. The size is variable, from smaller than 1 cm to an entire area in the anogenital region. Because EMPD can have many clinical characteristics in common with eczema, bacterial and fungal infections, and nonspecific dermatitis, the diagnosis is often made by biopsy of lesions not responding to standard therapies. In most cases, EMPD is confined to the epidermis and is well controlled with excision. When invasion of the deeper structures occurs, the disease becomes increasingly difficult to control, and the mortality rate approaches 50%. Because EMPD is also associated with an increased risk for simultaneous internal malignant neoplasms in the genitourinary and gastrointestinal tracts, a complete workup includes a survey of these locations via endoscopy. Standard treatment is surgical resection extending to histologically negative margins, which may require a number of procedures to achieve because the histologic changes are best seen on permanent section. Patients require close clinical follow-up because local recurrences are common. Radiation therapy may reduce the incidence of local recurrence after excision.

SELECTED REFERENCES

Amaria RN, Prieto PA, Tetzlaff MT, et al. Neoadjuvant plus adjuvant dabrafenib and trametinib versus standard of care in patients with high-risk, surgically resectable melanoma: a single-centre, open-label, randomised, phase 2 trial. *Lancet Oncol.* 2018;19:181–193.

This randomized phase 2 study established the safety and efficacy of a neoadjuvant therapy approach to BRAF-mutant, resectable stage III melanoma. Expect more trials in the future to build off of this study design, in which on-treatment biopsies and pathologic response to therapy are endpoints to neoadjuvant immunotherapy studies.

Faries MB, Thompson JF, Cochran AJ, et al. Completion dissection or observation for sentinel-node metastasis in melanoma. *N Engl J Med.* 2017;376:2211–2222.

The published results of MSLT-II, which establishes level I evidence that a completion lymphadenectomy after a positive sentinel lymph node biopsy does not improve survival. This is a practice-changing study that has altered the way micrometastatic stage III melanoma is treated.

Genomic Classification of cutaneous melanoma. *Cell.* 2015;161:1681–1696.

An important publication from The Cancer Genome Atlas Network, which defines four genomic subtypes of cutaneous melanoma. Potential markers of responsiveness to immunotherapies are reported as well.

Long GV, Hauschild A, Santinami M, et al. Adjuvant dabrafenib plus trametinib in stage III BRAF-mutated melanoma. *N Engl J Med.* 2017;377:1813–1823.

This randomized trial demonstrated a survival benefit with adjuvant dual BRAF-MEK inhibition in resected stage III BRAF-mutant melanoma.

Weber J, Mandala M, Del Vecchio M, et al. Adjuvant nivolumab versus ipilimumab in resected stage III or IV melanoma. *N Engl J Med.* 2017;377:1824–1835.

A randomized, multicenter clinical trial that has established the efficacy of adjuvant nivolumab for resected stage III and IV melanoma.

REFERENCES

1. Number of new cases per 100,000 persons by race/ethnicity & sex: melanoma of the skin. *J Natl Cancer Inst.* 2016;108.
2. Vogel RI, Ahmed RL, Nelson HH, et al. Exposure to indoor tanning without burning and melanoma risk by sunburn history. *J Natl Cancer Inst.* 2014;106.
3. Hodis E, Watson IR, Kryukov GV, et al. A landscape of driver mutations in melanoma. *Cell.* 2012;150:251–263.
4. Genomic classification of cutaneous melanoma. *Cell.* 2015;161:1681–1696.
5. Kim CC, Berry EG, Marchetti MA, et al. Risk of subsequent cutaneous melanoma in moderately dysplastic nevi excisionally biopsied but with positive histologic margins. *JAMA Dermatol.* 2018;154:1401–1408.
6. Lawrence MS, Stojanov P, Polak P, et al. Mutational heterogeneity in cancer and the search for new cancer-associated genes. *Nature.* 2013;499:214–218.
7. Egger ME, Huber KM, Dunki-Jacobs EM, et al. Incidence of sentinel lymph node involvement in a modern, large series of desmoplastic melanoma. *J Am Coll Surg.* 2013;217:37–44; discussion 44–35.
8. Holtkamp LHJ, Read RL, Emmett L, et al. Futility of imaging to stage melanoma patients with a positive sentinel lymph node. *Melanoma Res.* 2017;27:457–462.
9. Thomas JM, Newton-Bishop J, A'Hern R, et al. Excision margins in high-risk malignant melanoma. *N Engl J Med.* 2004;350:757–766.
10. Gillgren P, Drzewiecki KT, Niin M, et al. 2-cm versus 4-cm surgical excision margins for primary cutaneous melanoma thicker than 2 mm: a randomised, multicentre trial. *Lancet.* 2011;378:1635–1642.
11. Gershenwald JE, Scolyer RA, Hess KR, et al. Melanoma staging: evidence-based changes in the American Joint Committee on Cancer eighth edition cancer staging manual. *CA Cancer J Clin.* 2017;67:472–492.
12. Sinnamon AJ, Neuwirth MG, Yalamanchi P, et al. Association between patient age and lymph node positivity in thin melanoma. *JAMA Dermatol.* 2017;153:866–873.
13. Egger ME, Stevenson M, Bhutiani N, et al. Should sentinel lymph node biopsy be performed for all T1b Melanomas in the new 8(th) edition American Joint Committee on Cancer Staging System? *J Am Coll Surg.* 2019;228:466–472.
14. Morton DL, Thompson JF, Cochran AJ, et al. Sentinel-node biopsy or nodal observation in melanoma. *N Engl J Med.* 2006;355:1307–1317.
15. Egger ME, Bower MR, Czyszczon IA, et al. Comparison of sentinel lymph node micrometastatic tumor burden measurements in melanoma. *J Am Coll Surg.* 2014;218:519–528.
16. van der Ploeg AP, van Akkooi AC, Haydu LE, et al. The prognostic significance of sentinel node tumour burden in melanoma patients: an international, multicenter study of 1539 sentinel node-positive melanoma patients. *Eur J Cancer.* 2014;50:111–120.
17. Leiter U, Stadler R, Mauch C, et al. Complete lymph node dissection versus no dissection in patients with sentinel lymph node biopsy positive melanoma (DeCOG-SLT): a multicentre, randomised, phase 3 trial. *Lancet Oncol.* 2016;17:757–767.
18. Faries MB, Thompson JF, Cochran AJ, et al. Completion dissection or observation for sentinel-node metastasis in melanoma. *N Engl J Med.* 2017;376:2211–2222.
19. Long GV, Hauschild A, Santinami M, et al. Adjuvant Dabrafenib plus trametinib in stage III BRAF-mutated melanoma. *N Engl J Med.* 2017;377:1813–1823.
20. Eggermont AM, Chiarion-Sileni V, Grob JJ, et al. Adjuvant ipilimumab versus placebo after complete resection of high-risk stage III melanoma (EORTC 18071): a randomised, double-blind, phase 3 trial. *Lancet Oncol.* 2015;16:522–530.
21. Eggermont AM, Chiarion-Sileni V, Grob JJ, et al. Prolonged survival in stage III melanoma with ipilimumab adjuvant therapy. *N Engl J Med.* 2016;375:1845–1855.

22. Weber J, Mandala M, Del Vecchio M, et al. Adjuvant nivolumab versus ipilimumab in resected stage III or IV melanoma. *N Engl J Med.* 2017;377:1824–1835.
23. Eggermont AMM, Blank CU, Mandala M, et al. Adjuvant pembrolizumab versus placebo in resected stage III melanoma. *N Engl J Med.* 2018;378:1789–1801.
24. Henderson MA, Burmeister BH, Ainslie J, et al. Adjuvant lymph-node field radiotherapy versus observation only in patients with melanoma at high risk of further lymph-node field relapse after lymphadenectomy (ANZMTG 01.02/TROG 02.01): 6-year follow-up of a phase 3, randomised controlled trial. *Lancet Oncol.* 2015;16:1049–1060.
25. Lee AY, Droppelmann N, Panageas KS, et al. Patterns and timing of initial relapse in pathologic stage II melanoma patients. *Ann Surg Oncol.* 2017;24:939–946.
26. Vogel RI, Strayer LG, Engelman L, et al. Sun exposure and protection behaviors among long-term melanoma survivors and population controls. *Cancer Epidemiol Biomarkers Prev.* 2017;26:607–613.
27. van der Leest RJ, Flohil SC, Arends LR, et al. Risk of subsequent cutaneous malignancy in patients with prior melanoma: a systematic review and meta-analysis. *J Eur Acad Dermatol Venereol.* 2015;29:1053–1062.
28. Beasley GM, Hu Y, Youngwirth L, et al. Sentinel lymph node biopsy for recurrent melanoma: a multicenter study. *Ann Surg Oncol.* 2017;24:2728–2733.
29. Andtbacka RH, Kaufman HL, Collichio F, et al. Talimogene laherparepvec improves durable response rate in patients with advanced melanoma. *J Clin Oncol.* 2015;33:2780–2788.
30. Chesney J, Puzanov I, Collichio F, et al. Randomized, open-label phase II Study evaluating the efficacy and safety of talimogene laherparepvec in combination with ipilimumab versus ipilimumab alone in patients with advanced, unresectable melanoma. *J Clin Oncol.* 2018;36:1658–1667.
31. Puzanov I, Milhem MM, Minor D, et al. Talimogene laherparepvec in combination with ipilimumab in previously untreated, unresectable stage IIIB–IV melanoma. *J Clin Oncol.* 2016;34:2619–2626.
32. Sun L, Funchain P, Song JM, et al. Talimogene laherparepvec combined with anti-PD-1 based immunotherapy for unresectable stage III-IV melanoma: a case series. *J Immunother Cancer.* 2018;6:36.
33. Amaria RN, Prieto PA, Tetzlaff MT, et al. Neoadjuvant plus adjuvant dabrafenib and trametinib versus standard of care in patients with high-risk, surgically resectable melanoma: a single-centre, open-label, randomised, phase 2 trial. *Lancet Oncol.* 2018;19:181–193.
34. Robert C, Thomas L, Bondarenko I, et al. Ipilimumab plus dacarbazine for previously untreated metastatic melanoma. *N Engl J Med.* 2011;364:2517–2526.
35. Schachter J, Ribas A, Long GV, et al. Pembrolizumab versus ipilimumab for advanced melanoma: final overall survival results of a multicentre, randomised, open-label phase 3 study (KEYNOTE-006). *Lancet.* 2017;390:1853–1862.
36. Wolchok JD, Chiarion-Sileni V, Gonzalez R, et al. Overall survival with combined nivolumab and ipilimumab in advanced melanoma. *N Engl J Med.* 2017;377:1345–1356.
37. Long GV, Stroyakovskiy D, Gogas H, et al. Combined BRAF and MEK inhibition versus BRAF inhibition alone in melanoma. *N Engl J Med.* 2014;371:1877–1888.
38. Robert C, Karaszewska B, Schachter J, et al. Improved overall survival in melanoma with combined dabrafenib and trametinib. *N Engl J Med.* 2015;372:30–39.
39. Jones MS, Lee J, Stern SL, et al. Is pregnancy-associated melanoma associated with adverse outcomes? *J Am Coll Surg.* 2017;225:149–158.
40. Bichakjian CK, Olencki T, Aasi SZ, et al. *NCCN Guidelines Version 2.2018: Squamous cell skin cancer.* The National Comprehensive Cancer Network; 2017. Accessed May 31, 2019. https://oncolife.com.ua/doc/nccn/Squamous_Cell_Skin_Cancer.pdf.
41. Maubec E, Petrow P, Scheer-Senyarich I, et al. Phase II study of cetuximab as first-line single-drug therapy in patients with unresectable squamous cell carcinoma of the skin. *J Clin Oncol.* 2011;29:3419–3426.
42. Foote MC, McGrath M, Guminski A, et al. Phase II study of single-agent panitumumab in patients with incurable cutaneous squamous cell carcinoma. *Ann Oncol.* 2014;25:2047–2052.
43. Gold KA, Kies MS, William Jr WN, et al. Erlotinib in the treatment of recurrent or metastatic cutaneous squamous cell carcinoma: a single-arm phase 2 clinical trial. *Cancer.* 2018;124:2169–2173.
44. Migden MR, Rischin D, Schmults CD, et al. PD-1 Blockade with cemiplimab in advanced cutaneous squamous-cell carcinoma. *N Engl J Med.* 2018;379:341–351.
45. Sekulic A, Migden MR, Oro AE, et al. Efficacy and safety of vismodegib in advanced basal-cell carcinoma. *N Engl J Med.* 2012;366:2171–2179.
46. Sekulic A, Migden MR, Basset-Seguin N, et al. Long-term safety and efficacy of vismodegib in patients with advanced basal cell carcinoma: final update of the pivotal ERIVANCE BCC study. *BMC Cancer.* 2017;17:332.
47. Migden MR, Guminski A, Gutzmer R, et al. Treatment with two different doses of sonidegib in patients with locally advanced or metastatic basal cell carcinoma (BOLT): a multicentre, randomised, double-blind phase 2 trial. *Lancet Oncol.* 2015;16:716–728.
48. MacDonald M, You J. Merkel cell polyomavirus: a new DNA virus associated with human cancer. *Adv Exp Med Biol.* 2017;1018:35–56.
49. Nghiem PT, Bhatia S, Lipson EJ, et al. PD-1 blockade with pembrolizumab in advanced Merkel-cell carcinoma. *N Engl J Med.* 2016;374:2542–2552.
50. Kaufman HL, Russell J, Hamid O, et al. Avelumab in patients with chemotherapy-refractory metastatic Merkel cell carcinoma: a multicentre, single-group, open-label, phase 2 trial. *Lancet Oncol.* 2016;17:1374–1385.
51. Hodi FS, O'Day SJ, McDermott DF, et al. Improved survival with ipilimumab in patients with metastatic melanoma. *N Engl J Med.* 2010;363:711–723.
52. Robert C, Long GV, Brady B, et al. Nivolumab in previously untreated melanoma without BRAF mutation. *N Engl J Med.* 2015;372:320–330.
53. Postow MA, Chesney J, Pavlick AC, et al. Nivolumab and ipilimumab versus ipilimumab in untreated melanoma. *N Engl J Med.* 2015;372:2006–2017.

32 CHAPTER

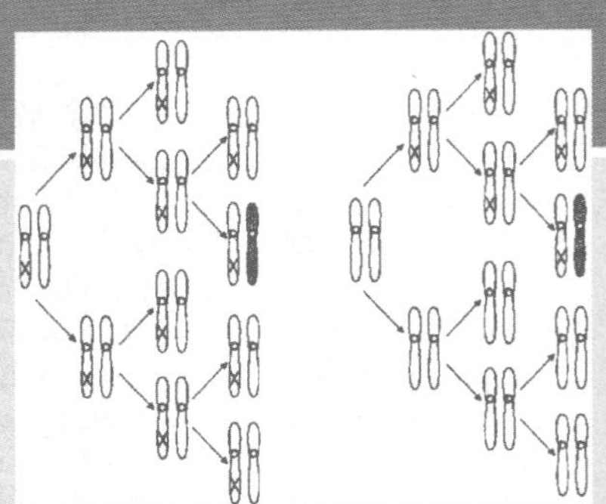

Soft Tissue Sarcoma

Carlo M. Contreras, Marty J. Heslin

OUTLINE

EPIDEMIOLOGY

Soft tissue sarcoma (STS) is a diverse group of more than 60 neoplasms that can arise from virtually any anatomic site and can affect the very young as well as the elderly. The tissue types of STS origin include skeletal muscle, adipose cells, blood and lymphatic vessels, and connective tissue or those cells with a common mesoderm origin (Fig. 32.1 and Table 32.1). Also included are peripheral nerves derived from the neuroectoderm. Clinical behaviors of mesodermal tumors occupy a wide spectrum from indolent low-grade neoplasms, such as benign lipomas, to tumors with aggressive tumor biology, such as metastatic angiosarcoma. STS is relatively rare, with 12,020 estimated new cases and an estimated 4,740 deaths for the year 2014. Whereas this accounts for 1% of cancer incidence in the United States, it accounts for 2% of cancer-related deaths. The diagnosis of patients with STS is challenging because, although it is rare in the general population, a number of common, non-neoplastic conditions can mimic STS (see Box 32.1).

Although there is a great deal of overlap between the various STS subtypes, the most traditional categorization separates trunk and extremity STS from retroperitoneal sarcomas. Before these varieties are discussed in detail, this chapter first reviews core concepts that are relevant to all STS. These core concepts include STS etiology, STS staging, consideration of the lipomatous tumor spectrum, and the STS category previously referred to as malignant fibrous histiocytoma (MFH). A more detailed discussion of trunk and extremity STS and retroperitoneal sarcoma follows. Other specific and relevant STS subtypes are addressed in more detail throughout the chapter as well.

Large published series demonstrate that extremity and trunk STS is more common than intraperitoneal and retroperitoneal STS.[1] Among extremity STS, the proximal limb is more commonly affected than the distal portion, with the thigh the most common location, accounting for 44% of patients. The age at diagnosis and the histologic STS subtype are often closely linked. Rhabdomyosarcoma, hemangioma, neurofibroma, and alveolar sarcoma tend to disproportionately affect children and young adults. Most STS occurs sporadically, but other well-documented causes include germline mutations, radiation exposure, and environmental exposure.

CORE CONCEPTS

Germline Mutations

Neurofibromatosis Type 1

Neurofibromatosis type 1 (NF1) is an autosomal dominant condition caused by mutations of the *NF1* gene, which is located at chromosome 17q11.2. *NF1* codes for a protein called neurofibromin, which acts as a tumor suppressor of the *ras* oncogene signaling pathway. In addition to the ubiquitous development of multiple cutaneous neurofibromas, these patients have a 10% risk for development of a malignant peripheral nerve sheath tumor (MPNST; which is covered in more detail later in this chapter). NF1 is also related to a variety of other tumors, including schwannomas and gliomas.

Li-Fraumeni Syndrome

The Li-Fraumeni syndrome is a rare autosomal dominant disorder caused by mutations of the *TP53* gene, which is located at chromosome 17p13.1. The *TP53* gene codes for p53, a protein that acts as a tumor suppressor. Wild-type p53 functions to facilitate the clearance of damaged cellular DNA and to prevent the clonal propagation of these mutated sequences. *TP53* mutations, therefore, contribute to an increased risk of various malignant neoplasms. In order of decreasing prevalence, these include breast cancer, STS (especially rhabdomyosarcoma, undifferentiated pleomorphic sarcoma, and pleomorphic sarcoma), adrenocortical carcinoma, brain cancer, osteosarcoma, and hematologic malignant neoplasms. Patients affected by the Li-Fraumeni syndrome exhibit a range of phenotypes, depending on the types of mutations involved, with some patients developing rhabdomyosarcoma before 4 years of age. Annual whole-body magnetic resonance imaging (MRI) has been advocated for patients with the Li-Fraumeni syndrome, in addition to dedicated breast imaging and colonoscopy.[2]

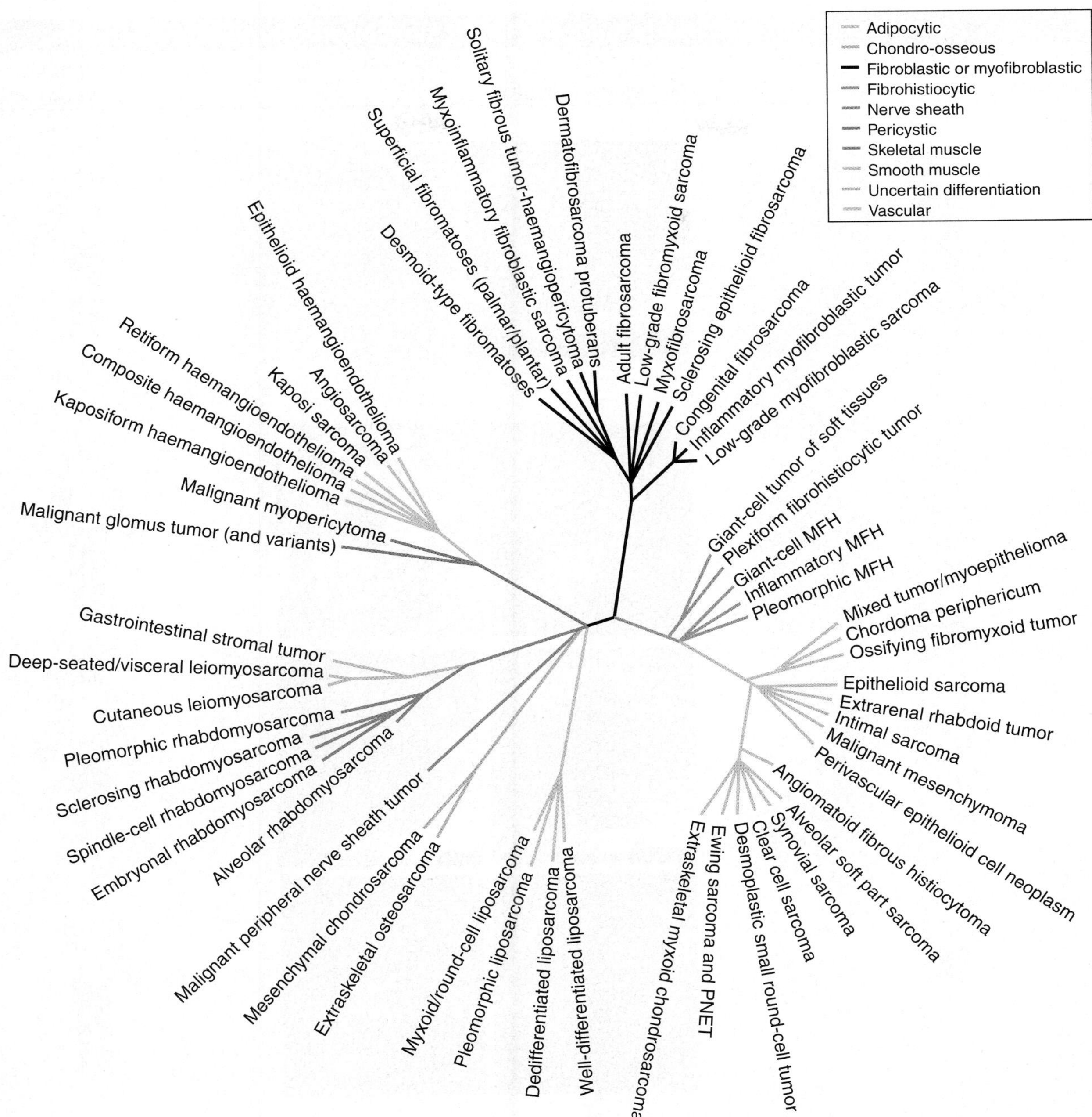

FIG. 32.1 Taxonomy of soft tissue sarcoma. This unrooted phylogeny shows about 60 sarcoma subtypes, as originally defined by the World Health Organization International Agency for Research on Cancer, amended and updated on the basis of current knowledge. The classification reflects relationships among lineage, prognosis (malignant, intermediate or locally aggressive, intermediate or rarely metastasizing), driver alterations, and additional parameters. Branch lengths are determined by nearest neighbor joining of a discretized distance matrix based on the aforementioned variables. Initial branching reflects differences in lineage, with associated lineages appearing closer in distance (such as skeletal and smooth muscle). Subsequent branching denotes similarity in prognosis, whether they are translocation associated, and, if so, the genes shared among distinct fusions (in this order). Although incomplete, as many subtypes lack sufficient global molecular profiling data on which to base a phylogeny, this initial formulation minimally reflects the relationships among lineage and major molecular lesions in the subtypes. The illustration excludes 52 benign types of tumor. (From Taylor BS, Barretina J, Maki RG, et al. Advances in sarcoma genomics and new therapeutic targets. *Nat Rev Cancer*. 2011;11:541–557.) *MFH*, Undifferentiated pleomorphic sarcoma; *PNET*, primitive neuroectodermal tumor.

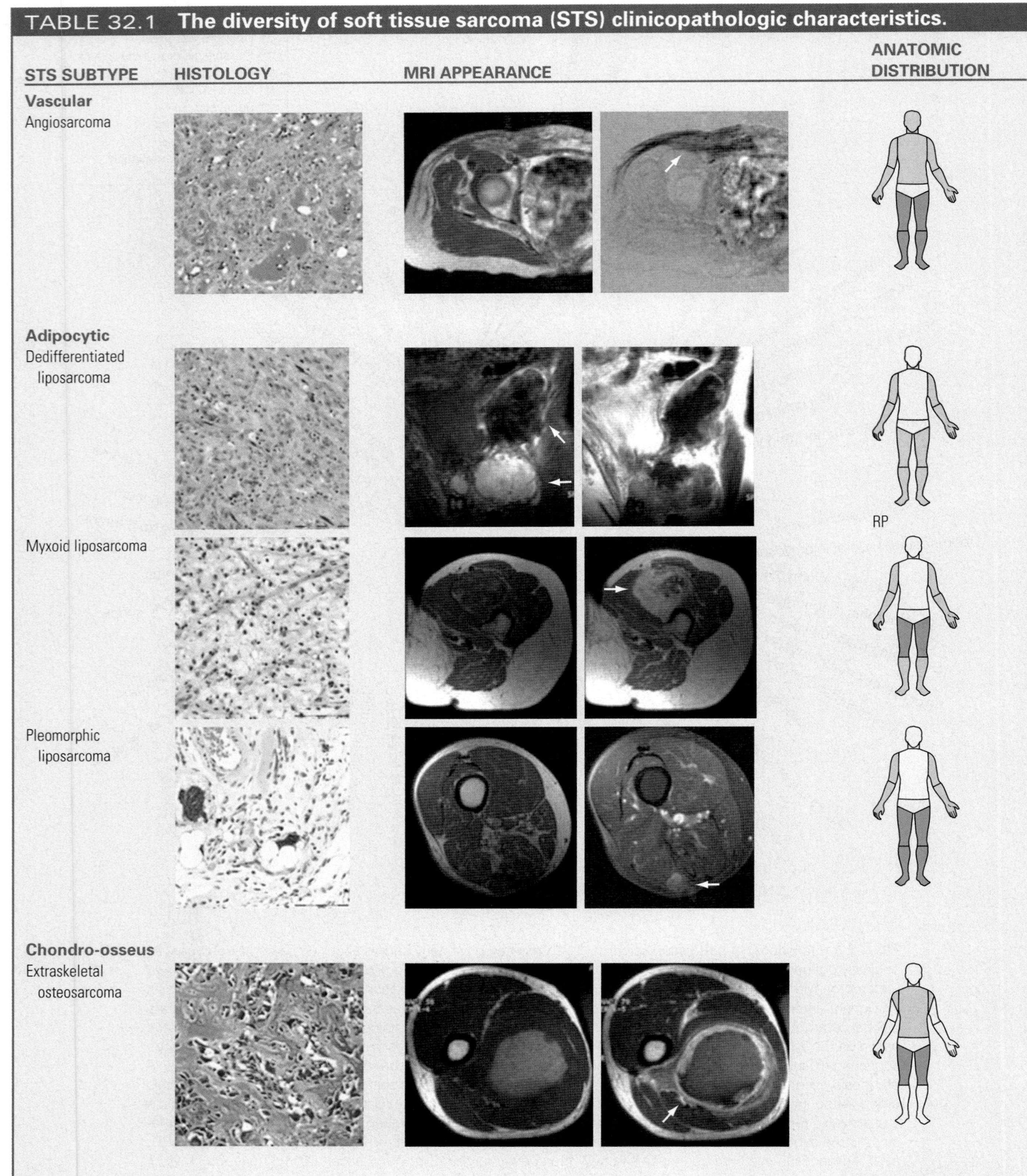

TABLE 32.1 **The diversity of soft tissue sarcoma (STS) clinicopathologic characteristics.**

STS SUBTYPE	HISTOLOGY	MRI APPEARANCE	ANATOMIC DISTRIBUTION
Vascular			
Angiosarcoma			
Adipocytic			
Dedifferentiated liposarcoma			RP
Myxoid liposarcoma			
Pleomorphic liposarcoma			
Chondro-osseus			
Extraskeletal osteosarcoma			

TABLE 32.1 **The diversity of soft tissue sarcoma (STS) clinicopathologic characteristics.—cont'd**

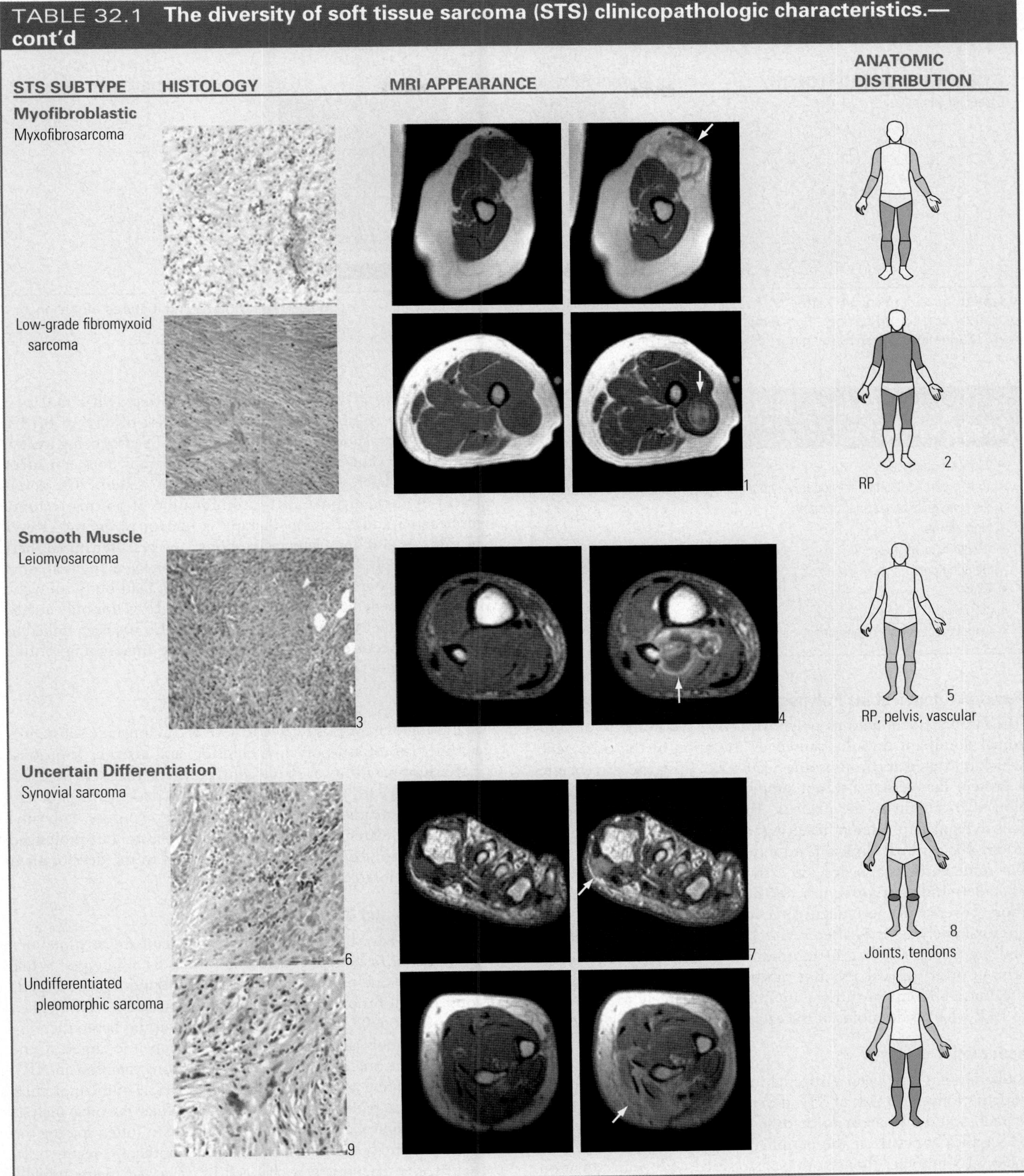

STS SUBTYPE	HISTOLOGY	MRI APPEARANCE	ANATOMIC DISTRIBUTION
Myofibroblastic			
Myxofibrosarcoma			
Low-grade fibromyxoid sarcoma		1	2 RP
Smooth Muscle			
Leiomyosarcoma	3	4	5 RP, pelvis, vascular
Uncertain Differentiation			
Synovial sarcoma	6	7	8 Joints, tendons
Undifferentiated pleomorphic sarcoma	9		

Continued

TABLE 32.1 The diversity of soft tissue sarcoma (STS) clinicopathologic characteristics.—cont'd

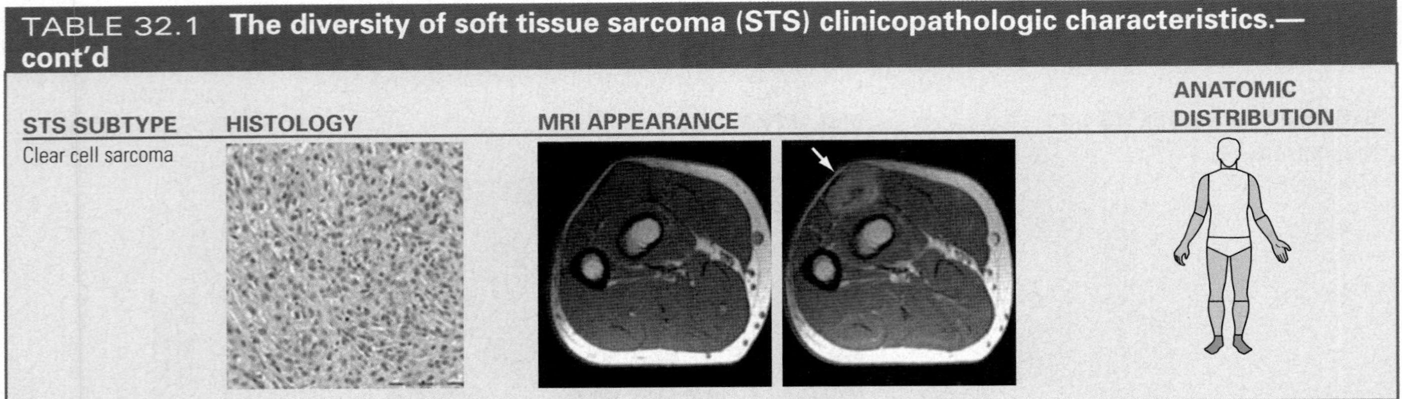

STS SUBTYPE	HISTOLOGY	MRI APPEARANCE	ANATOMIC DISTRIBUTION
Clear cell sarcoma			

Adapted from van Vliet M, Kliffen M, Krestin G, et al. Soft tissue sarcomas at a glance: clinical, histological, and MR imaging features of malignant extremity soft tissue tumors. *Eur Radiol.* 2009;19:1499–1511.
MRI, Magnetic resonance imaging; *RP*, retroperitoneum.

BOX 32.1 Entities that may mimic soft tissue sarcoma.

- Hypertrophic scar
- Retroperitoneal lymphadenopathy: lymphoma, germ cell tumor, or metastasis from gastrointestinal primary
- Hematoma
- Myositis ossificans
- Benign lipoma
- Cyst
- Abscess
- Cutaneous malignant neoplasms, including melanoma

Familial Adenomatous Polyposis and Gardner Syndrome

The familial adenomatous polyposis (FAP) syndrome is an autosomal dominant disorder caused by mutation of the *APC* gene, which is located at chromosome 5q21-q22. This gene also encodes a protein that acts as a tumor suppressor, inhibiting the localization of β-catenin to the nucleus. The truncated mutant protein fails to regulate β-catenin, resulting in unchecked cellular proliferation. The cardinal clinical feature is innumerable colonic polyps, but some patients also develop extracolonic manifestations, such as epidermoid cysts, osteomas, and desmoid tumors. Desmoid tumors, covered in more detail later in this chapter, typically arise approximately 5 years after FAP-related prophylactic colectomy and are a major source of morbidity and mortality. They often arise in prior surgical sites but can be manifested at virtually any site. Intra-abdominal tumors are much more likely to be related to FAP, whereas desmoids of the extremities are typically sporadic.

Radiation

Radiation has long been suspected to significantly contribute to a patient's long-term risk of STS development. Whereas the effects of radiation are thought to be dose dependent, radiation-related STS typically occurs at the periphery of the radiation field. The main STS subtypes thought to be associated with prior radiation exposure include unclassified pleomorphic sarcoma, angiosarcoma, leiomyosarcoma, fibrosarcoma, and MPNST.[3] Compared with sporadic forms of these same STS subtypes, those arising after radiation exposure tend to have a shorter disease-specific survival. In the setting of adjuvant radiation therapy for breast cancer, a large cohort of 122,991 women demonstrated that radiation contributes to an absolute increase in the risk of STS of 0.13% during 10 years. Patients who later develop STS after being treated as children for cancers requiring radiation therapy do so a median of 11.8 years later, also in a dose-dependent fashion. The development of angiosarcoma after a combination of postmastectomy lymphedema and radiation therapy is known as Stewart-Treves syndrome; it also has a latency of about 10 years after initial therapy. Interestingly, Stewart-Treves syndrome–related angiosarcoma usually occurs outside the previous radiation field but within the zone of lymphedema. An increased risk of STS is not only attributable to therapeutic doses of radiation but also has been linked to lower doses encountered by pediatric patients undergoing routine computed tomography (CT) scan.

Carcinogens

Hepatic angiosarcoma is related to several carcinogenic substances including Thorotrast, polyvinyl chloride, and arsenic. Thorotrast is a thorium-based intravenous contrast agent that was used between the years 1930 and 1955. In affected patients, hepatic angiosarcoma is diagnosed 20 to 30 years after exposure. Polyvinyl chloride is an extremely common form of plastic, but prolonged and unprotected exposures have been linked to the development of hepatic angiosarcoma.

Gene Fusions and Molecular Testing

Gene fusions have been identified as important driver mutations in a number of tissue types, including various STS subtypes. While approximately one-third of STS have been found to harbor gene fusions, not all fusion products are pathogenetically relevant (i.e., "driver mutations"). Thus, the utility of gene fusions lies in their use as diagnostic tools, and also as potential therapeutic targets. Gene fusions are but one example of how mutations manifest in STS. An ever-expanding array of platforms are available in the molecular analysis of these patients. In one study, molecular sarcoma analysis changed the clinical diagnosis in 13% of patients, often sparing the patient the toxicity of a nontherapeutic chemotherapy regimen. In particular, the diagnosis was changed in 23% of patients initially suspected to have dedifferentiated liposarcoma.[4] The routine use of molecular analysis is likely to grow in this field as additional gene mutations and fusion events predictive of response to specific chemotherapy agents are discovered. For example, a platform called Complex INdex in SARComas (CINSARC) consists of a group of

TABLE 32.2 American Joint Committee on Cancer staging for soft tissue sarcomas.

Primary Tumor (T)	
Primary tumor cannot be assessed	TX
No evidence of primary tumor	T0
Tumor 5 cm or less in greatest dimension	T1
Tumor more than 5 cm and less than or equal to 10 cm in greatest dimension	T2
Tumor more than 10 cm and less than or equal to 15 cm in greatest dimension	T3
Tumor more than 15 cm in greatest dimension	T4
Regional Lymph Nodes (N)	
Regional lymph nodes cannot be assessed	NX
No regional lymph node metastasis	N0
Regional lymph node metastasis	N1
Distant Metastasis (M)	
No distant metastasis	M0
Distant metastasis	M1

TABLE 32.3 Anatomic stage and prognostic groups for soft tissue sarcomas.

GROUP	T	N	M	GRADE
Stage IA	T1	N0	M0	G1, GX
Stage IB	T2–4	N0	M0	G1, GX
Stage II	T1	N0	M0	G2, G3
Stage IIIA	T2	N0	M0	G2, G3
Stage IIIB	T3, T4	N0	M0	G2, G3
Stage IV	Any T	N1*	M0	Any grade
	Any T	Any N	M1	Any grade

*For retroperitoneal sarcoma, N1 disease is designated as stage IIIB, not stage IV.

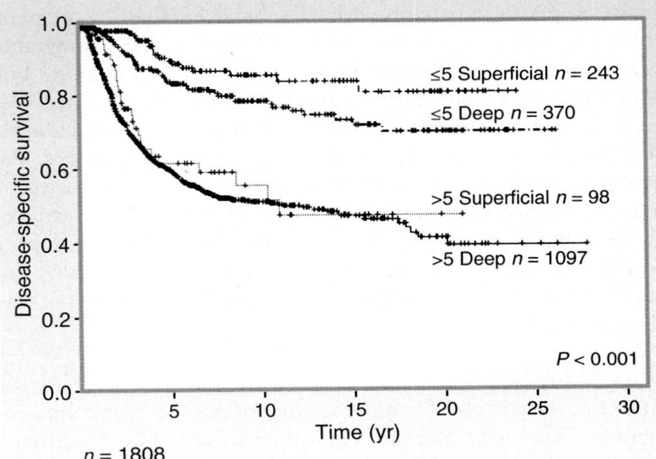

FIG. 32.2 Importance of size and depth among primary high-grade soft tissue sarcoma tumors. (From Brennan MF, Antonescu CR, Moraco N, et al: Lessons learned from the study of 10,000 patients with soft tissue sarcoma. *Ann Surg* 260:416–422, 2014.)

67 genes that have been demonstrated to predict metastasis-free survival. These genes, which are associated with mitosis and chromosome management, show promise in being able to predict prognosis more effectively than histologic grade, even in patients with grade 1 tumors. While these early data have not been prospectively validated, they do give a glimpse into the future of how STS patients may be evaluated in the future.

Staging

Tumor Grade

The inclusion of tumor grade into the American Joint Committee on Cancer (AJCC) staging system for STS distinguishes it from most other types of cancer. Internationally, the two most widely applied grading systems are the French Fédération Nationale des Centres de Lutte Contre le Cancer (FNCLCC) system and the National Institutes of Health (NIH) system. The FNCLCC is a score based on the sum of three categories: tumor differentiation, rate of mitoses, and amount of tumor necrosis. The NIH system is similar but for certain STS subtypes requires that the pathologist state the degree of tumor cellularity and pleomorphism, which can limit its reproducibility. The FNCLCC and the NIH systems were compared, and the FNCLCC was found to be superior in estimating the risk of distant metastasis and survival.

Beyond sarcoma type, tumor grade, the other important staging parameters include tumor size, nodal involvement, and involvement of distant sites. The schema for the eighth edition AJCC staging system is a significant update over the seventh edition (see Tables 32.2 and 32.3). The AJCC staging system states that the FNCLCC is preferred over the NIH system.[5]

The eighth edition has separate staging definitions for the following anatomic sarcoma locations: head and neck, trunk and extremities, abdomen and visceral organs, and the retroperitoneum. The separate schemas for gastrointestinal stromal tumor (GIST), bone sarcoma, uterine sarcoma, Kaposi sarcoma, and dermatofibrosarcoma protuberans (DFSP) are maintained. These changes are in response to criticism that grouping heterogeneous tumors decreases the prognostic power compared with a schema in which separate subtypes are individually considered. As the AJCC eighth edition does not stage tumors based on histologic sarcoma subtype, Anaya and colleagues[6] demonstrated that a more descriptive and clinically relevant method of estimating prognosis involves segregating patients into three histologic groups: well-differentiated liposarcoma, dedifferentiated or pleomorphic liposarcoma, and all other retroperitoneal sarcoma histologic types.

Based largely on two publications, the eighth edition size thresholds defining the tumor category have changed. T1 tumors are defined as 5 cm or less, T2 tumors are >5 to ≤10 cm, T3 tumors are >10 to ≤15 cm, and T4 tumors are >15 cm.[7] The superficial versus deep anatomic designation of the tumor with respect to the investing fascia has been eliminated. Compared with extremity STS, visceral and retroperitoneal STS appears to have a lower disease-specific survival. In the case of visceral STS, this decreased disease-specific survival is driven by the likelihood for distant metastasis; but for retroperitoneal STS, the low disease-specific survival is driven by the risk of local recurrence.[1]

The importance of the size of the primary STS to prognosis is well described (Fig. 32.2), but the current size thresholds specified by the AJCC eighth edition have been challenged. Greater prognostic discrimination is proposed by designating all low grade tumors as stage I, high-grade tumors less than 7.5 cm as stage II, high-grade tumors greater than 7.5 cm as stage III, and metastatic as stage IV.[8]

Overall, regional lymph node involvement for STS is uncommon (2% to 10%). The most common STS subtypes undergoing lymphadenectomy for nodal metastases are angiosarcoma, rhabdomyosarcoma, MFH (recently reclassified as undifferentiated pleomorphic sarcoma), epithelioid sarcoma, clear cell sarcoma, and liposarcoma. Although regional nodal involvement is an important prognosticator of survival, patients with a single lymph node, multiple positive nodes, and distant metastatic disease all have similar survival.[1] Some groups have proposed the use of sentinel lymph node dissection for epithelioid sarcoma, clear cell sarcoma, and rhabdomyosarcoma in the pediatric population, but the accuracy is generally unacceptable, and the technique has never been successfully applied to STS in a well-designed clinical trial.

Nomograms have been developed in response to the fact that standard staging systems, like the AJCC, do not adequately consider the relevant parameters and therefore may not accurately estimate prognosis of patients with STS. No fewer than 13 different nomograms have been published for STS alone. The nomograms were developed to address a number of oncologic outcomes but most typically predict local recurrence or overall survival (Fig. 32.3). In general, the nomograms are reported to more accurately prognosticate outcome than traditional staging systems, but few have been validated in a data set beyond that which was used to generate the nomogram. Nonetheless, they can provide meaningful information that, when used appropriately, can have an impact on the care of patients with STS. It remains to be seen how the proliferation of these nomograms will affect future editions of traditional staging systems.

Clinical Evaluation

There are dozens of STS subtypes that affect the trunk and extremities. The most common clinical presentation is of a patient with a painless mass without prior evaluation. If STS is included in the differential diagnosis, appropriate oncologic staging should be undertaken. This staging starts by performing a detailed history and physical examination. These are important in determining the likelihood of STS versus other more common mimicking diagnoses, such as hypertrophic scar, myositis ossificans, hematoma, or cyst (Box 32.1). Small, superficial, and mobile masses highly suggestive of STS that are separate from skeletal or neurovascular structures may be taken to the operating room for resection with wide gross margins, depending on the location relative to vital structures. Tumors close to vital structures may be referred to a center with expertise treating STS. In these patients, a preoperative biopsy is unnecessary. The undesirable consequences of an unnecessary preoperative biopsy include a pathology report that provides the incorrect non-STS diagnosis because of an insufficient specimen, a nonideal placement of the biopsy site leading to a larger incision than otherwise necessary, and delay in therapy.

Larger or otherwise more complicated lesions require additional oncologic staging. The extent of staging is highly individualized and adapted to each patient. In general, the indications for preoperative imaging and biopsy include the following;

- Inability to determine the extent of the mass on physical examination.
- Suspected neurovascular involvement.
- Suspicion for regional or distant metastasis.
- Need for operation that would likely result in a significant functional deficit.
- Suspicion that the mass is unresectable or resectable with questionable surgical margins at presentation.

Rigorous studies evaluating the utility of MRI versus CT are dated. Whereas MRI is generally considered the most informative imaging modality for trunk and extremity STS, there are important roles for the use of contrast-enhanced CT and ultrasound. In addition to imaging of the primary STS site, a chest

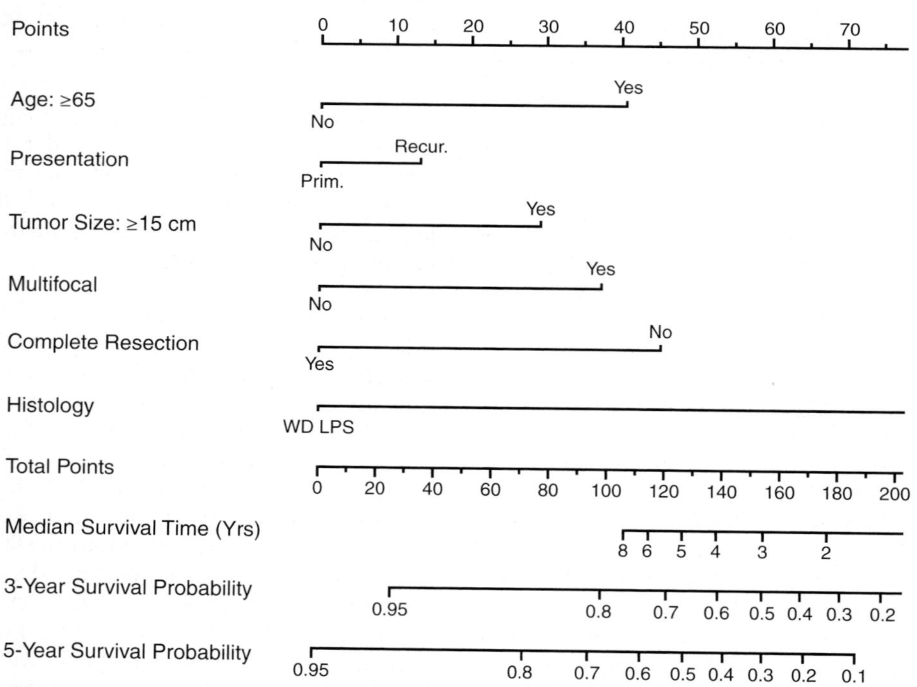

FIG. 32.3 Postoperative nomogram for median, 3- and 5-year overall survival prediction in patients with non-metastatic, resectable, retroperitoneal sarcoma. *WD LPS*, Well-differentiated liposarcoma. (From Anaya DA, Lahat G, Wang X, et al. Postoperative nomogram for survival of patients with retroperitoneal sarcoma treated with curative intent. *Ann Oncol.* 2010;21:397–402. Oxford University Press, European Society of Medical Oncology.)

CT scan should generally be obtained as this is the most frequent site of metastasis. When they are available, the biopsy results may prompt consideration of additional imaging. For example, a CT scan of the abdomen and pelvis should be considered for patients with more aggressive histologic types, such as myxoid or round cell liposarcoma, epithelioid sarcoma, angiosarcoma, and leiomyosarcoma. Brain imaging may be considered to exclude metastasis from alveolar soft part sarcoma, clear cell sarcoma, and angiosarcoma.

The surgeon may choose from a variety of biopsy methods. Given the rarity of STS and the scant amount of tissue procured, a fine-needle aspirate is generally unsatisfactory except in the diagnosis of a local recurrence. An image-guided core needle biopsy is more likely to provide a reliable diagnosis, but when it is applied to large cystic lesions or lesions with a considerable myxoid component, a core needle biopsy may still be nondiagnostic. To decrease the risk of local recurrence, the core biopsy approach should be planned so that the entire needle trajectory can be easily incorporated into the forthcoming surgical resection volume. If the core needle biopsy attempts are still nondiagnostic, an incisional biopsy may be necessary. Here, again, it is critical to plan the incision so that the entire biopsy trajectory is ultimately included within the resection volume.

Armed with radiographic and pathologic information, a multidisciplinary team at a high-volume STS center, with representatives from surgical oncology, medical oncology, diagnostic radiology, pathology, and radiation oncology in attendance, ideally discusses the case. The goal of this discussion is to assess which treatment modalities are most appropriate for each patient and in what sequence each modality should be implemented (Fig. 32.4). Up to 74% of patients who undergo an unplanned trunk or extremity sarcoma resection have residual disease at the time of re-resection. Thirty-day mortality, rates of limb preservation, and overall survival have been linked to care delivered at high-volume STS centers.[9]

Because of the considerable risk for recurrence, close postoperative surveillance is important for STS patients. In general, these patients should undergo a physical examination every 3 to 6 months for 2 or 3 years, then every 6 months for the next 2 years, and then annually. Radiographic surveillance of the chest,

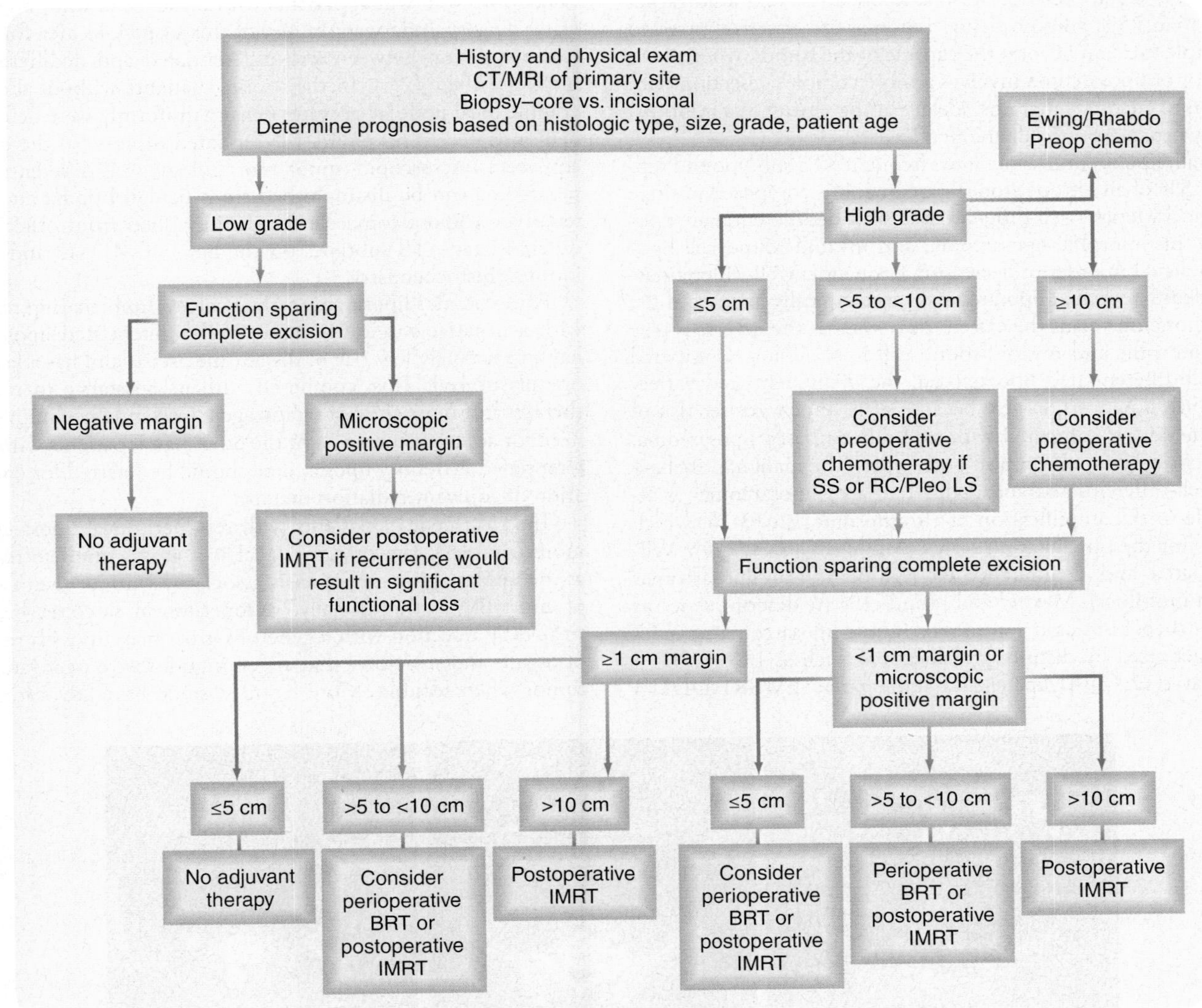

FIG. 32.4 Algorithm for the management of primary (with no metastases) extremity or trunk soft tissue sarcoma using a biologic rationale (i.e., size and grade of tumor). *BRT*, Brachytherapy; *CT*, computed tomography; *EBRT*, external beam radiation therapy; *IMRT*, intensity-modulated radiation therapy; *MRI*, magnetic resonance imaging; *RC/Pleo LS*, round cell–pleomorphic liposarcoma; *SS*, synovial sarcoma.

abdomen, and pelvis should also be undertaken at regular intervals. The modality (CT vs. MRI) and the frequency should be individualized to the patient and the tumor characteristics. The most informative preoperative imaging modality is favored, but consideration should also be given to avoiding unnecessary radiation exposure by ultrasound or MRI. The imaging frequency for STS patients has not been rigorously studied, but a shorter imaging frequency may be appropriate for a patient with close surgical margins or a patient with a particularly ominous histologic type.

Lipomatous Tumors

Lipomas are adipocytic tumors that can arise from any part of the body. By definition, they are benign neoplasms, but they can cause symptoms as a consequence of the adjacent structures that the lipoma displaces. Lipomas are encapsulated and devoid of nodularity or thick internal septations. They are generally homogeneous but may contain calcifications or hemorrhage as a result of trauma. There can be a great deal of clinical overlap between lipoma and the malignant liposarcoma. The CT and MRI features that have been demonstrated to be associated with liposarcoma over lipoma include tumor size larger than 10 cm, presence of thick (more than 2 mm) septa, presence of nonadipose areas, and lesions that are less than 75% adipose tissue. Lipomas are effectively treated by a simple excision beyond the capsule of the tumor, whereas the treatment of liposarcoma involves a more complex resection with attention to adequate margins, ideally in the setting of a multidisciplinary care team specializing in STS.

Overall, liposarcoma is the most frequent STS subtype and represents 45% of all retroperitoneal sarcoma; it is composed of three histologic varieties: well-differentiated and dedifferentiated liposarcoma, pleomorphic liposarcoma, and myxoid/round cell liposarcoma, listed in order of decreasing frequency. Well-differentiated and dedifferentiated liposarcomas more typically arise from the retroperitoneum versus the extremities, whereas the inverse is true for pleomorphic and myxoid/round cell liposarcoma. Compared with well-differentiated liposarcoma, the dedifferentiated variety has a worse prognosis, largely because of its much greater risk of distant metastasis compared with well-differentiated liposarcoma. Local recurrence is common in both types. The malignant behavior of well-differentiated and dedifferentiated liposarcomas is attributable to the amplification of chromosome 12q13-15, which accounts for the upregulation of MDM2 and CDK4. Both well-differentiated and dedifferentiated retroperitoneal liposarcomas are often multifocal. Myxoid and round cells are descriptive terms based on their histologic appearance. These liposarcoma varieties are characterized by distinct translocations such as FUS-DDIT3 located at t(12;16)(q13;p11) and more rarely EWSR1-DDIT3 located at t(12;22)(q13;q12). Multiple tumor-promoting pathways including MET, RET, and PI3K/Akt are activated as a result of these translocations. Myxoid liposarcoma is unusual in its relative sensitivity to radiation and chemotherapy, resulting in a 10-year disease-specific survival of 87%. Considered a poorly differentiated form of the myxoid variety, the round cell variety has a worse outcome than myxoid liposarcoma, with metastasis developing in 21% of patients in one large series. Pleomorphic liposarcoma is another example of a poorly differentiated liposarcoma with a poor outcome. It displays a variety of genetic abnormalities, none as reliable as those described for the preceding liposarcoma varieties.

In routine practice, one of the key preoperative distinctions is between well-differentiated and dedifferentiated retroperitoneal liposarcomas because of differences in natural history and management. MRI and CT scan are useful in making this distinction but can be difficult because a given tumor may contain elements of both. The imaging characteristics that raised suspicion of a dedifferentiated histology in a cohort of 78 patients with retroperitoneal liposarcoma included tumor hypervascularity, areas of necrosis or cystic change, adjacent organ invasion, and areas of focal nodular or water density.[10] These authors proposed a clinical algorithm in which patients with evidence of focal nodular or water density underwent biopsy of this suspicious area for definitive distinction between well-differentiated and dedifferentiated histology (Fig. 32.5). In their series, patients without the radiographic focal nodular or water density uniformly were definitively demonstrated to have well-differentiated tumors. In the event of equivocal microscopic tumor morphology, well-differentiated liposarcoma can be distinguished from benign lipoma and dedifferentiated liposarcoma can be distinguished from other poorly differentiated STS subtypes on the basis of MDM2 and CDK4 immunohistochemistry.

For extremity liposarcoma, the goal is a limb-sparing resection with a negative surgical margin. Well-differentiated liposarcoma has an extremely low risk of distant metastasis and has a favorable overall survival. This, combined with its resistance to radiation therapy and most chemotherapy agents, essentially eliminates the need for adjuvant therapy. On the other hand, patients with dedifferentiated extremity liposarcoma should be referred for consideration of adjuvant radiation therapy.

The treatment of patients with retroperitoneal liposarcoma is more complex. The principal goal is a gross complete resection as incomplete gross resection is associated with an increased risk of mortality.[11] Traditionally, retroperitoneal sarcoma has been treated by resection with a generous gross margin, with resection of organs and structures that are contiguous with or invading the tumor when feasible. More recently, some have advocated for a

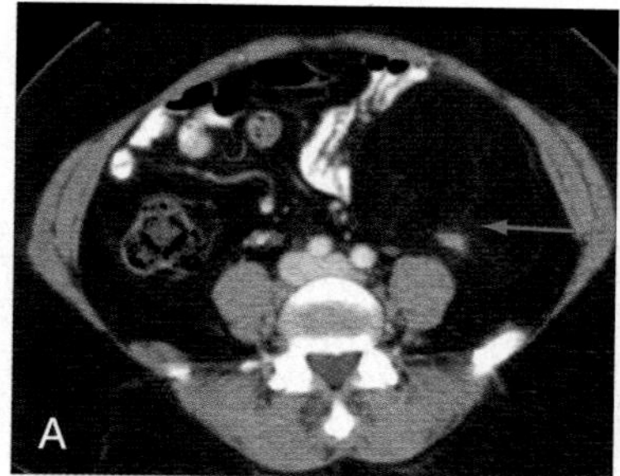

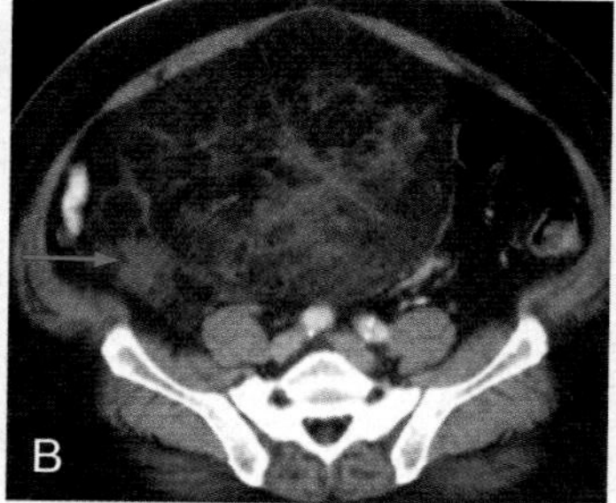

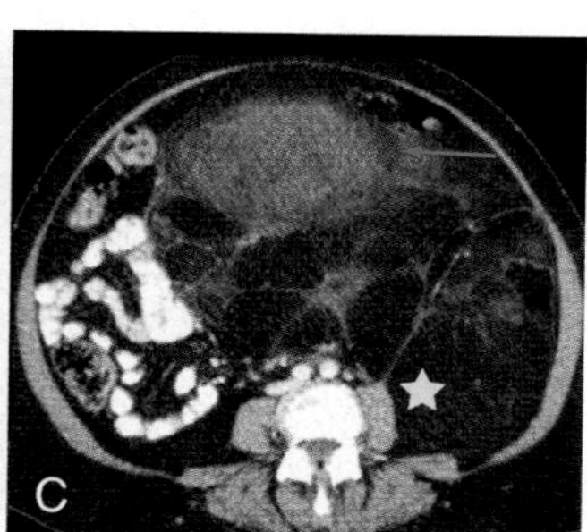

FIG. 32.5 Variability in computed tomography appearance of retroperitoneal liposarcoma. (A) Simple, predominantly fatty, well-differentiated tumor; the *arrow* marks the inferior mesenteric vein. Thin septa are appreciable within the tumor. (B) A hypercellular well-differentiated tumor with a focal nodular or water density area *(arrow)*. (C) This tumor contains well-differentiated areas *(star)* as well as dedifferentiated elements *(arrow)*.

"complete compartmental resection," which mandates the resection of adjacent organs, even if they are not directly involved with the tumor.[12] Although it is controversial, the concept that "the resection is only as good as the closest margin" is an important one. This takes into account the relationships between vital structures on one side of the tumor and not resecting contiguous but uninvolved organs. Understanding of the patterns of retroperitoneal liposarcoma recurrence is important in planning the optimal approach. For patients with well-differentiated retroperitoneal liposarcoma, a unifocal versus multifocal presentation does not appear to confer an adverse prognosis, but patients with dedifferentiated disease multifocality have a worse overall survival.[13] Patients who develop recurrence after initial resection are likely to develop multifocal disease. This appears to be reflective of the tumor biology because an initial resection with positive margins does not appear to affect whether a patient develops a unifocal versus multifocal recurrence. The complete compartmental resection approach results in frequent multivisceral resections, with the following organs resected in more than 50% of cases: spleen, pancreas, diaphragm, adrenal gland, and kidney.[12] Proponents of a more traditional approach in which only tumor-contiguous organs are removed point out that 15% of patients who have recurrence after undergoing standard resection do so beyond the compartmental bounds of their initial tumor.[13] These out-of-field recurrences are unlikely to have been prevented with an aggressive complete compartmental resection strategy, and patients who may eventually benefit from nephrotoxic systemic chemotherapy are adversely affected by a potentially unnecessary complete compartmental resection–related nephrectomy.

Although grossly incomplete resections are to be avoided, a margin-negative resection is not possible in some situations. At times, this can be predicted on the basis of the preoperative imaging, but at other times, the difficulty of the resection is not appreciated until during the operation. A single-institution retrospective study compared the outcome of patients with retroperitoneal liposarcoma who underwent an incomplete resection versus patients who underwent exploration and biopsy without tumor resection. Even incomplete resection provides a statistically significant improvement in survival compared with no resection, 26 versus 4 months. In addition, 75% of patients undergoing incomplete resection reported palliation of their presenting symptoms. In the setting of recurrent retroperitoneal liposarcoma, the rate of recurrent tumor growth is associated with prognosis. Patients whose recurrence grows less than 0.9 cm/mo benefitted from complete resection of the recurrence, whereas recurrent tumor growth of more than 0.9 cm/mo was associated with poor outcome.[14] Palliative chemotherapy options are emerging for patients with unresectable recurrence who have already failed chemotherapy. A subgroup analysis of a randomized phase 3 trial comparing eribulin versus dacarbazine for either extremity or retroperitoneal liposarcoma showed that eribulin was associated with an improvement in overall survival (15.6 vs. 8.4 months). Based on these data, single-agent eribulin is approved in the palliative setting for patients with liposarcoma. Together, these observations contribute to the complexity of developing an individualized treatment plan for retroperitoneal liposarcoma.

Malignant Fibrous Histiocytoma Reclassification

In past decades, MFH was considered the most common STS in adults. Improvements and innovations in the pathologic review of STS have drastically altered the definition of MFH. Various authors have retrospectively reevaluated tumors originally classified as MFH and found that the majority merited reclassification. In one seminal manuscript, 63% were reclassified, and only 13% truly met pathologic criteria for MFH. These data shifted the diagnosis of MFH to one of exclusion, and this movement culminated in the 2013 World Health Organization classification of soft tissue tumors that completely eliminated the term. Tumors that still meet pathologic criteria for MFH are now referred to as unclassified or undifferentiated pleomorphic sarcoma. Careful histologic, immunohistochemical, and molecular analysis by a pathologist with STS expertise is crucial in the accurate diagnosis and treatment of these patients. With precise pathologic review, patients with tumors originally classified as MFH have demonstrably different prognoses based on the actual line of STS differentiation.[15]

TRUNK AND EXTREMITY SARCOMA

Extremity STS poses a particular challenge with respect to balancing the degree of limb function with tumor control. Historically, surgeons had a much lower threshold to recommend extremity amputation for STS. Data from clinical trials have prompted a shift toward limb preservation in these patients. The ability to offer limb preservation is a result of improvements in the multidisciplinary care of these patients. One of the seminal trials conducted at the National Cancer Institute (NCI) proposed that extremity STS resection might be addressed by a limb-sparing approach instead of amputation.[16] Forty-three patients with high-grade extremity STS were randomized to undergo a limb-sparing operation followed by adjuvant radiation therapy versus amputation alone; both groups received adjuvant chemotherapy. This approach resulted in no statistical significant difference in local recurrence in the limb-sparing group as compared with the amputation group. Disease-free and overall survival rates were also equivalent between the two groups. These results were supported by a similar contemporary trial that compared 126 patients who were randomized to limb-sparing STS resection with or without adjuvant brachytherapy. In this trial, brachytherapy was associated with improved local recurrence, but subset analysis suggests that this result may have been driven by the favorable response in patients with high-grade tumors. In a later NCI study, patients demonstrated a decrease in local recurrence regardless of tumor grade with the addition of external beam radiation therapy. The STS literature lacks a randomized trial to identify in which patients adjuvant radiation therapy can be safely omitted because of the large sample size required to satisfy the accompanying power calculation.[17] Retrospective data indicate that adjuvant radiation therapy may be omitted for T1 extremity STS that is resected with negative surgical margins, even considering that 58% of these patients had high-grade tumors.[18] A large retrospective Scandinavian study of 1093 patients found that whereas a narrow or involved surgical margin does increase the risk of local recurrence, adjuvant radiation therapy improved local control independent of tumor grade, tumor depth (superficial or deep), or margin status. In the event that adjuvant radiation therapy is indicated, the surgeon should consider two technical maneuvers. The first is placement of a few metallic clips at the boundaries of the resection bed in the event that adjuvant radiation therapy is indicated; the second is that when a surgical drain is necessary, the skin exit site should be placed near the incision as the entire surgical drain track is usually included in the radiation field. Metallic clips within the resection bed will assist with radiation planning, and careful drain placement reduces an otherwise unnecessary expansion of the radiation field.

Above and beyond the established local control benefits of adjuvant radiation, delivery of neoadjuvant radiation for STS offers a number of conceptual advantages. Before surgical resection, the target tissue oxygenation is superior, which facilitates the generation of intratumoral free radicals and ultimately tumor cell destruction. When neoadjuvant radiation is administered, the radiation field includes a smaller volume of adjacent nontumor tissue compared with the radiation field after surgical resection.[19] When radiation is delivered with the tumor in situ, a lower preoperative dose is required versus in the postoperative setting. If radiation is delivered preoperatively, patients would be predicted to complete all components of their therapy more promptly as delayed wound healing can delay initiation of postoperative radiation therapy. In contrast to other tumors, administration of neoadjuvant radiation therapy rarely results in measurable tumor shrinkage but may cause varying degrees of histologic tumor necrosis.[20] A complete pathologic response after neoadjuvant therapy is an important prognostic factor in a variety of malignant neoplasms including breast cancer, esophageal cancer, and rectal cancer. Unfortunately, this relationship does not appear to hold true for STS. When most of the resected tumor is nonviable after neoadjuvant radiation therapy or chemoradiotherapy, patients with STS do not have improvements in overall survival or local recurrence.[21] Patients with a positive surgical margin after undergoing preoperative radiation therapy do not appear to derive a significant reduction in local recurrence by administration of a postoperative radiation boost.

Only one clinical trial has randomized patients with extremity STS to receive either neoadjuvant or postoperative radiation therapy. In this trial, neoadjuvant external beam radiation therapy was associated with an increased risk of wound complications.[19] Although the authors reported a statistically significant difference in overall survival favoring the neoadjuvant arm, survival was a secondary end point, and the trial was not properly powered to evaluate this parameter. One would expect that another conceptual advantage of choosing a neoadjuvant approach would be to decrease the incidence and consequences of positive surgical margins by delivering tumoricidal doses preoperatively to the areas most at risk. In actuality, the existing randomized trial showed equivalent rates of negative surgical margins in patients receiving preoperative versus postoperative radiation therapy (83% and 85%, respectively).[19] Using the existing retrospective data to explore this question is problematic as there are clear selection biases in which patients receive neoadjuvant therapy and their subsequent risk for positive surgical margins. Finally, the definition of a positive or negative surgical margin differs among manuscripts, which contributes to the difficulty in interpreting the reported data. The long-term implications of a positive margin are independent of whether radiation therapy is delivered preoperatively or postoperatively; positive margins are associated with an increased risk for local recurrence, whereas overall survival is generally unchanged.

Preoperative regimens combining chemotherapy and radiation therapy have also been investigated. A retrospective review of 112 patients undergoing either neoadjuvant chemoradiation or neoadjuvant radiation versus surgery alone found equivalent oncologic outcomes among the three approaches. When stratified by size, the overall survival of patients with tumors larger than 5 cm was improved in treatment with either neoadjuvant chemoradiation or neoadjuvant radiation therapy compared with surgery alone. Preoperative chemoradiation therapy followed by surgical resection and additional chemotherapy was shown to be associated with an increased overall survival. This was suggested in a retrospective study of 48 patients whose chemotherapy included a combination of doxorubicin, ifosfamide, and dacarbazine. All 48 patients had high-grade extremity STS measuring at least 8 cm, and additional postoperative radiation therapy was delivered in the event of positive surgical margins.[22] Patients undergoing this intensive preoperative and postoperative chemotherapy regimen were matched to historical controls. In this study, the resection margin status was similar between the two groups. The outcomes of this preoperative and postoperative chemoradiation treatment schema were verified in radiation therapy oncology group (RTOG) 9514, a single-arm, multi-institutional phase 2 trial.[23]

The use of chemotherapy in the adjuvant setting for STS is controversial. European Organisation for Research and Treatment Center (EORTC) 62931 was a randomized multi-institutional trial that randomized 351 patients to receive adjuvant chemotherapy (doxorubicin, ifosfamide, and the hematopoietic growth factor lenograstim) versus no chemotherapy. The overall and relapse-free survivals were equivalent in both groups. A meta-analysis of 1953 patients who had participated in 18 trials showed that those patients who received adjuvant doxorubicin had statistically significant improvements in local, distant, and overall recurrence. A randomized phase 2 study of 150 patients showed that neoadjuvant chemotherapy (doxorubicin and ifosfamide) was not associated with improvements in disease-free or overall survival. Because of the abundance of conflicting data, consensus guidelines such as those of the National Comprehensive Cancer Network and the European Society for Medical Oncology remain guarded in their recommendation for adjuvant chemotherapy.

Another treatment strategy that has been employed in patients with locally advanced extremity STS is regional chemotherapy, namely, limb perfusion. More commonly used in the treatment of locally advanced melanoma, this involves placement of both intravenous and intraarterial catheters that are positioned within the affected limb proximal to the tumor. The combination of the limb vasculature and the intravascular catheters completes a circuit through which hyperthermic chemotherapy is circulated. A tourniquet proximal to the tips of the catheters separates the limb circulation from the systemic circulation to minimize systemic chemotherapy toxicity. The most common perfusion agents used are melphalan, tumor necrosis factor-α, and interferon-γ. Isolated limb perfusion is often combined with other modalities, namely, surgical resection. The technical demands and potential for local toxicities limit the application of this therapy. Currently, only one randomized trial has compared regional chemotherapy with other standard STS therapies. Overall, the published data are insufficient to conclusively establish the role of regional chemotherapy in the care of extremity STS.

The question as to what constitutes an adequate STS resection margin is complex, but the following is clear: the volume of tissue that is resected has clear implications as to the postoperative function of the limb, and a quantitative definition of an adequate surgical margin has never been defined in a randomized, prospective format. Whereas advances in rehabilitation medicine and prosthetic construction have significantly improved the functional capacity of patients who undergo extremity STS resection, the aforementioned data demonstrate that the goal of effective tumor extirpation with the smallest functional deficit is possible. Unlike in the melanoma literature, patients with extremity STS have never been randomized to compare surgical margin widths. Retrospectively, the local recurrence rate after resection of extremity STS with a microscopic margin of 1 cm or more is superior to when the margin is less than 1 cm.[24] However, in a different retrospective study, the only factor associated with an increased risk of local recurrence was tumor at the margin of resection.[25]

Because reresection has been associated with improvements in local recurrence, patients with positive margins should be offered re-resection to achieve margins of 1 cm.[26] In difficult anatomic situations, pursuit of clear surgical margins should be weighed against the natural history of extremity STS and the risk of an increased functional deficit. Even in the setting of multimodality therapy, the risk of distant metastasis consistently outweighs the risk of local recurrence in high-grade tumors.

The gross morphology of STS is such that during resection, the plane of least resistance is usually along a tumor pseudocapsule. The pseudocapsule is a characteristic plane of thickened tissue that radiographically and during intraoperative palpation gives the impression of representing the interface between tumor and normal tissue. Resections that proceed along the pseudocapsule plane are generally enucleations with involved margins. Traditionally, a 1- to 2-cm grossly negative margin beyond the pseudocapsule is recommended, but this may be difficult or impossible to achieve in certain anatomic sites and may be unnecessary in dealing with low-grade tumors. Neoadjuvant therapy may be associated with formation of a more robust tumor pseudocapsule populated by fewer tumor cells.[27] Ultimately, as discussed in the section on retroperitoneal sarcoma, the resection margin is only as good as the closest margin in any region of the tumor, so that extending resections to increase morbidity in one region is not necessary if a closer margin exists in another region.

STS tumors tend to metastasize hematogenously principally not only to the lungs but also to the liver and bone. Tumor grade is the most important predictor of metastasis, with a 43% rate of metastasis-free survival in patients with high-grade tumors.[28] Other important predictors of metastasis include tumor size, bone or neurovascular involvement, and tumor depth (superficial vs. deep). The prevalence of pulmonary metastases among patients previously treated for extremity STS is approximately 19%. Isolated pulmonary metastases should be resected whenever feasible.[29] A prolonged disease-free interval between initial STS treatment and development of lung metastasis is generally a favorable prognostic factor. In the absence of effective systemic therapies, repeated pulmonary metastasectomy is also a consideration. Patients who are not candidates for metastasectomy should be evaluated for ablative or systemic therapies. Many types of STS are relatively chemoresistant; notable exceptions include angiosarcoma and synovial sarcoma. Typical agents for metastatic STS include doxorubicin, dacarbazine, ifosfamide, gemcitabine, docetaxel, eribulin, pazopanib, regorafenib, and olaratumab.

Malignant Peripheral Nerve Sheath Tumors

MPNSTs occur in roughly equal frequency sporadically and as part of NF1. These tumors are the malignant form of the benign schwannoma. Although they arise from a peripheral nerve or the nerve sheath, they are often painless on presentation. The most common age at presentation is 20 to 50 years. Historically, other names have been applied to MPNST, such as malignant schwannoma, neurogenic sarcoma, and neurofibrosarcoma. The term *malignant schwannoma* is avoided because not all MPNSTs actually arise from Schwann cells. These are generally aggressive tumors; recent large series have shown a local recurrence rate of about 20% and a 10-year disease-specific survival of more than 40%. The key prognostic factors include tumor size at presentation and tumor grade. There is no consensus in the literature as to whether MPNST in the setting of NF1 carries a worse prognosis than spontaneous cases. Treatment of these tumors is similar to that of other STS subtypes, with a focus on margin-negative resection. Although it has not been studied prospectively in the MPNST population, most retrospective reports agree that adjuvant radiation therapy is indicated to decrease the rate of local recurrence in extremity and superficial trunk lesions.

Desmoid Tumor

Desmoid tumors, also known as aggressive fibromatosis, are an uncommon group of fibroblastic tumors that have a curious natural history in that distant metastases are extremely rare. Approximately 75% to 85% of cases arise sporadically; the others are related to FAP. Among the sporadic cases, recent pregnancy and antecedent trauma are recognized associations. These tumors are two to three times more common in women than in men and are most commonly diagnosed in patients aged 30 to 40 years. Approximately 20% of FAP patients develop desmoid tumors, and a common presentation involves a desmoid at the prior colectomy scar. Desmoid tumors are usually preceded by colonic polyposis in FAP patients and represent the second leading cause of death in FAP patients. A detailed family history should be obtained from patients presenting with desmoid tumors to rule out unappreciated FAP, and consideration should also be given to screening colonoscopy.

The molecular underpinnings of desmoids, regardless of sporadic or syndromic association, are related to the Wingless and Int-1 (WNT) signaling pathway. In sporadic cases, *CTNNB1* mutations result in the expression of a stabilized form of β-catenin, which ultimately accumulates and is transported to the nucleus, where it exerts its proliferative effects through activation of transcription factors. In the setting of FAP, *APC* mutations also cause β-catenin stabilization, which also activates nuclear transcription and cellular proliferation. Specific *APC* codon mutations appear to confer a higher desmoid risk than other codon mutations.

Clinically, the most common areas of origin include the extremity, intraperitoneal, abdominal wall, and chest wall. Affected patients may present with a painful versus asymptomatic firm mass, bowel obstruction, or bowel ischemia. Desmoid tumors are usually slow-growing but on occasion do grow aggressively. On radiographic evaluation, these tumors are generally homogeneous and solid in appearance. They may have either a distinct or an infiltrating boundary. Both CT scan and MRI are useful imaging modalities. Especially in sporadic cases, desmoid tumors are indistinguishable from a variety of other STS subtypes based on imaging alone. Core needle biopsy is indicated in situations in which treatment recommendations will be altered on the basis of tumor histology.

Treatment of these tumors can be challenging. When tumors are large or infiltrating crucial anatomic structures, surgical resection with widely negative margins may not be possible. Even when the tumors are adequately resected, especially in the FAP population, desmoid tumors show a high likelihood of local recurrence. These observations have prompted various recommendations for consideration of active surveillance for desmoid tumors rather than reflexive resection on diagnosis. In addition, the role of radiation may be appropriate, especially in recurrent extremity tumors. When considering that many desmoids are indolent and show very little growth after presentation and that resection may mandate significant functional deficits, an active surveillance strategy may be appropriate for selected patients. A small German trial enrolled 38 patients with progressive desmoid tumors and showed that 65% of patients treated with imatinib achieved progression arrest after 6 months, and 45%, after 24 months.[30]

Angiosarcoma

Angiosarcoma is a malignant tumor that arises from the endothelial lining of blood vessels and therefore can arise from almost any site. Overall, it accounts for 2% of all STS, but approximately 40% of all angiosarcomas are radiation associated.[3] In decreasing order of frequency, the most important primary sites are the trunk, head, and neck (particularly the scalp) and the viscera. Within the head and neck, the scalp is often the site of angiosarcoma origin. Angiosarcoma typically is diagnosed in the seventh and eighth decades. Although most angiosarcoma is sporadic, risk factors include previous therapeutic radiation exposure and lymphedema (see previous section). Angiosarcoma, in contrast to other STS, does have a higher frequency of involved regional lymph nodes. Approximately 20% of patients present with metastasis, most frequently to the lung.[31] On histologic evaluation, these tumors range from extremely well differentiated, mimicking hemangioma, to very poorly differentiated. Consistent with this, there is a wide variety of cytogenetic changes. On immunohistochemical examination, CD31 and FLI-1 are the most consistent markers.

The primary therapy for these lesions is surgical resection with negative margins. On microscopic examination, these tumors often infiltrate well beyond the area of gross involvement. For patients with head and neck angiosarcoma, this can present a reconstructive challenge. Angiosarcoma that arises within the breast after breast-conserving therapy is managed with mastectomy. Even after surgical resection, the outcome is poor, with a 5-year disease-specific survival of 53%.[31] In the cohort with resectable disease, tumor size larger than 5 cm and histologic evidence of an epithelioid component are indicators of poor prognosis. After resection, distant failure predominates over local failure, although both are common. These tumors are often locally advanced and unresectable at presentation; fortunately, these tumors are responsive to chemotherapy and radiation therapy, and a neoadjuvant approach may be feasible.

The median survival of stage IV angiosarcoma is 8 to 12 months. Unlike other STS, metastatic angiosarcoma may be manifested with hemopneumothorax. Breast angiosarcoma may metastasize to the liver. The most typical agents employed in the unresectable or metastatic setting include paclitaxel and doxorubicin, followed by radiation therapy, except perhaps in patients whose tumor was incited by previous radiation therapy. A host of ongoing trials including angiosarcoma patients are underway that are exploring the utility of a range of agents including tyrosine kinase inhibitors and combination therapy of angiogenesis inhibitors with cytotoxic agents (https://clinicaltrials.gov/).

Dermatofibrosarcoma Protuberans

DFSP is an uncommon STS that affects approximately 1 in 4.2 million patients in the United States. This tumor affects men and women equally and appears to be more common in African American patients than in whites. The typical range of presentation is between the fourth and seventh decades. The trunk, upper extremity, and lower extremity are equally frequent sites of DFSP, followed by the head and neck. On physical examination, these are firm, indurated nodules that are reddish or brown in appearance. On histologic evaluation, DFSP is a dermal or subdermal tumor without penetration into the epidermis. Cytogenetically, the majority of DFSP displays the t(17;22)(q22;q13) translocation, which fuses the *COL1A1* and platelet-derived growth factor B genes and accounts for its platelet-derived growth factor B overexpression. In difficult cases, this gene fusion can be detected by fluorescence in situ hybridization. Because of its somewhat bland visual appearance and the lack of associated pain, it can often be large at presentation, having been mistaken for a hypertrophic scar or a keloid.

DFSP frequently recurs locally, and consequently, the treatment is surgical resection with wide margins. As is true with most STS, there are no well-designed clinical trials to define an adequate margin. Recurrence can be successfully treated with resection. The 5-year survival is 99.2%. DFSP rarely metastasizes, but when it does, it often implies degeneration to fibrosarcoma. Because of the platelet-derived growth factor B upregulation, patients with unresectable disease may be treated with neoadjuvant imatinib.

RETROPERITONEAL AND VISCERAL SARCOMA

Retroperitoneal sarcoma represents approximately 15% of all STS. The sequestered location of the retroperitoneum probably accounts for the fact that the average tumor size at presentation is 15 cm.[32] The most frequent retroperitoneal sarcoma subtypes are liposarcoma, leiomyosarcoma, and MFH undifferentiated pleomorphic sarcoma. The predominant intraperitoneal STS subtypes are GIST and leiomyosarcoma, which are discussed separately. The average age at presentation is 54 years, and there is an equal male-to-female distribution. In most series, the overall survival of patients presenting with retroperitoneal sarcoma is 33% to 39%. Even after optimal surgical resection, at least 70% of patients will relapse. In one large retrospective series, approximately 12% of patients presented with metastatic disease, predominantly pulmonary or hepatic.

The presentation of retroperitoneal sarcoma is variable, depending on the size and location of the tumor. Some are asymptomatic and incidentally discovered. Symptomatic tumors may be manifested with abdominal pain, weight loss, early satiety, nausea, emesis, back or flank pain, paresthesias, and weakness. CT and MRI are widely used for the evaluation of retroperitoneal sarcoma because of their excellent spatial resolution and reproducible axial image acquisition. The advantages of CT scan include rapid image acquisition, nearly universal availability, and a concise image set that can be more intuitive for the nonradiologist to interpret. The advantages of MRI include a wider range of soft tissue differentiation, but the disadvantages include an increased susceptibility to claustrophobia and motion artifact, the more limited availability, and a greater number of implant-related contraindications compared with CT scan. These modalities can be complementary, and at times, both provide useful information. The patient must be carefully evaluated along with the imaging studies to verify that the retroperitoneal mass does not represent an unappreciated lymphoma, germ cell tumor, or metastasis from another primary tumor as the management of these tumors is quite different from that of retroperitoneal sarcoma.

A number of consensus guidelines strongly recommend performing a preoperative biopsy, but as previously discussed with extremity STS, biopsy for retroperitoneal sarcoma is not mandatory and has drawbacks in certain situations. By definition, a surgical biopsy ruptures the tumor, seeding the operative field and potentially reducing the possibility of a margin-negative resection. Preoperative biopsy can be particularly misleading in patients with large tumors as the biopsy is susceptible to a significant degree of sampling bias. This sampling bias can provide inappropriately reassuring information. The preoperative CT scan often contains enough information to proceed with treatment without a preoperative biopsy as long as the other basic considerations in the differential diagnosis are considered excluded. This includes lymphoma, germ cell tumors, and other metastatic disease (see Box 32.1). In a retrospective study from a large, single, tertiary care institution, the initial staging CT scan was sufficient in assessing the need for preoperative biopsy and assigning a treatment approach for those tumors for which biopsy is not indicated; this approach is discussed in greater detail in the lipomatous tumor section.[10] For this reason, if preoperative biopsy is obtained from a heterogeneous mass, the specimen should be obtained from the most concerning region under image guidance.

When possible, treatment should proceed with a complete gross resection. In the retroperitoneal sarcoma literature, the concept of margin status is different from that for extremity STS. Because extremity STS tumors are usually smaller than retroperitoneal sarcoma tumors, microscopic evaluation of the entire surgical specimen margin is often feasible. Given the much larger tumor dimensions of most retroperitoneal sarcomas, it is not practical and often impossible to microscopically evaluate 100% of the surgical specimen margin surface area. Consequently, most of the retroperitoneal sarcoma literature refers to complete gross resection. In one large series, complete gross resection was achieved in 80% of initial sarcoma resections, 57% of operations for first recurrence, 33% of operations at second recurrence, and 14% of operations at third recurrence. In 75% of patients, achieving complete gross resection may mean resecting contiguous or inseparable adjacent organs, such as the kidney, bowel, or pancreas and vascular structures. Resection requiring pancreaticoduodenectomy, major vascular resection, or splenectomy was more likely to result in a major postoperative complication, but a major postoperative complication does not appear to adversely affect long-term survival or recurrence.[33]

Predicting histologic invasion on the basis of gross intraoperative findings can be inaccurate. Before the era of modern CT technology, patients who underwent nephrectomy because of intraoperative evidence of suspected involvement during retroperitoneal sarcoma resection were further evaluated for histologic evidence of sarcoma invasion. In 73% of cases, the nephrectomy specimen did not contain STS. Improvements in the quality of preoperative imaging probably decrease the rate of adjacent organ resection based solely on intraoperative suspicion. As expected, predictors of poor prognosis include gross residual disease after resection, unresectable disease (either metastatic or locally advanced), and high tumor grade. Patients with a complete gross resection have a median survival of 103 months compared with 18 months for patients with incomplete resections. Even with optimal chemotherapy and radiation therapy, the median survival of patients with unresectable disease is 10 months.[34] Patients who undergo complete resection should undergo active surveillance, as the risk of local recurrence and distant metastasis after 5 years is 23% and 21%, respectively. Although palliative resection may often be the only meaningful option in patients who develop recurrence, reresection of the recurrent disease was of limited value, resulting in 17% 3-year disease-free survival.[35]

In contrast to extremity sarcoma, the role of multimodality therapy is more controversial in retroperitoneal sarcoma. Given the success of adjuvant radiation in extremity STS, this approach has been applied to retroperitoneal sarcoma, but with fewer randomized data to support its efficacy. The 60- to 70-Gy dose that is considered sarcoma lethal and typically used for extremity STS is not feasible in the adjuvant setting for retroperitoneal sarcoma because of bowel toxicity. Even dose reduction to 50 to 55 Gy results in significant enteritis. These tolerability issues prompted consideration of neoadjuvant radiation for retroperitoneal sarcoma. An advantage of neoadjuvant radiation is that the in situ tumor displaces the bowel anteriorly, thus facilitating the delivery of a higher radiation dose posteriorly, which is the most likely site of a positive histologic margin (Fig. 32.6). This approach delivers 45 Gy to the planned target volume, and the projected at-risk margins are boosted up to 65 Gy. Two separate studies have demonstrated that the neoadjuvant approach is well tolerated and that long- and short-term oncologic outcomes are favorable compared with historical cohorts treated with resection alone.[36,37]

For patients with metastatic retroperitoneal sarcoma, there are few effective chemotherapeutic options. Single or combination therapy with anthracyclines can be used as first-line therapy. A second-line regimen is gemcitabine and docetaxel. Thus far, the experience with immunotherapy agents in STS patients has been disappointing. One encouraging finding is that patients with undifferentiated pleomorphic sarcoma or dedifferentiated liposarcoma have a somewhat more promising objective response rate than those with other STS subtypes when treated with pembrolizumab, a programmed death-1 inhibitor.[38] In an open-label phase 2 trial, combined programmed death-1 inhibitor and cytotoxic T-lymphocyte (CTLA-4) inhibition showed very poor response rates in patients with metastatic sarcoma.[39] Novel agents undergoing further study include trabectedin, tyrosine kinase inhibitors, MDM2 antagonists, peroxisome proliferator-activated receptor gamma agonists, and CDK4 antagonists.

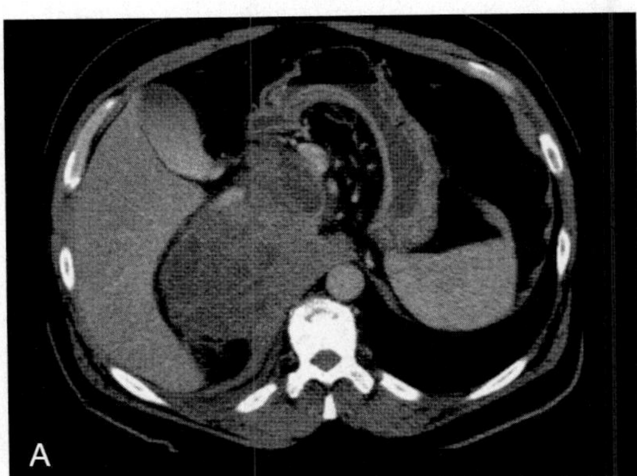

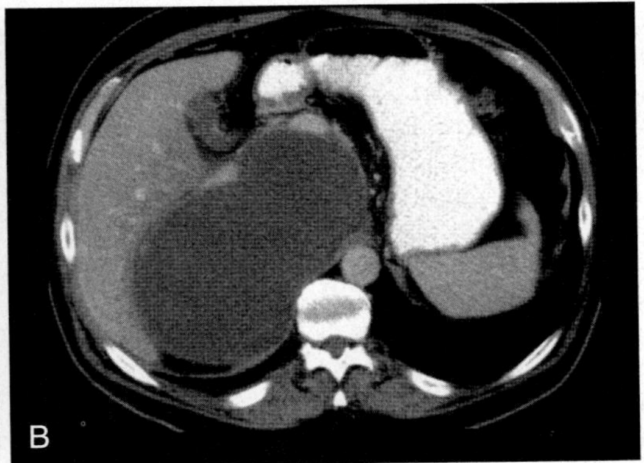

FIG. 32.6 Liquefaction of a high-grade retroperitoneal sarcoma before (A) and after (B) administration of 60-Gy preoperative radiation therapy. The tumor was subsequently resected with negative surgical margins, and no viable tumor was histologically identifiable.

Gastrointestinal Stromal Tumor

GIST is the most common variety of visceral STS. These tumors are believed to originate from the interstitial cells of Cajal within the gastrointestinal myenteric plexus and emanate from nearly any part of the alimentary tract, from esophagus to anus. The most prevalent GIST sites are the stomach, the small bowel, and the rectum. Cajal cells are thought to function as pacemaker cells in the viscera, mediating contractions. Cajal cells and GIST share common markers for CD117 and a calcium-activated chloride channel called DOG1. CD117 is another name for the *KIT* gene, which codes for a tyrosine kinase transmembrane receptor called c-kit. These molecular descriptions led to dramatic refinements in the diagnosis and treatment of patients with GIST. In morphologic appearance, GIST is classically a spindle cell neoplasm of smooth muscle origin. Although these tumors were previously described as leiomyoma or leiomyosarcoma, GISTs are differentiated on the basis of CD34, CD117, and DOG1 expression and the lack of smooth muscle staining.

The c-kit receptor is a proto-oncogene that belongs to the platelet-derived growth factor receptor (PDGFR) superfamily. The natural c-kit ligand is a stem cell factor, and its binding causes tyrosine kinase receptor homodimerization, autophosphorylation, and activation of multiple pathways, including RAS, RAF, MAPK, AKT, and STAT3. Certain mutations of the c-kit receptor confer constitutive activation of the receptor, which ultimately results in cellular proliferation. The other relevant gene, also found on chromosome 4, that bears striking similarity to c-kit is the PDGFRα. Overall, about 70% of GISTs have *KIT* gene mutations, approximately 7% have *PDGFRα* mutations, and 15% have wild-type *KIT* and *PDGFRα* genotypes. These GISTs are characterized by a number of other mutations affecting succinate dehydrogenase *(SDH)*, *BRAF*, *KRAS*, and *NF1*. *SDH* mutations are related to GIST in patients affected by the Carney-Stratakis syndrome, and *NF1* mutations drive GIST formation in patients with NF1.

The clinical presentation of these tumors is variable, ranging from incidental to symptomatic with respect to pain, nausea, vomiting, or, more rarely, gastrointestinal blood loss. On endoscopic examination, GIST usually appears as a smooth submucosal tumor that extrinsically impinges on the visceral lumen as opposed to an ulcerated mucosal mass. The endoscopic differential diagnosis of an intramural visceral mass includes GIST, neuroendocrine tumor, intramural lipoma, and lymphoma. Some GISTs are serosally pedunculated and do not contribute to intestinal obstruction. CT imaging shows that these tumors are well encapsulated and generally have heterogeneous contrast enhancement because of regions of necrosis within the tumor. Metastasis is not rare, but affected sites include the liver and peritoneal surface. The majority of GISTs are sporadic, but there are notable examples of syndromic involvement. These include NF1, germline SDH mutations, the Carney-Stratakis syndrome, von Hippel-Lindau disease, and other minor familial GIST syndromes.

Because these are submucosal tumors, endoscopic forceps biopsies are often nondiagnostic. Tumors situated between the ligament of Treitz and the ileocecal valve can be localized by double-balloon enteroscopy or capsule endoscopy. Blood loss related to GIST may indicate that the tumor has ulcerated through the mucosa. An endoscopic ultrasound-guided needle biopsy generally shows a spindle cell neoplasm; if sufficient tissue is available, this can be submitted for CD117 evaluation. Preoperative biopsy for suspected GIST is not mandatory, but preoperative histologic verification of GIST obviates the need for empirical lymphadenectomy at the time of resection, which would be crucial for neuroendocrine tumor or intestinal adenocarcinoma. Appropriate preoperative staging for GIST includes a contrast-enhanced CT scan of the chest, abdomen, and pelvis. Localized lesions are taken to the operating room for resection with grossly negative surgical margins. Obtaining wide surgical margins has not been demonstrated to improve local recurrence rates or overall survival. Given the rarity of lymph node involvement, lymphadenectomy is not mandatory for GIST. Care should be taken not to compromise the capsule of the tumor as rupture can seed the exposed tissues and adversely affect the prognosis of the patient. As long as the risk of tumor rupture is not elevated, consideration of minimally invasive surgical resection techniques is appropriate and may accelerate the recovery. The operative note should clearly document the integrity of the tumor capsule as it can profoundly affect recommendations for adjuvant therapy.

Ideally, the pathology report follows a synoptic guideline to ensure that all relevant parameters are communicated to the multidisciplinary team. The key parameters include the tumor site organ of origin, tumor size, tumor focality, mitotic rate, immunohistochemical CD117 status, margin status, and results of molecular genetic studies, if performed. The mitotic rate is defined as the total count of mitoses per 5 mm^2 on the glass slide section and is reported in the most proliferative area of the tumor. In GISTs, the mitotic rate parameter is synonymous with the tumor grade that is included with most other STS subtypes. Entities that can mimic GIST microscopically include melanoma, paraganglioma, neuroendocrine tumors, and nerve sheath tumors.

Distinct from other STS subtypes, the AJCC eighth edition staging system has a schema that separates GISTs based on anatomic site of origin; gastric and omental tumors versus nongastric tumors (Tables 32.4 to 32.6). The anatomic site of origin

TABLE 32.4 American Joint Committee on Cancer staging for gastrointestinal stromal tumor.

Primary Tumor (T)	
TX	Primary tumor cannot be assessed
T0	No evidence for primary tumor
T1	Tumor 2 cm or less
T2	Tumor >2 cm, ≤5 cm
T3	Tumor >5 cm, ≤10 cm
T4	Tumor >10 cm
Regional Lymph Nodes (N)	
N0	No regional lymph node metastasis
N1	Regional lymph node metastasis
Distant Metastasis (M)	
M0	No distant metastasis
M1	Distant metastasis
Histologic Grade (G)	
GX	Grade cannot be assessed
G1	Low grade; mitotic rate ≤5 per 5 mm^2
G2	High grade; mitotic rate >5 per 5 mm^2

From Amin MB, Edge SB, Greene FL, et al. *AJCC Cancer Staging Manual.* 8th ed. New York: Springer; 2017.

TABLE 32.5 Anatomic stage and prognostic groups for gastric and omental gastrointestinal stromal tumor.

GROUP	T	N	M	GRADE
Stage IA	T1 or T2	N0	M0	Low
Stage IB	T3	N0	M0	Low
Stage II	T1	N0	M0	High
	T2	N0	M0	High
	T4	N0	M0	Low
Stage IIIA	T3	N0	M0	High
Stage IIIB	T4	N0	M0	High
Stage IV	Any T	N1	M0	Any rate
	Any T	Any N	M1	Any rate

From Amin MB, Edge SB, Greene FL, et al. *AJCC Cancer Staging Manual*. 8th ed. New York: Springer; 2017.

TABLE 32.6 Anatomic stage and prognostic groups for nongastric* gastrointestinal stromal tumor.

GROUP	T	N	M	GRADE
Stage IA	T1 or T2	N0	M0	Low
Stage II	T3	N0	M0	Low
Stage IIIA	T1	N0	M0	High
	T4	N0	M0	Low
Stage IIIB	T2	N0	M0	High
	T3	N0	M0	High
	T4	N0	M0	High
Stage IV	Any T	N1	M0	Any rate
	Any T	Any N	M1	Any rate

From Amin MB, Edge SB, Greene FL, et al. *AJCC Cancer Staging Manual*. 8th ed. New York: Springer; 2017.
*Nongastric includes small bowel, colorectal, esophageal, mesentery, and peritoneal.

is important from a surgical planning standpoint, and from a prognostic standpoint. In order of decreasing prognosis are the following sites of tumor origin: gastric, jejunal/ileal, and colorectal GIST. A number of tools available to predict prognosis after resection can then be used on the basis of these pathologic and clinical parameters. The Memorial Sloan-Kettering Cancer Center (MSKCC) group developed a nomogram based on the size of the resected GIST, the mitotic rate, and the anatomic site of origin, which is validated to predict the probabilities of 2- and 5-year recurrence-free survival.[37] The nomogram was developed using data from 127 patients treated at MSKCC and then validated in two independent GIST populations from other institutions. The target population of this nomogram is patients undergoing complete GIST resection who did not receive adjuvant therapy. Another prognostic tool is the Armed Forces Institute of Pathology criteria, designed to predict the risk of progressive disease after resection and based on data from more than 1900 patients with resected GIST who also did not receive adjuvant therapy. Inputs into this schema include mitotic rate, size, and anatomic site of origin. This series has not been validated to the same degree as the MSKCC nomogram but was developed using a more robust sample size. The modified NIH criteria were established on the basis of several data sets, including the Armed Forces Institute of Pathology criteria, and have subsequently been validated (Table 32.7).[40,41]

TABLE 32.7 Assessing the prognosis of resected gastrointestinal stromal tumor.

TUMOR SIZE	MITOTIC RATE (MITOSES/ MM^2)	RISK OF TUMOR PROGRESSION, WITHOUT ADJUVANT THERAPY: GASTRIC ORIGIN	SMALL BOWEL ORIGIN
≤2 cm	≤5	0%	0%
	>5	0%*	50%*
>2 cm, ≤5 cm	≤5	1.9%	4.3%
	>5	16%	73%
>5 cm, ≤10 cm	≤5	3.6%	24%
	>5	55%	85%
>10 cm	≤5	12%	52%
	>5	86%	90%

Adapted from Miettinen M, Lasota J. Gastrointestinal stromal tumors: review on morphology, molecular pathology, prognosis, and differential diagnosis. *Arch Pathol Lab Med.* 2006;130:1466–1478.
*These values are based on small sample sizes, which limits their clinical applicability.

As predictors of outcome after surgical resection, these risk assessment tools are routinely used to also assess the need for adjuvant therapy. Although none of these risk assessment tools includes it as an input parameter, the success of adjuvant therapy is dependent on the GIST molecular phenotype. Specific *KIT* mutations differentially affect long-term prognosis and response to therapy. The specific *KIT* exon in which the GIST mutation resides affects the molecular and clinical phenotype. For example, a *KIT* mutation in exon 13 resides within the tyrosine kinase domain and confers susceptibility to imatinib therapy. Exon 9 mutations correspond to the extracellular domain of the c-kit receptor, are observed principally in small bowel or colon GIST, and are less sensitive to imatinib. Routine genetic analysis at GIST diagnosis to determine the precise mutated exon is strongly recommended by consensus guidelines as this information may alter treatment recommendations and patient outcome.[42]

Systemic therapy is indicated for adjuvant therapy after GIST resection, for the treatment of metastatic GIST, and for the neoadjuvant therapy of unresectable or locally advanced tumors. Imatinib, the best studied of these systemic agents, is an oral tyrosine kinase inhibitor of c-kit. In general, the presence of a *KIT* mutation is highly associated with response to this oral medication. Again, because of the similarities to the c-kit and *PDGFRαs*, some patients with wild-type *KIT* are sensitive to imatinib. Dasatinib was associated with progression-free survival in patients with imatinib-resistant GIST, including the PDGFRα D842V mutation.[43] Other available agents capable of GIST-related tyrosine kinase inhibition include sunitinib and regorafenib. The third major molecular GIST group is characterized by *SDH* mutations. Patients with these mutations are generally younger, have multiple gastric GISTs, and have a poor response to imatinib. Although it is not universally accepted as standard of care, advanced molecular analysis should be considered for all patients. This may affect the choice and dose of tyrosine kinase inhibitor for patients with *KIT* or *PDGFRα* mutations and in patients with wild-type *KIT* and *PDGFRα* GISTs; further molecular evaluation may identify clinically relevant *SDH* or *BRAF* mutations.

Imatinib was first developed to treat Philadelphia chromosome–positive chronic myelogenous leukemia. Soon after, its efficacy was demonstrated in the setting of metastatic GIST, adjuvant therapy for resected GIST, and neoadjuvant therapy for unresectable GIST. Imatinib was demonstrated to be associated with a dramatic improvement in the median overall survival of metastatic GIST from 20 months to 57 months.[44] In the adjuvant setting after complete surgical resection, two randomized studies have demonstrated improved disease-free recurrence.[45,46] Because these trials vary in their clinicopathologic inclusion criteria and study design, there remains debate as to which patients should receive imatinib and for what duration.

The ACOSOG Z9001 was a double-blind trial that randomized patients with a grossly negative GIST resection to receive imatinib versus placebo for 1 year. All tumors were larger than 3 cm, and all were c-kit positive by immunohistochemistry. One year of adjuvant imatinib was associated with a statistically significant improvement in the recurrence-free survival versus placebo (98% vs. 83%, respectively).[45] A subsequent Z9001 follow-up study demonstrated a persistent improvement in recurrence-free survival but did not demonstrate any improvement in overall survival.[47] In a separate trial, patients were randomized to 1 versus 3 years of adjuvant imatinib after resection of c-kit–positive GIST. This trial stipulated that patients must have high-risk disease per the NIH consensus criteria. The 3-year duration of therapy was associated with improvements not only in recurrence-free survival but also in overall survival.

Joensuu and colleagues[48] published the first data describing the parameters associated with tumor recurrence after resection in patients already treated with adjuvant imatinib. Data sets from two of the aforementioned three randomized trials were used to construct and to validate a risk stratification score. Two such scores were developed. The five-parameter score includes mitotic count, organ of origin, size, tumor rupture, and duration of imatinib therapy; the two-parameter score includes mitotic count and organ of origin. These data support a 3-year duration of imatinib therapy and indicate that nongastric organ of origin and a high mitotic count adversely affect recurrence-free survival. Because the previous risk assessment schemas were developed using patient cohorts who had never been treated with adjuvant imatinib, this stratification score may prove to be clinically relevant. More recently, a single arm, phase 2 clinical trial (Postresection Evaluation of Recurrence-free Survival for Gastrointestinal Stromal Tumors with 5 Years of Adjuvant Imatinib [PERSIST-5]) showed that of the 46 patients who completed 5 years of adjuvant imatinib, no patient with sensitive mutations experienced tumor recurrence.[49]

Leiomyosarcoma

Leiomyosarcoma is a malignant smooth muscle tumor that can originate from virtually any part of the body. The most common sites affected are the retroperitoneum and the peritoneal cavity, namely, the uterus; about 25% rise from the trunk and extremities. Overall, after liposarcoma, leiomyosarcoma is the second most frequent STS subtype.[1] The peak incidence of leiomyosarcoma is in the sixth and seventh decades. Retroperitoneal and uterine leiomyosarcoma is more common in women, but there is a male predominance in other leiomyosarcoma sites. Predisposing risk factors for leiomyosarcoma include prior radiation exposure and immunosuppression combined with Epstein-Barr virus–related tumor promotion. Leiomyosarcoma does not arise from a degenerated leiomyoma, a common benign soft tissue tumor.

Leiomyosarcoma is generally a heterogeneous, well-circumscribed tumor with an often cystic or necrotic central area. This tumor stains positive for desmin and smooth muscle actin. It has a wide variety of cytogenetic aberrations but no reliable or pathognomonic markers. Before the description of *KIT* mutations, tumors that are now appreciated to represent GIST were described as leiomyosarcoma.

First-line therapy for leiomyosarcoma is surgical resection with negative margins. For uterine leiomyosarcoma, a total abdominal hysterectomy and bilateral oophorectomy is indicated. Resection of tumors that invade or are intimately associated with the inferior vena cava (IVC) require special planning. Depending on the size and position of the tumor, an approach including neoadjuvant radiation therapy may be a consideration. The intraoperative options include tumor resection with IVC ligation, patching of the IVC, and interposition graft of the IVC. Tumors involving the IVC typically have a great deal of collateralization already in place. For a tumor that requires segmental resection of the infrahepatic IVC, if the collaterals can be preserved, ligation without reconstruction may be an acceptable maneuver as postoperative lower extremity edema is well tolerated. Because of the rarity of IVC leiomyosarcoma, a future randomized trial further evaluating these maneuvers is unlikely.

Regardless of the organ of origin, adjuvant therapy is not currently recommended, although this is the subject of ongoing trials, especially for uterine leiomyosarcoma. Affecting 44% of patients, metastasis is usually hematogenous in nature, mainly to the lung and liver. Historically, doxorubicin, ifosfamide, docetaxel, and gemcitabine have been used in the metastatic setting but recently olaratumab with doxorubicin was approved for advanced, unresectable STS. Olaratumab is a recombinant human monoclonal antibody that binds PDGFRα. In combination with doxorubicin, it showed an improvement in overall and progression-free survival for patients with advanced, unresectable STS. In subgroup analysis, the improvement in survival was greater for patients with leiomyosarcoma versus other histologic subtypes.[50]

SUMMARY

STS is a fascinating aspect of surgical oncology that requires an understanding of multiple tumor types. To effectively treat STS patients, the surgeon must have a strong understanding of tumor biology, the physiologic consequences of various resection strategies, and the ability to effectively work within the context of a multidisciplinary oncology team. Recent discoveries relating to the molecular and genetic underpinnings demonstrate that, although they are rare, these tumors may offer opportunities in the development of novel targeted therapies.

SELECTED REFERENCES

Anya DA, Lahat G, Wang X, et al. Postoperative nomogram for survival of patients with retroperitoneal sarcoma treated with curative intent. *Ann Oncol.* 2010;21:397–402.

A thoughtful, pragmatic, and easily applicable approach to the management of retroperitoneal sarcomas.

Brennan MF, Antonescu CR, Moraco N, et al. Lessons learned from the study of 10,000 patients with soft tissue sarcoma. *Ann Surg.* 2014;260:416–421; discussion 421–422.

The largest surgical series of soft tissue sarcoma demonstrates a number of key concepts that relate to natural history and management of patients with this disease.

Fletcher CD, Gustafson P, Rydholm A, et al. Clinicopathologic re-evaluation of 100 malignant fibrous histiocytomas: prognostic relevance of subclassification. *J Clin Oncol.* 2001;19:3045–3050.

This illustrates the concept that the historical term malignant fibrous histiocytoma is pathologically imprecise and fails to accurately predict outcome.

Heslin MJ, Lewis JJ, Nadler E, et al. Prognostic factors associated with long-term survival for retroperitoneal sarcoma: implications for management. *J Clin Oncol.* 1997;15:2832–2839.

An important manuscript demonstrating the natural history of patients undergoing resection for retroperitoneal sarcoma.

Joensuu H, Eriksson M, Hall KS, et al. Risk factors for gastrointestinal stromal tumor recurrence in patients treated with adjuvant imatinib. *Cancer.* 2014;120:2325–2333.

Whereas most retrospective reviews focus on gastrointestinal stromal tumor (GIST) prognosis after resection alone, this paper describes a methodology to stratify the risk of GIST recurrence in patients treated with adjuvant imatinib.

Joensuu H, Eriksson M, Sundby Hall K, et al. One vs three years of adjuvant imatinib for operable gastrointestinal stromal tumor: a randomized trial. *JAMA.* 2012;307:1265–1272.

In demonstrating superior recurrence-free and overall survival, this trial established the duration of adjuvant imatinib for patients with a high risk for gastrointestinal stromal tumor following resection.

O'Sullivan B, Davis AM, Turcotte R, et al. Preoperative versus postoperative radiotherapy in soft-tissue sarcoma of the limbs: a randomised trial. *Lancet.* 2002;359:2235–2241.

The National Cancer Institute of Canada/Canadian Sarcoma Group SR2 clinical trial represents the only prospective randomized comparison of preoperative versus postoperative radiation therapy for extremity sarcoma.

Pisters PW, Pollock RE, Lewis VO, et al. Long-term results of prospective trial of surgery alone with selective use of radiation for patients with T1 extremity and trunk soft tissue sarcomas. *Ann Surg.* 2007;246:675–681.

Compelling data supporting the selective use of adjuvant radiation for early-stage soft tissue sarcoma.

Rosenberg SA, Tepper J, Glatstein E, et al. The treatment of soft-tissue sarcomas of the extremities: prospective randomized evaluations of (1) limb-sparing surgery plus radiation therapy compared with amputation and (2) the role of adjuvant chemotherapy. *Ann Surg.* 1982;196:305–315.

This phase 3 National Cancer Institute (NCI) study paved the way for a generation of studies examining the role for limb-sparing surgery in the setting of multimodal therapy.

Taylor BS, Barretina J, Maki RG, et al. Advances in sarcoma genomics and new therapeutic targets. *Nat Rev Cancer.* 2011;11:541–557.

A unique perspective on the taxonomy and classification of soft tissue sarcoma, driven by the molecular genetics of this diverse tumor family.

van Vliet M, Kliffen M, Krestin GP, et al. Soft tissue sarcomas at a glance: clinical, histological, and MR imaging features of malignant extremity soft tissue tumors. *Eur Radiol.* 2009;19:1499–1511.

This manuscript is a concise atlas of soft tissue sarcoma that correlates the natural history of the disease to the imaging and histologic characteristics.

REFERENCES

1. Brennan MF, Antonescu CR, Moraco N, et al. Lessons learned from the study of 10,000 patients with soft tissue sarcoma. *Ann Surg.* 2014;260:416–421; discussion 421–412.
2. Ballinger ML, Goode DL, Ray-Coquard I, et al. Monogenic and polygenic determinants of sarcoma risk: an international genetic study. *Lancet Oncol.* 2016;17:1261–1271.
3. Gladdy RA, Qin LX, Moraco N, et al. Do radiation-associated soft tissue sarcomas have the same prognosis as sporadic soft tissue sarcomas? *J Clin Oncol.* 2010;28:2064–2069.
4. Italiano A, Di Mauro I, Rapp J, et al. Clinical effect of molecular methods in sarcoma diagnosis (GENSARC): a prospective, multicentre, observational study. *Lancet Oncol.* 2016;17:532–538.
5. Amin MB, Edge SB, Greene FL, et al. *AJCC Cancer Staging Manual.* 8th ed. New York: Springer; 2017.
6. Anaya DA, Lahat G, Wang X, et al. Establishing prognosis in retroperitoneal sarcoma: a new histology-based paradigm. *Ann Surg Oncol.* 2009;16:667–675.
7. Lahat G, Anaya DA, Wang X, et al. Resectable well-differentiated versus dedifferentiated liposarcomas: two different diseases possibly requiring different treatment approaches. *Ann Surg Oncol.* 2008;15:1585–1593.
8. Johnson AC, Ethun CG, Liu Y, et al. A novel, simplified, externally validated staging system for truncal/extremity soft tissue sarcomas: an analysis of the US Sarcoma Collaborative database. *J Surg Oncol.* 2018;118:1135–1141.
9. Gutierrez JC, Perez EA, Moffat FL, et al. Should soft tissue sarcomas be treated at high-volume centers? An analysis of 4205 patients. *Ann Surg.* 2007;245:952–958.
10. Lahat G, Madewell JE, Anaya DA, et al. Computed tomography scan–driven selection of treatment for retroperitoneal liposarcoma histologic subtypes. *Cancer.* 2009;115:1081–1090.
11. Heslin MJ, Lewis JJ, Nadler E, et al. Prognostic factors associated with long-term survival for retroperitoneal sarcoma: implications for management. *J Clin Oncol.* 1997;15:2832–2839.

12. Bonvalot S, Rivoire M, Castaing M, et al. Primary retroperitoneal sarcomas: a multivariate analysis of surgical factors associated with local control. *J Clin Oncol.* 2009;27:31–37.
13. Tseng WW, Madewell JE, Wei W, et al. Locoregional disease patterns in well-differentiated and dedifferentiated retroperitoneal liposarcoma: implications for the extent of resection? *Ann Surg Oncol.* 2014;21:2136–2143.
14. Park JO, Qin LX, Prete FP, et al. Predicting outcome by growth rate of locally recurrent retroperitoneal liposarcoma: the one centimeter per month rule. *Ann Surg.* 2009;250:977–982.
15. Fletcher CD, Gustafson P, Rydholm A, et al. Clinicopathologic re-evaluation of 100 malignant fibrous histiocytomas: prognostic relevance of subclassification. *J Clin Oncol.* 2001;19:3045–3050.
16. Rosenberg SA, Tepper J, Glatstein E, et al. The treatment of soft-tissue sarcomas of the extremities: prospective randomized evaluations of (1) limb-sparing surgery plus radiation therapy compared with amputation and (2) the role of adjuvant chemotherapy. *Ann Surg.* 1982;196:305–315.
17. Pisters PW, O'Sullivan B, Maki RG. Evidence-based recommendations for local therapy for soft tissue sarcomas. *J Clin Oncol.* 2007;25:1003–1008.
18. Pisters PW, Pollock RE, Lewis VO, et al. Long-term results of prospective trial of surgery alone with selective use of radiation for patients with T1 extremity and trunk soft tissue sarcomas. *Ann Surg.* 2007;246:675–681; discussion 681–672.
19. O'Sullivan B, Davis AM, Turcotte R, et al. Preoperative versus postoperative radiotherapy in soft-tissue sarcoma of the limbs: a randomised trial. *Lancet.* 2002;359:2235–2241.
20. Canter RJ, Martinez SR, Tamurian RM, et al. Radiographic and histologic response to neoadjuvant radiotherapy in patients with soft tissue sarcoma. *Ann Surg Oncol.* 2010;17:2578–2584.
21. Mullen JT, Hornicek FJ, Harmon DC, et al. Prognostic significance of treatment-induced pathologic necrosis in extremity and truncal soft tissue sarcoma after neoadjuvant chemoradiotherapy. *Cancer.* 2014;120:3676–3682.
22. Mullen JT, Kobayashi W, Wang JJ, et al. Long-term follow-up of patients treated with neoadjuvant chemotherapy and radiotherapy for large, extremity soft tissue sarcomas. *Cancer.* 2012;118:3758–3765.
23. Kraybill WG, Harris J, Spiro IJ, et al. Phase II study of neoadjuvant chemotherapy and radiation therapy in the management of high-risk, high-grade, soft tissue sarcomas of the extremities and body wall: Radiation Therapy Oncology Group Trial 9514. *J Clin Oncol.* 2006;24:619–625.
24. Baldini EH, Goldberg J, Jenner C, et al. Long-term outcomes after function-sparing surgery without radiotherapy for soft tissue sarcoma of the extremities and trunk. *J Clin Oncol.* 1999;17:3252–3259.
25. Heslin MJ, Woodruff J, Brennan MF. Prognostic significance of a positive microscopic margin in high-risk extremity soft tissue sarcoma: implications for management. *J Clin Oncol.* 1996;14:473–478.
26. Zagars GK, Ballo MT, Pisters PW, et al. Surgical margins and reresection in the management of patients with soft tissue sarcoma using conservative surgery and radiation therapy. *Cancer.* 2003;97:2544–2553.
27. Grabellus F, Podleska LE, Sheu SY, et al. Neoadjuvant treatment improves capsular integrity and the width of the fibrous capsule of high-grade soft-tissue sarcomas. *Eur J Surg Oncol.* 2013;39:61–67.
28. Coindre JM, Terrier P, Guillou L, et al. Predictive value of grade for metastasis development in the main histologic types of adult soft tissue sarcomas: a study of 1240 patients from the French Federation of Cancer Centers Sarcoma Group. *Cancer.* 2001;91:1914–1926.
29. Blackmon SH, Shah N, Roth JA, et al. Resection of pulmonary and extrapulmonary sarcomatous metastases is associated with long-term survival. *Ann Thorac Surg.* 2009;88:877–884; discussion 884–875.
30. Kasper B, Gruenwald V, Reichardt P, et al. Imatinib induces sustained progression arrest in RECIST progressive desmoid tumours: final results of a phase II study of the German Interdisciplinary Sarcoma Group (GISG). *Eur J Cancer.* 2017;76:60–67.
31. Lahat G, Dhuka AR, Hallevi H, et al. Angiosarcoma: clinical and molecular insights. *Ann Surg.* 2010;251:1098–1106.
32. Stoeckle E, Coindre JM, Bonvalot S, et al. Prognostic factors in retroperitoneal sarcoma: a multivariate analysis of a series of 165 patients of the French Cancer Center Federation Sarcoma Group. *Cancer.* 2001;92:359–368.
33. MacNeill AJ, Gronchi A, Miceli R, et al. Postoperative morbidity after radical resection of primary retroperitoneal sarcoma: a report from the Transatlantic RPS Working Group. *Ann Surg.* 2018;267:959–964.
34. Lewis JJ, Leung D, Woodruff JM, et al. Retroperitoneal soft-tissue sarcoma: analysis of 500 patients treated and followed at a single institution. *Ann Surg.* 1998;228:355–365.
35. Gronchi A, Miceli R, Allard MA, et al. Personalizing the approach to retroperitoneal soft tissue sarcoma: histology-specific patterns of failure and postrelapse outcome after primary extended resection. *Ann Surg Oncol.* 2015;22:1447–1454.
36. Pawlik TM, Pisters PW, Mikula L, et al. Long-term results of two prospective trials of preoperative external beam radiotherapy for localized intermediate- or high-grade retroperitoneal soft tissue sarcoma. *Ann Surg Oncol.* 2006;13:508–517.
37. Gold JS, Gonen M, Gutierrez A, et al. Development and validation of a prognostic nomogram for recurrence-free survival after complete surgical resection of localised primary gastrointestinal stromal tumour: a retrospective analysis. *Lancet Oncol.* 2009;10:1045–1052.
38. Tawbi HA, Burgess M, Bolejack V, et al. Pembrolizumab in advanced soft-tissue sarcoma and bone sarcoma (SARC028): a multicentre, two-cohort, single-arm, open-label, phase 2 trial. *Lancet Oncol.* 2017;18:1493–1501.
39. D'Angelo SP, Mahoney MR, Van Tine BA, et al. Nivolumab with or without ipilimumab treatment for metastatic sarcoma (Alliance A091401): two open-label, non-comparative, randomised, phase 2 trials. *Lancet Oncol.* 2018;19:416–426.
40. Rutkowski P, Bylina E, Wozniak A, et al. Validation of the Joensuu risk criteria for primary resectable gastrointestinal stromal tumour—the impact of tumour rupture on patient outcomes. *Eur J Surg Oncol.* 2011;37:890–896.
41. Joensuu H, Vehtari A, Riihimaki J, et al. Risk of recurrence of gastrointestinal stromal tumour after surgery: an analysis of pooled population-based cohorts. *Lancet Oncol.* 2012;13:265–274.
42. Soft tissue sarcoma. NCCN Evidence Blocks. National Comprehensive Cancer Network. 2018, Accessed December 28, 2018. https://www.nccn.org/professionals/physician_gls/pdf/sarcoma_blocks.pdf.
43. Schuetze SM, Bolejack V, Thomas DG, et al. Association of dasatinib with progression-free survival among patients with advanced gastrointestinal stromal tumors resistant to imatinib. *JAMA Oncol.* 2018;4:814–820.

44. Blanke CD, Demetri GD, von Mehren M, et al. Long-term results from a randomized phase II trial of standard- versus higher-dose imatinib mesylate for patients with unresectable or metastatic gastrointestinal stromal tumors expressing KIT. *J Clin Oncol.* 2008;26:620–625.
45. Dematteo RP, Ballman KV, Antonescu CR, et al. Adjuvant imatinib mesylate after resection of localised, primary gastrointestinal stromal tumour: a randomised, double-blind, placebo-controlled trial. *Lancet.* 2009;373:1097–1104.
46. Joensuu H, Eriksson M, Sundby Hall K, et al. One vs three years of adjuvant imatinib for operable gastrointestinal stromal tumor: a randomized trial. *JAMA.* 2012;307:1265–1272.
47. Corless CL, Ballman KV, Antonescu CR, et al. Pathologic and molecular features correlate with long-term outcome after adjuvant therapy of resected primary GI stromal tumor: the ACOSOG Z9001 trial. *J Clin Oncol.* 2014;32:1563–1570.
48. Joensuu H, Eriksson M, Hall KS, et al. Risk factors for gastrointestinal stromal tumor recurrence in patients treated with adjuvant imatinib. *Cancer.* 2014;120:2325–2333.
49. Raut CP, Espat NJ, Maki RG, et al. Efficacy and tolerability of 5-year adjuvant imatinib treatment for patients with resected intermediate- or high-risk primary gastrointestinal stromal tumor: the PERSIST-5 Clinical Trial. *JAMA Oncol.* 2018;4:e184060.
50. Tap WD, Jones RL, Van Tine BA, et al. Olaratumab and doxorubicin versus doxorubicin alone for treatment of soft-tissue sarcoma: an open-label phase 1b and randomised phase 2 trial. *Lancet.* 2016;388:488–497.

33 CHAPTER

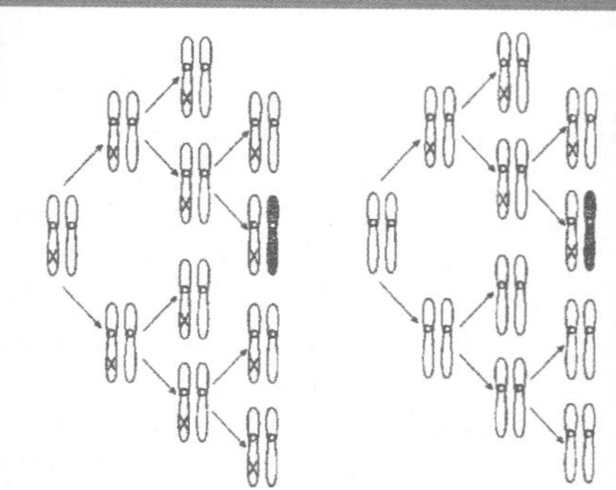

Bone Tumors

Herbert S. Schwartz, Ginger E. Holt, Jennifer L. Halpern

OUTLINE

OVERVIEW

Orthopedic oncology is a complex surgical discipline that involves the diagnosis, management, and surveillance of primary mesenchymal malignancies (sarcomas), benign bone and soft tissue masses, and secondary neoplasms of bone and soft tissue. The unique structural qualities of bone, along with its complex microenvironment, must be considered when formulating strategies for management of bone tumors. This chapter reviews the complex biology of the bone microenvironment as it relates to tumor progression, skeletal stability, and potential treatment options. It also presents a general approach to the diagnosis, management, and appropriate triage of primary and secondary bone tumors, both benign and malignant. Although making a diagnosis is paramount, the restoration of function in the setting of skeletal compromise/instability is also critical in the management of bone tumors. Therefore, a complex understanding of what the tumor is doing to the bone, what the bone is doing to the tumor, where the lesion is, and what the lesion is making impacts how bone tumors are managed (Table 33.1).

BONE MICROENVIRONMENT

An understanding of the bone microenvironment impacts the macroscopic management of skeletal tumors. In the absence of tumor, bone is a dynamic and symbiotic organ, actively maintained by cells that respond to stimuli such as injury, stress, or metabolic need. Osteoblasts represent a terminal differentiation of a mesenchymal stem cell. They generate a collagen matrix, which is then mineralized. When osteoblasts become surrounded by the matrix they create, they are deemed osteocytes—and serve to maintain the bony environment. Osteoclasts are multinucleated cells derived from a hematopoietic lineage (macrophages), which resorb bone. The constant interplay of those cells (osteoblast, osteocyte, osteoclast) is necessary to maintain bone health. The marrow space is also home to other significant cell populations, such as mesenchymal stem cells. The active and ongoing homeostasis of bone and its intramedullary inhabitants generate a microenvironment rich in growth factors and signaling molecules, making it an ideal soil for osteophilic tumors.

In the setting of metastatic to bone neoplasms, intravascular tumor cells are attracted to the microenvironment of bone because it is both preconditioned for tumor cell arrival by circulating factors and because it is inherently attractive due to the proteins, signaling molecules, and cells that it contains (Fig. 33.1). That concept was first coined the "seed and soil" theory by Dr. Stephen Paget in 1889.[1] For example, mesenchymal stem cells return (in part) to the bone marrow due to a signaling pathway involving the CXCL12 chemokine and the CXCR4 receptor. Intramedullary mesenchymal stem cells secrete CXCL12, and circulating stem cells that express the correlating CXCR4 receptor are recruited to the marrow space. Similarly, in the setting of metastatic breast cancer as an example, tumor cells express CXCR4 receptor and therefore can also be recruited to the marrow space via the chemokine CXCL12.[2] In general, cell signaling molecules produced in the marrow space are recognized by tumor-based receptors and represent one example of how the bone microenvironment influences tumor deposition. Other players involved in homing of tumor cells to bone include, but are not limited to, exosomes/oncosomes, adhesion molecules, platelets, and circulating stem cells.[3]

Once in the bone microenvironment, in what is deemed the "vicious cycle," tumor cells hijack the endogenous cells of bone to create an environment that fosters their own growth. Normally, the balance of lysis and bone formation in bone is maintained through the strategic production of signaling proteins. For

TABLE 33.1 Four questions asked to evaluate bone tumors.

	QUESTION	ANSWER	CLINICAL SIGNIFICANCE	EXAMPLE
1	Where is the lesion—which bone and what part of that bone?	Which bone? (e.g., femur)	Some lesions occur most often in a specific bone.	Chondromyxoid fibroma—tibia
		Where is the bone? (e.g., epiphyseal, metaphyseal, diaphyseal)	There is a specific differential for lesions that occur in specific regions of the bone.	Differential diagnosis of epiphyseal lesions is giant cell tumor, chondroblastoma, infection, and ganglion.
2	What is the lesion doing to the bone?	Destructive	If a lesion essentially erases the bone, it implies that the lesion is aggressive and therefore likely to be malignant.	Metastatic lung carcinoma essentially erases the cortex, destabilizing the bone.
		No change in overall morphology	If the lesion does not deform, distort, or destroy the bone, it suggests that the lesion is benign.	An enchondroma is an eccentric cartilage deposit within the intramedullary canal. If covered up, the bone would look normal.
3	What is the bone doing to the lesion?	Failing to contain it	If the bone cannot respond to the assault of a tumor, the tumor is aggressive.	Osteosarcoma breaks out of the bone and elevates periosteum.
		Expanding and thinning	If the lesion is growing but the bone is trying to contain it, the bone may appear expanded and thinned. It may fall into the benign aggressive differential.	Aneurysmal bone cysts, giant cell tumors
		Creating a sclerotic border around the lesion	When the bone forms a sclerotic rim around a lesion, the lesion is typically benign.	Nonossifying fibroma, intraosseous ganglion
4	What is the lesion making?	Matrix-cartilage, bone, fibrous tissue	The matrix a tumor produces is part of its inherent classification.	Bone forming—osteoid osteoma, osteoblastoma, osteosarcoma

example, receptor activator of nuclear factor-κB ligand (RANKL) is generated by osteoblasts, and recognized by its osteoclast receptor (RANK). When bound, RANKL stimulates osteoclastogenesis.[4] Osteoprotegerin is a decoy receptor secreted by osteoblasts, which inhibits RANKL binding and therefore inhibits osteoclastogenesis.[5] Tumor cells can disturb bone homeostasis in a variety of ways. Tumor cells can directly stimulate osteoblasts to generate RANKL, which is the most prominent cytokine inducer of osteoclastogenesis.[6,7] Alternatively, tumor-secreted matrix metalloproteinase-7 can cleave extracellular matrix where bound and inactive RANKL resides, thereby releasing the active form of RANKL.[8] Once overactive osteoclastogenesis is initiated, tumor growth is fueled by this aggressive bone degradation, which frees an abundance of growth factors that can drive tumor proliferation.

This chapter is not intended to cover all aspects of the microenvironment tumor-native bone interplay. However, an appreciation of those complex relationships is important. Medical therapies can target not only tumor cells (the seed) but also the soil—essentially preventing tumor growth by making the environment less favorable. In patients with bone metastases, and even in the setting of benign but locally aggressive lytic/osteoclast filled tumors, systemic medications designed to limit osteoclast function are now utilized. The goal of those medicines is to reduce the number of skeletally related events (SREs), which include hypercalcemia of malignancy, bone pain, pathologic fracture, spinal cord compression, or the need for palliative radiation.

Drug Therapies

Bisphosphonates are a class of drugs that inhibits bone resorption and can decrease the number of SREs.[9] Nitrogen-containing bisphosphonates bind to and inhibit key enzymes of the intracellular mevalonate pathway, thereby preventing the prenylation and activation of small guanosine triphosphatases that are essential for the bone-resorbing activity and survival of osteoclasts. Bisphosphonates are only taken up by active osteoclasts. Zoledronic acid (Zometa) is commonly used for oncology patients as a means of preventing SREs.[10]

Denosumab (Xgeva) is a monoclonal antibody generated against RANKL. This drug mimics the natural action of osteoprotegerin, which prevents RANKL binding to RANK, thereby preventing osteoclast maturation. However, it does not also block the tumor necrosis factor-related apoptosis-inducing ligand, which is the principal mediator of tumor cell death by the human host cells.[11] Denosumab inhibits osteoclast recruitment, maturation, and function and ultimately induces apoptosis of activated osteoclasts and therefore stops bone resorption.[12] Examination of denosumab-treated bone shows an absence of osteoclasts.[13] Denosumab has been compared to zoledronic acid through a randomized double blind trial in men with metastatic prostate cancer and shown to be more effective in preventing SREs than zoledronic acid.[14] Denosumab was also found to be superior to zoledronic acid in delaying time to SRE in patients with metastatic breast cancer.[15] Although the aforementioned studies suggest that denosumab is superior to zoledronic acid in treatment of metastatic bone lesions in the case of breast and prostate cancer, denosumab is not universally used at this time for treatment of bone metastases. That fact likely relates to economic and availability issues, as well as the need for studies to assess longer term follow and ideal dosing protocols.[13]

BONE MACROENVIRONMENT

Primary tumors of bone, both benign and malignant, tend to form in specific geographic regions of bone (Fig. 33.2). The primary differential diagnosis of epiphyseal tumors includes giant cell tumor, chondroblastoma, infection, or intraosseous ganglion. Clear

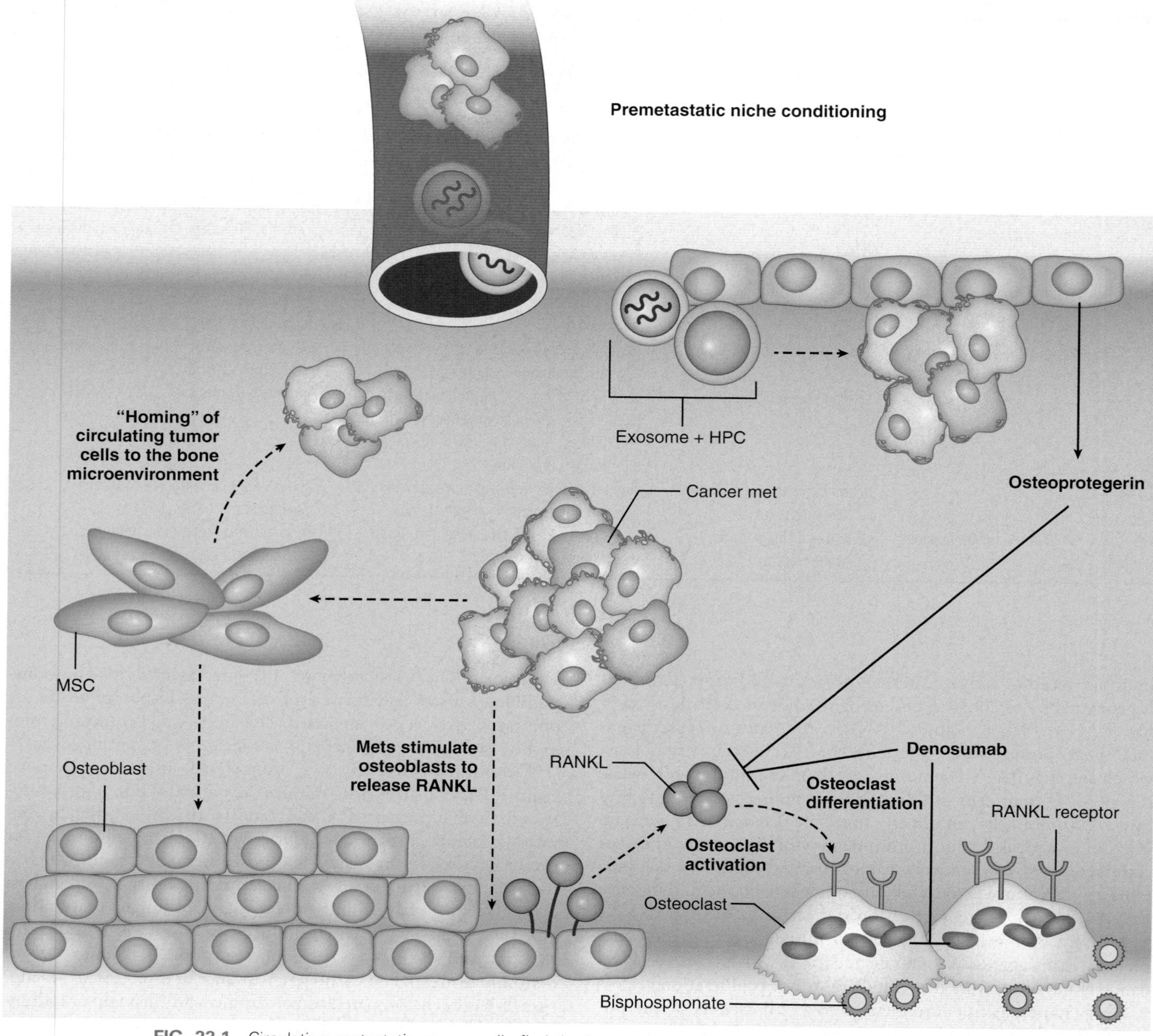

FIG. 33.1 Circulating metastatic cancer cells find the bone microenvironment through a complex series of steps. Prior to their arrival, circulating factors optimize the bone (premetastatic niche conditioning). Cells are then recruited to the bone by signaling molecules called chemokines (homing). Once in the bone, tumor cells hijack normal bone metabolism (the vicious cycle). Medical therapies used in the treatment of metastatic bone cancers exploit the understanding of the vicious cycle. Denosumab is a human monoclonal antibody that binds the receptor activator of nuclear factor-κB ligand (*RANKL*) and directly inhibits osteoclastogenesis. Zoledronic acid is a bisphosphonate that is taken up by and then inhibits activated osteoclasts. (Adapted from Cook LM, Shay G, Araujo A, et al. Integrating new discoveries into the "vicious cycle" paradigm of prostate to bone metastases. *Cancer Metastasis Rev.* 2014;33:511–525.) *HPC*, Hematopoietic progenitor cell; *MSC*, mesenchymal stem cell.

cell chondrosarcoma is a less common epiphyseal lesion. Common diaphyseal lesions include adamantinoma, Ewing sarcoma, infection, osteoid osteoma/osteoblastoma, and fibrous dysplasia. Osteosarcoma most commonly forms in metaphyseal bone of the distal femur, proximal tibia, and proximal humerus. Metastatic bone disease can occur in all regions of the bone, although certain sites are considered more typical for specific cancers. Acral metastases and intracortical metastases are typically lung carcinomas. The common locations of tumors and the structural integrity and demands of the bone in those locations are important facts to consider when formulating plans for biopsy and reconstruction. For example, biopsy of an intraosseous, diaphyseal femoral lesion through a transcortical approach, even with a large bore needle (core biopsy), can increase the risk of fracture at the site of

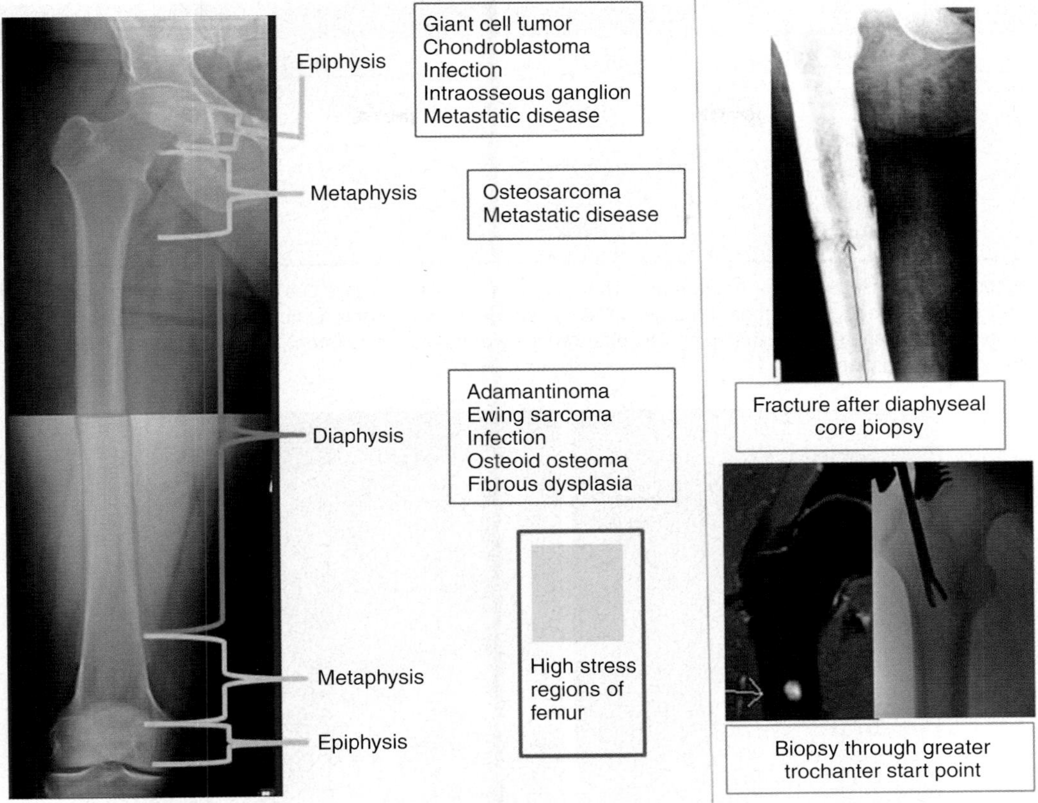

FIG. 33.2 The location of tumors helps to narrow the differential diagnosis. Biopsy in certain locations can increase the risk of fracture in long bones. Pictured is an example of a fracture created in the diaphyseal femur following a core-biopsy needle. Biopsy through the greater trochanter, an intramedullary nail starting point, is a biomechanically safer option.

biopsy (Fig. 33.2). An alternative, depending upon the proximity of the lesion to the greater trochanter, is to perform an intramedullary biopsy through a greater trochanteric starting point, using pituitary rongeurs to grab intramedullary bone at a predetermined location (Fig. 33.2). That biopsy entrance site does not destabilize the bone, and it still can be resected as part of a wide tumor resection if needed. Alternatively, lesions at the metaphyseal flare can often be biopsied directly, because the biomechanical stress in that area places it at much lower risk for fracture, even if a small bone window is created to obtain tissue.

The relevance of tumor location is reflected in Mirels' criteria, which allow for a more objective assessment of pathologic fracture risk in patients with bone tumors (Table 33.2). In that system, a numeric score is assigned to observed metastatic lesions in bone.[16] Lesions are categorized by location, size, and nature (lytic vs. blastic). Based on a total score, recommendations can be made for operative prophylaxis. This classification/scoring system is designed to assist with decision making but in no way replaces clinical judgments made in consideration of each patient. However, it does capture the fact that lesions in high-stress, weight-bearing areas of the skeleton, such as the trochanteric femur, are at highest risk of fracture.

BIOPSY

Biopsy is a complex cognitive skill in the skeleton for two primary reasons. First, as previously mentioned, one must be aware of what approaches might further destabilize the bone in question. Second, one must place the biopsy tract in a location that accommodates future wide resection. Specifically, if a diagnosis of primary malignancy is rendered, a wide resection must include the biopsy tract, which harbors malignant cells. If a significant hematoma forms after bone biopsy, then larger resection may be needed to obtain adequate margins (Fig. 33.3).

There are different modalities of bone biopsy. Fine-needle aspirate is rarely used unless there is a significant extraosseous soft tissue component that is accessible or significant bony lysis. Core biopsy, often performed with computed tomography (CT) scan guidance, can be performed through intact cortices (with adjunct use of a combined biopsy/drill system) or through areas of soft tissue extension. Incisional biopsy is a surgical procedure during which a carefully planned small incision is made in line with the tumor, with respect to neurovascular structures and bone biomechanics. Open biopsy allows for acquisition of the most tissue as compared to other techniques. If the cortex is intact, a high-speed burr is often used to create a less than dime-sized window into the bone. Meticulous hemostasis must be obtained to prevent contamination of surrounding tissues. Often, Surgicel and Gelfoam are packed into defects created in the soft tissue extraosseous component of the tumor, and then the tumor capsule and superficial layers are closed meticulously. If the cortex has been violated, often bone wax or a small plug of bone cement is used to prevent intramedullary extravasation of blood and tumor into the biopsy tract.

Inappropriately placed biopsy tracts can change the nature of surgery required—even changing a potential limb salvage candidate into a patient requiring an amputation. Biopsy placement and execution are critical. It has been conclusively shown in several studies that surgeons inexperienced in musculoskeletal oncology principles have a three to four times increased rate of complication from a poorly placed biopsy site.[17–19]

TABLE 33.2 Mirels scoring system.

SCORE	SITE OF LESION	SIZE OF LESION	LESION TYPE	PAIN
1	Upper limb	$>\frac{1}{3}$ cortex	Blastic	Mild
2	Lower limb	$\frac{1}{3}$-$\frac{2}{3}$ cortex	Mixed	Moderate
3	Trochanteric	$>\frac{2}{3}$ cortex	Lytic	Functional

The Mirels scoring system allows assessment of fracture risk. There are four factors (site, size, lesion type, pain) that are assigned a numeric score of 1 to 3. The four scores are added together. If the overall score is more than 9, prophylactic fixation is indicated. A score of less than 7 can often be treated with radiation and medical therapies. Despite the utility of the scoring system, clinical judgment must always be taken into consideration regarding a specific patient.[16]

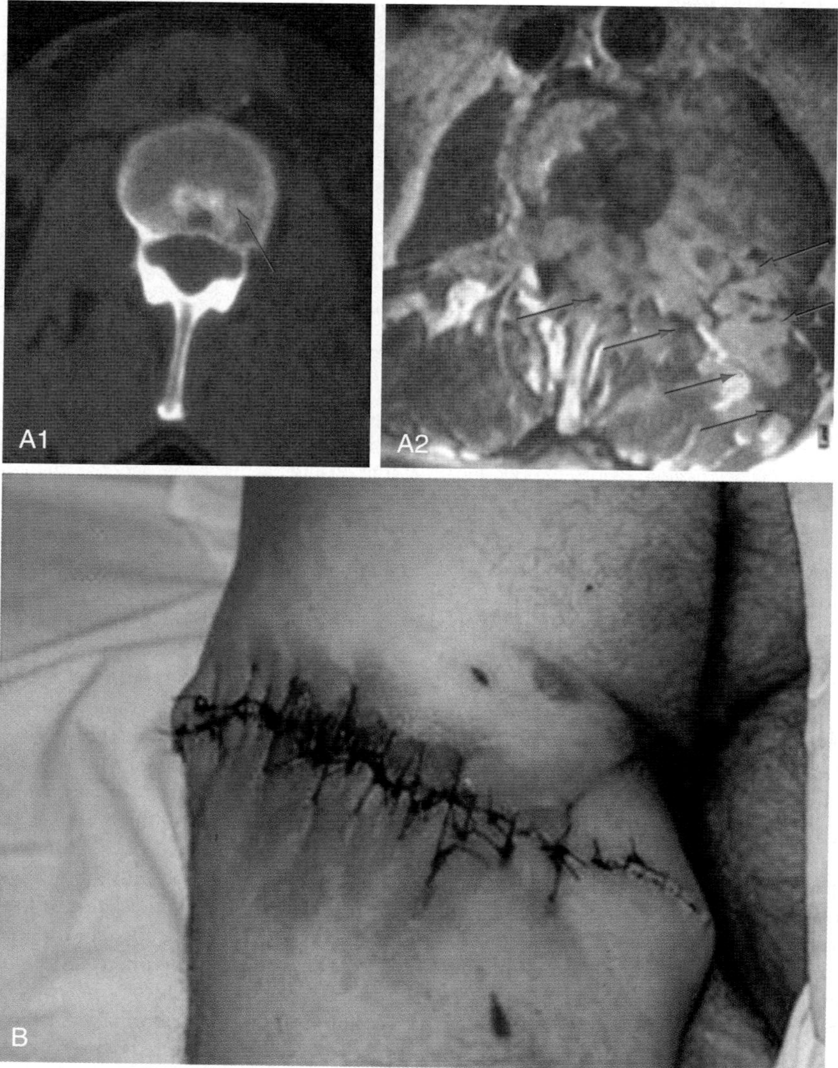

FIG. 33.3 When planning a biopsy location, one must consider that the biopsy tract will be contaminated and, in the case of malignant tumors, will require resection. In panel A1, a computed tomography–guided biopsy tract into the vertebral body is demonstrated by the arrow. In panel A2, the arrows indicate the extent of biopsy tract recurrence. Panel B is an excellent example of an inappropriate biopsy, which mandated an otherwise unnecessary amputation in the patient. Biopsies must be performed in line with the incision that will eventually be required to resect a tumor. The entire biopsy tract must be resected. Therefore, a biopsy incision is typically small and strategically placed.

The biopsy result is the most important factor driving a patient's care. The tissue obtained allows one to render a diagnosis and build a treatment pathway. As such, when a biopsy is performed, it is critical that the surgeon has a basic understanding of how to make a correct diagnosis. Surgical pathology tissue review includes histologic evaluation and immunohistochemistry. The challenge in sarcoma care has previously been interobserver reliability with regard to diagnosis. The molecular pathology of bone tumors—identification of genetic signatures that correlate to skeletal neoplasia—allows for consistency in diagnoses and is emerging as a powerful tool in the care of bone tumor patients. Table 33.3 documents the pathognomonic mutations associated with various bone tumors.[20]

STAGING

A critical part of biopsy planning includes a global understanding of the nature of a tumor—whether it is localized or part of a more systemic process. Patient history and physical examination are vital parts of evaluation. Physical examination must include chaperoned breast examination or prostate examination in patients who potentially may have a metastatic to bone process. A series of radiologic studies are then performed to characterize the scope of the disease process. When a patient presents with an isolated bone lesion that may represent a malignancy, especially without antecedent history of cancer, the following studies or labs are typically obtained:

1. Magnetic resonance imaging (MRI) of the entire affected bone with contrast—identifies a soft tissue component of the tumor that, if present, may be easier to sample and also helps to identify skip metastases.
2. CT scan of the chest, abdomen, and pelvis with and without intravenous and oral contrast—screens for common osteophilic carcinomas including breast, lung, renal, thyroid, and prostate and also helps to establish whether solid organ metastases are present.
3. CT with two-dimensional reconstructions of the affected bone—allows a better three-dimensional understanding of how the tumor has affected the bone.
4. Whole body bone scan—identifies other possible osseous sites/metastases.
5. Plain radiographs of the affected bone—show where in the bone the tumor is located (epiphyseal, metaphyseal, diaphyseal), show what the tumor is doing to the bone (lytic, blastic), show what the bone is doing to the tumor (containment vs. failure to contain) and show the matrix of the lesion (bone, cartilage, fibrous, etc.) (Table 33.1).
6. Laboratory evaluation to include prostate-specific antigen, serum electrophoresis, calcium to rule out hypercalcemia of malignancy, lactate dehydrogenase, alkaline phosphatase, complete blood count with differential, comprehensive metabolic panel, sedimentation rate, and C-reactive.

There are two primary staging systems used to describe skeletal sarcoma. In the Musculoskeletal Tumor Society Staging System, or Enneking system,[21] Stage I refers to a low-grade skeletal sarcoma, Stage II refers to a high-grade skeletal sarcoma, and Stage III represents metastatic disease, either regional or distant. The letter A refers to intracompartmental tumor localization, whereas the letter B refers to extracompartmental extension. An example of extracompartmental extension would include an osteosarcoma with extraosseous soft tissue mass or a pathologic fracture through an osteosarcoma, resulting in hematoma contamination. The American Joint Committee on Cancer staging system has been updated.[22] Tumors are described by grade (I, low; II, high; III, tumor of any grade with skip metastasis; IV, tumor of any grade with distant metastasis) and size (<8 cm, A; >8 cm, B). Staging systems in general are designed to reflect prognosis and therefore guide treatment algorithms.

Enneking also developed a staging system for benign bone tumors.[23] In the Enneking system, tumors are characterized as latent (1), active (2), or aggressive (3). Aggressive benign tumors often have a higher risk of local recurrence. Although aggressive benign tumors still can be technically resected in an intralesional fashion, resection must be meticulous, often utilizing high-speed burrs and other adjuvants. The most important factor in preventing recurrence is likely to be adequacy of resection.[24]

ONCOLOGIC RESECTION

There are four types of surgical resection: (1) intralesional, (2) marginal, (3) wide, and (4) radical. The type of margin reflects the surgical dissection plane relative to the tumor or capsule of the tumor. Intralesional resections involve an incision made into the substance of tumor. Intralesional resections in bone are typically exemplified by curettage or debulking. They are used in the setting of benign bone tumors and metastatic to bone tumors. Marginal resections theoretically involve resection of the tumor around its capsule and by definition leave microscopic disease behind. Wide resections involve resection of the tumor with a surrounding rim of normal tissue, designed to remove the entirety of a tumor. Radical resections include not only the tumor and a rim of normal tissue but also the entirety of the compartment in which the tumor

TABLE 33.3 Skeletal neoplasia DNA alterations.

TUMOR	SUPPRESSOR GENE	ONCOGENE	TRANSLOCATIONS	CHROMOSOME LOSS	CHROMOSOME GAIN	PROTEIN CHANGE
Osteosarcoma	*RB, p53* *INK4A, INK2A*	*CDK4, FOS, cMYC* *MDM2, MET*		6q, 13q, 15q, 17p, 18q	1q, 5p, 6p, 7q, 8q, 12q, 17p, 19q	
Ewing sarcoma	*KCMF1*	*CD99*	t(11;22)(q24;q12) EWS-FLI1 t(21;22)(q22;q12) EWS-ERG			
Chondrosarcoma		*IDH1, IDH2*		1p, 5q, 6p, 9p, 14q, 22q	7p, 12q, 21q	
Osteochondroma	*EXT1, EXT2*					
Enchondroma					12q	IHH-PTHrP
Aneurysmal bone cyst			t(16;17)(q22;p13) CDH11-USP6			
Fibrous dysplasia		*GNAS1*		20q		G_S
Giant cell tumor		*TPX2* *H3F3*	Telomeric fusions	1q	20q	RANKL Histone

G_s, Mutation in alpha-subunit of the G_S stimulatory protein leading to activation and inappropriate cyclic adenosine monophosphate production (cAMP); *IHH-PTHrP*, Indian hedge-hog-PTH-related protein; *RANKL*, receptor activator of nuclear factor-κB ligand.

resides. Wide resections are more commonly utilized in the treatment of skeletal sarcomas, as opposed to radical resections.

SKELETAL RECONSTRUCTION

The type of reconstruction needed often depends upon the type of resection that is indicated. It also depends greatly on the reparative potential of the bone. For example, children can regenerate bone at a higher rate than adults, and therefore in the setting of benign tumors like aneurysmal bone cyst, bone graft might be utilized in a child, whereas in an adult bone, cement might be used. Another important factor is the posttreatment impact of a tumor on bone. For example, a lytic lesion caused by multiple myeloma has a better chance of healing following medical therapies that a lytic lesion caused by lung cancer. The potential for bone regeneration at the site of tumor relates in many ways to the stromal content of the tumor. Lymphoma of bone is predominantly cellular, whereas lung carcinoma in bone has a significant stromal component. The footprint of the tumor cannot be erased in stromal-heavy tumors.

Skeletal Stabilization Utilized in Intralesional Resections

Skeletal stabilization/reconstruction comes in many forms. Plates and screws that span defects can be used following curettage of lesions. Bone strength can be augmented through the insertion of polymethylmethacrylate (bone cement) into skeletal defects along with plates and screws (rebar) (Fig. 33.4). Intramedullary nail fixation is a common strategy for prophylaxis of diaphyseal lesions, especially in the femur (Fig. 33.5). In the setting of metastatic disease with palliation as a goal, the reconstruction strategy selected should impart immediate stability and immediate full weight-bearing potential whenever possible.

Skeletal Reconstruction Utilized in Wide Resections

In the case of wide resection (skeletal sarcomas), large segments of bone are resected (Fig. 33.5B and C). In those cases, reconstruction often involves the use of intercalary allografts or metal components, osteoarticular allografts, allograft-prosthetic composites, arthroplasty utilizing megaprosthesis, or arthrodesis. Autologous vascularized free tissue transfer, such as vascularized free fibulas, can also be an option. Amputation is also always an alternative in select cases.

Allograft

When a patient is identified who will require a large bulk allograft, templated x-rays of the bone needed (or the contralateral bone if there is too much deformity) are obtained. Approved tissue banks harvest materials with meticulous sterility, and then can assess whether any in-stock cadaveric allografts match the bone being requested.[25] Allografts can be harvested with soft tissue attachments, and in that case, the host tendons can be sewn into the allograft attachment sites. Allografts can be fortified with cement augmentation, if possible, and then secured to the native bone utilizing plates and screws (Fig. 33.6). Allografts are obviously nonviable scaffolds, and therefore, ultimate healing at the native bone-allograft interface depends upon the native bone use of the allograft as a scaffold through which new bridging bone is formed. Intercalary allografts are essentially bony place holders

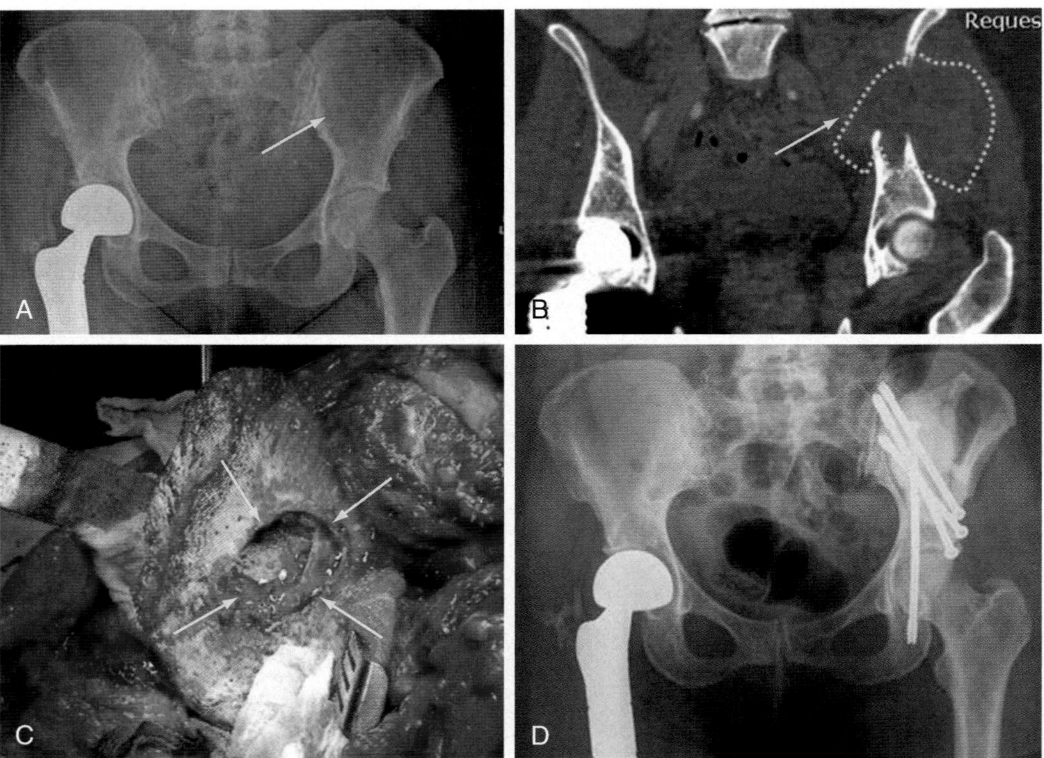

FIG. 33.4 The patient had a prior right proximal femur metastatic lesion treated with proximal femur resection and megaprosthesis. She then developed a large, lytic, painful left iliac wing lesion, which required intralesional resection and reconstruction utilizing cement and 7.3 mm cannulated screws. (A) Anteroposterior pelvis x-ray shows the lytic defect *(arrow)*. (B) Computed tomography scan two-dimensional coronal reconstruction view shows not only the bony defect, but also the associated soft tissue mass *(arrow and dotted line)*. (C) Intraoperative view of the bony defect *(arrows)*. (D) Postoperative anteroposterior pelvis.

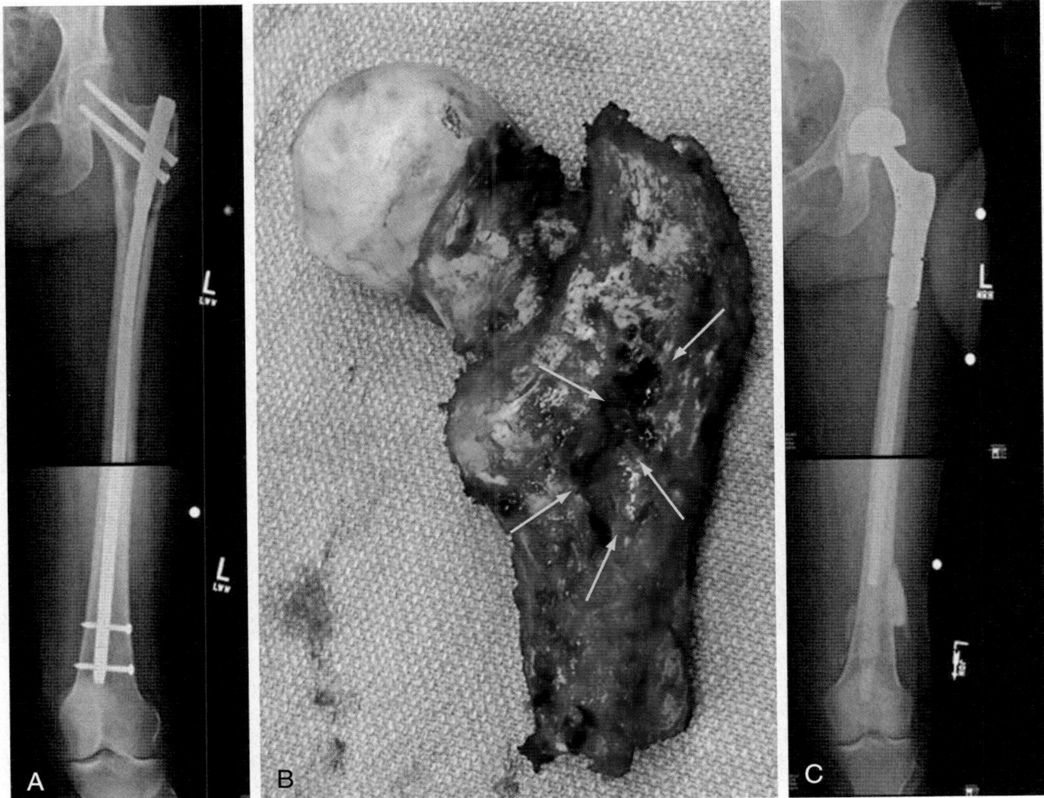

FIG. 33.5 This patient had intramedullary nail stabilization and palliative radiation of the left femur for treatment of a peritrochanteric metastatic renal cell carcinoma lesion. (A) Despite appropriate attempt at stabilization and adjuvant therapies, she had persistent pain. A left proximal femoral resection and proximal femur megaprosthesis was performed. (B) Gross specimen revealed persistent lysis of the bone *(arrows)*. (C) A long-cemented stem proximal femur endoprosthesis was used for reconstruction.

and can often be secured in situ through the use of intramedullary stabilization. Osteoarticular allografts include implantation of a new joint surface. In weight-bearing joints, osteoarticular allograft fracture and collapse over time are common. However, especially in the growing child, they allow for delay of arthroplasty and generation of additional bone stock.

The means of reconstruction is often dictated by the weight-bearing demands of the bone in question. For example, an osteoarticular allograft is a good option for the proximal humerus—a technically non–weight-bearing limb. An allograft with soft tissue attachments allows the rotator cuff tendons to be sewn to the implant, thereby potentiating some overhead mobility. An osteoarticular allograft in the distal femur may be more problematic because of weight-bearing demands. Therefore, arthroplasty may be preferred.

Arthroplasty

Arthroplasty is a common reconstruction strategy utilized following tumor resections that include portions of a joint (Fig. 33.7) The so-called megaprosthesis is named such because large modular metal implants are combined to restore length to the limb and replace large bone defects. Those metal replacements are either potted into the bone using bone cement or press fit into the long bone canal. Bone cement offers immediate stability, but increased chance of aseptic loosening over time.[26] Press fit stems require ingrowth or ongrowth of host bone over time around the stem periphery. In the case of the proximal humerus and proximal femur, no additional resurfacing of the acetabulum or glenoid is typically done. For distal femur or proximal tibia tumors, the tumor-unaffected side of the joint requires resurfacing to accommodate a hinge mechanism.

Amputation

Amputation is indicated in the setting of primary tumors when an adequate margin cannot be obtained through the use of limb salvage or when the functional result achieved through limb salvage is worse than that achieved by amputation. Amputation may be indicated in the setting of metastatic or advanced cancers for the purposes of palliation.

BENIGN BONE TUMORS

The incidence of benign bone tumors far exceeds that of skeletal sarcomas. In these authors' clinical experience, there are at least five benign bone tumors for every primary malignant bone neoplasm. Fifty-four percent of benign bone tumors are chondrogenic (enchondroma or osteochondroma).[27] The true prevalence of these tumors is unknown because many go undetected and unreported. Aggressive benign bone tumors, such as giant cell tumor and aneurysmal bone cysts, have a local recurrence rate as high as 30% and require meticulous intralesional resection utilizing high-speed burr resection and other adjuvants.[28]

Enchondroma

Enchondromas are benign proliferations of hyaline cartilage typically found in the appendicular skeleton, less likely detected in the

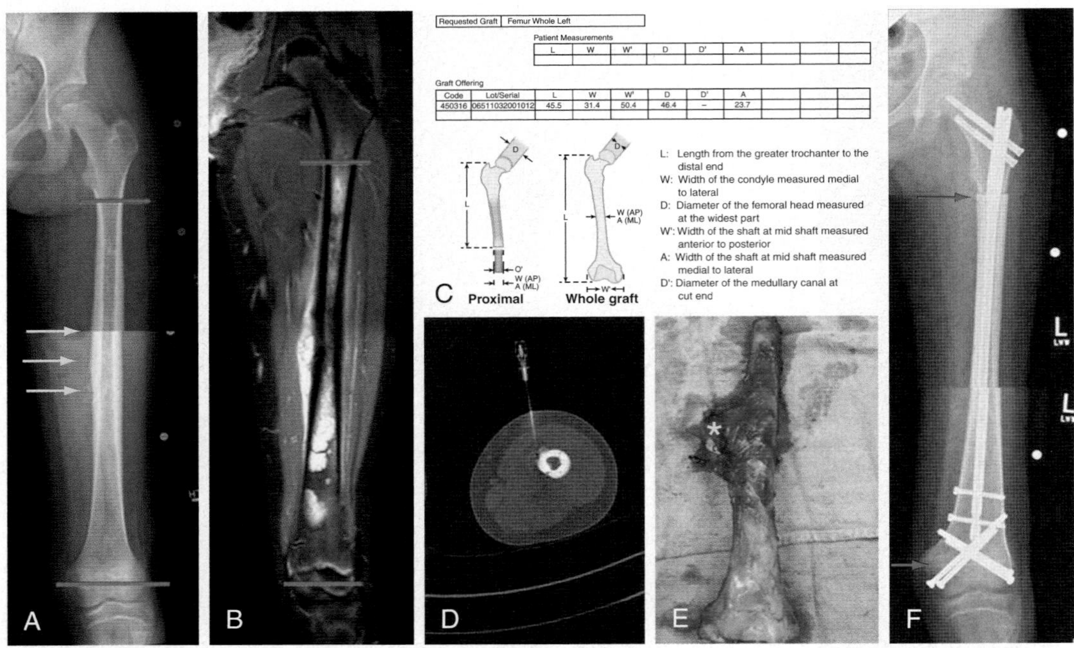

FIG. 33.6 Allograft reconstruction can be used in osteoarticular, intercalary, or allograft-prosthetic composite reconstructions. An 11 year old with an extensive left femoral diaphyseal osteosarcoma with multiple skip metastases. (A) Anteroposterior femur x-ray demonstrates periosteal reaction *(yellow arrows)*. Anticipated resection is denoted with *red lines*. (B) Magnetic resonance imaging (MRI) shows the extent of tumor, which does not extend distal to the physis. Proximal extent of tumor extends to the inferior aspect of lesser trochanter. MRI allows planning of intercalary femoral resection. (C) Allograft matched. (D) Biopsy tract. (E) Resection performed with negative margins and includes the medial biopsy tract (*). (F) Anteroposterior femur x-ray postresection. *Red arrows* indicate allograft–native bone interfaces.

axial skeleton, which are centered in the metaphysis. They typically are incidental findings discovered during radiographic evaluations for other symptoms, except in the phalanges, where they can cause pathologic fracture (Fig. 33.8A). Enchondromas represent lobular cartilage islands, which retain chondroid features and continue to grow until skeletal maturity, at which time they begin to undergo calcification. Their long-term physiologic activity is the reason that they remain scintigraphically active decades later on a bone scan. Isolated lesions do not cause progressive deformity of the bone. Malignant transformation is rare.

However, in patients with multiple enchondromas, such as Ollier disease or Maffucci syndrome (Ollier with subcutaneous hemangiomas), the risk of progressive bone deformity is higher, as is the risk of malignant transformation into a secondary chondrosarcoma. Interestingly, individuals with Maffucci syndrome also have a higher risk of developing occult carcinomas.[29]

Treatment of enchondromas remains conservative, and serial radiographic evaluation is the primary means of punctuated surveillance. Surgical intervention is only required if there is a question of malignant transformation. In that setting, albeit rare, the entire lesion is often curetted and submitted to surgical pathology. Cartilage lesions have areas of heterogeneity, therefore, in the case of malignant transformation, often only a small portion of the lesion appears malignant. The histopathologic interpretation of cartilage lesions depends on radiographic information and clinical information. For example, an enchondroma biopsied from the finger will look hypercellular but, because of its location, will be called an enchondroma. The same material, however, if biopsied from the pelvis, would be called a higher-grade chondrosarcoma. Clinical context is vital for proper evaluation of cartilage lesions (Fig. 33.8). If there is a question surrounding the diagnosis of enchondroma and open biopsy is performed, the biopsy entrance site, along with the lesion, is often packed with bone cement and the bone is stabilized with a plate and screws. Bone grafting of the resected lesion is also an option. If lesions are called chondrosarcoma, then, depending on the grade of the tumor, further resection or wide resection may be indicated.

Osteochondroma

Although discussed as a benign bone tumor, an osteochondroma is better described as a hamartoma of bone. It develops from aberrant growth cartilage and radiographically is a "cartilage capped bony projection on the external surface of the bone" according to the World Health Organization (Fig. 33.9). It is typically detected in the second decade of life. It presents as a painless mass, or a mass associated with pain due to mechanical symptoms. There are two distinct radiographic types of osteochondroma—pedunculated and sessile. On three-dimensional imaging analysis, the intramedullary component of an osteochondroma should be confluent with the intramedullary canal of the affected bone. The lesion itself is capped by cartilage, and therefore, the lesion grows through skeletal development and stops growing at skeletal maturity. If a lesion continues to grow after skeletal maturity, or if radiographically a cartilage cap exceeds 2 cm in thickness after skeletal maturity, then there is concern for potential malignant transformation. The majority of osteochondromas are solitary, and in those cases, the chance of malignant transformation is less than 1%.

However, osteochondromas can develop in a polyostotic fashion—as in hereditary multiple osteochondral exostosis or osteochondromatosis. Hereditary multiple osteochondral exostosis is an autosomal dominant condition. Three separate loci are implicated in its development: 1) *EXT1* (8q24.1), 2) *EXT2*

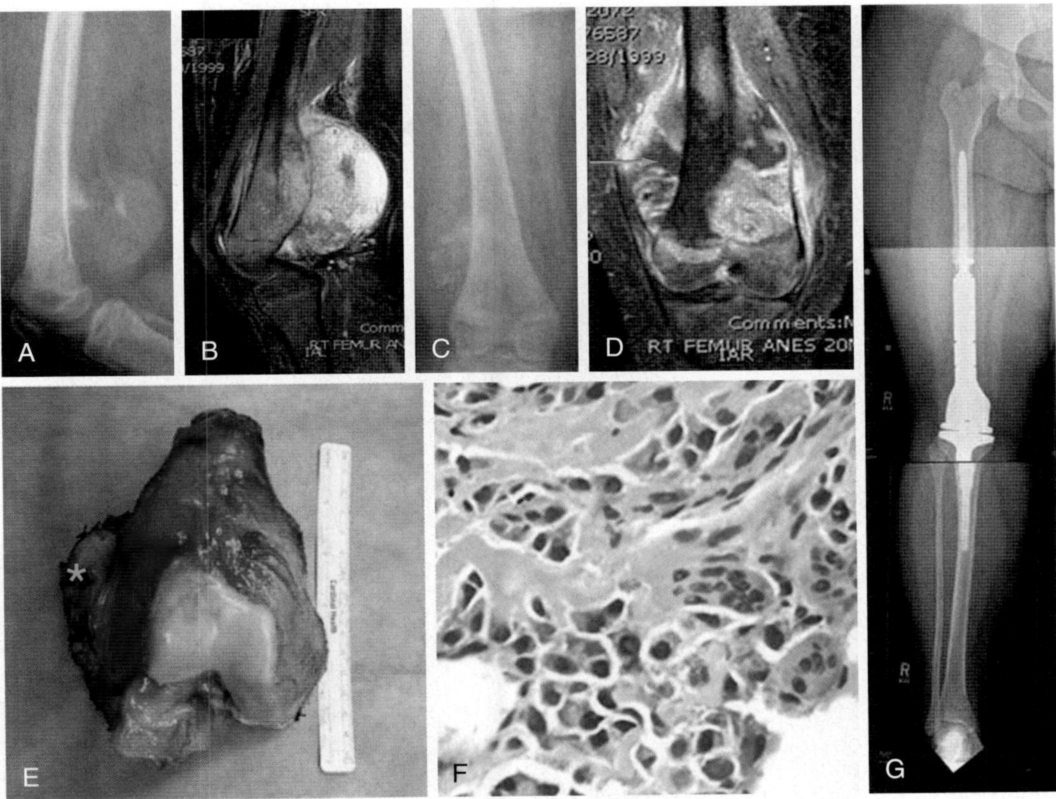

FIG. 33.7 Endoprostheses are used to reconstruct periarticular malignant tumors. (A) Lateral x-ray distal femur shows aggressive bone tumor with large soft tissue extension. (B) Magnetic resonance imaging (MRI) T2 sagittal shows true extent of bone involvement and soft tissue mass. (C) Anteroposterior distal femur x-ray demonstrates osteoblastic matrix. (D) MRI T2 coronal shows planned biopsy trajectory—lateral to access soft tissue mass *(arrow)*. (E) Resection specimen with biopsy tract (*). (F) Histology analysis shows malignant cells with lace-like osteoid matrix. (G) Right distal femur endoprosthesis utilizing press-fit fixation into the femoral canal.

(11p11-12), and 3) *EXT3* (19p).[30,31] Affected children present with mass lesions and skeletal growth anomalies, including short stature, limb length discrepancies, angular deformity of knees and ankles, radial bowing and wrist deviation, and subluxation of the radiocapitellar joint.[32] The risk over time of malignant transformation of an osteochondroma in this scenario ranges from 10% to 30%. Osteochondromas that transform are called secondary chondrosarcomas.

Osteoid Osteoma

Osteoid osteoma is a benign osteoblastic tumor (Fig. 33.10). Although self-limited, the symptoms generated by this less than 1 cm in diameter lesion can be debilitating. Osteoid osteomas typically occur in the diaphysis of long bones, but can occur anywhere, such as the posterior elements of the spine. Osteoblastomas are essentially giant osteoid osteomas that occur primarily in the spine. Both conditions can lead to scoliosis if in the spine—related to pain and muscle spasm or joint pain and sympathetic effusion if in the proximity of a joint. Radiographically, these lesions show a radiolucent nidus, surrounded by an area of thickened cortical bone and sclerosis. On MRI, there is often extensive edema surrounding the lesions. The patient's history elicited is classic, in that pain is worse at night and relieved with nonsteroidal anti inflammatory drugs. Although these self-limited lesions can be managed for a period of years with nonsteroidal anti inflammatory drug therapy, watchful waiting, given the profound associated symptoms, is unacceptable to most patients. Osteoid osteoma can be treated with radiofrequency ablation using CT-guided percutaneous techniques. In that scenario, a lesion can be localized in three dimensions, biopsied to obtain definitive tissue for diagnosis, and then ablated using high-frequency radio waves that essentially heat the surrounding tissue around the probe. In areas not amenable to radiofrequency ablation, such as those that are too subcutaneous or near vital structures like the spinal cord, surgical resection of the lesion including the nidus is still performed.

Giant Cell Tumor

Giant cell tumor, which represents approximately 20% of benign bone tumors, is the most aggressive benign bone tumor (Fig. 33.11). Giant cell tumor occurs in the epiphyseal portion of a long bone or flat bones like the pelvis or sacrum in individuals between 20 and 40 years of age. Patients present with pain, which usually results from periarticular subchondral pathologic fractures. Along with eventual biopsy to rule out malignancy, preoperative evaluation also includes chest imaging and local site imaging. Surgical management requires exposure of the affected bone and creation of a large bony window allowing access to the entirety of the tumor cavity. Local recurrence rates after treatment of giant cell tumor in a bone can be as high as 40%, and, therefore, resection must be meticulous and often includes the use of adjuvants. Following gross resection through the use of curettage, a high-speed burr is used to resect tumor from characteristic bony pits. Additional adjuvants, such as polymethyl

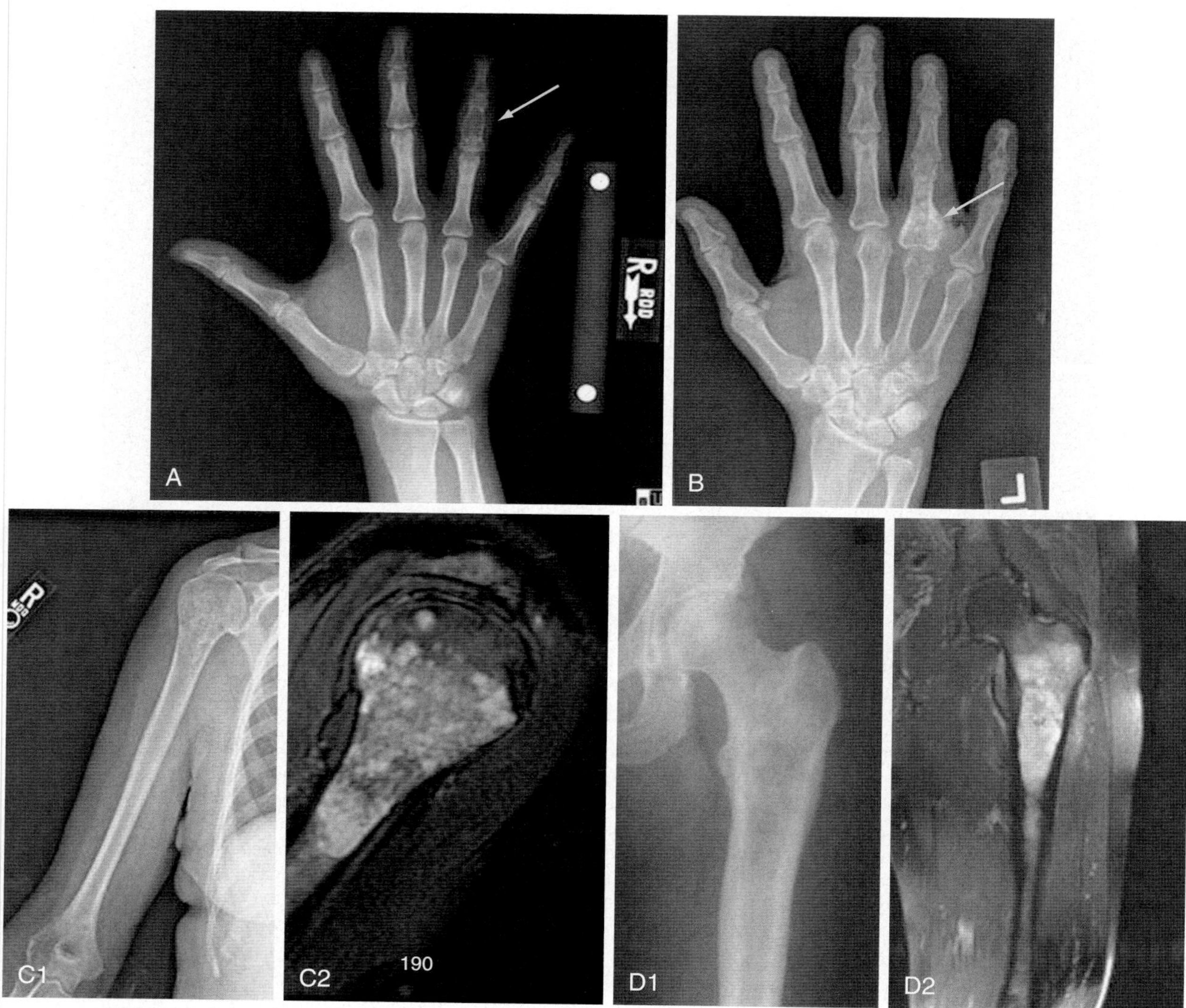

FIG. 33.8 The differential diagnosis of cartilage lesions depends upon clinical and radiographic information. (A) Middle phalanx expansile lesion with internal calcification presenting as pathologic fracture is a typical presentation for enchondroma. (B) Although the more distal a cartilage lesion is, the less likely it is malignant, another patient presented with an aggressive proximal phalanx lesion, marked by pain, periosteal reaction, and internal calcification, and she was diagnosed with chondrosarcoma. (C) Patient has a proximal humerus cartilage lesion with expected calcification on anteroposterior proximal humerus x-ray without destruction of surrounding cortex (C1). The lesion is lobular in nature as apparent on MRI (C2). The patient is being followed radiographically. (D) In comparison, another patient had an aggressive appearing lesion in the left proximal femur, causing bony distortion (D1), which on MRI was associated with surrounding bone edema (D2). The patient was diagnosed with a high-grade chondrosarcoma and treated with proximal femoral resection, megaprosthesis.

methacrylate bone cement, liquid nitrogen, phenol, or argon beam laser, are then used to try to decrease recurrence rates.[28] Finally, periarticular stabilization is performed, typically with a combination of cement and hardware. Bone grafting in those cases is often inadequate to restore stability. Periarticular cement offers immediate stability but may be associated with thermal damage to articular cartilage.[33] Giant cell tumors in the spine, sacrum, and pelvis present greater surgical challenges. Oftentimes, preoperative embolization is required because intraoperative tumor hemorrhage can be significant if the tumor has an aneurysmal bone cyst component.

Despite its benign description, there are instances of giant cell tumor lung metastases, which occur in approximately 1% to 2% of cases.[34] In those cases, the metastatic focus in the lung does not histopathologically meet the criterion for malignancy and is identical in appearance to the benign bone tumor in the skeleton. Survival rates are approximately 80% with aggressive treatment. Patients require long-term follow-up because recurrences may develop several years postoperatively. Medical therapies, such as bisphosphonates and human monoclonal RANKL antibodies (denosumab), can be useful in refractory giant cell tumor as well.[35,36] Those medicines target the role of osteoclasts in tumor development and decrease osteoclast function. However, their efficacy is not complete, as denosumab does not affect neoplastic stromal cell proliferation.[37] Radiation treatment may have a role in primary giant cell tumors of the axial skeleton or in recurrent refractory giant cell tumors in a long bone. There is strong evidence, however, that irradiation of giant cell tumors

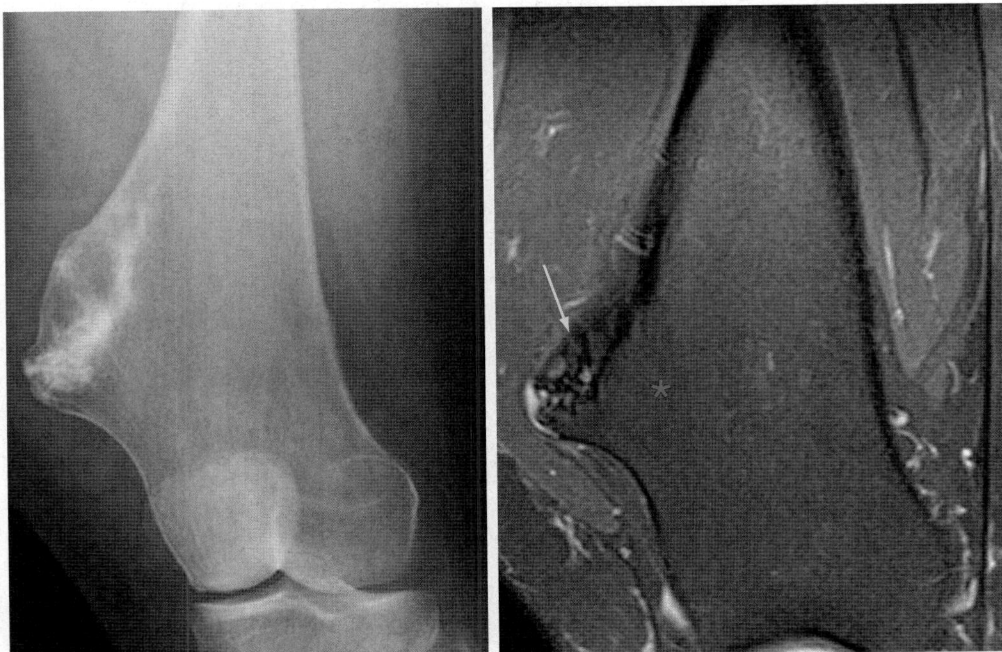

FIG. 33.9 Osteochondromas are considered more a growth aberrancy than a tumor. Typical features in a skeletally mature individual are small cartilage cap less than 2 cm *(arrow)* and intramedullary canal of lesion confluent with intramedullary canal of the affected bone (*).

increases the chance for malignant transformation to a frank giant cell sarcoma decades later.[38]

SKELETAL SARCOMAS

The American Cancer Society estimates that 3500 new cases of primary bone cancers will be diagnosed in 2019.[39] In adults, 40% of primary bone cancers are chondrosarcomas, 28% are osteosarcomas, 10% are chordomas, 8% are Ewing sarcomas, and 4% are skeletal sarcomas of bone not otherwise specified. In children, osteosarcoma is the most common primary bone tumor (56%), followed by Ewing sarcoma (28%) and chondrosarcoma (6%). The incidence of skeletal sarcomas is approximately equal in the pediatric and adult populations.

The modern-day algorithm for treatment of bone sarcomas, which includes neoadjuvant chemotherapy, wide surgical resection, and adjuvant chemotherapy, was a serendipitous discovery in the 1970s.[40] During that time, intensive chemotherapy was administered to many teenagers with nonmetastatic osteosarcoma of the extremities after biopsy, while they awaited fabrication of a custom endoprosthesis. After several months, the tumor was surgically removed and the implant inserted to preserve the limb. The resected bone was then examined histopathologically for evidence of chemotherapy effect. A survival benefit was noted in children who had received chemotherapy. That observation evolved into the modern day treatment algorithm for skeletal sarcoma, which includes neoadjuvant chemotherapy, wide surgical resection, and subsequent adjuvant chemotherapy.

Wide surgical resections are mandated for skeletal sarcomas. The surgical goal is a local recurrence rate of less than 7%. Early studies by Simon et al.[41] and Link et al.[42] documented equivalent local recurrence and survival rates between limb salvage and amputation for distal femoral osteosarcoma. Cure rates are approximately 67% for extremity sarcomas, whereas axial tumors in the pelvis or spine have a worse prognosis (33%) for a similar tissue type.[43,44]

It has been demonstrated that limb salvage is more cost-effective over a period of decades than immediate amputation in the teenage population.[45] Implant survival is complicated in the short-term by infection (allografts) and in the long-term by aseptic loosening (metal).[46] Ten-year implant survival rates for metallic prostheses range from 50% to 80% in the proximal tibia, distal femur, and proximal femur, respectively.[47] Wound healing, especially while administering chemotherapy, is enhanced with healthy local flaps. Rotational flaps are often used around the knee to improve prosthetic coverage. For example, in proximal tibia resections, a medial gastrocnemius flap is needed to cover the prosthesis and to reconstruct the extensor mechanism.

Osteosarcoma

Osteosarcoma, or osteogenic sarcoma, is defined as a malignant tumor that produces neoplastic osteoid. Neoplastic cartilage or fibrous tissue may be present. There are many types of osteosarcoma and they vary by location (intraosseous, surface, or extraskeletal), grade, or etiology. Spontaneous osteosarcomas are most common, but some osteosarcomas occur in the genetic syndromes of Li-Fraumeni, hereditary retinoblastoma, and in postradiation scenarios. There is a bimodal age of tumor occurrence. Conventional osteosarcomas occur in the first two decades of life, whereas posttreatment or secondary (malignant transformation) osteosarcomas occur much later. Survival is best predicted by the degree of chemotherapy-induced necrosis.[48] Nonmetastatic extremity osteosarcoma with greater than 90% chemotherapy-induced necrosis has survival rates of 80% at 5 years. Pelvic osteosarcoma with less than 90% chemotherapy-induced necrosis has a survival rate of approximately 30%.[43,44]

Ewing Sarcoma

Ewing sarcoma and primitive neuroectodermal tumor are small blue cell (microscopic appearance) malignancies of bone that cytogenetically represent the same entity. They share a common

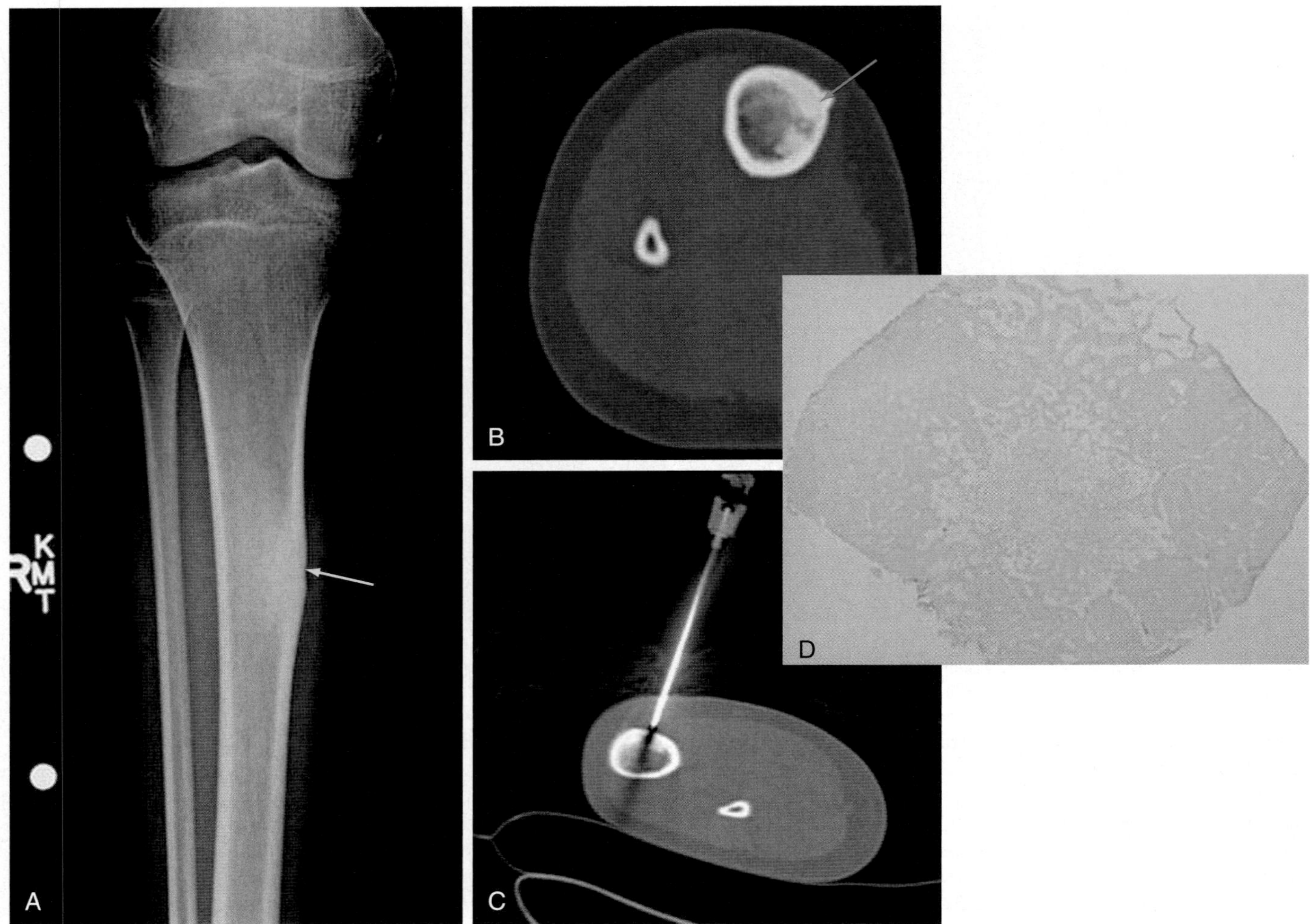

FIG. 33.10 Osteoid osteomas are benign bone-forming lesions, which, despite their small size, can cause significant pain. (A) Anteroposterior tibia x-ray shows new bone formation and cortical thickening *(arrow)*. (B) Axial computed tomography scan shows thickened cortex with a central nidus *(arrow)*. (C) In appropriate lesions, computed tomography–guided biopsy for diagnosis can be followed by radiofrequency ablation for definitive treatment. (D) An excised osteoid osteoma with a cherry red nidus and surrounding bone.

translocation, t(11;22)(q24;q12), in 85% of cases. Molecular cloning of the translocation reveals fusion between the 5′ end of the *EWS* gene from the 22q12 chromosome and the 3′ end of the 11q24 *FLI1* gene.[49] This tumor is exquisitely sensitive to chemotherapy and radiation treatment. Neither modality alone or in combination is sufficient to maximize the cure rate, however. Surgical extirpation in conjunction with chemotherapy is the preferred treatment. Reconstruction options follow those of other skeletal sarcomas.

Chondrosarcoma

Chondrosarcoma is a malignant skeletal neoplasm that produces hyaline cartilage (Fig. 33.8D1 and D2). Several pathologic subtypes exist in which the neoplastic cells produce unusual matrices. Histopathology alone does not predict biologic behavior. Rather, a combination of histopathology, age, location, and radiographic appearance yields the best predictor of tumor aggressiveness. A low-grade cartilage tumor of the phalanx may have the same microscopic appearance as a pelvic chondrosarcoma. It would be exceedingly rare to die of a phalanx cartilage tumor. However, local control is notoriously difficult to achieve in pelvic chondrosarcomas, and long-term cure rates require massive resection. Secondary chondrosarcomas occur after malignant transformation of benign cartilage tumors such as enchondroma or osteochondroma.

BONE METASTASES

Skeletal metastases are approximately 500 times more common than skeletal sarcomas; 1.2 million new cases of carcinoma are diagnosed each year in the United States. The most common osteophilic carcinomas include prostate, thyroid, breast, lung, bladder, and renal carcinoma.

As cancer therapeutics improve, the prevalence of patients living with metastatic cancer also increases. Displaced pathologic fractures and impending pathologic fractures represent common problems for the orthopedic oncologist. The workup for a metastatic skeletal carcinoma of unknown primary origin includes a detailed physical exam, including breast and prostate exam. The radiographic studies ordered include a computed axial tomographic scan of the chest, abdomen, and pelvis; a whole body bone scan; serum protein electrophoresis; and assay for prostate-specific

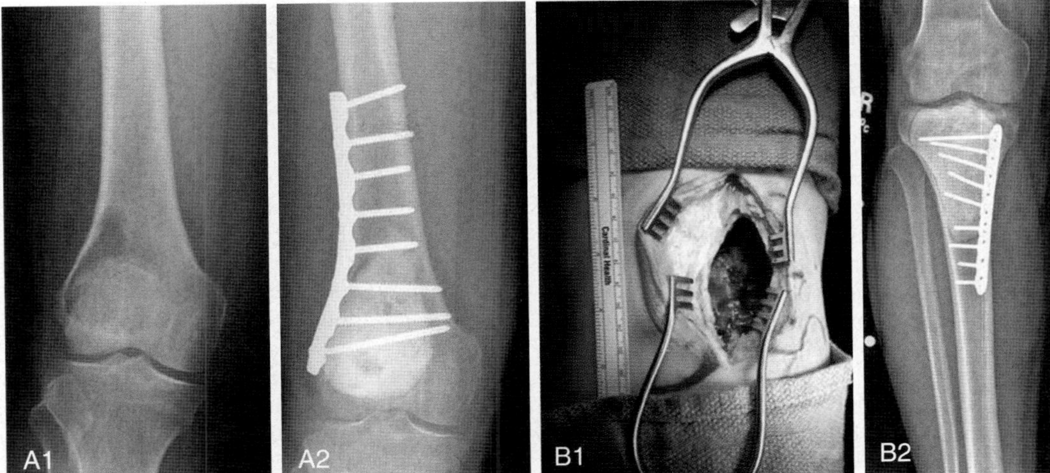

FIG. 33.11 Giant cell tumors are destructive epiphyseal lesions that can cause articular surface compromise. (A1) They present as lytic lesions in the epiphyseal bone as on this anteroposterior distal femur x-ray. (A2) Intralesional resection and adjuvant treatment are performed and followed by cement, plate, and screw reconstruction. (B1) Although adjuvants are used, the most important part of limiting recurrence is meticulous resection. To accomplish that goal, a bony window often as large as the lesion itself must be created so that all aspects of the lesion can be addressed. (B2) Cement reconstruction allows for immediate stability as well as a means of radiographic monitoring for signs of recurrence.

antigen.[50] If a diagnosis of metastatic to bone carcinoma is established, then there are certain medical therapies that can be used to decrease the number of SREs in a patient (or clinically significant bone metastases).

Intralesional resection after tissue confirmation of the diagnosis and stabilization of bone lesions can provide excellent palliation of symptoms and improvements in quality of life. When considering surgical stabilization, often whole bone prophylaxis is performed utilizing metal implants and cement augmentation. Postoperative radiation therapy must include delivery to the entire bone from joint to joint. A surgical goal of a local recurrence rate less than 15% is preferred. Isolated metastases such as from renal cell carcinoma or melanoma can be treated aggressively if they are indeed isolated and occur after a long hiatus (several years) from initial diagnosis. Cures, in such instances, are not rare.

Reconstructive goals consist of choosing an implant durable enough to outlive the patient and understanding what, if any, healing capacity the bone may have. A variety of surgical techniques are used to reconstruct the skeleton (Figs. 33.5 and 33.6). Palliative relief of pain and maximization of function are the goals of surgery.

CONCLUSION

The management of bone tumors requires an expertise and understanding of the bone microenvironment combined with a knowledge of macroscopic bone biomechanics. Tumor resections in the skeleton mandate concurrent plans for stable skeletal reconstruction. In the case of primary malignant bone tumors, studies demonstrate that patients have better outcomes when treated in a tertiary care facility with orthopedic oncology expertise. With regard to the management of secondary malignancies of bone, multiple factors—the nature of the tumor, the location of the lesion, and the demands of specific bone locations—may affect decisions regarding resection and reconstruction. Benign bone tumors often do not require surgical intervention, only surveillance. Aggressive benign tumors can be resected in an intralesional fashion, but that resection must be meticulous, and those patients must be followed for evidence of recurrence. Skeletal sarcomas are treated with wide excision and appropriate reconstruction. An evolving understanding of the bone microenvironment has translated into better pharmaceutical options for the treatment of bone tumor lesions and a better understanding of the bone-specific and tumor-specific demands in tumor reconstruction.

SELECTED REFERENCES

Baumhoer D, Amary F, Flanagan AM. An update of molecular pathology of bone tumors. Lessons learned from investigating samples by next generation sequencing. *Genes Chromosomes Cancer*. 2019;58:88–99.

A majority of primary bone tumors, excluding high-grade osteosarcoma, can now be defined by molecular genetic alterations. The ability to identify distinct molecular markers in bone sarcoma allows one to more reliably determine definitive diagnosis. The right diagnosis has ramifications for developing appropriate treatment pathways and for generating meaningful research study groups.

Enneking WF, Spanier SS, Goodman MA. A system for the surgical staging of musculoskeletal sarcoma. *Clin Orthop Relat Res*. 1980;153:106–120.

This surgical staging system for musculoskeletal sarcomas stratifies bone and soft-tissue tumors of any by the grade of biologic aggressiveness, by the anatomic setting, and by the presence of metastasis. It consists of three stages: I—low grade; II—high grade; and III—presence of metastases. These stages are subdivided by whether the lesion is anatomically confined (a) within a compartment or (b) beyond a compartment in ill-defined fascial planes and spaces. It has proven to be the most correlative system for predicting sarcoma outcomes.

Fizazi K, Carducci M, Smith M, et al. Denosumab versus zoledronic acid for treatment of bone metastases in men with castration-resistant prostate cancer: a randomised, double-blind study. *Lancet.* 2011;377:813–822.

In this phase 3 randomized controlled trial, denosumab was shown to be better than zoledronic acid in the prevention of skeletally related events. The results reflect the importance of understanding the bone microenvironment in which tumors proliferate. Denosumab is a human monoclonal antibody targeted against receptor activator of nuclear factor κB ligand Zoledronic acid is a bisphosphonate that inhibits the activated osteoclasts.

Mankin HJ, Mankin CJ, Simon MA. The hazards of the biopsy, revisited. Members of the Musculoskeletal Tumor Society. *J Bone Joint Surg Am.* 1996;78:656–663.

This investigation reviewed the hazards associated with biopsies of primary malignant musculoskeletal sarcomas and demonstrated that there were troubling rates in errors in diagnosis and technique, which adversely affected patient care. In addition, it was noted that patients had a decreased incidence of biopsy-related complications or adverse change in outcome when biopsy was performed in a sarcoma care center. On the basis of those observations, whenever possible, musculoskeletal tumor biopsies should be done in a tertiary-type sarcoma center by an orthopedic oncologist or collaborating musculoskeletal radiologist.

Rougraff BT, Kneisl JS, Simon MA. Skeletal metastases of unknown origin. A prospective study of a diagnostic strategy. *J Bone Joint Surg Am.* 1993;75:1276–1281.

In 85% of patients, the primary site of metastatic origin was identified with the use of a computed tomography (CT) scan of the chest, abdomen, and pelvis. This diagnostic strategy was simple and highly successful for the identification of the site of an occult malignant tumor before biopsy in patients who had skeletal metastases of unknown origin. In a patient presenting with a skeletal lesion suspicious for a metastatic lesion with an unknown primary, CT scan is the test of choice to identify the primary lesion. In an era when insurance approval of such tests is increasingly more difficult, it is important to advocate for patients to receive this standard of care examination.

Simon MA, Aschliman MA, Thomas N, et al. Limb-salvage treatment versus amputation for osteosarcoma of the distal end of the femur. *J Bone Joint Surg Am.* 1986;68:1331–1337.

This study compared three groups of patients who had a limb-sparing procedure, an above-the-knee amputation, or disarticulation of the hip for osteosarcoma of the distal femur. The use of a limb-salvage procedure for osteosarcoma of the distal end of the femur did not shorten the disease-free interval or compromise long-term survival.

REFERENCES

1. Paget S. The distribution of secondary growths in cancer of the breast. *Lancet.* 1889;1:571–573.
2. Kang Y, Siegel PM, Shu W, et al. A multigenic program mediating breast cancer metastasis to bone. *Cancer Cell.* 2003;3:537–549.
3. Cook LM, Shay G, Araujo A, et al. Integrating new discoveries into the "vicious cycle" paradigm of prostate to bone metastases. *Cancer Metastasis Rev.* 2014;33:511–525.
4. Boyle WJ, Simonet WS, Lacey DL. Osteoclast differentiation and activation. *Nature.* 2003;423:337–342.
5. Morony S, Capparelli C, Sarosi I, et al. Osteoprotegerin inhibits osteolysis and decreases skeletal tumor burden in syngeneic and nude mouse models of experimental bone metastasis. *Cancer Res.* 2001;61:4432–4436.
6. Mundy GR. Metastasis to bone: causes, consequences and therapeutic opportunities. *Nat Rev Cancer.* 2002; 2:584–593.
7. Weilbaecher KN, Guise TA, McCauley LK. Cancer to bone: a fatal attraction. *Nat Rev Cancer.* 2011;11:411–425.
8. Lynch CC, Hikosaka A, Acuff HB, et al. MMP-7 promotes prostate cancer-induced osteolysis via the solubilization of RANKL. *Cancer Cell.* 2005;7:485–496.
9. Pavlakis N, Schmidt R, Stockler M. Bisphosphonates for breast cancer. *Cochrane Database Syst Rev.* 2005:CD003474.
10. Aapro M, Abrahamsson PA, Body JJ, et al. Guidance on the use of bisphosphonates in solid tumours: recommendations of an international expert panel. *Ann Oncol.* 2008;19:420–432.
11. Sheridan JP, Marsters SA, Pitti RM, et al. Control of TRAIL-induced apoptosis by a family of signaling and decoy receptors. *Science.* 1997;277:818–821.
12. Body JJ, Facon T, Coleman RE, et al. A study of the biological receptor activator of nuclear factor-kappaB ligand inhibitor, denosumab, in patients with multiple myeloma or bone metastases from breast cancer. *Clin Cancer Res.* 2006;12:1221–1228.
13. Rordorf T, Hassan AA, Azim H, et al. Bone health in breast cancer patients: a comprehensive statement by CECOG/ SAKK Intergroup. *Breast.* 2014;23:511–525.
14. Fizazi K, Carducci M, Smith M, et al. Denosumab versus zoledronic acid for treatment of bone metastases in men with castration-resistant prostate cancer: a randomised, double-blind study. *Lancet.* 2011;377:813–822.
15. Stopeck AT, Lipton A, Body JJ, et al. Denosumab compared with zoledronic acid for the treatment of bone metastases in patients with advanced breast cancer: a randomized, double-blind study. *J Clin Oncol.* 2010;28:5132–5139.
16. Mirels H. Metastatic disease in long bones. A proposed scoring system for diagnosing impending pathologic fractures. *Clin Orthop Relat Res.* 1989;249:256–264.
17. Mankin HJ, Mankin CJ, Simon MA. The hazards of the biopsy, revisited. Members of the Musculoskeletal Tumor Society. *J Bone Joint Surg Am.* 1996;78:656–663.
18. Randall RL, Bruckner JD, Papenhausen MD, et al. Errors in diagnosis and margin determination of soft-tissue sarcomas initially treated at non-tertiary centers. *Orthopedics.* 2004;27:209–212.
19. Trovik CK. Scandinavian Sarcoma Group Project. *Acta Orthop Scand Suppl.* 2001;300:1–31.
20. Baumhoer D, Amary F, Flanagan AM. An update of molecular pathology of bone tumors. Lessons learned from investigating

samples by next generation sequencing. *Genes Chromosomes Cancer*. 2019;58:88–99.
21. Enneking WF, Spanier SS, Goodman MA. A system for the surgical staging of musculoskeletal sarcoma. *Clin Orthop Relat Res*. 1980;153:106–120.
22. American Joint Committee on Cancer. Bone. In: Edge SB, Greene FL, Byrd DR, et al., eds. *AJCC Cancer Staging Manual*. 7th ed. New York: Springer-Verlag; 2010:281–287.
23. Enneking WF. *Staging Musculoskeletal Tumors in Musculoskeletal Tumor Surgery*. New York: Churchill Livingstone; 1983.
24. Blackley HR, Wunder JS, Davis AM, et al. Treatment of giant-cell tumors of long bones with curettage and bone-grafting. *J Bone Joint Surg Am*. 1999;81:811–820.
25. Joyce MJ. Safety and FDA regulations for musculoskeletal allografts: perspective of an orthopaedic surgeon. *Clin Orthop Relat Res*. 2005;435:22–30.
26. Myers GJ, Abudu AT, Carter SR, et al. The long-term results of endoprosthetic replacement of the proximal tibia for bone tumours. *J Bone Joint Surg Br*. 2007;89:1632–1637.
27. Unni KK. *Dahlin's Bone Tumors: General Aspects and Data on 11,087 Cases*. ed 5. Philadelphia: Lippincott-Raven; 1996.
28. Turcotte RE, Wunder JS, Isler MH, et al. Giant cell tumor of long bone: a Canadian Sarcoma Group study. *Clin Orthop Relat Res*. 2002;397:248–258.
29. Altay M, Bayrakci K, Yildiz Y, et al. Secondary chondrosarcoma in cartilage bone tumors: report of 32 patients. *J Orthop Sci*. 2007;12:415–423.
30. Wuyts W, Van Hul W. Molecular basis of multiple exostoses: mutations in the EXT1 and EXT2 genes. *Hum Mutat*. 2000;15:220–227.
31. Le Merrer M, Legeai-Mallet L, Jeannin PM, et al. A gene for hereditary multiple exostoses maps to chromosome 19p. *Hum Mol Genet*. 1994;3:717–722.
32. Vanhoenacker FM, Van Hul W, Wuyts W, et al. Hereditary multiple exostoses: from genetics to clinical syndrome and complications. *Eur J Radiol*. 2001;40:208–217.
33. Radev BR, Kase JA, Askew MJ, et al. Potential for thermal damage to articular cartilage by PMMA reconstruction of a bone cavity following tumor excision: a finite element study. *J Biomech*. 2009;42:1120–1126.
34. Dominkus M, Ruggieri P, Bertoni F, et al. Histologically verified lung metastases in benign giant cell tumours—14 cases from a single institution. *Int Orthop*. 2006;30:499–504.
35. Chawla S, Henshaw R, Seeger L, et al. Safety and efficacy of denosumab for adults and skeletally mature adolescents with giant cell tumour of bone: interim analysis of an open-label, parallel-group, phase 2 study. *Lancet Oncol*. 2013;14:901–908.
36. Balke M, Campanacci L, Gebert C, et al. Bisphosphonate treatment of aggressive primary, recurrent and metastatic giant cell tumour of bone. *BMC Cancer*. 2010;10:462.
37. Mak IW, Evaniew N, Popovic S, et al. A translational study of the neoplastic cells of giant cell tumor of bone following neoadjuvant denosumab. *J Bone Joint Surg Am*. 2014;96:e127.
38. Rock MG, Sim FH, Unni KK, et al. Secondary malignant giant-cell tumor of bone. Clinicopathological assessment of nineteen patients. *J Bone Joint Surg Am*. 1986;68:1073–1079.
39. Cancer Facts and Figures 2019. American Cancer Society, Accessed July 30, 2019. https://www.cancer.org/cancer/bone-cancer/about/key-statistics.html.
40. Rosen G, Marcove RC, Caparros B, et al. Primary osteogenic sarcoma: the rationale for preoperative chemotherapy and delayed surgery. *Cancer*. 1979;43:2163–2177.
41. Simon MA, Aschliman MA, Thomas N, et al. Limb-salvage treatment versus amputation for osteosarcoma of the distal end of the femur. *J Bone Joint Surg Am*. 1986;68:1331–1337.
42. Link MP, Goorin AM, Miser AW, et al. The effect of adjuvant chemotherapy on relapse-free survival in patients with osteosarcoma of the extremity. *N Engl J Med*. 1986;314:1600–1606.
43. Pakos EE, Nearchou AD, Grimer RJ, et al. Prognostic factors and outcomes for osteosarcoma: an international collaboration. *Eur J Cancer*. 2009;45:2367–2375.
44. Goorin AM, Schwartzentruber DJ, Devidas M, et al. Presurgical chemotherapy compared with immediate surgery and adjuvant chemotherapy for nonmetastatic osteosarcoma: pediatric Oncology Group Study POG-8651. *J Clin Oncol*. 2003;21:1574–1580.
45. Grimer RJ, Carter SR, Pynsent PB. The cost-effectiveness of limb salvage for bone tumours. *J Bone Joint Surg Br*. 1997;79:558–561.
46. Mankin HJ, Hornicek FJ, Raskin KA. Infection in massive bone allografts. *Clin Orthop Relat Res*. 2005;432:210–216.
47. Jeys LM, Kulkarni A, Grimer RJ, et al. Endoprosthetic reconstruction for the treatment of musculoskeletal tumors of the appendicular skeleton and pelvis. *J Bone Joint Surg Am*. 2008;90:1265–1271.
48. Picci P, Bacci G, Campanacci M, et al. Histologic evaluation of necrosis in osteosarcoma induced by chemotherapy. Regional mapping of viable and nonviable tumor. *Cancer*. 1985;56:1515–1521.
49. Aurias A, Rimbaut C, Buffe D, et al. Chromosomal translocations in Ewing's sarcoma. *N Engl J Med*. 1983;309:496–498.
50. Rougraff BT, Kneisl JS, Simon MA. Skeletal metastases of unknown origin. A prospective study of a diagnostic strategy. *J Bone Joint Surg Am*. 1993;75:1276–1281.

SECTION VI

HEAD AND NECK

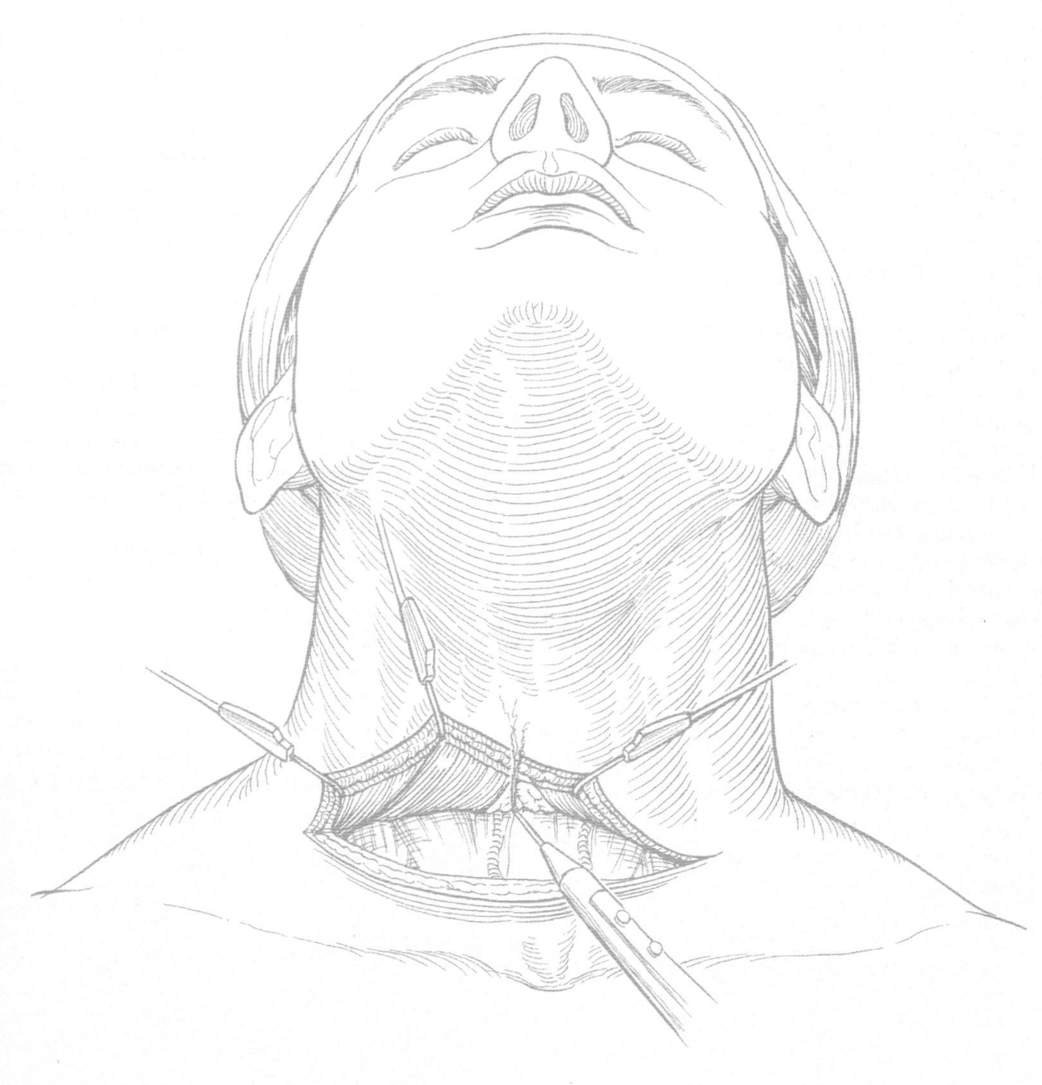

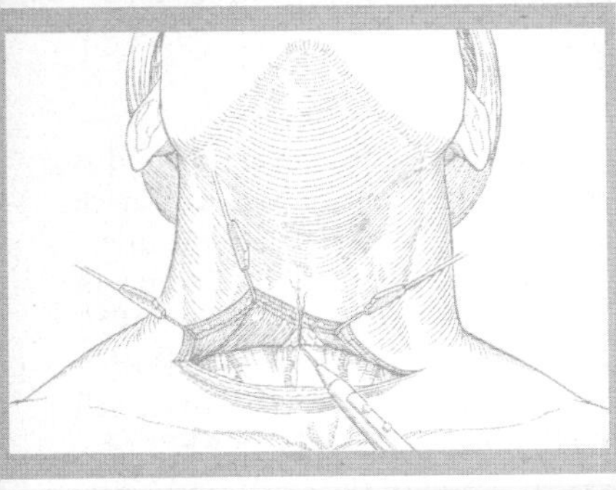

CHAPTER 34

Head and Neck

Wendell G. Yarbrough, Adam Zanation, Samip Patel, Saral Mehra

OUTLINE

Please access Elsevier eBooks for Practicing Clinicians to view the videos for this chapter https://expertconsult.inkling.com/.

NORMAL HISTOLOGY

The normal histology of the upper aerodigestive tract varies based on the cells, tissues, and function required of each site. A complete review of the thyroid and parathyroid glands is beyond the scope of this chapter. The upper aerodigestive tract can be conceptualized to start with the openings to the nose and mouth. The shape of the nasal vestibule is maintained by underlying septal, upper lateral, and lower lateral cartilages and is a cutaneous structure lined by keratinizing squamous epithelium that has sebaceous and sweat glands, as well as hair follicles. The limen nasi, or mucocutaneous junction, is where the epithelium changes to a ciliated pseudostratified columnar (respiratory) epithelium that lines the sinus and nasal cavities with the exception of the olfactory epithelium at the roof of the nasal cavity. The olfactory epithelium is a specialized tissue composed of supporting cells and bipolar olfactory neural cells with odorant receptors on cilia that face the nasal cavity and axons that coalesce to form the olfactory nerve (CN I) and pass through the cribriform plate on the deep surface. As with the nasal cavity, the paranasal sinuses are also lined by respiratory epithelium, but it tends to be thinner and less vascular than that of the nasal cavity. The nasopharyngeal lining varies from squamous to respiratory epithelium in an inconsistent manner. The adenoidal pad is a lymphoid tissue containing germinal centers without capsules or sinusoids and, like the palatine and lingual tonsils, contains a specialized lymphoepithelium with discontinuous basement membrane and intermixing of stromal, immune, and epithelial cells. The oral cavity is lined by nonkeratinized, stratified squamous epithelium with minor salivary glands throughout the submucosa and within the muscular tissue of the tongue. The oral cavity transitions to the oropharynx at the junction between the hard and soft palates and at the anterior tonsillar pillar. Waldeyer ring is formed by lymphoid tissues of the palatine tonsils, adenoids, lingual tonsils, and adjacent submucosal lymphatics. Similar to the adenoids, the palatine tonsils contain germinal centers without capsules or sinusoids, but, in contrast to the adenoids, the tonsils have crypts lined by stratified squamous epithelium with the lymphoepithelial cells residing at the base of the crypts. The junction between the oropharynx and hypopharynx is a horizontal line at the top of the hyoid bone. The hypopharynx is lined by nonkeratinizing, stratified squamous epithelium. Seromucous glands are found throughout the submucosa of the hypopharynx, in the lower two-thirds of the epiglottis and in the potential space between the true and false vocal folds known as the ventricle. The lining of the larynx transitions from nonkeratinizing, stratified squamous epithelium of the epiglottis and true vocal folds to pseudostratified, ciliated respiratory epithelium of the false vocal fold, ventricle, and subglottis. The thyroid, cricoid, and arytenoid cartilages are composed of hyaline cartilage, whereas the epiglottis, cuneiform, and corniculate cartilages are composed of elastic-type cartilage.

The external ear is a cutaneous structure lined with keratinizing squamous epithelium and associated adnexal structures. The external third of the external auditory canal is unique in that it contains modified apocrine glands that produce cerumen. The middle ear is lined with respiratory epithelium.

Numerous noncancerous changes in squamous epithelium can be seen in the upper aerodigestive tract. *Leukoplakia*, which describes any white mucosal lesion, and *erythroplakia,* which describes

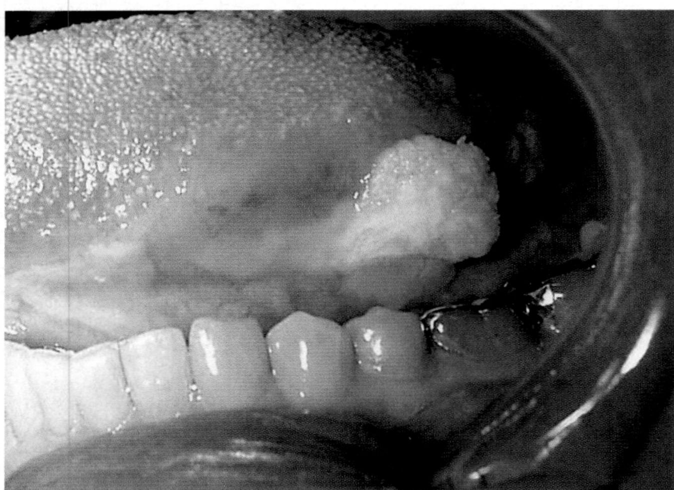

FIG. 34.1 Leukoplakic lesion on the left mobile tongue. On biopsy, this lesion was determined to be hyperkeratosis without invasive cancer.

any red mucosal lesion, are clinical descriptions and should not be used as diagnostic terms (Fig. 34.1). *Erythroplakia* is more concerning than leukoplakia, since it is more often associated with an underlying malignant lesion. *Hyperplasia* refers to thickening of the epithelium, while *parakeratosis* is an abnormal presence of nuclei in the keratin layers, and *dyskeratosis* refers to any abnormal keratinization of epithelial cells and is found in dysplastic lesions.

EPIDEMIOLOGY

The American Joint Committee on Cancer (AJCC) staging system divides sites of malignancies originating in the upper aerodigestive tract (i.e., head and neck) into eight major sites: lip and oral cavity, oropharynx, hypopharynx, larynx, nasal cavity and ethmoid sinus, maxillary sinus, major salivary glands, and thyroid.[1] Excluding salivary and thyroid, these cancers historically have been tightly associated with exposure to causative tobacco carcinogenesis. In the latter part of the twentieth century, the human papillomavirus (HPV) was identified as a cause of oropharyngeal and nasopharyngeal cancers and is also associated with a portion of sinonasal and nasopharyngeal cancers. Epstein-Barr virus (EBV) is responsible for a subset of nasopharyngeal cancers. While there remains a male preponderance in smoking-associated aerodigestive tract malignancies, the male-to-female ratio has been decreasing because of the direct association between tobacco as a causative agent and the increased incidence of female smokers. For reasons that are not totally understood, HPV-associated head and neck squamous cell carcinoma (HNSCC) has a 4:1 male preponderance.[2] The increased risk associated with combined abuse of alcohol and tobacco is multiplicative. By 2012, HPV caused more oropharyngeal cancers than uterine cervical cancers, and by 2015, HPV-associated oropharyngeal cancers accounted for more than 40% of all HPV-associated cancers in the United States.[2] HPV-associated cancer of the oropharynx affects younger individuals and is not associated with alcohol or tobacco use.

According to the National Cancer Database, squamous cell carcinoma (SCC) is the most common head and neck tumor of the major head and neck sites (88.9%), adenocarcinoma is the most common of the major salivary glands (56.4%), SCC is the most common of the sinonasal tract (43.6%), and lymphoma is the most common of the sites classified as "other" (82.5%).[4]

CARCINOGENESIS

Tobacco exposure is associated with many human cancers and is the major dose-dependent carcinogen that causes head and neck cancers (HNCs) that are not associated with HPV. HPV infection is now the primary cause of oropharyngeal carcinoma in the United States. Evidence has amassed mandating that HPV-positive and HPV-negative HNSCCs be considered two distinct cancers.[5] High-risk HPV types suppress apoptosis and activate cell growth through actions of the HPV oncogenes, E6 and E7. Malignant transformation requires expression of the HPV oncogenic proteins E6 and E7 that inactivate the p53 and retinoblastoma tumor suppressors, respectively.[6] E6 binds the cellular E6-associated protein and this complex targets p53 for ubiquitination and degradation contributing to unregulated cell growth. Likewise, E7 associates with retinoblastoma and targets retinoblastoma for proteasomal degradation.[6]

The Cancer Genome Atlas (TCGA) has added immensely to understanding of carcinogenesis. Mutation profiles have been assigned based on mutation type, and analysis of HNCs has revealed that there are two major patterns. HPV-negative HNSCCs are associated with mutational profiles associated with tobacco carcinogens and those associated activity of apolipoprotein B mRNA-editing enzyme catalytic polypeptide (APOBEC), while HPV-positive cancers have mutational profiles associated with APOBEC.[7] APOBECs are DNA editing enzymes that deaminate cytosine to form uracil in single-stranded DNA, thus creating a DNA mismatch. APOBECs, especially APOBEC3B, are important in innate immunity and A3B is upregulated in response to HPV, likely contributing to higher levels of APOBEC mutations in HPV-associated HNSCCs. APOBEC activity in HPV-positive HNSCC has been associated with the increased percentage of PIK3CA mutations in these tumors.[8]

Many years after Slaughter proposed field cancerization, the molecular basis of HNSCC began to be defined. Chromosomal gain and loss were initially studied, revealing that loss of heterozygosity at 9p21 and 3p21 was among the earliest detectable events leading to dysplasia, with further genetic alteration in 11q, 13q, and 14q being associated with carcinoma in situ.[9] The high rate of recurrence, in part, results from histopathologically benign squamous cell epithelium harboring a clonal population with genetic alterations. Patients with HNSCC have a 3% to 7% annual incidence of secondary lesions in the upper aerodigestive tract, esophagus, or lung. A synchronous second primary lesion is defined as a tumor detected within 6 months of the index tumor. The occurrence of a second primary lesion more than 6 months after the initial lesion is referred to as metachronous. A second primary develops in the aerodigestive tract of 14% of patients with HNSCC over the course of their lifetime, with more than half of these lesions occurring within the first 2 years of the index tumor.

Many individual studies identified important genetic defects that drive HNSCC or tumor maintenance. These studies culminated in a National Cancer Institute–led effort—TCGA—to molecularly characterize more than 500 HNSCCs through RNA sequencing, whole exome sequencing, methylation analysis, and reverse-phase protein analysis.[10] TCGA characterization of HNSCC clearly identified that HPV-associated and HPV-negative HNSCCs were molecularly distinct. Despite this distinction, many copy number alterations were shared between HPV-positive and HPV-negative HNSCCs, including losses of 3p and 8p and gains of 3q and 8q. Some copy number variants were unique to HPV-negative HNSCC, such as amplification of CCND1 (cyclin

D1) and loss of CDKN2A (p16INK4a), while amplification of FGFR 3 was observed primarily in HPV-associated SCC. Compared to many other tumor types, the number of structural alterations was high in HNSCC, averaging 141 amplifications or deletions and 62 chromosomal fusions per tumor genome. Gene mutation analysis confirmed defects in many known tumor suppressors and oncogenes, including p53, CDKN2A, PIK3CA, EGFR, and HRAS. While targeting of some frequently mutated oncogenes (MYC, HRAS) and tumor suppressor genes (*TP53, CDKN2A, NOTCH*) has not yet been successful for HNSCC, combined mutation and copy number analysis revealed that several receptor tyrosine kinases for which there are inhibitors (EGFR, FGFR1, ERBB2, IGF1R, FGFR2, FGFR3, MET) were altered in HPV-negative cancers. Unfortunately, these potential therapeutic targets in HNSCC have not advanced to clinical use.

A novel finding of the TCGA was identification of deletions and truncating mutations of the tumor necrosis factor (TNF) receptor–associated factor 3 (TRAF3) that previously was found only in hematologic malignancies. These defects were only found in HPV-positive HNSCC, and further analysis of TCGA data revealed that a portion of HPV-positive HNSCCs also harbored defects in CYLD (cylindromatosis lysine 63 deubiquitinase), with close to 30% of these tumors having a defect in one of these genes. TRAF3 and CYLD share common functions to inhibit the nuclear factor-κB (NF-κB) and activate innate immunity, and HPV-positive HNSCCs containing defects and TRAF3 or CYLD had increased expression of NF-κB regulated genes and downregulation of immune genes.[11] HNSCC with TRAF3 or CYLD defects lacked integrated HPV and had distinct methylation, HPV gene expression, and somatic gene expression profiles. Interestingly, no other solid tumors carry such high levels of inactivating defects in TRAF3 or CYLD except for nasopharyngeal cancer associated with EBV.[11] It is surprising that uterine cervical cancers, which are also caused by HPV, do not harbor a defect in these genes and that somatic mutations are largely not shared between HPV-associated HNSCC and uterine cervical cancer.[12] Clinical differences between uterine and cervical cancer and HPV-positive HNSCC are highlighted by treatment response and cure rate, which are higher in HNCs. Together, these data suggest that uterine cervical cancer and HPV-associated HNC are distinct. The high rate of episomal HPV, coupled with defects in innate immunity found in HNSCC, suggests that HPV integration, as described in uterine cervical cancer, is not required in HNSCC, suggesting that HPV may cause cancer through a different mechanism in the oropharynx. The Centers for Disease Control and Prevention reported that by 2012, HNCs were more common than uterine cervical cancer and was the most common HPV-associated cancer reported in the United States,[2] highlighting that HNSCC is a public health concern on par with uterine cervical cancer.

Alterations in immune recognition are common in both HPV-positive and HPV-negative HNSCCs with defects in human leukocyte antigen (HLA)-A/B noted in both tumor types, and it is becoming clear that tumors alter many normal processes to evade immune recognition. Over the last several years, drugs targeting the programmed cell death receptor 1 (PD-1)/PD-1 ligand (PD-L1) axis have been approved for use in recurrent and metastatic HNSCC. Response rates in these initial trials were approximately 20%, and promisingly, some responses persisted for years. There was a higher response rate in patients with a higher percentage of tumor cells or inflammatory cells in the tumor that expressed PD-L1. Other markers associated with response to PD-axis inhibitors include mutational load, immune cell infiltrate, and neoantigen expression.[13] Harnessing the immune system to control HNSCC has garnered great enthusiasm with many new and combination immune therapies emerging and being tested.

Understanding of mutational drivers of HPV-associated and HPV-negative HNSCC, as well as modulators of immune recognition, provides great promise for future advances in treatment. We currently lack adequate tools to pair ideal treatments with each patient's tumor. This shortcoming highlights the urgent need for identification of reliable prognostic biomarkers as we move toward personalized therapy of HNSCC.

STAGING

The AJCC creates criteria for tumor staging based on characteristics of the primary tumor (T) and nodal metastases (N), as well as the presence of distant metastases (M), accumulatively TNM. All tumors can have clinical TNM (cTNM) staging, and cancers that are treated surgically can have pathologic staging–designated pTNM.[1] The T classification refers to the extent of the primary tumor and is specific to each of the six sites of origin, with subclassifications within each site. The N classification identifies the pattern of lymphatic spread within the neck nodes. Clinical staging of the neck is based on palpation for enlarged nodes and radiographic evaluation of the neck. Using the computed tomography (CT) criteria for identification of nodal metastases, central necrosis or size larger than 1.0 cm (>1.5 cm for level II), 7% of pathologically positive lymph nodes are misclassified as negative based on CT imaging, and these smaller nodes are most often found in necks with more extensive disease. ^{18}F-fluorodeoxyglucose positron emission tomography (^{18}F-FDG PET)/CT scanning and advanced informatics techniques are being explored to improve detection of nodal metastases of HNSCC, especially for the clinically N0 (cN0) necks. Metastatic disease is reported as Mx (cannot be assessed), M0 (no distant metastases are present), or M1 (metastases present). The most common sites of distant spread are the lungs, whereas hepatic, bone, and brain metastases occur less frequently. The risk for distant metastases depends more on nodal staging than on primary tumor size.

Classification of nodal metastases for thyroid, nasopharynx, mucosal melanoma, and skin has consistently differed from HNSCC because of differences in behavior of these distinct tumor types. Until the eighth edition of the AJCC staging manual, HPV-positive and HPV-negative cancers used identical criteria for TNM classification and had the same staging grid. As an acknowledgement that HPV-positive and HPV-negative HNSCC are distinct diseases, they now have distinct T and N classification in the eighth edition of the AJCC staging manual (Figs. 34.2 and 34.3). For the first time, the pathologic and clinical T and N classifications of HNSCC are based on different criteria (data not shown and Tables 34.1 and 34.2). Finally, HPV-positive and HPV-negative HNSCCs have different staging criteria, with one example being that stage IV in HPV-positive HNSCC applies only to patients with distant metastases, whereas in HPV-negative HNSCC, stage IV also encompasses all patients with T4, N2, or N3 disease (Figs. 34.2 and 34.3).

In the eighth edition of the *AJCC Cancer Staging Manual*,[1] a descriptor has been added as ECS+ or ECS–, depending on the presence or absence of nodal extracapsular spread (ECS).

After complete resection of the primary and nodal disease, pathologic staging may be reported as pTNM. Pathologic T and N classification allows occult spread or microscopic disease to be considered and is useful in determining prognosis.

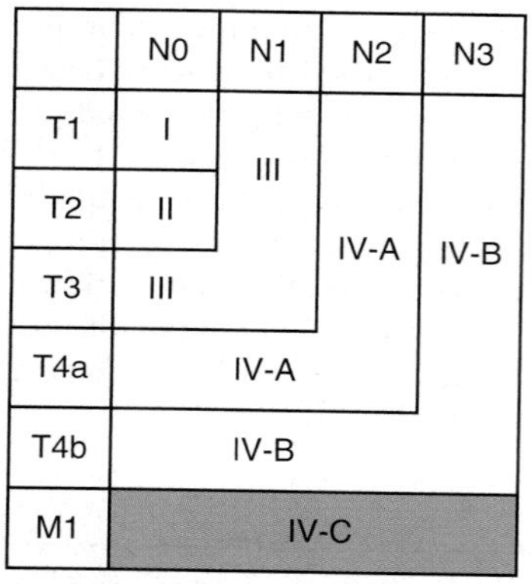

<table>
<tr><th></th><th>N0</th><th>N1</th><th>N2</th><th>N3</th></tr>
<tr><td>T1</td><td>I</td><td rowspan="2">III</td><td rowspan="3">IV-A</td><td rowspan="4">IV-B</td></tr>
<tr><td>T2</td><td>II</td></tr>
<tr><td>T3</td><td colspan="2">III</td></tr>
<tr><td>T4a</td><td colspan="3">IV-A</td></tr>
<tr><td>T4b</td><td colspan="4">IV-B</td></tr>
<tr><td>M1</td><td colspan="4">IV-C</td></tr>
</table>

FIG. 34.2 Standard staging (human papillomavirus–negative head and neck squamous cell carcinoma) pathologic and clinical are identical.

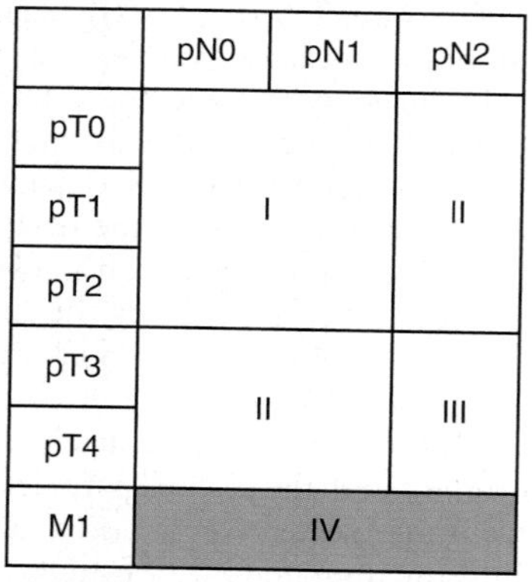

<table>
<tr><th></th><th>pN0</th><th>pN1</th><th>pN2</th></tr>
<tr><td>pT0</td><td colspan="2" rowspan="3">I</td><td rowspan="3">II</td></tr>
<tr><td>pT1</td></tr>
<tr><td>pT2</td></tr>
<tr><td>pT3</td><td colspan="2" rowspan="2">II</td><td rowspan="2">III</td></tr>
<tr><td>pT4</td></tr>
<tr><td>M1</td><td colspan="3">IV</td></tr>
</table>

FIG. 34.3 Human papillomavirus–positive pathologic staging.

Staging of HNCs changes as we more accurately identify determinants of outcome. The eighth edition of the *AJCC* Cancer Staging Manual highlights that the TNM classification system for HNCs is constantly evolving as new therapies and knowledge impacting outcome advance.

CLINICAL OVERVIEW

Evaluation

Proper treatment of HNC requires careful evaluation of tumor and patient characteristics, as well as accurate clinical and radiographic staging. Patients with HNC are initially evaluated in a similar manner, regardless of the site of tumor. Patient histories focus on manifestations of the tumor, including the duration of symptoms, detection of masses, location of pain, and presence of referred pain. Special attention is paid to numbness, cranial nerve weakness, dysphagia, odynophagia, hoarseness, airway compromise, trismus, nasal obstruction, and bleeding. Alcohol and tobacco use histories are elicited. Office examination includes direct visual inspection of the oral cavity and upper oropharynx, fiberoptic visualization of the nasopharynx, lower oropharynx, larynx, and hypopharynx, as well as palpation of accessible tumors and neck to detect potential nodal spread. The examiner should be especially vigilant for second primary tumors and should not be preoccupied by the obvious primary lesion. Contrast-enhanced CT and/or magnetic resonance imaging (MRI) of the head and neck are performed for evaluation of the tumor and detection of clinically undetected lymphadenopathy. CT scanning is best at evaluating bony destruction, whereas MRI can determine soft tissue involvement and neural spread and is excellent at evaluating parotid and parapharyngeal space tumors. Chest CT scanning is

TABLE 34.1 Clinical metastatic classification of regional lymph nodes (cN).

	DESCRIPTION	
CATEGORY	**HPV POSITIVE**	**HPV NEGATIVE**
cNX	Regional lymph nodes not assessed	Regional lymph nodes not assessed
cN0	No regional lymph node	No regional lymph node
cN1	1+ ipsilateral lymph node, ≤6 cm	Single ipsilateral lymph node, ≤3 cm
cN2	Bilateral lymph node all ≤6 cm	
cN2a		Single ipsilateral lymph node >3–6 cm
cN2b		Multiple ipsilateral lymph nodes ≤6 cm
cN2c		Bilateral/contralateral lymph nodes with all ≤6 cm
cN3	Any lymph node >6 cm	
cN3a		Any lymph node >6 cm
cN3b		Any lymph node over and ENE+

ENE, Extranodal extension; *HPV*, human papillomavirus

TABLE 34.2 Pathologic metastatic classification of regional lymph nodes (pN).

	DESCRIPTION	
CATEGORY	**HPV POSITIVE**	**HPV NEGATIVE**
pNX	Regional lymph nodes not assessed	Regional lymph nodes not assessed
pN0	No regional lymph node	No regional lymph node
pN1	Up to four lymph nodes with metastasis	Single ipsilateral lymph node, ≤3 cm
pN2	≥5 lymph nodes with metastasis	
pN2a		Single ipsilateral lymph node >3–6 cm or single ipsilateral lymph node ≤3 cm, ENE+
pN2b		Multiple ipsilateral lymph nodes ≤6 cm
pN2c		Bilateral/contralateral lymph nodes with all ≤6 cm
pN3a		Any lymph node >6 cm
pN3b		Any non pN1 lymph node, ENE+

ENE, Extranodal extension; *HPV*, human papillomavirus.

performed to rule out synchronous lung lesions, be they second primaries of metastatic lesions. Alternatively, ^{18}F-FDG PET imaging can be used for staging and detection of distant metastases, but anatomic detail at the primary site and nodal metastases frequently is not adequate to determine the extent of tumor spread. For HNC, excluding thyroid cancers, there are currently no blood markers that are used for diagnosis or prognosis of HNC. Circulating EBV DNA is used to follow tumor response for EBV-positive nasopharyngeal cancers and HPV DNA is being tested as a potential marker for following tumor response in HPV-positive HNSCC.

Direct laryngoscopy and examination under anesthesia are commonly performed as part of the evaluation of HNC. These procedures allow the physician to evaluate tumors without patient discomfort and

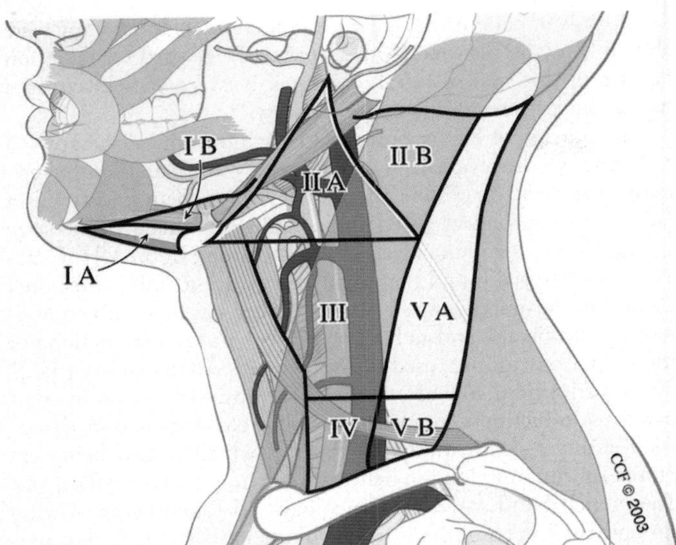

FIG. 34.4 Diagram of cervical lymph node levels I through V. Level II is divided into regions A and B by the spinal accessory nerve. (Courtesy Cleveland Clinic Foundation, 2003.)

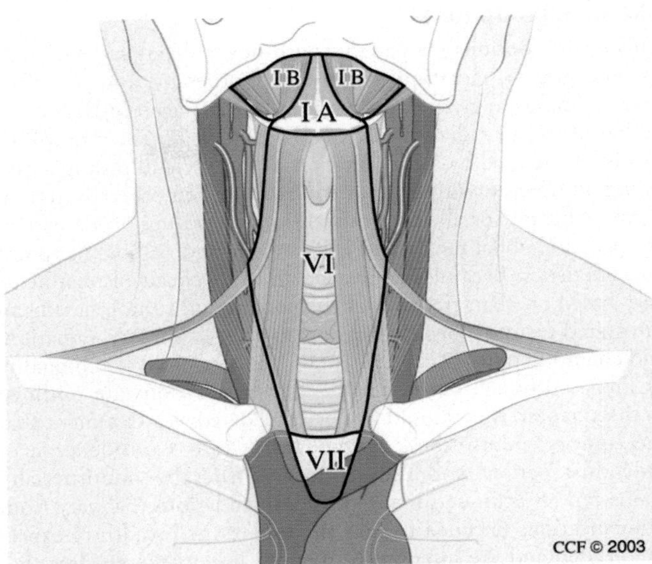

FIG. 34.5 Diagram of anterior lymph node levels I, VI, and VII. Although large in area, most level VI lymph nodes are confined to the paratracheal region. (Courtesy Cleveland Clinic Foundation, 2003.)

with muscle paralysis that aids in detection of tumors in areas that are difficult to palpate or visualize. Exam under anesthesia improves evaluation of the oropharynx, hypopharynx, and larynx and eases the ability to obtain biopsy samples. Pathologic confirmation of cancer is mandatory before initiating treatment, but this can be done by a biopsy with frozen section during the same anesthetic before a planned complete resection. Concurrent bronchoscopy and esophagoscopy have historically been recommended for the detection of synchronous second primaries of the aerodigestive tract, which occur in 4% to 8% of patients who have one head and neck malignancy. With a normal CT or PET scan, bronchoscopy and esophagoscopy have a low yield for discovering second primaries but are useful for determining direct tumor spread to the upper esophagus, subglottis, or trachea.

Increases in HPV-positive HNSCC have increased the portion of patients presenting without an obvious primary site. These *carcinomas of unknown primary* typically present with cancer in neck nodes, but the primary site cannot be identified clinically or radiographically. Since excisional biopsies should be a last resort for diagnosis for neck nodes, fine-needle aspirations (FNAs) and cytology can identify SCC in cervical nodes. HPV testing of FNA from neck nodes can be very useful, both for identification of nodal metastasis when the specimen is acellular and for directing the search for the primary cancer site, the oropharynx.

Lymphatic Spread

The cervical lymphatic nodal basins contain 50 to 70 lymph nodes per side and are divided into seven levels (Figs. 34.4 and 34.5).

Level I is subdivided:

- Level IA is bounded by the anterior belly of the digastric muscle, hyoid bone, midline, and mandible.
- Level IB is bounded by the anterior and posterior bellies of the digastric muscle and the inferior border of the mandible. Level IB contains the submandibular gland.

Level II is bounded superiorly by the skull base, anteriorly by the stylohyoid muscle, inferiorly by a horizontal plane extending posteriorly from the hyoid bone, and posteriorly by the posterior edge of the sternocleidomastoid muscle. Level II is further subdivided:

- Level IIA is anterior to the spinal accessory nerve.
- Level IIB, or the so-called submuscular triangle, is posterior to the nerve.

Level III begins at the inferior edge of level II and is bounded by the laryngeal strap muscles anteriorly, by the posterior border of the sternocleidomastoid muscle posteriorly, and by a horizontal plane extending posteriorly from the inferior border of the cricoid cartilage.

Level IV begins at the inferior border of level III and is bounded anteriorly by the strap muscles, posteriorly by the posterior edge of the sternocleidomastoid muscle, and inferiorly by the clavicle.

Level V is posterior to the posterior edge of the sternocleidomastoid muscle, anterior to the trapezius muscle, superior to the clavicle, and inferior to the base of the skull.

Level VI is bounded by the hyoid bone superiorly, the common carotid arteries laterally, and the sternum inferiorly. Although level VI is large in area, the few lymph nodes that it contains are mostly in the paratracheal regions near the thyroid gland.

Level VII (superior mediastinum) lies between the common carotid arteries and is superior to the aortic arch and inferior to the upper border of the sternum.

Lymphatic drainage usually occurs in a superior to inferior direction and follows predictable patterns based on the primary site. Primary tumors of the lip and oral cavity generally metastasize first to nodes in levels I, II, and III. The upper lip primarily metastasizes ipsilaterally, whereas the lower lip has ipsilateral and contralateral drainage. Tumors of the oropharynx, hypopharynx, and larynx usually metastasize to ipsilateral levels II, III, and IV with the exception of supraglottic larynx and base-of-tongue subsites that can spread bilaterally. Tumors of the nasopharynx spread to the retropharyngeal and parapharyngeal lymph nodes as well as to levels II through V. Other sites that metastasize to the retropharyngeal lymph nodes are the soft palate, posterior and lateral oropharynx, and hypopharynx. Scalp, ear, and posterior facial skin cancers can also metastasize to level V. Tumors of the subglottis, thyroid, hypopharynx, and cervical esophagus spread to levels VI and VII.

Therapeutic Options

Therapeutic options for patients with newly diagnosed HNSCC include surgery, radiation therapy, chemotherapy, and combination regimens. In general, early-stage disease (stage I or II) is treated by surgery or radiation therapy. Late-stage disease (stage III or IV) is best treated by a combination of surgery and postoperative radiation therapy, with upfront concurrent chemotherapy and radiation therapy, or all three modalities, depending on the site of the primary, nodal metastasis, HPV status, and pathologic tumor characteristics. Because the benefits and side effects of treatments vary based on characteristics of the patient and tumor, having an integrated team of specialists with expertise in surgery, radiation, and chemotherapy is critical to attain the best survival and quality of life.[14] Although current practice generalizations are outlined in this chapter, they should not be considered as a statement that the authors endorse these as standard of care. Consideration of individual patient and tumor characteristics by multispecialty teams can result in personalized recommendations that vary from generalizations outlined herein. Because of the breadth of expertise needed and the intensity of therapy, it has become clear that outcome is improved when patients are treated at centers that treat large numbers of patients with HNSCC.[14]

Since the highest risk of failure for HNSCC is by recurrence at the primary site or in regional cervical lymphatics, characteristics of the primary tumor and nodal metastases must be considered for therapeutic decisions. The neck is generally treated when there are clinically positive nodes or the historical risk for occult disease in an N0 neck approaches or is more than 20%, based on the location and classification of the primary lesion. The nodal basins at risk can be treated with neck dissection, radiation, or concurrent chemotherapy and radiation. If nonoperative therapy is recommended, addition of chemotherapy to radiation is influenced by the tumor's HPV status and the T and N classification with larger tumors or more advanced neck disease more frequently treated with concurrent radiation and chemotherapy, and early-stage disease with low T and low N classification more often treated with radiation alone. For surgically treated primary lesions, neck dissection is commonly performed if nodal disease is present or if the historical risk of occult nodal disease approaches or is more than 20%. For oral cancers, nodal dissection can be recommended for all patients or with consideration of depth of the primary tumor, which modifies the risk of nodal spread.[15,16]

Photon irradiation is effective for eradicating microscopic SCC and is an alternative to surgery for many early-stage, low-volume lesions. Subsets of tonsil, tongue base, and nasopharyngeal primary tumors are especially responsive to photon irradiation, particularly those driven by oncogenic viruses. Neutron and proton irradiation are used much less often in the head and neck, although experience has grown with their role in salivary gland malignancies (neutron irradiation) and skull base cancers (proton irradiation). Electrons are not commonly used in the head and neck for noncutaneous tumors. Intensity-modulated radiation therapy, which can reduce the photon dosage to surrounding normal tissue through computer three-dimensional (3D) planning, has been widely implemented in the head and neck in attempts to minimize the side effects of radiation. Radiation therapy is not as effective in treating large-volume, low-grade neoplasms or tumors involving bone or cartilage or in close proximity to the mandible.

A landmark chemotherapy trial for HNSCC was the Department of Veterans Affairs larynx trial, published in 1991.[17] This study established that response to induction chemotherapy in laryngeal cancer could be used to predict sensitivity to radiation. Two-thirds of patients treated with induction chemotherapy were able to keep their larynx. With surgical salvage used for radiation failures in this trial, survival was equal between patients treated with laryngectomy and radiation therapy.

This success of larynx preservation by nonsurgical therapy led to further studies evaluating chemotherapy and radiation for primary treatment of HNC. The idea of using chemotherapy as a radiation sensitizer was tested by the Radiation Therapy Oncology Group (RTOG) and the Head Neck Intergroup in the RTOG 91-11 trial. This trial found that organ preservation and locoregional control for advanced-stage laryngeal cancer was best with concurrent chemotherapy and radiation compared to radiation alone or the induction regimen used in the Veterans Affairs larynx trial.[18] The superiority of concurrent chemotherapy with radiation compared to induction chemotherapy followed by radiation dampened enthusiasm for induction therapy, which is now being explored for tumor reduction before surgery to preserve vital organs. The French Head and Neck Oncology and Radiotherapy Group strengthened the argument for chemotherapy as a radiation sensitizer by finding that concomitant chemotherapy with radiation improved overall survival and locoregional control compared to radiation alone for advanced oropharyngeal cancer.[19] Combined, these studies and others established cisplatin and radiation therapy as an alternative to surgery, followed by radiation therapy for primary treatment of SCC of the head neck.

Short-term improvement in progression-free survival, locoregional control, and overall survival contributed to the establishment of concurrent platinum-based chemotherapy with radiation as a standard therapeutic option for previously untreated head neck cancer therapy. Ten-year results from the RTOG 91-11 trial revealed that while concurrent chemotherapy with radiation-maintained superiority for locoregional control, long-term laryngectomy-free and overall survival were better for patients treated with induction chemotherapy followed by radiation.[20] Similarly, analyses using nationwide databases have indicated that relative to nonoperative therapy, total laryngectomy improves survival for advanced-stage larynx cancer.[14] These findings indicate that for some head and neck tumors, concurrent chemotherapy and radiation may be associated with worse outcome due to less adequate therapy or long-term mortality unrelated to cancer recurrence. The balance between organ preservation, survival, and side effects of therapeutic modalities is another reason for personalization of therapy and further supports the multidisciplinary team model that is employed at high volume centers.

The efficacy of chemotherapy as a radiation sensitizer for primary treatment of HNSCC led to testing the addition of chemotherapy to postoperative radiation. Because of the increased short-term morbidity, concurrent chemotherapy and radiation were reserved for postoperative patients at high risk for recurrence based on T and N classification or poor pathologic features such as perineural spread, positive margins, or extracapsular extension of lymphatic metastasis. The European Organization for Research and Treatment of Cancer (EORTC) Trial 22931 and the RTOG Trial 9501 compared postoperative treatment of advanced-stage, high-risk HNSCC with radiation alone or concurrent cisplatin and radiation therapy. In the RTOG, the 2-year locoregional control rate was 82% for the group receiving chemoradiation therapy versus 72% for the radiation therapy–alone group. Disease-free survival was significantly longer in the patients who received chemoradiation therapy, although overall survival was not significantly different between the groups. In the EORTC trial, locoregional control, disease-free survival, and overall survival were superior for patients treated with postoperative concurrent chemotherapy and radiation compared to radiation alone. As expected, more toxicity and treatment morbidity were seen in the combined-treatment group, and further prognostic indicators to determine which patients are at high risk for failure are needed to predict which groups warrant this more intensive adjuvant therapy.

Standard therapy for recurrent or metastatic HNSCC has been cytotoxic chemotherapy, and the EXTREME trial established the combination of cisplatin, 5-fluorouracil, and the anti-EGFR antibody cetuximab as the most effective of the cytotoxic regimens.[21] Although the response rate of the EXTREME regimen is close to 40%, median overall survival of patients with EXTREME was approximately 10 months and the regimen is very toxic, with high percentages of patients experiencing severe toxicities. Despite reasonable activity, the toxicity and relatively modest increase in survival have limited the adoption of the EXTREME regimen and led investigators to search for alternatives. The success of therapy to reactivate the immune system in an array of solid tumors prompted testing of immune therapy in HNSCC. Inhibition of the PD-1/PD-L1 axis, which normally inhibits the adaptive immune response, was initially tested for second-line therapy of recurrent/metastatic HNSCC after failure of platin-containing regimens. In these trials, antibodies targeting PD-1 have improved overall survival with a near doubling of the response rate compared to a single agent EGFR inhibitor, methotrexate, or taxane therapy.[22] As compared to other therapies for recurrent or metastatic HNSCC, some patients treated with immunotherapy maintained long-term tumor-free status. Unfortunately, response in the recurrent or metastatic patient population to this promising therapy has been low, 13% to 20%, indicating that better prognostic markers or additional therapies are needed. Prognostic markers including immune infiltrate, PD-L1 expression in tumor cells, PD-L1 expression in tumor infiltrating immune cells, and mutational load are all currently being explored.

PD-1–axis antibodies are now being tested in first-line therapy for patients with recurrent/metastatic head and neck cell carcinoma both as a single agent and in combination with standard cytotoxic chemotherapy or other therapies. Early results are promising, with response rates to immunotherapy slightly lower than that observed with EXTREME, but in patients with even modest PD-L1 expression in tumor or immune cells, overall survival was superior with immune therapy.[23] When data are fully analyzed, immunotherapy may become the preferred first-line treatment for recurrent and metastatic HNSCC.

ANATOMIC SITES

Neck

The neck is not an anatomic site for primary tumors within the upper aerodigestive tract; however, cervical lymph nodes must be treated if involved by metastatic HNC and are typically treated if the risk of metastatic lymphadenopathy is predicted to be greater than 20%. HNSCC has a relatively low propensity for distant metastatic spread but commonly spreads to lymph nodes within the anterior cervical chains, making treatment of local and regional disease of utmost importance for cure. Neck dissections have been categorized based on nonlymphatic structures that are removed and based on the levels of lymph nodes that are excised. Radical neck dissection (RND) is the most comprehensive procedure with removal of levels I to V, as well as the jugular vein, sternocleidomastoid muscle, and spinal accessory nerve (cranial nerve XI). Lateral neck dissections remove lymphatic tissue from levels II to IV, while lymphatic tissue excised with supraomohyoid neck dissection is limited to levels I to III. The anterior neck is a compact area packed with somatic and cranial nerves, named and unnamed vessels, lymphatics including the specialized thoracic duct, salivary glands, endocrine organs, and structures of the respiratory, digestive, and combined aerodigestive tracts. Excision of cervical lymph nodes requires identification of the many nerves, vessels, and other structures that can and should be preserved unless characteristics of the tumor mandate their removal.

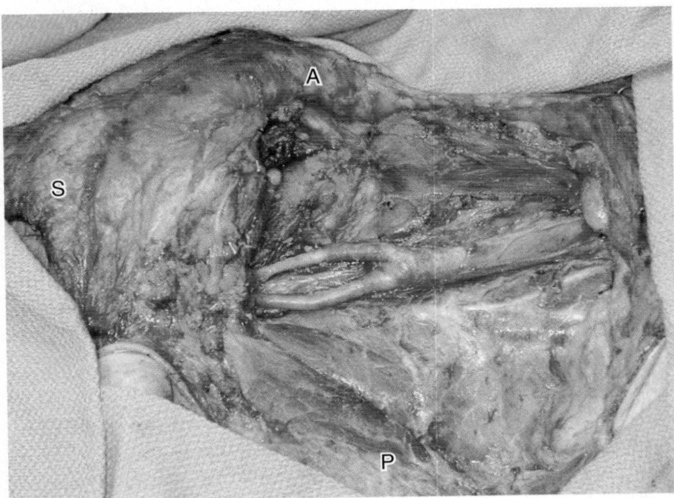

FIG. 34.6 Proper appearance of the right neck after a radical neck dissection. In addition to all lymphatic tissue, the three structures of the internal jugular vein, sternocleidomastoid muscle, and spinal accessory nerve have been resected. *A*, Anterior; *P*, posterior; *S*, superior.

The RND was attributed to Crile in 1906 and, for many years, was the only described technique for oncologic removal of nodal metastases (Fig. 34.6). All modifications of neck dissection are described in relation to the standard RND, which removes nodal levels I through V and the sternocleidomastoid muscle, internal jugular vein, cranial nerve XI, cervical plexus, and submandibular gland. Preservation of the sternocleidomastoid muscle, internal jugular vein, or cranial nerve XI in any combination is referred to as a modified RND, and the structures preserved are specified for nomenclature. A modified neck dissection may also be referred to as a Bocca neck dissection, named after the surgeon who demonstrated that not only is modified RND equally as effective in controlling neck disease as RND, but also the functional outcomes of patients after modified RND are superior to functional outcomes after RND.[24] Although resection of the sternocleidomastoid muscle or one internal jugular vein is relatively nonmorbid, loss of cranial nerve XI leaves a denervated trapezius muscle, which can cause a painful chronic frozen shoulder; however, physical therapy can prevent or limit pain and maximize mobility. Documentation that tumor control was equivalent with modified RND while sparing uninvolved structures within the neck has led to a wider adoption of modified RND and selective neck dissections for HNC.

Selective neck dissection is a neck dissection that preserves any level (I–V) and is based on the knowledge of the patterns of regional metastatic spread to the cervical lymphatics. Oral cavity cancers mostly likely involve levels I to III, while pharyngeal and laryngeal most likely involve levels II to IV. Selective neck dissections are frequently used for clinically negative (cN0) necks to spare nodal groups carrying less than a 20% chance of being involved with metastatic disease. Postoperative neck radiation or concurrent chemotherapy with radiation may be added based on pathologic staging of excised nodes removed during selective neck dissection. The movement toward more minimal surgery for clinically negative necks (cN0) has progressed to exploration of sentinel lymph node biopsy, which attempts to predict the disease status of the neck based on removal and pathologic examination of the first echelon of tumor-draining nodes. Although sentinel lymph node biopsy has been used extensively with melanoma, its use in HNSCC has been hindered by technical issues, including difficulties with injection of the primary site and proximity of the primary cancer to nodes of interest. A study by the American College of Surgeons Oncology Group examined stages I and II oral SCCs, with findings that sentinel lymph node biopsy and enhanced pathologic examination of sentinel nodes from N0 necks correctly predicted pathologically negative cervical metastasis in 96% of patients.[25] Sentinel node technology continues to advance, with more specific detection now being explored in HNSCC.

The neck is the site of metastases of HNSCC and is anatomically complex with many critical structures. Neck dissections are used to clear nodal disease or to stage the neck to determine if postoperative therapy is needed. If the neck contains no metastatic disease or only a single neck node is involved, and if there are no poor prognostic features, then the patient may be spared postoperative therapy.

Oral Cavity

There are many diseases of the oral cavity, and a number of systemic diseases can manifest with lesions in the oral cavity. Persistent oral lesions should be appropriately evaluated with history, possible biopsy, and/or follow-up to assess for premalignant or malignant oral lesions. Lesions that come and go, or move to different locations, are less worrisome for cancer. Biopsy to establish a diagnosis should be a relatively small in-office pinch, punch, or incisional biopsy, to allow appropriate work-up if carcinoma is identified. Oral leukoplakia is a white patch in the oral cavity that has a low, but clinically significant, risk of either being cancer or progressing to cancer. The risk of a red lesion (erythroplakia) in the mouth being malignant is higher compared to leukoplakia.[26]

Mucosal lesions in the oral cavity can be diagnosed on biopsy as dysplasia, which is a histopathologic diagnosis based on a number of architectural and cellular changes. Grading of dysplasia includes mild, moderate, severe, and carcinoma in situ. Severe dysplasia and carcinoma in situ are premalignant lesions and treated similarly by complete surgical excision while mild and moderate dysplasia may be observed or excised. There are a number of oral mucosal lesions that can look like carcinoma but are either self-limited or treated medically, such as lichen planus, midline glossitis, pseudoepitheliomatous hyperplasia, and necrotizing sialometaplasia.

In addition to the stratified squamous epithelium lining the oral cavity, the mouth has nearly 1000 submucosal minor salivary glands, two sublingual salivary glands, bone, teeth, and neurovascular structures, all of which can lead to congenital, infectious, inflammatory, and neoplastic pathology. Examples of some rare but destructive or deforming oral cavity lesions that must be distinguished from oral cavity cancer include lymphovascular malformations (Fig. 34.7), granular cell tumors (with tongue as the most common site), hemangiomas, neuromas, neurofibromas, and leiomyomas. There are also a number of benign bone or dental tumors and cysts such as ameloblastoma, keratocystic odontogenic tumor, and dentigerous cyst that are treated surgically by either curettage or segmental mandibular or maxillary resection depending on various factors.

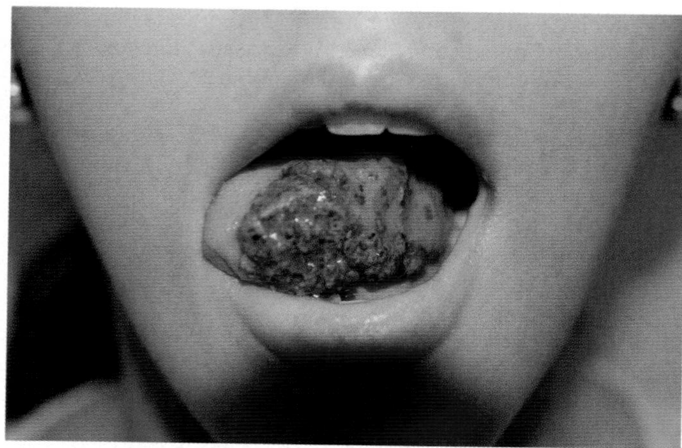

FIG. 34.7 Vascular malformation of the tongue.

Oral Cavity Malignancy

The oral cavity is the most common site of head and neck malignancy, and over 90% of oral cavity cancers are SCCs. Additional types of malignancies include minor salivary gland, mucosal melanoma, sarcomas (including Kaposi sarcoma), and lymphoma. Risk factors specific for oral cavity squamous cell cancer include tobacco products, alcohol, areca nut (also known as betel nut), and (for lip cancer) ultraviolet light exposure. Familial predisposition to HNSCC, including oral cavity cancers, occurs in patients with CDKN2A ($p16^{INK4a}$) mutations that are also predisposed to melanoma and in patients with Fanconi anemia, who are approximately 700 times more likely to develop HNSCC and can do so at a younger age.[27,28]

Staging of oral cavity cancer is based on tumor size and depth of invasion (DOI) beyond the basement membrane: T1, less than 2 cm and DOI less than 5 mm; T2, 2 to 4 cm and DOI less than 10 mm or less than 2 cm and DOI 5 to 10 mm; T3, greater than 4 cm or any size DOI greater than 10 mm; T4a, invading adjacent structures, such as mandible/maxilla bone (superficial erosion alone of bone or tooth socket by gingival primary does not count as bone invasion), deep muscle of tongue, or facial skin; and T4b, invading masticator space, pterygoid plates, skull base, encases internal carotid artery. For lip cancer, T4a is defined as invasion through the cortical bone and involvement of the inferior alveolar nerve, floor of mouth, or skin of the face.[1] Minor salivary gland malignancies are staged according to the site of tumor origin.

Oral Cavity Cancer Treatment

Upfront surgery remains the preferred initial treatment for oral cavity carcinoma [29] Surgery for oral cavity malignancy should include wide local resection of the primary tumor with negative margins. In most cases, positive margins in the oral cavity on final pathology should be re-resected if feasible. Reconstructive surgery should be an integral part of the treatment decision, as most oral cavity tumors are resectable, with suitable functional and cosmetic outcome if all reconstructive options are considered.

Management of the neck for oral cavity cancer depends on the presence or risk of regional metastases; in general, for early-stage oral cavity SCC, when the DOI is larger than 3 mm, an elective neck dissection is indicated. The extent of neck dissection can be either a selective supraomohyoid neck dissection (levels I–III) for

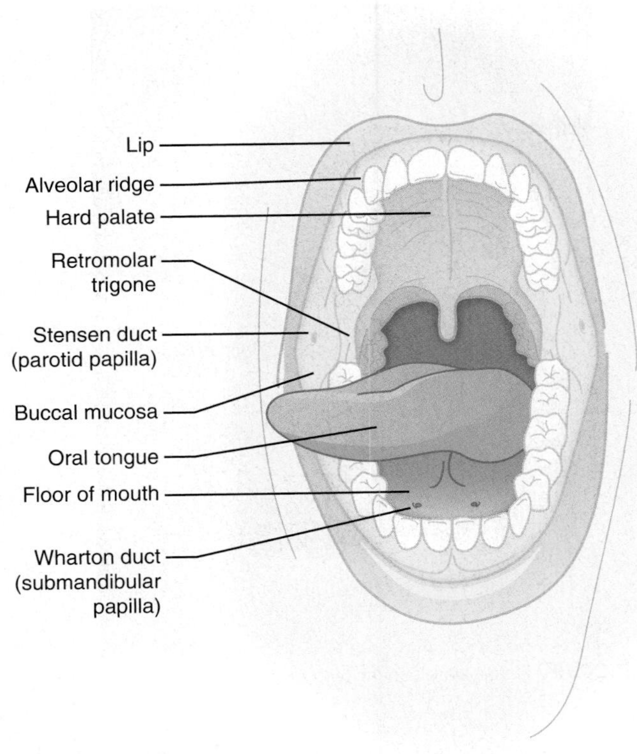

FIG. 34.8 Anatomy of the oral cavity and its subsites.

a clinically N0 neck or up to a modified RND (sparing all muscular and neurovascular structures if possible) for cN+ disease. If the primary tumor crosses the midline, bilateral neck treatment should be performed. Although not common practice in the United States for early-stage oral cancer, there are data to support elective neck dissection in all patients with T1 to T2 lateralized oral cavity SCC[15] and sentinel lymph node biopsy in early-stage oral cavity cancer.[25] The recommendation for adjuvant radiotherapy depends on particular pathologic factors, including the presence of perineural or lymphovascular invasion, T-stage, and regional nodal disease. Advanced-stage tumors are generally treated with adjuvant radiotherapy; chemotherapy is reserved for extranodal extension, close or positive margins (that cannot be re-resected), and, in some cases, high node burden or advanced T stage.

Subsites of the Oral Cavity

There are seven subsites to the oral cavity (Fig. 34.8), and each should be understood separately because the surgical and reconstructive considerations can be quite distinct. Importantly, the base of tongue, tonsils, tonsillar pillars, soft palate, and posterior pharynx wall are all part of the oropharynx (not the oral cavity) and have distinct functions and often pathology than the oral cavity. While HPV-related cancers of the head and neck have seen a remarkable increase in incidence, HPV is not thought to contribute significantly to oral cavity SCC at this time.

Lip. The lip starts at the junction of the facial skin and vermillion border and ends at the point where the upper and lower lips meet when the mouth is closed. The oral commissures are the lateral-most aspects of the lip and are important anatomic considerations as size and position are important for oral competence and mouth opening. In the United States, rates of lip cancer have decreased over the last 40 years, stabilizing at approximately 0.7 per 100,000 population, with white males having the highest incidence per person.[30] The incidence of lip cancer is much higher in countries that have higher rates of skin cancer (such as Australia) and in countries where tobacco use is more prevalent. Risk factors for lip cancer are similar to other oral cavity cancer sites, with the addition of ultraviolet exposure from sunlight and tanning beds (similar to skin cancers). Approximately 90% of lip tumors involve the lower lip (Fig. 34.9), and the most common type of lip cancer is SCC, but other cancers can include basal cell carcinoma (BCC), melanoma, and minor salivary gland tumors. In the United States, 5-year overall survival for cancers of the lip from 2008 to 2014 was 88.4%.[30] The main reconstructive considerations following lip surgery are maintenance of oral competence and appearance. Reconstructive methods for the lips can range from primary closure, mucosal advancement flaps, lip-switch staged flaps, adjacent tissue transfer, nasolabial flaps, and free flaps for cases of total lip reconstruction.

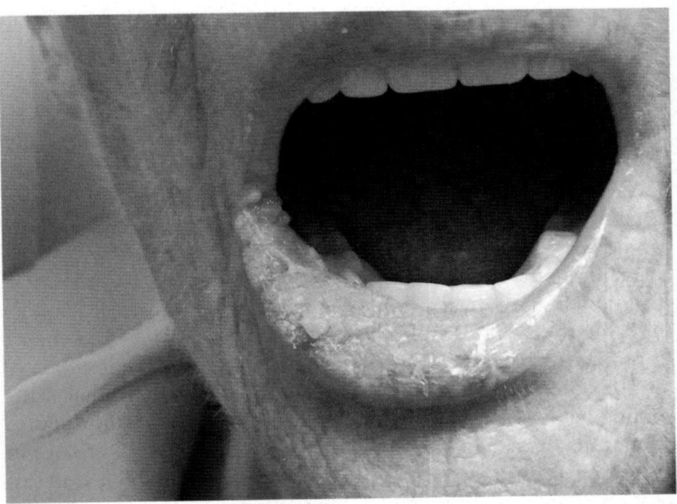

FIG. 34.9 Lip cancer.

Oral tongue. The oral tongue extends from the floor of mouth to the circumvallate papillae posteriorly. The base of tongue (and lingual tonsils) is not anatomically part of the oral tongue or the oral cavity. The tongue is a muscular organ made of four intrinsic muscles and four extrinsic muscles, which are anchored to bone and/or aponeurosis. Lesions in the tongue can be described by location, including lateral border, dorsal tongue, or ventral tongue. The oral tongue plays a critical function in speech articulation and the oral phase of swallowing. Partial glossectomy is appropriate surgery for tongue malignancy, and larger tumors can require resection of adjacent subsites such as the floor of mouth, alveolar mucosa, mandible, or maxilla. If bilateral lingual arteries and/or hypoglossal nerves are sacrificed as part of tumor extirpation, vascularity and function will be compromised; therefore, if the tumor extent allows, effort should be made to maintain neurovascular integrity to one side of the tongue. If total glossectomy is required for adequate tumor extirpation, the risk of aspiration is greatly increased and patients may require a total laryngectomy to avoid aspiration pneumonia. Reconstruction following glossectomy considers optimizing tongue mobility for speech and swallowing, maintenance of adequate oral bulk for propulsion of food boluses, and minimizing the risk of aspiration. In cases where the extrinsic tongue muscles are separated from the hyoid bone, a hyoid and/or laryngeal suspension procedure should be considered to decrease risk of aspiration.

Floor of the mouth. The floor of mouth extends from the lingual surface of the mandible to the ventral tongue anteriorly, and to the glossotonsillar sulcus (or anterior tonsillar pillars) posteriorly. The left and right sides are separated by the lingual frenulum, and lateral to the frenulum on each side is the papilla of the submandibular duct (Wharton duct). The submandibular duct papilla should be cannulated and protected in surgeries involving the floor of mouth whenever possible, and redirection with sialodochoplasty can be performed to maintain submandibular gland salivary flow. The submandibular duct in the floor of mouth is also the most common site of salivary stones, which can oftentimes be successfully removed endoscopically.[31] In addition, the lingual nerve (a branch of trigeminal V3 cranial nerve) travels in the floor of mouth quite superficially and is crossed by the duct. Finally, the sublingual gland lies in the floor of mouth and can be the source of a ranula or malignancy. The floor of mouth plays an important role in separating the tongue from the mandible, which is necessary for tongue mobility and a major consideration in oral cavity reconstruction.

Buccal mucosa. The buccal mucosa extends from the inner surfaces of the upper and lower lips to the labial aspect of the maxilla and mandible. Chewing tobacco, including snuff dipping, is especially associated with dysplasia and carcinoma of the buccal mucosa. Additionally, oral submucosal fibrosis commonly involves the buccal mucosa and is associated with consumption of areca nut (commonly referred to as betel nut), which is a fruit of areca palm. Oral submucosal fibrosis is an inflammatory, premalignant condition that leads to significant scarring and fibrosis in this region and resultant trismus. Surgical considerations for the buccal mucosa include the parotid duct (Stensen duct) and parotid papilla, which opens in the buccal mucosa adjacent to the upper second molar. Maintaining adequate mouth opening to avoid trismus is a major reconstructive consideration following ablative surgery of the buccal mucosa, and the use of mouth opening exercises and physical therapy as surgical adjuncts can help to improve function.

Palate. The hard palate is the area medial to the maxillary alveolar ridges and extends posteriorly to the soft palate (which is part of the oropharynx). The hard palate forms the roof of the mouth separating the mouth from the nose. Deep to the mucosal lining, the hard palate is formed by the palatine process of the maxillary bone and the palatine bone. For erosive, submucosal, and invasive lesions of the hard palate, the nasal cavity and sinuses should be examined because a small hard palate lesion could be just the tip of more substantial nasal or paranasal sinus pathology (Fig. 34.10). For example, in immunocompromised patients, invasive fungal sinusitis can present as a palatal erosion, and although not a cancer, it carries a high mortality and must be dealt with expeditiously. There are several benign conditions of the palate with some that mimic a mass or cancer. Torus palatini is a common and benign bone growth in the center hard palate, which only requires surgical removal if it interferes with function such as adequate fitting of upper dentures. Necrotizing sialometaplasia is a self-limited ulcerative inflammatory lesion of minor salivary glands that can mimic carcinoma on physical examination and requires clinical suspicion for appropriate diagnosis and avoidance of inappropriate treatment.

Tumors of the hard palate can arise from the stratified squamous mucosa, with the most frequent malignancy being SCC or from minor salivary glands. Due to a thick mucoperichondrium that is fixed to the bone, hard palate malignancies typically require removal of bone for adequate margin, and surgical approaches include infrastructure maxillectomy or total maxillectomy depending on extent of tumor. The main reconstructive considerations are separation of the oral and nasal cavities for optimization of speech and swallowing, dental restoration for mastication and appearance, as well as upper alveolar arch reconstruction for midface form. Reconstruction of maxillectomy defects can include dental obturation, soft tissue regional/free flaps for posterolateral defects, or bone-containing free flaps with the possibility of subsequent dental implantation.

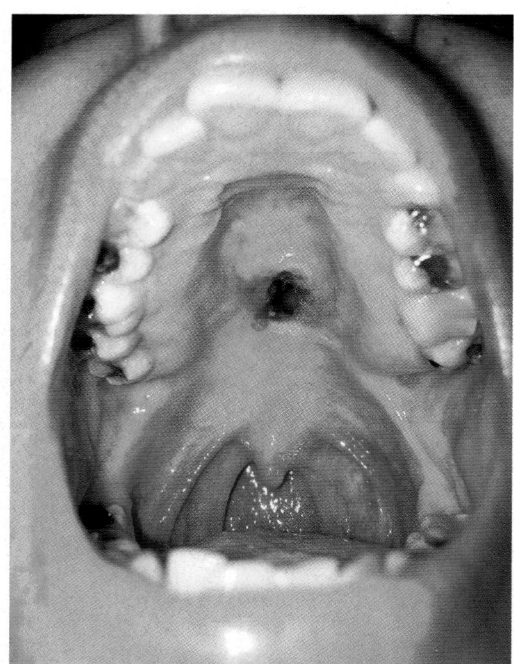

FIG. 34.10 Hard palate cancer with erosion into the nasal cavity.

Alveolus. The alveolus (or alveolar ridge) and the accompanying gingiva extend from the gingivobuccal sulcus laterally to the floor of mouth and hard palate and make up the dental surfaces of the maxilla and mandible. SCC is the most common malignancy of the alveolus and is much more common at the lower gingiva. Upper gingival primaries often extend onto the hard palate and many surgical considerations are the same for both. Adequate tumor resection requires resection of the alveolar ridge mucosa and underlying periosteum. The periosteum of the mandible is a strong tumor barrier, and tumors that abut the bone may be resected along with the adjacent periosteum only. Tumors adherent to the periosteum should undergo excision with marginal mandibulectomy, which involves resection of the superior or inner cortical portions of the mandible, with preservation of a continuous rim. If there is more than superficial cortical erosion of the mandible, the marrow space is at risk of harboring malignancy, and thus, a segmental mandibulectomy is required for adequate margin control. In many cases of alveolar primary tumors, dental extraction is required for both exposure and osteotomies. Reconstructive considerations of the alveolus include maintaining tongue mobility if adjacent floor of mouth is also resected, vestibule height if adjacent buccal mucosa/inner lip is resected, and dental restoration with prosthesis or implants if possible. For marginal mandibulectomy defects involving adjacent floor of mouth, in many cases, lowering the mandible height can allow for closure by undermining and mobilizing floor of mouth without tethering the tongue. For segmental mandible defects (Fig. 34.11), obturation is not a

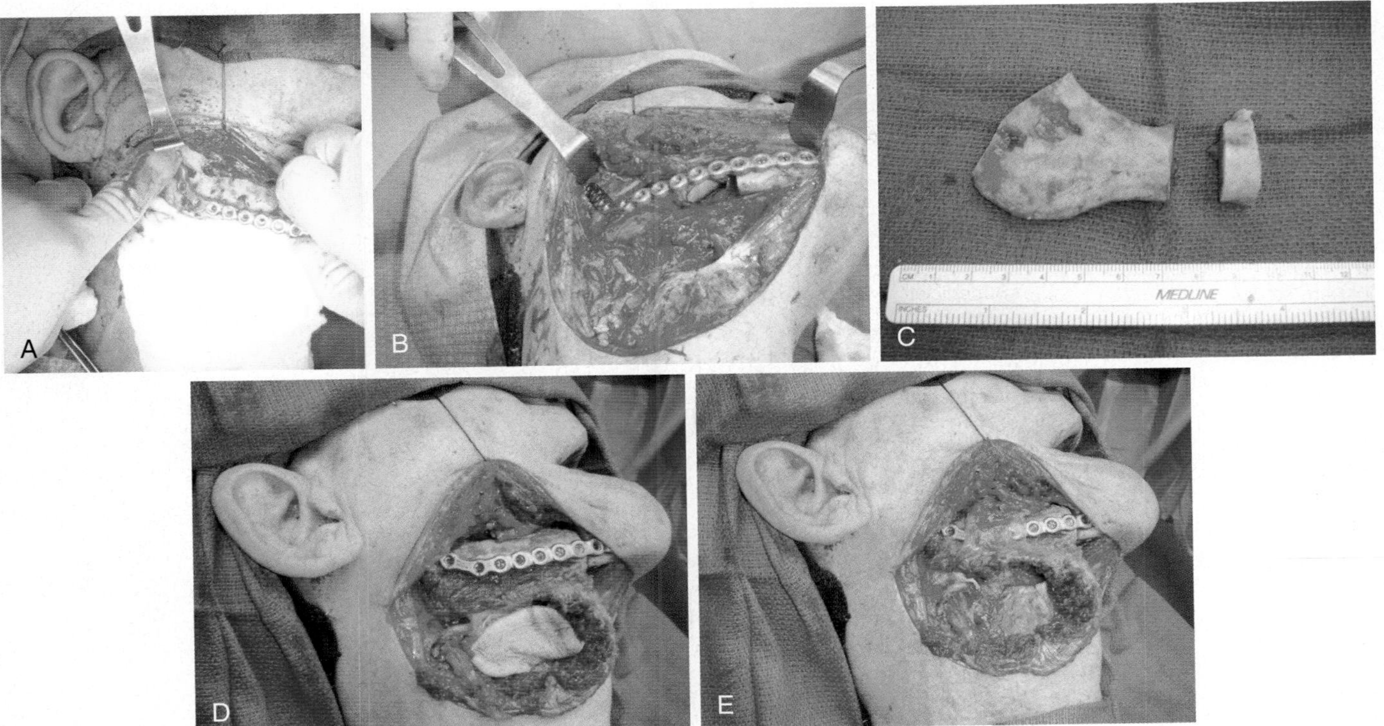

FIG. 34.11 Segmental mandible resection and osseocutaneous fibula free flap reconstruction for alveolar ridge primary carcinoma. (A) Mandible exposure with prebending of plate prior to resection. (B) Defect showing mandible resected along with floor of mouth defect into oral cavity. (C) Resected right mandible with additional piece for improved margin. (D) Fibula free flap in place under titanium plate prior to turning skin inside mouth. (E) Skin paddle flipped over plate for closure of intraoral defect.

suitable reconstructive option and vascularized osseocutaneous (or bone only) free flaps are the preferred reconstruction.

Retromolar trigone. The retromolar trigone is the region defined by the ascending ramus of the mandible starting on each side just posterior to the last molar tooth and ending adjacent to the tuberosity of the maxilla. Numerous adjacent subsites of the oral cavity (buccal mucosa, upper and lower alveolar ridge) and oropharynx (anterior tonsil pillar and soft palate) are immediately adjacent to the retromolar trigone, making exact identification of the primary site difficult. In addition, the attached gingiva in this region is extremely thin, and the inferior alveolar nerve enters the mandible through the mandibular foramen near this region of the mandible. For these reasons, tumors in the retromolar trigone have a higher propensity for bone invasion, and the inferior alveolar nerve is at greater risk when performing marginal mandibulectomy in this region. Reconstructive considerations are the same as those for mandibular or lower alveolar ridge reconstruction, issues inherent to multiple subsite involvement, and trismus. The buccal fat flap can be quickly and easily harvested to reconstruct defects of the retromolar trigone with vascularized tissue.

Oropharynx

Anatomy

Until the epidemic of HPV-associated HNC hit the United States, the oropharynx was a low-volume site for HNSCC, with laryngeal cancer and oral cavity cancers far outnumbering those of the oropharynx. Since the epidemic, HPV-positive oropharyngeal SCC (OPSCC) has increased ~225%, while HPV-negative OPSCC has decreased 50%. Likewise, the 1990s to the present have seen a steadily decreasing incidence of oral cavity and larynx cancers.[32] Since 2012, the incidence of HPV-positive OPSCC has been greater than the incidence of uterine cervical cancer, making oropharyngeal cancer the most commonly diagnosed HPV-associated cancer in the United States.[2] In 2015, HPV-positive OPSCC was more common than HPV-associated vulvar, vaginal, anal, and penile cancers combined.[33]

Anatomic borders of the oropharynx include the circumvallate papillae anteriorly, plane of the superior surface of the soft palate superiorly, plane of the hyoid bone inferiorly, pharyngeal constrictors laterally and posteriorly, and medial aspect of the mandible laterally. Subsites within the oropharynx include the base of the tongue, inferior surface of the soft palate and uvula, anterior and posterior tonsillar pillars, glossotonsillar sulci, pharyngeal tonsils, and lateral and posterior pharyngeal walls. Unlike other sites within the upper aerodigestive tract and other subsites within the oropharynx, the tonsil and base of tongue are predisposed to develop HPV-associated cancers. The selectivity of HPV for the base of tongue and tonsil likely relates to the specialized reticular epithelium that is closely associated with lymphatic tissue that is designated lymphoepithelium. Lymphoepithelial cells are specialized for antigen presentation, and related to this function, they reside in the depths of tonsillar crypts, where they directly contact and intermingle with lymphatic and professional antigen-presenting cells in an area where there is a discontinuous basement membrane (Fig. 34.12). Although poorly understood, it has been suggested that unique molecular characteristics of lymphoepithelial cells or signaling with surrounding lymphatic cells permits or accelerates HPV carcinogenesis. Regardless, the pharyngeal and lingual tonsils within the oropharynx are sites that account for the vast majority of HPV-positive HNSCCs.

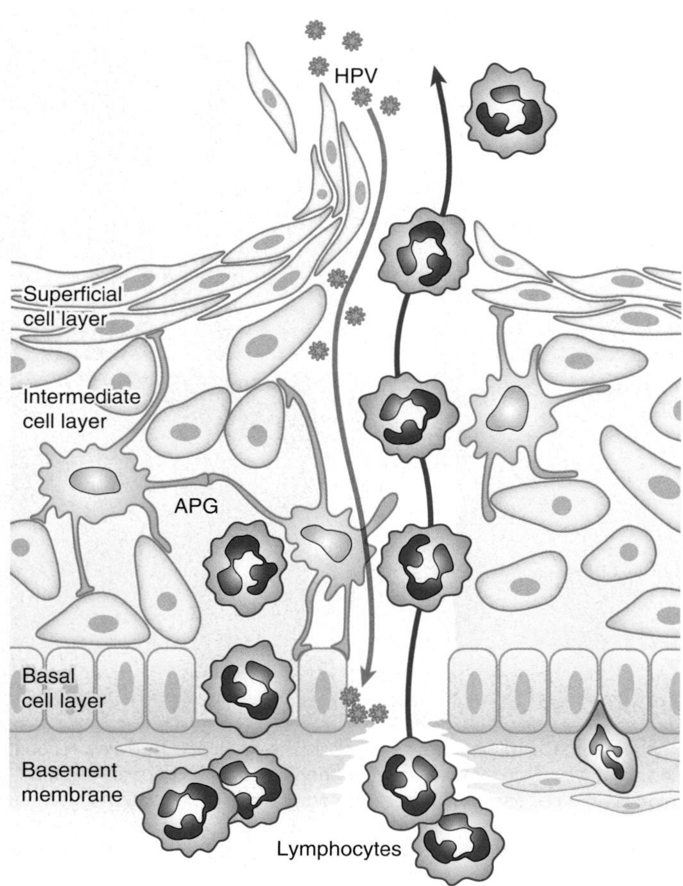

FIG. 34.12 The specialized reticulated epithelium lining the tonsillar crypts. The basal, intermediate, and superficial layers are interrupted by migrating nonepithelial cells including lymphocytes and antigen-presenting cells. Destruction to the basement membrane causes contact to viral particles (Drawing by T. Phelps). *APG*, Antigen-presenting group; *HPV*, human papillomavirus.

Oropharyngeal Cancer and Treatment

Of tumors of the oropharynx, 90% are SCCs. Other tumors include lymphoma of the pharyngeal tonsils or lingual tonsils at the tongue base or salivary gland neoplasms arising from minor salivary glands in the soft palate, tongue base, or less frequently the pharyngeal walls. Initial symptoms of oropharyngeal cancer include sore throat, bleeding, dysphagia and odynophagia, referred otalgia, globus sensation, and voice changes including a muffled quality or "hot potato" voice. HPV-positive cancers are more likely to be asymptomatic and present with a neck mass as the only sign. Trismus suggests spread outside of the oropharynx with involvement of the pterygoid musculature. For treatment decision-making, imaging studies are obtained to evaluate invasion through the pharyngeal constrictors, bony involvement of the pterygoid plates or mandible, invasion of the parapharyngeal space, relationship of the tumor to the carotid artery, relationship of the carotid artery to the pharyngeal wall, involvement of the prevertebral fascia and laryngeal extension. If present, lymph node metastases generally occur in levels II to IV of the jugular chain of nodes. Cystic metastatic nodes are frequently seen with HPV-positive OPSCC, and bilateral metastases are more common with tongue base involvement, especially as cancers approach the midline.

Standard concurrent chemotherapy and radiation provide excellent local control and overall survival for nonsmokers with HPV-positive OPSCC, even for patients with regional lymphatic metastases. For similar patients with HPV-positive OPSCC who have more than 10-pack years of smoking, survival following chemoradiation is not as favorable as patients with minimal smoking history, but still equivalent to patients with early-stage HPV-negative cancer.[34] HPV-associated SCC accounts for more than 75% of oropharyngeal cancers in the United States, and the high rate of cure coupled with the toxicity of therapy in these patients has sparked interest in deintensification of therapy. The reasons and support for de-escalation approaches are that response and survival are high with standard therapies, but aggressive therapies currently used for treatment of HNSCC were developed to improve the survival of patients with HPV-negative HNSCC and carry significant morbidity. Patients with HPV-positive OPSCC are healthier, smoke less, are younger, and have longer expected survival compared to HPV-negative HNSCC patients, spurring investigators to seek less aggressive therapies with the goal of decreasing long-term morbidities. In addition to deintensification through limiting chemotherapy or decreasing radiation fields or dosage, transoral robotic surgery (TORS) has a role for de-escalation with excellent results as a single modality for early-stage disease. TORS can also be used to avoid concurrent chemotherapy and is being explored as a means to decrease radiation dosage. A cooperative group trial used pathologic stratification after TORS and neck dissection to assign deintensified radiation for HPV-associated

OPSCC, but results are not yet mature. Other de-escalation trials for untreated advanced-stage HPV-positive HNSCC used response to induction chemotherapy to stratify patients to lower radiation doses, but results are not mature to determine if this strategy is advantageous.[35] A randomized cooperative group trial (RTOG 1016) compared concurrent radiation and cetuximab versus cisplatin for patients with HPV-positive OPSCC and nodal metastasis.[36] The trial's goal was to determine if side effects and morbidity associated with cisplatin could be safely avoided by substitution of cetuximab. Unfortunately, the trial found that cetuximab and radiation were inferior to the standard, but more toxic, therapy of cisplatin and radiation. Exploratory trials targeting advanced-stage HPV-positive HNSCC have tested the efficacy of lower radiation doses combined with concurrent weekly cisplatin and found a high rate of pathologic complete response.[37] Many of these early de-escalation studies for HPV-positive OPSCC have been promising, with results suggesting that therapy for HPV-positive HNSCC can be deintensified, but the results of the only randomized trial (RTOG 1016) are cautionary showing that some strategies designed to decrease side effects will also decrease efficacy and adversely impact survival. One central issue that hinders de-escalation studies is inability to select patients with low-risk HPV-positive HNSCC.

The lone marker used clinically to predict response and survival in patients with HPV-associated HNSCC is patients' tobacco smoking history. Those with more extensive smoking history have worse response and survival than those who smoked less. Why smoking history correlates with survival for HPV-positive HNSCC is unknown, especially since smoking is not a risk factor for this subset of HNSCC. New predictive biomarkers, especially molecular markers, are needed to appropriately choose low-risk patients with HPV-associated OPSCC for therapeutic deintensification while simultaneously identifying patients who need aggressive therapy. Recently, defects in *TRAF3* and *CYLD*, genes that regulate innate immunity and NF-κB, were found in approximately 30% of HPV-positive, but not in HPV-negative, HNSCCs.[11] Patients whose tumors harbored defects in these genes had improved survival compared to patients whose tumors lacked these defects. These results suggest that defects in *TRAF3* or *CYLD* may be used as a predictive biomarker; however, additional confirmatory studies and trials are needed before they can be used for clinical decision-making.

Regardless of HPV status, surgery is generally recommended for primary disease that involves bony structures such as the mandible or pterygoid plates, as well as for recurrent disease after radiation failure. However, some centers are individualizing treatment and recommending nonsurgical therapy for early bony invasion. Radiation, chemoradiation, and surgery with or without adjuvant treatment each have a role for management of OPSCC and therapy is commonly personalized based on the tumor characteristics, risk of recurrence, patient age and comorbidities, and expected side effects of therapy. Extensive surgery of the tongue base can significantly impair swallowing and in cases requiring excision of more than half of the base of tongue, chemoradiation is frequently recommended as the initial therapy. On the other hand, lateral cancers of the base of tongue, pharyngeal walls, or tonsil typically have good recovery of swallow and speech functions after surgical excision and secondary healing or reconstruction. Similar outcomes and functional recovery after surgery or nonsurgical therapy for lateralized oropharyngeal cancers makes either surgical and nonsurgical treatments reasonable.

The development and adoption of TORS have revitalized surgical therapies of OPSCC. Scopes with angled or flexible optics, combined with articulated or flexible instruments, is the innovation allowing surgeons to feel secure and adopt transoral resection of pharyngeal cancers. Wide-angle and high-quality visualization, coupled with retractors and instruments for exposure and retraction in the confined area of the pharynx, was required to assure margin negative resections for most pharyngeal tumors. With TORS, an assistant is at the head of the bed with the surgeon controlling the robot from a console (Fig. 34.13). The major advantage of TORS relative to traditional mandibular splitting approaches is that TORS avoids division and repair of soft tissues and bone and therefore has advantages for cosmesis, functional recovery, healing time, and complication rate. On the other hand, flap reconstruction is difficult without wider exposure provided by traditional lip and mandible splitting approaches, and following most TORS excisions, healing is by secondary intent. As surgeons have become more familiar with TORS, its utility has expanded, with it now being used or tested for excision of larger tumors, as well as for identification of the site of unknown primaries.

Hypopharynx

Anatomy

The hypopharynx is posterior and lateral to the larynx and extends inferiorly from the horizontal plane of the top of the hyoid bone to a horizontal plane extending posteriorly from the inferior border of the cricoid cartilage. The hypopharynx is composed of three distinct subsites and includes bilateral piriform sinuses, posterior hypopharyngeal wall, and the postcricoid space. The postcricoid area extends inferiorly from the two arytenoid cartilages to the inferior border of the cricoid cartilage, connecting the piriform sinuses and forming the anterior hypopharyngeal wall. The piriform sinuses are inverted, pyramid-shaped potential spaces medial to the thyroid lamina; they begin at the pharyngoepiglottic folds and extend to the cervical esophagus at the inferior border of the cricoid cartilage.

Hypopharyngeal Cancer and Therapy

Hypopharyngeal cancer is a rare cancer of the head and neck, with approximately 2500 to 3000 new cases diagnosed yearly in the United States. It is more common in older men with a history of alcohol abuse and smoking. The exception is in the postcricoid area in which cancers are more common worldwide in women; this is related to Plummer-Vinson syndrome, a combination of dysphagia, hypopharyngeal and esophageal webs, weight loss, and iron deficiency anemia usually occurring in middle-aged women. In patients who fail to undergo treatment consisting of dilation, iron replacement, and vitamin therapy, postcricoid carcinoma may develop just proximal to the web. Over 95% of all cancers arising in the hypopharynx are SCCs, and hypopharynx cancers are frequently diagnosed at later stages and have the poorest prognosis of all head and neck squamous cell cancers.

The role of HPV in carcinogenesis of hypopharyngeal cancer is unclear, with HPV detected in fewer than 30% of tumors; however, a recent large population-based cohort study analyzing the National Cancer Database data revealed a large survival benefit for patients with the HPV-positive hypopharyngeal cancer (52.2% vs. 28.8%) similar to the benefit for HPV-positive oropharyngeal patients, suggesting that HPV is etiologic in a portion of these cancers.[38]

Hypopharyngeal tumors manifest most commonly with dysphagia, hoarseness, neck mass, weight loss, sore throat, referred otalgia, and hemoptysis, in descending order. A high index of suspicion should be maintained because similar symptoms may

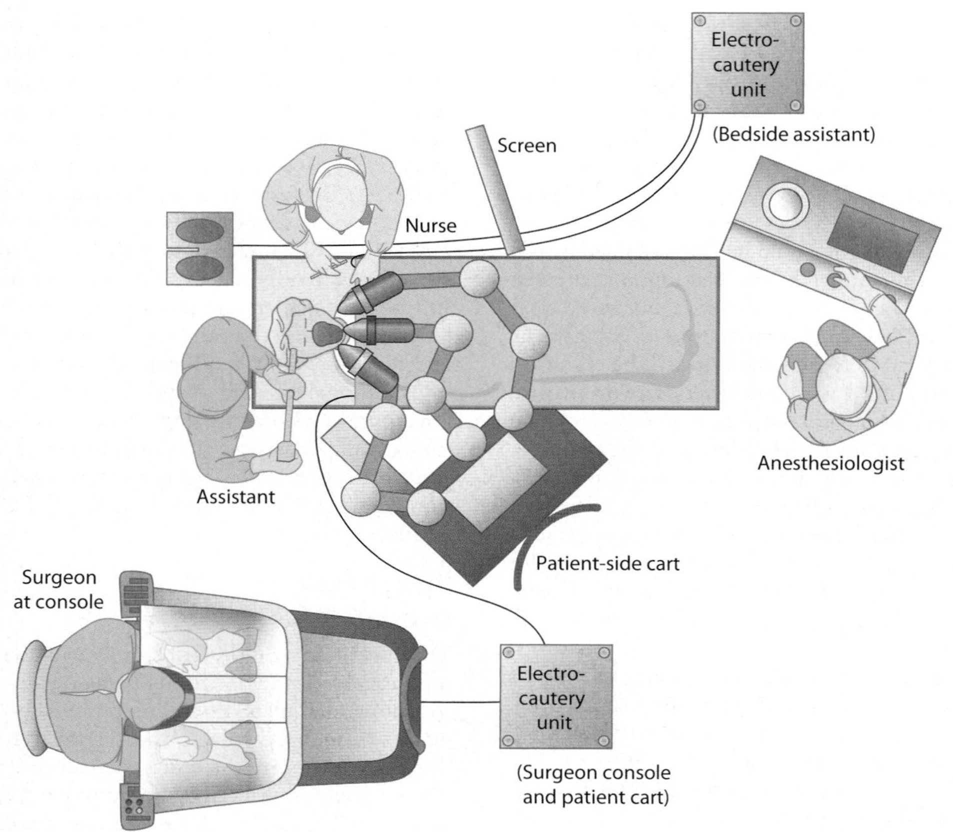

FIG. 34.13 Operating room setup for da Vinci transoral robotic surgery.

be seen with the more common gastroesophageal reflux disease. In advanced disease, hoarseness may develop from direct involvement of the arytenoid cartilages, recurrent laryngeal nerves, or paraglottic spaces. The rich lymphatics that drain the hypopharyngeal region contribute to early lymphatic metastasis, with 70% of patients having palpable lymphadenopathy upon presentation. Patients with hypopharyngeal cancer have the highest rate of synchronous malignancies and the highest rate of development of second HNSCC primaries of any of the head and neck sites. Staging for hypopharyngeal cancer is based on the number of involved subsites or size of the tumor.

Physical examination for hypopharyngeal lesions includes in-office fiberoptic flexible endoscopy. Having the patient blow against closed lips and closing the palate or pinching the nose inflates the potential spaces of the piriform sinuses and can assist in visualization of the tumor. Moving the larynx back and forth while pressing it against the spine may demonstrate a loss of laryngeal crepitus, and a fixed larynx suggests posterior extension into the prevertebral fascia and indicates that the tumor may not be resectable. Barium swallow may demonstrate mucosal abnormalities associated with an exophytic tumor and is useful for determining the extent of involvement of the cervical esophagus if esophagoscopy is not possible. It also assists in determining the presence and amount of aspiration present. CT or MRI is commonly performed to determine the local extent of the tumor, the presence of thyroid cartilage invasion, extralaryngeal spread, direct extension into the neck, and pathologic lymphadenopathy (Fig. 34.14). Direct laryngoscopy and biopsy under general anesthesia are usually required to obtain diagnostic material, and esophagoscopy can directly determine the inferior tumor extent.

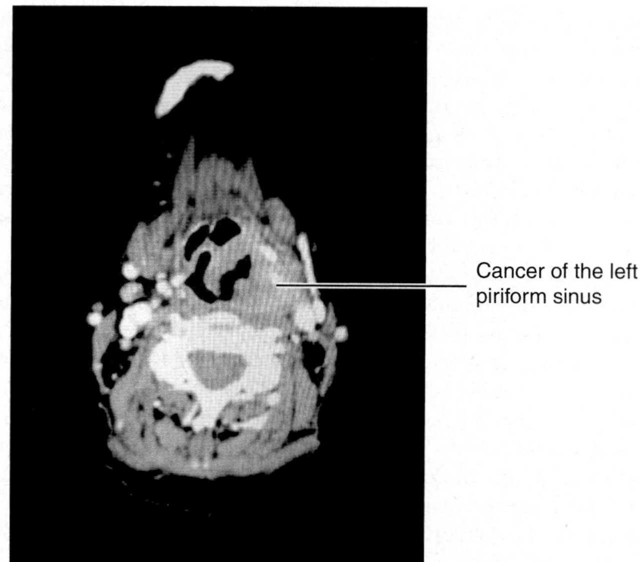

FIG. 34.14 Computed tomography scan to review the local extent of the tumor, presence of thyroid cartilage invasion, extralaryngeal spread, direct extension into the neck, and pathologic lymphadenopathy.

The most common area for lymphatic spread is the upper jugular nodes, even with inferior tumors. Other lymphatic regions at risk are the lateral nodes and paratracheal and retropharyngeal nodes. The presence of contralateral cervical metastases or level V involvement is a poor prognostic indicator. With the exception of HPV-associated hypopharyngeal tumors, outcomes for hypopharyngeal cancers are worse than outcomes for other sites in the head and neck. It is unclear how molecular alterations of the tumor, differences in lymphatic density, or other anatomic characteristics of the hypopharynx contribute to the relatively poor prognosis for hypopharyngeal SCC. For early lesions confined to the medial wall of the piriform or posterior pharyngeal wall, radiation or chemoradiation therapy is effective as a primary treatment modality. Because of the high incidence of postoperative aspiration, laryngeal-sparing partial pharyngectomy is rarely possible for hypopharyngeal cancer. Small tumors of the medial piriform wall or pharyngoepiglottic fold may be amenable to conservation surgery, but they should not involve the piriform apex, and the patient must have mobile vocal cords and adequate pulmonary reserve.

Concurrent chemotherapy with radiation for hypopharyngeal cancer is now the most common initial treatment and has resulted in decreased rates of laryngopharyngectomy.[39] Surgery is recommended for advanced tumor stage when laryngeal function is already compromised or when posttreatment aspiration is expected. Hypopharyngeal cancer surgery usually requires laryngopharyngectomy, bilateral neck dissection, and central neck dissection, followed by adjuvant radiation plus or minus concomitant chemotherapy. Survival for patients whose initial therapy was chemoradiation or surgery followed by postoperative radiation or chemoradiation is less than 40% at 5 years.[39]

After total laryngectomy and partial pharyngectomy, primary closure may be possible if at least 4 cm of viable pharyngeal mucosa remains. Primary closure using less than 4 cm of mucosa generally leads to stricture and an inability to swallow effectively. A pedicled regional flap, such as a pectoralis major myocutaneous flap or supraclavicular fasciocutaneous flap, or free flaps can be used to augment any remaining mucosa in these cases. When total laryngopharyngectomy with esophagectomy has been performed, a gastric pull-up may be used for reconstruction, but more contemporary methods to reconstruct the total pharyngectomy defect include free flap reconstruction with enteric (jejunum) flaps or tubed cutaneous flaps.

Larynx

Anatomy

The larynx serves critical functions for breathing, airway protection, and voice. To understand the pathology and surgical approaches to the larynx, thorough knowledge of the 3D anatomy of the larynx and its subsites is needed (Fig. 34.15). Using the cartilage framework of the larynx as the boundaries, the concept of a "voice box" becomes apparent. The anterior border of the larynx is composed of the lingual surface of the epiglottis, thyrohyoid membrane, anterior commissure, and anterior wall of the subglottis (which consists of the thyroid cartilage, cricothyroid membrane, and anterior arch of the cricoid cartilage). The posterior and lateral limits of the larynx are the arytenoids, interarytenoid region, aryepiglottic folds, and posterior wall of the subglottis (which is the mucosa covering the surface of the cricoid cartilage). The superior limit anteriorly is the tip and lateral borders of the epiglottis, laterally is the aryepiglottic folds, and posteriorly is the arytenoids and interarytenoid area. The inferior limit is defined as the plane passing through the inferior edge of the cricoid cartilage.

The superior laryngeal nerve provides innervation to the larynx with an external branch that supplies the cricothyroid and inferior constrictor muscles and an internal branch with afferent sensory fibers from the mucosa of the false vocal folds and piriform sinuses. The recurrent laryngeal nerve supplies motor innervation to all the intrinsic muscles of the larynx and sensation to the mucosa of the true vocal folds, subglottic region, and adjacent esophageal mucosa.

The normal functions of the larynx are to provide airway patency, protect the tracheobronchial tree from aspiration, provide resistance for Valsalva maneuvers and coughing, and facilitate phonation. Therefore, laryngeal pathology is usually manifest with voice, breathing, and sometimes swallowing complaints. Tumors that involve the larynx impair these functions to a variable degree, depending on location, size, and DOI. Dysphonia that persists more than 4 to 6 weeks should be evaluated by direct or indirect laryngoscopy (Fig. 34.16).

Vocal cord immobility is identified on flexible laryngoscopy and can be related to central pathology or peripheral pathology along the course of the recurrent laryngeal nerve extending from the skull base into chest and back to the larynx. Evaluation of vocal paralysis should be done before attributing this to viral or idiopathic causes. In addition to primary laryngeal pathology, primary malignancies of the thyroid, thymus, lung, and skull base can manifest as vocal cord paralysis. Metastatic cancers to the lungs, mediastinum, and central or lateral neck can also present with vocal cord paralysis. Benign pathology of the larynx includes respiratory papillomatosis, laryngeal cysts, vocal fold nodules and polyps, contact ulcers, subglottic stenosis, and systemic diseases such as amyloidosis and sarcoidosis. Benign neoplasms such as granular cell tumors, minor salivary gland neoplasms, and chondromas also affect the larynx. Exposure to carcinogens (e.g., tobacco) can cause a series of mucosal changes in the epithelium of the larynx, clinically referred to as leukoplakia (any white lesion of the mucosa) or erythroplakia (a red lesion), that consist of hyperplasia, metaplasia, or variable degrees of dysplasia, which are diagnosed by biopsy.

Laryngeal Cancer and Therapy

While the most common malignant lesion of the larynx is SCC derived from the epithelial lining, mucous glands within the mucosa can give rise to malignant histologies associated with those of minor salivary gland origin such as adenocarcinoma, adenoid cystic carcinoma, and mucoepidermoid carcinoma. Other tumors found in the larynx include neuroendocrine carcinoma, adenosquamous carcinoma, chondrosarcoma, synovial sarcoma, and, rarely, distant metastases from other organ systems. Invasive thyroid cancers can also be associated with direct laryngeal invasion.

For classification and staging of cancers, the larynx is separated into the supraglottis, glottis, and subglottis, reflecting differences in metastatic potential, treatment, and prognosis.[39a] The supraglottis includes all structures superior to the laryngeal ventricle, including the suprahyoid and infrahyoid epiglottis, aryepiglottic fold, arytenoids, and false vocal cords. The glottic larynx is formed by the true vocal cords, including the anterior and posterior commissures. The subglottis extends from the glottis to the bottom of the cricoid cartilage. Flexible laryngoscopy is commonly performed in the clinic to assess the extent of tumor involvement and vocal cord motion. Biopsy is frequently performed in the operating room under general anesthesia via direct laryngoscopy, where the tumor extent is determined for accurate clinical staging, and to plan for surgical excision. The extent and location of the tumor determine if partial laryngectomy is possible and if transoral endoscopic approaches are feasible. For T1 tumors with high suspicion of cancer preoperatively, patients can be counseled on the possibility of biopsy with frozen section diagnosis followed by transoral excision during the same anesthetic.

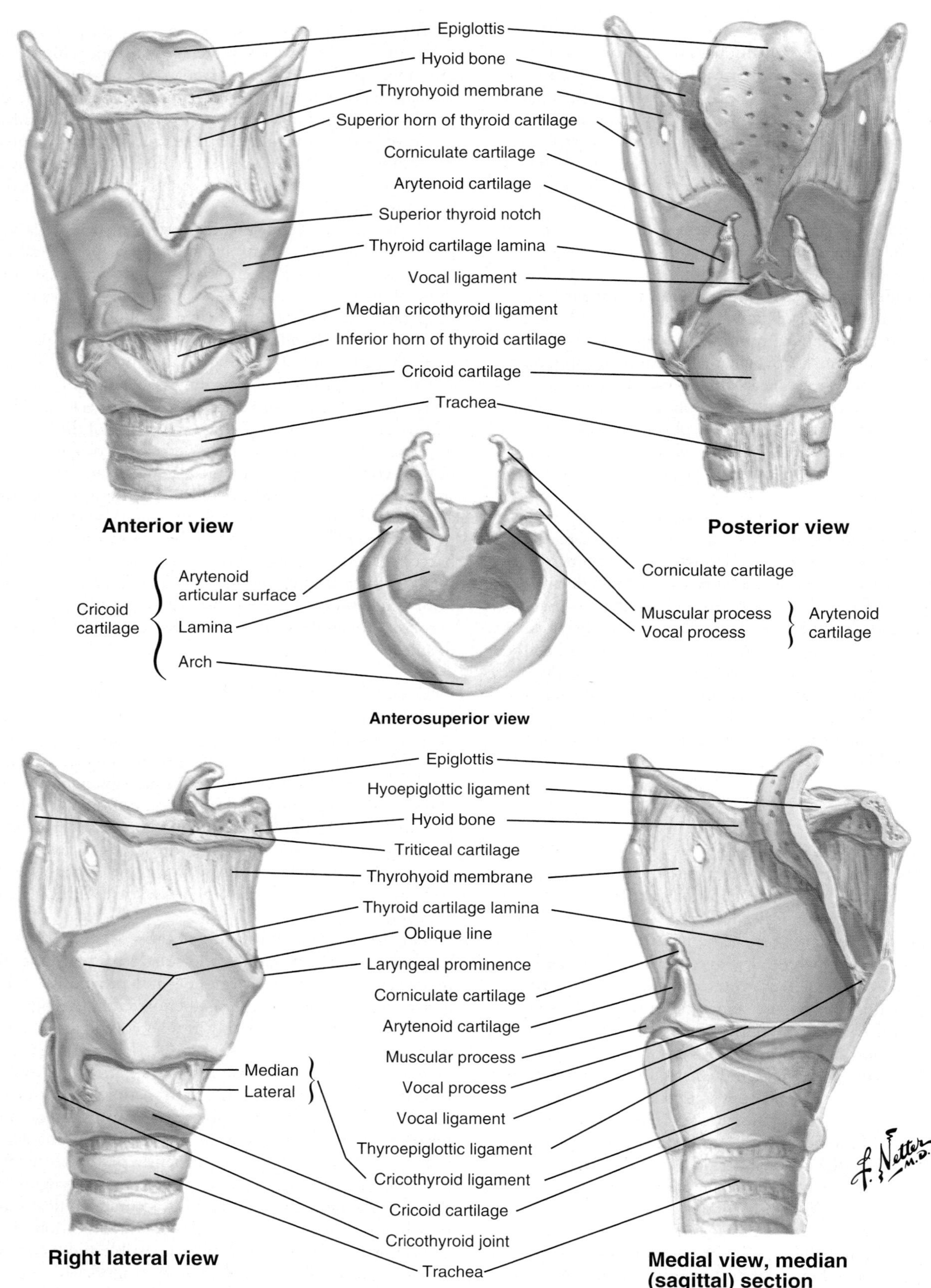

FIG. 34.15 Framework anatomy of the larynx demonstrating the boundaries.

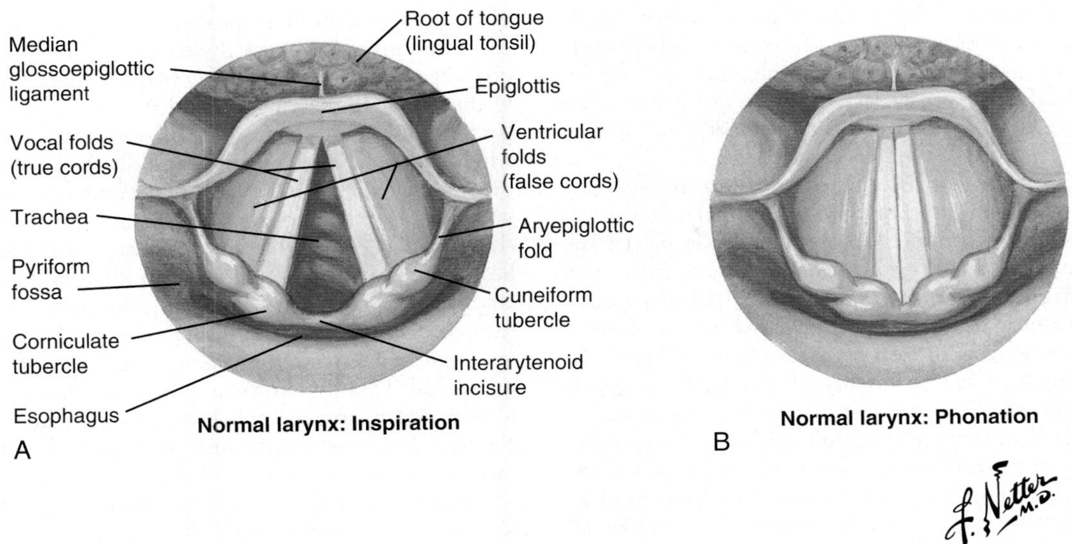

FIG. 34.16 Endoscopic view of larynx during inspiration (A) and phonation (B).

CT or MRI with thin-cut slices through the larynx is useful to determine the extent of local and regional disease. Chest imaging is performed to identify second primary cancers and metastatic disease. If larynx-conserving surgeries are being considered, the patient should have adequate pulmonary reserve given the increased risk of aspiration after partial laryngectomy. Formal pulmonary function testing (PFT) can be performed, but guidelines have not been validated, so the need for PFTs is considered individually.

Treatment of Larynx Cancer

Treatment decision-making in larynx cancer is complex because competing options can produce similar oncologic outcomes and because the risks to speech and swallow function with different therapies can be hard to predict. Therefore, treatment recommendations are best made with multidisciplinary evaluation taking into account functional outcomes, patient preference, surgical experience, and a number of patient and tumor characteristics. For example, poor pulmonary function may decrease enthusiasm for partial laryngectomy procedures, while a nonfunctional larynx on presentation (e.g., gastric tube and tracheotomy dependent) suggests that larynx preserving treatment options may not benefit the patient.

There are many treatment options for tumors not requiring total laryngectomy for surgical management. For early-stage larynx cancer (T1–T2 N0, stage I–II), there is debate as to the difference in voice and swallowing outcomes following surgical versus nonsurgical treatment. T1 to T2 N0 (and select T3 tumors) can be treated with either radiation therapy or partial laryngectomy (+/- neck dissection) with adjuvant treatment guided by pathologic features or presence of nodal disease.

T1 to T2 N+ (and select T3N1) tumors can be treated with surgery, radiation therapy, or concurrent chemoradiotherapy. For T3 tumors that would require total laryngectomy for tumor extirpation, an organ-preserving approach with chemotherapy and radiation is frequently recommended, reserving total laryngectomy for treatment failures. Induction chemotherapy options can also be considered in specific circumstances, assessing response to therapy as a harbinger for definitive treatment as surgical versus nonsurgical.

Cartilage invasion or extralaryngeal involvement (i.e., T4a tumors) suggests that the function of the larynx cannot be preserved, indicating that total laryngectomy may be preferred as initial therapy with adjuvant radiation or chemoradiation guided by pathology results.

Complications and Morbidity following Nonsurgical Treatment

While the advantages of organ-preserving treatment for certain stage III to IV larynx cancers are obvious, there are a number of posttreatment issues. Standard concurrent chemoradiation regimens are based on cisplatin that is associated with hearing loss and renal injury, and failure of chemoradiation as a primary treatment usually excludes larynx preservation for salvage surgery. In addition, chemotherapy with high-dose radiation can cause laryngeal dysfunction due to chondronecrosis, fibrosis, or extensive lymphedema, even in the absence of recurrent tumor. Pharyngoesophageal stenosis is another complication of nonsurgical treatment of laryngeal cancer. Partial stenosis can be treated with serial dilations, while the rare patient with total stenosis requires anterograde/retrograde rendezvous procedures, open surgical procedures with lumen augmentation, or open surgical procedures with circumferential pharyngoesophageal reconstruction with tubed skin flaps, visceral flaps such as jejunum, or gastric pull-up.

Surgical Therapy

Partial laryngectomy. If characteristics of the cancer allow laryngeal preservation surgery, patient factors such as pulmonary function and cardiovascular status are assessed because these patients often have to tolerate some amount of aspiration or airway compromise.

Modern partial laryngectomy procedures include open and endoscopic approaches. In the current era, endoscopic (or transoral) laryngeal procedures are far more common than open partial laryngectomy procedures. Transoral laryngeal surgery is typically done with microsuspension laryngoscopy and use of the CO_2 laser, called transoral laser microsurgery. TORS is also a promising tool for partial laryngectomy, but with current instrumentation, exposure, and access issues, TORS is limited given excellent results with transoral laser microsurgery. Currently, most partial laryngectomy procedures are performed endoscopically, but the surgeon should be aware of open partial laryngectomy procedures since there are specific situations in which these remain good options for patients.

For T1 tumors of the glottis, a microsuspension laryngoscopy and tumor resection to negative margins with either cold steel or CO_2 laser are the most common approaches. Open partial laryngectomy procedures for T1 glottic tumors can include open cordectomy and open anterior frontolateral partial laryngectomy, while larger glottic tumors can be excised with open vertical hemilaryngectomy. Reconstruction of vertical hemilaryngectomy requires strap muscle or fascial free flap to provide bulk against which with unaffected vocal cord can contact to prevent aspiration and for voice. Contraindications to vertical partial laryngectomy include subglottic extension greater than 10 mm anteriorly or 5 mm posteriorly, most T3 glottic cancers, involvement of an entire vocal cord, and more than one third of the contralateral vocal cord.

For supraglottic tumors, open horizontal laryngectomy procedures can be done, including supraglottic horizontal partial laryngectomy and supracricoid horizontal partial laryngectomy for supraglottic tumors extending onto the glottis. Each of these procedures requires reconstruction with cricohyoidoepiglottopexy or cricohyoidopexy to suspend the larynx as high as possible to decrease the risk of postoperative aspiration. Open horizontal partial laryngectomies have a greater impact on swallowing, and prolonged rehabilitation is necessary to maximize postoperative recovery. Perioperative tracheotomy is a necessity for the more extensive open approaches, with the goal of decannulation within 2 to 4 weeks of surgery.

Near-total laryngectomy is an uncommonly performed procedure, leaving patients dependent on tracheotomy for breathing, but gives them laryngeal voice ability via a tracheoesophageal conduit. There may be a value in parts of the world where speech rehabilitation following total laryngectomy is difficult to obtain.

Total laryngectomy. Total laryngectomy requires removal of the entire larynx (Fig. 34.17) and creation of a permanent tracheostoma by circumferentially sewing the superior trachea to the neck skin. Preservation of pharyngeal mucosa enables primary closure

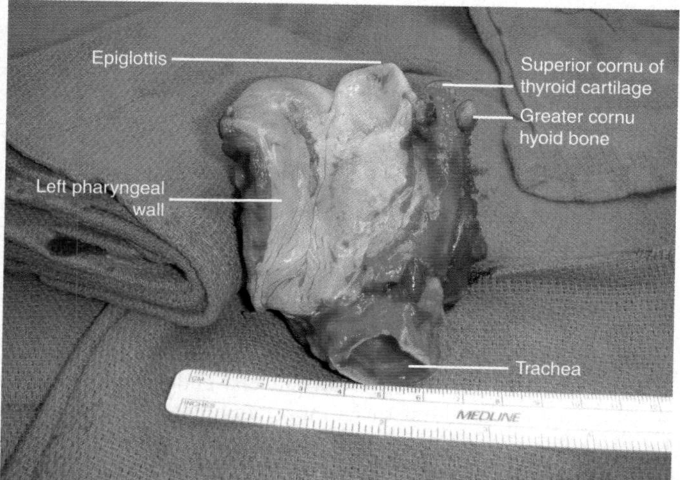

FIG. 34.17 Total laryngectomy specimen with left piriform sinus and pharyngeal wall also removed

of the pharynx. Adjunct procedures at the time of total laryngectomy can include neck dissection, cricopharyngeal myotomy, pharyngeal plexus neurectomy, hemithyroidectomy on the side of the tumor (preserving the contralateral thyroid to protect the parathyroid glands), primary tracheoesophageal puncture (with or without prosthesis placement), and dividing the sternal heads of the sternocleidomastoid muscle to prevent a deep stoma and assist with postoperative appliance placement. Immediate postoperative risks include pharyngocutaneous fistula and hypocalcemia. All healthcare providers should be aware that patients who have had laryngectomy cannot be intubated transorally; the airway can be secured or intubated only through the tracheostoma in patients who have had laryngectomy. Long-term issues after laryngectomy can include hypothyroidism and perceived loss of taste and smell. Stomal and pharyngoesophageal stenosis is increased if postoperative radiation or chemoradiation is required but can usually be managed with stomaplasty and pharyngeal dilation, respectively.

Total laryngectomy can also be performed in the salvage setting for persistent/recurrent tumor after radiotherapy, chemoradiation, or for a nonfunctional larynx. In the setting of prior treatment with radiation with or without chemotherapy, there is a higher risk of pharyngocutaneous fistula and pharyngoesophageal stenosis, and these risks can be improved with use of on-lay or augmentation free or pedicled flaps (e.g., anterior lateral thigh, radial forearm, or pectoralis major flap).

Speech and Swallowing Rehabilitation

Speech and swallowing rehabilitation is an integral part of laryngeal cancer treatment requiring preoperative planning. Prior to performing total laryngectomy, speech rehabilitation should be explained by surgeons and/or a speech language pathologist, and if possible, patients can discuss lifestyle implications of a permanent neck tracheostoma and changes in communication with a laryngectomy patient.

There are currently a number of speech rehabilitation options following total laryngectomy. The creation of speech requires an air generator (e.g., pulmonary or esophageal exhalation), a sound source (e.g., a vibratory surface), and a set of resonator and articulators within a cavity to transform the sound into intelligible speech (e.g., vocal tract including tongue, mouth, nasal cavity). The main speech rehabilitation options after total laryngectomy include electrolarynx, esophageal speech, and tracheoesophageal puncture with prosthesis.

With the electrolarynx, a vibratory sound wave generator is placed directly on the submandibular area, cheek, or oral cavity and the sound generated in this way is transformed in the vocal tract to create speech. The patient mouths words to produce a monotone, electronic-sounding speech that can take considerable time, coaching, and practice to maximize speech intelligibility.

Esophageal speech is produced by swallowing air into the esophagus and expulsing the air back through the pharynx, which vibrates as the air passes. The ability to master esophageal speech requires a motivated patient who can control the release of air through the upper esophageal sphincter.

Finally, tracheoesophageal puncture is a surgically created conduit between the tracheal stoma and pharynx that is made at the time of laryngectomy or secondarily. This conduit is fitted with a one-way valve that allows passage of air posteriorly from the trachea to the pharynx but prevents food and liquid from passing into the airway. By occluding the stomal opening with the thumb during exhalation, the patient can pass air from the trachea into the pharynx, which vibrates and allows remarkable clarity of speech. Hands-free mechanisms that do not require manual occlusion of the stoma are preferred by many patients. There are cost and maintenance associated with cleaning and changing the prosthesis on a regular basis.

Salivary

Anatomy

There are three paired major salivary glands: the parotid glands, submandibular glands, and sublingual glands. There are also up to 1000 minor salivary glands located submucosally throughout the oral cavity, pharynx, and larynx as depicted (Fig. 34.18). Given the widespread location of salivary glands, tumors and lesions of salivary glands can be found almost anywhere in the head and neck region and upper aerodigestive tract.

The parotid glands are the largest salivary glands, and salivary secretions are directed into the oral cavity via the parotid (Stensen) duct opening in the buccal mucosa next to the second maxillary molar. Although there is no capsular or fascial separation, the parotid gland is practically separated into superficial and deep lobes with the separation defined as the plane of the facial nerve. A feature unique to the parotid among the major salivary glands is the presence of lymph nodes within the fascial envelop. Treatment of intraparotid nodes must be considered for parotid cancers as well as for skin cancers of the face, temple, eyelid, ear, and scalp. The submandibular glands are the second largest salivary glands and secrete saliva through the submandibular (Wharton) duct, which opens in the anterior floor of mouth adjacent to the lingual frenulum. The final pair of major salivary glands, the sublingual glands, are found in the floor of mouth, superficial to the lingual nerve and mylohyoid muscle, and drain into the floor of mouth via the ducts of Rivinus, some of which also drain into the Wharton duct. Minor salivary glands drain individually through the mucosa without named ducts.

Nonneoplastic Salivary Disease

Nonneoplastic diseases of salivary glands are most commonly obstructive, infectious, or inflammatory and typically manifest as enlargement and tenderness of the affected gland(s). Viruses and or aerobic/anaerobic bacteria are the most common infectious causes and are associated with acute onset and rapid resolution following appropriate therapy. More persistent and indolent granulomatous infections can be caused by typical or atypical tuberculosis, toxoplasmosis, actinomycosis, and Bartonella henselae (cat-scratch disease). Bacterial sialadenitis is typically unilateral and painful, and purulence can often be expressed from the ductal opening with deep palpation and sometimes skin changes are evident (Fig. 34.19). Bacterial salivary gland infections are associated with dehydration (or ductal obstruction) and are more common in elderly or infirm patients who may be on dehydrating medication. Sudden and acute swelling of a single major salivary gland typically indicates ductal obstruction and can be caused by salivary stones, strictures, thick saliva, or bacterial infection. Viral sialadenitis is typically bilateral and can be caused by the mumps virus as well a number of other more common viral infections that impact the upper aerodigestive tract. Multiple, large, bilateral cysts of the parotid glands (lymphoepithelial cysts) can be seen in poorly controlled HIV infection.

A major cause of salivary obstruction is salivary stones (sialolithiasis) that cause gland swelling upon eating. Small stones in the parotid or submandibular duct can be managed with salivary endoscopy (Video 34.3). Obstructive or inflammatory sialadenitis can also be manifestations of systemic diseases such as Sjogren syndrome, sarcoidosis, or immunoglobulin G4 (IgG4)-related disease. In addition, patients treated with radioactive iodine for thyroid cancer are much more prone to developing obstructive sialadenitis that can be immediately associated with treatment or up to 1 year following completion of therapy.

Neoplasms of the Salivary Glands

Salivary neoplasms manifest as masses either within one of the major salivary glands or submucosally when arising from a minor salivary gland. Deep lobe parotid tumors can present as what appears to be unilateral tonsil hypertrophy or soft palate bulge, which is actually caused by mass effect within the parapharyngeal space pushing the palatine tonsil medially within the oropharynx. Deep lobe parotid tumors may have no outward signs or symptoms and are frequently found incidentally on imaging. Warthin tumors are the second most common benign salivary neoplasm and are ^{18}F-FDG avid by PET imaging because of the high mitochondrial content of oncocytes within the tumor. When Warthin tumors are found by staging or restaging PET imaging of cancer patients, they raise concern for metastasis or second primary malignancy.

Benign salivary neoplasms. Pretreatment evaluation of salivary gland masses may include cross-sectional imaging (CT or MRI) and/or FNA. FNA either with direct palpation or under image guidance (ultrasound or CT) can help identify benign versus malignant salivary tumors. The benefit of FNA in the work-up of salivary gland tumors is controversial since cytologic accuracy varies based on experience of the cytologist and is not definitive with the sensitivity of distinguishing benign from malignant tumors being approximately 80%.[40] In addition, most parotid tumors are benign, and surgical removal is recommended for almost all regardless of pathology. Advocates of FNA tout the value of identifying a malignancy prior to surgery for improved patient counseling, patient expectations, and surgical planning (i.e., the likelihood of facial nerve sacrifice, the extent of parotidectomy, and the need for concomitant neck dissection). In addition, intraoperative frozen section pathologic analysis of the tumor can help the guide extent of surgery and avoid the need for reoperation following pathologic diagnosis.

Most salivary neoplasms (~75%) are found in the parotid gland, and the majority of parotid salivary tumors are benign. As a general rule, the larger the salivary gland, the more likely a tumor within that gland is benign; for example, the probability of a tumor being malignant in the parotid, submandibular, and sublingual/minor salivary glands is approximately 25%, 50%, and 75%, respectively. The most common benign neoplasm is pleomorphic adenoma, followed by Warthin tumor (also known as papillary cystadenoma lymphomatosum).

Treatment for benign salivary tumors is surgical removal, either parotidectomy, submandibular gland excision, or wide local excision of the minor salivary gland with margin control. Removal of benign salivary gland tumors upon detection improves the accuracy of histopathologic diagnosis, avoids more difficult dissection, and lowers the risk of patient morbidity (e.g., facial nerve injury, aesthetic concerns) by removal of the tumor before it enlarges. Removal of benign tumors also prevents malignant transformation that can occur with some histologies, particularly transformation of pleomorphic adenoma to an aggressive cancer, carcinoma ex

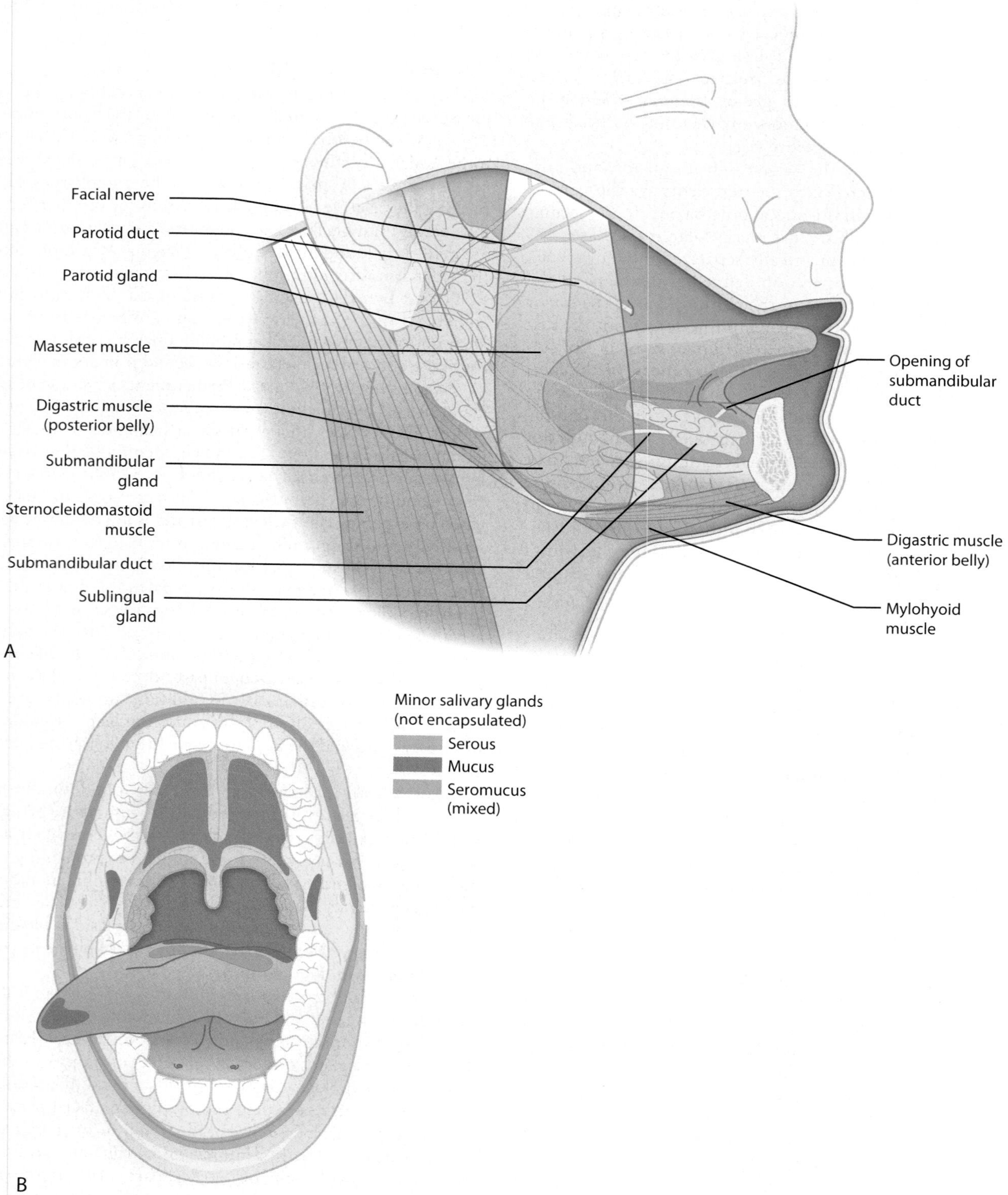

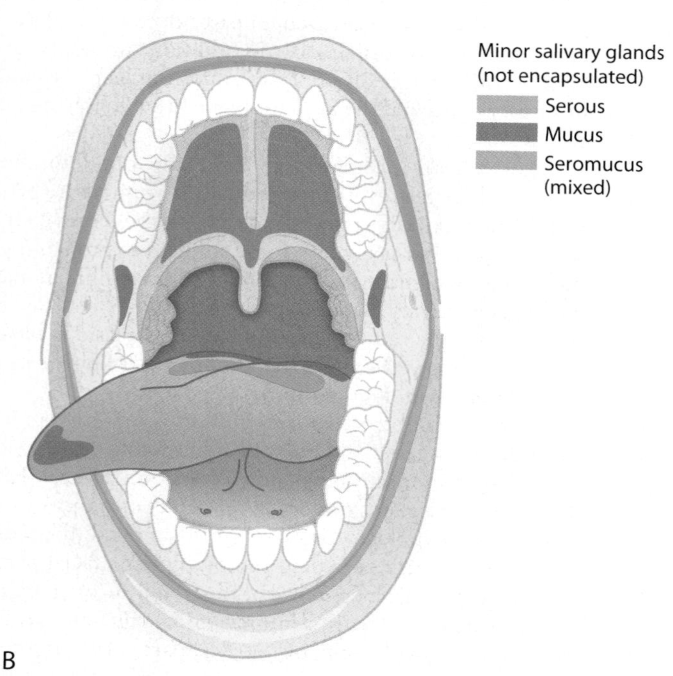

FIG. 34.18 Anatomic distribution of the major salivary glands (A) and minor salivary glands (B).

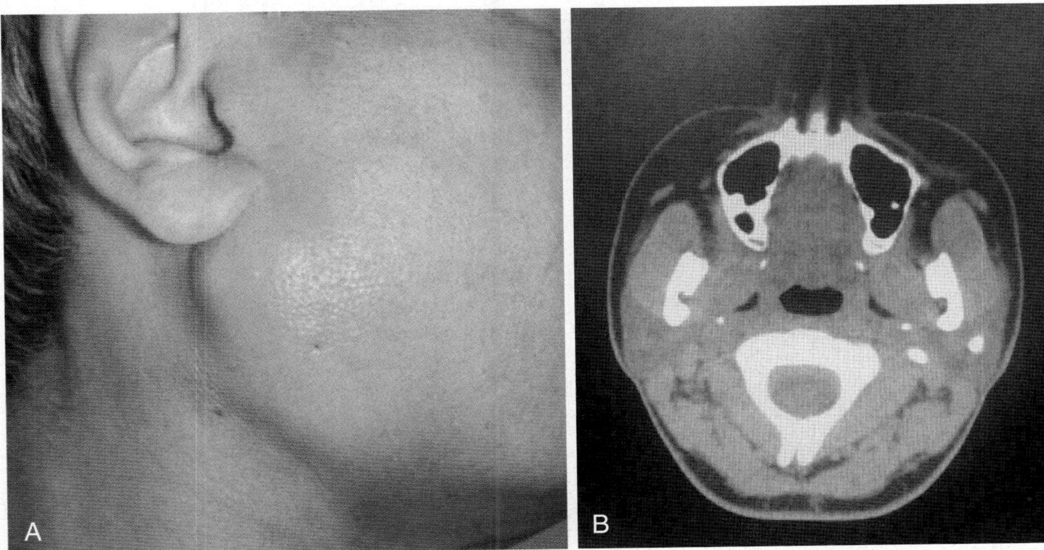

FIG. 34.19 (A) Acute right parotitis with infection caused by obstruction of Stensen duct by a salivary stone. (B) Computed tomography scan showing parotid stone within the left duct (not during active infection).

pleomorphic adenoma. On the other hand, some benign tumors may be observed based on patient preference, patient suitability for surgery, patient life expectancy, and histopathology. Patients with Warthin tumors that are not enlarging or that were incidentally found or that occur in patients with metastatic cancer or in patients with contraindications to surgery may be appropriate for observation since this tumor has no malignant potential.

Salivary Cancer and Therapy

Salivary malignancy is rare but can be found almost anywhere in the head and neck due to the diverse location of the major and minor salivary glands. The most common presentation is a mass in the location of the salivary gland. Symptoms such as a facial nerve paralysis can indicate a parotid malignancy in the setting of a parotid mass and/or a history of head and neck skin cancers. Population studies have identified an increased relative risk of salivary gland cancer in patients with a history of thyroid cancer, particularly those treated with radioactive iodine.[41]

The most common primary salivary gland malignancies are mucoepidermoid carcinoma, adenoid cystic carcinoma, adenocarcinoma, carcinoma ex-pleomorphic adenoma, and acinic cell carcinoma. Secretory carcinoma (previously mammary-analog secretory carcinoma) is a recently described salivary malignancy with a translocation mutation that results in the fusion gene ETV6-NTRK3.[42] In the past, secretory carcinoma was categorized as other carcinomas, most commonly acinic cell carcinoma. Lymph nodes within the parotid gland are common sites of metastasis of the ear, face, and scalp SCC or melanoma. Lymphoma and metastases from other sites (kidney, lung, breast, prostate) can also be seen in the parotid salivary gland. A complete list of salivary tumors (malignant and benign) based on the 2017 World Health Organization (WHO) Classification of salivary gland tumors is shown in Table 34.3.[43]

Primary salivary malignancy is staged according to the location of the salivary glands. T-stage for the major salivary glands (parotid, submandibular, and sublingual) is based primarily on size: T1, less than 2 cm; T2, 2 to 4 cm; T3, more than 4 cm and/or extraparenchymal extension; T4a, invading skin, mandible, ear canal, and/or facial nerve; and T4b, invading the skull base, pterygoid plates, and/or encasing carotid artery.[1] Staging of minor salivary gland malignancy is based on the staging systemic of the anatomic location of the minor salivary gland; for example, a salivary carcinoma of the hard palate is staged using the oral cavity cancer staging system.

Following appropriate staging work-up, treatment for almost all primary salivary gland cancer is surgery with complete tumor resection. There is some controversy as to the extent of parotidectomy that should be performed for the treatment of malignant tumors. At a minimum, gross total tumor resection is the goal. For deep lobe parotid malignancy, a total parotidectomy (superficial and deep lobe) is usually required and includes removal of all parotid lymph nodes and mobilization of the facial nerve branches. For other malignant parotid tumors, total superficial parotid lobectomy and total parotidectomy have each been advocated. If possible, the facial nerve and its branches should be preserved except in cases of gross tumor invasion (Fig. 34.20). Radical parotidectomy, or extended radical parotidectomy to include resection of skin, facial nerve, or temporal bone, may be required for gross total tumor extirpation. For submandibular, sublingual, and minor salivary gland tumors, gross total tumor resection with negative margins is also the goal. Once again, major nerves whose sacrifice would cause functional deficits (lingual, hypoglossal, marginal mandibular branch of the facial, etc.) should be spared unless the tumor cannot be completely removed without removal of the nerves.

Neck dissection is usually recommended for the clinically node positive necks, high-grade primary tumors, and T3 to T4 tumors. For incompletely resected tumors or those with gross residual disease, surgical re-resection should be offered if possible. Adjuvant radiation therapy is typically recommended for gross residual disease and/or adverse features such as intermediate or high-grade, close or positive margins, neural/perineural invasion, lymph node metastases, lymphatic/vascular invasion, and T3 to T4 tumors. Radiation therapy is typically recommended following removal of adenoid cystic carcinomas with radiation fields extended to cover adjacent or involved nerves due to its high propensity for perineural invasion and spread. The role of systemic therapy in salivary malignancy is less studied but can be considered for cases of gross residual disease or adverse pathologic features.

TABLE 34.3 2017 WHO classification of primary salivary gland tumors.

MALIGNANT TUMORS	BENIGN TUMORS
Acinic cell carcinoma	Pleomorphic adenoma
Secretory carcinoma	Myoepithelioma
Mucoepidermoid carcinoma	Basal cell adenoma
Adenoid cystic carcinoma	Warthin tumor
Polymorphous adenocarcinoma	Oncocytoma
Epithelial-myoepithelial carcinoma	Lymphadenoma
Clear cell carcinoma	Cystadenoma
Basal cell adenocarcinoma	Sialadenoma papilliferum
Sebaceous adenocarcinoma	Ductal papillomas
Intraductal carcinoma	Sebaceous adenomas
Cystadenocarcinoma	Canalicular adenoma and other ductal adenomas
Adenocarcinoma, NOS	
Salivary duct carcinoma	**Soft Tissue Tumors**
Myoepithelial carcinoma	Hemangioma
Carcinoma ex pleomorphic adenoma	Lipoma/sialolipoma
Carcinosarcoma	Nodular fasciitis
Poorly differentiated carcinoma	
Neuroendocrine and nonneuroendocrine undifferentiated carcinoma	**Hematolymphoid Tumors**
Large cell neuroendocrine carcinoma	Extranodal marginal zone lymphoma of MALT
Small cell neuroendocrine carcinoma	
Lymphoepithelial carcinoma	**Other Epithelial Lesions**
Squamous cell carcinoma	Sclerosing polycystic adenosis
Oncocytic carcinoma	Nodular oncocytic hyperplasia
Sialoblastoma (borderline tumor)	Lymphoepithelial lesions
	Intercalated duct hyperplasia

From El-Naggar AK, Chan JKC, Takata T, et al. The fourth edition of the head and neck World Health Organization blue book: editors' perspectives. *Hum Pathol.* 2017;66:10–12.

MALT, Mucosa-associated lymphoid tissue; *NOS*, not otherwise specified; *WHO*, World Health Organization.

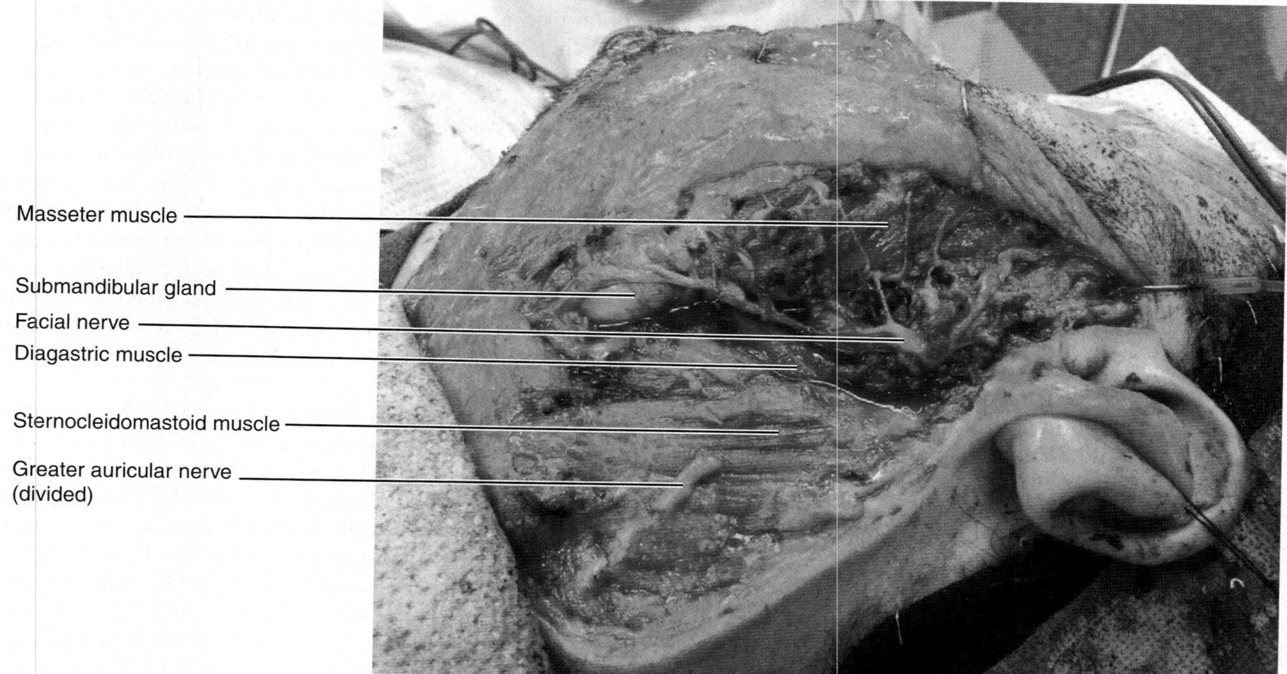

FIG. 34.20 Total parotidectomy field with identification, mobilization, and preservation of all branches of facial nerve.

Surgical Technique

Submandibular gland excision is classically performed via a transcervical incision, raising subplatysmal flaps, and protecting the marginal mandibular branch of the facial nerve. The Hayes-Martin maneuver of dividing the facial vein at the inferior aspect of the gland and raising it with the gland fascia can protect the facial nerve branch because it travels superficial to this vein. The superior aspect of the gland is then dissected free (with division of the facial artery) and the inferior aspect of the gland is dissected off the anterior belly of the digastric muscle, and the gland is freed from the posterior border of the mylohyoid muscle, which is retracted medially-superiorly, revealing the lingual nerve, submandibular ganglion, and the submandibular duct. The hypoglossal nerve can be identified with medial-inferior retraction of the mylohyoid muscle. Finally, the gland is dissected free posteriorly, and the facial artery is once again divided along the posterior aspect of the gland.

Parotidectomy is demonstrated in Video SALIV-2. The most common incision is a cervicomastoid incision as described by Blair in 1912 and modified by Bailey in 1941. Skin flaps are raised in a subplatysmal plane in the neck and over the parotid fascia in the face. The parotid gland is freed from the sternocleidomastoid muscle, often requiring division of the greater auricular nerve and external jugular vein, and the posterior belly of the digastric muscle is identified. Next, the parotid gland is dissected from the tragal cartilage proceeding deep to the tympanic and mastoid bones and the lateral aspect of the tympanomastoid suture line. The tissue between the digastric dissection and mastoid dissection is carefully divided, and the parotid gland retracted medially. The main trunk of the facial nerve is identified at the tympanomastoid suture line, at the level of the digastric muscle approximately 1 cm anterior, inferior, deep to the tragal pointer. The nerve and its branches are followed distally, dividing the overlying parotid tissue to expose the nerve. The tumor is removed en bloc with visualization and dissection of the nerve branches. Mobilization of nerve branches is required for large or deep lobe tumors as shown in Fig. 34.21. Facial nerve electromyographic monitoring can be used if available per surgeon preference.

The parotidectomy defect, which can be deforming depending on the extent of parotidectomy the need for resection of skin, temporal bone, or facial nerve, can be reconstructed with considerations being tumor characteristics and patient wishes. For standard parotidectomy defects, the main goals of reconstruction are to cover the facial nerve, avoid contact of parotid parenchyma with sweat glands of the facial skin, and fill contour defects. Since most reconstructive methods create a barrier between the remaining parotid tissue and the skin, they reduce the risk of Frey syndrome (gustatory sweating). Reconstructive options include the use of acellular dermal matrix, free fat grafting, sternocleidomastoid muscle flap, digastric muscle flap, other regional buried flaps, or buried free flaps. The latter two are more typically used in the case of total parotidectomy defects, especially if a neck dissection is performed concomitantly.

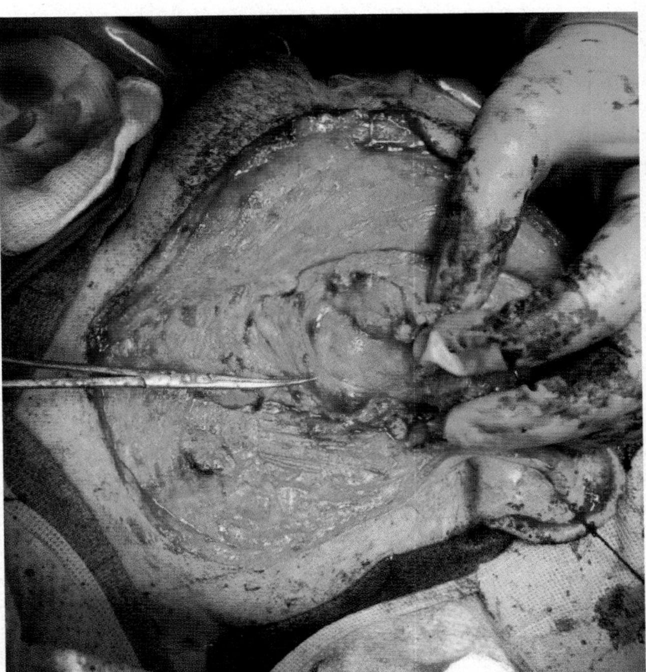

FIG. 34.21 Deep lobe parotid tumor with mobilization of the facial nerve inferiorly to expose and remove the tumor.

Nasal Cavity and Paranasal Sinuses

Anatomy

The nasal cavity and paranasal sinuses comprise a complex 3D structure that abuts critical structures including the orbit, cranium, and skull base. The anatomic boundaries are the palate and oral cavity inferiorly, the soft tissue of the face or nose anteriorly, and the cranial base or orbits laterally, superiorly, and posteriorly. The nasal cavity begins at the anterior nasal vestibules and contains the bony and cartilaginous nasal septum, structures of the lateral nasal wall, and the olfactory cleft. The paranasal sinuses are divided into paired maxillary and ethmoid sinuses and the central sphenoid and frontal sinuses that are usually completely separated by septae into right and left halves. Structures of the lateral nasal wall include the inferior, middle, and superior turbinates and the superior, middle, and inferior meatus named for the turbinate superior to them. The maxillary, anterior ethmoid, and frontal sinuses drain via the infundibulum into the middle meatus, while the nasolacrimal duct drains into the inferior meatus.

The four paired paranasal sinuses lie lateral and superior to the nasal cavity. The frontal sinuses are the most anterior and superior air cavities that lie within the frontal bone and drain into the nasal cavity via the frontal recesses into the middle meatus. The ethmoid sinuses are a honeycomb-like bony labyrinth that are located medial to the orbits and inferior to the anterior cranial fossa. The lamina papyracea is the thin lateral wall of the ethmoid sinus that constitutes the medial wall of the orbit. The anterior and posterior ethmoid cavities are separated by the basal lamella of the middle turbinate with the anterior ethmoids draining into the middle meatus and the posterior ethmoids draining via the sphenoethmoidal recess into the posterior nasal cavity. The sphenoid sinus lies in the middle of the sphenoid bone and is the most posterior and central of the sinuses. The vital structures of the optic nerves, carotid arteries, and cavernous sinuses are immediately adjacent to the lateral walls of the sphenoid sinus, whereas the sella turcica and optic chiasm are immediately superior to the central and posterior superior sinus roof. Additionally, the very lateral boundaries of the sphenoid sinus are adjacent to the second division of the trigeminal nerves (V2) and the vidian nerves. The maxillary sinuses drain into the middle meatus and are bound posteriorly by the pterygopalatine fossa, laterally by the zygomatic process of the maxilla, superiorly by the orbital floor, and inferiorly by the palate.

Pathology of the Nasal Cavity and Paranasal Sinuses

The most common diseases of the nasal cavity and paranasal sinuses are inflammatory in nature related to allergies or infections with viruses or bacterial. Although these inflammatory diseases can cause severe symptoms or even be life-threatening, most frequently, they are intermittent, mild, or self-limited when treated with anti inflammatory drugs and/or antibiotics. The majority of sinus infections resolve with no treatment or a short course of antibiotics; however, some infections require several weeks of antibiotic therapy combined with systemic steroids. On rare occasions, sinus infections can spread into the orbit or intracranially, resulting in the need for intravenous antibiotics and surgical procedures to open and drain the infected sinus.

Tumors of the nasal cavity and paranasal sinuses most frequently present at late stages because common associated symptoms of nasal congestion, headache, and facial pain are attributed to more common diseases such as allergies and sinusitis. Tumors can also present with involvement of structures surrounding the paranasal sinuses such as the orbits, the infratemporal fossa, and the cranial fossa. Proptosis, orbital pain, diplopia, epiphora, and vision loss are symptoms of orbital invasion, whereas sensory nerve involvement is heralded by facial numbness in the distribution of the infraorbital nerve or the palate. Tumors that involve the infratemporal fossa often present with trismus from involvement of pterygoid muscles and numbness in the distribution of the third division of the trigeminal nerve (V3). Finally, tumors involving the anterior cranial fossa can cause various central nervous system symptoms such as seizure, personality changes, or meningitis.

Both benign and malignant tumors arise within the sinonasal cavity with most arising from the epithelial lining. Schneiderian papilloma (also call sinonasal papilloma) is the most common benign tumor of the nasal cavity,[44] and patients present with unilateral nasal congestion and/or epistaxis. This benign tumor is associated with local destruction and has potential for malignant transformation. Schneiderian papilloma should be on the differential diagnosis for any unilateral sinonasal mass (Fig. 34.22). Sinonasal papilloma is classified into three groups:

1. Septal papilloma. These tumors usually began growing on the septum; they are exophytic and not associated with malignant degeneration.
2. Inverted papilloma (most common). Tumors usually arise along the lateral nasal wall and have an inverted growing pattern with local destruction. Inverted papillomas have an approximately 10% to 15% malignant degeneration rate.
3. Cylindrical cell papilloma (very rare). An oncocytic variant, and like inverted papilloma, these tumors most commonly originate from the lateral nasal wall. These tumors have equal or slightly higher potential for malignant transformation compared to inverted papilloma.

The treatment of choice for sinonasal papillomas is complete resection with negative margins. In the case of inverted papilloma and cylindrical papilloma, removal of bone at the base of the tumor is important to prevent recurrence. With complete removal of sinonasal papilloma, recurrence rates are low. Open and endoscopic approaches are safe and effective for resection of these tumors; however, endonasal endoscopic approaches are preferred when possible since they avoid the lateral rhinotomy and associated facial scar.

Other benign nasal lesions include hemangioma, benign fibrous histiocytoma, fibromatosis, leiomyoma, ameloblastoma, myxoma, fibromyxoma, and fibro-osseous and osseous lesions, such as fibrous dysplasia, ossifying fibroma, and osteoma. Growth of tumors, weakness of the skull base, or the combination can allow intracranial tumors or normal tissues to extend into the nasal cavity presenting as encephaloceles, meningoceles, dermoids, or pituitary tumors.

CT and MRI are each important imaging studies to obtain for evaluation of sinonasal and skull base tumors, since they provide complimentary information. Together, these imaging studies help clinicians narrow the potential differential diagnoses as they also assist in the identification of intracranial connections, involvement or impingement on critical structures (e.g., orbit, cranial nerves), and tumor vascularity. T2-weighted MRI images are more sensitive to differentiate tumors from obstructed secretions within the nasal or sinus cavities (Fig. 34.22), while CT images help identify bony destruction. Identification of structures involved by or adjacent to the tumor assists with diagnostic, treatment, and surgical planning. It is particularly important to determine if the tumor breeches the skull base, since intracranial involvement can increase the risk of cerebrospinal fluid (CSF) leak, even with diagnostic biopsy.

Malignancies of the sinonasal cavity are extremely rare, accounting for less than 1% of all cancers and less than 5% of HNCs. There is a slight male predominance and the peak incidence varies by tumor histology, but patient age most frequently ranges from the 40s to the 60s. Because respiratory epithelium can differentiate into squamous or glandular histology, SCC and adenocarcinoma represent two of the most common sinonasal cancers.[45] Risk factors for sinonasal cancer are woodworking or exposure to wood dust or metal/nickel most commonly from commercial smelting. Other sinonasal malignancies include olfactory neuroblastoma, neuroendocrine carcinoma, sinonasal undifferentiated carcinoma (SNUC), malignant fibrous histiocytoma, osteosarcoma, chondrosarcoma, mucosal melanoma, lymphoma, fibrosarcoma, leiomyosarcoma, angiosarcoma, teratocarcinoma, hemangiopericytoma, and metastases from other organ systems (e.g., renal cell carcinoma). In addition to tumor that arises in the nasal and sinus cavities, tumors of the central nervous system and primary skull base tumors such as chordomas, invasive pituitary adenomas, chondrosarcomas, and meningiomas can breech anatomic barriers to present in the sinonasal cavity.

In the eighth edition of the AJCC staging manual, the nasal cavity, ethmoid, and maxillary sinuses are distinguished as separate primary sites. The staging system applies only to epithelial carcinomas excluding neuroendocrine and primary skull base pathologies. Additionally, staging currently does not include frontal or sphenoid sinus as separate sites. Primary site staging (T stage) depends on tumor extent, with a key distinction being invasion into adjacent sinonasal structures versus invasion into the orbit, soft tissues of the face, palate, or cribriform plate/brain.

Lymph node metastases are uncommon (5%–15%), and elective neck dissection for primary sinonasal carcinomas is generally not recommended. However, if a carcinoma arising in the nasal or sinus cavity extends to the oral cavity or there is concern that the tumor arose in the oral cavity before extending into the sinonasal cavities, then a I through IV elective neck dissection should be considered. Additionally, neck dissection may be performed if neck surgery is needed for vessel control or to identify vessels for free flap reconstruction. Primary elective radiation to the upper neck nodal basins is often included with postoperative adjuvant therapy. Involved nodal groups may include the retropharyngeal, parapharyngeal, submental, and upper jugulodigastric nodes.

Evaluation and Treatment of Sinonasal Cancer

Sinonasal cancers can involve or closely approximate the orbits, cranial base, carotid arteries, cavernous sinus, multiple cranial

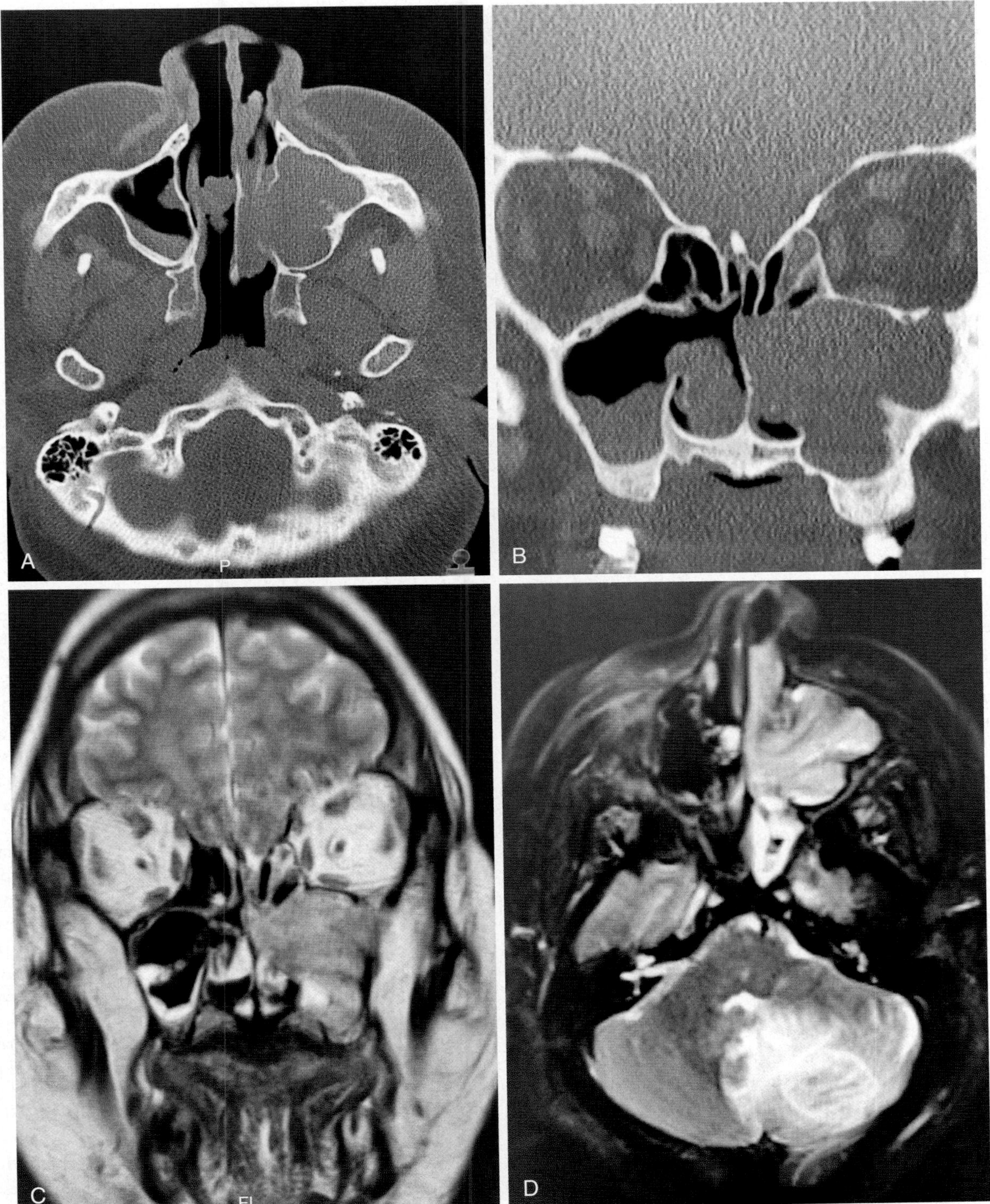

FIG. 34.22 (A) Axial computed tomography (CT) of an inverted papilloma showing base of the tumor in the lateral maxillary wall with hyperostosis noted. (B) Coronal CT of an inverted papilloma showing base of the tumor in the lateral maxillary wall with hyperostosis noted. (C) Coronal T1 magnetic resonance imaging (MRI) showing soft tissue boundaries of the tumor filling the maxillary sinus, abutting the orbital wall but without orbital soft tissue invasion. (D) Axial T2 MRI showing the soft tissue tumor filling the maxillary sinus but with T2 hyperintense signal in the sphenoid sinus showing mucous instead of tumor in the sphenoid.

nerves, palate, brain, or other critical structures. The complexity of resection, reconstruction, and radiation planning is hard to overstate speaking to the advantage of experienced multidisciplinary teams for treatment, reconstruction, and rehabilitation.

Preoperative workup consists of primary site imaging often with CT scans and MRI scans as well as local, regional, and distant staging with either CTs or PET/CTs. Biopsy of the primary site is required to establish pathologic diagnosis. Once a diagnosis

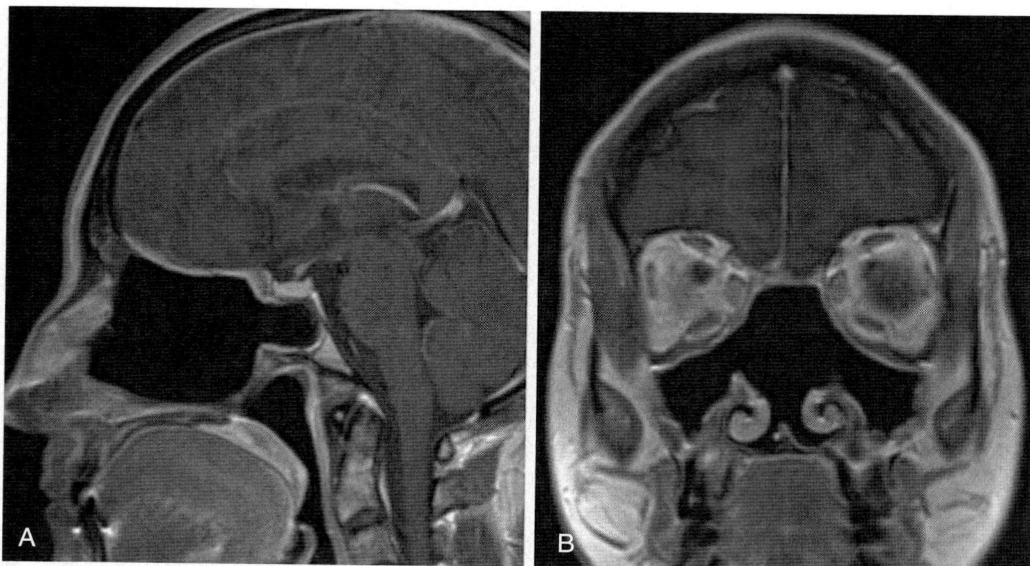

FIG. 34.23 Postoperative (5 year) endoscopic craniofacial T1 magnetic resonance imaging showing no evidence of recurrent disease and a healthy nasoseptal flap skull base reconstruction

is established and staging completed, a multidisciplinary treatment plan is established.

Treatment of most sinonasal malignancies relies on a negative margin surgical resection. Postoperative radiation is considered for high-stage disease or high-grade pathologies. For most sinonasal cancers, the utility of chemotherapy as a postoperative radiation sensitizer is unclear; however, concurrent chemotherapy with radiation is considered for treatment of tumors with high-risk pathologic features (e.g., positive margins, nodal disease, extracapsular nodal extension) or for those with high-grade histology (e.g., SNUC or small cell carcinoma). Clinical trials are currently underway to evaluate the utility of neoadjuvant preoperative chemotherapy to shrink tumors before surgery to aid with preservation of critical structures.

Preoperative planning is particularly important for sinonasal tumors to identify structures involved or adjacent to the tumor, to plan reconstruction, to assemble the surgical team, and to inform patients of surgical risks that may alter appearance or function. Preoperative studies also identify highly vascular tumors allowing preoperative embolization to decrease intraoperative blood loss and aid with complete tumor removal. Identification of tumors that transgress the dura alerts the treatment team of the potential need for perioperative lumbar drainage and for dural repair. Placement of a tracheotomy for craniofacial surgery to reduce the risk for postoperative pneumocephalus is controversial; however, depending on the planned reconstruction, it can be considered if there is risk of oral swelling, large skull base defects, or in patients who are obese or have obstructive sleep apnea.

Endoscopic techniques continue to evolve and allow for control of resection margins for many primary ethmoid as well as anterior skull base malignancies. Primary maxillary carcinoma involving the medial wall can also be performed endoscopically; however, if the palate or lateral maxilla is involved, then a radical maxillectomy with traditional approaches is preferred. Endoscopic techniques have evolved beyond dissection within the sinonasal cavities and now include dissection of the orbital lamina, periorbital, and intraorbital tumors. Additionally, resections of the bony skull base, dura, and intradural olfactory tracts can be performed via an endoscopic endonasal route (Fig. 34.23). Sinonasal cancers that involve the skin, palate, or intraconal orbit and that have far lateral extent or excessive intracranial extent are not ideal for endoscopic resection. Advancement in reconstruction using endoscopic techniques has been a driver of more aggressive endoscopic resections and has increasingly relied on the pedicled nasoseptal flap.[46] This flap is based on the posterior nasal artery that is a reliable branch of the sphenopalatine artery. Increased use of the posteriorly based nasoseptal flap has resulted in a marked decrease of CSF leak rates to less than 5% following endoscopic resection of intracranial pathologies such as craniopharyngiomas, meningiomas, and other primary neural tumors. However, the nasal septum is often involved with sinonasal carcinomas, and margins should not be compromised to preserve the blood supply to the nasal septal flap. In situations that the pedicled nasoseptal flap cannot be used, a tunneled pericranial flap can be used for endonasal skull base reconstruction. This flap is harvested with either a coronal incision or with endoscopic techniques before tunneling it through the nasion.[47] For more lateral defects, tunneled temporoparietal fascial flaps are also useful. Endoscopic resection and reconstruction techniques have been remarkably advanced and now offer a less morbid treatment option with outcomes comparable to open surgery for many sinonasal cancers.

Primary radiation therapy with concurrent chemotherapy for sinonasal malignancies continues to be studied, and these nonsurgical therapies are used for unresectable tumors and tumors whose excision would cause unacceptable morbidity. In addition, neoadjuvant chemotherapy or chemoradiation therapy plays an integral role for some aggressive histologies (e.g., SNUC, rhabdomyosarcoma, and midline reticulocytosis). Recent data suggest that chemoselection may be used to identify patients with sinonasal undifferentiated cancers who are best treated surgically or nonsurgically.

Given the low incidence of sinonasal cancer, trials to advance therapy for this orphan disease have been difficult to complete; however, molecular analysis of these tumors is providing insight into sinonasal carcinogenesis that is changing tumor categorization with future treatment implications. Retrospective analysis of sinonasal cancers has revealed that as many as one in five are associated with high-risk HPV. Most HPV-associated tumors are SCCs, but HPV is also detected in tumors with adenoid cystic-like features. Identification of HPV in sinonasal tumors is associated with improved overall and disease-free survival, possibly related to increased sensitivity to DNA damaging agents.[48] Analysis of SNUCs or nonkeratinizing SCC found loss of SMARCB1 (SWI/SNF related, matrix associated, actin dependent regulator of chromatin, subfamily B, member 1) expression. These tumors have poor outcomes, and currently, there is no therapy targeting loss of SMARCB1. Poor prognosis is also characteristic of undifferentiated or poorly differentiated squamous cell sinonasal tumors that contain fusions genes of NUT (nuclear protein in testis gene) and BRD4 or BRD3 (bromodomain containing 4 or 3). Although there are currently no targeted therapies for NUT carcinoma, bromodomain inhibitors are a logical choice for patients who fail standard therapy. Finally, IDH2 (isocitrate dehydrogenase 2) hotspot mutations have been identified in a significant portion (~50%) of SNUCs. Identification of this mutation in a large portion of SNUCs has therapeutic implications since inhibitors of mutant IDH are available.

Nasopharynx

Anatomy

The nasopharynx is positioned at the posterior aspect of the nasal cavity and at the superior aspect of the pharynx, is anatomically distinct from the nasal cavity and sinuses, and unlike the sinonasal complex, it contains lymphatic tissue and lymphoepithelial cells. Superiorly, the nasopharynx is defined by the mucosally covered bony choana and sphenoid rostrum. From this superior border, the nasopharynx extends inferiorly to the soft palate comprised largely by the adenoid pad bounded posteriorly by the clivus and upper spine. The lateral walls include the fossae of Rosenmuller, as well as the eustachian tube orifices.

Pathology of the Nasopharynx

Inflammatory disease of the nasopharynx is primarily centered on the lymphatic tissue and lymphoepithelial cells of the adenoids. Bacterial and viral infections that cause tonsillitis also infect the adenoids that can lead to nasal obstruction. Persistently enlarged adenoids can contribute to obstructive sleep apnea in pediatric patients, and because of the proximity of adenoids to the eustachian tube orifices, infected adenoids contribute to eustachian tube dysfunction resulting in otitis media with effusion, acute, or chronic otitis media. Treatment of recurrent acute or chronic otitis media may include removal of adenoid tissue in addition to pressure equalization tube insertion.

Tumors of the nasopharynx arise from the structures it comprises, including the epithelium, the adenoids (lymphoid and epithelial tissues), and deeper tissues, including fascia, cartilage, bone, and muscle. Although all tumors of the nasopharynx are rare, papillomas, teratomas, and fibromas are among the most commonly diagnosed benign tumors in this area. Angiofibroma, a benign vascular tumor that affects young male patients, is the most common benign tumor of the nasopharynx in children (Fig. 34.24). Although these tumors frequently involved the nasopharynx, juvenile nasopharyngeal angiofibromas (JNAs) originate from the cells surrounding the sphenopalatine artery and extend into the pterygomaxillary space, pushing the posterior wall of the maxillary sinus anteriorly. Molecular analysis of JNA shows frequent activating mutations in beta-catenin, and mutations in the adenomatous polyposis coli (APC) gene are also described by possibly explaining why these tumors occur up to 25 times more frequently in adolescents affected by familial adenomatous polyposis. Thornwaldt cyst is a midline mass of the inferior nasopharynx that originates from a remnant of the caudal notochord containing a jelly-like material that can become chronically inflamed. Rarely tumors of the central nervous system and upper spine can also involve the nasopharynx.

Nasopharyngeal tumors cause symptoms of nasal obstruction, serous otitis with effusion (often unilateral), and associated conductive hearing loss, epistaxis, and nasal drainage. Findings such as cervical lymphadenopathy, pain, trismus, and cranial nerve involvement suggest malignancy. Diagnosis is aided by clinic examination of the nasopharynx using flexible or rigid nasopharyngoscopes under topical anesthesia. If the mass is easily visualized, exophytic, and not vascular or pulsatile, then in-clinic biopsies can be considered with epistaxis being the primary risk. Otherwise, biopsy is performed in the operating room. CT scanning can identify widening of cranial nerve foramina, indicating nerve involvement, and bony destruction, especially around the clivus and upper spine, and contrast can give an indication of the vascularity of the tumor. MRI is complimentary to assess soft tissue involvement, intracranial extension, perineural spread, cavernous sinus extension, and carotid involvement.

Surgery is the primary treatment for benign tumors of the nasopharynx. Endoscopic techniques have evolved to allow for complete negative margin resections of most benign nasopharyngeal pathology without the need for palatal splitting or facial incisions. JNA is a prime example of tumors whose treatment has shifted from open to endoscopic approaches (Fig. 34.24). If tumors are embolized, excision of JNAs is performed 1 to 2 days after embolization of the arterial supply, which most frequently arises from the internal maxillary artery.

In addition to benign tumors, cancers arise in the nasopharynx, including nasopharyngeal carcinoma, low-grade nasopharyngeal papillary adenocarcinoma, lymphoma, plasmacytoma, rhabdomyosarcoma, malignant schwannoma, liposarcoma, chondrosarcoma, and chordoma. The staging system of malignant tumors of the nasopharynx only applies to epithelial tumors and is based on confinement of the tumor within the nasopharynx or spread to surrounding structures.[1] Although nasopharyngeal carcinoma accounts for much less than 1% of cancers diagnosed in North America, it represents between 15% and 20% of all malignancies in China and Sub-Saharan Africa. There is a strong correlation with EBV in these countries, but the association of EBV and nasopharyngeal carcinoma in the United States is less frequent. The WHO histopathologic grading system describes three types of nasopharyngeal cancer:

I. Keratinizing SCC
II. Nonkeratinizing SCC
III. Undifferentiated carcinoma (most common subtype)

WHO type I accounts for 20% of tumors in the United States and is associated with tobacco and alcohol exposure rather than EBV. WHO types II and III represent the remainder of cases in the United States, as well as the endemic form seen in Southeast Asia. In addition to EBV, another virus, HPV, has been found in up to 20% of nasopharyngeal cancers. HPV-positive nasopharyngeal tumors have a trend toward improved overall survival, but analyses have been difficult due to inability to control for EBV status of these tumors.

The most common presenting sign of a primary nasopharyngeal cancer is cervical node metastases, particularly to level

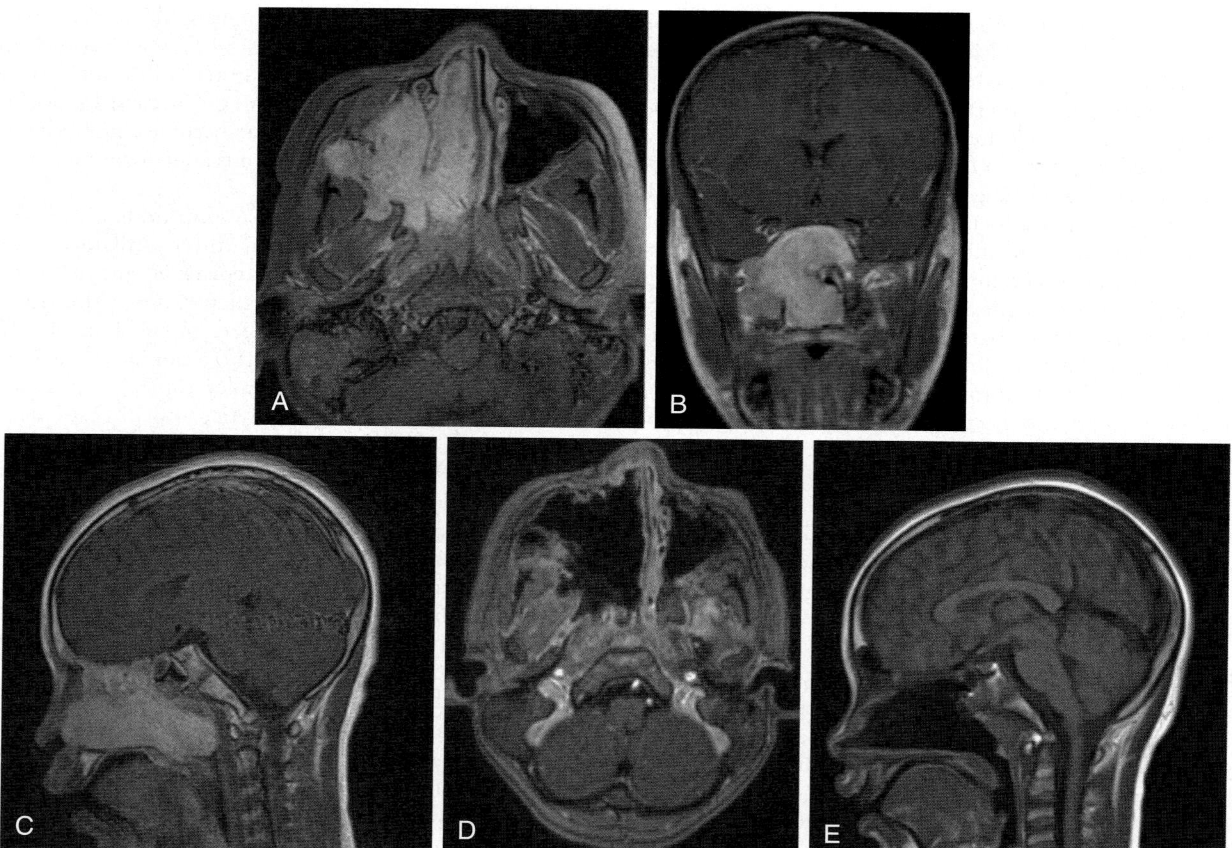

FIG. 34.24 (A) Axial T1 magnetic resonance imaging (MRI) of a juvenile nasopharyngeal angiofibromas (JNAs) showing infratemporal fossa involvement. (B) Coronal T1 MRI of a JNA showing infratemporal fossa involvement. (C) Sagittal MRI of a JNA showing clival and nasopharyngeal involvement. (D) Postoperative axial T1 MRI of a JNA after infratemporal fossa resection. (E) Postoperative sagittal T1 MRI of a JNA after clival and nasopharyngeal resection.

V and to the posterior cervical triangle. High-dose radiation therapy with concurrent chemotherapy to the primary tumor and bilateral necks including the retropharyngeal nodal basins is the primary treatment. Intensity-modulated radiation therapy has become a standard for nasopharyngeal carcinoma treatment since it results in a lower incidence of xerostomia and may provide a better quality of life compared to conventional 3D or 2D radiation therapy. A phase II RTOG study (RTOG-0225) showed the feasibility of intensity-modulated radiation therapy in a multi-institutional setting with a positive impact on xerostomia marked by low rates of grade III and IV xerostomia rates.[49]

Surgery is most commonly used for persistent neck disease and for selected cases of local recurrence. Surgery for small and/or midline recurrent tumors can be performed via endonasal endoscopic techniques; however, endoscopic techniques can be limited by inability to control feeding vessels, inability to obtain adequate margins, and limited access the infratemporal fossa (see below). Additionally, vascularized reconstructive options after radiation and/or reirradiation are limited within the nose. Transfacial maxillary swing-type operations are preferred for larger or lateral tumors since they provide much broader access for tumor excision and reconstruction with unirradiated free tissue transfer.

A nasopharyngeal mass in pediatric patients should be aggressively pursued since the nasopharynx is the second most common site for rhabdomyosarcoma. Rhabdomyosarcoma is the most frequent soft tissue sarcoma in pediatric patients and is the most common sarcoma occurring in the head and neck. Radiotherapy plus multiagent chemotherapy is the cornerstone of treatment, with surgery being reserved for recalcitrant or recurrent lesions.

Although surgery of the nasopharynx is performed primarily for benign pathologies, numerous open approaches are described for excision of malignant tumors of the nasopharynx and surrounding skull base region. Transoral transpalatal and transfacial with lateral rhinotomy are direct approaches that may be extended to swing of the anterior face of the maxilla and palate or mobilization of the orbit. As adjuncts to the transoral approach, transmandibular or LeFort I osteotomies with midfacial degloving and palatal drop can increase access and visualization. Lastly, lateral approaches that include transmandibular and transparotid as well as far lateral approaches through the temporal bone and jugular fossa can be used for tumors involving the clivus, petroclival synchondrosis, and petrous apex.

Endoscopic skull-based tumor surgery of the nasopharynx has evolved significantly over the last decade and indications for its use continue to expand. Endoscopic approaches have advantages of illumination and magnified visualization, allowing curative resections of benign nasopharyngeal and control rates for malignant pathologies that frequently equal open approaches. A key for control of benign and malignant nasopharyngeal tumors with endoscopic approaches is adherence to oncologic principles of obtaining negative margins.

Parasellar and Pituitary Skull Base Surgery

In the late twentieth and early twenty-first century, approaches to the pituitary and pituitary tumor extirpation evolved from transseptal/transsphenoid with microscopic visualization to endonasal transsphenoid with endoscopic visualization. The endoscopic approaches are quicker and less invasive, with less morbidity. Highly functioning skull base programs rely on multidisciplinary collaboration between otolaryngology and neurosurgery to manage diseases of the sellar and parasellar areas. Primary pathologies involving the sella and parasellar region are pituitary adenomas, Rathke cleft cyst, craniopharyngioma, and meningiomas. In addition to being less invasive, the endoscopic techniques provide better visualization of the suprasellar and cavernous sinus areas. Reconstruction using vascularized tissue, such as the nasal septal flap, has reduced postoperative CSF leak rates following sellar or parasellar endoscopic surgery to less than 3%.[50] With appropriate otolaryngology follow-up and postoperative care, sinonasal function can be maintained equivalent to baseline.

Ear and Temporal Bone

Anatomy

The external ear is made up of the skin and cartilage of the auricle or pinna and the cartilaginous and bony external auditory canal to the tympanic membrane. The middle ear is a space that starts medial to the tympanic membrane and goes to the labyrinthine structures and eustachian tube orifice. It contains the ossicular chain and the facial nerve. The inner ear is contained within the petrous portion of the temporal bone and consists of the cochlea, semicircular canals, and balance organs. The inner ear spans to the internal auditory canal through which cranial nerves VII and VIII pass to the midbrain.

Pathology of the Ear and Temporal Bone

Inflammatory and infectious ear disease is very common particularly in the pediatric population due to the frequency of eustachian tube dysfunction and recurrent viral infections. Viral and bacterial infections cause otitis media and are usually self-limited or easily treated with available antibiotics; however, more resistant community-acquired bacteria are becoming more common. Resistant, recurrent, or chronic infections are managed with tympanostomy tube insertion that can be accompanied by adenoidectomy for recalcitrant infections. Guidelines for placement of tympanostomy tubes in children are published by the American Academy of Otolaryngology-Head and Neck Surgery (https://www.entnet.org/sites/default/files/July2013_TubesFactSheet.pdf).

Tumors of the ear can involve the external ear, ear canal, middle ear, or inner ear structures. Progressively, the tumors become higher stage and are associated with worse survival as they involve deeper more internal structures. Primary neoplasms of the pinna and external ear are most often skin cancers, with sun exposure being the primary risk factor. SCCs have a worse overall prognosis than BCCs. In the external auditory canal, ceruminous gland adenocarcinomas and minor salivary gland carcinomas can also arise but are rare.

Within the temporal bone, benign neoplasms include adenoma, bony tumors, schwannomas, paragangliomas, acoustic neuroma, and meningioma. Squamous cell cancer is the most common primary cancer of the temporal bone, with other histologies being adenocarcinoma of middle ear or endolymphatic sac origin, and osteosarcomas. The temporal bone can also be invaded by adjacent parotid cancers and metastatic disease from distant sources.

Evaluation of Ear and Temporal Bone Tumors

Evaluation of primary cancers of the ear and temporal bone usually includes pathologic analysis and imaging for anatomic staging. When evaluating skin cancers of the external ear, the external auditory canal should be evaluated for involvement. Evaluation of ear cancers frequently includes audiometric analysis of hearing function in both the affected and nonaffected ears since treatments such as surgery, chemotherapy, and radiation can adversely affect hearing. Fine-cut CT scans including the ears and temporal bones are excellent for determining bony involvement, and MRIs with gadolinium can detect perineural spread and intracranial involvement. Although only 10% of primary ear and temporal bone tumors present with lymph node or distant metastasis, staging with either parotid, neck and chest CT scans, or PET/CT scans is standard. Depending on the location and extent of the cancer within the ear or temporal bone, primary echelon nodal drainage can be to the parotid lymph nodes and/or the upper neck.

Treatment of Ear and Temporal Bone Tumors

Primary treatment of ear and temporal bone tumors involves surgery with surgical goals of obtaining negative soft tissue and bony margins while maintaining functional preservation of the facial nerve and potential hearing structures. Involvement of the ear canal by an external ear tumor usually changes the surgical planning from auriculectomy to an auriculectomy with a primary lateral temporal bone resection, but minimal involvement or well-circumscribed ear canal involvement can be safely removed with a sleeve resection. Parotidectomy and neck dissection or postoperative radiation should be considered for extensive SCCs involving the tragus or anterior external auditory canal to control direct or lymphatic spread to the parotid or parotid lymph nodes and to gauge the need for adjuvant therapy.

Radiation therapy is less frequently used as primary treatment for primary ear and temporal bone malignancies; however, it is effective for skin malignancies of the pinna without bone involvement. Postoperative adjuvant radiotherapy should be considered for stage III and IV disease, as well as for poor pathologic prognosticators of perineural spread or metastatic spread to multiple lymph nodes. Chemoradiation can be considered for patients with positive margins or ECS of their involved lymph nodes.

Reconstruction of ear and temporal bone defects ranges from local primary closures to pedicled temporoparietal fascial or temporalis flaps to extensive microvascular free flap reconstructions. If the facial nerve has to be sacrificed, primary reconstruction as well as facial reanimation goals should be considered. The paramount consideration after sacrifice of the facial nerve is to protect the patient's ipsilateral eye from corneal abrasions. Planning for reconstruction must include coverage of exposed bone and neurovascular structures, potential CSF leak closure, and cosmesis.

HEAD AND NECK RECONSTRUCTION

Reconstructive surgery for the head and neck (upper aerodigestive tract and soft tissues) presents unique surgical challenges, although one that has shown great improvement over the last several decades. Advancements in technology, skills, and training have given surgeons more leeway in ablative procedures for locoregional control of head and neck neoplasms and in performing salvage procedures after failure of radiation therapy.

The goals of reconstructive surgery for defects created by oncologic head and neck surgery, in order of priority, are 1) separation of upper aerodigestive tract contamination from other critical compartments, such as intradural, mediastinal, and deep neck contents; 2) maximization of function, including breathing, speech, swallowing, vision, and hearing; and 3) optimization of form or cosmesis.

Reconstructive Goal 1: Separation of Upper Aerodigestive Tract From Sterile Compartments

Without thoughtful and advanced reconstructive surgery, contamination from the upper aerodigestive tract after tumor extirpation can lead to life-threatening complications such as meningitis, encephalitis, mediastinitis, persistent deep neck infection, hemorrhage, pharyngocutaneous fistula, and carotid artery blowout. Therefore, reconstruction of the upper aerodigestive tract should prioritize watertight closure of mucosal wounds and, in some cases (especially areas at high risk of leak), second layer onlay coverage.

Reconstructive Goal 2: Optimizing Function

Of these three major reconstructive goals, perhaps the most challenging is planning a reconstructive method that maximizes function. The most common functional problems following HNC extirpation are related to speech and swallowing. Resection of tissues of the oral cavity, oropharynx, hypopharynx, larynx, or cervical esophagus frequently alters swallowing function. Surgery for oral cancer or pharyngeal cancers can impede tongue motion, mouth opening, and oral competence. Loss of innervation—sensory or motor, locally or at the skull base—can also severely impair swallowing. Complicating matters further is that swallowing and speech rehabilitation are very closely related to airway (including patency of airway and aspiration). Other issues such as orbital position, patency of the external auditory canal, flow of tears into the nose, and eustachian tube patency are functional issues that must also be considered.

Reconstructive Goal 3: Optimization of Form/Cosmesis

The third important goal of head and neck reconstruction is to restore form and appearance. Resection of some HNCs causes cosmetic disfigurement that can have a major impact on patients' quality of life. Understanding all available reconstruction options, including free tissue transfer, allows the reconstructive surgeons to choose a donor site that optimizes all three goals.

Prioritization of reconstructive goals assists in optimizing reconstructive plans. Of course, the size, shape, and location of the expected defect are important in decision-making; however, patient comorbidities, surgeon experience, and the need for postoperative treatment also factor into reconstructive decision-making. For example, reconstruction of a scalp defect with exposed bone resulting from excision of an aggressive malignancy may be optimally reconstructed with hair bearing coverage by tissue expansion with delayed adjacent tissue transfer; however, the reconstructive surgeon must be aware of the impact that this may have in delaying adjuvant treatment such as radiation therapy and thus potentially oncologic outcomes. Thus, reconstructive surgeons should be an integral part of the multidisciplinary team involved in treatment planning for patients with HNC.

Reconstructive Options in Head and Neck Surgery

For reconstruction in many parts of the body, the simplest method is usually the best. Functional implications inherent to head and neck reconstruction frequently mandate that the simplest reconstructive method may not be the best option. The framework of the reconstructive ladder and reconstructive elevator systematically organize various reconstructive options. The concept of the elevator is particularly important for planning reconstruction of head and neck defects, purporting that more advanced reconstructive techniques that lead to improved function or oncologic outcome may be preferred.[51]

Secondary Intention

Healing by secondary intention is an excellent option in several clinical scenarios in the head and neck. Mucosal defects with an underlying layer of vascularized muscle, fat, or bone that will not contract to the point of impeding function may be left to close by secondary intention. One major advantage of many transoral procedures, including transoral laser microsurgery and TORS, is that significant defects of the larynx and pharynx heal by secondary intention with good functional results. If healing by secondary intent is planned following resection of oropharyngeal tumors, major vessels including internal and external carotid arteries and major branches should be covered. In addition, there should be no connections between the pharynx and neck if a concomitant neck dissection is performed. Healing by secondary intention is frequently used for small to moderate size defects of the lateral pharyngeal wall, hard palate, base of tongue, superficial tongue, external nose, scalp, and larynx.

Primary Closure

Primary closure is an option for reconstruction of cutaneous defects and select oral cavity and pharyngeal defects. For facial reconstruction with primary closure, attempts should be made to keep incisions within the relaxed skin tension lines. Incisions that parallel these lines respect facial esthetic units and can be closed with the less tension to decrease scarring. Z-plasty can be used to reorient an unfavorable line of closure into a relaxed skin tension line. For oral cavity and oropharynx reconstruction, attention must be given to risk of dehiscence associated with mobility and muscular forces. Avoiding decreased tongue motion is a primary concern with oral reconstruction since it can lead to difficulties with swallowing or speech. In addition to skin, primary closure can be used for tongue-wedge resections without any significant floor of mouth involvement, minimal lateral tongue defects, and alveolar resections particularly if mandibular height is decreased by a marginal mandibulectomy.

Nonvascularized Grafts

Nonvascularized grafts including split-thickness and full-thickness skin grafts, cartilage grafts, and bone grafts can be used in select situations where there is underlying or surrounding healthy vascularized tissue. Prior radiation therapy to the recipient area limits the use of some nonvascularized grafts, particularly bony and cartilaginous grafts.

Skin grafts are completely dependent for nutrition from the underlying tissue bed and can heal well over muscle, perichondrium, and periosteum. They do not take well over bone or cartilage or on tissue that has been irradiated or that is infected or hypovascular. Skin grafts are generally used for superficial oral cavity, ear, or maxillectomy defects.

Split-thickness skin grafts contain the epidermis and a portion of the dermis and are harvested with a dermatome at approximately 0.012-inch to 0.018-inch thickness. Thinner grafts require fewer nutrients to remain viable but also contract more when healing. A nonadherent antibiotic-impregnated bolster is commonly used to maintain stability between the split-thickness skin graft and recipient bed for 5 days to allow transmission of nutrients and capillary ingrowth while healing. Harvest sites include the anterior and lateral aspects of the thighs and buttocks.

Full-thickness skin grafts are characterized by a better color match, texture, contour and less contracture, but success rates are lower than with split-thickness skin grafts due to increased thickness needed for diffusion. Commonly used donor sites include the postauricular, upper eyelid, neck, and supraclavicular fossa skin.

Composite grafts are occasionally needed for cartilage and skin reconstruction of the nasal ala and may be harvested from the conchal bowl without significantly affecting the appearance of the pinna. Similarly, nonvascularized bone grafts from the hip or rib can be used in highly selected laryngeal, nasal, or mandibulomaxillary augmentation but not typically in the setting of previous or anticipated radiation therapy. Acellular cadaveric human dermis that has been prepared by removing immunogenic cells while leaving the collagen matrix intact can be used as a skin graft substitute and avoids donor site morbidity.

Adjacent Tissue Transfer and Local Flaps

Local skin flaps can have an excellent tissue match because of their proximity to the defect. Commonly used designs include advancement, rotation, transposition, rhomboid, and bilobed flaps (Fig. 34.25). Similar to primary closure, local flaps should be designed to be incorporated into the lines of relaxed skin tension. Although most local flaps depend on the subdermal plexus of capillaries, there are axial based interpolated local flaps such as the paramedian forehead flap, nasolabial flap, facial artery myomucosal, and nasoseptal flaps that can be used for a variety of defects of the face, nose, oral cavity, and skull base.

Regional Flaps

Regional flaps are based on axial blood flow and are located at a significant distance from the donor site. Harvest of the flap requires maintenance of the axial blood supply and reaching the defect frequently requires creation of a subcutaneous tunnel. The degree of dissection of the feeding vessels depends on mobility and reach required and care should be taken to avoid kinking or compression of the blood supply.

Despite many advances in head and neck reconstruction over the past 40 years, the pectoralis major myocutaneous regional flap first described for head and neck reconstruction in 1979 remains an important reconstructive option due to its ease of harvest, long reach to many parts of the head and neck, and healthy muscle and skin components. The pectoralis flap can be harvested as a musculocutaneous flap or muscle only flap and is based on the pectoral branch of the thoracoacromial artery which enters the muscle from the deep surface and skin perforators through the muscle to supply the skin. Following flap harvest, a subcutaneous tunnel is created from the donor site, over the clavicles, to the defect. Division of the pectoral nerve branches ensures atrophy of the muscle to reduce the bulge over the clavicle over time.

Regional flaps commonly used in head and neck reconstruction are shown in Table 34.4, some of which are also depicted in Fig. 34.26. Currently, less commonly used regional flaps in head and neck reconstruction include the deltopectoral flap, infraclavicular artery island flap, trapezius flap, and platysma flap, among others.

Free Tissue Transfer

Free tissue transfer entails removal of composite tissue from a distant site, along with its blood supply, and revascularization through microvascular anastomosis of one or more arteries and veins within or near the reconstructive field. Contemporary head and neck microvascular free flap success rates are over 95% at high-volume centers, reflecting incremental improvements in technology, surveillance, training, and experience. Free tissue transfer allows for reconstruction of essentially any head and neck defect, and the choice for the donor site depends on the characteristic of the tissue needed for reconstruction (e.g., size, bone, bulk, epithelial lining) as well as patient and surgeon considerations.

Commonly used free flaps used in head and neck reconstruction are the radial forearm, lateral arm, and anterolateral thigh when soft tissue and epithelial lining is needed. Fibula and

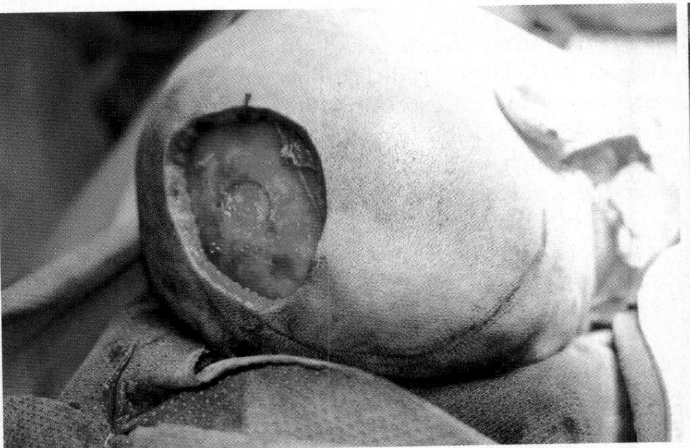

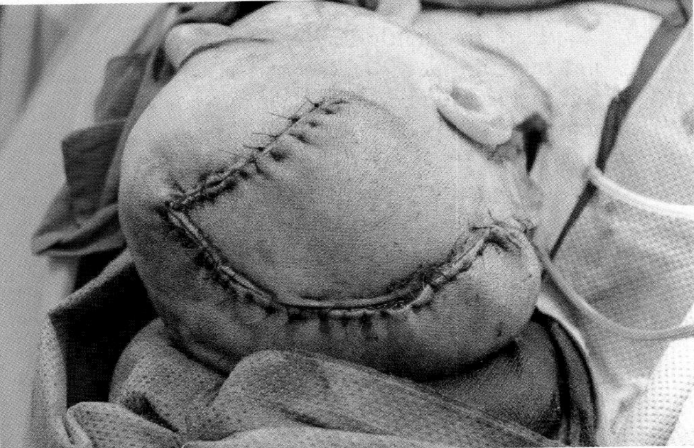

FIG. 34.25 Adjacent tissue transfer used for large scalp defect in a young, unirradiated patient.

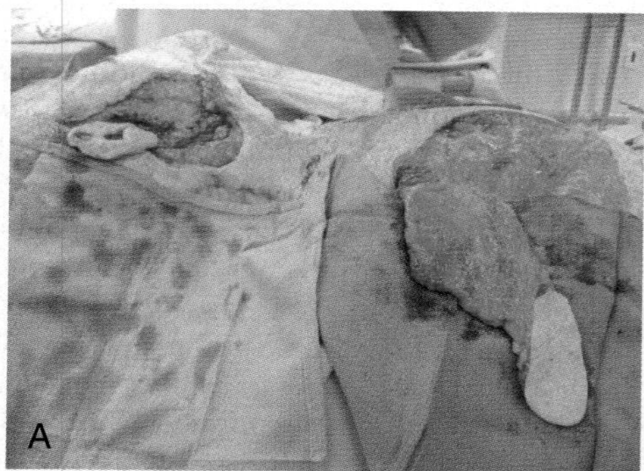

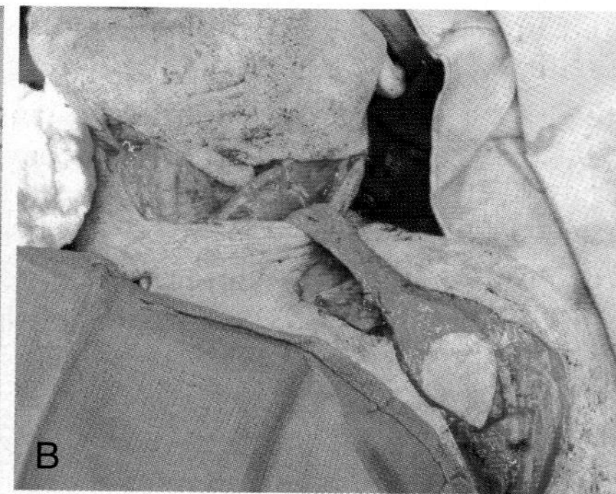

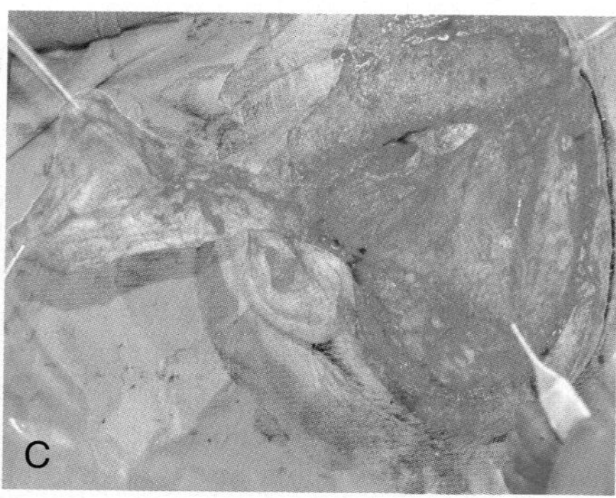

FIG. 34.26 Example of regional flaps used in head and neck reconstruction. (A) Pectoralis major myocutaneous flap. (B) Supraclavicular artery island flap. (C) Temporoparietal fascia flap and temporalis muscle flap.

TABLE 34.4 Commonly used regional flaps in head and neck reconstruction.

FLAP NAME	VASCULAR SUPPLY	COMPONENTS
Pectoralis major	Pectoral branch of thoracoacromial artery	Muscle Musculocutaneous
Supraclavicular artery island	Supraclavicular branch of transverse cervical artery	Fasciocutaneous
Submental artery island	Submental branch of facial artery	Fasciocutaneous
Temporalis	Deep temporal artery	Muscle
Temporoparietal fascia	Superficial temporal artery	Fascia Fasciocutaneous
Latissimus dorsi	Thoracodorsal artery	Muscle Musculocutaneous
Deltopectoral flap	Intercostal perforators of the internal mammary artery	Fasciocutaneous

TABLE 34.5 Commonly used free flaps in head and neck reconstruction.

FASCIAL AND/OR FASCIOCUTANEOUS	MUSCLE AND/OR MYOCUTANEOUS	BONE-CONTAINING FREE FLAPS	VISCERAL
Radial forearm	Rectus abdominis	Fibula	Jejunal
Anterolateral thigh	Latissimus dorsi	Scapula (lateral border or tip)	Omentum
Lateral arm	Gracilis	Radial forearm	Gastro-omentum
Ulnar forearm	Anterolateral thigh with vastus lateralis	Iliac crest/external oblique	
Temporoparietal fascia			
Lateral thigh			

scapula free flaps are frequently used when soft tissue, epithelial lining, and bone are needed. Rectus and latissimus can be useful for large defects requiring muscle only or muscle with skin. Because of the complexity of reconstruction in the head and neck and because the first choice for free flap reconstruction of a defect may not be possible due to previous therapy or patient considerations, the reconstructive surgeon should have a grasp of many potential donor sites as indicated in Table 34.5. Figs. 34.27 and 34.28 depict some of the commonly used flaps and insets. Additional flaps have also been described in case series such as the medial sural artery perforator free flap, the anterolateral thigh osteomyocutaneous free flap, and a number of perforator-type skin flaps.

In addition to the characteristics and composition of the defect that will guide flap selection, patient and donor site considerations include previous surgeries, preoperative testing (such as Allen test for radial forearm free flap, and arterial imaging for the fibula free flap), pedicle length, pedicle caliber, donor site morbidity, patient preference, and the expectation for osseointegrated implants into bone. Age itself is not a contraindication to free flap reconstruction, although a history of prior failed free flaps, clotting disorders, or of vascular disease should raise caution.

Perhaps the most versatile donor site for head and neck free flap reconstruction is the system of flaps from the subscapularis vascular system.[52] The subscapularis artery, from the axillary artery, has a number of branches and can thus allow for multiple soft and hard tissue components that have a good amount of independent mobility yet a single arterial and single venous anastomosis (Fig. 34.29). From the pedicled subscapularis artery and vein, the reconstructive surgeon can obtain a large number of flaps based on branches: thoracodorsal artery and circumflex scapular artery (Table 34.6). This system of flaps has further

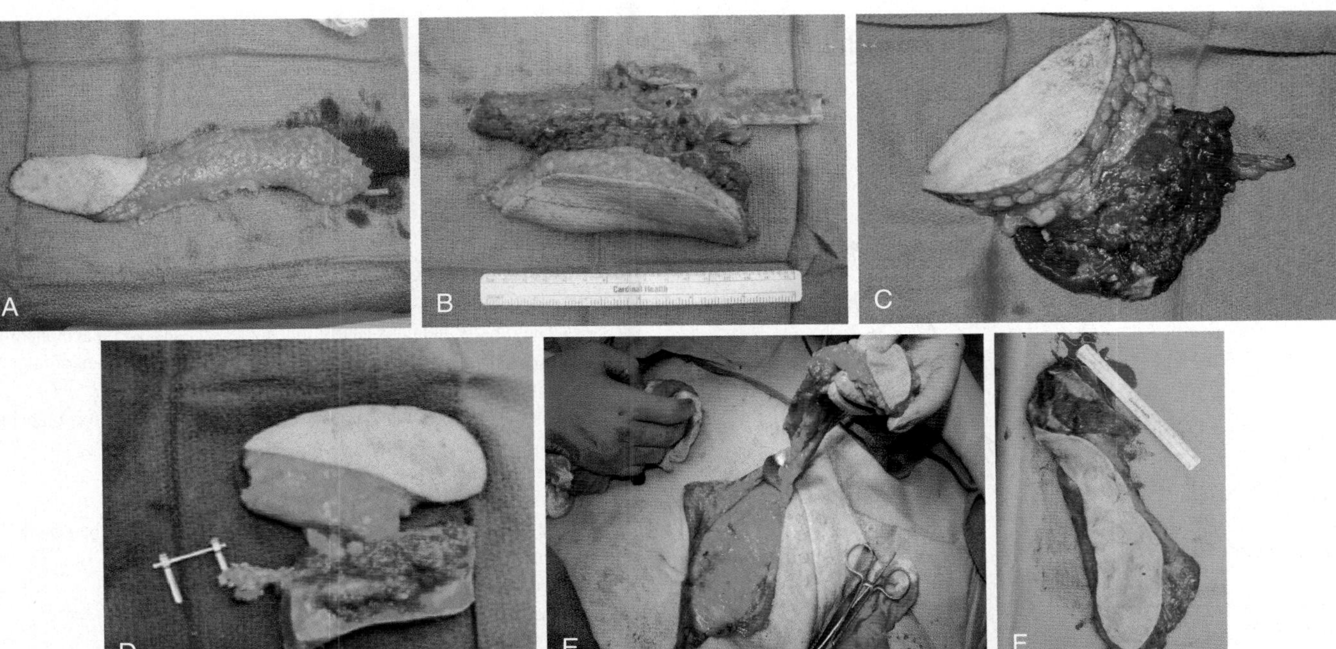

FIG. 34.27 Commonly used free flaps in head and neck reconstruction. (A) Radial forearm free flap. (B) Fibula free flap. (C) Anterolateral thigh free flap (in this case with a large cuff of vastus lateralis muscle). (D) Scapula free flap. (E) Rectus abdominis free flap. (F) Scapula and latissimus dorsi free flap.

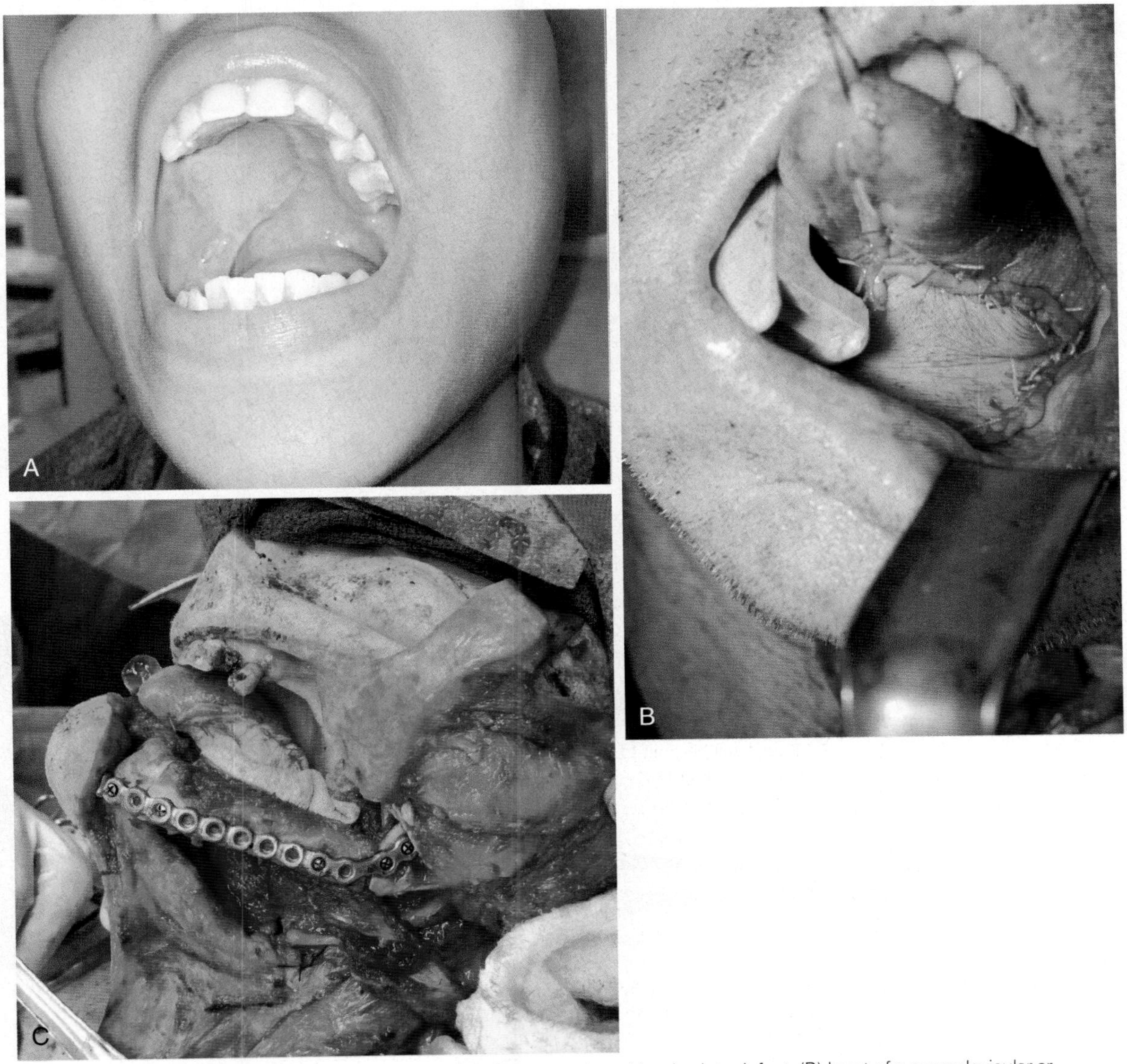

FIG. 34.28 (A) Inset of radial forearm free flap for posterolateral hard palate defect. (B) Inset of a supraclavicular artery island flap (regional) for floor of mouth and tongue. (C) Inset of a fibula-free flap and floor-of-mouth/tongue defect.

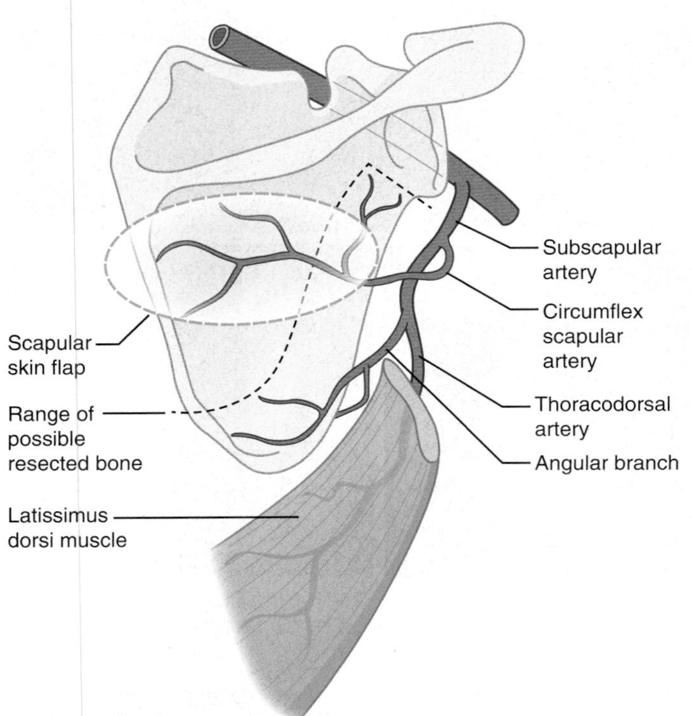

FIG. 34.29 Subscapularis system of flaps.

TABLE 34.6 Individual flaps based on the subscapular artery and vein.

FLAP COMPONENTS	BLOOD SUPPLY (ALL FROM THE SUBSCAPULARIS ARTERY)
Scapular fasciocutaneous flap	Circumflex scapular (transverse branch)
Parascapular fasciocutaneous flap	Circumflex scapular (vertical branch)
Scapular-parascapular osteofasciocutaneous flap	Circumflex scapular (bone perforators)
Scapula tip osteofasciocutaneous flap	Thoracodorsal (angular artery branch)
Latissimus dorsi muscle or myocutaneous flap	Thoracodorsal
Latissimus dorsi osteomusculocutaneous flap	Thoracodorsal and bone component
Serratus anterior muscular flap	Thoracodorsal
Serratus anterior musculocutaneous flap	Thoracodorsal
Serratus anterior with rib flap	Thoracodorsal

These individual flaps can be combined into a mega-flap with multiple components revascularized with a single arterial and single venous anastomosis of the subscapularis artery and vein.

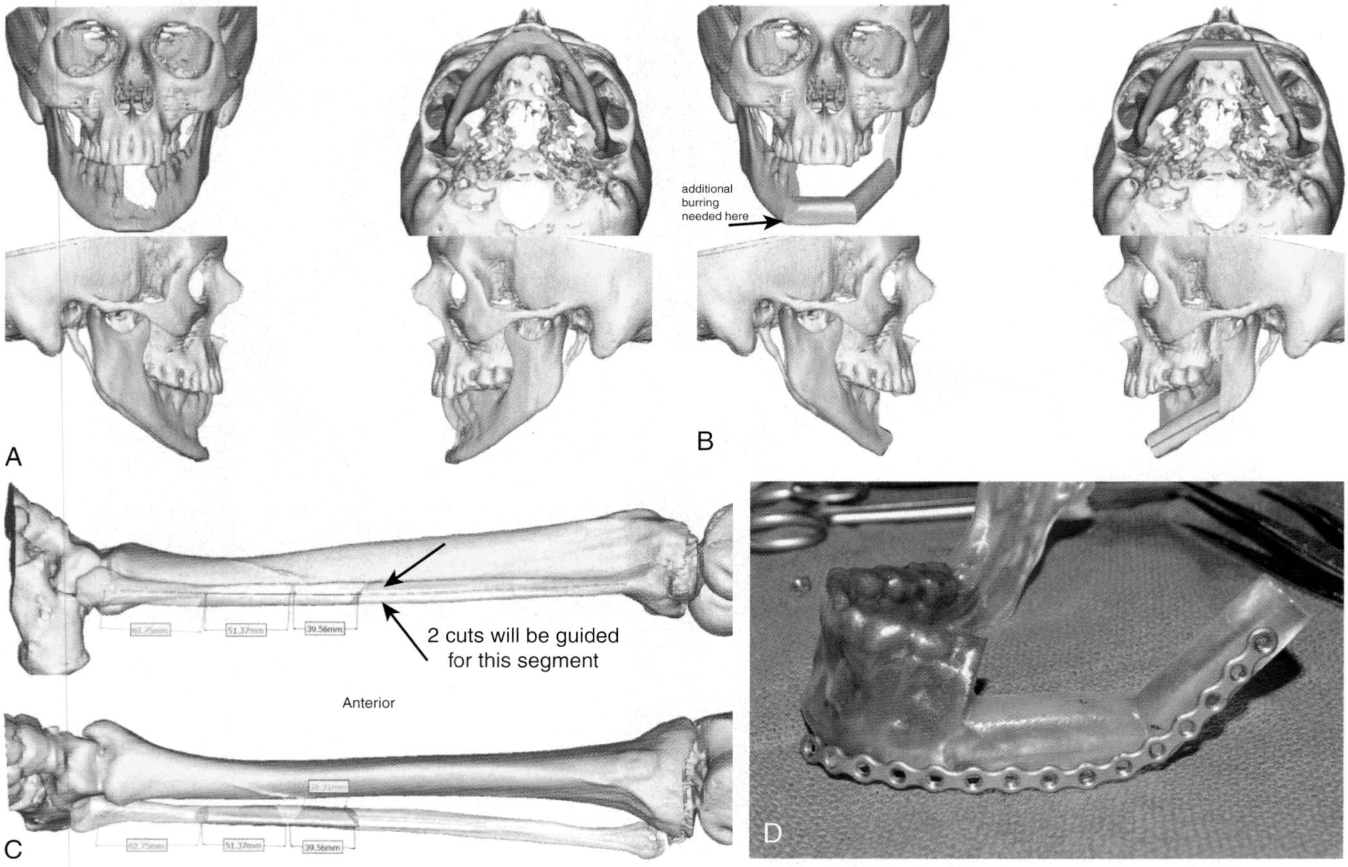

FIG. 34.30 A virtual surgical plan for mandible reconstruction. (A) Plan for surgical resection. (B) Plan for fibula reconstruction. (C): Patient-specific fibula cutting plan for ostectomy and osteotomies. (D) Three-dimensional model and prebent plate ready prior to surgery (different case).

advantages of rarely being affected by atherosclerosis and minimal donor site morbidity especially in the lame, very elderly, or frail population, in which fibula harvest could severely impact early ambulation and is important for a healthy postoperative recovery.

Virtual Surgical Planning for Reconstruction of the Facial Skeleton

Virtual surgical planning (VSP) for maxillomandibular reconstruction is increasingly used, although the exact indications, advantages, and disadvantages are still debated. There is general consensus of value for reconstruction of facial skeletal defects if they are too distorted from trauma or pathology to prebend a plate. In these cases, VSP optimizes occlusion and projection by either prebending or 3D printing reconstruction plates and providing osteotomy cutting guides. The value of 3D planning has been extolled for all maxillomandibular reconstruction to decrease operative time and increased accuracy in occlusion and bone-bone contact. The main disadvantages for VSP are the added cost and, in cases of malignancy, the increased time required to plan the surgery as well as the possibility of not adhering to the preoperative plan because of intraoperative findings related to unrecognized tumor extent and/or margin status. Fig. 34.30 depicts VSP for mandibular reconstruction.

SELECTED REFERENCES

Ang KK, Harris J, Wheeler R, et al. Human papillomavirus and survival of patients with oropharyngeal cancer. *N Engl J Med.* 2010;363(1):24–35.

This classic article used results of a randomized clinical trial (Radiation Therapy Oncology Group [RTOG] 0129) to analyze survival in the subset of patients with oropharyngeal squamous cell carcinoma (OPSCC) based on human papillomavirus (HPV) status. Findings clarified that patients with HPV-associated OPSCC have improved overall and progression-free survival. The study also identified smoking history of greater than 10 pack-years as a negative prognostic factor in HPV-positive OPSCC.

Chen AY, Fedewa S, Pavluck A, et al. Improved survival is associated with treatment at high-volume teaching facilities for patients with advanced stage laryngeal cancer. *Cancer.* 2010;116:4744–4752.

This article was amongst the earliest to identify the type of treatment center as a significant factor that impacts patient survival. Analysis of patients from the National Cancer Database with advanced laryngeal cancer revealed improved survival for patients treated at high volume teaching/research facilities compared to low volume teaching/research facilities, community facilities, or community cancer centers. The value of multidisciplinary care was implied since high volume for surgical treatment and nonsurgical treatment for laryngeal cancer independently correlated with improved survival.

Ferris RL, Blumenschein Jr G, Fayette J, et al. Nivolumab for recurrent squamous-cell carcinoma of the head and neck. *N Engl J Med.* 2016;375:1856–1867.

The U.S. Food and Drug Administration (FDA) approval of the first immune therapy for head and neck squamous cell carcinoma (HNSCC) was based on this study. The randomized phase 3 trial of recurrent HNSCC after platinum therapy revealed that overall survival was improved in patients treated with nivolumab compared to the standard of care single-agent therapy. Response rate and 6-month progression-free survival were approximately doubled in patients treated with nivolumab, whereas high-grade toxicity was decreased.

Forastiere AA, Zhang Q, Weber RS, et al. Long-term results of RTOG 91-11: a comparison of three nonsurgical treatment strategies to preserve the larynx in patients with locally advanced larynx cancer. *J Clin Oncol.* 2013;31:845–852.

Long-term results of a phase 3 clinical trial (Radiation Therapy Oncology Group [RTOG] 91-11) in advanced laryngeal cancer were used to compare survival between patients in the three treatment arms: (1) induction cisplatin/fluorouracil (PF) followed by radiation therapy (RT), (2) concomitant cisplatin/RT, and (3) RT alone. Short-term results of this trial revealed superior laryngeal preservation and locoregional control for patients in the concomitant treatment arm; however, long-term results revealed no difference in laryngectomy-free survival (at 10 years) with a strong trend toward improved overall survival at 10 years in patients treated in the induction arm compared to concurrent cisplatin/RT. This report shows that early and long-term results of trials may conflict and that delayed analysis may alter impressions about optimal therapy.

Marur S, Li S, Cmelak AJ, et al. E1308: phase II trial of induction chemotherapy followed by reduced-dose radiation and weekly cetuximab in patients with HPV-associated resectable squamous cell carcinoma of the oropharynx—ECOG-ACRIN Cancer Research Group. *J Clin Oncol.* 2017;35:490–497.

This article describes a phase 2 trial (E1308) that used response to induction chemotherapy as a marker to select patients for lower dose radiation therapy in advanced stage human papillomavirus (HPV)<en dash>associated oropharyngeal squamous cell carcinoma (OPSCC). The trial revealed significantly improved swallowing function for patients treated with deintensified radiation therapy and identified a low-risk group (<T4, <N2C, <10 pack-year smoking) with excellent 2-year progression-free and overall survival when treated with lower dose radiation.

REFERENCES

1. Amin M, Edge SB, Greene FL, et al. *AJCC Cancer Staging Manual*. 8th ed. Chicago: Springer; 2018.
2. Viens LJ, Henley SJ, Watson M, et al. Human papillomavirus-associated cancers—United States, 2008–2012. *MMWR Morb Mortal Wkly Rep*. 2016;65:661–666.
3. Centers for Disease Control and Prevention. Prevention 2018 #5231. Accessed; 2019, https://www.cdc.gov/cancer/hpv/basic_info/hpv_oropharyngeal.htm.
4. Cooper JS, Porter K, Mallin K, et al. National Cancer Database report on cancer of the head and neck: 10-year update. *Head Neck*. 2009;31:748–758.
5. Gillison ML. Current topics in the epidemiology of oral cavity and oropharyngeal cancers. *Head Neck*. 2007;29:779–792.
6. McLaughlin-Drubin ME, Munger K. Oncogenic activities of human papillomaviruses. *Virus Res*. 2009;143:195–208.
7. Alexandrov LB, Nik-Zainal S, Wedge DC, et al. Signatures of mutational processes in human cancer. *Nature*. 2013;500:415–421.
8. Zhang Z, Lopez-Giraldez F, Townsend JPLOX. inferring level of expression from diverse methods of census sequencing. *Bioinformatics*. 2010;26:1918–1919.
9. Califano J, van der Riet P, Westra W, et al. Genetic progression model for head and neck cancer: implications for field cancerization. *Cancer Res*. 1996;56:2488–2492.
10. National Cancer Institute. *The Cancer Genome Atlas Program*; 2015. Accessed; 2019, https://seer.cancer.gov/statfacts/html/lip.html.
11. Hajek M, Sewell A, Kaech S, et al. TRAF3/CYLD mutations identify a distinct subset of human papillomavirus–associated head and neck squamous cell carcinoma. *Cancer*. 2017;123:1778–1790.
12. Rusan M, Li YY, Hammerman PS. Genomic landscape of human papillomavirus–associated cancers. *Clin Cancer Res*. 2015;21:2009–2019.
13. Topalian SL, Taube JM, Anders RA, et al. Mechanism-driven biomarkers to guide immune checkpoint blockade in cancer therapy. *Nat Rev Cancer*. 2016;16:275–287.
14. Chen AY, Fedewa S, Pavluck A, et al. Improved survival is associated with treatment at high-volume teaching facilities for patients with advanced stage laryngeal cancer. *Cancer*. 2010;116:4744–4752.
15. D'Cruz AK, Vaish R, Kapre N, et al. Elective versus therapeutic neck dissection in node-negative oral cancer. *N Engl J Med*. 2015;373:521–529.
16. Almangush A, Coletta RD, Bello IO, et al. A simple novel prognostic model for early stage oral tongue cancer. *Int J Oral Maxillofac Surg*. 2015;44:143–150.
17. Wolf GT, Fisher SG, Hong WK, et al. Induction chemotherapy plus radiation compared with surgery plus radiation in patients with advanced laryngeal cancer. *N Engl J Med*. 1991;324:1685–1690.
18. Adelstein DJ, Li Y, Adams GL, et al. An intergroup phase III comparison of standard radiation therapy and two schedules of concurrent chemoradiotherapy in patients with unresectable squamous cell head and neck cancer. *J Clin Oncol*. 2003;21:92–98.
19. Denis F, Garaud P, Bardet E, et al. Final results of the 94-01 French Head and Neck Oncology and Radiotherapy Group randomized trial comparing radiotherapy alone with concomitant radiochemotherapy in advanced-stage oropharynx carcinoma. *J Clin Oncol*. 2004;22:69–76.
20. Forastiere AA, Zhang Q, Weber RS, et al. Long-term results of RTOG 91-11: a comparison of three nonsurgical treatment strategies to preserve the larynx in patients with locally advanced larynx cancer. *J Clin Oncol*. 2013;31:845–852.
21. Rapidis AD, Vermorken JB, Bourhis J. Targeted therapies in head and neck cancer: past, present and future. *Rev Recent Clin Trials*. 2008;3:156–166.
22. Ferris RL, Blumenschein Jr G, Fayette J, et al. Nivolumab for recurrent squamous-cell carcinoma of the head and neck. *N Engl J Med*. 2016;375:1856–1867.
23. Lheureux S, Butler MO, Clarke B, et al. Association of ipilimumab with safety and antitumor activity in women with metastatic or recurrent human papillomavirus–related cervical carcinoma. *JAMA Oncol*. 2018;4:e173776.
24. Bocca E, Pignataro O. A conservation technique in radical neck dissection. *Ann Otol Rhinol Laryngol*. 1967;76:975–987.
25. Civantos FJ, Zitsch RP, Schuller DE, et al. Sentinel lymph node biopsy accurately stages the regional lymph nodes for T1–T2 oral squamous cell carcinomas: results of a prospective multi-institutional trial. *J Clin Oncol*. 2010;28:1395–1400.
26. Warnakulasuriya S, Ariyawardana A. Malignant transformation of oral leukoplakia: a systematic review of observational studies. *J Oral Pathol Med*. 2016;45:155–166.
27. Alter BP. Fanconi anemia and the development of leukemia. *Best Pract Res Clin Haematol*. 2014;27:214–221.
28. Yu KK, Zanation AM, Moss JR, et al. Familial head and neck cancer: molecular analysis of a new clinical entity. *Laryngoscope*. 2002;112:1587–1593.
29. National Comprehensive Cancer Network. *Head and Neck Cancer*. 2nd ed. Accessed; 2018, https://www.nccn.org/store/login/login.aspx?ReturnURL=https://www.nccn.org/professionals/physician_gls/pdf/head-and-neck.pdf.
30. National Cancer Institute. Surveillance, Epidemiology, and End Results Program. Accessed; 2015, https://seer.cancer.gov/statfacts/html/lip.html.
31. Rahmati R, Gillespie MB, Eisele DW. Is sialendoscopy an effective treatment for obstructive salivary gland disease? *Laryngoscope*. 2013;123:1828–1829.
32. Pytynia KB, Dahlstrom KR, Sturgis EM. Epidemiology of HPV-associated oropharyngeal cancer. *Oral Oncol*. 2014;50:380–386.
33. Van Dyne EA, Henley SJ, Saraiya M, et al. Trends in human papillomavirus–associated cancers—United States, 1999–2015. *MMWR Morb Mortal Wkly Rep*. 2018;67:918–924.
34. Ang KK, Harris J, Wheeler R, et al. Human papillomavirus and survival of patients with oropharyngeal cancer. *N Engl J Med*. 2010;363:24–35.
35. Marur S, Li S, Cmelak AJ, et al. E1308: phase II trial of induction chemotherapy followed by reduced-dose radiation and weekly cetuximab in patients with HPV-associated resectable squamous cell carcinoma of the oropharynx—ECOG-ACRIN Cancer Research Group. *J Clin Oncol*. 2017;35:490–497.
36. Gillison ML, Trotti AM, Harris J, et al. Radiotherapy plus cetuximab or cisplatin in human papillomavirus–positive oropharyngeal cancer (NRG Oncology RTOG 1016): a randomised, multicentre, non-inferiority trial. *Lancet*. 2019; 393:40–50.
37. Chera BS, Amdur RJ, Tepper J, et al. Phase 2 Trial of de-intensified chemoradiation therapy for favorable-risk human papillomavirus–associated oropharyngeal squamous cell carcinoma. *Int J Radiat Oncol Biol Phys*. 2015;93:976–985.

38. Li H, Torabi SJ, Yarbrough WG, et al. Association of human papillomavirus status at head and neck carcinoma subsites with overall survival. *JAMA Otolaryngol Head Neck Surg*. 2018;144:519–525.
39. Kuo P, Sosa JA, Burtness BA, et al. Treatment trends and survival effects of chemotherapy for hypopharyngeal cancer: analysis of the National Cancer Data Base. *Cancer*. 2016;122:1853–1860.
39a. Mahul B, Edge SB, Greene FL, et al. AJCC Cancer Staging Manual 8/e, Chicago, Springer, 2018.
40. Zbaren P, Triantafyllou A, Devaney KO, et al. Preoperative diagnostic of parotid gland neoplasms: fine-needle aspiration cytology or core needle biopsy? *Eur Arch Otorhinolaryngol*. 2018;275:2609–2613.
41. Sharma E, Dahal S, Sharma P, et al. Secondary salivary gland malignancy in thyroid cancer: a United States population based study. *J Clin Med Res*. 2018;10:601–605.
42. Skalova A, Vanecek T, Sima R, et al. Mammary analogue secretory carcinoma of salivary glands, containing the ETV6-NTRK3 fusion gene: a hitherto undescribed salivary gland tumor entity. *Am J Surg Pathol*. 2010;34:599–608.
43. El-Naggar AK, Chan JKC, Takata T, et al. The fourth edition of the head and neck World Health Organization blue book: editors' perspectives. *Hum Pathol*. 2017;66:10–12.
44. Lisan Q, Laccourreye O, Bonfils P. Sinonasal inverted papilloma: from diagnosis to treatment. *Eur Ann Otorhinolaryngol Head Neck Dis*. 2016;133:337–341.
45. Svider PF, Setzen M, Baredes S, et al. Overview of sinonasal and ventral skull base malignancy management. *Otolaryngol Clin North Am*. 2017;50:205–219.
46. Klatt-Cromwell CN, Thorp BD, Del Signore AG, et al. Reconstruction of skull base defects. *Otolaryngol Clin North Am*. 2016;49:107–117.
47. Zanation AM, Snyderman CH, Carrau RL, et al. Minimally invasive endoscopic pericranial flap: a new method for endonasal skull base reconstruction. *Laryngoscope*. 2009; 119:13–18.
48. Alos L, Moyano S, Nadal A, et al. Human papillomaviruses are identified in a subgroup of sinonasal squamous cell carcinomas with favorable outcome. *Cancer*. 2009;115:2701–2709.
49. Lee N, Harris J, Garden AS, et al. Intensity-modulated radiation therapy with or without chemotherapy for nasopharyngeal carcinoma: Radiation Therapy Oncology Group Phase II trial 0225. *J Clin Oncol*. 2009;27:3684–3690.
50. Patel MR, Taylor RJ, Hackman TG, et al. Beyond the nasoseptal flap: outcomes and pearls with secondary flaps in endoscopic endonasal skull base reconstruction. *Laryngoscope*. 2014; 124:846–852.
51. Gottlieb LJ, Krieger LM. From the reconstructive ladder to the reconstructive elevator. *Plast Reconstr Surg*. 1994;93:1503–1504.
52. Gibber MJ, Clain JB, Jacobson AS, et al. Subscapular system of flaps: an 8-year experience with 105 patients. *Head Neck*. 2015;37:1200–1206.

SECTION VII

Breast

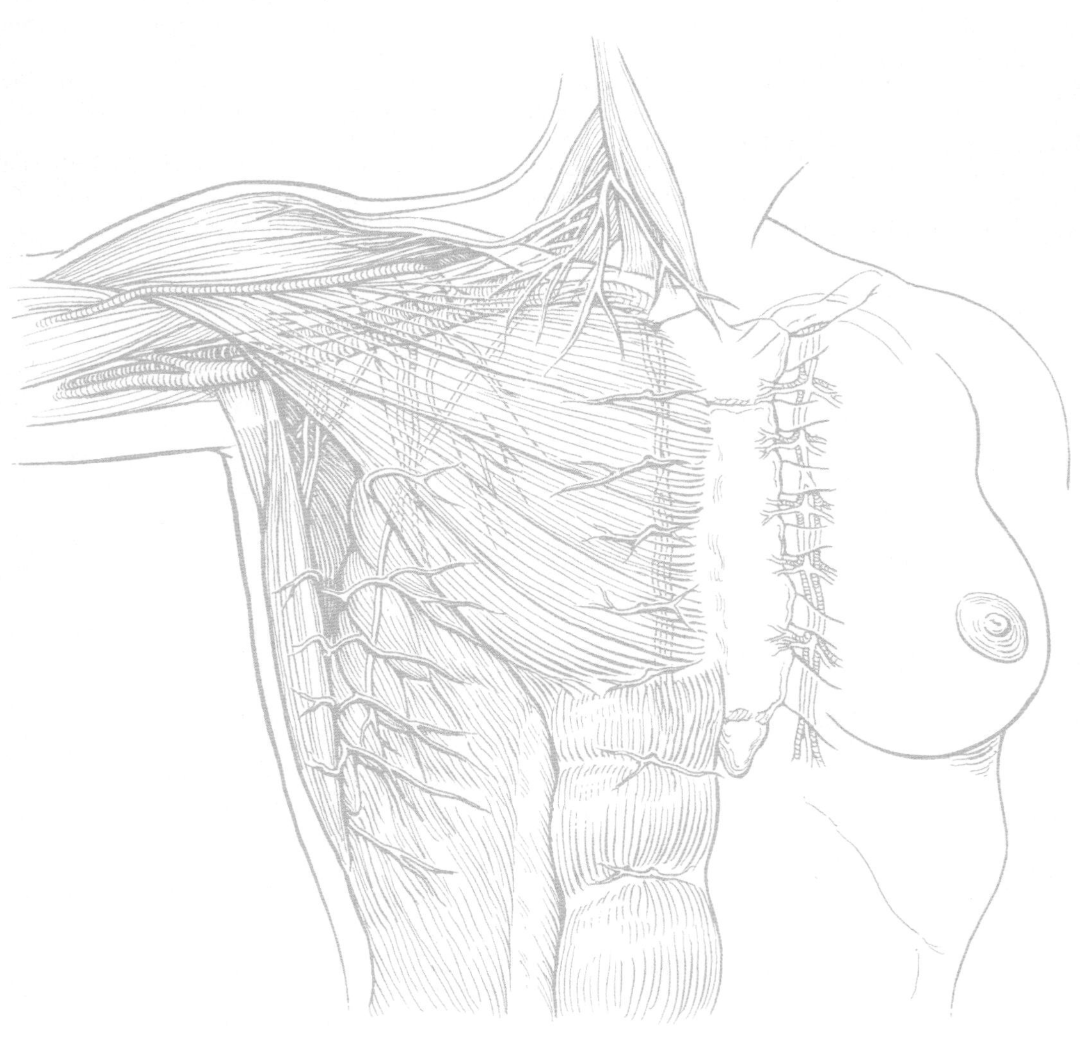

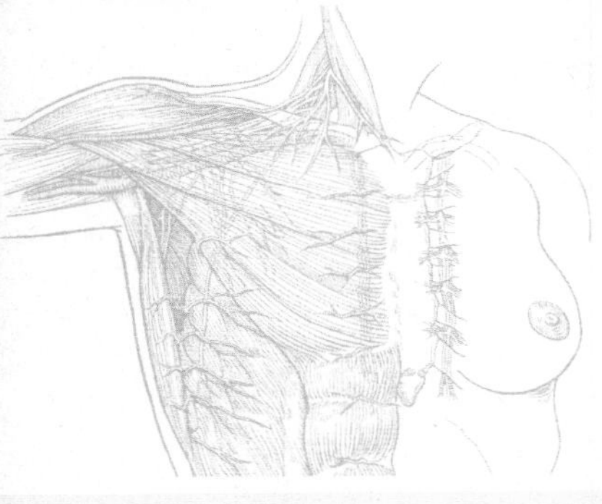

CHAPTER 35

Diseases of the Breast

V. Suzanne Klimberg, Kelly K. Hunt

OUTLINE

ANATOMY

The breast lies between the subdermal layer of adipose tissue and the superficial pectoral fascia (Fig. 35.1). The breast parenchyma is composed of lobes that comprise multiple lobules. Multiple fibrous bands termed the *suspensory ligaments of Cooper* provide structural support and run from the chest wall to the dermis. The retromammary fat pad is a relatively avascular space that lies between the breast and pectoralis major muscle. Located deep to the pectoralis major muscle, the pectoralis minor muscle is enclosed in the clavipectoral fascia, which extends laterally to fuse with the axillary fascia.

The axillary lymph nodes, grouped by location, are shown in Fig. 35.2. Axillary nodes are typically described as three anatomic levels defined by their relationship to the pectoralis minor muscle. Level I nodes are located lateral to the lateral border of the pectoralis minor muscle. Level II nodes are located posterior to the pectoralis minor muscle as well as anterior to the pectoralis minor and posterior to the pectoralis major (Rotter or interpectoral nodes).

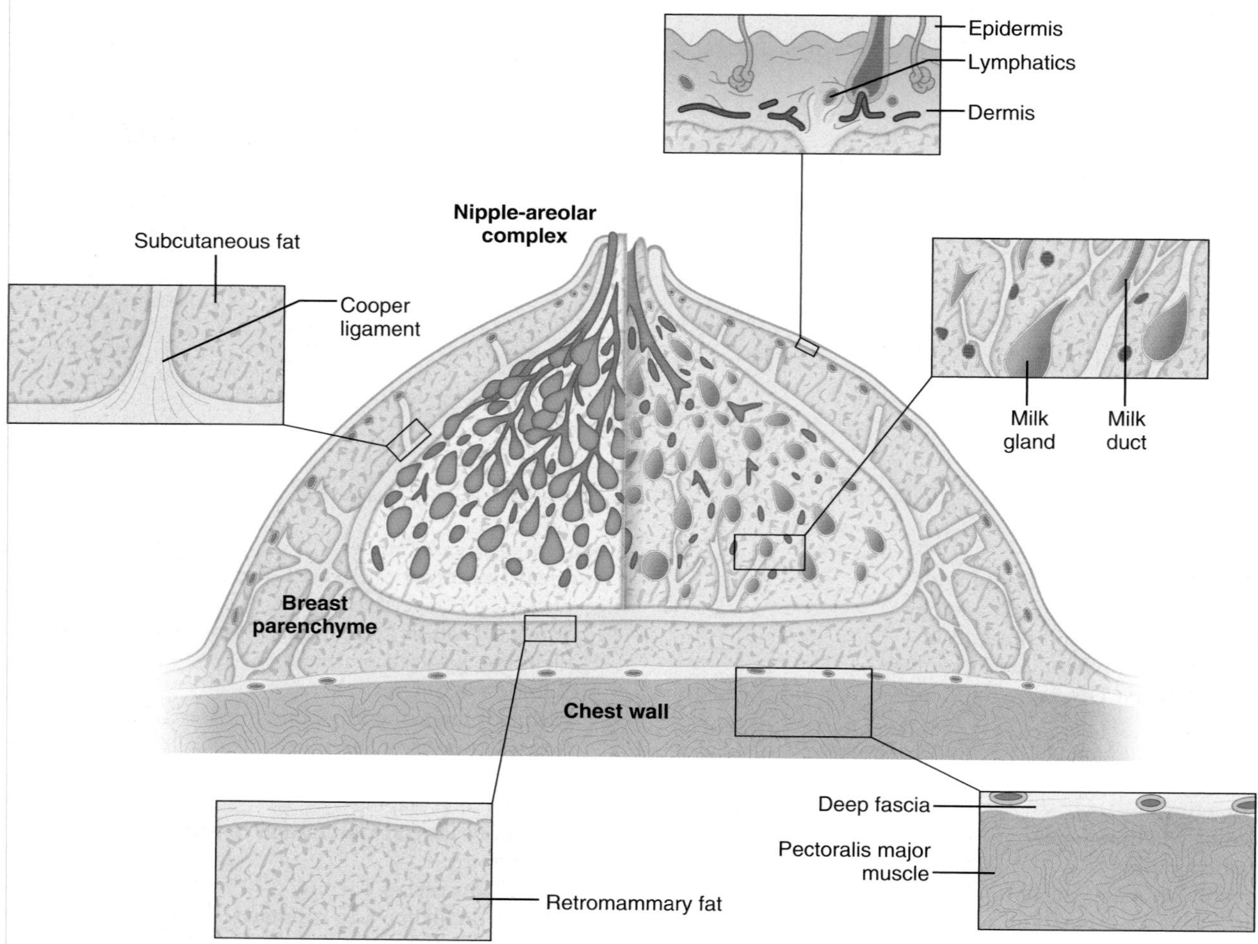

FIG. 35.1 Cut-away diagram of a mature resting breast. The breast lies cushioned in fat between the overlying skin and pectoralis major muscle. The skin and the retromammary space under the breast are rich with lymphatic channels. Cooper ligaments, the suspensory ligaments of the breast, fuse with the overlying superficial fascia just under the dermis, coalesce as the interlobular fascia in the breast parenchyma, and then join with the deep fascia of breast over the pectoralis muscle. The system of ducts in the breast is configured like an inverted tree, with the largest ducts just under the nipple and successively smaller ducts in the periphery. After several branching generations, small ducts at the periphery enter the breast lobule, which is the milk-forming glandular unit of the breast.

Level III nodes are located medial to the pectoralis minor muscle and include the subclavicular nodes. The apex of the axilla is defined by the costoclavicular ligament (Halsted ligament), at which point the axillary vein passes into the thorax and becomes the subclavian vein. However, functionally, the lymph nodes of the axilla are made up of lymphatics from the upper extremity, the back, and the breast. Boneti and colleagues[1] described the anatomic drainage of the lymphatics from the arm within the axilla (Fig. 35.3), including the traditional position just below the vein, above the vein or going directly into the subclavian, a sling pattern that comes well below the axilla, a medial or lateral apron pattern, and a twine pattern. Four percent of the time, the nodes from the breast merge with those draining the upper extremity within Level I. The functional anatomy of these lymph nodes is important in preventing lymphedema during lymphadenectomy for breast cancer.

Lymphatic channels are abundant in the breast parenchyma and dermis. Specialized lymphatic channels collect under the nipple and areola and form Sappey plexus, named for the anatomist who described them in 1885. Lymph flows from the skin to the subareolar plexus and then into the interlobular lymphatics of the breast parenchyma. Appreciation of lymphatic flow is important for performing successful sentinel lymph node surgery (see “Lymph Node Staging” later on). Of the lymphatic flow from the breast, 75% is directed into the axillary lymph nodes. A minor amount of the lymphatic flow from the breast goes through the pectoralis muscle and into more medial lymph node groups (see Fig. 35.2). Lymphatic drainage also occurs through the internal mammary lymph nodes as the predominant drainage in 5% of patients and as a secondary route in combination with axillary drainage in approximately 20% of patients. A major route of breast cancer metastasis is through lymphatic channels; an understanding of the patterns of regional spread of cancer is important to provide optimal locoregional control of the disease.

Coursing deep and close to the chest wall on the medial side of the axilla is the long thoracic nerve (see Fig. 35.2), also known as the external respiratory nerve of Bell, which innervates the serratus anterior muscle. This muscle is important for fixing the scapula to the chest wall during adduction of the shoulder and extension of the arm. Division of this nerve may result in the winged scapula deformity. For this reason, the long thoracic nerve is preserved during axillary surgery. The second major nerve encountered during axillary dissection is the thoracodorsal nerve, which innervates

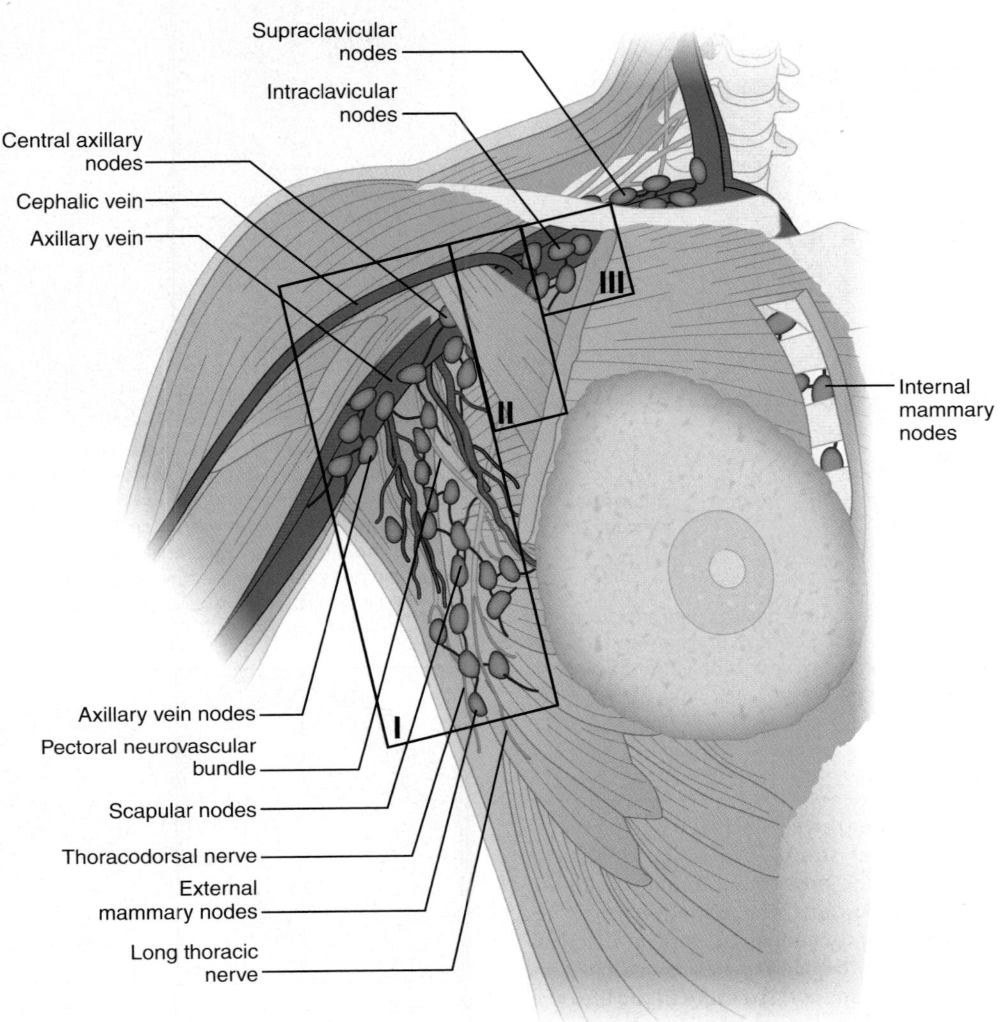

FIG. 35.2 Contents of the axilla. In this diagram, there are five named and contiguous groupings of lymph nodes in the full axilla. Complete axillary dissection, as done in the historical radical mastectomy, removes all these nodes. However, the subclavicular nodes in the axilla are continuous with the supraclavicular nodes in the neck and nodes between the pectoralis major and minor muscles, called the *interpectoral nodes* in this diagram (also known as *Rotter lymph nodes*). The sentinel lymph node is functionally the first node in the axillary chain and, anatomically, is usually found in the external mammary group. The relative positions of the long thoracic, thoracodorsal, and medial pectoral nerves are shown. These major nerves along with the pectoral neurovascular bundle should be preserved during surgery.

the latissimus dorsi muscle. This nerve arises from the posterior cord of the brachial plexus and enters the axillary space under the axillary vein, close to the entrance of the long thoracic nerve. The thoracodorsal nerve crosses the axilla to the medial surface of the latissimus dorsi muscle. The thoracodorsal nerve and vessels are preserved during dissection of the axillary lymph nodes. The medial pectoral nerve, named for its derivation from the medial cord of the brachial plexus, innervates the pectoralis major muscle and lies within a neurovascular bundle that wraps around the lateral border of the pectoralis minor muscle. The pectoral neurovascular bundle is a useful landmark because it indicates the position of the axillary vein, which is just cephalad and deep (superior and posterior) to the bundle. This neurovascular bundle should be preserved, if possible, during any lymphadenectomy.

There are three to five sensory intercostal brachial or brachial cutaneous nerves that cross the axilla horizontally and supply sensation to the undersurface of the upper inner surface of the arm and skin of the chest wall along the posterior margin of the axilla. Lymphatics run along these nerves as well. Dividing these nerves results in cutaneous anesthesia in these areas, and the possibility of this outcome should be explained to patients before axillary dissection. Denervation of the areas supplied by these sensory nerves causes chronic and uncomfortable pain syndromes in a small percentage of patients. Preservation of the most superior nerve maintains sensation to the posterior aspect of the upper part of the arm without compromising the axillary dissection in most patients. Taking these nerves with their associated lymphatics may lead to lymphedema of the chest wall.

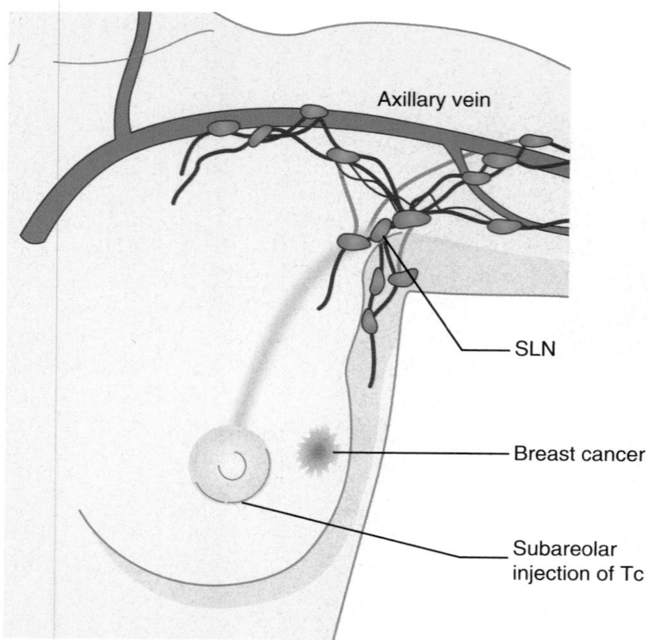

FIG. 35.3 Axillary anatomy of lymphatics draining the arm. (Adapted from Boneti C, Korourian S, Diaz Z, et al. Scientific Impact Award: axillary reverse mapping (ARM) to identify and protect lymphatics draining the arm during axillary lymphadenectomy. *Am J Surg.* 2009;198:482–487.) *SLN*, Sentinel lymph node.

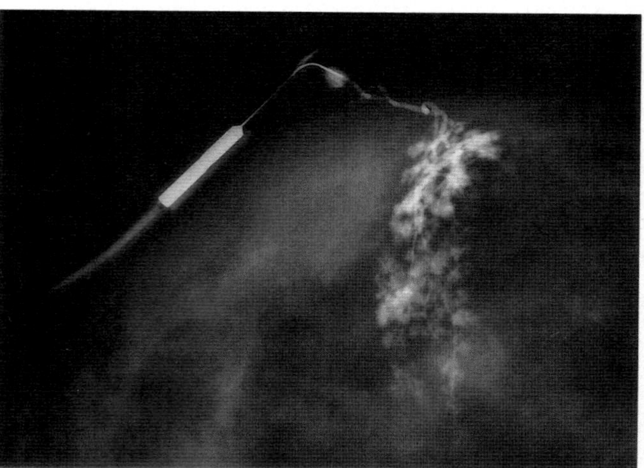

FIG. 35.4 Injection of contrast material into a single ductal system (ductogram). Occasionally used to evaluate surgically significant nipple discharge, ductography is performed by cannulation of an individual duct orifice and injection of contrast material. This ductogram opacifies the entire ductal tree, from the retroareolar duct to the lobules at the end of the tree. It also demonstrates the functional independence of each duct system; there is no cross-communication between independent systems.

MICROSCOPIC ANATOMY

The mature breast is composed of three principal tissue types: (1) glandular epithelium, (2) fibrous stroma and supporting structures, and (3) adipose tissue. The breast also contains lymphocytes and macrophages. In adolescents, the predominant tissues are epithelium and stroma. In postmenopausal women, the glandular structures involute and are largely replaced by adipose tissue. Cooper ligaments provide shape and structure to the breast as they course from the overlying skin to the underlying deep fascia. Because these ligaments are anchored into the skin, infiltration of these ligaments by carcinoma commonly produces tethering, which can cause dimpling or subtle deformities on the otherwise smooth surface of the breast.

The glandular apparatus of the breast is composed of a branching system of ducts, organized in a radial pattern spreading outward from the nipple-areolar complex (see Fig. 35.1). It is possible to cannulate individual ducts and visualize the lactiferous ducts with contrast agents. Fig. 35.4 shows the arborization of branching ducts, which end in terminal lobules. The contrast dye opacifies only a single ductal system and does not enter adjacent and intertwined branches from functionally independent ductal branches. Each major duct has a dilated portion (lactiferous sinus) below the nipple-areolar complex. These ducts converge through a constricted orifice into the ampulla of the nipple.

Each of the major ducts has progressive generations of branching and ultimately ends in the terminal ductules or acini (Fig. 35.5). The acini are the milk-forming glands of the lactating breast and, together with their small efferent ducts or ductules, are known as *lobular units* or *lobules*. The terminal duct lobular units are invested in a specialized loose connective tissue that contains capillaries, lymphocytes, and other migratory mononuclear cells. This intralobular stroma is clearly

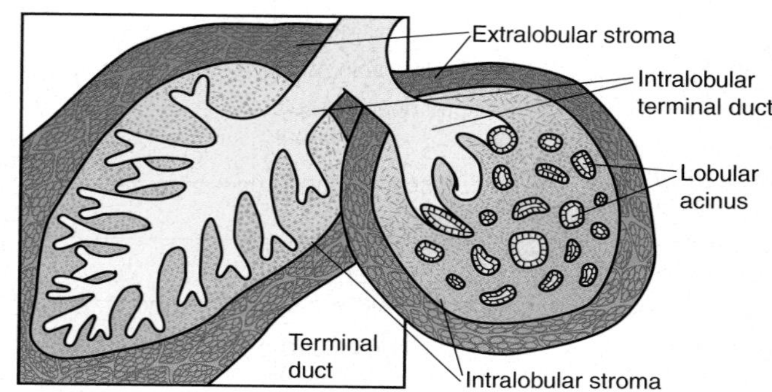

FIG. 35.5 Mature resting lobular unit. At the distal end of the ductal system is the lobule, which is formed by multiple branching events at the end of terminal ducts, each ending in a blind sac or acini, and is invested with specialized stroma. The lobule is a three-dimensional structure but is seen in two dimensions in a histologic thin section, shown in the *lower right*. The intralobular terminal ductule and acini are invested in loose connective tissue containing a modest number of infiltrating lymphocytes and plasma cells. The lobule is distinct from the denser interlobular stroma, which contains larger breast ducts, blood vessels, and fat.

distinguished from the denser and less cellular interlobular stroma and from the adipose tissue within the breast.

The entire ductal system is lined by epithelial cells, which are surrounded by specialized myoepithelial cells that have contractile properties and serve to propel milk formed in the lobules toward the nipple. Outside the epithelial and myoepithelial layers, the ducts of the breast are surrounded by a continuous basement membrane containing laminin, type IV collagen, and proteoglycans. The basement membrane layer is an important boundary in differentiating in situ from invasive breast cancer. Continuity of this layer is maintained in ductal carcinoma in situ (DCIS), also termed *noninvasive breast cancer* (see "Pathology" later on). Invasive breast cancer is defined by penetration of the basement membrane by malignant cells invading the stroma. Invasion or infiltration of the wall of the duct gives tumor cells access to the lymphatics and blood vessels that twine around the outside of the ducts.

BREAST DEVELOPMENT AND PHYSIOLOGY

Normal Development and Physiology

In utero, the milk bud develops from the ectodermal thickening in the pectoral area and extends as the milk streak (mammary ridge) from the axilla to the inguinal area. At 9 weeks of gestation, the milk streak begins to atrophy to normally form a single pair of bilateral glands. When less than the normal atrophy of the milk streak occurs, then polymastia and/or polythelia occurs. Rarely, congenital amastia occurs as a result of failure of the milk bud.

Ninety percent of newborns will have a breast secretion that is commonly referred to as "witches milk" that is the result of elevated maternal hormones and prolactin levels. If the secretion sequesters within the nipple, it can cause a mass or lactocele that will resolve on its own in 3 to 4 weeks, as will the discharge.

Before puberty, the breast is composed primarily of dense fibrous stroma and scattered ducts lined with epithelium. In the United States, puberty, as measured by breast development and the growth of pubic hair, begins between the ages of 9 and 12 years, and menarche (onset of menstrual cycles) begins at approximately 11 to 14 years of age. These events are initiated by low-amplitude pulses of pituitary gonadotropins, which increase serum estradiol concentrations. In the breast, this hormone-dependent maturation (thelarche) entails increased deposition of fat, the formation of new ducts by branching and elongation, and the first appearance of lobular units. This process of growth and cell division is under the control of estrogen, progesterone, adrenal hormones, pituitary hormones, and the trophic effects of insulin and thyroid hormone. There is evidence that local growth factor networks are also important. The exact timing of these events and the coordinated development of both breast buds may vary from the average in individual patients. The term *prepubertal gynecomastia* refers to symmetrical enlargement and projection of the breast bud in a girl before the average age of 12 years, unaccompanied by the other changes of puberty. This process, which may be unilateral, should not be confused with neoplastic growth and is not an indication for biopsy.

The postpubertal mature or resting breast contains fat, stroma, lactiferous ducts, and lobular units. During phases of the menstrual cycle or in response to exogenous hormones, the breast epithelium and lobular stroma undergo cyclic stimulation. The dominant process appears to be hypertrophy and alteration of morphology rather than hyperplasia. In the late luteal (premenstrual) phase, there is an accumulation of fluid and intralobular edema. This edema can produce pain and breast engorgement.

These physiologic changes can lead to increased nodularity and may be mistaken for a malignant tumor. Ill-defined masses in premenopausal women are generally observed through the course of the menstrual cycle before any intervention is undertaken. With pregnancy, there is diminution of the fibrous stroma and the formation of new acini or lobules, termed *adenosis of pregnancy.* After birth, there is a sudden loss of placental hormones, which, combined with continued high levels of prolactin, is the principal trigger for lactation. The actual expulsion of milk is under hormonal control and is caused by contraction of the myoepithelial cells that surround the breast ducts and terminal ductules. There is no evidence for innervation of these myoepithelial cells; their contraction appears to occur in response to the pituitary-derived peptide oxytocin. Stimulation of the nipple appears to be the physiologic signal for continued pituitary secretion of prolactin and acute release of oxytocin. When breastfeeding ceases, the prolactin level decreases and there is no stimulus for release of oxytocin. The breast returns to a resting state and to the cyclic changes induced when menstruation resumes.

Menopause is defined by cessation in menstrual flow for at least 1 year; in the United States, it usually occurs between the ages of 40 and 55 years, with a median age of 51 years. Menopause may be accompanied by symptoms such as vasomotor disturbances (hot flashes), vaginal dryness, urinary tract infections, and cognitive impairment (possibly secondary to interruption of sleep by hot flashes). Menopause results in involution and a general decrease in the epithelial elements of the resting breast. These changes include increased fat deposition, diminished connective tissue, and the disappearance of lobular units. The persistence of lobules, hyperplasia of the ductal epithelium, and cyst formation all can occur under the influence of exogenous ovarian hormones, usually in the form of postmenopausal hormone replacement therapy (HRT). Physicians should inquire about the menstrual history, age at onset of menses, and cessation of menses and record the use of HRT because all of these factors can influence a woman's risk of developing breast cancer. HRT can lead to increased breast density, which may decrease the sensitivity of mammography.

Fibrocystic Changes and Breast Pain

The condition previously referred to as *fibrocystic disease* represents a spectrum of clinical, mammographic, and histologic findings and is common during the fourth and fifth decades of life, generally lasting until menopause. An exaggerated response of breast stroma and epithelium to various circulating and locally produced hormones and growth factors is frequently characterized by the constellation of breast pain, tenderness, and nodularity. Symptomatically, the condition manifests as premenstrual cyclic mastalgia, with pain and tenderness to touch. This mastalgia can be worrisome to many women; however, breast pain is not usually a symptom of breast cancer. Pain without other signs or symptoms of breast cancer is uncommon, occurring in only approximately 7% of patients with breast cancer. In women with breast pain and an associated palpable mass, the presence of the mass is the focus of evaluation and treatment. Normal ovarian hormonal influences on breast glandular elements frequently produce cyclic mastalgia, pain generally in phase with the menstrual cycle. Noncyclic mastalgia is more likely idiopathic and difficult to treat. Women 30 years and older with noncyclic mastalgia should undergo breast imaging with mammography and ultrasonography in addition to a physical examination. If examination reveals a mass, this should become the focus of subsequent evaluation (see "Biopsy" later on). Occasionally, a simple cyst may cause cyclical or noncyclic breast pain, and aspiration of the cyst usually resolves the pain. In the case of large cysts, which will quickly recur after aspiration, percutaneous excision with a vacuum-assisted device will be definitive. Most patients with simple cysts do not require further evaluation. Patients with complex cysts with solid intracystic components require additional evaluation including biopsy of the solid components. Treatment with danocrine, lupron, and tamoxifen are effective but with significant side effects. Referred pain can be a significant cause of breast pain, the most common source of which is scapulothoracic bursitis. It can be cyclical but is most often noncyclical. Because of the confluence of afferent signals from the shoulder and the dorsal horn of the spinal cord, one can get referred pain from the shoulder in the distribution of the intercostal nerves along the axilla, the breast, and the arm. Trigger point injection along the medial scapular border in order to access the scapulothoracic bursa are both diagnostic and therapeutic for this malady. Heat and nonsteroidal antiinflammatory drugs will aid in alleviating the inflammation.[2]

Patients with fibrocystic changes have clinical breast findings that range from mild alterations in texture to dense, firm breast tissue with palpable masses. The appearance of large palpable cysts completes the picture. Fibrocystic changes are usually seen on mammography as diffuse or focal radiologically dense tissue. On ultrasonography, cysts are seen in one-third of all women 35 to 50 years old; most of these cysts are nonpalpable. Palpable cysts or multiple small cysts are typical of fibrocystic disease. Cysts with or without fibrocystic disease are uncommon in postmenopausal women.

Histologically, in addition to macrocysts and microcysts, women with fibrocystic changes may have identified solid elements, including adenosis, sclerosis, apocrine metaplasia, stromal fibrosis, and epithelial metaplasia and hyperplasia. Depending on the presence of epithelial hyperplasia, fibrocystic changes are classified as nonproliferative, proliferative without atypia, or proliferative with atypia. All three types of changes can occur alone or in combination and to a variable degree, and in the absence of epithelial atypia, these changes represent the histologic spectrum of normal breast tissue. However, epithelial atypia (atypical ductal hyperplasia [ADH]) is a risk factor for the development of breast cancer. Atypical proliferations of ductal epithelial cells confer increased risk for breast cancer; however, fibrocystic change is not itself a risk factor for the development of breast malignancy.

Abnormal Development and Physiology

Absent or Accessory Breast Tissue

Absence of breast tissue (amastia) and absence of the nipple (athelia) are rare anomalies. Unilateral rudimentary breast development is more common, as is adolescent hypertrophy of one breast with lesser development of the other. Poland syndrome is thought to be a genetic disorder that presents as a unilateral variable loss of the breast tissue, pectoralis major and minor, and serratus anterior muscles as well as several ribs.

Accessory breast tissue (polymastia) and accessory nipples (supernumerary nipples) are common as a result of persistence of the mammary ridge. Supernumerary nipples are usually rudimentary and occur along the milk line from the axilla to the pubis in males and females. They may be mistaken for a small mole. Accessory nipples are usually removed only for cosmetic reasons. True polythelia refers to more than one nipple serving a single breast, which is rare. Accessory breast tissue is commonly located above the breast in the axilla. Rudimentary nipple development may be present, and lactation is possible with more complete development. Accessory breast tissue may be seen as an enlarging mass in the axilla during pregnancy and persists as excess tissue in the axilla after lactation is complete. The accessory mammary tissue may be removed surgically if it is large or cosmetically deforming or to prevent enlargement during future pregnancy. Care should be taken to avoid removing axillary lymph nodes.

Gynecomastia

Hypertrophy of breast tissue in men is a clinical entity for which there is frequently no identifiable cause. Pubertal hypertrophy occurs in boys between age 13 years and early adulthood, and senescent hypertrophy is diagnosed in men older than 50 years. Gynecomastia in teenage boys is common and may be bilateral or unilateral. Unless it is unilateral or painful, it may pass unnoticed and regress with adulthood. Pubertal hypertrophy is generally treated by observation without surgery. Surgical excision may be discussed if the enlargement is unilateral, fails to regress, or is cosmetically unacceptable. Hypertrophy in older men is also common. The enlargement is frequently unilateral, although the contralateral breast may enlarge with time. Many commonly used drugs, such as digoxin, thiazides, estrogens, phenothiazines, theophylline, and cannabis, may exacerbate senescent gynecomastia. In addition, gynecomastia may be a systemic manifestation of hepatic cirrhosis, renal failure, or malnutrition. In pubertal and senescent gynecomastia, the mass is smooth, firm, saucer shaped, and symmetrically distributed beneath the areola. It is frequently tender, which is often the reason for seeking medical attention. Pubertal and senescent gynecomastia may be managed nonoperatively and can be fully characterized with ultrasonography. There is little confusion with carcinoma occurring in the breast. Carcinoma is not usually tender, is asymmetrically located beneath or beside the areola, and may be fixed to the overlying dermis or to the deep fascia. A dominant mass suspicious for carcinoma should be examined with core needle biopsy (CNB). Mammography and ultrasonography can also be useful tools to discriminate between gynecomastia and a suspected malignancy of the breast in older men. A nipple-sparing mastectomy can be performed to remove the enlarged breast. A donut of deepithelized skin around the nipple is then enfolded to remove the excess skin as one would do for a Benelli reduction mammoplasty.[3]

Nipple Discharge

The appearance of discharge from the nipple (Fig. 35.6A) of a nonlactating woman is a common condition and is rarely associated with an underlying carcinoma. In one review of 270 subareolar biopsies for discharge from one identifiable duct and without an associated breast mass, carcinoma was found in only 16 patients (5.9%). In these cases, the fluid was bloody or tested strongly positive for occult hemoglobin. In another series of 249 patients with discharge from a single identifiable duct, breast carcinoma was found in 10 patients (4%). In eight of these patients, a mass lesion was identified in addition to the discharge. In the absence of a palpable mass or suspicious findings on mammography, discharge is rarely associated with cancer.

It is important to establish whether the discharge comes from one breast or from both breasts, whether it comes from multiple duct orifices or from just one, and whether the discharge is grossly bloody or contains blood. A milky discharge from both breasts is termed *galactorrhea*. In the absence of lactation or a history of recent lactation, galactorrhea may be associated with increased production of prolactin. Radioimmunoassay for serum prolactin is diagnostic. However, true galactorrhea is rare and is diagnosed only when the discharge is milky (contains lactose, fat, and milk-specific proteins). Unilateral discharge from one duct orifice is often treated surgically when there is a significant amount of discharge. However, the underlying cause is rarely a breast malignancy.

The most common cause of spontaneous nipple discharge from a single duct is a solitary intraductal papilloma (60%–80%) in one of the large subareolar ducts under the nipple. Subareolar duct ectasia producing inflammation and dilatation of large collecting ducts under the nipple is common (20%) and usually involves discharge from multiple ducts. Cancer is a very unusual cause of discharge in the absence of other signs. However, papillomas that are located away from the nipple-areolar complex are at higher risk of malignancy (20%). A papilloma is the most common benign tumor to develop breast cancer, primarily DCIS.

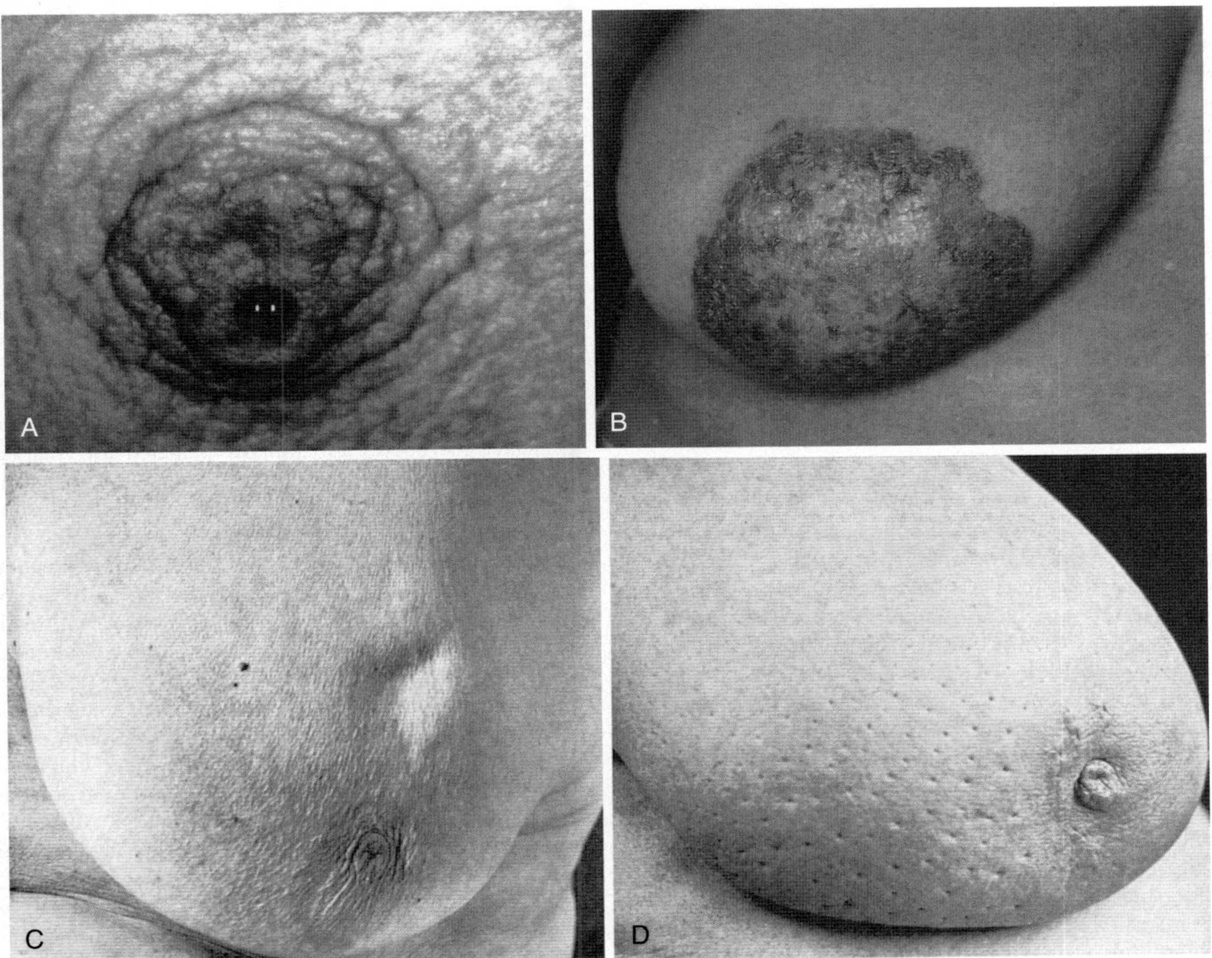

FIG. 35.6 Common physical findings during breast examination. (A) Nipple discharge. Discharge from multiple ducts or bilateral discharge is a common finding in healthy breasts. In the case shown, the discharge is from a single duct orifice and may signify underlying disease in the discharging duct. In this patient, a papilloma was the source of her symptoms. (B) Paget disease of the nipple. Malignant ductal cells invade the epidermis without traversing the basement membrane of the subareolar duct or epidermis. The disease appears as a psoriatic rash that begins on the nipple and spreads off onto the areola and into the skin of the breast. (C) Skin dimpling. Traction on Cooper ligaments by a scirrhous tumor is distorting the surface of the breast and producing a dimple best seen with angled indirect lighting during abduction of the arms upward. (D) Peau d'orange (skin of the orange) or edema of the skin of the breast. This finding may be caused by dependency of the breast, lymphatic blockage (from surgery or radiation), or mastitis. The most feared cause is inflammatory carcinoma, in which malignant cells plug the dermal lymphatics—the pathologic hallmark of the disease.

Nipple discharge that is bilateral and comes from multiple ducts is not usually a cause for surgery. Bloody discharge from a single duct often requires surgical excision to establish a diagnosis and control the discharge. Bilateral bloody spontaneous discharge is likely endocrine in nature and is associated with pregnancy and hypothyroidism.

Galactocele

A galactocele is a milk-filled cyst that is round, well circumscribed, and easily movable within the breast. A galactocele generally occurs after the cessation of lactation or when feeding frequency has declined significantly, although galactoceles may occur 6 to 10 months after breastfeeding has ceased. The pathogenesis of galactocele is unknown, but inspissated milk within ducts is thought to be responsible. The cyst is usually located in the central portion of the breast or under the nipple. Needle aspiration produces thick, creamy material that may be tinged dark green or brown. Although it appears purulent, the fluid is sterile. Treatment is large bore needle aspiration, and withdrawal of thick milky secretion confirms the diagnosis; surgery is reserved for cysts that cannot be aspirated or that become infected.

DIAGNOSIS OF BREAST DISEASE

Patient History

In a woman in whom breast disease is suspected, it is important for the examiner to determine the patient's age and to obtain a reproductive history, including age at menarche, age at menopause, and history of pregnancies including age at first full-term pregnancy. A previous history of breast biopsies should be obtained, including the pathologic findings. If the patient has had a hysterectomy, it is important to determine whether the ovaries were removed. In premenopausal women, a recent history of pregnancy and lactation should be noted. The history should include any use of HRT or use of hormones for contraception. The family history should detail any known genetic abnormalities as well as any cancer, but especially of the breast and ovaries and the menopausal status of any affected relatives.

With respect to the specific breast complaint, the patient should be asked about history of a mass, breast pain, nipple discharge, and any skin changes. If a mass is present, the patient should be asked how long it has been present and whether it has grown or changes with the menstrual cycle. If a cancer diagnosis is suspected, inquiry about constitutional symptoms, bone pain, weight loss, respiratory changes, and similar clinical indications can direct investigations that could reveal evidence of metastatic disease.

Physical Examination

The physical examination begins with the patient in the upright sitting position. The breasts are visually inspected for obvious masses, asymmetries, and skin changes. The nipples are examined and compared for the presence of retraction, nipple inversion, or excoriation of the superficial epidermis such as that seen with Paget disease (Fig. 35.6B). The use of indirect lighting can unmask subtle dimpling of the skin or nipple caused by a carcinoma that places Cooper ligaments under tension (Fig. 35.6C). Simple maneuvers such as stretching the arms high above the head or tensing the pectoralis muscles may accentuate asymmetries and dimpling. If carefully sought, dimpling of the skin or nipple retraction is a sensitive and specific sign of underlying cancer.

Edema of the skin produces a clinical sign known as *peau d'orange* (Fig. 35.6D). Peau d'orange and tenderness, warmth, and swelling of the breast are the hallmarks of inflammatory carcinoma but may be mistaken for acute mastitis. The inflammatory changes and edema are caused by obstruction of dermal lymphatic channels by emboli of carcinoma cells. Occasionally, a bulky tumor may produce obstruction of lymph channels that results in overlying skin edema. This is not typically the case with inflammatory carcinoma, where there is usually no discrete palpable mass but diffuse changes throughout the breast parenchyma. In 40 patients with inflammatory carcinoma described by Haagensen, erythema and edema of the skin were present in all cases, a palpable mass or localized induration was noted in 19 patients, and no localized tumor was present in 21 patients. Inflammatory cancer also has a rapid onset (less than 3 months) as compared to a similar presentation for locally advanced cancer, which may have been present for years and neglected.

Involvement of the nipple and areola can occur with carcinoma of the breast, especially when the primary tumor is located in the subareolar position. Direct involvement may result in retraction of the nipple. Flattening or inversion of the nipple can be caused by fibrosis in certain benign conditions, especially subareolar duct ectasia. In these cases, the finding is frequently bilateral, and the history confirms that the condition has been present for many years. Unilateral retraction or retraction that develops over weeks or months is more suggestive of carcinoma. Centrally located tumors that go undetected for a long time may directly invade and ulcerate the skin of the areola or nipple. Peripheral tumors may distort the normal symmetry of the nipples by traction on Cooper ligaments.

Paget disease is a condition of the nipple that is commonly associated with an underlying breast cancer. First described by Paget in 1874, Paget disease produces histologically distinct changes within the dermis of the nipple. There is often an underlying intraductal carcinoma in the large sinuses just under the nipple (see Fig. 35.6B). Carcinoma cells invade across the junction of epidermal and ductal epithelial cells and enter the epidermal layer of the skin of the nipple. Clinically, dermatitis occurs that may appear eczematoid and moist or dry and psoriatic. It begins in the nipple, although it can spread to the skin of the areola. Many benign skin conditions affecting the breast, such as eczema, frequently begin on the areola, whereas Paget disease originates on the nipple and secondarily involves the areola.

Visual inspection should be followed by palpation of the regional lymph nodes and breast tissue. While the patient is still in the sitting position, the examiner supports the patient's arm and palpates each axilla from a posterior approach to detect the presence of enlarged axillary lymph nodes. The supraclavicular and infraclavicular spaces are similarly palpated for enlarged nodes. Then the patient lies down, and the breast is palpated. Palpation of the breast is always done with the patient lying supine on a solid examining surface, with the arm stretched above the head. Palpation of the breast while the patient is sitting often leads to inaccurate interpretation because the overlapping breast tissue may feel like a mass or a mass may go undetected within the breast tissue. The breast is best examined with compression of the tissue toward the chest wall, with palpation of each quadrant and the tissue under the nipple-areolar complex. Palpable masses are characterized according to their size, shape, consistency, and location and whether they are fixed to the skin or underlying musculature. Benign tumors, such as fibroadenomas and cysts, can be as firm as carcinomas; usually, these benign entities are distinct, well circumscribed, and movable. Carcinoma is typically firm but less circumscribed, and moving a carcinoma produces a drag of adjacent tissue. Cysts and fibrocystic changes can be tender with palpation of the breast; however, tenderness is rarely a helpful diagnostic sign. Most palpable masses are self-discovered by patients during casual or intentional self-examination. Ultrasonography can be used as an extension of your physical exam delineating normal ridges from worrisome masses and cystic from solid (see Ultrasonography section).

Biopsy

Fine-Needle Aspiration

Historically, fine-needle aspiration (FNA) was a common tool used in the diagnosis of breast masses. FNA can be done with a 22-gauge needle, an appropriately sized syringe, and an alcohol preparation pad. The needle is repeatedly inserted into the mass while constant negative pressure is applied to the syringe. In this way, multiple areas of a mass could be sampled. Suction is released, and the needle is withdrawn. The fluid and cellular material within the needle are submitted in physiologically buffered saline or fixed immediately on slides in 95% ethyl alcohol. The slides are submitted for cytologic evaluation of the aspirated material. A limitation of FNA in evaluating solid masses is that cytologic evaluation does not differentiate noninvasive lesions from invasive lesions if malignant cells are identified. If FNA demonstrates malignancy, a CNB is still required for definitive histologic diagnosis before surgical intervention.

One clinical scenario in which FNA still has utility is in the evaluation of a second suspicious lesion in the ipsilateral breast of a patient with a known malignancy. In this case, FNA can be used to determine if the second lesion is malignant and confirm a diagnosis of multifocal breast cancer. This information can aid in determining the appropriate surgical plan. A second clinical scenario in which

FNA is commonly used is in the evaluation of lymph nodes that are suspicious on either physical examination or imaging, particularly high-resolution ultrasonography of the regional nodal basins. Suspicious lymph nodes can be evaluated by FNA to determine whether metastatic disease is present. In this situation, FNA has a reported sensitivity of approximately 90% and a specificity of up to 100%. Determining whether the tumor has spread to the lymph nodes is an important step in the initial staging of breast cancer that provides prognostic information and helps determine appropriate management strategies. In the setting where neoadjuvant therapy is to be utilized, a clip must be placed in the positive node.

Core Needle Biopsy

CNB is the method of choice to sample breast lesions. Biopsies can be performed with trigger devices requiring multiple entries or with vacuum-assisted devices that require only single insertion. The size of a CNB ranges from 8 to 14 gauge. CNB can be performed under mammographic (stereotactic), ultrasound, or magnetic resonance imaging (MRI) guidance. Mass lesions that are visualized on ultrasonography can be sampled under ultrasound guidance; calcifications and densities that are best seen on mammography are sampled under stereotactic guidance. During stereotactic CNB, the breast is compressed, most often with the patient lying prone on the stereotactic CNB table. A robotic arm and biopsy device are positioned by computed analysis of triangulated mammographic images. After local anesthetic is injected, a small skin incision is made, and a core biopsy needle is inserted into the lesion to obtain the tissue sample with vacuum assistance. There are standards for the appropriate number of core samples to be obtained for each type of abnormality being sampled. A clip should be placed to mark the site of the lesion, particularly for small lesions that may be difficult to find after extensive sampling or when neoadjuvant therapy is to be performed. The specimens should be imaged to confirm that the targeted lesion has been adequately sampled. A similar approach is used for ultrasound-guided and MRI-guided biopsy of lesions.

Specimen radiography of excised cores is performed to confirm that the targeted lesion has been sampled and to direct pathologic assessment of the tissue. A mammogram obtained after biopsy confirms that a defect has been created within the target lesion and that the marking clip is in the correct position. Image-guided localization and surgical excision are required if the lesion cannot be adequately sampled by CNB or if there is discordance between the imaging abnormality and pathologic findings.

The small samples obtained by CNB necessitate proper interpretation of the pathology results. Most patients undergoing CNB have benign findings and may return to routine screening with no other intervention required. If a malignancy is detected, histologic subtype, grade, and receptor status should be determined from the CNB specimen. The patient may proceed to definitive treatment of the cancer if it is an early-stage breast cancer. Patients with aggressive, locally advanced, or inflammatory breast cancer should be treated with systemic chemotherapy before surgical intervention. Depending on the size and grade of the imaging abnormality, approximately one-third of patients with a diagnosis of DCIS on CNB are found to have some invasive carcinoma at definitive surgery.

Excisional Biopsy

Use of a minimally invasive procedure, such as CNB, is the preferred approach for diagnosis of breast lesions. The use of excisional breast biopsy as a diagnostic procedure increases costs and results in delays of definitive surgery for patients with cancer.[4] Less than 10% of patients who undergo CNB have inconclusive results and require surgical biopsy for definitive diagnosis. Biopsy results that are not concordant with the targeted lesion (e.g., a spiculated mass on imaging and normal breast tissue on CNB) necessitate surgical excision. When ADH is found on CNB, surgical excision reveals DCIS or invasive carcinoma in 20% to 30% of cases because of the difficulty of distinguishing ADH and DCIS in a limited tissue sample. A finding of a cellular fibroadenoma on CNB requires excision to rule out a phyllodes tumor.

BREAST IMAGING

Breast imaging techniques are used to detect small, nonpalpable breast abnormalities, evaluate clinical findings, and guide diagnostic procedures. The primary imaging modality for screening asymptomatic women is mammography. During mammography, the breast is compressed between plates to reduce the thickness of the tissue through which the radiation must pass, separate adjacent structures, and improve resolution. On screening mammography, two views of each breast are obtained, mediolateral oblique and craniocaudal and ready at a later time usually in batches. For further evaluation of abnormalities identified on a screening mammogram or of clinical findings or symptoms, diagnostic mammography is indicated, which is read at the time of performance so additional views may be performed. Magnification views are obtained to evaluate calcifications, and compression views are used to provide additional detail for mass lesions.

Sensitivity of mammography is limited by breast density, and 10% to 15% of clinically evident breast cancers have no visible abnormality on mammography. Digital mammography acquires digital images and stores them electronically, allowing manipulation and enhancement of images to facilitate interpretation. Digital mammography appears to be superior to traditional film-screen mammography for detecting cancer in younger women and women with dense breasts. Mammography in women younger than 30 years, whose breast tissue is dense with stroma and epithelium, may produce an image without much definition. As women age, the breast tissue involutes and is replaced by fatty tissue. On mammography, fat absorbs relatively little radiation and provides a contrasting background that favors detection of small lesions. Computer-assisted diagnosis has been shown to increase the sensitivity and specificity of mammography and ultrasonography over review by the radiologist alone.

Screening Mammography

Screening mammography is performed in asymptomatic women with the goal of detecting occult breast cancer. This approach assumes that breast cancers identified through screening will be smaller, have a better prognosis, and require less aggressive treatment than cancers identified by palpation. The potential benefits of screening are weighed against the cost of screening and the number of false-positive studies that prompt additional workup, biopsies, and patient anxiety.

Eight prospective randomized trials of screening mammography have been performed, with almost 500,000 women participating. In these trials, among women 39 to 49 years old, screening mammography reduced the risk for breast cancer death by 15% (relative risk [RR], 0.85; credible interval [CrI], 0.75–0.96). In the six trials that included women 50 to 59 years old, screening mammography reduced the risk for breast cancer death in this age group by 14% (RR, 0.86; CrI, 0.75–0.99). Two trials included

TABLE 35.1 Effect on breast cancer mortality and false-positive mammograms by age group in breast cancer screening trials.

AGE GROUP (YEARS)	NO. TRIALS	BREAST CANCER MORTALITY, RR (95% CrI)	NO. NEEDED TO INVITE FOR SCREENING TO PREVENT ONE BREAST CANCER DEATH (95% CrI)	FALSE-POSITIVE MAMMOGRAMS/ SCREENING ROUND*
39–49	8	0.85 (0.75–0.96)	1904 (929–6378)	97.8
50–59	6	0.86 (0.75–0.99)	1339 (322–7455)	86.6
60–69	2	0.68 (0.54–0.87)	377 (230–1050)	79.0
70–74	1	1.12 (0.73–1.72)	NA	68.8

Adapted from Nelson HD, Tyne K, Naik A, et al, U.S. Preventive Services Task Force: Screening for breast cancer: systematic evidence review update for the U.S. Preventive Services Task Force. *Ann Intern Med.* 2009;151:727.
CrI, Credible interval; *NA*, not available; *RR*, relative risk.
*Per 1000 screened.

women 60 to 69 years old, and screening mammography reduced the risk for breast cancer death in this age group by 32% (RR, 0.68; CrI, 0.54–0.87). Only one trial included women older than 70 years, and data were insufficient to recommend routine screening in this age group. On the basis of these results, the most recent U.S. Preventive Services Task Force report recommended biennial screening mammography for women 50 to 74 years old and recommended against screening for women 40 to 49 years old or older than 75 years.[4] The recommendations were based on the risk reduction, number of women needed to invite for screening to prevent one breast cancer death, and potential for harm from additional testing and biopsies (Table 35.1).

At the present time, the American Cancer Society continues to recommend annual screening mammography for women older than 40 years and suggests that this practice should continue as long as the woman is in good health. Younger women with a previous breast cancer, significant family history of breast cancer, or histologic risk factors for breast cancer equal to a 20% lifetime risk are recommended for screening with MRI. Although the randomized trials of screening mammography did not enroll women older than 74 years, breast cancer risk increases with age, and the sensitivity and specificity of mammography are highest in older women, whose breast tissue has usually been replaced by fat. It is reasonable to continue mammographic screening in older women who are in good general health who would be considered appropriate candidates for surgery.

Recent advances with breast cancer screening include tomosynthesis (three-dimensional [3D] mammography). Tomosynthesis acquired thin sections of tissue with its main advantage being to separate overlapping breast tissues, decrease callbacks, and find smaller significant disease. The Screening With Tomosynthesis or Standard Mammography-2 (STORM-2) prospective trial compared two-dimensional (2D) and 3D mammography. In this trial, 9672 patients were randomized and showed a significantly higher detection of breast cancer but a slightly higher false positive recall.[5] Tomosynthesis excels in delineating small and multiple masses, microcalcifications, and distortion due to ducts and vessels. The question is whether it should be used for screening in a risk-adjusted manner due to the modest increase in radiation dose to the patient.

Ultrasonography

Ultrasonography is useful in determining whether a lesion detected by mammography is solid or cystic. Ultrasonography can also be useful for discriminating lesions in patients with dense breasts. However, it has not been found to be useful as a breast cancer screening tool because it is highly dependent on the operator performing the freehand screening and there are no standardized screening protocols. The American College of Radiology Imaging Network (ACRIN) performed a trial (ACRIN 6666) in high-risk women in whom mammography and ultrasonography were performed and were randomized in order to compare the sensitivity, specificity, and diagnostic yield of ultrasonography plus mammography compared with mammography alone.[6] The investigators found that the combination of mammography plus ultrasonography resulted in detection of an additional 4.2 cancers per 1000 women. However, the use of ultrasonography resulted in more false-positive events and required more callbacks and biopsies. There are no data available showing that the use of screening ultrasonography can reduce mortality caused by breast cancer. Automated breast ultrasound overcomes some of the issues of freehand ultrasonography, but randomized trials are forthcoming.

Magnetic Resonance Imaging

MRI is increasingly being used for the evaluation of breast abnormalities. It is useful for identifying the primary tumor in the breast in patients who present with axillary lymph node metastases without mammographic evidence of a primary breast tumor (unknown primary tumor) or in patients with Paget disease of the nipple without radiographic evidence of a primary tumor. MRI may also be useful for assessing the extent of the primary tumor, particularly in young women with dense breast tissue; extent of residual disease after lumpectomy with positive margins; for evaluating for the presence of multifocal or multicentric cancer; for screening of the contralateral breast; and for evaluating invasive lobular cancers. Some surgeons use MRI preoperatively to determine eligibility for breast conservation; however, there are no high-level data showing that use of MRI to guide decision-making about local therapy improves local recurrence rates or survival. Other diagnostic indications include assessment of treatment response after neoadjuvant chemotherapy. It can also be used for assessing implant rupture or assessing the breast when silicone injections have been used.

The sensitivity of MRI is greater than 90% for the detection of invasive cancer but only 60% or less for the detection of DCIS. The specificity of MRI is only moderate as compared to mammography or ultrasound; there is significant overlap in the appearance on MRI of benign and malignant lesions. A meta analysis of 22 studies reporting the detection of contralateral breast cancer by MRI revealed a mean incremental cancer detection rate of 4.1% and a positive predictive value of 47.9%. This high rate of detection may result partly from selection bias; however, it is of significant concern that more than 50% of the abnormalities detected on MRI represented false-positive findings, resulting in the need for additional imaging studies and biopsies.

BOX 35.1 American Cancer Society

Women at High Lifetime Risk (Risk Criteria for Breast Magnetic Resonance Imaging Screening. ≈20%–25% or Greater) of Breast Cancer

- Known *BRCA1* or *BRCA2* gene mutation
- First-degree relative with *BRCA1* or *BRCA2* gene mutation, but have not had genetic testing themselves
- Lifetime risk of breast cancer of ≈20%–25% or greater
- Radiation therapy to the chest between the ages of 10 and 30
- Li-Fraumeni syndrome or Cowden syndrome or a first-degree relative with one of these syndromes

Women at Moderately Increased (15%–20%) Lifetime Risk

- Lifetime risk of breast cancer of 15%–20% according to risk assessment tools based mainly on family history
- Personal history of breast cancer, ductal carcinoma in situ, lobular carcinoma in situ, atypical ductal hyperplasia, or atypical lobular hyperplasia
- Extremely dense breasts or unevenly dense breasts when viewed by mammograms

The Comparative Effectiveness of MRI in Breast Cancer (COMICE) trial was a multicenter trial that recruited 1623 women aged 18 years or older with newly diagnosed breast cancer to assess the clinical efficacy of contrast-enhanced MRI.[7] Patients had standard clinical and radiologic examinations and were randomly assigned to undergo MRI or no further imaging. The primary end point was the proportion of patients undergoing another surgical procedure (reexcision or mastectomy) within 6 months. There was no statistically significant difference in reoperation rates between patients who did or did not undergo MRI. The contralateral breast cancer detection rate in the COMICE trial was 1.6%, significantly lower than that reported in other trials. This trial was criticized because MRI-guided biopsy was not available at all centers to assess suspicious findings identified on MRI. This situation led to numerous mastectomies without pathologic verification that the additional findings were malignancy.

With respect to using MRI for routine screening, the American Cancer Society has recommended a risk-adjusted model. Annual MRI screening is recommended beginning at age 30 years for women at high lifetime risk for breast cancer development (approximately 20%–25% or greater) (Box 35.1). Women at moderately increased lifetime risk (15%–20%) are advised to discuss with their physicians the benefits and limitations of adding MRI screening. MRI is not recommended for women with a lifetime risk of developing breast cancer of less than 15%. When MRI is used for screening, it should be used in addition to screening mammography. Although MRI is more sensitive than mammography, it may still miss some malignancies that a mammogram would detect.

Nonpalpable Mammographic Abnormalities

Mammographic abnormalities that cannot be detected by physical examination include clustered microcalcifications and areas of abnormal density (e.g., masses, architectural distortions, asymmetries) that have not produced a palpable finding (Fig. 35.7). The Breast Imaging Reporting and Data System (BI-RADS) is used to categorize the degree of suspicion of malignancy for a mammographic abnormality (Table 35.2). To avoid unnecessary biopsies for low-suspicion mammographic findings, probably benign lesions are designated BI-RADS 3 and are monitored with 6-month interval mammograms over a 2-year period. Biopsy is performed only for lesions that progress during follow-up. Because 75% to 80% of patients for whom diagnostic biopsy of a nonpalpable mammographic lesion is recommended have benign findings, the less invasive and less costly image-guided CNB approach is preferred whenever feasible.

Image-Localized Surgical Excision of Nonpalpable Breast Lesions

Nonpalpable breast lesions should be assessed with image-guided CNB, as appropriate, according to the type of abnormality. If the diagnosis is not concordant with imaging findings or there is ADH in a field of microcalcifications that may represent DCIS, most patients should proceed to excisional biopsy for definitive diagnosis.

To ensure that the abnormality is completely excised, it should be localized with any of a number of different methods. If visible with ultrasonography, then intraoperative ultrasonography can avoid the preoperative pain, vasovagal events and delays of the old standard needle localization breast biopsy. If a wire is used to localize the lesion, it is placed through an introducer needle and has a hook that engages within the breast parenchyma at or near the abnormality to hold it in position after the introducer is withdrawn. Images with the wire in place are made available in the operating room to guide the surgeon. Depending on the size of the breast and length of the localization wire, the hook may be a long distance from the skin entry site. The surgical excision can be performed directly over the lesion or via a number of oncoplastic techniques for better cosmesis. Depending on the size of the lesion and the degree of suspicion of malignancy, some surgeons will excise shaved margins around the resection cavity to ensure a better chance of complete removal with a negative margin.[8] After excision, a specimen radiography confirms that the targeted lesion has been excised. Patients who have a diagnosis of benign findings on excision should undergo new baseline mammogram 4 to 6 months after the surgical procedure.

Other techniques have been developed to facilitate resection of nonpalpable lesions, including radioactive seed localization, which involves positioning a 4.5-mm ^{125}I seed in the breast tissue, most of which require a second procedure. Radioactive seeds are preloaded into needles that are advanced under mammographic or ultrasound guidance into the lesion of interest, after which the seeds are deployed. Images with the seed in place are made available in the operating room to guide the surgeon. In the operating room, a gamma probe, which detects technetium-99m (^{99m}Tc), commonly used for sentinel lymph node dissection (SLND), and ^{125}I can be used to guide the breast resection. After excision, the specimen is sent for specimen radiography to confirm that the targeted lesion and radioactive seed have been excised. A newer technique, fluoroscopic intraoperative neoplasm or node detection, utilizes fluoroscopy to find the radio-opaque clip placed at the time of the original CNB. It avoids any other procedures while the patient is awake and can be used interactively at the time of surgery.

IDENTIFICATION AND CARE OF HIGH-RISK PATIENTS

Risk Factors for Breast Cancer

Identification of factors associated with an increased incidence of breast cancer development is important in general health screening for women (Box 35.2). Risk factors for breast cancer can be

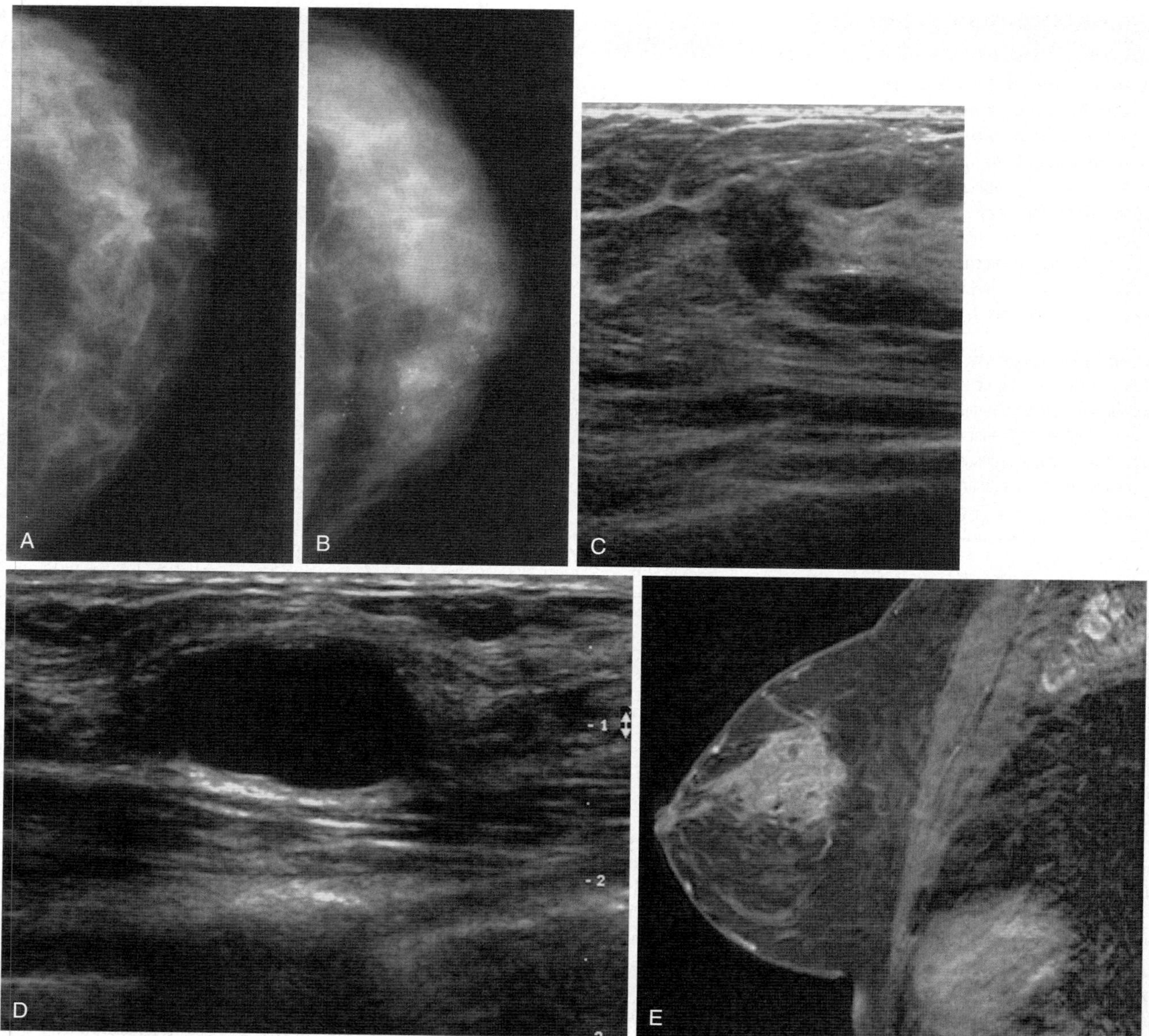

FIG. 35.7 Mammography, ultrasound, and magnetic resonance imaging (MRI) findings in breast disease. (A) Stellate mass in the breast. The combination of density with spiculated borders and distortion of surrounding breast architecture suggests a malignancy. (B) Clustered microcalcifications. Fine, pleomorphic, and linear calcifications that cluster together suggest the diagnosis of ductal carcinoma in situ. (C) Ultrasound image of breast cancer. The mass is solid, contains internal echoes, and displays an irregular border. Most malignant lesions are taller than they are wide. (D) Ultrasound image of a simple cyst. On ultrasound, the cyst is round with smooth borders, there is a paucity of internal sound echoes, and there is increased through-transmission of sound with enhanced posterior echoes. (E) Breast MRI showing gadolinium enhancement of a breast cancer. Rapid and intense gadolinium enhancement reflects increased tumor vascularity. Lesion contour and size may also be assessed by MRI.

divided into seven broad categories—age and gender, personal history of breast cancer, histologic risk factors, family history of breast cancer and genetic risk factors, reproductive risk factors, and exogenous hormone use.

Age and Gender

Age is probably the most important risk factor for breast cancer development. The age-adjusted incidence of breast cancer continues to increase with advancing age of the female population. Breast cancer is rare in women younger than 20 years and constitutes less than 2% of the total cases. Thereafter, the incidence increases to 1 in 225 from ages 30 to 39 years, 1 in 69 from ages 40 to 49, 1 in 44 from ages 50 to 59, 1 in 29 from ages 60 to 69, and 1 in 8 by age 80 years (American Cancer Society, Breast Cancer Facts & Figures). Stated another way, women now have an average risk of 12.2% of being diagnosed with breast cancer at some time during their lives.

Gender is also an important risk factor because most breast cancers occur in women. Breast cancer does occur in men; however, the incidence in men is less than 1% of the incidence in women. Of 235,030 cases of invasive breast cancer anticipated in 2014, 2360 cases were expected to occur in men. Masses in

TABLE 35.2 Breast Imaging Reporting and Data System final assessment category.

CATEGORY	DEFINITION
0	Incomplete assessment—need additional imaging evaluation or prior mammograms for comparison
1	Negative—nothing to comment on; usually recommend annual screening
2	Benign finding—usually recommend annual screening
3	Probably benign finding (<2% malignant)—initial short-interval follow-up suggested
4	Suspicious abnormality (2%–95% malignant)—biopsy should be considered
5	Highly suggestive of malignancy (>95% malignant)—appropriate action should be taken
6	Known biopsy—proven malignancy

Adapted from Liberman L, Abramson AF, Squires FB, et al. The Breast Imaging Reporting and Data System: positive predictive values of mammographic feature and final assessment categories. *AJR Am J Roentgenol.* 1998;171:35; and Liberman L, Menell JH. Breast Imaging Reporting and Data System (BI-RADS). *Radiol Clin North Am.* 2002;40:409.

BOX 35.2 Risk factors for breast cancer.

Risk Factors That Cannot Be Modified

Increasing age
Female sex
Menstrual factors
Early age at menarche (onset of menses before age 12 years)
Older age at menopause (onset beyond age 55 years)
Nulliparity
Family history of breast cancer
Genetic predisposition (*BRCA1* and *BRCA2* mutation carriers)
Personal history of breast cancer
Race, ethnicity (white women have increased risk compared with women of other races)
History of radiation exposure

Risk Factors That Can Be Modified

Reproductive factors
Age at first live birth (full-term pregnancy after age 30 years)
Parity
Lack of breastfeeding
Obesity
Alcohol consumption
Tobacco smoking
Use of hormone replacement therapy
Decreased physical activity
Shift work (night shifts)

Histologic Risk Factors

Proliferative breast disease
Atypical ductal hyperplasia
Atypical lobular hyperplasia
Lobular carcinoma in situ

the breast of a man are more likely to be benign and the result of gynecomastia (see earlier) or other noncancerous tumors rather than breast cancer.

Personal History of Cancer

A history of cancer in one breast increases the likelihood of a second primary cancer in the contralateral breast. The magnitude of risk depends on the age at diagnosis of the first primary cancer, estrogen receptor (ER) status of the first primary cancer, and use of adjuvant systemic chemotherapy and endocrine therapy. In absolute terms, the actual risk varies from 0.5% to 1% per year in younger patients to 0.2% per year in older patients.[6] In patients with other cancers requiring mantle irradiation, especially before the age of 30, the risk of breast cancer is estimated at twofold to fourfold.

Histologic Risk Factors

Histologic abnormalities diagnosed by breast biopsy constitute an important category of breast cancer risk factors. These abnormalities include lobular carcinoma in situ (LCIS) and proliferative changes with atypia. LCIS is an uncommon condition that is observed predominantly in younger premenopausal women. It is typically an incidental finding at biopsy for another condition and does not manifest as a palpable mass or suspicious microcalcifications on mammography. In a report on more than 5000 biopsies performed for benign disease, LCIS was found in 3.6% of cases. In a review of 297 patients with LCIS treated by biopsy and careful observation, it was determined that the actuarial probability of carcinoma developing at the end of 35 years was 21.4%. Using data from the Connecticut Tumor Registry, it was determined that the risk ratio for patients with LCIS (ratio of expected to observed cases of invasive breast cancer) was 7:1. Significantly, 40% of the carcinomas that subsequently developed in patients with LCIS were purely in situ lesions. The invasive carcinomas that developed were predominantly ductal and not lobular in histology, and 50% of the carcinomas occurred in the contralateral breast. LCIS is not considered a breast cancer but rather a histologic marker for increased breast cancer risk, which is estimated at slightly less than 1% per year, longitudinally.

For most patients with a diagnosis of LCIS, a conservative approach is favored. The three options that can be discussed with the patient are close observation; chemoprevention with tamoxifen, raloxifene, or arimidex; or bilateral mastectomy. LCIS predisposes to subsequent carcinoma, and the risk is lifelong and equal for both breasts. A 5-year course of tamoxifen provides a 56% reduction in breast cancer risk.[9] For patients who elect surgery rather than observation, bilateral total nipple skin-sparing mastectomy is the procedure of choice.

Benign breast disease produces a spectrum of histologic lesions that are broadly divided into nonproliferative and proliferative epithelial changes. Nonproliferative changes include mild to moderate hyperplasia of luminal cells within breast ducts; these changes do not significantly increase a woman's lifetime risk for development of breast cancer. Proliferative changes within the breast ductal system are associated with an increased risk of developing breast cancer. Dupont and Page divided proliferative lesions into lesions with atypia and lesions without atypia; proliferative lesions without atypia sometimes are termed *severe hyperplasia*.

TABLE 35.3 Histologic risk factors for development of breast cancer.

HISTOLOGIC DIAGNOSIS	ESTIMATES, RR*
Nonproliferative disease†	1.0
Proliferative disease without atypia‡	1.3–1.9
Proliferative disease with atypia§	3.7–4.2
and strong family history	4–9
LCIS	>7

Data from Hartmann LC, Sellers TA, Frost MH, et al. Benign breast disease and the risk of breast cancer. *N Engl J Med.* 2005;353:229; London SJ, Connolly JL, Schnitt SJ, et al. A prospective study of benign breast disease and the risk of breast cancer. *JAMA.* 1992;267:1780; and Dupont WD, Parl FF, Hartmann WH, et al. Breast cancer risk associated with proliferative breast disease and atypical hyperplasia. *Cancer.* 199371:1258.

LCIS, Lobular carcinoma in situ; *RR*, relative risk.

*Ratio of observed incidence over the incidence in women without proliferative disease.

†Fibrocystic change with no, usual, or mild hyperplasia.

‡Fibrocystic change with hyperplasia greater than mild or usual, papilloma, papillomatosis, sclerosing adenosis, radial scar, and other findings.

§Any diagnosis of atypical ductal or lobular hyperplasia, or both.

Subsequent studies adopted this classification scheme—nonproliferative lesions, proliferative changes without atypia (severe hyperplasia), and proliferative changes with atypia. ADH and atypical lobular hyperplasia (ALH) are categorized as proliferative changes with atypia. The risk for development of breast cancer in women with ADH or ALH is approximately four to five times the risk in the general population. A family history of breast cancer and atypical hyperplasia increases the risk to almost nine times that of the general population. The annual risk for development of breast cancer in a woman with ADH or ALH is 0.5% to 1% per year. The estimates of breast cancer risk according to histologic risk factors are influenced by age at diagnosis, menopausal status, and family history. Histologic risk factors are listed in Table 35.3.

Family History of Breast Cancer and Genetic Risk Factors

Many studies have examined the relationship between family history of breast cancer and the risk for breast cancer. First-degree relatives (mothers, sisters, and daughters) of patients with breast cancer have a twofold to threefold excess risk for development of the disease. Risk is much higher if affected first-degree relatives of the mother or father had premenopausal-onset and bilateral breast cancer. In families with multiple affected members, particularly with bilateral and early-onset cancer, the absolute risk in first-degree relatives approaches 50%, consistent with an autosomal-dominant mode of inheritance in these families.

Genetic factors are estimated to be responsible for 5% to 10% of all breast cancer cases, but they may account for 25% of cases in women younger than 30 years. In 1990, King and colleagues identified a region on the long arm of chromosome 17 (17q21) that contained a cancer susceptibility gene. The *BRCA1* gene was discovered in 1994; it is now known that mutations in *BRCA1* account for up to 40% of familial breast cancers. A second susceptibility gene, *BRCA2*, was discovered in 1995. In addition to being at increased risk for breast cancer, women with mutations in *BRCA1* or *BRCA2* are at increased risk for ovarian cancer (45% lifetime risk for *BRCA1* carriers).

Deleterious mutations in *BRCA1* or *BRCA2* are rare in the general population. The frequency of mutations is approximately 1 in 1000 (0.1%) in the U.S. population. Certain relatively closed populations may have higher prevalence rates and show preference for certain mutations, termed *founder mutations,* including the 185delAG and 5382insC mutations in *BRCA1*, which are found in 1.0% of the Ashkenazi Jewish population (Jews of Eastern European descent), and the C4446T mutation found in French Canadian families. *BRCA1* is a large gene with 22 coding exons and more than 500 mutations; many of these are unique and limited to a given family, which makes genetic testing technically difficult. *BRCA1* is a tumor suppressor gene with disease susceptibility inherited in an autosomal dominant fashion. Germline mutations inactivate a single inherited allele of *BRCA1* in every cell, and this precedes a somatic event in breast epithelial cells that eliminates the remaining allele and causes the cancer. The gene product may provide negative regulation of cell growth and is involved in recognition and repair of genetic damage. If a patient presents with a triple-negative breast cancer, there is a ~20% risk of a BRAC1 mutation. If there is a family history of breast and ovarian cancer in different relatives of a breast cancer patient, then there is ~40% risk of a BRAC gene. If a relative has both breast and ovarian cancer, the risk can be as high as 80%.

The *BRCA2* gene is located on chromosome 13 and accounts for 30% of familial breast cancers; in contrast to *BRCA1*, *BRCA2* is associated with increased breast cancer risk in men. Women with a mutation in *BRCA2* also have a 20% to 30% lifetime risk for ovarian cancer. Founder mutations of *BRCA2* include the 617delT mutation, present in 1.4% of the Ashkenazi population; 8765delAG mutation, present in the French Canadian population, and 999del15 mutation, found in the Icelandic population. In Iceland, 7% of unselected women with breast cancer and 0.6% of individuals in the general population carry the 999del15 mutation.

The penetrance of a gene refers to the chance that carriers of mutations in the gene will actually develop breast cancer. The initial estimates of the penetrance of *BRCA1* and *BRCA2* mutations were high, but the penetrance of *BRCA1* and *BRCA2* mutations more recently has been estimated to be 56% (95% confidence interval [CI], 40%–73%). It is reasonable to quote lifetime rates of breast cancer between 50% and 70% for carriers of *BRCA1* or *BRCA2* mutations.

The histopathology of *BRCA1*-associated breast cancer is unfavorable compared with *BRCA2*-associated cancer and includes tumors that are high grade, hormone receptor–negative, and aneuploid, with an increased S phase fraction. There is a strong association between the basal-like breast cancer subtype and *BRCA1* mutations. Women who carry a *BRCA1* mutation and develop breast cancer are highly likely to have basal-like breast cancer, and 10% of basal-like tumors arise in women with a *BRCA1* mutation. The same is not true for *BRCA2*-associated cancers, which are more commonly hormone receptor–positive. Overall mortality rates in patients with *BRCA1*-associated or *BRCA2*-associated breast cancer are similar to mortality rates in women with sporadic breast cancer. Because the risk for development of breast cancer is high in carriers of a *BRCA* gene mutation, prophylactic surgery is considered to be the most rational approach. MRI is encouraged for women who prefer intensive screening rather than prophylactic surgery. The efficacy of chemoprevention in *BRCA* mutation carriers is unclear, especially in women with *BRCA1* mutations, who tend to develop ER-negative breast cancers.

Reproductive Risk Factors

Reproductive milestones that increase a woman's lifetime estrogen exposure are thought to increase her breast cancer risk. These include onset of menarche before 12 years of age, first live childbirth after age 30 years, nulliparity, and menopause after age 55 years. There is a 10% reduction in breast cancer risk for each 2-year delay in menarche; the risk doubles with menopause after age 55. A first full-term pregnancy before age 18 years is associated with half the risk for development of breast cancer of a first full-term pregnancy after age 30 years. Induced abortion is not associated with increased breast cancer risk. Breastfeeding has been reported to reduce breast cancer risk, and this effect may be secondary to a decrease in the number of lifetime menstrual cycles. Compared with gender, age, histologic risk factors, and genetics, reproductive risk factors are relatively mild in terms of their contribution to risk (RR, 0.5–2.0). However, in contrast to family history or histologic factors, reproductive risk factors have a large influence on breast cancer prevalence in populations.

Exogenous Hormone Use

Therapeutic or supplemental estrogen and progesterone are taken for various conditions, with the two most common scenarios being contraception in premenopausal women and HRT in postmenopausal women. Other indications for use of exogenous hormones include menstrual irregularities, polycystic ovaries, fertility treatment, and hormone insufficiency states. Studies have suggested that breast cancer risk is increased in current or past users of oral contraceptives but that the risk decreases as the interval after cessation of use increases.

The use of HRT was studied in the Women's Health Initiative, a prospective, randomized controlled trial in which healthy postmenopausal women 50 to 79 years old received various dietary and vitamin supplements and postmenopausal HRT. The study assessed the benefits and risks associated with HRT, a low-fat diet, and calcium and vitamin D supplementation and their effects on rates of cancer, cardiovascular disease, and osteoporosis-related fractures. During the period from 1993 to 1998 at 40 centers in the United States, 16,608 women were randomly assigned to receive combined conjugated equine estrogens (e.g., Premarin, 0.625 mg/day) plus medroxyprogesterone acetate (2.5 mg/day) or placebo. Screening mammography and clinical breast examinations were performed at baseline and yearly thereafter. The study reached a stopping rule at 5.2 years of follow-up, at which time there were 245 cases of breast cancer (invasive and noninvasive) in the combined HRT group versus 185 cases in the placebo group. Compared with placebo, the combination of estrogen and progesterone, specifically Prempro, increased the risk of developing breast cancer in postmenopausal women with an intact uterus. Of greater concern was that breast cancer was more likely to be diagnosed at a more advanced stage in women receiving estrogen plus progesterone, and these women were substantially more likely to have abnormal mammograms.

Also in the Women's Health Initiative, 10,739 women who had had a hysterectomy were randomly assigned to conjugated equine estrogens (e.g., Premarin) at a dose of 0.625 mg daily or a placebo. After 7 years of follow-up, the two groups had similar rates of breast cancer (RR for the estrogen group, 0.80; 95% CI, 0.62–1.04). There was a statistically significant difference between the treatment and control groups in the need for short-interval mammographic follow-up examinations, which was higher in the group that received Premarin (36.2% vs. 28.1%).

These data show that women receiving combination HRT with estrogen and progesterone for 5 years have approximately a 20% increased risk for the development of breast cancer. Women who take estrogen-only formulations (because of previous hysterectomy) do not appear to be at significant increased risk for breast cancer.

Risk Assessment

A model for assessing breast cancer risk, known as the *Gail model*, was developed from case-control data in the Breast Cancer Detection Demonstration Project. (This model is available for clinical use at http://www.cancer.gov/bcrisktool.) In developing the model, factors influencing the risk for breast cancer were identified as age, race, age at menarche, age at first live birth, number of previous breast biopsies, presence of proliferative disease with atypia, and number of first-degree female relatives with breast cancer. The model does not include detailed information about genetic factors and may underestimate the risk for *BRCA1* or *BRCA2* mutation carriers and overestimate the risk for noncarriers. The model should not be used in women with a diagnosis of LCIS or DCIS. The Gail model for breast cancer risk was used in the design of the Breast Cancer Prevention Trial, which randomly assigned women at high risk (>1.67%) to receive tamoxifen or a placebo, and in the design of Study of Tamoxifen and Raloxifene (STAR), which randomly assigned women at high risk to receive tamoxifen or raloxifene.

The Gail model assesses population risk using nongenetic factors, whereas hereditary and familial models assess genetic and familial factors of breast cancer. The Gail model is not accurate for African Americans and a specific model, CARE, was developed. The Claus model is based on assumptions about the prevalence of high-penetrance breast cancer susceptibility genes. The Claus model provides individual estimates of breast cancer risk according to decade of life based on knowledge of first-degree and second-degree relatives with breast cancer and their ages at diagnosis. Many other models have been developed for specific populations, all with similar discriminatory power as compared with the nonspecific traditional models. Mammographic density is associated with high risk for breast cancer. However, models including breast density have only minimal discriminatory power. Other well-known risk factors not included in most if not all risk assessment tools are alcohol consumption, body weight, and physical activity.

Several models have been designed to assess the risk for harboring a mutation in *BRCA1* or *BRCA2*. These models can be useful in determining whether genetic testing is needed. The Couch model predicts risk for a mutation in the *BRCA1* gene. The BRCAPro model, developed by Myriad Genetics Laboratories, estimates the risk of *BRCA1* and *BRCA2* mutations. The Tyrer-Cuzick model incorporates personal risk factors and genetic analysis to give a more comprehensive and individual risk assessment. Such models have estimated that the incidence of clinically significant *BRCA1* or *BRCA2* mutations in the general population is approximately 1 in 300 to 500. Indications for consideration of genetic testing include breast cancer diagnosed before age 50, bilateral breast cancer, breast and ovarian cancer in the same individual, and breast cancer in men. Other factors that may be indications for testing are a family history (maternal or paternal) of two or more individuals with breast and ovarian cancer, a close male relative with breast cancer, a close relative with early-onset (<50 years) breast or ovarian cancer, and known *BRCA1* or *BRCA2* mutation in the family. Online risk calculators are available.

In addition to BRCA1 and 2, there are many other recognized genes and familial syndromes with lesser but significant risk of breast cancer. The development and reduced cost of multiple gene panel testing make screening for these other genes meaningful. These include evaluation for Li-Fraumeni syndrome (TP53 mutation), Cowden syndrome (PTEN mutation), and PALB2, CHEK2, CDH1, STK-11, NF1, and ATM carriers. The American Society of Breast Surgeons developed recommendations for screening and treatment of the lesser-known genes in the Consensus Guidelines on Hereditary Genetic Testing for Patients With and Without Breast Cancer (https://www.breastsurgeons.org/docs/statements/Consensus-Guideline-on-Genetic-Testing-for-Hereditary-Breast-Cancer.pdf, accessed December 27, 2018). In the process of genetic testing, individuals with Variant of Uncertain Significance will be identified but should not be acted upon.

Care of High-Risk Patients

In practice, clinicians assess risk factors and consider the factors that are important to individual patients in making recommendations about breast cancer screening and prevention. Increased risk for breast cancer is defined as a 5-year calculated risk of 1.66% or higher using the National Cancer Institute (NCI) risk calculator, which is based on the Gail model. This is the average risk for a woman who is 60 years old; it has been used in the design of the U.S. prevention trials. This risk calculator is not applicable to women with a history of invasive breast cancer, DCIS, or LCIS or African-Americans. The model does not make adjustments for a first-degree relative with premenopausal or bilateral breast cancer and does not consider genetic mutations. The clinician must understand that risk may be significantly underestimated if these factors are present, and risk should be calculated within the context of the patient's overall personal and family history. However, even with these limitations, the Gail model provides a valuable starting point for the evaluation of breast cancer risk assessment. This risk assessment can provide a context for recommendations for primary prevention strategies and screening appropriate to the individual's risk level. For women found to be at high risk for the development of breast cancer, options include close surveillance with clinical breast examination, mammography, and breast MRI (with a lifetime risk of >20%) and interventions to reduce risk, such as chemoprevention or a bilateral prophylactic mastectomy and/or salpingo-oophorectomy.

Close Surveillance

Surveillance guidelines for individuals at high risk for breast cancer were established in 2002 by the National Comprehensive Cancer Network and the Cancer Genetics Studies Consortium. These guidelines are based primarily on expert opinion; screening guidelines for high-risk individuals are not established by prospective trials. Recommendations for women in a family with a breast and ovarian cancer syndrome include monthly breast self-examination beginning at age 18 to 20 years, semiannual clinical breast examination beginning at age 25 years, and annual mammography beginning at age 25 years or 10 years before the earliest age at onset of breast cancer in a family member. Nonetheless, studies of women with known *BRCA1* or *BRCA2* mutations found that 50% of the detected breast cancers were diagnosed as interval cancers; that is, they occurred between screening episodes and not during the course of routine screening. This observation prompted many groups to add annual screening MRI to screening mammography, with some groups recommending doing the two examinations simultaneously and others recommending staggering the two examinations. For women with a strong family history of early-onset breast and ovarian cancer who have not undergone genetic counseling, genetic counseling is offered; this includes a discussion of genetic testing of multiple gene panel testing.

Chemoprevention for Breast Cancer

Drugs currently approved for reducing breast cancer risk are the selective ER modulators tamoxifen and raloxifene and the aromatase inhibitors (AIs). Tamoxifen has proven beneficial for the treatment of ER-positive breast cancer (see "Endocrine Therapy" later on). Tamoxifen has been used as adjuvant treatment for breast cancer for several decades and is known to reduce the incidence of a second primary breast cancer in the contralateral breast of women who receive the drug as adjuvant therapy for a first primary breast cancer. The largest comprehensive analysis of the benefits of tamoxifen was done by the Early Breast Cancer Trialists' Collaborative Group (EBCTCG). This group meets every 5 years to review outcome data from breast cancer trials conducted worldwide. Findings from the EBCTCG overview analysis demonstrated that adjuvant tamoxifen reduces the risk for a second breast cancer in the unaffected breast by 47%. Four prospective randomized trials were completed that evaluated tamoxifen for chemoprevention in healthy women at increased risk for breast cancer.

In the National Surgical Adjuvant Breast and Bowel Project (NSABP) P-1 trial, 13,388 women who were 35 to 59 years old and had a diagnosis of LCIS, who had a moderately increased risk for breast cancer (RR, 1.66 over a 5-year period), or who were 60 years old or older were randomly assigned to tamoxifen or placebo. The risk estimates were based on the Gail model of risk (see earlier). In this study, tamoxifen reduced the risk for invasive breast cancer by 49% through 69 months of follow-up; the risk reduction was 59% in women with LCIS and 86% in women with ADH or ALH. The reduction in risk was noted only for ER-positive cancers. Tamoxifen treatment for 5 years was not without side effects and complications. In the tamoxifen treatment arm, endometrial cancers resulting from estrogen-like effects of the drug on the endometrium were increased by a factor of approximately 2.5. Pulmonary embolism (RR, 3) and deep venous thrombosis (RR, 1.7) were also more common in women who received tamoxifen. Data on the efficacy of tamoxifen for reduction of breast cancer risk in *BRCA1* and *BRCA2* mutation carriers were limited because mutation testing was not routinely performed on P-1 study participants. Tamoxifen is most effective at reducing the incidence of ER-positive breast cancers, so its role in *BRCA1* mutation carriers (who more often develop ER-negative breast cancers) is questionable.

Three other tamoxifen prevention trials were conducted approximately the same time as the NSABP P-1 trial, including the Italian Tamoxifen Prevention Study, Royal Marsden Hospital Pilot Tamoxifen Chemoprevention Trial, and International Breast Cancer Intervention Study-I (IBIS-I). The Italian and Royal Marsden studies did not show any benefit of tamoxifen over placebo in terms of reduced incidence of breast cancer.

There were some differences in the study populations and trial designs, which may explain the negative results compared with the P-1 trial. The IBIS-I trial showed a 33% reduction in the incidence of breast cancer with tamoxifen, slightly lower than the risk reduction in P-1 but confirming the risk reduction benefit of tamoxifen. Subsequently, a meta analysis of all the tamoxifen prevention trials found that tamoxifen reduced the risk of breast cancer by 38%. This analysis also confirmed the increased risks of endometrial cancer and venous thromboembolic events seen with tamoxifen use.

The NSABP P-2 trial (STAR trial) compared tamoxifen with raloxifene in postmenopausal women. This comparison was based on the findings from the MORE trial, which included more than 10,000 women who received placebo versus raloxifene for the prevention and treatment of osteoporosis. In the MORE trial, at an average of 3 years of follow-up, there was a 54% reduction in the incidence of breast cancer and no increase in uterine cancer. The STAR trial enrolled 19,747 women at increased risk for breast cancer and demonstrated that tamoxifen and raloxifene each reduced the risk for invasive breast cancer by approximately 50%. Raloxifene had a more favorable toxicity profile. The number of uterine cancers was reduced by 36% in the raloxifene group compared with the tamoxifen group, and women taking raloxifene had 29% fewer episodes of venous thrombosis and a reduced incidence of pulmonary embolism compared with the tamoxifen group.

Because studies showed that AIs prevent more contralateral breast cancers than tamoxifen in postmenopausal women with early-stage breast cancer, AIs have been evaluated for chemoprevention. The NCI of Canada Clinical Trials Group completed the Mammary Prevention 3 (MAP.3) trial investigating the AI exemestane. In this study, 4560 postmenopausal women who had at least one of several breast cancer risk factors (≥60 years old; Gail model 5-year risk score >1.66%; prior ADH, ALH, or LCIS; or prior DCIS with mastectomy) were randomly assigned to exemestane or placebo. After a median follow-up of 35 months, exemestane was associated with a 65% relative reduction in the annual incidence of invasive breast cancer, with 11 invasive cancers detected in the exemestane group and 32 detected in the placebo group. Adverse events occurred in 88% of subjects in the exemestane group and 85% of subjects in the placebo group ($P = 0.003$), with significant differences noted in the development of endocrine, gastrointestinal, and musculoskeletal symptoms. Exemestane has not been approved by the U.S. Food and Drug Administration as a chemopreventive agent; however, it has a category 1 recommendation for breast cancer prevention in the National Comprehensive Cancer Network clinical practice guidelines.

Prophylactic Mastectomy

Prophylactic mastectomy has been shown to reduce the chance of breast cancer development in high-risk women by 90%. Hartmann and colleagues performed a retrospective review of 639 women with a family history of breast cancer who underwent prophylactic mastectomy. The women were divided into high-risk (n = 214) and moderate-risk (n = 425) groups, with women at high risk defined as women with a family history suggestive of an autosomal-dominant predisposition to breast cancer. For women at moderate risk, the number of expected breast cancers was calculated according to the Gail model. On the basis of this model, 37.4 breast cancers were expected to develop, but only 4 cancers occurred, for an incidence risk reduction of 89%. For women in the high-risk cohort, the Gail model would underestimate the risk for development of breast cancer. The expected number of breast cancers was calculated by using three different statistical models from a control study of the high-risk probands (sisters). Three breast cancers developed after prophylactic mastectomy, for an incident risk reduction of at least 90%.

Several groups reported on prospective studies in *BRCA1* and *BRCA2* mutation carriers treated with prophylactic mastectomy versus surveillance and showed that mastectomy is highly effective in preventing breast cancers. More recently, results of risk-reducing mastectomy and risk-reducing salpingo-oophorectomy were reported in *BRCA1* and *BRCA2* mutation carriers followed in 22 centers as part of the PROSE consortium. None of the participants who underwent risk-reducing mastectomy developed a subsequent breast cancer compared with 7% of the women who did not undergo this surgery. The use of risk-reducing salpingo-oophorectomy reduced the incidence of ovarian cancers from 5.8% to 1.1% and the incidence of breast cancers from 19.2% to 11.4%. Risk-reducing salpingo-oophorectomy was associated with a significant reduction in breast cancer–specific mortality, ovarian cancer–specific mortality, and all-cause mortality. The available data suggest that *BRCA* mutation carriers should be counseled to consider risk-reducing surgeries as a strategy to reduce cancer incidence and improve survival.

Women who undergo annual mammographic screening have an overall 80% chance of surviving breast cancer after it has been detected. Given the penetrance in the range of 50% to 60% for *BRCA1* or *BRCA2* mutation carriers, the chance of a *BRCA1* or *BRCA2* mutation carrier dying of breast cancer is approximately 10% if she chooses not to undergo risk-reducing surgery.

The use of risk-reducing surgery in women who are not known to have deleterious mutations in *BRCA1* or *BRCA2* is controversial. Trends have suggested that more women with newly diagnosed breast cancer are choosing to undergo contralateral prophylactic mastectomy as a strategy for reducing the risk of contralateral breast cancer, but it also reduces quality of life. The American Society of Breast Surgeons does not recommend the routine use of contralateral mastectomy in the sporadic cancer patient, but as many women request such procedures, it favors a shared-decision model.[10]

Summary: Risk Assessment and Management

Understanding risk factors for the development of disease provides clues to pathogenesis and identifies patients likely to benefit from risk-reducing strategies. Although breast cancer can develop in both sexes, the risk of breast cancer development is much higher in women; breast cancer in men is uncommon. Age is a strong determinant of risk and is part of the NCI risk assessment tool. Family history is most significant when breast cancer affects first-degree relatives (mothers, sisters, and daughters) at a young age and when cases of ovarian cancer are found on the same side of the family. This type of family history may preclude the use of the NCI tool for accurate risk assessment. The most significant histologic risk factors for the development of breast cancer are LCIS, ADH, and ALH. A personal history of breast cancer predisposes to contralateral breast cancer, although adjuvant therapy (endocrine therapy and chemotherapy) reduces this risk.

BENIGN BREAST TUMORS AND RELATED DISEASES

Breast Cysts

Cysts within the breast parenchyma are fluid-filled, epithelial-lined cavities that vary in size from microscopic to large palpable masses containing 20 to 30 mL of fluid. A palpable cyst develops in at least 1 in every 14 women, and 50% of cysts are multiple or recurrent. The pathogenesis of cyst formation is not well understood; however, cysts appear to arise from destruction and dilatation of lobules and terminal ductules. Microscopic studies showed that fibrosis at or near the lobule, combined with continued secretion, results in unfolding of the lobule and expansion of an epithelial-lined cavity containing fluid.

Cysts are influenced by ovarian hormones, a fact that explains their variation with the menstrual cycle. Most cysts occur in women older than 35 years; the incidence steadily increases until menopause and sharply declines thereafter. New cyst formation in older women is generally associated with exogenous HRT.

Intracystic carcinoma is exceedingly rare. Rosemond reported that only three cancers were identified in more than 3000 cyst aspirations (0.1%). Other investigators confirmed this low incidence. There is no evidence of increased risk for breast cancer associated with cyst formation.

A palpable mass can be confirmed to be a cyst by direct aspiration or ultrasonography. Cyst fluid can be straw-colored, opaque, or dark green and may contain debris. Given the low risk for malignancy within a cyst if it appears to be a simple cyst without internal perturbation and smooth borders an aspiration is not necessary. If the mass is complex, then aspiration may be necessary. If the cyst resolves after aspiration and the cyst contents are not grossly bloody, the fluid does not need to be sent for cytologic analysis. If the cyst recurs multiple times (more than twice is a reasonable rule), CNB should be performed to evaluate any solid elements. The entire cystic structure can be percutaneously removed with a vacuum-assisted core needle device.[11] Surgical removal of a cyst is usually not indicated but may be required if the cyst recurs multiple times or if needle biopsy reveals findings of atypia, incompletely removes the mass, or if the cyst is large and painful for the patient.

Fibroadenomas and Other Benign Tumors

Fibroadenomas are benign solid tumors composed of stromal and epithelial elements. Fibroadenoma is the second most common tumor in the breast (after carcinoma) and is the most common tumor in women younger than 30 years. In contrast to cysts, fibroadenomas most often arise during the late teens and early reproductive years. Fibroadenomas are rarely seen as new masses in women after age 40 or 45 years. Clinically, fibroadenomas manifest as firm masses that are easily movable and may increase in size over several months and wax and wane with the menstrual cycle. They slide easily under the examining fingers and may be lobulated or smooth. On excision, fibroadenomas are well-encapsulated masses that may detach easily from surrounding breast tissue. Mammography is of little help in discriminating between cysts and fibroadenomas; however, ultrasonography can readily distinguish between them because each has specific characteristics.

Fibroadenomas are benign tumors, although neoplasia may develop in the epithelial elements within them. Cancer in a newly discovered fibroadenoma is exceedingly rare (0.2%); 50% of findings in fibroadenomas are LCIS, which is no longer considered stage 0 breast cancer in the eighth edition of the American Joint Committee on Cancer (AJCC) staging system but signifies a high risk for developing breast cancer, 35% are invasive carcinomas, and 15% are intraductal carcinoma. When a tissue diagnosis confirms that the breast mass is a fibroadenoma, the patient can be reassured, and surgical excision is not needed. If the patient is bothered by the mass or it continues to grow, the mass can be removed with open excisional biopsy or via percutaneous approach.[11]

Two subtypes of fibroadenoma are recognized. *Giant fibroadenoma* is a descriptive term applied to a fibroadenoma that attains an unusually large size (typically >5 cm). The term *juvenile fibroadenoma* refers to a large fibroadenoma that occasionally occurs in adolescents and young adults and histologically is more cellular than the usual fibroadenoma. Although these lesions may display remarkably rapid growth, surgical removal is curative.

Hamartomas and Adenomas

Hamartomas and adenomas are benign proliferations of variable amounts of epithelium and stromal supporting tissue. A hamartoma is a discrete nodule that contains closely packed lobules and prominent, ectatic extralobular ducts. On physical examination, mammography, and gross inspection, a hamartoma is indistinguishable from a fibroadenoma. Page and Anderson described an adenoma or tubular adenoma as a benign cellular neoplasm of ductules packed closely together so that they form a sheet of tiny glands without supporting stroma. During pregnancy and lactation, adenomas may increase in size, and histologic examination shows secretory differentiation. Biopsy is required to establish the diagnosis.

Breast Infections and Abscess

There are two general categories of infections of the breast: lactational infections and chronic subareolar infections associated with duct ectasia. Lactational infections are thought to arise from entry of bacteria through the nipple into the duct system and are characterized by fever, leukocytosis, erythema, and tenderness. Infections of the breast are most often caused by *Staphylococcus aureus* and may manifest as cellulitis with breast parenchymal inflammation and swelling, termed *mastitis*, or as abscesses. Treatment requires antibiotics and frequent emptying of the breast. True abscesses require drainage. Initial attempts at drainage should include needle aspiration; surgical incision and drainage should be reserved for abscesses that do not resolve after aspiration and treatment with antibiotics. In such cases, abscesses are generally multiloculated. Ultrasound evaluation can assist in characterizing a breast abscess and help to guide needle aspiration.

In women who are not lactating, a chronic relapsing form of infection may develop in the subareolar ducts of the breast that is variously known as *periductal mastitis* or *duct ectasia*. This condition appears to be associated with smoking and diabetes. The infections are most often mixed infections that include aerobic and anaerobic skin flora. A series of infections with resulting inflammatory changes and scarring may lead to retraction or inversion of the nipple, masses in the subareolar area, and occasionally a chronic fistula from the subareolar ducts to the periareolar skin. Palpable masses and mammographic changes may result from the infection and scarring; these can make surveillance for breast cancer more challenging.

Subareolar infections may initially manifest as subareolar pain and mild erythema. Warm soaks and oral antibiotics may be effective treatment at this stage. Antibiotic treatment generally requires coverage for aerobic and anaerobic organisms. If an abscess has developed, needle aspiration is required in addition to antibiotics. Surgical incision and drainage are reserved for abscesses that do not resolve with these more conservative measures. Repeated infections are treated by excision of the entire subareolar duct complex after the acute infection has resolved completely, together with intravenous antibiotic coverage. Rarely, patients have recurrent infections requiring excision of the nipple and areola.

A presumed infection of the breast generally clears promptly and completely with antibiotic therapy. If erythema or edema persists, a diagnosis of inflammatory carcinoma should be considered and biopsy of the skin as well as underlying breast tissue will be needed.

Papillomas and Papillomatosis

Solitary intraductal papillomas are true polyps of epithelial-lined breast ducts. Solitary papillomas are most often located close to the areola but may be present in peripheral locations. Most papillomas are smaller than 1 cm but can grow to 4 or 5 cm. Larger papillomas may appear to arise within a cystic structure, probably representing a greatly expanded duct. Papillomas are the benign tumor most associated with the development of DCIS.

Papillomas located close to the nipple are often accompanied by bloody nipple discharge. Less frequently, they are discovered as a palpable mass under the areola or as a density seen on a mammogram. Treatment is excision through a circumareolar incision. For peripheral papillomas, the differential diagnosis is between papilloma and invasive papillary carcinoma.

It is important to distinguish papillomatosis from solitary or multiple papillomas. Papillomatosis refers to epithelial hyperplasia, which commonly occurs in younger women or is associated with fibrocystic change. Papillomatosis is not composed of true papillomas but rather consists of hyperplastic epithelium that may fill individual ducts similar to a true polyp but has no stalk of fibrovascular tissue.

Sclerosing Adenosis

Adenosis refers to an increased number of small terminal ductules or acini. Adenosis is frequently associated with a proliferation of stromal tissue that produces a histologic lesion, sclerosing adenosis, which can be confused with carcinoma grossly and histologically. Sclerosing adenosis can be associated with deposition of calcium, which can be seen on a mammogram in a pattern indistinguishable from the microcalcifications of intraductal carcinoma. In many series, sclerosing adenosis is the most common pathologic diagnosis in patients undergoing needle-directed biopsy of microcalcifications. Sclerosing adenosis is frequently listed as one of the component lesions of fibrocystic disease; it is common and is not believed to have significant malignant potential.

Radial Scars

Radial scars belong to a group of abnormalities known as *complex sclerosing lesions*. Radial scars can appear similar to carcinomas mammographically because they create irregular spiculations in the surrounding stroma. Radial scars contain microcysts, epithelial hyperplasia, and adenosis and have a prominent display of central sclerosis. The gross abnormality is rarely more than 1 cm in diameter. Larger lesions may form palpable tumors and appear as spiculated masses with prominent architectural distortion on a mammogram. These tumors can cause skin dimpling by producing traction on surrounding tissues. Radial scars generally require excision to rule out an underlying carcinoma. Radial scars are associated with a modestly increased risk for breast cancer.

Fat Necrosis

Fat necrosis can mimic cancer on mammography by producing a palpable mass or density that may contain calcifications. Fat necrosis may follow an episode of trauma to the breast or be related to a prior surgical procedure or radiation therapy. Calcifications are characteristic of fat necrosis and can often be visualized on ultrasonography as well. Histologically, fat necrosis is composed of lipid-laden macrophages, scar tissue, and chronic inflammatory cells. This lesion has no malignant potential.

EPIDEMIOLOGY AND PATHOLOGY OF BREAST CANCER

Epidemiology

It has been estimated that 266,120 cases of invasive breast cancer and 63,960 cases of in situ breast cancer would be diagnosed in 2018 in the United States. Breast cancer is the second leading cause of cancer-related deaths, second to lung cancer, with approximately 40,920 deaths caused by breast cancer annually. Breast cancer is also a global health problem, with more than 2 million cases of breast cancer diagnosed worldwide each year. The overall incidence of breast cancer was increasing until approximately 1999 because of increases in the average life span, lifestyle changes that increase the risk for breast cancer, and improved survival rates for other diseases. Breast cancer incidence decreased from 1999 to 2006 by approximately 2% per year. This decrease may be attributed to a reduction in the use of HRT after the initial results of the Women's Health Initiative were published but may also be the result of a reduction in the use of screening mammography (70.1% of women ≥40 years old were screened in 2000 vs. 66.4% in 2005). During the years 2006 to 2010, breast cancer incidence rates were stable.

Survival rates in women with breast cancer have steadily improved over the last several decades, with 5-year survival rates of 63% in the early 1960s, 75% during the years 1975 to 1977, 79% during 1984 to 1986, and 90% during 1995 to 2005. The largest decreases in death rates from breast cancer have been in women younger than 50 years (decreases of 3.2% per year), although breast cancer death rates have also decreased in women older than 50 years (by 2% per year). The decreased mortality from breast cancer is thought to be the result of earlier detection via mammographic screening, a decreased incidence of breast cancer, and improvements in therapy. The survival rate for stage I breast cancer is 98.7%. The current treatment of breast cancer is guided by pathology, staging, and more recent insights into breast cancer biology. There is an increased emphasis on defining disease biology and status in individual patients, with the subsequent tailoring of therapies.

Pathology

Noninvasive Breast Cancer

Noninvasive neoplasms of the breast were previously broadly divided into two major types, LCIS and DCIS (Box 35.3). LCIS is no longer regarded as a neoplasm of the breast in the eighth edition of the AJCC staging system but is regarded as a risk factor for the development of breast cancer. LCIS is recognized by its conformity to the outline of the normal lobule, with expanded and filled acini (Fig. 35.8A). One variant of LCIS, pleomorphic LCIS, has been recognized more recently as a distinct, more aggressive histopathologic subtype. Pleomorphic LCIS shows marked nuclear pleomorphism compared with classic LCIS. One or more lobules are distended by discohesive cells with irregularly shaped, high-grade nuclei. Pleomorphic LCIS may or may not be associated with comedonecrosis and calcifications. If pleomorphic LCIS is associated with calcifications, it may be detected mammographically. The natural history of pleomorphic LCIS is unknown, and there is debate regarding treatment; many experts

BOX 35.3 Classification of primary breast cancer.

Noninvasive Epithelial Cancers

Lobular carcinoma in situ

Ductal carcinoma in situ or intraductal carcinoma

- Papillary, cribriform, solid, and comedo types

Invasive Epithelial Cancers (Percentage of Total)

Invasive lobular carcinoma (10%)

Invasive ductal carcinoma

- Invasive ductal carcinoma, not otherwise specified (50%–70%)
- Tubular carcinoma (2%–3%)
- Mucinous or colloid carcinoma (2%–3%)
- Medullary carcinoma (5%)
- Invasive cribriform carcinoma (1%–3%)
- Invasive papillary carcinoma (1%–2%)
- Adenoid cystic carcinoma (1%)
- Metaplastic carcinoma (1%)

Mixed Connective and Epithelial Tumors

Phyllodes tumors, benign and malignant

Carcinosarcoma

Angiosarcoma

Adenocarcinoma

suggest that pleomorphic LCIS be treated with surgical excision similar to DCIS.

DCIS is more morphologically heterogeneous than LCIS, and pathologists recognize four broad types of DCIS: papillary, cribriform, solid, and comedo. The latter three types are shown in Fig. 35.8. DCIS is recognized as discrete spaces filled with malignant cells, usually with a recognizable basal cell layer composed of presumably normal myoepithelial cells. The four morphologic types of DCIS are rarely seen as pure lesions; DCIS lesions are usually of mixed morphology. The papillary and cribriform types of DCIS are generally lower-grade lesions and may take longer to transform to invasive cancer. The solid and comedo types of DCIS are generally higher-grade lesions.

As the cells inside the ductal membrane grow, they have a tendency to undergo central necrosis. The necrotic debris in the center of the duct undergoes coagulation and finally calcifies, leading to the tiny, pleomorphic, and frequently linear forms of microcalcifications that can be seen on mammograms. In some patients, an entire ductal tree may be involved in the malignancy, and the mammogram shows typical calcifications that can span from the nipple extending posteriorly into the interior of the breast (termed *segmental calcifications*).If not treated, DCIS can transform into an invasive cancer, usually recapitulating the morphology of the cells inside the duct. In other words, low-grade cribriform DCIS tends to be associated with low-grade invasive lesions that retain some cribriform features. DCIS frequently coexists with invasive cancers, and when this is the case, the two phases of the malignancy are usually morphologically similar.

Invasive Breast Cancer

Invasive breast cancers are recognized by their lack of overall organized architecture with infiltration of cells haphazardly into a variable amount of stroma, or formation of sheets of continuous and monotonous cells without respect for form and function of a glandular organ. Pathologists broadly divide invasive breast cancer into ductal and lobular histologic types, which probably does not reflect histogenesis and imperfectly predicts clinical behavior. Invasive ductal cancer tends to grow as a cohesive mass; it appears as discrete abnormalities on mammograms and is often palpable as a discrete lump in the breast. Invasive lobular cancer tends to permeate the breast in a single-file nature, which explains why it remains clinically occult and often escapes detection on mammography or physical examination until the disease is extensive. The growth patterns of invasive ductal and lobular carcinomas are shown in Fig. 35.9.

Invasive ductal cancer, also known as *infiltrating ductal carcinoma*, is the most common form of breast cancer; it accounts for 50% to 70% of invasive breast cancers. Invasive lobular carcinoma accounts for 10% of breast cancers, and mixed ductal and lobular cancers have been increasingly recognized and described in pathology reports. When invasive ductal carcinomas take on differentiated features, they are named according to the features that they display. If the infiltrating cells form small glands lined by a single row of bland epithelium, they are called *infiltrating tubular carcinoma* (see Fig. 35.9C). The infiltrating cells may secrete copious amounts of mucin and appear to float in this material. These lesions are called *mucinous* or *colloid tumors* (see Fig. 35.9D). Tubular and mucinous tumors are usually low-grade (grade I) lesions; these tumors each account for approximately 2% to 3% of invasive breast carcinomas.

Medullary cancer is characterized by bizarre invasive cells with high-grade nuclear features, many mitoses, and lack of an in situ component (see Fig. 35.9E). The malignancy forms sheets of cells in an almost syncytial fashion, surrounded by an infiltrate of small mononuclear lymphocytes. The borders of the tumor push into the surrounding breast rather than infiltrate or permeate the stroma. In its pure form, medullary cancer accounts for only approximately 5% of breast cancers; however, some pathologists have described a so-called *medullary variant* that has some features of the pure form of the cancer. These tumors are uniformly high grade, ER and progesterone receptor (PR) negative, and negative for the human epidermal growth factor receptor 2 (HER-2/neu; HER-2) cell surface receptor.

Another rare subtype of breast cancer that is typically high grade and negative for ER, PR, and HER-2 is metaplastic carcinoma. Most metaplastic carcinomas are node negative, but they have high potential for metastatic spread, and 10% of patients present with de novo metastatic disease. Even patients presenting with localized metaplastic carcinoma have a poor prognosis: Approximately 50% experience local or distant relapse.

Tumors that lack expression of ER, PR, and HER-2 are often called *triple-negative breast cancers*. Gene expression profiling and microarray analysis of breast cancers have revealed that triple-negative breast cancers are distinctly different from other ductal breast cancers and may also express molecular markers found in basal or myoepithelial cells. There may be some overlap between triple-negative breast cancer and *basal-like breast cancer*, but these categories were developed using differing technologies, and the two categories do not exactly overlap. The term *basal-like breast cancer* describes a specific subtype of breast cancer defined by microarray analysis, whereas triple-negative breast cancer is defined by lack of immunohistochemical detection of ER, PR, and HER-2.

The different histologic subtypes of breast cancer have some relationship with prognosis, although this is influenced by tumor size, histologic grade, hormone receptor status, HER-2 status, lymph node status, and other prognostic variables. The prognosis

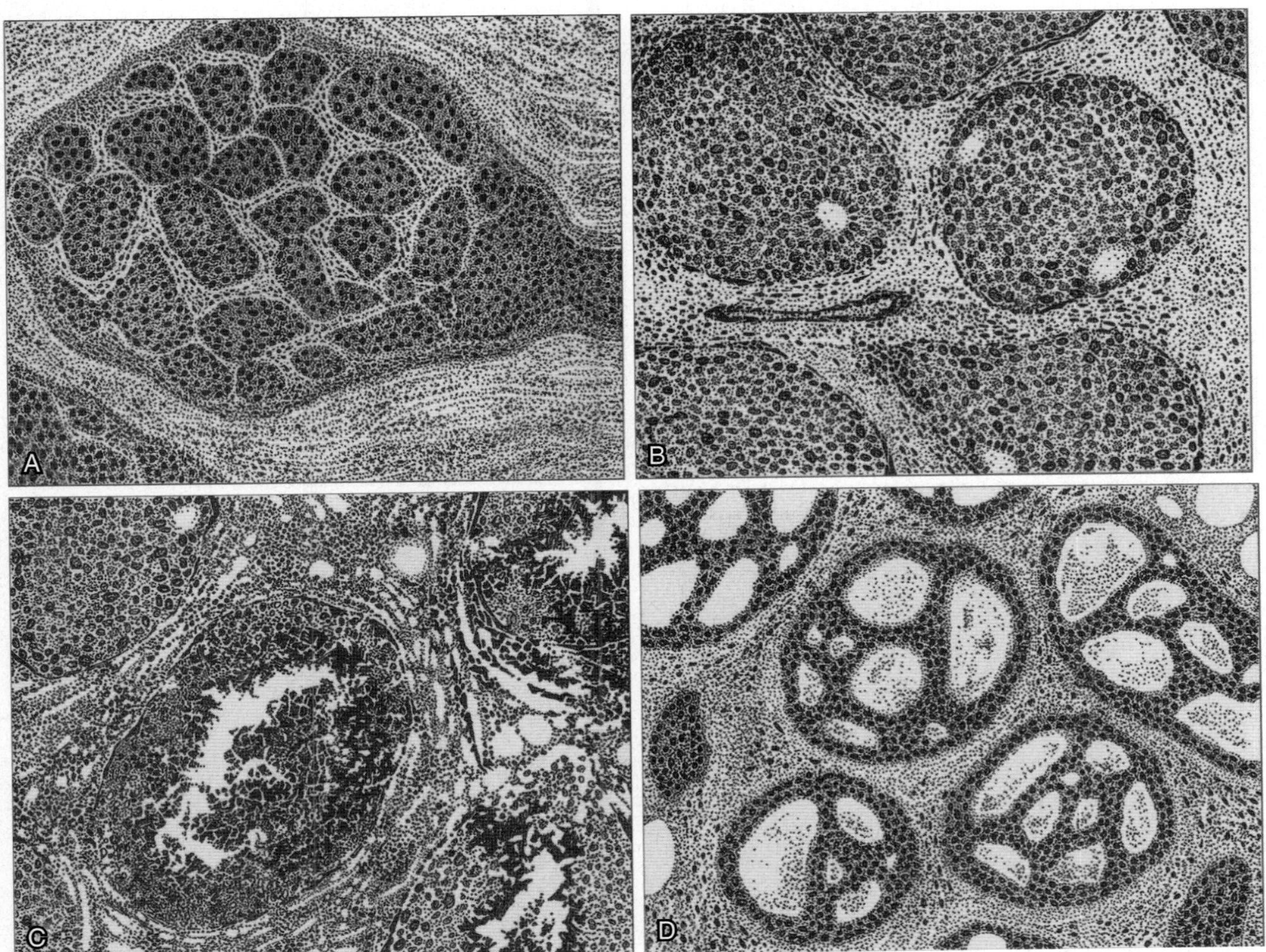

FIG. 35.8 Noninvasive breast cancer. (A) Lobular carcinoma in situ (LCIS). The neoplastic cells are small with compact, bland nuclei and are distending the acini but preserving the cross-sectional architecture of the lobular unit. (B) Ductal carcinoma in situ (DCIS), solid type. The cells are larger than in LCIS and are filling the ductal rather than the lobular spaces. However, the cells are contained within the basement membrane of the duct and do not invade the breast stroma. (C) DCIS, comedo type. In comedo DCIS, the malignant cells in the center undergo necrosis, coagulation, and calcification. (D) DCIS, cribriform type. In this type, bridges of tumor cells span the ductal space and leave round, punched-out spaces.

of invasive ductal carcinoma, not otherwise specified, is variable, modified by histologic grade and expression of molecular markers. Basal-like breast cancer is commonly aggressive, and because it is triple receptor negative, there are no targeted treatments for this form of cancer. Invasive lobular breast cancers carry an intermediate prognosis, and tubular and mucinous cancers have the best overall prognosis. These generalizations about the prognosis associated with different histologic subtypes are useful only in the context of tumor size, grade, and receptor status. Modern classification schemes based on determination of molecular markers and breast cancer subtype by microarray analysis are replacing these older morphologic descriptions.

Molecular Markers and Breast Cancer Subtypes

Numerous molecular markers have been reported to affect breast cancer outcomes, including molecules in the steroid hormone receptor pathway (ER and PR), molecules in the HER pathway (HER family), angiogenesis-related molecules, cell cycle–related molecules (e.g., cyclin-dependent kinases), apoptosis modulators, proteasomes, cyclooxygenase-2, peroxisome-proliferator-activated receptor γ, insulin-like growth factors (insulin-like growth factor family), transforming growth factor-γ, platelet-derived growth factor, and *p53*. Most of these markers are not routinely tested on breast cancer specimens at the time of diagnosis; such testing would not be feasible. Categorizing breast cancer according to the expression of molecular targets of treatments is practical, and the resulting classifications appear to agree with nonbiased classifications based on gene expression. Classification schemes reflect biology and predict treatment efficacy.

Incorporating predictive markers into the routine testing of breast cancers can help predict which patients would be most likely to benefit from therapies directed at those markers. The best example of this is testing for ER. Before the discovery of ER, all breast cancers were considered potentially sensitive to endocrine therapy. Pathologic assessment of ER is now performed on all primary tumors and predicts which patients may benefit from and should receive endocrine therapy. Patients whose tumors are ER negative can be spared endocrine therapy.

A second important predictive factor in breast cancer, discovered in 1985, is HER-2. This protein is the product of the *erb-B2* gene and is amplified in approximately 20% of human breast cancers. The extracellular domain of the receptor is present on the surface

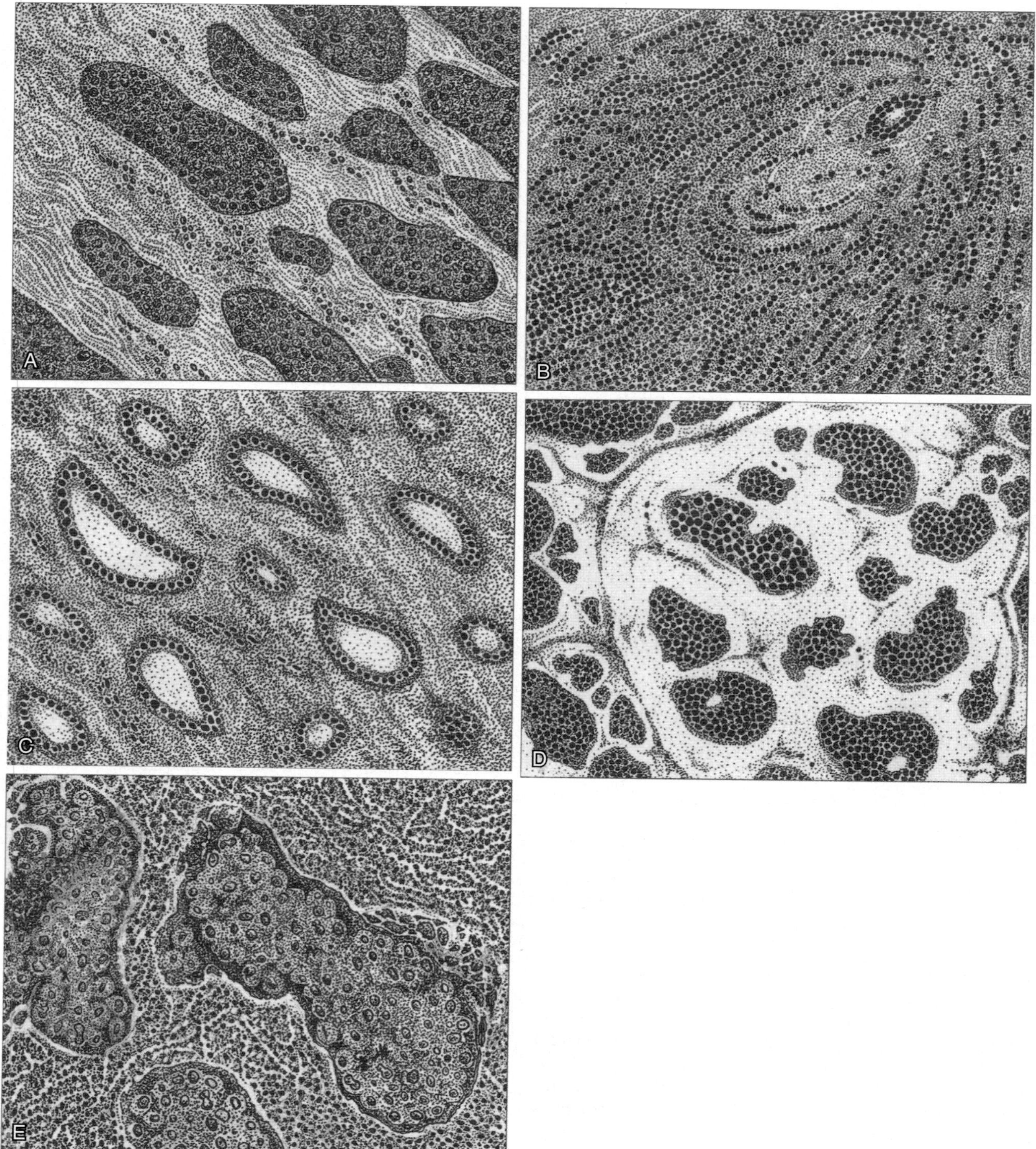

FIG. 35.9 Invasive breast cancer. (A) Invasive ductal carcinoma, not otherwise specified. The malignant cells invade in haphazard groups and singly into the stroma. (B) Invasive lobular carcinoma. The malignant cells invade the stroma in a characteristic single-file pattern and may form concentric circles of single-file cells around normal ducts (targetoid pattern). (C) Invasive tubular carcinoma. The cancer invades as small tubules, lined by a single layer of well-differentiated cells. (D) Mucinous or colloid carcinoma. The bland tumor cells float like islands in lakes of mucin. (E) Medullary carcinoma. The tumor cells are large and very undifferentiated with pleomorphic nuclei. The distinctive features of this tumor are the infiltrate of lymphocytes and the syncytium-appearing sheets of tumor cells.

of breast cancer cells, and an intracellular tyrosine kinase enzyme links the receptor to the internal machinery of the cell. HER-2 is a member of the epidermal growth factor receptor family of receptor tyrosine kinases. The tyrosine kinase of HER-2 is activated when the HER-2 receptor heterodimerizes with other members of the family that have been bound by growth factors or when the HER-2 receptor homodimerizes. There is no known ligand that binds to the HER-2 receptor. HER-2 protein overexpression is measured clinically by immunohistochemistry and scored on a scale from 0 to 3+. Alternatively, fluorescence in situ hybridization, which directly detects the number of HER-2–gene copies, can be used to detect gene amplification. Inhibiting the function of the HER-2 receptor slows the growth of HER-2–positive tumors in laboratory models and in clinical trials. Trastuzumab and pertuzumab are antibodies directed against the extracellular domain of the HER-2 surface receptor and are effective treatment for HER-2–positive breast cancer (see "HER-2–Based Targeted Therapy" later on). HER-2 testing is now a standard part of pathologic reporting on the primary tumor and is a predictive marker for HER-2–directed therapies.

A logical classification scheme for invasive breast cancer is based on the expression of ER status and HER-2. This classification has the advantage of directing treatment choices. Patients with ER-positive tumors receive endocrine therapies, and patients with HER-2–positive tumors receive HER-2–targeted therapy generally with systemic chemotherapy. However, breast cancer is a heterogeneous disease, and different breast cancers behave in different ways. For example, some ER-positive tumors are indolent and not life-threatening, whereas other ER-positive tumors are very aggressive. In an attempt to subclassify the disease further, investigators are turning to global assessment of gene expression using microarrays; these are composed of oligonucleotide probes to almost every known expressed sequence of DNA in the human genome. Similar technologies based on single-nucleotide polymorphisms in the cancer DNA and profiles of expressed proteins are being developed to subclassify cancers and direct treatment.

A typical microarray experiment, commonly known as a *heat map*, is shown in Fig. 35.10; the colors indicate levels of gene expression. Such a portrayal of the disease shows how different ER-positive tumors are from ER-negative tumors and underscores the modern concept that subclassification is needed not only to define different groups of breast cancer but also to guide treatment. In Fig. 35.10, HER-2–positive tumors form two clusters (*in green at the top*), although these clusters are fused together in many depictions. HER-2–positive tumors cluster similarly and are responsive to inhibitors of the HER-2 receptor (e.g., trastuzumab and pertuzumab). An unexpected finding is the uniqueness of tumors that are both ER negative and HER-2 negative. These tumors, also negative for PR, are called *triple-negative cancers*. They express proteins in common with myoepithelial cells at the base of mammary ducts and are also called *basal-like cancers* (see earlier). Women who carry a deleterious mutation in *BRCA1* (but not *BRCA2*) are much more likely to contract a basal-like cancer (triple-negative) than other subtypes.

In addition to being used to classify breast cancer subtypes, molecular markers are used to select patients for systemic treatment (e.g., chemotherapy, endocrine therapy) and to predict the tumor response to these pharmacologic treatments. The simplest example is the use of ER or HER-2 status to predict the response to endocrine treatment or trastuzumab. Microarray experiments use thousands of gene transcripts (messenger RNAs) to provide a snapshot of the molecular phenotype of an individual cancer. To adapt this technology for clinical application, investigators selected critical assemblies of gene products that provide the same predictive ability as a nonbiased, genome-wide analysis. The most utilized in the United States is a 21-gene test that can be used on paraffin-embedded tumor material from breast surgical specimens (Oncotype DX assay, a 21-gene recurrence score assay). Originally designed to predict the recurrence of ER-positive, node-negative breast cancer treated with adjuvant endocrine therapy, the 21-gene recurrence score assay provides a recurrence score for ER-positive breast cancer that is used clinically to determine whether

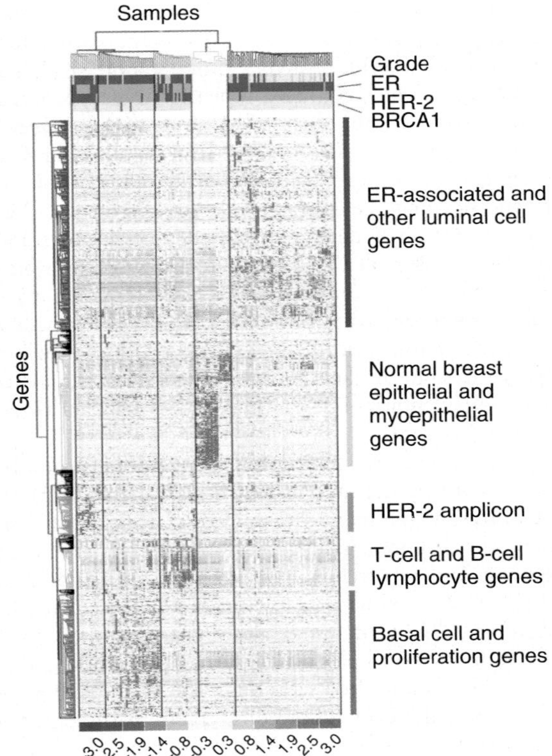

FIG. 35.10 Microarray representation of human breast cancer. This portrayal of global gene expression is called a *heat map*, with shades of red indicating high gene expression and shades of blue indicating low gene expression relative to a mean across tissue samples. Tissue samples are present across the top in columns, and individual genes are in rows down the side; the intersection is an individual gene in a particular sample. A computer-clustering algorithm aligns samples with similar gene expression and genes with similar expression patterns in the samples (two-way clustering). This illustration provides an unbiased look at breast cancer according to gene expression. The dendrogram at the top depicts the degree of similarity of the tissue samples: *yellow*, normal breast epithelium; *blue*, predominantly ER-positive cancers; *red*, basal-like or triple-negative cancers; and *green*, HER-2–positive cancers (in two clusters defined by the degree of lymphocytic infiltrate). The *stripes* at the top indicate grade (shades of darker purple are higher grades), ER expression (purple is positive; green is negative), and HER-2 (purple is positive; green is negative). *BRCA1* mutation was determined for other reasons in this experiment. (Courtesy Dr. Andrea Richardson, Department of Pathology, Brigham and Women's Hospital, Boston, MA.) *ER*, Estrogen receptor; *HER-2*, human epidermal growth factor receptor 2.

women with high-risk ER-positive breast cancer should receive adjuvant chemotherapy in addition to tamoxifen or other endocrine therapies (see "Endocrine Therapy" later on). Another multigene assay for determining prognosis is the MammaPrint assay. The MammaPrint assay analyzes data from 70 genes to develop a risk profile. The test provides a simple readout of low-risk or high-risk disease. This tool can be used for risk assessment in patients with ER-positive or ER-negative tumors. Tests based on critical combinations of genes will likely increasingly be used to guide clinical decision-making regarding breast cancer treatment.

Other Tumors of the Breast

Phyllodes tumors. Tumors of mixed connective tissue and epithelium constitute an important group of unusual primary breast tumors. On one end of the spectrum are benign fibroadenomas, which are characterized by a proliferation of connective tissue and a variable component of ductal elements that may appear compressed by the swirls of fibroblastic growth. Clinically more challenging are phyllodes tumors, which contain a biphasic proliferation of stroma and mammary epithelium. First called *cystosarcoma phyllodes*, these tumors are now called *phyllodes tumors* in recognition of their usually benign course. However, with increasing cellularity, an invasive margin, and sarcomatous appearance, these tumors may be classified as malignant phyllodes tumors. Benign phyllodes tumors are firm lobulated masses that can range in size, with an average size of approximately 5 cm (larger than average fibroadenomas). Histologically, benign phyllodes tumors are similar to fibroadenomas, but the whorled stroma forms larger clefts lined by epithelium that resemble clusters of leaf-like structures. The stroma is more cellular than in a fibroadenoma, but the fibroblastic cells are bland, and mitoses are infrequent.

Phyllodes tumors are seen on mammography as round densities with smooth borders and are indistinguishable from fibroadenomas. Ultrasonography may reveal a discrete structure with cystic spaces. The diagnosis is suggested by the larger size, history of rapid growth, and occurrence in older patients. Cytologic analysis is unreliable in differentiating a low-grade phyllodes tumor from a fibroadenoma. CNB is preferred, although it is difficult to classify phyllodes tumors with benign or intermediate malignant potential on the basis of a limited sampling. The final diagnosis is best made by excisional biopsy followed by careful pathologic review.

Local excision of a benign phyllodes tumor, similar to local excision of a fibroadenoma, is curative. Intermediate tumors, also called *borderline phyllodes tumors*, are tumors to which it is difficult to assign a benign classification. These tumors are treated by excision with negative margins (often suggested to be at least 1 cm) to prevent local recurrence. Affected patients are at some risk for local recurrence, most often within the first 2 years after excision. Close follow-up with examination and imaging allows early detection of recurrence.

At the other end of the spectrum of tumors of mixed connective tissue and epithelium are frankly malignant stromal sarcomas. Malignant phyllodes tumors are characterized by features such as cellular atypia, high number of mitoses, and stromal overgrowth, the extent of which is the main predictor of survival. These tumors are treated similarly to soft tissue sarcomas that occur on the trunk or extremities. Complete surgical excision of the entire tumor with a margin of normal tissue is advised. When the tumor is large with respect to the size of the breast, total mastectomy may be required. If mastectomy is performed and the margins are negative, radiation therapy is not recommended. If the margins are concerning or close, if the tumor involves the fascia or chest wall, or if the tumor is very large (>5 cm), irradiation of the chest wall is considered. If only wide local excision is performed, adjuvant radiation therapy is recommended. As with other soft tissue sarcomas, regional lymph node dissection is not required for staging or locoregional control. Metastases from malignant phyllodes tumors occur via hematogenous spread; common sites of metastasis include lung, bone, abdominal viscera, and mediastinum. Systemic therapeutic agents used for sarcomas have resulted in minimal success.

Angiosarcoma. Angiosarcoma, a rare vascular tumor (1% of all breast tumors), may occur de novo in the breast parenchyma or within the dermis of the breast after irradiation for breast cancer. Angiosarcoma has also been seen to develop in the upper extremity of patients with lymphedema, historically 10 to 15 years after radical mastectomy and irradiation. Angiosarcomas arising in the absence of previous radiation therapy or surgery (primary angiosarcomas) generally form an ill-defined mass within the parenchyma of the breast. In contrast, angiosarcomas caused by prior radiation therapy (secondary angiosarcomas) arise in the irradiated skin as purplish vascular proliferations that may go unrecognized for a period of time. The development of angiosarcoma in the ipsilateral arm to surgery is called Stewart-Treves syndrome and is secondary to long-standing lymphedema. The differential diagnosis is frequently between malignant angiosarcoma and atypical vascular proliferations in irradiated skin. Histologically, angiosarcoma is composed of an anastomosing tangle of blood vessels in the dermis and superficial subcutaneous fat. The atypical and crowded vessels invade through the dermis and into subcutaneous fat. These tumors are graded by the appearance and behavior of the associated endothelial cells. Pleomorphic nuclei, frequent mitoses, and stacking of the endothelial cells lining neoplastic vessels are features seen in higher-grade lesions. Necrosis, rarely seen in hemangiomas, is common in high-grade angiosarcomas. Clinically, radiation-induced angiosarcoma is identified as a reddish brown to purple raised rash within the radiation portals and on the skin of the breast or chest wall. As the disease progresses, tumors protruding from the surface of the skin may predominate.

Mammography is unrevealing in most cases of angiosarcoma. In the absence of metastatic disease at initial evaluation, surgery is performed to secure negative skin margins and usually involves a total mastectomy. A split-thickness skin graft or myocutaneous flap may be needed to replace a large skin defect created by the resection. Metastasis to regional nodes is extraordinarily rare, and axillary dissection is not required.

Patients remain at high risk for local recurrence after resection of angiosarcoma. For patients who present with primary angiosarcoma of the breast, radiation therapy is beneficial in locoregional treatment. Metastatic spread occurs hematogenously, most commonly to the lungs and bone and less frequently to the abdominal viscera, brain, and contralateral breast. Adjuvant chemotherapy is generally recommended and may improve outcomes of patients with angiosarcoma. Angiosarcomas can be divided into low-, intermediate-, and high-grade lesions with the commensurate survival being 91%, 68%, and 14%, respectively

STAGING OF BREAST CANCER

Breast cancer stage is determined clinically by physical examination and imaging studies before treatment, and breast cancer stage is determined pathologically by pathologic examination of the primary tumor and regional lymph nodes after definitive surgical treatment. Staging is performed to group patients into risk categories that define prognosis and guide treatment recommendations for patients with a similar prognosis. Breast cancer is classified with the tumor-node-metastasis (TNM) classification system, which groups patients into four stage groupings based on the size of the primary tumor (T), status of the regional lymph nodes (N), and presence or absence of distant metastasis (M). The most widely used system is that of the AJCC. This system is updated every 6 to 8 years to reflect current understanding of tumor behavior. The TNM classification is shown in Table 35.4.[12] Staging with the eighth edition of the AJCC has become much more complex as it includes T, N, and M as well as biologic markers (ER, PR, and HER-2), histologic grade, and, where applicable, Oncotype Dx score. For example, a tumor with the same TNM staging and molecular markers but with different Oncotype Dx scores can have different stages. A staging website is best utilized to determine stage (https://cancerstaging.org/About/news/Pages/

TABLE 35.4 **TNM classification for breast cancer (pathologic staging).**

Primary Tumor (T)	
TX	Primary tumor cannot be assessed
T0	No evidence of primary tumor
Tis	Carcinoma in situ
Tis (DCIS)	DCIS
Tis (LCIS)	LCIS
Tis (Paget)	Paget disease of the nipple not associated with invasive carcinoma or carcinoma in situ (DCIS and/or LCIS) in underlying breast parenchyma
T1	Tumor ≤20 mm in greatest dimension
T1mi	Tumor ≤1 mm in greatest dimension
T1a	Tumor >1 mm but ≤5 mm in greatest dimension
T1b	Tumor >5 mm but ≤10 mm in greatest dimension
T1c	Tumor >10 mm but ≤20 mm in greatest dimension
T2	Tumor >20 mm but ≤50 mm in greatest dimension
T3	Tumor >50 mm in greatest dimension
T4	Tumor of any size with direct extension to the chest wall and/or to the skin
T4a	Extension to the chest wall, not including only pectoralis muscle adherence or invasion
T4b	Ulceration and/or ipsilateral satellite nodules and/or edema of the skin
T4c	Both T4a and T4b
T4d	Inflammatory carcinoma
Regional Lymph Nodes (N)	
pNX	Regional lymph nodes cannot be assessed
pN0	No regional lymph node metastasis
pN0(i–)	No regional lymph node metastasis histologically, negative IHC
pN0(i+)	Malignant cells in regional lymph nodes no greater than 0.2 mm
pN0(mol–)	No regional lymph node metastasis histologically, negative molecular findings (IHC)
pN0(mol+)	Positive molecular findings (RT-PCR), but no metastasis detected by histology or IHC
pN1	Micrometastases; or metastases in one to three axillary nodes and/or in internal mammary nodes with metastases detected by sentinel lymph node biopsy but not clinically detected
pN1mi	Micrometastases (>0.2 mm and/or >200 cells but none >2.0 mm)
pN1a	Metastases in one to three axillary nodes; at least one metastasis >2.0 mm
pN1b	Metastases in internal mammary nodes with micrometastasis or macrometastases detected by sentinel lymph node biopsy (not clinically detected)
pN1c	Metastases in one to three axillary nodes and in internal mammary nodes with micrometastases or macrometastases detected by sentinel lymph node biopsy but not clinically detected
pN2	Metastases in four to nine axillary nodes or in clinically detected internal mammary lymph nodes in the absence of axillary lymph node metastases
pN2a	Metastases in four to nine axillary nodes (at least one tumor deposit >2.0 mm)
pN2b	Metastases in clinically detected internal mammary lymph nodes in the absence of axillary lymph node metastases
pN3	Metastases in ≥10 axillary nodes; or in infraclavicular (level III axillary nodes) or in clinically detected ipsilateral internal mammary lymph nodes in the presence of one or more positive level I, II axillary nodes; or in >3 axillary lymph nodes and internal mammary lymph nodes, with micrometastases or macrometastases detected by sentinel lymph node biopsy but not clinically detected; or in ipsilateral supraclavicular lymph nodes
Distant Metastases (M)	
M0	No clinical or radiographic evidence of distant metastases
cM0(i+)	No clinical or radiographic evidence of distant metastases, but deposits of molecularly or microscopically detected tumor cells in circulating blood, bone marrow, or other nonregional nodal tissue that are no larger than 0.2 mm in a patient without symptoms or signs of metastases
M1	Distant detectable metastases as determined by classic clinical and radiographic means and/or histologically proven larger than 0.2 mm

DCIS, Ductal carcinoma in situ; *IHC*, immunohistochemistry; *LCIS*, lobular carcinoma in situ; *RT-PCR*, reverse transcriptase polymerase chain reaction.
From Edge SB, Byrd DR, Compton CC, et al, eds. *AJCC Cancer Staging Manual*. 7th ed. New York: Springer-Verlag; 2010.

Updated-Breast-Chapter-for-8th-Edition.aspx). Metastasis to ipsilateral axillary nodes predicts outcome after surgical treatment more powerfully than tumor size. Before the incorporation of systemic therapies in the management of breast cancer, when treatment was with surgery alone, the survival rate decreased almost linearly with increasing nodal involvement.

Although staging is an important part of the initial assessment of breast cancer patients, it has traditionally been based on anatomic variables without other important prognostic factors. The new staging form has a place to record other variables, including tumor grade, ER status, PR status, HER-2 status, circulating tumor cells, disseminated tumor cells (in bone marrow), multigene recurrence score, and response to chemotherapy.

Some prefixes and suffixes are used with the cTNM (clinical) and pTNM (pathologic) staging systems to designate special cases. These do not affect the stage group but indicate that they must be analyzed separately. These prefixes and suffixes include the "m" suffix, which signifies multiple primary tumors, pT(m) NM; the "y" prefix, which denotes patients who have received systemic therapy before surgery, ypTNM; and the "r" prefix, which indicates a recurrent tumor, rTNM. In clinical practice, physicians use the anatomic stage grouping in addition to important biologic factors to determine risk and guide treatment recommendations.

SURGICAL TREATMENT OF BREAST CANCER

Historical Perspective

Through the mid-twentieth century, breast cancer was thought to arise in the breast and progress to other sites largely via centrifugal spread. In this model, more extensive surgical procedures were expected to reduce mortality by resecting locoregional disease before it could spread to distant sites. This model was supported, in part, by the results of the Halsted radical mastectomy, which was the first procedure that demonstrated improvements in breast cancer survival relative to the local excision of tumors. Introduced in the 1890s, the radical mastectomy included removal of the breast, overlying skin, and underlying pectoralis muscles in continuity with the regional lymph nodes along the axillary vein up to the costoclavicular ligament. The procedure often required a skin graft to cover the large skin defect that was created. This approach was well suited to breast cancer biology of the time, when most tumors were locally advanced, frequently with chest wall or skin involvement and extensive axillary nodal disease. Radical mastectomy provided improved local control and led to an increasing population of long-term survivors. Radical mastectomy continued to be the mainstay of surgical therapy into the 1970s.

Numerous women continued to die of metastatic breast cancer after radical mastectomy and even after more extensive surgical procedures, including radical mastectomy with en bloc resection of the internal mammary and supraclavicular nodes. This situation eventually led to a shift in the theory of primary centrifugal spread to the more modern theory that breast cancer spreads centrifugally to adjacent structures and via lymphatics and blood vessels to distant sites.

In the modern era, breast cancer treatment includes local and regional approaches (surgery and radiation therapy) in addition to medical therapies designed to treat systemic disease. Multimodality treatment approaches were the first to show significant improvements in locoregional control and survival. As breast cancer was being recognized at earlier stages, radical mastectomy was abandoned in favor of more conservative surgical approaches in combination with radiation therapy. The result was dramatic reductions in the extent of surgery required for local control of breast cancer and decreases in treatment-related morbidity. Breast cancer is a heterogeneous disease, and current treatment is guided by molecular properties of the individual patient's tumor as well as the size and location of the tumor.

Surgical Trials of Local Therapy for Operable Breast Cancer

Radical Mastectomy Versus Total Mastectomy With or Without Radiation Therapy

In the NSABP B-04 trial, patients with clinically negative nodes were randomly assigned to radical mastectomy, total mastectomy with irradiation of the chest wall and regional nodes, or total mastectomy alone with delayed axillary dissection if nodes became clinically enlarged. Patients did not receive systemic therapy. Patients with clinically positive nodes were randomly assigned to radical mastectomy or total mastectomy with irradiation of the chest wall and regional lymphatics. At 25 years of follow-up, overall survival (OS) and disease-free survival (DFS) were equivalent in all treatment arms within the node-positive and node-negative groups. Of the patients with clinically node-negative disease who underwent radical mastectomy, 38% were found to have nodal metastases at surgery, yet only 18% of patients undergoing total mastectomy without axillary dissection or radiation therapy developed axillary recurrence requiring delayed dissection. Those individuals with axillary bed recurrences and delayed axillary node resection did very poorly. However, OS was equivalent in all three groups.

Mastectomy Versus Breast-Conserving Therapy

Six prospective clinical trials that included more than 4500 patients compared mastectomy versus breast-conserving therapy (Table 35.5). In all these trials, there was no survival advantage for the use of mastectomy over breast preservation. The largest of these trials, NSABP B-06, enrolled 1851 patients with tumors up to 4 cm in diameter and clinically negative lymph nodes. Patients were randomly assigned to undergo modified radical mastectomy, lumpectomy alone, or lumpectomy with postoperative irradiation of the breast without an extra boost to the lumpectomy site. All patients with histologically positive axillary nodes received chemotherapy. At 20 years of follow-up, OS and DFS were the same in all three treatment groups.

NSABP B-06 provided valuable information about rates of ipsilateral breast cancer recurrence after lumpectomy, with or without breast irradiation. At 20 years of follow-up, local recurrence rates were 14.3% in women treated with lumpectomy and radiation therapy and 39.2% in women treated with lumpectomy alone ($P < 0.001$). For patients with positive nodes who received chemotherapy, the local recurrence rate was 44.2% for lumpectomy alone and 8.8% for lumpectomy plus radiation therapy.

Another important trial that evaluated breast-conserving therapy was the Milan I trial. This trial enrolled patients with smaller tumors and used more extensive surgery and radiation therapy than the NSABP B-06 trial. There were 701 women with tumors up to 2 cm and clinically negative nodes randomly assigned to undergo radical mastectomy or quadrantectomy with axillary dissection and postoperative irradiation. Patients with pathologically positive nodes received chemotherapy. OS at 20 years did not differ between the two groups. Locoregional failure rates differed between the groups: Chest wall recurrence occurred in 2.3% of women who underwent radical mastectomy, and ipsilateral breast tumor recurrence occurred in 8.8% of women who underwent quadrantectomy and radiation therapy (20-year follow-up). After quadrantectomy, local failure rates were higher in younger women, with rates of 1% per year in women younger than 45 years and 0.5% per year in older women.

TABLE 35.5 **Randomized trials comparing breast conservation versus mastectomy.**

TRIAL	NO. PATIENTS	MAXIMUM TUMOR SIZE (CM)	SYSTEMIC THERAPY	FOLLOW-UP (YEARS)	% SURVIVAL LUMPECTOMY + XRT	% SURVIVAL MASTECTOMY	LOCAL RECURRENCE (BCT) (%)
NSABP B-06[a]	1851	4	Yes	20	47	46	14*
Milan Cancer Institute[b]	701	2	Yes	20	44	43	8.8*
Institute Gustave-Roussy[c]	179	2	No	14	73	65	13
National Cancer Institute[d]	237	5	Yes	10	77	75	16
EORTC[e]	868	5	Yes	10	65	66	17.6
Danish Breast Cancer Group[f]	905	None	Yes	6	79	82	3

BCT, Breast-conserving therapy; *EORTC*, European Organization for Research and Treatment of Cancer; *NSABP*, National Surgical Adjuvant Breast and Bowel Project; *XRT*, radiation therapy.

*Includes only women whose excision margins were negative.

[a]Fisher B, Anderson S, Bryant J, et al. Twenty-year follow-up of a randomized trial comparing total mastectomy, lumpectomy, and lumpectomy plus irradiation for the treatment of invasive breast cancer. *N Engl J Med.* 2002;347:1233.

[b]Veronesi U, Cascinelli N, Mariani L, et al. Twenty-year follow-up of a randomized study comparing breast-conserving surgery with radical mastectomy for early breast cancer. *N Engl J Med.* 2002;347:1227.

[c]Arriagada R, Le M, Rochard F, et al. Conservative treatment versus mastectomy in early breast cancer: Patterns of failure with 15 years of follow-up data. *J Clin Oncol.* 1996;14:1558.

[d]Jacobson J, Danforth D, Cowan K, et al. Ten-year results of a comparison of conservation with mastectomy in the treatment of stage I and II breast cancer. *N Engl J Med.* 1995;332:907.

[e]van Dongen J, Voogd A, Fentiman I, et al. Long-term results of a randomized trial comparing breast-conserving therapy with mastectomy: European Organization for Research and Treatment of Cancer 10801 Trial. *J Natl Cancer Inst.* 2000;92:1143.

[f]Blichert-Toft M, Rose C, Andersen J, et al: Danish randomized trial comparing breast conservation therapy with mastectomy: six years of life-table analysis. Danish Breast Cancer Cooperative Group. *J Natl Cancer Inst Monogr.* 1992;11:19.

Three other randomized trials in patients with operable breast cancer found no survival benefit of mastectomy over breast-conserving therapy. In the European Organization for Research and Treatment of Cancer (EORTC) Trial 10801, in which 868 women were randomly assigned to modified radical mastectomy or lumpectomy and irradiation, there was no difference in survival at 10 years. This trial included patients with tumors up to 5 cm, and 80% of women enrolled had tumors larger than 2 cm. Positive margins were allowed, and the results showed lower rates of local recurrence with clear versus involved margins.

In the Institut Gustave-Roussy trial, 179 women with tumors smaller than 2 cm were randomly assigned to modified radical mastectomy or lumpectomy with a 2-cm margin of normal tissue around the cancer. No differences were observed between the two surgical groups in risk for death, metastases, contralateral breast cancer, or locoregional recurrence at 15 years of follow-up.

In the U.S. NCI trial, 237 women with tumors 5 cm or smaller were randomly assigned to lumpectomy with axillary dissection and radiation therapy or modified radical mastectomy. No differences were seen in OS or DFS rates at 10 years.

Planning Surgical Treatments

It is critical to establish the diagnosis of breast cancer firmly before initiation of definitive surgical treatment. CNB of a palpable or image-detected lesion is the preferred approach for diagnosis. Open surgical biopsy is reserved for lesions not amenable to CNB and cases in which CNB has proved nondiagnostic. Examination of biopsy material should provide information about tumor histologic type and grade, ER and PR status, and HER-2 status. Oncotype DX is indicated for patients with ER-positive, node-negative disease.

A history and physical examination, in addition to appropriate imaging studies, are important to establish the extent of disease and assign a clinical stage. The most common sites of distant metastases from breast cancer are the bone, liver, and lungs followed by brain. The National Comprehensive Cancer Network provides guidelines regarding the use of laboratory and radiologic testing in patients at initial diagnosis based on clinical stage. Computed tomography scans, bone scans, and other imaging studies are generally reserved for patients with clinically positive nodes, abnormalities on blood chemistry tests or chest radiographs, and for patients with locally advanced or inflammatory breast cancer. Thorough imaging of the ipsilateral and contralateral breast is performed to look for areas of concern other than the index lesion. Breast MRI may be used in selected cases to define the extent of tumor and look for additional breast lesions or to document response to neoadjuvant chemotherapy; however, there is no high-level evidence demonstrating that use of MRI to guide decisions regarding local therapy improves local recurrence rates or survival.

In the absence of metastatic disease, the first intervention for patients with early-stage breast cancer is surgery for excision of the tumor and surgical staging of the regional lymph nodes. Assessment of the primary tumor size and regional lymph nodes defines the pathologic stage and provides an estimate of the prognosis to inform decisions about systemic therapy. Patients with locally advanced and inflammatory breast cancers should receive systemic therapy before surgery (see "Neoadjuvant Systemic Therapy for Operable Breast Cancer" later on).

The selection of surgical procedures takes into account patient characteristics and other clinical and pathologic variables. Patient characteristics, including age, family history, menopausal status, and overall health, are assessed. Some patients may undergo

BOX 35.4 Contraindications to radiation.

Absolute
- Pregnancy

Relative
- Systemic scleroderma*
- Active systemic lupus erythematosus*
- Prior radiation to breast or chest wall
- Severe pulmonary disease
- Severe cardiac disease (if tumor is left sided)
- Inability to lie supine
- Inability to abduct arm on affected side
- *p53* mutation†

*Other collagen vascular diseases are not contraindications to radiation, although patients should not be taking immunosuppressants such as methotrexate because they are radiosensitizers.

†Patients with p53 mutations are highly susceptible to radiation-induced cancers.

genetic testing for *BRCA* or other gene mutations at the time of diagnosis. Patients with a known BRCA mutation are generally counseled toward bilateral mastectomy for treatment of the index breast and reduction of the risk of contralateral breast cancer. The location of the tumor within the breast and tumor size relative to breast size are evaluated. Patient preferences for breast preservation versus mastectomy are determined. For patients considering mastectomy, options for immediate reconstruction are discussed.

Selection of Surgical Therapy

Mastectomy and breast-conserving therapy have been shown to be equivalent in terms of patient survival, and the choice of surgical treatment is individualized. Patients who desire breast-conserving surgery must be willing to attend postoperative radiation therapy sessions and to undergo postoperative surveillance of the treated breast. Consultation with a radiation oncologist may be arranged before the planned surgery. Patients are advised about the risks and long-term sequelae of radiation therapy. A mastectomy is generally recommended for patients who have contraindications to radiation therapy (Box 35.4). Although pregnancy is an absolute contraindication to radiation therapy, many patients pregnant at diagnosis can complete their pregnancy and receive radiation therapy after delivery.

A significant factor in determining whether breast-conserving therapy is feasible is the relationship between tumor size and breast size. In general, the tumor must be small enough in relation to the breast size so that the tumor can be resected with adequate margins and acceptable cosmesis. In patients with large tumors for whom adjuvant (postoperative) systemic chemotherapy will likely be recommended, the use of preoperative chemotherapy may be considered. Chemotherapy administered before surgery may decrease the tumor size sufficiently to permit breast-conserving surgery in patients who would not otherwise appear to be good candidates. Another strategy is to consider oncoplastic breast surgery with local tissue rearrangement or pedicled myocutaneous flaps (latissimus dorsi) to fill the defect resulting from breast-conserving surgery.[13] Patients with multicentric tumors are usually served best by mastectomy because it is difficult to perform more than one breast-conserving surgery in the same breast with acceptable cosmesis, although clinical trials are ongoing to determine the feasibility of multiple resections followed by radiation therapy. Although high nuclear grade, presence of lymphovascular invasion, and negative steroid hormone receptor status all have been linked to increased local recurrence rates, none of these factors are considered contraindications to breast conservation.

Factors Influencing Eligibility for Breast Conservation

Randomized trials have demonstrated the efficacy of breast-conserving therapy for a wide variety of breast cancers and have defined eligibility criteria for breast conservation. With these criteria and current surgical and radiation therapy approaches, local recurrence rates after lumpectomy and radiation therapy are less than 5% at 10 years at many large centers.

Tumor Size

Tumors smaller than 5 cm tumors with clinically positive nodes, and tumors with lobular and ductal histology were included in the randomized trials of mastectomy versus breast-conserving therapy. In current practice, lumpectomy is considered when the tumor, regardless of size, can be excised with clear margins and an acceptable cosmetic result.

Margins

The appropriate margin width for lumpectomy specimens has been debated. Although the NSABP B-06 trial defined a negative margin as "no ink on tumor," other trials evaluating breast-conserving therapy did not specify a required margin width or did not evaluate microscopic margins. The optimal margin width has been open to interpretation, resulting in substantial variability in treatment and recommendations regarding the need for reexcision for wider margins. The Society of Surgical Oncology and American Society for Radiation Oncology convened a multidisciplinary panel to address the question of what margin width is required to minimize the risk of ipsilateral breast tumor recurrence.[14] The panel used a meta analysis of margin width and ipsilateral breast tumor recurrence from a systematic review of 33 studies including 28,162 patients. They found that positive margins, defined as ink on invasive carcinoma or DCIS, were associated with a twofold increase in ipsilateral breast tumor recurrence risk compared with negative margins. The risk was not affected by any specific clinicopathologic features, including favorable biology, use of endocrine therapy, or administration of a radiation boost. In addition, more widely clear margins than no ink on tumor did not significantly decrease the ipsilateral breast tumor recurrence risk, including in patients with unfavorable biology, lobular cancers, or cancers with an extensive intraductal component. The panel concluded that "no ink on tumor" should be used as the standard for an adequate margin in invasive breast cancer. European consensus groups vary on their recommendations for margin width ranging from 2 mm to 5 mm.

Histology

Invasive lobular cancers and cancers with an extensive intraductal component can be treated with lumpectomy if clear margins can be achieved. Atypical hyperplasia (ductal and lobular) and LCIS at resection margins do not increase local recurrence rates.

Patient Age

Local recurrence rates after breast-conserving surgery are higher for younger women than for older women. Local recurrence rates are reduced in patients of all ages with the use of radiation therapy. A radiation boost to the tumor bed has been shown to reduce local

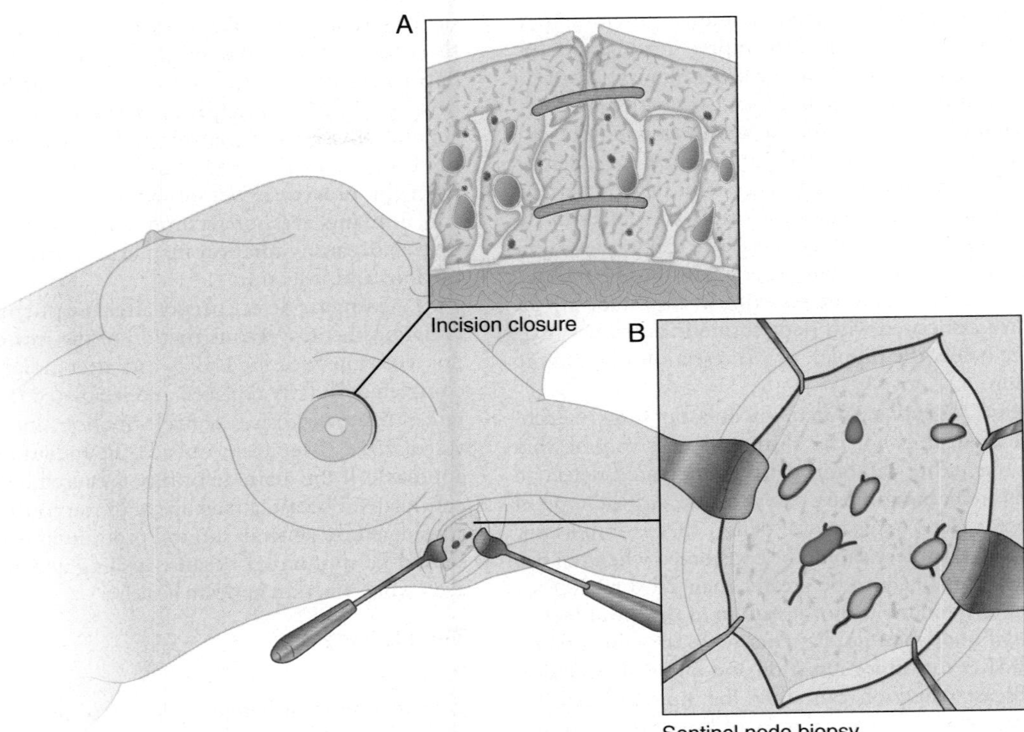

FIG. 35.11 Breast-conserving surgery. (A) Incisions to remove malignant tumors are placed directly over the tumor or around the areola. After the partial mastectomy has been completed, the parenchymal defect is closed *(inset)* to prevent a cosmetic deformity. (B) A transverse incision below the axillary hairline is used for sentinel node biopsy or axillary dissection. The boundaries of the axillary dissection are the axillary vein superiorly, the latissimus dorsi muscle laterally, and the chest wall medially. The inferior dissection enters the tail of Spence (the axillary tail of the breast). In sentinel node biopsy, a similar transverse incision is made, which may be located by percutaneous mapping with the gamma probe to detect a hot spot from the radiolabeled colloid. It is extended through the clavipectoral fascia, and the true axilla is entered. The sentinel node is located by staining with blue dye *(inset)*, radioactivity, or both and is dissected free as a single specimen.

failures after lumpectomy with negative margins, particularly in younger women.

Breast-Conserving Surgery

Technical Aspects

Excision of the primary tumor with preservation of the breast has been referred to by many terms, including *lumpectomy*, *partial mastectomy*, *segmental mastectomy*, *segmentectomy*, *tylectomy*, and *wide local excision*. Breast-conserving surgery removes the malignancy with a surrounding rim of grossly normal breast parenchyma. This procedure is depicted in Fig. 35.11, which shows the completed lumpectomy and skin incision for the axillary component of the procedure.

The breast specimen that is removed is oriented and its edges are inked before sectioning. Specimen radiography should be performed for all nonpalpable lesions or if there are microcalcifications associated with the palpable tumor. If a margin appears to be close or is positive histologically on intraoperative assessment, reexcision to remove more tissue frequently achieves a clear margin and allows conservation of the breast. Orientation of the surgical specimen allows focal reexcision of involved margins rather than global reexcision and improves the cosmetic result by reducing the amount of normal breast parenchyma that is excised.

There is level I evidence that shaved margins at the time of the lumpectomy reduces the need for reexcision.[15] The larger the volume of excision, the better the margin clearance, but the poorer the cosmetic result. The surgical defect created after lumpectomy is closed in cosmetic fashion. There is increasing interest in the use of advancement flap closure and other oncoplastic surgical techniques to maximize the cosmetic result.

Surgical staging of the axilla is performed through a separate incision in most patients undergoing breast conservation. SLND (see Fig. 35.11) has replaced anatomic axillary node dissection in patients with clinically negative axillary nodes. For patients who require axillary dissection, the extent of the dissection is identical to the axillary component of the modified radical mastectomy (see Fig. 35.11).

Cosmetic Challenges

The term *oncoplastic surgery* has been popularized to stress the importance of achieving the best possible esthetic result in the context of resecting the tumor with adequate oncologic margins. The goal is to retain as much of the natural breast size and contour as possible to provide optimal cosmesis and symmetry with the opposite breast. When the primary tumor is resected using an incision directly over the tumor and closure of the skin without reapproximation of any breast tissue, several deformities can occur, including volumetric deformity from a large parenchymal resection (retraction deformity when the seroma resorbs at the operative site); skin–pectoral muscle adherence deformity, in which the skin adheres to the underlying pectoral muscle; and lower pole deformity with downward turning of the nipple (bird beak deformity) caused by excision of a tumor in the lower hemisphere of the breast. These deformities can make it difficult for patients to wear tight-fitting clothing because significant asymmetry may be evident. It is important to correct these deformities before radiation therapy because the irradiation may further accentuate any asymmetry and make it more challenging to correct the defect in the future. The surgeon should consider oncoplastic techniques in the following situations: (1) a significant area of skin is to be resected with the tumor, (2) a large-volume resection is expected, (3) the tumor is in an area associated with poor cosmetic outcomes (e.g., lower hemisphere below the nipple), or (4) resection may lead to nipple malposition.

Extent of breast resection. When oncoplastic surgery techniques are considered, it is not the absolute breast volume that will be resected but rather the ratio of the anticipated defect to the volume of the remaining breast parenchyma and the type of parenchyma present (fatty replaced vs. dense) that is important. In general, oncoplastic surgery should be considered when the size of the surgical defect is likely to be greater than 20% to 30% of the breast volume and for any tumor resection in the lower breast.

Breast size and body habitus. Patients with large breasts are often good candidates for tumor resection and bilateral reduction mammaplasty. Breast reduction can allow for improved esthetic outcomes after resection of large volumes of breast tissue at any location. Obese patients should be considered for this approach because they are often poor candidates for autologous tissue reconstruction after mastectomy, and implants are often not large enough to recreate a breast proportional in size to the contralateral breast. Breast reduction surgery is a good option because this can relieve the symptoms of macromastia and allow for improved outcomes after breast irradiation.

Tumor location. Tumors lying directly under the nipple-areolar complex and tumors located between the nipple-areolar complex and inframammary fold require special attention to avoid nipple-areolar complex distortion and contour deformity. In general, the skin and well-vascularized breast parenchyma must be adjusted to correct for the removal of breast tissue in these areas. As noted, deformities in the contour will be exacerbated by radiation and may be more challenging to correct at a later date. Fig. 35.12 shows the various incisions for tumors located in different parts of the breast. Upper pole lesions can be served by a variety of techniques (Fig. 35.12A), including round block (one or more lesion in any quadrant but especially nice for upper inner quadrant lesions), crescent mastopexy (for those who need a minor lift), and batwing or hemi-batwing (for those who need more of a lift).

Lower pole lesions (Fig. 35.12B) may use techniques that require a mastopexy based on a superior pedicle flap. Lower outer lesions may require a J or V plasty to retain the shape of the breast. A Benelli includes a deepithelization circumferentially around the areola and is especially useful for the lower inner quadrant of the breast as well as a minor reduction in breast volume.

These techniques can also be used to correct defects left from previous surgeries.

Short-term follow-up shows that oncoplastic techniques have greater patient satisfaction, less complications, and less local recurrence.[16]

Timing of Oncoplastic Surgery

Immediate repair of a partial mastectomy defect is almost always preferred to a delayed approach. Oncoplastic techniques such as tissue advancement and local tissue rearrangement at the time of the initial surgical procedure tend to provide the optimal solution. This approach has not been associated with delay in delivery of adjuvant systemic therapy or radiation. In general, local tissue transfer and breast reduction surgery cannot be performed on the irradiated breast; it is preferable to perform the procedure before radiation therapy. Tissue expanders and implants are not recommended to fill partial mastectomy defects because radiation may lead to capsular contracture, distortion, and infection.

If a cosmetic defect occurs after breast-conserving surgery and radiation therapy, reconstruction of the treated breast is generally not recommended for 1 to 2 years after radiation therapy has been completed. In fatty replaced and irradiated tissue, there is a higher rate of tissue necrosis, seroma formation, and infection. The use of vascularized tissue from outside the radiation field is the favored approach. If the main deformity is caused by asymmetry with the contralateral breast, a mastopexy of the contralateral breast can be considered. In general, surgical procedures on the irradiated breast should be minimized because healing and recovery are impaired even when the skin appears healthy.

Mastectomy

Indications

Certain tumors still require mastectomy, including tumors that are large relative to breast size, tumors with extensive calcifications on mammography, tumors for which clear margins cannot be obtained on wide local excision, and tumors in patients with contraindications to breast irradiation (see Box 35.4). Patient preference for mastectomy or a desire to avoid radiation is also a valid indication for mastectomy.

Postmastectomy Breast Reconstruction

Breast reconstruction may be performed immediately—that is, the same day as mastectomy—or as delayed reconstruction, months or years later. Immediate reconstruction has the advantages of preserving the maximum amount of breast skin for use in reconstruction, combining the recovery period for both procedures, and avoiding a period of time without a breast mound. Immediate reconstruction does not have a detrimental effect on long-term survival, local recurrence rates, or detection of local recurrence. Reconstruction may or may not be delayed in patients who might require postmastectomy radiation therapy. Reconstruction options include tissue expander/implant and autologous tissue reconstructions, most often with transverse rectus abdominis muscle flaps, latissimus dorsi flaps, or muscle-preserving perforator abdominal flaps.

Technical Details

Simple or total mastectomy refers to complete removal of the mammary gland, including the nipple and areola. Modified radical mastectomy refers to removal of the mammary gland, nipple, and areola, with the addition of a complete axillary lymph node dissection (ALND) (Fig. 35.13). For either a total mastectomy or a modified radical mastectomy, an elliptical skin incision is planned to include the nipple and areola and usually any previous excisional biopsy scars (see Fig. 35.13). Skin flaps are raised to separate the underlying gland from the overlying skin along the subdermal plexus (see Fig. 35.13). If immediate reconstruction is not planned, sufficient skin is taken to allow smooth closure of skin flaps without redundant skin folds; this facilitates comfortable use of a breast prosthesis.

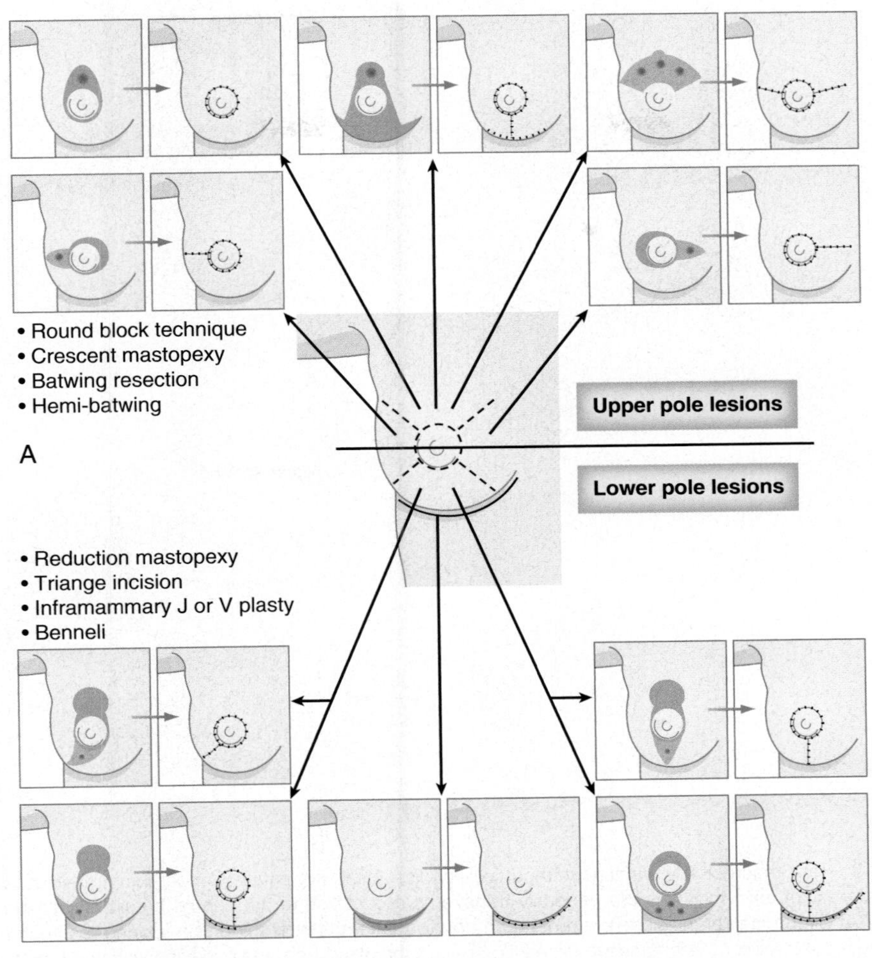

FIG. 35.12 The various incisions for tumors located in different parts of the breast. (A) Upper pole lesions can be served by a variety of techniques, including round block, crescent mastopexy, and batwing or hemi-batwing. (B) Lower pole lesions may use techniques that require a mastopexy based on a superior pedicle flap. Including reduction mastopexy, triangle insision, J or V plasty, and Benneli. (Adapted from Fitoussi A, Berry MG, Couturaud B, et al. *Oncoplastic and reconstructive surgery for breast cancer: The Institut Curie Experience.* Paris: Springer; 2008.)

If immediate reconstruction is planned, a skin-sparing mastectomy may be performed in which only the nipple-areola complex is removed and the maximum amount of skin is left for use in the reconstruction. Nipple-areola–sparing mastectomy has been used with increasing frequency for selected patients with breast cancer. Multiple studies have shown the safety and feasibility of this approach, with many series showing comparably low recurrence rates in patients undergoing nipple-areola–sparing mastectomy (Table 35.6). Nipple-areola–sparing mastectomy has also been demonstrated to be safe in patients undergoing prophylactic mastectomy for risk reduction, including *BRCA1* and *BRCA2* gene mutation carriers.[17]

Breast tissue is separated from the underlying pectoralis muscle, and the pectoral fascia is generally taken with the breast specimen. In a total mastectomy (see Fig. 35.13), breast tissue is separated from the axillary contents, and all breast tissue superficial to the fascia of the axilla is removed. In a modified radical mastectomy, the level I and II axillary lymph nodes are taken with the axillary breast tissue (see Fig. 35.13). Level I nodes are nodes inferior to the axillary vein and lateral to the pectoralis minor muscle, and level II nodes are nodes anterior or posterior to the pectoralis minor.

Lymph Node Staging

The pathologic status of the axillary lymph nodes is one of the most important prognostic factors in patients with breast cancer. Identification of metastatic tumor deposits in the axillary nodes indicates a poorer prognosis and often prompts a recommendation for more aggressive systemic and locoregional therapies.

Historical Perspective

Historically, ALND was a routine component of the surgical management of breast cancer. It provides prognostic information about axillary nodal status and plays a therapeutic role in

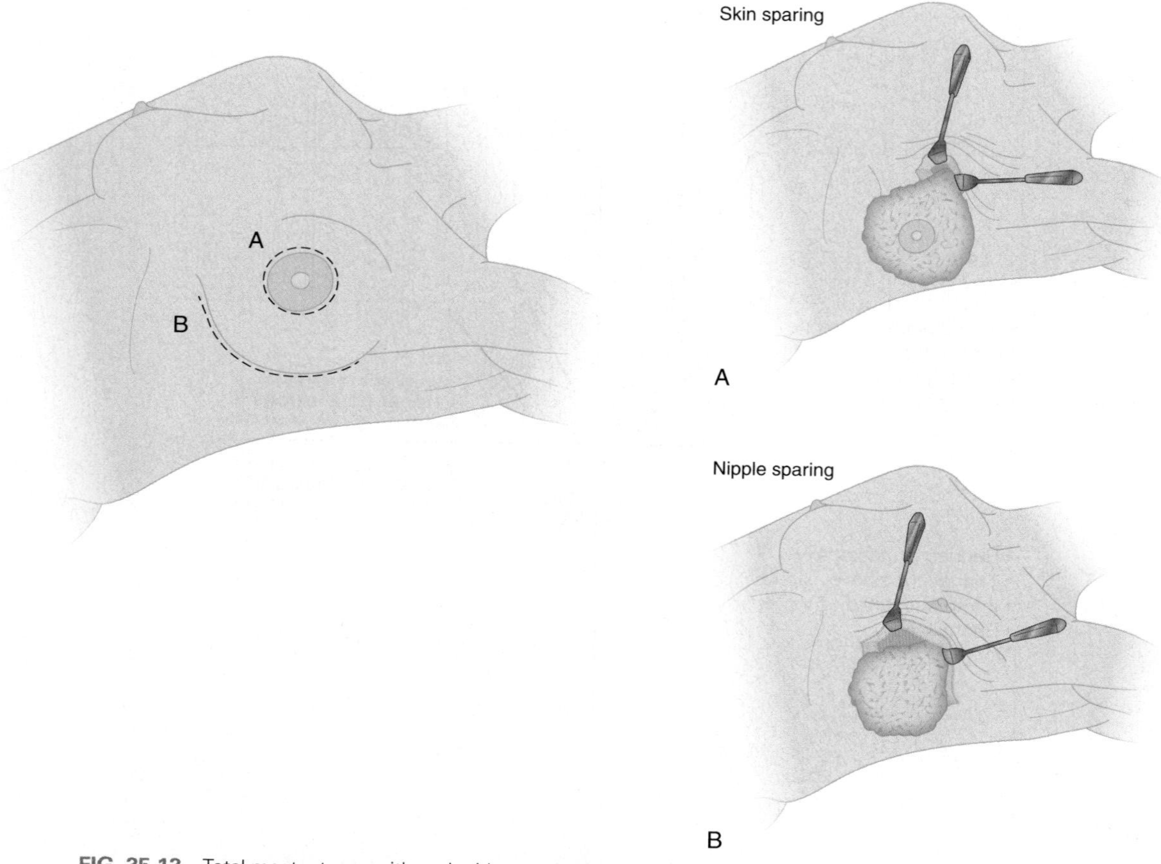

FIG. 35.13 Total mastectomy with and without axillary dissection. For patients undergoing mastectomy without reconstruction, skin incisions are generally transverse and surround the central breast and nipple-areolar complex. (A) Circumareolar incisions are most common for patients undergoing skin-sparing mastectomy with immediate reconstruction. Skin flaps are raised to separate the gland from the overlying skin and then the gland from the underlying muscle. Simple mastectomy divides the breast from the axillary contents and stops at the clavipectoral fascia. If axillary staging is planned, this is generally performed through a separate transverse axillary incision. (B) An inframammary incision is shown for nipple-areolar–sparing mastectomy.

removing axillary disease in patients with positive nodes. The surgical procedure includes clearance of node-bearing tissue between the pectoralis major and latissimus dorsi muscles from the edge of the breast tissue in the low axillary region to the axillary vein and removal of the nodes posterior to the pectoralis minor muscle. Axillary dissection is the main source of morbidity in patients with early-stage breast cancer. The immediate problems include acute pain and paresthesias, need for hospitalization, reduced range of motion at the shoulder joint, and need for a drain in the surgical bed for 7 to 10 days. Long-term problems resulting from axillary dissection include lymphedema of the ipsilateral arm, numbness, chronic pain, and reduced range of motion at the shoulder joint.

Sentinel Lymph Node Dissection

Identification of the first, or sentinel, node draining the area of the primary tumor in the breast allows for a more selective approach to the axilla. The sentinel node is the most likely node to contain metastatic disease, if present, and the pathologist can focus the examination on the sentinel node(s) without the added cost and time required to examine the full axillary contents. The technique of SLND was developed to reduce the morbidity associated with axillary surgery, while still providing accurate staging information. Many patients now present with clinically node-negative disease, and SLND can identify those patients with node-positive disease who may benefit from completion of ALND. Patients with negative sentinel lymph nodes can avoid the morbidity of axillary dissection. In sentinel node surgery, radiolabeled colloid, blue dye, or both are injected into breast tissue at the site of the primary tumor; the material passes through the lymphatics to the first draining node(s), where it accumulates. The procedure can also be performed with injection of the mapping agents that can be injected subareolar position or in a subdermal location overlying the site of the primary tumor. The sentinel node is identified as a blue, radioactive, fluorescent, or magnetic node or a combination of these. If the pathologic analysis of the sentinel node is negative for evidence of metastasis, the likelihood that other nodes are involved is sufficiently low that ALND is not required.

The NSABP B-32 trial was a critical study evaluating SLND.[18] In that study, 5611 patients with clinically node-negative breast cancer were randomly assigned to undergo SLND plus ALND or SLND with ALND only if the sentinel node was positive. The sentinel node was positive in 26% of patients in both groups. For patients with a pathologically negative sentinel node ($n = 3986$), in whom the primary analysis was performed, there was no difference in OS, DFS, or regional control rates, demonstrating that when the sentinel node is negative, SLND alone without further ALND is appropriate for patients with clinically negative lymph nodes. A randomized trial conducted at the European Institute of Oncology

TABLE 35.6 **Studies on nipple and local recurrence rates in patients undergoing nipple-areola–sparing mastectomy.**

AUTHOR	YEAR	PROCEDURES N	FOLLOW-UP (MONTHS)	NAC RECURRENCE (%)	LOCAL RECURRENCE (%)
Crowe[a]	2004	54	NA	10*	NA
Margulies[b]	2005	50	7.9	0	0
Boneti[c]	2011	281	25.3	0	7
Filho[d]	2011	157	10	0	0
Jenson[e]	2011	127	60	0	0
Peled[f]	2012	412	28	0	2
Loshiriwat[g]	2012	934	64	0	0
Coopey[h]	2013	156	22	0	2.6
Krajewski[i]	2015	226	24	0	1.7
Orzalesi[j]	2016	755	36	0.6	2.9
Smith[k]	2017	2182	51	0	3.7
Radovanovic[l]	2018	441	108	5.4*	7.3
Galimberti[m]	2018	1989	94	1.8	5.3

*Nipple-areolar complex involved at the time of surgery and excised.
[a]Crowe JP Jr, Kim JA, Yetman R, et al. Nipple-sparing mastectomy: technique and results of 54 procedures. *Arch Surg.* 2004;139:148–150.
[b]Margulies AG, Hochberg J, Kepple J, et al. Total skin-sparing mastectomy without preservation of the nipple-areola complex. *Am J Surg.* 2005;190:907–912.
[c]Boneti C, Yuen J, Santiago C, et al. Oncologic safety of nipple skin-sparing or total skin-sparing mastectomies with immediate reconstruction. *J Am Coll Surg.* 2011;212:686–693; discussion 693–685.
[d]de Alcantara Filho P, Capko D, Barry JM, et al. Nipple-sparing mastectomy for breast cancer and risk-reducing surgery: the Memorial Sloan-Kettering Cancer Center experience. *Ann Surg Oncol.* 2011;18:3117–3122.
[e]Jensen JA, Orringer JS, Giuliano AE. Nipple-sparing mastectomy in 99 patients with a mean follow-up of 5 years. *Ann Surg Oncol.* 2011;18:1665–1670.
[f]Warren Peled A, Foster RD, Stover AC, et al. Outcomes after total skin-sparing mastectomy and immediate reconstruction in 657 breasts. *Ann Surg Oncol.* 2012;19:3402–3409.
[g]Lohsiriwat V, Martella S, Rietjens M, et al. Paget's disease as a local recurrence after nipple-sparing mastectomy: clinical presentation, treatment, outcome, and risk factor analysis. *Ann Surg Oncol.* 2012;19:1850–1855.
[h]Coopey SB, Tang R, Lei L, et al. Increasing eligibility for nipple-sparing mastectomy. *Ann Surg Oncol.* 2013;20:3218–3222.
[i]Krajewski AC, Boughey JC, Degnim AC, et al. Expanded indications and improved outcomes for nipple-sparing mastectomy over time. *Ann Surg Oncol.* 2015;22:3317–3323.
[j]Orzalesi L, Casella D, Santi C, et al. Nipple sparing mastectomy: surgical and oncological outcomes from a national multicentric registry with 913 patients (1006 cases) over a six year period. *The Breast.* 2016;25:75–81.
[k]Smith BL, Tang R, Rai U, et al. Oncologic safety of nipple-sparing mastectomy in women with breast cancer. *J Am Coll Surg.* 2017;225:361–365.
[l]Radovanovic Z, Ranisavljevic M, Radovanovic D, et al. Nipple-sparing mastectomy with primary implant reconstruction: surgical and oncological outcome of 435 breast cancer patients. *Breast Care (Basel).* 2018;13:373–378.
[m]Galimberti V, Morigi C, Bagnardi V, et al. Oncological outcomes of nipple-sparing mastectomy: a single-center experience of 1989 patients. *Ann Surg Oncol.* 2018;25:3849–3857.

and numerous single-institution reports confirmed the findings from the NSABP B-32 trial showing that the technique is accurate. Identification of the sentinel node allows for a more detailed analysis of the lymph node most likely to have a positive yield.

In general, pathologists section the sentinel node along its short axis and submit all the sections for paraffin embedding of the tissues. The paraffin blocks can be sectioned and examined with hematoxylin-eosin staining of sections from each block. Some pathologists perform more detailed analysis of the sentinel nodes with step-sectioning of the paraffin blocks and immunohistochemical staining for cytokeratin, which enhances sensitivity by allowing detection of micrometastases. However, the clinical relevance of these micrometastases and small tumor deposits detected by immunohistochemical techniques has been questioned. The NSABP B-32 trial provided an opportunity to investigate the clinical significance of occult metastatic disease. For patients with negative sentinel nodes by hematoxylin-eosin staining, additional sections were evaluated by immunohistochemistry to identify occult metastases. The 5-year DFS rate was 86.4% for patients with occult metastases compared with 89.2% for patients without occult metastases (absolute difference = 2.8%), and the 5-year OS rate was 94.6% for patients with occult metastases compared with 95.8% for patients without occult metastases (absolute difference = 1.2%). These differences were statistically significant given the large number of patients enrolled in the study; however, because the absolute differences were small, the NSABP investigators concluded that the presence of occult metastases was not clinically significant. This conclusion was confirmed by the American College of Surgeons Oncology Group (ACOSOG) Z0010 trial, which was designed to evaluate the significance of sentinel node and bone marrow micrometastases in patients with early-stage breast cancer undergoing breast-conserving therapy.[19] In that study, the 5-year DFS rates for patients with immunohistochemistry-positive and immunohistochemistry-negative sentinel nodes were 90% and 92%, respectively ($P = 0.82$), whereas the 5-year OS rates were 95% and 96%, respectively ($P = 0.64$).

Lymphatic Mapping Technique and Selection of Patients for Sentinel Lymph Node Dissection

Lymphatic mapping can be performed with a combination of ^{99m}Tc-labeled sulfur colloid and a vital blue dye, isosulfan blue (Lymphazurin), fluorescence, magnetic particles, or with a single agent for localization of the sentinel node(s). Studies indicate that using the combination technique may result in the lowest possible false-negative rate. Preoperative lymphoscintigraphy can provide information on the specific nodal basins draining the primary tumor. Using a peritumoral injection technique, approximately 70% of patients have drainage to the axilla, 20% have drainage to the axilla and the internal mammary nodal basin, 2% to 3% have drainage to the internal mammary nodal basin alone, and 8% do not show any drainage to the regional nodal basins. If a subareolar or subdermal injection technique is used, drainage is seen almost exclusively in the axillary nodal basins. A dose of 2.5 mCi of ^{99m}Tc-labeled sulfur colloid can be injected on the day before surgery for preoperative lymphoscintigraphy; this allows for adequate activity to remain in the sentinel nodes for the intraoperative lymphatic mapping procedure the following day without the need for reinjection. Alternatively, for surgeons not using preoperative lymphoscintigraphy, 0.5 to 1.0 mCi of ^{99m}Tc-labeled sulfur colloid can be injected in the operating suite and avoids the preoperative pain and vasovagal events.

In the operating suite, 3 to 5 mL of blue dye can be injected peritumorally, and the injection site is massaged to facilitate passage of the dye through the lymphatics. A handheld gamma probe is used to localize transcutaneously the area of increased radioactivity; this helps to guide placement of the incision for the sentinel node procedure. After the incision is made, an area of increased radioactivity is localized with the handheld gamma probe, and the surgeon visualizes blue lymphatic channels leading to the sentinel node. Dissection is performed to avoid prematurely disrupting the afferent lymphatics. If a blue-stained lymphatic channel or a specific area of radioactivity ("hot spot") cannot be identified, the primary tumor can be resected to remove the site of injection, decreasing the background shine-through radioactivity. The sentinel node may be identified and removed, after which the nodal basin is checked again to confirm that the level of radioactivity has decreased. If the level of radioactivity remains high, additional sentinel nodes may remain in the nodal basin, and additional dissection should be completed to remove all sentinel nodes. Published studies have demonstrated an average of two or three sentinel nodes per patient.

Surgeons experienced in SLND can identify a sentinel node in more than 95% of patients. The false-negative rate for sentinel node surgery ranges from 0% to 11%, as reported in the NSABP B-32 trial.[18] Surgeons should be trained in SLND before using this procedure as a staging tool. Patients who present with clinically palpable lymph nodes should be evaluated with axillary ultrasonography and fine-needle aspiration biopsy (FNAB) of the nodes. If axillary metastasis is confirmed, patients can proceed directly to standard axillary node dissection or be considered for preoperative chemotherapy. If axillary metastasis is not confirmed by FNAB, patients can proceed to sentinel node surgery for staging.

Some studies have shown that patients who have undergone previous excisional biopsy of the primary tumor are more likely to have a false-negative sentinel node.[18] The lymphatics may be disrupted by the biopsy, which can affect drainage patterns of the area surrounding the excisional biopsy site. To avoid this scenario, CNB is the preferred diagnostic approach in patients suspected to have breast cancer.

In older studies, SLND was reported to be less accurate in patients treated with preoperative chemotherapy. A meta analysis of the published studies on sentinel node surgery after chemotherapy suggested that this technique is accurate; a more recent comparison showed that false-negative rates after chemotherapy compared favorably with false-negative rates observed in patients who undergo surgery first.[20]

Outcomes of Sentinel Lymph Node Dissection

Morbidity rates are substantially lower with SLND than with ALND. Another advantage is that SLND can be performed as an outpatient procedure and does not require a drain. Patients have more rapid return to full mobility and are able to return to work and other activities weeks sooner than after axillary dissection. Long-term morbidity, including lymphedema, numbness, and chronic pain, is greatly reduced.

SLND has been shown to provide reliable pathologic staging of the axilla, with false-negative rates generally less than 5% in experienced hands. Axillary recurrence rates have been shown to be extremely low after a negative sentinel node biopsy without axillary dissection. A negative sentinel node is now widely accepted as sufficient to establish node-negative disease in a patient, with no further axillary treatment required.[18]

When the sentinel node contains metastatic disease, the likelihood of additional involved nodes is directly proportional to the size of the primary breast tumor, presence of lymphatic vascular invasion, and size of the lymph node metastasis. Although ALND has been standard practice for patients with positive sentinel nodes, the need for ALND in all patients with a positive sentinel node has been called into question because many patients have small-volume metastases, and the sentinel node is often the only positive node. A meta analysis of studies evaluating patients with positive sentinel nodes showed that 53% of patients have additional positive nodes at ALND. In the case of micrometastatic disease in the sentinel nodes, the rate of nonsentinel node involvement is 20%, and for patients with isolated tumor cells, it is less than 12%. These findings led to a trend of omitting ALND in selected patients with positive sentinel nodes. An analysis of SEER data from the years 1998 to 2004 revealed that 16% of patients with sentinel node–positive disease did not undergo ALND. These patients were more commonly older patients with low-grade, ER-positive tumors. During this time period, the proportion of patients with micrometastasis in the sentinel node who did not undergo ALND increased from 21% to 38%. A review of the National Cancer Data Base data from the years 1998 to 2005 revealed similar findings, with 20.8% of patients with sentinel node–positive disease avoiding ALND. There were no differences in axillary recurrence rates or survival between patients who had sentinel node surgery only and patients who underwent ALND.

The ACOSOG initiated a prospective randomized trial in 1999 designed specifically to evaluate the impact of ALND on locoregional recurrence and survival in patients with early-stage breast cancer.[21,22] The trial now with 10-year follow-up, ACOSOG Z0011, enrolled patients with clinical T1 or T2 breast cancer with one or two positive sentinel nodes who were planning to undergo breast-conserving surgery and whole breast irradiation (WBI). Patients were randomly assigned to undergo completion ALND or no further surgery (sentinel node surgery alone). The primary end point of the Z0011 study was OS; secondary end points were locoregional recurrence and lymphedema. Patients enrolled in the Z0011 study had relatively favorable disease characteristics: The median age was 55 years, 70% of patients had T1 tumors, 82% had ER-positive tumors, 71% had only one positive sentinel node, and 44% had micrometastases. At a median follow-up of 9.3 years, the 10-year OS was 86.3% in the SLND-alone group and 83.6% in the ALND group (P = 0.02). The 10-year DFS was 80.2% in the SLND-alone group and 78.2% in the ALND group (P = 0.32). Ten-year regional recurrence did not differ significantly between the two groups. The Z0011 study investigators concluded that ALND may be safely omitted in patients with early-stage breast cancer with a positive sentinel node who are undergoing breast-conservation surgery (BCS), have one to two positive nodes, and receive whole breast radiation and systemic therapy. This study did not include mastectomy patients. Trials are ongoing to determine the feasibility of omitting ALND in mastectomy patients. It should be noted, however, that there was no significant difference in lymphedema seen between the groups. This may be because this trial included WBI, which in most patients included the Level I axilla or higher.

Conventional wisdom teaches that the lymphatics reside juxtaposed to the vein, and if the surgeon can avoid skeletonizing the vein, then the risk of lymphedema could be minimized or avoided (Fig. 35.2). If this were the case, then SLND should have cured the problem of surgical lymphedema. In fact, lymphatics are seen from the SLN incision nearly one-third of the time. In the more than 10 randomized studies of SLND versus ALND for breast cancer, the lymphedema rate varies between 0% and 13% for SLND and 7% and 77% for ALND. From these varying rates, it is obvious that not everyone is performing the same procedure. Klimberg and colleagues developed the axillary reverse mapping (ARM) procedure to intraoperatively recognize the lymphatic drainage of the upper extremity and preserve it. The procedure consists of radioactivity in the breast and blue dye in the arm (split mapping) in order to identify and protect the lymphatics draining the upper extremity. In a 26-month median follow-up of a phase II trial of 654 patients receiving SLND or ALND with ARM, the rate of lymphedema was less than 1% and 6%, respectively.[23] When any cut lymphatics were reapproximated, the rate of lymphedema was nil for either group. Alliance 221702 is a randomized trial that will further determine the efficacy of ARM.

ALND remains the standard of care for patients with locally advanced breast cancer or inflammatory breast cancer, patients with a positive sentinel node who are scheduled for mastectomy, patients with a positive sentinel node who are scheduled for accelerated partial breast irradiation (PBI), and patients with clinically positive nodes as well as a positive sentinel node after neoadjuvant chemotherapy.

TREATMENT OF DUCTAL CARCINOMA IN SITU

DCIS, or intraductal cancer, accounts for approximately 25% of all newly diagnosed breast cancers. It was anticipated that more than 63,960 new cases of DCIS would be diagnosed in 2016. Most cases of DCIS are detected as an area of clustered calcifications on a screening mammogram without an associated palpable abnormality. Rarely, DCIS manifests as a palpable mass or as unilateral, single-duct nipple discharge.

Findings on mammography in patients with DCIS include clustered calcifications without an associated density in 75% of patients, calcifications coexisting with an associated density in 15%, and a density alone in 10%. The calcifications seen on a mammogram generally correspond to areas within the central involved duct in which there is often necrosis and debris. DCIS calcifications tend to cluster closely together, are pleomorphic, and may be linear or branching, suggesting their ductal origin.

DCIS is viewed as a precursor to invasive ductal cancer, and treatment aims to remove the DCIS to prevent progression to invasive disease. Because the prevalence of metastatic disease in patients with DCIS without demonstrable invasion is low (<1%), systemic chemotherapy is not required. Hormonal therapy may be used for prevention of new primary tumors and to improve local control after breast-conserving therapy but is generally recommended only when the DCIS is positive for ER on immunohistochemistry.

Treatment recommendations for a patient with DCIS are based on the extent of disease within the breast, histologic grade, ER status, and presence of microinvasion as well as patient age and preference. Treatment options for DCIS include mastectomy, breast-conserving surgery with irradiation, and breast-conserving surgery alone. When the patient is treated with breast conservation or unilateral mastectomy, there is also the option of adjuvant hormonal therapy with tamoxifen to reduce the risk of local recurrence or contralateral breast cancer.

Mastectomy

Local recurrence of DCIS is ~1% to 2% per year when treated with BCS versus 1% to 2% lifetime when treated with mastectomy. The survival rates with either treatment are the same, 98% to 99%.

Reasons to select total mastectomy for treatment of DCIS include the following:

1. Diffuse suspicious mammographic calcifications suggestive of extensive disease
2. Inability to obtain clear margins with breast-conserving surgery
3. Likelihood of a poor cosmetic result after breast-conserving surgery
4. Patient not motivated to comply with follow-up surveillance imaging
5. Patient choice
6. Contraindications to radiation therapy (see Box 35.4)

Breast-Conserving Therapy

As for invasive breast cancer, breast-conserving therapy for DCIS requires resection to microscopically clear margins. The Consensus Conference on DCIS[24] that more widely clear margins do not significantly decrease ipsilateral breast tumor recurrence compared with 2-mm margins was based on a meta analysis of 20 studies.[25] The use of adjuvant whole breast radiation therapy has been demonstrated in prospective randomized trials to decrease the risk for local recurrence. The use of hormonal therapy in patients with ER-positive DCIS can decrease further the risk for local recurrence and reduces the risk for development of new contralateral and ipsilateral breast cancers.

The use of radiation therapy after lumpectomy was investigated in four prospective randomized trials (Table 35.7), the results of which are remarkably consistent. In the NSABP B-17 trial, 818 women with DCIS were randomly assigned to lumpectomy alone versus lumpectomy plus 50 Gy of postoperative WBI. The addition of radiation to surgery decreased the ipsilateral recurrence rate from 30.8% to 14.9% ($P < 0.000005$), as shown by 12-year actuarial recurrence data. The addition of radiation also decreased the incidence of invasive breast cancer, from 16.4% to 7.1% ($P < 0.00001$), and produced a smaller decrease in the incidence of in situ recurrence, from 14.1% to 7.8% ($P < 0.001$) (see Table 35.7). In the EORTC 10853 trial, 1010 women with DCIS were randomly assigned to lumpectomy alone versus lumpectomy plus 50 Gy of radiation therapy. Radiation reduced the 10-year breast recurrence rate from 26% to 15% ($P < 0.0001$) and reduced the rate of invasive recurrences from 13% to 8% (P = 0.0011). The UK ANZ (United Kingdom, Australia, and New Zealand) trial, which included 1701 patients, was a large randomized trial

TABLE 35.7 Randomized trials of lumpectomy for ductal carcinoma in situ: impact of radiation therapy and tamoxifen.

			LOCAL RECURRENCE RATES (%)			
TRIAL	NO. PATIENTS	FOLLOW-UP (YEAR)	LUMPECTOMY	LUMPECTOMY + XRT	LUMPECTOMY + XRT + TAMOXIFEN	*P* VALUE
NSABP B-17[a]	818	12	30.8	14.9		<.000005
EORTC 10853[b]	1010	4.25	16	9		<.005
UK ANZ	1701	5	20	8	6	<.0001
SweDCIS	1067	5	7	22		<.0001
NSABP B-24[c]	1804	7		9	6	.04

EORTC, European Organization for Research and Treatment of Cancer; *NSABP*, National Surgical Adjuvant Breast and Bowel Project; *SweDCIS*, Swedish Ductal Carcinoma In Situ trial; *UK ANZ*, United Kingdom, Australia, and New Zealand; *XRT*, radiation therapy.

[a]Fisher B, Dignam J, Wolmark N, et al. Lumpectomy and radiation therapy for the treatment of intraductal breast cancer: findings from National Surgical Adjuvant Breast and Bowel Project B-17. *J Clin Oncol*. 1998;16:441.

[b]Julien JP, Bijker N, Fentiman IS, et al. Radiotherapy in breast-conserving treatment for ductal carcinoma in situ: first results of the EORTC randomised phase III trial 10853. EORTC Breast Cancer Cooperative Group and EORTC Radiotherapy Group. *Lancet*. 2000;355:528.

[c]Fisher B, Land S, Mamounas E, et al. Prevention of invasive breast cancer in women with ductal carcinoma in situ: an update of the National Surgical Adjuvant Breast and Bowel Project experience. *Semin Oncol*. 2001;28:400.

that simultaneously evaluated the benefits of radiation therapy and tamoxifen after breast-conserving surgery for patients with DCIS. This trial also demonstrated that radiation therapy reduced the risk of breast cancer recurrence (hazard ratio [HR], 0.38; $P < 0.0001$) and invasive breast cancer recurrence (HR, 0.45; $P = 0.01$). Finally, the SweDCIS trial included 1067 patients with DCIS. After a median follow-up of 5 years, the cumulative incidence of breast recurrence was 22% in the group that underwent surgery only versus 7% in the group that underwent surgery plus radiation therapy ($P < 0.0001$).

Attempts have been made to identify subsets of DCIS for which wide excision without irradiation would provide sufficient local control. Silverstein[26] derived the Van Nuys criteria for classifying DCIS from a series of patients with DCIS treated by wide excision with and without radiation therapy. A system was proposed to identify patients who do not need radiation therapy because they have a low DCIS nuclear grade, a small lesion (<1.4 cm), older age (>60), and wide surgical margins (>1 cm). Silverstein reported low breast recurrence rates with surgery alone for patients with favorable Van Nuys scores. However, in a prospective trial testing this approach, investigators from Harvard enrolled 158 patients from the most favorable Van Nuys subset (low-grade or intermediate-grade DCIS <2.5 cm, with a minimum 1-cm margin on excision) and were unable to reproduce the results; the Harvard investigators stopped the trial early because the rates of recurrence exceeded the predefined stopping rules. More recently, Eastern Cooperative Oncology Group investigators reported the first result of a relatively large prospective single-arm study of surgery with negative margins of at least 3 mm without radiation therapy for patients with favorable subsets of DCIS.[27] Patients with low-grade or intermediate-grade DCIS measuring 2.5 cm or smaller had a 5-year rate of ipsilateral breast recurrence of only 6.1%. In contrast, patients with high-grade disease had a much higher 5-year ipsilateral breast recurrence rate of 15.3%.

Taken together, the data from these trials of treatment for DCIS suggest that WBI after lumpectomy should be recommended for most patients with DCIS. The one subgroup that appears to have favorable outcomes without radiation are patients with small-grade, low-grade or intermediate-grade lesions.

Role of Tamoxifen and Aromatase Inhibitors

The use of tamoxifen has been shown to reduce the risk for development of new breast cancers in high-risk women, including women with a previous breast cancer (see "Chemoprevention for Breast Cancer" earlier). The NSABP B-24 protocol evaluated the benefit of tamoxifen for patients with DCIS. In this trial, 1804 women who had undergone lumpectomy and radiation therapy for DCIS were randomly assigned to 5 years of tamoxifen or placebo. Study criteria allowed enrollment of patients with positive margins, and ER was not measured. At 7 years of follow-up, the addition of tamoxifen to lumpectomy and radiation therapy decreased the incidence of recurrent ipsilateral breast cancers from 9% to 6% and reduced the risk for a new contralateral breast cancer by 47% (an absolute reduction of 2%) (see Table 35.7).

For the NSABP B-17 and NSABP B-24 trials combined, at 7 years of follow-up, the total (ipsilateral plus contralateral) breast cancer recurrence rate was 30% for excision alone; 17% for excision with radiation therapy; and 10% for excision, irradiation, and tamoxifen. Subsequent analyses demonstrated that the benefit from tamoxifen is seen only in women with ER-positive DCIS. Patients at highest risk for local recurrence—and most likely to benefit from tamoxifen—were patients with positive margins, comedonecrosis, a mass on physical examination, and age younger than 50 years. For individual patients, the benefits of tamoxifen are weighed against its side effects, including risk for endometrial carcinoma, thromboembolic events, hot flashes, and cataracts.

IBIS-II enrolled 2980 postmenopausal women in a randomized trial comparing tamoxifen versus arimidex. There were no differences between the groups in recurrence rates or side effects.[28]

Sentinel Node Surgery

DCIS, by definition, represents breast cancer contained within an intact basement membrane and without access to lymphatic or vascular channels. However, when ALND was performed during mastectomy for DCIS, positive nodes were found in 3.6% of cases, as indicated by a review of more than 10,000 patients in the National Cancer Data Base. These positive nodes probably result from microinvasive disease in the primary tumor that was not detected on routine pathologic analysis.

Sentinel node surgery is currently recommended in patients undergoing mastectomy for DCIS because 20% to 30% of patients with DCIS on a diagnostic CNB are found to have invasive cancer on detailed evaluation of the mastectomy specimen. The addition of sentinel node surgery to mastectomy adds minimal morbidity and avoids the need for ALND if invasive cancer is identified (sentinel node mapping is not possible after mastectomy). For patients undergoing breast-conserving surgery for DCIS, sentinel node surgery may be considered for patients with larger areas of DCIS, particularly patients with high-grade histology or with high suspicion of microinvasion.

RADIATION THERAPY FOR BREAST CANCER

Radiation Therapy after Breast-Conserving Surgery

For patients with invasive breast cancer treated with breast-conserving surgery, adjuvant irradiation of the breast has been conclusively demonstrated to reduce the probability of a breast recurrence and improve outcome. The EBCTCG published a meta analysis of the data from 7300 women who participated in randomized trials of breast-conserving surgery with or without WBI therapy. In this analysis, radiation was found to reduce the 10-year rate of in-breast recurrence from 29% to 10% for patients with negative lymph nodes and from 47% to 13% for patients with positive lymph nodes. This improvement in local control led to a reduction in the 15-year breast cancer mortality rate and overall death rate. On the basis of these data, radiation therapy after breast-conserving surgery should be considered as a standard. Most trials attempting to define subgroups of patients who could potentially avoid radiation after lumpectomy have been unsuccessful. The only group identified that might have been able to avoid irradiation safely is patients older than 70 years who undergo lumpectomy and adjuvant hormonal therapy for a stage I ER-positive breast cancer. However, at 10 years, 98% of patients receiving tamoxifen and radiation compared with 90% of those receiving tamoxifen alone were free from local and regional recurrences.[29]

Historically, radiation therapy after lumpectomy has consisted of a 6- to 8-week treatment course, which can be a hardship for patients. An important Canadian trial successfully compared this historical schedule with a more abbreviated WBI schedule. On the basis of long-term outcome results from this study, it is reasonable to treat a postmenopausal patient with a non–high-grade, ER-positive, stage I breast cancer with a 16-fraction course of treatment, which shortens the overall treatment time to approximately 3 weeks.

There has also been significant interest in shortening the treatment course to 1 week or less through an approach that focuses the radiation exclusively on the area around the tumor bed. This approach, called *partial breast irradiation*, may be performed with brachytherapy catheters, balloon catheters, or external-beam radiation.

The NRG (NSABP B-39/RTOG 0413) trial randomly assigned 4216 women who had recently undergone lumpectomy to receive either WBI or accelerated PBI. Women enrolled in the study had zero to three positive axillary nodes on study entry. Twenty-five percent of the group had DCIS, 65% had stage I breast cancer, and 10% had stage II disease. The majority of women also had hormone receptor–positive tumors. Women who were assigned to the WBI arm following adjuvant chemotherapy received daily treatment with 2.0 Gy/fraction of radiation totaling 50 Gy with a sequential boost to the surgical site.

Those assigned to accelerated PBI prior to adjuvant chemotherapy received a total of 10 treatments given twice-daily treatment with 3.4 to 3.85 Gy given as either brachytherapy or 3D external-beam radiation. The 10-year cumulative incidence of ipsilateral breast tumor recurrence was very low in both groups, at 4.6% for patients in the accelerated PBI arm versus 3.9% for those in the WBI arm but did not meet equivalence. There were no differences in distant disease-free interval, OS, or DFS.

The American Society for Radiation Oncology published a consensus statement highlighting appropriate selection criteria that should be considered if patients are to be treated with PBI outside the context of a clinical trial (Table 35.8).[30]

Postmastectomy Radiation Therapy

For patients with T1N0 or T2N0 breast cancer, mastectomy and SLND provide effective local control, and radiation therapy is not required. In contrast, patients with stage III breast cancer have high rates of locoregional recurrence after treatment with a modified radical mastectomy and adjuvant or neoadjuvant chemotherapy. Clinical trial data indicate that postmastectomy radiation therapy can significantly improve the outcome of patients who would be expected to have a 20% to 40% risk of locoregional recurrence without radiation therapy.

Three prospective randomized trials addressed the role of postmastectomy irradiation. In the Danish Trials, premenopausal women with stage II or III breast cancer were randomly assigned to chemotherapy alone or chemotherapy plus chest wall and nodal irradiation (protocol 82b); postmenopausal women were randomly assigned to tamoxifen alone or tamoxifen plus radiation therapy (protocol 82c). In the British Columbia study, premenopausal women with node-positive breast cancer were randomly assigned to chemotherapy alone or chemotherapy plus chest wall and nodal irradiation.[31] In addition to reducing locoregional recurrences, as expected, postmastectomy irradiation significantly improved OS in all three trials (Table 35.9).

In 2005, the EBCTCG published the results of a meta analysis of trials of postmastectomy radiation therapy, which included data from 9933 patients treated with mastectomy or axillary clearance with or without postmastectomy radiation. Postmastectomy radiation therapy decreased the 15-year isolated locoregional recurrence rate for patients with lymph node–positive disease from 29% to 8% and reduced the 15-year breast cancer mortality rate from 60% to 55%. The most recent analysis from this group suggested that benefits of postmastectomy radiation therapy are similar for patients with one to three positive lymph nodes and patients with four or more positive lymph nodes.[32]

There is consensus that patients with four or more positive lymph nodes or other features characteristic of stage III disease should be counseled to undergo radiation therapy. However, the use of postmastectomy radiation therapy for patients with stage II disease is controversial because many U.S. series indicated that locoregional recurrence rates after a standard modified radical mastectomy and adjuvant chemotherapy are only 12% to 15%, much lower than rates reported in the clinical trials of postmastectomy irradiation and the EBCTCG meta analysis. On the basis of this disparity, it is reasonable to consider postmastectomy radiation therapy only for selected patients with stage II disease, such as patients with extracapsular extension, lymphovascular invasion, age 40 years or younger, close/positive surgical margins, or a nodal positivity ratio (ratio of positive nodes to total nodes examined) of 20% or greater and patients who have undergone less than a standard level I or II axillary dissection.

SYSTEMIC THERAPY FOR BREAST CANCER

Despite advances in locoregional therapy, a significant proportion of women with breast cancer develop metastatic disease within 5 to 10 years after diagnosis. Most patients who develop metastatic

TABLE 35.8 American Society for Radiation Oncology guidelines for accelerated partial breast irradiation.

FACTOR	"SUITABLE" GROUP	"CAUTIONARY" GROUP	"UNSUITABLE" GROUP
Patient Factors			
Age (years)	≥60	50–59	<50
Tumor Factors			
Tumor size (cm)	≤2	2.1–3.0	>3
T stage	T1	T0 or T2	T3 or T4
Margins	Negative by at least 2 mm	Close (<2 mm)	Positive
Histology	Invasive ductal carcinoma or other favorable subtypes	Invasive lobular carcinoma	NA
Pure DCIS	Not allowed	≤3 cm	>3 cm
Grade	Any	NA	NA
LVI	None	Limited/focal	Extensive
ER status	Positive	Negative	NA
Multicentricity	Unicentric	NA	If present
Multifocality	Clinically unifocal with total size ≤2 cm	Clinically unifocal with total size 2.1–3 cm	Clinically multifocal or microscopically multifocal >3 cm
Nodal factors			
N stage	pN0	NA	pN1-3
Treatment factors			
Neoadjuvant chemotherapy	Not allowed	NA	If used

Adapted from Smith BD, Arthur DW, Buchholz TA, et al. Accelerated partial breast irradiation consensus statement from the American Society for Radiation Oncology (ASTRO). *J Am Coll Surg.* 2009;209:269.
DCIS, Ductal carcinoma in situ; *ER*, estrogen receptor; *LVI*, lymphovascular invasion; *NA*, not available.

TABLE 35.9 Trials of systemic therapy with or without irradiation after mastectomy.

	NO. PATIENTS			LOCAL RECURRENCE RATE (%)			OS (%)		
TRIAL	SYSTEMIC THERAPY + XRT	SYSTEMIC THERAPY ALONE	TOTAL	SYSTEMIC THERAPY + XRT	SYSTEMIC THERAPY ALONE	*P* VALUE	SYSTEMIC THERAPY + XRT	SYSTEMIC THERAPY ALONE	*P* VALUE
DBCG 82b (10 years; chemo)[a]	852	856	1708	9	32	<0.001	54	45	<0.001
DBCG 82c (10 years; tamoxifen)[b]	686	689	1375	8	35	<0.001	45	38	0.03
DBCG 82c (combined 18 years)[b]	1538	1545	3083	14	49	<0.001	37	27	
British Columbia Trial (20 years)[c]	164	154	318	13	25	0.003*	64	54	0.003*

chemo, Chemotherapy; *DBCG*, Danish Breast Cancer Group; *OS*, overall survival; *XRT*, radiation therapy.
*Aggregate *P* value for comparisons at various follow-up intervals; this is the 10-year result.
[a]Overgaard M, Hansen Per S, Overgaard J, et al. Postoperative radiotherapy in high-risk premenopausal women with breast cancer who receive adjuvant chemotherapy. *N Engl J Med.* 1997;337:949.
[b]Overgaard M, Jensen M-B, Overgaard J, et al. Postoperative radiotherapy in high-risk postmenopausal breast cancer patients given adjuvant tamoxifen: Danish Breast Cancer Cooperative Group DBCG 82c randomized trial. *Lancet.* 1999;353:1641.
[c]Ragaz J, Jackson S, Le N, et al. Adjuvant radiotherapy and chemotherapy in node-positive premenopausal women with breast cancer. *N Engl J Med.* 1997;337:956.

breast cancer die of their disease. Metastatic disease is the principal cause of death from breast cancer.

Systemic therapy is used to treat and prevent recurrence of microscopic metastatic breast cancer. For women with stage IV breast cancer, systemic therapy is given to palliate symptoms from cancer and potentially prolong survival. Current thinking is that metastasis occurs early in the progression of breast cancer, probably before initial clinical evaluation in most patients. This concept argues for administration of systemic therapy for breast cancer in concert with local treatment. What is missing at the present time is the ability to detect occult metastatic disease accurately and select appropriate patients to receive systemic treatment.

The first prospective trials of systemic therapy for breast cancer combined oophorectomy, to deprive patients of estrogens, with radical mastectomy. Since these early trials, hundreds of prospective studies of systemic therapy have been conducted involving thousands of women. Medications used to treat early breast cancer have their foundation as treatment for advanced disease. In general, treatments that are used effectively to improve outcome for patients with incurable breast cancer are estimated to have an increased impact on outcomes for patients with earlier stages of breast cancer, who have smaller volumes of disease and potentially less resistance to therapy. When medications are identified that improve outcomes for patients with incurable stage IV breast cancer, they are often brought forward into clinical studies for earlier stages of disease.

Goals of Therapy and Assessment of Potential Benefits and Risks from Therapy

For patients with stage I to III invasive breast cancer, the goal of treatment is cure. In selecting treatment, the potential benefits of therapy (reduction in the risk of recurrence) are considered together with the potential harms of treatment. Patient preferences, particularly preferences regarding adjuvant therapy, are carefully considered. Some patients believe that the reduction in risk of recurrence with adjuvant therapy is not worth the adverse effects of the therapy, particularly in the case of chemotherapy. Often, several long discussions with the patient are essential to determine the treatment that best suits that patient.

The risk of systemic recurrence increases with increasing stage of disease. The biologic characteristics of an individual tumor also influence the risk of systemic recurrence. The most commonly used breast cancer biomarkers—ER, PR, and HER-2—not only affect prognosis but also predict response to different systemic therapies. In general terms, tumors that have no ER or PR expression and tumors with high levels of HER-2 are associated with worse cancer outcomes than tumors that are strongly positive for ER and PR and have negative or normal levels of HER-2. For most patients, risk of recurrence is estimated on the basis of population-based statistics. Current federal and international guidelines use stage and biologic characteristics in the development of treatment recommendations to guide decisions regarding systemic therapy for breast cancer (Table 35.10).

Multigene assays, such as the 21-gene recurrence score assay (Oncotype DX Breast Cancer Assay, Genomic Health, Inc., Redwood City, CA), have been developed in an attempt to identify a specific molecular phenotype of a tumor in an individual patient and use the phenotype to predict the response to therapy or provide information regarding prognosis. The Oncotype DX assay was developed from a candidate pool of 250 genes and narrowed to a specific 21-gene panel on the basis of three independent studies of the candidate genes. This assay was validated first in patients with ER-positive, lymph node–negative breast cancer (NSABP B-14). The Oncotype DX assay was found to be prognostic for OS and predictive of the benefits of different systemic therapies, with higher recurrence scores predicting increased benefit from chemotherapy and lower scores predicting lesser benefit from chemotherapy and increased benefit from endocrine therapy. This assay was validated in subsequent studies. The Oncotype DX assay can help clinicians estimate the benefits of therapy for patients with lymph node–negative, ER-positive breast cancer. For patients with low recurrence scores, chemotherapy appears to have marginal benefit in terms of reducing the risk of distant recurrence, but for patients with high recurrence scores, chemotherapy offers marked benefit. A cooperative group trial, TAILORx, was conducted to determine the benefit from chemotherapy in patients with intermediate recurrence scores. This trial was recently reported involving 9719 women with hormone receptor–positive, HER-2–negative, axillary node–negative breast cancer.[33] Patients with a recurrence scores less than 11 received endocrine therapy. Patients with a recurrence scores greater than 25 received chemotherapy. There were 6711 patients who had midrange recurrence scores of 11 to 25 and were randomly assigned to receive either chemoendocrine therapy or endocrine therapy alone. Endocrine therapy was noninferior to chemoendocrine therapy in the analysis of invasive DFS, invasive disease recurrence, second primary cancer, and OS at 9-year follow-up. Some benefit of chemotherapy was found in women 50 years of age or younger with a recurrence score of 16 to 25. Therefore, chemotherapy is not recommended for patients with hormonal receptor–positive, HER-2–negative and node-negative disease and recurrence scores of less than 25 for women over 50 years of age or recurrence scores of less than 16. This represents a majority of the patients presenting for breast cancer treatment today.

Chemotherapy

The main classes of chemotherapeutics used to treat early-stage breast cancer include anthracyclines (e.g., doxorubicin, epirubicin) and taxanes (e.g., paclitaxel, docetaxel). The anthracyclines, which act as topoisomerase II inhibitors and antimetabolites, have high levels of activity in the treatment of breast cancer. When anthracyclines are delivered as single agents for the treatment of metastatic breast cancer, responses to therapy are generally seen in 45% to 80% of patients. The 2005 EBCTCG analysis[32] noted that compared with nonanthracycline, CMF (cyclophosphamide, methotrexate, 5-fluorouracil)-type therapies, anthracyclines are associated with a 16% reduction in the risk of death and an 11% reduction in the risk of recurrence. Anthracyclines are associated with the potential long-term toxic effect of cardiomyopathy, which may lead to congestive heart failure, often many years after treatment. The risk of cardiac dysfunction resulting from anthracyclines is dose dependent, and current anthracycline-containing chemotherapy regimens are associated with a risk of cardiac dysfunction of 1.5% to 3%. An additional dangerous risk of anthracycline-based chemotherapy is the risk of development of leukemia (<1%).

Taxanes (microtubule inhibitors) have significant activity in the treatment of metastatic breast cancer and are active not only in tumors previously unexposed to chemotherapy but also in anthracycline-resistant tumors. Numerous clinical trials have evaluated the use of taxanes for treatment of early-stage breast cancer. A meta analysis of the use of taxanes in 13 different studies from the Intergroup Trial C9741/Cancer and Leukemia Group B (CALGB) trial 9741 found improvement in DFS (HR, 0.83; 95% CI, 0.79–0.87; $P < 0.0001$) and OS (HR, 0.85; 95% CI, 0.79–0.91; $P < 0.0001$). The antitumor activity of paclitaxel depends on the timing of treatment: More frequent administration of paclitaxel improves outcomes. The activity of docetaxel depends less on the timing of treatment, and docetaxel is generally administered on an every-3-week schedule. The two taxanes, when given at their optimal dose and schedule, produce equivalent outcomes. The taxanes are associated with the potential permanent toxic effect of peripheral neuropathy but do not cause long-term increased risk of cardiac dysfunction or second cancers.

TABLE 35.10 **Decision-making for systemic therapy.**

STAGE	SYSTEMIC THERAPY	COMMENTS
I (<1 cm)		
Hormone receptor–positive	Endocrine therapy ± chemotherapy	Consider genomic testing
Hormone receptor–negative	Consider chemotherapy	
HER-2–positive	Strongly consider trastuzumab and chemotherapy	
I (>1 cm)		
Hormone receptor–positive	Endocrine therapy ± chemotherapy	Consider genomic testing
Hormone receptor–negative	Chemotherapy	
HER-2–positive	Trastuzumab and chemotherapy	
II (Lymph Node–Negative)		
Hormone receptor–positive	Endocrine therapy ± chemotherapy	Consider genomic testing
Hormone receptor–negative	Chemotherapy	
HER-2–positive	Trastuzumab and chemotherapy	
II (Lymph Node–Positive), III		
Hormone receptor–positive	Chemotherapy + endocrine therapy	Endocrine therapy should be recommended for all patients
Hormone receptor–negative	Chemotherapy	Decision-making for chemotherapy may be influenced by results from ongoing clinical trials
HER-2–positive	Trastuzumab and chemotherapy	Consider neoadjuvant chemotherapy with dual HER-2–targeted therapy

HER-2, Human epidermal growth factor receptor 2.

Chemotherapy is generally administered with combinations of medications in an effort to take advantage of nonoverlapping toxic effects and to maximize different mechanisms of action in targeting tumor cells. The largest comprehensive analysis to date of the benefits of polychemotherapy for breast cancer is the EBCTCG analysis published in 2012. This analysis summarized data from randomized trials that were initiated between 1973 and 2003. The authors presented individual patient data from trials comparing a taxane-plus-anthracycline–based regimen versus a nontaxane-containing regimen with the same or higher cumulative doses of each nontaxane component (n = 44,000), trials comparing one anthracycline-based regimen versus another (n = 7000) or versus CMF (n = 18,000), and trials comparing polychemotherapy versus no chemotherapy (n = 32,000). On the basis of the drug dosages and the anthracycline used (either doxorubicin [Adriamycin; A] or epirubicin [E]), regimens were defined as including standard CMF, standard Adriamycin/Cytoxin (AC), Cytoxin/Adriamycin/fluorouracil (CAF), or Cytoxin/epirubicin/fluorouracil (CEF). A meta analysis showed that compared with no chemotherapy, use of CMF or standard AC reduced the recurrence rate by one-third at 8 years and produced a 20% to 25% reduction in breast cancer mortality. The addition of more chemotherapy (i.e., CAF or CEF compared with CMF or AC) resulted in an additional proportional reduction of 15% to 20% in breast cancer mortality. On average, the taxane-plus-anthracycline–based control regimens were superior to standard AC but were not superior to anthracycline regimens with extra cycles (i.e., CAF or CEF). In analyses comparing taxane-based and anthracycline-based regimens, the proportional risk reductions were not significantly affected by age, tumor size, nodal status, tumor grade, or ER status. Taken together, these data suggest that independent of age or tumor characteristics, a chemotherapy regimen that include a taxane or anthracycline regimens with higher cumulative dosages reduced breast cancer mortality by approximately one third.

HER-2–Based Targeted Therapy

HER-2 gene amplification or protein overexpression occurs in approximately 20% to 25% of breast cancers. Amplification leads to protein overexpression, measured clinically by immunohistochemistry and scored on a scale from 0 to 3+. Alternatively, fluorescence in situ hybridization directly detects the quantity of HER-2 gene copies; the normal copy number is two (see "Molecular Markers and Breast Cancer Subtypes" earlier).

Trastuzumab is a humanized monoclonal antibody developed to target the extracellular domain of the HER-2 receptor. When trastuzumab is used as a single agent for treatment of metastatic breast cancer, response is seen in approximately 30% of patients. Trastuzumab combined with chemotherapy is even more effective, with synergy seen with multiple agents. Trastuzumab-based chemotherapy regimens improve DFS and OS for patients with metastatic disease. Given the promising activity of trastuzumab against metastatic disease, numerous trials of trastuzumab for adjuvant and neoadjuvant therapy have been conducted; these trials demonstrated improved outcomes for patients with stage I to III breast cancer. The HERA (HERceptin Adjuvant) trial (N = 5090) enrolled patients with HER-2–positive breast cancer and randomly assigned them to trastuzumab treatment (for 1 or 2 years) versus observation after completion of chemotherapy. In a comparison of 1-year of trastuzumab treatment versus observation, trastuzumab reduced the risk of a breast cancer–related event by 46% (HR, 0.54; 95% CI, 0.43–0.67; $P < 0.001$) and improved OS by 34% (HR, 0.66; 95% CI, 0.47–0.91; $P < 0.0115$). Treatment with trastuzumab for 2 years was not more effective than 1 year of treatment and 6 months was inferior, which established 1 year of treatment as standard of care.

Long-term follow-up of the NSABP B-31 and NCCTG-N9831 adjuvant trials, which were similar in study design, demonstrate that the initial benefit seen with adjuvant trastuzumab persist with an improvement in 10-year OS from 75.2% to 84%.[34] Patients receiving trastuzumab-based therapy in NSABP B-31 (AC followed by paclitaxel-trastuzumab) had an increased risk of cardiac dysfunction, with a 3-year event rate of 4.1% versus 0.8% in the control arm.[34] Patients with lower ejection fraction at the initiation of therapy, older age, or hypertension were at highest risk of cardiac dysfunction.

The BCIRG 006 trial used a nonanthracycline-containing regimen as one of its treatment groups and showed equivalence in outcome between AC followed by docetaxel-trastuzumab (AC-TH) and docetaxel combined with carboplatin and trastuzumab (TCH).[35] Both trastuzumab-containing treatments were superior in terms of DFS to the control treatment of AC followed by docetaxel, with HR of 0.61 (95% CI, 0.48–0.76; $P < 0.001$) for the AC-TH group and HR of 0.67 for the TCH group (95% CI, 0.54–0.83). Rates of cardiac toxic effects were markedly lower in the TCH group (0.37%) than in the AC-TH group (1.87%).

Additional drugs targeting HER-2 in combination with trastuzumab are being evaluated, including the tyrosine kinase inhibitor lapatinib; the trastuzumab drug conjugate trastuzumab emtansine; neratinib and pertuzumab, a monoclonal antibody that inhibits dimerization of HER-2 with other HER-2 receptors. The combination of trastuzumab and pertuzumab is approved in all disease settings, while trastuzumab/neratinib is approved in the adjuvant setting and trastuzumab/lapatinib in metastatic disease. Trials are ongoing with further combinations with PI3/AKT/mTOR inhibitors, CDK4/6 inhibitors, anti-PD(L)1 antibodies, endocrine therapy, and new anti-HER-2 agents.[36]

Endocrine Therapy

One of the original targeted therapy approaches was the use of oophorectomy to reduce systemic estrogen production as a treatment for breast cancer. Most breast cancers (>60%) express ER or PR or both; interruption of the production of estrogen or the ability of estrogen to interact with the ER has been associated with improved DFS and OS for women with metastatic breast cancer. This therapeutic approach is associated with a generally favorable adverse effect profile compared with the adverse effects of chemotherapy.

Tamoxifen

Tamoxifen is a selective ER modulator that has antagonistic and weak agonistic effects. It is generally well tolerated; the most common side effect is hot flashes or vasomotor symptoms, which occur in less than 50% of patients. Potentially serious but rare effects include increased risk of thromboembolic disease and uterine cancer.

Clinical trials of tamoxifen as treatment for early-stage breast cancer began in the 1970s. In 2005, the EBCTCG meta analysis reported data of more than 80,000 women treated in clinical studies.[32] Tamoxifen administered for 5 years was found to reduce the risk of recurrence of breast cancer for patients with hormone receptor–positive disease by 41% (recurrence rate ratio, 0.59; SE, 0.03). The risk of death from breast cancer was reduced by approximately one third (death rate ratio, 0.66; SE, 0.04). Tamoxifen was shown to be beneficial for premenopausal and postmenopausal women and had a similar magnitude of benefit for patients with lymph node–positive and lymph node–negative disease. The duration of therapy with tamoxifen was also evaluated; 5 years of therapy was found to be superior to only 1 to 2 years of therapy in terms of breast cancer recurrence (15.2% proportionate reduction; $P < 0.001$) and death from breast cancer (7.9% proportionate reduction; $P = 0.01$).

Tamoxifen therapy for more than 5 years has been investigated, and results from the two largest studies with the longest follow-up were recently reported. The Adjuvant Tamoxifen: Longer Against Shorter (ATLAS) trial showed an approximately 25% reduction in the rate of recurrence and approximately 3% reduction in mortality risk in women taking 10 years of tamoxifen versus 5 years, with the benefit being most pronounced after year 10.[37] These findings were confirmed in the Adjuvant Tamoxifen–to Offer MDore? (aTTom) trial, in which patients were also randomly assigned to 5 years versus 10 years of tamoxifen. There was a decrease in breast cancer recurrence rates and breast cancer mortality rates in patients treated for a longer duration. In light of these findings, the American Society of Clinical Oncology (ASCO) updated their guidelines regarding adjuvant endocrine therapy. For premenopausal or perimenopausal women, tamoxifen for 5 years is recommended. After 5 years, if the patient is still premenopausal, she should be offered an additional 5 years of tamoxifen therapy.[38]

Aromatase Inhibitors

AIs block the conversion of the hormone androstenedione into estrone by inhibition of the aromatase enzyme. This enzyme is present in adipose tissue, breast tissue, breast tumor cells, and other sites. Multiple generations of medications that block the aromatase enzyme have been evaluated, less specific agents such as aminoglutethimide also suppress production of other hormones, and this is associated with unacceptable side effects. Selective or third-generation AIs purely block the final step of conversion of hormones into estrogen and are not associated with the broad hormone suppression seen with earlier AIs. Selective AIs, which include anastrozole, exemestane, and letrozole, are unable to suppress ovarian function completely in a premenopausal or perimenopausal woman and are restricted for use in postmenopausal women. Selective AIs as a group have similar adverse effects, including hot flashes, vasomotor symptoms, joint symptoms, myalgias, bone loss, and vaginal dryness.

Several different trial designs have been used to evaluate AIs as adjuvant therapy. Direct comparisons of 5 years of a selective AI versus 5 years of tamoxifen demonstrated improvement in cancer outcomes for anastrozole and letrozole.[39] The Arimidex, Tamoxifen, Alone or in Combination (ATAC) trial demonstrated that 5 years of anastrozole significantly improved DFS by 17% compared with 5 years of tamoxifen (HR, 0.83; 95% CI, 0.73–94; $P = 0.05$). In addition to reducing the risk of distant recurrence (distant DFS HR, 0.86; 95% CI, 0.74–0.99; $P = 0.04$), anastrozole reduced the risk of development of contralateral breast cancers by 42%.[39]

Administration of selective AIs for 2 to 3 years after tamoxifen for 2 to 3 years has been compared with 5 years of tamoxifen treatment.[40] The use of all three modern AIs after 2 to 3 years of tamoxifen was associated with better cancer outcomes than the use of tamoxifen alone. In addition, extended adjuvant therapy with 5 years of the AI letrozole after 5 years of tamoxifen was shown to improve outcome compared with placebo after 5 years of tamoxifen. The use of letrozole versus placebo reduced the risk of breast cancer events by 43% ($P < 0.008$). In the most recent ASCO guidelines, if women are pre- or perimenopausal and have received 5 years of adjuvant tamoxifen, they should be offered 10-years total duration of tamoxifen. If women are postmenopausal and have received 5 years of adjuvant tamoxifen, they should be offered the choice of continuing tamoxifen or switching to an AI for 10-years total adjuvant endocrine therapy.[41]

Ovarian Ablation

The EBCTCG meta analysis evaluated premenopausal women who were treated with ovarian ablation or suppression and found that this treatment reduced the risk of relapse and death from breast cancer.[32] Compared with the use of CMF chemotherapy, the use of ovarian ablation with goserelin as treatment for lymph node–positive, stage II breast cancer in premenopausal women resulted in equivalent outcomes in terms of DFS (HR, 1.01; P = 0.94) and OS (HR, 0.99; P = 0.94). Even with this high level of activity, the optimal role for addition of ovarian ablation is unknown.

Results were reported from two phase III trials that evaluated use of an AI with ovarian suppression in premenopausal patients with hormone receptor–positive early breast cancer. These trials were Tamoxifen and Exemestane Trial (TEXT) and Suppression of Ovarian Function Trial (SOFT).[42] TEXT was designed to evaluate 5 years of the AI exemestane plus ovarian suppression with a gonadotropin-releasing hormone agonist versus tamoxifen plus the gonadotropin-releasing hormone agonist. SOFT was designed to evaluate 5 years of the AI exemestane plus ovarian suppression versus tamoxifen plus ovarian suppression versus tamoxifen alone. The initial combined analysis looked at AI plus ovarian suppression versus tamoxifen plus ovarian suppression; the tamoxifen-alone arm from SOFT was not included. After a median follow-up of 68 months, the addition of ovarian suppression to hormone suppression did not show an overall clinical benefit but did show a benefit in those with the highest risk disease. Therefore, the consensus guidelines state that if the patient has high-risk disease, then ovarian suppression should be considered in addition to hormonal suppression.[43]

Neoadjuvant Systemic Therapy for Operable Breast Cancer

Chemotherapy is most commonly administered as adjuvant therapy after completion of surgery. Neoadjuvant therapy, the administration of systemic chemotherapy or endocrine therapy before surgery, can result in a significant reduction in tumor size and convert inoperable tumors to operable ones, make tumors that would require mastectomy amenable to lumpectomy, and shrink larger tumors to allow an improved cosmetic outcome with breast-conserving surgery.

Several prospective randomized trials evaluated the efficacy of chemotherapy and endocrine therapy administered as neoadjuvant (before surgery) versus adjuvant (after surgery) therapy. These studies all demonstrated increased rates of breast conservation with the use of neoadjuvant systemic therapy. The NSABP B-18 trial included 1523 patients and found no survival advantage (or detriment) in patients who received preoperative doxorubicin and cyclophosphamide chemotherapy versus the same regimen delivered postoperatively. The breast conservation rate was higher in women completing neoadjuvant chemotherapy, and the rate of in-breast recurrence in women who underwent neoadjuvant therapy followed by lumpectomy was not significantly different from the rate of in-breast recurrence in women who underwent lumpectomy before adjuvant chemotherapy.

Delivering chemotherapy before surgery has other theoretical advantages, including the potential to lower the volume of microscopic metastatic disease, decrease drug resistance by treating tumors before resistance has developed, increase the efficacy of treatment because the vascular system has not been disrupted by surgery, and permit evaluation of the response to treatment in vivo. In theory, the ability to evaluate response to therapy in vivo may help avoid administration of ineffective therapy and allow the clinician to tailor therapy to the individual patient. In addition, it has been shown that response to neoadjuvant chemotherapy correlates with survival outcomes. In the NSABP B-18 trial, after 9 years of follow-up, the DFS rate in patients achieving a complete pathologic response in the neoadjuvant therapy arm (no evidence of tumor at surgery) was 75% compared with 58% in patients who had any residual invasive disease after chemotherapy. A meta-analysis of 12 randomized trials evaluating neoadjuvant chemotherapy found that 18% of patients had a pathologic complete response, defined as no residual invasive disease in the breast or axilla, and 13% had a pathologic complete response defined as no residual invasive or in situ disease. A pathologic complete response by either definition was associated with improved event-free survival and OS.[44] The association between pathologic complete response and long-term outcomes was strongest in patients with aggressive tumor subtypes, including patients with triple-negative breast cancer and patients with HER-2–positive, hormone receptor–negative breast cancer who received trastuzumab as part of their neoadjuvant regimen.

There are several surgical considerations for patients receiving neoadjuvant chemotherapy. By the end of systemic therapy, a percentage of patients has complete resolution of their tumors by clinical examination and imaging but might have microscopic residual disease. This percentage ranges from 10% to 15% in patients with hormone receptor–positive tumors to approximately 50% in patients with HER-2–positive tumors receiving trastuzumab in combination with chemotherapy as neoadjuvant therapy. Consequently, a metallic clip is placed at the primary tumor site under image guidance before neoadjuvant chemotherapy is initiated to allow identification of the original tumor site for excision after therapy.

Management of the axilla in patients undergoing neoadjuvant therapy has evolved. The timing of SLND has been debated, with some centers performing SLND before neoadjuvant therapy in patients with clinically negative nodes to inform decisions about systemic and radiation therapy. Advocates of SLND before neoadjuvant chemotherapy cite concerns about lower successful mapping rates and higher false-negative rates after neoadjuvant therapy. Other centers favor SLND after neoadjuvant therapy for any patient whose axilla is clinically negative after therapy to obtain more information about the status of the nodes after neoadjuvant therapy. Two meta analyses of single-institution and multicenter studies were conducted and concluded that SLND is feasible and accurate after neoadjuvant chemotherapy, resulting in sentinel node identification rates of approximately 91%.[45] Both of these meta analyses included patients with clinically node-negative and node-positive disease. In one, the authors evaluated studies that included only patients with clinically node-negative disease and found a pooled sentinel node identification rate of 93%. These two meta analyses also examined the accuracy of SLND in patients receiving neoadjuvant chemotherapy and reported false-negative rates of 10.5% to 12%.

In addition, neoadjuvant chemotherapy eradicates microscopic disease in the regional nodes in 40% of patients, reducing the need for complete ALND at the time of surgical intervention. Complete ALND remains the standard for all patients receiving neoadjuvant therapy who have biopsy-proven, node-positive disease at initial presentation; however, there is significant interest in identifying patients in whom SLND might be appropriate after neoadjuvant chemotherapy. The ACOSOG reported the results of the Z1071 trial, a phase II study in which patients with clinically node-positive disease (clinical N1 disease) receiving neoadjuvant chemotherapy underwent SLND followed by planned completion ALND. This study allowed for determination of the false-negative rate for SLND, which was 12.6%—higher than the prespecified end point of 10%.[46] The false-negative rate was lower when dual tracers were used for mapping (false-negative rate, 10.8%) and when three or more sentinel nodes were identified (false-negative rate, 9.1%). These data are consistent with two other trials that evaluated SLND in patients with clinically node-positive disease, the Sentinel Neoadjuvant (SENTINA) trial and the Sentinel Node Biopsy Following Neoadjuvant Chemotherapy (SN FNAC) trial (in biopsy-proven, node-positive breast cancer). The results of these studies suggest that surgical technique is critical in reducing the false-negative rate for SLND in patients with clinically node-positive disease receiving neoadjuvant chemotherapy. If a clip is left in the positive axillary node prior to chemotherapy and that clip and the SLN are retrieved at the time of axillary surgery (targeted axillary dissection), then the false-negative rate was lowered in a single institution trial to 1.4%.[47] Trials are ongoing to determine if, in the neoadjuvant setting, it is safe to omit ALND if the sentinel lymph node is negative.

Some key concepts have been gleaned from the results of neoadjuvant therapy trials. The use of neoadjuvant chemotherapy as a research platform has led to the identification of patient and tumor characteristics that can predict response to therapy. This information allows clinicians to define better the population of patients who are most likely to benefit from neoadjuvant chemotherapy. Targeted therapies, such as trastuzumab, can be safely administered in combination with chemotherapy for neoadjuvant treatment in patients with HER-2–positive breast cancer, resulting in markedly increased rates of pathologic complete response. More recently, studies showed the benefit of dual HER-2 targeting. In the NeoSphere trial, patients with operable, HER-2–positive breast cancer were randomly assigned to one of four neoadjuvant regimens: (1) trastuzumab plus docetaxel, (2) pertuzumab and trastuzumab plus docetaxel, (3) pertuzumab and trastuzumab, or (4) pertuzumab plus docetaxel.[48] The study included 417 patients, and the primary end point was pathologic complete response, which was seen in 46% of patients in the pertuzumab and trastuzumab plus docetaxel arm versus 29% of patients in the trastuzumab plus docetaxel arm. On the basis of these results, the Food and Drug Administration granted pertuzumab accelerated approval as the first drug approved for the neoadjuvant treatment of breast cancer. A pathologic complete response was shown in 17% of patients in the trastuzumab plus pertuzumab arm, suggesting that some patients with HER-2–positive breast cancer could be treated with targeted therapy alone without chemotherapy.

In the context of targeted therapy, patients with ER-positive disease can be treated with endocrine therapy as neoadjuvant therapy, and this approach produces significant response rates and increased rates of breast-conserving surgery. This approach is optimal in postmenopausal women with ER-positive tumors for whom endocrine therapy provides more protection than standard chemotherapy against risk of recurrence and death caused by breast cancer. Finally, because new and more targeted regimens have led to an increasing population of patients with a clinical complete response to neoadjuvant therapy, accurately assessing the residual tumor burden in the breast and regional nodes will become increasingly important in terms of defining prognosis and determining what further therapy is needed. Neoadjuvant chemotherapy has potential disadvantages in terms of loss of prechemotherapy prognostic information (e.g., axillary lymph node status, actual invasive tumor size), which may have an impact on decision-making with respect to postmastectomy radiation therapy.

TREATMENT OF LOCALLY ADVANCED AND INFLAMMATORY BREAST CANCER

Patients with locally advanced breast cancer include patients with large primary tumors (>5 cm), tumors involving the chest wall, skin involvement, ulceration or satellite skin nodules, inflammatory carcinoma, bulky or fixed axillary nodes, and clinically apparent internal mammary or supraclavicular nodal involvement (stages IIB, IIIA, and IIIB disease). Central to treatment is the concept that the disease is advanced on the chest wall, in regional lymph nodes, or both with no evidence of metastasis to distant sites. These patients are recognized to be at significant risk for the development of subsequent metastases, and treatment must address the risk for local and systemic relapse. Experience before the 1970s demonstrated that surgery alone provided poor local control, with local relapse rates of 30% to 50% and mortality rates of 70%. Similar results were reported when radiation therapy was the sole modality of treatment. Current management includes surgery, radiation therapy, and systemic therapy, with the sequence and extent of treatment determined by specifics of the patient's circumstance.

Although inflammatory breast cancer is rare, accounting for approximately 1% to 5% of all breast tumors, it is the most aggressive subtype of breast cancer. The hallmark of inflammatory breast cancer is diffuse tumor involvement of the dermal lymphatic channels within the breast and overlying skin, often without a discrete underlying tumor mass. Inflammatory breast cancer manifests clinically as erythema, edema, and warmth of the breast as a result of lymphatic obstruction. There may be no abnormality on mammography beyond skin thickening, and a palpable mass is not required for the diagnosis. The term *peau d'orange* is used to describe the orange-peel appearance of the skin resulting from edema and dimpling at sites of hair follicles (see Fig. 35.6D). The history should reveal a rapid onset of the disease, with progression over weeks to 3 months. Neglected primary breast tumors that lead to secondary inflammatory changes within the breast should not be categorized as inflammatory breast cancer. Inflammatory cancer is a clinical diagnosis and can occur with tumors of ductal or lobular histology. The pathologic hallmark of inflammatory cancer is the presence of tumor cells within dermal lymphatics, but this is often missed because of sampling error and is not a prerequisite for diagnosis. Axillary nodal metastases are common, and there is a significant risk for distant metastases. Sentinel lymph node biopsy is not performed for inflammatory breast cancer as ALND should always be performed.

Current treatment approaches emphasize aggressive use of combined-modality treatment, including neoadjuvant chemotherapy, mastectomy, and radiation therapy, with endocrine therapy for ER-positive tumors and trastuzumab for HER-2–positive tumors. With multimodality treatment, relapse-free survival rates are 50% or higher at 5 years; in contrast, a single-institution historical series showed a 5-year survival rate of 7% in patients receiving less aggressive treatment.[49]

TREATMENT OF SPECIAL CONDITIONS

Breast Cancer in Older Adults

Several studies have explored options that reduce the extent of surgery and radiation therapy for older women with breast cancer. In two trials, older women were randomly assigned to lumpectomy with or without irradiation. In the CALGB 9343 trial, 636 women 70 years or older with ER-positive tumors 2 cm or smaller and clinically negative nodes received lumpectomy and tamoxifen and were randomly assigned to irradiation or no irradiation.[29] At 10 years, the in-breast recurrence rate was 9% in the no-radiation arm versus 2% in the radiation arm. This difference in in-breast recurrence did not translate into a survival benefit: The 10-year breast cancer–specific survival estimates were 98% in the no-radiation arm and 97% in the radiation arm.

Fyles and colleagues reported the results of a Canadian trial with more inclusive eligibility criteria in which 769 women 50 years or older with tumors up to 5 cm and positive or negative ER status were enrolled. All patients underwent wide excision and received tamoxifen and were randomly assigned to irradiation or no irradiation. Recurrence rates were significantly higher overall in patients who did not receive radiation therapy. However, in an unplanned analysis of a subset of 193 women older than 60 years, the local recurrence rate was only 1.2% without radiation therapy, and there were no recurrences with radiation therapy. These low rates of local recurrence and the significant rates of death from other comorbid conditions led to the acceptance of wide excision and endocrine therapy without irradiation for selected older patients with small ER-positive tumors and clinically negative axillary nodes. Axillary surgery was omitted in such patients in the past; however, SLND can easily be incorporated, with minimal morbidity.

Paget Disease

Paget disease accounts for 1% or less of breast malignancies. It is characterized clinically by nipple erythema and irritation with associated pruritus and may progress to crusting and ulceration. The condition may spread outward from the nipple and onto the areola and surrounding skin of the breast (see Fig. 35.6). The differential diagnosis of scaling skin and erythema of the nipple-areola complex includes eczema, contact dermatitis, postradiation dermatitis, and Paget disease. A biopsy of the skin of the nipple should be performed; a specimen containing Paget cells confirms the diagnosis.

Pathologically, a Paget cell is a large, pale-staining cell with round or oval nuclei and large nucleoli located between the normal keratinocytes of the nipple epidermis. Paget cells spread into the lactiferous sinuses under the nipple and upward to invade the overlying epidermis of the nipple. Paget cells do not invade through the dermal basement membrane and are categorized as carcinoma in situ. More than 95% of patients with Paget disease have an underlying breast carcinoma. Paget disease may be accompanied by a palpable mass in slightly more than 50% of patients. Invasive breast cancer is identified in more than 90% of patients with a palpable mass and Paget disease.

Treatment of Paget disease includes mastectomy with axillary staging or wide local excision of the nipple and areola to achieve clear margins, axillary staging, and radiation therapy. For many patients, lumpectomy and irradiation provide an acceptable cosmetic appearance and obviate the need for mastectomy and breast reconstruction. Nipple-areolar reconstruction can be performed 4 to 6 months after radiation therapy or via 3D tattoo (Fig. 35.14). For patients considering lumpectomy, thorough preoperative evaluation is required to rule out occult multicentric disease.

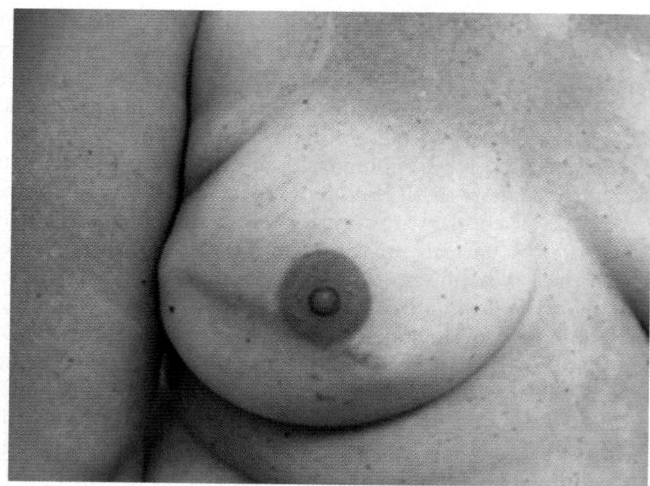

FIG. 35.14 Three-dimensional tattoo of the nipple-areolar complex.

Breast Cancer in Men

Breast cancer occurring in the mammary gland of men is infrequent; it accounts for 0.8% of all breast cancers, less than 1% of all newly diagnosed cancers in men, and 0.2% of cancer deaths in men. In the United States, 1500 new cases of breast cancer in men and 400 deaths from this disease are reported annually. The median age at diagnosis is 68 years, 5 years older than in women. Risk factors include increasing age; radiation exposure; and factors related to abnormalities in estrogen and androgen balance, including testicular disease, infertility, obesity, and cirrhosis. Risk factors related to a genetic predisposition include Klinefelter syndrome (47,XXY karyotype); family history; and *BRCA* gene mutations, particularly *BRCA2* mutations. Gynecomastia is not a risk factor.

Histologically, 90% of breast cancers in men are invasive ductal carcinomas. Approximately 80% are ER positive, 75% are PR positive, and 35% overexpress HER-2. The remaining 10% are DCIS. Given the absence of terminal lobules in the normal breast in men, invasive and in situ lobular carcinoma is rarely seen.

Most men with breast cancer have a breast mass. The differential diagnosis includes gynecomastia, primary breast carcinoma, metastasis to the breast from carcinoma at another site, sarcoma, and breast abscess. In addition to local pain and axillary adenopathy, initial symptoms may include nipple retraction, ulceration, bleeding, and discharge. Evaluation includes breast imaging studies and diagnostic CNB. Prognostic factors for breast cancer in men are the same as prognostic factors for breast cancer in women and include nodal involvement, tumor size, histologic grade, and receptor status. Survival in men with breast cancer is similar to survival in women with breast cancer matched for age and stage.

Treatment of breast carcinoma in men depends on the stage and local extent of the tumor, with treatment options similar to the options for women. Small tumors may be treated by local excision and irradiation or by mastectomy. Sentinel node biopsy has been shown to be effective for staging breast cancer in men. Breast tumors in men more commonly involve the pectoralis major muscle, probably because breast tissue in men is scant. If the underlying pectoral muscle is involved, modified radical mastectomy with excision of the involved portion of muscle is adequate treatment, but it may be combined with postoperative radiation therapy. Adjuvant systemic therapy for breast cancer in men is the same as adjuvant therapy for breast cancer in women. Most breast cancers in men are hormone receptor positive. Adjuvant endocrine therapy with tamoxifen or AIs is indicated for patients with node-positive disease and high-risk patients with node-negative disease. Adjuvant chemotherapy is used in men at substantial risk for metastatic disease.

SELECTED REFERENCES

Barnard K, Klimberg VS. An update on randomized clinical trials in breast cancer. *Surg Oncol Clin N Am*. 2017;26:587–620.

This paper reviews some of the most important clinical trials in the past 5 years.

Clarke M, Collins R, Darby S, et al. Early Breast Cancer Trialists' Collaborative Group (EBCTCG): effects of radiotherapy and of differences in the extent of surgery for early breast cancer on local recurrence and 15-year survival: an overview of the randomized trials. *Lancet*. 2005;366:2087–2106.

This overview analysis by the Early Breast Cancer Trialists' Collaborative Group showed the benefit of radiotherapy on survival in patients with breast cancer.

Domchek S, Friebel TM, Singer CF, et al. Association of risk-reducing surgery in BRCA1 or BRCA2 mutation carriers with cancer risk and mortality. *JAMA*. 2010;304:967–975.

This was the first trial to demonstrate the survival benefit of risk-reducing surgery in BRCA1 and BRCA2 mutation carriers.

Early Breast Cancer Trialists' Collaborative Group (EBCTCG). Effects of chemotherapy and hormonal therapy for early breast cancer on recurrence and 15-year survival: an overview of the randomised trials. *Lancet*. 2005;365:1687–1717.

This overview analysis by the Early Breast Cancer Trialists' Collaborative Group showed the benefit of chemotherapy and hormonal therapy on survival based on stage of disease and hormone receptor status.

Fisher B, Anderson S, Bryant J, et al. Twenty-year follow-up of a randomized trial comparing total mastectomy, lumpectomy, and lumpectomy plus irradiation for the treatment of invasive breast cancer. *N Engl J Med*. 2002;347:1233–1241.

This randomized trial showed no difference in survival between total mastectomy and breast-conserving surgery with or without radiation.

Fisher B, Costantino JP, Wickerham DL, et al. Tamoxifen for prevention of breast cancer: Report of the National Surgical Adjuvant Breast and Bowel Project P-1 Study. *J Natl Cancer Inst*. 1998;90:1371–1388.

In this first randomized trial for breast cancer prevention in a high-risk population, patients were assessed for risk based on the Gail model and randomly assigned to receive 5 years of tamoxifen or placebo. The use of tamoxifen reduced breast cancer incidence by approximately 50%.

Fisher B, Jeong JH, Anderson S, et al. Twenty-five-year follow-up of a randomized trial comparing radical mastectomy, total mastectomy, and total mastectomy followed by irradiation. *N Engl J Med*. 2002;347:567–575.

This report showed no difference in survival between radical mastectomy and total mastectomy with or without radiation.

Giuliano AE, Ballman KV, McCall L, et al. Effect of axillary dissection vs no axillary dissection on 10-year overall survival among women with invasive breast cancer and sentinel node metastasis: the ACOSOG Z0011 (Alliance) Randomized Clinical Trial. *JAMA*. 2017;318:918–926.

This randomized trial showed no benefit to completion of axillary lymph node dissection in selected patients with early-stage breast cancer and positive sentinel lymph nodes.

Krag DN, Anderson SJ, Julian TB, et al. Sentinel-lymph-node resection compared with conventional axillary-lymph-node dissection in clinically node negative patients with breast cancer: overall survival findings from the NSABP B-32 randomised phase 3 trial. *Lancet Oncol*. 2010;11:927–933.

In this randomized trial of sentinel lymph node dissection versus axillary dissection in early-stage breast cancer, there was no difference in overall survival or locoregional recurrence among patients undergoing sentinel node surgery versus standard axillary surgery.

Perou CM, Sorlie T, Eisen MB, et al. Molecular portraits of human breast tumours. *Nature*. 2000;406:747–752.

This article provided the first description of molecular subtypes of breast cancer using microarray analysis.

Rossouw JE, Anderson GL, Prentice RL, et al. Risks and benefits of estrogen plus progestin in healthy postmenopausal women: principal results from the Women's Health Initiative randomized controlled trial. *JAMA*. 2002;288:321–333.

In this long-term follow-up study of participants in the Women's Health Initiative, the risks and benefits of hormone replacement therapy in postmenopausal women were demonstrated.

REFERENCES

1. Boneti C, Korourian S, Diaz Z, et al. Scientific Impact Award: Axillary reverse mapping (ARM) to identify and protect lymphatics draining the arm during axillary lymphadenectomy. *Am J Surg*. 2009;198:482–487.
2. Boneti C, Arentz C, Klimberg VS. Scapulothoracic bursitis as a significant cause of breast and chest wall pain: underrecognized and undertreated. *Ann Surg Oncol*. 2010;17(suppl 3):321–324.
3. Mancino AT, Young ZT, Bland KI. Gynecomastia. In: Bland KI, Copeland EM, Klimberg VS, et al, eds. *The Breast: Comprehensive Management of Benign and Malignant Disease*. 5th ed. Philadelphia: Elsevier; 2018:104–115.
4. Nelson HD, Tyne K, Naik A, et al. Screening for breast cancer: an update for the U.S. Preventive Services Task Force. *Ann Intern Med*. 2009;151:727–737; W237–W742.
5. Bernardi D, Macaskill P, Pellegrini M, et al. Breast cancer screening with tomosynthesis (3D mammography) with acquired or synthetic 2D mammography compared with 2D mammography alone (STORM-2): a population-based prospective study. *Lancet Oncol*. 2016;17:1105–1113.
6. Berg WA, Blume JD, Cormack JB, et al. Combined screening with ultrasound and mammography vs mammography alone in women at elevated risk of breast cancer. *JAMA*. 2008;299:2151–2163.
7. Turnbull L, Brown S, Harvey I, et al. Comparative effectiveness of MRI in breast cancer (COMICE) trial: a randomised controlled trial. *Lancet*. 2010;375:563–571.
8. Chagpar AB, Killelea BK, Tsangaris TN, et al. A randomized, controlled trial of cavity shave margins in breast cancer. *N Engl J Med*. 2015;373:503–510.
9. Fisher B, Costantino JP, Wickerham DL, et al. Tamoxifen for prevention of breast cancer: report of the National Surgical adjuvant Breast and bowel Project P-1 Study. *J Natl Cancer Inst*. 1998;90:1371–1388.
10. Boughey JC, Attai DJ, Chen SL, et al. Contralateral prophylactic mastectomy consensus statement from the american Society of breast surgeons: additional considerations and a framework for shared decision making. *Ann Surg Oncol*. 2016;23:3106–3111.
11. Johnson AT, Henry-Tillman RS, Smith LF, et al. Percutaneous excisional breast biopsy. *Am J Surg*. 2002;184:550–554; discussion 554.
12. Giuliano AE, Edge SB, Hortobagyi GN. Eighth edition of the AJCC cancer staging manual: Breast cancer. *Ann Surg Oncol*. 2018;25:1783–1785.
13. Hu J, Rainsbury RM, Segaran A, et al. Objective assessment of clinical, oncological and cosmetic outcomes following volume replacement in patients undergoing oncoplastic breast-conserving surgery: protocol for a systematic review. *BMJ Open*. 2018;8:e020859.
14. Moran MS, Schnitt SJ, Giuliano AE, et al. Society of Surgical Oncology–American Society for radiation oncology consensus guideline on margins for breast-conserving surgery with whole-breast irradiation in stages I and II invasive breast cancer. *Ann Surg Oncol*. 2014;21:704–716.
15. Harrigan M, Cartmel B, Loftfield E, et al. Randomized trial comparing telephone versus in-person weight loss counseling on body composition and circulating biomarkers in women treated for breast cancer: the Lifestyle, Exercise, and Nutrition (LEAN) Study. *J Clin Oncol*. 2016;34:669–676.
16. Losken A, Dugal CS, Styblo TM, et al. A meta-analysis comparing breast conservation therapy alone to the oncoplastic technique. *Ann Plast Surg*. 2014;72:145–149.
17. Weber WP, Haug M, Kurzeder C, et al. Oncoplastic breast Consortium consensus conference on nipple-sparing mastectomy. *Breast Cancer Res Treat*. 2018;172:523–537.
18. Krag DN, Anderson SJ, Julian TB, et al. Sentinel-lymph-node resection compared with conventional axillary-lymph-node dissection in clinically node-negative patients with breast cancer: Overall survival findings from the NSABP B-32 randomised phase 3 trial. *Lancet Oncol*. 2010;11:927–933.
19. Giuliano AE, Hawes D, Ballman KV, et al. Association of occult metastases in sentinel lymph nodes and bone marrow with survival among women with early-stage invasive breast cancer. *JAMA*. 2011;306:385–393.
20. Hunt KK, Yi M, Mittendorf EA, et al. Sentinel lymph node surgery after neoadjuvant chemotherapy is accurate and reduces the need for axillary dissection in breast cancer patients. *Ann Surg*. 2009;250:558–566.
21. Giuliano AE, Ballman KV, McCall L, et al. Effect of axillary dissection vs no axillary dissection on 10-year overall survival among women with invasive breast cancer and sentinel node metastasis: the ACOSOG Z0011 (Alliance) Randomized Clinical Trial. *JAMA*. 2017;318:918–926.
22. Giuliano AE, Hunt KK, Ballman KV, et al. Axillary dissection vs no axillary dissection in women with invasive breast cancer and sentinel node metastasis: a randomized clinical trial. *JAMA*. 2011;305:569–575.
23. Tummel E, Ochoa D, Korourian S, et al. Does axillary reverse mapping prevent lymphedema after lymphadenectomy? *Ann Surg*. 2017;265:987–992.
24. Morrow M, Van Zee KJ, Solin LJ, et al. Society of Surgical Oncology–American society for radiation oncology–American society of clinical oncology consensus guideline on margins for breast-conserving surgery with whole-breast irradiation in ductal carcinoma in situ. *J Clin Oncol*. 2016;34:4040–4046.
25. Marinovich ML, Azizi L, Macaskill P, et al. The association of surgical margins and local recurrence in women with ductal carcinoma in situ treated with breast-conserving therapy: a meta-analysis. *Ann Surg Oncol*. 2016;23:3811–3821.
26. Silverstein MJ. The University of Southern California/Van Nuys prognostic index for ductal carcinoma in situ of the breast. *Am J Surg*. 2003;186:337–343.
27. Hughes LL, Wang M, Page DL, et al. Local excision alone without irradiation for ductal carcinoma in situ of the breast: a trial of the Eastern Cooperative Oncology Group. *J Clin Oncol*. 2009;27:5319–5324.
28. Forbes JF, Sestak I, Howell A, et al. Anastrozole versus tamoxifen for the prevention of locoregional and contralateral breast cancer in postmenopausal women with locally excised ductal carcinoma in situ (IBIS-II DCIS): a double-blind, randomised controlled trial. *Lancet*. 2016;387:866–873.
29. Hughes KS, Schnaper LA, Bellon JR, et al. Lumpectomy plus tamoxifen with or without irradiation in women age 70 years or older with early breast cancer: long-term follow-up of CALGB 9343. *J Clin Oncol*. 2013;31:2382–2387.
30. Smith BD, Arthur DW, Buchholz TA, et al. Accelerated partial breast irradiation consensus statement from the American society for radiation oncology (ASTRO). *Int J Radiat Oncol Biol Phys*. 2009;74:987–1001.
31. Ragaz J, Olivotto IA, Spinelli JJ, et al. Locoregional radiation therapy in patients with high-risk breast cancer receiving

adjuvant chemotherapy: 20-year results of the British Columbia randomized trial. *J Natl Cancer Inst.* 2005;97:116–126.
32. Effects of chemotherapy and hormonal therapy for early breast cancer on recurrence and 15-year survival: an overview of the randomised trials. *Lancet.* 2005;365:1687–1717.
33. Sparano JA, Gray RJ, Makower DF, et al. Adjuvant chemotherapy guided by a 21-gene expression assay in breast cancer. *N Engl J Med.* 2018;379:111–121.
34. O'Sullivan CC, Bradbury I, Campbell C, et al. Efficacy of adjuvant trastuzumab for patients with human epidermal growth factor receptor 2-positive early breast cancer and tumors </= 2 cm: a meta-analysis of the randomized trastuzumab trials. *J Clin Oncol.* 2015;33:2600–2608.
35. Slamon D, Eiermann W, Robert N, et al. Adjuvant trastuzumab in HER2-positive breast cancer. *N Engl J Med.* 2011;365:1273–1283.
36. Ocana A, Amir E, Pandiella A. Dual targeting of HER2-positive breast cancer with trastuzumab emtansine and pertuzumab: understanding clinical trial results. *Oncotarget.* 2018;9:31915–31919.
37. Davies C, Pan H, Godwin J, et al. Long-term effects of continuing adjuvant tamoxifen to 10 years versus stopping at 5 years after diagnosis of oestrogen receptor-positive breast cancer: ATLAS, a randomised trial. *Lancet.* 2013;381:805–816.
38. Burstein HJ, Prestrud AA, Seidenfeld J, et al. American Society of Clinical Oncology clinical practice guideline: update on adjuvant endocrine therapy for women with hormone receptor-positive breast cancer. *J Clin Oncol.* 2010;28:3784–3796.
39. Howell A, Cuzick J, Baum M, et al. Results of the ATAC (Arimidex, Tamoxifen, Alone or in Combination) trial after completion of 5 years' adjuvant treatment for breast cancer. *Lancet.* 2005;365:60–62.
40. Boccardo F, Rubagotti A, Aldrighetti D, et al. Switching to an aromatase inhibitor provides mortality benefit in early breast carcinoma: pooled analysis of 2 consecutive trials. *Cancer.* 2007;109:1060–1067.
41. Burstein HJ, Temin S, Anderson H, et al. Adjuvant endocrine therapy for women with hormone receptor-positive breast cancer: American Society of Clinical Oncology clinical practice guideline focused update. *J Clin Oncol.* 2014;32:2255–2269.
42. Pagani O, Regan MM, Walley BA, et al. Adjuvant exemestane with ovarian suppression in premenopausal breast cancer. *N Engl J Med.* 2014;371:107–118.
43. Burstein HJ, Lacchetti C, Anderson H, et al. Adjuvant endocrine therapy for women with hormone receptor-positive breast cancer: American Society of Clinical Oncology clinical practice guideline update on ovarian suppression. *J Clin Oncol.* 2016;34:1689–1701.
44. Cortazar P, Zhang L, Untch M, et al. Pathological complete response and long-term clinical benefit in breast cancer: the CTNeoBC pooled analysis. *Lancet.* 2014;384:164–172.
45. van Deurzen CH, Vriens BE, Tjan-Heijnen VC, et al. Accuracy of sentinel node biopsy after neoadjuvant chemotherapy in breast cancer patients: a systematic review. *Eur J Cancer.* 2009;45:3124–3130.
46. Boughey JC, Suman VJ, Mittendorf EA, et al. Sentinel lymph node surgery after neoadjuvant chemotherapy in patients with node-positive breast cancer: the ACOSOG Z1071 (Alliance) clinical trial. *JAMA.* 2013;310:1455–1461.
47. Caudle AS, Yang WT, Krishnamurthy S, et al. Improved axillary evaluation following neoadjuvant therapy for patients with node-positive breast cancer using selective evaluation of clipped nodes: implementation of targeted axillary dissection. *J Clin Oncol.* 2016;34:1072–1078.
48. Gianni L, Pienkowski T, Im YH, et al. Efficacy and safety of neoadjuvant pertuzumab and trastuzumab in women with locally advanced, inflammatory, or early HER2-positive breast cancer (NeoSphere): randomised multicentre, open-label, phase 2 trial. *Lancet Oncol.* 2012;13:25–32.
49. Cristofanilli M, Gonzalez-Angulo AM, Buzdar AU, et al. Paclitaxel improves the prognosis in estrogen receptor negative inflammatory breast cancer: The M. D. Anderson Cancer Center experience. *Clin Breast Cancer.* 2004;4:415–419.

36 CHAPTER

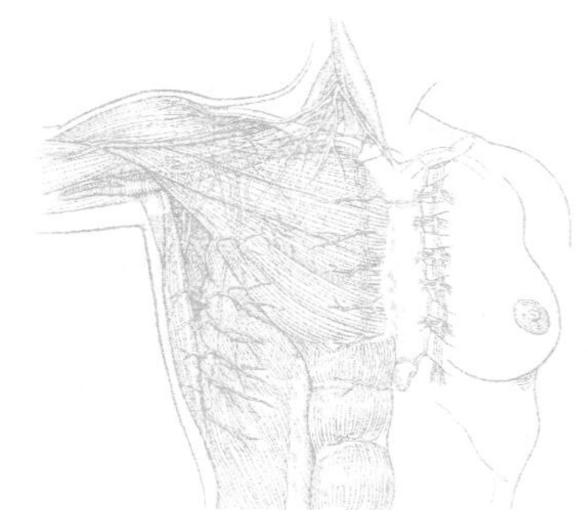

Breast Reconstruction

Stefanos Boukovalas, Shana S. Kalaria, Julie E. Park

OUTLINE

In women in the United States, breast cancer is the most common cancer and the second most common cause of death from cancer. From the 1980s to 2015, breast cancer mortality rates have declined, and 5-year survival has increased to almost 90%.[1] The American Cancer Society (ACS) adjusted its breast cancer screening guidelines in 2015 and now strongly recommends annual mammograms from age 45 and older. Women aged 40 to 44 should be given the opportunity to begin screening earlier according to the qualified recommendation. Women 55 and older may switch to biennial screening but should be given the option to continue annual screening if they prefer. The ACS recommendation is that screening mammography should continue so long as a woman is healthy and life expectancy is 10 years or longer.[2]

The American Joint Committee on Cancer (AJCC) published its latest *Eighth Edition Cancer Staging Manual*, which describes a novel breast cancer staging system that combines the traditional anatomic staging system of tumor size, nodal status, and metastasis (TNM staging) with biologic markers—estrogen receptor, progesterone receptor, human epidermal growth factor receptor 2, grade, and multigene assays. Treatment is dependent on the clinical diagnosis and stage of the breast cancer and is usually designed to address the local cancer with breast-conserving therapy with radiation or mastectomy and address the systemic cancer with chemotherapy and endocrine therapy.

BREAST CONSERVATION THERAPY—ONCOPLASTIC TECHNIQUES

While lumpectomy combined with adjuvant radiation therapy confers the same survival benefits as mastectomy, postradiation contracture can cause contour deformities of the breast and nipple areolar deviation toward the location of the lumpectomy. Oncoplastic breast reconstruction, a term coined in the 1980s, prevents these deformities and offers lower morbidity, higher quality of life, and a more natural aesthetic outcome than traditional breast reconstruction techniques following mastectomies.[3] It gives women multiple conservative options if they choose breast-conserving therapy but also offers them contralateral breast surgery to achieve a symmetric result or if they are unhappy with the unaffected breast. Careful coordination and communication between the breast oncologic surgeons and reconstructive surgeons is important for the optimal preoperative planning of incisions to achieve both oncologic and aesthetic outcomes.

The goals of oncoplastic breast reconstruction are obliteration of dead space, vascular support of the nipple, and tailoring the local tissues to place the nipple areolar complex and the remaining skin and parenchyma in an aesthetically acceptable shape such that postradiation contractile forces will be concentric so as to prevent distortion. It encompasses three main techniques: reduction/mastopexy, intrinsic tissue rearrangement, and adjacent tissue transfer/locoregional flaps.

Certain considerations regarding adjuvant radiation therapy affect surgical planning and technique. Whether or not the patient requires a boost during radiation therapy can affect which type of reconstruction is performed, in order to minimize the degree to which the margins of the lumpectomy cavity are rearranged within the breast. Since the dead space is obliterated, there will not be seroma formation to guide the radiation therapist about the lumpectomy margins. Therefore, either the surgical oncologist or the plastic surgeon must clearly define the margins with clips prior to any rearrangements. It is also preferable to avoid using clips for hemostasis to avoid confusion. Electrocautery or suture ties/ligations are other options for hemostatic control. Consideration should also be given to the amount of tissue rearrangement that will be required in case positive or close margins requires reexcision. Likewise, all tissue excised, especially around the lumpectomy margins, should be oriented and clearly labeled. There are several strategies to deal with the issue of margin status, including staging the oncoplastic reconstruction portion to after the final margins are known or proceeding with immediate reconstruction and the possibility of radiation therapy. Multidisciplinary breast conference is an ideal place to discuss these options.

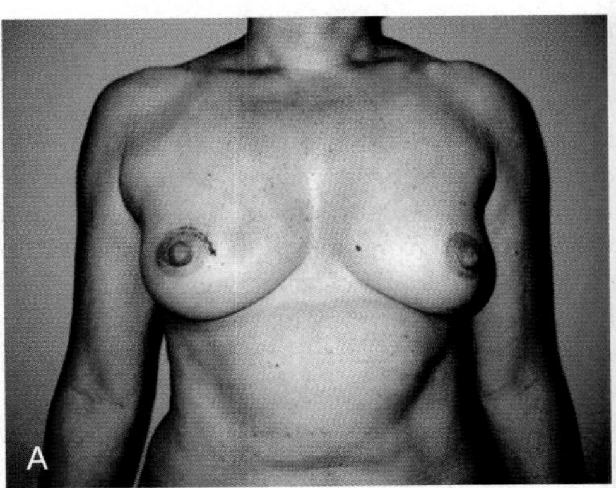

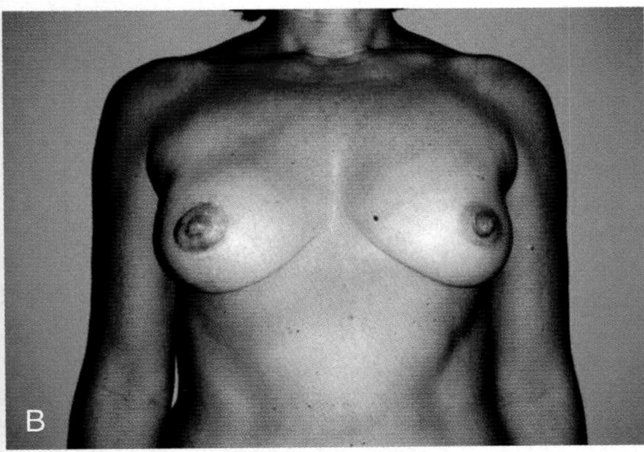

FIG. 36.1 Patient with right breast cancer before (A) and after (B) unilateral right breast reconstruction using a transverse upper gracilis flap. (A) Before reconstruction. (B) 33 months after reconstruction. (From Schoeller T, Huemer GM, Wechselberger G. The transverse musculocutaneous gracilis flap for breast reconstruction: guidelines for flap and patient selection. *Plast Reconstr Surg.* 2008;122:29–38.)

Breast reduction strategies are used to treat patients with large and/or ptotic breasts with unifocal disease in which breast-conserving therapy is appropriate. Various breast reduction strategies can be used, but there must be a discussion with the breast surgeon prior to surgery regarding the planned segmental mastectomy incisions. Wise-pattern skin reductions afford more flexibility in incision planning for the breast surgeon but have a larger scar burden that the patient must be counseled on. They can be used in combination with various pedicles depending on the location and size of the tumor as well as the planned area and amount of resection. Likewise, vertical breast reductions can be used to accomplish the combined goals of reconstruction and reduction in smaller, less ptotic breasts and are especially effective for lesions in the 6 o'clock region. Regardless the specific technique chosen, the underlying principles are the same as previously stated, with the lumpectomy location incorporated into the tissue that would be resected in a regular reduction (Fig. 36.1).

When adjacent tissue must be recruited into the defect without decreasing the size of the breast or lifting the nipple local and regional flaps can be used to recreate the shape of the breast. Local flaps include intrinsic parenchymal flaps to support nipple areolar complex vascularity or to fill in dead space. Regional flaps include lateral, medial, and anterior intercostal artery perforator flaps (LICAP, MICAP, and AICAP), as well as the lateral thoracic artery perforator (LTAP), thoracodorsal artery perforator (TDAP), and internal mammary artery perforator (IMAP) flaps.[3] These flaps can be chosen and tailored based on patient breast size, location of the tumor, planned size of resection/anticipated defect, and understanding of radiation effects on this local flap, which mainly includes knowledge of the radiation effects on autologous tissue, which mainly includes fat necrosis.[4]

Fat grafting has become a popular adjunct technique in breast reconstruction given its low complication profile, readily available donor site, option to be performed in the outpatient setting, and ability to improve the skin and dermal quality especially in radiated fields.[5] The concern for local recurrence of breast cancer after fat grafting arose after it was shown that a subset group of women younger than 50, with in situ tumors, Ki-67 ≥14, and quadrantectomy had an increased risk of developing a local recurrence event after fat grafting.[6] While several studies have shown there is no increased risk of recurrent breast cancer when compared with breasts that are not fat grafted,[7,8] they are not sufficiently powered to answer the questions regarding this particular subset. Therefore, it is important to have a careful discussion with the patient while obtaining full consent and long-term oncologic surveillance and follow-up. Typical complications following fat grafting include oil cysts, infection, resorption, and fat necrosis.[8]

BOX 36.1 Options for breast reconstruction.

Autogenous
- Abdominal-based flaps
- Transverse rectus abdominis muscle (TRAM)
- Single pedicle
- Double pedicle
- Free flap*
- Deep inferior epigastric perforator flap*

Latissimus dorsi musculocutaneous flap
Gluteal flap*
- Superiorly based
- Inferiorly based

Rubens flap*
Thoracoepigastric flap
Lateral thigh flap*
Breast-splitting procedure†
Alloplastic
- Silicone gel implant
- Silicone implant with saline fill
- Smooth wall
- Textured wall
- Round
- Anatomic shaped

Combination procedures
- Latissimus dorsi flap with implant
- TRAM flap with implant

*Requires microsurgical procedure.
†Historical note only.

RECONSTRUCTION AFTER MASTECTOMY

Breast reconstruction after mastectomy typically utilizes an alloplastic device (tissue expander or implant), autologous tissue, or combination of the two. The different methods of breast reconstruction are further described in the following paragraphs and are summarized in Box 36.1. Each technique presents with

BOX 36.2 Implant reconstruction.

Indications
Bilateral reconstruction
Patient requesting augmentation in addition to reconstruction
Patient not suited for long surgery
Lack of adequate abdominal tissue
Patient unwilling to have additional scars on back or abdomen
Small breast mound with minimal ptosis

Relative Contraindications
Young age (may need implant replaced multiple times)
Patient unwilling to adhere to follow-up
Very large breast
Very ptotic breast
Silicon allergy
Implant fear
Previous failed implants
Need for adjuvant radiation therapy

advantages and disadvantages, and the final choice must take into account the extent of skin resection, need for neoadjuvant or adjuvant radiation and chemotherapy, patient body habitus, aesthetic desires, and activity level (Box 36.2).

Blondeel and colleagues[9] described a method for approaching the breast in both aesthetic and reconstructive surgery by analyzing the breast footprint or interface with the thoracic wall, conus or the shape and volume of the breast gland, and envelope or the skin and subcutaneous tissue. These factors should be critically analyzed in deciding on reconstructive options. Symmetry should be addressed with the patient and assumed to be a paramount expectation as it leads to better patient reported outcomes, higher satisfaction, and more self-confidence.

Contralateral Breast

Breast reconstruction should not be limited to focusing on the affected breast and attaining symmetry to the native breast but must consider patient goals and satisfaction for both breasts.[10] The Women's Health and Cancer Rights Act of 1998 (WHCRA) requires by federal law that group and individual health insurance plans pay for all stages of breast reconstruction on the mastectomy side as well as reconstruction of the contralateral breast, prostheses, and treatment of complications of mastectomy including lymphedema. Some women are primarily concerned with eradication of cancer and may opt for the more aggressive surgical option, including contralateral prophylactic mastectomies, especially in patients at high lifetime risk of contralateral breast cancer, for example, those with a pathogenic germline *BRCA* gene mutation. In the preoperative assessment, patients should be asked if they are comfortable with the contralateral breast being operated on and what if anything bothers them about that breast. Then they should be thoroughly counseled regarding the timing options, scars, risks, benefits, and complications of operating on the contralateral breast. Among patients undergoing unilateral autologous or implant-based reconstruction, the most common contralateral procedure is breast reduction followed by mastopexy and augmentation.[11]

Radiation

Any discussion about oncoplastic breast surgery would be incomplete without explaining the effects of radiation on both implant-based and autologous reconstruction and timing effects of radiation therapy. Preoperative radiation damages the recipient field and intramammary vessels increasing the risk of intraoperative vascular complications, minor complications, skin loss, and infection in autologous reconstruction.[12] The higher risk of reconstructive failure (reported to be as high 50%), total complications, capsular contracture, infection, mastectomy flap necrosis, and seroma have led implant-based reconstruction to fall out of favor in the setting of prior radiation.[12] Autologous reconstruction is the ideal method of reconstruction in a patient with prior chest wall irradiation. Although radiation after completion of implant-based reconstruction has lower complications than radiation before implant-based reconstruction, it is never advised to delay cancer treatment for reconstructive purposes. The effects of radiation are more profound on tissue expanders over implants and studies have shown higher reconstructive failure rates when tissue expanders are radiated compared to permanent implants.[12–14] Finally, adjuvant radiation effects on autologous reconstruction are minor and include an increased risk of fat necrosis, but no additional flap complications or increase in number of revision surgeries, making postoperative radiation of autologous reconstruction more favorable than radiation of implant-based reconstruction.[4]

Quality Measurements and Outcomes

Women undergoing breast reconstruction after mastectomy have been shown to have significantly increased satisfaction scores compared to women with no reconstruction. Beugels and colleagues[15] evaluated quality of life after immediate or delayed reconstruction with abdominal-based free flaps using the BREAST-Q. The results of their study demonstrated high and comparable satisfaction rates after 1-year postreconstruction, regardless of timing of reconstruction. In a different study, Santosa and colleagues[16] compared quality of life of 2013 women from 11 centers across the United States after autologous and implant-based reconstruction. Satisfaction rates were assessed using the BREAST-Q, and it was found that 2 years after reconstruction, women who underwent free flap reconstruction had greater psychosocial and sexual well-being, reporting higher satisfaction rates. When comparing satisfaction rates among different autologous techniques, deep inferior epigastric perforator (DIEP) flap reconstruction seems to provide the highest rates of well-being.[17] Cost-effective analyses have been performed to compare autologous and implant-based techniques. Matros and colleagues[18] suggest that DIEP flap reconstruction is cost-effective when compared with implants, especially in unilateral cases. Given the higher cost of the index procedure, the cost-effectiveness is maximized in younger patients with good prognosis and longer life expectancy. There are some data supporting that pedicled transverse rectus abdominis muscle (TRAM) flap reconstruction is associated with lower total hospital charges; however, long-term outcomes and potential need for revision surgery or abdominal wall reconstruction make this comparison less reliable.[19]

Alloplastic Reconstruction

Implant-based breast reconstruction popularized in the 1970s involves either tissue expansion or implant placement and can be performed either in an immediate or delayed fashion. It is generally a better option in thin women with small breasts who desire bilateral reconstruction and have satisfactory tissue coverage of the implants.[20] It is not a first choice option in a patient who has had or will need radiation.[12,21] These procedures are quicker, less morbid, and have less recovery time compared to autologous reconstruction (Box 36.2).

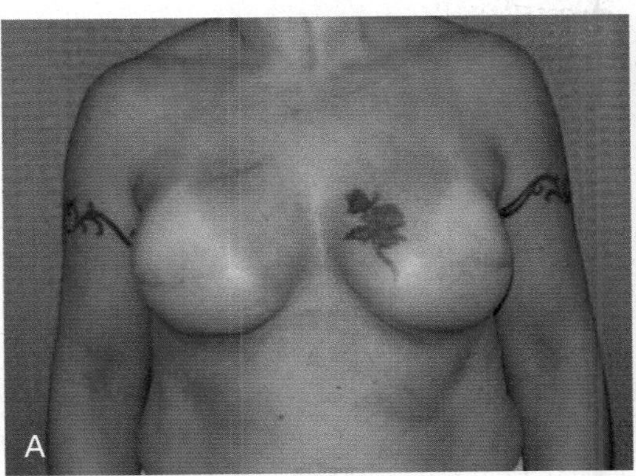

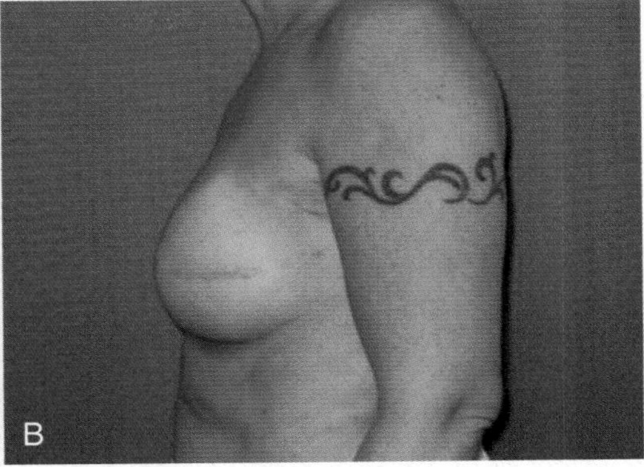

FIG. 36.2 A 41-year-old woman with left breast cancer who underwent bilateral mastectomy with immediate placement of bilateral tissue expanders with bioprosthetic slings. Final reconstruction was carried out with the exchange of expanders for 533-mL silicone gel breast prostheses. (From Roehl KR. Breast reconstruction. *Open Breast Cancer J.* 2010;2:25–37. Photos courtesy John D. Bauer, MD.)

Timing—Immediate Versus Delayed

The timing of breast reconstruction surgery has evolved from delayed to immediate to delayed-immediate options. The optimal timing for breast reconstruction after mastectomy remains a controversial topic and difficult decision given added factors such as radiation and various adjunct reconstructive options such as fat grafting and use of acellular dermal matrix. Factors that weigh heavily to patients in this decision are final reconstructive outcome, number of surgeries involved in the reconstruction, and postoperative complications.

Delayed

In the past, breast reconstruction was typically performed in a delayed manner after the mastectomy flaps healed. Delayed reconstruction in the setting of implant-based reconstruction is classically accomplished with two stages using a tissue expander to gradually expand the mastectomy flaps and breast pocket followed by exchange for permanent implant. Use of a tissue expander requires weekly visits for expansion and requires a compliant patient who preferably lives close to the clinic. This method traditionally includes use of acellular dermal matrix to support the tissue expander or implant and can be performed in the subpectoral or, more recently, prepectoral plane. Many surgeons delay reconstruction until 6 months after the completion of radiation to minimize the chance for wound healing problems.

Immediate

Immediate breast reconstruction, a newer concept, means that the final reconstructive modality is done at the time of the mastectomy. The advantages of direct-to-implant breast reconstruction are the "breast in a day" concept, with fewer number of surgeries, quicker return to work, better cosmetic outcome, and psychological benefit.[22] Immediate breast reconstruction does not delay detection of a chest wall recurrence or change oncologic outcomes and is thus considered a safe method of reconstruction.[23] Many surgeons are reluctant to place the added weight and stress of direct expansion on already compromised mastectomy skin particularly in the cases of thin or bruised mastectomy flaps and when the need for radiation is not definitively known. Additionally, the direct-to-implant method has risks of skin necrosis, nipple necrosis, seroma, infection, and implant exposure, leading to increased costs particularly in older patients with large implants.[22] This may be the appropriate choice of reconstruction for a young, thin, healthy, nonsmoker with small breasts, who desires to be approximately the same size, who has thick and well-perfused mastectomy skin flaps.[20]

Delayed-Immediate

Delayed-immediate reconstruction was first described in 2004 and referred to the immediate placement of tissue expanders at the time of skin-sparing mastectomies followed by delayed reconstruction in the case of radiation and immediate reconstruction (implants or autologous) in the case of no radiation (Fig. 36.2).[24] Because radiation makes such a profound difference on the complication rates and aesthetic outcomes especially when using implants, the delayed-immediate method of reconstruction is generally preferred. The delayed-immediate method allows those who do not require radiation to achieve aesthetic outcomes similar to those undergoing immediate reconstruction and allows those who require radiation to avoid complications associated with radiating an implant that is placed immediately.[24]

Location of Implant—Prepectoral Versus Subpectoral

Traditional two-stage implant-based breast reconstruction involved maximization of muscular coverage in a total musculofascial pocket and has evolved to partial subpectoral coverage with use of acellular dermal matrix as a sling at the inferior border of the pectoralis major.[25,26] The thought was that muscle coverage of the tissue expander and final implant was necessary in a radiated field to protect against wound dehiscence, infection, and wound healing complications (Figs. 36.3 and 36.4).

As the pendulum has swung from subglandular to subpectoral and now potentially back to subglandular breast augmentation, so has implant position in breast reconstruction. Prepectoral breast augmentation, first used in 1971, has been modified due to advances in surgical technique and mainly in refinements of newer generation tissue expanders and implants. The focus on enhanced recovery after surgery protocols and limiting pain and prescription of narcotics further pushes surgeons away from more invasive subpectoral dissection, which carries with it increased risks of animation deformity, muscle spasms, postoperative pain, and longer operative times. Prepectoral breast reconstruction carries a higher risk of surgical-site infection when compared to subpectoral in the irradiated breast but also has a lower risk of overall complications, capsular contracture, hematoma, and reconstructive failure.[27] Prepectoral reconstruction is performed by creating a new pocket anterior to the pectoralis muscle and can be done immediately

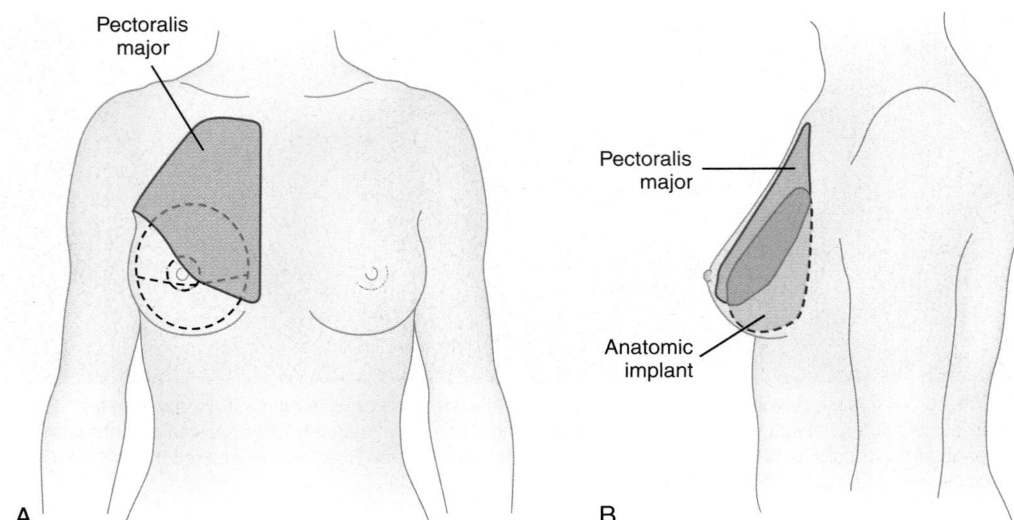

FIG. 36.3 (A, B) Schematic representation of implant position, pectoralis position, and chest wall. The pectoralis muscle cannot cover the inferior pole of the breast, and bioprosthetic material is needed in the area of greatest expansion. (From Breuing KH, Warren SM. Immediate bilateral breast reconstruction with implants and inferolateral AlloDerm slings. *Ann Plast Surg.* 2005;55:232–239.)

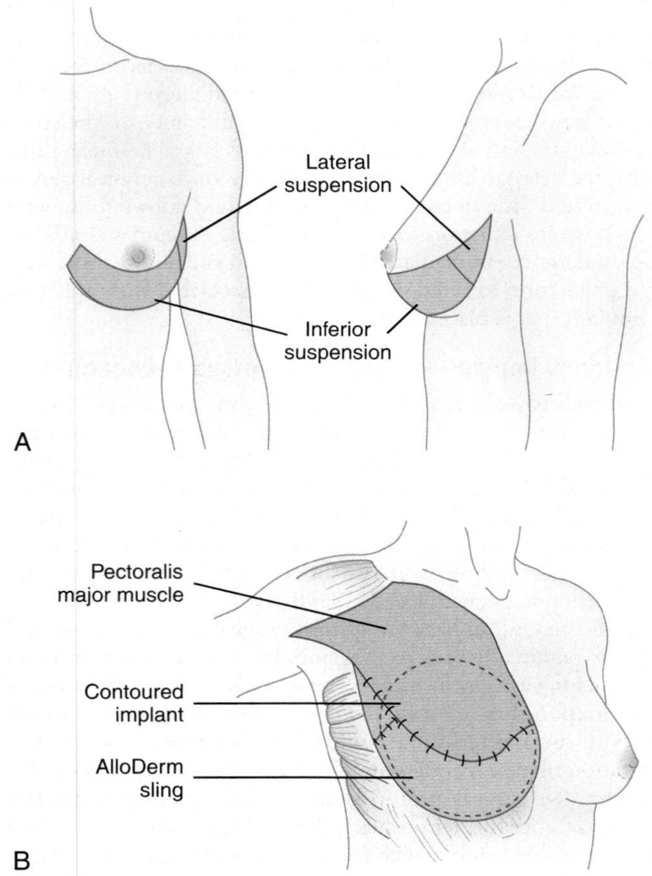

FIG. 36.4 (A, B) Schematic representation of chest wall, breast, pectoralis muscle, bioprosthetic sling, and implant. Bioprosthetic material is sutured to the inferior border of the pectoralis muscle superiorly, the inframammary fold inferiorly, and curved laterally along the chest wall to recreate the footprint of the breast for expansion. (From Breuing KH, Warren SM. Immediate bilateral breast reconstruction with implants and inferolateral AlloDerm slings. *Ann Plast Surg.* 2005;55:232–239.)

or delayed, in one or two stages, with saline or air in the tissue expander, and with or without acellular dermal matrix (Fig. 36.5). Prepectoral reconstruction should be discouraged in patients with a high risk of infection or those with thin poorly perfused mastectomy skin flaps.[28] The advantages of decreased pain, muscle spasm, and overall complications with prepectoral reconstruction should be weighed against the disadvantages of increased surgical site infection when compared to subpectoral reconstruction.[27]

Complications

Complications in implant-based reconstruction include hematoma, wound dehiscence, malposition, deflation, adverse scarring, capsular contracture, mastectomy skin flap necrosis, infection, seroma, extrusion, reconstructive failure, and venous thromboembolic events.[12,29] The total complication risk is increased particularly in the setting of preoperative radiation (25% complication rate vs. 13.9% complication rate without radiation), postoperative radiation (odds ratio 6.4), obesity (odds ratio 1.8), larger breast size (odds ratio 2.89) and smoking (odds ratio 2.2–3.07).[12,29] Many patients are still under the impression that implants should be exchanged every 10 years. These patients should be counseled that this is not necessary, but complications should be explained thoroughly so they can promptly address any problems with their tissue expanders or implants. Smoking and obesity (body mass index [BMI] > 25) have proven increased risk of complications and reconstructive failure especially in implant-based reconstruction and may preclude surgery.[29] Complications in breast reconstruction are extremely important to avoid and address promptly because in addition to added financial burden on the patient, they can cause a delay in chemotherapy treatments, affecting oncologic outcomes. Poor cosmetic outcome and need for revision surgeries are additional risks that can be limited by meticulous surgical planning and patient selection.

Autologous Breast Reconstruction

Autologous breast reconstruction utilizes the patient's own tissue instead of prosthetic devices. This offers the advantages of no tissue rejection and ability to resurface the skin envelope if deficient, damaged, or absent. Additionally, it provides a more natural shape and

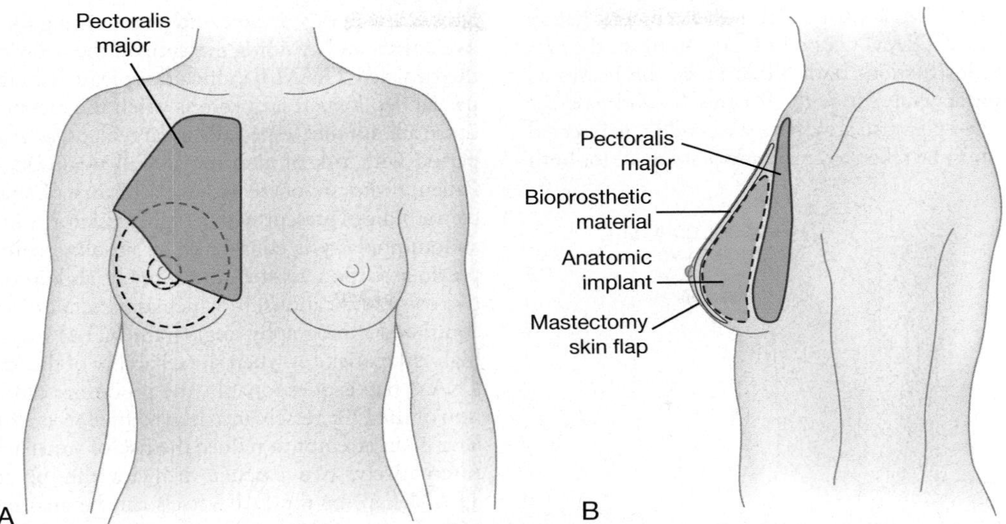

FIG. 36.5 Schematic representation of implant position, pectoralis position, and chest wall. The pectoralis muscle remains attached to the chest wall and the implant is placed in the prepectoral plane, with or without bioprosthetic material reinforcement. (Adapted from Breuing KH, Warren SM. Immediate bilateral breast reconstruction with implants and inferolateral AlloDerm slings. *Ann Plast Surg*. 2005;55:232–239.)

BOX 36.3 Transverse rectus abdominis muscle flap reconstruction.

Indications
Breasts of all sizes
Breast ptosis

Relative Contraindications
Smoking
Abdominal liposuction
Previous abdominal surgery
Pulmonary disease
Obesity

Contraindications
Previous abdominoplasty
Patient unable to tolerate 4- to 6-week recovery period
Patient unable to tolerate longer procedure

BOX 36.4 Latissimus dorsi reconstruction.

Indications
Small breast
Minor breast ptosis
Abdominal donor site unavailable (e.g., scars, lack of tissue)
Salvage of previous breast reconstruction

Relative Contraindications
Planned postoperative radiation therapy
Bilateral reconstruction
Significant breast ptosis

Contraindications
Previous lateral thoracotomy
Very large breast in patient who does not desire reduction

texture, proportional changes in size and contour of the breast with the rest of the body following weight changes, as well as potential improvement in the contour of other parts of the body that serve as donor sites. History of radiation and/or infection is a common indication for autologous breast reconstruction given the often-extensive radiation injury to skin and soft tissues. On the other hand, autologous breast reconstruction often requires longer operative time, involves additional surgical sites, and is associated with the potential risk of partial or complete flap loss (Boxes 36.3 and 36.4).

Pedicled Flaps (TRAM, Latissimus)

Pedicled flaps maintain their blood supply as they remain attached to the donor site, in contrast with free flaps, in which the vascular pedicle is being divided and reconnected to the recipient vessels in the chest using microsurgical technique. Pedicled flaps offer the advantages of autologous tissue reconstruction utilizing tissue adjacent to the breast. The most reliable pedicled flaps include the TRAM flap and the latissimus dorsi (LD) muscle flap.

The first description of the rectus abdominis muscle (RAM) flap for breast reconstruction was published in 1979 by Robbins, which included a vertical skin paddle. The technique evolved and a transverse skin paddle was first described by Hartrampf in 1982.[30] TRAM flap places the scar in a more acceptable location similar to an abdominoplasty scar. The lower abdominal area provides soft tissue of similar consistency to the breast with favorable results. In this setting, the TRAM flap is receiving blood supply from the superior epigastric vessels. These connect with the deep inferior epigastric (DIE) vessels via a rich circuit known as choke vessels, usually above the level of the umbilicus. The entire TRAM flap with various skin paddles can be reliably harvested based on the superior epigastric vessels after ligating the inferior epigastric system. For unilateral breast reconstruction, usually the contralateral TRAM is used to facilitate inset by decreasing the arc of rotation and subsequently the risk of vascular compromise from pressure on the pedicle. The perfusion of the TRAM flap's skin paddle has been evaluated by several studies. There are four distinct zones: perfusion is most reliable over the TRAM on the side of the pedicle (Zone I), followed by the area of the contralateral TRAM (Zone II). Following is the region lateral to the ipsilateral TRAM (Zone III) and, lastly, the region lateral to the contralateral TRAM (Zone IV) (Fig. 36.6). In the case of bilateral breast reconstruction, both TRAMs can be harvested and used for the contralateral side with the muscles and vascular pedicles crossing in the epigastric area. The skin paddle is bisected in the midline. Care must be taken to create adequate space for both

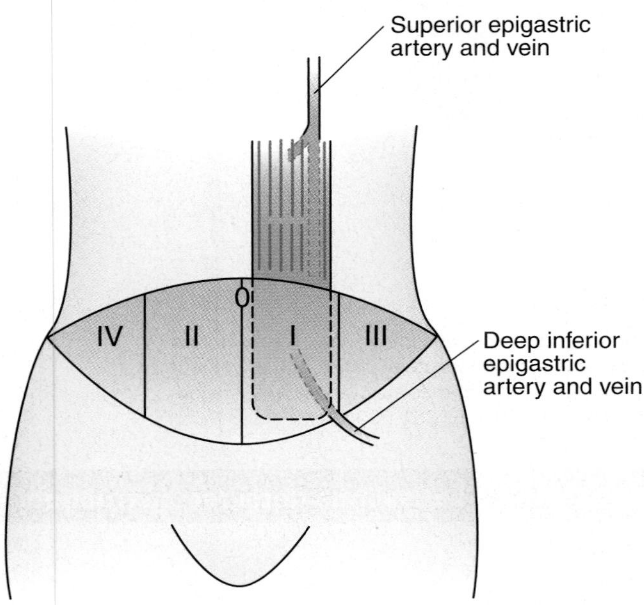

FIG. 36.6 Vascular territories of the abdominal wall provided by a unilateral pedicled transverse rectus abdominis muscle flap (as determined by Moon and Taylor). Blood flow is best in zone I, followed by zones II, III, and IV. (Moon HK, Taylor GI. The vascular anatomy of rectus abdominis musculocutaneous flaps based on the deep superior epigastric system. *Plast Reconstr Surg*. 1988;82:815–832.)

flaps in the epigastric area, often accounting for possible postoperative edema and avoiding pressure on the pedicles. Disadvantages of the pedicled TRAM flap include epigastric bulge, the potential for partial flap loss, or fat necrosis when the metabolic demands of the tissue are not met, especially in large flaps, as well as longer recovery period with risk of abdominal wall weakness, bulge, or hernia.[31] Patients who are obese or have a history of smoking and multiple comorbidities present with a higher risk for complications. Previous abdominoplasty is considered an absolute contraindication, while previous suction assisted lipectomy or abdominal surgeries are relative contraindications, in which assessment of vascular supply with computed tomography angiogram (CTA) may be warranted. In a high-risk patient or when the reliability of the vascular supply of the TRAM flap is questionable, the procedure can be staged with ligation of the DIE vessels and delayed final reconstruction 2 to 3 weeks later in an attempt to reduce the risk of vascular complications.[32,33] Alternatively, two vascular pedicles can be used (supercharged TRAM flap) or the DIE vessels can be anastomosed in the chest with the internal mammary or thoracodorsal vessels using microsurgical technique (turbocharged TRAM flap), improving vascular supply of the flap (Box 36.3).[34]

The LD muscle or myocutaneous flap is another alternative for autologous reconstruction using a pedicled flap. It was first described by Tansini in the late 1800s for coverage of radical mastectomy defects, and since then, several modifications have been developed to improve reliability and volume of the flap.[31,35,36] The LD is a broad flat muscle on the back with attachments to the spine medially and the posterior iliac crest inferiorly and inserts into the humerus. The LD flap is based on the thoracodorsal vessels, branching off the subscapular axis. A large skin paddle can be included in the flap, allowing resurfacing of the breast skin envelope. The skin paddle is often centered over the muscle and designed at an oblique or horizontal orientation to allow for tension-free closure but also placement within the bra line (Fig. 36.7). The LD flap

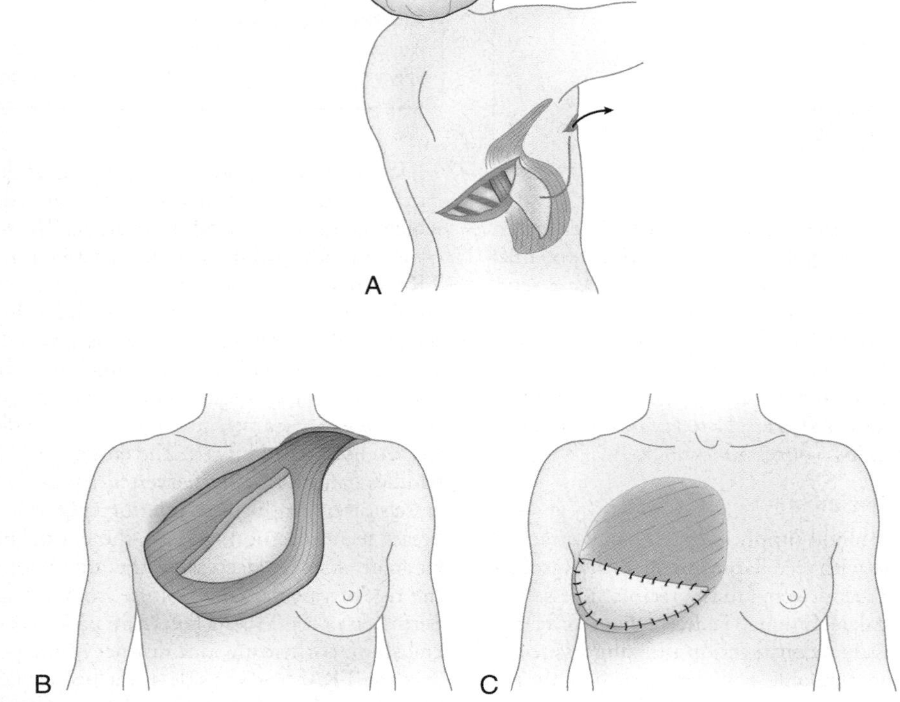

FIG. 36.7 Schematic representation of latissimus dorsi flap. (A) Flap elevation. (B) Flap transposition. (C) Flap inset.

provides adequate coverage of the anterior chest and can be used alone for reconstruction of women who desire a small size breast. Several techniques have been described to increase the volume of the LD flap, including harvesting of the supramuscular and subscapular fat (known as extended latissimus flap), fat grafting in a one-stage or multiple-stage procedure, or addition of an implant (see later; combined reconstruction).[36,37] Advantages of the LD flap include reliable anatomy and favorable location in close proximity to the breast. Axillary dissection of the muscular insertion and pedicle can be challenging in patients with previous radiation in the area and should be performed with caution. Additionally, limiting dissection in the axillary and lateral chest region is essential for a pleasing aesthetic outcome and avoiding lateral chest fullness from prominent pedicle. Regarding donor site morbidity, seroma is a commonly reported complication; its risk can be minimized with the use of quilting sutures and drains. Postoperative animation deformity from muscular contractions can be prevented or treated at a later stage by deinnervating the LD muscle and/or disinserting it from the humerus (Box 36.4). In case the thoracodorsal pedicle has been divided accidentally or during the axillary lymph node dissection, the flap can be converted to a free flap or raised on the serratus muscle branches of the thoracodorsal pedicle, if the injury is more proximal. The muscle sparing TDAP flap has been described as an alternative to the traditional LD myocutaneous flap, in which case the muscle is split but not harvested with the flap, minimizing donor site morbidity and risk of seroma.[38]

Free Flaps (ms-TRAM, DIEP, SIEA, PAP/TUG, SGAP, IGAP, Preoperative Planning, SPY, and Postoperative Monitoring)

Abdominal-based flaps. Lower abdominal soft tissue and skin can be utilized for breast reconstruction as free tissue transfer.[31] The dominant blood supply of the region is the DIE pedicle off the external iliac system, including the DIE artery (DIEA) with its venae comitantes. The DIEA provides robust blood supply to the RAM and overlying soft tissue, which decreases the risk of partial flap necrosis and fat necrosis when the tissue is harvested as free flap compared to pedicled. Additionally, free tissue transfer avoids the epigastric bulge that is often a result of the rotation of the pedicle in a TRAM flap. Experience with this flap has allowed for significant advances in the surgical technique the last 20 years. Instead of harvesting the entire RAM, plastic surgeons are now aiming for muscle-sparing techniques. The internal mammary vessels are commonly used as recipient vessels, even though axillary vessels, such as the thoracodorsal, can be reliably utilized. The topography of DIEA perforators has been analyzed extensively, illustrating medial and lateral row vessels. The perfusion zones are different compared to the pedicled TRAM flap. Blood supply is more reliable over the muscle on the side ipsilateral to the pedicle (Zone I), followed by the area lateral to the ipsilateral muscle (Zone II). Following is the region of the contralateral RAM (Zone III) and, lastly, the area lateral to the contralateral muscle (Zone IV) (Fig. 36.8). The dominance of these perforators varies among patients, but studies have demonstrated that reliable perforators are expected to be encountered 5 cm around the umbilicus.[31,39] In an attempt to minimize donor site morbidity, the muscle-sparing TRAM (ms-TRAM) free flap was developed. In this approach, only muscle around the perforators is harvested, preserving part of the RAM and rectus fascia. Recent advances in microsurgical techniques and perforator dissection have allowed refined harvest of abdominal flaps based off multiple perforators or even a single-dominant perforator, making this a true perforator flap (also known as DIEP flap).[31,39] This approach allows for muscle- and

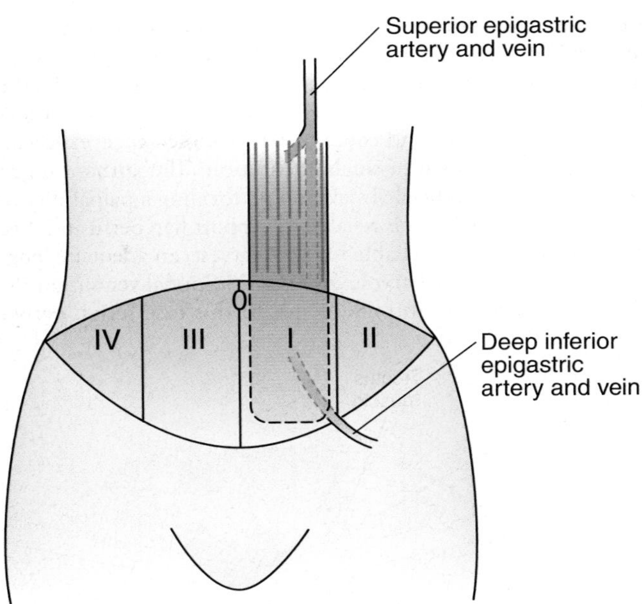

FIG. 36.8 Vascular territories of the abdominal wall provided by a unilateral free transverse rectus abdominis muscle or unilateral deep inferior epigastric artery flap (as determined by Moon and Taylor). Blood flow is best in zone I, followed by zones II, III, and IV. (Adapted from Holm C, Mayr M, Höfter E, et al. Perfusion zones of the DIEP flap revisited: a clinical study. *Plast Reconstr Surg.* 2006;117(1):37–43.)

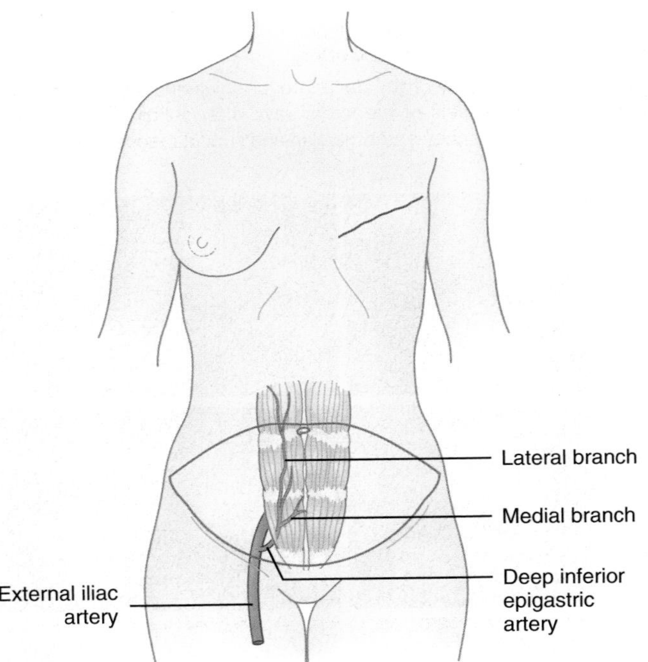

FIG. 36.9 Schematic of lower abdomen markings for autologous reconstruction based on the medial and lateral row of perforators, which are based on the deep inferior epigastric artery system.

fascia-sparing flap harvest, also preserving innervation, minimizing the risk for abdominal wall weakness or postoperative bulge and hernia, often avoiding the use of mesh during the donor site repair (Figs. 36.9 to 36.11).

An alternative option is utilizing the superficial inferior epigastric artery and vein (SIEA and SIEV) flaps or the superficial circumflex iliac vein, branching off the common femoral vessels. This pedicle exists in approximately 30% of patients and is prone to vasospasms; however, it allows for flap harvest without violating the rectus sheath, eliminating the risk of abdominal wall weakening (Fig. 36.12). Park and colleagues[40] presented their experience with 145 SIEA flaps in a single institution. The authors suggest identifying the superficial vessels and performing a palpability test to determine if the SIEA is reliable to support flap perfusion. Even when the SIEA is not reliable for flap harvest, an adequate length of the SIEV should be harvested in case additional venous outflow is required, especially in bulky flaps. In this case series, patients who suffered postoperative arterial thrombosis or required intraoperative anastomotic revisions had low chances of flap salvage. The total flap loss rate was 8%, with 4.8% secondary to anastomotic complication. 10.3% of flaps had partial necrosis, and there were no hernias or bulges in 31 months of average follow-up.[40]

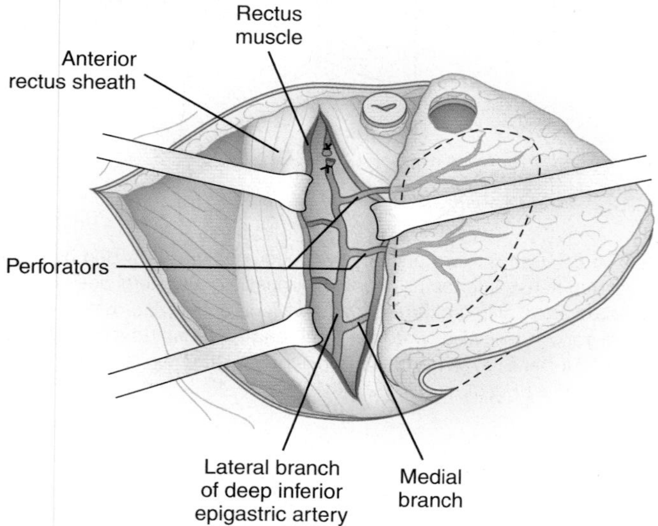

FIG. 36.10 Anatomy of the deep inferior epigastric artery flap. Shown are perforating vessels of the lateral row, after splitting the rectus abdominis muscle, as they enter the skin and subcutaneous tissue.

As a general guide, in cases where a reliable SIEA is identified, the flap can be based on the SIEA and SIEV. If the robust DIEA perforators are identified with good caliber and dissection can be performed without dividing the muscle, a DIEP flap is preferred. Otherwise, if small-caliber perforators are encountered and not aligned over the medial or lateral row, a ms-TRAM flap is performed to ensure flap viability.

A recent meta analysis performed by the American Society of Plastic Surgeons (ASPS) Breast Reconstruction Work Group demonstrated that pedicled TRAM flaps have a higher rate of hernias compared to DIEP flaps (3.50% vs. 0.74%) but slightly lower rates of bulging (3.50% vs. 4.62%).[39] The latter may be explained by the higher probability of mesh use in pedicle TRAM flap reconstruction. In pedicled TRAM flaps, the total flap loss rate ranged from 0 to 0.2% and partial flap loss rate up to 8.5%, whereas DIEP flaps had a total flap loss rate of 0 to 4.7% and a partial flap loss rate of 1.8% to 4.7%.[39] In a different study analyzing 3310 abdominally based flaps for immediate unilateral breast reconstruction, the rates for of reoperation for the revision of a vascular anastomosis for pedicled TRAM, free TRAM, DIEP, and SIEA flaps were 0.0%, 1.72%, 2.66%, and 5.64%, respectively.[19] Other studies agree with these results.[17,31] Chang and colleagues[41] compared the outcomes of bilateral autologous breast reconstruction at a single institution. Bilateral reconstruction had a higher flap loss rate but equivalent complication rates compared to unilateral. Patients undergoing bilateral immediate/delayed reconstruction had increased rates of revision surgery on the contralateral side of prophylactic mastectomy to achieve symmetry.

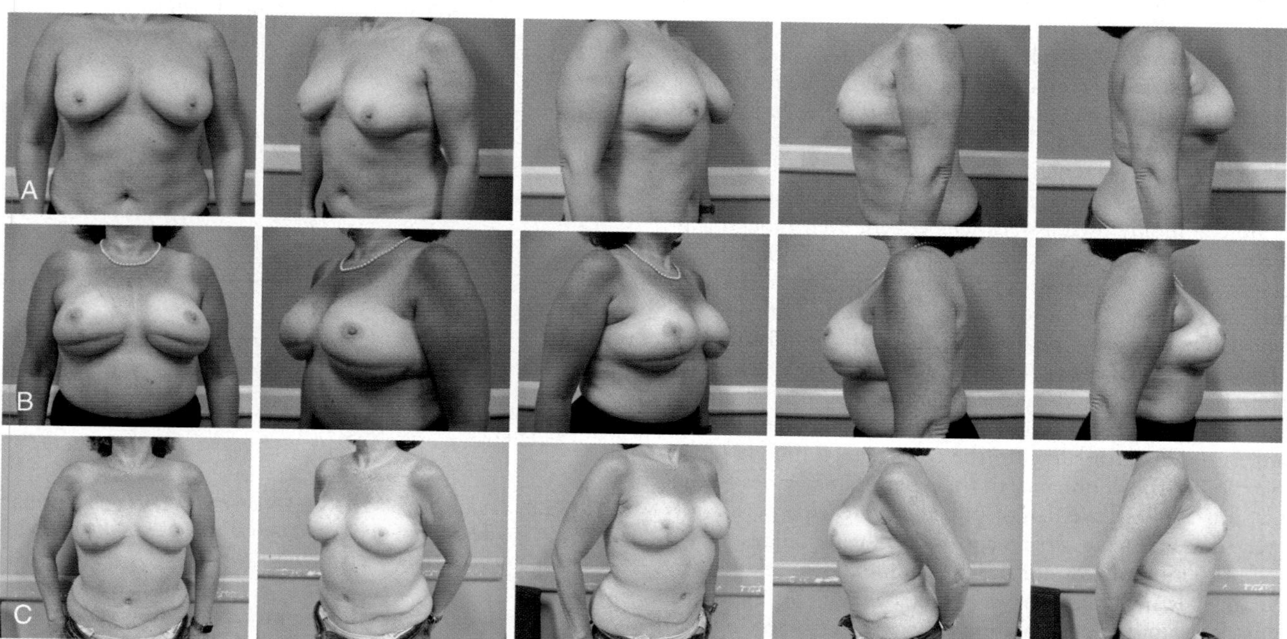

FIG. 36.11 (A) Preoperative pictures of a patient with right breast cancer who underwent nipple-sparing mastectomy with lymph node dissection and contralateral prophylactic nipple-sparing mastectomy followed by immediate reconstruction with bilateral deep inferior epigastric perforator flaps. (B) Patient as presented 3 months after initial reconstruction. (C) Postoperative pictures 6 weeks after bilateral breast revision, fat grafting, and abdominal donor site revision.

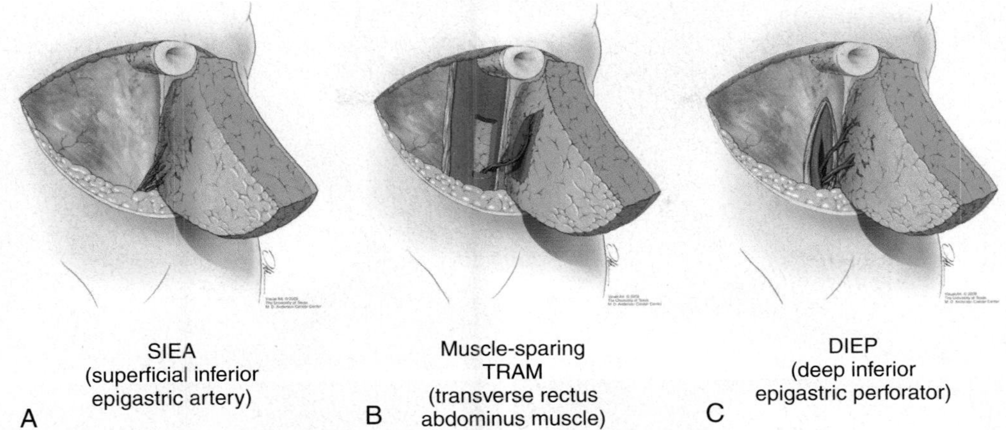

FIG. 36.12 Schematic representation of the superficial inferior epigastric artery flap in which abdominal wall fascia is undisturbed (A); deep inferior epigastric perforator flap, in which all muscle is spared (B); and muscle-sparing transverse rectus abdominis muscle flap, in which a small window of muscle is taken around the supplying perforators (C). (©2009 The University of Texas M.D. Anderson Cancer Center.)

Patients with a history of abdominoplasty or absence of excess lower abdominal tissue are not candidates for this procedure. For patients undergoing bilateral breast reconstruction, realistic counseling should be provided regarding expected postoperative reconstructed breast size, often limited by the amount of tissue available.

Thigh-based flaps. The medial thigh donor site is another option for free tissue transfer for breast reconstruction that has received more popularity recently.[42–44] It is usually considered for women with previous abdominal scars or inadequate lower abdominal tissue. These flaps can be based on the gracilis vascular supply, harvested as a myocutaneous or as a true perforator flap based on the profunda femoris artery perforator (PAP). The orientation of the skin paddle can be transverse (a transverse upper gracilis [TUG]), a vertical (VUG), or a diagonal (DUG) flap (Figs. 36.1 and 36.13). The scar of the TUG flap is hidden in the upper inner thigh, compared to the PAP flap, which results in a more posterior scar. Bilateral thighs can be used for unilateral or bilateral breast reconstruction, depending on the amount of available tissue. In unilateral breast reconstruction requiring large volume to match the contralateral side, stacked flaps from both thighs can be utilized with excellent results. Microvascular anastomoses are being performed either to separate recipient vessels (i.e., antegrade and retrograde to internal mammary vessels) or by connecting one flap to the other as flow-through design. Complications include wound healing problems, visible scar, and lymphedema, which could be minimized with careful patient selection and flap design.[44]

Gluteal-based flaps. Gluteal tissue can be utilized alternatively for autologous breast reconstruction based on the superior and inferior gluteal artery and vein.[43] It is considered for patients who have had previous abdominal surgery including abdominoplasty or inadequate abdominal tissue to support breast reconstruction. The lateral thighs or buttocks often provide enough adipose tissue and scar placement is favorable, hidden at the waist or the inferior gluteal crease. The consistency of the fat in the area is firm, which results in a reconstructed breast that is less soft but with significant projection that is often maintained over time. These flaps were initially described as myocutaneous flaps, with significant donor site morbidity. More recently, these flaps are harvested as muscle-sparing or true superior or inferior gluteal artery perforator (SGAP or IGAP) flaps, which limits contour deformity, muscle weakness, and sciatica (Figs. 36.14 to 36.17). Disadvantages include difficulty in flap harvest, the need for intraoperative positioning changes, short pedicle length, size discrepancy between the gluteal vein and the commonly used recipient vessels in the chest or the axilla, as well as potential buttock contour deformity. Despite the technical difficulties, in experienced hands, these flaps can provide sufficient tissue for reconstruction with reasonable donor site morbidity. In the case of bilateral reconstruction, this is often staged given the necessary positioning changes that can prolong operative time significantly.

Preoperative imaging. CTA has been proposed to facilitate preoperative planning, even though it is not considered standard of care and recommended to be used on a case-by-case basis or upon surgeon experience. It provides information regarding the location and intramuscular course of perforators. In a recent study, Vargas and colleagues[45] assessed the impact of preoperative CTA on the outcomes of abdominal perforator–based autologous breast reconstruction at a single institution for a 10-year period. The use of CTA significantly increased with time and was found to be associated with high BMI, history of previous abdominal surgery, and bilateral reconstruction. Ischemia-related complications were decreased in the CTA group, but this was not statistically significant. Given the associated costs, radiation exposure, and questionable impact on patient outcomes, it should be reserved for select patients. Similarly, preoperative imaging is not necessary for myocutaneous gracilis–based flaps (TUG, VUG, DUG), even though it is recommended for PAP flaps, which are truly perforator based.[44] CTA for planning of perforator flap reconstruction (DIEP, SIEA, or PAP) should be ordered according to the recommended protocol which obtains 1-mm slices instead of the typical 3-mm slices of a regular computed tomography of the abdomen and pelvis. Magnetic resonance angiography (MRA), even though more costly, is an alternative modality that has been shown to provide accurate visualization of abdominal or thigh perforators, avoiding ionizing radiation.[46]

Monitoring. Postoperatively, the flap can be monitored by assessing color, turgor, temperature, and capillary refill. A cool, pale flap with minimal or no bleeding from the wound edges and

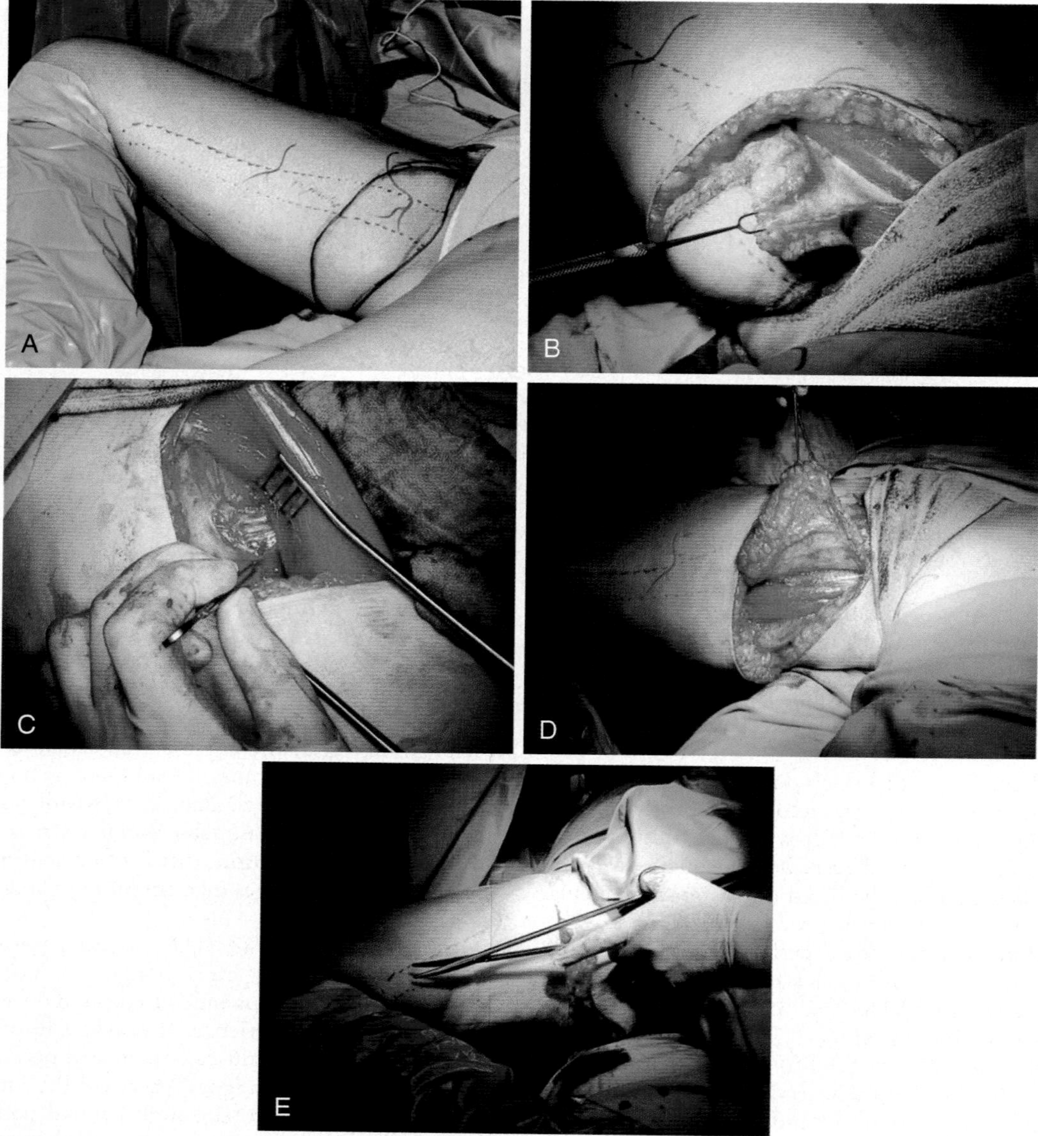

FIG. 36.13 (A) Typical marking of the transverse upper gracilis flap. (B) The anterior portion of the flap is dissected first off the underlying adductor longus. The pedicle, medial circumflex femoral artery, is identified at the dorsal border of this muscle. (C) Posterior portion of the skin island is lifted off the underlying muscle. The overlying skin is supplied by multiple perforators arising from within the gracilis. (D, E) After complete skin dissection, the gracilis muscle is cut at its tendinous junction. (From Schoeller T, Huemer GM, Wechselberger G. The transverse musculocutaneous gracilis flap for breast reconstruction: guidelines for flap and patient selection. *Plast Reconstr Surg.* 2008;122:29–38.)

delayed capillary refill of more than 2 to 3 seconds is likely suffering from arterial insufficiency. A hyperemic or purple, edematous, warm flap with rapid capillary refill of less than 2 seconds and/or rapid, dark oozing from wound edges is indicative of venous congestion. Both scenarios require attention and reexploration. A handheld Doppler device is very useful to assess for arterial and venous signals and can provide valuable information.

Fluorescent angiography can also be utilized intraoperatively to assess vascular supply of the flap. In this technique, indocyanine green is injected intravenously and a probe is used to assess perfusion of the cutaneous territory of the flap. The device is linked to a computer screen, which displays flap perfusion in real-time. This technique is also useful to evaluate the perfusion of the mastectomy flaps or the nipple-areola complex in nipple-sparing mastectomy.

Postoperatively, close flap monitoring by experienced personnel is critical and can predict successful outcomes. Physical exam remains the most reliable method of monitoring. Skin color, turgor, temperature, capillary refill, and Doppler signals evaluated in a unit allowing for hourly nurse checks is key for early detection of flap failure. Transferred tissue is susceptible to ischemia due to venous congestion or arterial insufficiency, leading to fat necrosis, partial or complete flap loss unless immediate intervention is pursued.

Near-infrared spectroscopy is a continued method to monitor the flap, usually used in conjunction with physical exam and flap checks. A probe is applied on the flap skin paddle and measures oxygenation of the superficial tissue, no more than 2 cm in depth. The readings of the probe are displayed on a screen bedside with continuous readings,

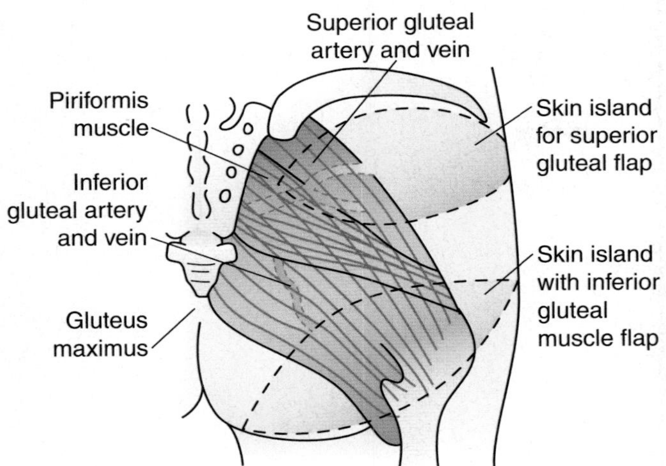

FIG. 36.14 Skin island location of superior gluteal artery perforator (GAP) and inferior GAP flaps. The skin paddle can be oriented over the superior or inferior gluteal artery.

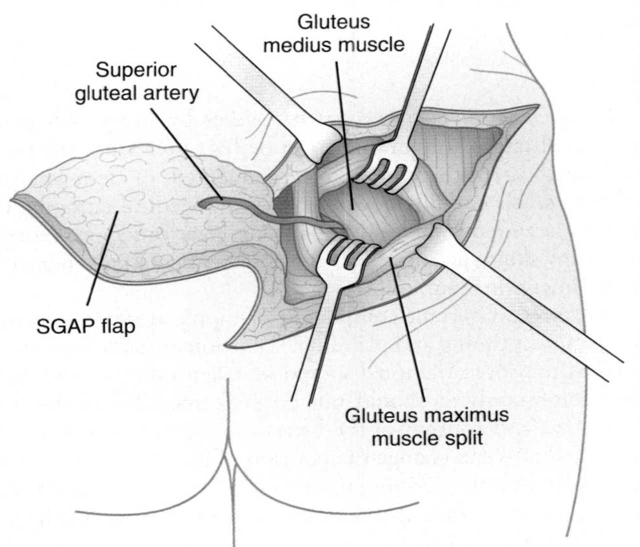

FIG. 36.15 Superior gluteal vessel dissection through the retracted gluteus maximus muscle. *SGAP,* Superior gluteal artery perforator.

correlating to blood flow and tissue perfusion. A sudden and persistent drop in tissue oxygenation indicates an acute event affecting perfusion of the flap, which can precede changes in physical examination, allowing for timely intervention. The readings of the monitor can now be wirelessly transmitted to the surgeon's computer or cell phone, allowing for remote flap monitoring.

Implantable Doppler devices can be used to monitor free flaps that are completely buried and do not have an external skin paddle. A Doppler probe is being attached to the vascular pedicle at the level or just distal to the anastomosis and is connected to an external device which continuously monitors the flow of the microvascular anastomosis. For example, in patients who undergo nipple-sparing mastectomy, no skin paddle is required for breast envelope resurfacing. In that case, the flap can be completely buried under the mastectomy flaps and implantable Doppler devices can be used for flap monitoring. Frey and colleagues[47] compared outcomes of reconstruction with buried free flap versus free flap with skin paddle after nipple-sparing mastectomy. Comparing the two groups, there were no differences in flap loss rates or reoperation rates; however, the mean number of revisions was higher in the buried flap reconstruction group.

Complications

Complications associated with autologous breast reconstruction include partial or total flap loss and problems related to the donor site. Fat necrosis can present later as a firm nodule. Free ms-TRAM or DIEP flaps have lower rates of partial flap loss, fat necrosis, and abdominal wall weakness, bulge, or hernia compared to pedicled TRAM flaps. On the other hand, free flaps, in general, have relatively higher rates of complete flap loss.

Chemotherapy has little effect on the outcomes of breast reconstruction, as long as surgical procedures are delayed after neoadjuvant therapy and adjuvant chemotherapy is not performed before surgical sites are healed and the patient has recovered from surgery. On the other hand, radiation therapy can impact autologous reconstruction. Reconstruction after completion of radiotherapy is associated with higher rates of complications compared to no radiation, and patients should be counseled appropriately. However, autologous reconstruction after radiation is still the preferred method of reconstruction when compared to no reconstruction or immediate autologous reconstruction with postoperative adjuvant radiation as the complication rates are acceptable and the aesthetic outcomes are superior. On the other hand, immediate autologous reconstruction followed by radiation has complication rates up to 50% and aesthetic outcomes are significantly inferior due to the effects of ionizing radiation to soft tissues, causing cellular injury and fibrosis, with subsequent wound healing complications, contour deformities, and tissue firmness.[12,39] Data support that immediate breast reconstruction typically does not delay initiation of adjuvant treatments including radiation and chemotherapy; however, all surgical sites need to be healed to avoid further complications.[39,48]

Combination of Reconstruction Techniques With or Without Implants

In patients who desire large-size reconstructed breasts or have lower amounts of subcutaneous fat, a combination of autologous and implant-based breast reconstruction can be considered. Often, the amount of tissue available in the lower abdomen, inner thighs, or gluteal region is not sufficient to provide the desired result. In these cases, a combination of free flaps can be utilized, anastomosed with separate recipient vessel in the chest and the axilla or anastomosed in continuity, performing intraflap anastomosis (also known as "stacked flaps").[42–44] This technique requires technical expertise, an experienced team, and a two-surgeon approach and the patient must be medically fit for a prolonged operation as well as agreeable to multiple donor sites. Secondary fat grafting can be performed to increase volume if the tissue to reconstruct the envelope is sufficient. Alternatively, autologous tissue breast reconstruction can be combined with implant placement, with or without acellular dermal matrix support. The implant placement can be performed immediately or in a delayed fashion, depending on the size of the flap and the desired size of the implant. The acellular dermal matrix can be used as a sling attached laterally, inferiorly, and medially or circumferentially, to provide more fixed support, preventing displacement or pressure on the flap. The cost of reconstruction should be considered in these cases with judicious utilization of that technique when necessary.

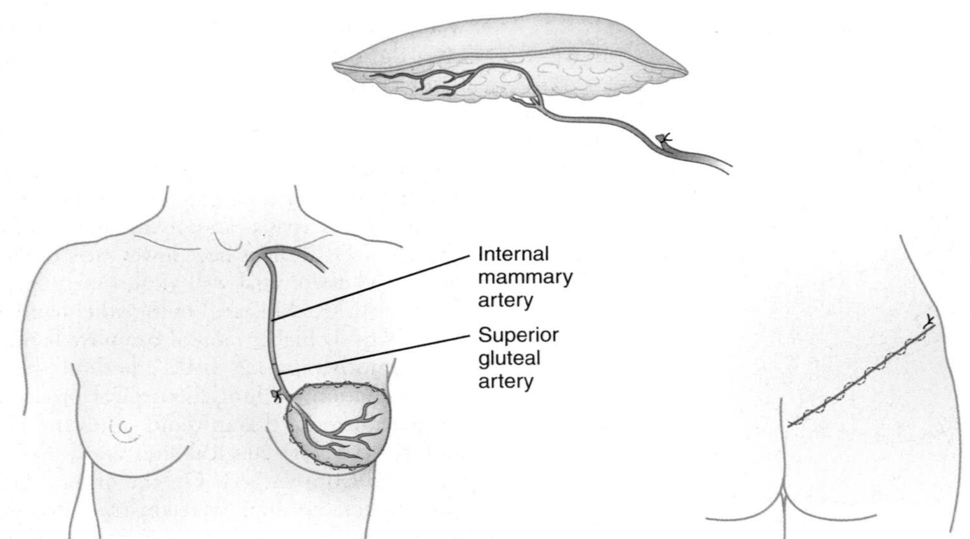

FIG. 36.16 Schematic of the gluteal perforator flap, inset into the defect via the internal mammary vessels, and donor site closure. (From Granzow JW, Levine JL, Chiu ES, et al. Breast reconstruction with gluteal artery perforator flaps. *J Plast Reconstr Aesthet Surg.* 2006;59:614–621)

NIPPLE-AREOLA RECONSTRUCTION

Nipple-areola reconstruction is an important part of breast reconstruction. The goal is to create symmetric nipples and areolas on both breasts of appropriate size, location, shape, color, and texture, providing an aesthetically pleasing result. Nipple projection is important at this stage. In unilateral breast reconstruction, the optimal technique depends on the size and position of the contralateral breast. Commonly, a nipple-areola reduction technique enhances the aesthetics of the contralateral breast, offering tissue that can be utilized for reconstruction of the affected breast. Simple triangulation measurements may not be applicable, since the shape of the reconstructed breast is often different compared to the contralateral native breast, even if symmetry mastopexy has been performed.

The nipple can be reconstructed with multiple techniques, including local flaps, grafts, injectable fillers, engineered tissue substitutes, or combinations of the these.[49] Several local flaps have been described utilizing the skin of the breast mound, such as the T-, S-, skate, star, wrap, H-, propeller, C-V, arrow, cigar roll, V-V, and rolled triangular dermal-fat flap. Postoperative contraction is to be anticipated so the reconstructed nipple is designed 25% to 50% larger than the desired final size. Local flap techniques have similar outcomes and complication rates, and the selection process depends on the presence of previous scars and surgeon preference. Loss of projection, partial flap loss, and need for minor revisions are potential complications to be considered. In an attempt to avoid loss of projection and contraction, the use of augmentation grafts has been described. Autografts (i.e., costal, auricular cartilage, or fat) do not undergo rejection; however, they add donor site and may still undergo degradation with loss of projection over time. Allogenic grafts (i.e., acellular dermal matrix) incorporate to local tissues and provide adequate maintenance of projection with reproducible results, no donor site morbidity, and low complication rates. Synthetic grafts have been used in the past, including silicone, Teflon, and hydroxyapatite-based materials with high extrusion and overall complication rates. The contralateral nipple can be used as donor site in women with large nipples. Part of the nipple and potentially areola complex are used as composite grafts providing excellent color and texture match. Despite the additional donor site morbidity, studies have shown satisfactory long-term nipple projection with minimal complications.

The areola can be reconstructed either by using skin grafts or medical tattoo.[49] Skin grafts can be harvested from the groin area, which is naturally more hyperpigmented, or from the contralateral areola combined with mastopexy. Medical tattooing has demonstrated remarkable advances, with great variety in colors to match any skin type and ability to simulate the natural areola in a three-dimensional fashion.

The most important component of nipple-areola reconstruction is correct timing and planning.[49] Previous radiation, scarring, or failed previous attempted should be taken into consideration. Most importantly, it should not be performed before the final shape, size, and contour of the breast mound are finalized, since major revisions can change the position of the reconstructed nipple areolar complex. Nipple reconstruction is usually performed as an office procedure after breast reconstruction is complete. It could be performed in the operating room in conjunction with other minor revision procedures, provided these will not affect the construct of the reconstructed breast.

REVISION SURGERY—AESTHETICS OF BREAST RECONSTRUCTION

Revision surgery after the initial reconstruction has become a common part of the reconstructive pathway for women undergoing mastectomy. Regardless of the type of reconstruction, implant-based versus autologous breast revisions can optimize the final outcomes and refine the results, achieving the goal of breast reconstruction—offering back the feeling of "whole" and providing an aesthetically and functionally pleasing result. Available techniques include fat grafting, scar revision, suction-assisted lipectomy, and mastopexy for symmetry, especially in unilateral cases. Specifically for patients with history of implant-based reconstruction, implant exchange, capsulotomy, capsulectomy, and capsulorrhaphy are commonly performed procedures. Clarke-Pearson and colleagues[50] demonstrated similar revision rates of approximately 21% in immediate direct-to-implant breast reconstruction compared to tissue expander/implant reconstruction in a single-institution retrospective review. For patients with a history of autologous-based reconstruction, flap repositioning or debulking, suction-assisted lipectomy, and donor site revision surgery

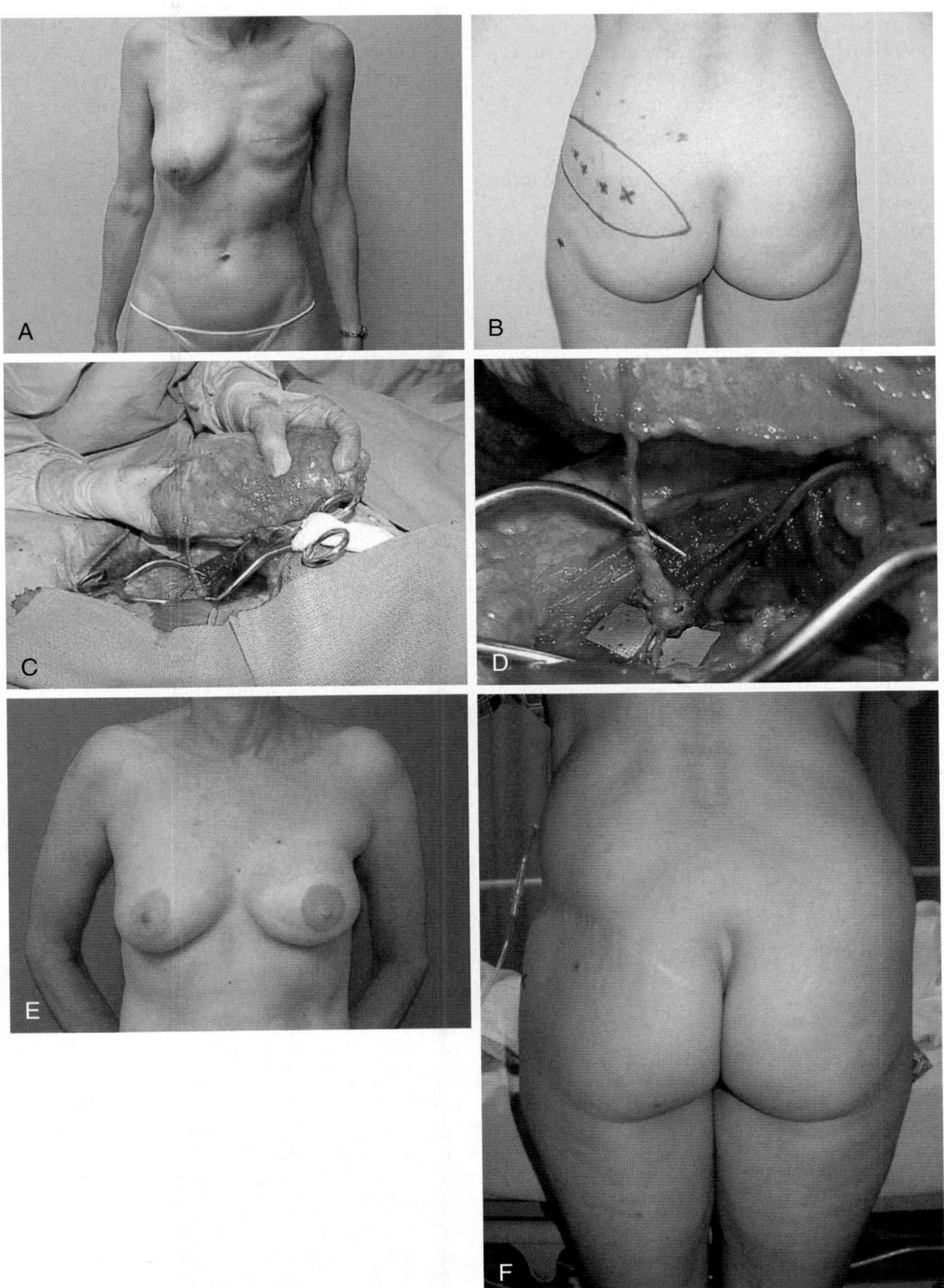

FIG. 36.17 (A, B) Preoperative view and markings. (C, D) Intraoperative views of flap and superior gluteal artery perforator vessels. (E, F) Postoperative views (anterior and posterior) 21 months after surgery. (From Granzow JW, Levine JL, Chiu ES, et al. Breast reconstruction with gluteal artery perforator flaps. *J Plast Reconstr Aesthet Surg.* 2006;59:614–621.)

are common procedures. Hanson and colleagues[51] performed a retrospective analysis of 139 patients who underwent autologous breast reconstruction with either an abdominal-based free flap or a pedicled LD muscle flap. The revision rates were significantly higher in the latissimus group (92% vs. 67%), even though complication rates were similar. In a different study comparing revision rates in unilateral and bilateral breast free flap reconstruction, younger patients and smokers were more likely to undergo revision surgery.[41] Patients who underwent bilateral reconstruction had higher rates of revisions compared to those who underwent unilateral reconstruction (69% vs. 64%, $P = 0.03$), with those undergoing bilateral immediate/delayed reconstruction demonstrating the highest rates of revision surgery. The rates of revisions are higher in the close postoperative period for autologous reconstruction; however, implant-based reconstruction often requires multiple revision operations later because of capsular contracture, implant displacement, and changes in the patient's body habitus. In general, revision procedures should be offered to the patients no sooner than 3 months after their initial procedure or previous revision surgery.

CONCLUSION

Breast reconstruction is a vital component in the treatment of breast cancer for many women. It is often the optimistic portion of a devastating diagnosis. Reconstruction lessens the psychological and physical burden of the diagnosis. When possible, immediate reconstruction is preferred because it does not increase oncologic risk or delay adjuvant therapies, provides improved aesthetic outcomes, and results in less depression, since patients do not experience the results of mastectomy. Planning and decision-making for reconstruction must be individualized to each patient to achieve her desires in the safest and most reasonable fashion. There are advantages and disadvantages of each procedure; decision-making should be individualized for the patient and her reconstructive surgeon to determine the most rational treatment plan. In the era of changing healthcare policies and increased healthcare costs, the surgeon must take into consideration the parameter of cost-effectiveness to ensure high-quality care with reasonable utilization of available resources.

SELECTED REFERENCES

Jabo B, Lin AC, Aljehani MA, et al. Impact of breast reconstruction on time to definitive surgical treatment, adjuvant therapy, and breast cancer outcome. *Ann Surg Oncol.* 2018;25:3096–3105.

This article investigates time to treatment and survival outcomes in breast cancer patients undergoing immediate breast reconstruction.

Lee BT, Agarwal JP, Ascherman JA, et al. Evidence-based clinical practice guideline: autologous breast reconstruction with DIEP or pedicled TRAM abdominal flaps. *Plast Reconstr Surg.* 2017;140:651e–664e.

This article presents the available evidence collected by the American Society of Plastic Surgeons Work Group aiming to develop recommendations on autologous breast reconstruction with the deep inferior epigastric perforator and pedicled transverse rectus abdominis muscle flaps.

Macadam SA, Zhong T, Weichman K, et al. Quality of life and patient-reported outcomes in breast cancer survivors: a multicenter comparison of four abdominally based autologous reconstruction methods. *Plast Reconstr Surg.* 2016;137:758–771.

This article compares outcomes and patient satisfaction among different methods of abdominally based autologous breast reconstruction using the BREAST-Q.

Momoh AO, Ahmed R, Kelley BP, et al. A systematic review of complications of implant-based breast reconstruction with prereconstruction and postreconstruction radiotherapy. *Ann Surg Oncol.* 2014;21:118–124.

This article provides a systematic review on outcomes of allogenic breast reconstruction with radiation therapy before or after reconstruction.

Rochlin DH, Jeong AR, Goldberg L, et al. Postmastectomy radiation therapy and immediate autologous breast reconstruction: integrating perspectives from surgical oncology, radiation oncology, and plastic and reconstructive surgery. *J Surg Oncol.* 2015;111:251–257.

This article evaluates the evidence from all fields involved in care of the breast cancer patients in order to develop recommendations on therapeutic sequences of postmastectomy radiation therapy on immediate autologous reconstruction.

REFERENCES

1. Howlader N, Noone AM, Krapcho M, et al. *Seer Cancer Statistics Review, 1975–2012.* National Cancer Institute; 2015. https://seer.cancer.gov/archive/csr/1975_2012/. Accessed June 12, 2019.
2. Smith RA, Andrews KS, Brooks D, et al. Cancer screening in the United States, 2018: a review of current American Cancer Society guidelines and current issues in cancer screening. *CA Cancer J Clin.* 2018;68:297–316.
3. Macmillan RD, McCulley SJ. Oncoplastic breast surgery: what, when and for whom? *Curr Breast Cancer Rep.* 2016;8:112–117.
4. Rochlin DH, Jeong AR, Goldberg L, et al. Postmastectomy radiation therapy and immediate autologous breast reconstruction: integrating perspectives from surgical oncology, radiation oncology, and plastic and reconstructive surgery. *J Surg Oncol.* 2015;111:251–257.
5. Largo RD, Tchang LA, Mele V, et al. Efficacy, safety and complications of autologous fat grafting to healthy breast tissue: a systematic review. *J Plast Reconstr Aesthet Surg.* 2014;67:437–448.
6. Petit JY, Rietjens M, Botteri E, et al. Evaluation of fat grafting safety in patients with intraepithelial neoplasia: a matched-cohort study. *Ann Oncol.* 2013;24:1479–1484.
7. Kronowitz SJ, Mandujano CC, Liu J, et al. Lipofilling of the breast does not increase the risk of recurrence of breast cancer: a matched controlled study. *Plast Reconstr Surg.* 2016;137:385–393.
8. Cohen O, Lam G, Karp N, et al. Determining the oncologic safety of autologous fat grafting as a reconstructive modality: an institutional review of breast cancer recurrence rates and surgical outcomes. *Plast Reconstr Surg.* 2017;140:382e–392e.
9. Blondeel PN, Hijjawi J, Depypere H, et al. Shaping the breast in aesthetic and reconstructive breast surgery: an easy three-step principle. *Plast Reconstr Surg.* 2009;123:455–462.
10. Barone M, Cogliandro A, Signoretti M, et al. Analysis of symmetry stability following implant-based breast reconstruction and contralateral management in 582 patients with long-term outcomes. *Aesthetic Plast Surg.* 2018;42:936–940.
11. Nahabedian MY. Managing the opposite breast: contralateral symmetry procedures. *Cancer J.* 2008;14:258–263.
12. Nelson JA, Disa JJ. Breast reconstruction and radiation therapy: an update. *Plast Reconstr Surg.* 2017;140:60S–68S.
13. Momoh AO, Ahmed R, Kelley BP, et al. A systematic review of complications of implant-based breast reconstruction with prereconstruction and postreconstruction radiotherapy. *Ann Surg Oncol.* 2014;21:118–124.
14. El-Sabawi B, Sosin M, Carey JN, et al. Breast reconstruction and adjuvant therapy: a systematic review of surgical outcomes. *J Surg Oncol.* 2015;112:458–464.

15. Beugels J, Kool M, Hoekstra LT, et al. Quality of life of patients after immediate or delayed autologous breast reconstruction: a multicenter study. *Ann Plast Surg.* 2018;81:523–527.
16. Santosa KB, Qi J, Kim HM, et al. Long-term patient-reported outcomes in postmastectomy breast reconstruction. *JAMA Surg.* 2018;153:891–899.
17. Macadam SA, Zhong T, Weichman K, et al. Quality of life and patient-reported outcomes in breast cancer survivors: a multicenter comparison of four abdominally based autologous reconstruction methods. *Plast Reconstr Surg.* 2016;137:758–771.
18. Matros E, Albornoz CR, Razdan SN, et al. Cost-effectiveness analysis of implants versus autologous perforator flaps using the BREAST-Q. *Plast Reconstr Surg.* 2015;135:937–946.
19. Kwok AC, Simpson AM, Ye X, et al. Immediate unilateral breast reconstruction using abdominally based flaps: analysis of 3,310 cases. *J Reconstr Microsurg.* 2019;35:74–82.
20. Rodriguez-Feliz J, Codner MA. Embrace the change: incorporating single-stage implant breast reconstruction into your practice. *Plast Reconstr Surg.* 2015;136:221–231.
21. Cordeiro PG, Pusic AL, Disa JJ, et al. Irradiation after immediate tissue expander/implant breast reconstruction: outcomes, complications, aesthetic results, and satisfaction among 156 patients. *Plast Reconstr Surg.* 2004;113:877–881.
22. Choi M, Frey JD, Alperovich M, et al. "Breast in a day": examining single-stage immediate, permanent implant reconstruction in nipple-sparing mastectomy. *Plast Reconstr Surg.* 2016;138:184e–191e.
23. Langstein HN, Cheng MH, Singletary SE, et al. Breast cancer recurrence after immediate reconstruction: patterns and significance. *Plast Reconstr Surg.* 2003;111:712–720; discussion 721–712.
24. Kronowitz SJ. State of the art and science in postmastectomy breast reconstruction. *Plast Reconstr Surg.* 2015;135:755e–771e.
25. Gruber RP, Kahn RA, Lash H, et al. Breast reconstruction following mastectomy: a comparison of submuscular and subcutaneous techniques. *Plast Reconstr Surg.* 1981;67:312–317.
26. Cordeiro PG, Jazayeri L. Two-stage implant-based breast reconstruction: an evolution of the conceptual and technical approach over a two-decade period. *Plast Reconstr Surg.* 2016;138:1–11.
27. Elswick SM, Harless CA, Bishop SN, et al. Prepectoral implant-based breast reconstruction with postmastectomy radiation therapy. *Plast Reconstr Surg.* 2018;142:1–12.
28. Nahabedian MY. Current approaches to prepectoral breast reconstruction. *Plast Reconstr Surg.* 2018;142:871–880.
29. American Society of Plastic Surgeons. *Evidence-Based Clinical Practice Guideline: Breast Reconstruction With Expanders and Implants*; 2003. https://www.plasticsurgery.org/documents/medical-professionals/quality-resources/guidelines/guideline-2013-breast-recon-expanders-implants.pdf. Accessed June 12, 2019.
30. Hartrampf CR, Scheflan M, Black PW. Breast reconstruction with a transverse abdominal island flap. *Plast Reconstr Surg.* 1982;269:216–225.
31. Macadam SA, Bovill ES, Buchel EW, et al. Evidence-based medicine: autologous breast reconstruction. *Plast Reconstr Surg.* 2017;139:204e–229e.
32. Cederna PS, Chang P, Pittet-Cuenod BM, et al. The effect of the delay phenomenon on the vascularity of rabbit rectus abdominis muscles. *Plast Reconstr Surg.* 1997;99:194–205.
33. Codner MA, Bostwick 3rd J. The delayed TRAM flap. *Clin Plast Surg.* 1998;25:183–189.
34. Lee JW, Lee YC, Chang TW. Microvascularly augmented transverse rectus abdominis myocutaneous flap for breast reconstruction—reappraisal of its value through clinical outcome assessment and intraoperative blood gas analysis. *Microsurgery.* 2008;28:656–662.
35. Schneider WJ, Hill Jr HL, Brown RG. Latissimus dorsi myocutaneous flap for breast reconstruction. *Br J Plast Surg.* 1977;30:277–281.
36. Mushin OP, Myers PL, Langstein HN. Indications and controversies for complete and implant-enhanced latissimus dorsi breast reconstructions. *Clin Plast Surg.* 2018;45:75–81.
37. Johns N, Fairbairn N, Trail M, et al. Autologous breast reconstruction using the immediately lipofilled extended latissimus dorsi flap. *J Plast Reconstr Aesthet Surg.* 2018;71:201–208.
38. Saint-Cyr M, Nagarkar P, Schaverien M, et al. The pedicled descending branch muscle-sparing latissimus dorsi flap for breast reconstruction. *Plast Reconstr Surg.* 2009;123:13–24.
39. Lee BT, Agarwal JP, Ascherman JA, et al. Evidence-based clinical practice guideline: autologous breast reconstruction with DIEP or pedicled TRAM abdominal flaps. *Plast Reconstr Surg.* 2017;140:651e–664e.
40. Park JE, Shenaq DS, Silva AK, et al. Breast reconstruction with SIEA flaps: a single-institution experience with 145 free flaps. *Plast Reconstr Surg.* 2016;137:1682–1689.
41. Chang EI, Soto-Miranda MA, Zhang H, et al. Evolution of bilateral free flap breast reconstruction over 10 years: optimizing outcomes and comparison to unilateral reconstruction. *Plast Reconstr Surg.* 2015;135:946e–953e.
42. Park JE, Alkureishi LW, Song DH. TUGs into VUGs and friendly BUGs: transforming the gracilis territory into the best secondary breast reconstructive option. *Plast Reconstr Surg.* 2015;136:447–454.
43. Opsomer D, van Landuyt K. Indications and controversies for nonabdominally-based complete autologous tissue breast reconstruction. *Clin Plast Surg.* 2018;45:93–100.
44. Dayan JH, Allen Jr RJ. Lower extremity free flaps for breast reconstruction. *Plast Reconstr Surg.* 2017;140:77S–86S.
45. Vargas CR, Koolen PG, Ho OA, et al. Preoperative CT-angiography in autologous breast reconstruction. *Microsurgery.* 2016;36:623–627.
46. Agrawal MD, Thimmappa ND, Vasile JV, et al. Autologous breast reconstruction: preoperative magnetic resonance angiography for perforator flap vessel mapping. *J Reconstr Microsurg.* 2015;31:1–11.
47. Frey JD, Stranix JT, Chiodo MV, et al. Evolution in monitoring of free flap autologous breast reconstruction after nipple-sparing mastectomy: is there a best way? *Plast Reconstr Surg.* 2018;141:1086–1093.
48. Jabo B, Lin AC, Aljehani MA, et al. Impact of breast reconstruction on time to definitive surgical treatment, adjuvant therapy, and breast cancer outcomes. *Ann Surg Oncol.* 2018;25:3096–3105.
49. Gougoutas AJ, Said HK, Um G, et al. Nipple-areola complex reconstruction. *Plast Reconstr Surg.* 2018;141:404e–416e.
50. Clarke-Pearson EM, Lin AM, Hertl C, et al. Revisions in implant-based breast reconstruction: how does direct-to-implant measure up? *Plast Reconstr Surg.* 2016;137:1690–1699.
51. Hanson SE, Smith BD, Liu J, et al. Fewer revisions in abdominal-based free flaps than latissimus dorsi breast reconstruction after radiation. *Plast Reconstr Surg Glob Open.* 2016;4:e866.

SECTION VIII

Endocrine

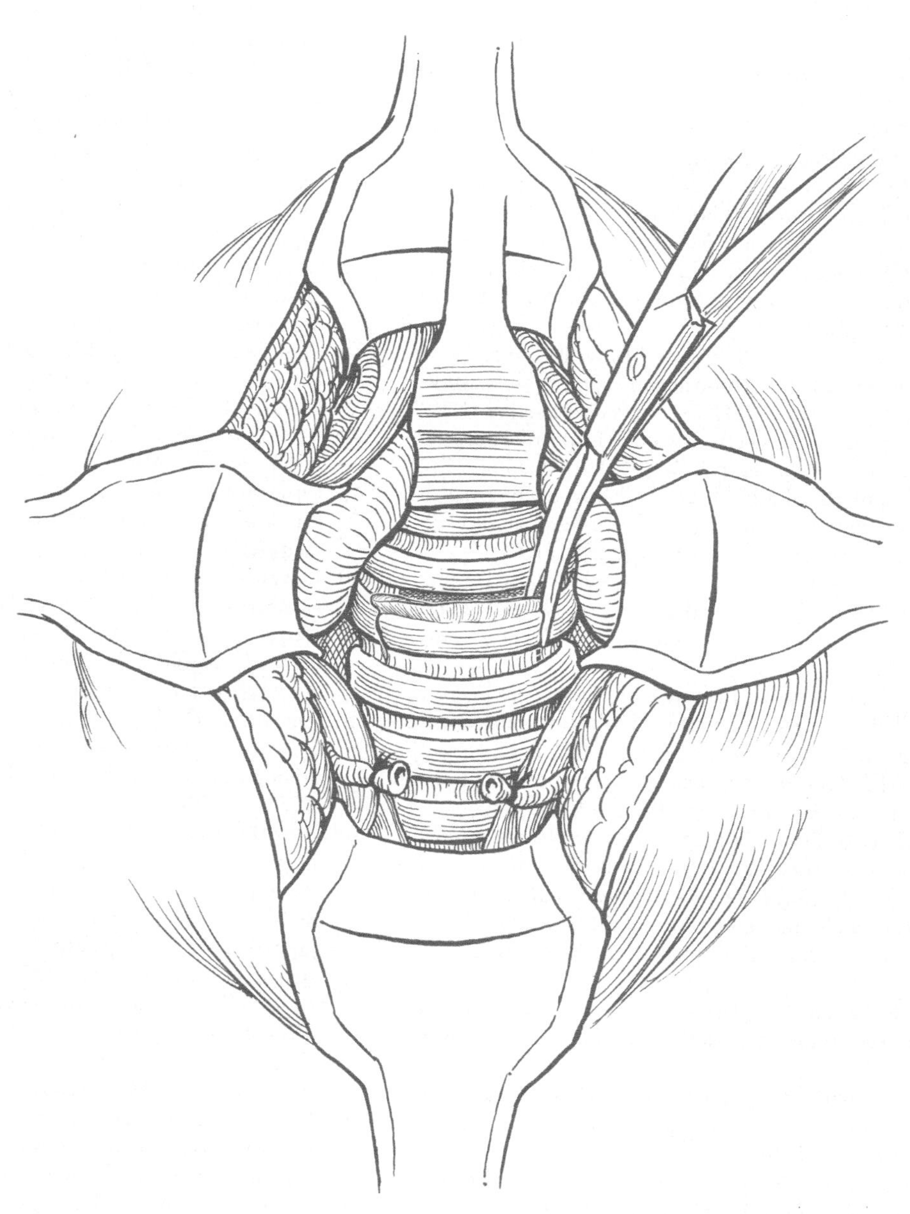

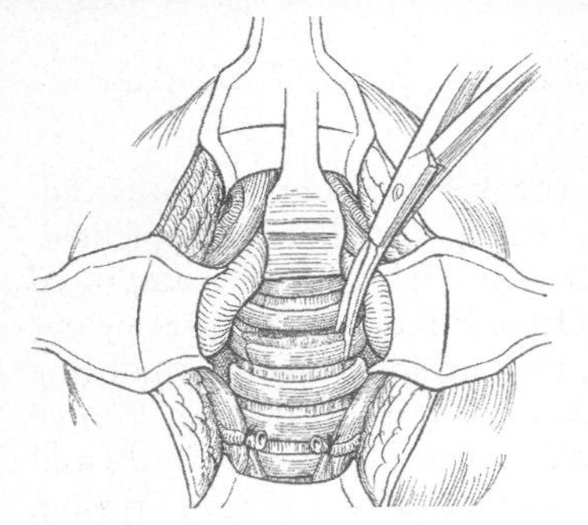

CHAPTER 37

Thyroid

Insoo Suh, Julie Ann Sosa

OUTLINE

DISCLOSURES

IS is a consultant for Medtronic and Prescient Surgical.

JAS is a member of the Data Monitoring Committee of the Medullary Thyroid Cancer Consortium Registry supported by GlaxoSmithKline, Novo Nordisk, Astra Zeneca, and Eli Lilly.

HISTORY OF THYROID SURGERY

The history of thyroid surgery began more than 1000 years ago.[1] Most records agree that the first thyroidectomy was performed for endemic goiter by the legendary surgeon Abu al-Qasim in 952 ad, although the patient was said to have barely survived due to torrential blood loss during the procedure. The majority of the ensuing millennium did not see encouraging advancements in either the understanding of the thyroid gland's function or its safe extirpation. In the twelfth century, Roger Frugardii of the Italian Salerno school described a morbid method of thyroid removal involving the insertion of hot iron setons through the skin and into the gland, with gradual superficialization of the gland until the seton and thyroid tissue penetrated through the skin and were removed. This type of procedure exemplified what the early Catholic Church deemed to be the brutality and uncouthness of surgery, which led to a retreat of surgery from the mainstream of medicine and science during much of medieval European history.

The anatomy of the thyroid was first described in the early sixteenth century by Leonardo da Vinci; unfortunately, he did not understand the thyroid gland's function beyond its filling in an empty space in the neck between muscle layers in order to protect the trachea from the sternum. As the study of anatomy and surgery became more culturally acceptable during the Renaissance, additional incremental advancements in the understanding of thyroid anatomy occurred. The term *thyroid* was first coined by the anatomist Thomas Wharton in 1646; it was a derivation of the Greek word *thyreos*, or "shield."

Advancements in thyroid surgery, however, were relatively few and far between until well into the nineteenth century. Wilhelm Fabricius described a case in the mid-1600s of a "rash" and "audacious doctor" who performed the first thyroidectomy using scalpels for a goiter in a 10-year-old girl who died on the operating table; this surgeon was reported to have been imprisoned as a result. The first well-documented successful partial thyroidectomy was performed in 1791 by Pierre Joseph Desault during the French Revolution, and other surgeons reported small case series of successful thyroidectomies over the ensuing 50 years. Notable among them was the German surgeon Johann Hedenus, whose zero percent mortality rate following the removal of six "suffocating" goiters was considered remarkable for the time. Despite this, thyroid surgery was still associated with (at minimum) a 40% mortality rate in the early to mid-1800s, such that the leading surgical figures and professional associations of the time emphatically advised against performing thyroidectomy. Thyroid surgery was deemed by Liston "a proceeding by no means to be thought of," by Diffenbach as "most thankless, most perilous…foolhardy performances," and by Gross as "horrid butchery. No honest and sensible surgeon would ever engage in it." The French Academy of Medicine frankly banned thyroid surgery during this time.

Starting in the mid-nineteenth century and continuing on into the early twentieth century, the course of thyroid surgery rapidly evolved from a dangerous and morbid endeavor into a safe, elegant, and modern practice. The practice of surgery as a whole advanced due to the triple developments of anesthesia, antisepsis/infection prophylaxis, and instrumentation for hemostasis. Thanks in large part to these innovations, the surgical giants of the day were able to more carefully study and refine surgical thyroidology. Theodor Billroth's foray into thyroid surgery was initially marked by 16 deaths among 36 thyroidectomies; however, he was able to dramatically reduce his mortality rate to 8% after introducing newer methods of hemostasis and antisepsis in his surgical practice. Theodor Kocher, Billroth's pupil, is widely regarded as the "father of modern thyroid surgery." He performed more than 5000 thyroidectomies during his career, with an associated mortality rate of 0.5%, which was widely attributed to his extreme meticulousness in antisepsis and hemostatic techniques. His remarkable surgical results as well as his seminal research contributions to the understanding of thyroid function led to his receiving the Nobel Prize in Medicine and Physiology in 1909, the first Nobel ever awarded to a surgeon. The Australian surgeon Thomas Dunhill is credited for his excellent results pioneering a safe bilateral operation of unilateral complete thyroid lobectomy with contralateral subtotal thyroid lobe resection for thyrotoxicosis, an operation that still bears his name today.

William Stewart Halsted's stature as the "father of modern surgery" and creator of the contemporary American surgical residency program makes it sometimes easy to overlook his many contributions to thyroid surgery. His research elucidated parathyroid blood supply as well as "ultraligation" of the distal thyroid artery branches to avoid parathyroid gland devascularization and avoid postoperative tetany. He also performed experiments that supported the mechanistic connection between hypoparathyroidism and tetany and its reversal with either calcium supplementation or parathyroid transplantation. Halsted further improved upon the techniques he learned from Billroth and Kocher by improving surgical instrumentation for hemostasis and introducing surgical gloves for sterile technique. Two of his trainees, George Crile and Frank Lahey, went on to become luminaries in thyroid surgery. Ultimately, Halsted wrote that thyroid surgery "typifies perhaps better than any other operation the supreme triumph of the surgeon's art."

Charles Mayo and his medical colleague Henry Plummer demonstrated the safe conduct of thyroidectomy for Graves disease with preoperative iodine preparation. Mayo's surgical volume and superlative outcomes far exceeded other contemporaries and led to his reputation for being the "father of American thyroid surgery."

Additional innovations over the past century have undoubtedly improved the conduct of modern thyroid surgery, but the influence around the turn of the twentieth century of the abovementioned luminaries, and particularly Kocher, remain unmatched.

THYROID EMBRYOLOGY AND ANATOMY

Embryology

The thyroid gland originates from the median and lateral thyroid anlages—embryologic precursor tissues—which follow separate embryologic paths prior to fusing and forming a single gland.

Median Thyroid Anlage

The primitive pharynx begins to form the median thyroid anlage starting at the second week of gestation. This structure appears as an epithelial proliferation in the floor of the pharynx between the tuberculum impar and the copula, arising at the level of the second branchial arch. As it descends toward the primitive heart, the median thyroid anlage becomes a bilobed diverticulum with a median tubal structure called the thyroglossal duct, which keeps the structure connected to the tongue. The thyroglossal duct becomes a solid structure in the fifth week, after which it fragments and disappears. The obliteration of this structure leaves the foramen cecum at the base of the tongue superiorly and, when present, the pyramidal lobe inferiorly. The thyroid continues to descend to its final position anterior to the trachea by the seventh week. The cells derived from the median thyroid anlage arrange to form follicles and produce thyroid hormone by the tenth week of gestation.

Lateral Thyroid Anlage

The lateral thyroid anlage arises from the pharyngeal endoderm and fuses to the median anlage in the fifth week during its embryologic descent. The lateral thyroid anlage is comprised in part from cells of the ultimobranchial bodies, which originate from the fourth and fifth pharyngeal pouches. It is from these ultimobranchial bodies that the calcitonin-secreting parafollicular C cells arise (the median anlage does not carry these cells). The lateral thyroid anlage comprises approximately one-third of the total mass of the eventual developed thyroid gland.

Anomalies in the embryologic development of the thyroid gland can lead to a variety of conditions, some of which can be pathologic (Fig. 37.1).

Thyroglossal Duct Cyst

The normal development and subsequent obliteration of the thyroglossal duct are connected to that of the hyoid bone, which forms starting at the seventh week of gestation and functionally

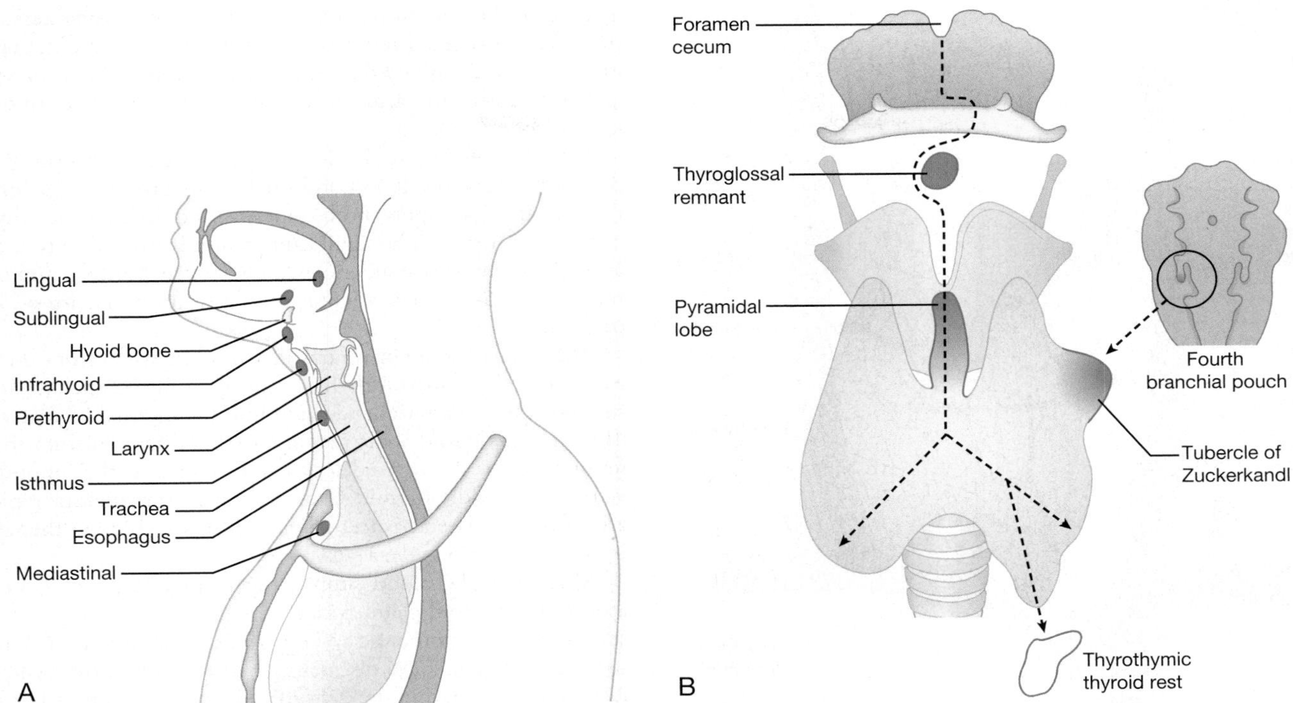

FIG. 37.1 (A) Schema illustrating some common sites for midline ectopic thyroid masses. (B) A summary of the major medial and lateral embryologic elements of the thyroid gland and their potential adult anatomic consequences. (From Agarwal A, Mishra AK, Lomardi CP, et al: Applied embryology of the thyroid and parathyroid glands. In: Randolph GW, ed. *Surgery of the Thyroid and Parathyroid Glands.* 2nd ed. Philadelphia: Elsevier Saunders; 2013:18.)

divides the thyroglossal tract into superior and inferior aspects. When the thyroglossal duct does not completely obliterate and the epithelial duct cells remain, a thyroglossal duct cyst may arise from a persistent connection between the thyroid gland and the foramen cecum. This scenario typically presents as a painless midline neck mass at or near the level of the hyoid, although it can be found near the base of the tongue or at the thyroid gland proper. Occasionally, these cysts can become infected from oral bacteria from the tongue, and can also form fistulous sinuses to the skin.

The Sistrunk procedure, originally described in 1920, is the surgical treatment of choice for thyroglossal duct cysts that become chronically infected. A number of modifications have been described, but the key component of the procedure involves excision of the entirety of the cyst and surrounding thyroglossal duct tract, including the central portion of the hyoid bone. Resection of a small portion of the tongue is no longer thought to be necessary in the majority of cases.

Ectopic Thyroid Tissue

Aberrant thyroid tissue can be found anywhere along the normal path of development and descent of the thyroid gland, from the foramen cecum down to the anterior mediastinum. The development of an undescended thyroid can lead to the formation of a lingual thyroid gland near the base of the foramen cecum. This abnormal thyroid tissue is often associated with inadequate thyroid hormone production with subsequent goitrous enlargement, which in turn can lead to local compressive symptoms of the upper neck, such as airway obstruction and dysphagia. Surgical excision is occasionally necessary for these cases.

The other common locations for ectopic thyroid tissue are along the path of the thyrothymic tract, which originates from the third pharyngeal pouch and pulls along the inferior parathyroid glands and lower poles of the thyroid lobes along the descending path of the thymus gland. Foci of normal thyroid tissue along this tract are typically referred to as thyroid rests. These rests can occur in up to 50% of people and are typically not thought to be pathologic findings in and of themselves, although they may occasionally be mistaken for pathologic lymph nodes or parathyroid glands. Rests either can be connected to the thyroid gland proper by a thin stalk or can exist as completely separate structures. Primary intrathoracic goiters are thought to arise from enlargement of intrathoracic thyroid rests. Surgical treatment of thyroid rest tissue may occasionally be indicated if clinically relevant; examples of this include thyroid cancer requiring resection of a thyroid rest as a part of thyroidectomy or local compressive symptoms from an intrathoracic goiter.

Anatomy

The normal thyroid gland is reddish-brown in color and rubbery in texture, with an adult gland typically weighing about 20 g. The thyroid gland typically is situated behind the sternohyoid and sternothyroid strap muscles and the superficial and middle layers of the deep cervical fascia.

When viewed in an anteroposterior plane, the shape of the thyroid resembles the silhouette of a butterfly, with two lateral lobes connected by an isthmus draped over the upper trachea just caudal to the cricoid cartilage. A normal-sized thyroid lobe is typically 4 to 6 cm in height and 1.3 to 1.8 cm in both transverse and anteroposterior dimensions. The isthmus typically has a thickness of 2 to 3 mm. In half to three-quarters of people, a pyramidal lobe extends superiorly from the isthmus and represents the caudal remnant of the thyroglossal duct. The right and left thyroid

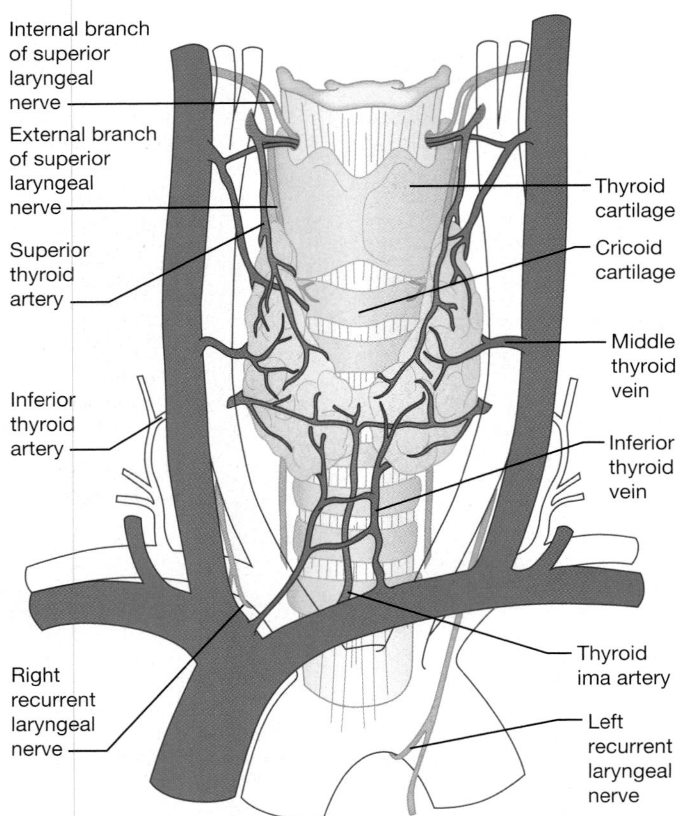

FIG. 37.2 Anatomy of the thyroid gland and surrounding structures. (From McHenry CR: Thyroidectomy for nodules or small cancers. (From McHenry CR. Thyroidectomy for nodules or small cancers. In: Duh QY, Clark OH, Kebebew E, eds. *Atlas of Endocrine Surgical Techniques*. Philadelphia: Elsevier Saunders; 2010:7.)

lobes make up the majority of the gland's volume. Each lobe's height extends from the level of the mid to upper aspect of the thyroid cartilage down to the fifth to sixth tracheal rings. Laterally, the lobe extends to the sternocleidomastoid muscle and carotid artery, with a small posterolateral projection or lump known as the tubercle of Zuckerkandl. The capsule enveloping the thyroid also form separate "pseudolobules" within the parenchyma of the gland itself; these coalesce into a solid ligamentous structure at the posterolateral aspect of the upper trachea called the suspensory ligament of Berry. The tubercle of Zuckerkandl and Berry ligament are relatively constant anatomic landmarks for identification of the distal recurrent laryngeal nerve (RLN), which typically runs just posterior to these structures.

Blood and Lymphatic Supply

The thyroid is a highly vascular gland with abundant and redundant blood supply (Fig. 37.2). The arterial supply to the thyroid gland generally derives from two bilateral pairs of arteries. The superior thyroid arteries originate from the external carotid arteries, and divide as they enter the superior poles of the thyroid lobes. The inferior thyroid arteries are branches from the thyrocervical trunks of the subclavian arteries. Because they branch fairly proximally from the thyrocervical trunk, their course runs cephalad and posterior to the carotid sheath before making a turn and entering the mid thyroid lobes. In about 2% of people, a third artery called the thyroid ima artery arises directly from the aorta or innominate artery. This artery follows a midline path and enters the thyroid isthmus or the inferior poles of the thyroid lobes. The direction of the inferior thyroid artery as it enters the thyroid gland is another important landmark used for the identification of the RLN, which typically crosses the artery perpendicularly as it travels into the larynx (see below).

Branches of the inferior and superior arteries also supply the parathyroid glands. It is traditionally thought that the inferior thyroid arteries supply both superior and inferior parathyroid glands, but there can be significant anatomic variation around the arterial supply to the superior glands, which can be supplied by the inferior thyroid artery alone, the superior thyroid artery alone, or both.

There are three main venous drainage pathways from the thyroid gland. The superior thyroid veins typically run parallel to the superior thyroid arteries and drain into the internal jugular veins. The inferior thyroid veins run in a caudal direction from the inferior poles of the thyroid lobes and drain into the innominate veins. The middle thyroid veins are highly variable but typically arise from the lateral aspect of the mid thyroid lobes; they drain into the internal jugular veins.

Much like the blood supply, the lymphatic network in and around the thyroid gland is rich and extensive. A proper understanding of the lymphatic system is of critical importance in the surgical management of diseases such as thyroid cancer. Lymphatic vessels course within the thyroid and drain into regional cervical lymph nodes. There is a standardized method and nomenclature for organizing the cervical lymph nodes into seven discrete "levels" (Fig. 37.3). An understanding of the pattern of lymphatic drainage from the thyroid is particularly important for understanding the surgical management of thyroid cancer (see "Thyroid Cancer" section below). The bulk of lymphatic drainage from the thyroid first goes to the perithyroidal lymph nodes in the central neck collectively grouped as level VI, which includes the lymph nodes between the two carotid arteries and bounded by the hyoid bone superiorly and the sternal notch inferiorly. The lateral neck jugular lymph nodes (IIa, III and IV) as well as those in the posterior triangle of the neck (particularly level Vb) also drain lymphatics from the thyroid, typically in transit from the central neck lymph nodes. Skip metastases that avoid Level VI and extend directly from the primary tumor (typically in the superior pole of the thyroid) to the lateral neck are exceptional cases that occur in less than 15% of cases. Other levels of the neck are rarely associated with regional thyroid cancer metastases.

Nerves Associated With the Thyroid Gland

The thyroid is directly supplied by a network of tiny autonomic nerves arising from the superior and middle cervical sympathetic ganglia and parasympathetic fibers derived from the vagus nerve. The two most important nerves associated with the thyroid gland for the surgeon are the RLN and the external branch of the superior laryngeal nerve (EBSLN). It is critical that the thyroid surgeon have a thorough understanding of the normal and anomalous paths of these nerves, such that these structures can be better preserved during thyroidectomy.

The RLN and EBSLN are the main nerves responsible for the function of the larynx. Each nerve is paired, with a right and left side. The RLN is by far the more important nerve and innervates the motor function of all of the intrinsic laryngeal muscles except for the cricothyroid. It carries sensory fibers from the lower larynx, as well as minor motor and sensory fibers from the trachea and esophagus. Unilateral injury to the RLN leads to paralysis of the ipsilateral vocal fold, with typical symptoms ranging from voice

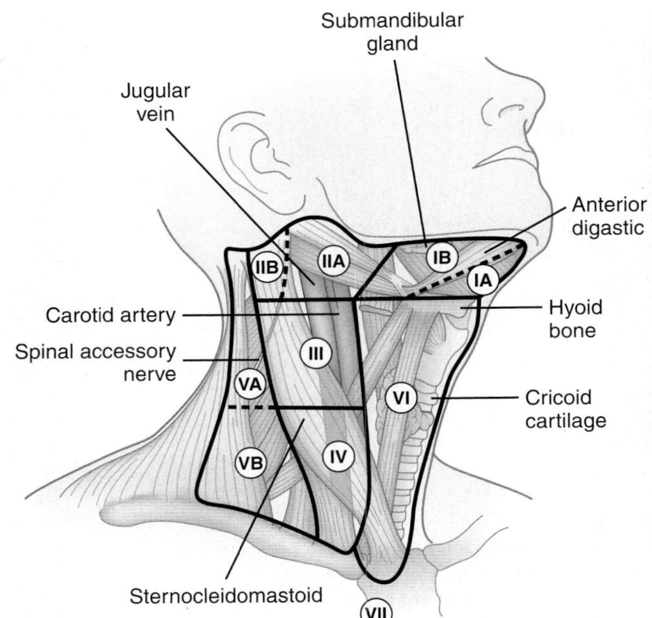

FIG. 37.3 Lymph node compartments separated into levels and sublevels. Level VI contains the thyroid gland and the adjacent nodes bordered superiorly by the hyoid bone, inferiorly by the innominate (brachiocephalic) artery, and laterally on each side by the carotid sheaths. Level II, III, and IV nodes are arrayed along the jugular veins on each side, bordered anteromedially by level VI and laterally by the posterior border of the sternocleidomastoid muscle. Level III nodes are bounded superiorly by the level of the hyoid bone and inferiorly by the inferior aspect of the cricoid cartilage; levels II and IV are above and below level III, respectively. The level I node compartment includes the submental and submandibular nodes above the hyoid bone and anterior to the posterior edge of the submandibular gland. Level V nodes are in the posterior triangle, lateral to the lateral edge of the sternocleidomastoid muscle. Levels I, II, and V can be further subdivided as noted in the figure. The inferior extent of level VI is defined as the suprasternal notch. Many authors also include the pretracheal and paratracheal superior mediastinal lymph nodes above the level of the innominate artery (sometimes referred to as level VII) in central neck dissection.

complaints such as hoarseness and vocal fatigue to aspiration. Bilateral RLN injury with subsequent bilateral vocal fold paralysis may require tracheostomy for airway control if the paralyzed vocal folds rest in a median position preventing adequate air exchange; alternatively, the risk of persistent aspiration and respiratory tract infections is high if the resting vocal folds remain in an abducted position. The EBSLN innervates the cricothyroid muscles, and it contributes to vocal fold tone and tension. EBSLN injury leads to difficulties with achieving high pitch and vocal projection and volume. The nerve became a historical focus of attention after the famous opera singer Amelita Galla-Curci developed difficulty singing high notes after thyroidectomy; this was thought to be due to its injury during surgery, although subsequent historical reports dispute this claim.

The anatomy of the left and right RLN differs based on their embryologic development (Fig. 37.4). Both RLNs are derived from the sixth branchial arches below the sixth aortic arches. As the fifth and sixth aortic arches above the RLNs subsequently regress in embryogenesis, the two nerves then anchor to and follow the right and left fourth aortic arch structures, which develop into differing arteries—the right subclavian artery and the aortic arch, respectively. Both nerves loop back, or "recur," into the neck due to the heart and great vessels descending into the thorax, bringing the RLNs down with them. The left RLN loops under the ligamentum arteriosum at the aortic arch and travels in the tracheoesophageal groove until it reaches the thyroid. The right RLN loops under the right carotid-subclavian artery junction and migrates to the cricothyroid joint at the insertion into the larynx. Because of the lateral location of the right carotid-subclavian junction and the shorter length of the course of the right RLN, this nerve can be identified traveling in a slightly anterior plane and an oblique direction compared to the left RLN, which tends to stay relatively deep and straight in the tracheoesophageal groove.

There are a number of anatomic landmarks that can aid in identification and characterization of the RLN. The tubercle of Zuckerkandl typically lies just anterior and lateral to the nerve. There is an intimate relationship between the nerve, Berry ligament, and the inferior thyroid artery at the level of the cricoid cartilage. Here, the nerve crosses the artery (usually posteriorly) and typically curves anteriorly toward the ligament before diving posteriorly again into the laryngeal insertion point at the cricothyroid joint. There are numerous anatomic variations of the course of the nerve and its relationship with the three structures, particularly with respect to how anteriorly the nerve can be positioned. In addition, the RLN may branch more proximally in up to 20%–30% of cases, and preservation of all of the branches is important to preserve nerve function; this is particularly true for the anterior branches, which predominantly provide motor innervation.

The RLN also may course in a nonrecurrent fashion, instead branching in a direct path from the cervical vagus (Fig. 37.4). On the right side, this is associated with and likely secondary to an aberrant right subclavian artery arising directly from the aortic arch instead of the innominate artery (called the "lusoria artery"). This artery arises distal to the left subclavian artery and crosses the midline posterior to the esophagus. Because of the absence of a normal right subclavian-carotid junction to pull down the right RLN during embryologic development, the right RLN follows a straight path from the vagus to the larynx. A right-sided non-RLN occurs in up to 1% of people. A left-sided nonrecurrent nerve can occur in the extremely rare scenarios of a patient with situs inversus and a right-sided aortic arch.

Like the RLN, the superior laryngeal nerves arise from the vagus nerve. The EBSLN branches off at the hyoid bone and runs along the inferior pharyngeal constrictor muscle before running parallel to the upper aspect of the superior pole thyroid vessels and then terminating in the cricothyroid muscle. Although the EBSLN is typically fairly high above the thyroid lobe, care must be taken when ligating and dividing the superior pole vessels during thyroidectomy, as the anatomic variations in the EBSLN can run quite close to the vessels and the upper thyroid lobe and must be dissected away as the superior pole of the gland is taken down (Fig. 37.5).

THYROID HISTOLOGY AND PHYSIOLOGY

Histology

The thyroid is comprised mainly of two epithelial cell types. The first and predominant type is the follicular cell, which is responsible for the production and secretion of thyroid hormone (Fig. 37.6). The second type is the parafollicular C cell, which secretes calcitonin. The histologic architecture of the thyroid is arranged into spherical follicles containing colloid. Colloid is made up of thyroglobulin (Tg), which is the noniodinated precursor to active thyroid hormone and acts as a reservoir. The parafollicular

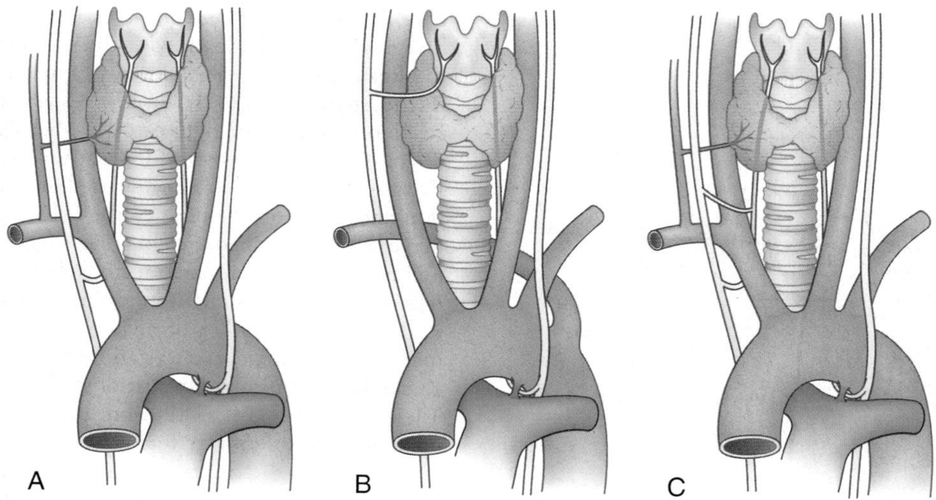

FIG. 37.4 Anomalous variations in the course of the right recurrent laryngeal nerve. (A) The normal course of the recurrent laryngeal nerve arises from the vagus after it passes beneath the subclavian artery. A nonrecurrent laryngeal nerve arises from the vagus and courses medially into the larynx in the setting of an aberrant origin of the right subclavian artery. (B) A nonrecurrent laryngeal nerve arises from the vagus and courses medially into the larynx in the setting of an aberrant origin of the right subclavian artery. (C) The unusual coexistence of a nonrecurrent laryngeal nerve and the recurrent laryngeal nerve forms a common distal nerve.

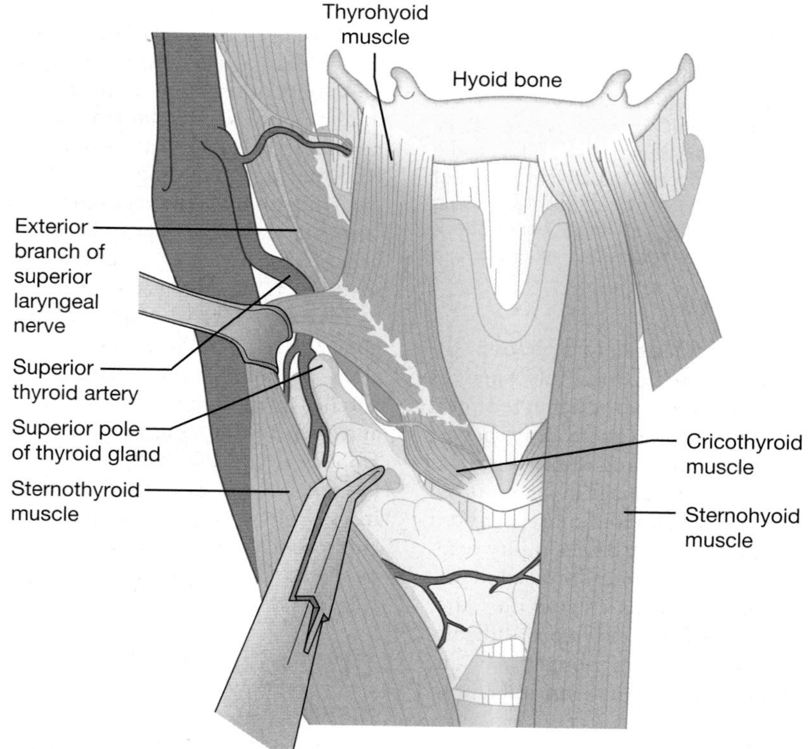

FIG. 37.5 Dissection and ligation of the superior pole thyroid vessels should be performed as far caudally on the thyroid gland as possible to avoid injury to the external branch of the superior laryngeal nerve (EBSLN). (From Randolph GW. Surgical anatomy, intraoperative neural monitoring, and operative management of the RLN and SLN. In: Duh QY, Clark OH, Kebebew E, eds. *Atlas of Endocrine Surgical Techniques*. Philadelphia: Elsevier Saunders; 2010:105.)

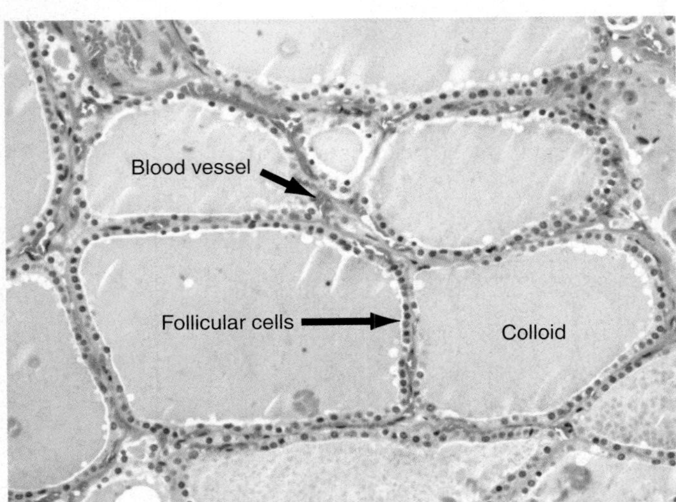

FIG. 37.6 Photomicrograph of normal thyroid parenchyma with hematoxylin and eosin staining. The follicular unit contains colloid at the center, and each follicle is surrounded by a single layer of well-ordered, cytologically normal follicular cells. The parafollicular spaces contain blood vessels and parafollicular cells.

C cells are located within the interfollicular stroma, and are mainly found in the lateral aspect of the mid and upper thyroid lobes.

Normal Thyroid Physiology

Thyroid Hormone

The synthesis of thyroid hormones is a complex multistep process that occurs within the thyroid follicle unit. The process is dependent upon the presence of iodine and is outlined below:

- Follicular cells actively transport iodide anion across the cell membrane from the bloodstream into the cytoplasm via the Na/I symporter membrane protein. The concentration of iodine within the follicular cells is normally many-fold higher than that of the systemic circulation due to this active transport.
- Iodide then moves toward the follicular cell border with the colloid stores, and the anions are oxidized to form the neutral I_2 molecule. This form of iodine can pass through the cell membrane into the colloid.
- Colloid stores Tg, which contains a multitude of tyrosine residues. Colloid also contains the enzyme thyroid peroxidase (TPO), which catalyzes the next major step in thyroid hormone synthesis, which is the iodination of tyrosine residues on Tg. A tyrosine residue iodinated by a single iodine molecule leads to the formation of the molecule monoiodotyrosine, and that iodinated by two iodine molecules leads to diiodotyrosine (DIT).
- The DIT and monoiodotyrosine molecules form covalent bonds with one another to constitute the active forms of thyroid hormone tetraiodothyronine or thyroxine (T_4), formed by two DITs and carrying four iodine molecules) and triiodothyronine (T_3), formed by a DIT and monoiodotyrosine and carrying three iodine molecules). When stimulated by thyroid-stimulating hormone (TSH), the follicular cells transport the activated thyroid hormones from the colloid center into the bloodstream (Fig. 37.7).

Once in the bloodstream, greater than 99% of circulating thyroid hormones are bound to transport proteins such as albumin and T_4-binding globulins; less than 1% exists in free form. This allows a relatively tight degree of control of thyroid hormone diffusion into target cells in that the bound hormones will be released if circulating free levels decrease. Although there is normally a higher concentration of T_4 compared to T_3, T_3 is the more potent form, and in fact many target organs such as the brain, liver, gut, skeletal muscle, and thyroid are able to convert T_4 to T_3 through the deiodinase system that removes one of the iodine molecules.

Iodine plays a primary role in thyroid hormone physiology, and it is predicated on there being an adequate supply in the body. The average daily iodine requirement for adult humans is 0.1 mg, and this is entirely derived from dietary intake. The thyroid is the target for the overwhelming majority of the body's iodine stores. Seafood such as fish, shrimp, and seaweed are rich in iodine stores. Since 1924, the United States has iodized salt, which effectively has eliminated iodine deficiency in this country. Many regions of the world remain at risk for iodine deficiency despite worldwide efforts to improve access to iodized salt; the World Health Organization estimates that 54 countries remain iodine-deficient.

Thyroid hormone is critical for normal bodily function. On a cellular level, T_4 and T_3 bind to mitochondrial receptors, leading to increased ATP production, oxygen consumption, and glucose oxidation in a calorigenic process that releases heat. Therefore, thyroid hormone function is often referred to shorthand as the primary driver of the basal metabolic rate. It is hypothesized that virtually all cells in the body are end-targets for thyroid hormone, mostly through their actions with regard to stimulating lipid and carbohydrate metabolism. Thyroid hormone is critical for normal in utero and childhood growth and development, especially with respect to neurologic function. The cardiovascular system is an important target of thyroid hormone, which increases cardiac output and vasodilatation. Normal reproductive function is highly dependent on thyroid hormone (see below).

The regulation of thyroid hormone production is tightly controlled by interactions between the hypothalamus, pituitary, and thyroid glands. Low circulating levels of T_4 and T_3 stimulate the hypothalamus to release thyrotropin-releasing hormone, which in turn stimulates the release of TSH from the anterior pituitary. TSH stimulates the formation of thyroid hormones by binding to its receptor on the thyroid follicular cells, leading to both increased transport of iodine as well as transport and release of T_4 and T_3 from the colloid into the bloodstream. Conversely, elevated circulating thyroid hormone levels lead to a negative feedback loop, with downregulation of thyrotropin-releasing hormone and TSH from the hypothalamus and pituitary, respectively.

Calcitonin

The thyroid gland also produces calcitonin from the parafollicular C cells, but the production of calcitonin is not regulated by the same processes that govern that of thyroid hormone. The primary known function of calcitonin is to decrease the serum concentration of calcium through its end effect actions on bone (increasing osteoblast and decreasing osteoclast activity), gut (decreasing calcium absorption), and kidney (increasing urinary calcium excretion), and its release is stimulated by elevated serum calcium levels. However, the absence of calcitonin does not lead to a noticeable change in calcium homeostasis—as it would for parathyroid hormone (PTH)—and so its ultimate importance for normal physiologic function remains poorly understood.

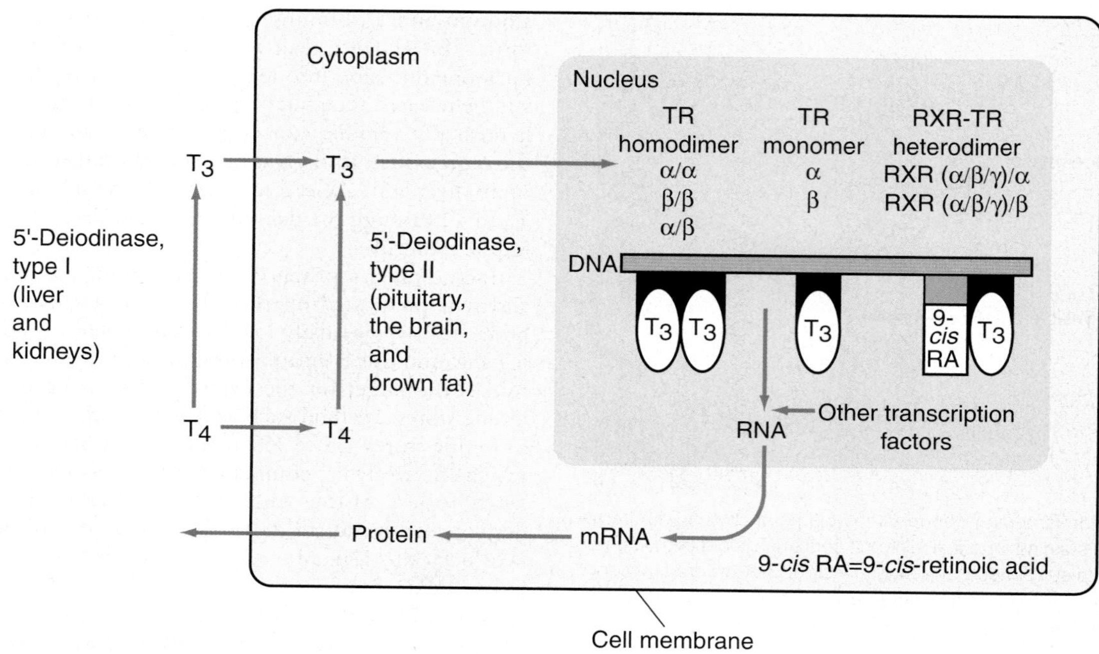

FIG. 37.7 Cellular and molecular events involved in thyroid hormone function. Thyroxine *(T_4)* is converted in the periphery and in the cytoplasm of the cell into triiodothyronine *(T_3)*. T_3 travels to the nucleus, where it binds to a thyroid hormone receptor *(TR)*(homodimer, monomer, or heterodimer). TR binding leads to RNA transcription in association with other transcription factors; messenger RNA is subsequently expressed and then translated into protein.

Thyroid Physiology in Pregnancy

Normal pregnancy induces significant changes in thyroid hormone function due to its critical importance for early fetal development. Although multiple fetal processes depend on thyroid hormone, including overall growth, metabolic regulation, and bone maturation, neuronal and brain development are the most critical, as evidenced by the finding of severe neurocognitive deficits in babies born to mothers with untreated hypothyroidism.

During the first trimester, maternal thyroid hormone production rises significantly, with total T_4 concentrations increasing up to 1.5 times that of the nonpregnant state. Although the details are not completely elucidated, it is thought that this rise is at least in part due to the rapidly increasing levels of human chorionic gonadotropin, which shares a common alpha subunit with TSH and acts as a TSH agonist. This can occasionally lead to a phenomenon known as transient gestational thyrotoxicosis occurring only in the first trimester and resolving spontaneously.

The rise in T_4 concentration is also accompanied by a concomitant increase in T_4-binding globulin concentration in the bloodstream, which results in greater binding of the circulating T_4 and relative stability in free T_4 levels. Because of the increased demands for thyroid hormone production, the daily recommended iodine intake during pregnancy also rises. Maternal T_4 is transported to the fetal circulation via specialized thyroid hormone transporters in the placenta.

Maternal thyroid hormone production increases and peaks during the first trimester of pregnancy and declines steadily afterward; this likely coincides with the development and early function of the fetal thyroid. Measurable levels of fetal thyroid hormone can be detected by the eleventh week of gestation, but maturation of the entire hypothalamic-pituitary-thyroid feedback axis does not occur until the mid-second trimester; thus, it is thought that properly regulated maternal thyroid function remains important at least until this stage.

Thyroid dysfunction is associated with adverse maternal and fetal outcomes. As a result, regular monitoring of thyroid function is a standard component of routine prenatal care. Hypothyroidism is the most common type of thyroid dysfunction in pregnancy, occurring in up to 0.5% of pregnant women. Iodine deficiency is the most common cause of hypothyroidism in iodine-deficient regions, whereas autoimmune thyroiditis is the most common cause in iodine-replete areas. Maternal hypothyroidism is associated with an increased risk of infertility and perinatal complications. Fetal/neonatal hypothyroidism from iodine deficiency leads to cretinism, a syndrome presenting with severe growth and cognitive deficits, deafness, and failure of sexual development. Hyperthyroidism, most commonly due to Graves disease, occurs in about 0.3% of pregnant women; left untreated, this leads to an increased risk of maternofetal complications, including miscarriage, preeclampsia, preterm delivery, and abruptio placentae.

Thyroid Physiology in Nonthyroidal Illness (Euthyroid Sick Syndrome)

Many acute and chronic nonthyroidal disease states can affect thyroid function measurement. This phenomenon, commonly called "euthyroid sick syndrome" or "nonthyroidal illness syndrome," leads to the finding of abnormal thyroid function tests in the setting of nonthyroidal illness in a patient without preexisting thyroid disease. The most common finding is low serum T_3 concentrations, with decreases in T_4 also seen in more severe disease states. TSH concentrations remain relatively normal to slightly elevated, but not to the degree of true hypothyroidism. Patients do not exhibit any signs of clinical thyroid dysfunction.

The pathophysiology behind euthyroid sick syndrome remains poorly understood, although several theories exist. Some believe that conversion of T_4 to T_3 in the target tissues is impaired during nonthyroidal illness due to decreased activity of peripheral deiodinase enzymes (in particular, deiodinase type 2). Others have investigated the role of cytokines such as tumor necrosis factor-α, interleukin 1, and interleukin 6 in decreasing thyroid hormone production at the level of the thyroid follicular cell. Others hypothesize that the inhibition of thyroid hormone binding to various thyroid binding proteins may lead to inaccurate measurement of true free hormone levels. Regardless of theory, it is generally believed that patients with this phenomenon are in fact euthyroid and do not have intrinsic thyroid dysfunction.

Common states associated with euthyroid sick syndrome in surgical patients include sepsis, fasting/starvation, trauma, thermal injury, and myocardial infarction. Many medications such as corticosteroids and amiodarone also can affect thyroid function measurement. There is no treatment for euthyroid sick syndrome other than treating the underlying condition, which resolves the thyroid function test abnormalities.

THYROID BIOMARKERS

Thyroid-Stimulating Hormone

TSH is a 28-kDa glycoprotein secreted from the anterior pituitary gland in a pulsatile fashion; it follows a circadian rhythm. Its actions on the TSH receptor on thyroid follicular cells as a part of the hypothalamic-pituitary-thyroid axis make it a primary regulatory driver of thyroid hormone secretion. Measurement of serum TSH is the most common and reliable test for screening for thyroid dysfunction. This is because the negative feedback loop from T_4 and T_3 onto pituitary TSH secretion follows a log-linear relationship, resulting in more significant changes in TSH concentrations relative to smaller changes in thyroid hormone levels.

TSH is currently measured using third- and fourth-generation ultrasensitive radioimmunoassays, with associated degrees of precision to less than 0.002 μIU/mL and sensitivity up to 97%. The currently accepted normal range of serum TSH for adults is 0.4 to 4.12 mIU/L, with minor variation depending on the specific assay used. TSH measurement is indicated as a part of evaluation of suspected thyroid dysfunction, as well as for screening and surveillance in high-risk settings such as pregnancy. Despite its overall high yield as a screening test, TSH values should be interpreted with caution in a number of nonthyroidal health states that can affect its measurement, such as pregnancy, nonthyroidal illness (euthyroid sick syndrome), and medications such as glucocorticoids, furosemide, anticonvulsants, and metformin.

Tetraiodothyronine and Triiodothyronine

Serum measurement of T_4 and T_3 is an important confirmatory component in the evaluation of thyroid dysfunction. The vast majority of both thyroid hormones in systemic circulation are bound to plasma proteins such as T_4-binding globulins, with less than 0.2% of the hormones available in the free, biologically active states. Because of this, measurement of free T_4 and free T_3 levels are more accurate in reflecting thyroid function compared to measuring total hormone levels, which can be falsely affected by the presence of various circulating transporter proteins.

The measurement of TSH and free T_4 are the most commonly paired thyroid function tests because of their accurate interpretability in the majority of scenarios, including the diagnosis and treatment monitoring of thyroid dysfunction. Free T_3 is not as useful for the diagnosis of hypothyroidism, but it can be useful for the confirmation of other conditions such as hyperthyroidism and euthyroid sick syndrome. All forms of thyroid hormones are measured using modern competitive immunoassays, with mild variations in normal ranges depending on the method and manufacturer. Normal reference ranges are also age dependent, with different standards for pediatric and adult populations.

Thyroid Autoantibodies

The measurement of serum thyroid autoantibodies is useful in the diagnosis of various autoimmune thyroid diseases, although their variable sensitivities and specificities require caution in test interpretation. The three most commonly measured autoantibodies today are anti-TPO (TPOAb), anti-Tg (TgAb), and anti-TSH receptor (TRAb).

Measurement of TPOAb is the most accurate and commonly used screening test for autoimmune thyroiditis. TPOAb is positive in over 90% of patients with autoimmune thyroiditis, as well as 80% of patients with Graves disease. However, it also has a false-positive rate of 10% to 15%. Measurement of TgAb is commonly performed, with 80% sensitivity for autoimmune thyroiditis and 30% sensitivity for Graves disease, and a similar false-positive rate as TPOAb. Importantly, the presence of TgAb interferes with the interpretation of Tg measurement for the surveillance of differentiated thyroid cancer ([DTC] see below). TPOAb is usually measured by ultrasensitive immunoradiometric assays; TgAb also can be measured with this method, although other techniques such as radioimmunoassay or enzyme-linked immunosorbent assay are also acceptable. These two tests are often ordered together and are generally readily available in most clinical laboratories.

Measurement of TRAb is typically reserved for diagnostic confirmation of Graves disease, as it is positive in over 90% of patients with the diagnosis. TRAb measurement is typically performed in one of two ways: 1) a TSH receptor-binding inhibitory immunoglobulin bioassay, which detects immunoglobulins inhibiting the binding of TSH to the recombinant TSH receptor, and 2) a thyroid-stimulating immunoglobulin (TSI) bioassay, which more specifically detects the stimulatory subtype of TRAb that activates the TSH receptor on the thyroid follicular cells. TSI measurement has been hypothesized to more closely correlate with the severity of active Graves disease. Both of these tests are currently more resource-intensive and costly; as such, their additional utility beyond other diagnostic methods for Graves—namely, history and physical exam, thyroid function tests, and measurement of the other thyroid autoantibodies, neck ultrasound, and thyroid uptake scan—remains unclear. Most agree about their utility in special situations, such as diagnostic challenges in patients with nodular goiter and hyperthyroidism, eye disease, and diagnosis and surveillance during pregnancy.

Thyroglobulin

Tg is a large 660-kDa glycosylated protein that acts as a precursor protein for the active iodinated forms of thyroid hormone. Although the majority of Tg is stored in colloid within the thyroid follicles, a small amount of Tg escapes into the systemic circulation during the conversion process to T_4 and T_3 and is thus detectable in peripheral blood. Tg can be particularly elevated in patients with DTC, although with low diagnostic utility for routine measurement or prior to total thyroidectomy. On the other hand, postoperative serum Tg measurement after total thyroidectomy for DTC remains among the most sensitive cancer biomarkers in existence today, with the caveat that its accuracy depends on the absence of TgAb.

Current widely used immunoassay methods for Tg measurement include enzyme-linked immunosorbent assay, enzyme multiplied immunoassay, fluorescence polarization immunoassay, and immunochemiluminometric assay. All of these immunoassay methods have made Tg measurement highly sensitive and specific, such that it is possible to detect Tg down to the 0.1 ng/mL level. For postoperative surveillance of DTC, the sensitivity of Tg measurement can be augmented further with TSH stimulation, either following withdrawal of thyroid hormone or after injection of recombinant human TSH. A stimulated Tg of more than 1 to 2 ng/mL is considered higher risk for persistent or recurrent disease in the post thyroidectomy setting.

The accuracy of serum Tg testing is highly dependent upon the absence of TgAb, which must be obtained at the same time. TgAb is present in 10% to 15% of the general population and can limit the interpretability of postoperative Tg measurement. Even in these scenarios, TgAb often can be used as a crude surrogate biomarker, since autoantibodies can disappear over time after the successful treatment of thyroid cancer; in addition, an increase in TgAb levels can signify disease recurrence. Newer Tg assays that employ mass spectrometry offer reasonable detection capability even in the presence of TgAb, with sensitivities down to 0.5 ng/mL, approaching those of the immunoassays.

Calcitonin

Calcitonin is a 32–amino acid protein secreted by the parafollicular C cells. Normally, serum calcitonin levels are highest in infancy, decline rapidly in early childhood, then remain relatively stable through adulthood (although absolute levels can fluctuate minute to minute). Calcitonin does not appear to play a significant role in calcium homeostasis despite its known mechanisms of action at the level of the bone, gut, and kidney. Serum calcitonin is the most sensitive biomarker for the detection and surveillance of medullary thyroid cancer (MTC), which is a malignancy of the parafollicular C cells. This test is performed in patients with—or family members at risk for—MTC or multiple endocrine neoplasia type 2 (MEN2; see below). There is controversy around the utility of measuring serum calcitonin as a routine screening test in the evaluation of a thyroid nodule.[2] Calcitonin is currently measured using a variety of methods, including radioimmunoassays, enzyme-linked immunosorbent assay, and immunochemiluminometric assay, with differing sensitivities, specificities, and reference ranges.

THYROID IMAGING

Neck Ultrasound

Neck ultrasonography is the preferred modality for routine radiographic evaluation of the thyroid gland, as it offers the most accurate visualization of thyroid nodular disease and allows for the concomitant ability to perform percutaneous fine-needle aspiration (FNA) biopsy of thyroid lesions (see below). Neck ultrasound provides information about overall thyroid size and vascularity, presence and risk stratification of thyroid nodules, and presence of suspicious cervical lymphadenopathy; in addition, it can be used to localize parathyroid disease. Advantages of ultrasound include the fact that it is noninvasive and portable for the clinic and it is not associated with radiation exposure.

One potential disadvantage of neck ultrasound is that the study quality is highly dependent on having a skilled operator; this issue is amplified by practice- and institution-specific variations on what specialties perform ultrasound, since radiologists, surgeons, pathologists, and medical endocrinologists all may be trained to perform the procedure. Efforts to standardize the quality of neck ultrasound have included common ultrasound training and credentialing pathways regardless of specialty, as well as standardized templates for neck ultrasound reporting.

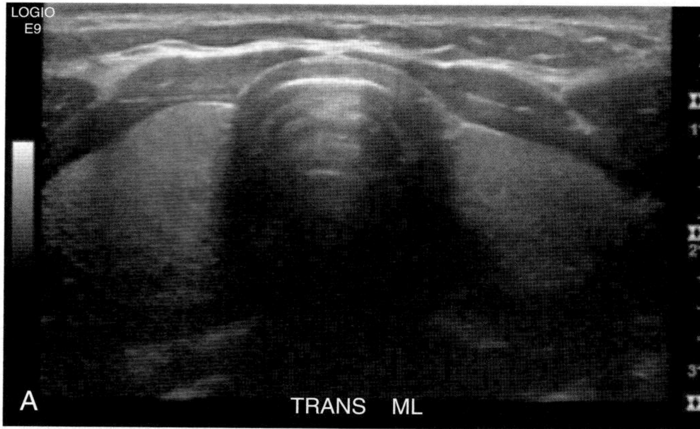

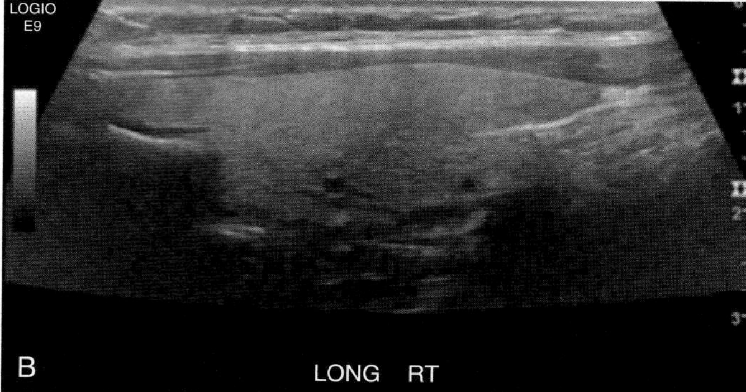

FIG. 37.8 Normal appearance of the thyroid gland on neck ultrasound. Note the homogeneous echogenicity with uniform echotexture of the gland. (A) Transverse midline view with the two lobes on either side of the trachea. (B) Longitudinal view of the right thyroid lobe.

The normal sonographic appearance of the thyroid is homogeneously echogenic with a uniform echotexture (Fig. 37.8). Pathologic findings on thyroid ultrasound are described in the appropriate sections below.

Nuclear Scintigraphy

Thyroid scintigraphy is performed using either technetium-99m pertechnetate or a radiolabeled iodine nuclide (typically ^{123}I or ^{131}I). Depending on the specific study, the tracer can be administered intravenously, orally, or via inhalation, and images are obtained anywhere from 30 minutes (for intravenous [IV] injection) to 24 hours (for oral administration) afterward. The thyroid normally displays symmetric uptake bilaterally. Nodular disease can be classified into whether there is increased focal uptake (the so-called "hot" nodule, Fig. 37.9) or not (the "cold" nodule). Classically, "hot" nodules in the setting of hyperthyroidism are thought to be benign toxic nodules with extremely low risk of malignancy, whereas "cold" nodules carry a 15% risk of malignancy.

Improvements in ultrasonography and cross-sectional imaging over the past few decades have rendered thyroid scintigraphy obsolete in all but a few scenarios. A thyroid uptake scan is useful for the differential diagnosis of hyperthyroidism by determining

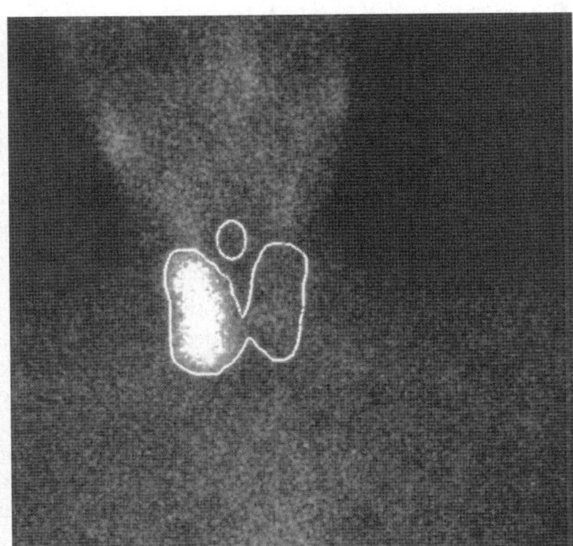

FIG. 37.9 ^{131}I scan demonstrating an area of increased uptake in the right lobe of a 32-year-old woman with increased thyroid function test values and a palpable nodule. This scan is consistent with a toxic or hyperfunctioning nodule.

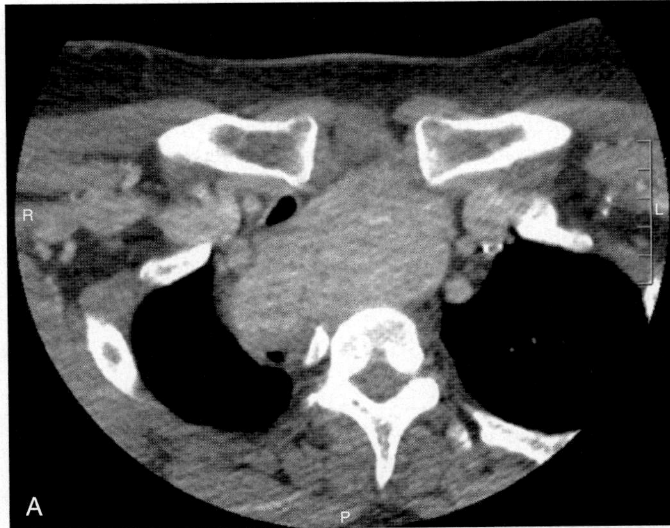

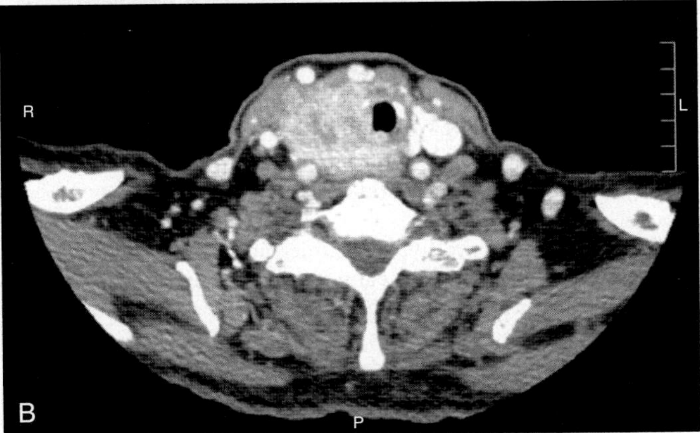

FIG. 37.10 Computed tomography (CT) scans provide useful anatomic information about the thyroid in selected scenarios. (A) Contrast-enhanced CT scan demonstrating a left-sided substernal goiter extending into the posterior mediastinum and crossing over to the right side with tracheal compression and deviation of both the trachea and esophagus. (B) Contrast-enhanced CT scan of a bulky locally advanced follicular thyroid cancer originating in the right lobe with invasion into the lateral tracheal wall and esophagus and obliteration of the right internal jugular vein.

whether increased radiotracer uptake occurs diffusely throughout the gland as in the case of Graves disease or in more discrete "hot" nodules in cases of solitary toxic adenoma or toxic multinodular goiter (TMG). In addition, radiolabeled iodine scans (usually referred to as radioactive iodine [RAI] scans) are commonly performed to assess for, and treat, persistent/recurrent or metastatic disease in the setting of DTC (see below).

Cross-Sectional Imaging

Computed tomography (CT) or magnetic resonance imaging (MRI) scans can be useful adjuncts to ultrasound for specific indications, as they can provide precise cross-sectional anatomic assessment of the thyroid gland relative to the other structures in the neck, including the larynx and trachea, esophagus, muscles, and major vascular structures. These modalities are helpful particularly for two scenarios: substernal (intrathoracic) goiter and advanced thyroid cancer (Fig. 37.10). CT and MRI have improved ability over ultrasound in visualizing the infraclavicular mediastinum. In addition, cross-sectional imaging more readily detects vascular anomalies such as the lusoria artery that can alert the surgeon to complex anatomic situations (e.g., presence of nonrecurrent laryngeal nerve) and assist with perioperative planning. Many surgeons prefer CT over MRI due to its greater ease of interpretation, as well as its superiority over MRI in the detection of cervical lymph node metastases.

If ordered, cross-sectional thyroid imaging should evaluate not just the neck but a wide craniocaudal dimension from the skull base to the tracheal bifurcation in order to accurately assess the extent of intrathoracic goiter or malignancy. Both CT and MRI can be performed with or without IV contrast, depending on the clinical scenario. For evaluation of substernal goiter, a noncontrast CT or MRI is sufficient. On the other hand, IV contrast is indicated for clinical suspicion of advanced thyroid cancer such as locally advanced tumors or those with multiple and/or bulky lymph node metastases. Contrast-enhanced images are best for assessing local invasion into neighboring structures, particularly the aerodigestive tract.

On noncontrast CT scan, the thyroid appears homogeneous and mildly hyperattenuating compared to the surrounding muscles, whereas iodinated contrast administration leads to fairly bright diffuse enhancement. On MRI, the thyroid can be mildly hyperintense on both T1- and T2-weighted images, with bright enhancement on gadolinium contrast administration. Incidental thyroid nodules can be found in up to 9% of neck CT or MRI scans. Iodine is generally cleared within 4 to 8 weeks after iodinated contrast administration, which generally does not cause a clinically significant delay in postoperative RAI administration for DTC.

Positron Emission Tomography

Positron emission tomography (PET, typically coupled with CT or MRI) is most frequently performed with the administration of [^{18}F]-fluorodeoxyglucose radiotracer, which is taken up in tissues with elevated metabolism of glucose. The normal thyroid takes up [^{18}F]-fluorodeoxyglucose to a similar level as surrounding skeletal muscle. The role of [^{18}F]-fluorodeoxyglucose PET is limited to selected cases of higher-risk thyroid cancers, such as for surveillance and staging for RAI-refractory DTC.

PET is not recommended for the routine evaluation of thyroid disease. However, with greater use of these scans, along with other cross-sectional modalities for cancer surveillance purposes, incidental thyroid nodular disease is being detected by PET scans with increasing frequency. Up to 3% of PET scans identify incidental thyroid nodules. PET-positive nodules are generally associated with an elevated risk of malignancy (up to 35% on average), but this fact does not supersede the need for standard evaluation with neck ultrasound and FNA biopsy prior to consideration of surgical management.

HYPOTHYROIDISM

Hypothyroidism is a disorder characterized by inadequate thyroid hormone production and/or availability in peripheral target tissues. Hypothyroidism is a common disorder in the world, although the specific causes differ depending on geography. The most common cause overall is iodine deficiency, which is primarily encountered in the developing world due to lack of sufficient dietary iodine; the same pathophysiology leads to an elevated risk of developing endemic goiter. In the developed world, the most common causes include autoimmune thyroiditis and iatrogenic hypothyroidism as a result of thyroidectomy or RAI treatment with insufficient thyroid hormone supplementation or replacement.

With respect to the hypothalamic-pituitary-thyroid axis, the overwhelming majority of causes of hypothyroidism are primary—that is, the lack of thyroid hormone production is due to causes at the level of the thyroid. A small percentage of cases may be due to inadequate secretion of TSH from the pituitary or thyrotropin-releasing hormone from the hypothalamus, which are referred to as secondary or tertiary hypothyroidism, respectively.

The symptoms and signs of hypothyroidism can range from mild to no symptoms, to the classic presentation of cold intolerance, fatigue, puffiness and weight gain, dry skin, and hair loss. Myxedema represents an extreme of symptomatic hypothyroidism in which patients develop a constellation of severe findings, such as altered mental status or coma, hypothermia, bradycardia, and electrolyte abnormalities, with an increased risk of cardiomegaly, pericardial effusion and ascites, and shock. Myxedema typically occurs as a decompensation of chronic hypothyroidism due to an acute physiologic stressor, such as trauma, infection, or an acute cardiovascular event.

Thyroid function tests and particularly TSH are highly sensitive for screening for hypothyroidism. In adults, primary hypothyroidism is generally suspected when serum TSH levels are above 4.12 mIU/L, although normal ranges differ depending on age as well as pregnancy.[3] Further testing typically includes measurement of thyroid hormones, including free T_4 and T_3 levels. Elevated TSH levels with decreased free T_4 and T_3 levels are diagnostic of primary hypothyroidism. Elevated TSH levels with relatively normal levels of thyroid hormones are considered to be subclinical or mild hypothyroidism.

Hypothyroidism is fortunately easily treatable with pharmacologic agents such as levothyroxine (LT_4) or liothyronine (LT_3), which are synthetic versions of T_4 and T_3, respectively. LT_4 is recommended as the first-line therapy in most patients for the treatment of hypothyroidism and is available in oral, intramuscular, and IV forms. The rationale for LT_4 lies in the body's ability to convert the exogenously administered T_4 into T_3 by deiodinases in the peripheral tissues. Other therapeutic strategies include a combination of LT_4 and LT_3, LT_3 alone, and desiccated thyroid extracts; all strategies were developed under the hypothesis that LT_4 administration alone may be insufficient to replicate the normal euthyroid state, whether due to inadequate in vivo conversion to T_3 or the absence of some other heretofore undescribed molecule(s). None of these options is recommended currently as routine first-line therapy. Regarding combination LT_4 and LT_3 therapy, multiple randomized controlled trials have failed to demonstrate superiority over LT_4 monotherapy in various outcomes, including achievement of target TSH and thyroid-specific symptoms and thyroid-specific health outcomes; further research is needed to study the possible benefit of combination therapy in selected patients with low serum T_3 levels or persistent symptoms on monotherapy. Both LT_3 monotherapy and thyroid extract regimens have some preliminary supporting evidence on short-term outcomes and preference, but high-quality long-term data on safety and equivalent efficacy are lacking.

Autoimmune Thyroiditis

Autoimmune thyroiditis is the most frequent cause of hypothyroidism in iodine-replete populations. The most common type is chronic lymphocytic thyroiditis, otherwise known as Hashimoto thyroiditis. This disorder is found predominantly in females at up to a 10:1 female-to-male incidence ratio. In addition, there is a strong hereditary component, with first-degree relatives of Hashimoto's patients having a nine-fold risk of also developing the disease. The etiology of Hashimoto thyroiditis is due to the presence of circulating autoantibodies to thyroid antigens, resulting in a chronic autoimmune destructive process involving the formation of immune complexes and complement in the basement membrane of follicular cells. This leads to the infiltration of lymphocytes into the thyroid follicles and eventually results in fibrosis, which decreases the effective number of follicles needed to produce thyroid hormones.

The biochemical workup for Hashimoto thyroiditis includes measurement of thyroid function tests as well as circulating thyroid autoantibodies, including TPOAb and TgAb (see above), which are present in 95% and 60% of patients, respectively. Euthyroid and subclinically hypothyroid patients with elevated autoantibody titers are at greater risk of progressing to overt hypothyroidism. In addition, thyroid autoantibody measurement is recommended in patients at higher risk of developing hypothyroidism, including those with other autoimmune diseases or taking drugs such as lithium or amiodarone.[3]

There is typically no role for imaging studies in the workup and diagnosis of Hashimoto thyroiditis. However, patients with Hashimoto thyroiditis will frequently have symptoms of neck discomfort, pain, and globus sensation, necessitating neck ultrasound for diagnostic workup. Sonographic characteristics of Hashimoto thyroiditis include coarse, heterogeneous, and hypoechoic parenchymal echotexture with increased vascularity, often with the presence of fine echogenic septae producing a pseudonodular appearance that can sometimes be confused with discrete thyroid nodules (Fig. 37.11). The size of the thyroid may range from diffusely or focally enlarged to small and atrophic, and there may be mildly enlarged and more numerous perithyroidal lymph nodes from the autoimmune inflammatory process. Hashimoto thyroiditis has been associated with an increased risk of papillary thyroid cancer (PTC) but possibly with a slight improvement in prognosis based on a number of single-institution surgical series, so any suspicious thyroid nodules or lymph nodes in the setting of

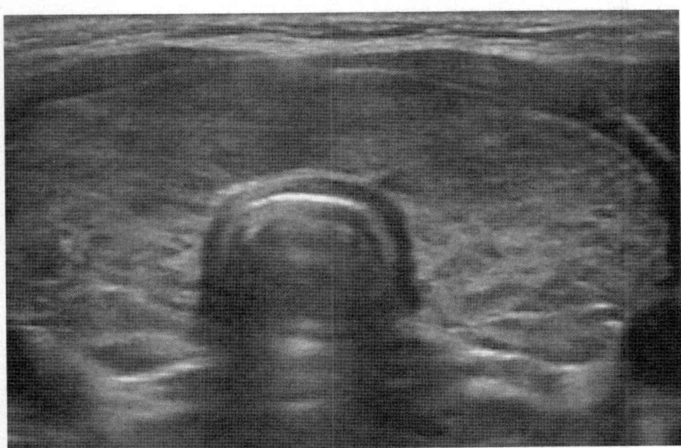

FIG. 37.11 Sonographic features of Hashimoto thyroiditis. In this image, the thyroid gland is enlarged, predominantly hyperechoic, and diffusely heterogeneous, with irregular echotexture and poorly defined hyperechoic regions separated by fibrous strands. (From Andrioli M, Valcavi R. Sonography of normal and abnormal thyroid and parathyroid glands. *Front Horm Res.* 2016;45:1–15.)

Hashimoto thyroiditis should be appropriately worked up with FNA biopsy.

Cytologic features of Hashimoto thyroiditis include a moderately cellular specimen with aggregates of follicular cells with oncocytic/Hürthle cell changes, minimal colloid, and infiltration of mature lymphocytes. Giant cells, plasma cells, macrophages, histiocytes, and eosinophils also may be seen. Primary thyroid lymphoma, a rare thyroid malignancy with an annual incidence of 2 per 1 million, is associated with Hashimoto thyroiditis and can often be difficult to distinguish based on cytology due to similarities around having large numbers of lymphoid cells and lymphoid follicles with decreased colloid.

The second most common type of autoimmune thyroiditis is postpartum thyroiditis, which can occur in up to 10% of women within the first 2 to 12 months of the postpartum period. The pathogenesis of postpartum thyroiditis appears to have similarities and parallels to that of Hashimoto thyroiditis in that 1) hypothyroidism may be preceded by a short thyrotoxic state; 2) it is often associated with the presence of circulating TPOAb; and 3) postpartum thyroiditis is associated with a ten-fold risk of ultimately developing Hashimoto thyroiditis. Postpartum thyroiditis is typically short-lived, with resolution in 2 to 4 months. A short course of exogenous thyroid hormone supplementation/replacement may be necessary.

Subacute Thyroiditis

Subacute thyroiditis, also known as de Quervain disease or subacute granulomatous thyroiditis, is a relatively uncommon disease found primarily in the developed world. It has a female preponderance, with a 2:1 female-to-male ratio, and typically occurs in the fourth decade of life. The pathogenesis remains poorly understood, but the disease often occurs after a viral prodrome such as an upper respiratory infection. The hallmark of the clinical presentation for de Quervain thyroiditis is pain and swelling in the thyroid region, along with low-grade fevers, dysphagia, and severe fatigue. Biochemical findings may include an elevated erythrocyte sedimentation rate, which is diagnostic. As with autoimmune thyroiditis, de Quervain thyroiditis can be associated with transient hyperthyroidism followed by hypothyroidism. Cytopathologic characteristics from FNA biopsy include the presence of multinucleated giant cell granulomas. Histopathology shows evidence of granulomatous changes in the thyroid follicles. The follicles are enlarged, with infiltration by mononuclear cells, neutrophils, and lymphocytes.

The time course of de Quervain thyroiditis is typically 2 to 5 months, and the vast majority of patients return to a euthyroid state spontaneously. Because of its self-limited course, no specific treatments are indicated except for symptomatic relief of pain and/or temporary treatment of clinical hypothyroidism. The pain associated with de Quervain thyroiditis can be treated with nonsteroidal antiinflammatory drugs; more severe cases can be treated with a course of corticosteroids. Surgery is not typically indicated for treatment of de Quervain thyroiditis, and reassurance and emotional counseling are often necessary, particularly during the painful phase of the disease.

Riedel Thyroiditis

Riedel thyroiditis, also known as Riedel struma or chronic fibrous thyroiditis, is an extremely rare and poorly understood inflammatory process causing diffuse destruction and fibrosis of the thyroid. The primary theories for the etiology of this disease are that it is either an autoimmune process or a specific fibrotic disorder related to multifocal fibrosclerosis. The most relevant finding in Riedel thyroiditis is the presence of an extremely firm and constricting gland that can be very uncomfortable for patients. The fibrotic process often extends into surrounding structures, including the aerodigestive tract and RLN, which may cause clinically significant airway obstruction, dysphagia, and dysphonia.

Patients with Riedel thyroiditis have the biochemical markers of hypothyroidism. Imaging is necessary to rule out other causes of the dramatic local symptoms. Ultrasound characteristics often demonstrate a diffusely hypoechoic gland with ill-defined borders. FNA cytology reveals dense fibrotic changes but cannot be reliably distinguished from fibrotic changes often associated with anaplastic thyroid cancer (ATC).

Medical treatment to treat the inflammatory component of Riedel thyroiditis traditionally consists of corticosteroids and tamoxifen. Other agents such as mycophenolate and rituximab also have been used. Thyroid hormone supplementation/replacement is used to treat the associated hypothyroidism. Surgical resection is often indicated to rule out malignancy such as ATC or primary thyroid lymphoma or to treat aerodigestive tract obstruction. Surgery is usually extremely challenging due to the firmness of the gland and obliteration or normal planes and landmarks. Partial resection of only the affected components is recommended, with simple wedge resection of the isthmus being the most common surgical therapy for relief of tracheal compression. There is no evidence to suggest that Riedel thyroiditis is associated with an increased risk of thyroid malignancy.

Acute Suppurative Thyroiditis

Acute suppurative thyroiditis is rare and defined as an acute pyogenic infection of the thyroid gland. The most common underlying cause is infection of a congenital pyriform sinus fistula which tracks and communicates with the thyroid. The clinical presentation of acute thyroiditis is that of a bacterial infection: fever, severe unilateral pain and swelling at the thyroid gland (typically left-sided), and cervical lymphadenopathy. The most common organisms include the *Staphylococcus* and *Streptococcus* species, but other aerobic or anaerobic species also may be involved. The thyroiditis can also lead to thyroid abscess formation; rarely, it can lead to even more serious sequelae, including retropharyngeal abscess, tracheal obstruction, mediastinitis, and jugular venous thrombosis.

Thyroid function tests are rarely useful in the diagnosis of acute suppurative thyroiditis; rather, other biochemical findings of acute systemic illness and sepsis are more useful, such as a complete blood count marked by a leukocytosis with a left shift. Ultrasound with FNA biopsy can be useful for bacterial culture and speciation of any abscess fluid. Treatment consists of appropriate-spectrum antibiotics, as well percutaneous drainage of any identified abscess. Acute thyroiditis does not generally lead to long-term hypothyroidism requiring thyroid hormone supplementation therapy.

Iatrogenic Hypothyroidism

Aside from postthyroidectomy hypothyroidism due to the absence of sufficient thyroid parenchyma, pharmacotherapy is the primary cause of iatrogenic hypothyroidism. The number and variety of medications and therapies that are associated with hypothyroidism are extensive (Box 37.1). The most common medications associated with hypothyroidism include RAI (^{131}I), antithyroid thionamides (such as methimazole and propylthiouracil [PTU]), amiodarone, lithium, immune modulators, and kinase inhibitors.

The etiology of drug-induced hypothyroidism depends on the specific agent. In the case of RAI therapy, the often-expected hypothyroidism is due to direct destruction of the thyroid follicular cells by the delivered radioactive agent. Thionamides such as methimazole and PTU directly inhibit T_4 and T_3 synthesis (as well as block peripheral conversion of T_4 to T_3 in the case of PTU). The antiarrhythmic agent amiodarone can lead to both hypothyroidism and hyperthyroidism due to a number of mechanisms, including inability to escape from the Wolff-Chaikoff effect from the drug's high iodine content, inhibition of deiodinase activity, inhibition of thyroid hormone entry into the periphery, and direct cytotoxic thyroiditis (see below). Lithium may act by directly inhibiting the cAMP-dependent pathway, leading to thyroid hormone formation in the thyroid follicle. Tyrosine kinase inhibitors such as sunitinib and vandetanib cause hypothyroidism in different ways, including direct destructive autoimmune thyroiditis, reduction in vascular endothelial growth factor (VEGF)–related thyroid vasculature, and reduction of thyroid iodine uptake.

Treatment of drug-related hypothyroidism usually consists of removal of the offending agent if possible, as well as thyroid hormone supplementation/replacement as necessary.

BOX 37.1 Medications that may cause iatrogenic hypothyroidism.

Inhibition of Thyroid Hormone Synthesis or Secretion
Aminoglutethimide
Lithium
Perchlorate
Thalidomide
Thionamides (methimazole, propylthiouracil)
Iodine-containing medications
- Amiodarone
- Iodinated IV contrast
- Guaifenesin
- Kelp
- Potassium iodide
- Topical antiseptics

Immune Dysregulation
Interferon alfa
Interleukin-2
Alemtuzumab
Ipilimumab
Nivolumab
Pembrolizumab

TSH Suppression
Dopamine

Destructive Thyroiditis
Sunitinib

Increased Type 3 Deiodinase Activity
Sorafenib

Increased T_4 Clearance and TSH Suppression
Bexarotene

IV, Intravenous; *T_4*, tetraiodothyronine or thyroxine; *TSH*, thyroid-stimulating hormone.

HYPERTHYROIDISM

Hyperthyroidism is defined as a clinical state of elevated thyroid hormone action in tissues, usually due to inappropriately high constitutive secretion of thyroid hormone from the thyroid. The degree of severity of hyperthyroidism is typically divided into two groups: overt (suppressed TSH levels with concomitant elevations in free T_4 or T_3) and subclinical (suppressed TSH with normal free T_4 and T_3). Both overt and subclinical hyperthyroidism can lead to clinically significant symptoms or signs, although subclinical disease is more likely to be milder in presentation.

The clinical symptoms and signs of hyperthyroidism are broad, reflecting the fact that thyroid hormone exerts an effect on nearly every organ system. Overt hyperthyroidism can cause a litany of effects, including tremor, heat intolerance, tachycardia and atrial fibrillation, increased gastrointestinal motility, muscle weakness, anxiety, and embolic events. Uncontrolled hyperthyroidism can rarely cause severe cardiovascular complications, including cardiomyopathy and congestive heart failure that can even progress to cardiovascular collapse and death. Subclinical hyperthyroidism typically has milder manifestations along this same disease symptomatology.

The prevalence of hyperthyroidism in the United States is approximately 1.2%. The most common causes of hyperthyroidism—Graves disease, TMG, and solitary toxic adenoma—are all those in which thyroidectomy plays an important, if not primary, role in management. These three disease states are discussed in further detail below. Other causes of hyperthyroidism are listed in Box 37.2, and amiodarone-induced thyrotoxicosis (AIT) is also discussed below.

Graves Disease

Graves disease, named after Dr. Robert J. Graves from the 1830s, is an autoimmune disease characterized by the constitutive activation of the TSH receptor by TRAb, which results in increased synthesis and secretion of thyroid hormone. Graves disease is the most common cause of hyperthyroidism in the United States, with an estimated incidence of 30 cases per 100,000 persons per year. The disease has a female predominance, with an 8:1 female-to-male

BOX 37.2 Causes of hyperthyroidism.

Associated With Normal/Elevated RAI Uptake
Graves disease
Toxic multinodular goiter
Toxic adenoma
Trophoblastic disease
TSH-producing pituitary adenoma
Thyroid hormone resistance

Associated With No/Minimal RAI Uptake
Painless thyroiditis
Amiodarone-induced thyroiditis
Subacute thyroiditis
Iatrogenic thyrotoxicosis
Struma ovarii
Acute thyroiditis
Follicular thyroid cancer metastases
Palpation thyroiditis

RAI, Radioactive iodine; *TSH*, thyroid-stimulating hormone.

ratio, and typically presents during younger adult life, with a typical patient age range of between 20 and 40 years.

Because of its autoimmune etiology, Graves disease can have other manifestations in addition to the classic symptoms and signs of hyperthyroidism. The most common is Graves orbitopathy, which occurs in up to 25% to 30% of patients. In this process, autoimmune reactions at the orbital and periorbital soft tissues lead to proptosis, eyelid retraction, chemosis, periorbital edema, and diminished ocular muscle motility (Fig. 37.12); if left untreated, the orbitopathy can lead to vision loss from corneal lesions or optic nerve compression. Skin manifestations also can occur, including pretibial myxedema and acropachy (edema at the digits). Other autoimmune conditions that have been associated with Graves disease include Hashimoto thyroiditis, lupus, rheumatoid arthritis, pernicious anemia, and Addison disease, among others.

The biochemical workup for Graves disease typically includes thyroid function tests, including TSH, free T_4 and T_3, as well as measurement for TRAb (typically with TSI but also with TSH receptor-binding inhibitory immunoglobulin in selected scenarios). The presence of TRAb is diagnostic for Graves disease. Imaging may consist of neck ultrasound and/or nuclear medicine thyroid uptake scan, depending on the indications. Sonographic features may include a diffusely hypervascular gland, often with heterogeneous echogenicity; thyroid nodular disease may also be identified. Nuclear scintigraphy using either ^{99m}technetium pertechnetate or ^{123}I may help differentiate TSI-negative Graves disease from toxic nodular disease based on diffuse versus nodular uptake pattern. Cross-sectional imaging of the head may be useful for the evaluation of orbitopathy.

The three management options for Graves hyperthyroidism include antithyroid medications, RAI ablation, and thyroidectomy. In the United States, RAI is the most common employed treatment option, although antithyroid medication is being used more frequently as a first option; nearly one-third of patients may be able to achieve long-term remission with medication alone. In truth, each of the three treatment options comes with its own unique set of advantages and disadvantages, as well as indications and contraindications, which must be tailored according to individual patient values and preferences. The 2016 American Thyroid Association (ATA) guidelines on the management of hyperthyroidism provide a helpful evidence-based summary of the clinical scenarios that would most favor a particular option for treatment (Table 37.1).[4]

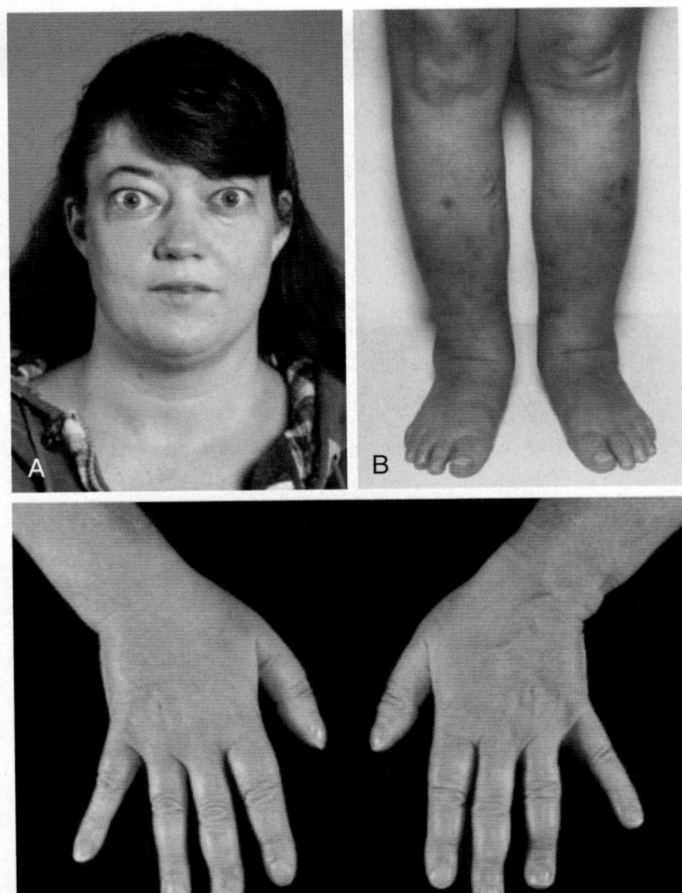

FIG. 37.12 Extrathyroidal manifestations of Graves disease. (A) Orbitopathy. (B) Dermopathy (pretibial myxedema). (C) Acropachy. (From Al-Shoumer KAS, Gharib H. Hyperthyroidism: toxic nodular goiter and Graves' disease. In: Randolph GW, ed. *Surgery of the Thyroid and Parathyroid Glands 2*. Philadelphia: Elsevier Saunders; 2013:53.)

In general, thyroidectomy is the preferred modality in the following situations: presence of severe eye disease, failure or contraindications to other treatment options, need or desire for rapid reversal of hyperthyroidism, presence of concomitant suspicious thyroid nodules, large goiters with locally compressive symptoms, and pregnancy or postpartum/breastfeeding states. Although thyroidectomy is a first-line treatment option, in practice, it is often relegated to a secondary role due to perceived risks associated with general anesthesia and surgery.

For patients choosing surgical management, the recommended extent of surgery is a total or near-total thyroidectomy, which is associated with a nearly 0% risk of recurrent hyperthyroidism. In contrast, subtotal thyroidectomy is associated with a 5% to 10% risk of recurrence from the presence of residual thyroid tissue. Although the risk of thyroidectomy-specific complications (including permanent hypoparathyroidism, RLN injury, and neck hematoma) is higher in Graves disease than for other indications, the absolute risks remain low particularly in the hands of higher-volume surgeons and are no different between total/near-total and

TABLE 37.1 Clinical situations that favor a particular modality as treatment for Graves hyperthyroidism.

CLINICAL SITUATIONS	RADIOACTIVE IODINE	ANTITHYROID DRUG	SURGERY
Pregnancy	×	√√/!	√/!
Comorbidities with increased surgical risk and/or limited life expectancy	√√	√	×
Inactive Graves ophthalmopathy	√	√	√
Active Graves ophthalmopathy	!	√√	√√
Liver disease	√√	!	√
Major adverse reactions to antithyroid drugs	√√	×	√
Patients with previously operated or externally irradiated necks	√√	√	!
Lack of access to a high-volume thyroid surgeon	√√	√	!
Patients with high likelihood of remission (especially women, with mild disease, small goiters, and negative or low-titer TRAb)	√	√√	√
Patients with periodic paralysis	√√	√	√√
Patients with right pulmonary hypertension or congestive heart failure	√√	√	!
Elderly with comorbidities	√	√	!
Thyroid malignancy confirmed or suspected	×	-	√√
One or more large thyroid nodules	-	√	√√
Coexisting primary hyperparathyroidism requiring surgery	-	-	√√

From Ross DS, Burch HB, Cooper DS, et al. 2016 American Thyroid Association guidelines for diagnosis and management of hyperthyroidism and other causes of thyrotoxicosis. *Thyroid*. 2016;26:1343–1421.
√√ = Preferred therapy; √ = acceptable therapy; ! = cautious use; - = not first-line therapy but may be acceptable depending on the clinical circumstances; × = contraindication.

subtotal thyroidectomy groups. The rate of permanent RLN injury is 0% to 2%, permanent hypoparathyroidism is 0.6% to 6%, and neck hematoma is 0.3% to 0.7% for total thyroidectomy performed in the setting of Graves disease. The risk of complications from remedial thyroidectomy is up to ten-fold higher than initial thyroidectomy, which further underscores why subtotal thyroidectomy with its risk of recurrent disease is no longer favored.

Preoperatively, patients should ideally be rendered euthyroid prior to thyroidectomy with antithyroid medications; typically, today, this is methimazole since PTU was found to be associated with liver failure resulting in the need for transplantation. Beta blockers may be added for patients who remain hyperthyroid and/or tachycardic. High-concentration potassium iodide solutions including Lugol solution for super saturate potassium iodide (SSKI) can be given for 7 to 10 days prior to surgery; they are thought to be beneficial for decreasing thyroid blood flow and vascularity of the gland as well as rapidly achieving a euthyroid state via the Wolff-Chaikoff effect, although their use may not be needed in selected situations. All other associated medical and surgical comorbidities should be optimized. Lastly, preoperative optimization of calcium and vitamin D status, including preoperative supplementation with calcitriol, has been shown to decrease the postoperative risk of transient hypocalcemia.

Thyroid storm is a rare state of life-threatening physiologic decompensation in patients with severe, uncontrolled hyperthyroidism, which often occurs after an inciting stressor event (including thyroidectomy). The symptoms can be dramatic and severe, including fever; cardiac effects, including hypertension, tachycardia, arrhythmia, and congestive heart failure; mental status changes, including agitation, stupor, and coma; and hepatic failure. Treatment is multimodal and consists of beta blockade, antithyroid medications, potassium iodide, corticosteroids, mechanical cooling therapies, and intensive supportive care.

Toxic Multinodular Goiter

TMG is an enlarged nodular thyroid containing one or more autonomously functioning nodules leading to a state of hyperthyroidism. This condition is also known as Plummer disease, so named after Henry Plummer of the Mayo Clinic in 1913. TMG is the second most common cause of hyperthyroidism in the United States after Graves disease. Among the elderly as well as those who live in iodine-deficient regions, TMG is the most common cause of hyperthyroidism. TMG has a female predominance, with an approximately 5:1 female-to-male ratio, and typically affects adults above the age of 50 years.

Autonomously functioning nodules in TMG often result from mutations in the TSH receptor gene leading to constitutive synthesis and secretion of thyroid hormones. These "warm" or "hot" nodules are rarely malignant and typically do not require biopsy. However, these nodules can coexist with other nonfunctioning nodules in the same gland, which should be evaluated independently (see "Thyroid Nodule" section below).

The workup of TMG consists of both biochemical and radiographic testing. As with Graves disease, thyroid function tests are mandatory in order to diagnose hyperthyroidism. In addition, a survey of thyroid antibodies (including TRAb) is necessary to identify coexisting autoimmune thyroiditis and rule out Graves disease. Nuclear scintigraphy is a first-line imaging study and, in the case of TMG, can identify the location and distribution of autonomously functioning nodules and/or regions. In addition, ultrasound is highly recommended as a correlative study to assess overall thyroid size and characterize any nonfunctioning nodules that may require biopsy.

The three management options for TMG—antithyroid medication, RAI, and thyroidectomy—are the same as those for Graves disease, but with some differences. First, antithyroid medication is generally not advocated as a long-term management strategy except for patients in whom the other two options are absolutely contraindicated, such as in some elderly or otherwise ill or frail patients with limited life expectancy. Because this disease state is not autoimmune in nature, autonomous nodules do not undergo remission with medical therapy. Second, RAI with ^{131}I is the most common definitive treatment for TMG in the United States;

however, the dose of radiation is typically higher (and by extension the risk of treatment failure and need for retreatment) than in Graves disease because of lower uptake of iodine in TMG. Third, both RAI and surgery should be preceded by optimal preoperative treatment of the hyperthyroid state, which typically includes methimazole with or without beta blockade; however, SSKI and Lugol solutions are not indicated for TMG as they are for Graves disease, since the high iodine concentration may not achieve a temporary euthyroid state from the Wolff-Chaikoff effect. They induce hyperthyroidism from the Jod-Basedow phenomenon.

Near-total or total thyroidectomy is the generally recommended surgical treatment of TMG. As in the case of Graves disease, complete extirpation can be performed with a similar low rate of complications as subtotal thyroidectomy while at the same time virtually eliminating the risk of disease recurrence.

Solitary Toxic Adenoma

A toxic adenoma is a single autonomously functioning nodule existing within an otherwise normal or nontoxic nodular thyroid gland. The main theory around its pathogenesis focuses on constitutively activating mutations in the TSH receptor gene, although the prevalence of these mutations is not universal and varies widely by geography. Toxic adenoma affects women at a median age of 50 to 60 years, with a mild female predominance. Toxic adenoma shares many if not most of the diagnostic approach and workup with TMG; in fact, the ATA guidelines on the management of hyperthyroidism combine the two groups together in their treatment recommendations.

The treatment philosophy for toxic adenoma generally follows the same principles as those for TMG—namely, that antithyroid medications are not effective for long-term remission and that either RAI or thyroidectomy is the preferred method for definitive treatment. Thyroidectomy is typically limited to unilateral lobectomy addressing the side of the toxic adenoma; this strategy is associated with a near-universal cure for the hyperthyroidism. Near-total or total thyroidectomy is indicated only in the presence of other factors, such as bilateral nodules with suspicion for cancer or a large and/or symptomatic goiter.

More recently, percutaneous ultrasound-guided ablative techniques have been described as an alternative treatment option for toxic adenoma and some TMG. These techniques involve either the injection of ethanol or application of radiofrequency or other destructive energy sources into a nodule of interest. The majority of the published experiences are in Europe and Asia, with limited adoption currently in the United States. These ablative techniques have the theoretical benefit of targeting only the target lesion and reducing the risk of hypothyroidism inherent with RAI or surgery; however, in practice, drawbacks have been reported, including patient pain and unusual complications such as transient thyrotoxicosis and necrosis of neighboring structures. Currently, these techniques require further study, as the lack of high-volume robust evidence precludes their widespread recommendation outside of experienced centers.

Amiodarone-Induced Thyrotoxicosis

Amiodarone is an antiarrhythmic medication used frequently for atrial or ventricular tachyarrythmias. Molecularly, amiodarone is an iodine-rich compound with structural similarities to T_4 that contains 37% iodine content by molecular weight; a normal dosing schedule can deliver over 100 times the daily dietary iodine requirement. AIT occurs in up to 6% of patients taking this medication.

There are two distinct mechanisms proposed in the development of AIT. Type 1 AIT is caused by the Jod-Basedow phenomenon, in which the high iodine load potentiates excess thyroid hormone synthesis and release. Type 1 AIT is more common in patients with preexisting hyperthyroid disease. Type 2 AIT usually occurs in patients with preexisting normal thyroids and is caused by a destructive thyroiditis from direct drug toxicity on follicular cells leading to release of preformed thyroid hormone. Mixed forms of AIT also can occur.

Medical treatment of AIT typically consists of methimazole, with corticosteroids added to address the thyroiditis in type 2 AIT. The decision to halt amiodarone treatment must be determined carefully on an individual basis in consultation with the treating cardiologist in order to ensure continuity of adequate antiarrhythmic therapy in these often high-risk patients. Total thyroidectomy is recommended for patients who are unresponsive to aggressive medical therapy. Although thyroidectomy is associated with more risks for AIT compared to most other indications (with perioperative mortality of 9%–10%), delay in surgery carries an even higher risk of mortality.

NONTOXIC GOITER

A nontoxic goiter is defined as any benign, noninflammatory enlargement of the thyroid gland that is not associated with hyperthyroidism. The causes of nontoxic goiter can be broadly divided into diffuse and nodular enlargement, which roughly lead to the respective entities of endemic/diffuse and sporadic multinodular goiter, each with their own pathogenesis, risk factors, and management strategies.

Endemic (Diffuse) Goiter

Strictly defined, endemic goiter occurs in more than10% of a given population; however, the only known cause of endemic goiter is dietary iodine deficiency, which predisposes people predominantly to diffuse goiter from persistent TSH stimulation, leading to diffuse follicular epithelial hyperplasia. In effect, the terms "endemic goiter" and "diffuse goiter" have functionally become synonymous.

It is estimated that more than 2 billion people worldwide are exposed to iodine-deficient diets. In iodine-deficient populations, a palpable goiter can be detected in up to 40% to 90% of individuals, and hypothyroidism can be found in up to 50%. The risk of goiter and hypothyroidism increases proportionally to the severity of iodine deficiency. There is a female predominance in the prevalence of endemic goiter (approximately 2–3 times higher than in men), and its incidence increases by age group due to its environmental etiology.

The morbidity and mortality from endemic goiter are due to its association with chronic untreated hypothyroidism and cretinism as much as—if not more than—the local effects on the neck due to its size. Instituting proper iodine supplementation in iodine-deficient populations has been shown to be an effective strategy for decreasing the incidence of these diseases.

Nontoxic Multinodular Goiter

Sporadic multinodular goiter is the most common cause of nontoxic goiter in the United States and other developed nations with iodine-rich diets, with an incidence of approximately 5%. Although there is a known stepwise pathophysiologic process in which iodine deficiency can first cause diffuse follicular hyperplasia and subsequently stimulate nodule formation, the causes of the majority of sporadic multinodular goiter remain unknown.

The incidence of multinodular goiter increases with age, probably paralleling the age-related incidence of thyroid nodules in general.

Substernal Goiter

Substernal (or retrosternal) goiter is defined broadly as a goiter with a significant proportion of the gland extending inferiorly through the thoracic inlet and into the mediastinum. The incidence of substernal goiter is estimated at 0.02% in the general population, with 60% occurring among patients who are over the age of 60 years. There are a number of subtypes of substernal goiter. The most common subtype extends into the anterior mediastinum. The second subtype extends posteriorly to the great vessels, trachea, and/or RLN, sometimes crossing over to the contralateral neck. The third and least common subtype is the isolated mediastinal goiter with no connection to the normal cervical orthotopic gland and with unique blood supply from the chest.

Substernal goiters are more likely than cervical goiters to be associated with local compressive symptoms including shortness of breath/orthopnea and dysphagia. This is because the mediastinal extension of the goiter pushes against and compresses the normal thoracic inlet structures (trachea, esophagus, vascular structures) within a fixed bony space bound by the ribs and vertebrae. Tracheal compression is of particular concern, as minor degrees of goiter enlargement and resultant narrowing of tracheal diameter can lead to dramatic reductions in ventilatory flow (Poiseuille law) in a relatively short period of time. In contrast, primarily cervical goiters are often capable of dramatic growth without causing significant compressive symptoms due to the expandability of the surrounding cervical soft tissues. Interestingly, vocal cord paralysis from RLN compression is extremely rare, and the presence of vocal cord dysfunction should raise the concern for malignancy harbored within the goiter.

Workup

The workup of nontoxic goiter consists of thyroid function testing to rule out hyperthyroidism and imaging studies to assess for goiter extent and presence of nodules. The mainstay for thyroid imaging is neck ultrasound, which offers the highest resolution description of thyroid size/volume, presence or absence of significant thyroiditis, and characterization of thyroid nodules. As stated in the ATA guidelines, every nodule at least 1 cm should be evaluated for suspicious sonographic features on an individual basis, and FNA should be performed preferentially based on suspicion for malignancy.

Cross-sectional imaging with either CT or MRI is essential for the assessment of and preoperative planning for substernal goiter and is indicated for any patient with significant compressive symptoms and/or sonographic evidence of inferior extension past the clavicle (Figs. 37.10A and 37.13). Cross-sectional imaging is useful because it provides information about the degree of tracheoesophageal deviation/compression, laterality of dominant substernal lobe, inferior-most extent, anterior versus posterior pattern of extension, presence of cross-over to the contralateral chest, and presence of a separate intrathoracic "rest." Unless there is concern for malignancy, the need for contrast enhancement is typically unnecessary.

Management

The management options for nontoxic goiter generally consist of nonoperative surveillance, TSH suppression with thyroid hormone supplementation, RAI ablation, and thyroidectomy. Small nontoxic goiters generally can be followed expectantly with periodic thyroid function testing and neck imaging. TSH-suppressive therapy with LT_4 is often employed by endocrinologists as a first-line treatment option, particularly for smaller goiters. The results of several large-scale trials are somewhat mixed but do appear to show goiter size reductions in about 30% of patients; however, these results must be balanced against the drawbacks of therapy, including the need for lifelong suppression and the long-term effects of subclinical hyperthyroidism on the heart and bone. RAI ablation can reduce goiter size by up to 50% over a 1-year period, and it is an increasingly popular treatment option in many developing countries where access to thyroidectomy is limited. However, the effect of RAI is gradual; acute transient thyroiditis can occur, which may exacerbate local symptoms, and it is ineffective for larger goiters.

The absolute indications for thyroidectomy in nontoxic goiter include local compressive symptoms, substernal extension (which often present with compressive symptoms), presence of nodules suspicious or diagnostic for malignancy in which prolonged ultrasound surveillance would be hampered, and patient preference (assuming that the patient is otherwise an acceptable surgical candidate). The extent of thyroidectomy, specifically unilateral lobectomy versus total thyroidectomy, can be tailored to the individual patient and goiter scenario. Total or near-total thyroidectomy is typically the procedure of choice; subtotal thyroidectomy is associated with an unacceptably high rate of recurrence in the long-term (>50% in some studies). However, unilateral lobectomy may suffice in certain scenarios, such as a single-side dominant goiter with a relatively normal contralateral lobe and in patients predicted to have poor adherence to daily thyroid hormone replacement.

Thyroidectomy for substernal goiter presents a unique challenge depending on the amount and pattern of intrathoracic extension, specifically in relation to the probability of requiring partial or complete sternotomy. Most substernal goiters can be resected via standard cervical thyroidectomy incision because the majority of substernal goiters are anterior and extend inferiorly to a point no lower than the superior aspect of the aortic arch on cross-sectional imaging. These goiters can readily be retrieved via cervicotomy with proper neck extension and patient positioning. On the other hand, goiters extending further inferiorly than the aortic arch, extending posteriorly, and/or crossing the midline from the dominant side are significantly more difficult and likely require sternal split and partial or even total median sternotomy. Thoracic surgery assistance is useful, especially for the more difficult substernal goiters requiring sternotomy or other mediastinal access.

THYROID NODULE

A thyroid nodule is a commonly identified discrete lesion within the thyroid gland. Up to 5% of women and 1% of men in iodine-replete areas have palpable thyroid nodules, and with the advent of ever-improving high-resolution ultrasound, the frequency of thyroid nodules has been estimated to be as high as 19% to 68% due to imaging's ability to pick up nonpalpable, incidentally discovered thyroid nodules, or "incidentalomas." Although thyroid nodules are quite common, the majority do not require extensive (or any) workup, and the vast majority do not require surgical intervention. The primary reasons for surgical intervention for thyroid nodules include 1) concern for malignancy, 2) hyperfunction, and 3) local compressive symptoms.

The management of thyroid nodules (and thyroid cancer) is the subject of much active research and controversy. Multiple

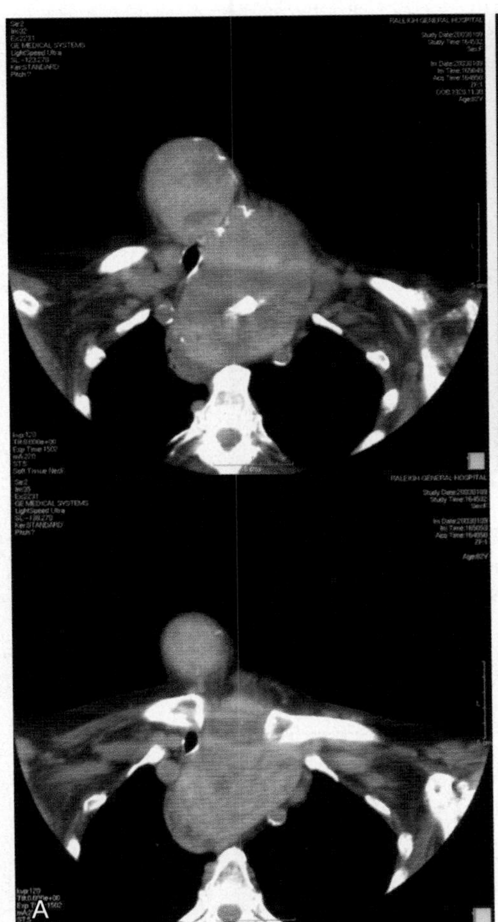

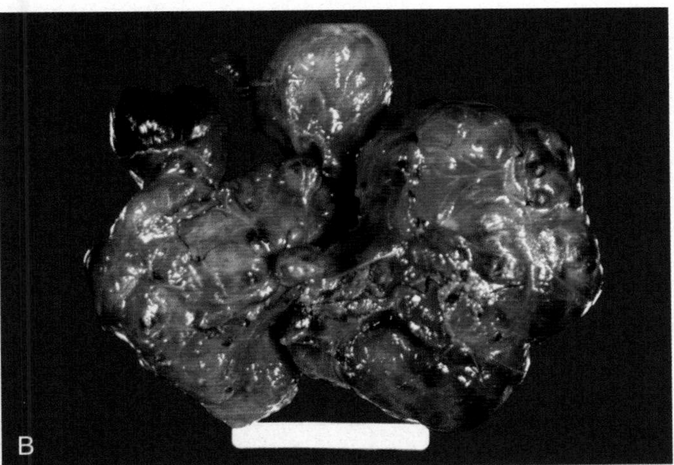

FIG. 37.13 (A) Computed tomography scan at the level of the thoracic inlet demonstrating a heterogeneous, large thyroid mass that involves both lobes of the thyroid and displaces the trachea. It has extended into the anterior mediastinum. This patient ultimately proved to have a large multinodular goiter. (B) Gross picture of the resected multinodular goiter.

organizations have published clinical practice guidelines over the past 25 years. The ATAs guidelines were first published in 1996 and updated over the years, most recently in 2006, 2009, and 2015, and arguably remain the most comprehensive, current, and cited among thyroidologists.[5] Much of this section will reflect the evidence and recommendations contained in the most recent iteration of the ATA guidelines.

Clinical Presentation and Workup

The majority of thyroid nodules are benign and asymptomatic, and as mentioned above, many are now diagnosed as "incidentalomas." Several clinical findings on history or physical exam raise the suspicion for thyroid cancer. These include patient age younger than 20 years or older than 70 years, male sex, local compressive or infiltrative symptoms such as hoarseness or dysphagia, firm and/or immobile nodule, nodules larger than 3 to 4 cm, cervical lymphadenopathy, history of neck irradiation, and history of thyroid cancer in first-degree family members. In addition, although less common, the suspicion for a hyperfunctioning nodule or toxic adenoma is raised when there are symptoms or signs of thyrotoxicosis, including palpitations, atrial fibrillation, anxiety, insomnia, weight loss, heat intolerance, diaphoresis, and increased defecation.

The workup of thyroid nodules typically includes assessment of thyroid function with serum TSH as a screening test, as well as neck ultrasound (Fig. 37.14). The finding of a suppressed TSH level also may trigger further workup of hyperthyroidism as detailed above, including thyroid antibody workup and thyroid nuclear medicine scintigraphy. Further workup for malignancy always includes FNA biopsy (see below) and, depending on the concern for locally advanced or metastatic behavior, may include cross sectional imaging.

The majority of thyroid nodules are benign neoplasms and include colloid nodules, degenerative cysts, nodular hyperplasia, and follicular or Hürthle cell adenomas. The most common malignant diagnosis is PTC and in decreasing order of frequency also includes follicular thyroid cancer (FTC), Hürthle cell cancer (HCC), MTC, poorly differentiated thyroid cancer (PDTC), and ATC; other rare malignancies including primary thyroid lymphoma and metastasis to the thyroid gland can occur (see the "Thyroid Cancer" section below for more details).

Ultrasound Evaluation of Thyroid Nodules

Neck ultrasound is the most important radiographic study for the evaluation of thyroid nodules. Ultrasound offers the

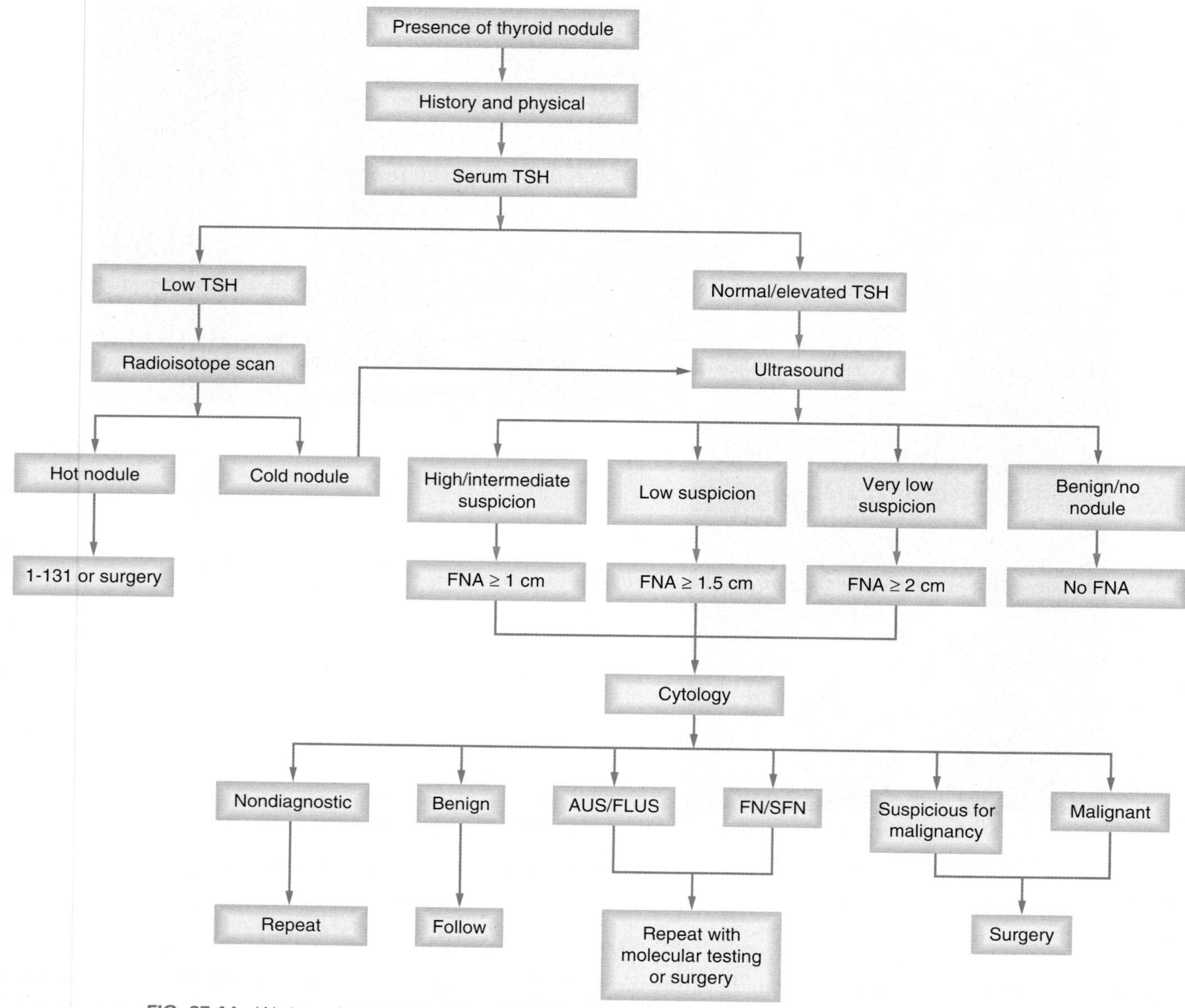

FIG. 37.14 Workup of a thyroid nodule. *AUS*, Atypia of undetermined significance; *FLUS*, follicular lesion of undetermined significance; *FN*, follicular neoplasm; *FNA*, fine-needle aspiration biopsy; *SFN*, suspicious for follicular neoplasm; *TSH*, thyroid-stimulating hormone.

highest-resolution image of the thyroid gland by well characterizing parenchymal and nodular abnormalities; it also provides the most sensitive radiographic assessment of cervical lymphadenopathy. Ultrasound is also an essential adjunct for the performance of image-guided FNA biopsy of suspicious nodules and lymph nodes (see below). Other advantages of ultrasound include its portability, absence of the need for ionizing radiation, and overall cost-effectiveness in the initial evaluation and longer-term management of thyroid nodules. Lastly, neck ultrasound has been shown in selected patients to be a useful tool for noninvasive assessment of vocal cord function, which is important for informing surgical management.

For patients with hyperthyroidism and thyroid nodules, both nuclear medicine thyroid scintigraphy and ultrasound are recommended, in order to determine concordance in the presence of a possible toxic nodule, as well as to assess for other "cold" or nonfunctioning nodules.

As neck ultrasound has become more accessible to clinicians and viewed as an extension of the physical exam, it has become more widely used by surgeons and endocrinologists in addition to radiologists. However, because the operator dependence of this modality greatly affects the quality of ultrasound exam, efforts have been made on the national level to provide standardized educational and certification pathways for ultrasound expertise. For surgeons, the American College of Surgeons offers a two-step advanced neck ultrasound training program.

The need for proper education and standardization is especially apparent considering the number and degree of findings that one must assess for and document in every ultrasound. These findings include, at minimum, the following: 1) parenchymal pattern and overall thyroid gland size; 2) presence, size, location, and characteristics of any nodules; and 3) presence/absence, size, location, and characteristics of any suspicious cervical lymph nodes. Survey of the cervical lymph nodes is particularly specialized and

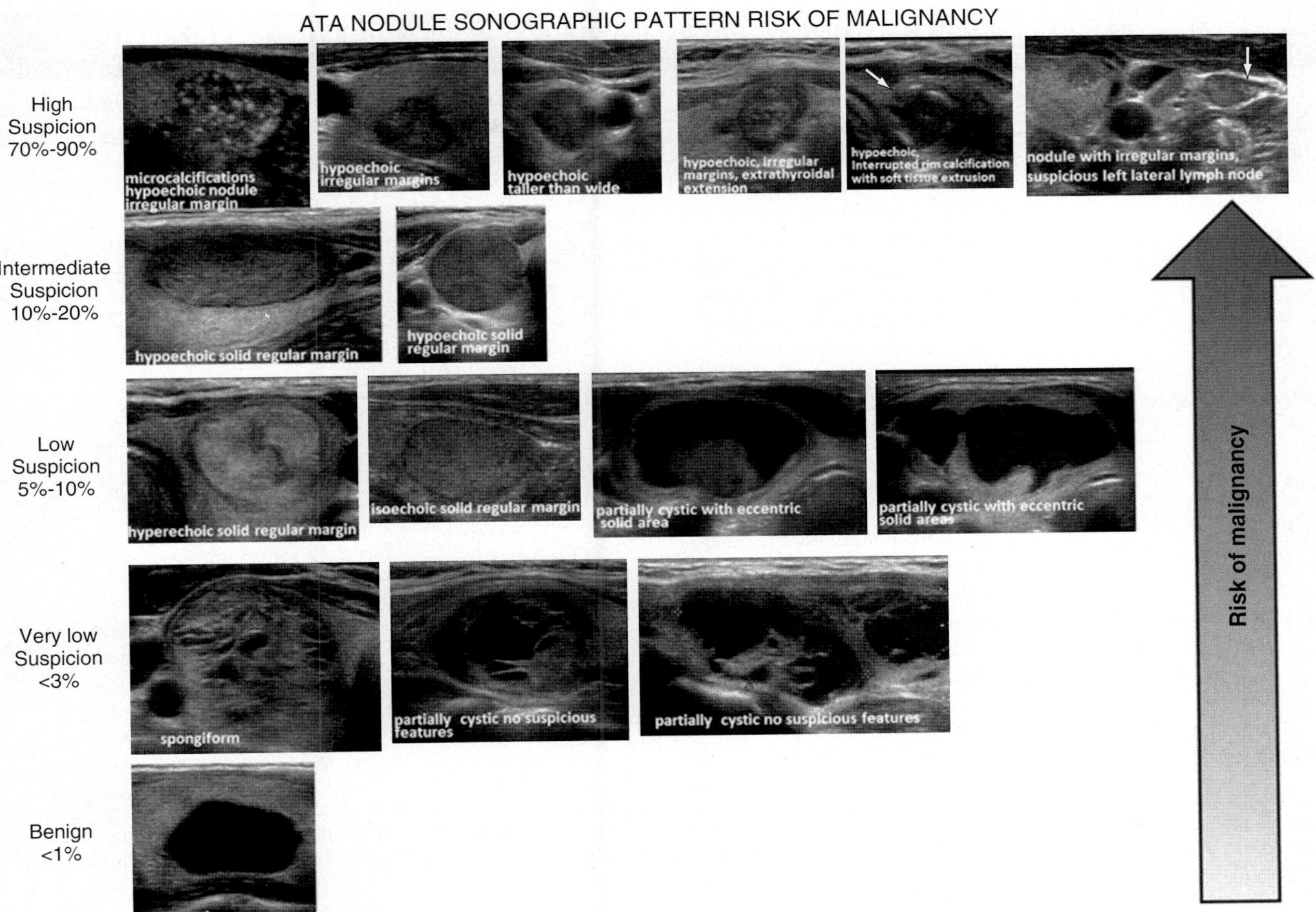

FIG. 37.15 American Thyroid Association *(ATA)* nodule sonographic patterns and risk of malignancy. (From Haugen BR, Alexander EK, Bible KC, et al. 2015 American Thyroid Association management guidelines for patients with thyroid nodules and differentiated thyroid cancer. *Thyroid.* 2016;26:1–133.)

important in the evaluation of thyroid nodules. Fig. 37.3 shows the levels of the nodal stations in the neck, with the accepted numerical nomenclature initially created for neck dissection for head and neck cancers. Thorough examination must be performed particularly of the pretracheal and paratracheal nodes of the central neck and mediastinum (levels VI and VII, respectively), as well as the lateral jugular chain nodes (levels IIa/IIb, III, IV, and Vb).

Sonographic Risk Stratification of Thyroid Nodules

The sonographic characteristics in thyroid nodules that appear to confer the highest risk of malignancy—specifically PTC—include 1) the presence of microcalcifications, 2) hypoechogenicity, 3) irregular margins, and 4) a taller-than-wide nodule shape. Size is also thought to be a predictor and is clinically relevant, although whether size is an independent predictor is controversial. Intranodular vascularity has historically been thought to also be predictive of malignancy but is likely more correlated with FTC than PTC. Although each individual ultrasound characteristic is relatively unreliable in isolation for predicting malignancy, the combination provides improved specificity. On the opposite end of the spectrum, features such as spongiform pattern or a purely cystic appearance dramatically decrease the risk of malignancy.

Because the sonographic interpretation for malignancy is based on synthesizing a constellation of features, large-scale efforts have been made to create graduated risk stratification systems, with higher sonographic risk nodules recommended to undergo FNA biopsy at a smaller size threshold. In the 2015 guidelines, the ATA proposed a five-grade sonographic classification system, which is graphically summarized in Fig. 37.15. Only those nodules in the higher-risk categories—called high, intermediate, and low suspicion—have associated definitive recommendations regarding FNA biopsy, whereas the two lower-risk categories—called very low suspicion and benign—can usually be safely observed. Table 37.2 summarizes the sonographic categories, their estimated risks of malignancy, and size-based recommendations for biopsy.

Despite the prominence of the ATA's guidelines for clinical practice, other organizations and societies also have proposed sonographic risk stratification systems for thyroid nodules. Probably the most commonly used alternative is the Thyroid Imaging, Reporting and Data System (TI-RADS), which was originally described in 2005 but formalized by the American College of Radiology in 2015. TI-RADS stratifies nodule characteristics into five risk levels, from TR1 (benign) to TR5 (highly suspicious); however, the categorization method differs in that it converts feature patterns into a discrete number of points along five feature dimensions—nodule composition, echogenicity, shape, margin, and echogenic foci—and the total accumulated points determines the ultimate TI-RADS level.[6] The TI-RADS level, in turn, determines

TABLE 37.2 Sonographic patterns, estimated risk of malignancy, and fine-needle aspiration guidance for thyroid nodules.

SONOGRAPHIC PATTERN	SONOGRAPHIC FEATURES	ESTIMATED RISK OF MALIGNANCY	FNA SIZE CUTOFF (LARGEST DIMENSION)
High suspicion	Solid hypoechoic nodule or solid hypoechoic component of a partially cystic nodule *with* one or more of the following features: irregular margins (infiltrative, microlobulated), microcalcifications, taller than wide shape, rim calcifications with small extrusive soft tissue component, evidence of ETE	>70%–90%	Recommend FNA at ≥1 cm
Intermediate suspicion	Hypoechoic solid nodule with smooth margins *without* microcalcifications, ETE, or taller than wide shape	10%–20%	Recommend FNA at ≥1 cm
Low suspicion	Isoechoic or hyperechoic solid nodule or partially cystic nodule with eccentric solid areas *without* microcalcification, irregular margin or ETE, or taller than wide shape	5%–10%	Recommend FNA at ≥1.5 cm
Very low suspicion	Spongiform or partially cystic nodules *without* any of the sonographic features described in low, intermediate, or high suspicion patterns	<3%	Consider FNA at ≥2 cm; observation without FNA also reasonable
Benign	Purely cystic nodules (no solid component)	<1%	No biopsy; aspiration reasonable for symptomatic or cosmetic drainage

From Haugen BR, Alexander EK, Bible KC, et al. 2015 American Thyroid Association Management guidelines for adult patients with thyroid nodules and differentiated thyroid cancer: the American Thyroid Association Guidelines Task Force on Thyroid Nodules and Differentiated Thyroid Cancer. *Thyroid*. 2016;26:1–133.
ETE, Extrathyroidal extension; *FNA*, fine-needle aspiration.

size-based recommendations for biopsy or surveillance; the size thresholds also vary somewhat from those of the ATA. Fig. 37.16 shows a summary schematic of the TI-RADS system. Comparative studies to date would suggest that the ATA and TI-RADS systems perform with high sensitivity and negative predictive value (NPV) and represent a significant improvement in standardization and completeness in ultrasound reporting.[7]

Neither system recommends routine FNA biopsy of nodules less than 1 cm. This strategy accepts the tradeoff of not diagnosing all thyroid cancers smaller than 1 cm against the current reality of many countries (including the United States) experiencing dramatic increases in overdiagnosis of clinically insignificant papillary thyroid microcarcinomas (see below). However, other factors such as the location of the nodule in the thyroid, presence of lymphadenopathy, genetic or environmental risk factors, patient age, and patient preference may take precedence in influencing whether a subcentimeter thyroid nodule is biopsied.

Ultrasound elastography is a technique that measures the stiffness of a thyroid nodule and that was originally developed with the promise of incrementally improving ultrasound's noninvasive risk assessment of malignancy. Initial results were promising, although follow-up results have been mixed on validation studies.[8] Elastography is a highly specialized technique with unique equipment, and it is most effective for only a small subset of nodules. Currently, elastography is not recommended for routine use in the evaluation of thyroid nodules, but it may be useful for selected cases in specialized centers.

FNA Cytology

FNA biopsy is the most accurate and cost-effective invasive procedure in the workup of thyroid nodules. For all thyroid nodules, FNA has a mean sensitivity of over 80% and a mean specificity of over 90%. Although FNA can technically be performed without ultrasound guidance for palpable nodules, the accuracy overall with ultrasound assistance is superior. FNA is performed with a small-gauge needle (typically 23–27 gauge), and it may be performed with capillary or suction techniques. Ideally, the adequacy of the specimen can be confirmed at the time of the procedure with on-site cytopathologic evaluation. The excellent discriminatory ability and extremely low complication rate of FNA have rendered biopsy methods with larger bore needles such as core needle biopsy obsolete.

The indications for FNA biopsy are described in greater detail above and are largely dependent upon the risk profile of the thyroid nodule on ultrasound. For example, FNA would be recommended for higher-risk pattern nodules classified as ATA high-suspicion or TI-RADS TR5; in other words, solid hypoechoic nodules with microcalcifications that are at least 1 cm should be considered for biopsy while very low-risk nodules that are spongiform have higher size cutoffs for biopsy or can be observed. Risk factors other than sonographic profile can reduce the threshold for performing FNA biopsy, including positive family history of thyroid cancer, history of significant radiation exposure, and PET-positivity. FNA should only be performed if the results would influence patient

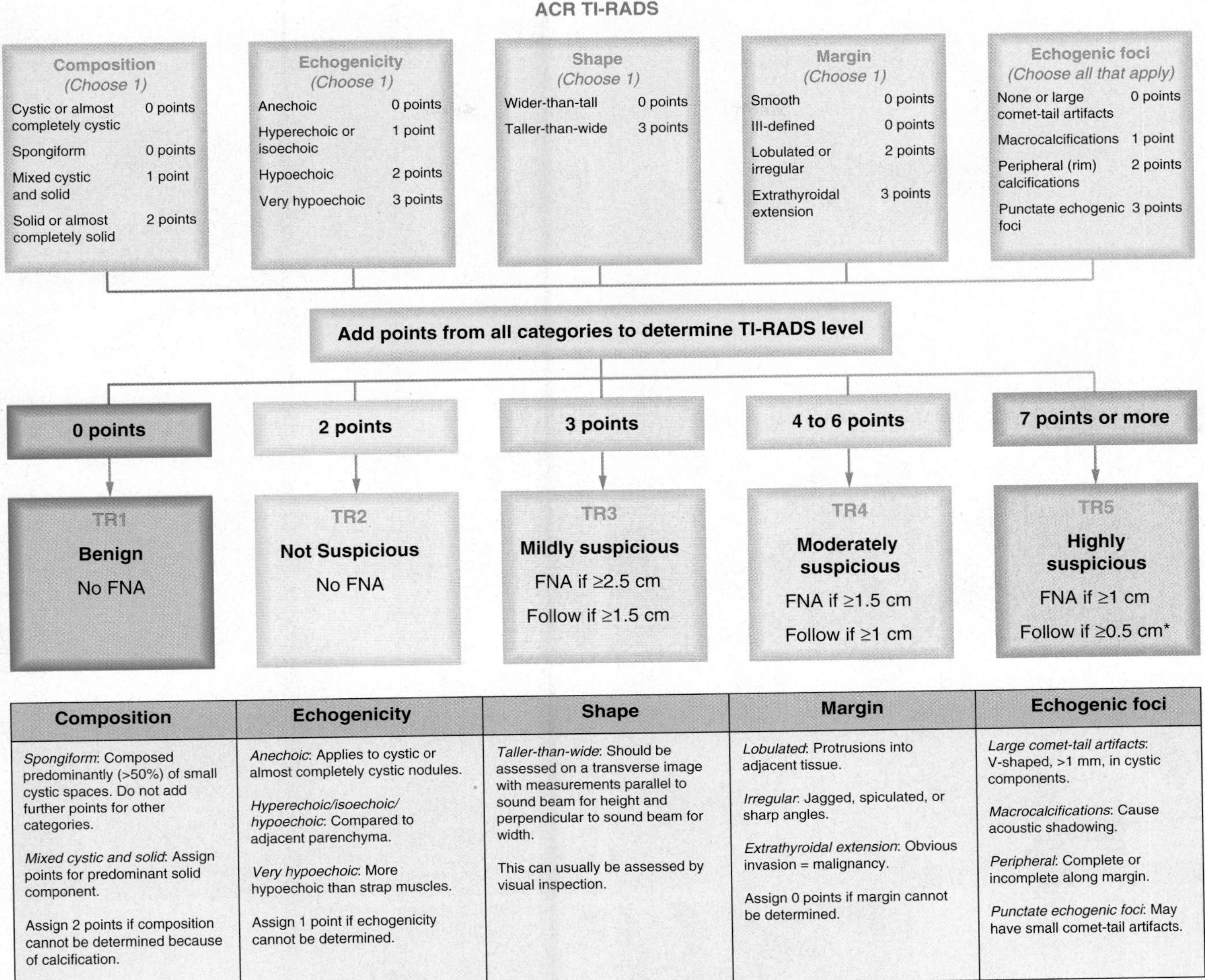

Composition	Echogenicity	Shape	Margin	Echogenic foci
Spongiform: Composed predominantly (>50%) of small cystic spaces. Do not add further points for other categories. *Mixed cystic and solid*: Assign points for predominant solid component. Assign 2 points if composition cannot be determined because of calcification.	*Anechoic*: Applies to cystic or almost completely cystic nodules. *Hyperechoic/isoechoic/hypoechoic*: Compared to adjacent parenchyma. *Very hypoechoic*: More hypoechoic than strap muscles. Assign 1 point if echogenicity cannot be determined.	*Taller-than-wide*: Should be assessed on a transverse image with measurements parallel to sound beam for height and perpendicular to sound beam for width. This can usually be assessed by visual inspection.	*Lobulated*: Protrusions into adjacent tissue. *Irregular*: Jagged, spiculated, or sharp angles. *Extrathyroidal extension*: Obvious invasion = malignancy. Assign 0 points if margin cannot be determined.	*Large comet-tail artifacts*: V-shaped, >1 mm, in cystic components. *Macrocalcifications*: Cause acoustic shadowing. *Peripheral*: Complete or incomplete along margin. *Punctate echogenic foci*: May have small comet-tail artifacts.

**Refer to discussion of papillary microcarcinomas for 5–9 mm TR5 nodules.*

FIG. 37.16 The American College of Radiology *(ACR)* Thyroid Imaging, Reporting and Data System (TI-RADS) lexicon, TR levels, and criteria for fine-needle aspiration biopsy. (From Tessler FN, Middleton WD, Grant EG, et al. ACR Thyroid Imaging, Reporting and Data System (TI-RADS): white paper of the ACR TI-RADS Committee. *J Am Coll Radiol.* 2017;14:587–595.)

management. For instance, small- to moderate-sized thyroid nodules in the extreme elderly or those with prohibitive surgical risk, or in patients without other concerning features who are already proceeding with thyroidectomy, do not require FNA.

Historically, cytological findings from FNA were broadly categorized into three categories: benign, malignant, and indeterminate. Although this system was generally helpful for the majority of thyroid nodules with highly predictive benign and malignant features, its drawbacks included 1) significant variability in pathology evaluation and reporting and 2) inability to more finely discriminate features within the broadly termed "indeterminate" category. To address these limitations, the National Cancer Institute convened a State of the Science conference in 2007 to develop a consensus for cytologic terminology known as the Bethesda System for Reporting Thyroid Cytopathology; an updated second version was published in 2017 and is described here.[9] This system formalized six diagnostic categories of FNA cytology, with an estimation of cancer risk associated with each category based on literature review and expert opinion. These categories, in increasing numerical order, are 1) nondiagnostic/unsatisfactory; 2) benign; 3) atypia of undetermined significance/follicular lesion of undetermined significance (AUS/FLUS); 4) follicular neoplasm/suspicious for follicular neoplasm (FN/SFN), which also encompasses Hürthle cell neoplasm; 5) suspicious for malignancy; and 6) malignant (Fig. 37.17). Table 37.3 provides a breakdown of these categories and their associated malignancy risk, in addition to the possible changes in malignancy risk if the new histopathologic diagnosis of noninvasive follicular thyroid neoplasm with papillary-like nuclear features (NIFTP, see below) were no longer to be included as a malignancy.

The broad institution of the Bethesda classification system across virtually all major centers has led to significant improvements in

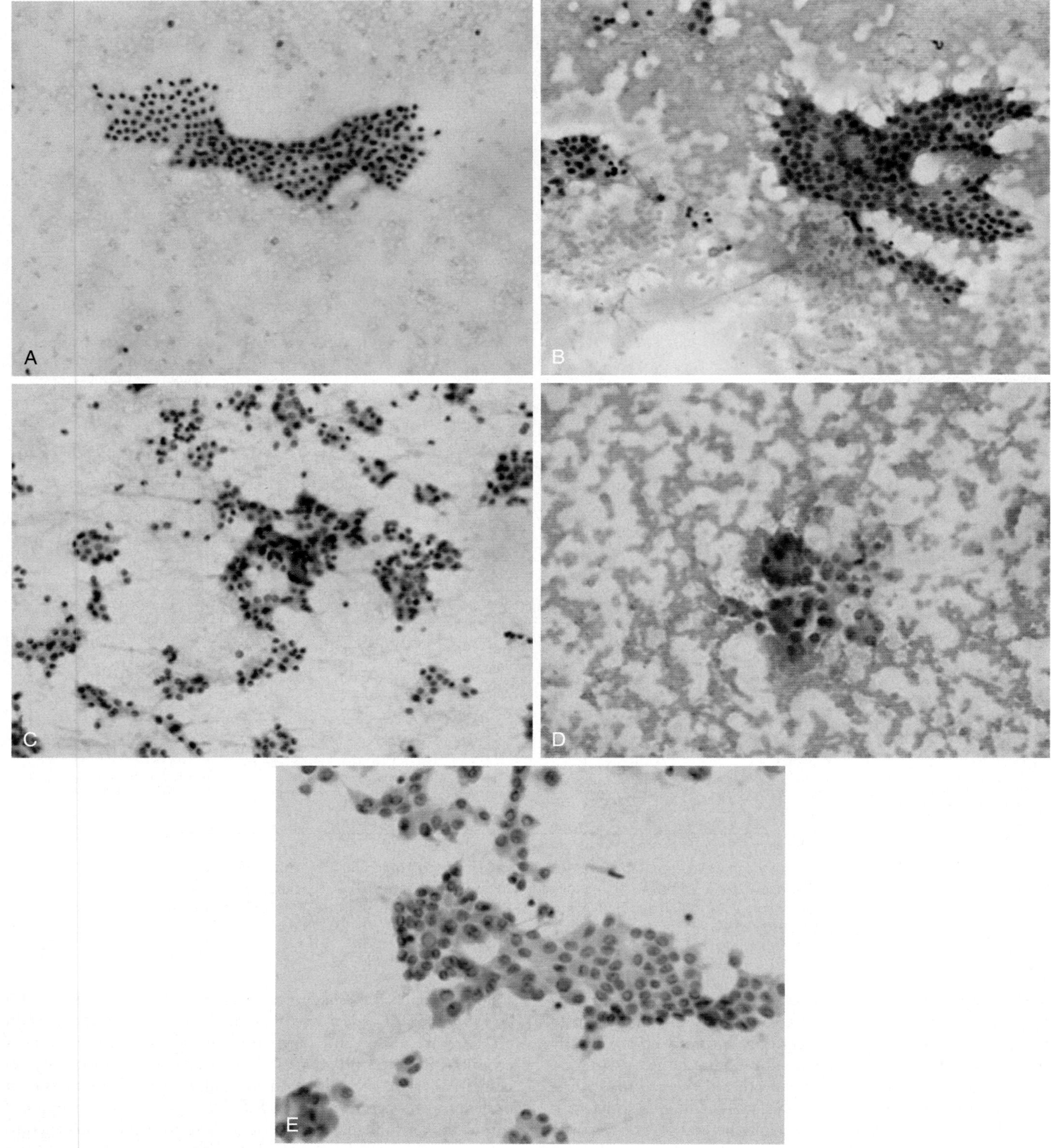

FIG. 37.17 Representative cytologic features of thyroid fine-needle aspiration specimens arranged according to the Bethesda classification for prediction of malignancy. (A) Category II: benign colloid nodule with bland-appearing follicular cells arranged in a macrofollicular pattern and abundant colloid in the background. (B) Category III: atypia of undetermined significance; follicular cells show nuclear enlargement of most nuclei with occasional intranuclear grooves. (C) Category IV: follicular neoplasm with highly cellular aspirate composed of uniform follicular cells arranged in microfollicles. (D) Category V: suspicious for papillary thyroid cancer; these representative microfollicular groups show nuclear enlargement and pale chromatin and rare intranuclear grooves and pseudoinclusions. (E) Category VI: papillary thyroid cancer demonstrating a large sheet of neoplastic cells with enlarged oval "Orphan Annie eye" nuclei; multiple intranuclear pseudoinclusions are also present. (Courtesy of Elham Khanafshar, MD, MS, Department of Pathology and Laboratory Medicine, University of California, San Francisco.)

TABLE 37.3 **The 2017 Bethesda system for reporting thyroid cytopathology implied risk of malignancy and recommended clinical management.**

DIAGNOSTIC CATEGORY (BETHESDA NUMBER)	RISK OF MALIGNANCY IF NIFTP ≠ CANCER	RISK OF MALIGNANCY IF NIFTP = CANCER	USUAL MANAGEMENT
Nondiagnostic or unsatisfactory (I)	5%–10%	5%–10%	Repeat FNA with ultrasound guidance
Benign (II)	0%–3%	0%–3%	Clinical and sonographic follow-up
AUS/FLUS (III)	6%–18%	~10%–30%	Repeat FNA, molecular testing, or lobectomy
FN/SFN (IV)	10%–40%	25%–40%	Molecular testing or lobectomy
Suspicious for malignancy (V)	45%–60%	50%–75%	Near-total thyroidectomy or lobectomy
Malignant (VI)	94%–96%	97%–99%	Near-total thyroidectomy or lobectomy

From Cibas ES, Ali SZ. The 2017 Bethesda system for reporting thyroid cytopathology. *Thyroid.* 2017; 27:1341–1346.
AUS/FLUS, Atypia of undetermined significance or follicular lesion of undetermined significance; *FN/SFN,* follicular neoplasm or suspicious for follicular neoplasm; *FNA,* fine-needle aspiration; *NIFTP,* noninvasive follicular thyroid neoplasm with papillary-like nuclear features.

standardization of care, communication of cancer risk with other providers and patients, and research efforts. Validation studies in large numbers of patients have shown overall good concordance in the FNA reporting patterns and malignancy rates. However, there is significant variability in the risk of malignancy in each category, particularly in the atypia of undetermined significance or follicular lesion of undetermined significance category.[10] This has led to the recommendation for each individual institution to define its own patient population's malignancy risks for each of the Bethesda categories by correlating cytology to surgical histopathology from surgical specimens.

Molecular Testing of FNA Specimens

Although no FNA cytology can completely rule out or rule in malignancy in a thyroid nodule, the cytologic diagnoses of benign (Bethesda category II) and malignant (Bethesda VI) are highly accurate with an error rate of less than 3%. On the other hand, the remaining "indeterminate" categories—particularly atypia of undetermined significance or follicular lesion of undetermined significance and follicular neoplasm (Bethesda III and IV, respectively)—are associated with a cancer risk anywhere from 6% to 40%, with Bethesda III nodules falling in the 6% to 30% range and the Bethesda IV nodules in the 10% to 40% range. Bethesda V lesions (suspicious for malignancy) are also technically indeterminate, but since these are associated with a 50% to 75% risk of malignancy, they are typically managed similarly to malignant (Bethesda VI) cytology.

Traditionally, the malignancy risk associated with Bethesda III or IV cytology in a thyroid nodule led to the recommendation of diagnostic thyroid lobectomy, but since the majority of these nodules are still ultimately benign on final pathology, efforts have been made in molecular genetics to improve prediction capability and reduce the number of unnecessary thyroidectomies. Advancements in molecular genetics have enabled the creation of relatively affordable high-throughput DNA or RNA-based assays for creating molecular profiles or signatures of cytology samples that would provide more accurate assessment of malignancy risk in thyroid nodules. There are multiple commercial providers for these tests, but the two most prominent tests are the Afirma (Veracyte, San Francisco, CA) and ThyroSeq (CBLPath, Rye Brook, NY).

The Afirma product was the first molecular test commercially available in this space. Its first generation assay, the Gene Expression Classifier, employed proprietary machine learning algorithms on a 167-gene mRNA microarray to separate nodules' gene expression signatures into "benign" and "suspicious" categories. The Gene Expression Classifier test's accuracy was first evaluated in 2012 in a study of surgically excised thyroid nodule specimens, and it was found to demonstrate excellent sensitivity and NPV (90% and ~95%, respectively), but with relatively poor specificity and positive predictive value (PPV, ~50% and 38%, respectively) for Bethesda III and IV nodules. Subsequent studies have largely validated the original study's findings, but many of them have been limited by the lack of a true negative (i.e., benign) reference standard.[10]

To address its limitations as a "rule-in" test due to its poor specificity and PPV, the newest Afirma product, the Genomic Sequence Classifier (GSC), improved the core machine learning algorithm for its larger gene expression array of 10,196 genes and also included seven other upstream components evaluating for a number of genetic mutations highly specific for malignancy. The performance of the GSC was recently evaluated in a multi-institutional blinded validation study on 191 cytology samples from 183 patients. For Bethesda III and IV lesions, the GSC demonstrated incremental improved performance compared to the Gene Expression Classifier, with sensitivity, specificity, NPV, and PPV of 91%, 68%, 96%, and 47%, respectively, based on a 24% cancer prevalence. Hürthle cell neoplasms remained an area of weakness in the GSC; it accurately predicted Hürthle cell adenoma and carcinoma in only 10/17 and 1/9 specimens, respectively.[11]

The ThyroSeq product approaches molecular classification differently from Afirma, in that it employs next-generation DNA sequencing technology to detect the presence or absence of a discrete list of known gene mutations and gene fusions associated with thyroid cancer. This technology is based on work described by Nikiforov and colleagues[12] at the University of Pittsburgh, and the second version of the product (termed "v2") evaluating 13 mutations and 42 fusions demonstrated promising results in their single-institution studies, with sensitivities and specificities in the low 90% range, PPV in the high 60% to 80% range, and NPV over 95%. These initial data originally generated excitement that perhaps the ThyroSeq v2 would offer ideal accuracy characteristics because the PPV appeared to approximate that of Bethesda V cytology while maintaining excellent NPV; however, subsequent validation studies showed less impressive results.[12]

The newest generation ThyroSeq product (termed "v3") improves the number of genes in its mutational panel and incorporates other genetic information such as changes in gene copy number, as well as some gene expression data. Steward and colleagues[13] conducted a prospective blinded multicenter study of the ThyroSeq v3 in 286 cytologically indeterminate FNA samples with known surgical pathology results. In Bethesda III and IV nodules, the test had a sensitivity and specificity of 94% and 82%, respectively, and an NPV and PPV of 97% and 66%, respectively, based on a cancer/NIFTP prevalence of 28%. Importantly, the test correctly predicted Hürthle cell adenoma and carcinoma in 62% and 100% of cases, respectively.[13]

The early data for both the Afirma GSC and ThyroSeq v3 suggest promising improvements over previous-generation products and subsequent management guidelines for thyroid nodules will likely incorporate molecular testing to a greater degree. Ultimately, the decision whether or not to use molecular testing needs to be placed in the context of other variables that go into clinical decision-making. First, whether to proceed with thyroidectomy may rest on factors other than the results of an FNA biopsy, let alone molecular testing. Second, the price of these assays is not insignificant, and their institutional setting-specific incremental value and cost-effectiveness must be taken into account. Third, patients should be counseled about the inherent uncertainties in the therapeutic and long-term clinical implications of pursuing molecular testing.

THYROID CANCER

Thyroid cancers are generally classified into DTC, PDTC, MTC, and ATC. Other thyroid malignancies including primary thyroid lymphoma, thyroid sarcoma, and metastases to the thyroid gland are rare. DTCs—consisting of the PTC, FTC, and HCC—are considered "differentiated" because they arise from the thyroid follicular epithelial cells and generally retain the ability to organify iodine. PDTC and ATC are also thought to arise from follicular cells but are more clinically aggressive compared to DTC due to their loss of differentiation. MTC, unlike the other tumors described, arise from the neuroendocrine parafollicular C cells.

DTC makes up the vast majority of thyroid cancers, with PTC and FTC representing 84% and 11%, respectively, of all thyroid cancer diagnoses. MTC represents 2%, and ATC occurs in 1% of all cases. Thyroid cancer overall carries an excellent prognosis, primarily due to the predominance of PTC, whereas ATC is among the most aggressive and lethal solid tumors with a nearly 100% mortality rate.

Incidence

Approximately 54,000 new cases of thyroid cancer are diagnosed each year in the United States, with over 2000 annual deaths. There is a more than threefold female predominance in incidence, and thyroid cancer has now become the fastest growing cancer in American women. Over the past three decades, the incidence of thyroid cancer has tripled in incidence in the United States and has seen similar dramatic increases in other developed and developing countries throughout the world.[14] The vast majority of the increase in diagnoses has been the result of the changing epidemiology of PTC. In a study using the Surveillance, Epidemiology, and End Results (SEER) database of thyroid cancer trends from 1975 to 2009, Davies and Welch found that overall mortality remained stable at 0.5 deaths per 100,000 despite the tripling of incidence, leading the investigators to conclude that the new epidemic of thyroid cancer was primarily one that resulted from the overdiagnosis of smaller and clinically insignificant tumors.

Other authors, however, have advised caution in attributing these increases solely to overdiagnosis. An independent analysis of the SEER database revealed substantial increases in the incidence of larger and advanced-stage PTC concomitant with the increase in the smaller and likely more indolent tumors. Lim and colleagues[15] found in another SEER analysis that the incidence-based mortality actually increased both overall in all PTCs and particularly in the advanced-stage tumors, suggesting that there was in fact a true increase in the occurrence of thyroid cancer over the past several decades. The implications of these opposing conclusions will be important in determining both how to optimize screening and diagnosis thresholds for thyroid nodules, as well as how to individualize effective treatment regimens that account for both indolent and aggressive tumors.

Differentiated Thyroid Cancer

The primary cancers arising from the thyroid follicular epithelial cells are PTC, FTC, and HCC. Despite some differences in biologic and clinical behavior, DTCs are generally approached and managed similarly.

PTC, as mentioned above, is the most common type of thyroid cancer overall, comprising 84% of all incident cases. There is a female predominance with a 3:1 female-to-male ratio, and peak incidence is in the third to fifth decades of life. PTC disseminates primarily via the lymphatic route and affects the cervical lymph nodes in the central and lateral compartments (see below); however, distant metastases do occur in up to 3% to 5% of patients, typically to lung and bone. Histologically, PTC is characterized by complex branching papillae with pseudoinclusions, nuclear grooving, and psammoma bodies (Fig. 37.18A). The so-called follicular variant of PTC (fvPTC) has a similar prognosis to classical PTC and histologically has well-defined follicles with minimal papillary projections. Other less common but more aggressive histologic subtypes of PTC include tall cell (Fig. 37.18B), hobnail, diffuse sclerosing, and columnar variants, which together comprise less than 1% of all PTCs.

FTC is the second most common type of DTC. FTC occurs in older adults, with peak incidence in the fourth and sixth decades. As in the case of PTC, the incidence of FTC is female-predominant, with a 3:1 female-to-male ratio. In contrast to that of PTC, the pattern of spread of FTC is hematogenous, typically to the lungs and bone (Fig. 37.19). Regional nodal metastases occur in less than 10% of cases. Cytologically, FTC can range from having virtually normal-appearing follicular cells to those with various abnormal features, including nuclear atypia, discohesion, hypercellularity, and microfollicles; thus, FTC cannot be reliably diagnosed by FNA. FTC can only be definitively diagnosed on histologic examination based on the presence of capsular and vascular invasion (Fig. 37.20A).

HCC is a less common type of DTC with distinct and more aggressive behavior. HCC occurs in older adults, with peak incidence in the sixth and seventh decades. Metastases can occur both via lymphatic and hematogenous route, and they are present in up to 20% of patients at initial diagnosis. HCC is less RAI-avid compared to other DTCs, with 38% of primary tumors being RAI avid. Nevertheless, RAI treatment is associated with improved survival in patients with HCCs that are 2 to 4 cm. HCC is distinguished from FTC histologically by the presence of oxyphilic Hürthle (or oncocytic) cells; these cells show a characteristic cellular enlargement with abundant eosinophilic granular cytoplasm due to an increased number of mitochondria (Fig. 37.20B).

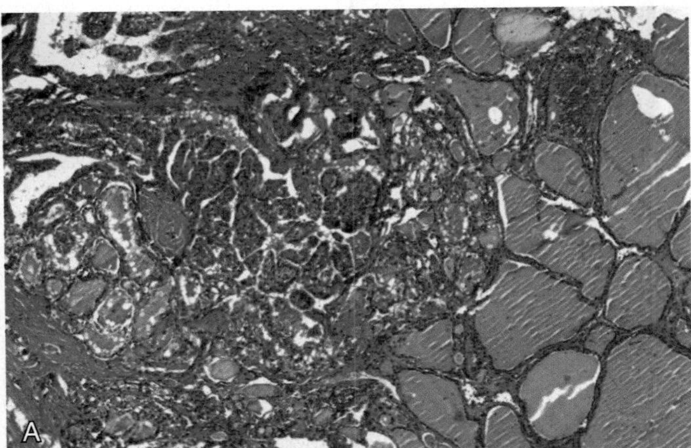

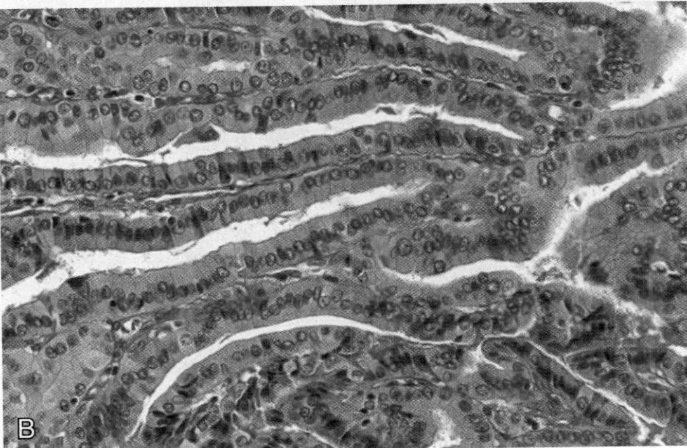

FIG. 37.18 (A) Hematoxylin and eosin (H&E) staining of a thyroid mass reveals papillary projections consistent with papillary thyroid cancer (PTC). (B) H&E staining of PTC shows cells with an increased height-to-width ratio in a single row of cells. This is the so-called tall cell variant of PTC, which is associated with a poorer prognosis than well-differentiated PTC.

A New Entity: Noninvasive Follicular Thyroid Neoplasm With Papillary-Like Nuclear Features

fvPTC entered the pathology nomenclature in the 1970s. It is a term that has been used to describe a tumor of neoplastic follicles without papillary structures but with nuclear features characteristic of PTC, such as enlargement, crowding/overlapping, elongation, irregular contours, grooves, pseudoinclusions, and chromatin clearing. Traditionally, two main subtypes of fvPTC were described: encapsulated and invasive (unencapsulated). The encapsulated subtype had been a subject of contentious debate in the pathology community, because, in the absence of capsular invasion, the diagnosis of cancer was wholly dependent upon nuclear findings that are highly subjective and variable. In addition, the clinical behavior and prognosis of encapsulated fvPTC were extremely indolent and clearly distinct from those of its invasive counterpart.

To address this problem, in 2016, a multidisciplinary group of international thought leaders in thyroidology performed a pivotal retrospective analysis of 109 patients with the encapsulated variant and 101 patients with invasive fvPTC; patients had a median follow-up period of 13 years (range, 10–26 years) for the encapsulated variant group and 3.5 years (range, 1–18 years) in the invasive fvPTC group. The authors found that none of the patients with encapsulated fvPTC had died or had evidence of disease after treatment, compared to a 12% rate of adverse oncologic outcomes in the invasive fvPTC cohort. Based on these findings, the authors proposed a change in terminology from encapsulated fvPTC to "noninvasive follicular thyroid neoplasm with papillary-like nuclear features," or NIFTP (Fig. 37.21), with the goal being to more accurately reflect the indolent nature of this tumor as well as to deemphasize the connotations of malignancy from the name.[16]

Recategorization of these tumors as NIFTP has potentially far-reaching implications, in that it changes the estimated risk of malignancy from FNA cytology specimens and could also lead to modification in the aggressiveness of treatment and surveillance for affected patients. NIFTPs appear to be increasing in frequency; some estimate that the incidence of this tumor type (whether it is called NIFTP or encapsulated fvPTC) has increased up to threefold over the past three decades. Overall, most would agree that NIFTPs are far more indolent and less concerning than their invasive counterpart, but several authors have cautioned against reclassifying NIFTP as a truly "benign" tumor, based on a low but real risk of metachronous disease recurrence and metastasis.[17] Further study with longer follow-up around NIFTP is needed in real-world practice.

Thyroid Follicular Cell Neoplasia and Oncogenesis

The two major molecular mechanisms governing thyroid follicular cell oncogenesis are the mitogen-activated protein kinase (MAPK) signaling and the phosphatidylinositol 3-kinase/protein kinase B (PI3K/AKT) pathways (Fig. 37.22). Together, these mechanisms govern normal thyroid cell survival and function; perturbations at multiple points in these pathways have been directly linked to the pathogenesis of thyroid cancer.

The MAPK signaling pathway is activated by growth factors binding to cell-surface transmembrane tyrosine kinase receptors. This triggers an intracellular signaling cascade that ultimately regulates the intranuclear transcription of genes responsible for cellular growth/proliferation, differentiation, migration, and survival. Mutations in the major intracellular MAPK pathway genes—BRAF, RET/PTC, RAS, and neurotrophic tropomyosin receptor kinase (NTRK)—have been directly linked to the development of DTC.

The PI3K/AKT pathway, like the MAPK pathway, involves a series of phosphorylation reactions starting with a transmembrane protein kinase; ultimately, this leads to the activation of AKT, which in turn phosphorylates proteins both in the cytosol and the nucleus. Downstream targets of AKT regulate apoptosis, proliferation, cell-cycle progression, cytoskeletal integrity, and energy metabolism. This pathway is in part mediated and is thought to be particularly relevant to the development of FTC; further supporting this theory is the finding that mutations in PTEN, an inhibitor of AKT activation, are found in both sporadic FTC and FTC associated with Cowden syndrome, a hereditary disorder characterized by multiple hamartomas, particularly of the skin and mucous membranes, macrocephaly, and an increased risk of other solid organ cancers such as breast cancer, endometrial cancer, and colorectal cancer.

In 2014, The Cancer Genome Atlas project consortium published its results from a comprehensive multiplatform next-generation genomic sequencing analysis of 496 PTCs. This seminal study confirmed the dominant and mutually exclusive roles of driving somatic genetic alterations in the MAPK and PI3K/AKT pathways in PTC, with distinct signaling differences in RAS- and BRAF V600E-driven tumors. In addition, The Cancer Genome Atlas project identified several new alterations, including new

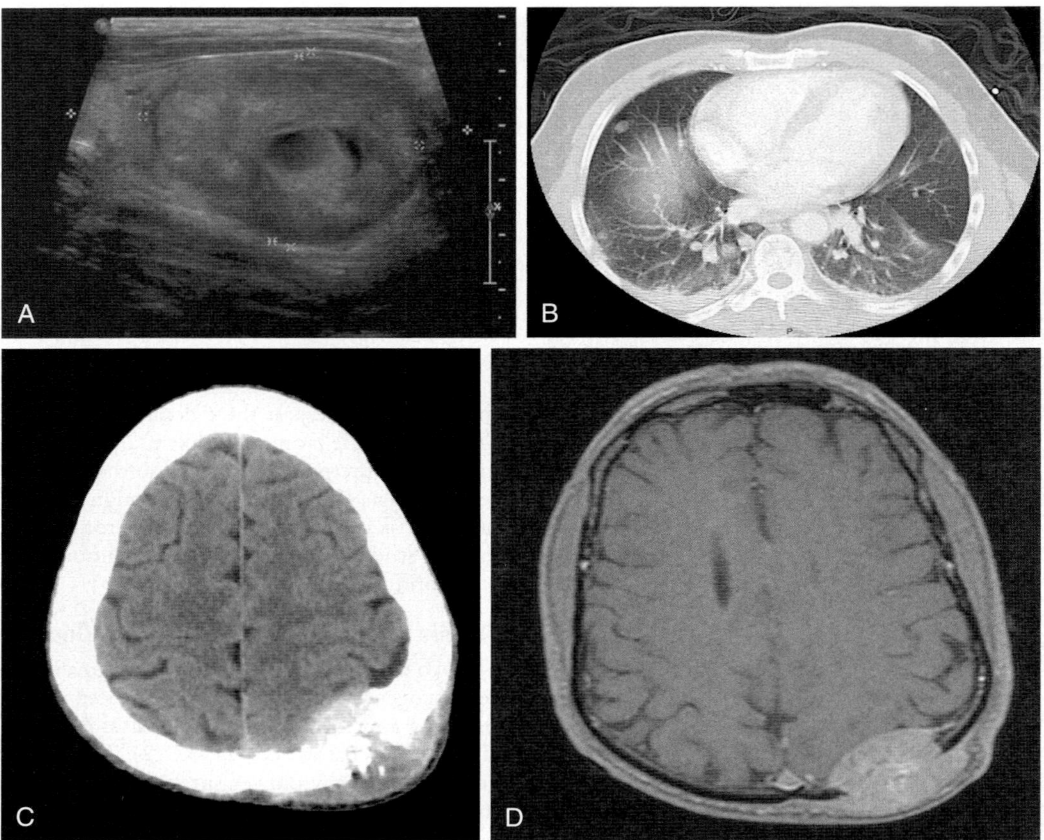

FIG. 37.19 Metastatic follicular cancer; all images are from the same patient. (A) Preoperative ultrasound demonstrates a 6.7-cm mass in the left lobe of the thyroid; pathology demonstrated follicular cancer. (B) Computed tomography (CT) image of the chest demonstrates multiple pulmonary metastases. (C) CT image of the head demonstrates left parietal bone metastasis. (D) Magnetic resonance imaging of the head demonstrates left parietal bone metastasis with an epidural component and mass effect on the brain.

driver mutations in EIF1AX; individual genes such as CHEK2, ATM, and TERT promoter; functionally related genes related to chromatin remodeling; and altered micro-RNA expression patterns (particularly in miR-21 and miR-146b) that contribute to distinct clinical subtypes of PTC. Altogether, the results of the Cancer Genome Atlas are estimated to have increased the proportion of PTCs that can be identified based on molecular signature using current genome sequencing technology from 75% to over 96%.[18] This has translated into improved molecular testing methods to facilitate the preoperative diagnosis of thyroid cancer (see above).

Risk Factors

The two most studied and validated risk factors for PTC include a history of ionizing radiation exposure and a family history of DTC.

The association of ionizing radiation exposure in childhood and adolescence in particular is clear for PTC and perhaps ATC.[19] Acute environmental exposures from catastrophic occurrences, such as the Chernobyl nuclear accident and nuclear bombings in Hiroshima and Nagasaki, have dramatically validated the impact of radiation on thyroid follicular cell oncogenesis. Atomic bomb survivors in Japan have been found to have an increased risk of thyroid nodules and PTC up to 50 years after the incident, with a linear radiation dose response. Medical sources of irradiation, such as external beam radiation therapy to the head and neck as well as historical practices such as radiation therapy in the 1950s and 1960s for acne and tonsillitis, also have been linked to the subsequent development of PTC. Children and adolescents are particularly vulnerable, with even low dose radiation exposure (e.g., equivalent to a single chest X-ray) increasing PTC risk in a dose-dependent fashion.

A strong family history of DTC has also been shown to increase the risk of DTC. This may be in the setting of known hereditary cancer syndromes with specific single gene mutations such as Gardner syndrome (which predisposes to PTC), Cowden syndrome (FTC and occasionally PTC), Carney complex (PTC and FTC), and Werner syndrome (PTC and FTC). In addition, a separate entity known as familial non-MTC was coined to describe families with two or more first-degree relatives diagnosed with DTC in the absence of other hereditary cancer syndromes. Familial non-MTC tumors are thought to be more aggressive and portend a worse prognosis than their sporadic counterparts.[20] However, the exact inheritance pattern and genetics underlying familial non-MTC remain poorly understood.

Obesity has also consistently been identified as a risk factor for DTC.[19] There has been a close parallel increase in the trends of obesity prevalence and the incidence of thyroid cancer. A pooled analysis of 22 prospective studies found that thyroid cancer risk was associated with multiple markers of obesity including waist circumference, body mass index (BMI), and BMI gain between

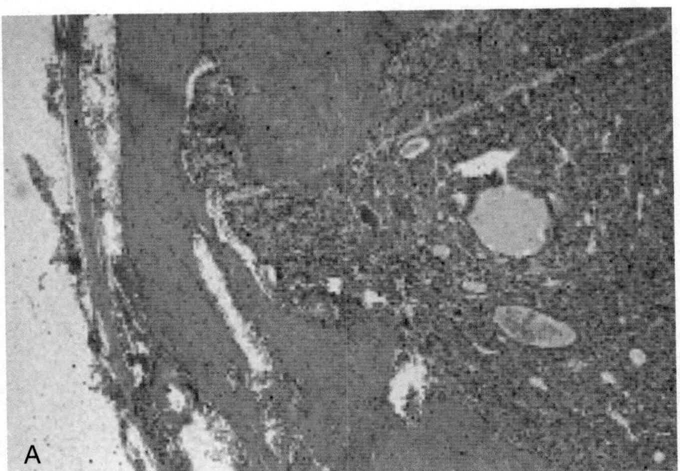

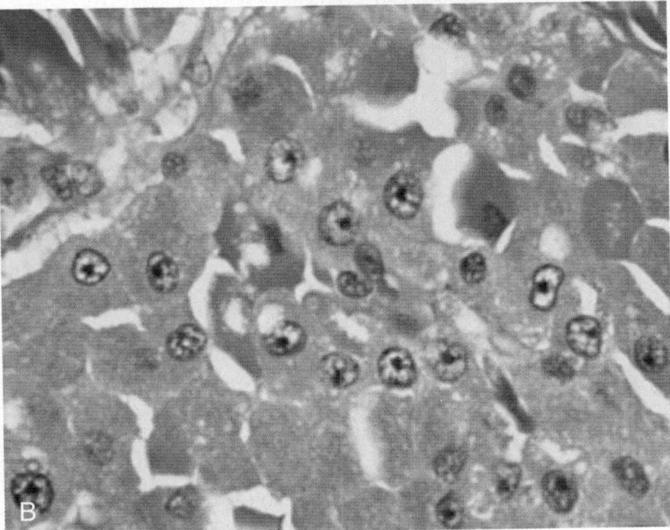

FIG. 37.20 (A) Hematoxylin and eosin (H&E) staining of a follicular lesion. High-power examination reveals capsular invasion by follicular cells, which is consistent with a diagnosis of follicular thyroid cancer. (B) H&E staining of Hürthle cell cancer showing vesicular nuclei with irregular macronucleoli. (From Freeman JL, Kim DS. Hürthle cell tumors of the thyroid. In Randolph GW, ed. *Surgery of the Thyroid and Parathyroid Glands 2*. Philadelphia: Elsevier Saunders; 2013:207)

young adulthood and study baseline. In addition, PTCs in obese patients have been associated with more aggressive tumor characteristics.

Other environmental exposures have been hypothesized to increase the risk of DTC. Hoffman and colleagues[21] recently published a case-control study of patients with PTC and demonstrated a link between the levels at home of certain common flame retardant chemicals to increased odds of PTC, particularly decabromodiphenyl ether and tris(2-chloroethyl) phosphate. An increased risk of DTC also has been reported in clusters of volcanic areas around the world, including Hawaii, Iceland, French Polynesia, New Caledonia, and Sicily; this may be due, in part, to exposure to heavy metals and other toxic compounds from gas, ash, and lava emissions from volcanoes that contaminate ground water and food sources.[22] The underlying mechanisms for all of these potential environmental carcinogens remain unclear and require further study.

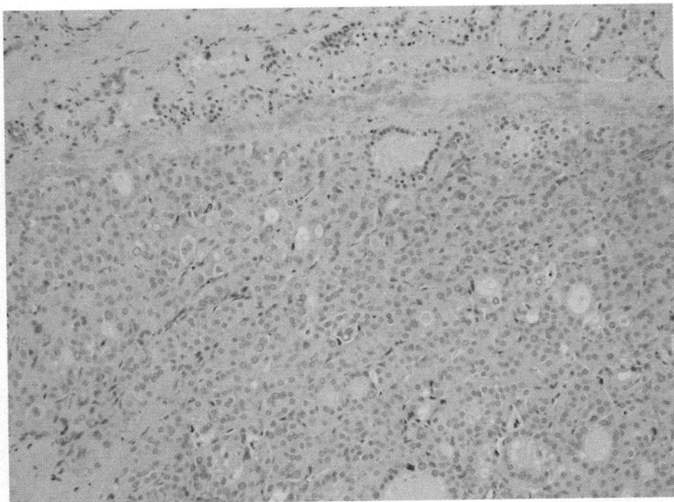

FIG. 37.21 Noninvasive follicular thyroid neoplasm with papillary-like nuclear features (NIFTP) is a well-circumscribed/encapsulated microfollicular-pattern neoplasm with no capsular or vascular invasion. The neoplastic cells show nuclear features similar to those of papillary thyroid cancer. (Courtesy of Elham Khanafshar, MD, MS, Department of Pathology and Laboratory Medicine, University of California, San Francisco.)

Clinical Presentation

The classic presentation of DTC is that of an asymptomatic, palpable thyroid nodule discovered by either patients or physicians during routine examination. Palpable thyroid nodules are present in approximately 5% of the population, the majority of which are benign. With the improvements in high-resolution ultrasonography and other imaging modalities, thyroid nodules—and by extension thyroid cancer—have become more commonly diagnosed in asymptomatic individuals, as described above.

DTCs are typically slow growing, painless, and often asymptomatic. Acute pain is more typical of a benign process such as thyroiditis or an acute bleed into a benign cyst; however, pain can also be indicative of less common and more aggressive thyroid cancers such as MTC, primary thyroid lymphoma, and ATC. Concerning features include rapid growth of the nodule and symptoms such as hoarseness, coughing, or dysphagia, which could signal local invasion into surrounding structures such as the RLN and aerodigestive tract (Fig. 37.23).

On physical exam, palpable DTC can vary from soft to firm in texture on palpation. Firm and fixed masses may suggest locally advanced disease. Patients may have palpable or imaging-detected cervical lymphadenopathy.

Imaging Workup

To adequately inform initial surgical treatment, the quality of preoperative imaging is paramount. The most important imaging modality for surgical planning is comprehensive thyroid ultrasound with lymph node mapping of the bilateral central and lateral neck lymph nodes. Preoperative ultrasound is the most sensitive test for the characterization of thyroid nodules as well as identification of pathologic lymphadenopathy, with its results affecting the extent of initial surgical therapy in over 30% of patients.

Cross-sectional imaging (contrast-enhanced CT or MRI of the neck and chest) and intraluminal imaging (laryngoscopy, bronchoscopy, or esophagoscopy) may be required in patients with potentially more advanced local and regional disease. Clinical manifestations that may lead the clinician to obtain

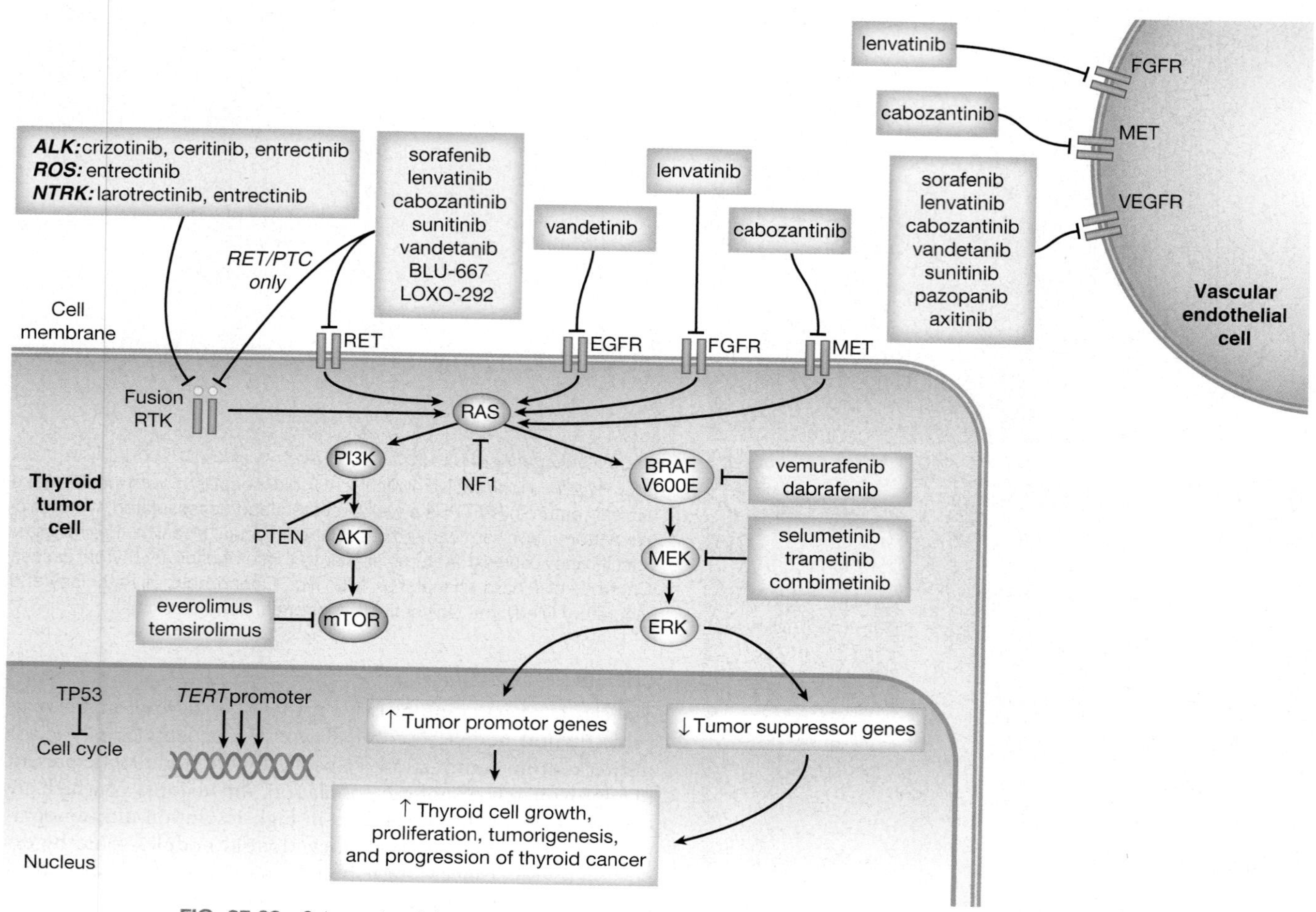

FIG. 37.22 Schematic of the two most common pathways and genetic alterations associated with thyroid follicular cell oncogenesis, the MAPK and the PI3K-AKT pathways. Also shown are the current targeted therapies studied in thyroid cancer. (From Rao SN, Cabanillas ME. Navigating systemic therapy in advanced thyroid carcinoma: from standard of care to personalized therapy and beyond. *J Endocr Soc.* 2018;2:1109–1130.) *AKT,* Protein kinase B; *ALK,* anaplastic lymphoma kinase; *ERK,* extracellular signal–regulated kinase; *EGFR,* epidermal growth factor receptor; *FGFR,* fibroblast growth factor receptor; *MAPK,* mitogen-activated protein kinase; *mTOR,* mammalian target of rapamycin; *NTRK,* neurotrophic tropomyosin receptor kinase; *PI3K,* phosphatidylinositol 3-kinase; *PTC,* papillary thyroid cancer; *RTK,* receptor tyrosine kinase; *TERT,* telomerase reverse transcription; *VEGFR,* vascular endothelial growth factor receptor.

these additional studies include concerning symptoms such as voice changes, dysphagia, respiratory symptoms such as cough or hemoptysis, as well as palpable evidence of rapidly enlarging, bulky, and/or fixed disease on physical exam. Sonographic indications include evidence of bulky disease, disease extending into the chest or extending posteriorly, and extrathyroidal extension.

The routine use of PET scanning in preoperative planning is not recommended.

Staging

There have been many proposed staging systems over the years for estimating disease-specific mortality from DTC, but the American Joint Committee on Cancer (AJCC) and Union for International Cancer Control Tumor, Node, Metastasis (TNM) classification has emerged as the most widely accepted and easily understood. The current eighth edition of the TNM system, which took effect in early 2018, is summarized in a tables in Ref. 22a The eighth edition has made a number of major changes that better optimize prediction and stratification of patient survival. These include the following:

1. The age cutoff for staging, which was originally established to reflect the survival benefit of younger age, was increased from 45 to 55 years at diagnosis.
2. Minimal extrathyroidal extension detected only on histologic examination—as opposed to gross extrathyroidal extension—was removed from the definition of T3 disease, effectively eliminating this factor from staging.
3. N1 (regional nodal) disease no longer upstages a patient 55 years of age or older to stage III.
4. T3a is a new category for tumors larger than 4 cm confined to the thyroid gland.
5. T3b is a new category for tumors of any size, demonstrating gross extrathyroidal extension into the strap muscles.

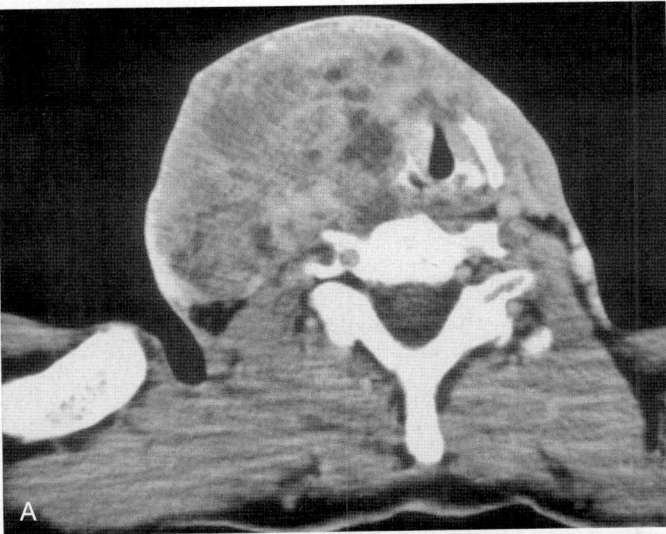

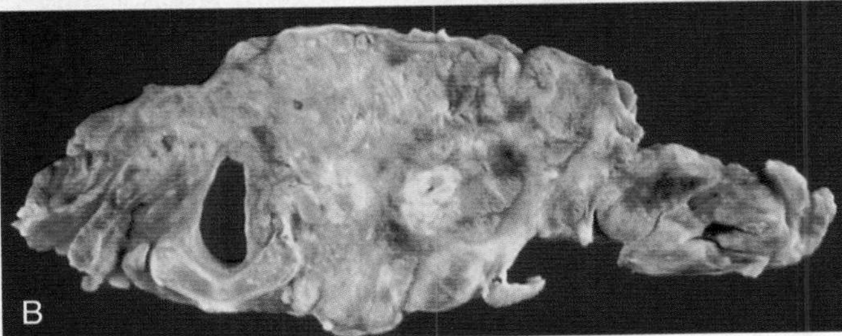

FIG. 37.23 (A and B) Rapidly enlarging thyroid mass in a 70-year-old man. Computed tomography image demonstrates displacement of the larynx and lateral involvement of both jugular veins. The patient died within 6 months of rapidly progressing follicular cancer.

6. Level VII lymph nodes were reclassified as central neck lymph nodes (N1a) as opposed to lateral neck lymph nodes to be more anatomically consistent.
7. The presence of distant metastases in patients 55 years of age or older was reclassified from stage IVC to stage IVB.

The downstream effect of the changes made to the eighth edition is to downstage many patients into lower stages; as a result, patients with higher-stage disease experience a worse prognosis in the new system, thus better discriminating prognosis between stages and more accurately reflecting the overall lower risk of thyroid cancer mortality. Under the eighth edition, the estimated disease-specific survival in younger patients is expected to be 98% to 100% for stage I and 85% to 95% for stage II, and in older patients over 55 years 98% to 100%, 85% to 95%, 60% to 70%, and less than 50% for stage I, II, III, and IV, respectively.[23]

Although systems such as TNM are important for making initial estimates of disease-specific mortality, the fact remains that the vast majority of patients will have excellent long-term survival. Therefore, what is arguably more clinically relevant to patients with DTC is the risk of disease recurrence, which is an outcome that systems such as TNM are not designed to measure. In response, the ATA proposed in its 2009 guidelines a system for estimating the initial risk of recurrence based on a number of clinicopathologic features, with a three-tiered risk classification that stratified patients into low-risk (~3%), intermediate-risk (~21%), and high-risk (~68%) categories.[24] In the 2015 updated guidelines, it was acknowledged that even within these three tiers, the level of risk depends on many individual tumor characteristics and actually exists on a continuum (Fig. 37.24). Molecular testing and profiling will likely enhance clinical staging systems.

The ATA guidelines have proposed a system that dynamically changes the initial risk estimates based on the clinical course of disease and response to therapy.[5] The four response-to-initial-therapy categories in this system include the following:

1. "Excellent response": no clinical, biochemical, or structural evidence of disease (translating to a 1%–4% risk of recurrence).
2. "Biochemical incomplete response": abnormal Tg or rising anti-Tg antibody levels in the absence of localizable disease (translating to 50% achieving no-evidence-of-disease status either spontaneously or with additional therapy and a 20% risk of developing structural disease).
3. "Structural incomplete response": persistent or newly identified locoregional or distant metastases (disease-specific mortality as high as 11% with locoregional disease and 50% with distant metastases).
4. "Indeterminate response": nonspecific biochemical or structural findings that cannot be confidently classified as either benign or malignant, including patients with stable or declining anti-Tg antibody levels without definitive structural evidence of disease (15%–20% will have structural disease identified during follow-up).

Surgical Management

Surgery is the mainstay of therapy for DTC. With the appropriate choice of operation and in the hands of a high-volume surgeon (see below), thyroidectomy is extremely safe and effective. The appropriate extent of thyroidectomy depends on multiple factors, including the extent of disease and the patient's perioperative risk, with official recommendations evolving over the past several years.

In the past, total thyroidectomy was the traditionally recommended treatment for the majority of DTCs at least 1 cm. However, ipsilateral thyroid lobectomy has become an acceptable alternative to total thyroidectomy for low-risk unilateral DTCs between 1 and 4 cm without extrathyroidal extension or evidence of metastatic disease, and it is the recommended surgical option for DTCs that are less than1 cm. This shift in recommendations resulted from newer data in large observational database studies demonstrating equivalent survival between selected patients undergoing either total thyroidectomy or lobectomy for DTCs between 1 and 4 cm.[25] Thus, total thyroidectomy is now the preferred evidence-based approach only for those DTCs at higher risk for recurrence and/or disease-specific mortality. Such scenarios include the following:

- Tumor at least 4 cm
- Gross extrathyroidal extension
- Evidence of metastatic disease
- Radiation-induced DTC
- Familial nonmedullary thyroid cancer
- Multifocal bilateral DTC.

For DTCs with clinical and/or radiographic evidence of cervical lymph node metastases, therapeutic compartment-based lymph node dissection is recommended. The lymph node compartments in the neck follow a standardized nomenclature, which is shown in Fig. 37.3. The most relevant nodal stations for thyroid cancer include the central compartment (level VI and VII), which consists of the perithyroidal lymphoadipose tissue bounded by the carotid arteries laterally, the hyoid bone superiorly, and the innominate artery inferiorly, and the lateral compartments containing the jugular groups (levels II, III, and IV) and the inferior posterior triangle (level Vb). Therapeutic lymph

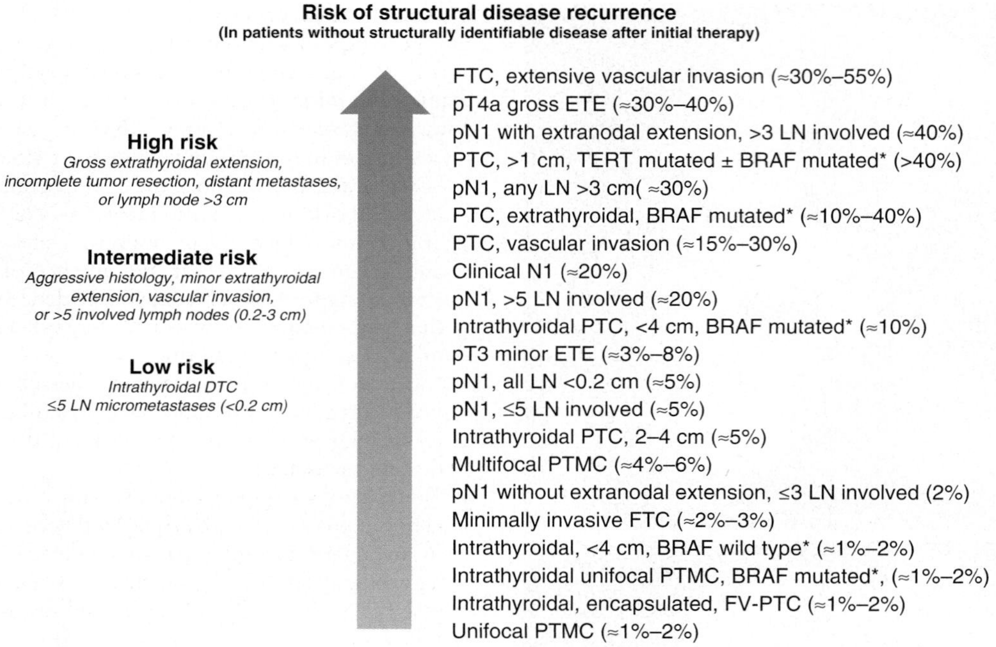

Risk of structural disease recurrence
(In patients without structurally identifiable disease after initial therapy)

High risk
Gross extrathyroidal extension, incomplete tumor resection, distant metastases, or lymph node >3 cm

Intermediate risk
Aggressive histology, minor extrathyroidal extension, vascular invasion, or >5 involved lymph nodes (0.2-3 cm)

Low risk
Intrathyroidal DTC ≤5 LN micrometastases (<0.2 cm)

FTC, extensive vascular invasion (≈30%–55%)
pT4a gross ETE (≈30%–40%)
pN1 with extranodal extension, >3 LN involved (≈40%)
PTC, >1 cm, TERT mutated ± BRAF mutated* (>40%)
pN1, any LN >3 cm(≈30%)
PTC, extrathyroidal, BRAF mutated* (≈10%–40%)
PTC, vascular invasion (≈15%–30%)
Clinical N1 (≈20%)
pN1, >5 LN involved (≈20%)
Intrathyroidal PTC, <4 cm, BRAF mutated* (≈10%)
pT3 minor ETE (≈3%–8%)
pN1, all LN <0.2 cm (≈5%)
pN1, ≤5 LN involved (≈5%)
Intrathyroidal PTC, 2–4 cm (≈5%)
Multifocal PTMC (≈4%–6%)
pN1 without extranodal extension, ≤3 LN involved (2%)
Minimally invasive FTC (≈2%–3%)
Intrathyroidal, <4 cm, BRAF wild type* (≈1%–2%)
Intrathyroidal unifocal PTMC, BRAF mutated*, (≈1%–2%)
Intrathyroidal, encapsulated, FV-PTC (≈1%–2%)
Unifocal PTMC (≈1%–2%)

FIG. 37.24 The risk of structural disease recurrence for differentiated thyroid cancer after initial therapy exists on a continuum of risk estimates. The three-tiered American Thyroid Association modified initial risk stratification system is shown on the left-hand column. (From Haugen BR, Alexander EK, Bible KC, et al. 2015 American Thyroid Association Management guidelines for adult patients with thyroid nodules and differentiated thyroid cancer: the American Thyroid Association Guidelines Task Force on Thyroid Nodules and Differentiated Thyroid Cancer. *Thyroid.* 2016;26:1–133.)

node dissection should be performed in patients with radiographic or clinical evidence of metastatic disease as determined either preoperatively or intraoperatively. The presence of ipsilateral central compartment nodal involvement warrants a level VI (+/-VII) dissection. The presence of lateral neck nodal metastases warrants both a central and lateral compartment-based neck dissection, even in the 12% of patients with skip metastases to the lateral neck (i.e., bypassing the central neck nodes). Radical neck dissection causes significant patient morbidity and is rarely necessary for oncologic purposes.

Because microscopic lymph node metastases may occur in up to 80% of patients with PTC, some investigators have suggested routine prophylactic central neck dissection during the index thyroidectomy procedure. However, because microscopic nodal disease is rarely of clinical significance, the role of prophylactic central neck dissection remains controversial. The evidence is largely based on observational data and decidedly mixed, with some studies showing a modest benefit of prophylactic central neck dissection in reducing long-term locoregional recurrence. However, central neck dissection has been associated with a higher risk of temporary and permanent hypoparathyroidism, although this effect is blunted when the operation is performed by experienced surgeons.[26] Currently, the ATA guidelines suggest that prophylactic central neck dissection should be considered for certain higher risk patients with cN0 papillary thyroid carcinomas with more advanced primary tumors (T3 or T4) and clinically involved lateral neck nodes and/or if the information would be helpful in guiding additional therapy.

For locally invasive primary tumors involving structures such as the strap muscles, trachea, esophagus, larynx, and RLN, careful preoperative planning with cross-sectional imaging and (rarely) endoscopic studies is critical (see above). Consultation and assistance from allied specialties including thoracic surgery and otolaryngology are recommended for complex tumors requiring segmental laryngotracheal or esophageal resection. The oncologically ideal goal of gross total resection of all visible tumor should be balanced against the potential life-changing morbidity of radical resections.

Active Nonoperative Surveillance of PTC

Despite advances in the management of higher-risk cancers as described above, arguably the most striking advance in the management of DTC in the past decade has been the dramatic de-escalation of treatment for smaller thyroid cancers, which now includes nonoperative active surveillance for papillary thyroid microcarcinomas smaller than 1 cm.

This treatment option has been best studied in the Japanese population. The initial report published in 2010 by Ito and colleagues[27] studied 340 patients with unilateral papillary thyroid microcarcinomas who underwent once- or twice-yearly ultrasound and observation/surveillance over a mean period of 74 months. The proportion of patients in whom the tumors grew by 3 mm or more was 16% at 10 years and in whom new cervical nodal metastases were detected was 3.4% at 10 years.[27] A subsequent report by the same group of 1235 patients undergoing observation showed that patients older than 60 years had extremely slow progression to any form of clinical disease, with an overall rate of 2.5% at 10 years. In contrast, up to 23% of younger patients progressed to clinical disease at 10 years. Importantly, those patients who initially underwent observation and eventually had surgical resection had no detectable negative perioperative or oncologic consequences from having waited for surgical rescue.

Based on the results of these landmark studies from Japan, centers in other countries have begun to study the role of active surveillance in their specific patient populations. The largest ongoing prospective trial in the United States is at the Memorial Sloan-Kettering Cancer Center, where highly selected patients with no more than 1.5 cm unifocal PTCs and papillary thyroid microcarcinomas are enrolled into a regimented active surveillance program. A multicenter prospective cohort study is also currently underway in Korea.

When considering whether active surveillance is appropriate for a specific patient and treatment venue, several attributes must be evaluated, including tumor features and risk profile; patient demographics, long-term compliance, and patient preferences; and the experience of the medical/surgical team running the surveillance program. In addition, a significant and controversial concern in the current health care climate is the geography-specific cost-effectiveness implications of long-term surveillance versus surgery.[28] Further research is needed to better identify those lowest-risk patients in whom active surveillance would benefit the most, possibly with the incorporation of molecular testing.

Postoperative Thyroid-Stimulating Hormone Suppression

In many patients after thyroidectomy for DTC, TSH suppressive doses of thyroid hormone medication are recommended to prevent hypothyroidism and to reduce the risk of TSH-stimulated tumor growth and recurrence. TSH suppression has been shown to improve overall survival in stage II, III, and IV patients; however, the degree of suppression required for survival benefit remains a point of controversy, and overall, there has been a trend toward less aggressive suppression over time.[29]

The TSH goals depend on both the risk of recurrence after initial treatment, as well as the presence of comorbid conditions that may increase the risks of hyperthyroidism, such as older age, atrial fibrillation, and osteoporosis. For patients with low- to intermediate-risk tumors, serum TSH can initially be maintained between 0.1 and 0.5 mU/L, whereas patients with high-risk tumors should be kept initially at a TSH level of less than 0.1 mU/L if possible. The TSH level also may be allowed to increase closer to the normal range in patients who have an excellent response to therapy.

Radioactive Iodine

RAI therapy with ^{131}I for DTC is based on the fact that thyroid follicular cells have a unique ability to take up iodine (see Thyroid Physiology, above). DTC is generally very iodine avid, at least initially, albeit at a lesser degree than normal thyroid follicular cells due to reduced expression of the sodium-iodide transporter. Thus, RAI is a useful adjunct in the treatment of PTC and FTC—as well as certain cases of HCC despite its relative iodine nonavidity, whereas it plays no role in cancers that do not take up iodine, such as PDTC, MTC, and ATC.

In DTC, RAI is typically administered after thyroidectomy. There are generally two broad indications for RAI. The first indication is to ablate any residual normal thyroid tissue remaining after thyroidectomy. The rationale for this is threefold: 1) the elimination of normal thyroid tissue increases the specificity of both postoperative serum Tg and subsequent ^{131}I scanning for detection of recurrent disease; 2) remnant ablation prevents subsequent de novo thyroid cancer formation in the remnant tissue; and 3) it can be used at higher doses to treat microscopic disease as adjuvant therapy to prevent clinical recurrences. The second indication for RAI is to treat clinically detectable disease that cannot be addressed by surgery.

The role for postthyroidectomy RAI has become much more selective in the past decade, largely due to convincing evidence of the lack of benefit of RAI in low-risk DTC patients. These patients include those with intrathyroidal tumors smaller than 4 cm without high-risk histologic features or small multifocal cancers. Multiple large database studies and systematic reviews have demonstrated no benefit of RAI in these patients with respect to either disease recurrence or mortality. The literature suggests some benefit of RAI for intermediate-risk patients. For example, a 21,870 patient study from the National Cancer Database demonstrated a 29% reduction in the risk of death in intermediate-risk thyroid cancer, with an even greater benefit in younger patients.[30] However, further research is necessary to determine the specific subgroups in the intermediate-risk category that would benefit the most. RAI is routinely recommended for high-risk cancers.

RAI should be administered in patients in a low-iodine state, and in a setting of high TSH levels to stimulate maximal iodine uptake by thyroid tissue. Two methods of TSH stimulation exist: administration of recombinant human TSH, and thyroid hormone withdrawal. The dose of RAI administered depends on the risk profile of the thyroid cancer and the indication(s) for RAI. Generally, remnant ablation doses of RAI fall in the 30 to 50 mCi range, whereas treatment-level doses are typically in the 100 to 150 mCi range. As long as there is evidence that thyroid cancer remains iodine avid, repeated treatments with RAI are appropriate assuming acceptable toxicity profiles. Dosimetry also can be used to help guide dosing regimens that optimize therapeutic activity while minimizing toxicity. The adverse effects of RAI include sialadenitis, nasolacrimal duct obstruction, transient tumor/thyroid swelling, infertility, and development of secondary malignancies (particularly leukemia); the risks of all of these occurrences are dose dependent. The maximal cumulative lifetime exposure to RAI is somewhat controversial but generally approximates 600 mCi. Pregnancy and breastfeeding are absolute contraindications to RAI.

Adjuvant Therapies

External beam radiotherapy (EBRT) plays a limited but important palliative role for selected situations in DTC. There are no randomized clinical trials, and EBRT practice patterns vary, so many of the recommendations rely on expert opinion and single-institution studies. The main indications for EBRT include local control of unresectable locally advanced macroscopic or microscopic residual disease after thyroidectomy (particularly in tumors thought to be RAI nonavid and affecting the aerodigestive tract), as well as treatment of symptomatic distant metastatic foci that are RAI nonavid.

Other treatment options for local control of recurrent and/or metastatic disease exist in a limited number of centers. These include percutaneous ethanol or radiofrequency ablation for cervical nodal metastases, radiofrequency ablation of lung or bone metastases, and palliative embolization of bone metastases. In addition, there is much research activity around newer targeted systemic therapies for RAI-refractory disease (see below).

Medullary Thyroid Cancer

MTC is an uncommon thyroid malignancy, comprising only 2% of all incident thyroid cancers in the United States.[15] Hazard and colleagues first coined the term "medullary" in 1959 to describe a unique thyroid tumor with nonfollicular characteristics and amyloid-containing stroma. Unlike DTC, MTC arises from the neuroendocrine parafollicular C cells which secrete the polypeptide calcitonin (Fig. 37.25). MTC usually occurs as a sporadic tumor, but 25% of cases, on average, occur in the

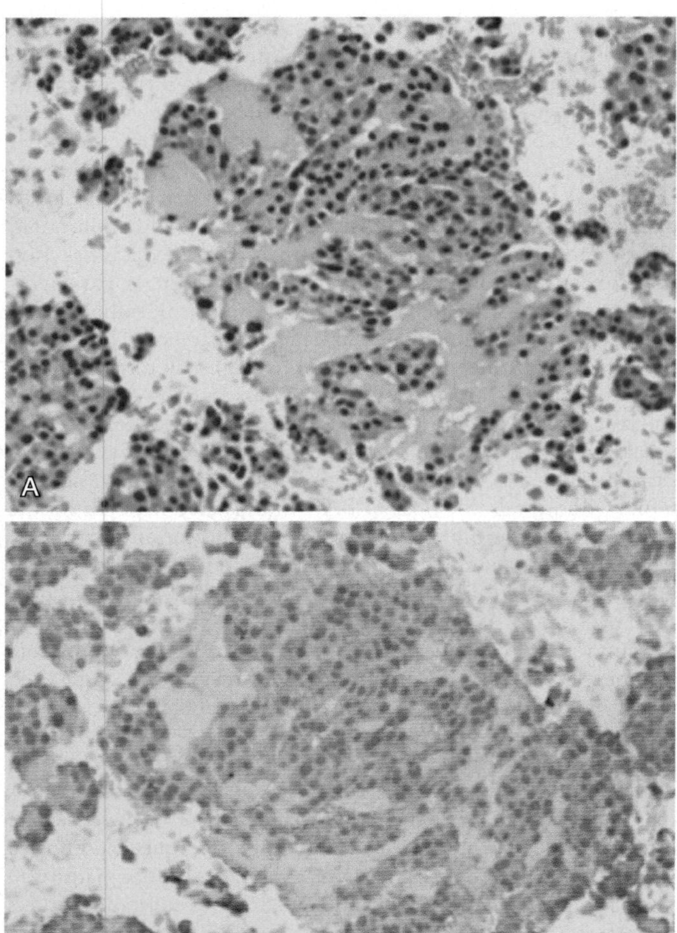

FIG. 37.25 Medullary thyroid cancer (MTC). (A) Hematoxylin and eosin staining of an MTC specimen showing plasmacytoid morphology with eccentric round nuclei, "salt-and-pepper" chromatin, small nucleoli, and amyloid infiltrate. (B) MTC exhibits cytoplasmic positivity on calcitonin staining. (Courtesy of Elham Khanafshar, MD, MS, Department of Pathology and Laboratory Medicine, University of California, San Francisco.)

context of hereditary syndromes linked to germline mutations in the *RET* proto-oncogene, such as MEN types 2A and 2B (MEN2A and MEN2B, respectively), as well as familial MTC syndrome.

Clinical Presentation

The typical clinical presentation of MTC depends on whether the disease is sporadic or hereditary. Sporadic MTC usually presents between the fourth and sixth decades of life; the most common presentation (occurring in up to 50% of cases) is a palpable neck mass from the primary tumor itself or from associated lymphadenopathy. These tumors are usually unifocal and, based on the distribution of C cells in the thyroid, often arise in the superior lateral thyroid lobes. In sporadic MTC patients with a palpable thyroid nodule, cervical nodal metastases are present in up to over 70% of cases and distant metastases in 10% to 15% of cases. The most common locations of distant metastasis are the liver, mediastinum, lungs, and bone.

Hereditary MTC presents at a younger age compared to sporadic MTC; patients with familial MTC or MEN2A typically present in the third decade of life, and patients with MEN2B present prior to the second decade. Depending on the specific *RET* mutation, hereditary MTC can present very early in life within the first months to year (see below). Unlike in sporadic MTC, hereditary MTC often presents as multifocal disease. Fortunately, most patients with hereditary MTC are now identified at an earlier age by genetic screening of at-risk family members (see below). Hereditary MTC also can present during the diagnosis and workup of an associated disease, such as pheochromocytoma or primary hyperparathyroidism.

In both sporadic and hereditary MTC, elevated levels of circulating calcitonin can lead to diarrhea, flushing, and weight loss. Uncommonly, MTC also can produce a number of other hormones, such as carcinoembryonic antigen (CEA), adrenocorticotrophic hormone, chromogranin, and somatostatin, which can lead to paraneoplastic syndromes such as Cushing and carcinoid syndromes.

RET and MTC

The RET proto-oncogene is the most important gene associated with MTC. RET is located on chromosome 10q11.2 and encodes a transmembrane tyrosine kinase receptor with regulatory effects on cell growth and survival. Virtually all patients with a hereditary form of MTC have one of over 100 described germline mutations in RET, with each mutation portending a unique profile of MTC aggressiveness and frequency of other syndromic manifestations (e.g., pheochromocytoma, primary hyperparathyroidism, cutaneous lichen amyloidosis, and Hirschsprung disease). Mutations in codon C634 are the most common.

The 2015 revised ATA guidelines around the management of MTC proposed a modified risk classification system for hereditary MTC aggressiveness based mainly on the type of *RET* mutation identified in order to better inform the timing of prophylactic thyroidectomy in affected family members.[2] This classification has three risk categories: "highest risk," "high risk," and "moderate risk." The highest-risk category includes patients with MEN2B and the codon M918T mutation in whom macroscopic MTC and nodal metastases can present within the first year of life; in these patients, total thyroidectomy is recommended as soon as possible in the first few months of life. The high-risk category comprises patients with the codon C634 and A883F mutations in whom thyroidectomy is recommended by the age of 5 years or sooner in the presence of elevated serum calcitonin levels. The moderate-risk category includes patients with all other mutations in whom either annual surveillance or thyroidectomy may be pursued. Fig. 37.26 shows the ATA management algorithm for patients with a *RET* germline mutations.

RET testing in sporadic MTC is also important in two respects. First, apparently sporadic MTCs may in fact be the initial manifestation of a hereditary syndrome. Therefore, all patients with a diagnosis of MTC or C cell hyperplasia should undergo genetic testing to rule out hereditary disease. Second, approximately 50% of sporadic MTCs have somatic *RET* mutations, which are associated with a higher incidence of nodal metastases, persistent disease, and disease-specific mortality. Therefore, they warrant more aggressive surveillance and treatment.

Workup

MTC is definitively diagnosed by FNA biopsy, from which cytology can demonstrate the presence of stromal amyloid and absence

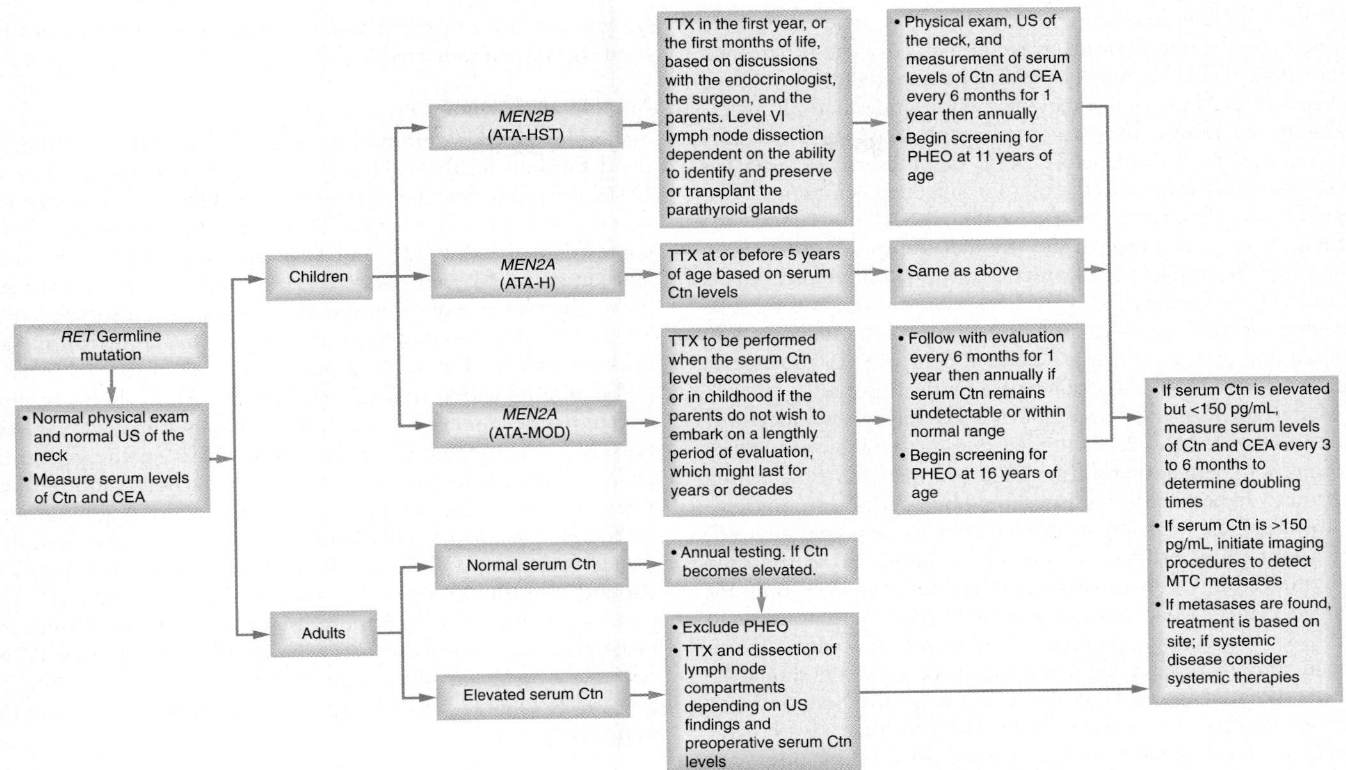

FIG. 37.26 Recommended management of patients at risk for hereditary medullary thyroid cancer *(MTC)* based on positive *RET* germline mutation detected on genetic screening. (From Wells SA Jr, Asa SL, Dralle H, et al. Revised American Thyroid Association guidelines for the management of medullary thyroid carcinoma. *Thyroid.* 2015;25:567–610.)

of thyroid follicular cells. Measurement of elevated calcitonin levels in the FNA washout fluid increases the accuracy of FNA to 98%. Once MTC is diagnosed, measurement of serum calcitonin and CEA is recommended to establish a pretreatment baseline. Measurement of serum calcitonin and CEA as a screening test in the absence of cytologically confirmed MTC, on the other hand, is controversial. ATA guidelines recommend that a serum calcitonin of at least 100 pg/mL should be considered suspicious for MTC. In addition, a calcitonin value at least 500 pg/mL prior to treatment should raise the suspicion for distant metastases. Notably, serum calcitonin can be elevated due to multiple states other than MTC, including autoimmune thyroiditis, hyperparathyroidism, lung cancer, and age younger than 3 years. Serum CEA is not a specific biomarker for MTC and thus is more useful as an adjunctive test. CEA is often elevated in more aggressive MTCs that have lost calcitonin secretory function, thus acting as a marker for dedifferentiation. Measurement of both serum calcitonin and CEA is recommended to establish a pretreatment baseline and to track disease progression.

Neck ultrasound is the most important preoperative imaging study in MTC in that it provides sensitive characterization of thyroid lesions and cervical lymph nodes. Cross-sectional imaging of the neck and chest (preferably CT with IV contrast) may be indicated depending on the suspicion for bulky or locally advanced disease. In higher-risk patients such as those with high-burden cervical disease, symptoms suspicious for distant metastases, or serum calcitonin levels at least 500 pg/mL, radiographic survey for distant metastases should be performed. The most common tests include multiphase CT or MRI of the liver, axial MRI, and bone scintigraphy.

All patients with hereditary MTC should be biochemically screened for pheochromocytoma and primary hyperparathyroidism. If a pheochromocytoma is identified, then treatment for the pheochromocytoma should precede that of MTC in virtually all cases. Primary hyperparathyroidism can be surgically managed at the time of thyroidectomy for MTC, if present concurrently.

Surgical Treatment

The surgical treatment for MTC is divided into that for clinically evident disease versus that performed as a prophylactic measure at an early age in hereditary MTC syndromes.

Clinically evident MTC is treated with at minimum total thyroidectomy and bilateral central neck dissection, as central nodal metastases are present in more than 70% of cases with palpable tumors regardless of tumor size. The role of routine lateral neck dissection (levels II–V) is controversial. One school of thought advocates for prophylactic lateral neck dissection on at least the side ipsilateral to the primary tumor, as several single-institution series have demonstrated not only a more than 70% incidence of ipsilateral lateral neck metastases, but also a more than 40% incidence in the contralateral lateral neck. The opposing opinion cites the morbidity of lateral neck dissection, along with the fact that over 65% of patients with MTC have evidence of systemic disease even after bilateral central and lateral neck dissections. Recognizing this controversy, the current ATA guidelines recommend that prophylactic ipsilateral and contralateral lateral neck dissection be considered based on serum calcitonin levels; for example, in patients with ipsilateral lateral neck metastases noted on preoperative ultrasound, prophylactic contralateral lateral neck dissection should be considered if the basal serum calcitonin level is at least 200 pg/mL.

For at-risk children with hereditary MTC syndromes, prophylactic total thyroidectomy is recommended. The progression of hereditary MTC generally proceeds sequentially from C cell hyperplasia to MTC to locoregional lymph nodes and ultimately to distant metastases. The purpose of prophylactic thyroidectomy is to remove the thyroid before MTC develops, or if cancer has developed, it is confined to the thyroid, such that central neck dissection is unnecessary and cure is secured. As described above, the optimal timing for prophylactic thyroidectomy depends largely on the specific germline *RET* mutation, which can predict typical age of MTC onset as well as aggressiveness of disease. This must be balanced with the risk of complication rates of thyroidectomy in children and infants, which are elevated compared to adolescents and adults even in the hands of experienced surgeons.[31]

Management of the parathyroid glands during thyroidectomy in patients with MEN2A is unique due to the 20% penetrance of primary hyperparathyroidism. As mentioned above, screening for primary hyperparathyroidism should be done prior to thyroidectomy. For biochemically diagnosed primary hyperparathyroidism, a four-gland exploration should be performed at the time of thyroidectomy with intentional resection performed only for enlarged glands. Most cases of primary hyperparathyroidism in MEN2 involve a single parathyroid adenoma. If a normal parathyroid gland is devascularized during surgery, then it should be autotransplanted into a heterotopic site (e.g., the nondominant forearm) for ease of access due to the risk of primary hyperparathyroidism developing in the transplanted tissue later in life.

For patients with familial MTC, MEN2B, or sporadic MTC undergoing thyroidectomy, devascularized parathyroids may be autotransplanted into the sternocleidomastoid because these patients are not at increased risk for primary hyperparathyroidism.

Postoperative Surveillance and Adjuvant Therapies

MTC is associated with an overall 50% rate of disease recurrence; therefore, close postoperative surveillance should begin as soon as 3 months after surgery with a check of serum calcitonin and CEA levels. If these values are negative or in the normal range, they should be repeated at every 6-month intervals for the first year, and then annually thereafter. The doubling time of calcitonin (and to a lesser extent CEA) is an accurate estimate of MTC growth as well as a prognostic indicator. A calcitonin doubling time of less than 6 months is associated with a 5-year survival rate of 25%, compared to 92% if the doubling times is greater than or equal to 6 months.[32] Elevated calcitonin levels raise the suspicion of recurrence and should be further evaluated with physical exam and neck ultrasound; significantly elevated calcitonin levels (>150 pg/mL) should prompt additional imaging workup for recurrent or persistent distant disease, including chest CT, multiphase CT or MRI of the liver, bone scintigraphy, and MRI of the pelvis and axial skeleton.

Adjuvant therapies play important but limited roles in MTC management. Traditional systemic chemotherapy regimens are generally ineffective, and RAI is not taken up by the parafollicular cells. Two tyrosine kinase receptor therapies are currently approved in the United States for the treatment of advanced MTC (see below). EBRT to the neck and mediastinum is effective for locoregional control in patients with incompletely resected tumors or those at high risk of local recurrence, although there is no benefit to overall survival. Isolated distant metastases to the liver, bone, and brain may be addressed with local therapies, such as surgical resection, ablation, and EBRT. Patients with significant tumor burden and distant metastases at initial presentation can be considered for up-front systemic therapy in conjunction with local therapies if indicated.

Staging and Prognosis

Staging of MTC is summarized in a tables in Ref. [22a]; although the definitions for the T, N, and M categories are the same as for DTC, the prognostic stage groupings are different. The overall 10-year survival of patients with MTC is approximately 80%. Disease confined to the thyroid gland at presentation confers an excellent long-term prognosis with 5-year overall survival approaching 95%. The presence of cervical nodal metastases is associated with a reduction in survival to approximately 75%, and distant metastases are associated with compromised survival further to 35%.

Despite its widespread use, the current AJCC TNM staging system has been modeled largely after that used for DTC. However, MTC is inherently distinct from DTC, so the generalizability of one staging system to another is likely not appropriate. Adam and colleagues proposed a revision in the staging groups based on a recursive partitioning analysis using the National Cancer Data Base and the SEER databases to better divide MTC patients into four groups with more similar overall survival. The proposed revision led to a more useful and stepwise downward progression of survival estimates compared to the existing TNM system, with 5-year overall survival of 92% to 94%, 86% to 87%, 69% to 81%, and 33% to 35% for stages I, II, III, and IV, respectively.

Anaplastic Thyroid Cancer

ATC is an extremely aggressive undifferentiated tumor of follicular cell origin. ATC is uncommon, comprising approximately 1% of all thyroid cancers. The mean age at diagnosis is 65 years, with a 2:1 female-to-male incidence ratio; a history multinodular goiter and previous thyroidectomy exists in up to 50% of patients. ATC is thought to arise from DTC of follicular cell origin (particularly PTC), based on the coexistence of PTC in at least 30% of cases, as well as longitudinal case studies demonstrating dedifferentiation and transformation from differentiated cancer to ATC over time. On a molecular level, the dedifferentiation event in ATC may involve mutations in the p53, 16p, catenin, beta 1, and PIK3CA genes.

Patients with ATC typically present with a rapidly enlarging neck mass. Unlike in other thyroid tumors, local cervical symptoms are frequent and severe and include neck pain, dyspnea, cough/hemoptysis, dysphagia, and hoarseness. Over half of patients have cervical lymphadenopathy, and 15% to 50% of patients have distant metastases at the time of presentation. The most common sites of distant metastases include the lungs, bone, and brain; other sites may include the skin, liver, kidneys, pancreas, heart, and adrenal glands.

Diagnosis is confirmed with FNA, which is associated with a 95% diagnostic accuracy for malignancy overall and a 90% accuracy specifically for ATC. Incisional biopsy is typically not required. Cytologic features of ATC include mixed patterns of spindled, pleomorphic giant, and squamoid cells with mitotic figures, atypical mitoses, and extensive necrosis. ATCs typically do not secrete or stain for Tg, although differentiated components of tumors may retain the ability to make Tg (Fig. 37.27).

Workup and management of ATC should proceed expeditiously because of the rapid progression of disease. Workup includes neck ultrasound and cross-sectional imaging of the neck and mediastinum to assess the extent of locoregional disease. Unlike in DTCs or MTCs, PET scan is recommended for a metastatic

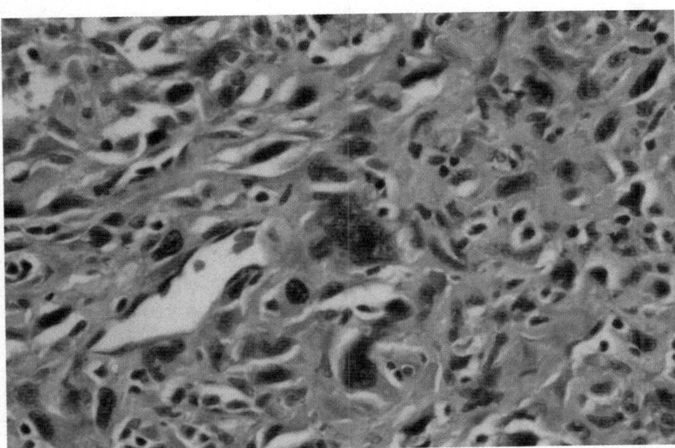

FIG. 37.27 Anaplastic thyroid cancer. Hematoxylin and eosin staining showing marked nuclear pleomorphism, oval to spindle-shaped cells, and multinucleated tumor cell. (From Baloch ZW, Livolsi VA. Surgical pathology of the thyroid gland. In: Randolph GW, ed. *Surgery of the Thyroid and Parathyroid Glands 2*. Philadelphia: Elsevier Saunders; 2013:420.)

survey in the initial evaluation of ATC due to its intense PET-avidity.

According to the AJCC TNM system, all ATCs are considered stage IV disease, and overall prognosis is dismal, with nearly 100% disease-specific mortality. Median survival in patients without distant metastases at the time of diagnosis is 6 months. Because of rapid lethality and relative rarity of ATC, there are few randomized trials of treatment strategies, and treatment recommendations are largely based on single-institution case series and clinical experience. There is equipoise around the benefit of thyroidectomy, chemotherapy, and radiotherapy for these tumors, and the specific treatment regimen is usually decided based on a case-by-case basis. Multimodal treatment with EBRT and systemic therapy is indicated for locally advanced and metastatic disease. Newer mutation-directed systemic therapies hold some promise (see below); if possible, mutational analysis of the tumor should be performed to optimize therapy selection. Thyroidectomy may be pursued for resectable localized disease confined to the thyroid, and for formerly unresectable tumors that have been downstaged with other therapies. RAI is typically not indicated except in selected scenarios in which a large DTC component exists. All patients with ATC should have initial consultations with palliative and end-of-life care specialists, and all treatment options should be weighed carefully to balance the morbidity of treatment versus that of the natural course of disease.

Systemic Therapies for Advanced Thyroid Cancers

Although the majority of thyroid cancer is made up of DTC, which is indolent and carries an excellent prognosis, less than 10% of cases demonstrate more aggressive behavior and are more challenging to treat. This grouping of advanced thyroid cancers actually consists of a number of different tumors, including locally advanced, rapidly progressive, or metastatic DTC/PDTC and MTC, as well as ATC. These cancers require a multimodal treatment strategy with alternative systemic therapies as a component.

There are currently four Food and Drug Administration (FDA)–approved systemic multitargeted tyrosine kinase inhibitor drugs for the treatment of advanced thyroid cancer in the United States.[33] Lenvatinib and sorafenib are approved for the treatment of RAI-refractory DTC, and vandetanib and cabozantinib are approved for progressive and advanced MTC. Each agent has a unique profile of multikinase targets; for example, lenvatinib targets VEGF receptor 1 to 3, fibroblast growth factor receptor 1 to 4, platelet-derived growth factor receptor-α, RET, and c-Kit signaling pathways, whereas vandetanib selectively targets RET, VEGF receptor, and epidermal growth factor receptor signaling. Sorafenib and vandetanib were the first FDA-approved agents for the treatment of advanced RAI-refractory DTC and MTC, respectively. Their approved uses were based on phase 3 open-label randomized controlled trials showing significant improvement in progression-free survival, as evaluated by Response Evaluation Criteria in Solid Tumors (RECIST) criteria and defined as the time from date of randomization to the date of radiologic progression or death. Adverse reactions are common for these agents, occurring in up to 70% of patients. Because of their multitargeted mechanisms, each of these four agents is (or has been) studied for their efficacy in advanced thyroid cancers other than the specific ones for which they are approved. The ATA guidelines recommend the use of these kinase inhibitors for advanced metastatic, rapidly progressive, symptomatic, and/or imminently threatening disease that is not otherwise amenable to local control using other approaches; however, the guidelines also advise that patients be thoroughly counseled about the risks versus benefits of these drugs, considering its significant side effect profile and the current lack of evidence of benefit in overall survival or quality of life.

There are a number of promising new drugs that more selectively inhibit molecules and pathways specific to thyroid oncogenesis. The selective BRAF and MEK inhibitors dabrafenib and trametinib were FDA approved as combination therapy for BRAF V600E mutated advanced and unresectable ATC based on a phase 2 international open-label trial in 16 ATC patients, which demonstrated a 69% overall response rate, with 80% survival at 1 year. They also have been studied in advanced DTC. One mechanism behind these drugs' efficacy may be in their ability to redifferentiate thyroid cancer cells so that they may once again respond to RAI treatment. The first to demonstrate this effect was selumetinib in 2013, although subsequent trials have failed to demonstrate benefit, leading to withdrawal of the drug from further clinical trials in DTC. Nevertheless, multiple preclinical and early-phase clinical studies have shown tumors' ability to take up RAI after treatment with other BRAF or MEK inhibitors.

Another selective inhibitor class of drugs that has been studied is the mammalian target of rapamycin, including everolimus and temsirolimus. These agents block the PI3K/Akt pathway, which is downstream of RAS. Everolimus has been studied in a trial of advanced thyroid cancers, including DTC, MTC, and ATC. It appears to be highly effective in selected patients, although the overall response rate is low. Other selective inhibitors that are currently in preclinical or early clinical evaluation include those inhibiting RET, NTRK, ALK, and ROS1. Loxo-292, a selective RET inhibitor, has recently been granted a breakthrough therapy designation by the FDA, and it is currently in clinical trials under expedited review. Lastly, based on successful implementation in melanoma and other solid organ cancers, immunotherapy is currently under active clinical investigation in advanced thyroid cancers. Pembrolizumab, spartalizumab, and nivolumab are immunotherapy agents currently on the market, all of which are inhibitors of the programmed cell death protein 1 on T cells.

Doxorubicin is the only FDA-approved cytotoxic chemotherapy agent for thyroid cancer in the United States. It appears to have a modest benefit in ATC but has not shown consistent evidence of benefit in advanced DTC or MTC. Anecdotal evidence exists around its potential benefit in selected patients who are unresponsive to other therapies.

THYROIDECTOMY

Indications and Nomenclature

Broadly speaking, the indications for thyroidectomy include the following:

1. Hyperthyroidism for which nonsurgical management has failed or is not preferred,
2. Goiters with or without local compressive symptoms, and
3. Thyroid nodules and thyroid cancer.

The extent of thyroid resection was a topic of much discussion historically, but in modern practice, the vast majority of thyroid resections fall under two categories: *total thyroidectomy*, in which all or nearly all of the visible thyroid gland is excised, and *thyroid lobectomy* (also referred to as hemithyroidectomy), in which all of the visible thyroid on one side is excised along with the isthmus and, if present, the pyramidal lobe. *Near-total thyroidectomy*, in which less than 1 g of remnant thyroid tissue is left at the ligament of Berry, is also commonly performed. *Subtotal thyroidectomy*, in which 3 to 5 g of thyroid tissue is left, is less commonly performed today. The rationale for these lesser-extent lobar resections has been to protect the RLN and blood supply to the parathyroids, as well as to preserve thyroid function without the need for thyroid hormone replacement. Lastly, *isthmusectomy* is resection of only the thyroid isthmus and pyramidal lobe.

Thyroidectomy Outcomes

There are over 130,000 thyroidectomies performed annually in the United States, making thyroidectomy one of the most common surgical procedures. The rate of thyroidectomy is likely to increase in pace with the increased number of thyroid biopsies and diagnoses of thyroid cancer.[34] Thyroidectomy has evolved from a dangerous and morbid operation historically (see above) to a generally safe procedure, many of which can be performed in the outpatient setting.

Despite its safety, thyroidectomy is associated with a risk of complications such as RLN and EBSLN injury, hypoparathyroidism, and neck hematoma (see below), which, although rare, can nevertheless lead to significant patient morbidity and disability when they occur. Various efforts to minimize these complications and optimize thyroidectomy outcomes exist. One approach is to standardize the teaching and performance of thyroidectomy technique, such as that found in the *Operative Standards for Cancer Surgery* initiative by the American College of Surgeons, in an effort to minimize the potentially harmful effects of significant deviations of technique from evidence-based norms.[35]

Other efforts to study and improve thyroidectomy have focused on concentrating expertise and referral patterns into more experienced hands, as surgeon experience as measured by operative volume has been clearly established as an important and modifiable determinant of thyroidectomy outcomes. A large body of literature has demonstrated that higher-volume surgeons have fewer complications, shorter hospital stays, and lower costs. The threshold for what qualifies as a "high-volume" surgeon has been studied extensively; a recent study of 16,954 patients undergoing total thyroidectomy between 1998 and 2009 in the Nationwide Inpatient Sample database demonstrated on restricted cubic splines analysis that patient outcomes improved with increasing surgeon volume up to a threshold of 26 cases per year.[36] Data such as these will be important for setting minimum case volume thresholds for professional society credentialing and volume-based referral initiatives.

Preoperative Preparation

All patients undergoing thyroidectomy should have biochemical assessment of thyroid function, as well as appropriate imaging studies, particularly neck ultrasound. As described in more detail above, thyroid nodular disease or malignancy should be assessed with appropriate FNA biopsy. For operations performed for hyperthyroidism, patients should ideally be rendered euthyroid by the time of operation with antithyroid medication with or without beta blockade; for Graves disease, Lugol solution or SSKI also can be administered within 10 days of surgery per surgeon preference for rapid correction of thyroid function. Measurement of serum calcium levels should be performed in patients at risk for concurrent primary hyperparathyroidism, such as those with MEN2A.

Assessment of Voice and Laryngeal Function

Voice assessment is critical prior to thyroidectomy, as vocal cord dysfunction is one of the most important complications of thyroid surgery. Vocal cord dysfunction can lead to significant decrement in quality of life, and it is one of the most frequent causes of medicolegal action. All preoperative voice assessments include a thorough patient history around voice changes and abnormalities, prior history of surgery that may have been associated with the risk injury to the vagus verve or the RLN, and the surgeon's objective assessment of the voice.

Laryngoscopy is an indispensable tool in the objective preoperative assessment of vocal cord function and must be performed in patients at higher risk for vocal cord paralysis, including those with a history of voice changes or prior relevant surgical history, or thyroid cancers with fixed masses, posteriorly extending extrathyroidal extension, or bulky metastases. The role of routine preoperative laryngoscopy for all patients regardless of risk assessment is controversial. Proponents of routine laryngoscopy in all patients cite 1) its ability to confirm preoperative vocal cord dysfunction in up to 3.5% of patients with benign thyroid disease and in up to 8% of patients with thyroid cancer; 2) its ability to definitively diagnose preoperative dysfunction is important for operative management in these cases, and 3) vocal cord paralysis can be associated with a normal voice in up to 20% of cases.[37] On the other hand, proponents of selective laryngoscopy state that the true incidence of preoperative vocal cord dysfunction in patients with a truly negative risk assessment by history and physical exam is closer to 0.5% and that subjecting all thyroid surgery patients to laryngoscopy is not cost-effective.[38]

Transcutaneous laryngeal ultrasound has emerged recently as a noninvasive alternative to laryngoscopy for assessment of vocal cord function in selected patients undergoing thyroidectomy. Studies in both Asian and Western patients have demonstrated high accuracy of laryngeal ultrasound for the detection of vocal cord paralysis (sensitivity and specificity 93%–100% and 97%–100%, respectively), as well as broad applicability in thyroid surgery practices with over 74% of examinations able to adequately visualize the vocal cords for assessment.[39] In addition to its noninvasiveness, other advantages of this modality include its low cost, rapid learning curve, and increased efficiency if performed as part of another ultrasound examination.

It is less reliable in older and male patients largely due to inability of the transducer to penetrate beyond thyroid cartilage calcification.

Current ATA guidelines recommend that all patients undergoing thyroid surgery should have noninvasive preoperative voice assessment as a part of the physical examination, with the selective use of laryngoscopy for patients with preoperative voice abnormalities, history of cervical or upper chest surgery, or known thyroid cancer with posterior extrathyroidal extension or extensive nodal metastases. Laryngeal ultrasound is not incorporated into the current ATA guidelines, although its use is recommended for selected patients in other surgical guidelines.

Technique

Anesthesia and Positioning

Most thyroidectomies are performed under general endotracheal anesthesia. A neuromonitoring-specific endotracheal tube with contact electrodes for the vocal cords can be used if intraoperative neuromonitoring (IONM) is planned (see below). The patient is placed supine with both arms tucked. The back is raised 20 degrees and the neck is extended by placing a soft roll behind the scapulae, with the head resting on a foam or gel ring; this brings the thyroid up to a more anterior and superior position in the neck, which is particularly helpful for glands that have substernal extension. The head is well supported to prevent neck hyperextension and postoperative posterior neck pain.

Intraoperative preincision neck ultrasound can be useful for confirming the findings of preoperative imaging and identifying any possible new findings, as well as for assessing the overall anatomy of the thyroid to facilitate incision placement and operative planning.

Incision and Initial Exposure of the Thyroid

A centrally placed transverse incision is made between the sternal notch and the cricoid cartilage, with effort made to place the incision in a normal skin line of the neck for cosmetic purposes (Fig. 37.28). The length of the incision is typically 4 to 5 cm but should be appropriately sized based on the volume of the gland being excised as well as patient factors such as body habitus and degree of neck extension. The incision is extended through the platysma muscle, and subplatysmal flaps are raised up to the thyroid cartilage superiorly and down to the sternal notch inferiorly. Care is taken to identify the anterior jugular veins draped between platysma and the strap muscles.

The strap muscles are separated in the midline via an incision through the superficial layer of the deep cervical fascia starting at the sternal notch and extending cephalad to the thyroid cartilage. For a cancer operation, dissection of the thyroid gland is generally begun on the side of the suspected tumor. The sternohyoid, which is the more superficial of the strap muscles, is separated from the deeper sternothyroid muscle by blunt dissection. This dissection can be taken as far laterally until the ansa cervicalis is visible at the lateral border of the sternothyroid; this maneuver is useful for thyroid mobilization, particularly for larger goiters. The sternothyroid is then dissected off of the underlying thyroid capsule, and with the thyroid steadily retracted and rotated anteromedially, the carotid sheath is identified laterally (Fig. 37.29). For mobilization of larger glands, the sternothyroid may be partially or completely divided near its superior attachment to the thyroid cartilage, to be reapproximated during closure. The middle thyroid vein is identified laterally, and ligated and divided.

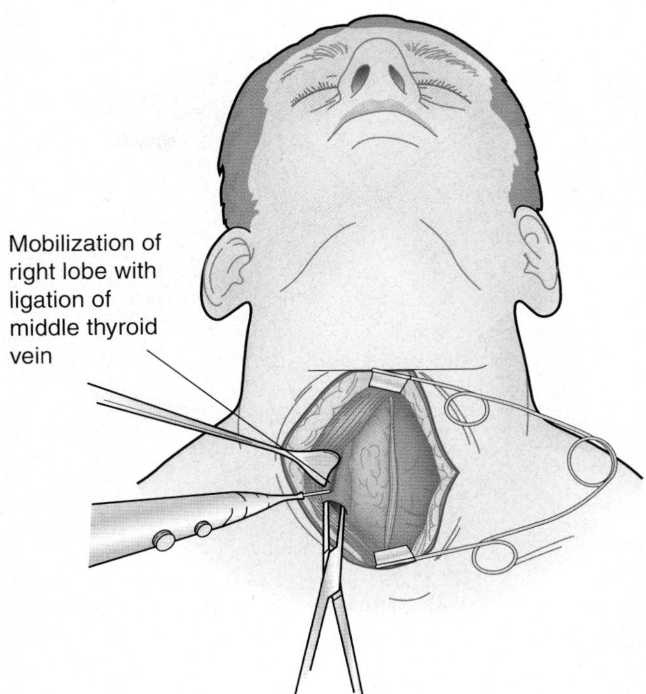

FIG. 37.28 Image depicting a cervicotomy incision to facilitate exposure. After creation of a subplatysmal plane, the strap muscles (sternohyoid and sternothyroid) are separated by dividing the tissues in the avascular midline plane from the thyroid cartilage to the suprasternal notch. The thyroid lobe is exposed by mobilizing the strap muscles away from the lobe by means of lateral retraction on the muscles. The middle vein is exposed, divided, and ligated. (From Sabiston DC Jr, ed. *Atlas of General Surgery*. Philadelphia: Saunders; 1995.)

Dissection and Release of the Superior Pole

The superior pole attachments are separated from the surrounding muscles and exposed mostly in a blunt fashion with a small peanut sponge. These exposure maneuvers are carried out superolaterally and posteriorly, with downward and lateral countertraction of the thyroid using large Kelly or Allis clamps (Fig. 37.30). This exposes the superior pole thyroid vessels, as well as some connective tissue lateral to the superior pole. These lateral tissues are carefully mobilized to below the level of the cricothyroid muscle, as the RLN passes through Berry ligament and dives deep into the laryngeal insertion point at the level of the cricoid cartilage.

The superior pole is similarly separated from the cricothyroid muscle medially with gentle blunt dissection. There is an avascular space between the medial superior pole and the cricothyroid muscle, often referred to as the space of Reeves, which is helpful for progressive dissection of the superior pole vessels. These vessels are individually isolated, ligated, and divided; the use of energy-sealing devices may replace or augment manual ligation. Care must be taken to divide these vessels close to the surface of the thyroid in order to prevent injury to the EBSLN; neuromonitoring can also assist in its identification and preservation (see below). Division and release of the superior pole vessels allow for easy sweeping of the remaining filmy tissues away from the posterior aspect of the superior pole via blunt dissection. At this point in the dissection, the superior parathyroid gland is often identified behind the mid-superior pole at the approximate level of the cricoid cartilage.

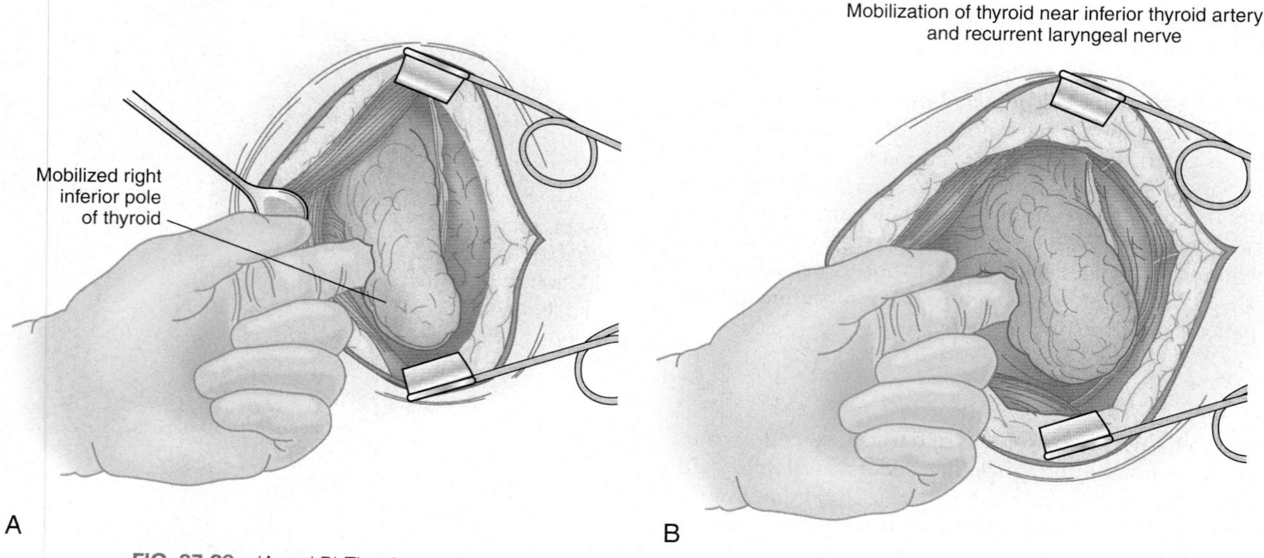

FIG. 37.29 (A and B) The thyroid lobe is retracted medially to allow the posterolateral surface of the thyroid to be exposed. (From Sabiston DC Jr, ed. *Atlas of General Surgery*. Philadelphia: Saunders; 1995.)

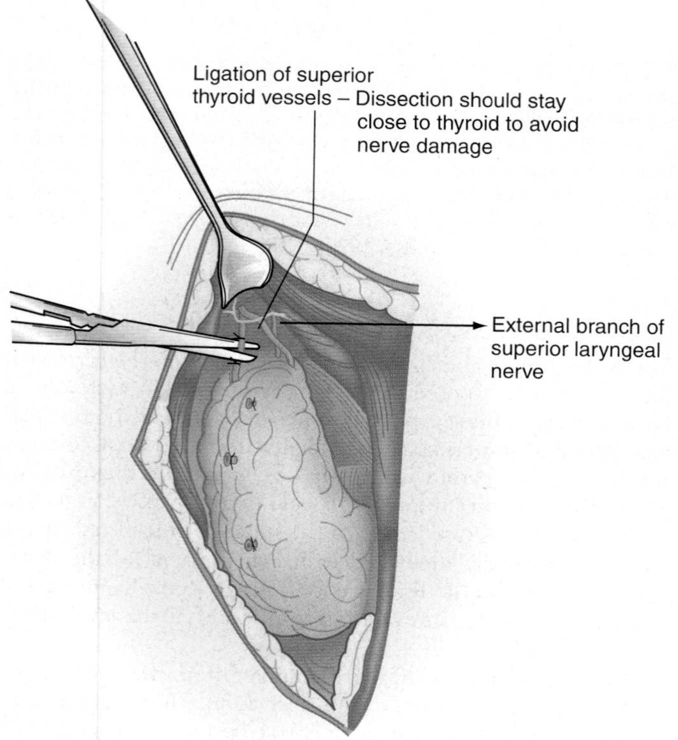

FIG. 37.30 Downward and lateral traction exposes the superior pole vessels, including branches of the superior thyroid artery. The external branch of the superior laryngeal nerve courses along the cricothyroid muscle just medial to the superior pole vessels. To avoid injury to this nerve, the superior pole vessels are divided individually as close as possible to the point where they enter the thyroid gland. (From Sabiston DC Jr, ed. *Atlas of General Surgery*. Philadelphia: Saunders; 1995.)

Mobilization of Inferior Pole and Medial Rotation of the Thyroid Lobe

The mobilization of the lateral and inferior aspects of the thyroid lobe includes identification of the inferior parathyroid gland. With the inferior thyroid lobe grasped with an Allis or large Kelly clamp and retracted anteromedially, the inferior pole vessels entering anterolateral to the tracheal surface are ligated and divided. Retraction of the strap muscles exposes the carotid artery laterally, and the thyroid is progressively rotated and delivered from the wound in an anteromedial direction. The lymphoadipose tissues immediately adjacent to the lateral aspect of the thyroid are dissected off with a combination of sharp dissection with fine-tipped dissectors and ligation of small vessels, as well as blunt sweeping with the peanut sponge.

The inferior parathyroid is usually encountered during these maneuvers as the posterolateral thyroid is exposed. The location of the inferior parathyroid gland is less constant than that of the superior gland, but it is invariably located on a plane anterior to the RLN and inferior to the inferior thyroid artery as this blood vessel crosses the RLN. In its typical location, the inferior gland is often adherent to the posterolateral surface of the inferior thyroid lobe. All normal parathyroid glands should be carefully dissected and swept away from the thyroid on as broad a vascular pedicle as possible in order to prevent devascularization.

Identification of the RLN and Completion of Lobectomy

Once the superior and inferior attachments of the thyroid lobe are freed, the majority of the gland aside from its tracheal attachments can be delivered from the incision with anteromedial rotation and retraction. Judicious retraction is performed with either a peanut sponge or with a finger wrapped with gauze. Care must be taken not to use excessive force when retracting the thyroid at this point, as this may stretch the RLN at its tethering points at Berry ligament and the larynx, which can increase the risk of neuropraxic injury.

The course of the right and left RLN varies considerably. The left RLN is typically situated deeper and more medially and runs in a straighter cephalocaudad direction along the tracheoesophageal groove, whereas the right RLN takes a more superficial and oblique course and may pass either anterior or posterior to the inferior thyroid artery (Fig. 37.31). Two commonly used rules of thumb are used for RLN identification: 1) it is located within 1 cm anteromedial to the superior parathyroid, at the level where nerve crosses the inferior thyroid artery; and 2) its course through Berry ligament is also situated just underneath and medial to the

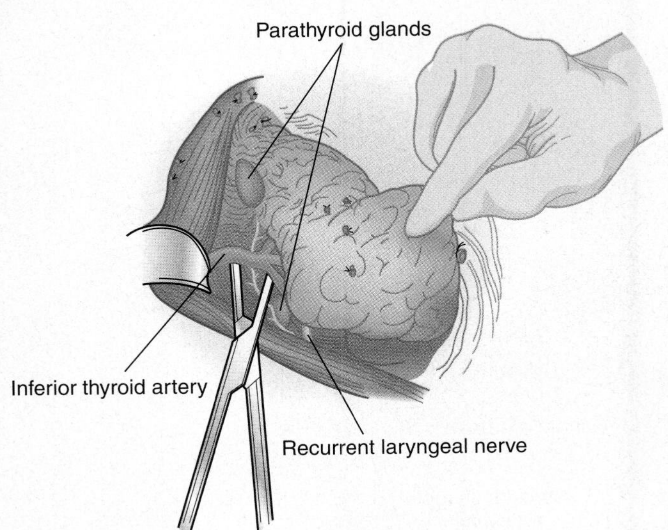

FIG. 37.31 As the thyroid is retracted medially, gentle dissection is used to expose the parathyroid glands, inferior thyroid artery, and recurrent laryngeal nerve. The recurrent nerve usually passes deep to the inferior thyroid artery but may lie anterior to it. It is best found by careful dissection just inferior to the artery. The nerve can then be traced upward, and its position in relation to the thyroid can be determined. Parathyroid glands that lie on the thyroid surface can be mobilized with their vascular supply and preserved. (From Sabiston DC Jr, ed. *Atlas of General Surgery*. Philadelphia: Saunders; 1995.)

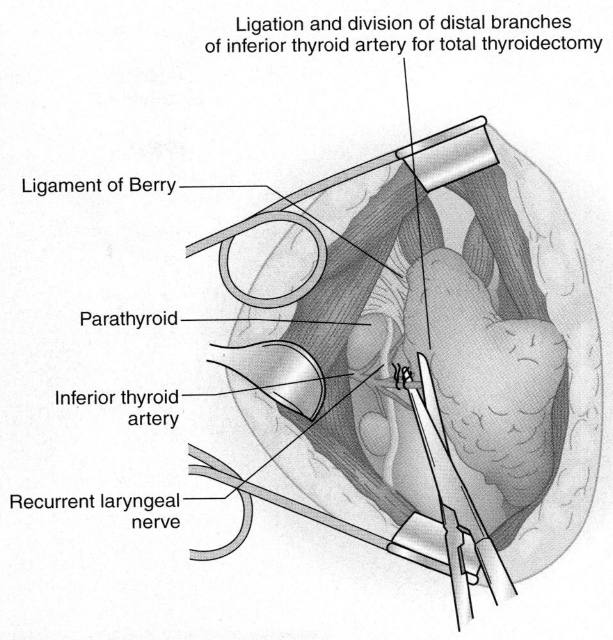

FIG. 37.32 To complete the lobectomy, branches of the inferior thyroid artery are divided at the surface of the thyroid gland. The inferior thyroid veins can then be ligated and divided. Superiorly, the connective tissue (ligament of Berry), which binds the thyroid to the tracheal rings, is carefully divided. Several small accompanying vessels are usually present, and the recurrent nerve is closest to the thyroid and most vulnerable at this point. Division of the ligament allows the thyroid to be mobilized medially. (From Sabiston DC Jr, ed. *Atlas of General Surgery*. Philadelphia: Saunders; 1995.)

tubercle of Zuckerkandl, the small posterior protuberance of the mid-thyroid lobe. Utmost care must be taken not to transect any substantial structures or tissues in this area until the RLN, inferior thyroid artery, and blood supply to the parathyroid glands are dissected and confidently identified (Fig. 37.32).

Once the parathyroids and RLN are identified and preserved, the remainder of the thyroid may be dissected in a more superficial plane off of the trachea, including Berry ligament. The course of the RLN here can vary such that it travels just under, within, or even anterior to Berry ligament; this requires careful mobilization of the nerve while the thyroid is peeled off of this area (Fig. 37.33). Fine dissection of tissues with the judicious use of manual pressure, small clips, ties, and bipolar forceps is encouraged, as this area contains tiny vessels that can nevertheless bleed and obscure the operative field. Occasionally, it may be appropriate to leave a tiny amount of thyroid tissue in the interest of protecting the nerve. The rest of the attachments to the anterior trachea are then divided, and the entire thyroid lobe should now be completely mobilized and freed (Fig. 37.34).

If a unilateral lobectomy is planned, the isthmus is divided lateral to the midline in order to minimize the risk of subsequent hypertrophy of the remaining gland (alternatively, the isthmus also can be divided early on prior to dissection of the lobe per the surgeon's preference to facilitate mobilization). The gland can be divided either with an energy sealing device or clamped and oversewn depending on the surgeon's preference (Fig. 37.35). The pyramidal lobe, present in up to 80% of patients, drapes cephalad from the isthmus just to the right or (more commonly) left of midline and may extend as high as to the hyoid bone. This must be dissected until thyroid tissue tapers into a fibrous band before division and ligation.

The specimen is properly oriented with sutures and checked to ensure that no parathyroid tissue was inadvertently removed before passing it off for pathologic examination.

Closure

Meticulous hemostasis is necessary prior to closure in order to minimize the risk of postoperative neck hematoma (see below). Some surgeons utilize a Valsalva maneuver performed by anesthesia as a confirmation of hemostasis under increased intrathoracic and cervical pressure. For closure, the sternothyroid and sternohyoid muscles are reapproximated with 3-0 absorbable sutures, with a small opening left in the lower midline to facilitate any blood to exit the deeper resection bed and into the superficial spaces. The platysma is reapproximated with similar sutures, and the skin is closed with a 5-0 subcuticular suture. No drain is required in the majority of cases.

Postoperative Care and Complications

Postoperatively, patients are positioned in a low Fowler position with the head and shoulders elevated at least 10 to 20 degrees in order to maintain low venous pressure in the neck. Diet is advanced quickly as the patient emerges from the effects of anesthesia. For patients who have undergone total thyroidectomy, serum calcium levels can be tracked periodically during the hospital stay. Prophylactic oral calcium supplementation can be administered, and additional supplementation may be given for symptomatic hypocalcemia. Prophylactic calcitriol also may be started preoperatively in patients at higher risk of postoperative hypocalcemia, such as those with Graves disease. Some practitioners measure preclosure intraoperative PTH or 4-hour postoperative intact PTH levels to help guide the dosing of calcium/calcitriol supplementation. There are several variations of these strategies with evidence-based literature, and any one of them would be helpful in the prevention and treatment of

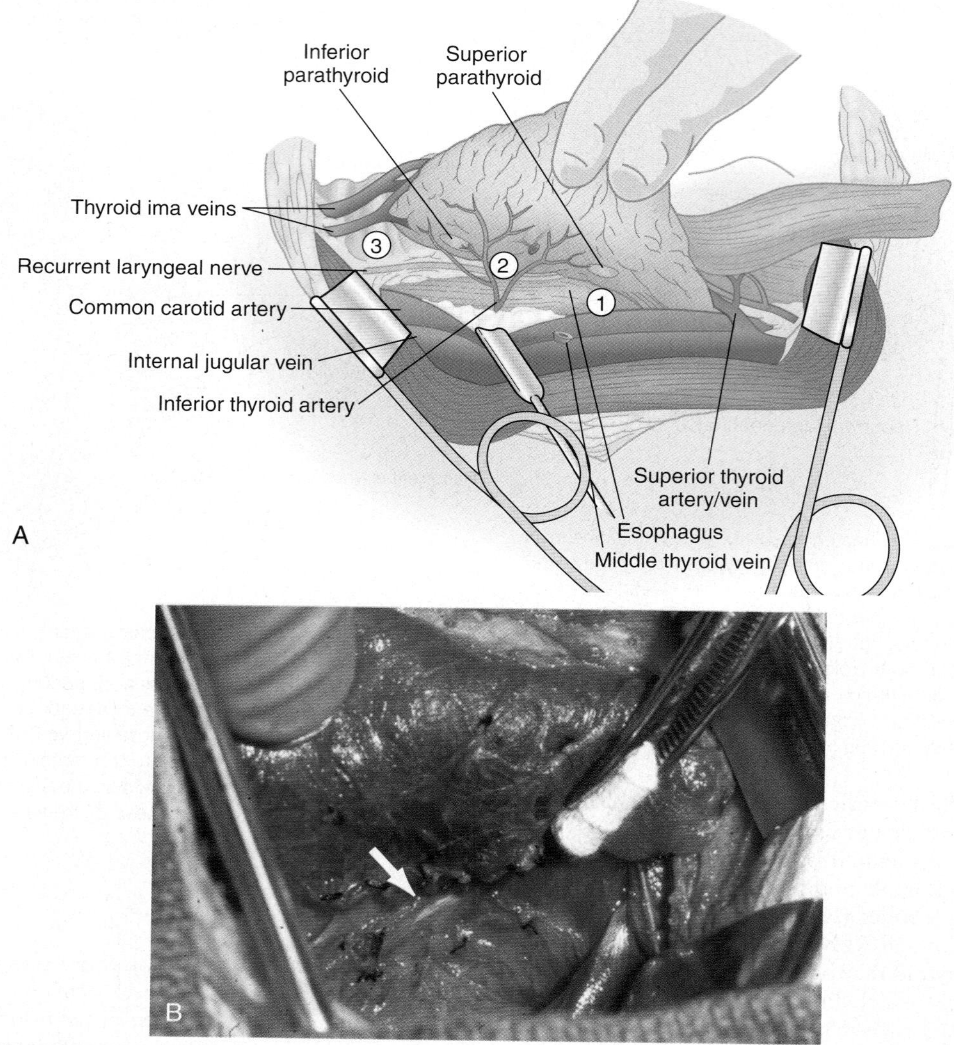

FIG. 37.33 (A) During thyroidectomy, the recurrent laryngeal nerve is at greatest risk for injury at the ligament of Berry *(1)* during ligation of branches of the inferior thyroid artery *(2)* and at the thoracic inlet *(3)*. (B) Intraoperative photo of the recurrent laryngeal nerve in the tracheoesophageal groove *(arrow)*. (A, From Kahky MP, Weber RS. Complications of surgery of the thyroid and parathyroid glands. *Surg Clin North Am.* 1993;73:307–321.)

postoperative hypocalcemia. Patients who had undergone first-time unilateral lobectomy do not require any biochemical evaluation or calcium supplementation.

The vast majority of patients are discharged within 2 to 24 hours after surgery, with most procedures being performed in the outpatient setting. Patients having undergone total thyroidectomy are prescribed thyroid hormone replacement at a weight-based dose. Some practitioners prescribe a time-limited course of prophylactic calcium supplementation. Opioid analgesics are virtually never needed upon discharge. Most patients can return to work or full activity within 1 week and are typically seen for a postoperative check and pathology review within 2 weeks.

The length of hospital stay following thyroidectomy has evolved. Historically, patients undergoing thyroidectomy have been observed overnight so that complications, particularly neck hematoma (see below), could be identified and managed expeditiously. Over the past decade, however, outpatient thyroidectomy has become a safe alternative for many selected patients undergoing routine thyroidectomy, as the rate and sequelae of neck hematoma have been shown to be acceptable and similar to those undergoing thyroidectomy with at least one overnight stay in the hospital. We would suggest that outpatient thyroidectomy is appropriate for patients who 1) live within driving distance to the hospital, 2) have reliable transportation and adult support at home for at least 24 hours, 3) do not have significant perioperative comorbidities or take anticoagulants, and 4) do not have Graves disease.

Complications

Thyroidectomy is associated with three major complications: vocal cord paralysis from RLN injury, hypoparathyroidism, and postoperative neck hematoma.

Vocal cord paralysis. Rates of temporary and permanent RLN injury during thyroidectomy are in the 4% to 10% and 0.5% to 2% ranges, respectively[40]; rates in the pediatric population are estimated to be up to fourfold higher.[31] Unilateral injury to the RLN and resultant vocal cord paralysis can cause a spectrum of problems with the voice or swallowing, due to the mixed motor

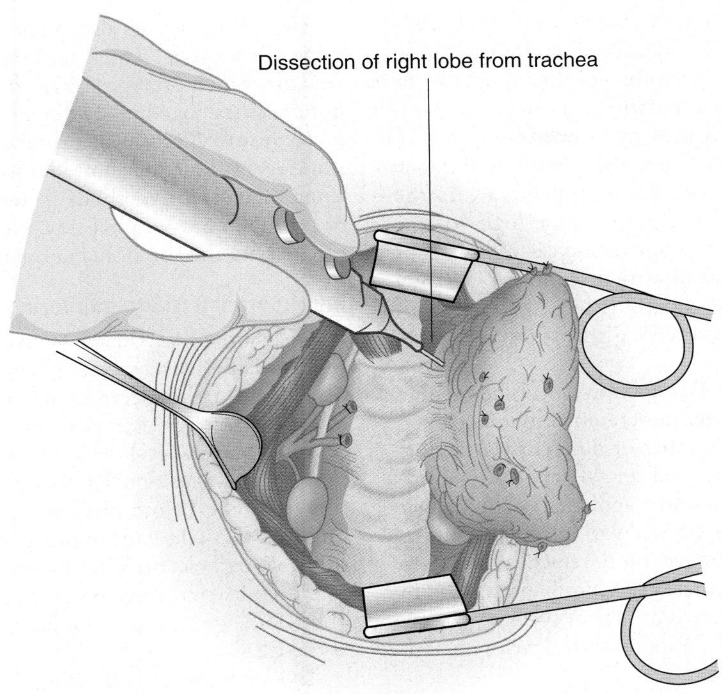

FIG. 37.34 Dissection of the medial tracheal attachments is minimally vascular. Dissection is extended under the isthmus, and the specimen is divided so that the isthmus is included with the resected lobe. The pyramidal lobe also is included if present. (From Sabiston DC Jr, ed. *Atlas of General Surgery*. Philadelphia: Saunders; 1995.)

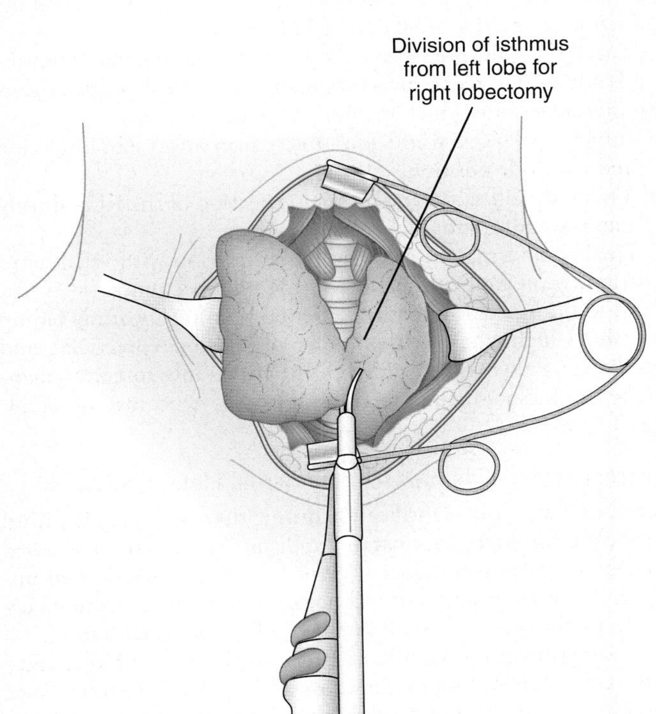

FIG. 37.35 The thyroid can now be divided with an energy device so that the isthmus is included in the specimen. (From Sabiston DC Jr, ed. *Atlas of General Surgery*. Philadelphia: Saunders; 1995.)

and sensory fibers within the nerve. Symptoms can include hoarse and breathy voice, vocal fatigue, dysphagia, and aspiration. Rarely, bilateral RLN injury with resultant resting vocal cord position in the midline can lead to airway compromise and can potentially require temporary or permanent tracheostomy. Risk factors for RLN injury include low surgeon volume, reoperative thyroid surgery, more extensive surgery for malignancy, Graves disease, and large substernal goiter.

Injury to the EBSLN also can lead to postoperative voice abnormalities due to its innervation of the cricothyroid muscle and contribution to vocal cord muscle tone. Symptoms of EBSLN injury include vocal fatigue, decreased ability to reach higher pitch, and decreased ability to project the voice. Definitive diagnosis of EBSLN injury is challenging as laryngoscopy is often normal and may require electromyographic studies; as such, estimates of the rate of injury are imperfect and range from 2.5% to 28%.[40]

Hypoparathyroidism. Hypoparathyroidism is the most common complication of thyroid surgery. The rate of temporary hypoparathyroidism is estimated to be as high as 5% to 15%, but the vast majority of these cases resolve within 6 months, leading to a rate of permanent hypoparathyroidism of 1% to 3%.[41] The wide variation in rates is in part due to differences in the definition of hypoparathyroidism in the published literature, which can be based on biochemical evidence of decreased serum calcium and/or PTH levels, or symptomatic hypocalcemia requiring calcium or vitamin D supplementation. Risk factors for hypoparathyroidism include bilateral neck exploration, extensive central neck dissection, reoperative surgery, thyroidectomy for Graves disease, and pediatric patients.

The blood supply to the parathyroid glands is extremely delicate and easily injured, so meticulous dissection and preservation of the glands is critical. All thyroidectomy specimens should be checked for inadvertently resected parathyroid tissue; if parathyroid tissue is present and confirmed by either frozen section or intraoperative PTH aspiration, then the parathyroid tissue can be preserved on ice, minced, and autotransplanted into the sternocleidomastoid muscle prior to closure. Some high-volume endocrine surgical units administer prophylactic calcium with or without calcitriol supplementation in patients undergoing total thyroidectomy, with higher-risk populations (e.g., patients with Graves disease, pediatric patients) receiving preoperative administration as well.[41]

Postoperative neck hematoma. Postoperative neck hematoma occurs in 0.1% to 1.1% of patients undergoing thyroidectomy. Various studies have identified a number of different risk factors for hematoma, particularly male sex, advanced age, bilateral operation, Graves disease, and use of anticoagulants.[42] The danger lies not in the effect of blood loss on circulating blood volume, but rather on the local compressive effect on the trachea leading to rapid airway compromise. Neck hematoma typically presents with pain, oozing from the incision, ecchymosis, firm swelling overlying the resection bed and incision. Patients can develop stridor with rapid airway collapse.

The vast majority of hematomas occur within the first 6 hours after the operation, 20% of cases occur between 6 and 24 hours, and very few cases occur afterward.[43] The key to management is early recognition and management. Depending on the clinical status of the patient, the patient can be transported immediately back to the operating room for opening of the incision under a controlled setting with anesthesia availability; however, if the patient exhibits signs of impending airway collapse, the incision should be opened immediately wherever the patient may be. Because of this possibility, instruments for emergent opening of the incision should be present at the bedside at all times. When opening the incision, all three layers to the thyroidectomy bed—the skin, platysma, and strap muscles—must be opened to allow for maximal decompression.

Adjunctive Technologies During Thyroidectomy

Energy Sealing Devices and Hemostatic Agents

Technologies for minimizing the risk of bleeding after thyroidectomy generally fall under two categories: energy sealing devices, which are used as adjuncts or replacements for traditional clamp/tie or clipping methods for ligation of bleeding vessels; and hemostatic agents, which are typically placed on the thyroid resection bed as adjuvant methods mainly for controlling oozing-type bleeding. Energy sealing devices clamp down with force on blood vessels and apply one of two different types of energy—bipolar radiofrequency or ultrasonic vibration—to fuse the clamped tissues together. These devices are used for ligation of major structures such as the superior pole vessels, and some practitioners use them also for dissection of finer vessels around the RLN and the parathyroid glands; however, because their primary limitation is the radial spread of thermal energy and potential for damage to neighboring structures, care must be taken when using them around these critical structures. Multiple metaanalyses have demonstrated that energy sealing devices are associated with equivalent outcomes compared to traditional clamp-tie methods with respect to operative blood loss and rate of postoperative neck hematoma, along with improved operative times.[43]

Hemostatic agents also fall under multiple mechanistic groups: topical hemostats, which facilitate clotting at a bleeding surface; sealants, which prevent leakage from vessels; and adhesives, which bond tissues together. Different products can have overlapping mechanisms. A recent metaanalysis grouping studies of all hemostatic agents together showed improvements compared to conventional hemostatic methods in terms of drain output and length of postoperative hospital stay, but no significant differences were observed in the risk of hematoma formation.[44]

Intraoperative Neuromonitoring

IONM systems for the RLN involve the use of electrical stimulator probes to deliver electrical current to the vagus nerve or RLN, which leads to an electromyographic signal at the vocal cord detected by contact electrodes embedded on the surface of the endotracheal tube. All IONM systems use intermittent direct stimulation of the vagus and RLN with electrical current delivered via contact probe before, during, and after thyroid resection; some surgeons also add continuous stimulation of the vagus nerve via a flexible cuff electrode to monitor for fluctuations in the quality and integrity of the nerve signal in real time during the dissection. The IONM systems can also be used to stimulate and test integrity of the EBSLN.

The adoption of IONM has increased over the past 15 years, and in some countries, the routine use of IONM is mandatory. Despite the widespread adoption, the added benefit of IONM for reducing the risk of RLN injury remains controversial. Multiple systematic reviews and metaanalyses have failed to demonstrate a significant benefit of routine IONM in reducing RLN injury rates during thyroidectomy, although these conclusions have been limited by the quality of data coming largely from nonrandomized observational studies.[45] Proponents of IONM cite its benefit in higher-risk operative scenarios, such as reoperative surgery, surgery for malignancy, thyrotoxicosis, or substernal goiter,[46] and the reduction in the risk of bilateral RLN injury.

The 2018 guidelines from the International Neural Monitoring Study Group recommend standardized IONM practices during thyroidectomy, which include the following steps:

1. Initial vagal nerve stimulation to confirm intact RLN function and electrode position;
2. Visual identification and direct stimulation of the RLN during the course of thyroid lobectomy, and
3. Final reconfirmation of intact RLN function with vagal nerve stimulation after completion of thyroid lobectomy.

In addition, the International Neural Monitoring Study Group guidelines highlight the importance of surgeons' practicing and familiarizing themselves with IONM to be able to comprehensively troubleshoot equipment issues from true loss of RLN-signaling events.[47]

Fluorescent Imaging Aids for Parathyroid Identification

Because parathyroid identification during thyroidectomy is critical for the prevention of hypoparathyroidism, there has been renewed interest in newer technologies for intraoperative parathyroid imaging. The most prominent technologies under investigation currently are those that detect fluorescence from the parathyroid.

Parathyroid tissue autofluorescence in the near-infrared spectrum when exposed to a laser at a wavelength of 285 nm. Since this discovery in 2011, subsequent studies have demonstrated that parathyroid autofluorescence can be reliably detected both ex and en vivo. Detection can either be done by spectroscopy using a contact probe or specialized near-infrared spectrum cameras, with parathyroid glands that can be located in 76% to 100% of cases.[48] The potential advantages of this technology are its noninvasiveness and avoidance of an exogenously administered fluorophore. Current disadvantages include its limited penetration to up to only a few millimeters' depth, subtle and subjective fluorescence images with current-generation cameras and image processing software, and requirement for white (visible-spectrum) light to be turned off or minimized for the signal to be detected.

Exogenously administered fluorophores can aid in identification by more dramatically fluorescing the parathyroid glands. The fluorophore of greatest interest currently is indocyanine green, a water-soluble tricarbocyanine dye that rapidly binds to proteins in plasma following IV injection. Indocyanine green is a commonly used dye with low toxicity and a variety of clinical uses in other surgical procedures, and its use has been studied in both thyroidectomy and parathyroidectomy.

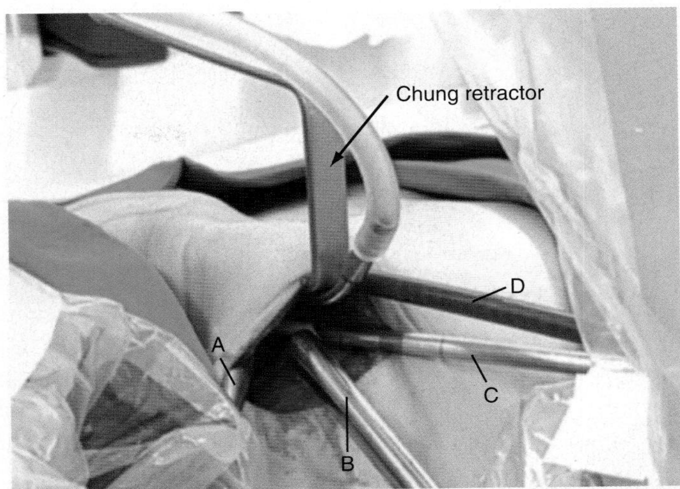

FIG. 37.36 Transaxillary robotic right thyroidectomy with a single incision and gasless approach. The Chung retractor lifts the tunneled working space from the axilla to the neck. The camera is placed in *port B*, and robotic instruments are placed in *ports A, C,* and *D*. (From Chang EHE, Kim HY, Koh YW, et al. Overview of robotic thyroidectomy. *Gland Surg*. 2017;6:218–228.)

Alternative Approaches to Thyroidectomy

The techniques detailed above describe conventional thyroidectomy via an open, anterior cervicotomy approach that has become the standard of care worldwide. As techniques have been refined and technologies have improved, various efforts to minimize the cosmetic effect of a visible neck incision have been investigated. From a historical perspective, the most direct and straightforward means to this end was to decrease the length of the standard cervicotomy incision from 6 to 8 cm down to 3 to 4 cm using traditional instruments and 1.5 to 2.5 cm with the aid of endoscopic instruments. A number of variations have been described with differing terminology, including *minimally invasive*, *video-assisted*, *videoscopic/endoscopic*, and *mini-open*, all of which have demonstrated reasonable feasibility and safety in carefully selected patients.

In addition, various investigators have described nontraditional techniques that place incisions in hidden places away from the visible part of the neck, with subcutaneous and/or subplatysmal dissection using minimally invasive surgical instruments to the thyroidectomy area of interest. These so-called "remote access" approaches have largely been developed and widely adopted in Asia and have subsequently established a small but growing niche in the United States and Europe. All require the use of either laparoscopic or robotic instruments, and virtually all can be performed using insufflation of a closed space with CO_2 gas or with a gasless technique using custom long tunneled retractors.

There are several different remote access approaches described in the literature differentiated by where the "hidden" incision is placed; the most common sites are the axilla, nipple-areolar complex or chest, retroauricular area at the hairline (the so-called "face-lift" approach), and the oral cavity. The most common approaches in the United States are the axillary and transoral approaches.

Transaxillary thyroidectomy using laparoscopic instruments via three small port incisions was first described in Japan in 2000 but first gained traction in the United States in 2007 based on excellent results from South Korea using a robotic, gasless technique with a single incision in the axilla (Fig. 37.36). The initial American experience was marked by an upsurge of complications, including brachial plexus injury, tracheoesophageal injury, lymph leak, and hematoma, which was exacerbated by a combination of inadequate surgeon training and aggressive marketing by the medical device industry. After issuance of warnings by the U.S. FDA in 2013, the manufacturers of the da Vinci surgical robotic system (Intuitive Surgical, Sunnyvale, CA) withdrew active support for robotic thyroidectomy, which led to an abrupt plateau in the adoption of robotic thyroidectomy cases. Since this initial turbulent experience, robotic transaxillary thyroidectomy has benefited from systematic study and steadier reintroduction in only a handful of more experienced centers. A recent experience of 301 cases in the United States revealed excellent technical feasibility (one conversion to open thyroidectomy) and safety (1.3% permanent RLN injury, 1.1% permanent hypoparathyroidism, 0.3% neck hematoma), with only one patient with an approach-specific complication (arm lymphedema which resolved with conservative management) and no recurrences among the 133 patients who had cancer identified histologically.[49]

Among all of the remote-access approaches, only the transoral route offers the potential of avoiding an incision at the skin altogether. However, there were many theoretical concerns around removing the thyroid through the mouth, not least of which was introducing a new risk of infection from oral flora as well as injury to other structures in the oral cavity as well as at the chin. The most adopted technique was popularized in Thailand and uses laparoscopic instruments and gas insufflation via three small port incisions in the oral vestibule (Fig. 37.37). The largest published experience is a 425-patient case series from Thailand revealing zero cases of permanent RLN injury or permanent hypoparathyroidism, one case of neck hematoma requiring open thyroidectomy, and three intraoperative conversions to open thyroidectomy. With respect to approach-specific complications, three patients (0.7%) had transient mental nerve palsy and no patients experienced a postoperative infection.[50] Other groups have replicated these results.

These excellent results have led to early adoption of the technique in the United States. However, with lessons learned from prior experiences around the rollout of transaxillary thyroidectomy, greater efforts are in place to introduce this technique in a more organized and responsible manner. Greater emphasis now exists on ensuring proper training, credentialing, and outcomes-tracking procedures for surgeons, and adoption is mainly occurring in larger, high-volume institutions at this time. Based on broad consensus, the selection criteria for transoral thyroidectomy have remained relatively constrained in the early phase

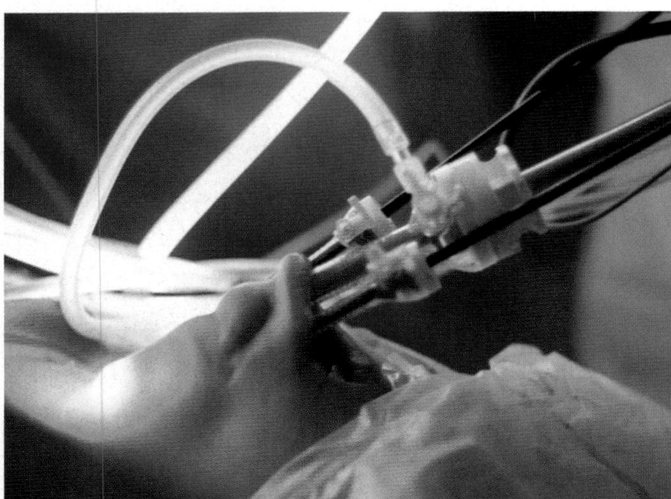

FIG. 37.37 Transoral endoscopic thyroidectomy vestibular approach. Three laparoscopic ports are placed in the oral vestibule, and dissection is carried out down to the subplatysmal plane in the neck *(picture-left)*.

of its adoption. It is with these quality-control efforts that transoral thyroidectomy—and other future innovations—will be introduced in a manner that both fosters innovation and protects patient safety.

SELECTED REFERENCES

Adam MA, Pura J, Gu L, et al. Extent of surgery for papillary thyroid cancer is not associated with survival: an analysis of 61,775 patients. *Ann Surg*. 2014;260:601–605.

This analysis from the National Cancer Database showing that lobectomy for selected papillary thyroid cancers was not associated with worse survival was an important paper that changed treatment guidelines.

Cibas ES, Ali SZ. The 2017 Bethesda system for reporting thyroid cytopathology. *Thyroid*. 2017;27:1341–1346.

This paper on the current Bethesda classification system for reporting thyroid cytopathology provides updated data on risk of malignancy in light of the new histologic diagnosis of noninvasive follicular neoplasm with papillary-like nuclear features.

Haugen BR, Alexander EK, Bible KC, et al. American Thyroid Association Management guidelines for adult patients with thyroid nodules and differentiated thyroid cancer: the American Thyroid Association Guidelines Task Force on Thyroid Nodules and Differentiated Thyroid Cancer. *Thyroid*. 2015;26:1–133; 2016.

The 2015 American Thyroid Association guidelines are arguably the most comprehensive and widely used evidence-based guidelines on the management of thyroid nodules and differentiated thyroid cancer.

Ito Y, Miyauchi A, Inoue H, et al. An observational trial for papillary thyroid microcarcinoma in Japanese patients. *World J Surg*. 2010;34:28–35.

This landmark paper from Japan was the first to demonstrate the safety and feasibility of nonoperative surveillance of papillary thyroid microcarcinomas.

Lim H, Devesa SS, Sosa JA, et al. Trends in thyroid cancer incidence and mortality in the United States, 1974–2013. *JAMA*. 2017;317:1338–1348.

This updated analysis from the Surveillance, Epidemiology, and End Results database demonstrated that mortality from advanced stage papillary thyroid cancer rose in parallel with the increasing incidence of thyroid cancer overall, suggesting that the rise in cancer incidence could not be fully attributed to overdiagnosis.

REFERENCES

1. Giddings AE. The history of thyroidectomy. *J R Soc Med.* 1998;91(suppl 33):3–6.
2. Wells Jr SA, Asa SL, Dralle H, et al. Revised American Thyroid Association guidelines for the management of medullary thyroid carcinoma. *Thyroid.* 2015;25:567–610.
3. Garber JR, Cobin RH, Gharib H, et al. Clinical practice guidelines for hypothyroidism in adults: cosponsored by the American Association of Clinical Endocrinologists and the American Thyroid Association. *Thyroid.* 2012;22:1200–1235.
4. Ross DS, Burch HB, Cooper DS, et al. American Thyroid Association Guidelines for diagnosis and management of hyperthyroidism and other causes of thyrotoxicosis. *Thyroid.* 2016;26:1343–1421; 2016.
5. Haugen BR, Alexander EK, Bible KC, et al. American Thyroid Association Management guidelines for adult patients with thyroid nodules and differentiated thyroid cancer: the American Thyroid Association Guidelines Task Force on Thyroid Nodules and Differentiated Thyroid Cancer. *Thyroid.* 2015;26:1–133; 2016.
6. Tessler FN, Middleton WD, Grant EG, et al. ACR thyroid imaging, reporting and data system (TI-RADS): white paper of the ACR TI-RADS Committee. *J Am Coll Radiol.* 2017;14:587–595.
7. Yoon JH, Lee HS, Kim EK, et al. Malignancy risk stratification of thyroid nodules: comparison between the thyroid imaging reporting and data system and the 2014 American Thyroid Association Management Guidelines. *Radiology.* 2016;278:917–924.
8. Azizi G, Keller JM, Mayo ML, et al. Thyroid nodules and shear wave elastography: a new tool in thyroid cancer detection. *Ultrasound Med Biol.* 2015;41:2855–2865.
9. Cibas ES, Ali SZ. The 2017 Bethesda System for reporting thyroid cytopathology. *Thyroid.* 2017;27:1341–1346.
10. Duh QY, Busaidy NL, Rahilly-Tierney C, et al. A systematic review of the methods of diagnostic accuracy studies of the Afirma gene expression classifier. *Thyroid.* 2017;27:1215–1222.
11. Patel KN, Angell TE, Babiarz J, et al. Performance of a genomic sequencing classifier for the preoperative diagnosis of cytologically indeterminate thyroid nodules. *JAMA Surg.* 2018;153:817–824.
12. Nikiforov YE, Carty SE, Chiosea SI, et al. Highly accurate diagnosis of cancer in thyroid nodules with follicular neoplasm/suspicious for a follicular neoplasm cytology by ThyroSeq v2 next-generation sequencing assay. *Cancer.* 2014;120:3627–3634.
13. Steward DL, Carty SE, Sippel RS, et al. Performance of a multigene genomic classifier in thyroid nodules with indeterminate cytology: a prospective blinded multicenter study. *JAMA Oncol.* 2019;5:204–212.
14. Wiltshire JJ, Drake TM, Uttley L, et al. Systematic review of trends in the incidence rates of thyroid cancer. *Thyroid.* 2016;26:1541–1552.
15. Lim H, Devesa SS, Sosa JA, et al. Trends in thyroid cancer incidence and mortality in the United States, 1974–2013. *JAMA.* 2017;317:1338–1348.
16. Nikiforov YE, Seethala RR, Tallini G, et al. Nomenclature revision for encapsulated follicular variant of papillary thyroid carcinoma: a paradigm shift to reduce overtreatment of indolent tumors. *JAMA Oncol.* 2016;2:1023–1029.
17. Parente DN, Kluijfhout WP, Bongers PJ, et al. Clinical safety of renaming encapsulated follicular variant of papillary thyroid carcinoma: is NIFTP truly benign? *World J Surg.* 2018;42:321–326.
18. Cancer Genome Atlas Research Network. Integrated genomic characterization of papillary thyroid carcinoma. *Cell.* 2014;159:676–690.
19. Kitahara CM, Sosa JA. The changing incidence of thyroid cancer. *Nat Rev Endocrinol.* 2016;12:646–653.
20. Alsanea O, Wada N, Ain K, et al. Is familial non-medullary thyroid carcinoma more aggressive than sporadic thyroid cancer? A multicenter series. *Surgery.* 2000;128:1043–1050; discussion 1050–1041.
21. Hoffman K, Lorenzo A, Butt CM, et al. Exposure to flame retardant chemicals and occurrence and severity of papillary thyroid cancer: a case-control study. *Environ Int.* 2017;107:235–242.
22. Nettore IC, Colao A, Macchia PE. Nutritional and environmental factors in thyroid carcinogenesis. *Int J Environ Res Public Health.* 2018;15:1735.

22a. Amin MB, Edge SB, Greene, Fl, et al. *AJCC Cancer Staging Manual*, 8th edition, American College of Surgeons, New York: Springer; 2018.

23. Tuttle RM, Haugen B, Perrier ND. Updated American Joint Committee on Cancer/Tumor-Node-Metastasis Staging System for Differentiated and Anaplastic Thyroid Cancer (Eighth Edition): what changed and why? *Thyroid.* 2017;27:751–756.
24. Tuttle RM, Tala H, Shah J, et al. Estimating risk of recurrence in differentiated thyroid cancer after total thyroidectomy and radioactive iodine remnant ablation: using response to therapy variables to modify the initial risk estimates predicted by the new American Thyroid Association staging system. *Thyroid.* 2010;20:1341–1349.
25. Adam MA, Pura J, Gu L, et al. Extent of surgery for papillary thyroid cancer is not associated with survival: an analysis of 61,775 patients. *Ann Surg.* 2014;260:601–605; discussion 605–607.
26. Shan CX, Zhang W, Jiang DZ, et al. Routine central neck dissection in differentiated thyroid carcinoma: a systematic review and meta-analysis. *Laryngoscope.* 2012;122:797–804.
27. Ito Y, Miyauchi A, Inoue H, et al. An observational trial for papillary thyroid microcarcinoma in Japanese patients. *World J Surg.* 2010;34:28–35.
28. Venkatesh S, Pasternak JD, Beninato T, et al. Cost-effectiveness of active surveillance versus hemithyroidectomy for micropapillary thyroid cancer. *Surgery.* 2017;161:116–126.
29. Jonklaas J, Sarlis NJ, Litofsky D, et al. Outcomes of patients with differentiated thyroid carcinoma following initial therapy. *Thyroid.* 2006;16:1229–1242.
30. Ruel E, Thomas S, Dinan M, et al. Adjuvant radioactive iodine therapy is associated with improved survival for patients with intermediate-risk papillary thyroid cancer. *J Clin Endocrinol Metab.* 2015;100:1529–1536.
31. Sosa JA, Tuggle CT, Wang TS, et al. Clinical and economic outcomes of thyroid and parathyroid surgery in children. *J Clin Endocrinol Metab.* 2008;93:3058–3065.

32. Barbet J, Campion L, Kraeber-Bodere F, et al. Prognostic impact of serum calcitonin and carcinoembryonic antigen doubling-times in patients with medullary thyroid carcinoma. *J Clin Endocrinol Metab*. 2005;90:6077–6084.
33. Rao SN, Cabanillas ME. Navigating systemic therapy in advanced thyroid carcinoma: from standard of care to personalized therapy and beyond. *J Endocr Soc*. 2018;2:1109–1130.
34. Sosa JA, Hanna JW, Robinson KA, et al. Increases in thyroid nodule fine-needle aspirations, operations, and diagnoses of thyroid cancer in the United States. *Surgery*. 2013;154:1420–1426; discussion 1426–1427.
35. American College of Surgeons Clinical Research Program, Alliance for Clinical Trials in Oncology, Nelson HD, Hunt KK. *Operative Standards for Cancer Surgery. Volume I Breast, Lung, Pancreas, Colon*. Philadelphia: Wolters Kluwer Health; 2015.
36. Adam MA, Thomas S, Youngwirth L, et al. Is there a minimum number of thyroidectomies a surgeon should perform to optimize patient outcomes? *Ann Surg*. 2017;265:402–407.
37. Randolph GW, Kamani D. The importance of preoperative laryngoscopy in patients undergoing thyroidectomy: voice, vocal cord function, and the preoperative detection of invasive thyroid malignancy. *Surgery*. 2006;139:357–362.
38. Zanocco K, Kaltman DJ, Wu JX, et al. Cost effectiveness of routine laryngoscopy in the surgical treatment of differentiated thyroid cancer. *Ann Surg Oncol*. 2018;25:949–956.
39. Wong KP, Au KP, Lam S, et al. Lessons learned after 1000 cases of transcutaneous laryngeal ultrasound (TLUSG) with laryngoscopic validation: is there a role of TLUSG in patients indicated for laryngoscopic examination before thyroidectomy? *Thyroid*. 2017;27:88–94.
40. Deniwar A, Kandil E, Randolph G. Electrophysiological neural monitoring of the laryngeal nerves in thyroid surgery: review of the current literature. *Gland Surg*. 2015;4:368–375.
41. Kazaure HS, Sosa JA. Surgical hypoparathyroidism. *Endocrinol Metab Clin North Am*. 2018;47:783–796.
42. Dehal A, Abbas A, Hussain F, et al. Risk factors for neck hematoma after thyroid or parathyroid surgery: ten-year analysis of the nationwide inpatient sample database. *Perm J*. 2015;19:22–28.
43. Materazzi G, Ambrosini CE, Fregoli L, et al. Prevention and management of bleeding in thyroid surgery. *Gland Surg*. 2017;6:510–515.
44. Khadra H, Bakeer M, Hauch A, et al. Hemostatic agent use in thyroid surgery: a meta-analysis. *Gland Surg*. 2018;7:S34–S41.
45. Pisanu A, Porceddu G, Podda M, et al. Systematic review with meta-analysis of studies comparing intraoperative neuromonitoring of recurrent laryngeal nerves versus visualization alone during thyroidectomy. *J Surg Res*. 2014;188:152–161.
46. Wong KP, Mak KL, Wong CK, et al. Systematic review and meta-analysis on intra-operative neuro-monitoring in high-risk thyroidectomy. *Int J Surg*. 2017;38:21–30.
47. Schneider R, Randolph GW, Dionigi G, et al. International neural monitoring study group guideline 2018, part I: staging bilateral thyroid surgery with monitoring loss of signal. *Laryngoscope*. 2018;128(suppl 3):S1–S17.
48. Abbaci M, De Leeuw F, Breuskin I, et al. Parathyroid gland management using optical technologies during thyroidectomy or parathyroidectomy: a systematic review. *Oral Oncol*. 2018;87:186–196.
49. Stang MT, Yip L, Wharry L, et al. Gasless transaxillary endoscopic thyroidectomy with robotic assistance: a high-volume experience in North America. *Thyroid*. 2018;28:1655–1661.
50. Anuwong A, Ketwong K, Jitpratoom P, et al. Safety and outcomes of the transoral endoscopic thyroidectomy vestibular approach. *JAMA Surg*. 2018;153:21–27.

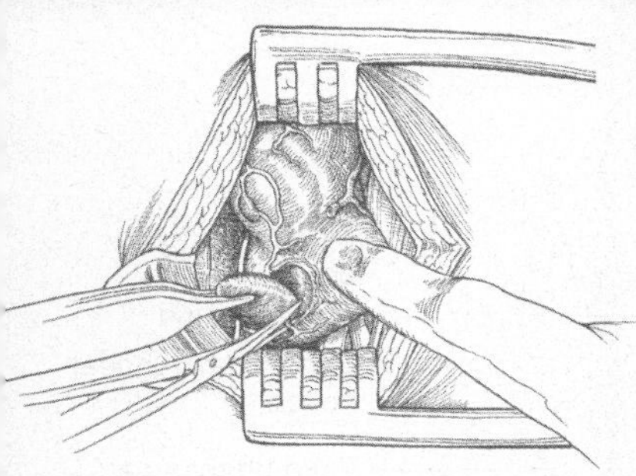

CHAPTER 38

The Parathyroid Glands

Iuliana Bobanga, Christopher R. McHenry

OUTLINE

HISTORY OF THE PARATHYROID GLANDS

The parathyroid glands were the last endocrine glands to be discovered. The earliest reference to the parathyroid glands is Sir Richard Owen's description of a small compact yellow glandular body that was attached to the thyroid gland in the Indian rhinoceros.[1] Ivar Victor Sandstrom, a 25-year-old Swedish medical student at the University of Uppsala, has been credited with first identifying the parathyroid glands in human cadavers in 1880, naming them "glandulae parathyreoideae" and providing a detailed gross anatomic and microscopic description.[2]

Anton Wolfer first described postoperative tetany in 1879 in Theodore Billroth's first survivor of total thyroidectomy.[3] Eugene Gley, a professor of physiology at the College de France in Paris, was the first to recognize the association of tetany with the parathyroid glands. In 1891, he reported tetany and death in rabbits and rats following thyroidectomy and removal of the glands described by Sandstrom.[3,4]

Also in 1891, Friedrich von Recklinghausen, Professor of Pathology in Strasbourg, reported a patient with multiple fractures, bending of the long bones, fibrosis, cystic changes, and brown tumors. This constellation of findings was termed *osteitis fibrosa cystica of von Recklinghausen.*[3,5] In 1904, the association of osteitis fibrosa cystica and parathyroid disease was identified by Max Askanazy, a German-Swiss pathologist who reported two patients with severe bone changes and a parathyroid tumor.[6] At that time it was hypothesized that the changes in the parathyroid glands were the result of primary bone disease, and patients with severe bone disease were treated with parathyroid extract.

It was not until 1915 that the severe bone disease was considered to be the result of changes in the parathyroid glands. Dr. Friedrich Schlagenhaufer, a professor of pathology in Vienna, reported autopsy results in two patients with osteomalacia who were found to have a solitary parathyroid tumor.[4] It was then that enlargement of the parathyroid gland was considered to be the primary event in the development of bone disease and Schlagenhaufer suggested that some patients may benefit from parathyroid tumor excision.[3]

In 1905, William MacCallum, a pathologist at Johns Hopkins Hospital, demonstrated that administration of calcium or parathyroid extract could reverse or prevent postoperative tetany.[7] Likely influenced by the work of MacCallum, William Halstead used intravenous calcium gluconate to treat tetany in patients following thyroidectomy and emphasized the importance of preventing injury to the parathyroid glands at the time of thyroidectomy to prevent tetany.[3] However, the prevailing view at the time was that the primary function of the parathyroid glands was to detoxify the blood, much like the liver.

It was not until 1925 when James B. Collip, a Canadian biochemist at the University of Alberta, used hot acid extraction to produce parathyroid hormone (PTH) extracts that were used to successfully reverse tetany in parathyroidectomized animals.[3–5] Collip and colleagues also reported that repeated injections of parathyroid extract in dogs produced hypercalcemia, vomiting, dehydration, atony, and eventually death. Collip suggested that the function of the parathyroid glands was to regulate calcium metabolism.

One of the most important events in the history of the parathyroid glands occurred in Vienna in 1925, when Felix Mandl, a Viennese surgeon, treated Albert Jahne, a 38-year-old tramcar conductor who had severe bone disease from primary hyperparathyroidism (HPT). Mandl, influenced by Friedrich Schlagenhaufer's finding of a single parathyroid tumor in two patients with osteitis fibrosa cystica, performed a neck exploration on Albert Jahne under local anesthesia on July 30, 1925, and excised a 2.5-cm parathyroid gland that resulted in dramatic improvement of his bone disease.[3] This was an epic event because it established the relationship of osteitis fibrosa cystica to enlargement of a parathyroid gland and helped dispel the belief that the severe bone disease was the result of parathyroid deficiency.

In the United States, Captain Charles Martell was the first and most well-recognized case of primary HPT.[8] He was a merchant marine sea captain who presented with severe progressive bone disease manifested by loss of height, multiple fractures, generalized demineralization, and cysts. He also had kidney stones, lethargy, and fatigue and was found to have elevated serum calcium, low serum phosphorus, and hypercalciuria. Martell underwent six unsuccessful cervical explorations before Edward Churchill, with the assistance of Oliver Cope, performed a mediastinal exploration at the Massachusetts General Hospital in 1932 and removed a 3-cm parathyroid tumor just medial to the superior vena cava.[3]

In 1929, Barr, Bulger, and Dixon from Barnes Hospital in St. Louis introduced the term *hyperparathyroidism* to describe a syndrome characterized by rarefaction of bone and cystic bone tumors, kidney stones, muscle weakness, hypotonia, and high levels of calcium in the serum and urine.[9] This was the direct result of their care of Elva Dawkins, who was diagnosed with HPT and underwent the first successful parathyroidectomy in the United States by Isaac Y. Olch at Barnes Hospital in St. Louis on August 1, 1928.[3]

In the 1930s, Fuller Albright, a Harvard physician, noted that 80% of patients with osteitis fibrosa cystica had nephrocalcinosis and nephrolithiasis, which were the hallmarks for primary HPT.[5] He further defined primary HPT as "a condition in which PTH is higher than needed" and identified single adenoma, multiple adenomas, diffuse hyperplasia, and cancer as causes for primary HPT. He also described secondary and tertiary HPT and distinguished them from primary HPT.

The modern era of parathyroid history began with the invention of the autoanalyzer in 1951 by Leonard Skeggs, an American biochemist.[5] Multichannel autoanalyzers were introduced into clinical use in the 1970s, and this eventually led to rapid serum analysis and diagnosis of hypercalcemia. Over time, more and more patients with HPT were incidentally diagnosed with hypercalcemia on routine blood work and were less likely to have the severe bone disease.

A second major development was the successful purification and isolation of PTH by Auerbach and later by Rasmussen and Craig.[8] More effective measurement of serum PTH followed in the second half of the twentieth century and resulted in an improvement in the diagnosis of HPT. In 1963, Berson and colleagues reported the use of an immunoassay to measure human PTH.[7] This was followed by the successful sequencing and synthesis of PTH in the early 1970s by Potts and colleagues at Harvard University.[3] Further refinement in the diagnosis of HPT occurred as a result of the development of radioimmunoassays by Rosalyn Yalow for measurement of peptide hormones for which she won the Nobel Prize in 1977.[3,4,7] In 1987, Nussbaum and colleagues developed a two-site immunoradiometric assay that measured the active intact PTH.[7]

Initially, a minimum of 24 hours was required for measurement of intact PTH using the two-site immunoradiometric assay. Recognizing that the half-life of PTH was on average 3 to 5 minutes, it was not long until a "quick" intraoperative PTH (IOPTH) assay was developed by modifying reagents and reducing incubation time that could produce an intact PTH result in 10 minutes. This led to the development and use of IOPTH monitoring for determining curative parathyroidectomy, which was championed by Irvin and colleagues in the early 1990s.[10] This, in combination with advances in parathyroid localization paved the way for minimally invasive or focused parathyroidectomy.

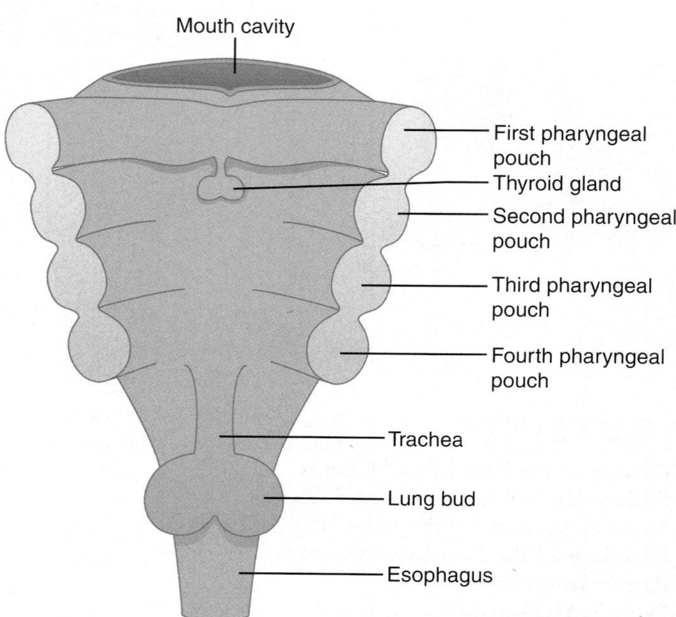

FIG. 38.1 The four pharyngeal pouches at the fourth week of embryologic development. The thyroid gland can be seen as an endodermal outpouching originating from the foramen cecum.

EMBRYOLOGY OF THE PARATHYROID GLANDS

The pharyngeal pouches in the human embryo give rise to the face, neck, and surrounding structures (Fig. 38.1). The two pairs of parathyroid glands develop from the endoderm of the third and fourth branchial pouches and neural crest mesenchyme. The paired inferior parathyroid glands and the thymus develop from the third branchial pouch. The paired superior parathyroid glands develop from the fourth branchial pouch along with the lateral lobes of the thyroid gland and the ultimobranchial bodies (Fig. 38.2).

In the fifth week of embryologic development, the dorsal and ventral aspects of the third pharyngeal pouch differentiate into the inferior parathyroid glands and the thymus, respectively. At the sixth week of embryologic development, the inferior parathyroid glands and the primordia of the thymus lose their attachment with the pharynx and migrate caudally. The inferior parathyroid glands eventually locate on the dorsal surface of the inferior poles of the thyroid gland.

The dorsal aspect of the fourth pharyngeal pouch forms the superior parathyroid glands. The fourth pharyngeal pouch is also thought to give rise to the lateral lobes of the thyroid gland. When the superior parathyroid glands lose their attachment with the pharynx, they are thought to attach themselves to the thyroid, which descends caudally.

The more extensive embryologic migration of the inferior parathyroid glands is the explanation for their more frequent ectopic location. The embryologic migration of the superior parathyroid glands is more limited and, as a result, they are more likely to be found in the predictable anatomic location.

The mammalian homolog of drosophila glial cell missing gene (*GCM2*) has been identified as a key regulatory gene in parathyroid differentiation and development. *GCM2* has been shown to regulate the expression of key functional genes including PTH and may also be involved with the regulation of PTH gene expression. The factors involved in the upregulation of *GCM2*, as well as

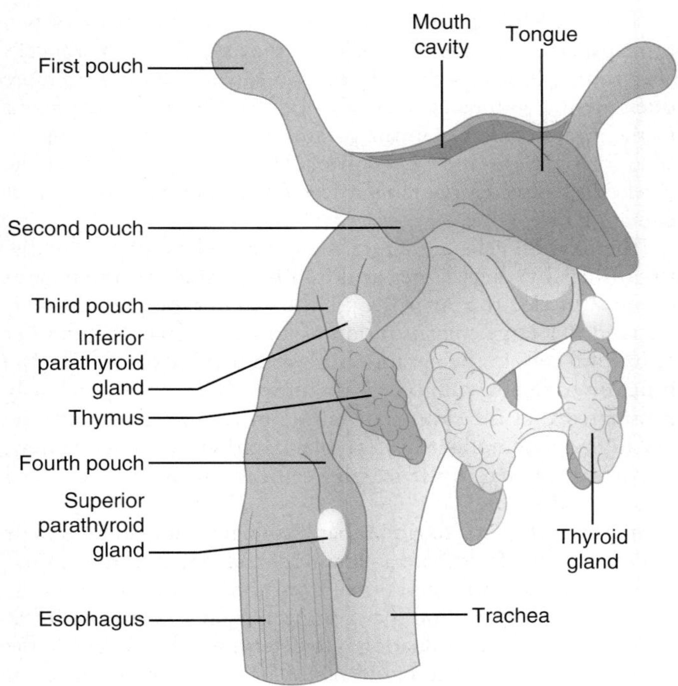

FIG. 38.2 The pharynx and adjacent structures are depicted between the sixth and seventh weeks of embryologic development. The thyroid gland has descended to its normal location in the neck. The inferior parathyroid glands and thymus are seen arising from the third pharyngeal pouches. The superior parathyroid glands are seen arising from the fourth pharyngeal pouches.

the transcription factors and signaling pathways that are involved in the embryologic development of the parathyroid glands, have yet to be elucidated.[11] Mutations in the *GCM2* gene have also been associated with familial isolated HPT and a higher risk of parathyroid cancer.

SURGICAL ANATOMY OF THE PARATHYROID GLANDS

Most individuals have paired superior and inferior parathyroid glands, although supernumerary and less than four glands have been reported in autopsy studies. Approximately 84% of individuals have four glands, 13% have more than four glands, and 3% have three glands. Normal parathyroid glands are oval, spherical, or bean shaped; they vary in color from yellow-tan to reddish brown, and on average are 5 × 3 × 2 mm in size and weigh 35 to 40 mg (Fig. 38.3).[12,13] Parathyroid glands are typically surrounded by adipose tissue anteriorly, laterally, and posteriorly and the vascular pedicle is medial in location.

The inferior thyroid artery is the predominant vascular supply for both the superior and inferior parathyroid glands in 80% of cases. The inferior thyroid artery is a branch of the thyrocervical trunk that originates from the subclavian artery. Alternatively, the parathyroid glands may receive their blood supply from the superior thyroid artery or from small arterial branches directly from the thyroid gland. Each parathyroid gland has one or more fine end arterial branches that are sensitive to devascularization during parathyroid and thyroid surgery. In 70% to 80% of cases, the ipsilateral and contralateral parathyroid glands are located in symmetrical positions in the neck. Approximately 16% of patients with primary HPT will have parathyroid glands in an ectopic location.[14]

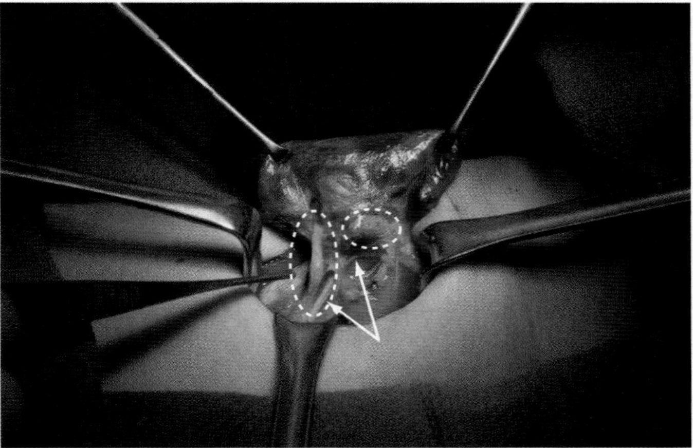

FIG. 38.3 Intraoperative photograph demonstrating normal left superior and inferior parathyroid glands surrounded by adipose tissue and their relationship to the thyroid and the recurrent laryngeal nerve (right side of image is rostral, left side is caudal; dashed lines encircle the parathyroid glands and the arrows point to the left recurrent laryngeal nerve).

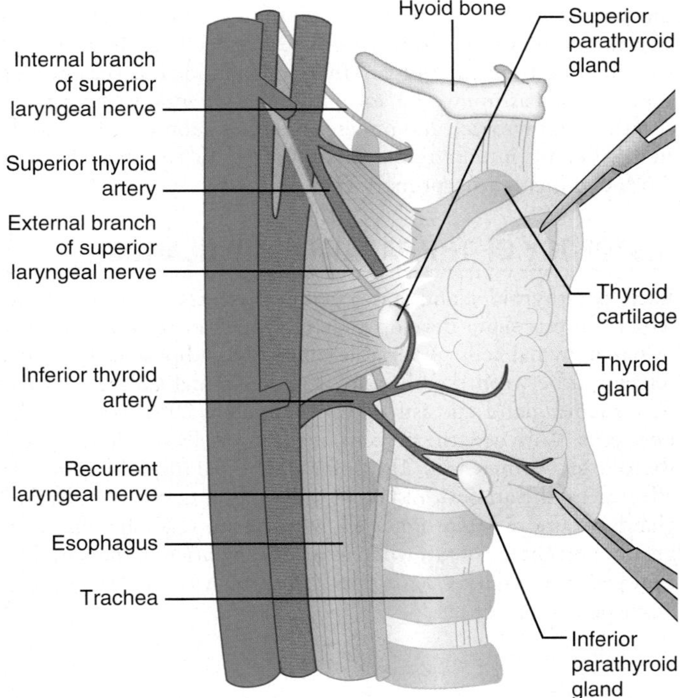

FIG. 38.4 The superior and inferior parathyroid glands and their normal anatomic relationships are depicted with the right lobe of the thyroid gland retracted anteriorly and medially.

The parathyroid glands are usually found within 5 mm of the superior and inferior margins of the tubercle of Zuckerkandl along the posterior capsule of the lateral lobes of the thyroid gland. The superior parathyroid glands are most commonly located on the posterior surface of the upper pole of the thyroid gland, posterior and superior to the recurrent laryngeal nerve (Fig. 38.4). Because of their shorter embryologic migration compared to the inferior parathyroid glands, they have a more predictable anatomic location and are less likely to be ectopic. Eighty percent of the superior glands are found in their expected anatomic location, approximately 1 cm superior to the junction of the inferior thyroid artery and the recurrent laryngeal nerve at the level of the cricoid cartilage where the recurrent laryngeal nerve enters the larynx. The superior parathyroid glands are often found within the capsule of the thyroid gland.

The challenge in identifying the superior parathyroid glands at the time of surgery is usually due to a lack of adequate mobilization and anteromedial rotation of the thyroid lobe to access their posterior location. In such a situation, ligation and division of the superior pole vessels may be helpful in optimizing exposure of an abnormal superior parathyroid gland. Ectopic locations of the superior parathyroid glands include the tracheoesophageal groove, behind the esophagus or the pharynx, in the posterior mediastinum and intrathyroidal.[13]

The inferior parathyroid glands are most commonly found 1 cm inferior to the junction of the inferior thyroid artery and the recurrent laryngeal nerve, anterior and medial to the recurrent laryngeal nerve on the posterolateral aspect of the inferior pole of the thyroid lobe (Fig. 38.4). The inferior parathyroid glands are less often found in a subcapsular location. Due to their more extensive embryologic migration, the inferior parathyroid glands are more commonly ectopic and can be found anywhere from the angle of the mandible to the pericardium. The most common ectopic location for an inferior gland is within the thymus (Fig. 38.5). Other sites for an ectopic inferior parathyroid gland include the anterior superior mediastinum, the aortopulmonary window, the carotid sheath, intrathyroidal, and undescended in a submandibular location.[13] Ectopic intrathyroidal parathyroid glands occur in 0.7% to 3.6% of patients with primary HPT.[12]

HISTOLOGY OF THE PARATHYROID GLANDS

Each parathyroid gland has a connective tissue capsule from which fibrous septa develop that support and separate clusters of parenchymal cells. A variable number of adipose cells are interspersed between the clusters of parenchymal cells. A normal parathyroid gland consists of approximately 25% to 40% adipose cells. With age, the percent of adipose cells within the parathyroid gland increases. The color of the parathyroid glands is affected by the amount of fat. In older patients, the parathyroid glands are more often light yellow or tan in color because of a greater percentage of fat, whereas in young patients, the parathyroid glands are darker with a reddish-brown color because of a lesser percentage of fat.

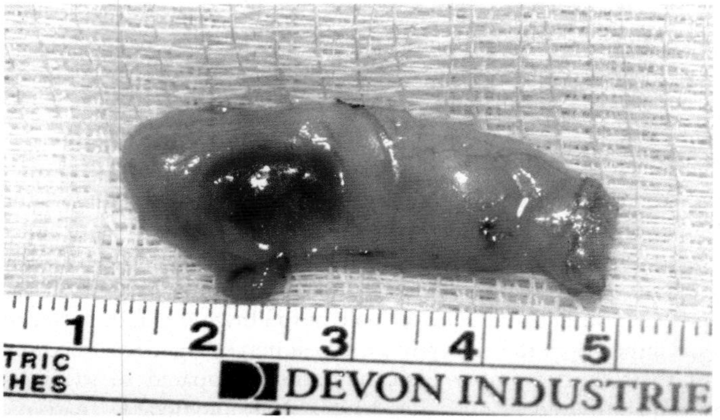

FIG. 38.5 Ectopic intrathymic parathyroid adenoma.

The parenchymal cells of the parathyroid gland consist of two principal cell types: the chief cells and the oxyphil cells. Clear cells are a third cell type, which may occasionally be seen and are more often present with parathyroid hyperplasia. Chief cells are present in the greatest number in the parathyroid gland and are responsible for synthesis and secretion of PTH. The cytoplasm of the chief cells has secretory granules seen on electron microscopy that contain PTH.

The oxyphil cells are larger than chief cells and can be distinguished by their large, acidophilic granules in their cytoplasm. On electron microscopy, the acidophilic granules correspond to a large concentration of mitochondria. The number of oxyphil cells in the parathyroid gland increases with age. The function of the oxyphil cells is unknown. It has been previously postulated that the success or failure of technetium-99m-sestamebi imaging in identification of a parathyroid adenoma may, in part, be related to the oxyphil cell content of the abnormal parathyroid tissue.

It is important to recognize that histologic evaluation is unable to definitively differentiate a parathyroid adenoma from parathyroid hyperplasia and even normal from abnormal parathyroid tissue. The only expectation that a surgeon should have from intraoperative pathologic evaluation is to determine whether or not the tissue submitted is parathyroid tissue. It is sometimes important to ensure that excised tissue, presumed to be parathyroid, is not thyroid, nodal, or thymic tissue. Intraoperative pathologic examination of an excised parathyroid gland is usually unnecessary if IOPTH monitoring is used.

PARATHYROID PHYSIOLOGY

Extracellular calcium concentration is the predominant regulator of PTH synthesis and secretion by the chief cells of the parathyroid glands. Calcium binds to calcium-sensing receptors (CaSRs) on the surface of the chief cells and inhibits PTH secretion and PTH gene expression. High calcium also enhances PTH degradation into fragments. Conversely, when calcium is reduced, PTH gene expression and secretion are increased. 1,25-Dihydroxyvitamin D (1,25[OH]$_2$D), the active form of vitamin D, binds to vitamin D receptors on chief cells and inhibits PTH gene expression and parathyroid cell proliferation. Other regulators of PTH secretion include lithium, transforming growth factor-alpha, prostaglandins, inorganic phosphate, and fibroblast growth factor 23.[15]

PTH synthesis begins with the production of a 115-amion acid pre-pro-PTH polypeptide, which is cleaved in the chief cells to the active 84–amino acid intact-PTH peptide. The NH2 terminus, a 34-amino acid residue and the biologically active part of the intact-PTH peptide, which binds to the G-protein-coupled PTH/PTHrP receptor type 1 (PTHR1). PTHR1 is highly expressed in bone and kidney.

PTH is essential in the regulation of calcium and phosphate metabolism. Extracellular calcium concentration is the principal stimulus regulating PTH secretion. A reverse sigmoidal relationship exists between extracellular calcium concentration and PTH secretion (Fig. 38.6). Maximum PTH secretion occurs at low extracellular calcium concentrations and maximal suppression occurs at high extracellular calcium concentrations. Extracellular calcium levels are tightly maintained at a calcium set point, which is defined as the extracellular calcium concentration where PTH secretion is half-maximally suppressed. The calcium set point occurs on the steep portion of the PTH curve such that large increases in PTH secretion occur in response to small reductions in extracellular calcium concentration and large reductions in PTH secretion occur with small increases in extracellular calcium concentration detected by the CaSR on parathyroid chief cells.

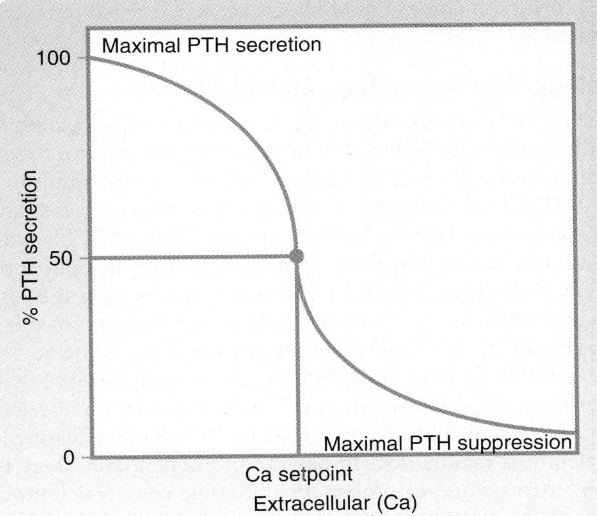

FIG. 38.6 The inverse sigmoidal relationship of parathyroid hormone *(PTH)* to changes in extracellular calcium concentration and the calcium set point. *Ca*, Calcium.

PTH acts on the ascending limb of the loop of Henle and the distal convoluted tubule of the kidneys to enhance calcium reabsorption, inhibit phosphate reabsorption, and increase phosphate excretion causing phosphaturia. Also in the kidneys, PTH stimulates the conversion of 25-hydroxyvitamin D (25[OH]D) to the active metabolite 1,25[OH]$_2$D by activating the gene that encodes for 25-hydroxyvitamin D-1α hydroxylase enzyme (Fig. 38.7). 1,25[OH]$_2$D increases intestinal absorption of dietary calcium in the small intestine (Fig. 38.7). PTH increases bone remodeling and release of calcium and phosphate from the skeleton. The PTH-mediated renal effects to maintain calcium homeostasis are rapid, taking minutes to hours, compared to the skeletal effects, which take hours to days.

PTH has a complex effect on bone remodeling, with both anabolic and catabolic effects. PTH binds to the PTHR1 receptor that is found on cells of the osteoblastic lineage, which ultimately leads to the formation of new bone matrix and mineralization. However, osteoblast-lineage cells also produce regulators of osteoclast formation, such as the receptor activator of nuclear factor-κB, receptor activator of nuclear factor-κB ligand, and osteoprotegerin. PTH increases osteoclast activity indirectly through the effects of receptor activator of nuclear factor-κB ligand and osteoprotegerin, leading to increased bone resorption with calcium and phosphate ion release from hydroxyapatite, the major mineral component of bone. The net effect of PTH on bone varies based on the severity and chronicity of PTH excess.[15] In patients with chronically elevated PTH levels, such as primary and secondary HPT, the net effect is

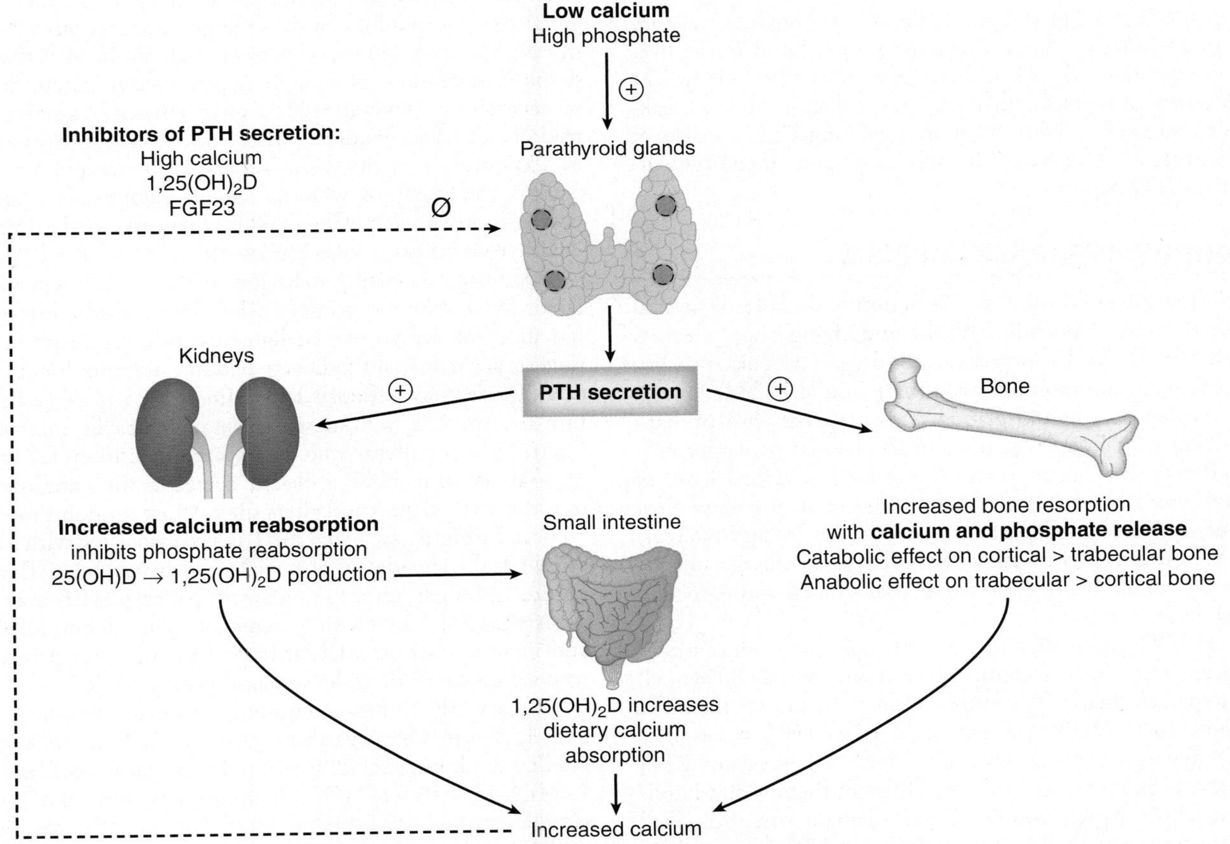

FIG. 38.7 Regulators of parathyroid hormone *(PTH)* secretion and PTH effects on calcium homeostasis. *FGF23*, Fibroblast growth factor 23; *25(OH)D*, 25-hydroxyvitamin D; *1,25(OH)$_2$D*, 1,25-dihydroxyvitamin D.

TABLE 38.1 Causes of hypercalcemia.

Endocrine	Primary hyperparathyroidism
	Tertiary hyperparathyroidism
	Familial hypocalciuric hypercalcemia
	Hyperthyroidism
Malignancy	Tumors producing PTHrP (SCC of lung, bladder cancer, renal cell cancer)
	Osteolytic bone metastasis
	Hematologic malignancies (lymphoma, leukemia, multiple myeloma)
Granulomatous Disease	Sarcoidosis
	Tuberculosis
	Fungal infection
Medications	Calcium
	Thiazide diuretics
	Lithium
	Vitamin A and D intoxication
	Milk alkali syndrome
Miscellaneous	Paget and other bone diseases with prolonged immobilization

PTHrP, Parathyroid hormone–related peptide; *SCC*, squamous cell carcinoma.

bone resorption leading to osteopenia and osteoporosis. However, intermittent administration of recombinant human PTH has been shown to stimulate bone formation more than resorption and is currently in clinical use for treatment of osteoporosis.[16]

The half-life of PTH is 3 to 5 minutes, although it can vary from 1 to 21 minutes. PTH fragments are produced in the liver and in the parathyroid cells and are excreted by the kidney. The renal clearance of PTH fragments is slower than the PTH breakdown into fragments. Thus, 80% of circulating PTH consists of fragments that are inactive, while only 20% is the intact biologically active PTH peptide.

PRIMARY HYPERPARATHYROIDISM

HPT refers to excess synthesis and secretion of PTH by abnormal parathyroid glands. Depending on the underlying cause of excess PTH, HPT is classified as primary, secondary, or tertiary. Primary HPT is caused by autonomous overproduction of PTH by one or more abnormal parathyroid glands. Most patients with primary HPT present with hypercalcemia and an elevated or inappropriately high-normal (nonsuppressed) PTH level. It affects 1 out of every 500 women and 1 out of every 2000 men. It occurs most commonly in postmenopausal women between 50 and 60 years of age. The incidence of primary HPT increases with age and the prevalence is about 1% in postmenopausal women and 0.86% in the general population.[17]

Primary HPT and malignancy are the most common causes of hypercalcemia in adults, accounting for approximately 80% of all cases of hypercalcemia. Less common causes account for the other 20% (Table 38.1). Unlike primary and tertiary HPT, most other causes of hypercalcemia are associated with a low serum PTH level, with the exception of prolonged lithium therapy and familial hypocalciuric hypercalcemia (FHH). Patients on prolonged lithium therapy may develop lithium-induced HPT.

FHH is a rare autosomal dominant disorder affecting the renal CaSR that results in a higher set point for renal calcium excretion, hypocalciuria, asymptomatic hypercalcemia, and normal or mildly elevated PTH levels. Patients with FHH have none of the clinical manifestations of primary HPT. Because FHH has a high penetrance, patients typically develop chronically elevated serum calcium levels before the age of 30, and thus, it is uncommon for a postmenopausal woman to be newly diagnosed with FHH without a history of chronic mild hypercalcemia.[18,19] No treatment is required for FHH.

Etiology, Pathophysiology, and Risk Factors

Primary HPT occurs when one or more abnormal parathyroid glands enlarge and secrete PTH inappropriately relative to serum calcium levels. The three pathologic conditions that result in primary HPT are parathyroid adenoma, hyperplasia, and carcinoma. Increased serum calcium levels occur as a result of PTH-induced increases in bone resorption, renal calcium reabsorption, and indirectly by increased dietary calcium absorption from the gastrointestinal tract. Under normal conditions, a high serum calcium level should inhibit excess PTH production (Figs. 38.6 and 38.7). However, the parathyroid cells in a parathyroid adenoma have a lower-than-normal sensitivity to the inhibitory action of calcium, with a higher calcium set point, such that a higher circulating level of calcium is maintained. In parathyroid hyperplasia, there is an overall increase in the number of parathyroid cells, which produce excess PTH but maintain their normal sensitivity to calcium.[20] Both conditions give rise to primary HPT and cause hypercalcemia.

The frequency of multigland disease (double adenoma or four gland hyperplasia) is variable and is dependent on how it is defined. Historically, multigland disease has been defined based on gland size, morphology, and histology. More recently, multigland disease has been defined as persistent elevation of IOPTH levels despite the removal of a single hypersecreting parathyroid gland or persistent postoperative HPT after removal of a single parathyroid gland. Multiglandular disease occurs in approximately 10% to 15% of all patients with primary HPT, ranging from 4% to 33% in the literature, whereas a single parathyroid adenoma occurs in approximately 85% to 90% of patients with primary HPT. Parathyroid cancer is found in less than 1% of cases.[18,19]

Exposure to ionizing radiation in the cervical region is a risk factor for developing primary HPT. This includes external beam radiation for benign and malignant conditions, exposure during nuclear accidents and radioactive iodine ablation for thyroid disease. The latency period is approximately 25 to 40 years.[17] Lithium therapy is a well-known cause of hypercalcemia and HPT. Up to 15% of patients who are on chronic lithium for more than 10 years develop HPT. Lithium decreases the parathyroid cells' sensitivity to calcium and alters the calcium set point for PTH secretion. Lithium-associated HPT is also associated with a comparatively higher incidence of parathyroid hyperplasia. Thiazide diuretics, although not a risk factor for primary HPT, may unmask preexisting HPT by causing increased renal calcium reabsorption and increased serum calcium levels. Patients with primary HPT who are taken off thiazides remain hypercalcemic.[19]

Primary HPT is most commonly a sporadic disease. In approximately 3% to 5% of patients, primary HPT occurs as part of a familial syndrome including multiple endocrine neoplasia (MEN) 1, MEN2A, MEN4, HPT-jaw tumor syndrome (HPT-JT), and familial isolated HPT (Table 38.2). Some of the mutations that cause sporadic primary HPT overlap with mutations found in familial HPT. Patients with inherited HPT are typically younger, may have a family history of endocrinopathies, and may exhibit

TABLE 38.2 **Genetic abnormalities associated with sporadic and inherited forms of primary HPT: disorder, genes, inheritance, phenotype, and recommended surgical approach.**

DISORDER	GENES	INHERITANCE	PHENOTYPE	AGE*	SURGICAL APPROACH†
Sporadic					
Parathyroid adenoma and hyperplasia	*PRAD1, CCND1* (20%–40%), *MEN1* (12%–35%), *CDC73, CDKN1B, AIP*	Sporadic	Isolated pHPT with single adenoma, double adenoma or four-gland hyperplasia	>45	Minimally invasive parathyroidectomy with IOPTH or bilateral exploration
Parathyroid carcinoma	*RB1, CDC73, MEN1, microRNA-296*	Sporadic	pHPT secondary to parathyroid carcinoma	>45	En bloc resection
Inherited					
MEN1	*MEN1*	AD	pHPT (95%) in third decade, pNETs (40%), pituitary adenomas (30%), adrenocortical and thyroid tumors, meningioma, facial angiofibromas, lipomas	25–45	Subtotal parathyroidectomy and transcervical thymectomy
MEN2A	*RET*	AD	pHPT (15%–35%), MTC (99%), pheochromocytoma (50%), lichen planus, amyloidosis, Hirschsprung disease	38	Resection of only visibly enlarged parathyroid glands. Address or rule out pheochromocytoma first
MEN4	*CDKN1B*	AD	pHPT (80%), pituitary adenoma (40%), pNETs, adrenal, thyroid, gonadal and renal tumors	50	Same as MEN1
Familial isolated HPT	*MEN1, CDC73, CASR, GCM2, CDKN1B*	AD	Isolated pHPT, parathyroid carcinoma (*GCM2* mutation)	39	Bilateral neck exploration with resection of enlarged glands only versus subtotal parathyroidectomy En bloc resection for parathyroid cancer
HPT-JT	*CDC73*	AD	pHPT in second or third decade, parathyroid carcinoma (35%), ossifying fibromas of mandible and maxilla, renal cysts, hamartomas and Wilms tumor, and uterine tumors	32	Minimally invasive parathyroidectomy with IOPTH or bilateral exploration En bloc resection for parathyroid cancer

Adapted from Silva BC, Cusano NE, Bilezikian JP. Primary hyperparathyroidism. *Best Pract Res Clin Endocrinol Metab.* 2018;32:593–607; Bilezikian JP, Cusano NE, Khan AA, et al. Primary hyperparathyroidism. *Nat Rev Dis Primers.* 2016;2:16033; Wilhelm SM, Wang TS, Ruan DT, et al. The American Association of Endocrine Surgeons guidelines for definitive management of primary hyperparathyroidism. *JAMA Surg.* 2016;151:959–968; and El Lakis M, Nockel P, Gaitanidis A, et al. Probability of positive genetic testing results in patients with family history of primary hyperparathyroidism. *J Am Coll Surg.* 2018;226:933–938.
AD, Autosomal dominant; *HPT*, hyperparathyroidism; *HPT-JT*, hyperparathyroidism-jaw tumor syndrome; *IOPTH*, intraoperative parathyroid hormone; *MEN*, multiple endocrine neoplasia; *MTC*, medullary thyroid cancer; *pHPT*, primary hyperparathyroidism; *PTH*; parathyroid hormone; *pNET*, pancreatic neuroendocrine tumors.
*Age = mean age at presentation of primary HPT in years.
†Surgical approach to HPT associated with the disorder.

other associated findings of a particular syndrome (see "Familial Primary HPT" section).

Clinical Manifestations

Up to 80% of patients with primary HPT are diagnosed as a result of incidental hypercalcemia found on routine bloodwork. However, patients with primary HPT can have diverse symptoms, which are the result of calcium effects on multiple organ systems, including the renal, skeletal, gastrointestinal, cardiac, and neuromuscular systems (Table 38.3). In a recent cohort study of over 9000 patients, 35% of patients had objective findings of end-organ effects at the time of diagnosis, including osteoporosis, nephrolithiasis, or hypercalciuria. In addition, 62% of patients developed end-organ effects within 5 years of diagnosis.[21] Up to 20% of patients with primary HPT have symptomatic nephrolithiasis, 10% of patients have recurrent kidney stones, and up to 12% of patients have "silent nephrolithiasis" when they are screened with abdominal imaging.[17,18]

Primary HPT results in loss of bone mass, which is most pronounced at sites of cortical bone in the distal third of the radius and the femoral neck. However, recent studies using high-resolution peripheral quantitative CT (HRpQCT) have demonstrated that both cortical and trabecular bone are affected by primary HPT, with increased fractures seen in the vertebral bodies in patients with primary HPT compared to a control population.[19,20] Up to 15% of patients with HPT have osteopenia in the lumbar spine.[18] In a longitudinal observational study, patients with untreated primary HPT followed for 15 years had a decline in bone mineral density of 35% at the distal radius and 10% at the femoral neck.[22] All patients with primary HPT should be screened for osteopenia and osteoporosis with measurement of bone mineral density of the distal third of the radius, the lumbar spine, the femoral neck, and the hip.

TABLE 38.3 Signs and symptoms of primary hyperparathyroidism.

TARGET ORGAN OR SYSTEM	SYMPTOMS	COMMENTS
Renal	Nephrolithiasis, nephrocalcinosis, polyuria, polydipsia, renal insufficiency	15%–20% of patients have kidney stones
Skeletal	Fragility fractures	Unrelated to significant trauma
	Osteopenia/osteoporosis	Cortical bone > trabecular bone (distal third of radius most affected)
	Bone pain	Common
	Osteitis fibrosa cystica	Rare, but may occur with advanced disease, characterized by bone pain and multiple skeletal deformities including salt and pepper appearance of the skull, bone cysts, and brown tumors of bone
Neuromuscular	Proximal muscle weakness, muscular atrophy, gait disturbance	Rare
	Easy fatigability, generalized weakness	Common
Gastrointestinal	Gastroesophageal reflux, constipation, abdominal pain, peptic ulcer disease	Common Rare
	Nausea, vomiting, acute pancreatitis	Rare, can be seen in cases of severe hypercalcemia
Neuropsychiatric	Fatigue, depression, anxiety, emotional lability, sleep disturbances, lethargy, memory loss, inability to concentrate,	Often reported
	mental status change, psychosis, obtundation, and coma	Rare, can be seen with severe hypercalcemia
Cardiovascular	Exacerbation of hypertension, valvular disease, myocardial calcifications, premature atherosclerosis, left ventricular hypertrophy, shortened QT interval, conduction abnormalities, and heart block	Conflicting data on improvement of cardiac parameters after parathyroidectomy

Neuromuscular and neuropsychiatric symptoms are often reported by patients with primary HPT. Many of these symptoms may improve with surgical intervention, and include easy fatigability, generalized weakness, depression, anxiety, memory loss, and inability to concentrate. Three randomized controlled trials show neurocognitive benefits of surgery when compared with observation in patients with primary HPT.[17]

Diagnosis and Evaluation

The diagnostic evaluation of primary HPT should include measurements of serum total calcium, intact PTH, creatinine, and 25(OH)D levels (Table 38.4). Serum phosphorus, alkaline phosphatase, and 24-hour urine calcium and creatinine levels may also be of value. Classic primary HPT is defined by hypercalcemia associated with an elevated intact PTH level or an inappropriately normal intact PTH level. Patients with hypercalcemia from most other causes have a low (suppressed) PTH level. In a patient with hypercalcemia, if the PTH level is greater than 25 pg/mL, primary HPT remains a consideration. These patients should be asked about biotin supplementation, which should be stopped a few weeks prior to PTH testing, as biotin can falsely lower PTH test results.[19] Calcium measurements should be repeated to ensure persistent elevation. Total serum calcium levels should be corrected for abnormal serum albumin using the following equation: corrected calcium (mg/dL) = (0.8[4.0 – patient's albumin (g/dL)] + total calcium (mg/dL).[17]

In patients with primary HPT, vitamin D deficiency is associated with more significant hypercalcemia, more severe bone disease, and increased parathyroid adenoma weight.[17] Measurement of blood urea nitrogen, serum creatinine, and glomerular filtration rate (GFR) is essential because renal insufficiency is a known complication of primary HPT and to rule out chronic kidney disease, which is associated with a secondary increase in PTH levels. A 24-hour urine calcium and creatinine measurements are checked to evaluate for elevated urine calcium greater than 400 mg, which is associated with an increased risk of nephrolithiasis and is an established indication for parathyroidectomy, and to help rule out FHH, which can mimic primary HPT. Patients with FHH have a 24-hour urine calcium less than 100 mg and a calcium creatinine clearance ratio (CCCR) less than 0.01 (Table 38.4). The usefulness of routine measurement of CCCR to differentiate primary HPT from FHH has recently been called into question by a large study of 1000 patients with surgically confirmed primary HPT. Nineteen percent of patients with primary HPT had CCCR less than 0.01, 63% had a CCCR less than 0.02%, and none of them had FHH. Thus, calculating CCCR to differentiate FHH from primary HPT should not be prioritized in the workup of primary HPT unless there is high clinical suspicion of FHH.[23]

Normocalcemic primary HPT is a recognized variant of primary HPT that presents with high PTH levels and normal total and ionized serum calcium levels in the absence of secondary causes for HPT. Most patients with normocalcemic primary HPT are diagnosed as a result of evaluation for kidney stones or osteoporosis. There is increased recognition of this variant, particularly in centers where all patients with osteopenia or osteoporosis are screened for primary HPT.[19] Up to 16% of patients may progress over time to hypercalcemic primary HPT.[17] An ionized calcium level should be obtained in all patients with suspected normocalcemic primary HPT but it is not necessary to make the diagnosis of primary HPT in hypercalcemic patients. In patients with a normal serum calcium level and an elevated PTH level, other causes for an increased PTH level should be investigated, including, vitamin D deficiency, renal insufficiency, primary hypercalciuria, malabsorption syndromes, and medications such as bisphosphonates and denosumab. Normocalcemic primary HPT is associated with complications similar to those of hypercalcemic HPT, and thus, the management is no different for normocalcemic primary HPT than for classical primary HPT.[24]

Normohormonal primary HPT is another variant of primary HPT characterized by hypercalcemia and normal but inappropriately high intact PTH levels (>30 pg/mL). Rarely, patients with normohormonal primary HPT may have PTH levels less than 30 pg/

TABLE 38.4 Evaluation of patients with suspected or confirmed primary HPT.

TESTS	COMMENTS
Lab Tests	
Serum total calcium Intact PTH Creatinine, GFR 25-hydroxyvitamin D	Baseline laboratory tests for diagnosis of primary HPT and to rule out the most common causes of secondary HPT
Ionized calcium	For patients with normocalcemic primary HPT
Albumin	If low, calculate corrected calcium (mg/dL) = (0.8 [4.0-patient's albumin (g/dL)] + total calcium (mg/dL)
Serum phosphate	Low in approximately 50% of patients with primary HPT
Alkaline phosphatase	Marker of bone turnover, indicates extent of bone disease
Urine Tests	
24-hour urine calcium and creatinine	Screen for increased risk of kidney stones and for familial hypocalciuric hypercalcemia
If urine calcium <100 mg/24 hours, calculate CCCR	CCCR = (24-hour calcium urine/calcium serum)/(24-hour creatinine urine/creatinine serum)
Imaging	
DXA	Measurements of bone mineral density at the lumbar spine, hip femoral neck, and distal radius
Abdominal imaging for kidney stones or nephrocalcinosis	Plain abdominal x-ray, abdominal ultrasound, or noncontrasted CT
Vertebral spine assessment	Plain x-ray, CT, or DXA
Genetic Testing	
Indications	Patients with pHPT less than 40 years with multigland disease and patients with a family history of pHPT or syndromes associated with pHPT

CCCR, Calcium creatinine clearance ratio; *GFR*, glomerular filtration rate; *CT*, computed tomography; *DXA*, dual-energy x-ray absorptiometry; *HPT*, hyperparathyroidism; *pHPT*, primary hyperparathyroidism; *PTH*; parathyroid hormone.

mL, which is thought to be due to fragments of PTH not detected by current PTH assays or an early form of primary HPT.[17] Other theories on the lack of PTH elevation include a higher calcium set point, pulsatile PTH secretion, and presence of unmeasured but active PTH fragments.[25] The incidence of normohormonal HPT ranges from 0.3% to 18% in the literature,[25] but overall, it is uncommon in most surgeons' experience. A definitive diagnosis of normohormonal primary HPT is challenging and it is often a diagnosis of exclusion, as other causes of hypercalcemia need to be ruled out. Obtaining biochemical measurements at multiple time points may be helpful. It can be a challenging patient population to decide whom to operate on. Localizing studies, when positive, add an extra level of support in recommending surgery for these patients. Despite the atypical range of PTH values, patients with normohormonal primary HPT have the same signs and symptoms as expected for typical primary HPT, with similar cure rates after surgery.[25]

BOX 38.1 Established indications for parathyroidectomy in patients with primary hyperparathyroidism.

- All symptomatic patients (renal, bone, neurocognitive, or neuropsychiatric symptoms)
- Serum calcium >1 mg/dL above the upper limit of normal
- Age <50 years
- BMD T score <-2.5 (osteoporosis) or significant reduction in BMD
- Vertebral compression fracture on spine imaging
- Impaired renal function with GFR <60 mL/min
- Nephrolithiasis or nephrocalcinosis
- Hypercalciuria with increased stone risk (urine calcium >400 mg/24 hours)
- When active surveillance and routine long-term follow-up is not a good option

BMD, Bone mineral density; *GFR*, glomerular filtration rate.

All patients with primary HPT should undergo bone mineral density measurement with dual-energy x-ray absorptiometry. The World Health Organization defines osteopenia as a T score of −1.0 to −2.5 and osteoporosis as having a T score of less than −2.5. The distal third of the radius is most significantly affected by primary HPT, which is cortical bone. The lumbar spine, which is primarily trabecular bone, is the least affected.[17] Due to the association of primary HPT with vertebral fractures and silent nephrolithiasis, renal and spine imaging should be considered in the evaluation of patients with primary HPT (Table 38.4). Genetic counseling and genetic testing should be considered in patients with a diagnosis of primary HPT who are less than 40 years of age with multigland disease and those with a strong family history of syndromic manifestations.

Management

Indications for Parathyroidectomy

Parathyroidectomy is the only curative treatment for primary HPT, and for this reason, all patients with primary HPT should be presented with the option for definitive surgical treatment. Osteoporosis, nephrolithiasis, nephrocalcinosis, impaired renal function (GFR <60 mL/min), urine calcium greater than 400 mg/24 hours, and vertebral compression factures on spine imaging or a fragility fracture are established indications for parathyroidectomy (Box 38.1). Age less than 50 years, a serum total calcium level greater than 1 mg/dL above the upper limit of normal or inability, and unwillingness to participate in long-term active surveillance are other established indications for parathyroidectomy in patients with primary HPT regardless of the presence or absence of signs or symptoms.

Patients who are less than 50 years of age and decline surgical intervention will need long-term monitoring and are more likely to develop progression of primary HPT with complications over the course of their lifetime.[17,26] Parathyroidectomy is more cost-effective when compared to long-term observation for progression of disease in patients with asymptomatic primary HPT. Patients with neurocognitive symptoms and even those considered to have asymptomatic primary HPT have been reported to have improvement in quality of life indexes following parathyroidectomy.[27]

Parathyroid Localization

Parathyroid imaging has no role in confirming or excluding the diagnosis of HPT. Parathyroid imaging is reserved for patients with

TABLE 38.5 Characteristic of preoperative imaging studies in patients with hyperparathyroidism.

IMAGING	IMAGING FINDINGS	SENSITIVITY, PPV	ADVANTAGES	LIMITATIONS	UPDATES
US	Hypoechoic nodule with well-defined hypervascular echogenic capsule	76%, 93%	Noninvasive, inexpensive, can be performed rapidly by the surgeon with simultaneous evaluation of the thyroid	Unable to see ectopic mediastinal, retroesophageal, or retropharyngeal glands; decreased sensitivity in multigland disease and small glands; thyroid nodules and lymph nodes can cause false-positives	US elastography
Sestamibi-SPECT	Increased focal uptake and prolonged retention of the technetium-99m sestamibi	79%, 90%	Detects ectopic and posterior glands; lower radiation than 4D-CT, operator-independent	Long duration of time for the exam; more expensive than US and 4D-CT, radiation exposure; decreased sensitivity for multigland disease and small glands; false-positives (lymph nodes, thyroid tissue, granulomatous disease)	PET scanning with various radiopharmaceuticals under investigation
4D-CT	Soft tissue nodule with peaked enhancement in arterial phase and washout in venous phase with polar vessel	81%–89%, 93%	Rapid acquisition time, superior anatomic information, superior sensitivity than other techniques, more successful in localizing small adenomas and multigland disease	High radiation dose, intravenous contrast use, some contrast artifact in neck veins can occur	Protocols with fewer phases or less contrast, to diminish radiation and contrast dose
MRI	Homogeneous or marbled appearance with high intensity on T2-weighed images, intermediate to low intensity on T1-weighed images	43%–94%	No radiation, contrast not necessary, superior anatomic information	Expensive, long duration of study acquisition, cannot use in patients with metal implants, low specificity	Dixon fat suppression method
^{18}F-fluorocholine PET/CT	Focal tracer uptake	93%, 90%	Decreased radiation and acquisition time compared to some sestamibi protocols, higher sensitivity	Limited data on new tracer, limited availability	Ability to differentiate between parathyroid adenoma and hyperplasia preoperatively based on maximal standardized uptake values

CT, Computed tomography; *4D-CT*, four-dimensional CT; *MRI*, magnetic resonance imaging; *PET/CT*, positron emission tomography/CT; *SPECT*, single photon emission CT; *US*, ultrasound.

an established diagnosis of HPT to localize abnormal parathyroid glands for operative planning. The goal of parathyroid imaging is to help focus the exploration and to identify ectopic parathyroid glands. Negative imaging studies do not alter the recommendation for surgical exploration. In a recent study, surgical cure was achieved in greater than 97% of patients with nonlocalizing preoperative studies, despite a greater incidence of multigland disease and requirement for more extensive surgery.[28] Parathyroid imaging is significantly less accurate for multigland disease compared to single or double adenoma, likely due to the smaller gland size and different pathophysiology of those glands.

The most common imaging modalities used for localization of abnormal parathyroid glands are ultrasound and sestamibi scintigraphy (Table 38.5). There is no clear algorithm for parathyroid imaging, and the choice for one or a combination of studies depends on their availability, preferences, and institutional expertise. Ultrasound is often used as the initial imaging modality because it is readily available, inexpensive, and noninvasive and can be performed by surgeons in their office. On ultrasound, an abnormal parathyroid gland appears as a round or oval hypoechoic mass with a well-defined hypervascular echogenic capsule, typically located posterior to the superior or inferior pole of the lobe of the thyroid gland (Fig. 38.8). Cervical ultrasound is performed with a high-frequency probe, and both the central and lateral compartments of the neck are imaged, with evaluation for thyroid and parathyroid abnormalities. The accuracy of ultrasound is dependent on the skill and experience of the sonographer. A recent meta analysis documented an overall sensitivity of 76% for ultrasound, with a sensitivity of only 35% for identification of multigland disease (Table 38.5).[29,30] The disadvantages of ultrasound include its inability to detect ectopic parathyroid glands in the mediastinum, retropharyngeal, or retroesophageal locations and its decreased sensitivity in multigland disease. Another challenge is discerning differences in appearance between lymph nodes, thyroid nodules, and abnormal parathyroid glands on ultrasound. Recent studies have evaluated the method of ultrasound

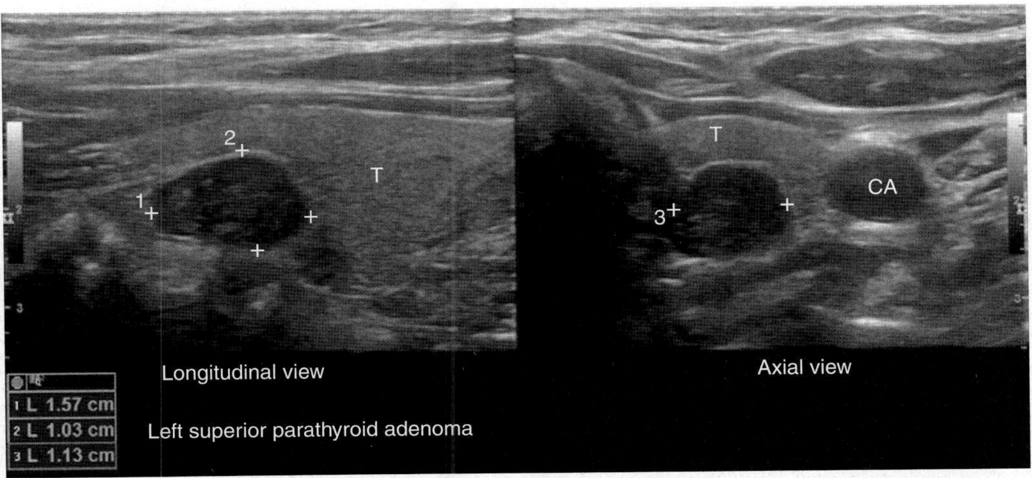

FIG. 38.8 High-resolution ultrasound images demonstrating a 1.57 × 1.03 × 1.13 cm hypoechoic mass posterior to the superior pole of the left lobe of the thyroid gland in longitudinal and axial views, which corresponded to a left superior parathyroid adenoma. Parathyroid gland marked by measuring points. *CA*, Carotid artery; *T*, thyroid.

elastography as a technique to quantify the stiffness of tissues. Malignant thyroid nodules have greater stiffness than parathyroid adenomas, which are stiffer than thyroid nodules and hyperplastic parathyroid glands. Initial data suggest that it might be a useful adjunct to parathyroid ultrasound imaging, but additional studies will be necessary.[31]

Sestamibi is the dominant radioisotope used for parathyroid imaging; sestamibi imaging relies on the differential uptake and retention of radiotracer in mitochondria-rich cells of metabolically active tissues. Hyperfunctioning parathyroid glands preferentially take up and retain the radiotracer. Sestamibi scintigraphy can be performed with dual-phase technique using a single isotope or single-phase technique using dual isotopes. Both techniques can be combined with single photon emission CT (SPECT) and SPECT/CT imaging. There are advantages and disadvantages for the various nuclear medicine protocols. SPECT provides three-dimensional (3D) imaging and improves parathyroid lesion localization, while the addition of CT images provides additional anatomic detail.[29] The main benefits of sestamibi imaging include its ability to identify ectopic glands in the mediastinum or deep cervical region and provide anatomic details of abnormal glands (Fig. 38.9). The sensitivity of sestamibi-SPECT is 79% for localization of a parathyroid adenoma and 44% for multigland disease.[29,30] The combination of ultrasound and sestamibi imaging improves the accuracy of parathyroid localization, with the combined sensitivity significantly higher than either imaging technique alone. This is a commonly employed practice by a majority of clinicians.

Dynamic four-dimensional CT (4D-CT) is a newer modality used to identify abnormal parathyroid glands (Table 38.5). Approximately 10% of institutions have adopted it as the initial imaging modality for parathyroid localization.[29] The four dimensions refer to a noncontrast phase, an early arterial phase (45 seconds after intravenous contrast injection), a delayed phase (75 seconds after contrast injection), and an assessment of the change in perfusion over time. A parathyroid adenoma has a lower attenuation value compared to the thyroid gland on unenhanced images; an average of 45 Hounsfield units compared to 90 Hounsfield units, respectively. On the early arterial phase, a parathyroid adenoma demonstrates rapid contrast enhancement with maximum attenuation values of approximately 130 Hounsfield units. On the delayed phase, there is rapid washout of the contrast material. An overall 81% to 89% sensitivity has been reported for 4D-CT imaging and 55% sensitivity for multigland disease. 4D-CT has been suggested to be particularly useful in localizing small adenomas and abnormal glands in reoperative cases. Limitations of 4D-CT include a high radiation dose and use of intravenous contrast.[29]

Magnetic resonance imaging (MRI) is seldom used in parathyroid imaging and is usually reserved as a second- or third-line modality in challenging or reoperative cases. It has a lower sensitivity than other modalities, with a range of 43% to 94% reported in the literature. Adenomas have a homogenous or marbled appearance with high intensity on T2-weighed images and intermediate to low intensity on T1-weighed images. There is ongoing investigation to try to develop new fat suppression sequences that may improve the usefulness of MRI in parathyroid imaging.[29]

Recently, the role of positron emission tomography/CT (PET/CT) has been evaluated for localization of abnormal parathyroid glands using specific PET tracers. PET/CT using the tracer ^{18}F-fluorocholine, a marker of cellular proliferation, has shown promising results in parathyroid localization.[32] It is a hybrid imaging technique, which combines metabolic data with anatomic localization to enhance spatial resolution. In a recent study comparing ^{18}F-fluorocholine PET/CT with ^{99m}Tc-MIBI/tetrofosmin SPECT/CT in 100 patients that underwent both studies, ^{18}F-fluorocholine PET/CT was superior to SPECT/CT, with sensitivities of 93% and 61%, respectively. In addition, ^{18}F-fluorocholine PET/CT was able to detect a parathyroid adenoma in 23 patients in whom sestamibi SPECT/CT was negative. It was also effective in localizing small parathyroid adenomas.[33] While still under investigation, this is a potentially promising technique for parathyroid localization. Other modalities such as selective venous PTH sampling, preoperative bilateral jugular vein PTH sampling, and ultrasound-guided fine-needle aspiration biopsy may have a role in highly selected cases of persistent or recurrent HPT requiring reoperation.

Surgical Options and Intraoperative Adjuncts

Definitive treatment of primary HPT consists of removal of all hyperfunctioning parathyroid glands and this may be

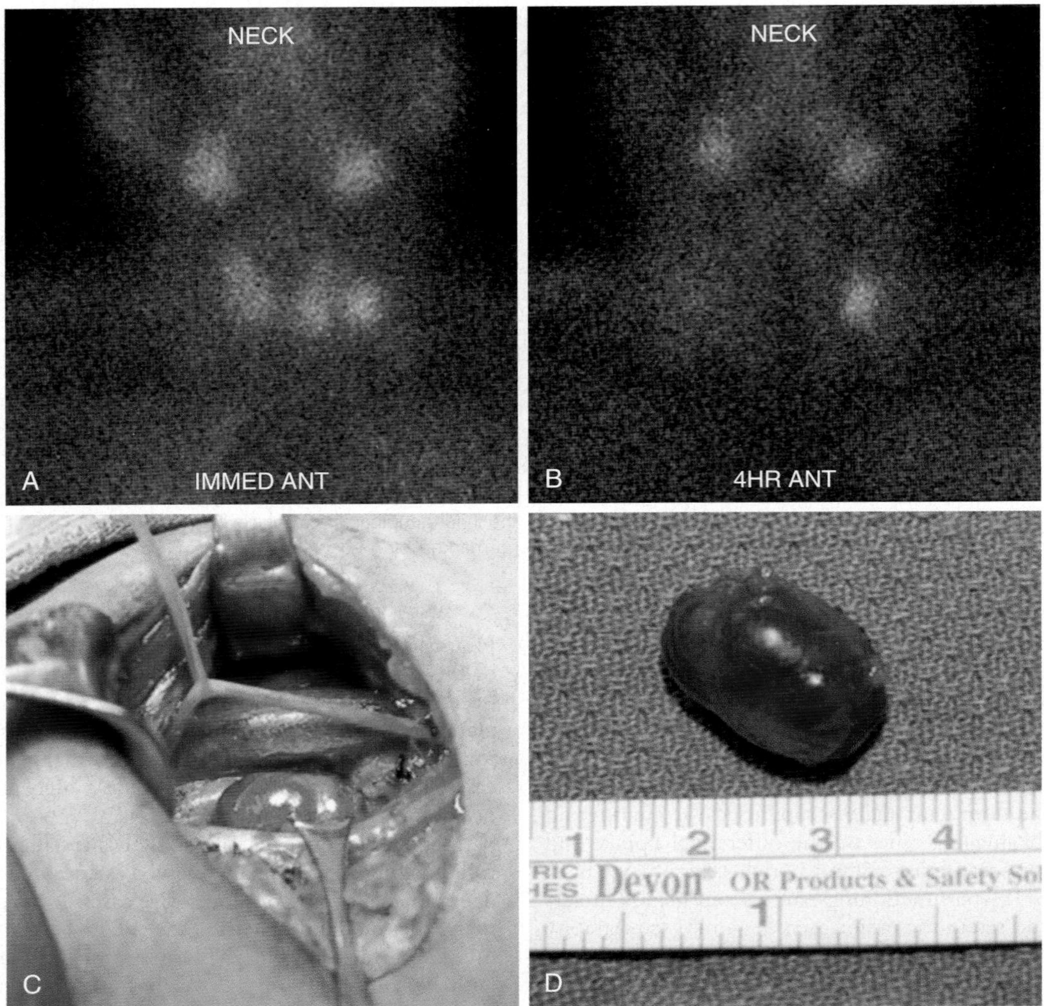

FIG. 38.9 (A) A focal area of abnormal radiotracer accumulation lateral to the thyroid gland on an immediate technetium 99m sestamibi image. (B) A 4-hour delayed image. (C) An intraoperative photograph of an ectopic parathyroid gland in the left carotid sheath present between the internal jugular vein and common carotid artery. The vagus nerve is retracted with a vessel loop anteromedially, and the common carotid artery is retracted laterally. (D) Ex vivo ectopic parathyroid adenoma excised from the left carotid sheath.

accomplished by performing a focused parathyroidectomy or a bilateral neck exploration. A focused parathyroidectomy, often referred to as MIP, is typically an outpatient procedure, which can be performed under local or general anesthesia through a small incision (3–4 cm), and consists of a focused dissection usually limited to only one gland that has been localized on preoperative imaging. Visualization of the other ipsilateral parathyroid gland depends on surgeon preference and practice. Bilateral neck exploration is performed to visualize all four parathyroid glands with subsequent removal of one or more abnormal glands.

IOPTH monitoring is a commonly used adjunct, which guides the surgeon on when to stop the parathyroid exploration. It helps confirm that there is no residual hyperfunctioning parathyroid tissue. IOPTH improves cure rates in patients with primary HPT and well-localized disease undergoing MIP from 96% without IOPTH to 97% to 99%.[17] Blood is drawn from a peripheral vein, arterial line, anterior jugular vein, or internal jugular vein at specific time points before and during the operation based on the protocol followed. The PTH level is expected to drop after the pathologic gland(s) are excised due to the short half-life of PTH (3–5 minutes). While local practices vary, PTH levels are drawn at the following time points: (1) preincision (at a date prior to surgery or prior to starting the operation on the day of surgery); (2) preexcision (after exposing an abnormal gland but prior to ligating the blood supply to the gland); (3) 5 minutes after gland removal; and (4) 10 minutes after gland removal. Based on the Miami Criteria, a more than 50% decline in PTH at 10 minutes following parathyroid gland removal compared to the highest baseline level, either the preincision or preexcision, suggests cure and the procedure can be terminated. Dual criteria are commonly used to decide when to stop parathyroid exploration, which requires a more than 50% PTH decrease from the preincision level plus a final PTH that is within the normal range. Studies reporting on both of these well-validated protocols report cure rates of 97% to 99% with recurrence rates less than 3%.[17,34,35] Additional PTH levels may be obtained if the 10-minute PTH level does not decline by more than 50% or does not fall into the normal range as expected (at 15 or 20 minutes after gland excision) and/or after further dissection and other gland(s) excision is carried out. The advantages of a MIP include a smaller incision, shorter operative time, and a dissection that is limited to one side of the neck, with lower rates of transient hypocalcemia compared to bilateral exploration.

Indications for a bilateral exploration include surgeon preference, failure of a focused exploration (PTH does not drop per expected protocol), known or intraoperatively identified parathyroid hyperplasia, high suspicion of multigland disease (secondary and tertiary HPT, lithium-induced HPT, familial HPT), and discordant or negative preoperative localization studies. During a bilateral exploration, all glands are identified and compared to decide if the patient has a single adenoma, double adenoma, or four-gland hyperplasia. Ectopic parathyroid glands can pose a challenge, as approximately 16% of patients have ectopic glands and 13% of patients have supernumerary parathyroid glands.[14] Ectopic locations should be evaluated when an abnormal parathyroid gland cannot be identified. The most common ectopic location for a missing inferior gland is in the thymus (Fig. 38.5). Other ectopic sites for a missing inferior gland are the thyrothymic ligament, the anterior superior mediastinum, the aortopulmonary window, undescended in a submandibular location, the carotid sheath (Fig. 38.9), and intrathyroidal. The most common ectopic location for a missing superior parathyroid gland is in the tracheoesophageal groove. Other ectopic sites for a missing superior parathyroid gland include retroesophageal, retropharyngeal, the posterior mediastinum, and intrathyroidal.

If all four glands appear to be abnormal, a subtotal parathyroidectomy is performed, which entails the removal of three glands entirely and part of the fourth, leaving a remnant that is approximately 1 to 2 times a normal gland. The remnant should be fashioned prior to removal of the remaining glands, marked with a surgical clip and should be rechecked for viability prior to removing the other parathyroid glands. A transcervical thymectomy is also performed because the thymus is the most common site for a supernumerary parathyroid gland, which occurs in 13% of patients. The adjunctive use of IOPTH can be considered and is sometimes routinely used during bilateral neck exploration to confirm cure, particularly when all four parathyroid glands are not able to be identified. While complication rates are similar to MIP, bilateral neck exploration is associated with a higher rate of transient hypocalcemia.

Because parathyroid tissue can resemble fat, lymph nodes, thyroid tissue, or thymus, intraoperative identification can be confirmed with frozen section analysis or rarely by ex vivo aspiration and PTH measurement. Aspiration is performed by taking a small amount of parathyroid tissue with a fine needle and rinsing it into 1 cc of normal saline, followed by measuring PTH in the sample. Neither frozen section exam nor tissue PTH measurement is necessary when the results of IOPTH measurement confirm that all hypersecreting parathyroid tissue has been removed.

An additional intraoperative adjunct to help improve parathyroid gland visualization is the use of indocyanine green dye and near-infrared autofluorescence. Other adjuncts that can aid in intraoperative parathyroid gland localization include ultrasound, bilateral jugular venous sampling, and radio-guided parathyroidectomy using a gamma probe. Recurrent laryngeal nerve monitoring is used less often in parathyroid compared to thyroid surgery, but can be considered in reoperative cases.

Unique surgical approaches to the central neck have surfaced in the last decade. A few specialized centers offer endoscopic or robotic parathyroidectomies for select patients who wish to avoid a neck incision. Access to the central neck is gained through an axillary incision or through a transoral vestibular approach. Operative times are longer with increased technical difficulty and limited long-term outcome data.[36]

During parathyroid surgery, meticulous dissection should be carried out to prevent disruption of the capsule of an abnormal parathyroid gland, which can lead to parathyromatosis. Parathyromatosis refers to multiple parathyroid implants in the soft tissue of the neck, which cause chronic intractable hypercalcemia. Also, care should be taken to prevent devascularization of the normal parathyroid glands. If a normal parathyroid gland is devascularized, it should be autotransplanted in the ipsilateral sternocleidomastoid muscle, a strap muscle, or the forearm and its location marked with clips for future identification.

Postoperative Management

After parathyroidectomy, patients are observed for neck hematoma and signs or symptoms of hypocalcemia. Depending on the extent of surgery and surgeon preference, patients are discharged after a normal recovery in the postanesthesia care unit or are admitted for overnight observation. Neck hematoma is a rare but life-threatening complication, with a rate of 0.3% after parathyroidectomy.[37] Patients at an increased risk for postoperative bleeding such as those on anticoagulation or hemodialysis or with a known coagulopathy should be considered for overnight observation. Hypocalcemia is uncommon after removal of a single adenoma and patients typically do not need calcium supplementation. Hypocalcemia is more common following subtotal parathyroidectomy. Symptoms of hypocalcemia include acral and perioral numbness and paresthesias, muscle cramping, and weakness, and are treated with intravenous calcium gluconate and/or oral calcium carbonate with or without vitamin D supplementation, postoperatively. Patients with profound hypocalcemia may experience tetany with carpopedal spasm or trismus. Patients are educated on the symptoms of hypocalcemia preoperatively and instructed to have calcium and vitamin D supplements available at home if a specific prescription is not given.

Patients with primary HPT who have vitamin D deficiency should receive vitamin D supplementation postoperatively with reevaluation of 25(OH)D levels at 3 months. Calcium levels are typically checked on postoperative day 1, at 2 weeks after surgery, and again at 6 months after surgery to confirm cure of primary HPT, which is defined as eucalcemia at 6 months after surgery.

Medical Management of Primary Hyperparathyroidism

Patients with primary HPT who do not undergo parathyroidectomy should be monitored for signs and symptoms of disease progression. Guidelines recommend annual measurements of serum calcium, creatinine, and GFR. Bone mineral density should be monitored every 1 to 2 years at the spine, hip, and forearm. Vertebral fracture evaluation should be performed if there is clinical suspicion due to new back pain or loss of height. Similarly, reevaluation for kidney stones should be performed if suggestive symptoms emerge.[20,26] During the surveillance period, patients who were originally asymptomatic should be referred for surgical evaluation if serum calcium concentration becomes more than 1 mg/dL above the upper limit or normal, if GFR falls below 60 mL/min, for significant bone mineral density reduction or development of osteoporosis, or if patients develop new kidney stones or vertebral fractures.[26]

The goals of medical management of primary HPT are to control hypercalcemia and hypercalciuria and prevent progression of renal and bone disease. Hydration should be encouraged to prevent progression of hypercalcemia and nephrolithiasis. Cinacalcet is an allosteric activator of the CaSR, and has been used for treatment of hypercalcemia in patients with recurrent or metastatic parathyroid cancer, hypercalcemic crisis (HC), and secondary HPT. It sensitizes the CaSR to serum calcium, which suppresses the secretion of PTH. It has not been approved for routine use in patients with primary HPT who are surgical candidates, but has been approved by the FDA for patients with severe primary HPT who are unable to undergo surgery.[20] In a randomized controlled trial, after a year of treatment with cinacalcet, both calcium and PTH values were reduced in 19% of patients with primary HPT who received cinacalcet compared to placebo. However, cinacalcet has no effect on bone loss, which continues at the same rate without surgery.[18] For patients with primary HPT, surgery is more effective at treating and preventing complications of HPT and is more cost-effective compared to medical therapy.[17]

Bisphosphonate therapy can be used to improve bone mass in patients with primary HPT and osteoporosis. Bisphosphonates do not change calcium or PTH levels. In patients with primary HPT who require both a reduction in serum calcium levels and improvement in bone mineral density but cannot undergo parathyroidectomy, the combination of cinacalcet and bisphosphonate therapy can be considered, but studies are limited and retrospective.[20] Thiazide diuretics can be used to decrease the urine calcium levels in patients with primary HPT and hypercalciuria, which can reduce the risk of calcium stone disease.[18]

Outcomes After Surgery

When parathyroidectomy is performed by an experienced surgeon, cure rates for sporadic primary HPT are 95% to 99%. Complications include transient hypocalcemia (5%–47%), permanent hypoparathyroidism (0%–3%), recurrent laryngeal nerve injury (<1%), neck hematoma (0.3%), and wound infection.[17,37] Surgical cure of primary HPT is followed by an increase in bone mass in increments of 2% to 4% in the first postoperative year.[18] Patients with normal, osteopenic, or osteoporotic bones will have improvement in bone mineral density with a deceased fracture rate. In a 15-year retrospective study, rates of hip and wrist fracture decrease by 50% to 64% at 10 years in patients who underwent curative parathyroidectomy compared to a matched cohort who did not undergo surgery.[38] Following curative parathyroidectomy, patients have a decreased risk of recurrent kidney stones and a decrease in urinary calcium levels. While there may be no improvement in nephrocalcinosis and renal insufficiency, further decline in renal function will be prevented.[18] Neurocognitive symptoms attributed to primary HPT have shown variable degrees of improvement after curative surgery.[17]

SECONDARY AND TERTIARY HYPERPARATHYROIDISM

Secondary Hyperparathyroidism

Secondary HPT initially occurs as a physiologic response of parathyroid glands to hypocalcemia. It is characterized by elevated PTH levels with low or normal serum calcium levels. Secondary HPT is most commonly due to chronic kidney disease, vitamin D deficiency, and intestinal calcium malabsorption. Additional causes of secondary HPT are listed in Box 38.2. Vitamin D deficiency and hypocalcemia worsen secondary HPT by causing increased secretion of PTH and must be treated with vitamin D and calcium supplementation. Patients should receive 1000 to 1200 mg of calcium per day (from diet or supplementation) and vitamin D supplementation to maintain a serum 25(OH)D of more than 30 ng/mL.[18]

BOX 38.2 Causes of secondary hyperparathyroidism.

- Chronic renal failure
- 25-Hydroxyvitamin D deficiency
- Malabsorption syndromes
  - Celiac disease
  - Cystic fibrosis
  - Short gut syndrome
  - Bariatric procedures
- Medications
  - Lithium
  - Diuretics (e.g., hydrochlorothiazide, furosemide)
- Metabolic abnormalities
  - Hypermagnesemia
  - Hyperphosphatemia
- Congenital disorders
  - Transient neonatal hyperparathyroidism
  - DiGeorge syndrome

Chronic renal failure causes secondary HPT by multiple mechanisms. Patients with chronic renal failure have reduced phosphate excretion and increased serum phosphate, which binds to calcium and reduces serum-free calcium levels. They also have reduced 1-hydroxylase activity in the kidney, which results in decreased renal conversion of 25 (OH) vitamin D to 1, 25, $(OH)_2$ vitamin D (the biologically active form of vitamin D) and decreased intestinal absorption of calcium. The net effect of hyperphosphatemia and low levels of the biologically active form of vitamin D is chronic hypocalcemia, which causes: (1) down-regulation of the *CaSR* on the parathyroid cells and shift in the calcium set point; (2) down-regulation of the vitamin D receptor on parathyroid cells; and (3) alterations in cell cycle regulation—all leading to PTH hypersecretion, parathyroid cell proliferation, and parathyroid gland hyperplasia.[39]

An estimated 90% of patients with chronic renal insufficiency develop secondary HPT, most of whom can be managed medically with dietary phosphate reduction, phosphate binders, oral calcium and calcitriol supplementation, intravenous vitamin D analogues, and dialysis. In addition, cinacalcet, a calcimimetic agent, is used to alter the sensitivity of the *CaSR* of the parathyroid cells and reduce PTH secretion helping to restore calcium-phosphate homeostasis.[39,40] International guidelines from The Kidney Disease Improving Global Outcomes work group recommend lowering serum phosphorus levels into the normal range and maintaining intact-PTH levels between 2 and 9 times the upper limit of the normal range.[41]

Parathyroidectomy is indicated for patients with medically refractory or complicated renal HPT, accounting for 1% to 2% of patients with renal HPT per year.[40] A consensus report from the European Society of Endocrine Surgeons recommends the following indications for parathyroidectomy in patients with renal HPT: (1) a PTH greater than 800 pg/mL, (2) sustained hypercalcemia, (3) refractory hyperphosphatemia, (4) elevation of calcium-phosphorous product greater than 55 mg^2/dL^2, (5) severe symptomatic bone disease, and 6) calciphylaxis.[40] Other potential indications include symptomatic ectopic extraosseous calcification (calcinosis), intolerance to cinacalcet, profound muscle weakness, and intractable pruritus. Parathyroidectomy is important because of the evidence for increased mortality from cardiovascular complications and ectopic calcifications in patients with medically refractory renal HPT. Kidney transplantation remains the best option for treatment of the metabolic derangements associated with refractory renal HPT.

The standard surgical options for treatment of renal HPT are subtotal parathyroidectomy or total parathyroidectomy with autotransplantation. Both surgical options include a transcervical thymectomy to remove potential supernumerary glands, which are most often found in the thymus. When performing a subtotal parathyroidectomy, an in-situ, 40- to 80- mg well-vascularized, parathyroid remnant is fashioned initially, followed by removal of all remaining parathyroid glands after confirming the viability of the remnant. The remnant is marked with a large clip or a nonabsorbable suture to help facilitate identification in the event of a future remnant recurrence.

In patients who undergo total parathyroidectomy and autotransplantation, the autotransplant is preferably performed in the brachioradialis muscle of the nondominant forearm. This may help avoid reoperation in the neck and allows for differential measurement of PTH in the graft-bearing and non–graft-bearing forearms to help differentiate the remnant from the neck as the site for recurrence. Proponents for subtotal or total parathyroidectomy and autotransplantation suggest that there are higher rates of recurrence for subtotal parathyroidectomy versus higher rates of hypoparathyroidism for total parathyroidectomy and autotransplantation. Median recurrence rates after either surgical technique is 7%, with a 2% rate of permanent hypoparathyroidism.[40]

Tertiary Hyperparathyroidism

Tertiary HPT refers to autonomous overproduction of PTH with the development of hypercalcemia in patients with chronic renal failure and preexisting secondary HPT. Tertiary HPT is also used to define HPT that persists or occurs after successful renal transplantation.[40] Patients with tertiary HPT have elevated serum calcium and intact-PTH levels. While secondary HPT resolves in many patients after transplantation, up to 25% of patients with secondary HPT will have persistent HPT (tertiary HPT) 1 year after transplantation in the form of diffuse and nodular hyperplasia.[42] Prolonged PTH increase in kidney transplant recipients is associated with increases risk of bone loss, decreased allograft survival, and decreased patient survival.

The two treatment options for tertiary HPT are medical therapy with cinacalcet and parathyroidectomy. Surgery has been shown to be superior to cinacalcet in normalizing calcium and PTH levels at 1 year after surgery as well as lower rates of allograft failure.[42] Despite improved outcomes with surgery, only 7% of patients with tertiary HPT end up undergoing parathyroidectomy.[42] Indications for parathyroidectomy in tertiary HPT include persistent hypercalcemia or hypercalciuria, renal phosphorous wasting, low bone mineral density, nephrocalcinosis, symptomatic disease, and enlarged parathyroids on imaging.[42] In patients who are allograft candidates and have tertiary HPT with high PTH and calcium levels, pretransplant parathyroidectomy should be considered, as it has been associated with improved graft function.[40]

Profound postoperative hypocalcemia is common after parathyroidectomy for renal HPT. Postoperative hypocalcemia is attributed to renal osteodystrophy and "hungry bone syndrome" and occurs due to the sudden decline in circulating PTH levels after surgery, causing a surge in bone uptake of calcium as a result of remineralization.[43] Cinacalcet may also contribute to postoperative hypocalcemia. Patients may or may not experience symptoms related to hypocalcemia, which include acral and perioral numbness and paresthesias, muscle cramping, neuromuscular irritability with carpopedal spasm or trismus, and cardiac arrhythmias. Patients usually require admission for 3 to 5 days after parathyroidectomy for treatment of hypocalcemia with oral and intravenous calcium replacement and calcitriol administration. Correction of associated hypomagnesemia also often is required. Because calcitriol may take up to 48 hours to work, recent studies have evaluated the utility of preoperative calcitriol loading. Preoperative calcitriol treatment starting 5 days prior to surgery resulted in a reduction in intravenous calcium requirement postoperatively and a 50% reduction in the length of hospital stay.[43]

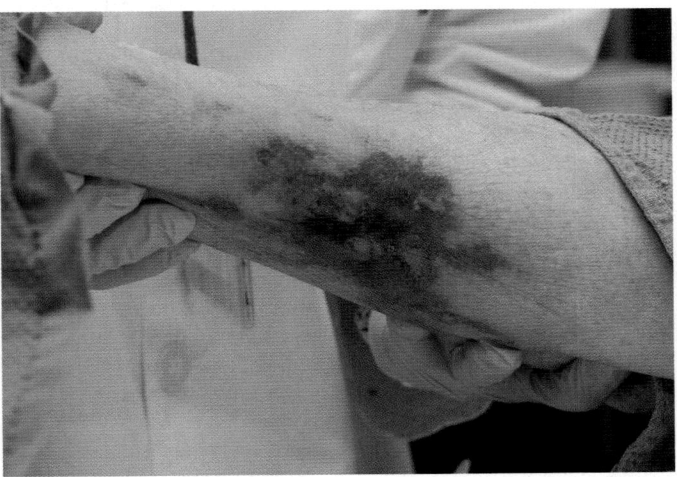

FIG. 38.10 A violaceous skin lesion with ischemia and eschar formation resulting from calciphylaxis.

Calciphylaxis

Calciphylaxis, also referred to as calcific uremic arteriolopathy, is a rare disease manifested by painful violaceous skin lesions with associated ulceration, ischemia, necrosis, and eschar formation (Fig. 38.10). Calciphylaxis is characterized by microvascular calcification, intimal proliferation, fibrosis, and thrombotic occlusion of small subcutaneous vessels. It predominantly affects patients with end-stage renal disease and secondary HPT but may also occur in renal transplant recipients and rarely in patients with primary HPT. Painful nonhealing wounds with areas of skin necrosis develop in these patients with secondary infection, gangrene, sepsis, and death. Mortality rates of 50% to 80% are reported in patients with calciphylaxis. Factors that have been implicated in the pathogenesis of calciphylaxis include medically-refractory hyperphosphatemia, a high calcium-phosphate product, high PTH levels, use of warfarin, protein C and protein S deficiency, and other causes of thrombophilia. A diagnosis of calciphylaxis is made in a patient with chronic kidney disease and secondary HPT who has the combination of painful, violaceous, tender cutaneous skin lesions, and a skin biopsy demonstrating vascular and extravascular calcifications in the absence of histologic findings of vasculitis.

The relationship between HPT and calciphylaxis is not fully understood, as most patients with severe HPT do not develop calciphylaxis and many patients with end-stage renal disease and calciphylaxis do not have HPT. However, in small studies, patients with elevated PTH levels and calciphylaxis have been found to benefit from parathyroidectomy. Treatment options for calciphylaxis include sodium thiosulfate, phosphate binders, low calcium dialysate bath, bisphosphonates, calcimimetics, and parathyroidectomy. Because of the high mortality associated with calciphylaxis and the potential for progression after subtotal parathyroidectomy, total parathyroidectomy with transcervical thymectomy is the preferred operation. Debridement may be necessary for control of wound sepsis, but debridement of dry eschar should be avoided since this can lead to progression of calciphylaxis.

The role of urgent parathyroidectomy is controversial in the management of calciphylaxis, due to only a limited number of small studies that demonstrate a survival advantage in parathyroidectomy patients, but were likely affected by selection bias. One retrospective case-control study failed to show a survival advantage among end-stage renal disease patients with calciphylaxis who had parathyroidectomy compared to those who did not.[44] In contrast, several small series have shown a survival benefit in patients with end-stage renal disease, calciphylaxis, and severe HPT (PTH >400) who underwent parathyroidectomy compared to those without surgery.[45] Further studies are needed to further delineate the pathophysiology and optimal treatment of calciphylaxis.

HYPERPARATHYROIDISM-INDUCED HYPERCALCEMIC CRISIS

HC is a rare, potentially life-threatening condition. HPT and advanced malignancy are the two most common causes, accounting for 90% or more of all cases. HPT-induced HC (HIHC) is one of the few endocrine emergencies. In 1932, Lowenburg and Ginsburg reported a case of HC in a boy who was receiving parathyroid extract for treatment of purpura hemorrhagica.[46] In 1939, Hanes described the clinical syndrome of HIHC and reported the first death from HIHC. More recently, in 2001, Ziegler reported asystole intraoperatively and death from asystole postoperatively following removal of an 8.3-g parathyroid adenoma in a patient with HIHC.[47]

The definition of HIHC has not been standardized, and various definitions exist in the medical and surgical literature. A clinically useful definition is an albumin-corrected serum calcium level of 14 mg/dL or greater with associated organ dysfunction. As a result of the various definitions that have been used to define HIHC, its incidence among all patients with HPT is variable. Rates of 2% to 7% for HIHC are reported in the literature.

HIHC is usually characterized by an acute onset following some intercurrent illness or precipitating event with dehydration. Patients often present with symptoms related to dysfunction of the gastrointestinal, renal, cardiac, and central nervous systems, some of which may be life-threatening. Gastrointestinal manifestations include anorexia, nausea, vomiting, acute pancreatitis, and severe peptic ulcer disease. Acute pancreatitis is more common in patients with HIHC than in patients with HPT without crisis. Renal manifestations include nephrocalcinosis, nephrolithiasis, polyuria and polydipsia, acute kidney injury, oliguria, and anuria. Cardiac manifestations include shortening of the QT interval, bradycardia, complete heart block, myocardial calcinosis, and development of ventricular tachyarrhythmias. Neurocognitive derangements are common, such as exacerbation of underlying psychiatric illness, lethargy, somnolence, confusion, obtundation, and coma.

Patients with HIHC are more likely to have a palpable neck mass than patients with HPT without HC. The laboratory evaluation in patients with HIHC, in addition to higher calcium levels, is notable for significantly higher intact PTH, chloride, and alkaline phosphatase levels and significantly lower phosphorus levels than their counterparts with HPT without HC. Patients may also have evidence for volume depletion, hypokalemia, and acute kidney injury.

The management of HIHC consists of interventions to rapidly reduce serum calcium levels followed by expeditious parathyroidectomy. Large well-designed clinical studies assessing the appropriate management of HIHC are lacking. The rationale for lowering serum calcium levels prior to operation is to reduce the potential for life-threatening cardiac arrhythmias, multiorgan system failure, and refractory shock, which have been documented as causes for perioperative mortality in patients with HIHC.

Patients with HIHC should undergo rapid expansion of their extracellular fluid volume with intravenous isotonic sodium chloride solution to promote calciuresis. Once their volume deficit has been corrected, furosemide may be given to further increase calciuresis. Bisphosphonate drugs, which inhibit osteoclast function, are regarded as first line therapy of HIHC in combination with intravenous volume expansion. Either pamidronate or zoledronic acid is highly effective in reducing serum calcium levels. Zoledronic acid is preferable because of its greater potency and ease of administration. Four milligrams of zoledronic acid administered as an intravenous infusion over 5 to 15 minutes produces a reduction of serum calcium in 24 to 48 hours. While awaiting a response to the bisphosphonate agent, calcitonin, which also inhibits osteoclast function, may be given as a temporizing agent. It has a rapid onset of action, within 12 to 24 hours, and can be effectively used in combination with bisphosphonates. Its effect on serum calcium is modest, reducing calcium by approximately 1 mg/dL. However, its effect is transient and tachyphylaxis develops within 48 hours. In selected circumstances, other modalities may be used for treatment of HIHC refractory to bisphosphonate, including: (1) denosumab, a monoclonal antibody which inhibits osteoclast function; (2) cinacalcet, a calcimimetic agent, which binds to the calcium receptor on the parathyroid cell and reduces PTH secretion; and (3) low calcium hemodialysis or continuous venovenous hemodiafiltration, especially for patients with renal failure who cannot tolerate volume loading.

Rapid reduction in serum calcium levels and optimization of organ function with extracellular fluid volume expansion using intravenous isotonic sodium chloride, furosemide-induced calciuresis, and the combination of calcitonin and a bisphosphonate agent to inhibit osteoclast function is a highly effective bridge to parathyroidectomy. It allows time for correction of fluid and electrolyte abnormalities and treatment of other medical problems. Parathyroidectomy should be performed expeditiously, but only after the patient's condition has been optimized.

Parathyroid localization with ultrasound and sestamibi with SPECT imaging should be performed once the patient is medically stabilized and can be performed concomitantly with correction of hypercalcemia. Sestamibi with SPECT imaging is important because patients with HIHC are more likely to have an ectopic parathyroid adenoma.

Patients with HIHC have significantly larger parathyroid glands and are more likely to have ectopic mediastinal glands. Parathyroid cancer occurs in 5% of patients with HIHC. Postoperatively, patients with HIHC may develop symptomatic hypocalcemia requiring intravenous and oral calcium, vitamin D therapy, and inpatient calcium monitoring. "Bone hunger" is the primary cause for the hypocalcemia, but bisphosphonates and calcimimetic agents also may contribute to the postoperative hypocalcemia.

PARATHYROID CANCER

Fritz DeQuervain reported the first case of parathyroid cancer in 1909. Parathyroid cancer is one of the rarest human cancers, with a prevalence 0.005% and an estimated incidence of 11 cases per 10 million population per year.[48] It accounts for less than 1% of all patients with primary HPT. In contrast to all patients with primary HPT, with a female-to-male ratio of 4:1, parathyroid cancer affects men and women in an equal distribution. Parathyroid cancer most often occurs sporadically but may also occur in patients with familial HPT, most notably the HPT-JT and familial isolated HPT. Inactivating mutations in the cell division cycle 73 (CDC73) tumor suppressor gene (also known as HRPT2) and CGM2 mutations are frequently seen in patients with familial parathyroid cancer associated with HPT-JT and familial isolated HPT, respectively. Somatic mutations in the CDC73 tumor suppression gene also occur in sporadic parathyroid cancer.

Parathyroid cancer is almost a uniformly functional tumor. Patients with parathyroid cancer typically present with severe primary HPT and the median age at diagnosis is 57 years. Most patients are symptomatic, with a high prevalence of skeletal manifestations, nephrolithiasis, and renal insufficiency in contrast to other patients with primary HPT, where it is rare to have nephrolithiasis and bone disease occur concomitantly. Patients with parathyroid cancer are also more likely to present with HC.

Up to 50% of patients with parathyroid cancer present with a palpable neck mass. Parathyroid cancer should be suspected in patients with HPT, hoarseness, and unilateral vocal cord paralysis. Patients with parathyroid cancer often present with serum calcium levels greater than 14 mg/dL, serum intact PTH levels that are 3 to 10 times normal, and increased alkaline phosphatase levels.

There are rare reports of nonfunctional parathyroid cancers. Most patients with nonfunctional parathyroid cancer present with a palpable neck mass. Calcium and PTH levels are normal. The prognosis is typically worse because of detection at an advanced stage.

The definitive diagnosis of parathyroid cancer is made on the basis of invasion of adjacent tissue or regional or systemic metastases. As a result, parathyroid cancer is usually diagnosed at the time of operation and may be unsuspected preoperatively. Microscopic features associated with parathyroid cancer, including thick fibrous trabeculae, nuclear atypia and pleomorphism, mitoses, a trabecular growth pattern, and capsular invasion, are nonspecific and may also be seen in patients with a benign parathyroid adenoma. Parathyroid cancers are large tumors that are most often more than 3 cm in maximum dimension.

At operation, a parathyroid cancer is identified as a solid firm mass with a grayish white appearance and a firm consistency. The normal tissue planes between the parathyroid mass and the thyroid lobe are absent and there is invasion of surrounding structures, most commonly the thyroid gland and the strap muscles, but the recurrent laryngeal nerve, trachea, and esophagus may be also be involved. In contrast, a benign parathyroid adenoma is a soft tumor that has a definite connective tissue plane separating it from the thyroid gland, allowing for easy dissection of the tumor from surrounding tissues.

Treatment of patients with parathyroid cancer consists of medical management of severe hypercalcemia prior to operation in patients with HC to reduce the risk of cardiac arrhythmias and other organ dysfunction. Operative therapy consists of an en bloc resection of the cancer and any adjacent involved structures, including the recurrent laryngeal nerve when it is invaded by cancer. Care should be taken to not disrupt the capsule of the tumor. If the recurrent laryngeal nerve is resected, immediate reconstruction with a primary repair or an ansa cervicalis graft can be considered. Tracheal invasion is managed by local en bloc resection and either tracheostomy, primary repair or muscle coverage to deal with the defect in the trachea. For esophageal invasion confined to the muscle layers, partial resection of the esophageal wall is completed. A small full-thickness esophageal resection with muscle flap reinforcement may be necessary.

Cervical lymph node metastases are uncommon, occurring in approximately 3% of patients with parathyroid cancer.[48] Cervical lymph node dissection, either in the central or lateral compartments of the neck, is reserved for patients with lymph node metastases identified on preoperative physical examination, sonographic evaluation, or at operation. Compartment-oriented lymph node dissection is only necessary when lymph nodes are involved with metastatic disease. There is no role for prophylactic central or lateral compartment neck dissection, which is associated with increased morbidity and has not resulted in improved survival.

Recurrence rates are high, occurring in an estimated 40% to 70% of patients, usually within 2 to 5 years of initial surgery. Positive margins are correlated with higher recurrence rates, underscoring the importance of achieving clear margins and avoiding disruption of the capsule of the tumor. Locoregional recurrence is most common, but systemic metastases are not infrequent, most commonly affecting the lung and bone. Local and regional recurrences and systemic metastases should be resected when possible. This is important to help control hypercalcemia.

In general, parathyroid cancer is radioresistant and chemotherapy is ineffective. The median disease specific survival is 75 months for all patients with parathyroid cancer; the overall cancer specific survival is 89% at a median 4.5-year follow-up and the 5- and 10-year overall survival rates for parathyroid cancer are 82% and 66%, respectively.[48] Patients with persistent metastases have a median survival of only 2.5 months.

Patients with parathyroid cancer die of either metastatic disease or complications of chronic intractable hypercalcemia. The medical management of hypercalcemia from parathyroid cancer usually consists of a bisphosphonate agent or cinacalcet. Calcimimetic agents were approved by the Food and Drug Administration in 2004 for treatment of hypercalcemia secondary to parathyroid cancer.

FAMILIAL PRIMARY HYPERPARATHYROIDISM

Primary HPT is familial in 3% to 5% of patients.[17,19] The syndromic forms of primary HPT include MEN1, MEN2A, MEN4, and HPT-JT. The nonsyndromic familial form of primary HPT is familial isolated HPT (Table 38.2). To screen for familial HPT, all patients should be asked about a family history of HPT and other endocrinopathies that make up the syndromic forms of primary HPT, as well as previous neck surgery and kidney stones in other family members.[17]

The American Association of Endocrine Surgeons (AAES) parathyroidectomy guidelines recommend genetic counseling and testing in patients with primary HPT younger than 40 years of age with multigland disease and in patients with clinical manifestations or a family history that is suggestive of a familial syndrome.[17] The European Society of Endocrine Surgeons recommends MEN 1 genetic testing in primary HPT patients younger than 40 years old with multigland disease or persistent or recurrent primary HPT. A recent study evaluating the probability of positive genetic testing in patients with family history of primary HPT recommends genetic testing in patients with a family history of primary HPT and male sex, age younger than 45 years, or presence of multigland disease.[49]

MEN1 is the most common familial form of primary HPT, affecting 2% to 4% of patients with primary HPT. MEN1 is an autosomal dominant disorder that occurs because of a germline, loss-of-function mutation in the *MEN1* tumor suppression gene. HPT is the most common feature of MEN1, with most MEN1 patients developing HPT in their third decade.[17] Almost all MEN1 patients develop primary HPT by 50 years of age and are most likely to develop multigland disease. Primary HPT occurs in association with a microadenoma of the anterior pituitary and pancreatic neuroendocrine tumors, and less commonly, adrenocortical and thyroid tumors; neuroendocrine tumors of the thymus, bronchus, and stomach; meningioma; facial angiofibroma; and multiple lipomas (Table 38.2).[49] MEN4 is a rare inherited syndrome with clinical manifestations similar to MEN1, but patients lack the *MEN1* gene mutation and instead have mutations in the *CDKN1B* gene.[17] Subtotal parathyroidectomy (or total parathyroidectomy and heterotopic autotransplantation) and transcervical thymectomy is recommended for treatment of primary HPT in patients with MEN1 or MEN4 because of the high incidence of multigland disease.

MEN2A occurs due to a gain-of-function germline mutation in the *RET* proto-oncogene. Primary HPT in MEN2A has a penetrance of 15% to 35%, compared to >90% for medullary thyroid cancer and 40% to 50% for pheochromocytoma.[17,49] Primary HPT in MEN2A occurs as a single adenoma (30% to 50%) or diffuse hyperplasia. Specific *RET* mutations correspond to different rates of primary HPT. In patients with a known RET mutation, screening for primary HPT and pheochromocytoma should occur annually. In patients with *RET* mutations in codons 634 and 883 ("high risk"), evaluation should occur by age 11, whereas in patients with other *RET* mutations ("moderate risk"), evaluation for primary HPT should occur by age 16.[17]

The surgical management of HPT in MEN2A is challenging due to the heterogeneity of the parathyroid glands and frequently more difficult operations related to prior thyroidectomy and central neck dissection for medullary thyroid cancer. The surgical options include (1) resection of visibly enlarged parathyroid glands, (2) subtotal parathyroidectomy, or (3) total parathyroidectomy with immediate heterotopic autotransplantation. The AAES parathyroidectomy guidelines preferentially recommend resection of only visibly enlarged glands in MEN2-associated HPT.[17] Pheochromocytoma must be ruled out or addressed prior to surgery for MEN2-associated primary HPT.

HPT-JT is an autosomal dominant disorder consisting of primary HPT, ossifying fibromas of the mandible and maxilla, renal cysts, hamartomas, Wilms tumors, and uterine tumors. It is caused by a mutation in the *CDC73* gene. Primary HPT occurs in the second or third decade and is due to single gland disease in approximately 90% of patients. Parathyroid carcinoma develops in 15% to 20% of patients with HPT-JT.[17,49] Because of the predominance of single gland disease, patients with HPT-JT can be treated with focused parathyroidectomy guided by IOPTH measurement when the tumor is localized preoperatively. Patients with parathyroid cancer are treated with an en bloc resection of the tumor and anything that the tumor is invading. Genetic evaluation and testing for the *CDC73* gene are recommended for all patients with parathyroid carcinoma, for patients with primary HPT and ossifying fibromas of the mandible and maxilla, and young patients with primary HPT and multigland disease in the absence of a *MEN1* gene mutation.[17]

Familial isolated HPT is an autosomal dominant disorder characterized by a family history of primary HPT and a lack of syndromic manifestations. There are multiple potential causative genetic mutations (Table 38.2), including the *MEN1* gene, which is more likely to be associated with multigland disease and the *CDC73* gene, which is most often associated with single gland disease. Approximately 18% of patients with familial isolated HPT have a mutation in the *GCM2* proto-oncogene, which is also associated with multigland disease and a higher risk of parathyroid cancer.[49] The extent of parathyroidectomy in patients with familial isolated HPT is controversial. Because of the high incidence of multigland disease, consideration should be given to bilateral neck exploration. It is our preference to proceed with a bilateral neck exploration and only resect enlarged glands and use IOPTH monitoring as an adjunct, whereas others have advocated for routine subtotal parathyroidectomy or total parathyroidectomy and autotransplantation.

In contrast to sporadic primary HPT, familial primary HPT is associated with a higher rate of recurrence following parathyroidectomy and a lower overall cure rate. Recurrence rates following parathyroidectomy vary from 17% to 46% in MEN1, 6% to 11% in MEN2A, 15% to 20% in HPT-JT, and 11% in familial isolated HPT, with an expected 5- to 15-year interval of normocalcemia before recurrence.[17] Because of the higher incidence of recurrence, patients with syndromic and nonsyndromic familial HPT require lifelong follow-up.

REOPERATIVE NECK SURGERY FOR PERSISTENT OR RECURRENT HYPERPARATHYROIDISM

Operative failure resulting in persistent HPT occurs in 1% to 5% of cases of sporadic primary HPT and higher in familial and renal HPT.[17] Persistent HPT is defined as failure to achieve normocalcemia within 6 months of parathyroidectomy. Recurrent primary HPT is defined as recurrent hypercalcemia after an interval of normal calcium levels for at least 6 months following parathyroidectomy. A cervical exploration that is performed in a patient who has had a prior parathyroidectomy, thyroidectomy, tracheostomy, carotid endarterectomy, or a cervical fusion via an anterior approach constitutes reoperative neck surgery. Reoperation for persistent or recurrent HPT is challenging due to scarring, loss of normal tissue planes, and distortion of normal anatomy. Rates of hypoparathyroidism and recurrent laryngeal nerve injury are higher after parathyroid reexploration.

Prior to reoperation, the diagnosis of primary HPT should be confirmed, and a thorough history should be obtained to determine the extent and severity of the patient's symptoms. A family history is important to help understand whether the patient is more likely to have single or multigland disease. Previous imaging studies and the operative and pathology reports should be reviewed to determine the extent of the prior surgery and the location of the glands that were removed and that remain. Patients are more likely to have multiple abnormal glands if two abnormal parathyroid glands were removed at the initial surgery or if less than three abnormal parathyroid glands were removed for secondary, tertiary, or familial HPT.

Preoperative localizing studies for reoperative parathyroidectomy are important for operative success. It is useful to have two positive imaging studies that are concordant, but it is essential to have at least one positive imaging study before reoperation is recommended. Two or more standard noninvasive imaging studies are obtained initially including ultrasound, sestamibi, or 4D-CT. 4D-CT has been shown to have higher sensitivity (88%) than sestamibi imaging (54%) prior to reoperation. MRI and PET/CT may also be obtained when necessary.[50] Selective venous sampling is reserved when noninvasive imaging localization is unsuccessful. Selective venous sampling is done by interventional radiologists via a catheter placed in the femoral vein, which allows for cervical and mediastinal venous blood sampling and testing for PTH levels. Mapping the PTH levels to the corresponding veins helps determine a gradient that suggests the location of the abnormal gland. If there is failure of localization of abnormal glands, nonoperative management and continued surveillance is recommended.

In most cases, reoperation for persistent or recurrent HPT consists of a focused exploration based on review of the operative and pathology reports from the initial operation and/or the site localized preoperatively to minimize the risk of complications. IOPTH monitoring and nerve monitoring are useful adjuncts during reoperation. In addition, cryopreservation of the removed glands can be performed at centers where this is available. Resected parathyroid tissue is frozen with liquid nitrogen and stored; it can be thawed and autotransplanted in the rare cases when permanent hypoparathyroidism occurs. Besides reoperative parathyroidectomy, cryopreservation is also used at the time of initial surgery when subtotal or total parathyroidectomy is performed and there is a higher risk of permanent hypoparathyroidism. However, it is a labor intensive process that is available at few specialized centers, and the use of cryopreserved parathyroid tissue for reimplantation is infrequent.[17]

SELECTED REFERENCES

Bilezikian JP, Brandi ML, Eastell R, et al. Guidelines for the management of asymptomatic primary hyperparathyroidism: summary statement from the Fourth International Workshop. *J Clin Endocrinol Metab*. 2014;99:3561–3569.

The management of asymptomatic primary hyperparathyroidism (HPT) remains controversial, with wide variation in management between clinicians. This summary statement paper provides guidance and outlines the indications for parathyroidectomy in patients with asymptomatic primary HPT.

El Lakis M, Nockel P, Gaitanidis A, et al. Probability of positive genetic testing results in patients with family history of primary hyperparathyroidism. *J Am Coll Surg*. 2018;226:933–938.

This is a large retrospective analysis of patients with primary hyperparathyroidism (HPT) and a family history of HPT, which identified factors associated with positive genetic testing. It emphasizes the importance of identifying patients who are at increased risk for familial primary HPT and who will benefit from genetic testing and counseling. It further emphasizes how genetic testing affects the management of patients with familial HPT and optimizes their chance of cure after initial parathyroid exploration.

Lo WM, Good ML, Nilubol N, et al. Tumor size and presence of metastatic disease at diagnosis are associated with disease-specific survival in parathyroid carcinoma. *Ann Surg Oncol*. 2018;25:2535–2540.

Parathyroid cancer is rare but has been reported to be increasing in incidence. This is the largest retrospective analysis of parathyroid cancer patients to date, including 520 patients from the Surveillance Epidemiology and End Results (SEER) database, which outlines factors associated with parathyroid cancer-specific survival.

Lorenz K, Bartsch DK, Sancho JJ, et al. Surgical management of secondary hyperparathyroidism in chronic kidney disease—a consensus report of the European Society of Endocrine Surgeons. *Langenbecks Arch Surg*. 2015;400:907–927.

The extent of parathyroidectomy and other controversial issues related to the operative management of renal hyperparathyroidism (HPT) are discussed. While the majority of patients with renal HPT are medically treated with calcimimetics, this consensus report gives evidence-based recommendations on the surgical management of this complex group of patients.

Wilhelm SM, Wang TS, Ruan DT, et al. The American Association of Endocrine Surgeons guidelines for definitive management of primary hyperparathyroidism. *JAMA Surg*. 2016;151:959–968.

Evidence-based recommendations are provided to assist clinicians with the optimal management of patients with primary hyperparathyroidism (HPT). The emphasis of the guidelines is on the detailed operative management of primary HPT to help ensure appropriate, effective, and safe parathyroidectomy.

REFERENCES

1. Owen R. On the anatomy of the Indian Rhinoceros (Th. Unicornis). *Trans Zool Soc Lond*. 1862;4:31–58.
2. IV S. On a new gland in man and several mammals (glanduloe parathyroid). English translation by Carl M Seipel. *Bull Hist Med*. 1938;6:192–222.
3. Thompson NW. The history of hyperparathyroidism. *Acta Chir Scand*. 1990;156:5–21.
4. Giddings CE, Rimmer J, Weir N. History of parathyroid gland surgery: an historical case series. *J Laryngol Otol*. 2009;123:1075–1081.
5. Sethi N, England RJA. Parathyroid surgery: from inception to the modern day. *Br J Hosp Med (Lond)*. 2017;78:333–337.
6. Johansson H. The Uppsala anatomist Ivar Sandstrom and the parathyroid gland. *Ups J Med Sci*. 2015;120:72–77.
7. Toneto MG, Prill S, Debon LM, et al. The history of the parathyroid surgery. *Rev Col Bras Cir*. 2016;43:214–222.
8. Potts Jr JT. A short history of parathyroid hormone, its biological role, and pathophysiology of hormone excess. *J Clin Densitom*. 2013;16:4–7.
9. Barr DP, Bulger HA, Dixon HH. Hyperparathyroidism. *JAMA*. 1929;92:951–952.
10. Irvin 3rd GL, Dembrow VD, Prudhomme DL. Clinical usefulness of an intraoperative "quick parathyroid hormone" assay. *Surgery*. 1993;114:1019–1022; discussion 1022–1013.
11. Peissig K, Condie BG, Manley NR. Embryology of the parathyroid glands. *Endocrinol Metab Clin North Am*. 2018;47:733–742.
12. Mohebati A, Shaha AR. Anatomy of thyroid and parathyroid glands and neurovascular relations. *Clin Anat*. 2012;25:19–31.
13. Fancy T, Gallagher 3rd D, Hornig JD. Surgical anatomy of the thyroid and parathyroid glands. *Otolaryngol Clin North Am*. 2010;43:221–227; vii.
14. Phitayakorn R, McHenry CR. Incidence and location of ectopic abnormal parathyroid glands. *Am J Surg*. 2006;191:418–423.
15. Goltzman D. Physiology of parathyroid hormone. *Endocrinol Metab Clin North Am*. 2018;47:743–758.

16. Leder BZ. Parathyroid hormone and parathyroid hormone-related protein analogs in osteoporosis therapy. *Curr Osteoporos Rep*. 2017;15:110–119.
17. Wilhelm SM, Wang TS, Ruan DT, et al. The American Association of Endocrine Surgeons guidelines for definitive management of primary hyperparathyroidism. *JAMA Surg*. 2016;151:959–968.
18. Insogna KL. Primary hyperparathyroidism. *N Engl J Med*. 2018;379:1050–1059.
19. Silva BC, Cusano NE, Bilezikian JP. Primary hyperparathyroidism. *Best Pract Res Clin Endocrinol Metab*. 2018;32:593–607.
20. Bilezikian JP, Cusano NE, Khan AA, et al. Primary hyperparathyroidism. *Nat Rev Dis Primers*. 2016;2:16033.
21. Assadipour Y, Zhou H, Kuo EJ, et al. End-organ effects of primary hyperparathyroidism: a population-based study. *Surgery*. 2019;165:99–104.
22. Rubin MR, Bilezikian JP, McMahon DJ, et al. The natural history of primary hyperparathyroidism with or without parathyroid surgery after 15 years. *J Clin Endocrinol Metab*. 2008;93:3462–3470.
23. Moore EC, Berber E, Jin J, et al. Calcium creatinine clearance ratio is not helpful in differentiating primary hyperparathyroidism from familial hypercalcemic hypocalciuria: a study of 1000 patients. *Endocr Pract*. 2018;24:988–994.
24. Pierreux J, Bravenboer B. Normocalcemic primary hyperparathyroidism: a comparison with the hypercalcemic form in a tertiary referral population. *Horm Metab Res*. 2018;50:797–802.
25. Wallace LB, Parikh RT, Ross LV, et al. The phenotype of primary hyperparathyroidism with normal parathyroid hormone levels: how low can parathyroid hormone go? *Surgery*. 2011;150:1102–1112.
26. Bilezikian JP, Brandi ML, Eastell R, et al. Guidelines for the management of asymptomatic primary hyperparathyroidism: summary statement from the Fourth International Workshop. *J Clin Endocrinol Metab*. 2014;99:3561–3569.
27. Pasieka JL, Parsons L, Jones J. The long-term benefit of parathyroidectomy in primary hyperparathyroidism: a 10-year prospective surgical outcome study. *Surgery*. 2009;146:1006–1013.
28. Vuong C, Frank E, Simental AA, et al. Outcomes of parathyroidectomy for primary hyperparathyroidism with nonlocalizing preoperative imaging. *Head Neck*. 2019;41:666–671.
29. Kuzminski SJ, Sosa JA, Hoang JK. Update in parathyroid imaging. *Magn Reson Imaging Clin N Am*. 2018;26:151–166.
30. Cheung K, Wang TS, Farrokhyar F, et al. A meta-analysis of preoperative localization techniques for patients with primary hyperparathyroidism. *Ann Surg Oncol*. 2012;19:577–583.
31. Batur A, Atmaca M, Yavuz A, et al. Ultrasound elastography for distinction between parathyroid adenomas and thyroid nodules. *J Ultrasound Med*. 2016;35:1277–1282.
32. Hocevar M, Lezaic L, Rep S, et al. Focused parathyroidectomy without intraoperative parathormone testing is safe after preoperative localization with (18)F-fluorocholine PET/CT. *Eur J Surg Oncol*. 2017;43:133–137.
33. Beheshti M, Hehenwarter L, Paymani Z, et al. (18) F-Fluorocholine PET/CT in the assessment of primary hyperparathyroidism compared with (99m)Tc-MIBI or (99m)Tc-tetrofosmin SPECT/CT: a prospective dual-centre study in 100 patients. *Eur J Nucl Med Mol Imaging*. 2018;45:1762–1771.
34. Irvin 3rd GL, Dembrow VD, Prudhomme DL. Operative monitoring of parathyroid gland hyperfunction. *Am J Surg*. 1991;162:299–302.
35. Wharry LI, Yip L, Armstrong MJ, et al. The final intraoperative parathyroid hormone level: how low should it go? *World J Surg*. 2014;38:558–563.
36. Russell JO, Clark J, Noureldine SI, et al. Transoral thyroidectomy and parathyroidectomy—a North American series of robotic and endoscopic transoral approaches to the central neck. *Oral Oncol*. 2017;71:75–80.
37. Talutis SD, Drake FT, Sachs T, et al. Evacuation of postoperative hematomas after thyroid and parathyroid surgery: an analysis of the CESQIP Database. *Surgery*. 2019;165:250–256.
38. Vestergaard P, Mosekilde L. Parathyroid surgery is associated with a decreased risk of hip and upper arm fractures in primary hyperparathyroidism: a controlled cohort study. *J Intern Med*. 2004;255:108–114.
39. Mizobuchi M, Ogata H, Koiwa F. Secondary hyperparathyroidism: pathogenesis and latest treatment. *Ther Apher Dial*. 2019;23:309–318.
40. Lorenz K, Bartsch DK, Sancho JJ, et al. Surgical management of secondary hyperparathyroidism in chronic kidney disease—a consensus report of the European Society of Endocrine Surgeons. *Langenbecks Arch Surg*. 2015;400:907–927.
41. KDIGO clinical practice guideline for the diagnosis, evaluation, prevention, and treatment of chronic kidney disease-mineral and bone disorder (CKD-MBD). *Kidney Int Suppl*. 2009:S1–130.
42. Finnerty BM, Chan TW, Jones G, et al. Parathyroidectomy versus cinacalcet in the management of tertiary hyperparathyroidism: surgery improves renal transplant allograft survival. *Surgery*. 2019;165:129–134.
43. Alsafran S, Sherman SK, Dahdaleh FS, et al. Preoperative calcitriol reduces postoperative intravenous calcium requirements and length of stay in parathyroidectomy for renal-origin hyperparathyroidism. *Surgery*. 2019;165:151–157.
44. Weenig RH, Sewell LD, Davis MD, et al. Calciphylaxis: natural history, risk factor analysis, and outcome. *J Am Acad Dermatol*. 2007;56:569–579.
45. McCarthy JT, El-Azhary RA, Patzelt MT, et al. Survival, risk factors, and effect of treatment in 101 patients with calciphylaxis. *Mayo Clin Proc*. 2016;91:1384–1394.
46. Lowenburg H, Ginsburg TM. Acute hypercalcemia: report of a case. *JAMA*. 1932;99:1166.
47. Ziegler R. Hypercalcemic crisis. *J Am Soc Nephrol*. 2001;12(suppl 17):S3–S9.
48. Lo WM, Good ML, Nilubol N, et al. Tumor size and presence of metastatic disease at diagnosis are associated with disease-specific survival in parathyroid carcinoma. *Ann Surg Oncol*. 2018;25:2535–2540.
49. El Lakis M, Nockel P, Gaitanidis A, et al. Probability of positive genetic testing results in patients with family history of primary hyperparathyroidism. *J Am Coll Surg*. 2018;226:933–938.
50. Mortenson MM, Evans DB, Lee JE, et al. Parathyroid exploration in the reoperative neck: improved preoperative localization with 4D-computed tomography. *J Am Coll Surg*. 2008;206:888–895; discussion 895–886.

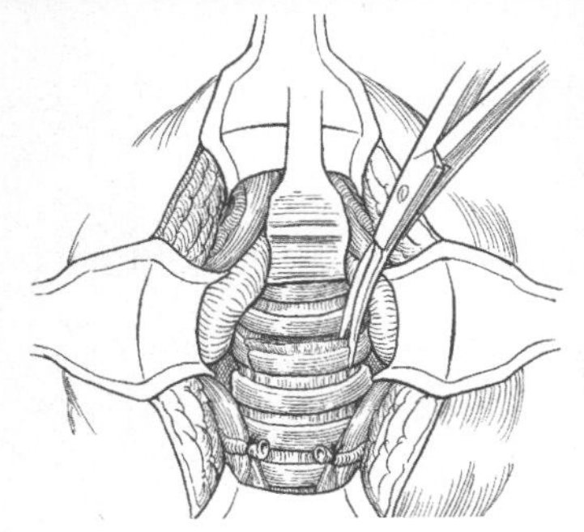

CHAPTER 39

Endocrine Pancreas

Amanda K. Arrington, Taylor S. Riall

OUTLINE

First identified over 400 years ago by Greek anatomists, the pancreas is located in the retroperitoneum with the head of the pancreas lying in the C loop of the duodenum (Fig. 39.1A and B). The pancreas has distinct hormonal (endocrine) and digestive (exocrine) functions. Endocrine cells are organized in discrete clusters throughout the pancreas. First described in 1869 by then medical student Paul Langerhans, these islets of Langerhans (Fig. 39.1C) secrete hormones directly into the bloodstream.

The primary physiologic function of the endocrine pancreas is glucose/insulin regulation through secretion of insulin and glucagon directly into the bloodstream in response to blood glucose levels. In 1889, through a landmark study in dogs, Minkowski and von Mering made the connection between diabetes and the pancreas. While studying fat absorption in dogs after total pancreatectomy, they noted that surgical removal of the pancreas led to glucosuria, ketonuria, coma, and eventual death. On the heels of this discovery, Frederick Banting and Charles Best identified the hormone insulin in 1922 in studies where atrophied pancreas in an iatrogenic diabetic dog was extracted, homogenized, and injected back into the animal, temporarily reversing the diabetic condition.

In this chapter, we will cover the histomorphology, embryology, physiology, and pathophysiology of the endocrine pancreas. We will focus on the diagnosis and management of diseases relevant to surgeons, including tumors of the endocrine pancreas, diabetes, and the endocrine complications of surgical therapy.

EMBRYOLOGY OF THE ENDOCRINE PANCREAS

In the human fetus, pancreatic islets initially comprise approximately one third of the pancreatic mass. Pancreatic formation begins during the fifth week of gestation as separate dorsal and ventral endodermal pancreatic buds, which form at the junction of the foregut and the midgut. The dorsal and ventral buds are comprised of endoderm covered in splanchnic mesoderm. Both the acinar and islet cells differentiate from the endodermal cells found in the embryonic buds while the splanchnic mesoderm eventually develops into the dorsal and ventral mesentery. The first glucagon-producing cells (A cells) appear in 3-week-old embryos and the first organized islets appear at approximately 10 weeks. B cell formation primarily occurs before birth with a burst of proliferation up to the first 2 years of life. The B-to-A-cell ratio doubles neonatally, reflecting increased growth of B cells.

HISTOMORPHOLOGY OF ISLETS

The adult pancreas consists of endocrine cells organized in islets of Langerhans (Fig 39.1C) and digestive acinar cells contained in clusters and draining into a centralized ductal system. Endocrine cells comprise less than 2% of the overall pancreatic mass in the adult pancreas. The adult pancreas contains approximately 1 million islets, with each islet containing approximately 3000 cells and ranging in diameter from 40 μm to 1 mm. Pancreatic islets have complex architecture and are composed of four cell types: A (alpha), B (beta), D, and F cells. The four cell types are not evenly distributed within the islets or throughout the pancreas. Table 39.1 describes the cell types, their hormonal products, and their location within the islet and the pancreas.

The A cells, located in the periphery, secrete glucagon and constitute approximately 10% of the islet cell mass. Islets largely (up to 70%) consist of B cells which secrete the hormone insulin and are located centrally within the islet. In comparison, F cells constitute approximately 15% of islet cell mass and secrete the hormone pancreatic polypeptide (PP). The D cells are evenly distributed throughout the islet and constitute approximately 5% of the islet cell mass. D cells secrete somatostatin and D2 cells secrete vasoactive intestinal peptide (VIP). Within the actual pancreas, B and D

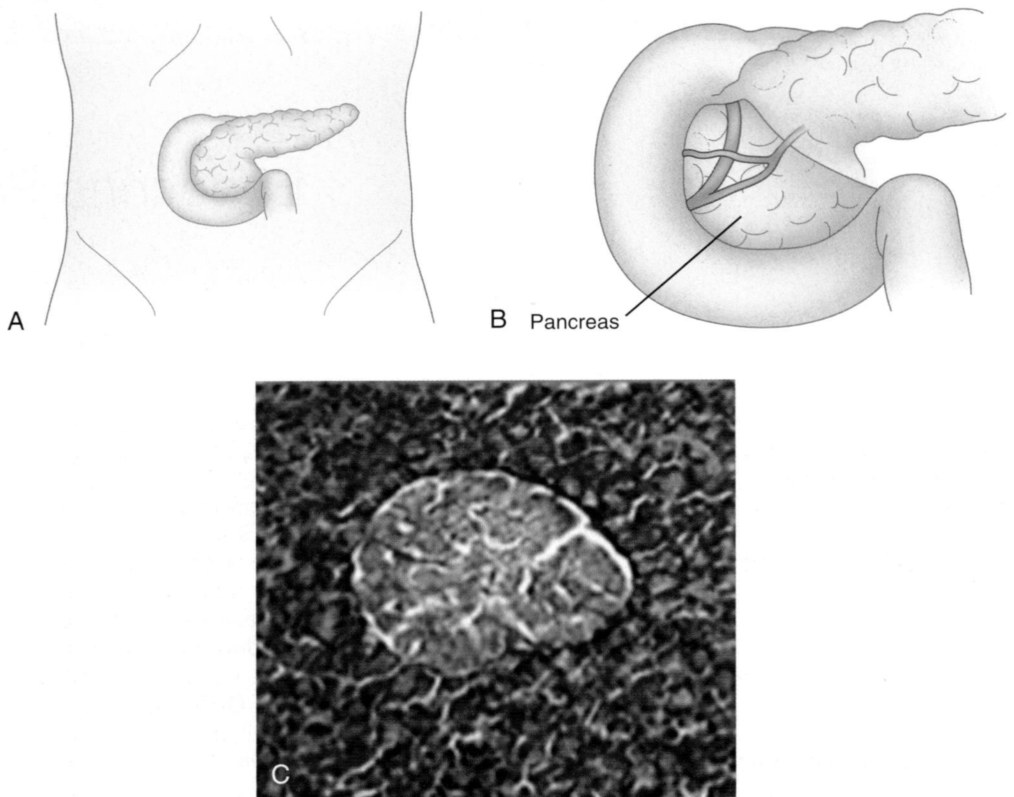

FIG. 39.1 (A) The pancreas is noted in its retroperitoneal position at the level of the second lumbar vertebra. (B) Relationship of the head of the pancreas in the C loop of the duodenum, with the pancreatic duct and common bile duct emptying into the ampulla of Vater. (C) On microscopic view, the endocrine cells are located in nests, called islets of Langerhans, which are distributed throughout the pancreas (trichrome stain, ×10).

cells are concentrated in the body and tail of the pancreas, while F cells are heavily concentrated in the uncinate process, and A cells are evenly distributed throughout the gland.

The rich portal microcirculation of the pancreatic islets allows for the endocrine-to-endocrine cell signaling necessary for hormonal regulation. Afferent arterioles enter the islet on the periphery into the center of the islet, which consists of B cells. The order of islet cellular perfusion and interaction is from this B cell core outward to the mantle, first to A cells and then to the more distal/peripheral D cells. This allows B cells to inhibit A cell secretion and A cells to stimulate D cell secretion.

Pancreatic endocrine secretion regulates pancreatic exocrine secretion through the islet-acinar axis of the pancreas. Although islets constitute less than 2% of pancreatic volume, the arterial blood supply to the pancreas predominantly flows first to the islets and then via the islets to the exocrine portion of the gland. The distribution of blood flow is relevant to the potential physiologic interactions. The B cells' insulin stimulates pancreatic exocrine secretion, amino acid transport, and synthesis of protein and enzymes. On the other hand, the islets A cells' glucagon acts in a counterregulatory fashion, inhibiting the same processes.

ENDOCRINE PHYSIOLOGY

Glucose Homeostasis: Insulin and Glucagon

The primary function of the endocrine pancreas is regulation of glucose homeostasis. In response to blood glucose levels, the secretion of insulin and glucagon is tightly regulated through a variety of feedback and regulatory mechanisms. Secreted by B cells within the islets of Langerhans, insulin functions to store energy by promoting glucose transport into cells, inhibiting glycogenolysis and fatty acid breakdown, and stimulating protein synthesis. Glucagon is the major counterregulatory hormone to insulin, increasing blood glucose levels through stimulation of glycogenolysis, lipolysis, and gluconeogenesis.

Insulin

Insulin is an anabolic hormone that promotes glucose transport into all cells except B cells, hepatocytes, and central nervous system cells. Insulin is a 56–amino acid polypeptide with a molecular weight of 6 kDa, which is synthesized as proinsulin, its precursor peptide. In response to pancreatic B cell stimulation by glucose, proinsulin is synthesized in the endoplasmic reticulum and transported to the Golgi complex, where it is cleaved into insulin and the residual C-peptide (Fig. 39.2). The resulting insulin molecule consists of two polypeptide chains (A and B) joined by two disulfide bridges. C-peptide and insulin are secreted in equimolar amounts. After cleavage of C-peptide, insulin is moved via microtubules into secretory granules, where it is released directly into the bloodstream via exocytosis.

The B cell is highly sensitive to changes in glucose concentration and is maximally stimulated at concentrations of 400 to 500 mg/dL. In response to glucose, the islets of Langerhans immediately react with a short burst of stored insulin (4–6 minutes), followed by a sustained secretion of insulin, which requires active synthesis of the hormone within the islet cell. Insulin binds to a specific 300-kDa glycoprotein cell surface receptor, and stimulation of this insulin receptor is dependent on insulin concentration.

TABLE 39.1 **Endocrine cells of the pancreas and tumor syndromes.**

CELL TYPE	% ISLET CELL MASS	LOCATION WITHIN ISLET	LOCATION WITHIN PANCREAS	MAJOR (MINOR) HORMONE SECRETED	ASSOCIATED TUMOR SYNDROME	DIAGNOSTIC HORMONE LEVELS
A (alpha)	10%	Peripheral	Evenly distributed	Glucagon (glicentin, TRH, CCK, endorphin, PP, pancreastatin)	Glucagonoma: necrolytic migratory erythema, diabetes, hypoaminoacidemia	Normal = <150 pg/mL Tumor = fasting glucagon >1000 pg/mL
B (beta)	70%	Central	Body/tail	Insulin (TRH, CGRP, amylin, pancreastatin, prolactin)	Insulinoma: hypoglycemia and associated symptoms	>5 μU/mL in the face of hypoglycemia
D	5%*	Evenly distributed	Evenly distributed	Somatostatin (met-encephalon)	Somatostatinoma: diabetes, gallstones, steatorrhea	Normal = 10–25 pg/mL Tumor = >160 pg/mL
D_2	5%*	Evenly distributed	Evenly distributed	VIP	VIPoma: high-volume secretory diarrhea, hypokalemia, metabolic acidosis, hypochlorhydria	Normal = <200 pg/mL Tumor = 225–2000 pg/mL
F	15%	Peripheral	Head and uncinate process	PP	Treatment directed at presenting symptoms	NA
E C	<1%	Evenly distributed	Evenly distributed	Substance P, serotonin	None	NA
G	Not present in normal physiologic state	Not applicable	Head, uncinate process, duodenum	Gastrin, ACTH-related peptides	Gastrinoma: acid hypersecretion, gastric/duodenal ulcers, diarrhea	Normal <100 pg/mL Suspicious = >1000 pg/mL with secretin test, an increase of >200 pg/mL diagnostic

Adapted from Bonner-Weir S. Anatomy of the islet of Langerhans. In: Samols E, ed. *The Endocrine Pancreas*. New York: Raven Press; 1991:16; and Marx M, Newman JB, Guice KS, etal. Clinical significance of gastrointestinal hormones. In: Thompson JC, Greeley GH Jr, Rayford PL, etal, eds. *Gastrointestinal Endocrinology*. New York: McGraw-Hill; 1987:416.

ACTH, Adrenocorticotropic 2 hormone; *CCK*, cholecystokinin; *CGRP*, calcitonin gene–related peptide; *NA*, not applicable; *PP*, pancreatic polypeptide; *TRH*, thyrotropin-releasing hormone; *VIP*, vasoactive intestinal peptide; *VIPoma*, XXX.

*Combined D and D2 islet cell mass.

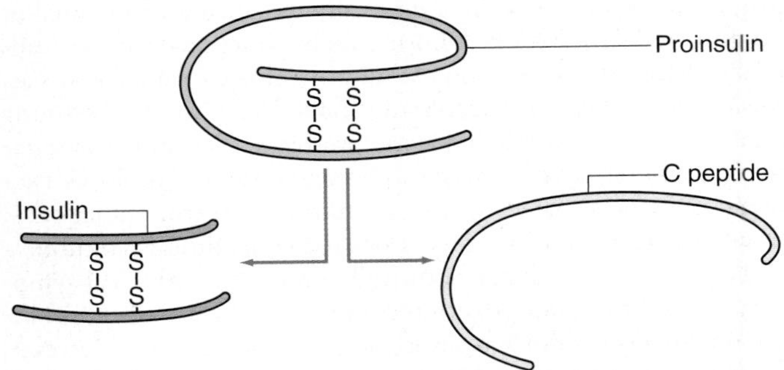

FIG. 39.2 Diagram of insulin synthesis. Proinsulin, synthesized by the endoplasmic reticulum, is packaged within secretory granules of the beta cell, where it is cleaved to insulin and C-peptide. Equimolar amounts of insulin and C-peptide are secreted into the bloodstream. (From Andersen DK, Brunicardi FC. Pancreatic anatomy and physiology. In: Greenfield LJ, Mulholland MW, Oldham KT, et al, eds. *Surgery: Scientific Principles and Practice*. 2nd ed. Philadelphia: Lippincott-Raven; 1997:869.)

After insulin receptor stimulation, glucose is actively transported across cell membranes throughout the body by membrane-bound glucose transporters. There are several classes of glucose transporters, with varying affinities for glucose. Insulin resistance, present in type 2 diabetes, can be the result of decreased numbers of receptors or a decreased affinity of receptors for insulin.

Glucagon

Glucagon is a 29–amino acid, straight chain polypeptide with a molecular weight of 3.5 kDa. Secreted by A cells within islets, the primary function of glucagon is to elevate blood glucose levels through stimulation of glycogenolysis and gluconeogenesis in the hepatocytes. Islet A and B cells respond primarily to serum glucose concentration, but in a reciprocal fashion. Like epinephrine, cortisol, and growth hormone, glucagon is considered a stress hormone because it increases metabolic fuel in the form of glucose during stress. Glucose has a strong suppressive effect on glucagon secretion. Excess glucagon can lead to hyperglycemia, whereas insufficient glucagon can lead to profound hypoglycemia. Dysfunctional secretion of glucagon may play a role in the elevation of blood glucose levels in diabetes.

Other Influences on Glucose Homeostasis

Enteric peptide hormones released from the proximal gastrointestinal tract also influence glucose homeostasis through the enteroinsular axis. Therefore, orally administered glucose has a greater effect on insulin secretion than an equivalent amount of glucose administered intravenously, even though blood glucose levels might be similar. Insulinotropic factors, called incretins, act directly on the B cells to stimulate insulin release. Incretins such as glucose-dependent insulinotropic polypeptide and glucagon-like peptide 1 are intestinal hormones that are released in response to ingestion of nutrients, particularly carbohydrates. They have a number of important biological effects, which include release of insulin, inhibition of glucagon and somatostatin, maintenance of beta-cell mass, delay of gastric emptying, and inhibition of feeding. In comparison to incretins' stimulation of insulin, humoral inhibitors of insulin secretion include somatostatin, amylin, leptin, and pancreastatin.

Ghrelin is a 28–amino acid peptide hormone produced by ghrelin cells of the gastrointestinal tract. Discovered in 1999, ghrelin was found to exert a series of metabolic effects, including the regulation of glucose metabolism. Ghrelin primarily inhibits insulin release from the pancreas, increases hepatic glucose production, and prevents glucose disposal in muscle and adipose tissues, which collectively leads to hyperglycemia and impaired glucose tolerance. In diet-induced obesity, ghrelin exacerbates hyperglycemia; in starvation or severe calorie restriction, ghrelin increases blood glucose concentrations in order to maintain glucose homeostasis.

Leptin is a peptide hormone produced in adipose cells. Leptin is released into the circulatory system based on energy stores and functions as a feedback mechanism that signals to regulatory centers in the brain to inhibit food intake and to regulate body weight. In response to adequate fat stores, leptin inhibits insulin secretion. In obese humans, leptin levels are increased, exacerbating hyperglycemia. In the obese state, there is thought to be leptin resistance, with lack of inhibition of food intake.

Both insulin and glucagon secretions are also under neuronal control. Vagal (cholinergic) stimulation leads to the release of insulin. Insulin release is stimulated by the autonomic peptidergic nerve release of gastrin-releasing peptide, cholecystokinin (CCK), gastrin, enkephalin, and VIP, as well as β-sympathetic nerve stimulation. On the other hand, insulin release is inhibited by neurotensin, substance P, somatostatin, and α-sympathetic nerve stimulation. In comparison, glucagon secretion is stimulated by sympathetic neural transmitters, epinephrine, and the amino acids arginine and alanine.

Somatostatin

Somatostatin is a 14–amino acid polypeptide weighing 1.6 kDa secreted by islet D cells. Although exogenous administration of somatostatin has been shown to inhibit the release of insulin, glucagon, and PP, and to inhibit gastric, pancreatic, and biliary secretion, endogenous somatostatin has not been proven to influence the secretion of other islet hormones directly. Both long- and short-acting synthetic octapeptides that mimic the pharmacologic action of somatostatin have been developed. These synthetic peptides have a longer half-life in the serum than endogenous somatostatin and are more potent inhibitors of growth hormone, glucagon, and insulin secretion than the natural hormone. The potent inhibitory effect of synthetic somatostatin analogues has been used to treat exocrine and endocrine disorders of the pancreas, including secretory diarrhea, bowel fistulas, pancreatic fistulas, and endocrine hypersecretory syndromes.

Pancreatic Polypeptide

PP is a 36–amino acid, 4.2-kDa polypeptide secreted by the islet F cells. PP belongs to the peptide YY/neuropeptide Y family of polypeptides. Infusion of PP in humans caused loss of appetite and reduced food intake. As its true physiologic role remains unclear, PP's clinical usefulness is limited to its role as a marker for other endocrine tumors of the pancreas. As cholinergic innervation predominantly regulates PP secretion, surgical vagotomy ablates the increased PP response normally observed after meals. In diabetes and normal aging, PP secretion is increased, resulting in increased circulating PP levels. Absence of PP may play a role in the diabetes observed after total pancreatectomy or after chronic atrophic pancreatitis.

Other Peptide Hormones

In addition to the main hormones secreted by islets cells, other peptide hormones secreted includes VIP, amylin, galanin, and serotonin. VIP is a 28–amino acid, 3.3-kDa polypeptide that stimulates insulin release and inhibits gastric secretion at physiologic level. It is found not only throughout the gastrointestinal tract but also in the respiratory tract, where it causes vasodilatation and bronchodilation. Amylin, a 36–amino acid polypeptide, is secreted by B cells and inhibits the secretion and uptake of insulin. Amylin deposits in the pancreas of patients with type 2 diabetes have been implicated in the pathogenesis of the disease. Pancreastatin is part of a larger ubiquitous molecule, chromogranin A, which inhibits insulin secretion. Gastrin-producing cells are present in the fetal pancreas, but not in the normal adult pancreas. Many additional peptides, including thyrotropin-releasing hormone, glicentin, CCK, peptide YY, gastrin-releasing factor (GRF), calcitonin gene–related peptide, prolactin, adrenocorticotropic hormone (ACTH), parathyroid hormone–related protein, and ghrelin have been reported in normal islets and in islet cell tumors.

PANCREATIC NEUROENDOCRINE TUMORS

Overview and History

Pancreatic neuroendocrine tumors (PNETs) account for less than 3% of pancreatic neoplasms. The incidence of PNETs has increased more than sevenfold in the last two decades. In a study using the Surveillance, Epidemiology, and End Results database, the overall incidence of gastroenteropancreatic neuroendocrine tumors (NETs) was 1.00 case per 100,000 between 1973 and 1977 and increased to 3.65 cases per 100,000 between 2003 and 2007.[1] PNETs comprised 7% of all gastroenteropancreatic NETs. The observed increase in incidence is likely multifactorial and includes increased awareness among physicians, more frequent use of computed tomography (CT) and magnetic resonance imaging (MRI), and improved sensitivity of immunohistochemical and radiologic diagnostic testing.[1] PNETs are broadly classified as functional or nonfunctional. Secretion of hormones by functional tumors leads to the characteristic syndromes and physiologic derangements associated with these rare neoplasms (Table 39.1). Immunostaining often identifies multiple hormone products, even in the absence of clinically relevant hormone secretion. Although multiple hormones may be secreted by a single tumor, the term "functional" should be reserved for tumors associated with clinical symptoms.

Nonfunctional tumors historically presented with local symptoms related to tumor growth including pain, mass effect, or biliary obstruction, similar to exocrine pancreatic cancer. However, more frequently, nonfunctional tumors are being identified incidentally on imaging done for other purposes and are asymptomatic at the time of diagnosis.

Histopathology and Staging

The incidence of malignancy in these tumors varies from approximately 10% in insulin-secreting PNETs (insulinoma) to almost 100% in glucagon- or somatostatin-secreting tumors (Table 39.1). However, unlike most other solid tumors, which are classified as benign or malignant based on histopathology of the primary tumor, malignancy in PNETs can only definitely be determined by the presence of metastasis.

The 2010 World Health Organization (WHO) staging system is the most widely used staging system for NETs.[2] It includes all NETs regardless of site of origin or functional hormone secretion and classifies based on differentiation and grade. The tumor grade for NETs is categorized as low grade (grade 1, G1), intermediate grade (grade 2, G2), or high grade (grade 3, G3) based on appearance, mitotic

TABLE 39.2 World Health Organization staging system for neuroendocrine tumors.

	WELL DIFFERENTIATED		POORLY DIFFERENTIATED
	LOW GRADE (G1)	INTERMEDIATE GRADE (G2/G3)	HIGH GRADE (G3)
Appearance	Homogeneous small, round cells with abundant expression of neuroendocrine markers		Pleomorphic cells with nuclear irregularity, necrosis
Mitotic rate	<2 mitoses/10 HPF	G2 2–20 mitoses/10 HPF G3 >20 mitoses/10 HPF	>20 mitoses/10 HPF
Ki-67 Index	<3%	G2 3%–20% G3 >20%	>20%
Behavior	Indolent		Aggressive

HPF, High-power field.

TABLE 39.3 American Joint Committee on Cancer (AJCC) and European Neuroendocrine Tumor Society (ENETS) staging for pancreatic neuroendocrine tumors.

	AJCC 8TH EDITION	ENETS
Primary Tumor (T)		
T1	Maximum tumor diameter <2 cm	Tumor limited to the pancreas <2 cm
T2	Maximum tumor diameter >2 but <4 cm	Tumor limited to the pancreas, 2–4 cm
T3	Maximum tumor diameter >4 cm	Tumor limited to the pancreas, >4 cm, or invading the duodenum or common bile duct
T4	Tumor involves the celiac axis or superior mesenteric artery	Tumor invades adjacent structures
Nodal Metastases (N)		
N0	No regional lymph node metastases	No regional lymph node metastasis
N1	Metastasis in one to three regional lymph nodes	Regional lymph node metastasis
N2	Metastasis in four or more regional lymph nodes	
Metastatic Disease (M)		
M0	No distant metastasis	No distant metastasis
M1	Distant metastasis	Distant metastasis
Stage		
I	T1, N0, M0 (Ia) T2, N0, M0 (Ib)	T1, N0, M0 (Ia) T2, N0, M0 (Ib)
II	T3, N0, M0 (IIa) T1-3, N2, M0 (IIb)	T3, N0, M0 (IIa) T1-3, N2, M0 (IIb)
III	Any T, N2, M0 T4, any N, M0	T4, any N, M0
IV	Any T, any N, M1	Any T, any N, M1

Adapted from Li X, Gou S, Liu Z, et al. Assessment of the American Joint Commission on Cancer 8th edition staging system for patients with pancreatic neuroendocrine tumors: a surveillance, epidemiology, and end results analysis. *Cancer Med.* 2018;7:626–634.

rates, invasion of other organs, angioinvasion, and the Ki-67 proliferative index (Table 39.2). G1 and G2 tumors are considered well differentiated, and G3 tumors are poorly differentiated and is by far the most important prognostic indicator. High-grade/poorly differentiated PNETs are sometimes referred to as "neuroendocrine carcinoma" and account for fewer than 3% of PNETs. However, it is important to emphasize that well-differentiated tumors do still have malignant potential, but that the differences in behavior persist, even for patients with metastatic disease.

The American Joint Committee on Cancer (AJCC) and European Neuroendocrine Tumor Society (ENETS) also have proposed staging schemes for PNETs. Neither system includes tumor grade, and both apply staging similar to that of exocrine pancreatic cancers to PNETs (Table 39.3). In another study, a tumor, grade, metastases (TGM) staging system was proposed as a more accurate prognostic tool.[3] In a recent study using the Surveillance, Epidemiology, and End Results databases, the 8th edition AJCC staging system exhibited good prognostic discrimination across stages in both resected and unresected patients.[4]

Molecular Genetics of PNETs

Although most PNETs occur sporadically, others can be associated with genetic syndromes. The most common genetic syndrome associated with PNETs is multiple endocrine neoplasia type 1 (MEN1), characterized by PNETs, parathyroid adenomas or hyperplasia, and pituitary adenomas. MEN1 is caused by mutations or allelic deletions in the tumor suppressor gene, menin, on chromosome 11q13 and is inherited in an autosomal dominant fashion. Menin is a component of the histone methyltransferase complex and is involved in control of G1 to S phase cell cycle

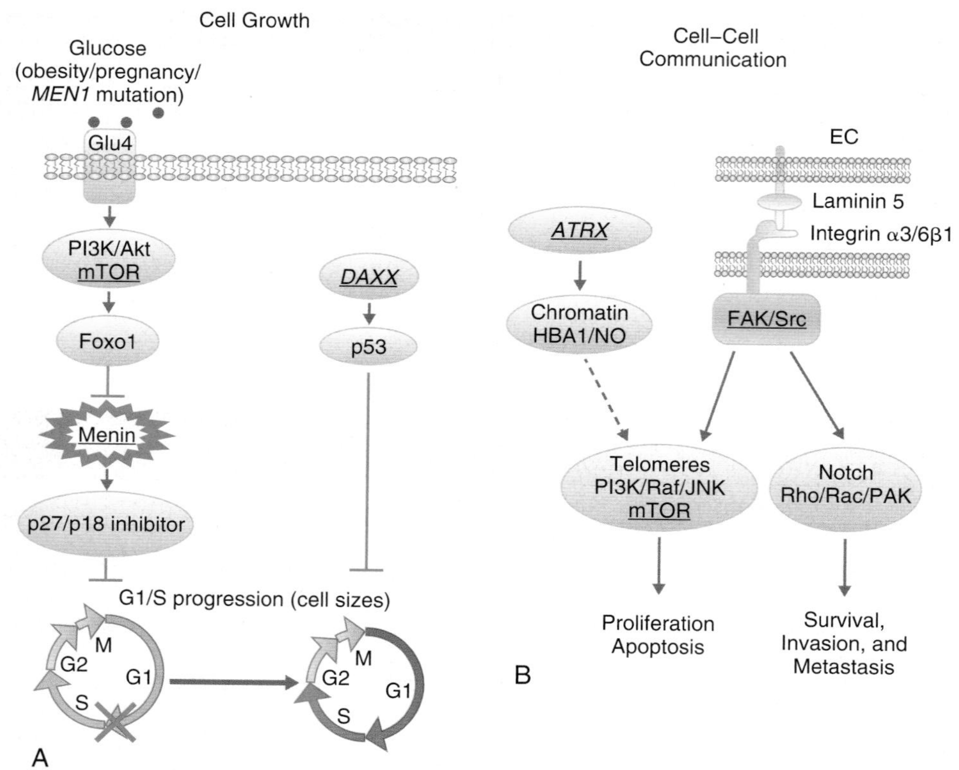

FIG. 39.3 Common genetic mutations and impacted signal transduction pathways in pancreatic neuroendocrine tumors (PNETs). (A) Cell growth. MEN1 mutations decrease Menin-regulated p27/p18 expression, which abrogates the glucose sensor. DAXX mutations decrease p53 levels, diminishing the checkpoint for cellular/DNA damages. Both MEN1 and DAXX mutations promote cell cycle progression from the G1 to S phase, regardless of glucose levels and damage. (B) Cell–cell communications. Endocrine cells, such as beta or alpha cells, relay on the endothelium to provide extracellular matrix, which disables the attachment requirement needed for cancer cells to invade and migrate. ATRX mutation-modulated chromatin modification may play a role in the abnormal activation of FAK/Src and mTOR pathways in PNET. Underlines indicate the mutated genes or activated protein. (With permission from Zhang J, Francois R, Iyer R, et al. Current understanding of the molecular biology of pancreatic neuroendocrine tumors. *J Natl Cancer Inst.* 2013;105:1005–1017, p 1008.) *EC*, Endothelial cell; *FAK*, focal adhesion kinase; *HBA1*, hemoglobin-α; *JNK*, c-Jun N-terminal kinase; *MEN1*, multiple endocrine neoplasia type 1; *mTOR*, mammalian target of rapamycin; *NO*, nitric oxide; *PAK*, p21-activated kinase; *PI3K/Akt*, phosphoinositide-3-kinase/protein kinase B.

progression. Mutation or allelic deletion causes loss of tumor suppressor function and predisposes patients to neoplastic growth in the parathyroid, pituitary, and pancreatic endocrine tissue.

Von Hippel-Lindau (VHL) syndrome is also associated with PNETs. Patients with inherited mutations of the VHL gene are at risk for the development of renal cell carcinoma, pheochromocytoma, benign tumors of the central nervous system, retina, epididymis, and inner ear and pancreatic lesions, including NETs, microcystic adenomas, and simple cysts. Similar to MEN1, the management of PNETs can be challenging, since they are often multifocal and associated with tumors in other locations. PNETs associated with VHL generally behave in an indolent fashion, and it has been suggested that these tumors can be observed until they reach at least 2 3 cm in size. However, specific germline mutations in exon 3 of the VHL gene may be associated with a more aggressive phenotype and warrant earlier treatment and closer surveillance.[5]

Most PNETs, however, are not associated with a known genetic syndrome and occur sporadically. Other than family history, risk factors for PNETs are not well defined. As in other neoplastic processes, tumorigenesis of PNETs involves an accumulation of a number of genetic events. The common genetic mutations and impacted signal transduction pathways in PNETs is shown in Fig. 39.3. Complete exomic sequencing of a discovery set of 10 sporadic PNETs revealed mutations in 149 genes, of which 6 were selected for further analysis in a validation set of 58 PNETs.[6] Inactivating mutations in MEN1 were seen in 44% of sporadic tumors. Mutations in death-domain associated protein (DAXX) and alpha thalassemia-mental retardation syndrome X-linked (ATRX), whose protein products are involved in p53-mediated DNA damage repair, were seen in 25% and 18%, respectively. Patients with mutations in MEN1 or DAXX/ATRX had prolonged survival compared to those who did not. Previous expression analyses had suggested dysregulation of the mammalian target of rapamycin (mTOR) pathway in a large proportion of tumors.[7,8] The mTOR protein is serine/threonine kinase and a key component of a cellular pathway playing an important role in the regulation of cell growth and proliferation. mTOR is upregulated in several tumors, including PNETs. This has potential clinical implications since the mTOR inhibitor everolimus has been U.S. Food and Drug Administration (FDA) approved for advanced NETs. Potentially, mutational testing will allow selection of patients most likely to benefit from this targeted therapy. Overall,

TABLE 39.4 Comparison of commonly mutated genes in PNET and PDAC.

GENES	PNET	PDAC
MEN1	44%	0%
DAXX, ATRX	43%	0%
Genes in mTOR pathway	15%	0.8%
TP53	3%	85%
KRAS	0%	100%
CDKN2A	0%	25%
TGFBR1, SMAD3, SMAD4	0%	38%

Adapted from Jiao Y, Shi C, Edil BH, et al. DAXX/ATRX, MEN1, and mTOR pathway genes are frequently altered in pancreatic neuroendocrine tumors. *Science*. 2011;331:1199–1203.
mTOR, Mammalian target of rapamycin; *PDAC*, pancreatic ductal adenocarcinoma; *PNET*, pancreatic neuroendocrine tumor.

the mutational analysis was most remarkable for how distinct the genetic abnormalities were from those observed in a similar study of pancreatic adenocarcinoma (Table 39.4).[9] Mutations in KRAS were not seen in PNETs and mutations in P53 were seen only rarely, at least not in these well-differentiated tumors.

In a separate study comparing well- and poorly differentiated PNETs, MEN1 and DAXX/ATRX expression by immunohistochemistry was abnormal in approximately half of well-differentiated tumors. In contrast, staining of DAXX/ATRX was normal in poorly differentiated tumors, but there was a high incidence of abnormal p53 and retinoblastoma expression as well as overexpression of the antiapoptotic protein Bcl2, implicating it as a target for therapy in these tumors.[10]

General Principles of Diagnosis and Treatment of PNETs

Diagnosis and Evaluation

The diagnosis and evaluation of PNETs are dependent on the history, symptoms, and imaging available at the time of presentation. Patient presentation can vary widely and include an incidental finding in an asymptomatic patient: functional hormonal syndromes, abdominal symptoms due to mass effect or metastatic disease such as abdominal or back pain, jaundice, anorexia, and weight loss. Until nonfunctional tumors grow large enough to cause symptoms related to mass effect, they often have no or vague symptoms and present at a more advanced stage. Finally, with the increase in the number of incidentally found PNETs on imaging done for other reasons, patients may be completely asymptomatic. All patients with suspected PNETs, regardless of presentation, need, at minimum, 1) a careful history screening for functional tumor symptoms, with biochemical confirmation if indicated, 2) cross-sectional or more advanced imaging when necessary to localize the PNET, 3) evaluation for metastatic disease, and 4) a thorough family history to rule out associated genetic syndromes. A general algorithm for the management of patient with suspected PNET is shown in Fig. 39.4.

Screening for Functional Tumors

The diagnosis of functional PNETs can be detected by elevated serum levels of the suspected peptide based on symptoms (Table 39.1). In patients presenting with a hyperenhancing pancreatic mass on cross-sectional imaging suggestive of PNET, the history should screen for neuroglycopenic symptoms, diarrhea, ulcer diathesis, rash, and other symptoms suggestive of a classic hormonal syndrome. A family history should also be obtained to rule out the possibility of MEN1-associated PNET. In the absence of symptoms, a full hormonal screen is not necessary.

PNETs often produce distinct gastrointestinal peptides including chromogranin A, neurotensin, and PP. While these peptides are not associated with clinical symptoms or syndromes, they can aid in the confirmation of the diagnosis. Chromogranin A levels have been shown to correlate with tumor presence in both functional and nonfunctional PNETs. Similar to other biomarkers, chromogranin A is useful for both confirmation of the diagnosis in a patient with suspected PNET on imaging as well as posttreatment surveillance for recurrence. Chromogranin A levels can also be elevated in patients on proton pump inhibitors (PPIs), with atrophic gastritis, and in patients with hepatic or renal insufficiency.

Localization

The vast majority of noninsulinoma or nongastrinoma pancreatic endocrine tumors will be identified on cross-sectional imaging. Once the diagnosis of a functional PNET is made, cross-sectional imaging with CT or MRI is the first step in localization. Because of their rich vascular supply, PNETs are hyperattenuating when compared with surrounding pancreatic tissue on contrast-enhanced multidetector CT (MDCT; Figs. 39.5A and 39.6A–D). Insulinomas and gastrinomas, which are smaller at presentation, can be more difficult to localize. CT technique, including thinner collimation (1.25-mm cuts) and multiple-phase imaging, is critical to improving sensitivity of CT for these small lesions. Capturing the vascular blush in the arterial phase is critical for identification and differentiation from other types of pancreatic tumors, which is less pronounced in the venous phase. In addition, the use of water instead of oral contrast may assist in identifying small duodenal gastrinomas. The sensitivity of MDCT in the localization of PNETs, in general, is 73% to 96% and is directly related to the size and location of the tumor.[11]

MRI can also be used for localization (Fig. 39.5B). Pancreatic endocrine tumors demonstrate low-signal intensity on T1-weighted images and high-signal intensity on T2-weighted images. As with CT, size is directly related to sensitivity. In one large series of insulinomas, contrast-enhanced MRI identified all lesions larger than 3 cm, 50% of lesions 1 to 2 cm, and no lesions smaller than 1 cm.[12] The overall sensitivity of MRI for detecting PNETs is between 80% and 90%.[11,13]

If unable to localize a pancreatic endocrine tumor on CT or MRI, endoscopic ultrasound (EUS) should be performed. EUS has an overall sensitivity of approximately 90% for tumors of all sizes and better sensitivity for detecting tumors smaller than 3 cm than CT or MRI.[13] EUS has the best diagnostic performance in detection and localization of insulinoma. However, EUS has a limited ability to detect small duodenal tumors, with a sensitivity of only 50% in this setting. EUS also allows for fine-needle aspiration of tumors for a pathologic diagnosis. This is especially useful for nonfunctional tumors without a classic CT appearance of pancreatic endocrine tumors (Fig. 39.6A–D).

The abundance of somatostatin receptors on most PNETs makes somatostatin receptor scintigraphy (SRS) a useful adjunct in localization, if tumors are not evident on CT or MRI. The sensitivity for SRS is over 80% for all pancreatic endocrine tumors excluding insulinomas. SRS has an overall sensitivity of 80% to 100% and specificity higher than 90% for gastrinomas, as somatostatin receptors are present in more than 90% of gastrin-secreting PNETs. Somatostatin receptors are also present in a significant

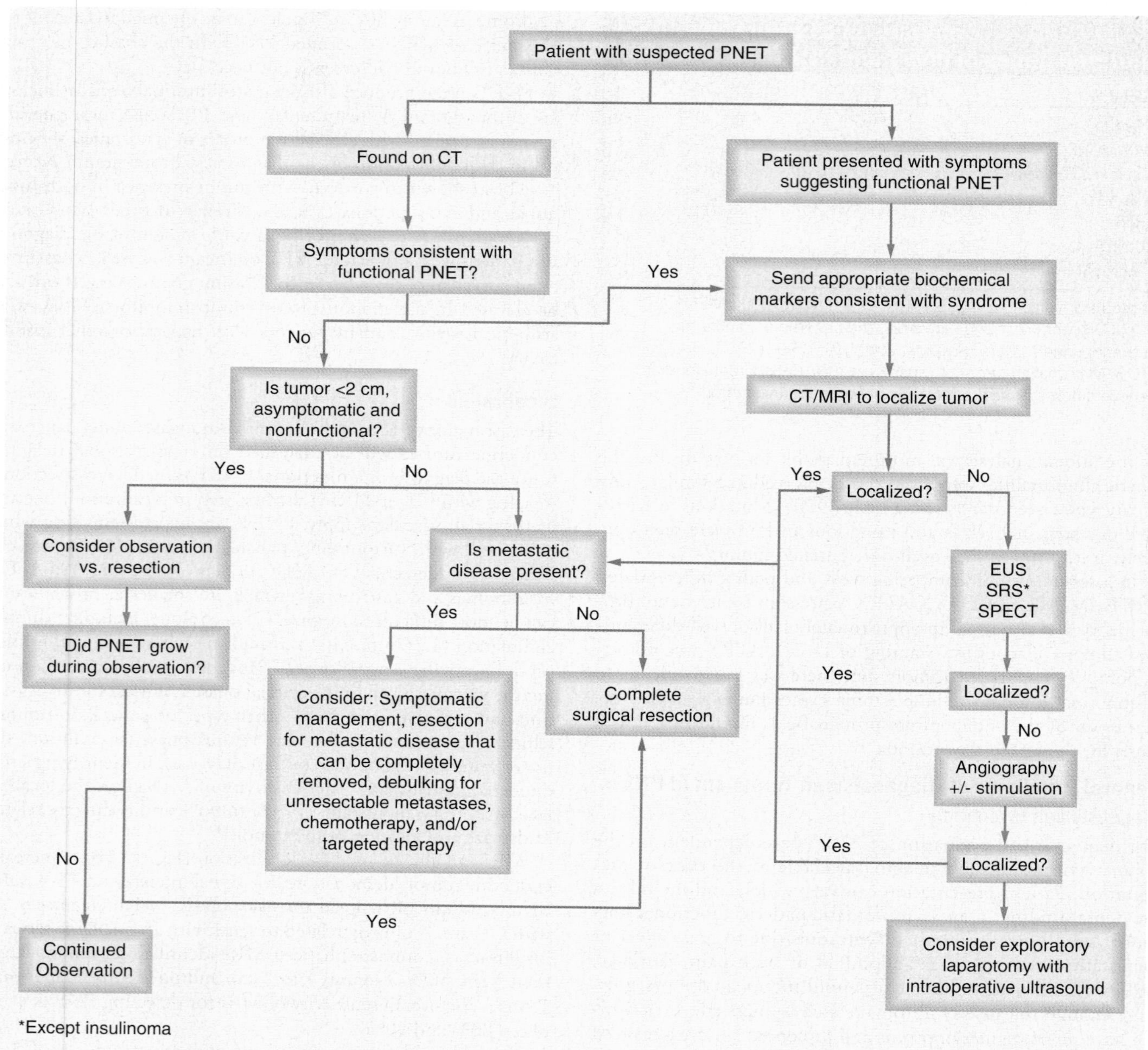

FIG. 39.4 General diagnosis, localization, and treatment algorithm for a patient with suspected pancreatic neuroendocrine tumor *(PNET)*. *CT*, Computed tomography; *EUS*, endoscopic ultrasound; *MRI*, magnetic resonance imaging; *SPECT*, single-photon emission computed tomography; *SRS*, somatostatin receptor scintigraphy.

portion of glucagon-secreting and nonfunctioning PNETs. In contrast, insulin-secreting PNETs and pancreatic adenocarcinomas do not possess somatostatin receptors. SRS is also useful for detecting hepatic metastases from noninsulinoma PNETs.

SRS is limited by physiologic sites or benign conditions that may show tracer uptake and lacks anatomic precision in localization (Fig. 39.5C). Although sensitive, SRS may not show the exact location of a tumor but only indicates its general vicinity within a few centimeters. The shortcomings of SRS, especially those linked to the limited spatial resolution and the lack of anatomical landmarks, may be overcome by the use of hybrid single-photon emission CT (SPECT)/CT imaging. SPECT/CT provides incremental diagnostic value over SRS, mainly because of a precise anatomical localization that helps discriminate between tumor lesions and physiologic uptake (Fig. 39.5D).[14] In a recent study of 281 patient G1 and G2 PNET, SPECT/CT had a sensitivity of 96% and a specificity of 97% for initial diagnosis and staging as well as follow-up.[15]

If the previous studies are unsuccessful in localizing the tumor, angiography can be useful. For insulinomas, often the hardest to localize, angiography detects approximately 70% of insulinomas larger than 5 mm, showing a characteristic vascular blush that corresponds to the highly vascular nature of insulinomas (Fig. 39.7). If standard radiographic techniques are unsuccessful, portal venous sampling for insulin or gastrin levels may allow localization to a region of the pancreas (head, body, or tail) to aid in operative planning. Portal venous sampling does not absolutely localize the tumor but provides accurate information on the region of the pancreas from which the high levels of hormones are released.

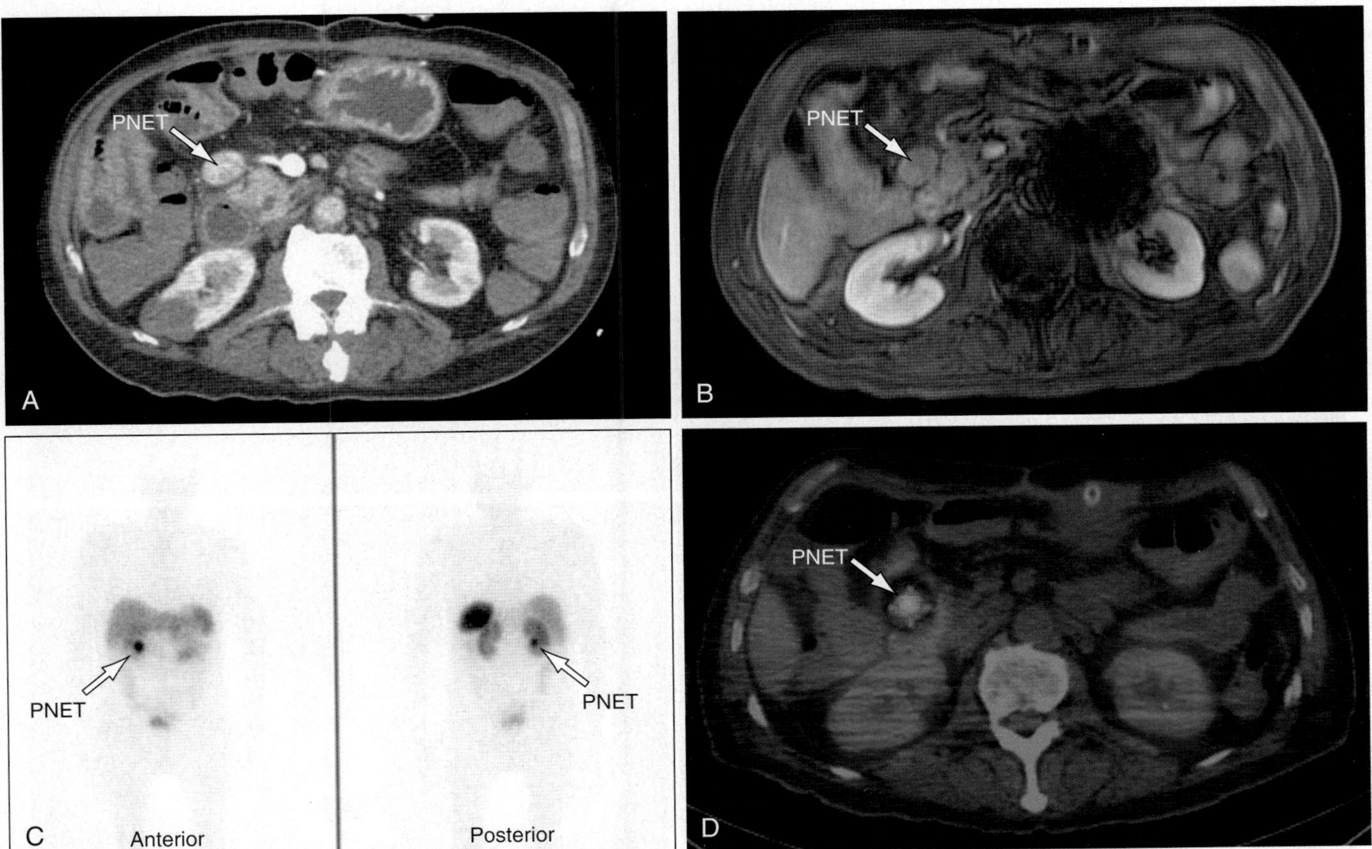

FIG. 39.5 Patient with a pancreatic neuroendocrine tumor *(PNET)*. (A) Computed tomography (CT) scan demonstrating a hyperenhancing lesion adjacent to the head of the pancreas *(arrow)*. (B) Same lesion shown on magnetic resonance imaging. (C) Same lesion shown on somatostatin receptor scintigraphy, anterior and posterior view; note the nonprecise anatomic localization and the physiologic uptake of tracer in the kidneys, liver, and spleen. (D) Same lesion on single-photon emission CT/CT; note the better anatomic localization and clear identification of nonphysiologic tracer uptake.

Calcium stimulates insulin release from insulinomas, whereas secretin stimulates gastrin release from gastrinomas. Arterial stimulation by injecting calcium or secretin into the celiac and superior mesenteric arteries can further increase the likelihood of localization with simultaneous portal venous sampling for appropriate hormone levels. Arterial stimulation venous sampling has a sensitivity of higher than 90%. However, with modern localization techniques, this is rarely necessary.

Treatment of Nonmetastatic, Symptomatic PNETs Localized Preoperatively

In the absence of metastatic disease, the primary treatment of symptomatic or functional PNETs is surgical resection. The approach and extent of resection are dictated by the functional status or tumor type, location, stage, grade, and patient factors. In most cases, a partial pancreatic resection is performed (i.e., pancreatic head resection, distal pancreatic resection, or enucleation), which can be performed with an open or minimally invasive approach. The goal of the procedure in most patients is to remove the primary tumor and regional lymph nodes. In most PNETs, the surrounding normal pancreas has a soft texture, increasing the risk of pancreatic fistula after partial pancreatectomy. Although generally less problematic than leaks after pancreaticoduodenectomy, leaks after distal pancreatectomy and enucleation are more common.

While enucleation preserves pancreatic parenchyma, one of the theoretical disadvantages of enucleation over the more radical procedures is that regional lymph nodes are not sampled. Knowledge of lymph node status allows for a better determination of prognosis, although there is no proven therapeutic value to lymph node removal. Similarly, the importance of splenectomy with distal pancreatectomy is controversial, as spleen-preserving techniques have lower lymph node yields.

Incidentally Found, Small, Nonfunctional PNETs

Historically, all PNETs were thought to have malignant potential, and, when identified, resection was recommended. However, the increasing use of high-resolution diagnostic imaging in the United States has led to increased identification of incidental, asymptomatic PNETs, with potential overdiagnosis and overtreatment. In autopsy series, PNETs occur with a prevalence of 1% to 10%, depending on the number of sections performed. Much lower than the documented worldwide disease prevalence, this suggests that the majority of PNETs may never become clinically relevant and would not progress to cause symptoms or death. Given the high morbidity associated with pancreatic resection, many recent studies have evaluated the role of observation in small nonfunctional PNETs. Significant controversy remains regarding observation of small nonfunctional PNETs.

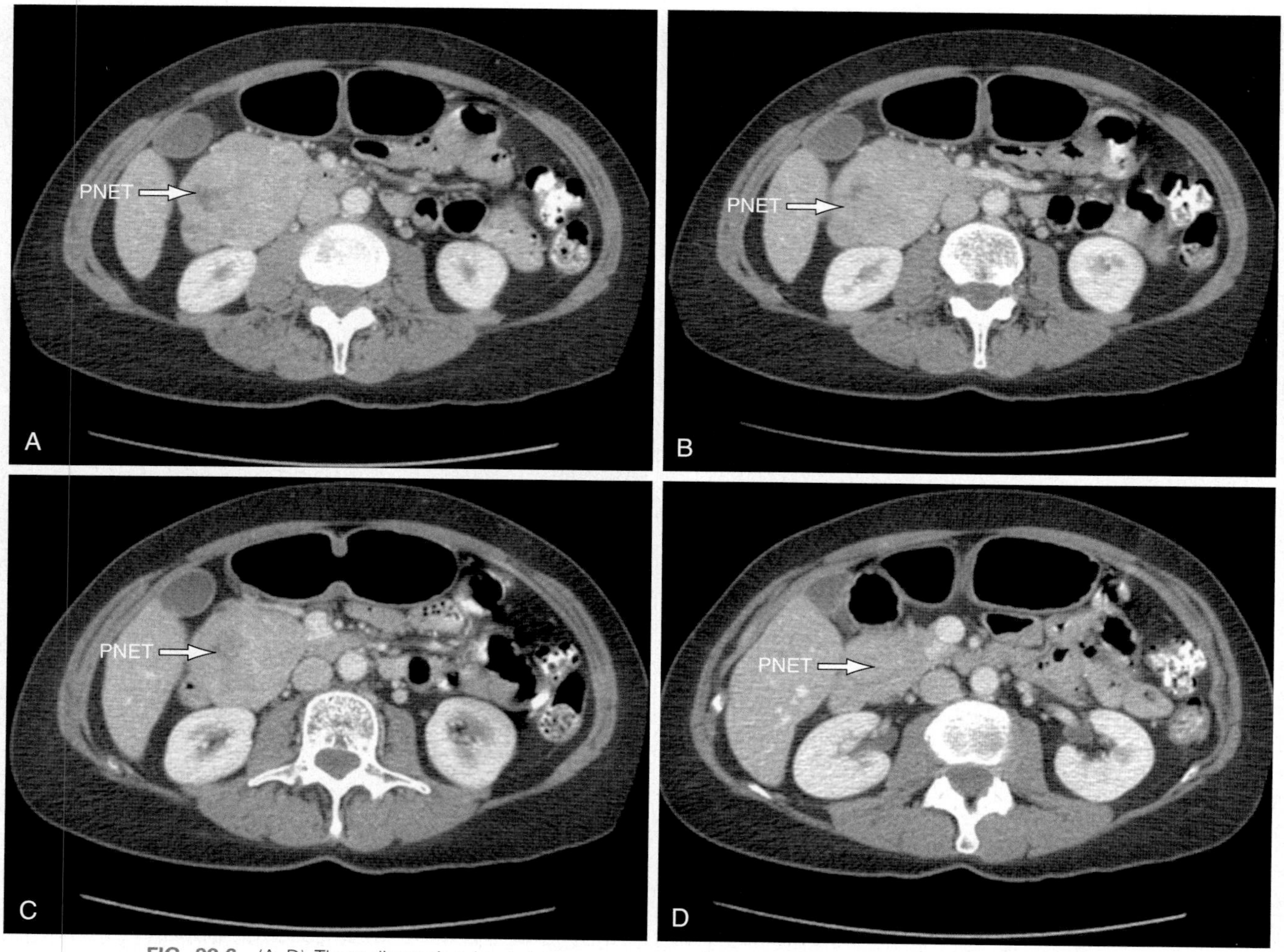

FIG. 39.6 (A–D) Three-dimensional spiral, pancreas protocol computed tomography scan demonstrating a hyperattenuating 5.0-cm lesion in the head of the pancreas *(arrow)* in a patient with a 7-year history of episodic symptomatic hypoglycemia. On a 72-hour monitored fast, the patient demonstrated symptomatic hypoglycemia and associated high insulin and C-peptide levels. *PNET*, Pancreatic neuroendocrine tumor.

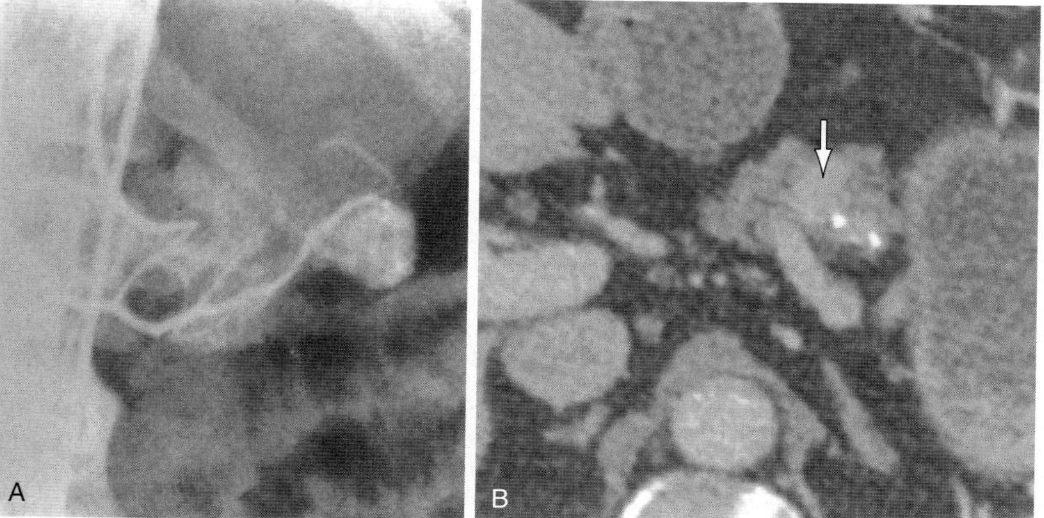

FIG. 39.7 Arteriographic demonstration of an insulinoma. (A) Selective injection into the specific dorsal pancreatic artery demonstrates the tumor precisely. (B) Insulinoma with triphasic enhancement on computed tomography. The mass in the pancreatic body *(arrow)* demonstrates early and prolonged enhancement with washout during the portal venous phase; note that the maximal difference in enhancement between the tumor and normal pancreas occurs during the pancreatic phase (shown).

According to the ENETS 2016 guidelines for the management of PNETs, observation of tumors less than 2 cm is safe in the setting of WHO G1 and low G2 tumors (Ki-67 index <10%) and absence of malignant findings on staging imaging.[16] Likewise, the most recent National Comprehensive Cancer Network (NCCN) guidelines offer observation as a treatment option for nonfunctional PNETs less than 2 cm.[17] ENETS recommends mandatory EUS and MRI repeated every 6 months if observation is chosen, with a lengthening of the interval to 12 months if no changes in size are demonstrated. If an increase of 0.5 cm (or more) in the size of the lesion occurs, patients should be reevaluated for surgery.[16] The NCCN surveillance recommendation interval is similar at 6 to 12 months and they recommend history and physical, CT or MRI of the abdomen, and CT of the chest when indicated.

These guidelines are based on data from multiple observational studies. A review of 143 PNETs demonstrated that incidentally found tumors had a 5-year progression-free survival rate of 86% compared to 59% for symptomatic tumors (P = 0.007). The improved survival was true across stages, supporting nonoperative management for incidentally found lesions.[18] Lee and colleagues[19] reviewed 131 patients with small, asymptomatic nonfunctional PNETs, 77 were observed; the median tumor size (1 cm; range, 0.3–3.2 cm) did not change over the mean 45-month follow-up, and there was no disease progression or disease-specific mortality. Additionally, in the operative group (n=56; median tumor size, 1.8 cm; range, 0.5–3.6 cm), 46% had a complication, most due to a clinically significant pancreatic leak.[19] Sadot and colleagues[20] performed a retrospective observational study comparing 104 patients with PNETs smaller than 3 cm to 77 resected patients matched on size. All patients had stage I and II disease and were diagnosed between 1993 and 2013. At last follow-up, no patients in the observational group developed metastatic disease or had a change in tumor size. While 25% of patients underwent resection, only eight patients were resected for an increase in tumor size, with rest being primarily patient or surgeon choice. Several studies support observation in tumors less than 2 cm.[21–24] Gaujoux and colleagues[21] followed 46 patients with asymptomatic PNETs less than 2 cm. At a median follow-up of 38 months, no patients developed distant or nodal metastases. Six patients developed an increase in tumor size of 20%, with a median tumor growth of 0.12 mm/year.[21] A smaller study by Rosenberg and colleagues[23] with 35 patients also demonstrated no progression in patients followed a median follow-up of 28 months. A single-institution study by Zhang and colleagues[24] demonstrated that resection of PNETs larger than 1.5 cm improved survival, but the value of resection in PNETs smaller than 1.5 cm was not clear. The study by Sadot and colleagues[20] had higher rates of salvage surgery, possibly due to the larger size cutoff but also because the majority of resections in initially observed patients were patient or physician choice.

These data support observation in patients with incidental tumors smaller than 2 cm. However, when conservative management is chosen, careful surveillance must be undertaken per NCCN or ENETS guidelines. Careful observation allows for observation of the natural history and intervention in the case of more aggressive tumors (Fig. 39.4).

Nonmetastatic Pancreatic Neuroendocrine Tumors—Unlocalized Preoperatively

With modern imaging, this should be a rare occurrence. However, in cases where the PNET cannot be localized preoperatively, intraoperative ultrasonography is essential and several reports have attested to the high degree of accuracy. To perform adequate ultrasound in the setting of an unlocalized tumor, the entire pancreas needs to be mobilized. Higher resolution (7.5- to 10-MHz) transducers are used for the pancreas; because of its greater depth of penetration, a 5-MHz transducer is better for the liver. Islet tumors are detected as sonolucent masses, generally of uniform consistency. The color Doppler attachment allows the detection of adjacent vessels and aids in the identification of the pancreatic ductal system, which shows up as a lucent tube without flow. Identification of the ductal system is useful to prevent pancreatic fistula formation after enucleation.

Metastatic Disease

Metastases are detected at diagnosis in approximately 40% to 80% of patients with PNETs, with the liver being the most frequent site. Although the presence of distant metastases is poor prognostic indicator in PNETs, long-term outcomes for patients with neuroendocrine liver metastases are much more favorable than for patients with liver metastases from pancreatic adenocarcinoma or other gastrointestinal tumors. With advances in liver-directed therapy, cytotoxic chemotherapy, and targeted therapy, there is a wide variety of treatment options for these patients, and given the indolent nature of the disease even in the metastatic setting, aggressive therapy is warranted. Treatment for metastatic disease requires coordinated multidisciplinary care including surgeons, oncologists, and interventional radiologists. It is well summarized in a recent systematic review by Nigri and colleagues.[25] While the different treatment types are discussed below in isolation, combined approaches including aggressive surgical resection, ablative liver-directed therapy, and cytotoxic or targeted chemotherapy may be used to improve survival and quality of life.

Liver Surgery for Metastatic Disease

Liver resection in the setting of metastatic PNET can be either curative or palliative. Potentially curative surgery is possible in only 10% to 25% of patients with liver metastases. Resection is recommended if more than 90% of disease can be removed. Resection can be concurrent with the primary tumor or staged. Bilobar metastases may require a staged approach, with portal vein embolization to promote liver hypertrophy and staged resection of lesions on each side. Specific criteria portend a better prognosis and may aid in patient selection for curative or palliative resection; the factors include G1/G2 tumors, absence of distant lymph node metastases, and absence of extrahepatic or peritoneal metastases. After resection, even curative, the rates of recurrence at 5 years is 80%. However, despite this high recurrence rate, the overall 5-year survival is 85%.[25]

There have been no randomized trials comparing liver resection to other treatments for metastatic endocrine tumors. Long-term survival after surgical resection compared to other liver-directed therapies are better in observational studies. Elias and colleagues[26] reported a 5-year survival rate of 71% for 47 patients who underwent partial hepatectomy versus 31% for 65 patients treated with chemoembolization. Debulking for unresectable metastatic disease remains controversial but is reasonable in the setting of G1/G2 disease localized to the liver in a good surgical candidate. Current consensus is that debulking is warranted if more than 90% of tumor can be resected. This was disputed more recently with Morgan and colleagues,[27] suggesting a threshold of 70%, as long-term outcomes were similar when 70%, 90%, and 100% were resected. In addition, debulking surgery improves the effect of the subsequent locoregional treatment.[28]

Liver-Directed Therapy for Metastatic Disease

Alternatives to liver resection include other liver-directed therapies such as radiofrequency ablation, cryoablation, transarterial embolization, transarterial chemoembolization, and radioembolization. These modalities are not considered curative and can be associated with significant morbidity (e.g., abscess, cholecystitis, and liver failure). As such, they are generally reserved for patients with symptomatic disease that is not amenable to surgical resection.

Radiofrequency ablation is safe and can be used to treat unresectable metastases smaller than 5 cm and is effective in controlling symptoms related to hormone secretion. Given their often multifocal and highly vascular nature, endocrine liver metastases are particularly well suited to transcatheter transarterial therapies. Transarterial embolization uses lipiodol, gel foam particles, polyvinyl alcohol foam, or bland microspheres for embolization, while transarterial chemoembolization adds chemotherapeutic agents, which are most often doxorubicin, melphalan, and streptozocin. Intratumoral concentrations in transarterial chemoembolization exceed 20 times the concentration achieved with systemic chemotherapy. Intra arterial therapies have been associated with high partial response rates and even higher rates of symptomatic improvement in patients with functional tumors. Bland and chemoembolization techniques have been popular for years, but drug-eluting beads and yttrium-90 (Y90) microspheres are increasingly being used with the potential for more durable responses. Selective intra arterial radiotherapy consists of embolization with Y90 microspheres and has been shown to have a response rate of 55%, with an overall control rate of 88.9% at 3 months.[29]

Cytotoxic and Targeted Systemic Therapy

In parallel with advancements in liver-directed therapy, there have been significant improvements in the systemic therapy of metastatic NETs. Somatostatin analogues are effective in controlling both hormone secretion and stabilizing tumor growth in metastatic PNET. There are five different subtypes of somatostatin receptors (SSTR1, SSTR2, SSTR3, SSTR4, and SSTR5). Octreotide and lanreotide have high affinity for SSTR2 and bind to SSTR5, whereas pasireotide binds with high affinity for SSTR1, SSTR2, SSTR3, and SSTR5.[30] As such, knowing the type of somatostatin receptors expressed by the tumor can guide therapy. In the Placebo-Controlled, Double-Blind, Prospective, Randomized Study on the Effect of Octreotide LAR in the Control of Tumor Growth in Patients with Metastatic Neuroendocrine Midgut Tumors (PROMID) study, a long-acting somatostatin analog was demonstrated to increase time to progression in patients with metastatic well-differentiated PNETs.[31] This monthly injection is well tolerated, although cholelithiasis can develop with chronic use. For this reason, cholecystectomy should be considered in patients with advanced PNETs. However, the PROMID trial included only patients with limited liver involvement (≤10%) and already resected primary tumors.

The Controlled Study on Lanreotide Antiproliferative Response in Neuroendocrine Tumors (CLARINET) was a landmark study evaluating lanreotide autogel versus placebo in patients with metastatic G1/low G2 (proliferation index, Ki-67, up to 10%) somatostatin-receptor positive PNETs and other intestinal or unknown primary origin NETs with prior stable disease. Lanreotide prolonged progression-free survival over placebo. This was true regardless of hepatic tumor volume.[32]

Poorly differentiated neuroendocrine carcinomas behave more aggressively and respond better to cytotoxic chemotherapy than well-differentiated PNETs, but there is still a role for chemotherapy in unresectable low-grade PNETs, often in combination with other therapeutic modalities. Various cytotoxic agents are used to treat unresectable PNETs, including streptozotocin, cisplatin, dacarbazine, doxorubicin, and 5-fluorouracil. Response rates of 20% to 45% have been documented in G1/G2 PNETs with streptozotocin-based regimens with either 5-fluorouracil and/or epirubicin.[25,33] The alkylating agent temozolomide alone or in combination with capecitabine has been effective in G1/G2 PNETs with partial response rates of 70%, a median progression-free survival of 18 months, and 2-year survival of 92%.[34] For high-grade tumors with poor differentiation, platinum-based regimens are preferred. Response rates of 42% to 67% have been obtained combining cisplatin and etoposide.[35]

Recent understanding of the pathogenesis of PNETs has allowed for the development of targeted therapy. Everolimus is an oral inhibitor of mTOR, which is upregulated in many PNETs. In a randomized, placebo-controlled trial, the median overall survival was 44.0 months (95% confidence interval [CI], 35.6 to 51.8 months) for those randomly assigned to everolimus and 37.7 months (95% CI, 29.1 to 45.8 months) for those assigned to placebo (hazard ratio, 0.94; 95% CI, 0.73 to 1.20; $P = 0.30$). Patients in the everolimus group had a longer progression-free survival (11 months vs. 4.6 months) than patients receiving placebo.[36] Sunitinib is an inhibitor of the tyrosine kinases platelet-derived growth factor receptor (PDGFR), vascular endothelial growth factor receptor (VEGFR)-1, VEGFR-2, proto-oncogene CD117 (c-KIT), and CD135 (FLIT3). PNETs have frequent overexpression of vascular endothelial growth factor (VEGF) or VEFGR. Sunitinib has been shown to be well tolerated and effective in a randomized controlled phase III trial,[37] with a progression-free survival of 11.1 months in the group treated with sunitinib versus 5.5 months in the placebo group. Both of these targeted therapies have been approved by the FDA and—together with somatostatin analogs—have largely replaced cytotoxic chemotherapy in the management of advanced well-differentiated PNETs.

Radiolabeled somatostatin analogs represent a new treatment option in patients with strong radiotracer uptake in somatostatin receptors. Peptide receptor radionuclide therapy with radiolabeled somatostatin analogs allows administration of targeted radiotherapy to the tumor tissue and its metastases. The most used radiolabels are Y90 and ^{177}Lutetium. Complete tumor response is rare with this treatment (0%–6%), but results are encouraging, with partial tumor regression in 7% to 37% of patients and stabilization in 42% to 86% using Y90-labeled somatostatin analogues.[38] Peptide receptor radionuclide therapy is a promising therapeutic option, even if still investigational.

Liver Transplantation for Metastatic PNETs

PNETs tend to metastasize to the liver, and disease often does not spread beyond the liver. Even after treatment of liver metastases, most patients develop disease recurrence in the remnant liver within 2 years, demonstrating the strong predilection for PNETs to metastasize to the liver and the generally indolent nature of this disease. Therefore, total hepatectomy with liver transplantation has been proposed as a potentially curative treatment option for unresectable neuroendocrine metastases. In fact, unresectable neuroendocrine metastases is the only metastatic indication for transplantation. The same Milan group that created the commonly used criteria for transplantation in hepatocellular carcinoma also proposed criteria for transplantation in neuroendocrine metastases, which include age younger than 55 years, well-differentiated tumor status, Ki-67 proliferative marker index less than 5%, completely resected primary tumor with portal drainage, less than 50% liver involvement, and absence of extrahepatic disease.[39] Using these relatively strict criteria, 5-year overall survival rates of 90% were achieved. However, not all centers have adhered to these criteria, and results have been highly variable. In a multicenter study of 213 transplants for neuroendocrine metastases, the largest published to date, 5-year overall survival was 52%. The presence of hepatomegaly, high-grade tumors, and major or minor extrahepatic tumor resection at the time of liver transplantation were associated with worse outcomes in a multivariable model.[40] Although these survival rates are comparable to those for transplantation in hepatocellular carcinoma, they may not be significantly greater than survival rates for nonsurgical therapy of neuroendocrine metastases. Given the scarcity of organs, the role of transplantation in neuroendocrine metastases remains controversial.

Diagnosis and Treatment of Specific Functional Pancreatic Neuroendocrine Tumors

Insulin-Secreting Pancreatic Neuroendocrine Tumors (Insulinoma)

Insulinoma is the most common functioning PNET, with an incidence of 1 to 2 per million population annually in the United States. In 1935, Whipple and Frantz documented the clinical syndrome defined by 1) neuroglycopenic symptoms consistent with hypoglycemia, 2) a low plasma glucose concentration measured when symptoms were present, and 3) relief of symptoms with administration of glucose, which became known as Whipple's triad.

Symptoms may vary in patients with insulin-secreting PNETs. Some have symptoms related to sympathetic nervous system overactivity in response to hypoglycemia, including fatigue, weakness, fearfulness, hunger, tremor, diaphoresis, and tachycardia. In others, a central nervous system disturbance predominates with apathy, irritability, anxiety, confusion, excitement, loss of orientation, blurred vision, delirium, stupor, coma, and/or seizures. In many patients, symptoms have been present for years before diagnosis. Patients often report significant weight gain coinciding with the onset of symptoms, as they compensate by eating frequently to prevent hypoglycemia.

The average age at diagnosis is 45 years. Insulinomas are distributed equally throughout the pancreas despite predominance of beta cells in the body and tail. Rarely, they occur in the duodenum, splenic hilum, or gastrocolic ligament. Insulinomas are typically small, with an average size of 1.0 to 1.5 cm. Surgical resection of insulinoma is usually curative because most tumors tend to be small, benign (85%–95%), and solitary. While the majority of insulinomas are sporadic, 5% are associated with MEN1, and these are more likely to be multiple and malignant.

Diagnosis. In any patient in whom Whipple triad is documented, further evaluation is necessary to determine the underlying cause and guide appropriate management. The differential diagnosis of symptomatic hypoglycemia includes insulinoma, noninsulinoma pancreatogenous hypoglycemia syndrome (NIPHS), exogenous insulin or oral hypoglycemic agent administration (sulfonylureas, meglitinides), insulin autoimmune hypoglycemia, and insulin-like growth factor–mediated hypoglycemia (Table 39.5). In the setting of suspected hypoglycemia, blood glucose should be measured precisely and not using a home reflectance meter, as reflectance meters are not sufficiently reliable in the low range.

A critical first step is to review the patient's history in detail, particularly the timing of symptoms in relationship to meals, medications taken by the individual and by family members, family, and social history. The diagnosis of insulinoma requires demonstration of inappropriately high serum insulin concentrations during a spontaneous or induced episode of hypoglycemia. When hypoglycemia occurs, the clinician should measure plasma glucose, insulin, C-peptide, proinsulin, beta-hydroxybutyrate levels, and screen for oral hypoglycemic agents.

The gold standard for diagnosis of insulinoma is the 72-hour monitored fast. However, in cases where hypoglycemic episodes are observed and the above laboratory testing can be obtained, a monitored fast is not necessary. Testing should be guided by the history, especially in relation to the timing of symptoms. The 72-hour fast can be initiated at home after an evening meal, except for patients in whom hypoglycemia occurs after a short period of fasting. The date and time of the last meal should be noted. All nonessential medications should be stopped. Patients can drink calorie-free, caffeine-free beverages. Blood samples for measurement of plasma glucose, insulin, C-peptide, proinsulin, and beta hydroxybutyrate should be taken every 6 hours until the glucose concentration is below 60 mg/dL. After this, blood sampling should occur every 1 to 2 hours. Insulin, C-peptide, and proinsulin need only be measured in specimens corresponding to a plasma glucose concentration of 60 mg/dL or less. Insulin antibodies should be measured, but they do not have to be measured during hypoglycemia. The fast is stopped and glucose is administered when the blood glucose level is less than 55 mg/dL or the patient becomes symptomatic. During the fast, approximately two-thirds to three-quarters of patients with insulinomas will experience hypoglycemic symptoms in the first 24 hours, and 95% will experience symptoms by 72 hours.

When hypoglycemia is documented, plasma insulin, C-peptide, and proinsulin values are elevated in patients with insulinomas, but also elevated in other conditions. Oral hypoglycemic agent-induced hypoglycemia can be differentiated by documented sulfonylurea or meglitinides in the plasma. Insulin autoimmune hypoglycemia can be differentiated by the presence of insulin or insulin receptor antibodies. The differentiation of insulinoma and NIPHS can be difficult in the absence of a documented pancreatic tumor consistent with an insulinoma. The latter occurs more commonly in the postprandial setting. Evaluating the insulin-to-glucose ratio is also useful. A ratio higher than 0.3 occurs with insulinoma ([μU/mL of insulin/mg]/[dL of glucose]). Less commonly, a ratio of 0.3 can occur in the obese patient as a result of insulin resistance, but such patients should not be hypoglycemic. C-peptide levels higher than 1.2 μg/mL with a glucose level lower than 40 mg/dL are also highly suggestive of an insulinoma.

In patients who are surreptitiously administering insulin, plasma insulin values are higher than levels observed in insulinoma patients, but plasma C-peptide and proinsulin values are low or undetectable. Due to the antiketogenic effect of insulin, all patients with insulinoma should have serum beta hydroxybutyrate levels less than 2.7 mmol/L at the end of the fast. A plasma beta hydroxybutyrate level more than 2.7 and brisk plasma glucose response to intravenous glucagon support the diagnosis of insulinoma in cases of borderline insulin/C-peptide levels or suggest an insulin-like growth factor–mediated process when insulin levels are low. Hypoglycemia in the setting of low plasma concentrations of insulin, C-peptide, and proinsulin suggest noninsulin or insulin-like growth factor–mediated hypoglycemia, which is rare.

Localization and treatment. The general principles for treatment of PNETs apply to insulinomas. In patients with biochemical evidence of insulinoma, the localization and management algorithm are shown in Fig. 39.4. The only difference in insulinoma is that SRS is not indicated as they rarely express somatostatin receptors. Surgical resection is the mainstay of treatment and is the only curative option for insulinoma. Because more than 90% of insulinomas are benign, enucleation is usually preferred, when possible, to preserve functional pancreatic mass. Enucleation should not be performed if the tumor is within 2 mm of the main pancreatic duct, which can be identified on intraoperative ultrasound.

TABLE 39.5 Interpretation of laboratory results and differential diagnosis in patients with Whipple triad.

DIAGNOSIS	GLUCOSE (mg/dL)	INSULIN (mIU/mL)	C-PEPTIDE (nmol/L)	PROINSULIN (pmol/L)	ANTI INSULIN OR ANTI-INSULIN RECEPTOR ANTIBODY (+/–)	CIRCULATING ORAL HYPOGLYCEMIC AGENTS (SULFONYLUREAS, MEGLITINIDES)	BETA HYDOXY-BUTYRATE	PANCREATIC MASS (ISLET CELL TUMOR)	TIMING OF HYPOGLYCEMIA
Insulinoma	<55	≥3	≥0.2	≥5	–	No	≤2.7	Yes*	Fasting
NIPHS, post-gastric bypass hypoglycemia	<55	≥3	≥0.2	≥5	–	No	≤2.7	No	Postprandial
Surreptitious insulin administration	<55	>>>3	<0.2	<5	–	No	≤2.7	No	With administration of inappropriate insulin
Oral hypoglycemic administration	<55	≥3	≥0.2	≥5	–	Yes	≤2.7	No	With administration of oral agents
Insulin autoimmune hypoglycemia	<55	>>>3	>>>0.2	>>>5	+	No	≤2.7	No	Fasting
IGF mediated	<55	<3	<0.2	<5	–	No	≤2.7	No	Fasting
IGF mediated	<55	<3	<0.2	<5	–	No	>2.7	No	Fasting

IGF, Insulin-like growth factor; *NIPHS*, noninsulinoma pancreatogenous hypoglycemia syndrome.

*Laboratory findings consistent with insulinoma should prompt evaluation for islet cell tumor. In the minority of cases, the pancreatic islet cell tumor may be difficult to localize preoperatively.

Anatomic resection (i.e., distal pancreatectomy, central pancreatectomy, or pancreaticoduodenectomy) may be necessary for tumors abutting the main pancreatic duct or for large tumors.

Preoperatively, it is important to prevent severe hypoglycemic attacks. Glucose infusions must be used in the perioperative period, especially when patients are taking nothing by mouth. Administration of diazoxide decreases beta cell release of insulin (usually 3 mg/kg/day, divided into two or three daily doses) and should be used to prevent or attenuate symptoms of hypoglycemia prior to surgical intervention once the diagnosis is made.

With modern imaging capability, it is rare that preoperative imaging cannot localize the insulinoma. In this rare case, blind exploration with intraoperative ultrasound, combined with careful palpation and exploration of the entire pancreas and duodenum, will identify most tumors. Carrying out effective intraoperative pancreatic ultrasound requires complete mobilization of the pancreas. In the unlikely event in which the tumor cannot be localized with preoperative or intraoperative techniques, biopsies should be taken from the pancreatic tail to evaluate for nesidioblastosis. Distal pancreatectomy should be considered in this setting but remains controversial (see section on "Noninsulinoma Pancreatogenous Hypoglycemia Syndrome").

Life expectancy should be normal after the complete excision of a benign insulinoma. More extensive resections are required for complete excision of malignant insulinomas. Tumor debulking in the setting of metastatic insulinoma may result in a biochemical cure because some residual disease may not be functional. Persistent hyperinsulinism after surgery for metastatic islet cell tumors may be managed with somatostatin analogues, by hepatic artery tumor embolization, by diazoxide, or by streptozotocin plus 5-fluorouracil. Even with metastatic disease, the median survival following resection is approximately 5 years.

Gastrin-Secreting Pancreatic Neuroendocrine Tumor (Gastrinoma)

Gastrin-secreting PNET (gastrinoma) is the second most common functional pancreatic endocrine tumor, with an incidence of 1 per 2.5 million population, and first described in 1955 by Zollinger and Ellison. The mean age of patients at diagnosis is approximately 50 years. Gastrinomas are slightly more common in men (60%), are sporadic in 75% of patients, and are associated with MEN1 in 25%. The gastrin produced by islet cell tumors is not subject to the normal stimulation by amino acids and peptides in the stomach or by gastric distention. In addition, these tumors are not suppressed by a high luminal pH and can be stimulated (instead of inhibited) by secretin.

Patients with gastrinoma (or Zollinger-Ellison syndrome [ZES]) have a fulminant peptic ulcer disease, acid hypersecretion, and non–beta islet cell tumors of the pancreas. Hypergastrinemia results in peptic acid hypersecretion and refractory peptic ulcer disease. Duodenal ulcers are the most common, but jejunal ulceration may also occur; the presence of jejunal ulcers should raise suspicion for a gastrin-secreting PNET. Approximately 75% of patients present with abdominal pain; almost two thirds of these individuals have diarrhea, and in 10% to 20%, diarrhea is the only symptom. This acid-induced diarrhea is stopped by nasogastric aspiration of gastric secretions, differentiating it from other secretory diarrheas. Over one third of patients have signs and symptoms of gastroesophageal reflux disease, and this number appears to be increasing.

Ninety percent of gastrinomas are located within the gastrinoma triangle, bounded by the lines connecting the cystic duct, the junction between the second and third portions of the duodenum, and the junction between the neck and body of the pancreas (Fig. 39.8). Over 60% are located in the duodenum (Fig. 39.9A), with most arising in the first portion. Gastrinomas are occasionally localized to lymph nodes in this region, and it is unclear whether lymph nodes can be a true primary site for gastrinoma or whether they represent metastases from occult primary tumors in the duodenum or pancreas (Fig. 39.9B).

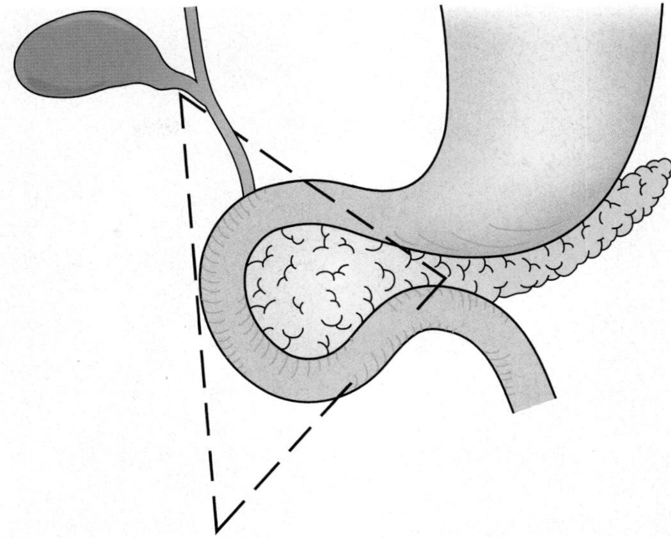

FIG. 39.8 The anatomic triangle in which approximately 90% of gastrinomas are found. The triangle is bounded by the lines connecting the cystic duct, the junction between the second and third portions of the duodenum, and the junction between the neck and body of the pancreas.

Diagnosis. Gastrin-secreting PNET (ZES) should be considered in all patients with intractable peptic ulcers (especially jejunal ulcers), severe esophagitis, or persistent secretory diarrhea. The diagnosis depends on the presence of hypergastrinemia and increased secretion of gastric acid. Most laboratories have an upper limit of normal of 100 pg/mL for fasting levels of gastrin. Levels of 100 to 1000 pg/mL are occasionally seen in nongastrinoma patients, and levels higher than 1000 pg/mL are highly suggestive of gastrinoma, provided that the patient demonstrated increased gastric acid secretion. Patients with pernicious anemia and those taking PPIs have very high gastrin levels in the abscess of gastric acid hypersecretion. In the work-up for ZES, all PPIs should be stopped 2 weeks prior to testing gastrin levels. An elevated serum gastrin level coupled with a pH lower than 2 in the gastric aspirate is diagnostic of gastrinoma. A gastric pH higher than 3 without acid-suppressing medications or prior acid-reducing operations strongly suggests that ZES is not the cause of hypergastrinemia.

If the diagnosis remains in doubt despite these measures, a secretin stimulation test can be helpful. In this test, the fasting gastrin level is measured before secretin (2 IU/kg) is administered intravenously, and subsequent samples are obtained 2, 5, 10, and 20 minutes after secretin administration. Gastrin levels greater than 200 pg/mL after administration of secretin is noted in 87% of patients, with no false-positive results. False-negative results may be caused by the presence of *Helicobacter pylori*. Other causes of hypergastrinemia must be excluded; the differential diagnosis can be further subdivided into hypergastrinemia associated with high and low gastric acid output (Table 39.6).

Localization and treatment. Once the diagnosis is established, the primary goal is to prevent acid secretion and relieve symptoms. The best results are achieved with PPIs; however, higher doses than that used for simple peptic ulcer or gastroesophageal reflux disease

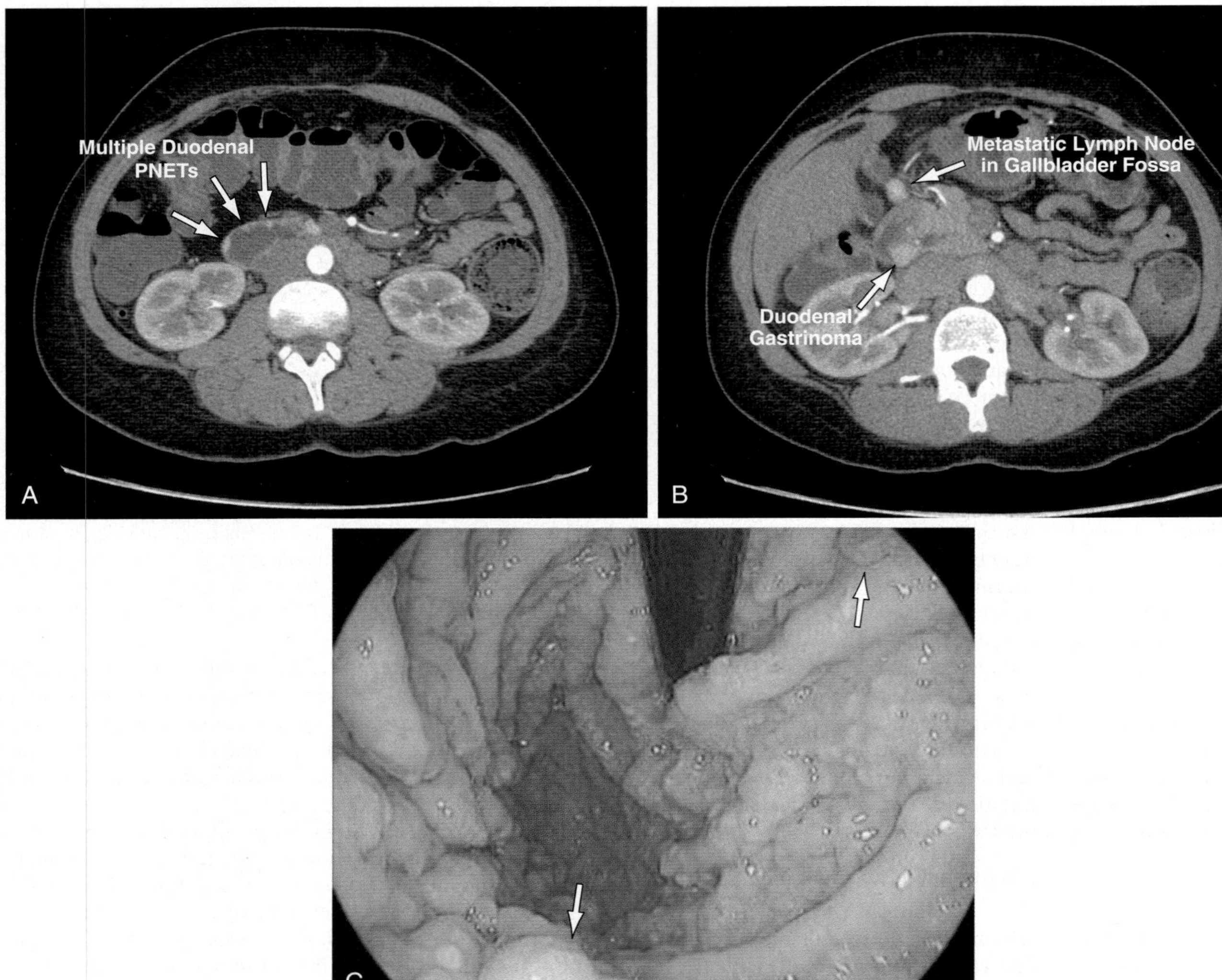

FIG. 39.9 (A) Computed tomography (CT) showing multiple small duodenal pancreatic neuroendocrine tumors *(PNETs)* in a patient with multiple endocrine neoplasia type 1 (MEN1). (B) CT showing metastatic gastrinoma to a lymph node in the gallbladder fossa and a large primary duodenal gastrinoma in the same patient. (C) Esophagogastroduodenoscopy showing multiple submucosal duodenal PNETs in a patient with MEN1; two large lesions *(arrows)* were removed endoscopically and consistent with PNET.

TABLE 39.6 Causes of hypergastrinemia.

HIGH GASTRIC ACID OUTPUT	NORMAL, LOW, OR NO GASTRIC ACID OUTPUT
ZES (gastrinoma)	H_2 receptor antagonist therapy
Gastric outlet obstruction	PPI therapy
G cell hyperplasia	Prior acid-reducing procedure
Retained gastric antrum	Atrophic gastritis, pernicious anemia, gastric cancer, vitiligo, achlorhydria, vagotomy, renal failure

PPI, Proton pump inhibitor; *ZES*, Zollinger-Ellison syndrome.

are often required. PPIs have been shown to be safe and effective at high doses and should be given at the dosage required to suppress gastric acid secretion.

Similar to all PNETs, for patients with biochemically confirmed ZES, the first step of the algorithm for localizing a gastrinoma should include CT or MRI. Water should be used as oral contrast on CT scans to allow for better visualization of hyperenhancing, small duodenal lesions. If the tumor is not localized by CT or MRI, SRS should be performed because almost all gastrinomas express somatostatin receptors. EUS may be useful to detect small pancreatic lesions. If localization has still not been accomplished, angiography with or without stimulation should be performed next. If all of these measures are unsuccessful and ZES is strongly suspected, it may be reasonable to proceed with operative exploration to localize and treat the tumor.

Operative treatment of gastrinomas is indicated when curative resection appears possible based on preoperative imaging or for palliative cytoreduction for symptom control. The presence or absence of malignant disease is the most important prognostic indicator. In 5% to 8% of cases, the surgeon is unable to localize a gastrinoma intraoperatively. If not localized preoperatively, finding tumors in the pancreas and duodenum may be difficult. Exploration includes the entire abdomen, from the undersurface of the diaphragm to the pelvic floor, with particular attention paid to the liver, right subhepatic and paraduodenal area, and pelvic cul-de-sac and ovaries. The entire small bowel and colon are examined carefully, with the surgeon looking for lymph nodes in the mesentery or attached to the wall of the bowel. The surgeon should carefully inspect the gastrinoma triangle (Fig. 39.8) to confirm the location of the tumor. Intraoperative ultrasound should be routinely performed to identify small pancreatic lesions or liver metastases. Transillumination of the duodenum with intraoperative endoscopy may help identify small submucosal lesions. After transillumination of the duodenum with intraoperative endoscopy, the duodenal wall can be gently palpated between the surgeon's fingers through a 3-cm duodenotomy on the anterolateral surface of the second portion of the duodenum, allowing for the detection of gastrinomas smaller than 1 cm. Duodenotomy will detect 25% to 30% of tumors not seen on preoperative imaging.

Most gastrinomas require segmental resection, including distal pancreatectomy or pancreaticoduodenectomy. Pancreaticoduodenectomy may increase disease-free survival in patients with MEN1 because, following local excision, recurrent tumors are most commonly found in the duodenum.[41] Detailed inspection of peripancreatic, periduodenal, and portohepatic lymph nodes should be performed because resection of grossly positive lymphatic spread may increase disease-free survival. Unfortunately, with long follow-up, almost 50% of patients initially free of disease show symptomatic or biochemical (i.e., a positive secretin test result) recurrence by 5 years.

Unfortunately, more than 50% of patients with gastrinomas have metastatic disease at the time of diagnosis. For patients with unresectable, symptomatic metastatic disease, treatment should focus on symptom control (i.e., reduction of acid production). Pharmacologic control of acid secretion with PPIs has rendered total gastrectomy, debulking, and other surgical acid-reducing procedures unnecessary. Symptoms are controlled in more than 90% of patients, starting with dosages of 60 to 80 mg pantoprazole daily, although higher dosages may be required. PPI dosage should be titrated to keep basal acid output lower than 10 mEq/hr (or <5 mEq/hr if the patient had a prior acid-reducing procedure). One of the few remaining indications for total gastrectomy in patients with ZES is the presence of gastric carcinoid tumors, which may arise from prolonged hypergastrinemia. Gastrectomy may also be indicated for patients who are unable to tolerate PPIs and cannot achieve acid secretion control through other means. Total gastrectomy cures all symptoms produced by excessive acid but has no effect on disease progression or survival for metastatic disease. Somatostatin analogues, used to decrease gastrin release and subsequent acid secretion, are rarely effective in suppressing acid without concurrent PPI use.

Aggressive surgical therapy is indicated, because patients have been known to live more than 20 years with residual disease. Gastrinoma may take an aggressive or relatively benign clinical course. The aggressive form, seen in about 25% of all patients, is associated with larger pancreatic tumors, liver metastases, and worse long-term survival; 90% of aggressive tumors are located in the pancreas. Ten-year survival rate is 30% in the aggressive form compared to greater than 90% in patients with the nonaggressive form. The best predictor of survival for patients with gastrinoma is the presence of liver metastases, whereas lymph node metastases are not predictive.[42] Resection of all gross disease and metastases may provide palliation of symptoms and has been associated with long-term survival rates of greater than 50%, but cures are rare.

Vasoactive Intestinal Peptide–Secreting Pancreatic Neuroendocrine Tumor

VIP is a small peptide normally found in the brain, G cells of the antrum, adrenal medulla, gut mucosa, pancreatic neurons, and D2 cells of the pancreas. First described by Verner and Morrison in 1958, VIP-secreting PNET (VIPomas) usually arise from pancreatic islet D2 cells and release high levels of VIP. This syndrome is also known as watery diarrhea, hypokalemia, achlorhydria (WDHA) syndrome or pancreatic cholera. Overall, these tumors are rare, with an incidence of 1 per 10 million population.

More than two thirds are malignant (Table 39.1), and at the time of presentation, over 70% of patients have metastatic disease. Ninety percent of lesions are found in the pancreas, and 10% have been described in the colon, bronchus, liver, adrenal gland, and sympathetic ganglia. Most patients are diagnosed with VIPomas at middle age, but approximately 10% of patients are diagnosed before the age of 10. Elevated VIP levels in these young patients are most commonly caused by ganglioneuromas, ganglioblastomas, or neuroblastomas, instead of pancreatic tumors.

Tumors are generally solitary, larger than 3 cm at diagnosis, and easily identified on cross-sectional imaging. VIPomas are found in the pancreatic body and tail in 75% of patients. Ninety-five percent are sporadic, and 5% are associated with MEN1.[43]

Diagnosis and treatment. VIP acts directly on intestinal epithelial cells to activate adenylate cyclase, thus increasing cyclic adenosine monophosphate levels within colonocytes, which stimulates the hypersecretion of fluid into the lumen, resulting in watery diarrhea. Profuse, watery, iso-osmotic secretory diarrhea is the most common presenting symptom and may exceed a volume of 3 to 5 L/day. The diagnosis of VIPoma is unlikely if the stool volume is less than 700 mL/day. The diarrhea is further exacerbated because cyclic adenosine monophosphate inhibits sodium reabsorption and stimulates chloride secretion, causing increased fluid and electrolyte shifts into the intestinal lumen. The diarrhea persists despite fasting, which qualifies it as a secretory diarrhea and, despite nasogastric aspiration, which differentiates it from the diarrhea seen with acid hypersecretion in ZES. Conditions to be considered in the differential diagnosis are laxative abuse, bacterial and parasitic diarrhea, carcinoid syndrome, which is associated with an elevated level of 5-hydroxyindoleacetic acid in the urine, and gastrinoma. The diagnosis is confirmed by VIP levels. Normal VIP levels are lower than 200 pg/mL; VIPoma patients have levels ranging from 225 to 2000 pg/mL. Levels of VIP should be measured after an overnight fast.

Weight loss, crampy abdominal pain, dehydration, electrolyte abnormalities, and metabolic acidosis (from fluid and bicarbonate loss) are common with VIPomas. Hypokalemia may be profound because patients can lose more than 400 mEq of potassium/day, which may lead to disturbances of cardiac rhythm and even sudden death in extreme cases. Almost 75% of patients have hypochlorhydria or achlorhydria, and decreased levels of magnesium and phosphorus are often present. The profound electrolyte abnormalities and dehydration need to be corrected prior to definitive surgical management.

The treatment of VIPomas begins with aggressive preoperative hydration and correction of electrolyte abnormalities and acid-base disturbances. Somatostatin analogues are commonly used preoperatively to reduce diarrhea volume and facilitate fluid and electrolyte replacement. If diarrhea persists despite somatostatin analogue therapy, addition of a glucocorticoid may be helpful. Given the high rate of malignant disease, formal anatomic resection (not enucleation) with negative margins and including lymphadenectomy is warranted in the setting of resectable disease. There is no evidence to support debulking in the setting of metastatic disease. Patients with VIPomas can expect a 5-year survival of approximately 68% after resection with the presence of metastatic disease representing a poor predictive factor.[43]

Glucagon-Secreting Pancreatic Neuroendocrine Tumor (Glucagonoma)

Glucagonomas are rare, with an estimated incidence of 1 per 20 million population.[44] They are two- to threefold more common in women. Compared with other pancreatic endocrine tumors, they tend to be larger, averaging 5 to 10 cm in size at the time of diagnosis. These tumors almost always arise in the pancreas, with 65% to 75% located in the body or tail, corresponding to the normal distribution of alpha cells in the pancreas. Glucagonomas are malignant in 50%–80% of cases; 80% of patients with malignant glucagonomas have liver metastases at the time of diagnosis. Most glucagonomas are sporadic; however, 5% to 17% are associated with MEN1.[44]

The glucagonoma syndrome is a rare syndrome, with a classic presentation of the "4Ds": diabetes, dermatitis, deep vein thrombosis, and depression. It is also characterized by a severe catabolic state with weight loss, depletion of fat and protein stores, and associated vitamin deficiencies. The characteristic skin lesion, a necrolytic migrating erythema (Fig. 39.10), is noted in approximately two thirds of patients and often appears before other symptoms of the syndrome. The cause is believed to be severe amino acid deficiency, although trace element deficiency and general malnutrition probably contribute. Parenteral administration of amino acids was found to result in the disappearance of the skin lesions. Diabetes develops in 76% to 94% of patients with glucagonoma at some point during their illness but is usually mild. The diagnosis of glucagonoma is established by measuring glucagon levels; normal fasting glucagon levels are less than 100 pg/mL. A fasting glucagon level higher than 1000 pg/mL is considered diagnostic.

Given their size and malignant behavior, glucagonomas are easily localized. Treatment begins with medical therapy to improve the nutritional status with supplemental enteral nutrition in excess of basic caloric needs. Octreotide is often required in conjunction with enteral nutrition to reverse the catabolic state. Intravenous infusions of amino acids may be required to reverse symptoms and improve dermatitis. Prophylaxis against thromboembolism should be instituted early during hospitalization to prevent perioperative deep vein thrombosis and pulmonary embolism, which occur commonly and are significant causes of morbidity and mortality in these patients. Like other PNETs, complete anatomic resection is indicated for resectable disease. Following resection, 5-year survival for patients with glucagonoma is almost 85% if no metastases are present. Five-year survival is approximately 60% in patients with metastatic disease.

Somatostatin-Secreting PNET (Somatostatin)

Somatostatinomas are exceedingly rare, with fewer than 100 cases reported in the literature. First described in 1977, the full syndrome of symptoms includes steatorrhea, diabetes mellitus, hypochlorhydria, and gallstones. Inhibition of pancreatic enzyme and hormone secretion by unregulated hypersecretion of somatostatin causes steatorrhea, diabetes, malabsorption, and cholelithiasis caused by reduced gallbladder emptying.[45] Because the symptoms are nonspecific, the diagnosis of somatostatinoma is rarely made preoperatively. In a patient with diabetes, gallstones, and steatorrhea, with or without the finding of a pancreatic or duodenal mass on radiographic studies, a fasting plasma somatostatin level should be measured. A concentration exceeding 160 pg/mL is suggestive of the diagnosis.

Somatostatinomas are usually solitary, and 85% are larger than 2 cm. More than 60% are found in the pancreas, usually the head, with the remainder in the duodenum or elsewhere in the small intestine. Patients are typically 50 to 60 years old at the time of diagnosis. Ninety percent are malignant, with metastases to the liver or lymph nodes commonly noted at the time of diagnosis. Somatostatinomas are rarely associated with MEN1 but are associated with von Recklinghausen's disease and pheochromocytomas. Given their rare nature, outcomes data are lacking, but 5-year survival is reported to be 30% to 60% for those with metastatic disease after resection.

Other Functional Pancreatic Endocrine Tumors

Pancreatic endocrine tumors that produce other hormones have been described but are also extremely rare. There have been case reports of pancreatic endocrine tumors that secrete GRF, parathyroid hormone–related peptide, PP, ACTH, calcitonin, enteroglucagon, CCK, gastric inhibitory peptide, luteinizing hormone, neurotensin, or ghrelin. GRFomas are invariably associated with MEN1 and only 30% arise in the pancreas. Patients with ACTH-secreting tumors have Cushing syndrome and usually have other endocrine syndromes, most commonly ZES. Usually malignant, neurotensinomas cause hypokalemia, weight loss, hypotension, cyanosis, flushing, and diabetes. PPomas are associated with high circulating levels of PP, but no associated clinical syndrome. Unless associated with MEN1, they are large and solitary. In addition, elevated PP levels are often seen in other endocrine tumor syndromes. PP, neurotensin, and calcitonin-secreting tumors are sometimes classified as nonfunctional because the hormone

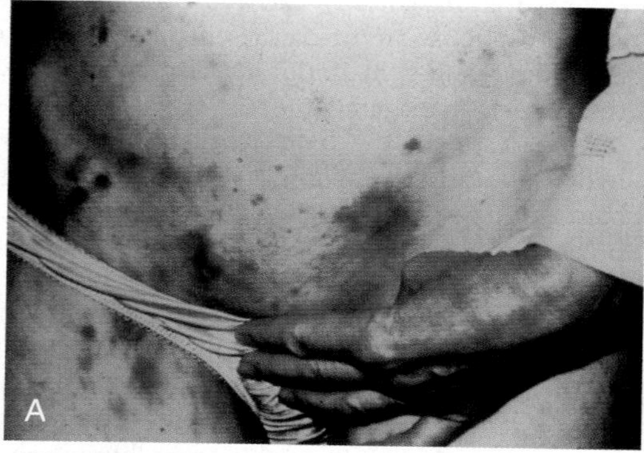

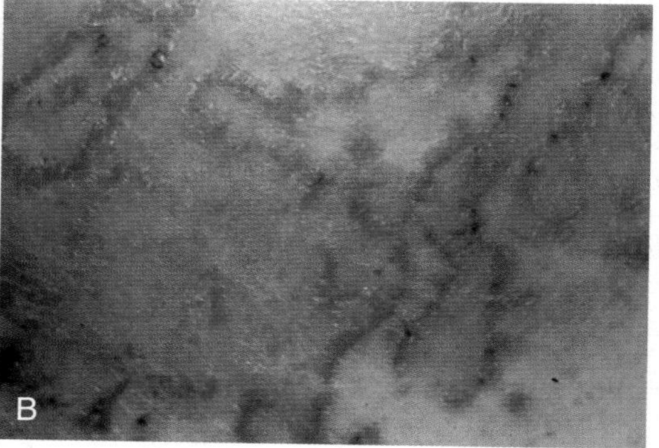

FIG. 39.10 The characteristic necrolytic migrating erythematous dermatitis of the glucagonoma syndrome. (A) Confluent patches with superficial necrosis. (B) Close-up showing serpiginous margins.

products have little biologic consequence and rarely cause symptoms.

Multiple Endocrine Neoplasia Type 1–Associated Pancreatic Neuroendocrine Tumor

Pancreatic endocrine tumors occur in 30% to 80% of patients with MEN1 and are the most common cause of tumor-related death in these patients. Patients with MEN1-associated pancreatic endocrine tumors tend to be younger, more likely to have malignant disease, and more likely to have multicentric disease than patients with sporadic tumors. Approximately 50% of patients with MEN1-associated NETs will present with metastatic disease.[22] The most common pancreatic endocrine syndrome seen in MEN1 patients is gastrinoma (54%), followed by insulinoma (21%), glucagonoma (3%), and VIPoma (1%). PPomas, which are not associated with a functional syndrome, occur most commonly in more than 80% of MEN1 cases.

Management of patients with MEN1 and pancreatic endocrine tumors requires recognition and staged treatment of associated tumors. Patients suspected of having MEN1 should undergo biochemical screening for gastrin, insulin and proinsulin, PP, glucagon, and chromogranin A (a tumor marker elaborated by most pancreatic endocrine tumors). All patients with suspected MEN1 should have a screening calcium level and, if elevated, a parathyroid hormone level. In the setting of hyperparathyroidism, sestamibi parathyroid scintigraphy should be performed to identify a parathyroid adenoma or hyperplasia (Fig. 39.11). Hyperparathyroidism, if present, should be treated first because correction of hyperkalemia will improve the outcome of treatment for the pancreatic endocrine tumor.

It is especially important to consider the diagnosis of MEN1 in patients with ZES because 20% of patients with ZES have MEN-associated disease. The average age at onset is usually 5 to 10 years earlier with MEN-associated gastrinomas. Gastrinomas in MEN1 patients are more likely to occur in the duodenum and are more likely to be multiple, complicating their management (Fig. 39.9B and C). Of MEN1 patients, 60% to 80% have duodenal gastrinomas, which are metastatic to the lymph nodes in 85% at presentation (Fig. 39.9B). They tend not to metastasize to the liver, whereas sporadic tumors larger than 3 cm tend to do so.

In patients with MEN1, careful surveillance is indicated with annual esophagogastroduodenoscopy and removal of larger duodenal lesions; surgical resection is indicated for lesions that appear malignant, as indicated by rapid growth or new appearance.

NONINSULINOMA PANCREATOGENOUS HYPOGLYCEMIA SYNDROME

Insulinoma is the most common cause of hyperinsulinemic hypoglycemia. However, NIPHS, or nesidioblastosis, can cause similar symptoms. NIPHS is characterized by excessive pancreatic B cell function, with associated pathologic changes including pancreatic islet hyperplasia and dysplasia, with histologic identification of B cells budding from and in apposition to pancreatic ductal structures. Nesidioblastosis is usually a disease of infancy, but in rare cases has been identified in adults. In the adult patient, it can be difficult to differentiate this NIPHS from insulinoma. However, it is critical to do so, as the surgical treatment is different.

Postprandial hypoglycemia, within 4 hours of a meal, is the hallmark of NIPHS and can help differentiate it from insulinoma, where this does not occur. However, like insulinoma, patients with NIPHS may have a positive 72-hour fast, with episodes of hypoglycemia associated with inappropriate elevation of insulin, C-peptide, and proinsulin levels. Nesidioblastosis is a clinical diagnosis of exclusion and is based on exclusion of insulinoma as described above. The final diagnosis can only be confirmed on pathologic examination of the pancreas and clinical response to treatment. The treatment of NIPHS includes pancreatectomy, most commonly 95% distal pancreatectomy, dietary control, and medical therapy with diazoxide and somatostatin analogues.

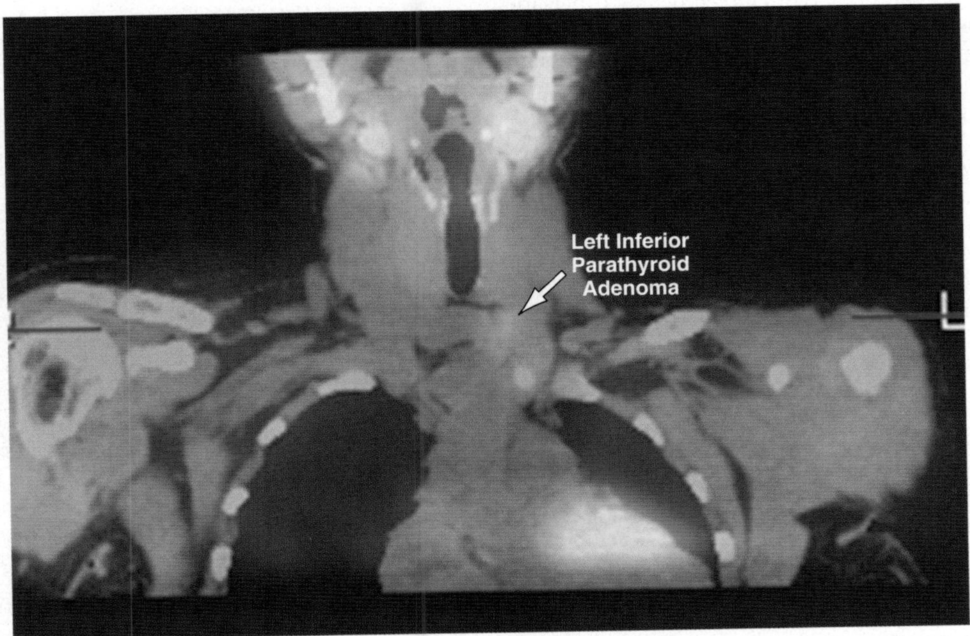

FIG. 39.11 Sestamibi scan in the patient with MEN1-associated gastrinoma in Fig. 39.9. The patient had an elevated calcium and parathyroid hormone level. Sestamibi shows a left inferior parathyroid adenoma.

ENDOCRINE COMPLICATIONS OF SURGICAL THERAPY

Postgastric Bypass Noninsulinoma Pancreatogenous Hypoglycemia Syndrome

NIPHS has been recognized as a complication of bariatric surgery, particularly with Roux-en-Y gastric bypass (RYGB). NIPHS includes a constellation of postprandial neuroglycopenic symptoms similar to insulinoma but in many cases more severe, with symptoms ranging from confusion, disorientation, unconsciousness, syncope, shakiness, tremors, abnormal behavior, anxiety, weakness, blurred vision, and seizures. Although relatively uncommon, given the increase in RYGB procedures and the fact that hypoglycemic events may actually be underestimated, recognition of this complication has clinical relevance. In the setting of RYGB, the actual etiology of nesidioblastosis is theorized to be due to obesity-induced B cell hypertrophy not reversed after RYGB, inappropriate growth factor release, or persistent altered gut hormonal signaling.

First-line treatment of post-RYGB NIPHS is dietary modifications and medication. With the addition of medical management strategies, including continuous glucose monitoring, acarbose, calcium channel blockade, diazoxide, and somatostatin analogues, hypoglycemic episodes are often controlled. Surgical intervention in the form of RYGB reversal or distal pancreatectomy should be considered in refractory cases in the context of the perioperative risk, long-term outcome, potential for weight regain, and the effects on obesity-related comorbidity. When surgical treatment is necessary, pancreatic resection is the most common surgical procedure used. However, the appropriate extent of resection is controversial and symptoms often recur.

Endocrine Insufficiency After Surgical Resection

Destruction or removal of 85% of islet cell mass is necessary before endocrine dysfunction becomes clinically apparent in the form of type 1 (insulin-dependent) diabetes. Approximately 20% to 50% of patients will develop diabetes after pancreatic resection. Pancreatectomy, most commonly performed for pancreatic/periampullary cancer or chronic pancreatitis, is often preceded by pancreatic endocrine insufficiency. It is difficult to predict who will develop pancreatic endocrine insufficiency after pancreatectomy, although studies suggest that hemoglobin A1c levels may be predictive.[46] In patients with existing chronic pancreatitis, diabetes is very common postoperatively. However, with pancreatic cancer surgery, the data are more polarized, with some studies reporting a high incidence of diabetes after resection for cancer while others report improvements in blood glucose control attributed primarily to relief of pancreatic ductal obstruction or other tumor-mediated factors.

Total pancreatectomy unquestionably leads to brittle diabetes. Due to the lack of endogenous glucagon to balance exogenously administered insulin, the resulting diabetes is very difficult to control. With the advent of longer-acting insulin formulations, the management of diabetes following total pancreatectomy has significantly improved.

SURGICAL TREATMENT OF DIABETES

Autologous Islet Cell Transplantation

Autologous islet cell transplantation has a role in patients with severe chronic pancreatitis. Surgical resection of all or part of the pancreas for this disease can significantly improve quality of life by eliminating or reducing intractable pain, allowing the return of a normal appetite with subsequent weight gain, and reducing the number of hospital admissions. Even without pancreatic resection, a significant number of patients with chronic pancreatitis will progress to develop diabetes or impaired glucose tolerance. Because of the loss of insulin, glucagon, and PP, the type of diabetes that develops in patients with chronic pancreatitis is similar to that following pancreatic resection.

Total or partial pancreatectomy with islet autotransplantation is being offered in several centers. This option has the potential to treat the symptoms of chronic pancreatitis definitively via resection of the pancreas while preventing the onset of diabetes in certain patients with the autotransplantation. Other patients remain or become insulin dependent but retain significant insulin and glucagon secretion and the benefits of endogenous C-peptide production, thus making the resulting diabetes easier to control. A diagrammatic representation of the islet isolation process is shown in Fig. 39.12. Patients undergo pancreatectomy; the pancreatic tissue is immediately digested with the use of enzyme solutions containing collagenase and neutral proteases and the islet cells are purified. The islet cells are then returned to the patient via infusion into the portal vein. This can be done at the time of pancreatectomy or percutaneously after resection. The islet cells engraft in the liver and produce insulin and C-peptide. Glucose levels are measured to evaluate the function of the transplanted islets.

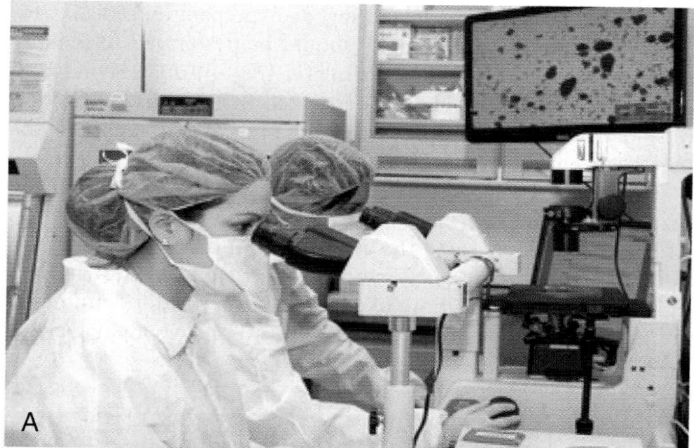

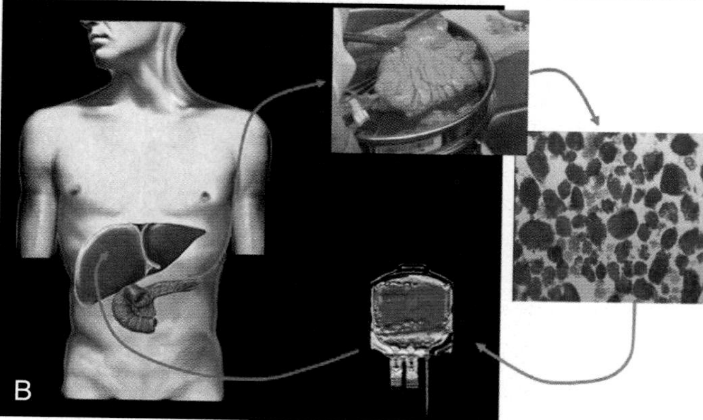

FIG. 39.12 (A) Dedicated islet isolation facility at the University of Texas Medical Branch. The screen in the upper right hand corner shows isolated islets stained red from a patient undergoing total pancreatectomy and islet autotransplantation. (B) This diagram depicts pancreatic islet autotransplantation. The patient undergoes partial or total pancreatectomy. The pancreatic tissue is immediately digested with the use of enzyme solutions containing collagenase and neutral proteases and the islet cells are purified. The islet cells are then returned to the patient via infusion into the portal vein.

Depending on center expertise and experience, variable results following pancreatic islet autotransplantation have been reported. With more than 1500 patients treated since 2000, insulin independence is as high as 40% to 80% initially in some patients, but there is a notable decline in islet function over time, with increased insulin requirements in the 10 years following transplantation. Only about 10% of patients remain insulin independent. Although insulin independence is not always achieved, most patients are C-peptide positive and have diabetes that is more manageable (i.e., less brittle). In addition, most studies demonstrate improvement in pain and other symptoms of chronic pancreatitis.[47–49] Success rates depend on the number of isolated and transplanted islets as well as the cause of the pancreatic disease. Patients who are not diabetic before autotransplantation, those who have not had prior pancreatic operations, and younger patients (especially preadolescents) achieve the best results. The most feared procedure-related complication is thrombosis of the portal vein, occurring in less than 1% of cases.

Pancreatic Transplantation and Islet Allotransplantation

Type 1 diabetes results from autoimmune destruction of pancreatic islets. For a select group of patients with difficult-to-manage type 1 diabetes who do not respond well to conventional approaches or insulin pumps, whole pancreas transplantation remains the gold standard for treatment. From 1966 through 2008, over 40,000 pancreas transplantations have been reported to the International Pancreas Transplant Registry. Recipients experience immediate normal fasting and postprandial glucose levels, and hemoglobin A1c levels return to normal. One-year graft survival rates in the United States have improved to 85% for simultaneous pancreas-kidney transplants, 78% for pancreas after kidney transplants, and 76% for pancreas-only transplants. With the observed decrease in morbidity and mortality, recipients who become insulin independent report a better quality of life, despite the need for immunosuppression. They also experience stabilization or improvements in retinopathy, nephropathy, neuropathy, and microvascular and macrovascular diseases normally associated with poor glucose control.

Compared to pancreatic transplantation, allogeneic islet transplantation is a less invasive, albeit less effective, method of achieving insulin independence. Currently, long-term insulin independence remains elusive for patients undergoing allogeneic islet transplantation. The data show that even with patients who receive multiple infusions, few remain normoglycemic over time. Data from the Collaborative Islet Transplant Registry (CITR) have demonstrated that 70% of patients achieve insulin independence within the first year (including patients with multiple infusions), but by the third year, the percentage of patients who remain insulin independent is closer to 35%.[50] The partial pancreatic endocrine function confers some benefit, with decreased occurrence of severe hypoglycemic events, abatement of hypoglycemic unawareness, persistent C-peptide levels, improvement in glycemic control, and stabilization of diabetic complications. In addition, islet cell transplantation requires two donors per recipient to maintain graft function. Stem cell therapy offers the potential of producing an unlimited source of cells, and a growing number of studies have demonstrated successful in vitro differentiation and expansion of embryonic cells of murine and human origin from pancreatic ducts that express insulin and respond to glucose stimulation.

SELECTED REFERENCES

Bilimoria KY, Talamonti MS, Tomlinson JS, et al. Prognostic score predicting survival after resection of pancreatic neuroendocrine tumors: analysis of 3851 patients. *Ann Surg*. 2008;247:490–500.

This large study utilizes the National Cancer Database to define prognostic factors after resection of pancreatic neuroendocrine tumors. The paper provides survival data for selected subgroups of patients as well as prognostic scoring system that can be applied to individual patients.

Caplin ME, Pavel M, Cwikla JB, et al. Lanreotide in metastatic enteropancreatic neuroendocrine tumors. *N Engl J Med*. 2014;371:224–233.

This multinational study of lanreotide in patients with advanced, well-differentiated or moderately differentiated, nonfunctioning, somatostatin receptor–positive neuroendocrine tumors of grade 1 or 2 (a tumor proliferation index [on staining for the Ki-67 antigen] of <10%) showed that lanreotide was associated with significantly prolonged progression-free survival among patients with metastatic enteropancreatic neuroendocrine tumors.

Jiao Y, Shi C, Edil BH, et al. DAXX/ATRX, MEN1, and mTOR pathway genes are frequently altered in pancreatic neuroendocrine tumors. *Science*. 2011;331:1199–1203.

This high impact original research study utilized high-throughput sequencing technology to characterize the most commonly mutated genes in sporadic pancreatic neuroendocrine tumors The findings helped to validate several gene products and pathways as potential targets for therapy.

Klimstra DS, Modlin IR, Coppola D, et al. The pathologic classification of neuroendocrine tumors: a review of nomenclature, grading, and staging systems. *Pancreas*. 2010;39:707–712.

This review clarifies the pathologic classification of neuroendocrine tumors, including the distinction between grade and differentiation and the prognostic significance of different pathologic factors. Guidance is also included on the minimum data that should be included in neuroendocrine pathology reports.

Krampitz GW, Norton JA. Pancreatic neuroendocrine tumors. *Curr Probl Surg*. 2013;50:509–545.

A comprehensive review by Dr. Jeffrey Norton, a world expert on pancreatic neuroendocrine tumors (PNETs). Particularly helpful are discussions on the diagnosis, localization, and management of functional PNETs with emphasis on differences between sporadic and multiple endocrine neoplasia type 1 (MEN1)-associated PNETs.

Mayo SC, de Jong MC, Bloomston M, et al. Surgery versus intra-arterial therapy for neuroendocrine liver metastasis: a multicenter international analysis. *Ann Surg Oncol*. 2011;18:3657–3665.

The management of neuroendocrine metastases is controversial and difficult to study due to the relative rarity of this disease and insufficient detail in national databases. This collaborative study pooled 753 patients to define prognostic factors after liver-directed therapy for neuroendocrine liver metastases.

Rinke A, Muller HH, Schade-Brittinger C, et al. Placebo-controlled, double-blind, prospective, randomized study on the effect of octreotide LAR in the control of tumor growth in patients with metastatic neuroendocrine midgut tumors: a report from the PROMID Study Group. *J Clin Oncol.* 2009;27:4656–4663.

Prior to this study, somatostatin analogs were known to be effective at controlling symptoms from functional tumors, but this study was the first to demonstrate a survival benefit for this approach, which has now become first-line therapy for unresectable disease.

REFERENCES

1. Lawrence B, Gustafsson BI, Chan A, et al. The epidemiology of gastroenteropancreatic neuroendocrine tumors. *Endocrinol Metab Clin North Am.* 2011;40:1–18, vii.
2. Klimstra DS, Modlin IR, Coppola D, et al. The pathologic classification of neuroendocrine tumors: a review of nomenclature, grading, and staging systems. *Pancreas.* 2010;39:707–712.
3. Martin RC, Kooby DA, Weber SM, et al. Analysis of 6,747 pancreatic neuroendocrine tumors for a proposed staging system. *J Gastrointest Surg.* 2011;15:175–183.
4. Li X, Gou S, Liu Z, et al. Assessment of the American Joint Commission on Cancer 8th Edition Staging System for Patients with Pancreatic Neuroendocrine Tumors: a surveillance, epidemiology, and end results analysis. *Cancer Med.* 2018;7:626–634.
5. Libutti SK, Choyke PL, Alexander HR, et al. Clinical and genetic analysis of patients with pancreatic neuroendocrine tumors associated with von Hippel-Lindau disease. *Surgery.* 2000;128:1022–1027; discussion 1027–1028.
6. Jiao Y, Shi C, Edil BH, et al. DAXX/ATRX, MEN1, and mTOR pathway genes are frequently altered in pancreatic neuroendocrine tumors. *Science.* 2011;331:1199–1203.
7. Missiaglia E, Dalai I, Barbi S, et al. Pancreatic endocrine tumors: expression profiling evidences a role for AKT-mTOR pathway. *J Clin Oncol.* 2010;28:245–255.
8. Zhang J, Francois R, Iyer R, et al. Current understanding of the molecular biology of pancreatic neuroendocrine tumors. *J Natl Cancer Inst.* 2013;105:1005–1017.
9. Jones S, Zhang X, Parsons DW, et al. Core signaling pathways in human pancreatic cancers revealed by global genomic analyses. *Science.* 2008;321:1801–1806.
10. Yachida S, Vakiani E, White CM, et al. Small cell and large cell neuroendocrine carcinomas of the pancreas are genetically similar and distinct from well-differentiated pancreatic neuroendocrine tumors. *Am J Surg Pathol.* 2012;36:173–184.
11. van Essen M, Sundin A, Krenning EP, et al. Neuroendocrine tumours: the role of imaging for diagnosis and therapy. *Nat Rev Endocrinol.* 2014;10:102–114.
12. Sheth S, Hruban RK, Fishman EK. Helical CT of islet cell tumors of the pancreas: typical and atypical manifestations. *AJR Am J Roentgenol.* 2002;179:725–730.
13. Fidler JL, Fletcher JG, Reading CC, et al. Preoperative detection of pancreatic insulinomas on multiphasic helical CT. *AJR Am J Roentgenol.* 2003;181:775–780.
14. Sainz-Esteban A, Olmos R, Gonzalez-Sagrado M, et al. Contribution of 111In-pentetreotide SPECT/CT imaging to conventional somatostatin receptor scintigraphy in the detection of neuroendocrine tumours. *Nucl Med Commun.* 2014.
15. Kolasińska-Ćwikła AD, Konsek SJ, Buscombe JR, et al. The value of somatostatin receptor scintigraphy (SRS) in patients with NETG1/G2 pancreatic neuroendocrine neoplasms (p-NENs) [published online ahead of print 2018]. *Nucl Med Rev Cent East Eur.*
16. Falconi M, Eriksson B, Kaltsas G, et al. ENETS consensus guidelines update for the management of patients with functional pancreatic neuroendocrine tumors and non-functional pancreatic neuroendocrine tumors. *Neuroendocrinology.* 2016;103:153–171.
17. National Comprehensive Cancer Network I. *Neuroendocrine and Adrenal Tumors, Version 2.2018*; 2018. https://www.nccn.org. Accessed December 20, 2018.
18. Cheema A, Weber J, Strosberg JR. Incidental detection of pancreatic neuroendocrine tumors: an analysis of incidence and outcomes. *Ann Surg Oncol.* 2012;19:2932–2936.
19. Lee LC, Grant CS, Salomao DR, et al. Small, nonfunctioning, asymptomatic pancreatic neuroendocrine tumors (PNETs): role for nonoperative management. *Surgery.* 2012;152:965–974.
20. Sadot E, Reidy-Lagunes DL, Tang LH, et al. Observation versus resection for small asymptomatic pancreatic neuroendocrine tumors: a matched case-control study. *Ann Surg Oncol.* 2016;23:1361–1370.
21. Gaujoux S, Partelli S, Maire F, et al. Observational study of natural history of small sporadic nonfunctioning pancreatic neuroendocrine tumors. *J Clin Endocrinol Metab.* 2013;98:4784–4789.
22. Kishi Y, Shimada K, Nara S, et al. Basing treatment strategy for non-functional pancreatic neuroendocrine tumors on tumor size. *Ann Surg Oncol.* 2014;21:2882–2888.
23. Rosenberg AM, Friedmann P, Del Rivero J, et al. Resection versus expectant management of small incidentally discovered nonfunctional pancreatic neuroendocrine tumors. *Surgery.* 2016;159:302–309.
24. Zhang IY, Zhao J, Fernandez-Del Castillo C, et al. Operative versus nonoperative management of nonfunctioning pancreatic neuroendocrine tumors. *J Gastrointest Surg.* 2016;20:277–283.
25. Nigri G, Petrucciani N, Debs T, et al. Treatment options for PNET liver metastases: a systematic review. *World J Surg Oncol.* 2018;16:142.
26. Elias D, Lasser P, Ducreux M, et al. Liver resection (and associated extrahepatic resections) for metastatic well-differentiated endocrine tumors: a 15-year single center prospective study. *Surgery.* 2003;133(4):375–382.
27. Morgan RE, Pommier SJ, Pommier RF. Expanded criteria for debulking of liver metastasis also apply to pancreatic neuroendocrine tumors. *Surgery.* 2018;163(1):218–225.
28. Tao L, Xiu D, Sadula A, et al. Surgical resection of primary tumor improves survival of pancreatic neuroendocrine tumor with liver metastases. *Oncotarget.* 2017;8(45):79785–79792.
29. Jia Z, Paz-Fumagalli R, Frey G, et al. Single-institution experience of radioembolization with yttrium-90 microspheres

for unresectable metastatic neuroendocrine liver tumors. *J Gastroenterol Hepatol.* 2017;32(9):1617–1623.
30. Appetecchia M, Baldelli R. Somatostatin analogues in the treatment of gastroenteropancreatic neuroendocrine tumours, current aspects and new perspectives. *J Exp Clin Cancer Res.* 2010;29:19.
31. Rinke A, Muller HH, Schade-Brittinger C, et al. Placebo-controlled, double-blind, prospective, randomized study on the effect of octreotide LAR in the control of tumor growth in patients with metastatic neuroendocrine midgut tumors: a report from the PROMID Study Group. *J Clin Oncol.* 2009;27(28):4656–4663.
32. Caplin ME, Pavel M, Cwikla JB, et al. Lanreotide in metastatic enteropancreatic neuroendocrine tumors. *N Engl J Med.* 2014;371(3):224–233.
33. Kouvaraki MA, Ajani JA, Hoff P, et al. Fluorouracil, doxorubicin, and streptozocin in the treatment of patients with locally advanced and metastatic pancreatic endocrine carcinomas. *J Clin Oncol.* 2004;22(23):4762–4771.
34. Strosberg JR, Fine RL, Choi J, et al. First-line chemotherapy with capecitabine and temozolomide in patients with metastatic pancreatic endocrine carcinomas. *Cancer.* 2011;117(2):268–275.
35. Yamaguchi T, Machida N, Morizane C, et al. Multicenter retrospective analysis of systemic chemotherapy for advanced neuroendocrine carcinoma of the digestive system. *Cancer Sci.* 2014;105:1176–1181.
36. Yao JC, Shah MH, Ito T, et al. Everolimus for advanced pancreatic neuroendocrine tumors. *N Engl J Med.* 2011;364:514–523.
37. Raymond E, Dahan L, Raoul JL, et al. Sunitinib malate for the treatment of pancreatic neuroendocrine tumors. *N Engl J Med.* 2011;364:501–513.
38. Filice A, Fraternali A, Frasoldati A, et al. Radiolabeled somatostatin analogues therapy in advanced neuroendocrine tumors: a single centre experience. *J Oncol.* 2012;2012:320198.
39. Mazzaferro V, Pulvirenti A, Coppa J. Neuroendocrine tumors metastatic to the liver: how to select patients for liver transplantation? *J Hepatol.* 2007;47:460–466.
40. Le Treut YP, Gregoire E, Klempnauer J, et al. Liver transplantation for neuroendocrine tumors in Europe-results and trends in patient selection: a 213-case European liver transplant registry study. *Ann Surg.* 2013;257:807–815.
41. Gibril F, Schumann M, Pace A, et al. Multiple endocrine neoplasia type 1 and Zollinger-Ellison syndrome: a prospective study of 107 cases and comparison with 1009 cases from the literature. *Medicine (Baltimore).* 2004;83:43–83.
42. Krampitz GW, Norton JA. Pancreatic neuroendocrine tumors. *Curr Probl Surg.* 2013;50:509–545.
43. Soga J, Yakuwa Y. Vipoma/diarrheogenic syndrome: a statistical evaluation of 241 reported cases. *J Exp Clin Cancer Res.* 1998;17:389–400.
44. Kindmark H, Sundin A, Granberg D, et al. Endocrine pancreatic tumors with glucagon hypersecretion: a retrospective study of 23 cases during 20 years. *Med Oncol.* 2007; 24:330–337.
45. Krejs GJ, Orci L, Conlon JM, et al. Somatostatinoma syndrome. Biochemical, morphologic and clinical features. *N Engl J Med.* 1979;301:285–292.
46. Hamilton L, Jeyarajah DR. Hemoglobin A1c can be helpful in predicting progression to diabetes after Whipple procedure. *HPB (Oxford).* 2007;9:26–28.
47. Argo JL, Contreras JL, Wesley MM, et al. Pancreatic resection with islet cell autotransplant for the treatment of severe chronic pancreatitis. *Am Surg.* 2008;74(6):530–536; discussion 536–537.
48. Dixon J, DeLegge M, Morgan KA, et al. Impact of total pancreatectomy with islet cell transplant on chronic pancreatitis management at a disease-based center. *Am Surg.* 2008;74(8):735–738.
49. Morgan K, Owczarski SM, Borckardt J, et al. Pain control and quality of life after pancreatectomy with islet autotransplantation for chronic pancreatitis. *J Gastrointest Surg.* 2012;16(4):129–133; discussion 133–124.
50. Alejandro R, Barton FB, Hering BJ, et al. 2008 Update from the collaborative Islet Transplant Registry. *Transplantation.* 2008;86:1783–1788.

40 CHAPTER

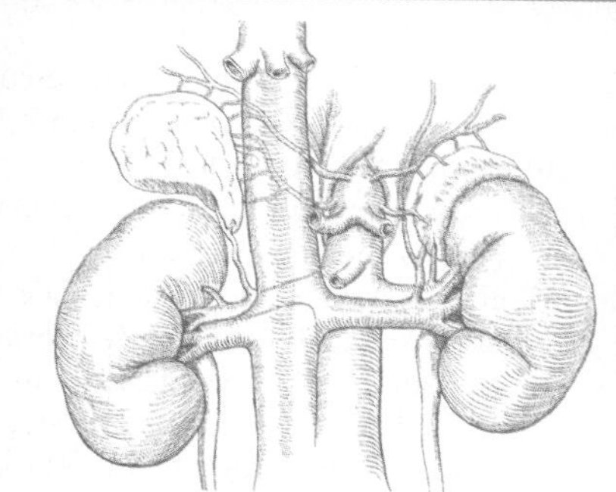

The Adrenal Glands

Michael W. Yeh, Masha Livhits, Quan-Yang Duh

OUTLINE

HISTORY

The adrenal glands were first described by the Italian anatomist Bartolomeo Eustachi in 1563. The German comparative anatomist Albert von Kölliker (1817–1905), who noted the presence of the adrenals in a number of vertebrate species, is credited with first identifying two distinct portions of the adrenal gland, the cortex and the medulla. Although Thomas Addison described the clinical features of primary adrenal failure in 1855, it was not until nearly a century later that the adrenal hormones were fully isolated and characterized. Adrenaline (or epinephrine) was first isolated from adrenal extract at the turn of the century. Steroid hormones were crystallized from cortical extract ("cortin") by Swiss and American investigators in the 1930s, but their highly similar chemical structures made isolation of the individual compounds challenging. Edward Kendall, Tadeus Reichstein, and Philip Hench jointly received the 1950 Nobel Prize in Physiology or Medicine for their groundbreaking work on the adrenocortical hormones. The Austrian-born endocrinologist Hans Selye first described the stress response in mammals in 1936 and made major contributions to the understanding of the hypothalamic-pituitary-adrenal (HPA) axis. Roger Guillemin, Andrew Schally, and Rosalyn Yalow were awarded the Nobel Prize in 1977 for characterizing the peptide hormones of the brain that underlie the HPA axis as we now understand it.[1,2]

ANATOMY AND EMBRYOLOGY

General and Developmental Aspects

The adrenal glands are paired, mustard-colored structures that are positioned superior and slightly medial to the kidneys in the retroperitoneal space (Fig. 40.1). They are flattened and roughly pyramidal (right) or crescent shaped (left), weighing approximately 4 g each. The adrenals are among the most highly perfused organs in the body, receiving 2000 mL/kg/min of blood, after only the kidney and thyroid. In most respects, the cortex and medulla can be considered two completely distinct organs that happen to colocalize during development. The two portions have disparate embryologic origins. The primordial cortex arises from the coelomic mesodermal tissue near the cephalic end of the mesonephros during the fourth to fifth week of gestation. Biosynthetic activity can be detected as early as the seventh week. Cortical cell mass dominates the fetal adrenal at 4 months of development, and steroidogenesis is maximum during the third trimester. The adrenal medulla arises from the ectodermal tissues of the embryonic neural crest. It develops in parallel with the sympathetic nervous system, beginning in the fifth to sixth week of gestation. From their original position adjacent to the neural tube, neural crest cells migrate ventrally to assume a para-aortic position near the developing adrenal cortex. There, they differentiate into chromaffin cells that make up the adrenal medulla.

This course of embryologic development yields certain surgically relevant sequelae. Both cortical and medullary tissue can be found at extra-adrenal sites (Fig. 40.2). The range of potential sites is wider for chromaffin tissue than for cortical tissue. Pheochromocytomas may arise in extra-adrenal sites more commonly than previously believed. When they are extra-adrenal, pheochromocytomas are also termed "paragangliomas."

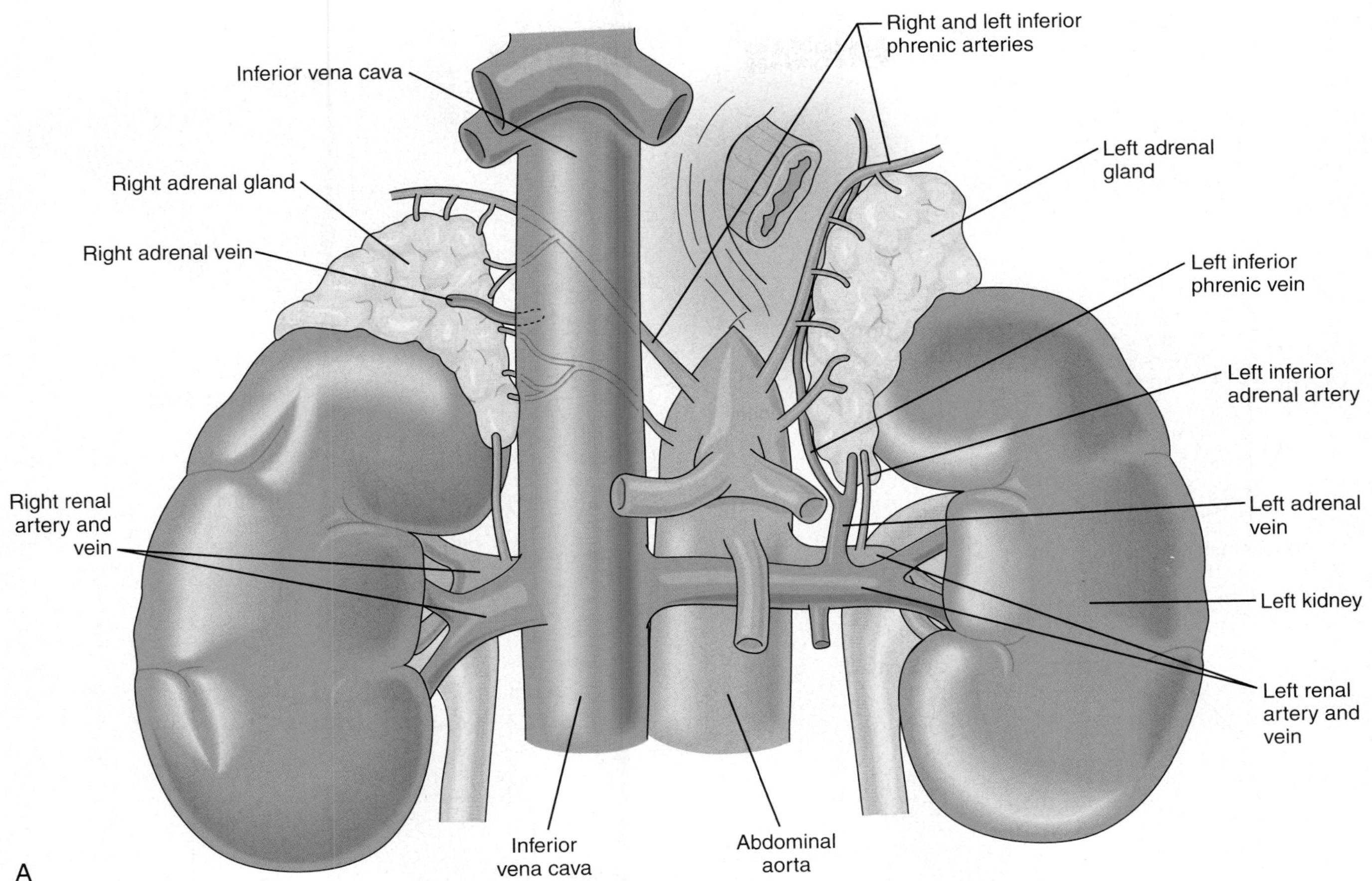

FIG. 40.1 Anatomy of the adrenal glands. (A) Left and right adrenal glands in situ.

(Continued)

Relationships

The right adrenal gland abuts the posterolateral surface of the retrohepatic vena cava. The right adrenal fossa is bounded by the right kidney inferolaterally, diaphragm posteriorly, and bare area of the liver anterosuperiorly. The left adrenal gland lies between the left kidney and aorta, with its inferior limb extending farther caudad toward the renal hilum than the right adrenal. The other relationships of the left adrenal gland are the diaphragm posteriorly and the tail of the pancreas and splenic hilum anteriorly. Each adrenal gland is enveloped by its proper capsule, in addition to sharing Gerota fascia with the kidneys. The adrenal capsules are immediately associated with the perirenal fat.

Vasculature

Knowledge of the macroscopic vascular anatomy of the adrenal glands is essential to proper surgical management. It is important to conceptualize that although the arterial supply is *diffuse*, the venous drainage of each gland is usually *solitary*. The arterial supply arises from three distinct vessels—superior adrenal arteries from the inferior phrenic arteries, small middle adrenal arteries from the juxtaceliac aorta, and inferior adrenal arteries from the renal arteries. Of these, the inferior is the most prominent and is commonly a single identifiable vessel. The left adrenal vein is approximately 2 cm long and drains into the left renal vein after joining the inferior phrenic vein.[3] The right adrenal vein is typically as short as it is wide (0.5 cm) and drains directly into the vena cava. This configuration presents a surgical challenge that is discussed in more detail later in this chapter. In up to 20% of individuals, the right adrenal vein may drain into an accessory right hepatic vein or into the vena cava, at or near the confluence of such a vein. Vigilance about this variant and others (Fig. 40.3) may reduce the likelihood of intraoperative venous hemorrhage during right adrenalectomy.

NORMAL HISTOPATHOLOGY

The cortex is approximately 2 mm thick and composes more than 80% of the mass of the gland. It is made up of three layers (Fig. 40.4). The outer *zona glomerulosa* is a thin layer of relatively small cells with moderately eosinophilic, lipid-poor cytoplasm. It has an undulating inner border and normally does not form a complete circumferential layer. Most of the adrenal cortex is formed by the *zona fasciculata*, a middle layer composed of long radial columns of large, clear, lipid-laden cells. The inner *zona reticularis* is made up of small nests of compact, eosinophilic cells. The adrenal medulla consists of clusters and short cords of chromaffin cells, which are large, polyhedral, and packed with basophilic secretory granules. Catecholamines within these granules yield a brown reaction when treated with chromium salts, giving the cells their name. In contrast to the cortex, the adrenal medulla is richly endowed with autonomic nerve fibers and ganglion cells. Sympathetic fibers synapse directly with the chromaffin cells, constituting an interface between the nervous and endocrine systems.

The microvasculature of the adrenal gland functionally unifies the cortex and medulla. The adrenal arteries arborize extensively before entering the capsule to form a subcapsular plexus. Blood

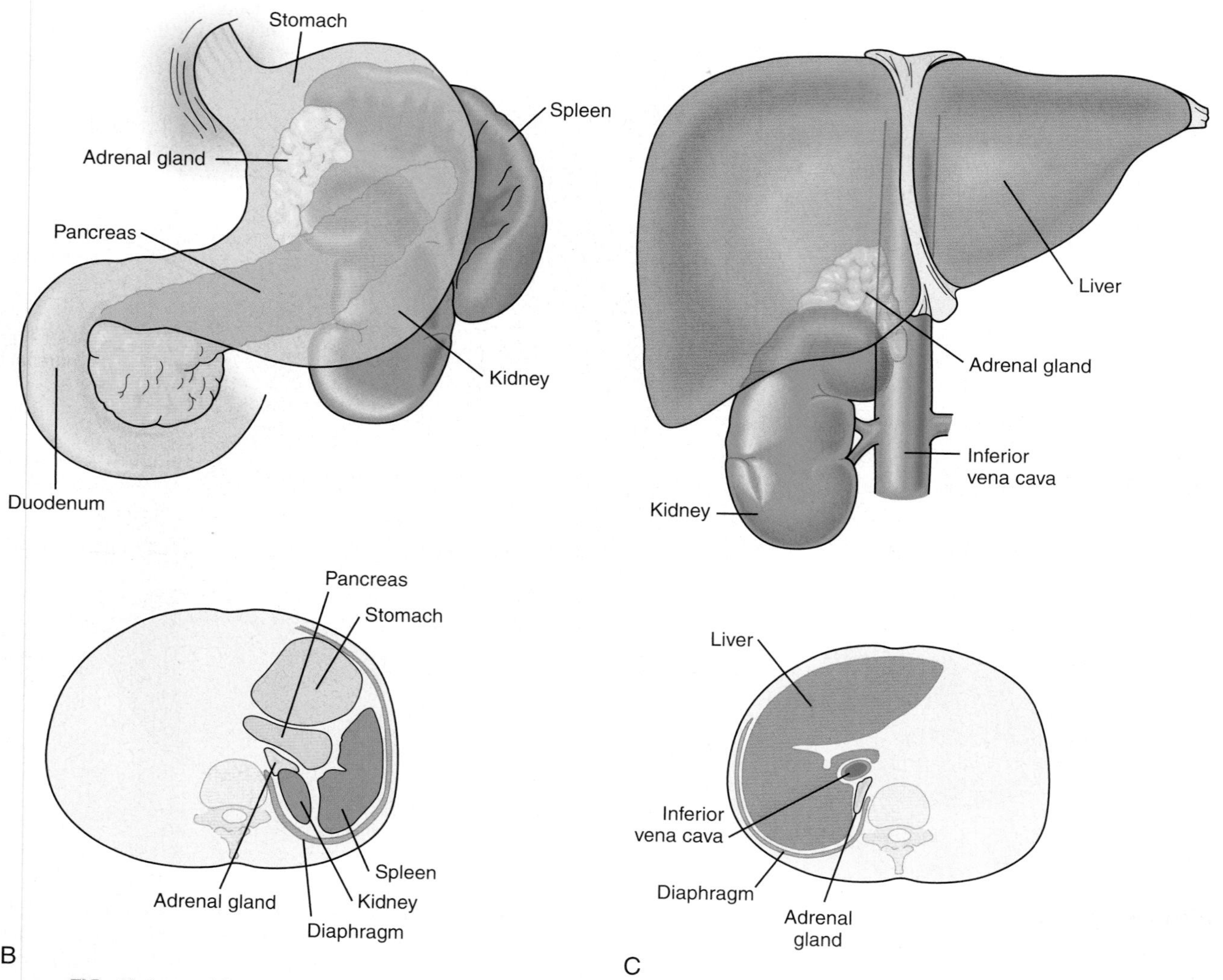

FIG. 40.1, cont'd (B) Relationships of the left adrenal gland. (C) Relationships of the right adrenal gland.

flows centripetally through capillaries in the zona glomerulosa and zona fasciculata before forming a deep plexus within the zona reticularis. From there, steroid-enriched postcapillary blood enters the medulla, where cortisol drives the expression of phenylethanolamine *N*-methyltransferase. Phenylethanolamine *N*-methyltransferase is responsible for the conversion of norepinephrine to epinephrine. This microvascular arrangement is essentially a portal system between the cortex and medulla.

BIOCHEMISTRY AND PHYSIOLOGY

Adrenal Steroid Biosynthesis

Adrenal steroid biosynthesis begins with the transport of cholesterol to the inner mitochondrial membrane by the steroidogenic acute regulatory protein (Fig. 40.5). Cholesterol then undergoes a series of oxidative reactions catalyzed predominantly by membrane-associated enzymes belonging to the cytochrome P450 (CYP) family. Cleavage of the cholesterol side chain yields the hormonally inactive compound pregnenolone, the immediate precursor to the adrenal steroid hormones. Serial oxidation by CYP17 converts pregnenolone and progesterone into the major adrenal sex steroids dehydroepiandrosterone (DHEA) and androstenedione. Additional enzymatic steps confined to the gonads generate testosterone, estrone, and estradiol from androstenedione. Oxidation of 17-hydroxypregnenolone by 3β-hydroxysteroid dehydrogenase followed by action of CYP21A2 and CYP11B1 yields cortisol, the active glucocorticoid hormone in humans. Aldosterone is generated by the oxidation of corticosterone by CYP11B2 within the zona glomerulosa. CYP17 expression is confined to the zona fasciculata and zona reticularis, accounting for the synthesis of glucocorticoids and adrenal sex steroids in these regions.

Steroid Hormone Physiology and Metabolism

Steroid hormones belong to a general class of low-molecular-weight, lipophilic signaling molecules that act by entering cells and binding to intracellular receptors. This group of hormones also includes thyroid hormone, retinoids, and vitamin D. Hormone binding results in alterations in gene expression that show a delayed and prolonged response compared with changes induced by peptide hormones, which act by binding to cell surface receptors. In the circulation, endogenous steroid hormones are largely bound to highly specific binding globulins. Serum levels of these proteins—and hence free hormone levels—can be altered by certain physiologic and disease states, such as pregnancy,

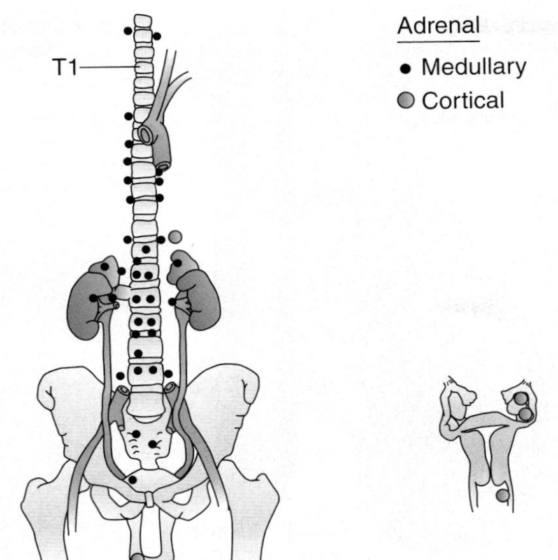

FIG. 40.2 Sites of extra-adrenal cortical and medullary tissue.

nephrotic syndrome, and cirrhosis. Metabolism of both endogenous and pharmacologic steroids generally proceeds through hydroxylation, sulfonation, or conjugation to glucuronic acid in the liver, followed by urinary excretion. The regulation and physiologic actions of individual steroid hormones are discussed here.

Glucocorticoids

The release of corticotropin-releasing factor into the hypothalamic-pituitary portal system by hypothalamic neurons results in adrenocorticotropic hormone (ACTH) secretion by the anterior pituitary. ACTH binds to a G protein–coupled receptor on the adrenocortical cell surface and stimulates glucocorticoid secretion. Steroidogenesis is acutely upregulated by increased steroidogenic acute regulatory protein-mediated cholesterol transport and pregnenolone synthesis by CYP11A1. ACTH is released in a pulsatile fashion that normally displays a circadian rhythm. The highest levels of ACTH and, thus, of cortisol are generally detected on waking, with levels gradually declining throughout the day to reach a nadir in the early evening. This pattern must be considered in evaluating patients for glucocorticoid deficiency or excess.

Glucocorticoid hormones have broad-ranging effects on almost all organ systems in the body. As a rule, they generate a catabolic state that characterizes the body's response to stress. The hormones are so named because they cause alterations in carbohydrate, protein, and lipid metabolism that have the net effect of increasing blood glucose concentrations. Hepatic glucose output is elevated by the upregulation of gluconeogenesis, and net glycogen deposition occurs. Glucose uptake by peripheral tissues is directly inhibited. Glucocorticoids stimulate lipolysis with release of free fatty acids into the circulation, and a general state of insulin resistance is induced, resulting in protein catabolism. Fatty acids and amino acids serve as energy sources and substrates for gluconeogenesis. In the cardiovascular system, glucocorticoids exert a permissive and enhancing effect on catecholamine signaling by sensitizing arterial smooth muscle cells to β-adrenergic stimulation and increasing catecholamine concentrations in neuromuscular junctions. Cardiac contractility and peripheral vascular tone are thus maintained, explaining why the hemodynamic collapse that accompanies acute adrenal insufficiency can be remedied by glucocorticoid administration.

Glucocorticoids are potent antiinflammatory and immunosuppressive agents. Acutely, glucocorticoids reduce circulating lymphocyte and eosinophil counts while increasing neutrophil counts. Lymphocyte apoptosis is promoted, cytokine and immunoglobulin production is decreased, and histamine release is suppressed. Glucocorticoids also reduce prostaglandin synthesis through inhibition of phospholipase A2.

Mineralocorticoids

Aldosterone release from the zona glomerulosa is principally regulated by angiotensin II and the blood potassium level. The renin-angiotensin-aldosterone axis is responsive to sodium delivery to the distal convoluted tubule of the kidney. Low sodium delivery, which occurs in states such as hypovolemia, shock, renal artery vasoconstriction, and hyponatremia, stimulates the release of renin from the juxtaglomerular apparatus. The prohormone angiotensinogen is synthesized by the liver and is cleaved to inactive angiotensin I by renin. Further cleavage of angiotensin I by angiotensin-converting enzyme in the lungs and elsewhere yields angiotensin II, a potent vasoconstrictor and stimulator of aldosterone release. Hypokalemia reduces aldosterone release by suppressing renin secretion and also by acting directly at the zona glomerulosa. Hyperkalemia has the opposite effect.

Aldosterone regulates circulating fluid volume and electrolyte balance by promoting sodium and chloride retention by the distal tubule. Potassium and hydrogen ions are secreted into the urine. Acutely, expansion of the extracellular fluid volume and a rise in blood pressure are observed after aldosterone infusion. Negative feedback occurs primarily through an increase in sodium delivery to the distal tubule, suppressing renin release.

Adrenal Sex Steroids

Secretion of the adrenal androgens androstenedione, DHEA, and DHEA-S (the sulfonated derivative of DHEA, synthesized in the adrenal and liver) is regulated by ACTH and other incompletely understood mechanisms. Of the three, androstenedione is produced in the smallest quantities. The physiologic effects of adrenal sex steroids are generally weak in comparison to the gonadal sex steroids, particularly in males. In females, peripheral conversion of DHEA and DHEA-S to more potent androgens, including androstenedione, testosterone, and dihydrotestosterone, supports normal pubic and axillary hair growth and may play a role in maintaining libido and a sense of well-being.

Catecholamine Biosynthesis and Physiology

Synthesis of catecholamines in the adrenal medulla begins with the hydroxylation of tyrosine, a rate-limiting step that generates dihydroxyphenylalanine (L-dopa) in the cytosol (Fig. 40.6). Decarboxylation of L-dopa generates dopamine, which is then β-hydroxylated to form norepinephrine. Epinephrine is created by the action of phenylethanolamine *N*-methyltransferase, which, unlike the other enzymes involved in catecholamine synthesis, is localized to the chromaffin cells of the adrenal medulla and organ of Zuckerkandl. Sympathetic stimulation of the adrenal medulla results in the release of stored catecholamines into the circulation. Basal levels of adrenal catecholamine secretion are normally low, although large (up to fifty fold) increases in levels may be observed in response to major physiologic or psychological stressors. Target tissue responses are mediated by α- and β-adrenergic receptors. α-Adrenergic receptors display greater affinity for norepinephrine compared with epinephrine, and the opposite is true for β-adrenergic receptors. Stimulation of β_1-adrenergic receptors in

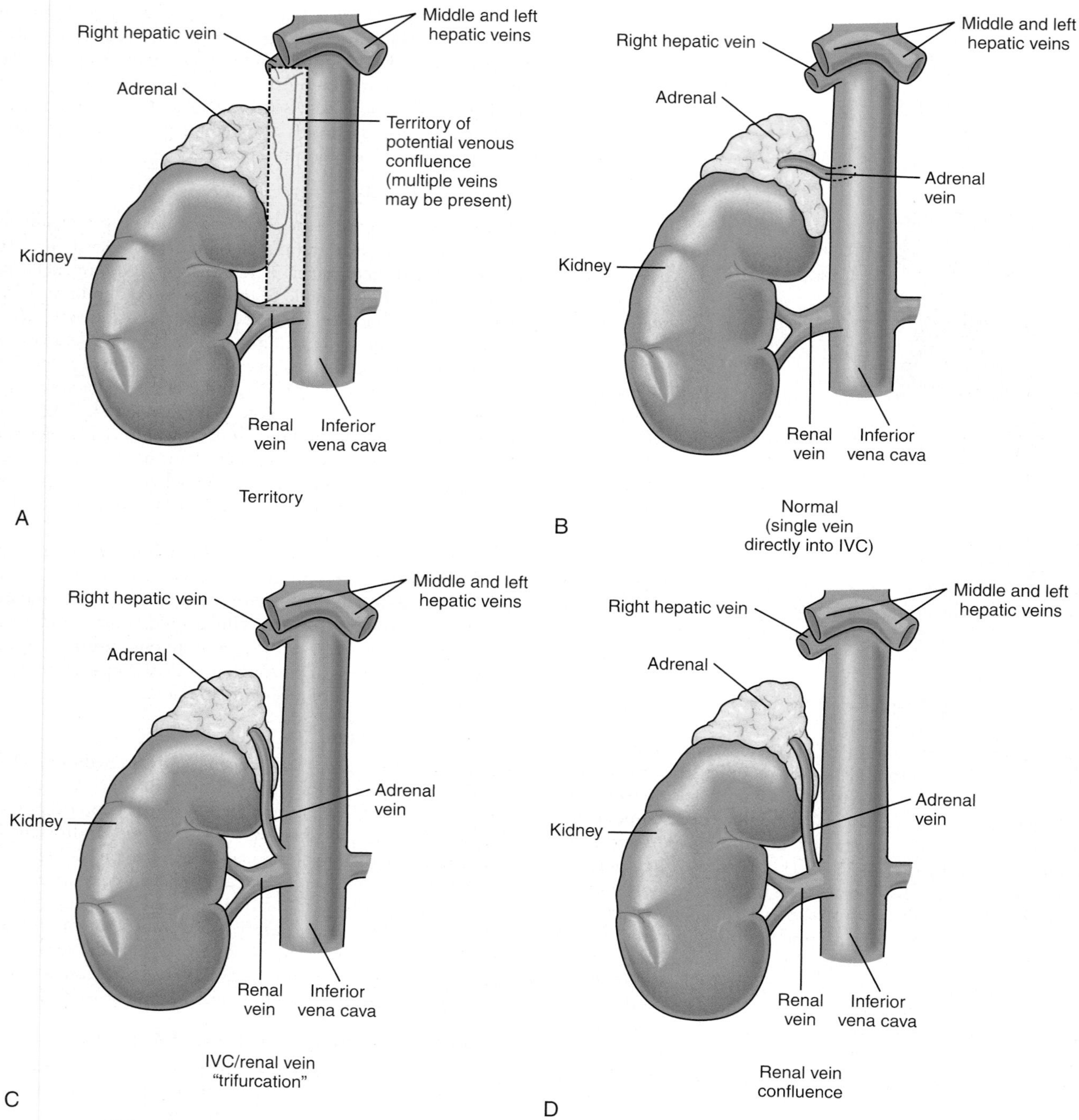

FIG. 40.3 Variations in right adrenal vein anatomy. (A) Territory of potential right adrenal vein confluence. (B) Normal (>80%); single vein directly into the inferior vena cava (*IVC*). (C) IVC–renal vein trifurcation. (D) Renal vein confluence.

(Continued)

the myocardium results in increased heart rate and contractility. Stimulation of β_2-adrenergic receptors results in smooth muscle relaxation in tissues such as the uterus, bronchi, and skeletal muscle arterioles. α_1-Adrenergic receptors mediate vasoconstriction in tissues such as the skin and gastrointestinal tract. α_2-Adrenergic receptors exist in presynaptic locations in the central nervous system, where they mediate attenuation of sympathetic outflow. The net effect of adrenal catecholamine release is to augment blood flow and oxygen delivery to the brain, heart, and skeletal muscle, which are essential to the fight-or-flight response, at the expense of other organ systems.

Catecholamine Clearance

Catecholamines are potent and short-acting compounds, with a plasma half-life on the order of 1 minute. Their presence in synapses and the circulation exhibits tight negative regulation by both reuptake and degradation. Degradation pathways merit some discussion because they generate the metabolites commonly measured

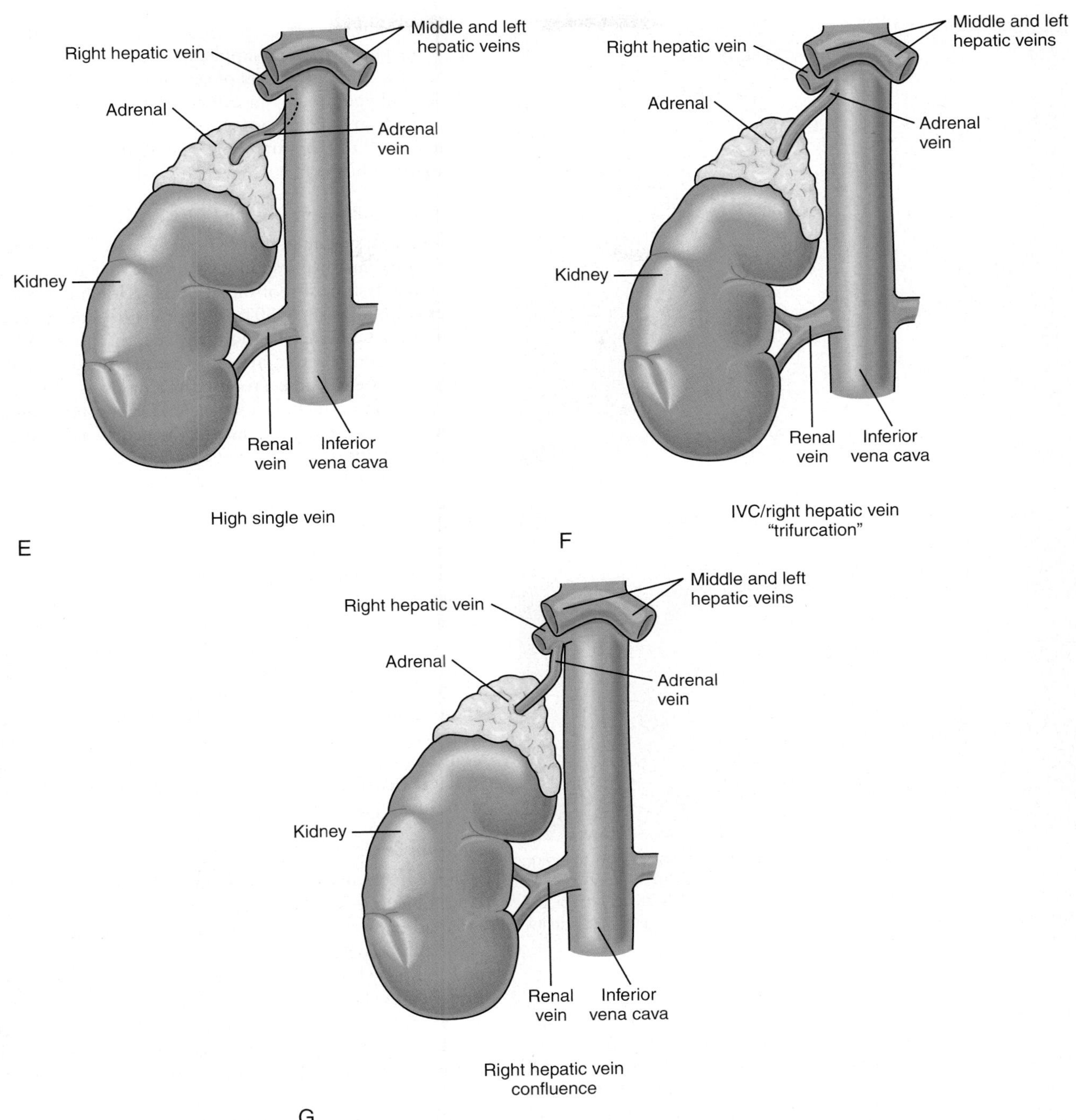

FIG. 40.3, cont'd (E) High single vein into the IVC. (F) IVC–right hepatic vein trifurcation. (G) Right hepatic vein confluence.

in the biochemical evaluation of pheochromocytoma (see later). Epinephrine and norepinephrine are inactivated by one or both of the enzymes monoamine oxidase and catechol-*O*-methyltransferase (see Fig. 40.6). Initial methylation by catechol-*O*-methyltransferase yields metanephrine and normetanephrine, which can be detected in plasma and urine. Their relatively stable plasma levels, which contrast with the high-amplitude fluctuations seen in plasma epinephrine and norepinephrine levels, make them attractive diagnostic markers.[4] The sequential action of monoamine oxidase and catechol-*O*-methyltransferase generates the major final product, vanillylmandelic acid. Catecholamine metabolites are excreted in the urine, sometimes after sulfonation or conjugation to glucuronic acid in the liver.

ADRENAL INSUFFICIENCY

Types of Adrenal Insufficiency

Primary Adrenal Insufficiency (Addison Disease)

Originally described in patients with tuberculous destruction of the adrenal glands, Addison disease is a rare disease that is manifested with weakness and fatigue, anorexia, nausea or vomiting, weight loss, hyperpigmentation, hypotension, and electrolyte disturbances (hyponatremia and hyperkalemia). Hyperpigmentation, previously believed to be caused by elevated levels of pro-opiomelanocortin and its cleavage product α-melanocyte-stimulating hormone, is now believed to result from ACTH-induced melanogenesis.[5]

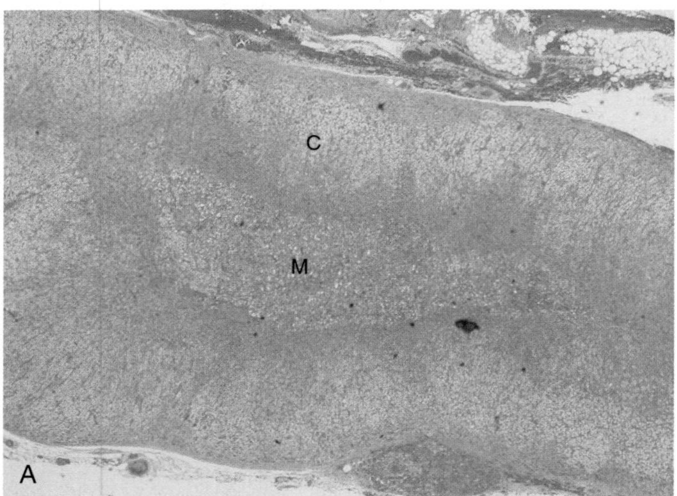

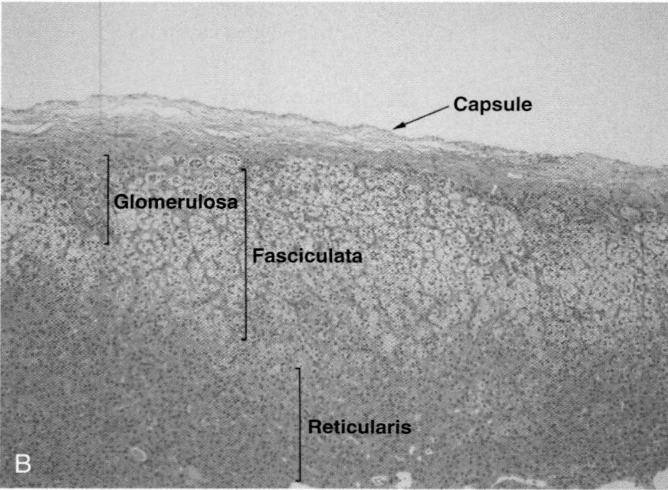

FIG. 40.4 Normal adrenal histopathology. (A) Low-power view showing the adrenal cortex *(C)* and medulla *(M)*. (B) Medium-power view demonstrating individual layers of the adrenal cortex. The thickness of the zona glomerulosa varies along its length (hematoxylin and eosin stain). (Courtesy Dr. Anthony Gill.)

Hormonal insufficiency caused by intrinsic adrenal disease arises from three general mechanisms—congenital adrenal dysgenesis/hypoplasia, defective steroidogenesis, and adrenal destruction. Of these, adrenal destruction from autoimmune causes is the most common, followed by infectious adrenalitis (e.g., tuberculous, fungal, viral), adrenal replacement by metastatic tumor, and adrenal hemorrhage (Waterhouse-Friderichsen syndrome). The last occurs in the setting of septicemia caused by meningococcal or other organisms and is more common in pediatric and asplenic patients.

Secondary Adrenal Insufficiency

Secondary adrenal insufficiency is a relatively common disorder resulting from ACTH deficiency, often occurring in the setting of pharmacologic steroid withdrawal. Patients receiving high supraphysiologic doses of glucocorticoids (more than the equivalent of 20 mg of prednisone daily; Table 40.1) for more than 5 days and those receiving low supraphysiologic doses for more than 3 weeks are at risk for HPA axis suppression. Surgical cure of Cushing syndrome likewise results in glucocorticoid withdrawal. The rate of recovery from HPA axis suppression varies in accordance with the duration and severity of previous glucocorticoid excess, and the need for glucocorticoid supplementation may last several years.[6] Other less common causes of secondary adrenal insufficiency include panhypopituitarism caused by neoplastic or infiltrative replacement, granulomatous disease, and pituitary hemorrhage or infarction. Pituitary infarction may occur in the setting of severe postpartum hemorrhage (Sheehan syndrome).

Adrenal Insufficiency in the Critically Ill

Studies have suggested that critically ill patients with sepsis or systemic inflammatory response syndrome may be affected by acute reversible dysfunction of the HPA axis. The incidence of the disorder is approximately 30% in critically ill patients, although this figure may be higher in those with septic shock. Whether these patients incur increased mortality because of adrenal insufficiency remains to be defined. Proposed mechanisms of reversible HPA axis dysfunction include adrenal ACTH resistance and decreased responsiveness of target tissues to glucocorticoids. Glucocorticoid supplementation in septic patients has been the topic of at least 42 randomized controlled trials. Among these studies, corticosteroid administration was associated with a small reduction in 30-day mortality (1.8% absolute risk reduction) and faster shock reversal. There appears to be an inverse relationship between survival benefit and glucocorticoid dose, with physiologic (i.e., replacement) doses yielding a possible benefit and high supraphysiologic doses demonstrating significant harm. Adverse effects of corticosteroid administration in this patient population include hypernatremia, hyperglycemia, and muscle weakness. Earlier trials suggested that patients with severe septic shock, particularly those requiring vasopressors, may benefit from 5- to 7-day courses of glucocorticoids up to 300 mg/day or less of hydrocortisone or equivalent. As more recent data have not confirmed a significant survival benefit, glucocorticoid use should be individualized in critically ill patients.[7]

Adrenal Crisis

Acute adrenal insufficiency, or adrenal crisis, is a life-threatening condition that typically occurs in individuals with already marginal adrenocortical function who are subjected to a significant acute physiologic stressor, such as infection or trauma. Sudden and complete loss of adrenal function, as occurs with Waterhouse-Friderichsen syndrome and certain hypercoagulable states, can also be manifested with adrenal crisis. Clinical findings include shock, abdominal pain, fever, nausea and vomiting, electrolyte disturbances, and occasionally hypoglycemia. Mineralocorticoid deficiency, resulting in an inability to maintain sodium and intravascular volume, is the primary pathogenic mechanism, although diminished cardiovascular responsiveness to catecholamines caused by glucocorticoid deficiency also plays a role. Treatment for suspected adrenal crisis should not be delayed while awaiting the results of diagnostic testing. The treatment of adrenal crisis centers around large-volume (1–2 L) intravenous resuscitation with isotonic saline and glucocorticoid administration in the form of hydrocortisone (100 mg intravenous bolus followed by 75 mg every 8 hours) or dexamethasone (4 mg intravenously every 24 hours). Dexamethasone is long acting and carries the advantage of not interfering with biochemical assays of endogenous glucocorticoid production. Ironically, mineralocorticoid replacement is not an early priority because the sodium- and fluid-retaining effects of mineralocorticoids are not manifested until several days after administration. Fluid and electrolyte balance can be rapidly achieved by saline infusion.

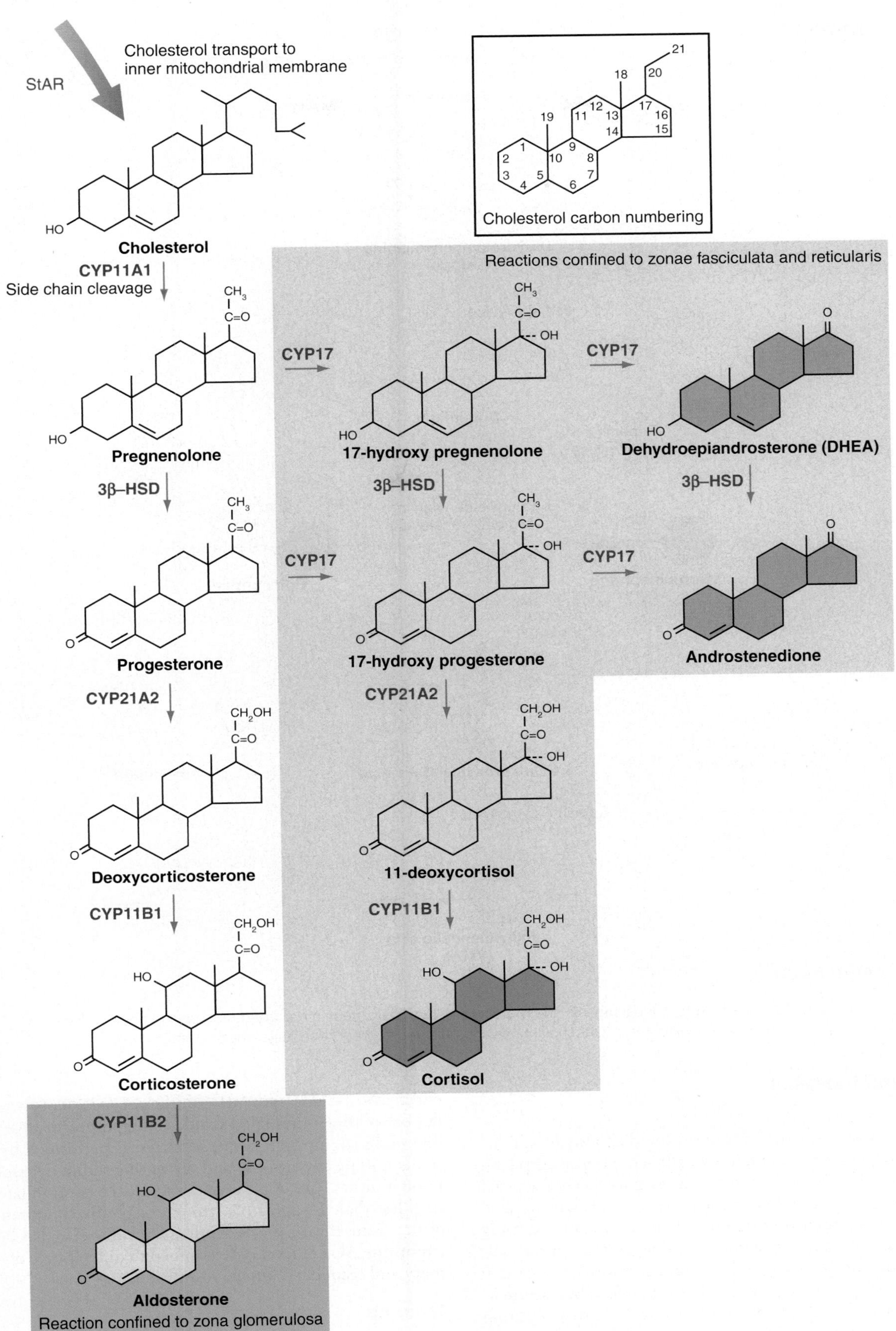

FIG. 40.5 Adrenal steroid biosynthesis. Reactions confined to the zona glomerulosa are shaded *turquoise*, and those confined to the zonae fasciculata and reticularis are shaded *orange*. Human mineralocorticoids are indicated in *yellow*, glucocorticoids in *green*, and sex steroids in *blue*. *3β-HSD*, 3β-Hydroxysteroid dehydrogenase; *StAR*, steroidogenic acute regulatory protein.

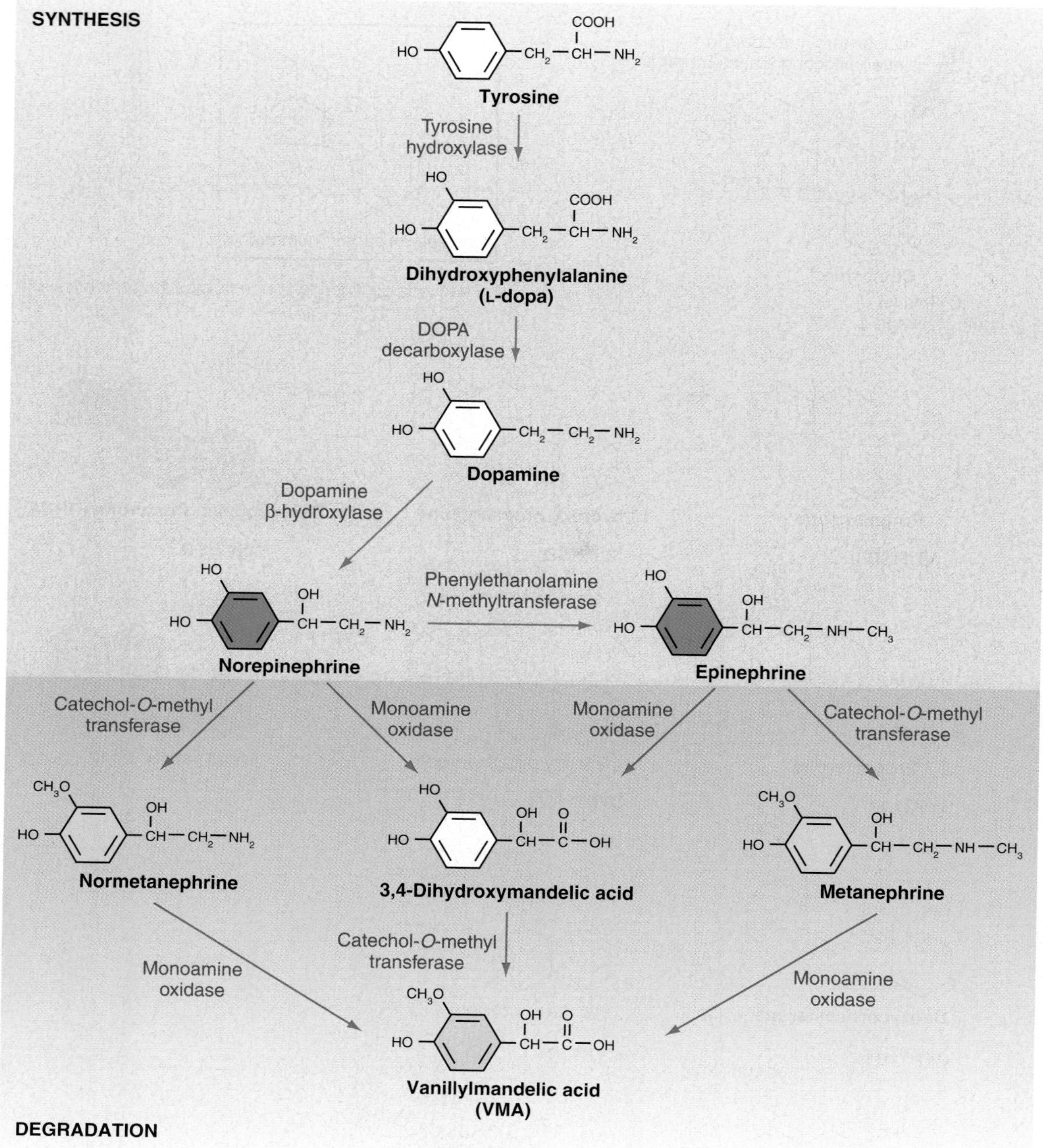

FIG. 40.6 Catecholamine biosynthesis and metabolism. Synthetic steps are shaded *orange*, and degradative steps are shaded *turquoise*. Major catecholamines are indicated in *green*, and major metabolites, in *yellow*.

Diagnosis and Treatment

Diagnosis

As is true for most endocrine disorders, the diagnosis of adrenal insufficiency depends on maintaining sufficient clinical suspicion for the disease. The clinical manifestations have been discussed earlier. Surgeons are most likely to encounter patients with adrenal insufficiency in the intensive care unit, trauma suite, or operating room when treating patients with steroid-dependent chronic illnesses. Routine and provocative biochemical testing is necessary to confirm the diagnosis (Fig. 40.7). The first step is to document inadequate cortisol production, which can be done by measuring morning levels of cortisol in the serum or saliva. In most patients, morning serum cortisol concentration higher than 15 μg/dL or morning salivary cortisol concentration higher than 5.8 ng/mL effectively excludes adrenal insufficiency. Patients whose levels fall below these thresholds should undergo provocative testing. A high-dose cosyntropin stimulation test is performed by administering 250 μg cosyntropin and measuring serum cortisol levels 30 to 60 minutes later. A positive test result (i.e., a stimulated cortisol level less than 18 μg/dL) is strongly suggestive of adrenal insufficiency. After the diagnosis of adrenal insufficiency has been made, a morning ACTH level is determined to differentiate between primary and secondary adrenal insufficiency.

Treatment

The treatment of adrenal crisis has been discussed. The goal of maintenance therapy for chronic adrenal insufficiency is to replace physiologic glucocorticoid and mineralocorticoid levels.

TABLE 40.1 Properties of endogenous and commonly used pharmacologic glucocorticoids.

COMPOUND	IV/PO*	COMMON TRADE NAME	RELATIVE POTENCY	DAILY PHYSIOLOGIC DOSE	DOSING INTERVAL
Cortisol = hydrocortisone	Both	Cortef (PO) Solu-Cortef (IV)	1×	20 mg	q8–12h
Cortisone	PO	—	0.8×	25 mg	q8–12h
Prednisone	PO	—	4×	5 mg	q24h
Prednisolone	PO	—	4×	5 mg	q24h
Methylprednisolone	Both	Medrol (PO) Solu-Medrol (IV)	5×	4 mg	q24h
Dexamethasone†	Both	Decadron	25×	1 mg	q24h

IV, Intravenous; *PO*, orally.
*Oral and intravenous dosages are similar.
†Does not cross-react with the cortisol assay.

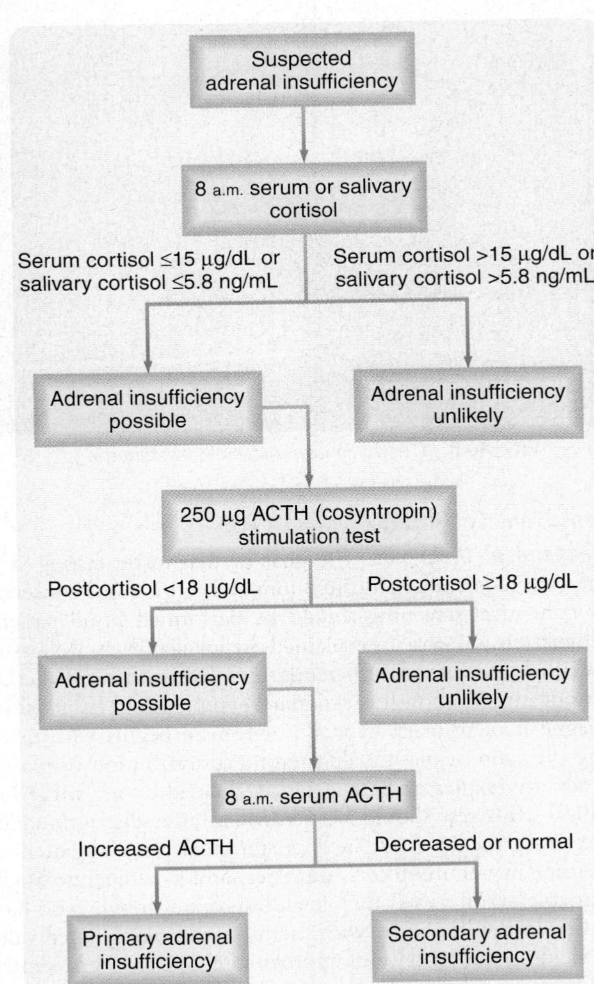

FIG. 40.7 Algorithm for the diagnosis of adrenal insufficiency. The adequacy of cortisol production is initially assessed with morning cortisol level measurement. Patients with low or borderline values undergo provocative adrenocorticotropic hormone *(ACTH)* stimulation testing, with serum cortisol levels measured before and 30 to 60 minutes after the administration of ACTH. Failure to mount an adequate response to ACTH usually establishes the diagnosis of adrenal insufficiency. The cause of adrenal insufficiency is then investigated with a morning ACTH level measurement.

Daily adult cortisol production is in the range of 10 to 20 mg, which can be replaced by the long-acting, orally bioavailable agent prednisone at a dosage of 5 mg/day. Typical mineralocorticoid replacement consists of fludrocortisone, 0.1 mg/day. Commensurate increased dosages of glucocorticoids are needed during periods of minor and major physiologic stress, such as mild infections (minor) and trauma, significant infections, burns, or elective surgery (major).

Perioperative Steroid Administration

Recommendations concerning glucocorticoid administration during elective surgery have been based primarily on uncontrolled retrospective studies. The need for supraphysiologic doses of glucocorticoids in this setting has generally been overstated. Patients with primary adrenal insufficiency (Addison disease) are at increased risk for perioperative adrenal crisis because of their inability to increase endogenous cortisol production in response to stress. They generally require hydrocortisone 100 mg intravenously just before induction of anesthesia. Patients with secondary adrenal insufficiency caused by chronic glucocorticoid treatment for autoimmune or inflammatory conditions have only a 1% to 2% risk of hypotensive crisis without perioperative glucocorticoid coverage. To prevent this rare but hazardous complication, chronic glucocorticoid users should, at the least, be maintained on their usual glucocorticoid dosage throughout the perioperative period. Supplementation above this level should be given in short courses according to the guidelines listed in Table 40.2.[8] Patients undergoing unilateral adrenalectomy should be given supplemental glucocorticoids only if the underlying diagnosis is Cushing syndrome.

DISEASES OF THE ADRENAL CORTEX

Primary Hyperaldosteronism

Epidemiology and Clinical Features

Primary hyperaldosteronism, the unregulated release of excess aldosterone from one or both adrenal glands, was first described by Jerome Conn in 1954. Primary hyperaldosteronism classically is manifested with resistant hypertension and hypokalemia, although studies have revealed that most patients may be normokalemic, depending on the population screened. Hypokalemia is likely a manifestation of severe or late-stage disease. The prevalence of primary hyperaldosteronism has been the topic of considerable debate. It was generally believed to affect approximately 1% of hypertensives. Widespread application of the aldosterone-to-renin

TABLE 40.2 Perioperative glucocorticoid regimens for patients with secondary adrenal insufficiency.*

DEGREE OF SURGICAL STRESS	EXAMPLES	INTRAOPERATIVE GLUCOCORTICOID DOSAGE	GLUCOCORTICOID TAPER
Minor	Procedures under local anesthetic, most outpatient procedures, inguinal hernia repair	None (take usual morning steroid dosage)	None (continue to take usual dosage)
Moderate	Routine abdominal, peripheral vascular, or orthopedic surgery	Hydrocortisone 50 mg or equivalent before procedure	Hydrocortisone 25 mg every 8 hours for 24 hours, then resume usual dosage
Major	Resection of gastrointestinal cancer, cardiopulmonary bypass	Hydrocortisone 100 mg or equivalent before procedure	Hydrocortisone 50 mg every 8 hours for 24 hours, then taper by half every day to usual dosage

*Caused by chronic pharmacologic steroid use.

ratio as a screening test in certain centers led to reports of a 10% to 40% prevalence of primary hyperaldosteronism among hypertensive patients. There is some consensus that these higher figures reflect strong referral bias and that the actual prevalence in unselected hypertensive patients is likely to be 7% or less.[9] Nonselective use of the aldosterone-to-renin ratio to identify patients with primary hyperaldosteronism is known to decrease the fraction of patients with surgically correctible disease (unilateral aldosteronoma) significantly, although the absolute number of surgically treatable cases has increased.

The mean age at diagnosis for primary hyperaldosteronism is approximately 50 years, and the disease has a slight male predilection. Most patients are asymptomatic, although patients with significant hypokalemia may complain of muscle cramps, weakness, or paresthesias. Patients typically have moderate to severe hypertension that is refractory to medical therapy. It is common for them to require two to four antihypertensive medications. Responsiveness to spironolactone may be seen, a feature that is predictive of a good response to surgical treatment.

Primary hyperaldosteronism is a potentially curable cause of significant cardiovascular disease. A study comparing 270 subjects with biochemically confirmed primary hyperaldosteronism with case-matched hypertensive controls has revealed that primary hyperaldosteronism is associated with a significantly increased risk of stroke, myocardial infarction, arrhythmias including atrial and ventricular fibrillation, and heart failure.[10] These results add to existing evidence indicating that the adverse cardiovascular sequelae of primary hyperaldosteronism are more pronounced than those caused by blood pressure elevation alone. Successful removal of an aldosteronoma leads to regression of many of these adverse physiologic changes.

The most common causes of primary hyperaldosteronism are unilateral aldosterone-producing adenomas (aldosteronomas; Fig. 40.8) and bilateral adrenal hyperplasia (also termed idiopathic hyperaldosteronism; Table 40.3). In the past, aldosteronoma was present in more than 60% of cases, but this number has decreased substantially as nonselective screening with the aldosterone-to-renin ratio has been applied. This phenomenon may reflect increased detection of hyperplasia, which is characterized by milder biochemical abnormalities than aldosteronoma. Recent sequencing of aldosterone-producing adrenal nodules has revealed somatic mutations in the potassium channel gene, which may be the cause of up to 40% of aldosteronomas.[11]

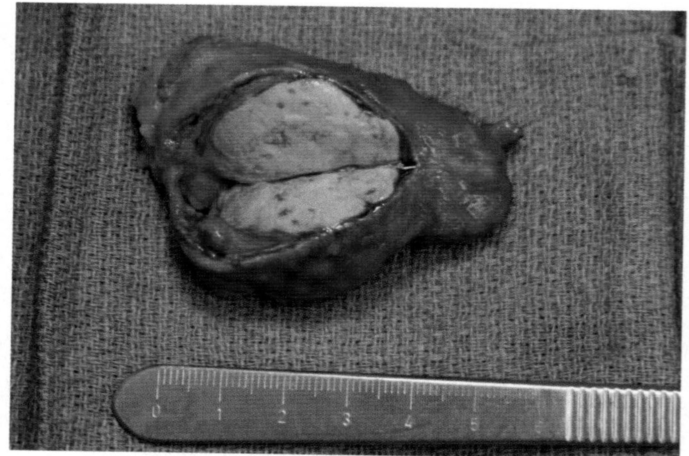

FIG. 40.8 Classic canary-yellow aldosteronoma.

Diagnosis and Localization

Biochemical Diagnosis. The goal of diagnostic testing is to identify and to lateralize aldosteronomas. There is some consensus that biochemical screening should be performed in all patients with hypertension and unexplained hypokalemia as well as in those with hypertension sufficiently resistant to medical therapy to warrant investigation for secondary hypertension. Establishing the diagnosis of primary hyperaldosteronism begins with determining the ratio of plasma aldosterone concentration to plasma renin activity (expressed here as ng/dL divided by ng/[mL • hr]; Fig. 40.9). This test should be performed after discontinuation of interfering medications, such as spironolactone, angiotensin-converting enzyme inhibitors, diuretics, and β-adrenergic blockers. Variable cutoff values for the aldosterone-to-renin ratio have been used in the literature, with the most commonly cited value of 30 yielding a sensitivity of approximately 90%. Some centers have advocated a lower threshold of 20; this increases sensitivity at some cost to specificity and conceptually reflects appreciation of the clinical gravity of failing to diagnose surgically correctable hyperaldosteronism.[12] A subset of patients with essential hypertension will have suppressed renin levels, which may result in false elevations of the aldosterone-to-renin ratio. Thus, the inclusion of an absolute aldosterone concentration higher than 15 mg/dL increases the specificity of initial screening. Patients who test positive and are younger than 30 years should be genetically screened

TABLE 40.3 Causes of primary hyperaldosteronism.

CAUSE	SCREENING*	
	SELECTIVE (%)	NONSELECTIVE (%)
Aldosterone-producing adenoma	60	30
Bilateral adrenal hyperplasia (idiopathic hyperaldosteronism)	35	65
Aldosterone-producing adrenocortical carcinoma	<1	<1
Familial hyperaldosteronism		
Type I (glucocorticoid-remediable aldosteronism)	<1	<1
Type II (non–glucocorticoid-remediable aldosteronism)	<1	<1

*Rates of specific pathologic processes are highly dependent on the pattern of screening (selective vs. nonselective).

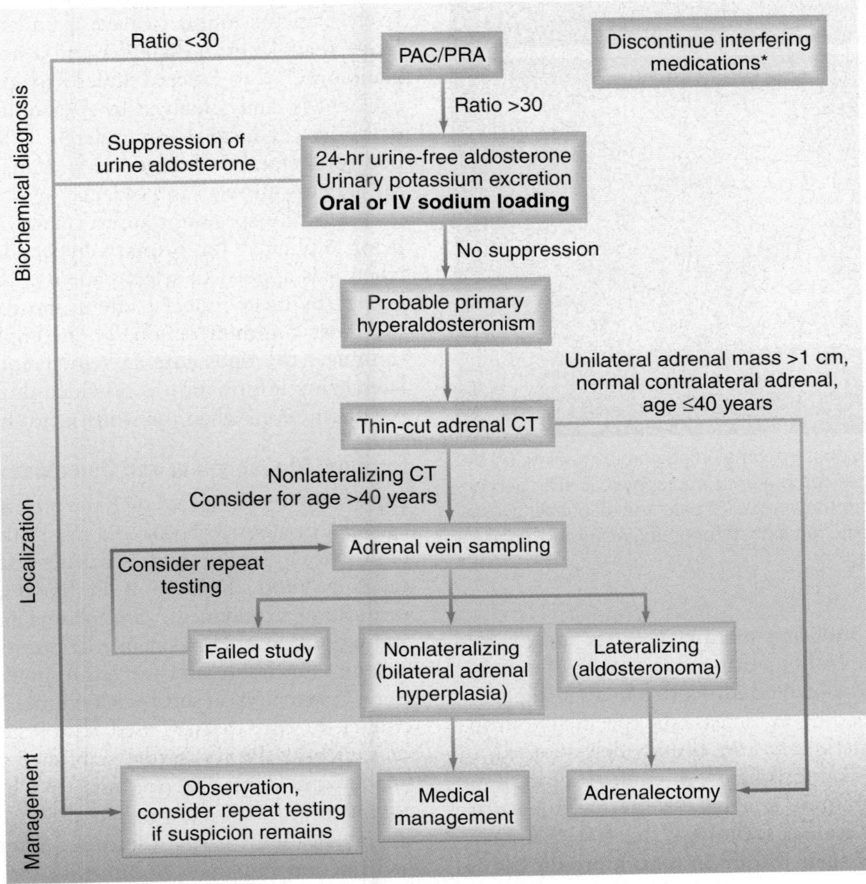

FIG. 40.9 Algorithm for diagnosis, localization, and management of primary hyperaldosteronism. Initial screening is done with determination of the PRA/PAC ratio, followed by confirmatory testing with sodium loading. After the biochemical diagnosis has been established, noninvasive localization is attempted with computed tomography *(CT)*. Patients with clear CT evidence of a unilateral abnormality can proceed to adrenalectomy with a more than 90% cure rate. Adrenal vein sampling is done in patients with equivocal CT findings and older patients, especially those older than 60 years, because nonfunctional cortical adenomas are found in 4% or more of this population and can cause false-positive CT localization. *ACE*, Angiotensin-converting enzyme; *PAC*, plasma aldosterone concentration, in ng/dL; *PRA*, plasma renin activity, in ng/(mL • hr).

for glucocorticoid-remediable aldosteronism (familial hyperaldosteronism type I), especially if they have a family history of early-onset hypertension. This rare autosomal dominant condition results in abnormal regulation of aldosterone synthesis by ACTH and can be medically treated.

Confirmatory biochemical testing is aimed at demonstrating inappropriately high (nonsuppressible) aldosterone levels by creating a state of hypervolemia-sodium excess. This is done with intravenous saline loading (2–3 L of isotonic saline given during 4–6 hours, followed by measurement of plasma aldosterone) or oral

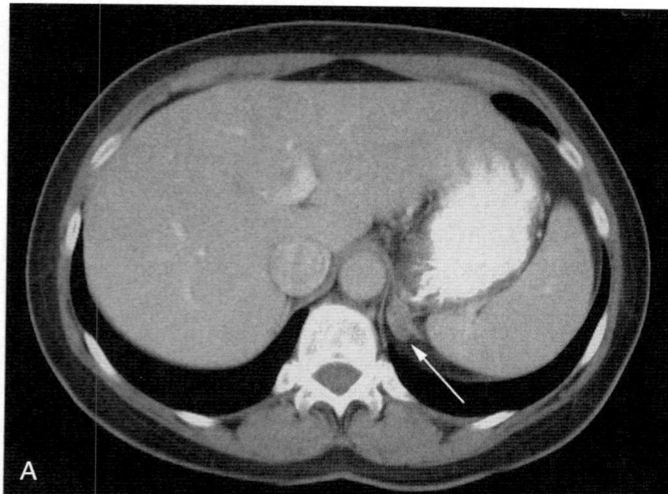

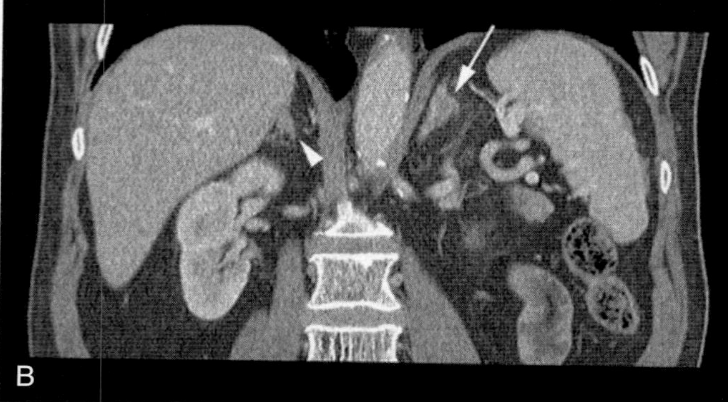

FIG. 40.10 Appearance of aldosteronoma on anatomic imaging. (A) Venous phase, contrast-enhanced computed tomography (CT) scan demonstrating a 2-cm left aldosteronoma *(arrow)*. (B) Late arterial phase, coronal CT scan demonstrating a 1.7-cm left aldosteronoma *(arrow)* and a normal right adrenal gland *(arrowhead)*.

salt loading (200 mEq = 5000 mg sodium daily for 3 days, followed by measurement of 24-hour urine aldosterone excretion). Some centers administer high-dose fludrocortisone (0.1 mg every 6 hours) during oral salt loading to increase the specificity of suppression testing, but this method has not been widely adopted.

Localization. After the diagnosis has been confirmed, localization is performed with anatomic imaging, selective venous sampling, and sometimes functional scanning. The fact that most aldosteronomas are smaller than 15 mm in maximum dimension poses some challenges to localization. Thin-cut (3 mm) adrenal computed tomography (CT) scanning is the preferred initial localization test (Fig. 40.10).

The next step in the localization algorithm is selective adrenal vein sampling (AVS). This test relies on the simultaneous measurement of cortisol and aldosterone levels in the peripheral circulation and left and right adrenal veins (Fig. 40.11). More than a fivefold elevation of the cortisol concentration in a sample relative to peripheral blood indicates successful cannulation of an adrenal vein (positive control). Lateralization is indicated by an unbalanced ratio of aldosterone to cortisol in the left and right adrenal veins, with the ratio on one side being fourfold higher than the other to identify the culprit gland. Considerable controversy exists about which patients should undergo AVS, an invasive procedure with a 90% technical success rate in experienced hands. There is consensus that AVS should be applied in all cases in which the biochemical diagnosis of primary hyperaldosteronism has been confirmed and thin-cut adrenal CT reveals no abnormalities or bilateral abnormalities. Of the remaining patients who have a unilateral mass on CT scan, a small but not insignificant fraction (2%–10%) will represent false-positive localization and have persistent hyperaldosteronism after unilateral adrenalectomy. In these patients, the adrenal mass represents a nonfunctioning cortical adenoma, and the true underlying diagnosis is a contralateral microaldosteronoma or bilateral adrenal hyperplasia, the latter of which is not surgically remediable.

Because patients 40 years and older are more likely to possess nonfunctioning adrenal cortical adenomas, some authors have advocated AVS in all older patients, and others have recommended universal application of this test in the workup of primary hyperaldosteronism.[12] It has been our practice to perform AVS selectively. Patients found to have a unilateral cortical adrenal mass larger than 1 cm in diameter and a normal contralateral adrenal gland on CT can proceed directly to adrenalectomy, as their management is rarely changed by AVS results, whereas those without definitive CT localization undergo AVS.[13] In consideration of the body of literature, we advocate for more liberal application of AVS for patients 40 years and older.

Practically speaking, approximately 30% to 40% of patients being evaluated for primary hyperaldosteronism undergo AVS when it is applied to select patients. The usefulness of the test is limited by its low success rate in most reports (40%–80%), with the most common reason for incomplete AVS being failure to cannulate the right adrenal vein. Frequently, however, sufficient lateralizing information is provided during AVS to guide surgical treatment, even when the study is not bilaterally selective.[14]

Surgical Management and Outcomes

Laparoscopic adrenalectomy is the preferred procedure for the management of aldosteronoma and most other adrenal tumors.[15] Cure of primary hyperaldosteronism is defined by clinical and biochemical end points. Reductions in blood pressure, antihypertensive medication requirements, and plasma and urine aldosterone levels and resolution of hypokalemia (if previously present) are observed as soon as 24 hours after successful surgery. Overall cure rates range from 75% to 95% at subspecialty centers, depending on the specific criteria for cure that are used. The Primary Aldosteronism Surgical Outcome (PASO) study established an international consensus for outcomes after adrenalectomy.[15] Clinical success is defined as complete (normalization of blood pressure without antihypertensive medication), partial (decrease in antihypertensive medication or reduction in blood pressure with same medication), or absent. Biochemical success is defined as complete (correction of hypokalemia and normalization of aldosterone to renin ratio), partial (correction of hypokalemia and ≥50% decrease in plasma aldosterone but persistently elevated aldosterone to renin ratio), or absent. In general, more than 80% of patients can expect either normalization of blood pressure or a significant reduction in antihypertensive medication requirements (typically, from three to four medications down to one). In some patients, depending on the degree of preoperative sodium overload, blood pressure may take several weeks to improve. Our practice is to stop all antihypertensive medications immediately after surgery, with the exception of beta blockers and clonidine, which must be tapered to avoid a rebound phenomenon. For those patients who continue to be hypertensive in the short term, medications may be added back temporarily, as needed, until the blood pressure gradually reaches a new equilibrium over time.

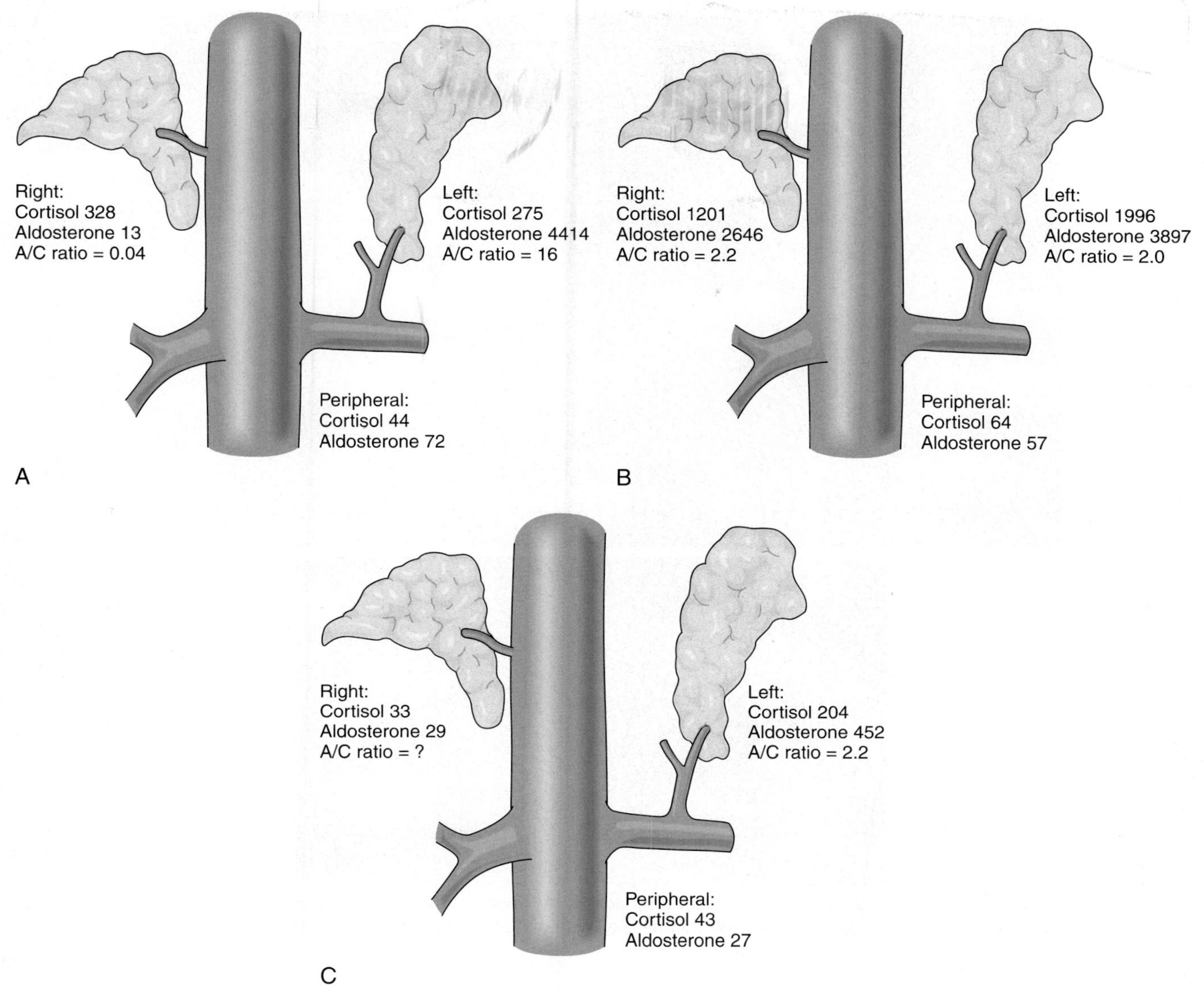

FIG. 40.11 Possible outcomes of adrenal vein sampling for primary hyperaldosteronism. Aldosterone is expressed in ng/dL, cortisol in μg/dL. (A) Successful study lateralizing strongly to the left adrenal. (B) Successful study, nonlateralizing. Stimulation with adrenocorticotropic hormone yielded high adrenal vein cortisol levels. (C) Failed study. The right adrenal vein was not cannulated.

Patients with hyperaldosteronism have a higher incidence of chronic kidney disease compared to hypertensive controls. Glomerular hyperfiltration caused by hyperaldosteronism can artificially raise creatinine clearance and mask renal insufficiency. After adrenalectomy, the decrease in aldosterone levels can lower glomerular filtration and unmask the true degree of chronic kidney disease. In addition, hyperkalemia due to transient suppression of the contralateral adrenal gland may occur in 5%–10% of patients following adrenalectomy for hyperaldosteronism.[16] Renal insufficiency and suppression of aldosterone secretion from the contralateral adrenal gland at AVS are predictors of hyperkalemia. Hyperkalemia occurs within 1 to 3 weeks after surgery; therefore, patients should be monitored with weekly serum potassium levels for 1 month postresection. Persistent hyperkalemia can be treated with mineralocorticoid replacement therapy (fludrocortisone).

A subset of patients with the following preoperative features display reduced benefit from surgical treatment and continue to require antihypertensive medications after operation: men older than 45 years, family history of hypertension, long-standing hypertension, requirement of more than two antihypertensive medications, and nonresponse to spironolactone. These indicate a component of essential hypertension and, in some cases, irreversible cardiovascular alterations caused by chronic disease. On the basis of these features, patients should be appropriately counseled as to what they should expect to gain from surgery.

Cushing Syndrome

Epidemiology and Clinical Features

The clinical features of glucocorticoid excess were first documented by Harvey Cushing in 1912. He described a young woman of "extraordinary appearance" who developed obesity, hirsutism, amenorrhea, easy bruising, and extreme muscle weakness. The principal differential diagnosis to be considered in evaluating patients for Cushing syndrome is obesity, an increasingly common

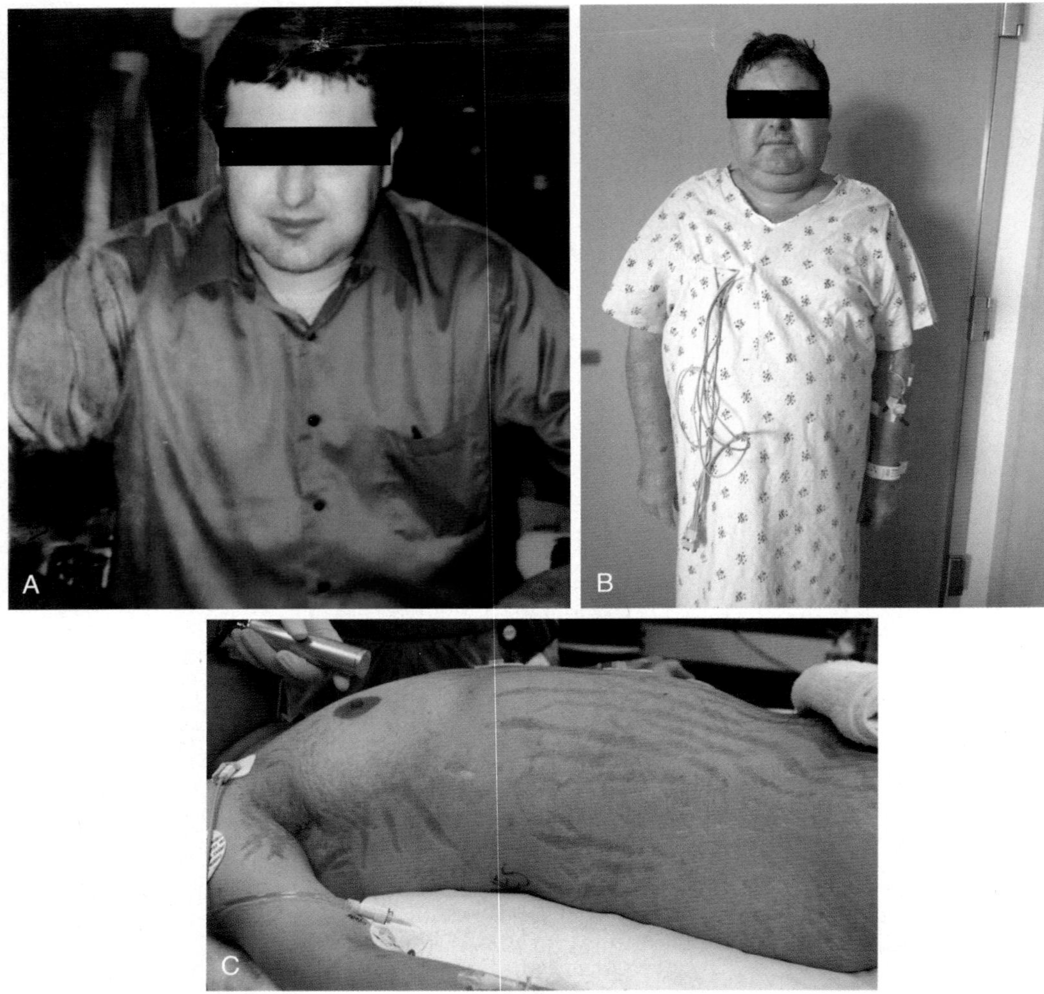

FIG. 40.12 Clinical manifestations of Cushing syndrome. (A) Appearance of a man before development of Cushing syndrome. (B) Same man 1 year after development of Cushing syndrome. (C) Purple abdominal and axillary striae in a man with Cushing syndrome.

condition. A subset of signs and symptoms, including easy bruising, muscle weakness, hypertension, plethora (a red facial appearance caused by thinning of the skin), and hirsutism, may allow discrimination between Cushing syndrome and obesity based on clinical features (Fig. 40.12). The genetic pathogenesis of cortisol-producing adrenal adenomas is not well understood. Recent next-generation sequencing on whole exome DNA has revealed a specific mutation of protein kinase A that is present in cortisol-producing adenomas, particularly in patients with overt Cushing syndrome.[17]

The most common cause of Cushing syndrome is pharmacologic glucocorticoid use for the treatment of inflammatory disorders. Endogenous Cushing syndrome is rare, affecting 5 to 10 individuals/million. Of these, most affected individuals (75%) will have Cushing *disease,* that is, glucocorticoid excess caused by an ACTH-hypersecreting pituitary adenoma. The remainder will be split between primary adrenal Cushing syndrome (15%) and ectopic ACTH syndrome (<10%), the latter of which usually is caused by neuroendocrine tumors or bronchogenic malignant neoplasms arising in the thorax.

Cushing syndrome is a lethal disease. The physiologic derangements resulting from glucocorticoid excess, including hypertension (present in >70% of cases), hyperglycemia, and truncal obesity, ultimately yield a fivefold excess mortality, primarily because of cardiovascular complications.[18] Thus, all efforts should be made to identify and appropriately treat patients with Cushing syndrome.

Biochemical Diagnosis and Localization

The diagnosis of Cushing syndrome is reliant on demonstration of inappropriate cortisol secretion or the loss of physiologic negative feedback. Normally, cortisol release follows a predictable circadian rhythm, peaking approximately 1 hour after waking and reaching a nadir around midnight. Thus, inappropriate cortisol secretion can be detected as elevated cortisol release during a 24-hour period or as a higher-than-expected level in the late evening. Traditionally, lack of negative feedback has been assessed with dexamethasone suppression testing and other types of provocative tests, many of which are cumbersome and require inpatient hospitalization. The 1-mg overnight dexamethasone suppression test is commonly used to diagnose Cushing syndrome, but its poor specificity results in a substantial number of false-positive tests. The development of late evening salivary cortisol testing has provided an attractive and feasible alternative to suppression testing.

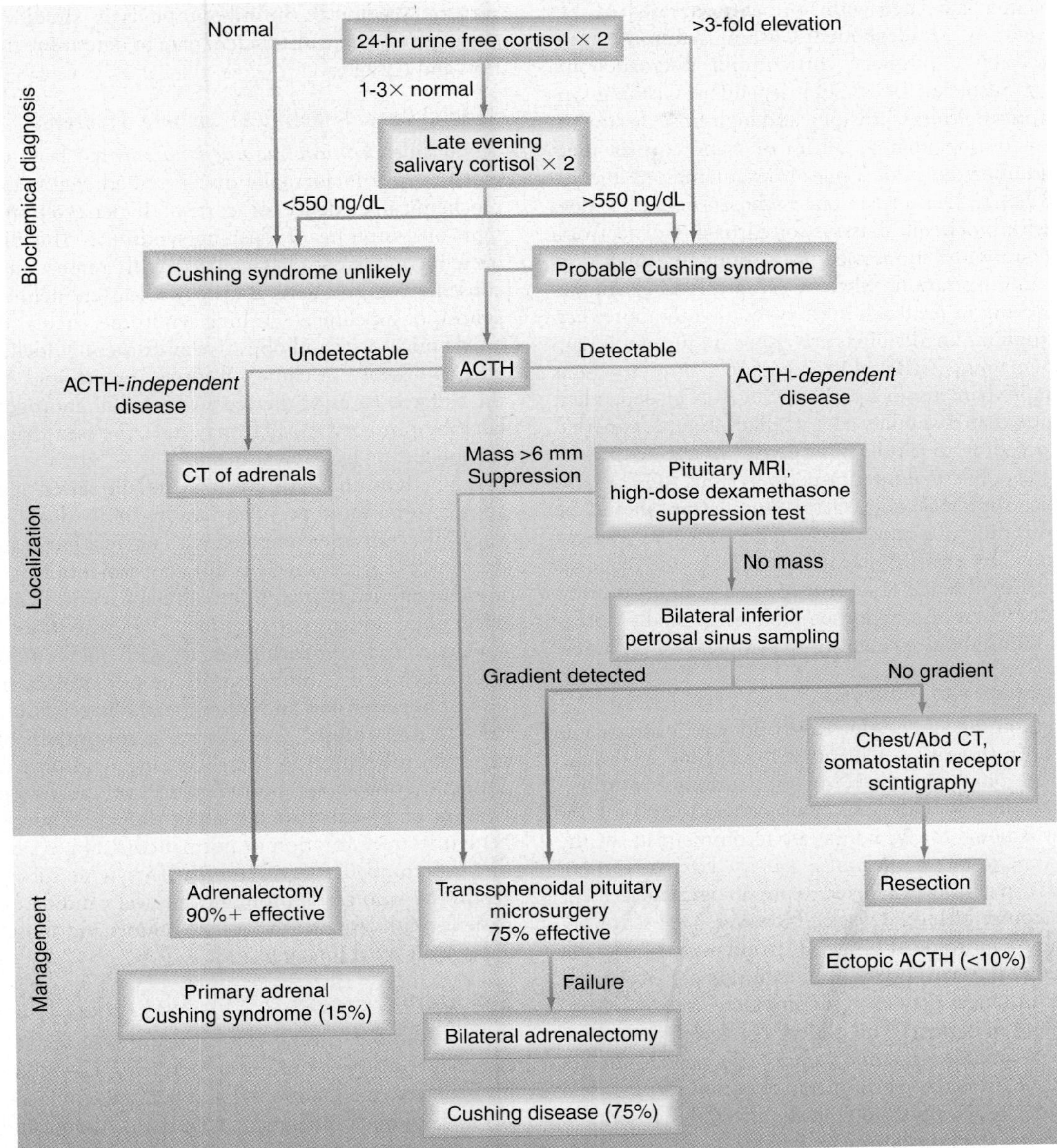

FIG. 40.13 Algorithm for the diagnosis, localization, and management of endogenous Cushing syndrome. A biochemical diagnosis can be established with an unequivocally elevated 24-hour urine-free cortisol level (greater than a threefold elevation) or an elevated late evening salivary cortisol level. Most cases of Cushing syndrome are caused by Cushing disease (pituitary corticotroph microadenoma) in which the plasma adrenocorticotropic hormone *(ACTH)* level is elevated. An undetectable ACTH level establishes the diagnosis of ACTH-independent Cushing syndrome and prompts adrenal imaging. Bilateral adrenalectomy is considered for patients with Cushing disease not cured by transsphenoidal surgery. *Abd,* Abdomen; *CT,* computed tomography; *MRI,* magnetic resonance imaging.

More than 90% of circulating cortisol is bound to plasma proteins. Unbound cortisol can be detected in the urine and saliva, and assessment of these body fluids forms the basis of biochemical screening for Cushing syndrome (Fig. 40.13); 24-hour urine collection for urine-free cortisol should be performed at least twice for initial screening. Unequivocally elevated levels should prompt immediate further testing to determine the cause and subtype of Cushing syndrome (i.e., primary adrenal cause, pituitary cause, and having ectopic ACTH syndrome). Patients with moderately elevated 24-hour urine cortisol levels should undergo confirmatory testing with two late evening (bedtime) cortisol measurements. A high cutoff value of 550 ng/mL has a sensitivity of 93% and specificity of 100%.[19]

Primary adrenal Cushing syndrome, also termed *ACTH-independent Cushing syndrome,* is caused by autonomous adrenal cortisol production and therefore is generally associated with an undetectable ACTH level (<5 pg/mL) because of feedback inhibition. The underlying pathologic process is variable, with solitary adrenal adenoma found in approximately 90% of cases, adrenocortical carcinoma in less than 10%, and bilateral micronodular or macronodular hyperplasia in less than 1%. Almost all these lesions, except micronodular hyperplasia, are readily apparent on CT scans.

Hypercortisolemia associated with normal or elevated ACTH levels is indicative of ACTH-dependent Cushing syndrome, most commonly caused by a pituitary corticotroph microadenoma (Cushing disease). Suspicion for ACTH-dependent Cushing syndrome should prompt pituitary imaging and high-dose dexamethasone suppression testing, that is, serum or urine cortisol measurement after administration of 2 mg of dexamethasone every 6 hours during 48 hours. Dexamethasone is chosen because it does not cross-react with biochemical assays for cortisol. Corticotroph adenomas are commonly suppressed in response to high-dose dexamethasone administration, whereas ectopic ACTH sources are completely lacking in feedback inhibition. Slightly more than 50% of corticotroph microadenomas are visible on pituitary magnetic resonance imaging (MRI). Detection of a pituitary mass larger than 6 mm in diameter in a patient with ACTH-dependent Cushing syndrome that is suppressed with high-dose dexamethasone justifies proceeding to pituitary surgery.[20] In the absence of a demonstrable mass, bilateral inferior petrosal sinus ACTH sampling with corticotropin-releasing factor stimulation should be pursued. Demonstration of a central to peripheral ACTH gradient in a study performed by a skilled physician is sufficient to diagnose Cushing disease. The absence of a clear gradient should prompt CT imaging of the chest and abdomen and, occasionally, somatostatin receptor scintigraphy to identify an ectopic ACTH source.

Surgical Management and Outcomes

Perioperative and postoperative glucocorticoid administration is obviously essential in the care of patients with Cushing syndrome. For patients undergoing adrenalectomy for Cushing syndrome, perioperative stress dose steroids (e.g., hydrocortisone 100 mg intravenously every 8 hours for 24 hours) are recommended. In the most common scenario of resection of a solitary adrenal Cushing adenoma, steroids can usually be tapered to physiologic replacement levels during the course of several weeks. However, a subset of patients with Cushing syndrome of longer duration and severity will demonstrate lasting HPA axis suppression, requiring glucocorticoid supplementation for longer periods, sometimes longer than 1 year.

The management of patients who undergo pituitary surgery for Cushing disease is variable. In some centers, glucocorticoids are withheld during the immediate postoperative period to provide a window during which early remission may be assessed.[21] A subnormal morning cortisol level on postoperative day 1 or 2 is indicative of cure. Glucocorticoid supplementation is then resumed until the HPA axis recovers, usually for at least 6 months. Because of the significant risk of postoperative adrenal crisis in patients with Cushing syndrome of all subtypes, glucocorticoid management is ideally done in conjunction with an experienced endocrinologist.

Adrenalectomy is more than 90% effective in the treatment of primary adrenal Cushing syndrome. Resolution of symptoms typically takes months to years, and certain deleterious physiologic effects regarding bone density, body composition, and inflammation are extremely persistent.[22] Failures may result from local and occasionally distant tumor recurrence in the case of malignant disease. Pituitary microsurgery for Cushing disease, typically performed through a transnasal transsphenoidal approach, is approximately 90% successful in expert hands. Remission rates may be improved by reoperation or pituitary irradiation for patients whose basal cortisol levels do not fall appropriately after initial surgery. Laparoscopic bilateral adrenalectomy should be considered for patients in whom pituitary surgery has failed. Patients with Cushing syndrome are hypercoagulable and carry a risk of venous thromboembolism of up to 5% after pituitary or adrenal surgery. Chemical thromboprophylaxis should be considered, although there are insufficient data to determine the optimal duration and dosage.[23]

Special Case: Subclinical Cushing Syndrome

The term *subclinical Cushing syndrome* has been used to describe patients with incidentally discovered adrenal masses who display biochemical evidence of cortisol hypersecretion without overt signs or symptoms of Cushing syndrome. This disease entity has been incompletely characterized with respect to its physiologic consequences and natural history. Clear-cut definitions for the diagnosis of subclinical Cushing syndrome, such as cutoff values for biochemical tests and objective assessment guidelines for the presence or absence of clinical features, are lacking. A low DHEA-S, the sulfated form of the secreted adrenal androgen DHEA regulated by pituitary ACTH, may have the best diagnostic accuracy for subclinical hypercortisolism.[24]

Hypertension, dyslipidemia, and impaired glucose tolerance appear to be more prevalent among individuals with subclinical Cushing syndrome compared with normal individuals. Retrospective studies suggest that this subset of patients experience improvement in obesity, hypertension, glycemic control, and dyslipidemia when they are treated surgically.[25] Furthermore, a randomized controlled trial comparing surgery with observation in 45 patients with subclinical Cushing syndrome noted more frequent resolution of hypertension and other metabolic conditions in the surgically treated group.[26] We observe a continuum of disease ranging from subclinical to overt Cushing syndrome, which arises as a function of both symptom severity and the perceptiveness of the treating physician. Patients along the entire spectrum appear to benefit from restoration of normal cortisol physiology. We therefore recommend surgery for patients with subclinical Cushing syndrome who are appropriate surgical candidates, especially for patients with larger (3- to 4-cm) tumors and those whose tumors enlarge on serial imaging studies.

Sex Steroid Excess

Adrenal tumors causing clinical features of sex steroid excess are rare. Most of these tumors are virilizing (as opposed to feminizing) and may be manifested at a late stage in association with an advanced adrenal malignant neoplasm. Almost all feminizing tumors are malignant, whereas approximately one third of virilizing tumors are malignant. Of adrenocortical carcinomas, 20% cause virilization, with most of these cases occurring in children. An additional 24% of adrenocortical carcinomas will display mixed features of Cushing syndrome and virilization.[27] Virilizing tumors may be biochemically detected by measurements of 24-hour urine testosterone, DHEA, and DHEA-S. Although laparoscopic adrenalectomy remains the preferred procedure for most sex steroid–secreting tumors, the high probability of malignancy merits close radiographic and intraoperative inspection for evidence of invasion or metastasis. Open adrenalectomy should be performed for obviously malignant tumors.

Adrenocortical Carcinoma

Adrenocortical carcinoma is a rare tumor with an annual incidence of approximately 1/million. Almost all cases occur in patients aged 40 to 50 years, although there is a minor peak in occurrence among children younger than 5 years. It demonstrates no significant gender predilection. At the time of presentation, adrenocortical carcinomas tend to be very large (mean tumor size, 9–13 cm) and have usually spread beyond the confines of the adrenal gland.[28]

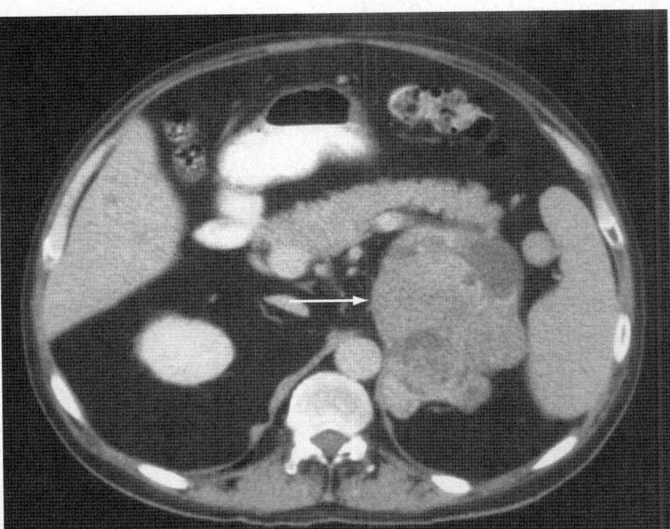

FIG. 40.14 Computed tomography scan demonstrating a 10-cm left adrenocortical carcinoma. Note the area of central necrosis *(arrow)*.

Historically, overall 5-year survival rates have been in the 15% to 20% range. Among patients who undergo surgical resection, 5-year survival is approximately 40%, a figure that has essentially remained unchanged during the past two decades.[29] A higher risk of death is associated with increasing age of the patient, poorly differentiated or high-grade tumors, positive surgical margins, and presence of distant metastases. More than 50% of adrenocortical carcinomas are functional. Cushing syndrome is most commonly seen, followed by virilization. Radiographic evaluation is primarily performed with CT, which typically reveals a heterogeneous mass with irregular or indistinct borders, central necrosis, and invasion of adjacent structures (Fig. 40.14). Metastases to lymph nodes, liver, and lungs may be found.

Treatment of adrenocortical carcinoma requires radical resection, which is achieved by an open approach. Complete resection can be achieved in up to 70% of patients in experienced hands. This frequently involves en bloc resection of adjacent organs or regional lymphadenectomy. Particular care must be taken in dealing with right-sided adrenocortical carcinomas larger than 9 cm because direct tumor extension into the inferior vena cava and sometimes the right side of the heart may be observed. Tumors demonstrating intravascular extension may need to be resected while the patient is on cardiopulmonary bypass to reduce the likelihood of lethal intraoperative tumor embolization.[30]

Patients who undergo incomplete resection of adrenocortical carcinomas have extremely limited life expectancy (median survival <1 year). Even those who undergo successful surgery are prone to development of local recurrence and metastases, which typically occur within 2 years. The principal chemotherapeutic agent for the treatment of adrenocortical carcinoma is mitotane [*o,p*-DDD, or 1,1-dichloro-2-(*o*-chlorophenyl)-2-(*p*-chlorophenyl)ethane], a derivative of the insecticide DDT that is a direct adrenocortical toxin. Mitotane has been used clinically as an adjuvant to surgery and as primary therapy in individuals with unresectable or metastatic disease. A multinational retrospective study examining the efficacy of adjuvant mitotane after radical surgery has demonstrated a significant improvement in recurrence-free survival.[31] The use of mitotane is limited by significant, dose-dependent gastrointestinal and neurologic toxicity. The multinational First International Randomized Trial in Locally Advanced and Metastatic Adrenocortical Carcinoma Treatment (FIRM-ACT) trial randomized 304 patients with locally advanced or metastatic adrenocortical carcinoma to receive etoposide, doxorubicin, cisplatin, and mitotane or streptozotocin and mitotane. There was a significantly improved response rate and progression-free survival in the former group, but median overall survival remained poor in both groups (14.8 vs. 12.0 months).[32] A number of other trials are examining targeted agents such as epidermal growth factor inhibitors, insulin-like growth factor I inhibitors, antiangiogenic agents, and broad-spectrum tyrosine kinase inhibitors. There is also an emerging interest in individualized therapy based on genomic and expression profiling of tumors.

DISEASES OF THE ADRENAL MEDULLA

Pheochromocytoma

Epidemiology and Clinical Features

The first account of pheochromocytoma was published in 1886 by Felix Frankel, who described a young woman suffering from intermittent attacks of palpitations, anxiety, vertigo, and headache. Autopsy revealed bilateral adrenal tumors that stained brown when treated with chromium salts. Because of the characteristic positive chromaffin reaction, these adrenomedullary tumors are termed *pheochromocytoma* (dusky-colored tumor, from the Greek *phaios*, dusky). Successful surgical management of pheochromocytoma was initially described in 1926 by both César Roux and Charles Mayo.[33]

Pheochromocytoma affects approximately 0.2% of hypertensive individuals. Men and women are affected equally. The peak incidence in sporadic cases is between the ages of 40 and 50 years, whereas familial cases tend to be manifested earlier. A subset of patients present with the classic triad of headache, diaphoresis, and palpitations, although almost all patients will display at least one of these symptoms. Hypertension is present in 90% of cases and may be episodic or sustained. The principal challenge in making the diagnosis of pheochromocytoma arises from the fact that essential hypertension is common and the clinical features suggestive of pheochromocytoma are nonspecific. In fact, only 0.5% of patients with hypertension and suggestive features will ultimately prove to have the disease. The differential diagnosis of pheochromocytoma is wide, encompassing diverse processes such as hyperthyroidism, hypoglycemia, coronary artery disease, heart failure, stroke, drug-related effects, and panic disorder. Pheochromocytoma has been described as a biologic time bomb because of the potentially lethal cardiovascular effects of the bioactive compounds secreted by these tumors. Thus, despite the challenges in diagnosis, clinicians should screen for this disease aggressively and seek appropriate treatment for affected patients.

Previously, pheochromocytoma was termed the *10% tumor*, suggesting that 10% are bilateral, 10% malignant, 10% extra-adrenal, and 10% familial. Discoveries regarding the genetic underpinnings of pheochromocytoma have challenged these old axioms.

Special Case: Pheochromocytoma in Pregnancy

Pheochromocytoma during pregnancy, although very rare, is potentially fatal for the mother and child. When diagnosed in the antenatal period, pheochromocytoma results in 12% fetal mortality. However, if the diagnosis is delayed until labor or postpartum, the rate of fetal and maternal mortality increase to 29%.[34] If the diagnosis is made within the first 24 weeks of pregnancy, adrenalectomy is recommended in the second trimester, while surgery should be postponed until after delivery if the diagnosis is made in the third trimester.

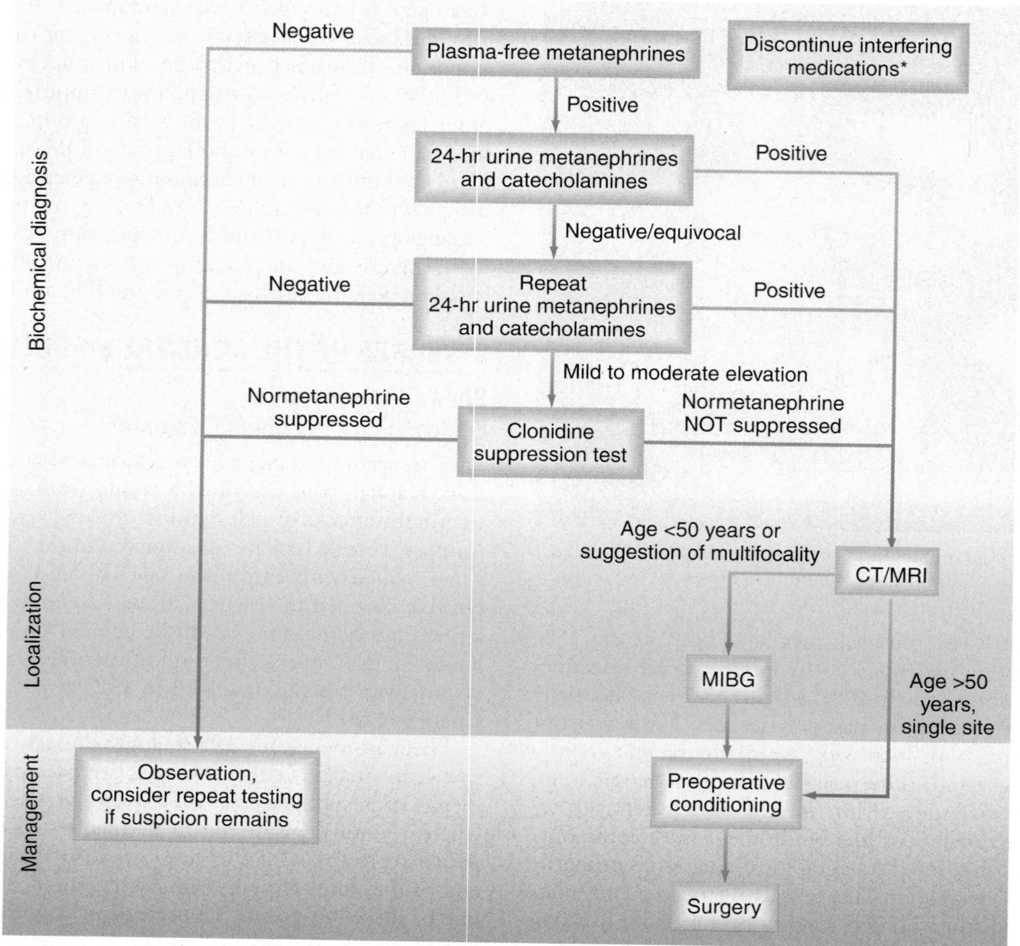

*Including sympathomimetics, phenoxybenzamine, acetaminophen, many psychotropic drugs.

FIG. 40.15 Algorithm for the diagnosis, localization, and management of pheochromocytoma. Initial plasma-free metanephrine testing can effectively exclude the diagnosis if the result is negative. A 24-hour urine collection for catecholamines and their metabolites is generally performed twice, with cutoffs approximately twice the upper limit of normal being criteria for positivity (see Table 40.4). Clonidine suppression testing can be used for the small fraction of patients in whom the diagnosis remains uncertain after urine testing. Localization with computed tomography *(CT)* or magnetic resonance imaging *(MRI)* follows biochemical confirmation of the diagnosis, with metaiodobenzylguanidine *(MIBG)* scanning performed for younger patients and those otherwise at risk for multifocal disease. Phenoxybenzamine is given in escalating doses for at least 2 weeks before surgery.

Biochemical Diagnosis and Localization

Establishing the biochemical diagnosis of pheochromocytoma is based on the detection of elevated levels of catecholamines and their metabolites in body fluids. Measurements of 24-hour urine levels of these compounds have long been the cornerstone of biochemical testing and are still the most reliable tests available today. In 2002, measurement of free (unconjugated) metanephrines in plasma was introduced as an alternative screening tool for pheochromocytoma. Plasma free metanephrine testing carries an extremely high sensitivity, approaching 99%, and being a one-time blood test, it is more convenient than 24-hour urine testing. However, the specificity of plasma free metanephrine testing is 89% at best, with specificities at most laboratories likely to be in the 85% range or below. Given that pheochromocytoma is a rare diagnosis that is sought within a large pool of hypertensive individuals, false-positive test results are a major problem. It has been estimated that false-positive test results outnumber true-positive test results by as much as 30:1 when plasma free metanephrine testing is used as a principal screening tool.[35]

Therefore, the primary usefulness of plasma free metanephrine testing is to exclude pheochromocytoma when the test result is negative (Fig. 40.15). When the test result is positive, confirmatory testing with 24-hour urine levels of catecholamines and their metabolites is recommended. Many drugs and conditions are capable of confounding catecholamine-based testing, contributing further to the problem of false-positive results. These include sympathomimetics (present in many cold remedies), phenoxybenzamine (frequently initiated when suspicion for pheochromocytoma is raised), acetaminophen (which interferes with the plasma free metanephrine assay), many psychotropic drugs (notably tricyclic antidepressants), and major physical or psychological stressors. Results of tests performed during episodes of acute pain, critical illness, or urgent hospitalization may be misleading. The presence of confounding factors is extremely common in the population being screened because they represent manifestations or treatments of competing diagnoses. Clearly, biochemical testing should be ideally performed when the patient is as free as practically possible of all confounding factors.

TABLE 40.4 Cutoff values for biochemical diagnosis of pheochromocytoma.

TEST*	CUTOFF VALUE MOL	CUTOFF VALUE G	DEFINITIONS	SENSITIVITY (%)	SPECIFICITY (%)
Plasma-free metanephrine	0.3 nmol/L	59 µg/L	Paired test, positive result if either or both values are elevated	99	85–89
Plasma-free normetanephrine	0.6 nmol/L	110 µg/L			
Urinary total metanephrines	6.6 µmol/day	1.3 mg/day		71	99.6
Urinary epinephrine	191 nmol/day	35 µg/day		29	99.6
Urinary norepinephrine	1005 nmol/day	170 µg/day		50	99.6
Urinary dopamine	4571 nmol/day	700 µg/day		8	100
Urinary total metanephrines and catecholamines	—		Grouped test, positive result if any one of the following three urinary values is elevated: total metanephrines, epinephrine, norepinephrine, dopamine	88	99
Urinary vanillylmandelic acid	40 µmol/day	7.9 mg/day		64	95
Clonidine suppression test			Positive result = elevated level after clonidine and fall of <40	96	100
Plasma-free normetanephrine	0.61 nmol/L	112 µg/L			

*When it is performed twice, 24-hour urine testing of urinary total metanephrines and catecholamines (grouped test) is highly sensitive and highly specific.

The operating characteristics of catecholamine-based plasma and urine tests are listed, along with corresponding cutoff values, in Table 40.4. Cutoff values for 24-hour urine tests are deliberately set high to maximize specificity; these values are approximately double the upper 95% reference range in most laboratories. A urine collection may be considered positive if total metanephrines or any single catecholamine fraction (e.g., epinephrine, norepinephrine, and dopamine) is elevated above its cutoff value. This approach maintains high specificity and yields an acceptable sensitivity of 88%.[36] Importantly, it takes into account the fact that pheochromocytomas synthesize and metabolize catecholamines and that tumors may possess heterogeneous secretory profiles, depending on their relative expression of synthetic and degradative enzymes (see Fig. 40.6).

Two 24-hour urine collections for catecholamines and their metabolites are sufficient to make (or to exclude) the diagnosis of pheochromocytoma in almost all cases. Clonidine suppression testing, the measurement of plasma free normetanephrine levels after the oral administration of 0.3 mg clonidine, may help clarify equivocal test results but is rarely used. Anatomic localization may be performed with MRI or CT. MRI is slightly more sensitive, but CT often yields better anatomic definition for operative planning (Fig. 40.16). The specificity of either modality is only 70% because of the high prevalence of incidental adrenal nodules. Scintigraphy with ^{131}I- or ^{123}I-labeled metaiodobenzylguanidine (MIBG; Fig. 40.17) can be performed in select patients in whom multifocal or malignant disease is suspected. MIBG scanning is highly specific for pheochromocytoma but carries a sensitivity of only 77% to 90%. Positron emission tomography (PET) and PET/CT using novel radionuclides such as ^{18}F-L-dihydroxyphenylalanine (^{18}F-DOPA; Fig. 40.18) and ^{18}F-dopamine are highly sensitive and superior to MIBG scanning in the imaging of pheochromocytoma.[37] Currently, the best PET/CT radiopharmaceutical for the localization of pheochromocytoma is ^{68}Ga-DOTATATE, which has a rate of lesion detection compared to ^{18}F-fluorodeoxyglucose (FDG) PET/CT (49%) and ^{18}F-FDOPA PET/CT (75%).[38] However, the availability of these techniques remains confined to a small number of academic centers worldwide.

Perioperative Care

Throughout the first half of the twentieth century, perioperative mortality rates in the treatment of pheochromocytoma ranged from 26% to 50%. Currently, the mortality rate in most specialty centers is approximately 1%. This dramatic improvement can largely be ascribed to advances in pharmacology, physiology, anesthesia, and perioperative medical care. The adverse perioperative hemodynamic changes most commonly observed with pheochromocytoma are intraoperative hypertension and postoperative hypotension. Intraoperative hypertension may be caused by stimulation of catecholamine release by anesthetic induction agents as well as by direct manipulation of the tumor. Postoperative hypotension may be profound. It results from a state of hypovolemia created by the presence of excess circulating catecholamines. Sudden withdrawal of this stimulus after tumor removal leads to peripheral arteriolar vasodilatation and a dramatic increase in venous capacitance, which together may precipitate cardiovascular collapse. In their early report of a large successful case series, investigators at the Mayo Clinic described the use of intraoperative α-adrenergic blockade followed by aggressive volume repletion and the administration of α-adrenergic agonists in the immediate postoperative period.[39]

The principles of perioperative care remain much the same. As soon as the biochemical diagnosis of pheochromocytoma has been confirmed, α-adrenergic blockade should be initiated to protect against hemodynamic lability. Our practice is to start with phenoxybenzamine 10 mg twice daily. The dosage can be titrated upward every 2 to 3 days to a maximum of 40 mg three times daily to achieve normalization of heart rate and blood pressure. The period of preoperative conditioning should last at least 2 weeks to allow adequate reversal of α-adrenergic receptor downregulation. This restores sensitivity to vasopressor agents, which can then be used to treat the patient postoperatively. Phenoxybenzamine is a nonspecific, noncompetitive (irreversible), long-acting (half-life of 24 hours) α-adrenergic antagonist. Although its use is associated with the side effects of postural hypotension and significant nasal congestion, it is generally favored over α_1-adrenergic selective agents, such as prazosin and doxazosin. Nasal congestion can actually serve as a useful indicator of adequate blockade. Furthermore, phenoxybenzamine provides the most complete alpha blockade among available agents, and its pharmacokinetics permit serum

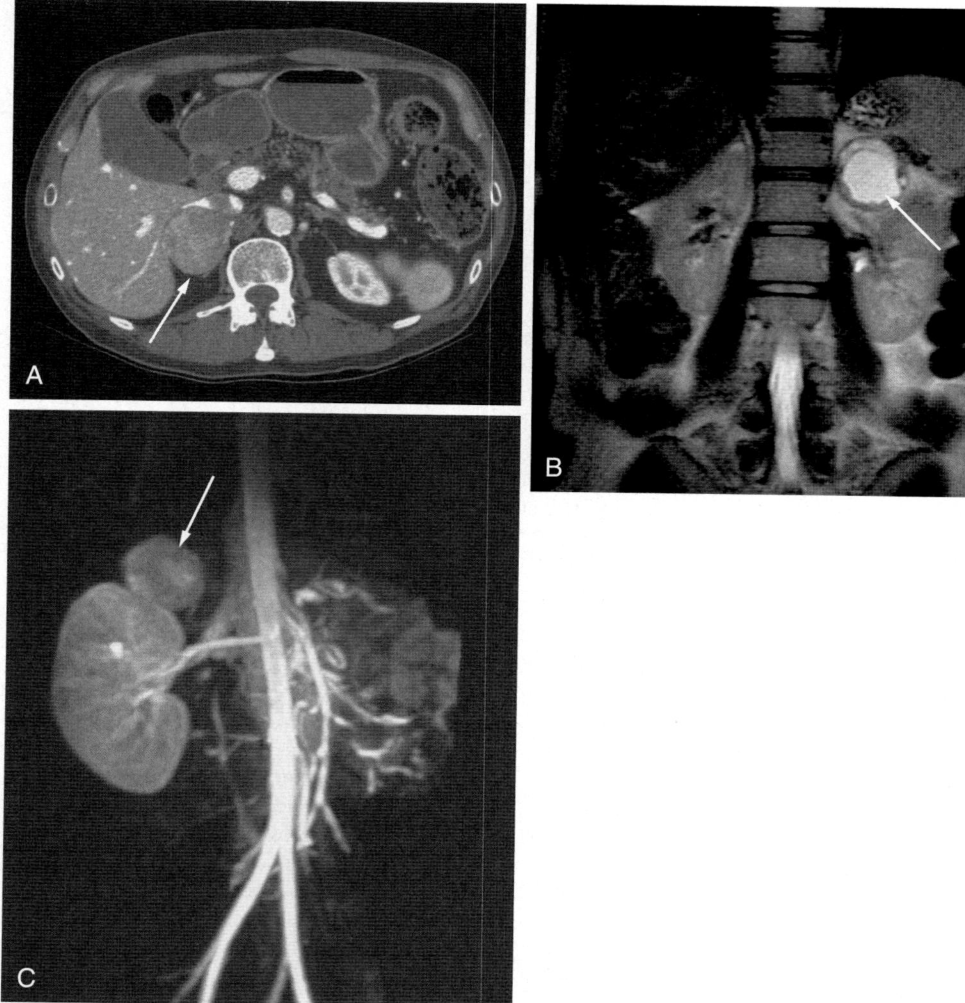

FIG. 40.16 Appearance of pheochromocytoma on anatomic imaging. (A) Venous phase, contrast-enhanced computed tomography scan demonstrating a right adrenal pheochromocytoma *(arrow)*. The heterogeneity in the inferior vena cava represents swirling of contrast material, not tumor thrombus or invasion. (B) Coronal T2-weighted magnetic resonance imaging scan demonstrating a left adrenal pheochromocytoma with central cystic change *(arrow)*. (C) Left anterior oblique magnetic resonance angiographic reconstruction demonstrating a right adrenal pheochromocytoma *(arrow)*.

drug levels to decay in parallel with catecholamine levels postoperatively. Calcium channel blockers may be added for patients who have inadequate blood pressure control after titration of an alpha blocker. The cost and availability of phenoxybenzamine in the United States have become highly variable in recent years, making it an impractical choice for a significant number of patients. For this reason, selective alpha blockers have gained popularity as the preferred medication for preoperative conditioning in some centers. Due to the possibility of increased intraoperative hemodynamic fluctuation with this approach, the experience and communication between the anesthesia and surgical teams are critical to ensure patient safety.

Beta blockers may be administered after adequate alpha blockade has been achieved for the subset of patients with persistent tachycardia, who often have predominantly epinephrine-secreting tumors. Beta blockers should never be the first agent administered because a decrease in peripheral vasodilatory beta receptor stimulation results in unopposed α-adrenergic tone, which may exacerbate hypertension. Preoperative volume expansion with isotonic fluids has been advocated in the past. However, in our experience, the need for this is significantly reduced when aggressive preoperative alpha blockade has been achieved because the resultant increase in venous capacitance restores euvolemia gradually by stimulating thirst. Clinical suspicion for hypovolemia should remain high in the postoperative period, and patients should be resuscitated aggressively if they become hypotensive or oliguric. Some patients may require vasopressors after tumor removal, especially if preoperative alpha blockade is incomplete.

Surgical Management and Outcomes

Successful operative treatment of pheochromocytoma is dependent on close communication between the surgeon and anesthesiologist. Invasive hemodynamic monitoring is required, and fluid management must be meticulous. Manipulation of the tumor should be minimized, and the anesthetic team should be prepared to administer supplemental intravenous alpha and beta blockers as well as vasopressors when necessary.

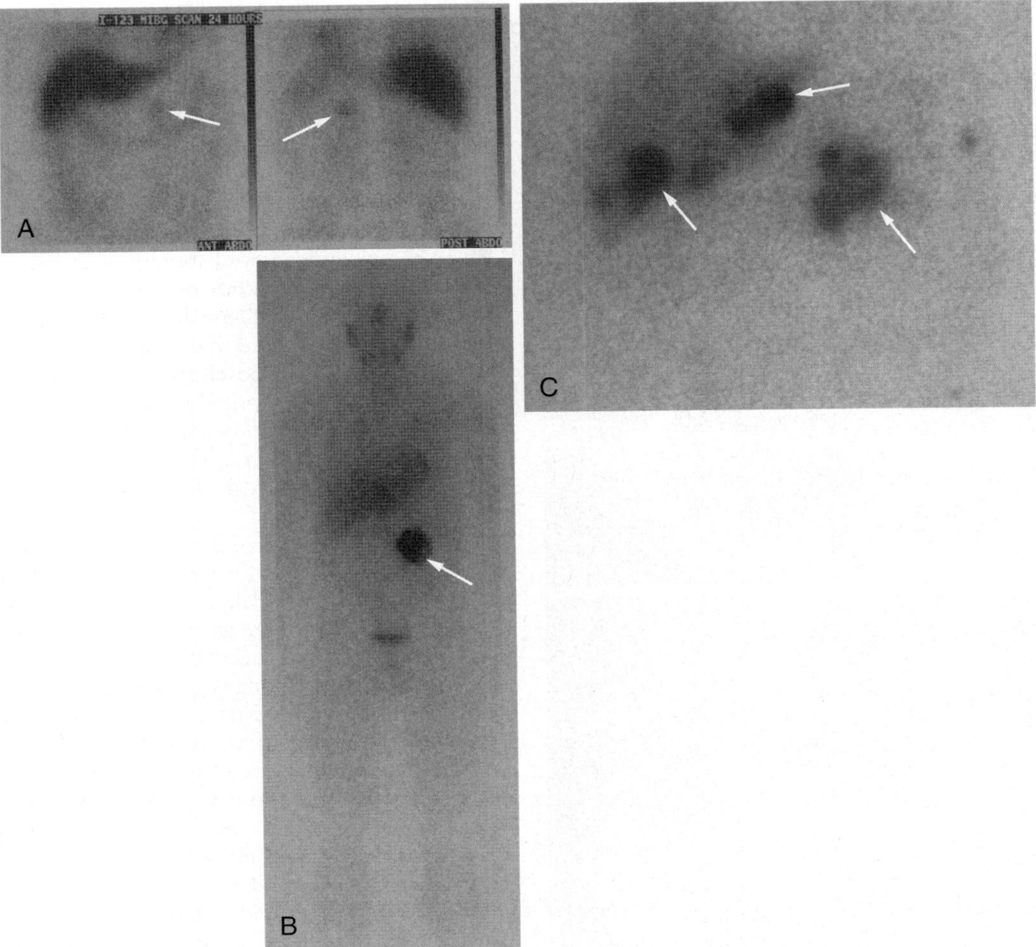

FIG. 40.17 Appearance of pheochromocytoma on functional imaging (metaiodobenzylguanidine [MIBG] scanning). (A) ^{123}I-MIBG scan of the abdomen demonstrating an isolated left adrenal pheochromocytoma *(arrows)*. Physiologic radiotracer uptake is noted in the liver, right colon, and transverse colon. (B) Whole-body ^{131}I-MIBG scan demonstrating a large, left, para-aortic extra-adrenal pheochromocytoma *(arrow)*. Physiologic radiotracer uptake is noted in the liver, salivary glands, and bladder. (C) ^{131}I-MIBG scan of the abdomen demonstrating malignant pheochromocytoma, with local recurrence in the left adrenal bed and liver metastases *(arrows)*.

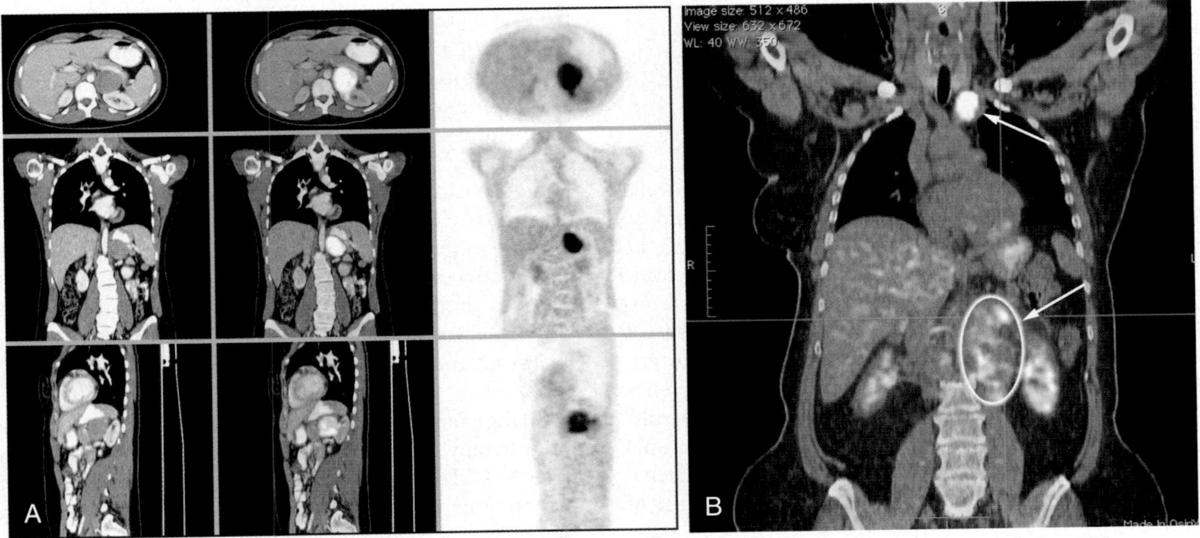

FIG. 40.18 (A) Appearance of pheochromocytoma on functional imaging (^{18}F-L-dihydroxyphenylalanine [^{18}F-DOPA]). (B) ^{18}F-DOPA positron emission tomography/computed tomography scan in a patient with malignant multifocal pheochromocytoma. Diffuse uptake above background is seen in the region of the left adrenal gland and left periaortic region, where a locally invasive tumor was found at surgery *(arrow)*. A second area of intense tracer uptake is seen in the left paratracheal region, where a carotid sheath paraganglioma was found *(arrow)*. The patient is an *SDHB* mutation carrier.

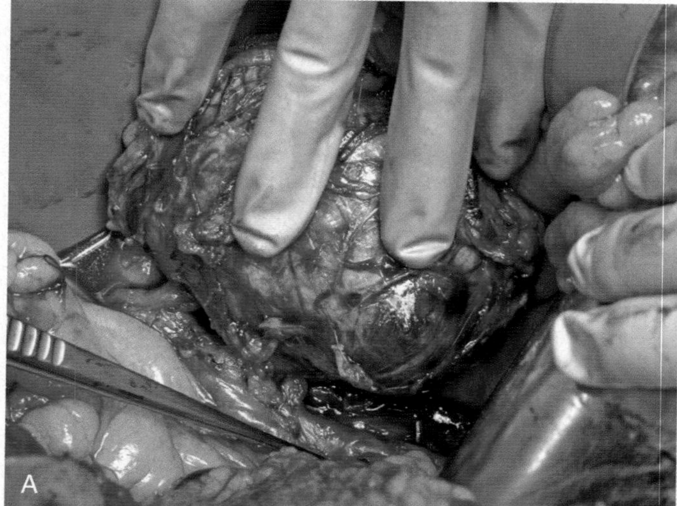

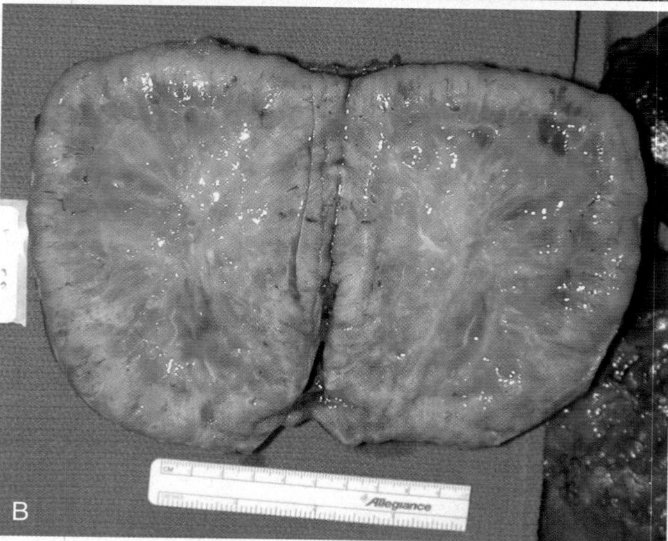

FIG. 40.19 Gross appearance of pheochromocytoma. (A) Open resection of a left para-aortic extra-adrenal pheochromocytoma (depicted in Fig. 40.17B) through an infracolic approach. The patient's head is to the right. The tumor is being rotated medially by the surgeon's hand to reveal the left ureter, indicated by forceps. (B) Left adrenal pheochromocytoma. (A, Courtesy Dr. Stan Sidhu.)

Surgery is curative in more than 90% of pheochromocytoma cases. Although these tumors are highly vascular and tend to adhere to adjacent structures (Fig. 40.19), most of them can be removed successfully by a laparoscopic approach. Laparoscopic resection is contraindicated when preoperative imaging demonstrates local invasion. Open resection should be considered for larger (>6 cm) pheochromocytomas depending on surgeon experience to prevent tumor rupture, which can lead to local recurrence even in benign cases.[40] Advances in surgical technique have resulted in reduced operative complication rates. Specifically, functional image-guided focused exploration has replaced bilateral adrenal and retroperitoneal exploration, leading to diminished rates of solid organ injury.

Molecular Genetics of Pheochromocytoma

A number of reports describing novel germline mutations have demonstrated that familial pheochromocytomas are much more common than previously believed. Before 2000, pheochromocytoma was known to be associated with multiple endocrine neoplasia type 2 syndromes (40%–50% penetrant), von Hippel-Lindau syndrome (10% to 20% penetrant), and neurofibromatosis type 1 (1%–5% penetrant). The discovery that neuroendocrine cells of the carotid body proliferate in response to hypoxic stimuli has led to the identification of mutations in the succinate dehydrogenase gene family in kindreds affected with pheochromocytoma or paraganglioma. Succinate dehydrogenase, which is made up of four subunits, is localized to the mitochondria and catalyzes essential steps in oxidative phosphorylation. Germline mutations in the B and D subunits, inherited in an autosomal dominant fashion, have been identified in approximately 10% of apparently sporadic pheochromocytoma cases. Thus, there is consensus that at least one third of patients with pheochromocytoma have a germline mutation.[41]

Familial cases are manifested at an earlier age and are more likely to be multifocal (Table 40.5). Succinate dehydrogenase B mutation carriers have high rates of extra-adrenal (abdominal or thoracic) pheochromocytomas and malignant disease, whereas succinate dehydrogenase D carriers tend to present with multiple tumors and hormonally inactive paragangliomas of the head and neck. The lifetime penetrance of succinate dehydrogenase mutations is estimated at more than 75%. Genetic counseling should be considered in all patients, particularly those younger than 45 years and those with multiple tumors, extra-adrenal location, and previous head and neck paraganglioma. The discovery of a germline mutation may influence prognosis and surveillance, prompt additional investigations, and enable early identification of affected family members. Cortical-sparing adrenalectomy should be considered in cases of familial pheochromocytoma where the risk of contralateral pheochromocytoma is high. Preservation of at least one third of one adrenal gland is necessary to allow for adequate cortical function without the need for exogenous steroids.[40]

Malignant Pheochromocytoma

Depending on the underlying genotype, 2.5% to 40% of pheochromocytomas are malignant. Survival at 5 years ranges from 20% to 45%.[42] No histopathologic criteria for determining malignancy have demonstrated the ability to predict the clinical course accurately. Thus, malignancy is defined by the development of metastases (i.e., tumor implants distant from the primary mass in locations in which neuroectodermal tissues are not normally found). The latter criterion distinguishes metastatic disease from possible multifocal primary disease. The most common sites of metastasis are the axial skeleton, lymph nodes, liver, lung, and kidney. Treatment of primary and recurrent disease centers on surgical resection, which, even in the absence of cure, may have significant palliative benefits in terms of managing mass effect in critical anatomic locations and reducing the systemic impact of catecholamine excess.[43]

Malignant pheochromocytomas are minimally responsive to radiotherapy and chemotherapy. In a recent phase 2 study, high-dose ^{131}I-MIBG radionuclide therapy was shown to achieve a complete or partial response rate of 22% in select patients with metastatic pheochromocytoma.[44] Significant hematologic toxicities were observed, and long-term benefit remains uncommon. Chronic medical management of catecholamine excess should be performed with α_1-adrenergic selective blockers because of their favorable side-effect profile.

TABLE 40.5 **Hereditary syndromes associated with pheochromocytoma.**

SYNDROME	GENE MUTATION	PHENOTYPE
Multiple endocrine neoplasia type 2A	*RET*	Medullary thyroid cancer, primary hyperparathyroidism
Multiple endocrine neoplasia type 2B	*RET*	Medullary thyroid cancer, marfanoid habitus, mucosal neuromas
Neurofibromatosis type 1 (von Recklinghausen disease)	*NF1*	Neurofibromas, café au lait spots, Lisch nodules (benign iris hamartomas)
von Hippel-Lindau	*VHL*	Retinal angioma, central nervous system hemangioblastoma, renal cell cancer, primitive neuroectodermal tumor, pancreatic and renal cysts
Familial paraganglioma syndrome	*SDHA, SDHB, SDHC, SDHD, SDHAF2*	Gastrointestinal stromal tumor *SDHB* may be associated with renal cell cancer
Hereditary pheochromocytoma	*TMEM127*	Possibly other tumors
Hereditary pheochromocytoma	*MAX*	Possibly other tumors
Hereditary pheochromocytoma	*HIF2A*	Familial polycythemia, somatostatinomas

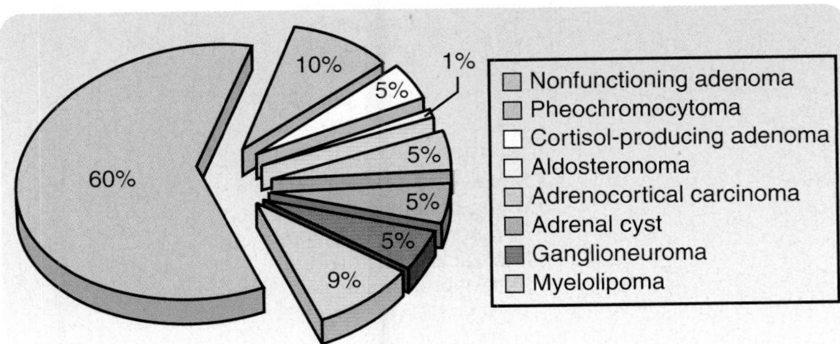

FIG. 40.20 Differential diagnosis of adrenal incidentaloma in patients without a history of malignant disease. Approximate proportions of the various pathologic processes are shown.

OTHER ADRENAL DISEASES

Incidentally Discovered Adrenal Mass (Incidentaloma)

Epidemiology and Differential Diagnosis

Incidentally discovered adrenal masses, also termed *clinically inapparent adrenal masses* or *incidentalomas*, are discovered through imaging performed for unrelated nonadrenal disease. Their existence as a clinical entity is a byproduct of advanced medical imaging. Incidentalomas were first described in the early 1980s, when CT scanners became more prevalent in developed nations, and they have become a common clinical problem as the use of CT and MRI has become widespread. Incidentalomas have been found in up to 8% of autopsies and 1% to 4% of abdominal imaging studies. The prevalence increases to as high as 10% in patients older than 60 years.[45]

The differential diagnosis of adrenal incidentaloma is wide and includes secreting and nonsecreting neoplasms (Fig. 40.20). In patients with a history of malignant disease, metastatic disease is the most likely cause of adrenal masses, particularly when they are bilateral (see later, "Metastases to the Adrenal Gland"). In those without a clear history of malignant disease, at least 80% of incidentalomas will turn out to be nonfunctioning cortical adenomas or other benign lesions that do not require surgical management. Thus, in most patients, the most important aspect of management is to distinguish the subset of adrenal masses that are likely to have a clinical impact from the large proportion that are not.

Clinical Evaluation and Surgical Management

The workup of the adrenal incidentaloma integrates hormonal evaluation with size criteria. The principles and methods of hormonal evaluation have been discussed in the tumor-specific sections (see earlier) and are generally applicable to incidentalomas. However, one conceptual difference is that the biochemical thresholds that prompt operative treatment are somewhat lower in patients with an initial radiographic presentation (incidentalomas) compared with those with an initial clinical presentation. This is because tumor size, which correlates strongly with risk of malignancy, contributes an additive effect in favor of surgical management.

Evaluation begins with history taking, with a focus on prior malignant disease, hypertension, and symptoms of glucocorticoid or sex steroid excess. Biochemical investigations for hormonally active tumors are followed by consideration of size criteria (Fig. 40.21). In a general sense, surgery is recommended for hormonally active tumors and those that carry a significant risk of malignancy. Adrenocortical carcinomas represent less than 2% of adrenal tumors measuring 4 cm or smaller and roughly 6% of those measuring 4 to 6 cm. Tumors larger than 6 cm carry a more than 25% risk of malignancy. Because studies have consistently found that CT and MRI underestimate adrenal tumor size by approximately 20%, an effect that is exaggerated in smaller tumors, our practice is to remove all incidentalomas measuring 4 cm or larger in low-risk surgical patients. We strongly consider removal of those measuring 3 to 4 cm, particularly in younger patients who wish to avoid the burden of surveillance imaging.

Factors that should be considered in surgical decision-making for this latter group include suspicious imaging characteristics, the patient's age and surgical risk, growth on interval imaging, and the patient's preference. Characteristics suggestive of a benign lesion on CT scan include homogeneous appearance, well-defined borders, high lipid content, rapid washout of contrast material,

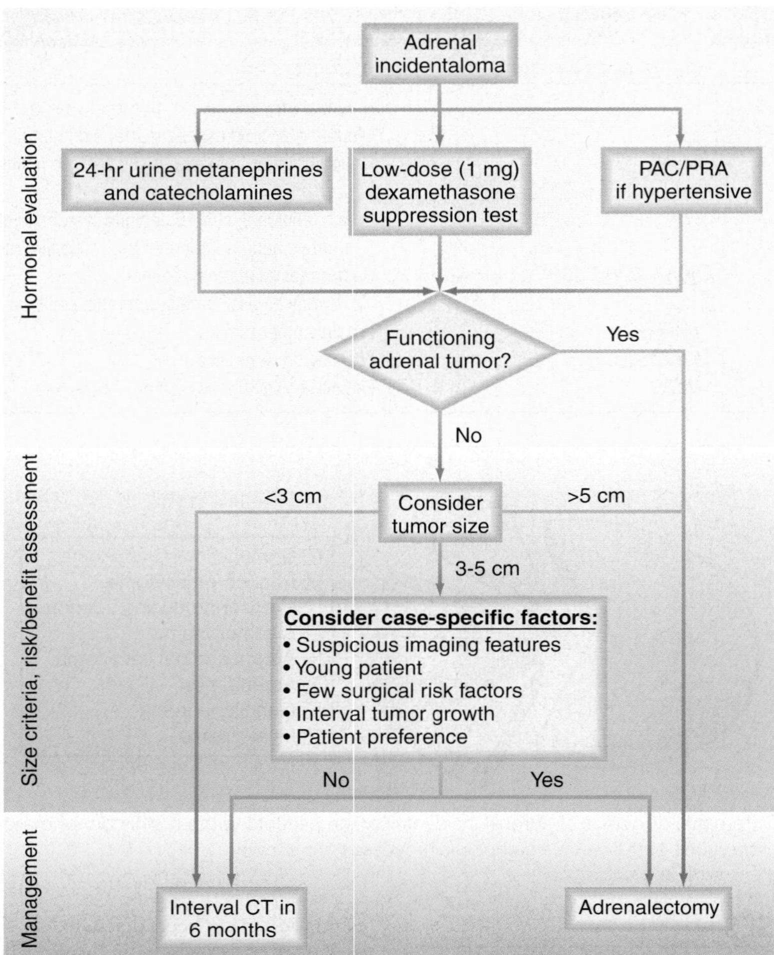

FIG. 40.21 Algorithm for the management of an adrenal incidentaloma. Adrenalectomy is recommended for all patients with functional tumors. For nonfunctioning tumors, the risk for malignancy is assessed according to size. Tumors larger than 5 cm on computed tomography carry a more than 25% risk for malignancy and need to be removed. Those smaller than 3 cm can be safely observed. Case-specific factors must be considered for intermediate-sized tumors. *CT*, Computed tomography; *PAC*, plasma aldosterone concentration, in ng/dL; *PRA*, plasma renin activity, in ng/(mL • hr).

and low degree of vascularity. Features that are concerning for malignancy include irregular or ill-defined borders, necrosis, internal calcifications or hemorrhage, and high vascularity. ^{18}F-FDG PET is usually reserved for suspicious cases and has high sensitivity and specificity for distinguishing between benign and malignant adrenal lesions, although it cannot differentiate between a metastasis and primary adrenocortical carcinoma. If observation is chosen, patients should undergo repeated imaging in 6 to 12 months and then on an annual basis for a few more years, given the fact that 5% to 25% of adrenal masses may increase in size.

It must be emphasized that CT-guided fine-needle aspiration is rarely helpful in the evaluation of adrenal masses and may be hazardous. The diagnosis of primary adrenal malignancy cannot reliably be made on the basis of cytologic criteria alone. Therefore, the use of fine-needle aspiration is generally confined to patients with a history of extra-adrenal malignancy in whom the clinician seeks to establish the diagnosis of metastatic disease. In all cases, pheochromocytoma must be excluded before attempting such a procedure to avoid precipitating potentially fatal hypertensive crisis.

As with the other disease processes that have been discussed, most adrenal incidentalomas can be removed laparoscopically, except for those displaying obvious malignant features on imaging. No upper size limit to this approach has been established, and tumors measuring 15 cm have been successfully removed laparoscopically by experienced surgeons. Our usual threshold is about 8 cm for the right and 10 cm for the left adrenal gland.

Metastases to the Adrenal Gland

Epidemiology and Clinical Features

The adrenal glands are common sites of metastasis because of their rich vascular supply. Autopsy studies have revealed that approximately 25% of patients with carcinomas eventually develop adrenal involvement. In 50% of these cases, metastatic disease is bilateral. The primary cancers that most often spread to the adrenals are those of the lung, gastrointestinal tract, breast, kidney, pancreas, and skin (melanoma). Patients with isolated adrenal metastases represent a very small subset of the total. However, these individuals are of particular interest to the surgeon and oncologist because resection of isolated adrenal metastases may improve survival. Depending on the underlying disease, 5-year survival rates of approximately 25% can be achieved after adrenalectomy for metastasis.

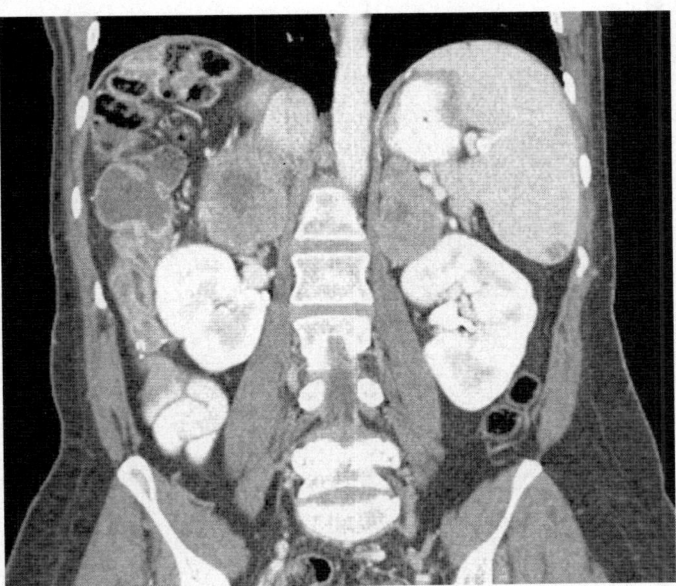

FIG. 40.22 Isolated bilateral 7-cm adrenal metastases from colorectal cancer causing adrenal insufficiency. The patient had undergone previous right colectomy and right hepatectomy. Bilateral adrenal metastasectomy was performed laparoscopically.

Clinical Evaluation and Surgical Management

Evaluation of patients presenting with isolated adrenal metastases must involve careful exclusion of extra-adrenal disease with CT or MRI (including the head in cases of breast cancer or melanoma, and triphasic contrast-enhanced CT evaluation of the liver plus 3-mm slices through the lungs for gastrointestinal malignant neoplasms) as well as bone and PET scans, when appropriate. Patients presenting with isolated bilateral adrenal metastases (Fig. 40.22) must be evaluated for adrenal insufficiency because of replacement of all normal adrenal tissue with tumor, which may occur in up to 30% of these patients. This is best performed with measurement of morning cortisol and ACTH levels. Cortical insufficiency should be adequately treated before operation to avoid perioperative adrenal crisis.

Most adrenal metastases are well encapsulated and are thus amenable to laparoscopic resection. Complete adrenal metastasectomy has yielded mean survival rates of up to 3 years compared with 12 months for patients undergoing incomplete resection and 6 months for patients not undergoing surgical therapy.[46]

TECHNICAL ASPECTS OF ADRENALECTOMY

Choice of Operative Approach

In our practice, approximately 90% of adrenalectomies are performed laparoscopically. Laparoscopic adrenalectomy affords many advantages, including reduced length of hospitalization, reduced pain, decreased operative blood loss, and lower rate of postoperative complications, compared with conventional open surgery. Similar degrees of benefit are observed with laparoscopic transabdominal and posterior retroperitoneoscopic approaches. One randomized controlled trial demonstrated reduced postoperative pain and faster recovery after the posterior retroperitoneoscopic approach.[47] We currently employ both techniques and favor the retroperitoneoscopic approach for tumors smaller than 6 cm, for bilateral tumors, and in patients with a history of extensive prior abdominal surgery. The retroperitoneoscopic approach is more challenging in older, obese male patients because of increased retroperitoneal fat, making initial entry and orientation more difficult. Severe obesity (body mass index >35) results in compression of the retroperitoneum by the abdominal viscera when the patient is in the prone position and is a relative contraindication to the retroperitoneoscopic approach, depending on the surgeon's experience. The lateral transabdominal technique offers a wider operative field and greater versatility, and it is well suited for larger tumors and obese patients. The overall conversion rate to open adrenalectomy is less than 5% with either technique in large series.[48]

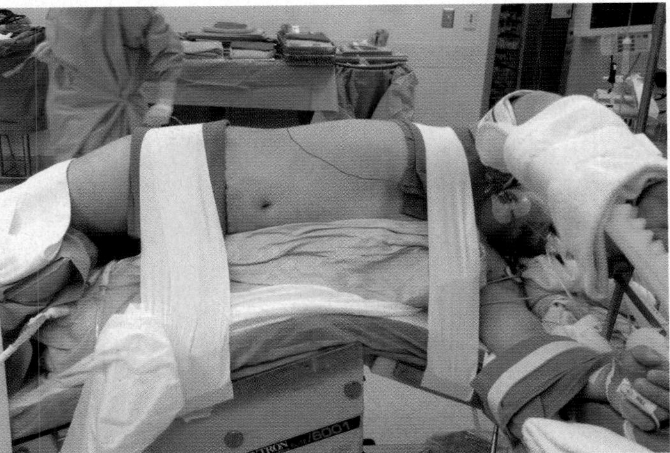

FIG. 40.23 Positioning of the patient for left lateral transabdominal laparoscopic adrenalectomy.

As noted, open adrenalectomy should be performed for primary adrenal tumors demonstrating features suggestive of malignancy, such as large size (>8 cm), clinical feminization, hypersecretion of multiple steroid hormones, or any of the following imaging attributes: local or vascular invasion, regional adenopathy, and metastases. For open adrenalectomy, we prefer a transabdominal approach, which is performed through a subcostal incision (see later).

Laparoscopic Lateral Transabdominal Adrenalectomy

Patient Preparation and Positioning

Draw sheets and a full-length beanbag are placed on the operating table in advance. It is important that the table be capable of flexion and have a kidney rest that can be elevated. The patient is initially positioned supine for induction of anesthesia and placement of a urinary catheter. Intermittent pneumatic compression devices are applied to the legs. The placement of an orogastric or nasogastric tube for gastric decompression is frequently helpful, particularly in treating left-sided lesions. The patient is then turned on his or her side (80-degree lateral decubitus position), with the side of the lesion facing upward (Fig. 40.23). At this point, the patient is carefully positioned cephalocaudally so that the 10th rib is directly over the break point in the table. The table is flexed and the beanbag rigidified in a position that supports the buttocks and back while leaving the umbilicus, an important surface landmark, exposed. Flexing the table and raising the kidney rest serve to widen the space between the costal margin and iliac crest and to drop the iliac crest away from the plane of the laparoscopic instruments. Wide cloth tape is used to secure the patient to the table at the chest, hips, and lower extremities. Great care must be taken to protect bone prominences and points of potential peripheral

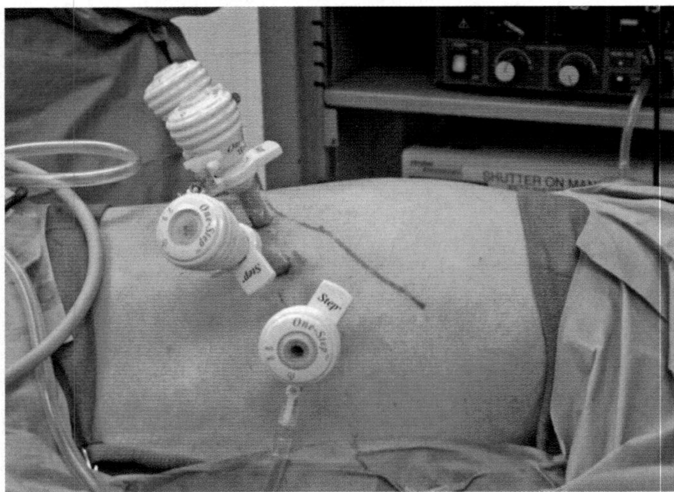

FIG. 40.24 Port placement for right laparoscopic adrenalectomy. The patient is lying right-side up, with the head toward the right. The *marked line* denotes the costal margin. Ports are placed approximately 2 cm inferior to the costal margin, spaced about four fingerbreadths apart.

nerve compression in the extremities. The surgical preparation is carried from the nipple line to the pubis and from the umbilicus to the midline of the back.

Careful positioning is essential for technical success in laparoscopic adrenalectomy. As will be discussed, the surgeon is reliant on gravity to serve as a retractor for providing the necessary exposure. Having the patient securely fixed to the table permits the often extreme positioning with respect to pitch (Trendelenburg, reverse Trendelenburg) and roll (tilting left, right) that is necessary during the operation.

Technique

Left adrenal. Initial peritoneal access is achieved 2 cm inferior to the costal margin in the midclavicular line (Palmer point). This can be performed with the Veress technique or using an optical trocar in most cases. We generally use three radially dilating trocars, and a fourth may be added in cases in which the spleen and pancreatic tail require additional retraction. The ports are equally distributed along the costal margin, with the posterior port placed as far lateral-posterior as permitted by the position of the colon (Fig. 40.24). It is advisable to leave at least 5 cm (4 fingerbreadths) between each port to minimize external interference of the laparoscopic instruments. For tissue dissection, we employ the hook monopolar cautery and an energy-based tissue sealing or dividing device.

The lateral attachments of the spleen are taken down first, with the goal of rotating the left upper quadrant viscera anteromedially. Care must be taken to avoid a capsular tear of the spleen, which may arise from undue tension on a congenital or acquired adhesive band. Splenic mobilization is continued until the greater curvature of the stomach becomes visible at its apex, at which point the spleen and tail of the pancreas are allowed to fall anteriorly with rightward tilting of the table and gentle use of the fan retractor, if necessary. It is critical to achieve the correct plane of dissection precisely during this part of the procedure because the tail of the pancreas and splenic vessels are potentially vulnerable to injury. In patients with large or inferiorly positioned tumors, the splenic flexure of the colon must be mobilized caudally by dividing the splenocolic ligament. We use an open book technique, which involves developing the cleft-like plane just medial to the

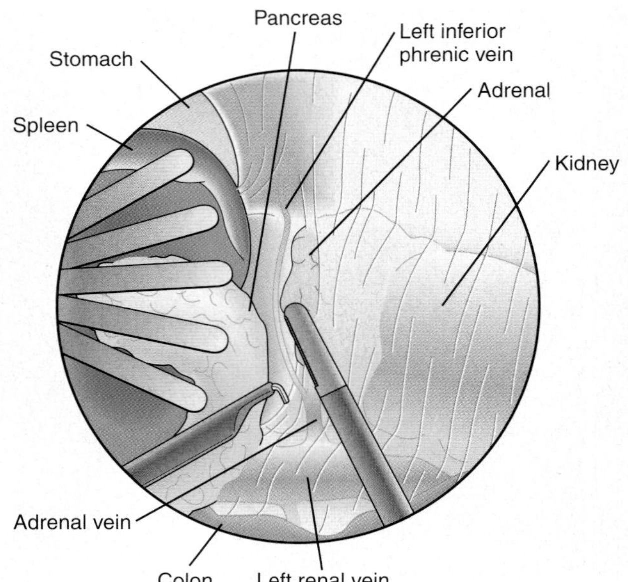

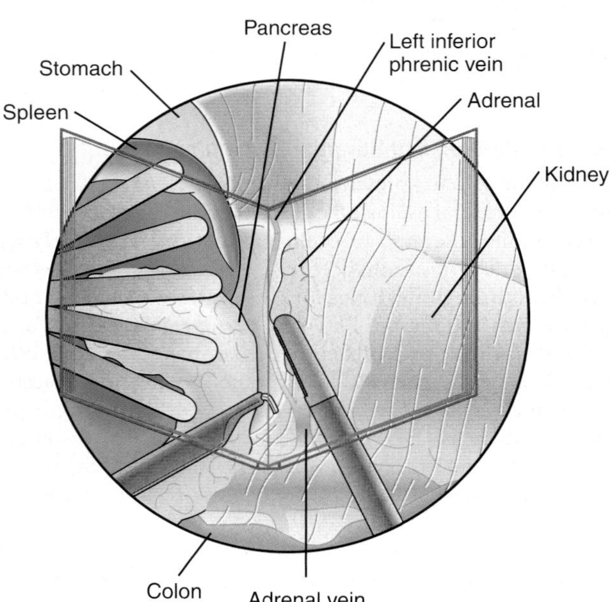

FIG. 40.25 Technique of left laparoscopic adrenalectomy. The spleen and pancreatic tail have been mobilized and retracted anteromedially to expose the adrenal gland. The cleft of the open book is developed in a superior to inferior direction to identify the inferior phrenic vein and adrenal vein.

adrenal gland and lateral to the aorta (Fig. 40.25). The left-hand page of the book is composed of the spleen, tail of the pancreas, and greater curvature of the stomach. The right-hand page of the book is made up by the kidney and adrenal tumor. The left crus of the diaphragm is a useful landmark that leads the surgeon to the left inferior phrenic vein.

As mentioned in the anatomy section of this chapter, the left inferior phrenic vein courses along the medial aspect of the left adrenal gland before joining with the left adrenal vein. By developing the cleft of the open book, moving from superior to inferior, the adrenal vein is encountered at the inferomedial aspect of the adrenal gland. The small adrenal arteries that lie within this plane can be handled with energy-based coagulation. The left adrenal

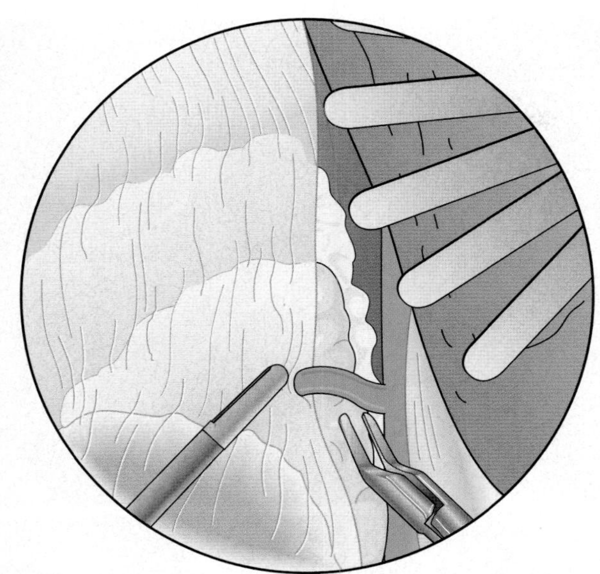

FIG. 40.26 Technique of right laparoscopic adrenalectomy. The liver has been mobilized and retracted medially to expose the adrenal gland and inferior vena cava. The space just medial to the adrenal gland is developed to identify the adrenal vasculature.

vein is carefully dissected out, aggressively coagulated or clipped, and divided. The inferior tip of the left adrenal gland may extend low, approaching the renal hilum within millimeters. However, because the left adrenal vein is rather long (2 cm), it is generally not necessary to expose the renal vasculature during left adrenalectomy. Many patients have a superior pole renal artery branch that approaches the inferior aspect of the left adrenal gland. Injury to this structure must be carefully avoided by keeping dissection close to the adrenal capsule while the specimen is elevated away from the medial aspect of the superior pole of the left kidney.

The adrenal gland is liberated by completing dissection circumferentially and posteriorly, taking the specimen off of the superior pole of the kidney and posterior abdominal wall. These attachments are deliberately divided last because they aid in suspending the adrenal gland on the lateral-superior wall of the operative field, providing exposure of the medial vascular plane during the critical initial portion of the procedure. The tumor is placed into a resilient catchment device, morcellated, and extracted. If noncutting trocars are used, only the skin will need to be closed.

Right Adrenal. Laparoscopic right adrenalectomy is, in some respects, a mirror image of the procedure just described. During right adrenalectomy, the left-hand page of the open book is made up by the kidney and adrenal tumor and the right-hand page is composed of the bare area of the liver (Fig. 40.26). To gain access to the appropriate plane, the right triangular ligament of the liver must first be completely mobilized and the liver allowed to rotate anteromedially. On the right side, the colon usually lies well inferior to the operative field. When developing the space between the adrenal gland and inferior vena cava from superior to inferior, the surgeon must be mindful of adrenal vein variants, as illustrated in the anatomy section of this chapter (see Fig. 40.3). The right adrenal vein is a potentially perilous structure to manage because it is short, wide, variable, and confluent with thin-walled, large-capacitance vessels (the inferior vena cava in more than 80% of cases, followed by the renal vein and, uncommonly, the right hepatic vein) that can bleed briskly if directly injured (e.g., by the cautery), lacerated from undue traction on adjacent structures, or

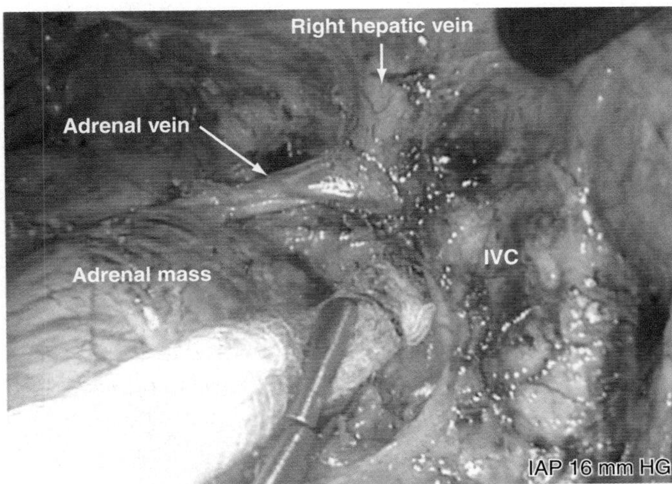

FIG. 40.27 Right adrenal vein variant. This solitary adrenal vein arises from the superior apex of the gland and drains into the confluence of the inferior vena cava *(IVC)* and right hepatic vein, as shown in Fig. 40.3F.

sheared by clips. A significant second adrenal vein may be found in up to 10% of patients. By methodically dissecting one layer at a time and moving from superior to inferior, all potential adrenal vein variants can be encountered in a controlled fashion (Fig. 40.27). The adrenal vein must be dissected out delicately, definitively ligated (usually with two clips on the patient's side), and then divided. Loss of control of the adrenal vein stump should be avoided; should this occur, conversion to an open procedure may be necessary. A conceptual contrast between left and right adrenalectomy is that left adrenalectomy centers on identification of the correct plane of dissection and right adrenalectomy centers on the avoidance of venous bleeding.

Of note, the junction of the inferior vena cava and right renal vein is frequently difficult to identify. In vivo, the transition is a gradual curve rather than the 90-degree takeoff depicted in anatomy texts. Therefore, it cannot be used as a reliable anatomic landmark for identification of the adrenal vein. After control of the vein, the remaining mobilization of the right adrenal gland is straightforward because the inferomedial limb generally does not reach as far down toward the renal hilum as on the left side.

Posterior Retroperitoneoscopic Adrenalectomy

Posterior retroperitoneoscopic adrenalectomy was popularized in 1994 by Walz and associates.[49] The technique has undergone a series of refinements so that now a subset of lean patients with tumors smaller than 4 cm in diameter can be managed by a novel single-access technique.[50] The retroperitoneal approach has several advantages, including avoidance of mobilization of the solid organs that is necessary with transabdominal approaches, elimination of the need for repositioning during bilateral adrenalectomy, and avoidance of anterior adhesions in patients with extensive prior abdominal surgery. One disadvantage is the relatively small working space, which makes the retroperitoneal technique best suited for tumors smaller than 7 cm in diameter.

A prone position is used, with supports placed under the lower chest and pelvic girdle so that the abdomen is allowed to hang anteriorly (Fig. 40.28A). Three ports are placed inferior to the twelfth rib (Fig. 40.28B) using a direct cut-down technique for initial access. Relatively high insufflation pressures of 20 to 28 mm Hg are used and have caused no complications in regard to air emboli,

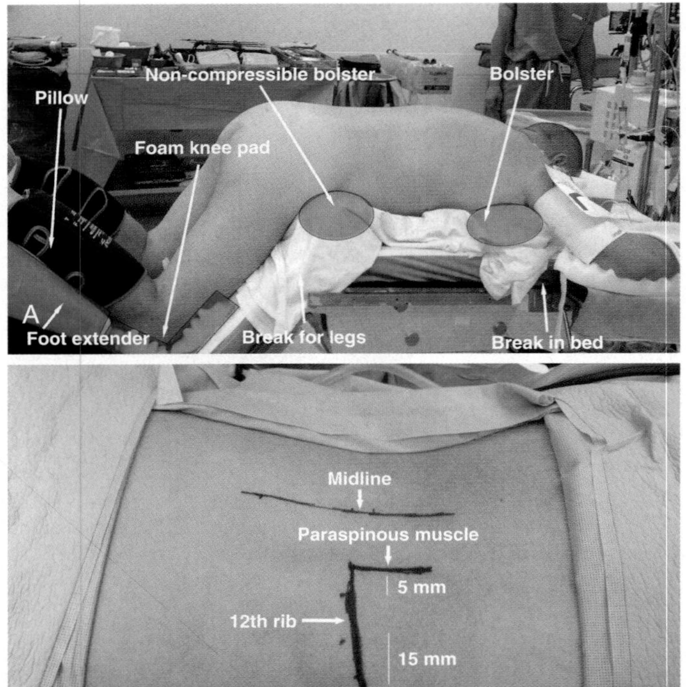

FIG. 40.28 (A) Positioning of the patient for posterior retroperitoneoscopic adrenalectomy. (B) Port placement for posterior retroperitoneoscopic adrenalectomy.

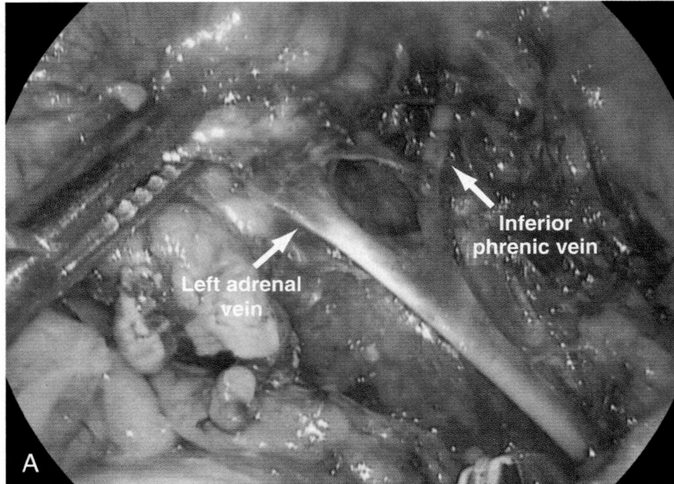

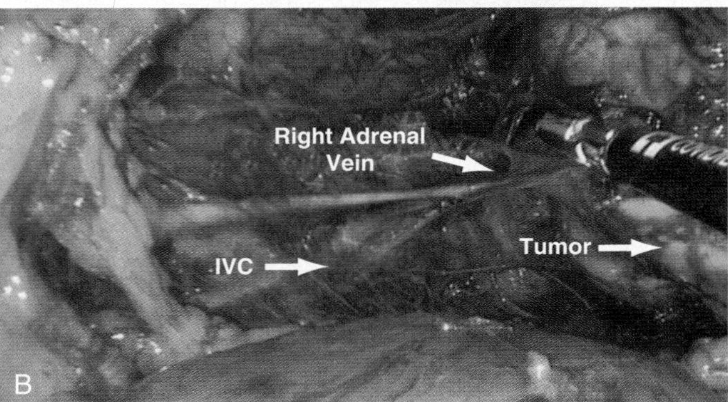

FIG. 40.29 (A) Posterior view of the left adrenal vein. (B) Posterior view of the right adrenal vein. *IVC*, Inferior vena cava.

hypercapnia, or clinically significant soft tissue emphysema. The working space is initially created by bluntly dissecting the retroperitoneal contents anteriorly away from the ports. The upper pole of the kidney is mobilized and reflected inferiorly to expose the adrenal gland. Mobilization of the adrenal gland begins near the paraspinous muscles, at the inferomedial aspect of the gland. This is where the left adrenal vein is almost always encountered early in the procedure (Fig. 40.29A). On the right side, the vein is encountered slightly later as dissection proceeds superiorly (Fig. 40.29B). The small adrenal arteries that run within the medial vascular space are coagulated. After the superior apex of the adrenal gland is mobilized, dissection proceeds circumferentially to include the periadrenal fat.

Complications and Postoperative Care

Potential technical complications include venous hemorrhage and bleeding from solid organ capsular injuries. Small amounts of bleeding can often be managed with coagulation or direct pressure using a rolled Kittner gauze. Hollow viscus injuries are uncommon but may be associated with procedures performed in patients with prior major abdominal surgery. Pancreatic injuries and fistulas have been reported with left-sided procedures; these are rare complications, as are port site hernias and port site metastases in cases of malignant disease. Violation of the tumor capsule and tumor spillage can lead to tumor recurrence, especially in the case of pheochromocytoma. Patients undergoing laparoscopic adrenalectomy for Cushing syndrome are at risk for surgical site infections because of their catabolic and immunosuppressed state. These include port site infections in 5% of patients and, rarely, subphrenic abscesses requiring catheter drainage. One complication specific to the retroperitoneal approach is injury of the subcostal nerve causing relaxation or hypoesthesia of the abdominal wall, which occurs in 8% of cases and is usually temporary.

Patients who undergo laparoscopic adrenalectomy recover rapidly. Most patients, including approximately 50% of those treated for pheochromocytoma, can leave the hospital on the first postoperative day. In the treatment of adrenal tumors, successful outcomes hinge on excellent perioperative medical management as much as technical skill, particularly in cases of pheochromocytoma and Cushing syndrome. These considerations were discussed earlier.

Open Anterior Transabdominal Adrenalectomy

Patient Preparation and Positioning

Neuraxial blockade (use of an epidural catheter) is routinely used for intraoperative and postoperative anesthetic or analgesic management. The patient is positioned supine, with the ipsilateral side slightly elevated on a bolster (Fig. 40.30). A urinary catheter, orogastric or nasogastric tube, and intermittent pneumatic compression devices are placed. The surgical preparation is carried from the nipple line to the pubis and down to the table on either side.

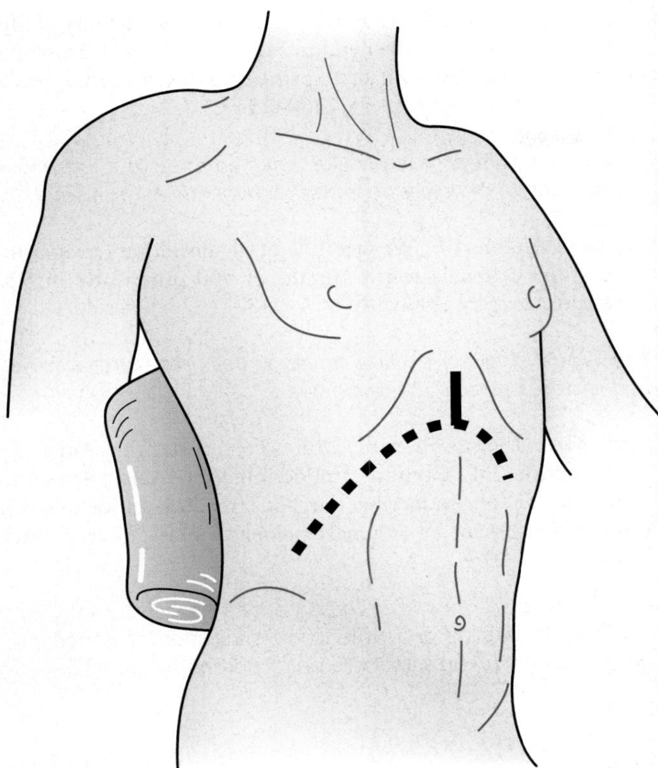

FIG. 40.30 Positioning of the patient for open right adrenalectomy.

Technique

Left Adrenal. We prefer to use a subcostal incision, which may be extended across the midline (chevron), with or without a vertical upper midline extension, to achieve wide exposure. The left adrenal can be exposed by entering the lesser sac through the gastrocolic ligament and incising the retroperitoneum inferior to the tail of the pancreas or by rotating the spleen, pancreatic tail, and stomach anteromedially, as described earlier in the section on laparoscopic adrenalectomy. We use the latter approach in our practice. The splenic flexure of the colon is mobilized inferiorly, and the plane medial to the adrenal gland is developed. The adrenal vein is isolated, tied in continuity, and divided. The small adrenal arteries can be ligated or electrocoagulated and the specimen removed after circumferential dissection is completed.

Right Adrenal. Open right adrenalectomy begins with complete mobilization of the right lobe of the liver, including the lateral attachments and the falciform ligament. The adrenal can be exposed by rotating the liver medially or, more commonly, retracting the inferoposterior segments cephalad using long padded retractors (liver, renal vein, Deaver, or Harrington types). The retroperitoneum is entered by performing a Kocher maneuver (Fig. 40.31), and the inferior vena cava is exposed by medial reflection of the duodenum. The plane between the adrenal gland and inferior vena cava is developed first. Vascular structures, which may be numerous in highly angiogenic tumors, are ligated sequentially. The adrenal vein is isolated, securely tied, and divided. Loss of control of the adrenal vein stump may be managed with the application of a side-biting (Satinsky) vascular clamp. As noted, open adrenalectomy is generally performed in cases of suspected or known malignant disease (Fig. 40.32). Locally invasive right-sided adrenal tumors can be challenging to manage, given their frequent invasion of adjacent venous structures (Fig. 40.33A). It is our practice to involve an experienced vascular or liver surgeon in the management of tumors with extensive venous invasion. Locally invaded organs, most commonly the kidney, should be resected en bloc with the primary mass. Complete radical resection is a critical determinant of survival in patients with malignant adrenal tumors; in some cases, this can be achieved only if immediate venous reconstruction is performed (Fig. 40.33B).

Complications and Postoperative Care

Technical complications of open adrenalectomy include venous hemorrhage, tumor embolization in cases with intravascular tumor extension, and solid-organ injury. Postoperative complications are similar to those associated with other major abdominal procedures. Most patients experience return of bowel function within 3 to 4 days and are able to leave the hospital on postoperative day 5 to 7.

SELECTED REFERENCES

Benn DE, Gimenez-Roqueplo AP, Reilly JR, et al. Clinical presentation and penetrance of pheochromocytoma/paraganglioma syndromes. *J Clin Endocrinol Metab*. 2006;91:827–836.

International SDH Consortium study elucidating genotype–phenotype associations in patients with pheochromocytoma/paraganglioma.

Chen Y, Scholten A, Chomsky-Higgins K, et al. Risk factors associated with perioperative complications and prolonged length of stay after laparoscopic adrenalectomy. *JAMA Surg*. 2018;153:1036–1041.

The largest single-institution series on laparoscopic transperitoneal adrenalectomy.

Fassnacht M, Terzolo M, Allolio B, et al. Combination chemotherapy in advanced adrenocortical carcinoma. *N Engl J Med*. 2012;366:2189–2197.

Until recently, mitotane has been the only accepted systemic therapy for patients with adrenocortical cancer. This randomized study of 304 patients in Europe showed improved progression-free survival in patients treated with multidrug chemotherapy in addition to mitotane.

Gifford Jr RW, Kvale WF, Maher FT, et al. Clinical features, diagnosis and treatment of pheochromocytoma: a review of 76 cases. *Mayo Clin Proc*. 1964;39:281–302.

A landmark account of the biochemical, pharmacologic, and physiologic advances that allowed collaborators at the Mayo Clinic to treat 76 patients with pheochromocytoma while experiencing only one death.

Lenders JW, Duh QY, Eisenhofer G, et al. Pheochromocytoma and paraganglioma: an Endocrine Society clinical practice guideline. *J Clin Endocrinol Metab*. 2014;99:1915–1942.

Consensus guidelines from the Endocrine Society recommending the appropriate biochemical, imaging, and genetic evaluations as well as treatment for patients with pheochromocytoma and paraganglioma.

Lectures Nobel. *Physiology or Medicine 1942–1962*. Amsterdam: Elsevier Publishing Company; 1964.

An account of the clinical discoveries and advances in organic chemistry that led to the identification, isolation, and artificial synthesis of adrenal cortical hormones. A full transcript can be found at http://nobelprize.org.

Lectures Nobel. *Physiology or Medicine 1971–1980*. Amsterdam: Elsevier Publishing Company; 1992.

Documents the formidable challenges surmounted in the identification of peptide hormones found in such minute concentrations and the development of the radioimmunoassay necessary for their detection. A full transcript can be found at http://nobelprize.org.

Sukor N, Kogovsek C, Gordon RD, et al. Improved quality of life, blood pressure, and biochemical status following laparoscopic adrenalectomy for unilateral primary aldosteronism. *J Clin Endocrinol Metab*. 2010;95:1360–1364.

This prospective pilot study examines an array of short-term outcomes after surgical treatment of hyperaldosteronism.

Walz MK, Alesina PF, Wenger FA, et al. Posterior retroperitoneoscopic adrenalectomy—results of 560 procedures in 520 patients. *Surgery*. 2006;140:943–948.

The largest single-institution series on this procedure, written by the developers of the technique.

Zeiger MA, Thompson GB, Duh QY, et al. The American Association of Clinical Endocrinologists and American Association of Endocrine Surgeons medical guidelines for the management of adrenal incidentalomas. *Endocr Pract*. 2009;15:1–20.

Consensus guidelines from the American Association of Clinical Endocrinologists and American Association of Endocrine Surgeons on workup and treatment of adrenal incidentalomas.

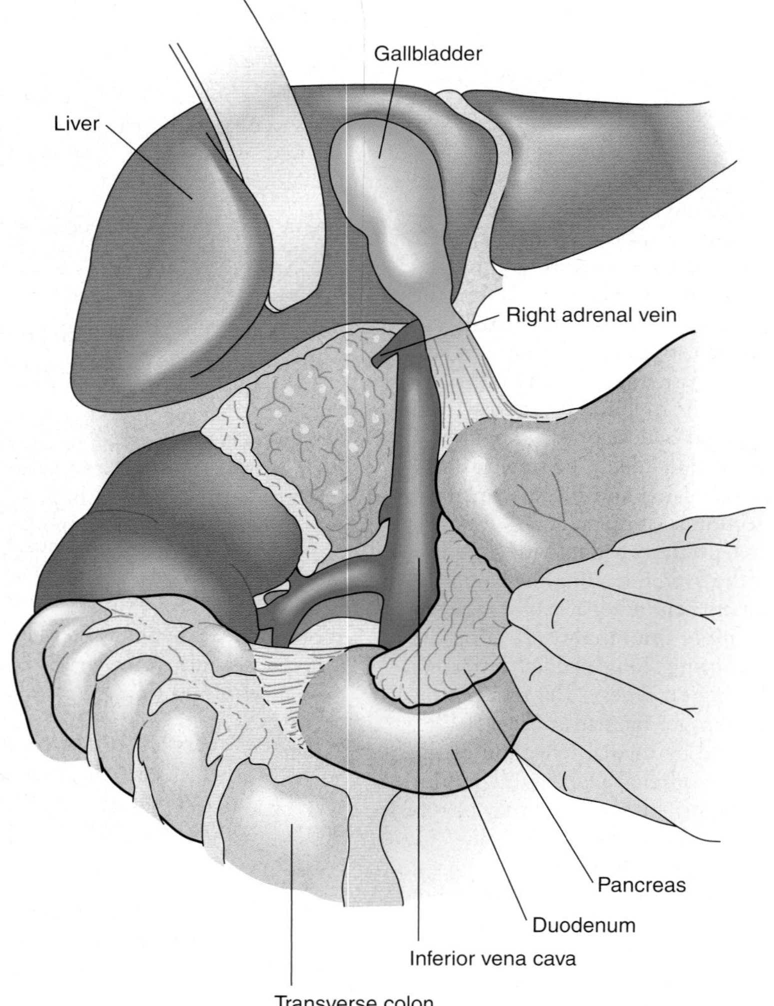

FIG. 40.31 Open right adrenalectomy. The right lobe of the liver and the hepatic flexure of the colon have been completely mobilized. The retroperitoneum is entered, and the duodenum and head of the pancreas are reflected medially (Kocher maneuver) to expose the adrenal gland and inferior vena cava.

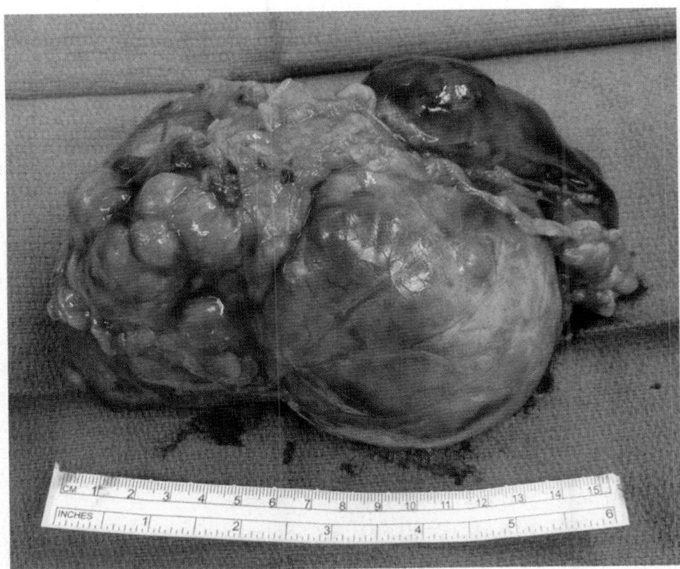

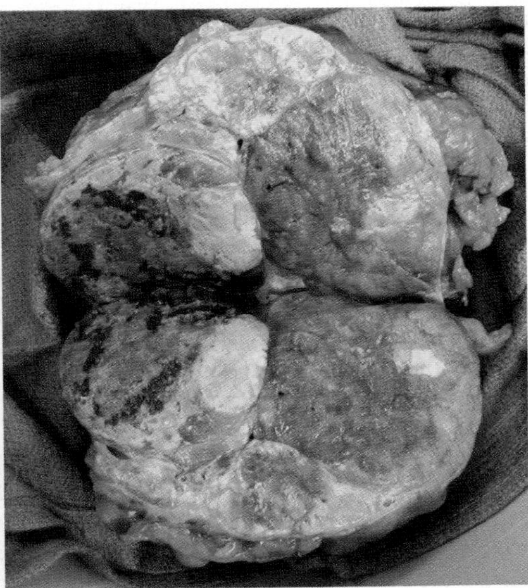

FIG. 40.32 Gross appearance of adrenocortical carcinoma.

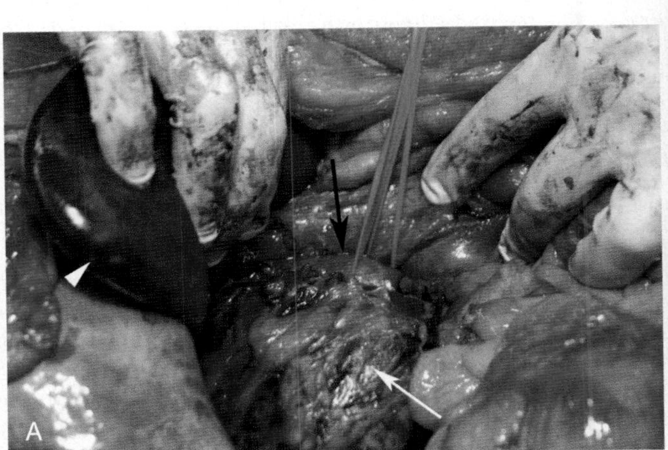

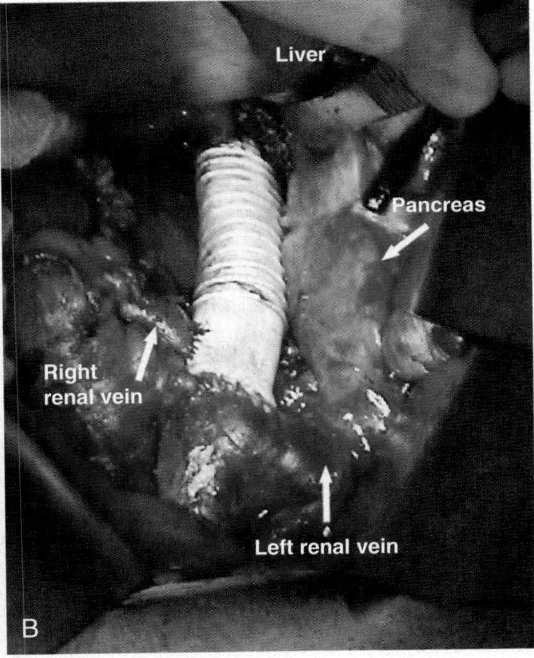

FIG. 40.33 (A) Open resection of a right adrenocortical carcinoma invading the inferior vena cava. The patient's head is to the left. The liver (*arrowhead*) is retracted cephalad. The *white arrow* indicates the tumor; the *black arrow* indicates the inferior vena cava, which is encircled with vessel loops. (B) The infrahepatic inferior vena cava has been replaced with a polytetrafluoroethylene graft.

REFERENCES

1. Lectures Nobel. *Physiology or Medicine 1942–1962*. Amsterdam: Elsevier Publishing Company; 1964.
2. Lectures Nobel. *Physiology or Medicine 1971–1980*. Amsterdam: Elsevier Publishing Company; 1992.
3. Scholten A, Cisco RM, Vriens MR, et al. Variant adrenal venous anatomy in 546 laparoscopic adrenalectomies. *JAMA Surg*. 2013;148:378–383.
4. Lenders JW, Pacak K, Walther MM, et al. Biochemical diagnosis of pheochromocytoma: which test is best? *JAMA*. 2002;287:1427–1434.
5. Bornstein SR, Allolio B, Arlt W, et al. Diagnosis and treatment of primary adrenal insufficiency: an Endocrine Society clinical practice guideline. *J Clin Endocrinol Metab*. 2016;101:364–389.

6. Di Dalmazi G, Berr CM, Fassnacht M, et al. Adrenal function after adrenalectomy for subclinical hypercortisolism and Cushing's syndrome: a systematic review of the literature. *J Clin Endocrinol Metab*. 2014;99:2637–2645.
7. Rochwerg B, Oczkowski SJ, Siemieniuk RAC, et al. Corticosteroids in sepsis: an updated systematic review and meta-analysis. *Crit Care Med*. 2018;46:1411–1420.
8. Marik PE, Varon J. Requirement of perioperative stress doses of corticosteroids: a systematic review of the literature. *Arch Surg*. 2008;143:1222–1226.
9. Kayser SC, Dekkers T, Groenewoud HJ, et al. Study heterogeneity and estimation of prevalence of primary aldosteronism: a systematic review and meta-regression analysis. *J Clin Endocrinol Metab*. 2016;101:2826–2835.
10. Mulatero P, Monticone S, Bertello C, et al. Long-term cardio- and cerebrovascular events in patients with primary aldosteronism. *J Clin Endocrinol Metab*. 2013;98:4826–4833.
11. Boulkroun S, Beuschlein F, Rossi GP, et al. Prevalence, clinical, and molecular correlates of KCNJ5 mutations in primary aldosteronism. *Hypertension*. 2012;59:592–598.
12. Funder JW, Carey RM, Mantero F, et al. The management of primary aldosteronism: case detection, diagnosis, and treatment: an Endocrine Society clinical practice guideline. *J Clin Endocrinol Metab*. 2016;101:1889–1916.
13. Dekkers T, Prejbisz A, Kool LJS, et al. Adrenal vein sampling versus CT scan to determine treatment in primary aldosteronism: an outcome-based randomised diagnostic trial. *Lancet Diabetes Endocrinol*. 2016;4:739–746.
14. Pasternak JD, Epelboym I, Seiser N, et al. Diagnostic utility of data from adrenal venous sampling for primary aldosteronism despite failed cannulation of the right adrenal vein. *Surgery*. 2016;159:267–273.
15. Williams TA, Lenders JWM, Mulatero P, et al. Outcomes after adrenalectomy for unilateral primary aldosteronism: an international consensus on outcome measures and analysis of remission rates in an international cohort. *Lancet Diabetes Endocrinol*. 2017;5:689–699.
16. Shariq OA, Bancos I, Cronin PA, et al. Contralateral suppression of aldosterone at adrenal venous sampling predicts hyperkalemia following adrenalectomy for primary aldosteronism. *Surgery*. 2018;163:183–190.
17. Beuschlein F, Fassnacht M, Assie G, et al. Constitutive activation of PKA catalytic subunit in adrenal Cushing's syndrome. *N Engl J Med*. 2014;370:1019–1028.
18. Lindholm J, Juul S, Jorgensen JO, et al. Incidence and late prognosis of Cushing's syndrome: a population-based study. *J Clin Endocrinol Metab*. 2001;86:117–123.
19. Elias PC, Martinez EZ, Barone BF, et al. Late-night salivary cortisol has a better performance than urinary free cortisol in the diagnosis of Cushing's syndrome. *J Clin Endocrinol Metab*. 2014;99:2045–2051.
20. Lacroix A, Feelders RA, Stratakis CA, et al. Cushing's syndrome. *Lancet*. 2015;386:913–927.
21. Esposito F, Dusick JR, Cohan P, et al. Clinical review: early morning cortisol levels as a predictor of remission after transsphenoidal surgery for Cushing's disease. *J Clin Endocrinol Metab*. 2006;91:7–13.
22. Raffaelli M, De Crea C, D'Amato G, et al. Outcome of adrenalectomy for subclinical hypercortisolism and Cushing syndrome. *Surgery*. 2017;161:264–271.
23. Nieman LK, Biller BM, Findling JW, et al. Treatment of Cushing's syndrome: an Endocrine Society clinical practice guideline. *J Clin Endocrinol Metab*. 2015;100:2807–2831.
24. Dennedy MC, Annamalai AK, Prankerd-Smith O, et al. Low DHEAS: a sensitive and specific test for the detection of subclinical hypercortisolism in adrenal incidentalomas. *J Clin Endocrinol Metab*. 2017;102:786–792.
25. Chiodini I, Morelli V, Salcuni AS, et al. Beneficial metabolic effects of prompt surgical treatment in patients with an adrenal incidentaloma causing biochemical hypercortisolism. *J Clin Endocrinol Metab*. 2010;95:2736–2745.
26. Toniato A, Merante-Boschin I, Opocher G, et al. Surgical versus conservative management for subclinical Cushing syndrome in adrenal incidentalomas: a prospective randomized study. *Ann Surg*. 2009;249:388–391.
27. Puglisi S, Perotti P, Pia A, et al. Adrenocortical carcinoma with hypercortisolism. *Endocrinol Metab Clin North Am*. 2018;47:395–407.
28. Else T, Williams AR, Sabolch A, et al. Adjuvant therapies and patient and tumor characteristics associated with survival of adult patients with adrenocortical carcinoma. *J Clin Endocrinol Metab*. 2014;99:455–461.
29. Kim Y, Margonis GA, Prescott JD, et al. Curative surgical resection of adrenocortical carcinoma: determining long-term outcome based on conditional disease-free probability. *Ann Surg*. 2017;265:197–204.
30. Yeh MW, Lisewski D, Campbell P. Virilizing adrenocortical carcinoma with cavoatrial extension. *Am J Surg*. 2006;192:209–210.
31. Berruti A, Grisanti S, Pulzer A, et al. Long-term outcomes of adjuvant mitotane therapy in patients with radically resected adrenocortical carcinoma. *J Clin Endocrinol Metab*. 2017;102:1358–1365.
32. Fassnacht M, Terzolo M, Allolio B, et al. Combination chemotherapy in advanced adrenocortical carcinoma. *N Engl J Med*. 2012;366:2189–2197.
33. Welbourn RB. Early surgical history of phaeochromocytoma. *Br J Surg*. 1987;74:594–596.
34. Biggar MA, Lennard TW. Systematic review of phaeochromocytoma in pregnancy. *Br J Surg*. 2013;100:182–190.
35. Sawka AM, Prebtani AP, Thabane L, et al. A systematic review of the literature examining the diagnostic efficacy of measurement of fractionated plasma free metanephrines in the biochemical diagnosis of pheochromocytoma. *BMC Endocr Disord*. 2004;4:2.
36. Perry CG, Sawka AM, Singh R, et al. The diagnostic efficacy of urinary fractionated metanephrines measured by tandem mass spectrometry in detection of pheochromocytoma. *Clin Endocrinol (Oxf)*. 2007;66:703–708.
37. Timmers HJ, Chen CC, Carrasquillo JA, et al. Comparison of 18F-fluoro-L-DOPA, 18F-fluoro-deoxyglucose, and 18F-fluorodopamine PET and 123I-MIBG scintigraphy in the localization of pheochromocytoma and paraganglioma. *J Clin Endocrinol Metab*. 2009;94:4757–4767.
38. Janssen I, Chen CC, Millo CM, et al. PET/CT comparing (68)Ga-DOTATATE and other radiopharmaceuticals and in comparison with CT/MRI for the localization of sporadic metastatic pheochromocytoma and paraganglioma. *Eur J Nucl Med Mol Imaging*. 2016;43:1784–1791.
39. Gifford Jr RW, Kvale WF, Maher FT, et al. Clinical features, diagnosis and treatment of pheochromocytoma: a review of 76 cases. *Mayo Clin Proc*. 1964;39:281–302.

40. Lenders JW, Duh QY, Eisenhofer G, et al. Pheochromocytoma and paraganglioma: an endocrine society clinical practice guideline. *J Clin Endocrinol Metab*. 2014;99:1915–1942.
41. Nockel P, El Lakis M, Gaitanidis A, et al. Preoperative genetic testing in pheochromocytomas and paragangliomas influences the surgical approach and the extent of adrenal surgery. *Surgery*. 2018;163:191–196.
42. Hamidi O, Young Jr WF, Iniguez-Ariza NM, et al. Malignant pheochromocytoma and paraganglioma: 272 patients over 55 years. *J Clin Endocrinol Metab*. 2017;102:3296–3305.
43. Strajina V, Dy BM, Farley DR, et al. Surgical treatment of malignant pheochromocytoma and paraganglioma: retrospective case series. *Ann Surg Oncol*. 2017;24:1546–1550.
44. Gonias S, Goldsby R, Matthay KK, et al. Phase II study of high-dose [131I]metaiodobenzylguanidine therapy for patients with metastatic pheochromocytoma and paraganglioma. *J Clin Oncol*. 2009;27:4162–4168.
45. Fassnacht M, Arlt W, Bancos I, et al. Management of adrenal incidentalomas: European Society of Endocrinology Clinical Practice Guideline in collaboration with the European Network for the Study of Adrenal Tumors. *Eur J Endocrinol*. 2016;175:G1–G34.
46. Russo AE, Untch BR, Kris MG, et al. Adrenal metastasectomy in the presence and absence of extraadrenal metastatic disease. *Ann Surg*. 2019;270:373–377.
47. Barczynski M, Konturek A, Nowak W. Randomized clinical trial of posterior retroperitoneoscopic adrenalectomy versus lateral transperitoneal laparoscopic adrenalectomy with a 5-year follow-up. *Ann Surg*. 2014;260:740–747; discussion 747–748.
48. Chen Y, Scholten A, Chomsky-Higgins K, et al. Risk factors associated with perioperative complications and prolonged length of stay after laparoscopic adrenalectomy. *JAMA Surg*. 2018;153:1036–1041.
49. Walz MK, Alesina PF, Wenger FA, et al. Posterior retroperitoneoscopic adrenalectomy—results of 560 procedures in 520 patients. *Surgery*. 2006;140:943–948; discussion 948–950.
50. Sho S, Yeh MW, Li N, et al. Single-incision retroperitoneoscopic adrenalectomy: a North American experience. *Surg Endosc*. 2017;31:3014–3019.

41 CHAPTER

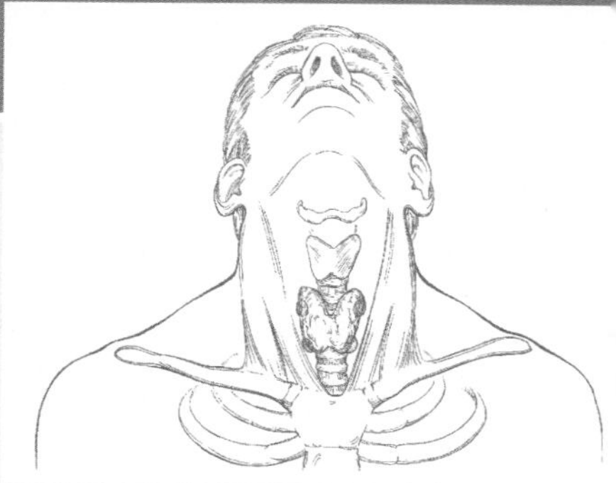

The Multiple Endocrine Neoplasia Syndromes

Amanda M. Laird, Steven K. Libutti

OUTLINE

The multiple endocrine neoplasia (MEN) syndromes occur as a result of a genetic change leading to the development of tumors in endocrine organs and tissues. Alterations in the menin gene, a tumor suppressor gene, results in MEN type 1 (MEN1), while MEN type 2 (MEN2) occurs as a result of changes in the *RET* proto-oncogene. This results in both benign and malignant endocrine tumors, and the individual possessing a mutation in either is at lifelong risk of development of these tumors. Each of the MEN syndromes is clinically characterized by the phenotypic expression of specific tumors. Strategies for management include screening for the presence of a mutation in some cases as well as follow-up and management directed specifically at the involved structure or organ. This may include prophylactic surgery, in the case of medullary thyroid cancer (MTC) in the setting of MEN2, or surveillance, for example, for pancreatic neuroendocrine tumors (PNETs) in MEN1.

The type of endocrine tumors that develop follows a pattern specific to each syndrome. *MEN1* is characterized by the presence of parathyroid adenomas in multiple glands, neuroendocrine tumors (NETs) of the gastrointestinal system and pancreas, and adenomas of the pituitary gland. While these are the most frequently occurring tumors within the syndrome, carriers may also develop carcinoid tumors of the thymus, facial angiofibromas, adrenal adenomas, lipomas, and collagenomas.[1] MEN2 is further subdivided into types A and B. Patients with MEN2A have MTC or thyroid C-cell hyperplasia, pheochromocytomas, and parathyroid tumors. Those with MEN2B also have MTC or thyroid C-cell hyperplasia and pheochromoctyomas, as well as mucosal neuromas, ganglioneuromatosis of the gastrointestinal tract, and a distinct appearance referred to as marfanoid.

MULTIPLE ENDOCRINE NEOPLASIA TYPE 1

Incidence and Epidemiology

Like other genetic syndromes, MEN1 is relatively rare among the general population, occurring in 1 of 30,000 people. In patients with primary hyperparathyroidism (PHPT), it occurs in 1% to 18%, while patients with pituitary adenomas have MEN1 less than 3% of the time. The presence of MEN1 varies in patients with NETs depending on type.[1] It is distributed across all ages, ranging from 9 to 77. Typically, the clinical manifestations of MEN1 will have developed by age 29. Overall survival in carriers is 82% with a disease-specific survival of 88% at 30 years with a mean age at death of 50 to 55 years.[2]

Genetics

MEN1 is a hereditary cancer syndrome inherited in an autosomal dominant manner. Prior to the discovery of the genetic abnormality responsible for development of the MEN1 syndrome, also called Wermer syndrome, the diagnosis was made clinically. Commercial testing for the mutation has now been available for a little over 30 years. The syndrome MEN1 develops as a result of a germline mutation and loss of heterozygosity in the *MEN1* gene in target tissue, leading to the development of tumors. The gene encodes the protein menin, which functions as a tumor suppressor in target tissues. By definition, tumor suppressor genes encode for proteins that regulate cell growth and proliferation. Loss of function of a tumor suppressor gene results in cell proliferation and, in turn, neoplastic transformation. Menin would normally participate in transcriptional regulation, DNA repair, and cell signaling, and mutations lead to a nonfunctioning protein. In the "two-hit" hypothesis of tumor development, a mutation is inherited as a

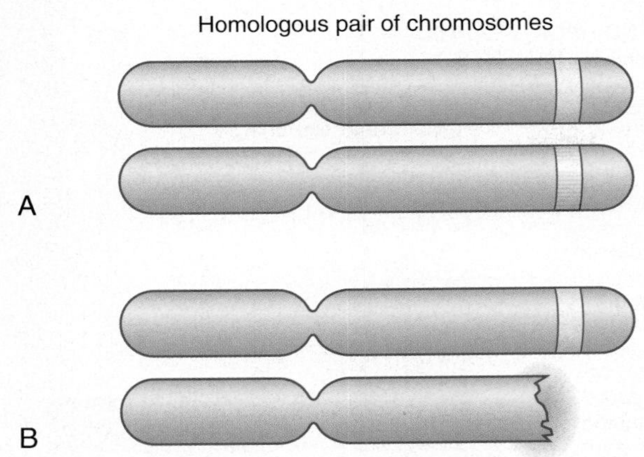

FIG. 41.1 Illustration of somatic mutation leading to loss of function of the menin gene in heterozygous individuals. (A) Normal allele. (B) Somatic mutation affects normal allele.

germline mutation, thereby making involved tissues or organs susceptible to growth of neoplasms. The remaining normal or functional gene then undergoes a somatic mutation, or a "second hit," thus resulting in cancer development (Fig. 41.1). This process is described as loss of heterozygosity whereby a cell with the germline mutation receives a second hit to the functional copy becoming homozygous and resulting in disruption of the function of the normally produced protein.

In order to identify the specific mutation, *MEN1* families underwent genetic analysis, and *MEN1*-associated tumors were specifically studied ultimately localizing the tumor suppressor gene on chromosome 11q13.[3] Gene cloning led to the identification of the protein product of the gene, menin, a 610-amino acid protein.[4] Menin is expressed in endocrine and nonendocrine cells, with varying levels of expression, and is located primarily in the cell nucleus. Through protein-protein interaction methods, the function of menin has been elucidated. These studies indicate that menin has multiple functions in transcription regulation as either a corepressor or coactivator, DNA repair, cell signaling, cytoskeletal structure, cell division, cell adhesion, or cell motility. In addition to its role in endocrine tissues, menin has been identified as playing a role as a pro-oncogenic factor in mixed lineage leukemia (*MLL*) by interacting with *MLL-1* fusion proteins to cause leukemia. It has also been identified as having a role in estrogen receptor regulation, and women with *MEN1* are at increased risk for the development of breast cancer.[5]

A database of known *MEN1* mutations was published in 2008, with just over 1300 mutations identified.[6] An additional 208 were identified after review of the literature and existing gene databases. The distribution of *MEN1* mutations includes 20% to 25% missense mutations, 14% to 23% nonsense mutations, 42% frameshift mutations, 10.5% exon region deletion, 9% RNA splice mutations, and 1% to 2.5% large deletions.[7] Genetic changes occur throughout the coding sequence. Somatic mutations occur frequently in nonsyndromic endocrine tumors.

Somatic *MEN1* mutations are reported in 60% of glucagonomas, 57% of VIPomas, 44% of nonfunctioning PNETs, 38% of gastrinomas, 35% of bronchial carcinoids, 35% of parathyroid adenomas, up to 19% of insulinomas, 3.5% of anterior pituitary tumors, and 2% of adrenocortical tumors otherwise believed to be sporadic. This suggests that loss of the *MEN1* gene plays a role in the development of nonhereditary endocrine tumors as well.

DNA testing of persons who have relatives known to have MEN1 may be performed in order to identify the presence of the mutation and inform surveillance and intervention for the endocrine tumors known to affect these patients. Clinical practice guidelines recommend genetic testing for index patients with MEN1 as well as their first-degree relatives.[1] *MEN1* germline mutation testing should also be offered to asymptomatic relatives as manifestations may begin as early as age 5. Given the chance of inheriting the mutation is 50%, identification of a mutation avoids potential unnecessary screening in individuals without a mutation. Newly identified families with *MEN1* should undergo testing; however, 10% to 20% will not have a mutation identifiable by conventional testing.[7] For this reason, the diagnosis of MEN1 is made either clinically in patients with two or more MEN1-associated tumors or in a patient with one MEN1-associated tumor and a first-degree relative with *MEN1*, a scenario that occurs in 5% to 10% of patients,[6] or in an individual with a known *MEN1* mutation but no clinical manifestations.[1] All patients with a diagnosis of MEN1 either clinically or via genetic testing should be offered combined clinical, biologic, and radiologic screening periodically.[1] No genotype-phenotype correlations have been established for MEN1. There are, however, some data that identify mutations targeting the JunD interacting domain of the gene as being associated with an increased risk of death.[8] Additionally, some alterations may predispose the patient to familial PHPT only. Despite more recent identification of these specific mutations, genetic testing cannot be used to predict disease course or severity in affected patients.

Recently, germline mutations of the *CDKN1B* gene have been associated with the development of parathyroid adenomas, pituitary adenomas, and PNETs, known as MEN4.[9] Clinically similar to MEN1, this may account for persons who meet clinical criteria for MEN1 without possessing a known mutation of the *MEN1* gene. Thus far, few pathogenic mutations of the *CDKN1B* gene have been found and its prevalence remains unknown.

Clinical Features and Management

Parathyroid adenomas occur in 95% of MEN1 patients, and PHPT is the first clinical manifestation of MEN1 in 90% of patients. Individuals with MEN1 also develop tumors of the pancreas and duodenum, bronchial and thymic carcinoids, and adenomas of the anterior pituitary gland. In addition, patients are more likely to develop adrenal adenomas and nonendocrine tumors such as angiofibromas, collagenomas, and meningiomas.[1] In patients with MEN1 who undergo postmortem examination, there is involvement of all endocrine tissue in essentially all patients.

MEN1 occurs equally in male and female patients with an autosomal dominant pattern of inheritance without apparent racial predilection. Untreated patients with MEN1 have a decreased life expectancy, with a 50% probability of death by age 50 years. The cause of death is either progression and spread of a malignant tumor that occurs within the syndrome, most often a gastroenteropancreatic NET or thymic carcinoids, or other sequelae of the disease. Historically, ulcer disease as a result of Zollinger-Ellison syndrome (ZES) leads to significant morbidity and mortality; however, this has improved with the introduction of acid-suppression treatment.

The signs and symptoms of MEN1 are attributed to the involvement of a specific endocrine gland or other tissue. These are as a direct result of either hormone overproduction or local effect of tumor or malignant progression of tumors. Most typically, PHPT is the first clinical manifestation, followed by pancreatic

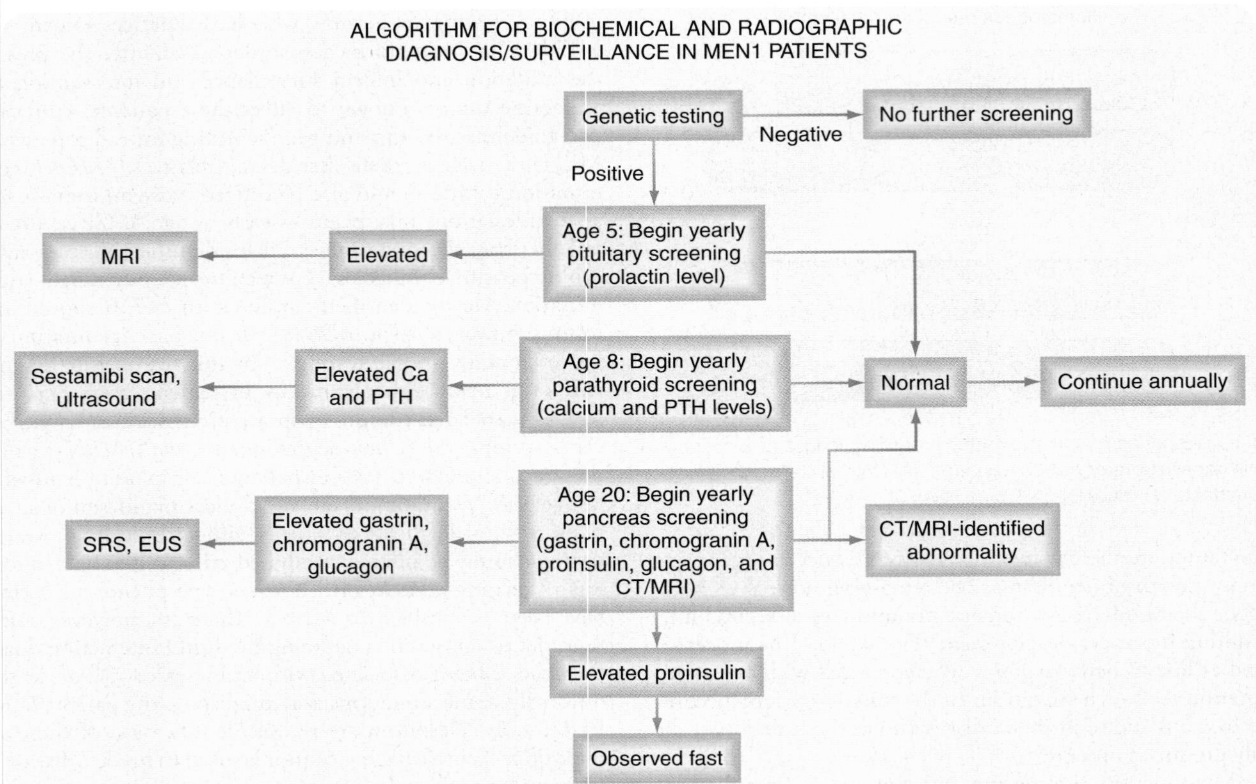

FIG. 41.2 Algorithm for screening and management in multiple endocrine neoplasia type 1 (*MEN1*) syndromes.

islet cell tumors and other NETs. Screening is offered to known kindreds and to those with known mutations, with surgical intervention offered to those with known tissue involvement and hormone excess. An algorithm for diagnosis and surveillance is demonstrated in Fig. 41.2. The goals of therapy, therefore, are management of hormone excess and prevention of tumor spread.

Parathyroid Glands

PHPT is the most common feature of MEN1, occurring in more than 90% of patients, and it is the experience of these authors that all patients with MEN1 have PHPT. Like sporadic PHPT, patients may have asymptomatic disease, osteoporosis, nephrolithiasis, or symptoms including fatigue, malaise, polyuria, polydipsia, and constipation. The diagnosis is made biochemically with an elevated calcium and an inappropriately nonsuppressed parathyroid hormone (PTH) level. Compared to sporadic cases, PHPT occurs in the setting of MEN1 at an earlier age (20–25 years vs. 55 years) and an equal female:male ratio (1:1 vs. 3:1). One of the hallmarks of PHPT in MEN1 versus its sporadic form is the presence of multiglandular disease; that is, all parathyroid glands are equally at risk for involvement and asymmetric hyperplasia (Fig. 41.3). Affected parathyroid glands in the setting of MEN1 are typically benign, although rare cases of parathyroid carcinoma are reported.

Surgery is the treatment of choice for PHPT in MEN1. While preoperative imaging has been employed in the management of sporadic PHPT, including ultrasound, sestamibi parathyroid scintigraphy, and four-dimensional computed tomography (CT), it may have less utility in familial PHPT. Sestamibi parathyroid scintigraphy may be useful to screen for parathyroid glands that are ectopic from the expected anatomic location in the neck. The recommended surgical approach from the 2012 MEN1 Clinical Practice Guidelines is to explore both sides of the neck via a standard open approach with the goal of identifying all four parathyroid glands.[1] This is the appropriate operation because all four glands are typically affected.

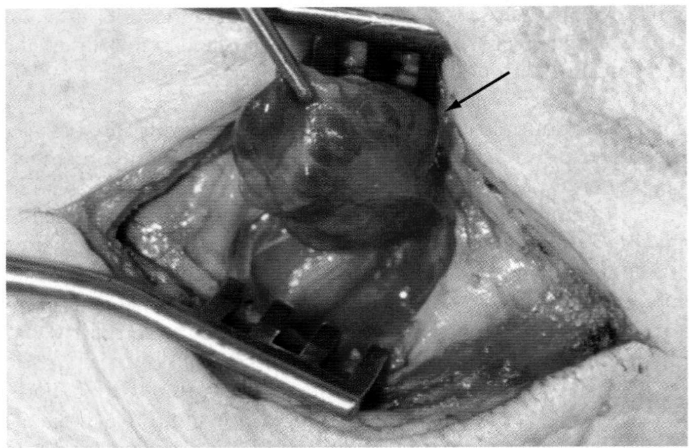

FIG. 41.3 Parathyroid adenoma with asymmetric hyperplasia, indicated by *arrow*.

Two operative procedures are options for management: subtotal parathyroidectomy with removal of 3.5-parathyroid glands versus total parathyroidectomy with removal of all four glands along with an autotransplantation of the patient's own parathyroid tissue into a location outside of the neck, typically the brachioradialis muscle of the forearm. Intraoperative PTH testing may also be used to guide extent of surgery in less than total operations. The goal of surgery is management of hormone levels within a normal range for the longest period of time with limited morbidity. The advantage of a subtotal or 3.5-gland parathyroidectomy is that a period of postoperative hypocalcemia is less likely. Approximately 20% to 30% of patients have either recurrent or persistent hypercalcemia following this procedure within 10 to 12 years, with a rate of hypoparathyroidism of 26% to 45%.[10] The advantage of a total parathyroidectomy with parathyroid autotransplantation is that recurrence rates are lower, ranging from 4% to 20%, but permanent hypoparathyroidism is more likely at 40% to 60%.[10] With either, initial biochemical cure rate is high when performed in experienced groups at 98%, comparable to surgical results in patients with sporadic PHPT.[10] A randomized prospective trial of 32 MEN1 patients undergoing operation for PHPT compared subtotal parathyroidectomy to total parathyroidectomy and autotransplantation. Rates of recurrence were statistically similar, although slightly higher in the subtotal parathyroidectomy group, rates of hypoparathyroidism were similar, and rates of reoperation were similar.[11] Both procedures therefore yield excellent results, but the overall advantage of subtotal parathyroidectomy may be avoiding an initial postoperative period of hypocalcemia. However, if followed long enough, all MEN1 patients will ultimately recur, and, therefore, MEN1-related hyperparathyroidism is never cured, and patients with recurrent disease may need reoperation.

In sporadic PHPT, preoperative imaging is used to guide focused reoperations, but due to the etiology of PHPT in MEN1, focused reexplorations may not be feasible. Using a combination of intraoperative PTH and preoperative imaging, normocalcemia can be achieved in 92%. A strategy to manage hypoparathyroidism after either approach is to cryopreserve a portion of the patient's parathyroid tissue at the time of initial operation. The cryopreserved autograft may then be transplanted with 60% of delayed grafts, demonstrating some evidence of function with normal PTH levels, and 40% fully functioning off all calcium and vitamin D supplementation.[12] Those patients with recurrence and failed operations or in whom surgery is contraindicated may be treated with calcimimetics as a last option. Vital transplantation may also achieve improved or normal postoperative calcium levels, avoiding hypocalcemia. It may be necessary in cases where a total parathyroidectomy is done at initial operation, or a patient undergoes reoperation and all remaining parathyroid tissue is removed from the neck. Autotransplantation to the brachioradialis muscle of the forearm yields full function in a third of autografts, while an additional 20% are at least partially functional.

Enteropancreatic NETs

Following parathyroid disease, the next most common tumor type to occur in MEN1 patients are enteropancreatic NETs. They occur in between 30% and 80% of patients depending on the study.[1] They may be functional or nonfunctional, that is, some tumors may secrete hormones in excess, yielding symptoms unique to the tumor type, while some do not. Either type has malignant potential, and surgical management, depending on the situation, is aimed at controlling hormone excess, preventing potential metastatic progression, and preventing local invasion. Tumors may secrete gastrin, insulin, or vasoactive intestinal peptide (VIP) and are termed according to the type of hormone secreted, for example, gastrinoma. Hormones also prove to be useful markers for follow-up. While nonfunctional tumors may not secrete hormones in excess, tumor markers such as chromogranin A or pancreatic polypeptide may be useful for follow-up. In contrast to sporadic NETs, MEN1-associated NETs may more often be multiple, and any treatment and follow-up must take this into consideration. Guidelines suggest screening in individuals with a known diagnosis of MEN1 biochemically with gastrin, fasting glucose, insulin, chromogranin A, pancreatic polypeptide, glucagon, and VIP measurements at 6- to 12-month intervals.[1] Any elevation of one of these would then require further investigation with radiographic studies.

There have been many improvements in the imaging of enteropancreatic NETs in recent years, not only as the quality of CT and magnetic resonance imaging (MRI) has improved, but also with the use of alternative imaging methods such as somatostatin receptor scintigraphy (SRS) and the recent introduction of gallium-68 somatostatin analog positron emission tomography (^{68}GaSA-PET). In addition to making an initial diagnosis, imaging also is critical to surgical planning to determine the resectability and appropriateness of surgery in the setting of metastases to lymph nodes and distant organs. Endoscopic ultrasound (EUS) is useful for obtaining a tissue diagnosis and allowing for proper grading of the tumor but may also play a role in follow-up. There is variability of sensitivity and specificity of each modality, but all play an important role in evaluation and treatment.

SRS is nuclear scintigraphy that was once the gold standard for the imaging of NETs. The somatostatin analog octreotide is administered as indium-labeled octreotide, which binds to somatostatin receptors. Sensitivity ranges from 70% to 90%, with a specificity approaching 100%.[13] In contrast to anatomic imaging, SRS has the advantage of being whole-body imaging, and it is also widely available but is limited by resolution and ability to detect lesions smaller than 1 cm.[13] CT is probably the most widely used imaging modality, with similar sensitivity to SRS in the detection of both primary lesions as well as metastases while being slightly better than SRS at detecting extrahepatic metastases. In patients suspected of having an enteropancreatic NET, CT should be done as an early arterial-phase CT. This demonstrates the typical imaging characteristics, where lesions are isodense on precontrast images, then enhance in the arterial phase, with contrast washout on portal venous phase. Compared to other modalities, however, CT has provided the most information with respect to the tumor's relationship to surrounding structures and aids in surgical planning. MRI is similar to CT in that anatomic relationships are demonstrated but has the advantage of not exposing the patient to ionizing radiation, which may be of concern over a long period of follow-up. MRI done with gadolinium with precontrast, arterial phase, and portal venous phase imaging is similar in sensitivity to CT. On MRI, enteropancreatic NETs are hypo- or isodense on precontrast T1 images and are hyperdense on T2 images with enhancement postcontrast administration. EUS can be very useful in the evaluation of PNETs. A fine-needle aspiration done at the time of EUS provides information to confirm tumor type and establishes grade by obtaining tissue that can be stained and a Ki-67 index determined. While EUS does not provide information regarding distant metastatic disease, it may demonstrate additional detail not seen on either CT or MRI to help determine resectability as it allows for improved visualization of margins with the superior mesenteric artery and other adjacent structures. Duodenal gastrinomas are difficult to see on EUS, and in this situation, traditional visual endoscopy has an advantage.

^{68}GaSA administered as part of PET is the latest addition for imaging of NETs. ^{68}GaSA-PET images are also fused with CT to improve sensitivity. Sensitivity is approximately 80% with a specificity of 90%,[14] and specificity approaches 100% for metastases

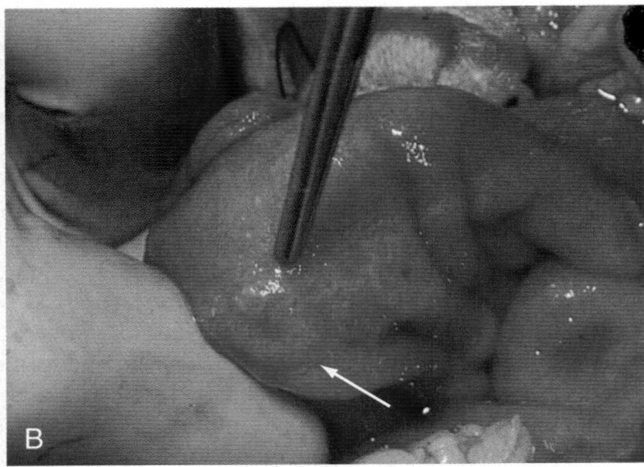

FIG. 41.4 Gastrinoma, intraoperative findings. (A) Duodenotomy and palpation of the duodenal wall. (B) Typical appearance of a gastrinoma in the duodenal wall, indicated by *arrow*.

when used to evaluate for disease beyond the pancreas. ^{68}GaSA-PET/CT detects a greater number of primary and metastatic lesions compared to SRS. In addition to providing useful anatomic information, ^{68}GaSA may also inform therapeutic decision-making, as PNETs that take up ^{68}GaSA may predict patients who respond to somatostatin analogs. Sensitivity may be limited by the accumulation of ^{68}GaSA in the uncinate process of the pancreas or inflammation, which can lead to false-positive studies.

Approximately 50% of enteropancreatic NETs that develop in the setting of MEN1 are gastrin-secreting tumors called gastrinomas. Conversely, 20% of patients with gastrinomas will have MEN1.[15] This produces a clinical syndrome termed ZES, and patients present with recurrent multiple peptic ulcers, abdominal pain, and esophagitis. The disease should be suspected in patients with multiple ulcers that occur in atypical locations, fail to respond to usual therapy, and/or recurrent, or occur in the setting of PHPT. This should prompt evaluation for a gastrinoma. Hypergastrinemia attributed to a gastrinoma is diagnosed by elevated fasting serum gastrin levels greater than 10 times the normal obtained after at least 2 weeks off of a proton-pump inhibitor. If fasting gastrin levels are not diagnostic, provocative testing can be done with secretin stimulation, which is more sensitive and specific than calcium stimulation. Up to 90% of gastrinomas diagnosed within the setting of MEN1 are malignant, and more than half have lymph node metastases.[16] The development of either hepatic metastases and/or lymph node metastases tends to be size dependent, with a greater likelihood of either as the primary tumor is larger.[16] Survival in patients with MEN1 approaches 100% at 15 years regardless of primary tumor size and nodal status, but this is reduced to 52% in the setting of liver metastases.

There is no consensus for the role of surgery in the management of ZES in MEN1 patients. Patients with gastrinomas in this setting rarely achieve long-term eugastrinemia, as evidenced by a review of a series of patients with the disease managed surgically.[17] Further, the availability of proton-pump inhibitors has made medical therapy for control of symptoms possible given that the disease is not curable. In patients with PHPT, surgical correction improves fasting gastrin levels and reduces basal acid output. Therefore, the remaining controversy surrounds the utility of surgery given the malignant potential of the tumor despite the likelihood of long-term biochemical cure. Because most gastrinomas are duodenal, recommendations for management include endoscopic gastroduodenoscopy, duodenotomy and transduodenal exploration, and resection of any malignant-appearing lymph nodes. The typical appearance of a gastrinoma and duodenotomy with palpation of the duodenal wall is demonstrated in Fig. 41.4. Liver metastases are rare when tumor size is less than 2 cm.[17] Clinical guidelines recommend the surgical approach be tailored to the individual situation incorporating patient preference into the decision-making.[1] The rationale for this approach is based on the likelihood of recurrence given the presence of metastases at diagnosis as well as the potential for development of multiple tumors as well as the high morbidity associated with major pancreas resection. Patients are also at risk for type 1 gastric carcinoids, which develop due to hypergastrinemia and stimulation of enterochromaffin cells. They are present in up to a third of patients with ZES and may be managed expectantly with observation and endoscopic resection, although long-term endoscopic surveillance is necessary.

Insulinomas, which are β-islet cell tumors that secrete insulin, represent up to 30% of PNETs in patients with MEN1, while 4% of patients with an insulinoma have MEN1. They present with a constellation of symptoms known as "Whipple triad" including fasting glucose levels less than 50 mg/dL, symptoms of hypoglycemia, and resolution of symptoms upon administration of glucose. These symptoms include sweating, dizziness, confusion, and syncope. Historically, the diagnosis was made during a monitored 72-hour supervised fast where plasma glucose, insulin, and C-peptide levels are measured at 6-hour intervals. An elevated insulin level with a low glucose level is diagnostic.[1] However, data now suggest that a 48-hour fast is adequate and as accurate and should replace the 72-hour fast. Use of oral hypoglycemic agents should be excluded during the duration of the supervised fast. Insulinomas may be multifocal and occur throughout the pancreas and are best imaged by CT and EUS, although they can be difficult to locate and may ultimately be identified at operative exploration with or without intraoperative ultrasound. Anatomic imaging such as CT, MRI, and EUS have varying sensitivities all less than 50%. Calcium arterial stimulation exceeds 90% and is useful in regionalizing the lesion before surgery, and is more accurate than anatomic imaging when used intraoperatively.[18] Intraoperative ultrasound employed in a traditional open or laparoscopic exploration is then used to guide intraoperative exploration with success rates of 86%. Once the suspected insulinoma is identified intraoperatively, aspiration of the lesion and use of a rapid assay for insulin confirm or eliminate the identified lesion as an insulinoma and may be used

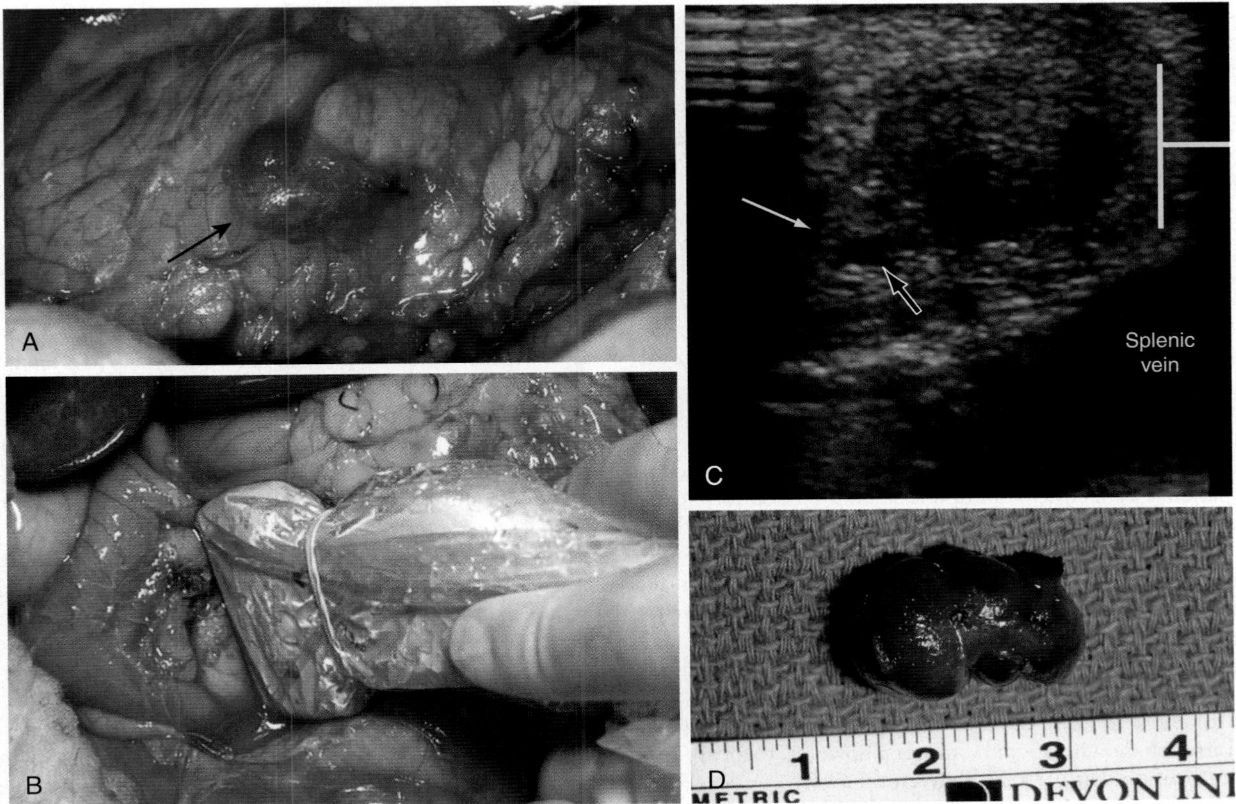

FIG. 41.5 Insulinoma. (A) Insulinoma, reddish in appearance, posterior body of pancreas, indicated by *arrow*. (B) Intraoperative ultrasound used to identify insulinoma and define relationship to vessels and pancreatic duct. (C) Ultrasound image of insulinoma. (D) Resected insulinoma.

in addition.[19] Many lesions are amenable to enucleation, but larger tumors or those that appear to be malignant with invasion of adjacent structures may require anatomic pancreatic resection,[17] although approximately 10% are malignant. Fig. 41.5 demonstrates the application of intraoperative ultrasound to surgical exploration in the identification and resection of an insulinoma on the posterior body of the pancreas. Patients with unresectable disease due to either a locally invasive tumor or, more likely, distant metastases may be treated with chemotherapy including somatostatin analogs.

Other functional tumors include glucagonomas, VIPomas, and somatostatinomas, although these comprise fewer than 5% of functional PNETs in MEN1. Symptoms of glucagonomas include a skin rash known as necrolytic migratory erythema, weight loss, anemia, and stomatitis, although a glucagonoma may be present in the absence of symptoms. They most often occur in the tail of the pancreas and surgery is the treatment of choice. They are frequently malignant and 50% to 80% have metastases at the time of diagnosis.[1] VIPomas are infrequent and present with symptoms of severe intermittent watery diarrhea, hypokalemia, achlorhydria, acidosis, flushing, and hypotension. They are often located in the tail of the pancreas and are nearly always malignant. When feasible, they are best managed with surgery. Somatostatinomas also occur infrequently and present with symptoms of cholelithiasis, diabetes, and steatorrhea. They are diagnosed biochemically and treatment is surgical.

The majority of enteropancreatic NETs in MEN1 patients are nonfunctional PNETs, which are hormonally inactive. They are not associated with a clinical syndrome and therefore are diagnosed on surveillance imaging or investigation performed due to the development of symptoms related to local effects of tumor. Screening for enteropancreatic NETs in general should begin at age 10 in patients with known *MEN1* mutations.[1] More recent data indicate a correlation between exon 2 mutations and development of nonfunctional PNETs at an earlier age, potentially identifying a group who would benefit from more frequent, earlier screening.[20] Recommendations for surgical intervention are made incorporating two issues into decision-making: the potential for the development of multiple tumors and, therefore, need for multiple operations and the malignant potential of PNETs. Much like recommendations for management of sporadic nonfunctional PNETs, management of familial nonfunctional PNETs is based on size and grade based on mitotic index and Ki-67 index. Observational studies reveal an increasing rate of presence of metastases as tumor size increases. In a group of 108 MEN1 patients with nonfunctional PNETs managed surgically, those with tumors smaller than 1 cm had metastases 4% of the time, tumors 1.1 to 2 cm had metastases 10% of the time, tumors 2.1 to 3 cm had metastases 18% of the time, and if more than 3 cm, metastases were present in 43%.[21] A more recent evaluation of a population of MEN1 patients indicate a relatively increased risk of metastases in tumors exceeding 2 cm.[22] In patients with tumors larger than 3 cm, observation is associated with increased mortality and development of metastases compared to those who had surgery, while the benefit for those with tumors 2 to 3 cm was less clear. Those with tumors less than 2 cm had no clear benefit from surgery.[23] The current consensus recommendation is that tumors less than 2 cm should be observed with imaging at regular intervals.[24] A decision to proceed with surgery should also be made in patients with tumors that demonstrate significant growth after interval imaging, apparent development of metastases, or if patient-specific factors make observation less desirable. Observation and expectant management for patients with tumors smaller than 2 cm should be recommended given the morbidity surrounding pancreatic surgery.

Pituitary Gland

The presence of an anterior pituitary adenoma in patients with MEN1 varies from 15% to 50% and typically occurs between the ages of 20 and 40.[1] Approximately 1% of patients with pituitary adenomas have MEN1. Pituitary adenomas are not frequently the initial manifestation of the disease. Pituitary tumors may cause symptoms either as a result of hormone secretion or from local effects of the tumor, which may result in visual field defects. The majority secrete hormones including prolactin, growth hormone, or corticotropin. Further, they tend to be benign and unifocal. In a group of Dutch patients, pituitary adenomas identified in MEN1 patients were either nonfunctional and tended to remain stable in size over time or, if functional, responded to medical therapy.[25] Biochemical screening for pituitary adenomas should begin at age 5, with MRI evaluation done every 3 years.[1] Treatment of pituitary tumors in MEN1 utilizes therapies similar to those used for sporadic adenomas. This includes both medical and surgical therapy. Medical therapy is aimed at controlling hormone excess, much like with other endocrine tumors. There are data that suggest that the severity of disease may be worse in patients with MEN1 versus those with sporadic tumors; however, there are few series that focus on comparisons between the two.

Other Tumors

A variety of other tumors may occur in the setting of MEN1. These include carcinoids of the thymus, bronchi, and gastrointestinal tract; adrenocortical tumors; and cutaneous tumors such as lipomas, facial angiofibromas, and collagenomas. Thymic carcinoid tumors are the most likely to be malignant, tend to be aggressive, and have a poor prognosis. They occur twice as often in men and have a 45% 10-year survival as well as an association with smoking.[26] There is not an optimum method of screening; however, CT and MRI are recommended every 1 to 2 years for earlier detection.[1] Surgery is the preferred treatment when feasible. Transcervical thymectomy has been used in the past as a way to remove additional parathyroid tissue and once was thought to prevent thymic carcinoids. However, in a series of patients operated on for PHPT with total parathyroidectomy and planned transcervical thymectomy, no thymic carcinoids were identified. Thus, preventative transcervical thymectomy is not recommended. Adrenal tumors are common, with approximately 20% of patients having some type of adrenal hyperplasia.[27] In a large cohort of MEN1 patients, a variety of adrenal tumors were identified, both functional and nonfunctional, benign and malignant. Compared to sporadic adrenal tumors, MEN1 patients had adrenocortical carcinoma and primary hyperaldosteronism more frequently.[27] There are no established guidelines for management of adrenal tumors in this setting; therefore, the suggested management follows that for adrenal masses diagnosed outside of the setting of MEN1. Tumors 4 cm or greater in size, tumors that exhibit radiologic features suspicious for malignancy, those that produce hormones in excess, and those that demonstrate significant growth over at least a 6-month imaging interval should be managed surgically. The remaining tumors including lipomas, facial angiofibromas, and collagenomas may be useful in aiding in the diagnosis of MEN1, but they occur infrequently and generally do not require any treatment.

MULTIPLE ENDOCRINE NEOPLASIA TYPE 2

MEN2 syndromes include MEN2A and familial MTC (FMTC). They all have in common MTC, which occurs in almost 100% of patients. FMTC is an entity within MEN2A, but different in that patients will only have the potential for development of MTC. Clinically, MEN2A and MEN2B, like MEN1, are defined by the occurrence of other tumor types (Fig. 41.6). In both, patients have adrenal medullary hyperplasia and develop pheochromocytomas. In MEN2A, patients may also develop PHPT. Patients with MEN2B may possess other conditions that give them a distinct physical appearance. MEN2 syndromes are due to mutations in the *RET* proto-oncogene, which is inherited in an autosomal dominant fashion, although some are acquired as new mutations. The penetrance of tumors except MTC depend on the type of *RET* mutation carried. Unlike MEN1, there is a distinct genotype-phenotype correlation based on the type of *RET* mutation identified; therefore, this becomes a useful predictor of tumor behavior and can inform both surveillance and intervention. Thus, treatment is based on identification of the specific *RET* mutation and tailoring care according to its known characteristics and behavior. Further, early thyroidectomy in known carriers can prevent MTC and improve survival. Its prevalence is estimated at 1/35,000 persons.[28] In the following sections, the genetics, clinical features, and management are detailed.

RET Proto-oncogene

The *RET* (*RE*arranged during *T*ransfection) proto-oncogene is named after its original transfection assay and codes for a membrane receptor with tyrosine kinase activity. It is located on chromosome 10q11.2. Each of the MEN2 syndromes as well as FMTC occurs as a result of a *RET* mutation, inherited in an autosomal dominant pattern. Mutations that result in the development of MTC are missense mutations that change a single amino acid. This causes an activating, or gain-of-function mutation. The *RET* protein is formed by an extracellular ligand-binding domain, a transmembrane domain, and a cytoplasmic tyrosine kinase domain. The intracellular tyrosine kinase subdomains are involved in intracellular signal transduction pathways. This ultimately plays a role in cell growth and survival, and mutations in the *RET* gene, thus, results in unregulated cell growth.

RET participates in a number of cell signaling pathways and is expressed in multiple tissues that arise from the neural crest, including thyroid parafollicular cells (C cells), parathyroid glands, adrenal chromaffin cells, enteric ganglia, and peripheral and central neurons. Mice with mutated *RET* genes have renal agenesis and a lack of neurons throughout the digestive tract, suggesting that *RET* also plays a role in development of both structures. Ultimately, inactivating mutations in *RET* were found to be associated with Hirschsprung disease in humans, a defect in the development of enteric neurons resulting in megacolon and constipation in infancy.

Unlike MEN1, strong genotype–phenotype correlations exist in MEN2. Therefore, the presence or absence of specific *RET* mutations can predict disease course. Anticipated age at disease onset can be estimated and disease aggressiveness can be predicted, and prophylactic surgery is then offered in an effort to improve survival. Patients with apparently sporadic MTC may carry *RET* mutations, and they should all be offered testing.

Multiple Endocrine Neoplasia Type 2A and Familial Medullary Thyroid Cancer

The syndrome of MEN2 was first described by Sipple and Steiner in the 1960s upon recognition of the association of thyroid cancer

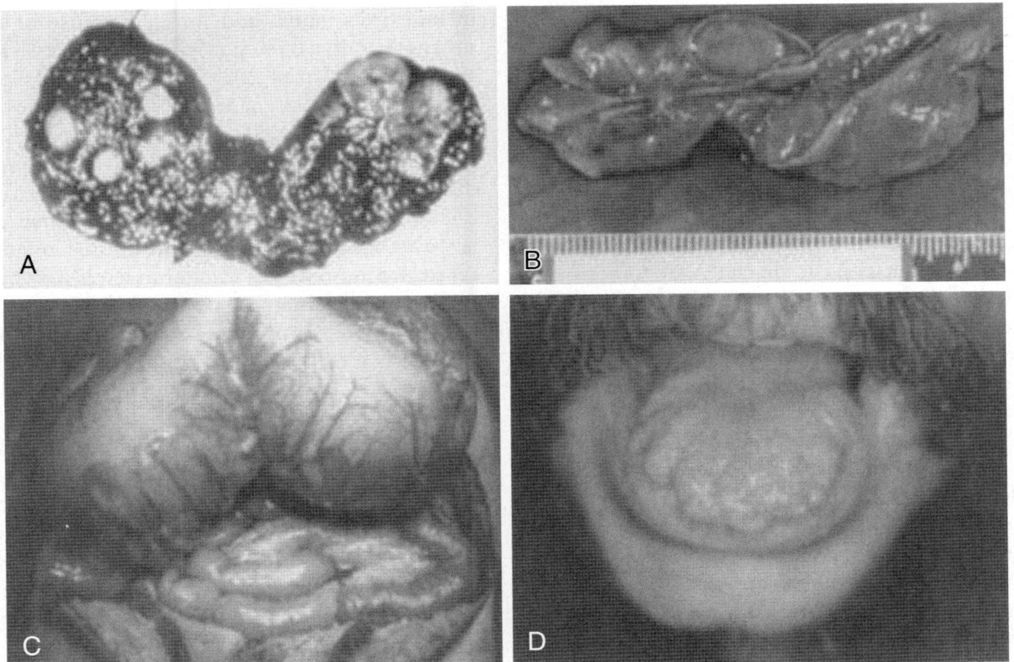

FIG. 41.6 Clinical manifestations of multiple endocrine neoplasia type 2 (MEN2) syndromes. (A) Multifocal medullary thyroid cancer. (B) Adrenal medullary hyperplasia. (C) Megacolon in Hirschprung disease. (D) Mucosal neuromas found in MEN2B.

with pheochromocytoma and PHPT.[29] MEN2A is the most common subtype of the MEN2 syndromes, comprising the majority of cases. The hallmark characteristic of MEN2A is the development of MTC, with a greater than 90% penetrance. In addition to MTC, pheochromocytoma develops in 50% to 60% of patients and PHPT in up to 30% with both adrenal glands and all parathyroid glands at risk.[30] The degree of penetrance of each tumor type is associated with specific codon mutations, and all patients are at risk for the development of multiple tumors within each endocrine organ, including multifocal MTC. Patients with MEN2A have a normal physical appearance and body habitus, unlike those with MEN2B that are associated with a Marfanoid habitus and neurofibromas of the tongue.

Other conditions that occur within MEN2A include cutaneous lichen amyloidosis and Hirschsprung disease. Cutaneous lichen amyloidosis is uncommon and typically occurs with codon 634 mutations. It is characterized by the symptom of pruritus and it is thought that repeated scratching then leads to amyloid deposition in the papillary dermis of the skin. As a result, patients develop cutaneous plaques, often located on the back. Hirschsprung disease may also occur in patients with either MEN2A or FMTC. The disease is characterized by the congenital absence of ganglion cells within the myenteric and submucosal plexus of the distal colon. Symptoms in the newborn include abdominal distention and constipation with megacolon as a result of the relative distal obstruction that occurs due to aganglionosis. Most often, there are mutations in codons 609, 618, and 620 in MEN2A/Hirschsprung disease patients. In these kindreds, nearly 20% will have Hirschsprung disease, and patients with MEN2A should be counseled regarding the possibility of the disease in offspring. Hirschsprung disease occurring outside of the setting of MEN2A is as a result of inactivating, or loss-of-function, *RET* mutations. Hirschsprung disease affects approximately 7% of MEN2A patients overall, while between 2% and 5% of patients with Hirschsprung disease will have MEN2A.[31]

FMTC is considered to be a variant of MEN2A rather than a separate clinical entity. It was first characterized in 1986 within kindreds of patients with FMTC but no evidence of pheochromocytoma or PHPT. FMTC is characterized by the identification of a *RET* mutation in families with MTC with no history of pheochromocytoma or PHPT. While all patients ultimately developed MTC, on average, they are diagnosed in their mid-40s, approximately 20 years later than MTC associated with MEN2A. Thus, FMTC may be a less aggressive entity than the MTC that develops within MEN2A kindreds.[32] The clinician should be cautioned, however, to carefully categorize those with FMTC rather than MEN2A as an incorrect diagnosis could lead to overlooking the presence of a pheochromocytoma.

The majority of patients with MEN2A have *RET* mutations in codons 609, 611, 618, or 602 of exon 10 or codon 634 of exon 11. Nearly all develop MTC, but there is variable penetrance of the presence of pheochromocytoma or PHPT depending on the mutation.[31] As in MEN1, a clinical diagnosis of MEN2A can be made in families with features of the syndrome but who have no identifiable *RET* mutation.

Multiple Endocrine Neoplasia Type 2B

As in MEN2A, the hallmark characteristic of MEN2B is the development of MTC. Approximately 50% of MEN2B patients develop pheochromocytomas, but unlike MEN2A patients, PHPT is not part of the syndrome. Further, they have a characteristic appearance with elongated facies and a Marfanoid body habitus, everted eyelids, ophthalmologic abnormalities, skeletal abnormalities including pectus excavatum and scoliosis, and mucosal neuromas of the lips and tongue.[31] Patients also have ganglioneuromatosis throughout the gastrointestinal tract leading to esophageal dysmotility, abdominal bloating, intermittent constipation, and diarrhea. In contrast to MEN2A, the MTC in MEN2B often develops as early as infancy and tends to be aggressive with early metastasis, and early thyroidectomy in these patients is critical. The majority of MEN2B patients have germline mutations in exon 16, codon 918, while fewer than 5% have mutations in codon A883F. Those with A883F mutations may have a milder, less aggressive form of MTC.[33] Approximately 50% of cases are due to de novo mutations.

Genetic Testing for Multiple Endocrine Neoplasia Type 2

Prior to the identification of the *RET* gene, the diagnosis of MEN2 was made clinically in patients with the characteristic tumor types present as well as with screening via pentagastrin-stimulated calcitonin testing. The standard of care now is with sequencing of the *RET* gene to identify germline mutations. The recommendation for testing is sequencing of the anticipated involved coding regions related to the MEN2 type known to the kindred or suspected based on clinical findings. All offspring of known kindreds should be offered genetic counseling and genetic testing ideally in infancy as should first-degree relatives of those with FMTC.[31]

In some cases, the presenting tumor known to occur within MEN2 may be the first evidence of the syndrome. Up to 7% of patients with apparently sporadic MTC have *RET* mutations and should therefore be offered genetic counseling and genetic testing.[34] Further, they may occur as de novo mutations, and the absence of family history should not preclude testing. Nearly a quarter of patients with apparently nonsyndromic pheochromocytoma will have an identified genetic mutation, with approximately 5% of those due to a *RET* mutation.[35] Additional recommendations for testing include infants or young children with Hirschsprung disease, parents whose infants or children have the physical phenotype of MEN2B, and patients with cutaneous lichen amyloidosis.[31]

Medullary Thyroid Cancer

MTC represents fewer than 2% of all thyroid cancers based on current data from the Surveillance, Epidemiology, and End Results database.[36] Unlike papillary and follicular thyroid cancers, MTC arises from the parafollicular C-cells, which produce calcitonin; therefore, traditional treatments such as suppression of thyroid stimulating hormone and radioactive iodine (RAI) are not used as C-cells are not sensitive to these therapies. Approximately 25% of MTC is familial and C-cell hyperplasia precedes the development of MTC. While MTC is a relatively indolent malignancy, there are distinct differences in outcomes between sporadic MTC and MTC in the setting of MEN2A and MEN2B. In an Italian database of MTC patients, overall 10-year survival was 84.4%; however, survival was worse in MEN2B patients at 60% compared to sporadic MTC and MEN2A at 80.4% and 94%, respectively. Independent predictors of worse outcomes were male sex, tumor size larger than 1 cm, and lateral neck lymph node metastases.[37]

Once clinically apparent, MTC may present as a central neck mass. Symptoms from local effects such as compression or hoarseness may be present due to tumor invasion. FMTC tends to be multifocal, necessitating total thyroidectomy in all cases. Diagnosis can be made with fine-needle aspiration biopsy, and in addition to the presence of parafollicular cells and staining for calcitonin, the tissue has staining properties similar to amyloid, a hallmark feature. Nearly half of patients have lymph node metastases if the diagnosis is made clinically rather than based on calcitonin levels. Evaluation for lymph node disease should be done, including the central compartment (level VI) and the lateral compartment (levels II, III, IV, and V). MTC with distant metastases (outside of the neck) is incurable, and metastases may be occult, with elevations of serum calcitonin as the only sign.[31] Frequent sites of metastases include liver, bone, and lungs. Presence of metastases worsens prognosis with a 51% survival at 1 year, 26% at 5 years, and 10% at 10 years.[38] Up to 20% of MTC patients with a clinically evident, palpable neck mass, will have metastases at diagnosis.

C-cells secrete calcitonin, which becomes a useful surrogate marker for both diagnosis and recurrence as calcitonin is produced by virtually all MTC. Historically, provocative testing for calcitonin with pentagastrin was performed as a screening test; however, it is no longer available in the United States. After surgical treatment of MTC, calcitonin levels may be used to determine presence of persistent or recurrent disease, both regional and distant. Some MTCs produce carcinoembryonic antigen (CEA), and while it is less useful for diagnosis, once an individual is known to have MTC, it is helpful for monitoring patients for recurrence postthyroidectomy.[31]

Ultrasound is the most sensitive method of imaging the neck in patients with primary, persistent, or recurrent MTC and is useful for obtaining fine-needle aspiration biopsies of either thyroid nodules or suspicious-appearing lymph nodes in the neck. CT of the neck may be useful in planning surgery with apparently bulky disease as the iodinated contrast does not pose an issue for MTC as RAI is not used in treatment. CT may be more useful in imaging for metastatic disease for the chest and abdomen. MRI is helpful to determine the presence or absence of liver metastases or to better characterize liver lesions identified on CT. In some cases of MTC, the tumor expresses somatostatin receptors, and ^{68}GaSA-PET/CT has been proposed as an adjunct to traditional imaging not only for lesion detection but potentially for therapeutic planning.[39]

Surgery for Medullary Thyroid Cancer

Surgery for MTC in patients with MEN2 occurs in one of two settings. It is done either for already clinically apparent disease diagnosed by the finding of a thyroid nodule or cervical lymphadenopathy on physical exam or imaging, or it is done as a preventative measure in an effort to limit potential tumor spread and improve survival.

For those with clinically evident disease, preparation for surgery includes a biochemical evaluation as well as imaging to determine the extent of tumor involvement not only in the neck but, depending on preoperative calcitonin level, may also include cross-sectional imaging of the chest, abdomen, and pelvis to evaluate for distant metastases. Guidelines recommend obtaining preoperative calcitonin and CEA measurements to which postoperative tumor markers obtained can be compared to assess completeness of resection.[31] In addition, a critical element of preoperative planning for surgery for MTC is obtaining plasma or 24-hour urine metanephrines to exclude the possibility of a concomitant pheochromocytoma. Ultrasound of the neck is the most sensitive modality of imaging for both primary tumors of the thyroid as well as of the lateral neck nodal basins, although it is less sensitive for central neck lymph nodes due to the overlying thyroid. Contrast-enhanced CT of the neck may be helpful in the setting of either a large primary tumor or bulky lateral node metastases to gauge extension into the mediastinum and invasion of vascular structures. MRI with contrast or CT including arterial and portal venous phase imaging is recommended in patients with calcitonin levels exceeding 500 pg/mL to evaluate for distant metastatic disease,[31] although this may not impact the decision to resect the primary tumor and regional metastases to lymph nodes.

At a minimum, total thyroidectomy should be performed in all patients with MTC as nearly 90% of patients with a familial

TABLE 41.1 **Summary of recommendations for prophylactic thyroidectomy and screening in MEN2.**

RET MUTATION	CLINICAL SYNDROME	ATA RISK CATEGORY	AGE AT TT	PHEO	PHPT	AGE TO INITIATE SCREENING, YEARS	OTHER CONDITIONS
M918T	MEN2B	HST	<12 months	Y	N	11	-
C634	MEN2A	H	<5 years	Y	Y	11	CLA
A883F	MEN2A	H	<5 years	Y	Y	11	-
G533C	MEN2A	MOD	>5 years*	Y	N	16	-
C609	MEN2A	MOD	>5 years*	Y	Y	16	HD
C611	MEN2A	MOD	>5 years*	Y	Y	16	HD
C618	MEN2A	MOD	>5 years*	Y	Y	16	HD
C620	MEN2A	MOD	>5 years*	Y	Y	16	HD
C630	MEN2A	MOD	>5 years*	Y	Y	16	-
D631	MEN2A	MOD	>5 years*	Y	N	16	-
K666E	MEN2A	MOD	>5 years*	Y	N	16	-
E768D	FMTC	MOD	>5 years*	N	N	16	-
L790F	MEN2A	MOD	>5 years*	Y	N	16	-
V804L	MEN2A	MOD	>5 years*	Y	Y	16	-
V804M	MEN2A	MOD	>5 years*	Y	Y	16	CLA
S891A	MEN2A	MOD	>5 years*	Y	Y	16	-
R912P	FMTC	MOD	>5 years*	N	N	16	-

Adapted from Wells SA Jr, Asa SL, Dralle H, et al. Revised American Thyroid Association guidelines for the management of medullary thyroid carcinoma. *Thyroid.* 2015;25:567–610.
ATA categories: *HST*, ATA highest; *H*, ATA high; *MOD*, ATA moderate; *CLA*, Cutaneous lichen amyloidosis; *HD*, Hirschprung disease; *MEN2*, multiple endocrine neoplasia type 2 syndromes; *Pheo*, pheochromocytoma; *PHPT*, rimary hyperparathyroidism; *TT*, prophylactic thyroidectomy.
p*Screening begins at age 5 and timing of TT may be based on calcitonin levels.

form of MTC will have bilobar, multifocal disease. Initial operation should also always include a compartment-oriented bilateral central (level VI) lymph node dissection, that is, removal of all lymph node tissue en bloc in the compartment bounded by the hyoid bone superiorly, the innominate vein inferiorly, the carotid sheaths laterally, and anterior to the trachea, recurrent laryngeal nerves, and deepest layer of cervical fascia whether or not they appear to be clinically involved. The rate of lymph node metastases to level VI is excessively high, found in both the ipsilateral and contralateral compartments ranging from 50% to 80%.[40] Even nodes that are apparently normal should be removed as intraoperative surgeon-performed inspection has a low sensitivity and specificity for detection of involved nodes at 65% and 47%, respectively.[41] Both the ipsilateral and contralateral lateral nodal compartments, levels II to V, are also frequently involved. The occurrence rates of lateral node metastases depend on primary tumor size as well as extent of involvement of the central compartment, and preoperative calcitonin and CEA levels positively correlate with the presence of lateral node metastases.[31] Ideally, the central compartment should be addressed at the time of the initial operation as reoperations in level VI are higher risk, with increased rates of both recurrent laryngeal nerve injury and permanent hypoparathyroidism in reoperations. Ultrasound has a high sensitivity and specificity, 83.5% and 97.7%, respectively, for the lateral neck compartment. Further, the lateral neck compartments are anatomically separate from the central neck and the implications of increased rates of both recurrent nerve injury and hypoparathyroidism do not apply as they do in the central compartment. Therefore, guidelines recommend a patient-tailored approach when considering lateral neck dissection at the time of the initial operation. Careful attention should be paid to the identification of the parathyroid glands at operation in order to maintain function. Ideally, they should be maintained in situ, but in situations where this is not possible, they may be autotransplanted into either sternocleidomastoid muscle or to the brachioradialis muscle of the forearm depending on the familial setting and likelihood of developing PHPT.

The goal of preventative surgery in those known to carry *RET* mutations is to limit the potential for metastatic spread of MTC and to improve overall survival as essentially all MEN2 patients will develop MTC at some point in their lifetime. Improved survival is linked to performing thyroidectomy and central node dissection when calcitonin levels are either undetectable or very low and when there is no clinically apparent MTC. Therefore, preventative or "prophylactic" thyroidectomy is recommended in infants, children, and adolescents, and recommendations are stratified according to mutation present.

With the publication of the 2015 American Thyroid Association guidelines, the management of MTC was updated. In previous editions, categories A, B, C, and D were used to define risk, where risk is related to the aggressiveness of MTC, A being the lowest and D being the highest. With the revised edition, these have been changed to moderate (ATA-MOD), high (ATA-H), and highest (ATA-HST) risk categories. Patients with MEN2B all fall into the ATA-HST risk, previously D, category due to the early onset of MTC in these patients and the more aggressive course of the disease. Category C is now ATA-H and includes patients with codon C634 and A883F mutations. Categories A and B are now merged into the category ATA-MOD and include patients with all other *RET* mutations, excluding M918T, C634, and A883F.[31] Recommendations for management are then stratified based on risk category, summarized in Table 41.1. Recommendations are similar to those published by other societies.

Carriers in the ATA-MOD risk category should begin annual screening with physical and ultrasound examination as well as calcitonin measurements done at 6- to 12-month intervals beginning at the age of 5. The timing of thyroidectomy can then be determined using calcitonin levels.[31] In one database series of young patients, those operated on with calcitonin levels less than 30 pg/mL had no persistent or recurrent disease at follow-up.[42] In another series of patients who underwent preventative surgery, the mean age at detection of no nodal metastases was age 10.[43] Therefore, for this category, the type of operation may be individualized based on calcitonin levels and age at the time of operation and the extent of surgery may only need to be total thyroidectomy rather than total thyroidectomy with a central lymph node dissection. The follow-up period in this group may extend for several years and there is potential for loss of continuity, and these factors should be considered when timing preventative surgery.[31]

Those in the ATA-H risk category should have a preventative thyroidectomy performed at the age of 5 years or earlier if serum calcitonin levels dictate otherwise. Inclusion of central lymph node dissection at the time of total thyroidectomy is based on preoperative calcitonin levels as well as intraoperative inspection of lymph nodes.[31]

The recommendation for children in the ATA-HST risk category, limited to those with MEN2B and an M918T mutation, should have a total thyroidectomy in the first year of life. The decision to perform central lymph node dissection at the time of operation is dictated based on the presence of clinically suspicious level VI lymph nodes and the ability of the surgeon to identify and preserve parathyroid glands.[31] Children operated on at an earlier age are more likely to have a biochemical cure, with undetectable calcitonin levels, and improved survival. Most will develop MTC by age 16 and are likely to possess physical characteristics associated with MEN2B. Therefore, screening for MEN2B or MTC should be considered in children with the typical physical phenotype.

Outcomes of the familial forms of MTC are largely dependent on the age and stage at the time of surgical management. In a population of patients with MEN2-associated MTC, overall survival at 5 and 10 years was 100% and 94%, respectively, and disease-free survival at 5 and 10 years was 92.9% and 71.6%, respectively, with a mean age at diagnosis of 43.9 years. Age, preoperative calcitonin levels, and presence of vascular invasion were all predictors of survival.[44] In another series of patients, approximately one third of patients achieved biochemical cure, or normalization of calcitonin, with appropriate surgical management,[45] which has been linked to improved survival. Ultimately, though, carriers of *RET* mutations require lifelong follow-up not only for detection of recurrent MTC, but following total thyroidectomy, patients require thyroid hormone replacement to physiologic levels. Calcitonin and CEA levels should be measured every 3 months postoperatively, or, if undetectable after surgery, the interval can be lengthened to 6 to 12 months.

Recurrent and Metastatic Disease

Approximately 50% of patients with MTC will have either persistent or recurrent disease after initial operation. These patients are identified by either a palpable neck mass following surgery or as evidenced by calcitonin levels. Depending on the degree to which calcitonin is elevated or if it is rising, distant metastatic disease should be considered and evaluated as previously stated. Regional recurrences, that is, those limited to the neck, are best managed with repeat operation. Benefits of reoperation in the neck include potential for achieving biochemical cure, known to correlate with survival, as well as potentially identifying patients who may have calcitonin elevations as a result of distant metastasis once the neck is free of disease. Reoperative neck surgery should be focused on treating compartments with imageable or biopsy-proven disease, with the operation done in a compartment-oriented fashion. Beyond surgery, limited options exist for management. Postoperative RAI is not indicated as C-cells do not take up iodine. External beam radiation therapy is of little benefit for the management of recurrent disease in the neck and does not improve survival. It may play a role in the palliation of bone metastases. Single-agent or combination cytotoxic chemotherapies have a low response to treatment and are typically not used as first-line therapy.[31] Understanding the genetics of MTC has allowed for the development of targeted therapies primarily falling into the class of agents known as tyrosine kinase inhibitors. Vandetanib is the primary agent used, and in clinical trials, both partial and complete responses have been observed. It has also been demonstrated to improve progression-free survival and its use in metastatic MTC is Food and Drug Administration approved.[46]

Pheochromocytoma

Pheochromocytomas are tumors arising from the chromaffin cells of the adrenal medulla. These cells secrete catecholamines, which are produced in excess in the setting of a pheochromocytoma. Typical symptoms of pheochromocytoma include sweating, tremulousness, headache, flushing, palpitations, and anxiety. Typical age at diagnosis is in the 30s or 40s, although they may also be identified in children and adolescents. Identification of a pheochromocytoma prior to surgical management of MTC is critical to avoid intraoperative hypertensive crisis and death, and evaluation is done by measuring plasma or timed urinary metanephrines prior to surgery. If a pheochromocytoma is identified prior to thyroidectomy, then in almost all situations, an adrenalectomy would be done first to normalize catecholamine levels.

Compared to patients with sporadic pheochromocytoma, MEN2-pheochromocytoma occur in younger patients, are often bilateral, and have higher baseline metanephrine levels. In one series of patients, MEN2-pheochromocytoma patients were more than 10 years younger on average and had bilateral tumors approximately 50% of the time.[47] In another series of patients, pheochromocytoma was diagnosed synchronously with MTC in 34% of patients, highlighting the importance of screening for pheochromocytoma prior to thyroidectomy. In the same group, survival was equivalent in patients with MTC with and without pheochromocytoma.[48] The most common mutation identified in patients with pheochromocytoma is a codon 634 mutation followed by codon 918 mutations.[47,48] In patients with a codon 634 mutation, penetrance is 25% by age 30, 52% by age 50, and 88% by age 77, while all patients with a codon 918 mutation (MEN2B) developed a pheochromocytoma by age 56 years. In all other mutations, the penetrance is 32%.

MEN2-pheochromocytoma tend to be benign, but given the potential for recurrence and bilaterality, patients require lifelong monitoring. They can be malignant, but it is uncommon, occurring less than 5% of the time.

All patients with MEN2A or MEN2B should be screened for pheochromocytoma. Recommendations for screening are stratified according to the ATA risk categories where HST, H, and

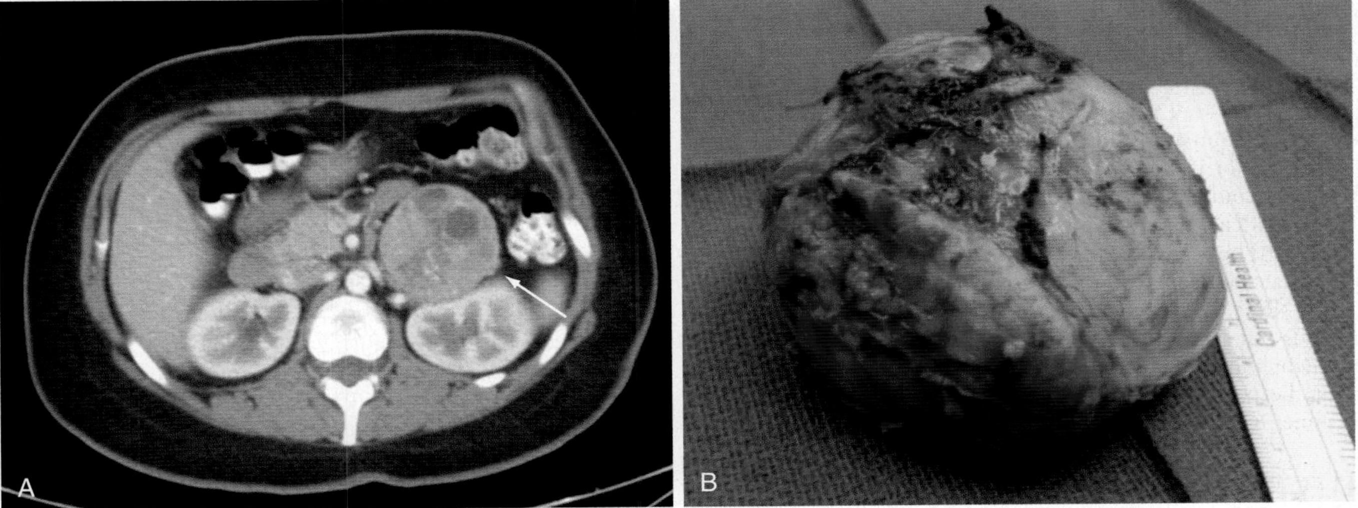

FIG. 41.7 (A) Typical computed tomography appearance of pheochromocytoma, indicated by *arrow*. (B) Resected adrenal pheochromocytoma.

MOD risk patients begin screening at the ages of 11, 11, and 16, respectively.[31] Measurements of plasma free metanephrines and normetanephrines or 24-hour urinary metanephrines and normetanephrines should be done at a minimum annually. If there is any abnormality with testing, that is, elevated levels of either, further investigatory imaging should be done with either CT or MRI of the abdomen to evaluate for the presence of an adrenal mass.

Patients confirmed to have a pheochromocytoma should undergo surgical resection. The procedure of choice for operative management is either a laparoscopic or retroperitoneoscopic adrenalectomy, and the selection of the procedure depends on the expertise of the surgeon (Fig. 41.7). The safety of either of these procedures is well established, and they are comparable to one another. Minimally invasive adrenalectomies are associated with a shorter hospital stay and less postoperative pain compared to open adrenalectomy. Laparoscopic transabdominal adrenalectomy may be better for larger lesions; however, and it is still an appropriate choice for pheochromocytoma that are larger as well. If there is any radiologic evidence of invasion of adjacent organs or structures, the pheochromocytoma would then be presumed to be malignant, and an open adrenalectomy is preferred.

A major concern surrounding operation for MEN2-pheochromocytoma is that they are likely to either be bilateral or recur over time, and patients will potentially need multiple operations. Because of this, when feasible, a cortical-sparing or partial adrenalectomy should be performed. The safety of this procedure is established, and it is done in an effort to avoid adrenal insufficiency. Situations where cortical-sparing adrenalectomy is preferred include patients who have had the contralateral adrenal gland removed and small tumors where there is a portion of normal-appearing adrenal gland that could potentially be left in situ. Approximately 90% of patients after cortical-sparing adrenalectomy will remain steroid-independent.[49] The decision to perform a cortical-sparing adrenalectomy should be weighed against the risks of developing another pheochromocytoma over the lifetime of the patient, and treatment decisions should be individualized based on patient-specific details. All patients undergoing surgery for a pheochromocytoma should receive appropriate preoperative preparation with an alpha-blocker or calcium-channel blocker.

Primary Hyperparathyroidism

Up to a third of patients with MEN2A can develop PHPT, and the likelihood of development is predictable based on which mutation is present. PHPT is not found in patients with MEN2B or with FMTC; therefore, screening and surveillance are not indicated. PHPT tends to occur earlier and is most commonly found in patients with codon 634 mutations, ATA-H category.[50] The recommended age at which screening and annual surveillance should begin follows the recommendations for pheochromocytoma. ATA-H and ATA-MOD category patients should begin annual testing of calcium levels and PTH at the ages of 11 and 16 years, respectively.[31]

Options for surgical management include subtotal parathyroidectomy, leaving a portion of one gland in situ, total parathyroidectomy with autotransplantation into the brachioradialis muscle of the forearm, or parathyroidectomy with removal of only abnormal-appearing glands guided by intraoperative PTH measurements in order to establish that the patient has been biochemically cured. Over time, the surgical management of PHPT in the setting of MEN2A has evolved to the latter procedure, where only abnormal-appearing glands are removed at the time of surgery. The rate of both persistent and recurrent disease is low even with focused or image-guided parathyroidectomy. In planning for a focused parathyroidectomy, preoperative imaging should be obtained based on surgeon comfort and experience with interpretation of the study. Patients who develop PHPT following a thyroidectomy for MTC should have imaging prior to undergoing reoperative neck surgery in order to localize the abnormal gland or glands.[31]

CONCLUSION

Management of MEN has evolved over time and has been greatly impacted by both better understanding of the natural history of the disease, as well as discovery and characterization of the related genetic mutations. Identification of a mutation in either the *MEN1* gene or in the *RET* gene offers a way for the clinician to predict the course of the disease over time and tailor care to the individual patient. Patients with MEN2 may be offered preventative surgery and be cured of MTC. Those with MEN1 can be offered appropriate surveillance to avoid sequelae of malignant progression of NETs. Exclusion of the presence of a mutation in known kindreds can avoid lifelong unnecessary testing. Surveillance and treatment will continue to be tailored over time as more is learned about the pathogenesis of these diseases, resulting in improved outcomes in those affected.

SELECTED REFERENCES

Alesina PF, Hinrichs J, Meier B, et al. Minimally invasive cortical-sparing surgery for bilateral pheochromocytomas. *Langenbecks Arch Surg*. 2012;397:233–238.

This report of a single-institution experience of patients undergoing bilateral cortical-sparing adrenalectomy for pheochromocytoma demonstrates that patients undergoing this procedure have a low recurrence rate and few have adrenal insufficiency postoperatively.

Elaraj DM, Skarulis MC, Libutti SK, et al. Results of initial operation for hyperparathyroidism in patients with multiple endocrine neoplasia type 1. *Surgery*. 2003;134:858–864; discussion 864–855.

This is a single-institution series evaluating the outcomes of parathyroidectomy and patient characteristics in patients undergoing parathyroidectomy for primary hyperparathyroidism with a known diagnosis of multiple endocrine neoplasia type 1.

Nell S, Verkooijen HM, Pieterman CRC, et al. Management of MEN1 related nonfunctioning pancreatic NETs: a shifting paradigm: results from the DutchMEN1 Study Group. *Ann Surg*. 2018;267:1155–1160.

Using a prospectively collected database of patients known to have multiple endocrine neoplasia type 1, these data compare the outcomes and characteristics of patients with nonfunctional pancreatic neuroendocrine tumors (NETs) stratified by size managed with surgery versus observation.

Neumann HP, Bausch B, McWhinney SR, et al. Germ-line mutations in nonsyndromic pheochromocytoma. *N Engl J Med*. 2002;346:1459–1466.

These data evaluated a population of patients with apparent nonsyndromic pheochromocytoma and found that up to 25% possess a previously unknown genetic mutation.

Wells Jr SA, Asa SL, Dralle H, et al. Revised American Thyroid Association guidelines for the management of medullary thyroid carcinoma. *Thyroid*. 2015;25:567–610.

These are the most recently published management guidelines for medullary thyroid carcinoma written by a consensus group of experts in the field.

REFERENCES

1. Thakker RV, Newey PJ, Walls GV, et al. Clinical practice guidelines for multiple endocrine neoplasia type 1 (MEN1). *J Clin Endocrinol Metab*. 2012;97:2990–3011.
2. Ito T, Igarashi H, Uehara H, et al. Causes of death and prognostic factors in multiple endocrine neoplasia type 1: a prospective study: comparison of 106 MEN1/Zollinger-Ellison syndrome patients with 1613 literature MEN1 patients with or without pancreatic endocrine tumors. *Medicine (Baltimore)*. 2013;92:135–181.
3. Larsson C, Skogseid B, Oberg K, et al. Multiple endocrine neoplasia type 1 gene maps to chromosome 11 and is lost in insulinoma. *Nature*. 1988;332:85–87.
4. Chandrasekharappa SC, Guru SC, Manickam P, et al. Positional cloning of the gene for multiple endocrine neoplasia-type 1. *Science*. 1997;276:404–407.
5. Dreijerink KM, Goudet P, Burgess JR, et al. Breast-cancer predisposition in multiple endocrine neoplasia type 1. *N Engl J Med*. 2014;371:583–584.
6. Lemos MC, Thakker RV. Multiple endocrine neoplasia type 1 (MEN1): analysis of 1336 mutations reported in the first decade following identification of the gene. *Hum Mutat*. 2008;29:22–32.
7. Marini F, Giusti F, Brandi ML. Genetic test in multiple endocrine neoplasia type 1 syndrome: an evolving story. *World J Exp Med*. 2015;5:124–129.
8. Thevenon J, Bourredjem A, Faivre L, et al. Higher risk of death among MEN1 patients with mutations in the JunD interacting domain: a Groupe d'etude des Tumeurs Endocrines (GTE) cohort study. *Hum Mol Genet*. 2013;22:1940–1948.
9. Pardi E, Mariotti S, Pellegata NS, et al. Functional characterization of a CDKN1B mutation in a Sardinian kindred with multiple endocrine neoplasia type 4 (MEN4). *Endocr Connect*. 2015;4:1–8.
10. Elaraj DM, Skarulis MC, Libutti SK, et al. Results of initial operation for hyperparathyroidism in patients with multiple endocrine neoplasia type 1. *Surgery*. 2003;134:858–864; discussion 864–855.
11. Lairmore TC, Govednik CM, Quinn CE, et al. A randomized, prospective trial of operative treatments for hyperparathyroidism in patients with multiple endocrine neoplasia type 1. *Surgery*. 2014;156:1326–1334; discussion 1334–1325.
12. Cohen MS, Dilley WG, Wells Jr SA, et al. Long-term functionality of cryopreserved parathyroid autografts: a 13-year prospective analysis. *Surgery*. 2005;138:1033–1040; discussion 1040–1031.
13. Kwekkeboom DJ, Krenning EP. Somatostatin receptor imaging. *Semin Nucl Med*. 2002;32:84–91.
14. Haug AR, Cindea-Drimus R, Auernhammer CJ, et al. The role of 68Ga-DOTATATE PET/CT in suspected neuroendocrine tumors. *J Nucl Med*. 2012;53:1686–1692.

15. Fendrich V, Langer P, Waldmann J, et al. Management of sporadic and multiple endocrine neoplasia type 1 gastrinomas. *Br J Surg*. 2007;94:1331–1341.
16. Norton JA. Surgical treatment and prognosis of gastrinoma. *Best Pract Res Clin Gastroenterol*. 2005;19:799–805.
17. Norton JA, Jensen RT. Resolved and unresolved controversies in the surgical management of patients with Zollinger-Ellison syndrome. *Ann Surg*. 2004;240:757–773.
18. Guettier JM, Kam A, Chang R, et al. Localization of insulinomas to regions of the pancreas by intraarterial calcium stimulation: the NIH experience. *J Clin Endocrinol Metab*. 2009;94:1074–1080.
19. Albright SV, McCart JA, Libutti SK, et al. Rapid measurement of insulin using the Abbott IMx: application to the management of insulinoma. *Ann Clin Biochem*. 2002;39:513–515.
20. Christakis I, Qiu W, Hyde SM, et al. Genotype-phenotype pancreatic neuroendocrine tumor relationship in multiple endocrine neoplasia type 1 patients: a 23-year experience at a single institution. *Surgery*. 2018;163:212–217.
21. Triponez F, Dosseh D, Goudet P, et al. Epidemiology data on 108 MEN 1 patients from the GTE with isolated nonfunctioning tumors of the pancreas. *Ann Surg*. 2006;243: 265–272.
22. Vinault S, Mariet AS, Le Bras M, et al. Metastatic potential and survival of duodenal and pancreatic tumors in multiple endocrine neoplasia type 1: a GTE and AFCE cohort study (Groupe d'etude des Tumeurs Endocrines and Association Francophone de Chirurgie Endocrinienne) [published online ahead of print 2018]. *Ann Surg*.
23. Nell S, Verkooijen HM, Pieterman CRC, et al. Management of MEN1 related nonfunctioning pancreatic NETs: a shifting paradigm: results from the DutchMEN1 Study Group. *Ann Surg*. 2018;267:1155–1160.
24. Falconi M, Eriksson B, Kaltsas G, et al. ENETS consensus guidelines update for the management of patients with functional pancreatic neuroendocrine tumors and non-functional pancreatic neuroendocrine tumors. *Neuroendocrinology*. 2016; 103:153–171.
25. de Laat JM, Dekkers OM, Pieterman CR, et al. Long-term natural course of pituitary tumors in patients with MEN1: results from the DutchMEN1 Study Group (DMSG). *J Clin Endocrinol Metab*. 2015;100:3288–3296.
26. Christakis I, Qiu W, Silva Figueroa AM, et al. Clinical features, treatments, and outcomes of patients with thymic carcinoids and multiple endocrine neoplasia type 1 syndrome at MD Anderson Cancer Center. *Horm Cancer*. 2016;7:279–287.
27. Gatta-Cherifi B, Chabre O, Murat A, et al. Adrenal involvement in MEN1. Analysis of 715 cases from the Groupe d'etude des Tumeurs Endocrines database. *Eur J Endocrinol*. 2012;166:269–279.
28. Callender GG, Rich TA, Perrier ND. Multiple endocrine neoplasia syndromes. *Surg Clin North Am*. 2008;88:863–895, viii.
29. Steiner AL, Goodman AD, Powers SR. Study of a kindred with pheochromocytoma, medullary thyroid carcinoma, hyperparathyroidism and Cushing's disease: multiple endocrine neoplasia, type 2. *Medicine (Baltimore)*. 1968;47: 371–409.
30. Eng C, Clayton D, Schuffenecker I, et al. The relationship between specific RET proto-oncogene mutations and disease phenotype in multiple endocrine neoplasia type 2. International RET Mutation Consortium analysis. *JAMA*. 1996;276:1575–1579.
31. Wells Jr SA, Asa SL, Dralle H, et al. Revised American Thyroid Association guidelines for the management of medullary thyroid carcinoma. *Thyroid*. 2015;25:567–610.
32. Farndon JR, Leight GS, Dilley WG, et al. Familial medullary thyroid carcinoma without associated endocrinopathies: a distinct clinical entity. *Br J Surg*. 1986;73:278–281.
33. Jasim S, Ying AK, Waguespack SG, et al. Multiple endocrine neoplasia type 2B with a RET proto-oncogene A883F mutation displays a more indolent form of medullary thyroid carcinoma compared with a RET M918T mutation. *Thyroid*. 2011;21:189–192.
34. Elisei R, Romei C, Cosci B, et al. RET genetic screening in patients with medullary thyroid cancer and their relatives: experience with 807 individuals at one center. *J Clin Endocrinol Metab*. 2007;92:4725–4729.
35. Neumann HP, Bausch B, McWhinney SR, et al. Germ-line mutations in nonsyndromic pheochromocytoma. *N Engl J Med*. 2002;346:1459–1466.
36. Noone AM, Howlader N, Krapcho M, et al. *SEER Cancer Statistics Review, 1975–2015*. National Cancer Institute; 2018. https://seer.cancer.gov/archive/csr/1975_2015/. Accessed June 13, 2019.
37. Torresan F, Cavedon E, Mian C, et al. Long-term outcome after surgery for medullary thyroid carcinoma: a single-center experience. *World J Surg*. 2018;42:367–375.
38. Wells Jr SA, Pacini F, Robinson BG, et al. Multiple endocrine neoplasia type 2 and familial medullary thyroid carcinoma: an update. *J Clin Endocrinol Metab*. 2013;98: 3149–3164.
39. Castroneves LA, Coura Filho G, de Freitas RMC, et al. Comparison of 68Ga PET/CT to other imaging studies in medullary thyroid cancer: superiority in detecting bone metastases. *J Clin Endocrinol Metab*. 2018;103: 3250–3259.
40. Moley JF, DeBenedetti MK. Patterns of nodal metastases in palpable medullary thyroid carcinoma: recommendations for extent of node dissection. *Ann Surg*. 1999;229:880–887; discussion 887–888.
41. Laird AM, Gauger PG, Miller BS, et al. Evaluation of postoperative radioactive iodine scans in patients who underwent prophylactic central lymph node dissection. *World J Surg*. 2012;36:1268–1273.
42. Rohmer V, Vidal-Trecan G, Bourdelot A, et al. Prognostic factors of disease-free survival after thyroidectomy in 170 young patients with a RET germline mutation: a multicenter study of the Groupe Francais d'Etude des Tumeurs Endocrines. *J Clin Endocrinol Metab*. 2011;96:E509–518.
43. Machens A, Niccoli-Sire P, Hoegel J, et al. Early malignant progression of hereditary medullary thyroid cancer. *N Engl J Med*. 2003;349:1517–1525.
44. Jayakody S, Reagh J, Bullock M, et al. Medullary thyroid carcinoma: survival analysis and evaluation of mutation-specific immunohistochemistry in detection of sporadic disease. *World J Surg*. 2018;42:1432–1439.

45. Cupisti K, Wolf A, Raffel A, et al. Long-term clinical and biochemical follow-up in medullary thyroid carcinoma: a single institution's experience over 20 years. *Ann Surg.* 2007;246:815–821.
46. Wells Jr SA, Robinson BG, Gagel RF, et al. Vandetanib in patients with locally advanced or metastatic medullary thyroid cancer: a randomized, double-blind phase III trial. *J Clin Oncol.* 2012;30:134–141.
47. Rajan S, Zaidi G, Agarwal G, et al. Genotype-phenotype correlation in Indian patients with MEN2-associated pheochromocytoma and comparison of clinico-pathological attributes with apparently sporadic adrenal pheochromocytoma. *World J Surg.* 2016;40:690–696.
48. Thosani S, Ayala-Ramirez M, Palmer L, et al. The characterization of pheochromocytoma and its impact on overall survival in multiple endocrine neoplasia type 2. *J Clin Endocrinol Metab.* 2013;98:E1813–E1819.
49. Alesina PF, Hinrichs J, Meier B, et al. Minimally invasive cortical-sparing surgery for bilateral pheochromocytomas. *Langenbecks Arch Surg.* 2012;397:233–238.
50. Schuffenecker I, Virally-Monod M, Brohet R, et al. Risk and penetrance of primary hyperparathyroidism in multiple endocrine neoplasia type 2A families with mutations at codon 634 of the RET proto-oncogene. Groupe D'etude des Tumeurs a Calcitonine. *J Clin Endocrinol Metab.* 1998;83:487–491.

SECTION IX

Esophagus

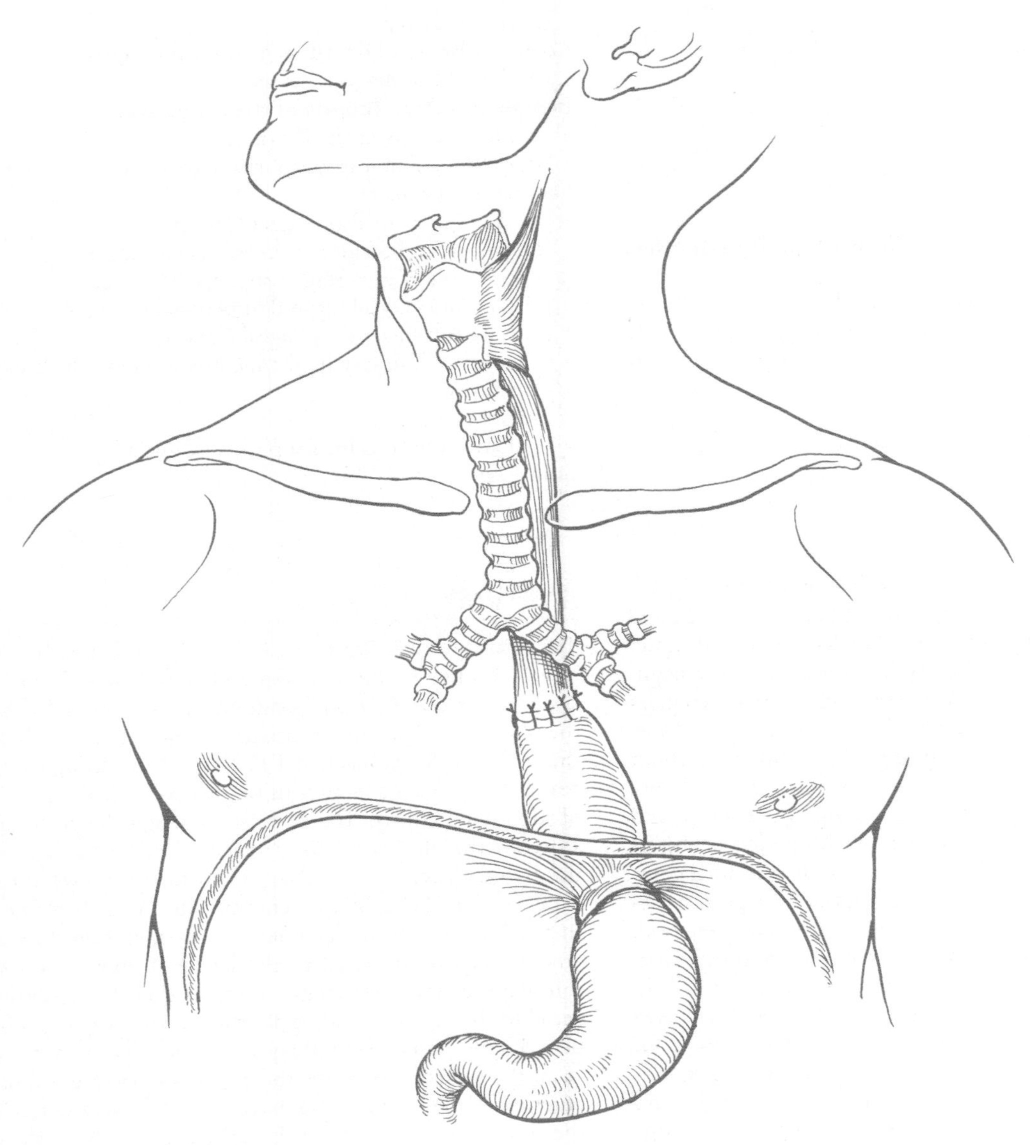

42 CHAPTER

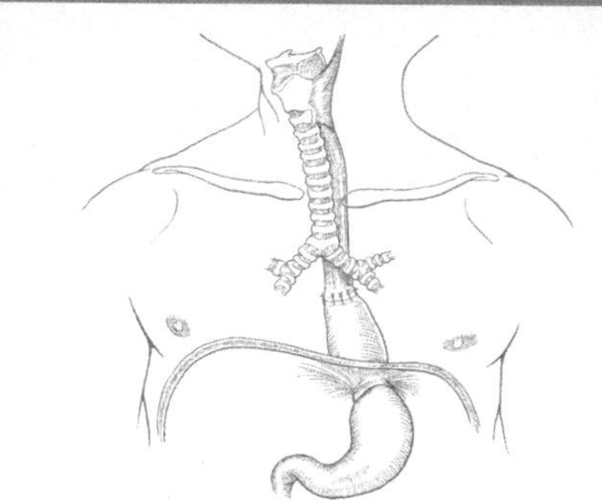

Esophagus

Ravi Rajaram, Jonathan D. Spicer, Rajeev Dhupar, Jae Y. Kim, Boris Sepesi, Wayne L. Hofstetter

OUTLINE

An organ that spans the distance of neck to stomach, the esophagus for all of its tube-like simplicity is in actuality a complex and relatively durable organ. It traverses the outside world and passes through precious territory in the mediastinum. The esophagus functions within areas that transition through pressure changes ranging from atmospheric to vacuum. Yet, the precision of a normal esophagus is virtually unrecognized. We swallow without effort, pain, or thought; but introduce disease within the organ, and we incur various degrees of malady, some quite severe and invariably chronic. We have yet to come up with perfect solutions for most of the dysfunction that is described in the forthcoming section, and replacement of the esophagus at this point is accomplished only by substitution of tissues rather than a renewal. Ultimately, among the "fixes" that are described, nothing functions as well as the original healthy organ. However, advances in perioperative care, surgical safety, and minimally invasive as well as endoscopic techniques have improved patient outcomes for many esophageal pathologies. Nevertheless, future generations of esophagologists have the opportunity to further innovate and contribute to the management of this complex organ. Our hope is that this chapter serves as an introduction to the esophagus and its various forms of function and dysfunction. One could literally spend a lifetime delving into each of these areas.

ANATOMY

The esophagus is a two-layered, mucosa-lined muscular tube that travels through the neck, chest, and abdomen and rests unobtrusively in the posterior mediastinum. It commences at the base of the pharynx at C6 and terminates in the abdomen, where it joins the cardia of the stomach at T11 (Fig. 42.1). Along its 25- to 30-cm course, it winds its way through a path yielding to structures of more vital efforts. The cervical esophagus begins as a midline structure that deviates slightly to the left of the trachea as it passes through the neck into the thoracic inlet. At the level of the carina, it deviates to the right to accommodate the arch of the aorta. It then winds its way back under the left mainstem bronchus and remains slightly deviated to the left as it enters the diaphragm through the esophageal hiatus at the level of the eleventh thoracic vertebra. In the neck and upper thorax, the esophagus is secured between the vertebral column posteriorly and the trachea anteriorly. At the level of the carina, the heart and pericardium lie directly anterior to the thoracic esophagus. Immediately before entering the abdomen, the esophagus is pushed anteriorly by the descending thoracic aorta that accompanies the esophagus through the diaphragm into the abdomen separated by the median arcuate ligament.

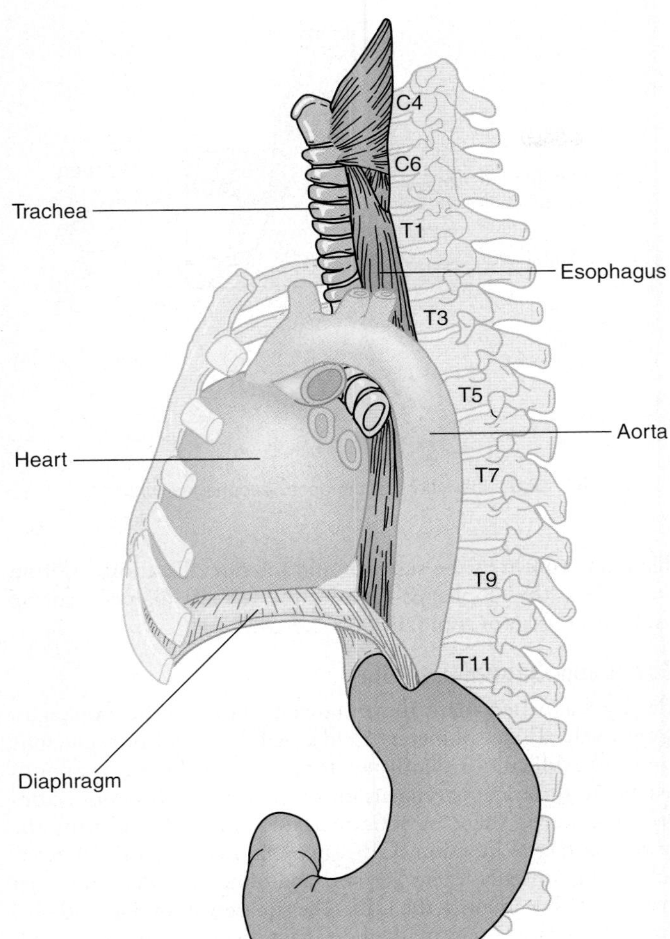

FIG. 42.1 Course of the esophagus.

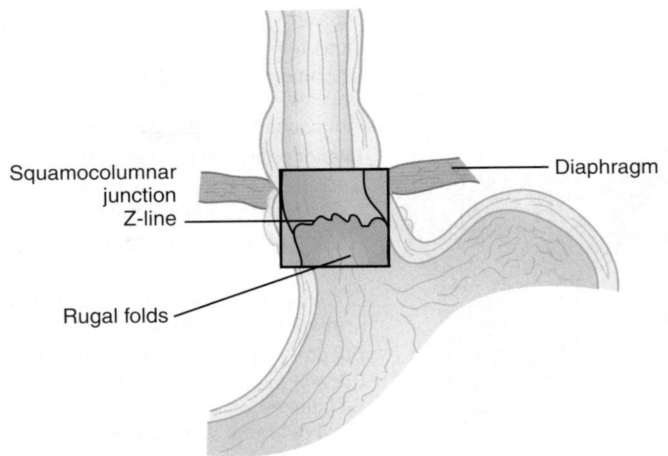

FIG. 42.2 Z-line.

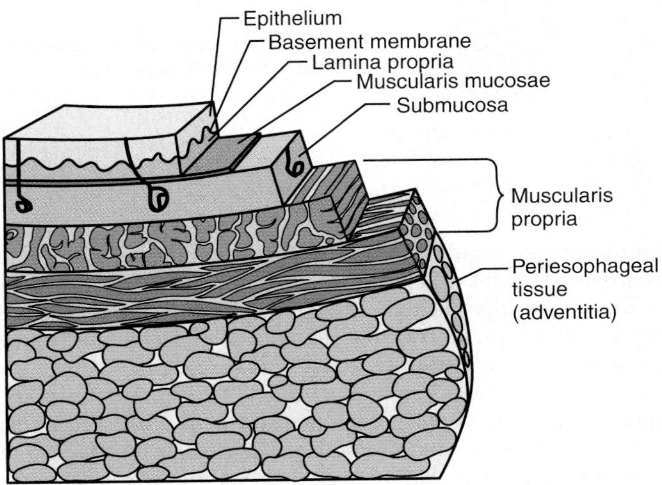

FIG. 42.3 Layers of the esophagus. (Adapted from Pearson FG, Cooper JD, Deslauriers J, et al. *Esophageal surgery*. 2nd ed. New York, NY: Churchill Livingstone; 2002:124.)

The journey through the muscular esophagus begins and ends with two distinct high-pressure zones, the upper (UES) and lower esophageal sphincter (LES). After passing through the UES, four esophageal segments are encountered: the pharyngeal, cervical, thoracic, and abdominal esophagus. The LES is the outlet through which passage into the stomach is then facilitated.

Esophageal Inlet

The high-pressure zone at the inlet of the esophagus is the UES, which anatomically marks the end of a complex configuration of muscles that begins in the larynx and posterior pharynx and ends in the neck. The pharyngeal constrictor muscles are three consecutive muscles that begin at the base of the palate and end at the crest of the esophagus. The superior and middle pharyngeal constrictor muscles, as well as the oblique, transverse, and posterior cricoarytenoid muscles, are immediately proximal to the UES and serve to anchor the pharynx and larynx to structures in the mouth and palate. These muscles also aid in deglutition and speech but are not responsible for the high pressures noted in the UES. The inferior pharyngeal constrictor muscle is the final bridge between the pharyngeal and esophageal musculature.

Inserting into the median pharyngeal raphe, the inferior pharyngeal constrictor muscle is composed of two consecutive muscle beds—the thyropharyngeus and cricopharyngeus muscles—that originate bilaterally from the lateral portions of the thyroid and cricoid cartilages, respectively. The transition between the oblique fibers of the thyropharyngeus muscle and the horizontal fibers of the cricopharyngeus muscle creates a point of potential weakness, known as Killian triangle (site of a Zenker diverticulum). The cricopharyngeus muscle is responsible for generating a high-pressure zone that marks the position of the UES and esophageal introitus. Its distinctive bowing array of muscle fibers is unique and serves to transition into the circular esophageal musculature. This point of transition is flanked by the longitudinal esophageal muscles that extend superiorly to attach to the midportion of the posterior surface of the cricoid cartilage and form the V-shaped area of Laimer.

Esophageal Layers

The esophagus is comprised of two proper layers, the mucosa and muscularis propria. It is distinguished from the other layers of the alimentary tract by its lack of a serosa. The mucosa is the innermost layer and consists of squamous epithelium for most of its course. The distal 1 to 2 cm of esophageal mucosa transitions to cardiac mucosa or junctional columnar epithelium at a point known as the Z-line (Fig. 42.2). Within the mucosa, there are four distinct layers: the epithelium, basement membrane, lamina propria, and muscularis mucosae. Deep to the muscularis mucosae lays the submucosa (Fig. 42.3). Within it is a plush network of

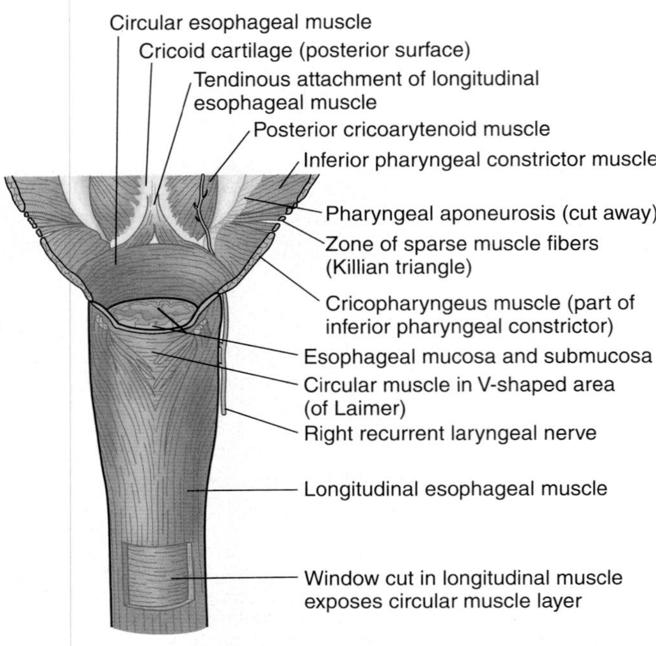

FIG. 42.4 Muscles of the esophagus.

lymphatic and vascular structures, as well as mucous glands and Meissner neural plexus.

Enveloping the mucosa, directly abutting the submucosa, is the muscularis propria. Below the cricopharyngeus muscle, the esophagus is composed of two concentric muscle bundles: an inner circular and outer longitudinal (Fig. 42.4). Both layers of the upper third of the esophagus are striated, whereas the layers of the lower two-thirds are smooth muscle. The circular muscles are an extension of the cricopharyngeus muscle and traverse through the thoracic cavity into the abdomen, where they become the middle circular muscles of the lesser curvature of the stomach. The collar of Helvetius marks the transition of the circular muscles of the esophagus to oblique muscles of the stomach at the incisura (cardiac notch). Between the layers of esophageal muscle is a thin septum comprised of connective tissue, blood vessels, and an interconnected network of ganglia known as Auerbach plexus. Enshrouding the inner circular layer, the longitudinal muscles of the esophagus begin at the cricoid cartilage and extend into the abdomen, where they join the longitudinal musculature of the cardia of the stomach. The esophagus is then wrapped by a layer of fibroalveolar adventitia.

Anatomic Narrowing

The esophageal silhouette resembles an hourglass. There are three distinct areas of narrowing that contribute to its shape. Measuring 14 mm in diameter, the cricopharyngeus muscle is the narrowest point of the gastrointestinal tract and marks the superiormost portion of the hourglass-shaped esophagus. Located just below the carina, where the left mainstem bronchus and aorta abut the esophagus, the bronchoaortic constriction at the level of the fourth thoracic vertebra creates the center narrowing and measures 15 to 17 mm. Finally, the diaphragmatic constriction, measuring 16 to 19 mm, marks the inferior portion of the hourglass and is located where the esophagus passes through the diaphragm. Between these three distinct areas of anatomic constriction are two areas of

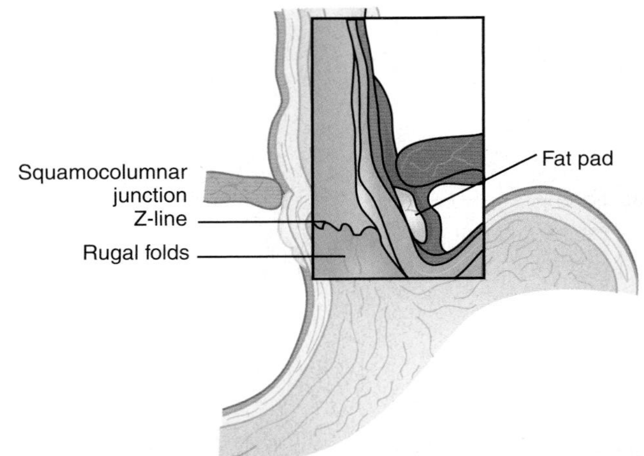

FIG. 42.5 Identifiers of the gastroesophageal junction.

dilatation known as the superior and inferior dilatations. Within these areas, the esophagus resumes the normal diameter for an adult and measures approximately 2.5 cm.

Gastroesophageal Junction

The UES and LES mark the entrance and exit to the esophagus, respectively. These sphincters are defined by a high-pressure zone but can be difficult to identify anatomically. The UES corresponds reliably to the cricopharyngeus muscle, but the LES is more complex to discern. There are four anatomic points that identify the gastroesophageal junction (GEJ): two endoscopic and two external. Endoscopically, there are two anatomic considerations that may be used to identify the GEJ. The squamocolumnar epithelial junction (Z-line) may mark the GEJ provided that the patient does not have a distal esophagus replaced by columnar-lined epithelium, as seen with Barrett esophagus. The transition from the smooth esophageal lining to the rugal folds of the stomach may also identify the GEJ accurately. Externally, the collar of Helvetius (or loop of Willis), where the circular muscular fibers of the esophagus join the oblique fibers of the stomach, and the gastroesophageal fat pad are consistent identifiers of the GEJ (Fig. 42.5).

Vasculature

The rich vascular and lymphatic structures that nourish and drain the esophagus serve as a surgical safety net and a highway for metastases. The vasculature is divided into three segments: cervical, thoracic, and abdominal. The cervical esophagus receives most of its blood supply from the inferior thyroid arteries, which branch off of the thyrocervical trunk on the left and the subclavian artery on the right (Fig. 42.6). The cricopharyngeus muscle, which marks the inlet of the esophagus, is supplied by the superior thyroid artery. The thoracic esophagus receives its blood supply directly from four to six esophageal arteries coming off the aorta, as well as esophageal branches off the right and left bronchial arteries. It is supplemented by descending branches off the inferior thyroid arteries, intercostal arteries, and ascending branches of the paired inferior phrenic arteries. The abdominal esophagus receives its blood supply from the left gastric artery and paired inferior phrenic arteries. All the arteries that supply blood to the esophagus terminate in a fine capillary network before they penetrate the muscular wall of the esophagus. After penetrating and supplying the muscular layers, the capillary network continues the length of the esophagus within the submucosal layer.

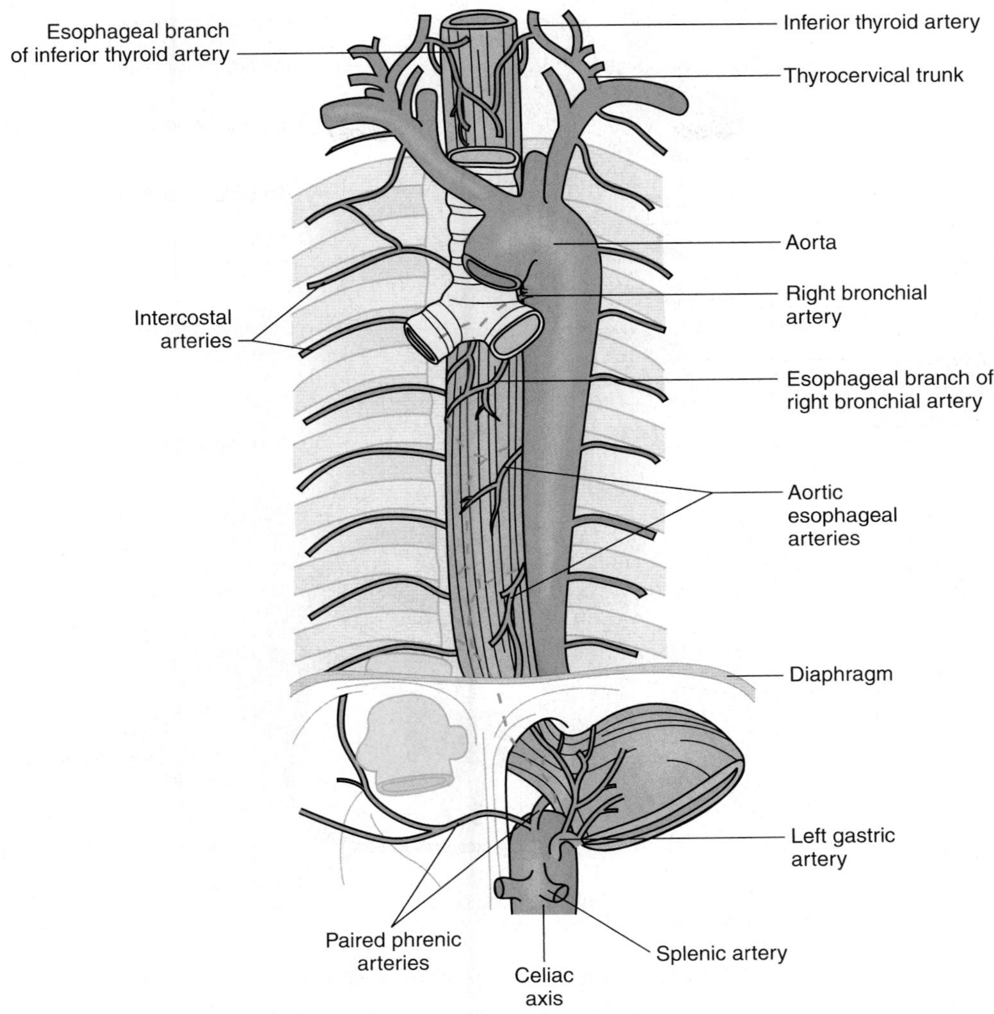

FIG. 42.6 Arterial supply to the esophagus.

The venous drainage parallels the arterial vasculature and is just as complex. In all parts of the esophagus, the rich submucosal venous plexus is the first basin for venous drainage of the esophagus. In the cervical esophagus, the submucosal venous plexus drains into the inferior thyroid veins, which are tributaries of the left subclavian vein and right brachiocephalic vein (Fig. 42.7). The drainage of the thoracic esophagus is more intricate. The submucosal venous plexus of the thoracic esophagus joins with the more superficial esophageal venous plexus and the venae comitantes that envelop the esophagus at this level. This plexus, in turn, drains into the azygos and hemiazygos veins on the right and left sides of the chest, respectively. The intercostal veins also drain into the azygos venous system. The abdominal esophagus drains into the systemic and portal venous systems through the left and right phrenic veins and left gastric (coronary) vein and short gastric veins, respectively.

Lymphatics

The lymphatic drainage of the esophagus is extensive; it consists of two interconnecting lymphatic plexuses arising from the submucosa and muscularis layers. The submucosal lymphatics penetrate the muscularis propria and drain into the plexus that runs longitudinally in the esophageal wall. They then egress and drain into regional lymph node beds. In the upper two-thirds of the esophagus, lymphatic flow is upward, whereas in the distal third, flow tends to be downward. Esophageal lymphatics begin in the neck with drainage to the paratracheal lymph nodes anteriorly and deep lateral cervical and internal jugular nodes laterally and posteriorly. Once inside the chest, the lymphatics form a matrix of interconnecting channels that drain into the mediastinal lymph nodes and thoracic duct. Anteriorly, the paratracheal and subcarinal lymph nodes and the paraesophageal, retrocardiac, and infracardiac nodes all drain the esophagus.

Other mediastinal stations, such as the para-aortic and inferior pulmonary ligament nodes, can also receive drainage from the thoracic esophagus. Posteriorly, nodes along the esophagus and azygos veins are the primary sites of drainage (Fig. 42.8). The intricate lymphatic network of the esophagus allows for rapid spread of infection and tumor into three body cavities. It stands to reason that the rich arterial supply to the esophagus makes it one of the more durable organs in the body with respect to surgical manipulation, whereas its comprehensive venous and lymphatic drainage create an oncologic challenge to controlling cellular migration. These anatomic complexities lead to surgical challenges when treating esophageal cancer and other esophageal diseases.

Innervation

The innervation to the esophagus is sympathetic and parasympathetic (Fig. 42.9). The cervical sympathetic trunk arises from the

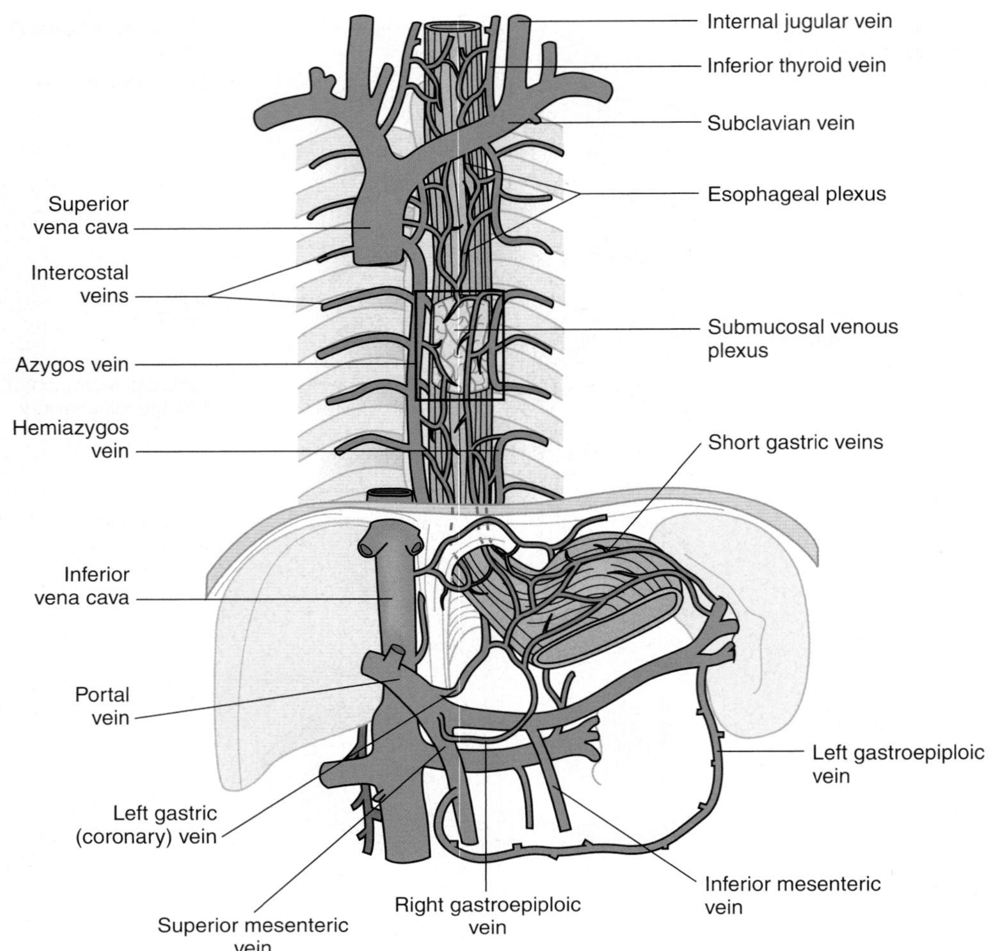

FIG. 42.7 Venous drainage of the esophagus.

superior ganglion in the neck. It extends next to the esophagus into the thoracic cavity, where it terminates in the cervicothoracic (stellate) ganglion. Along the way, it gives off branches to the cervical esophagus. The thoracic sympathetic trunk continues on from the stellate ganglion, giving off branches to the esophageal plexus, which envelops the thoracic esophagus anteriorly and posteriorly. Inferiorly, the greater and lesser splanchnic nerves innervate the distal thoracic esophagus. In the abdomen, the sympathetic fibers lay posteriorly alongside the left gastric artery.

The parasympathetic fibers arise from the vagus nerve, which gives rise to the superior and recurrent laryngeal nerves. The superior laryngeal nerve branches into the external and internal laryngeal nerves that supply motor innervation to the inferior pharyngeal constrictor muscle and cricothyroid muscle and sensory innervation to the larynx, respectively (Fig. 42.10). The right and left recurrent laryngeal nerves come off the vagus nerve and loop underneath the right subclavian artery and aortic arch, respectively. They then travel upward in the tracheoesophageal groove to enter the larynx laterally underneath the inferior pharyngeal constrictor muscle. Along the way, they innervate the cervical esophagus, including the cricopharyngeus muscle. Unilateral injury to the superior or recurrent laryngeal nerve results in hoarseness and aspiration from laryngeal and UES dysfunction. In the thorax, the vagus nerve sends fibers to the striated muscle and parasympathetic preganglionic fibers to the smooth muscle of the esophagus. A weblike nervous plexus envelops the esophagus throughout its thoracic extent. These sympathetic and parasympathetic fibers penetrate through the muscular wall, forming networks between the muscle layers to become Auerbach plexus and within the submucosal layer to become Meissner plexus (Fig. 42.11). They provide an intrinsic autonomic nervous system within the esophageal wall that is responsible for peristalsis. The parasympathetic fibers coalesce 2 cm above the diaphragm into the left (anterior) and right (posterior) vagus nerves, which descend anteriorly onto the fundus and lesser curvature and posteriorly onto the celiac plexus, respectively.

PHYSIOLOGY

Chicago architect Louis Sullivan is well known for his progressive philosophy that form should follow function. In anatomy this is demonstrated often, and there is no better illustration of this principle in the human body than the esophagus. The primary function of the esophagus is to transport material from the pharynx to the stomach. Secondarily, the esophagus needs to constrain the amount of air that is swallowed and the amount of material that is refluxed. Its form has evolved nicely to enable it to function seamlessly. The esophagus usually measures 30 cm, extending from the pharynx down onto the cardia of the stomach. Under ideal physiologic conditions, the concentric muscular configuration permits effortless unidirectional flow of material from the top to the bottom of the esophagus. The UES, 4 to 5 cm in length, remains in

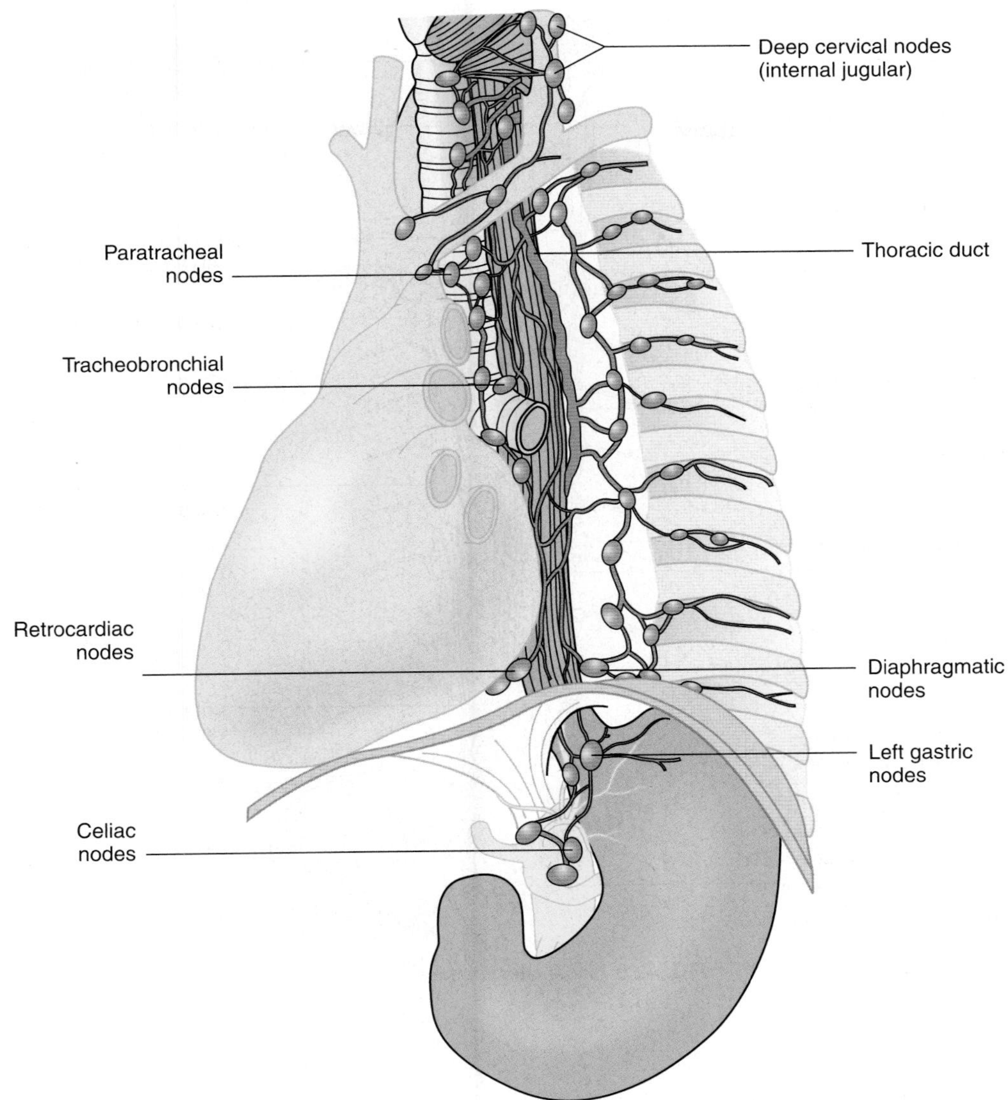

FIG. 42.8 Lymphatic drainage of the esophagus.

a constant state of tone (mean, 60 mm Hg), preventing a steady flow of air into the esophagus, whereas the tone in the LES (mean, 24 mm Hg) remains elevated just enough to prevent excessive material from refluxing back up into the esophagus (Table 42.1). Transport of a food bolus from the mouth through the esophagus into the stomach begins with swallowing and ends with postrelaxation contraction of the LES, requiring coordinated peristaltic contractions in transit. The material in transit can move easily because the esophageal neuromuscular form provides all functions necessary to power the food bolus through three body cavities.

Swallowing

There are three phases to swallowing: oral, pharyngeal, and esophageal. Six events occur during the oropharyngeal phase of swallowing (Fig. 42.12). These rapid series of events last about 1.5 seconds and, once initiated, are completely reflexive.

1. Elevation of the tongue. Food is taken into the mouth and mixed with saliva to prepare a soft bolus for transport. The tongue pushes the bolus into the posterior oropharynx.
2. Posterior movement of the tongue. The tongue moves posteriorly and thrusts the food bolus into the hypopharynx.
3. Elevation of the soft palate. Simultaneously, as the tongue moves the food bolus into the hypopharynx, the soft palate is elevated to close off the passage into the nasopharynx.
4. Elevation of the hyoid. To help bring the epiglottis under the tongue, the hyoid bone moves anteriorly and upward.
5. Elevation of the larynx. The change in position of the hyoid elevates the larynx and opens up the retrolaryngeal space, further facilitating the movement of the epiglottis under the tongue.
6. Tilting of the epiglottis. Finally, the epiglottis tilts back, covering the opening of the larynx to prevent aspiration.

Esophageal Phase

Upper esophageal sphincter. The esophageal phase of swallowing is initiated by the actions during the pharyngeal phase. To allow passage of the food bolus, the UES relaxes and the peristaltic contractions of the posterior pharyngeal constrictors propel the bolus into the esophagus. The pressure differential generated between the positive pressure in the cervical esophagus and the negative intrathoracic pressure sucks the bolus into the thoracic esophagus. Within 0.5 second of the initiation of swallowing, the UES closes, reaching close to 90 mm Hg. This postrelaxation

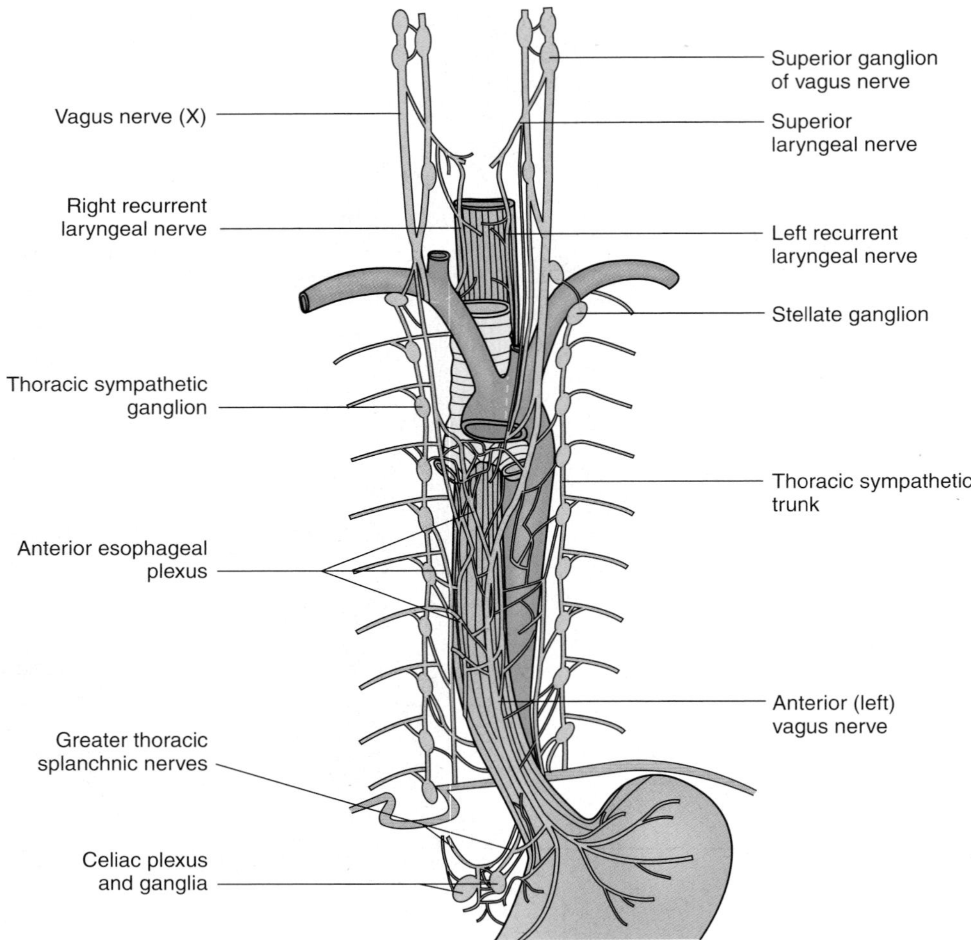

FIG. 42.9 Innervation of the esophagus.

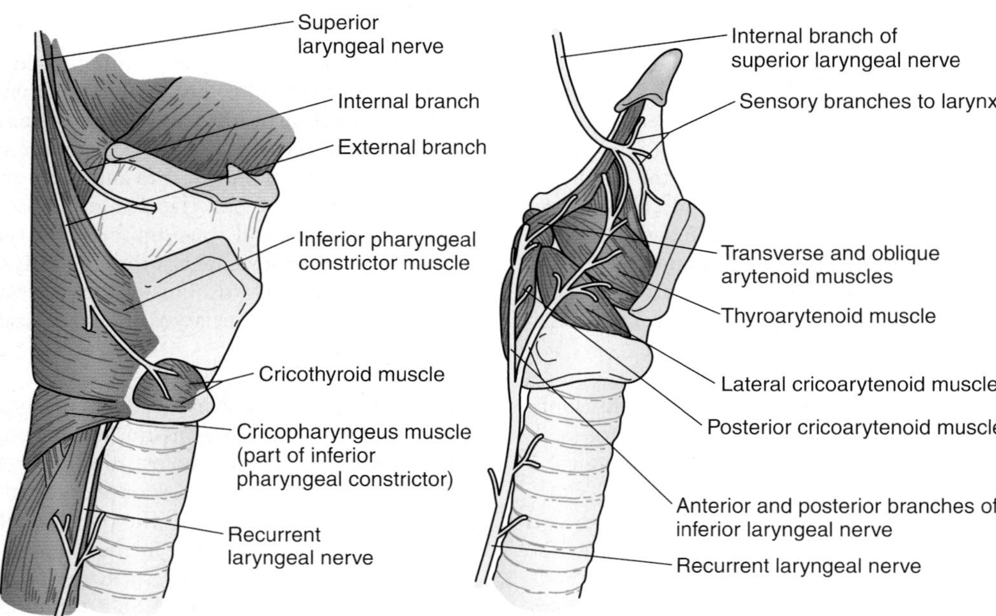

FIG. 42.10 Innervation of the larynx.

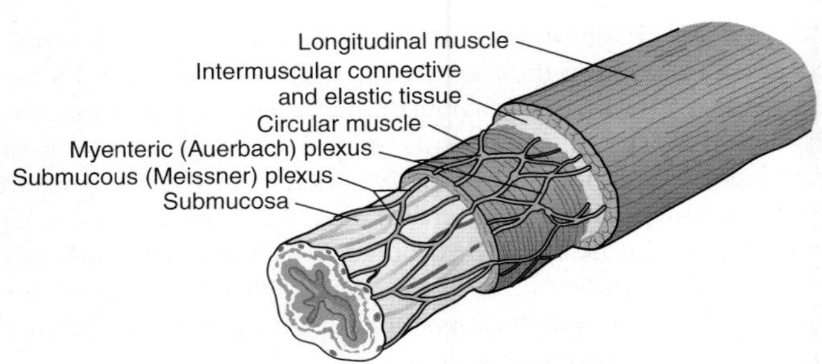

FIG. 42.11 Intrinsic esophageal innervation.

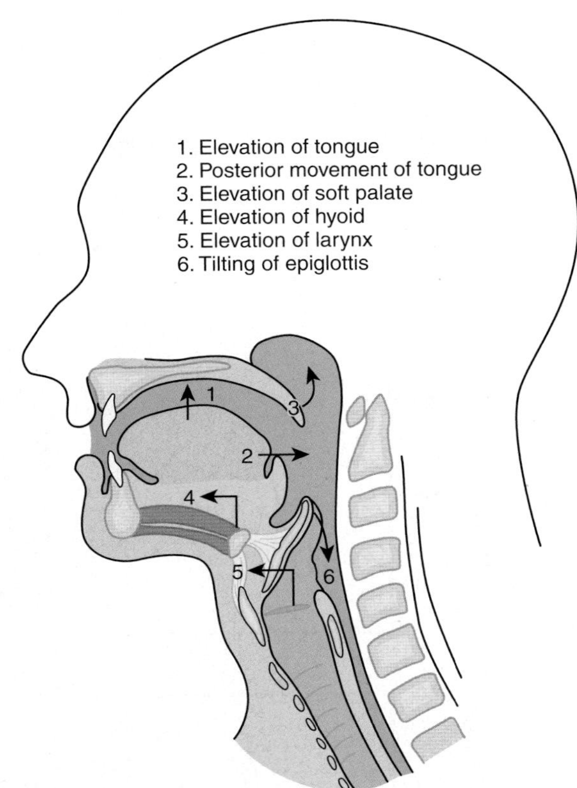

FIG. 42.12 Phases of oropharyngeal swallowing. (Adapted from Zuidema GD, Orringer MB. *Shackelford's surgery of the alimentary tract.* 3rd ed. Philadelphia, PA: WB Saunders; 1991:95.)

TABLE 42.1 Normal manometric values.

PARAMETER	VALUE
Upper Esophageal Sphincter	
Total length	4.0–5.0 cm
Resting pressure	60.0 mm Hg
Relaxation time	0.58 sec
Residual pressure	0.7–3.7 mm Hg
Lower Esophageal Sphincter	
Total length	3–5 cm
Abdominal length	2–4 cm
Resting pressure	6–26 mm Hg
Relaxation time	8.4 sec
Residual pressure	3 mm Hg
Esophageal Body Contractions	
Amplitude	40–80 mm Hg
Duration	2.3–3.6 sec

contraction lasts 2 to 5 msec, initiates peristalsis, and prevents reflux of the bolus back into the pharynx. The UES pressure returns to resting pressure (60 mm Hg) as the wave travels into the mid-esophagus (Fig. 42.13).

Peristalsis. There are three types of esophageal contractions: primary, secondary, and tertiary. Primary peristaltic contractions are progressive and move down the esophagus at a rate of 2 to 4 cm/sec and reach the LES about 9 seconds after the initiation of swallowing (Fig. 42.14). They generate an intraluminal pressure from 40 to 80 mm Hg. Successive swallows will follow with a similar peristaltic wave unless swallowing is repeated rapidly, at which time the esophagus will remain relaxed until the last swallow occurs, and peristalsis will follow. Secondary peristaltic contractions are also progressive but are generated from distention or irritation of the esophagus rather than voluntary swallowing. They can occur as an independent local reflex to clear the esophagus of material that was left behind after the progression of the primary peristaltic wave. Tertiary contractions are nonprogressive, nonperistaltic, monophasic or multiphasic, simultaneous waves that can occur after voluntary swallowing or spontaneously between swallows throughout the esophagus. They represent uncoordinated contractions of the smooth muscle that are responsible for esophageal spasm.

Lower esophageal sphincter. The final phase of esophageal bolus transit occurs through the LES. Although this is not a true sphincter, there is a distinct high-pressure zone that measures 2 to 5 cm in length and generates a resting pressure of 6 to 26 mm Hg. The LES is located in the chest and abdomen. A minimum total length of 2 cm, with at least 1 cm of intraabdominal length, is required for normal LES function. The transition from the intrathoracic to the intraabdominal sphincter is noted on a manometric tracing and is known as the respiratory inversion point (RIP; Fig. 42.15). At this point, the pressure of the esophagus changes from negative to positive with inspiration and positive to negative with expiration.

Peristaltic contractions alone do not generate enough force to open up the LES. Vagal-mediated relaxation of the LES occurs 1.5 to 2.5 seconds after pharyngeal swallowing and lasts 4 to 6 seconds. This flawlessly timed relaxation is needed to allow efficient transport of a food bolus out of the esophagus and into the stomach. A postrelaxation contraction of the LES occurs after the peristaltic wave has passed through the esophagus, allowing the LES to return to its baseline pressure (Fig. 42.16), reestablishing a barrier to reflux.

Reflux Mechanism

Not all reflux is abnormal. Healthy individuals have occasional episodes of gastroesophageal reflux that is a result of spontaneous opening of the LES. The competence of the LES and its ability to establish a barrier to reflux depends on several factors: adequate pressure and length, radial symmetry, and motility of the esophagus and stomach. A competent sphincter is at least 2 cm and carries a pressure between 6 and 26 mm Hg. Radial asymmetry and abnormal peristalsis prevent proper closure and allow free refluxing of gastric material into the distal esophagus. Abnormal esophageal motility and poor gastric emptying result in inadequate esophageal clearance that also encourages reflux. Finally,

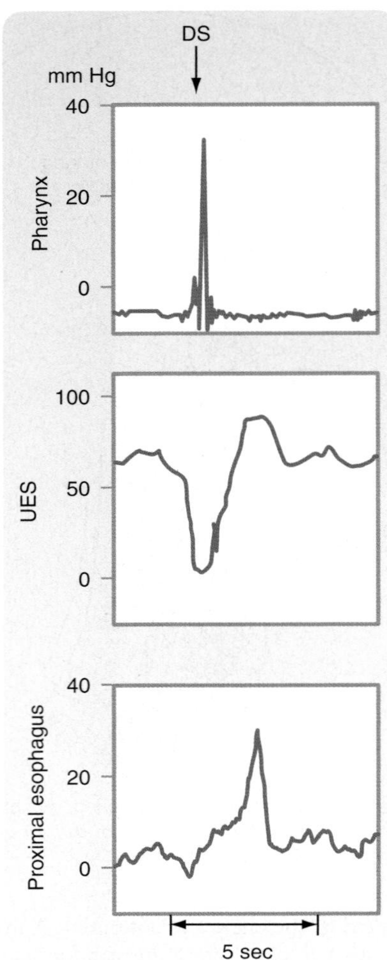

FIG. 42.13 Manometry of the upper esophageal sphincter *(UES)*. (Adapted from Pearson FG, Cooper JD, Deslauriers J, et al. *Esophageal surgery*. 2nd ed. New York, NY: Churchill Livingstone;2002:480.)

neurotransmitters, hormones, and peptides that regulate the LES can increase or decrease tone. All these anatomic and physiologic disruptions can result in reflux through the LES and are implicated in the development of gastroesophageal reflux disease (GERD).

DIAGNOSIS AND MANAGEMENT OF ESOPHAGEAL MOTILITY DISORDERS

Diagnosis

Esophageal motility disorders constitute a relatively rare group of conditions, the underlying causes of which remain poorly understood. Patients with these conditions will present with a variety of symptoms including dysphagia, chest pain, heartburn, regurgitation, and weight loss. By definition, esophageal motility disorders are diagnosed when manometric findings exceed two standard deviations from normal. Unfortunately, symptom severity does not always correlate well with manometry, which is of critical importance in planning for surgical intervention in these generally complicated patients. Esophageal motility disorders are best classified by the Chicago classification, which was derived from data obtained by high-resolution manometry (HRM) with esophageal pressure topography (Table 42.2).[1] Because this classification is purely based on differentiating patterns of manometric findings, the exact clinical utility of this classification remains under investigation. Nevertheless, the findings from these ultramodern diagnostic modalities correlate well with those from conventional, water-perfused manometry. From a practical standpoint, the primary difference between HRM and conventional manometry is that in HRM, the pressure sensors are no more than 1 cm apart rather than every 3 to 5 cm. Up to 36 sensors can be found distributed radially and longitudinally, allowing a three-dimensional spatial pressure map to be drawn during deglutition. The graphic representation of this is what is referred to as esophageal pressure topography.

Whereas manometry is diagnostic for patients with named esophageal motility disorders, their presenting complaints are frequently vague and nonspecific. Hence, a complete workup including careful exclusion of other organ systems (cardiac, respiratory, peptic ulcer disease, and pancreaticobiliary disease) as the source of symptoms is paramount. In addition, attention to systemic symptoms of connective tissue disorders such as scleroderma is key as the surgical management of such patients requires specific modifications to avoid disastrous outcomes. With respect to the esophageal portion of the workup, a barium esophagram continues to be a highly useful road map to guide further investigations. A timed barium esophagram in which images are taken at 1, 2, and 5 minutes after the initial swallow may further characterize esophageal emptying and be particularly helpful in evaluating a patient with suspected achalasia. When the esophagus is thought to be the cause of the patient's symptoms, upper endoscopy is necessary to rule out mucosal abnormalities and to provide improved visualization of the defects in question (stricture, hernia, diverticulum, esophagitis, masses). A computed tomography (CT) scan of the chest and abdomen is not uniformly required but may be helpful, particularly when there is suspicion of an extrinsic cause for the presenting symptoms. The addition of pH testing in the context of a documented esophageal motility disorder is necessary only when the motility disorder is thought to be the result of end-stage GERD as a means of documenting this.

Classically, esophageal motility disorders have been classified into primary and secondary causes. Primary disorders fall into five categories of motor disorders: achalasia, diffuse esophageal spasm (DES), nutcracker (jackhammer) esophagus, hypertensive LES, and ineffective esophageal motility (IEM). Secondary conditions result from progressive damage induced by an underlying collagen vascular or neuromuscular disorder; they include scleroderma, dermatomyositis, polymyositis, lupus erythematosus, Chagas disease, and myasthenia gravis. Whereas such a classification is rooted in the basic etiology of this collection of diseases, it does not help much with interpreting manometric results, nor is it helpful as a guide to treatment strategies. For this reason, we suggest an anatomic approach to classifying esophageal motility disorders based on involvement of the esophageal body or LES as this is the basis for understanding basic esophageal manometry and often the key to guide surgical therapy.

Motility Disorders of the Esophageal Body

Diffuse Esophageal Spasm

DES is a poorly understood hypermotility disorder of the esophagus. Under the Chicago classification, this is now called *distal esophageal spasm*. Although it is manifested in a similar fashion to achalasia, it is five times less common. It is seen most often in women and is often found in patients with multiple medical complaints. The cause of the neuromuscular physiology is unclear. The basic pathology is related to a motor abnormality

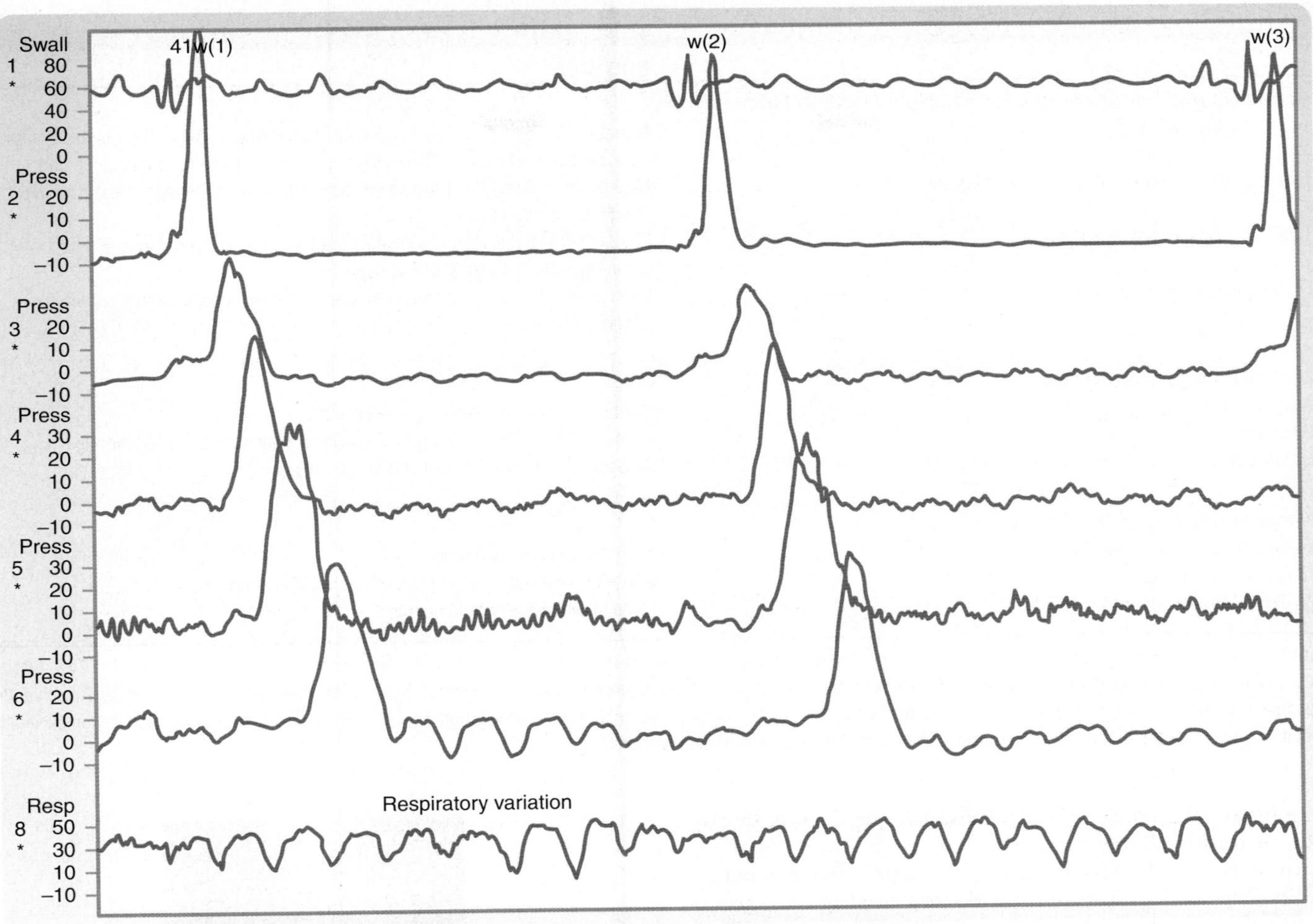

FIG. 42.14 Normal esophageal peristalsis. (From Bremner CG, DeMeester TR, Bremner RM, et al. *Esophageal motility testing made easy*. St Louis: Quality Medical Publishing; 2001:35.)

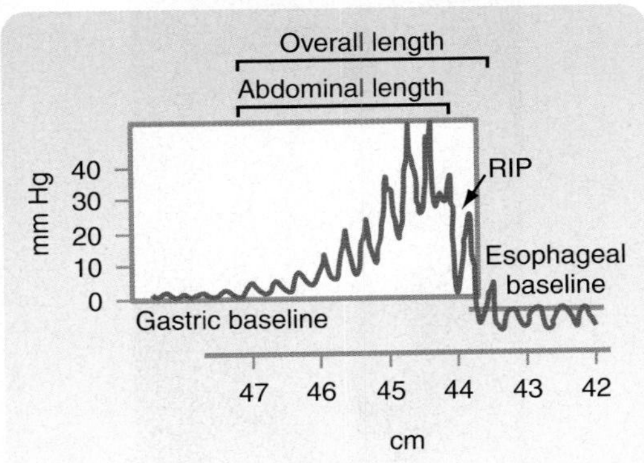

FIG. 42.15 Normal lower esophageal sphincter. (From Bremner CG, DeMeester TR, Bremner RM, et al. *Esophageal motility testing made easy*. St Louis: Quality Medical Publishing; 2001:15.) *RIP*, Respiratory inversion point.

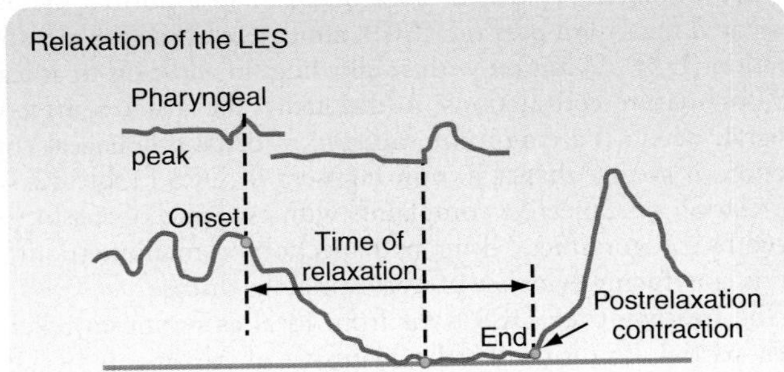

FIG. 42.16 Relaxation of the lower esophageal sphincter *(LES)*. (From Bremner CG, DeMeester TR, Bremner RM, et al. *Esophageal motility testing made easy*. St Louis: Quality Medical Publishing; 2001:24.)

of the esophageal body that is most notable in the lower two-thirds of the esophagus. Muscular hypertrophy and degeneration of the branches of the vagus nerve in the esophagus have been observed. As a result, unlike the normally organized peristaltic contractions typically seen with swallowing (Fig. 42.14), DES esophageal contractions are repetitive, simultaneous, and of high amplitude.

The clinical presentation of DES is typically that of chest pain and dysphagia. These symptoms may be related to eating or exertion and may mimic those of angina. Patients will complain of a squeezing pressure in the chest that may radiate to the jaw, arms, and upper back. The symptoms are often pronounced during times of heightened emotional stress. Regurgitation of esophageal contents and saliva is common, but acid reflux is not. However, acid reflux can aggravate the symptoms, as can cold liquids. Other functional gastrointestinal complaints, such as irritable bowel syndrome and pyloric spasm, may accompany DES, whereas other

TABLE 42.2 **The Chicago classification of esophageal motility, v3.0.**

	CRITERIA
Achalasia and Esophagogastric Junction Outflow Obstruction	
Type I achalasia (classic)	Median IRP >15 mm Hg, 100% failed peristalsis (DCI <100 mm Hg·s·cm); premature contractions with DCI <450 mm Hg·s·cm satisfy criteria for failed peristalsis
Type II achalasia (with esophageal compression)	Median IRP >15 mm Hg; 100% failed peristalsis, panesophageal pressurization with ≥20% of swallows
Type III achalasia (spastic achalasia)	Median IRP >15 mm Hg; no normal peristalsis, spastic contractions with DCI >450 mm Hg·s·cm with ≥20% of swallows
Esophagogastric junction outflow obstruction (achalasia in evolution)	Median IRP >15 mm Hg; sufficient evidence of peristalsis such that criteria for types I-III are not met
Major Disorders of Peristalsis	
Absent contractility	Normal median IRP, 100% failed peristalsis
Distal esophageal spasm	Normal median IRP; ≥20% premature contractions with DCI >450 mm Hg·s·cm
Hypercontractile esophagus (nutcracker or jackhammer)	At least 2 swallows with DCI >8000 mm Hg·s·cm
Minor Disorders of Peristalsis	
Ineffective esophageal motility	≥50% ineffective swallows
Fragmented peristalsis	≥50% fragmented contractions with DCI >450 mm Hg·s·cm
Normal esophageal motility	None of the above criteria are met

Data from Roman S, Gyawali CP, Xiao Y, et al. The Chicago classification of motility disorders. *Gastrointest Endosc Clin N Am.* 2014; 24:545–561.
Integrated relaxation pressure *(IRP)* is the mean of the 4 seconds of maximal deglutitive relaxation in the 10-second window beginning at the upper esophageal sphincter relaxation referenced to gastric pressure; distal contractile integral *(DCI)* is the amplitude × duration × length (mm Hg·s·cm) of the distal esophageal contraction exceeding 20 mm Hg from the transition zone to the proximal margin of the lower esophageal sphincter.

gastrointestinal problems, such as gallstones, peptic ulcer disease, and pancreatitis, all trigger DES.

The diagnosis of DES is made by radiographic and manometric studies. The classic picture of the corkscrew esophagus or pseudodiverticulosis on an esophagram is caused by the presence of tertiary contractions and indicates advanced disease (Fig. 42.17). A distal bird beak narrowing of the esophagus and normal peristalsis can also be noted. HRM findings in DES are a normal median integrated relaxation pressure (IRP), a measure of esophagogastric junction (EGJ) relaxation with swallowing, in addition to at least 20% premature contractions. Additionally, the distal contractile integral, which is a composite measure of distal esophageal contraction, is greater than 450 mm Hg·s·cm in DES (Table 42.2).[1] Correlation of subjective complaints with evidence of spasm (induced by a vagomimetic drug, bethanechol) on manometric tracings is convincing evidence of this capricious disease.

The treatment for DES is far from ideal as symptom relief is often partial. Traditionally, the mainstay of treatment for DES is nonsurgical, and pharmacologic or endoscopic intervention is preferred. All patients are evaluated for psychiatric conditions, including depression, psychosomatic complaints, and anxiety. Control of these disorders and reassurance of the esophageal nature of the chest pain that the patient is experiencing is often alleviating to distressed patients. If dysphagia is a component of a patient's symptoms, steps must be taken to eliminate trigger foods or drinks from the diet. Similarly, if reflux is a component, acid suppression medications are helpful. Nitrates, calcium channel blockers, sedatives, and anticholinergics may be effective in some cases, but the relative efficacy of these medicines is not known. Peppermint may also provide temporary symptomatic relief. Bougie dilatation of the esophagus up to 50 or 60 Fr provides relief for severe dysphagia and is 70% to 80% effective. Botulinum toxin injections have also been tried with some success, but the results are not sustainable.

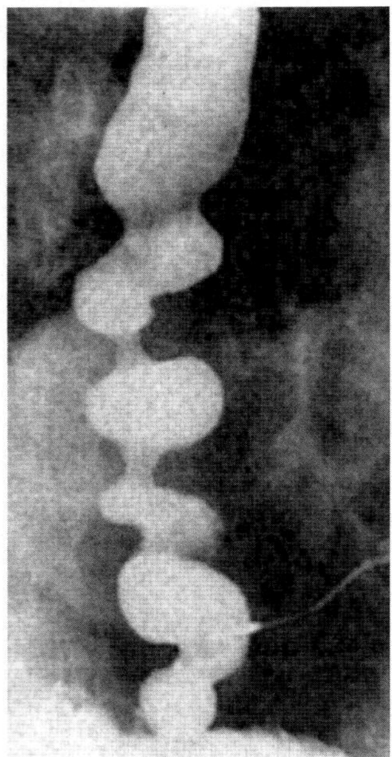

FIG. 42.17 Barium esophagram of diffuse esophageal spasm. (Adapted from Peters JH, DeMeester TR. Esophagus and diaphragmatic hernia. In: Schwartz SI, Fischer JE, Spencer FC, et al, eds. *Principles of surgery.* 7th ed. New York, NY: McGraw-Hill;1998.)

Surgery is indicated for patients with incapacitating chest pain or dysphagia who have failed to respond to medical and endoscopic therapy or in the presence of a pulsion diverticulum of the thoracic esophagus. Historically, a long esophagomyotomy is performed either through the abdomen or a left thoracotomy or video-assisted thoracoscopic approach in the chest is used. While some surgeons advocate extending the myotomy up into the thoracic inlet, most agree that the proximal extent generally should be high enough to encompass the entire length of the abnormal motility, as determined by manometric measurements. The distal extent of the myotomy is extended down onto the LES, but the need to include the stomach is not agreed on uniformly. A Dor fundoplication is recommended to provide reflux protection as the surgery itself interrupts the phrenoesophageal ligament and encourages reflux. Results of a long esophagomyotomy for DES are variable, but it is reported to provide relief of symptoms in up to 80% of patients.

Recently, several authors have reported their experience with the use of peroral endoscopic myotomy (POEM) in the treatment of motility disorders of the esophageal body. In this natural orifice approach, an operating endoscope is used to perform a mucosotomy and a submucosal tunnel is created. Through this tunnel, the circular muscular layer of the esophagus is visualized and divided, effectively performing an endoscopic myotomy. In one series, 73 patients with medically refractory motility disorders of the esophageal body, including nine with DES, underwent POEM and had a clinical response rate of 93%.[2] Furthermore, in the 44 patients with repeat manometry available after POEM, all demonstrated resolution of the abnormal manometric findings seen on initial testing. Though POEM has most often been described in motility disorders of the LES, in particular achalasia (see Achalasia section below), this technology represents a novel surgical approach for performing a long esophagomyotomy in DES patients with early promising results.

Nutcracker Esophagus

Recognized in the late 1970s as a distinct entity and known as hypercontractile esophagus in the Chicago classification, nutcracker or jackhammer esophagus is a disorder characterized by excessive contractility. It is described as an esophagus with hypertensive peristalsis or high-amplitude peristaltic contractions. It is seen in patients of all ages, with equal gender predilection and is the most common of all esophageal hypermotility disorders. Like DES, the pathophysiologic process is not well understood. It is associated with hypertrophic musculature that results in high-amplitude contractions of the esophagus and is the most painful of all esophageal motility disorders.

Patients with nutcracker esophagus present in a similar fashion to those with DES and frequently complain of chest pain and dysphagia. Odynophagia is also noted, but regurgitation and reflux are uncommon. An esophagram may or may not reveal any abnormalities, depending on how well "behaved" the esophagus is during the examination. The Chicago classification characterizes the diagnosis of nutcracker esophagus as the subjective complaint of chest pain with at least two swallows showing a distal contractile integral greater than 8000 mm Hg·s·cm with single or multipeaked contractions on HRM. The LES pressure is normal, and relaxation occurs with each wet swallow. Ambulatory monitoring can help distinguish this disorder from DES.

Similar to DES, the primary initial treatment of nutcracker esophagus is medical. Calcium channel blockers, nitrates, and antispasmodics may offer temporary relief during acute spasms. Bougie dilatation may offer some temporary relief of severe discomfort but has no long-term benefits. Patients with nutcracker esophagus may have triggers and are counseled to avoid caffeine, cold, and hot foods. Although surgery was not historically included in the management of this disease, early results from POEM demonstrating excellent clinical responses have led gastroenterologists and surgeons to rethink this conventional wisdom.[2]

Motility Disorders of the Lower Esophageal Sphincter

Hypertensive Lower Esophageal Sphincter

Hypertensive LES has been renamed in the Chicago classification as EGJ outflow obstruction and is defined on HRM as a median IRP greater than 15 mm Hg (ineffective EGJ relaxation with swallowing). Thought by some to be achalasia in evolution, the diagnosis differs by evidence of effective peristalsis that is not present in achalasia. Hypertensive LES may be observed in patients presenting with dysphagia, chest pain, and, less frequently, heartburn and regurgitation. The diagnosis is made by manometry with a hypertensive, poorly relaxing sphincter. Localization of the LES may be aided by identification of the RIP (Fig. 42.15). Motility of the esophageal body may be hyperperistaltic or normal. An esophagram may show narrowing at the GEJ with delayed emptying and abnormalities of esophageal contraction; however, these are nonspecific findings. About 50% of the time, peristalsis in the esophageal body is normal. In the remainder, abnormal contractions are noted to be hypertensive peristaltic or simultaneous waveforms. The pathogenesis is not well understood.

The treatment of hypertensive LES is with endoscopic and surgical intervention. Botox injections alleviate symptoms temporarily, and hydrostatic balloon dilatation may provide long-term symptomatic relief. Surgery is indicated for patients who fail to respond to interventional treatments and those with significant symptoms. Historically, a laparoscopic Heller esophagomyotomy is the operation of choice. In patients with normal esophageal motility, a partial antireflux procedure (e.g., Dor or Toupet fundoplication) is added to prevent postoperative reflux. Additionally, the use of POEM for such patients has also been described with several studies supporting its use.

Motility Disorders Affecting Both Body and Lower Esophageal Sphincter

Achalasia

The literal meaning of the term *achalasia* is "failure to relax." It is the best understood of all esophageal motility disorders. The incidence is 6/100,000 persons/year with a predilection to affect young women. Its pathogenesis is presumed to be idiopathic or infectious neurogenic degeneration. Severe emotional stress, trauma, drastic weight reduction, and Chagas disease (parasitic infection with *Trypanosoma cruzi*) have also been implicated. Regardless of the cause, the muscles of the esophagus and LES are affected. Prevailing theories support the model that the destruction of the nerves to the LES is the primary pathologic process and that degeneration of the neuromuscular function of the body of the esophagus is secondary. This degeneration results in hypertension of the LES and failure of the LES to relax on pharyngeal swallowing as well as pressurization of the esophagus, esophageal dilatation, and resultant loss of progressive peristalsis.

The classic triad of presenting symptoms of achalasia consists of dysphagia, regurgitation, and weight loss. Heartburn, postprandial choking, and nocturnal coughing are commonly seen. The dysphagia that patients experience often begins with liquids and progresses to solids. Most patients describe eating as a laborious process during which they must pay special attention to the process. They eat slowly and use large volumes of water to help wash the food down into the stomach. As the water builds up pressure, retrosternal chest pain is experienced and can be severe

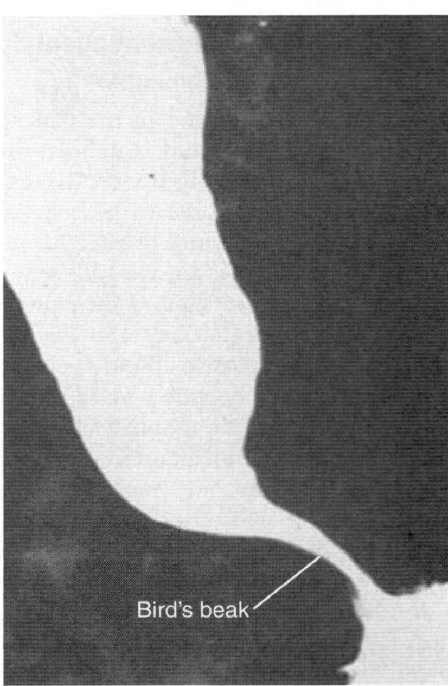

FIG. 42.18 Barium swallow showing achalasia. (Adapted from Dalton CB. Esophageal motility disorders. In: Pearson FG, Cooper JD, Deslauriers J, et al, eds. *Esophageal surgery*. 2nd ed. New York, NY: Churchill Livingstone; 2002.)

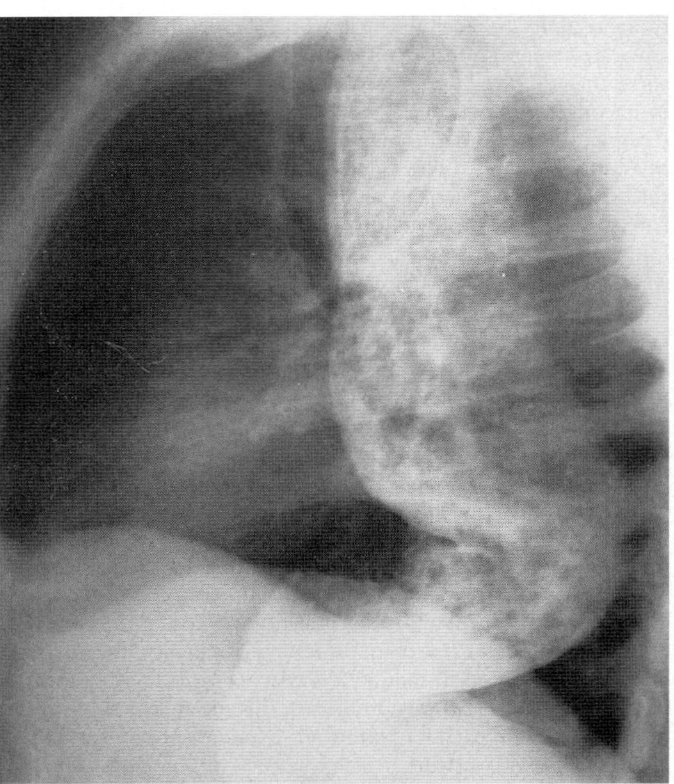

FIG. 42.19 Barium swallow showing megaesophagus. (From Orringer MB. Disorders of esophageal motility. In: Sabiston DC, ed. *Textbook of surgery*. 15th ed. Philadelphia, PA: WB Saunders; 1997.)

until the LES opens, which provides quick relief. Regurgitation of undigested, foul-smelling food is common, and with progressive disease, aspiration can become life-threatening. Pneumonia, lung abscess, and bronchiectasis often result from long-standing achalasia. The dysphagia progresses slowly during years, and patients adapt their lifestyle to accommodate the inconveniences that accompany this disease. Patients often do not seek medical attention until their symptoms are advanced and will present with marked distention of the esophagus.

Achalasia is also known to be a premalignant condition of the esophagus. During a 20-year period, a patient will have up to an 8% chance for development of carcinoma. Squamous cell carcinoma (SCC) is the most common type identified and is thought to be the result of long-standing retained undigested fermenting food in the body of the esophagus, causing mucosal irritation. If the histology is adenocarcinoma, it tends to appear in the middle third of the esophagus, below the air-fluid level, where the mucosal irritation is the greatest. In contrast to these theories of carcinogenesis, it appears that, even in patients with treated achalasia, there is an ongoing cancer incidence risk. Although no specific surveillance program for patients with treated achalasia has yet been endorsed by any of the gastroenterology societies, long-term surveillance is strongly recommended to monitor for recurrent achalasia and cancer.

The diagnosis of achalasia is usually made from an esophagram and a motility study. The findings may vary, depending on the degree to which the disease has advanced. The esophagram will often show a dilated esophagus with a distal narrowing referred to as the classic bird beak appearance of the barium-filled esophagus (Fig. 42.18). Sphincter spasm and delayed emptying through the LES as well as dilatation of the esophageal body are observed. A lack of peristaltic waves in the body and failure of relaxation of the LES (the sine qua non of this disease) are noted. Lack of a gastric air bubble is a common finding on the upright portion of the esophagram and is a result of the tight LES not allowing air to pass easily into the stomach. In the more advanced stage of disease, massive esophageal dilatation, tortuosity, and sigmoidal esophagus (megaesophagus) are seen (Fig. 42.19).

Manometry is the "gold standard" test for diagnosis and distinguishes achalasia from other potential esophageal motility disorders (Fig. 42.20). Achalasia is defined by a median IRP greater than 15 mm Hg (failure of LES relaxation with deglutition) and absence of normal peristalsis. Additional manometric findings associated with achalasia include esophageal body pressurization from incomplete air evacuation, simultaneous mirrored contractions without evidence of progressive peristalsis, and low-amplitude waveforms indicating a lack of muscle tone. The Chicago classification further subdivides achalasia into three types based on characteristic HRM findings (Table 42.2).[1] In type I (classic) achalasia, the median IRP greater than 15 mm Hg and there is 100% failed peristalsis with minimal esophageal pressurization. In type II achalasia, the median IRP greater than 15 mm Hg, 100% failed peristalsis, and panesophageal pressurization with at least 20% of swallows. In type III (spastic or vigorous) achalasia, the median IRP greater than 15 mm Hg without normal peristalsis and there are spastic contractions (distal contractile integral >450 mm Hg·s·cm) with at least 20% of swallows (Fig. 42.20). The amplitude of the contractions in response to swallowing is normal or high and patients oftentimes present with chest pain. It is postulated that patients in the early phases of achalasia may not have abnormalities in the esophageal body that are seen in later stages of the disease. Patients presenting with spastic achalasia may be in this early phase and will go on to develop abnormal esophageal body contractions predicated on the presence of outflow obstruction of the esophagus. Endoscopy must also be performed in

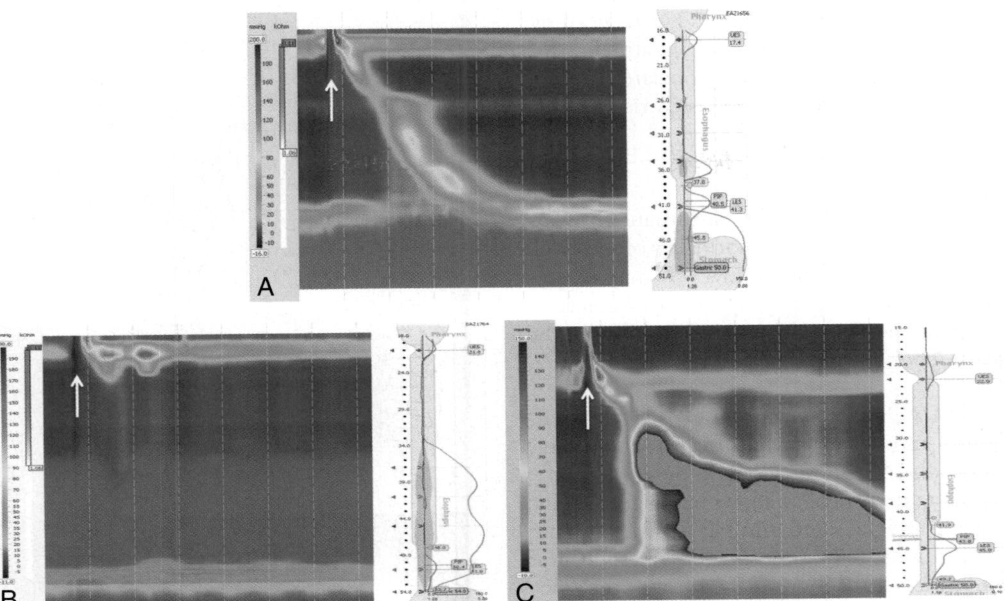

FIG. 42.20 High-resolution esophageal manometry. (A) A normal swallowing pattern. (B) and (C) Classic (type I) achalasia and atypical spastic or vigorous achalasia (type III). The *arrows* denote initiation of swallowing.

all suspected achalasia patients to evaluate the mucosa for esophagitis and rule out secondary causes of distal esophageal narrowing ("pseudoachalasia") such as GEJ tumors, neuropathy, and strictures.

There are surgical and nonsurgical treatment options for patients with achalasia; all are directed toward relieving the obstruction caused by the LES. Because none of them are able to address the issue of decreased motility in the esophageal body, they are all palliative treatments. Nonsurgical treatment options include medications and endoscopic interventions but usually are only a short-term solution to a lifelong problem. In the early stage of the disease, medical treatment with sublingual nitroglycerin, nitrates, or calcium channel blockers may offer hours of relief from chest pressure before or after a meal. Pneumatic dilatation has been shown to provide excellent relief of symptoms although frequently requiring multiple interventions and with a risk of esophageal perforation. Injection of botulinum toxin (Botox) directly into the LES blocks acetylcholine release, prevents smooth muscle contraction, and effectively relaxes the LES. With repeated treatments, Botox may offer symptomatic relief for years, but symptoms recur more than 50% of the time within six months. In comparing balloon dilatation to Botox injections, remission of symptoms occurred in 89% versus 38% of patients at one year, respectively.

Surgical esophagomyotomy offers excellent results that are durable. The current technique is a modification of the Heller myotomy that was described originally through a laparotomy in 1913. Various changes have been made to the originally described procedure, but the modified laparoscopic Heller myotomy is now the operation of choice. A robotic-assisted approach may also be performed. The decision to perform an antireflux procedure remains controversial. Most patients who have undergone a myotomy will experience some amount of reflux, either symptomatic or not. The addition of a partial antireflux procedure, such as a Toupet or Dor fundoplication, will restore a barrier to reflux and decrease postoperative symptoms. Studies done to compare balloon dilatation versus surgery have shown perforation rates of 4% and 1% and mortality rates of 0.5% and 0.2%, respectively. Results were historically considered excellent in 60% of patients undergoing balloon dilatation and in 85% of those undergoing surgery. However, in a randomized controlled trial of the European Achalasia Trial Investigators, pneumatic dilatation was found to be equivalent to laparoscopic Heller myotomy and Dor fundoplication with therapeutic success rates of 86% versus 90% at two years.[3] Perforation occurred in 4% of the patients during pneumatic dilatations and mucosal tears occurred in 12% during laparoscopic Heller myotomy, but all were repaired intraoperatively. Notably, patients in the pneumatic dilatation cohort had a 25% rate of redilation to achieve treatment success. Clinicians need to remain wary and vigilant with achalasia patients, even after "successful" intervention. Continued asymptomatic outflow obstruction will lead to dilatation. Close monitoring of these patients is appropriate.

The use of POEM in the treatment of achalasia has been well described. Through the submucosal tunnel, the muscular layer of the distal esophagus, LES, and cardia is visualized and divided. Although concern for the lack of an antireflux procedure and the possibility of symptomatic reflux remains, results thus far have been encouraging. This is a promising new technique and outcomes thus far suggest equivalency with Heller myotomy in the short-term.[4] However, it remains to be seen if POEM outcomes will compare favorably in the long-term to the excellent results reported in multiple large series of Heller myotomy patients.

Esophagectomy is considered in any symptomatic patient with a tortuous dilated esophagus (megaesophagus), sigmoid esophagus, failure of more than one myotomy, or reflux stricture that is not amenable to dilatation. Less than 60% of patients undergoing repeated myotomy benefit from surgery, and fundoplication for treatment of reflux strictures has even more dismal results. In addition to definitively treating the end-stage achalasia patient, esophageal resection also eliminates the risk for carcinoma in the resected area. A transhiatal esophagectomy with or without preservation of the vagus nerve offers a good long-term result. However, in the setting of megaesophagus, a total esophagectomy incorporating a transthoracic dissection may be safest, given the difficulty in palpating the borders of the esophagus through a transhiatal approach. Notably, POEM in end-stage achalasia patients with sigmoid esophagus has also been reported. In a recent study, two-year outcomes after POEM demonstrated treatment success in 96.8% of patients.[5] Use of POEM may obviate the need for esophagectomy in this malnourished, often high-risk, patient population.

Ineffective Esophageal Motility

IEM was first recognized as a distinct motility disturbance by Castell in 2000. It is defined as a contraction abnormality of the distal esophagus and is usually associated with GERD. It may be secondary to inflammatory injury of the esophageal body because of increased exposure to gastric contents. Dampened motility of the esophageal body leads to poor acid clearance in the lower esophagus.

The symptoms of IEM are mixed, but patients usually present with symptoms of reflux and dysphagia. Heartburn, chest pain, and regurgitation are noted. Diagnosis is made by manometry. IEM is defined by greater than 50% of swallows being deemed ineffective (distal contractile integral <450 mm Hg·s·cm). A barium esophagram demonstrates nonspecific abnormalities of esophageal contraction but will not further distinguish IEM from other motor disorders.

The best treatment of IEM is prevention, which is associated with effective treatment of GERD. Once altered motility occurs, it appears to be irreversible. Similarly, scleroderma may manifest on HRM as IEM and is best treated by addressing the underlying condition. In cases in which the motility disorder has become irreversible and intractable, the surgical approach must be tailored to the manometric findings. However, great caution must be taken in approaching surgical therapy in this cohort of patients as the likelihood of a favorable result remains low.

DIVERTICULAR DISORDERS

It is now well established that most diverticula are a result of a primary motor disturbance or an abnormality of the UES or LES. Diverticula were originally classified according to their location, and as a convention, these are classifications to which we still adhere. The three most common sites of occurrence are pharyngoesophageal (Zenker), parabronchial (midesophageal), and epiphrenic (supradiaphragmatic). True diverticula involve all layers of the esophageal wall, including mucosa, submucosa, and muscularis. A false diverticulum consists of mucosa and submucosa only. Pulsion diverticula are false diverticula that occur because of elevated intraluminal pressures generated from abnormal motility disorders. These forces cause the mucosa and submucosa to herniate through the esophageal musculature. Both a Zenker diverticulum and an epiphrenic diverticulum fall under the category of false pulsion diverticula. Traction, or true, diverticula result from external inflammatory mediastinal lymph nodes adhering to the esophagus as they heal and contract, pulling the esophagus during the process. Over time, all layers of the esophageal wall herniate, forming an outpouching, and a true diverticulum ensues. These are more common in the midesophageal region around the carinal lymph nodes.

Pharyngoesophageal (Zenker) Diverticulum

Originally described by Zenker and von Ziemssen, the pharyngoesophageal diverticulum (Zenker diverticulum) is the most common esophageal diverticulum found today (Fig. 42.21). It is usually manifested in older patients in the seventh decade of life and has been postulated to be a result of loss of tissue elasticity

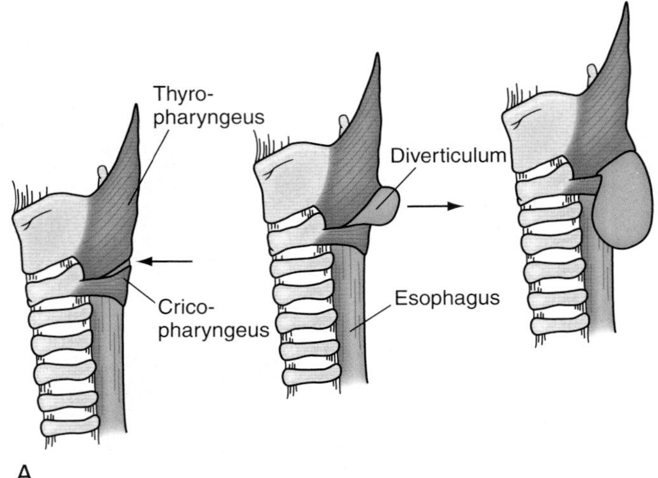

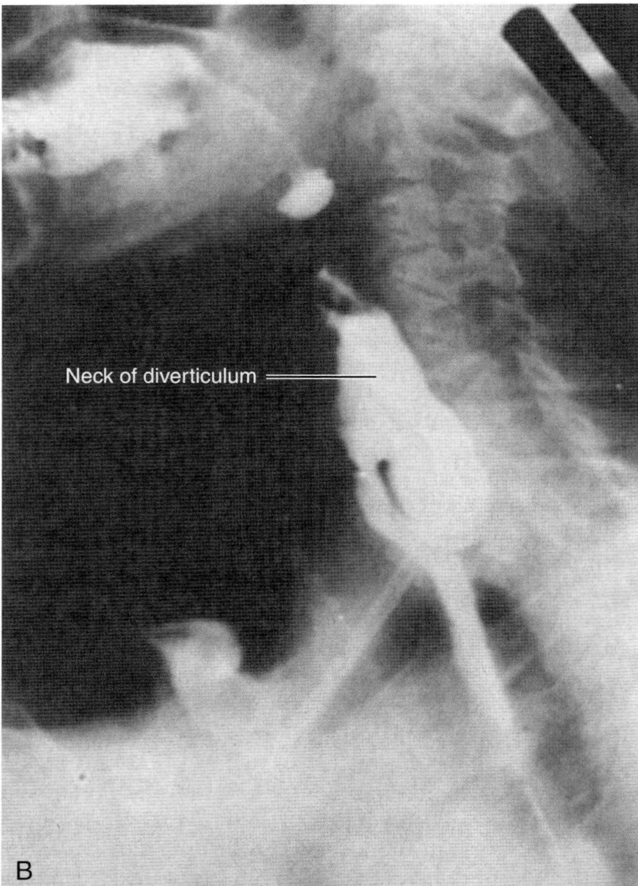

FIG. 42.21 (A) Zenker diverticulum. (B) Barium swallow showing Zenker diverticulum. (Adapted from Trastek VF, Deschamps C. Esophageal diverticula. In: Shields TW, Locicero J III, Ponn RB, eds. *General thoracic surgery*. 5th ed. Philadelphia, PA: Lippincott Williams & Wilkins; 1999.)

and muscle tone with age. It is specifically found herniating from Killian triangle, between the oblique fibers of the thyropharyngeus muscle and the horizontal fibers of the cricopharyngeus muscle. As the diverticulum enlarges, the mucosal and submucosal layers dissect down the left side of the esophagus into the superior mediastinum, posteriorly along the prevertebral space. Zenker diverticulum is often referred to as cricopharyngeal achalasia and is managed accordingly.

Until the Zenker diverticulum begins to enlarge, patients are often initially asymptomatic. Commonly, patients complain of a sticking in the throat. A nagging cough, excessive salivation, and intermittent dysphagia often are signs of progressive disease. As the sac increases in size, regurgitation of foul-smelling, undigested material is common. Halitosis, voice changes, retrosternal pain, and respiratory infections are especially common in older adults. The most serious complication from an untreated Zenker diverticulum is aspiration pneumonia or lung abscess. In an older patient, this can be morbid and sometimes fatal.

Diagnosis is made by barium esophagram. At the level of the cricothyroid cartilage, the diverticulum can be seen filled with barium resting posteriorly alongside the esophagus (the "cricopharyngeal bar"). Lateral views are critical because this is usually a posterior structure. Neither esophageal manometry nor endoscopy is needed to diagnose Zenker diverticulum.

Surgical or endoscopic repair of a Zenker diverticulum is the gold standard of treatment. Traditionally, an open repair through the left side of the neck was advocated. However, endoscopic exclusion has gained popularity in many centers. Two types of open repair are performed: resection or surgical fixation of the diverticulum. The diverticulectomy and diverticulopexy are performed through an incision in the left side of the neck. In all cases, a myotomy of the proximal and distal thyropharyngeus and cricopharyngeus muscles is performed. In cases of a small diverticulum (<2 cm), a myotomy alone is often sufficient. In most patients with good tissue or a large sac (>5 cm), excision of the sac is indicated. Should a diverticulopexy be performed, it is important to suture the diverticulum to the posterior pharynx as opposed to the prevertebral fascia to allow free vertical movement of the pharynx during deglutition. The postoperative stay is approximately 2 or 3 days, during which the patient remains unable to eat or to drink.

An alternative to open surgical repair is the endoscopic Dohlman procedure, which has become more popular. Endoscopic division of the common wall between the esophagus and diverticulum using a laser, electrocautery, or stapler device has been similarly successful. Because of the configuration of the inline-stapling device, this approach has been advocated for larger diverticula. The risk for an incomplete myotomy increases with diverticula smaller than 3 cm. This method divides the distal cricopharyngeus muscle while obliterating the sac. The esophagus and diverticulum ultimately form a common channel. The technique requires maximal extension of the neck and can be difficult to perform in older patients with cervical stenosis. For this reason, many have advocated the use of the needle knife by flexible endoscopy to perform the myotomy. Overall, the postoperative course is slightly shorter for transoral approaches, with patients taking liquids the following day and requiring only a single overnight hospital stay. Thus, these techniques have gained favor and are advocated for patients with diverticula between 2 and 5 cm. A recent metaanalysis demonstrated endoscopic treatment of Zenker diverticulum is well-tolerated, with low adverse event and recurrence rates.[6] Regardless of the method of repair, patients do well and the results are excellent.

Midesophageal Diverticula

Midesophageal diverticula were first described in the nineteenth century. Historically, inflamed mediastinal lymph nodes from an infection with tuberculosis accounted for most cases. Infections with histoplasmosis and resultant fibrosing mediastinitis have now become more common. Inflammation of the lymph nodes exerts traction on the wall of the esophagus and leads to the formation of a true diverticulum in the midesophagus. This continues to be an important mechanism for these traction diverticula, but it is now believed that some may also be caused by a primary motility disorder, such as achalasia, DES, or other esophageal motility disorders.

Most patients with a midesophageal diverticulum are asymptomatic. They are often incidentally found during a workup for some other complaint (Fig. 42.22). Dysphagia, chest pain, and regurgitation can be present and are usually indicative of an underlying primary motility disorder. Patients presenting with a chronic cough are under suspicion for development of a bronchoesophageal fistula. Rarely, hemoptysis can be a presenting symptom, indicating infectious erosion of lymph nodes into major vasculature and the bronchial tree. In this case, the diverticulum is an incidental finding of lesser importance.

The diagnosis of the anatomic structure as well as of the size and location of an esophageal diverticulum is made through barium esophagram. Midesophageal diverticula typically are on the right because of the overabundance of structures in the midthoracic region of the left side of the chest. A CT scan is helpful to identify any mediastinal lymphadenopathy and may help lateralize the sac. Endoscopy is important to rule out mucosal abnormalities, including cancer that may be hidden in the sac. In addition, endoscopy may aid in identifying a fistula. Manometric studies are undertaken in all patients, symptomatic or not, to identify a primary motor disorder. Treatment is guided by the results of the manometric findings.

Determining the cause for midesophageal diverticula is critical for guiding treatment. In asymptomatic patients who have inflamed mediastinal lymph nodes, treatment of the underlying cause is the management of choice. If the diverticulum is smaller than 2 cm, it can be observed. If patients progress to become symptomatic or if the diverticulum is 2 cm or larger, surgical intervention is indicated. Usually, midesophageal diverticula have a wide mouth and rest close to the spine. Therefore, a diverticulopexy can be performed, whereby the diverticulum is suspended from the thoracic vertebral fascia. Alternatively, a diverticulectomy may be performed with care taken not to narrow the esophageal lumen. In patients with severe chest pain or dysphagia and a documented motor abnormality, a long esophagomyotomy is also indicated.

Epiphrenic Diverticula

Epiphrenic diverticula are found adjacent to the diaphragm in the distal third of the esophagus, within 10 cm of the GEJ. They are most often related to thickened distal esophageal musculature or increased intraluminal pressure. They are pulsion, or false, diverticula that are often associated with DES, achalasia, or hypertensive LES disorders. In patients in whom a motility abnormality cannot be identified, a congenital (Ehlers-Danlos syndrome) or traumatic cause is considered. As with midesophageal diverticula, epiphrenic diverticula are more common on the right side and tend to be wide-mouthed.

Most patients with epiphrenic diverticula present asymptomatically. They may present with dysphagia or chest pain, which is indicative of a motility disturbance. The diagnosis is often made during the workup for a motility disorder, and the diverticulum is found incidentally. Other symptoms, such as regurgitation, epigastric pain, anorexia, weight loss, chronic cough, and halitosis, are indicative of an advanced motility abnormality resulting in a sizable epiphrenic diverticulum.

A barium esophagram is the best diagnostic tool to detect an epiphrenic diverticulum (Fig. 42.23). The size, position, and proximity of the diverticulum to the diaphragm can all be clearly delineated. The underlying motility disorder is often identified as well;

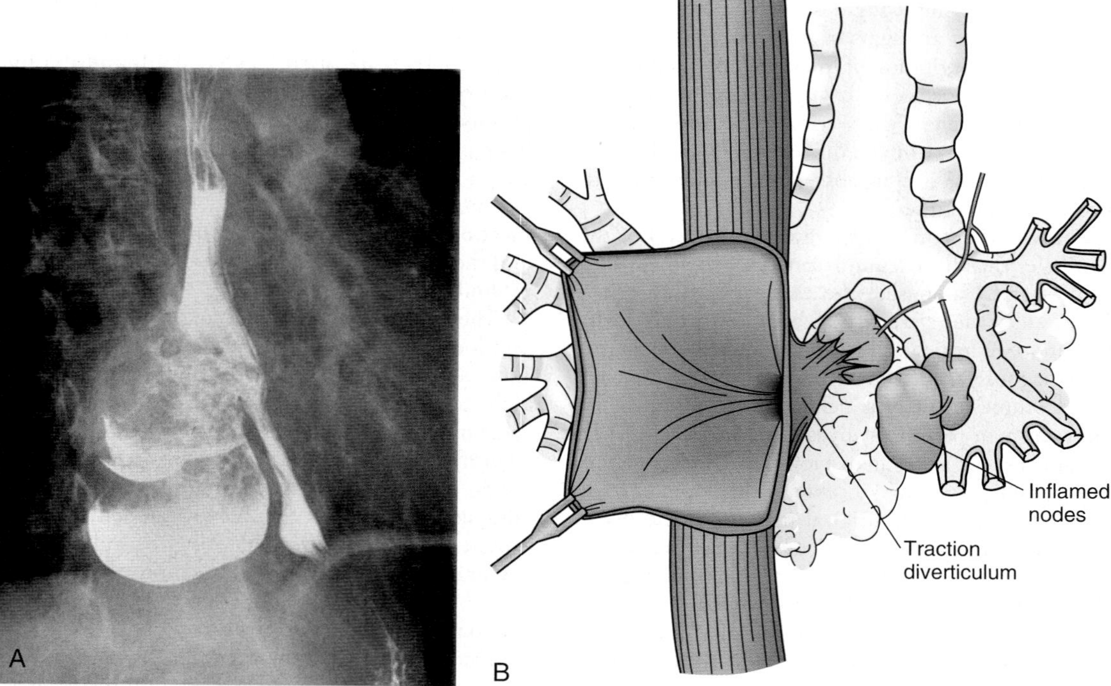

FIG. 42.22 (A) Barium esophagram demonstrating a giant midesophageal diverticulum. (B) Midesophageal diverticulum. (Courtesy Dr. Lorenzo E. Ferri); Adapted from Peters JH, DeMeester TR. Esophagus and diaphragmatic hernia. In: Schwartz SI, Fischer JE, Spencer FC, et al, eds. *Principles of surgery*. 7th ed. New York, NY: McGraw-Hill; 1998.)

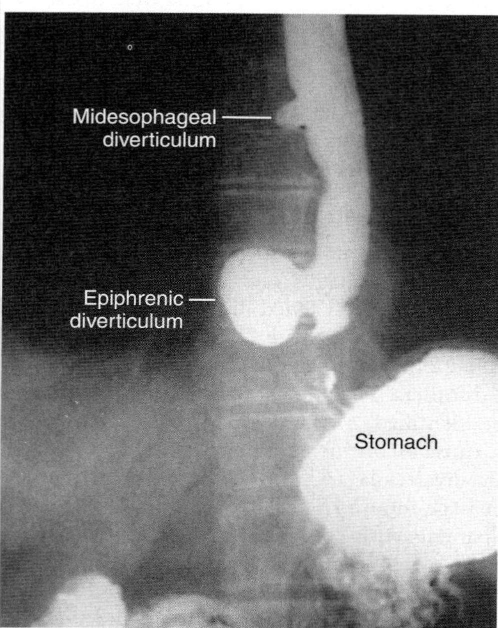

FIG. 42.23 Barium swallow showing mid and distal esophageal diverticula. (Adapted from Pearson FG, Cooper JD, Deslauriers J, et al. *Esophageal surgery*. 2nd ed. New York, NY: Churchill Livingstone; 2002.)

however, manometric studies need to be undertaken to evaluate the overall motility of the esophageal body and LES. Endoscopy is performed to evaluate for mucosal lesions, including esophagitis, Barrett esophagus, and cancer.

The treatment of an epiphrenic diverticulum is similar to that of a midesophageal diverticulum. These types of diverticula also have a wide mouth and rest close to the spine. Small (<2 cm) diverticula can also be suspended from the vertebral fascia and need not be excised. If a diverticulopexy is performed, a myotomy is begun at the neck of the diverticulum and extended onto the LES. If a diverticulectomy is pursued, a vertical stapling device is placed across the neck and the diverticulum is excised. It is essential during this process to have an esophageal bougie in place to avoid narrowing the esophageal lumen while stapling. The muscle is closed over the excision site, and a long myotomy is performed on the opposite esophageal wall, extending from the level of the diverticulum onto the LES. If a large hiatal hernia is also present, the diverticulum is excised, a myotomy performed, and the hiatal hernia repaired. Failure to repair the hernia results in a high incidence of postoperative reflux. It is essential to relieve outflow obstruction in patients with diverticula; failure to do so can result in significant complications of leak or recurrence. Recent experience has demonstrated that thoracic esophageal diverticula, particularly epiphrenic diverticula, may be safely approached using minimally invasive techniques (laparoscopy and thoracoscopy) with excellent outcomes including significant improvements in patient quality of life.

GASTROESOPHAGEAL REFLUX DISEASE

GERD is the most common benign condition of the esophagus, affecting millions of people worldwide. It occurs when there is retrograde flow of gastric contents through the LES with the typical symptoms of this disease including heartburn most commonly, in addition to regurgitation and dysphagia. The disease is characterized by progressive worsening of symptoms until they are frequent, persistent, and troublesome and possibly result in primary or secondary complications. Some of these complications include strictures, ulcers, metaplasia, dysplasia, carcinoma, and pulmonary disease (asthma, chronic cough, fibrosis).

The treatment of GERD has evolved significantly in the last several decades with the improved efficacy of antisecretory medications and refinement of surgical procedures. For many, the symptoms can be managed with medication and lifestyle modification alone. However, some people will experience symptoms that are refractory to these treatments or complications that are not medically treatable and require surgical intervention. The following sections explore the workup and surgical management of GERD in the context of failed medical management.

Medical Management

Although some patients wish to have antireflux surgery to avoid taking medication, most referrals to a surgeon are because of uncontrolled, persistent symptoms of heartburn or regurgitation despite medication. Commonly, patients will have tried proton pump inhibitors (PPIs) once daily and have progressed to twice daily. Frequently, patients will have tried several brands of PPI and have mixed multiple antacid medications. Cessation of PPIs will often result in heartburn or regurgitation that is prohibitive to normal function. Patients for whom medical therapy never relieved symptoms or who demonstrate atypical symptoms, such as chronic cough, hoarseness, asthma, or chest pain, should be further investigated for other causes before surgery is offered. It has been observed that the patients with the greatest likelihood of successful surgical therapy are those who have typical symptoms and good response to antisecretory therapy.

Lifestyle modifications will rarely eliminate GERD symptoms, but they can decrease severity and duration and result in greater efficacy of medication. The modifications include weight loss (if overweight), smoking cessation, elimination of inciting foods, smaller and more frequent meals, alcohol cessation, and elimination of constipation. Medical therapy is usually maximal with twice-daily PPI therapy.

Workup

There are several components to the workup for surgical management of GERD that will promote successful selection of therapy. They allow tailoring of the surgical procedure to the patient's needs and avoidance of unanticipated events during surgery. The standard studies include pH testing, esophageal manometry, video esophagram, and upper endoscopy with biopsy. Additional tests may include a gastric emptying study or CT scan.

Because gastric contents are acidic, measurement of pH acts as a surrogate for acid reflux. Not only will it document exposure of the lower esophagus to gastric refluxate, but it will also correlate symptoms with this exposure. The test is performed by placing a disposable probe in the distal esophagus (commonly by endoscopy) and allowing a remote recorder to collect data for 24 to 48 hours. It is critical to document abnormal refluxate exposure because other disease processes can have GERD-like symptoms. In addition, several studies have correlated abnormal pH testing with successful surgical outcomes. The patient should be off of antisecretory and antacid medications at the time of testing (usually cease medications 5 days to 2 weeks prior). A DeMeester score greater than 14.72 confirms pathologic GERD.

Esophageal motility testing allows the surgeon to evaluate if peristaltic contractions are strong and effective, if there is a motility disorder, and if there is an incompetent LES. Not only is this important in distinguishing GERD from other disorders (such as achalasia or scleroderma), but it can allow tailoring of surgery for patients with coexistent GERD and motility disorder. For example, a patient with mildly impaired motility in the setting of positive pH testing might be suited to a floppy or partial fundoplication procedure rather than a full wrap. Often, patients with long-standing GERD will have esophageal dysmotility, and they must be counseled about postoperative dysphagia after fundoplication. Patients with severe dysmotility should be considered for further workup or nonsurgical therapy.

Video esophagram shows both structure and function. It will diagnose abnormalities that would modify surgical treatment, such as strictures, masses, hiatal hernia, foreshortened esophagus, or diverticula. Functionally, video esophagram confirms reflux and can be suggestive of motility disorders or achalasia. It is considered the "road map" before surgery, can be obtained immediately after surgery, and is useful in long-term follow-up.

Finally, endoscopy allows the surgeon to evaluate the shape and course of the esophagus, to evaluate for signs of reflux such as esophagitis and metaplasia, and to rule out masses and strictures as a cause of symptoms. A particularly dilated and tortuous esophagus can be indicative of motility disorders, and hiatal hernias not seen on esophagram can be seen on retroflexed views in the stomach. Biopsy of abnormal findings will evaluate for metaplasia, dysplasia, and carcinoma, which might alter plans for surgery and surveillance.

If there are inconsistencies between the findings on workup and the patient's symptoms, it is important to revise the diagnosis, to continue investigation, or to obtain second opinions. Surgical procedures when the diagnosis is incorrect can result in additional new symptoms without resolution of the initial complaint, leading to a dissatisfying outcome. In patients with atypical symptoms or a history of not responding to PPI, the surgeon should be especially wary. We recommend confirmation of pathologic acid reflux with at least two objective tests prior to offering antireflux surgery in these individuals. Adjunct studies to consider include CT scan of the chest and abdomen, small bowel follow-through, gastric emptying study, and colonoscopy.

Surgical Therapy

Several operations termed "antireflux" procedures have been developed over the years as surgeons have tailored them to the symptoms of patients. This section will not discuss transthoracic approaches because these are rarely indicated as primary procedures for reflux. Rather, it outlines the basic concepts of the most commonly performed transabdominal fundoplication procedure and some variations.

After it is verified that the patient's symptoms are due to acid reflux (see earlier) and the patient is deemed a safe surgical candidate, the surgeon has several options. Regardless of the procedure chosen, the basic tenets of antireflux surgery remain constant: (1) preserve natural tissue planes and linings, (2) identify and preserve both vagus nerves, (3) identify the true EGJ for placement of the wrap, (4) have sufficient length of intraabdominal esophagus, and (5) reestablish the angle of His.

The Nissen fundoplication, first described in the 1950s, has become a standard in antireflux surgery (Fig. 42.24A). Conceptually, it is the recreation of a sphincter around the EGJ, done by a full 360-degree wrap of the fundus around the distal esophagus.

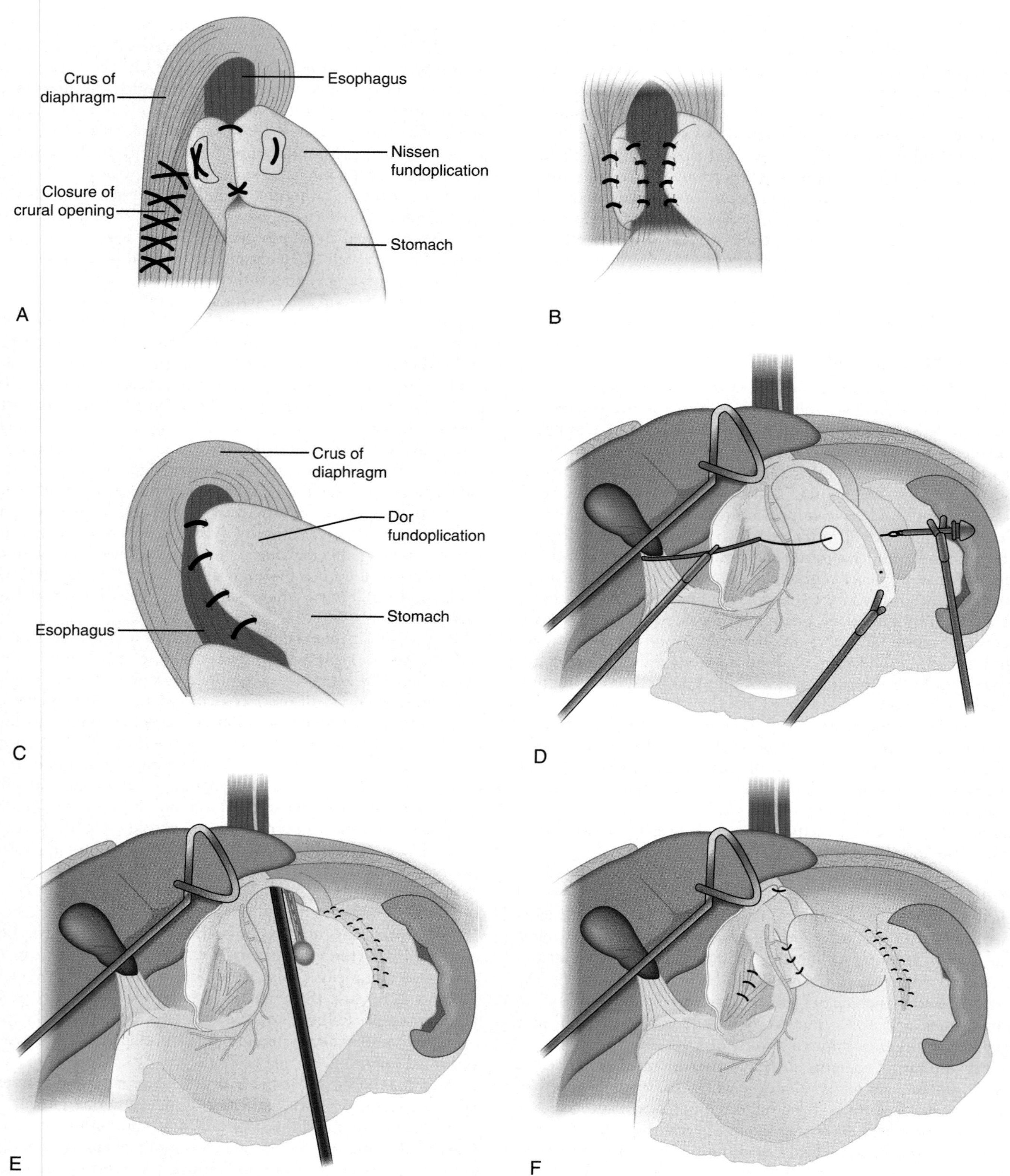

FIG. 42.24 (A) Nissen fundoplication. (B) Toupet fundoplication. (C) Dor fundoplication. (D-F) Collis gastroplasty.

Whether by laparoscopy or laparotomy, the procedure is the same. The gastrohepatic ligament is incised until the phrenoesophageal ligament is visualized, with care taken to avoid replaced hepatic arteries. The esophagus is circumferentially mobilized, with great care to preserve both vagus nerves and the peritoneal lining along the crura. Short gastric vessels are taken, and the gastrosplenic ligament is mobilized to meet the dissection along the left crus, with care taken to remain far from the splenic hilum. Any hiatal hernia will require dissection in the mediastinum to bring down sufficient esophageal length. The fat pad is then mobilized from the anterior stomach or esophagus to visualize the true EGJ and to be able to exclude both vagus nerves from the wrap. At least 2 to 3 cm of intraabdominal esophagus should be present to minimize the likelihood of postoperative hiatal hernia. The diaphragmatic hiatus is assessed and crura closed with nonabsorbable suture anterior and posterior to the esophagus, ensuring not to kink or impinge on the esophagus. Usually, the passage of instruments easily through the hiatus ensures that it is not too tight.

With sufficient esophageal and gastric mobilization as well as exposure of the true EGJ, the fundic tip along the line of the short gastrics can be passed posterior to the esophagus (excluding the vagus nerves in the fat pad) to create the wrap. A "shoeshine maneuver" ensures adequate mobility and lack of tension. A 50 to 54 Fr bougie is usually in the esophagus while the edges of the wrap are sutured together with incorporation of a portion of the anterior esophagus. After the bougie is removed, the crural closure and wrap are reassessed to ensure appropriate tension. Postoperatively, it is important that antiemetics are administered liberally to avoid retching or emesis as this may disrupt the repair.

Some surgeons have advocated the use of mesh at the hiatus as "reinforcement" or if there is excessive tension at the crural closure. Mesh is not usually necessary if the natural peritoneal linings are preserved along the crus. If there is tension on closure, the amount of carbon dioxide insufflation can be reduced, which will reduce the cephalad displacement of the diaphragm and usually allows tension-free closure. Additionally, relaxing incisions on the diaphragm, typically just lateral to the right crus, have also been described.

The wrap can be individualized to the patient's symptoms. Complete 360-degree wraps are particularly important when reflux causes respiratory compromise, such as the lung transplant population. Even in complete wraps, there should be space for the passage of an instrument between the stomach and esophagus to reduce postoperative dysphagia and gas bloat.

Variations on this classic procedure exist that allow an operation to be individualized to the patient's needs. Toupet fundoplication involves posterior partial wrap of 270 degrees, with additional tacking sutures to fix the stomach to the crura in the abdomen (Fig. 42.24B). Dor fundoplication is most commonly used in the setting of esophageal myotomy but consists of an anterior 180 to 200 degree wrap (Fig. 42-24C). As postoperative dysphagia is a major cause of reoperation in Nissen patients, partial wraps are preferred in patients with a history of preoperative dysphagia or poor peristalsis on manometry. Regardless of the choice of wrap, the rate of recurrent GERD is not insignificant, with one recent population study reporting reflux recurrence in 17.7% of patients at median follow-up of 5.6 years.[7] These findings highlight the critical importance of appropriate patient selection and medical therapy prior to entertaining antireflux surgery.

A newer device named LINX can be used in patients with minimal or no hiatal hernia.[8] It is a series of magnetic beads that are placed around the EGJ that will stretch with slight pressure in the esophagus, thereby mimicking the natural LES. In a prospective study, nearly two-thirds of LINX patients had significant reductions in esophageal acid exposure at 1 year and over 90% experienced significant improvements in their quality of life and reductions in PPI use.[8] In a follow-up study reporting 5-year outcomes, no device erosions or migrations were found and patients continued to have excellent control of their reflux symptoms.[9] In another recent multicenter trial, LINX patients had similar improvements in postoperative GERD-health–related quality of life as fundoplication patients and experienced significantly less regurgitation, gas bloat, and PPI use at one year.[10] Additionally, use of this device has been reported in patients with hiatal hernias greater than 3 cm with excellent outcomes. Long-term studies are needed to further characterize outcomes in LINX patients with or without large hiatal hernias as well as define the role fundoplication plays in light of this new technology.

A consideration for patients with bile or gastric reflux, morbid obesity, diabetes, or esophageal dysmotility is Roux-en-Y reconstruction. A near-esophagojejunostomy (with small gastric pouch) allows the passage of almost all gastric and biliary contents far downstream from the esophagus, thereby preventing symptoms related to reflux. In this population, there will be additional benefits of impact on obesity and diabetes. This is also an option in revisional surgery in which there is a lot of scarring or the integrity of the vagus nerves is questionable.

Finally, the patient undergoing fundoplication in whom there is less than adequate intraabdominal esophagus may require an esophageal lengthening procedure, or Collis gastroplasty (Fig. 42.24D–F). This involves stapling the fundus of the stomach ("wedge fundectomy") with a bougie in the esophagus to create a few centimeters of additional neoesophageal length around which the stomach can be wrapped. Both transthoracic and transabdominal approaches have been described, and although this technically difficult maneuver should be approached with caution, it is imperative to realize when it should be done. Collis patients should be continued on PPIs postoperatively in the short-term due to the presence of acid-secreting gastric mucosa above the wrap.

Complicated GERD

Long-standing reflux will cause complications to the esophagus, which require management that extends beyond antireflux surgery. In the patient with esophagitis, biopsy specimens from endoscopy can reveal medically treatable problems, such as candidiasis or eosinophilic infiltrative processes. Often, these patients can have relief of symptoms without surgical intervention, and surgical intervention may not relieve their symptoms. All strictures should be biopsied to rule out malignant processes and can frequently be managed with dilatation if they are benign. Intestinal metaplastic changes (Barrett esophagus) should be biopsied in four quadrants every centimeter to evaluate for dysplasia and cancer. Fundoplication procedures can still be performed in this setting and some evidence suggests histologic regression of Barrett in the long-term, though this is controversial.[11] Regardless, surveillance must continue at regular intervals by experienced endoscopists in the majority of patients with Barrett esophagus to evaluate for progression to malignancy.[12]

Some patients with heartburn or dysphagia will have a partial or complete intrathoracic stomach. The workup and surgical therapy for these patients can be significantly different from that for standard GERD, depending on the degree of hiatal herniation. Small hernias where the GEJ is above the diaphragmatic hiatus can be manifested with classic GERD symptoms, and the workup and therapy can be the same. When there is a moderate to large hiatal hernia, consideration must be given to the degree of symptoms related to the mechanical component versus the reflux. This can be a confusing picture because patients often have symptoms from both, but if the main complaints are dysphagia, food sticking, early satiety, regurgitation, chest pain, and vomiting, the mechanical component may be the dominant pathologic process. This is particularly true of intrathoracic stomachs. Workup may include pulmonary function tests because of compromised lung function and thorough cardiac evaluation because of overlapping symptoms. Manometry testing is often not possible with large hernias.

During reduction of the hernia, the esophagus might be foreshortened, and the options of gastropexy versus fundoplication or Collis gastroplasty/fundoplication will have to be weighed. With dominant mechanical symptoms, patients have relief with return of the stomach to the abdominal cavity with gastropexy. However, they may subsequently suffer from reflux symptoms and require antisecretory medication thereafter. Most patients would likely benefit from a partial fundoplication procedure, keeping in mind that esophageal motility will likely be unknown. Further review on GERD and hiatal hernia are covered elsewhere in this textbook.

ACQUIRED BENIGN DISORDERS OF THE ESOPHAGUS

Acquired Esophageal Disease

Perforation

Esophageal perforation is a potentially lethal condition that can have poor outcomes if there is a delay in diagnosis or improper treatment. Historically, most series have reported overall mortality between 15% and 30%, frequently with strong correlations to etiology and time interval from event to intervention.[13,14] The most commonly recognized causes are iatrogenic perforation during endoscopy and forceful retching (Boerhaave syndrome), with others being traumatic injury, foreign body ingestion, and tumor perforation.[13] In a recent multicenter series, perforation was found to be isolated to the thoracic esophagus in nearly two-thirds of patients with the remaining patients having an abdominal component.[13] It is generally regarded that better outcomes are possible if the intervention is within 24 hours of the event, and poor outcomes are associated with cancer-related perforations. The key to management and patient survival is early recognition with timely diagnosis and therapy.

Suspicion of esophageal perforation begins with symptoms of epigastric or chest pain, neck or throat pain, and dysphagia. Physical examination findings might include crepitus on the chest, neck, or face; neck swelling; epigastric tenderness; nasal voice; or sometimes normal examination findings. Other early evidence might include a chest radiograph with mediastinal or cervical air, free abdominal air, or pleural effusion. A CT scan may show mediastinal air and periesophageal air or fluid. Of course, the mechanism of injury can be the greatest clue that would initiate further workup.

Once there is suspicion, the diagnostic workup must proceed on the basis of the index of suspicion. Barium esophagram is the standard for diagnosis (Fig. 42.25), but CT scan with oral administration of contrast material may also be acceptable if an esophagram cannot be obtained. If the results of these studies are normal but the level of suspicion is high, patients may require evaluation by direct laryngoscopy or endoscopy, depending on the clinical circumstance. Of note, procedural evaluation can convert a small or partial perforation into a more clinically significant process, so caution must be used with these procedures. Once the diagnosis is made, there are several therapeutic options that must be considered on an individual basis by a team of experienced surgeons as the subtleties of management preclude algorithmic treatment. Determining severity of injury to prognosticate morbidity and mortality can be done with a clinical severity score proposed by the Pittsburgh group (Table 42.3).[15] This score has been correlated with morbidity, mortality, and hospital stay and can be used to guide treatment (Table 42.4).[15,16]

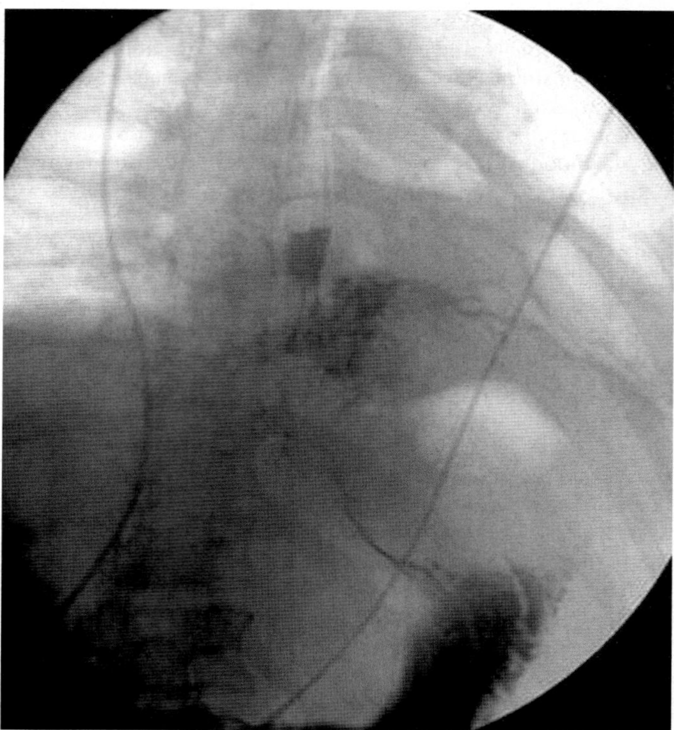

FIG. 42.25 Barium esophagram demonstrating an esophageal perforation.

TABLE 42.3 Criteria in the Pittsburgh esophageal perforation severity score.

VARIABLE	SCORE
Age >75 years	1
Tachycardia (>100 beats/min)	1
Leukocytosis (>10,000 white blood cells/mL)	1
Pleural effusion	1
Fever (>38.5°C)	2
Noncontained leak (barium swallow or CT scan)	2
Respiratory compromise (respiratory rate >30, increasing oxygen requirement, or mechanical ventilation)	2
Time to diagnosis >24 hours	2
Presence of cancer	3
Hypotension	3

CT, Computed tomography.
Score ranges 0 to 18 with higher scores indicating greater morbidity with worse prognosis.
Data From Abbas G, Schuchert MJ, Pettiford BL, Pennathur A, Landreneau J, Landreneau J, et al. Contemporaneous management of esophageal perforation. Surgery. 2009;146:749–755.

The principles of management after diagnosis include (1) treatment of contamination, (2) wide local drainage, (3) source control, and (4) enteral feeding access. In the circumstance of small perforations with contained leaks and no fluid collections in the mediastinum or chest, contamination might be minimal. In general, though, perforation is treated with broad-spectrum antibiotics, including antifungals, with duration that will vary on the basis of control of infection and the patient's condition. Drainage of the area with chest tubes is most common, with the number, location, and duration to vary by the degree of leak. In select cases, radiologically guided drains can be

TABLE 42.4 Pittsburgh esophageal perforation severity score.

SCORE	<3	3–5	>5
Morbidity (%)	53	65	81
Mortality (%)	2	6	27
Median length of stay (days)	10	16	28

Score ranges 0 to 18 with higher scores indicating greater morbidity with worse prognosis.
Data from Abbas G, Schuchert MJ, Pettiford BL, et al. Contemporaneous management of esophageal perforation. Surgery. 2009;146:749–755.

used as well. Video-assisted thoracoscopic surgery (VATS) or open thoracic washout with decortication may be necessary, depending on the duration of the leak and amount of pleural space soiling.

Source control will also depend on the patient's condition, the severity and location of perforation, and the surgeon's experience. Endoluminal therapy with covered stents has become more widely popularized and can give good results when it is used in the appropriate patient population.[17] Stent migration is a concern, however, and frequent chest X-rays are typically performed to evaluate the position of the stent. In a systematic review, plastic stents had higher rates of migration and required more reinterventions, albeit with lower stricture rates, when compared to metallic stents.[17] Although the criteria are still debated, stents can be considered in patients with early, small perforations, with minimal contamination in a location amenable to stenting. Additionally, if there is a delay between injury and diagnosis then stents are still an option given the poor tissue quality likely to be found if approached surgically. However, in these patients, VATS is also often used for drainage and decortication of the lung in addition to chest tube placement. Use of stents, with or without VATS, in esophageal perforation may be as effective as open surgery with evidence suggesting less morbidity, shorter lengths of stay, and less costs associated with an endoluminal approach.

If the decision is made to intervene surgically, the approach depends on the location of the leak. In general, high perforations are approached through a left-sided neck incision, midesophageal through a right thoracotomy, and distal esophageal through a left thoracotomy or thoracoabdominal approach. Radiographic studies that demonstrate a right- or left-sided leak may modify the approach. Minimally invasive approaches are reasonable, depending on the surgeon's preference.

After the area of perforation is identified, assessment continues with myotomy to expose the full extent of mucosal injury, debridement of devitalized tissues, assessment of injury, and considerations for repair. Any sign of obstruction (achalasia, stricture, tumor) must be remedied at the time of the initial operation, else the perforation will not heal. In the setting of achalasia or a hypertensive LES, a contralateral myotomy should be performed to relieve the distal obstruction. Small injuries with healthy tissues can be repaired primarily in two layers with tissue flap coverage (intercostal muscle, pericardial fat, pleura, omentum), but extensive injuries with devitalized areas can be managed with controlled fistulization by T-tube. Very large or devitalized defects will require esophageal exclusion with creation of a cervical esophagostomy and gastrostomy tube, with plans for future reconstruction by esophagectomy with typically a substernal gastric, colon, or small bowel conduit. Gastrostomy and jejunostomy tubes at the first operation are important to provide decompression and drainage near the perforation as well as enteral access for nutrition.

Recently, endoscopic vacuum therapy (EVT) has emerged as an option for surgeons in the management of esophageal perforation.[18] Borrowing traditional principles of wound healing in vacuum therapy for skin and soft tissue defects, EVT has been described for both esophageal perforation and anastomotic leak after esophagectomy. This technique involves endoscopic placement of a sponge into the site of esophageal injury. Tubing from the sponge is connected externally to a vacuum device with continuous negative pressure applied to the site of perforation. Serial endoscopies are then performed every several days to weeks to examine the site of injury and to evaluate for appropriate granulation tissue and for exchange of the sponge. Once the mucosa has sufficiently healed, the sponge is removed and diet liberalized. Another recent endoscopic option for esophageal perforation, particularly those identified acutely, is placement of over-the-scope clips to seal the site of injury.[18] Use of EVT and over-the-scope clips still mandates that basic principles of esophageal perforation are adhered to, namely wide local drainage, decortication, and feeding access. However, early evidence suggests these therapies may be safe and viable options with good outcomes in appropriately selected patients.[18]

Mortality from esophageal perforation may be decreasing over time.[14] Use of minimally invasive and endoluminal techniques, in addition to improved imaging and perioperative care, are important contributing factors. Additionally, regionalization of esophageal perforation to high-volume centers may also translate into improved survival.[14]

Caustic Ingestion

The majority of caustic ingestion is accidental small-volume drinking of household products by young children. In adults, it is more commonly a suicide attempt with large volumes, and therefore more extensive injury is usually present. The injury pattern can vary from short-segment superficial injury to full-thickness necrosis of the proximal gastrointestinal tract. There are many factors that affect the extent of injury (pH, volume, duration of exposure), and the evaluation and management after the ingestion are challenging and require experience and sound judgment.

The initial evaluation should involve a surgeon immediately. Physical examination findings of upper airway compromise (dyspnea, drooling, stridor, hoarseness) will likely require endotracheal intubation. However, this should be done with bronchoscopic guidance and preparation to perform cricothyroidotomy as there is danger of inability to secure a safe airway or iatrogenic perforation. Nasogastric and orogastric tubes should not be inserted blindly. Subsequent evaluation should include radiographic studies to guide the first procedure, ideally a CT scan of chest and abdomen with intravenous and oral administration of contrast material, followed by a barium swallow study.

Evaluation continues in the operating room. With rare exception, most patients should have an endoscopic evaluation of the degree and extent of injury. It is recommended that this be done early in the hospital course as the risk of perforation increases after 48 hours. Pediatric endoscopes are useful to minimize insufflation and mechanical stresses. The traditional teaching is that endoscopy should not proceed past an area of circumferential injury; however, an experienced endoscopist can cautiously proceed to complete the evaluation if it is thought that management will change with additional information. It is important to note the severity and degree of injury at all locations because subsequent evaluations are frequently necessary. A classification system for endoscopic grading of injuries from caustic ingestions has been described (Table 42.5).

TABLE 42.5 Classification scheme for caustic ingestion.

ENDOSCOPIC FINDING	GRADE
Normal	0
Superficial edema/erythema	1
Mucosal/submucosal ulceration	2
Superficial edema/erythema	2A
Deep or circumferential	2B
Transmural ulcerations with necrosis	3
Focal necrosis	3A
Extensive necrosis	3B
Perforation	4

Data from Zargar SA, Kochhar R, Mehta S, et al. The role of fiberoptic endoscopy in the management of corrosive ingestion and modified endoscopic classification of burns. *Gastrointest Endosc.* 1991;37:165–169.

All patients should be treated with broad-spectrum antibiotics. Depending on the clinical course, patients may benefit from repeated endoscopy 48 to 72 hours after the event to assess for signs of worsening injury. Of paramount importance is frequent clinical reassessment as deterioration at any time should prompt resumption of workup and surgical intervention as indicated. Surgical intervention can vary from endoscopy only to placement of gastrostomy or jejunostomy tubes or esophagectomy, gastrectomy, and small bowel resection with proximal diversion and feeding tube. Reconstruction can be complicated, sometimes requiring several months of recovery and the use of colon or small bowel conduits. In the long term, patients may develop strictures that require repeated dilatation or eventual resection, fistulas that require surgical interventions, or esophageal cancer (>1000 times increased risk). The use of routine corticosteroids is no longer advocated. Early dilatation, esophageal stents, and other adjunctive measures must be considered on a case-by-case basis.

Foreign Body Ingestion, Benign Tracheoesophageal Fistula, and Schatzki Ring

The patient with foreign body ingestion can require technical expertise to prevent iatrogenic perforation. If the object is lodged in the esophagus, careful endoscopy under general anesthesia is preferred. Forceful pushing to move the object into the stomach can result in perforation. Full relaxation, lubrication with water, and gentle pressure can sometimes be enough. Bringing the object proximally requires special large endoscopic graspers, nets, or lassoes along with patience and full visualization as the object is removed to prevent injury in the esophagus and oropharynx. Over-tubes are frequently useful in this setting, as is rigid esophagoscopy. If the object is not retrievable, laparoscopy or laparotomy with gastrotomy may be necessary. Evaluation of the full gastrointestinal tract is recommended with radiographs and CT scan before an intervention. For patients with repeat foreign body ingestions, or those ingesting objects for the purpose of self-harm, inpatient psychiatric evaluation is warranted.

Benign tracheoesophageal fistula can be seen in patients with multiple procedures or foreign bodies in the upper mediastinum. A classic example of benign tracheoesophageal fistula is in the patient with endotracheal tube (or tracheostomy) and nasogastric tube. It is manifested most commonly with recurrent or persistent respiratory infection and bilious or salivary contents emanating from the tracheostomy. CT scan and barium swallow can be helpful in determining the diagnosis. Further evaluation is done with bronchoscopy and endoscopy, ensuring that bronchoscopy is performed such that the entire airway is evaluated. The tracheostomy balloon will have to be deflated and usually temporarily removed during the evaluation for visualization. If tracheoesophageal fistula is identified, treatment principles are (1) discontinuation of the causative agent, (2) consideration of exclusion of the fistula by stent or diversion, and finally (3) repair or delayed healing. In a stable patient, definitive repair may preclude the need for temporary exclusion or diversion. If the fistula was caused by a tracheostomy balloon, a longer or cuffless tracheostomy will be required. Antibiotics are usually employed as well. Enteral access and gastric decompression can be achieved with gastrostomy and jejunostomy tubes. Repair can be undertaken when the patient is medically suitable by either thoracotomy or cervical approach with resection of the fistula, possible primary repair or resection, and vascularized tissue interposition. Attempts at definitive repair in a compromised patient are not optimal. Delayed healing can occur if the offending agents are removed and diversion is successful. Esophageal stents can occasionally be used in this setting as well, although this must be determined on a case-by-case basis. Placement of simultaneous esophageal and airway stents ("kissing stents") is typically reserved for only the most moribund patients as they have the potential to worsen the size of the fistula due to radial forces. EVT has also been described in the management of tracheoesophageal fistula, though clinical experience with this application is still relatively new.

A Schatzki ring is a concentric, nonmalignant, fibrous thickening and narrowing of the GEJ with squamous epithelium above and columnar cells below (Fig. 42.26). The cause is unknown, with correlations to reflux disease. The majority of patients with a Schatzki ring have a concomitant finding of hiatal hernia. Presence of a ring is not pathologic, but these can be seen in patients suffering from dysphagia or obstruction. In the symptomatic patient, whether the diagnosis is by esophagram or endoscopy, treatment is usually with dilatation (bougie or balloon). The area should always be biopsied to rule out malignancy. Repeated dilatation is often necessary and is a reasonable way to manage symptomatic rings as there are few permanent surgical options. Persistent strictures should always raise suspicion for malignant disease.

BENIGN AND RARE TUMORS OF THE ESOPHAGUS

Benign Tumors of the Esophagus

Benign tumors of the esophagus are less common than esophageal cancer. Among benign lesions, tumors of the submucosa and muscularis propria occur more frequently than mucosal tumors. Most of these lesions are asymptomatic and are identified incidentally on endoscopy. Barium esophagram characteristically demonstrates a smooth defect in the lumen.

Benign mucosal tumors include granular cell tumors and fibrovascular polyps. Granular cell tumors may be found in a variety of locations, including the skin, respiratory tract, gastrointestinal tract, breast, and tongue. These tumors derive from Schwann cells of nerve sheath origin and most often emanate from the mucosa or submucosa.[19] Within the gastrointestinal tract, the distal third of the esophagus is the most common location. They can appear as either sessile or bulging whitish-grey lesions with often normal-appearing mucosa. Up to 11% of patients may have multiple tumors.[19] On endoscopic ultrasound (EUS), lesions typically have regular borders and arise within the first and second sonographic layers. Because these lesions are usually covered by a layer of normal squamous

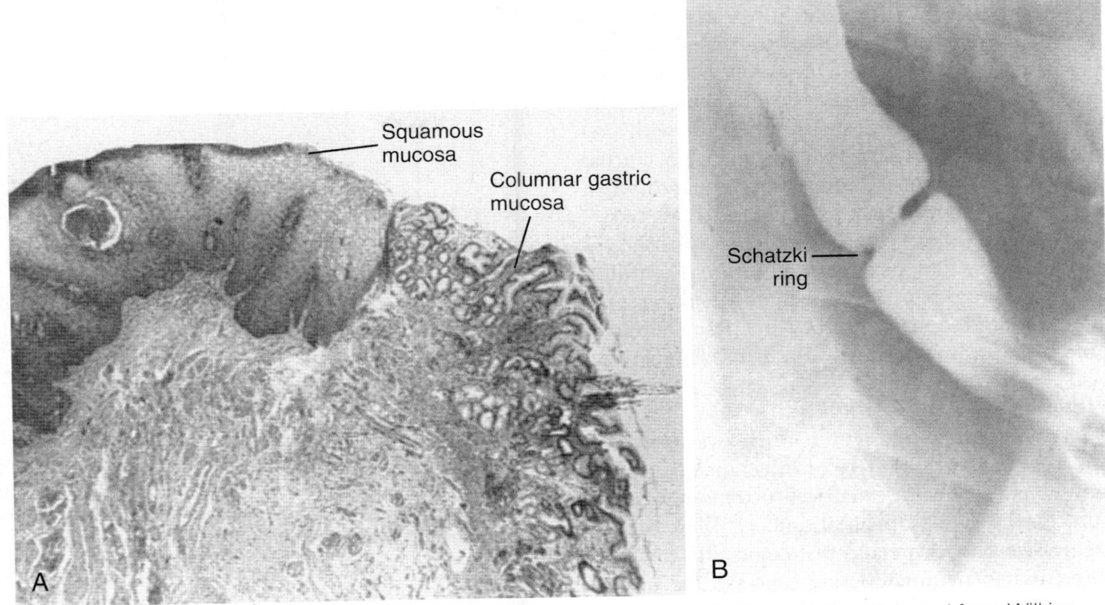

FIG. 42.26 (A) Histology of a Schatzki ring. (B) Barium esophagram of a Schatzki ring. (Adapted from Wilkins EW Jr. Rings and webs. In: Pearson FG, Cooper JD, Deslauriers J, et al, eds. *Esophageal surgery*. 2nd ed. New York, NY: Churchill Livingstone; 2002.)

epithelium, standard biopsies may be nondiagnostic. Tunneled biopsies will reveal eosinophilic granules. The tumors stain positive for S100, further supporting their origin from Schwann cells. Granular cell tumors are largely benign lesions, with only 1% to 2% having been described as malignant. Atypical features on EUS, large size (>2 cm), and presence of symptoms are reasonable indications for excision. Endoscopic resection is a valuable tool for these lesions when diagnosis is in question and to rule out malignancy.

Fibrovascular polyps are a heterogeneous group of soft tissue tumors most often found in the cervical esophagus at or near the cricopharyngeus. They appear cylindrical or elongated, with a stalk. Symptoms are rare, but large tumors may cause dysphagia and some may even prolapse into the hypopharynx, causing airway obstruction. Even large tumors can usually be resected endoscopically after securing the airway.

Squamous papillomas most often occur in the distal esophagus and are usually associated with some underlying inflammation. They appear as colorless, exophytic projections, with a wart-like projection.[20] Additionally, they are often seen with a crossing vessel on the surface of the lesion. There is also evidence suggesting a link between squamous papillomas and human papillomavirus (HPV).[20] Complete excision is warranted to rule out carcinoma and can usually be performed endoscopically with little morbidity.

Benign submucosal tumors include lipomas, hemangiomas, and neural tumors. Lipomas have a characteristic, homogeneous, hyperechoic, smooth appearance on EUS. Symptoms are rare even with large tumors. Resection is seldom warranted. Hemangiomas typically appear as a purple or reddish nodule. EUS will demonstrate a smooth, hypoechoic, submucosal mass. Most tumors are asymptomatic. Lesions causing either dysphagia or bleeding can usually be treated endoscopically. Neural tumors including neurofibromas and schwannomas are rare in the esophagus. The majority are benign, with a handful of case reports on malignant esophageal schwannoma.[21] Symptomatic tumors can usually be resected by enucleation. Large tumors may require esophagectomy.

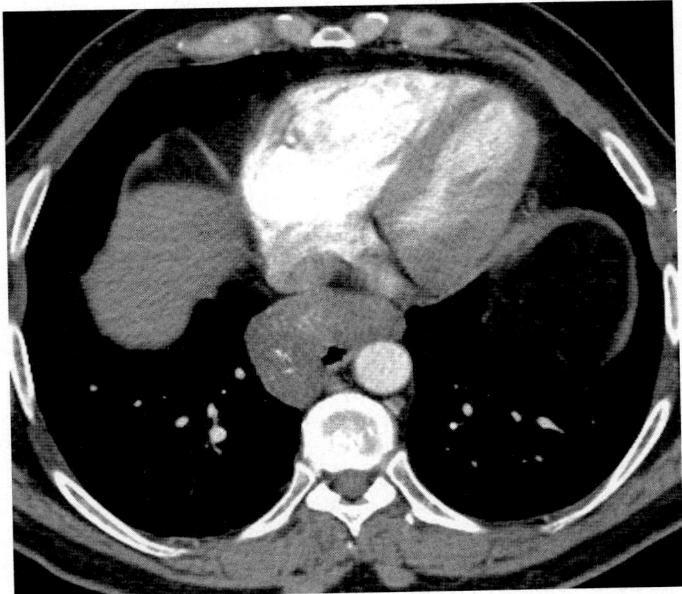

FIG. 42.27 Computed tomography image of an 8-cm leiomyoma that was causing dysphagia. The lesion was enucleated thoracoscopically, and the patient's dysphagia resolved.

Leiomyomas are the most common benign tumors of the esophagus. They have a 2:1 male predominance. Although they are usually asymptomatic, large tumors may cause dysphagia or discomfort (Fig. 42.27). The tumors arise in the muscularis propria and are usually found in the mid to distal esophagus. Like most other benign esophageal tumors, they will demonstrate a smooth filling defect on barium esophagram. The endoscopic appearance is a round protrusion into the lumen of the esophagus with smooth, normal mucosa. On EUS, leiomyomas are hypoechoic, have regular borders, and arise from the fourth endosonographic layer. Tumors with EUS characteristics suggestive of a leiomyoma should not be biopsied as this will complicate subsequent attempts at enucleation. Small, asymptomatic lesions with this appearance may be safely observed without biopsy. Symptomatic lesions may be enucleated, and even large lesions can usually be removed with a VATS approach. Additionally, endoscopic resection with creation of a submucosal tunnel for leiomyomas up to 5.5 cm has been described. Oncologic outcomes appear to be similar to VATS with the added benefits of shorter lengths of stay and less cost.[22] As technology continue to improve, many benign esophageal tumors may be approached endoscopically in the future. Regardless of the surgical approach, one must keep in mind the differential diagnosis of a large smooth esophageal tumor, including leiomyosarcoma, gastrointestinal stromal tumor (GIST), and leiomyoma.

Rare Malignant Tumors of the Esophagus

Although SCC and adenocarcinoma represent the overwhelming majority of esophageal cancers, a variety of other malignant histologic types may be encountered. Small cell carcinomas of the esophagus account for 0.6% of esophageal cancers. These tumors have the same aggressive phenotype and histologic appearance of other poorly differentiated neuroendocrine cancers. The tumors typically present with lymph node involvement and at an advanced stage.[23] Long-term survival is possible in earlier stage tumors treated with surgery, although the overall prognosis is poor. Systemic chemotherapy is often used to impact survival. Stage at diagnosis is the most important prognostic factor.[23]

Primary melanoma of the esophagus is even rarer than small cell carcinoma, accounting for 0.1% to 0.2% of esophageal malignant neoplasms. Similar to small cell carcinoma, most tumors are manifested at a late stage, and prognosis is generally poor.

Sarcomas and GISTs of the esophagus are far less common than benign leiomyomas. Although well-differentiated leiomyosarcomas may be difficult to distinguish from leiomyomas, these are rare tumors that often erode through the mucosa, appearing as an ulcerated or exophytic mass on endoscopy. EUS may show more irregular borders or a heterogeneous appearance that is uncharacteristic for leiomyoma. In general, esophagectomy with radical lymphadenectomy is the treatment of choice for leiomyosarcomas.[24] GISTs have similar appearance to leiomyomas but can be distinguished histologically by CD117 (c-kit) and CD34 stain positivity. Additionally, compared to leiomyomas, GISTs tend to be larger, with uptake of IV contrast on CT, and often have significant positron emission tomography (PET) avidity.[25] GISTs may be enucleated provided that negative margins can be obtained. However, if concerns about margin status or tumor recurrence persist, formal esophagectomy should be performed.[26] Imatinib should be considered for any GIST larger than 3 cm or with other high-risk features. Imatinib may also be considered in the neoadjuvant setting for locally advanced tumors. Lymph node metastasis is an unusual event in these mesenchymal tumors. Compared to the more commonly found gastric GISTs, esophageal GISTs tend to have worse disease-free and overall survival.[26] Other sarcomas of the esophagus have been reported but are much rarer.

ESOPHAGEAL CANCER

Epidemiology of Esophageal Cancer

Nearly 18,000 cases of esophageal cancer occur annually in the United States and about 572,000 cases occur worldwide.[27,28] Unfortunately, esophageal cancer is typically manifested at an advanced stage and current 5-year survival is only approximately 19%, with the majority of patients dying of their disease.[28] Adenocarcinoma is the most common histology in Westernized counties, including the United States. During the last several decades there has been a concomitant decline in the incidence of SCC both worldwide and in the United States (Fig. 42.28).[29] These histologic changes are thought to reflect the increasing obesity epidemic and GERD contributing to adenocarcinoma in conjunction with global reductions in cigarette smoking, a key risk factor for SCC.[27] This appears to be a true increase in incidence of adenocarcinoma rather than overdiagnosis as the overall stage distribution has not significantly shifted during this time. Other types of esophageal tumors, including mesenchymal tumors, neuroendocrine cancers, and benign tumors, are much rarer.

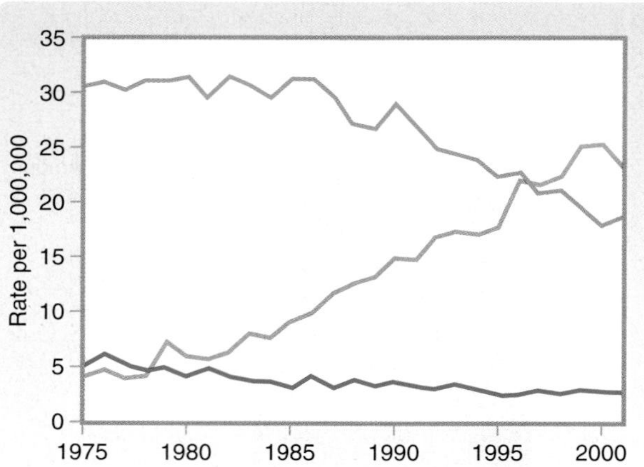

FIG. 42.28 Trends in incidence of esophageal cancer histologic types (1975-2001). *Red line,* Adenocarcinoma; *blue line,* squamous cell carcinoma; *green line,* not otherwise specified. (From Pohl H, Welch HG. The role of overdiagnosis and reclassification in the marked increase of esophageal adenocarcinoma incidence. *J Natl Cancer Inst.* 2005;97:142–146.)

Tobacco and alcohol are strong risk factors for SCC, and they have a synergistic effect on risk.[27] The disease is three to four times more prevalent in men, and race also appears to be a factor.[28] The incidence of SCC is much higher amongst African Americans compared with their white counterparts, even after adjusting for socioeconomic status, tobacco, and alcohol use. Worldwide, parts of the Middle East, central Asia, and China have the highest rates of SCC, after adjusting for tobacco and alcohol use, indicating that there may be some genetic predisposition or other environmental factors. The recognition of the importance of HPV in the pathogenesis of SCC in other organs has spurred an interest in its role in esophageal SCC. Currently, it appears that HPV-related SCC represents only a small subset of esophageal SCC. For those tumors that are HPV related, the clinical implications of HPV association are unclear. SCC is associated with certain intrinsic disorders of the esophagus, such as Plummer-Vinson syndrome and achalasia. Other hereditary cancer syndromes associated with esophageal SCC include tylosis and Fanconi anemia. Patients with a history of caustic ingestion or achalasia are at significantly increased risk for SCC.

The incidence of esophageal adenocarcinoma has increased dramatically in the last four decades, amongst the highest of any cancer in the United States. It is now the most common histologic type of esophageal cancer in the United States.[30] Though overall incidence rates of adenocarcinoma have stabilized to decreased in the last 10 to 15 years, within the subpopulation of younger non-Hispanic whites, the incidence is increasing.[30] It continues to be relatively uncommon in African Americans. Adenocarcinoma often arises in the setting of Barrett esophagus. The frequency and duration of GERD symptoms is significantly associated with the risk of developing adenocarcinoma. As with SCC, there is a male predominance. There are also familial forms of Barrett esophagus that increase the risk of adenocarcinoma.

SCC may arise in any part of the esophagus, but the majority of cases arise in the proximal and middle esophagus. In contrast, the majority of adenocarcinomas arise in the distal esophagus or GEJ. Under current American Joint Committee on Cancer (AJCC) and National Comprehensive Cancer Network (NCCN) staging guidelines, GEJ adenocarcinomas are staged and classified as esophageal cancers, with the exception of Siewert III tumors (tumors with an epicenter 2–5 cm below the GEJ) which are classified with gastric cancers.[31,32]

The majority of esophageal cancers are symptomatic at the time of diagnosis. Dysphagia is the most common symptom, with the majority of patients reporting difficulty in swallowing at the time of presentation. Often, patients will report progressive dysphagia, beginning with an initial episode after eating solid food. After the initial episode of dysphagia, many patients will adapt by chewing more thoroughly, avoiding hard foods, or drinking liquids with swallows. Thus, it is only after the dysphagia has worsened significantly that patients seek medical attention, by which point the majority have weight loss. Many patients with adenocarcinoma will endorse a long history of reflux symptoms including heartburn and regurgitation. Other associated findings may include fatigue, retrosternal pain, and anemia. Locally advanced tumors may be manifested with laryngeal nerve involvement causing hoarseness or with tracheoesophageal fistula. A careful physical examination should be performed with particular attention to cervical and supraclavicular lymph nodes. Early-stage tumors are often asymptomatic and are sometimes discovered during endoscopy done for Barrett esophagus.

Diagnosis and Staging of Esophageal Cancer

Barium esophagram may demonstrate irregular narrowing or ulceration (Fig. 42.29). The classic "apple-core" filling defect is seen only if there is symmetrical, circumferential narrowing. Instead, there is often an asymmetric bulge seen with an infiltrative appearance.

The diagnosis of esophageal cancer is almost always made by endoscopic biopsy. Endoscopy should be performed in any patient with dysphagia, even if the barium esophagram is suggestive of a motility disorder. Classically, esophageal cancers appear as friable, ulcerated masses, but the endoscopic appearance can be varied. Early-stage tumors may appear as ulcerations or small nodules. More advanced tumors are more likely to be friable masses but may also appear as strictures or ulcerations. In many cases, the initial endoscopist may not recognize the presence of cancer and a single biopsy may not be diagnostic. Therefore, multiple biopsies should be performed for any suspicious lesions. During endoscopy, the location of the tumor relative to the incisors and GEJ should be noted, as well as the length of the tumor and degree of obstruction. The most proximal extent and circumferential extent of any Barrett esophagus should also be noted according to the Prague criteria.[12] For small tumors or nodules, an experienced endoscopist should perform endoscopic mucosal resection (EMR) to provide a specimen that accurately assesses depth of invasion.

Once a diagnosis of esophageal cancer is made, accurate staging is essential to guide appropriate therapy and to predict prognosis. The eighth edition AJCC staging system acknowledges differences

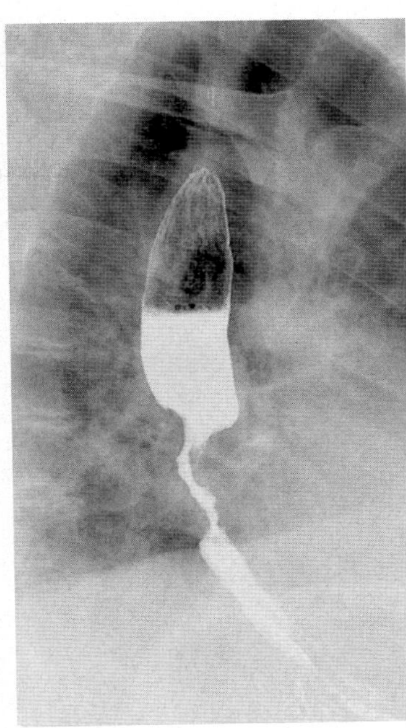

FIG. 42.29 Barium esophagram demonstrating advanced carcinoma with abrupt, irregular narrowing in the distal esophagus with more proximal dilatation and air-fluid level.

in the biology of adenocarcinoma and SCC by creating separate stage groupings for the two histologic types (Tables 42.6 to 42.11). Additionally, this is the first edition to separate staging into clinical, pathologic, and postneoadjuvant staging groups.[32] The inclusion of postneoadjuvant tumor, node, metastasis stage (ypTNM) is a response to the increasing proportion of operable patients undergoing induction therapy prior to resection. Pathologic stage is included for those patients undergoing resection that did not have neoadjuvant therapy. Tumor location affects pathologic stage for SCC but not for adenocarcinoma (Fig. 42.30). The cervical esophagus begins at the hypopharynx and extends to the thoracic inlet, which is the level of the sternal notch. On endoscopy, this corresponds to approximately 15 to 20 cm from the incisors. The upper thoracic esophagus begins at the thoracic inlet and extends to the azygos vein. This is approximately 20 to 25 cm from the incisors. Midthoracic tumors arise from the lower border of the azygos vein to the inferior pulmonary vein. This is approximately 25 to 30 cm from the incisors. Lower tumors arise distal to the lower border of the inferior pulmonary vein to the GEJ. This is usually more than 30 cm from the incisors. Tumor grade is included in pathologic stage classification for earlier stage tumors for both adenocarcinoma and SCC.[32] In both histologies, clinical and postneoadjuvant staging includes only the TNM classification without use of tumor location or grade.

Nodal classification is based on the total number of involved nodes. The eighth edition staging system introduces an esophagus-specific regional lymph node map for descriptive purposes.[32]

The depth of invasion of the tumor defines the T-status (Fig. 42.31). High-grade dysplasia includes malignant cells confined to the epithelium by the basement membrane and is by definition noninvasive (Tis). T1a tumors invade the lamina propria or muscularis mucosa, whereas T1b tumors invade into the submucosa. T2 tumors invade the muscularis propria, and T3 tumors invade the adventitia but not surrounding structures. T4a tumors invade adjacent structures that are usually

TABLE 42.6 Esophageal carcinoma stage classifications.

Primary Tumor (T)	
TX	Tumor cannot be assessed
T0	No evidence of tumor
Tis	High-grade dysplasia
T1a	Tumor invades the lamina propria or muscularis mucosa
T1b	Tumor invades the submucosa
T2	Tumor invades into but not beyond the muscularis propria
T3	Tumor invades the adventitia
T4a	Tumor invades adjacent structures that are usually resectable (diaphragm, pleura, azygos vein, peritoneum, or pericardium)
T4b	Tumor invades structures that are usually unresectable (aorta, vertebral body, or trachea)
Regional Lymph Nodes (N)	
NX	Regional lymph nodes cannot be assessed
N0	No regional lymph node metastasis
N1	Metastasis in 1–2 regional lymph nodes
N2	Metastasis in 3–6 regional lymph nodes
N3	Metastasis in ≥ 7 regional lymph nodes
Distant Metastasis (M)	
M0	No distant metastasis
M1	Distant metastasis
Histologic Grade (G)	
GX	Grade cannot be assessed
G1	Well differentiated
G2	Moderately differentiated
G3	Poorly differentiated or undifferentiated
Location (L) – Applicable to Squamous Cell Carcinoma Only	
LX	Location unknown
Upper	Cervical esophagus to lower border of azygos vein
Middle	Lower border of azygos vein to lower border of inferior pulmonary vein
Lower	Lower border of inferior pulmonary vein to stomach, including esophagogastric junction

Adapted from Rice TW, Ishwaran H, Ferguson MK, et al. Cancer of the esophagus and esophagogastric junction: An eighth edition staging primer. *J Thorac Oncol.* 2017;12:36–42.

TABLE 42.7 Clinical stage groupings (cTNM) for esophageal adenocarcinoma.

	T	N	M
Stage 0	Tis	N0	M0
Stage I	T1	N0	M0
Stage IIA	T1	N1	M0
Stage IIB	T2	N0	M0
Stage III	T2	N1	M0
	T3	N0-1	M0
	T4a	N0-1	M0
Stage IVA	T1-4a	N2	M0
	T4b	N0-2	M0
	Any T	N3	M0
Stage IVB	Any T	Any N	M1

Adapted from Rice TW, Ishwaran H, Ferguson MK, et al. Cancer of the esophagus and esophagogastric junction: An eighth edition staging primer. *J Thorac Oncol.* 2017;12:36–42.
T, Tumor status; *N,* lymph node status; *M,* metastasis.

resectable (diaphragm, pleura, and pericardium). T4b tumors invade adjacent structures that are typically unresectable (trachea and aorta).

Small, superficial lesions that are evaluated by an experienced endoscopist may be resected by EMR. In this setting, EMR often provides accurate staging for depth of penetration (T-status) and may provide additional information about the risk of nodal metastasis such as finding of lymphovascular invasion. EUS has less accuracy for superficial disease and will seldom obviate the need for EMR.[33] For T1a tumors resected by EMR, the risk of lymph node metastasis is very low, and additional staging studies are not required.

Most tumors, however, will be manifested as larger lesions. For these, further staging with a contrast-enhanced CT scan of the chest and abdomen and PET/CT to evaluate for distant metastatic disease should be performed. If there is no evidence of distant metastatic disease, EUS should be done to assess T-status and regional lymph nodes. Coupling EUS with fine needle aspiration of any suspicious nodes further increases the accuracy of this test.[31] Obtaining the PET/CT scan before EUS has several advantages.

TABLE 42.8 Pathologic stage groupings (pTNM) for esophageal adenocarcinoma.

	T	N	M	G
Stage 0	Tis	N0	M0	N/A
Stage IA	T1a	N0	M0	G1
	T1a	N0	M0	GX
Stage IB	T1a	N0	M0	G2
	T1b	N0	M0	G1-2
	T1b	N0	M0	GX
Stage IC	T1	N0	M0	G3
	T2	N0	M0	G1–2
Stage IIA	T2	N0	M0	G3
	T2	N0	M0	GX
Stage IIB	T1	N1	M0	Any
	T3	N0	M0	Any
Stage IIIA	T1	N2	M0	Any
	T2	N1	M0	Any
Stage IIIB	T2	N2	M0	Any
	T3	N1–2	M0	Any
	T4a	N0–1	M0	Any
Stage IVA	T4a	N2	M0	Any
	T4b	N0–2	M0	Any
	Any T	N3	M0	Any
Stage IVB	Any T	Any N	M1	Any

T, Tumor status; N, lymph node status; M, metastasis; G, grade.
Adapted from Rice TW, Ishwaran H, Ferguson MK, et al: Cancer of the esophagus and esophagogastric junction: An eighth edition staging primer. J Thorac Oncol 12:36-42, 2017.

TABLE 42.9 Clinical stage groupings (cTNM) for esophageal squamous cell carcinoma.

	T	N	M
Stage 0	Tis	N0	M0
Stage I	T1	N0–1	M0
Stage II	T2	N0–1	M0
	T3	N0	M0
Stage III	T3	N1	M0
	T1–3	N2	M0
Stage IVA	T4	N0–2	M0
	Any T	N3	M0
Stage IVB	Any T	Any N	M1

T, Tumor status; N, lymph node status; M, metastasis.
Adapted from Rice TW, Ishwaran H, Ferguson MK, et al: Cancer of the esophagus and esophagogastric junction: An eighth edition staging primer. J Thorac Oncol 12:36-42, 2017.

The PET/CT scan may demonstrate distant metastatic disease, eliminating the need for the patient to undergo EUS. The PET/CT scan may also identify a suspicious lymph node that can be specifically examined and sampled during the EUS procedure (Fig. 42.32). EUS is superior to CT or PET for assessment of both T and N-status. It is highly accurate for celiac nodal status, though slightly lower for other regional lymph nodes due to difficulty accessing the node without traversing the tumor. Obstructing lesions may preclude EUS assessment. In these cases, dilatation to perform EUS is associated with a risk of perforation. These risks must be weighed against the benefits of obtaining additional staging information. Most tumors with such tight stenoses are locally advanced and should likely be treated with multimodality therapy. Although EUS provides information about invasion of adjacent structures, bronchoscopy should also be performed for proximal and middle third esophageal tumors to assess for direct tracheal invasion. It is important to remember that for more superficial tumors (T1a–T2), the accuracy of EUS is significantly diminished and EMR provides the most accurate staging information.[31,33]

Appropriate staging is critical for treatment decisions. Superficial T1a tumors can usually be treated with EMR. Locally advanced tumors (T3 tumors or T2 tumors with nodal involvement) require multimodality therapy. Stage IV disease requires systemic or palliative therapy. Without accurate staging, patients are likely to be either undertreated or overtreated, leading to decreased survival and quality of life.

Approach to Early-Stage Esophageal Cancer

In the last 15 years, there has been a significant shift in the way early-stage esophageal cancers are treated. Improved endoscopic technology as well as a better understanding of the biology of early-stage tumors has led to the increased use of endoscopic therapies for the diagnosis, staging, and treatment of early-stage esophageal cancers. It is likely that surgery will play a smaller role for superficial cancers as endoscopic and ablative therapies continue to evolve and biomarkers of prognosis are refined. Given the changing nature of these treatments, multidisciplinary care with surgeons, gastroenterologists, and pathologists is essential to providing patients with the best long-term outcomes.

High-Grade Dysplasia and Superficial Cancers

Barrett esophagus is a significant risk factor for the development of esophageal adenocarcinoma. However, the absolute annual risk of developing cancer in a patient with Barrett has been estimated to be as low as 0.12%.[34] Thus, increasing attention has been paid towards those with findings of dysplasia and eradication therapies to prevent the development of invasive malignancy in this subpopulation. Dysplasia arising in Barrett esophagus is characterized by cytologic malignant changes including atypical nuclei, increased mitoses, and lack of surface maturation. High-grade dysplasia is distinguished from low-grade dysplasia by more prominent cytologic or architectural derangements. As long as the cells are confined to the epithelium without invasion of the basement membrane, the pathology should be described as dysplasia regardless of the degree of abnormality. This encompasses what was previously referred to as carcinoma in situ. Historically, esophagectomy was often recommended for patients with high-grade dysplasia for a number of reasons. In the past, endoscopic biopsies were relatively inaccurate, and up to 50% of patients who underwent esophagectomy for high-grade dysplasia were found to have invasive cancer in the surgical specimen. Also, therapies to reverse or to halt the progression of dysplasia to invasive cancer were unavailable. Although esophagectomy had very high rates of cure for high-grade dysplasia, it was associated with significant morbidity.

Overtreatment has also been a concern. Despite the historical data that many patients with high-grade dysplasia have invasive cancer found on esophagectomy, there is evidence from other groups reporting that only a minority of patients with flat high-grade dysplasia develop invasive cancer on follow-up endoscopy. Some of the conflict may be due to interobserver

TABLE 42.10 Pathologic stage groupings (pTNM) for esophageal squamous cell carcinoma.

	T	N	M	G	L
Stage 0	Tis	N0	M0	N/A	Any
Stage IA	T1a	N0	M0	G1	Any
	T1a	N0	M0	GX	Any
Stage IB	T1a	N0	M0	G2–3	Any
	T1b	N0	M0	G1–3	Any
	T1b	N0	M0	GX	Any
	T2	N0	M0	G1	Any
Stage IIA	T2	N0	M0	G2–3	Any
	T2	N0	M0	GX	Any
	T3	N0	M0	Any	Lower
	T3	N0	M0	G1	Upper/middle
Stage IIB	T3	N0	M0	G2–3	Upper/middle
	T3	N0	M0	GX	Any
	T3	N0	M0	Any	Location X
	T1	N1	M0	Any	Any
Stage IIIA	T1	N2	M0	Any	Any
	T2	N1	M0	Any	Any
Stage IIIB	T2	N2	M0	Any	Any
	T3	N1–2	M0	Any	Any
	T4a	N0–1	M0	Any	Any
Stage IVA	T4a	N2	M0	Any	Any
	T4b	N0–2	M0	Any	Any
	Any T	N3	M0	Any	Any
Stage IVB	Any T	Any N	M1	Any	Any

G, grade; L, Location; M, metastasis; N, lymph node status; T, Tumor status.
Adapted from Rice TW, Ishwaran H, Ferguson MK, et al. Cancer of the esophagus and esophagogastric junction: An eighth edition staging primer. J Thorac Oncol. 2017;12:36–42.

TABLE 42.11 Postneoadjuvant therapy stage groupings (ypTNM) for esophageal adenocarcinoma and squamous cell carcinoma.

	T	N	M
Stage I	T0–2	N0	M0
Stage II	T3	N0	M0
Stage IIIA	T0–2	N1	M0
Stage IIIB	T3	N1	M0
	T0–3	N2	M0
	T4a	N0	M0
Stage IVA	T4a	N1–2	M0
	T4a	NX	M0
	T4b	N0–2	M0
	Any T	N3	M0
Stage IVB	Any T	Any N	M1

T, Tumor status; N, lymph node status; M, metastasis.
Adapted from Rice TW, Ishwaran H, Ferguson MK, et al. Cancer of the esophagus and esophagogastric junction: An eighth edition staging primer. J Thorac Oncol. 2017;12:36–42.

variation in the diagnosis of high-grade dysplasia versus invasive adenocarcinoma on biopsy specimens and the practice of diligent search for cancer at some institutions. Any biopsy specimens with high-grade dysplasia or invasive adenocarcinoma should be reviewed by a specialty pathologist experienced with Barrett esophagus and esophageal cancer. In contrast to the high rates of cancer development in patients with high-grade dysplasia, the incidence of cancer with nondysplastic Barrett esophagus appears to be low. The largest study of endoscopic surveillance in patients with Barrett esophagus found that the annual risk for development of cancer was 0.39% in patients with no dysplasia versus 0.77% in patients with low-grade dysplasia.[35]

The Seattle biopsy protocol is still widely accepted for mapping of Barrett esophagus with high-grade dysplasia. This involves four-quadrant biopsies at 1-cm intervals along the entire length of Barrett esophagus in addition to targeted biopsies of all visible lesions. Emerging endoscopic imaging techniques increase the sensitivity for detection of dysplasia. Many specialty centers routinely use high-resolution endoscopy and some sort of chromoendoscopy or simulated chromoendoscopy, such as narrow-band imaging (Olympus), to evaluate Barrett esophagus. Narrow-band imaging uses light filters to allow more narrow wavelengths of light. The wavelengths penetrate only superficially and are absorbed well by hemoglobin, better revealing irregular mucosal vascular patterns (Fig. 42.33). Use of narrow-band imaging is associated with high accuracy is diagnosing dysplasia.[36] Additional technologies include autofluorescence endoscopy and optical coherence tomography. Notably, confocal endomicroscopy was shown in a randomized trial to reduce the need for random biopsies and improve the diagnostic yield and accuracy of identifying dysplasia in patients with Barrett esophagus.[37] These techniques hold promise for even greater resolution but require more specialized training and equipment compared with the relatively user-friendly technology of high-resolution endoscopy and narrow-band imaging.

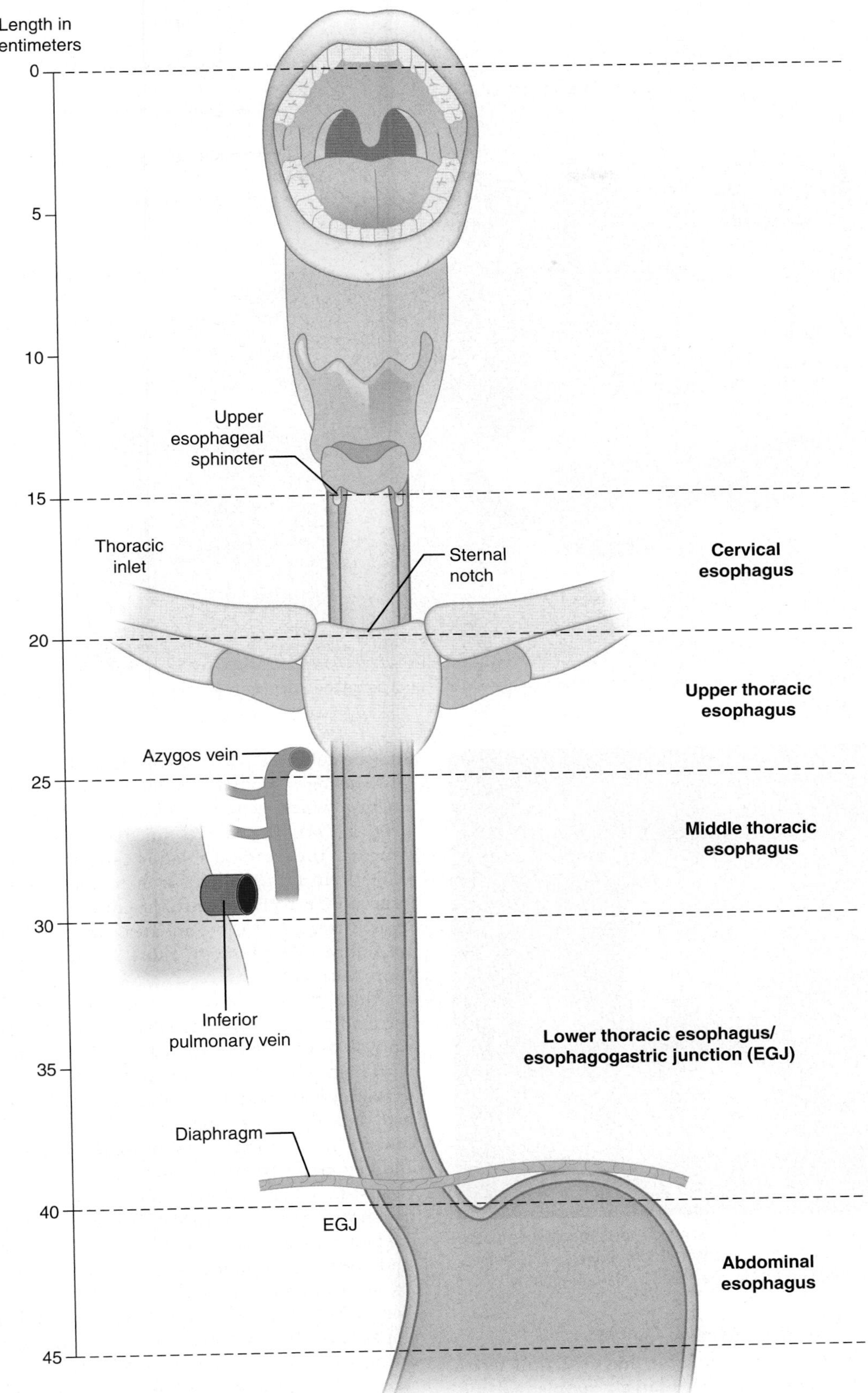

FIG. 42.30 Regions of the esophagus. The cervical esophagus extends from the upper esophageal sphincter to the thoracic inlet. The upper thoracic esophagus extends from the thoracic inlet to the azygos vein. The mid-thoracic esophagus extends from the lower border of the azygos vein to the inferior pulmonary vein. The lower thoracic esophagus extends from the lower border of the inferior pulmonary vein to the gastroesophageal junction.

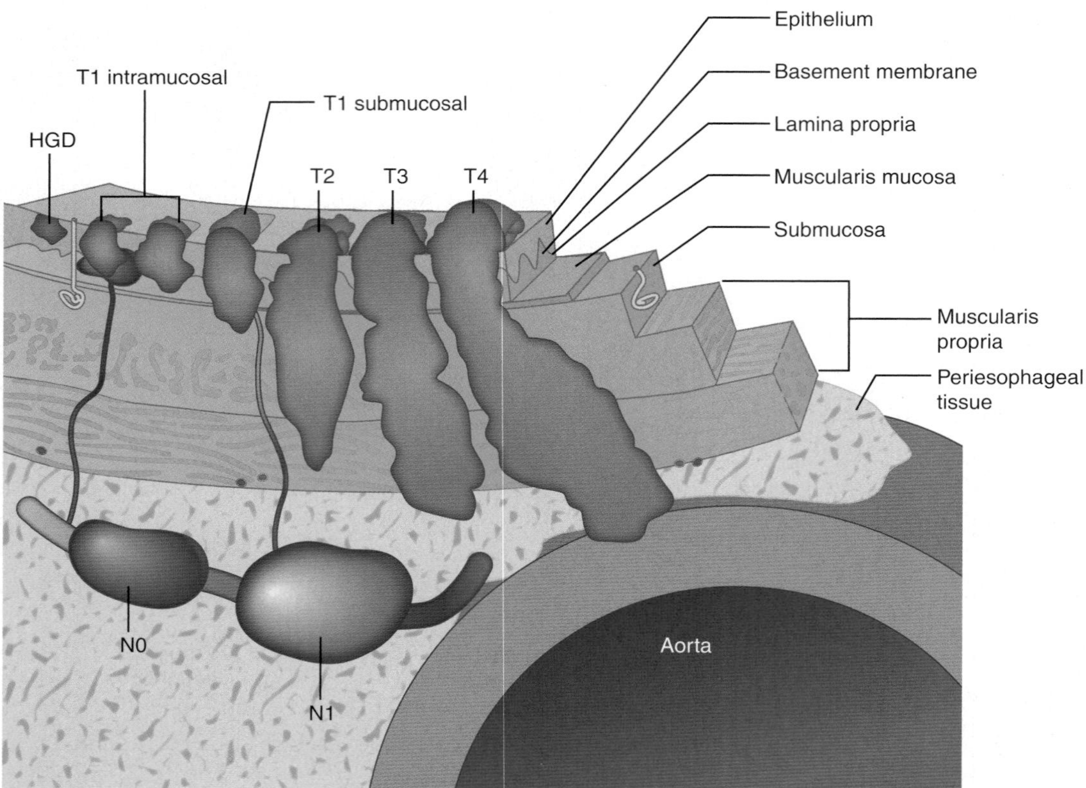

FIG. 42.31 Tumor classification for esophageal carcinoma as defined by depth of invasion. *HGD*, High-grade dysplasia.

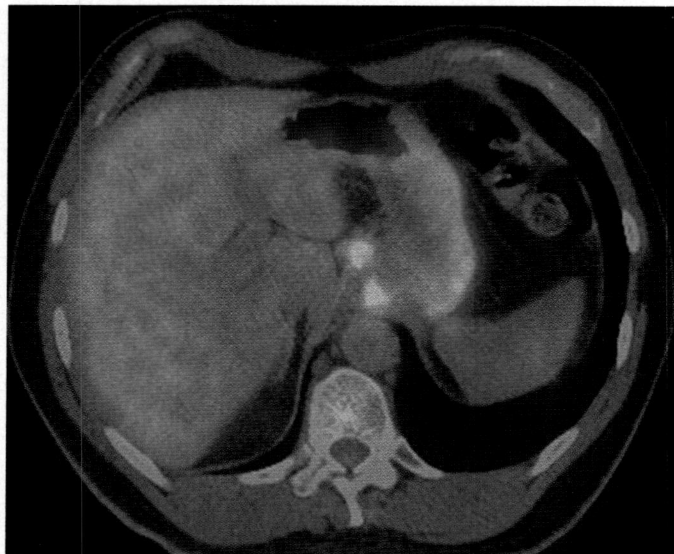

FIG. 42.32 Fused transaxial positron emission tomography/computed tomography image demonstrating increased fluorodeoxyglucose activity in a gastroesophageal junction tumor and celiac lymphadenopathy.

Therapeutic Approaches to Esophageal Cancer

Ablation. Various endoscopic ablative and resection techniques have been developed that have largely supplanted the role of esophagectomy for high-grade dysplasia. The most commonly used technology today is radiofrequency ablation (RFA). RFA is much more effective than photodynamic therapy with a lower stricture (and overall complication) rate. RFA may be delivered with a circumferential balloon or an electrical plate using a bipolar electrode that transmits radiofrequency energy, which generates heat and destroys superficial tissue (Fig. 42.34). The treated mucosa is replaced by neosquamous mucosa. The standard ablation program uses two double pulses of 12 J/cm^2. The balloon is then repositioned distally, and the procedure is repeated until the entire segment of Barrett esophagus is treated. If there are areas of residual Barrett esophagus on follow-up endoscopy, those segments may be treated with more focal ablation.

Multiple studies have demonstrated the effectiveness of RFA for eradicating Barrett esophagus and dysplasia. In the Ablation of Intestinal Metaplasia (AIM-II) trial, 81% of patients with high-grade dysplasia and 90% of patients with low-grade dysplasia had eradication of dysplasia.[38] Only 4% of patients had their dysplasia progress to a higher grade of dysplasia or cancer. In a European trial of patients with Barrett esophagus and low-grade dysplasia, 136 patients were randomized to RFA versus surveillance. Only 1.5% of ablated patients progressed to cancer versus 8.8% in the surveillance arm.[39] RFA was able to eradicate dysplasia in 92.6% of patients. Finally, in a registry study of patients undergoing RFA for Barrett esophagus, only 2% developed cancer and only 0.2% died of their disease.[40] American College of Gastroenterology guidelines recommend all patients with low-grade dysplasia undergo endoscopic eradication therapy, with yearly endoscopic surveillance being an acceptable alternative.[12] All patients with high-grade dysplasia should undergo endoscopic therapy if medically able to tolerate the procedure.

Cryotherapy. Cryotherapy is an alternative ablative technique that uses extreme cold rather than heat to destroy tissue

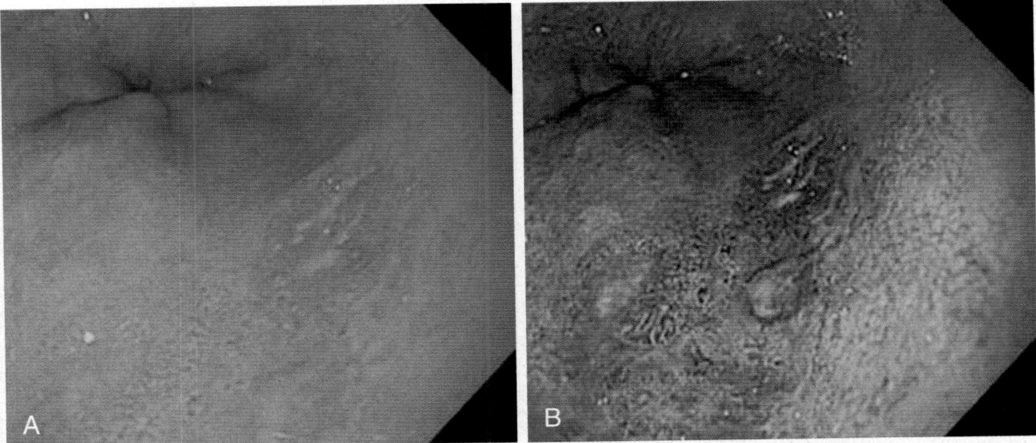

FIG. 42.33 Traditional, white light view of Barrett esophagus with high-grade dysplasia *(A)* and narrow-band imaging of the same area *(B)*.

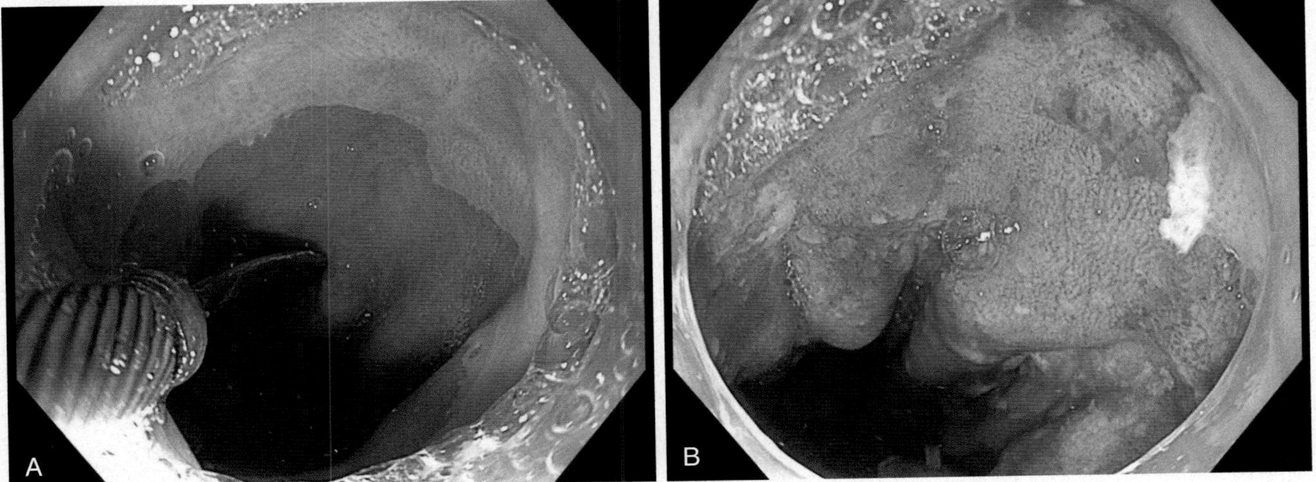

FIG. 42.34 Radiofrequency ablation performed in a patient with Barrett esophagus. (A) Preablation with catheter seen adjacent to area of metaplastic disease. (B) Posttreatment after radiofrequency ablation. (From Rajaram R, Hofstetter WL. Mucosal ablation techniques for Barrett's esophagus and early esophageal cancer. *Thorac Surg Clin.* 2018;28:473–480.)

(Fig. 42.35). Cryotherapy is generally well tolerated with little pain and low stricture rates. One advantage of cryotherapy compared with RFA is that cryotherapy does not require a probe to be in contact with the tissue. Endoscopists typically use either an endoscopic spray catheter or in some cases, an endoscopic balloon, to deliver cold liquid nitrogen (–196°C). A decompression tube is typically required to prevent overdistention of the stomach and intestine with gas. In a large registry series, cryotherapy eradicated low- and high-grade dysplasia in 91% and 81% of patients, respectively.[41] In another study, use of cryotherapy, in conjunction with EMR, for patients with high-grade dysplasia and intramucosal adenocarcinoma resulted in eradication rates of dysplasia of nearly 90% at five years.[42] Additionally, cryotherapy has been used as salvage therapy after prior failed RFA. There have been no head-to-head comparisons between cryotherapy and RFA, but reports indicate similar efficacy to RFA.

Regardless of what ablation technology is used, patients should have close surveillance and long-term acid suppression after ablation. In patients with high-grade dysplasia, a repeat endoscopy should be performed three months after ablative therapy has completely eradicated their dysplasia/Barrett esophagus, preferably with high-resolution endoscopy and some form of chromoendoscopy.[12] In those with low-grade dysplasia, the first surveillance endoscopy should be performed 6 months after their Barrett esophagus/dysplasia is completely eradicated.[12] Many patients will require more than one ablation session to eradicate all Barrett esophagus. There is also a small risk that areas of Barrett epithelium could be hidden beneath areas of the new squamous epithelium, known as buried glands. Malignancy can arise within these buried glands, and these cancers may be more difficult to identify during endoscopy. The clinical significance of this phenomenon is unknown, and the incidence of malignancy developing within these areas of buried glands appears to be very low. Nevertheless, the potential implications of unrecognized incomplete eradication justifies future surveillance of ablated patients.

Endoscopic mucosal resection. One limitation of ablative therapies is the limited depth of penetration. Another

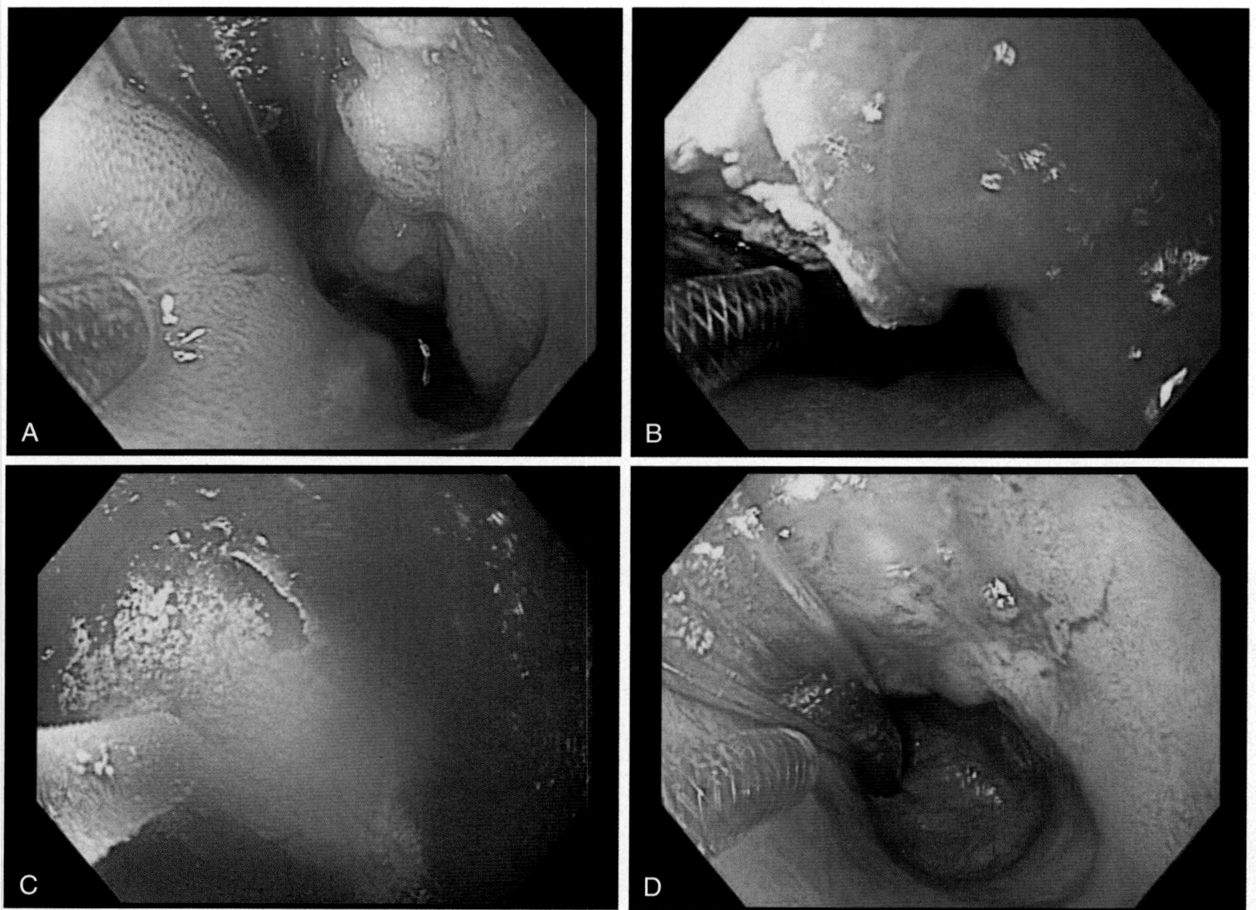

FIG. 42.35 Liquid nitrogen spray cryotherapy performed in a patient with Barrett esophagus and dysplasia. (A) Dysplastic segment in background of Barrett esophagus seen anteriorly. (B) and (C) Targeted delivery of liquid nitrogen spray cryotherapy. (D) Posttreatment after liquid nitrogen spray cryotherapy. (From Rajaram R, Hofstetter WL: Mucosal ablation techniques for Barrett's esophagus and early esophageal cancer. *Thorac Surg Clin.* 2018;28:473–480.)

disadvantage is the lack of definitive pathologic analysis. Therefore, patients with nodular or raised Barrett esophagus or other abnormalities suggestive of superficial invasive cancer should undergo EMR rather than ablation. EMR provides larger specimens to accurately determine the depth of invasion. EMR resects the full thickness of the mucosa, down into the submucosa (Fig. 42.36). Thus, it is a good therapeutic option for superficial lesions with a low risk of nodal metastases. In a study of 1000 patients with mucosal adenocarcinoma, use of EMR was found to achieve long-term eradication rates of 93.8% at near 5-year median follow-up.[43]

However, use of EMR needs to be individualized as it does not address the potential for nodal disease. Depending on the size of the lesion (>2 cm), degree of differentiation (intermediate/high-grade), and lymphovascular invasion, the overall risk of nodal metastasis for lesions confined to the mucosa (T1a) ranges from less than 2% to more than 15% (Table 42.12).[44] For selected T1a lesions, EMR is highly effective (Fig. 42.37). Although EMR can technically remove lesions involving the submucosa (T1b), the risk of lymph node involvement increases with depth of submucosal invasion. Therefore, EMR is generally not considered adequate for tumors involving the deeper submucosa. However, lesions involving only the most superficial third of the submucosa (SM1) have relatively low rates of nodal metastases, possibly less than 10%. On the other hand, lesions involving the deepest two-thirds of the submucosa (SM2/SM3) may have nodal involvement in nearly 40% of cases, with some studies finding significantly higher rates of nodal disease.[45] T1b cancers with squamous cell histology also appear to have a higher risk of nodal metastasis compared with adenocarcinoma (45% vs. 26%).[46] EUS has low accuracy for assessing T-status for superficial tumors, so patients with suspected T1 lesions should have EMR performed by a qualified endoscopist to obtain accurate staging. Thorough and accurate pathologic assessment is critical to formulating treatment plans. NCCN guidelines currently recommend use of EMR ± ablation in patients with Tis and T1a tumors as a preferred therapy over esophagectomy.[31] Additionally, in superficial T1b (SM1) patients with adenocarcinomas and low-risk features, endoscopic eradication is a reasonable alternative to surgery.

Complications of EMR include bleeding, stricture, pain, and perforation. The stricture risk is increased for patients requiring circumferential resection. In a study of EMR use in high-grade dysplasia and early esophageal cancer, approximately one-third of patients required dilatation though very few had long-term dysphagia.[47] Although EMR may be performed for the entire segment

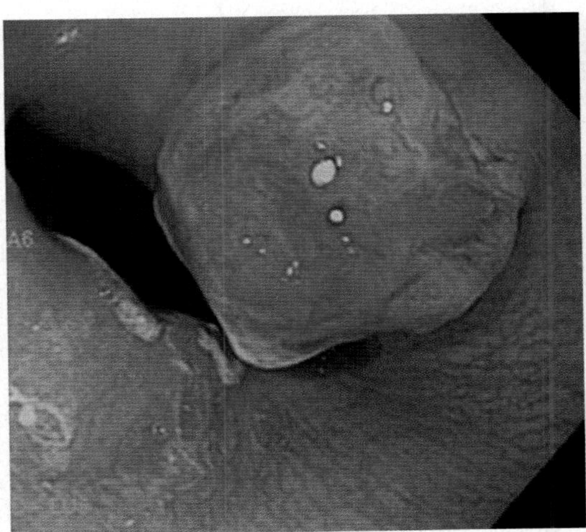

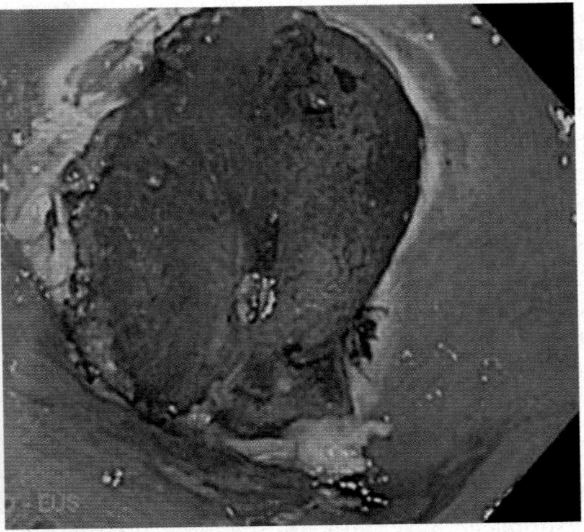

FIG. 42.36 A superficial T1a adenocarcinoma arising in the setting of Barrett esophagus *(left)* and submucosal defect after endoscopic mucosal resection *(right)*.

TABLE 42.12 Nomogram for prediction of lymph node metastases in early-stage esophageal cancer.

VARIABLE	POINTS
Size, per cm	+ 1 (per cm)
Depth	
T1a	+ 0
T1b	+ 2
Differentiation	
Well	+ 0
Moderate	+ 3
Poor	+ 3
Lymphovascular invasion	+ 6

RISK CATEGORY	POINTS	PREDICTED RISK OF LYMPH NODE METASTASES (%)
Low	0-1	≤ 2
Moderate	2–4	3–6
High	5+	≥ 7

Adapted from Lee L, Ronellenfitsch U, Hofstetter WL, et al. Predicting lymph node metastases in early esophageal adenocarcinoma using a simple scoring system. *J Am Coll Surg*. 2013;217:191–199.

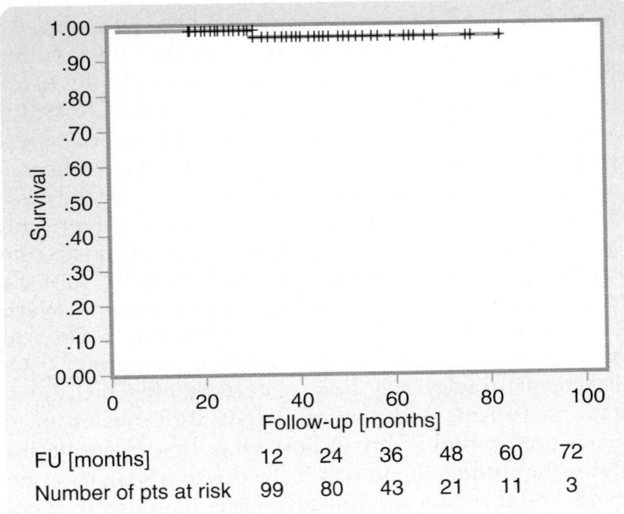

FIG. 42.37 Survival curve of patients undergoing endoscopic mucosal resection for low-risk, superficial esophageal adenocarcinoma. (From Ell C, May A, Pech O, et al. Curative endoscopic resection of early esophageal adenocarcinomas [Barrett's cancer]. *Gastrointest Endosc*. 2007;65:3–10.)

of Barrett esophagus, complication rates are lower if EMR is focused on specific areas combined with ablation for residual Barrett esophagus.

EMR may be performed with a submucosal lifting technique, which raises the target lesion by injecting fluid into the submucosa beneath the lesion. This allows the lesion to be suctioned more easily into a cap, creating a pseudopolyp, allowing resection with a snare. Another technique uses suction to raise the lesion, allowing a band to be placed at the base of the pseudopolyp that is created and then using a snare to resect. One drawback of EMR is that larger lesions are typically removed piecemeal. Reports describe the efficacy of endoscopic submucosal dissection using an endoscopic needle knife that allows greater submucosal dissection and en-bloc resection of larger lesions.[48] The safety of this technique outside a few specialized centers is unknown.

Surveillance is an important component of the treatment for superficial esophageal cancers. Patients should receive high-dose acid suppression therapy with a PPI to help EMR and ablation sites to heal. Many patients require multiple procedures to completely eradicate Barrett epithelium. Short-interval follow-up endoscopy should be performed three months after endoscopic treatment is completed. Any residual Barrett epithelium may be focally ablated at that time. Surveillance endoscopies should be performed frequently (i.e., every three months) for the first year after endoscopic treatment for high-grade dysplasia or intramucosal cancer, after which time the frequency of endoscopic surveillance may be spaced out.[12] For superficial lesions treated endoscopically, radiologic imaging, such as fluorodeoxyglucose (FDG) PET, has no value.

Esophagectomy. The role of esophagectomy as a single-modality treatment for esophageal cancer is diminishing. Most tumors are found after symptoms develop, at which point they are usually locally advanced or metastatic. Locally advanced tumors should be treated with multimodality therapy. Asymptomatic tumors are usually found during surveillance for Barrett esophagus. These are typically superficial and can be treated with EMR with lower complication rates than with esophagectomy. This leaves a relatively narrow subset of tumors that are treated appropriately with surgery only. As discussed earlier, T1b tumors have significant risk for nodal metastasis and, with exception of some SM1 tumors, most should be treated with esophagectomy. High-risk T1a lesions (larger tumors or lesions with lymphovascular invasion) could also be considered for esophagectomy. Extensive, multifocal lesions and ulcerated tumors may also be difficult to eradicate endoscopically and would be appropriate candidates for esophagectomy.

An area of controversy is the optimal treatment for clinical T2N0 tumors. Esophagectomy with an adequate lymphadenectomy would be expected to confer an overall 5-year survival of anywhere between 40% and 65% for a pathologic T2N0 cancer, depending on histology, grade, and location of tumor.[31] Unfortunately, a clinical stage of T2N0 is inaccurate in the majority of cases, and many patients are found to have node-positive disease on final pathology after esophagectomy.[49] Clinical T2N0 patients were included in the Chemoradiotherapy for Oesophageal Cancer Followed by Surgery Study (CROSS) trial, which compared neoadjuvant chemoradiation followed by surgery versus surgery alone for esophageal and GEJ cancer. Although the trial demonstrated a survival benefit for the neoadjuvant chemoradiation arm, clinical T2N0 patients represented only a small subset of the study cohort, and it is unclear how much benefit these patients in particular received.[50] It is clear that many patients with clinical T2N0 disease are understaged, but retrospective analyses indicate that there may not be a survival advantage for neoadjuvant therapy in this group.[51] One management strategy may be to selectively offer neoadjuvant therapy to patients with clinical T2N0 disease based on the patient's pretest probability of upstaging. In a recent decision analysis, the authors found that if the risk of upstaging is more than 48.1%, there is a survival advantage to induction chemoradiation.[52] Furthermore, they identified long tumors (>3 cm), presence of lymphovascular invasion, and high-grade as clinical factors associated with meeting this threshold and benefiting from induction therapy. It is important to also note that an equal number of patients with cT2N0 are actually overstaged, so liberal use of diagnostic EMR is appropriate.[49]

The advent of EMR also influences the type of esophagectomy that should be performed in early-stage esophageal cancer. Because of the potential for decreased complication and improved physiologic outcomes, vagal-sparing esophagectomy has been advocated by some for intramucosal adenocarcinoma and high-grade dysplasia. However, most low-risk lesions are now resected by EMR.

Regarding surgical technique, a randomized trial of transhiatal esophagectomy compared to an extended transthoracic approach with en-bloc lymphadenectomy found lower perioperative morbidity in the transhiatal group with a trend towards increased overall and disease-free survival in transthoracic patients.[53] The benefit of a transthoracic approach is the ability to perform an extensive lymphadenectomy, with some suggesting a minimum of 23 lymph nodes should be removed to maximize survival benefit.[54] Minimally invasive esophagectomy (MIE) is also an approach gaining favor. Use of MIE is associated with shorter lengths of stay with similar 30-day mortality and 3-year survival outcomes as open esophagectomy.[55] While MIE involves a completely minimally invasive approach, a hybrid esophagectomy is one in which the abdominal portion is approached laparoscopically and an open right thoracotomy is performed (Ivor Lewis esophagectomy). In a recent randomized controlled trial, hybrid Ivor Lewis esophagectomy was associated with almost half as many major complications as open surgery with differences in pulmonary events being a driving factor.[56] Additionally, 3-year overall and disease-free survival was similar in the two groups. Surgeons have also reported using a robotic-assisted approach for MIE with excellent oncologic outcomes, albeit with a significant learning curve associated with this technology.

Perioperative outcomes after esophagectomy have been reported from the Society of Thoracic Surgeons General Thoracic Surgery Database.[57] Postoperative 30-day mortality was 3.4% and major morbidity was 33.1%, and included return to the operating room (15.6%), anastomotic leaks (12.9%), reintubation (12.2%), and pneumonia (12.2%). In an attempt to address perioperative morbidity, several centers have implemented enhanced recovery or fast-track programs with results suggesting less ICU days, shorter lengths of stay, reduced costs, and fewer postoperative complications.[58]

Patients have increasing endoscopic and surgical options for the treatment of early-stage esophageal cancers. Care needs to be individualized so patients may make informed decisions, balancing the effectiveness of therapies with their risks and impact on quality of life.

Locally Advanced Esophageal Cancer

Despite improved awareness of the increasing trend in esophageal adenocarcinoma and more frequent detection of early esophageal adenocarcinoma on surveillance endoscopies, the majority of patients with esophageal cancer still present with locally advanced or metastatic disease. Usually, it is not until patients experience dysphagia, which generally signifies transmural tumor involvement (T3), that an esophageal cancer is diagnosed. In this setting, the probability of lymph node metastases reaches 80%, so the majority of patients present with clinical stage T3N1–3 according to the eighth edition (AJCC) of esophageal cancer staging. It should be reiterated that the eighth edition staging criteria includes not only clinical and pathologic stage, but also ypTNM stage.[32] Inclusion of post-neoadjuvant therapy stage reflects the significant survival benefit patients with locally advanced esophageal cancer have experienced from multimodality therapy in the current era.[50]

Current staging recognizes the prognostic value in the number of metastatic lymph nodes and groups patients into three categories: N1 (one to three positive nodes), N2 (four to six positive nodes), and N3 (seven or more positive nodes). The anatomic location of the regional nodal disease relative to the primary tumor is not a factor involved in staging. However, recent evidence suggests that nodal location, such as celiac axis or upper mediastinum, may significantly affect survival.[59] In clinical practice, nodal disease location continues to influence treatment decisions. This confusion is partly due to the lack of consensus and definition of which nodal stations represent regional versus distant metastatic disease. In the era of multimodality therapy and selective surgery, the rigorous definition of locally advanced esophageal cancer is necessary to guide pretreatment therapeutic decisions before committing to either aggressive locoregional therapy or initiating systemic treatment.

For esophageal adenocarcinoma, mostly located in the distal esophagus or GEJ, we consider nodal disease located in the area from the celiac axis up to the paratracheal region to represent regional disease; nodal disease located outside of these boundaries is regarded as distant disease. For esophageal SCC, which mostly arises in the mid or proximal esophagus, periesophageal cervical lymphadenopathy is still considered a regional disease. Whereas the current staging system takes the tumor differentiation into account, it is mainly the disease burden that dictates the decisions about the treatment strategy, and therapeutic decisions are best discussed in a multidisciplinary setting.

Principles of Multimodality Therapy for Locally Advanced Esophageal Cancer

Surgical resection of the esophagus was the mainstay of esophageal cancer treatment in the past. However, we have learned that even the most radical resections with extensive lymph node dissections are not adequate to cure locoregionally advanced disease in the majority of cases. Distant recurrence or metastatic disease continues to be the main cause of death in patients with esophageal cancer.

Our understanding and treatment of esophageal cancer have evolved significantly during the last 100 years. The initial recognition that a localized esophageal cancer may be cured with surgical resection dates back to the first successful esophagectomy performed by Franz Torek in 1913. Despite rather poor perioperative outcomes at that time, surgery became a supplement to radiation as the treatment of choice for localized esophageal cancer in the early twentieth century. Over time, more extensive en-bloc esophageal resections and lymphadenectomy became favored with the hope that radical resection of disease would result in a cure more frequently. However, similar to Halstead radical mastectomy, we have learned that whereas extended esophagectomy may lead to better locoregional control, it fails to achieve cure in patients destined to die of metastatic disease. Today, technical aspects of esophagectomy are still passionately debated as the technological advances enable us to perform these procedures safely even with less invasive or robotically assisted techniques. From an oncologic standpoint, however, surgical therapy has its limits in what it can contribute to the cure rate of esophageal cancer. Moreover, there continues to be a tremendous variability in the performance of surgical resection of the esophagus among surgeons, with some favoring transthoracic and some transabdominal approaches with varied extents of lymph node dissections. This lack of procedural standardization confounds the analysis of esophageal cancer treatment outcomes.

Increased understanding of cancer biology led to the development of nonsurgical treatment strategies for solid organ malignant neoplasms, including esophageal carcinoma. Chemotherapy was combined concomitantly with radiation therapy to improve the local-regional efficacy and potentially for systemic effect. Intuitively, this strategy targets both local disease and systemic micrometastases. The demonstrated efficacy of this treatment paradigm subsequently stimulated interest in combining surgery, radiation, and chemotherapy to maximize the treatment effect. The combination of these treatment modalities became the focus of several clinical trials investigating the role and timing of each method.

Treatment Modalities Used in Locally Advanced Esophageal Cancer

Radiation therapy. Radiation was employed as the first treatment modality for esophageal cancer. Early experiences with radium bougies and external beam radiation demonstrated esophageal tumor regression with occasional complete tumor responses. With the evolution of surgical care, radiation became a part of a multidisciplinary approach to esophageal cancer therapy with the goal of sterilizing areas within or around the operative field. Early randomized trials of neoadjuvant radiation administered doses of 20 to 40 Gy before resection in an attempt to decrease local recurrence and to improve survival rates. With one exception, all of these trials included patients with SCC only, and none of the trials demonstrated significant benefits of adding radiation therapy to resection.

Although the lower radiation doses (20–40 Gy) may have been inadequate, clinicians were wary of combining higher dose radiation before surgery, given the toxicity risks (note that radiation delivery and particles used in therapy were very different in the past compared with current therapy). Nonetheless, high rates of locoregional recurrence after surgery led to the consideration of adjuvant radiation therapy for esophageal cancer. The rationale for this approach was the ability to deliver higher doses (40–60 Gy) of radiation postoperatively without worsening perioperative complications. Postoperative radiation therapy for esophageal cancer appeared to be potentially beneficial in several trials, although the data are conflicting and subject to selection bias.

Chemotherapy. The cause of death from esophageal cancer is mainly due to metastatic disease. Intuitively, systemic chemotherapy has the potential to target micrometastatic deposits. Even in the setting of a seemingly localized disease, it usually downstages marginally resectable tumors, allowing improved complete (R0) resection rates, and decreases the incidence of locoregional recurrence. The synergistic effect of chemotherapy with radiation strengthens the argument for its use. Importantly, when it is administered preoperatively, the biologic response can be evaluated and quantified pathologically in terms of pathologic tumor histoviability, and the degree of this response has been correlated as an indicator of outcome. Current chemotherapeutic regimens are based on platinum compounds (cisplatin and carboplatin) in combination with 5-fluorouracil or taxanes as a doublet. In several prospective randomized trials, researchers compared chemotherapy followed by surgery with surgery alone for both esophageal adenocarcinoma and SCC (Table 42.13).[60] The landmark trial by Roth and colleagues demonstrated longer median survival durations in patients with major or complete response to chemotherapy, which highlighted the biologic diversity of esophageal cancers and their varied susceptibility to chemotherapy.[61] In a phase 3 study run by the Medical Research Council (MRC) in the United Kingdom, patients with locally advanced esophageal cancer randomized to chemotherapy plus surgery, versus surgery alone, experienced a survival benefit.[62] The largest trial of its kind, the MRC trial included 802 patients randomized to receive chemotherapy plus esophagectomy versus esophagectomy alone. The survival benefit of chemotherapy persisted at the updated median follow-up duration of six years, with 5-year survival rates of 23% with chemotherapy plus surgery and 17% with surgery alone (P = 0.03). Both adenocarcinoma and SCC patients experienced benefit. Another commonly referenced trial that demonstrated survival advantage and better R0 resection rate of neoadjuvant chemotherapy and surgery over surgery alone was the MRC Adjuvant Gastric Infusional Chemotherapy (MAGIC) trial by Cunningham and

TABLE 42.13 **Randomized trials comparing chemotherapy and surgery versus surgery alone.**

TRIAL	N	HISTOLOGY	CHEMOTHERAPY	R0 (%)	SURVIVAL
MRC		SCC, ADC	Cisplatin, 5-FU		Median (months)
CT-Sx	400			60	17
Sx	402			54	13
RTOG 8911		SCC, ADC	Cisplatin, 5-FU		Median (months)
CT-Sx	213			63	14.9
Sx	227			59	16.1
MAGIC		ADC	Epirubicin, cisplatin, 5-FU	NA	5 years (%)
CT-Sx	250				36*
Sx	253				23
FFCD		ADC	Cisplatin, 5-FU		5 years (%)
CT-Sx	113			84	38*
Sx	111			74	24

**P* < 0.05.*
ADC, Adenocarcinoma; CT, chemotherapy; 5-FU, 5-fluorouracil; MRC, Medical Research Council; SCC, squamous cell carcinoma; Sx, surgery.
Adapted from Cools-Lartigue J, Spicer J, Ferri LE. Current status of management of malignant disease: Current management of esophageal cancer. J Gastrointest Surg. 2015; 19:964–972.

colleagues.[63] The majority of the enrolled patients had gastric carcinoma, with only a subgroup having esophageal or GEJ tumors.

In the adjuvant setting, the results of chemotherapy have not been convincing. The majority of trials were in the esophageal SCC setting, such as a phase 3 multicenter Japan Clinical Oncology Group trial (JCOG 9907), which randomized 330 patients comparing the effects of neoadjuvant (164 patients) and adjuvant (166 patients) chemotherapy for stage II and stage III esophageal SCC.[64] Patients received two cycles of cisplatin and 5-fluorouracil before or after radical resection. The interim analysis demonstrated a significantly better ($P = 0.044$) median progression-free survival duration in the neoadjuvant group (three years) than in the adjuvant group (two years) and the difference in estimated 5-year overall survival rate of 60% versus 38% in the neoadjuvant and adjuvant arms, respectively ($P = 0.013$). On the basis of these findings, it was recommended to terminate the trial.

Definitive chemoradiation. Chemoradiation may be administered in a preoperative or postoperative setting, as definitive bimodality therapy, or as part of trimodality therapy when combined with surgery. Concomitant administration of chemotherapy and radiation has a synergistic effect with increased tumor cytotoxicity at low doses. The validity of chemoradiation use for all locations of esophageal cancer is based on encouraging results of definitive chemoradiation for cervical esophageal SCC. Randomized trials of chemoradiation versus radiation alone include RTOG 85-01 by Herskovic and colleagues, which established that a group of patients with esophageal SCC or adenocarcinoma could be cured with bimodality therapy alone. To improve on the favorable outcomes observed in the RTOG 85-01 trial, researchers attempted to increase locoregional disease control rates in the subsequent Intergroup 0123/RTOG 94-05 trial by modifying the intensity of radiation therapy to high-dose 64.8 Gy given concurrently with chemotherapy. Unfortunately, at a median follow-up duration of 16 months, the survival and locoregional disease control rates with the higher radiation dose did not differ significantly from those in the RTOG 85-01 trial, but the toxicity and treatment-related deaths were worse in the high-dose radiation therapy group. This study established that 50.4 Gy of radiation used concomitantly with chemotherapy is both a neoadjuvant and potentially definitive dose.[65]

Chemoradiation and surgery. When used alone, each cancer treatment modality has its limitations, ranging from inadequate therapeutic effect to excessive toxicity. The synergistic effect of chemoradiation combined with surgical resection maximizes the chances of effectively treating both locoregional disease and potential undetectable metastases (Table 42.14). Early clinical trials testing a trimodality treatment paradigm did not demonstrate a survival advantage over surgery alone. Many of these trials were underpowered and mixed SCC and esophageal adenocarcinoma histology as well as varied radiation and chemotherapy regimens. Some trials suffered from poor patient accrual or inconsistent surgical outcomes.

However, in locally advanced esophageal cancer the effect of trimodality therapy in well-selected patient populations appears to be significant. The most notable and frequently quoted trial that compared chemoradiation followed by surgery with surgery alone for esophageal and EGJ cancer was the CROSS trial.[50] This trial enrolled an impressive 368 patients during a 4-year period, and 366 patients were included in the final analysis. The surgery-alone group consisted of 188 patients, whereas 178 underwent chemoradiation followed by surgery. The majority (75%) of the patients had adenocarcinoma, and 22% had SCC. The chemoradiation regimen consisted of a 5-week course of carboplatin and paclitaxel administered concurrently with radiation therapy at a dose of 41.4 Gy given in 23 fractions five days a week. Esophagectomy was performed within 4 to 6 weeks in the treatment group and immediately after randomization in the control group. The completeness (R0) of resection was higher in the trimodality group than in the surgery-alone group (92% vs. 69%; $P < 0.001$). Patients undergoing trimodality therapy with SCC experienced complete pathologic response (ypT0N0M0) significantly more than patients with adenocarcinoma (49% vs. 29%; $P < 0.001$). Expectedly, nodal positivity was higher in patients with surgery alone compared with the trimodality group (75% vs. 31%; $P < 0.001$). At a median follow-up duration of 45 months, patients receiving the trimodality therapy had significantly longer median overall survival duration (49.4 months) than did patients undergoing surgery alone (24 months; hazard ratio [HR], 0.65; 95% confidence interval [CI], 0.49–0.87; $P = 0.003$). The estimated 5-year survival rate in the trimodality therapy group was 47%

TABLE 42.14 Randomized trials comparing chemoradiation and surgery versus surgery alone.

TRIAL	N	HISTOLOGY	CHEMOTHERAPY	RT (GY)	PCR (%)	R0 (%)	SURVIVAL
Walsh		ADC	Cisplatin, 5-FU	40	25	NA	3 years (%)
CT-RT-Sx	58						32*
Sx	55						6
Bosset		SCC	Cisplatin	37	26	NA	Median (months)
CT-RT-Sx	143						18.6
Sx	149						18.6
Urba		SCC, ADC	Cisplatin, 5-FU, vinblastine	45	28	90	3 years (%)
CT-RT-Sx	50					90	30*
Sx	50						16
Lee		SCC	Cisplatin, 5FU	45.6	43		Median (months)
CT-RT-Sx	51					100	27.3
Sx	50					87.5	28.2
Burmeister		SCC, ADC	Cisplatin, 5-FU	35	16		Median (months)
CT-RT-Sx	128					80*	22.2
Sx	128					59	19.3
Tepper		SCC, ADC	Cisplatin, 5-FU	50.4	33	NR	5 years (%)
CT-RT-Sx	30						39*
Sx	26						16
CROSS		SCC, ADC	Carboplatin, paclitaxel	41.4	29		5 years (%)
CT-RT-Sx	178					92*	47*
Sx	188					69	34
Mariette		SCC, ADC	Cisplatin, 5-FU	45	33.3		3 years (%)
CT-RT-Sx	98					93.8	47.5
Sx	97					92.1	53
Yang		SCC	Cisplatin, vinorelbine	40	43.2		Median (months)
CT-RT-Sx	224					98.4*	100.1*
Sx	227					91.2	66.5

*$P < 0.05$.
ADC, Adenocarcinoma; CROSS, chemoradiotherapy for Oesophageal Cancer Following Surgery Study; CT, chemotherapy; 5-FU, 5-fluorouracil; NA, not available; NR, not reported; pCR, pathologic complete response; RT, radiotherapy; SCC, squamous cell carcinoma; Sx, surgery.
Edited and adapted from Cools-Lartigue J, Spicer J, Ferri LE. Current status of management of malignant disease: Current management of esophageal cancer. J Gastrointest Surg. 2015;19:964–972.

compared with 34% (HR, 0.65; 95% CI, 0.49–0.87; $P = 0.003$) in the surgery group. Interestingly, trimodality therapy did not significantly benefit patients with adenocarcinoma histology (HR, 0.74; 95% CI, 0.53–1.02; $P = 0.07$) in the initial analysis. However, in a subsequent study with longer follow-up, the survival benefit of trimodality therapy in both SCC and adenocarcinoma was confirmed.[50,66]

The Role of Surgery in Trimodality Therapy and Salvage Surgery

Subsequent to the CROSS trial report, many Western centers adopted the trimodality therapy as the standard of care for the treatment of esophageal carcinoma. However, this trial still left many questions unanswered about the treatment strategy for locoregional esophageal carcinoma. Whereas we have observed that neoadjuvant chemoradiation improves R0 resection and locoregional recurrence rates and results in pathologic complete responses in many patients, other subgroups of patients clearly derive no benefit from neoadjuvant therapy over surgery alone. Equally, patients who are "cured" by neoadjuvant chemoradiation derive no additional survival benefit from further surgical extirpation of the esophagus. We are currently unable to identify these groups of patients and must search for simple, reproducible, and validated surrogate markers predictive of treatment outcome. So far, only histopathologic tumor response after neoadjuvant therapy has emerged as a predictor of survival in esophageal cancer patients.[67] Surgical resection and evaluation of histopathologic tumor response will therefore continue to play a role in the treatment of esophageal cancer in upcoming years.

Studies have been published comparing preoperative chemotherapy versus preoperative chemoradiation. In a randomized trial of patients with adenocarcinoma of the EGJ, trimodality therapy had significantly higher pathologic complete response rates and higher probability of tumor-free lymph nodes compared to induction chemotherapy.[68] Additionally, trimodality patients had much higher survival at 3-years compared to induction chemotherapy patients (47.4% vs. 27.7%, $P = 0.07$). However, these results did not meet statistical significance due to poor accrual and early trial closure. A metaanalysis inclusive of 24 trials and 4188 patients focusing on survival after neoadjuvant chemotherapy or chemoradiotherapy for resectable esophageal carcinoma provided strong evidence for survival benefit of multimodality therapy versus surgery alone.[69] The results of this metaanalysis also suggested a reduction in mortality with trimodality therapy compared to induction chemotherapy, although this did not meet statistical significance (HR, 0.88; 95% CI, 0.76–1.01; $P = 0.07$).

Some authors have debated the value of surgery after bimodality therapy. Murphy and colleagues subsequently showed that surgical resection and tumor differentiation were the only independent predictors of survival in a retrospective analysis.[70]

Clearly, impeccable perioperative outcomes are necessary to demonstrate oncologic benefit of surgical therapy. Hence, one strategy is to use esophageal resection selectively, only in the setting of disease persistence or recurrence after definitive chemoradiation. This treatment paradigm was the focus of the RTOG 0246 phase 2 trial by Swisher and colleagues.[71] The study was designed to detect improvement in 1-year survival in patients undergoing selective or salvage esophagectomy. More than 70% of enrolled patients had T3 or N1 disease stage. Forty-one patients were included in the analysis and underwent chemoradiation. Subsequently, 21 (51%) underwent salvage esophagectomy because of residual or recurrent disease; one patient requested resection. Patients with complete clinical response after definitive chemoradiation had overall survival of 53%, with clinical incomplete response of 33% and clinical incomplete response salvaged by surgery of 41%. The estimated one-year survival was 71% and the study failed to achieve the prespecified 77.5% survival at one year. However, more recent studies suggest that salvage esophagectomy may confer survival that approaches planned trimodality therapy, albeit with higher postoperative morbidity and mortality.[72] Differences in outcomes appear to exist for whether salvage surgery is undertaken for persistent versus recurrent disease, likely reflecting tumor biology. The role of salvage esophagectomy after definitive chemoradiation may be a potentially feasible treatment strategy and prospective studies are needed to identity patients best suited for this approach.

Surveillance

Patients who have received definitive chemoradiation therapy (bimodality therapy) for esophageal cancer continue to suffer from the fear that the disease may reappear again either as locoregional or distant metastatic recurrence. The purpose behind the periodic surveillance of patients who completed definitive bimodality therapy is to potentially implement salvage therapy for locoregional failure. High-level evidence-based surveillance algorithms are not available. However, per NCCN guidelines and expert opinion, providers should consider observing patients every three to six months with clinical examination, endoscopy studies, and a variety of imaging studies (CT chest/abdomen ± PET).[31] This strategy is often costly and anxiety-provoking for patients, and it may not change the ultimate outcome for the patient. Considering the fact that more than 98% of local recurrences occur in the first 36 months, most authors suggest vigilant surveillance during this time after bimodality therapy to potentially catch recurrences early enough to render salvage surgery a feasible strategy.

Palliative Options for Esophageal Cancer

Patients with poor performance status or distant metastatic disease at the time of diagnosis are not candidates for aggressive locoregional therapy. The goal of treatment in these circumstances is either to palliate existing symptoms or potentially to avoid future complications related to the disease extent. Metastatic esophageal carcinoma may be manifested with a variety of symptoms, depending on the disease spread; however, dysphagia, odynophagia, chest pain, fatigue, and weight loss are likely to be among the most common symptoms. Palliative treatment is always individualized on the basis of a patient's physiologic status, symptoms, disease extent, and wishes. Options for palliation range from best supportive care for symptom control to the use of chemotherapy or radiation, esophageal stent placement, and enteral nutrition support. With advancements in image-guided percutaneous and endoscopic procedures, surgical procedures for palliation of esophageal carcinoma have become exceedingly rare. Recently, immunotherapy in the form of checkpoint inhibitors has been used in patients with advanced esophageal carcinoma and demonstrated promising results.[73] Further investigational use of immunotherapy is ongoing and may represent a novel treatment approach in patients with metastatic disease.

SUMMARY

Multimodality therapy using a combination of neoadjuvant chemotherapy typically with concurrent radiation followed by surgery is presently regarded as the standard of care for either locally advanced esophageal adenocarcinoma or SCC. Whereas some patients benefit from this aggressive locoregional treatment strategy, many patients continue to develop distant metastatic disease, which is presently incurable. As the search for molecular predictors and targeted therapies for this cancer continues, we will have to rigorously test novel agents to determine their places in the therapeutic armamentarium. Standardized perioperative care in well-designed clinical trials will be imperative so the potential therapeutic benefit of surgery is not offset by unacceptably high perioperative mortality rates. Minimally invasive and hybrid approaches to esophagectomy may further mitigate perioperative risk while preserving the oncologic benefits of surgical resection. The heterogeneity of esophageal cancer will require novel treatment strategies to personalize and improve upon treatment outcomes for future patients.

ANNOTATED REFERENCES

Gu Y, Swisher SG, Ajani JA, et al. The number of lymph nodes with metastasis predicts survival in patients with esophageal cancer or esophagogastric junction adenocarcinoma who receive preoperative chemoradiotherapy. *Cancer*. 2006;106:1017–1025.

This paper discusses the notion that, in addition to location and response to neoadjuvant therapy, the number of lymph nodes may be one of the most significant predictors of outcome.

Hulscher JB, van Sandick JW, de Boer AG, et al. Extended transthoracic resection compared with limited transhiatal resection for adenocarcinoma of the esophagus. *N Engl J Med*. 2002;347:1662–1669.

This randomized trial evaluated two different approaches for esophagectomy and demonstrated: (1) less morbidity with a transhiatal approach and (2) a trend towards improved long-term survival in the transthoracic group with en-bloc lymphadenectomy.

Kahrilas PJ, Bredenoord AJ, Fox M, et al. The Chicago classification of esophageal motility disorders, v3.0. *Neurogastroenterol Motil*. 2015;27:160–174.

The Chicago classification has provided a framework to understand and categorize esophageal motility disorders through the use of precise definitions involving high-resolution manometry.

Orringer MB, Sloan H. Esophagectomy without thoracotomy. *J Thorac Cardiovasc Surg*. 2002;76:643–654.

This landmark paper was the first to describe the transhiatal esophagectomy and to document the outcomes in detail.

Park W, Vaezi MF. Cause and pathogenesis of achalasia: the current understanding. *Am J Gastroenterol*. 2006;101:202–203.

This concise review of achalasia gives a thorough overview of the evolution of the cause and pathogenesis of this disease.

Shaheen NJ, Sharma P, Overholt BF, et al. Radiofrequency ablation in Barrett's esophagus with dysplasia. *N Engl J Med*. 2009;360:2277–2288.

This randomized trial demonstrated that endoscopic ablation of dysplastic Barrett esophagus not only could eradicate intestinal metaplasia, but also could significantly reduce the likelihood of disease progression and subsequent invasive cancer from developing.

van Hagen P, Hulshof MC, van Lanschot JJ, et al. Preoperative chemoradiotherapy for esophageal or junctional cancer. *N Engl J Med*. 2012;366:2074–2084.

This landmark randomized controlled study (Chemoradiotherapy for Oesophageal Cancer Following Surgical Study [CROSS] trial) is one of the most cited papers demonstrating a significant survival benefit from induction chemoradiotherapy prior to surgical resection.

Yammamoto S, Kawahara K, Maekawa T. Minimally invasive esophagectomy for stage I and II esophageal cancer. *Ann Thorac Surg*. 2005;80:2070–2075.

This is one of the largest series of esophageal cancer patients undergoing a minimally invasive procedure to treat early-stage disease. It has become an important study, suggesting that minimally invasive surgery may be a viable option in these patients.

REFERENCES

1. Kahrilas PJ, Bredenoord AJ, Fox M, et al. The Chicago classification of esophageal motility disorders, v3.0. *Neuro Gastroenterol Motil*. 2015;27:160–174.
2. Khashab MA, Messallam AA, Onimaru M, et al. International multicenter experience with peroral endoscopic myotomy for the treatment of spastic esophageal disorders refractory to medical therapy (with video). *Gastrointest Endosc*. 2015;81:1170–1177.
3. Boeckxstaens GE, Annese V, des Varannes SB, et al. Pneumatic dilation versus laparoscopic Heller's myotomy for idiopathic achalasia. *N Engl J Med*. 2011;364:1807–1816.
4. Bhayani NH, Kurian AA, Dunst CM, et al. A comparative study on comprehensive, objective outcomes of laparoscopic Heller myotomy with per-oral endoscopic myotomy (POEM) for achalasia. *Ann Surg*. 2014;259:1098–1103.
5. Hu JW, Li QL, Zhou PH, et al. Peroral endoscopic myotomy for advanced achalasia with sigmoid-shaped esophagus: long-term outcomes from a prospective, single-center study. *Surg Endosc*. 2015;29:2841–2850.
6. Ishaq S, Hassan C, Antonello A, et al. Flexible endoscopic treatment for Zenker's diverticulum: a systematic review and meta-analysis. *Gastrointest Endosc*. 2016;83:1076–1089. e1075.
7. Maret-Ouda J, Wahlin K, El-Serag HB, et al. Association between laparoscopic antireflux surgery and recurrence of gastroesophageal reflux. *JAMA*. 2017;318:939–946.
8. Ganz RA, Peters JH, Horgan S, et al. Esophageal sphincter device for gastroesophageal reflux disease. *N Engl J Med*. 2013;368:719–727.
9. Ganz RA, Edmundowicz SA, Taiganides PA, et al. Long-term outcomes of patients receiving a magnetic sphincter augmentation device for gastroesophageal reflux. *Clin Gastroenterol Hepatol*. 2016;14:671–677.
10. Riegler M, Schoppman SF, Bonavina L, et al. Magnetic sphincter augmentation and fundoplication for GERD in clinical practice: one-year results of a multicenter, prospective observational study. *Surg Endosc*. 2015;29:1123–1129.
11. Knight BC, Devitt PG, Watson DI, et al. Long-term efficacy of laparoscopic antireflux surgery on regression of Barrett's esophagus using BRAVO wireless pH monitoring: a prospective clinical cohort study. *Ann Surg*. 2017;266:1000–1005.
12. Shaheen NJ, Falk GW, Iyer PG, et al. ACG clinical guideline: diagnosis and management of Barrett's esophagus. *Am J Gastroenterol*. 2016;111:30.
13. Ali JT, Rice RD, David EA, et al. Perforated esophageal intervention focus (PERF) study: a multi-center examination of contemporary treatment. *Dis Esophagus*. 2017;30:1–8.
14. Markar SR, Mackenzie H, Wiggins T, et al. Management and outcomes of esophageal perforation: a national study of 2,564 patients in England. *Am J Gastroenterol*. 2015;110:1559–1566.
15. Abbas G, Schuchert MJ, Pettiford BL, et al. Contemporaneous management of esophageal perforation. *Surgery*. 2009;146:749–755; discussion 755–756.
16. Schweigert M, Sousa HS, Solymosi N, et al. Spotlight on esophageal perforation: a multinational study using the pittsburgh esophageal perforation severity scoring system. *J Thorac Cardiovasc Surg*. 2016;151:1002–1009.
17. Dasari BV, Neely D, Kennedy A, et al. The role of esophageal stents in the management of esophageal anastomotic leaks and benign esophageal perforations. *Ann Surg*. 2014;259:852–860.
18. Mennigen R, Senninger N, Laukoetter MG. Novel treatment options for perforations of the upper gastrointestinal tract: endoscopic vacuum therapy and over-the-scope clips. *World J Gastroenterol*. 2014;20:7767–7776.
19. Thumallapally N, Ibrahim U, Kesavan M, et al. Esophageal granular cell tumor: a case report and review of literature. *Cureus*. 2016;8:e782.
20. Wong MW, Bair MJ, Shih SC, et al. Using typical endoscopic features to diagnose esophageal squamous papilloma. *World J Gastroenterol*. 2016;22:2349–2356.
21. Murase K, Hino A, Ozeki Y, et al. Malignant schwannoma of the esophagus with lymph node metastasis: literature review of schwannoma of the esophagus. *J Gastroenterol*. 2001;36:772–777.
22. Tan Y, Lv L, Duan T, et al. Comparison between submucosal tunneling endoscopic resection and video-assisted thoracoscopic surgery for large esophageal leiomyoma originating from the muscularis propria layer. *Surg Endosc*. 2016;30:3121–3127.

23. Deng HY, Ni PZ, Wang YC, et al. Neuroendocrine carcinoma of the esophagus: clinical characteristics and prognostic evaluation of 49 cases with surgical resection. *J Thorac Dis*. 2016;8:1250–1256.
24. Mege D, Depypere L, Piessen G, et al. Surgical management of esophageal sarcoma: a multicenter European experience. *Dis Esophagus*. 2018;31:dox146.
25. Winant AJ, Gollub MJ, Shia J, et al. Imaging and clinicopathologic features of esophageal gastrointestinal stromal tumors. *AJR Am J Roentgenol*. 2014;203:306–314.
26. Lott S, Schmieder M, Mayer B, et al. Gastrointestinal stromal tumors of the esophagus: evaluation of a pooled case series regarding clinicopathological features and clinical outcome. *Am J Cancer Res*. 2015;5:333–343.
27. Bray F, Ferlay J, Soerjomataram I, et al. Global cancer statistics 2018: GLOBOCAN estimates of incidence and mortality worldwide for 36 cancers in 185 countries. *CA Cancer J Clin*. 2018;68:394–424.
28. Siegel RL, Miller KD, Jemal A. Cancer statistics, 2019. *CA Cancer J Clin*. 2019;69:7–34.
29. Pohl H, Welch HG. The role of overdiagnosis and reclassification in the marked increase of esophageal adenocarcinoma incidence. *J Natl Cancer Inst*. 2005;97:142–146.
30. Islami F, DeSantis CE, Jemal A. Incidence trends of esophageal and gastric cancer subtypes by race, ethnicity, and age in the United States, 1997-2014. *Clin Gastroenterol Hepatol*. 2018.
31. Esophageal and Esophagogastric Junction Cancers - Version 2.2018. *National Comprehensive Cancer Network - Clinical Practice Guidelines in Oncology*; 2018. www.nccn.org. Accessed December, 2018.
32. Rice TW, Ishwaran H, Ferguson MK, et al. Cancer of the esophagus and esophagogastric junction: an eighth edition staging primer. *J Thorac Oncol*. 2017;12:36–42.
33. Dhupar R, Rice RD, Correa AM, et al. Endoscopic ultrasound estimates for tumor depth at the gastroesophageal junction are inaccurate: implications for the liberal use of endoscopic resection. *Ann Thorac Surg*. 2015;100:1812–1816.
34. Hvid-Jensen F, Pedersen L, Drewes AM, et al. Incidence of adenocarcinoma among patients with Barrett's esophagus. *N Engl J Med*. 2011;365:1375–1383.
35. de Jonge PJ, van Blankenstein M, Looman CW, et al. Risk of malignant progression in patients with Barrett's oesophagus: a dutch nationwide cohort study. *Gut*. 2010;59:1030–1036.
36. Song J, Zhang J, Wang J, et al. Meta-analysis of the effects of endoscopy with narrow band imaging in detecting dysplasia in Barrett's esophagus. *Dis Esophagus*. 2015;28:560–566.
37. Canto MI, Anandasabapathy S, Brugge W, et al. In vivo endomicroscopy improves detection of Barrett's esophagus-related neoplasia: a multicenter international randomized controlled trial (with video). *Gastrointest Endosc*. 2014;79:211–221.
38. Shaheen NJ, Sharma P, Overholt BF, et al. Radiofrequency ablation in Barrett's esophagus with dysplasia. *N Engl J Med*. 2009;360:2277–2288.
39. Phoa KN, van Vilsteren FG, Weusten BL, et al. Radiofrequency ablation vs endoscopic surveillance for patients with Barrett esophagus and low-grade dysplasia: a randomized clinical trial. *JAMA*. 2014;311:1209–1217.
40. Wolf WA, Pasricha S, Cotton C, et al. Incidence of esophageal adenocarcinoma and causes of mortality after radiofrequency ablation of Barrett's esophagus. *Gastroenterology*. 2015;149:1752–1761. e1751.
41. Ghorbani S, Tsai FC, Greenwald BD, et al. Safety and efficacy of endoscopic spray cryotherapy for Barrett's dysplasia: results of the National Cryospray Registry. *Dis Esophagus*. 2016;29:241–247.
42. Ramay FH, Cui Q, Greenwald BD. Outcomes after liquid nitrogen spray cryotherapy in Barrett's esophagus-associated high-grade dysplasia and intramucosal adenocarcinoma: 5-year follow-up. *Gastrointest Endosc*. 2017;86:626–632.
43. Pech O, May A, Manner H, et al. Long-term efficacy and safety of endoscopic resection for patients with mucosal adenocarcinoma of the esophagus. *Gastroenterology*. 2014;146:652–660. e651.
44. Lee L, Ronellenfitsch U, Hofstetter WL, et al. Predicting lymph node metastases in early esophageal adenocarcinoma using a simple scoring system. *J Am Coll Surg*. 2013;217:191–199.
45. Manner H, Wetzka J, May A, et al. Early-stage adenocarcinoma of the esophagus with mid to deep submucosal invasion (pT1b sm2-3): the frequency of lymph-node metastasis depends on macroscopic and histological risk patterns. *Dis Esophagus*. 2017;30:1–11.
46. Gockel I, Sgourakis G, Lyros O, et al. Risk of lymph node metastasis in submucosal esophageal cancer: a review of surgically resected patients. *Expert Rev Gastroenterol Hepatol*. 2011;5:371–384.
47. Bahin FF, Jayanna M, Hourigan LF, et al. Long-term outcomes of a primary complete endoscopic resection strategy for short-segment Barrett's esophagus with high-grade dysplasia and/or early esophageal adenocarcinoma. *Gastrointest Endosc*. 2016;83:68–77.
48. Hirasawa K, Kokawa A, Oka H, et al. Superficial adenocarcinoma of the esophagogastric junction: long-term results of endoscopic submucosal dissection. *Gastrointest Endosc*. 2010;72:960–966.
49. Crabtree TD, Kosinski AS, Puri V, et al. Evaluation of the reliability of clinical staging of T2 N0 esophageal cancer: a review of the society of thoracic surgeons database. *Ann Thorac Surg*. 2013;96:382–390.
50. van Hagen P, Hulshof MC, van Lanschot JJ, et al. Preoperative chemoradiotherapy for esophageal or junctional cancer. *N Engl J Med*. 2012;366:2074–2084.
51. Speicher PJ, Ganapathi AM, Englum BR, et al. Induction therapy does not improve survival for clinical stage T2N0 esophageal cancer. *J Thorac Oncol*. 2014;9:1195–1201.
52. Semenkovich TR, Panni RZ, Hudson JL, et al. Comparative effectiveness of upfront esophagectomy versus induction chemoradiation in clinical stage T2N0 esophageal cancer: a decision analysis. *J Thorac Cardiovasc Surg*. 2018;155:2221–2230. e2221.
53. Hulscher JB, van Sandick JW, de Boer AG, et al. Extended transthoracic resection compared with limited transhiatal resection for adenocarcinoma of the esophagus. *N Engl J Med*. 2002;347:1662–1669.
54. Peyre CG, Hagen JA, DeMeester SR, et al. The number of lymph nodes removed predicts survival in esophageal cancer: an international study on the impact of extent of surgical resection. *Ann Surg*. 2008;248:549–556.
55. Yerokun BA, Sun Z, Yang CJ, et al. Minimally invasive versus open esophagectomy for esophageal cancer: a population-based analysis. *Ann Thorac Surg*. 2016;102:416–423.
56. Mariette C, Markar SR, Dabakuyo-Yonli TS, et al. Hybrid minimally invasive esophagectomy for esophageal cancer. *N Engl J Med*. 2019;380:152–162.

57. Raymond DP, Seder CW, Wright CD, et al. Predictors of major morbidity or mortality after resection for esophageal cancer: a society of thoracic surgeons general thoracic surgery database risk adjustment model. *Ann Thorac Surg.* 2016;102:207–214.
58. Shewale JB, Correa AM, Baker CM, et al. Impact of a fast-track esophagectomy protocol on esophageal cancer patient outcomes and hospital charges. *Ann Surg.* 2015;261:1114–1123.
59. Anderegg MC, Lagarde SM, Jagadesham VP, et al. Prognostic significance of the location of lymph node metastases in patients with adenocarcinoma of the distal esophagus or gastroesophageal junction. *Ann Surg.* 2016;264:847–853.
60. Cools-Lartigue J, Spicer J, Ferri LE. Current status of management of malignant disease: current management of esophageal cancer. *J Gastrointest Surg.* 2015;19:964–972.
61. Roth JA, Pass HI, Flanagan MM, et al. Randomized clinical trial of preoperative and postoperative adjuvant chemotherapy with cisplatin, vindesine, and bleomycin for carcinoma of the esophagus. *J Thorac Cardiovasc Surg.* 1988;96:242–248.
62. Medical Research Council Oesophageal Cancer Working G. Surgical resection with or without preoperative chemotherapy in oesophageal cancer: a randomised controlled trial. *Lancet.* 2002;359:1727–1733.
63. Cunningham D, Allum WH, Stenning SP, et al. Perioperative chemotherapy versus surgery alone for resectable gastroesophageal cancer. *N Engl J Med.* 2006;355:11–20.
64. Ando N, Kato H, Igaki H, et al. A randomized trial comparing postoperative adjuvant chemotherapy with cisplatin and 5-fluorouracil versus preoperative chemotherapy for localized advanced squamous cell carcinoma of the thoracic esophagus (JCOG9907). *Ann Surg Oncol.* 2012;19:68–74.
65. Minsky BD, Pajak TF, Ginsberg RJ, et al. INT 0123 (Radiation Therapy Oncology Group 94-05) phase III trial of combined-modality therapy for esophageal cancer: high-dose versus standard-dose radiation therapy. *J Clin Oncol.* 2002;20:1167–1174.
66. Shapiro J, van Lanschot JJB, Hulshof M, et al. Neoadjuvant chemoradiotherapy plus surgery versus surgery alone for oesophageal or junctional cancer (CROSS): long-term results of a randomised controlled trial. *Lancet Oncol.* 2015;16:1090–1098.
67. Davies AR, Gossage JA, Zylstra J, et al. Tumor stage after neoadjuvant chemotherapy determines survival after surgery for adenocarcinoma of the esophagus and esophagogastric junction. *J Clin Oncol.* 2014;32:2983–2990.
68. Stahl M, Stuschke M, Lehmann N, et al. Chemoradiation with and without surgery in patients with locally advanced squamous cell carcinoma of the esophagus. *J Clin Oncol.* 2005;23:2310–2317.
69. Sjoquist KM, Burmeister BH, Smithers BM, et al. Survival after neoadjuvant chemotherapy or chemoradiotherapy for resectable oesophageal carcinoma: an updated meta-analysis. *Lancet Oncol.* 2011;12:681–692.
70. Murphy CC, Correa AM, Ajani JA, et al. Surgery is an essential component of multimodality therapy for patients with locally advanced esophageal adenocarcinoma. *J Gastrointest Surg.* 2013;17:1359–1369.
71. Swisher SG, Winter KA, Komaki RU, et al. A phase II study of a paclitaxel-based chemoradiation regimen with selective surgical salvage for resectable locoregionally advanced esophageal cancer: initial reporting of RTOG 0246. *Int J Radiat Oncol Biol Phys.* 2012;82:1967–1972.
72. Markar S, Gronnier C, Duhamel A, et al. Salvage surgery after chemoradiotherapy in the management of esophageal cancer: is it a viable therapeutic option? *J Clin Oncol.* 2015;33:3866–3873.
73. Shah MA, Kojima T, Hochhauser D, et al. Efficacy and safety of pembrolizumab for heavily pretreated patients with advanced, metastatic adenocarcinoma or squamous cell carcinoma of the esophagus: the Phase 2 KEYNOTE-180 Study. *JAMA Oncol.* 2018.

43 CHAPTER

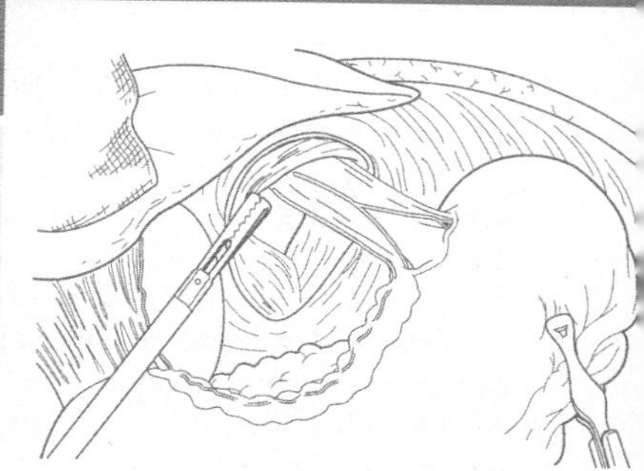

Gastroesophageal Reflux Disease and Hiatal Hernia

Robert B. Yates, Brant K. Oelschlager

OUTLINE

Please access Elsevier eBooks for Practicing Clinicians to view the videos for this chapter https://expertconsult.inkling.com/.

Gastroesophageal reflux disease (GERD) is the most common benign medical condition of the stomach and esophagus. In patients with GERD who experience persistent life-limiting symptoms despite maximal medical therapy, antireflux surgery should be strongly considered. The application of laparoscopy to antireflux surgery has decreased perioperative morbidity, hospital length of stay, and cost compared with open operations. Conceptually, laparoscopic antireflux surgery (LARS) is straightforward; however, the correct construction of a fundoplication requires significant operative experience and skills in complex laparoscopy. In patients who present with late complications of antireflux surgery, including recurrent GERD and dysphagia, reoperative antireflux surgery can be effectively performed. Compared with first-time operations, however, reoperative antireflux surgery is technically more challenging, is associated with higher risk of perioperative complications, and results in less durable symptom improvement. Consequently, surgeons should have a higher threshold for performing reoperative antireflux surgery, and reoperations should be performed by experienced, high-volume gastroesophageal surgeons. To decrease perioperative risk and to maximize long-term relief of GERD symptoms, surgeons must be familiar with all aspects of preoperative evaluation and operative management of patients with GERD.

Hernias at the esophageal hiatus span the spectrum from a small sliding hiatal hernia to a large paraesophageal hernia (PEH). Similarly, the symptoms of PEH can vary from mild GERD and gastroesophageal obstructive symptoms to severe, acute complications, including gastric volvulus, which requires immediate evaluation by a surgeon. The repair of a large PEH is challenging, but when it is performed at high-volume centers by experienced surgeons, hiatal hernia and PEH can be repaired safely and provide patients with long-lasting control of gastroesophageal symptoms.

Technologic advancements in the surgical management of benign gastroesophageal disease include the application of robotic assisted laparoscopic surgery and the use of magnetic sphincter augmentation devices (MSADs) at the lower esophageal sphincter (LES). These options hold promise for further advancement of the care of patients with these conditions; however, they do not supplant the need for comprehensive understanding of these disease processes, perioperative patient management, and technical expertise in operative correction of these conditions.

GASTROESOPHAGEAL REFLUX DISEASE

Pathophysiology

Endogenous antireflux mechanisms include the LES and spontaneous esophageal clearance. GERD results from the failure of these endogenous antireflux mechanisms.

The LES has the primary role of preventing reflux of gastric contents into the esophagus. Rather than a distinct anatomic structure, the LES is a zone of high pressure located in the lower end of the esophagus. The LES can be identified with esophageal manometry.

The LES is made up of four anatomic structures:

1. The *intrinsic musculature of the distal esophagus* is in a state of tonic contraction. Within 500 milliseconds of the initiation of a swallow, these muscle fibers relax to allow passage of liquid or food into the stomach, and then they return to a state of tonic contraction.
2. *Sling fibers of the gastric cardia* are oriented diagonally from the cardia-fundus junction to the lesser curve of the stomach. Located at the same anatomic depth as the circular muscle fibers of the esophagus, the sling fibers contribute significantly to the high-pressure zone of the LES (Fig. 43.1).
3. The *crura of the diaphragm* surround the esophagus as it passes through the esophageal hiatus. During inspiration, intrathoracic pressure decreases relative to intra abdominal pressure, favoring the movement of intra abdominal gastric contents into the esophagus located in the posterior mediastinum of the thorax. To counteract this pressure differential during inspiration,

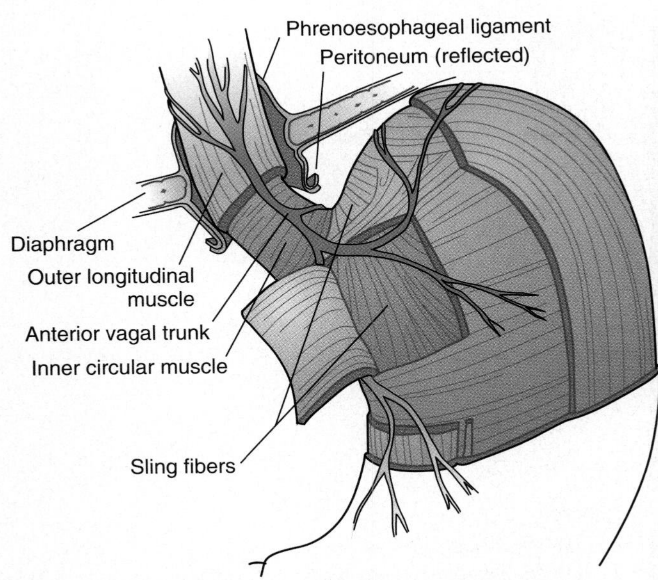

FIG. 43.1 Schematic drawing of the muscle layers at the gastroesophageal junction. The intrinsic muscle of the esophagus, diaphragm, and sling fibers contribute to lower esophageal sphincter pressure. The circular muscle fibers of the esophagus are at the same depth as the sling fibers of the cardia.

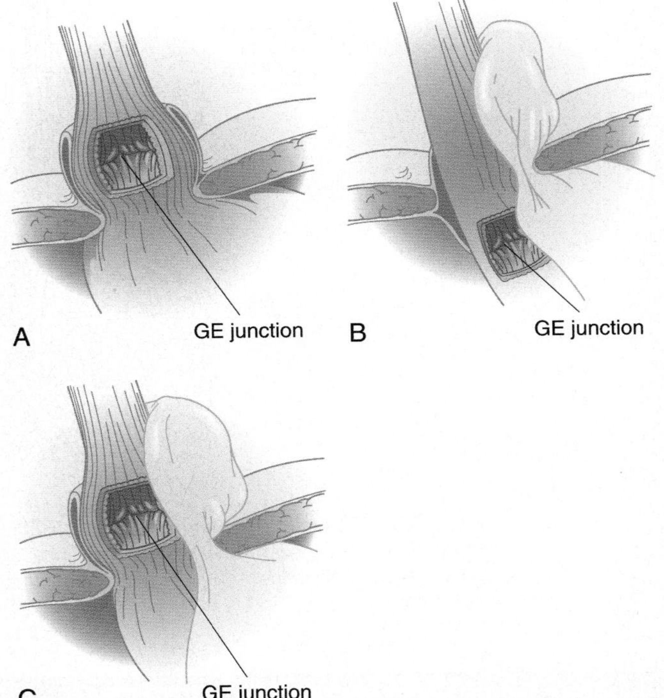

FIG. 43.2 The three types of hiatal hernia. (A) Type I is also called a sliding hernia. (B) Type II is known as a rolling hernia. (C) Type III is referred to as a mixed hernia. *GE*, Gastroesophageal.

the anteroposterior diameter of the crural opening is decreased, compressing the esophagus and increasing the measured pressure at the LES. Because of this fluctuation in LES pressure, it is important to measure the LES pressure at mid-expiration or end-expiration.

4. When the gastroesophageal junction (GEJ) is firmly anchored in the abdominal cavity, *increased intra abdominal pressure* is transmitted to the GEJ, which increases the pressure on the distal esophagus and prevents spontaneous reflux of gastric contents.

Gastroesophageal reflux (GER) occurs when intragastric pressure is greater than the high-pressure zone of the distal esophagus. This can develop under two conditions: the LES resting pressure is too low (i.e., hypotensive LES) and the LES with normal resting pressure inappropriately relaxes in the absence of peristaltic contraction of the esophagus (i.e., spontaneous LES relaxation). Hypotensive LES is frequently associated with hiatal hernia because of displacement of the GEJ into the posterior mediastinum. However, hypotensive LES can occur in its normal anatomic position, and even small changes in this high-pressure zone can compromise its effectiveness.

Not all GER is pathologic—in fact, it is a normal physiologic process that occurs even in the setting of a normal LES. Physiologic GER provides us the ability to rapidly evacuate swallowed air from the stomach that would otherwise cause unwanted bloating and flatus. The distinction between physiologic reflux (i.e., GER) and pathologic reflux (i.e., GERD) hinges on the total amount of esophageal acid exposure, the patient's symptoms, and the presence of mucosal damage of the esophagus.

Hiatal hernias are often associated with GERD because their abnormal anatomy compromises the efficacy of the LES. Hiatal hernias are classified into four types (I to IV). Type I hiatal hernia (Fig. 43.2A), also called a sliding hiatal hernia, is the most common. A type I hernia is present when the GEJ migrates cephalad into the posterior mediastinum. This occurs because of laxity of the phrenoesophageal membrane, a continuation of the endoabdominal peritoneum that reflects onto the esophagus at the hiatus (Fig. 43.3). A small sliding hernia does not necessarily imply an incompetent LES, but the larger its size, the greater the risk for abnormal GER. Furthermore, the presence of a type I sliding hiatal hernia alone does not constitute an indication for operative repair. In fact, many patients with small type I hiatal hernias do not have symptoms and do not require treatment.

Hiatal hernia types II to IV, also referred to as PEH, are frequently associated with gastroesophageal obstructive symptoms (e.g., dysphagia, early satiety, and epigastric pain). However, they can also be associated with GERD. A type II hernia (Fig. 43.2B) occurs when the GEJ is anchored in the abdomen, and the gastric fundus migrates into the mediastinum through the hiatal defect. A type III hernia (Fig. 43.2C) is characterized by both the GEJ and fundus located in the mediastinum. Finally, a type IV hernia occurs when the stomach and any other visceral structure (e.g., colon, spleen, pancreas, or small bowel) migrates cephalad to the esophageal hiatus and into the mediastinum. For more information on PEH, refer to the last section of this chapter.

Clinical Presentation

Typica Symptoms of GERD

The prevalence of symptoms among 1000 patients with GERD is presented in Table 43.1. Heartburn, regurgitation, and water brash are the three typical esophageal symptoms of GERD. Heartburn and regurgitation are the most common presenting symptoms. Heartburn is specific to GERD and described as an epigastric or retrosternal caustic or stinging sensation. Typically, it does not radiate to the back and is not described as a pressure sensation, which are more characteristic of pancreatitis and acute coronary syndrome, respectively. It is important to ask the patient about

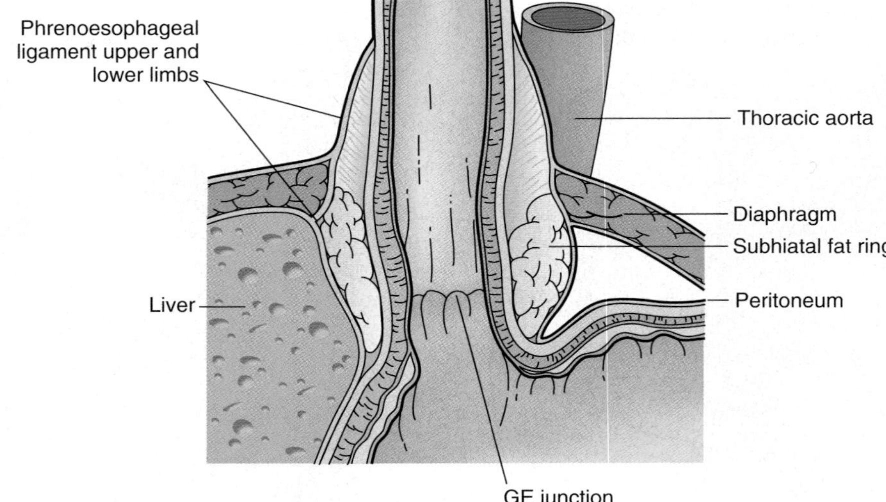

FIG. 43.3 Section of the gastroesophageal *(GE)* junction demonstrates the relationship of the peritoneum to the phrenoesophageal membrane. The phrenoesophageal membrane continues as a separate structure into the posterior mediastinum. The parietal peritoneum continues as the visceral peritoneum as it reflects onto the stomach.

TABLE 43.1 Prevalence of symptoms occurring more frequently than once per week in 1000 patients with gastroesophageal reflux disease.

SYMPTOM	PREVALENCE (%)
Heartburn	80
Regurgitation	54
Abdominal pain	29
Cough	27
Dysphagia for solids	23
Hoarseness	21
Belching	15
Bloating	15
Aspiration	14
Wheezing	7
Globus	4

BOX 43.1 Extraesophageal symptoms of gastroesophageal reflux disease.

Laryngeal Symptoms of Reflux
Hoarseness or dysphonia
Throat clearing
Throat pain
Globus
Choking
Postnasal drip
Laryngeal and tracheal stenosis
Laryngospasm
Contact ulcers

Pulmonary Symptoms of Reflux
Cough
Shortness of breath
Wheezing
Pulmonary disease (asthma, idiopathic pulmonary fibrosis, chronic bronchitis, and others)

his or her symptoms in detail to differentiate typical heartburn from symptoms of peptic ulcer disease, cholelithiasis, or coronary artery disease.

The presence of regurgitation often indicates progression of GERD. In severe cases, patients will be unable to bend over or lie supine without experiencing an episode of regurgitation. Regurgitation of gastric contents to the oropharynx and mouth can produce a sour taste that patients will describe as either acid or bile. This phenomenon is referred to as water brash. In patients who report regurgitation as a frequent symptom, it is important to distinguish between regurgitation of undigested food and regurgitation of digested food. Regurgitation of undigested food is not common in GERD and suggests the presence of a different pathologic process, such as an esophageal diverticulum or achalasia.

Extraesophageal Symptoms of GERD

Extraesophageal symptoms of GERD arise from the respiratory tract and include both laryngeal and pulmonary symptoms (Box 43.1). Two mechanisms may lead to extraesophageal symptoms of GERD. First, proximal esophageal reflux and microaspiration of gastroduodenal contents cause direct caustic injury to the larynx and lower respiratory tract; this is the most common mechanism. Second, distal esophageal acid exposure triggers a vagal nerve reflex that results in bronchospasm and cough. The latter mechanism is due to the common vagal innervation of the trachea and esophagus.

Unlike typical GERD symptoms (i.e., heartburn and regurgitation), extraesophageal symptoms of reflux are not specific to GERD. Before LARS is considered for a patient with primarily extraesophageal symptoms, it is necessary to determine whether those symptoms are due to abnormal GER or a primary laryngeal, bronchial, or pulmonary cause. This can be challenging. A lack of response of extraesophageal symptoms to proton pump inhibitor (PPI) therapy cannot reliably refute GERD as the cause of these symptoms.

Although PPI therapy can improve or completely resolve *typical* GERD symptoms, patients with *extraesophageal symptoms* experience variable response to medical treatment. This may be explained by recent evidence suggesting that acid is not the only underlying caustic agent resulting in laryngeal and pulmonary injury.[1] PPI therapy will suppress gastric acid production, but microaspiration of nonacid refluxate, which contains caustic bile salts and pepsin, can cause ongoing injury and symptoms. Therefore, in patients with extraesophageal symptoms of GERD, a mechanical barrier to reflux (i.e., esophagogastric fundoplication) may be necessary to prevent ongoing laryngeal, tracheal, or bronchial injury.

In patients who present with abnormal GER and bothersome extraesophageal symptoms, a thorough evaluation must be completed to rule out a primary disorder of the upper or lower respiratory tract. This should be completed whether or not typical GERD symptoms are also present. At the University of Washington Center for Esophageal and Gastric Surgery, we frequently refer patients with GERD and extraesophageal symptoms to a laryngologist or a pulmonologist to determine if a nongastrointestinal condition is causing these symptoms. If a nonreflux cause of the extraesophageal symptoms cannot be identified, then proceeding with an antireflux operation is acceptable. We counsel these patients a 70% likelihood of improvement in extraesophageal symptoms after LARS.[2] If a patient's laryngeal or pulmonary symptoms are not due to abnormal GER, an antireflux operation is not performed.

Pulmonary Disease, GERD, and Antireflux Surgery

Increasing evidence suggests that GERD is a contributing factor to the pathophysiologic mechanism of several pulmonary diseases. In their extensive review, Bowrey and colleagues[3] examined medical and surgical antireflux therapy in patients with GERD and asthma. In these patients, the use of antisecretory medications is associated with improved respiratory symptoms in only 25% to 50% of patients with GERD-induced asthma. Furthermore, less than 15% of these patients experience objective improvement in pulmonary function. One explanation for these results is that most of these studies lasted 3 months or less, which is potentially too short to see any improvement in pulmonary function. In addition, in several trials, gastric acid secretion was incompletely blocked by acid suppression therapy, and patients experienced ongoing GERD.

In patients with asthma and GERD, antireflux surgery appears to be more effective than medical therapy at managing pulmonary symptoms. Antireflux surgery is associated with improvement in respiratory symptoms in nearly 90% of children and 70% of adults with asthma and GERD. Several randomized trials have compared histamine 2 receptor antagonists and antireflux surgery in the management of GERD-associated asthma. Compared with patients treated with antisecretory medications, patients treated with antireflux surgery were more likely to experience relief of asthma symptoms, to discontinue systemic steroid therapy, and to improve peak expiratory flow rate.

Idiopathic pulmonary fibrosis (IPF) is a severe, chronic, and progressive lung disease that generally results in death within 5 years of diagnosis. Proximal esophageal reflux with microaspiration of acid and nonacid gastric contents has been implicated as one possible cause of alveolar epithelial injury that can lead to IPF. The incidence of GERD in patients with IPF has been reported to be as high as 94%.[4] Because typical symptoms of GERD are not sensitive for abnormal reflux in patients with IPF, the threshold for testing patients with IPF for GERD should be low.

Medical treatment of GERD in patients with IPF is associated with longer survival and slower pulmonary decline.[5] Whereas this is promising, PPI therapy does not prevent reflux of nonacid gastroduodenal contents, which may contribute to ongoing pulmonary injury in some patients. Therefore, in IPF patients with significant GERD, the argument can be made that a mechanical barrier to both acid and nonacid reflux (i.e., LARS) is more appropriate than PPI therapy. Although very little literature exists on LARS in patients with IPF, it appears to be safe and to provide effective control of distal esophageal acid exposure, and it may mitigate decline in pulmonary function.[6]

Laparoscopic antireflux surgery for the treatment of idiopathic pulmonary fibrosis (WRAP-IPF) is a multicenter controlled phase 2 trial and the only randomized study comparing LARS to PPI therapy in patients with IPF and GERD confirmed by 24-hour pH probe.[7] Of 72 eligible patients, 58 were equally randomized into surgery and no surgery groups (29 each group). The primary endpoint was change in forced vital capacity (FVC) at 48 weeks of treatment. Even in this patient population with severe systemic disease, LARS was deemed generally safe and well tolerated. Intention-to-treat analysis failed to show a difference between the two groups for FVC at 48 weeks ($P = 0.28$), which was the primary endpoint. However, a more nuanced analysis of the data is necessary. The surgery group had one death and the no surgery group had four deaths, and all deaths were preceded by acute IPF exacerbation. The specified statistical analytic method assumes that any missing data (those from patients who died during the trial) is random. However, given that these deaths appeared directly due to progression of the underlying pulmonary disease, this missing data did not appear random. Consequently, a post hoc analysis was performed using an approach to this data (Lachin's worst-rank analysis) that assumes missing data are not random and may be informative to the outcome of the study. Performing the analysis with this approach revealed a significant difference in FVC decline ($P = 0.017$) that favored the LARS group. Furthermore, the surgery group showed less pulmonary disease progression as measured by 10% FVC decline, acute exacerbation, or death ($P = 0.048$). Taken together, these results suggest that LARS may still play an important role in the mitigation of pulmonary decline in IPF patients with GERD. The failure to show a statistically significant difference in the intention to treat analysis may have resulted from an underpowered study, inappropriate choice of statistical analytic tool, or placing too much emphasis on decline of FVC. Future efforts to elucidate the role of LARS in IPF should take these considerations into account during study design and analysis.

Physical Examination

Except in patients with severely advanced disease, the physical examination rarely contributes to confirmation of the diagnosis of GERD. In such patients, several observations may suggest the presence of GERD. For example, a patient who constantly drinks water during the interview may be facilitating esophageal clearance, which can suggest frequent reflux. Other patients with advanced disease will sit leaning forward and carry out the interview with their lungs inflated to almost vital capacity. This maneuver flattens the diaphragm, narrows the anteroposterior diameter of the hiatus, and increases the LES pressure to counteract GER. Patients who have severe proximal esophageal reflux and regurgitation of gastric contents into the mouth may develop erosion of their dentition (revealing yellow teeth caused by the loss of dentin), injected oropharyngeal mucosa, or signs of chronic sinusitis.

Although physical examination findings are generally not specific for GERD, the physical examination may be helpful in determining the presence of other disease processes. For example, supraclavicular lymphadenopathy in a patient with heartburn and dysphagia may suggest esophageal or gastric cancer. Similarly, if the patient's retrosternal pain is reproducible with palpation, a musculoskeletal source of the pain should be investigated. Short of these extreme presentations, the physical examination is generally not helpful in confirming or excluding GER as a pathologic entity.

Preoperative Diagnostic Testing

Frequently, the diagnosis of GERD is based on the presence of typical symptoms and improvement in those symptoms with PPI therapy. However, when a surgeon evaluates a patient for antireflux surgery, four diagnostic tests are useful to establish the diagnosis of GERD and to identify abnormalities in gastroesophageal anatomy and function that may have an impact on the performance of LARS.

Ambulatory pH and Impedance Monitoring

Ambulatory pH monitoring quantifies distal esophageal acid exposure and is the "gold standard" test to diagnose GERD. A 24-hour pH monitoring is conducted with a thin catheter that is passed into the esophagus through the patient's nares. The simplest catheter is a dual-probe pH catheter, which contains two solid-state electrodes that are spaced 10 cm apart and detect fluctuations in pH between 2 and 7. To ensure valid study results, the distal electrode must be placed 5 cm proximal to the LES; the location of the LES is identified on esophageal manometry (see next section). Alternatively, 48-hour ambulatory pH monitoring can be performed using an endoscopically placed wireless pH monitor.

Ambulatory pH monitoring generates a large amount of data concerning esophageal acid exposure, including total number of reflux episodes (pH <4), longest episode of reflux, number of episodes lasting longer than 5 minutes, and percentage of time spent in reflux in the upright and supine positions. A formula assigns each of these data points a relative weight according to its capacity to cause esophageal injury, and the composite DeMeester score is calculated. Abnormal distal esophageal acid exposure is defined by a DeMeester score of 14.7 or higher.

In addition to these objective data, the patient can keep track of reflux-related symptoms by pressing a button on an electronic data recorder. During the interpretation of the pH study, symptom index and symptom-associated probability are calculated on the basis of the temporal relationship between the symptom event and episodes of distal esophageal acid exposure (Fig. 43.4). A symptom episode that occurs within 2 minutes of a reflux episode is defined as a close temporal relationship and suggests, but does not confirm, a cause and effect relationship between GER and the patient's symptoms. When interpreting these studies, it should be remembered that patients often do not maintain their normal activities and eating patterns when they have the catheter in place. Consequently, their symptoms may not be as prevalent during the study period. Whereas the decision to perform LARS should not hinge on symptom correlation, it can help predict symptom improvement after LARS.[8]

Esophageal impedance monitoring identifies episodes of nonacid reflux. Similar to 24-hour pH monitoring, esophageal impedance is performed with a thin, flexible catheter placed through the patient's nares into the esophagus. Impedance catheters use electrodes placed at 1-cm intervals to detect changes in the resistance to flow of an electrical current (i.e., impedance). Impedance increases in the presence of air and decreases in the presence of a liquid bolus. Therefore, this technology can detect both gas and liquid movement in the esophagus.

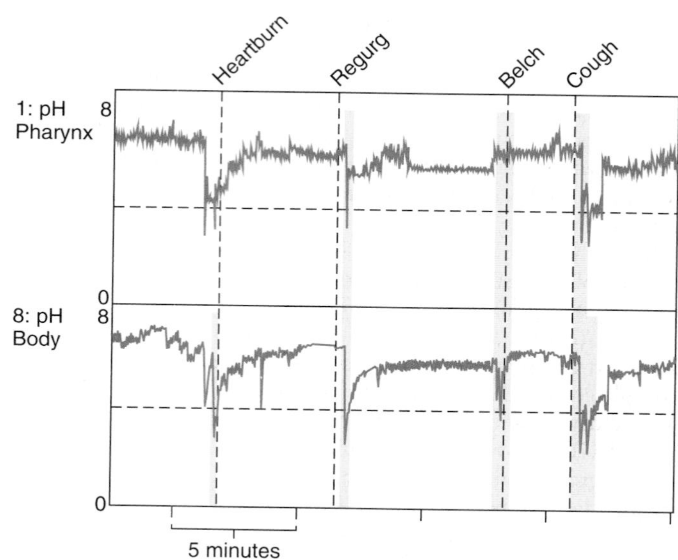

FIG. 43.4 A 1-hour segment from a 24-hour ambulatory pH study. Time is marked on the x-axis, and pH is marked on the y-axis. Symptom events are marked along the top of the tracing. (Courtesy University of Washington Center for Esophageal and Gastric Surgery, Seattle.)

Some impedance catheters also have one or more pH sensors, allowing the simultaneous detection of acid and nonacid reflux. When pH-impedance catheters are used, it is possible to determine the direction of movement of esophageal acid exposures and therefore to differentiate between an antegrade event (as in a swallow) and a retrograde event (as in GER). There also exists a specialized pH-impedance catheter with a very proximal pH sensor that detects pharyngeal acid reflux. This catheter can be useful in the evaluation of patients with extraesophageal symptoms, such as cough, throat clearing, hoarseness, and wheezing. One disadvantage of impedance technology, however, is that the automated analytic software is very sensitive and tends to overestimate the number of nonacid reflux episodes, mandating that these studies be manually reviewed and edited, which can be time-consuming.

Combined impedance-pH monitoring has been shown to identify reflux episodes with greater sensitivity than pH testing alone.[9] Although there is no consensus on whether impedance-pH testing should be performed on or off acid-suppression therapy, our practice is to perform all pH and impedance-pH testing off acid suppression. Furthermore, how impedance-pH monitoring should guide the management of GERD is unknown. Patel and colleagues[10] attempted to determine the parameters on esophageal impedance-pH monitoring that predict response of GERD symptoms to both medical and surgical treatment. They showed that acid exposure time, and not the number of nonacid reflux events, best predicted symptom improvement with both medical and surgical therapy. Although the addition of impedance monitoring increased the sensitivity of the study, nonacid reflux measurements alone were unable to accurately predict symptom response to medical or surgical therapy for GERD.

Esophageal Manometry

Esophageal manometry is the most effective way to assess function of the esophageal body and the LES. Standard esophageal manometry provides linear tracings of pressure waves of the esophageal body and LES (Fig. 43.5). High-resolution esophageal manometry gathers data using a 32-channel flexible catheter with pressure-sensing devices arranged at 1-cm intervals, placed into the esophagus through the nares; the study is conducted in approximately 15 minutes, during which time the patient performs 10 swallows. A color-contour plot is generated and shows the response of the upper esophageal sphincter and LES as well as of the esophageal body; time is on the x-axis, esophageal length is on the y-axis, and pressure is represented by a color scale (Fig. 43.6). In patients undergoing evaluation for GERD, esophageal manometry can exclude achalasia and identify patients with ineffective esophageal body peristalsis. Repeated exposure of the esophagus to gastric reflux can lead to esophageal motility disorders; in one study, 25% of patients with mild esophagitis demonstrated esophageal dysmotility, whereas 48% of patients with severe esophagitis had impaired motility on manometry.[11] In patients with significant esophageal dysmotility who are undergoing LARS, the surgeon should consider a partial fundoplication to decrease the likelihood of postoperative dysphagia. A full discussion of the implications of esophageal dysmotility on the type of fundoplication is presented in a later section of this chapter. Esophageal manometry also measures the LES resting pressure and assesses the LES for appropriate relaxation with deglutition. Because the LES is the major barrier to GER, a defective LES is common in patients with GERD.

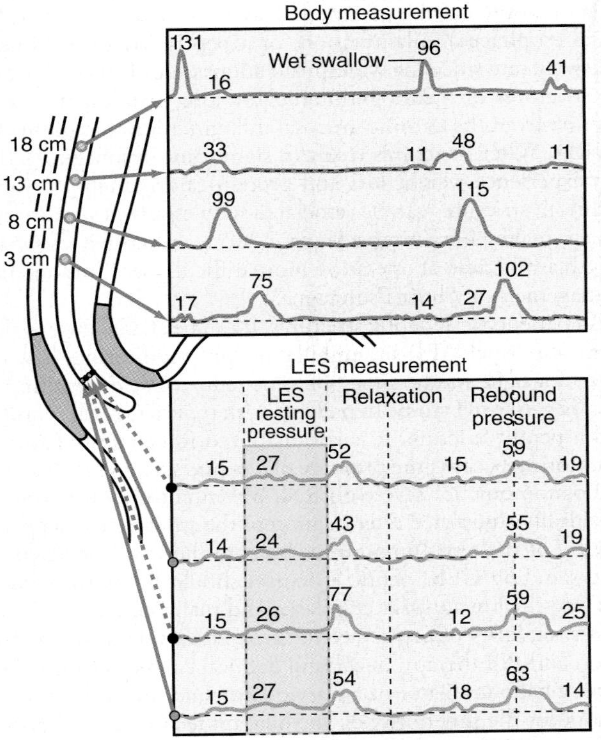

FIG. 43.5 Representative linear tracings from standard esophageal manometry. A wet swallow initiates both esophageal peristalsis and lower esophageal sphincter *(LES)* relaxation.

Esophagogastroduodenoscopy

Endoscopy is an essential step in the evaluation of patients with GERD who are being considered for LARS. The esophagus should be examined for evidence of mucosal injury due to GER, including ulcerations, peptic strictures, and Barrett esophagus. Esophagitis can be reported according to several scoring systems, including the Savary-Miller and Los Angeles (LA) classifications.[12] Both peptic strictures and LA class C and D esophagitis can be considered pathognomonic for GERD. Consequently, ambulatory pH monitoring is unnecessary in these patients. However, because of significant interobserver variability in LA class A and B esophagitis, these forms of mild esophagitis cannot be considered reliable markers of GERD.[13] As such, patients found to have LA class A and B esophagitis should undergo pH testing to confirm abnormal distal esophageal acid exposure.

Endoscopic evaluation should also include an assessment of the GEJ flap valve. To do this, the endoscope is retroflexed 180 degrees in the stomach to visualize the GEJ from below. The flap valve is graded 1 to 4, according to the length of the valve and how tightly it adheres to the endoscope. The endoscopist should make note of the presence of a hiatal hernia, and the hernia should be measured in both cranial-caudal and lateral dimensions. In patients who are being evaluated for persistent or recurrent gastroesophageal symptoms after an antireflux operation or PEH repair, it is recommended that the surgeon who is evaluating the patient perform

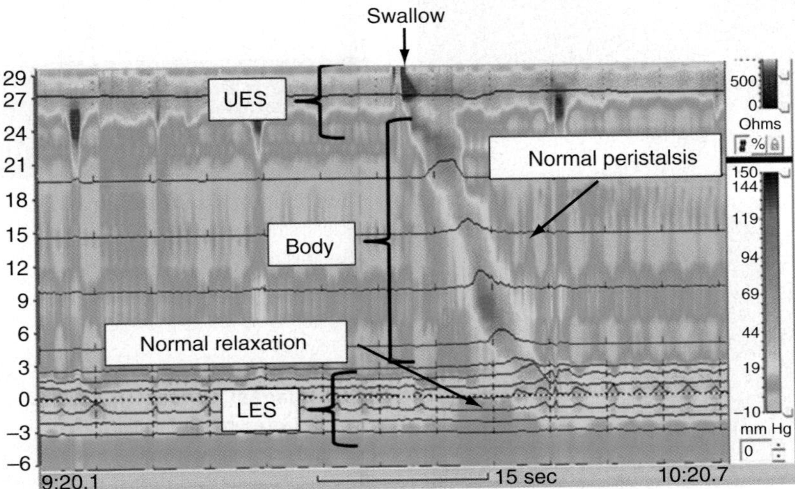

FIG. 43.6 High-resolution esophageal manometry. The initiation of a swallow is associated with simultaneous relaxation of the upper esophageal sphincter *(UES)* and lower esophageal sphincter *(LES)* and onset of peristalsis in the esophageal body.

the endoscopy. This allows the operating surgeon to correlate endoscopic findings with the patient's symptoms and data obtained on 24-hour pH monitoring, esophageal manometry, and upper gastrointestinal (UGI) series to determine if a functional or anatomic abnormality exists that can be corrected with reoperation.

Barium Esophagram

Barium esophagram provides a detailed anatomic evaluation of the esophagus and stomach that is useful during preoperative evaluation of patients with GERD. Of particular importance are the presence, size, and anatomic characteristics of a hiatal hernia or PEH (Fig. 43.7). For example, a GEJ that is fixed in the posterior mediastinum on esophagography can suggest a more difficult operation that may require a more extensive intrathoracic esophageal mobilization. Despite its ability to identify episodes of GER, which can occur spontaneously or in response to positioning of the patient during the study, barium esophagram cannot confirm or refute the diagnosis of GERD. On occasion, patients presenting to the surgical clinic for evaluation of GERD may have already undergone computed tomography scan of the chest or abdomen to evaluate atypical symptoms of GERD (e.g., chest or abdominal pain). Horizontal images as well as coronal and sagittal reconstructions can provide information concerning the anatomic relationship of the stomach and esophagus to other abdominal and thoracic structures. However, we still prefer to obtain a barium esophagram as computed tomography scan frequently fails to identify important anatomic and functional gastroesophageal disease.

Additional gastroesophageal conditions that can be identified on barium esophagram are esophageal diverticula, tumors, peptic strictures, achalasia, dysmotility, and gastroparesis. If any one of these is found in a patient undergoing evaluation for GERD, LARS should be delayed until appropriate evaluation of the unexpected findings is completed.

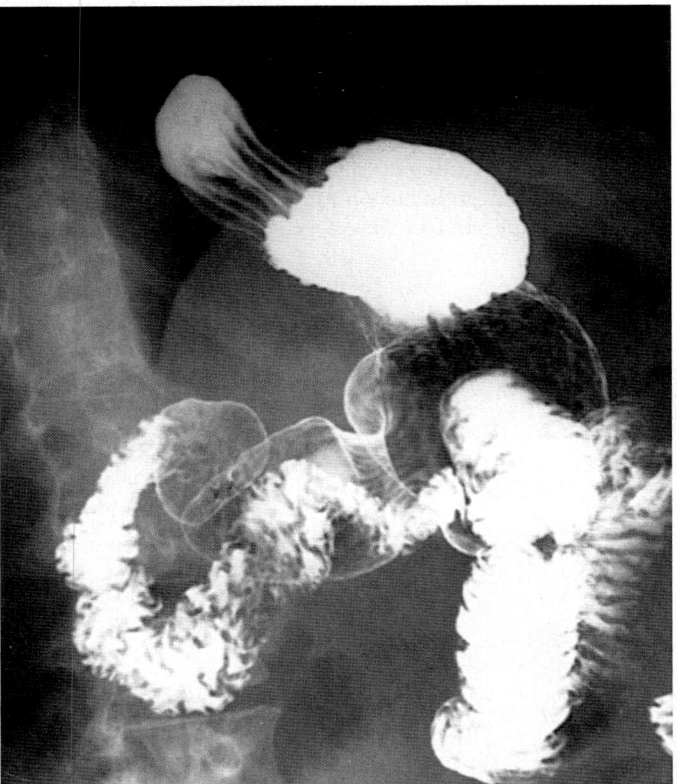

FIG. 43.7 Upper gastrointestinal series demonstrating a large hiatal hernia. The rugal folds of the stomach clearly transgress the shadow of the left hemidiaphragm.

Additional Preoperative Considerations

Dysphagia

Patients with GERD will occasionally experience dysphagia. The causes of dysphagia are listed in Box 43.2. In patients with GERD, the most common cause of dysphagia is a reflux-associated inflammatory process of the esophageal wall. This inflammation can be manifested as a Schatzki ring, a diffuse distal esophageal inflammation, or a peptic stricture. Although relatively rare since the widespread adoption of PPI therapy, peptic strictures are pathognomonic for long-standing reflux and develop from the chronic mucosal inflammation that occurs with GERD. When strictures result in significant dysphagia, patients can experience weight loss and protein-calorie malnutrition. In addition, strictures can be associated with esophageal shortening, which makes obtaining adequate intra abdominal esophageal length at the time of operation more difficult (see "Intraoperative Management of Short Esophagus").

In patients with peptic strictures, it can be challenging to document abnormal GER on ambulatory pH monitoring. The presence of a tight stricture may prevent reflux of acid, resulting in a false-negative pH study. In patients with typical GERD symptoms and a peptic stricture, it is reasonable to forego ambulatory pH monitoring because the presence of a peptic stricture is considered pathognomonic for severe GER. If pH monitoring is performed, it is ideally completed after dilation of the stricture to increase the validity of the test. Importantly, because they are associated with long-standing GER, peptic strictures should be biopsied to rule out intestinal metaplasia, dysplasia, and malignancy.

The majority of peptic strictures are effectively treated with dilation and PPI therapy. Successful dilation can be performed with either a balloon dilator or Savary dilator, and no strong data exist to support the superiority of one dilation technique over another. Refractory peptic strictures are defined as strictures that recur despite dilation and PPI therapy. Although rare, refractory strictures can pose a significant challenge to surgeons and gastroenterologists. In these patients, LARS should strongly be considered. For patients who are unfit for or do not wish to undergo an operation,

BOX 43.2 Potential causes of dysphagia in patients undergoing evaluation for gastroesophageal reflux disease.

Esophageal Obstruction
Peptic strictures
Schatzki ring
Malignant neoplasm
Benign neoplasm
Foreign body

Esophageal Motility Disorders
Ineffective esophageal motility
Diffuse esophageal spasm
Hypercontractile ("Jackhammer") esophagus
Fragmented peristalsis
Achalasia

steroid injections of the stricture have been shown to result in fewer dilations.[14]

Another cause of dysphagia in patients with GERD is a Schatzki ring. Similar to peptic strictures, these are located in the distal esophagus. However, Schatzki rings are submucosal fibrotic bands (as opposed to mucosal strictures). Typically, peptic strictures and Schatzki rings can be differentiated on endoscopy. Both should be dilated to relieve obstruction, but Schatzki rings develop in the submucosal space, so in the absence of other endoscopically identified mucosal abnormalities, biopsies do not need to be performed. Furthermore, Schatzki rings are not pathognomonic for GERD, so abnormal distal esophageal acid exposure must be documented on ambulatory pH monitoring to confirm the presence of abnormal GER before LARS is performed.

Dysphagia in patients with GERD may not have a clear anatomic cause, and mild dysphagia in these patients may simply be due to the esophageal inflammation that results from persistent GER. This type of dysphagia tends to resolve after abnormal reflux is controlled. In patients who present with dysphagia and GERD, other causes of dysphagia must be excluded, including tumors, diverticula, and esophageal motor disorders. Although these conditions are much less common than peptic stricture and Schatzki ring, they require dramatically different treatments. In patients who report simultaneous onset of dysphagia to liquids and solids, one must have a high suspicion for a neuromuscular or autoimmune disorder as the etiology. Finally, some patients with severe GERD experience dysphagia without exhibiting an anatomic or physiologic abnormality of the esophagus. This is believed to be caused by inflammation associated with reflux, and we have found that such patients typically experience improvement in dysphagia after LARS.

Obesity

GERD is a common comorbid condition with obesity. Compared with patients of normal weight, obese patients have several factors that place them at increased risk for GERD, including increased intra abdominal pressure, decreased LES pressure, impaired esophageal body peristalsis, and more frequent transient LES relaxations. Importantly, in obese patients, symptom assessment alone is inadequate to determine the presence of GERD. Up to 45% of patients undergoing assessment for bariatric surgery have evidence of silent (asymptomatic) reflux.[15] Obese patients with GERD recalcitrant to medical therapy present a challenge to surgeons. Whereas it is clear that LARS can be performed safely in obese patients, the literature is mixed on the ability of LARS to provide long-term control of GERD-related symptoms. In appropriately selected patients, laparoscopic Roux-en-Y gastric bypass (RYGB) is a durable method of weight loss, controls obesity-related comorbidities, and provides durable improvement in GERD. RYGB is extremely effective treatment for GERD for two reasons: first, it excludes the vast majority of acid-producing parietal cells from continuity with the esophagus; and second, the long Roux limb prevents reflux of nonacid duodenal contents into the esophagus. For these reasons, in severely obese patients with GERD, serious consideration should be given to performing a laparoscopic RYGB instead of a fundoplication; however, the decision to pursue gastric bypass instead of fundoplication must include a careful balance of the patient's interest in bariatric surgery, the presence of other medical comorbidities, and the availability of a surgeon to perform the operation. Fundoplication in patients with a body mass index (BMI) above 40 should rarely be considered.

Ineffective Esophageal Motility

Ineffective esophageal motility is defined by the Chicago Classification of Esophageal Motility Disorders v3.0 as at least 50% weak or failed peristaltic swallows on high-resolution manometry.[16] In patients with GERD and ineffective esophageal motility, it has been suggested that partial (Toupet or Dor) fundoplication should be performed out of concern that a Nissen fundoplication will lead to greater postoperative dysphagia. Despite randomized clinical trials[14,15] and two meta analyses,[16,17] there still remains conflicting evidence about the fundoplication that provides the most durable control of reflux and the best side-effect profile. This is likely due to the heterogeneity of these studies related to patient characteristics, patient selection, and operative technique. Currently, the only consistent finding in these studies is that anterior fundoplication provides less durable control of GERD than posterior partial and total fundoplication. Total fundoplication results in more dysphagia in the first year. Beyond 1 year, the incidence of dysphagia is similar between the two techniques. The same trend seems to occur with bloating, belching, and bothersome flatus. It also appears that GERD control in the long run (5 years and beyond) favors total fundoplication. Taken together, the trade-off appears to be increased incidence of short-term side effects versus superior long-term control of GERD symptoms. The point at which the esophageal motility is poor enough for changing from a total to partial fundoplication is still the judgment of the surgeon, although almost all surgeons do a partial fundoplication when esophageal motility demonstrates absence of esophageal body contractility (100% failed swallows).

Barrett Esophagus

Long-standing acid and alkaline reflux can result in histologic change of the distal esophageal mucosa from its normal squamous epithelium to a columnar configuration. This histologic alteration is called intestinal metaplasia or Barrett esophagus. On endoscopic evaluation, Barrett esophagus appears as velvety-red "tongues" of mucosa that extend cephalad from the GEJ. Based on endoscopic measurements, it can be classified into long segment (≥3 cm) and short segment (<3 cm). If Barrett esophagus is suspected on the basis of endoscopic appearance of the esophageal mucosa, multiple biopsy specimens should be taken to histologically evaluate for intestinal metaplasia and the presence of dysplasia. When dysplasia is present, there is an increased risk for development of adenocarcinoma. Although the incidence of adenocarcinoma in patients with Barrett esophagus is about 40 times greater than that in the general population, the overall incidence of cancer in these patients is still very low.

Because Barrett esophagus is the result of repeated injury of the mucosa due to GER, it would be expected that antireflux surgery should result in resolution of intestinal metaplasia. However, in our experience at the University of Washington and in another study,[18] regression of intestinal metaplasia following antireflux surgery occurred in just over 50% of patients. One of the reasons for these variable results may relate to the durability of the antireflux operation. Knight and colleagues[19] evaluated 50 patients with a preoperative diagnosis of Barrett esophagus at a mean of nearly 12 years following LARS. Endoscopic regression of Barrett esophagus was found in 32 (64%) of patients, and histologic regression of Barrett esophagus was found in 20 (40%) of patients. Compared to patients without regression in Barrett esophagus, patients with either endoscopic or pathologic regression were found to have reduced distal esophageal acid exposure on 48-hour BRAVO pH evaluation. Furthermore, patients without Barrett regression at follow-up had higher incidence of hiatal hernia and endoscopic evidence of absent fundoplication, both of which may contribute to GER and esophageal injury.

Because of the variability in regression in Barrett esophagus following antireflux surgery, it should not be considered an indication for antireflux surgery. Further, it is important to continue endoscopic surveillance postoperatively according to the accepted guidelines.

Treatment of GERD

Medical Management

For patients who present with typical symptoms of GERD, an 8-week course of PPI therapy is recommended.[20] However, before empirically prescribing a PPI, it is necessary to ensure that the patient does not have symptoms that may indicate the presence of a gastroesophageal malignant neoplasm or other non-GERD diagnosis, including rapidly progressive dysphagia, regurgitation of undigested food, anemia, extraesophageal symptoms of GERD, and weight loss. If the symptoms improve with PPI therapy, the trial is considered both diagnostic and therapeutic. If the symptoms persist after a trial of medical therapy, a more extensive evaluation, as described earlier, is indicated. Although lifestyle modification has been advocated before or as an adjunct to medical therapy, the efficacy of such changes in the treatment of esophagitis has not been proved.[21]

PPIs have revolutionized the pharmacologic treatment of GERD. As one of the most widely prescribed drugs worldwide, the annual expenditure on PPI therapy has reached approximately $24 billion.[19] These drugs stop gastric acid production by irreversibly binding the proton pump in the parietal cells of the stomach. The maximal pharmacologic effect occurs approximately 4 days after initiation of therapy, and the effect lasts for the life of the parietal cell. For this reason, patients must stop PPI therapy 1 week before ambulatory pH monitoring to avoid a false-negative test result.

PPIs are well-tolerated medications. Immediate side effects of PPI therapy are relatively rare and generally mild, including headache, abdominal pain, flatulence, constipation, and diarrhea. This relatively safe side-effect profile and their effectiveness at controlling GERD symptoms have led to overprescription of these medications in both the outpatient and inpatient settings.[22] Although there are published evidence-based recommendations that might limit this practice of overprescription, including on-demand dosing and step-down therapy, clinicians frequently do not follow these guidelines.

Despite their short-term safety, several recent studies using very large patient data sets have generated concern about the long-term effects of PPI use.[23] Specifically, PPI use has been associated with the following: loss of bone density and risk of fracture, dementia, myocardial infarction, micronutrient (magnesium, iron, B-12) deficiencies, *Clostridioides difficile* infection, kidney disease, and interactions with antiplatelet medications. These findings have garnered attention of patients and the media, and frequently, clinicians engage in lengthy and nuanced discussions with patients regarding the potential risks of PPI use. However, careful assessment of the quality of these studies demonstrates most are low or very low (according to the GRADE system), and the number of patients needed to harm is high. In the case of *Clostridioides difficile* infection, for example, a systematic review of 51 studies found that the overall relative risk of infection in the setting of PPI use was increased to 1.51 and the number needed to harm was 3935.[24] In comparison, the number needed to harm for patients completing a 2-week course of antibiotics was 50. While broad sweeps of these data sets have identified statistically significant associations, these associations do not equate to causation, and confounding explanations may exist. For example, patients prescribed PPI therapy have more comorbid conditions than the general population. The most applicable take-away from this literature is that while PPIs are generally safe, no therapy is without risk, and judicious prescription of PPIs for well-established indications is prudent.

Surgical Management

For patients who exhibit elevated distal esophageal acid exposure and persistent typical GERD symptoms despite maximal medical therapy, antireflux surgery should be strongly considered. The application of laparoscopy to antireflux surgery has decreased patient morbidity and hospital length of stay, and several studies have shown that LARS is cost-effective compared with prolonged PPI therapy.[12]

Operative Technique

We perform all laparoscopic antireflux operations with the patient in low lithotomy position. This provides the surgeon improved ergonomics by standing between the patient's legs; the assistant stands at the patient's left. In addition, the patient is placed in steep reverse Trendelenburg position, which allows improved visualization of the esophageal hiatus. The patient is appropriately padded to prevent pressure ulcers and neuropathies. Preoperative antibiotics are administered to reduce the risk of surgical site infection, and subcutaneous heparin and sequential compression devices are used to reduce the risk of venous thromboembolic events.

Access to the abdomen is obtained with a Veress needle at Palmer point in the left upper quadrant of the abdomen. Three additional trocars are placed. The surgeon operates through the two most cephalad ports, and the assistant operates through the two caudad ports. A Nathanson liver retractor does not require a trocar and is placed through a small epigastric incision (Fig. 43.8).

We begin our dissection at the left crus by dividing the phrenogastric membrane and then enter the lesser sac at the level of the inferior edge of the spleen. This allows early ligation of the short

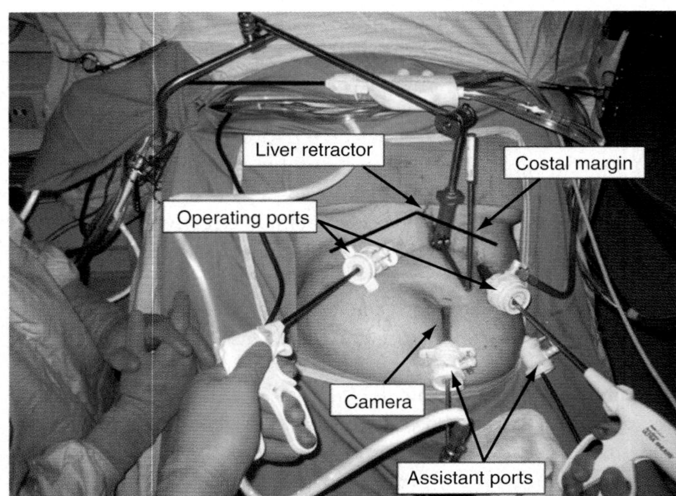

FIG. 43.8 Port placement for laparoscopic antireflux surgery. The surgeon operates through the two cephalad ports, and the assistant operates through the two caudad ports.

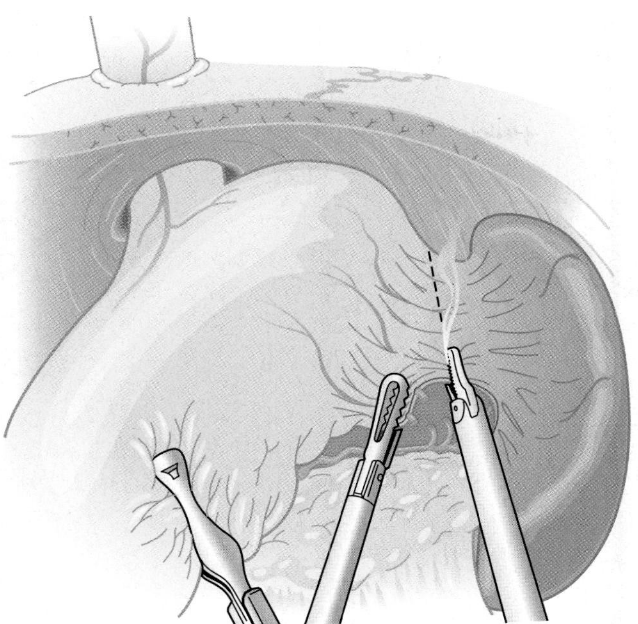

FIG. 43.9 In the left crus approach to the esophageal hiatus, the fundus of the stomach is mobilized early during the operation to provide early visualization of the spleen, which helps prevent splenic injury.

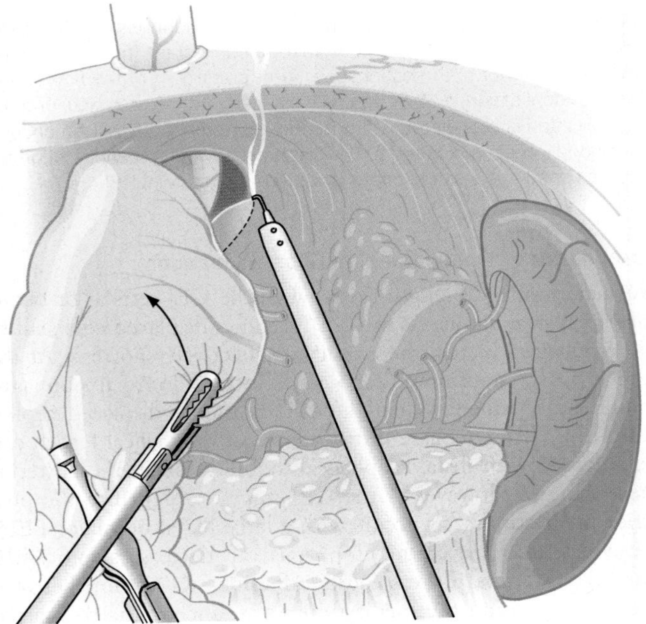

FIG. 43.10 After the fundus has been mobilized, the phrenoesophageal membrane is incised at the left crus, with care taken to avoid injury to the esophagus, posterior vagus nerve, and aorta.

gastric vessels and mobilization of the gastric fundus (Fig. 43.9). After the fundus is mobilized, the phrenoesophageal membrane is divided to expose the entire length of the left crus (Fig. 43.10).

Right crural dissection is then performed. The gastrohepatic ligament is divided, and the right phrenoesophageal membrane is opened to expose the right crus (Fig. 43.11). A retroesophageal window is created. Care is taken to preserve the anterior and posterior vagus nerves during this mobilization. A Penrose drain is placed around the esophagus to facilitate the posterior mediastinal dissection and to assist with the creation of the fundoplication.

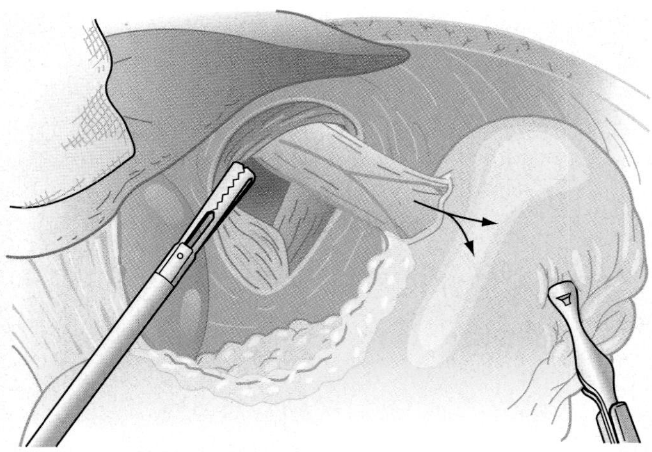

FIG. 43.11 The phrenoesophageal membrane is incised at the right crus to complete the exposure of the hiatus. Performing the dissection immediately adjacent to the crura decreases the likelihood of injury to adjacent structures.

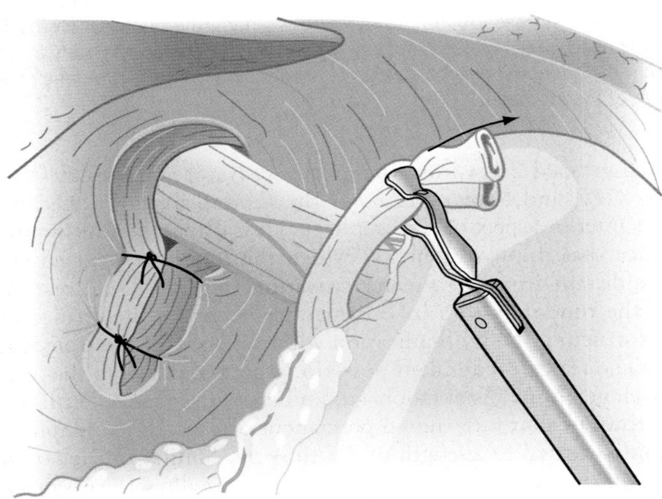

FIG. 43.12 Posterior crural closure is performed with heavy permanent suture. Note how the peritoneum overlying the crura is incorporated into the closure. The exposure is facilitated by displacement of the esophagus anteriorly and to the left.

The esophagus is mobilized in the posterior mediastinum to obtain a minimum of 3 cm of intra abdominal esophagus. Then, the crura are approximated posteriorly with permanent sutures (Fig. 43.12). The esophagus should maintain a straight orientation without angulation, and a 52-Fr bougie should easily pass beyond the esophageal hiatus and into the stomach. At this point, the fundoplication is created.

Creation of a 360-Degree Fundoplication

The most common technical failure in performing a Nissen fundoplication is failure to create appropriate fundoplication anatomy. The description that follows clearly explains our method of performing a correct, effective, and reproducible Nissen fundoplication. To maintain appropriate orientation of the fundus during the creation of the fundoplication, the posterior aspect of the fundus is marked with a suture 3 cm distal to the GEJ and 2 cm off the greater curvature (Fig. 43.13). The posterior fundus is then passed behind the esophagus from the patient's left to right. The anterior fundus on the left side of the esophagus is

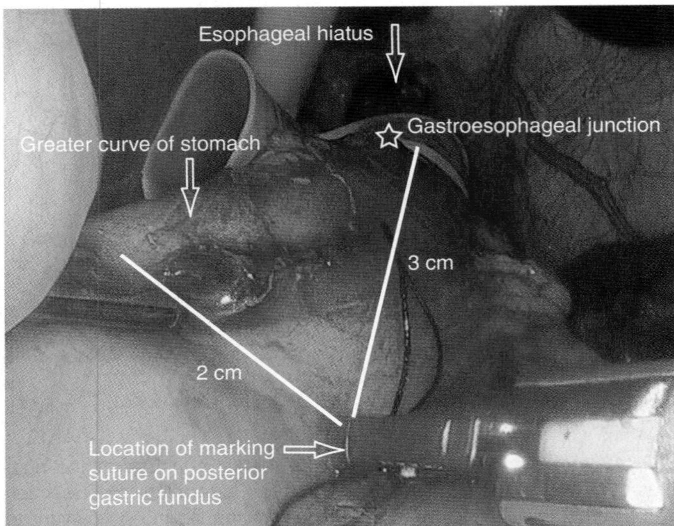

FIG. 43.13 A posterior gastric marking suture is helpful to ensure proper geometric configuration of the fundoplication. With the greater curvature of the stomach rotated to the patient's right, the posterior stomach is exposed, and a marking stitch is placed on the posterior fundus 3 cm from the gastroesophageal junction (☆) and 2 cm from the greater curvature of the stomach.

then grasped 2 cm from the greater curvature and 3 cm from the GEJ, and both portions of the fundus are positioned on the anterior aspect of the esophagus. It is of paramount importance that the two points at which the fundus is grasped are equidistant from the greater curvature (Fig. 43.14). Creation of the fundoplication in this manner decreases the chance of constructing the fundoplication with the body of the stomach, which creates a redundant posterior aspect of the wrap that can impinge on the distal esophagus and cause dysphagia. With use of three or four interrupted permanent sutures, the fundoplication is created to a length of 2.5 to 3 cm. Similar to the crural repair, the completed fundoplication should allow the easy passage of a 52 Fr bougie. After removal of the bougie, the wrap is anchored to the esophagus and crura (Fig. 43.14, inset) to help prevent herniation into the mediastinum and slipping of the fundoplication over the body of the stomach. The suture line of the fundoplication should lie parallel to the right anterior aspect of the esophagus.

Creation of a Partial Fundoplication

There are several types of partial fundoplications. The most commonly performed is the Toupet fundoplication. In this operation, the gastric and esophageal dissections as well as the repair of the crura are the same as for a 360-degree fundoplication. In addition, the fundoplication must be created with the fundus, not the body, of the stomach. The key difference is that the stomach is wrapped 180 to 270 degrees (compared with 360 degrees) around the posterior aspect of the esophagus (Fig. 43.15A and C). On both sides of the esophagus, the most cephalad sutures of the fundoplication incorporate the fundus, crus, and esophagus; the remaining sutures anchor the fundus to either the crura or the esophagus.

If an anterior fundoplication is to be performed (e.g., Thal or Dor), there is no need to disrupt the posterior attachments of the esophagus, and the fundus is folded over the anterior aspect of the esophagus and anchored to the hiatus and esophagus (Fig. 43.15B).

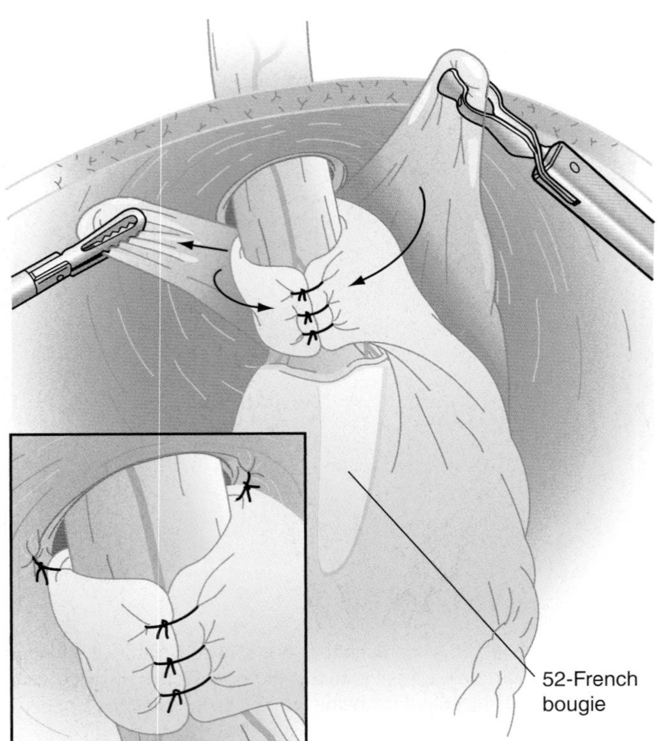

FIG. 43.14 Creation of a 360-degree Nissen fundoplication. The anterior and posterior fundus must be grasped equidistant from the greater curvature posterior to the esophagus. After placement of the first suture of the fundoplication, a 52 Fr bougie is passed into the stomach, and the fundoplication is completed. With the bougie removed from the patient, the fundoplication is secured to the diaphragm with right and left coronal sutures (*inset*) and a single posterior suture (not shown).

Intraoperative Management of Short Esophagus

Normal esophageal length exists when the GEJ rests at or below the esophageal hiatus. As the GEJ becomes displaced cephalad to the esophageal hiatus, the esophagus effectively shortens. At the time of LARS, a minimum of 3 cm of intra abdominal esophagus should be obtained. When the GEJ is mildly displaced cephalad to the GEJ, adequate intra abdominal esophageal length can be obtained with distal esophageal mobilization in the posterior mediastinum. However, if the GEJ migrates high into the posterior mediastinum, as occurs with a large hiatal hernia or PEH, the effective length of the esophagus can decrease significantly. Furthermore, this process causes adhesions to develop between the esophagus and the mediastinum that anchor the contracted esophagus in the chest. When this occurs, extensive mobilization of the esophagus must be undertaken, sometimes to the level of the inferior pulmonary veins. Even in the case of a large hiatal hernia or PEH, in most patients, mediastinal dissection alone can return the GEJ to the abdominal cavity.

In some cases, despite extensive mediastinal mobilization of the esophagus, intra abdominal esophageal length still appears inadequate. In these rare cases, a unilateral vagotomy can result in an additional 1 to 2 cm of esophageal length, and division of both vagus nerves typically yields 3 to 4 cm of additional esophagus. Many surgeons hesitate to electively transect the vagus nerves because of concern for the development of postoperative delayed gastric emptying. However, we have shown this not to be the case. In our study of 102 patients who underwent reoperative LARS

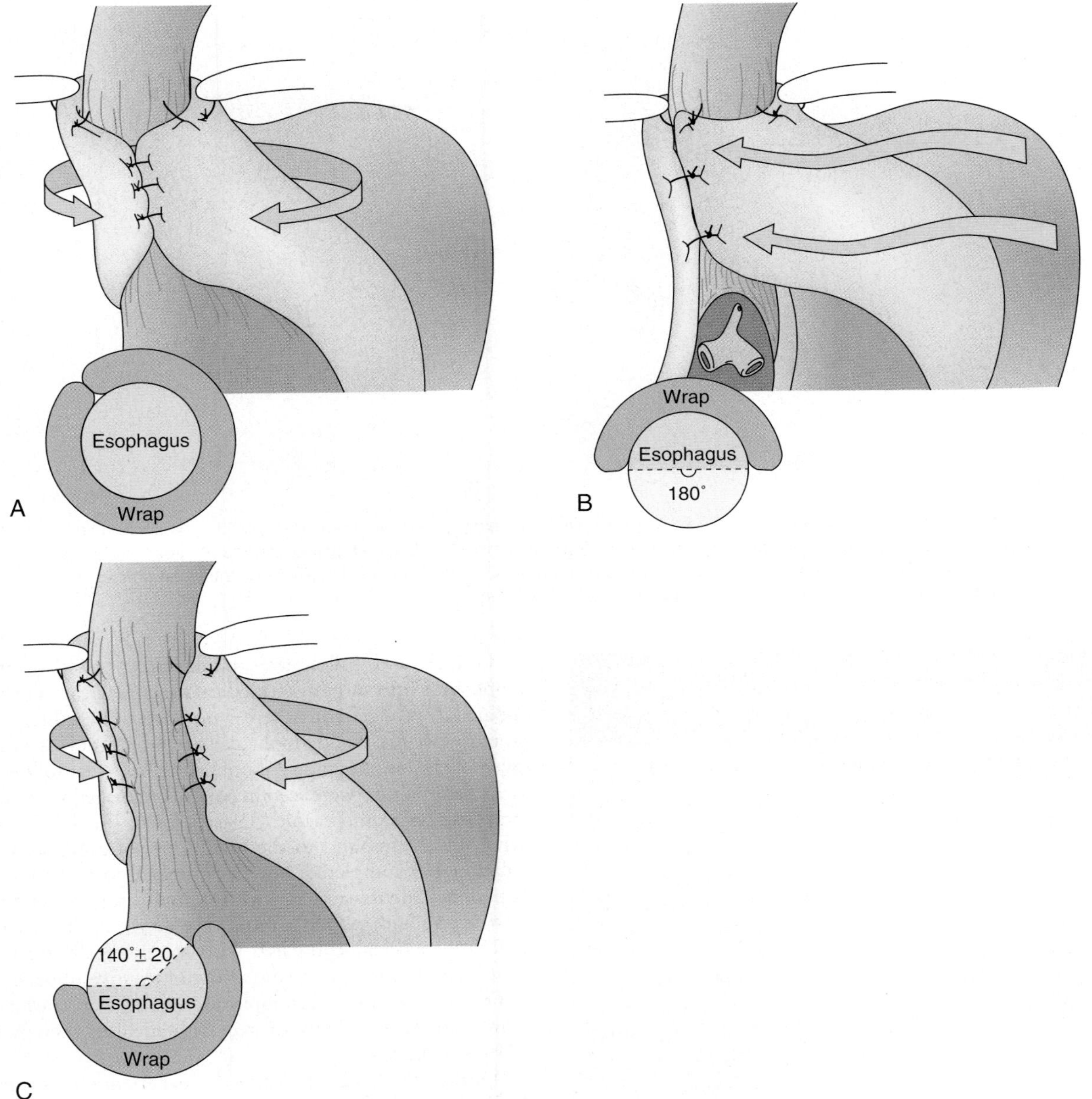

FIG. 43.15 Three types of fundoplication. (A) A 360-degree fundoplication. (B) Partial anterior fundoplication. (C) Partial posterior fundoplication.

(n = 50) or PEH repair (n = 52), we performed a vagotomy in 30 patients (29%) to increase intra abdominal esophageal length after extensive mediastinal mobilization.[25] Compared with patients who did not undergo vagotomy, patients who underwent vagotomy reported similar severity of abdominal pain, bloating, diarrhea, and early satiety.

The other option for achieving adequate intra abdominal esophageal length is a stapled wedge gastroplasty (Fig. 43.16). Since the widespread adoption of laparoscopy in the management of GERD and PEH, wedge gastroplasty has generally supplanted the traditional Collis gastroplasty that used a double-staple technique (circular and linear stapler). It should be noted, however, that the aforementioned techniques of esophageal lengthening (posterior mediastinal mobilization of the esophagus and, if necessary, vagotomy) achieve adequate intraabdominal esophageal length in all but a very small number of patients. Therefore, stapled wedge gastroplasty is reserved for use only in patients in whom these other techniques fail to achieve adequate intraabdominal esophageal length.

Postoperative Care and Recovery

Except when the patient's comorbid medical conditions dictate otherwise, patients are admitted postoperatively to a general surgical ward without cardiac or pulmonary monitoring. Patients are given a clear liquid diet the evening of the operation and are advanced to a full liquid diet on postoperative day 1. Discharge requirements include tolerance of a diet to maintain hydration and nutrition, adequate pain control with oral analgesics, and ability to void without a Foley catheter. After discharge from the hospital, patients can slowly introduce soft foods into their diet, and they should expect to resume a diet without limitations in about 4 to 6 weeks.

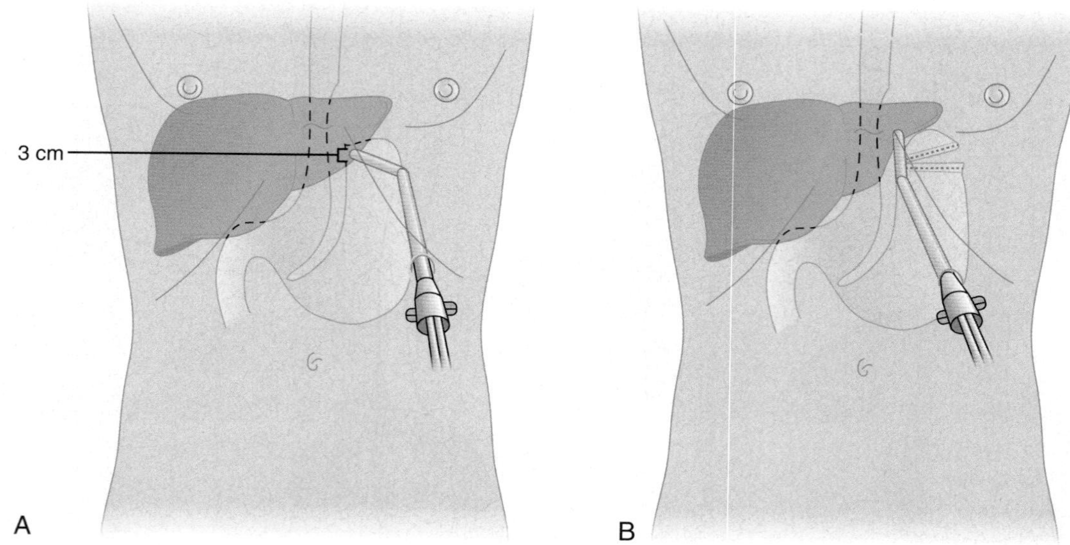

FIG. 43.16 Laparoscopic stapled wedge gastroplasty for esophageal lengthening. (A) With a 48-Fr bougie placed beyond the gastroesophageal junction and into the stomach, a linear stapler is used to transect the fundus perpendicular to the bougie approximately 3 to 4 cm distal to the angle of His. (B) A second linear stapler is used to resect the portion of gastric fundus parallel to the bougie.

TABLE 43.2 Randomized controlled trials comparing surgical and medical therapies for gastroesophageal reflux disease.

STUDY	STUDY GROUPS	FOLLOW-UP	OUTCOME
Anvari, 2011	PPI, $n = 52$ ARS, $n = 52$	3 years	ARS and PPI provided equal symptom control; ARS provided more heartburn-free days
Grant, 2008	PPI, $n = 179$ ARS, $n = 178$	1 year	Reflux score: PPI, 73; ARS, 85; $P < 0.05$
Lundell, 2009	Omeprazole, $n = 71$ ARS, $n = 53$	12 years	Treatment failure: omeprazole, 55%; ARS, 47%; $P = 0.022$
Lundell, 2007	Omeprazole, $n = 119$ ARS, $n = 99$	7 years	Treatment failure: omeprazole, 53%; ARS, 33%; $P = 0.002$

ARS, Antireflux surgery; *PPI*, proton pump inhibitor.

Clinical Outcomes of Antireflux Surgery

The success of antireflux surgery can be measured by relief of symptoms, improvement in esophageal acid exposure, complications, and failures. Several randomized trials with long-term follow-up have compared medical and surgical therapy for GERD (Table 43.2). LARS is a safe operation that provides durable improvement in typical symptoms of GERD that are refractory to medical management.

Spechler and colleagues[26] found that surgical therapy results in good symptom control after 10-year follow-up. Although 62% of patients in the surgical group were taking antisecretory medications at long-term follow-up, GERD symptoms were not the indication for this medication use in all patients, and reflux symptoms did not change significantly when these patients stopped taking these medications.

Lundell and colleagues[27] randomized patients with erosive esophagitis into surgical or medical therapy. Treatment failure was defined as moderate or severe symptoms of heartburn, regurgitation, dysphagia, or odynophagia; recommencement of PPI therapy; reoperation; or grade 2 esophagitis. At 7-year follow-up, fewer treatment failures were seen in patients managed with fundoplication than with omeprazole (33% vs. 53%; $P = 0.002$). In patients who did not respond to the initial dose of omeprazole, dose escalation was completed; however, surgical intervention remained superior. Patients treated with fundoplication experienced more obstructive and gas-bloat symptoms (e.g., dysphagia, flatulence, inability to belch) compared with the medically treated cohort. At 12-year follow-up, the durability of these results remained; patients who underwent fundoplication had fewer treatment failures compared with patients treated with medical therapy (47% vs. 55%; $P = 0.022$).[28]

During the past 25 years, the experience of surgeons with LARS has increased dramatically. With increased experience, the durability of symptom improvement has increased, and perioperative complications have decreased. This is especially true in high-volume centers. In one single-institution study that observed 100 patients for 10 years after LARS, 90% of patients remained free of GERD symptoms.[29] We published our experience in a cohort of 288 patients undergoing LARS. With median follow-up of more than 5 years, symptom improvement was 90% for heartburn and 92% for regurgitation.[30] These results confirm that LARS can provide excellent durable relief of GERD when patients are appropriately selected and excellent technique is employed. It is important to keep in mind that these result from experienced gastroesophageal surgeons with significant expertise in the management and treatment of GERD.

Operative Complications and Side Effects of Antireflux Surgery

LARS is a safe operation when it is performed by experienced surgeons. Using the American College of Surgeons National Surgical Quality Improvement Program, Niebisch and colleagues[31]

TABLE 43.3 Complications in 400 laparoscopic antireflux procedures at the University of Washington.

COMPLICATION	NO. OF PATIENTS (%)
Postoperative ileus	28 (7)
Pneumothorax	13 (3)
Urinary retention	9 (2)
Dysphagia	9 (2)
Other minor complications	8 (2)
Liver trauma	2 (0.5)
Acute herniation	1 (0.25)
Perforated viscus	1 (0.25)
Death	1 (0.25)
Total	72 (17.25)

reviewed more than 7500 patients who underwent laparoscopic fundoplication between 2005 and 2009. Overall, 30-day mortality was rare (0.19%). In patients older than 70 years, mortality was statistically significantly higher (0.8%; $P < 0.0001$). Complications were also more frequent in older patients (2.2% in patients <50 years and 7.8% in patients >70 years; $P < 0.0001$) and in patients with higher American Society of Anesthesiologists classification (2% in class 2 and 14% in class 4).

Complications of LARS are typically minor and not related specifically to antireflux surgery; they include urinary retention, wound infection, venous thrombosis, and ileus. Complications that are specific to antireflux surgery include pneumothorax, gastric or esophageal injury, and splenic or liver injury. In addition, LARS can result in postoperative side effects, including bloating and dysphagia. Complications in 400 patients who have undergone LARS at the University of Washington are listed in Table 43.3.

Operative Complications

Pneumothorax. Pneumothorax is one of the most common intraoperative complications, yet it is reported to occur in less than 2% of patients.[32] Although postoperative chest radiographs are not obtained in all patients, pneumothorax should rarely be missed as intraoperative identification of pleural violation that causes pneumothorax should be identified. The pleural violation results in intrathoracic infusion of carbon dioxide, which is absorbed rapidly. Because no underlying lung injury exists, the lung will reexpand without incident. When violation of the pleura is identified intraoperatively, the pleura should be closed with a suture, and a postoperative radiograph should be obtained. If a pneumothorax is identified on this radiograph, the patient may be maintained on oxygen therapy to facilitate its resolution. Unless the patient experiences shortness of breath or persistent oxygen therapy to maintain normal hemoglobin oxygenation saturation, no further radiographs are obtained.

Gastric and esophageal injuries. Gastric and esophageal injuries have been reported to occur in approximately 1% of patients undergoing LARS.[32] Typically, these injuries result from overaggressive manipulation of these organs or at the time the bougie is passed into the stomach. Gastric and esophageal injuries are more likely to occur in reoperative cases and should be rare during initial operations. If they are identified at the time of operation, these injuries can be repaired with suture (more commonly) or stapler (if the injury involves the stomach) without sequelae. If the injury is not identified intraoperatively, the patient will likely need a second operation to repair the viscus, unless the leak is small and contained.

Splenic and liver injuries or bleeding. The incidence of bleeding from splenic parenchymal injury during antireflux surgery is about 2.3%; major liver injury is rarely reported.[33] Most commonly, splenic injury occurs during mobilization of the fundus and greater curvature of the stomach. For this reason, we prefer beginning laparoscopic fundoplication with the "left crus approach" to provide early and direct visualization of the short gastric vessels and the spleen. Care must be taken during mobilization of the fundus to avoid excessive traction on the splenogastric ligament. If bleeding does occur, it generally can be controlled with direct pressure and hemostatic agents, as electrosurgical current is ineffective. Very rarely is splenectomy required due to bleeding. A second type of injury is a partial splenic infarction, which can occur during transection of the short gastric vessels and inadvertent coagulation of superior pole branch of the main splenic artery.[33] Partial splenic infarction rarely causes any symptoms. Finally, lacerations and subcapsular hematomas of the left lateral section of the liver can be avoided by carefully retracting it out of the operative field with a fixed retractor.

Side Effects

Bloating. The normal act of air swallowing is the main factor leading to gastric distention, and the physiologic mechanism for venting this air is belching. Gastric belching occurs through vagus nerve–mediated transient LES relaxation. After antireflux surgery, patients experience fewer transient LES relaxations and, therefore, decreased belching. Consequently, patients can experience abdominal bloating. Kessing and colleagues[34] investigated the impact of gas-related symptoms on the objective and subjective outcomes of both Nissen and Toupet fundoplications. Interestingly, they demonstrated that preoperative belching and air swallowing were not predictive of postoperative gas-related symptoms, including bloating. They concluded that gas-related symptoms are, in part, due to gastrointestinal hypersensitivity to gaseous distention. In this study, all patients experienced postoperative normalization of esophageal acid exposure. However, these authors found that patients who developed postoperative gas symptoms were less satisfied with LARS compared with patients who did not experience these symptoms.

During the early postoperative period, patients who report persistent nausea and demonstrate inadequate intake of a liquid diet should undergo abdominal radiography. If significant gastric distention is identified, a nasogastric tube can safely be placed to decompress the stomach for 24 hours. Few patients require further intervention for gastric bloating.

Dysphagia. It is expected that patients will experience mild, temporary dysphagia during the first 2 to 4 weeks postoperatively. This is thought to be a result of postoperative edema at the fundoplication and esophageal hiatus. In the majority of these patients, this dysphagia spontaneously resolves. A second but less common cause of dysphagia in the early postoperative period is the presence of a hematoma of the stomach or esophageal wall that develops during the placement of the sutures to create the fundoplication. Although this may create more severe dysphagia, it typically resolves in several days. In both these situations, surgeons should ensure that the patient can maintain nutrition and hydration on a liquid or soft diet; however, additional interventions are rarely needed. If the patient cannot tolerate liquids, a UGI series should be obtained to ensure that no anatomic abnormality, such as an early hiatal hernia, exists. Assuming that there is no early recurrent hiatal hernia and the patient can tolerate liquids, patience should be employed for 3 months. If the patient cannot maintain hydration or dysphagia persists beyond 3 months, a UGI series should be obtained to ensure no anatomic abnormality that could explain the dysphagia. If the UGI series demonstrates an appropriately positioned fundoplication below the diaphragm, esophagogastroduodenoscopy with empirical dilation of the GEJ should be performed.

Failed antireflux surgery. Patients who have undergone antireflux surgery may present back to the physician with recurrent, persistent, or completely new foregut symptoms. The most common symptoms of failed LARS are typical symptoms of GERD (i.e., heartburn, regurgitation, and water brash sensation) and dysphagia. During the first 2 months after the operation, most symptoms, particularly when they are mild, are of little significance, and the majority of these will abate with time. One large retrospective review of more than 1700 patients who underwent antireflux surgery found that only 5.6% of patients ultimately required a reoperation for symptoms of recurrent GERD or dysphagia.[35] Persistent symptoms should be investigated by the surgeon to evaluate for functional and anatomic problems associated with the fundoplication or the hiatal closure. Anatomic problems after a fundoplication that can cause symptoms include persistent or recurrent hiatal hernia, slipped fundoplication, and incorrectly constructed fundoplication.

All patients who present with recurrent or persistent symptoms of GERD should be evaluated with esophageal manometry and ambulatory pH study. If the pH study demonstrates elevated distal esophageal acid exposure, an esophagram and upper endoscopy should be performed. Once the diagnosis of persistent or recurrent GERD is made, PPI therapy should be instituted. Most of these patients experience resolution of their symptoms with resumption of PPI therapy. If the patient's symptoms are not effectively managed by medical therapy, reoperation should be performed to create an effective antireflux valve.

The late development of dysphagia after LARS suggests esophageal obstruction. In this setting, esophageal obstruction most frequently results from a recurrent hiatal hernia or a slipped fundoplication. A UGI series and esophagogastroduodenoscopy should be the initial studies obtained in these patients. If a clear anatomic abnormality is visualized (Fig. 43.17), reoperation can be performed without further investigation. If concurrent GERD symptoms are present, ambulatory pH testing and manometry should be performed. To achieve resolution of symptoms, reoperation is almost always necessary in these patients.

Some patients experience no improvement or even worsened symptoms after initial LARS. In these patients, one ought to examine the indication for the original procedure and the technique of the operation as these are the two most important factors associated with success or failure. An incorrectly constructed fundoplication (generally created out of the body of the stomach and not the fundus) can do nothing to prevent GER and cause new-onset gastroesophageal obstructive symptoms. Failure to completely excise the sac of a hiatal hernia or PEH frequently leads to an early recurrence of hiatal hernia. In our experience, patients who present with persistent symptoms or early recurrence of symptoms after LARS typically require operative management. After appropriate evaluation with pH testing, manometry, UGI series, and esophagogastroduodenoscopy, the patient should undergo operative correction of the anatomic problem with creation of an appropriately constructed fundoplication.

It is important to understand that reoperative antireflux surgery comes with higher stakes than first-time antireflux surgery. Tissues are less pliable, making it more challenging for surgeons

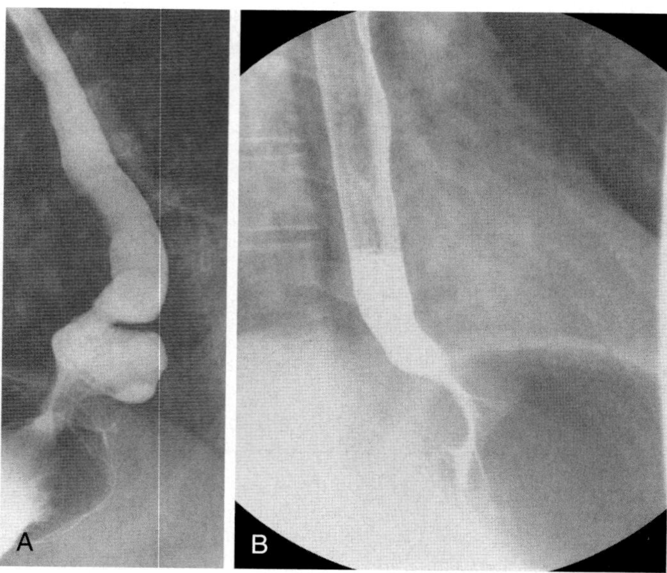

FIG. 43.17 An upper gastrointestinal series provides invaluable anatomic information in patients with persistent or recurrent postoperative symptoms. (A) Upper gastrointestinal series demonstrating a 360-degree fundoplication that has both slipped down around the stomach and herniated into the mediastinum. (B) Normal anatomic appearance of 360-degree fundoplication. Note the smooth tapering of the distal esophagus.

to construct an effective antireflux valve. In addition, adhesions and less visible tissue planes contribute to increased rates of intraoperative injury of the stomach and esophagus. Consequently, we have a higher threshold to perform reoperative antireflux surgery. With the exceptions described before, we reserve reoperation for patients with significant symptoms despite maximal nonoperative management.

GERD in the setting of previous bariatric surgery. RYGB can provide excellent control of GERD; however, patients who have undergone RYGB can still develop symptomatic reflux. In 10,766 patients who underwent surgery at 1 year following RYGB, 43.8% continued preoperative acid suppression medications and 19.2% had started acid suppression medication during the year following RYGB.[32] GERD following RYGB can result from an overly large gastric pouch, gastrogastric fistula, and development of hiatal hernia.

Sleeve gastrectomy (SG) is a safe and effective alternative to RYGB for the control of obesity and its related conditions. In the current literature, the relationship between SG and GERD is inconsistent; however, there is evidence that SG can worsen preexisting GERD and even cause de novo development of GERD. The mechanisms underlying GERD following SG are multiple: decreased gastric compliance, proximal gastric pouch dilation, weakened distal esophageal contractility, disruption of the gastric sling fibers, and compromise of the phrenoesophageal membrane.

The initial evaluation of patients with a history of bariatric surgery who present with symptoms of GERD should follow the same paradigm previously described for patients who have not undergone bariatric surgery. Similarly, initial treatment should include a trial of acid suppression therapy for a minimum of several months with close assessment of symptom control. In patients who have undergone bariatric surgery and have GERD that is unresponsive to maximal medical therapy, operative management strategies should be considered.

Operative management strategies for GERD in patients following SG and RYGB are limited due to the lack of gastric fundus for creation of a fundoplication. For patients following RYGB, operations target the underlying mechanism of GERD and include closure of gastrogastric fistula, correction of hiatal hernia, and revision of large gastric pouch. In patients following SG, options include conversion to RYGB and correction of hiatal hernia. While these strategies can be effective at controlling GERD in this population, they are complex reoperative gastroesophageal operations and are associated with risks of anastomotic leak, gastroesophageal injury, and conversion to open operation. In one series, conversion of SG to RYGB was associated with a 31.5% risk of early (<30 day) postoperative complications, including anastomotic leak, surgical site infection, deep organ space infection, inadvertent enterotomy, and gastric remnant staple line leak.[33]

An alternative to these aforementioned operations is the implantation of a MSAD. Currently, the only device available on the market (LINX, Torax Medical, Shoreview, MN) is comprised of a series of interconnected magnetic beads that is positioned around the distal esophagus to augment LES resting pressure. (For more information on MSAD, see next section in this chapter, "Alternative Operative Therapies for GERD"). Although one stated contraindication to MSAD implantation is prior esophageal or gastric surgery, some surgeons have been using the device off-label, including in patients with GERD recalcitrant to medical therapy who are status post bariatric surgery.

There are two reports of LINX use in patients with GERD enterotomy following RYGB. In one case report, the patient was 8 years status post RYGB with typical symptoms of GERD not alleviated by medications.[36] She had elevated distal esophageal acid exposure, normal esophageal motility, and a small hiatal hernia. Following uneventful laparoscopic hiatal hernia repair and LINX placement, the patient was discharged on postoperative day 1 and PPI therapy was discontinued at 1 week. Six weeks following operation, her gastroesophageal reflux disease health-related quality of life (GERD-HQOL) score decreased from 21/75 preoperatively to 0/75, and repeat pH study showed normalization of DeMeester score.

Munoz-Largacha and colleagues[37] reported their experience with two patients status post RYGB with GERD. Both patients exhibited typical and extraesophageal symptoms of GERD with confirmed reflux on pH-impedance monitoring. LINX implantation was performed laparoscopically and patients were discharged on postoperative day 1. GERD-HRQL improved in the first patient from 38/75 (preoperatively) to 4/75 (6 months) and in the second patient from 22/75 (preoperatively) to 2/75 (11 months). Additionally, the patient reported extraesophageal symptoms and dysphagia also improved following LINX implantation.

Magnetic sphincter implantation also appears to be an acceptable treatment for GERD following SG. In the largest series to date, Hawasli and colleagues[38] retrospectively reviewed charts of 13 patients who presented with medically refractory GERD following SG who also refused conversion to RYGB. All patients underwent thorough gastroesophageal evaluation and were found to have abnormal reflux on pH study. Mean BMI was 33 ± 6 kg/m^2. All operations were performed laparoscopically and included posterior cruroplasty. No intraoperative complications occurred, and mean hospital length of stay was 1.1 ± 0.3 days. One patient was lost to follow-up and one patient demanded removal of the LINX postoperative day 18 due to dysphagia. For the remaining 11/13 (91.7%) patients, mean follow-up was 26 ± 12 months, and GERD-HRQL improved significantly from 47/75 ± 17/75 to 12/75 ± 14/75 (P = 0.0003). However, 6/11 (54.5%) of patients had some recurrent GERD symptoms; three patients required intermittent PPI, and three patients required daily PPI, beginning 7 ± 6 months post-LINX implantation. Greater than 50% GERD recurrence notwithstanding, LINX was associated with significant patient reported GERD symptoms. One contributing factor to this disappointing GERD recurrence rate could be the patient BMI at time of LINX placement.

Kuckelman and colleagues[39] compared outcomes for management of GERD with LINX for patients with standard U.S. Food and Drug Administration (FDA) indications and patients with GERD status post bariatric surgery. Out of 28 patients, 10 had undergone prior bariatric surgery (8 SG, 1 RYGB, and 1 biliopancreatic diversion following SG). All patients had GERD confirmed on pH study. All operations were performed laparoscopically, and no intraoperative or immediate postoperative complications occurred. Prolonged dysphagia (>3 months) was reported by four patients; one patient who previously had bariatric surgery required removal of the LINX due to dysphagia. Endoscopic dilation was successful at managing dysphagia in the other three patients. Both groups showed significant improvement in GERD-HRQL with no significant differences in dysphagia (10% post bariatric; 12.5% standard), satisfaction (100% post bariatric; 94% standard), and PPI use (10% post bariatric; 6% standard). Overall, this small retrospective observational study suggests that use of LINX to manage GERD in patients following bariatric surgery provides similar outcomes to patients that satisfy the standard FDA indications for the device.

Alternative Operative Therapies for GERD

Despite the fact that LARS provides durable symptom relief with an excellent safety profile, the last decade has seen a drive to develop new therapies for GERD. These efforts have focused on augmenting the LES by modalities such as radiofrequency energy (Mederi Therapeutics Inc., Greenwich, CN), injection of inert biopolymers (Enteryx; Boston Scientific, Natick, MA), creation of gastroplications (EndoCinch, Bard, Warwick, RI; EsophyX, EndoGastric Solutions, Redmond, WA; Plicator, NDO Surgical, Mansfield, MA), and implantation of a MSAD (LINX, Torax Medical, Shoreview, MN). The two most studied therapies that are currently available clinically are endoscopic transoral incisionless fundoplication (TIF) and MSAD.

Transoral Incisionless Fundoplication

TIF is performed with a flexible, multichannel endoluminal device that uses fasteners to construct a full-thickness gastric plication and to create an antireflux valve at the GEJ. The endoluminal fundoplication can be created up to 4 cm in length and 270 degrees. The procedure is performed under general anesthesia; the device is inserted over a gastroscope, and because multiple fasteners are loaded on the end of the device, the entire antireflux valve can be created during a single device insertion.

Since the initial studies evaluating the safety of TIF were published in 2008, additional investigation has demonstrated that TIF improves GERD-related quality of life, results in patient satisfaction with GERD symptom control, is associated with reduced PPI use, and is associated with few side effects.[40] However, whereas it appears that TIF is associated with significant *reduction* in acid exposure and improvement in GERD symptoms, *normalization* of esophageal acid exposure and complete cessation of PPI use have not been demonstrated in these short-term studies. In a long-term (3-year) follow-up study, Muls and colleagues[41] demonstrated similar results. Patients reported durable improvement in GERD-related quality of life and significant reduction in PPI use; however, 48% of patients had normalization of pH study results. Furthermore, 12 of 66 patients required revisional procedures (11 redo TIF and 1 Nissen) because of inadequate control of GERD symptoms associated with esophagitis (92%), PPI use (83%), and Hill grade III or IV antireflux valve (92%).

The TIF 2.0 versus Medical PPI Open label (TEMPO) trial reported 5-year follow-up data on TIF versus PPI therapy in 44/63 (70%) randomized at the beginning of the study.[42] The primary symptom assessed was regurgitation, which was present in 43/44 (98%) of patients. At 5 years following TIF, elimination of regurgitation was achieved in 37/43 (86%) of patients, and significant improvement was seen in Reflux Symptom Index Score (6.3 vs. 22.2 at baseline), average regurgitation score (0.7 vs. 3 at baseline), and GERD-HRQL score (6.8 vs. 26.4 at baseline). Importantly, these symptom scores were assessed with patients on acid suppression therapy they were using at 5-year follow-up, and 54% of patients were using PPI therapy on a daily basis (34%) or occasionally (20%). A total of 3/60 (5%) required reoperation (1 Dor and 2 Nissen) for recurrent GERD symptoms despite PPI therapy.

Magnetic Sphincter Augmentation

The MSAD is a series of magnetic beads that is positioned around the distal esophagus to increase LES resting pressure to counteract GER. During peristaltic swallows, the propagated bolus of liquid or food separates the beads, opening the GEJ and allowing the bolus to pass into the stomach, after which the beads return to their original position to augment the LES resting pressure. Laparoscopic placement of the MSAD is more easily reproducible than creating a fundoplication, which may reduce variability in operative technique among surgeons.

In 2016, Ganz and colleagues reported 5-year outcomes on 85 patients who underwent MSAD placement.[41] Significant improvements were seen in patient-reported heartburn (89%–11.9%; $P < 0.001$), regurgitation (57%–1.2%; $P < 0.001$), and dissatisfaction with their GERD (95%–7.1%; $P < 0.001$). Further, daily PPI use was present in 15.3% of patients at 5 years (compared to 100% at baseline), while 75.3% of patients reported complete cessation of PPI. Improvements in esophagitis were also seen in this cohort. Complete healing was seen in 26 of 34 patients with preoperative esophagitis; of the remaining 8 patients, 6 had Grade A and 2 had Grade B esophagitis. Further, these improvements occurred in the absence of significant side effects. All patients reported the ability to belch or vomit if needed, and dysphagia was no worse at 5-year follow-up compared to baseline (6% vs. 5%; $P = 0.739$). Lastly, one early concern for MSAD was device erosion, migration, and malfunction. In this study, no such events were reported. A total of seven patients had the device removed for dysphagia (four patients), and one patient each for vomiting, chest pain, and persistent reflux symptoms.

Bell and colleagues[43] completed a prospective randomized controlled study to compare the effectiveness of twice-daily (BID) PPI therapy to MSAD in patients with moderate to severe regurgitation recalcitrant to once daily PPI therapy. One hundred fifty-two patients with GERD and regurgitation despite once daily PPI therapy were randomized to BID PPI (102 patients) or MSAD (50 patients). At 6 month follow-up, compared to patients who took BID PPI, patients who underwent MSAD showed significantly greater resolution of regurgitation (89% vs. 10%; $P < 0.001$), greater improvement in GERD-HRQL scores (24–6 vs. 25–24; $P < 0.002$), and greater overall satisfaction with their current condition (81% vs. 2%). When assessed by 24-hour pH-impedance study, the MSAD group showed fewer total number of reflux events, greater likelihood of normal number of reflux episodes, and more frequent normalization of total distal esophageal acid exposure and DeMeester composite score compared to patients who took BID PPI therapy. Dysphagia was the most common side effect (15 patients, 32%) reported by patients who underwent MSAD implantation. Nine patients required no treatment; endoscopic dilation (3 patients), systemic corticosteroid (3 patients), and hiatal hernia repair (1 patient) were used to the remaining patients.

Better control of regurgitation with MSAD compared to PPI therapy is not surprising. Regurgitation results from an ineffective mechanical barrier to reflux, whereas heartburn results from acidic gastric contents contacting the esophageal mucosa. While PPI therapy alkalinizes the gastric contents and is very effective at controlling heartburn, it does nothing to counteract reflux itself; therefore, regurgitation is frequently no better improved with PPI therapy. On the other hand, MSAD creates a mechanical barrier to reflux, counteracting regurgitation. Compared with PPI use, improvement in regurgitation following MSAD implantation is not surprising, as PPI therapy only reduces the acidity of regurgitated contents and does nothing to counteract GER. A more balanced comparison of therapies would be MSAD versus the gold standard for surgical reflux, a therapy that effectively controls both heartburn and regurgitation: fundoplication.

Aiolfi and colleagues[44] published the only systemic review and meta analysis on MSAD compared to laparoscopic fundoplication. They identified seven studies published between 2014 and 2017 with a total of 1211 patients (sample size 24–415); all studies were observational, cohort studies. Ultimately, both laparoscopic fundoplication and MSAD appear to be safe and effective at controlling GERD symptoms, improving GERD-HRQL scores and distal esophageal acid exposure up to 1-year follow-up. The most significant advantage of MSAD was preservation of the ability to belch and vomit as well as reduction in gas-bloat. Dysphagia requiring dilation and reoperation was equally common in each group. Although the heterogeneity of studies was low and overall robustness of these analyses was high, it would benefit surgeons to have a randomized study comparing MSAD to fundoplication to gain a better understanding of the advantages and weaknesses of each therapy.

Postoperative rates of dysphagia appear similar between MSAD and Nissen fundoplication; however, the need for dilation is more frequent with MSAD. This is likely due to extrinsic compression of the device on the esophagus or formation of a fibrotic band around the distal esophagus.

Device erosion is a feared complication of MSAD implantation. Alicuben and colleagues[45] found 29 reported cases of MSAD erosion out of 9453 devices placed (0.31%). Erosion was more common among smaller (12 magnet) devices (18 erosions in 365 devices implanted; 4.93% incidence). This suggests that size mismatch or undersizing the device is a risk factor for erosion due to excessive compression of the distal esophagus by an undersized device.

Patients with device erosion present most commonly years following device placement with new onset chest pain or dysphagia. While barium esophagram can rule out alternative causes of these symptoms, endoscopy confirms the diagnosis of device erosion. When erosion is identified, removal of the device can be done safely with minimal morbidity. Most devices were removed initially with an endoscopic approach followed by delayed laparoscopic removal of the remainder of the device.

PARAESOPHAGEAL HERNIA

The anatomic definitions of PEH are discussed in a previous section and can be reviewed in Fig. 43.2. PEH is frequently associated with obstructive symptoms and, less frequently, typical symptoms of GERD. On occasion, a PEH is identified incidentally on imaging performed for another purpose, and the patient's PEH is asymptomatic. An indication for operative repair of PEH is based on the size of the hernia and the presence and severity of symptoms. To prevent acute gastric volvulus and gastric strangulation, a case can be made for operative repair of a large but minimally symptomatic PEH. Otherwise, the presence of a small asymptomatic hiatal hernia or PEH does not constitute an indication for operative correction.

Pathophysiology

The two key events that facilitate the formation of a PEH are the widening of the diaphragmatic crura at the esophageal hiatus and stretching of the phrenoesophageal membrane. As the hernia enlarges, the phrenoesophageal membrane balloons into the posterior mediastinum like a parachute. After repeated episodes of the viscera entering the hernia sac, adhesions develop between the wall of the sac and the surrounding thoracic structures, thus preventing the herniated abdominal contents from returning to their normal position in the peritoneal cavity. The most common structure to herniate through the esophageal hiatus is the fundus of the stomach; however, the entire stomach as well as other abdominal organs, including the spleen, colon, pancreas, small bowel, and omentum, can migrate into the chest.

Gastric volvulus develops because of laxity in the stomach's peritoneal attachments and subsequent rotation of the gastric fundus on the organoaxial or mesenteric axis of the stomach (Fig. 43.18). The frequency with which this occurs is a matter of debate. Historically, surgeons believed that a large PEH would inevitably result in volvulus, become incarcerated, and result in gastric strangulation; the mere presence of a PEH was an indication for operative repair. However, more recent evidence suggests that the risk for acute strangulation is approximately 1% per year.[46] We recommend operative repair of completely asymptomatic large hernias only in young (<60 years) and otherwise healthy patients.

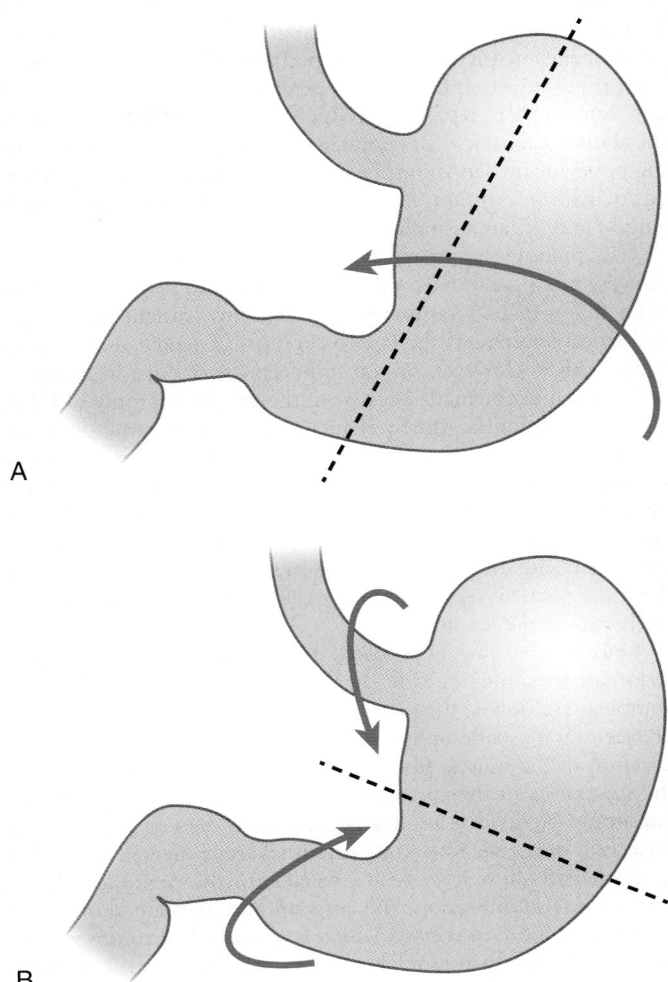

FIG. 43.18 Gastric volvulus develops because of laxity in the stomach's peritoneal attachments and subsequent rotation of the gastric fundus on the (A) organoaxial or (B) mesenteric axis of the stomach.

Clinical Presentation

The symptoms of PEH are diverse and nonspecific. The most common symptoms attributed to PEH are gastroesophageal obstructive symptoms, including dysphagia, odynophagia, and postprandial chest pain, as well as early satiety. When intermittent visceral torsion and distention occur, epigastric and chest pain can develop due to the resulting ischemia of the hernia contents. Spontaneous reduction then provides relief of these symptoms. Gastrointestinal bleeding can result from mucosal ischemia or mechanical ulceration of the gastric mucosa. Respiratory symptoms, primarily shortness of breath, can be explained by the mass effect of the hernia contents in the chest. Finally, heartburn and regurgitation are also reported by patients with PEH. These symptoms can be present individually or in combination. Because of these varied symptoms, the diagnosis of PEH is often made only after performance of a barium esophagram or UGI endoscopy.

Preoperative Evaluation

The clinical investigations obtained in patients with PEH are similar to those of patients undergoing workup for GERD. A barium esophagogram provides the operating surgeon the most accurate image of the gastroesophageal anatomy (Fig. 43.19). Endoscopy evaluates the gastric and esophageal mucosa for mechanical gastric mucosal erosions (i.e., Cameron ulcers) that can result in gastrointestinal blood loss and Barrett's esophagus, which require postoperative endoscopy for surveillance. Manometry is necessary to determine the motor function of the esophageal body, which can affect the type of antireflux operation performed at the time of PEH repair. Even if a large PEH prevents the passage of the manometry catheter through the LES, it is generally possible to determine the degree of esophageal peristalsis. Finally, in patients with typical symptoms of GERD, ambulatory pH monitoring is indicated to document the presence of abnormal distal esophageal acid exposure. Although the results of ambulatory pH monitoring rarely change the decision for operative repair of PEH, preoperative documentation of GERD is particularly useful as a baseline for comparison in patients who have recurrent symptoms postoperatively.

Operative Repair

PEH can be repaired through the left side of the chest or the abdomen and with open or minimally invasive techniques. Laparoscopy has decreased perioperative morbidity associated with elective

PEH repair, and most PEH repairs are currently performed by a laparoscopic approach. This is of particular importance because PEH occurs frequently in older patients with multiple medical comorbidities. Regardless of the operative approach, there are four key steps to PEH repair: (1) reduction of the hernia contents to the abdominal cavity; (2) complete excision of the hernia sac from the posterior mediastinum; (3) mobilization of the distal esophagus to achieve a minimum of 3 cm of intra abdominal esophageal length; and (4) an antireflux operation.

Our preferred approach is laparoscopic PEH repair. Only in the very rare patient have we found the need to perform either an open abdominal operation or a thoracotomy. Patient positioning and trocar placement for laparoscopic PEH repair are the same as for LARS. However, several important variations in operative technique must be made because of the unique anatomy of PEH.

The operation begins by reducing the hernia contents to the abdominal cavity using gentle traction and only to the extent that the contents can be easily reduced. Frequently, however, the hernia contents cannot be fully reduced because adhesions develop between the hernia sac and the posterior mediastinum. This prevents clear visualization of the left crus. Consequently, we divide the short gastric vessels to mobilize the fundus of the stomach and safely expose the left crus.

Once the left crus is exposed, it is necessary to enter the posterior mediastinum outside the hernia sac, which will facilitate complete excision of the hernia sac from the chest. This plane lies between the phrenoesophageal membrane and the left crus. Visualization of the muscle fibers of the left crus is confirmation that the surgeon is in the correct plane. At this point, the peritoneal sac should be divided anteriorly, parallel to the left crus. Further dissection of the sac from its mediastinal attachments will free the stomach and allow it to be delivered into the peritoneal cavity. During this mobilization, the surgeon and assistant must avoid vigorous traction on the sac, which is still attached to the esophagus and can result in esophageal tears. After the hernia contents are returned to the peritoneal cavity, the hernia sac must be transected circumferentially at the hiatus.

The most challenging aspect of the sac dissection is encountered during the mobilization of the posterior sac. The esophagus and posterior vagus nerve are intimately associated with the sac posteriorly and can be easily injured during this dissection. A lighted bougie helps identify the exact location of the esophagus. Once the esophagus is clearly identified, the bougie should be pulled back to avoid unnecessarily thinning of the esophageal wall and maximizing the posterior mediastinal space to facilitate further dissection. After the sac is freed at the hiatus, a concerted effort is made to remove as much of the hernia sac from the mediastinum as possible. However, the pleura, esophagus, pericardium, aorta, and inferior pulmonary veins are intimately related to the hernia sac, and these vital structures may be injured during this dissection. The surgeon's desire to remove the entire sac must be tempered by the possibility of injuring these vital structures. Once the sac is excised from the mediastinum, the esophagus is further mobilized to obtain a minimum of 3 cm of intra abdominal length. Then, the crura are reapproximated with interrupted nonabsorbable suture.

Tension-free closure of the esophageal hiatus is a key step in the repair of PEH. In some patients, lack of pliability of the diaphragmatic crura makes a tension-free closure of the hiatus impossible. In our experience, the size of the hernia does not accurately predict the ability to close the hiatus without tension. However, scarred and poorly pliable crura are frequently encountered during repair of recurrent hiatal hernias. If a tension-free closure is not possible, two options are available: (1) close the hiatus under tension and reinforce the closure with biologic mesh; and (2) perform a diaphragmatic relaxing incision to allow primary tension-free closure of the hiatus and reinforce the relaxing incision and hiatal closure with biologic mesh. Importantly, permanent synthetic mesh should never be used at the esophageal hiatus as it is associated with esophageal erosion and stenosis.

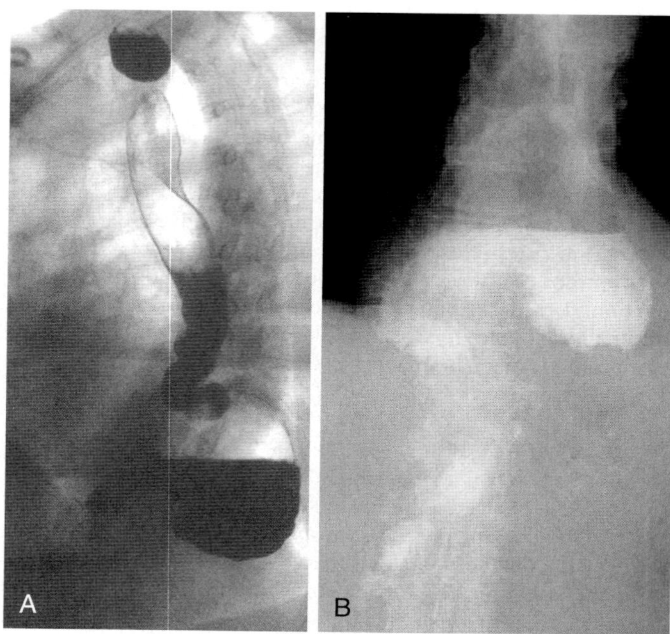

FIG. 43.19 Upper gastrointestinal series is essential to understand the anatomy of a paraesophageal hernia. (A) Oblique view demonstrating a distended stomach with an air-fluid level anterior to the esophagus and well into the mediastinum. (B) Anteroposterior view demonstrating complete organoaxial volvulus with a completely intrathoracic stomach and the pylorus at the hiatus.

If the hiatus can be closed primarily but under some tension, biologic mesh should be placed to reinforce this closure. To do this, a 7 × 10-cm piece of biologic mesh is cut into the shape of a horseshoe. The mesh is then placed at the hiatus. This can be done in a U configuration, with the base overlying the posterior hiatal closure, or in a C configuration, with the base overlying the right crus and limbs of the mesh lying anterior and posterior to the esophagus. The C configuration has the advantage of reinforcing the anterior and posterior hiatus. The orientation of the mesh placement should be according to the surgeon's preference. The mesh is sutured to the diaphragm, and fibrin glue is used to reinforce the mesh placement (Fig. 43.20).

Several studies have investigated the use of mesh to reinforce hiatal closure in PEH repair (Table 43.4). A multi-institutional randomized clinical trial compared primary hiatal closure and reinforcement of primary closure with biologic mesh. At 6 months of follow-up, hiatal hernia recurrence rate was significantly lower when the hiatus was reinforced with biologic mesh compared with primary closure alone (9% vs. 24%; $P = 0.04$).[47] However, at 5-year follow-up, there was no significant difference in hiatal hernia recurrence rates between patients with and without mesh.[48] This suggests that biologic mesh reinforcement of the hiatal closure in PEH repair decreases early but not late recurrent hiatal hernias. In this randomized trial using biologic mesh, there were no mesh-related complications.

On occasion, the pliability of the crura is so poor that the hiatus cannot be closed primarily. In this situation, a crural relaxing incision is performed to facilitate closure. Relaxing incisions have been described on the right and left crura. We prefer to perform a relaxing incision on the right crus (Fig. 43.21) and to patch the defect with a U-shaped biologic mesh, as described before. In very few patients, when the hiatus will not close with a right-sided relaxing incision, a left-sided relaxing incision is performed, which facilitates medialization of the left crus and primary closure. In our experience, coverage of the left-sided relaxing incision with biologic mesh is associated with the development of diaphragmatic hernias and need for reoperation. Therefore, we now patch this defect with permanent synthetic polytetrafluoroethylene mesh (Fig. 43.22). We have not encountered any complications with permanent mesh placement in this location.

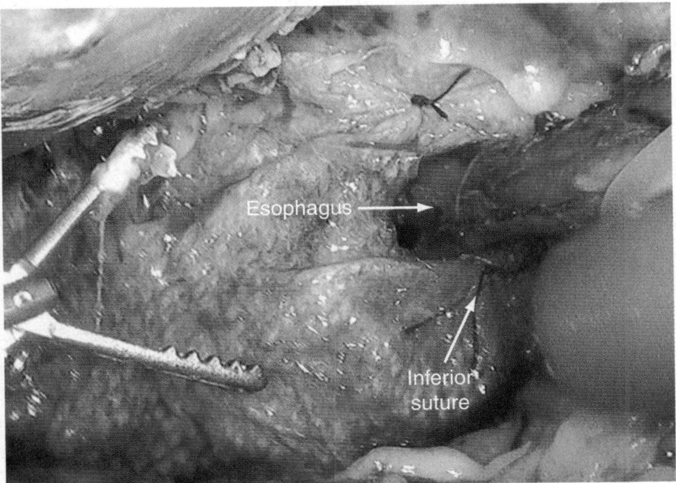

FIG. 43.20 When the closure of the esophageal hiatus is met with mild to moderate tension, we place a 7 × 10-cm piece of biologic mesh to reinforce the hiatal closure.

After the hiatus is closed, an antireflux procedure is performed. A Nissen fundoplication is performed in all patients except those with severely ineffective motility or aperistaltic esophagus. In such patients, a Toupet fundoplication is performed. Although the need for an antireflux procedure is controversial, many patients with PEH have abnormal reflux, and the fundoplication will seal the hiatus, preventing access by other viscera. Postoperative care is the same as for patients who have undergone LARS.

Acute Gastric Volvulus

A relatively rare occurrence, acute gastric volvulus is a clinical emergency. Patients present with sudden onset of chest or epigastric pain associated with retching without the production of emesis. The development of fever, tachycardia, and leukocytosis suggests gastric strangulation and impending perforation. Gastric volvulus is necessary but not sufficient for gastric ischemia to develop. More often, patients present with subacute or chronic recurrent gastric volvulus, which causes gastroesophageal obstructive symptoms but never results in gastric ischemia.

Initial management of acute gastric volvulus should include placement of a nasogastric tube for gastric decompression. If bedside placement of a nasogastric tube is not possible, esophagoscopy can facilitate gastric decompression and nasogastric tube placement. On occasion, endoscopic reduction of volvulus is possible. Endoscopy also allows assessment of the gastric mucosa; if gastric ischemia is present, emergent operation is indicated.

TABLE 43.4 Studies of biologic mesh in patients undergoing paraesophageal hernia repair.

STUDY	STUDY DESIGN	ARMS	MEDIAN FOLLOW-UP	RECURRENCE
Oelschlager, 2011[48]	RCT	Surgisis, $n = 26$; no mesh, $n = 34$	59 months	Surgisis, 54%; no mesh, 59%; $P = 0.7$
Oelschlager, 2006[47]	RCT	Surgisis, $n = 51$; no mesh, $n = 57$	6 months	Surgisis, 9%; no mesh, 24%; $P = 0.04$
Ringley, 2006	Retrospective	Alloderm, $n = 22$; no mesh, $n = 22$	7 months	Alloderm, 0%; no mesh, 9%; $P < 0.05$
Jacobs, 2007	Retrospective	Surgisis, $n = 127$; no mesh, $n = 93$	38 months	Surgisis, 3%; no mesh, 20%; $P < 0.01$

RCT, Randomized controlled trial.

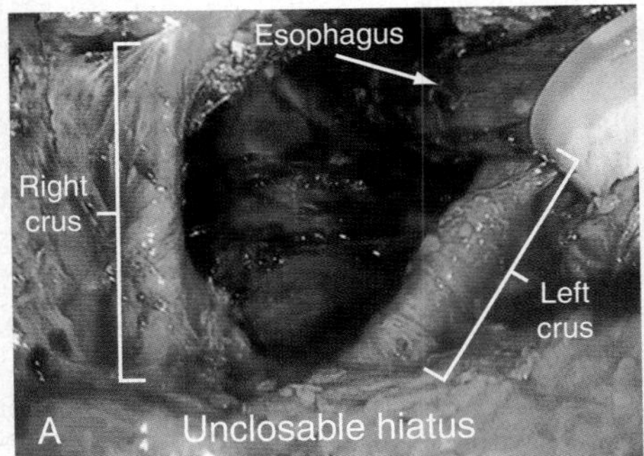

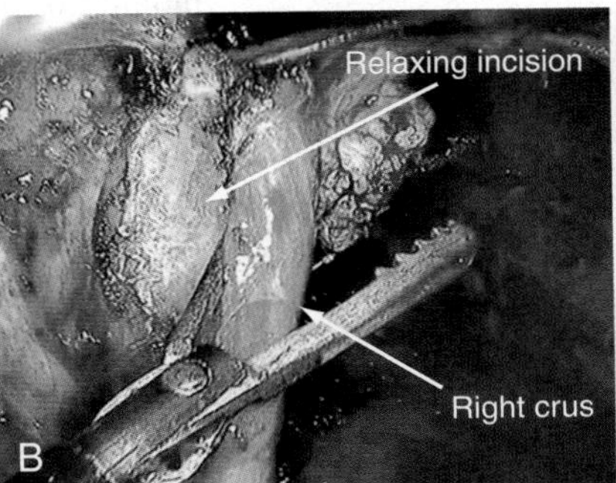

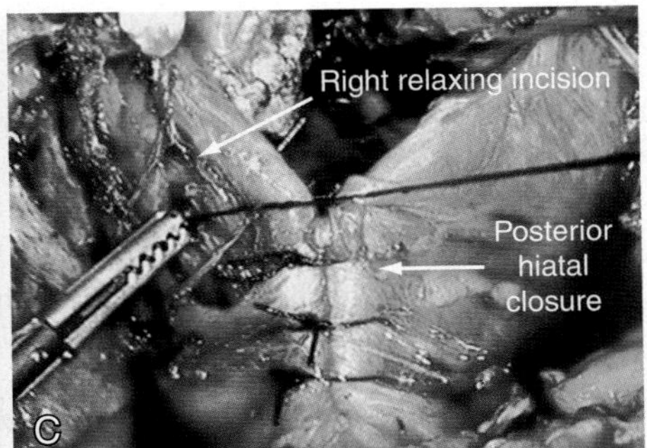

FIG. 43.21 When poorly pliable crura prevent primary closure of the esophageal hiatus (A), a relaxing incision is placed on the right crus (B) to facilitate closure (C).

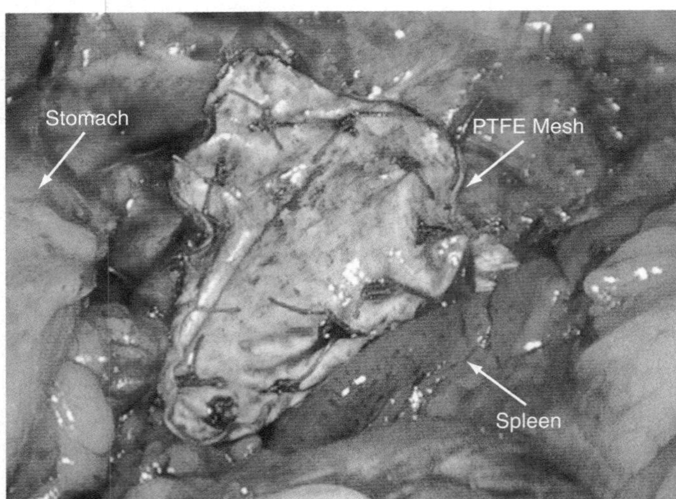

FIG. 43.22 When bilateral relaxing incisions are necessary to facilitate hiatal closure, the left-sided relaxing incision is covered with permanent mesh to prevent the development of a diaphragmatic hernia. *PTFE*, Polytetrafluoroethylene.

The operative management of acute gastric volvulus should follow the same tenets as for PEH repair. In otherwise healthy patients, a formal laparoscopic PEH repair should be performed. In high-operative-risk patients who may not tolerate a prolonged general anesthetic necessary for PEH repair, consideration should be given to laparoscopic reduction of the gastric volvulus and anterior abdominal wall gastropexy.

SUMMARY

Operative treatment of GERD and PEH has become more common in the era of laparoscopic procedures. Careful selection of patients based on symptom assessment, response to medical therapy, and preoperative testing will optimize chances for effective and durable postoperative control of symptoms. Complications of LARS and repair of PEH are rare and generally can be managed without reoperation. When reoperation is necessary for operative failures, it should be performed by high-volume surgeons.

SELECTED REFERENCES

Jobe BA, Richter JE, Hoppo T, et al. Preoperative diagnostic workup before antireflux surgery: an evidence and experience-based consensus of the esophageal diagnostic advisory panel. *J Am Coll Surg*. 2013;217:586–597.

A consensus statement from experienced surgeons and gastroenterologists in the field of gastroesophageal reflux disease (GERD) on the preoperative diagnostic testing of patients with GERD.

Oelschlager BK, Petersen RP, Brunt LM, et al. Laparoscopic paraesophageal hernia repair: defining long-term clinical and anatomic outcomes. *J Gastrointest Surg*. 2012;16:453–459.

A multicenter randomized trial that evaluated the symptomatic response to laparoscopic paraesophageal hernia repair as well as the relationship between recurrent symptoms and recurrent hiatal hernia.

Rickenbacher N, Kotter T, Kochen MM, et al. Fundoplication versus medical management of gastroesophageal reflux disease: systematic review and meta-analysis. *Surg Endosc*. 2014;28:143–155.

Meta analysis of trials comparing surgical fundoplication with medical management of gastroesophageal reflux disease.

Weltz PA, Sanford Z, Addo A, et al. Laparoscopic antireflux surgery (LARS) is highly effective in the treatment of select patients with chronic cough. *Surgery*. 2019;166:34–40.

A retrospective review of laparoscopic antireflux surgery for management of extraesophageal symptoms of gastroesophageal reflux disease that offers guidance in patient selection.

Worrell SG, Greene CL, DeMeester TR. The state of surgical treatment of gastroesophageal reflux disease after five decades. *J Am Coll Surg*. 2014;219:819–830.

A clear, concise, and thorough description of the approach to the surgical management of patients with gastroesophageal reflux disease, including selection of the appropriate operation and avoidance of operative technical pitfalls.

Yadlapati H, Whitsett M, Thuluvath AJ, et al. Review of antireflux procedures for proton pump inhibitor nonresponsive gastroesophageal reflux disease. *Dis Esophagus*. 2017;30:1–14.

A thorough review of operative and endoscopic procedures to manage gastroesophageal reflux disease that is recalcitrant to proton pump inhibitor therapy.

Yadlapati R, Hungness E, Pandolfino J. Complications of antireflux surgery. *Am J Gastroenterology*. 2018;113:1137–1147.

A comprehensive review offering classification of complications of antireflux surgery.

REFERENCES

1. Mainie I, Tutuian R, Shay S, et al. Acid and non-acid reflux in patients with persistent symptoms despite acid suppressive therapy: a multicentre study using combined ambulatory impedance-pH monitoring. *Gut*. 2006;55:1398–1402.
2. Worrell SG, DeMeester SR, Greene CL, et al. Pharyngeal pH monitoring better predicts a successful outcome for extraesophageal reflux symptoms after antireflux surgery. *Surg Endosc*. 2013;27:4113–4118.
3. Bowrey DJ, Peters JH, DeMeester TR. Gastroesophageal reflux disease in asthma: effects of medical and surgical antireflux therapy on asthma control. *Ann Surg*. 2000;231:161–172.
4. Raghu G, Freudenberger TD, Yang S, et al. High prevalence of abnormal acid gastro-oesophageal reflux in idiopathic pulmonary fibrosis. *Eur Respir J*. 2006;27:136–142.
5. Lee JS, Ryu JH, Elicker BM, et al. Gastroesophageal reflux therapy is associated with longer survival in patients with idiopathic pulmonary fibrosis. *Am J Respir Crit Care Med*. 2011;184:1390–1394.

6. Raghu G, Yang ST, Spada C, et al. Sole treatment of acid gastroesophageal reflux in idiopathic pulmonary fibrosis: a case series. *Chest.* 2006;129:794–800.
7. Raghu G, Pellegrini CA, Yow E, et al. Laparoscopic anti-reflux surgery for the treatment of idiopathic pulmonary fibrosis (WRAP-IPF): a multicentre, randomised, controlled phase 2 trial. *Lancet Respir Med.* 2018;6:707–714.
8. Campos GM, Peters JH, DeMeester TR, et al. Multivariate analysis of factors predicting outcome after laparoscopic Nissen fundoplication. *J Gastrointest Surg.* 1999;3:292–300.
9. Bredenoord AJ, Weusten BL, Timmer R, et al. Addition of esophageal impedance monitoring to pH monitoring increases the yield of symptom association analysis in patients off PPI therapy. *Am J Gastroenterol.* 2006;101:453–459.
10. Patel A, Sayuk GS, Gyawali CP. Parameters on esophageal pH-impedance monitoring that predict outcomes of patients with gastroesophageal reflux disease. *Clin Gastroenterol Hepatol.* 2015;13:884–891.
11. Kahrilas PJ, Dodds WJ, Hogan WJ, et al. Esophageal peristaltic dysfunction in peptic esophagitis. *Gastroenterology.* 1986;91:897–904.
12. Armstrong D. Endoscopic evaluation of gastro-esophageal reflux disease. *Yale J Biol Med.* 1999;72:93–100.
13. Epstein D, Bojke L, Sculpher MJ. Laparoscopic fundoplication compared with medical management for gastro-oesophageal reflux disease: cost effectiveness study. *BMJ.* 2009;339:b2576.
14. Wong RK, Hanson DG, Waring PJ, et al. ENT manifestations of gastroesophageal reflux. *Am J Gastroenterol.* 2000;95:S15–S22.
15. Borbely Y, Schaffner E, Zimmermann L, et al. De novo gastroesophageal reflux disease after sleeve gastrectomy: role of preoperative silent reflux. *Surg Endosc.* 2019;33:789–793.
16. Kahrilas PJ, Bredenoord AJ, Fox M, et al. The Chicago Classification of esophageal motility disorders, v3.0. *Neurogastroenterol Motil.* 2015;27:160–174.
17. Booth MI, Stratford J, Jones L, et al. Randomized clinical trial of laparoscopic total (Nissen) versus posterior partial (Toupet) fundoplication for gastro-oesophageal reflux disease based on preoperative oesophageal manometry. *Br J Surg.* 2008;95:57–63.
18. Oleynikov D, Eubanks TR, Oelschlager BK, et al. Total fundoplication is the operation of choice for patients with gastroesophageal reflux and defective peristalsis. *Surg Endosc.* 2002;16:909–913.
19. Knight BC, Devitt PG, Watson DI, et al. Long-term efficacy of laparoscopic antireflux surgery on regression of Barrett's esophagus using BRAVO wireless pH monitoring: a prospective clinical cohort study. *Ann Surg.* 2017;266:1000–1005.
20. Shan CX, Zhang W, Zheng XM, et al. Evidence-based appraisal in laparoscopic Nissen and Toupet fundoplications for gastroesophageal reflux disease. *World J Gastroenterol.* 2010;16:3063–3071.
21. Kaufman JA, Houghland JE, Quiroga E, et al. Long-term outcomes of laparoscopic antireflux surgery for gastroesophageal reflux disease (GERD)-related airway disorder. *Surg Endosc.* 2006;20:1824–1830.
22. Katz PO, Gerson LB, Vela MF. Guidelines for the diagnosis and management of gastroesophageal reflux disease. *Am J Gastroenterol.* 2013;108:308–328; quiz 329.
23. Brisebois S, Merati A, Giliberto JP. Proton pump inhibitors: review of reported risks and controversies. *Laryngoscope Investig Otolaryngol.* 2018;3:457–462.
24. Tleyjeh IM, Bin Abdulhak AA, Riaz M, et al. Association between proton pump inhibitor therapy and clostridium difficile infection: a contemporary systematic review and meta-analysis. *PLoS One.* 2012;7:e50836.
25. Oelschlager BK, Yamamoto K, Woltman T, et al. Vagotomy during hiatal hernia repair: a benign esophageal lengthening procedure. *J Gastrointest Surg.* 2008;12:1155–1162.
26. Spechler SJ, Lee E, Ahnen D, et al. Long-term outcome of medical and surgical therapies for gastroesophageal reflux disease: follow-up of a randomized controlled trial. *JAMA.* 2001;285:2331–2338.
27. Lundell L, Miettinen P, Myrvold HE, et al. Seven-year follow-up of a randomized clinical trial comparing proton-pump inhibition with surgical therapy for reflux oesophagitis. *Br J Surg.* 2007;94:198–203.
28. Lundell L, Miettinen P, Myrvold HE, et al. Comparison of outcomes twelve years after antireflux surgery or omeprazole maintenance therapy for reflux esophagitis. *Clin Gastroenterol Hepatol.* 2009;7:1292–1298; quiz 1260.
29. Dallemagne B, Weerts J, Markiewicz S, et al. Clinical results of laparoscopic fundoplication at ten years after surgery. *Surg Endosc.* 2006;20:159–165.
30. Oelschlager BK, Eubanks TR, Oleynikov D, et al. Symptomatic and physiologic outcomes after operative treatment for extra-esophageal reflux. *Surg Endosc.* 2002;16:1032–1036.
31. Niebisch S, Fleming FJ, Galey KM, et al. Perioperative risk of laparoscopic fundoplication: safer than previously reported-analysis of the American College of Surgeons National Surgical Quality Improvement Program 2005 to 2009. *J Am Coll Surg.* 2012;215:61–68; discussion 68–69.
32. Bizekis C, Kent M, Luketich J. Complications after surgery for gastroesophageal reflux disease. *Thorac Surg Clin.* 2006;16:99–108.
33. Odabasi M, Abuoglu HH, Arslan C, et al. Asymptomatic partial splenic infarction in laparoscopic floppy Nissen fundoplication and brief literature review. *Int Surg.* 2014;99:291–294.
34. Kessing BF, Broeders JA, Vinke N, et al. Gas-related symptoms after antireflux surgery. *Surg Endosc.* 2013;27:3739–3747.
35. Lamb PJ, Myers JC, Jamieson GG, et al. Long-term outcomes of revisional surgery following laparoscopic fundoplication. *Br J Surg.* 2009;96:391–397.
36. Varban OA, Hawasli AA, Carlin AM, et al. Variation in utilization of acid-reducing medication at 1 year following bariatric surgery: results from the Michigan Bariatric Surgery Collaborative. *Surg Obes Relat Dis.* 2015;11:222–228.
37. Munoz-Largacha JA, Hess DT, Litle VR, et al. Lower esophageal magnetic sphincter augmentation for persistent reflux after Roux-en-Y gastric bypass. *Obes Surg.* 2016;26:464–466.
38. Hawasli A, Tarakji M, Tarboush M. Laparoscopic management of severe reflux after sleeve gastrectomy using the LINX((R)) system: technique and one year follow up case report. *Int J Surg Case Rep.* 2017;30:148–151.
39. Kuckelman JP, Phillips CJ, Derickson MJ, et al. Esophageal magnetic sphincter augmentation as a novel approach to post-bariatric surgery gastroesophageal reflux disease. *Obes Surg.* 2018;28:3080–3086.
40. Hawasli A, Sadoun M, Meguid A, et al. Laparoscopic placement of the LINX((R)) system in management of severe reflux after sleeve gastrectomy. *Am J Surg.* 2019;217:496–499.

41. Muls V, Eckardt AJ, Marchese M, et al. Three-year results of a multicenter prospective study of transoral incisionless fundoplication. *Surg Innov*. 2013;20:321–330.
42. Bell RC, Mavrelis PG, Barnes WE, et al. A prospective multicenter registry of patients with chronic gastroesophageal reflux disease receiving transoral incisionless fundoplication. *J Am Coll Surg*. 2012;215:794–809.
43. Bell R, Lipham J, Louie B, et al. Laparoscopic magnetic sphincter augmentation versus double-dose proton pump inhibitors for management of moderate-to-severe regurgitation in GERD: a randomized controlled trial. *Gastrointest Endosc*. 2019;89:14–22e11.
44. Aiolfi A, Asti E, Bernardi D, et al. Early results of magnetic sphincter augmentation versus fundoplication for gastroesophageal reflux disease: systematic review and meta-analysis. *Int J Surg*. 2018;52:82–88.
45. Alicuben ET, Bell RCW, Jobe BA, et al. Worldwide experience with erosion of the magnetic sphincter augmentation device. *J Gastrointest Surg*. 2018;22:1442–1447.
46. Stylopoulos N, Gazelle GS, Rattner DW. Paraesophageal hernias: operation or observation? *Ann Surg*. 2002;236:492–500; discussion 500–491.
47. Oelschlager BK, Pellegrini CA, Hunter J, et al. Biologic prosthesis reduces recurrence after laparoscopic paraesophageal hernia repair: a multicenter, prospective, randomized trial. *Ann Surg*. 2006;244:481–490.
48. Oelschlager BK, Pellegrini CA, Hunter JG, et al. Biologic prosthesis to prevent recurrence after laparoscopic paraesophageal hernia repair: long-term follow-up from a multicenter, prospective, randomized trial. *J Am Coll Surg*. 2011;213:461–468.

SECTION X

Abdomen

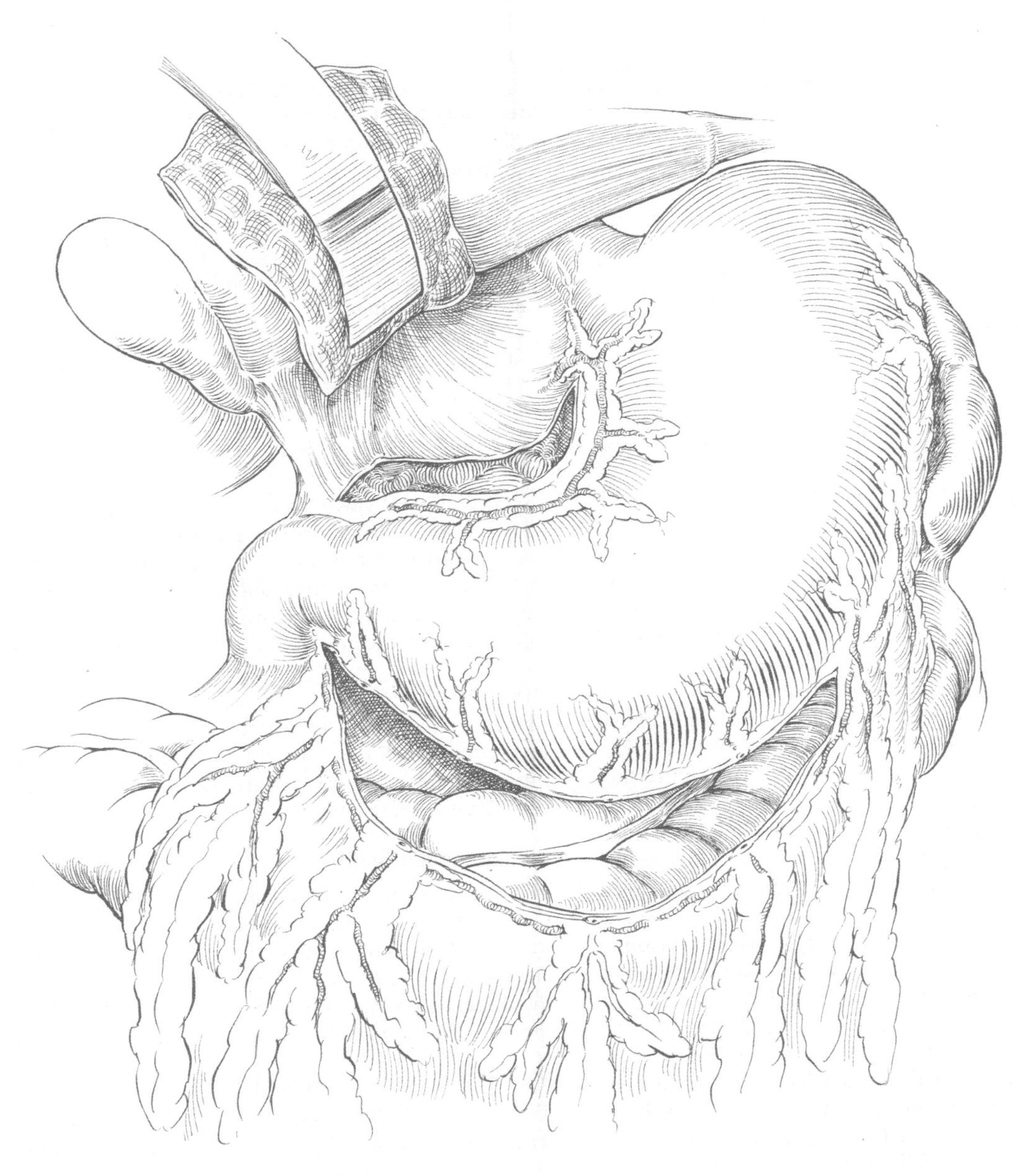

44 CHAPTER

Abdominal Wall, Umbilicus, Peritoneum, Mesenteries, Omentum and Retroperitoneum

Anna M. Privratsky, Juan Camilo Barreto, Richard H. Turnage

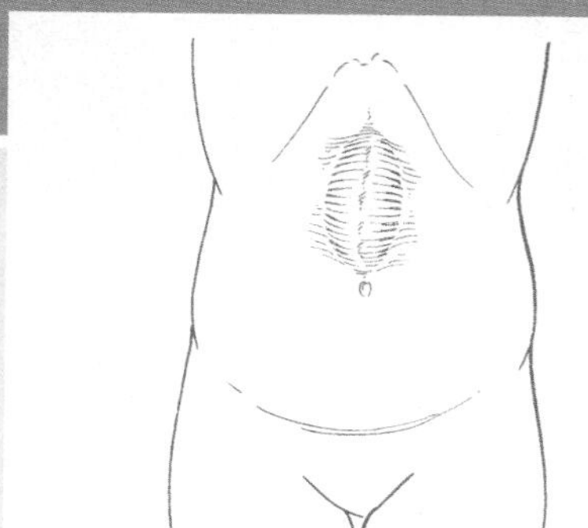

OUTLINE

ABDOMINAL WALL AND UMBILICUS

Embryology

The abdominal wall begins to develop in the earliest stages of embryonic differentiation from the lateral plate of the embryonic mesoderm. At this stage, the embryo consists of three principal layers—an outer protective layer termed the *ectoderm*; an inner nutritive layer, the *endoderm*; and the *mesoderm*.

The mesoderm becomes divided by clefts on each side of the lateral plate that ultimately develop into somatic and splanchnic layers. The splanchnic layer with its underlying endoderm contributes to the formation of the viscera by differentiating into muscle, blood vessels, lymphatics, and connective tissues of the alimentary tract. The somatic layer contributes to the development of the abdominal wall. Proliferation of mesodermal cells in the embryonic abdominal wall results in the formation of an inverted U–shaped tube that in its early stages communicates freely with the extraembryonic coelom.

As the embryo enlarges and the abdominal wall components grow toward one another, the ventral open area, bounded by the edge of the amnion, becomes smaller. This results in the development of the umbilical cord as a tubular structure containing the omphalomesenteric duct, allantois, and fetal blood vessels, which pass to and from the placenta. By the end of the third month of gestation, the body wall has closed, except at the umbilical ring. Because the alimentary tract increases in length more rapidly than the coelomic cavity increases in volume, much of the developing gut protrudes through the umbilical ring to lie within the umbilical cord. As the coelomic cavity enlarges to accommodate the intestine, the intestine returns to the peritoneal cavity so that only the omphalomesenteric duct, allantois, and fetal blood vessels pass through the shrinking umbilical ring. At birth, blood no longer courses through the umbilical vessels, and the omphalomesenteric duct has been reduced to a fibrous cord that no longer communicates with the intestine. After division of the umbilical cord, the umbilical ring heals rapidly by scarring.

Anatomy

There are nine layers to the abdominal wall: skin, subcutaneous tissue, superficial fascia, external oblique muscle, internal oblique muscle, transversus abdominis muscle, transversalis fascia, preperitoneal adipose and areolar tissue, and peritoneum (Fig. 44.1).

Subcutaneous Tissues

The subcutaneous tissue consists of Camper and Scarpa fasciae. Camper fascia is the more superficial adipose layer that contains the bulk of the subcutaneous fat. Scarpa fascia is a deeper, denser layer of fibrous connective tissue contiguous with the fascia lata of the thigh. Approximation of Scarpa fascia aids in the alignment of the skin after surgical incisions in the lower abdomen.

Muscle and Investing Fasciae

The muscles of the anterolateral abdominal wall include the external and internal oblique and transversus abdominis. These flat muscles enclose much of the circumference of the torso and give rise anteriorly to a broad flat aponeurosis investing the rectus abdominis muscles, termed the *rectus sheath*. The external oblique muscles are the largest and thickest of the flat abdominal wall

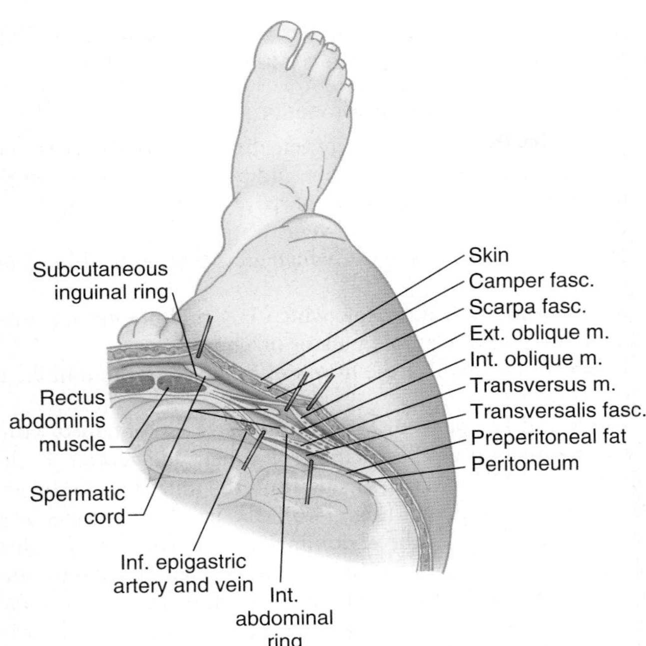

FIG. 44.1 The nine layers of the anterolateral abdominal wall. (From Thorek P. *Anatomy in Surgery*. 2nd ed. Philadelphia: JB Lippincott; 1962:358.)

muscles. They originate from the lower seven ribs and course in a superolateral to inferomedial direction. The most posterior of the fibers run vertically downward to insert into the anterior half of the iliac crest. At the midclavicular line, the muscle fibers give rise to a flat, strong aponeurosis that passes anteriorly to the rectus sheath to insert medially into the linea alba (Fig. 44.2). The lower portion of the external oblique aponeurosis is rolled posteriorly and superiorly on itself to form a groove on which the spermatic cord lies. This portion of the external oblique aponeurosis extends from the anterior superior iliac spine to the pubic tubercle and is termed the *inguinal* or *Poupart ligament.* The inguinal ligament is the lower free edge of the external oblique aponeurosis posterior to which pass the femoral artery, vein, and nerve and the iliacus, psoas major, and pectineus muscles. A femoral hernia passes posterior to the inguinal ligament, whereas an inguinal hernia passes anterior and superior to this ligament. The shelving edge of the inguinal ligament is used in various repairs of inguinal hernia such as the Bassini and the Lichtenstein tension-free repairs (see Chapter 45).

The internal oblique muscle originates from the iliopsoas fascia beneath the lateral half of the inguinal ligament, from the anterior two thirds of the iliac crest and lumbodorsal fascia. Its fibers course in a direction opposite to those of the external oblique (i.e., inferolateral to superomedial). The uppermost fibers insert into the lower five ribs and their cartilages (Figs. 44.2A and 44.3). The central fibers form an aponeurosis at the semilunar line, which, above the semicircular line (of Douglas), is divided into anterior and posterior lamellae that envelop the rectus abdominis muscle. Below the semicircular line, the aponeurosis of the internal oblique muscle courses anteriorly to the rectus abdominis muscle as part of the anterior rectus sheath. The lowermost fibers of the internal oblique muscle pursue an inferomedial course, paralleling that of the spermatic cord, to insert between the symphysis pubis and pubic tubercle. Some of the lower muscle fascicles accompany the spermatic cord into the scrotum as the cremasteric muscle.

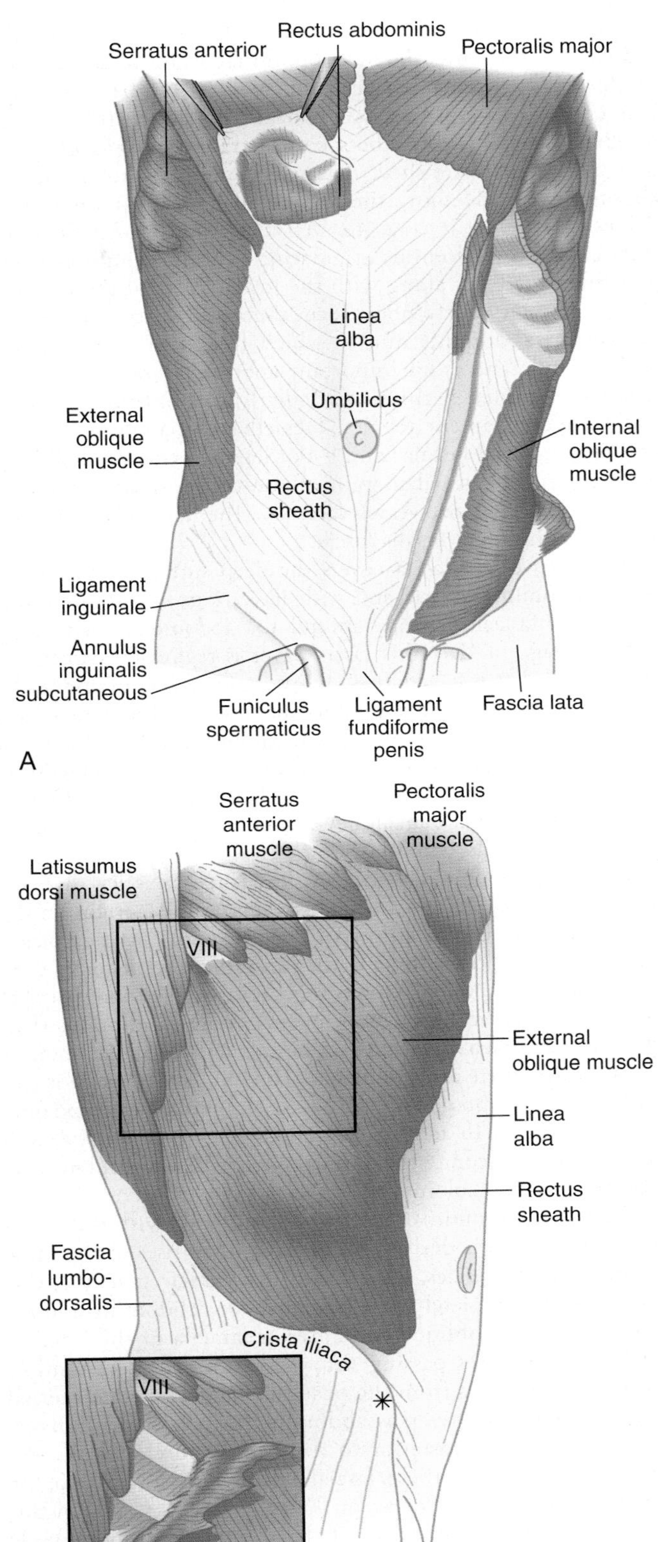

FIG. 44.2 (A) External oblique, internal oblique, and rectus abdominis muscles and anterior rectus sheath. (B) Lateral view of the external oblique muscle and its aponeurosis as it enters the anterior rectus sheath. *Inset,* Origin of the external oblique muscle fibers from the lower ribs and their costal cartilages. (From McVay C. *Anson and McVay's Surgical Anatomy.* 6th ed. Philadelphia: WB Saunders; 1984:477–478.) *Anterior superior iliac spine.

The transversus abdominis muscle is the smallest of the muscles of the anterolateral abdominal wall. It arises from the lower six costal cartilages, spines of the lumbar vertebrae, iliac crest, and iliopsoas fascia beneath the lateral third of the inguinal ligament. The fibers course transversely to give rise to a flat aponeurotic sheet that passes posterior to the rectus abdominis muscle above the semicircular line and anterior to the muscle below it (Fig. 44.4A). The inferiormost fibers of the transversus abdominis originating from the iliopsoas fascia pass inferomedially along with the lower fibers of the internal oblique muscle. These fibers form the aponeurotic arch of the transversus abdominis muscle which lies superior to Hesselbach triangle and is an important anatomic landmark in the repair of inguinal hernias, particularly the Bassini operation and Cooper ligament repairs. Hesselbach triangle is the site of direct inguinal hernias and is bordered by the inguinal ligament inferiorly, lateral margin of the rectus sheath medially, and inferior epigastric vessels laterally. The floor of Hesselbach triangle is the transversalis fascia.

The transversalis fascia covers the deep surface of the transversus abdominis muscle and with its various extensions forms a complete fascial envelope around the abdominal cavity (Fig. 44.5; see Fig. 44.4B). This fascial layer is regionally named for the muscles that it covers (e.g., iliopsoas fascia, obturator fascia, and inferior fascia of the respiratory diaphragm). The transversalis fascia binds together the muscle and aponeurotic fascicles into a continuous layer and reinforces weak areas where the aponeurotic fibers are sparse. This layer is responsible for the structural integrity of the abdominal wall, and by definition, a hernia results from a defect in the transversalis fascia.

The rectus abdominis muscles are paired muscles that appear as long, flat, triangular ribbons wider at their origin on the anterior surfaces of the fifth, sixth, and seventh costal cartilages and the xiphoid process than at their insertion on the pubic crest and pubic symphysis. Each muscle is composed of long parallel fascicles interrupted by three to five tendinous inscriptions (Fig. 44.5), which attach the rectus abdominis muscle to the anterior rectus sheath. There is no similar attachment to the posterior rectus sheath. These muscles lie adjacent to each other, separated only by the linea alba. In addition to supporting the abdominal wall and protecting its contents, contraction of these powerful muscles flexes the vertebral column.

The rectus abdominis muscles are contained within the rectus sheath, which is derived from the aponeuroses of the three flat abdominal muscles. Superior to the semicircular line, this fascial sheath completely envelops the rectus abdominis muscle with the external oblique and anterior lamella of the internal oblique aponeuroses passing anterior to the rectus abdominis and the aponeuroses from the posterior lamella of the internal oblique muscle, transversus abdominis muscle, and transversalis fascia passing posterior to the rectus muscle. Below the semicircular line, all these fascial layers pass anterior to the rectus abdominis muscle except the transversalis fascia. In this location, the posterior aspect of the rectus abdominis muscle is covered only by transversalis fascia, preperitoneal areolar tissue, and peritoneum.

The rectus abdominis muscles are held closely in apposition near the anterior midline by the linea alba. The linea alba consists of a band of dense, crisscrossed fibers of the aponeuroses of the broad abdominal muscles that extends from the xiphoid to the pubic symphysis. It is much wider above the umbilicus than below, thus facilitating the placement of surgical incisions in the midline without entering the right or left rectus sheath.

Preperitoneal Space and Peritoneum

The preperitoneal space lies between the transversalis fascia and parietal peritoneum and contains adipose and areolar tissue. Coursing through the preperitoneal space are the following:

- Inferior epigastric artery and vein
- Medial umbilical ligaments, which are the vestiges of the fetal umbilical arteries
- Median umbilical ligament, which is a midline fibrous remnant of the fetal allantoic stalk or urachus
- Falciform ligament of the liver, extending from the umbilicus to the liver

The round ligament, or ligamentum teres, is contained within the free margin of the falciform ligament and represents the obliterated umbilical vein coursing from the umbilicus to the left branch of the portal vein (Fig. 44.6). The parietal peritoneum is the innermost layer of the abdominal wall. It consists of a thin layer of dense, irregular connective tissue covered on its inner surface by a single layer of squamous mesothelium. The anatomy and physiology of the peritoneum are covered in greater depth later in this chapter.

Vessels and Nerves of the Abdominal Wall

Vascular Supply

The anterolateral abdominal wall receives its arterial supply from the last six intercostal and four lumbar arteries, superior and inferior epigastric arteries, and deep circumflex iliac arteries (Fig. 44.7). The trunks of the intercostal and lumbar arteries, together with the intercostal, iliohypogastric, and ilioinguinal nerves, course between the transversus abdominis and internal oblique muscles. The distal-most extensions of these vessels pierce the lateral margins of the rectus sheath at various levels and communicate with branches of the superior and inferior epigastric arteries. The superior epigastric artery, one of the terminal branches of the internal mammary artery, reaches the posterior surface of the rectus abdominis muscle through the costoxiphoid space in the diaphragm. It descends within the rectus sheath to anastomose with branches of the inferior epigastric artery. The inferior epigastric artery, derived from the external iliac artery just proximal to the inguinal ligament, courses through the preperitoneal areolar tissue to enter the lateral rectus sheath at the semilunar line of Douglas. The deep circumflex iliac artery, arising from the lateral aspect of the external iliac artery near the origin of the inferior epigastric artery, gives rise to an ascending branch that penetrates the abdominal wall musculature just above the iliac crest, near the anterior superior iliac spine.

The venous drainage of the anterior abdominal wall follows a relatively simple pattern in which the superficial veins above the umbilicus empty into the superior vena cava by way of the internal mammary, intercostal, and long thoracic veins. The veins inferior to the umbilicus, the superficial epigastric, circumflex iliac, and pudendal veins, converge toward the saphenous opening in the groin to enter the saphenous vein and become a tributary to the inferior vena cava (Fig. 44.8). The numerous anastomoses between the infraumbilical and supraumbilical venous systems provide collateral pathways whereby venous return to the heart may bypass an obstruction of the superior or inferior vena cava. The paraumbilical vein, which passes from the left branch of the portal vein along the ligamentum teres to the umbilicus,

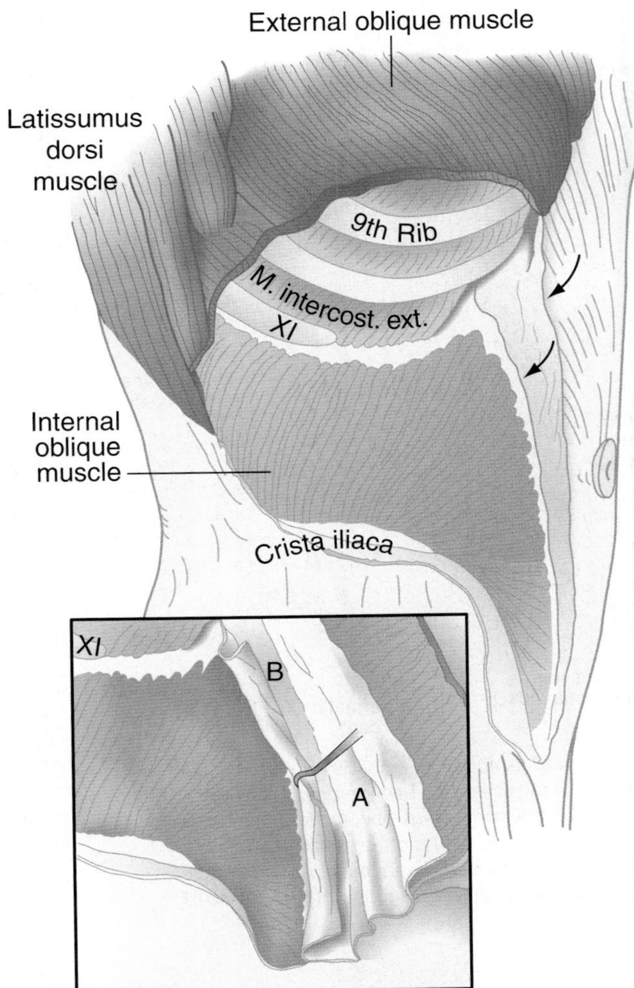

FIG. 44.3 Lateral view of the internal oblique muscle. The external oblique muscle has been removed to show the underlying internal oblique muscle originating from the lower ribs and costal cartilages. (From McVay C. *Anson and McVay's Surgical Anatomy*. 6th ed. Philadelphia: WB Saunders; 1984:479.)

provides important communication between the veins of the superficial abdominal wall and portal system in patients with portal venous obstruction. In this setting, portal blood flow is diverted away from the higher pressure portal system through the paraumbilical veins to the lower pressure veins of the anterior abdominal wall. In this setting, dilated superficial paraumbilical veins are termed *caput medusae*.

The lymphatic supply of the abdominal wall follows a pattern similar to the venous drainage. Those lymphatic vessels arising from the supraumbilical region drain into the axillary lymph nodes, whereas those arising from the infraumbilical region drain toward the superficial inguinal lymph nodes. The lymphatic vessels from the liver course along the ligamentum teres to the umbilicus to communicate with the lymphatics of the anterior abdominal wall. It is from this pathway that carcinoma in the liver may spread to involve the anterior abdominal wall at the umbilicus (Sister Mary Joseph node or nodule).

Innervation

The anterior rami of the thoracic nerves follow a curvilinear course forward in the intercostal spaces toward the midline of the body (see Fig. 44.7). The upper six thoracic nerves end near the sternum as anterior cutaneous sensory branches. Thoracic nerves 7 to 12 pass behind the costal cartilages and lower ribs to enter a plane between the internal oblique muscle and the transversus abdominis. The seventh and eighth nerves course slightly upward or horizontally to reach the epigastrium, whereas the lower nerves have an increasingly caudal trajectory. As these nerves course medially, they provide motor branches to the abdominal wall musculature. Medially, they perforate the rectus sheath to provide sensory innervation to the anterior abdominal wall. The anterior ramus of the tenth thoracic nerve reaches the skin at the level of the umbilicus, and the twelfth thoracic nerve innervates the skin of the hypogastrium.

The ilioinguinal and iliohypogastric nerves often arise in common from the anterior rami of the twelfth thoracic and first lumbar nerves to provide sensory innervation to the hypogastrium and lower abdominal wall. The iliohypogastric nerve runs parallel to the twelfth thoracic nerve to pierce the transversus abdominis muscle near the iliac crest. After coursing between the transversus abdominis muscle and internal oblique for a short distance, the nerve pierces the internal oblique to travel under the external oblique fascia toward the external inguinal ring. It emerges through the superior crus of the external inguinal ring to provide sensory innervation to the anterior abdominal wall in the hypogastrium. The ilioinguinal nerve courses parallel to the iliohypogastric nerve but closer to the inguinal ligament than the iliohypogastric nerve. Unlike the iliohypogastric nerve, the ilioinguinal nerve courses with the spermatic cord to emerge from the external inguinal ring with its terminal branches providing sensory innervation to the skin of the inguinal region and scrotum or labium. The ilioinguinal nerve, iliohypogastric nerve, and genital branch of the genitofemoral nerve are commonly encountered during the performance of inguinal herniorrhaphy.

Abnormalities of the Abdominal Wall

Congenital Abnormalities

Umbilical hernias. Umbilical hernias may be classified into three distinct forms: omphalocele and gastroschisis, infantile umbilical hernia, and acquired umbilical hernia.

Omphalocele. An omphalocele is a funnel-shaped defect in the central abdomen through which the viscera protrude into the base of the umbilical cord. It is caused by failure of the abdominal wall musculature to unite in the midline during fetal development. The umbilical vessels may be splayed over the viscera or pushed to one side. In larger defects, the liver and spleen may lie within the cord, along with a major portion of the bowel. There is no skin covering these defects, only peritoneum and, more superficially, amnion. Of infants who are born with an omphalocele, 50% to 60% will have concomitant congenital anomalies of the skeleton, gastrointestinal (GI) tract, nervous system, genitourinary (GU) system, or cardiopulmonary system.

Gastroschisis. Gastroschisis is a congenital defect of the abdominal wall in which the umbilical membrane has ruptured in utero allowing the intestine to herniate outside the abdominal cavity. The defect is almost always to the right of the umbilical cord, and the intestine is not covered with skin or amnion. Typically, the intestine has not undergone complete mesenteric rotation and fixation; hence, the infant is at risk for mesenteric volvulus with resultant intestinal ischemia and necrosis. Concomitant congenital anomalies occur in about 10% of these patients. Both omphalocele and gastroschisis are discussed in greater detail in Chapter 67.

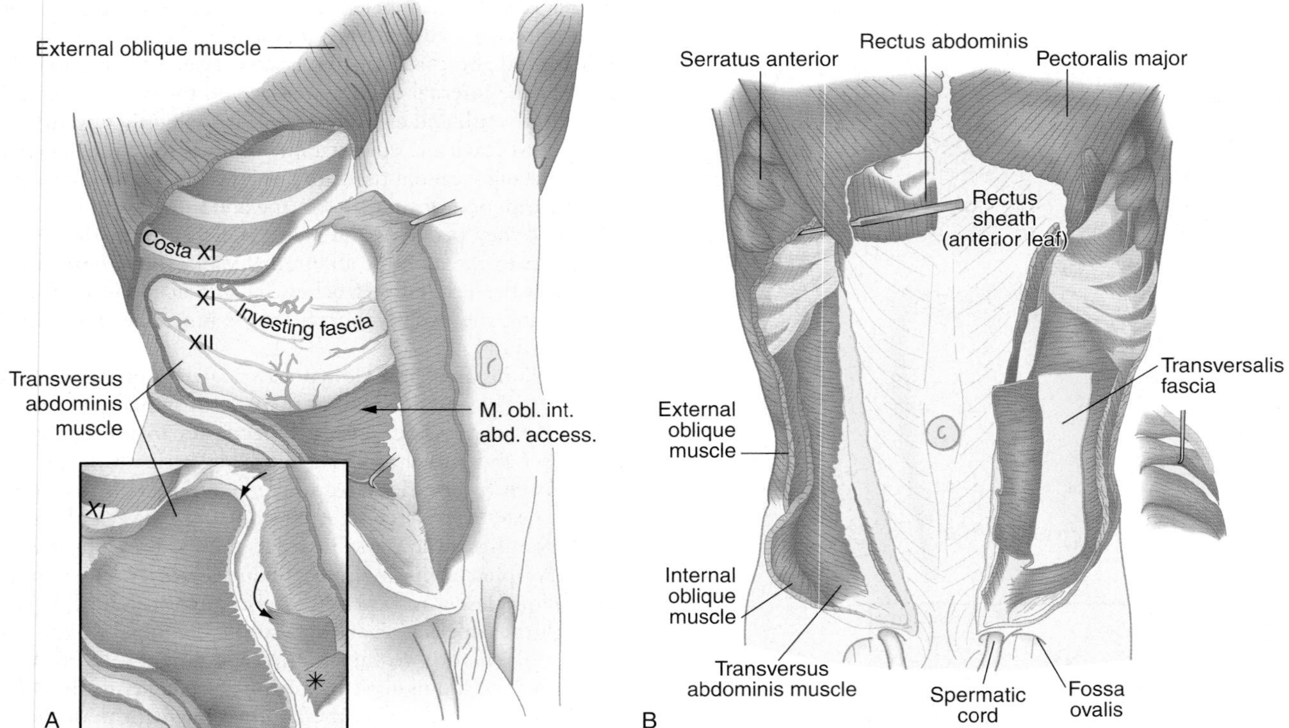

FIG. 44.4 (A) Anterolateral view of the investing fascia of the transversus abdominis muscle and the muscle itself with the fascia removed *(inset)*. The external and internal oblique muscles have been removed. Also note the appearance of the intercostal nerves lying between the fascia of the transversus abdominis muscle and internal oblique muscle. (B) Anterior view of the transversus abdominis muscle *(left)* and the transversalis fascia *(right)*. Note that the transversalis fascia is shown by reflecting the overlying transversus abdominis muscle medially. (From McVay C. *Anson and McVay's Surgical Anatomy*. 6th ed. Philadelphia: WB Saunders; 1984:480–481.)

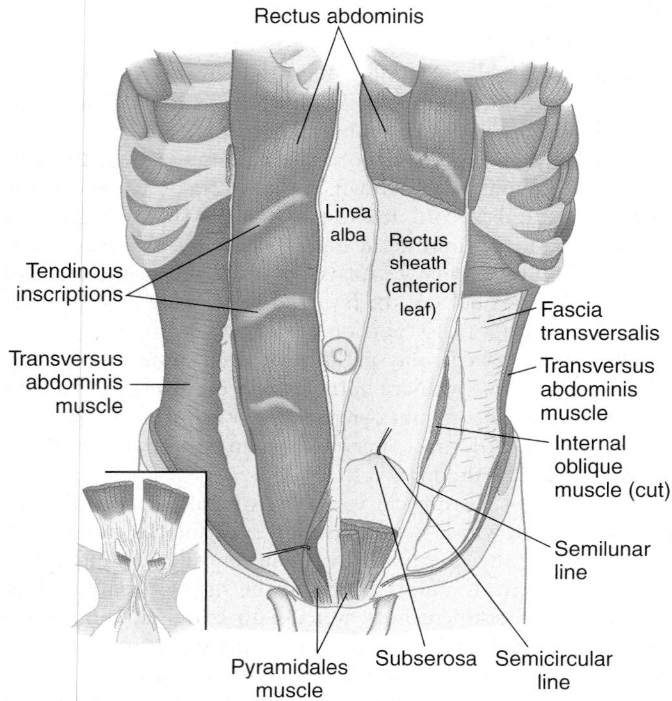

FIG. 44.5 Rectus abdominis muscle and contents of the rectus sheath. Note the semicircular line, below which the posterior rectus sheath is absent; the rectus abdominis muscle overlies the transversalis fascia, preperitoneal areolar tissue, and peritoneum. (From McVay C. *Anson and McVay's Surgical Anatomy*. 6th ed. Philadelphia: WB Saunders; 1984:482.)

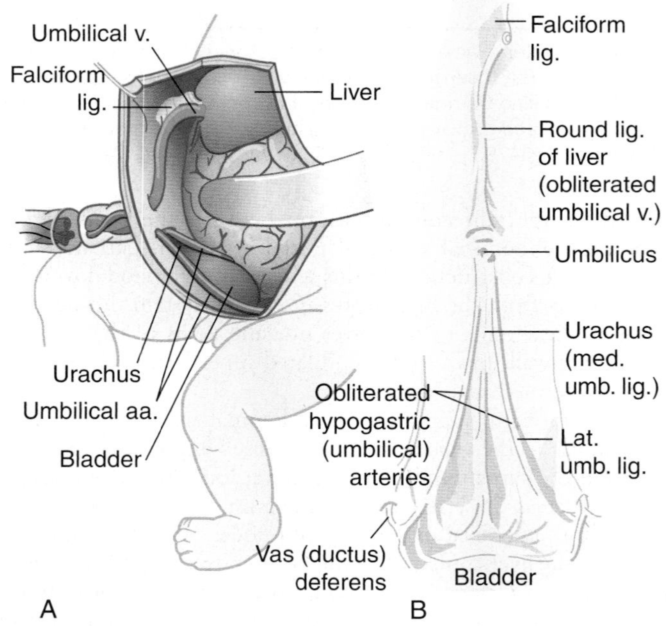

FIG. 44.6 Umbilicus. (A) In the fetus, the umbilical vein superiorly and the two umbilical arteries and urachus inferiorly radiate from the umbilicus. (B) View of the umbilicus from within the peritoneal cavity showing the round ligament of the liver (derived from the obliterated umbilical vein) superiorly and the median umbilical ligament (derived from the obliterated urachus) and medial umbilical ligaments (also called the lateral umbilical ligaments, derived from the obliterated umbilical arteries). (From Thorek P. *Anatomy in Surgery*. 2nd ed. Philadelphia: JB Lippincott; 1962:375.)

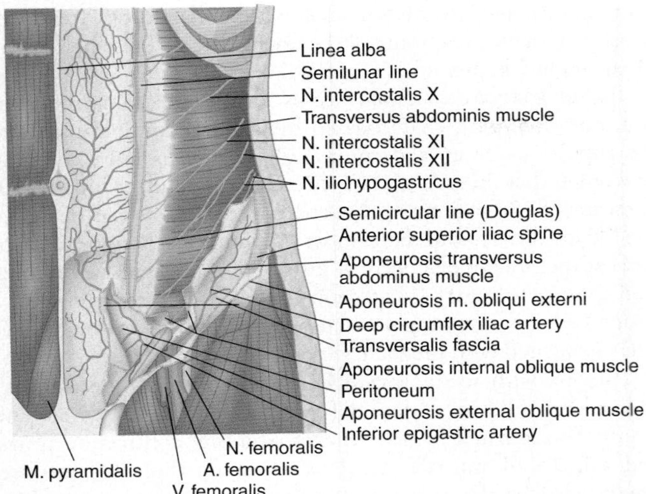

FIG. 44.7 Arteries and nerves of the anterolateral abdominal wall. (From McVay C. *Anson and McVay's Surgical Anatomy.* 6th ed. Philadelphia: WB Saunders; 1984:501.)

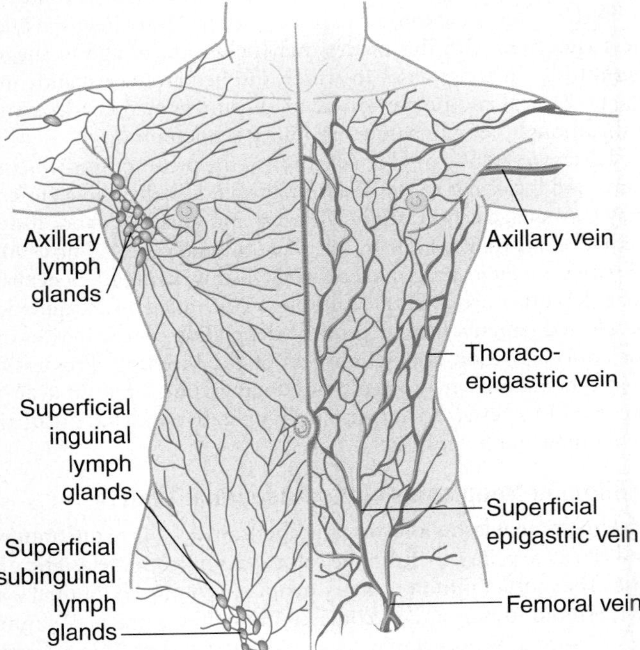

FIG. 44.8 Venous and lymphatic drainage of the anterolateral abdominal wall. (From Thorek P. *Anatomy in Surgery.* 2nd ed. Philadelphia: JB Lippincott; 1962:345.)

Infantile umbilical hernia. Infantile umbilical hernia appears within a few days or weeks after the stump of the umbilical cord has sloughed. It is caused by a weakness in the adhesion between the scarred remnants of the umbilical cord and umbilical ring. In contrast to omphalocele, the infantile umbilical hernia is covered by skin. In general, these small hernias occur in the superior margin of the umbilical ring. They are easily reducible and become prominent when the infant cries. Most of these hernias resolve within the first 24 months of life and complications such as strangulation are rare. Operative repair is indicated for those children in whom the hernia persists beyond the age of 3 or 4 years. This condition and its management are discussed further in Chapters 45 and 67.

Acquired umbilical hernia. In this condition, an umbilical hernia develops at a time remote from closure of the umbilical ring. This hernia occurs most commonly at the upper margin of the umbilicus and results from weakening of the cicatricial tissue that normally closes the umbilical ring. This weakening can be caused by excessive stretching of the abdominal wall, which may occur with pregnancy, vigorous labor, or ascites. In contrast to infantile umbilical hernias, acquired umbilical hernias do not spontaneously resolve but gradually increase in size. The dense fibrous ring at the neck of this hernia makes strangulation of herniated intestine or omentum an important complication.

Abnormalities resulting from persistence of the omphalomesenteric duct. During fetal development, the midgut communicates widely with the yolk sac through the vitelline or omphalomesenteric duct. As the abdominal wall components approximate one another, the omphalomesenteric duct narrows and comes to lie within the umbilical cord. Over time, communication between the yolk sac and intestine becomes obliterated, and the intestine resides free within the peritoneal cavity. Persistence of part or all of the omphalomesenteric duct results in a variety of abnormalities related to the intestine and abdominal wall (Fig. 44.9).

Persistence of the intestinal end of the omphalomesenteric duct results in Meckel diverticulum. These true diverticula arise from the antimesenteric border of the small intestine, most often the ileum. A rule of 2s may be applicable to these lesions in that they are found in approximately 2% of the population, are within 2 feet of the ileocecal valve, are often 2 inches in length, and contain two types of ectopic mucosa (gastric and pancreatic). Meckel diverticula may be complicated by inflammation, perforation, hemorrhage, or obstruction. GI bleeding is caused by peptic ulceration of adjacent intestinal mucosa from hydrochloric acid secreted by ectopic parietal cells located within the diverticulum. Intestinal obstruction associated with Meckel diverticulum is usually caused by intussusception or volvulus around an abnormal fibrous connection between the diverticulum and posterior aspect of the umbilicus. These lesions are discussed in Chapter 50.

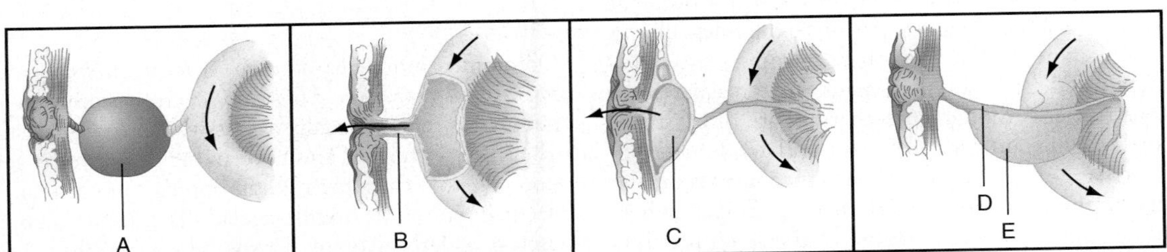

FIG. 44.9 Abnormalities resulting from persistence of the omphalomesenteric duct. (A) Omphalomesenteric duct cyst. (B) Persistent omphalomesenteric duct with an enterocutaneous fistula. (C) Omphalomesenteric duct cyst and sinus. (D) Fibrous cord between the small intestine and the posterior surface of the umbilicus. (E) Meckel diverticulum. (From McVay C. *Anson and McVay's Surgical Anatomy.* 6th ed. Philadelphia: WB Saunders; 1984:576.)

The omphalomesenteric duct may remain patent throughout its course, producing an enterocutaneous fistula between the distal small intestine and umbilicus. This condition is manifested with the passage of meconium and mucus from the umbilicus in the first few days of life. Because of the risk for mesenteric volvulus around a persistent omphalomesenteric duct, these lesions are promptly treated with laparotomy and excision of the fistulous tract. Persistence of the distal end of the omphalomesenteric duct results in an umbilical polyp, which is a small excrescence of omphalomesenteric ductal mucosa at the umbilicus. Such polyps resemble umbilical granulomas except that they do not disappear after silver nitrate cauterization. Their presence suggests that a persistent omphalomesenteric duct or umbilical sinus may be present, and hence they are most appropriately treated by excision of the mucosal remnant and underlying omphalomesenteric duct or umbilical sinus, if present. Umbilical sinuses result from the persistence of the distal omphalomesenteric duct. The morphology of the sinus tract can be delineated by a sinogram. Treatment involves excision of the sinus. Finally, the accumulation of mucus in a portion of a persistent omphalomesenteric duct may result in the formation of a cyst, which may be associated with the intestine or umbilicus by a fibrous band. Treatment consists of excision of the cyst and associated persistent omphalomesenteric duct.

Abnormalities resulting from persistence of the allantois. The allantois is the cranial-most component of the embryologic ventral cloaca. The intraabdominal portion is termed the *urachus* and connects the urinary bladder with the umbilicus, whereas the extraabdominal allantois is contained within the umbilical cord. At the end of gestation, the urachus is converted into a fibrous cord that courses between the extraperitoneal urinary bladder and umbilicus as the median umbilical ligament. Persistence of part or all of the urachus may result in the formation of a vesicocutaneous fistula with the appearance of urine at the umbilicus, an extraperitoneal urachal cyst presenting as a lower abdominal mass, or an urachal sinus with the drainage of a small amount of mucus. Because of the risk of complications, including transformation into malignancy, treatment is excision of the urachal remnant with closure of the bladder if necessary.

Acquired Abnormalities

Diastasis recti. Diastasis recti refers to a thinning of the linea alba in the epigastrium and is manifested as a smooth midline protrusion of the anterior abdominal wall. The transversalis fascia is intact, and hence this is not a hernia. There are no identifiable fascial margins and no risk for intestinal strangulation. The presence of diastasis recti may be particularly noticeable to the patient on straining or when lifting the head from the pillow. Appropriate treatment consists of reassurance of the patient and family about the innocuous nature of this condition.

Anterior abdominal wall hernias. Epigastric hernias occur at sites through which vessels and nerves perforate the linea alba to course into the subcutaneum. Through these openings, extraperitoneal areolar tissue and, at times, peritoneum may herniate into the subcutaneous tissue. Although these hernias are often small, they may produce significant localized pain and tenderness because of direct pressure of the hernia sac and its contents on the nerves emerging through the same fascial opening. Spigelian hernias occur through the fascia in the region of the semilunar line and are manifested with localized pain and tenderness. The hernia sac is only rarely palpable because it is often small and tends to remain beneath the external oblique aponeurosis. Ultrasonography of the abdominal wall or computed tomography (CT) with thin cuts through the abdomen should be diagnostic. Treatment consists of operative closure of the fascial defect. These hernias are discussed in Chapter 45.

Rectus sheath hematoma. Rectus sheath hematoma is an uncommon condition characterized by acute abdominal pain and the appearance of an abdominal wall mass. It is more common in women than in men and in older than in younger individuals. A review of 126 patients with rectus sheath hematomas treated at the Mayo Clinic found that almost 70% were receiving anticoagulants at the time of diagnosis. A history of nonsurgical abdominal wall trauma or injury is common (48%), as is the presence of a cough (29%).[1] In young women, rectus sheath hematomas have been associated with pregnancy.

Patients with rectus sheath hematomas usually present with the sudden onset of abdominal pain, which may be severe and is often exacerbated by movements requiring contraction of the abdominal wall musculature. Physical examination demonstrates tenderness over the rectus sheath often with voluntary guarding. An abdominal wall mass may be noted in some patients, 63% in the Mayo Clinic series.[1] Abdominal wall ecchymosis, including periumbilical ecchymosis (Cullen sign) and blue discoloration in the flanks (Grey Turner sign), may be present if there is a delay from the onset of symptoms to presentation. The pain and tenderness associated with this process may be severe enough to suggest peritonitis. In those cases in which the hematoma expands into the perivesical and preperitoneal spaces, the hematocrit level may fall, although hemodynamic instability is uncommon.

Ultrasonography or CT will confirm the presence of the hematoma and localize it to the abdominal wall. Usually, these patients may be managed successfully with rest and analgesics and, if necessary, blood transfusion. In the Mayo Clinic series, almost 90% of patients were managed successfully in this manner.[1] In general, coagulopathies are corrected, although continued anticoagulation of selected patients may be prudent depending on the indications for anticoagulation and seriousness of the bleeding. Progression of the hematoma may necessitate angiographic embolization of the bleeding vessel or uncommonly operative evacuation of the hematoma and hemostasis.

Malignant Neoplasms of the Abdominal Wall

Malignant neoplasms affecting the abdominal wall are uncommon and can arise primarily from the soft tissues or from metastatic disease. The most common primary neoplasms of the abdominal wall are desmoid tumors and sarcomas. Although it is unusual, a number of common cancers may metastasize through the bloodstream to the soft tissue of the abdominal wall. Melanoma, in particular, may metastasize in this manner. Finally, transperitoneal seeding of the abdominal wall by intraabdominal malignant neoplasms may complicate transabdominal biopsies or operative procedures.

Desmoid Tumor

Desmoid tumors, also known as *fibromatosis*, *aggressive fibromatosis*, or *desmoid-type fibromatosis*, are uncommon mesenchymal neoplasms that are locally aggressive but lack metastatic potential. They are rare tumors and have an incidence in the general population of 2 to 4 cases per million population per year. These tumors occur in young or middle-age adults and are uncommon in children or elderly patients. In sporadic cases, there is a female predominance of two to one. Ten to 15% of cases occur in patients with familial adenomatous polyposis (FAP), Gardner syndrome (FAP, desmoid tumor, and osteomas of the skull and mandible, sebaceous cysts, and cutaneous and subcutaneous fibromas), or

Turcot syndrome (FAP and brain tumor). Males are affected as commonly as females in these instances.

Desmoid tumors encompass at least two distinct clinicopathological entities based on their underlying molecular biology. Sporadic desmoid tumors are most commonly associated with somatic mutations of the *CTNNB1* gene, causing an abnormal stabilization of β-catenin, accumulation of β-catenin within the nucleus, and activation of the Wnt signaling pathway. This results in dysregulated gene transcription, the activation of oncogenes, and tumor production.[2] Desmoid tumors associated with FAP are caused by germline mutations of the adenomatous polyposis coli *(APC)* gene.[3,4] Normally *APC* regulates cellular β-catenin levels by participating in the phosphorylation, ubiquitination, and degradation of β-catenin in the proteasome. Patients with FAP possess a truncated, inactive form of the APC protein, causing the accumulation of nuclear β-catenin and the overexpression of target oncogenes.[4]

Typically, desmoid tumors present as a firm, nonpainful, nontender mass in the abdominal wall, shoulder, hip, limbs, mesentery, or pelvis. About 10% to 15% of patients with FAP will develop a desmoid tumor, most of which are located within the mesentery or abdominal wall.[3] Desmoids infiltrate surrounding structures and spread along tissue planes and muscles. They have been associated with trauma, pregnancy, and oral contraceptive use. Surgical history is a particularly important risk factor for the occurrence of a desmoid tumor. A metaanalysis of five European FAP registries of 2260 patients identified prior surgery as an independent risk factor for the development of a desmoid tumor.[3]

Magnetic resonance imaging (MRI) is the preferred imaging modality for diagnosis, local staging, and follow-up of patients with desmoid tumors. On T1-weighted MRI images, these tumors appear as a homogeneous mass, isointense compared with muscle. T2-weighted images show a hyperintense lesion with greater heterogeneity and a signal that is slightly less intense than fat (Fig. 44.10).

The diagnosis is usually established by core needle biopsy. Histologically, desmoids are characterized by well-differentiated bundles of spindle cells with abundant collagenous matrix. The nuclear overexpression of β-catenin may be a useful diagnostic feature, although some nondesmoid soft tissue neoplasms may also exhibit this staining pattern.[5]

Traditionally, resection of the tumor with a wide margin of normal tissue was the standard of care. The locally aggressive, infiltrative nature of these tumors often required large soft tissue resections with complex reconstructive techniques to achieve tumor-free surgical margins. Local recurrence is common despite this aggressive treatment.[6] A number of retrospective studies have shown progression-free survival rates of 50% at 5 years for patients managed with a "watchful waiting" approach.[5] Spontaneous regression occurs in as many as 30% of cases.[7] These observations made "watchful waiting" the preferred strategy for managing most patients with desmoid tumors that are not causing severe symptoms or close to critical structures.[8] This approach requires close observation with physical examination and MRI to identify tumor progression as early as possible. Patients with progression of the tumor or the appearance of tumor-related complications are treated with complete resection.

Radiation therapy has been used principally as adjuvant therapy after surgical resection with positive or close resection margins.[9] It has also been used to treat patients who develop recurrent disease following resection.[10] The applicability of radiation therapy to treat young patients with abdominal wall desmoid tumors is limited by the long-term potential for radiation-induced secondary malignancies, most notably sarcoma.

Systemic treatment options for patients with desmoid tumors include antihormonal therapies, nonsteroidal antiinflammatory drugs (NSAIDs), low-dose chemotherapy, tyrosine kinase inhibitors, and full-dose chemotherapy. Antihormonal agents, such as tamoxifen, have been used either alone or in combination with NSAIDs as first-line medical therapy. Advantages to their use include limited toxicity, rare adverse events, and low cost. Observational studies have demonstrated the arrest of tumor progression with combination therapy.[11] Cytotoxic chemotherapy has also been used to treat patients with aggressively growing, symptomatic, or life-threatening desmoid tumors who are not surgical candidates and have failed treatment with antihormonal therapies and NSAIDs. Recommended regimens have included "low-dose" methotrexate with or without vinblastine/vinorelbine or conventional dose chemotherapy with anthracycline-based regimes, such as doxorubicin. Lastly, phase II studies have shown that tyrosine kinase inhibitors such as imatinib and sorafenib may produce 1-year progression-free survival rates of 66%.[5] Unfortunately, the

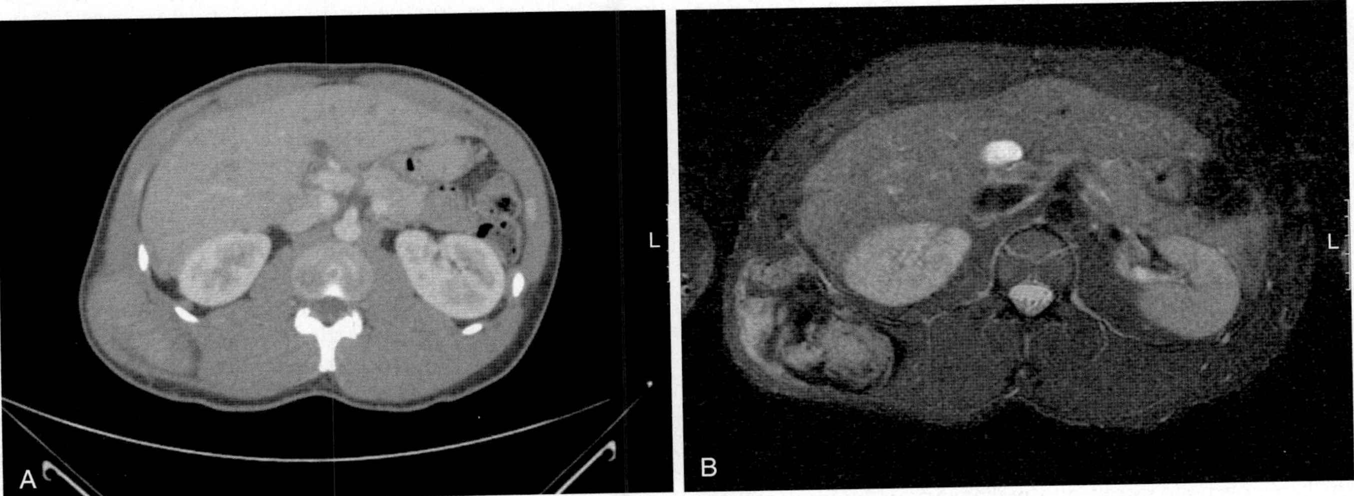

FIG. 44.10 Large posterolateral abdominal wall desmoid tumor. (A) Computed tomography scan shows a homogeneous mass to surrounding muscle. (B) Magnetic resonance imaging shows more heterogeneous appearance with areas of less intense signal.

absence of internal controls or randomization of patients in these studies of systemic therapy makes it difficult to attribute observed slowing of tumor progression to the real activity of systemic treatment versus the natural history of the disease.

Abdominal Wall Sarcoma

Soft tissue sarcomas are a diverse group of mesenchymal malignancies that account for less than 1% of malignancies. The classification of sarcomas is based on the cell type they resemble histologically and immunohistochemically. The most common subtypes of sarcoma are liposarcoma, myxofibrosarcoma, leiomyosarcoma, rhabdomyosarcoma, and undifferentiated pleomorphic sarcomas. Less than 5% of soft tissue sarcomas affect the abdominal wall.

Patients present most commonly with a firm, painless, poorly circumscribed soft tissue mass that is fixed to the surrounding skeletal muscle and fascia. Radiation exposure and genetic syndromes (i.e., neurofibromatosis and Li-Fraumeni syndrome) are important predisposing factors. Cross-sectional imaging with CT or MRI will characterize the morphology of the tumor and define its anatomic site of origin and its relationship to surrounding structures. MRI provides better definition of the soft tissues. CT of the chest can document the presence of pulmonary metastases. The diagnosis is best established by core needle biopsy. Deep lesions can be biopsied using CT guidance. Open biopsy of the tumor should be avoided because of the risk of compromising the curative resection by inappropriate orientation of the incision and promoting local extension of the tumor by raising tissue flaps or the development of a postoperative hematoma. If an open biopsy is required, it should be performed by the surgeon who will perform the definitive resection.

Standard treatment of localized disease is resection of the tumor with margins that are free of microscopic disease. Most surgeons attempt to obtain at least a 2-cm margin of normal tissue around the tumor. Less than 5% of sarcomas metastasize to lymph nodes; therefore, lymphadenectomy is not performed unless there is evidence of lymphatic spread. Resection of these tumors often results in a large soft tissue defect that requires reconstruction with a myocutaneous flap or synthetic mesh prosthesis. Radiation therapy has been used in patients with large, high-grade sarcomas either before or after resection. Much of the evidence for this approach has come from clinical trials enrolling patients with extremity sarcomas.

The prognosis of these tumors depends upon the grade and stage of the tumor and the adequacy of resection. The grade of the tumor is based on tumor differentiation, mitotic count, and the presence or absence of necrosis. The American Joint Committee on Cancer staging system combines the size of the tumor, the involvement of lymph nodes, the presence of metastases, the type and grade of the sarcoma.[12] There are no large series that address the outcomes after resection of sarcomas located in the abdominal wall exclusively. In studies that include other anatomic sites, local recurrence rates after resection with negative margins average 10% to 15%. Depth, size, positive margin status, and high tumor grade are associated with increased risk of recurrence.[13] Soft tissue sarcomas are discussed in greater detail in Chapter 32.

Metastatic Disease

Metastases from advanced malignancies may also present as soft tissue masses of the abdominal wall. These tumors may result from hematogenous spread of a malignancy or by implantation of tumor during biopsy or resection of an intraabdominal malignancy. Almost always, abdominal wall metastases occur in the setting of advanced malignancy. Malignancies most commonly associated with hematogenous metastasis to the abdominal wall include lung, colon, renal carcinoma, as well as melanoma.[14] The incidence of tumor implantation after laparoscopic colon resection for colorectal adenocarcinoma is about 1%, similar to the risk of tumor recurrence in the wound after open colectomy.[15] This occurs most frequently in the setting of peritoneal carcinomatosis.

Similar to desmoid tumors and sarcomas, these patients present with a firm abdominal wall mass that may or may not be associated with pain or tenderness. Cross-sectional imaging will characterize the mass and distinguish it from an incarcerated abdominal wall hernia. The diagnosis is established by core needle biopsy. Immunohistochemistry staining of the tumor may allow identification of the type of primary tumor and facilitate differentiation from primary sarcomas of the abdominal wall.

The treatment of abdominal wall metastases is dictated by the biology or natural history of the primary tumor, by symptoms, and by the presence of other sites of disease. The vast majority of patients will have disseminated disease, and treatment should be either palliative systemic therapy or directed toward symptom relief. Asymptomatic patients with multiple sites of disease will not need a change to this approach. Patients with symptomatic tumors not responsive to systemic therapy can benefit from selective use of radiation therapy for palliative purposes or resection if it does not cause excessive morbidity.

Symptoms of Intraabdominal Disease Referred to the Abdominal Wall

Abdominal pain may be categorized as visceral, somatoparietal, and referred. Visceral pain is caused by stimulation of visceral nociceptors by inflammation, distention, or ischemia. The pain is dull in nature and poorly localized to the epigastrium, periumbilical regions, or hypogastrium, depending on the embryonic origin of the organ involved. Inflammation of the stomach, duodenum, and biliary tract (derivatives of the embryonic foregut) localizes visceral pain to the epigastrium. Stimulation of nociceptors in midgut-derived organs (small intestine, appendix, right colon, proximal transverse colon) causes the sensation of pain in the periumbilical region, whereas inflammation or distention of hindgut-derived organs (distal transverse colon, left colon, and rectum) causes hypogastric pain. The pain is felt in the midline because these organs transmit sympathetic sensory afferents to both sides of the spinal cord. The pain is poorly localized because the innervation of most viscera is multisegmental and contains fewer nerve receptors than highly sensitive organs such as the skin. The pain is often characterized as cramping, burning, or gnawing and may be accompanied by secondary autonomic effects such as sweating, restlessness, nausea, vomiting, perspiration, and pallor.

Somatoparietal pain arises from inflammation of the parietal peritoneum; it is more intense and more precisely localized than visceral pain. The nerve impulses mediating parietal pain travel within the somatosensory spinal nerves and reach the spinal cord from the peripheral nerves corresponding to the cutaneous dermatomes from the T6 to the L1 region. Lateralization of parietal pain is possible because only one side of the nervous system innervates a given part of the parietal peritoneum.

The difference between visceral and somatoparietal pain is well illustrated by the pain associated with acute appendicitis, in which the early, vague, periumbilical visceral pain is followed by the localized somatoparietal pain at McBurney point. The visceral pain is produced by distention and inflammation of the appendix, whereas the localized somatoparietal pain in the right lower quadrant of the abdomen is caused by extension of the inflammation to the parietal peritoneum.

Referred pain is felt in anatomic regions remote from the diseased organ. This phenomenon is caused by convergence of visceral afferent neurons innervating an injured or inflamed organ with somatic afferent fibers arising from another anatomic region. This occurs within the spinal cord at the level of second-order neurons. Well-known examples of referred pain include shoulder pain on irritation of the diaphragm, scapular pain associated with acute biliary tract disease, and testicular or labial pain caused by retroperitoneal inflammation.

PERITONEUM AND PERITONEAL CAVITY

Anatomy

The peritoneum consists of a single sheet of simple squamous epithelium of mesodermal origin, termed *mesothelium,* lying on a thin connective tissue stroma. The surface area is 1.0 to 1.7 m^2, approximately that of the total body surface area. In males, the peritoneal cavity is sealed, whereas in females, it is open to the exterior through the ostia of the fallopian tubes. The peritoneal membrane is divided into parietal and visceral components. The parietal peritoneum covers the anterior, lateral, and posterior abdominal wall surfaces and the inferior surface of the diaphragm and the pelvis. The visceral peritoneum covers most of the surface of the intraperitoneal organs (i.e., stomach, jejunum, ileum, transverse colon, liver, and spleen) and the anterior aspect of the retroperitoneal organs (i.e., duodenum, left and right colon, pancreas, kidneys, adrenal glands).

The peritoneal cavity is subdivided into interconnected compartments or spaces by 11 ligaments and mesenteries. The peritoneal ligaments or mesenteries include the coronary, gastrohepatic, hepatoduodenal, falciform, gastrocolic, duodenocolic, gastrosplenic, splenorenal, and phrenicocolic ligaments and the transverse mesocolon and small bowel mesentery (Fig. 44.11). These structures partition the abdomen into nine potential spaces: right and left subphrenic, subhepatic, supramesenteric and

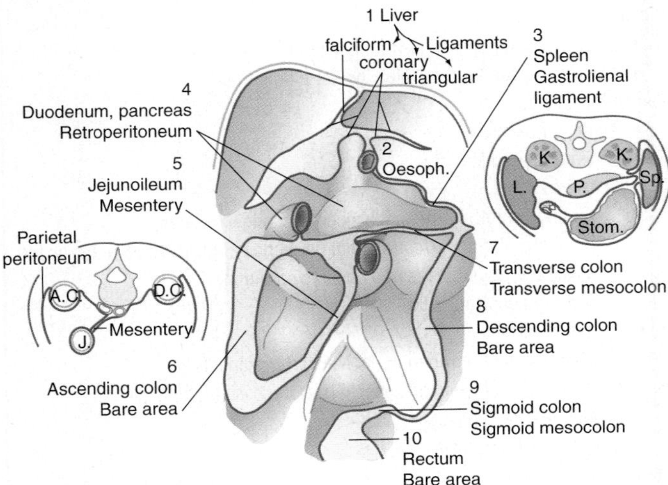

FIG. 44.11 Peritoneal ligaments and mesenteric reflections in the adult. These attachments partition the abdomen into nine potential spaces: right and left subphrenic, subhepatic, supramesenteric, and inframesenteric spaces; and right and left paracolic gutters, pelvis, and omental bursa *(inset, right).* (From McVay C. *Anson and McVay's Surgical Anatomy.* 6th ed. Philadelphia: WB Saunders; 1984:589.)

inframesenteric, right and left paracolic gutters, pelvis, and lesser space. These ligaments, mesenteries, and peritoneal spaces direct the circulation of fluid in the peritoneal cavity and thus may be useful in predicting the route of spread of infectious and malignant diseases. For example, perforation of the duodenum from peptic ulcer disease may result in the movement of fluid (and the development of abscesses) in the subhepatic space, right paracolic gutter, and pelvis. The blood supply to the visceral peritoneum is derived from the splanchnic blood vessels, whereas the parietal peritoneum is supplied by branches of the intercostal, subcostal, lumbar, and iliac vessels. The innervation of the visceral and parietal peritoneum is discussed earlier.

Physiology

The peritoneum is a bidirectional, semipermeable membrane that controls the amount of fluid in the peritoneal cavity, promotes the sequestration and removal of bacteria from the peritoneal cavity, and facilitates the migration of inflammatory cells from the microvasculature into the peritoneal cavity. Normally, the peritoneal cavity contains less than 100 mL of sterile serous fluid. Microvilli on the apical surface of the peritoneal mesothelium markedly increase the surface area and promote the rapid absorption of fluid from the peritoneal cavity into the lymphatics and portal and systemic circulations. The amount of fluid in the peritoneal cavity may increase to many liters in some diseases, such as cirrhosis, nephrotic syndrome, and peritoneal carcinomatosis.

The circulation of fluid in the peritoneal cavity is driven in part by the movement of the diaphragm. Intercellular pores in the peritoneum covering the inferior surface of the diaphragm (termed *stomata*) communicate with lymphatic pools in the diaphragm. Lymph flows from these diaphragmatic lymphatic channels through subpleural lymphatics to the regional lymph nodes and, ultimately, the thoracic duct. Relaxation of the diaphragm during exhalation opens the stomata, and the negative intrathoracic pressure draws fluid and particles, including bacteria, into the stomata. Contraction of the diaphragm during inhalation propels the lymph through the mediastinal lymphatic channels into the thoracic duct. It is postulated that this so-called diaphragmatic pump drives the movement of peritoneal fluid in a cephalad direction toward the diaphragm and into the thoracic lymphatic vessels. This circulatory pattern of peritoneal fluid toward the diaphragm and into the central lymphatic channels is consistent with the rapid appearance of sepsis in patients with generalized intra-abdominal infections as well as the perihepatitis of Fitz-Hugh-Curtis syndrome in patients with acute salpingitis.

The peritoneum and peritoneal cavity respond to infection in five ways:

1. Bacteria are rapidly removed from the peritoneal cavity through the diaphragmatic stomata and lymphatics.
2. Peritoneal macrophages release proinflammatory mediators that promote the migration of leukocytes into the peritoneal cavity from the surrounding microvasculature.
3. Degranulation of peritoneal mast cells releases histamine and other vasoactive products causing local vasodilation and the extravasation of protein-rich fluid containing complement and immunoglobulins into the peritoneal space.
4. Protein in the peritoneal fluid opsonizes bacteria, which along with activation of the complement cascade promotes neutrophil- and macrophage-mediated bacterial phagocytosis and destruction.
5. Bacteria become sequestered within fibrin matrices, thereby promoting abscess formation and limiting the generalized spread of the infection.

Peritoneal Disorders

Ascites

Pathophysiology and cause. Ascites is the pathologic accumulation of fluid in the peritoneal cavity. The principal causes of ascites formation are listed in Box 44.1 according to underlying pathophysiology. Cirrhosis is the most common cause of ascites in the United States, accounting for approximately 85% of cases. Ascites is the most common complication of cirrhosis, with approximately 50% of compensated cirrhotic patients developing ascites within 10 years of diagnosis. The onset of ascites is an important prognostic factor in patients with cirrhosis because of its association with the occurrence of spontaneous bacterial peritonitis (SBP), renal failure, worsened quality of life, and increased likelihood of death within 2 to 5 years.

In cirrhotic patients, the two principal factors underlying the formation of ascites are renal sodium and water retention and portal hypertension. Renal sodium retention is driven by activation of the renin-angiotensin-aldosterone and sympathetic nervous systems, which cause proximal and distal renal tubule sodium reabsorption. It is postulated that the abnormal release of nitric oxide within the splanchnic circulation causes vasodilation and a decrease in the effective circulating blood volume. Renin, aldosterone, and other hormones are generated as a counterregulatory mechanism to restore the effective circulating blood volume to normal. Portal hypertension is produced by postsinusoidal vascular obstruction from the deposition of collagen in the cirrhotic liver. Increased hydrostatic pressure within the hepatic sinusoids and splanchnic vasculature drives the extravasation of fluid from the microvasculature into the extracellular compartment. Ascites results when the capacity of the lymphatic system to return this fluid to the systemic circulation is overwhelmed.

Obstruction of portal venous blood flow (e.g., portal vein thrombosis) or hepatic venous blood flow (e.g., Budd-Chiari syndrome) also causes ascites formation by increasing hydrostatic pressure within the splanchnic microvasculature. A similar pressure-based mechanism contributes to ascites formation in patients with heart failure, although the release of vasopressin and renin-angiotensin-aldosterone also promotes sodium and water retention in these patients. Patients with malignant neoplasms develop ascites by one of three mechanisms:

1. Multiple hepatic metastases cause portal hypertension by narrowing or occluding branches of the portal venous system.
2. Malignant cells scattered throughout the peritoneal cavity release protein-rich fluid into the peritoneal cavity, as in peritoneal carcinomatosis.
3. Obstruction of retroperitoneal lymphatics by a tumor, such as lymphoma, causes rupture of major lymphatic channels and the leakage of chyle into the peritoneal cavity.

Finally, ascites may result from the leakage of pancreatic fluid, bile, or lymph into the peritoneal cavity after iatrogenic or inflammatory disruption of a major pancreatic, bile, or lymphatic duct.

Clinical presentation and diagnosis. The diagnosis of ascites is made on the basis of the medical history and appearance of the abdomen. Obviously, risk factors for hepatitis or cirrhosis are sought, as is evidence of cardiac disease, renal disease, or malignant disease. A full bulging abdomen with dullness of the flanks on percussion is suggestive of the presence of ascites. Approximately 1.5 L of fluid must be present before dullness can be detected by percussion. Physical evidence of cirrhosis is also sought such as palmar erythema, dilated abdominal wall collateral veins, and multiple spider angiomas. Patients with cardiac ascites have impressive jugular venous distention and other evidence of congestive heart failure.

BOX 44.1 Principal causes of ascites formation categorized by underlying pathophysiology.

Portal Hypertension

Cirrhosis

Noncirrhotic

- Prehepatic portal venous obstruction
  - Chronic mesenteric venous thrombosis
  - Multiple hepatic metastases
- Posthepatic venous obstruction: Budd-Chiari syndrome

Cardiac

Congestive heart failure

Chronic pericardial tamponade

Constrictive pericarditis

Malignant Disease

Peritoneal carcinomatosis

- Primary peritoneal malignant neoplasms
  - Primary peritoneal mesothelioma
  - Serous carcinoma
- Metastatic carcinoma
  - Gastrointestinal carcinomas (e.g., gastric, colonic, pancreatic cancer)
  - Genitourinary carcinomas (e.g., ovarian cancer)

Retroperitoneal obstruction of lymphatic channels

- Lymphoma
- Lymph node metastases (e.g., testicular cancer, melanoma)

Obstruction of the lymphatic channels at the base of the mesentery

- Gastrointestinal carcinoid tumors

Miscellaneous

Bile ascites

- Iatrogenic after operations of the liver or biliary tract
- Traumatic after injuries to the liver or biliary tract

Pancreatic ascites

- Acute pancreatitis
- Pancreatic pseudocyst

Chylous ascites

- Disruptions of retroperitoneal lymphatic channels
  - Iatrogenic during retroperitoneal dissections: retroperitoneal lymphadenectomy, abdominal aortic aneurysmorrhaphy
  - Blunt or penetrating trauma
- Malignant disease
  - Obstruction of retroperitoneal lymphatic channels
  - Obstruction of lymphatic channels at the base of the mesentery
- Congenital lymphatic abnormalities

Primary lymphatic hypoplasia

Peritoneal infections

- Tuberculous peritonitis
- Myxedema
- Nephrotic syndrome
- Serositis in connective tissue disease

Ascitic fluid analysis. Paracentesis with ascitic fluid analysis is the most rapid and cost-effective method of determining the cause of ascites and should be performed for patients with new-onset ascites. Another important indication for early paracentesis in a patient with ascites is the occurrence of signs and symptoms of infection, such as abdominal pain or tenderness, fever, encephalopathy, hypotension, renal failure, acidosis, and/or leukocytosis. Paracentesis can be performed safely in most patients, including those with cirrhosis and mild coagulopathy. It is usually performed in the lower abdomen with the left lower quadrant preferred to the right. Ultrasound guidance may be useful in obese patients and in those with a history of laparotomy. Runyon[16] has suggested that only ongoing disseminated intravascular coagulation or clinically evident fibrinolysis is a contraindication to paracentesis in patients with ascites. In this study, no cases of hemoperitoneum, death, or infection occurred after more than 229 paracenteses performed in 125 cirrhotic patients; abdominal hematomas occurred in 2% of cases with only 50% of these requiring blood transfusion.

Examination of the ascitic fluid begins with its gross appearance. Normal ascitic fluid is slightly yellow and transparent. The presence of more than 5000 leukocytes/mm^3 will cause the fluid to be cloudy; ascitic fluid with fewer than 1000 cells/mm^3 is almost clear. Blood in the ascitic fluid may be caused by a traumatic tap, in which case the fluid may be blood streaked and will often clot unless it is immediately transferred to a tube containing an anticoagulant. Nontraumatic blood-tinged ascitic fluid does not clot because the required factors have been depleted by previous clotting in the peritoneal cavity. Lipid in the ascitic fluid, such as that which accompanies chylous ascites, causes the fluid to appear opalescent, ranging from cloudy to completely opaque. If it is placed in the refrigerator for 48 to 72 hours, the lipids layer out.

The most valuable laboratory tests on ascitic fluid are the cell count, differential, and determination of ascitic fluid albumin and total protein concentrations. Ascitic fluid from patients with uncomplicated cirrhosis will have a total leukocyte count less than 250 cell/mm^3 with approximately half of these cells will be neutrophils. An increased polymorphonuclear neutrophil count (>250 cells/mm^3) suggests an acute inflammatory process, the most common of which is SBP.

The serum-ascites albumin gradient (SAAG) is the most reliable method to differentiate causes of ascites due to portal hypertension from those due to other causes. The SAAG is calculated by measuring the albumin concentration of serum and ascitic fluid specimens and subtracting the ascitic fluid value from the serum value. If the SAAG is 1.1 g/dL or more, the patient has portal hypertension; a SAAG of less than 1.1 g/dL is consistent with the absence of portal hypertension. Examples of high- and low-gradient causes of ascites are shown in Table 44.1. The accuracy of this measurement in predicting the presence or absence of portal hypertension is approximately 97%.[17]

Treatment of ascites in cirrhotic patients. The standard treatment protocol for patients with ascites caused by portal hypertension is a stepwise approach beginning with sodium restriction, diuretic therapy, and paracentesis. The initial goal of medical therapy is to induce a state in which renal sodium excretion exceeds sodium intake, a situation that will reduce the extracellular volume and improve ascites. A reasonable dietary sodium restriction for most cirrhotic patients with ascites is 88 mEq (2 g) per day. Patient compliance may be assessed by measuring the 24-hour urinary sodium excretion. Patients who are compliant with their dietary restriction and excrete more than 78 mmol/day of sodium in their urine lose weight. However, most patients will require a combination of sodium restriction and diuretics. Spironolactone and furosemide, when given in a dosing ratio of 100:40, will promote natriuresis while maintaining normokalemia. In general, spironolactone (100 mg/day) and furosemide (40 mg/day) are begun initially. If this regimen is ineffective in increasing urinary sodium excretion and decreasing body weight, the dosages of these drugs may be increased while maintaining the 100:40 ratio.

Large-volume paracentesis, in which more than 5 L of ascites fluid is removed from the peritoneal cavity, may be useful for patients with ascites that has been unresponsive to sodium restriction and diuretic treatment; this occurs in less than 10% of patients. The intravenous infusion of albumin (6–8 g/L of ascitic fluid removed) at the time of paracentesis will minimize the symptoms of intravascular volume depletion and renal insufficiency, which may accompany the removal of more than 5 L of ascitic fluid. The continuation of diuretics and salt restriction will prevent or delay the reaccumulation of ascites after paracentesis. Others have suggested that weekly albumin administration, independent of large-volume paracentesis, may be a useful adjunct to salt restriction and diuretic therapy in patients with refractory ascites. Transjugular intrahepatic portosystemic shunt and, ultimately, hepatic transplantation have been used to manage ascites refractory to simpler, less invasive options. These modalities are discussed in Chapter 54.

Chylous ascites. Chylous ascites is the collection of chyle in the peritoneal cavity and may result from one of three mechanisms: (1) obstruction of major lymphatic channels at the base of the mesentery or the cisterna chyli with exudation of chyle from dilated mesenteric lymphatics; (2) direct leakage of chyle through a lymphoperitoneal fistula caused by abnormal or injured retroperitoneal lymphatic vessels; and (3) exudation of chyle through the walls of retroperitoneal megalymphatics without a visible fistula or thoracic duct obstruction.

The most common cause of chylous ascites in adults is an intra-abdominal malignancy obstructing the lymphatic channels at the base of the mesentery or in the retroperitoneum. Lymphoma is the most common malignant neoplasm associated with chylous ascites, although chylous ascites has also been associated with ovarian, colon, renal, prostate, pancreatic, and gastric malignant neoplasms. Carcinoid tumors may cause chylous ascites by obstructing the lymphatics at the base of the mesentery through direct invasion and the dense fibrosis characteristic of this neoplasm. Chylous ascites may also result from injury to the retroperitoneal lymphatics during surgical procedures, such as operations on the

TABLE 44.1 Classification of ascites by serum-ascites albumin gradient.

HIGH GRADIENT (≥1.1 g/dL)	LOW GRADIENT (<1.1 g/dL)
Cirrhosis	Peritoneal carcinomatosis
Alcoholic hepatitis	Tuberculous peritonitis
Cardiac failure	Pancreatic ascites
Massive liver metastases	Biliary ascites
Fulminant hepatic failure	Nephrotic syndrome
Budd-Chiari syndrome	Postoperative lymphatic leak
Portal vein thrombosis	Serositis in connective tissue diseases
Myxedema	

From Runyon B. Ascites: spontaneous bacterial peritonitis. In: Sleisenger MH, Feldman M, Friedman LS, eds. *Sleisenger and Fordtran's Gastrointestinal and Liver Disease: Pathophysiology, Diagnosis, Management.* 7th ed. Philadelphia: WB Saunders; 2002:1523.

abdominal aorta and retroperitoneal lymph node dissections. Blunt and penetrating traumatic injuries may also cause chylous ascites. In children, chylous ascites may result from trauma or be caused by congenital lymphatic abnormalities such as primary lymphatic hypoplasia, which results in lower extremity lymphedema, chylothorax, and chylous ascites.

Patients with chylous ascites most often present with painless abdominal distention. Malnutrition and dyspnea occur in approximately 50% of cases. Paracentesis yields a characteristic milky fluid with a high protein and fat content. The SAAG will be less than 1.1 mg/dL, and the triglyceride level will be two to eight times higher than that of plasma. CT, lymphoscintigraphy, and lymphangiography may provide information about the site of obstruction.

Although large studies are lacking on ideal practices, management of patients with chylous ascites includes the maintenance or improvement of nutrition, reduction in the rate of chyle formation, and correction of the underlying disease process. Most patients will be successfully treated with either a high-protein, low-fat diet and diuretics or fasting with total parenteral nutrition with or without somatostatin. A low-fat, medium-chain triglyceride diet combined with diuretics has been used successfully to treat adults with chylous ascites complicating retroperitoneal lymph node dissections. It is postulated that reducing the intake of long-chain triglycerides will reduce the rate of chyle flow because their metabolites are transported through the splanchnic lymphatics as chylomicrons. In contrast, medium-chain triglycerides are directly absorbed by enterocytes and transported to the liver through the splanchnic blood vessels as free fatty acids and glycerol. Paracentesis may temporarily relieve the dyspnea and abdominal discomfort associated with chylous ascites; however, repeated paracentesis leads to hypoproteinemia and malnutrition. Experience with peritoneovenous shunts to treat chylous ascites has generally been disappointing. Surgical exploration of the abdomen and retroperitoneum is generally reserved for patients who fail to improve with nonoperative management. In rare cases, the application of fibrin glue has been a beneficial adjunct to surgical exploration of the retroperitoneum.

Peritonitis. Peritonitis is inflammation of the peritoneum and peritoneal cavity usually caused by a localized or generalized infection. Primary peritonitis results from bacterial, chlamydial, fungal, or mycobacterial infection in the absence of perforation or inflammation of the GI or GU tract. Secondary peritonitis occurs in the setting of GI or GU perforation or inflammation with common causes including acute appendicitis, colonic diverticulitis, and pelvic inflammatory disease.

Spontaneous bacterial peritonitis. SBP is defined as a bacterial infection of ascitic fluid in the absence of an intraabdominal source of infection, such as visceral perforation, abscess, acute pancreatitis, or cholecystitis. Although it is usually associated with cirrhosis, SBP may also occur in patients with nephrotic syndrome and, less commonly, congestive heart failure. It is extremely rare for patients with ascitic fluid containing a high protein concentration to develop SBP, such as patients with peritoneal carcinomatosis. The most common pathogens in adults with SBP are the aerobic enteric flora *Escherichia coli* and *Klebsiella pneumoniae.* In children with nephrogenic or hepatogenic ascites, group A streptococcus, *Staphylococcus aureus*, and *Streptococcus pneumoniae* are common isolates. SBP is seldom produced by anaerobic microorganisms because of their inability to translocate through the intestinal mucosa and the high volume of oxygen in the intestinal wall and surrounding tissues.[18]

Bacterial translocation from the GI tract is thought to be an important step in the pathogenesis of SBP. Impaired GI motility in cirrhotics alters normal gut microflora, and impaired local and systemic immune function prevents the effective clearance of translocated bacteria from mesenteric lymphatics and bloodstream. The low protein concentration in ascitic fluid prevents effective opsonization of bacteria and, hence, clearance by macrophages and neutrophils.

The diagnosis of SBP is made initially by demonstrating more than 250 neutrophils/mm^3 of ascitic fluid in a clinical setting consistent with this diagnosis, for example, abdominal pain, fever, or leukocytosis in a patient with low-protein ascites. In addition, cultured fluid can be only monomicrobial as polymicrobial infections, particularly with gram-negative enteric organisms, raise the suspicion of secondary peritonitis. It is unusual to document bacterascites on Gram staining of ascitic fluid, and delay of appropriate antibiotic management until the ascitic fluid cultures grow bacterial isolates risks the development of overwhelming infection and death. Bedsides screening of ascitic fluid for leukocyte esterase, using colorimetric leukocyte esterase reagent strips has been used to shorten the time from paracentesis to treatment, although its widespread use remains controversial.[19]

Broad-spectrum antibiotics, such as a third-generation cephalosporin, are started immediately in patients suspected of having ascitic fluid infection. These agents cover about 95% of the bacteria most commonly associated with SBP and are the antibiotics of choice for patients thought to have SBP.[18,20] The spectrum of the antibiotic coverage may be narrowed once the results of antibiotic sensitivity tests are known. Repeated paracentesis with ascitic fluid analysis is not needed when there is typical rapid improvement in response to antibiotic therapy. If the setting, symptoms, ascitic fluid analysis, and response to therapy are atypical, repeated paracentesis may be helpful for detecting secondary peritonitis. The immediate mortality risk caused by SBP is low, particularly if it is recognized and treated expeditiously. However, the development of other complications of hepatic failure, including GI hemorrhage and hepatorenal syndrome, contributes to the death of many of these patients during the hospitalization in which SBP is detected. The occurrence of SBP is an important landmark in the natural history of cirrhosis, with 1- and 2-year survival rates of approximately 30% and 20%, respectively. Several studies, including a randomized controlled trial, have shown that plasma expansion with albumin improves circulatory function and reduces the risk of hepatorenal syndrome and hospital mortality in patients with SBP.

Tuberculous peritonitis. Tuberculosis is common in impoverished areas of the world and is encountered in the United States and other developed countries in patients with human immunodeficiency virus infection and receiving chronic immunosuppressive medications. Others have described an association between peritoneal tuberculosis and alcoholic cirrhosis and chronic renal failure.[21] Peritoneal tuberculosis is the sixth most common site of extrapulmonary tuberculosis, after lymphatic, GU, bone and joint, miliary, and meningeal. Most cases result from reactivation of latent peritoneal disease that had been previously established hematogenously from a primary pulmonary focus. Only approximately 17% of cases are associated with active pulmonary disease.

The illness often is manifested insidiously with patients having had symptoms for several weeks to months at the time of presentation. Its clinical presentation mimics inflammatory conditions such as Crohn disease and malignant diseases, so obtaining a diagnosis can be problematic at times. Abdominal swelling caused by ascites formation is the most common symptom, occurring in more than 80% of cases. Most patients complain of a poorly localized, vague abdominal pain. Constitutional symptoms such as low-grade fever and night sweats, weight loss, anorexia, and malaise are reported in approximately 60% of patients. The concomitant presence of other chronic conditions, such as uremia, cirrhosis, and AIDS, makes these symptoms difficult to interpret. Abdominal tenderness is present in approximately 50% of patients with peritoneal tuberculosis.[21]

A positive tuberculin skin test response is present in most cases of tuberculous peritonitis. Only approximately 50% of these patients will have an abnormal chest radiograph. The ascitic fluid SAAG is less than 1.1 g/dL, consistent with a high protein concentration in the ascitic fluid. Microscopic examination of the ascites shows erythrocytes and an increased number of leukocytes, most of which are lymphocytes. Measurement of ascitic fluid adenosine deaminase activity and polymerase chain reaction assays have been used as rapid, noninvasive diagnostic tests for tuberculous peritonitis. Ascitic fluid adenosine deaminase activity, in particular, appears to be highly sensitive and specific for tuberculous peritonitis.

Abdominal imaging with ultrasound or CT may suggest the diagnosis but lacks the sensitivity and specificity to be diagnostic. Ultrasound may demonstrate the ascitic fluid containing echogenic material, seen as fine mobile strands or particulate matter. CT will document a thickened and nodular mesentery with mesenteric lymphadenopathy and omental thickening.

The diagnosis is usually made by laparoscopy with directed biopsy of the peritoneum. In more than 90% of cases, laparoscopy demonstrates a number of whitish nodules (<5 mm) scattered over the visceral and parietal peritoneum; histologic examination demonstrates caseating granulomas. Multiple adhesions are commonly present between the abdominal organs and parietal peritoneum. The gross appearance of the peritoneal cavity is similar to that of peritoneal carcinomatosis, sarcoidosis, and Crohn disease, thus reiterating the importance of biopsy. Blind percutaneous peritoneal biopsy has a much lower yield than directed biopsy, and laparotomy with peritoneal biopsy is reserved for cases in which laparoscopy has been nondiagnostic or cannot be safely performed. Microscopic examination of ascitic fluid for acid-fast bacilli identifies the organism in less than 3% of cases, and culture results are positive in less than 20% of cases. The diagnostic usefulness of mycobacterial cultures is further limited by the time it may take for the cultures to yield definitive information, up to 8 weeks.

Treatment of peritoneal tuberculosis consists of antituberculous drugs. Drug regimens useful in treating pulmonary tuberculosis are also effective for peritoneal disease; a commonly used and effective regimen is isoniazid and rifampin daily for 9 months. The presence of associated alcoholic cirrhosis may complicate the use of these agents because of hepatotoxicity.

Peritonitis associated with chronic ambulatory peritoneal dialysis. In the United States, approximately 6% of patients with chronic renal failure undergo chronic ambulatory peritoneal dialysis (CAPD). Peritonitis is one of the most common complications of CAPD, occurring with an incidence of approximately one episode every 1 to 3 years. A study of all patients undergoing peritoneal dialysis in Scotland between 1999 and 2002 found that one episode of peritonitis occurred in every 19.2 months of peritoneal dialysis. Importantly, refractory or recurrent peritonitis was the most common cause of technical failure, accounting for 43% of all cases of technique failure.[22]

Patients present with abdominal pain, fever, and cloudy peritoneal dialysate containing more than 100 leukocytes/mm^3, with more than 50% of the cells being neutrophils. Gram staining detects organisms only in approximately 10% to 40% of cases. Approximately 75% of infections are caused by gram-positive organisms, with *Staphylococcus epidermidis* accounting for 30% to 50% of cases. *S. aureus*, gram-negative bacilli, and fungi are also important causes of CAPD-associated peritonitis.[22]

Peritoneal dialysis–associated peritonitis is treated by the intraperitoneal administration of antibiotics, usually a first-generation cephalosporin. Overall, 75% of infections are cured by culture-directed antibiotic therapy. The cure rate for peritonitis using antibiotics without catheter removal varies according to the causative organism; one study showed rates of 90% with coagulase-negative staphylococcus compared with rates of 66%, 56%, and 0% for *S. aureus*, gram-negative bacilli, and fungi, respectively.[22] Recurrent or persistent peritonitis requires removal of the dialysis catheter and resumption of hemodialysis.

Malignant Neoplasms of the Peritoneum

Most malignant neoplasms that involve the peritoneum are transperitoneal metastases originating from carcinomas of the GI tract (especially the stomach, colon, and pancreas) and the GU tract (usually ovarian). *Carcinomatosis* is the term used to describe the diffuse coating of the visceral and parietal peritoneum by peritoneal metastases from an intraabdominal or pelvic malignancy. Primary malignant neoplasms of the peritoneum are rare; they include malignant mesothelioma and primary peritoneal carcinoma. Sarcomas, especially angiosarcoma, may also originate from the peritoneum.

Pseudomyxoma peritonei. Pseudomyxoma peritonei is a rare disease characterized by mucinous ascites and peritoneal implants that arise most often from a perforated mucinous tumor of the appendix. The mucus, and the cells contained within it, are distributed throughout the peritoneal cavity and are particularly prominent in the pelvis, paracolic gutters, omentum, and subdiaphragmatic spaces. Similar clinical features may occur in patients with mucinous tumors of the ovary, colon, and pancreas. The discussion in this chapter is limited to pseudomyxoma peritonei associated with epithelial neoplasms of the appendix.

A recent international consensus group has standardized the pathologic classification of pseudomyxoma peritonei and the associated appendiceal mucinous neoplasm.[23] The grading of these tumors is based upon the presence or absence of infiltrative invasion, high cytologic grade, high tumor cellularity, angiolymphatic invasion, perineural invasion, and signet ring cells.[24] Appendiceal mucinous neoplasms are categorized by the presence or absence of infiltrative invasion of the appendiceal wall and the degree of cellular atypia into low-grade, high-grade, and mucinous adenocarcinoma.[23] The histology of appendiceal tumors is an important predictor of survival; adenomucinosis has the best survival rate (75% at 5 years), and peritoneal mucinous carcinomatosis, the worst (14% at 5 years).[25]

Pseudomyxoma peritonei occurs most commonly in individuals 40 to 50 years of age, with a similar frequency in men and women. Patients are often asymptomatic until late in the course of their disease. On presentation, they will often describe a global deterioration in their health, long before the diagnosis is made. Symptoms of abdominal pain and distention and nonspecific complaints are common. Physical examination may reveal a new hernia, ascites, abdominal distention with nonshifting dullness, and on occasion a palpable abdominal mass.

CT of the chest, abdomen, and pelvis may demonstrate ascites, loculated pools of fluid, peritoneal-based tumor nodules, a thickened omentum, scalloping of the liver margins, and evidence of invasion of the mesentery, porta hepatis, and small intestine. The amount and distribution of disease provide important information regarding the ability to achieve complete cytoreduction, which is often limited by diffuse involvement of the small bowel or porta hepatis by tumor. Preoperative colonoscopy will differentiate a mucinous neoplasm of the appendix from that arising from the colon. On occasion, the diagnosis is made at laparotomy when an unsuspecting surgeon encounters tenacious, semisolid mucus and large, loculated cystic masses upon entering or exploring the peritoneal cavity. In this setting, the best approach is to establish the diagnosis by the least invasive procedure possible and to relieve intestinal obstruction, if present. The patient can then be referred to a center experienced in the management of this rare disease.

The current treatment of patients with pseudomyxoma peritonei involves resection of as much of the tumor as possible (cytoreduction) and hyperthermic intraperitoneal chemotherapy (HIPEC). Operative management includes lesser and greater omentectomy, stripping of involved parietal peritoneum, resection of involved organs, and appendectomy or ileocolectomy. The goal is to leave no visible disease or, if this is not feasible, to leave no nodules larger than 2 mm in diameter. The latter facilitates penetration of the chemotherapy into the residual disease. HIPEC can be performed using an open technique in which the abdomen is left open to ensure adequate chemotherapy distribution throughout the peritoneal cavity or a closed technique in which the abdomen is closed after inflow and outflow cannulas are placed. The closed technique allows easier maintenance of hyperthermia (Fig. 44.12). The most commonly used drugs for intraperitoneal chemotherapy are mitomycin C and oxaliplatin.

Patients with low-grade tumors who undergo complete cytoreduction with HIPEC have 5-year survival rates of 60% to 90%. Even patients with high-grade mucinous tumors may achieve 5-year survival rates of 50% if complete cytoreduction can be achieved.[26]

Cytoreduction and HIPEC is an extensive surgical procedure, and appropriate candidates must have a good performance status. Even at experienced centers, the 30-day postoperative mortality rate is 2% to 3%. Of patients, 25% to 35% will develop a serious complication, most commonly prolonged ileus and pulmonary complications. Hemorrhage, intraabdominal infections, enterocutaneous fistula, pancreatitis, and bone marrow suppression are also reported.

Carcinomatosis from colorectal cancer. About 8% of patients with colorectal cancer develop peritoneal metastases. In half of these the peritoneum is the only site of disease. Untreated, metastatic disease is uniformly fatal.

Cytoreductive surgery with HIPEC has been performed in highly selected patients with isolated peritoneal metastases from colorectal cancer that is amenable to cytoreduction. A randomized trial in the Netherlands showed improved survival compared to systemic chemotherapy, particularly in patients with limited involvement of the peritoneum and in whom complete cytoreduction was feasible.[27] A recent multicenter trial of highly selected patients compared cytoreduction versus cytoreduction and HIPEC using oxaliplatin. It demonstrated a remarkable median overall survival of 41 months in both groups; interestingly, the use intraperitoneal chemotherapy did not have an additional benefit over cytoreduction alone.[28] Current research is focused on determining optimal patient selection and treatment regimens.

Peritoneal mesothelioma. The most common primary malignant neoplasm of the peritoneum is mesothelioma. This tumor results from the malignant transformation of the simple squamoid epithelium covering the peritoneal cavity. There are three histologic subtypes (epithelioid, sarcomatoid, and biphasic), of which the epithelioid subtype is the most common and has the best prognosis.

This is a rare tumor, with approximately 800 new cases diagnosed per year in the United States. It occurs with similar frequency in men as in women. The median age at presentation is 50 years.[29] A history of asbestos exposure is elicited in only about one third of patients, significantly less than the association between asbestos exposure and pleural mesothelioma.[30]

Peritoneal mesothelioma tends to involve all peritoneal surfaces, producing hard, white masses, and plaques of tumor. In contrast to pseudomyxoma peritonei, which tends to spare the small bowel initially, mesothelioma is associated with local invasion of intraabdominal organs. Encasement of the small bowel may create a bowel obstruction and eventually death.

Peritoneal mesothelioma has a variable rate of progression and tends to remain confined to the abdominal cavity until very late in the course of the disease. Direct extension of the tumor into one or both pleural cavities is more likely than hematogenous dissemination. The most important other disease in the differential diagnosis is carcinomatosis from a malignancy of an intraabdominal or pelvic organ such as the stomach, ovaries, colon, or pancreas.

Most patients with peritoneal mesothelioma present with abdominal pain and weight loss. Ascites is common and is often intractable. The omentum may become diffusely involved with tumor and present as an epigastric mass. Abdominal CT

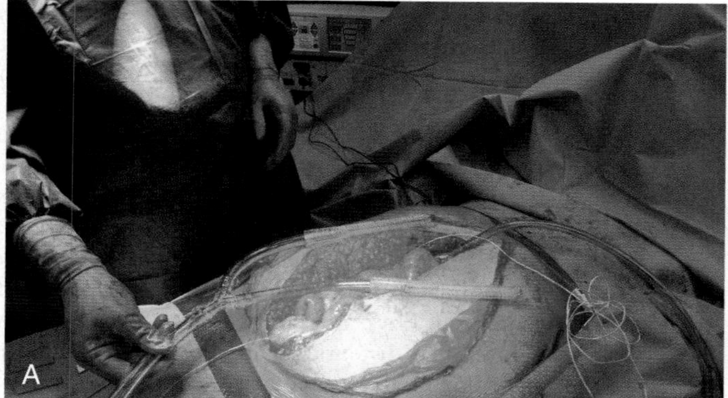

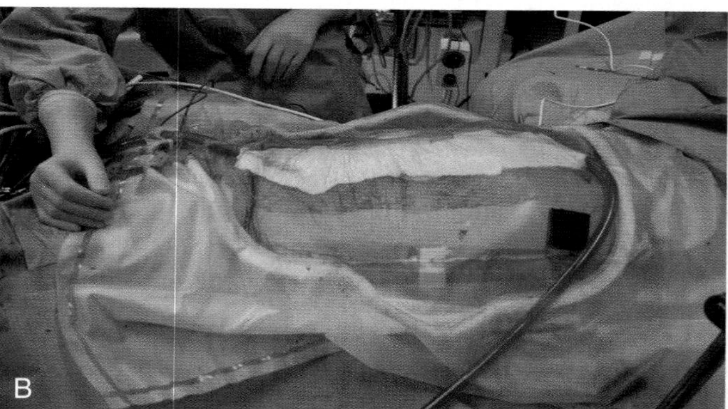

FIG. 44.12 Hyperthermic intraperitoneal chemotherapy, closed technique. (A) Placement of cannulas and temperature probes in the abdomen. (B) Temporary abdominal closure for perfusion.

demonstrates mesenteric thickening, peritoneal studding, hemorrhage within the tumor, and ascites. Paracentesis has a low diagnostic yield, and either image-guided core needle biopsy of a visible implant or diagnostic laparoscopy is often required to establish the diagnosis.

As with pseudomyxoma peritonei, combined-modality approaches using cytoreductive surgery and HIPEC offers better survival rates when compared with historical controls. Several retrospective series report median survival rates of 30 to 60 months for patients with peritoneal mesothelioma undergoing cytoreductive surgery and HIPEC. A metaanalysis and systematic review found that 67% of selected patients were able to undergo complete cytoreduction, and the 5-year survival for these patients was 42%.[31] Factors associated with improved outcomes include complete or near complete cytoreduction, low histologic tumor grade, epithelioid histology, and use of cisplatin for HIPEC.[31] Some authors consider sarcomatoid or biphasic histologies to be contraindications for surgical resection.[32] The rate of postoperative complications from cytoreduction and HIPEC in treating patients with peritoneal mesothelioma is similar to that of patients undergoing this treatment for pseudomyxoma peritonei. A multi-institutional report of 405 patients reported a postoperative mortality rate of 2%, with 46% of patient sustaining a complication.[33] Together, these reports demonstrate that there can be a role for aggressive surgical treatment of patients with peritoneal mesothelioma. Systemic chemotherapy with cisplatin and pemetrexed has a modest benefit on survival and is used for palliative treatment of patients who are not surgical candidates.

MESENTERY AND OMENTUM

Embryology and Anatomy

The greater and lesser omenta are complex peritoneal folds that pass from the stomach to the liver, transverse colon, spleen, bile duct, pancreas, and diaphragm. They originate from the dorsal and ventral midline mesenteries of the embryonic gut. In the very early stages of development, the alimentary canal traverses the future coelomic cavity as a straight tube, suspended posteriorly by an uninterrupted dorsal mesentery and anteriorly by a ventral mesentery in the cranial portion of its extent. The embryonic stomach rotates 90 degrees on its longitudinal axis so that the lesser curvature faces to the right and the greater curvature to the left. Much of the embryonic ventral mesentery is resorbed; however, the portion extending from the fissure of the ligamentum venosum and porta hepatis to the proximal duodenum and lesser curvature of the stomach (gastrohepatic ligament) persists as the lesser omentum. The right border of the lesser omentum is a free edge that forms the anterior border of the opening into the lesser sac, termed the *foramen of Winslow*. Between the layers of the lesser omentum, and at its right border, are the common hepatic duct, portal vein, and hepatic artery.

The embryonic dorsal mesogastrium grows as a sheet of peritoneum extending from the greater curvature of the stomach over the anterior surface of the small intestine. After passing inferiorly almost to the pelvis, the peritoneal membrane turns up on itself to pass upward to a line of attachment on the transverse colon slightly above that of the transverse mesocolon. Fat is laid down in this omental apron and provides an insulating layer of protection of the abdominal viscera.

Early in its development, the small intestine elongates to form an anteriorly oriented intestinal loop, which then rotates counterclockwise so that the cecum and ascending colon move to the right side of the peritoneal cavity, and the descending colon assumes a vertical position on the left wall of the peritoneal cavity. The jejunum and ileum are supported by the peritoneum-covered dorsal mesentery carrying the mesenteric blood vessels and lymphatics. The posterior line of attachment of the mesentery extends obliquely from the duodenojejunal junction at the left side of the second lumbar vertebra toward the right iliac fossa to terminate anterior to the sacroiliac articulation.

Physiology

The omentum and intestinal mesentery are rich in lymphatics and blood vessels. The omentum contains areas with high concentrations of macrophages, which may aid in the removal of foreign material and bacteria. Furthermore, the omentum becomes densely adherent to intraperitoneal sites of inflammation, often preventing diffuse peritonitis during cases of intestinal gangrene or perforation, such as acute diverticulitis or acute appendicitis.

Diseases of the Omentum

Omental Cysts

Omental cysts are unilocular or multilocular cysts containing serous fluid that are thought to arise from congenital or acquired obstruction of omental lymphatic channels. They are lined by a lymphatic endothelium similar to that of cystic lymphangiomas. These lesions are most common in children and young adults, in whom small cysts are usually asymptomatic and discovered incidentally. Larger cysts may present as a palpable abdominal mass. Uncomplicated cysts usually lie in the lower mid-abdomen and are freely movable, smooth, and nontender. Complications are more common in children and include torsion, infection, and rupture.

Plain radiographs of the abdomen may show a well-circumscribed soft tissue density in the midabdomen, and contrast studies of the intestine may show displacement of intestinal loops and extrinsic compression on adjacent bowel. Ultrasound or CT will show a fluid-filled, complex cystic mass with internal septations. The differential diagnosis includes cysts and solid tumors of the mesentery, peritoneum, and retroperitoneum, including desmoid tumors. Ultimately, the diagnosis is made by excision of the cyst and histologic examination of the wall. Local excision, either laparoscopically or open, is curative.

Omental Torsion and Infarction

Torsion of the greater omentum is defined as the axial twisting of the omentum along its long axis. If the twist is tight enough or the venous obstruction is of sufficient duration, arterial inflow will become compromised, leading to infarction and necrosis. Omental torsion is classified as primary when no coexisting causative condition is identified or secondary when the torsion occurs in association with a causative condition such as a hernia, tumor, or adhesion. Primary omental torsion usually involves the right side of the omentum.

Omental torsion occurs twice as often in men as in women and is most frequent in patients in their fourth or fifth decade of life. Patients often present with the acute onset of severe abdominal pain localized to the right side of the abdomen. Nausea and vomiting may be present but are not predominant findings. The patient's temperature is usually normal. Palpation of the abdomen demonstrates localized abdominal tenderness with guarding suggesting peritonitis. A mass may be palpable if the involved omentum is sufficiently large.

The differential diagnosis includes any disease associated with right-sided abdominal pain and tenderness, most notably acute appendicitis, acute cholecystitis, and torsion of an ovarian cyst. CT often demonstrates an omental mass with signs of inflammation.

Usually, the patient's clinical presentation justifies laparotomy or laparoscopy at which time a segment of the omentum appears congested and acutely inflamed. Serosanguineous fluid is often present in the peritoneal cavity. Treatment consists of resection of the involved omentum and correction of any related condition.

Omental Neoplasms

Primary malignant neoplasms of the omentum are extremely rare and are usually of soft tissue origin (sarcomas). The omentum is often involved by metastatic tumor that has spread transperitoneally from intraabdominal or pelvic malignancies.

Omental Grafts and Transpositions

The arterial and venous blood supplies to the greater omentum are derived from omental branches of the right and left gastroepiploic arteries, which course along the greater curvature of the stomach. Division of the right or left gastroepiploic artery and vasa recta along the greater curvature of the stomach, with mobilization of the omentum from the transverse colon, allows the development of a vascularized omental pedicle flap. This graft may be used to cover chest and mediastinal wounds after chest wall resections and to prevent the small intestine from entering the pelvis after abdominal perineal resection, thus preventing radiation enteritis during radiation therapy for rectal carcinoma. Finally, the formation of dense adhesions between the omentum and sites of perforation or inflammation facilitates its use as a patch for duodenal perforations from peptic ulcer disease (termed a Graham patch; Fig. 44.13).

Diseases of the Mesentery

Mesenteric Cysts

The most common non-neoplastic mesenteric cysts are termed *mesothelial cysts* on the basis of the ultrastructure of the cells lining the cyst. The cysts contain chyle or a clear serous fluid and occur in the mesentery of the small intestine (60%) or colon (40%). These cysts usually occur in adults, with a mean age of 45 years, and are twice as common in women as in men. Depending on the size of the cyst, patients may present with abdominal pain, fever, and emesis. A midabdominal mass may be palpable on physical examination. The diagnosis can usually be made preoperatively with ultrasonography or CT. Enucleation of the cyst at laparotomy is curative and can generally be accomplished because the mesenteric blood vessels and intestinal wall are usually not adherent to the cyst wall. Internal drainage of the cyst into the peritoneal cavity has also been successfully used in the treatment of very large cysts. Aspiration alone has a high rate of cyst recurrence. In those cases in which the cyst is not completely excised, the contents of the cyst and the internal architecture of the cyst wall must be carefully inspected and the cyst wall examined histologically to rule out a neoplastic etiology.

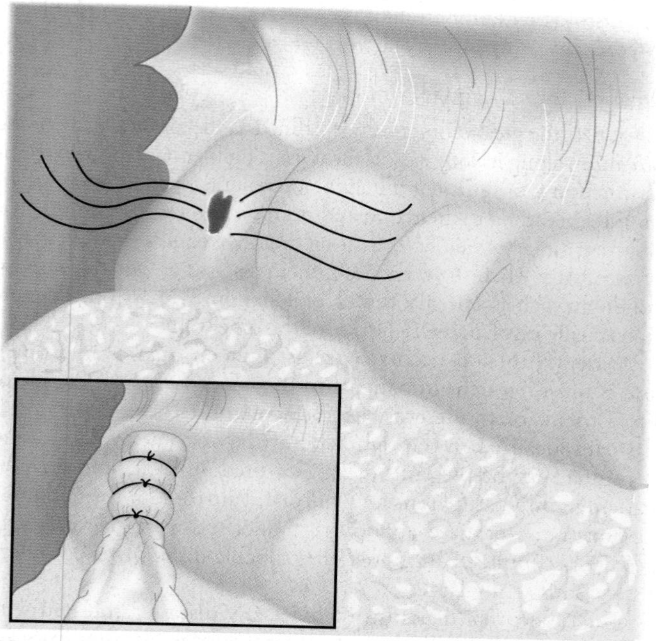

FIG. 44.13 Closure of a perforated duodenal ulcer with an omental (Graham) patch. (From Graham RR. The treatment of perforated duodenal ulcers. *Surg Gynecol Obstet.* 1937;64:235–238.)

Acute Mesenteric Lymphadenitis

Acute mesenteric lymphadenitis is a syndrome of acute right lower quadrant abdominal pain associated with mesenteric lymph node enlargement and a normal appendix. Historically, the diagnosis was made on exploration of the abdomen of a patient suspected of having acute appendicitis, at which time a normal appendix and enlarged mesenteric lymph nodes were discovered. With the increasing use of abdominal ultrasound in the diagnosis of acute appendicitis in children, acute mesenteric lymphadenitis is now most often diagnosed through imaging as well. This syndrome occurs most commonly in children and young adults with equal frequency in males and females.

Numerous causative agents have been implicated in the pathobiology of acute mesenteric lymphadenitis including viral, bacterial, parasitic, and fungal infections. *Yersinia enterocolitica* in particular has been associated with this syndrome in children. Culture and histologic examination of the enlarged lymph nodes, stool culture, and antibody titers have been used to identify causative agents but are not routinely used in the evaluation or management of these patients.

The symptom complex associated with acute mesenteric lymphadenitis includes the acute onset of periumbilical pain which shifts to the right lower quadrant over time. Physical examination demonstrates right lower quadrant tenderness with abdominal wall muscle rigidity and rebound tenderness. Nausea, vomiting, diarrhea, and anorexia may also be present, along with fever and elevated white blood cell count.[34] Because the symptom complex of acute mesenteric lymphadenitis is so similar to that of acute appendicitis in children, it is recommended that abdominal ultrasound be obtained for definitive diagnosis. Definitive diagnosis of acute mesenteric lymphadenitis will prevent unnecessary surgical intervention for a disease that is self-limiting.

Sclerosing Mesenteritis

Sclerosing mesenteritis is a rare inflammatory disease of the mesentery characterized histologically by sclerosing fibrosis, fat necrosis with lipid-laden macrophages, chronic inflammation with germinal centers, and focal calcification. Early in the course of the disease, sclerosing mesenteritis has a loose myxomatous appearance that progresses to chronic inflammation and dense sclerosis. This condition is characterized grossly by marked thickening of the mesentery of the small intestine with irregular areas of discoloration suggesting fat necrosis. There may also be multiple discrete nodules on the mesentery or the disease may appear as a single matted mass. The process most often involves the root of the small bowel mesentery and frequently encompasses the mesenteric vessels. It affects the small bowel by retraction and shortening of the mesentery without direct invasion. In advanced cases, mesenteric venous and lymphatic obstructions are present. The mesocolon may also be affected but less commonly than the small bowel mesentery.

Sclerosing mesenteritis is twice as common in men as in women and usually occurs in the fifth decade of life. Most patients are asymptomatic, and the diagnosis is discovered incidentally on imaging for an unrelated condition. When symptoms are present, abdominal pain or symptoms of intestinal obstruction with nausea, vomiting, and abdominal distention are most common. An abdominal mass is palpable in more than 50% of patients. Laboratory studies are usually normal except that the erythrocyte sedimentation rate and C-reactive protein levels may be elevated.

The differential diagnosis of sclerosing mesenteritis includes a heterogeneous group of conditions that alter the density of the mesenteric fat including inflammatory and neoplastic causes. Differentiation from peritoneal carcinomatosis, carcinoid tumor, and mesenteric and retroperitoneal sarcomas is particularly important. The CT characteristics of sclerosing mesenteritis are well described[35] and include the following:

- A fatty mass arising from the base of the mesentery that has well-delineated margins separating it from normal mesentery, a feature described as a *tumoral pseudocapsule*
- The presence of normal adipose tissue surrounding mesenteric vessels, termed *fat ring sign*
- The presence of normal mesenteric vessels coursing through the fatty mass, without evidence of vascular involvement or deviation
- An intraabdominal mass that displaces adjacent bowel loops without invading them.

Laparotomy or laparoscopy with biopsy of the involved mesentery remains necessary for definitive diagnosis.

Most patients with mesenteric panniculitis experience spontaneous resolution of their symptoms. If patients do not improve, corticosteroids and other antiinflammatory and immunosuppressive agents have been found to improve the symptoms and radiographic findings. Operative management is indicated only for patients in whom there is confusion about the diagnosis and for the treatment of intestinal obstruction.

Intraabdominal (Internal) Hernias

Internal Hernias Caused by Developmental Defects

There are three general mechanisms whereby developmental abnormalities result in the formation of internal hernias: (1) abnormal retroperitoneal fixation of the mesentery resulting in anomalous positioning of the intestine (e.g., mesocolic or paraduodenal hernia); (2) abnormally large internal foramina or fossae (e.g., foramen of Winslow, supravesical hernia); and (3) incomplete mesenteric surfaces with the presence of an abnormal opening through which the intestine herniates (e.g., mesenteric hernia). The anatomic and radiographic features of acquired and congenital internal hernias have been reviewed by Martin and associates.[36]

Mesocolic (paraduodenal) hernias. Mesocolic hernias are unusual congenital hernias in which the small intestine herniates behind the mesocolon. They result from abnormal rotation of the midgut and have been categorized as right or left. A right mesocolic hernia occurs when the prearterial limb of the midgut loop fails to rotate around the superior mesenteric artery. This results in most of the small intestine remaining to the right of the superior mesenteric artery. Normal counterclockwise rotation of the cecum and proximal colon into the right side of the abdomen and fixation to the posterolateral peritoneum cause the small intestine to become trapped behind the mesentery of the right colon. The ileocolic, right colic, and middle colic vessels lie within the anterior wall of the sac, and the superior mesenteric artery courses along the medial border of the neck of the hernia (Fig. 44.14A).

Left mesocolic hernias are thought to be caused by in utero herniation of the small intestine between the inferior mesenteric vein and posterior parietal attachments of the descending mesocolon to the retroperitoneum. The inferior mesenteric artery and vein are integral components of the hernia sac (Fig. 44.14B). Approximately 75% of mesocolic hernias occur on the left side.

Patients with paraduodenal hernias usually present with symptoms of acute or chronic small bowel obstruction. Barium radiographs will demonstrate displacement of the small intestine to the left or right side of the abdomen. CT with intravenous contrast may demonstrate displacement of the mesenteric vessels and evidence of intestinal obstruction, if present.

The operative treatment of patients with a right mesocolic hernia involves incision of the lateral peritoneal reflections along the right colon with reflection of the right colon and cecum to the left. The entire gut then assumes a position simulating that of nonrotation of the prearterial and postarterial segments of the midgut. Opening the neck of the hernia will injure the superior mesenteric vessels and fails to free the herniated bowel (Fig. 44.14C).

The operative treatment of patients with a left mesocolic hernia consists of incision of the peritoneal attachments and adhesions along the right side of the inferior mesenteric vein, with reduction of the herniated small intestine from beneath the inferior mesenteric vein. The vein is then allowed to return to its normal position to the left of the base of the mesentery of the small intestine. The neck of the hernia may be closed by suturing the peritoneum adjacent to the vein to the retroperitoneum (Fig. 44.14D).

Mesenteric hernias. Mesenteric hernias occur when the intestine herniates through an abnormal orifice in the mesentery of the small intestine or colon. The most common location for these hernias is near the ileocolic junction, although defects in the sigmoid mesocolon have also been described. Patients present with intestinal obstruction resulting from compression of the loops of bowel at the neck of the hernia or torsion of the herniated segment. Treatment involves reduction of the hernia and closure of the mesenteric defect.

Acquired Internal Hernias

Acquired internal hernias result from the creation of abnormal mesenteric defects after operative procedures or trauma. These usually result from inadequate closure (or dehiscence) of mesenteric defects created during the performance of gastrojejunostomy, colostomy, ileostomy, or bowel resection. The creation of a small space allows the herniation of the small intestine through the mesenteric rent and the development of intestinal obstruction. Depending on the type of surgery performed, variation exists in routine closure of the mesenteric defect. For instance, herniation after laparoscopic colectomy is uncommon (approximately 1%), so the defect is usually not closed. However, hernia rates after laparoscopic Roux-en-Y gastric bypass (i.e., Peterson hernia) are reported as high as 9%, so the defect is usually closed.[37] Treatment of these patients is operative reduction of the hernia and closure of the peritoneal defect.

Malignant Neoplasms of the Mesentery

Similar to the peritoneum and omentum, the most common neoplasm affecting the mesentery is metastatic disease from an intraabdominal adenocarcinoma. This may result from direct

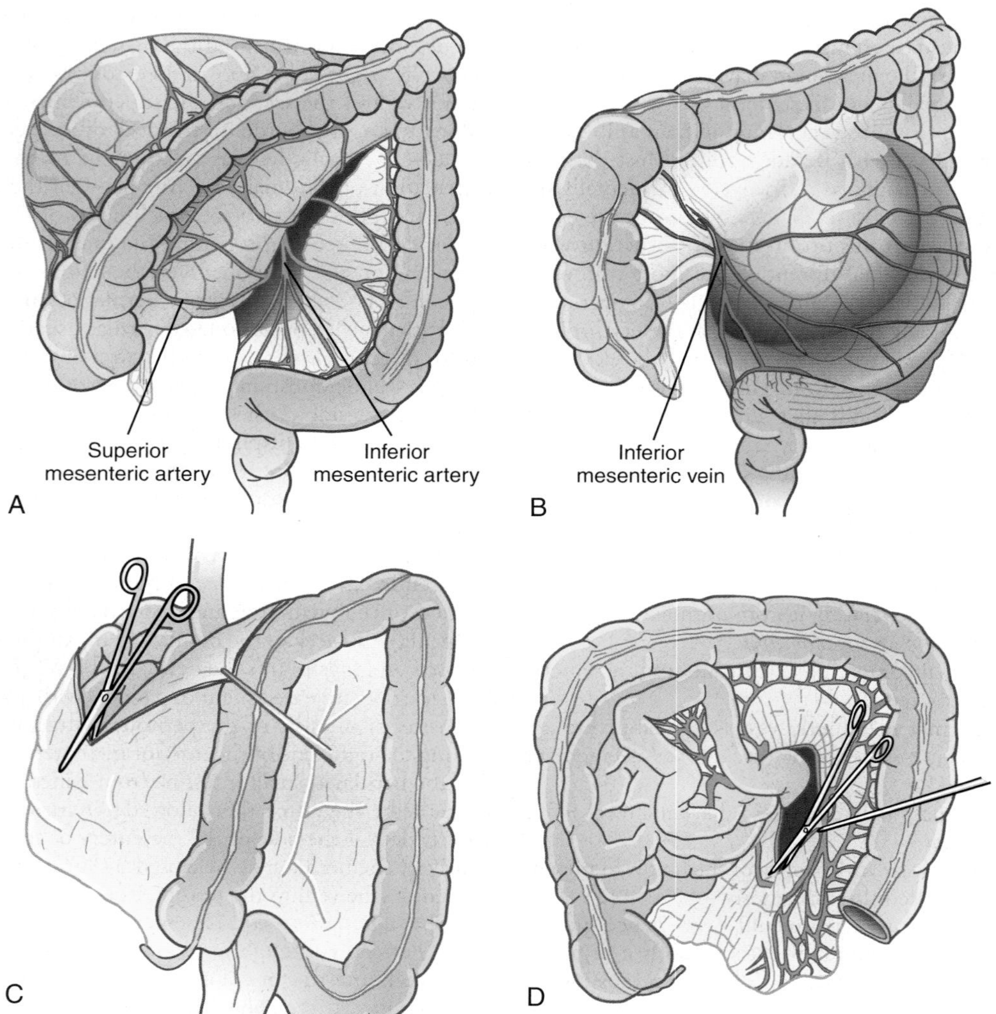

FIG. 44.14 (A) Right mesocolic (paraduodenal) hernia. Note that the anterior wall of a right mesocolic hernia is the ascending mesocolon. The hernia orifice lies to the right of the midline, and the superior mesenteric artery and ileocolic artery course along the anterior border of the hernia neck. (B) Left mesocolic (paraduodenal) hernia. The hernia orifice is to the left of the midline, and the herniated intestine lies behind the anterior wall of the descending mesocolon. (C) A right mesocolic hernia is repaired by division of the lateral peritoneal attachments of the ascending colon, reflecting it toward the left side of the abdomen. The small and large intestine then assume a position simulating that of nonrotation of the prearterial and postarterial segments of the midgut. Opening the neck of the hernia will injure the superior mesenteric vessels and fail to free the herniated bowel. (D) A left mesocolic hernia is reduced by incising the hernia sac along an avascular plane immediately to the right of the inferior mesenteric vessels. (A, B, From Brigham RA, d'Avis JC. Paraduodenal hernia. In: Nyhus LM, Condon RE, eds. *Hernia*. 3rd ed. Philadelphia: JB Lippincott; 1989:484–485. C, D, From Brigham R, Fallon WF, Saunders JR, et al. Paraduodenal hernia: diagnosis and surgical management. *Surg*. 1984;96:498–502.)

invasion of the primary tumor (or its lymphatic metastases) into the mesentery or from the transperitoneal spread of the malignant neoplasm into the mesentery. Distortion and fixation of the mesentery by the tumor itself or by the resultant desmoplastic reaction may cause intestinal obstruction. Small bowel carcinoid tumors in particular can cause bulky mesenteric lymphadenopathy and retraction with consequent small bowel obstruction.

Mesenteric and Intraabdominal Desmoid Tumors

The most common primary malignant tumor of the mesentery is a desmoid. In contrast to sporadic desmoids caused by a mutation of the CTNNB1 gene, most desmoid tumors occurring in patients with FAP are located within the abdominal (80%).[4,38] Patients with Gardner syndrome are especially likely to have intraabdominal desmoid tumors.

As mentioned earlier, surgical procedures play an important role in the induction and progression of desmoid tumors. This is particularly important in patients with FAP who undergo preventative proctocolectomy. In these patients, desmoid tumors are an important cause of long-term morbidity and mortality. The risk of desmoid tumor is lower in patients undergoing laparoscopic proctocolectomy compared to open procedures (4% vs. 16%, respectively).[39,40]

Intraabdominal desmoids are more lethal than those that occur at other anatomic sites because of the possibility of bowel obstruction, bowel ischemia, hydronephrosis, and vascular involvement.

Complete resection is less feasible and associated with greater risk to critical structures than that associated with extraabdominal sites. Resection of mesenteric desmoids may require sacrifice of significant lengths of intestine, thus leaving the patient with an inadequate GI absorptive capacity. Ureteral involvement by the tumor may require resection and reconstruction.

As with desmoid tumors at other locations, the biologic behavior of mesenteric desmoids is highly variable and includes periods of quiescence and even regression. This, combined with a high likelihood of recurrence following resection, has made the strategy of "watchful waiting" preferable for patients with stable intraabdominal desmoid tumors.[41] As with other desmoids, systemic therapy, with antiestrogens and NSAIDs for slow-growing lesions and cytotoxic chemotherapy for lesions with more aggressive behavior, may be a useful therapeutic strategy. Overall the 10-year survival rate for patients with intraabdominal desmoid tumors is 60% to 70%.

RETROPERITONEUM

Anatomy

The retroperitoneal space lies between the peritoneum and posterior parietal wall of the abdominal cavity extending from the diaphragm to the pelvis. This space contains the contiguous lumbar and iliac fossae. The lumbar fossa extends from the twelfth thoracic vertebra and lateral lumbocostal arch superiorly to the base of the sacrum, iliac crest, and iliolumbar ligament inferiorly. The floor of the space is formed by the fascia overlying the quadratus lumborum and psoas major muscles. This space contains varying amounts of fatty areolar tissue and the adrenal glands, kidneys, ascending and descending colon, pancreas, and duodenum. It is also traversed by the ureter, renal vessels, gonadal vessels, inferior vena cava, and aorta. The iliac fossa is contiguous with the lumbar fossa superiorly, lateral and anterior preperitoneal spaces of the abdominal wall, and pelvis inferiorly. The iliacus muscle with its investing fascia is the floor of the iliac fossa, which contains the iliac vessels, ureter, genitofemoral nerve, gonadal vessels, and iliac lymph nodes.

Operative Approaches

The aorta, vena cava, iliac vessels, kidneys, and adrenal glands may be approached operatively through the retroperitoneal space. Specific operative procedures performed through the retroperitoneum include adrenalectomy, nephrectomy, and renal transplantation. The advantages to this approach over a transabdominal approach include less postoperative ileus facilitating a more rapid resumption of a normal diet and earlier discharge from the hospital; no intraabdominal adhesions, reducing the likelihood of subsequent small bowel obstruction; less intraoperative evaporative fluid losses with less dramatic perioperative intravascular fluid shifts; and fewer respiratory complications such as atelectasis and pneumonia.

Retroperitoneal Disorders

Retroperitoneal Abscesses

Retroperitoneal abscesses may be classified as primary if the infection results from hematogenous spread or secondary if it is related to infection in an adjacent organ. The conditions associated with the development of retroperitoneal abscesses are shown in Box 44.2. The anatomic relationship of retroperitoneal abscesses to surrounding structures is shown in Fig. 44.15.

BOX 44.2 Causes of retroperitoneal abscesses.

Cause

Renal diseases, such as pyelonephritis
Gastrointestinal diseases, such as diverticulitis, appendicitis, and Crohn disease
Hematogenous spread from remote infections
Abscesses complicating operative procedures
Bone infections, such as tuberculosis of the spine
Trauma
Malignant neoplasms
Miscellaneous causes

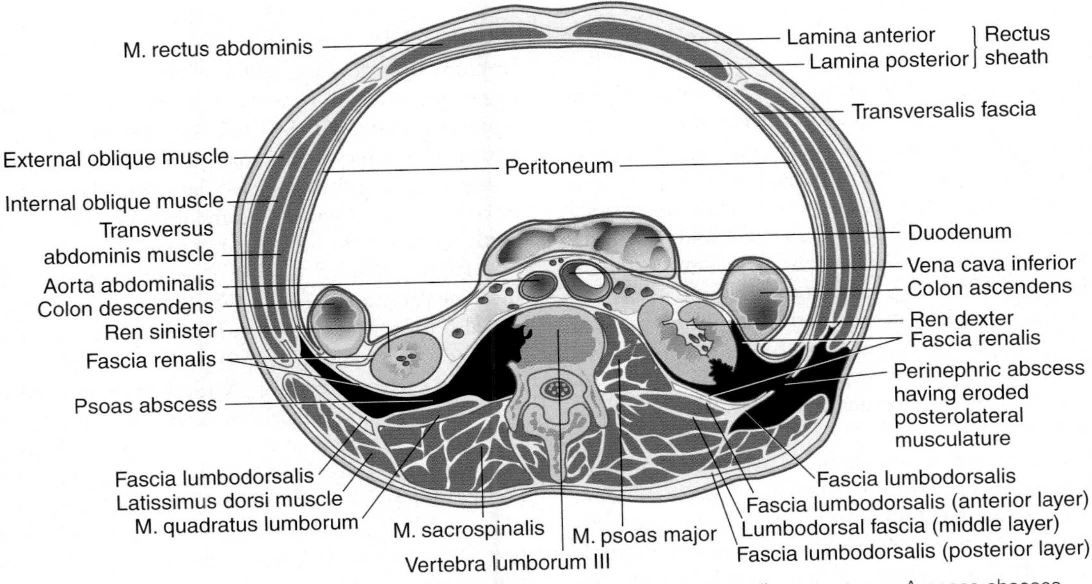

FIG. 44.15 Anatomic relationships of retroperitoneal abscesses to surrounding structures. A psoas abscess *(left)* and perinephric abscess *(right)* are shown. (From McVay C. *Anson and McVay's Surgical Anatomy*. 6th ed. Philadelphia: WB Saunders; 1984:735.)

Most retroperitoneal abscesses originate as inflammatory processes in the kidney and GI tract. Renal causes include infections related to renal lithiasis or previous urologic operative procedures. GI causes include appendicitis, diverticulitis, pancreatitis, and Crohn disease. In one series from an urban center, tuberculosis of the spine was a common cause of retroperitoneal abscesses, with *Mycobacterium tuberculosis* being the second most common bacterial isolate after *E. coli*.[42]

The bacteriology of retroperitoneal abscesses is related to the underlying etiology. Infections originating from the kidney are usually monomicrobial and involve gram-negative bacilli such as *Proteus mirabilis* and *E. coli*. Abscesses associated with diseases of the GI tract involve *E. coli*, *Enterobacter* spp., enterococci, and anaerobic species such as *Bacteroides*. These infections are multimicrobial. Infections from hematogenous sources are usually monomicrobial and most often staphylococcal species. As alluded to earlier, tuberculosis of the spine is an important cause of retroperitoneal abscesses in immunocompromised individuals and in those immigrating from underdeveloped countries.

The most common symptoms of retroperitoneal abscesses include abdominal or flank pain (60%–75%), fever and chills (30%–90%), malaise (10%–22%), and weight loss (12%). Patients with psoas abscesses may have referred pain to the hip, groin, or knee. The duration of symptoms is usually longer than 1 week. Patients with retroperitoneal abscesses often have concurrent, chronic illnesses such as renal lithiasis, diabetes mellitus, HIV infection, or malignancies.

CT will demonstrate a low-density mass in the retroperitoneum with surrounding inflammation. Gas is present in as many as one third of these lesions.[42] CT provides important information about the location of the abscess and its relationship to contiguous organs and hence likely sources of the infection.

Treatment of retroperitoneal abscesses includes appropriate antibiotics and adequate drainage. Many reports have demonstrated the efficacy of CT-guided drainage in managing this aspect of treatment. Operative drainage through a retroperitoneal approach is indicated for lesions not amenable to percutaneous drainage or those that fail percutaneous drainage. The mortality rate for patients with retroperitoneal abscesses is related in large part to the presence of significant medical comorbidities.

Retroperitoneal Hematomas

Retroperitoneal hematomas usually occur after blunt or penetrating injuries, in the setting of ruptured abdominal aortic or visceral artery aneurysms, or after acute or chronic anticoagulation or fibrinolytic therapy. The diagnosis and management of retroperitoneal hematomas occurring in the setting of trauma or aneurysmal rupture are considered in detail in Chapters 17, 62, and 64. Bleeding into the retroperitoneum may also complicate anticoagulant therapy for atrial fibrillation, deep venous thrombosis, or arterial catheterization during cardiac catheterization and endovascular procedures. Retroperitoneal hematomas have also been described in patients undergoing fibrinolytic therapy for peripheral or coronary arterial thrombosis and in patients with bleeding diatheses such as hemophilia.

Patients present with abdominal or flank pain that may radiate into the groin, labia, or scrotum. Clinical evidence of acute blood loss may be present depending on the volume of blood lost and the rapidity with which the patient bled. A palpable abdominal mass as well as physical evidence of ileus may be present. As many as 20% to 30% of patients will develop signs of a femoral neuropathy.[43] The complete blood count may provide evidence of subacute or chronic blood loss or platelet deficiency. The prothrombin and partial thromboplastin times may demonstrate a coagulopathy. Microscopic hematuria is a common finding on urinalysis. CT establishes the diagnosis by demonstrating a high-density mass in the retroperitoneum with surrounding stranding in the retroperitoneal tissue planes. These findings are readily distinguishable from the low-density mass characteristic of retroperitoneal abscesses.

Patients who develop retroperitoneal hematomas as a result of anticoagulation are best managed by the restoration of circulating blood volume and correction of the underlying coagulopathy. In rare circumstances, arteriography with embolization of a bleeding artery or operative exploration is required to stop the bleeding.

Retroperitoneal Fibrosis

Retroperitoneal fibrosis is characterized by chronic inflammation and fibrosis surrounding the abdominal aorta and iliac arteries that extend laterally to envelop surrounding structures especially the ureters. Seventy percent of cases are idiopathic (Ormond disease), whereas 30% are associated with various drugs (most notably ergot alkaloids or dopaminergic agonists), infections, trauma, retroperitoneal hemorrhage, retroperitoneal operations, radiation therapy, or primary or metastatic neoplasms. Many idiopathic cases are associated with inflammatory abdominal aortic aneurysms. Thus, idiopathic retroperitoneal fibrosis might best be categorized with inflammatory abdominal aortic aneurysms and perianeurysmal retroperitoneal fibrosis as a form of chronic periaortitis.[44] The fibrosis is usually confined to the central and paravertebral spaces between the renal arteries and sacrum and tends to encase the aorta, inferior vena cava, and ureters. The process usually begins at the level of the aortic bifurcation and spreads cephalad. In 15% of cases, the fibrotic process extends outside the retroperitoneum to involve the peripancreatic and periduodenal spaces, pelvis, and mediastinum.

There is considerable evidence to suggest that idiopathic retroperitoneal fibrosis is a manifestation of a systemic autoimmune disease. A case-control study of 35 patients found that the disease is associated with HLA-DRB1*03, an allele linked to various autoimmune diseases including type 1 diabetes mellitus, myasthenia gravis, and systemic lupus erythematosus. In some patients, the disease will develop in the setting of a well-defined systemic autoimmune disorder (e.g., systemic lupus erythematosus) or so-called organ-specific autoimmune diseases (e.g., Hashimoto thyroiditis, sclerosing cholangitis). There are also histologic similarities between idiopathic retroperitoneal fibrosis and other systemic inflammatory conditions such as large-vessel vasculitides.[44] Systemic or constitutional symptoms are often present such as fatigue, low-grade fever, weight loss, and myalgias.

Men are affected two to three times as often as women. The mean age at presentation is 50 to 60 years, although the condition has also been reported in children and older adults. Patients may present with localized symptoms of side, back, or abdominal pain or lower extremity edema. Scrotal swelling is common as is the occurrence of a varicocele or hydrocele. In most patients, localized symptoms are preceded by or coexist with systemic or constitutional symptoms. Laboratory tests may demonstrate azotemia, and 80% to 100% of patients will have elevated concentrations of acute-phase reactants (e.g., erythrocyte sedimentation rate, C-reactive protein). The nonspecific nature of the clinical features of this disease contributes to the considerable delay between the onset of symptoms and the diagnosis. As such, ureteral involvement is present in 80% to 100% of cases.[44]

Evaluation of patients thought to have retroperitoneal fibrosis often starts with a CT scan. Without intravenous contrast, the CT scan will demonstrate a homogeneous fibrous plaque surrounding the lower abdominal aorta and the iliac arteries, which is usually isodense to surrounding muscle. MRI of early benign retroperitoneal fibrosis may show areas of high signal intensity on T2-weighted images due to the abundant fluid content and hypercellularity associated with acute inflammation. In the mature and quiescent stages of benign retroperitoneal fibrosis, there is a low signal intensity on T1- and T2-weighted images, similar to that of psoas muscle.

The primary goals of treatment for patients with idiopathic retroperitoneal fibrosis are to stop the progression of retroperitoneal inflammation and fibrosis, to prevent or relieve ureteral obstruction, to inhibit the systemic inflammatory response, and to improve the constitutional manifestations of the disease. The mainstay of treatment has been the administration of corticosteroids, which suppress the synthesis of proinflammatory cytokines and inhibit collagen synthesis and maturation. This will often result in prompt improvement in symptoms, reduction in the size of the retroperitoneal mass, and relief of ureteral obstruction. The optimal dose and duration of treatment have not been well established. Immunosuppressants such as mycophenolate mofetil, cyclophosphamide, azathioprine, methotrexate, cyclosporine, and tamoxifen have also been used to treat patients with idiopathic retroperitoneal fibrosis, particularly those whose disease is unresponsive to steroids. Operative management is generally performed to relieve ureteral obstruction by open ureterolysis with intraperitoneal transposition and omental wrapping of the ureters. In most cases, when the clinical findings and imaging suggest the diagnosis of retroperitoneal fibrosis, the temporary placement of ureteral stents followed by medical therapy is the recommended course of action. Operative ureterolysis is reserved for patients with refractory disease.

When retroperitoneal fibrosis is associated with an abdominal aortic aneurysm, repair of the aneurysm is warranted when the aortic diameter exceeds 4.5 to 5 cm. The effect of aneurysm repair on the periaortic fibrosis is unclear, with some reports documenting resolution of the fibrosis and others reporting persistence or even progression of the inflammatory process.

Retroperitoneal Malignant Neoplasms

Malignant neoplasms in the retroperitoneum can be broadly categorized as primary or secondary. The most common primary malignant neoplasm of the retroperitoneum is a sarcoma (see Chapter 32). Other primary retroperitoneal malignancies are lymphoma and extragonadal germ cell tumors. Secondary retroperitoneal neoplasms include extracapsular growth of a malignant tumor in a retroperitoneal organ, such as the kidney, adrenal, colon, or pancreas, or metastases from a remote primary tumor, such as GU lymph node metastases.

Retroperitoneal Sarcoma

Approximately 15% of soft tissue sarcomas arise within the retroperitoneum. In this location, the most common histologic subtypes are liposarcoma and leiomyosarcoma. Most patients present with a large abdominal mass. Abdominal pain is present in about 50% of the patients. Other symptoms are related to organ compression from the tumor and include early satiety, nausea, vomiting, constipation, weight loss, and lower extremity edema. Symptoms due to nerve compression by the tumor, such as lower extremity paresthesia and paresis, are also reported.

Cross-sectional imaging with CT or MRI will provide important information about the size and precise location of the tumor and its relationship to major vascular structures (Fig. 44.16). These studies will also document the presence or absence of metastatic disease in the lungs or liver. Retroperitoneal sarcomas generally present as a large, well-circumscribed mass that displaces rather than invades intraabdominal organs. They tend to be solid, but higher-grade tumors may be heterogeneous or partially cystic due to areas of necrosis. Liposarcomas show variable areas of fat density. The appearance of these tumors on CT or MRI will usually obviate the need for image-guided biopsy.

The differential diagnosis of a retroperitoneal mass includes bulky lymphadenopathy associated with lymphoma or testicular

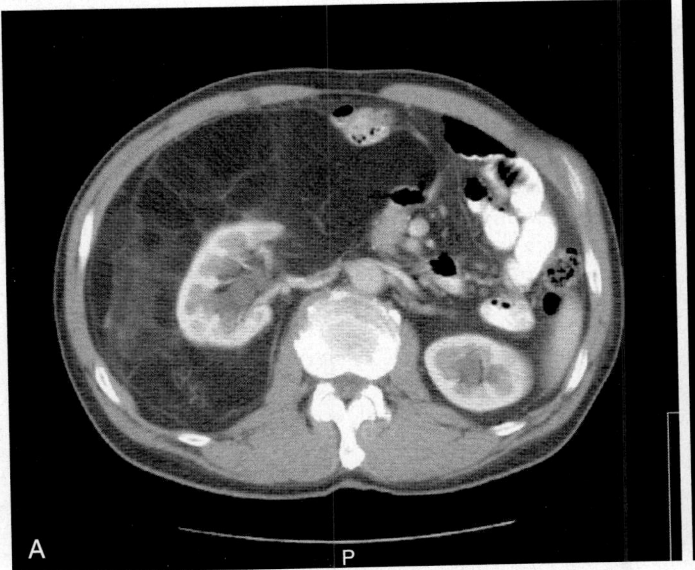

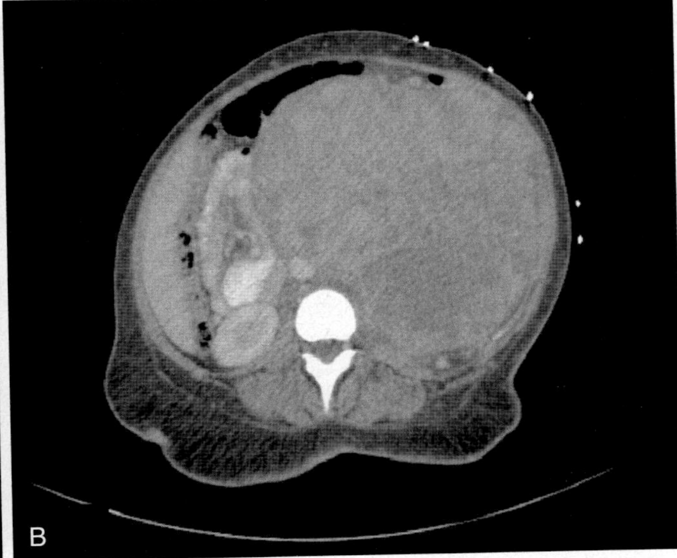

FIG. 44.16 Retroperitoneal sarcomas shown on computed tomography scans. (A) Large well-differentiated liposarcoma involving right kidney, displacing abdominal contents to the left. Tumor density is similar to mature fat. (B) High-grade leiomyosarcoma in left abdomen, demonstrated as a hyperdense, heterogeneous mass.

cancer as well as direct extension of primary malignancies of retroperitoneal organs, especially adrenal, renal, or pancreatic carcinoma. Constitutional symptoms of fevers, night sweats, and weight loss may suggest lymphoma as would peripheral lymphadenopathy. The evaluation of male patients should include careful testicular examination and serologic testing for alpha-fetoprotein and human chorionic gonadotropin.

The goal of surgical therapy for patients with retroperitoneal sarcoma is the removal of all gross disease (macroscopically negative margin) with en bloc resection of adherent organs. The large size of these tumors and their proximity to critical retroperitoneal structures make microscopically negative (R0) margins difficult to document and to achieve. Extension of the resection margin to include adjacent uninvolved organs is associated with increased morbidity without a clear survival benefit.[45,46] Lymph node metastases by sarcoma are rare (<5%); therefore, lymphadenectomy is not required unless there is evidence of lymph node involvement. The large size of these tumors and their proximity to critical retroperitoneal structures frequently requires complex, multiorgan resections, best performed in referral centers that are experienced in treating patients with these rare tumors.

The completeness of resection is an important prognostic factor for patients with retroperitoneal sarcomas.[47] Complete resection is achieved in 50% to 67% of cases depending upon the size and location of the tumor and the experience of the surgeon.[48] Patients undergoing an incomplete gross resection (R2) have the same survival rates as patients who are unresectable. Incomplete resection (R2) should be undertaken only for palliative purposes for all histologic types of sarcoma except liposarcoma.[47] The incomplete resection of well-differentiated liposarcomas has been shown to not only improve symptoms but may prolong survival as well.[49]

Of patients undergoing a complete resection, 25% to 50% will develop local recurrence of their tumor. Patients with an isolated local recurrence will benefit from complete resection. Lewis and colleagues[47] at Memorial-Sloan Kettering Cancer Center was able to achieve complete resection in 35 of 61 patients with recurrent retroperitoneal sarcoma. The 5-year disease-specific survival for these patients was 60% compared with 18% for those patients undergoing incomplete resection ($P = 0.01$).

Radiation therapy has proven effective in increasing local control for extremity sarcomas. However, retroperitoneal sarcomas pose a challenge due to their larger size and toxicity to adjacent organs (e.g., kidney, spine, liver, or small bowel), which limits its use in the adjuvant setting. There is also a lack of prospective trials that have shown a benefit in survival. For these reasons, some experts do not recommend routine use of adjuvant radiation therapy after resection. However, a large case-control study using a national database found an association with improved survival with the use of radiation therapy, either pre- or postoperatively, compared to resection alone. Preoperative radiation therapy has the benefits of less toxicity, since the tumor displaces sensitive organs, requires a lower dose, and has more accurate targets. An ongoing phase 3 randomized trial is assessing the benefit of preoperative radiation therapy compared to curative surgery alone and will help determine its role.[50]

SELECTED REFERENCES

Carr NJ, Cecil TD, Mohamed F, et al. A consensus for classification and pathologic reporting of pseudomyxoma peritonei and associated appendiceal neoplasia. The results of the Peritoneal Surface Oncology Group International (PSOGI) modified Delphi process. *Am J Surg Pathol.* 2016;40:14–26.

This consensus, written by the most renowned experts in hyperthermic intraperitoneal chemotherapy, establishes and clarifies in detail the previously confusing terminology of pseudomyxoma peritonei and appendiceal neoplasms.

Helm JH, Miura JT, Glenn JA, et al. Cytoreductive surgery and hyperthermic intraperitoneal chemotherapy for malignant peritoneal mesothelioma: a systematic review and meta-analysis. *Ann Surg Oncol.* 2015;22:1686–1693.

This systematic review provides a recent report of the outcomes of treatment for this rare disease.

Koulaouzidis A, Bhat S, Saeed AA. Spontaneous bacterial peritonitis. *World J Gastroenterol.* 2009;15:1042–1049.

This is a well-written and thorough review of the pathophysiology, bacteriology, and treatment of spontaneous bacterial peritonitis.

Martin LC, Merkle EM, Thompson WM. Review of internal hernias: radiographic and clinical findings. *AJR Am J Roentgenol.* 2006;186:703–717.

This is a thorough and well-illustrated review of the types of congenital and acquired internal hernias.

Runyon BA, Montano AA, Akriviadis EA, et al. The serum-ascites albumin gradient is superior to the exudate-transudate concept in the differential diagnosis of ascites. *Ann Intern Med.* 1992;117:215–220.

This well-written paper established the use of serum-ascites albumin gradient in the elucidation of the pathophysiology of ascites formation.

Smith K, Desai J, Lazarakis S, et al. Systematic review and clinical outcomes following various treatment options for patients with extraabdominal desmoid tumors. *Ann Surg Oncol.* 2018;25:1544–1554.

This recent systematic review provides an analysis of multiple treatment modalities for desmoid tumors, including observation with a "wait and see" approach.

Trans-Atlantic RPS Working Group. Management of primary retroperitoneal sarcoma (RPS) in the adult: a consensus approach from the Trans-Atlantic RPS Working Group. *Ann Surg Oncol.* 2015;22:256–263.

This paper provides updated consensus statements on the management of retroperitoneal sarcoma.

Verwaal VJ, Bruin S, Boot H, et al. 8-year follow-up of randomized trial: cytoreduction and hyperthermic intraperitoneal chemotherapy versus systemic chemotherapy in patients with peritoneal carcinomatosis of colorectal cancer. *Ann Surg Oncol.* 2008;15:2426–2432.

This is a follow-up of a classic randomized trial showing the potential benefit of cytoreduction and hyperthermic intraperitoneal chemotherapy in carcinomatosis from colorectal cancer.

REFERENCES

1. Cherry WB, Mueller PS. Rectus sheath hematoma: review of 126 cases at a single institution. *Medicine (Baltim).* 2006;85:105–110.
2. Li J, Wang CY. TBL1-TBLR1 and beta-catenin recruit each other to Wnt target-gene promoter for transcription activation and oncogenesis. *Nat Cell Biol.* 2008;10:160–169.
3. Nieuwenhuis MH, Lefevre JH, Bulow S, et al. Family history, surgery, and APC mutation are risk factors for desmoid tumors in familial adenomatous polyposis: an international cohort study. *Dis Colon Rectum.* 2011;54:1229–1234.
4. De Marchis ML, Tonelli F, Quaresmini D, et al. Desmoid tumors in familial adenomatous polyposis. *Anticancer Res.* 2017;37:3357–3366.
5. Kasper B, Baumgarten C, Garcia J, et al. An update on the management of sporadic desmoid-type fibromatosis: a European consensus Initiative between sarcoma PAtients EuroNet (SPAEN) and European Organization for research and treatment of cancer (EORTC)/Soft tissue and bone sarcoma group (STBSG). *Ann Oncol.* 2017;28:2399–2408.
6. Crago AM, Denton B, Salas S, et al. A prognostic nomogram for prediction of recurrence in desmoid fibromatosis. *Ann Surg.* 2013;258:347–353.
7. Bonvalot S, Ternes N, Fiore M, et al. Spontaneous regression of primary abdominal wall desmoid tumors: more common than previously thought. *Ann Surg Oncol.* 2013;20:4096–4102.
8. Smith K, Desai J, Lazarakis S, et al. Systematic review of clinical outcomes following various treatment options for patients with extraabdominal desmoid tumors. *Ann Surg Oncol.* 2018;25:1544–1554.
9. Janssen ML, van Broekhoven DL, Cates JM, et al. Meta-analysis of the influence of surgical margin and adjuvant radiotherapy on local recurrence after resection of sporadic desmoid-type fibromatosis. *Br J Surg.* 2017;104:347–357.
10. Keus RB, Nout RA, Blay JY, et al. Results of a phase II pilot study of moderate dose radiotherapy for inoperable desmoid-type fibromatosis—an EORTC STBSG and ROG study (EORTC 62991-22998). *Ann Oncol.* 2013;24:2672–2676.
11. Quast DR, Schneider R, Burdzik E, et al. Long-term outcome of sporadic and FAP-associated desmoid tumors treated with high-dose selective estrogen receptor modulators and sulindac: a single-center long-term observational study in 134 patients. *Fam Cancer.* 2016;15:31–40.
12. Soft tissue sarcoma of the trunk and extremities. In: Amin MB, Edge SB, Greene FL, et al., eds. *AJCC Cancer Staging Manual.* 8th ed. New York: Springer; 2018:507–516.
13. Biau DJ, Ferguson PC, Chung P, et al. Local recurrence of localized soft tissue sarcoma: a new look at old predictors. *Cancer.* 2012;118:5867–5877.
14. Plaza JA, Perez-Montiel D, Mayerson J, et al. Metastases to soft tissue: a review of 118 cases over a 30-year period. *Cancer.* 2008;112:193–203.
15. Fleshman J, Sargent DJ, Green E, et al. Laparoscopic colectomy for cancer is not inferior to open surgery based on 5-year data from the COST Study Group Trial. *Ann Surg.* 2007;246:655–662; discussion 662–654.
16. Runyon BA. Paracentesis of ascitic fluid. A safe procedure. *Arch Intern Med.* 1986;146:2259–2261.
17. Runyon BA, Montano AA, Akriviadis EA, et al. The serum-ascites albumin gradient is superior to the exudate-transudate concept in the differential diagnosis of ascites. *Ann Intern Med.* 1992;117:215–220.
18. Koulaouzidis A, Bhat S, Saeed AA. Spontaneous bacterial peritonitis. *World J Gastroenterol.* 2009;15:1042–1049.
19. Nguyen-Khac E, Cadranel JF, Thevenot T, et al. Review article: the utility of reagent strips in the diagnosis of infected ascites in cirrhotic patients. *Aliment Pharmacol Ther.* 2008;28:282–288.
20. Chavez-Tapia NC, Soares-Weiser K, Brezis M, et al. Antibiotics for spontaneous bacterial peritonitis in cirrhotic patients. *Cochrane Database Syst Rev.* 2009:CD002232.
21. Sanai FM, Bzeizi KI. Systematic review: tuberculous peritonitis—presenting features, diagnostic strategies and treatment. *Aliment Pharmacol Ther.* 2005;22:685–700.
22. Kavanagh D, Prescott GJ, Mactier RA. Peritoneal dialysis-associated peritonitis in Scotland (1999–2002). *Nephrol Dial Transplant.* 2004;19:2584–2591.
23. Carr NJ, Cecil TD, Mohamed F, et al. A consensus for classification and pathologic reporting of pseudomyxoma peritonei and associated appendiceal neoplasia: the results of the Peritoneal Surface Oncology Group International (PSOGI) Modified Delphi Process. *Am J Surg Pathol.* 2016;40:14–26.
24. Davison JM, Choudry HA, Pingpank JF, et al. Clinicopathologic and molecular analysis of disseminated appendiceal mucinous neoplasms: identification of factors predicting survival and proposed criteria for a three-tiered assessment of tumor grade. *Mod Pathol.* 2014;27:1521–1539.
25. Ronnett BM, Yan H, Kurman RJ, et al. Patients with pseudomyxoma peritonei associated with disseminated peritoneal adenomucinosis have a significantly more favorable prognosis than patients with peritoneal mucinous carcinomatosis. *Cancer.* 2001;92:85–91.
26. Votanopoulos KI, Shen P, Skardal A, et al. Peritoneal metastases from appendiceal cancer. *Surg Oncol Clin N Am.* 2018;27:551–561.
27. Verwaal VJ, Bruin S, Boot H, et al. 8-year follow-up of randomized trial: cytoreduction and hyperthermic intraperitoneal chemotherapy versus systemic chemotherapy in patients with peritoneal carcinomatosis of colorectal cancer. *Ann Surg Oncol.* 2008;15:2426–2432.
28. Quenet F, Elias D, Roca L, et al. A UNICANCER phase III trial of hyperthermic intra-peritoneal chemotherapy (HIPEC) for colorectal peritoneal carcinomatosis. PRODIGE 7. *Eur J Surg Oncol.* 2019;45:E17.
29. Teta MJ, Mink PJ, Lau E, et al. US mesothelioma patterns 1973–2002: indicators of change and insights into background rates. *Eur J Cancer Prev.* 2008;17:525–534.
30. Mirarabshahii P, Pillai K, Chua TC, et al. Diffuse malignant peritoneal mesothelioma—an update on treatment. *Cancer Treat Rev.* 2012;38:605–612.
31. Helm JH, Miura JT, Glenn JA, et al. Cytoreductive surgery and hyperthermic intraperitoneal chemotherapy for malignant peritoneal mesothelioma: a systematic review and meta-analysis. *Ann Surg Oncol.* 2015;22:1686–1693.
32. Sugarbaker PH. Update on the management of malignant peritoneal mesothelioma. *Transl Lung Cancer Res.* 2018;7:599–608.
33. Yan TD, Deraco M, Baratti D, et al. Cytoreductive surgery and hyperthermic intraperitoneal chemotherapy for malignant peritoneal mesothelioma: multi-institutional experience. *J Clin Oncol.* 2009;27:6237–6242.

34. Gross I, Siedner-Weintraub Y, Stibbe S, et al. Characteristics of mesenteric lymphadenitis in comparison with those of acute appendicitis in children. *Eur J Pediatr*. 2017;176:199–205.
35. Levy AD, Rimola J, Mehrotra AK, et al. From the archives of the AFIP: benign fibrous tumors and tumorlike lesions of the mesentery: radiologic-pathologic correlation. *Radiographics*. 2006;26:245–264.
36. Martin LC, Merkle EM, Thompson WM. Review of internal hernias: radiographic and clinical findings. *AJR Am J Roentgenol*. 2006;186:703–717.
37. Cabot JC, Lee SA, Yoo J, et al. Long-term consequences of not closing the mesenteric defect after laparoscopic right colectomy. *Dis Colon Rectum*. 2010;53:289–292.
38. Gurbuz AK, Giardiello FM, Petersen GM, et al. Desmoid tumours in familial adenomatous polyposis. *Gut*. 1994;35:377–381.
39. Vitellaro M, Sala P, Signoroni S, et al. Risk of desmoid tumours after open and laparoscopic colectomy in patients with familial adenomatous polyposis. *Br J Surg*. 2014;101:558–565.
40. Sinha A, Burns EM, Latchford A, et al. Risk of desmoid formation after laparoscopic versus open colectomy and ileorectal anastomosis for familial adenomatous polyposis. *BJS Open*. 2018;2:452–455.
41. Guillem JG, Wood WC, Moley JF, et al. ASCO/SSO review of current role of risk-reducing surgery in common hereditary cancer syndromes. *J Clin Oncol*. 2006;24:4642–4660.
42. Paley M, Sidhu PS, Evans RA, et al. Retroperitoneal collections—aetiology and radiological implications. *Clin Radiol*. 1997;52:290–294.
43. Loor G, Bassiouny H, Valentin C, et al. Local and systemic consequences of large retroperitoneal clot burdens. *World J Surg*. 2009;33:1618–1625.
44. Vaglio A, Salvarani C, Buzio C. Retroperitoneal fibrosis. *Lancet*. 2006;367:241–251.
45. Gronchi A, Lo Vullo S, Fiore M, et al. Aggressive surgical policies in a retrospectively reviewed single-institution case series of retroperitoneal soft tissue sarcoma patients. *J Clin Oncol*. 2009;27:24–30.
46. Pisters PW. Resection of some—but not all—clinically uninvolved adjacent viscera as part of surgery for retroperitoneal soft tissue sarcomas. *J Clin Oncol*. 2009;27:6–8.
47. Lewis JJ, Leung D, Woodruff JM, et al. Retroperitoneal soft-tissue sarcoma: analysis of 500 patients treated and followed at a single institution. *Ann Surg*. 1998;228:355–365.
48. Mendenhall WM, Zlotecki RA, Hochwald SN, et al. Retroperitoneal soft tissue sarcoma. *Cancer*. 2005;104:669–675.
49. Shibata D, Lewis JJ, Leung DH, et al. Is there a role for incomplete resection in the management of retroperitoneal liposarcomas? *J Am Coll Surg*. 2001;193:373–379.
50. European Organisation for Research and Treatment of Cancer. *EORTC: Surgery with or without Radiation Therapy in Untreated Nonmetastatic Retroperitoneal Sarcoma (STRASS)*. NIH U.S. National Library of Medicine; 2016. https://clinicaltrials.gov/ct2/show/NCT01344018. Accessed July 2, 2019.

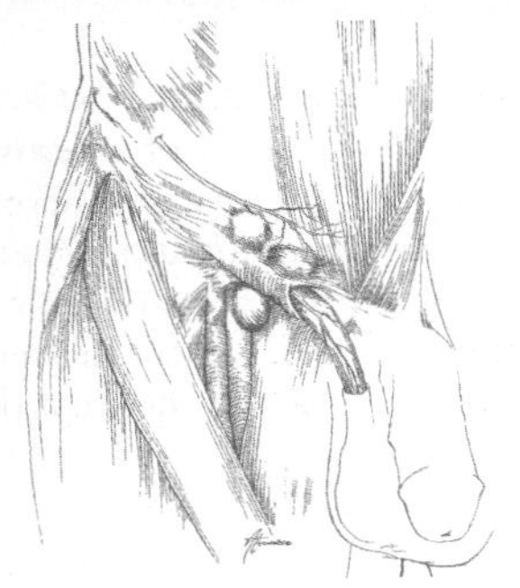

CHAPTER 45

Hernias

Benjamin K. Poulose, Alfredo Maximiliano Carbonell, Michael J. Rosen

OUTLINE

Nearly 1 million hernias are repaired annually in the United States, making hernia repair one of the most common operations performed by general surgeons. Despite the frequency of this procedure, no surgeon has ideal results, and complications such as postoperative pain, nerve injury, and surgical site infection remain. The chance of recurrence, especially after ventral hernia repair, generally increases with time, suggesting that hernia is a chronic disease process affecting patients over their lifetime.

General surgeons care for many diseases affecting the abdominal wall, including intrinsic diseases (hernia, diastasis, athletic pubalgia/core muscle injury, benign and malignant tumors) and extrinsic diseases (prosthetic- and intervention-related complications, benign and malignant tumors). The field of Abdominal Core Health has been recognized as encompassing the stability, function, and quality of life involving the abdominal core. The abdominal core is defined as the circumferential soft tissues of the diaphragm superiorly, the pelvic floor inferiorly, and the abdominal wall and flank anterolaterally, excluding the abdominopelvic viscera. Maintenance of abdominal core health may include exercise, physical therapy, medical therapy (including compression garment or truss use), alternative medical therapies (including acupuncture or yoga), surgical intervention, and measures to prevent disease (e.g., hernia prophylaxis). Rebranding this area of surgery is reflective of the care actually provided to patients and may provide new avenues for clinical care and research that are badly needed to help determine optimal treatments and to identify methods of prevention. The management of hernia is an integral component of maintaining abdominal core health.

Hernia is derived from the Latin word for rupture. A hernia is defined as an abnormal protrusion of an organ or tissue through a defect in its surrounding walls. Although a hernia can occur at various sites of the body, these defects most commonly involve the abdominal wall, particularly the inguinal region. Abdominal wall hernias occur only at sites at which the aponeurosis and fascia are not covered by striated muscle (Box 45.1). These sites most commonly include the inguinal, femoral, and umbilical areas; linea alba; lower portion of the semilunar line; and sites of prior incisions (Fig. 45.1). The so-called neck or orifice of a hernia is located at the innermost musculoaponeurotic layer, whereas the hernia sac is lined by peritoneum and protrudes from the neck. There is no consistent relationship between the area of a hernia defect and the size of a hernia sac.

A hernia is reducible when its contents can be replaced within the surrounding musculature, and it is irreducible or incarcerated when it cannot be reduced. A strangulated hernia has compromised blood supply to its contents, which is a serious and potentially fatal complication. Strangulation occurs more often in large hernias that have small orifices. In this situation, the small neck of the hernia obstructs arterial blood flow, venous drainage, or both to the contents of the hernia sac. Adhesions between the contents of the hernia and peritoneal lining of the sac can provide a tethering point that entraps the hernia contents and predisposes to intestinal obstruction and strangulation. A more unusual type of strangulation is a Richter hernia. In a Richter hernia, a small portion of the antimesenteric wall of the intestine is trapped within the hernia, and strangulation can occur without the presence of intestinal obstruction.

BOX 45.1 Primary abdominal wall hernias.

Groin
Inguinal
  Indirect
  Direct
  Combined
Femoral

Anterior
Umbilical
Epigastric
Spigelian

Pelvic
Obturator
Sciatic
Perineal

Posterior
Lumbar
  Superior triangle
  Inferior triangle

An external hernia protrudes through all layers of the abdominal wall, whereas an internal hernia is a protrusion of intestine through a defect in the peritoneal cavity. An interparietal hernia occurs when the hernia sac is contained within a musculoaponeurotic layer of the abdominal wall. In broad terms, most abdominal wall hernias can be separated into inguinal and ventral hernias. This chapter focuses on the specific aspects of each of these conditions individually.

INGUINAL HERNIAS

Inguinal hernias are classified as direct or indirect. The sac of an indirect inguinal hernia passes from the internal inguinal ring obliquely toward the external inguinal ring and ultimately into the scrotum. In contrast, the sac of a direct inguinal hernia protrudes outward and forward and is medial to the internal inguinal ring and inferior epigastric vessels. As indirect hernias enlarge, it sometimes can be difficult to distinguish between indirect and direct inguinal hernias. This distinction is of little importance because the operative repair of these types of hernias is similar. A pantaloon-type hernia occurs when there is both an indirect and a direct hernia component.

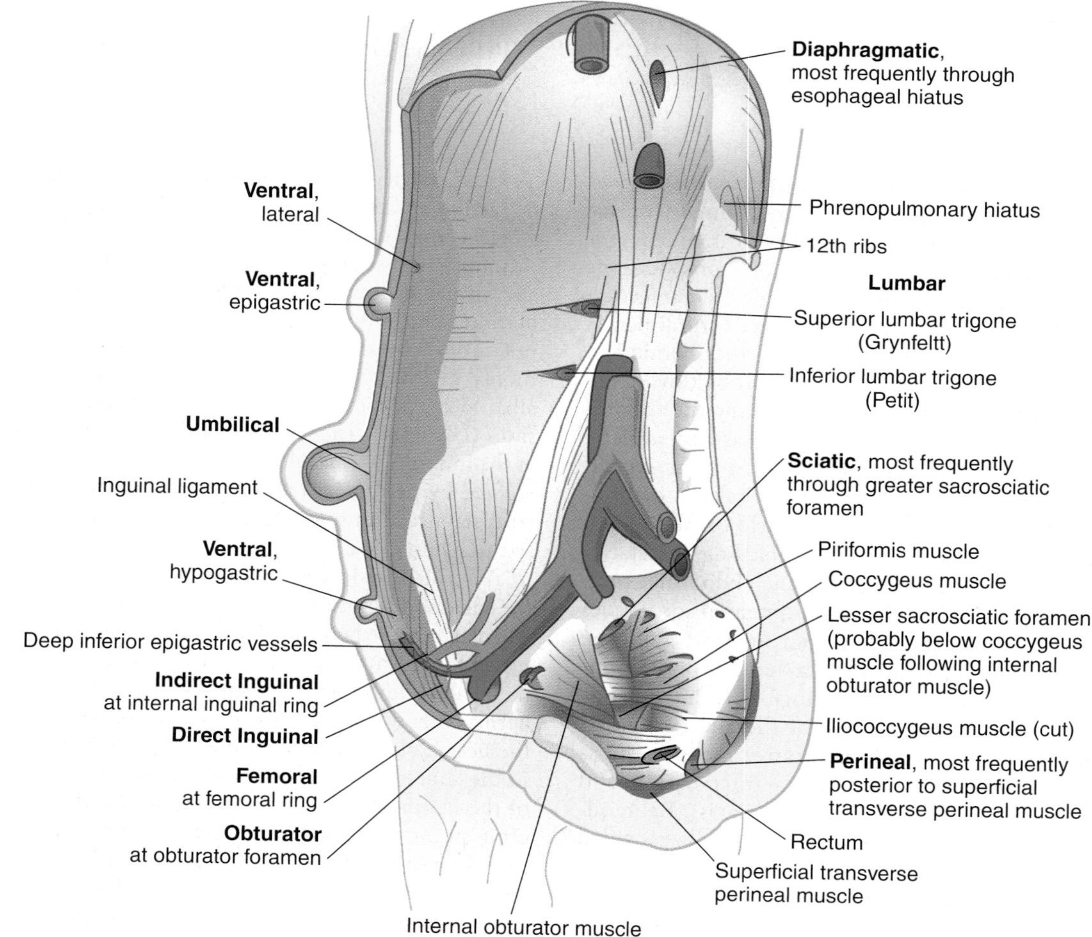

FIG. 45.1 Types of abdominal wall hernias. (From *Dorland's Illustrated Medical Dictionary*. 31st ed. Philadelphia: WB Saunders; 2007: Plate 21.)

Incidence

Hernias are a common problem; however, their true incidence is unknown. It is estimated that 5% of the population will develop an abdominal wall hernia, but the prevalence may be even higher. About 75% of all hernias occur in the inguinal region. Two-thirds of these are indirect and the remainder are direct inguinal hernias. Femoral hernias represent only 3% of all groin hernias.

Men are 25 times more likely to have a groin hernia than women. An indirect inguinal hernia is the most common hernia, regardless of gender. In men, indirect hernias predominate over direct hernias at a ratio of 2:1. Indirect hernias are by far the most common type of hernia in women. The female-to-male ratio for femoral and umbilical hernias, however, is about 10:1 and 2:1, respectively. Although femoral hernias occur more frequently in women than in men, inguinal hernias remain the most common hernia in women. Femoral hernias are rare in men. Ten percent of women and 50% of men who have a femoral hernia have or will develop an inguinal hernia.

Indirect inguinal and femoral hernias occur more commonly on the right side. This is attributed to a delay in atrophy of the processus vaginalis after the normal slower descent of the right testis to the scrotum during fetal development. The predominance of right-sided femoral hernias is thought to be caused by the tamponading effect of the sigmoid colon on the left femoral canal.

The prevalence of hernias increases with age, particularly for inguinal, umbilical, and femoral hernias. The likelihood of strangulation and need for hospitalization also increase with aging. Strangulation, the most common serious complication of a hernia, occurs in only 1% to 3% of groin hernias and is more common at the extremes of life. Most strangulated hernias are indirect inguinal hernias; however, femoral hernias have the highest rate of strangulation (15%–20%) of all hernias, and it is therefore recommended that all femoral hernias be repaired at the time of discovery.

Anatomy of the Groin

The surgeon must have a comprehensive understanding of the anatomy of the groin to select and to use various options for hernia repair properly. In addition, the relationships of muscles, aponeuroses, fascia, nerves, blood vessels, and spermatic cord structures in the inguinal region must be completely understood to obtain the lowest incidence of recurrence and to avoid complications. These anatomic considerations must be understood from the anterior and posterior approaches because both are useful in different situations (Figs. 45.2 and 45.3).

From anterior to posterior, the groin anatomy includes the skin and subcutaneous tissues, below which are the superficial circumflex iliac, superficial epigastric, and external pudendal arteries and accompanying veins. These vessels arise from and drain to the proximal femoral artery and vein, respectively, and are directed superiorly. If encountered during operation, these vessels can be retracted or even divided when necessary.

External Oblique Muscle and Aponeurosis

The external oblique muscle is the most superficial of the lateral abdominal wall muscles; its fibers are directed inferiorly and medially and lie deep to the subcutaneous tissues. The aponeurosis of the external oblique muscle is formed by a superficial and deep layer. This aponeurosis, along with the bilaminar aponeuroses of the internal oblique and transversus abdominis, forms the anterior rectus sheath and, finally, the linea alba by linear decussation. The external oblique aponeurosis serves as the superficial boundary of

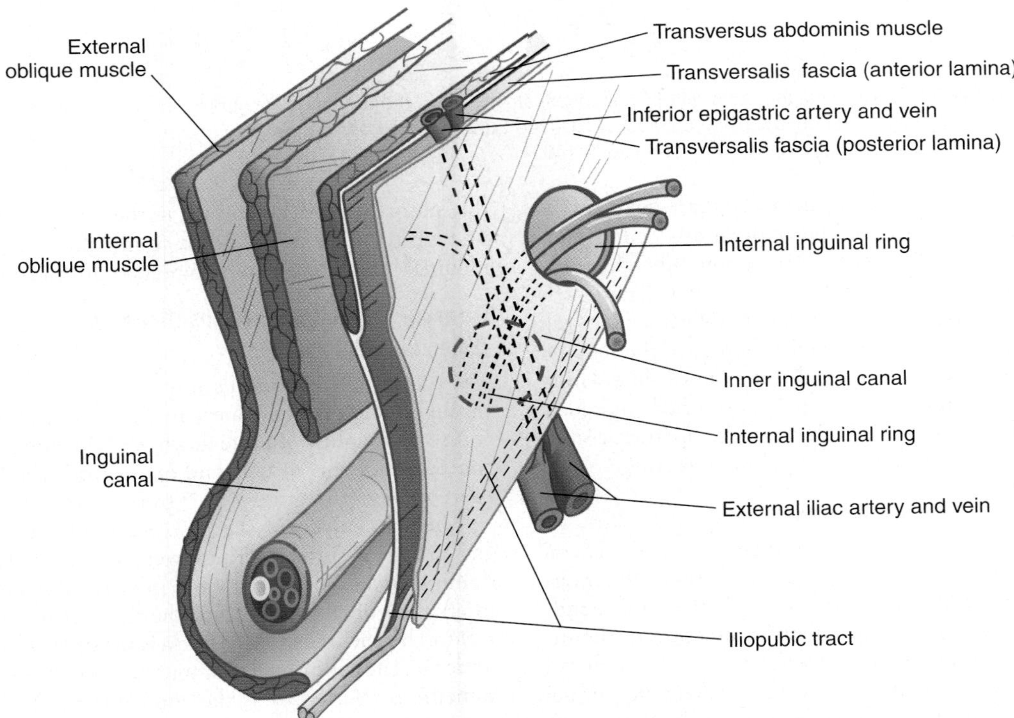

FIG. 45.2 Nyhus's classic parasagittal diagram of the right midinguinal region illustrating the muscular aponeurotic layers separated into anterior and posterior walls. The posterior laminae of the transversalis fascia have been added, with the inferior epigastric vessels coursing through the abdominal wall medially to the inner inguinal canal. (From Read RC. The transversalis and preperitoneal fasciae: a re-evaluation. In: Nyhus LM, Condon RE, eds. *Hernia*. 4th ed. Philadelphia: JB Lippincott; 1995:57–63.)

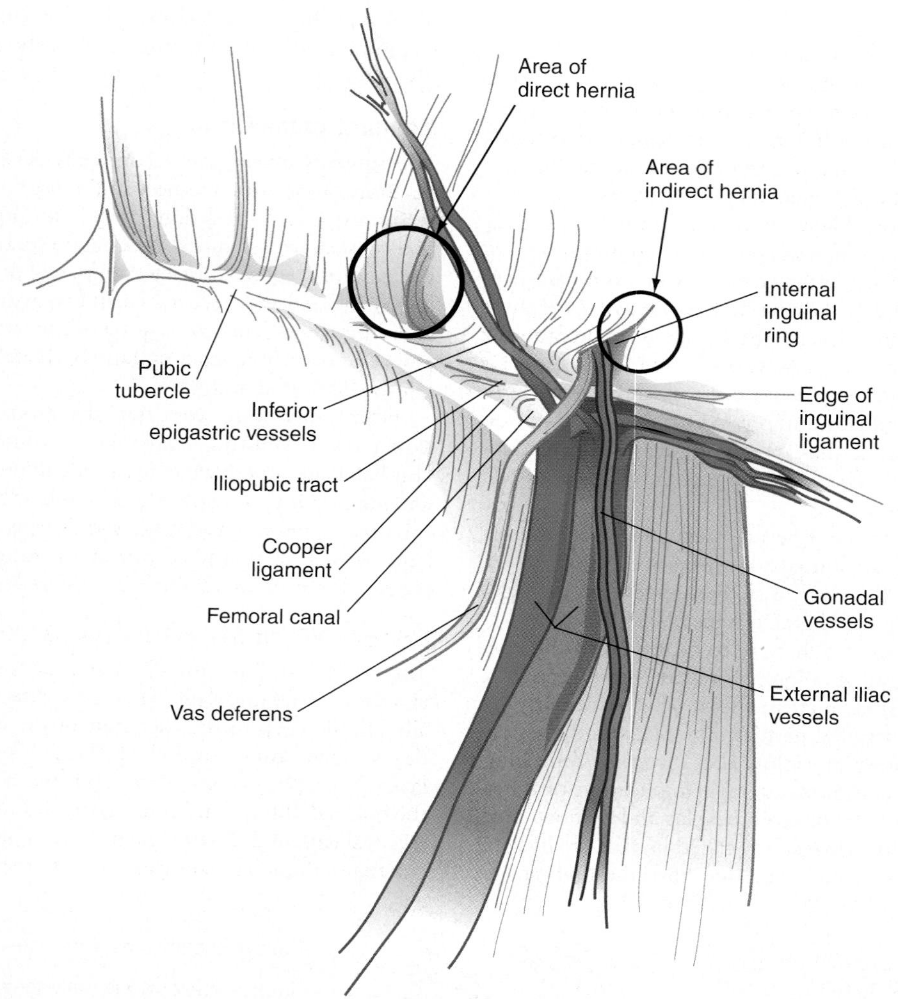

FIG. 45.3 Anatomy of the important preperitoneal structures in the right inguinal space. (From Talamini MA, Are C. Laparoscopic hernia repair. In: Zuidema GD, Yeo CJ, eds. *Shackelford's Surgery of the Alimentary Tract.* 5th ed. Vol. 5. Philadelphia: WB Saunders; 2002:140.)

the inguinal canal. The inguinal ligament (Poupart ligament) is the inferior edge of the external oblique aponeurosis and extends from the anterior superior iliac spine to the pubic tubercle, turning posteriorly to form a shelving edge. The lacunar ligament is the fan-shaped medial expansion of the inguinal ligament, which inserts into the pubis and forms the medial border of the femoral space. The external (superficial) inguinal ring is an ovoid opening of the external oblique aponeurosis that is positioned superiorly and slightly laterally to the pubic tubercle. The spermatic cord exits the inguinal canal through the external inguinal ring.

Internal Oblique Muscle and Aponeurosis

The internal oblique muscle forms the middle layer of the lateral abdominal musculoaponeurotic complex. The fibers of the internal oblique are directed superiorly and laterally in the upper abdomen; however, they run in a slightly inferior direction in the inguinal region. The internal oblique muscle serves as the cephalad (or superior) border of the inguinal canal. The medial aspect of the internal oblique aponeurosis fuses with fibers from the transversus abdominis aponeurosis to form a conjoined tendon. This structure actually is present in only 5% to 10% of patients and is most evident at the insertion of these muscles on the pubic tubercle. The cremaster muscle fibers arise from the internal oblique, encompass the spermatic cord, and attach to the tunica vaginalis of the testis. These muscle fibers should be minimally disrupted during open inguinal hernia repair to help reduce chronic groin pain.

Transversus Abdominis Muscle and Aponeurosis and Transversalis Fascia

The transversus abdominis muscle layer is oriented horizontally throughout most of its area; in the inguinal region, these fibers course in a slightly oblique downward direction. The strength and continuity of this muscle and aponeurosis are important for the prevention and treatment of inguinal hernia.

The aponeurosis of the transversus abdominis covers anterior and posterior surfaces. The lower margin of the transversus abdominis arches along with the internal oblique muscle over the internal inguinal ring to form the transversus abdominis aponeurotic arch. The transversalis fascia is the connective tissue layer that underlies the abdominal wall musculature. The transversalis fascia, sometimes referred to as the endoabdominal fascia, is a component of the inguinal floor. It tends to be denser in this area but still remains relatively thin.

The iliopubic tract is an aponeurotic band that is formed by the transversalis fascia and transversus abdominis aponeurosis and fascia. The iliopubic tract is located posterior to the inguinal ligament and crosses over the femoral vessels and inserts on the anterior superior iliac spine and inner lip of the wing of the ilium.

The inferior crus of the deep inguinal ring is composed of the iliopubic tract; the superior crus of the deep ring is formed by the transversus abdominis aponeurotic arch. The lateral border of the internal ring is connected to the transversus abdominis muscle, which forms a shutter mechanism to limit the development of an indirect hernia.

The iliopubic tract is an extremely important structure in the repair of hernias from the anterior and posterior approaches. It composes the inferior margin of most anterior repairs. The portion of the iliopubic tract lateral to the internal inguinal ring serves as the inferior border below which staples or tacks are not placed during a laparoscopic repair because the femoral, lateral femoral cutaneous, and genitofemoral nerves are located inferior to the iliopubic tract. Although it cannot always be visualized during posterior repairs, if the tacking device cannot be palpated on the anterior abdominal wall, one must assume it is below the iliopubic tract.

Pectineal (Cooper) Ligament

The pectineal (Cooper) ligament is formed by the periosteum and aponeurotic tissues along the superior ramus of the pubis. This structure is posterior to the iliopubic tract and forms the posterior border of the femoral canal. In approximately 75% of patients, there will be a vessel that crosses the lateral border of Cooper ligament that is a branch of the obturator artery. If this vessel is injured, troublesome bleeding can result. Cooper ligament is an important landmark for open and laparoscopic repairs and is a useful anchoring structure, particularly in laparoscopic repairs.

Inguinal Canal

The inguinal canal is about 4 cm in length and is located just cephalad to the inguinal ligament. The canal extends between the internal (deep) inguinal and external (superficial) inguinal rings. The inguinal canal contains the spermatic cord in men and the round ligament of the uterus in women.

The spermatic cord is composed of the cremaster muscle fibers, testicular artery and accompanying veins, genital branch of the genitofemoral nerve, vas deferens, cremasteric vessels, lymphatics, and processus vaginalis. These structures enter the cord at the internal inguinal ring, and vessels and vas deferens exit the external inguinal ring. The cremaster muscle arises from the lowermost fibers of the internal oblique muscle and encompasses the spermatic cord in the inguinal canal. The cremasteric vessels are branches of the inferior epigastric vessels and pass through the posterior wall of the inguinal canal through their own foramen.

The inguinal canal is bounded superficially by the external oblique aponeurosis. The internal oblique and transversus abdominis musculoaponeuroses form the cephalad wall of the inguinal canal. The inferior wall of the inguinal canal is formed by the inguinal ligament and lacunar ligament. The posterior wall, or floor of the inguinal canal, is formed by the aponeurosis of the transversus abdominis muscle and transversalis fascia.

Hesselbach triangle refers to the margins of the floor of the inguinal canal. The inferior epigastric vessels serve as its superolateral border, the rectus sheath as the medial border, and the inguinal ligament and pectineal ligament as the inferior border. Direct hernias occur within Hesselbach triangle, whereas indirect inguinal hernias arise lateral to the triangle. It is not uncommon, however, for medium and large indirect inguinal hernias to involve the floor of the inguinal canal as they enlarge.

The iliohypogastric and ilioinguinal nerves and genital branch of the genitofemoral nerve are the important sensory nerves in the groin area (Fig. 45.4). The iliohypogastric and ilioinguinal nerves provide sensation to the skin of the groin, base of the penis, and ipsilateral upper medial thigh. The iliohypogastric and ilioinguinal nerves lie beneath the internal oblique muscle to a point just medial and superior to the anterior superior iliac spine, where they penetrate the internal oblique muscle and course beneath the external oblique aponeurosis. The main trunk of the iliohypogastric nerve runs on the anterior surface of the internal oblique muscle and aponeurosis medial and superior to the internal ring. The iliohypogastric nerve may provide an inguinal branch that joins the ilioinguinal nerve. The ilioinguinal nerve runs anterior to the spermatic cord in the inguinal canal and branches at the superficial inguinal ring. The genital branch of the genitofemoral nerve innervates the cremaster muscle and skin on the lateral side of the scrotum and labia. This nerve lies on the iliopubic tract and accompanies the cremaster vessels to form a neurovascular bundle. In women, this branch generally follows the course of the round ligament.

Preperitoneal Space

The preperitoneal space contains adipose tissue, lymphatics, blood vessels, and nerves. The nerves of the preperitoneal space of specific concern to the surgeon include the lateral femoral cutaneous nerve and genitofemoral nerve. The lateral femoral cutaneous nerve originates as a root of L2 and L3 and is occasionally a direct branch of the femoral nerve. This nerve courses along the anterior surface of the iliac muscle beneath the iliac fascia and passes under or through the lateral attachment of the inguinal ligament at the anterior superior iliac spine. This nerve runs beneath or occasionally through the iliopubic tract, lateral to the internal inguinal ring.

The genitofemoral nerve usually arises from the L2 or L1–L2 nerve roots. It divides into genital and femoral branches on the anterior surface of the psoas muscle. The genital branch enters the inguinal canal through the deep ring, whereas the femoral branch enters the femoral sheath lateral to the artery.

The inferior epigastric artery and vein are branches of the external iliac vessels and are important landmarks for laparoscopic hernia repair. These vessels course medial to the internal inguinal ring and eventually lie beneath the rectus abdominis muscle, immediately superficial to the transversalis fascia. The inferior epigastric vessels serve to define the types of inguinal hernia. Indirect inguinal hernias occur lateral to the inferior epigastric vessels, whereas direct hernias occur medial to these vessels.

The deep circumflex iliac artery and vein are located below the lateral portion of the iliopubic tract in the preperitoneal space. These vessels are branches of the inferior epigastric or external iliac artery and vein. It is important to dissect only above the iliopubic tract during a laparoscopic hernia repair to avoid injury to these vessels.

The vas deferens courses through the preperitoneal space from caudad to cephalad and medial to lateral to join the spermatic cord at the deep inguinal ring.

Femoral Canal

The boundaries of the femoral canal are the iliopubic tract anteriorly, Cooper ligament posteriorly, and femoral vein laterally. The pubic tubercle forms the apex of the femoral canal triangle. This canal usually contains connective tissue and lymphatic tissue. A femoral hernia occurs through this space and is medial to the femoral vessels.

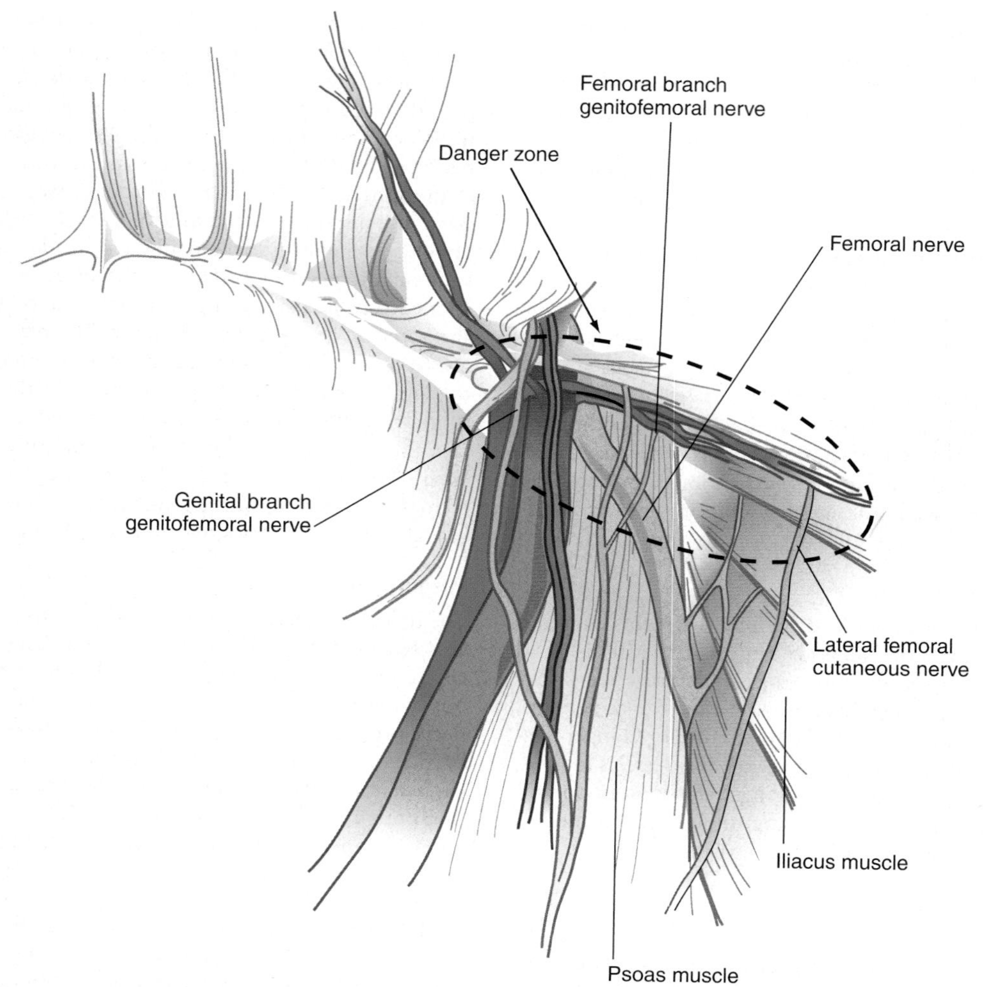

FIG. 45.4 Important nerves and their relationship to inguinal structures (the right side is illustrated). (From Talamini MA, Are C. Laparoscopic hernia repair. In: Zuidema GD, Yeo CJ, eds. *Shackelford's Surgery of the Alimentary Tract*. 5th ed. Vol. 5. Philadelphia: WB Saunders; 2002:140.)

Diagnosis

A bulge in the inguinal region is the main diagnostic finding in most groin hernias. Most patients will have associated pain or vague discomfort in the region, but one-third of patients will have no symptoms. Groin hernias are usually not extremely painful unless incarceration or strangulation has occurred. In the absence of physical findings, alternative causes for pain need to be considered. On occasion, patients may experience paresthesias related to compression or irritation of the inguinal nerves by the hernia. Masses other than hernias can occur in the groin region. Physical examination alone often differentiates between a groin hernia and these masses (Box 45.2).

The inguinal region is examined with the patient in the supine and standing positions. The examiner visually inspects and palpates the inguinal region, looking for asymmetry, bulges, or a mass. Having the patient cough or perform a Valsalva maneuver can facilitate identification of a hernia. The examiner places a fingertip over the inguinal canal and repeats the examination. Finally, a fingertip is placed into the external inguinal ring by invaginating the scrotum to detect a small hernia. A bulge moving lateral to medial in the inguinal canal suggests an indirect hernia. If a bulge progresses from deep to superficial through the inguinal floor, a direct hernia is suspected. This distinction is not critical because repair is approached the same way, regardless of the type of hernia. A bulge identified below the inguinal ligament is consistent with a femoral hernia.

A bulge of the groin described by the patient that is not demonstrated on examination presents a dilemma. Having the patient stand or ambulate for a time may allow an undiagnosed hernia to become visible or palpable. If a hernia is strongly suspected but undetectable, repeated examination at another time may be helpful.

Ultrasonography also can aid in the diagnosis. There is a high degree of sensitivity and specificity for ultrasound in the detection of occult direct, indirect, and femoral hernias.[1] On occasion, laparoscopy can be diagnostic and therapeutic for particularly challenging cases.

Classification

There are numerous classification systems for groin hernias. One simple and widely used system is the Nyhus classification (Box 45.3). The European Hernia Society Groin Hernia Classification has gained acceptance as a simple scheme that is easy to apply clinically. Hernias are characterized as femoral hernias, or hernias that are medial or lateral to the epigastric vessels. Each of these

BOX 45.2 Differential diagnosis of groin and scrotal masses.

- Inguinal hernia
- Hydrocele
- Varicocele
- Ectopic testis
- Epididymitis
- Testicular torsion
- Lipoma
- Hematoma
- Sebaceous cyst
- Hidradenitis of inguinal apocrine glands
- Inguinal lymphadenopathy
- Lymphoma
- Metastatic neoplasm
- Femoral hernia
- Femoral lymphadenopathy
- Femoral artery aneurysm or pseudoaneurysm

BOX 45.3 Nyhus classification of groin hernia.

Type I
Indirect inguinal hernia: internal inguinal ring normal (e.g., pediatric hernia)

Type II
Indirect inguinal hernia: internal inguinal ring dilated but posterior inguinal wall intact; inferior deep epigastric vessels not displaced

Type III
Posterior wall defect
A. Direct inguinal hernia
B. Indirect inguinal hernia: internal inguinal ring dilated, medially encroaching on or destroying the transversalis fascia of Hesselbach triangle (e.g., scrotal, sliding, or pantaloon hernia)
C. Femoral hernia

Type IV
Recurrent hernia
A. Direct
B. Indirect
C. Femoral
D. Combined

three possibilities is then further characterized according to the size of the orifice (1 for <1.5 cm, 2 for 1.5 cm to 3 cm, 3 for >3 cm). Though their purpose is to promote a common language and understanding for communication of physicians and to allow appropriate comparisons of therapeutic options, these classifications are incomplete and contentious. Most surgeons continue to describe hernias by their type, location, and volume of the hernia sac.

Treatment

Nonoperative Management

Most surgeons recommend operation on discovery of a symptomatic inguinal hernia because the natural history of a groin hernia is that of progressive enlargement and weakening, with a small potential for incarceration and strangulation. However, in patients with minimal symptoms, the clinician is often faced with balancing the risk for hernia-related complications, such as incarceration and bowel strangulation, with the potential for complications in the short and long term. Fitzgibbons and colleagues[2] reported a prospective randomized trial of a watchful waiting strategy for men with asymptomatic or minimally symptomatic inguinal hernias. These investigators randomized more than 700 men to a watchful waiting or open tension-free hernia repair. At 2 years of follow-up, there were no deaths attributed to the study, and the risk for hernia incarceration in the watchful waiting group was extremely low, 0.3% of study participants or 1.8 events/1000 patient-years. Almost 25% of patients assigned to watchful waiting crossed over to the surgical group, usually for pain related to the hernia that limited activity. In a later report, the crossover rate had increased to 68% at 10 years, with nearly 80% of men older than 65 years having an operation.[3] Patients who later had surgery did not have increased surgical site infections or higher recurrence rates than those who were initially assigned to early repair. These studies provide conclusive evidence that a strategy of watchful waiting is safe for older patients with asymptomatic or minimally symptomatic inguinal hernias and that even though most patients eventually undergo repair, when they do, the operative risks and complication rates are no different from those of patients undergoing immediate repair. Watchful waiting can be a cost-effective management strategy for selected patients with no or minimal symptoms or who have suboptimal risk for operation. These results should not be applied to women, as women have not been included in these studies, or to patients with femoral hernias, which have a greater risk of strangulation than inguinal hernias.

Patients electing nonoperative management can occasionally have symptomatic improvement with the use of a truss. This approach is more commonly used in Europe. Spring trusses are more versatile than elastic ones, although most information on their use has been anecdotal. Correct measurement and fitting are important. Symptom control has been reported in about 30% of patients. Complications associated with the use of a truss include testicular atrophy, ilioinguinal or femoral neuritis, and hernia incarceration.

It is generally agreed that nonoperative management is not used for femoral hernias because of the high incidence of associated complications, particularly strangulation.

Operative Repair

Anterior Repairs. Anterior repairs are the most common operative approach for inguinal hernias. Tension-free repairs are now standard, and there are a variety of different types. Older tissue types of repair are rarely indicated, except for patients with simultaneous contamination or concomitant bowel resection, when placement of a mesh prosthesis may be contraindicated.

There are some technical aspects of the operation common to all anterior repairs. Open hernia repair is begun by making a transversely oriented linear or slightly curvilinear incision above the inguinal ligament and a fingerbreadth below the internal inguinal ring. The internal inguinal ring is located topographically at the midpoint between the anterior superior iliac spine and ipsilateral pubic tubercle. Dissection is continued through the subcutaneous tissues and Scarpa fascia. The external oblique fascia and external inguinal ring are identified. The external oblique fascia is incised through the superficial inguinal ring to expose the inguinal canal. The genital branch of the genitofemoral nerve and the ilioinguinal and ilioh ypogastric nerves are identified and avoided or mobilized to prevent transection and entrapment. The spermatic cord is mobilized at the pubic tubercle by a combination of blunt and sharp dissection. Improper mobilization of the spermatic cord too lateral to the pubic tubercle can cause confusion in the identification of tissue planes and essential structures and may result in injury to the spermatic cord structures or disruption of the floor of the inguinal canal.

The cremaster muscle of the mobilized spermatic cord is separated parallel to its fibers from the underlying cord structures. The cremaster artery and vein, which join the cremaster muscle near the inguinal ring, can usually be avoided but may need to be cauterized or ligated and divided. In general, minimal disruption of the cremasteric fibers and vasculature are recommended to minimize chronic groin pain. When an indirect hernia is present, the hernia sac is located deep to the cremaster muscle and anterior and superior to the spermatic cord structures. Incising the cremaster muscle in a longitudinal direction usually suffices to expose an indirect sac. The hernia sac is carefully separated from adjacent cord structures and dissected to the level of the internal inguinal ring. The sac is opened and examined for visceral contents if it is large; however, this step is unnecessary in small hernias. The sac can be mobilized and placed within the preperitoneal space, or the neck of the sac can be ligated at the level of the internal ring and any excess sac excised. If a large hernia sac is present, it can be divided with use of electrocautery to facilitate ligation. It is not necessary to excise the distal portion of the sac. If the sac is broad based, it may be easier to displace it into the peritoneal cavity rather than to ligate it. Direct hernia sacs protrude through the floor of the inguinal canal and can be reduced below the transversalis fascia before repair. To accomplish this, the weakened floor (transversalis fascia) is incised, exposing the preperitoneal fat below. This fat is mobilized from the neck of the direct defect and any other component of the direct hernia is reduced. The redundant transversalis fascia is excised and the floor can often be reapproximated using a running absorbable suture. A "lipoma" of the cord actually represents retroperitoneal fat that has herniated through the deep inguinal ring; this should be suture ligated and removed.

A sliding hernia presents a special challenge in handling the hernia sac. With a sliding hernia, a portion of the sac is composed of visceral peritoneum covering part of a retroperitoneal organ, usually the colon or bladder. In this situation, the grossly redundant portion of the sac (if present) is excised and the peritoneum reclosed. The organ and sac then can be reduced below the transversalis fascia, similar to the procedure for a direct hernia.

Tissue Repairs. Although tissue repairs have largely been abandoned because of unacceptably high recurrence rates, they remain useful in certain situations. In strangulated hernias, for which bowel resection is necessary, mesh prostheses are contraindicated and a tissue repair is necessary. Available options for tissue repair include iliopubic tract, Shouldice, Bassini, and McVay repairs.

The iliopubic tract repair approximates the transversus abdominis aponeurotic arch to the iliopubic tract with the use of interrupted sutures (Fig. 45.5). The repair begins at the pubic tubercle and extends laterally past the internal inguinal ring. This repair was initially described using a relaxing incision (see later); however, many surgeons who use this repair do not perform a relaxing incision.

The Shouldice repair emphasizes a multilayer imbricated repair of the posterior wall of the inguinal canal with a continuous running suture technique. After completion of the dissection, the posterior wall of the inguinal canal is reconstructed by superimposing running suture lines progressing from deep to more superficial layers. The initial suture line secures the transversus abdominis aponeurotic arch to the iliopubic tract. Next, the internal oblique and transversus abdominis muscles and aponeuroses are sutured to the inguinal ligament. The Shouldice repair is associated with a very low recurrence rate and a high degree of patient satisfaction in highly selected patients.

The Bassini repair is performed by suturing the transversus abdominis and internal oblique musculoaponeurotic arches or conjoined tendon (when present) to the inguinal ligament. This once popular technique is the basic approach to nonanatomic hernia repairs and was the most popular type of repair done before the advent of tension-free repairs.

Cooper ligament repair, also known as the McVay repair, has traditionally been popular for the correction of direct inguinal hernias, large indirect hernias, recurrent hernias, and femoral hernias. Interrupted nonabsorbable sutures are used to approximate the edge of the transversus abdominis aponeurosis to Cooper ligament. When the medial aspect of the femoral canal is reached, a transition suture is placed to incorporate Cooper ligament and the iliopubic tract. Lateral to this transition stitch, the transversus abdominis aponeurosis is secured to the iliopubic tract. An important principle of this repair is the need for a relaxing incision. This incision is made by reflecting the external oblique aponeurosis cephalad and medial to expose the anterior rectus sheath. An incision is then made in a curvilinear direction, beginning 1 cm above the pubic tubercle throughout the extent of the anterior sheath to near its lateral border. This relieves tension on the suture line and results in decreased postoperative pain and hernia recurrence. The fascial defect is covered by the body of the rectus muscle, which prevents herniation at the relaxing incision site. The McVay repair is particularly suited for strangulated femoral hernias because it provides obliteration of the femoral space without the use of mesh.

Tension-free Anterior Inguinal Hernia Repair. Tension-free repair has become the dominant method of inguinal hernia repair (Fig. 45.6). Recognizing that tension in a repair is the principal cause of recurrence, current practices in hernia management use a synthetic mesh prosthesis to bridge the defect, a concept popularized by Lichtenstein. There are several options for placement of mesh during anterior inguinal herniorrhaphy, including the Lichtenstein approach, plug and patch technique, and sandwich technique, with both an anterior and preperitoneal piece of mesh.

In the Lichtenstein repair,[4] a piece of prosthetic nonabsorbable mesh is fashioned to fit the canal. A slit is cut into the distal lateral edge of the mesh to accommodate the spermatic cord. There are various preformed, commercially available prostheses available for use. The periosteum overlying the pubic tubercle is exposed and this dissection is extended medially toward the midline of the pubis for at least 15 to 20 mm. Fixation of mesh to the pubic tubercle itself should be avoided to minimize the risk of chronic groin pain. The inferolateral edge of the mesh is sutured to the shelving edge of the inguinal ligament starting just adjacent (but not into) the pubic tubercle) using a nonabsorbable suture. The medial aspect of the mesh is allowed to generously overlap the pubic tubercle by at least 15 mm. This suture is taken to a point just lateral and superior to the internal inguinal ring and tied. Interrupted sutures are then placed affixing the superomedial aspect of the mesh to the conjoined tendon. Great care is taken to visualize the ilioinguinal and iliohypogastric nerves to avoid injury or entrapment. In addition, adequate medial overlap of the mesh medial to the pubic tubercle is ensured. At this point, the tails created by the slit are sutured together around the spermatic cord, snugly

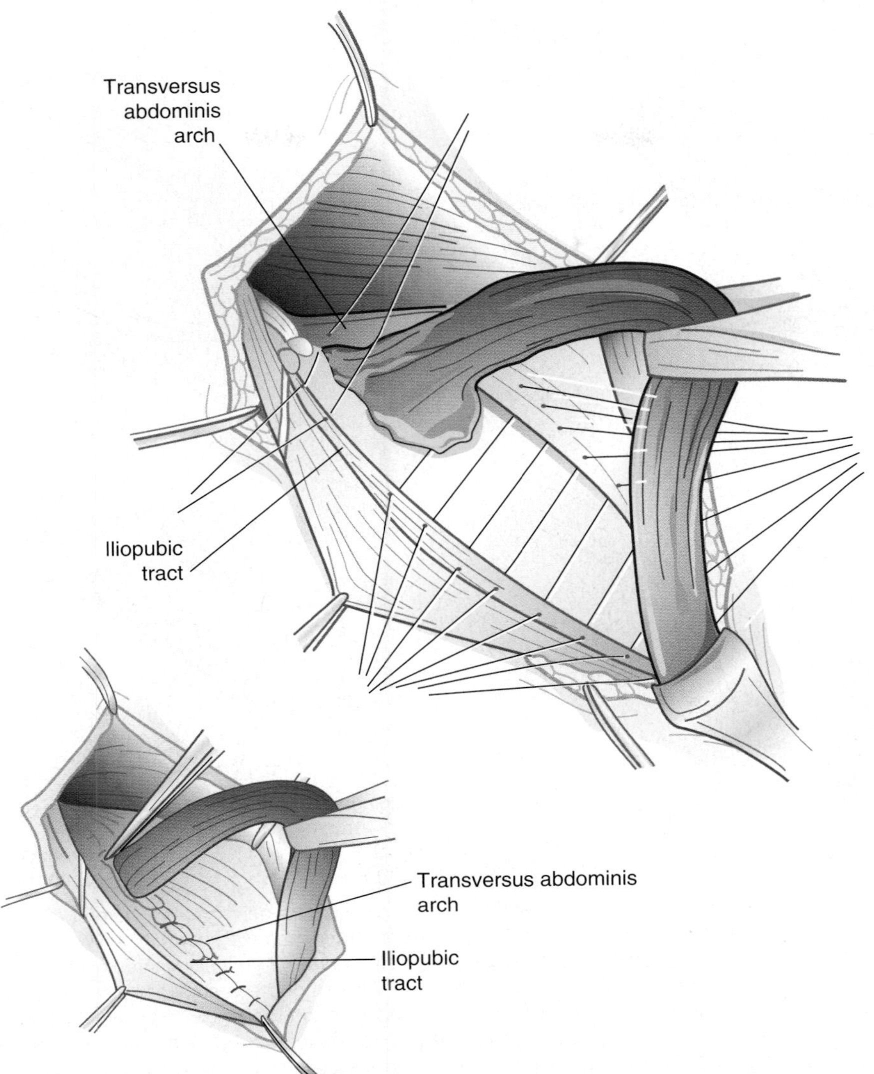

FIG. 45.5 Iliopubic tract repair. *Top*, Sutures lateral to the cord complete reconstruction of the deep inguinal ring. These sutures encompass the transversus abdominis arch above and the cremaster origin and iliopubic tract below. *Bottom*, The complete repair is ready for wound closure. The reconstruction of the deep ring should be snug but also loose enough to admit the tip of a hemostat. (From Condon RE. Anterior iliopubic tract repair. In: Nyhus LM, Condon RE, eds. *Hernia*. 2nd ed. Philadelphia: JB Lippincott; 1974:204.)

forming a new internal inguinal ring. It is important to protect the ilioinguinal nerve and genital branch of the genitofemoral nerve from entrapment by placing them with the cord structures as they are passed through this newly fashioned internal inguinal ring or avoiding their enclosure in the repair.

Adapting the principles of tension-free repair, Gilbert[5] has reported using a cone-shaped plug of polypropylene mesh that, when inserted into the internal inguinal ring, would deploy like an upside-down umbrella and occlude the hernia. This plug is sewn to the surrounding tissues and held in place by an additional overlying mesh patch. This patch may not need to be secured by sutures; however, to do so requires dissection to create a sufficient space between the external and internal oblique muscles for the patch to lie flat over the inguinal canal. This so-called plug and patch repair, an extension of the Lichtenstein original mesh repair, has now become the most commonly performed primary anterior inguinal hernia repair. Although this repair can be done without suture fixation by some experienced surgeons, most secure plug and patch with several monofilament nonabsorbable sutures, especially for very weak inguinal floors or large defects.

The sandwich technique involves a bilayered device, with three polypropylene components. An underlay patch provides a posterior repair similar to that of the laparoscopic approach, a connector functions similar to a plug, and an onlay patch covers the posterior inguinal floor. The use of interrupted fixating sutures is not mandatory, but most surgeons place three or four fixation sutures in this repair.

Another option for a tension-free mesh repair involves a preperitoneal approach using a self-expanding polypropylene patch.[6] A pocket is created in the preperitoneal space by blunt dissection, and then a preformed mesh patch is inserted into the hernia defect, which expands to cover the direct, indirect, and femoral spaces. The patch lies parallel to the inguinal ligament. It can remain without suture fixation, or a tacking suture can be placed.

The Stoppa-Rives repair uses a subumbilical midline incision to place a large mesh prosthesis into the preperitoneal space.[7] Blunt

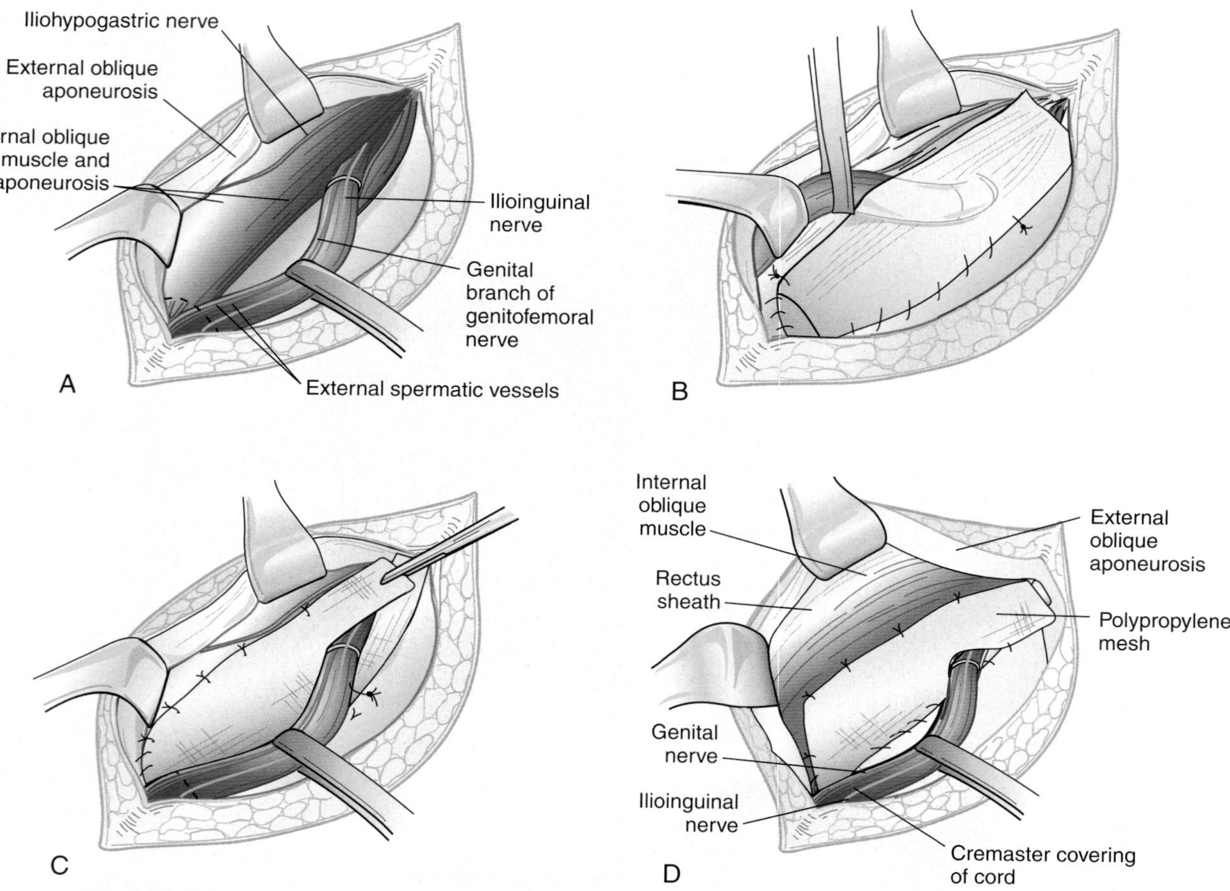

FIG. 45.6 Lichtenstein tension-free hernia repair. (A) This procedure is performed by careful dissection of the inguinal canal. High ligation of an indirect hernia sac is performed, and the spermatic cord structures are retracted inferiorly. The external oblique aponeurosis is separated from the underlying internal oblique muscle high enough to accommodate a 6- to 8-cm-wide mesh patch. Overlap of the internal oblique muscle edge by 2 to 3 cm is necessary. A sheet of polypropylene mesh is fashioned to fit the inguinal canal. A slit is made in the lateral aspect of the mesh, and the spermatic cord is placed between the two tails of the mesh. (B) The spermatic cord is retracted in the cephalad direction. The medial aspect of the mesh overlaps the pubic bone by approximately 2 cm. The mesh is secured to the aponeurotic tissue overlying the pubic tubercle by a running suture of nonabsorbable monofilament material. The suture is continued laterally by suturing the inferior edge of the mesh to the shelving edge of the inguinal ligament to a point just lateral to the internal inguinal ring. (C) A second monofilament suture is placed at the level of the pubic tubercle and continued laterally by suturing the mesh to the internal oblique aponeurosis or muscle approximately 2 cm from the aponeurotic edge. (D) The lower edges of the two tails are sutured to the shelving edge of the inguinal ligament to create a new internal ring made of mesh. The spermatic cord structures are placed within the inguinal canal overlying the mesh. The external oblique aponeurosis is closed over the spermatic cord. (From Arregui ME, Nagan RD, eds. *Inguinal Hernia: Advances or Controversies?* Oxford, England: Radcliffe Medical; 1994.)

dissection is used to create an extraperitoneal space that extends into the prevesical space, beyond the obturator foramen, and posterolateral to the pelvic brim. This technique has the advantage of distributing the natural intra abdominal pressure across a broad area to retain the mesh in a proper location. The Stoppa-Rives technique is particularly useful for large, recurrent, or bilateral hernias.

Preperitoneal Repair. The open preperitoneal approach is useful for the repair of recurrent inguinal hernias, sliding hernias, femoral hernias, and some strangulated hernias.[8] A transverse skin incision is made 2 cm above the internal inguinal ring and is directed to the medial border of the rectus sheath. The muscles of the anterior abdominal wall are incised transversely, and the preperitoneal space is identified. If further exposure is needed, the anterior rectus sheath can be incised and the rectus muscle retracted medially. The preperitoneal tissues are retracted cephalad to visualize the posterior inguinal wall and the site of herniation. The inferior epigastric artery and veins are generally beneath the midportion of the posterior rectus sheath and usually do not need to be divided. This approach avoids mobilization of the spermatic cord and injury to the sensory nerves of the inguinal canal, which is particularly important for hernias previously repaired through an anterior approach. If the peritoneum is incised, it is sutured closed to avoid the evisceration of intraperitoneal contents into the operative field. The transversalis fascia and transversus abdominis aponeurosis are identified and sutured to the iliopubic tract with permanent sutures. Femoral hernias repaired by this approach require closure of the femoral canal by securing the repair to Cooper ligament. A mesh prosthesis is frequently used to obliterate the defect in the femoral canal, particularly with large hernias.

Laparoscopic Repair. Laparoscopic inguinal hernia repair is another method of tension-free mesh repair based on a preperitoneal approach. The laparoscopic approach provides the mechanical advantage of placing a large piece of mesh behind the defect, covering the myopectineal orifice, and using the natural forces of the abdominal wall to disperse intra abdominal pressure over a larger area to support the mesh in place. Proponents have touted quicker recovery, less pain, better visualization of anatomy, and usefulness for fixing all inguinal hernia defects. Critics have emphasized longer operative times, technical challenges, increased risk of recurrence, and increased cost. Laparoscopic repair is also associated with an approximately 0.3% risk of visceral or vascular injury.[9] Although controversy exists about the usefulness of laparoscopic repair for primary unilateral inguinal hernias, most agree that this approach has advantages for patients having bilateral or recurrent hernia repairs.[10] Adopting practice guidelines for the performance of laparoscopic hernia repairs could help control costs.

When considering the laparoscopic approach for repair of inguinal hernias, the surgeon has several options. The most popular techniques are totally extraperitoneal (TEP) and transabdominal preperitoneal (TAPP) approaches. The main difference between these two techniques is the sequence of gaining access to the preperitoneal space. In the TEP approach, the dissection begins in the preperitoneal space using a balloon dissector. With the TAPP repair, the preperitoneal space is accessed after initially entering the peritoneal cavity. Each approach has its merits. With the TEP approach, the preperitoneal dissection is quicker, and the potential risk for intraperitoneal visceral damage is minimized. However, the use of dissection balloons is costly, the working space is more limited, and it may not be possible to create a working space if the patient has had a prior preperitoneal operation. Also, if a large tear in the peritoneum is created during a TEP approach; the potential working space can become obliterated, necessitating conversion to a TAPP approach. For these reasons, knowledge of the transabdominal technique is essential in performing laparoscopic inguinal hernia repairs. The transabdominal approach allows identification of the groin anatomy before extensive dissection and disruption of natural tissue planes. The larger working space of the peritoneal cavity can make early experience with the laparoscopic approach easier.

There are no absolute contraindications to laparoscopic inguinal hernia repair other than the patient's inability to tolerate general anesthesia. Patients who have had extensive prior lower abdominal surgery can require significant adhesiolysis and may be best approached anteriorly. In particular, in patients who have had a radical retropubic prostatectomy with the preperitoneal space previously dissected, accurate and safe dissection can be challenging.

In the TEP approach, an infraumbilical incision is used. The anterior rectus sheath is incised, the ipsilateral rectus abdominis muscle is retracted laterally, and blunt dissection is used to create a space beneath the rectus. A dissecting balloon is inserted deep to the posterior rectus sheath, advanced to the pubic symphysis, and inflated under direct laparoscopic vision (Fig. 45.7). After it is opened, the space is insufflated, and additional trocars are placed. A 30-degree laparoscope provides the best visualization of the inguinal region (see Fig. 45.3). The inferior epigastric vessels are identified along the lower portion of the rectus muscle and serve as a useful landmark. Cooper ligament must be cleared from the pubic symphysis medially to the level of the external iliac vein. The iliopubic tract is also identified. Care must be taken to avoid injury to the femoral branch of the genitofemoral nerve and lateral femoral cutaneous nerve, which are located lateral to and below the iliopubic tract (see Fig. 45.4). Lateral dissection is carried out to the anterior superior iliac spine. Finally, the testicular vessels and vas deferens are identified and mobilized away from the peritoneum.

In the TAPP approach, an infraumbilical incision is used to gain access to the peritoneal cavity directly. Two 5-mm ports are placed lateral to the inferior epigastric vessels at the level of the umbilicus. A peritoneal flap is created high on the anterior abdominal wall, extending from the median umbilical fold to the anterior superior iliac spine. The remainder of the operation proceeds similar to a TEP procedure.

A direct hernia sac and associated preperitoneal fat are gently reduced by traction if not already reduced by balloon expansion of the peritoneal space. A small, indirect hernia sac is mobilized from the cord structures and reduced into the peritoneal cavity. A large sac may be difficult to reduce. In this case, the sac is divided with cautery near the internal inguinal ring, leaving the distal sac in situ. The proximal peritoneal sac is closed with a loop ligature or clips to prevent pneumoperitoneum from occurring. After all hernias are reduced, a 12 × 14-cm piece of polypropylene mesh is inserted through a trocar and unfolded. It covers the direct, indirect, and femoral spaces and rests over the cord structures. It is imperative that the peritoneum be dissected at least 4 cm off the cord structures to prevent the peritoneum from encroaching beneath the mesh, which can lead to recurrence. The mesh is carefully secured with a fixation device to Cooper ligament medially, anteriorly to the posterior rectus musculature and transversus abdominis aponeurotic arch at least 2 cm above the hernia defect, and laterally to the iliopubic tract. The mesh extends beyond the pubic symphysis and below the spermatic cord and peritoneum (Fig. 45.8). The mesh is not fixed in this area and tacks are not placed inferior to the iliopubic tract beyond the external iliac artery. Fixation placed in this area may injure the femoral branch of the genitofemoral nerve or lateral femoral cutaneous nerve. Fixation is also avoided in the so-called triangle of doom, bounded by the ductus deferens medially and spermatic vessels laterally, to avoid injury to the external iliac vessels and femoral nerve. As long as one can palpate the tip of the tacking device, these structures are not likely to be injured.

Robotic Repair. The TAPP technique can also be performed robotically, with a similar trocar configuration, similar steps for dissection, mesh positioning, and similar outcomes to laparoscopy.[11] An advantage of the robotic approach is the three-dimensional optics and wristed instrumentation. This allows for improved visualization of the anatomy compared to the two-dimensional view of laparoscopy. The wristed instruments provide improved mobility for dissection and suturing. Another advantage is the simplicity of fixating the mesh to the abdominal wall utilizing sutures rather than a penetrating mechanical fixation device with tacks or staples. Similarly, the peritoneal flap can also be sutured closed. Although unproven, this may confer a slight pain advantage compared to tacks or staples.

Complications and Results of Inguinal Hernia Repair

The best information on the results of hernia repair is available from large prospective randomized trials, meta analyses of clinical trials, and two large national registries: the Danish Hernia Database and the Swedish Hernia Register. The Danish Hernia Database includes more than 98% of inguinal hernia repairs; the capture rate of the Swedish Hernia Register is approximately 80%.[12,13] In spite of the randomized nature of some trials, caution must be used in interpreting the results. Many of these patients

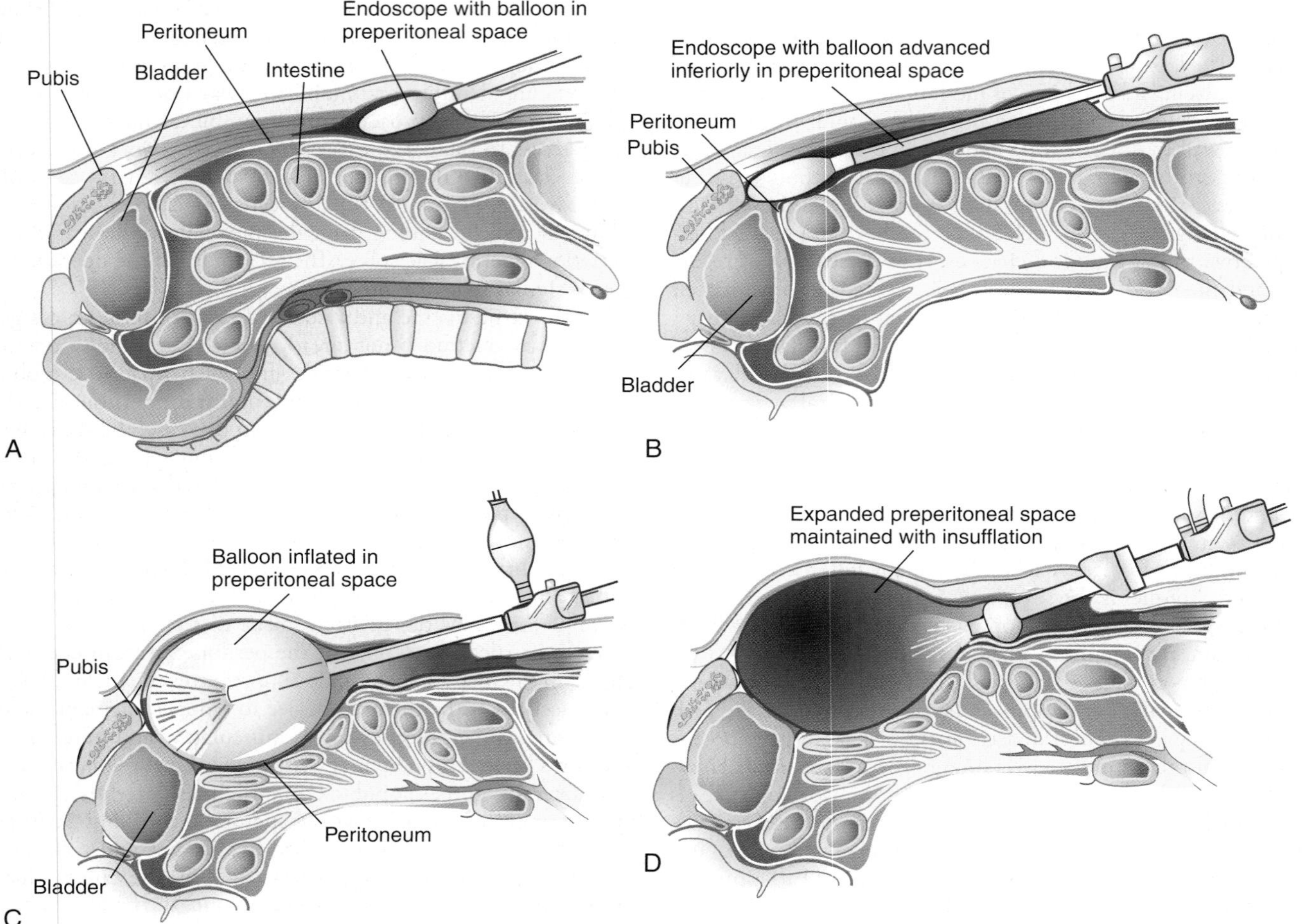

FIG. 45.7 Totally extraperitoneal laparoscopic hernia repair. (A) Access to the posterior rectus sheath is gained in the periumbilical region. A balloon dissector is placed on the anterior surface of the posterior rectus sheath. (B) The balloon dissector is advanced to the posterior surface of the pubis in the preperitoneal space. (C) The balloon is inflated, thereby creating an optical cavity. (D) The optical cavity is insufflated by carbon dioxide, and the posterior surface of the inguinal floor is dissected.

were highly selected, and most trials excluded recurrent hernias, obese individuals, and large inguinal hernias. Also, some follow-up results were completed by telephone interviews and not by physical examination. The national registries collect information only on operations, so the incidence of recurrence is lower than if all patients had been interviewed and examined.

The mortality of all types of repair is low, and there are no significant differences reported among the various techniques. There is a greater mortality associated with the repair of strangulated hernias. Otherwise, the risk of death is related to individual comorbid conditions and should be evaluated in each patient. The type of anesthetic does not affect the recurrence rate.[13] Open repairs can be performed under local anesthesia, which can be an advantage in operating on high-risk patients.

There are important differences in the results of primary hernia repair. Hernia recurrence is the primary outcome assessed by most studies. Large series, including multiple types of repairs, have suggested that recurrence ranges from 1.7% to 10%.[12–14]

The results of tissue repairs were often based on reports consisting of personal or single institutional series that were not prospective or randomized and had erratic follow-up periods. Not surprisingly, recurrence was variable.

Tension-free repairs have a lower rate of recurrence than tissue repairs.[13,15,16] Results from the Danish Hernia Database have demonstrated that hernia recurrence resulting in reoperation after the Lichtenstein repair is only 25% that of nonmesh repairs.[12] A Cochrane review reported that prosthetic mesh repairs have a 50% to 75% lower risk of hernia recurrence, a lower risk of chronic postherniorrhaphy groin pain, and an earlier return to work than open repairs.[15] The Shouldice repair has a higher recurrence rate than mesh repairs unless mesh is used.[16] A meta analysis comparing the Lichtenstein, mesh plug, and bilayered repairs has reported no significant differences in the rate of recurrence, chronic groin pain, other complications, or time to return to work.[17] Approximately 50% of recurrences are found within 3 years after primary repair. Recurrence continues to occur after this time in nonmesh-based repairs but is uncommon with tension-free repairs.

An extensive systematic review of randomized controlled trials was published in 2002 by the European Union Hernia Trialists Collaboration.[18] The authors reported a meta analysis of 4165 patients in 25 studies. Based on the available data, the laparoscopic repair resulted in a more rapid return to normal activity and decreased persistent postoperative pain. The recurrence rate for the laparoscopic repair was lower compared with open nonmesh

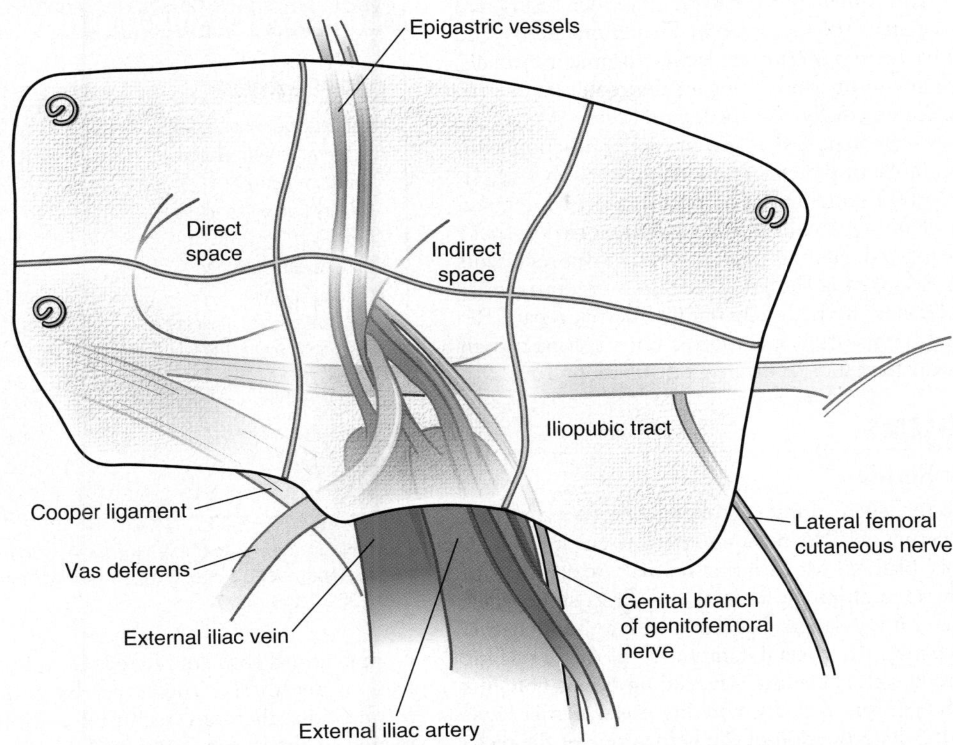

FIG. 45.8 Prosthetic mesh placement for totally extraperitoneal hernia repair. (From Corbitt J. Laparoscopic transabdominal transperitoneal patch hernia repair. In: Ballantyne GH, ed. *Atlas of Laparoscopic Surgery*. Philadelphia: WB Saunders; 2000:511.)

repairs; however, open and laparoscopic mesh repairs had similar recurrence rates.

A prospective trial sponsored by the Veterans Administration randomized 1983 patients to undergo an open Lichtenstein repair or laparoscopic repair, of which 90% were TEP repairs.[14] Most surgeons in this study may have had a suboptimal experience with the laparoscopic approach; only 25 prior repairs were necessary to be eligible to enroll patients, which is consistent with the seemingly high conversion rate of 5%. Despite these factors, the investigators found a twofold higher incidence of recurrence after laparoscopic repair (10%) than after open repair (5%). This difference in recurrence remained for primary hernias (10% laparoscopic vs. 4% open); however, recurrent hernias repaired by the laparoscopic approach tended to have fewer re-recurrences (10% vs. 14%). In another study by this group, surgeon inexperience with laparoscopy and surgeon age older than 45 years were both predictors of recurrence after laparoscopic repair.[17] What can be concluded from these results? These results demonstrate that the laparoscopic repair of inguinal hernias has a definite learning curve to achieve an acceptably low recurrence rate.

In a Cochrane review of more than 1000 patients in eight nonrandomized trials, there was no difference in hernia recurrence between TAPP and TEP repairs.[19] TAPP procedures were associated with more port site hernias and vascular injuries, whereas the TEP approach had a greater conversion rate.

FEMORAL HERNIAS

A femoral hernia occurs through the femoral canal, which is bounded superiorly by the iliopubic tract, inferiorly by Cooper ligament, laterally by the femoral vein, and medially by the junction of the iliopubic tract and Cooper ligament (lacunar ligament). A femoral hernia produces a mass or bulge below the inguinal ligament. On occasion, some femoral hernias will present over the inguinal canal. In this case, the femoral hernia sac still exits inferior to the inguinal ligament through the femoral canal but ascends in a cephalad direction. Approximately 50% of men with a femoral hernia will have an associated direct inguinal hernia, whereas this relationship occurs in only 2% of women.

A femoral hernia can be repaired by the standard Cooper ligament repair, a preperitoneal approach, or a laparoscopic approach. The essential elements of femoral hernia repair include dissection and reduction of the hernia sac and obliteration of the defect in the femoral canal, either by approximation of the iliopubic tract to Cooper ligament or by placement of prosthetic mesh to obliterate the defect. The incidence of strangulation in femoral hernias is high; therefore, all femoral hernias should be repaired, and incarcerated femoral hernias should have the hernia sac contents examined for viability. In patients with a compromised bowel, the Cooper ligament approach is the preferred technique because mesh is contraindicated. When the incarcerated contents of a femoral hernia cannot be reduced, dividing the lacunar ligament can be helpful. A useful method of identifying and repairing femoral hernias during an anterior approach is to dissect the subcutaneous fat from the external oblique aponeurosis, exposing the anterior reflection of inguinal ligament. The femoral artery is easily palpated and the potential space for femoral hernia medial to the vein can be digitally and visually inspected. Should a femoral hernia be discovered, the sac and contents are mobilized and reduced. The inguinal ligament often needs to be divided for a small length to facilitate reduction. The medial aspect of the femoral vein is not skeletonized, leaving a generous amount of tissue medial to the vein itself. A small prosthetic plug can then be inserted into the empty space previously occupied by the femoral hernia and sutured to Cooper ligament posterior, the lacunar ligament medially, and the inguinal ligament superiorly using an absorbable suture. No suture fixation is placed medially near the femoral vein.

Femoral hernias were reported to occur in conjunction with inguinal hernias in 0.3% of patients in a large national hernia database of almost 35,000 patients.[20] The occurrence of a femoral hernia after repair of an inguinal hernia has been reported to be 15 times the normal expected rate. It is unclear whether this represents a femoral hernia overlooked at the prior operation or a propensity to development of a new hernia after inguinal hernia repair. Recurrence of femoral hernia after operation is only 2%. Recurrent femoral hernia repairs have a re-recurrence rate of about 10%.

SPECIAL PROBLEMS

Sliding Inguinal Hernia

A sliding hernia occurs when an internal organ composes a portion of the wall of the hernia sac. The most common viscus involved is the colon or urinary bladder. Most sliding hernias are a variant of indirect inguinal hernias, although femoral and direct sliding hernias can occur. The primary danger associated with a sliding hernia is the failure to recognize the visceral component of the hernia sac before injury to the bowel or bladder. The sliding hernia contents are reduced into the peritoneal cavity, and any excess hernia sac is ligated and divided. After reduction of the hernia, one of the techniques described earlier can be used for repair of the inguinal hernia.

Recurrent Inguinal Hernia

The repair of recurrent inguinal hernias is challenging, and results are associated with a higher incidence of secondary recurrence. Recurrent hernias almost always require placement of prosthetic mesh for successful repair. The exception is when infected mesh is associated with a recurrent hernia. Recurrences after anterior hernia repair using mesh are best managed by a laparoscopic or open posterior approach, with placement of a second prosthesis.

Strangulated Inguinal Hernia

Repair of a suspected strangulated hernia is most easily done using a preperitoneal approach (see earlier). With this exposure, the hernia sac contents can be directly visualized and their viability assessed through a single incision. The constricting ring is identified and can be incised to reduce the entrapped viscus with minimal danger to the surrounding organs, blood vessels, and nerves. If it is necessary to resect strangulated intestine, the peritoneum can be opened and resection done without the need for a second incision.

Bilateral Inguinal Hernias

The approach to repair of bilateral inguinal hernias is based on the extent of the hernia defect. Simultaneous repair of bilateral hernias has a similar recurrence rate to unilateral repair, regardless of whether the open or laparoscopic technique is used.[21] The use of a giant prosthetic reinforcement of the visceral sac (Stoppa repair)[7] or the laparoscopic repair is preferred for simultaneous repair of bilateral inguinal hernias.

COMPLICATIONS AND RESULTS

There are myriad complications related to open and laparoscopic inguinal hernia repair (Table 45.1). Some are general complications that are related to underlying diseases and the effects of anesthesia. These vary by patient population and risk. In addition, there are technical complications that are directly related to the repair. Technical complications are affected by the experience of the surgeon and are more frequent during and after the repair of recurrent hernias. There is increased scarring and disturbed anatomy with hernia recurrence that can result in an inability to identify important structures at operation. This is the principal reason that we recommend using a different approach for recurrent hernias.

Although the overall complication rate from hernia repair has been estimated to be approximately 10%, many of these complications are transient and can be easily addressed. More serious complications from a large experience are listed in Table 45.1.

TABLE 45.1 Complications after open and laparoscopic inguinal hernia repair (%).

COMPLICATION	OPEN REPAIR (*N* = 994)	LAPAROSCOPIC REPAIR (*N* = 989)
Intraoperative complications	1.9	4.8
Postoperative complications	19.4	24.6
Urinary retention	2.2	2.8
Urinary tract infection	0.4	1.0
Orchitis	1.1	1.4
Surgical site infection	1.4	1.0
Neuralgia, pain	3.6	4.2
Life-threatening complications	0.1	1.1
Long-term complications	17.4	18.0
Seroma	3.0	9.0
Orchitis	2.2	1.9
Infection	0.6	0.4
Chronic pain	14.3	9.8
Recurrence	4.9	10.1

From Neumayer L, Giobbie-Hurder A, Jonassen O, et al. Open mesh versus laparoscopic mesh repair of inguinal hernias. *N Engl J Med.* 2004;350:1819–1827.

Surgical Site Infection

The risk for surgical site infection is estimated to be 1% to 2% after open inguinal hernia repair and slightly less with laparoscopic repairs. These are clean operations, and the risk for infection is primarily influenced by associated patient diseases. Most would agree that there is no need to use routine antimicrobial prophylaxis for hernia repair.[18] Prospective randomized clinical trials have not supported the routine use of perioperative antimicrobial prophylaxis for inguinal hernia repair for patients at low risk for infection.[22] Patients who have significant underlying disease, as reflected by an American Society of Anesthesiology score of 3 or more, receive perioperative antimicrobial prophylaxis with cefazolin, 2 to 3 g, given intravenously 30 to 60 minutes before the incision. Clindamycin, 900 mg intravenously, can be used for patients allergic to penicillin. Only a single dose of antibiotic is necessary. The placement of prosthetic mesh does not increase the risk for infection and does not affect the need for prophylaxis. Superficial surgical site infections are treated by opening the incision, local wound care, and healing by secondary intention. Some mesh infections will be manifested as a chronic draining sinus that tracks to the mesh or occurs with extruded mesh. Deep surgical site infections usually involve the prosthetic mesh, which should be explanted.

The risk for infection can be decreased by using proper operative technique, preoperative antiseptic skin preparation, and appropriate hair removal. There is an increased risk for infection for patients who have had prior hernia incision infections, chronic skin infections, or infection at a distant site. These infections are treated before elective surgery.

Nerve Injuries and Chronic Pain Syndromes

Nerve injuries are an infrequent and underrecognized complication of inguinal hernia repair. Injury can occur from traction, electrocautery, transection, and entrapment. The use of prosthetic mesh can result in dysesthesias, which are usually temporary. The nerves most commonly affected during open hernia repair are the ilioinguinal, genital branch of the genitofemoral, and iliohypogastric nerves. During laparoscopic repair, the lateral femoral cutaneous and genitofemoral nerves can be affected. Rarely, the main trunk of the femoral nerve can be injured during open or laparoscopic inguinal hernia repair.

Transient neuralgias involving sensory nerves can occur and are usually self-limited and resolve within a few weeks after surgery. Persistent neuralgias usually result in pain and hyperesthesia in the area of distribution. Symptoms are often reproduced by palpation over the point of entrapment or hyperextension of the hip and may be relieved by flexion of the thigh. Transection of a sensory nerve usually results in an area of numbness corresponding to the distribution of the involved nerve.

With more attention to patient outcomes, chronic groin pain has replaced recurrence as the primary complication after open inguinal hernia repair. Approximately 10% of patients will have chronic postherniorrhaphy pain, defined as pain persisting more than 3 months after operation, and pain has been reported to interfere with activities of daily living in 2% to 4%.[23] Strategies of routine nerve division in open surgery have not been associated with a reduction in chronic pain in mesh-based anterior repairs. In contrast, routine ilioinguinal nerve division is associated with significantly more sensory disturbances. In laparoscopic repairs, by operating in a remote area to the commonly injured nerves and with judicious use of appropriately placed tacks, chronic groin pain intuitively is less common. Some reports comparing laparoscopic and open repairs have reported lower rates of chronic postoperative inguinal pain, but this observation remains controversial. Measures to reduce chronic groin pain during open repair include identification and preservation of all three major nerves leaving them in situ (ilioinguinal, iliohypogastric, genital branch of the genital nerve), avoidance of fixation directly to the pubic tubercle, minimal disruption of cremasteric fibers, and utilization of absorbable interrupted suture fixation superomedially. The latter is employed to avoid impingement or entrapment of nervous structures.

Various approaches to management of residual neuralgia have been described. Early symptoms are treated with antiinflammatory agents, analgesics, and local anesthetic nerve blocks. A programmatic approach in specialized centers should be utilized to maximize the chance of positive outcome and minimize the chance of making a difficult situation even worse. In general, operative approaches for chronic groin pain are divided into local interventions (mesh or tack excision, mesh debulking) near the operative site and nerve-related interventions away from the immediate hernia repair site. At present, the extent and approach for local interventions are poorly understood, but some patients do benefit from an aggressive approach. Neurectomy can often be performed open or in a minimally invasive fashion (laparoscopically or robotically), often trading chronic pain for chronic anesthesia or paresthesia. In many patients with debilitating pain, this is a welcome tradeoff. Identifying patients in whom these approaches would be successful is in its infancy. Much data are needed to help with decision making in this complex population.

Ischemic Orchitis and Testicular Atrophy

Ischemic orchitis usually occurs from thrombosis of the small veins of the pampiniform plexus within the spermatic cord. This results in venous congestion of the testis, which becomes swollen and tender 2 to 5 days after surgery. The process may continue for an additional 6 to 12 weeks and usually results in testicular atrophy. Ischemic orchitis also can be caused by ligation of the testicular artery. It is treated with antiinflammatory agents and analgesics. Orchiectomy is rarely necessary.

The incidence of ischemic orchitis can be minimized by avoiding unnecessary dissection within the spermatic cord. The incidence increases with dissection of the distal portion of a large hernia sac and in patients who have anterior operations for hernia recurrence or for spermatic cord disease. In these situations, the use of a posterior approach is preferred.

Testicular atrophy is a consequence of ischemic orchitis. It is more common after repair of recurrent hernias, particularly when an anterior approach is used. The incidence of ischemic orchitis increases by a factor of three or four with each subsequent hernia recurrence.

Injury to the Vas Deferens and Viscera

Injury to the vas deferens and intraabdominal viscera is unusual. Most of these injuries occur in patients with sliding inguinal hernias when there is failure to recognize the presence of intraabdominal viscera in the hernia sac. With large hernias, the vas deferens can be displaced in an enlarged inguinal ring before its entry into the spermatic cord. In this situation, the vas deferens is identified and protected.

Inguinal Hernia Recurrence

Hernia recurrences are usually caused by technical factors, such as excessive tension on the repair, missed hernias, failure to include an adequate musculoaponeurotic margin in the repair, and improper mesh size and placement. Recurrence also can result from failure to close a patulous internal inguinal ring, the size of which is always assessed at the conclusion of the primary surgery. Other factors that can cause hernia recurrence are chronically elevated intraabdominal pressure, a chronic cough, deep incisional infections, and poor collagen formation in the wound. Recurrences are more common in patients with direct hernias and usually involve the floor of the inguinal canal near the pubic tubercle, where suture line tension is greatest. The use of a relaxing incision when there is excessive tension at the time of primary hernia repair is helpful to reduce recurrence. A femoral hernia is found in approximately 5% to 10% of patients with an inguinal hernia recurrence and should always be investigated at surgery.[12]

Most recurrent hernias require the use of prosthetic mesh for successful repair. Choosing a different approach (usually posterior) avoids dissection through scar tissue, improves visualization of the defect and reduction of the hernia, and decreases the incidence of complications, particularly ischemic orchitis and injury to the ilioinguinal nerve. Recurrences after initial prosthetic mesh repairs can be caused by displaced prostheses or the use of a prosthetic of inadequate size. Recurrences are best managed by placing a second prosthesis through a different approach.

A metaanalysis of 58 reports comparing synthetic mesh techniques with nonmesh repairs has demonstrated an almost 60% reduction in recurrence with the use of mesh.[18] This report concluded that there was no difference in the rate of hernia recurrence between laparoscopic and open approaches that used mesh. A recent metaanalysis of recurrent hernia repairs reported no difference between open and laparoscopic mesh repairs in re-recurrence or chronic groin pain.[24]

Recurrence is more common after repair of recurrent hernias and is directly related to the number of previous attempts at repair. Large population-based studies have reported a re-recurrence rate of 4% to 5% in the first 24 months, which increases to 7.5% at 5 years.[25] Tension-free and mesh-based repairs have the lowest rates of reoperation after recurrence and result in a reduction in recurrence of approximately 60% compared with more traditional repairs.

There is a successive decrease in the time to hernia recurrence with each subsequent repair.[25] Re-recurrences are associated with increased operative times and a greater rate of complications.

Quality of Life

The major quality indicators that have been assessed for hernia repair are postoperative pain and return to work. Tension-free and laparoscopic mesh-based approaches have been demonstrated to be less painful than nonmesh repairs. Laparoscopic repairs have the least amount of postoperative pain and have been shown to provide a marginal advantage in reducing time off work.[10]

VENTRAL HERNIAS

A ventral hernia is defined by a protrusion through the anterior abdominal wall. These defects can be categorized as spontaneous or acquired or by their location on the abdominal wall. Epigastric hernias occur from the xiphoid process to the umbilicus, umbilical hernias occur at the umbilicus, and hypogastric hernias are rare spontaneous hernias that occur below the umbilicus in the midline. Acquired hernias typically occur after surgical incisions and are therefore termed incisional hernias. Although not a true hernia, diastasis recti can present as a midline bulge. In this condition, the linea alba is stretched, resulting in bulging at the medial margins of the rectus muscles. Abdominal wall diastasis can occur at other sites in addition to the midline. There is no fascial ring or hernia sac, and unless it is significantly symptomatic, surgical correction is generally avoided.

Incidence

Based on national operative statistics, incisional hernias account for 15% to 20% of all abdominal wall hernias; umbilical and epigastric hernias constitute 10% of hernias. Incisional hernias are twice as common in women as in men and can occur up to 41% of the time 2 years after oncologic resection. An estimated 350,000 to 500,000 ventral hernia repairs are performed each year. Several technical and patient-related factors have been linked to the occurrence of incisional hernias. There is no conclusive evidence demonstrating that the type of suture at the primary operation affects hernia formation.[26] Patient-related factors linked to ventral hernia formation include obesity, older age, male gender, sleep apnea, emphysema, and prostatism. It has been proposed that the same factors associated with destruction of the collagen in the lung result in poor wound healing, with increased hernia formation. Wound infection has been linked to hernia formation. Recent data suggest that the surgical technique used to close a midline laparotomy is highly associated with incisional hernia formation. The use of a suture to wound length ratio of 4:1 has been shown to significantly reduce incisional hernia formation compared with the 1-cm bites and 1-cm advancement suturing technique typically employed by most surgeons.[27]

Whether the type of initial abdominal incision influences the incisional hernia rate remains controversial. As noted, the incidence of ventral herniation after midline laparotomy ranges from 3% to 20% and doubles if the operation is associated with a surgical site infection. A metaanalysis of 11 studies examining the incidence of ventral hernia formation after various types of abdominal incisions has concluded that the risk is 10.5% for midline, 7.5% for transverse, and 2.5% for paramedian incisions.[28] Given the likely similar rates of incisional hernia formation after transverse and midline incisions, the surgeon should plan the incision on the basis of the operative exposure desired to complete the procedure safely.

Few data are available about the natural history of untreated ventral hernias. As noted, asymptomatic or minimally symptomatic inguinal hernias purposely observed during 2 years have a low incidence of complications.[2] Whether this paradigm applies for asymptomatic ventral or incisional hernias is unclear. Because there is no prospective cohort available to determine the natural history of untreated ventral hernias, most surgeons recommend that these hernias be repaired when discovered.

Anatomy

The anatomy of the anterior abdominal wall is straightforward and considerably easier to grasp than the anatomy of the inguinal area. However, a clear understanding of the blood supply and innervation of the abdomen is important in performing advanced abdominal wall reconstruction. The lateral musculature is composed of three layers, with the fascicles of each directed obliquely at different angles to create a strong envelope for the abdominal contents. Each of these muscles forms an aponeurosis that inserts into the linea alba, a midline structure joining both sides of the abdominal wall. The external oblique is the most superficial muscle of the lateral abdominal wall. Deep to the external oblique lies the internal oblique muscle. The fibers of the external oblique course in an inferomedial direction (like hands in pockets), whereas those of the internal oblique muscle run deep to and opposite the external oblique. The deepest muscle layer of the abdominal wall is the transversus abdominis muscle. Its fibers course in a horizontal direction. These three lateral muscles give rise to aponeurotic layers lateral to the rectus, which contribute to the anterior and posterior layers of the rectus sheath.

The medial extension of the external oblique aponeurosis forms the anterior layer of the rectus sheath. The transversus abdominis muscle and aponeurosis extend medial to the linea semilunaris, contributing components to the posterior rectus sheath. At the midline, the two anterior rectus sheaths form the tendinous linea alba. On either side of the linea alba are the rectus abdominis muscles, whose fibers are directed longitudinally and run the length of the anterior abdominal wall. Below each rectus muscle lies the posterior layer of the rectus sheath, which also contributes to the linea alba.

Another important anatomic structure of the anterior abdominal wall is the arcuate line, which is located 3 to 6 cm below the umbilicus. The arcuate line delineates the point below which the posterior rectus sheath is absent. Above the arcuate line, the aponeurosis of the internal oblique muscle contributes to the anterior and posterior rectus sheaths, and the aponeurosis of the transversus abdominis muscle passes posterior to the rectus muscle to form the posterior rectus sheath. Below the arcuate line, the internal oblique and transversus abdominis aponeuroses pass completely anterior to the rectus muscle (Fig. 45.9). The posterior rectus sheath below the arcuate line is composed of the transversalis fascia and peritoneum only.

The abdominal wall receives most of its innervation from intercostal nerves 7 through 12 and the first and second lumbar nerves. These rami provide innervation to the lateral abdominal muscles and the rectus muscle and overlying skin. The nerves traverse through the lateral abdominal wall between the transversus abdominis and internal oblique muscles and penetrate the posterior rectus sheath just medial to the linea semilunaris.

The lateral abdominal muscles receive their blood supply from the lower three or four intercostal arteries, deep circumflex iliac artery, and lumbar arteries. The rectus abdominis has a more complex blood supply derived from the superior epigastric artery (a terminal branch of the internal mammary artery), inferior epigastric artery (a branch of the external iliac artery), and lower intercostal arteries. The superior and inferior epigastric arteries anastomose near the umbilicus. The periumbilical area provides critical perforator vessels that, if preserved, can decrease skin flap necrosis during extensive skin undermining (Fig. 45.10).

Diagnosis

The evaluation of abdominal wall hernias requires diligent physical examination. As with the inguinal region, the anterior abdominal wall is evaluated with the patient in standing and supine positions, and a Valsalva maneuver is also useful to demonstrate the site and size of a hernia. Imaging modalities may play a greater role in the diagnosis of more unusual hernias of the abdominal wall. Computed tomography (CT) evaluation and surgeon-performed ultrasound (dynamic abdominal sonography for hernia [DASH]) are the most useful adjuncts to physical examination.

Classification

Umbilical Hernia

The umbilicus is formed by the umbilical ring of the linea alba. Intraabdominally, the round ligament (ligamentum teres) and paraumbilical veins join into the umbilicus superiorly and the median umbilical ligament (obliterated urachus) enters inferiorly. Umbilical hernias in infants are congenital and are common. They close spontaneously in most cases by the age of 2 years. Those that persist after the age of 5 years are frequently repaired surgically, although complications related to these hernias in children are unusual. There is a strong predisposition toward the development of these hernias in individuals of African descent. In the United

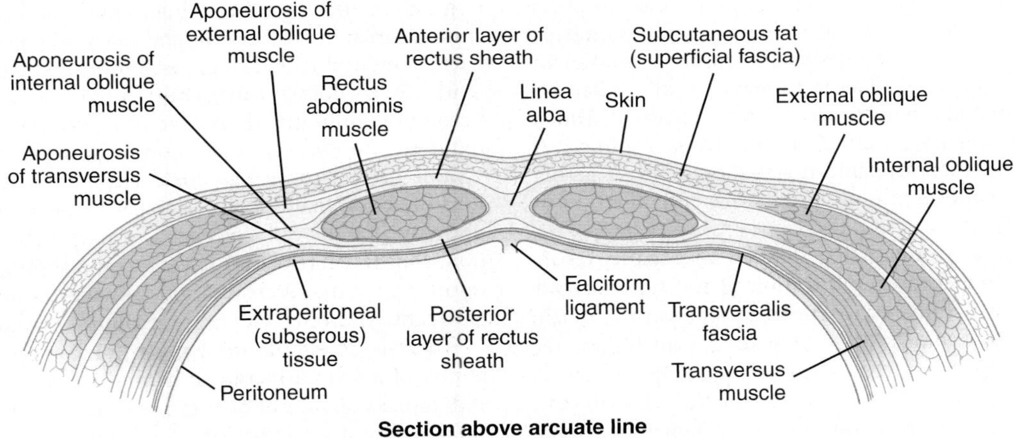

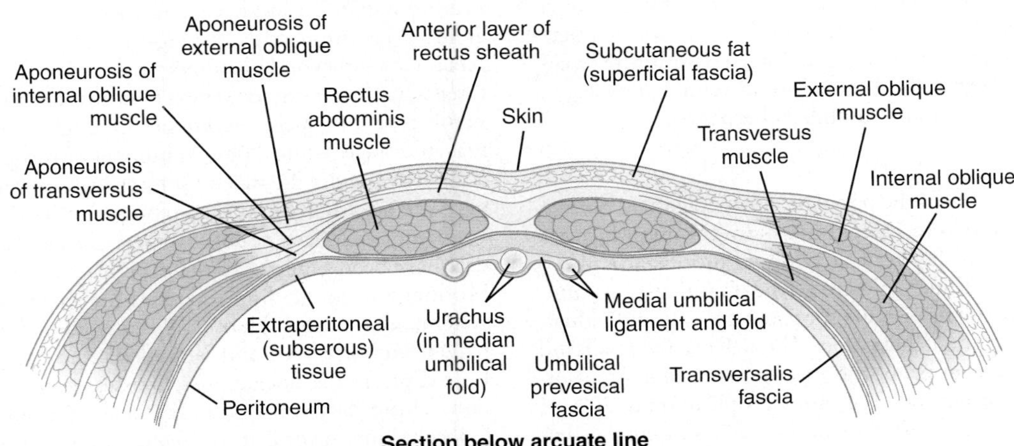

FIG. 45.9 Cross-sections of the rectus abdominis muscle and aponeurosis above and below the arcuate line. (From Netter FT. *Atlas of Human Anatomy*. Summit, NJ: Ciba-Geigy; 1989: Plate 235.)

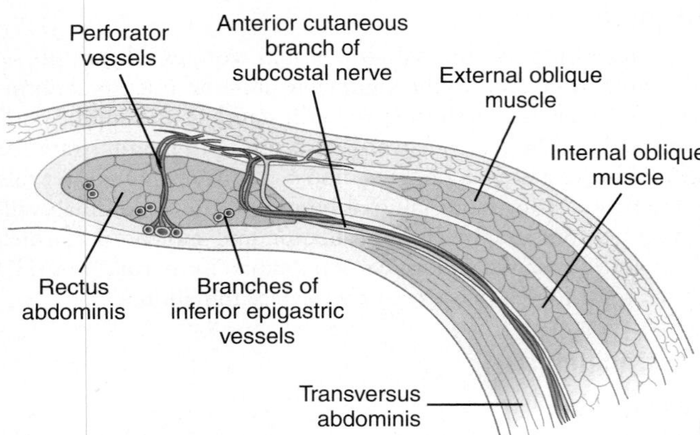

FIG. 45.10 Cross-section of the lateral abdominal wall detailing location of intercostal neurovascular bundle traveling between the transversus abdominis and internal oblique muscles.

States, the incidence of umbilical hernia is eight times higher in African American than in white infants.

Umbilical hernias in adults are largely acquired. These hernias are more common in women and in patients with conditions that result in increased intraabdominal pressure, such as pregnancy, obesity, ascites, or chronic abdominal distention. Umbilical hernia is more common in those who have only a single midline aponeurotic decussation compared with the normal decussation of fibers from all three lateral abdominal muscles. Strangulation is unusual in most patients; however, strangulation or rupture can occur in chronic ascitic conditions. Small asymptomatic umbilical hernias barely detectable on examination need not be repaired. Adults who have symptoms, a large hernia, incarceration, thinning of the overlying skin, or uncontrollable ascites should have a hernia repair. Spontaneous rupture of umbilical hernias in patients with ascites can result in peritonitis and death.

Classically, repair was done using the vest over pants repair proposed by Mayo, which uses imbrication of the superior and inferior fascial edges. Because of increased tension on the repair and recurrence rates of almost 30% with long-term follow-up, however, the Mayo repair is rarely performed today. Instead, small defects are closed primarily after separation of the sac from the overlying umbilicus and surrounding fascia. Defects larger than 3 cm are closed using prosthetic mesh.[29] There are a number of techniques to place this mesh, and no prospective data have conclusively found clear advantages of one technique over another. Options for mesh implantation include bridging the defect, placing a preperitoneal underlay of mesh reinforced with suture repair, and placing it laparoscopically. There is no universal consensus on the most appropriate method of umbilical hernia repair.

Epigastric Hernia

Approximately 3% to 5% of the population has epigastric hernias. Epigastric hernias are two to three times more common in men. These hernias are located between the xiphoid process and umbilicus and are usually within 5 to 6 cm of the umbilicus. Like umbilical hernias, epigastric hernias are more common in individuals with a single aponeurotic decussation. The defects are small and often produce pain out of proportion to their size because of incarceration of preperitoneal fat. They are multiple in up to 20% of patients, and approximately 80% are in the midline. Repair usually consists of excision of the incarcerated preperitoneal tissue and simple closure of the fascial defect, similar to that for umbilical hernias. Small defects can be repaired under local anesthesia. Uncommonly, these defects can be sizable, can contain omentum or other intraabdominal viscera, and may require mesh repairs. Epigastric hernias are better repaired anteriorly because the defect is small and fat that has herniated from within the peritoneal cavity is difficult to reduce.

Incisional Hernia

Of all hernias encountered, incisional hernias can be the most challenging and difficult to treat. Incisional hernias occur as a result of excessive tension and inadequate healing of a previous incision, which may be associated with surgical site infection. These hernias enlarge over time, leading to pain, bowel obstruction, incarceration, and strangulation. Obesity, advanced age, malnutrition, ascites, pregnancy, and conditions that increase intraabdominal pressure are factors that predispose to the development of an incisional hernia. Obesity can cause an incisional hernia to occur because of increased tension on the abdominal wall from the excessive bulk of a thick pannus and large omental mass. Chronic pulmonary disease and diabetes mellitus have also been recognized as risk factors for the development of incisional hernia. Medications such as corticosteroids and chemotherapeutic agents and surgical site infection can contribute to poor wound healing and increase the risk for development of an incisional hernia.

Large hernias can result in loss of abdominal domain, which occurs when the abdominal contents no longer reside in the abdominal cavity. These large abdominal wall defects also can result from the inability to close the abdomen primarily because of bowel edema, abdominal packing, peritonitis, and repeated laparotomy. With loss of domain, the natural rigidity of the abdominal wall becomes compromised and the abdominal musculature is often retracted. Respiratory dysfunction can occur because these large ventral defects cause paradoxic respiratory abdominal motion. Loss of abdominal domain can also result in bowel edema, stasis of the splanchnic venous system, urinary retention, and constipation. Return of displaced viscera to the abdominal cavity during repair may lead to increased abdominal pressure, abdominal compartment syndrome, and acute respiratory failure.

There is no simple mechanism for communicating the complexity of a ventral incisional hernia. Defect size, location on the abdominal wall, loss of domain, patient comorbidities, presence of contamination, necessity for an ostomy, acuity of the presentation, and history of prior repairs with or without a prosthetic allow an infinite number of permutations. The absence of a universal classification system has hindered comparisons within the literature and at meetings, indirectly delaying meaningful conversations about repair techniques and prosthetic choice. The tumor, node, and metastasis model for cancer staging is an enviable model to strive for in hernia repair. As such, a recent group sought to stratify ventral hernias into stages using a limited number of preoperative variables to accurately predict the two most meaningful surgical outcomes: surgical site occurrence (SSO) and long-term hernia recurrence rates.

Two of the most popular ventral hernia classification tools to date have been generated from expert opinion: the Ventral Hernia Working Group grading scale and the European Hernia Society system. The Ventral Hernia Working Group grading scale uses patient comorbidities and wound class to predict SSO risk. The European Hernia Society system assesses hernia width and location. Using data from 333 ventral hernia repairs with no filter for technique, investigators presented a multivariate analysis that identified hernia width (<10 cm, 10–20 cm, ≥20 cm) and the presence of contamination as the two variables associated with

TABLE 45.2 Incisional hernia staging system.

Stage I Risk: low recurrence, low SSO	<10 cm, clean
Stage II Risk: moderate recurrence, moderate SSO	<10 cm, contaminated 10–20 cm, clean
Stage III Risk: high recurrence, high SSO	≥10 cm, contaminated Any ≥20 cm

SSO, Surgical site occurrence.

wound morbidity (SSO) and hernia recurrence. Hernia location and patient comorbidities were not significant in this model for either outcome measure. Hernias could be grouped into stages (I to III) using width and wound class alone (Table 45.2), with ordinal increments in both outcome measures. Stage I hernias are smaller than 10 cm/clean and associated with low SSO and recurrence risk. Stage II hernias are 10 to 20 cm/clean or smaller than 10 cm/contaminated and carry an intermediate risk of SSO and recurrence. Stage III hernias are either 10 cm and larger/contaminated or any hernia 20 cm or larger, and these are associated with high SSO and recurrence risk. Table 45.3 demonstrates the reported rates for SSO and recurrence using this system.

The staging system is simple but comprehensive in its ability to stratify patients by risk of wound morbidity and recurrence, the two chief outcome parameters of repair. Importantly, this system does not include intraoperative details, such as approach (open vs. laparoscopic), mesh choice (biologic vs. synthetic), or mesh position (onlay vs. sublay). It is hoped that this platform can be the basis of future inclusion and exclusion criteria for studies regarding technique.

Treatment: Operative Repair

Primary repair of incisional hernias can be done when the defect is small (≤2–3 cm in diameter) and there is viable surrounding tissue or in cases in which the hernia was clearly a result of a technical error at the initial operation, such as a suture fracturing. Larger defects (>2–3 cm in diameter) have a high recurrence rate if closed primarily and are repaired with a prosthesis. In general, recurrence rates seem to increase with time. This suggests that incisional hernia is likely a chronic disease and an array of management options will need to be utilized to care for a patient throughout the course of their life. Prosthetic material may be placed as an onlay patch to buttress a tissue repair, interposed between the fascial defect, sandwiched between tissue planes, or put in a sublay position. Depending on its location, several important properties of the mesh must be considered.

Prosthetic Materials for Ventral Hernia Repair

Permanent Synthetic Materials. Various synthetic mesh products are available. Desirable characteristics of a synthetic mesh include its being chemically inert, resistant to mechanical stress while maintaining compliance, sterilizable, and noncarcinogenic; it should incite minimal inflammatory reaction and be hypoallergenic. The ideal mesh has yet to be defined. When selecting the appropriate mesh, the surgeon must consider the position of the mesh, whether it will be in direct contact with the viscera, and the presence or risk of infection. Mesh constructs can be classified on the basis of weight of the material, pore size, water angle (hydrophobic or hydrophilic), and whether there is an antiadhesive barrier present. In placing a mesh in the extraperitoneal position without the risk of bowel erosion, a macroporous unprotected mesh is appropriate. Both polypropylene and polyester mesh have been successfully placed in the extraperitoneal position. Polypropylene mesh is a hydrophobic macroporous mesh that allows the ingrowth of native fibroblasts and incorporation into the surrounding fascia. It is semirigid, somewhat flexible, and porous. Recently, lighter weight polypropylene mesh has been introduced to address some of the long-term complications of heavyweight polypropylene mesh. The definition of lightweight mesh was arbitrarily chosen at less than 40 g/m^2; medium weight mesh, 40 to 60 g/m^2; and intermediate weight mesh, 60 to 75 g/m^2 with heavyweight mesh weighing more than 75 g/m^2. These lightweight mesh products often have an absorbable component of material that provides initial handling stability, typically composed of Vicryl (polyglactin 910) or Monocryl (poliglecaprone 25; Ethicon, Somerville, NJ).

TABLE 45.3 Surgical site occurrence (SSO) and recurrence rates.

	SSO RATE	RECURRENCE RATE
Stage I Risk: low recurrence, low SSO <10 cm, clean	7/77 (10%)	7/77 (10%)
Stage II Risk: moderate recurrence, moderate SSO <10 cm, contaminated 10–20 cm, clean	30/151 (20%)	22/151 (15%)
Stage III Risk: high recurrence, high SSO ≥10 cm, contaminated Any ≥20 cm	44/105 (42%)	27/105 (26%)

Whether lightweight mesh results in improved patient outcomes is controversial. Two prospective randomized trials evaluating the incidence of postoperative pain after open inguinal hernia repair have shown mixed results. In a recent randomized controlled trial, heavyweight mesh has been shown to exhibit less recurrence and chronic pain 2 years after laparoscopic TEP inguinal repair compared to lightweight mesh.[30] The inverse has been shown in a large registry study evaluating patients undergoing open anterior mesh repair for inguinal hernia. In this study, long-term recurrence was no different using lightweight polypropylene mesh compared to heavyweight mesh.[31] Given the lightweight polypropylene mesh had less overall mesh-related issues compared to heavyweight mesh in this setting, lightweight mesh is favored. Notably, these advantages were not observed for lightweight mesh with a partially absorbable component. In a randomized controlled trial evaluating lightweight versus heavyweight polypropylene mesh for ventral hernia repair, the recurrence rate in the lightweight group was more than twice that in the heavyweight group (17% for lightweight mesh vs. 7% for heavyweight mesh), which approached statistical significance (P = 0.052).[32] Several investigators have reported concerning rates of central mesh failures with ultra-lightweight polypropylene mesh and lightweight polyester mesh.[33] Another recent finding with regard to large-pore lightweight mesh is its ability to resist bacterial contamination. Several animal studies have reported high rates of bacterial clearance with large-pore synthetic mesh when it is exposed to gastrointestinal flora and methicillin-resistant *Staphylococcus aureus*.[34] A large multicenter retrospective experience with 100 cases of large-pore polypropylene mesh used in clean-contaminated and contaminated ventral hernia repairs was reported.[35] These authors noted excellent medium-term results with a 7% recurrence rate. Longer-term data to verify the safety and durability of this approach are needed.

Polyester mesh is composed of polyethylene terephthalate and is a hydrophilic, heavyweight, macroporous mesh. This mesh has several different weaves that can yield a two-dimensional flat screen-like mesh and a three-dimensional multifilament weave. When it is placed in the preperitoneal position in complex ventral hernia repairs, complication rates are comparable to other products.[7,36] Long-term surveillance data are needed to ensure that long-term infection rates with polyester mesh are no worse than that for other products.

When mesh is placed in an intraperitoneal position, several options are available. A single sheet of mesh with both sides constructed to reduce adhesions and a composite-type mesh with one side made to promote tissue ingrowth and the other to resist adhesion formation are available composed of expanded polytetrafluoroethylene (ePTFE). This prosthetic has a visceral side that is microporous (3 μm) and an abdominal wall side that is macroporous (17–22 μm) and promotes tissue ingrowth. This product differs from other synthetic meshes in that it is flexible and smooth. Some fibroblast proliferation occurs through the pores, but PTFE is impermeable to fluid. Unlike polypropylene, PTFE is not incorporated into the native tissue. Encapsulation occurs slowly, and infection can occur during the encapsulation process. When it is infected, PTFE almost always must be removed.

To promote better tissue integration, composite mesh was developed. This product combines the attributes of polypropylene and PTFE by layering the two substances on top of one another. The PTFE surface serves as a permanent protective interface against the bowel and the polypropylene side faces superficially to be incorporated into the native fascial tissue. These materials have variable rates of contraction and, when placed together, can result in buckling of the mesh and visceral exposure to the polypropylene component. Other composite meshes recently have been developed that combine a macroporous mesh with a temporary, absorbable antiadhesive barrier. Basic constructs of these mesh materials include heavyweight or lightweight polypropylene or polyester. Absorbable barriers are typically composed of oxidized regenerated cellulose, omega-3 fatty acids, or collagen hydrogels. A number of small animal studies have validated the antiadhesive properties of these barriers, but currently, no human trials exist evaluating the ability of these composite materials to resist adhesion formation.

Biologic Materials. Biologic prostheses for ventral hernia repair are nonsynthetic, natural tissue mesh. There are numerous biologic grafts available for abdominal wall reconstruction (Table 45.4). These products can be categorized on the basis of the source material (e.g., human, porcine, bovine), postharvesting processing techniques (e.g., cross-linked, non–cross-linked), and sterilization techniques (e.g., gamma radiation, ethylene oxide gas sterilization, nonsterilized). These products are largely composed of acellular collagen and theoretically provide a matrix for neovascularization and native collagen deposition. These properties may provide advantages in infected or contaminated cases in which synthetic mesh is thought to be contraindicated. Ideal placement techniques are yet to be defined for these relatively new products; however, some general principles apply. These products function best when used as a fascial reinforcement rather than as a bridge or interposition repair. The long-term durability of biologic mesh has recently been questioned in the largest series of biologic mesh use in a contaminated setting.[37] Biologic mesh has found increased use in very challenging contaminated situations where permanent prosthetic use would be ill advised and native tissue coverage is difficult or impossible. In these unique situations, biologic mesh used in a bridge configuration can be used to minimize evisceration and provide a barrier separating viscera from atmosphere. There are no prospective randomized data comparing the effectiveness of these natural tissue alternatives with that of synthetic mesh repairs in various settings of complex hernia repairs.

Absorbable Synthetic Materials. Given the challenges observed with permanent synthetic meshes and biologic meshes, the use of absorbable synthetic materials for ventral hernia repair has gained popularity. The original absorbable synthetic material used for repair, polyglactin, remains a mainstay of managing challenging situations in contaminated fields. This material can be placed in any plane typically used for repair, ideally with soft tissue coverage anterior to the mesh. It is rapidly absorbable and hydrolyzes completely in 8 to 9 weeks. Variations of this material have been produced, resulting in slower hydrolysis and better handling characteristics at the time of implantation. In a prospective case series, slowly resorbable polyglactin mesh was found to have an acceptable recurrence rate of 17% when placed in a retromuscular position during contaminated complex ventral hernia repair.[38] Another material based on poly-4-hydroxybutyrate has shown promise in a prospective case series with recurrence rate of 9% 18 months after implantation in class I (clean) wounds. Multiple techniques were used and the bare mesh was not placed in the intraperitoneal space. This product resorbs completely between 12 and 18

TABLE 45.4 Biologic mesh for abdominal wall reconstruction and postharvesting processing techniques.

PRODUCT	SOURCE	CROSS-LINKED	STERILIZATION METHOD
AlloDerm (LifeCell, Branchburg, NJ)	Human dermis	No	Ionic
AlloMax (Davol, Warwick, RI)	Human dermis	No	E beam
FlexHD (Ethicon, Sommerville, NJ)	Human dermis	No	Ethanol
Strattice (LifeCell, Branchburg, NJ)	Porcine dermis	No	Gamma irradiation
Permacol (Covidien, Norwalk, CT)	Porcine dermis	Yes	Ethanol
CollaMend (Davol, Warwick, RI)	Porcine dermis	Yes	Ethanol
XenMatrix (Davol, Warwick, RI)	Porcine dermis	No	Gamma irradiation
SurgiMend (TEI Biosciences, Boston, MA)	Bovine fetal dermis	No	Ethanol
Veritas (Synovis, St. Paul, MN)	Bovine	No	
Peri-Guard (Synovis, St. Paul, MN)	Bovine	Yes	
Surgisis (Cook, Bloomfield, IN)	Porcine intestine	No	Ethanol

months. Use of these longer-term absorbable heavyweight meshes should be avoided in contaminated situations as 30-day infections can be increased even when compared to the use of midweight polypropylene.[39]

Operative Technique

Ventral Hernias. It is generally agreed that all but the smallest incisional hernias can be repaired with mesh, and the surgeon has various options for placing the mesh. The onlay technique involves primary closure of the fascia defect and placement of a mesh over the anterior fascia. The major advantage of this approach is that the mesh is placed outside the abdominal cavity, avoiding direct interaction with the abdominal viscera. However, disadvantages include the large subcutaneous dissection, the increased likelihood of seroma formation, the superficial location of the mesh (which places it in jeopardy of contamination if the incision becomes infected), and the repair is usually under tension. Prospective analysis of this technique is not available, but a retrospective review has reported recurrence rates of 28%.[40] Modifications of the traditional onlay repair in highly selected patients using midweight polypropylene mesh and fibrin glue fixation have shown comparable infection rates compared to permanent synthetic mesh placed in the sublay position.[41] Interposition prosthetic repairs involve securing the mesh to the fascial edge without overlap. This results in a predictably high recurrence rate; the synthetic often pulls away from the fascial edge because of increased intra abdominal pressure. A sublay technique involves placing the prosthetic below the fascial components. The mesh can be placed intraperitoneally, preperitoneally, or in the retrorectus (retromuscular) space. It is highly desirable to have the mesh placed beneath the fascia. With a wide overlap of mesh and fascia, the natural forces of the abdominal cavity act to hold the mesh in place and prevent migration. This can be accomplished by several techniques (Fig. 45.11).

Intraperitoneal mesh placement. After reopening of the prior incision and with the use of available dual-type mesh or composite mesh, the mesh can be placed in an intraperitoneal position at least 4 cm beyond the fascial margin and secured with interrupted mattress sutures. This technique requires raising subcutaneous flaps, and the mesh may be in direct contact with the abdominal contents.

The laparoscopic approach for ventral hernia repair relies on the same principles as the retrorectus repair; however, the mesh is placed within the peritoneal cavity. This repair is useful, particularly for hernia repair in patients with high wound risk. Trocars are placed as far laterally as feasible based on the size and location of the hernia. The hernia contents are reduced, and adhesions are lysed. The surface area of the defect is measured, and a barrier-coated mesh is fashioned with at least 4 cm of overlap around the defect. The mesh is rolled, placed into the abdomen, and deployed. It is secured to the anterior abdominal wall with pre-placed mattress sutures that are passed through separate incisions; a fixation device is used to further secure the mesh to the anterior abdominal wall. A minimum 4-cm overlap should be utilized beyond the edge of the fascial defect. For smaller defects, primary repair can be performed with passage of transabdominal sutures prior to mesh repair. There are fewer wound complications with the laparoscopic approach because large incisions and subcutaneous undermining are avoided.

Myofascial releases. One of the underlying principles of abdominal wall reconstruction is to reestablish the linea alba. Restoring the linea alba to the midline provides the advantage of a

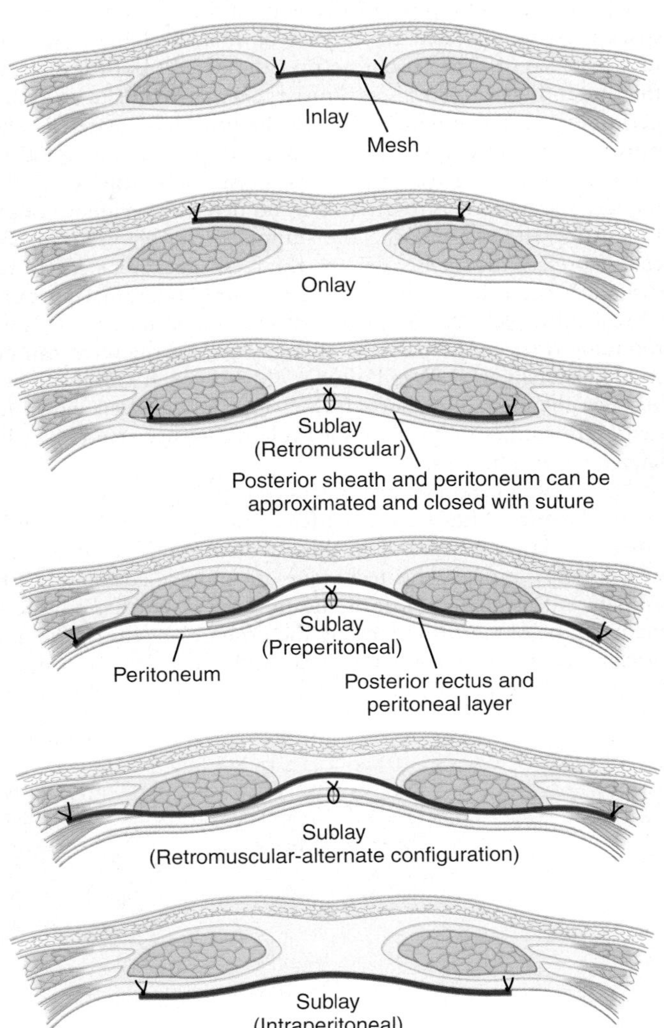

FIG. 45.11 Mesh placement options for abdominal wall reconstruction.

functional abdominal wall, often protects the mesh from superficial wound issues, and might result in a more durable repair. Myofascial release techniques are utilized to achieve these goals. In general, a myofascial release is defined as a fascial layer being separated from a muscular layer in the abdominal wall. In larger hernias, there are several options to provide the myofascial release necessary to reconstruct the midline and to restore contour to the abdominal wall. The basic tenets of these procedures are that the abdominal wall and rectus muscle are bounded by several different myofascial compartments, and by releasing one or more fascial bundles, advancement of the rectus muscle to the midline is possible. In essence, each of these procedures creates a local advancement flap of the rectus muscle. Great care should be taken to identify and to preserve the neurovascular structures to the rectus muscle to ensure a functional well-vascularized graft.

Posterior rectus sheath incision with retromuscular mesh placement. This technique involves placing prosthetic mesh in the extraperitoneal position in the preperitoneal space or retrorectus position. This technique was initially described by Stoppa.[7] A large piece of mesh is placed in the retromuscular space on top of the posterior rectus sheath or peritoneum. The compartment is accessed through an incision in the posterior rectus sheath approximately 1 cm from the medial edge of the rectus muscle. This space must be dissected laterally on both sides of the linea alba to a distance of 8 to 10 cm beyond the defect. Both leaflets of the posterior sheath are then sutured together to create an extraperitoneal pocket in which to place the prosthetic material. The prosthetic mesh extends 5 to 6 cm beyond the superior and inferior borders of the defect. The use of transfascial sutures to secure the mesh remains controversial, and no definitive evidence exists supporting either approach. The authors selectively use transfascial sutures. With smaller defects, the mesh does not need to be sutured because it is held in place by intra abdominal pressure (Pascal principle), allowing eventual incorporation into the surrounding tissues. Alternatively, in larger defects, the mesh can be secured laterally with several sutures. This approach avoids contact between the mesh and abdominal viscera and has been shown in long-term studies to have a respectable recurrence rate (14%) in large incisional hernias.

Posterior component separation/transversus abdominis release. The retrorectus space is bordered laterally by the linea semilunaris. In larger hernias or in those patients with atrophic narrowed rectus muscles, this technique can provide adequate mesh overlap and facilitate posterior sheath closure. Further advancement can be obtained by incising the posterior rectus sheath approximately 1 cm medial to the linea semilunaris. At this location, the posterior leaflet of the internal oblique and the transversus abdominis muscle are incised to gain access to either the pretransversalis plane or the preperitoneal space. These planes can be extended to the retroperitoneum and eventually to the psoas muscle if necessary. Very large sheets of prosthetic mesh can be placed in this location with wide defect coverage.[42] In one comparative analysis of posterior and anterior component separation, similar amount of fascial advancement was reported with a significant reduction in wound morbidity with use of the posterior approach.[42] Additional experience with a posterior component separation/transversus abdominis release (TAR) has shown excellent durability with acceptable short-term morbidity in expert hands.[43]

Anterior component separation. Another option for the repair of complex or large ventral defects is the anterior component separation technique (Fig. 45.12). This involves separating the lateral muscle layers of the abdominal wall to allow their advancement. Primary fascial closure at the midline is often possible. The procedure is performed by raising large subcutaneous flaps above the external oblique fascia. These flaps are carried laterally past the linea semilunaris. This lipocutaneous dissection itself can provide some advancement of the abdominal wall. Large perforating subcutaneous vessels can be preserved to prevent ischemic necrosis of the skin flaps. A relaxing incision is made 2 cm lateral to the linea semilunaris on the lateral external oblique aponeurosis from several centimeters above the costal margin to the pubis. The external oblique is then bluntly separated in the avascular plane, away from the internal oblique, allowing its advancement. Further

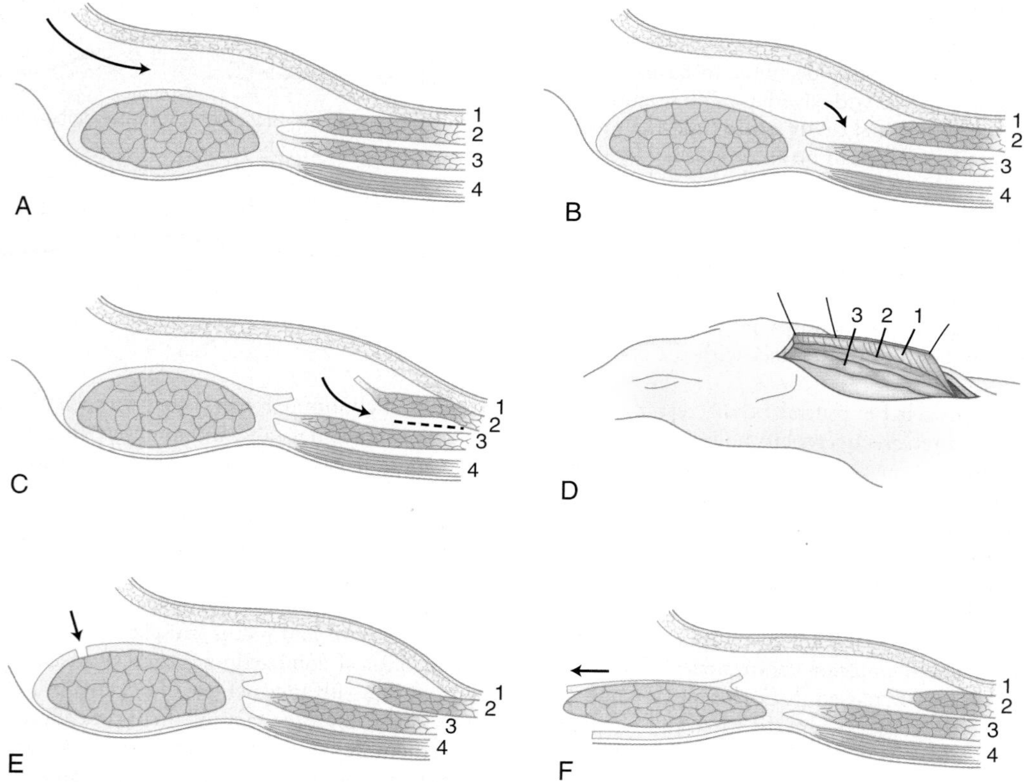

FIG. 45.12 Component separation technique. (A) The skin and subcutaneous fat are dissected free from the anterior sheath of the rectus abdominis muscle and the aponeurosis of the external abdominal oblique muscle. (B) The external abdominal oblique is incised 1 to 2 cm lateral to the rectus abdominis muscle. (C) The external abdominal oblique is separated from the internal abdominal oblique. (D) The dissection is carried to the posterior axillary line. (E) Additional length can be achieved by incising the posterior rectus sheath above the arcuate line. (F) Care must be taken to avoid damaging the nerves and blood supply that enter the rectus abdominis posteriorly. (From de Vries Reilingh TS, van Goor H, Rosman C, et al. Components separation technique for the repair of large abdominal wall hernias. *J Am Coll Surg.* 2003;196:32–37.)

relaxing incisions have been described to the aponeurotic layers of the internal oblique or transversus abdominis, but this can result in problematic lateral bulges or herniation at this site. Additional release can be safely achieved by incising the posterior rectus sheath. These techniques, when applied to both sides of the abdominal wall, can yield up to 20 cm of mobilization. Although this technique often allows tension-free closure of these large defects, recurrence rates as low as 20% have been reported with the use of prosthetic reinforcement in large hernias.[44] It is important that patients understand that a lateral bulge can occur after release of the external oblique aponeurosis. Recognizing the high recurrence rates with component separation alone, several authors have reported small series of biologic mesh reinforcement of these repairs. To date, no randomized controlled trials have supported a lower recurrence rate with biologic prosthetic reinforcement. If a bioprosthetic is placed, it can be secured with an underlay or onlay technique. No comparative data exist demonstrating the superiority of either repair technique.

Robotic approaches to ventral hernia repair. Robotic surgery can be used to perform several different types of ventral hernia repairs such as TAPP repair, intraperitoneal mesh placement, and retromuscular repair techniques with and without posterior component separation.

Robotic intraperitoneal mesh placement. Indications for the robotic approach are similar to laparoscopy and begin by port placement in the lateral abdomen. Once the robot is docked, adhesiolysis proceeds as usual. After identification of the entire hernia defect, it is closed with a continuous barbed suture. A tissue-separating mesh is chosen and typically sized to overlap the size of the original hernia defect by 4 to 5 cm on each side. The mesh is introduced and then fixated circumferentially to the abdominal wall with a continuous barbed suture. Two suturing techniques may be used for mesh fixation. The "baseball" stitch alternates between the edge of the mesh and the adjacent peritoneum/posterior fascia. The "dolphin" stitch is a horizontal mattress-type suture placed just inside the edge of the mesh, where the suture passes through the mesh, through the tissue and back through the mesh.

The robotic intraperitoneal onlay of mesh (IPOM) technique is near identical to the standard laparoscopic IPOM but avoids the need for mechanical mesh fixation. This may result in less postoperative pain. A large study of the Americas Hernia Society Quality Collaborative registry compared 454 patients undergoing standard laparoscopic IPOM procedures to 177 undergoing robotic IPOM utilizing a propensity score analysis. Although operative time greater than 2 hours was more common in the robotic cohort (47% vs. 31%), the length of stay (0 vs. 1 day) and the SSO rate (5% vs. 14%) were lower than laparoscopy.[45]

Robotic retromuscular repair with TAR. Patient selection for the robotic TAR is critical in ensuring a successful hernia repair. Patients with risk factors for increased wound morbidity, such as smoking, diabetes, and obesity, appear to be well suited for robotic hernia repair. A robotic approach is ideal as the surgeon can replicate the steps of an open repair, with the benefit of decreased wound complications seen with laparoscopic surgery. Compared to the open approach, the robotic retromuscular repair technique has demonstrated a significantly shorter length of hospital stay with no difference in 30-day readmissions.[46] An increased SSO rate was noted with the robotic approach, which were mostly seromas. Large mid-line defects, up to 20 cm in width, have been closed robotically; however, defects 10 to 15 cm in widest dimension seem to be best suited for the robotic TAR technique with good cosmetic results.

Three robotic ports are placed in the lateral abdomen on one side. Similar to the open approach, the contralateral posterior rectus sheath is incised vertically, immediately lateral to the hernia edge or linea alba. The dissection is extended at least 5 to 7 cm above and below the hernia to allow for sufficient mesh overlap. The posterior rectus sheath is subsequently peeled away from the posterior aspect of the rectus muscle, and dissection carried laterally until the neurovascular bundles which innervate the rectus muscle are encountered. The posterior rectus sheath and transversus abdominis muscle are incised dorsally, approximately 1 cm medial to the neurovascular bundles, exposing the transversalis fascia. The dissection then proceeds in either the pretransversalis fascia or preperitoneal planes laterally, peeling the peritoneum or transversalis fascia away from the posterior aspect of the cut transversus abdominis muscle. This space is dissected, lateral, until the peritoneal flap, with the attached posterior sheath, rests without tension, upon the visceral contents below.

Next, a similar configuration of ports is placed on the contralateral side, and the robot is undocked from the original side, the patient bed is rotated 180 degrees, and the robot is redocked on the contralateral side. The retrorectus and TAR dissection is now carried out, identically, on the contralateral side.

The posterior rectus sheaths are now suture-approximated in the midline, utilizing a barbed suture, completely closing the visceral sac. The anterior rectus sheath and hernia defect are subsequently suture-approximated with a barbed suture as well. Decreasing the intraabdominal pressure to 8 to 10 mm Hg helps facilitate the fascial closure. Once the defect is closed, the robot is undocked, and the laparoscope is inserted to measure the dissected space for mesh placement. A standard flat piece of permanent synthetic mesh is deployed into the retromuscular pocket and not fixated, as it conforms to the space. The ports are then removed and the procedure ended. The port sites do not require fascial closure, since the mesh extends beyond the fascial incisions in the retromuscular plane.

Robotic extended TEP technique. The robotic extended TEP technique replicates the posterior rectus sheath incision with retromuscular mesh placement technique previously described but avoids the need for laparotomy, thus obviating any adhesiolysis, and can be performed as a same-day surgical procedure.[47] Patient selection is important, and a preoperative CT scan may aid in surgical planning. This technique is best employed on patients with wide rectus muscles and hernia defects less than 10 to 12 cm in width.

The first step requires laparoscopic entry through the rectus muscle, into the retrorectus space on one side utilizing an optical port. This is performed either far above or far below the level of the hernia defect. Once in position, the retrorectus space is insufflated and additional ports are placed to facilitate the dissection. If the retrorectus space is wide enough, the robot can be docked at this point; if not, it is docked once ports have been placed into the contralateral retrorectus space. Next, the posterior rectus sheath is incised immediately lateral to its insertion on the linea alba, allowing access to the preperitoneal plane, dorsal to the linea alba. The dissection is carried out in the preperitoneal plane, toward the contralateral side. Once the contralateral posterior rectus sheath is identified, it is incised, allowing entrance into the contralateral retrorectus plane, where additional robotic trocars are placed. If the robot was not docked before, it is docked now. Dissection then commences, dividing the insertion of both posterior rectus sheaths on either side of the linea alba, all the while maintaining the peritoneal layer in the midline intact, thus avoiding peritoneal entry. Once the hernia sac is encountered, it is either reduced intact if possible, or it is incised circumferentially around the hernia defect

TABLE 45.5 Comparative randomized studies between open and laparoscopic ventral hernia repair.

STUDY	NO. OF PATIENTS		MESH USED		INTRAOPERATIVE COMPLICATIONS (%)		LOS (DAYS)		POSTOPERATIVE COMPLICATIONS (%)		FOLLOW-UP (MONTHS)		RECURRENCE (%)	
	LAP	OPEN	LAP	OPEN	LAP	OPEN	LAP	OPEN	LAP	OPEN	LAP	OPEN	LAP	OPEN
McGreevy et al. (2003)[49]	65	71	ePTFE or polyester + collagen	PP	N/A	N/A	1.1	1.5	7.70	21.10	N/A	N/A	N/A	N/A
Lomanto et al. (2006)[50]	50	50	Polyester + collagen	ePTFE	2	2	2.74	4.7	26	40	19.6	21	2	10
Bingener et al. (2007)[51]	127	233	ePTFE, PP, or ePTFE	PP	N/A	N/A	N/A	N/A	33.10	43.30	36	36	13	9
Olmi et al. (2007)[48]	85	85	Polyester + collagen	PP	N/A	N/A	2.7	9.9	16.50	29.40	24	24	2	4
Pring et al. (2008)*	31	27	PTFE	PTFE	N/A	N/A	1	1	33	49	28	28	3.30	4.20
Asencio et al. (2009)†	45	39	PTFE or PP	PP	6.70	0	3.46	3.33	5.20	33.30	12	12	9.70	7.90

ePTFE, Expanded polytetrafluoroethylene; *LAP*, laparoscopic; *LOS*, length of stay; *N/A*, not available; *PP*, polypropylene.
*Pring CM, Tran V, O'Rourke N, et al. Laparoscopic versus open ventral hernia repair: a randomized controlled trial. *ANZ J Surg*. 2008;78:903–906.
†Asencio F, Aguilo J, Peiro S, et al. Open randomized clinical trial of laparoscopic versus open incisional hernia repair. *Surg Endosc*. 2009;23:1441–1448.

and the fenestration closed at a later time. Further division of the posterior rectus sheath insertions on either side of the linea alba is performed caudal or cephalad to the hernia defect, depending upon where the initial trocars were placed. Any tears in the posterior sheath or peritoneum are repaired, and the hernia defect is closed with a running barbed suture. A posterior component separation or TAR technique can easily be performed at this point, if deemed necessary to facilitate midline abdominal wall reconstruction. The robot is undocked, and the laparoscope is inserted to measure the retrorectus dissected space for mesh placement. A standard flat piece of permanent synthetic mesh is deployed into the retromuscular pocket and not fixated, as it conforms to the space.

Results of Incisional Hernia Repairs

Several prospective randomized trials have compared laparoscopic and open ventral hernia repairs (Table 45.5).[48–51] Although most of these studies were small, with fewer than 100 patients, the results tend to favor a laparoscopic approach for small to medium-sized defects. The incidence of postoperative complications and recurrence were less in hernias repaired laparoscopically. Several retrospective reports have demonstrated similar advantages for a laparoscopic approach. Until an appropriately powered prospective randomized trial is performed, the ideal approach will largely be based on surgeon expertise and preference. In addition, these trials will need to provide guidance on the most appropriate hernia size to be repaired by either an open or a laparoscopic approach.

UNUSUAL HERNIAS

There are a number of hernias that occur infrequently, of various types.

Types

Spigelian Hernia

A spigelian hernia occurs through the spigelian fascia, which is composed of the aponeurotic layer between the rectus muscle medially and semilunar line laterally. Almost all spigelian hernias occur at or below the arcuate line. The absence of posterior rectus fascia may contribute to an inherent weakness in this area. These hernias are often interparietal, with the hernia sac dissecting posterior to the external oblique aponeurosis. Most spigelian hernias are small (1–2 cm in diameter) and develop during the fourth to seventh decades of life. Patients often present with localized pain in the area without a bulge because the hernia lies beneath the intact external oblique aponeurosis. Ultrasound or CT of the abdomen can be useful to establish the diagnosis.

A spigelian hernia is repaired because of the risk for incarceration associated with its relatively narrow neck. The hernia site is marked before operation; the DASH technique is very useful to localize the hernia prior to anesthetic induction and can minimize the size of open incision. A transverse incision is made over the defect and carried through the external oblique aponeurosis. The hernia sac is opened, dissected free of the neck of the hernia, and excised or inverted. The defect is closed transversely by simple suture repair of the transversus abdominis and internal oblique muscles, followed by closure of the external oblique aponeurosis. Larger defects are repaired with a mesh prosthesis. A laparoscopic approach can also be used (especially in those with higher wound risk), but care should be undertaken to completely reduce all contents prior to repair. Recurrence is uncommon.

Obturator Hernia

The obturator canal is formed by the union of the pubic bone and ischium. This canal is covered by a membrane pierced at the medial and superior border by the obturator nerve and vessels. Weakening of the obturator membrane may result in enlargement of the canal and formation of a hernia sac, which can lead to intestinal incarceration and strangulation. The patient can present with evidence of compression of the obturator nerve, which causes pain in the anteromedial aspect of the thigh (Howship-Romberg sign) that is relieved by thigh flexion. Almost 50% of patients with obturator hernia present with complete or partial bowel obstruction. An abdominal CT scan can establish the diagnosis, if necessary.

A posterior approach, open or laparoscopic, is preferred. This approach provides direct access to the hernia. After reduction of the hernia sac and contents, any preperitoneal fat within the obturator canal is reduced. If necessary, the obturator foramen is opened posterior to the nerve and vessels. The obturator nerve can be manipulated gently with a blunt nerve hook to facilitate reduction of the fat pad. The obturator foramen is repaired with prosthetic mesh, with care taken to avoid injury to the obturator nerve and vessels. Patients with compromised bowel usually require laparotomy.

Lumbar Hernia

Lumbar hernias can be congenital or acquired after an operation on the flank and occur in the lumbar region of the posterior abdominal wall. Hernias through the superior lumbar triangle (Grynfeltt triangle) are more common. The superior lumbar triangle is bounded by the twelfth rib, paraspinal muscles, and internal oblique muscle. Less common are hernias through the inferior lumbar triangle (Petit triangle), which is bounded by the iliac crest, latissimus dorsi muscle, and external oblique muscle. Weakness of the lumbodorsal fascia through either of these areas results in progressive protrusion of extraperitoneal fat and a hernia sac. Lumbar hernias are not prone to incarceration. Small lumbar hernias are frequently asymptomatic. Larger hernias may be associated with back pain. CT is useful for diagnosis.

Both open and laparoscopic repairs are useful. Satisfactory suture repair is difficult because of the immobile bone margins of these defects. Repair is best done by placement of prosthetic mesh, which is sutured beyond the margins of the hernia. There is usually sufficient fascia over the bone to anchor the mesh.

Interparietal Hernia

Interparietal hernias are rare and occur when the hernia sac lies between layers of the abdominal wall. These hernias most frequently occur in previous incisions. Spigelian hernias are almost always interparietal.

The correct preoperative diagnosis of interparietal hernia can be difficult. Many patients with complicated interparietal hernias present with intestinal obstruction. Abdominal CT can assist in the diagnosis. Large interparietal hernias usually require placement of prosthetic mesh for closure. When this cannot be done, the component separation technique may be useful to provide natural tissues to obliterate the defect.

Sciatic Hernia

The greater sciatic foramen can be a site of hernia formation. These hernias are extremely unusual and difficult to diagnose and frequently are asymptomatic until intestinal obstruction occurs. In the absence of intestinal obstruction, the most common symptom is the presence of an uncomfortable or slowly enlarging mass in the gluteal or intragluteal area. Sciatic nerve pain can occur, but sciatic hernia is a rare cause of sciatic neuralgia.

A transperitoneal approach is preferred if bowel obstruction or strangulation is suspected. Hernia contents can usually be reduced with gentle traction. Prosthetic mesh repair is usually preferred. A transgluteal approach can be used if the diagnosis is certain and the hernia is reducible, but most surgeons are not familiar with this approach. With the patient prone, an incision is made from the posterior edge of the greater trochanter across the hernia mass. The gluteus maximus muscle is opened, and the sac is visualized. The muscle edges of the defect are reapproximated with interrupted sutures, or the defect is obliterated with mesh.

Perineal Hernia

Perineal hernias are caused by congenital or acquired defects and are uncommon. These hernias may also occur after abdominoperineal resection or perineal prostatectomy. The hernia sac protrudes through the pelvic diaphragm. Primary perineal hernias are rare, occur most commonly in older multiparous women, and can be quite large. Symptoms are usually related to protrusion of a mass through the defect that is worsened by sitting or standing. A bulge is frequently detected on bimanual rectal-vaginal examination.

Perineal hernias are generally repaired through a transabdominal approach or combined transabdominal and perineal approaches. After the sac contents are reduced, small defects may be closed with nonabsorbable suture, whereas large defects are repaired with prosthetic mesh.

Loss of Domain Hernias

Loss of domain implies a massive hernia in which the herniated contents have resided for so long outside the abdominal cavity that they cannot simply be replaced into the peritoneal cavity. We typically classify loss of domain hernias into patients with and without preoperative contamination. Each group is then subcategorized into two groups. Patients with a small hernia defect and a massive hernia sac (e.g., large inguinoscrotal hernias) require restoration of peritoneal cavity domain, whereas patients with a large defect and a massive hernia sac (open abdomen with skin graft) require restoration of peritoneal domain and complex reconstruction of the abdominal wall.

Before repair of these complex defects, the patient must undergo careful preoperative evaluation. A clear understanding of the morbidity and mortality associated with these reconstructive procedures is critical. Weight reduction, smoking cessation, optimization of nutrition, and glucose control are all important aspects of complex abdominal wall reconstruction. Previously, methods to stretch the abdominal wall gradually were used to allow the restoration of abdominal domain and closure. This was accomplished by insufflation of air into the abdominal cavity to create a progressive pneumoperitoneum. Repeated administrations of increasing volumes of air during 1 to 3 weeks allowed the muscles of the abdominal wall to become lax enough for primary closure of the defect. This technique is particularly suited for small defects and massive hernia sacs.[52] For large defects, some authors have also described a staged approach using ePTFE dual mesh for patients with loss of abdominal domain and lateral retraction of the abdominal wall musculature. The initial stage involves reduction of the hernia and placement of a large sheet of ePTFE dual mesh secured to the fascial edges with a running suture. Subsequent stages involve serial elliptical excision of the mesh until the fascia can be approximated in the midline without tension. Finally, the mesh is completely excised, and the fascia is reapproximated with component separation and a biologic underlay patch, if necessary.[53] This approach is technically feasible but does require multiple operations and long hospital stays, and it is associated with a fairly high morbidity rate.

Parastomal Hernia Repair

Parastomal hernia is a common complication of stoma creation. In fact, the creation of a stoma by strict definition is an abdominal wall hernia. The incidence of parastomal hernias is highest for colostomies and occurs in up to 50% of stomas. Fortunately, most patients remain asymptomatic, and life-threatening complications, such as bowel obstruction and strangulation, are rare. Unlike midline incisional hernia repair, routine repair of parastomal hernias is not recommended. Surgical repair should be reserved for patients experiencing symptoms of bowel obstruction, problems with pouch fit, or cosmetic issues.

Three general approaches are available for parastomal hernia repair. These techniques include primary fascial repair, stoma relocation, and prosthetic repair. Primary fascial repair involves hernia reduction and primary fascial reapproximation through a peristomal incision. This technique carries a predictably high recurrence rate. The advantage of this approach is that the abdomen often is not entered, making the operation less complex. Because of the high recurrence rate with this technique, it should be reserved for patients who will not tolerate a laparotomy. Stoma relocation improves results; however, it requires a laparotomy and predisposes to another parastomal hernia in the future.

Prosthetic repairs of parastomal hernias can provide excellent long-term results with a lower rate of hernia recurrence, but a higher rate of prosthetic complications must be accepted. Regardless of the technique, a permanent foreign body placed in apposition to the bowel can result in erosion, obstruction, and disastrous complications. Several approaches to prosthetic mesh placement have been described. The mesh can be placed as an onlay patch, intra abdominally, or in the retrorectus position. When the mesh is placed intraperitoneally, a keyhole is fashioned around the stoma site or placed as a flat sheet, lateralizing the stoma as it exits the abdomen, as described by Sugarbaker (Fig. 45.13).[54] A retromuscular repair that takes advantage of many of the advanced reconstructive techniques described in this chapter has recently been reported. In this approach, a laparotomy is performed, and the stoma is taken down and eventually resited to the contralateral side of the abdomen. A posterior component separation is then performed; a large mesh is deployed in the retromuscular space to cover the old stoma site and the entire midline incision, and it is used to prophylactically reinforce the new stoma site. The stoma is eventually brought out through a keyhole incision in the mesh and matured.[55] All these series are fairly small, with fewer than 100 patients, and have reported only short-term to medium-term follow-up, limiting our ability to make clear recommendations for this difficult problem.

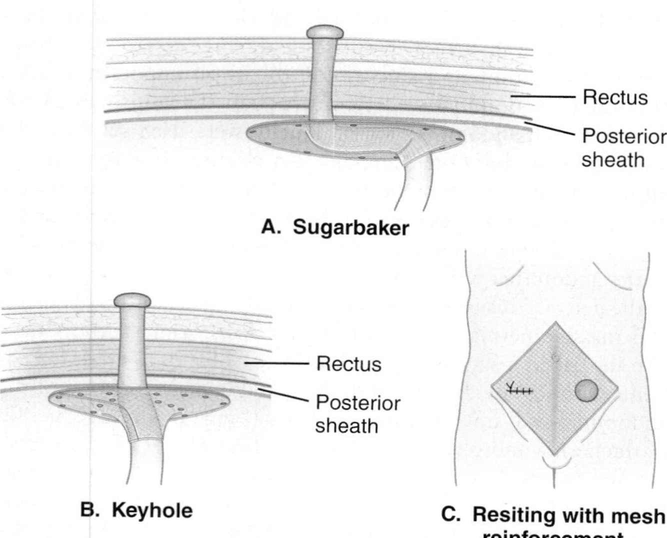

FIG. 45.13 Surgical approaches for parastomal hernia repair.

Complications

General Considerations

Increased attention has been placed on mesh-related complications after hernia repair. As an increased population of patients are exposed to longer periods of indwelling mesh, a higher group of patients will exist with long-term mesh-related complications. The rate of these complications, which can be potentially harmful, is not well characterized. Kokotovic and colleagues[56] found that in a healthy Danish population, the rate of mesh-related complications requiring operative removal at 5 years was 4.9%. The lack of an effective postmarket surveillance system in the United States makes it extremely difficult to determine the rate of serious long-term mesh-related complications.

Mesh Infection

Mesh infections are serious complications that can be difficult to treat. Infections can generally be divided into acute situations where abdominal wall sepsis is present resulting in a system inflammatory response and chronic indolent infections in which no sepsis is present. In acute with sepsis, the patients are emergently and aggressively treated including monitored admission to the hospital, intravenous antibiotics, and early debrided and mesh removal. Mesh salvage can often be employed with chronic mesh infections. This approach employs percutaneous drainage of any fluid collection and antibiotic suppression based on culture results. As drainage diminishes, a repeat CT scan is performed to assess resolution of the fluid collection and the drain is removed if minimal output. Continued antibiotic suppression is continued based on clinical judgment. The success in managing chronic infections depends largely on patient factors and prosthetic type. All efforts to eliminate nicotine use and control diabetes and excess weight are employed. If ePTFE becomes infected, it requires removal with the resultant morbidity of another defect, which often must be closed under tension, leading to inevitable recurrence. Infected polyester mesh often requires at least partial removal; areas of mesh that are still clearly well incorporated at the time of operation can usually be left in place taking into consideration the morbidity of complete removal. Polypropylene products tend to be the most successful in terms of mesh salvage. Use of the laparoscopic technique and placement of a large piece of mesh without undermining large subcutaneous tissue flaps avoid wound complications. In a series of almost 1000 patients who had laparoscopic ventral hernia repair, mesh infections occurred in less than 1% of cases.[57] Perhaps the greatest advantage of the laparoscopic approach for repairing ventral hernias is this reduction in infectious complications. However, higher rates of missed enterotomy have been noted with minimally invasive approaches to ventral hernia.

Seromas

Seroma formation can occur after laparoscopic and open ventral hernia repair. In open ventral hernia repair, drains are often placed in an attempt to obliterate the dead space caused by the hernia and tissue dissection. These drains can cause mesh contamination, and seromas can form after drain removal. With laparoscopic repair, the hernia sac is not resected, and a seroma cavity will result. Most of these seromas will resolve over time as the mesh becomes incorporated on the hernia sac. Preoperative discussions with the patient describing the expectations of a temporary seroma are imperative before laparoscopic ventral hernia repair. We reserve aspiration for symptomatic or persistent seromas after 6 to 8 weeks.

Enterotomy

Intestinal injury during adhesiolysis can be catastrophic. Management of an enterotomy during a hernia repair is controversial and depends on the segment of intestine injured (small vs. large bowel) and amount of spillage. Options include aborting the hernia repair, using a primary tissue or biologic tissue repair, and performing a delayed repair with prosthetic mesh in 3 to 4 days. When there is gross contamination, the use of synthetic mesh is contraindicated.

SELECTED REFERENCES

Anson BJ, McVay CB. Inguinal hernia: the anatomy of the region. *Surg Gynecol Obstet.* 1938;66:186–191.

Condon RE. Surgical anatomy of the transversus abdominis and transversalis fascia. *Ann Surg.* 1971;173:1–5.

Nyhus LM. An anatomic reappraisal of the posterior inguinal wall, with special consideration of the iliopubic tract and its relation to groin hernias. *Surg Clin North Am.* 1960;44:1305.

These three references are classic descriptions of the anatomy of the groin. All are well illustrated.

Bisgaard T. Bay-Nielsen M, Kehlet H. Re-recurrence after operation for recurrent inguinal hernia. A nationwide 8-year follow-up study on the role of type of repair. *Ann Surg.* 2008;247:707–711.

This long-term population-based study provides useful information about the results of recurrent inguinal hernia repairs.

de Vries Reilingh TS, van Goor H, Charbon JA, et al. Repair of giant midline abdominal wall hernias: "Components separation technique" versus prosthetic repair: interim analysis of a randomized controlled trial. *World J Surg.* 2007;31:756–763.

This is a prospective randomized trial evaluating outcomes of open ventral hernia repair with synthetic mesh versus component separation without reinforcement.

Fitzgibbons Jr RJ, Forse RA. Clinical practice. Groin hernias in adults. *N Engl J Med.* 2015;372:756–763.

Recent review of the diagnosis and management of groin hernias in adults.

Forbes SS, Eskicioglu C, McLeod RS, et al. Meta-analysis of randomized controlled trials comparing open and laparoscopic ventral and incisional hernia repair with mesh. *Br J Surg.* 2009;96:851–858.

This is a meta analysis evaluating eight prospective randomized trials comparing laparoscopic with open ventral hernia repair.

Itani KM, Hur K, Kim LT, et al. Veterans Affairs Ventral Incisional Hernia Investigators: comparison of laparoscopic and open repair with mesh for the treatment of ventral incisional hernia: a randomized trial. *Arch Surg.* 2010;145:322–328.

This is a prospective randomized trial evaluating laparoscopic versus open ventral hernia repairs.

Neumayer L, Giobbie-Hurder A, Jonasson O, et al. Open mesh versus laparoscopic mesh repair of inguinal hernia. *N Engl J Med.* 2004;350:1819–1827.

Excellent prospective randomized trial comparing these two types of hernia repairs in Veterans Administration hospitals.

Zhao G, Gao P, Ma B, et al. Open mesh techniques for inguinal hernia repair: a meta-analysis of randomized controlled trials. *Ann Surg.* 2009;250:35–42.

Excellent meta analysis of various techniques of tension-free repairs.

REFERENCES

1. Bradley M, Morgan D, Pentlow B, et al. The groin hernia—an ultrasound diagnosis? *Ann R Coll Surg Engl.* 2003;85:178–180.
2. Fitzgibbons Jr RJ, Giobbie-Hurder A, Gibbs JO, et al. Watchful waiting vs repair of inguinal hernia in minimally symptomatic men: a randomized clinical trial. *JAMA.* 2006;295:285–292.
3. Fitzgibbons Jr RJ, Ramanan B, Arya S, et al. Long-term results of a randomized controlled trial of a nonoperative strategy (watchful waiting) for men with minimally symptomatic inguinal hernias. *Ann Surg.* 2013;258:508–515.
4. Lichtenstein IL, Shulman AG, Amid PK, et al. The tension-free hernioplasty. *Am J Surg.* 1989;157:188–193.
5. Gilbert AI. Sutureless repair of inguinal hernia. *Am J Surg.* 1992;163:331–335.
6. Kugel RD. Minimally invasive, nonlaparoscopic, preperitoneal, and sutureless, inguinal herniorrhaphy. *Am J Surg.* 1999;178:298–302.
7. Stoppa RE. The treatment of complicated groin and incisional hernias. *World J Surg.* 1989;13:545–554.
8. Malangoni MA, Condon RE. Preperitoneal repair of acute incarcerated and strangulated hernias of the groin. *Surg Gynecol Obstet.* 1986;162:65–67.
9. Ahmad G, Duffy JM, Phillips K, et al. Laparoscopic entry techniques. *Cochrane Database Syst Rev.* 2008:CD006583.
10. Voyles CR, Hamilton BJ, Johnson WD, et al. Meta-analysis of laparoscopic inguinal hernia trials favors open hernia repair with preperitoneal mesh prosthesis. *Am J Surg.* 2002;184:6–10.
11. Muysoms F, Van Cleven S, Kyle-Leinhase I, et al. Robotic-assisted laparoscopic groin hernia repair: observational case-control study on the operative time during the learning curve. *Surg Endosc.* 2018;32:4850–4859.
12. Bisgaard T, Bay-Nielsen M, Kehlet H. Re-recurrence after operation for recurrent inguinal hernia. A nationwide 8-year

follow-up study on the role of type of repair. *Ann Surg*. 2008;247:707–711.

13. Nordin P, Haapaniemi S, van der Linden W, et al. Choice of anesthesia and risk of reoperation for recurrence in groin hernia repair. *Ann Surg*. 2004;240:187–192.
14. Neumayer L, Giobbie-Hurder A, Jonasson O, et al. Open mesh versus laparoscopic mesh repair of inguinal hernia. *N Engl J Med*. 2004;350:1819–1827.
15. McCormack K, Scott NW, Go PM, et al. Laparoscopic techniques versus open techniques for inguinal hernia repair. *Cochrane Database Syst Rev*. 2003:CD001785.
16. Amato B, Moja L, Panico S, et al. Shouldice technique versus other open techniques for inguinal hernia repair. *Cochrane Database Syst Rev*. 2012:CD001543.
17. Zhao G, Gao P, Ma B, et al. Open mesh techniques for inguinal hernia repair: a meta-analysis of randomized controlled trials. *Ann Surg*. 2009;250:35–42.
18. Repair of groin hernia with synthetic mesh: meta-analysis of randomized controlled trials. *Ann Surg*. 2002;235:322–332.
19. Wake BL, McCormack K, Fraser C, et al. Transabdominal pre-peritoneal (TAPP) vs totally extraperitoneal (TEP) laparoscopic techniques for inguinal hernia repair. *Cochrane Database Syst Rev*. 2005:CD004703.
20. Mikkelsen T, Bay-Nielsen M, Kehlet H. Risk of femoral hernia after inguinal herniorrhaphy. *Br J Surg*. 2002;89:486–488.
21. Kald A, Fridsten S, Nordin P, et al. Outcome of repair of bilateral groin hernias: a prospective evaluation of 1,487 patients. *Eur J Surg*. 2002;168:150–153.
22. Aufenacker TJ, van Geldere D, van Mesdag T, et al. The role of antibiotic prophylaxis in prevention of wound infection after Lichtenstein open mesh repair of primary inguinal hernia: a multicenter double-blind randomized controlled trial. *Ann Surg*. 2004;240:955–960; discussion 960–951.
23. Simons MP, Aufenacker T, Bay-Nielsen M, et al. European Hernia Society guidelines on the treatment of inguinal hernia in adult patients. *Hernia*. 2009;13:343–403.
24. Karthikesalingam A, Markar SR, Holt PJ, et al. Meta-analysis of randomized controlled trials comparing laparoscopic with open mesh repair of recurrent inguinal hernia. *Br J Surg*. 2010;97:4–11.
25. Sevonius D, Gunnarsson U, Nordin P, et al. Repeated groin hernia recurrences. *Ann Surg*. 2009;249:516–518.
26. Rucinski J, Margolis M, Panagopoulos G, et al. Closure of the abdominal midline fascia: meta-analysis delineates the optimal technique. *Am Surg*. 2001;67:421–426.
27. Muysoms FE, Antoniou SA, Bury K, et al. European Hernia Society guidelines on the closure of abdominal wall incisions. *Hernia*. 2015;19:1–24.
28. Carlson MA, Ludwig KA, Condon RE. Ventral hernia and other complications of 1,000 midline incisions. *South Med J*. 1995;88:450–453.
29. Luijendijk RW, Hop WC, van den Tol MP, et al. A comparison of suture repair with mesh repair for incisional hernia. *N Engl J Med*. 2000;343:392–398.
30. Burgmans JP, Voorbrood CE, Simmermacher RK, et al. Long-term results of a randomized double-blinded prospective trial of a lightweight (Ultrapro) versus a heavyweight mesh (Prolene) in laparoscopic total extraperitoneal inguinal hernia repair (TULP-trial). *Ann Surg*. 2016;263:862–866.
31. Melkemichel M, Bringman SAW, Widhe BOO. Long-term comparison of recurrence rates between different lightweight and heavyweight meshes in open anterior mesh inguinal hernia repair: a nationwide population-based register study. *Ann Surg*. 2019.
32. Conze J, Kingsnorth AN, Flament JB, et al. Randomized clinical trial comparing lightweight composite mesh with polyester or polypropylene mesh for incisional hernia repair. *Br J Surg*. 2005;92:1488–1493.
33. Petro CC, Nahabet EH, Criss CN, et al. Central failures of lightweight monofilament polyester mesh causing hernia recurrence: a cautionary note. *Hernia*. 2015;19:155–159.
34. Diaz-Godoy A, Garcia-Urena MA, Lopez-Monclus J, et al. Searching for the best polypropylene mesh to be used in bowel contamination. *Hernia*. 2011;15:173–179.
35. Carbonell AM, Criss CN, Cobb WS, et al. Outcomes of synthetic mesh in contaminated ventral hernia repairs. *J Am Coll Surg*. 2013;217:991–998.
36. Rosen MJ. Polyester-based mesh for ventral hernia repair: is it safe? *Am J Surg*. 2009;197:353–359.
37. Rosen MJ, Krpata DM, Ermlich B, et al. A 5-year clinical experience with single-staged repairs of infected and contaminated abdominal wall defects utilizing biologic mesh. *Ann Surg*. 2013;257:991–996.
38. Rosen MJ, Bauer JJ, Harmaty M, et al. Multicenter, prospective, longitudinal study of the recurrence, surgical site infection, and quality of life after contaminated ventral hernia repair using biosynthetic absorbable mesh: the COBRA Study. *Ann Surg*. 2017;265:205–211.
39. Sahoo S, Haskins IN, Huang LC, et al. Early wound morbidity after open ventral hernia repair with biosynthetic or polypropylene mesh. *J Am Coll Surg*. 2017;225:472–480.e471.
40. de Vries Reilingh TS, van Geldere D, Langenhorst B, et al. Repair of large midline incisional hernias with polypropylene mesh: comparison of three operative techniques. *Hernia*. 2004;8:56–59.
41. Haskins IN, Voeller GR, Stoikes NF, et al. Onlay with adhesive use compared with sublay mesh placement in ventral hernia repair: was Chevrel right? An Americas Hernia Society quality Collaborative analysis. *J Am Coll Surg*. 2017;224:962–970.
42. Krpata DM, Blatnik JA, Novitsky YW, et al. Posterior and open anterior components separations: a comparative analysis. *Am J Surg*. 2012;203:318–322; discussion 322.
43. Novitsky YW, Fayezizadeh M, Majumder A, et al. Outcomes of posterior component separation with transversus abdominis muscle release and synthetic mesh sublay reinforcement. *Ann Surg*. 2016;264:226–232.
44. de Vries Reilingh TS, van Goor H, Charbon JA, et al. Repair of giant midline abdominal wall hernias: "components separation technique" versus prosthetic repair: interim analysis of a randomized controlled trial. *World J Surg*. 2007;31:756–763.
45. Prabhu AS, Dickens EO, Copper CM, et al. Laparoscopic vs robotic intraperitoneal mesh repair for incisional hernia: an Americas Hernia Society Quality Collaborative analysis. *J Am Coll Surg*. 2017;225:285–293.
46. Carbonell AM, Warren JA, Prabhu AS, et al. Reducing length of stay using a robotic-assisted approach for retromuscular ventral hernia repair: a comparative analysis from the Americas Hernia Society Quality Collaborative. *Ann Surg*. 2018;267:210–217.
47. Belyansky I, Reza Zahiri H, Sanford Z, et al. Early operative outcomes of endoscopic (eTEP access) robotic-assisted retromuscular abdominal wall hernia repair. *Hernia*. 2018;22:837–847.

48. Olmi S, Scaini A, Cesana GC, et al. Laparoscopic versus open incisional hernia repair: an open randomized controlled study. *Surg Endosc*. 2007;21:555–559.
49. McGreevy JM, Goodney PP, Birkmeyer CM, et al. A prospective study comparing the complication rates between laparoscopic and open ventral hernia repairs. *Surg Endosc*. 2003;17:1778–1780.
50. Lomanto D, Iyer SG, Shabbir A, et al. Laparoscopic versus open ventral hernia mesh repair: a prospective study. *Surg Endosc*. 2006;20:1030–1035.
51. Bingener J, Buck L, Richards M, et al. Long-term outcomes in laparoscopic vs open ventral hernia repair. *Arch Surg*. 2007;142:562–567.
52. McAdory RS, Cobb WS, Carbonell AM. Progressive preoperative pneumoperitoneum for hernias with loss of domain. *Am Surg*. 2009;75:504–508; discussion 508–509.
53. Lipman J, Medalie D, Rosen MJ. Staged repair of massive incisional hernias with loss of abdominal domain: a novel approach. *Am J Surg*. 2008;195:84–88.
54. Sugarbaker PH. Peritoneal approach to prosthetic mesh repair of paraostomy hernias. *Ann Surg*. 1985;201:344–346.
55. Raigani S, Criss CN, Petro CC, et al. Single-center experience with parastomal hernia repair using retromuscular mesh placement. *J Gastrointest Surg*. 2104;18:1673–1677.
56. Kokotovic D, Bisgaard T, Helgstrand F. Long-term recurrence and complications associated with elective incisional hernia repair. *JAMA*. 2016;316:1575–1582.
57. Heniford BT, Park A, Ramshaw BJ, et al. Laparoscopic repair of ventral hernias: nine years' experience with 850 consecutive hernias. *Ann Surg*. 2003;238:391–399; discussion 399–400.

46 CHAPTER

Acute Abdomen

Alessandra Landmann, Morgan Bonds, Russell Postier

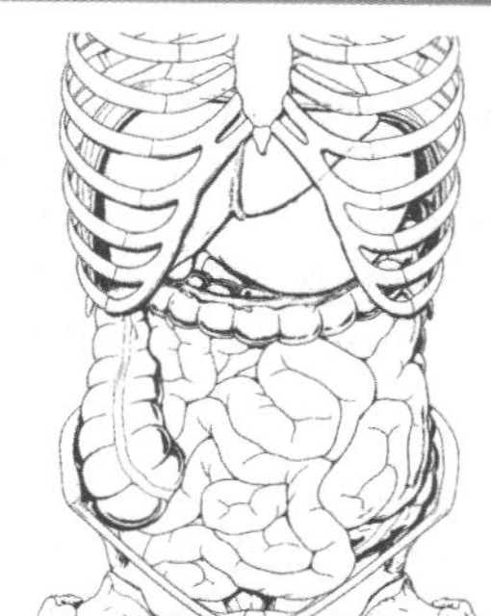

OUTLINE

The term *acute abdomen* refers to the signs and symptoms of abdominal pain and tenderness. This situation often represents an underlying surgical problem that requires prompt diagnosis and surgical treatment. While the ready availability of diagnostic studies such as computed tomography (CT) scans or magnetic resonance imaging (MRI) has added greatly to our ability to accurately diagnose most of the conditions responsible for the acute abdomen, the mainstay for diagnosis remains a good history and physical exam complemented by laboratory and radiologic studies as appropriate. In addition, many conditions that are not surgical or even centered in the abdomen can also cause this presentation.[1] A prompt and accurate diagnosis is necessary in order to select the appropriate therapy, which may be a laparoscopy or laparotomy.

Age, gender, and a history of prior abdominal surgical procedures are associated with different problems causing the acute abdomen. Certain diseases like appendicitis and mesenteric adenitis are more common in the young while biliary tract disease, diverticulitis, and intestinal ischemia are more common in older populations.[2] Chapter 67 deals with abdominal pain in children.

Numerous problems that are not surgical may also present as an acute abdomen. These include endocrine and metabolic issues, hematologic problems, and disorders caused by toxins or drugs (Box 46.1).[3,4] Endocrine and metabolic diagnoses include uremia, diabetic or Addisonian crisis, acute intermittent porphyria, hyperlipoproteinemia, and hereditary Mediterranean fever. Hematologic disorders include sickle cell crisis and acute leukemia. Toxins and drugs that can cause acute abdominal pain are lead and other heavy metal intoxications, narcotic withdrawal, and black widow spider bites. All of these need to be considered when evaluating a patient with sudden onset abdominal pain.

The need for prompt surgical treatment of those causes of the acute abdomen that require operation mandates an expeditious evaluation so that the proper therapy can be carried out (Box 46.2). A focused history and physical examination and indicated laboratory and imaging studies will then allow for the correct diagnosis and guide appropriate therapy. While imaging studies have added greatly to the accuracy of the diagnosis of causes of the acute abdomen, a thorough history and careful physical examination remain the mainstays of evaluation.

ANATOMY AND PHYSIOLOGY

Abdominal pain is visceral, parietal, or referred. The presentation for each helps determine the source of the pain. Visceral pain is vague and localized to the epigastrium, periumbilical region, or lower abdomen, depending on whether it originates from the foregut, midgut, or hindgut. Visceral pain is usually due to the distention of a hollow viscus. Parietal pain is sharper and better localized than visceral pain and corresponds to the nerve roots that supply the peritoneum. Referred pain is perceived at a site distant from the source of the pain. Common sites of referred pain and their sources are listed in Box 46.3. Determining whether the pain is visceral, parietal, or referred can usually be accomplished with a careful history.

Whenever bacteria or visceral contents from a perforation are introduced into the peritoneal cavity, an outpouring of fluid from the peritoneal surface ensues. The peritoneum responds to such insults by increasing blood flow, increasing permeability, and forming a fibrinous exudate on its surface. A generalized or localized loss of intestinal motility usually results. Adhesions between loops or bowel, bowl and omentum, or bowel and abdominal wall then occur, which help to localize the inflammatory insult. As a result, an abscess may cause sharp, localized pain but with normal peristalsis whereas a diffuse process such as a duodenal perforation generally results in generalized abdominal pain with absent bowel sounds.

BOX 46.1 Nonsurgical causes of the acute abdomen.

Endocrine and Metabolic Causes
Acute intermittent porphyria
Addisonian crisis
Diabetic crisis
Hereditary Mediterranean fever
Uremia

Hematologic Causes
Acute leukemia
Sickle cell crisis

Toxins and Drugs
Black widow spider poisoning
Lead poisoning
Other heavy metal poisoning
Narcotic withdrawal

BOX 46.2 Surgical acute abdominal conditions.

Hemorrhage
Aortoduodenal fistula after aortic vascular graft
Arteriovenous malformation of the gastrointestinal tract
Bleeding gastrointestinal diverticulum
Hemorrhagic pancreatitis
Intestinal ulceration
Leaking or ruptured arterial aneurysm
Mallory-Weiss syndrome
Ruptured ectopic pregnancy
Solid organ trauma
Spontaneous splenic rupture

Infection
Appendicitis
Cholecystitis
Diverticulitis
Hepatic abscess
Meckel diverticulitis
Psoas abscess

Ischemia
Buerger disease
Ischemic colitis
Mesenteric thrombosis or embolism
Ovarian torsion
Strangulated hernia
Testicular torsion

Obstruction
Cecal volvulus
Gastrointestinal malignancy
Incarcerated hernias
Inflammatory bowel disease
Intussusception
Sigmoid volvulus
Small bowel obstruction

Perforation
Boerhaave syndrome
Perforated diverticulum
Perforated gastrointestinal cancer
Perforated gastrointestinal ulcer

Peritonitis is recognized on physical examination by severe tenderness, with or without rebound tenderness, and guarding. It is due to peritoneal inflammation of any cause. It is usually due to an inflammatory insult, commonly gram-negative infection with either an enteric organism or anaerobe.[5] It can also be caused by inflammation that is not due to infection, such as pancreatitis. Another form of peritonitis that occurs in children and is caused by *Pneumococcus* or hemolytic *Streptococcal* species and occurs in adults on peritoneal dialysis is called *primary peritonitis.* The organisms most often seen in the adult, peritoneal dialysis population are *Escherichia coli* and *Klebsiella.*

HISTORY

Despite advances in laboratory studies and imaging, a detailed and focused history is essential to formulating an accurate differential diagnosis in the patient with an acute abdomen. The history should focus on the onset and nature of the pain, any associated symptoms such as nausea or anorexia, whether they began before or after the pain, and the progression of the pain. A history of inflammatory bowel disease, prior abdominal procedures, either open or laparoscopic is important in constructing a differential diagnosis. Often, additional information may be obtained by observing how the patient describes the pain that is experienced. Pain identified with one finger is more localized and typical of parietal innervation or peritoneal inflammation as compared to indicating the area of discomfort with the palm of the hand, which is more typical of the visceral discomfort of bowel or solid organ disease. The intensity and severity of the pain are related to the underlying tissue damage. Sudden onset of excruciating pain suggests conditions such as intestinal perforation or arterial embolization with ischemia, although other conditions, such as biliary colic, can present suddenly as well. Pain that develops and worsens over several hours is typical of conditions of progressive inflammation or infection such as cholecystitis, colitis, or bowel obstruction. The history of progressive worsening versus intermittent pain can help differentiate infectious process from the spasmodic colicky pain associated with bowel obstruction, biliary colic from cystic duct obstruction, or genitourinary obstruction (Fig. 46.1).

The location, character, and radiation of the pain are important to elicit. Tissue injury or inflammation can result in visceral and somatic pain. Solid organ visceral pain in the abdomen is generalized in the quadrant of the involved organ, such as liver pain across the right upper quadrant of the abdomen. Small bowel pain is perceived as poorly localized periumbilical pain, whereas pain from a colonic origin is centered between the umbilicus and pubic symphysis. As inflammation expands to involve the peritoneal surface, parietal nerve fibers from the spine allow for a focal and intense sensation. This combination of innervation is responsible for the classic diffuse periumbilical pain of early appendicitis that later shifts to become an intense focal pain in the right lower abdomen at McBurney point. Further, the pain may also extend well beyond the diseased site. For example, the liver shares some of its innervation with the diaphragm. Thus, liver inflammation may create referred pain to the right shoulder from the C3–C5 nerve roots. Also, genitourinary pain commonly has a radiating pattern.

BOX 46.3 Locations and causes of referred pain.

Left Shoulder
Heart
Left hemidiaphragm
Spleen
Tail of pancreas

Right Shoulder
Gallbladder
Liver
Right hemidiaphragm

Scrotum and Testicles
Ureter

Symptoms are primarily in the flank region, originating from the splanchnic nerves of T11–L1, but the pain often radiates to the scrotum or labia via the hypogastric plexus of S2–S4.

Determining what factors, if any, worsen or lessen the pain is important. Eating will often worsen the pain of bowel obstruction, biliary colic, pancreatitis, diverticulitis, or bowel perforation. Food can lessen the pain from peptic ulcer disease or gastritis. Patients with peritonitis will avoid any activity that stretches or moves the abdomen. Those patients will describe worsening of the pain with any sudden body movement and realize that there is less pain if their knees are flexed. Anything that causes movement of the abdomen, such as the car ride to the hospital, can be agonizing.

Associated symptoms and their timing are important diagnostic clues. Nausea, vomiting, constipation, diarrhea, pruritus, melena, hematochezia, and hematuria are all helpful symptoms if present. Vomiting may occur because of severe abdominal pain of any cause or as a result of either mechanical bowel obstruction or ileus. Vomiting is more likely to precede the onset of significant abdominal pain in many nonsurgical conditions, whereas in the

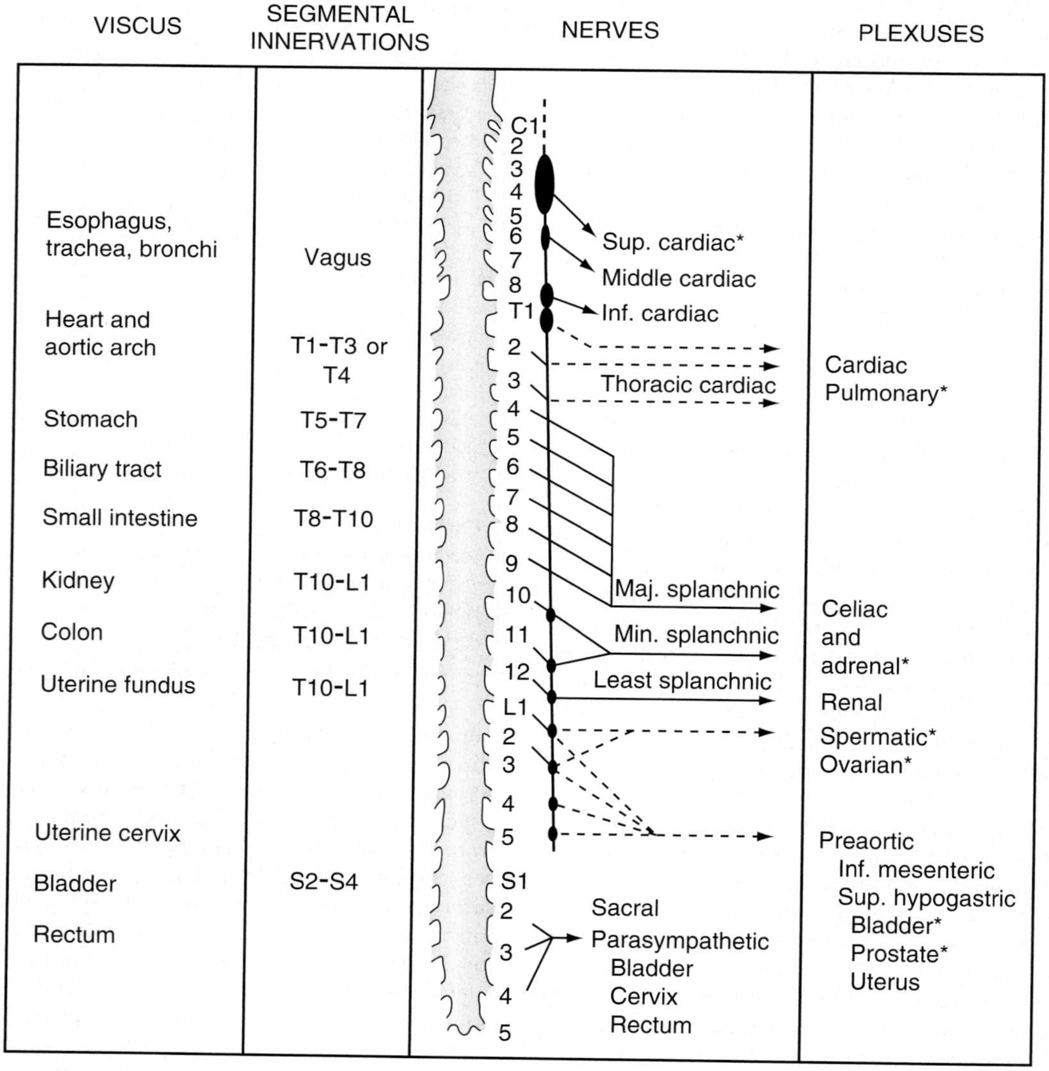

VISCUS	SEGMENTAL INNERVATIONS
Esophagus, trachea, bronchi	Vagus
Heart and aortic arch	T1-T3 or T4
Stomach	T5-T7
Biliary tract	T6-T8
Small intestine	T8-T10
Kidney	T10-L1
Colon	T10-L1
Uterine fundus	T10-L1
Uterine cervix	
Bladder	S2-S4
Rectum	

NERVES
Sup. cardiac*
Middle cardiac
Inf. cardiac
Thoracic cardiac
Maj. splanchnic
Min. splanchnic
Least splanchnic
Sacral Parasympathetic
Bladder
Cervix
Rectum

PLEXUSES
Cardiac
Pulmonary*
Celiac and adrenal*
Renal
Spermatic*
Ovarian*
Preaortic
Inf. mesenteric
Sup. hypogastric
Bladder*
Prostate*
Uterus

* No known sensory fibers in sympathetic rami.

FIG. 46.1 Sensory innervation for viscera.

pain of an acute abdomen with an underlying surgical cause, the pain will precede the vomiting. Constipation or obstipation can be the result of mechanical obstruction or decreased peristalsis. It may either be the primary problem and can be treated with laxatives or prokinetic agents or it may be merely a symptom of an underlying more serious condition. Knowing whether or not the patient continues to pass flatus or have bowel movements is thus important. A complete obstruction, with the absence of flatus or bowel movements is more likely to be associated with subsequent bowel ischemia or perforation caused by the significant distention that can occur. Diarrhea is associated with several conditions that are not treated with operations. These include infectious enteritis, inflammatory bowel disease, or parasitic infections. Bloody diarrhea can be seen in these medical conditions as well as in colonic ischemia.

A careful past history can be exceedingly helpful in making the correct diagnosis of the patient with acute abdominal pain. Previous illness or diagnoses can greatly increase or decrease the likelihood of certain conditions that may not otherwise be thought of. For example, patients may report that the current pain is similar to the pain experienced during the passage of a renal stone several years previously. A prior history of appendectomy, pelvic inflammatory disease, or cholecystectomy can significantly limit the differential diagnosis. Any abdominal scars present on the abdomen during the physical exam need to be accounted for in the history that is obtained.

Certain medications can both create and mask the symptoms of an acute abdominal condition. High dose narcotics can interfere with bowel motility and lead to obstipation and obstruction. Narcotics can also contribute to spasm of the sphincter of Oddi and exacerbate biliary or pancreatic pain. They can also suppress pain sensations and alter mental status. Both of these impair the ability of the surgeon to diagnose the condition accurately. Nonsteroidal antiinflammatory drugs are associated with upper gastrointestinal inflammation and perforation. Steroids can block protective gastric mucous production by chief cells and reduce the inflammatory reaction to infection, including significant peritonitis. The class of agents that are immunosuppressive increase a patient's risk of acquiring various bacterial or viral illnesses and also blunt the inflammatory response, diminishing the pain that should be present and limiting the overall physiologic response. Anticoagulant drugs use is common in our elderly population and may be the cause of gastrointestinal bleeding, retroperitoneal hemorrhage, or rectus sheath hematomas. They can also complicate the preoperative preparation of the patient and be the cause of substantial morbidity if their use goes unrecognized. Finally, recreational drugs can also be the cause of acute abdominal pain. Cocaine and methamphetamine use can create an intense vasospasm that can cause life-threatening cardiac or intestinal ischemia as well as severe hypertension.

The differential diagnosis of the acute abdomen in women includes many more conditions than are found in the male population. In the past, the negative laparotomy or laparoscopy rate in women with acute abdominal pain was significant and substantially higher than that seen in men. Improvements in, and the widespread availability of, advanced imaging such as MRI and CT scans have improved the diagnostic accuracy of the evaluation of acute abdominal pain in this population. A careful gynecologic history remains important in the evaluation of abdominal pain in young women. The likelihood of ectopic pregnancy, pelvic inflammatory disease, mittelschmerz, and severe endometriosis are all dependent upon the details elicited in the gynecologic history.

PHYSICAL EXAMINATION

The physical examination remains an essential component in the evaluation of the acute abdomen. You will be able to garner valuable information from this step to better inform the next steps in the diagnostic pathway. Physical examination will generate a more precise differential diagnosis, and this will allow for the initiation of necessary therapy in a timely manner. Despite wider availability of advanced diagnostic imaging, it cannot replace an organized and thorough physical examination.

The initial evaluation of all patients should begin with general inspection. Information regarding the severity of the illness can quickly be assessed upon walking into the room. Symptoms such as diaphoresis, pallor, dyspnea, and decreased alertness can be assessed rapidly and will forewarn the examiner that a serious issue is at hand. For an acute abdomen, the general inspection will be the first evidence of whether the patient has peritoneal inflammation. These patients tend to be very still as movement aggravates their abdominal pain. In contrast, patients with abdominal pain without peritoneal inflammation will fidget in attempts to find a comfortable position.

Inspection of the abdomen is the next step. Attention is focused on the contour of the abdomen and skin abnormalities. Abdominal wall distension occurs in several abdominal processes such as intestinal obstruction, development of ascites, or presence of a growing mass. Surgical scars should be identified and correlated to the history taken prior to the physical examination. Other skin findings, such as erythema or blistering, can alert the examiner to the possibility of soft tissue infections that may require immediate debridement. Ecchymosis can also be an indication of a fascial necrotizing infection; additionally, it may alert the examiner to accidental or nonaccidental trauma and may warrant further social investigation.

Historically, the next step in evaluation is auscultation. This maneuver should be done prior to percussion or palpation as bowel activity can be affected by manual manipulation. Vascular abnormalities, such as arterial stenosis or arteriovenous fistulas, can be detected by auscultating bruits within the abdomen. Auscultation for bowel activity is controversial. It has been taught that the quantity and quality of bowel sounds heard correlate with the motility of the bowel. Ileus is associated with hearing fewer than one bowel sounds every 15 seconds per quadrant. Conversely, high-pitched tinkling sounds are associated with mechanical bowel obstruction. Many argue that history of flatus and bowel movements are more accurate at determining whether the patient is having a bowel motility issue than auscultation. A recent review article cited low sensitivity and positive predictive values for auscultating bowel sounds in normal volunteers, patients with bowel obstruction, and patients with postoperative ileus. They also noted poor interobserver reliability for bowel auscultation, recording it at 54%.[6] Auscultation can be useful but must be correlated with history and other exam findings.

Percussion is capable of eliciting a wealth of information. Dull resonance in the right upper quadrant identifies the liver; measuring the superior-inferior range of this dullness will give the examiner a rough estimate of liver size. Percussion is useful in determining whether abdominal distension is due to excess air or fluid. The presence of localized dullness elsewhere in the abdomen should raise concern for an intraabdominal mass. Tympany, or hyperresonance, is consistent with gas-filled structure deep to the abdominal wall. If tympany is heard in the right upper quadrant, where the liver is located, this indicates there is air between

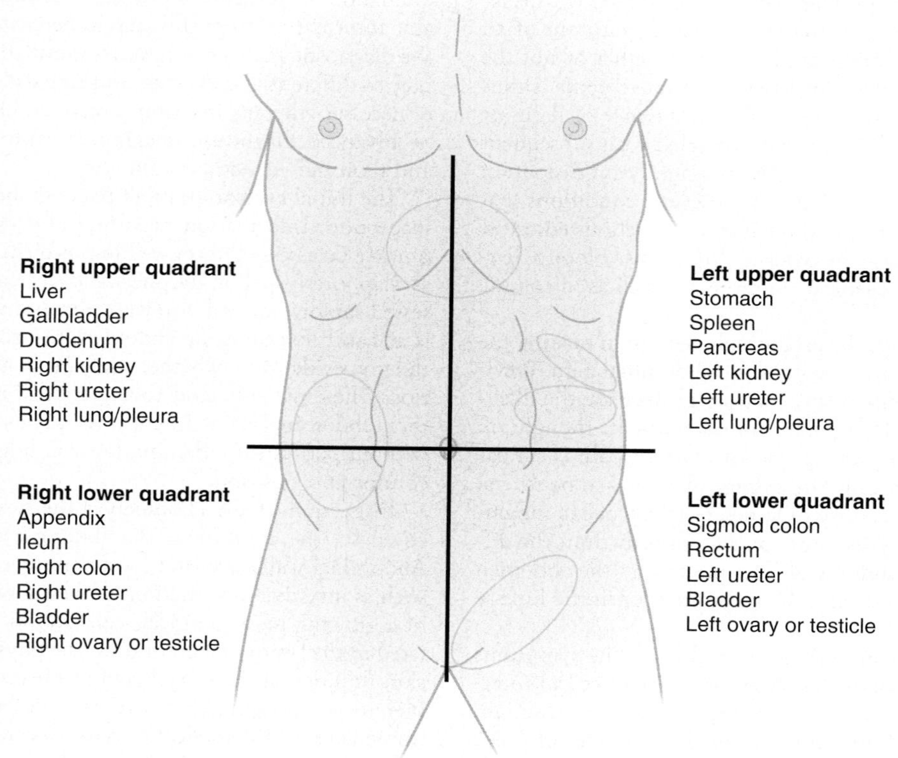

FIG. 46.2 Abdominal structures by palpations quadrants.

the abdominal wall and liver, and intraperitoneal free air should be suspected. Diffuse dullness to percussion raises suspicion for a fluid-filled abdomen. A fluid wave can be created by a quick firm compression of the lateral abdominal wall; a wave should then travel medially across the abdominal wall.

Percussion can also be useful identifying the presence of peritonitis. A patient with peritonitis will have exquisite tenderness during percussion of the abdomen and may not be able to withstand the maneuver. Jostling the abdominal viscera by percussing the flank, iliac crest, or the heel of an extended lower extremity will illicit the characteristic signs of peritonitis. These maneuvers are more reliable for detecting inflammation of the peritoneal lining than the historical technique of deep palpation followed by quick withdrawal of pressure and asking whether the pressure or release was most painful. This can be very painful, regardless of the presence of peritonitis, and leaves room for subjective interpretation by the patient.

The final portion of the abdominal exam is palpation. Generally, this is the most informative portion of the examination. It provides details that help you localize the source of pain as well as abnormalities within the abdomen. The examiner should begin with superficial palpation away from the area with the most significant pain; superficial palpation allows for assessment of masses or fluid collections anterior to the abdominal wall and whether the pain is associated with these abnormalities. More pressure should then be applied to perform deep palpation. Deep palpation allows the examiner to assess pain from an intraabdominal source as well as the presence of any intraabdominal masses or organomegaly. Diffuse tenderness to palpation suggests extensive inflammation or delayed presentation of an ongoing disease process. Identifying the region of maximum tenderness will give the examiner the likely source of abdominal pain. By identifying the quadrant causing the pain, a differential diagnosis can be developed based on the structures within that quadrant (Fig. 46.2).

Guarding can be encountered while performing abdominal palpation. It is necessary to differentiate between voluntary and involuntary guarding. Voluntary guarding occurs when the patient anticipates painful stimuli and tenses their abdominal wall muscles. To prevent this, have the patient lie supine on the exam table and bend his or her legs to place the soles of their feet flat on the bed. Instruct them to take a deep breath while you palpate. These maneuvers result in relaxation of the abdominal wall as well as distracting the attention of the patient, preventing voluntary guarding. If the abdominal wall tenses despite the above techniques, the patient has involuntary guarding which is a sign of peritonitis.

There are several named exam maneuvers associated with different disease processes. These can be seen in Table 46.1. Murphy sign for acute cholecystitis which involves deeply palpating the right subcostal region while the patient inspires deeply. If cholecystitis is present, the inspiration will be cut short due to pain as the gallbladder encounters the anterior abdominal wall. The obturator and psoas signs can be useful identifying the relative position of an inflamed appendix. Rovsing sign suggests right lower quadrant peritonitis.

TABLE 46.1 **Abdominal examination signs.**

History		
Danforth sign	Shoulder pain on inspiration	Hemoperitoneum
Inspection		
Cruveilhier sign	Varicose veins at umbilicus	Portal hypertension
Cullen sign	Periumbilical bruising	Hemoperitoneum
Grey Turner sign	Local areas of discoloration near umbilicus and flanks	Acute pancreatitis
Ransohoff sign	Yellow discoloration of umbilical region	Ruptured common bile duct
Palpation		
Aaron sign	Pain or pressure in epigastrium or anterior chest with persistent firm pressure applied to McBurney point	Acute appendicitis
Bassler sign	Sharp pain created by compressing appendix between abdominal wall and iliacus	Chronic appendicitis
Blumberg sign	Transient abdominal wall rebound tenderness	Peritoneal inflammation
Carnett sign	Loss of abdominal tenderness when abdominal wall muscles contracted	Intraabdominal source of abdominal pain
Chandelier sign	Extreme pelvic pain with movement of the cervix	Pelvic inflammatory disease
Courvoisier sign	Palpable gallbladder when jaundice is present	Periampullary mass
Fothergill sign	Abdominal wall mass that does not cross midline and is palpable when rectus is contracted	Rectus muscle hematoma
Iliopsoas sign	Elevation of extended leg against resistance is painful	Retrocecal acute appendicitis
Murphy sign	Pain caused by inspiration while applying pressure to right upper abdomen	Acute cholecystitis
Obturator sign	Flexion and external rotation of right thigh creates hypogastric pain	Pelvic abscess or inflammatory mass (appendicitis)
Rovsing sign	Pain at McBurney point when palpating the left lower quadrant	Acute appendicitis
ten Horn sign	Pain caused by gentle traction of right testicle	Acute appendicitis

Additional exams often provide useful information. Digital rectal exam provides information about hollow viscus bleeding and sources of distal obstruction causing constipation and obstipation. In women, results of pelvic exam will help include or exclude gynecologic sources of lower abdominal pain. A 2014 study found that of 290 women of reproductive age with right lower quadrant pain thought to have acute appendicitis 37 (12.8%) had gynecologic pathology with a normal appendix.[7] Pelvic examination may identify this pathology earlier and allow for appropriate counseling prior to surgery.

LABORATORY STUDIES

Laboratory studies can narrow the differential diagnosis of abdominal pain. Box 46.4 contains a complete list of laboratory tests that can assist the workup an acute abdomen. A complete blood count gives several important data points. The white blood cell count can be elevated or decreased in the setting of an acute abdomen. The best evidence of an acute infection is an elevated absolute number or percentage of band cells, so it is ideal to send for a complete blood cell count with a white blood cell differential. Low hemoglobin and hematocrit alert the care team to a source of bleeding that may be associated with the source of abdominal pain. If the hemoglobin and hematocrit are higher than normal, one should evaluate the patient for signs of dehydration.

Patients with abdominal pain should also have a complete metabolic panel sent. Electrolytes such as sodium, potassium, and calcium are evaluated as well as renal function tests such as blood urea nitrogen and creatinine. Alterations in these values will alert the physician to fluid losses from diarrhea or vomiting as well as possible endocrine sources of abdominal pain (i.e., hyperparathyroidism). The complete metabolic panel contains "liver function tests" that, when elevated, should lead to further assessment of the hepatic and biliary systems. Viral hepatitis panels should be sent when a source for elevated liver enzymes cannot be identified. Amylase and lipase are indicated when pancreatitis is a suspected source of abdominal pain.

BOX 46.4 **Laboratory tests for abdominal pain.**

- White blood cell count with differential
- Hemoglobin
- Platelets
- Electrolytes
- Creatinine and blood urea nitrogen
- Amylase and lipase
- Total and fractionated serum bilirubin
- Serum lactate levels
- Viral hepatitis panel
- Urinalysis
- Urine human chorionic gonadotropin
- *Clostridium difficile* culture and toxin assay

Arterial blood gas with serum lactate measurements are valuable tests when evaluating any severely ill patient. In the setting of the acute abdomen, lactic acidemia is a sign of hypoperfusion and depending on the circumstances raises the concern for mesenteric ischemia. Mesenteric ischemia is a serious condition with significant mortality despite improvements in critical care and can be tricky to diagnose in some patients. Attempts to identify additional markers specific to mesenteric ischemia are underway but not yet available for clinical use.[8]

Urine studies should be a standard laboratory test sent in a patient with abdominal pain. A urinalysis can give several points of information. The presence of bacteria, white blood cells, and leukocyte esterase in the sample raises concern for a urinary tract infection and possibly pyelonephritis; this would account for suprapubic pain or flank pain, respectively. Nephrolithiasis and nephritic syndromes can be detected by noting red blood cells in urine. Casts within the urine should also raise concern for a renal source of abdominal pain. Finally, in women of childbearing age, a urine human chorionic gonadotropin level should be sent as her symptoms may be due to complications of pregnancy.

Additional tests should be sent in select cases. Patients with diarrhea should have stool samples sent for culture and ova assessment. Importantly, *Clostridium difficile* culture and toxin measurements should be performed as the incidence of this infection is increasing within the community.[9] Women in the third trimester of pregnancy with right upper quadrant pain, elevated liver enzymes, and low platelets should be assessed for HELLP syndrome; expedient diagnosis is necessary to get the patient lifesaving plasma exchange therapy.[10]

DIAGNOSTIC IMAGING

Diagnostic imaging should be the final step in the work up of a patient with an acute abdomen. It is imperative that, prior to ordering any diagnostic imaging, a working differential diagnosis has been formulated so that the appropriate modality is chosen. There is a wide range of options. Many are expensive and can expose patients to ionizing radiation, so it is important to choose the most useful modality for the patient being worked up.

Ultrasound is a relatively cheap and expedient imaging modality that can be very useful in evaluating the acute abdomen. It remains the best modality for evaluating right upper quadrant pain, especially pain that is suspected to emanate from the gallbladder. Ultrasound sensitivity and specificity are high for detecting pericholecystic fluid, gallbladder wall thickening, and gallstones.[11] It is also a useful modality for diagnosing appendicitis in patients where avoiding ionizing radiation is desired, such as the pediatric population and early pregnancy.[12,13] When ruling out gynecologic sources of acute abdominal pain, transvaginal ultrasound should be utilized as it is more accurate than transabdominal ultrasound. Ultrasonography can have limitations with visualization due to abdominal wall thickness, bowel gas contents and operator experience.

Plain films of the abdomen can provide useful information in certain patients. When concerned for hollow viscus perforation, an upright plain film taken at the level of the diaphragm will reveal free air under the diaphragm which is diagnostic and should prompt surgical exploration (Fig. 46.3). It has been shown that time to surgical consultation and time to the operating room is shorter if diagnosis can be made with plain film as opposed to CT. However, CT can provide more information regarding location of perforation and specific cause.[14] Historically, upright and supine radiographs of the abdomen have been used to diagnosis bowel obstructions. Small bowel obstruction is suspected on plain film when air-fluid levels are seen in the upright position and paucity of gas in the distal colon with distended bowel loops in the supine position. Haustral markings from the teniae coli will help differentiate small bowel gas from colonic gas (Fig. 46.4). However, the diagnostic accuracy of plain films to diagnose mechanical bowel obstruction or paralytic ileus in a patient with abdominal pain is low.[15] Colonic volvulus can be diagnosed on plain films as well. Cecal volvulus typically appears as a comma shape loop of bowel with the concavity facing inferiorly and to the right. Sigmoid volvulus presents as the "bent inner tube" or "coffee bean" sign, where the apex of the dilated colon points into the right upper quadrant (Fig. 46.5).

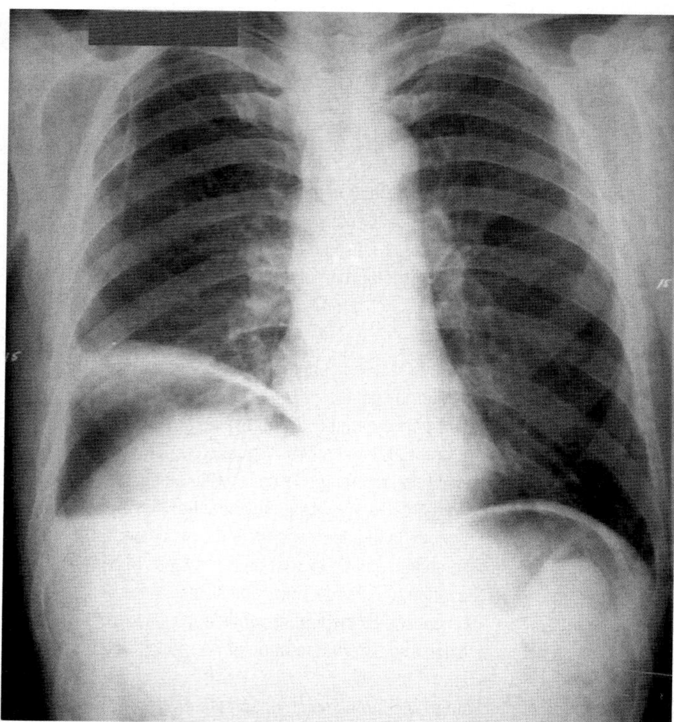

FIG. 46.3 Upright plain abdominal film demonstrating pneumoperitoneum, a finding consistent with perforated hollow viscus.

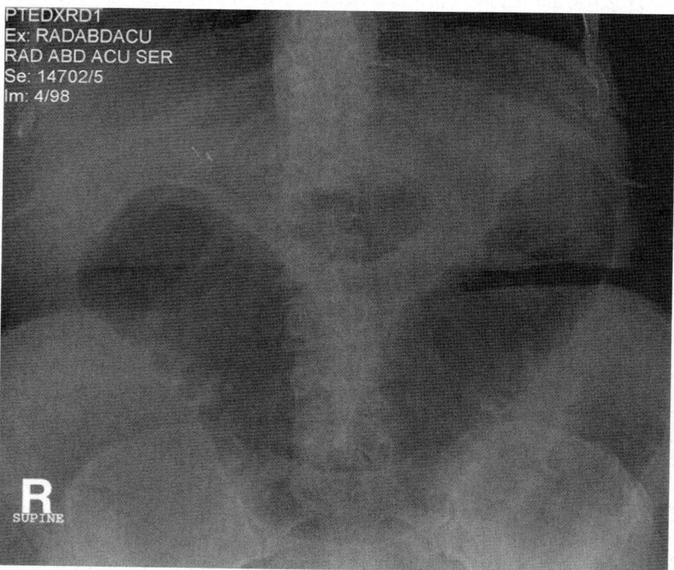

FIG. 46.4 An abdominal film of a patient with large bowel obstruction. The dilated loop of bowel can be identified as transverse colon by the haustral markings.

CT has become the primary diagnostic tool in patients with abdominal pain over the past decades. It is readily available, provides detailed information about the entire abdomen and pelvis, and can be performed relatively quickly. The quality of the CT images is less dependent on operator skill than ultrasound and provides more detail than plain films. A differential diagnosis will guide the CT technique needed. For example, if nephrolithiasis is suspected the imaging will be done without contrast but if a small bowel obstruction is suspected the CT should be ordered with

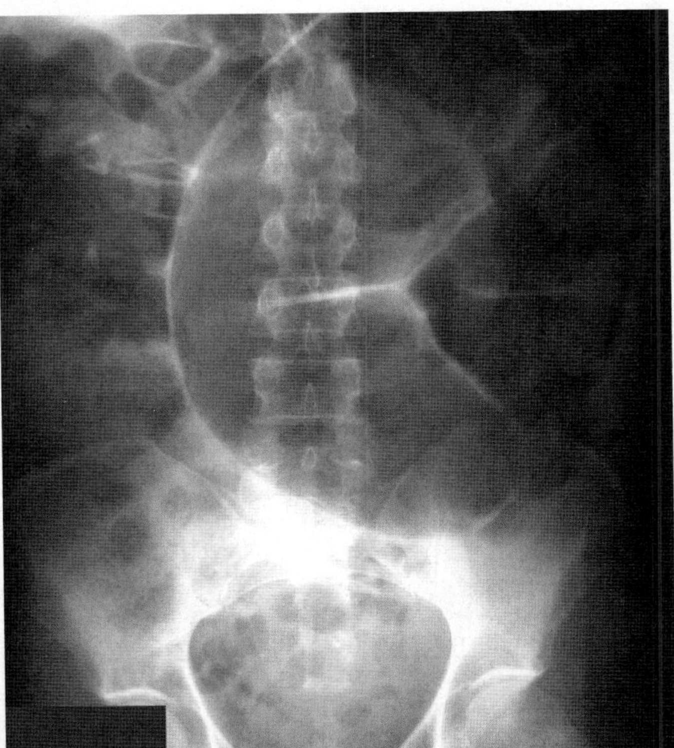

FIG. 46.5 Abdominal plain film showing sigmoid volvulus. Note the distended sigmoid colon in the right upper quadrant; this is the classic "coffee bean" or "bent inner tube" sign.

oral and intravenous contrast. These considerations are essential to provide the most diagnostic images.

Many studies have shown the improved diagnostic accuracy of CT over other imaging modalities. It has been shown that using CT as part of an imaging pathway will result in earlier diagnosis, though it will not decrease hospital stay or morbidity.[16] This is particularly true for appendicitis (Fig. 46.6). A recent evidence-based review reported that the sensitivity and specificity of CT for identifying appendicitis were 98.5% and 98%, respectively. Several studies included in this review showed a decrease in the negative appendectomy rate with the use of CT.[17] A retrospective study sought to determine the effect of CT imaging on diagnosis and disposition in patients over age 80. They found that their diagnosis changed in 43% of patients after obtaining a CT; this difficulty with diagnosis was particularly prominent in the presence of small bowel obstruction, colonic obstruction, and diverticulitis. Clinically, the findings on CT resulted in a statistically significant change in disposition.[18] These findings demonstrate the usefulness of CT.

Due to the radiation exposure associated with CT, studies have sought whether low-dose imaging retains diagnostic accuracy. In one recent study, two radiologists compared high-dose and low-dose CT images in patients with nontraumatic abdominal pain. They reported high confidence in their interpretation for both radiation doses despite there being slightly more image noise in the low-dose images. Diagnostic accuracy was not statistically significant between radiation doses; the low-dose CT had a sensitivity and specificity of 93.7% and 88.2%, respectively, while the high-dose CT had a sensitivity and specificity of 95.8% and 94.1%, respectively.[19] Low-dose CT should be considered in children and patients who undergo frequent imaging.

Diagnostic Laparoscopy

Diagnostic laparoscopy can be used as a final diagnostic adjunct should other tests prove equivocal; the advantage is that it may also prove therapeutic. A study of patients over 70 years old compared laparoscopic versus open exploration and intervention for the acute abdomen. The laparoscopic group showed no difference in morbidity or mortality.[20] Laparoscopy can be safely used in patients with sepsis if measures to reduce the negative hemodynamic effects of pneumoperitoneum are employed; these include keeping the intraabdominal pressure under 12 mm Hg and making sure appropriate antibiotics have been given prior to insufflation. Diagnostic laparoscopy should not be used when irreversible sepsis is present or if the operator is uncomfortable with laparoscopy. An emergency situation is not the appropriate time to learn new skills. A relative contraindication to diagnostic laparoscopy is extremely dilated bowel as visualization can limit complete exploration, but this would depend on the surgeon's comfort with laparoscopy.[21] While it should not be used routinely, diagnostic laparoscopy can assist determining the cause of the acute abdomen in select cases.

INTRAABDOMINAL PRESSURE MONITORING

The acute abdomen can either cause or be due to increased intraabdominal pressure. If the intraabdominal pressure is sustained above 20 mm Hg it is defined as abdominal compartment syndrome (ACS). This is a life-threatening condition as the elevated pressure results in decreased venous return and tidal volumes from elevated inspiratory pressures. It can also lead to visceral ischemia due to poor perfusion.

Normal intraabdominal pressure should be between 5 to 7 mm Hg. Abdominal obesity, accessory muscle respiration, and upright positioning will all artificially increase intraabdominal pressure. Bladder catheter pressure monitoring is used to measure intraabdominal pressures. The World Society of the Abdominal Compartment Syndrome (WSACS) recommends measuring bladder pressures after instilling 25 mL of room temperature saline into the bladder. The patient should be supine with the transducer at zeroed at the midaxillary line. Pressure measurements should be taken at the end of expiration or with the patient paralyzed with the ventilator paused if unable to participate in exam.[22] Grades of intraabdominal hypertension can be seen in Table 46.2.

Treatment of intraabdominal hypertension and ACS depends on the cause and severity. Primary ACS is due to a disease process within the abdomen that is best treated with decompressive laparotomy and correction of the inciting disease process. Abdominal closure may not be possible without causing recurrent ACS which should prompt use of a temporary abdominal closure maneuvers. Secondary ACS is a condition that arises from a condition not located in the abdomen or pelvis. Initial management of secondary ACS without evidence of end organ damage should be treated medically. Medical management includes correcting a positive fluid balance, evacuating intraluminal contents via a nasogastric tube, Foley and enemas, relaxing the abdominal wall with adequate sedation and pain control, and drainage of peritoneal fluid.[22] A low threshold should be held for decompressive laparotomy to limit morbidity and mortality from this condition.

DIFFERENTIAL DIAGNOSIS

Formulation of the differential diagnosis for an acute abdomen should be a continuous process throughout every step of evaluation. The list developed after history and physical examination

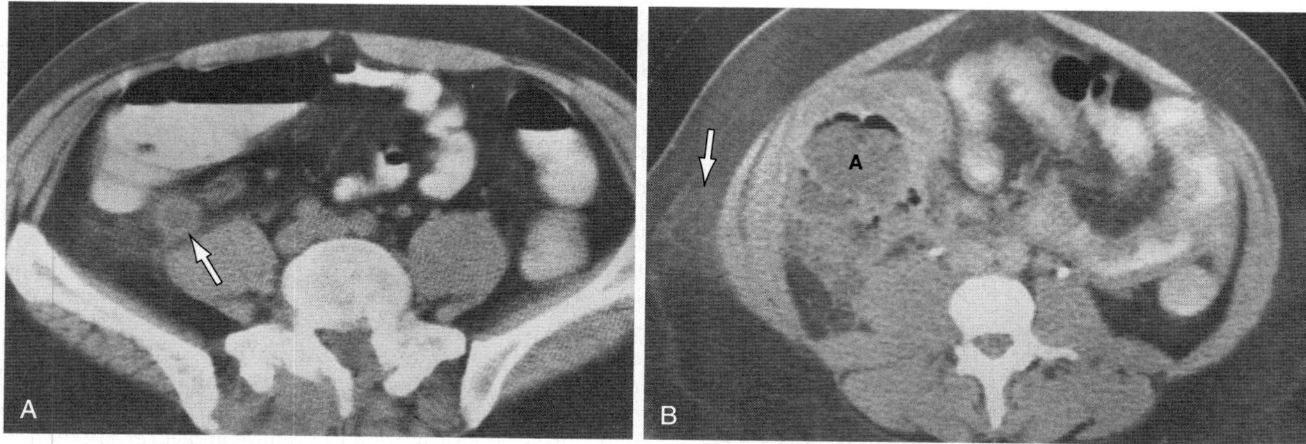

FIG. 46.6 (A) Computed tomography demonstrating a dilated retrocecal appendix *(arrow)* with periappendiceal stranding. (B) This image represents a pelvic abscess *(A)* caused by perforated appendicitis. The *arrow* shows the inflammatory process extending into subcutaneous tissues.

TABLE 46.2 Abdominal hypertension and treatment by grade.

	INTRAABDOMINAL PRESSURE	TREATMENT
Normal pressure	5–7 mm Hg	None
Grade 1 hypertension	12–15 mm Hg	Maintain euvolemia
Grade 2 hypertension	16–20 mm Hg	Nonsurgical decompression (diuresis, etc.)
Grade 3 hypertension	21–25 mm Hg	Surgical decompression via laparotomy
Grade 4 hypertension	>25 mm Hg	Surgical decompression; explore for cause

should guide the laboratory and imaging tests you order. By the end of the evaluation, the list of potential diagnoses should be narrowed to one or two processes. The art of refining differential diagnoses requires extensive knowledge of the medical and surgical causes of acute abdominal pain. This knowledge must then be integrated with the demographics of the patient being evaluated.

It is imperative to determine early whether the disease process causing acute abdominal pain requires urgent surgical intervention. Many present with sepsis which must be managed expediently, even without a specific diagnosis. Box 46.5 presents examination, laboratory, and imaging findings associated with surgical disease. However, in real world situations, the patient may not be stable enough to be transported to another department for some of these tests. One option is to consider a test that can be performed at bedside such as ultrasonography or abdominal plain films. Another option is diagnostic peritoneal lavage. Using local anesthetic, a small incision is made in the midline near the umbilicus. A catheter is placed into the peritoneal cavity to infuse 1 L of normal saline, which is then siphoned out of the abdomen. The siphoned fluid is sent for cellular and biochemical analysis. Diagnostic peritoneal lavage can be used to detect hemoperitoneum and/or hollow viscous perforation.

Delays in surgical intervention should be avoided. Once you have diagnosed a patient with a surgical abdomen, there is no advantage to waiting for further diagnostic tests. Morbidity and mortality increase with unwarranted delays. Fluid resuscitation and stabilization of vital signs can continue in the operating room through multidisciplinary approach with anesthesia and nursing. Laparoscopy can assist in guiding placement of the laparotomy incision if forced to proceed to the operating room without a definitive diagnosis.

BOX 46.5 Findings that suggest need for surgical intervention.

Physical Exam Findings

Abdominal compartment pressure >25 mm Hg
Involuntary guarding
Rebound tenderness
Pain out of proportion to exam
Unexplained systemic sepsis
Transabdominal penetrating trauma

Laboratory Findings

Anemia from gastrointestinal hemorrhage requiring >4 units of blood transfusion
Evidence of hypoperfusion (acidosis, rising creatinine, rising liver function tests)

Diagnostic Imaging Findings

Pneumoperitoneum
Progressive dilatation of stationary loop of intestine (sentinel loop)
Evidence of bowel perforation (air or contrast near loop of bowel)
Fat stranding or thickened bowel wall with systemic sepsis
Bowel wall pneumatosis

Diagnostic Peritoneal Lavage Findings

Presence of feculent or particulate matter
>250 white blood cells per milliliter
>300,000 red blood cells per milliliter
Peritoneal bilirubin > serum bilirubin (bile leak)
Peritoneal creatinine > serum creatinine (urine leak)

Some patients are diagnosed with a medical cause of acute abdominal pain. This does not mean that a surgical process will not develop. These patients need close, careful observation in a monitored setting. Serial examinations and laboratories should be scheduled to ensure the patient is improving with medical therapy. Ideally, examinations are performed by the same examiner to avoid missing significant changes in the patient's condition or development of complications.

PREPARATION FOR EMERGENCY OPERATION

Patients with an acute abdomen vary greatly in their overall state of health at the time the decision to operate is made. Regardless of the patient's severity of illness, all patients require some degree of preoperative preparation. Intravenous access should be obtained, and any fluid or electrolyte abnormalities corrected. Nearly all patients will require antibiotic infusions. The bacteria common in acute abdominal emergencies are gram-negative enteric organisms and anaerobes. Infusions of antibiotics to cover these organisms should be begun once a presumptive diagnosis is made. Patients with generalized paralytic ileus or vomiting benefit from nasogastric tube placement to decrease the likelihood of vomiting and aspiration. Foley catheter bladder drainage to assess urine output, a measure of adequacy of fluid resuscitation, is indicated in most patients. Acidosis due to intestinal ischemia or infarction may be refractory to preoperative therapy. Significant anemia is uncommon, and preoperative blood transfusions are usually unnecessary, however cross-matched blood should be available at operation. The need for preoperative stabilization of patients must be weighed against the increased morbidity and mortality associated with a delay in the treatment. The underlying nature of the disease process, such as infarcted bowel, may require surgical correction before stabilization of the patient's vital signs and restoration of acid-base balance can occur. Resuscitation should be viewed as an ongoing process and continued after the surgery is completed. Deciding when the maximum benefit of preoperative therapy in these patients has been achieved requires good surgical judgment.

SPECIAL PATIENT POPULATIONS

Pregnancy

The workup and treatment of acute abdominal pain in the pregnant patient creates several unique diagnostic challenges. Providers often rely on imaging to differentiate between an urgent surgical problem from a nonsurgical or obstetric cause.[23] However, the greatest threat facing the pregnant patient with acute abdominal pain is the potential for delayed diagnosis and which have been proven to be far more morbid than the operations themselves.[24,25] Delays occur for several reasons: symptoms of abdominal pain, nausea, and vomiting are often attributed to the underlying pregnancy, pregnancy can alter the presentation of some disease processes and make the physical examination more challenging because of the enlarging uterus, and fear of exposure of a fetus to radiation or unnecessary procedures.[26] Laboratory studies such as white blood cell counts and other chemistries are also altered in pregnancy, making recognition of disease processes more difficult. These differences cause extra emphasis to be placed on other modalities, such as vital signs and laboratory studies, which can confuse or underestimate the extent of intraabdominal disease. Finally, physicians naturally tend to be more conservative in treating pregnant patients, especially in regard to imaging and surgical intervention.

Ultrasound is the initial imaging study of choice in the pregnant patient.[26,27] In addition to diagnosing the most common abdominal pathologies, appendicitis and cholelithiasis, this modality also adds the benefit of assessment of the fetus and evaluating for obstetrical pathology.[27] Radiation exposure should be avoided whenever possible, especially during the first trimester during organogenesis, and the next study of choice should be MRI.[26,27] If CT is the only imaging study available, risks and benefits should be weighed as a delay in diagnosis is often more morbid than a single imaging study. Studies have shown that up to 50 mGy of ionizing radiation, the equivalent of five abdominal plains films or one abdominal CT scan, results in no significant increase in teratogenic effects of radiation.[27] Whenever possible, such as during imaging of the brain, cervical spine, or chest x-ray, the fetus should be shielded with lead.

It is important to remember that pregnancy is a highly controlled process that involves almost every organ system in a self-regulated environment that is extremely sensitive to maternal volume loss and catecholamine response.[26] Maternal hemorrhage is often compensated by decreased uterine flow, and marked fetal distress is often the first manifestation of an acute surgical pathology, even before maternal hypotension or tachycardia is identified.[26] The presence of peritoneal signs is not a normal finding in pregnancy, and the development of peritonitis can often be delayed by abdominal laxity and an enlarged uterus. Its presence should prompt an immediate search for its cause to avoid additional morbidity and mortality.[28]

The differential diagnosis of acute abdomen in pregnancy can be broad; however, the presentation does not differ much from that of the adult patient if one pays special attention to patient symptomatology and history. The most common pathologies and the recommended screening imaging studies are listed in Table 46.3. In addition to gastrointestinal pathology, it is important to include gynecologic and obstetrical causes of acute abdomen in the patient's workup, including uterine rupture, ectopic pregnancy, ruptured corpus luteum cyst, adnexal torsion, placenta percreta, among others.[27] Ovarian torsion can often be distinguished from other abdominal pathology with its characteristic presentation of waxing and waning abdominal pain.[28]

Acute appendicitis is the most common nonobstetric abdominal emergency requiring surgery with an overall incidence of 101 cases per 100,000 pregnancies.[23] Diagnostic findings on ultrasound are a dilated, blind-ending, thickened, tubular, and noncompressible structure 6 mm or larger in size.[29] Ultrasound can have its limitations and should be followed by advanced imaging if the diagnosis is in question. MRI and CT findings are similar to ultrasound and also include periappendiceal inflammation, presence of an appendicolith, or the presence of an established abscess.[29] Twenty percent of patients will have peritonitis or established intraabdominal abscess at presentation, with an associated higher risk of complications including a 20% to 35% rate of fetal loss for perforated appendicitis.[23] The added difficulties in evaluating the pregnant patient with right lower quadrant abdominal pain have resulted in significantly higher negative appendectomy rate compared with nonpregnant patients in the past. Although this diagnostic error rate would be unacceptable in a typically young healthy woman, it is widely accepted because of the fetal mortality risk when appendicitis progresses to perforation before surgery.

General anesthesia is considered safe in all stages of pregnancy and patients should be considered a high aspiration risk for induction. Pregnant women should be treated as though they have

TABLE 46.3 **Differential diagnosis of abdominal pain in pregnancy and recommended imaging studies.**

SITE	PREFERRED IMAGING MODALITY FOR DIAGNOSIS
Gallbladder disease	US > MRI
Hepatitis	US > MRI
Pancreatitis	US > MRI > CT
Bowel obstruction	US > MRI > CT
Perforated ulcer	Plain films > CT
Appendicitis	US > MRI > CT
Nephrolithiasis	US > MRI > CT
Inflammatory bowel disease	MRI > CT
Gynecologic causes	US > MRI
Diverticulitis	MRI > CT
Trauma	US > CT> MRI

Adapted from Baheti AD, Nicola R, Bennett GL, et al. Magnetic resonance imaging of abdominal and pelvic pain in the pregnant patient. *Magn Reson Imaging Clin N Am.* 2016;24:403–417.
CT, Computed tomography; *MRI*, magnetic resonance imaging; *US*, ultrasound.

a full stomach whenever intubation is planned.[28] Intraoperative care during pregnancy is focused on optimal care of the mother. If the fetus is previable, fetal heart tones should be measured before and after the surgery. If the fetus is viable, fetal heart tones should be measured throughout the surgery with a provider capable of performing an intervention available. The safety of laparoscopic surgery in pregnancy has been extensively studied and established. Laparoscopy allows for decreased manipulation of the uterus, and as a result, less uterine irritability with lower risk of contractions, spontaneous abortions, preterm labor, and premature delivery.[30] In order to safely enter the abdomen, the open Hassen technique is considered standard, with care to avoid injury to the enlarging uterus.[31]

Additional causes of acute abdomen include biliary disease, bowel obstruction, and pancreatitis, among others. Biliary disease is common, as sex steroids interfere with gallbladder emptying resulting in bile stasis.[28] Ultrasound is the diagnostic test of choice. Treatment is recommended in the second trimester to avoid complications of biliary disease as the pregnancy progresses. Gallstone pancreatitis and acute cholecystitis should be managed more carefully. Gallstone pancreatitis has been associated with a fetal loss as high as 60%. If a woman does not respond quickly to conservative treatment with hydration, bowel rest, analgesia, and judicious use of antibiotics, further evaluation should be performed as surgical intervention may be indicated. Endoscopic retrograde cholangiopancreatography is considered safe and low radiation risk to the fetus, should the patient present with cholangitis or choledocholithiasis.

Small bowel obstruction is often confused with the normal nausea and vomiting associated with pregnancy. It is important to remember that peritoneal signs in the presence of nausea and vomiting is never considered normal and should prompt further workup.[28] Abdominal distention with colic should key the clinician to the diagnosis.

Pediatrics

Evaluating a child with an acute abdomen can be difficult for the clinician not accustomed to performing an abdominal exam in children. In contrast to performing an examination on an adult who is able to communicate with the clinician and give feedback when abdominal pain is elicited, much of the examination on a child occurs through observation. Children can be poor historians because of their age, being afraid of the situation, and being unable to verbalize their symptoms. Clues to the extent of peritoneal irritation include a child's willingness or unwillingness to stand or move about the hospital bed freely. Children with peritonitis will demonstrate abdominal pain with standing, jumping, or coughing.[3] The abdominal exam should be performed thoughtfully and only to the extent to identify the presence of abdominal wall spasm in response to intraabdominal pathology.

The most common cause of acute surgical abdomen in the pediatric population remains acute appendicitis and occurs most commonly in older children and adolescents with a presentation of anorexia, low-grade fever, and right-lower quadrant pain similar to adult patients.[32] Younger children may present differently and pose a challenge to the clinician with reports from parents of a vague onset of symptoms. Their inability to characterize their pain, nonspecific signs, and difficulty in eliciting a physical exam results in imaging playing a crucial role in diagnosis. Almost all children, 99% in some reports, with appendicitis will have preoperative imaging before surgical intervention.[32–34] Ultrasound often demonstrates pathologic concordance when performed in the hands of an experience ultrasonographer, especially those performed at a free-standing children's hospital.[34] Children presenting to a nonchildren's hospital are more likely to have a CT scan diagnosis of appendicitis, despite the recommendations from multiple pediatric societies on the risks of radiation.[34]

Additional causes of acute abdomen are broken down by age and listed in Table 46.4. Intussusception should be considered in the differential of abdominal pain in children less than 3 years old. Gastroenteritis, Meckel diverticulitis, and *C. difficile* colitis are among other causes of abdominal pain, and presentation is similar to adult patients. Inconsolable crying and lethargy in small infants can be ominous. Any history of emesis in a newborn should prompt careful questioning regarding the character and timing of emesis episodes; bilious emesis is a surgical emergency and prompts urgent evaluation for midgut volvulus. A history of fever, passage of currant jelly stools, and lower gastrointestinal track bleeding should prompt further workup.[35]

Critical Illness

Establishing a diagnosis of an acute abdomen in the critically ill can be challenging. The clinician must navigate an environment of deep-sedation, multiple etiologies of sepsis, multiorgan failure,

TABLE 46.4 **Differential diagnosis of abdominal pain in children by age.**

< 2-YEARS OLD	2- TO 5-YEARS OLD	5- TO 12-YEARS OLD	>12-YEARS OLD
Intussusception	Intussusception	Appendicitis	Appendicitis
Gastroenteritis	Appendicitis	Gastroenteritis	Gastroenteritis
Constipation	Gastroenteritis	Constipation	Constipation
Infantile colic	Constipation	Mesenteric adenitis	Ovarian/testicular torsion
Malrotation with midgut volvulus	Mesenteric adenitis	Functional abdominal pain	Dysmenorrhea
Incarcerated inguinal hernia	Malrotation with midgut volvulus	Pneumonia	Pelvic inflammatory disease
Obstruction due to Hirschsprung disease	Sickle cell crisis	Sickle cell crisis	Ectopic pregnancy
UTI	Henoch-Schonlein purpura	Henoch-Schonlein purpura	
Meckel diverticulum	UTI	UTI	
	Trauma	Trauma	
	Meckel diverticulum		

Adapted from Yang WC, Chen CY, Wu HP. Etiology of non-traumatic acute abdomen in pediatric emergency departments. *World J Clin Cases*. 2013;1:276–284.
UTI, Urinary tract infection.

TABLE 46.5 **Differential diagnosis of acute abdomen in transplant patients.**

LIVER[37]	LUNG[38]	HEMATOPOIETIC STEM CELL[39]
Biliary complications of transplant	Gastroesophageal reflux	Acute graft versus host disease
Vascular complications of transplant	Infectious enterocolitis	Cholangitis
Small bowel obstruction	Peptic ulcer disease	Neutropenic enterocolitis
Acute appendicitis	Gastroparesis	Infectious enterocolitis
Urinary tract infection	Diverticulitis	Pneumatosis
Acute diverticulitis	Pancreatitis	
Acute pancreatitis	Gastrointestinal bleed	

and absent or subtle clinical exam findings. Unrecognized abdominal pathology can cause patients to persist in their critical state or even progress to their demise. Critically ill patients may not be able to demonstrate the typical signs and symptoms of acute abdomen due to narcotic analgesia, blunting of the inflammatory response due to antibiotics or immunosuppression, and nutritional deficiency.

Imaging is often necessary to establish a diagnosis as multiple causes for abdominal distention, sepsis, or organ failure may be at play in the intensive care unit (ICU) patient.[36] Some patients, will be unstable for transport and the clinician will be challenged with the risks and benefits of obtaining advancing imaging, such as CT, versus operative exploration with the potential of a nontherapeutic laparotomy. Determining which patients are stable enough to survive an operation, potentially a nontherapeutic intervention, can be unpredictable.[37] A small cohort of clinicians advocate for diagnostic laparoscopy in the ICU as a mode of both diagnosis and treatment of the acute abdomen in the critically ill patient. However, this is coupled with the difficulties of performing bedside laparoscopic surgery, the invasive nature of procedure, and the costs of the equipment and anesthesia.[37] As technology continues to advance, this is an area where change is likely to occur.

Immunocompromised

Transplant patients often present to the emergency room with abdominal complaints. In one study, researchers found that 33% to 60% of transplant patients sought care in the emergency room after their procedure.[38] Inflammation is necessary in the pathophysiology of abdominal pain and peritonitis, and this may be blunted in the transplant patient. This can result in unreliable leukocytosis, delayed development of fever, and subjectively decreased abdominal symptoms. They may also present in a delayed fashion, which may be very quickly followed by overwhelming systemic collapse. As a result, although the abdominal pathology is similar to that seen in healthy adult patients, the immunosuppressed may have atypical presentations with very minimal symptoms.

In one study of over 70,000 transplant patients, the incidence of emergency surgery was found to be 2.5%. The indications for surgical intervention were biliary disease (80%), gastrointestinal perforation (9%), complicated diverticulitis (6%), small bowel obstruction (2%), and appendicitis (2%). Overall mortality in this patient cohort was 5.5%.[38] A differential diagnosis of abdominal pathology is listed in Table 46.5 broken down by type of transplant.

Routine blood work should be performed in addition to checking serum levels of immunosuppressive drugs. These medications can cause many side effects that may cloud the presentation of acute abdomen, including loss of gastrointestinal mucosal integrity and regeneration, alterations in gastric acidity, and impaired immune response to illness. This often presents as diarrhea, abdominal pain, nausea, vomiting, and weight loss.[38] Transplant patients may not mount an inflammatory response to illness, and serum markers may not be elevated despite ongoing abdominal pathology.

Pseudomembranous colitis has increasingly been seen in the immunocompromised patient, independent of a recent association with broad-spectrum antibiotics. Typical presentations include diarrhea, abdominal pain, fever, and leukocytosis; however, this may not be seen in this patient cohort. A high index of suspicion, reliance on CT imaging and stool assays should be considered early.

Cytomegalovirus infection is another important pathogen to consider in the transplant patient. The presentation can vary, including diarrhea, dysphagia, nausea, vomiting, abdominal pain, gastrointestinal bleeding, and intestinal perforation. Cytomegalovirus is diagnosed by biopsy demonstrating virus in the gastric or intestinal mucosa and is treated with antivirals.

Atypical infections, including peritoneal tuberculosis, fungal infections, and endemic mycoses, can also be seen in this group. Due to the decreased inflammatory response, an abdominal infection may not present with a typically walled off abscess and CT scan imaging may not demonstrate classic findings.[39] Immunosuppressed patients with suspicious abdominal pathology should have inpatient monitoring with a low threshold for operative intervention if an atypical infection that is not improving despite adequate therapy.

Cardiac Patients

Abdominal emergencies in the cardiac patient can be easily masked by their postoperative recovery, ongoing management of their cardiac dysfunction, mechanical ventilation, arrhythmias, hemodynamic instability, and sedation.[40] Risk factors are associated with the procedure performed, such as length of cardiopulmonary bypass, interventions on valvular heart disease, and need for intraaortic balloon pump. In addition, the patient's preoperative physiology also has some effect, such as arrhythmias, hypertension, hypercholesterolemia, diabetes, renal disease, and need for preoperative inotropic support.[41] Patients undergoing an open abdominal aortic aneurysm repair have the highest incidence, especially those repaired through a transabdominal approach. The highest mortality is seen in patients with intestinal ischemia and in those patients who required a valve repair.[40]

The pathophysiology of gastrointestinal complications is thought to be associated with disturbances in the superior mesenteric artery blood flow during cardiopulmonary bypass.[42] The most common gastrointestinal diagnoses are ileus, pancreatitis, mesenteric ischemia, bowel obstruction, acute cholecystitis, and perforation.[41] Risk factors for development of an abdominal complication after cardiothoracic surgery are listed in Box 46.6.

BOX 46.6 Risk factors for the development of gastrointestinal complications after cardiothoracic surgery.

- Age >70
- Low cardiac output
- Peripheral vascular disease
- Need for reoperation due to hemorrhage
- Acute/chronic renal failure
- Cardiopulmonary bypass time >150 minutes
- Intraaortic balloon pump
- Preoperative inotropic support
- Active smoker
- Chronic obstructive pulmonary disease
- Prolonged ventilation
- Valve surgery
- Sepsis/sternal wound infections
- Liver failure
- Myocardial infarction

From Buczacki SJA, Davies J. The acute abdomen in cardiac intensive care unit. In: Valchanov K, Jones N, Hogue CW, eds. *Core topics in cardiothoracic critical care*. 2nd ed. Cambridge: Cambridge University Press; 2018:294–300.

Morbidly Obese

The classic presentation of an acute abdomen is not a reliable indicator of intraabdominal pathology in the morbidly obese. The presentation is often subtle, leading to rapid progression to sepsis, organ failure, and death.[42] In contrast to normal weight patients, the morbidly obese can mask the signs of peritonitis, even in the setting of abdominal catastrophes, such as anastomotic leaks, until very late in the disease process, leading to a high incidence of complications and increased mortality.[42] Physical examination findings are difficult to interpret. Abdominal sepsis may only be associated with malaise, shoulder pain, hiccups, and shortness of breath.[43] Severe abdominal pain is uncommon. Appreciation of abdominal distention or a mass is difficult because of their increased abdominal girth. The presence of anorexia is also highly unpredictable, and their reported symptoms or abdominal complaints can be exceedingly vague. With an unreliable physical exam, clinicians must rely on laboratory exams, tachycardia, x-ray imaging findings, and subtle clinical symptoms to make the diagnosis of an abdominal problem.[42] Abdominal x-rays have reduced clarity and may require multiple films to image the entire abdomen. CT may be limited due to weight restrictions on the examination table, although this is increasingly becoming less of an issue due to the increasing numbers of morbidly obese patients. Early laparoscopy, especially in the postoperative bariatric patient, is often used for both diagnosis and treatment. Examples of concerning CT imaging findings are listed in Box 46.7.

BOX 46.7 Concerning CT imaging findings in the postbariatric surgery patient.

- Dilated alimentary limb
- Dilated excluded stomach
- Dilated biliopancreatic limb
- Transition between dilated and nondilated bowel
- Mesenteric swirl sign
- Cluster of small bowel loops
- Horizontal position of the superior mesenteric artery

From Karila-Cohen P, Cuccioli F, Tammaro P, et al. Contribution of computed tomographic imaging to the management of acute abdominal pain after gastric bypass: correlation between radiological and surgical findings. *Obes Surg*. 2017;27:1961–1972.
CT, Computed tomography.

Elderly

The diagnosis of an acute abdomen in the elderly patient is no different from that of the adult patient. This patient population, however, is unique in that they often suffer from delay in surgical treatment as a result of their age due to biases regarding the morbidity of the proposed intervention. This often occurs despite data to suggest that increased age does not independently affect mortality, morbidity, or length of hospital stay.[44] With an aging population, surgeons and clinicians are now challenged with how to care for this patient cohort, and they must let go of their strong-held beliefs that patients can be "too old," "too high risk,"

BOX 46.8 Differential diagnosis of acute abdomen in the elderly patient.

- Peptic ulcer disease
- Gastrointestinal bleed
- Biliary disease
- Pancreatitis
- Bowel obstruction (large and small)
- Volvulus
- Diverticulitis
- Appendicitis
- Abdominal aortic aneurysm
- Mesenteric ischemia

From Rubinfeld I, Thomas C, Berry S, et al. Octogenarian abdominal surgical emergencies: not so grim a problem with the acute care surgery model? *J Trauma*. 2009;67:983–989; and Magidson PD, Martinez JP. Abdominal pain in the geriatric patient. *Emerg Med Clin North Am*. 2016;34:559–574.

or "nonsurvivable."[45] Approaching these patients with a "damage-control" mentality of aggressive resuscitation and careful attention to hypothermia, coagulopathy, acidosis, or hypotension and returning after adequate resuscitation are suggested to improve outcomes.[45] Box 46.8 lists the most common indications for surgical intervention in the elderly patient population.

Advanced Disease

Surgery in patients with advanced or disseminated cancer can be fraught with complications with little chance of prolonging their survival. Emergency procedures, such as for perforation or obstruction, are performed in this patient population with grave risks, as their disseminated disease has little chance of cure. One study demonstrated that those that undergo an operation for perforation have an approximate 1 in 3 chance of mortality; this is only slightly improved to 1 in 6 for those undergoing an operation for obstruction.[46] These complications may occur as a side effect of cancer treatment or it may represent disease progression. Regardless the cause, frank discussion with patients and their families are fundamental, and decisions regarding the patient's goals of care, overall survival, and prolonged institutionalization should be discussed with respect to the patient's wishes.[46] Emergency surgery in patients with advanced disease often heralds an inflection point in their care and these patients are unlikely to obtain their goal of discharge home.[46] Box 46.9 lists the differential diagnosis of acute abdomen in the oncologic patient.

SUMMARY

Despite improvements in laboratory examinations and imaging, the evaluation and management of the patient with acute abdominal pain remains a challenging part of a surgeon's practice. However, a careful history and thorough physical examination continue to remain the most important part of the evaluation of the patient with acute abdominal pain. The surgeon continues to be required to make the decision to perform laparoscopy or laparotomy with some degree of uncertainty as to the expected findings. The increased morbidity and mortality associated with a delay in the treatment of many of the surgical causes of the acute abdomen argue for an aggressive and expeditious surgical approach.

BOX 46.9 Differential diagnosis of acute abdomen in the oncology patient.

- Tumor infiltration
- Gastrointestinal bleed
- Bowel obstruction
- Biliary disease
- Appendicitis
- Neutropenic enterocolitis
- Invasive aspergillosis
- Digestive tract graft versus host disease
- Mesenteric ischemia
- Diverticulitis

From Mokart D, Penalver M, Chow-Chine L, et al. Surgical treatment of acute abdominal complications in hematology patients: outcomes and prognostic factors. *Leuk Lymphoma*. 2017;58:2395–2402; and Cauley CE, Panizales MT, Reznor G, et al. Outcomes after emergency abdominal surgery in patients with advanced cancer: Opportunities to reduce complications and improve palliative care. *J Trauma Acute Care Surg*. 2015;79:399–406.

SELECTED REFERENCES

Bouyou J, Gaujoux S, Marcellin L, et al. Abdominal emergencies during pregnancy. *J Visc Surg*. 2015;152:S105–115.

This paper reviews the presentations of abdominal emergencies in pregnant patients as well as the best way to approach these conditions.

de Burlet KJ, Ing AJ, Larsen PD, et al. Systematic review of diagnostic pathways for patients presenting with acute abdominal pain. *Int J Qual Health Care*. 2018;30:678–683.

An excellent resource for systematic evaluation and diagnosis in a patient with an acute abdomen.

Malbrain ML, Cheatham ML, Kirkpatrick A, et al. Results from the international conference of experts on intra-abdominal hypertension and abdominal compartment syndrome. I. Definitions. *Intensive Care Med*. 2006;32:1722–1732.

A consensus statement that defines abdominal compartment syndrome and provides evidence-based algorithm on its diagnosis and treatment.

Navez B, Navez J. Laparoscopy in the acute abdomen. *Best Pract Res Clin Gastroenterol*. 2014;28:3–17.

This paper highlights the usefulness of minimally invasive surgery in approaching the acute abdomen.

Steinheber FU. Medical conditions mimicking the acute surgical abdomen. *Med Clin North Am*. 1973;57:1559–1567.

This classic article nicely reviews the various medical conditions that can manifest as an acute abdomen. It is well written and remains pertinent to the evaluation of these patients.

REFERENCES

1. Al-Mane N, Al-Mane F, Abdalla Z, et al. Acute surgical abdomen: an unusual presentation of pulmonary embolus. *J Investig Med High Impact Case Rep*. 2014;2:1–4.
2. Hijaz NM, Friesen CA. Managing acute abdominal pain in pediatric patients: current perspectives. *Pediatric Health Med Ther*. 2017;8:83–91.
3. Nakayama DK. Examination of the acute abdomen in children. *J Surg Educ*. 2016;73:548–552.
4. Medford-Davis L, Park E, Shlamovitz G, et al. Diagnostic errors related to acute abdominal pain in the emergency department. *Emerg Med J*. 2016;33:253–259.
5. Maraolo AE, Gentile I, Pinchera B, et al. Current and emerging pharmacotherapy for the treatment of bacterial peritonitis. *Expert Opin Pharmacother*. 2018;19:1317–1325.
6. Van Bree SW, Prins MC, Juffermans NP. Auscultation for bowel sounds in patients with ileus: an outdated practice in the ICU. *Neth J Crit Care*. 2018;26:142–146.
7. Hatipoglu S, Hatipoglu F, Abdullayev R. Acute right lower abdominal pain in women of reproductive age: clinical clues. *World J Gastroenterol*. 2014;20:4043–4049.
8. Treskes N, Persoon AM, van Zanten ARH. Diagnostic accuracy of novel serological biomarkers to detect acute mesenteric ischemia: a systematic review and meta-analysis. *Intern Emerg Med*. 2017;12:821–836.
9. Reveles KR, Pugh MJV, Lawson KA, et al. Shift to community-onset clostridium difficile infection in the national veterans health administration, 2003-2014. *Am J Infect Control*. 2018;46:431–435.
10. Erkurt MA, Berber I, Berktas HB, et al. A life-saving therapy in Class I HELLP syndrome: therapeutic plasma exchange. *Transfus Apher Sci*. 2015;52:194–198.
11. Hanbidge AE, Buckler PM, O'Malley ME, et al. From the RSNA refresher courses: imaging evaluation for acute pain in the right upper quadrant. *Radiographics*. 2004;24: 1117–1135.
12. Binkovitz LA, Unsdorfer KM, Thapa P, et al. Pediatric appendiceal ultrasound: accuracy, determinacy and clinical outcomes. *Pediatr Radiol*. 2015;45:1934–1944.
13. Drake FT, Kotagal M, Simmons LE, et al. Single institution and statewide performance of ultrasound in diagnosing appendicitis in pregnancy. *J Matern Fetal Neonatal Med*. 2015;28:727–733.
14. Park J, Young-Hoon Y, Horeczko T, et al. Changes of clinical practice in gastrointestinal perforation with the increasing use of computed tomography. *J Korean Soc Traumatol*. 2017;30:25–32.
15. Geng WZM, Fuller M, Osborne B, et al. The value of the erect abdominal radiograph for the diagnosis of mechanical bowel obstruction and paralytic ileus in adults presenting with acute abdominal pain. *J Med Radiat Sci*. 2018;65:259–266.
16. de Burlet KJ, Ing AJ, Larsen PD, et al. Systematic review of diagnostic pathways for patients presenting with acute abdominal pain. *Int J Qual Health Care*. 2018;30:678–683.
17. Shogilev DJ, Duus N, Odom SR, et al. Diagnosing appendicitis: evidence-based review of the diagnostic approach in 2014. *West J Emerg Med*. 2014;15:859–871.
18. Gardner CS, Jaffe TA, Nelson RC. Impact of CT in elderly patients presenting to the emergency department with acute abdominal pain. *Abdom Imaging*. 2015;40:2877–2882.
19. Othman AE, Bongers MN, Zinsser D, et al. Evaluation of reduced-dose CT for acute non-traumatic abdominal pain: evaluation of diagnostic accuracy in comparison to standard-dose CT. *Acta Radiol*. 2018;59:4–12.
20. Cocorullo G, Falco N, Tutino R, et al. Open versus laparoscopic approach in the treatment of abdominal emergencies in elderly population. *G Chir*. 2016;37:108–112.
21. Navez B, Navez J. Laparoscopy in the acute abdomen. *Best Pract Res Clin Gastroenterol*. 2014;28:3–17.
22. Malbrain ML, Cheatham ML, Kirkpatrick A, et al. Results from the international conference of experts on intra-abdominal hypertension and abdominal compartment syndrome. I. Definitions. *Intensive Care Med*. 2006;32:1722–1732.
23. Abbasi N, Patenaude V, Abenhaim HA. Management and outcomes of acute appendicitis in pregnancy-population-based study of over 7000 cases. *BJOG*. 2014;121: 1509–1514.
24. Kort B, Katz VL, Watson WJ. The effect of nonobstetric operation during pregnancy. *Surg Gynecol Obstet*. 1993;177:371–376.
25. Sadot E, Telem DA, Arora M, et al. Laparoscopy: a safe approach to appendicitis during pregnancy. *Surg Endosc*. 2010;24:383–389.
26. Skubic JJ, Salim A. Emergency general surgery in pregnancy. *Trauma Surg Acute Care Open*. 2017;2:e000125.
27. Bouyou J, Gaujoux S, Marcellin L, et al. Abdominal emergencies during pregnancy. *J Visc Surg*. 2015;152:S105–S115.
28. Kilpatrick CC, Monga M. Approach to the acute abdomen in pregnancy. *Obstet Gynecol Clin North Am*. 2007;34:389–402, x.
29. Baheti AD, Nicola R, Bennett GL, et al. Magnetic resonance imaging of abdominal and pelvic pain in the pregnant patient. *Magn Reson Imaging Clin N Am*. 2016;24:403–417.
30. Kirshtein B, Perry ZH, Avinoach E, et al. Safety of laparoscopic appendectomy during pregnancy. *World J Surg*. 2009;33:475–480.
31. Chung JC, Cho GS, Shin EJ, et al. Clinical outcomes compared between laparoscopic and open appendectomy in pregnant women. *Can J Surg*. 2013;56:341–346.
32. Aydin D, Turan C, Yurtseven A, et al. Integration of radiology and clinical score in pediatric appendicitis. *Pediatr Int*. 2018;60:173–178.
33. Kotagal M, Richards MK, Flum DR, et al. Use and accuracy of diagnostic imaging in the evaluation of pediatric appendicitis. *J Pediatr Surg*. 2015;50:642–646.
34. Yang WC, Chen CY, Wu HP. Etiology of non-traumatic acute abdomen in pediatric emergency departments. *World J Clin Cases*. 2013;1:276–284.
35. Fui SL, Lupinacci RM, Tresallet C, et al. How to avoid non-therapeutic laparotomy in patients with multiple organ failure of unknown origin. The role of CT scan revisited. *Int Surg*. 2015;100:466–472.
36. Gagne DJ, Malay MB, Hogle NJ, et al. Bedside diagnostic minilaparoscopy in the intensive care patient. *Surgery*. 2002;131:491–496.
37. Cesaretti M, Dioguardi Burgio M, Zarzavadjian Le Bian A. Abdominal emergencies after liver transplantation: presentation and surgical management. *Clin Transplant*. 2017;31: e13102.
38. de'Angelis N, Esposito F, Memeo R, et al. Emergency abdominal surgery after solid organ transplantation: a systematic review. *World J Emerg Surg*. 2016;11:43.

39. Grass F, Schafer M, Cristaudi A, et al. Incidence and risk factors of abdominal complications after lung transplantation. *World J Surg*. 2015;39:2274–2281.
40. Chaudhry R, Zaki J, Wegner R, et al. Gastrointestinal complications after cardiac surgery: a nationwide population-based analysis of morbidity and mortality predictors. *J Cardiothorac Vasc Anesth*. 2017;31:1268–1274.
41. Buczacki SJA, Davies J. The acute abdomen in cardiac intensive care unit. In: Valchanov K, Jones N, Hogue CW, eds. *Core Topics in Cardiothoracic Critical Care*. 2nd ed. Cambridge: Cambridge University Press; 2018:294–300.
42. Byrne TK. Complications of surgery for obesity. *Surg Clin North Am*. 2001;81:1181–1193, vii-viii.
43. Karila-Cohen P, Cuccioli F, Tammaro P, et al. Contribution of computed tomographic imaging to the management of acute abdominal pain after gastric bypass: correlation between radiological and surgical findings. *Obes Surg*. 2017;27:1961–1972.
44. Rubinfeld I, Thomas C, Berry S, et al. Octogenarian abdominal surgical emergencies: not so grim a problem with the acute care surgery model? *J Trauma*. 2009;67:983–989.
45. Magidson PD, Martinez JP. Abdominal pain in the geriatric patient. *Emerg Med Clin North Am*. 2016;34:559–574.
46. Mokart D, Penalver M, Chow-Chine L, et al. Surgical treatment of acute abdominal complications in hematology patients: outcomes and prognostic factors. *Leuk Lymphoma*. 2017;58:2395–2402.

47 CHAPTER

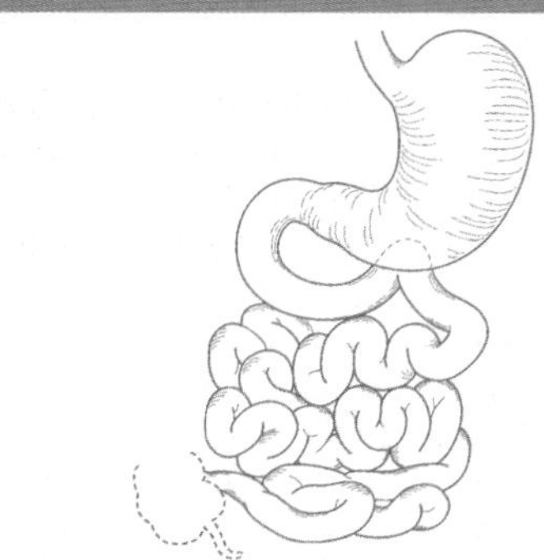

Acute Gastrointestinal Hemorrhage

Kevin J. Chiang, Noelle N. Saillant, Richard Hodin

OUTLINE

Gastrointestinal bleeding (GIB) is a term that describes the loss of blood from along the alimentary canal. GIB is classified by its anatomic location relative to the ligament of Treitz. Upper GIB (UGIB) is defined as being proximal to the ligament of Treitz. Upper intestinal hemorrhage is the most common presentation of GIB and is commonly from peptic ulcer disease (PUD) or esophageal varices. Pancreatic, liver, and other biliary origins of blood loss also are encompassed by this term.

Lower GIB (LGIB) accounts for 30% to 40% of all bleeds and is defined as distal to the ligament of Treitz. This most often originates from the colon from diverticular disease or angiodysplasias.

The term *massive GIB* refers to intestinal blood loss leading to hemodynamic instability or transfusion requirement, whereas *occult GIB* refers to anemia that persists or recurs after negative endoscopic evaluation and imaging workup.

Overall, bleeding is the most common cause of hospitalization from gastrointestinal (GI) disease in the United States, accounting for over 507,000 admissions annually with a total cost of over $5.8 billion.[1] The reported median length of hospital stay for GI hemorrhage is 3 to 6 days, with median cost ranging from $6700 to $20,370.[1–3] The peak incidence has steadily decreased by 1% annually since the mid-1990s due to the advent of proton pump inhibitors (PPIs), increased treatment of *Helicobacter pylori*, and avoidance of nonsteroidal antiinflammatory drugs (NSAIDs). Following this trend, mortality has dramatically decreased from the historical rates of 6% to 12% for UGIB to more contemporary rates of less than 2%.[1,3] While these advancements have steadily decreased hospital admissions for UGIB, admissions related to LGIB have increased.[4]

ACUTE MANAGEMENT OF PATIENTS WITH GASTROINTESTINAL HEMORRHAGE

Initial Evaluation

GIB may present in a subtle way as a diagnosis of unexplained microcytic anemia or the finding of a positive hemoccult stool study. In contrast, it may also present as massive life-threatening exsanguination. Depending on the manifestation, treatment may take place in the outpatient setting or be emergently managed. Regardless, a multidisciplinary approach is required to fully tend to the condition and to determine the location and best therapeutic approach for the blood loss.

Acute Exsanguination

Rapid triage of hemorrhaging patients while localizing the areas of blood loss is essential for resuscitation and prompt intervention.

Assessment should adhere to the ABCDEs: airway, breathing, circulation, disability, and exposure. Patency of the airway and adequacy of breathing are the priority. Severe hematemesis or decreased mental status from shock or hepatic encephalopathy may compromise oxygenation, ventilation, and airway protective reflexes. If an airway is needed, it should be secured with attention to the patient's hemodynamic status. Intravenous (IV) access with two large-bore (14- or 16- gauge) catheters should be obtained. Occasionally, in the massively hemorrhaging patient, central access with resuscitative lines is needed to maintain hemodynamic support. Invasive hemodynamic monitoring should also be considered in such patients. A urinary catheter should be placed to follow adequacy of resuscitation and preservation of renal function. The severity of hemorrhage can generally be determined quickly using simple clinical parameters. Tachypnea, tachycardia, hypotension, agitation, and mental status changes are all indicators of a severe degree of hemorrhage.

Hypotension is a harbinger of death. Systolic blood pressures under 90 mm Hg do not typically manifest until a patient has experienced a 30% to 40% blood loss. In well-compensated hosts, many of these signs may be absent or subtle, manifesting only as anxiety, tachypnea, or cool skin. The clinical response may be further blunted in patients taking beta blockers[5] or those patients who are at the extremes of age.

Additional management priorities include obtaining a type and crossmatch, complete blood count, metabolic panel, coagulation profile, and liver function tests. Serum lactate can be utilized as an endpoint of resuscitation when elevated. It is important to note that in acute severe blood loss, the serum hematocrit is not a reliable marker of the amount of blood loss as it may take hours to dilute as fluid shifts from the interstitium and the patient receives volume resuscitation.

The strategy for fluid resuscitation should be guided by the severity of hemorrhage. With large volume blood loss, the utilization of massive transfusion protocols can make universal donor blood products rapidly available in prespecified ratios with proven survival benefit in bleeding patients.[5] The ideal ratio of these products for GIB has not been well studied, although evidence suggests that a ratio of blood constituents (plasma and platelets) that approximates the whole blood (one unit fresh-frozen plasma per two units of packed red blood cells [RBCs] administered) lost during hemorrhage may be beneficial.[6,7] Furthermore, rapid blood loss can be complicated by preexisting or hemorrhage-related coagulopathy with deficiencies in both pro- and antithrombotic factors. Normalization of prothrombin time, partial thromboplastin time, fibrinogen levels, and platelet count are important adjuncts in management A role for viscoelastic tests such as thromboelastography or thromboelastometry has not been well studied in GIB but has shown benefit in other hemorrhage-related clinical scenarios.[8]

Use of a rapid infuser can be utilized to keep up with rapid blood loss and may help warm products to minimize hypothermia. These patients often require admission to the intensive care unit and urgent intervention to localize and control hemorrhage. Clinical response to volume to support mentation, radial pulse pressure, and at least a systolic blood pressure of 90 mm Hg, while following endpoints of resuscitation, such as lactate clearance and urine output, guides adequacy of resuscitation.

It is important to distinguish massively hemorrhaging patients from stable patients with GIB in whom a restrictive transfusion strategy should be employed. A landmark study by Villanueva compared a restrictive transfusion threshold of a hemoglobin level of 7 to 9 g/dL to a liberal threshold of 9 to 11 g/dL. This randomized controlled trial found lower rates of mortality, rebleeding, and other adverse outcomes with the restrictive strategy of 7 g/dL.[9] Importantly, this trial specifically excluded patients who were massively exsanguinating. In light of this study, such massively hemorrhaging patients should be considered a different patient population in terms of management strategy.

Localization

Running parallel with the active resuscitation of the patients is the equally important search to localize the site of blood loss (Fig. 47.1).

History and physical exam guide the assessment and may direct the examiner to a presumptive diagnosis. This information, combined with the characteristic of the blood loss, is helpful for determining an upper versus lower source.

Hematemesis is the emesis of blood or coffee ground gastric secretions, most commonly from a UGIB. Bleeding from the nasal or oropharyngeal space also may be swallowed or pool

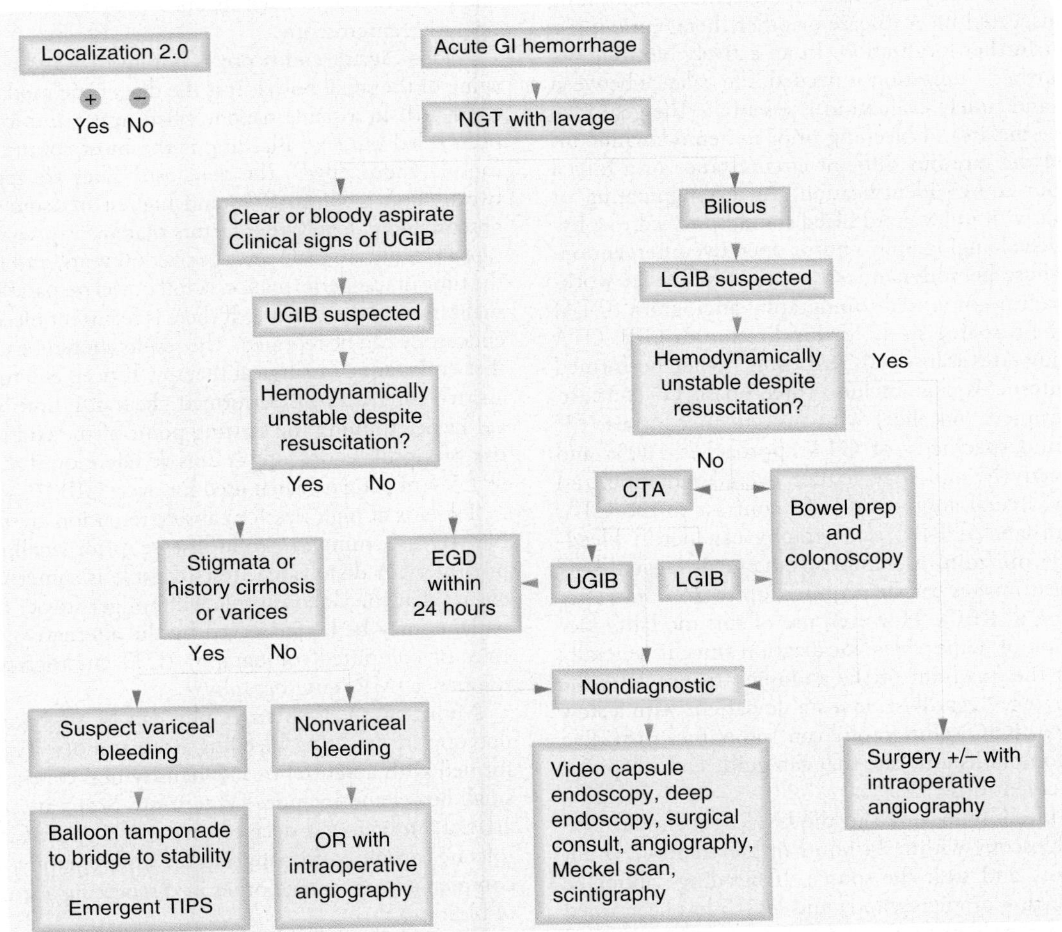

FIG. 47.1 Algorithm for the diagnosis of acute GI hemorrhage. *CTA*, Computed tomography angiogram; *EGD*, esophagogastroduodenoscopy; *GI*, gastrointestinal; *LGIB*, lower GI bleed; *NGT*, nasogastric tube; *TIPS*, transjugular intrahepatic portosystemic shunt; *UGIB*, upper GI bleed.

dependently in the stomach and thus lead to a non-GI source of hematemesis.

Melena, a malodorous, black stool with a tar-like quality, is also indicative of a proximal source of bleeding. Melena is the byproduct of hemoglobin degradation by digestive enzymes and intestinal bacterial flora. Hematin is produced from the degradation of hemoglobin, leading to a brownish blue coloration. Over 90% of melena arises from a UGIB, though it can originate from anywhere in the GI tract[10] if intestinal transit is slow. Hematochezia, the passage of bright red blood from the anus, is most commonly from hemorrhoidal disease. However, brisk UGIB with swift transit through the intestinal tract may also manifest as bright red blood per rectum and is an important etiology to rule out upon evaluation.

The first steps in differentiating a UGIB from a LGIB is aided by a nasogastric tube (NGT) lavage (Fig. 47.1). It can detect the presence of blood above the ligament of Treitz while also irrigating the stomach in preparation for an endoscopy. Aspiration of bile is required to assure sampling of postpyloric secretions. An aspiration, which is bilious and nonbloody, can effectively rule out an *active* UGIB. However, a nonactive upper GI (UGI) source is not definitively ruled out by a negative lavage if hemostasis occurred several hours prior.[10]

The next localization steps after NGT lavage is then based on clinical suspicion, patient stability, and bleeding rate.

Given enough clinical history or suspicion, one may target treatment to the most likely diagnosis, for instance, performing endoscopy for suspected ulcer disease or other therapeutic interventions without further localization. In an actively bleeding patient in whom further localization is needed, the balance between patient stability and timely evaluation is essential. The goal is to efficiently localize the area of bleeding prior to hemodynamic instability to avoid the rare but difficult circumstance of a forced procedure without source identification. An exsanguinating or moribund patient with unlocalized bleed should proceed to a hybrid room for visceral angiography and/or operative intervention.

In patients whose hemodynamics can support further workup, the multidetector computed tomography angiogram (CTA) is emerging as the first-line study for localization of GIB. CTA can detect bleeding rates as low as 0.3 mL/min[11] when performed under specific protocols that include three-phase IV contrast, multidetector scanners (64 slice) with no enteral contrast.[11,12] The sensitivity and specificity of CTA approaches 100% and over 90%, respectively, and may reduce overall radiation and IV contrast of a visceral angiogram.[12] In contrast to the CTA, technetium-99-m-labeled RBC scintigraphy can detect bleeding as low as 0.04 mL/min. A second advantage of tagged RBC scans is that repeat images can be acquired up to 24 hours after the initial labeling of RBCs. However, use of this modality sacrifices the precision of hemorrhage localization since it generally can only suggest the quadrant of the abdomen from where the bleeding is occurring. Regardless, in a stable patient with a slow intermittent bleed, RBC scintigraphy can sometimes provide a valuable estimation of bleeding site that can guide endoscopic or angiographic interventions.[11,13,14]

Patients with bleeding localized to the UGI tract should proceed to upper endoscopy within 24 hours of presentation, if not sooner, to diagnose and treat the source. If bleeding cannot be localized with imaging or angiography and UGIB has been ruled out, a colonoscopy should be performed if the patient is stable and can tolerate a full bowel preparation. A mechanical bowel prep assures a high-quality colonoscopy, as any stool or retained blood will often obscure the bleeding site. Diverticular bleeding is statistically the most common source of LGIB and visualization of bleeding within diverticula is severely impaired by the presence of stool and old blood. The exception to this is if a brisk bleed from the descending colon or rectum is suspected. In this case, a careful LGI endoscopy may be undertaken, as any colonoscopy without prep increases the risk of perforation.

To aid in the preparation of the colon to improve diagnostic accuracy, the patient should receive a "rapid prep," which is a minimum of 4 L of polyethylene glycol solution given within a period of approximately 4 hours, followed by colonoscopy within 1 to 2 hours.[14] This large volume of fluid is often difficult to tolerate, so administration through an NGT may be necessary. Administering prokinetics to improve gastric emptying can also reduce nausea and discomfort associated with the high volume of prep solution.

The colonoscopy should always include intubation of the terminal ileum to rule out a more proximal source of bleeding. A large working channel is highly recommended to facilitate suctioning of stool and clots. Water-jet irrigation should also be used to flush debris from the mucosa and improve visualization.

If UGI and colonic sources of bleeding have been excluded, the next most common location for bleeding is the small bowel, sometimes referred to as "middle GIB." This accounts for 5% of acute GIBs. CTA remains the first test of choice. In a stable patient, there are additional options for further localization of bleeding if the CTA is nondiagnostic. These include video capsule endoscopy and push, device-assisted (balloon or spiral enteroscopy), or intraoperative enteroscopy.

Video capsule endoscopy is noninvasive and is designed for imaging of the small bowel. It is the diagnostic modality of choice for overt GIB in a stable patient when upper and lower sources have been ruled out.[15,16] Bleeding is the most common indication for capsule endoscopy.[15] The diagnostic rates are reported to be between about 35% to 67% and highest in acute GIB rather than obscure blood loss. Other factors that are associated with a positive capsule study are male sex, age over 60 years, and hospitalization at the time of test performance. A full bowel preparation maximizes visualization of the mucosa. If there is recurrent bleeding, the capsule endoscopy can be repeated. The results should be used to guide further endoscopic or surgical therapy. If deep enteroscopy or device-assisted enteroscopy is performed, the transit time of the capsule can aid in determining the starting point of the endoscopy. The main risk of capsule endoscopy is capsule retention that can occur in up to 1.5% of patients when used for overt GIB.[15]

Patients at high risk for capsule retention are those with heavy NSAID use, tumors, Crohn disease, prior small bowel radiation, or surgery. A dissolvable "test" capsule is sometimes used first to ensure that the video capsule will not get stuck. These higher-risk patients may be better served by the alternative diagnostic strategies of computed tomography (CT) enterography or magnetic resonance (MR) enterography.[16]

Multiphase CT enterography can be superior to capsule endoscopy in detecting bleeding from tumors. Typically, it is performed with a neutral or low-density oral contrast to distend the small bowel and includes IV contrast. Scans are performed in the arterial, enteral, and delayed phase. If a patient is stable and can tolerate capsule endoscopy and CT enterography, these studies are complementary to each other in discovering a small bowel source of bleeding.[16]

A positive study with capsule endoscopy or CT/MR enterography should be followed with a push or device-assisted enteroscopy as these have therapeutic capability.

Push enteroscopy using a small-caliber colonoscope can reach about 50 to 70 cm past the ligament of Treitz and leads to successful diagnosis in 40% of patients with obscure small bowel bleeding.

Double-balloon endoscopy is quickly gaining favor in the diagnosis and treatment of small bowel lesions. The procedure uses the peristaltic "push/pull" motions from inflation and deflation of two balloons to course the small intestine along its length. This technique is capable of examining the entire small bowel, with successful identification of 77% to 85% of occult bleeding sources. Although technically challenging, it has a diagnostic efficacy greater than that of video capsule endoscopy.

Patients with altered anatomy, for example, Roux-en-Y bypasses, should undergo device-assisted endoscopy to evaluate the excluded portions of bowel. Intraoperative endoscopy, during laparotomy or laparoscopy, is a last resort when other modalities have failed to localize a source of small bowel bleeding and the patient continues to require transfusions or repeat hospitalizations. Surgery may also be necessary if a device-assisted enteroscopy cannot be performed without lysis of adhesions. This typically uses a sterile, small caliber colonoscope that is passed bidirectionally with the surgeon assisting to pass the bowel over the endoscope. Any suspicious areas are marked for possible resection or are dealt with endoscopically if feasible.[16]

Obscure Bleeding

The cause of obscure-overt bleeding is often a common lesion that is missed on initial evaluation. Repeated upper endoscopy and lower endoscopy should be performed and may identify lesions in up to 35% of patients. Tagged RBC scan and angiography can be helpful next steps but require ongoing hemorrhage. Small bowel enteroclysis, which uses barium, methylcellulose, and air to assist in image resolution, has been replaced largely in practice by CT enterography. CT enterography can identify gross lesions such as small bowel tumors and inflammatory conditions such as Crohn disease but cannot visualize angiodysplasias, the main cause of obscure small bowel hemorrhage.

Provocative angiographic testing, which involves administration of anticoagulants, fibrinolytics, or vasodilators to increase hemorrhage during angiography, has been employed in small series with favorable results, but reluctance to induce uncontrolled hemorrhage has limited its use. Surgical backup and the ability to salvage the patient in an operating room is essential to the planning of such a procedure.

SPECIFIC CAUSES OF UGIB

Due to the divergence in diagnostic and therapeutic maneuvers, UGIB is often further subdivided into either nonvariceal or variceal bleeding.

Nonvariceal Bleeding

Peptic Ulcer Disease

PUD is responsible for up to two-thirds of UGIBs and can develop in the stomach or duodenum.[17] Approximately 10% to 15% of patients with PUD will develop bleeding as part of their disease course.[18] PUD results from an imbalance between mucosal barriers and other aggravating factors. The major etiologic factors in PUD are *H. pylori* and NSAIDs, and in some patients, these can act synergistically in the development of ulcers through their additive insults to the gastroduodenal mucosa. Worldwide, it is estimated that up to 77% of duodenal ulcers are associated with *H. pylori* infection. The bacterium causes an inflammatory reaction within the mucosa that impairs mucosal defense and allows ulcer formation. NSAIDs also disrupt the mucosal barrier but via a different mechanism. NSAIDs inhibit cyclooxygenases (i.e., COX-1 and COX-2), thus impairing prostaglandin synthesis, enhancing neutrophil adherence and subsequent mucosal injury. NSAIDs additionally inhibit the release of nitric oxide (NO) and hydrogen sulfide (H_2S), further inhibiting protective mechanisms of the mucosa. In those patients with regular NSAID use, PUD has a prevalence of 15% to 20%.[17] Erosion of the mucosal surface leads to injury, ulceration, and chronic blood loss that can be further exacerbated by antiplatelet agents, anticoagulants, and selective serotonin reuptake inhibitors. Significant bleeding does not occur until the erosion reaches an artery of the submucosa or an even larger vessel in the case of a penetrating ulcer. The most significant hemorrhage occurs when duodenal or gastric ulcers penetrate branches of the gastroduodenal or left gastric arteries, respectively.[17]

Treatment of PUD begins with effective prophylaxis. Aggressive treatment of *H. pylori*, reduction of NSAIDs, and the use of alternative NSAIDS preparations such as COX-2 inhibitors for chronic therapy have further decreased the incidence of PUD. However, it has been the landmark discovery of PPIs that has most drastically impacted the treatment of PUD. Since their introduction in 1989, PPIs have become a mainstay in the treatment of acid-related disorders. Multiple randomized controlled trials have proven their efficacy in healing ulcers compared to placebo as well their superiority over H_2-inhibitors. PPIs inhibit the final common pathway of acid secretion by targeting the H^+/K^+-ATPase of parietal cells. Acid is suppressed until replacement pumps are synthesized (up to 36 hours), well beyond the required 18 to 20 hours of a pH greater than 3 required for effective ulcer healing.

Management. See localization algorithm for an outline of approach (Fig. 47.2). After initial resuscitation, patients should undergo esophagogastroduodenoscopy (EGD). Those with high clinical risk may benefit from EGD as soon as possible, with evidence supporting intervention within 12 hours of presentation,[19] rather than the more liberal time frame of 24 hours. While awaiting EGD, patients should be treated with a PPI.[20] Prokinetics should be considered, as a metaanalysis has supported erythromycin prior to endoscopy to reduce the need for second endoscopy, amount of blood transfusion, and hospital length of stay. An NGT can be helpful for diagnosis, but it is unlikely to clear enough clot to improve endoscopic visualization of the gastric mucosa.

The next steps after index endoscopy depend on the findings. The Forrest classification was developed to assess the risk of rebleeding based on endoscopic findings and groups patients into high, intermediate, and low risk of rebleeding (Table 47.1). Endoscopic therapy is recommended for ulcers with active bleeding as well as those with a visible ulcer (Forrest I–IIa). In cases with an adherent clot (Forrest IIb), the clot is removed and the ulcer evaluated. Ulcers with a clean base or black spot secondary to hematin deposition (Forrest IIc–III) do not require endoscopic treatment and are managed medically. Approximately 25% of patients undergoing EGD for UGIB will require an endoscopic intervention.[18] If the endoscopy is unable to achieve hemostasis, angiography should be performed. Surgery is the next step if angiography fails or is not available.

Medical management. All patients with confirmed peptic ulcer bleed should receive PPI therapy. Preendoscopic high-dose IV PPI therapy has been associated with decreased frequency of high-risk findings on endoscopy (Forrest Ia–IIa), leading to less

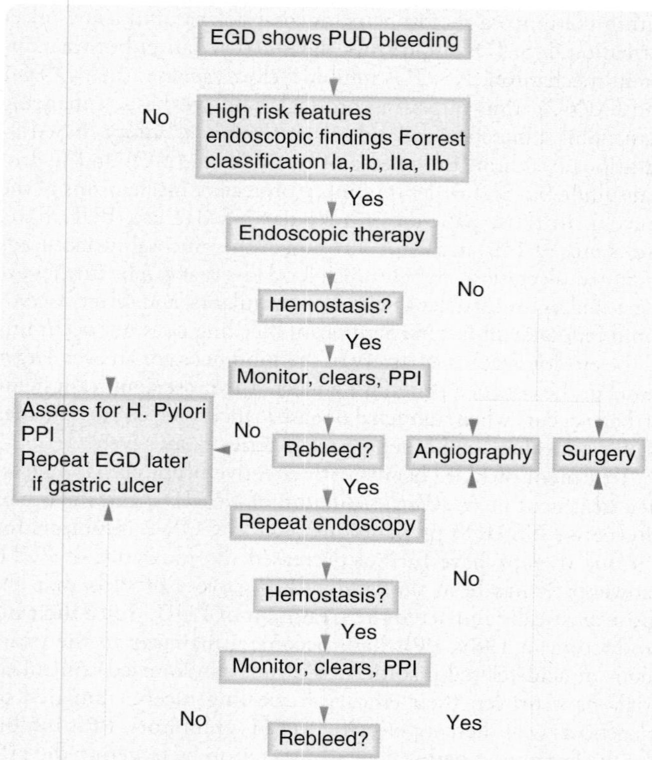

FIG. 47.2 Algorithm for the diagnosis and management of nonvariceal upper gastrointestinal bleeding. *EGD*, Esophagogastroduodenoscopy, *PPI*, proton pump inhibitor; *PUD*, peptic ulcer disease.

TABLE 47.1 The Forrest classification for endoscopic findings and rebleeding risks in peptic ulcer disease.

	CLASSIFICATION	REBLEEDING RISK
Grade Ia	Active, pulsatile bleeding	High
Grade Ib	Active, nonpulsatile bleeding	High
Grade IIa	Nonbleeding visible vessel	High
Grade IIb	Adherent clot	Intermediate
Grade IIc	Ulcer with black spot	Low
Grade III	Clean, nonbleeding ulcer bed	Low

need for endoscopic intervention. If PPI has not been started prior to endoscopy, a bolus of 80 mg should be given, followed by an infusion at 8 mg an hour for 72 hours. This approach has been shown to reduce risk of further bleeding, need for surgery, and mortality. Continuing PPI therapy postendoscopy also has been associated with reduced risk of further bleeding, need for surgery, and mortality.[19] Interestingly, no difference in these outcomes was established between oral and IV preparations in a recent meta-analysis. However, heterogeneity in the study design, PPI dosing, and endoscopic findings limit absolute conclusions in the absence of a well-designed noninferiority trial.

Eradication of *H. pylori* infection, if present, has been shown in multiple studies and metaanalysis to result in less rebleeding. Confirmation of successful therapy should be confirmed by breath or stool test or by biopsy on repeat endoscopy. Once *H. pylori* has been eradicated, there is no need for long-term acid suppression as it does not decrease the rebleed risk of 1.3%.[21]

All ulcerogenic medications such as NSAIDs or selective serotonin reuptake inhibitors should be discontinued in favor of alternatives. NSAIDs should be avoided as much as possible, although if they must be resumed, a combination of COX-2 selective NSAID and PPI should be used. Rebleeding rates with COX-2 inhibitors alone versus traditional NSAIDs plus a PPI are similar at 4% to 9%.[19] A double-blind trial showed that COX-2 inhibitors plus PPI has a much lower rebleed risk as compared to COX-2 selective NSAIDs alone (0% vs. 8.9%).[22] *H. pylori* eradication further improves the risk profile of NSAIDs.

The benefits of low-dose aspirin (ASA) for cardiovascular risk reduction are outweighed in some patients by the risk for GIB. The decision to continue ASA is based on its clinical indication for primary or secondary risk reduction. When used for primary risk reduction, the risk of recurrent GIB outweighs the benefit of ASA prophylaxis. A recent randomized controlled trial studied the benefits of ASA in primary prevention of cardiovascular events.[23] An analysis of secondary endpoints showed that ASA did not reduce cardiovascular events when compared to placebo but did increase the risk of significant hemorrhage in multiple areas of the body, including upper and lower GI.[23] However, ASA for secondary risk should be restarted in combination with a PPI within 1 to 7 days after bleeding cessation.[19] This recommendation is based on a randomized trial that compared patients who had high-risk features on endoscopy and resumed ASA immediately with those on placebo for 8 weeks. All patients received PPI infusion followed by oral therapy. At 30 days, the group receiving ASA did have a nonsignificant increased risk of bleeding. This risk was far outweighed by the notable finding that patients receiving ASA, compared to placebo, had a lower mortality at 30 days (1.3% vs. 9%) and 8 weeks (1.3% vs. 12.9%).[24]

Endoscopic management. Multiple endoscopic therapies have been used to treat PUD, including injection, thermal coagulation, plasma argon coagulation, mechanical clips, and fibrin glue. The recommended approach is to use thermal coagulation or clips, with or without epinephrine injection. This is based on meta-analysis showing that epinephrine monotherapy has a higher risk of rebleed compared to clipping or thermal coagulation. Injection therapy should be combined with other modalities such as heat or clipping.[25] Epinephrine is diluted 1:10,000 or 1:20,000 and is injected into all four quadrants of a bleeding lesion. The rate of initial hemostasis with epinephrine monotherapy is as high as 100%, although the risk of rebleeding remains high and thus mandates use of another modality. The ideal volume of injection is unknown, although generally, 0.2 to 2 mL is injected in each quadrant. Large volume injection (>13 mL) is associated with improved hemostasis, suggesting that part of the mechanism is by tamponade and compression of the bleeding vessel. In addition to injection, heat or mechanical therapy is usually added and together can achieve initial hemostasis in up to 90% of bleeding ulcers. Heat can be in the form of monopolar or bipolar cautery, heater probe, or argon plasma coagulation. All heat modalities have similar efficacy and are effective in achieving initial hemostasis, reducing recurrent bleeding, surgery, and mortality.[26]

Hemoclips are less effective than thermal therapy, although they may be advantageous in dealing with a spurting vessel for which they can provide immediate control of hemorrhage. Limitations of hemoclips are the difficulty in applying to fibrotic lesions and prolonged procedure time as only one clip can be applied at a time. It is important to properly place the first clip as improperly placed clips can impede placement of subsequent clips.[27] Clips can be useful if subsequent angiographic intervention is done, as they can assist in localizing the bleeding.

A less commonly used hemostatic therapy is sclerosant injection, such as absolute alcohol. This modality is effective but risks tissue damage, thus making it less attractive.

Rebleeding of an ulcer is associated with a significant increase in mortality. Patients at high risk of rebleeding should be identified early using previously described criteria and observed under higher levels of care such as in an intensive care unit. With rebleeding, a second attempt at endoscopic control is recommended and is successful in 75% of patients.

Angiographic management. Angiography is diagnostic as well as therapeutic and should be considered if a patient has failed endoscopic management or if the bleeding has not been localized. Access is obtained through the common femoral artery. The vessel interrogated first is based on clinical suspicion for location of the bleed. For suspected UGIB, the celiac artery and its branches are interrogated first as most UGIB is from gastric or duodenal ulcers supplied by branches of the celiac artery. The superior mesenteric artery and inferior mesenteric artery can also be evaluated if no bleeding is identified. The presence of clips or prior imaging can help guide further subselective catheterization.

In patients with repetitive, nondiagnostic workups, provocative maneuvers with systemic anticoagulation must be weighed against the risk of uncontrolled hemorrhage.

Transcatheter arterial embolization is effective at hemorrhage control when a bleeding source is found. Superselective embolization allows control of bleeding while maintaining adequate collateral flow to prevent bowel infarct. Examples include selective embolization of the left gastric artery or gastroduodenal artery for bleeding ulcers or the vasa recta or terminal branches of the inferior mesenteric artery for LGIB. There are various embolic agents such as coils, polyvinyl alcohol particles, Gelfoam, glue, and plugs. Coils and polyvinyl alcohol particles are most commonly used. Gelfoam is unique in that it is a temporary agent made of porcine adipose tissue and will recanalize over weeks to months, although the actual time course is often unpredictable. Success rates for UGIB embolization are cited at 44% to 100% and 88% to 93% for LGIB.[28]

Vasopressin infusion is less frequently used now that improved methods of transcatheter embolization are available. The mechanism of action is that vasopressin constricts arteries to reduce blood flow to the site of hemorrhage. Downsides to its use are cardiac side effects and high rates of rebleeding after cessation of infusion and the need to maintain vascular access in situ for 24 to 48 hours to continue the infusion. The cardiac effects can be mitigated to some degree with a nitroglycerin infusion to maintain coronary perfusion. Vasopressin infusion can be useful if there is diffuse bleeding or as a bridge to surgical intervention if superselective cannulation cannot be achieved.

Surgical management. Despite significant advances in endoscopic therapy, approximately 10% of patients with bleeding ulcers still require surgical intervention for effective hemostasis.[18] To assist in this decision making, several clinical and endoscopic parameters have been proposed that are thought to identify patients at high risk for failed endoscopic therapy. The Forrest classification is the best predictor of rebleeding (see Table 47.1). Other endoscopic factors associated with increased risk of rebleeding are active bleeding at time of endoscopy, large ulcer size (i.e., >2 cm), posterior duodenal wall ulcer, and lesser gastric curve ulcer.[29] Patients with these characteristics need closer monitoring and possibly earlier surgical intervention. Clearly, clinical judgment and local expertise must play a critical role in this decision.

Indications for surgery have traditionally been based on the blood transfusion requirements, success of endoscopic therapy, and recurrent bleeding after repeat endoscopy. Increased blood transfusions have been clearly associated with increased mortality. Although a less definitive criterion than it was in the past, most surgeons still consider an ongoing blood transfusion requirement more than 6 units as an indication for surgical intervention, particularly in the elderly, although an 8- to 10-unit loss may be more acceptable for the younger population. Current indications for surgery for peptic ulcer hemorrhage are summarized in Box 47.1. Secondary or relative indications include a rare blood type or difficult crossmatch, refusal of transfusion, shock on presentation, advanced age, severe comorbid disease, and a bleeding chronic gastric ulcer for which malignancy is a concern.

BOX 47.1 Indications for surgery in gastrointestinal hemorrhage.

- Hemodynamic instability despite vigorous resuscitation (>6-unit transfusion)
- Failure of endoscopic techniques to arrest hemorrhage
- Recurrent hemorrhage after initial stabilization (with up to two attempts at obtaining endoscopic hemostasis)
- Shock associated with recurrent hemorrhage
- Continued slow bleeding with a transfusion requirement exceeding 3 units/day

Surgical management of duodenal ulcers. The first step in the operative management for a duodenal ulcer is exposure of the bleeding site. Most of these lesions are in the duodenal bulb; stay sutures are placed on either side of a longitudinal duodenotomy or duodenopyloromyotomy. Hemorrhage typically can be controlled initially with pressure and then direct suture ligation with nonabsorbable suture. Anterior ulcers can be directly ligated. More commonly, a posterior ulcer erodes into the pancreaticoduodenal or gastroduodenal artery. Suture ligature of the vessel proximal and distally, typically in a superior and inferior orientation, as placement of medial-stitch to control the pancreatic branches typically arrests the bleed. The duodenotomy is closed transversely with an NGT above and a nasojejunal tube placed beyond the repair for distal enteral access. Omental buttressing of the suture line may assist in healing. A surgical drain can be left in place if there is significant concern for a potential leak.

Traditionally, a definitive acid-reducing operation was considered if the patient was hemodynamically stable. This practice has largely been abandoned in the era of *H. pylori* eradication and PPI therapy, such that there has been a dramatic reduction in the rates of definitive ulcer therapy (gastrectomy or vagotomy). The choice between various acid-reduction operations was guided by the hemodynamic condition of the patient and the presence or absence of long-standing history of refractory ulcer disease. The various operations for PUD are discussed in greater detail in Chapter 49. A pyloroplasty combined with truncal vagotomy is the most frequently performed acid-reduction surgery used in the setting of a bleeding duodenal ulcer. There is some evidence to suggest that a parietal cell vagotomy may represent a better therapy for a bleeding duodenal ulcer in the stable patient, although some of this benefit may be abrogated if the pylorus has been divided. In a patient who has a known history of refractory duodenal ulcer disease or who has failed to respond to more conservative surgery, antrectomy with truncal vagotomy may be more appropriate. However, this procedure is more complex and should generally not be done in a hemodynamically unstable patient.

Surgical management of gastric ulcer. Surgical control of a bleeding gastric ulcer begins with a gastrotomy and suture ligation.

This alone is associated with 30% risk of rebleeding. Gastric ulcer resection is generally indicated due to the 10% incidence of malignancy. Simple excision alone is associated with rebleeding in as many as 20% of patients, so distal gastrectomy is generally preferred. Alternatively, ulcer excision combined with vagotomy and pyloroplasty may be considered in high-risk patients. Bleeding ulcers of the proximal stomach near the gastroesophageal junction are more difficult to manage. Proximal or near-total gastrectomies are associated with a particularly high mortality in the setting of acute hemorrhage. Other options include distal gastrectomy combined with resection of a tongue of proximal stomach inclusive of the ulcer. Vagotomy and pyloroplasty combined with either wedge resection or a buttressed oversewing of the ulcer also may be appropriate. Again, the possibility of malignancy must be kept in mind, especially in gastric ulcers remote from the pylorus.

Esophagitis

The esophagus is an infrequent site of nonvariceal hemorrhage. When it does occur, it is most commonly the result of esophagitis. Esophageal inflammation secondary to repeated exposure of the esophageal mucosa to the acidic gastric secretions in gastroesophageal reflux disease leads to an inflammatory response that can result in chronic blood loss. Ulceration may accompany this, but the superficial mucosal ulcerations generally do not bleed acutely and are more commonly manifested as anemia or guaiac-positive stools. Various infectious agents may also cause esophagitis, particularly in the immune-compromised host (Fig. 47.3). With infection, hemorrhage can occasionally be massive. Other causes of esophageal bleeding include medications, Crohn disease, and radiation. Treatment typically includes acid suppressive therapy. Endoscopic control of the hemorrhage, usually with electrocoagulation or heater probe, is often successful. In patients with an infectious cause, targeted therapy is appropriate. Surgery is seldom necessary.

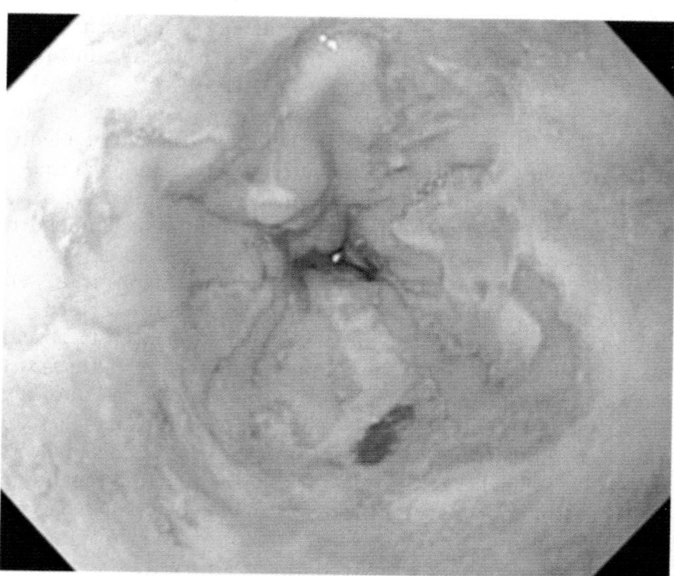

FIG. 47.3 Bleeding esophageal ulcer secondary to herpes esophagitis. (Courtesy Scott A. Hande, MD, Brigham and Women's Hospital.)

Gastritis

Stress-related gastritis is characterized by the appearance of multiple superficial erosions of the entire stomach, most commonly in the body. It is thought to result from the combination of acid and pepsin injury in the context of decreased mucosal protection from hypoperfusion, NSAIDs, chemotherapy, or other agents. Classically, gastritis commonly afflicted the critically ill. These lesions are different from the solitary ulcerations related to acid hypersecretion from severe head injury (i.e., Cushing ulcers). When stress ulceration is associated with major burns, these lesions are referred to as Curling ulcers. Significant hemorrhage from stress ulceration was common prior to improvements in the management of shock and prophylactic use of acid suppression in high-risk patients. In those who develop bleeding, acid suppressive therapy is often successful in controlling the hemorrhage. In rare cases when this fails, consideration should be given to the administration of octreotide or vasopressin, endoscopic therapy, or even angiographic embolization. Historically, such cases were more commonly seen and, at times, dealt with surgically. The surgical choices included vagotomy and pyloroplasty with oversewing of the hemorrhage or near-total gastrectomy. These procedures carried mortality rates as high as 60%. Fortunately, they are seldom necessary today.

Mallory-Weiss Tears

Mallory-Weiss tears are partial-thickness tears of the mucosa and submucosa that occur near the gastroesophageal junction. Classically, these lesions develop in alcoholic patients after a period of intense retching and vomiting following binge drinking, but they can occur in any patient who has a history of repeated emesis. The mechanism, proposed by Mallory and Weiss in 1929, is forceful contraction of the abdominal wall against an unrelaxed cardia, resulting in mucosal laceration of the cardia as a result of the increased intragastric pressure.

Such lesions account for 5% to 10% of cases of UGIB. They are usually diagnosed by history, and endoscopy is used to confirm the diagnosis. A retroflexion maneuver is necessary to view the area just below the gastroesophageal junction and should be performed routinely so as to not miss this diagnosis in UGIB patients. Most tears occur along the lesser curvature and can extend into the esophagus. Supportive therapy with acid suppression therapy is successful in 90% of bleeding episodes, the mucosa often healing within 72 hours.

In rare cases of severe ongoing bleeding, endoscopic therapy with injection or electrocoagulation may be effective. Angiographic embolization, usually with absorbable material such as a gelatin sponge, has been successfully employed in cases of failed endoscopic therapy. If these maneuvers fail, high gastrotomy and suturing of the mucosal tear are indicated. It is important to rule out the diagnosis of variceal bleeding in cases of failed endoscopic therapy by a thorough examination of the gastroesophageal junction. Recurrent bleeding from a Mallory-Weiss tear is uncommon.

Gastric Antral Vascular Ectasia

Gastric antral vascular ectasia is characterized by a collection of dilated venules that appear as a linear red streak converging on the antrum, giving the appearance of a watermelon. Severe hemorrhage is rare in gastric antral vascular ectasia, and most patients present with persistent, iron deficiency anemia from continued occult blood loss. Endoscopic therapy is indicated for persistent anemia or transfusion-dependent bleeding. The success rate is upward of 90% with argon plasma coagulation (Fig. 47.4). Patients failing to respond to endoscopic therapy should be considered for antrectomy.

Dieulafoy Lesion

Dieulafoy lesions are vascular malformations found primarily along the lesser curve of the stomach within 6 cm of the gastroesophageal junction, although they can occur elsewhere in the GI

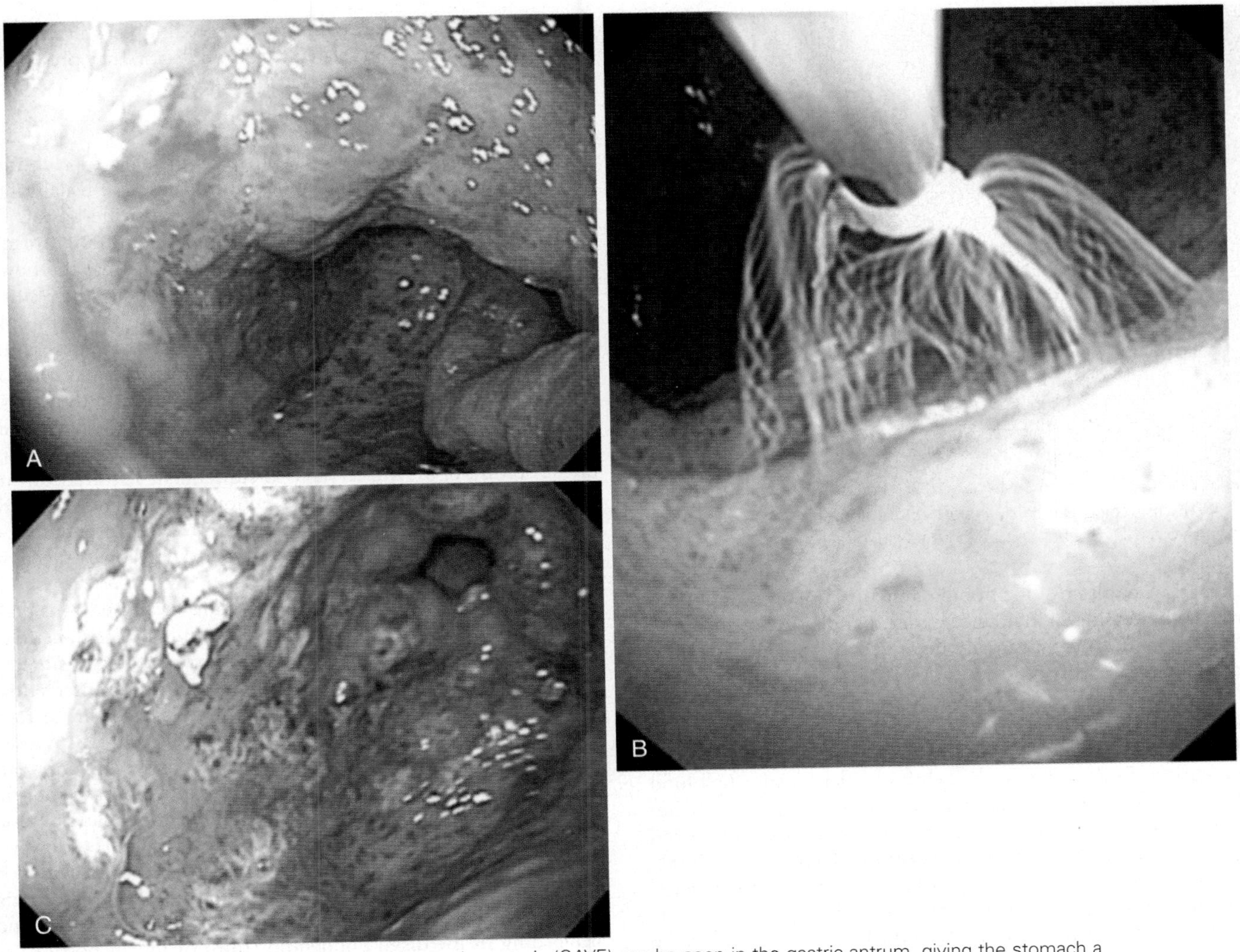

FIG. 47.4 (A) Gastric antral vascular ectasia (GAVE) can be seen in the gastric antrum, giving the stomach a watermelon appearance. (B) Argon plasma coagulation therapy of GAVE. (C) Posttherapy appearance of GAVE. (Courtesy David L. Carr-Locke, MD, Brigham and Women's Hospital.)

tract (Fig. 47.5). Erosion of the gastric mucosa overlying these sizable vessels (1 to 3 mm) found in the gastric submucosa leads to bleeding. The mucosal defect is usually small (2 to 5 mm), without an associated ulcer, thus making it difficult to identify.[30] Given the large size of the underlying artery, bleeding from a Dieulafoy lesion can be massive (Fig. 47.6).

Initial attempts at endoscopic control are often successful. Application of thermal or sclerosant therapy is effective in 80% to 100% of cases. In cases that fail endoscopic therapy, angiographic coil embolization can also be successful. If these approaches are unsuccessful, surgical intervention may be necessary; because of difficulties in visualization and palpation of these lesions, prior endoscopic tattooing or clipping can facilitate the procedure. A gastrotomy is performed, and attempts are made at identifying the bleeding source. The lesion can then be oversewn. In cases in which the bleeding point is not identified, a partial gastrectomy may be necessary.

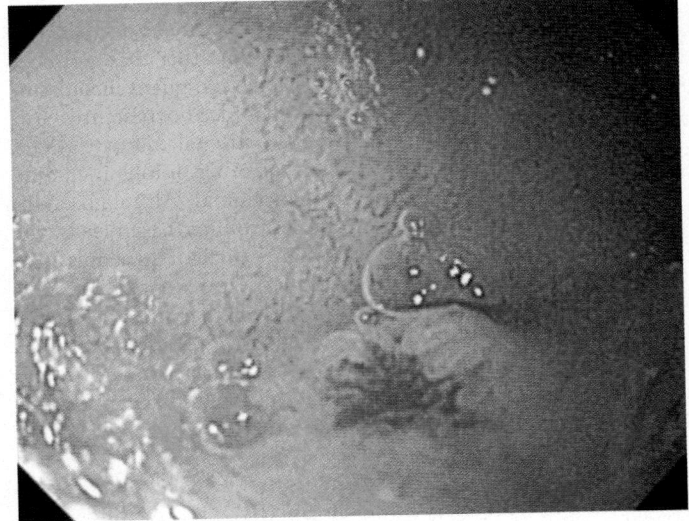

FIG. 47.5 Dieulafoy lesion of the stomach. (Courtesy Linda S. Lee, MD, Brigham and Women's Hospital.)

Hemobilia

Hemobilia is often a difficult diagnosis to make. It is typically associated with trauma, recent instrumentation of the biliary tree,

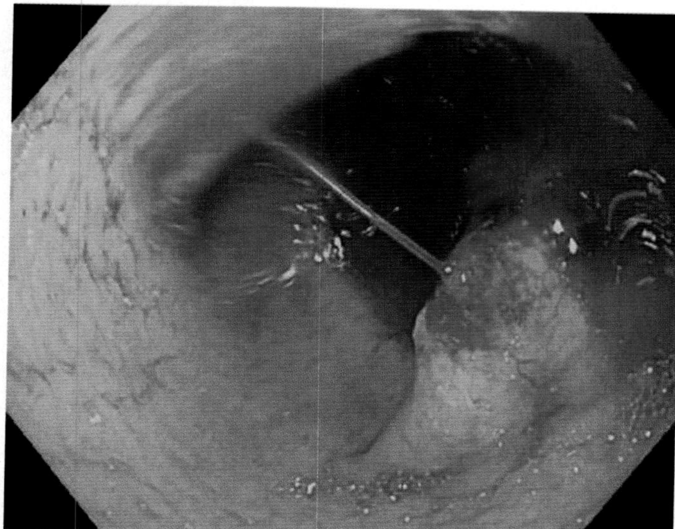

FIG. 47.6 Bleeding Dieulafoy lesion with a spurting vessel. (Courtesy Marvin Ryou, MD, Brigham and Women's Hospital.)

or hepatic neoplasms. Hemobilia remains uncommon but is gradually increasing in incidence with expanded use of advanced endoscopy and other minimally invasive hepatopancreaticobiliary procedures.[31] This unusual cause of GIB should be suspected in anyone with suggestive history or those with right upper quadrant pain and/or jaundice. CT with angiography protocol is the preferred modality for diagnosis in those with an equivocal presentation. Endoscopy can be helpful by demonstrating blood at the ampulla or other biliary abnormalities suggestive of hemobilia and can offer numerous therapeutic options. However, angiography remains the gold standard for diagnosis and intervention and should be considered as the first step in patients with swift bleeding and a suggestive history. If angiographic embolization is performed, the portal vein must be verified to be patent. Surgical intervention is rarely needed except when all other therapies have failed, although it is still used occasionally for infected pseudoaneurysms or compression of surrounding vascular structures.[31]

Malignancy

Malignant neoplasms of the UGI tract are usually associated with chronic anemia or hemoccult-positive stool rather than episodes of significant hemorrhage. On occasion, malignant neoplasms will be manifested as ulcerative lesions that bleed persistently. This is perhaps most characteristic of the GI stromal tumor (GIST), although it may occur with a variety of other lesions including adenocarcinoma, leiomyomas, and lymphomas. Although endoscopic therapy is often successful in controlling these bleeds, the rebleeding rate is high; therefore, when a malignant neoplasm is diagnosed, surgical resection is indicated. The extent of resection is dependent on the specific lesion and whether the resection is believed to be curative or palliative. Palliative resections for control of bleeding usually entail wedge resections. Standard cancer operations are indicated when possible, although this may depend on the hemodynamic stability of the patient.

Inflammatory Bowel Disease

UGIB from inflammatory bowel disease (IBD) is exceedingly rare, with a few reported cases of duodenal Crohn disease. This type of bleeding can be the result of an ulcer eroding into a vessel and is treated as such. More commonly, bleeding complications of IBD are self-limited and related to Crohn ileitis. They present as a LGIB that is responsive to medical therapy.

Aortoenteric Fistula

Aortoenteric fistulas can be classified as primary or secondary and most often involve the duodenum. These are usually fatal as they represent free rupture of the aorta into the bowel. Primary aortoenteric fistulas are rare and most commonly form as the result of an aortic aneurysm compressed against the bowel. Secondary fistulas are much more common and are the result of an aortic graft-enteric erosion and may develop in up to 0.4% to 4% of aortic graft cases. The interval between surgery and hemorrhage can be days to years, with the median interval about 3 years. The pathogenesis is poorly understood, although the sequence of formation is thought to involve the development of a pseudoaneurysm at the proximal anastomotic suture line in the setting of an infection with subsequent fistulization into the overlying duodenum. With endovascular stent-grafts, the mechanism may involve stent graft failure with an endoleak or fracture of the stent that allows aneurysm expansion or mechanical erosion into the adjacent bowel.

This diagnosis of an aortoenteric fistula should be considered in all bleeding patients with a known abdominal aortic aneurysm or any prior aortic reconstruction. Hemorrhage in this situation is often massive and fatal unless immediate surgical intervention is undertaken. Typically, patients with bleeding from an aortoenteric fistula will present first with a "sentinel bleed." This is a self-limited episode that heralds the subsequent massive and often fatal hemorrhage. These episodes can be separated by hours to months, and some patients may experience multiple sentinel bleeds. In stable patients, EGD is always the first-line test for UGIB. However, if the suspicion for an aortoenteric fistula is high, CTA should be the first-line study. One case series found CTA to have a sensitivity of 79%, whereas EGD had a sensitivity of 50%.[32] Any evidence of bleeding in the distal duodenum (third or fourth portion) on EGD in a patient at risk for an aortoenteric fistula should be considered diagnostic. A CT with IV contrast will often show air around the graft, which is suggestive of infection, possible pseudoaneurysm, and occasionally extravasation of IV contrast into the bowel lumen.

Therapy includes ligation of the aorta proximal to the graft, removal of the infected prosthesis with debridement of surrounding tissue, and extra-anatomic bypass. One must assume that the graft is infected, and treatment should include long-term antibiotics. Endovascular repair may be used as a bridge to definitive open repair.

Hemosuccus Pancreaticus

Bleeding from the pancreatic duct is one of the rarest causes of UGIB. Hemosuccus pancreaticus is bleeding from the pancreatic duct through the ampulla of Vater, most typically from a pancreatic source such as a malformation, ductal wall ulceration, or a pancreatic pseudocyst that erodes into a pseudoaneurysm. Angiography is the diagnostic gold standard and first therapeutic line of action due to high efficacy (75%–100%) and low-associated mortality. Operative interventions may occasionally be required to treat the pseudocyst and should be aided by intraoperative ultrasonography or pancreatoscopy to diagnose the site of hemorrhage to guide operative planning. Other surgical procedures such as pancreatic resection and/or arterial ligation have largely been replaced by endovascular intervention.[33]

Procedure-Related Bleeding

Percutaneous endoscopic gastrostomy tube placement is an increasingly common procedure that allows enteral nutrition in various acute and chronic disorders where patients are unable to have intake by mouth. Bleeding from percutaneous endoscopic gastrostomy placement is estimated to be as high as 3%. The bleeding most often occurs from puncture of a superficial vessel in the skin and is easily controlled with pressure. Bleeding from a punctured gastric vessel or mucosa is easily controlled by compression from traction on the bumper, although this should be temporary, with care taken to avoid pressure necrosis of the gastric wall. If these maneuvers are ineffective, then the tube may need to be removed and hemostasis achieved endoscopically.

Endoscopic sphincterotomy has similar bleeding rates to percutaneous endoscopic gastrostomy and represents another example of iatrogenic bleeding, with a bleeding complication rate of approximately 2%. Bleeding is often mild and self-limited. Delayed hemorrhage usually occurs within the first 48 hours and may require injection of the area with epinephrine. Surgical intervention is rarely required.

Hemobilia, as previously noted, may be iatrogenic in nature, particularly after percutaneous transhepatic procedures. Bleeding may also occur in any patient who has a suture or staple line from a gastric or intestinal resection and anastomosis. Risk factor reduction is largely based on the bariatric surgical literature and has revealed the following measures: maintaining systolic blood pressure control less than 140 mm Hg, staple line reinforcement with built-in pericardial strips or absorbable polymers, and intraoperative evaluation of resection lines at a reduced insufflation pressure (10 mm Hg) to diminish the tamponade effect of pneumoperitoneum during laparoscopic cases. Most surgical anastomotic bleeding resolves with nonoperative management In patients in whom bleeding persists, diagnostic and therapeutic endoscopy can be performed safely as long as insufflation is minimal and attention is paid to staple line stress. Reoperation for surgical anastomotic bleeding is rarely needed and has been estimated to occur in less than 1.4% of cases.[34]

Variceal Hemorrhage

Hypertension within the venous system of the GI tract can occur due to prehepatic (portal or splenic vein thrombus), intrahepatic (cirrhosis) or posthepatic (Budd-Chiari) pathology.

By far, the most common clinical scenario leading to variceal hemorrhage is portal hypertension from the sinusoidal fibrosis associated with cirrhosis. Portal hypertension is defined as a hepatic venous pressure gradient of more than 5 mm Hg; however, a pressure greater than 12 mm Hg is generally required to develop varices. Increased resistance to flow of the portal vein and its tributaries leads to engorgement of portacaval collaterals in the esophagus, stomach, and the hemorrhoidal plexus. This state is exacerbated by the hyperaldosteronism and expanded plasma volume, as well as splanchnic vasodilatation that congests the intestinal circulation. Due to the large capacitance of the venous system, veins may pathologically dilate to diameters upward of 1 to 2 cm with increased wall tension stressing the overlying mucosa. Catastrophic bleeding can occur with disruption of the overlying mucosa, which, despite medical advancement in the field, still has an associated 6-week mortality of 10% to 20%.[35]

Management of variceal hemorrhage begins with prevention. Identifying the at-risk population has been aided by the introduction of transient elastography. Liver stiffness measured by transient elastography values of more than 15 to 20 kPa suggests compensated advanced chronic liver disease and thus should prompt EGD to evaluate for gastric varices and measurement of hepatic venous pressure gradient. EGD findings then dictate the appropriate prophylaxis. Patients without varices should be surveyed every 2 years, whereas those with small varices should be scoped annually. If small varices are noted to have high-risk features such as red wale marks (longitudinal red streaking), patients may benefit from starting a nonselective beta blocker. Patients with medium or large varices benefit from treatment with nonselective beta blockade (propranolol, nadolol, and carvedilol) or prophylactic banding.[35]

In the acute hemorrhage, attention to the ABCDEs of resuscitation is of utmost importance and has been described earlier in the chapter. Bleeding from varices can be brisk and is often complicated by coagulopathy and thrombocytopenia. The goal of resuscitation is to maintain tissue perfusion. Transfusions should be based on hemodynamic status and tissue perfusion assessment, but a hemoglobin target between 7 and 8 g/dL is generally recommended to minimize increasing the hepatic venous pressure gradient.[9] Best evidence for reversal of coagulopathy has yet to be established, but the degree of hemostatic dysfunction may be belied by the international normalized ratio (INR) and partial thromboplastin time. Generally, attempts at an INR less than 2 and platelet count greater than 50,000 should be attempted. Vasoactive drugs such as terlipressin, somatostatin, octreotide, and vapreotide should be used prior to endoscopic evaluation and continued for up to 5 days. These medications decrease the flow to the mucosa and may decrease venous pressure. Importantly, antibiotics should be administered in any patient with UGIB and cirrhosis to guard against infection and spontaneous bacterial peritonitis. Current recommendations are for oral fluoroquinolones or IV Ceftriaxone (1 g every 24 hours) for patients with advanced disease or nil per os status.

In rare circumstances, patients may present with such severe instability that a device for mechanical tamponade of the esophageal varices must be placed to prevent imminent exsanguination. The Sengstaken-Blakemore tube is equipped with two inflatable balloons to provide mechanical pressure. The first balloon is a gastric balloon. With confirmed placement of the uninflated tube into the stomach, the gastric port is inflated and placed on tension by securing it to a fixed helmet. The tension is applied to the gastroesophageal junction and often may arrest hemorrhage. However, if bleeding continues, the second balloon (the esophageal port) may be inflated to further tamponade the lower esophageal venous plexus. These tubes are temporary measures reserved for pronounced hemodynamic instability as a bridge to more definitive therapy. It is estimated that over 50% of patients will rebleed with deflation. Furthermore, by virtue of the balloon tamponade, local esophageal trauma and ischemia may result from prolonged inflation. Recent trials using self-expanding esophageal stents to control massive variceal hemorrhage have been encouraging, and a randomized controlled trial is examining hemostasis failure and rebleeding rates with this approach, but as of now, their clinical use remains experimental.[36]

Endoscopy is the first recommended step in any patient with cirrhosis and UGIB. Endoscopic venous ligation is preferred over sclerotherapy for acute esophageal bleeding. Definitive long-term management with early transjugular intrahepatic portosystemic shunt (TIPS) should be performed within 24 hours for high-risk patients and within 72 hours for other patient populations. TIPS is a procedure that connects the hepatic vein with the portal vein via an image-guided deployment of a metal stent though the hepatic parenchyma. This effectively decreases the venous pressure and achieves definitive hemostasis in greater than 90% of patients.

Salvage therapy with this modality may be necessary in medically refractory or dying patients as this will immediately decrease the portal venous gradient. The incidence of encephalopathy is increased with TIPS, and there can be technical complications such as bleeding, arrhythmia, and stenosis. TIPS is contraindicated in patients with hepatocellular carcinoma (relative), heart failure, pulmonary hypertension, or tricuspid regurgitation. Failure of hemorrhage control is predicted by venous pressures greater than 20 mm Hg, Model for End-Stage Liver Disease (MELD) score greater than 20, Child-Pugh class C cirrhosis, and active bleeding at the time of intervention.

Surgical decompression of the portal system is accomplished by creating an anastomosis from the portal system to a caval tributary. Surgical intervention is an effective, oftentimes superior, long-term therapy for variceal hemorrhage but is associated with a mortality rate in excess of 50%. Shunts are characterized by the degree of diversion of flow. Shunts that decompress the entire portal tree are considered a nonselective shunt. Other surgical shunts, such as the distal splenorenal shunt, selectively decompress the gastroesophageal varices while leaving the superior mesenteric and portal veins intact.

Nonshunt operations are reserved for the moribund patients that are failing resuscitation efforts. These procedures include either esophageal transection in which the distal esophagus is transected and then a stapled reanastomosis performed in a delayed fashion after varices have been ligated or the Sugiura procedure, which entails devascularization of the gastroesophageal junction and splenectomy. Since the advent of TIPS, which similarly decompresses the portal system with less upfront mortality risk, operative interventions for variceal management are much less common and nonshunt operations are exceedingly rare.

ACUTE LOWER GASTROINTESTINAL HEMORRHAGE

LGIB is defined as bleeding originating distal to the ligament of Treitz, although, in some cases, it may refer specifically to bleeding distal to the ileocecal valve due to its unique nature when compared to small bowel bleeding.[14] The most common presentation is painless hematochezia, defined as bright red blood, clots, or burgundy stools. A brisk UGIB can also present in the same way, and initial evaluation of hematochezia should always begin by ruling out a UGIB, as discussed previously in this chapter. Melena, a common presentation of UGIB, can occasionally be a sign of LGIB. Information from a directed history and physical can suggest specific causes of LGIB. For example, abdominal pain with diarrhea suggests inflammatory, ischemic, or infectious-type colitis. Altered bowel habits, iron-deficiency anemia, or unexplained weight loss may suggest malignancy.[13]

LGIB is a less common reason for hospitalization in the United States when compared to UGIB and accounts for 30% to 40% of GIB[1] or an annual incidence of 35 per 100,000 persons.[37] The mortality rate associated with LGIB is slightly below that of UGIB at just below 2% and increases to about 5% in those individuals older than 85 years old. In patients with LGIB, more than 95% will have a source in the colon (Table 47.2). In general, the incidence of hospitalization, morbidity, and mortality for LGIB increases with age. The cause is also often related to age. Vascular lesions and diverticular disease affect all age groups but have an increasing incidence in middle-aged and elderly adults. In the pediatric population, intussusception is most commonly responsible, whereas Meckel diverticulum must be considered in the differential in the young adult. The clinical presentation of LGIB ranges from severe hemorrhage with diverticular disease or vascular lesions to a minor bleeding secondary to anal fissure or hemorrhoids.

TABLE 47.2 Differential diagnosis of lower gastrointestinal hemorrhage.

COLONIC BLEEDING	95%	SMALL BOWEL BLEEDING	5%
Diverticular disease	30%–40%	Angiodysplasias	
Anorectal disease	5%–15%	Erosions or ulcers (potassium, nonsteroidal antiinflammatory drugs)	
Ischemia	5%–10%	Crohn disease	
Neoplasia	5%–10%	Radiation	
Infectious colitis	3%–8%	Meckel diverticulum	
Postpolypectomy	3%–7%	Neoplasia	
Inflammatory bowel disease	3%–4%	Aortoenteric fistula	
Angiodysplasia	3%		
Radiation colitis or proctitis	1%–3%		
Other	1%–5%		
Unknown	10%–25%		

Diagnosis

Hemorrhage from the lower GI tract tends to be less severe and intermittent, often spontaneously resolving between attempts at localization with endoscopy or other modalities. Additionally, over 40% of patients with LGIB have multiple lesions identified as the potential source of bleeding. If more than one lesion is identified, it is critical to confirm the responsible lesion before initiating aggressive therapy. Due to these factors, there is no diagnostic modality as sensitive or specific in LGIB as endoscopy is in UGIB. Additionally, these patients may need longer observations and suffer several episodes of bleeding before a definitive diagnosis is made. In up to 25% of patients with LGIB, the source of bleeding is never accurately identified.

An algorithm for evaluation and management of LGIB is shown in Fig. 47.7. As always, one should begin with an initial evaluation and resuscitation as discussed previously. Anticoagulation should be reversed, and coagulation disorders treated aggressively. The exception to this rule is in the patient with high-risk cardiovascular disease in whom current guidelines support the continuation of ASA.

The first step in further workup is to rule out anorectal bleeding with a digital rectal examination and anoscopy or sigmoidoscopy and to provide appropriate treatment if positive. With significant bleeding, it is also important to eliminate a UGI source. Up to 15% of patients with hematochezia had a UGI source to account for the bleed.[37] A nasogastric aspirate that contains bile and no blood effectively rules out an active upper tract bleeding site. However, when emergent surgery for life-threatening hemorrhage is being contemplated, preoperative or intraoperative EGD can be appropriate even when LGIB is suspected.

Subsequent evaluation depends on the magnitude of the hemorrhage and can be classified as minor, major, or massive. Patients with minor LGIB are hemodynamically stable and generally can be evaluated as outpatients. The most common causes of minor LGIB are anorectal lesions such as hemorrhoids or fissures, although IBD, infectious colitis, arteriovenous malformations, polyps, and malignancy can also be potential sources. Major LGIB can be defined as hemorrhage associated with hemodynamic instability, altered mental status, or the need for two or more units

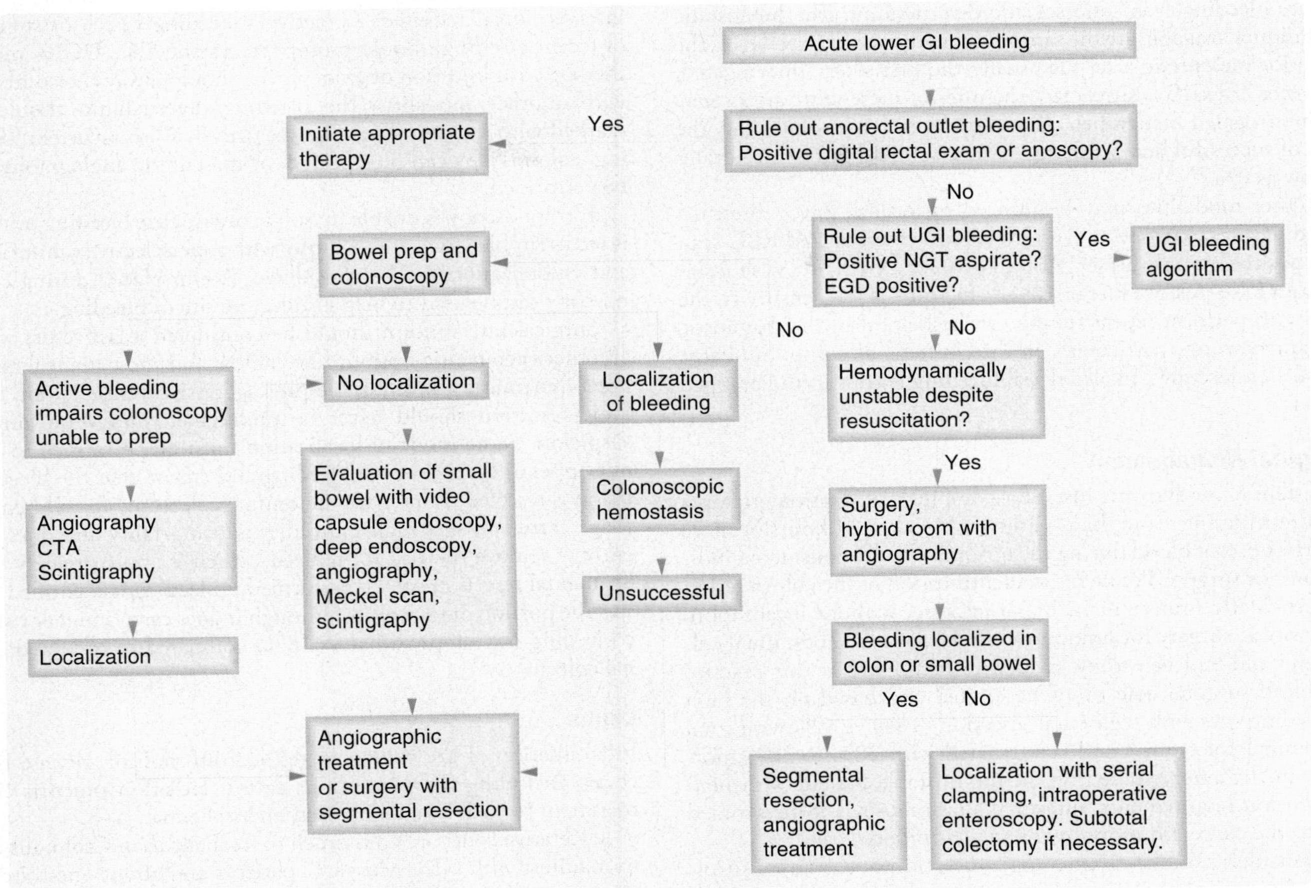

FIG. 47.7 Algorithm for diagnosis and management of lower GI hemorrhage. *CTA*, Computed tomography angiogram; *EGD*, esophagogastroduodenoscopy; *GI*, gastrointestinal; *NGT*, nasogastric tube; *UGI*, upper GI.

of blood. Massive LGIB is when a patient requires 10 or more units of blood products.

The truly unstable patient who continues to bleed and requires ongoing aggressive resuscitation belongs in the operating room for expeditious diagnosis and surgical intervention. In facilities equipped with hybrid operating rooms, angiography can be helpful to localize bleeding or attempt endovascular therapy in the presence of immediate surgical intervention. Intraoperative endoscopy is also a useful adjunct to identify a source of bleeding.

When the hemorrhaging patient responds to resuscitation and is hemodynamically stable, the evaluation and therapeutic intervention can be more directed. Colonoscopy is the mainstay here because it allows both visualization of the pathologic process and therapeutic intervention in colonic, rectal, and distal ileal sources of bleeding. CTA, mesenteric angiography, and tagged RBC scintigraphy are important components of the evaluation, provided there are no contraindications. If these modalities are nondiagnostic and UGIB has been ruled out, then the source of the hemorrhage is considered obscure and further evaluation is detailed previously the chapter.

Colonoscopy

For patients who are stable, colonoscopy is almost always the initial examination of choice for LGIB. Exceptions include patients who are unable to tolerate a bowel prep or if the bleeding is severe enough to limit the visualization through the colonoscope. Colonoscopy should only be performed after an adequate bowel prep, such as the "rapid prep" protocol described previously. Similar to endoscopy for UGIB, colonoscopy should be performed within 24 hours. The causes of LGIB most likely to have successful endoscopic treatment are diverticular, angioectasia, and postpolypectomy. Overall endoscopic success is good with one review showing a hemostasis rate of 92% and early and late rebleed rates of 8% and 12%, respectively.[38] The most common source of bleeding is diverticular, and even though an actively bleeding diverticulum may not be seen during endoscopy, certain features are predictive of high risk of rebleeding. Findings of active bleeding, a visible vessel, or adherent clot that cannot be dislodged by irrigation and suctioning are associated with a high risk of rebleed and should undergo endoscopic treatment.[39] An India ink tattoo should be placed to identify the area of bleeding in case repeat intervention is needed. Other endoscopic therapeutic interventions include polypectomy, epinephrine injection, direct contact thermal coagulation, argon plasma coagulation, application of metal clips to lesions, and band ligation of internal hemorrhoids or rectal varices

Angiography

When endoscopy is unable to localize a LGIB, angiography is an important diagnostic as well as therapeutic tool. Other imaging modalities that complement and help direct angiography are CTA and tagged RBC scintigraphy (see discussion above in "Localization"). When used prior to angiography, CTA and tagged RBC scans improve the localization of angiography.[11] Because it relies on active bleeding, angiography is most useful in the setting of brisk bleeding. Using superselective embolization, it is possible to isolate bleeding from one specific diverticulum. The hemostatic techniques available are the same as those discussed for UGIB. The superior mesenteric artery is usually the first artery interrogated; however, if LGIB is suspected, the inferior mesenteric artery may be interrogated first. When used to treat diverticular bleeding, the rate of successful hemostasis approaches 100%, with rebleed rates as low as 0%.[39]

Other modalities may be utilized to localize lower intestinal bleeding. In a retrospective review of 600 cases, tagged RBC scan was positive in only about 39% to 45% of LGIB,[40,41] with a significant false-positive rate of 10%.[41] Despite its low sensitivity, the ability to perform repeat testing can be helpful in the diagnostic armamentarium, particularly in intermittent bleeding. Similarly, capsule endoscopy can also reveal bleeding lesions in the prepped colon.

Surgical Management

Persistent hemodynamic instability despite resuscitation attempts or administering more than 4 units of blood in 24 hours or more than10 units of blood during the hospital stay are considered indications for surgery. Preoperative identification of the culprit lesion is particularly important in LGIB because, without localization, the empiric surgery for unlocalized LGIB is a total abdominal colectomy and end ileostomy. Evidence in support of this practice of "blind subtotal colectomy" is limited and based on the high rebleeding rate with segmental resection (18% vs. 4% with total abdominal colectomy) and is associated with 20% to 30% mortality in the emergent setting. In the unstable patient with high transfusion requirements, intestinal anastomosis is to be avoided due to the conferred mortality of an anastomotic leak.[42,43]

Consideration for an oncologic resection in scenarios suspicious for malignancy is important when hemodynamic stability allows. An alternative management strategy in the dying patient is a damage control operation with delayed definitive therapy in order to support the patient's physiology to "fight another day."

Specific Causes of Lower Gastrointestinal Tract Bleeding

Diverticula

In the United States, diverticula are the most common cause of significant LGIB. Among all with colonic diverticula, 3% to 15% will experience bleeding.[39] The incidence of diverticula increases with age, with 20% at age 40 and increasing to 60% and beyond at age 60.[44] In the past, diverticula were thought to be rare in patients younger than 40 years, but it is now an increasingly common diagnosis in this age group. Diverticula form at points of weakness in the bowel wall, where the vasa recta penetrate the circular muscle layer. As the dome of the diverticulum expands, the penetrating vessel is stretched and undergoes changes that can lead to vessel rupture and bleeding. In western countries, left-sided disease is far more common than right-sided disease; however, right-sided disease is responsible for over 50% of significant diverticular bleeding. Of those that bleed, more than 75% stop spontaneously, although approximately 10% will rebleed within a year and almost 50% within 10 years.[44]

Colonoscopy is the best modality for diagnosis and therapy. The endoscopic treatment options are similar to those for PUD and include injection, thermal coagulation, plasma argon coagulation, mechanical clips, and fibrin glue. Use of clips have an added advantage in that they can mark the location of bleeding if repeat intervention is required. An actively bleeding vessel, or stigmata of recent bleeding, should prompt treatment. Like UGIB, monotherapy with injection of epinephrine should always be combined with another modality. The bleeding diverticulum should be marked with a tattoo if no clip was placed. With recurrent bleeding, colonoscopy can be repeated, or mesenteric angiography can be performed.

If colonoscopy is unable to isolate or visualize bleeding or there is recurrent bleeding, angiography with superselective cannulation and embolization can be considered. A clip placed during colonoscopy can be used to help localize the site of bleeding.

Surgical intervention should be considered a last resort when all other therapeutic options have failed, and the patient remains hemodynamically unstable despite aggressive resuscitation. Colonic resection should never be undertaken purely on clinical suspicion. Some mode of localization must be performed to rule out upper and small bowel bleeding and ensure that the bleeding lesion is resected. Blind total abdominal colectomy for GI hemorrhage carries with it high morbidity and mortality and does not entirely remove the risk for rebleed, which is approximately 4%. Segmental resection can be performed if bleeding is identified at a specific portion of the colon, although it does carry a higher risk of rebleeding (i.e., approximately 18%) compared to total abdominal colectomy.[43]

Colitis

Inflammation of the colon can result from multiple disease processes, including IBD, infectious colitis, radiation proctitis after treatment for pelvic malignancies, and ischemia.

Ulcerative colitis (UC) is much more likely than Crohn disease to manifest with GIB. Most UC patients and about one-third of Crohn patients will experience gross bleeding at some point in their disease course.[45] Major acute hemorrhage from either form of IBD is rare. UC is a mucosal disease that begins in the rectum and can progress proximally to occasionally involve the entire colon. Patients typically present with diarrhea that may be bloody. Rectal inflammation results in small frequent bowel movements of up to 20 times a day, usually accompanied by crampy abdominal pain and tenesmus. Diagnosis is by careful history and colonoscopy with biopsy. The mainstays of treatment are supportive care with steroids, 5-aminosalicyclic acid compounds, immunomodulators, biologics, and antibiotics if indicated. Major hemorrhage from UC is rare. Bleeding will almost always be from a diffuse colitis with no discrete lesions amenable to endoscopic treatment. Urgent surgical therapy is occasionally needed because of ongoing bleeding but is more commonly indicated because of other complications of UC such as toxic megacolon or symptoms that are refractory to medical treatment.

Crohn disease is more typically associated with guaiac-positive diarrhea and mucous stools without gross blood. It can affect any portion of the GI tract and is characterized by skip lesions, transmural thickening and inflammation of the bowel wall, and granulomas. Diagnosis is by endoscopy, biopsy, and contrast studies. Medical management consists of steroids, 5-aminosalicylic acid compounds, antibiotics, immunomodulators, and biologics. Similar to UC, significant bleeding requiring intervention is rare in Crohn disease. In contrast, Crohn disease is more likely to have discrete lesions that can undergo endoscopic or angiographic intervention, usually in the form of an ulcer that has eroded into a vessel. These ulcers can occur anywhere in the upper or lower GI tract, including the small bowel.[45] Patients with long-standing disease may have strictures that impede passage of an endoscope.

Angiodysplasia/Arteriovenous Malformation

Angiodysplasias of the intestine are also referred to as arteriovenous malformations, angiectasias, and vascular ectasia. These are thought to be acquired degenerative lesions secondary to progressive dilatation of normal submucosal blood vessels due to venous obstruction and are distinct from true congenital arteriovenous malformations. They can be found anywhere in the GI tract, although typically they occur in the cecum, and accordingly, this is where they most often cause bleeding. Their prevalence increases with age, and they are associated with aortic stenosis and renal failure. There is no gender predilection. The presentation is similar to diverticular bleeding in that it is painless, usually self-limiting, and intermittent. Unlike diverticular bleeding, this tends to be venous bleeding, so it is less brisk and often occult and will present more often as chronic bleeding. Nevertheless, the hemorrhage can be significant in up to 15% of cases.

Diagnosis is by colonoscopy or angiography. CT scan is emerging as another reliable modality for diagnosis. On colonoscopy, these lesions appear as flat, bright-red, stellate lesions with a surrounding rim of pale mucosa. Angiography demonstrates dilated, slowly emptying veins and sometimes early venous filling. Incidentally discovered lesions do not require any further treatment. When treated endoscopically, noncontact thermal therapy with argon plasma coagulation is the preferred method. Angiographic techniques can also be used for hemostasis. If the bleeding has been localized and these attempts at hemostasis fail or bleeding recurs, segmental colon resection, most commonly right colectomy, is also effective.

Neoplasms

Colon cancer is an uncommon cause of significant LGIB, but it is essential to rule out the possibility of a colon malignancy in any patient with LGIB or iron-deficient anemia. The bleeding is usually painless, intermittent, and slow in nature. Colonoscopy is the gold standard for diagnosis, except in massive hemorrhage, where CTA, angiography, or emergent surgery may be necessary.

Another neoplastic cause for bleeding is GIST. GISTs are the most common soft tissue sarcoma in the digestive tract, with bleeding evident in 20% to 30% of cases. GISTs tend to present more frequently in the stomach and small intestine but can also affect the colon. Erosion into a blood vessel or alteration of the mucosal blood supply by local tumor growth leads to hemorrhage. Endoscopy is the best diagnostic tool. Oncologic resection based on the malignant risk of the tumor is needed to address this source.

Small bowel tumors are not common but can be sources of occult or frank GIB. Small bowel tumors are typically diagnosed by small bowel contrast series or spiral CT scan. Treatment involves surgical resection.

Intestinal polyps are rare sources of blood loss and more commonly present as an iatrogenic bled after polypectomy. In the pediatric population, they represent the second most common cause of bleeding. If the bleeding is attributable to a polyp, it can usually be treated with endoscopic therapy.

Ischemia

Insufficient blood flow to the intestinal tract may be due to cardiogenic shock or low flow states, mesenteric vascular disease, or diversion of flow from the splanchnic circulation (embolism, vasopressors, vascular surgery). Mesenteric ischemia should be considered in any patient with bleeding with a past medical history of cardiovascular disease, peripheral vascular disease, or vasculitis. Additionally, the diagnosis should be entertained in any patient with recent abdominal vascular surgery, shock, or hypercoagulable states or on high-dose vasopressors. Acute colonic ischemia is the most common form of mesenteric ischemia. It tends to occur in the watershed areas of the splenic flexure and the rectosigmoid colon but can be right sided in up to 40% of patients. Patients present with a characteristic "pain out of proportion to exam" and diarrhea that is often guaiac positive or bloody from mucosal degradation. CT may show thickened bowel wall, pneumatosis, or more subtle signs of vascular disease such as calcification of the takeoff of the mesenteric vasculature. The diagnosis is generally confirmed with flexible endoscopy, which reveals an abnormal mucosa. Treatment is supportive and consists of bowel rest, IV antibiotics, support of blood pressure, and correction of the low-flow state. In 85% of cases, the ischemia is self-limited and resolves without incident, although some patients develop a delayed colonic stricture. In the other 15% of cases, surgery is indicated because of progressive ischemia and gangrene. Marked leukocytosis, fever, ongoing resuscitation, lactic acidosis, or severe pain indicate ongoing ischemia and the likely need for surgical resection and an end ostomy creation.[46]

Infectious

Infectious colitis may present with bleeding. History, laboratory assessment, and culture data can inform the diagnosis. The two most notable organisms that can lead to LGIB are *Clostridium difficile* and cytomegalovirus. *C. difficile* colitis represents the overgrowth of a pathogenic clostridial bacterium that thrives after disruption of the normal gut microflora after antibiotic use. Explosive, voluminous, and, at times, bloody bowel movements can result from severe cases with associated mucosal sloughing. Profound leukocytosis is often observed as well as a characteristic foul smell. Treatment consists of stopping antibiotics, supportive care, and taking oral or IV metronidazole, oral vancomycin, or fidaxomicin.

Cytomegalovirus colitis should be suspected in any immunocompromised patient who presents with bloody diarrhea. Endoscopy with biopsy confirms the diagnosis; treatment is IV ganciclovir.

Diverticula

Meckel diverticula are congenital remnants of the vitelline duct that may contain either gastric or pancreatic ectopic tissue. Bleeding results from ulceration of the neighboring ileal tissue from irritation from an active focus of gastric mucosa. Bleeding is typically painless LGIB. Diagnosis can be made with capsule studies, CT, or with angiography in the setting of active bleeding. Angiographic findings aside from bleeding may include the presence of the vitelline artery, a superior mesenteric artery branch that is pathognomonic. A Meckel diverticulum scan, performed by administration of ^{99m}Tc-pertechnetate, can demonstrate ectopic gastric mucosa that can be localized with scintigraphy. Definitive treatment is surgical resection of the segment with care to incorporate the ulcerated ileal tissue, typically on the intestinal wall opposite the diverticulum.[47] Small bowel diverticula are also occasionally the source of bleeding, which is often occult. Diagnosis may be suspected based on a history of known small bowel diverticula, capsule endoscopy, or angiography. Definitive management is surgical resection.

Radiation Therapy

The use of radiation to treat pelvic cancers can be associated with bleeding-related complications. Bleeding from enteritis and, more commonly, proctitis complicates 1% to 5% of treated patients. Bleeding results from mucosal changes that, on endoscopy, reveal friability, angioectasias, and ulcerations. The American Society of Colon and Rectal Surgeons has published guidelines for therapy, which include strong recommendations for treatment with formalin 4% to 10%, sucralfate enemas, and hyperbaric oxygen. Endoscopic therapy with argon coagulation is additionally recommended as an effective treatment but is associated with fistula and stricture formation in 3% of patients.[48]

SELECTED REFERENCES

de Franchis R. Expanding consensus in portal hypertension: report of the Baveno VI Consensus Workshop: stratifying risk and individualizing care for portal hypertension. *J Hepatol.* 2015;63:743–752.

This consensus paper is the result of the most recent Baveno Consensus Workshop, a recurring meeting of international experts in the field of portal hypertension. The 2015 meeting focused on the topics of invasive and noninvasive methods for screening and surveillance of gastroesophageal varices and of portal hypertension, the impact of etiologic therapy for cirrhosis, the primary prevention of decompensation, the management of the acute bleeding episode, the prevention of recurrent hemorrhage and other decompensating events, and vascular diseases of the liver in cirrhotic and noncirrhotic patients.

Gurudu SR, Bruining DH, Acosta RD, et al. The role of endoscopy in the management of suspected small-bowel bleeding. *Gastrointest Endosc.* 2017;85:22–31.

Practice guidelines from the American Society for Gastrointestinal Endoscopy for the use of gastrointestinal endoscopy in small bowel bleeding.

Pasha SF, Leighton JA. Evidence-based guide on capsule endoscopy for small bowel bleeding. *Gastroenterol Hepatol (N Y).* 2017;13:88–93.

Capsule endoscopy is the test of choice to evaluate for small bowel bleeding when other gastrointestinal sources have been ruled out. This paper provides a comprehensive review of capsule endoscopy, covering topics a clinician should be familiar with when considering the use of this diagnostic tool.

Strate LL, Gralnek IM. ACG clinical guideline: management of patients with acute lower gastrointestinal bleeding. *Am J Gastroenterol.* 2016;111:755.

American College of Gastroenterology guidelines and literature review for management of acute lower gastrointestinal bleeding. It includes evidenced-based recommendations for resuscitation, risk stratification, diagnosis, and specific treatment modalities.

Tielleman T, Bujanda D, Cryer B. Epidemiology and risk factors for upper gastrointestinal bleeding. *Gastrointest Endosc Clin N Am.* 2015;25:415–428.

Describes historical as well as more recently identified risk factors for upper gastrointestinal bleeding.

Villanueva C, Colomo A, Bosch A, et al. Transfusion strategies for acute upper gastrointestinal bleeding. *N Engl J Med.* 2013;368:11–21.

Randomized trial comparing restrictive to liberal transfusion strategies in patients with acute upper gastrointestinal bleeding.

Wang YR, Richter JE, Dempsey DT. Trends and outcomes of hospitalizations for peptic ulcer disease in the United States, 1993 to 2006. *Ann Surg.* 2010;251:51–58.

This study describes the changes in epidemiology and outcomes of peptic ulcer disease as the approach to medical and surgical treatment has changed over time.

REFERENCES

1. Peery AF, Crockett SD, Barritt AS, et al. Burden of gastrointestinal, liver, and pancreatic diseases in the United States. *Gastroenterology.* 2015;149:1731–1741.e1733.
2. Nguyen NH, Khera R, Ohno-Machado L, et al. Annual burden and costs of hospitalization for high-need, high-cost patients with chronic gastrointestinal and liver diseases. *Clin Gastroenterol Hepatol.* 2018;16:1284–1292.e1230.
3. Abougergi MS, Travis AC, Saltzman JR. The in-hospital mortality rate for upper GI hemorrhage has decreased over 2 decades in the United States: a nationwide analysis. *Gastrointest Endosc.* 2015;81:882–888.e881.
4. Lanas A, Garcia-Rodriguez LA, Polo-Tomas M, et al. Time trends and impact of upper and lower gastrointestinal bleeding and perforation in clinical practice. *Am J Gastroenterol.* 2009;104:1633–1641.
5. Cannon JW. Hemorrhagic shock. *N Engl J Med.* 2018;378:370–379.
6. Etchill EW, Myers SP, McDaniel LM, et al. Should all massively transfused patients be treated equally? An analysis of massive transfusion ratios in the nontrauma setting. *Crit Care Med.* 2017;45:1311–1316.
7. Fabricius R, Svenningsen P, Hillingso J, et al. Effect of transfusion strategy in acute non-variceal upper gastrointestinal bleeding: a nationwide study of 5861 hospital admissions in Denmark. *World J Surg.* 2016;40:1129–1136.
8. Gonzalez E, Moore EE, Moore HB, et al. Goal-directed hemostatic resuscitation of trauma-induced coagulopathy: a pragmatic randomized clinical trial comparing a

viscoelastic assay to conventional coagulation assays. *Ann Surg*. 2016;263:1051–1059.

9. Villanueva C, Colomo A, Bosch A, et al. Transfusion strategies for acute upper gastrointestinal bleeding. *N Engl J Med*. 2013;368:11–21.
10. Cappell MS, Friedel D. Initial management of acute upper gastrointestinal bleeding: from initial evaluation up to gastrointestinal endoscopy. *Med Clin North Am*. 2008;92:491–509, xi.
11. Jacovides CL, Nadolski G, Allen SR, et al. Arteriography for lower gastrointestinal hemorrhage: role of preceding abdominal computed tomographic angiogram in diagnosis and localization. *JAMA Surg*. 2015;150:650–656.
12. Marti M, Artigas JM, Garzon G, et al. Acute lower intestinal bleeding: feasibility and diagnostic performance of CT angiography. *Radiology*. 2012;262:109–116.
13. Gralnek IM, Neeman Z, Strate LL. Acute lower gastrointestinal bleeding. *N Engl J Med*. 2017;376:1054–1063.
14. Strate LL, Gralnek IM. ACG clinical guideline: management of patients with acute lower gastrointestinal bleeding. *Am J Gastroenterol*. 2016;111:755.
15. Pasha SF, Leighton JA. Evidence-based guide on capsule endoscopy for small bowel bleeding. *Gastroenterol Hepatol (N Y)*. 2017;13:88–93.
16. Gurudu SR, Bruining DH, Acosta RD, et al. The role of endoscopy in the management of suspected small-bowel bleeding. *Gastrointest Endosc*. 2017;85:22–31.
17. Tielleman T, Bujanda D, Cryer B. Epidemiology and risk factors for upper gastrointestinal bleeding. *Gastrointest Endosc Clin N Am*. 2015;25:415–428.
18. Wang YR, Richter JE, Dempsey DT. Trends and outcomes of hospitalizations for peptic ulcer disease in the United States, 1993 to 2006. *Ann Surg*. 2010;251:51–58.
19. Laine L. Clinical practice. Upper gastrointestinal bleeding due to a peptic ulcer. *N Engl J Med*. 2016;374:2367–2376.
20. Sreedharan A, Martin J, Leontiadis GI, et al. Proton pump inhibitor treatment initiated prior to endoscopic diagnosis in upper gastrointestinal bleeding. *Cochrane Database Syst Rev*. 2010:CD005415.
21. Gisbert JP, Khorrami S, Carballo F. *H.pylori* eradication therapy vs. antisecretory non-eradication therapy (with or without long-term maintenance antisecretory therapy) for the prevention of recurrent bleeding from peptic ulcer. *Cochrane Database Syst Rev*. 2003:CD004062.
22. Chan FK, Wong VW, Suen BY, et al. Combination of a cyclo-oxygenase-2 inhibitor and a proton-pump inhibitor for prevention of recurrent ulcer bleeding in patients at very high risk: a double-blind, randomised trial. *Lancet*. 2007;369:1621–1626.
23. McNeil JJ, Wolfe R, Woods RL, et al. Effect of aspirin on cardiovascular events and bleeding in the healthy elderly. *N Engl J Med*. 2018;379:1509–1518.
24. Sung JJ, Lau JY, Ching JY, et al. Continuation of low-dose aspirin therapy in peptic ulcer bleeding: a randomized trial. *Ann Intern Med*. 2010;152:1–9.
25. Laine L, McQuaid KR. Endoscopic therapy for bleeding ulcers: an evidence-based approach based on meta-analyses of randomized controlled trials. *Clin Gastroenterol Hepatol*. 2009;7:33–47; quiz 31–32.
26. Lau JY, Sung JJ, Lam YH, et al. Endoscopic retreatment compared with surgery in patients with recurrent bleeding after initial endoscopic control of bleeding ulcers. *N Engl J Med*. 1999;340:751–756.
27. Kim JS, Park SM, Kim BW. Endoscopic management of peptic ulcer bleeding. *Clin Endosc*. 205;48:106–111.
28. Ramaswamy RS, Choi HW, Mouser HC, et al. Role of interventional radiology in the management of acute gastrointestinal bleeding. *World J Radiol*. 2014;6:82–92.
29. Elmunzer BJ, Young SD, Inadomi JM, et al. Systematic review of the predictors of recurrent hemorrhage after endoscopic hemostatic therapy for bleeding peptic ulcers. *Am J Gastroenterol*. 2008;103:2625–2632; quiz 2633.
30. Nguyen DC, Jackson CS. The Dieulafoy's lesion: an update on evaluation, diagnosis, and management. *J Clin Gastroenterol*. 2015;49:541–549.
31. Berry R, Han J, Girotra M, et al. Hemobilia: perspective and role of the advanced endoscopist. *Gastroenterol Res Pract*. 2018;2018:3670739.
32. Deijen CL, Smulders YM, Coveliers HME, et al. The Importance of early diagnosis and treatment of patients with aortoenteric fistulas presenting with Herald bleeds. *Ann Vasc Surg*. 2016;36:28–34.
33. Ferreira J, Tavares AB, Costa E, et al. Hemosuccus pancreaticus: a rare complication of chronic pancreatitis. *BMJ Case Rep*. 2015;2015.
34. Silecchia G, Iossa A. Complications of staple line and anastomoses following laparoscopic bariatric surgery. *Ann Gastroenterol*. 2018;31:56–64.
35. de Franchis R. Expanding consensus in portal hypertension: report of the Baveno VI Consensus Workshop: stratifying risk and individualizing care for portal hypertension. *J Hepatol*. 2015;63:743–752.
36. Zehetner J, Shamiyeh A, Wayand W, et al. Results of a new method to stop acute bleeding from esophageal varices: implantation of a self-expanding stent. *Surg Endosc*. 2008;22:2149–2152.
37. Laine L, Yang H, Chang SC, et al. Trends for incidence of hospitalization and death due to GI complications in the United States from 2001 to 2009. *Am J Gastroenterol*. 2012;107:1190–1195; quiz 1196.
38. Strate LL, Naumann CR. The role of colonoscopy and radiological procedures in the management of acute lower intestinal bleeding. *Clin Gastroenterol Hepatol*. 2010;8:333–343; quiz e344.
39. Niikura R, Nagata N, Shimbo T, et al. Natural history of bleeding risk in colonic diverticulosis patients: a long-term colonoscopy-based cohort study. *Aliment Pharmacol Ther*. 2015;41:888–894.
40. Zuckerman GR, Prakash C. Acute lower intestinal bleeding, part I: clinical presentation and diagnosis. *Gastrointest Endosc*. 1998;48:606–617.
41. Tabibian JH, Wong Kee, Song LM, et al. Technetium-labeled erythrocyte scintigraphy in acute gastrointestinal bleeding. *Int J Colorectal Dis*. 2013;28:1099–1105.
42. Bender JS, Wiencek RG, Bouwman DL. Morbidity and mortality following total abdominal colectomy for massive lower gastrointestinal bleeding. *Am Surg*. 1991;57:536–540; discussion 540–531.

43. Farner R, Lichliter W, Kuhn J, et al. Total colectomy versus limited colonic resection for acute lower gastrointestinal bleeding. *Am J Surg*. 1999;178:587–591.
44. Strate LL. Lower GI bleeding: epidemiology and diagnosis. *Gastroenterol Clin North Am*. 2005;34:643–664.
45. Pardi DS, Loftus Jr EV, Tremaine WJ, et al. Acute major gastrointestinal hemorrhage in inflammatory bowel disease. *Gastrointest Endosc*. 1999;49:153–157.
46. Walker AM, Bohn RL, Cali C, et al. Risk factors for colon ischemia. *Am J Gastroenterol*. 2004;99:1333–1337.
47. Hansen CC, Soreide K. Systematic review of epidemiology, presentation, and management of Meckel's diverticulum in the 21st century. *Medicine (Baltimore)*. 2018;97:e12154.
48. Paquette IM, Vogel JD, Abbas MA, et al. The American Society of Colon and Rectal Surgeons clinical practice guidelines for the treatment of chronic radiation proctitis. *Dis Colon Rectum*. 2018;61:1135–1140.

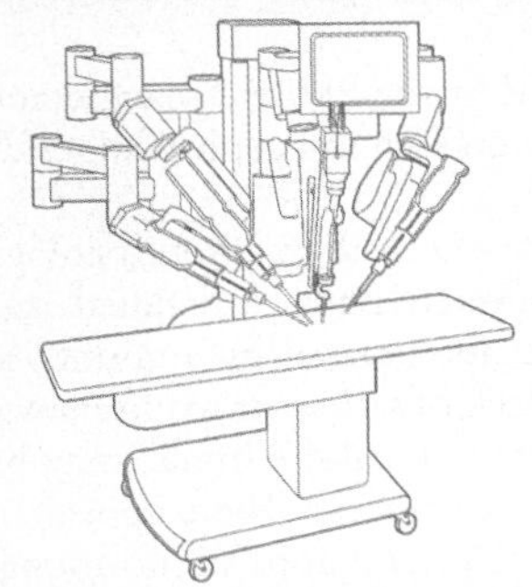

CHAPTER 48

Morbid Obesity

William O. Richards, Leena Khaitan, Alfonso Torquati

OUTLINE

Please access Elsevier eBooks for Practicing Clinicians to view the videos for this chapter https://expertconsult.inkling.com/.

OBESITY: THE MAGNITUDE OF THE PROBLEM

Until very recently, obesity was not recognized as a disease, which confounded the ability of physicians to be compensated for treatment they delivered and to treat the condition effectively. The American Medical Association (AMA) officially recognized obesity as a disease in 2013 and in 2014 voted to approve the resolution "that our AMA, advocate for patient access to the full continuum of care of evidence-based obesity treatment modalities (including surgical interventions)."

Morbid obesity is defined as being 100 lbs above ideal body weight, twice ideal body weight, or body mass index (BMI; measured as weight in kilograms divided by height in meters squared) of 40 kg/m^2. The last definition is more accepted internationally and has essentially replaced the former ones for all practical and scientific purposes. A consensus conference by the National Institutes of Health (NIH) in 1991 suggested that the term *severe obesity* is more appropriate for defining people of such size. This term is used interchangeably with *morbid obesity* in the remainder of this chapter.

The obesity epidemic in America continues to the point where nearly 40% of the U.S. adult population is obese, and prevalence of obesity in adolescents has increased to 18.5% in the most recent National Health and Nutrition Examination Survey (NHANES). The percentage of obese adults (BMI >30) in the United States increased 16 percentage points from 1980 to 2000, and increased by another 9 percentage points from 2000 to 2016.[1] There are also significant differences in the prevalence of obesity in adults by sex, race, and Hispanic origin. Non-Hispanic Asians (12.7%) had significantly lower rates of obesity than all other race and non-Hispanic origin groups. Non-Hispanic whites (37.9%) had a lower prevalence of obesity than non-Hispanic black (46.8%) and Hispanic adults (47%). Hispanic men (43.1%) had a greater prevalence of obesity compared to non-Hispanic Asian (10.1%) and non-Hispanic black men (36.9%).[1]

Worldwide, from 1975 to 2016, there has been a trend of increasing obesity in children and adolescents (age 5–19) in most regions of the world. The rate of increase in BMI has decreased in most high-income countries since 2000 albeit remaining at a high level. The rate of BMI increase, however, has accelerated in East, South, and Southeast Asia and is expected to surpass moderate to severe underweight children in those areas by 2022. Several countries (Nauru, Cook Islands, Palau, Niue, American Samoa) surpassed the United States in prevalence of obesity, while obesity was more than 20% or more in the United States, Polynesia, Micronesia, Middle East, and North Africa.[2]

The prevalence of morbidly obese adults (BMI >40) has increased to 6.3% of the adult United States population and is the second leading cause of preventable death in the United States. Morbid obesity is second only to smoking on the list of preventable factors responsible for increased health care costs. It is a sobering thought to realize that a 40-year-old morbidly obese man has a 12.4% reduction in life expectancy, or 9.1 years of life lost, compared with a normal-sized man. Moreover, the cost of care is staggering and may be as high as 9% of annual medical expenditures or $147 billion per year. There appears to be significant population heterogeneity between BMI and mortality that is attenuated by increasing age of the individual. Mortality also increases significantly even for individuals with minimal increases in BMI greater than 30.0. Thus, it appears that age, gender, race, and income level all play a role in the development of obesity and obesity-related mortality.[2]

PATHOPHYSIOLOGY AND ASSOCIATED MEDICAL PROBLEMS

The pathophysiology of severe obesity is multifactorial and has at its basis some genetic predisposition to obesity. There is a clear familial predisposition, and it is rare for a single-family member to have severe obesity. Scientists have identified specific genes that are associated with obesity, including the *FTO* gene (fat mass and obesity related) that plays a role in controlling feeding behavior and energy expenditure, the *MC4R* deficiency gene (melanocortin 4 receptor), which is associated with obesity, increased fat mass, and insulin resistance.[3]

Single gene mutations causing obesity are rare, and expressed during early childhood (Table 48.1). The most common single gene etiology of severe obesity is the MC4R, which induces appetite suppression (anorexigenic) effects on the hypothalamus in the regulation of energy homeostasis.[3] Recent studies have suggested that the cilium of MC4R neurons in the hypothalamus is the most common pathway underlying the genetic causes of human obesity (Table 48.1).[3]

Another theory suggests that bacteria within the gut, known as the microbiome, play an essential role in the metabolism and immune system. Simply giving subtherapeutic antibiotic treatment to mice for 4 weeks increases adiposity, plasma levels of insulin, leptin, and triglycerides when the mice are later fed a high-fat diet. The predilection to obesity is transferrable to other mice when the low-dose penicillin-selected gut bacteria are transferred to germ-free hosts, thus identifying that it is the action of the altered gut bacteria, not the antibiotics, that causes the obesity.[4] Recent studies have demonstrated that the gut microbiome circadian rhythm is disrupted by lifestyle differences in developed countries (shift work or jet lag), which provokes the development of altered microbial community, thus predisposing the host to obesity and glucose intolerance. Other studies have shown that degradation of dietary flavonoids through the altered microbiome results in diminished energy expenditure, which leads to obesity. It is fascinating to hypothesize that the current epidemic of obesity relates to changes in the microbiome created by the lifestyle changes and increased use of antibiotics in childhood seen in people who reside in developed countries.

Although there is no definitive answer to the pathophysiology of severe obesity, it is clear that a severely obese individual has, in general, persistent hunger that is not satiated by amounts of food that satisfy the nonobese. This lack of satiety or maintenance of hunger with corresponding increases in calorie intake may be the single most important factor in the process. There appear to be fundamental differences in the satiety and appetite hormonal control of eating that have created the current epidemic. This is hypothesized to occur when the brain's energy "set-point" rises to increase energy intake, through modulation of the individual's appetite.

We know that hormones, peptides, and vagal afferents to the brain have a major influence on satiety, appetite, and energy intake. Ghrelin, the only known orexigenic gut hormone, is also known as the hunger hormone and is secreted by P/D1 cells of the gastric fundus. Ghrelin stimulates release of various neuropeptides, such as neuropeptide Y (NPY) and growth hormone, from the hypothalamus, which creates an orexigenic or increased appetite state.[5] Increased levels of ghrelin produce increased food intake, and increased levels of ghrelin develop in individuals after low-calorie diets, thus suggesting that one possible mechanism for the failure of most diets after 6 months is the increase in the appetite hormone ghrelin.

One evolving concept is that the environment causes heritable change in gene function without modification of DNA sequences termed *gene-environment interactions*. The changes in the epigenome lead to the development of obesity and are much more common than either the monogenetic or the syndromic forms of obesity.[5]

Morbid obesity is a metabolic disease associated with numerous medical problems, some of which are virtually unknown in the absence of obesity. Box 48.1 lists the most common. These problems must be carefully considered when one is contemplating offering a patient weight reduction surgery. The most frequent problem is the combination of arthritis and degenerative joint disease, present in at least 50% of patients seeking surgery for severe obesity. The incidence of sleep apnea is high. Asthma is present in more than 25%, hypertension in more than 30%, diabetes in more than 20%, and gastroesophageal reflux in 20% to 30% of patients. The incidence of these conditions increases with age and the severity and duration of severe obesity.

The *metabolic syndrome* includes type 2 diabetes mellitus (insulin resistance), dyslipidemia, and hypertension. Patients with this constellation of problems are obese, with central body obesity being the primary essential feature (waist circumference >35 inches in women or >40 inches in men). The syndrome is characterized by impaired hepatic uptake of insulin, systemic hyperinsulinemia,

TABLE 48.1 Gene mutations associated with obesity.

GENE	EFFECT	ACTION ON	INHERITANCE	LINKED TO
Leptin/leptin receptor	Appetite stimulant	Hypothalamus	Autosomal recessive	Severe childhood obesity
Ghrelin receptor	Appetite stimulant	Hypothalamus	Autosomal recessive	Short stature and obesity
Melanocortin 4 receptor	Appetite inhibitor	Hypothalamus	Autosomal dominant	Increased fat mass, insulin resistance
Proopiomelanocortin (POMC)	Appetite inhibitor	Melanocortin 4 receptor in hypothalamus	Autosomal recessive	Severe early onset obesity by age 1 and excessive eating caused by insatiable hunger
Neuropeptide Y (NPY)	Appetite stimulant	Hypothalamus	Autosomal recessive	Hypertension, high low-density lipoprotein cholesterol, triglycerides, increased food intake and hunger

BOX 48.1 Medical conditions associated with severe obesity.

Cardiovascular
Hypertension
Sudden cardiac death myocardial infarction
Cardiomyopathy
Venous stasis disease
Deep venous thrombosis
Pulmonary hypertension
Right-sided heart failure

Pulmonary
Obstructive sleep apnea
Hypoventilation syndrome of obesity
Asthma

Metabolic
Metabolic syndrome (abdominal obesity, hypertension, dyslipidemia, insulin resistance)
Type 2 diabetes
Hyperlipidemia
Hypercholesterolemia
Nonalcoholic steatotic hepatitis (NASH) or nonalcoholic fatty liver disease (NAFLD)

Gastrointestinal
Gastroesophageal reflux disease
Cholelithiasis

Musculoskeletal
Degenerative joint disease
Lumbar disk disease
Osteoarthritis
Ventral hernias

Genitourinary
Stress urinary incontinence
End-stage renal disease (secondary to diabetes and hypertension)

Gynecologic
Menstrual irregularities

Skin/Integumentary System
Fungal infections
Boils, abscesses

Oncologic
Cancer of the thyroid, prostate, esophagus, kidney, stomach, colon, rectum, gallbladder, pancreas, female cancers of the breast, ovaries, cervix, and endometrium

Neurologic/Psychiatric
Pseudotumor cerebri
Depression
Low self-esteem
Stroke

Social/Societal
History of physical abuse
History of sexual abuse
Discrimination for employment
Social discrimination

and tissue resistance to insulin. Patients with metabolic syndrome are at high risk for early cardiovascular death.

Obesity has been shown to increase the risk of developing cancer of the thyroid, colon, rectum, esophagus, stomach, kidney, prostate, gallbladder, pancreas, breast (postmenopausal), endometrium, ovaries, and cervix.[5] There are several mechanisms that may be responsible for the increased risk of cancer. Obesity increases chronic inflammation, which is linked to the development of esophageal adenocarcinoma through chronic inflammation from gastroesophageal reflux disease (GERD). Fat produces excess levels of estrogen, which is linked to increased risk of endometrial, ovarian, and postmenopausal breast cancer. Increased levels of insulin and insulin-like growth factor 1 is hypothesized to be linked to the development of colon, prostate, kidney, endometrial, and postmenopausal breast cancer.[5]

Not listed in Box 48.1 are the associated societal discriminatory problems that severely obese individuals face. Public facilities in terms of seating, doorways, and restroom facilities often make access to events held in such settings unavailable to a severely obese person. Travel on public transportation is sometimes difficult, if not impossible. Employment discrimination clearly exists for these individuals. Finally, the combination of low self-esteem, a frequent history of sexual or physical abuse, and these social difficulties coalesce to create a very high incidence of depression in the population of morbidly obese patients.

MEDICAL VERSUS SURGICAL THERAPY

Medical therapy for severe obesity has limited short-term success and almost nonexistent long-term success. Once severely obese, the likelihood that a person will lose enough weight by dietary means alone and remain at a BMI below 35 kg/m^2 is estimated at 3% or less. The NIH consensus conference recognized that for this population of patients, medical therapy has been largely unsuccessful in treating the problem. Review of the clinical trials of lifestyle interventions for prevention of obesity demonstrated that the majority of trials were completely ineffective, and the few that were marginally effective had an extremely small impact on BMI.

One of the most remarkable stories in modern medicine has been the absolute superiority of bariatric surgery over medical therapy for the treatment of morbid obesity and its comorbidities. Multiple long-term follow-up trials comparing morbidly obese diabetics who underwent bariatric surgery with those who did not have shown decreased mortality long term after bariatric surgery as shown in Table 48.2.

The Swedish Obese Subjects (SOS) study is the first prospective controlled trial to provide long-term data on the effects of bariatric surgery on diabetes, cardiovascular events, cancer, and overall mortality. The study enrolled 2010 bariatric surgery subjects (gastric bypass, 13%; banding, 19%; vertical banded gastroplasty, 68%) and 2037 matched controls who received standard medical treatment and observed the subjects for 10 to 20 years. The SOS study was able to obtain follow-up on 98.9% of the subjects and found at 15 years after initiation that the surgery patients had lost 18% of their body weight, whereas the control group had only a 1% weight loss at 15 years. The long-term sustained weight loss and reduction in comorbid conditions after bariatric surgery resulted in a 29% reduction in mortality in the bariatric surgery patients (adjusted hazard ratio [HR], 0.71; 95% confidence interval, 0.54–0.92; $P = 0.01$), as shown in Fig. 48.1. The most common cause of death in the SOS study was cancer (47 in the control group and 29 in the surgery group). The incidence of myocardial infarction was significantly reduced in the surgery

TABLE 48.2 **Results of bariatric surgery compared to medically treated controls.**

STUDY	SURGERY MORTALITY RATE	MEDICAL MORTALITY RATE	ODDS RATIO OR HAZARD RATIO SURGICAL REDUCTION IN MORTALITY	NOTES
Swedish Obesity Study[6]	5.0%	6.3%	0.71 HR	Prospective trial of 2010 bariatric surgery and 2037 matched control patients, 15-year follow-up
Adams[7]	2.7%	4.1%	0.63 HR	Retrospective matched cohort of 7925 RYGB and 7925 severely obese control patients, mean follow-up 7.1 years
Guidry RYGB versus propensity-matched controls[9]	6.5%	12.7%	0.48 Odds ratio	Retrospective matched cohort of 401 RYGB and 401 matched control patients, 10-year follow-up
Arteburn[8]	13.8%	23.9%	0.47 HR	Veterans Affairs multisite cohort of 2500 bariatric surgery patients and 7462 matched control patients, 10-year follow-up
Kauppilia[10]	3.6%	15.2%	0.74 HR	5 Nordic countries, population-based study of 49,977 bariatric surgery patients and 494,842 who did not have surgery, 15-year follow-up

HR, Hazard ratio; *RYGB*, Roux-en-Y gastric bypass.

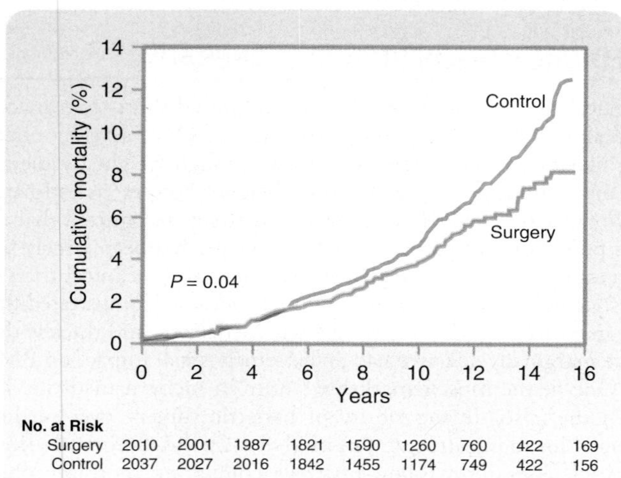

FIG. 48.1 Swedish obese subjects study weight loss for control and surgical subjects. (From Sjostrom L, Narbro K, Sjostrom CD, et al. Effects of bariatric surgery on mortality in Swedish obese subjects. *N Engl J Med.* 2007;357:741-752.)

group compared with the control group (HR, 0.56), and the surgery group had a lower number of first-time cardiovascular events (HR, 0.67) compared with the control group. Most strikingly, the SOS trial showed an 80% decrease in the annual mortality of diabetic individuals in the surgical weight loss group versus the matched control patients (9% mortality in the surgery group vs. 28% mortality in a control group).[6]

As can be seen in in Table 48.2, there are multiple studies with long-term follow-up comparing bariatric surgery to matched control groups and found the surgical groups have significant survival advantage (all cause, cancer, cardiovascular), associated with improvement in diabetes, obstructive sleep apnea, dyslipidemia, and hypertension.[6–10] These studies are convincing evidence that bariatric surgery provides long-term weight loss, resolution of comorbidities, and improvement in mortality. While the SOS study found improvement in all-cause mortality after 10 years of follow-up, the majority of procedures performed were vertical banded gastroplasty but Roux-en-Y gastric bypass (RYGB), a much more effective procedure comprised only 13% of the operations performed.[6] Since RYGB is a more effective procedure, it is not surprising that the Adams[7] and Guidry[9] studies, which compared RYGB to medical treatment, showed convincing mortality differences as early as 3 to 5 years after surgery, much earlier than the Swedish Obesity Study.[6] Similarly, Kauppila[10] studied 49,977 patients undergoing bariatric surgery, of which RYGB made up 73.4% of the operative procedures, and compared to a cohort of obese persons in five Nordic countries and found that all-cause mortality was reduced by 4 years and improved further at 15 years later.

Moreover, in the Adams study, the mortality for the first year was equal in the surgery and control groups (0.53% vs. 0.52%, respectively).[7] The Arterburn study[8] was from the Veterans Affairs (VA) hospitals in the United States, so it had a predominance of males (74% male) as opposed to all of the other reported trials having a majority of female subjects, but it also identified all-cause reduction in mortality at 5 years. The VA study is also remarkable for the higher first year mortality rate in the 2000 to 2005 period (HR, 1.66) than in the 2006 to 2011 period (HR, 0.88), which points to the improvements in surgical care occurring during this period. Despite the higher first year, mortality rate the all-cause mortality rate was lower for the surgery patients than the medical treated group after 5 to 14 years (HR, 0.47).[8]

Adams and colleagues[11] have recently updated the results of the trial reported in 2007 with outcomes measured 12 years after gastric bypass (N = 418) compared to 417 matched patients who sought but did not undergo surgery and to 321 patients who were matched but never sought to undergo surgery. The improvements in weight and comorbidity were continued at 12 years post-RYGB, as seen in Table 48.3.

The data from multiple studies comparing medical to surgical treatment strongly supports that bariatric surgery reduces long-term mortality. But does this long-term effect hold true for older patients who have a higher operative mortality and shorter time to see long-term benefits? Surprisingly, a cohort of 7925 morbidly

TABLE 48.3 Adjusted mean change from baseline at 12 years after RYGB in the Utah study.[11]

	RYGB	CONTROL GROUP 1	CONTROL GROUP 2
Weight loss	−26.9%	−2.0%	0.0%
Body mass index	−11.5	+0.1	+1.2
Glucose, mg/dL	−8.0	+14.4	+10.5
Systolic blood pressure	+0.1	+10.1	+8.3
LDL cholesterol	−11.0	+19.3	+16.5
HDL cholesterol	+12.9	−2.3	−3.3
Triglycerides	−62.8	+11.2	+11.7

HDL, High-density lipoprotein; *LDL*, low-density lipoprotein; *RYGB*, Roux-en-Y gastric bypass.

obese patients matched to an equal number of matched control patients not undergoing surgery showed that long-term mortality was lower in the surgery groups for patients age 35 and older. Patients younger than 35 had a significant increase in externally caused deaths (HR = 2.53, $P = 0.009$), which was even higher in young women (HR = 3.08, $P = 0.005$). Nevertheless, this study shows that older patients aged 55 to 74 years old had a significant reduction in long-term mortality and the highest reduction of long-term mortality was in men aged 55 to 74 years.[12]

One perception of bariatric surgery is that it may induce profound unalterable changes in eating that negatively affect the patients' health-related quality of life (HRQOL). A well-done 12-year prospective study evaluated HRQOL changes after gastric bypass surgery compared to two nonsurgical groups matched for similar demographics. The patients who underwent bariatric surgery had greatly improved QOL in the physical component from before surgery. There were also significant differences between the surgery patients and both nonsurgical groups for both the weight-related HRQOL and the physical HRQOL. The magnitude of improvement after 12 years after gastric bypass surgery from before surgery and between matched control groups supports the conclusion that bariatric surgery improves the patient's quality of life (QOL).[13] However, this study and the SOS study identified an increase in suicides and self-harm in patients undergoing bariatric surgery. The SOS study suicide and nonfatal health self-harm events were greater in the surgery group than in the matched controls ($N = 87$ and 49, respectively, out of 68,528 person-years, adjusted HR = 1.78). Analysis of the Utah long-term study[7] revealed that suicide and nonfatal self-harm events were more frequent after gastric bypass than in the intensive lifestyle group ($n = 341$ and 84, respectively, out of 149,582 person-years). The authors concluded that bariatric surgery, in particular gastric bypass, was associated with increased risk of suicide or self-harm, but the absolute risk and numbers of patients do not support not offering bariatric surgery to patients. They recommend that preoperative psychiatric mental health assessment and postoperative monitoring for mental health particularly substance abuse is needed.[14]

Metabolic Surgery Versus Medical Therapy for Diabetes

The Surgical Treatment and Medications Potentially Eradicate Diabetes Efficiently (STAMPEDE) trial[15] is 1 of 11 randomized controlled trials (RCTs) that have demonstrated the superiority of bariatric surgery over intensive medical therapy in type 2 diabetes. These trials have shown bariatric surgery to be more effective in glycemic control, weight loss, medication reduction, improvement in lipids, and in QOL, as shown in Fig. 48.2.[15–18] Metabolic surgery reduced hemoglobin A1c (HgbA1c) by 2% to 3.5% while medical therapy was only able to reduce HgbA1c by 1% to 1.5%. Short- and long-term (2- to 5- year) results shown in Table 48.4 demonstrate that a significant number of patients (28%–43%) undergoing laparoscopic RYGB (LRYGB) achieved HgbA1c levels less than 6 compared to only 5% to 7% of medically treated patients.[15–18] It is even more remarkable that the medically treated patients still required intensive medical therapy while the surgery patients had reduced or eliminated diabetic medications. Weight loss for both LRYGB and laparoscopic sleeve gastrectomy (LSG) was far superior to medical therapy. In the case of RYGB, the effect of duodenal bypass on the improvement in diabetes appears to be partially unrelated to weight loss, although in the STAMPEDE trial, the percentage weight loss attained at 1-year postoperative LRYGB was significantly associated with achieving HgbA1c less than 6 at 5 years postoperatively.[15] Thus, whereas there may be a benefit to bypassing the duodenum, the sustained long-term weight loss appears to be an essential element of the salutatory effects of RYGB on type 2 diabetes. LRYGB also improves the other associated medical conditions of the metabolic syndrome, including improvements in hypertension and high-density lipoprotein (HDL) cholesterol, as shown in Table 48.3, which results in reduced cardiovascular events/deaths. Specifically, diabetic patients who undergo bariatric surgery have a lower rate of incident microvascular disease (16.9% surgery vs. 34.7% medical), with an adjusted odds ratio (AOR) of 0.41. The reduced incidence rate of microvascular disease was largest in the reduction of nephropathy (59% reduction) but also present in diabetic neuropathy (63% reduction) and diabetic retinopathy (45% reduction).[19] The authors of this multi-institution study concluded that bariatric surgery not only improves glycemic control but also significantly reduced the incidence of microvascular disease, which improves survival. The authors argue that this additional evidence of improvement in microvascular disease should push primary care providers to talk to their obese diabetic patients about the benefits of bariatric surgery.[19]

BARIATRIC SURGERY MECHANISM OF ACTION

The first study reporting on the effectiveness of surgery in treating obesity and related comorbid conditions, published by Surgery, Gynecology & Obstetrics, in 1955 reported observing "the amelioration of diabetes mellitus following subtotal gastrectomy." A few decades later, the wide acceptance of bariatric surgery as treatment for severe obesity has given significant momentum to study the physiology of weight loss surgery. The initial prevailing theory behind bariatric surgery was based on two primary mechanisms for surgically induced weight loss: caloric restriction and nutrient malabsorption. There is little question that the reduction in caloric intake and resulting weight loss are responsible for much of the improvement in comorbidit-comorbidities after bariatric surgery. However, after taking into account the more recent scientific evidence, the concepts of restriction and malabsorption do not fully explain the metabolic effects of bariatric surgery. In fact, the mechanisms seem to extend beyond the magnitude of weight loss alone to include effects on central nervous system regulation of appetite and metabolism and improvements in insulin secretion and

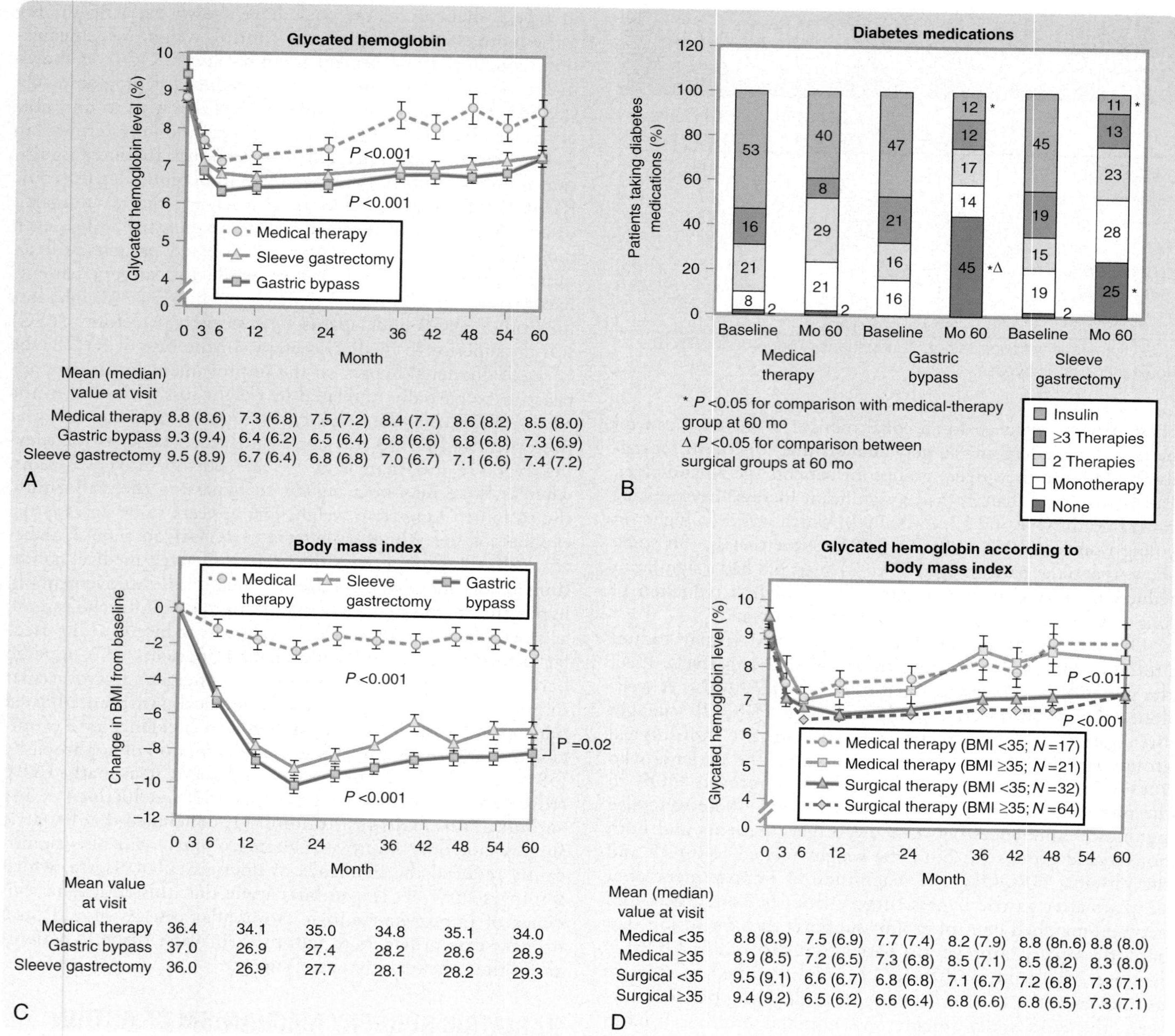

FIG. 48.2 *BMI*, Body mass index. (From Schauer PR, Bhatt DL, Kirwan JP, et al. Bariatric surgery versus intensive medical therapy for diabetes—5-year outcomes. *N Engl J Med.* 2017;376:641–651. Mean changes in measures of diabetes control from baseline to 5 years in medical and surgically treated subjects.)

insulin sensitivity. Long-term weight loss, improvement in glucose metabolism, and other metabolic effects clearly result from significant postoperative changes in the **enteroencephalic** and the **enteroinsular** endocrine axes, as shown in Table 48.5.

The Enteroencephalic Endocrine Axis

RYGB and LSG are known to increase satiety and reduce hunger. During the periprandial phase, the interplay between the gastrointestinal tract and the regulatory centers of the brain has been shown to activate complex neural networks to modulate food intake. In the central nervous system, the hypothalamus is the key area involved in the regulation of appetite. The hypothalamus regulates energy intake using a complex system of anorexic and orexigenic neuronal signaling. NPY is the dominant hormonal signal regulating energy intake. Release of NPY is modulated by hormones secreted into the circulation by gastrointestinal cells, such as ghrelin and peptide YY (PYY).

Ghrelin is secreted into the circulation by P/D1 cells located in the fundus of the stomach. Ghrelin levels increase significantly before a meal and levels quickly diminish postprandially. Ghrelin activates receptors in the arcuate nucleus and the lateral hypothalamus, stimulating the synthesis of NPY and agouti-related protein. This activation creates an orexigenic signal. The role of ghrelin in the postbariatric surgery regulation of appetite has been extensively studied, sometimes with controversial results. Most studies show that ghrelin levels fall significantly following LSG. In patients who undergo RYGB, the results of various studies are contradictory, especially when they compare fasting levels. A recent cross-sectional study performed by Svane and colleagues[20]

TABLE 48.4 Randomized prospective trials of bariatric surgery versus medical therapy in treatment of obese type 2 diabetics.

	SCHAUER[15] LRYGB	SCHAUER[15] LSG	IKRAMUDDIN[16] LRYGB	MINGRONE[17] LRYGB	SIMONSON[18] LRYGB
HgbA1c					
Medical therapy	5%*	5%*	7%	27%†	0%†
Surgery	29%*	23%*	38%	42%†	42%†
Change in Weight (Percentage or kg)					
Medical therapy	−5%	−5%	−7%	−6.9%	−5.2 kg
Surgery	−23%	−19%	−24%	−28.4%	−24.9 kg

HgbA1c, Hemoglobin A1c; *LRYGB*, laparoscopic Roux-en-Y gastric bypass; *LSG*, laparoscopic sleeve gastrectomy.
*HgbA1c <6.0%.
†HgbA1c <6.5%.

TABLE 48.5 Bariatric operations: mechanism of action.

	RESTRICTIVE	MALABSORPTION	ENTEROENCEPHALIC ENDOCRINE AXIS	ENTEROINSULAR AXIS
Vertical banded gastroplasty historical	++++	0	0	0
Lap adjustable gastric banding	++++	0	0	0
Laparoscopic sleeve gastrectomy	++++	+	++++	++
Roux-en-Y gastric bypass	++++	+++	++++	+++
Biliopancreatic diversion/duodenal switch	++	++++	+++	++++

has finally provided more definitive data regarding ghrelin levels during the periprandial period in postbariatric surgery patients. In this study, the postprandial areas under the curve (AUCs) for total and acylated ghrelin were significantly lower after LSG as compared with RYGB and controls. In addition, total ghrelin AUC was significantly lower after RYGB as compared with controls. This study provides significant evidence that anatomic changes after bariatric surgery reduce the postprandial secretion of ghrelin and thereby reduce hunger signals.

PYY is another hormone that acts on NPY neurons. L-cells found throughout the small and large intestines secrete PYY in response to the presence of nutrients within the lumen of the distal gut. PYY exerts an anorexigenic effect on NPY neurons. Svane and colleagues[20] showed that postprandial PYY levels are significantly affected by bariatric surgery. Patients after RYGB have significantly higher PYY peak and AUC than LSG and matched controls. No difference in PYY AUC was observed between LSG and matched obese controls.[20]

Enteroinsular Endocrine Axis

The remission/amelioration of type 2 diabetes mellitus is considered one of the major benefits after bariatric surgery. Although the mechanisms involved in type 2 diabetes mellitus remission are not completely understood, the improved insulin action, beta-cell function, and modulative effect of gut hormones in the enteroinsular axis appear to play a significant role. Among these hormones, glucagon-like peptide-1 (GLP-1) appears to be the major player. GLP-1 is released by L-cells in the distal gastrointestinal tract, and levels increase in response to the presence of nutrients in the lumen of the distal or hindgut intestines. In obese subjects, there is a delay in the postprandial release of GLP-1 and overall significantly reduced circulating levels of the peptide.[21] GLP-1 is known to exert anorexigenic effects in obese subjects secondary to a reduction in gastric emptying. However, GLP-1 action is more predominant in the enteroinsular axis. GLP-1 is part of a family of peptides involved in the synthesis, secretion, and regulation of insulin: the incretins. In the enteroinsular axis, GLP-1 has many physiologic functions, including the stimulation of insulin secretion by the pancreas, an increase in the insulin sensitivity of pancreatic cells (α-cells and β-cells), and inhibition of glucagon secretion. Many studies have shown that GLP-1 is a major driver of insulin secretion after bariatric surgery. GLP-1 has been found to be consistently elevated (peak and postprandial AUC) in response to both RYGB and LSG, with significant higher magnitude in RYGB than LSG. More important, the effect of both RYGB and LSG on postprandial GLP-1 secretion is not observed in subjects with an equivalent degree of weight loss achieved only by caloric restriction.[22] These results provide further evidence of a metabolic effect for bariatric surgery that it is independent of weight loss.

PREOPERATIVE EVALUATION AND SELECTION

Eligibility

Selection of patients for bariatric surgery is based on currently accepted NIH and American Heart Association/American College of Cardiology/The Obesity Society (AHA/ACC/TOS) guidelines. Patients must have a BMI greater than 40 kg/m^2 without associated comorbid medical conditions or a BMI greater than 35 kg/m^2 with an associated comorbid medical problem. They must have also failed dietary and behavioral therapy. Several criteria must also be used as guidelines for indications for surgery, including psychiatric stability, motivated attitude, and ability to comprehend the nature of the operation and its resultant changes in eating behavior and lifestyle. Criteria for eligibility for bariatric surgery are given in Box 48.2. An inability to fulfill these criteria is a contraindication to bariatric surgery.

One criterion not listed in Box 48.2 that unfortunately is often a significant issue for a severely obese patient is insurance coverage for the operation. The Affordable Care Act (ACA) mandates that patients covered under the ACA Marketplace health plans must receive obesity screening and counseling without charging of co-payment or coinsurance even if the patient has not met the yearly deductible. Remarkably, the ACA does not mandate coverage for bariatric surgery, and most Federal Marketplace insurance coverage does not cover bariatric surgery, despite that the writers of the ACA wanted to prevent bias against preexisting conditions and the overwhelming evidence that bariatric surgery is the only effective modality of long-term treatment in this population. Meanwhile, the medical societies recognize the need to refer severely obese individuals to bariatric surgeons particularly for the care of patients with type 2 diabetes. In the most recent guidelines, the ADA states: "Metabolic surgery should be recommended as an option to treat type 2 diabetes in appropriate surgical candidates with BMI >40 kg/m^2 (BMI >37.5 kg/m^2 in Asian Americans) who do not achieve durable weight loss and improvement in comorbidities (including hyperglycemia) with reasonable nonsurgical methods."[23]

The Centers for Medicare and Medicaid Services (CMS), the federal agency that sets Medicare guidelines, established criteria for coverage of bariatric surgery in 2006. The ruling required that only surgeons in hospitals that are designated Centers of Excellence perform bariatric surgery. The unique requirements for Medicare beneficiaries were at least partly due to concern by policymakers that the morbidity and mortality associated with bariatric surgery were high and that the explosive growth in the number of hospitals and surgeons performing the operations did not match the hospital oversight of these procedures and the resulting complications.

After the imposition of the CMS mandate in 2006, CMS removed the requirements for facility and surgeon certification to perform bariatric surgery in September 2013 partly based on improvements in bariatric surgery outcomes since the 2006 ruling. Today, greater than 88% of bariatric procedures are performed at Metabolic and Bariatric Accredited and Quality Improvement Programs (MBSAQIP).[24]

Accreditation, improvement in communication, and structured quality programs have been important in the improvements in quality of care. The American Society for Metabolic and Bariatric Surgery (ASMBS) has published recommendations on credentialing of bariatric surgeons by hospitals recently that include the need for active participation within a structured bariatric surgery program and quality improvement program. Although hospital-wide coordination of care, communication, and multidisciplinary teams must function well to achieve best results in bariatric surgery, the technical skill of the individual surgeon was highly correlated with significantly fewer complications, readmissions, reoperations, and visits to the emergency department.[25] There is considerable variation in serious complications within 30 days on the index bariatric procedure even among Bariatric Centers of Excellence. The differences in outcomes could not be totally explained by volume, case mix, or procedure type rates that the authors suggest are related to the skill of the individual surgeon and to inconsistent adherence to the pathways promulgated by the Centers of Excellence.[24] In summary, these studies show that the surgeon not only must achieve technical proficiency but also must engage the entire operative and hospital team to achieve excellent outcomes.

Bariatric operative mortality has declined around the world to remarkably low levels. In France, the mortality after 6056 laparoscopic adjustable gastric banding (LAGB) operations was zero in 2012 and LRYGB mortality has decreased threefold from 0.33% to 0.11% from 2008 to 2012.[26] In France, the independent factors associated with operative mortality were male sex (AOR, 1.94), age older than 50 (AOR, 3.69), BMI < 50 kg/m^2 (AOR, 2.05), and type 2 diabetes (AOR, 1.6). There was also a graded relationship between increased hospital volume and decreased operative mortality.[26]

BOX 48.2 Indications for bariatric surgery.

Patients must meet the following criteria for consideration for bariatric surgery:

- Body mass index (BMI) >40 kg/m^2 or BMI >35 kg/m^2 with an associated medical comorbidity worsened by obesity
- Failed dietary therapy
- Psychiatrically stable without alcohol dependence or illegal drug use
- Knowledgeable about the operation and its sequelae
- Motivated individual
- Medical problems not precluding probable survival from surgery

Medical contraindications to bariatric surgery are relative, and all patients with comorbid conditions are at greater risk. The surgeon must ensure that these risks are well understood by all patients before bariatric surgery, especially those at high risk. Ideally, several family members are included in these discussions. There are certain individuals who have end-stage organ dysfunction of the heart, lungs, or both. These patients are unlikely to gain the benefit of longevity and improved health.

Surgery is contraindicated in patients who are unable to ambulate because their level of debility precludes recovery during the rapid weight loss phase after surgery. Prader-Willi syndrome is another absolute contraindication because no surgical therapy affects the constant need to eat by these patients.

The U.S. Food and Drug Administration expanded the use of the LAP-BAND to include patients with BMI between 30 and 34 kg/m^2 who have an existing condition related to their obesity. Other contraindications to LAGB include cirrhosis, portal hypertension, autoimmune connective tissue disorders, chronic inflammatory conditions such as inflammatory bowel disease, and need for chronic administration of steroids.

Patients who weigh more than 500 lbs are at increased risk for mortality and have more complications. Many options for diagnostic testing, such as computed tomography (CT), are exceeded by this weight limit. At this weight, operating room tables, moving and lift equipment and teams, blood pressure cuffs, sequential compression device (SCD) boots, and any sort of invasive bedside procedures such as central venous catheters become extraordinarily difficult. It has been my practice to require patients weighing more than 500 lbs to lose weight down to that level by nonoperative methods.

Age is a controversial contraindication to bariatric surgery. For adolescents, most pediatric and bariatric surgeons recommend that the operation be performed after the major growth spurt (mid to late teens), thus allowing increased maturity on the part of the patient. The Teen–Longitudinal Assessment of Bariatric Surgery (Teen-LABS) demonstrated that severely obese teens (<19 years) had multiple comorbid conditions and could undergo one of three commonly performed operations (LRYGB, LSG, and LAGB) with no mortality and a favorable short-term complication profile. Three-year follow-up after LRYGB or LSG in Teen-LABS showed excellent and sustained weight loss and resolution of diabetes in 95% of patients who had type 2 diabetes at baseline, a figure far higher than the 50% to 70% of adult bariatric surgery patients. The authors hypothesize that adults accumulate pounds-years that are less reversible than in the adolescent population. They conclude LRYGB and LSG are effective at 3 years in adolescents.[27]

Although in our practice, we have generally set the age of 65 years as a rough cutoff for performing gastric bypass and 70 years for LSG, patients older than 70 years have been individually evaluated. Such evaluations focus on the patient's relative physiologic age and potential for longevity rather than chronologic age. The duration and degree of obesity are the most important factors in evaluating an older patient. In general, the duration and the severity of obesity and the number of comorbid medical problems that exist lower the potential for such individuals to benefit from bariatric surgery.

General Bariatric Preoperative Evaluation and Preparation

Preoperative assessment of a bariatric surgical patient involves two distinct areas. One is a specific preoperative assessment of candidacy for bariatric surgery and evaluation for comorbid conditions. The second is a general assessment and preoperative preparation as for any major abdominal surgery, which is discussed in depth in Chapter 10. A team approach is required for optimal care of a morbidly obese patient as shown in Box 48.3, and Box 48.4 summarizes the steps and tests routinely performed for the preoperative evaluation of bariatric patients in the author's clinics. Proper preoperative patient education is essential, and attendance at educational sessions is mandatory. After preoperative testing is completed, a final counseling session with the surgeon and an education session with the nurse educator and nutritionist are held.

Data support the use of preoperative antibiotics and deep venous thrombosis (DVT) prophylaxis. A first-generation cephalosporin, in a dose appropriate for weight, is given preoperatively, and antibiotics are continued for less than 24 hours. Bariatric surgery patients are at moderate to high risk for venous thromboembolism (VTE), and they should receive mechanical prophylaxis such as early ambulation and use of SCDs. Most patients are at moderate or high risk for VTE, and the preponderance of data suggests that both chemoprophylaxis and mechanical measures be used based on individual assessment of clinical judgment and risk of bleeding. The Michigan Bariatric Surgery Collaborative (MBSC) identified that preoperative and postoperative use of low-molecular-weight heparin was associated with significantly lower rates of VTE compared with patients given unfractionated heparin. High-risk patients (e.g., those with history of DVT, venous stasis ulcers, known or highly suspected pulmonary hypertension, hypoventilation syndrome of obesity, or need for reoperation during the initial hospitalization) are given low-molecular-weight heparin administered twice daily for a full 2-week course. The data are unclear about the use of prophylactic vena cava filters, and the ASMBS recommends their use only in combination with chemical and mechanical prophylaxis in extremely high-risk individuals in whom the risks of VTE are greater than filter-related complications.

BOX 48.3 The bariatric multidisciplinary team.

- Surgeon
- Assisting surgeon
- Nutritionist
- Anesthesiologist
- Operating room nurse
- Operating room scrub tech or nurse
- Nurse care coordinator or educator
- Secretary/administrator
- Psychiatrist/psychologist
- Primary care physician
- Medical specialists for cardiac, pulmonary, gastrointestinal, endocrine, musculoskeletal, and neurologic conditions as indicated

BOX 48.4 Preoperative evaluation and postoperative care.

Before the Clinic Visit
- Documented, medically supervised diet
- Counseling and referral from the primary care physician
- Reading a comprehensive written brochure and/or attendance at a seminar regarding operative procedures, expected results, and potential complications

Initial Clinic Visit
- Group presentation on information in the booklet
- Group presentation on preoperative and postoperative nutritional issues by the nutritionist
- Individual assessment by the surgeon's team
- Individual counseling session with the surgeon
- Individual counseling session with the nutritionist
- Screening blood tests

Subsequent Events/Evaluations
- Full psychological assessment and evaluation as indicated
- Medical specialist evaluations as indicated
- Insurance approval for coverage of the procedure
- Screening flexible upper endoscopy as indicated
- Screening ultrasound of the gallbladder (if present)
- Arterial blood gas analysis as indicated

Subsequent Clinic Visits
- Counseling session with the surgeon (including selection of the date for surgery)
- Education session with the nurse educator
- Preoperative evaluation by the anesthesiologist
- Final paperwork by the preadmissions center

Evaluation of Specific Comorbid Conditions

Cardiovascular evaluation of a bariatric patient must include a history of recent chest pain and functional assessment of activity in relation to cardiac function. Patients with a history of recent chest pain or a change in exercise tolerance need to undergo a formal cardiology assessment, including stress testing as indicated. We almost never resort to invasive central monitoring with a Swan-Ganz catheter because central venous and pulmonary hypertension is routinely present and must not be interpreted as volume overload.

The prevalence of obstructive sleep apnea diagnosed using sleep studies in the morbidly obese ranges between 35% and 94%, and the majority of the studies identified a prevalence of greater than 60%. A history of falling asleep while driving or while at work or a history of feeling tired after a night's sleep, coupled with a history of snoring or even witnessed apnea, is strongly suggestive of the condition. Patients with suggestive histories of clinically significant sleep apnea need to undergo preoperative sleep study testing. If the patient is found to have the condition, use of a continuous or bilevel positive airway pressure apparatus postoperatively while sleeping can eliminate the stressful periods of hypoxia that would otherwise result and has been found to reduce perioperative complications. Although tolerated under normal circumstances, these hypoxic episodes in the immediate postoperative period are more dangerous because of the enhanced effect of narcotic pain medications and postoperative fluid shifts that affect hemodynamic stability.

Reactive asthma is another common problem of the severely obese and one that is underrecognized. It requires less preoperative preparation in terms of testing than sleep apnea does and is less dangerous.

Hypoventilation syndrome of obesity (Pickwickian syndrome) is a diagnosis that should be suspected in the superobese (BMI >60) and by the patient's clinical appearance. Individuals with this diagnosis have plethoric faces, may appear clinically cyanotic, and clearly exhibit difficulty in normal respiratory efforts at baseline or with mild exertion. Arterial blood gas analysis reveals $Paco_2$ higher than Pao_2 and an elevated hematocrit. Pulmonary artery pressure is greatly elevated. These patients have significantly increased high cardiopulmonary morbidity and mortality and require significant preoperative weight loss and optimization of the patient's cardiopulmonary physiology before the operative procedure.

Because there is an increased incidence of hypertension or diabetes in patients with concomitant renal disease, the serum creatinine value is an excellent preoperative screening test for baseline renal function.

Musculoskeletal conditions, especially arthritis and degenerative joint disease, are the most common group of comorbid diseases found in severely obese patients. More than half the patients have some form of these conditions, often to an advanced degree. Limited ambulation, joint replacement, severe back pain, and other sequelae are not uncommon. Before surgery, it is important for patients to understand that any preexisting structural damage cannot be reversed by weight loss. Fortunately, significant weight loss often alleviates or even reverses the chronic pain or disability from such conditions. Significant weight loss after bariatric surgery will make subsequent knee and hip replacement surgery more effective and safer.

Metabolic problems are common in severely obese patients, particularly hyperlipidemia, hypercholesterolemia, and type 2 diabetes mellitus. All are easily screened for by simple blood tests. Twenty percent to 30% of severely obese patients undergoing bariatric surgery have clinically significant type 2 diabetes. Diabetes needs to be controlled preoperatively to reduce the incidence of perioperative morbidity.

The skin must be examined for fungal infection and venous stasis changes, which are associated with a greatly increased incidence of postoperative DVT. Umbilical or ventral hernias may be present. It has been our practice to postpone repair of ventral and incisional hernias until after significant weight loss. Repair of the hernias at the time of abdominoplasty enables the bariatric surgeon to complete physical reconstruction of the abdominal wall and to place prosthetic mesh to reinforce the abdominal wall, something that often cannot be accomplished during the initial bariatric procedure.

Cholelithiasis is the most prevalent of the several gastrointestinal conditions, and if gallstones are present, most surgeons agree that cholecystectomy needs to be performed simultaneously with the bariatric surgery. The incidence of gallstone or sludge formation after gastric bypass is approximately 30%. For patients undergoing malabsorptive operations, gallstone formation is so frequent that prophylactic cholecystectomy is a standard part of these procedures. However, for restrictive operations, screening ultrasound is recommended, particularly in patients undergoing LRYGB, because endoscopic retrograde cholangiopancreatography is not possible. Ursodeoxycholic acid, 300 mg twice daily for 6 months postoperatively, reduces the incidence of gallstone formation to 3% in patients who follow this treatment plan. Our current recommendations for patients undergoing laparoscopic bariatric surgery are simultaneous cholecystectomy if gallstones are present and ursodiol therapy for 6 months after surgery if the gallbladder is normal.

GERD is common in severely obese patients because of the increased abdominal pressure and shortened lower esophageal sphincter. Preoperative upper endoscopy is indicated in all patients who have GERD symptoms to detect Barrett esophagus and the presence of hiatal hernias and to evaluate the lower part of the stomach in patients undergoing RYGB.

A patient with nonalcoholic steatotic hepatitis (NASH) presents a potential problem. The size of the left lobe of the liver often inhibits the surgeon's ability to complete an operation laparoscopically. Patients with known enlarged fatty livers may benefit from calorie restriction, especially carbohydrate restriction, for a period of 5 to 10 days preoperatively. Bariatric surgery is beneficial for NASH; weight loss improves the prognosis. NASH is not a contraindication to bariatric surgery if there is no cirrhosis and portal hypertension or hepatocellular decompensation. Liver biopsy should be performed at the time of bariatric surgery in any patient whose liver appears abnormal.

Special Equipment

Clinic

The clinic for evaluating bariatric patients must be constructed with the needs of the patient in mind. The waiting area must contain comfortable benches with backs, not standard-size chairs. Doorways must be extra wide to accommodate wheelchairs. This is true for bathrooms as well, which must be equipped with toilets on the floor, not mounted on the wall. A scale that can weigh up to 800 lbs is necessary. Scales that use impedance to measure fat mass are useful in the evaluation and ongoing treatment of bariatric patients. The percentage of fat mass lost after surgery using the impedance scales is monitored to make sure that the patient is losing primarily fat mass and taking in enough protein to maintain muscle mass. Large-sized gowns, wide examining tables stable enough for large patients, and wide blood pressure cuffs are needed. A large room with appropriate seating is needed for the patient group education session.

Operating Room

The operating room needs to contain a hydraulically operated operating room table that can accommodate up to 800 lbs. Side attachments to widen the table as needed are required. Foam cushioning, extra-large SCD stockings, wide and secure padded straps for the abdomen and legs, and a footboard for the operating room table are all essential to safely secure the patient for placement in a steep reverse Trendelenburg position during surgery. Video telescopic equipment as used for any laparoscopic abdominal procedure is necessary. Two monitors, one near each shoulder, and high-flow insufflators able to maintain pneumoperitoneum are essential.

A 45-degree telescope, extra-long staplers, atraumatic graspers, extra-long trocars, and ultrasonic scalpel or other energy source instruments are essential for the laparoscopic operations. A fixed retractor device secured to the operating room table for clamping and holding the liver retractor is essential. This can pose one of the most difficult technical challenges in patients with a large, thick liver. Sometimes, two retractors may be necessary for a large liver.

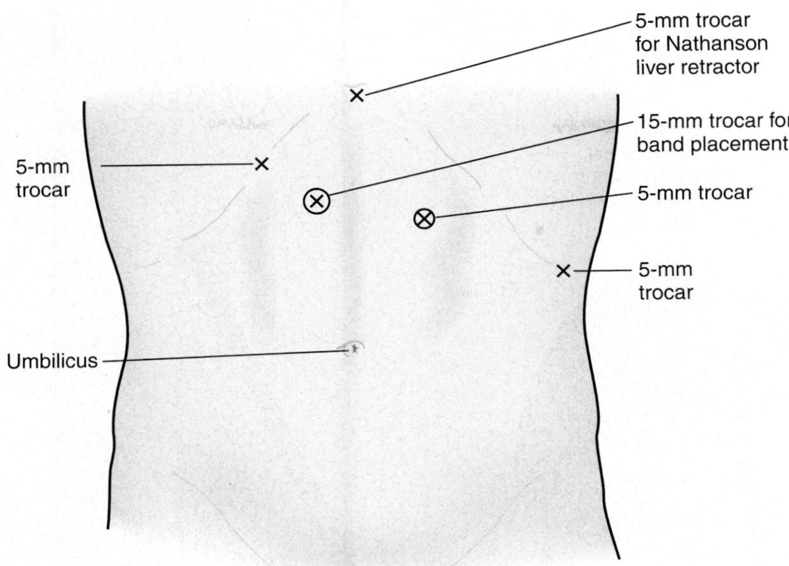

FIG. 48.3 Trocar location for adjustable gastric banding.

OPERATIVE PROCEDURES

Laparoscopic Adjustable Gastric Banding

The LAGB procedure may be performed with any of multiple types of adjustable bands. The techniques of placement of the bands are similar; only the locking mechanisms, band shape and configuration, and adjustment schedules vary somewhat for the different types of bands. Their advantage over other bariatric procedures is individualized adjustability and a markedly lower initial operative morbidity and mortality.

Trocar placement for LAGB is shown in Fig. 48.3. The surgeon stands to the patient's right; the assistant and the camera operator are to the patient's left. Most surgeons place the patient in the supine position, but some prefer to have the patient's legs spread so that the surgeon can stand between the legs. The peritoneum at the angle of His is divided to create an opening in the peritoneum between the angle of His and the top of the spleen (Fig. 48.4A). The laparoscope is placed through the left upper quadrant port for this part of the operation to maximally view the angle of His area.

The pars flaccida technique has become the approach of choice for placing the adjustable band; it begins with dividing the gastrohepatic ligament in its thin area just over the caudate lobe of the liver. The anterior branch of the vagus nerve is spared, and any aberrant left hepatic artery is preserved. The base of the right crus of the diaphragm is identified. Care must be taken to identify the crus because, occasionally, the vena cava can lie close to the caudate lobe. The surgeon gently follows the surface of the right crus posterior and inferior to the esophagus while aiming for the angle of His (Fig. 48.4B). A gentle spreading and pushing technique is used to create an avascular tunnel along this plane. Once the tip of the tunneling instrument is seen near the top of the spleen, it is gently pushed through any remaining peritoneal layers to complete the tunnel (Fig. 48.4C). The adjustable band has already been placed in the peritoneal cavity through the large 15-mm trocar located in the right upper quadrant before dissection of the pars flaccida. The narrow end of the band itself is grasped by the tunneling instrument and pulled through the tunnel from the greater to the lesser side of the stomach (Fig. 48.5). That end is then threaded through the locking mechanism of the band, after which the band is locked. Once the band has been locked in place, the buckle is adjusted to lie on the lesser curvature side of the stomach (Fig. 48.6). A 5-mm grasper inserted between the band and stomach ensures that the band is not too tight.

The anterior gastric wall is plicated over the band with three or four interrupted, nonabsorbable sutures (Fig. 48.7). There needs to be just enough stomach above the level of the band for incorporating that tissue into the suture. Suturing is carried as far posterolaterally as possible because this region has been the most frequent area of fundus herniation through the band. The band is thus ideally secured about 1 cm below the gastroesophageal junction with this technique.

The Silastic tubing leading from the band is pulled through the 15-mm trocar site in the right upper quadrant paramedian area to complete the laparoscopic portion of the operation. The trocar site incision is enlarged to reveal the anterior rectus fascia, which is exposed approximately 2 to 4 cm lateral to the existing fascial defect for the trocar, and the access port is connected to the inflation tubing. Four sutures inserted through the four holes on the access port are placed in the fascia, after which the port is tied to the fascia (Fig. 48.8). The redundant tubing is replaced in the abdominal cavity, with care taken to avoid kinking.

Roux-en-Y Gastric Bypass

The gastric bypass first described by Mason and Ito in 1969 incorporated a loop of jejunum anastomosed to a proximal gastric pouch. This operation proved unacceptable because of bile reflux, and RYGB, which eliminates bile reflux, has become one of the most commonly performed bariatric operations in the United States.

Described here is one technique that incorporates many of these modifications. There are certainly many variations of this technique, and many, if not most, will give excellent results. The essential principles of the operation are listed in Table 48.6.

The left subcostal region, near the midclavicular line, is an ideal location for the first trocar. Either a bladed trocar (United States Surgical Corporation, Norwalk, CT) or an optical trocar (Optiview, Ethicon Endo-Surgery) that dilates a tract under direct vision is placed. Subsequent trocars are placed under laparoscopic vision to achieve the configuration shown in Fig. 48.9.

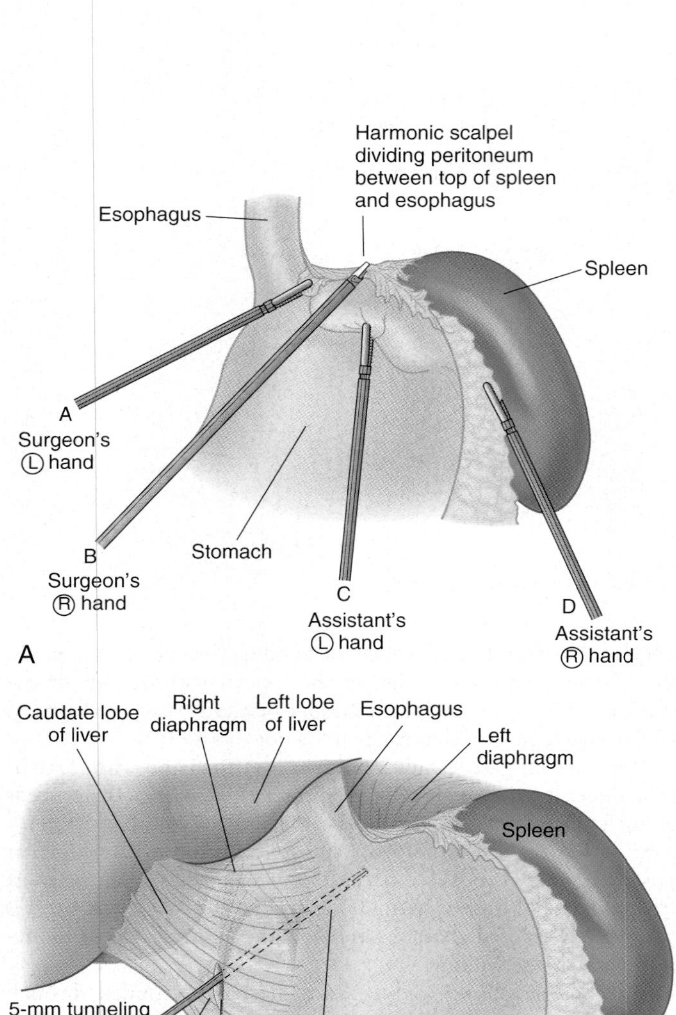

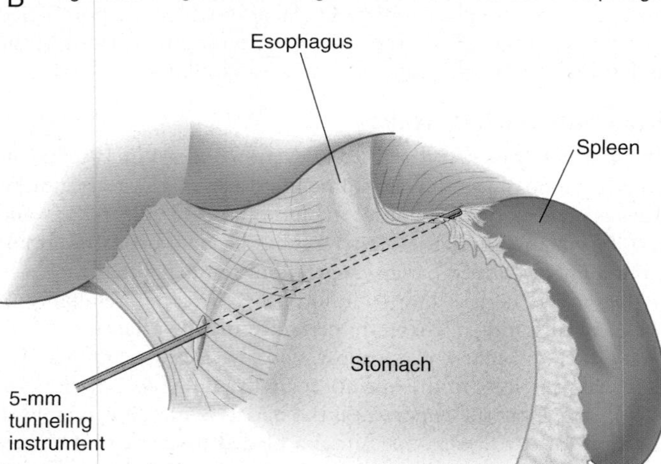

FIG. 48.4 (A) Dividing the peritoneum at the angle of His. (B) Pars flaccida technique in which the fat pad is divided at the base of the right crus. (C) Tunnel posterior to the stomach completed.

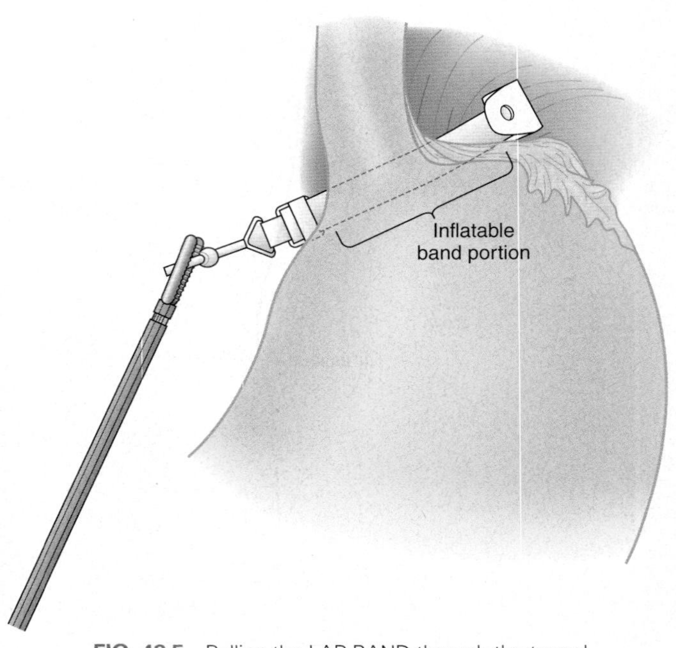

FIG. 48.5 Pulling the LAP-BAND through the tunnel.

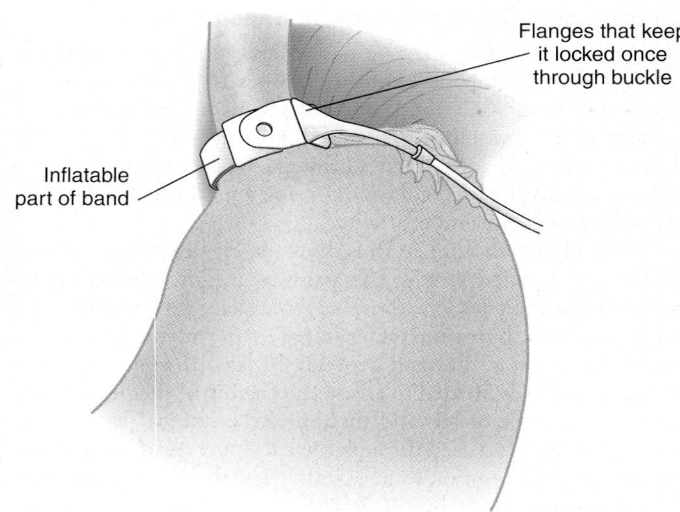

FIG. 48.6 Locking the LAP-BAND.

Once the omentum is mobilized, the ligament of Treitz is identified. A location approximately 30 to 40 cm distal to the ligament is chosen for division of the jejunum with an endoscopic stapler (Fig. 48.10). The mesentery is then further divided with staples or a harmonic scalpel.

The length of the Roux limb is influenced in our practices by the patient's weight. Patients with a BMI in the 40s will be well served with a Roux limb of 80 to 120 cm, whereas a Roux limb of approximately 150 cm is constructed for patients with a BMI in excess of 50. The proximal jejunum is left to lay to the patient's right side, and the Roux limb is lifted cephalad and coiled in the curve of the transverse colon mesentery (Fig. 48.11). This technique allows the proximal jejunum to be aligned directly alongside the designated point on the Roux limb for the distal anastomosis. The stapler is placed through the surgeon's right-hand port because the bowel segments are easily aligned to facilitate placement of the stapler into enterotomies created in each segment of bowel

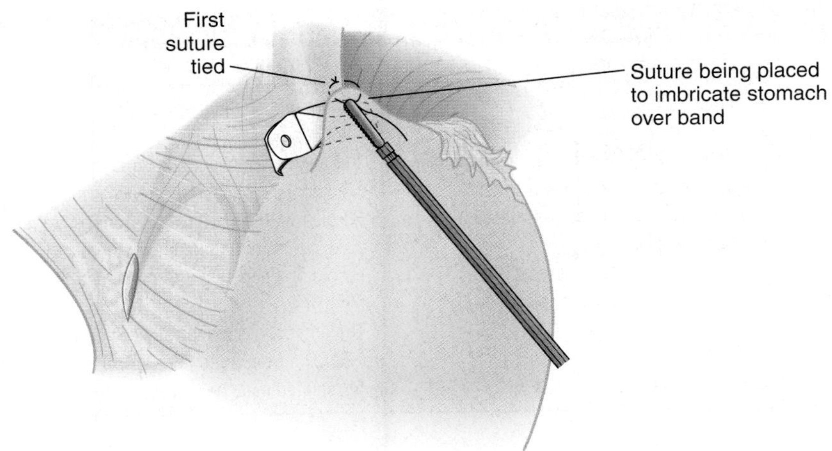

FIG. 48.7 Imbricating the anterior aspect of the stomach over the LAP-BAND.

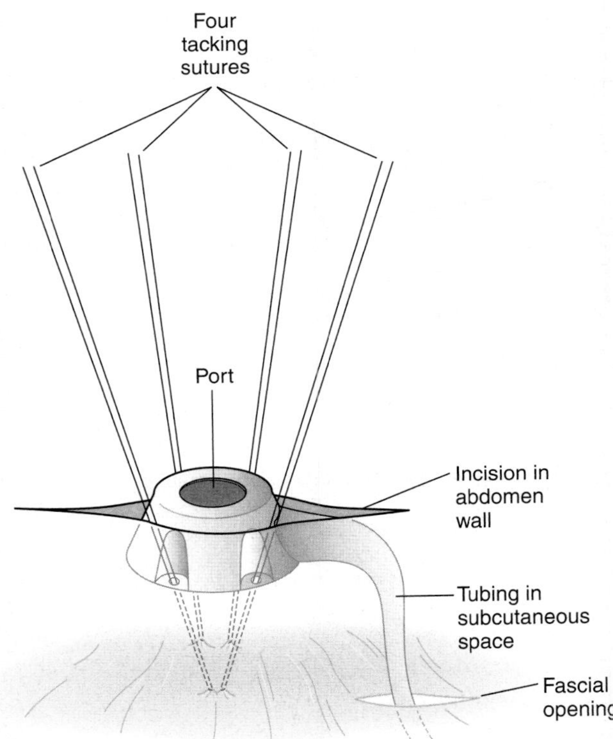

FIG. 48.8 Passing the inflation tubing through the abdominal wall sufficiently far from the port site to prevent acute kinking of the tubing.

at the desired location of the anastomosis (Fig. 48.12). Another firing of the stapler, this time from the left side of the patient, creates a large side-to-side anastomosis. Once the anastomosis is created, the stapler defect is closed with another fire of the stapler.

The left lobe liver retractor is now placed, and the patient is placed in the reverse Trendelenburg position. Exposure of the angle of His allows division of the peritoneum between the top of the spleen and the gastroesophageal junction with the ultrasonic scalpel. The lesser sac is entered through the gastrohepatic ligament, 3 to 4 cm below the gastroesophageal junction. The blue load of the linear stapler is now fired multiple times to create a 10- to 15-mL proximal gastric pouch based on the upper lesser curvature of the stomach (Fig. 48.13). Once the gastric pouch is created, the Roux limb may be passed toward the proximal gastric pouch through a retrocolic or antecolic pathway. The antecolic, antegastric approach is preferred to prevent the risk of an internal hernia through the transverse mesocolon or a hernia formed by the transverse mesocolon and the mesentery of the Roux limb in the retrocolic approach. The gastrojejunostomy may be performed with a circular stapler (Fig. 48.14) or a hand-sutured technique. The entire anastomosis is irrigated with saline, and a member of the operative team uses the endoscope to monitor occlusion of the Roux limb with an atraumatic 10-mm bowel clamp. Even the smallest leaks of air can be identified and closed with this technique. Studies have shown that use of this technique can dramatically reduce the incidence of postoperative leaks to very low levels. The mesenteric defect in the jejunojejunostomy is closed with a purse-string suture of 2-0 polypropylene that, combined with the antecolic Roux limb approach, has virtually eliminated a subsequent internal hernia (Fig. 48.15 and Table 48.6).

Biliopancreatic Diversion

Biliopancreatic diversion (BPD), like most bariatric operations that had been performed through an open approach, can be performed through a laparoscopic approach. BPD produces weight loss primarily based on malabsorption, but it does have a restrictive component as well.

The anatomic configuration of BPD is shown in Fig. 48.16. The intestinal tract is reconstructed to allow only a short, so-called common channel of the distal 50 cm of terminal ileum for absorption of fat and protein. The alimentary tract beyond the proximal part of the stomach is rearranged to include only the distal 200 cm of ileum, including the common channel. The proximal end of this ileum is anastomosed to the proximal end of the stomach after a distal hemigastrectomy is performed. The ileum proximal to the end that is anastomosed to the stomach is in turn anastomosed to the terminal ileum within the 50- to 100-cm distance from the ileocecal valve, depending on the surgeon's preference and the patient's size.

Duodenal Switch

The duodenal switch (DS) configuration is shown in Fig. 48.17. This modification was developed to help lessen the high incidence of marginal ulcers after BPD. The mechanism of weight loss is similar to that of BPD.

An appendectomy is followed by measurement of the terminal ileum. Notably, in the DS procedure, the common channel is 100

TABLE 48.6 Technical considerations during laparoscopic Roux-en-Y gastric bypass.

TECHNIQUE	RECOMMENDATION	RATIONALE
Pouch size	15–20 mL	Smaller pouch reduces marginal ulceration and is associated with improved long-term weight loss
Method of gastrojejunostomy	No difference in techniques between circular stapler, linear cutter, or hand sewn	Although the circular stapler is the most common technique, all have similar outcomes. Biggest difference is skill and efficiency of the surgeon.[25,29]
Operative time	Faster surgical procedures associated with reduced complications	Surgical skill and efficiency trump all other factors when comparing adjusting for patient characteristics.[42]
Mesenteric defects	Closure of all mesenteric defects with nonabsorbable sutures/staples	Marked reduction in internal hernia formation requiring surgical correction.[43]
Antecolic or retrocolic Roux limb	Antecolic	The antecolic is technically easier and reduces the number of mesenteric defects from three to one. The Roux limb is at least 75 cm in length.
Fibrin sealant	Use fibrin sealant	Associated in some studies with reduced leak rates.[29]

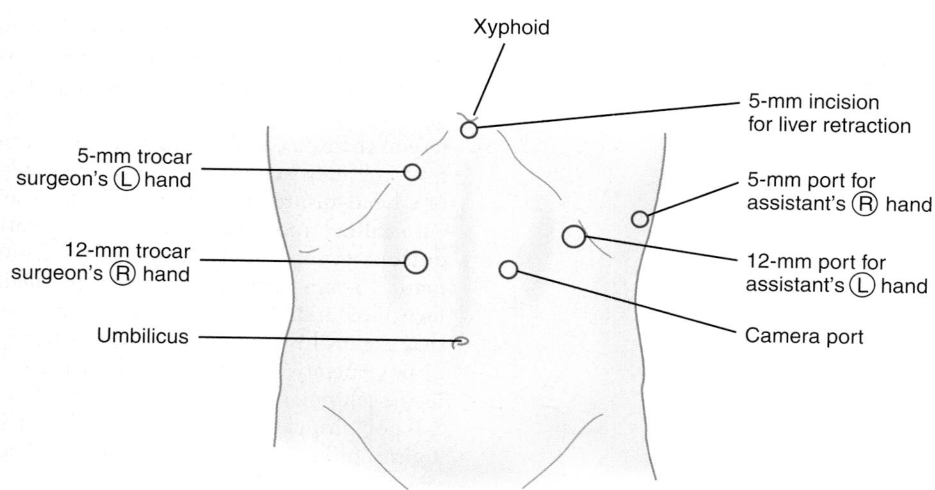

FIG. 48.9 Trocar configuration for laparoscopic Roux-en-Y gastric bypass and for laparoscopic sleeve gastrectomy.

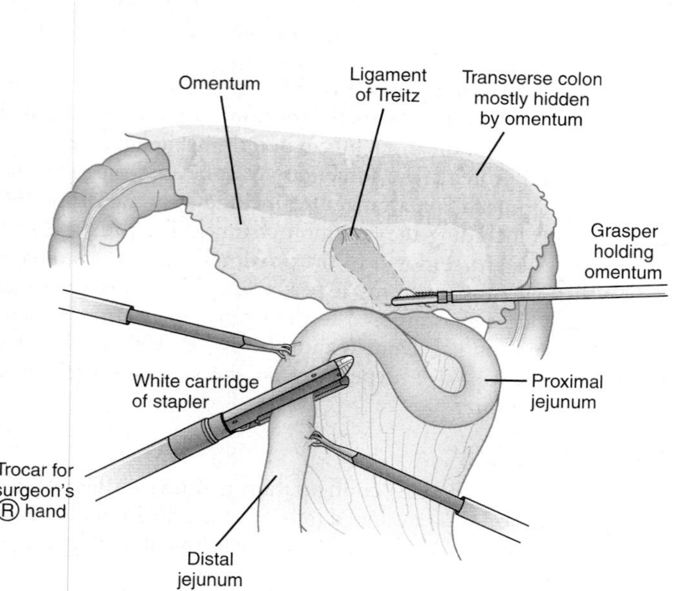

FIG. 48.10 Placing a stapler to divide the jejunum for creation of the Roux limb.

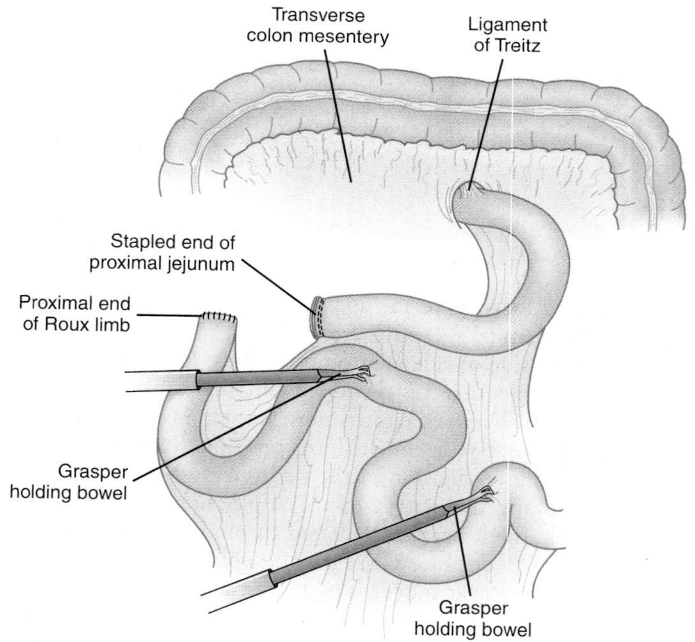

FIG. 48.11 Measuring and laying out the jejunum to set up a distal anastomosis for the length of the Roux-en-Y gastric bypass.

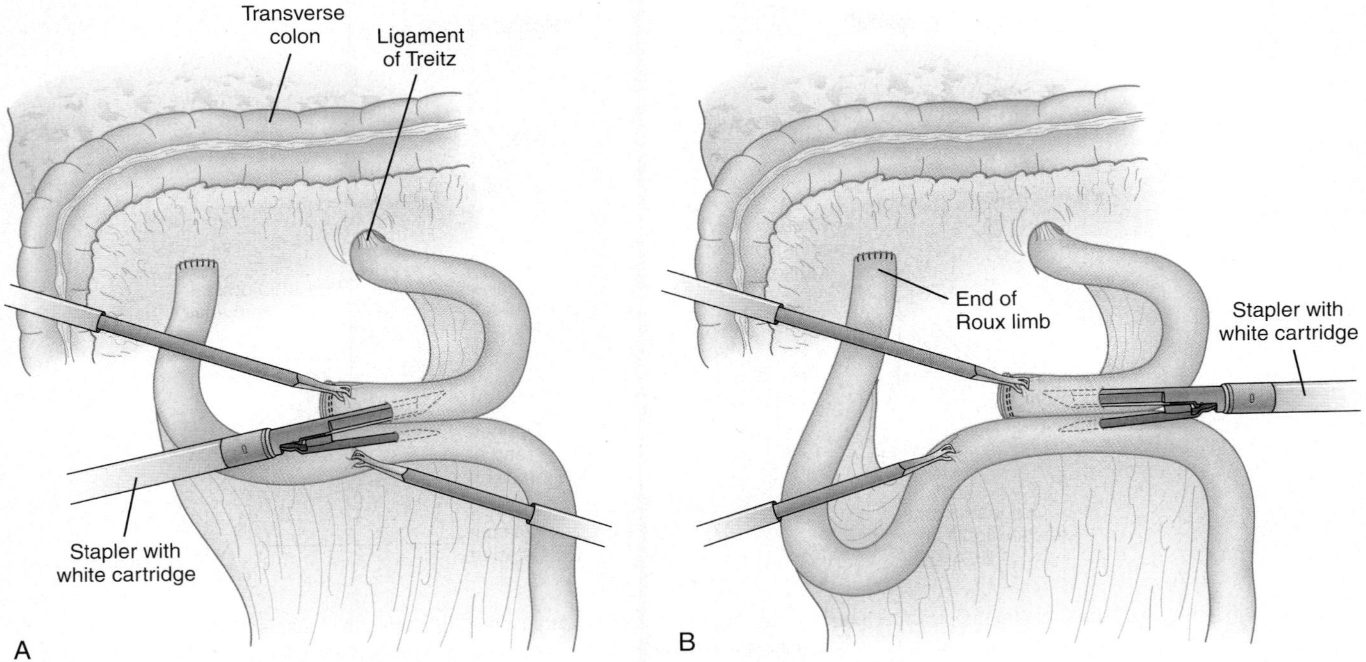

FIG. 48.12 Placing the stapler to create an enteroenterostomy. (A) The surgeon uses the 60-mm linear stapler to create the jejunojejunostomy between the biliopancreatic limb and the Roux limb. (B), The first assistant uses the 60-mm linear stapler to create a larger jejunojejunostomy. Not shown is the closure of the enterotomy using the 60-mm linear cutter as the final step.

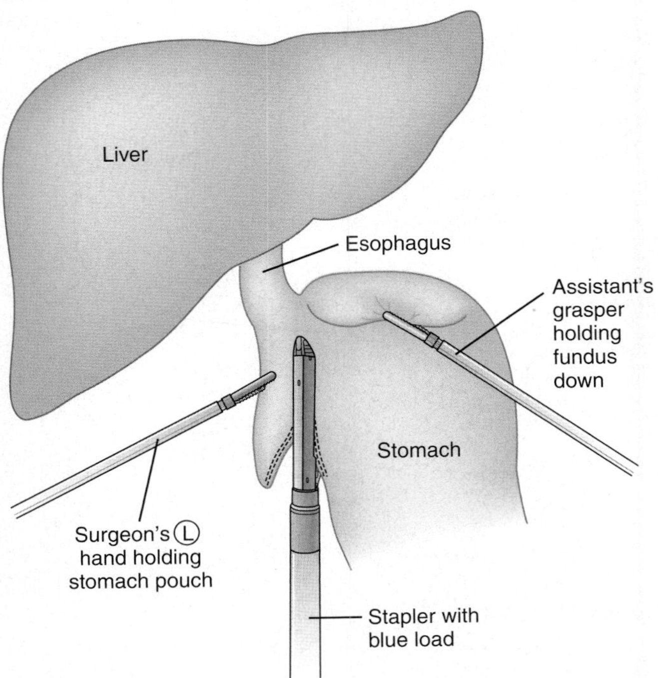

FIG. 48.13 Firing the stapler to create the proximal gastric pouch.

cm and the entire alimentary tract is 250 cm. However, the major difference between DS and BPD is the gastrectomy and the proximal anatomy. Instead of a distal hemigastrectomy, an LSG of the greater curvature of the stomach is performed. This procedure is done as the initial part of the operation because if the patient exhibits any intraoperative instability, the operation can be discontinued after the LSG alone. A two-stage DS has been used in patients who have an extremely high BMI and are high operative risks. The LSG alone usually produces enough weight loss to make the second stage of the operation technically easier. This approach lowers the mortality rate despite the need to undergo two operative procedures. The first step of a laparoscopic DS is to perform the LSG with a stapling technique that begins at the mid-antrum, and a staple line is created parallel to the lesser curvature of the stomach with a 40-Fr to 60-Fr Maloney dilator placed along the lesser curve to prevent narrowing. The staple line is created with multiple firings of the stapler until the angle of His is reached. The goal is to produce a lesser curvature gastric sleeve with a volume of 150 to 200 mL.

After LSG, the duodenum is divided with the stapler approximately 2 cm beyond the pylorus. The distal connections are performed as for BPD. The distal anastomosis is created at the 100-cm point proximal to the ileocecal valve. The proximal anastomosis is created between the proximal end of the 250 cm of terminal ileum and the first portion of the duodenum. The duodenoileostomy is an antecolic end-to-side anastomosis. This anastomosis is one of the most critical parts of the operation and either can be performed with a circular stapler or using a hand-sewn technique. If the EEA stapler is used, the anvil is directly inserted through the staple line of the duodenal stump through a gastrostomy under suture guidance or through an oral approach with a nasogastric tube.

Laparoscopic Sleeve Gastrectomy

LSG is now recognized as a primary procedure, and a *Current Procedural Terminology* code was assigned to the procedure in 2010. From 2008 to 2012, there was a precipitous increase in the number of LSG procedures (0.9%–36% of the total number of bariatric procedures), and by 2017, LSG made up 60% of the bariatric procedures performed in the United States (Table 48.7).[28] Advantages of LSG are the technical simplicity of the procedure, preservation of the pylorus (avoidance of dumping), metabolic reduction of ghrelin levels, no need for serial adjustments (as for LAGB), reduction in internal hernias (seen after LRYGB), reduction in malabsorption (seen with LRYGB), and ability to later modify the gastric sleeve to either an LRYGB or a

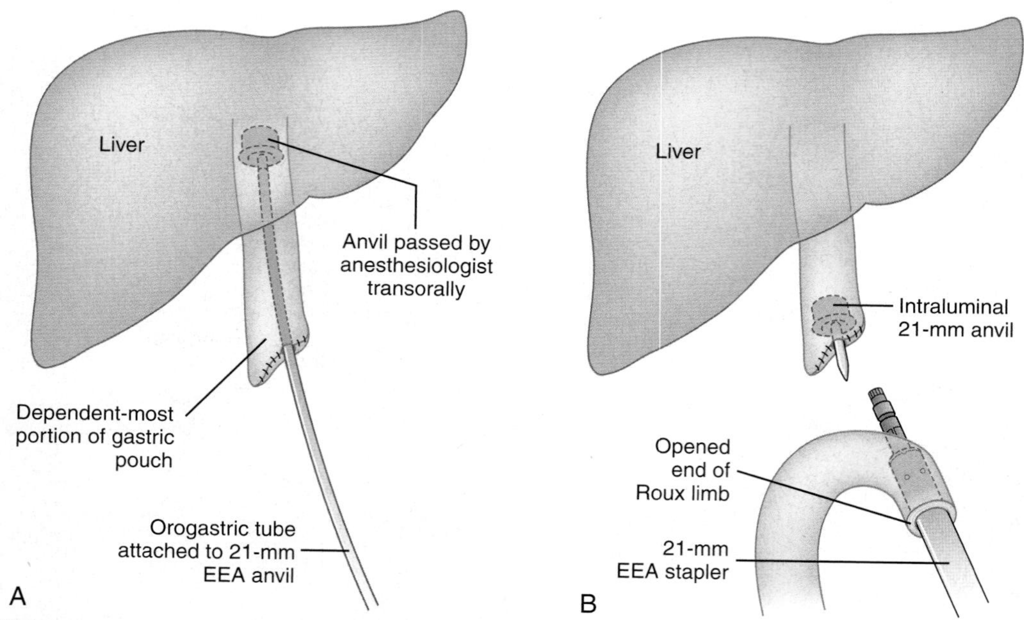

FIG. 48.14 Creating the proximal anastomosis. (A) Insertion of anvil transorally. (B) Insertion of stapler through Roux and creation of stapled anastomosis using the circular end-to-end anastomosis (EEA) stapler.Atest omnihil laccaepro

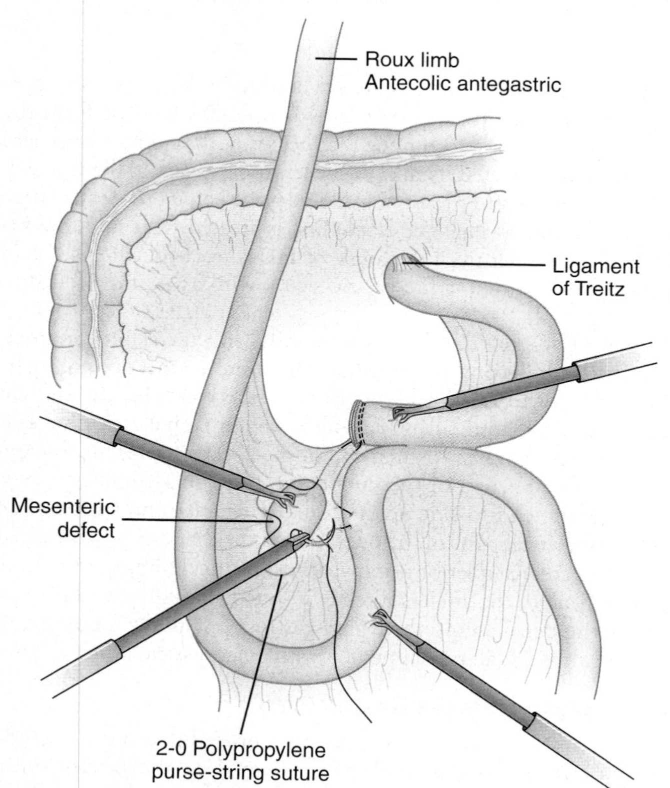

FIG. 48.15 Closure of mesenteric defect using purse-string suture of 2-0 polypropylene.

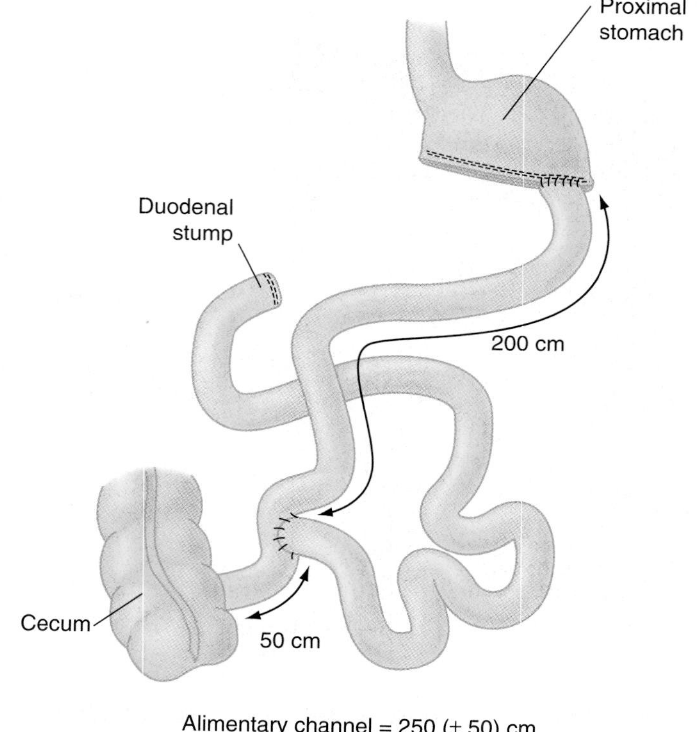

FIG. 48.16 Anatomic configuration of biliopancreatic diversion.

DS configuration in a second stage of the operation. The trocar placement is identical to that of LRYGB (see Fig. 48.9). As a primary procedure, the surgeon takes down the entire greater curvature, leaving intact the tissue within 3 cm of the pylorus and up to the angle of His and exposing the left crus of the diaphragm.

Then, with use of a 34-Fr to 40-Fr bougie, the stomach is divided from the antrum to the angle of His by sequential firings of the stapler (Fig. 48.18). It is vitally important in this procedure to preserve the left gastric vessels and lesser curve blood supply and to prevent twisting or spiraling of the gastric tube. Major controversy exists about techniques to reinforce the staple line to prevent bleeding or leaks from the staple line (Table 48.8).

POSTOPERATIVE CARE AND FOLLOW-UP

Laparoscopic Adjustable Gastric Banding

Patients undergoing LAGB experience an operation that may last as little as 1 hour in experienced hands. Discharge from the hospital after an overnight stay is the norm, with a few reports of same-day discharge. The band is initially placed without adding any saline to distend it. Saline is added in 1.0- to 1.5-mL increments to produce a desired weight loss of 1 to 2 kg/week. Excess weight loss (EWL) may lead to actual removal of a small amount of saline, whereas inadequate weight loss is an indication for the addition of more saline to the system to increase restriction of the band. The incidence of nutritional deficiencies is low after LAGB because there is no disruption of the normal gastrointestinal tract. Slippage of the lap band can result in acute strangulation of the stomach necessitating emergency surgical removal of the band but is more likely to present with symptoms of dysphagia, regurgitation, heartburn, and aspiration. Plain abdominal radiographs show the normally located 7 to 2 o'clock band position is either vertical or horizontal. Barium swallow demonstrates a slip of the band, which should be followed by either explantation or revision.

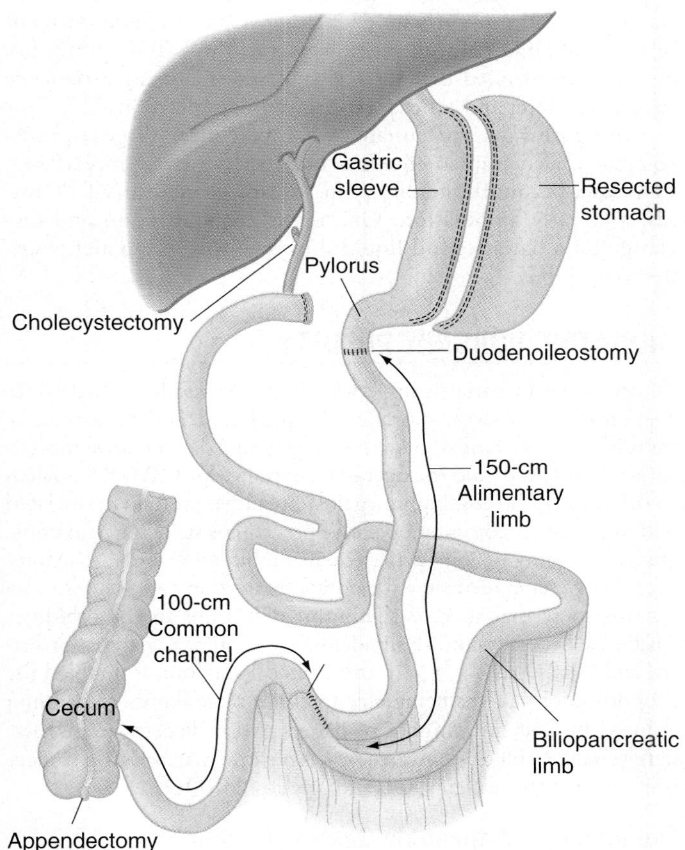

FIG. 48.17 Anatomic configuration of the duodenal switch.

Roux-en-Y Gastric Bypass, Biliopancreatic Diversion, Duodenal Switch, and Laparoscopic Sleeve Gastrectomy

Excellent surgical outcomes require the appropriate selection of patients, thorough preoperative preparation, technically well-performed operations, and attentive postoperative care. A bariatric patient requires particularly attentive and special postoperative care in several areas above and beyond that of the average surgical patient. The most dreaded complication after bariatric surgery is a leak from the gastrointestinal tract. Tachycardia, at times accompanied by tachypnea or agitation, is often the only manifestation of this severe intraabdominal problem. A severely obese patient may not be subject to the development of fever or signs of peritonitis, as would a patient with a normal body habitus. A high index of suspicion for leak must be present for postoperative patients who demonstrate sustained tachycardia, fever, or increased pain. If a leak is suggested, a CT scan with oral administration of a contrast agent or possibly laparoscopy may be needed to establish the diagnosis before overwhelming sepsis occurs.

Patients undergoing laparoscopic surgery usually have much less third space and operative blood loss than do patients undergoing open surgery and can be managed with 4 mL/kg/hour of intravenous fluids. Urine output intraoperatively is normally low because of the pneumoperitoneum and usually improves in the recovery room area. Some patients who have been taking diuretics chronically may not produce adequate urine output without diuretic use, but the surgeon must ensure that the patient is

TABLE 48.7 ASMBS total bariatric procedures performed in the United States, published June 2018.[28]

	2011	2012	2013	2014	2015	2016	2017
Total	**158,000**	**173,000**	**179,000**	**193,000**	**196,000**	**216,000**	**228,000**
Sleeve	17.80%	33.00%	42.10%	51.70%	53.61%	58.11%	**59.39%**
RYGB	36.70%	37.50%	34.20%	26.80%	23.02%	18.69%	**17.80%**
Band	35.40%	20.20%	14.00%	9.50%	5.68%	3.39%	**2.77%**
BPD-DS	0.90%	1.00%	1.00%	0.40%	0.60%	0.57%	**0.70%**
Revision	6.00%	6.00%	6.00%	11.50%	13.55%	13.95%	**14.14%**
Other	3.20%	2.30%	2.70%	0.10%	3.19%	2.63%	**2.46%**
Balloons	—	—	—	—	0.36%	2.66%	**2.75%**

From Estimate of Bariatric Surgery Numbers, 2011–2017. American Society of Metabolic and Bariatric Surgeons. 2018. https://asmbs.org/resources/estimate-of-bariatric-surgery-numbers. Accessed August 6, 2019.

ACS/MBSAQIP, American College of Surgeons/Metabolic and Bariatric Surgery Accreditation and Quality Improvement Program; *ASMBS*, American Society for Metabolic and Bariatric Surgery; *BPD-DS*, biliopancreatic diversion-duodenal switch; *Band*, adjustable gastric banding; *Sleeve*, sleeve gastrectomy; *RYGB*, Roux-en-Y gastric bypass.

The ASMBS total bariatric procedure numbers are based on the best estimation from available data (Bariatric Outcomes Longitudinal Database, ACS/MBSAQIP, National Inpatient Sample Data, and outpatient estimations).

adequately volume resuscitated before giving diuretics. Higher-than-expected fluid requirements, oliguria, and tachycardia are a constellation of postoperative findings suggesting intraabdominal problems.

Adequate pain control is essential. Narcotic requirements are decreased with a laparoscopic approach. A patient-controlled analgesia pump is appropriate and helpful. Non-narcotic intravenous pain medications have been extremely helpful in reducing postoperative pain, as have anesthetics injected locally in the incisions at the time of surgery.

Disadvantages of LSG seem to focus on the Achilles heel of the operation, which is a leak along the long gastric staple line. Whereas a leak after gastric bypass is one of the most feared complications, leaks after LSG appear between 1 and 4 weeks postoperative and present with an indolent infection/abscess but not in frank shock most of the time. There is conflicting evidence about the leak rate, and in some published series, leaks after LSG are more common than in LRYGB.[25,29] The most recent series show the leak rate is decreasing over time and less common in LSG than in LRYGB.[30–32] The leaks are most likely to be located in the proximal third of the stomach. Management of the leak includes adequate drainage, by either CT-guided percutaneous catheter placement or operative approaches, with institution of total parenteral nutrition, no oral intake, and antibiotics. Additionally, in most cases, endoscopic closure of fistula and endoscopic stenting to prevent ongoing contamination of the peritoneal cavity has been effective. The cause of leaks appears to be multifactorial, with early leaks (≤2 days postoperatively) related to stapler misfires or tissue trauma, whereas late leaks are related to ischemia and high intragastric pressure, particularly when there is distal stenosis, often at the incisura angularis.

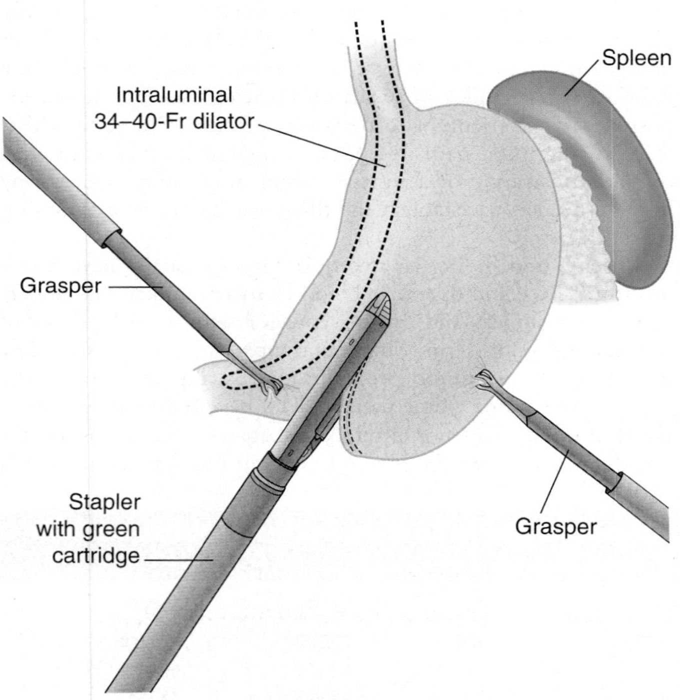

FIG. 48.18 Creation of the sleeve gastrectomy.

There is evidence that prevention of leaks after LSG can be accomplished as evidenced by the results of the MBSC, which demonstrated leak rates fell over a 5-year period (1.18%–0.36%).[29] Leak rates declined as case volume increased, and surgeons who performed more than 43 cases per year had a leak rate of less than1%. Decreased leak rates were associated with oversewing the staple line, and with higher case volume. In practice, the bariatric surgeon can support with data either staple line reinforcement or no staple line reinforcement; however, the MBSC group has clearly demonstrated that surgical skill and increasing experience reduce leak rates and other postoperative complications.[25]

Care pathways and enhanced recovery after surgery protocols have been implemented in bariatric surgery, emphasizing non-narcotic multimodality pain control, limitation of IV fluids, and early ambulation. One night hospitalization and discharge on a bariatric full liquid diet is routine for patients undergoing LSG.

BARIATRIC SURGERY RESULTS

Across the world, bariatric surgery has improved results, with declines over time in operative mortality, hospital stay, and postoperative morbidity. In the United States, Europe, and Asia, operative mortality is nil for LAGB and the operative mortality for LRYGB has fallen to 0.1% to 0.2%, coming up against operative mortality associated with many other common operative procedures such as laparoscopic cholecystectomy or joint replacement (Table 48.9).[26,30,31,33] Moreover, a large series reviewing the outcomes in countries or health care systems show that there is significant reductions in comorbidities (diabetes, hypertension, dyslipidemia, sleep apnea, asthma, arthritis, and GERD).[8,10,11,34,35] In the United Kingdom, it doubled the proportion of patients being able to climb three flights of stair and reduced by half the number of patients with diabetes related hyperglycemia.[35] Increasingly, studies also show that bariatric surgery improves weight-related QOL and physical HRQOL.[13]

Laparoscopic Adjustable Gastric Banding

As can be seen in Table 48.7, lap band operations rapidly increased in the early 2000s, peaked in 2011, and have now declined to 2.8% in 2017.[28] During the early 2000s, laparoscopic gastric bypass was associated with high mortality and complication rates, so a number of surgeons adopted the lap band procedure as a much simpler procedure with a dramatically lower morbidity and mortality rate. The early results with lap band were almost uniformly excellent with modest weight loss and very little morbidity or mortality. Results of the LAGB procedure show no 30-day mortality and reasonable weight loss as shown in Table 48.9 in select centers.[26,33]

TABLE 48.8 Technical considerations during laparoscopic sleeve gastrectomy.

TECHNIQUE	RECOMMENDATION	RATIONALE
Bougie size	34–40 French	Smaller bougie size associated with gastroesophageal reflux disease Larger associated with weight regain[45]
Staple line extent	Extend into antrum	Improved long-term weight loss
Staple line reinforcement	No staple line reinforcement	Some studies show increase in leak rate with staple line reinforcement[29]

TABLE 48.9 Results of the four major bariatric procedures.

	O'BRIEN[33]	LAZZATI[26]	BOLCKMANS[41]
LAGB			
EWL (%)	45.9	44	NR
Mortality (%)	0.0 Single center (8378 patients)	0.0 (6506 patients)	NR
LSG			
EWL (%)	53–62	56	NR
Mortality (%)	NR	0.08 (17,960 patients)	NR
RYGB			
EWL (%)	56.7	67%	NR
Mortality (%)		0.11% (10,526 patients)	NR
BPD/DS			
EWL	74.1	NR	65–70
Mortality (%)	NR	NR	1.9% Three deaths <6 months after surgery (153 patients)

BPD, Biliopancreatic diversion; *DS*, duodenal switch; *EWL*, excess weight loss; *LAGB*, laparoscopic adjustable gastric banding; *LSG*, laparoscopic sleeve gastrectomy; *NR*, not reported; *RYGB*, Roux-en-Y gastric bypass.

TABLE 48.10 Results of Roux-en-Y gastric bypass.

CRITERIA	COURCOULAS[34]	ADAMS[11]
Number of patients	1738	418
Age (years)	19-75 median 45	18–72
BMI (kg/m^2)	47%	45.9%
Follow-up (years)	7	12
Excess weight loss	52%	NR
Reduction in BMI (kg/m^2)	NR	−11.5
Percentage of baseline weight loss	−28.4% at 7 years	–
Diabetes	58.9% at 7 years	51%
Hypertension	39.3% at 7 years	36
Dyslipidemia	85.8% at 7 years*	59–94%†

BMI, Body mass index; *NR*, not reported.
*High triglycerides
†At 12 years after surgery for high triglyceride, low high-density lipoprotein cholesterol, and high low-density lipoprotein cholesterol levels.

Roux-en-Y Gastric Bypass

RYGB has an established record of accomplishment that is longer than that of any other bariatric operation. Its performance has been modified over the years, and the results presented in Table 48.10 reflect data from studies in the era of its performance as a laparoscopic procedure. Resolution of comorbid conditions after LRYGB has been excellent and sustained in long-term studies, as demonstrated in Tables 48.3 and 48.10.[7,11,33,34] It has been commonly thought that gastric bypass has been associated with higher morbidity and mortality in older individuals and that older individuals would not benefit from surgery long term. However, Davidson and colleagues[12] identified reduction in long-term mortality in older patients (55–74 years of age) when the patients were operated on at a center specializing in bariatric surgery. The demonstration of acceptable morbidity and mortality in older individuals, coupled with improvements in long-term survival, has led most bariatric surgeons to consider operating on older individuals if they meet criteria for operation.

Recovery After Roux-en-Y Gastric Bypass Is Improved After a Laparoscopic Approach

Another important advantage of LRYGB is a decrease in the incidence of wound complications and incisional hernia seen after open RYGB. Long-term follow-up of a prospective randomized trial comparing laparoscopic and open gastric bypass found a much higher rate of incisional hernias in the open surgery group. There was, however, no difference in the rate of resolution of comorbid conditions or weight loss between the two procedures. The duration of hospitalization has decreased in all patients undergoing RYGB. Patients undergoing LRYGB are usually hospitalized for about 2 days.

RYGB has also been shown to resolve the symptoms of pseudotumor cerebri as well as to cure the difficult problem of venous stasis ulcers. Immediate resolution of symptoms of GERD occurs in more than 90% of cases. The extremely small gastric pouch has a limited reservoir for holding gastric juice, and the cardia is a low acid-producing area of the stomach, so the Roux-en-Y reconstruction diverts gastric acid away from the esophagus immediately after surgery, thus accounting for its efficacy in alleviating heartburn.

Age has been shown previously to be an important determinant of operative morbidity and mortality. However, a matched pair analysis of the MBSAQIP database of 3371 patients older than age 60 years old matched to 3371 patients younger than 60 with similar BMI and comorbidities showed that there was comparable mortality between older individuals and younger individuals in both LSG and LRYGB. These data should not be misinterpreted to mean that older individuals have the same mortality risk as younger ones but to suggest that the surgeon can identify older patients who are qualified for bariatric surgery and can expect that operation can result in good short- and long-term outcomes.[30]

Biliopancreatic Diversion and Duodenal Switch

Most malabsorptive procedures performed in the United States are the DS modification of BPD, so this section discusses the results of both operations. EWL (65%–70%) after BPD/DS is the highest of the bariatric operations discussed in this chapter, with a mean percentage weight loss of 39% to 40% 10 years postoperative. BPD/DS has also been highly effective in treating comorbid conditions, including hypertension remission (81%), diabetes remission (87.5%), lipid disorders (triglycerides remission [89%], low-density lipoprotein [LDL] cholesterol remission [95%]), and obstructive sleep apnea.[41]

Thus, some surgeons argue that superobese patients fare better and maintain weight loss better in the long term after undergoing BPD/DS than after other bariatric operations. Others point out that serious complications such as deficiency in vitamin D (89%), vitamin K (65%), and zinc (65%); reoperation for correction of protein malnutrition (4%–10%); reoperation for treatment of incisional hernia or bowel obstruction (37%–42%); and morbidity are much higher with BPD/DS, and therefore, the incremental improvements in EWL are not justified.[41]

After BPD/DS, patients typically have between two and four bowel movements per day. Excessive flatulence and foul-smelling stools are the rule. Malabsorption of starch and fat provides the major mechanism of weight loss, and creates the vitamin deficiencies in fat-soluble vitamins (K, A, D, and E).

Surgeons caring for these patients must be alert to measure protein levels for confirmation of adequate absorption. When protein malnutrition does occur, the common channel may need to be lengthened with a reoperation. Patients must also be aware that their ability to absorb simple sugars, alcohol, and short-chain triglycerides is good and that overindulgence of sweets, milk products, soft drinks, alcohol, and fruit may produce excess weight gain.

Major considerations for achieving excellent results in patients offered BPD/DS include the ability to monitor these patients and to confirm that they are being compliant with the recommendations to take appropriate vitamin supplements. Supplements include multivitamins as well as at least 2 g of oral calcium per day. Supplemental fat-soluble vitamins, including D, K, and A, are indicated monthly as well.

TABLE 48.11 Results of laparoscopic sleeve gastrectomy.

CRITERIA	STAMPEDE[15]	SLEEVEPASS[37]	SM-BOSS[38]
Number of patients	49	121	107
Age (years)	Mean = 48	Mean = 48.5	Mean = 43
BMI (kg/m^2)	36.1	45.5	43.9
Follow-up (years)	5	5	5
Excess weight loss (%)	NR	49%	NR
Percentage BMI loss	NR	NR	61.1%
Percentage of baseline weight loss	−18.6%	NR	NR
Remission diabetes	23.4%	12%	61.5%
Remission hypertension	NR	29%	62.5%
Remission dyslipidemia	NR	20%	42.6%

BMI, Body mass index; *NR*, not reported.

Laparoscopic Sleeve Gastrectomy

Advantages of LSG are the technical ease of the procedure, induction of satiety through reduction in ghrelin levels, reduced need for postoperative adjustments as opposed to LAGB, preservation of the pylorus and avoidance of dumping, reduced risk of malabsorption, and apparent safety of the procedure in high-risk individuals. Use of LSG is advantageous for some populations of patients as outlined in Table 48.11.

LSG was developed because of a high incidence of morbidity and mortality (23% and 7%, respectively) in patients with a BMI greater than 60 kg/m^2 undergoing laparoscopic DS. Surgeons developed the two-stage DS, with SG alone performed as the first stage to decrease morbidity in this population of superobese patients. The Clinical Issues Committee of the ASMBS performed a comprehensive review of the subject, which demonstrated a lower rate of complications for DS in this population of high-risk patients (leak rate of 1.2%, bleeding rate of 1.6%, and mortality of 0.24%). The ASMBS concluded that LSG could be used in high-risk patients to reduce perioperative complications and also to induce weight loss as a standalone procedure. Modifications to LSG including reduced bougie size and extension of the LSG into the antrum all made LSG a primary bariatric procedure.

Five-year results after LSG in the STAMPEDE trial show good weight loss (−18.6% baseline) and remission of diabetes in 23.4% (Table 48.12).[15] O'Brien reported the collective series of LSG across the globe and reported a weighted mean of 58.3% EWL after LSG.[33] Two excellent RCTs give us comparative data on the outcomes 5 years after LSG and LRYGB, as shown in Table 48.12. The SLEEVEPASS trial shows that LRYGB has a greater percentage of weight loss than LSG (57% vs. 49%), but there was no statistical significant difference in HgbA1c (6.6% vs. 6.6%), dyslipidemia, QOL improvement, and late morbidity. There was a significant improvement in the resolution of hypertension based upon medication use in LRYGB (51% vs. 29% resolution).[37] The Swiss Multicentre Bypass or Sleeve Study (SM-BOSS) randomized trial found no significant difference in percentage of BMI loss (68.3% vs. 61.1%), complete remission of type 2 diabetes (67.9% vs. 61.5%), hypertension remission (70.3% vs. 62.5%), improvement in QOL, or in late complications (Table 48.12).[38]

COMPLICATIONS OF BARIATRIC SURGERY

The various procedures are associated with complications that can occur with any intraabdominal operation, such as pulmonary embolism. However, each operation has unique complications as well

TABLE 48.12 Comparison of laparoscopic sleeve gastrectomy versus laparoscopic Roux-en-Y gastric bypass: 5-year outcomes in the SLEEVEPASS[37] and SM-BOSS[38] randomized trials.

MEASURE	LSG	LRYGB	COMMENTS
Percent excess weight loss	49%	57%	LRYGB had more weight loss but not statistically significant
BMI at 5 years (kg/m^2)	31.6–36.5	32.5–35.4	No significant difference between procedures
Remission of type 2 diabetes	12%–61.5%	25%–67.9%	No significant differences
Remission of hypertension	29%–62.5%	51%–70.3%	LRYGB in the SLEEVEPASS trial had increased remission rate
LDL cholesterol (mg/dL)	104.3–116.1	96.5–101.1	LDL level significantly lower after LRYGB
Quality of life (QOL)	Improved	Improved	Both procedures improved QOL
Remission of GERD	25%	60.4%	LRYGB associated with greater remission of GERD. In the SLEEVEPASS trial, 7/10 reoperations were done for severe reflux
Late complications	14.9%–19%	17.3%–26%	No difference between techniques

BMI, Body mass index; *GERD*, gastroesophageal reflux disease; *LDL*, low-density lipoprotein; *LRYGB*, laparoscopic Roux-en-Y gastric bypass; *LSG*, laparoscopic sleeve gastrectomy. SM-BOSS Swiss Multicentre Bypass Or Sleeve Study.

as different incidences of some of the shared common complications seen after any abdominal operation.

It is now well accepted that laparoscopic and robotic procedures are much safer than open gastric bypass in 30-day mortality (e.g., overall complication rates, surgical site infection, and pulmonary complication). The benefits touted for laparoscopic surgery go beyond the cosmetic benefits and really do influence postoperative complication rates, which makes the laparoscopic technique our preferred approach in every patient, including remedial operations.

Laparoscopic Adjustable Gastric Banding

Although many centers have shown a very low (approaching zero) 30-day morbidity and mortality rate, long-term complications such as esophageal dilation, lap band slip, lap band erosion, and failure to lose weight have been the Achilles heel of this operation. High-resolution manometry of the esophagus in patients who present for LAGB removal have shown that 67% to 78% of patients have abnormal esophageal peristalsis, including simultaneous or failed peristalsis.[39] It has been noted that removal of the lap band in patients who have developed pseudoachalasia or megaesophagus will improve; therefore, surgeons should be vigilant regarding patients with lap bands who might have either a slip or significant esophageal motility disorders who need deflation and/or explantation of the band.

The 10-year outcomes of a prospective randomized trial of LAGB versus LRYGB demonstrated the Achilles heels of the LAGB procedure: poor long-term weight loss (LAGB 27.4 kg vs. LRYGB 42.4 kg), higher reoperation rate (LAGB 31.4% vs. LRYGB 8.1%), and lower rate of remission of comorbidities.[40] The natural history of LAGB was defined by a study of the French standardized national database of 53,000 patients, which demonstrated that 20% of the 52,868 patients underwent removal of the band, and by 7 years, 71% of the patients underwent revisional surgery. Many of the revisional procedures were conversions to either LSG or LRYGB for either lap band slippage or failure of weight loss with LAGB. The authors of the French study questioned whether the lap band was a viable procedure given the high rate of removal and complications.[41]

While a few centers who specialize in LAGB[33] have demonstrated much lower reoperation rates with much improved durable weight loss shown in (Table 48.13), the authors of this chapter no longer offer LAGB in their practices as the current surgical practice of LSG and LRYGB have low morbidity, much improved long-term weight loss, and improved resolution of comorbidity.

Roux-en-Y Gastric Bypass

The laparoscopic revolution has fundamentally changed the outcomes of many surgical procedures, but in particular, it has reduced operative mortality and morbidity significantly. The most recently reported mortality rates after LRYGB have generally been in the 0.1% to 0.3% range for a large series, as shown in Table 48.14. The MBSC identified 18 deaths (0.3%) in 6118 patients undergoing primary bariatric surgery in Centers of Excellence across the United States.[24] The most common cause of death was sepsis (33%), followed by cardiac (28%) and pulmonary embolism from 0.31% in 2009 to 0.11% in 2012.[26]

Mortality rates are influenced heavily by patient selection. Male gender was associated with an increased risk for morbidity and mortality in older series but not in the most recent experience. Almost all studies have identified BMI and history of VTE as independent predictors of complications. Complications specific to RYGB include anastomotic leaks from the proximal or distal anastomosis. Leaks from the gastrojejunostomy are more common and are generally the cause of a significant percentage of the life-threatening complications and deaths. Whereas the older studies found a leak rate of 2.2% in open and LRYGB, the more recent LRYGB studies report anastomotic leak rates of 0.5% to 1.5%.[29–31] These investigators found no difference in leak rates by type of anastomosis or stapling instrument used. They did find that the use of buttressing material was more common in patients who leaked.[29] Since there has been no study to conclude that buttressing material will prevent leaks and at least one study has shown an association, our practice has been to not utilize buttressing material for LRYGB or for LSG.

Data suggest that a surgeon's operative skill significantly influences the leak rate, with the most experienced surgeons recording the lowest complication rates.[25] The MBSC identified wide variation in complications after bariatric surgery among surgeons within Centers of Excellence across the United States.[24]

TABLE 48.13 Results of laparoscopic adjustable gastric banding procedures.

CRITERIA	O'BRIEN[33]	COURCOULAS[34]
Number of patients	714	610
Age (years)	Mean = 47	18–78
BMI (kg/m^2)	43.8	44
Follow-up (years)	10-15	7
Percentage of excess weight loss	47	NR
Reduction in BMI (kg/m^2)	NR	NR
Percentage of baseline weight loss	−21	−14.9%
Resolution of type 2 diabetes (%)	NR	20.3%

BMI, Body mass index; *NR*, not reported.

TABLE 48.14 Complications after laparoscopic Roux-en-Y gastric bypass.

CRITERIA	COURCOULAS[34]	KUMAR[31]	JANIK[30]	LAZZATI[26]
Number of patients	1738	41,080	3371	10,526
Age	19-75	Median = 45	>60	Mean = 41
Mortality	0.17%	0.2%	0.33%	0.11%
Leak/major wound complications	NR	1.6%	1.0%	NR
Surgical site infection	NR	0.9%	0.8%	NR
Pulmonary embolus/venous thromboembolism	NR	0.15	0.2%	NR
Reoperation	2.5%	3.2%	2.5%	NR
Revision	0.06%	NR	NR	NR
Reversal	0.02%	NR	NR	NR
Bleeding	NR	1.2%	1.5%	NR

NR, Not reported.

While Centers of Excellence certification has appeared to improve outcomes, it remains that surgeon skill is one of the most important determinant of early outcomes. Slow surgeons performing LRYGB (139 minutes) have greater odds of any complications, including VTE and prolonged length of stay, compared to a cohort of fast surgeons (86 minutes).[42] The study was able to exclude other factors such as volume, total number of cases performed, and gastrojejunostomy technique and found that shorter surgeon median time to perform LRYGB is independently associated with improved outcomes. Since surgeon-specific efficiency results in improved postoperative outcomes, improving surgical efficiency and surgical skill is an important part of quality improvement.[42]

Pulmonary embolism is one of the most feared complications after any form of bariatric surgery, and its incidence in large reported series of open RYGB sometimes exceeds 1%. Thrombotic complications such as DVT and pulmonary embolism are less frequently associated with laparoscopic surgery than with open gastric bypass but still account for 17% of deaths, and up to 80% of patients who die after bariatric surgery have evidence of VTE. Emphasis on DVT prophylaxis using SCDs, early ambulation, and low-molecular–weight heparin have reduced incidence of VTE to 0.23% in both LSG and LRYGB, evidenced by the latest reports from the MBSAQIP.[31]

Although nausea and vomiting are not unusual in isolated circumstances after RYGB, especially in relation to a patient's adaptation to food restriction, if persistent, these symptoms can lead to the obvious problem of dehydration. This must be aggressively treated in the postoperative period or in association with a viral or other gastrointestinal illness compounding the problem and further limiting oral intake. Intravenous fluids are indicated when in doubt. This is the case for all bariatric operations, not just RYGB.

One specific problem that may arise with persistent vomiting after *any* of the bariatric operations and that is *imperative* for the surgeon to treat is Wernicke's encephalopathy. This neurologic deficit is preventable with appropriate administration of parenteral thiamine (vitamin B_1) when the patient has persistent and severe vomiting. If the neurologic symptoms become significant, they may often not be fully reversed despite thiamine therapy.

Because depression is so frequent in the population of patients undergoing bariatric surgery, severe postoperative depression may develop after any of the bariatric operations as well. When it does occur, the patient may completely stop eating, thereby producing what at first seems like a wonderful response, but, if unrecognized, it can progress to loss of critical visceral and musculoskeletal protein mass, which can be life-threatening.

Another specific life-threatening complication that may result after RYGB is that of bowel obstruction. Patients who have a clinical or radiographic picture of small bowel obstruction after RYGB need a reoperation. The potential for internal hernias after this operation makes strangulation obstruction a frequent presentation. Patients with bowel obstruction are best diagnosed by an oral and intravenous contrast-enhanced CT scan of the abdomen to visualize the bypassed stomach and small bowel that may be obstructed or the mesenteric twist with volvulus of the Roux limb. These patients *must* be promptly treated before retrograde distention of the biliopancreatic limb and distal part of the stomach results in rupture of the distal gastric staple line with subsequent peritonitis. Closure of the mesenteric defects has been shown to reduce by more than fourfold the incidence of internal hernia associated bowel obstruction and added only 4 minutes to the operative time.[43] It is our practice to perform antecolic LRYGB and thus only have to close the jejunojejunostomy defect.

Stenosis of the gastrojejunostomy may occur after RYGB and has been reported in 2% to 14% of patients in various series. The higher incidence seems to be associated with a circular stapler versus sutured anastomoses. Postoperative anastomotic stenosis is usually manifested at 4 to 6 weeks postoperatively as progressive intolerance to solids and then liquids. The problem is successfully treated with endoscopic balloon dilation. Unless a marginal ulcer is associated with the stenosis, the problem does not require a reoperation.

A marginal ulcer occurs after 2% to 10% of RYGB procedures. The incidence can be decreased by preoperative treatment of patients for *Helicobacter pylori* colonization of the stomach. Patients with a marginal ulcer typically have continuous boring epigastric pain. Larger pouch size was associated with increased marginal ulceration in a study of Swedish procedures. The standard creation of the pouch entailed use of a 45-mm stapler to divide the stomach horizontally and one 60-mm and one 45-mm stapler to create the pouch. Each additional 1 cm added in the vertical stapling height increased the risk of marginal ulcer by 14%. Presumably, the additional size of the pouch had more parietal cells secreting acid, which increased the risk of marginal ulceration. The Swedish researchers also examined whether or not increased pouch size affected weight loss at 1 year. They found the slightly larger pouch had the same weight loss as the smaller pouch as long as the pouch is less than 25 mL.[44] Treatment of marginal ulcer consists of medical therapy with proton pump inhibitors and avoidance of nonsteroidal antiinflammatory drugs. Medical treatment resolves most of the marginal ulcers unless a fistula has formed to the lower part of the stomach, which creates an ongoing source of acid, thus exacerbating the ulcer. Surgery to divide the fistula is necessary to effect healing of the ulcer.

Iron and vitamin B_{12} deficiencies are the two most common long-term metabolic complications of RYGB. The incidence of iron insufficiency varies among reported series. Iron is preferentially absorbed in the duodenum and proximal jejunum. Hence, RYGB bypasses the area of maximal iron absorption in the gut. The iron deficiency, based on serum values, is between 15% and 40%, whereas actual iron deficiency anemia occurs in as many as 20% of patients after RYGB. This problem is treated in most cases with oral iron supplements. The gluconate form of iron is best absorbed in a nonacid environment.

The incidence of vitamin B_{12} deficiency after RYGB is reported as being 15% to 20%, although it rarely causes anemia. Vitamin B_{12} deficiency is due to inefficient absorption because of delayed mixing with intrinsic factor. Thus, B_{12} deficiency can develop despite plentiful oral administration. Several preparations include intrinsic factor, which maximizes absorption in the terminal ileum. Other routes of vitamin B_{12} administration include sublingual medication, nasal spray, and parenteral injections.

Biliopancreatic Diversion and Duodenal Switch

The most significant and specific long-term complication seen after BPD/DS is protein malnutrition, which occurs in 12% of patients. Treatment is hospitalization with 2 to 3 weeks of parenteral nutrition. This particular problem is usually manifested within the first few months after surgery, but it can occur sporadically, although less frequently, after surgery. In one series, 10.6% of patients eventually required a reoperation either to reverse the BPD completely or to lengthen the common channel.[41]

Malabsorption of fat-soluble vitamins is one of the major problems associated with BPD/DS. Two years after BPD, levels of vitamins D and A are significantly depressed, with vitamin D deficiency noted in 63% of patients and vitamin A deficiency in

69%. Lack of clinical correlation with these levels suggests that the problem may be more prevalent than originally reported or suspected from past series.

Although the complication of protein malnutrition and poor intake is theoretically most likely to occur soon after BPD/DS, the fact that late deaths occur from protein malnutrition and Wernicke encephalopathy suggests that these patients are always at risk for these problems. Marginal ulcers are a distinct problem of BPD, which has been addressed with the DS modification preserving the pylorus.

Perhaps it is the overall difficulty of the operation as well as the potential dangers of the operation that has relegated BPD to the least popular operation performed in the United States. Even the DS modification does not represent more than 1% of bariatric operations. Further studies are needed to evaluate the long-term consequences of BPD and DS to justify the performance of such operations as a primary procedure.

Laparoscopic Sleeve Gastrectomy

The mortality rate after LSG (0.08%–0.12%) is between that of LRYGB and LAGB as shown in Table 48.15. The morbidity associated with LSG, including infections, reoperation, and VTE, is below that of LRYGB but higher than that of LAGB. Malabsorption of vitamins and nutrients is much less for LSG compared with LRYGB or the laparoscopic DS and makes LSG ideally suited for patients with preexisting vitamin disorders or those who need full absorption of lifesaving medications as shown in Table 48.16. Moreover, studies of 30-day morbidity and mortality show that there has been a continual decline in postoperative complications associated with increased surgical experience.[25] Use of LSG is advantageous for some populations of patients, as outlined in Table 48.16.

The long-term morbidity of LSG is related to reoperation, primarily conversion to RYGB for severe GERD, which is exacerbated by the high-pressure system created by LSG. One report of the 10-year results after LSG showed that there was a high incidence of significant weight regain (21%) and intractable reflux (11%) leading to conversion to RYGB.[45] However, these long-term results were in a group of patients who underwent LSG prior to 2006 when a larger bougie was used and also did not include parts of the antrum. Felsenreich and colleagues[45] postulated that improved surgical technique using the recommended 34 to 40-Fr bougie and taking part of the antrum would improve long-term results. Indeed, both of the Sleeve versus Bypass randomized trials, which used a smaller bougie, did not show any significant weight regain requiring conversion, while in both randomized trials, there was a significant number of patients who developed more severe GERD or developed GERD de novo and required conversion to RYGB.[37,38]

TABLE 48.15 Complications after laparoscopic sleeve gastrectomy.

CRITERIA	LAZZATI[26]	KUMAR[31]	JANIK[30]
Number of patients	17,960	93,062	3371
Age	Mean = 40	Median = 44	>60
Mortality	0.08	0.1%	0.12%
Leak perforation	NR	0.8%	0.5%
Surgical site infection	NR	0.2%	0.2%
Pulmonary embolus/venous thromboembolism	NR	0.1%	0.1%
Reoperation	NR	1.2	0.9%
Bleeding	NR	0.6%	1.0%

REOPERATIVE SURGERY

A controversial topic is the appropriateness of performing repeated bariatric operations for a failed procedure. The absolute definition of a failed operation is unclear, but most surgeons would accept the criteria listed in Table 48.5 as appropriate when considering reoperation. If a patient has undergone an operation that has proved by experience to be ineffective, a repeated operation for failure of that procedure is appropriate. Complications of procedures, such as stenosis causing gastric outlet obstruction after vertical banded gastroplasty or metabolic complications after jejunoileal bypass, are obvious indications for revisional surgery. One mistake frequently made by a nonbariatric surgeon in correcting a complication of a bariatric operation is to perform a procedure that corrects the complication but does not provide for continued weight restriction. In these circumstances, a typical long-term course is for patients to slowly regain weight to their degree of obesity before the initial bariatric procedure and then to seek further surgical assistance.

In assessing a patient for the appropriateness of reoperative surgery, the surgeon must determine whether the original bariatric operation is intact and anatomically still appropriate for maintaining weight loss. If not, consideration for reoperation is appropriate. However, a patient who has failed an anatomically intact and well-constructed bariatric operation is, in our opinion, at high risk to fail a second or revisional bariatric operation. The incidence of infection, organ ischemia, anastomotic leakage, blood transfusion, and other severe intraabdominal complications is increased in revisional surgery.

All bariatric operations have some incidence of failure, which includes inadequate weight loss, inadequate resolution of medical comorbid conditions, development of side effects negatively influencing lifestyle and satisfaction, development of complications requiring medical or surgical intervention, and complications requiring alteration or reversal of the operation. Analysis of the 449,753 bariatric operations logged into the Bariatric Outcomes Longitudinal Database (BOLD) shows that 4.4% were corrective operations (i.e., operations that addressed complications or incomplete treatment effect of the primary bariatric operation) and 1.9% were conversions (i.e., operations in which the primary bariatric procedure was converted to another bariatric procedure).[46] Only 6.3% of bariatric operations needed reoperation and even fewer needed conversion to another bariatric procedure, which points out the relative efficacy of the commonly performed bariatric procedures being performed currently. Moreover, the reoperations had a low mortality rate of 0.12% to 0.21% and a 1-year EWL of 36% to 39%. The data suggest that reoperations for failure are not that common, the clinical results are comparable to those of primary operations, and they are associated with comparable mortality rates.[46]

ENDOSCOPIC PROCEDURES IN BARIATRIC SURGERY

Endoscopy has become an important part of management of complications after bariatric surgery, and in addition, a plethora of endoscopic weight loss procedures are being used or are in development.

Preoperative Use of Endoscopy

The Standards of Practice Committee of the American Society for Gastrointestinal Endoscopy, in conjunction with representatives

TABLE 48.16 **Potential role of laparoscopic sleeve gastrectomy in bariatric surgery.**

CONDITION	PROCEDURES CONTRAINDICATED	POTENTIAL ADVANTAGE OF LSG
Iron deficiency anemia	RYGB, BPD	Preservation of duodenum
Crohn small bowel disease	RYGB, DS, BPD, LAGB if taking steroids	Preservation of small bowel
Transplant patients taking immunosuppressive medications	LAGB if taking steroids; relative contraindication to RYGB, DS, and BPD	More stable absorption of antirejection medications
Cardiac failure patients	Malabsorption of medications by RYGB; DS and BPD a relative contraindication	More stable absorption of critically needed medications
Severe arthritis requiring nonsteroidal anti-inflammatory drugs	RYGB and BPD contraindicated because of ulcer risk	Preservation of stomach allows continued use of nonsteroidal antiinflammatory drugs
Patients who may not be able to comply with frequent follow-up	LAGB, RYGB, DS, BPD	Less risk of malabsorption and reduced need for LAGB adjustments
Patients with preexisting vitamin deficiencies (e.g., vitamin D, iron)	RYGB, DS, BPD	Preservation of entire small bowel reduces risk of vitamin deficiencies
Autoimmune connective tissue disorder	LAGB	LSG may be a good option

BPD, Biliopancreatic diversion; *DS*, duodenal switch; *LAGB*, laparoscopic adjustable gastric banding; *LSG*, laparoscopic sleeve gastrectomy; *RYGB*, Roux-en-Y gastric bypass.

from the Society of Gastrointestinal and Endoscopic Surgeons and the ASMBS, published guidelines on this topic in 2015. They concluded that the use of endoscopy should be based upon a close discussion between the patient and the surgeon. The ASMBS states endoscopy should be considered in the work up of patients if they have a history of GERD. The greatest unknown is the number of patients who do not have symptoms and yet have significant endoscopic findings. A comprehensive review of 28 studies and 6616 patients identified that the majority (92.4%) of preoperative endoscopic findings did not alter management; however, 7.6% of patients had findings that delayed or altered surgery.[47] This argues for the use of routine preoperative endoscopy to avoid any surprises at the time of surgery. Therefore, endoscopy for patients prior to bariatric surgery should be performed in symptomatic patients and consideration be given to preoperative endoscopy in asymptomatic patients.

Intraoperative Endoscopy

Many surgeons will do an intraoperative leak test in the operating room at the time of procedure to prevent complications after the procedure. The method of leak test varies from using methylene blue through an orogastric tube to air insufflation with a tube or an endoscope. When using an insufflation test, the staple line of the stomach and any proximal anastomosis is submerged under sterile saline and air is insufflated into the gastric pouch. One then looks for air bubbles to assess whether the staple lines are airtight under hyperdistention. The benefit of the endoscope is that is can be both diagnostic and therapeutic at the time of surgery. If a leak is noted, it may be able to be managed with endoscopic clips or externally placed sutures under endoscopic guidance. In addition, if bleeding is noted along any staple lines, it can be managed immediately rather than a potential return to the operating room later once the bleed becomes clinically evident. Finally, endoscopy allows the surgeon to assess the postsurgical anatomy more thoroughly to ensure it looks as intended.

Postoperative Endoscopy

Once a patient has had altered anatomy for a weight loss procedure, endoscopy is invaluable in evaluating patients who return with abdominal complaints, suffer from weight regain, or develop a complication of their procedure. Understanding the postsurgical anatomy after a bariatric procedure can be challenging, especially if the surgery was many years ago. The most common procedures one should recognize are the gastric bypass, vertical LSG, gastric banding, and vertical banded gastroplasty.

Endoscopic Management of Complications After Bariatric Surgery

Leaks after bariatric surgery are one of the most dreaded complications. These carry a high mortality and are the complications surgeons most want to avoid. One of the most commonly used interventions for a leak is the use of a fully covered stent. This endoscopically placed stent traverses the perforation, thereby decreasing ongoing contamination. This may allow the patient to continue oral intake through the postoperative period. One study describing the use of stents noted a healing period of 6 weeks and a 90% success rate. Migration of the stent was noted in 8/20 patients, which appears to be a major issue with these stents and the Achilles heel of this management approach.[48] To avoid migration, multiple methods of prevention have been described, including suturing it or clipping the stent in place. Clips are generally unsuccessful as they fall off quickly and the stents are left in place for 4 to 6 weeks. Sutures can be placed endoscopically, but these devices are sometimes bulky in this small space. Utilizing a suture, the stent can be bridled to the nose. Fluoroscopy is essential to ensure proper stent placement. Leaks after LSG can be particularly challenging, as the stents available in the United States are not long enough to traverse the entire sleeve. Many use two stents placed overlapping to mitigate this problem.

Another approach to leak management is the use of over-the-scope clips. This technology generally does not work for these leaks in the acute setting unless the hole is very small with fresh edges. Usually, this technology works better for chronic leaks that are small or fistulas that are less than 1 cm.

Endoscopic vacuum-assisted closure is now being used for the closure of large leaks. This technique involves placing the vacuum sponge on the end of an orogastric tube into the cavity external to the leak. Over time, this allows closure of this area. This works for encapsulated leaks. This technique is very labor intensive, as the device must be changed every few days, similar to any external wound vacuum device. Generally, patients will require 8 to 12 procedures over a period of weeks. The benefit is this can actually shorten the healing time compared to traditional methods.

If the hole is small but the external cavity of the leak is on the larger side, internal drainage with a double pigtail stent can also be used. This allows internal drainage of the extraluminal cavity. This is very helpful, particularly when the placement of an external drain is difficult. If the opening is small, an endoscopic septotomy has also been performed to allow better drainage of an extraluminal cavity.

Strictures After Bariatric Surgery

Strictures can occur at the outlet of a pouch after gastric bypass procedures or at the incisura angularis after LSG. After a gastric bypass, the anastomotic strictures can often be managed with through-the-scope balloons. These range from 5 mm to 20 mm in diameter. They are placed through the scope and across the stricture. If the scope cannot traverse the stricture, the balloon can be placed over a wire or with fluoroscopic guidance to avoid perforation. These strictures may require multiple dilations as one should not try to dilate the stricture more than 3 to 5 mm at any one sitting. In addition, the underlying cause of the stricture should be identified and addressed to avoid recurrence. Common causes include smoking and nonsteroidal medication use.

Strictures after LSG are most often at the incisura angularis. These have been managed with endoscopic balloon dilation and stent placement. Unfortunately, these methods are not always successful and conversion to a gastric bypass for management is necessary.

Weight Regain After Bariatric Surgery

Recidivism after bariatric surgery occurs around 10% to 15% of the time. Endoscopic suturing for pouch outlet reduction following gastric bypass procedure is the most commonly described procedure. An endoscopic suturing device that allows full-thickness bites is utilized to decrease the size of the gastrojejunostomy. The smaller diameter anastomosis allows for longer retention of food within the pouch, leading to greater satiety and reduced food intake. The endoscopic procedure is accompanied by lifestyle counseling to improve dietary and exercise habits and has been able to obtain weight loss at 6 months, but longer-term studies are needed to confirm the early success.

Primary Endoscopic Weight Loss Procedures

Currently, for those overweight, diet and exercise are recommended. For those with severe obesity, weight loss surgery is an option. For those in between, there are few interventions available. In addition, many patients do not wish to go as extreme as an anatomically altering weight loss surgery. Now there are several endoscopic options for weight loss. These work in various ways.

The most common endoscopic weight loss procedures are the space filling devices. They come in single- and multiple-balloon systems. The original gastric balloon was the Garren-Edwards balloon, but this was pulled from the market due to migrations and bowel obstructions. The modern balloons are more sophisticated and the most common is the Orbera balloon (Apollo Endosurgery, Inc.). Over 300,000 of these balloons have been placed with reasonable success. This balloon is placed endoscopically, remains in place for 6 months, and then is removed endoscopically. Throughout this time and the ensuing 6 months, the patient receives dietary and lifestyle counseling. Patients learn how much food they can live on while the balloon is in place, and the ongoing counseling is to help them maintain that lifestyle once the balloon is removed. Most patients lose 30 to 50 lbs. One of the largest series of Orbera placement comes from Brazil with a consensus statement after over 40,000 balloons. They note the balloon has reasonable success with minimal adverse events.[49] Other balloon systems are air filled or utilize multiple balloons to minimize the nausea that is encountered at initial placement. Newer balloons are on the horizon that do not require endoscopy for placement or removal. These are in trial currently.

The other endoscopic procedure that has gained popularity is the endoscopic sleeve gastroplasty. The stomach walls are sutured together to collapse the stomach utilizing an endoscopic suturing device. By doing so, the only lumen left behind emulates a sleeve gastroplasty. The weight loss reported in the short-term in small series is greater than medical therapy and long-term controlled trials are needed to evaluate the potential of this approach.

Other endoscopic procedures include liners that decrease absorption or by reducing gastric emptying, thereby inducing fullness in the patient. In addition, even magnets are being used to create bypasses endoscopically. All of these procedures have minimal data and their durability is unclear. These endoscopic procedures will never be as effective as surgery; however, they can provide a bridge to surgical procedures. They can also be an intervention that some patients can accept to facilitate weight loss that is less invasive than surgery.

CONTROVERSIES IN BARIATRIC SURGERY

Based upon the latest evidence, a few individuals have argued that guidelines for bariatric surgery based upon strict BMI cut-offs fail to identify some patients who would be most likely to benefit. For years, the criterion for bariatric surgery has been BMI, yet the evidence from the SOS study shows that BMI did not predict the beneficial effect of surgery on cardiovascular, diabetic, or cancer-related mortality.[50] On the other hand, fasting hyperinsulinemia, which is reflective of insulin resistance, was predictive of the positive bariatric surgery results in overall mortality, cardiovascular events, and incidence of diabetes. If the aim of bariatric surgery is not just weight loss but also to reduce mortality, prevent diabetes, and reduce cardiovascular events, Sjostrom[50] suggests preoperative insulin and glucose levels are better criteria to select those patients who will benefit most from bariatric surgery.

Level 1 evidence also demonstrates the efficacy of bariatric surgery (RYGB, LSG, and LAGB) over medical therapy in the treatment of type 2 diabetes in lower-BMI patients.[15–18] The concept that bariatric surgery is better than medical management of type 2 diabetes is new and very controversial. Although more medical societies[23] and internists are recognizing the benefits of bariatric surgery and even endorsing the referral to bariatric surgeons, it is unclear when and if insurance guidelines for bariatric surgery will endorse the use of surgery as a primary treatment of diabetes or use metabolic variables rather than BMI as primary criteria for surgery.

CONCLUSION

Surgical treatment of morbid obesity is no longer considered out of the mainstream of general surgery and is now a component of surgical residency training programs. It currently represents the fastest-growing area of general surgery. While patient demand for the procedure has vastly increased; at present, surgeons operate annually on less than 2% of the eligible patients who would benefit from bariatric surgery. This chapter has discussed all aspects of the performance of bariatric surgery in current surgical practice, including the most commonly performed procedures at this time. The disease process of morbid obesity is unfortunately incompletely understood but increasing in prevalence worldwide.

Surgical therapy has been shown to reduce long-term mortality and control of diabetes largely because surgery has proven to be a more effective intervention for weight loss than nonsurgical options. Recent randomized clinical trials of bariatric surgery versus medical treatment in obese diabetics have shown bariatric surgery to be more effective in the treatment of severe obesity, type 2 diabetes, hypertension, and dyslipidemia. With the positive results of bariatric surgery becoming more widely known, there has been movement by multiple medical societies to recognize the need for referral to bariatric surgeon for evaluation. It is hopeful that these data will also encourage the government and insurance companies to add bariatric and metabolic surgery coverage.

SELECTED REFERENCES

Adams TD, Gress RE, Smith SC, et al. Long-term mortality after gastric bypass surgery. *N Engl J Med.* 2007;357:753–761.

A retrospective cohort study determined the long-term mortality among 7925 patients who underwent Roux-en-Y gastric bypass (RYGB) matched by age, sex, and body mass index to 7925 severely obese persons who applied for driver's licenses. During a mean follow-up of 7.1 years, adjusted long-term mortality from any cause after RYGB decreased by 40% compared with that in the control group; cause-specific mortality in the surgery group decreased by 56% for coronary artery disease, by 92% for diabetes, and by 60% for cancer. They concluded that long-term total mortality after gastric bypass surgery was significantly reduced, particularly deaths from diabetes, heart disease, and cancer.

Adams TD, Davidson LE, Litwin SE, et al. Weight and metabolic outcomes 12 years after gastric bypass. *N Engl J Med.* 2017;377:1143–1155.

This follow-up study of the retrospective cohort study determined the long-term mortality among 7925 patients who underwent Roux-en-Y gastric bypass (RYGB) matched by age, sex, and body mass index to 7925 severely obese persons who applied for driver's licenses. The 2007 publication[7] identified reduced all-cause mortality in the surgery group, while the follow-up determined that the weight loss, fasting glucose level, systolic blood pressure, low-density lipoprotein cholesterol, high-density lipoprotein cholesterol, and triglycerides were all significantly improved 12 years after RYGB compared to matched control subjects. They concluded, "This study showed the long-term durability of weight loss and effective remission and prevention of type 2 diabetes, hypertension, and dyslipidemia after Roux-en-Y gastric bypass."

Birkmeyer JD, Finks JF, O'Reilly A, et al. Surgical skill and complication rates after bariatric surgery. *N Engl J Med.* 2013;369:1434–1442.

A study from the Michigan cooperative demonstrated that the surgeon's skill remains paramount in outcomes. The surgeons judged to be in the top quartile of technical skill on the basis of peer review of a video procedure showed significantly lower mortality (0.05% vs. 0.26%; P = 0.01) and lower morbidity (5.2% vs. 14.5%; P < 0.001) compared with the bottom quartile surgeons.

Courcoulas AP, King WC, Belle SH, et al. Seven-year weight trajectories and health outcomes in the Longitudinal Assessment of Bariatric Surgery (LABS) study. *JAMA Surg.* 2018;153:427–434.

A multicenter observational trial at 10 U.S. centers in 2348 subjects undergoing bariatric surgery. Weight loss was much greater for laparoscopic Roux-en-Y gastric bypass (LRYGB) than laparoscopic adjustable gastrointestinal banding (LAGB). Weight loss and remission of diabetes and lipids was durable following LRYGB. A high proportion of LAGB patients (26.2%) underwent reoperation in this 7-year trial supporting the observation that needs for band revisions, band removal, and conversion to another procedure limit the long-term effectiveness of the LAGB procedure.

Ikramuddin S, Korner J, Lee WJ, et al. Roux-en-Y gastric bypass vs intensive medical management for the control of type 2 diabetes, hypertension, and hyperlipidemia: the Diabetes Surgery Study Randomized Clinical Trial. *JAMA.* 2013;309:2240–2249.

A randomized prospective clinical trial comparing Roux-en-Y gastric bypass (RYGB) to intensive medical therapy in the control of type 2 diabetes, hypertension, and hyperlipidemia. At 24 months, 43% of the surgery group and only 14% of the intensive medical therapy group had achieved the primary end points (odds ratio 5.1). They concluded that in mild to moderately obese diabetic subjects, RYGB significantly improved the chances of achieving the composite end point. There were more serious adverse events (nutritional deficiencies and fractures) in the group undergoing surgery despite vitamin supplementation, and they cautioned potential benefits must be weighed against the risk of serious adverse events.

Kolotkin RL, Kim J, Davidson LE, et al. 12-year trajectory of health-related quality of life in gastric bypass patients versus comparison groups. *Surg Obes Relat Dis.* 2018;14:1359–1365.

This 12-year prospective study evaluated health-related quality of life (HRQOL) changes after gastric bypass surgery compared to two nonsurgical groups matched for similar demographics. The surgery group had greatly improved HRQOL in the physical component and in the weight-related component from baseline. Differences between the patient's undergoing gastric bypass in both nonsurgical groups were significant for both weight-related HRQOL and physical HRQOL. The magnitude of improvement 12 years after gastric bypass surgery supports the conclusion that bariatric surgery improves the patient's quality of life.

Nguyen NT, Kim E, Vu S, et al. Ten-year outcomes of a prospective randomized trial of laparoscopic gastric bypass versus laparoscopic gastric banding. *Ann Surg.* 2018;268:106–113.

Level 1 evidence that Roux-en-Y gastric bypass has better long-term weight loss, a lower rate of late reoperation, and improved remission of diabetes compared to laparoscopic adjustable gastrointestinal banding.

Peterli R, Wolnerhanssen BK, Peters T, et al. Effect of laparoscopic sleeve gastrectomy vs laparoscopic Roux-en-Y gastric bypass on weight loss in patients with morbid obesity: the SM-BOSS Randomized Clinical Trial. *JAMA*. 2018; 319:255–265.

Level 1 evidence from a randomized controlled trial demonstrating slightly better but not statistically significant weight loss, remission of diabetes after laparoscopic Roux-en-Y gastric bypass (LRYGB) compared to laparoscopic sleeve gastrectomy (LSG). Both procedures improved health-related quality of life and there was no difference in late complications. LRYGB was much better at remission of gastroesophageal reflux disease. The results of this trial and the SLEEVEPASS RCT show LSG to be an effective bariatric procedure that compares favorably to LRYGB at 5 years after surgery.

Salminen P, Helmio M, Ovaska J, et al. Effect of laparoscopic sleeve gastrectomy vs laparoscopic Roux-en-Y gastric bypass on weight loss at 5 years among patients with morbid obesity: the SLEEVEPASS Randomized Clinical Trial. *JAMA*. 2018;319:241–254.

Comparison of laparoscopic Roux-en-Y gastric bypass (LRYGB) to laparoscopic sleeve gastrectomy (LSG) in a randomized controlled trial demonstrated that weight loss was slightly better (57% vs. 49%, respectively) and resolution of hypertension was improved after LRYGB compared to LSG. The difference in weight loss between procedures did not have clinical significance. They also note both procedures had improved HRQOL and no difference in late complications. The majority (7/10) of reoperations after LSG were performed for severe reflux. The results of this trial and the SM-BOSS RCT show LSG to be an effective bariatric procedure that compares favorably to LRYGB at 5 years after surgery.

Schauer PR, Bhatt DL, Kirwan JP, et al. Bariatric surgery versus intensive medical therapy for diabetes—5-year outcomes. *N Engl J Med*. 2017;376:641–651.

The authors randomized 150 obese (body mass index 27–43) uncontrolled diabetics (HbA1c >7.0%) to intensive medical therapy or to laparoscopic sleeve gastrectomy or laparoscopic Roux-en-Y gastric bypass. Surgical groups had significant improvement in HbA1c, weight loss, and dyslipidemia and a reduction in the number of antihypertensive, lipid-lowering, and diabetic medications used at 1, 2, 3, and 5 years after randomization. The surgical patients also had a significant improvement in quality of life (QOL), whereas there was no change in the QOL for the medically treated patients. They concluded, "Bariatric surgery represents a potentially useful strategy for the management of type 2 diabetes, allowing many patients to reach and maintain therapeutic targets of glycemic control that otherwise would not be achievable with intensive medical therapy alone." This study, now with a 5-year follow-up showing sustained improvements for the surgical groups, adds to the strong evidence supporting bariatric surgery as a safe and effective therapy for treatment of type 2 diabetes.

Sjöström L. Review of the key results from the Swedish Obese Subjects (SOS) trial—a prospective controlled intervention study of bariatric surgery. *J Intern Med*. 2013;273: 219–234.

An excellent review of the results of the Swedish Obese Subjects trial. Bariatric surgery in 2010 obese subjects was associated with significant weight loss up to 20 years after surgery compared with a control group of 2037 who received standard medical care (18% vs. 1%). Long-term mortality was reduced in the bariatric surgery patients (adjusted hazard ratio, 0.71). The bariatric surgery group also had decreased incidence of diabetes, myocardial infarction, stroke, and cancer. Their analysis also showed that high insulin or high glucose levels at baseline predicted success, whereas the level of body mass index (BMI) did not, which leads the authors to suggest that the selection based on BMI needs reevaluation and that use of insulin and glucose values would better predict outcomes with bariatric surgery and therefore would be a better selection criterion.

Sjöström L, Narbro K, Sjöström CD, et al. Effects of bariatric surgery on mortality in Swedish obese subjects. *N Engl J Med*. 2007;357:741–752

This study compared a group of patients undergoing bariatric surgery with a group of matched control subjects and monitored them for 10.9 years. They had an unparalleled follow-up rate of 99.9% of the subjects in the study. They found a significant decrease in the weight and risk of death in individuals in the surgical weight loss group compared with control patients not undergoing surgery (unadjusted overall hazard ratio was 0.76 in the surgery group [P = 0.4] compared with the control group). This is the best long-term study indicating that bariatric surgery results in sustained weight loss, resolution of comorbid conditions, and increased survival in comparison to standard medical treatment.

REFERENCES

1. Hales CM, Carroll MD, Fryar CD, et al. Prevalence of obesity among adults and youth: United States, 2015–2016. *NCHS Data Brief.* 2017:1–8.
2. Ezzati M, Bentham J, De Cesare M, et al. Worldwide trends in body-mass index, underweight, overweight, and obesity from 1975 to 2016: a pooled analysis of 2416 population-based measurement studies in 128.9 million children, adolescents, and adults. *Lancet*. 2017;390:2627–2642.
3. Siljee JE, Wang Y, Bernard AA, et al. Subcellular localization of MC4R with ADCY3 at neuronal primary cilia underlies a common pathway for genetic predisposition to obesity. *Nat Genet*. 2018;50:180–185.
4. Mahana D, Trent CM, Kurtz ZD, et al. Antibiotic perturbation of the murine gut microbiome enhances the adiposity, insulin resistance, and liver disease associated with high-fat diet. *Genome Med*. 2016;8:48.
5. Singh RK, Kumar P, Mahalingam K. Molecular genetics of human obesity: a comprehensive review. *C R Biol*. 2017;340:87–108.

6. Sjostrom L, Narbro K, Sjostrom CD, et al. Effects of bariatric surgery on mortality in Swedish obese subjects. *N Engl J Med.* 2007;357:741–752.
7. Adams TD, Gress RE, Smith SC, et al. Long-term mortality after gastric bypass surgery. *N Engl J Med.* 2007;357: 753–761.
8. Arterburn DE, Olsen MK, Smith VA, et al. Association between bariatric surgery and long-term survival. *JAMA.* 2015;313:62–70.
9. Guidry CA, Davies SW, Sawyer RG, et al. Gastric bypass improves survival compared with propensity-matched controls: a cohort study with over 10-year follow-up. *Am J Surg.* 2015;209:463–467.
10. Kauppila JH, Tao W, Santoni G, et al. Effects of obesity surgery on overall and disease-specific mortality in a 5-country population-based study. *Gastroenterology.* 2019;157:119–127 e111.
11. Adams TD, Davidson LE, Litwin SE, et al. Weight and metabolic outcomes 12 years after gastric bypass. *N Engl J Med.* 2017;377:1143–1155.
12. Davidson LE, Adams TD, Kim J, et al. Association of patient age at gastric bypass surgery with long-term all-cause and cause-specific mortality. *JAMA Surg.* 2016;151:631–637.
13. Kolotkin RL, Kim J, Davidson LE, et al. 12-year trajectory of health-related quality of life in gastric bypass patients versus comparison groups. *Surg Obes Relat Dis.* 2018;14:1359–1365.
14. Neovius M, Bruze G, Jacobson P, et al. Risk of suicide and non-fatal self-harm after bariatric surgery: results from two matched cohort studies. *Lancet Diabetes Endocrinol.* 2018;6:197–207.
15. Schauer PR, Bhatt DL, Kirwan JP, et al. Bariatric surgery versus intensive medical therapy for diabetes—5-year outcomes. *N Engl J Med.* 2017;376:641–651.
16. Ikramuddin S, Billington CJ, Lee WJ, et al. Roux-en-Y gastric bypass for diabetes (the Diabetes Surgery Study): 2-year outcomes of a 5-year, randomised, controlled trial. *Lancet Diabetes Endocrinol.* 2015;3:413–422.
17. Mingrone G, Panunzi S, De Gaetano A, et al. Bariatric-metabolic surgery versus conventional medical treatment in obese patients with type 2 diabetes: 5 year follow-up of an open-label, single-centre, randomised controlled trial. *Lancet.* 2015;386:964–973.
18. Simonson DC, Halperin F, Foster K, et al. Clinical and patient-centered outcomes in obese patients with type 2 diabetes 3 years after randomization to Roux-en-Y gastric bypass surgery versus intensive lifestyle management: the SLIMM-T2D Study. *Diabetes Care.* 2018;41:670–679.
19. O'Brien R, Johnson E, Haneuse S, et al. Microvascular outcomes in patients with diabetes after bariatric surgery versus usual care: a matched cohort study. *Ann Intern Med.* 2018;169:300–310.
20. Svane MS, Bojsen-Moller KN, Martinussen C, et al. Postprandial nutrient handling and gastrointestinal hormone secretion after Roux-en-Y gastric bypass vs sleeve gastrectomy. *Gastroenterology.* 2019;156:1627–1641.e1621.
21. Evans S, Pamuklar Z, Rosko J, et al. Gastric bypass surgery restores meal stimulation of the anorexigenic gut hormones glucagon-like peptide-1 and peptide YY independently of caloric restriction. *Surg Endosc.* 2012;26:1086–1094.
22. Hutch CR, Sandoval D. The role of GLP-1 in the metabolic success of bariatric surgery. *Endocrinology.* 2017;158:4139–4151.
23. 8. Obesity management for the treatment of type 2 diabetes: standards of medical care in diabetes—2019. *Diabetes Care.* 2019;42:S81–S89.
24. Ibrahim AM, Ghaferi AA, Thumma JR, et al. Variation in outcomes at bariatric surgery centers of excellence. *JAMA Surg.* 2017;152:629–636.
25. Birkmeyer JD, Finks JF, O'Reilly A, et al. Surgical skill and complication rates after bariatric surgery. *N Engl J Med.* 2013;369:1434–1442.
26. Lazzati A, Audureau E, Hemery F, et al. Reduction in early mortality outcomes after bariatric surgery in France between 2007 and 2012: a nationwide study of 133,000 obese patients. *Surgery.* 2016;159:467–474.
27. Inge TH, Courcoulas AP, Jenkins TM, et al. Weight loss and health status 3 years after bariatric surgery in adolescents. *N Engl J Med.* 2016;374:113–123.
28. *Estimate of Bariatric Surgery Numbers, 2011–2017.* American Society of Metabolic and Bariatric Surgeons; 2018. https://asmbs.org/resources/estimate-of-bariatric-surgery-numbers. Accessed August 6, 2019.
29. Varban OA, Cassidy RB, Sheetz KH, et al. Technique or technology? Evaluating leaks after gastric bypass. *Surg Obes Relat Dis.* 2016;12:264–272.
30. Janik MR, Mustafa RR, Rogula TG, et al. Safety of laparoscopic sleeve gastrectomy and Roux-en-Y gastric bypass in elderly patients—analysis of the MBSAQIP. *Surg Obes Relat Dis.* 2018;14:1276–1282.
31. Kumar SB, Hamilton BC, Wood SG, et al. Is laparoscopic sleeve gastrectomy safer than laparoscopic gastric bypass? A comparison of 30-day complications using the MBSAQIP data registry. *Surg Obes Relat Dis.* 2018;14:264–269.
32. Stroh C, Kockerling F, Volker L, et al. Results of more than 11,800 sleeve gastrectomies: data analysis of the German Bariatric Surgery Registry. *Ann Surg.* 2016;263:949–955.
33. O'Brien PE, Hindle A, Brennan L, et al. Long-term outcomes after bariatric surgery: a systematic review and meta-analysis of weight loss at 10 or more years for all bariatric procedures and a single-centre review of 20-year outcomes after adjustable gastric banding. *Obes Surg.* 2019;29:3–14.
34. Courcoulas AP, King WC, Belle SH, et al. Seven-year weight trajectories and health outcomes in the longitudinal assessment of bariatric surgery (LABS) study. *JAMA Surg.* 2018;153:427–434.
35. Miras AD, Kamocka A, Patel D, et al. Obesity surgery makes patients healthier and more functional: real world results from the United Kingdom National Bariatric Surgery Registry. *Surg Obes Relat Dis.* 2018;14:1033–1040.
36. Bolckmans R, Himpens J. Long-term (>10 yrs) outcome of the laparoscopic biliopancreatic diversion with duodenal switch. *Ann Surg.* 2016;264:1029–1037.
37. Salminen P, Helmio M, Ovaska J, et al. Effect of laparoscopic sleeve gastrectomy vs laparoscopic Roux-en-Y gastric bypass on weight loss at 5 years among patients with morbid obesity: the SLEEVEPASS Randomized Clinical Trial. *JAMA.* 2018;319:241–254.
38. Peterli R, Wolnerhanssen BK, Peters T, et al. Effect of laparoscopic sleeve gastrectomy vs laparoscopic Roux-en-Y gastric bypass on weight loss in patients with morbid obesity: the SM-BOSS randomized clinical trial. *JAMA.* 2018;319:255–265.
39. Tchokouani L, Jayaram A, Alenazi N, et al. The long-term effects of the adjustable gastric band on esophageal

motility in patients who present for band removal. *Obes Surg.* 2018;28:333–337.
40. Nguyen NT, Kim E, Vu S, et al. Ten-year outcomes of a prospective randomized trial of laparoscopic gastric bypass versus laparoscopic gastric banding. *Ann Surg.* 2018;268:106–113.
41. Lazzati A, De Antonio M, Paolino L, et al. Natural history of adjustable gastric banding: lifespan and revisional rate: a nationwide study on administrative data on 53,000 patients. *Ann Surg.* 2017;265:439–445.
42. Reames BN, Bacal D, Krell RW, et al. Influence of median surgeon operative duration on adverse outcomes in bariatric surgery. *Surg Obes Relat Dis.* 2015;11:207–213.
43. Aghajani E, Nergaard BJ, Leifson BG, et al. The mesenteric defects in laparoscopic Roux-en-Y gastric bypass: 5 years follow-up of non-closure versus closure using the stapler technique. *Surg Endosc.* 2017;31:3743–3748.
44. Edholm D, Ottosson J, Sundbom M. Importance of pouch size in laparoscopic Roux-en-Y gastric bypass: a cohort study of 14,168 patients. *Surg Endosc.* 2016;30:2011–2015.
45. Felsenreich DM, Langer FB, Kefurt R, et al. Weight loss, weight regain, and conversions to Roux-en-Y gastric bypass: 10-year results of laparoscopic sleeve gastrectomy. *Surg Obes Relat Dis.* 2016;12:1655–1662.
46. Sudan R, Nguyen NT, Hutter MM, et al. Morbidity, mortality, and weight loss outcomes after reoperative bariatric surgery in the USA. *J Gastrointest Surg.* 2015;19:171–178; discussion 178–179.
47. Parikh M, Liu J, Vieira D, et al. Preoperative endoscopy prior to bariatric surgery: a systematic review and meta-analysis of the literature. *Obes Surg.* 2016;26:2961–2966.
48. Aryaie AH, Singer JL, Fayezizadeh M, et al. Efficacy of endoscopic management of leak after foregut surgery with endoscopic covered self-expanding metal stents (SEMS). *Surg Endosc.* 2017;31:612–617.
49. Neto MG, Silva LB, Grecco E, et al. Brazilian Intragastric Balloon Consensus Statement (BIBC): practical guidelines based on experience of over 40,000 cases. *Surg Obes Relat Dis.* 2018;14:151–159.
50. Sjostrom L. Review of the key results from the Swedish Obese Subjects (SOS) trial—a prospective controlled intervention study of bariatric surgery. *J Intern Med.* 2013;273:219–234.

49 CHAPTER

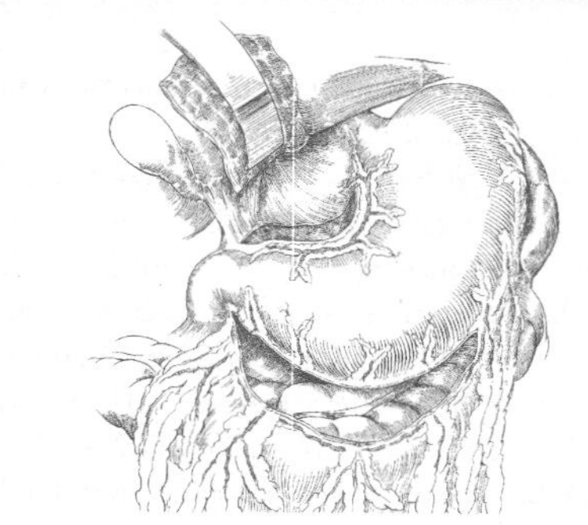

Stomach

David A. Mahvi, David M. Mahvi

OUTLINE

ANATOMY

Gross Anatomy

Divisions

The stomach is derived from the tubular embryonic foregut and begins as a dilation during the fifth week of gestation in the caudal portion. The embryonic stomach is invested by two mesenteries: dorsal (which becomes the gastrosplenic, gastrocolic, and gastrophrenic ligaments) and ventral (which becomes the hepatoduodenal and gastrohepatic ligaments of the lesser omentum and the falciform ligament). By the seventh week of gestation, the stomach descends, rotates, and further dilates with a disproportionate elongation of the greater curvature into its normal anatomic shape and position.

The most proximal region of the stomach is called the cardia and attaches to the esophagus. Immediately proximal to the cardia is the physiologically competent lower esophageal sphincter. The stomach is fixed at the gastroesophageal (GE) junction and pylorus, but its large midportion is mobile. The fundus represents the superior-most part of the stomach and is floppy and distensible. The angle of His is an important anatomic angle formed by the fundus with the left margin of the esophagus. The body of the stomach represents the largest portion and is also referred to as the corpus. The body is bounded on the right by the relatively straight lesser curvature and on the left by the longer greater curvature. At the angularis incisura, the lesser curvature abruptly angles to the right. The body of the stomach ends here and the antrum begins. Distally, the pylorus connects the distal stomach (antrum) to the proximal duodenum (Fig. 49.1).

The left lateral segment of the liver covers a large portion of the stomach anteriorly. Posteriorly, the stomach is bounded by the diaphragm, left kidney, pancreas, aorta, and celiac trunk. Inferiorly, the stomach is attached to the transverse colon via the gastrocolic ligament. Superiorly, the GE junction is found approximately 2 to 3 cm below the diaphragmatic esophageal hiatus in the horizontal plane of the seventh chondrosternal articulation, a plane only slightly cephalad to the plane containing the pylorus. The gastrosplenic ligament attaches the proximal greater curvature to the spleen.

Blood Supply

The celiac artery provides the majority of the blood supply to the stomach (Fig. 49.2). There are four main arteries—the left and right gastric arteries along the lesser curvature and the left and right gastroepiploic arteries along the greater curvature, with the left gastric artery being the largest. In addition, a substantial quantity of blood may be supplied to the proximal stomach by the inferior phrenic arteries and by the short gastric arteries from the spleen. Approximately 15% to 20% of patients have an aberrant left hepatic artery originating from the left gastric artery. Consequently, proximal ligation of the left gastric artery can result in acute left-sided hepatic ischemia. The right gastric artery arises

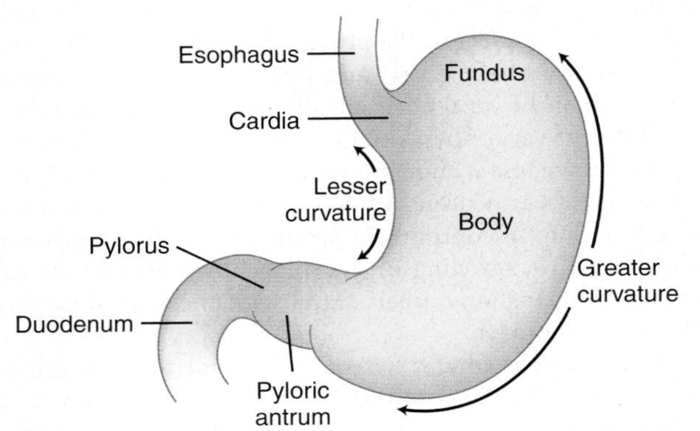

FIG. 49.1 Divisions of the stomach. (From Yeo C, Dempsey DT, Klein AS, et al, eds. *Shackelford's Surgery of the Alimentary Tract*. 6th ed. Philadelphia: Saunders; 2007.)

from the hepatic artery (or sometimes the gastroduodenal artery). The left gastroepiploic artery originates from the splenic artery, and the right gastroepiploic artery originates from the gastroduodenal artery. The extensive anastomotic connections between these major vessels ensures that, in most cases, the stomach will survive if three out of four arteries are ligated, provided that the arcades along the greater and lesser curvatures are not disturbed. In general, the veins of the stomach parallel the arteries. The left gastric (coronary) and right gastric veins usually drain into the portal vein. The right gastroepiploic vein drains into the superior mesenteric vein, and the left gastroepiploic vein drains into the splenic vein.

Lymphatic Drainage

The lymphatic drainage of the stomach parallels the vasculature and drains into four zones of lymph nodes (Fig. 49.3). The superior gastric group drains lymph from the upper lesser curvature into the left gastric and paracardial nodes. The suprapyloric group of nodes drains the antral segment on the lesser curvature of the stomach into the right suprapancreatic nodes. The pancreaticolienal group of nodes drains lymph high on the greater curvature into the left gastroepiploic and splenic nodes. The inferior gastric and subpyloric group of nodes drains lymph along the right gastroepiploic vascular pedicle. All four zones of lymph nodes drain into the celiac nodes and eventually into the thoracic duct. Although these lymph nodes drain different areas of the stomach,

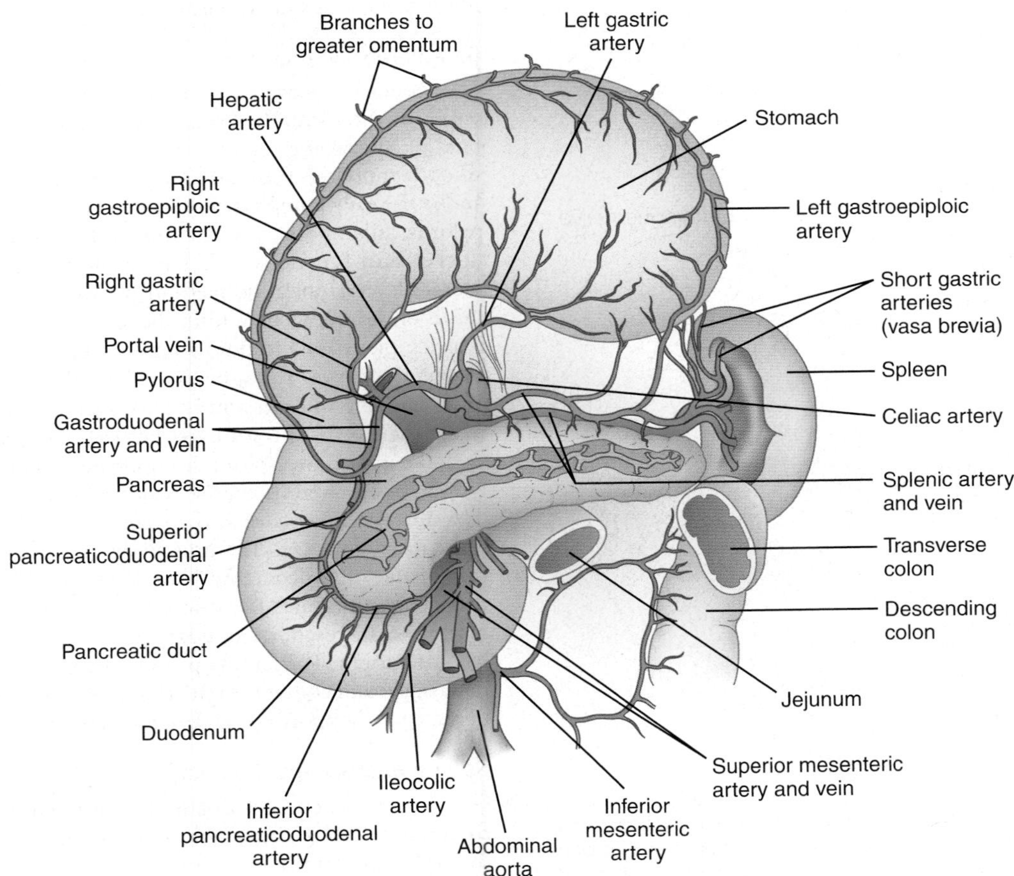

FIG. 49.2 Blood supply to the stomach and duodenum showing anatomic relationships to the spleen and pancreas. The stomach is reflected cephalad. (From Yeo C, Dempsey DT, Klein AS, et al, eds. *Shackelford's Surgery of the Alimentary Tract*. 6th ed. Philadelphia: Saunders; 2007.)

gastric cancers may metastasize to any of the four nodal groups, regardless of the cancer location. In addition, the extensive submucosal plexus of lymphatics accounts for the fact that there is frequently microscopic evidence of malignant cells several centimeters from gross disease.

Innervation

As shown in Fig. 49.4, the extrinsic innervation of the stomach is both parasympathetic (via the vagus nerve) and sympathetic (via the celiac plexus). The vagus nerve originates in the vagal nucleus in the floor of the fourth ventricle and traverses the neck in the carotid sheath to enter the mediastinum, where it divides into several branches around the esophagus. These branches coalesce above the esophageal hiatus to form the left and right vagus nerves. It is not uncommon to find more than two vagal trunks at the distal esophagus. At the GE junction, the left vagus is anterior, and the right vagus is posterior.

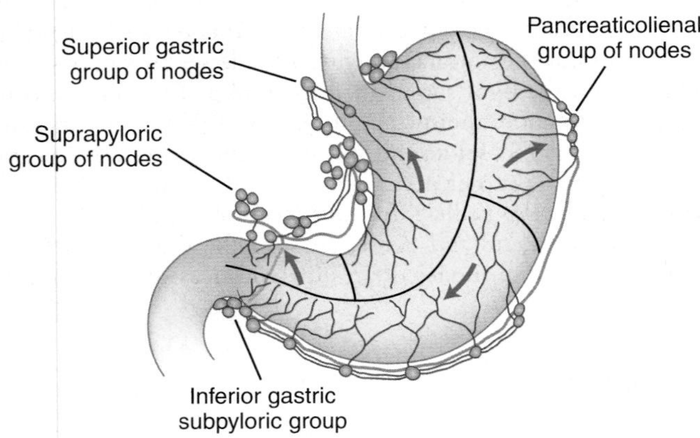

FIG. 49.3 Lymphatic drainage of the stomach.

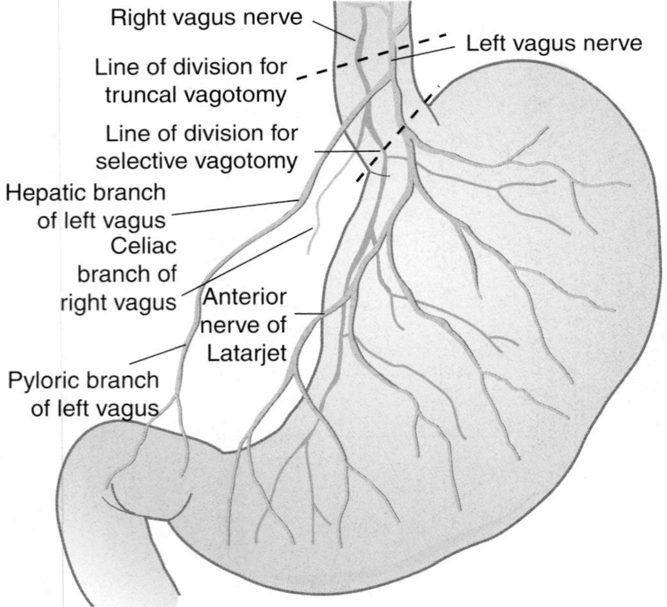

FIG. 49.4 Vagal innervation of the stomach. The line of division for truncal vagotomy is shown; it is above the hepatic and celiac branches of the left and right vagus nerves, respectively. The line of division for selective vagotomy is shown; this is below the hepatic and celiac branches. (From Mercer D, Liu T. Open truncal vagotomy. *Oper Tech Gen Surg.* 2003;5:8–85.)

The left vagus gives off the hepatic branch to the liver and continues along the lesser curvature as the nerve of Latarjet. The so-called criminal nerve of Grassi is the first branch of the right posterior vagus nerve; it is recognized as a potential cause of recurrent ulcers when left undivided. The right vagus nerve gives a branch off to the celiac plexus and continues posteriorly along the lesser curvature. A truncal vagotomy is performed above the celiac and hepatic branches of the vagi, whereas a selective vagotomy is performed below. A highly selective vagotomy is performed by dividing the crow's feet to the proximal stomach while preserving the innervation of the antral and pyloric parts of the stomach. Most (90%) of the vagal fibers are afferent, carrying stimuli to the brain. Efferent vagal fibers originate in the dorsal nucleus of the medulla and synapse with neurons in the myenteric and submucosal plexuses. These neurons influence gastric motor function and gastric secretion. In contrast, the sympathetic nerve supply comes from T5 to T10, traveling in the splanchnic nerve to the celiac ganglion. Postganglionic fibers travel with the arterial system to innervate the stomach.

The intrinsic or enteric nervous system of the stomach consists of neurons in Auerbach and Meissner autonomic plexuses. In these locations, cholinergic, serotoninergic, and peptidergic neurons are present. The exact function of these neurons is poorly understood. Nevertheless, numerous neuropeptides have been localized to these neurons, including acetylcholine, serotonin, substance P, calcitonin gene–related peptide, bombesin, cholecystokinin (CCK), and somatostatin.

Gastric Morphology

The stomach is covered by peritoneum, which forms the outer serosa of the stomach. Below this is the thicker muscularis propria, or muscularis externa, which is composed of three layers of smooth muscles. The middle layer of smooth muscle is circular and is the only complete muscle layer of the stomach wall. At the pylorus, this middle circular muscle layer becomes progressively thicker and functions as a true anatomic sphincter. The outer muscle layer is longitudinal and predominates in the distal two thirds of the stomach. Within the layers of the muscularis externa is a rich plexus of autonomic nerves and ganglia, called Auerbach myenteric plexus. The submucosa lies between the muscularis externa and the mucosa and is a collagen-rich layer of connective tissue that forms the strongest layer of the gastric wall. In addition, it contains the rich anastomotic network of blood vessels and lymphatics as well as the Meissner plexus of autonomic nerves. The mucosa consists of surface epithelium, lamina propria, and muscularis mucosae. The muscularis mucosae is on the luminal side of the submucosa and is probably responsible for the rugae that greatly increases the stomach's epithelial surface area. It also marks the microscopic boundary for invasive and noninvasive gastric carcinoma. The lamina propria represents a small connective tissue layer and contains capillaries, vessels, lymphatics, and nerves necessary to support the surface epithelium.

Gastric Microscopic Anatomy

Gastric mucosa consists of simple columnar epithelia interrupted by gastric pits containing one or more gastric glands. The cellular populations (and functions) of the cells forming this glandular epithelium vary based on their location in the stomach (Table 49.1). The glandular epithelium is divided into cells that secrete products into the gastric lumen for digestion (parietal

TABLE 49.1 Gastric cell types, location, and function.

CELL TYPE	LOCATION	FUNCTION
Parietal	Body	Secretion of acid and intrinsic factor
Mucus	Body, antrum	Mucus
Chief	Body	Pepsin
Surface epithelial	Diffuse	Mucus, bicarbonate, prostaglandins
Enterochromaffin-like	Body	Histamine
G	Antrum	Gastrin
D	Body, antrum	Somatostatin
Gastric mucosal interneurons	Body, antrum	Gastrin-releasing peptide
Enteric neurons	Diffuse	Calcitonin gene–related peptide, others
Endocrine	Body	Ghrelin

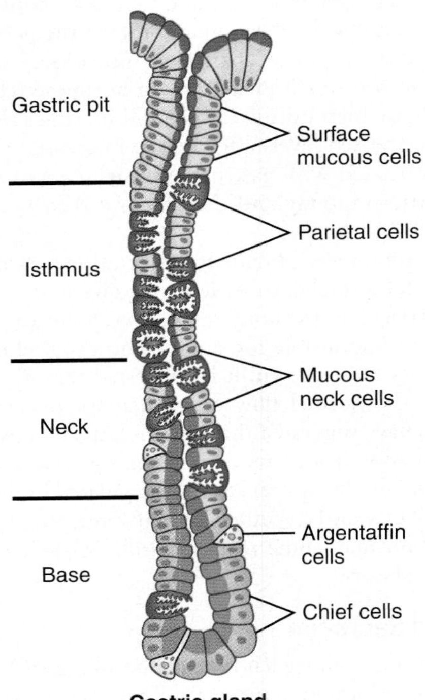

FIG. 49.5 Cells residing within a gastric gland. (From Yeo C, Dempsey DT, Klein AS, et al, eds. *Shackelford's Surgery of the Alimentary Tract.* 6th ed. Philadelphia: Saunders; 2007.)

cells, chief cells, mucus-secreting cells) and cells that control function (gastrin-secreting G cells, somatostatin-secreting D cells). In the cardia, the mucosa is arranged in branched glands, and the pits are short. In the fundus and body, the glands are more tubular, and the pits are longer. In the antrum, the glands are more branched. The luminal ends of the gastric glands and pits are lined with mucus-secreting surface epithelial cells, which extend down into the necks of the glands for variable distances. In the cardia, the glands are predominantly mucus-secreting. In the body, the glands are mostly lined from the neck to the base with parietal and chief cells (Fig. 49.5). There are a few parietal cells in the fundus and proximal antrum, but none in the cardia or prepyloric antrum. The endocrine G cells are present in greatest quantity in the antral glands.

PHYSIOLOGY

The principal function of the stomach is to prepare ingested food for digestion and absorption as it is propulsed into the small intestine. Receptive relaxation of the proximal stomach with ingestion of food enables the stomach to function as a storage organ. This relaxation enables liquids to pass easily from the stomach along the lesser curvature, whereas the solid food settles along the greater curvature of the fundus. In contrast to liquids, emptying of solid food is facilitated by the antrum, which propels solid food components into and through the pylorus. The antrum and pylorus function in a coordinated fashion, returning material to the proximal stomach until the size is suitable for delivery into the duodenum.

In addition to storing food, the stomach begins digestion of a meal. Starches undergo enzymatic breakdown through the activity of salivary amylase. Pepsin initiates protein digestion, although this hydrolysis is not completed in the stomach. The small intestine is primarily responsible for digestion of a meal and nutrient absorption.

Regulation of Gastric Function

Gastric function is under neural (sympathetic and parasympathetic) and hormonal control (peptides or amines that interact with target cells in the stomach). An understanding of the roles of endocrine and neural regulation of digestion is critical to understanding gastric physiology and the resultant physiologic effects of gastric surgical procedures on digestion. We initially focus here on peptide regulation of gastric function and then describe the interactions of these peptides with neural inputs in regard to acid secretion and gastric function.

Gastric Peptides

Gastrin

Gastrin is produced by G cells located in the gastric antrum and is the primary endocrine regulator of the secretory phase of a protein meal (see Table 49.1). It is synthesized as a prepropeptide and undergoes posttranslational processing by enzymatic cleavage in the rough endoplasmic reticulum and secretory vesicles to produce biologically reactive gastrin peptides. Several molecular forms of gastrin exist. The two major forms are G34 (big gastrin) and G17 (little gastrin). Ninety percent of antral gastrin is released as the 17–amino acid peptide, although G34 predominates in the circulation because its metabolic half-life is longer. The pentapeptide sequence contained at the carboxy terminus of gastrin is the biologically active component and is identical to that found on another gut peptide, CCK. CCK and gastrin differ by their tyrosine sulfation sites. Gastrin initiates its biologic actions by activation of surface membrane receptors. These receptors are members of the classic G protein–coupled receptor family and are classified as type A or B CCK receptors. The gastrin or CCK-B receptor has high affinity for gastrin and CCK, whereas type A CCK receptors have an affinity for sulfated CCK analogues and a low affinity for gastrin.

The release of gastrin is stimulated mostly by gastric distension, gastrin-releasing peptide (bombesin), and protein digestion products. Luminal acid inhibits the release of gastrin, specifically when the intragastric pH is below 3.0, via somatostatin release. In the antral location, somatostatin and gastrin release are functionally linked, and an inverse reciprocal relationship exists between these two peptides.

Gastrin is the major hormonal regulator of the gastric phase of acid secretion. Gastrin primarily does this by stimulating

TABLE 49.2 Causes of hypergastrinemia.

ULCEROGENIC CAUSES	NONULCEROGENIC CAUSES
Antral G cell hyperplasia or hyperfunction	Antisecretory agents (PPIs)
Retained gastric antrum	Atrophic gastritis
Zollinger-Ellison syndrome	Pernicious anemia
Gastric outlet obstruction	Acid-reducing procedure (vagotomy)
Short-gut syndrome	Gastric cancer
	Chronic renal failure

PPIs, Proton pump inhibitors.

enterochromaffin-like (ECL) cells to synthesize and release histamine. However, gastrin also exerts direct actions on the parietal cell to stimulate acid release. Gastrin also has considerable trophic effects on both parietal cells and ECL cells. Prolonged hypergastrinemia from any cause leads to mucosal hyperplasia and an increase in the number of ECL cells and, under some circumstances, is associated with the development of gastric carcinoid tumors.

The detection of hypergastrinemia may suggest a pathologic state of acid hypersecretion but most commonly is the result of treatment with agents to reduce acid secretion, such as proton pump inhibitors (PPIs). Table 49.2 lists common causes of chronic hypergastrinemia. Hypergastrinemia that results from the administration of acid-reducing drugs is an appropriate response caused by loss of feedback inhibition of gastrin release by luminal acid. Lack of acid causes a reduction in somatostatin release, which causes increased release of gastrin from antral G cells. Hypergastrinemia can also occur in the setting of pernicious anemia, uremia, or after surgical procedures such as vagotomy. In contrast, gastrin levels increase inappropriately in patients with gastrinoma (Zollinger-Ellison syndrome [ZES]). These gastrin-secreting tumors are not located in the antrum and secrete gastrin autonomously.

Somatostatin

Somatostatin is produced by delta cells and exists endogenously as either a 14–amino acid peptide or 28–amino acid peptide. The predominant molecular form in the stomach is somatostatin-14. It is produced by diffuse neuroendocrine cells located in the fundus and antrum. The principal stimulus for somatostatin release is antral acidification as well as gastrin-releasing peptide, whereas acetylcholine from vagal fibers inhibits its release. Somatostatin inhibits parietal cell acid secretion directly but also indirectly decreases acid secretion through inhibition of gastrin release from G cells and downregulation of histamine release from ECL cells.

Somatostatin receptors are also G protein–coupled receptors. Binding of somatostatin with its receptors is coupled to one or more inhibitory guanine nucleotide–binding proteins. Parietal cell somatostatin receptors appear to be a single subunit of glycoproteins with a molecular weight of 99 kDa, with equal affinity for somatostatin-14 and somatostatin-28. Somatostatin can inhibit parietal cell secretion through G protein–dependent and G protein–independent mechanisms. However, the ability of somatostatin to exert its inhibitory actions on cellular function is primarily thought to be mediated through the inhibition of adenylate cyclase, with a resultant reduction in cyclic adenosine monophosphate (cAMP) levels.

Histamine

Histamine (H_2) plays a prominent role in parietal cell stimulation. Administration of H_2-receptor antagonists almost completely abolishes gastric acid secretion in response to gastrin and acetylcholine, suggesting that histamine may be a necessary intermediary of these pathways. Histamine is stored in the acidic granules of ECL cells and in resident mast cells. ECL cells are located in the oxyntic mucosa in direct proximity to the parietal cell. Histamine release is stimulated by gastrin, vasoactive intestinal peptide, ghrelin, acetylcholine, and epinephrine through receptor-ligand interactions on ECL cells. In contrast, somatostatin inhibits gastrin-stimulated histamine release through interactions with somatostatin receptors located on the ECL cell, with other inhibitors including peptide YY and prostaglandins. The ECL cell plays an essential role in parietal cell activation, possessing stimulatory and inhibitory feedback pathways that modulate the release of histamine.

Ghrelin

Ghrelin is a 28–amino acid peptide predominantly produced by endocrine cells of the oxyntic glands in the stomach. Ghrelin appears to be under both endocrine and metabolic control, has a diurnal rhythm, and likely plays a major role in the neuroendocrine and metabolic responses to changes in nutritional status. Ghrelin has been shown to stimulate growth hormone release as well. Ghrelin levels are high during fasting and increases shortly before meals, with decreased levels after meals. Decreased ghrelin levels have been associated with gastritis. Within the stomach, ghrelin increases gastric emptying and motility and increases gastric acid secretion.

In human volunteers, ghrelin administration enhances appetite and increases food intake. In patients who have undergone a gastric bypass or sleeve gastrectomy, ghrelin levels are lower. Although the mechanism responsible for suppression of ghrelin levels after bariatric surgery is unknown, it is suggested that ghrelin may be responsive to the normal flow of nutrients across the stomach. Other studies have suggested that ghrelin leads to a switch toward glycolysis and away from fatty acid oxidation, which would favor fat deposition. Ghrelin appears to be upregulated in times of negative energy balance and downregulated in times of positive energy balance. Ghrelin may come to have a role in the treatment and prevention of obesity.

Gastric Acid Secretion

The hydrogen-potassium-adenosine triphosphatase (ATPase) acid-secreting pump is located in the parietal cell. Gastric acid secretion by the parietal cell is regulated mainly by three stimuli—acetylcholine, gastrin, and histamine. Acetylcholine is the principal neurotransmitter modulating acid secretion and is released from the vagus and parasympathetic ganglion cells; it mainly exerts effects on M3 receptors. Vagal fibers not only have a direct effect on parietal cells, but also modulate peptide release from G cells and ECL cells as well as inhibit somatostatin secretion. Gastrin has direct hormonal effects on the parietal cell and also stimulates histamine release. Histamine has paracrine-like effects on the parietal cell and, as shown in Fig. 49.6, plays a central role in the regulation of acid secretion by the parietal cell after its release from ECL cells. As depicted, somatostatin exerts inhibitory actions on gastric acid secretion. Release of somatostatin from antral D cells is stimulated in the presence of low intraluminal pH as well as vasoactive intestinal peptide and gastrin. After its release, somatostatin inhibits gastrin release through paracrine effects and modifies histamine release from ECL cells. Consequently, the precise state of acid secretion by the parietal cell depends on the overall influence of the positive and negative stimuli.

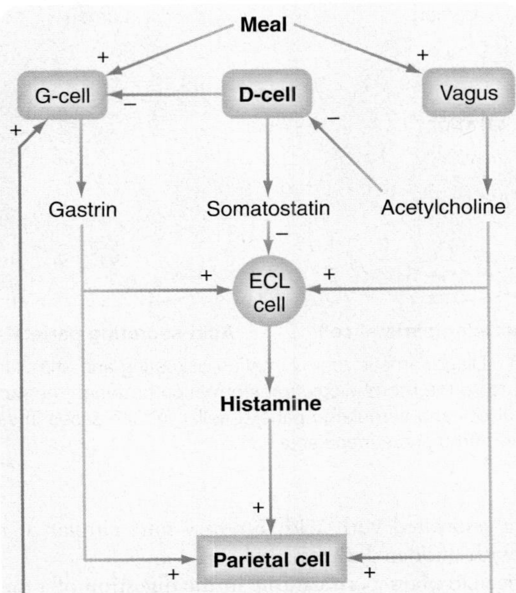

FIG. 49.6 Central role of the enterochromaffin-like *(ECL)* cell in regulation of acid secretion by the parietal cell. As shown, ingestion of a meal stimulates vagal fibers to release acetylcholine (cephalic phase). Binding of acetylcholine to M_3 receptors located on the ECL cell, parietal cell, and G cell results in the release of histamine, hydrochloric acid, and gastrin. Binding of acetylcholine to M_3 receptors on D cells results in the inhibition of somatostatin release. After a meal, G cells are also stimulated to release gastrin, which interacts with receptors located on ECL cells and parietal cells to cause the release of histamine and hydrochloric acid (gastric phase). Release of somatostatin from D cells decreases histamine release and gastrin release from ECL cells and G cells. In addition, somatostatin inhibits parietal cell acid secretion (not shown). The principal stimulus for the activation of D cells is antral luminal acidification (not shown). (From Yeo C, Dempsey DT, Klein AS, et al, eds. *Shackelford's Surgery of the Alimentary Tract.* 6th ed. Philadelphia: Saunders; 2007.)

In the absence of food, there is always a basal level of acid secretion that is approximately 10% of maximal acid output (1 to 5 mmol/hr). This is reduced after vagotomy or H_2-receptor blockade. Thus, it appears likely that basal acid secretion is caused by a combination of cholinergic and histaminergic input.

Stimulated Acid Secretion

Ingestion of food is the physiologic stimulus for acid secretion. Three phases of the acid secretory response to a meal have been described—cephalic, gastric, and intestinal. These three phases are interrelated and occur concurrently.

Cephalic phase. The cephalic phase originates with the sight, smell, thought, or taste of food, which stimulates neural centers in the hypothalamus. Although the exact mechanisms whereby senses stimulate acid secretion are not yet fully elucidated, it is hypothesized that several sites are stimulated in the brain. These higher centers transmit signals to the stomach via the vagus nerves, which release acetylcholine that activates muscarinic receptors located on target cells. Acetylcholine directly increases acid secretion by the parietal cells as well as stimulating ECL and G cells and inhibiting D cells. Although the intensity of the acid secretory response in the cephalic phase surpasses that of the other phases, it accounts for only 20% to 30% of the total volume of gastric acid produced in response to a meal because of its short duration.

Gastric phase. The gastric phase of acid secretion begins when food enters the gastric lumen. Protein products of ingested food interact with microvilli of antral G cells to stimulate gastrin release. Food also stimulates acid secretion by causing mechanical distention of the stomach. Gastric distention activates stretch receptors in the stomach to elicit the vagovagal reflex arc as well as local enteric nervous system acetylcholine release. The vasovagal reflex is abolished by proximal gastric vagotomy and is, at least in part, independent of changes in serum gastrin levels. Antral distention also causes gastrin release. The entire gastric phase accounts for most (60%–70%) of meal-stimulated acid output.

Intestinal phase. The intestinal phase of gastric secretion is initiated by entry of chyme into the duodenum, which initially stimulates gastrin release and suppresses gastric motility. It occurs after gastric emptying and lasts as long as partially digested food components remain in the proximal small bowel. It accounts for only 5% to 10% of the acid secretory response to a meal and does not appear to be mediated by serum gastrin levels. Chyme also stimulates release of CCK and secretin in the duodenum.

Activation and Secretion by the Parietal Cell

The two second messengers principally involved in stimulation of acid secretion by parietal cells are intracellular cAMP and calcium. These two messengers activate protein kinases and phosphorylation cascades. The intracellular events following ligand binding to receptors on the parietal cell are shown in Fig. 49.7. Histamine causes an increase in intracellular cAMP, which initiates a cascade of phosphorylation events that culminates in activation of proton pump (H^+, K^+-ATPase). In contrast, acetylcholine and gastrin stimulate phospholipase C, which converts membrane-bound phospholipids into inositol triphosphate to mobilize calcium from intracellular stores. Increased intracellular calcium activates other protein kinases that ultimately activate H^+, K^+-ATPase in a similar fashion to initiate the secretion of hydrochloric acid.

H^+, K^+-ATPase is the final common pathway for gastric acid secretion by the parietal cell. It is composed of two subunits, a catalytic α-subunit (100 kDa) and a glycoprotein β-subunit (60 kDa). During the resting state, gastric parietal cells store H^+, K^+-ATPase intracellularly. Cellular relocation of the proton pump subunits through cytoskeletal rearrangements must occur for acid secretion to increase in response to stimulatory factors. The subsequent heterodimer assembly of the H^+, K^+-ATPase subunits and insertion into the microvilli of the secretory canaliculus causes an increase in gastric acid secretion. A potassium chloride efflux pathway must exist to supply potassium to the extracytoplasmic side of the pump. Cytosolic hydrogen is secreted by H^+, K^+-ATPase in exchange for extracytoplasmic potassium (see Fig. 49.7), which is an electroneutral exchange and does not contribute to the transmembrane potential difference across the parietal cell. Secretion of chloride is accomplished through a chloride channel moving chloride from the parietal cell cytoplasm to the gastric lumen. The exchange of hydrogen for potassium requires energy in the form of adenosine triphosphate because hydrogen is being secreted against a gradient of more than a million fold. Because of this large energy requirement, the parietal cell has a mitochondrial compartment representing about one third of its cellular volume. In response to a secretagogue, the parietal cell undergoes a conformational change, and a several-fold increase in the canalicular surface area occurs (Fig. 49.8). In contrast to stimulated acid secretion, cessation of acid secretion requires endocytosis of H^+, K^+-ATPase, with regeneration of cytoplasmic tubulovesicles containing the subunits, and this occurs through

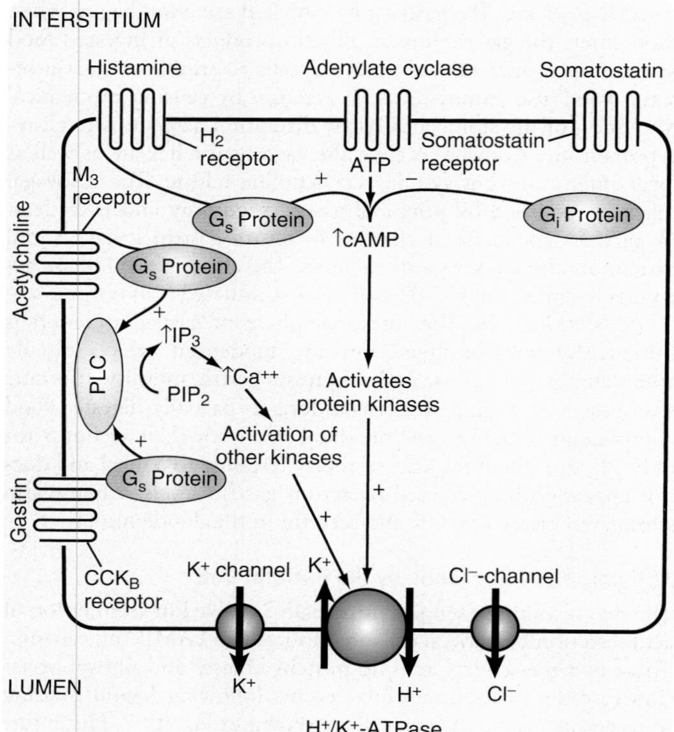

FIG. 49.7 Intracellular signaling events in a parietal cell. As shown, histamine binds to H_2 receptors, stimulating adenylate cyclase through a G protein–linked mechanism. Adenylate cyclase activation causes an increase in intracellular cAMP levels, which activates protein kinases. Activated protein kinases stimulate a phosphorylation cascade, with a resultant increase in levels of phosphoproteins that activate the proton pump. Activation of the proton pump leads to extrusion of cytosolic hydrogen in exchange for extracytoplasmic potassium. In addition, chloride is secreted through a chloride channel located on the luminal side of the membrane. Gastrin binds to type B CCK receptors, and acetylcholine binds to M_3 receptors. Following the interaction of gastrin and acetylcholine with their receptors, phospholipase C is stimulated through a G protein–linked mechanism to convert membrane-bound phospholipids into inositol triphosphate *(IP_3)*. IP_3 stimulates the release of calcium from intracellular calcium stores, leading to an increase in intracellular calcium that activates protein kinases, which activate the H^+/K^+-ATPase. (From Yeo C, Dempsey DT, Klein AS, et al, eds. *Shackelford's Surgery of the Alimentary Tract.* 6th ed. Philadelphia: Saunders; 2007.) *ATP*, Adenosine triphosphate; *ATPase*, adenosine triphosphatase; *CCK*, cholecystokinin; *G_i*, inhibitory guanine nucleotide protein; *G_s*, stimulatory guanine nucleotide protein; *PIP_2*, phosphatidylinositol 4,5-diphosphate; *PLC*, phospholipase C.

a tyrosine-based signal. The tyrosine-containing sequence is located on the cytoplasmic tail of the β-subunit and is highly homologous to the motif responsible for internalization of the transferrin receptor.

More than 1 billion parietal cells are found in the normal human stomach and are responsible for secreting approximately 20 mmol/hr of hydrochloric acid in response to a protein meal. There is a linear relationship between maximal acid output and parietal cell number. However, gastric acid secretory rates may be altered in patients with upper gastrointestinal (GI) disease. For example, gastric acid is often increased in patients with duodenal ulcer or gastrinoma, whereas it is decreased in patients with pernicious anemia or gastric atrophy. Patients with proximal gastric ulcers have lower secretory rates, whereas distal, antral, or prepyloric

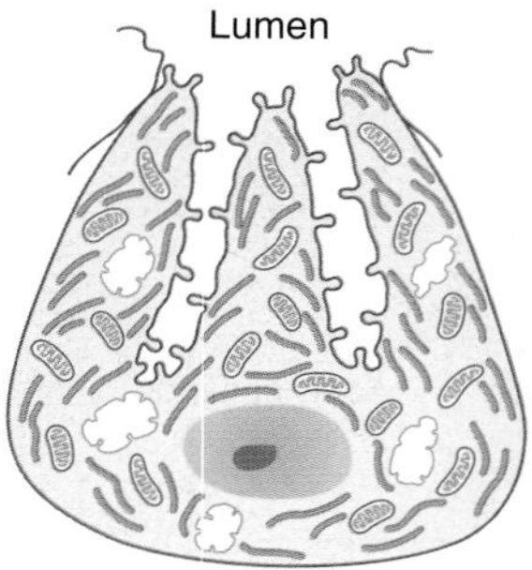

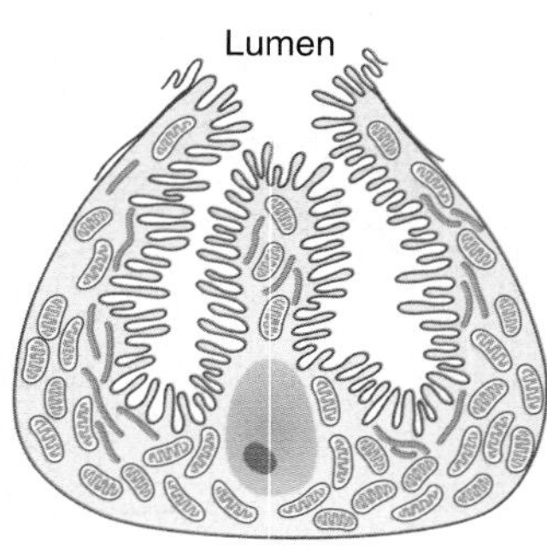

Nonsecreting parietal cell **Acid-secreting parietal cell**

FIG. 49.8 Diagrammatic representation of resting and stimulated parietal cells. Note the morphologic transformation between the nonsecreting parietal cell and stimulated parietal cell, with increases in secretory canalicular membrane surface area.

ulcers are associated with acid secretory rates similar to rates in patients with duodenal ulcers.

Gastric acid plays a critical role in the digestion of a meal. It is required to convert pepsinogen into pepsin, elicits the release of secretin from the duodenum, and limits colonization of the upper GI tract with bacteria.

Pharmacologic Regulation

Given the role stomach acid plays in many disease pathologies and the diversity of mechanisms that stimulate acid secretion, there has been much interest in the development of many site-specific drugs aimed at decreasing acid output by the parietal cell. The best-known site-specific antagonists are the group collectively known as the *H_2-receptor antagonists*, which inhibit the H_2-receptor on the parietal cell. The most potent of the H_2-receptor antagonists is famotidine, followed by ranitidine, nizatidine, and cimetidine.

PPIs block acid secretion more completely than H_2-receptor antagonists because of their irreversible inhibition of the H^+, K^+-ATPase proton pump. After oral administration, these agents are absorbed into the bloodstream as prodrugs and selectively concentrate in the secretory canaliculus of the parietal cell. At low pH, they become ionized and activated, with the formation of an active sulfur group. The cysteine residues on the α-subunit of the H^+, K^+-ATPase form a covalent disulfide bond with activated PPIs, which irreversibly inhibits the proton pump. Because of the covalent nature of this bond, these PPIs have more prolonged inhibition of gastric acid secretion than H_2 blockers. For recovery of acid secretion to occur, new protein pumps must be synthesized.

Antacids and sucralfate are two other medications with effects on gastric acid; however, they are both less potent. Antacids typically contain aluminum hydroxide, calcium carbonate, or magnesium trisilicate and can be used to neutralize gastric acid and decrease acid delivery to the duodenum, although the exact mechanism is unclear. Sucralfate is a sucrose octasulfate complexed with aluminum hydroxide and has been shown to bind to injured gastric tissue and stimulate angiogenesis and granulation tissue formation. Given the lower potency, the indications for antacids and sucralfate are limited to treatment of mild GE reflux disease.

Other Gastric Secretory Products

Gastric juice. Gastric juice is the combined result of secretion by the parietal cells, chief cells, and mucous cells, in addition to swallowed saliva and duodenal refluxate. The electrolyte composition varies with the rate of gastric secretion. Parietal cells secrete an electrolyte solution that is isotonic with plasma and contains 160 mmol/L. The pH of this solution is 0.8. The lowest intraluminal pH commonly measured in the stomach is 2 because of dilution of the parietal cell secretion by other gastric secretions, which also contain sodium, potassium, and bicarbonate.

Intrinsic factor. Intrinsic factor is a 50-kDa glycoprotein produced by the parietal cells that is essential for the absorption of vitamin B_{12} in the terminal ileum. It is secreted in amounts that far exceed the amounts necessary for vitamin B_{12} absorption. In general, secretion of intrinsic factor parallels gastric acid secretion, yet the secretory response is not linked to acid secretion. For example, PPIs do not block intrinsic factor secretion nor do not alter the absorption of vitamin B_{12}. Intrinsic factor deficiency can develop in the patients with pernicious anemia or in patients undergoing total gastrectomy; both groups of patients require vitamin B_{12} supplementation. Treatment typically consists of vitamin B_{12} supplementation via intramuscular injection of either cyanocobalamin or hydroxocobalamin, although oral administration may be similarly effective.

Pepsin. Pepsinogens are proteolytic proenzymes that are secreted by the glands of the gastroduodenal mucosa. Two types of pepsinogens are produced. Group 1 pepsinogens are secreted by chief cells and by mucous neck cells located in the glands of the acid-secreting portion of the stomach. Group 2 pepsinogens are produced by surface epithelial cells throughout the acid-secreting portion of the stomach, antrum, and proximal duodenum. In the presence of acid, both forms of pepsinogen are converted to pepsin by removal of a short amino-terminal peptide. Pepsin is an endopeptidase that preferentially hydrolyzes peptide linkages where one of the amino acids is aromatic and accounts for approximately 20% of the protein digestion in the GI tract. Pepsins have optimal function at a pH of 1.5 to 2.0 and become inactive at higher pH.

Mucus and bicarbonate. Mucus and bicarbonate combine to neutralize gastric acid at the gastric mucosal surface. They are secreted by the surface mucous cells and mucous neck cells located in the acid-secreting and antral portions of the stomach. Gastric mucin is a large glycoprotein and the mucus is a viscoelastic gel containing approximately 85% water and 15% mucin. It provides a mechanical barrier to injury, is relatively impermeable to pepsins, and also acts as an impediment to ion movement from the gastric lumen to the apical cell membrane. Mucus is in a constant state of flux because it is secreted continuously by mucosal cells while simultaneously being solubilized by luminal pepsin in the stomach. Mucus production is stimulated by vagal stimulation, cholinergic agonists, prostaglandins, and some bacterial toxins. In contrast, anticholinergic drugs and nonsteroidal antiinflammatory drugs (NSAIDs) inhibit mucus secretion. *Helicobacter pylori* secretes various proteases and lipases that break down mucin and impair the protective function of the mucous layer.

In the acid-secreting portion of the stomach, bicarbonate secretion is an active process, whereas in the antrum, active and passive secretion of bicarbonate occurs. However, the magnitude of bicarbonate secretion is considerably less than acid secretion. Although the luminal pH is 2, the pH observed at the surface epithelial cell is usually 7. The pH gradient found at the epithelial surface is a result of the unstirred layer of water in the mucus gel and of the continuous secretion of bicarbonate by the surface epithelial cells.

Gastric Motility

Gastric motility is regulated on three main levels: extrinsic neural control, intrinsic neural control, and myogenic control. The extrinsic neural controls are mediated through parasympathetic (vagus) and sympathetic pathways, whereas the intrinsic controls involve the enteric nervous system and interstitial cells of Cajal. In contrast, myogenic control resides in the excitatory membranes of the gastric smooth muscle cells.

Fasting Gastric Motility

The electrical basis of gastric motility begins with the depolarization of pacemaker cells located in the mid-body of the stomach along the greater curvature. Once initiated by the interstitial of Cajal, slow waves travel at 3 cycles/minute in a circumferential and antegrade fashion toward the pylorus. In addition to these slow waves, gastric smooth muscle cells are capable of producing action potentials, which are associated with larger changes in membrane potential than slow waves. Compared with slow waves, which are not associated with gastric contractions, action potentials are associated with actual muscle contractions. During fasting, the stomach goes through a cyclical pattern of electrical activity composed of slow waves and electrical spikes, which has been termed the migrating myoelectric complex. Each cycle of the migrating myoelectric complex lasts 90 to 120 minutes. The net effects of the myoelectric migrating complex are frequent clearance of gastric contents during periods of fasting. The exact regulatory mechanisms of myoelectric migrating complex activities are unknown, but these activities remain intact after vagal denervation.

Postprandial Gastric Motility

Ingestion of a meal results in a decrease in the resting tone of the proximal stomach and fundus, referred to as receptive relaxation and gastric accommodation, respectively. Because these reflexes are mediated by the vagus nerves, interruption of vagal innervation to the proximal stomach, such as by truncal vagotomy or proximal gastric vagotomy, can eliminate these reflexes, with resultant early satiety and rapid emptying of ingested liquids. In addition to its storage function, the stomach is responsible for the mechanical mixing of ingested solid food particles. This activity involves repetitive forceful contractions of the midportion and antral portion of the stomach, causing food particles to be propelled against a closed pylorus, with subsequent retropulsion of solids and liquids. The net effect is a thorough mixing of solids and liquids and sequential shearing of solid food particles to smaller than 1 mm prior to passage through the pylorus to the proximal duodenum.

The emptying of gastric contents is influenced by coordinated neural and hormonal mediators. Additionally, the chemical and mechanical properties and temperature of the intraluminal contents can influence the rate of gastric emptying. In general, liquids empty more rapidly than solids, and carbohydrates empty more readily than fats. In addition, hot and cold liquids tend to empty at a slower rate than ambient temperature fluids. These responses to luminal stimuli are regulated by the enteric nervous system. Osmoreceptors and pH-sensitive receptors in the proximal small bowel have also been shown to be involved in the activation of feedback inhibition of gastric emptying. Inhibitory peptides proposed to be active in this setting include CCK, vasoactive intestinal peptide, glucagon, and gastric inhibitory polypeptide.

Abnormal Gastric Motility

Symptoms of abnormal gastric motility are nausea/vomiting, postprandial fullness, early satiety, abdominal pain, and bloating. In the most severe cases, patients can suffer weight loss. The first steps in evaluating patients with suspected abnormal gastric motility after history and physical examination should be to exclude a mechanical obstruction with upper endoscopy and either a computed tomographic (CT) or magnetic resonance (MR) enterography or barium follow-through. The most common cause of gastroparesis is idiopathic, accounting for approximately half of patients. Other common causes include diabetes mellitus, viral infection (i.e., cytomegalovirus and Epstein-Barr virus), neurologic disease (i.e., multiple sclerosis, stroke, Parkinson disease), autoimmune disease, and certain medications such as tricyclic antidepressants, calcium channel blockers, and cyclosporine. Additionally, gastric motility can also be impaired after surgery due to either intentional or accidental vagotomy. Vagotomy results in loss of receptive relaxation and gastric accommodation in response to meal ingestion, with resultant early satiety, postprandial bloating, accelerated emptying of liquids, and delay in emptying of solids. Delayed gastric emptying is also seen after pancreatic surgery, most notably pancreaticoduodenectomy, where it is reported in 10% to 40% of patients postoperatively.

Clinical manifestations of diabetic gastropathy, which can occur in insulin-dependent or non–insulin-dependent patients, are thought to be related to a variety of factors. Impaired neural control via the vagus nerve, myenteric nervous system, interstitial cells of Cajal, and the underlying smooth muscle have been implicated. Additionally, hyperglycemia itself has been shown to cause a decrease in contractility of the gastric antrum, increase in pyloric contractility, relax the proximal stomach, and suppress the migrating myoelectric complexes. Hyperinsulinemia, which is often associated with non–insulin-dependent diabetes, may play a role in the gastroparesis seen in non–insulin-dependent diabetes because it also leads to suppression of migrating myoelectric complex activity.

Gastric-Emptying Studies

There are numerous ways to assess gastric emptying. The most common is a radionucleotide scan. This nuclear scintigraphy study is performed using a meal of radiolabeled food. Scans are obtained immediately after ingestion of the meal and at 1, 2, and 4 hours after the meal. Measurement of residual gastric contents at 4 hours provides the most sensitive means for diagnosing gastroparesis. At 4 hours, retention of 10% to 15% signifies mild gastroparesis, 15% to 35% is moderate, and greater than 35% is severe. More recently, some institutions include a clear liquid gastric-emptying study to detect patients with normal solid food emptying but delayed liquid emptying. There are multiple other diagnostic options; however, they are utilized less frequently. An upper abdominal x-ray series after barium swallow can provide information on gastric emptying and may reveal mechanical causes that could contribute to a delay, such as gastric outlet obstruction. An electrogastrogram or antroduodenal motility study assesses for nerve and muscle abnormalities; however, neither evaluates the actual functional significance. Wireless motility capsules have also been investigated as an alternative to scintigraphy, which can measure the pH, temperature, and pressure during its transit.

Treatment

Regardless of the cause of gastroparesis, initial first-line treatment of mild gastroparesis involves dietary modification.[1] Patients should be encouraged to eat multiple, small meals with little fat or insoluble fiber. Acidic and spicy foods should also be avoided. Medications that affect gastric motility, such as opioids, calcium channel blockers, tricyclic antidepressants, and dopamine agonists, should be stopped when possible. Glycemic control should be optimized in diabetic patients.

Pharmacologic therapy is necessary for persistent symptoms despite the above nonpharmacologic modifications. First-line medical therapy is metoclopramide (Reglan), a dopamine 2 receptor antagonist that stimulates antral contractions and decreases postprandial relaxation of the fundus. Outside of the United States, domperidone, another dopamine 2 antagonist, is available for patients who do not respond to metoclopramide or who experience side effects. Macrolide antibiotics (erythromycin and azithromycin) are motilin agonists that act by stimulating fundal contraction and have also shown benefit; they can be considered for second-line therapy.

Surgery for gastroparesis is rarely required and only indicated for refractory symptoms despite maximal medical therapy, partly because poor improvement in symptoms was observed historically after traditional open operations including gastrojejunostomy and subtotal gastrectomy. Surgical venting gastrostomy tubes can be placed (if unable to place endoscopically) for venting and jejunostomy tubes can be placed if needed for nutrition. Pyloromyotomy and pyloroplasty are options for the surgical management of gastroparesis that function by lowering outflow resistance at the pylorus and enhancing any remaining gastric contractility. Surgical implantation of gastric electrostimulators has also been used as a treatment for refractory idiopathic and diabetic gastroparesis. In this technique, electrical leads are placed onto the antrum laparoscopically and connected to a subcutaneously positioned simulator that delivers high-frequency, low-energy current. A recent systematic review reported that pyloric surgery improved nausea and abdominal pain more than gastric electrical stimulation[2]; however, robust comparative trials are lacking. Endoscopic therapies, such as the gastric peroral endoscopic myotomy, are also being explored. Retrospective series have shown durable improvement up to 1 year; however, prospective clinical trials are needed.[3] Endoscopic pyloric dilation and stenting can also be considered in select settings.

Gastric Barrier Function

The stomach's barrier function depends on multiple physiologic and anatomic factors. Blood flow plays a critical role in gastric mucosal defense by providing nutrients and delivering oxygen to ensure that the intracellular processes that underlie mucosal resistance to injury can proceed unabated. Decreased gastric mucosal blood flow has minimal effects on ulcer formation until it approaches 50% of normal. When blood flow is reduced by more than 75%, marked mucosal injury results, which is exacerbated in the presence of luminal acid. After damage occurs, injured surface epithelial cells are replaced rapidly by the migration of surface mucous cells located along the basement membranes. This process is referred to as restitution or reconstitution.

Exposure of the stomach to noxious agents causes a reduction in the potential difference across the gastric mucosa. In normal gastric mucosa, the potential difference across the mucosa is −30 to −50 mV and results from the active transport of chloride into the lumen and sodium into the blood by the activity of Na^+, K^+-ATPase. Disruption of the tight junctions between mucosal cells causes the epithelium to become leaky to ions (i.e., Na^+ and Cl^-) and a resultant loss of the high transepithelial electrical resistance normally found in gastric mucosa. In addition, agents such as NSAIDs or aspirin possess carboxyl groups that are nonionized at a low intragastric pH because they are weak acids. Consequently, they readily enter the cell membranes of gastric mucosal cells, whereas they will not penetrate the cell membranes at neutral pH because they are ionized. On entry into the neutral pH environment found in the cytosol, they become reionized, do not exit the cell membrane, and are toxic to the mucosal cells.

PEPTIC ULCER DISEASE

Peptic ulcers are erosions in the GI mucosa that extend through the muscularis mucosae. The most common symptom of peptic ulcer disease (PUD) is dyspepsia, although the majority of patients with peptic ulcers are asymptomatic. PUD can be complicated by bleeding, gastric outlet obstruction, fistulization, and perforation. The two predominant causes of PUD are *H. pylori* and NSAIDs. Many other less common mechanisms exist as well, including ZES, other medication and infectious exposures, radiation therapy, and gastric bypass surgery.

Epidemiology

The incidence and prevalence of PUD in developed countries, including the United States, have been declining in recent decades, as has the progression to complicated PUD. This change is likely due to a combination of increased detection and eradication of *H. pylori* infection, more rational NSAID use, and environmental factors. The lifetime prevalence of PUD is estimated to be 5% to 10%, with an annual incidence of 0.1% to 0.3%; however, both of these numbers are likely overestimations currently in developed countries.[4] In addition to declining incidence, epidemiological studies have shown decreased hospitalization and mortality related to PUD in the last two to three decades.[4] Much of this decline in ulcer incidence and the need for hospitalization have stemmed from increased knowledge of ulcer pathogenesis. Specifically, the role of *H. pylori* has been clearly defined, and the risks of long-term NSAID use have been better elucidated. The need for surgery in the treatment of ulcer disease has also decreased primarily as a result of a marked decline in elective surgical therapy for chronic disease.

Pathogenesis

Peptic ulcers are caused by decreased defensive factors, increased aggressive factors, or both. Protective (or defensive) factors include mucosal bicarbonate secretion, mucus production, adequate blood flow, growth factors, cell renewal, and endogenous prostaglandins. Damaging (or aggressive) factors include hydrochloric acid secretion, pepsins, ethanol ingestion, smoking, duodenal reflux of bile, ischemia, NSAIDs, hypoxia, and, most notably, *H. pylori* infection. Although it is now clear that most ulcers are caused by *H. pylori* infection or NSAID use, it is still important to understand all of the other protective and causative factors to optimize treatment and ulcer healing and prevent disease recurrence.

Helicobacter pylori Infection

It is estimated that half of the world's population is affected by *H. pylori*. While, previously, 80% to 95% of duodenal ulcers and approximately 75% of gastric ulcers were associated with *H. pylori* infection, its prevalence in peptic ulcers has fallen to 50% to 75% in developed countries more recently with improved diagnosis, treatment, and prevention. Infection with *H. pylori* has been shown to temporally precede ulcer formation, and when this organism is eradicated as part of ulcer treatment, ulcer recurrence is extremely rare. These observations have secured the place of *H. pylori* as a primary causative factor in the pathogenesis of PUD.

The interplay between bacterial and host factors determines the clinical outcome of *H. pylori* infection. *H. pylori* is a spiral-shaped, flagellate, gram-negative bacteria that resides in gastric-type epithelium within or beneath the mucus layer. Its shape and flagella aid its movement through the mucous layer, and it produces enzymes that help it adapt to this hostile environment. Mucolytic enzymes both facilitate passage through the mucus layer and protect the bacteria from mucin's antibiotic effects. Most notably, *H. pylori* is a potent producer of urease, which is capable of splitting urea into ammonia and bicarbonate, creating an alkaline microenvironment in the setting of an acidic gastric milieu, allowing for the bacteria's survival in the stomach. The bacteria attach to the gastric epithelial cells by binding to surface adhesions. *H. pylori* organisms are microaerophilic and can live only in gastric epithelium. Thus, *H. pylori* can also be found in heterotopic gastric mucosa in the proximal esophagus, in Barrett esophagus, in gastric metaplasia in the duodenum, within a Meckel diverticulum, and in heterotopic gastric mucosa in the rectum. The host response to *H. pylori* is at least partially determined genetically, with associations shown with interleukin 1β and toll-like receptors, both components of the inflammatory response.[5]

The exact mechanisms responsible for *H. pylori*–induced GI injury are still not fully understood, but the following four potential mechanisms have been proposed (and likely interact) to cause a derangement of normal gastric and duodenal physiology that leads to subsequent ulcer formation:

1. *Production of toxic products that cause local tissue injury.* Locally produced toxic mediators include breakdown products from urease activity (e.g., ammonia), cytotoxins, mucinase (which degrades mucus and glycoproteins), phospholipases that damage both epithelial and mucus cells, and platelet-activating factor (which is known to cause mucosal injury and thrombosis in the microcirculation).
2. *Induction of a local mucosal immune response. H. pylori* can cause a local inflammatory reaction in the gastric mucosa, attracting neutrophils and monocytes, which then produce numerous proinflammatory cytokines and reactive oxygen metabolites.
3. *Increased gastrin levels and changes in acid secretion.* In patients with antral *H. pylori* infection, basal and stimulated gastrin levels are significantly increased, presumably secondary to a reduction in somatostatin release from antral D cells because of infection with *H. pylori*. During the acute phase of *H. pylori* infection, acid secretion is decreased. With chronic infection, *H. pylori* has trophic effects on ECL and G cells, which can result in acid hypersecretion. A decrease in serum levels of somatostatin could also contribute to the gastric hyperacidity. However, if oxyntic glands are destroyed by the chronic infection, hypoacidity will result.
4. *Gastric metaplasia occurring in the duodenum.* Metaplastic replacement of areas of duodenal mucosa with gastric epithelium likely occurs as a protective response to decreased duodenal pH, resulting from the above-described acid hypersecretion; this allows for *H. pylori* to colonize these areas of the duodenum, which causes duodenitis and likely predisposes to duodenal ulcer formation. The presence of *H. pylori* in the duodenum is more common in patients with ulcer formation compared with patients with asymptomatic infections isolated to the stomach.

Peptic ulcers are also strongly associated with antral gastritis. Studies performed before the *H. pylori* era demonstrated that almost all patients with peptic ulcers have histologic evidence of antral gastritis. It is now known that most cases of histologic gastritis are caused by *H. pylori* infection. Of patients with NSAID-associated ulcers, 25% have evidence of a histologic antral gastritis compared with 95% of patients with non–NSAID-associated ulcers. In most cases, the infection tends to be confined initially to the antrum and results in antral inflammation. The causative role of *H. pylori* infection in the pathogenesis of gastritis and PUD was first elucidated by Marshall and Warren in Australia in 1984.[6] To prove this connection, Marshall himself ingested inocula of *H. pylori* after first confirming that he had normal gross and microscopic gastric mucosa. Within days, he developed abdominal pain, nausea, and halitosis as well as histologically confirmed presence of gastric *H. pylori* infection. Acute inflammation was observed histologically on days 5 and 10. By 2 weeks, acute inflammation had been replaced by chronic inflammation with evidence of a mononuclear cell infiltration. For their pioneering work, Marshall and Warren were jointly awarded the Nobel Prize in Medicine in 2005.

Evidence of infection is seen in childhood in developing countries and in adulthood in developed countries. Spontaneous remission is rare. There is an inverse relationship between infection rates and socioeconomic status. The reasons for this relationship are poorly understood, but it seems to be the result of factors such as sanitary conditions, familial clustering, lack of running water, and overcrowding. Such factors likely also explain why developing countries have a comparatively higher rate of *H. pylori* infection, especially in children. In the United States, *H. pylori* prevalence is higher in African Americans and Hispanics.

H. pylori infection is associated with many common upper GI disorders, but most infected individuals are asymptomatic. Healthy U.S. blood donors have an overall prevalence anywhere from 20% to 55%. *H. pylori* infection is almost always present in the setting of active chronic gastritis. In addition, most patients with gastric cancer have current or past *H. pylori* infection. Although the association between *H. pylori* and gastric cancer is strong, no causal relationship has been proven. However, *H. pylori*–induced chronic gastritis and intestinal metaplasia are thought to play a role. A meta analysis of case-control studies comparing *H. pylori*–positive and *H. pylori*–negative individuals found that infection was associated with a twofold increased risk of developing gastric cancer.[7] There is also a strong association between mucosa-associated lymphoid tissue (MALT) lymphoma and *H. pylori* infection. Regression of these lymphomas has been demonstrated after eradication of *H. pylori*.

Invasive Tests

Urease assay. Endoscopic biopsy specimens should be taken from the gastric body and the antrum and are then tested for urease. Sensitivity in diagnosing infection is greater than 90%, and specificity is 95% to 100%, meaning there are almost never false-positive results. However, the sensitivity of the test is lowered in patients who are taking PPIs, H_2-receptor antagonists, or antibiotics. Rapid urease test kits are commercially available and can detect urease in gastric biopsy specimens within 1 hour with a similar level of diagnostic accuracy.

Histology. Endoscopy can also be performed with biopsy samples of gastric mucosa, followed by histologic visualization of *H. pylori* using either routine hematoxylin-eosin stains or special stains (e.g., silver, Giemsa, Genta stains). Sensitivity is approximately 95% and specificity is 99%, making histology slightly more accurate than the urease assay testing. Similar to the urease assay, the sensitivity of histologic evaluation is lower in patients taking PPIs or H_2-receptor antagonists, but it remains the most accurate test available even in this setting. Histology additionally affords the ability to assess the severity of gastritis and confirm the presence or absence of the organism; however, it is a more expensive option for evaluation of biopsy samples than the urease assay.

Culture. Culturing of gastric mucosa obtained at endoscopy can also be performed to diagnose *H. pylori*. The sensitivity is approximately 80%, and specificity is 100%. However, culture requires laboratory expertise, is not widely available, is relatively expensive, and diagnosis requires 3 to 5 days. However, it does provide the opportunity to perform antibiotic sensitivity testing on isolates, if needed.

Noninvasive Tests

Urea breath test. The carbon-labeled urea breath test is based on the ability of *H. pylori* to hydrolyze urea as a result of its production of urease. Both sensitivity and specificity are greater than 95%. As with other testing modalities, the sensitivity of the urea breath test is reduced in patients taking antisecretory medications and antibiotics. It is recommended that patients discontinue antibiotics for 4 weeks and PPIs for 2 weeks to ensure optimal test accuracy. The urea breath test is less expensive than endoscopy and samples the entire stomach. In evaluating treatment efficacy, false-negative results can occur if the test is performed too soon after treatment, so it is usually best to perform this test 4 weeks after therapy is completed.

Stool antigen. *H. pylori* bacteria are present in the stool of infected patients, and several assays have been developed that use monoclonal antibodies to *H. pylori* antigens to test fecal specimens. These tests have demonstrated sensitivities of greater than 90% and sensitivities of 86% to 92%. Several studies have shown that stool antigen testing has an accuracy of greater than 90% in detecting eradication of infection after treatment, on par with invasive histology and noninvasive urea breath testing. Additionally, stool antigen testing is likely the most cost-effective method for assessing treatment efficacy.

Serology. There are various enzyme-linked immunosorbent assay laboratory-based tests available and some rapid office-based immunoassays that are used to test for the presence of IgG antibodies to *H. pylori*. Serology has a 90% sensitivity but a more variable specificity rate between 76% and 96%, and tests need to be locally validated based on the prevalence of specific bacterial strains. Antibody titers can remain high for 1 year or longer after eradication; consequently, this test cannot be used to assess response to therapy. For these reasons, stool antigen and urea breath tests are the preferred modalities for diagnosis and evaluation of treatment efficacy in patients with PUD and suspected *H. pylori* infection.

Nonsteroidal Antiinflammatory Drugs

NSAIDs, including aspirin, are absorbed through the stomach and small intestine and function as inhibitors of the cyclooxygenase enzymes. Cyclooxygenase enzymes form the rate-limiting step of prostaglandin synthesis in the GI tract. Prostaglandins (including thromboxane A2) promote gastric and duodenal mucosal protection from luminal acid and pepsin via numerous mechanisms, including increasing mucin and bicarbonate secretion and increasing blood flow to the mucosal endothelium and promoting epithelial cell proliferation and migration to the luminal surface. The presence of NSAIDs disrupts these naturally protective mechanisms, increasing the risk of peptic ulcer formation in the stomach and the duodenum.

The Food and Drug Administration estimates that NSAIDs are associated with a 1% to 4% risk per year of a clinically significant GI event, including bleeding, pyloric obstruction, and perforation. The risk for mucosal injury or ulceration is roughly proportional to the anti-inflammatory effect associated with each NSAID.

TABLE 49.3 Gastric ulcer types.

TYPE	LOCATION	ACID LEVEL
I	Lesser curve at incisura	Low to normal
II	Gastric body with duodenal ulcer	Increased
III	Prepyloric	Increased
IV	High on lesser curve	Normal
V	Anywhere	Normal, NSAID-induced

NSAID, Nonsteroidal antiinflammatory drug.

Compared with *H. pylori* ulcers, which are more frequently found in the duodenum, NSAID-induced ulcers are more often found in the stomach. *H. pylori* ulcers are also almost always associated with chronic active gastritis, whereas gastritis is not frequently found with NSAID-induced ulcers. When NSAID use is discontinued, the ulcers usually do not recur.

Gastric Ulcers

The modified Johnson anatomic classification system for gastric ulcers (i.e., types I through V, described in Table 49.3) was developed before the modern understanding that most ulcers are the consequence of *H. pylori* infection or NSAID usage. However, despite having an increased understanding of the mechanisms of how and why most ulcers develop, this historical classification system is still relevant to surgical treatment because it dictates what operation should be performed in the setting of complications of such ulcers.

Gastric ulcers can occur at any location in the stomach, although they usually manifest on the lesser curvature near the incisura. Approximately 60% of ulcers are in this location and are classified as type I gastric ulcers. These ulcers are generally not associated with excessive acid secretion and may occur with low to normal acid output. Most occur within 1.5 cm of the histologic transition zone between the fundic and antral mucosa and are not associated with duodenal, pyloric, or prepyloric mucosal abnormalities. In contrast, type II gastric ulcers (approximately 15%) are located in the body of the stomach in combination with a duodenal ulcer. These types of ulcers are usually associated with excess acid secretion. Type III gastric ulcers are prepyloric ulcers and account for approximately 20% of the lesions. They also behave similar to duodenal ulcers and are associated with hypersecretion of gastric acid. Type IV gastric ulcers occur high on the lesser curvature, near the GE junction. The incidence of type IV gastric ulcers is less than 10%, and they are not associated with excessive acid secretion. Type V gastric ulcers can occur at any location and are associated with long-term NSAID use. Finally, some ulcers may appear on the greater curvature of the stomach, but the incidence is less than 5%.

Gastric ulcers rarely develop before the age of 40 years, and the peak incidence occurs in individuals 55 to 65 years old. Gastric ulcers are more likely to occur in individuals in a lower socioeconomic class and are slightly more common in the non-white compared to the white population. Some clinical conditions that may predispose to gastric ulceration include chronic alcohol intake, smoking, long-term corticosteroid therapy, infection, and intra arterial therapy. With regard to acid and pepsin secretion, the presence of acid appears to be essential to the production of a gastric ulcer; however, the total secretory output appears to be less important. In contrast to the acidification of the duodenum leading to ulcer formation, patients with gastric ulcers caused by *H. pylori* can have normal or reduced gastric acid production. Ulcer formation is more likely due to an inflammatory response to the bacterial infection itself. Nevertheless, rapid healing follows antacid therapy, antisecretory therapy, or vagotomy even when the lesion-bearing portion of the stomach is left intact because in the presence of gastric mucosal damage, acid is ulcerogenic, even when present in normal or less than normal amounts.

Clinical Manifestations

One clinical challenge of gastric ulcer management is the differentiation between gastric carcinoma and a benign ulcer. This is in contrast to duodenal ulcers, in which malignancy is extremely rare. Similar to duodenal ulcers, gastric ulcers are also characterized by recurrent episodes of quiescence and relapse. They also cause pain, bleeding, and obstruction and can perforate. Occasionally, benign ulcers have also been found to result in spontaneous gastrocolic fistulas. Surgical intervention is required in patients who develop complications from gastric ulcer disease. Patients who develop significant bleeding from gastric ulcers usually are older, are less likely to stop bleeding spontaneously, and have higher morbidity and mortality rates than patients with bleeding from a duodenal ulcer. The most frequent complication of gastric ulceration is perforation. Most perforations occur along the anterior aspect of the lesser curvature. In general, older patients have increased rates of perforations, and larger ulcers are associated with higher morbidity and mortality. Similar to duodenal ulcers, gastric outlet obstruction can also occur in patients with type II or III gastric ulcers. However, one must carefully differentiate between benign obstruction and obstruction secondary to carcinoma.

Diagnosis and Treatment

The diagnosis and treatment of gastric ulceration generally mirror the diagnosis and treatment of duodenal ulcer disease. The significant difference is the possibility of malignancy in a gastric ulcer. This critical difference demands that cancer be ruled out in acute and chronic presentations of gastric ulcer disease. Acid suppression and *H. pylori* eradication are important aspects of any treatment.

As with duodenal ulcers, intractable nonhealing ulcers are becoming increasingly less common. It is important to ensure that adequate time has elapsed and appropriate therapy has been administered to allow healing of the ulcer to occur; this includes confirmation that *H. pylori* has been eradicated and that NSAIDs have been eliminated. The presentation of a nonhealing gastric ulcer in the *H. pylori* era should raise serious concerns about the presence of an underlying malignancy. These patients should undergo a thorough evaluation with multiple biopsies to exclude malignancy (Fig. 49.9). The approach for a complicated gastric ulcer varies depending on the type of ulcer and its association with pathophysiologic acid levels. Types I and IV ulcers, which are not associated with increased acid levels, do not require acid-reducing vagotomy. Fig. 49.10 is an algorithm for managing complicated gastric ulcers.

Duodenal Ulcer

Duodenal ulceration is a disease with numerous causes. The only requirements are acid and pepsin secretion in combination with infection by *H. pylori* or ingestion of NSAIDs.

Clinical Manifestations

Abdominal pain. Patients with duodenal ulcer disease can present in various ways. The most common symptom associated with duodenal ulcer disease is midepigastric abdominal pain that is usually well localized. The pain is generally tolerable and frequently relieved by food. The pain may be episodic, seasonal in the spring

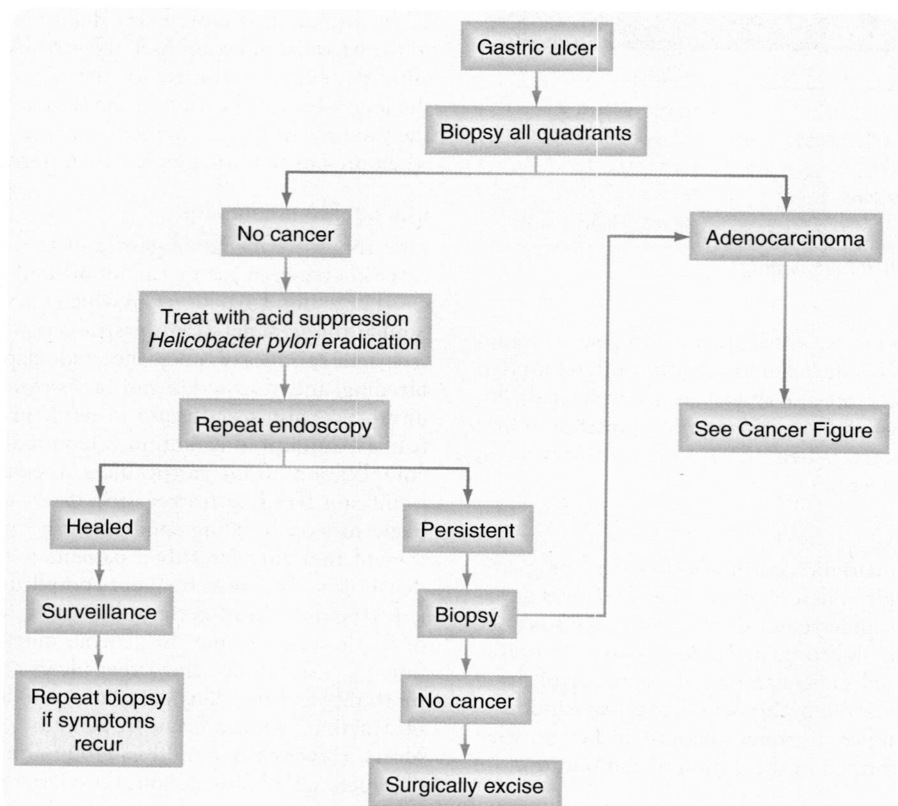

FIG. 49.9 Algorithm for evaluation, treatment, and surveillance of a patient with a gastric ulcer.

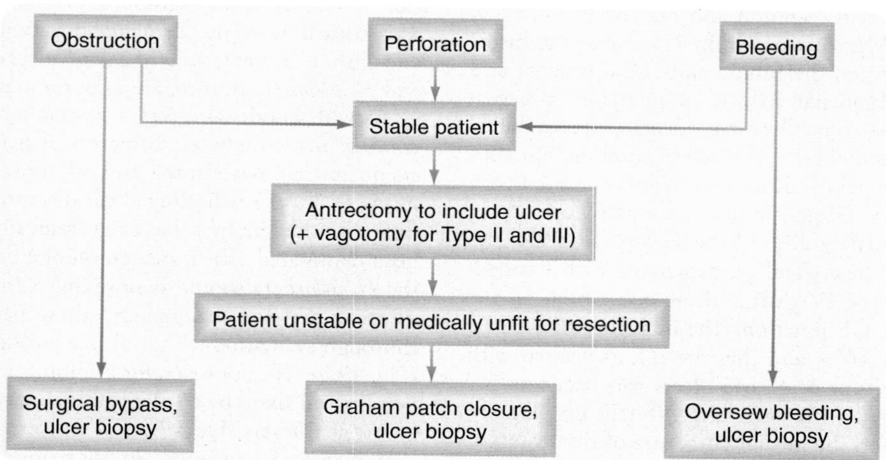

FIG. 49.10 Algorithm for the management of complicated gastric ulcer disease.

and fall, and worse during periods of emotional stress. Many patients do not seek medical attention until they have had the disease for many years. When the pain becomes constant, this suggests that there is deeper penetration of the ulcer. Referral of pain to the back is usually a sign of penetration into the pancreas, whereas diffuse peritoneal irritation is the result of free perforation.

Diagnosis

History and physical examination are of limited value in distinguishing between gastric and duodenal ulceration. Routine laboratory studies include complete blood count, liver chemistries, serum creatinine, serum amylase, and calcium levels. A serum gastrin level should also be obtained in patients with ulcers that are refractory to medical therapy or require surgery. The two principle means of diagnosing duodenal ulcers are upper GI radiography and flexible upper endoscopy.

Upper gastrointestinal radiography. Diagnosis of duodenal ulcer by upper GI radiography requires the demonstration of barium within the ulcer crater, which is usually round or oval and may or may not be surrounded by edema. This study is useful to

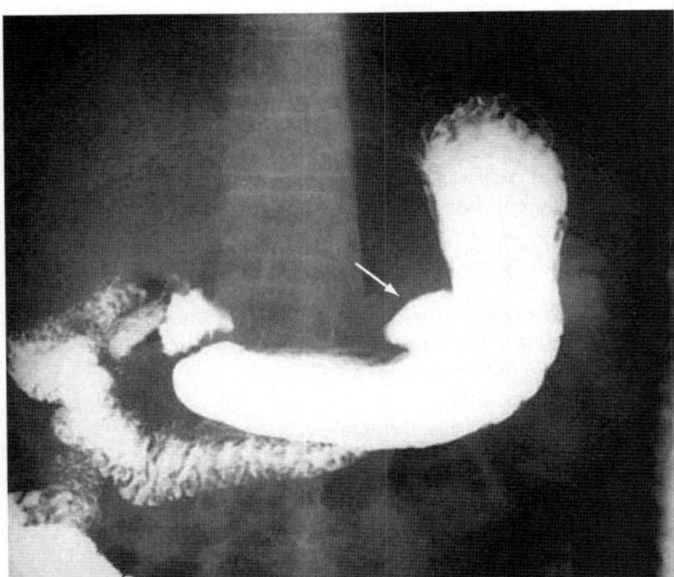

FIG. 49.11 A large, benign-appearing gastric ulcer protrudes medially from the lesser curvature of the stomach *(arrow)*, just above the gastric incisura. (Courtesy Dr. Agnes Guthrie, Department of Radiology, University of Texas Medical School, Houston, TX.)

determine the location and depth of penetration of the ulcer and the extent of deformation from chronic fibrosis. A characteristic barium radiograph of a peptic ulcer is shown in Fig. 49.11. The ability to detect ulcers on radiography requires the technical skills and abilities of the radiologist but also depends on the size and location of the ulcer. With single-contrast radiographic techniques, 50% of duodenal ulcers may be missed, whereas with double-contrast studies, 80% to 90% of ulcer craters can be detected. However, approximately 5% of ulcers that appear radiographically benign are malignant. Despite this increased accuracy with double-contrast techniques, upper GI radiography has largely been replaced by flexible upper endoscopy as the method of choice for diagnosis and evaluation of gastric and duodenal ulcers as this allows for biopsy to rule out malignancy and the ability to evaluate for other pathologies of the esophagus, stomach, and duodenum in addition to PUD that may be causing the patient's symptoms, such as esophagitis and gastritis.

Flexible upper endoscopy. Endoscopy is the most reliable method for diagnosing gastric and duodenal ulcers. In addition to providing a visual diagnosis, endoscopy provides the ability to sample tissue to evaluate for malignancy and *H. pylori* infection and may be used for therapeutic purposes in the setting of GI bleeding or obstruction.

Endoscopic evaluation of the stomach and duodenum has been shown to confirm a visual diagnosis of more than 90% of peptic ulcers, and this value is likely higher today with the use of high-definition endoscopes. When an ulcer has been detected endoscopically, biopsy is recommended in all cases to rule out malignancy. Larger ulcers and ulcers with irregular or heaped-up edges are more likely to harbor cancers. Multiple biopsy specimens should be taken of the ulcer for maximum diagnostic yield, preferably from all four quadrants if possible. An early study of the usefulness of endoscopic biopsy showed that the first biopsy sample taken of an ulcer had only a 70% sensitivity in detecting gastric cancer, whereas taking four biopsy specimens increased this yield to 95% and taking seven specimens increased it to 98%.

Helicobacter pylori testing. The gold standard for diagnosis of *H. pylori* is mucosal biopsy performed during upper endoscopy, but noninvasive tests offer an effective screening tool and do not require an endoscopic procedure. If endoscopy is to be performed, evaluation of biopsy samples with either a urease assay or histologic examination offers excellent diagnostic accuracy. Evaluation of serum antibodies is the test of choice for initial diagnosis when endoscopy is not required but has the drawback of remaining positive after treatment and eradication of infection. For monitoring treatment efficacy, stool antigen and urea breath testing are both adequate choices.

Medical Treatment

Antiulcer drugs fall into three broad categories—drugs targeted against *H. pylori*, drugs that reduce acid levels by decreasing secretion or chemical neutralization, and drugs that increase the mucosal protective barrier. In patients with PUD and *H. pylori* infection, the focus of therapy is on eradication of the bacteria. In addition to medications, lifestyle changes, such as smoking cessation, discontinuing NSAIDs and aspirin, and avoiding coffee and alcohol, help promote ulcer healing.

Antacids. Antacids are the oldest form of therapy for PUD. They reduce gastric acidity by reacting with hydrochloric acid, forming a salt, and raising the gastric pH. Antacids differ greatly in their buffering ability, absorption, and side effects. Magnesium antacids tend to be the best buffers but can cause significant diarrhea, whereas acids precipitated with phosphorus can occasionally result in hypophosphatemia and sometimes constipation. Aluminum hydroxide can bind growth factors and may increase their delivery to injured mucosa. The use of antacids has largely been replaced by the more efficacious antisecretory therapies (either H_2-receptor antagonists or PPIs) for the treatment of PUD.

Sucralfate. Sucralfate is structurally related to heparin but does not have any anticoagulant effects. It is an aluminum salt of sulfated sucrose that dissociates under the acidic conditions in the stomach. It is hypothesized that the sucrose polymerizes and binds to the ulcer crater to produce a protective coating that can last for 6 hours. It has also been suggested that it may bind and concentrate endogenous basic fibroblast growth factor, which appears to be important for mucosal healing. The efficacy and role of sucralfate in healing peptic ulcers caused by *H. pylori* infection has not been clearly established, and sucralfate is not currently included as part of initial treatment guidelines for PUD.

H_2-receptor antagonists. The H_2-receptor antagonists are structurally similar to histamine and function by inhibiting the H_2 receptors on parietal cells. Variations in ring structure and side chains cause differences in potency and side effects. Currently available H_2-receptor antagonists differ in their potency but only modestly in half-life and bioavailability. All undergo hepatic metabolism and are excreted by the kidney. Famotidine is the most potent, and cimetidine is the weakest. Continuous intravenous (IV) infusion of H_2-receptor antagonists has been shown to produce more uniform acid inhibition than intermittent administration. Many randomized controlled trials have indicated that all H_2-receptor antagonists result in duodenal ulcer healing rates of 70% to 80% after 4 weeks of therapy and 80% to 90% after 8 weeks.

Proton pump inhibitors. The most potent antisecretory agents are PPIs. These agents irreversibly bind and inhibit the hydrogen-potassium ATPase on the parietal cell. As a result, they provide a more complete and prolonged inhibition of acid secretion than H_2-receptor antagonists. PPIs have a healing rate of 85% at 4 weeks and 96% at 8 weeks and produce more rapid healing of ulcers than standard H_2-receptor antagonists. Because of this, PPIs have generally replaced H_2-receptor antagonists as primary therapy for PUD. PPIs require an acidic environment within the gastric lumen to become activated; thus, using antacids or H_2-receptor antagonists in combination with PPIs could have deleterious effects by promoting an alkaline environment. Maintenance PPI therapy is considered in patients with large (>2 cm) ulcers, refractory or frequent PUD, those with failed *H. pylori* eradication, or patients requiring continued NSAID use.

Treatment of Helicobacter pylori infection. After it became clear that the increased majority of cases were due to *H. pylori* infection, there was a paradigm shift that saw PUD as an infectious disease, rather than a consequence of pathologic acid secretion. Accordingly, treatment philosophy has shifted to focus on eradication of the infectious agent.

Current therapy is twofold in its approach, combining antibiotics against *H. pylori* with acid-reducing medications. The primary goal of the PPIs is to promote short-term healing by reducing pathologic acid levels and improve symptoms. *H. pylori* eradication helps with initial healing, but its primary efficacy is in preventing recurrence. There have been numerous trials comparing eradication therapy with ulcer-healing drugs alone or no treatment. Eradication of *H. pylori* has shown recurrence rates of 2%, with initial healing rates of 90%. Eradication rates after an initial course of therapy have been decreasing, likely as a result of increased prevalence of antibiotic-resistant strains of *H. pylori;* at the present time, approximately 20% of patients fail initial therapy. For this reason, monitoring for infection eradication with a urea breath test, stool antigen, or repeat endoscopy with biopsy at 4 to 6 weeks after therapy is important, and many patients will require further treatment with alternative regimens.

The treatment of *H. pylori*–positive peptic duodenal ulcer disease is triple or quadruple therapy aimed at the eradication of *H. pylori*, along with acid suppression (Box 49.1). This triple therapy includes a PPI and two antibiotics, with the addition of bismuth representing quadruple therapy. The choice of antibiotics should be guided by risk factors for macrolide resistance and the presence of a penicillin allergy. Risk factors for macrolide resistance are prior exposure to a macrolide antibiotic or local clarithromycin resistance rates of greater than 15%. Patients who do not have risk factors for macrolide resistance and are not allergic to penicillin should receive standard triple therapy, consisting of clarithromycin, amoxicillin, and a PPI. The amoxicillin can be replaced with metronidazole if the patient has a penicillin allergy. Patients who have a risk factor for macrolide resistance should be given bismuth quadruple therapy, which consists of bismuth, tetracycline, metronidazole, and a PPI.

Clinical guidelines generally recommend treatment with a 14-day course of triple therapy and a 10- to 14-day course of bismuth quadruple therapy.[8] Side effects, which are generally mild and resolve with cessation of treatment, include diarrhea, nausea and vomiting, rash, and altered taste. For the 20% of patients with refractory disease, a treatment course with new antibiotics, such as metronidazole and tetracycline, is initiated, and quadruple therapy with the addition of bismuth is recommended if not previously used. Levofloxacin and rifabutin triple therapies are also salvage therapeutic options.

Complicated Ulcer Disease

Ulcer surgery was previously a major part of general surgery practice. With the shift in understanding of PUD from one primarily of aberrant acid physiology to one of infectious disease, this situation has changed significantly, with most patients with ulcers being treated and cured medically. The surgeon's role now is primarily to treat the patients who have a complication from their disease, which includes hemorrhage, perforation, and obstruction (Box 49.2). Risk factors for complicated PUD include NSAIDs, *H. pylori*, and size of ulcer larger than 1 cm. Frequently included in discussions of complicated ulcer disease is an intractable ulcer. Although intractable disease no doubt exists, its definition is nebulous, and determining exactly when and what type of surgical intervention is required is primarily a matter of judgment. In the current era of excellent treatment options for *H. pylori* infection and acid suppression, few patients who are truly compliant with medical therapy develop intractable ulcer disease in the absence of malignancy. Early multidisciplinary management is imperative for patients with complicated PUD to ensure optimal patient outcomes.

Hemorrhage. Upper GI bleeding is a relatively common problem, with an annual incidence of approximately 19 to 57 cases per 100,000 individuals.[9] Patients with upper GI bleeding from PUD can present with hematemesis, melena, or both. The use of

BOX 49.1 First-line *Helicobacter pylori* treatment regimen.

Patients Without Penicillin Allergy, Prior Macrolide Exposure, or in Region With >15% Clarithromycin Resistance

- Bismuth quadruple therapy (PPI, bismuth, tetracycline, metronidazole)
- Clarithromycin triple therapy (PPI, clarithromycin, and amoxicillin or metronidazole)
- Concomitant regimen (PPI, clarithromycin, amoxicillin, nitroimidazole)

Patients Without Penicillin Allergy With Either Prior Macrolide Exposure or in a Region With >15% Clarithromycin Resistance

- Bismuth quadruple therapy
- Levofloxacin triple therapy (PPI, levofloxacin, amoxicillin)

Patients With a Penicillin Allergy But Without Prior Macrolide Exposure

- Bismuth quadruple therapy
- Clarithromycin triple therapy with metronidazole

Patients With Both a Penicillin Allergy and Either Prior Macrolide Exposure or in a Region With >15% Clarithromycin Resistance

- Bismuth quadruple therapy

From Chey WD, Leontiadis GI, Howden CW, Moss SF. Treatment of *Helicobacter pylori* Infection. *Am J Gastroenterol.* 2017;112:212–238.
PPI, Proton pump inhibitor.

BOX 49.2 Surgical treatment recommendations for complications related to peptic ulcer disease.

- Intractable: Parietal cell vagotomy ± antrectomy
- Bleeding: Oversewing of bleeding vessel with treatment of *Helicobacter pylori*
- Perforation: Patch closure with treatment of *H. pylori*
- Obstruction: Rule out malignancy and gastrojejunostomy with treatment of *H. pylori*

TABLE 49.4 Forrest classification of stigmata of recent hemorrhage on endoscopic examination of peptic ulcers and relative prevalence.

STIGMATA OF RECENT HEMORRHAGE	FORREST CLASSIFICATION	PREVALENCE	RISK OF REBLEEDING
Active bleeding			
Active spurting	IA	10%	90%
Active oozing	IB	10%	10%–20%
Recent hemorrhage			
Nonbleeding, visible vessel	IIA	25%	50%
Adherent clot	IIB	10%	25%–30%
Flat pigmented spot	IIC	10%	5%–10%
No signs of hemorrhage			
Clean-based ulcer	III	35%	3%–5%

Adapted from Katschinski B, Logan R, Davies J, et al. Prognostic factors in upper gastrointestinal bleeding. *Dig Dis Sci*. 1994. 39(4):706–712.

NSAIDs is the major risk factor for peptic ulcer bleeding, with relative risks reported from 2.7 to 33.9.[9] It should be noted that *H. pylori* testing can have decreased sensitivity both with active bleeding as well as PPI use, so its impact on bleeding may be underestimated. PUD hemorrhage is associated with an approximately 6% to 10% mortality rate.[9]

The initial approach to an upper GI bleed is similar to the approach to other patients presenting with acute hypovolemic blood loss. Large-bore IV access, rapid restoration of intravascular volume with fluid and blood products as the clinical situation dictates, and close monitoring of vital signs all are essential to effective management of these patients. Patients should be initiated on an IV PPI during their initial evaluation. The role of nasogastric (NG) lavage is controversial; however, it can be useful as a predictor of high-risk patients and as an aid for later endoscopic intervention. Patients with bright red blood on NG lavage, as opposed to clear or coffee-ground lavage, are at much higher risk for persistent bleeding or rebleeding. If the NG lavage returns bilious fluid without blood, indicating the duodenal as well as gastric contents have been sampled, a lower GI source of bleeding (i.e., one distal to the ligament of Treitz) should be considered. In addition to its diagnostic usefulness, the NG tube can be used to lavage the stomach and duodenum before endoscopy, removing clot and old blood that could obscure visualization of the source of bleeding.

Upper flexible endoscopy is the best initial procedure for diagnosis of the source of upper GI bleeding and for therapeutic intervention, including in the setting of bleeding ulcers. Almost all patients with a potentially substantial acute upper GI bleed should undergo endoscopy within 24 hours. Although the data are inconclusive, early endoscopy has been shown to be a cost-effective strategy by triaging patients to more rapid intervention, if warranted, and by identifying low-risk patients without the need for prolonged observation (and therefore earlier hospital discharge).

Patients who are noted on endoscopy to have active bleeding, via an arterial jet or oozing, an adherent clot, or a visible vessel within the ulcer, are at high risk, and intervention is required. Patients without active bleeding, no visible vessel, and a clean ulcer base are low risk and do not require further intervention. The most commonly used system for classifying the endoscopic appearance of bleeding ulcers is the Forrest classification (Table 49.4), which stratifies the risk of rebleeding based on observed "stigmata of recent hemorrhage." Lower-risk ulcers are much more frequently encountered than actively bleeding ones, even in the setting of inpatients undergoing endoscopy for diagnosis of upper GI bleeding. All patients undergoing endoscopic examination should be tested for *H. pylori* status.

For high-risk patients requiring intervention, the best initial approach is endoscopic control. The most recent consensus guidelines[10] for management of patients with peptic ulcer bleeding recommended endoscopic therapy for high-risk lesions and can consist of either thermal coagulation, hemoclips, or sclerosant injection. Epinephrine injection monotherapy is no longer recommended given the high rebleeding rates, but epinephrine can be added as a second modality to other endoscopic therapies. Patients with pigmented spots or clean ulcer bases should not receive endoscopic therapy and can receive standard PPI therapy (with *H. pylori* treatment if indicated). Routine second-look endoscopy is not recommended. Patients who have a second episode of bleeding after initially successful endoscopic therapy are typically treated with repeat endoscopy. Patients with recurrent bleeding can be considered for interventional angiography with transarterial embolization (Fig. 49.12) if they are hemodynamically stable and those resources are available. However, nonrandomized trials have shown higher rates of rebleeding with embolization compared to surgery. Embolization can still be useful, especially for patients who are poor surgical candidates based on other medical comorbidities.

All high-risk patients should be placed in a monitored setting. While prior consensus guidelines advocated for continuous IV PPI infusion, a more recent systematic review and meta analysis showed intermittent high-dose PPI therapy was comparable to continuous infusion for patients with endoscopically treated high-risk bleeding ulcers; intermittent high-dose IV PPI is now recommended in most cases.[11] Compared with a histamine blocker and placebo, IV PPI therapy showed lower rebleeding rates and a lower need for emergency surgery. Patients deemed high risk based on clinical factors should begin therapy immediately, even before endoscopy.

Despite the use of PPIs and improved methods of endoscopic control, 5% to 10% of patients have persistent bleeding that requires surgical intervention. Indications for surgical intervention in these patients include: failed endoscopic treatment (or recurrent hemorrhage after multiple endoscopic treatments), hemodynamic instability, or continued slow bleeding with transfusion requirement. The vessel most likely to be bleeding is the gastroduodenal artery because of erosion from a posterior ulcer. Although bleeding duodenal ulcers can be treated laparoscopically, the more typical approach is through an upper midline laparotomy, especially in patients who are hemodynamically unstable. A Kocher maneuver is performed to mobilize the duodenum. The anterior wall of

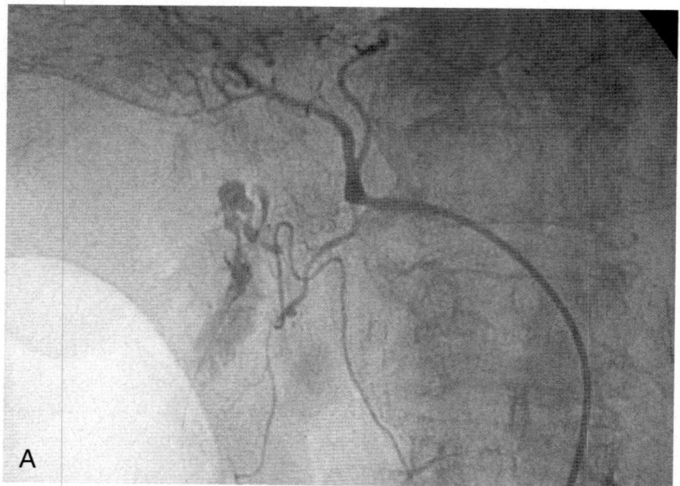

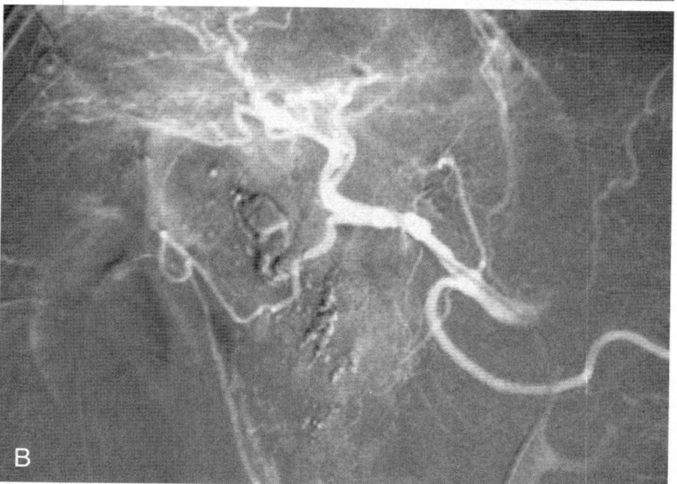

FIG. 49.12 Endovascular control of a bleeding duodenal ulcer. (A) An angiogram is obtained, which shows extravasation from a branch off of the gastroduodenal artery. (B) A completion angiogram after glue embolization of the vessel shows resolution of the bleed with preservation of flow through the gastroduodenal artery. (From Loffroy R, Guiu B, Cercueil JP, et al. Refractory bleeding from gastroduodenal ulcers: arterial embolization in high-operative-risk patients. *J Clin Gastroenterol.* 2008;42:361–367.)

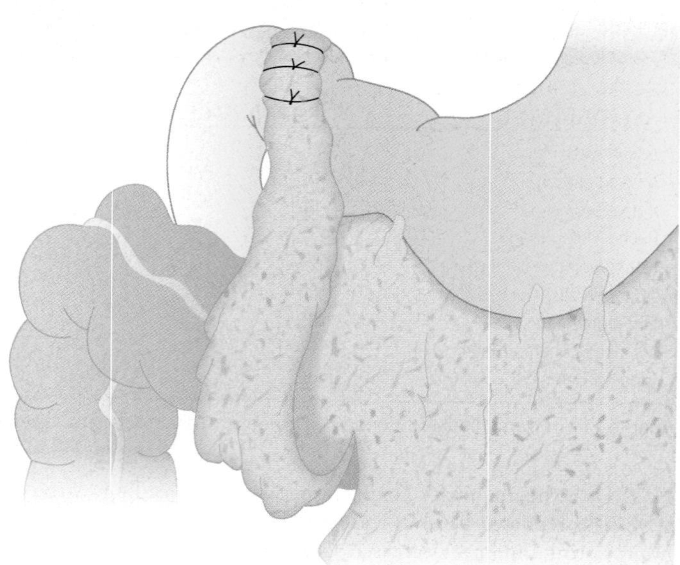

FIG. 49.13 Graham patch repair of a perforated duodenal ulcer. A "tongue" of omentum is brought up to cover the ulcer defect and secured in position with a series of interrupted sutures. In Graham's original description, the ulcer defect is not closed, but if the tissue edges are healthy and come together without undue tension, a primary closure can be performed and reinforced with an omental patch. (From Baker RJ. Operation for acute perforated duodenal ulcer. In Nyhus LM, Baker RJ, Fischer JE, eds. *Mastery of Surgery*. London: Little, Brown and Company; 1997.)

the duodenal bulb is opened longitudinally, and the incision can be carried across the pylorus, if needed. The gastroduodenal artery is oversewn, with a three-point U stitch technique, which effectively ligates the main vessel (superior and inferior stitches) and prevents back-bleeding from any smaller branches (medial stitch), such as the transverse pancreatic artery, that head to the patient's left toward the body of the pancreas. One must be careful to avoid incorporating the common bile duct into the stitch. The course of the common bile duct can be identified by inserting a probe through the ampulla of Vater transduodenally or performing an intraoperative cholangiogram. Hemostasis should be confirmed prior to duodenal closure. The duodenotomy is closed transversely to avoid narrowing.

Perforation. Patients with perforation typically complain of sudden-onset, severe epigastric pain, which can lessen a few hours after initial onset as the body tries to wall off the perforation. Patients frequently have free air visible on the chest radiograph and have localized peritoneal signs on examination. Patients with more widespread spillage have diffuse peritonitis. If there is no free air noted on x-ray, patients should undergo CT scan, preferably including oral contrast. For a small subset of patients, the perforation may seal spontaneously; however, operative intervention is required in almost all cases. Initial empiric antibiotic therapy should cover enteric gram-negative rods, anaerobes, and mouth flora and should be based on local susceptibility patterns. Perforation complicates 2% to 10% of PUD and has the highest mortality rate of any complication of ulcer disease, reported as high as 30%.

Perforation necessitates emergent surgical consultation. Patients with localized symptoms, in stable clinical condition, and with a water-soluble contrast study confirming a sealed leak can be considered for nonoperative management, although this must be considered with the knowledge that time of delay to surgery (when surgery is ultimately performed) has been shown to increase mortality.[12] Nonoperative management should consist of close hemodynamic monitoring, serial abdominal exams, nil per os, IV antibiotics, and IV PPI. Retrospective series have shown 50% to 75% of well-selected patients can avoid surgery in this setting.

The perforation usually can easily be accessed through an upper midline incision. Perforations smaller than 1 cm can generally be closed primarily and buttressed with a well-vascularized omentum. For larger perforations or ulcers with fibrotic edges that cannot be brought together without tension, a Graham patch repair with healthy omentum is performed. Multiple stay sutures are placed that incorporate healthy tissue on the proximal and the distal sides of the ulcer. The omentum is placed underneath these sutures, and they are tied to secure it in place and seal the perforation (Fig. 49.13). For very large perforations (>3 cm), control of the duodenal defect can be difficult. The defect should be closed by the application of healthy tissue, such as omentum or jejunal serosa from a Roux-en-Y type limb. In such cases, a pyloric exclusion is typically performed by oversewing the pylorus using absorbable suture or stapling across it using a noncutting linear stapler. A gastrojejunostomy is created to bypass the duodenum in a Billroth II or Roux-en-Y fashion. Over several weeks, the pyloric exclusion stitches or staples give way, restoring normal GI anatomy after the perforation site has been given time to heal. Alternatively, a duodenostomy tube can be placed through the perforation with wide peritoneal drainage. An alternative in this difficult situation is antrectomy and a Billroth II or Roux-en-Y reconstruction.

Perforations can also be treated laparoscopically. A meta analysis of seven randomized studies comparing laparoscopic repair versus open repair showed that laparoscopic surgery was associated with less postoperative morbidity, fewer wound infections, and shorter length of stay.[13] There was no difference shown in operative time, reoperation rates, leak rates, or mortality between open and laparoscopic repair. Based on these data, in experienced hands, laparoscopy appears to be the superior approach in patients with perforations who are hemodynamically stable.

For patients who are known to be negative for *H. pylori*, are taking long-term NSAIDs that they cannot discontinue, or have failed medical therapy in the past for their ulcer disease, an acid-reducing procedure can be added at the time of repair. These procedures are discussed elsewhere in this chapter and must be based on the clinical situation and comfort of the surgeon.

After repair, the stomach is decompressed with an NG tube. Drains should be kept in place until patients have eaten without a change in drain output or quality, which would suggest a leak. A routine contrast radiograph is not required before initiating eating but can be used to evaluate the security of the perforation closure should the patient exhibit symptoms or signs of enteric leak. All *H. pylori*–positive patients should undergo eradication with appropriate triple-therapy regimens. An elective upper endoscopy should be performed 6 to 8 weeks after surgery to assess for evidence of malignancy, ulcer healing, and to test for *H. pylori* if that diagnosis has not yet been established.

Gastric outlet obstruction. Acute inflammation of the duodenum or pylorus can lead to mechanical obstruction, with a functional gastric outlet obstruction manifested by early satiety, anorexia, weight loss, nausea, and vomiting. In cases of prolonged vomiting, patients often become dehydrated and develop a hypochloremic, hypokalemic metabolic alkalosis secondary to the loss of gastric juice rich in hydrogen and chloride. Chronic inflammation leads to recurrent episodes of injury and healing, ultimately leading to fibrosis, scarring, and stenosis of the outflow tract. The stomach can become massively dilated in this setting and lose its muscular tone. Marked weight loss and malnutrition are common.

Initial management should involve gastric decompression with NG tube placement and correction of fluid and electrolyte abnormalities. Nutritional status should be assessed as these patients often present malnourished. Gastric outlet obstruction from PUD is not a surgical emergency, and full diagnostic workup prior to any surgical intervention is necessary, especially as gastric cancer is the most common cause of this disorder. Upper endoscopy should be performed to rule out a malignancy and assess for *H. pylori* infection.

Endoscopic dilation (with or without stenting) and *H. pylori* eradication are the mainstays of initial therapy. Novel endoscopic techniques, including ultrasound-guided gastric bypass and peroral endoscopic myotomy, are also being explored.[14] Patients with refractory obstruction are best managed with primary antrectomy and reconstruction along with vagotomy. Another surgical option, especially when there is significant inflammation or scarring present, is vagotomy with a drainage procedure, typically either a Jaboulay gastroduodenostomy or a gastrojejunostomy.

Intractable peptic ulcer disease. Intractability is defined as failure of an ulcer to heal after an initial trial of 8 to 12 weeks of therapy or if patients relapse after therapy has been discontinued; it is estimated to occur in 5% to 10% of patients. Intractable PUD is unusual for duodenal ulcer disease in the *H. pylori* era. Benign gastric ulcers that persist must be evaluated for malignancy as well as other less common sources of ulceration such as ZES, Crohn disease, or sarcoid. For any intractable ulcer, adequate duration of antisecretory therapy, *H. pylori* eradication, and elimination of NSAID use must be confirmed. A fasting serum gastrin level should be obtained to rule out gastrinoma. Although rarely seen today, truly intractable ulcer disease that fails medical management should be treated with a vagotomy, with or without an antrectomy.

Surgical Procedures for Peptic Ulcers

Elective operative intervention for PUD has become rare as medical therapy has improved. The recognition of *H. pylori* and its eradication suggest that the intractability indication for surgery may apply only to patients in whom the organism cannot be eradicated, who cannot be taken off NSAIDs, or who have a rarer cause of PUD. Patients who are noncompliant with acid suppression therapy may also fall into this category, but this is more controversial.

The goal of operative ulcer therapy is to reduce gastric acid secretion. This can be accomplished by removing vagal stimulation via vagotomy, gastrin-driven secretion by performing an antrectomy, decreasing the number of parietal-cells with a subtotal gastrectomy, or a combination procedure. Vagotomy decreases peak acid output by approximately 50%, whereas vagotomy plus antrectomy decreases peak acid output by approximately 85%. These surgeries can be performed open or laparoscopically.

Truncal vagotomy. As seen in Fig. 49.4, truncal vagotomy is performed by division of the left and right vagus nerves above the hepatic and celiac branches, just above the GE junction. Most surgeons use some form of drainage procedure in association with truncal vagotomy to avoid gastric stasis. Pyloric relaxation is mediated by vagal stimulation, and a vagotomy without a drainage procedure can cause delayed gastric emptying. Truncal vagotomy in combination with a Heineke-Mikulicz pyloroplasty is shown in Fig. 49.14. When the duodenal bulb is scarred, a Finney pyloroplasty or Jaboulay gastroduodenostomy may be a useful alternative. Significant scarring or inflammation may necessitate a gastrojejunostomy. In general, there is little difference in the side effects associated with the type of drainage procedure performed, although bile reflux may be more common after gastroenterostomy, and diarrhea is more common after pyloroplasty. The incidence of dumping syndrome is similar for both.

Selective vagotomy. Selective vagotomy divides the main right and left vagus nerves just distal to the celiac and hepatic branches, and a pyloric drainage procedure is also performed. However, selective vagotomy results in higher ulcer recurrence rates than truncal vagotomy, with no advantage in terms of decreased postgastrectomy symptoms. For these reasons, selective vagotomy has largely been abandoned.

Highly selective vagotomy. Highly selective vagotomy is also called *parietal cell vagotomy* or *proximal gastric vagotomy*. This procedure was developed after recognition that truncal vagotomy, in

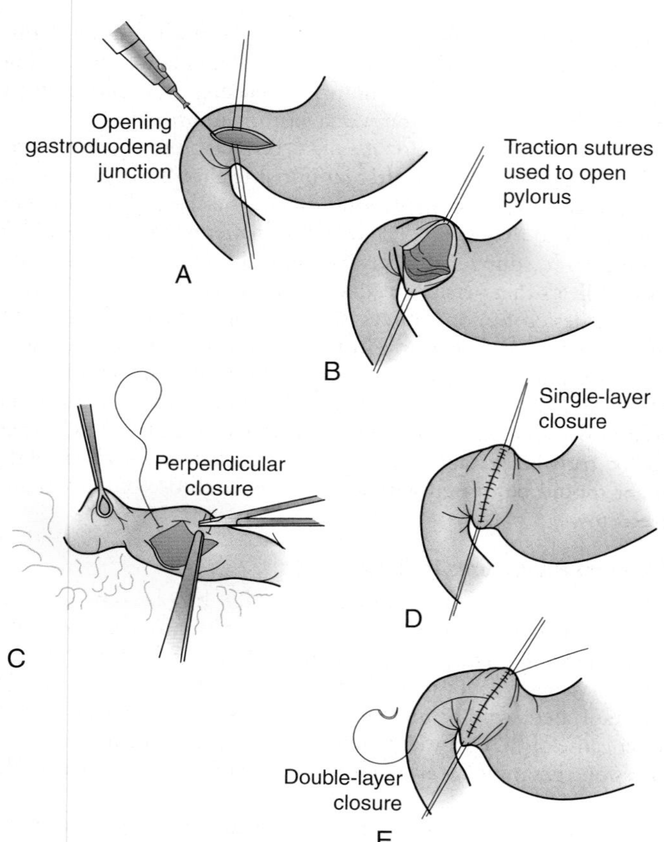

FIG. 49.14 (A–E) Heineke-Mikulicz pyloroplasty. (From Soreide JA, Soreide A. Pyloroplasty. *Oper Tech Gen Surg*. 2003;5:65–72.)

combination with a drainage procedure or gastric resection, adversely affects the pyloral antral pump function. A highly selective vagotomy divides only the vagus nerves supplying the acid-producing portion of the stomach within the corpus and fundus. This procedure preserves the vagal innervation of the gastric antrum and pylorus, so there is no need for routine drainage procedures. Consequently, the incidence of postoperative complications is lower. In general, the nerves of Latarjet are identified anteriorly and posteriorly, and the crow's feet innervating the fundus and body of the stomach are divided. These nerves are divided up until a point approximately 7 cm proximal to the pylorus, the area in the vicinity of the gastric antrum. Superiorly, division of these nerves is carried to a point at least 5 cm proximal to the GE junction on the esophagus (Fig. 49.15). Ideally, two or three branches to the antrum and pylorus should be preserved. The criminal nerve of Grassi represents a very proximal branch of the posterior trunk of the vagus, and great attention is needed to avoid missing this branch in the division process because it is frequently cited as a predisposition for ulcer recurrence if left intact.

The recurrence rates after highly selective vagotomy are variable and depend on the skill of the surgeon and duration of follow-up. Lengthy longitudinal follow-up is necessary to evaluate the results of this procedure because of the reported increase in recurrent ulceration with time. Recurrence rates of 10% to 15% have been reported for this procedure when performed by a skilled surgeon. These rates are slightly higher than the rates reported after truncal vagotomy in combination with pyloroplasty; however, highly selective vagotomy has lower rates of postvagotomy dumping syndrome and diarrhea.

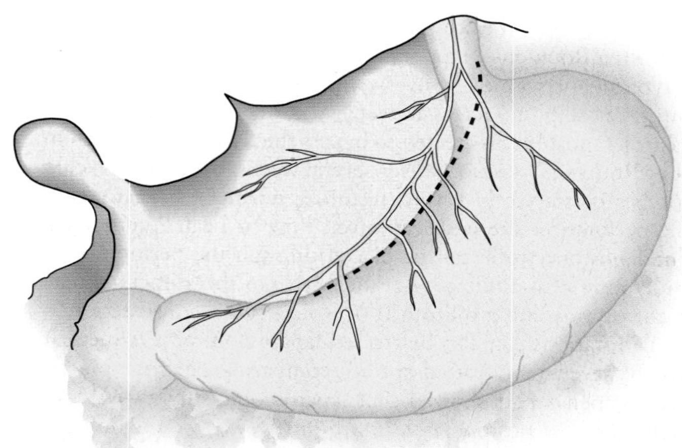

FIG. 49.15 Anterior view of the stomach and anterior nerve of Latarjet. Note the line of dissection for parietal cell or highly selective vagotomy *(dashed line)*. The last major branches of the nerve are left intact, and the dissection begins 7 cm from the pylorus. At the gastroesophageal junction, the dissection is well away from the origin of the hepatic branches of the left vagus. (From Kelly KA, Teotia SS. Proximal gastric vagotomy. In Baker RJ, Fischer JE, eds. *Mastery of Surgery*. Philadelphia: Lippincott Williams & Wilkins; 2001.)

Truncal vagotomy and antrectomy. Antrectomy is generally not performed for duodenal ulcers and is more commonly performed for gastric ulcers. Relative contraindications include cirrhosis; extensive scarring of the proximal duodenum that leaves a difficult or tenuous duodenal closure; and previous operations on the proximal duodenum. When done in combination with truncal vagotomy, it is more effective at reducing acid secretion and recurrence than truncal vagotomy in combination with a drainage procedure or highly selective vagotomy. The recurrence rate for ulceration after truncal vagotomy and antrectomy is 0% to 2%. However, this low recurrence rate needs to be balanced against the 20% rate of postgastrectomy and postvagotomy syndromes in patients undergoing antrectomy, longer operative times, and increased postoperative morbidity.

Antrectomy requires reconstruction of GI continuity that can be accomplished by a gastroduodenostomy (Billroth I procedure [Fig. 49.16]) or gastrojejunostomy (either Billroth II procedure [Fig. 49.17] or Roux-en-Y reconstruction). For benign disease, gastroduodenostomy is generally favored because it avoids the problem of retained antrum syndrome, duodenal stump leak, and afferent loop obstruction associated with gastrojejunostomy after resection. If the duodenum is significantly scarred, gastroduodenostomy may be technically more difficult, necessitating gastrojejunostomy. If a gastrojejunostomy is performed, the loop of jejunum chosen for anastomosis is usually brought through the transverse mesocolon in a retrocolic fashion. The gastric anastomosis is typically placed in a dependent portion of the stomach to facilitate drainage, often along the posterior wall of the greater curvature. The retrocolic anastomosis minimizes the length of the afferent limb and decreases the likelihood of twisting or kinking that could lead to afferent loop obstruction and predispose patients to the devastating complication of a duodenal stump leak. Although vagotomy and antrectomy are effective at managing ulcerations, they are used infrequently today in the treatment of patients with PUD. In general, operations of lesser magnitude are performed more frequently in the *H. pylori* era. The overall mortality rate for antrectomy is approximately 1% to 2% but is higher

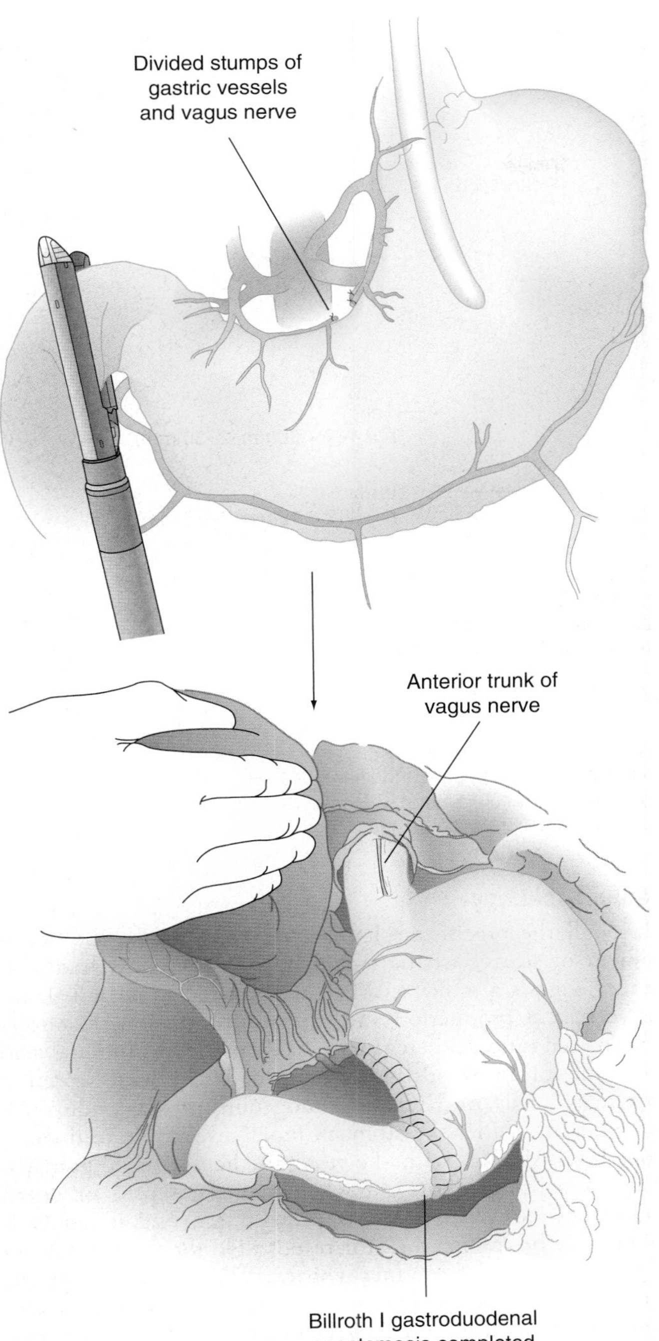

FIG. 49.16 Hemigastrectomy with a Billroth I (gastroduodenal) anastomosis. (From Dempsey D, Pathak A. Antrectomy. *Oper Tech Gen Surg.* 2003;5:86–100.)

in patients with comorbid conditions, such as insulin-dependent diabetes or immunosuppression.

Partial gastrectomy. Partial, or subtotal, gastrectomy removes both gastrin-producing and acid-secreting cells. Reconstruction is necessary following a subtotal gastrectomy, with Billroth II or Roux-en-Y being the most commonly used. Billroth I reconstruction is typically difficult due to the underlying inflammation.

Zollinger-Ellison syndrome. ZES is a clinical triad consisting of gastric acid hypersecretion, severe PUD, and gastrin-producing neuroendocrine tumors (NETs; gastrinomas). The islet cell tumor produces gastrin, and hypergastrinemia associated with ZES accounts for most, if not all, clinical symptoms experienced by patients. Abdominal pain and PUD are the hallmarks of the syndrome and typically occur in more than 80% of patients. Patients may also exhibit diarrhea, weight loss, steatorrhea, and esophagitis. Endoscopy frequently demonstrates prominent gastric rugal folds, reflecting the trophic effect of hypergastrinemia on the gastric fundus. Approximately 20% to 30% of patients have ZES as part of multiple endocrine neoplasia type 1, an autosomal dominant syndrome. Thus, any patient found to have ZES should have serum parathyroid hormone, ionized calcium, and prolactin levels checked.

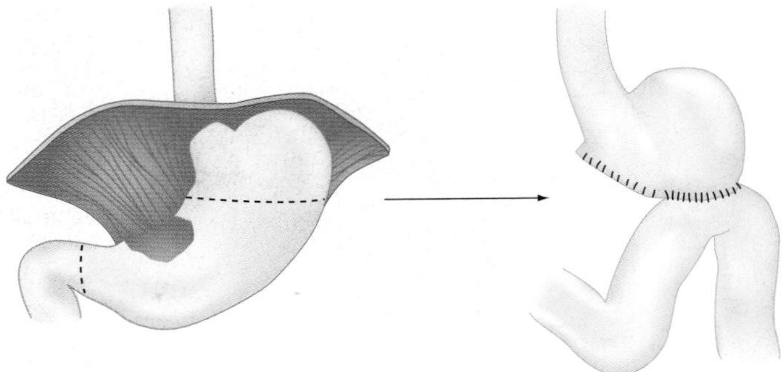

FIG. 49.17 Subtotal gastrectomy with a Billroth II anastomosis.

Provocative tests are generally not required to establish the diagnosis of ZES because fasting plasma gastrin levels are usually elevated. Most patients with gastrinoma have elevated fasting serum gastrin levels (>200 pg/mL), and values higher than 1000 pg/mL are diagnostic. Diagnosing ZES in patients with marginally elevated gastrin levels is difficult because PPI use, *H. pylori* infection, and renal failure all can cause an elevation of fasting serum gastrin. In patients with gastrin levels in this equivocal range, the most sensitive diagnostic test is the secretin-stimulated gastrin level. Serum gastrin samples are measured before and after IV secretin administration. An increase in the serum gastrin level of greater than 200 pg/mL above basal levels is suggestive of gastrinoma versus other causes of hypergastrinemia, which normally do not demonstrate this response.

After diagnosis of gastrinoma, acid suppression therapy is initiated, preferably with a high-dose PPI. Medical management is indicated preoperatively and for patients with metastatic or unresectable gastrinoma. The next step in management is localization and staging of the tumor. Most ZES gastrinomas are located in the duodenum or pancreas, within the "gastrinoma triangle"; the points of this triangle are made up of the cystic-common bile duct junction, the pancreas body-neck junction, and the junction between the second and third portions of the duodenum (Fig. 49.18). The best initial imaging study to localize the gastrin-secreting tumor is either triple-phase CT or MR imaging (MRI) of the abdomen. However, these imaging modalities have a relatively low sensitivity in detecting tumors that are less than 1 cm in diameter as well as small liver metastases. If initial imaging is nondiagnostic, localization can sometimes be achieved using somatostatin receptor scintigraphy or endoscopic ultrasound (EUS). If still unable to localize tumor, patients can be offered a surgical exploration.

Localized gastrinomas should be resected; however, long-term cure rates are only about 50%. Once the tumor is located intraoperatively, a resection according to oncologic principles should

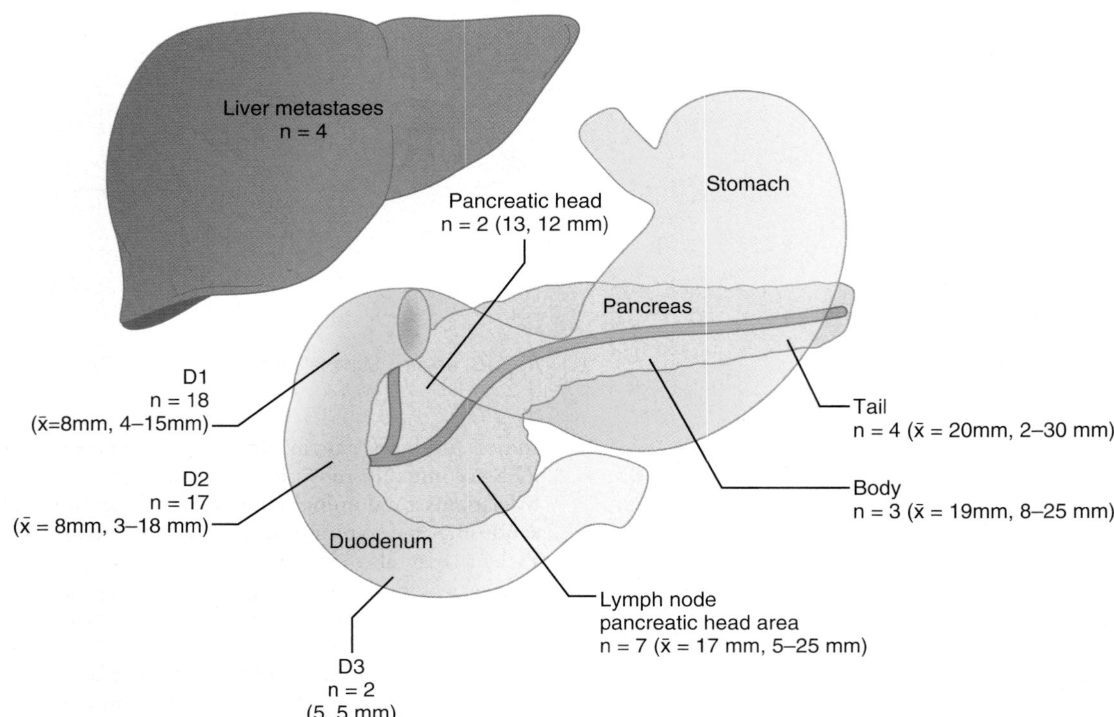

FIG. 49.18 The location of gastrinomas at surgery that were not detected on preoperative imaging. Most tumors were located in the first and second portions of the duodenum and the head of the pancreas, within the so-called gastrinoma triangle. (From Norton JA, Fraker DL, Alexander HR, et al. Value of surgery in patients with negative imaging and sporadic Zollinger-Ellison syndrome. *Ann Surg.* 2012;256:509–517.)

be performed (rather than a tumor enucleation) with at least 10 lymph nodes removed. Small case series suggest that patients who are not operative candidates may have symptom palliation and slower disease progression with radiation therapy. Patients with tumor recurrence or metastatic disease can be treated with a variety of treatments. The most commonly utilized are somatostatin analogs and/or chemotherapy (streptozocin/doxorubicin or temozolomide-based regimen). For patients with liver metastases, liver-directed therapies (radiofrequency ablation, cryoablation, embolization, resection, or transplantation) can be considered.

STRESS GASTRITIS

Stress gastritis can occur after physical trauma, shock, sepsis, hemorrhage, or respiratory failure and may lead to life-threatening gastric bleeding. Stress gastritis is characterized by multiple superficial (nonulcerating) erosions that typically begin in the proximal portion of the stomach and progress distally. They may also occur in the setting of a central nervous system disease elevating intracranial pressure with resultant vagal nerve stimulation (Cushing ulcer) or as a result of thermal burn injury involving more than 30% of the body surface area leading to gastric ischemia (Curling ulcer).

Stress gastritis lesions typically change with time. Early lesions are typically multiple and shallow, with discrete areas of erythema along with focal hemorrhage or an adherent clot. If the lesion erodes into the submucosa, which contains the blood supply, frank bleeding may result. They are almost always seen in the fundus of the stomach and only rarely in the distal stomach. Late lesions appear identical to regenerating mucosa around a healing gastric ulcer. Both types of lesions can be seen endoscopically.

Pathophysiology

Although the precise mechanisms responsible for the development of stress gastritis remain to be fully elucidated, evidence suggests a multifactorial cause related to an imbalance between acid production and mucosal protection. Examples of impaired mucosal defense mechanisms against luminal acid are reduction in blood flow, mucus, or bicarbonate secretion by mucosal cells, or decreased endogenous prostaglandins. All these factors render the stomach more susceptible to damage from luminal acid, with the resultant hemorrhagic gastritis. Stress is considered present when hypoxia, sepsis, or organ failure occurs. When stress is present, mucosal ischemia is thought to be the main factor responsible for the breakdown of these normal defense mechanisms. While increased gastric acid secretion rarely occurs in this situation, the presence of luminal acid appears to be a prerequisite for this form of gastritis to evolve.

Presentation and Diagnosis

Stress gastritis develops within 1 to 2 days after a traumatic event in more than 50% to 75% of patients, although the majority of patients have minimal or no related symptoms. The only clinical sign may be painless upper GI bleeding. The bleeding is usually slow and intermittent and may be detected by only a few flecks of blood in the NG tube or an unexplained decrease in hemoglobin level. Occasionally, there may be profound upper GI hemorrhage accompanied by hypotension and hematemesis. The stool is frequently guaiac-positive, although melena or hematochezia is rare. Endoscopy is required to confirm the diagnosis and differentiate stress gastritis from other sources of GI hemorrhage.

Prophylaxis

Because of the high mortality rate in patients with acute stress gastritis who develop hemodynamically significant upper GI hemorrhage, high-risk patients should be treated prophylactically, although the definition of what constitutes high risk is still debated. Because mucosal ischemia may alter many mucosal defense mechanisms that enable the stomach to withstand luminal irritants and protect itself from injury, every effort should be made to correct any perfusion deficits secondary to shock. The two strongest risk factors for developing clinically significant bleeding from gastric stress ulcers are coagulopathy and respiratory failure requiring prolonged mechanical ventilation (>48 hours). Other significant risk factors include a history of PUD or GI bleeding in the past year, central nervous system injury, significant burn injury, and sepsis. Enteral nutrition reduces the risk of stress ulcer formation and should be initiated as soon as possible. If prophylaxis is indicated, a PPI, rather than H_2-receptor antagonists or sucralfate, should be used, although the evidence supporting this is weak. Prophylaxis should be limited only to high-risk patients, as gastric acid suppression has been associated with increased rates of nosocomial pneumonia and *C. difficile* infection. Of note, a recent meta analysis showed that while prophylaxis did reduce the incidence of bleeding, the mortality rates were unaffected.[15] Larger randomized trials are still needed to determine which patients may benefit most from stress ulcer prophylaxis in the critical care setting.

Treatment

Any patient with significant upper GI bleeding requires fluid resuscitation with correction of any coagulation or platelet abnormalities. An NG tube should be placed if not already present and IV PPI therapy started promptly. Urgent endoscopy should be performed for diagnosis and treatment; however, the bleeding from stress ulcers is usually diffuse and the rebleeding rate is high. In experienced centers, vasopressin can be administered into the left gastric artery and can be embolized as well to help control bleeding. If the patient has underlying cardiac or liver disease, vasopressin should not be used.

Bleeding that results in hemodynamic instability or requires persistent transfusions is an indication for surgery. Because most lesions are in the proximal stomach or fundus, a long anterior gastrotomy should be made in this area. The gastric lumen is cleared of blood, and the mucosal surface is inspected for bleeding points. All bleeding areas are oversewn with figure-of-eight stitches taken deep within the gastric wall. Most superficial erosions are not actively bleeding and do not require ligation unless a blood vessel is seen at its base. In stable patients, the operation is completed by closing the anterior gastrotomy and performing a truncal vagotomy and pyloroplasty to reduce acid secretion. Less commonly, a partial gastrectomy combined with vagotomy is performed. Total gastrectomy should be performed rarely and only in patients with life-threatening hemorrhage refractory to other forms of therapy.

POSTGASTRECTOMY SYNDROMES

Gastric surgery can result in numerous physiologic derangements caused by loss of reservoir function, interruption of the pyloric sphincter mechanism, and vagal nerve transection. The GI and cardiovascular symptoms may result in disorders collectively referred to as *postgastrectomy syndromes*. Approximately 20% to 25% of patients who undergo surgery for PUD subsequently develop some degree of postgastrectomy syndrome, although this frequency is much lower in patients who undergo highly selective vagotomy. The physiologic changes are not specific to PUD and can occur after gastrectomy for resection of neoplasm or Roux-en-Y gastric bypass for treatment of severe obesity. Approximately 1% to 5% of patients become permanently disabled from their postgastrectomy symptoms.

Dumping Syndrome

Dumping syndrome is a combination of both GI and vasomotor symptoms due to rapid postprandial gastric emptying. GI symptoms include abdominal pain, early satiety, nausea/vomiting, diarrhea, and bloating. Vasomotor systemic symptoms include diaphoresis, tachycardia, palpitations, headache, and syncope. This symptom complex can develop after any operation on the stomach but is more common after partial gastrectomy with the Billroth II reconstruction. It is much less commonly observed after the Billroth I gastrectomy or after vagotomy and drainage procedures.

Dumping syndrome can be divided into two categories: early and late. Early dumping occurs within 30 minutes of a meal and is a result of rapid passage of high osmolarity food from the stomach into the small intestine. This occurs because gastrectomy, or any interruption of the pyloric sphincter mechanism, prevents the stomach from preparing its contents and delivering them to the proximal bowel in the form of small particles in isotonic solution. The resultant hypertonic food bolus passes into the small intestine, which induces a rapid shift of extracellular fluid into the intestinal lumen to achieve isotonicity. After this shift of extracellular fluid, luminal distention occurs and induces the resultant symptoms.

Late dumping occurs 1 to 3 hours after a meal and is less common. The basic defect of late dumping is also rapid gastric emptying; however, it is related specifically to carbohydrates being delivered rapidly into the proximal intestine. When carbohydrates are delivered to the small intestine, they are quickly absorbed, resulting in hyperglycemia, which triggers the release of large amounts of insulin to control the increasing blood sugar level. An overcompensation results so that profound hypoglycemia occurs in response to the insulin. This hypoglycemia activates the adrenal gland to release catecholamines, which results in diaphoresis, tremulousness, light-headedness, tachycardia, and confusion.

The symptoms associated with early dumping syndrome appear to be secondary to the release of several humoral agents, such as serotonin, bradykinin-like substances, neurotensin, and enteroglucagon. Dietary measures are usually sufficient to treat most patients. These include avoiding foods containing large amounts of sugar, frequent feeding of small meals rich in protein, fats, and fiber, and separating liquids from solids during a meal.

In some patients without a response to dietary measures, pharmacologic treatments directed at specific symptoms can be effective, such as tincture of opium or imodium for diarrhea and meclizine for nausea. Anticholinergics can slow gastric emptying and treat spasms. Octreotide can be given in either short-acting form immediately before a meal or via an intramuscular long-acting formulation. These peptides not only inhibit gastric emptying but also affect small bowel motility so that intestinal transit of the ingested meal is prolonged. Octreotide is the best studied medication for dumping syndrome and can be very effective. However, the peptides are expensive and are thus not considered first-line treatment typically. Patients with severe symptoms may require a reoperation if conservative management is unsuccessful. The choice of operation depends on the original gastric surgery. Pyloric reconstruction can sometimes be performed. For patients with a gastrojejunostomy without a gastrectomy, takedown of the gastrojejunostomy can be performed if the pylorus function is maintained. In patients with a prior distal gastrectomy, converting a loop gastrojejunostomy to a Roux-en-Y reconstruction is recommended.

Metabolic Disturbances

The most common metabolic defect appearing after gastrectomy is anemia. Anemia is related to iron deficiency (more common) or impairment in vitamin B_{12} metabolism. More than 30% of patients undergoing gastrectomy have iron deficiency anemia. The exact cause is not fully understood but appears to be related to a combination of decreased iron intake, impaired iron absorption, and chronic blood loss. In general, the addition of iron supplements to the patient's diet corrects this problem.

Megaloblastic anemia from vitamin B_{12} deficiency only rarely develops after partial gastrectomy but is dependent on the amount of stomach removed. Vitamin deficiency occurs secondary to poor absorption of dietary vitamin B_{12} because of the lack of intrinsic factor. Patients undergoing subtotal gastrectomy should be placed on lifelong vitamin B_{12} supplementation. If a patient develops a macrocytic anemia, serum vitamin B_{12} levels should be obtained and, if abnormal, treated with long-term vitamin B_{12} therapy.

Osteoporosis and osteomalacia have also been observed after gastric resection and appear to be caused by deficiencies in calcium. If fat malabsorption is also present, the calcium malabsorption is aggravated further because fatty acids bind calcium. The incidence of this problem also increases with the extent of gastric resection and is usually associated with a Billroth II gastrectomy. Bone disease generally develops approximately 4 to 5 years after surgery. Treatment of this disorder usually requires calcium supplements in conjunction with vitamin D. Patients with Billroth II or Roux-en-Y reconstruction that bypasses the duodenum should also receive supplementation of the fat-soluble vitamins (vitamins A, D, E, and K).

Afferent Loop Syndrome

The afferent loop is the duodenojejunal loop proximal to the gastrojejunal anastomosis after either a Billroth II reconstruction or gastrojejunostomy. Afferent loop syndrome occurs as a result of partial obstruction of the afferent limb, which is then unable to empty its contents. After obstruction of the afferent limb, pancreatic and hepatobiliary secretions accumulate within the limb, resulting in its distention, which causes epigastric discomfort and cramping. The intraluminal pressure eventually increases enough to empty the contents of the afferent loop forcefully into the stomach, resulting in projectile bilious vomiting that offers immediate relief of symptoms. If the obstruction has been present for a long time, it can also be aggravated by the development of blind loop syndrome. In this situation, bacterial overgrowth occurs in the static loop, and the bacteria bind with vitamin B_{12} and deconjugated bile acids; this results in a systemic deficiency of vitamin B_{12} (with the development of megaloblastic anemia), fat malabsorption, and deficiency in fat-soluble vitamins.

In contrast to the diagnosis of an acute bowel obstruction, the diagnosis of chronic afferent loop obstruction can be problematic. Failure to visualize the afferent limb on upper endoscopy is suggestive of the diagnosis. Radionuclide studies imaging the hepatobiliary tree have also been used with some success in diagnosing this syndrome. Normally, the radionuclides should pass into the stomach or distal small bowel after being excreted into the afferent limb. If this does not occur, the possibility of an afferent loop obstruction should be considered.

Surgical correction is indicated for this mechanical problem to prevent bowel necrosis or duodenal stump blowout. A long afferent limb is usually the underlying problem, so treatment involves the elimination of this loop. Remedies include conversion of the Billroth II construction into a Billroth I anastomosis, enteroenterostomy below the afferent and efferent loops, and conversion to a Roux-en-Y reconstruction.

Efferent Loop Obstruction

Obstruction of the efferent limb is rare. Efferent loop obstruction may occur at any time; however, more than 50% of cases do so within the first postoperative month. Establishing a diagnosis is difficult. Initial complaints may include left upper quadrant abdominal pain that is colicky in nature, bilious vomiting, and abdominal distention. The diagnosis is usually established by an upper GI series or CT with oral contrast, with failure of contrast to enter the efferent limb. Operative intervention is almost always necessary and consists of reducing the retroanastomotic hernia if this is the cause of the obstruction and closing the retroanastomotic space to prevent recurrence of this condition.

Alkaline Reflux Gastritis

After gastrectomy, reflux of bile is common. In a small percentage of patients, this reflux is associated with severe epigastric abdominal pain accompanied by bilious vomiting and weight loss. The diagnosis is typically made by careful history. A technetium biliary scan can be used to demonstrate reflux of bile into the stomach. Upper endoscopy demonstrates friable, beefy red mucosa.

Most patients with alkaline reflux gastritis have had gastric resection performed with a Billroth II anastomosis. Although bile reflux appears to be the inciting event, numerous issues remain unanswered with respect to the role of bile in its pathogenesis. For example, many patients have reflux of bile into the stomach after gastrectomy without any symptoms. Moreover, there is no clear correlation between the volume or composition of bile and the subsequent development of alkaline reflux gastritis. After a definitive diagnosis is made, therapy is directed at relief of symptoms. Most medical therapies that have been tried to treat alkaline reflux gastritis have not shown any consistent benefit. For patients with intractable symptoms, the surgical procedure of choice is conversion of the Billroth II anastomosis into a Roux-en-Y gastrojejunostomy, in which the Roux limb has been lengthened to more than 40 cm. In general, a Roux-en-Y procedure should be preferred over a Billroth II for reconstruction at the time of partial or subtotal distal gastrectomy to decrease the likelihood of alkaline reflux II.[16]

Gastric Atony

Gastric emptying is delayed after truncal and selective vagotomies but not after a highly selective vagotomy. With selective or truncal vagotomy, patients lose their antral pump function and have a reduction in the ability to empty solids. In contrast, emptying of liquids is accelerated due to the loss of receptive relaxation in the proximal stomach. Although most patients undergoing vagotomy and a drainage procedure manage to empty their stomach adequately, some patients have persistent gastric stasis that results in retention of food within the stomach for several hours. This condition may be accompanied by a feeling of fullness and, occasionally, abdominal pain. In still rarer cases, it may be associated with a functional gastric outlet obstruction.

The diagnosis of gastric atony is confirmed by scintigraphic assessment of gastric emptying. However, other causes of delayed gastric emptying, such as diabetes mellitus, electrolyte imbalance, drug toxicity, and neuromuscular disorders, must also be excluded. In addition, a mechanical cause of gastric outlet obstruction, such as postoperative adhesions, afferent or efferent loop obstruction, and internal herniation, must be ruled out. Endoscopic examination of the stomach also needs to be performed to rule out an anastomotic obstruction.

In patients with a functional gastric outlet obstruction and documented gastroparesis, pharmacotherapy is generally utilized. The agents most commonly used are prokinetic agents such as metoclopramide and erythromycin. Metoclopramide exerts its prokinetic effects by acting as a dopamine antagonist and has cholinergic-enhancing effects because of facilitation of acetylcholine release from enteric cholinergic neurons. In contrast, erythromycin markedly accelerates gastric emptying by binding to motilin receptors on GI smooth muscle cells, where it acts as a motilin agonist. In rare cases of persistent gastric atony refractory to medical management, gastrectomy may be required.

GASTRIC CANCER

Epidemiology

Incidence

Gastric cancer has the fourteenth highest cancer incidence and is the thirteenth highest cause of cancer death in the United States, with an estimated 26,240 new cases and more than 10,800 deaths in 2018.[17] The disease affects men disproportionately, with more than 60% of new cases and deaths occurring in men. It is a disease of older individuals, with peak incidence in the seventh decade of life. Among racial groups, the disease is more common and has a higher mortality in African Americans, Asian Americans, and Hispanics compared with whites.

Worldwide in 2018, gastric cancer is more prevalent; it is the fifth most common cancer and the second leading cause of cancer death.[18] Over half of new cases occur in developing countries. It is especially prevalent in East Asia, Eastern Europe, and Central and South America. Higher geographic latitudes are associated with higher gastric cancer risk. Among developed countries, Japan and Korea have the highest rates of the disease. Gastric cancer is the most common cancer in Japan. As a result, gastric cancer screening in Japan was started in the 1970s, with significant improvements in mortality.

Risk Factors

The major risk factors for gastric cancer are discussed here; they include both environmental and genetic factors (Box 49.3).

BOX 49.3 Factors associated with increased risk for developing stomach cancer.

Nutritional
Low fat or protein consumption
Salted meat or fish
High nitrate consumption
Obesity
High complex carbohydrate consumption

Environmental
Poor food preparation (smoked, salted)
Lack of refrigeration
Poor drinking water (e.g., contaminated well water)
Smoking and alcohol

Social
Low socioeconomic class

Medical
Prior gastric surgery
Helicobacter pylori and Epstein-Barr virus infection
Hereditary predisposition
Prior abdominal irradiation
Atrophic gastritis
Adenomatous polyps

Other
Male sex

Helicobacter pylori Infection

In 1994, the International Agency for Research on Cancer (IARC) labeled *H. pylori* a definite carcinogen; it is the most common cause of infection-related cancers.[19] Numerous longitudinal prospective studies have demonstrated its association with the development of gastric cancer. In epidemiological studies, *H. pylori* seropositivity has been associated with an approximately sixfold increased risk of developing gastric cancer. The primary mechanism is thought to be the presence of chronic inflammation. Long-term infection with the bacteria can lead to atrophic gastritis or chronic active gastritis. In some patients, gastritis progresses to intestinal metaplasia, dysplasia, and ultimately intestinal-type adenocarcinoma. A wide range of molecular alterations in intestinal metaplasia have been described and may affect the transformation into gastric cancer. These include overexpression of cyclooxygenase-2 and cyclin D2, *p53* mutations, microsatellite instability, decreased *p27* expression, and alterations in transcription factors such as CDX1 and CDX2.[19] Intestinal metaplasia is a risk factor for the development of gastric carcinoma; however, not every patient with intestinal metaplasia develops invasive cancer. Host inflammatory responses also play an important role in this process. Specifically, higher levels of interleukin-1β and tumor necrosis factor-α expression lead to an increased risk of gastric cancer development.

Some regional variances in the development of cancer may be attributed to the prevalence and virulence of *H. pylori*. It is more common in areas with less sanitation, and infection rates remain high in developing countries, with a concomitant increase in gastric cancer incidence. In contrast, the prevalence in more developed countries has been decreasing. The presence of the cytotoxin-associated gene A upregulates proinflammatory response, cellular migration, and elongation, leading to increased virulence and risk of gastric cancer. Countries with high levels of gastric cancer, such as Japan, have a much higher rate of cytotoxin-associated gene A–positive *H. pylori* infection than countries with lower rates of gastric cancer, such as the United States.

Dietary Factors

High-salt foods, particularly salted or smoked meats that contain high levels of nitrate, along with low intake of fruits and vegetables, are linked to an increased risk of gastric cancer. The mechanism is postulated to involve salt damaging the stomach mucosa. N-nitroso compounds are generated after nitrate ingestion. N-nitroso compounds are also found in tobacco smoke, another known risk factor for gastric cancer. Fresh fruits and vegetables

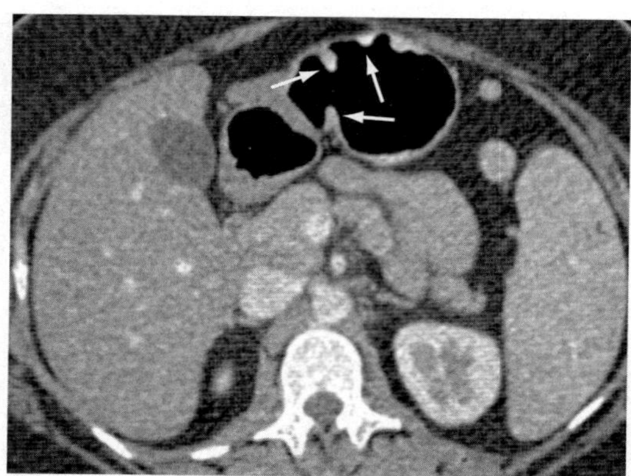
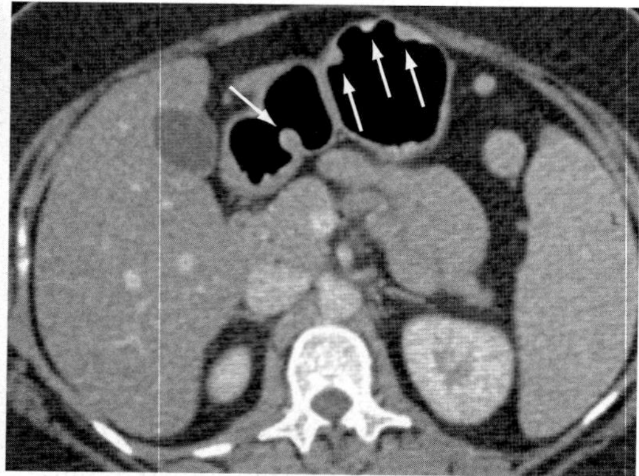

FIG. 49.19 Computed tomography scan of fundic gland polyps. (Courtesy Dr. David Bentrem, Department of Surgery, Northwestern University Feinberg School of Medicine, Chicago, IL.)

contain ascorbic acid, which can remove the carcinogenic N-nitroso compounds and oxygen free radicals.

Synergy between a high-salt diet and *H. pylori* infection has been shown, with the bacteria increasing carcinogen production and inhibiting its removal. *H. pylori* has been shown to promote the growth of the bacteria that generate the carcinogenic N-nitroso compounds. At the same time, *H. pylori* can inhibit the secretion of ascorbic acid, preventing effective scavenging of oxygen free radicals and N-nitroso compounds.

The increase in refrigeration over the past 70 years has likely contributed to the decrease in gastric cancer by reducing the amount of meat preserved by salting alone and allowing the increased storage and consumption of fresh fruits and vegetables. In 2015, the WHO IARC classified processed meats as a group 1 carcinogen.

Hereditary Risk Factors and Cancer Genetics

Gastric cancer is associated with several rare inherited disorders. Patients with hereditary diffuse gastric cancer, resulting from a gene mutation for the cell adhesion molecule E-cadherin (*CDH1*), have 60% to 70% lifetime incidence of developing gastric cancer. Prophylactic total gastrectomy should be considered for patients with this mutation prior to age 30. Notably, these patients are also at higher risk of lobular breast cancer and screening should begin by age 30, with consideration of prophylactic risk-reducing bilateral mastectomy. Two newer autosomal dominant disorders have been identified, gastric adenocarcinoma and proximal polyposis of the stomach and familial intestinal gastric cancer; the genetic causes of these have yet to be identified.

A number of hereditary cancer syndromes are associated with gastric cancer. In familial adenomatous polyposis, most patients have fundic or body sessile polyps, with 40% of these polyps having some degree of dysplasia. These polyps, combined with the much higher frequency of potentially malignant duodenal polyps, warrant upper GI surveillance. Li-Fraumeni syndrome is an autosomal dominant disorder caused by a mutation in the tumor suppressor gene *p53*, which puts patients at risk for gastric cancer as well as sarcoma, breast cancer, brain tumors, and adrenocortical carcinomas. Hereditary nonpolyposis colorectal cancer, or Lynch syndrome, is associated with microsatellite instability and increases risk of gastric and endometrial cancers.

Several genetic alterations have been identified that are associated with gastric adenocarcinoma. These changes can be classified as the activation of oncogenes, inactivation of tumor suppressor genes, reduction of cellular adhesion, reactivation of telomerase, and presence of microsatellite instability. The c-*met* proto-oncogene is the receptor for the hepatocyte growth factor and is frequently overexpressed in gastric cancer, as are the *K-ras* and *HER2* oncogenes. Inactivation of the tumor suppressor genes *p53* has been reported in diffuse and intestinal-type cancers, whereas adenomatous polyposis coli gene mutations tend to be more frequent in intestinal-type gastric cancers. Also, a reduction or loss in the cell adhesion molecule E-cadherin can be found in approximately 50% of diffuse-type gastric cancers. Microsatellite instability can be found in approximately 20% to 30% of intestinal-type gastric cancers. Aberrant epigenetic methylation can also play a role in carcinogenesis.

Polyps

Gastric polyps are a common incidental finding during upper endoscopy (seen in about 5% of procedures) and are usually asymptomatic. The malignancy risk and subsequent management largely are dependent on the polyp histopathology. Patients with an isolated polyp greater than 1 cm in size should have a complete polypectomy. For those with multiple polyps, the largest should be removed endoscopically, if possible, and remaining polyps should be biopsied. Biopsies of normal mucosa should be performed as well to assess for underlying dysplasia and *H. pylori* infection.[20]

Adenomatous polyps carry a distinct risk for the development of malignancy in the polyp and are felt to fall on the classic adenoma-carcinoma sequence. They are typically solitary lesions. Mucosal atypia is frequent, and progression from dysplasia to carcinoma in situ has been observed. The risk for the development of carcinoma is greater than 30% and increases with increasing size of the polyp.[20] Endoscopic removal is indicated for pedunculated lesions and is sufficient if the polyp is completely removed and there are no foci of invasive cancer on histologic examination. If the polyp is larger than 2 cm, is sessile, or has a proven focus of invasive carcinoma, operative excision is warranted.

Fundic gland polyps (Fig. 49.19) are benign lesions that are thought to result from glandular hyperplasia and decreased luminal flow. They are strongly associated with PPI use and occur in one third of patients by 1 year. Dysplasia, although common in patients whose polyps result from familial adenomatous polyposis, has been described only as individual case reports for patients whose polyps result from PPI therapy. Such cases do not require excision, regular surveillance, or cessation of therapy. Hyperplastic polyps are associated with *H. pylori* infection and chronic gastritis, with an associated malignancy rate of under 2%. Peutz-Jeghers syndrome also results in gastric polyps and has a 2% to 3% malignancy rate.[20]

Proton pump inhibitors

The use of PPIs has increased dramatically because they have been proven to be an effective treatment for patients with GE reflux disease and PUD. They are often prescribed empirically as first-line treatment for dyspepsia. The impact of prolonged PPI use on the incidence of gastric cancer is being actively explored.

Physiologically, PPIs, as their name suggests, block the hydrogen-potassium pump within the parietal cells, effectively blocking all acid secretion in the stomach. The potential for cancer is at the intersection between *H. pylori*, already considered a carcinogen for gastric cancer, and the physiologic changes that are a consequence of PPI use. In patients with *H. pylori* taking long-term PPIs, the low-acid environment allows the bacteria to colonize the gastric body, leading to corpus gastritis. One third of these patients develop atrophic gastritis, which is significantly more common in patients with *H. pylori* who are taking PPIs. While this atrophic gastritis quickly resolves after eradication of the *H. pylori*, atrophic gastritis is considered a major risk factor for the development of gastric cancer. Meta analyses of randomized trials have not shown clear evidence of elevated gastric cancer risk associated with PPI use. However, a recent study of over 63,000 patients in Hong Kong demonstrated an excess of 4.29 gastric cancers per 10,000 person-years and that long-term PPI use increased gastric cancer risk even after *H. pylori* eradication.[21] Other large observational studies have demonstrated increased risk of gastric cancer with prolonged PPI use, however, these studies are all prone to selection bias. Nonetheless, while PPIs are an effective first-line treatment for dyspepsia and remain an effective long-term therapy for patients with GE reflux disease, in patients with persistent symptoms after initiation of therapy or who require long-term therapy, surveillance for and eradication of *H. pylori* is warranted. Further research into potential gastric cancer risks is needed in order to make clinical guidelines for physicians considering long-term PPI therapy.

Other Risk Factors

Patients with pernicious anemia are at increased risk for developing gastric cancer. Achlorhydria is the defining feature of this condition; it occurs when chief and parietal cells are destroyed by an autoimmune reaction. Obesity was determined by the IARC to be a risk factor for gastric cardia cancers. Epstein-Barr virus infection is also associated with gastric cardia cancers. Smoking is associated with an approximately 1.5-fold increase in gastric cancer risk. Prior abdominal irradiation, most commonly after testicular cancer or Hodgkin lymphoma, increases gastric cancer risk.

Pathology

Numerous pathologic classification schemes of gastric cancer have been proposed. The Borrmann classification system was developed in 1926; it remains useful today for the description of gross appearance of endoscopic findings. This system divides gastric carcinoma into four types, type I for polypoid, type II for fungating, type III for ulcerating, and type IV for diffusely infiltrating growths (also referred to as linitis plastica in signet ring cell carcinoma) (Fig. 49.20). Other classification systems have been proposed, but the most useful and widely used system is the one proposed by Lauren in 1965. This system separates gastric adenocarcinoma into intestinal or diffuse types based on histology, with both types having distinct pathology, epidemiology, and prognosis (Table 49.5). Newer Japanese and Paris classification systems further subdivide lesions based on their level of elevation or depression.

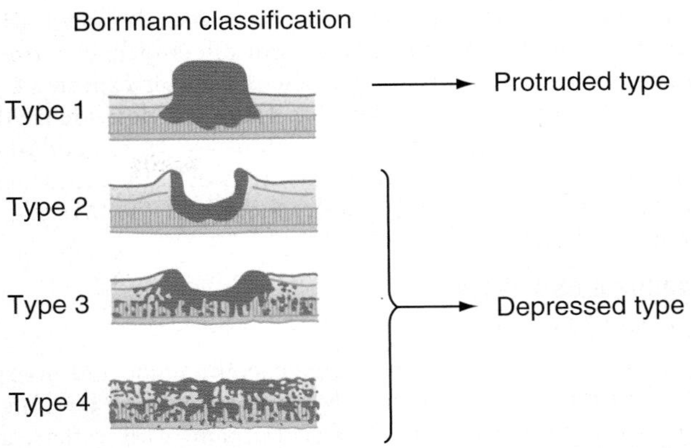

Borrmann classification

Type 1 → Protruded type

Type 2, Type 3, Type 4 → Depressed type

FIG. 49.20 Borrmann pathologic classification of gastric cancer based on gross appearance. (From Iriyama K, Asakawa T, Koike H, et al. Is extensive lymphadenectomy necessary for surgical treatment of intramucosal carcinoma of the stomach? *Arch Surg*. 1989;124:309–311.)

TABLE 49.5 Lauren classification system for gastric cancer.

INTESTINAL	DIFFUSE
Environmental	Familial
Gastric atrophy, intestinal metaplasia	Blood type A
Men > women	Women > men
Increasing incidence with age	Younger age group
Gland formation	Poorly differentiated, signet ring cells
Hematogenous spread	Transmural, lymphatic spread
Microsatellite instability	Decreased E-cadherin
APC gene mutations	
p53, p16 inactivation	*p53, p16* inactivation

APC, Adenomatous polyposis coli.

The intestinal variant is more well- differentiated and typically arises in the setting of a recognizable precancerous condition, such as gastric atrophy or intestinal metaplasia. Men are more commonly affected than women, and the incidence of intestinal-type gastric adenocarcinoma increases with age. These cancers have a tendency to form glands. The intestinal type is also the dominant histology in areas in which gastric cancer is epidemic, suggesting an environmental cause. Local rates of *H. pylori* prevalence likely play a large part in this increased environmental risk, as infection has been linked to the development of intestinal variant gastric cancer specifically.

The diffuse form of gastric adenocarcinoma consists of tiny clusters of small, uniform signet ring cells, is poorly differentiated, and lacks glands. It tends to spread submucosally, with early metastatic spread via transmural extension and lymphatic invasion. It is generally not associated with chronic gastritis, is equally frequent in both sexes, and affects a slightly younger age group. The diffuse form also has an association with blood type A and familial occurrence, suggesting an underlying genetic cause. Intraperitoneal metastases are frequent, and, in general, the prognosis is less favorable than for patients with intestinal-type cancers.

In 2010, the World Health Organization (WHO) revised their alternative classification system for gastric cancers based on morphologic features. In the WHO system, gastric adenocarcinoma is divided into five main categories—papillary, tubular, mucinous, poorly cohesive (including signet ring cell carcinoma), and uncommon histologic variants. Although widely used, the WHO classification system offers little in terms of patient management, although a new revision is expected soon that may be of greater clinical utility. There is little evidence that any of the above-mentioned classification systems can add to the prognostic information provided by the American Joint Cancer Commission (AJCC) tumor, node, metastasis (TNM) staging system (see later).

Diagnosis and Workup

Signs and Symptoms

The symptoms of gastric cancer are generally vague and nonspecific, contributing to its frequently advanced stage at the time of diagnosis. Symptoms include epigastric pain, early satiety, and weight loss. These symptoms are frequently mistaken for more common benign causes of dyspepsia including PUD and gastritis. The epigastric pain associated with gastric cancer tends to be constant and nonradiating and is generally not relieved by eating. More advanced lesions may manifest with either gastric outlet obstruction or dysphagia depending on the location of the tumor. Some degree of GI bleeding is common, with 40% of patients having some form of anemia.

A complete history and physical examination should be performed, with special attention to any evidence of advanced disease, including metastatic nodal disease. Presence of supraclavicular (Virchow node), axillary (Irish node), or periumbilical (Sister Mary Joseph node) adenopathy should be assessed, as well as any evidence of intra abdominal metastases such as hepatomegaly, jaundice, or ascites. Drop metastases to the ovaries (Krukenberg tumor) may be detectable on pelvic examination, and peritoneal metastases can be felt as a firm shelf (Blumer shelf) on rectal examination. Complete blood count, chemistry panel including liver function tests, and coagulation studies should be performed as well.

Screening

Gastric cancer screening has been implemented in some regions with high incidence, such as Japan, Korea, and Chile. The two primary modalities for screening are upper endoscopy and barium radiography, with upper endoscopy having better sensitivity. While there is evidence suggesting that screening in high-incidence populations improves oncologic outcomes, this has not been evaluated in a randomized trial. The optimal screening modality and interval have not been universally established and varies by region. Selective screening of patients with specific risk factors (see above) can be considered, including gastric polyps/adenomas, pernicious anemia, and certain genetic disorders. Of note, this should not include patients with hereditary diffuse gastric cancer as these tumors often arise beneath an intact mucosa and would be missed by routine screening.

Staging

The most widely used staging system is the AJCC TNM staging system. This system is based on the depth of tumor invasion (T), number of involved lymph nodes (N), and presence or absence of metastatic disease (M), with the 8th edition published in 2017 (Table 49.6). Before 1997, N stage was determined by the anatomic location of the nodes with respect to the primary tumor, rather than the absolute number of nodes. This staging, based on anatomy, was intimately related to the D1 versus D2 anatomic lymphadenectomy debate (see later). The revised system does not differentiate among the locations of positive nodes. In the current staging system, a minimum of 16 nodes must be evaluated for accurate staging. Some experts have suggested that other factors be included in the T and N assessment, such as the location of the primary (cardia compared with distal tumors) because this may independently predict survival and emphasis on the percentage of positive nodes (lymph node ratio) rather than the number of positive nodes. However, the current AJCC staging system does not reflect these factors. The most recent edition of TNM staging also includes a separate staging section for patients who received neoadjuvant therapy.

The Siewert classification system is used for adenocarcinomas that are in close proximity to the GE junction. This is an important distinction because such gastric cancers are more aggressive in nature and are treated in a similar manner to esophageal adenocarcinomas. There are three Siewert types: Type I tumors are tumors of the distal esophagus, within 1 to 5 cm above the GE junction; type II tumors have a tumor center located from 1 cm above the GE junction to 2 cm below; type III tumors are located between 2 and 5 cm caudad to the GE junction. In general, Siewert types I and II tumors are treated similar to esophageal adenocarcinoma, whereas type III tumors can be treated according to the guidelines for gastric adenocarcinoma described here, as long as the tumor does not extend into the GE junction; these distinctions are now reflected in the current AJCC TNM staging guidelines as well.

Although not part of the formal AJCC staging system, the term *R status*, first described by Hermanek in 1994, is used to describe tumor status after resection and is important for determining the adequacy of surgery. R0 describes a microscopically margin-negative resection, in which no gross or microscopic tumor remains in the tumor bed. R1 indicates removal of all macroscopic disease, but microscopic margins are positive for tumor. R2 indicates gross residual disease. Because the extent of resection can influence survival, some include this R designation to complement the TNM system. Long-term survival can be expected only after an R0 resection for patients with gastric cancer.

Staging Workup

The goals of preoperative staging are to gain information on prognosis, to counsel the patient effectively, and to determine the extent of disease to decide the most appropriate course of therapy. The three main treatment pathways are upfront resection (with or without subsequent adjuvant therapy), neoadjuvant therapy followed by resection, or treatment of systemic disease without resection (Fig. 49.21).

The main modalities for staging gastric adenocarcinoma are upper endoscopy; EUS; cross-sectional imaging such as CT, MRI, and/or positron emission tomography (PET); and diagnostic laparoscopy. Their roles are discussed here.

Endoscopy and endoscopic ultrasound. Flexible endoscopy is an essential tool for the diagnosis of gastric cancer. It allows visualization of the tumor, provides tissue for pathologic diagnosis, and can help treat patients with obstruction or bleeding (Fig. 49.22). On initial diagnostic endoscopy, if a suspicious mass or ulcer is encountered in the stomach, it is essential to obtain adequate tissue to confirm the correct diagnosis histologically. Current National Comprehensive Cancer Network (NCCN) guidelines recommend harvesting six to eight biopsy specimens from different areas of the lesion in order to maximize the diagnostic yield.[22] Small lesions (≤2 cm in diameter) can be resected at the time of initial diagnostic endoscopy using endoscopic mucosal resection (EMR) or endoscopic submucosal dissection (ESD,

TABLE 49.6 Tumor, node, metastasis classification of carcinoma of the stomach.

Primary Tumor (T)

TX	Primary tumor cannot be assessed
T0	No evidence of primary tumor
Tis	Carcinoma in situ; intraepithelial tumor without invasion of the lamina propria, high-grade dysplasia
T1	Tumor invades lamina propria, muscularis mucosae, or submucosa
T1a	Tumor invades lamina propria or muscularis mucosae
T1b	Tumor invades submucosa
T2	Tumor invades muscularis propria*
T3	Tumor penetrates subserosal connective tissue without invasion of visceral peritoneum or adjacent structures†
T4	Tumor invades serosa (visceral peritoneum) or adjacent structures†
T4a	Tumor invades serosa (visceral peritoneum)
T4b	Tumor invades adjacent structures

Regional Lymph Nodes (N)

NX	Regional lymph node(s) cannot be assessed
N0	No regional lymph node metastasis‡
N1	Metastasis in 1–2 regional lymph nodes
N2	Metastasis in 3–6 regional lymph nodes
N3	Metastasis in 7 or more regional lymph nodes
N3a	Metastasis in 7–15 regional lymph nodes
N3b	Metastasis in 16 or more regional lymph nodes

Distant Metastasis (M)

M0	No distant metastasis
M1	Distant metastasis

PATHOLOGIC STAGE	PROGNOSTIC GROUP		
0	Tis	N0	M0
IA	T1	N0	M0
IB	T1	N1	M0
	T2	N0	M0
IIA	T1	N2	M0
	T2	N1	M0
	T3	N0	M0
IIB	T1	N3a	M0
	T2	N2	M0
	T3	N1	M0
	T4a	N0	M0
IIIA	T2	N3a	M0
	T3	N2	M0
	T4a	N1	M0
	T4a	N2	M0
	T4b	N0	M0
IIIB	T1	N3b	M0
	T2	N3b	M0
	T3	N3a	M0
	T4a	N3a	M0
	T4b	N1	M0
	T4b	N2	M0
IIIC	T3	N3b	M0
	T4a	N3b	M0
	T4b	N3a	M0
	T4b	N3b	M0
IV	Any T	Any N	M1

From Amin MB, Edge SB, Greene FL, et al. *AJCC Cancer Staging Manual.* 8th ed. New York: Springer International Publishing; 2017.

*A tumor may penetrate the muscularis propria with extension into the gastrocolic or gastrohepatic ligaments, or into the greater or lesser omentum, without perforation of the visceral peritoneum covering these structures. In this case, the tumor is classified T3. If there is perforation of the visceral peritoneum covering the gastric ligaments or the omentum, the tumor should be classified T4.

†The adjacent structures of the stomach include the spleen, transverse colon, liver, diaphragm, pancreas, abdominal wall, adrenal gland, kidney, small intestine, and retroperitoneum.

‡A designation of pN0 should be used if all examined lymph nodes are negative, regardless of the total number removed and examined.

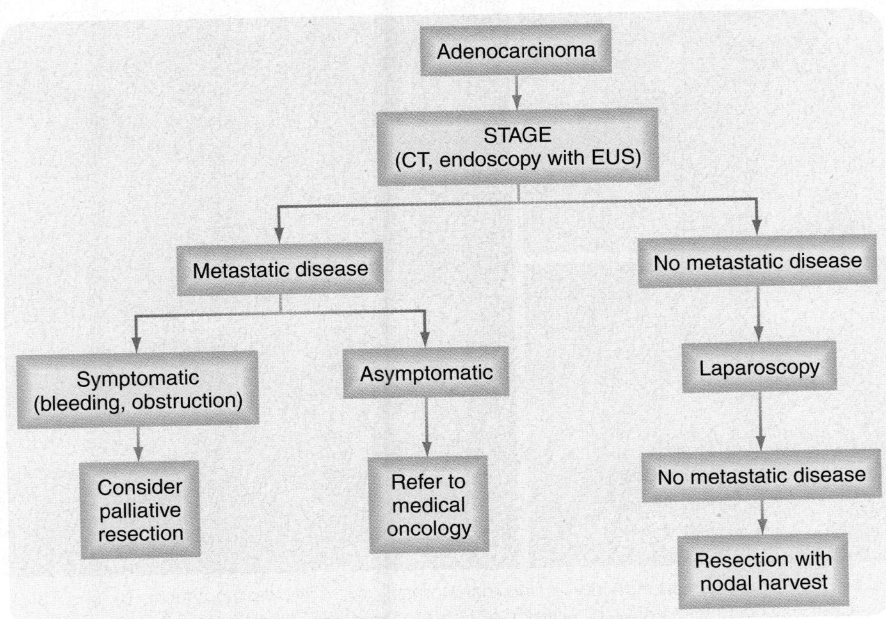

FIG. 49.21 General staging and treatment strategy for gastric adenocarcinoma. *CT*, Computed tomography; *EUS*, endoscopic ultrasound.

described in further detail later). This resection can provide a more complete specimen to aid the pathologist in obtaining an accurate diagnosis and can potentially be curative for early-stage cancers, obviating the need for invasive surgical intervention.

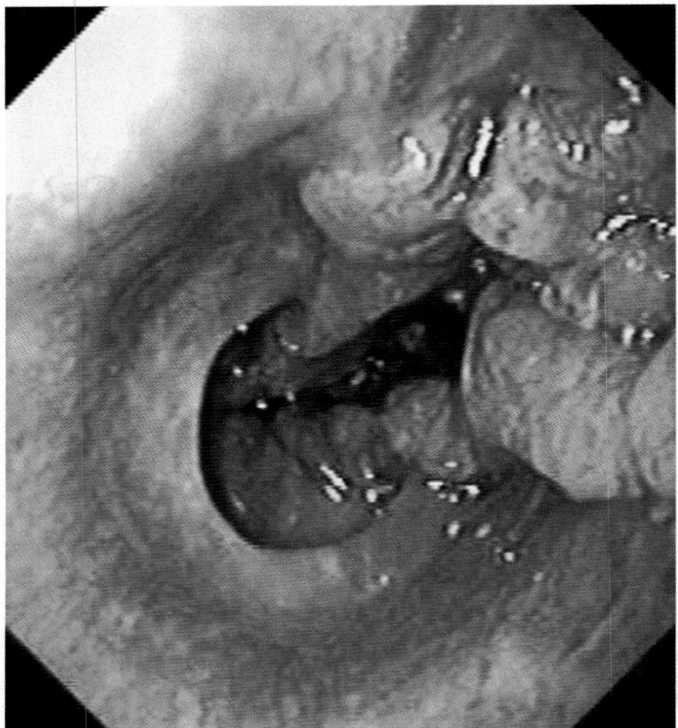

FIG. 49.22 Endoscopic view of intestinal-type adenocarcinoma of the gastric cardia. (Courtesy Dr. David Bentrem, Department of Surgery, Northwestern University Feinberg School of Medicine, Chicago, IL.)

EUS is recommended by NCCN guidelines as part of the staging workup for gastric cancer if there is no evidence of metastatic disease.[22] EUS provides the most accurate evaluation of the depth of tumor invasion, assessment of perigastric lymph node involvement, and can sometimes identify involvement of surrounding organs or the presence of ascites. EUS is performed using a flexible endoscope with a 7.5- to 12-MHz ultrasound transducer. The stomach is filled with water to provide an acoustic window, and the stomach wall is visualized as five alternating hypoechoic and hyperechoic layers (Fig. 49.23A). The mucosa and submucosa represent the first three layers (T1) (Fig. 49.23B). The fourth layer is the muscularis propria, invasion of which signifies a T2 tumor. Expansion of the tumor beyond the muscularis propria causing an irregular border correlates with expansion into the subserosa, or a T3 tumor (Fig. 49.23C). The serosa is the fifth layer, and loss of this bright line correlates with penetration through it, indicating a T4a tumor. Direct invasion of surrounding structures, including named vessels, indicates a T4b tumor. Nodes are evaluated based on their size and ultrasound appearance and can additionally be sampled using fine-needle aspiration (FNA) under EUS guidance. FNA can also be performed if ascites is present to evaluate for peritoneal spread.

The overall accuracy of EUS is operator dependent and ranges from 57% to 88% for T stage and 30% to 90% for N stage.[22] There is improved accuracy when T and N stages are grouped together to differentiate high-risk versus low-risk disease, defined by the presence of any subserosal or serosal (T3/T4) involvement or any nodal disease (>N0). From a prognostic and treatment standpoint, this classification may be more clinically relevant because an EUS finding indicative of advanced disease strongly correlates with decreased resectability and poorer disease-specific survival. A Cochrane meta analysis found that the summary sensitivity and specificity of EUS for discriminating T1/T2 versus T3/T4 disease were 86% and 90%, respectively.[23] The sensitivity and specificity for nodal involvement were 83% and 67%, respectively. EUS is becoming increasingly important in the workup of gastric cancer

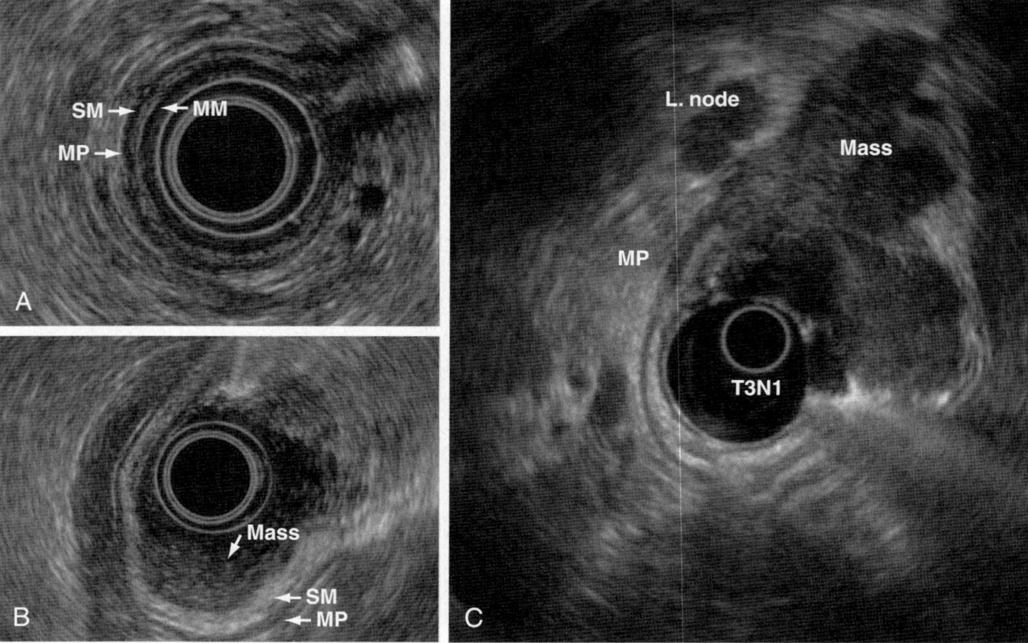

FIG. 49.23 Endoscopic ultrasound views of normal stomach (A), T1N0 gastric cancer (B), and T3N1 gastric cancer (C). (Courtesy Dr. Rajesh Keswani, Division of Gastroenterology, Department of Medicine, Northwestern University Feinberg School of Medicine, Chicago, IL.) *MM*, Mucosa; *MP*, muscularis propria; *SM*, submucosa.

to guide treatment decisions regarding neoadjuvant therapy and consideration for EMR (see below).

Computed tomography. CT of the chest, abdomen, and pelvis with oral and IV contrast agents is a mandatory component of the assessment of patients with gastric cancer to evaluate for metastatic disease. CT has also been used in locoregional staging but is less accurate than EUS. The overall accuracy of CT for T staging in 43% to 82%,[22] with tumors more often being understaged. Although improved technology may increase the role for CT in locoregional evaluation and for neoadjuvant therapy, its primary role remains the evaluation of metastatic disease.

Positron emission tomography. Combined PET/CT is more accurate in preoperative staging (68%) than either PET (47%) or CT (53%) alone.[22] The utility of PET/CT for initial staging of diffuse and mucinous cancers is limited due to low tracer accumulation. However, in patients with locally advanced disease and patients being considered for neoadjuvant therapy, there may be a role for PET/CT. PET/CT is slightly better than CT alone for detection of occult metastases. Further, patients with PET-avid tumors can be monitored for a response to neoadjuvant therapy, which strongly correlates with survival. Based on these data, the NCCN guidelines recommend considering PET/CT as part of staging for patients with greater than T1 disease without evidence of metastatic disease on initial CT.

Staging laparoscopy. Staging laparoscopy is an integral part of the standard workup for gastric cancer. The high rate of occult peritoneal metastatic disease makes laparoscopy an attractive staging modality given the low sensitivity of CT and PET/CT for detecting peritoneal metastases. Approximately 20% to 30% of patients undergoing staging laparoscopy for T2 or greater gastric cancer and no prior evidence of metastases will be found to have peritoneal disease; the NCCN recommends staging laparoscopic in this setting.[22] The overall sensitivity of laparoscopy for detecting metastatic disease is greater than 95%. Laparoscopy alters management in 9% to 60% of cases, depending on the series and patient population, and specifically allows patients to avoid an unnecessary laparotomy by detecting metastatic disease that was missed on preoperative staging. Positive peritoneal washing cytology without overt macroscopic evidence of metastatic disease is used by some as an indication for neoadjuvant therapy. Staging laparoscopy is a safe, low-risk procedure that can be planned as a single-stage procedure with resection. Meanwhile, there are many benefits of avoiding laparotomy, which include avoiding a delay in starting chemotherapy for patients with metastatic disease. Given the persistence of high rates of metastatic disease not detected by preoperative workup in many centers, even with improved imaging modalities, we believe that these benefits far outweigh the risk and that staging laparoscopy should be part of the workup for most patients with gastric cancer. An evolving research question is whether patients should undergo a repeat staging laparoscopy following neoadjuvant therapy for advanced disease. Retrospective series have shown a 5% to 15% rate of finding occult metastatic disease in this setting, even in those who had a negative staging laparoscopy prior to initiation of neoadjuvant therapy. While not currently standard of care, repeat staging laparoscopy after neoadjuvant therapy detects a nontrivial amount of occult metastatic disease and should be strongly considered prior to undergoing a laparotomy for curative intent.

Treatment

Surgical Therapy

Complete resection of a gastric tumor with a wide margin of normal stomach remains the standard of care for resection with curative intent. Patients without metastatic disease or invasion of unresectable vascular structures such as the aorta, celiac trunk, proximal common hepatic, or proximal splenic arteries are candidates for curative resection. The extent of resection depends on the location of the tumor in the stomach and size of the tumor. For T4 tumors, any organ with invasion needs to be removed en bloc with the gastrectomy specimen to achieve a curative resection. While worldwide the standard technique is via a laparotomy, minimally invasive techniques, including endoscopic resection for very early tumors and laparoscopy, have proven effective.

For cancers of the distal stomach, including the body and antrum, a distal gastrectomy is the appropriate operation. Because of propensity for intramural spread, the proximal stomach is transected at the level of the incisura at a margin of at least 2 to 3 cm for early cancers and at least 4 to 6 cm for advanced cancers. The distal margin is the proximal duodenum just distal to the pylorus. Frozen section analysis should be performed before reconstruction, and if positive, a wider excision should be performed when possible. The choice of reconstruction depends on the remnant anatomy with consideration of postgastrectomy physiology, although a Roux-en-Y reconstruction has been shown to result in less alkaline reflux gastritis and improved quality of life at 1 year compared to Billroth reconstruction.

In East Asian countries, where early gastric cancer is more common, a pylorus-preserving segmental gastrectomy can be performed for cT1N0M0 disease for cancers in the middle third of the stomach. The antral cuff length can range from 1.5 to 3 cm. A recent review showed that for early gastric cancers, the oncologic outcomes were similar between pylorus-preserving segmental gastrectomy and distal gastrectomy, with the former having lower rates of dumping syndrome, bile reflux, and malnutrition.[24] A randomized controlled trial in Korea (KLASS-04) is currently recruiting that will provide stronger evidence regarding the safety and oncologic equivalence of this newer technique.

For proximal lesions of the fundus or cardia that do not invade the GE junction, a total gastrectomy with a Roux-en-Y esophagojejunostomy and proximal gastrectomy are equivalent from an oncologic perspective. However, rates of anastomotic stenosis and reflux esophagitis are much higher after proximal gastrectomy and the lymph node harvest may be inadequate; thus, most surgeons prefer a total gastrectomy for these patients.

Minimally invasive techniques have been used for many GI malignancies, and gastric cancer is no exception. There is a learning curve to these procedures and a surgeon should be able to perform an equivalent oncologic resection and reconstruction. In systematic reviews, laparoscopic gastrectomy is associated with faster return of bowel function, shorter length of stay, and comparable lymph node retrieval, morbidity, and oncologic outcomes for early gastric cancers. The Japanese LOC-1 study propensity matched 1848 patients with stage I disease who underwent open and laparoscopic gastrectomy (n = 924 for both groups). They found that the 5-year overall survival and recurrence rates were similar between the two groups.[25] Smaller series have shown that laparoscopic gastrectomy is feasible for locally advanced gastric cancer (T2 or above); however, long-term oncologic data are currently lacking. Japanese and Korean trials are presently ongoing to address this issue. Similarly, multiple groups have reported on laparoscopic total gastrectomy, although this procedure is more technically demanding given the need for an esophagojejunostomy and most series are from high-volume centers with extensive laparoscopic experience. Robotic gastrectomy is also being explored and while there is currently no high-quality long-term oncologic data, there is a phase III trial

BOX 49.4 Standard criteria for endoscopic resection of gastric adenocarcinoma.

- Intestinal-type adenocarcinoma
- Tumor confined to the mucosa
- Absence of lymphovascular invasion
- Nonulcerated tumor
- Less than 2 cm in diameter

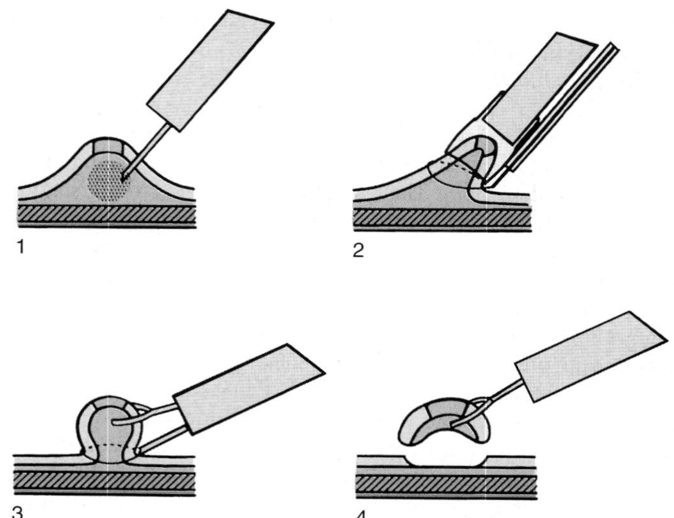

FIG. 49.24 Endoscopic mucosal resection by strip biopsy: Saline is injected into the submucosal layer, and the area is elevated *(1)*. The top of the mound is pulled upward with forceps, and the snare is placed at the base of the lesion *(2* and *3)*. Electrosurgical current is applied through the snare to resect the mucosa, and the lesion is removed *(4)*. (From Tanabe S, Koizumi W, Kokutou M, et al. Usefulness of endoscopic aspiration mucosectomy as compared with strip biopsy for the treatment of gastric mucosal cancer. *Gastrointest Endosc*. 1999;50:819–822.)

recruiting in Japan that randomizes patients between laparoscopic and robotic gastrectomy.

Similar to other GI surgeries, enhanced recovery after surgery (ERAS) protocols have been developed for perioperative care after gastrectomy. Specific recommendations from the ERAS society include no routine use of NG/nasojejunal decompression, avoiding perianastomotic drains, and using minimally invasive approaches when possible. A weak recommendation was also made for offering oral diet to patients undergoing a total gastrectomy starting on postoperative day 1. A recent updated meta analysis found that ERAS protocols resulted in similar rates of total complications, perioperative mortality, and reoperation. The incidence of pulmonary infections, length of stay, medical costs, and time to first flatus were all significantly lower and the quality of life was superior. However, the readmission rate was nearly tripled in the ERAS group.[26] ERAS and other fast-track protocols after gastrectomy are an area of active research interest and further optimization should elucidate ideal patient selection and balancing decreased length of stay with readmission rates.

Endoscopic Resection

For select patients with early gastric cancer, endoscopic tumor resection can be performed for curative intent with adequate oncologic outcomes. The two primary modalities are EMR and ESD. The most significant advantage of endoscopic resection is avoiding the need for gastrectomy, whether by laparotomy or laparoscopy. The major disadvantages are risk of incomplete resection and unrecognized lymph node metastases. The standard criteria for endoscopic resection consideration are intestinal type adenocarcinoma, tumor confined to the mucosa, absence of lymphovascular invasion, nonulcerated, and less than 2 cm in diameter (Box 49.4). A recent systematic review and meta analysis found that in 9800 patients, those who met these standard criteria had only a 0.2% rate of lymph node metastases.[27] Some centers in East Asia have proposed expanding criteria to include any differentiated mucosal tumor without ulceration, mucosal tumors up to 3 cm with ulceration, undifferentiated mucosal tumors up to 2 cm, and slight submucosal invasion. Risk of lymph node involvement in patients meeting this expanded criteria is higher at 0.7%, with undifferentiated histology and slight submucosal invasion having statistically significantly higher rates of lymph node metastases. Given that all these patients had early gastric cancer and were potentially curable with gastrectomy and lymphadenectomy, undertreatment in this group is not warranted unless part of a clinical trial or for patients with significant medical comorbidities who wish to avoid surgery.

The basic principle for EMR involves elevating the tumor using a saline injection, encircling the affected mucosa using a snare device, and then excising it with electrocautery. Perforation rates are low, and bleeding rates are approximately 15%; these can generally be controlled endoscopically without the need for further intervention (Fig. 49.24). En bloc resection is preferred, as piecemeal resection is associated with an increased risk of recurrence. Patients with positive lateral margins can be considered for repeat endoscopic therapy or close surveillance. Patients with positive vertical margins, lymphovascular invasion, or submucosal invasion should be referred for gastrectomy with lymphadenectomy.

ESD is mostly utilized in East Asia and allows for resection of larger tumors and those with limited submucosal involvement. This technique begins by marking the borders of the lesion using electrocautery. A submucosal injection of epinephrine with indigo carmine hydrodissects the lesion, and an insulation-tipped knife is used to remove the lesion by dissecting a submucosal plane deep to the tumor and removing it en bloc. Any bleeding is controlled with electrocautery (Fig. 49.25). There is a higher risk of perforation with ESD compared to EMR.

Endoscopic resection leads to similar survival outcomes in appropriately selected patients. A meta analysis comparing endoscopic resection to radical gastrectomy for early gastric cancer with standard endoscopic resection criteria found that endoscopic resection had higher rates of recurrence and metachronous lesions, but that 3-year and 5-year survival was similar. Further, the morbidity rate was significantly lower with endoscopic resection.[28]

Extent of Lymph Node Dissection

The stomach has a rich supply of lymphatics (Fig. 49.26). Number of positive lymph nodes correlates with survival in gastric cancer (Table 49.7). The extent of lymphadenectomy for gastric adenocarcinoma is a continuing area of ongoing debate. Historically, lymphadenectomy for gastric adenocarcinoma was defined by, and is still often discussed in terms of, the location of the nodes relative to the primary tumor. The extent of dissection ranges from the more local D1 lymphadenectomy involving only perigastric nodes

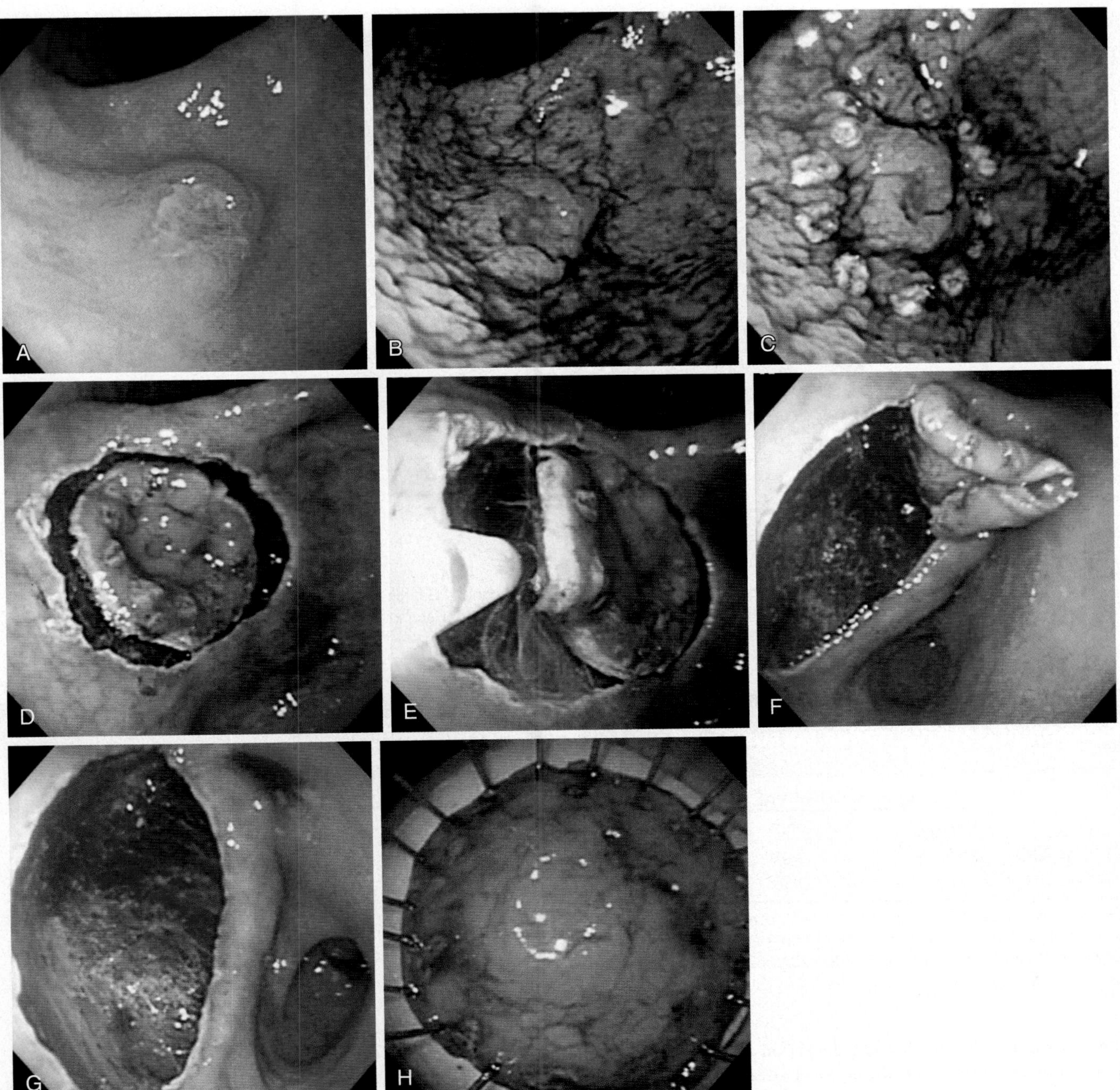

FIG. 49.25 Procedure of endoscopic submucosal dissection. (A) A type IIa + IIc early gastric cancer was located at the lesser curvature side of the antrum. (B) Indigo carmine dye was sprayed around the lesion to define the margin accurately. (C) Marking dots were made circumferentially at approximately 5 mm lateral to the margin of the lesion. (D) After a submucosal injection of saline with epinephrine mixed with indigo carmine, a circumferential mucosal incision was performed outside the marking dots to separate the lesion from the surrounding non neoplastic mucosa. (E and F) After an additional submucosal injection, the submucosal connective tissue just beneath the lesion was directly dissected using an electrosurgical knife instead of using a snare. (G) The lesion was completely resected, and the consequent artificial ulcer was seen. (H) The resected specimen with a central early gastric cancer. (From Min B-H, Lee JH, Kim JJ, et al. Clinical outcomes of endoscopic submucosal dissection (ESD) for treating early gastric cancer: comparison with endoscopic mucosal resection after circumferential precutting (EMR-P). *Dig Liver Dis.* 2009;41:201–209.)

(stations 1 to 7) to clearance of the celiac axis, with or without splenectomy, in an extended D2 dissection (stations 1 to 12a) to complete clearance of the celiac axis and periaortic nodes in a superextended D3 lymphadenectomy (stations 1 to 16) (Table 49.8).

Several randomized trials compared the outcomes of patients undergoing D1 versus D2 dissection, with conflicting results based on a combination of different patient populations, tumor biology, and surgical techniques. Earlier randomized trials showed

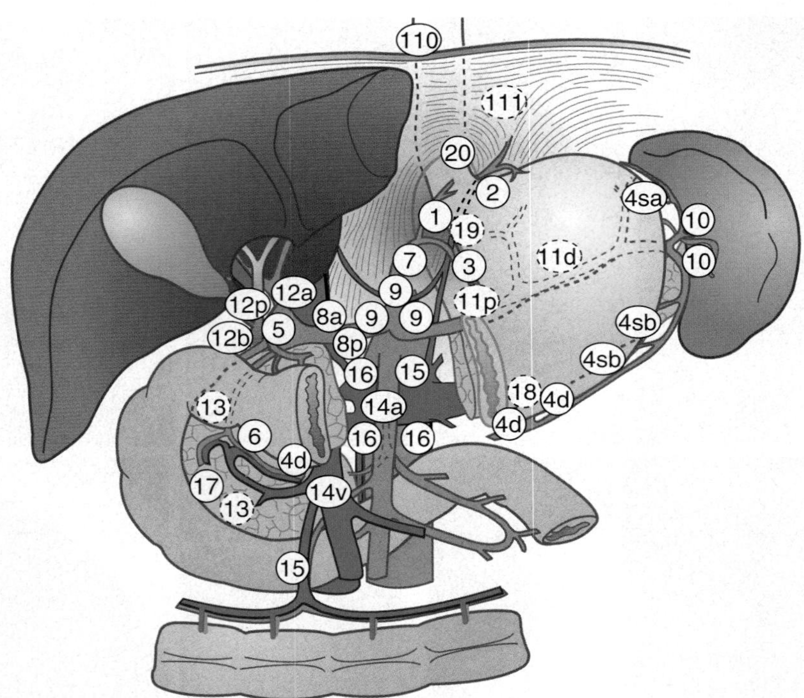

FIG. 49.26 Lymph node station numbers as defined by the Japanese Gastric Cancer Association. (From Japanese Gastric Cancer Association. Japanese Classification of Gastric Carcinoma, 2nd English edition. *Gastric Cancer*. 1998;1:10–24.)

TABLE 49.7 Median survival according to location of positive nodes versus number of positive nodes.

SIZE	MEDIAN SURVIVAL (MONTHS)		
	1–6 PNS	7–15 PNS	>15 PNS
<3 cm (*n* = 402)	38.8 (*n* = 311)	20.8 (*n* = 82)	9.5 (*n* = 9)
>3 cm (*n* = 233)	35.5 (*n* = 81)	19.7 (*n* = 96)	12.5 (*n* = 56)

Adapted from Karpeh MS, Leon L, Klimstra D, et al. Lymph node staging in gastric cancer: Is location more important than number? An analysis of 1038 patients. *Ann Surg*. 2000;232:362–371.
PN, Positive nodes.

either no survival benefit for D2 dissection or that while there was a significant disease-specific survival advantage that this was tempered by the increased perioperative mortality. More recently, it has been shown that the majority of this excess mortality was due to the routine use of splenectomy and distal pancreatectomy during D2 dissection, which is no longer standardly performed. A Cochrane review of five randomized trials comparing D2 to D1 dissection found a significantly improved hazard ratio of 0.81 in favor of D2 for disease-specific survival.[29] Given the improving perioperative mortality, the NCCN and European Society for Medical Oncology have recommended D2 dissection in patients undergoing surgery for curative intent. While there has been some study into the potential for sentinel lymph node mapping in cases of early gastric cancers, these results have been inconsistent and should be considered investigational at this time. On the other hand, a D3 dissection for more advanced disease has not been shown to offer a survival benefit but does increase morbidity and should not be considered standard.[29]

TABLE 49.8 Regional lymph nodes classification.

LYMPH NODE STATION (NO.)	DESCRIPTION
1	Right paracardial
2	Left paracardial
3	Lesser curvature
4sa	Short gastric
4sb	Left gastroepiploic
4d	Right gastroepiploic
5	Suprapyloric
6	Infrapyloric
7	Left gastric artery
8a	Anterior common hepatic
8p	Posterior common hepatic
9	Celiac artery
10	Splenic hilum
11p	Proximal splenic
11d	Distal splenic
12a	Left hepatoduodenal
12b, p	Posterior hepatoduodenal
13	Retropancreatic
14v	Superior mesenteric vein
14a	Superior mesenteric artery
15	Middle colic
16al	Aortic hiatus
16a2, b1	Paraaortic, middle
16b2	Paraaortic, caudal

From the Japanese Gastric Cancer Association. Japanese classification of gastric carcinoma. 2 English ed. *Gastric Cancer*. 1998;1:10–24.

The improvement in survival rates may be caused by stage migration. Patients who were previously understaged are now classified as having node-positive disease status, improving the prognosis of both groups. Regardless, better stage homogeneity and reducing understaging are critical to clinical decisions on potential treatments and prognosis. Recently, improved laparoscopic techniques have shown that laparoscopic lymph node dissection can achieve an adequate number of lymph nodes in experienced hands, and robotic-assisted surgery is also being actively explored to ensure oncologic equivalence.[30]

Locally Advanced Gastric Cancer

Patients with advanced disease that is deemed unresectable because of adjacent organ involvement, generally the pancreas or spleen, or extensive nodal disease, including the para-aortic nodes, are particularly challenging. Multiple studies have indicated that, unsurprisingly, multiorgan resection significantly increases morbidity and perioperative mortality. Underlying all these studies, and the objective of performing multiorgan resection in general, is the desire to achieve an R0 resection. Patients with proven T4 disease who achieve an R0 resection have a clinically and statistically significant survival benefit over patients undergoing palliative resection only, with the palliative resection group having survival rates similar to patients receiving chemotherapy alone.

In an effort to increase the number of patients for whom an R0 resection can be achieved, several investigators explored the role of neoadjuvant therapy in otherwise unresectable disease. A phase II trial treated 49 patients with clinically unresectable gastric cancer with cisplatin, docetaxel, and capecitabine and found an overall R0 resection rate of 63% compared with historical rates of 30% to 60%.[31] These patients were prospectively stratified according to which criteria made them unresectable—adjacent organ involvement, bulky para-aortic nodal disease, or limited peritoneal disease. For patients without peritoneal disease, the R0 resection rate was greater than 70%. Of all patients who achieved R0 resection, patients with only adjacent organ involvement had significantly better outcomes. At a median follow-up of 51 months, median progression-free and overall survival have yet to be reached, with a predicted 5-year overall survival of 54%. A separate Japanese phase II study of 55 patients with extensive lymph node metastases studied neoadjuvant irinotecan and cisplatin followed by gastrectomy with D3 lymphadenectomy.[32] The R0 resection rate was 65% and median OS was 14.6 months and 3-year survival was 27%, but with two chemotherapy-related deaths and one postoperative death.

All these data suggest that multiorgan resection is beneficial in a highly selected patient population and that neoadjuvant therapy followed by more extensive surgery may provide a chance for long-term survival, although with worse outcomes than patients with less advanced disease and higher treatment-associated morbidity and mortality. The difficulty is how to select these patients properly. As preoperative staging modalities improve in accuracy, so will the ability to select patients properly for various treatment modalities, including multiorgan resection. However, in patients who at the time of laparoscopy or laparotomy have clearly unresectable disease and who have no symptoms that would warrant resection, palliative resection should be avoided. Furthermore, any aggressive surgical intervention in these patients with locally advanced disease should be done within a multidisciplinary setting and preferably within the context of a clinical trial.

Adjuvant and Neoadjuvant Therapy

Gastric cancer remains a biologically aggressive cancer, with high recurrence and subsequent mortality rates. Recurrences are most commonly distant or peritoneal, but a large number of patients also have locoregional recurrence, with a subset of 10% to 20% having only a local recurrence. For patients who recur, the prognosis is dismal and there has been much focus on how to prevent recurrent disease with neoadjuvant and/or adjuvant therapies.

The Southwest Oncology Group (9008/INT-0116) reported a randomized controlled trial of 556 patients who underwent curative gastrectomy alone or gastrectomy combined with adjuvant 5-fluorouracil (5-FU) and radiotherapy.[33] This study demonstrated a significant benefit for adjuvant therapy for overall survival (41% vs. 50%) and recurrence-free survival (41% vs. 64%). However, several authors have criticized these results, noting a high rate of inadequate lymphadenectomy (54% of patients underwent a D0 resection). Given these findings, it is possible that some of the benefit from radiation was clearance of residual disease in the perigastric nodal basin. Also, treatment with a single-agent 5-FU does not perform as well as multiagent therapy. Furthermore, only 64% of patients randomly assigned to the treatment arm were able to complete therapy; 17% had to stop treatment because of toxic effects, and 5% progressed while on treatment.

Some of these study design deficiencies were addressed in the CLASSIC trial, which randomly assigned 1035 patients undergoing gastrectomy with D2 lymph node dissection to either surgery alone or surgery followed by eight 3-week cycles of capecitabine plus oxaliplatin. In the chemotherapy group, 67% of patients received all eight cycles as planned per protocol. At 5 years, the disease-free survival (68% vs. 53%) and overall survival (78% vs. 69%) were both significantly improved with adjuvant chemotherapy.[34]

Numerous other studies have been done and multiple meta-analyses support the survival benefit of adjuvant chemotherapy after complete oncologic resection for patients with greater than pathologic T2N0 disease. The optimal regimen has not been established. Common first-line regimens include ECF (epirubicin, cisplatin, and 5-FU), CAPOX (capecitabine and oxaliplatin), and FOLFOX (5-FU, leucovorin, and oxaliplatin).

The benefit of adjuvant radiotherapy is less clear and often debated but has theoretical benefits given the high rates of local recurrence and nodal disease. The previously mentioned INT-0116 trial did show a benefit to chemoradiation; however, this is at least in part due to inadequate lymphadenectomy. The ARTIST trial evaluated whether the addition of adjuvant radiotherapy would be beneficial by randomizing 458 patients undergoing gastrectomy with D2 dissection to adjuvant chemotherapy with capecitabine and cisplatin alone or with radiotherapy.[35] There was no difference in outcomes found between the adjuvant chemotherapy and adjuvant chemotherapy plus radiotherapy groups with 7-year follow-up. However, an initially unplanned subgroup analysis did show radiotherapy improved disease-free survival in patients who had lymph node metastases. A follow-up study (ARTIST 2) is ongoing to examine the benefit of radiotherapy in this patient subgroup alone. Based on presently available studies, adjuvant radiotherapy should be considered for patients with less than D2 lymphadenectomy and with positive nodal disease as part of multidisciplinary management.

Given the relatively high rate of failure to complete adjuvant treatment in these trials, there has been increased focus on neoadjuvant therapy for gastric cancer, rather than postoperative adjuvant therapy. The most significant results are those of the MAGIC trial, a randomized study of 503 patients with stage II or higher GE cancer (372 stomach, 58 GE junction, 73 lower esophagus) that compared perioperative chemotherapy with surgery alone.[36] The treatment group received three 3-week cycles of ECF preoperatively and three additional cycles postoperatively. More than 90% of patients who started the preoperative chemotherapy were able to complete it; however, only 65% of these patients went on to receive postoperative chemotherapy, and only 50% successfully completed both. The treatment group had significantly better pathologic results and long-term outcomes. The chemotherapy group had a higher percentage of T1 and T2 tumors in the final specimens, along with a higher proportion of limited (N0 and N1) nodal disease compared with the surgery alone arm. The rates of local recurrence, distant metastases, and 5-year overall survival were significantly improved in the chemotherapy group compared with the surgery-only group (14.4% vs. 20.6%, 24.4% vs. 36.8%, and 36.3% vs. 23%, respectively). Smaller trials and meta analyses have shown similar benefits with tumor downstaging and higher rates of R0 resection without significantly increased perioperative morbidity.

Recently, the FLOT4 study compared the regimen used in the MAGIC trial to four preoperative and four postoperative cycles of FLOT (docetaxel, oxaliplatin, leucovorin, and 5-FU). A total of 716 patients were randomized. They found that both median overall survival (50 vs. 35 months, $P = 0.012$) and progression-free survival (30 vs. 18 months, $P = 0.004$) significantly favored the FLOT regimen.[37]

The optimal chemotherapy regimen, timing of therapy, and addition of radiotherapy for patients with operable gastric cancer is an active and evolving area of research with numerous trials ongoing. Neoadjuvant and adjuvant therapy options and patient-specific recommendations are likely to change in the coming years based on further study and improved granularity. Furthermore, as discussed below, targeted treatments and immunotherapy have shown promise in advanced and systemic disease and may become a part of therapeutic regimens for patients with resectable gastric cancer as well.

Palliative Therapy and Systemic Therapy

Patients with unresectable or metastatic gastric cancer account almost 50% of patients presenting with the disease and have only a 3- to 5-month median survival with the best supportive therapy. While many patients with advanced disease are asymptomatic, a significant subset of patients with unresectable gastric cancer have debilitating symptoms and should be considered for palliative surgical therapy even in the setting of metastatic disease.

Common complications of locally advanced gastric cancer include bleeding, obstruction, pain, and nausea. Acute bleeding can be treatment related or a result of the tumor itself. Patients presenting with bleeding should undergo prompt endoscopic assessment with attempt at endoscopic control. However, the initial success rate and rate of recurrent bleeding are both suboptimal and patients should be considered for other potential interventions as well, such as angiographic embolization or external beam radiation therapy. Nausea and vomiting are common and should be treated with appropriate antiemetic therapy, but these patients should also be assessed for luminal obstruction. Obstructing gastric cancers can sometimes be symptomatically improved with the placement of an endoscopic enteral stent. Radiation therapy and systemic chemotherapy can be considered in an attempt to shrink the obstructing tumor. Surgical intervention can also be offered to patients fit to undergo surgery. The most common procedure in this setting is a gastrojejunostomy; however, a palliative gastrectomy can be considered in select patients. If the obstruction is unable to be alleviated, a venting gastrostomy tube can be placed either endoscopically, percutaneously, or surgically. Perforation of gastric cancer requires surgical intervention. Primary closure of perforated, frequently necrotic, tumor is not generally possible. Given the relatively poor functional status and prognosis for many of these patients, closure with healthy omentum is a reasonable approach. If it can be done without excess morbidity, gastrectomy can also be performed.

Chemotherapy improves survival in patients with unresectable tumors, although prognosis is still poor with a median survival of less than a year. Standard doublet regimens include 5-FU and a platinum agent (either cisplatin or oxaliplatin). There is a debate about the utility of adding a third agent (usually either a taxane or anthracycline), with possibly improved outcomes at the expense of increased toxicity.[38] NCCN guidelines recommend doublet regimens, with triplet regimens reserved for patients who are medically fit, have good performance status, and have access to frequent toxicity evaluation.[22]

Although better than supportive care alone, results of systemic treatments remain relatively poor. Investigators continue to evaluate for newer targeted therapeutic options. These include the epidermal growth factor receptor inhibitor cetuximab, vascular endothelial growth factor inhibitors ramucirumab and bevacizumab, and the human epidermal growth factor receptor 2 (HER2) antagonist trastuzumab. HER2 positivity has been reported about 20% of gastric cancers. Results of a phase III trial (ToGA trial) were first presented in 2009, evaluating 594 patients with HER2-overexpressing advanced gastric cancers. These patients were randomly assigned to receive capecitabine or 5-FU with cisplatin and trastuzumab or cisplatin alone. The trastuzumab group had a better median survival (13.8 vs. 11.1 months, $P = 0.0046$), and rates of severe complications did not differ between the groups.[39] HER2 testing is now recommended by the NCCN guidelines for all patients with metastatic disease at time of initial diagnosis.[22]

More recently, immunotherapy has been investigated as a potential adjunctive therapy for advanced gastric cancer. Approximately 40% of gastric tumors have the upregulated programmed death ligand.[38] Nivolumab and pembrolizumab have undergone trials, both with modest survival improvements in advanced disease.

Outcomes

The overall mortality rate and incidence of gastric cancer have been declining since 1930, likely because of changes in diet such as decreased sodium intake, changes in food storage and preparation, decreased smoking, and improved treatment options. Nonetheless, the overall 5-year survival remains poor, at approximately 30%. More than 63% of patients present with locally advanced or distant disease and are not candidates for surgery. For patients who undergo a potentially curative resection, overall 5-year survival rates range from of 25% to 75%; for the subset with early gastric cancer, cure rates are greater than 80%. For patients who present with distant disease, long-term survival is only 5% (Fig. 49.27).

Recurrence

Recurrence rates after gastrectomy are high, from 30% to 90%, depending on the series. Most recurrences occur within the first 2 years. Locoregional recurrence is seen in about 40% of these patients. The most common sites of locoregional recurrence are the gastric remnant at the anastomosis, in the gastric bed, and in the regional nodal basins. The predominant sites of systemic recurrence are the liver and peritoneum.

Surveillance. Although all patients should be followed systematically, the evidence for how this should occur is unclear and there is currently no evidence that follow-up improves long-term survival.[40] The NCCN recommends a complete history and physical examination every 3 to 6 months for 1 to 2 years, every 6 to 12 months for 3 to 5 years, and annually thereafter. Laboratory tests, including complete blood count and liver function tests, should be performed as clinically indicated. CT or PET/CT scans can be obtained if there is clinical suspicion of recurrence, although some perform these routinely in high-risk patients. Sensitivity for detecting peritoneal recurrence is low. Annual endoscopy can be considered for patients who have undergone a subtotal gastrectomy or endoscopic resection.

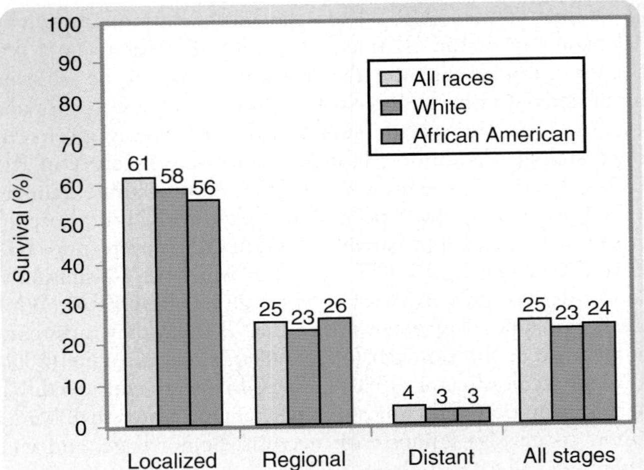

FIG. 49.27 The 5-year relative survival rates in patients with stomach cancers by race and stage at diagnosis, United States, 1996–2004. (From Jemal A, Siegel R, Ward E, et al. Cancer statistics. *CA Cancer J Clin.* 2009;59:225–249.)

Gastric Lymphoma

Epidemiology

The stomach is the most common site of extranodal lymphoma. However, primary gastric lymphoma is still relatively uncommon, accounting for approximately 3% of gastric cancers. Patients often present with vague symptoms, such as epigastric pain, early satiety, and fatigue. Constitutional B symptoms (i.e., fever, night sweats) occur in only about 10% of patients. Lymphomas occur in older patients, with the peak incidence in the sixth and seventh decades, and there is a slight male predominance. Gastric lymphomas usually occur in the gastric antrum, but can arise from any part of the stomach. Patients are considered to have primary gastric lymphoma if the stomach is the exclusive or predominant site of disease. Several conditions have been shown to be associated with gastric lymphoma, including *H. pylori* infection, certain autoimmune diseases (i.e., rheumatoid arthritis, systemic lupus erythematous), immunosuppression, and celiac disease.

Pathology

In the management of gastric lymphomas, as in the management of nodal lymphomas, it is important to determine not only the stage of disease but also the subtype of lymphoma. There are many classification systems for lymphomas (Table 49.9). The most common gastric lymphoma is diffuse large B cell lymphoma (DLBCL; 45%–60%), followed by gastric MALT lymphoma (40%–50%). Less commonly, peripheral T-cell lymphoma (1%–4%) and mantle cell and follicular lymphomas (both <1%) are seen.

DLBCLs are generally primary lesions; however, they may also occur from progression of less aggressive lymphomas, such as chronic lymphocytic leukemia, small lymphocytic lymphoma, follicular lymphoma, and MALT lymphoma. Immunodeficiency and *H. pylori* infection are risk factors for the development of primary DLBCL.

Evaluation and Staging

Endoscopy with biopsy is indicated for workup of patients with suspected gastric lymphoma. Occasionally, a submucosal growth pattern renders endoscopic biopsies nondiagnostic. EUS is useful to determine the depth of gastric wall invasion and to evaluate for regional lymph node involvement. Evidence of distant disease should be sought through upper airway examination to evaluate

TABLE 49.9 Comparison of gastrointestinal lymphoma classifications.

WHO CLASSIFICATION	REAL	WORKING	LUKES-COLLINS	KLEL	RAPPAPORT
Extranodal marginal zone lymphoma (MALT lymphoma)	—	Small-cleaved cell type	Small-cleaved cell type	Immunocytoma	Well-differentiated lymphocytic
Follicular lymphoma	Follicular center lymphoma	Small-cleaved cell type	Small-cleaved cell type	Centroblastic-centrocytic, follicular and diffuse	Nodular, poorly differentiated lymphocytic
Mantle cell lymphoma	–	–	–	Centrocytic	Intermediately or poorly differentiated lymphocytic, diffuse or nodular
Diffuse large B-cell lymphoma	Diffuse large B-cell lymphoma	Large-cleaved follicular center cell	Large-cleaved follicular center cell	Centroblastic, B-immunoblastic	Diffuse mixed lymphocytic and histiocytic
Burkitt lymphoma	Burkitt lymphoma	Small-noncleaved follicular center cell	Small-noncleaved follicular center cell	Burkitt lymphoma with intracytoplasmic immunoglobulin	Undifferentiated lymphoma, Burkitt type

MALT, Mucosa-associated lymphoid tissue; *WHO*, World Health Organization.

Waldeyer tonsillar ring, bone marrow biopsy, and CT of the chest and abdomen to detect lymphadenopathy. A PET/CT is often performed for patients with DLBCL as part of their initial assessment. Biopsies should be performed of enlarged lymph nodes. Histologic *H. pylori* testing should be performed and, if negative, confirmed by serology. Staging is important both for prognosis and treatment decision-making. The modified Lugano staging system is the most widely utilized for gastric lymphoma (Table 49.10).

Treatment

Oncologists utilize a multimodality treatment program for patients with gastric lymphoma. The most common chemotherapeutic combination is R-CHOP (rituximab, cyclophosphamide, hydroxydaunomycin [doxorubicin], Oncovin [vincristine], prednisone). A prospective randomized study evaluated several treatment strategies—surgical resection, resection plus radiation, resection plus chemotherapy, chemotherapy alone—in patients with early-stage (stage IE or II_1) disease.[41] The addition of chemotherapy was essential, with the surgery plus chemotherapy and chemotherapy-alone groups having significantly higher overall survival than the surgery-alone and surgery plus radiation groups. However, the addition of surgery to chemotherapy did not improve outcomes and increased morbidity. Thus, the primary role of surgery is currently limited to patients with symptomatic recurrence after treatment failure and patients who develop complications, such as bleeding, gastric outlet obstruction, or perforation. Chemotherapy for gastric lymphoma is associated with a 5% rate of gastric perforation and GI bleeding.

Mucosa-Associated Lymphoid Tissue Lymphomas

Gastric MALT lymphoma is lower grade than DLBCL and is usually preceded by *H. pylori*–induced gastritis.[42] Evidence of *H. pylori* infection can be found in almost every case of gastric MALT lymphoma. Genetically, MALT lymphoma is characterized by four chromosomic translocations t(1;14), t(3;14), t(11;18), and t(14;18). The t(1;14), t(11;18), and t(14;18) translocations result in increased nuclear factor-κB activity, with resultant enhanced cell survival. The t(3;14) translocation increases FOXP1 transcription factor levels, which has been shown to expand marginal zone B cells.

Treatment

Given the strong association with *H. pylori* and the low-grade MALT lymphoma, patients should be evaluated for active infection. Patients with early-stage MALT lymphomas and active *H. pylori* infection may be effectively treated by *H. pylori* eradication alone. Successful eradication results in remission in more than 75% of cases. However, careful follow-up is necessary, with repeat endoscopy in 2 months to document clearance of the infection and biannual endoscopy for 3 years to document regression. Some patients continue to demonstrate the lymphoma clone after *H. pylori* eradication, suggesting that the lymphoma became dormant rather than disappearing. The presence of transmural tumor extension, nodal involvement, transformation into a large cell phenotype, and nuclear *BCL-10* expression all predict failure after *H. pylori* eradication alone. Additionally, some patients with MALT lymphoma are *H. pylori*–negative. In these patients, consideration should be given to radiation therapy (if all the involved sites can be encompassed in a single field) and chemotherapy. A recent MALT lymphoma prognostic index was developed which identified three primary risk factors: age of 70 or above, stage IV disease, and elevated lactate dehydrogenase (LDH) level. The 5-year overall survival rates were 98.7% for no risk factors, 93.1% for one risk factor, and 64.3% for two to three risk factors ($P < 0.0001$).[43]

TABLE 49.10 Lugano staging system for gastrointestinal lymphoma.

STAGE	DESCRIPTION
I	Tumor confined to gastrointestinal tract
IE1	Involvement of mucosa +/- submucosa
IE2	Involvement of muscularis propria +/- serosa
II	Tumor extension into abdomen
II_1	Involvement of local nodes (paragastric for gastric lymphoma)
II_2	Involvement of distant nodes (paraaortic, paracaval, pelvic, or inguinal)
IIE	Serosa penetration to involve adjacent organs/tissues
IV	Disseminated extranodal involvement or supradiaphragmatic nodal involvement

Gastrointestinal Stromal Tumors

GI stromal tumors (GISTs) are the most common mesenchymal neoplasm of the GI tract. Originally thought to be a type of smooth muscle sarcoma, they are now known to be a distinct tumor derived from the interstitial cells of Cajal, a GI pacemaker cell. The incidence was difficult to assess previously given variable histologic definitions. However, since the discovery of KIT (CD117) and CD34 expression in GIST, more accurate estimates range from 7 to 15 cases per million per year. KIT is a receptor tyrosine kinase and approximately 95% of GISTs overexpress KIT. Most GISTs that lack a KIT mutation will have a mutation in platelet-derived growth factor receptor alpha (PDGFRA). While GISTs can appear anywhere within the GI tract, they most commonly arise in the stomach (40%–60%), small intestine (20%–40%), and colon/rectum (5%–15%). GISTs vary considerably in their presentation and clinical course, ranging from small benign tumors to massive lesions with necrosis, hemorrhage, and wide metastases. Their pathology, presentation, and management as they relate to the stomach are discussed here.

Gastric GISTs can manifest at any age, although most typically they manifest in patients older than 50 years. Approximately 5% of GISTs are associated with an underlying heritable mutation such as familial GIST syndrome (mutation in *KIT* or *PDGFRA*), neurofibromatosis 1, or Carney-Stratakis syndrome (GIST and paraganglioma with or without pulmonary chondroma). Most GISTs manifest with nonspecific symptoms, typically with early satiety, bloating, or vague abdominal pain. Bleeding can occur and is generally in the form of melena or, less frequently, frank hematemesis. Tumor rupture with intra abdominal hemorrhage is uncommon, but when it occurs, it frequently requires emergent surgical intervention. Many patients remain asymptomatic, and their tumors are discovered incidentally at the time of another surgery or, increasingly, during cross-sectional imaging performed for other indications.

Patients are evaluated with upper endoscopy, on which a smooth-appearing, round, submucosal tumor can be identified, occasionally containing an area of central ulceration. Because of the submucosal nature of the tumor, obtaining tissue for histologic analysis via conventional endoscopic biopsy results in a low diagnostic yield. EUS-directed FNA results in superior diagnostic accuracy, with a sensitivity of 82% and specificity of 100% in diagnosing GIST.[44] Given the expense and specialized expertise

BOX 49.5 Assessing malignant potential of gastric gastrointestinal stromal tumors of different sizes and mitotic activity.

Benign (No Tumor-Related Mortality)

- No larger than 2 cm, no more than 5 mitoses/50 HPF

Probably Benign (<3% With Progressive Disease)

- >2 cm but ≤5 cm; no more than 5 mitoses/50 HPF

Uncertain or Low Malignant Potential

- No larger than 2 cm; >5 mitoses/50 HPF

Low to Moderate Malignant Potential (12%–15% Tumor-Related Mortality)

- >10 cm; no more than 5 mitoses/HPF
- >2 cm but ≤5 cm; >5 mitoses/50 HPF

High Malignant Potential (49%-86% Tumor-Related Mortality)

- >5 cm but ≤10 cm; >5 mitoses/50 HPF
- >10 cm; >5 mitoses/50 HPF

From Miettinen M, Sobin L, Lasota J. Gastrointestinal stromal tumors of the stomach: a clinicopathologic, immunohistochemical, and molecular genetic study of 1765 cases with long-term follow-up. *Am J Surg Pathol.* 2005;29:52–58.
HPF, High-power field.

involved in performing EUS-directed FNA, in addition to the fact that most submucosal GI tumors require surgical resection regardless of histology, some experts have argued that routine preoperative pathologic diagnosis is not needed for such tumors. Presently, preoperative biopsy is not recommended if there is a high suspicion for GIST and the patient is otherwise operable, but is preferred to confirm presence of metastatic disease or if the patient is being considered for neoadjuvant imatinib therapy. CT of the abdomen and pelvis with oral and IV contrast is used to assess for metastatic disease. MRI is preferred in patients who cannot receive IV contrast or for rectal GISTs. Pathologically, GISTs can either have a spindle cell or epithelioid appearance. Immunohistochemical staining for CD117, CD34, and PDGFRA are used to confirm the diagnosis.

The mainstay of treatment is complete surgical resection. Tumors that are symptomatic or greater than 2 cm in diameter should be resected, but the treatment for smaller tumors is controversial. Tumors that are less than 2 cm but which have high-risk features on endoscopy and EUS, such as irregular borders, ulceration, echogenic foci, and heterogeneity, should be resected, whereas tumors without such features can be observed with repeat endoscopy and EUS at 6- to 12-month intervals. Depending on tumor size and location, resection can include wide local excision, enucleation, sleeve gastrectomy, or total gastrectomy, with or without en bloc resection of adjacent organs. No specific surgical margin other than an R0 resection is required, and an anatomic resection according to lymph node basins is not required, as lymph node metastases are rare. The tumor should be handled carefully intraoperatively to avoid rupture or spillage.

The two primary prognostic factors for gastric GISTs are tumor size and mitotic rate. Based on a long-term follow-up study of 1700 patients with gastric GISTs, malignant potential based on the combination of these two factors has been established (Box 49.5).[45] Most patients who experience recurrence demonstrate metastasis to the liver, with one-third having only isolated local recurrence. Recurrence can occur over 20 years after resection; thus, long-term follow-up is warranted.

Patients presenting with recurrent or metastatic disease are primarily treated with imatinib or a second-line tyrosine kinase inhibitor (see below), but a subset of patients may benefit from surgical intervention. A recent series of 323 patients found that response to neoadjuvant imatinib predicted clinical response after metastasectomy. Patients with responsive or stable disease had a median progression-free survival of 30 to 36 months, whereas those with unifocal or multifocal progressive disease had median progression-free survival of only 6 to 11 months.[46] The timing of surgery in this setting is typically 6 to 9 months after neoadjuvant therapy initiation. Patients who are not surgical candidates due to isolated liver metastases can be considered for radiofrequency ablation or hepatic arterial embolization, both of which have shown some benefit in nonrandomized series.

Adjuvant Therapy

Adjuvant therapy for GIST changed dramatically with the discovery of the tyrosine kinase inhibitor imatinib (Gleevec). Originally designed to treat chronic myelogenous leukemia, it has proven in randomized controlled trials to be an effective treatment modality for patients with GIST. The ACOSOG Z9001 phase III, placebo-controlled, randomized trial of 713 patients with *c-kit*–positive tumors 3 cm or larger who underwent complete resection found that patients treated with imatinib for 1 year had a significantly improved 1-year recurrence-free survival (98% vs. 83%, $P < 0.0001$).[47] This difference was even more pronounced for patients with larger tumors.

The Scandinavian Sarcoma Group XVIII trial compared an extended 36-month course of adjuvant imatinib to a 12-month course after resection for 400 patients with high-risk GISTs (defined as >10 cm tumor, mitotic count >10/50 HPF, both tumor >5 cm and mitotic count >5 per 50 HPF, or tumor rupture). In the second planned analysis of the trial, patients in the extended treatment arm had higher 5-year recurrence-free survival (71.1% vs. 52.3%, $P < 0.001$) and overall survival (91.9% vs. 85.3%, $P = 0.036$).[48] The results of this trial have established a 3-year course as the standard of care after surgical resection of high-risk GIST, though longer duration of therapy is being explored.

Imatinib has also been reported to be successful in the neoadjuvant treatment of patients with nonmetastatic but unresectable disease, although the exact indications are not yet fully defined. Currently, patients with locally advanced, borderline resectable disease or in whom tumor shrinkage would increase the likelihood of organ preservation should be considered for neoadjuvant therapy. As stated previously, patients with limited metastatic disease can be offered neoadjuvant imatinib followed by possible metastatectomy based on clinical response. Fig. 49.28 is an algorithm for using imatinib in the treatment of GISTs in the neoadjuvant, adjuvant, and palliative settings. Patients who progress on imatinib or are intolerant to the drug are typically offered second-line tyrosine kinase inhibitors such as sunitinib or regorafenib.

Other Neoplasms

Gastric Neuroendocrine Tumors

Gastric NETs, also referred to as carcinoid tumors, are a rare malignancy that arise from neuroendocrine precursor cells and can

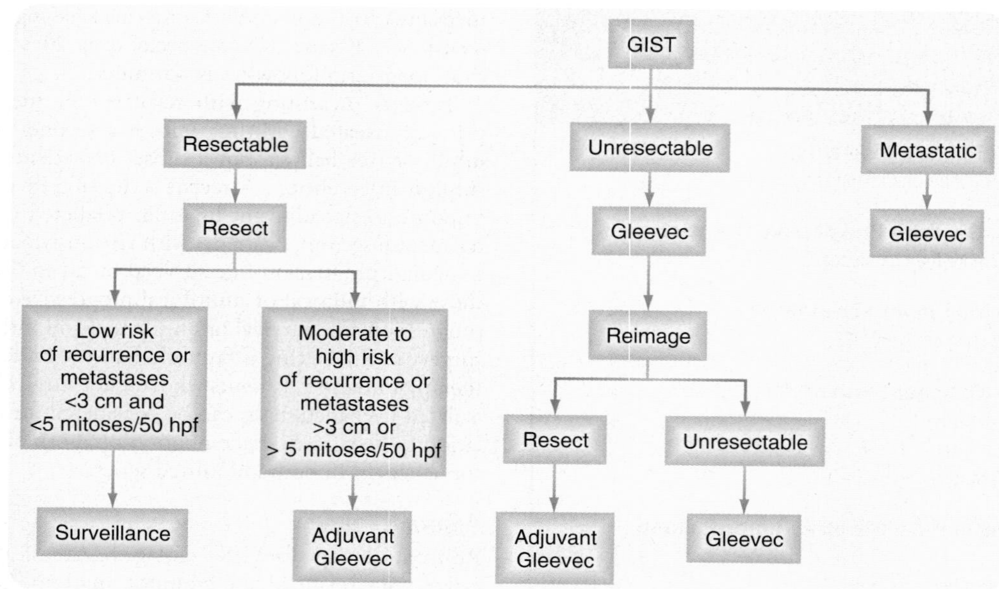

FIG. 49.28 Algorithm for the workup and treatment of gastrointestinal stromal tumors *(GISTs)*. *hpf*, High-power field.

TABLE 49.11 Gastric carcinoid types.

	TYPE 1	TYPE 2	TYPE 3
Percentage of gastric NETs	70%–80%	5%–10%	10%–15%
Associated pathology	Pernicious anemia	ZES, MEN1	n/a
Location	Fundus or body	Fundus, body, antrum	Fundus or antrum
Acid level	Low	High	Normal
Gastrin level	High	High	Normal
Prognosis	Excellent	Good	Poor

MEN, Multiple endocrine neoplasia; *n/a*, not applicable; *NETs*, neuroendocrine tumors; *ZES*, Zollinger-Ellison syndrome.

manifest at any site in the body. The most common sites in the GI tract are the small intestine, rectum, and appendix. The stomach is becoming an increasing common site of NETs, now representing 8% of tumors. This increasing incidence is thought to be due to a combination of improved surveillance and the widespread use of PPIs.[49] Unlike other GI tract NETs, gastric NETs are typically nonfunctioning and rarely cause carcinoid syndrome.

There are three distinct subtypes of gastric NETs (Table 49.11). Type I gastric NETs are the most common, accounting for 70%–80% of cases. They are associated with chronic achlorhydria from atrophic gastritis, pernicious anemia, or possibly prolonged PPI use.[49] Type 1 gastric NETs are typically seen as multiple small tumors confined to the mucosa and submucosa with a relatively benign course and favorable prognosis. Type II gastric NETs are associated with hypergastrinemia in the setting of gastrinomas and ZES. Similar to Type I, patients will have multiple small tumors. While the prognosis is still good, with long-term survival of 70% to 90%, Type II has a slightly higher risk of metastasis (5%–35% of patients have spread to regional lymph nodes). Type III tumors are sporadic lesions with no associated conditions and without hypergastrinemia. They typically present as a large solitary lesion and account for 15% to 20% of gastric NETs. Type III portends a more aggressive course, with higher rates of metastases resulting in a 5-year survival of 25% to 30%. The combined 5-year overall survival for all localized gastric NETs is 63%. While not universally adopted, neuroendocrine carcinoma has been referred to as Type IV gastric NET. These tumors are very aggressive, with most patients presenting with widespread metastatic disease. These patients are rarely candidates for curative resection but occasionally may require surgery to address bleeding, perforation, or obstruction.[49]

Diagnosis of gastric NET is established on esophagogastroduodenoscopy (EGD) with biopsy of the lesion. EUS can be performed to assess for depth of invasion subsequently. Either CT or MRI can be useful to evaluate for metastatic disease. Chromogranin A is often elevated and can serve as a biomarker for these tumors.

The treatment for localized NETs is complete removal. For small pedunculated lesions that do not invade beyond the submucosa, complete removal can be accomplished endoscopically. Larger (>1 cm) lesions may require wedge resection or partial gastrectomy. Some clinicians will perform an antrectomy for Type I NETs to remove the source of gastrin secretion. Patients with numerous gastric NETs may require total gastrectomy. In patients with type II NETs, gastrinoma resection should be performed as well, if possible. Patients with localized type III NETs should undergo oncologic resection with lymphadenectomy. For patients with recurrent or metastatic disease, somatostatin analogues or chemotherapy can be used to decrease the burden of disease and treat carcinoid syndrome.

Heterotopic Pancreas

Heterotopic pancreas (i.e., functioning pancreatic tissue is found in an abnormal anatomic location) is found in 0.5% to 14% of autopsy specimens. The most common location is within the stomach, typically along the antral greater curvature. Symptomatic patients generally present with vague abdominal pain. There have been reports of pancreatitis, islet cell tumors, and pancreatic adenocarcinoma within these lesions. On endoscopy and CT, they are frequently small submucosal masses and may be confused with a GIST or some other gastric neoplasm. The treatment is surgical excision, and the diagnosis is confirmed pathologically.

OTHER GASTRIC LESIONS

Hypertrophic Gastritis (Ménétrier Disease)

Ménétrier disease (hypoproteinemic hypertrophic gastropathy) is a rare disease characterized by massive gastric folds in the fundus and body of the stomach, giving the mucosa a cobblestone or cerebriform appearance. The antrum is typically spared. Histologic examination reveals foveolar hyperplasia (expansion of surface mucus cells), with decreased or absent parietal cells. The condition is also associated with protein loss from the stomach, excessive mucus production, and hypochlorhydria or achlorhydria. The cause of Ménétrier disease is unknown, but it has been associated with cytomegalovirus infection in children and *H. pylori* infection in adults. Also, increased levels of transforming growth factor-α have been noted in the gastric mucosa of patients with the disease, which can stimulate epithelial cell growth and inhibit gastric acid secretion. Patients often present with epigastric pain, vomiting, weight loss, decreased appetite, and peripheral edema. Typical gastric mucosal changes can be detected by radiographic or endoscopic examination. Biopsy should be performed to establish the diagnosis and to rule out gastric carcinoma or lymphoma. Medical treatment yields inconsistent results; however, some benefit has been shown with the use of acid suppression, octreotide, and cytomegalovirus or *H. pylori* eradication. Total gastrectomy should be performed in patients who continue to have massive protein loss despite optimal medical therapy and high-protein diet or if dysplasia or carcinoma develops. Given the increased risk of gastric neoplasms in patients with Ménétrier disease, patients should undergo endoscopic surveillance every 1 to 2 years.

Mallory-Weiss Tear

Mallory-Weiss tears are mucosal lacerations related to forceful vomiting, retching, coughing, or straining that cause disruption of the gastric mucosa high on the lesser curve at the GE junction. They account for 10% to 15% of acute upper GI hemorrhages and are rarely associated with massive bleeding. The overall mortality rate for the lesion is 3% to 5%, with the greatest risk for massive hemorrhage in alcoholic patients with preexisting portal hypertension. Most patients with active bleeding can be managed by endoscopic methods, such as multipolar electrocoagulation, epinephrine injection, endoscopic band ligation, or endoscopic hemoclipping. Angiographic transarterial embolization may be useful in patients who have persistent or recurrent bleeding after endoscopy. Operative intervention is rarely needed. If surgery is required, the lesion at the GE junction is approached through an anterior gastrotomy, and the bleeding site is oversewn with several deep 2-0 silk ligatures to reapproximate the gastric mucosa in an anatomic fashion.

Dieulafoy Gastric Lesion

Dieulafoy lesions account for 0.3% to 7% of nonvariceal upper GI hemorrhages. Bleeding from a gastric Dieulafoy lesion is caused by an abnormally large (1–3 mm), tortuous artery coursing through the submucosa without a primary ulcer. Erosion of the superficial mucosa overlying the artery occurs secondary to the pulsations of the large submucosal vessel. The artery is then exposed to the gastric contents, and further erosion and bleeding occur. Generally, the mucosal defect is 2 to 5 mm and is surrounded by normal-appearing gastric mucosa. The lesions generally occur near the GE junction along the lesser curvature. Dieulafoy lesions are more common in men (2:1), with associated comorbidities including cardiovascular disease, chronic kidney disease, and diabetes. Most patients present with hematemesis. The classic presentation of a patient with a Dieulafoy lesion is sudden onset of massive, painless hematemesis.

Detection and identification of the Dieulafoy lesion can be difficult. The diagnostic modality of choice is upper endoscopy, which correctly identifies the lesion in 80% of patients. Because of the intermittent nature of the bleeding, repeat endoscopies may be needed. If the lesion can be identified endoscopically and is actively bleeding, endoscopic modalities such as bipolar electrocoagulation, heater probe thermocoagulation, injection sclerotherapy, or endoscopic hemoclipping can be applied. Angiography can be useful in cases in which endoscopy is unable to definitely identify the source of bleeding. Angiographic findings may include a tortuous ectatic artery in the distribution of the left gastric artery, with accompanying contrast extravasation in the setting of acute bleeding. Embolization has been reported to control bleeding successfully in patients with Dieulafoy lesion, although the reported experience is limited.

Surgical therapy was once the only available treatment for Dieulafoy lesion, but it is now reserved for patients in whom other modalities have failed. Surgical management consists of gastric wedge resection to include the offending vessel. The difficulty at the time of exploration is locating the lesion, unless it is actively bleeding. The surgical procedure can be greatly facilitated by asking the endoscopist to tattoo the stomach when the lesion is identified or with intraoperative endoscopic localization. A wedge resection is performed with a linear stapling device using endoscopic transillumination to determine the resection margin.

Gastric Varices

Gastric varices are dilated submucosal veins commonly seen in patients with portal hypertension and cirrhosis. Gastric varices account for 10% to 30% of variceal hemorrhages. They are broadly classified into two types: isolated gastric varices and GE varices. Isolated gastric varices are subclassified into type 1 varices, located in the fundus of the stomach, and type 2, isolated ectopic varices located anywhere in the stomach. While GE varices are more common overall, isolated gastric varices are more prone to bleeding.

Gastric varices can develop secondary to portal hypertension, in conjunction with esophageal varices, or secondary to sinistral hypertension from splenic vein thrombosis. In generalized portal hypertension, the increased portal pressure is transmitted by the left gastric vein to esophageal varices and by the short and posterior gastric veins to the fundic plexus and cardia veins. Isolated gastric varices tend to occur secondary to splenic vein thrombosis, which is most commonly the result of pancreatitis. Splenic blood flows retrograde through the short and posterior gastric veins into the varices and then through the coronary vein into the portal vein. Left-to-right retrograde flow through the gastroepiploic vein to the superior mesenteric vein can explain the development of ectopic varices in the stomach.

The incidence of bleeding from gastric varices has been reported to be between 3% and 30%. However, the incidence of bleeding can be much higher in patients with splenic vein thrombosis and fundic varices. There are limited data on risk factors associated with hemorrhage in patients with gastric varices, although increasing size of the varices or decompensated cirrhosis increases the risk for bleeding.

Gastric varices in the setting of splenic vein thrombosis are readily treated by splenectomy. Patients with bleeding gastric varices should have an imaging study to document splenic vein thrombosis before a splenectomy is performed as gastric varices are more often associated with generalized portal hypertension.

Acutely bleeding gastric varices in the setting of portal hypertension should be managed similarly to esophageal varices. The patient should be volume-resuscitated, with attention paid to the correction of abnormal coagulation profiles. Temporary tamponade can be attempted with a Sengstaken-Blakemore tube. Endoscopy serves as the primary diagnostic and therapeutic tool. Endoscopic treatment options for gastric variceal bleeding include sclerotherapy, band ligation, glue, or thrombin injection. A major problem with gastric varices after endoscopic treatment is rebleeding, occurring in 10% to 35% of cases.[50] An emerging treatment modality is EUS-guided cyanoacrylate-lipiodol injection or coil embolization of perforating veins. Transjugular intrahepatic portosystemic shunting can be effective in controlling gastric variceal hemorrhage that does not respond to endoscopic treatments, with initial hemostasis rates over 90% and rebleeding rates of approximately 10% to 30%.[50] A gastrorenal shunt between gastric varices and the left renal vein is present in 60% to 85% of patients with gastric varices. This spontaneous shunt decompresses the portal system and lessens the efficacy of transjugular intrahepatic portosystemic shunting. A balloon catheter can be inserted into the gastrorenal shunt through the left renal vein, and the shunt can be occluded by inflating the balloon. A sclerosant (e.g., ethanolamine oleate iopamidol) is injected and left to remain until clots have formed within the varices. Balloon-occluded retrograde transvenous obliteration has a high success rate (75%–100%) with a low recurrence rate (0%–15%).[50] The major complication of this procedure is aggravation of esophageal varices secondary to an increase in portal pressure as a consequence of occluding the gastrorenal shunt.

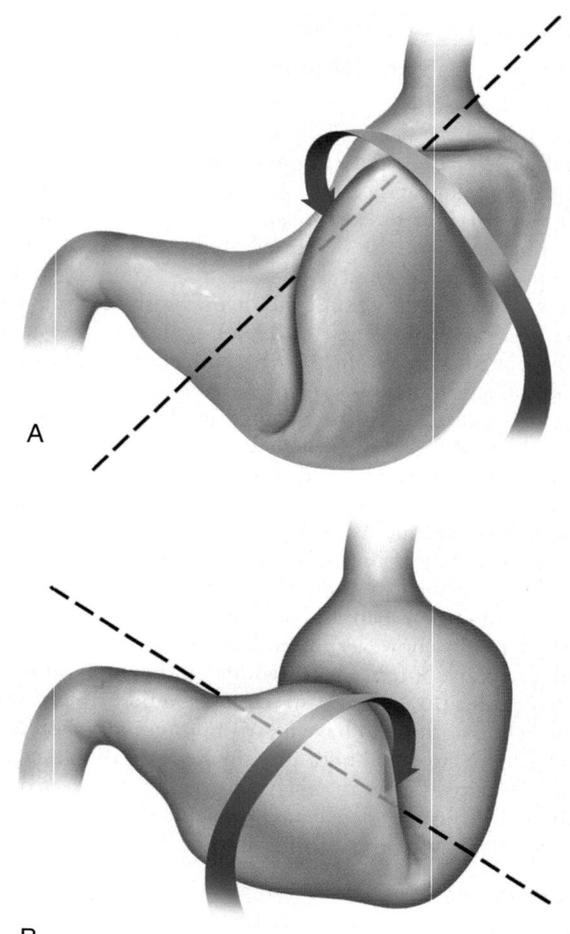

FIG. 49.29 Torsion of the stomach along the longitudinal axis (mesenteroaxial) (A) and along the vertical axis (organoaxial) (B). (From White RR, Jacobs DO. Volvulus of the stomach and small bowel. In Yeo CJ, Dempsey DT, Klein AS, et al, eds. *Shackelford's Surgery of the Alimentary Tract*. 6th ed. Philadelphia: Saunders; 2007.)

Gastric Volvulus

Gastric volvulus is an uncommon condition. Torsion occurs along the stomach's long longitudinal axis (organoaxial) in approximately two-thirds of cases and along the short vertical axis (mesenteroaxial) in one-third of cases (Fig. 49.29). Rotation more than 180 degrees causes gastric outlet obstruction and can lead to ischemia, necrosis, and potentially perforation if left uncorrected. Usually, organoaxial gastric volvulus occurs acutely and is associated with a diaphragmatic defect, whereas mesenteroaxial volvulus is partial (<180 degrees), recurrent, and not associated with a diaphragmatic defect. Rarely, a more complex form can occur with elements of both rotations. Primary gastric volvulus is due to abnormalities of the gastric ligaments (i.e., gastrocolic, gastrohepatic, etc.). Secondary gastric volvulus is due to other anatomic abnormalities, the most common being a paraesophageal hernia. In children, congenital defects such as the foramen of Bochdalek or diaphragmatic eventration are involved.

The classic symptoms at presentation are acute onset abdominal pain, distention, and vomiting. The sudden onset of constant and severe upper abdominal pain, recurrent retching with production of little vomitus, and the inability to pass an NG tube constitute the Borchardt triad. Plain films of the abdomen reveal a spherical gas-filled viscus in the chest or upper abdomen with an air-fluid level. The diagnosis can be confirmed by CT imaging. Acute volvulus is a surgical emergency. NG decompression should be performed immediately, which sometimes can cause the stomach to detorse spontaneously. Patients should then proceed with surgical intervention. For patients with acceptable surgical risk, an open or laparoscopic approach can be undertaken. The stomach is reduced and uncoiled through a transabdominal approach. The diaphragmatic defect is repaired, with consideration given to a fundoplication in the setting of a paraesophageal hernia. If strangulation has occurred, the compromised segment of stomach is resected. Spontaneous volvulus, without an associated diaphragmatic defect, is treated by detorsion and fixation of the stomach by gastropexy or tube gastrostomy. Patients with high surgical risk can instead undergo endoscopic detorsion with percutaneous endoscopic gastrostomy tube placement to fixate the stomach. Two percutaneous endoscopic gastrostomy tubes are used to prevent rotation. Percutaneous endoscopic gastrostomy tube placement can also be used as a temporizing measure in a hemodynamically unstable patient prior to definitive surgical repair.

Gastric Bezoars

Bezoars are collections of nondigestible materials, usually of vegetable origin (phytobezoar) but can also be composed of hair (trichobezoar), medications (pharmacobezoars), or other substances. Bezoars are most commonly found in patients who have underlying gastric dysmotility issues, such as prior gastric surgery, gastroparesis, or gastric outlet obstruction. The impaired grinding mechanism of the stomach and migrating motor complexes have been implicated as pathogenic causes of bezoars. Patients are often asymptomatic or have gradual symptom onset over years. The symptoms of gastric bezoars include early satiety, pain, nausea/vomiting, and weight loss. Physical exam is usually unremarkable, although sometimes a large mass may be palpable. Abdominal radiographs or CT scans can show a bezoar as a mass or filling defect within the stomach; diagnosis is confirmed by upper endoscopy. In 1959, Dan and coworkers were the first to suggest enzymatic therapy to attempt dissolution of the bezoar. Papain, found in Adolph's Meat Tenderizer, is given in a dose of 1 tsp in 150 to 300 mL water several times daily. The sodium concentration in Adolph's Meat Tenderizer is high, so hypernatremia may result if large quantities are administered. Alternative enzymes such as cellulase have been used with some success. Generally, enzymatic debridement is followed by aggressive Ewald tube lavage or endoscopic fragmentation. Failure of these therapies necessitates surgical removal.

Initial management of symptomatic bezoars is attempted chemical dissolution. There are a wide array of options, including soda, cellulose, papain, and acetylcysteine; no randomized trials exist to suggest superiority of one dissolving agent compared to others. Of note, trichobezoars are typically resistant to chemical dissolution. Pharmacobezoars may require decontamination depending on the medication involved. If chemical dissolution is ineffective or contraindicated, endoscopic fragmentation with a water jet, forceps, or direct suction can be performed and the fragments can either be removed via the endoscope, with an Ewald tube, or allowed to pass through the GI tract. Surgical removal is typically reserved for patients who fail more conservative management, present with a complication (i.e., perforation or excessive bleeding), or if other therapies are contraindicated based on the bezoar composition.

SELECTED REFERENCES

Abdelfatah MM, Barakat M, Lee H, et al. The incidence of lymph node metastasis in early gastric cancer according to the expanded criteria in comparison with the absolute criteria of the Japanese Gastric Cancer Association: a systematic review of the literature and meta-analysis. *Gastrointest Endosc.* 2018;87:338–347.

The purpose of this study was to quantify the rate of lymph node metastases in patients who would be eligible for endoscopic gastric cancer resection based on the established criteria of the Japanese Gastric Cancer Association via a meta analysis of 9798 patients. Among patients meeting the standard inclusion criteria, the incidence of lymph node metastasis was 0.2%. Two variables suggested for expanded endoscopic criteria, undifferentiated lesions and slight submucosal invasion, had significantly higher incidence of lymph node metastases.

Cheung KS, Chan EW, Wong AYS, et al. Long-term proton pump inhibitors and risk of gastric cancer development after treatment for *Helicobacter pylori*: a population-based study. *Gut.* 2018;67:28–35.

This is an epidemiological study from Hong Kong, which included 63,397 subjects who received clarithromycin-based triple therapy and compared proton pump inhibitor (PPI) versus H_2-receptor antagonist exposure with future gastric cancer development. They found that PPIs were associated with increased gastric cancer risk (hazard ratio, 2.44) and that the risk increased with longer duration of PPI therapy. The absolute risk difference for PPIs versus non-PPIs was 4.29 excess gastric cancers per 10,000 person-years.

Cunningham D, Allum WH, Stenning SP, et al. Perioperative chemotherapy versus surgery alone for resectable gastroesophageal cancer. *N Engl J Med.* 2006;355:11–20.

This major study showed a benefit to chemotherapy in gastric cancer. Patients underwent neoadjuvant treatment, and a much greater percentage were able to complete treatment compared with patients who completed the adjuvant trial. More patients had adequate lymphadenectomy than in the SWOG Intergroup 0116 trial.

DeMatteo RP, Ballman KV, Antonescu CR, et al. Adjuvant imatinib mesylate after resection of localized, primary gastrointestinal stromal tumour: a randomised, double-blind, placebo-controlled trial. *Lancet.* 2009;373:1097–1104.

Joensuu H, Eriksson M, Sundby Hall K, et al. Adjuvant imatinib for high-risk GI stromal tumor: analysis of a randomized trial. *J Clin Oncol.* 2016;34:244–250.

These two major randomized controlled trials established the role of adjuvant imatinib after surgical resection for the treatment of localized gastrointestinal stromal tumors (GISTs). The first study by DeMatteo and colleagues showed significantly less recurrence in patients who received imatinib compared with patients who did not; this was especially pronounced for patients at high risk of developing metastatic disease. The second trial by Joensuu and colleagues showed that a 36-month course of adjuvant imatinib was superior to a 12-month course in terms of disease-free and overall survival. These studies established long-term adjuvant treatment with imatinib as the standard of care for patients with GISTs.

Honda M, Hiki N, Kinoshita T, et al. Long-term outcomes of laparoscopic versus open surgery for clinical stage I gastric cancer: the LOC-1 study. *Ann Surg.* 2016;264:214–222.

This is a large propensity-matched retrospective study from Japan that included 1848 patients undergoing either laparoscopic or open gastrectomy for stage I gastric cancer to report oncologic outcomes (as long-term outcomes from multiple prospective randomized trials are awaited). The authors adjusted for 30 variables that may influence a surgeon's choice of operative approach. They found statistically equivalent 5-year overall survival and 3-year recurrence-free survival rates, suggesting oncologic equivalence for laparoscopic surgery in treatment of early gastric cancer.

Lanas A, Chan FKL. Peptic ulcer disease. *Lancet.* 2017;390: 613–624.

This is a Lancet Seminar that provides an excellent and comprehensive review of the current state of peptic ulcer disease. Specifically, the authors address current knowledge on the pathogenesis of peptic ulcer disease, updated guidelines for Helicobacter pylori *infection treatment, as well as how to approach treatment for patients with complications related to nonsteroidal antiinfalmmatory drugs (NSAIDs) and antithrombotic agents.*

Ning FL, Zhang CD, Wang P, et al. Endoscopic resection versus radical gastrectomy for early gastric cancer in Asia: a meta-analysis. *Int J Surg.* 2017;48:45–52.

This meta analysis compared patients from 15 retrospective series undergoing either endoscopic resection (n = 3737) or radical gastrectomy (n = 4246) for early gastric cancer. They found no difference in either 3-year or 5-year overall survival. Endoscopic resection was associated with a higher risk or recurrent or metachronous gastric cancers. However, radical gastrectomy was associated with a significantly higher complication rate.

Noh SH, Park SR, Yang HK, et al. Adjuvant capecitabine plus oxaliplatin for gastric cancer after D2 gastrectomy (CLASSIC): 5-year follow-up of an open-label, randomised phase 3 trial. *Lancet Oncol.* 2014;15:1389–1396.

Park SH, Sohn TS, Lee J, et al. Phase III trial to compare adjuvant chemotherapy with capecitabine and cisplatin versus concurrent chemoradiotherapy in gastric cancer: final report of the adjuvant chemoradiotherapy in stomach tumors trial, including survival and subset analyses. *J Clin Oncol.* 2015;33:3130–3136.

These are the long-term follow-ups to two large randomized controlled trials examined the role of adjuvant therapy after surgical resection for localized gastric cancer. The CLASSIC trial found that adjuvant chemotherapy (capecitabine plus oxaliplatin) improved long-term disease-free and overall survival compared with surgery alone. The ARTIST trial evaluated the addition of adjuvant radiotherapy plus chemotherapy and showed no improvement compared with adjuvant chemotherapy alone. However, radiotherapy did result in an improvement in outcomes in patients who had lymph node metastases on surgical resection.

REFERENCES

1. Camilleri M, Parkman HP, Shafi MA, et al. Clinical guideline: management of gastroparesis. *Am J Gastroenterol.* 2013;108:18–37; quiz 38.
2. Zoll B, Zhao H, Edwards MA, et al. Outcomes of surgical intervention for refractory gastroparesis: a systematic review. *J Surg Res.* 2018;231:263–269.
3. Su A, Conklin JL, Sedarat A. Endoscopic therapies for gastroparesis. *Curr Gastroenterol Rep.* 2018;20:25.
4. Lanas A, Chan FKL. Peptic ulcer disease. *Lancet.* 2017;390:613–624.
5. Datta De D, Roychoudhury S. To be or not to be: the host genetic factor and beyond in *Helicobacter pylori* mediated gastro-duodenal diseases. *World J Gastroenterol.* 2015;21:2883–2895.
6. Marshall BJ, Warren JR. Unidentified curved bacilli in the stomach of patients with gastritis and peptic ulceration. *Lancet.* 1984;1:1311–1315.
7. Eslick GD, Lim LL, Byles JE, et al. Association of *Helicobacter pylori* infection with gastric carcinoma: a meta-analysis. *Am J Gastroenterol.* 1999;94:2373–2379.
8. Chey WD, Leontiadis GI, Howden CW, et al. ACG clinical guideline: treatment of *Helicobacter pylori* infection. *Am J Gastroenterol.* 2017;112:212–239.
9. Lau JY, Sung J, Hill C, et al. Systematic review of the epidemiology of complicated peptic ulcer disease: incidence, recurrence, risk factors and mortality. *Digestion.* 2011;84:102–113.
10. Laine L, Jensen DM. Management of patients with ulcer bleeding. *Am J Gastroenterol.* 2012;107:345–360; quiz 361.
11. Sachar H, Vaidya K, Laine L. Intermittent vs continuous proton pump inhibitor therapy for high-risk bleeding ulcers: a systematic review and meta-analysis. *JAMA Intern Med.* 2014;174:1755–1762.
12. Søreide K, Thorsen K, Harrison EM, et al. Perforated peptic ulcer. *Lancet.* 2015;386:1288–1298.
13. Quah GS, Eslick GD, Cox MR. Laparoscopic repair for perforated peptic ulcer disease has better outcomes than open repair. *J Gastrointest Surg.* 2019;23:618–625.
14. Storm AC, Ryou M. Advances in the endoscopic management of gastric outflow disorders. *Curr Opin Gastroenterol.* 2017;33:455–460.
15. Reynolds PM, MacLaren R. Re-evaluating the utility of stress ulcer prophylaxis in the critically ill patient: a clinical scenario-based meta-analysis. *Pharmacotherapy.* 2019;39:408–420.
16. Yang D, He L, Tong WH, et al. Randomized controlled trial of uncut Roux-en-Y vs Billroth II reconstruction after distal gastrectomy for gastric cancer: which technique is better for avoiding biliary reflux and gastritis? *World J Gastroenterol.* 2017;23:6350–6356.
17. Siegel RL, Miller KD, Jemal A. Cancer statistics, 2018. *CA Cancer J Clin.* 2018;68:7–30.
18. Bray F, Ferlay J, Soerjomataram I, et al. Global cancer statistics 2018: GLOBOCAN estimates of incidence and mortality worldwide for 36 cancers in 185 countries. *CA Cancer J Clin.* 2018;68:394–424.
19. Wroblewski LE, Peek Jr RM, Wilson KT. *Helicobacter pylori* and gastric cancer: factors that modulate disease risk. *Clin Microbiol Rev.* 2010;23:713–739.
20. Schmocker RK, Lidor AO. Management of non-neoplastic gastric lesions. *Surg Clin North Am.* 2017;97:387–403.
21. Cheung KS, Chan EW, Wong AYS, et al. Long-term proton pump inhibitors and risk of gastric cancer development after treatment for *Helicobacter pylori*: a population-based study. *Gut.* 2018;67:28–35.
22. Ajani JA, D'Amico TA, Almhanna K, et al. Gastric cancer, version 3.2016, NCCN clinical practice guidelines in oncology. *J Natl Compr Canc Netw.* 2016;14:1286–1312.
23. Mocellin S, Pasquali S. Diagnostic accuracy of endoscopic ultrasonography (EUS) for the preoperative locoregional staging of primary gastric cancer. *Cochrane Database Syst Rev.* 2015:CD009944.
24. Oh SY, Lee HJ, Yang HK. Pylorus-preserving gastrectomy for gastric cancer. *J Gastric Cancer.* 2016;16:63–71.
25. Honda M, Hiki N, Kinoshita T, et al. Long-term outcomes of laparoscopic versus open surgery for clinical stage I gastric cancer: the LOC-1 study. *Ann Surg.* 2016;264:214–222.

26. Wang LH, Zhu RF, Gao C, et al. Application of enhanced recovery after gastric cancer surgery: an updated meta-analysis. *World J Gastroenterol.* 2018;24:1562–1578.
27. Abdelfatah MM, Barakat M, Lee H, et al. The incidence of lymph node metastasis in early gastric cancer according to the expanded criteria in comparison with the absolute criteria of the Japanese Gastric Cancer Association: a systematic review of the literature and meta-analysis. *Gastrointest Endosc.* 2018;87:338–347.
28. Ning FL, Zhang CD, Wang P, et al. Endoscopic resection versus radical gastrectomy for early gastric cancer in Asia: a meta-analysis. *Int J Surg.* 2017;48:45–52.
29. Mocellin S, McCulloch P, Kazi H, et al. Extent of lymph node dissection for adenocarcinoma of the stomach. *Cochrane Database Syst Rev.* 2015:CD001964.
30. Degiuli M, De Manzoni G, Di Leo A, et al. Gastric cancer: current status of lymph node dissection. *World J Gastroenterol.* 2016;22:2875–2893.
31. Sym SJ, Chang HM, Ryu MH, et al. Neoadjuvant docetaxel, capecitabine and cisplatin (DXP) in patients with unresectable locally advanced or metastatic gastric cancer. *Ann Surg Oncol.* 2010;17:1024–1032.
32. Yoshikawa T, Sasako M, Yamamoto S, et al. Phase II study of neoadjuvant chemotherapy and extended surgery for locally advanced gastric cancer. *Br J Surg.* 2009;96:1015–1022.
33. Macdonald JS, Smalley SR, Benedetti J, et al. Chemoradiotherapy after surgery compared with surgery alone for adenocarcinoma of the stomach or gastroesophageal junction. *N Engl J Med.* 2001;345:725–730.
34. Noh SH, Park SR, Yang HK, et al. Adjuvant capecitabine plus oxaliplatin for gastric cancer after D2 gastrectomy (CLASSIC): 5-year follow-up of an open-label, randomised phase 3 trial. *Lancet Oncol.* 2014;15:1389–1396.
35. Park SH, Sohn TS, Lee J, et al. Phase III trial to compare adjuvant chemotherapy with capecitabine and cisplatin versus concurrent chemoradiotherapy in gastric cancer: final report of the adjuvant chemoradiotherapy in stomach tumors trial, including survival and subset analyses. *J Clin Oncol.* 2015;33:3130–3136.
36. Cunningham D, Allum WH, Stenning SP, et al. Perioperative chemotherapy versus surgery alone for resectable gastroesophageal cancer. *N Engl J Med.* 2006;355:11–20.
37. Al Batran SE, Homann N, Schmalenberg H, et al. Perioperative chemotherapy with docetaxel, oxaliplatin, and fluorouracil/leucovorin (FLOT) versus epirubicin, cisplatin, and fluorouracil or capecitabine (ECF/ECX) for resectable gastric or gastroesophageal junction (GEJ) adenocarcinoma (FLOT4-AIO): a multicenter, randomized phase 3 trial. *J Clin Oncol.* 2017;35:4004.
38. Tan AC, Chan DL, Faisal W, et al. New drug developments in metastatic gastric cancer. *Therap Adv Gastroenterol.* 2018;11: 1756284818808072.
39. Bang YJ, Van Cutsem E, Feyereislova A, et al. Trastuzumab in combination with chemotherapy versus chemotherapy alone for treatment of HER2-positive advanced gastric or gastro-oesophageal junction cancer (ToGA): a phase 3, open-label, randomised controlled trial. *Lancet.* 2010;376:687–697.
40. Aurello P, Petrucciani N, Antolino L, et al. Follow-up after curative resection for gastric cancer: is it time to tailor it? *World J Gastroenterol.* 2017;23:3379–3387.
41. Aviles A, Nambo MJ, Neri N, et al. The role of surgery in primary gastric lymphoma: results of a controlled clinical trial. *Ann Surg.* 2004;240:44–50.
42. Hu Q, Zhang Y, Zhang X, et al. Gastric mucosa-associated lymphoid tissue lymphoma and *Helicobacter pylori* infection: a review of current diagnosis and management. *Biomark Res.* 2016;4:15.
43. Thieblemont C, Cascione L, Conconi A, et al. A MALT lymphoma prognostic index. *Blood.* 2017;130:1409–1417.
44. Watson RR, Binmoeller KF, Hamerski CM, et al. Yield and performance characteristics of endoscopic ultrasound–guided fine needle aspiration for diagnosing upper GI tract stromal tumors. *Dig Dis Sci.* 2011;56:1757–1762.
45. Miettinen M, Sobin LH, Lasota J. Gastrointestinal stromal tumors of the stomach: a clinicopathologic, immunohistochemical, and molecular genetic study of 1765 cases with long-term follow-up. *Am J Surg Pathol.* 2005;29:52–68.
46. Fairweather M, Balachandran VP, Li GZ, et al. Cytoreductive surgery for metastatic gastrointestinal stromal tumors treated with tyrosine kinase inhibitors: a 2-institutional analysis. *Ann Surg.* 2018;268:296–302.
47. DeMatteo RP, Ballman KV, Antonescu CR, et al. Adjuvant imatinib mesylate after resection of localized, primary gastrointestinal stromal tumour: a randomised, double-blind, placebo-controlled trial. *Lancet.* 2009;373:1097–1104.
48. Joensuu H, Eriksson M, Sundby Hall K, et al. Adjuvant imatinib for high-risk GI stromal tumor: analysis of a randomized trial. *J Clin Oncol.* 2016;34:244–250.
49. Corey B, Chen H. Neuroendocrine tumors of the stomach. *Surg Clin North Am.* 2017;97:333–343.
50. Wani ZA, Bhat RA, Bhadoria AS, et al. Gastric varices: classification, endoscopic and ultrasonographic management. *J Res Med Sci.* 2015;20:1200–1207.

50 CHAPTER

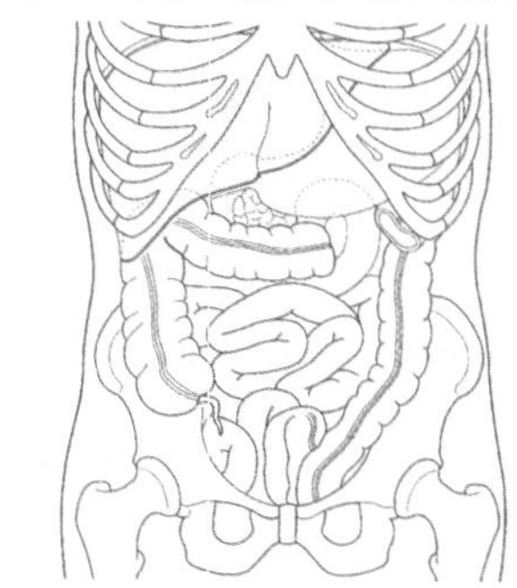

Small Intestine

Tong Gan, B. Mark Evers

OUTLINE

The small intestine is a marvel of complexity and efficiency. The primary role of the small intestine is the digestion and absorption of dietary components after they leave the stomach. This process depends on a multitude of structural, physiologic, endocrine, and chemical factors. Exocrine secretions from the liver and pancreas enable complete digestion of the ingested dietary components. The enlarged surface area of the small intestinal mucosa then absorbs these nutrients. In addition to its role in digestion and absorption, the small bowel is the largest endocrine organ in the body and one of the most important organs of immune function. Indeed, given its essential role and complexity, it is amazing that diseases of the small bowel are not more frequent. This chapter describes the normal anatomy and physiology of the small intestine as well as disease processes, including obstruction, inflammatory and infectious diseases, neoplasms, diverticular disease, and miscellaneous disorders.

EMBRYOLOGY

The primitive gut is formed from the endodermal lining, the yolk sac, which is enveloped by the developing embryo as a result of cranial and caudal folding during the fourth week of fetal human gestation.[1] The endodermal layer gives rise to the epithelial lining of the digestive tract, and the splanchnic mesoderm surrounding the endoderm gives rise to the muscular connective tissue and all the other layers of the intestine. The splanchnic mesoderm also wraps around the gut tube to form the mesenteries that suspend the gut within the body cavity; the mesoderm immediately adjacent to the endodermal tube also contributes to most of the wall of the gut tube. Nerves and neurons found in the wall are derived from the neural crest. Except for the duodenum, which is a primitive foregut structure, the small intestine is derived from the midgut. During the fifth week of fetal development, when the intestinal length is rapidly increasing, herniation of the midgut occurs through the umbilicus (Fig. 50.1). This midgut loop has a cranial and caudal limb, with the cranial limb developing into the distal duodenum, jejunum, and proximal ileum and the caudal limb becoming the distal ileum and proximal two thirds of the transverse colon. The juncture of the cranial and caudal limbs is where the vitelline duct joins to the yolk sac. This duct structure normally becomes obliterated before birth; however, it can persist as a Meckel diverticulum in approximately 2% of the population. As the gut tube develops, the endoderm proliferates rapidly and temporarily occludes the lumen of the tube around the fifth week of gestation. Growth and expansion of mesoderm components in

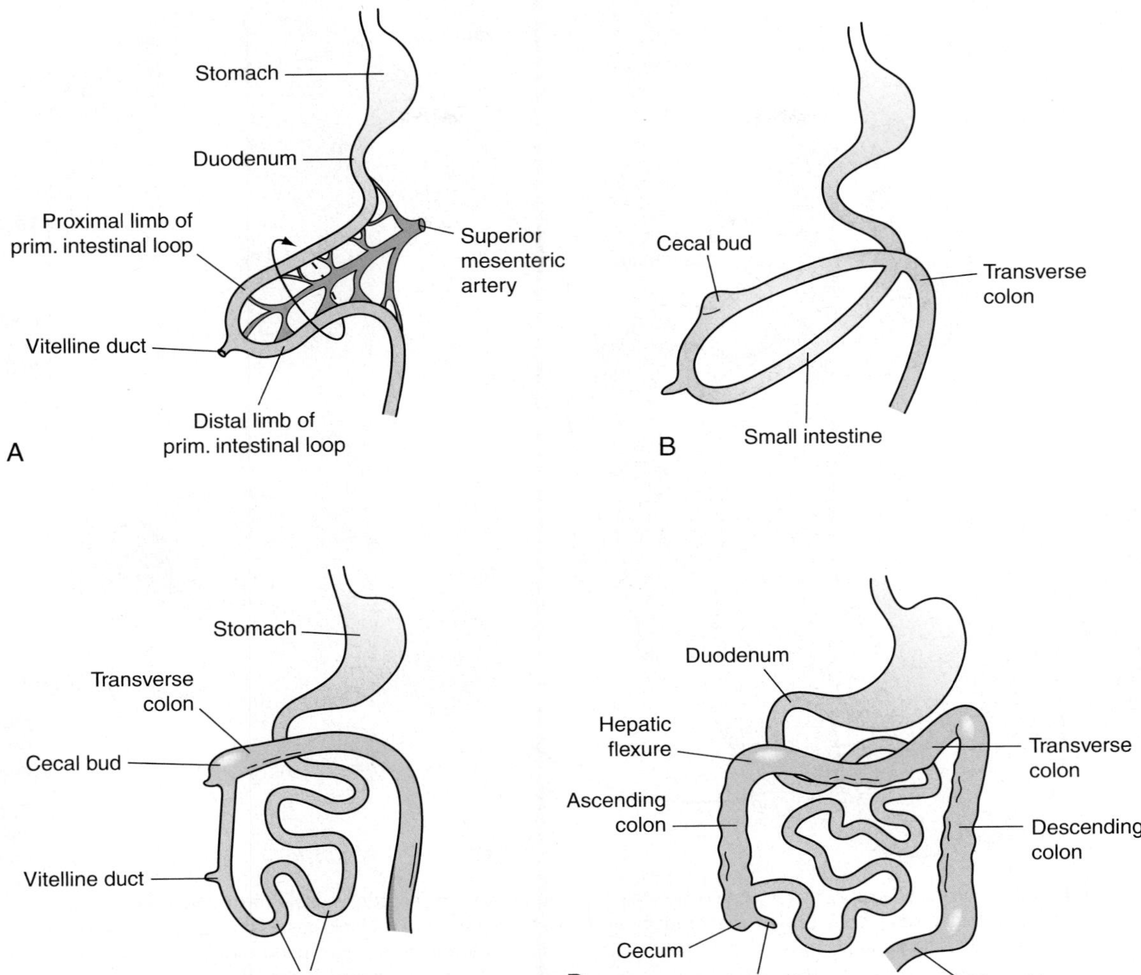

FIG. 50.1 Rotation of the Intestine. (A) The intestine after a 90-degree rotation around the axis of the superior mesenteric artery, the proximal loop on the right, and the distal loop on the left. (B) The intestinal loop after a further 180-degree rotation. The transverse colon passes in front of the duodenum. (C) Position of the intestinal loops after reentry into the abdominal cavity. Note the elongation of the small intestine, with formation of the small intestine loops. (D) Final position of the intestines after descent of the cecum into the right iliac fossa. (From Podolsky DK, Babyatshy MW. Growth and development of the gastrointestinal tract. In: Yamada T, ed. *Textbook of Gastroenterology*. Vol 2. Philadelphia: JB Lippincott; 1995.)

the wall, coupled with apoptosis of the endoderm during the seventh week, result in recanalization of the tube, and by the ninth week of gestation, the tube is again patent. Midgut herniation persists until about 10 weeks of fetal gestation, when the intestine returns to the abdominal cavity. After completing a 270-degree rotation from its initial starting point, the proximal jejunum reenters the abdomen and occupies the left side of the abdomen, with subsequent loops lying more to the right. The cecum enters last and is located temporarily in the right upper quadrant; however, with time, it descends to its normal position in the right lower quadrant.[1] Congenital anomalies of gut malrotation and fixation can occur during this process.

The primitive small bowel is lined by a sheet of cuboidal cells until about the ninth week of gestation, when villi begin to form in the proximal intestine and then proceed in a caudal fashion until the entire small bowel, and even the colon, for a time, is lined by these finger-like projections. Crypt formation begins in the 10th to 12th weeks of gestation. The crypt layer of the small bowel is the site of continual cell renewal and proliferation. As the cells ascend the crypt-villous axis, proliferation ceases, and cells differentiate into one of the four main cell types: absorptive enterocytes, which compose about 95% of the intestinal cell population; goblet cells; Paneth cells; and enteroendocrine cells. An important distinction regarding Paneth cells is that they remain in the crypt bases, where they protect intestinal stem cells from damage by releasing signaling molecules that affect the host tissues and influence the microbial populations to maintain homeostasis in the intestine.[2] The other differentiating cells ascending the crypt-villous axis are eventually extruded into the intestinal lumen. Amazingly, with the exception of Paneth cells, epithelial cell turnover occurs rapidly, with a life span of 3 to 5 days in humans.

ANATOMY

Gross Anatomy

The entire small intestine, which extends from the pylorus to the cecum, measures 270 to 290 cm, with duodenal length estimated at approximately 20 cm, jejunal length at 100 to 110 cm, and ileal

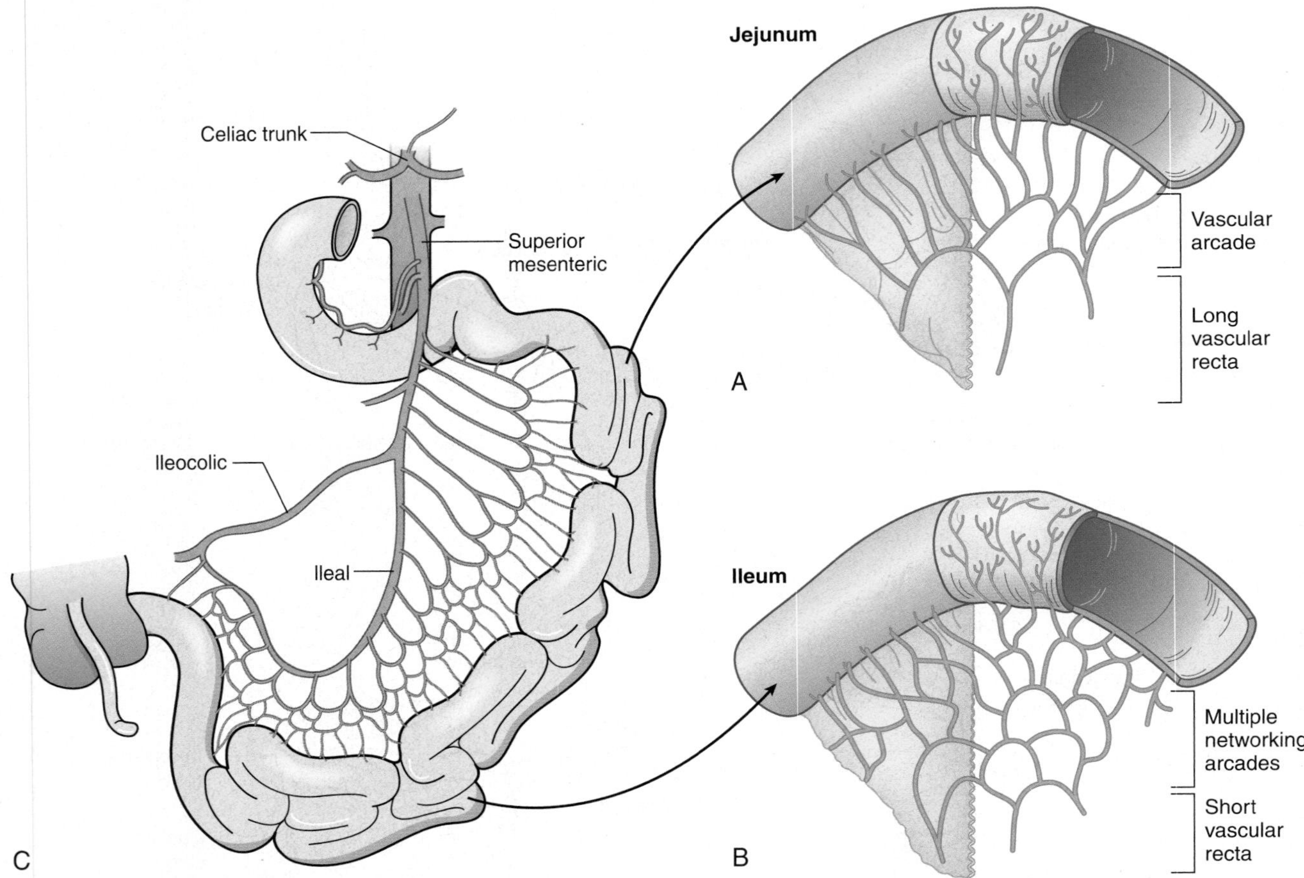

FIG. 50.2 Vascular supply of the small intestine. (A) The jejunal mesenteric vessels form only one or two arcades with long vasa recta. (B) The mesenteric vessels of the ileum form multiple vascular arcades with short vasa recta. (C) The superior mesenteric artery, which courses anterior to the third portion of the duodenum, provides blood supply to the jejunoileum and distal duodenum. The celiac artery supplies the proximal duodenum. (Adapted from Keljo DJ, Gariepy CE. Anatomy, histology, embryology, and developmental anomalies of the small and large intestine. In: Feldman M, Scharschmidt BF, Sleisenger MH, eds. *Sleisenger and Fordtran's Gastrointestinal and Liver Disease: Pathology, Diagnosis, Management*. Philadelphia: WB Saunders; 2002:1646; illustration courtesy Matt Hazzard, University of Kentucky Medical Center, Lexington, KY.)

length at 150 to 160 cm. The jejunum begins at the duodenojejunal angle, which is supported by a peritoneal fold known as the *ligament of Treitz*. There is no obvious demarcation between the jejunum and the ileum; by convention, the jejunum comprises the proximal two-fifths of the small intestine, and the ileum makes up the remaining three fifths. The jejunum has a somewhat larger circumference, is thicker than the ileum, and can be identified during surgery by examining mesenteric vessels (Fig. 50.2A). In the jejunum, only one or two arcades send out long, straight vasa recta to the mesenteric border, whereas the blood supply to the ileum may have four or five separate arcades with shorter vasa recta (Fig. 50.2B) The mucosa of the small bowel is characterized by transverse folds (plicae circulares), which are prominent in the distal duodenum and jejunum.

Neurovascular-Lymphatic Supply

The small intestine is served by rich vascular, neural, and lymphatic supplies, all traversing through the mesentery. The base of the mesentery attaches to the posterior abdominal wall to the left of the second lumbar vertebra and passes obliquely to the right and inferiorly to the right sacroiliac joint. The blood supply of the small bowel, except for the proximal duodenum, which is supplied by branches of the celiac axis, comes entirely from the superior mesenteric artery (Fig. 50.2C). The superior mesenteric artery courses anterior to the uncinate process of the pancreas and the third portion of the duodenum, where it divides to supply the pancreas, distal duodenum, entire small intestine, and ascending and transverse colons. There is an abundant collateral blood supply to the small bowel provided by vascular arcades coursing in the mesentery. Venous drainage of the small bowel parallels the arterial supply, with blood draining into the superior mesenteric vein, which joins the splenic vein behind the neck of the pancreas to form the portal vein.

The innervation of the small bowel is provided by parasympathetic and sympathetic divisions of the autonomic nervous system that, in turn, provide efferent nerves to the small intestine. The parasympathetic fibers derive from the vagus nerve; they traverse the celiac ganglion and influence secretion, motility, and probably all phases of bowel activity. Vagal afferent fibers are present but apparently do not carry pain impulses. The sympathetic fibers come from three sets of splanchnic nerves; their ganglion cells usually are located in a plexus around the base of the superior mesenteric artery. Motor impulses affect blood vessel motility and probably gut secretion and motility. Pain from the intestine is transmitted through general visceral afferent fibers of the sympathetic system.

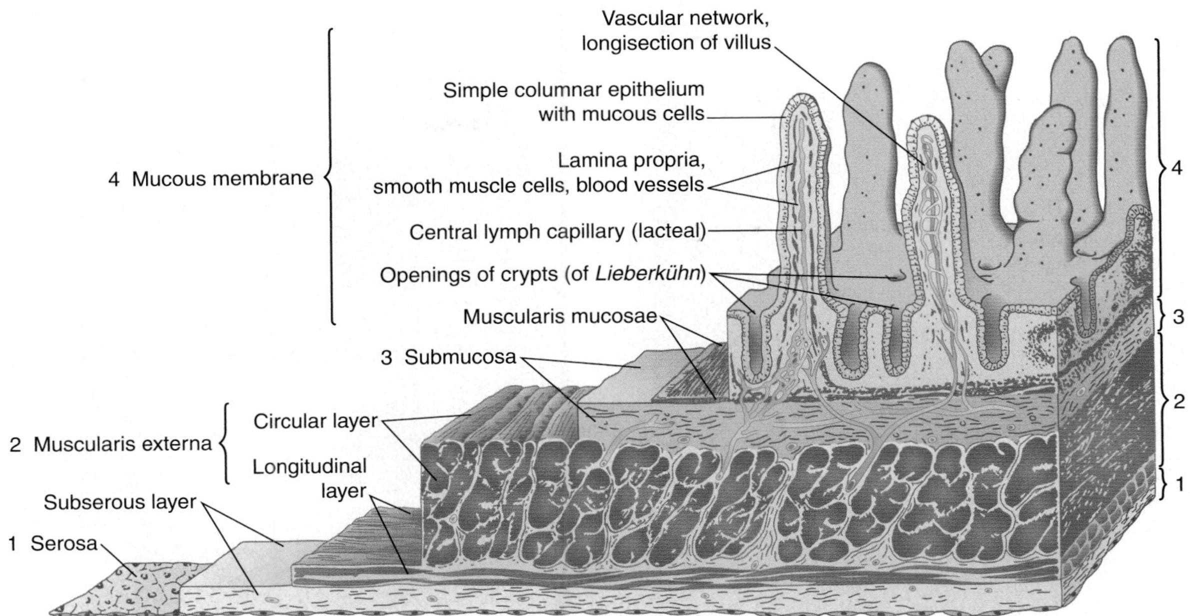

FIG. 50.3 Layers of the small intestine. A large surface is provided by villi for the absorption of required nutriments. The solitary lymph follicles in the lamina propria of the mucous membrane are not labeled. In the stroma of both sectioned villi are shown the central chyle (lacteal) vessels or villous capillaries. (From Sobotta J, Figge FHJ, Hild WJ. *Atlas of Human Anatomy*. New York: Hafner; 1974.)

Small intestine lymphatics are noted as major deposits of lymphatic tissue, particularly in the Peyer patches of the distal small bowel. Lymphatic drainage proceeds from the mucosa through the wall of the bowel to a set of nodes adjacent to the bowel in the mesentery. Drainage continues to a group of regional nodes adjacent to the mesenteric arterial arcades and then to a group at the base of the superior mesenteric vessels. From there, lymph flows into the cisterna chyli and then up the thoracic duct, ultimately to empty into the venous system at the confluence of the left internal jugular and subclavian veins. The lymphatic drainage of the small intestine plays a major role in immune defense, constitutes a major transport route of absorbed lipid into the circulation and also in the spread of cells arising from cancers of the gut.

Microscopic Anatomy

The small bowel wall consists of four layers: serosa, muscularis propria, submucosa, and mucosa (Fig. 50.3).

The serosa is the outermost layer of the small intestine and consists of visceral peritoneum, a single layer of flattened mesoepithelial cells that encircles the jejunoileum, and the anterior surface of the duodenum.

The muscularis propria consists of two muscle layers, a thin outer longitudinal layer and a thicker inner circular layer of smooth muscle. Ganglion cells from the myenteric (Auerbach) plexus are interposed between the muscle layers and send neural fibers into both layers, thus providing electrical continuity between the smooth muscle cells and permitting conduction through the muscle layer.

The submucosa consists of a layer of fibroelastic connective tissue containing blood vessels and nerves. It is the strongest component of the intestinal wall and therefore must be included in anastomotic sutures. It contains elaborate networks of lymphatics, arterioles, and venules and an extensive plexus of nerve fibers and ganglion cells (Meissner plexus). The nerves from the mucosa and submucosa muscle layers are interconnected by small nerve fibers; cross-connections between adrenergic and cholinergic elements have been described.

The mucosa has three layers: muscularis mucosae, lamina propria, and epithelial layers (Fig. 50.4). The muscularis mucosae is a thin layer of muscle that separates the mucosa from the submucosa. The lamina propria is a connective tissue layer between the epithelial cells and muscularis mucosae that contains a variety of cells, including plasma cells, lymphocytes, mast cells, eosinophils, macrophages, fibroblasts, smooth muscle cells, and noncellular connective tissue. The lamina propria, the base on which the epithelial cells lie, performs a protective role in the intestine; due to a rich supply of immune cells, it combats microorganisms that penetrate the overlying epithelium. Plasma cells actively synthesize immunoglobulins and other immune cells in the lamina propria and release mediators (e.g., cytokines, arachidonic acid metabolites, histamines) that can modulate the cellular functions of the overlying epithelium. The epithelial layer is a continual sheet of epithelial cells covering the villi and lining the crypts. The main functions of the crypt epithelium are cell renewal as well as exocrine, endocrine, water, and ion secretion; the main functions of the villous epithelium are digestion and absorption. Four main cell types are contained in the mucosal layer: (i) absorptive enterocytes; (ii) goblet cells, which secrete mucus; (iii) Paneth cells, which secrete lysozyme, tumor necrosis factor (TNF), and cryptdins, which are homologues of leukocyte defensin peptides thought to be related to the host mucosal defense system; and (iv) enteroendocrine cells, of which there are more than 15 distinct populations that produce the gastrointestinal hormones. The enteroendocrine cells also secrete a wide range of peptide hormones that, in a complex manner, control physiologic and homeostatic functions in the digestive tract, particularly postprandial secretion and motility.

The mucosa is designed for maximal absorptive surface area, with villi protruding into the lumen on microscopic examination. Villi are tallest in the distal duodenum and proximal jejunum and shortest in the distal ileum. Absorptive enterocytes represent the

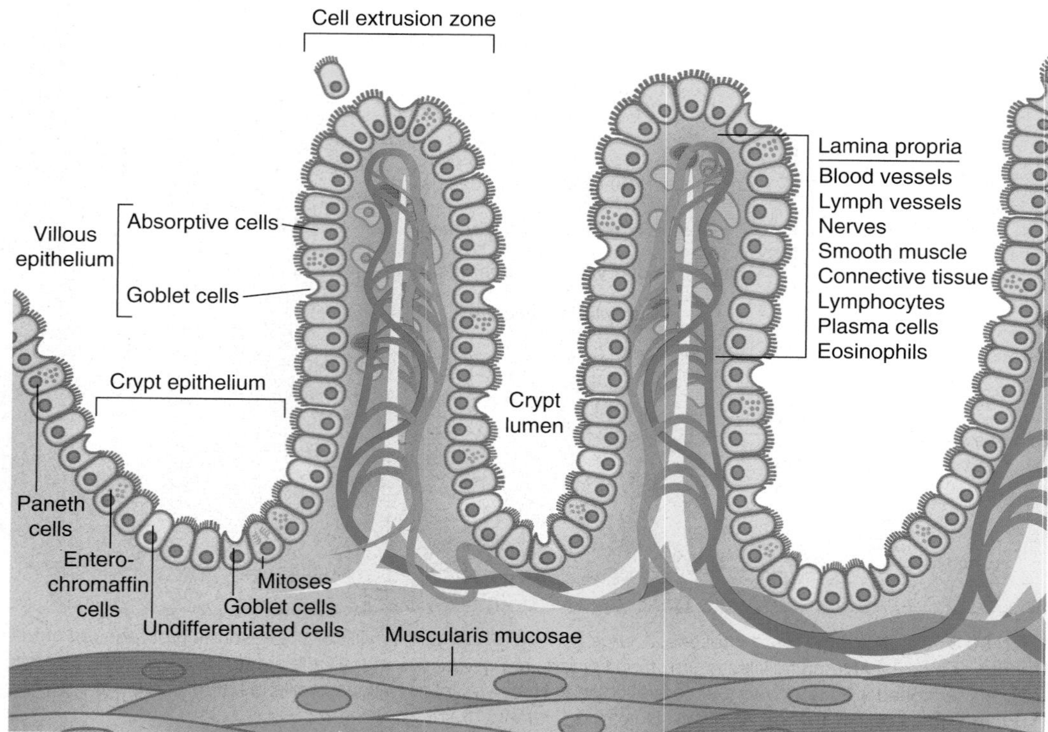

FIG. 50.4 Schematic diagram of the histologic organization of the small intestinal mucosa. (Adapted from Keljo DJ, Gariepy CE. anatomy, histology, embryology, and developmental anomalies of the small and large intestine. In: Feldman M, Scharschmidt BF, Sleisenger MH, eds. *Sleisenger and Fordtran's Gastrointestinal and Liver Disease: Pathology, Diagnosis, Management.* Philadelphia: WB Saunders; 2002:646.)

main cell type in the mucosa and are responsible for digestion and absorption. Their luminal surface is covered by microvilli that rest on a terminal web. The microvilli increase the absorptive capacity by 30-fold. To increase absorption further, the microvilli are covered by a fuzzy coat of glycoprotein called the glycocalyx.

PHYSIOLOGY

Digestion and Absorption

The complex process of digestion and eventual absorption of nutrients, water, electrolytes, and minerals is the main role of the small intestine. Liters of water and hundreds of grams of chyme are delivered to the small intestine daily, and with remarkable efficiency, almost all food is absorbed, except for indigestible cellulose. The stomach initiates the process of digestion with the breakdown of solids to particles 1 mm or smaller, which are then delivered to the duodenum, where pancreatic enzymes, bile, and brush border enzymes continue the process of digestion and eventual absorption through the small intestinal wall.[3] The small bowel is primarily responsible for absorption of the dietary components (carbohydrates, proteins, and fats) as well as trace elements, vitamins, and water.

Carbohydrates

An adult consuming a normal Western diet will ingest 300 to 350 g of carbohydrates a day, with about 50% consumed as starch, 30% as sucrose, 6% as lactose, and the remainder as maltose, trehalose, glucose, fructose, sorbitol, cellulose, and pectins.[3] Dietary starch is a polysaccharide consisting of long chains of glucose molecules. Amylose makes up about 20% of starch in the diet and is broken down at the α-1,4 bonds by salivary (i.e., ptyalin) and pancreatic amylases that convert amylose to maltotriose and maltose. Amylopectin constitutes about 80% of dietary starch and has branch points every 25 molecules along the straight glucose chains; the α-1,6 glucose linkages in amylopectin identify the end products of amylase digestion—maltose, maltotriose, and the residual branch saccharides, the dextrins. In general, the starches are almost totally converted into maltose and other small glucose polymers before they reach the duodenum or upper jejunum. The remainder of carbohydrate digestion occurs as a result of brush border enzymes of the luminal surface.

The brush border of the small intestine contains the enzymes lactase, maltase, sucrase-isomaltase, and trehalase, which split the disaccharides as well as other small glucose polymers into their constituent monosaccharides (Table 50.1). Lactase hydrolyzes lactose into glucose and galactose. Maltase hydrolyzes maltose to produce glucose monomers. Sucrase-isomaltase is a complex with two subunits; sucrase hydrolyzes sucrose to yield glucose and fructose, and isomaltase hydrolyzes the α-1,6 bonds in α-limit dextrins to yield glucose. Glucose represents more than 80% of the final product of carbohydrate digestion, with galactose and fructose usually representing no more than 10% of the products of carbohydrate digestion.

Carbohydrates are absorbed as monosaccharides. Transport of the released hexoses (glucose, galactose, and fructose) is by specific mechanisms involved in active transport. The major routes of absorption are by three membrane carrier systems (Fig. 50.5): sodium-glucose transporter 1 (SGLT-1), glucose transporter 5 (GLUT-5), and glucose transporter 2 (GLUT-2).[3] Glucose and galactose are absorbed by a carrier-mediated active transport mechanism, which involves the cotransport of sodium (SGLT-1 transporter). As sodium diffuses into the inside of the cell, it pulls

TABLE 50.1 Characteristics of brush border membrane carbohydrases.

ENZYME	SUBSTRATE	PRODUCTS
Lactase	Lactose galactose	Glucose
Maltase (glucoamylase)	α-1,4-Linked oligosaccharides, up to nine residues	Glucose
Sucrase-isomaltase (sucrose-α-dextrinase)		
Sucrase	Sucrose	Glucose Fructose
Isomaltase	α-Limit dextrin	Glucose
Both enzymes	α-Limit dextrin	
	α-1,4-Link at nonreducing end	Glucose
Trehalase	Trehalose	Glucose

From Marsh MN, Riley SA. Digestion and absorption of nutrients and vitamins. In: Feldman M, Scharschmidt BF, Sleisenger MH, eds. *Sleisenger and Fordtran's Gastrointestinal and Liver Disease: Pathophysiology, Diagnosis, Management.* Vol 2. Philadelphia: WB Saunders; 1998:1480.

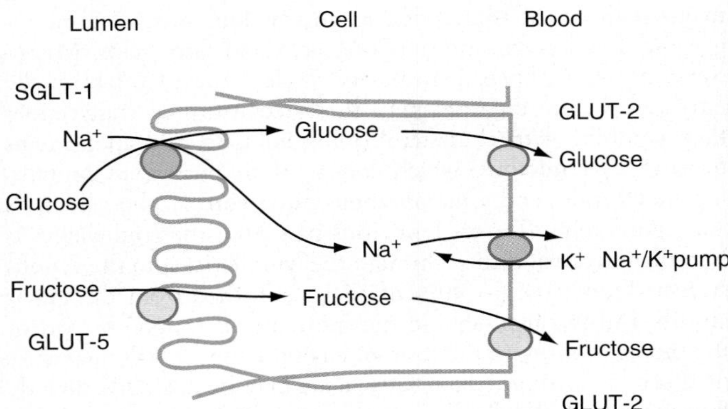

FIG. 50.5 Model for glucose, galactose, and fructose transport across the intestinal epithelium. Glucose and galactose are transported into the enterocyte across the brush border membrane by the sodium-glucose cotransporter *(SGLT-1)* and then transported out across the basolateral membrane down their concentration gradients by glucose transporter-2 *(GLUT-2)*. The low intracellular sodium concentration driving uphill sugar transport across the brush border is maintained by the Na^+,K^+ pump on the basolateral membrane. Glucose and galactose therefore stimulate sodium absorption across the epithelium. Fructose is transported across the cell down the concentration gradient across the brush border and basolateral membranes. Glucose transporter-5 *(GLUT-5)* is the brush border fructose transporter, whereas GLUT-2 handles fructose transport across the basolateral membrane. (From Wright EM, Hirayama BA, Loo DDF, et al. Intestinal sugar transport. In: Johnson LR, Alpers DH, Christensen J, et al, eds. *Physiology of the Gastrointestinal Tract.* 3rd ed, vol 2. New York: Raven Press; 1994:1752.)

the glucose or galactose along with it, thus providing the energy for transport of the monosaccharide. The exit of glucose from the cytosol into the intracellular space is achieved predominantly by a sodium-independent carrier (GLUT-2 transporter) located at the basolateral membrane of enterocytes. Fructose, the other significant monosaccharide, is also absorbed from the intestinal lumen through facilitated diffusion. This carrier, GLUT-5, is located in the apical membrane of the enterocytes. In contrast to SGLT-1, this transport process does not depend on sodium or energy. Fructose exits the basolateral membrane by another facilitated diffusion process involving the GLUT-2 transporter.

Protein

Protein digestion is initiated in the stomach, where gastric acid denatures proteins.[3] Digestion continues in the small intestine, where protein comes into contact with pancreatic proteases. Pancreatic trypsinogen is secreted in the intestine by the pancreas in an inactive form but becomes activated by the enzyme enterokinase, a brush border enzyme in the duodenum to an activated form of trypsin. Trypsin then activates the other pancreatic proteolytic enzyme precursors. The endopeptidases, which include trypsin, chymotrypsin, and elastase, act on peptide bonds at the interior of the protein molecule, producing peptides that are substrates for the exopeptidases (carboxypeptidases), which serially remove a single amino acid from the carboxyl end of the peptide (Table 50.2). This process results in splitting of the complex proteins into dipeptides, tripeptides, and some larger proteins, which are absorbed from the intestinal lumen by a sodium-mediated active transport mechanism and digested further by enzymes in the brush border and in the cytoplasm of enterocytes (Fig. 50.6). These peptidase enzymes include aminopeptidases and several dipeptidases, which split the remaining larger polypeptides into tripeptides and dipeptides and some amino acids. The amino acids, dipeptides, and tripeptides are easily transported through the microvilli into the epithelial cells, where, in the cytosol, additional peptidases hydrolyze the dipeptides and tripeptides into single amino acids; these molecules then pass through the epithelial cell membrane into the portal venous system. In normal humans, digestion and absorption of protein are usually 80% to 90% completed in the jejunum.

Fats

Emulsification. Most adults in North America consume 60 to 100 g/day of fat. Triglycerides, the most abundant fats, are composed of a glycerol nucleus and three fatty acids; small quantities of phospholipids, cholesterol, and cholesterol esters also are found in the normal diet. Essentially all fat digestion occurs in the small intestine, where the first step is the breakdown of fat globules into smaller sizes to facilitate further breakdown by water-soluble digestive enzymes, a process termed emulsification.[3] This process is facilitated by bile from the liver, which contains bile salts and the phospholipid lecithin. The polar regions of bile salts and the lecithin molecules are soluble in water, whereas the remaining portions are soluble in fat. Therefore, the fat-soluble portions interact with the surface layer of the fat globules, and the polar portions, projecting outward, are soluble in the surrounding aqueous fluids. This arrangement renders the fat globules more accessible to fragmentation by agitation in the small intestine. Therefore, a major function of bile salts, and especially lecithin, is to allow the fat globules to be fragmented by agitation in the intestinal lumen, which increases the fat globule surface area. With the increase in surface area, the fats are now readily attacked by pancreatic lipase,

TABLE 50.2 **Principal pancreatic proteases.**

ENZYME	PRIMARY ACTION
Endopeptidases	Hydrolyze interior peptide bonds of polypeptides and proteins
Trypsin	Attacks peptide bonds involving basic amino acids; yields products with basic amino acids at carboxyl-terminal end
Chymotrypsin	Attacks peptide bonds involving aromatic amino acids, leucine, glutamine, and methionine; yields peptide products with these amino acids at carboxyl-terminal end
Elastase	Attacks peptide bonds involving neutral aliphatic amino acids; yields products with neutral amino acids at carboxyl-terminal end
Exopeptidases	Hydrolyze external peptide bonds of polypeptides and protein
Carboxypeptidase A	Attacks peptides with aromatic and neutral aliphatic amino acids at carboxyl-terminal end
Carboxypeptidase B	Attacks peptides with basic amino acids at carboxyl-terminal end

From Castro GA. Digestion and absorption. In: Johnson LR, ed. *Gastrointestinal Physiology.* St. Louis: Mosby; 1991:108–130.

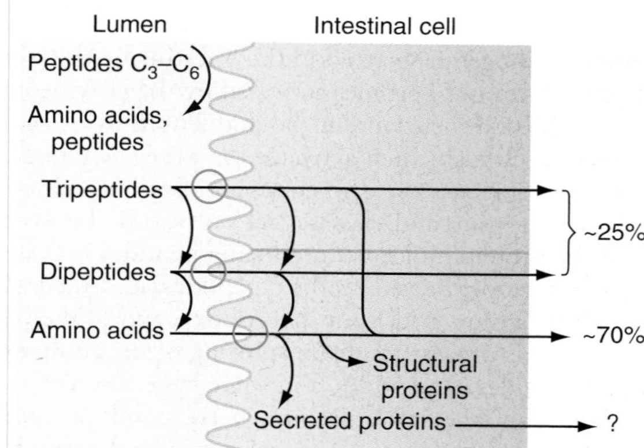

FIG. 50.6 Digestion and absorption of proteins. Endopeptidases and exopeptidases split complex proteins into dipeptides and tripeptides, which are absorbed from the intestinal lumen by a sodium-mediated active transport mechanism. These peptides are further digested by enzymes in the brush border and within enterocytes. (Adapted from Alpers DH. Digestion and absorption of carbohydrates and proteins. In: Johnson LR, Alpers DH, Christensen J, et al, eds. *Physiology of the Gastrointestinal Tract.* 3rd ed, vol 2. New York: Raven Press; 1994:1733.)

the most crucial enzyme in the digestion of triglycerides, which splits triglycerides into free fatty acids and 2-monoglycerides.

Micelle formation. Fat digestion is accelerated by bile salts, which, secondary to their amphipathic nature, can form micelles. Micelles are small spherical globules composed of 20 to 40 molecules of bile salts with a sterol nucleus that is highly fat soluble, and a hydrophilic polar group that projects outward. The mixed micelles thus formed are arrayed so that the insoluble lipid is surrounded by the bile salts oriented with their hydrophilic ends facing outward. Therefore, as quickly as the monoglycerides and free fatty acids are formed by lipolysis, they become dissolved in the central hydrophobic portion of the micelles, which then act to carry these products of fat hydrolysis to the brush borders of the epithelial cells, where absorption occurs.

Intracellular processing. The monoglycerides and free fatty acids, which are incorporated into the central lipid portion of the bile acid micelles, are absorbed through the brush border because of their highly lipid-soluble nature and simply diffuse into the interior of the cell.[3] After disaggregation of the micelle, bile salts remain within the intestinal lumen to repeat the process by the formation of new micelles and carry more monoglycerides and fatty acids to the epithelial cells. Inside the cell, the released fatty acids and monoglycerides reform into triglycerides. This reformation of a triglyceride occurs through the interactions of intracellular enzymes that are associated with the endoplasmic reticulum. The major pathway of triglyceride reconstruction involves 2-monoglycerides and coenzyme A (CoA)–activated fatty acids. Microsomal acyl-CoA lipase is necessary to cleave acyl-CoA from the fatty acid before esterification. These reconstituted triglycerides then combine with cholesterol, phospholipids, and apoproteins to form chylomicrons, which consist of an inner core containing triglycerides and a membranous outer core of phospholipids and apoproteins. The chylomicrons pass from the epithelial cells into the lacteals and then through the lymphatics into the venous system. From 80% to 90% of all fat absorbed from the gut is absorbed in this manner and transported to the blood by way of the thoracic lymph in the form of chylomicrons. Small quantities of short- to medium-chain fatty acids may be absorbed directly into the portal blood rather than being converted into triglycerides and absorbed into the lymphatics. These shorter-chain fatty acids are more water soluble, which allows direct diffusion into the bloodstream.

Enterohepatic circulation. The proximal intestine absorbs most of the dietary fat. Although unconjugated bile acids are absorbed into the jejunum by passive diffusion, the conjugated bile acids that form micelles are absorbed in the ileum by active transport, then reabsorbed from the distal ileum and pass through the portal venous system to the liver for secretion as bile. The total bile acid pool (approximately 2–3 g) recirculates about six times every 24 hours through the enterohepatic circulation.[3] Almost all the bile salts are reabsorbed, with only about 0.5 g lost in the stool every day; this loss is replaced by newly synthesized bile acids from cholesterol.

Water, Electrolytes, and Vitamins

Every day, 8 to 10 L of water enter the small intestine. Much of this is absorbed, with approximately 500 mL or less leaving the ileum and entering the colon (Fig. 50.7).[3] Water may be absorbed by the process of simple diffusion. In addition, water may be drawn in and out of the cell through a process of osmotic pressure, resulting from active transport of sodium, glucose, or amino acids into cells.

Electrolytes can be absorbed in the small bowel by active transport or by coupling to an organic solute.[3] Na^+ is absorbed by active transport through the basolateral membranes. Cl^- is absorbed in the upper part of the small intestine by a process of passive diffusion. Large quantities of HCO_3^- must be reabsorbed, which is accomplished in an indirect fashion. As Na^+ is absorbed, H^+ is secreted into the lumen of the intestine. Inside the lumen, H^+ combines with HCO_3^- to form carbonic acid, which then dissociates to form water and carbon dioxide. The water remains in the

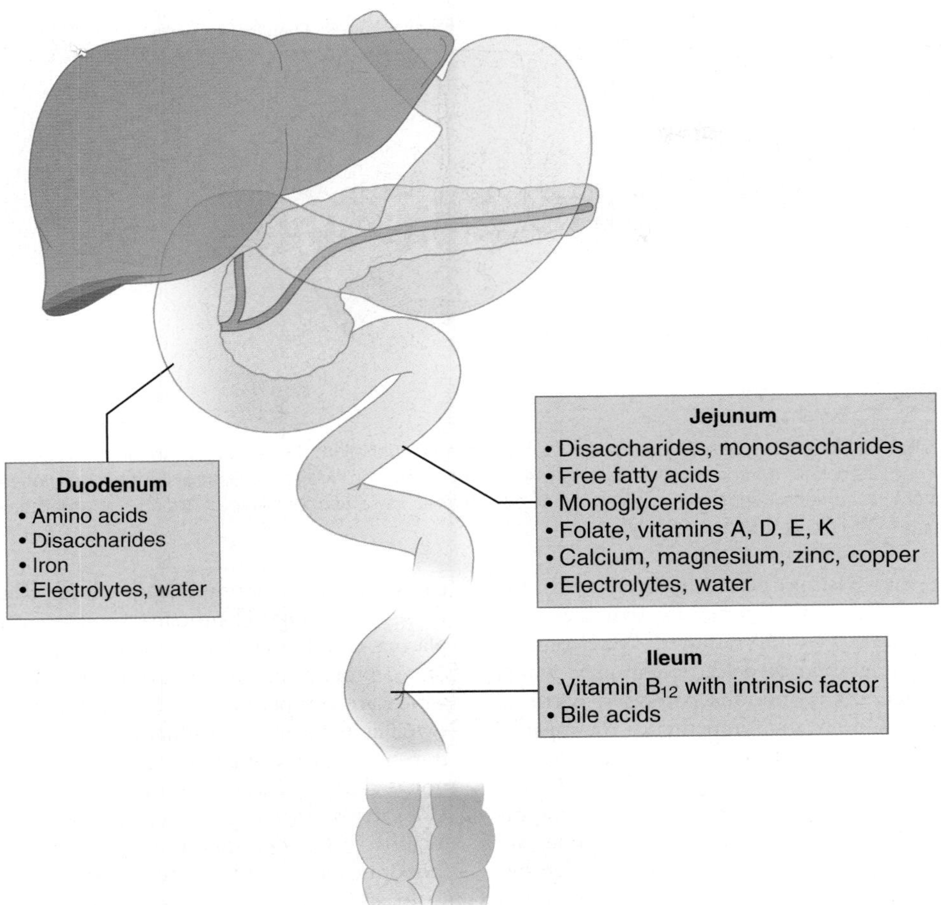

FIG. 50.7 Absorption of water, electrolytes, and nutrients in the small bowel. Each segment of small intestines play different roles in the absorption of micro and macronutrients. (Adapted from Westergaard H. Short bowel syndrome. In: Feldman M, Scharschmidt BF, Sleisenger MH, eds. *Sleisenger and Fordtran's Gastrointestinal and Liver Disease: Pathology, Diagnosis, Management*. Philadelphia: WB Saunders; 2002:1549.)

chyme, but the carbon dioxide is readily absorbed into the blood and is subsequently expired. Calcium is absorbed, particularly in the proximal intestine (duodenum and jejunum), by a process of active transport; absorption appears to be facilitated by an acid environment and is enhanced by vitamin D and parathyroid hormone. Iron is absorbed as a heme or nonheme component in the duodenum by an active process. The iron is then either deposited within the cell as ferritin or transferred to the plasma bound to transferrin. The total absorption of iron is dependent on body stores of iron and the rate of erythropoiesis; any increase in erythropoiesis increases iron absorption. Potassium, magnesium, phosphate, and other ions also can be actively absorbed throughout the mucosa.

Vitamins are fat soluble (e.g., vitamins A, D, E, and K) or water soluble (e.g., ascorbic acid [vitamin C], biotin, nicotinic acid, folic acid, riboflavin [vitamin B_2], thiamine [vitamin B_1], pyridoxine [vitamin B_6], and cobalamin [vitamin B_{12}]).[3] The fat-soluble vitamins are carried in mixed micelles and transported in chylomicrons of the lymph to the thoracic duct and into the venous system. The absorption of water-soluble vitamins appears to be more complex than originally thought. Vitamin C is absorbed by an active transport process that incorporates a sodium-coupled mechanism as well as a specific carrier system. Vitamin B_6 appears to be rapidly absorbed by simple diffusion into the proximal intestine. Vitamin B_1 is rapidly absorbed in the jejunum by an active process similar to the sodium-coupled transport system for vitamin C. Vitamin B_2 is absorbed in the upper intestine by facilitated transport. The absorption of vitamin B_{12} occurs primarily in the terminal ileum. Vitamin B_{12} is derived from cobalamin, which is freed in the duodenum by pancreatic proteases. The cobalamin binds to intrinsic factor, which is secreted by the stomach, and is protected from proteolytic digestion. Specific receptors in the terminal ileum take up the cobalamin–intrinsic factor complex, probably by translocation. In the ileal enterocyte, free vitamin B_{12} is bound to an ileal pool of transcobalamin II, which transports it into the portal circulation.

MOTILITY

Food particles are propelled through the small bowel by a complex series of muscle contractions.[3] Peristalsis consists of intestinal contractions passing aborally at a rate of 1–2 cm/sec. The major function of peristalsis is the movement of intestinal chyme through the intestine. Motility patterns in the small bowel vary greatly between the fed and fasted states. Pacesetter potentials, which are thought to originate in the duodenum, initiate a series of contractions in the fed state that propel food through the small bowel.

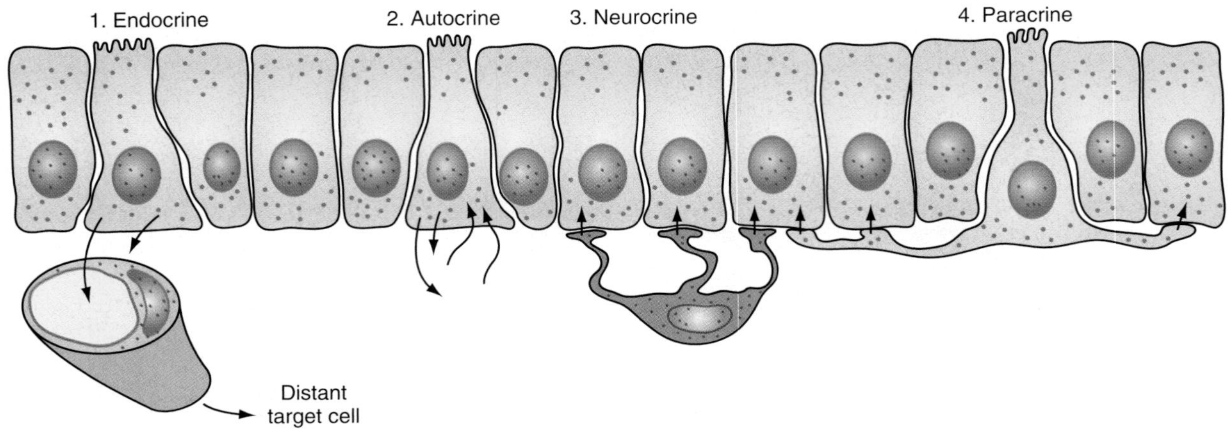

FIG. 50.8 Mechanisms of hormonal action in the intestinal epithelium. Intestinal hormones may act through endocrine, autocrine, neurocrine, or paracrine effects. (Adapted from Miller LJ. Gastrointestinal hormones and receptors. In: Yamada T, Alpers DH, Laine L, et al, eds. *Textbook of Gastroenterology.* 3rd ed, vol 1. Philadelphia: Lippincott Williams & Wilkins; 1999:37.)

During the interdigestive (fasting) period between meals, the bowel is regularly swept by cyclical contractions that move aborally along the intestine every 75 to 90 minutes. These contractions are initiated by the migrating myoelectric complex, which is under the control of neural and humoral pathways. Extrinsic nerves to the small bowel are vagal and sympathetic. The vagal fibers have two functionally different effects; one is cholinergic and excitatory, and the other is peptidergic and probably inhibitory. Sympathetic activity inhibits motor function, whereas parasympathetic activity stimulates it. Although intestinal hormones are known to affect small intestinal motility, the one peptide that has been clearly shown to function in this regard is motilin, which is found at its peak plasma level during phase III (intense bursts of myoelectrical activities resulting in regular, high-amplitude contractions) of migrating myoelectric complexes.

ENDOCRINE FUNCTION

Gastrointestinal Hormones

The gastrointestinal hormones are distributed along the length of the small bowel in a spatially specific pattern. In fact, the small bowel is the largest endocrine organ in the body. Although often classified as hormones, these agents do not always function in a true endocrine fashion (i.e., discharged into the bloodstream, where an action is produced at some distant site; Fig. 50.8). Sometimes, these peptides are discharged and act locally in a paracrine or autocrine manner. In contrast, some of these peptides may serve as neurotransmitters (e.g., vasoactive intestinal peptide). Gastrointestinal hormones play a major role in pancreaticobiliary and intestinal secretion, absorption, and motility. In addition, certain gastrointestinal hormones exert a trophic effect on normal and neoplastic intestinal mucosa and the pancreas. Moreover, recent studies show that certain hormones (e.g., neurotensin), when secreted in excess, can contribute to obesity, diabetes, and cardiovascular disease.[4] The location, major stimulants of release, and primary effects of the more important gastrointestinal hormones are summarized in Table 50.3. In addition, the diagnostic and therapeutic uses of gastrointestinal hormones are listed in Table 50.4.

Receptors

The gastrointestinal hormones interact with their cell surface receptors to initiate a cascade of signaling events that eventually culminate in their physiologic effects. These hormones primarily signal through G protein–coupled receptors that traverse the plasma membrane seven times and represent the largest group of receptors found in the body. The heterotrimeric G proteins, which are composed of α, β, and γ subunits, are the molecular switches for signal transduction. Agonist binding to the seven-transmembrane domain receptor is thought to cause a conformational change in the receptor that allows it to interact with the G proteins. Intracellular second messengers that are activated include cyclic adenosine monophosphate, Ca^{2+} cyclic guanosine monophosphate, and inositol phosphate.

In addition to the gastrointestinal hormones, receptors for a number of other peptides and growth factors are located in the gastrointestinal mucosa, including those for epidermal growth factor, transforming growth factor α and β, insulin-like growth factor (IGF), fibroblast growth factor, and platelet-derived growth factor (PDGF). These peptides play a role in cell growth and differentiation and act through tyrosine kinase receptors, which have a single membrane–spanning domain.

A third class of surface receptors, the ion channel–linked receptors, are found most commonly in cells of neuronal lineage and usually bind specific neurotransmitters. Examples include receptors for excitatory (acetylcholine and serotonin) and inhibitory (γ-aminobutyric acid and glycine) neurotransmitters. These receptors undergo a conformational change on binding of the mediator that allows passage of ions across the cell membrane and results in changes in voltage potential.

IMMUNE FUNCTION

During the course of a normal day, we ingest a number of bacteria, parasites, and viruses. The intestinal epithelium is a single layer of cells that serve as a major immunological barrier in addition to its important role in digestion and endocrine function. The small intestine has epithelial-lined villi that are absent in the colon; these villi significantly increase the surface area for the interaction with foreign pathogens. As a result of constant antigenic exposure, the intestine possesses abundant lymphoid cells (e.g., B and T lymphocytes) and myeloid cells (e.g., macrophages, neutrophils, eosinophils, mast cells). To deal with the constant barrage of potential toxins and antigens, the gut has evolved a highly organized and efficient mechanism for antigen processing, humoral

TABLE 50.3 Gastrointestinal hormones.

HORMONE	PRODUCED BY	MAJOR STIMULANTS OF PEPTIDE SECRETION	PRIMARY EFFECTS
Gastrin	Antrum, duodenum (G cells)	Peptides, amino acids, antral distention, vagal and adrenergic stimulation, gastrin-releasing peptide (bombesin)	Stimulates gastric acid and pepsinogen secretion Stimulates gastric mucosal growth
Cholecystokinin	Duodenum, jejunum (I cells)	Fats, peptides, amino acids	Stimulates pancreatic enzyme secretion Stimulates gallbladder contraction Relaxes sphincter of Oddi Inhibits gastric emptying
Secretin	Duodenum, jejunum (S cells)	Fatty acids, luminal acidity, bile salts	Stimulates release of water and bicarbonate from pancreatic ductal cells Stimulates flow and alkalinity of bile Inhibits gastric acid secretion and motility and inhibits gastrin release
Somatostatin	Pancreatic islets (D cells), antrum, duodenum	Gut: fat, protein, acid, other hormones (e.g., gastrin, cholecystokinin) Pancreas: glucose, amino acids, cholecystokinin	Universal "off" switch Inhibits release of gastrointestinal hormones Inhibits gastric acid secretion Inhibits small bowel water and electrolyte secretion Inhibits secretion of pancreatic hormones
Gastrin-releasing peptide (mammalian equivalent of bombesin)	Small bowel	Vagal stimulation	Universal "on" switch Stimulates release of all gastrointestinal hormones (except secretin) Stimulates gastrointestinal secretion and motility Stimulates gastric acid secretion and release of antral gastrin Stimulates growth of intestinal mucosa and pancreas
Gastric inhibitory polypeptide	Duodenum, jejunum (K cells)	Glucose, fat, protein adrenergic stimulation	Inhibits gastric acid and pepsin secretion Stimulates pancreatic insulin release in response to hyperglycemia
Motilin	Duodenum, jejunum	Gastric distention, fat	Stimulates upper gastrointestinal tract motility May initiate the migrating motor complex
Vasoactive intestinal peptide	Neurons throughout the gastrointestinal tract	Vagal stimulation	Primarily functions as a neuropeptide Potent vasodilator Stimulates pancreatic and intestinal secretion Inhibits gastric acid secretion
Neurotensin	Small bowel (N cells)	Fat	Stimulates growth of small and large bowel mucosa Facilitates absorption of fats in the intestine Stimulates growth of cancer with neurotensin receptors
Enteroglucagon	Small bowel (L cells)	Glucose, fat	Glucagon-like peptide 1 Stimulates insulin release Inhibits pancreatic glucagon release Glucagon-like peptide 2 Potent enterotrophic factor
Peptide YY	Distal small bowel, colon	Fatty acids, cholecystokinin	Inhibits gastric and pancreatic secretion Inhibits gallbladder contraction

Adapted from Rao JN, Wang JY. Regulation of gastrointestinal mucosal growth. In: *Role of GI Hormones on Gut Mucosal Growth*. 2nd ed. San Rafael, CA: Morgan & Claypool Life Sciences; 2010.

TABLE 50.4 Diagnostic and therapeutic uses of gastrointestinal hormones.

HORMONE	DIAGNOSTIC AND THERAPEUTIC USES
Gastrin	Pentagastrin (gastrin analogue) used to measure maximal gastric acid secretion
Cholecystokinin	Biliary imaging of gallbladder contraction
Secretin	Provocative test for gastrinoma Measurement of maximal pancreatic secretion
Glucagon	Suppresses bowel motility for endocrine spasm Relieves sphincter of Oddi spasm Provocative test for insulin, catecholamine, and growth hormone release Intraoperative relaxation of sphincter of Oddi to stimulate passage of common bile duct stone
Somatostatin analogs	Treat carcinoid diarrhea and flushing Decrease secretion from pancreatic and intestinal fistulas Ameliorate symptoms associated with hormone-overproducing endocrine tumors Treat esophageal variceal bleeding Used in imaging studies to localize somatostatin sensitive neuroendocrine tumors

Adapted from Townsend CM Jr, Thompson JC. The clinical use of gastrointestinal hormones for alimentary tract disease. *Adv Surg*. 1996;29:79–92; and Brubaker PL. Gut hormones fulfill their destiny: from basic physiology to the clinic. *Annu Rev Physiol*. 2-14;76:515-517.

immunity, and cellular immunity. The gut-associated lymphoid tissue is localized in four areas—Peyer patches, lamina propria lymphoid cells, Paneth cells, and intraepithelial lymphocytes.

Peyer patches are unencapsulated lymphoid nodules that constitute an afferent limb of the gut-associated lymphoid tissue, which recognizes antigens through a specialized sampling mechanism by the microfold (M) cells contained within the follicle-associated epithelium (Fig. 50.9). Antigens that gain access to Peyer patches activate and prime B and T cells in that site. The M cells cover the lymphoid follicles in the gastrointestinal tract and provide a site for selective sampling of intraluminal antigens. Activated lymphocytes from the intestinal lymphoid follicles then migrate into afferent lymphatics that drain into mesenteric lymph nodes. Furthermore, some of these cells migrate into the lamina propria to interact with intestinal epithelial cells to generate the mucosal immune response. The B lymphocytes become surface immunoglobulin A (IgA). IgA-bearing lymphoblasts also serve a critically important role in mucosal immunity.

B lymphocytes and plasma cells, T lymphocytes, macrophages, dendritic cells, eosinophils, and mast cells are scattered throughout the connective tissue of the lamina propria. Approximately 60% of the lymphoid cells are T cells. These T lymphocytes are a heterogeneous group of cells and can differentiate into one of several types of T effector cells. Cytotoxic T effector cells damage the target cells directly. Helper T cells are effector cells that help mediate the induction of other T cells or the induction of B cells to produce humoral antibodies. T suppressor cells perform just the opposite function. Approximately 40% of the lymphoid cells in the lamina propria are B cells, which are primarily derived from precursors in Peyer patches. These B cells and their progeny, plasma cells, are predominantly focused on IgA synthesis and, to a lesser extent, IgM, IgG, and IgE synthesis.

Paneth cells, like M cells, are unique to the small intestine. Paneth cells line the base of crypts and release antimicrobial factors to protect adjacent stem cells.[5] The intraepithelial lymphocytes are located in the space between the epithelial cells that line the mucosal surface and lie close to the basement membrane. Most of the intraepithelial lymphocytes are a unique subtype of T cells. On activation, the intraepithelial lymphocytes may acquire cytolytic functions that can contribute to epithelial cell death through apoptosis. These cells may be important in the immunosurveillance against abnormal epithelial cells.

As noted, one of the major protective immune mechanisms for the intestinal tract is the synthesis and secretion of IgA. The intestine contains more than 70% of the IgA-producing cells in the body. IgA is produced by plasma cells in the lamina propria and is secreted into the intestine, where it can bind antigens at the mucosal surface. The IgA antibody traverses the epithelial cell to the lumen by means of a protein carrier (the secretory component) that not only transports the IgA but also protects it against the intracellular lysosomes. IgA does not activate complement and does not enhance cell-mediated opsonization or destruction of infectious organisms or antigens, which is in sharp contrast to the role of other immunoglobulins. Secretory IgA inhibits the adherence of bacteria to epithelial cells and prevents their colonization and multiplication. In addition, secretory IgA neutralizes bacterial toxins and viral activity and blocks the absorption of antigens from the gut.

Recent studies demonstrated a symbiotic relationship between the intestinal microbiome and intestinal growth and function. The intestinal mucosa of germ-free mice has decreased epithelial proliferation, and a decreased production of mucin and immunological mediators that result in thinning of the mucosa with decreased tissue protection and repair. In addition, microbial metabolites from anaerobes generate much of the luminal butyrate, which is a fuel source for colonic cells, and luminal lactate, which promotes small intestinal stem cell proliferation and differentiation. Essentially, a functional molecular "crosstalk" occurs between intestinal epithelial cells and the gut microbiome. Disruption of this crosstalk can lead to adverse changes to the microbiome, a process called "dysbiosis." Enteric microbial dysbiosis has been identified in certain intestinal pathologies such as in inflammatory bowel disease.[5] Current studies focusing on the importance of the intestinal epithelium and crosstalk with the microbiome will lead to a better understanding of many small bowel diseases and is the source of many ongoing investigational efforts.

OBSTRUCTION

The description of patients presenting with small bowel obstruction dates back to the third or fourth century BC, when Praxagoras created an enterocutaneous fistula to relieve a bowel obstruction. Despite this success with operative therapy, the nonoperative management of these patients with attempted reduction of hernias, laxatives, ingestion of heavy metals (e.g., lead, mercury), and leeches to remove toxic agents from the blood was common practice until the late 1800s, when antiseptic and aseptic surgical techniques made operative intervention safer and more acceptable. A better understanding of the pathophysiologic process of bowel obstruction, surgical advances, antibiotics, intestinal tube decompression, and use of isotonic fluid resuscitation have greatly reduced the mortality rate for patients with a mechanical bowel obstruction. However, patients with a bowel obstruction still represent some of the most difficult and vexing problems that surgeons face with regard to accurate diagnosis, optimal timing of therapy, and appropriate treatment. Ultimately, a clinical decision about the management of these patients requires a thorough history and workup with a heightened awareness of potential complications.

Causes

Small bowel obstructions continue to be a significant cause of morbidity and mortality in the United States. The most common cause of intestinal obstruction in the Western countries is adhesive disease.[6] Other causes of small bowel obstruction are many (Fig. 50.10), but as a group, they can be effectively divided into three major categories:

1. Obstruction arising from extraluminal causes (e.g., adhesions, hernias, carcinomas, abscesses);
2. Obstruction intrinsic to the bowel wall (e.g., primary tumors); and
3. Intraluminal obturator obstruction (e.g., gallstones, enteroliths, foreign bodies, bezoars).

Adhesions, particularly after pelvic operations (e.g., gynecologic procedures, appendectomy, colorectal resection), are responsible for more than 60% of all causes of bowel obstruction in the United States. This preponderance of lower abdominal procedures to produce adhesions that result in obstruction is thought to occur because the bowel is more mobile in the pelvis and more tethered in the upper abdomen (Box 50.1).

Malignant tumors account for approximately 20% of the cases of small bowel obstruction. Most of these tumors are metastatic lesions that obstruct the intestine secondary to peritoneal implants that have spread from an intraabdominal primary tumor, such as

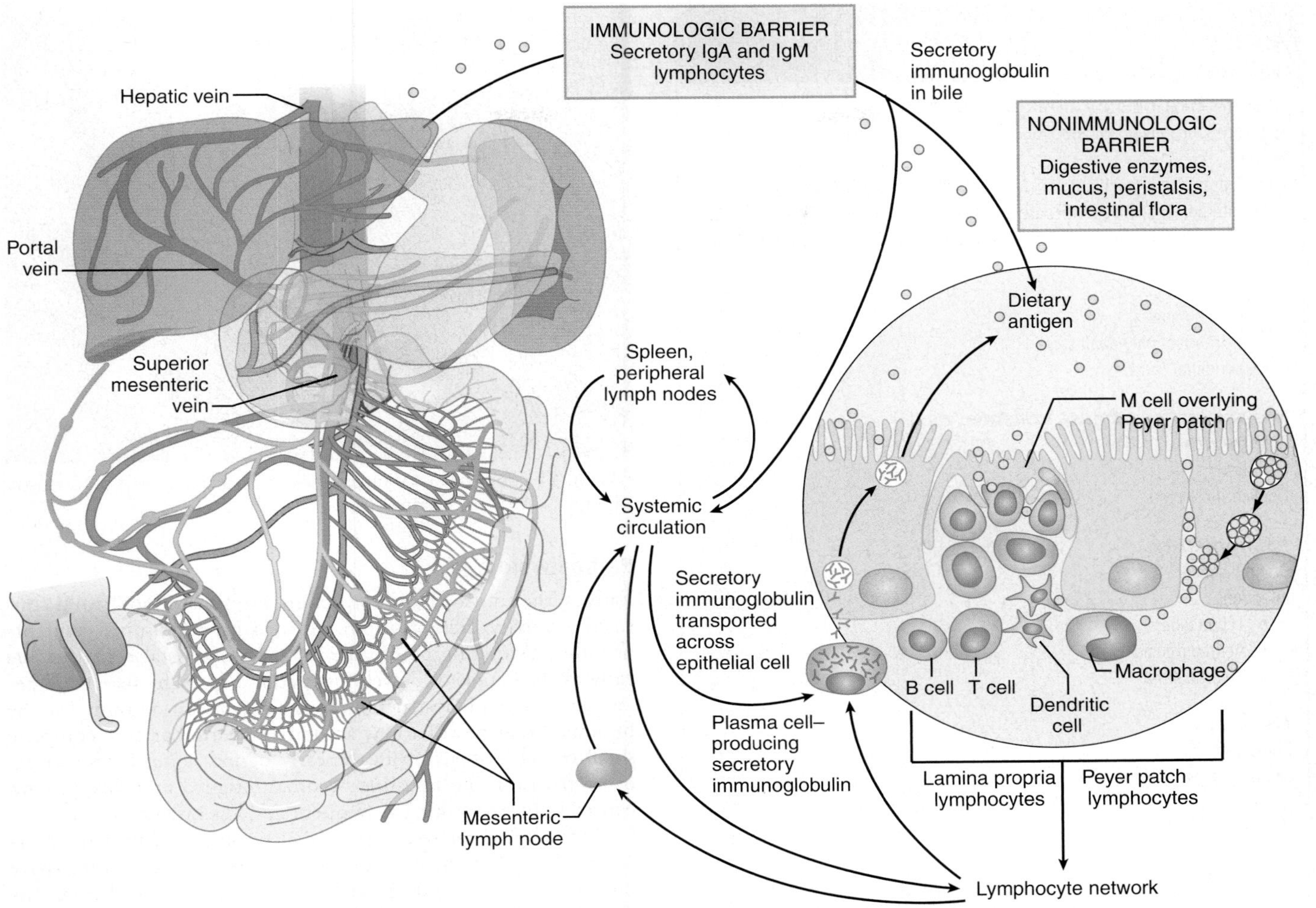

FIG. 50.9 Mucosal barrier of the gut. Antigens contact specialized microfold *(M)* cells that overlie Peyer patches, which then process and present the antigen to the immune system. When B lymphocytes are stimulated by antigenic material, the cells develop into antibody-forming cells that secrete various types of immunoglobulins, the most important of which is IgA. (Adapted from Duerr RH, Shanahan F. Food allergy. In: Targan SR, Shanahan F, eds. *Immunology and Immunopathology of the Liver and Gastrointestinal Tract.* New York: Igaku-Shoin; 1990:510; illustration courtesy Matt Hazzard, University of Kentucky Medical Center, Lexington, KY.) *IgA*, Immunoglobulin A; *IgM*, immunoglobulin M.

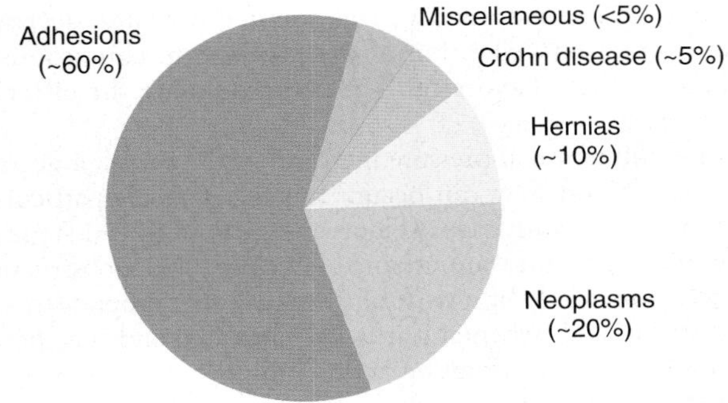

FIG. 50.10 Common causes of small bowel obstruction in industrialized countries.

ovarian, pancreatic, gastric, or colon cancer. Less often, malignant cells from distant sites, such as breast, lung, and melanoma, may metastasize hematogenously and account for peritoneal implants, resulting in an obstruction. Large intraabdominal tumors may also cause small bowel obstruction through extrinsic compression of the bowel lumen. Primary colonic cancers, particularly those arising from the cecum and ascending colon, may manifest as a small bowel obstruction. Primary small bowel tumors can cause obstruction but are exceedingly rare.

Hernias (typically ventral or inguinal hernias) represent the third leading cause of intestinal obstruction and account for approximately 10% of all cases. Internal hernias, generally related to prior abdominal surgery, can also result in small bowel obstruction. Less common hernias can also produce obstruction, such as femoral, obturator, lumbar, and sciatic hernias.

Crohn disease is the fourth leading cause of small bowel obstruction and accounts for approximately 5% of all cases. Obstruction can result from acute inflammation and edema, which may resolve with conservative management. In patients with longstanding Crohn disease, strictures can develop that may require resection and reanastomosis or strictureplasty.

An important cause of small bowel obstruction that is not routinely considered is obstruction associated with an intraabdominal

BOX 50.1 Causes of mechanical small intestinal obstruction in adults.

Lesions Extrinsic to the Intestinal Wall

Adhesions (usually postoperative)

Hernia

- External (e.g., inguinal, femoral, umbilical, or ventral hernias)
- Internal (e.g., congenital defects such as paraduodenal, foramen of Winslow, and diaphragmatic hernias or postoperative secondary to mesenteric defects)

Neoplastic

- Carcinomatosis
- Extraintestinal neoplasms

Intraabdominal abscess

Lesions Intrinsic to the Intestinal Wall

Congenital

Malrotation

Duplications, cysts

Inflammatory

Crohn disease

Infections

- Tuberculosis
- Actinomycosis
- Diverticulitis

Neoplastic

Primary neoplasms

Metastatic neoplasms

Traumatic

Hematoma

Ischemic stricture

Miscellaneous

Intussusception

Endometriosis

Radiation enteropathy/stricture

Intraluminal, Obturator Obstruction

Gallstone

Enterolith

Bezoar

Foreign body

Adapted from Tito WA, Sarr MG. Intestinal obstruction. In: Zuidema GD, ed. *Surgery of the Alimentary Tract*. Philadelphia: WB Saunders; 1996:375–416.

abscess, commonly from a ruptured appendix, diverticulum, or dehiscence of an intestinal anastomosis. The obstruction may be a result of a local ileus in the small bowel adjacent to the abscess. In addition, the small bowel can form a portion of the wall of the abscess cavity and become obstructed by kinking of the bowel at this point.

Miscellaneous causes of bowel obstruction account for 2% to 3% of all cases but should be considered in the differential diagnosis. These include intussusception of the bowel, which in the adult is usually secondary to a pathologic lead point, such as a polyp or tumor (Fig. 50.11); gallstones, which can enter the intestinal lumen by a cholecystoenteric fistula and cause obstruction; enteroliths originating from jejunal diverticula; foreign bodies; and phytobezoars.

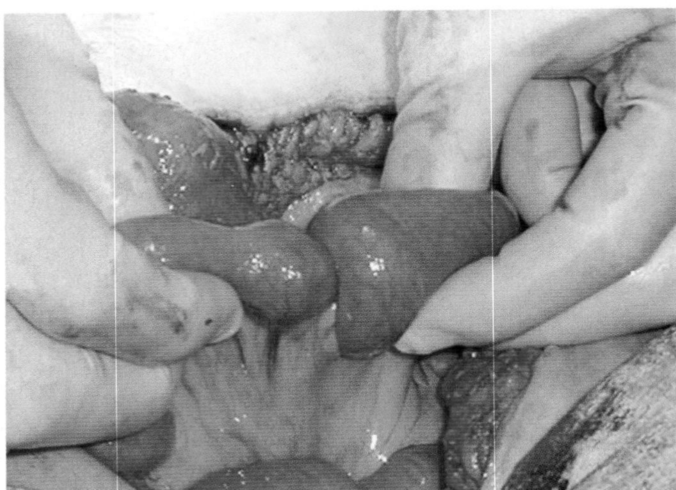

FIG. 50.11 Jejunojenunal intussusception in an adult patient. (Courtesy Dr. Steven Williams, Nampa, ID.)

Pathophysiology

Early in the course of an obstruction, intestinal motility and contractile activity increase in an effort to propel luminal contents past the obstructing point. The increase in peristalsis that occurs early in the course of bowel obstruction is present above and below the point of obstruction; this process can account for the finding of diarrhea that may accompany partial or even complete small bowel obstruction in the early period. Later in the course of obstruction, the intestine becomes fatigued and dilates, with contractions becoming less frequent and less intense.

As the bowel dilates, water and electrolytes accumulate intraluminally and in the bowel wall itself. This massive third-space fluid loss accounts for the dehydration and hypovolemia. The metabolic effects of fluid loss depend on the site and duration of the obstruction. With a proximal obstruction, dehydration may be accompanied by hypochloremia, hypokalemia, and metabolic alkalosis associated with increased vomiting. Distal obstruction of the small bowel may result in large quantities of intestinal fluid into the bowel; however, abnormalities in serum electrolyte levels are usually less dramatic. Oliguria, azotemia, and hemoconcentration can accompany the dehydration. Rarely, hypotension and shock can ensue. Other consequences of bowel obstruction include increased intraabdominal pressure, decreased venous return, and elevation of the diaphragm, compromising ventilation. These factors can serve to potentiate the effects of hypovolemia.

As the intraluminal pressure increases in the bowel, a decrease in mucosal blood flow can occur. This alteration is particularly noted in patients with a closed loop obstruction, in which greater intraluminal pressures are attained. A closed loop obstruction, produced commonly by a twist of the bowel, can progress to arterial occlusion and ischemia if it is left untreated and may potentially lead to bowel perforation and peritonitis.

In the absence of intestinal obstruction, the jejunum and proximal ileum have only 10^3 to 10^5 colony-forming units per milliliter (CFU/mL) of bacteria. With obstruction, however, the flora of the small intestine changes dramatically, in both the type of organism (most commonly *Escherichia coli*, *Streptococcus faecalis*, and *Klebsiella* spp.) and the quantity, with organisms reaching concentrations of 10^9 to 10^{10} CFU/mL. Studies have shown an increase in the number of indigenous bacteria translocating to mesenteric lymph nodes and even systemic organs. Bacterial translocation amplifies the local inflammatory response in the gut, leading to intestinal leakage and subsequent increase in systemic inflammation. This inflammatory cascade may result in systemic sepsis and multiorgan failure if it is unrecognized and untreated.

Clinical Manifestations and Diagnosis

The major challenge in the diagnosis of intestinal obstruction is the identification of bowel incarceration or strangulation. Although a thorough history and physical examination are important, neither is sensitive nor specific to the diagnosis of ischemia.[6] In some patients, a meticulous history and physical examination complemented by plain abdominal radiographs are all that is required to establish the diagnosis and to devise a treatment plan. More sophisticated radiographic studies, such as a computed tomography (CT) scan of the abdomen, represent invaluable tools in the identification of complications and potential causes.

History

The cardinal symptoms of intestinal obstruction include colicky abdominal pain, nausea, vomiting, abdominal distention, and obstipation. These symptoms may vary with the site and duration of obstruction. The typical crampy abdominal pain associated with intestinal obstruction occurs in paroxysms at 4- to 5-minute intervals and occurs less frequently with distal obstruction. Nausea and vomiting are more common with a higher obstruction and may be the only symptoms in patients with gastric outlet or high intestinal obstruction. An obstruction located distally is associated with less emesis; the initial and most prominent symptom is cramping abdominal pain. Abdominal distention occurs as the obstruction progresses and the proximal intestine becomes increasingly dilated. Obstipation is a later development. It must be reiterated that patients, particularly in the early stages of bowel obstruction, may relate a history of diarrhea that is secondary to increased peristalsis. Therefore, the important point to remember is that a complete bowel obstruction cannot be ruled out on the basis of a history of loose bowel movements. The character of the vomitus is also important to obtain in the history. As the obstruction becomes more complete with bacterial overgrowth, the vomitus becomes more feculent, indicating a late and established intestinal obstruction.

Physical Examination

The patient with intestinal obstruction may present with tachycardia and hypotension, demonstrating the severe dehydration that is present. Fever suggests the possibility of strangulation. Abdominal examination demonstrates a distended abdomen, with the amount of distention somewhat dependent on the level of obstruction. Previous surgical scars should be noted. Early in the course of bowel obstruction, peristaltic waves can be observed, particularly in thin patients, and auscultation of the abdomen may demonstrate hyperactive bowel sounds with audible rushes associated with vigorous peristalsis (borborygmi). Late in the obstructive course, minimal or no bowel sounds are noted. Mild abdominal tenderness may be present, with or without a palpable mass; however, localized tenderness, rebound, and guarding suggest peritonitis and the likelihood of strangulation. A careful examination must be performed to rule out incarcerated hernias in the groin, femoral triangle, and obturator foramen. A rectal examination should *always* be performed to rule out a distal colonic obstruction by intraluminal masses and to examine the stool for occult blood, which may be an indication of malignant disease, intussusception, or infarction.

BOX 50.2 Plain abdominal film signs of small bowel obstruction.

Supine or Prone
Dilated gas or fluid filled small bowel >3 cm
Dilated stomach
Small bowel dilated out of proportion to colon
Stretch sign
Absence of rectal gas
Gasless abdomen
Pseudotumor sign

Upright or Left Lateral Decubitus
Multiple air fluid levels
Air fluid levels longer than 2.5 cm
Air fluid levels in same loop of small bowel of unequal lengths
String of beads sign

Adapted from Paulson EK, Thompson WM. Review of small-bowel obstruction: the diagnosis and when to worry. *Radiology.* 2015;275:332–342.

Laboratory and Radiologic Studies

With a high suspicion of intestinal obstruction after a thorough history and physical examination, further studies are necessary to confirm the diagnosis. Laboratory tests are usually not helpful in the actual diagnosis of patients with small bowel obstruction but are extremely important in assessing the degree of dehydration. Patients with a bowel obstruction should routinely have laboratory measurements of serum sodium, chloride, potassium, bicarbonate, and creatinine levels. The serial determination of serum electrolyte levels should be performed to assess the adequacy of fluid resuscitation. Dehydration may result in hemoconcentration, as noted by an elevated hematocrit value. This level should be monitored because fluid resuscitation results in a decrease in the hematocrit, and some patients (e.g., those with intestinal malignant neoplasms) may require blood transfusions before surgery. In addition, the white blood cell count should be assessed. Leukocytosis may be found in patients with strangulation; however, an elevated white blood cell count does not necessarily denote strangulation. Conversely, the absence of leukocytosis does not eliminate strangulation as a possibility. Elevated lactic acid levels suggest intestinal ischemia or necrosis.

Radiographic studies can be very helpful in the diagnosis of small bowel obstruction. The accuracy of diagnosis of the small intestinal obstruction on plain abdominal radiographs is estimated to be approximately 86%, with an equivocal or a nonspecific diagnosis obtained in the remainder of cases. Characteristic findings on supine radiographs are dilated loops of small intestine, without evidence of colonic distention (Box 50.2). Upright radiographs demonstrate multiple air-fluid levels, which often layer in a stepwise pattern (Fig. 50.12). Paucity of gas when supine and small pockets of air appearing like a string of beads when upright is more concerning for high-grade or closed loop obstruction. Plain abdominal films (Fig. 50.13A) may also demonstrate the cause of the obstruction (e.g., foreign bodies, gallstones; Fig. 50.13B). In uncertain cases or when one is unable to differentiate partial from complete obstruction, further diagnostic imaging is required.

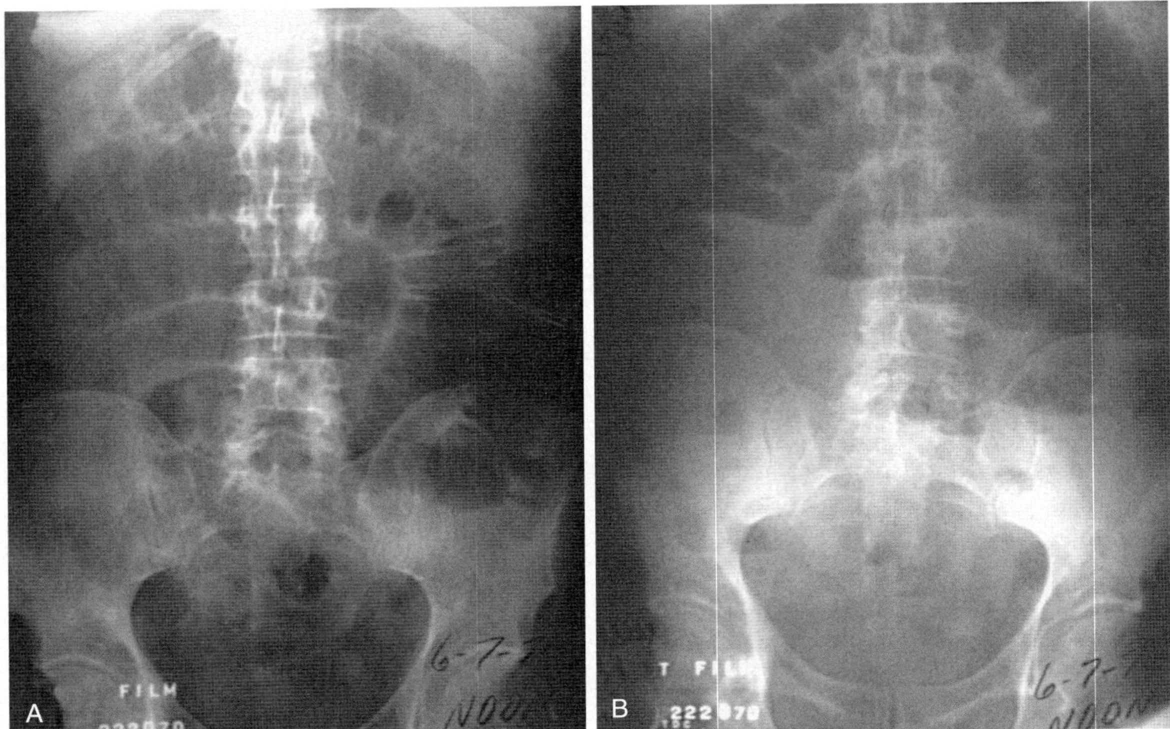

FIG. 50.12 Abdominal radiographs of a patient with a complete small bowel obstruction. (A) Supine film shows dilated loops of small bowel in an orderly arrangement, without evidence of colonic gas. (B) Upright film shows multiple, short air-fluid levels arranged in a stepwise pattern. (Courtesy Dr. Melvyn H. Schreiber, The University of Texas Medical Branch, Galveston, TX.)

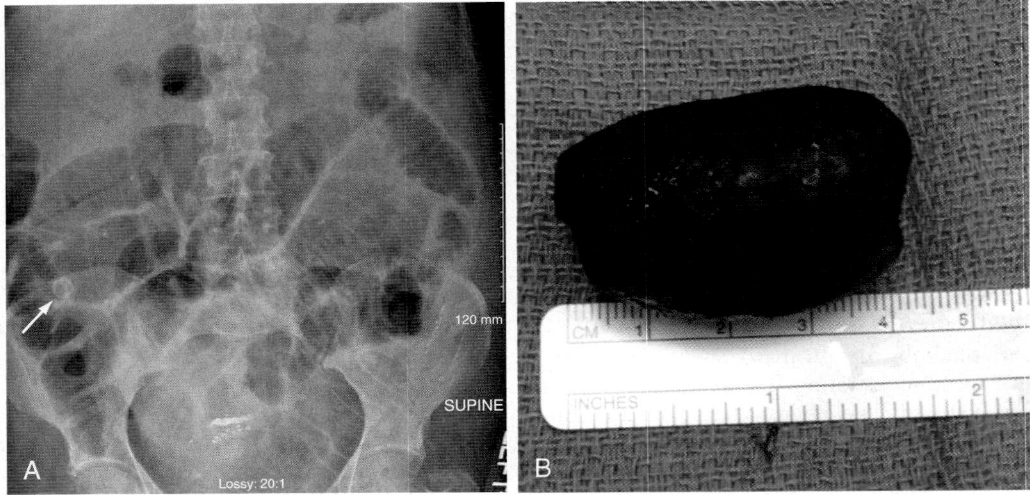

FIG. 50.13 Patient presents with gallstone ileus. (A) Plain abdominal film shows complete bowel obstruction caused by a large radiopaque gallstone *(arrow)* obstructing the distal ileum. (B) The large gallstone responsible for the obstruction seen in the corresponding plain abdominal film. (Courtesy Dr. Kristin Long, University of Kentucky Medical Center, Lexington, KY.)

In the more complex patient in whom the diagnosis is not readily apparent, an abdominal CT scan can be helpful and is often obtained. CT is particularly sensitive and specific (95% for both) for diagnosing complete or high-grade obstruction of the small bowel and for determining the location and cause of obstruction. However, a CT scan is less sensitive in patients with partial small bowel obstruction. A dilated bowel loop of more than 2.5 cm is very concerning for high-grade small bowel obstruction. In addition, CT is helpful to identify a transition zone in approximately 93% of cases. The CT scan is also helpful in the identification of an extrinsic cause of bowel obstruction (e.g., abdominal tumors, inflammatory disease, or abscess; Fig. 50.14). CT has also been described as useful for determining bowel strangulation, most commonly seen in the presence of

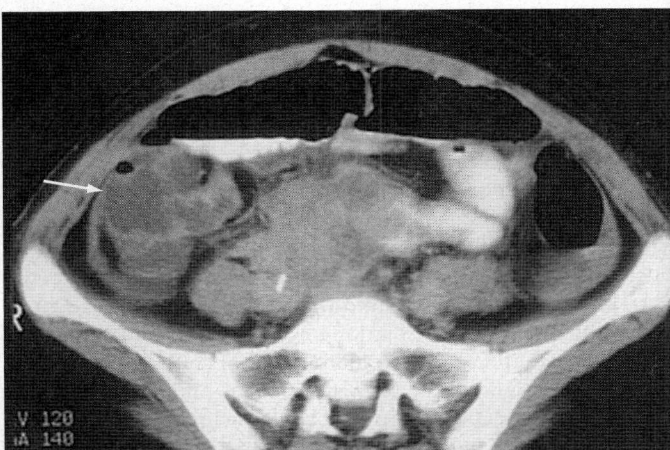

FIG. 50.14 Intraabdominal abscess causing small bowel obstruction. Computed tomography scan of the abdomen of a patient with a mechanical bowel obstruction secondary to an abscess in the right lower quadrant *(arrow)*. Multiple dilated and fluid-filled loops of small bowel are noted. (Courtesy Dr. Melvyn H. Schreiber, The University of Texas Medical Branch, Galveston, TX.)

hernia. Unfortunately, CT findings associated with strangulation are those of irreversible ischemia and necrosis. Importantly, the emergent surgical management of a toxic patient with a bowel obstruction identified by a thorough history and physical examination should not be delayed to perform unnecessary and costly radiographic studies.

Barium studies, namely, enteroclysis, have been used in certain patients with a presumed obstruction. This procedure involves the continued infusion of 500 to 1000 mL of thin barium sulfate and methylcellulose suspension into the intestine through a duodenal tube. The suspension is then viewed continuously with use of either fluoroscopy or standard radiographs taken at frequent intervals; therefore, this technique is a double-contrast procedure that allows detailed imaging of the entire small intestine. Enteroclysis has been advocated as a study to aid in the diagnosis of low-grade, intermittent, small bowel obstruction. In addition, barium studies can precisely demonstrate the level of the obstruction as well as the cause of the obstruction in certain cases (Fig. 50.15). The main disadvantages of enteroclysis are the need for nasoenteric intubation, slow transit of contrast material in patients with a fluid-filled hypotonic small bowel, and enhanced expertise required by the radiologist to perform this procedure.

Ultrasound has been reported to be useful for pregnant patients because radiation exposure is a concern. Magnetic resonance imaging (MRI) has been described in patients with obstruction; however, it appears to be no better diagnostically than CT.

To summarize, plain abdominal radiographs are usually diagnostic of bowel obstruction in up to 86% of the cases, but further evaluation (possibly by CT or barium radiography) may be necessary in 20% to 30% of cases. CT examination is particularly useful in patients with a history of abdominal malignant disease, postsurgical patients, and patients who have no history of abdominal surgery and present with symptoms of bowel obstruction. Barium studies may be helpful for patients with a history of recurring obstruction or low-grade mechanical obstruction to precisely define the obstructed segment and degree of obstruction.

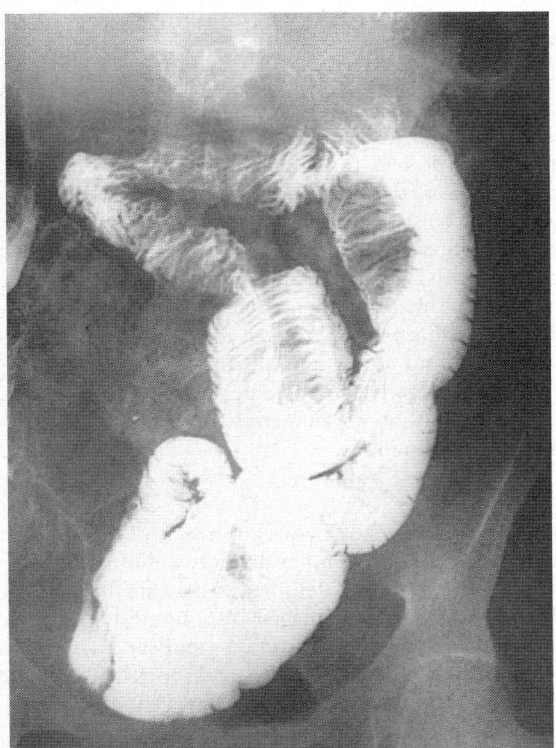

FIG. 50.15 Barium study demonstrates jejunojejunal intussusception. (Courtesy Dr. Melvyn H. Schreiber, The University of Texas Medical Branch, Galveston, TX.)

Simple Versus Strangulating Obstruction

Most patients with small bowel obstruction are classified as having simple obstructions that involve mechanical blockage of the flow of luminal contents without compromised viability of the intestinal wall. In contrast, a strangulated obstruction, which usually involves a closed loop obstruction with a compromised vascular supply to a segment of intestine, can lead to intestinal infarction. A strangulated obstruction is associated with an increased morbidity and mortality risk, and therefore, recognition of early strangulation is important. In differentiating from the simple intestinal obstruction, classic signs of strangulation have been described; these include tachycardia, fever, leukocytosis, and a constant, noncramping abdominal pain. However, a number of studies have convincingly shown that no clinical parameters or laboratory measurements can accurately detect or exclude the presence of strangulation in all cases. This reinforces the dictum that a careful history and physical examination are key for an accurate and timely diagnosis.

Closed loop obstructions occur when both ends of a segment of bowel are obstructed either by an adhesive band or from an internal hernia, which may result in ischemia and necrosis. Ischemia may worsen when this loop twists, creating a volvulus. CT examination is useful for detecting evidence of closed loop obstruction (U loop or coffee bean sign with tapering of both ends of bowel) and volvulus (mesenteric whirl). In addition, CT scans also demonstrate evidence of ischemia such as bowel wall thickening (>3 mm), mesenteric edema, fluid trapped in between loops, decreased bowel wall enhancement, pneumatosis intestinalis, and mesenteric or portovenous gas.[6] Serum levels, including lactate dehydrogenase, amylase, alkaline phosphatase, and ammonia levels, have been assessed with no real benefit. Previous reports described limited success in discriminating strangulation by measuring serum D-lactate, creatine kinase isoenzyme (particularly the BB isoenzyme), or intestinal fatty acid–binding protein; however, these studies were ultimately abandoned as they showed no significant diagnostic benefits. Finally, noninvasive determinations of mesenteric ischemia have been described using a superconducting quantum interference device (SQUID) magnetometer to detect mesenteric ischemia noninvasively. Intestinal ischemia is associated with changes in the basic electrical rhythm of the small intestine. This technique remains investigational and is not in widespread clinical use. Thus, it is important to remember that bowel ischemia and strangulation cannot be reliably diagnosed or excluded preoperatively in all cases by any known clinical parameter, combination of parameters, or current laboratory and radiographic examinations.

Treatment

Patients with symptoms of a bowel obstruction usually present to the emergency department for evaluation and often require a surgical consultation. Patients identified to have small bowel obstruction should be primarily managed by a surgical service. A large population-based study demonstrated significantly shorter length of stay, lower cost, readmission rate, and mortality rate when adhesive bowel obstruction was managed by a surgical service compared to being managed by a medicine service.[7]

Fluid Resuscitation and Antibiotics

Patients with intestinal obstruction are usually dehydrated and depleted of sodium, chloride, and potassium, requiring aggressive intravenous (IV) replacement with an isotonic saline solution such as lactated Ringer solution. Urine output should be monitored by the placement of a Foley catheter. After the patient has formed adequate urine, potassium chloride can be added to the infusion, if needed. Serial electrolyte level measurements as well as hematocrit and white blood cell count are performed to assess the adequacy of fluid repletion. Broad-spectrum antibiotics are given prophylactically by some surgeons on the basis of the reported findings of bacterial translocation occurring even in simple mechanical obstructions; however, there is no substantial evidence to support the use of antimicrobial therapy in nontoxic-appearing patients or those without suspected bacterial overgrowth of the small intestine. Antibiotics should only be administered preoperatively in the event that the patient requires surgery.

Tube Decompression

In addition to IV fluid resuscitation, another important adjunct to the supportive care of patients with intestinal obstruction is nasogastric suction. Suction with a nasogastric tube empties the stomach, reducing the hazard of pulmonary aspiration of vomitus and minimizing further intestinal distention from swallowed air. Nasogastric decompression in a patient with small bowel obstruction is still considered standard of care.

The use of long intestinal tubes (e.g., Cantor or Baker tube) has been advocated by some. However, prospective randomized trials have demonstrated no significant difference regarding the decompression achieved, success of nonoperative treatment, or incidence of postoperative morbidities compared with the use of nasogastric tubes. Furthermore, the use of these long tubes has been associated with a significantly longer hospital stay, duration of postoperative ileus, and postoperative complications in some series. Therefore, it appears that long intestinal tubes offer no benefit in the preoperative setting over nasogastric tubes.

Patients with a partial intestinal obstruction may be treated conservatively with resuscitation and tube decompression alone. Resolution of symptoms and discharge without the need for surgery have been reported in up to 85% of patients with a partial obstruction. Enteroclysis can assist in determining the degree of obstruction, with higher-grade partial obstructions requiring earlier operative intervention. Although an initial trial of nonoperative management of most patients with partial small bowel obstruction is warranted, clinical deterioration of the patient or increasing small bowel distention on abdominal radiographs during tube decompression warrants prompt operative intervention. The decision to continue to treat a patient nonoperatively with a presumed bowel obstruction is based on clinical judgment and requires constant vigilance to ensure that the clinical course has not changed.

Contrast Challenge

The use of a water-soluble contrast challenge in lower-grade obstructions (i.e., those that have not resolved from nasogastric suction management after 48 hours) has become a more common practice. The challenge requires 100 mL of water-soluble contrast given through the nasogastric tube and follow-up radiographs obtained after 8 and 24 hours. If contrast material still has not passed into the colon after 24 hours, conservative management will probably fail and surgical intervention is likely needed.[6]

Operative Management

As the management of intestinal obstruction has shifted more to conservative care with nasogastric tube decompression and rehydration, operative intervention is reserved for those who fail conservative management and have evidence of vascular compromise, strangulation, or perforation.[6] A nonoperative approach for selected patients with complete small intestinal obstruction has been proposed by some surgeons who argue that prolonged gastrointestinal decompression is safe in these patients, provided no fever, tachycardia, tenderness, or leukocytosis is noted. Nevertheless, one must weigh the risks and benefits of nonoperative management in overlooking an underlying strangulated obstruction. Retrospective studies report that a 12- to 24-hour delay is safe but that the incidence of strangulation and other complications increases significantly after this time period.

The nature of the problem dictates the approach for the obstructed patient. Patients with intestinal obstruction secondary to an adhesive band may be treated with lysis of adhesions. Great care should be used in the gentle handling of the bowel to reduce serosal trauma and to avoid unnecessary dissection and inadvertent enterotomies. Incarcerated hernias can be managed by manual reduction of the herniated segment of bowel and closure of the defect.

The treatment of patients with an obstruction and history of malignant tumors can be particularly challenging. In the terminal patient with widespread metastasis, nonoperative management, if successful, is usually the best course; however, only a small percentage of cases with complete obstruction can be successfully managed nonoperatively. In this case, an intestinal bypass of the obstructing lesion, by whatever means, may offer the best option rather than a long and complicated operation that might entail bowel resection.

An obstruction secondary to Crohn disease will often resolve with conservative management if the obstruction is acute. If a chronic fibrotic stricture is the cause of the obstruction, a bowel resection or strictureplasty may be required.

Patients with an intraabdominal abscess can present in a manner indistinguishable from those with mechanical bowel obstruction. CT is particularly useful in diagnosing the cause of the obstruction in these patients. Percutaneous drainage of the abscess may be sufficient to relieve the obstruction, but laparotomy and abdominal washout may be required for large and established abscesses. Laparoscopic drainage is also an option in cases not amenable to image-guided percutaneous drainage or for patients who would not otherwise tolerate a laparotomy; this procedure is associated with reduced wound morbidity and is also useful in multiloculated collections and allows a washout of the peritoneal cavity at the same time.

Radiation enteropathy, as a complication of radiation therapy for pelvic malignant neoplasms, may cause bowel obstruction. Most cases can be treated nonoperatively with tube decompression and the potential addition of corticosteroids, particularly during the acute setting. In the chronic setting, nonoperative management is rarely effective; laparotomy will be required with possible resection of the irradiated bowel or bypass of the affected area.

At the time of exploration, it can sometimes be difficult to evaluate bowel viability after the release of a strangulation. If intestinal viability is questionable, the bowel segment should be completely released and placed in a warm, saline-moistened sponge for 15 to 20 minutes and then reexamined. If normal color has returned and peristalsis is evident, it is safe to retain the bowel. A prospective controlled trial comparing clinical judgment with the use of a Doppler probe or the administration of fluorescein for intraoperative discrimination of viability found that the Doppler flow probe added little to the conventional clinical judgment of the surgeon. In difficult borderline cases, fluorescein fluorescence may supplement clinical judgment. Intraoperative near-infrared angiography to determine the presence of ischemic bowel has shown promising results, but this technique is currently not in wide clinical use. Another approach to the assessment of bowel viability is the so-called second-look laparotomy 18 to 24 hours after the initial procedure. This decision should be made at the time of the initial operation. A second-look laparotomy is clearly indicated for a patient whose condition deteriorates after the initial operation.

Multiple studies have evaluated the efficacy of laparoscopic management of acute small bowel obstruction. Laparoscopic treatment of small bowel obstruction appears to be effective and leads to a lower morbidity and mortality, shorter length of stay, shorter operating time, lower reoperation rate, and reduced overall complications in a select group of patients.[8] The patient profile appropriate for consideration of laparoscopic management include those with the following clinical presentation: mild abdominal distention proximal or partial obstruction; anticipated single-band obstruction, and those with low risk of strangulation or perforation.

In particular, laparoscopic treatment has been found to be of greatest benefit in patients who have undergone fewer than three previous operations, were seen early after the onset of symptoms, and were thought to have adhesive bands as the cause. Currently, patients with advanced, complete, or distal small bowel obstructions are not candidates for laparoscopic treatment. Similarly, patients with matted adhesions or carcinomatosis or those who remain distended after nasogastric intubation should be managed with conventional laparotomy. Therefore, the role of laparoscopic surgery in small bowel obstruction depends on clinical judgment and individualized treatment.[8]

Management of Specific Problems

Recurrent Intestinal Obstruction

All surgeons can readily remember the complicated patient with multiple previous abdominal operations and a frozen abdomen who presents with yet another bowel obstruction. An initial nonoperative trial is usually desirable and often safe. In those patients who do not respond conservatively, reoperation is required. This can often be a long and arduous procedure, with great care taken to prevent enterotomies or adjacent organ injury. In these difficult patients, various surgical procedures and pharmacologic agents have been tried in an effort to prevent recurrent adhesions and obstruction.

External plication procedures have been described in which the small intestine or its mesentery is sutured in large, gently curving loops. Common complications include the development of fistulas, gross leakage, peritonitis, and death. Because of frequent complications and low overall success rate, these procedures have largely been abandoned. Several series have reported moderate success with internal fixation or stenting procedures using a long intestinal tube inserted through the nose, a gastrostomy, or even a jejunostomy that is left in place for 2 weeks or longer. Complications associated with these tubes include prolonged drainage of bowel contents from the tube insertion site, intussusception, and difficult removal of the tube, which may require surgical reexploration.

Pharmacologic agents, including corticosteroids and other antiinflammatory agents, cytotoxic drugs, and antihistamines, have been used with limited success. The use of anticoagulants, such as heparin, dextran solutions, dicumarol, and sodium citrate, has modified the extent of adhesion formation, but their side effects far outweigh their efficacy. Intraperitoneal instillation of various proteinases (e.g., trypsin, papain, pepsin), which cause enzymatic digestion of the extracellular protein matrix, has been unsuccessful. Hyaluronidase has been of questionable value, and conflicting results were obtained with fibrinolytic agents such as streptokinase, urokinase, and fibrinolytic snake venoms. In a prospective multicenter trial, the use of a hyaluronate-based, bioresorbable membrane reduced the incidence and severity of postoperative adhesion formation. One study found that placement of this membrane reduced the severity but not the incidence of postoperative adhesions, and another study found that a multilayer approach has maximum effectiveness.[9] Longer term, prospective randomized studies are required to determine the efficacy of this material in preventing adhesions and ultimately preventing bowel obstructions.

To date, the most effective means of limiting the number of adhesions is a good surgical technique. This includes the gentle handling of the bowel to reduce serosal trauma, avoidance of unnecessary dissection, exclusion of foreign material from the peritoneal cavity (the use of absorbable suture material when possible, avoidance of excessive gauze sponge use, and the removal of starch from gloves), adequate irrigation and removal of infectious and ischemic debris, and preservation and use of the omentum around the site of surgery or in the denuded pelvis.

Acute Postoperative Obstruction

Small bowel obstruction that occurs in the immediate postoperative period presents a challenge with regard to diagnosis and treatment. Diagnosis is often difficult because the primary symptoms of abdominal pain and nausea or emesis may be attributed to a postoperative ileus. Electrolyte deficiencies, particularly hypokalemia, can be a cause of ileus and should be corrected. Plain abdominal films are usually not helpful to distinguish an ileus from obstruction. CT may be useful in this regard, and in particular, enteroclysis studies may be helpful in determining whether an obstruction exists and, if so, the level of the obstruction.[6] More than 90% of early postoperative obstructions are partial and will resolve spontaneously, given ample time. Conservative management in the form of bowel rest, fluid resuscitation, electrolyte replacement, and parenteral nutrition, if necessary, is routinely successful. However, the development of complete obstruction or signs of strangulation mandates reoperative intervention. Postoperative bowel obstruction after laparoscopic surgery is more commonly associated with a definitive obstruction point, such as a port site, hernia, or an internal hernia, and should prompt a high index of suspicion for the need for operative intervention.

Ileus

An ileus is defined as intestinal distention and the slowing or absence of passage of luminal contents without a demonstrable mechanical obstruction. An ileus can result from a number of causes, including those that are drug induced, or from metabolic, neurogenic, and infectious factors (Box 50.3).

Pharmacologic agents that can produce an ileus include anticholinergic drugs, autonomic blockers, antihistamines, and various psychotropic agents, such as haloperidol and tricyclic antidepressants. One of the more common causes of drug-induced ileus in the operative patient is the use of opiates, such as morphine or meperidine. Metabolic causes of ileus are common and include hypokalemia, hyponatremia, and hypomagnesemia. Other metabolic causes include uremia, diabetic coma, and hypoparathyroidism. Neurogenic causes of an ileus include postoperative ileus, which occurs after abdominal operations. Spinal injury, retroperitoneal irritation, and orthopedic procedures on the spine or pelvis can result in an ileus. Finally, infections can result in an ileus; common infectious causes include pneumonia, peritonitis, and generalized sepsis from a nonabdominal source.

Patients often present in a manner similar to those with a mechanical small bowel obstruction. Abdominal distention, usually without the colicky abdominal pain, is the typical and most notable finding. Nausea and vomiting may occur but may also be absent. Patients with an ileus may continue to pass flatus and diarrhea, which may help distinguish these patients from those with a mechanical small bowel obstruction.

BOX 50.3 Causes of ileus.

- After laparotomy
- Metabolic and electrolyte derangements (e.g., hypokalemia, hyponatremia, hypomagnesemia, uremia, diabetic coma)
- Drugs (e.g., opiates, psychotropic agents, anticholinergic agents)
- Intraabdominal inflammation
- Retroperitoneal hemorrhage or inflammation
- Intestinal ischemia
- Systemic sepsis

Adapted from Turnage RH, Bergen PC. Intestinal obstruction and ileus. In Feldman M, Scharschmidt FG, Sleisenger MH, eds. *Sleisenger and Fordtran's Gastrointestinal and Liver Disease: Pathophysiology, Diagnosis, Management*. Philadelphia: WB Saunders; 1998:1799–1810.

Radiologic studies may help distinguish ileus from small bowel obstruction. Plain abdominal radiographs may reveal distended small bowel as well as large bowel loops. In cases that are difficult to differentiate from obstruction, barium studies may be beneficial.

The treatment of an ileus is entirely supportive, with nasogastric decompression and IV fluids. The most effective treatment to correct the underlying condition may be aggressive treatment of the sepsis, correction of any metabolic or electrolyte abnormalities, and discontinuation of medications that may produce an ileus. Pharmacologic agents have been used but for the most part have been ineffective. Drugs that block sympathetic input (e.g., guanethidine) or stimulate parasympathetic activity (e.g., bethanechol, neostigmine) have been tried. Hormonal manipulation, using cholecystokinin or motilin, has been evaluated, but the results have been inconsistent. Erythromycin has been ineffective, and cisapride, although apparently beneficial in stimulating gastric motility, does not appear to alter intestinal ileus. Chewing gum has been suggested as an easy and inexpensive method to stimulate the cephalic phase of digestion (e.g., vagal cholinergic stimulation and the release of gastrointestinal hormones) and therefore a potential adjunct to prevent and to treat ileus. A more recent randomized trial demonstrated that chewing gum provides no benefit regarding return of bowel function or length of stay and even suggested that postoperative ileus may be further exacerbated by the use of sugared gum.

INFLAMMATORY AND INFECTIOUS DISEASES

Crohn Disease

Crohn disease is a chronic, transmural inflammatory disease of the gastrointestinal tract for which the definitive cause is unknown, although a combination of genetic and environmental factors has been implicated. Crohn disease can involve any part of the alimentary tract from the mouth to the anus but most commonly affects the small intestine and colon. The most common clinical manifestations are abdominal pain, diarrhea, and weight loss. Crohn disease can be complicated by intestinal obstruction or localized perforation with fistula formation. Medical and surgical treatments are palliative; however, operative therapy can provide effective symptomatic relief for patients with complications from Crohn disease and produces a reasonable long-term benefit.

History

The first documented case of Crohn disease was described by Morgagni in 1761. In 1913, the Scottish surgeon Dalziel described nine cases of intestinal inflammatory disease. However, it is the landmark paper by Crohn and colleagues in 1932 that provided, in eloquent detail, the pathologic and clinical findings of this inflammatory disease in young adults.[10] This classic paper crystallized the description of this inflammatory condition. Although many different (and sometimes misleading) terms have been used to describe this disease process, Crohn disease has been universally accepted as its name.

Incidence and Epidemiology

Crohn disease is the most common primary surgical disease of the small bowel. The annual incidence of Crohn disease, which is rising in the United States, is 3 to 20 cases per 100,000 individuals.[11] The total direct and indirect costs for Crohn disease in the United States have been estimated at more than $800 million when factoring both inpatient stays and outpatient visits. Crohn disease primarily attacks young adults in the second and third decades of life. However, a bimodal distribution is apparent, with a second smaller peak occurring in the sixth decade of life. Crohn disease is more common in urban dwellers, and although earlier reports suggested a somewhat higher female predominance, the two genders are affected equally. The risk for development of Crohn disease is about twice as high in smokers as in nonsmokers. Several studies indicate an increased incidence of Crohn disease in women using oral contraceptives; however, more recent studies have shown no differences. Worldwide, Crohn disease is relatively uncommon in African Americans; however, in the United States, the rates of Crohn disease in African Americans is similar to that seen in Caucasians. Certain ethnic groups, particularly Ashkenazi Jews, have a two- to four fold higher incidence of Crohn disease than age- and gender-matched control subjects. Individuals born during the spring months (e.g., April to June) are more likely to develop Crohn disease; there also appears to be a north-south gradient worldwide, and populations in higher latitudes have higher incidence rates than populations in lower latitudes. Of note, within one generation, migrants moving from a low-risk region to a high-risk region develop Crohn disease at similar rates to those in the high-risk region. There is a strong familial association, with the risk for development of Crohn disease increased about 30-fold in siblings and 14- to 15-fold for all first-degree relatives. Other analyses that support a genetic role for Crohn disease have shown a concordance rate of only 4% in dizygotic twins but a 20% to 50% rate in monozygotic twins. More recent studies evaluating twins with and without Crohn disease have used advanced genomic and proteomic techniques to show that intestinal microflora and epigenetic changes induced by environmental factors play an important role in disease development and progression in genetically susceptible individuals.[12]

Etiology

The cause(s) of Crohn disease remain unknown. A number of potential causes have been proposed, with the most likely possibilities being infectious, immunologic, and genetic. Other possibilities that have met with various levels of enthusiasm include environmental and dietary factors, smoking, and psychosocial factors. Although these factors may contribute to the overall disease process, it is unlikely that they represent the primary etiology for Crohn disease.

Infectious agents. Although a number of infectious agents have been proposed as potential causes of Crohn disease, the two that have received the most attention are mycobacterial infections, particularly *Mycobacterium paratuberculosis* and enteroadherent *E. coli*. The existence of atypical mycobacteria as a cause for Crohn disease was proposed by Dalziel in 1913. Subsequent studies using polymerase chain reaction (PCR) techniques have confirmed the presence of mycobacteria in intestinal samples of patients with Crohn disease. Transplantation of tissue from patients with Crohn disease has resulted in ileitis, but antimicrobial therapy directed against mycobacteria has not been effective in ameliorating the established disease process. Strains of enteroadherent *E. coli* are in higher abundance in patients with Crohn disease compared with the general population based on PCR analysis. More recent studies have used fluorescent in situ hybridization to demonstrate increased numbers of *E. coli* in the lamina propria of patients with active Crohn disease compared with those with inactive disease. Furthermore, an increased number of *E. coli* has been associated with a shorter time before relapse of the disease.

Immunologic factors. Humoral and cell-mediated immune reactions directed against intestinal cells in Crohn disease suggest an autoimmune phenomenon. Attention has focused on the role of cytokines, such as interleukin (IL)-1, IL-2, IL-8, and TNF-α, as contributing factors in the intestinal inflammatory response. The role of the immune response remains controversial in Crohn disease and may represent an effect of the disease process rather than an actual cause.

Genetic factors. Genetic factors play an important role in the pathogenesis of Crohn disease because the single strongest risk factor for development of disease is having a first-degree relative with Crohn disease. Several genome-wide association sequencing studies have been performed and have identified more than 200 alleles associated with Crohn disease (Table 50.5). The genes with the strongest and most frequently replicated associations with Crohn disease are *NOD2*, *MHC*, and *MST1* 3p21. Putative inflammatory bowel disease loci have been identified on chromosomes 16q, 5q, 19p, 7q, and 3p. The most important gene in Crohn disease development is *NOD2*. The *NOD2* gene is associated with a decreased expression of antimicrobial peptides by Paneth cells. Heterozygosity of one *NOD2* variant confers a 2- to 4-fold increase in risk of Crohn disease, while homozygosity confers a 17- to 40-fold increase in risk. In addition, *NOD2* has been identified as a genetic predictor of ileal disease, ileal stenosis, fistula, and Crohn-related surgery.[12] Another gene, *CARD15*, leads to impaired activation of the transcription factor nuclear factor kappa B (NF-κB) and also specifically codes for a protein expressed in monocytes, macrophages, dendritic cells, epithelial cells, and Paneth cells. *CARD15* is also helpful in distinguishing Crohn disease from ulcerative colitis as it is more strongly associated with Crohn disease, especially in patients of northern European descent. The *FHIT* gene located on 3p14.2 has been identified as a tumor suppressor gene and is suggested to play a role in the pathogenesis of Crohn disease as well as in the development and progression of Crohn disease–related cancers. A complex cellular and molecular crosstalk occurs between the genes *NOD2/CARD15* and the autophagy gene *ATG16L1*, which is associated with a synergistic increase in earlier onset and disease severity. Genetic profiling may be helpful in selecting patients who will benefit from intensified treatment with immunomodulators and anti-TNF therapy, thus decreasing medical nonresponse.

More recent genome-wide association sequencing studies in monozygotic twins have shown no reproducible differences within twin pairs in comparing whole genome sequences and tissue-specific variants in the intestinal mucosa directly affected by the inflammation of Crohn disease. These findings suggest that it is unlikely that somatic mutations have a substantial impact on the development of the disease, and simple Mendelian inheritance cannot account for the pattern of occurrence. Therefore, it is likely that multiple causes (e.g., environmental factors) contribute to the cause and pathogenesis of this disease.

Environmental factors. Low-risk countries in Asia that have adopted a more Western lifestyle have noted a significant rise in the incidence of Crohn disease. Smoking is the single largest environment factor, with a two fold increase in risk of Crohn disease. Single nucleotide polymorphisms associated with smoking increase the risk of Crohn disease in smokers, identifying a genetic disposition for an environmental risk factor.[13] In addition, other factors that increase the risk of Crohn disease include medications (oral contraceptives, aspirin, nonsteroidal antiinflammatory drugs

TABLE 50.5 Genetic polymorphisms related to Crohn disease.

Genes and the Diagnosis of Crohn Disease	
Genes related to innate pattern recognition receptors	NOD2/CARD15, OCTN, TLR
Genes related to epithelial barrier homeostasis	IBD5, DLG5
Genes related to molecular mimicry and autophagy	ATG16L1, IRGM, LRRK2
Genes related to lymphocyte differentiation	IL23R, STAT3
Genes related to secondary immune response and apoptosis	MHC, HLA
Genes and the Prognosis of Crohn Disease	
Genes related to age at Crohn disease onset	TNFRSF6B, CXCL9, IL23R, NOD2, ATG16L1, CNR1, IL10, MDR1, DLG5, IRGM
Genes Related to Crohn Disease Behavior	
Stenotic/structuring behavior	NOD2, TLR4, IL12B, CX3CR1, IL10, IL6
Penetrating/fistulizing behavior	NOD2, IRGM, TNF, HLADRB1, CDKAL1
Inflammatory behavior	HLA
Granulomatous disease	TLR4/CARD15
Genes Related to Crohn Disease Location	
Upper gastrointestinal	NOD2, MIF
Ileal	IL10, CRP, NOD2, ZNF365, STAT3
Ileocolonic	ATG16L1, TCF4 (TCF7L2)
Colonic	HLA, TLR4, TLR1, TLR2, TLR6
Other Genes Related to Crohn Disease	
Genes related to Crohn disease activity	HSP702, NOD2, PAI1, CNR1
Genes related to surgery	NOD2, HLAG
Genes related to dysplasia and cancer	FHIT
Genes related to extraintestinal manifestations	CARD15, FcRL3, HLADRB103, HLAB27, HLA-B44, HLA-B35, TNFa-308A, TNF-1031C, STAT3
Pharmacogenetics in Crohn Disease	CARD15, NAT, TPMT, MDR1, MIF, DLG5, TNF, LTA

Adapted from Tsianos EV, Katsanos KH, Tsianos VE. Role of genetics in the diagnosis and prognosis of Crohn's disease. *World J Gastroenterol.* 2012;18:105–118.

[NSAIDs]), decreased dietary fiber, and increase fat intake. In addition, dysbiosis with a decrease in intraluminal *Bacteroides* and *Firmicutes* and an increase in *Gammaproteobacteria* and *Actinobacteria* are associated with higher risk. Specifically, an increase of mucosal—adherent—invasive *E. coli* survive within macrophages and induce higher TNF-α production.[14] There are numerous studies evaluating the therapeutic benefits of microbiota manipulation.

Pathology

The most common sites of Crohn disease are the small intestine and colon. The location of disease involvement is biologically defined by the genetic variation. As such, a large multi-institutional study proposed a three-category model to better characterize inflammatory bowel disease into ileal Crohn disease, colonic Crohn disease, and ulcerative colitis. These categories provide risk stratification for surgical complications and genetic risk score based on location.[15] Ileal involvement has been shown with mutations of *IL10, CRP, NOD2, ZNF365*, and *STAT3*; ileocolonic involvement has been shown with mutations of *ATG16L1, TCF4*, and *TCF7L2*; and colonic involvement has been associated with mutations of *HLA, TLR4, TLR1, TLR2*, and *TLR6*. The involvement of the large and small intestine has been noted in about 55% of patients. Thirty percent of patients present with small bowel disease alone, and in 15%, the disease appears limited to the large intestine. The disease process is discontinuous and segmental. In patients with colonic disease, rectal sparing is characteristic of Crohn disease and helps distinguish it from ulcerative colitis. Perirectal and perianal involvement occurs in about one third of patients with Crohn disease, particularly those with colonic involvement. Crohn disease can also involve the mouth, esophagus, stomach, duodenum, and appendix. Involvement of these sites can accompany disease in the small or large intestine, but in only rare cases have these locations been the only apparent sites of involvement.

Gross pathologic features. At exploration, thickened gray-pink or dull purple-red loops of bowel are noted, with areas of thick gray-white exudate or fibrosis of the serosa. Areas of diseased bowel separated by areas of grossly appearing normal bowel, called *skip areas*, are commonly encountered. A striking finding of Crohn disease is the presence of extensive fat wrapping caused by the circumferential growth of the mesenteric fat around the bowel wall, also known as creeping fat (Fig. 50.16). As the disease progresses, the bowel wall becomes increasingly thickened, firm, rubbery, and almost incompressible (Fig. 50.17). The uninvolved proximal bowel may be dilated secondary to obstruction of the diseased segment. Involved segments often are adherent to adjacent intestinal loops or other viscera, with internal fistulas common in these areas. The mesentery of the involved segment is usually thickened, with enlarged lymph nodes often noted.

On opening of the bowel, the earliest gross pathologic lesion is a superficial aphthous ulcer noted in the mucosa. With increasing disease progression, the ulceration becomes pronounced, and complete transmural inflammation results. The ulcers are characteristically linear and may coalesce to produce transverse sinuses

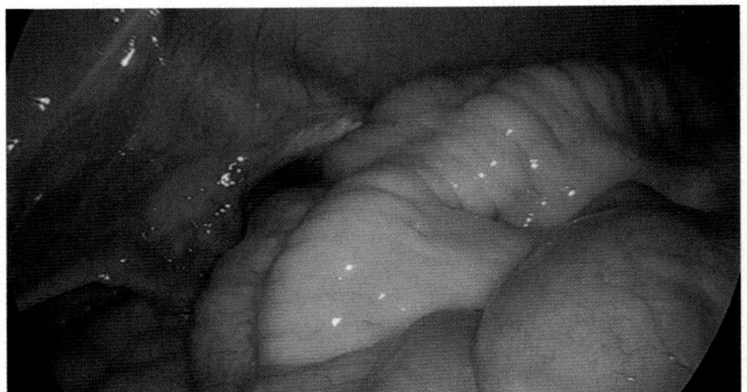

FIG. 50.16 Crohn disease with evidence of creeping fat. Laparoscopic evaluation of extensive fat wrapping caused by the circumferential growth of the mesenteric fat around the bowel wall. (Courtesy Dr. John Draus, University of Kentucky Medical Center, Lexington, KY.)

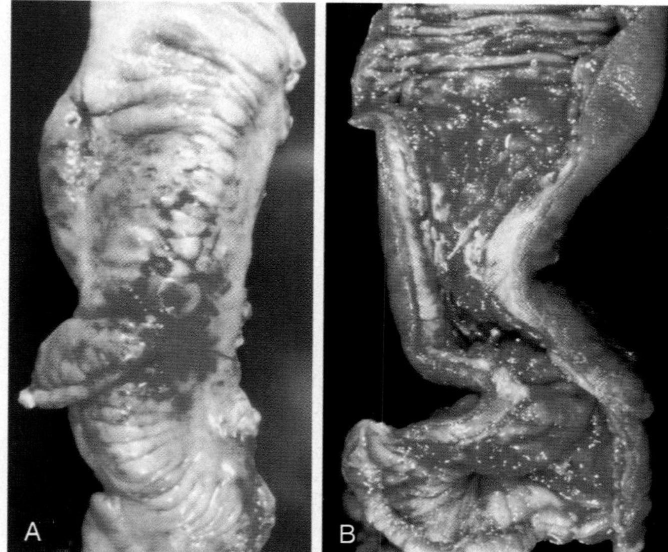

FIG. 50.17 Gross pathologic features of Crohn disease. (A) Serosal surface demonstrates extensive fat wrapping and inflammation. (B) Resected specimen demonstrates marked fibrosis of the intestinal wall, stricture, and segmental mucosal inflammation. (Courtesy Dr. Mary R. Schwartz, Baylor College of Medicine, Houston, TX.)

with islands of normal mucosa in between, thus giving the characteristic cobblestone appearance.

Microscopic features. Mucosal and submucosal edema may be noted microscopically before any gross changes. A chronic inflammatory infiltrate appears in the mucosa and submucosa and extends transmurally. This inflammatory reaction is characterized by extensive edema, hyperemia, lymphangiectasia, intense infiltration of mononuclear cells, and lymphoid hyperplasia. Characteristic histologic lesions of Crohn disease are noncaseating granulomas with Langerhans giant cells. Granulomas appear later in the course and are found in the wall of the bowel or in regional lymph nodes in 60% to 70% of patients (Fig. 50.18).

Clinical Manifestations

Crohn disease can occur at any age, but the typical patient is a young adult in the second or third decade of life. The onset of disease is often insidious, with a slow and protracted course. Characteristically, there are symptomatic periods of abdominal pain and diarrhea interspersed with asymptomatic periods of varying lengths. With time, the symptomatic periods gradually become more frequent, more severe, and longer lasting. The most common symptom of Crohn disease is chronic diarrhea, followed by intermittent and colicky abdominal pain, most commonly noted in the lower abdomen. The pain, however, may be more severe and localized in the right lower quadrant and may mimic the signs and symptoms of acute appendicitis.[16] In contrast to ulcerative colitis, patients with Crohn disease typically have fewer bowel movements, and the stools rarely contain mucus, pus, or blood. Systemic nonspecific symptoms include a low-grade fever present in about one third of the patients, weight loss, loss of strength, and malaise.

Clinically, Crohn disease is often classified on the basis of age at onset, behavior, and site of origin. The Montreal Classification (Table 50.6) divides all patients into distinct categories based on symptom onset (before or after the age of 40 years), disease behavior (nonstricturing/nonpenetrating, stricturing, or penetrating), and disease site (terminal ileum, colon, ileocolonic, upper gastrointestinal tract). This classification was developed to provide a reproducible staging of the disease, to help predict remission and relapse, and to direct therapy. The main intestinal complications of Crohn disease include obstruction and perforation. Obstruction can occur as a manifestation of an acute exacerbation of active disease or as the result of chronic fibrosing lesions, which eventually narrow the lumen of the bowel, producing partial or near-complete obstruction. Free perforations into the peritoneal cavity leading to a generalized peritonitis can occur in patients with Crohn disease, but this presentation is rare. More commonly, fistulas occur between the sites of perforation and adjacent organs, such as loops of small and large intestine, urinary bladder, vagina, stomach, and sometimes the skin, usually at the site of a previous laparotomy. Localized abscesses can occur near the sites of perforation. Patients with Crohn colitis may develop toxic megacolon and present with a marked colonic dilation, abdominal tenderness, fever, and leukocytosis. Bleeding is typically indolent and chronic, but massive gastrointestinal bleeding can occasionally occur, particularly in duodenal Crohn disease associated with chronic ulcer formation.

Long-standing Crohn disease predisposes to cancer of the small intestine and colon. These carcinomas typically arise at sites of chronic disease and more commonly occur in the ileum as a result of the chronic inflammation of the mucosa. Most are not detected until in advanced stages, and the prognosis is poor. Although the relative risk for small bowel cancer in Crohn disease is approximately 100-fold, the absolute risk is still small. Of greater concern is the development of colorectal cancer in patients with colonic involvement and a long duration of disease. Dysplasia is the putative precursor lesion for Crohn disease–associated cancer. Patients with long-standing Crohn disease should have an equally aggressive colonoscopic surveillance regimen as patients with extensive ulcerative colitis.[17] Small bowel adenocarcinoma associated with Crohn disease has an aggressive behavior and a strong probability of extracellular mucin. In surgical specimens from patients with Crohn disease, mucinous-appearing anal fistulas and ileal areas of adhesion/retraction should always be closely examined by a pathologist to evaluate for dysplasia or malignancy.

Extraintestinal cancer, such as squamous cell carcinoma of the vulva and anal canal and Hodgkin and non-Hodgkin lymphomas, may be more frequent in patients with Crohn disease, especially those treated with immunomodulators.

Perianal disease (fissure, fistula, stricture, or abscess) is common and occurs in 25% of patients with Crohn disease limited to the small intestine, 41% of patients with ileocolitis, and 48% of patients with colonic involvement alone. Perianal disease may be the sole presenting feature in 5% of patients and may precede the onset of intestinal disease by months or even years. Crohn disease should be suspected in any patient with multiple, chronic perianal fistulas.

Extraintestinal manifestations of Crohn disease may be present in 30% of patients. The most common symptoms are skin lesions (Fig. 50.19), which include erythema nodosum and pyoderma gangrenosum, arthritis and arthralgias, uveitis and iritis, hepatitis, pericholangitis, and aphthous stomatitis. In addition, amyloidosis, pancreatitis, and nephrotic syndrome may occur in these patients. These symptoms may precede, accompany, or appear independently of the underlying bowel disease.

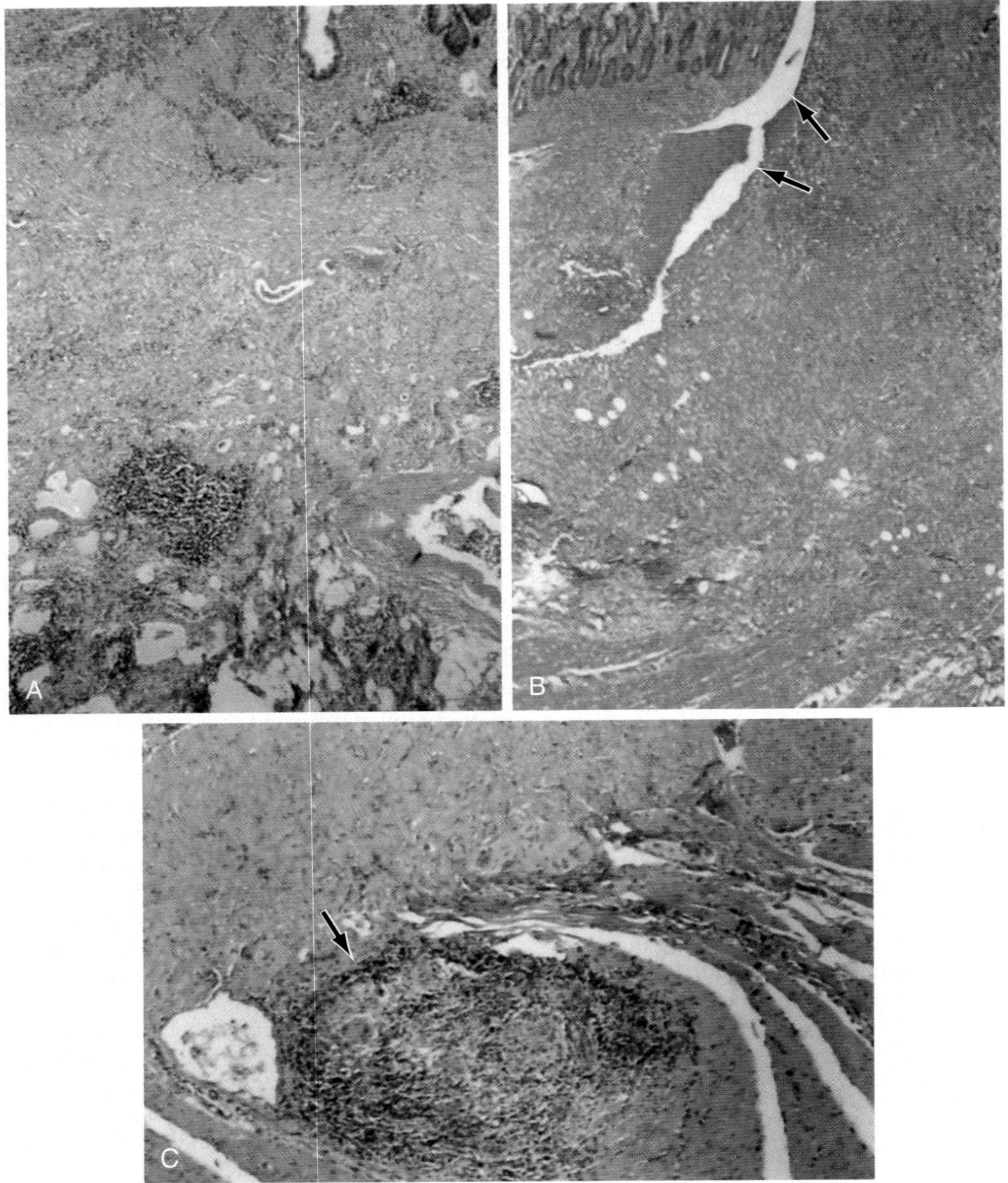

FIG. 50.18 Microscopic features of Crohn disease. (A) Transmural inflammation. (B) Fissure ulcer *(arrows)*. (C) Noncaseating granuloma located in the muscular layer of the small bowel *(arrow)*. (Courtesy Dr. Mary R. Schwartz, Baylor College of Medicine, Houston, TX.)

Diagnosis

A diagnosis of Crohn disease should be considered in patients with chronic recurring episodes of abdominal pain, diarrhea, and weight loss. However, there is not a single diagnostic test for Crohn disease; a multimodal approach of laboratory testing, endoscopy, radiology, and pathology is required.

Laboratory. Serologic markers may useful in the diagnosis of Crohn disease. In particular, perinuclear antineutrophil cytoplasmic antibody (and its target proteins bactericidal/permeability increasing protein [BPI], lactoferrin, cathepsin G and elastase), anti–*Saccharomyces cerevisiae* antibody (ASCA), outer membrane porin of flagellin (anti-CBir1), and outer membrane porin of *E. coli* (OmpC-IgG) can predict the development of inflammatory bowel disease even in patients thought to be at low risk for development of disease.[18] ASCA is also useful in differentiating Crohn disease from ulcerative colitis as well as playing a role in determining patients who will require surgery in the future.

Noninvasive inflammatory markers, historically C-reactive protein and erythrocyte sedimentation rate, were used to aid in the initial diagnosis, to rule out exacerbations, to monitor response to systemic therapy, and to predict relapse; however, these markers were generally nonspecific and have largely been abandoned. Stool lactoferrin, an iron-binding protein in the secretory granules of neutrophils, and fecal calprotectin, a protein with antimicrobial properties released by squamous cells in response to inflammation, are inflammatory markers specific to the intestine that have shown promising results for the detection and surveillance of Crohn disease. A prospective study showed that both calprotectin

TABLE 50.6 **Montreal classification of Crohn disease.**

Age at diagnosis (years)	A1: ≤16
	A2: 17–40
	A3: >40
Behavior	B1: Nonstricturing/nonpenetrating
	B2: Stricturing
	B3: Penetrating
	P: Perianal disease modifier (can add to B1-3)
Location	L1: Ileal
	L2: Colonic
	L3: Ileocolonic
	L4: Isolated upper gastrointestinal tract (can add to L1-3)

Adapted from Spekhorst LM, Visschedijk MC, Alberts R, et al. Performance of the Montreal classification for inflammatory bowel diseases. *World J Gastroenterol*. 2014;20:15374–15381.

and lactoferrin levels correlate well with CT enterography (CTE) images of small bowel inflammation (mucosal irregularity, hyperdensity, stenosis, prestenotic dilation and mesenteric hypervascularity [i.e., comb sign]). Fecal calprotectin levels greater than 140 ng/mL, predicted small bowel inflammation with a sensitivity of 69% and a specificity of 82%. Similarly, fecal lactoferrin (>6 ng/mL) predicted small bowel inflammation with a sensitivity of 69% and a specificity of 79%. Fecal calprotectin is associated with elevated C-reactive protein and erythrocyte sedimentation rate levels, whereas fecal lactoferrin is only associated with elevated C-reactive protein levels. Together, these findings identify fecal calprotectin and lactoferrin as helpful screening tools for detecting early small bowel Crohn disease.[19]

Radiology. CTE or magnetic resonance enterography (MRE) are often used as the initial assessment of Crohn disease to complement direct ileocolonoscopy. Imaging studies can provide information regarding severity of inflammation, length, and focality and identify complications (e.g., obstruction or fistula). In addition, these studies support surgical planning and the evaluation of response to medical therapy.[20] Previously, barium enema was commonly used to identify features of Crohn disease. For example, long lengths of narrowed terminal ileum (Kantor string sign) may be present with long-standing disease (Fig. 50.20). Segmental and irregular patterns of bowel involvement may be noted. Fistulas between adjacent bowel loops and organs may be apparent (Fig. 50.21).

CTE may be useful in demonstrating the marked transmural thickening; it can also greatly aid in diagnosing extramural complications of Crohn disease, especially in the acute setting (Fig. 50.22). Both MRE and CTE are equally accurate in assessing disease activity and bowel damage; however, MRE may be superior to CTE in detecting intestinal strictures and ileal wall enhancement.[20] Recent studies suggest limiting the use of CTE in patients with long-standing Crohn disease because of its significant radiation exposure and need for numerous studies during the course of the disease. MRE is a useful adjunct to determine intestinal strictures as well as fistulas and sinus tracks; however, the relatively high cost, prolonged examination time, and limited availability may preclude many patients from receiving this procedure. Ultrasonography has limited value in the evaluation of patients with Crohn disease and has an especially lower accuracy for detecting the disease proximal to the terminal ileum. One study determined that this modality failed to identify disease proximal to the terminal ileum in up to 67% of patients; however, ultrasound may be helpful in the assessment of undiagnosed right lower quadrant pain.

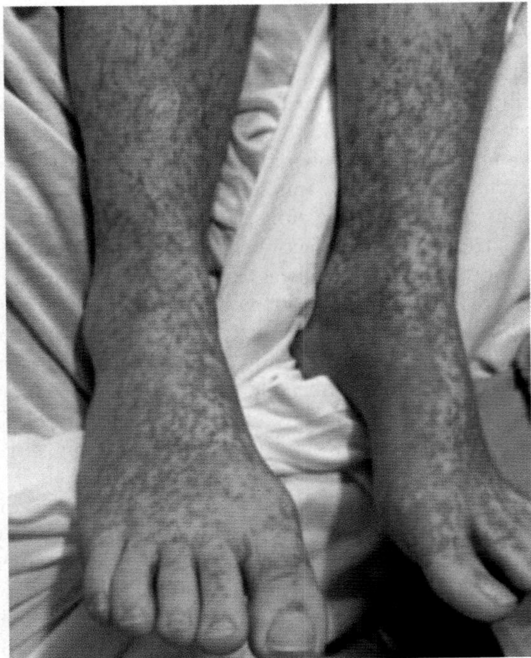

FIG. 50.19 Crohn disease patient with erythema nodosum. The most common extraintestinal presentations of Crohn disease are skin lesions, which include erythema nodosum and pyoderma gangrenosum.

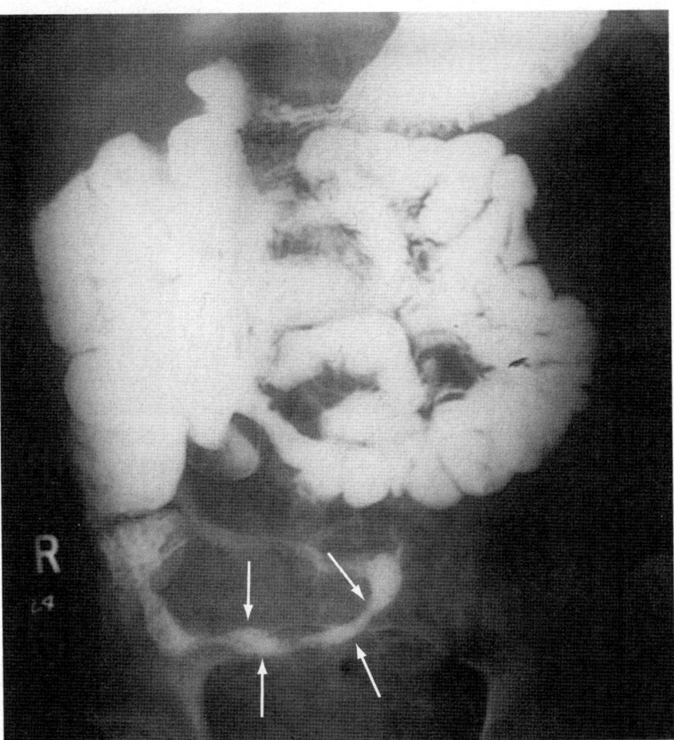

FIG. 50.20 Small bowel obstruction secondary to Crohn disease. Small bowel series in a patient with Crohn disease demonstrates a narrowed distal ileum *(arrows)* secondary to chronic inflammation and fibrosis. (Courtesy Dr. Melvyn H. Schreiber, The University of Texas Medical Branch, Galveston, TX.)

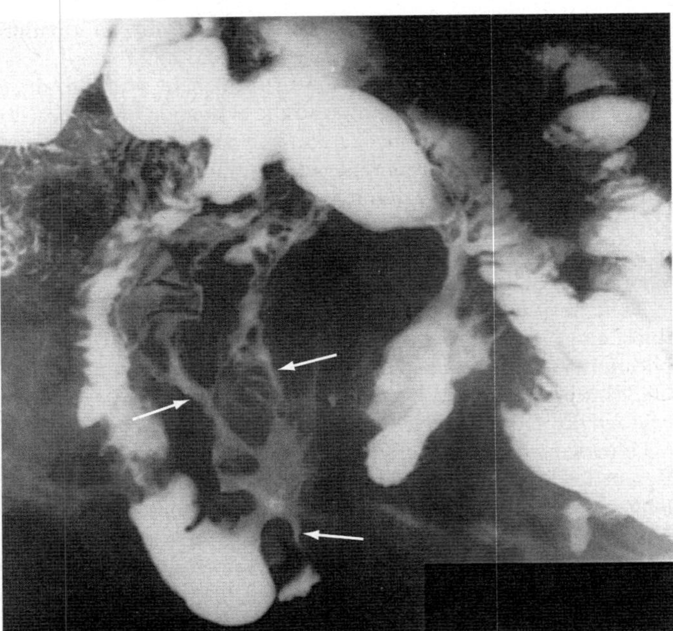

FIG. 50.21 Intraabdominal fistulas in Crohn disease. Multiple short fistulous tracts communicating between the distal loops of ileum and the proximal colon in a patient with Crohn disease *(arrows)*. (Courtesy Dr. Melvyn H. Schreiber, The University of Texas Medical Branch, Galveston, TX. Adapted from Evers BM, Townsend CM Jr, Thompson JC. Small intestine. In: Schwartz SI, ed. *Principles of Surgery*. 7th ed. New York: McGraw-Hill; 1999:1233.)

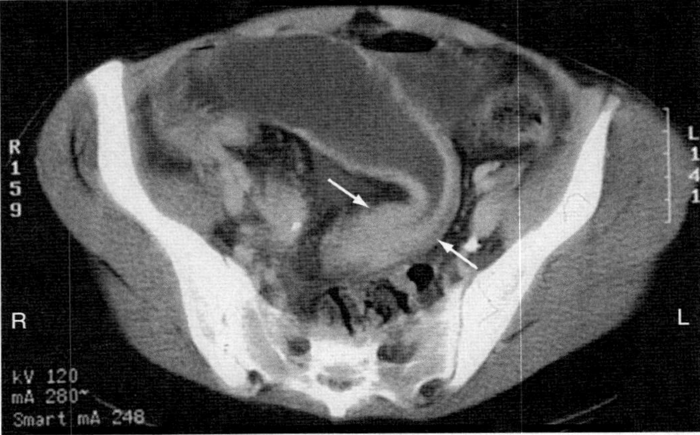

FIG. 50.22 Mechanical small bowel obstruction secondary to chronic structuring disease. Computed tomography enterography of a patient with Crohn disease demonstrates marked thickening of the bowel *(arrows)* with a high-grade partial small bowel obstruction and dilated proximal intestine. (Courtesy Dr. Melvyn H. Schreiber, The University of Texas Medical Branch, Galveston, TX. Adapted from Evers BM, Townsend CM Jr, Thompson JC. Small intestine. In: Schwartz SI, ed. *Principles of Surgery*. 7th ed. New York: McGraw-Hill; 1999:1233.)

Endoscopy. Ileocolonoscopy with biopsies of the terminal ileum are the gold standard for the diagnosis of Crohn disease. When the colon is involved, sigmoidoscopy or colonoscopy may reveal characteristic aphthous ulcers with granularity and a normal-appearing surrounding mucosa. Intubation of the ileocecal valve during colonoscopy allows examination and biopsy of the terminal ileum but fails to evaluate other segments of the small intestine. With more progressive and severe disease, the ulcerations involve progressively more of the bowel lumen, and it may be difficult to distinguish Crohn disease from ulcerative colitis. However, the presence of discrete ulcers and cobblestoning as well as the discontinuous segments of involved bowel favors a diagnosis of Crohn disease. Endoscopic advances that allow better evaluation of the small intestine include single-balloon enteroscopy, double-balloon enteroscopy, and spiral enteroscopy; the most well-established technique is double-balloon enteroscopy, which allows increased enteral intubation (240–360 cm) compared with push enteroscopy (90–150 cm) or ileocolonoscopy (50–80 cm). Limitations include specialized examiner skills and equipment, prolonged procedure times, and a 1% risk of complications (e.g., pancreatitis, perforation, or bleeding). After the diagnosis is confirmed, the Crohn Disease Endoscopic Index of Severity (CDEIS) or the Simple Endoscopic Score for Crohn Disease (SES-CD) is used to define extent of disease and severity.

Recently, capsule endoscopy was approved by the U.S. Food and Drug Administration (FDA) in 2001 and is helpful in the diagnosis of superficial mucosal abnormalities. The most commonly used criterion for an abnormal finding is the presence of three or more ulcers in the absence of NSAID use. The use of this modality is limited because of concern for capsule retention, defined as the presence of the capsule in the gastrointestinal tract for more than 2 weeks, which is of greater concern to patients with Crohn disease due to a significantly higher risk of retention (13%) compared with the general population (1%–2.5%). However, capsule endoscopy has been found to be superior to any other modality in the identification of intestinal ulceration. Severity is measured utilizing the Capsule Endoscopy Crohn Disease Activity Index (CECDAI or Niv score).[21] Further studies are needed to provide a more comprehensive evaluation of Crohn disease in the entire intestinal tract since new generations of capsule endoscopy devices will also provide visualization of colonic mucosa.

Histology

Differential diagnosis. The differential diagnosis of Crohn disease includes specific and nonspecific causes of intestinal inflammation. Bacterial inflammation (such as that caused by *Salmonella* and *Shigella*), intestinal tuberculosis, and protozoan infections (such as amebiasis) may manifest as an ileitis. In the immunocompromised host, rare infections, particularly mycobacterial and cytomegalovirus (CMV) infections, have become more common and may cause ileitis. Acute distal ileitis may be a manifestation of early Crohn disease, but it also may be unrelated, such as when it is caused by a bacteriologic agent (e.g., *Campylobacter*, *Yersinia*). Patients usually present in a similar fashion to those presenting with acute appendicitis, with a sudden onset of right lower quadrant pain, nausea, vomiting, and fever. These entities normally resolve spontaneously, and when they are noted during surgery, no biopsy or resection should be performed.

In most cases, Crohn disease of the colon can be readily distinguished from ulcerative colitis; however, in 5% to 10% of patients, the delineation between Crohn disease and ulcerative colitis may be difficult if not impossible to make (Table 50.7). Ulcerative colitis almost always involves the rectum most severely, with lessening inflammation from the rectum to the ileocolic area. In contrast, Crohn disease may be worse on the right side of the colon than on the left side, and sometimes the rectum is spared. Ulcerative colitis also demonstrates continuous involvement from

TABLE 50.7 **Diagnosis of Crohn colitis versus ulcerative colitis.**

PARAMETER	CROHN COLITIS	ULCERATIVE COLITIS
Symptoms and Signs		
Diarrhea	Common	Common
Rectal bleeding	Less common	Almost always
Abdominal pain (cramps)	Moderate to severe	Mild to moderate
Palpable mass	At times	No (unless large cancer)
Anal complaints	Frequent (>50%)	Infrequent (<20%)
Radiologic Findings		
Ileal disease	Common	Rare (backwash ileitis)
Nodularity, fuzziness	No	Yes
Distribution	Skip lesions	Rectum extending proximally and continuously
Ulcers	Linear, cobblestone, fissures	Collar-button
Toxic dilation	Rare	Uncommon
Proctoscopic Findings		
Anal fissure, fistula, abscess	Common	Rare
Rectal sparing	Common (50%)	Rare (5%)
Granular mucosa	No	Yes
Ulceration	Linear, deep, scattered	Superficial, universal

Adapted from Waugh N, Cummins E, Royle P, et al. Faecal calprotectin testing for differentiating amongst inflammatory and non-inflammatory bowel diseases: systematic review and economic evaluation. Southampton, UK: NIHR Journals Library; 2013 Nov. (Health Technology Assessment, No. 17.55. Appendix 1, Comparison of ulcerative colitis, Crohn's disease, irritable bowel syndrome and coeliac disease.

rectum to proximal segments, whereas Crohn disease is segmental. Although ulcerative colitis involves the mucosa of the large intestine, it does not extend deep into the wall of the bowel as does Crohn disease. Bleeding is a more common symptom in ulcerative colitis. Perianal involvement and rectovaginal fistulas are unusual in ulcerative colitis but are more common in Crohn disease. Other endoscopic features of Crohn disease are skip lesions, asymmetric involvement of bowel, and the cobblestone appearance that results from ulcerations interspersed with islands of edematous mucosa.

Management

Medical therapy. There is no cure for Crohn disease. Therefore, medical therapies are directed toward inducing and maintaining steroid-free remission as well as preventing acute exacerbations or complications of the disease. However, it is important to note that endoscopic healing has emerged as the therapeutic goal due to poor association of inflammation with symptoms.[14] Surgery is advocated for neoplastic and preneoplastic lesions, obstructing stenoses, suppurative complications, or medically intractable disease. Narcotic analgesia should be avoided except during the perioperative period because of the potential for tolerance and abuse in the setting of chronic disease. Drugs that have demonstrated efficacy in the induction or maintenance of remission in Crohn disease include aminosalicylates, such as sulfasalazine and mesalamine; corticosteroids; TNF antagonists, such as infliximab, adalimumab, and certolizumab; immunosuppressive agents, such as azathioprine (AZT), 6-mercaptopurine (6-MP), methotrexate (MTX), and tacrolimus (FK-506); antiadhesion molecules such as vedolizumab, etrolizumab, and natalizumab; the interleukin inhibitor ustekinumab; and antibiotics. The recent increase in the use of immunomodulators and biologic agents has significantly reduced surgery rates. The primary target of medical treatment is the reduction of the Crohn Disease Activity Index (CDAI), which uses eight major clinical factors to evaluate disease severity (Box 50.4).

BOX 50.4 **Crohn disease activity index (CDAI).**

Number of liquid or soft stools (each day for 7 days)
Abdominal pain, sum of 7 daily ratings (0 = none, 1 = mild, 2 = moderate, 3 = severe)
General well-being, sum of 7 daily ratings (0 = generally well, 1 = slightly under par, 2 = poor, 3 = very poor, 4 = terrible)
Number of listed complications (arthritis or arthralgia, iritis, uveitis, erythema nodosum or pyoderma gangrenosum, aphthous stomatitis, anal fissure, fistula or abscess, fever greater than 37.8°C [100°F]).
Use of diphenoxylate or loperamide for diarrhea (0 = no, 1 = year)
Abdominal mass (0 = no, 2 = questionable, 5 = definite)
Hematocrit (males >47%, or females >42%)
Body weight (1 - weight/standard weight) × 100 (add or subtract according to sign)

Adapted from Sandborn WJ, Feagan BG, Hanauer SB, et al. A review of activity indices and efficacy endpoints for clinical trials of medical therapy in adults with Crohn's disease. *Gastroenterology.* 2002;122:512–530.

Clinical remission is achieved when CDAI is below 150, and clinical response to therapy occurs with a drop of 100 points.[22] A score between 150 and 220 is considered mild to moderate disease and can be followed by outpatient visits; a score between 220 and 450 is considered moderate to severe disease and occurs after failure to first line therapy; a score greater than 450 is considered severe fulminant disease with failed medical therapy and complications of obstruction, peritonitis, and abscess. Other innovative therapies such as MadCAM-1 ([mucosal addressin cell adhesion molecule 1] inhibitor), tofacitinib (JAK3 pathway inhibitor), mongersen (SMAD7 inhibitor), and ozanimod (S1P1 inhibitor) are all currently under phase II/III clinical trials.

Aminosalicylates. Sulfasalazine (azulfidine) is an aminosalicylate with 5-aminosalicylic acid as the active moiety. Although a clear benefit has been noted in patients with colonic involvement, the effectiveness of sulfasalazine alone in the treatment of small bowel Crohn disease is controversial, and its use in maintenance therapy has fallen out of favor. Mesalamine, which is also an aminosalicylate, provides a slow release of 5-aminosalicylic acid with passage through the small bowel and colon. Clinical trials have demonstrated efficacy of mesalamine at a dosage of 4 g/day without an increase in side effects. However, 1% of patients will develop interstitial nephritis and renal function evaluation is needed periodically. If remission is achieved with mesalamine induction, then the medicine should be continued for maintenance.[11] Studies are currently being conducted to evaluate the efficacy of higher dosages of mesalamine to determine its continued utility as an appropriate first-line therapy.

Corticosteroids. Steroids are fast acting and effective at inducing remission but are not ideal as maintenance therapy. Budesonide, a corticosteroid, has a high first-pass hepatic metabolism, which allows targeted delivery to the intestine while mitigating the systemic effects of steroid therapy. Controlled ileal release budesonide (9 mg/day) is effective when active disease is confined to the ileum or right colon and has been shown to be more effective than either placebo or mesalamine.[23] Given a relatively good response and its relative safety, budesonide is recommended as the preferred primary treatment to mesalamine for patients with mild to moderately active Crohn disease with localized ileal disease.

An alternative corticosteroid, prednisone, can be beneficial in moderate to severe Crohn disease. Prednisone is not ideal for maintenance therapy as more than 50% of patients, particularly smokers, treated with corticosteroids become "steroid dependent," and chronic treatment is associated with osteoporosis and increased rates of Crohn disease relapse.[11] Patients with moderate to severe disease should be treated with high-dose (40–60 mg daily) prednisone until resolution of symptoms and resumption of weight gain. Parenteral corticosteroids are indicated for patients with severe disease once the presence of an abscess has been excluded. Steroids should be tapered once the patient experiences clinical improvement. Currently, there are no standards for corticosteroid taper, but doses are generally tapered by 5 to 10 mg/week until 20 mg, and then by 2.5 to 5 mg weekly until cessation. Dual-energy x-ray absorptiometry scan, calcium and vitamin D supplementation, and consideration of bisphosphonate therapy are warranted once corticosteroid therapy is initiated to identify baseline bone density and to prevent steroid-induced loss of bone mineral density.

Antibiotics. Certain antibiotics were found to be effective as a primary therapy for Crohn disease. Promising results were initially reported for metronidazole, but later studies determined that it was no more effective than placebo for inducing remission. Other antibiotics that have been used with varying success include ciprofloxacin, rifaximin, clofazimine, ethambutol, isoniazid, and rifabutin. Antibiotic therapy has a clear role in the septic complications associated with Crohn disease and is beneficial in perianal disease.[11] The mechanism of action of antibiotics in Crohn disease is unclear, and side effects of these antibiotics preclude their long-term use. Therefore, antibiotics may play an adjunctive role in the treatment of Crohn disease and, in selected patients, may be useful in treating perianal disease, enterocutaneous fistulas, or active colonic disease but should not be used in maintenance therapy or to induce remission.

Immunosuppressive agents. The immunosuppressive agents AZT, 6-MP, and MTX are effective in maintenance therapy and for the treatment of moderate to severe Crohn disease. AZT and 6-MP are effective for maintaining steroid-induced remission, and weekly IV MTX is effective for both induction and maintenance therapy.[11] Because of the slow onset of action of immunosuppressive agents and to prevent flares, steroids are needed for induction and continued until the transition to immunosuppressive agents is complete. Despite their potential toxicity, these drugs have proved to be relatively safe in patients with Crohn disease; the most common side effects are pancreatitis, hepatitis, fever, and rash. The more disconcerting complications of immunosuppressants include chronic liver disease, bone marrow suppression, and the potential for malignant transformation. No prospective controlled trial has evaluated dose escalation or initiation of therapy using these drugs. Genetic polymorphisms for thiopurine methyltransferase (TPMT), which is the primary enzyme that metabolizes AZT and 6-MP, have been identified and suggested for use to regulate therapy according to the measurement of their metabolites (6-thioguanine nucleotides). Patients with decreased TPMT activity have a significantly increased risk of fatal bone marrow suppression. Previous studies reported severe myelosuppression in patients who are wild-type or heterozygous carriers for TPMT variant alleles; these findings suggest that TPMT genotype testing may be a safe screening tool to determine which patients may have a genetic predisposition to adverse outcomes. MTX also has side effects of hepatotoxicity and can cause myelosuppression and should not be used in pregnant women.

Other immunosuppressive agents that have been used with some efficacy include cyclosporine and FK-506. FK-506 inhibits the production of IL-2 by helper T cells and was found to be effective for fistula improvement, but not fistula remission, in patients with perianal Crohn disease. Both of these agents have been used in patients with severe disease who do not respond to IV steroids. Low-dose cyclosporine was not found to be efficacious; however, in uncontrolled studies, FK-506 demonstrated some benefit in patients with steroid-refractory disease.

Anti-TNF therapy. The introduction of anti-TNF therapy for Crohn disease was considered a breakthrough in medical management. The first anti-TNF agent introduced was infliximab, a chimeric monoclonal antibody to TNF-α. Infliximab is efficacious and safe as a monotherapy in the treatment of moderate to severe Crohn disease and effective both an induction and maintenance agent. Multiple studies demonstrated that treatment with infliximab results in perineal fistula closure in approximately two-thirds of patients. Although it is highly effective in certain Crohn disease patients with penetrating and extraintestinal disease, not every patient responds to infliximab. Other FDA-approved TNF antagonists include adalimumab (humanized IgG1 monoclonal antibody), which is an effective maintenance agent that can be self-administered, and certolizumab (humanized antibody fragment), which is ideal in pregnant and nursing women as it is linked to a polyethylene glycol moiety and does not cross the placenta and is not excreted in breast milk. Safety profiles for these three anti-TNF medications are similar. There is an increased risk for tuberculosis reactivation, invasive fungal and other opportunistic infections, demyelinating central nervous system lesions, activation of latent multiple sclerosis, exacerbation of congestive heart failure, and concerns for increased risk of melanoma. Patients who develop a flare while on anti-TNF agents require measurement of serum drug concentrations and antidrug antibodies (antibodies binding to competitive and noncompetitive sites to inhibit drug function). Measured levels would indicate the need to increase dosage (if low drug concentration and low antibodies), switch to another anti-TNF agent (high antidrug antibodies), or switch to another drug class (normal drug concentration). Due to the potential for immunogenicity of monoclonal antibodies, the combination of an anti-TNF agent and an immunosuppressive provides optimal drug levels and low antidrug antibodies.[11]

Novel therapies. Other therapeutic agents for Crohn disease include leukocyte trafficking inhibitors, interleukin inhibitors, and antibodies to antiadhesion molecule. These agents are often used if the patient has failed or is unable to tolerate anti-TNF therapy. Natalizumab, a recombinant humanized monoclonal antibody against α_4 integrin, showed effectiveness in the induction and maintenance of remission in patients with active Crohn disease. It was removed from the market after several patients developed progressive multifocal leukoencephalopathy but was later reinstated for refractory Crohn disease and approved for use in 2008. Similarly, vedolizumab is a humanized monoclonal antibody that specifically binds to $\alpha_4\beta_7$ integrin and blocks its interaction with MadCAM-1; this action inhibits the translocation of memory T lymphocytes into inflamed gastrointestinal parenchymal tissues. Vedolizumab can be used for induction of remission, but it has a very slow onset of action. Because MadCAM-1 is preferentially expressed on blood vessels in the gastrointestinal tract, vedolizumab is more gut specific and therefore a more targeted form of immunosuppression. Also, vedolizumab prevents the gastrointestinal mucosal or transmural inflammation without the nonspecific neurologic side effects seen in less selective α_4 integrin inhibitors, such as natalizumab. Vedolizumab was approved for use in 2014 in those with a poor response to anti-TNF or immunosuppressants.[14] Ustekinumab is a humanized IgG1 monoclonal antibody that inhibits IL-12/23 through targeting of a shared p40 subunit. In two large trials, it was shown to be effective in severe Crohn disease that is refractory to anti-TNF therapies with similar efficacy. Ustekinumab was approved for use in 2016.[11] Compounds are also being evaluated that block certain signaling pathways (e.g., NF-κB, mitogen-activated protein kinases, and peroxisome proliferator-activated receptor-γ) in limited studies. Some compounds have shown clinical improvement, but results have varied, and these agents are still under development.

Nutritional therapy. Nutritional therapy in patients with Crohn disease has been used with varying success. The use of chemically defined elemental diets has been shown in some studies to reduce disease activity, particularly in patients with disease localized to the small bowel, and they can reduce corticosteroid-induced toxicities. Liquid polymeric diets may be as effective as elemental feedings and are more acceptable to patients. With few exceptions, standard elemental diets have not been effective to prevent relapse of Crohn disease. Total parenteral nutrition (TPN) was also useful in patients with active Crohn disease; however, complication rates exceed those for enteral nutrition. Although the primary role of nutritional therapy is questionable in patients with inflammatory bowel disease, there is definitely a secondary role for nutritional supplementation to replenish depleted nutrient stores, allowing intestinal protein synthesis and healing, and to prepare patients for surgery.

Smoking cessation. Although the implication of tobacco abuse as a causative factor in the development of Crohn disease has been difficult to prove, smoking clearly affects the disease course. Smoking is associated with the late bimodal onset of disease and has been shown to increase the incidence of relapse and failure of maintenance therapy. It also appears to be associated with the severity of disease in a linear dose-response relationship. Tobacco exposure is an independent predictor of the need for maintenance treatment, specifically biologic therapy. Therefore, smoking cessation therapy is an important component of medical therapy.

Surgical treatment. Although medical management is indicated during acute exacerbations of disease, most patients with chronic Crohn disease will require surgery at some time during the course of their illness. The goals are to preserve bowel length while minimizing postoperative complications and disease recurrence. Approximately 70% of patients will require surgical resection within 15 years after diagnosis. Indications for surgery include failure of medical treatment, bowel obstruction, fistula or abscess formation, steroid dependence, dysplasia or malignancy. Most patients can be treated with elective surgery, especially with the improvement of medical management in the past decade. However, patients with intestinal perforation, peritonitis, excessive bleeding, or toxic megacolon require urgent surgery.[24] Children with Crohn disease and resulting systemic symptoms, such as growth retardation, may benefit from resection. The extraintestinal complications of Crohn disease, although not primary indications for operation, often subside after resection of the involved bowel; exceptions are that problems may continue with ankylosing spondylitis and hepatic complications.

The aim of surgery for Crohn disease has shifted from a radical operation to one that achieves inflammation-free margins with minimal surgery, intended to remove just grossly inflamed tissue or to increase the luminal diameter of the bowel (i.e., dilation or strictureplasty). Even if adjacent areas of bowel are clearly diseased, they should be ignored. Fistulizing disease rarely requires operative intervention unless the fistula involves the bladder, vagina or skin. A bowel resection with fistulotomy may be needed. Early in the history of surgical therapy for Crohn disease, surgeons tended to perform wider resections with the hope of cure or significant remission. However, recurring wide resections resulted in neither cure nor a greater incidence of remissions and led to short bowel syndrome, a devastating surgical complication. Frozen sections to determine microscopic disease are unreliable and should be performed only when malignant disease is suspected. It must be emphasized that operative treatment of a complication must be limited to that segment of bowel involved with the complication, and no attempt should be made to resect more bowel, even though grossly evident disease may be apparent. However, often after removal of a diseased segment, endoscopic recurrence can occur up to 70% to 90% within 1 year after surgery in patients with Crohn disease.[24]

Laparoscopic surgery for patients with Crohn disease has been determined to be safe and feasible in appropriately selected patients, for example, those with localized abscesses, simple intra-abdominal fistulas, perianastomotic recurrent disease, and disease limited to the distal ileum. A large comparative study evaluating laparoscopic colectomy for Crohn colitis determined that the laparoscopic group had a significantly shorter median operative time, earlier return of bowel function, and shorter hospital stay.[25] Multiple randomized clinical trials verified that laparoscopic surgery is associated with a more rapid recovery of bowel function and shorter hospital stay; importantly, the rate of disease recurrence is similar when compared with open procedures. Randomized controlled trials with long-term follow-up have demonstrated that patients undergoing laparoscopic ileocolonic resection for Crohn disease had improved body image and satisfaction with cosmesis of surgery and less incidence of incisional hernia compared with the open surgery group. The potential for earlier recovery after laparoscopic resection has stimulated interest in extending the role of surgical resection to induce remission; the LIR!C trial is a randomized multicenter trial that found laparoscopic resection of uncomplicated ileocecal disease (terminal ileum <40 cm) that failed steroid treatment could be an alternative to anti-TNF therapy.[26]

Another difficult surgical decision important in Crohn disease involves performing a primary anastomosis versus initial ostomy formation with delayed reconstruction. Patients with Crohn disease are often malnourished, and receive intensive immunosuppressive therapy, or present with an element of intraabdominal sepsis. In general, standard surgical principles should direct this decision. Patients with adequate nutrition and minimal intraabdominal sepsis can safely undergo primary anastomosis at the initial operation, whereas malnourished and septic patients are best served by diversion, if possible. Although caution should be exercised in performing an anastomosis in the setting of high-dose immunosuppression, large series have confirmed that surgery is safe for patients with Crohn disease while they are receiving perioperative infliximab or immunosuppressive therapy. Regarding the anastomotic technique, several studies suggest that creating a wider anastomosis with a stapled functional end-to-end anastomosis may decrease fecal stasis and subsequent bacterial overgrowth, which are implicated in anastomotic recurrence in Crohn disease. However, a randomized controlled trial comparing side-to-side anastomosis versus end-to-end anastomosis determined that there was no difference in overall complication rates, anastomotic leak rates, or rates of symptomatic recurrence, with only a slight increase in endoscopic recurrence seen in the end-to-end anastomosis group (43% vs. 38%). Additionally, a new antimesenteric functional end-to-end hand-sewn anastomosis (known as Kono-S anastomosis) was created to minimize anastomotic restenosis in Crohn disease. This technique was demonstrated to have a significantly lower rate of stenosis and recurrence compared to conventional end to end anastomosis. Although further randomized control trials are needed, these findings demonstrate a promising novel surgical approach that may decrease the need for additional biologic therapy.[27]

Specific Problems

Acute ileitis (nonstricturing, nonpenetrating). Patients can present with acute abdominal pain localized to the right lower quadrant, signs and symptoms consistent with a diagnosis of acute appendicitis. At exploration, the appendix is found to be normal, but the terminal ileum is edematous and beefy red with a thickened mesentery and enlarged lymph nodes. This condition, known as *acute ileitis*, is a self-limited disease. Acute ileitis may be a manifestation of early Crohn disease but is most often unrelated. Bacteriologic agents such as *Campylobacter* and *Yersinia* may cause acute ileitis. Intestinal resection should not be performed. Although past management of the appendix was controversial, it is clear now that, in the absence of acute inflammatory involvement of the appendix or the cecum, appendectomy should be performed. This eliminates the appendix as a source of abdominal pain in the future.

Stricturing disease. Intestinal obstruction is the most common indication for surgical therapy in patients with Crohn disease. Obstruction in these patients is often partial, and nonoperative management is initially indicated. The success of nonoperative management can often be predicted on the basis of the chronicity of symptoms at the affected site. In patients for whom it is difficult to determine whether the site of obstruction is caused by an acute exacerbation or a chronically strictured segment, stool lactoferrin and calprotectin levels may help identify acute inflammation, whereas certain genetic markers (e.g., *NOD2*, *TLR4*, *CX-3CR1*) may predict potential success of medical therapy. In case of a chronic strictured segment, medical therapy is rarely effective. Operative intervention is required for patients with complete obstruction and partial obstruction whose condition does not resolve with nonoperative management. The treatment of choice for intestinal obstruction in patients with Crohn disease is segmental resection of the involved segment with primary reanastomosis. This may involve segmental resection and primary anastomosis of a short segment of ileum or an ileocecectomy if both the ileum and cecum are involved (Fig. 50.23).

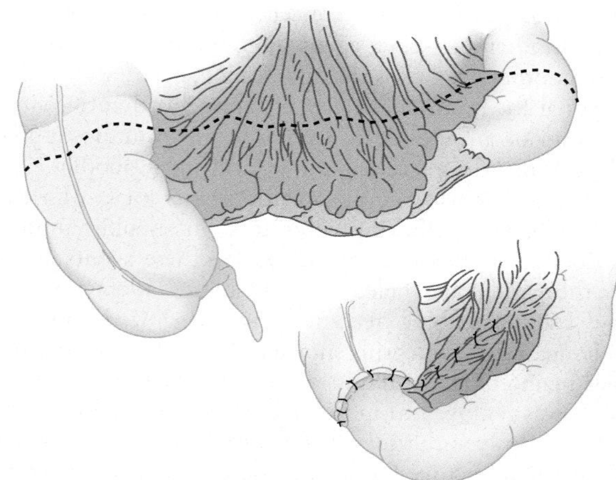

FIG. 50.23 Ileocecal resection secondary to Crohn disease. Resection of the ileum, ileocecal valve, cecum, and ascending colon for Crohn disease of the ileum. Intestinal continuity is restored by end-to-end anastomosis.

In selected patients with obstruction caused by strictures (single or multiple), one option is to perform a strictureplasty that effectively widens the lumen but avoids intestinal resection. Strictureplasty is performed by making a longitudinal incision through the narrowed area of the intestine, followed by closure in a transverse fashion in a manner similar to that for a Heineke-Mikulicz pyloroplasty (Fig. 50.24A). For longer diseased segments (>10 cm), the strictureplasty can be performed similar to a Finney pyloroplasty (Fig. 50.24B) or a side-to-side isoperistaltic strictureplasty.[24] Strictureplasty is best used in those patients with multiple short areas of narrowing present over long segments of intestine, in those who have already had several previous resections of the small intestine, and in those with chronic fibrous obstruction. This procedure preserves intestine and is associated with complication and recurrence rates comparable to those of resection and reanastomosis. Given the concerns for development of carcinoma at chronically strictured segments, full-thickness biopsy with frozen section of the stricture site has been advocated at the time of surgery to rule out malignant disease before strictureplasty is performed (Box 50.5).

In the past, bypass procedures were commonly used. There are two types of bypass operations: exclusion bypass and simple (continuity) bypass. For certain types of ileocecal disease associated with an abscess or phlegmon densely adherent to the retroperitoneum, the proximal transected end of the ileum is anastomosed to the transverse colon in an end-to-side fashion with or without construction of a mucous fistula using the distal transected end of the ileum (exclusion bypass), or an ileotransverse colonic anastomosis is made in a side-to-side fashion (continuity bypass). Currently, bypass with exclusion is used only in patients with severe gastroduodenal Crohn disease not amenable to strictureplasty, older poor-risk patients, patients who have had several prior resections and cannot afford to lose any more bowel, and those in whom

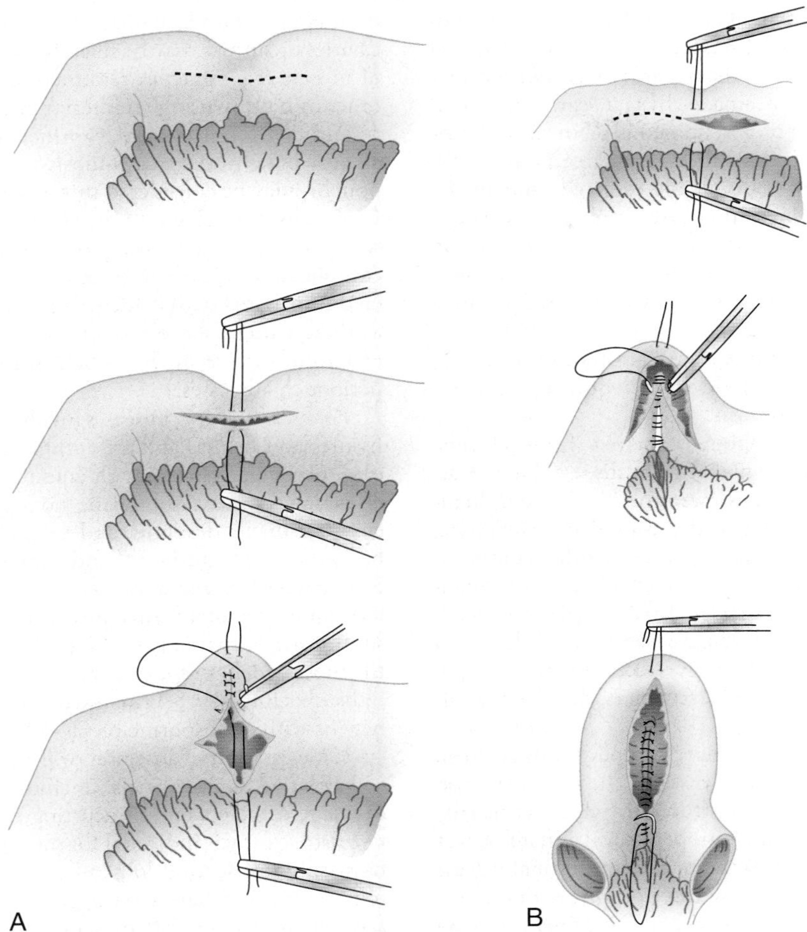

FIG. 50.24 Types of strictureplasty. (A) Technique of short strictureplasty in the manner of a Heineke-Mikulicz pyloroplasty. (B) For longer diseased segments, strictureplasty may be performed in a manner similar to Finney pyloroplasty. (Adapted from Alexander-Williams J, Haynes IG. Up-to-date management of small-bowel Crohn's disease. In: Mannick JA, ed. *Advances in Surgery*. St. Louis: Mosby; 1987:245–264.)

BOX 50.5 Contraindications to strictureplasty.

- Excessive tension due to rigid and thickened bowel segments
- Perforation of the intestine
- Fistula or abscess formation at the intended strictureplasty site
- Hemorrhagic strictures
- Multiple strictures within a short segment
- Malnutrition or hypoalbuminemia (<2.0 g/dL)
- Suspicion of cancer at the intended strictureplasty site

Adapted from Yamamoto T, Watanabe T. Surgery for luminal Crohn's disease. *World J Gastroenterol.* 2014;20:78–90.

resection would necessitate entering an abscess or endangering a normal structure.

Penetrating disease. Fistula and abscess in patients with Crohn disease are relatively common and usually involve adjacent small bowel, colon, or other surrounding viscera (e.g., bladder). The presence of a radiographically demonstrable enteroenteral fistula with no signs of sepsis or other complications is not in itself an indication for surgery. Furthermore, penetrating disease is particularly sensitive to anticytokine therapy, and a conservative, surgical approach to Crohn disease–related fistula is most appropriate.[24] Enterocutaneous fistulas may develop but are rarely spontaneous and are more likely to follow resection or drainage of intraabdominal abscesses. These fistulas may close spontaneously, and treatment should entail outflow reduction, preventing infection, maximizing nutrition and optimal skin care. If conservative management fails, excision of the fistula tract and primary anastomosis is preferred. Note that preoperative optimization is necessary, as Crohn patients with penetrating disease tend to have longer operative times, higher reoperation rates, increased length of stay, and postoperative complications. If the fistula forms between two or more adjacent loops of diseased bowel, the involved segments should be excised. Alternatively, if the fistula involves an adjacent normal organ, such as the bladder or colon, only the segment of the diseased small bowel and fistulous tract should be resected, and the defect in the normal organ should simply be closed. Most patients with ileosigmoid fistulas do not necessarily require resection of the sigmoid because the disease is usually confined to the small bowel. However, if the segment of sigmoid is also found to have Crohn disease, it should be resected along with the segment of diseased small bowel.

Perforation. Penetrating disease in the form of free perforation into the peritoneal cavity is uncommon in patients with Crohn disease. Typically, penetration is manifested with a localized abscess densely adherent to the diseased segment of bowel.

Patients who have an abscess smaller than 3 cm and have not been on biologics or have an associated fistula can be treated with antibiotics alone.[14] Abscesses that do not meet these criteria should undergo percutaneous drainage. In fact, early treatment of an abscess is key regardless of percutaneous or surgical drainage, in terms of time to resolution. In cases of free perforation, the segment of involved bowel should be resected, and in the presence of minimal contamination, a primary anastomosis can be performed. If generalized peritonitis is present, a safer option may be to create an ostomy until the intraabdominal sepsis is controlled and then have the patient return for restoration of intestinal continuity after a period of 4 to 6 weeks. Abscesses can be treated with percutaneous drainage and antibiotics; however, fistula or uncontrolled sepsis may develop, requiring resection with or without primary anastomosis.

Gastrointestinal bleeding. Although anemia from chronic blood loss is common in patients with Crohn disease, life-threatening gastrointestinal hemorrhage is rare. The incidence of hemorrhage is more common in patients with Crohn disease involving the colon rather than the small bowel. As with the other complications, the segment involved should be resected and intestinal continuity restored. Arteriography may be useful to localize the bleeding before surgery. In cases of bleeding associated with duodenal disease, endoscopic intervention is usually successful. However, in cases of failure, duodenotomy with oversewing of the bleeding ulcerative area is indicated.

Urologic complications. Genitourinary complications occur in up to one third of patients with Crohn disease. The most common urologic complication is ureteral obstruction, which is usually secondary to ileocolic disease with retroperitoneal inflammatory compression. Surgical treatment of the primary intestinal disease is adequate in most patients. In a few cases of long-standing inflammatory disease, periureteric fibrosis may be present and require ureterolysis with or without ureteral stenting.

Cancer. Patients with long-standing Crohn disease of the small bowel and, in particular, the colon have an increased incidence of cancer. The management of these patients is the same as that for any patient—resection of the cancer with appropriate margins, lymphadenectomy, and perioperative chemotherapy/radiation. Patients with cancer associated with Crohn disease commonly have a worse prognosis than those who do not have Crohn disease, largely because the diagnosis in these patients is often delayed. In addition, a strictureplasty should not be performed if malignant disease is suspected.

Colorectal disease. The same principle applies to patients with Crohn disease limited to the colon as to those with disease to the small bowel; that is, surgical resection should be limited to the main segment involved. Indications for surgery include a lack of response to medical management and complications of Crohn colitis, which include obstruction, hemorrhage, perforation, and toxic megacolon. Depending on the diseased segments, procedures commonly include segmental colectomy with colocolonic anastomosis, total abdominal colectomy with ileorectal anastomosis, total proctocolectomy with ileoanal anastomosis, and in patients with extensive perianal and rectal disease, abdominoperineal resection with end ileostomy. Strictureplasty has limited usefulness in colonic Crohn disease, and concerns of malignant transformation at an area of colonic obstruction should limit its application.

A particularly troubling problem after abdominoperineal resection in patients with Crohn disease is delayed healing of the perineal wound. More than half of perineal wounds are open 6 months after surgery in patients with Crohn disease. Persistent nonhealing wounds require excision with secondary closure. Large cavities or sinuses may be filled by using well-vascularized pedicles of muscle (e.g., gracilis, semimembranosus, rectus abdominis) or omentum or by using an inferior gluteal myocutaneous graft.

Although controversial, continence-preserving operations, such as ileal pouch–anal anastomosis or continent ileostomies (Kock pouch), may be considered in very carefully selected patients with Crohn disease isolated to the colon who undergo thorough counseling about the increased risk of anastomotic failure and wound complication. However, these procedures should never be considered in patients with evidence of terminal ileal or perianal disease as these patients have a significantly increased rate of recurrence of Crohn disease in the pouch, fistulas to the anastomosis, and peripouch abscesses.

Perianal disease. Diseases involving the perianal region include fissures and fistulas and are common in patients with Crohn disease, particularly those with colonic involvement. The treatment of perianal disease should be nonoperative unless an abscess or complex fistula develops, and even in these cases, surgery should be approached cautiously and limited to addressing the specific problem with minimal tissue loss. Nonsuppurative, chronic fistulization or perianal fissuring is treated with antibiotics, immunosuppressive agents (e.g., AZT or 6-MP), and infliximab, which is the most widely supported therapy as it has shown the best results in fistula closure.[11] Several uncontrolled studies have shown some benefit with cyclosporine or FK-506 treatment.

Wide excision of abscesses or fistulas is not indicated, but more conservative interventions, including the liberal placement of drainage catheters and noncutting setons, are preferable. Definitive fistulotomy is indicated for most patients with superficial, low trans-sphincteric, and low intersphincteric fistulas, although one must recognize that some degree of anal stenosis may occur as a result of chronic inflammation. High transsphincteric, suprasphincteric, and extrasphincteric fistulas are usually treated with noncutting setons. Fissures are usually lateral, relatively painless, large, and indolent and often respond to conservative management. Abscesses should be drained, but large excisions of tissue *should not* be performed. Advancement flap closure of perineal fistulas may be required in certain cases. Selective construction of diverting stomas has good results in combination with optimal medical therapy to induce remission of inflammation. Proctectomy is infrequent but required in a subset of patients who have persistent and unremitting disease despite conservative medical and surgical therapy.

Duodenal disease. Crohn disease of the duodenum occurs in less than 5% of patients with Crohn disease and occurs most commonly in the duodenal bulb.[14] Operative intervention is uncommon. The primary indication for surgery in these patients is duodenal obstruction that does not respond to medical therapy, with endoscopic balloon dilation and surgery being the mainstays of treatment. Gastrojejunostomy to bypass the disease rather than duodenal resection is the procedure of choice. Strictureplasties have been performed with success in selected patients and may avoid the marginal ulceration and diarrhea associated with gastrojejunostomy.

Prognosis

Crohn disease is a chronic inflammatory disorder that is not medically or surgically curable; therefore, therapeutic approaches are required to induce and to maintain symptomatic control, to improve quality of life, and to minimize long-term complications. It is estimated that approximately 71% of patients will require surgery within 10 years of diagnosis, and 50% require a second procedure within 20 years.[28] Symptomatic recurrence varies from 40% to 80%, and endoscopic recurrence is much higher, with up to 90% of patients having visible lesions within 5 years. The only clearly modifiable risk factor is smoking cessation. Surgery is generally indicated when the patient fails to respond to medical therapy or develops complications, and multiple studies have shown that patients report significant improvement in quality of life scores after surgical intervention. Although postsurgical recurrence is high, algorithms using careful endoscopic surveillance combined with maintenance immunomodulators, anti-TNF antibodies, anti-integrin therapy, and even investigational traditional Chinese medicine all play a role in the prevention of postoperative recurrence of Crohn disease (Fig. 50.25). Although there is currently no cure for this disease, advances in medical and surgical therapies have clearly increased quality of life and disease-free progression.

Standardized mortality rates in patients with Crohn disease show an increase in those whose disease began before the age of 20 years and in those who have had disease for longer than 13 years. Long-term survival studies suggest that patients with Crohn disease have a death rate approximately two to three times higher than that of the general population, which is most commonly related to chronic wound complications and sepsis. Gastrointestinal cancer remains the leading cause of disease-related deaths in patients with Crohn disease; other causes of disease-related deaths include sepsis, thromboembolic complications, and electrolyte disorders.

Typhoid Enteritis

Typhoid fever remains a significant problem in developing countries, most commonly in areas with contaminated water supplies and inadequate waste disposal. Roughly 21.6 million people worldwide develop typhoid fever with an estimated 200,000 deaths per year. Children and young adults are most often affected. Improvements in sanitation have decreased the incidence of typhoid fever in industrialized countries. Most cases of typhoid fever in the United States arise in international travelers; however, unrecognized and untreated typhoid fever is a life-threatening illness with significant long-term morbidity.

Typhoid enteritis is an acute systemic infection caused primarily by *Salmonella typhi*. The pathologic events of typhoid fever are initiated in the intestinal tract after oral ingestion of the typhoid bacillus. These organisms penetrate the small bowel mucosa, making their way rapidly to the lymphatics, and then spreading systemically. Hyperplasia of the reticuloendothelial system, including lymph nodes, liver, and spleen, is characteristic of typhoid fever. Peyer patches in the small bowel become hyperplastic and may subsequently ulcerate, complicated by hemorrhage or perforation.

The diagnosis of typhoid fever is confirmed by isolating the organism from blood (positive in 90% of the patients during the first week of the illness), bone marrow, and stool cultures. In addition, the finding of high titers of agglutinins against O and H antigens (Widal test) was used historically but is nonspecific and is no longer an acceptable clinical method. Assays for the diagnosis of *S. typhi* using PCR analysis are unpredictable. Combining blood and urine cultures achieved a sensitivity of 83% and reported specificity of 100%. Indirect hemagglutination, indirect fluorescent Vi antibody, and indirect enzyme-linked immunosorbent assay for IgM and IgG antibodies to *S. typhi* polysaccharide are promising, but the success rates of these assays vary greatly in the literature.

Typhoid fever and uncomplicated typhoid enteritis are treated by antibiotic administration. If a patient presents with clinical symptoms and has been in an endemic area, broad-spectrum empirical antibiotics should be started immediately. Treatment should not be delayed for confirmatory tests because prompt treatment drastically reduces the risk of complications and fatalities. Antibiotic therapy should be narrowed once more information is available. Chloramphenicol was initially the mainstay of treatment in the 1950s, but widespread antibiotic resistance occurred. Currently, the most widely used agents are fluoroquinolones and third-generation cephalosporins.

Complications requiring potential surgical intervention include hemorrhage and perforation. The incidence of hemorrhage

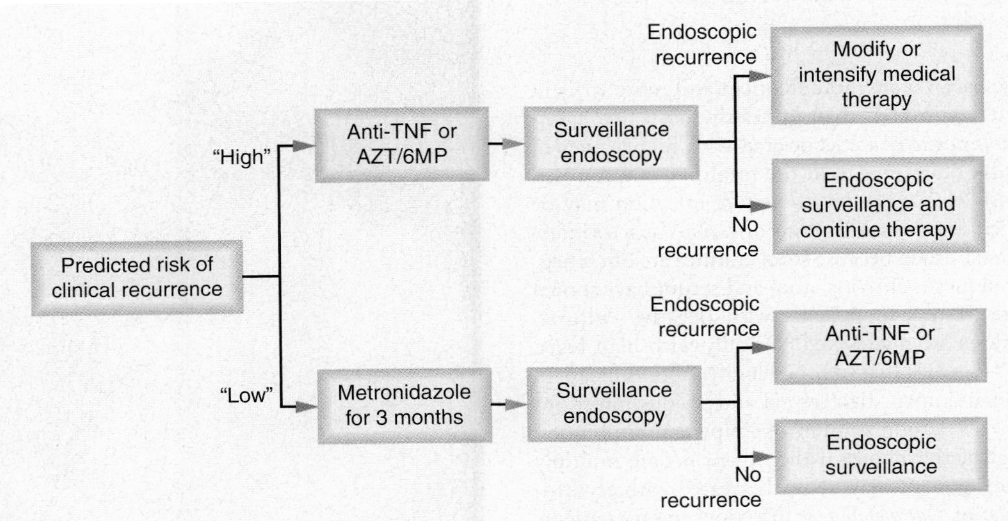

FIG. 50.25 Postoperative surveillance algorithm for Crohn disease. (Adapted from Vaughn BP, Moss AC. Prevention of post-operative recurrence of Crohn's disease. *World J Gastroenterol.* 2014;20:1147–1154; and Regueiro M, Feagan BG, Zou B, et al. Infliximab reduces endoscopic, but not clinical, recurrence of Crohn's disease after ileocolonic resection. *Gastroenterology.* 2016;150:1568–1578). *AZT*, Azathioprine; *6MP*, 6-mercaptopurine; *TNF*, tumor necrosing factor.

was reported to be as high as 20% in one series, but with the availability of antibiotics, this figure has decreased. When hemorrhage occurs, transfusion is indicated and usually suffices. Rarely, laparotomy must be performed for uncontrollable, life-threatening hemorrhage. Intestinal perforation through an ulcerated Peyer patch occurs in approximately 2% of cases. Typically, it is a single perforation in the terminal ileum, and simple closure of the perforation is the treatment of choice. Multiple perforations, which occur in about 25% of patients, may require resection with primary anastomosis or exteriorization of the intestinal loop.

Enteritis in the Immunocompromised Host

The acquired immunodeficiency syndrome (AIDS) epidemic, as well as the widespread use of immunosuppressive agents after organ transplantation, has resulted in a number of rare and exotic pathogens infecting the gastrointestinal tract. Almost all patients with AIDS have gastrointestinal symptoms during their illness, the most common of which is diarrhea. A surgeon may be asked to evaluate the immunocompromised patient with abdominal pain, acute abdomen, or gastrointestinal bleeding; a number of protozoal, bacterial, viral, and fungal organisms may be responsible.

Protozoa

Protozoa (e.g., *Cryptosporidium*, *Isospora*, and *Microsporidium*) are the most frequent class of pathogens causing diarrhea in patients with AIDS. The small bowel is the most common site of infection. Diagnosis may be established by acid-fast staining of the stool or duodenal secretions, and the introduction of specific antigen tests for stool examination has improved diagnostic capabilities. Immunochromatography cards for the rapid detection of protozoal proteins from a small sample of stool are available from several different commercial sources and are more sensitive and specific (>90%) than traditional microscopic examinations. Symptoms are most commonly related to diarrhea, which may be at times intractable. Current treatment regimens have not been entirely effective, but drugs such as prophylactic cotrimoxazole and a highly active antiretroviral therapy appear to elicit a response to human immunodeficiency virus (HIV)–related diarrheal illnesses.[29]

Bacteria

Infections by enteric bacteria are more frequent and more virulent in individuals infected with HIV than in healthy hosts. *Salmonella*, *Shigella*, and *Campylobacter* are associated with higher rates of bacteremia and antibiotic resistance in the immunocompromised patient. The diagnosis of *Shigella* or *Salmonella* infection may be established by stool cultures. The diagnosis of *Campylobacter* infection is not as easily established because stool cultures are often negative, but PCR techniques evaluating stool and serum have shown promising diagnostic results in patients with negative cultures. These enteric infections are manifested clinically with high fever, abdominal pain, and diarrhea that may be bloody. Abdominal pain may mimic an acute abdomen. Bacteremia and serious infections should be treated by IV administration of imipenem antibiotics; ciprofloxacin is an attractive choice if the organisms are multiply resistant; the pregnant patient may be safely treated with erythromycin. The incidence of *Campylobacter* infection among patients with AIDS who were treated with rifabutin prophylaxis was reported to be decreased compared with untreated controls.

Diarrhea caused by *Clostridium difficile* is more common in patients with AIDS because of the increased antibiotic use in this population compared with healthy hosts. Diagnosis is by standard assays of stool for *C. difficile* enterotoxin. Treatment with metronidazole or vancomycin is usually effective.

Mycobacteria

Mycobacterial infection is a frequent cause of intestinal disease in immunocompromised hosts. This can be secondary to *Mycobacterium tuberculosis* or *Mycobacterium avium complex* (MAC), which is an atypical mycobacterium related to the type that causes cervical adenitis (scrofula). The usual route of infection is by swallowed organisms that directly penetrate the intestinal mucosa. The luminal gastrointestinal tract is affected by MAC infection, with massive thickening of the proximal small intestine often noted (Fig. 50.26). Clinically, patients with MAC present with diarrhea, fever, anorexia, and progressive wasting.

The most frequent site of intestinal involvement of *M. tuberculosis* is the distal ileum and cecum, with approximately 90% of patients demonstrating disease at this site. The gross appearance can be ulcerative, hypertrophic, or ulcerohypertrophic. The bowel wall appears thickened, and an inflammatory mass often surrounds the ileocecal region. Acute inflammation is apparent, as are strictures and even fistula formation. The serosal surface is normally covered with multiple tubercles, and mesenteric lymph nodes are frequently enlarged and thickened; on sectioning, caseous necrosis is noted. The mucosa is hyperemic, edematous, and, in some cases, ulcerated. On histologic evaluation, the distinguishing lesion is a granuloma, with caseating granulomas found most commonly in the lymph nodes. Most patients complain of chronic abdominal pain that may be nonspecific, weight loss, fever, and diarrhea.

The diagnosis of mycobacterial infection is made by identification of the organism in tissue by direct visualization with an

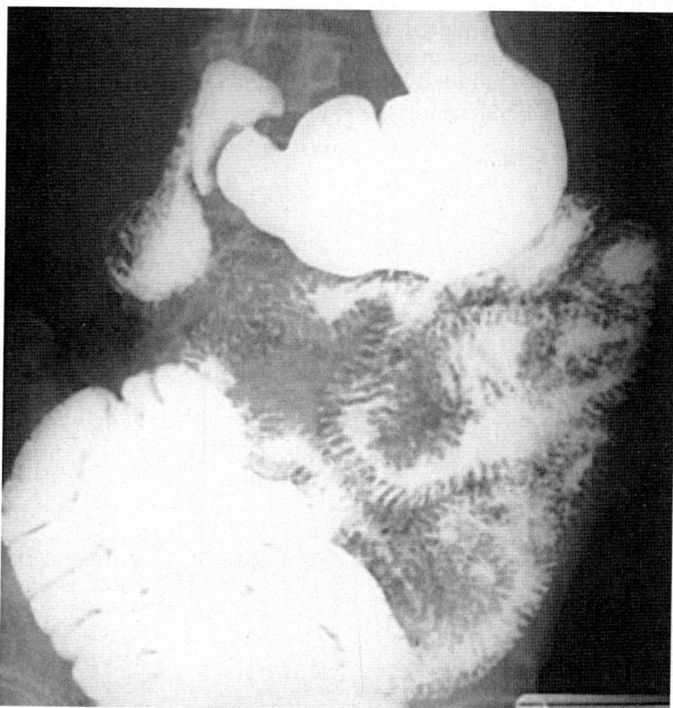

FIG. 50.26 Contrasted radiograph of thickened intestinal folds secondary to bacterial infection. A patient with acquired immunodeficiency syndrome shows thickened intestinal folds consistent with enteritis secondary to atypical mycobacterium. (Courtesy Dr. Melvyn H. Schreiber, The University of Texas Medical Branch, Galveston, TX.)

acid-fast stain, culture of the excised tissue, or PCR assay. Radiographic examinations usually reveal a thickened mucosa with distorted mucosal folds and ulcerations. CT may be useful and shows a thickening of the ileocecal valve and cecum.

The treatment of *M. tuberculosis* is similar in the immunocompromised or nonimmunocompromised host. The organism is usually responsive to multidrug antimicrobial therapy. The therapy for MAC infection is evolving; drugs that have been successfully used invivo and invitro include amikacin, ciprofloxacin, cycloserine, and ethionamide. Clarithromycin has also been successfully used in combination with other agents. Surgical intervention may be required for intestinal tuberculosis, particularly *M. tuberculosis*. Obstruction and fistula formation are the leading indications for surgery; however, with current treatment, most fistulas now respond to medical management. Surgery may be necessary for ulcerative complications when free perforation, perforation with abscess, or massive hemorrhage occurs. The treatment is usually resection with anastomosis.

Viruses

CMV is the most common viral cause of diarrhea in immunocompromised patients. Clinical manifestations include intermittent diarrhea accompanied by fever, weight loss, and abdominal pain. The manifestations of enteric CMV infection result from mucosal ischemic ulcerations, which account for the high rate of perforations noted with CMV. As a result of the diffuse ulcerating involvement of the intestine, patients may present with abdominal pain, peritonitis, or hematochezia. Diagnosis of CMV is made by demonstrating viral inclusions. The most characteristic form is an intranuclear inclusion, which is often surrounded by a halo, producing a so-called owl's eye appearance. There may also be cytoplasmic inclusions (Fig. 50.27). Cultures for CMV are usually positive when inclusion bodies are present, but these cultures are less sensitive and specific than histopathologic identification. Once CMV infection is diagnosed, treatment is usually effective with ganciclovir. An alternative to ganciclovir is foscarnet, a pyrophosphate analogue that inhibits viral replication. Infections with other less common viruses, including adenovirus, rotavirus, and novel enteric viruses such as astrovirus and picornavirus, have been reported.

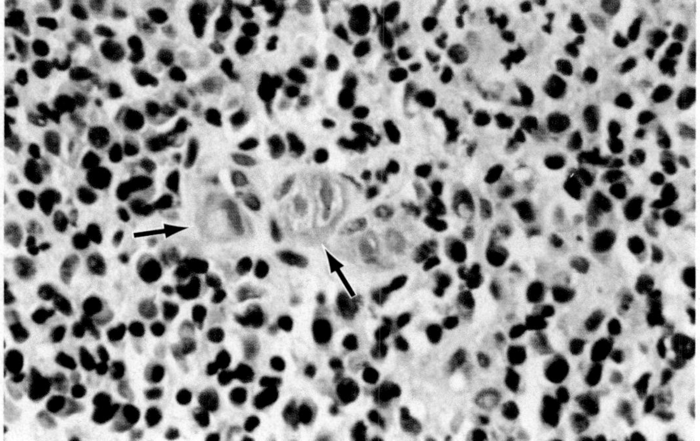

FIG. 50.27 Intestinal cytomegalovirus infection inclusions. Microscopic section of small bowel in a patient with acquired immunodeficiency syndrome who has cytomegalovirus enteritis. Multiple large cells with intranuclear and intracytoplasmic inclusions typical of cytomegalovirus are demonstrated *(arrows)*. (Courtesy Dr. Mary R. Schwartz, Baylor College of Medicine, Houston, TX.)

Fungi

Fungal infections of the intestinal tract have been recognized in patients with AIDS. Gastrointestinal histoplasmosis occurs in the setting of systemic infection, often in association with pulmonary and hepatic disease. Diagnosis is made by fungal smear and culture of infected tissue or blood. The infection is most commonly treated by the administration of amphotericin B. Coccidioidomycosis of the intestinal tract is rare and, like histoplasmosis, occurs in the context of systemic infection.

NEOPLASMS

General Considerations

Despite composing 75% of the length and 90% of the surface area of the gastrointestinal tract, the small bowel develops relatively few primary neoplasms and less than 2% of gastrointestinal malignant neoplasms. However, the incidence of small bowel cancer has increased an average of approximately 2% each year during the past 10 years. In 2018, an estimated 10,470 adults in the United States will be diagnosed with small bowel cancer, and approximately 1450 individuals will die of this disease. The 5-year survival for localized small bowel cancer is approximately 85%. Unfortunately, only 32% of patients are diagnosed with local disease; therefore, patients with regional and distant disease have 5-year survival rates of approximately 75% and 42%, respectively. This trend may be a reflection of the increase in incidence of small bowel carcinoids in the past decade.

The mean age at presentation is 62 years in the setting of benign tumors and approximately 57 years for malignant tumors. Similar to other cancers, there appears to be a geographic distribution, with the highest cancer rates found among the Maori of New Zealand and ethnic Hawaiians. The incidence of small bowel cancer is particularly low in India, Romania, and other parts of Eastern Europe. The incidence of small bowel neoplasia varies considerably, with benign lesions identified more often at autopsy. In contrast, malignant neoplasms account for 75% of symptomatic lesions that lead to surgery. This reflects the fact that most benign neoplasms are asymptomatic and often identified as an incidental finding. Stromal tumors and adenomas are the most frequent of the benign tumors and appear to be more common in the distal small bowel but may be somewhat misleading because of the relatively short length of the duodenum. Adenocarcinoma is the most common malignant neoplasm, accounting for 30% to 50% of malignant neoplasms of the small intestine; neuroendocrine tumors (NETs) account for 25% to 30% of small intestine malignant neoplasms. Adenocarcinomas are more prevalent in the proximal small bowel, whereas the other malignant lesions are more common in the distal small bowel.

The risk factors and associated conditions related to small bowel neoplasms have been described. These include patients with familial adenomatous polyposis (FAP), hereditary nonpolyposis colorectal cancer, Peutz-Jeghers syndrome, Crohn disease, gluten-sensitive enteropathy (i.e., celiac sprue), prior peptic ulcer disease, cystic fibrosis, and biliary diversion (i.e., previous cholecystectomy). Controversial factors that may contribute to small bowel neoplasms include smoking, heavy alcohol consumption (>80 g/day of ethanol), and consumption of red meat or salt-cured foods.

Although the molecular genetics of small bowel neoplasms have not been entirely characterized, similar to colorectal cancers, mutations of the *KRAS* gene are commonly identified. Allelic losses, particularly involving tumor suppressor genes at chromosome locations

5q (*APC* gene), 17q (*p53* gene), and 18q (*DCC* [deleted in *c*olon *c*ancer] and *DPC4* [*SMAD4*] genes), have been noted in some small bowel cancers. Recent findings demonstrate that in approximately 15% of small intestinal adenocarcinomas, DNA mismatch gene repair is inactivated and displays a high level of microsatellite instability (MSI-H). Interestingly, MSI-H is typical of small bowel carcinomas associated with celiac disease, which is potentially linked by an aberrant CpG island methylation. Furthermore, microarray analyses demonstrate a high percentage of small bowel tumors expressing both epidermal growth factor receptor and vascular endothelial growth factor (VEGF), which may contribute to carcinogenesis.

Clinical Manifestations

Symptoms associated with small bowel neoplasms are often vague and nonspecific and may include dyspepsia, anorexia, malaise, and dull abdominal pain, often intermittent and colicky. These symptoms may be present for months or years before diagnosis. Most patients with benign neoplasms remain asymptomatic, and the neoplasms are only discovered at autopsy or as incidental findings at laparotomy or upper gastrointestinal radiologic studies. Of the remainder, pain, most often related to obstruction, is the most frequent complaint. Usually, obstruction is the result of intussusception, and benign small tumors are the most common cause of this condition in adults. Hemorrhage is the next most common symptom. Bleeding is usually occult; hematochezia or hematemesis may occur, although life-threatening hemorrhage is uncommon.

Diagnosis

Because of the insidious nature of many small bowel neoplasms, a high index of suspicion must be present for these neoplasms to be diagnosed. In most series, a correct preoperative diagnosis is made in only 50% of symptomatic patients. Plain films may confirm the presence of an obstruction; however, for the most part, plain films are not helpful in making a diagnosis of small bowel neoplasms. An upper gastrointestinal tract series with small bowel follow-through yields an accurate diagnosis in 53% to 83% of patients with malignant neoplasms of the small intestine (Fig. 50.28). Ultrasonography has not proved effective for preoperative diagnosis of small bowel neoplasms. CT of the abdomen can prove particularly useful in detecting extraluminal tumors, such as malignant gastrointestinal stromal tumors (GISTs), and can provide helpful information about the staging of malignant cancers (Fig. 50.29). CT enteroclysis appears to be a more sensitive technique, with a diagnostic accuracy of approximately 95%, while MRI enteroclysis has a sensitivity and specificity of 98% and 97%, respectively.

Flexible endoscopy may be useful, particularly in diagnosing duodenal lesions, and the colonoscope can be advanced into the terminal ileum for visualization and biopsy of ileal neoplasms. Push enteroscopy has not been used routinely to evaluate lesions in the small bowel because this test may take up to 8 hours to perform and may not visualize the entire small bowel. Double-balloon enteroscopy can be a helpful adjunct; however, it should be reserved for cases in which biopsy or preoperative tattoo is required, as it carries a risk of perforation, and for cases where less invasive and more accurate diagnostic tools are unavailable. Lastly, more advanced capsule endoscopy may have a role in the diagnosis of intestinal lesions. The sensitivity and specificity for diagnosis of a small bowel tumor by capsule endoscopy in the setting of obscure bleeding are between 89% and 95% and between 75% and 95%, respectively. Angiography is of value in diagnosing and localizing tumors of vascular origin. Despite these sophisticated imaging and diagnostic modalities, diagnosis of a small bowel tumor is often achieved only at the time of surgical exploration.

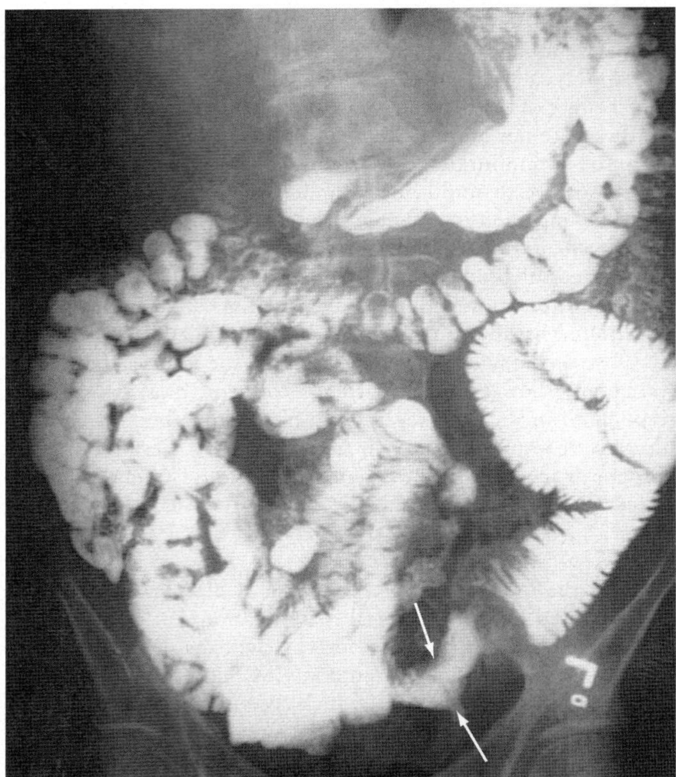

FIG. 50.28 Contrasted radiograph demonstrating a small bowel adenocarcinoma. Barium radiograph demonstrates a typical apple core lesion *(arrows)* caused by adenocarcinoma of the small bowel, producing a partial obstruction with dilated proximal bowel. (Courtesy Dr. Melvyn H. Schreiber, The University of Texas Medical Branch, Galveston, TX.)

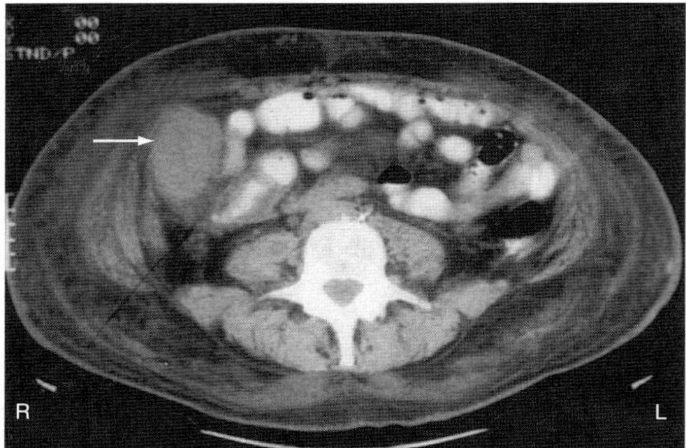

FIG. 50.29 Small bowel neoplasm. Computed tomography scan of the abdomen demonstrates a small bowel neoplasm *(arrow)*. (Courtesy Dr. Melvyn H. Schreiber, The University of Texas Medical Branch, Galveston, TX.)

Benign Neoplasms

The most common benign neoplasms include benign stromal tumors, adenomas, and lipomas. Adenomas are the most common benign tumors reported in autopsy series, but stromal tumors are the most common benign small bowel lesions that produce symptoms. In general, when a benign tumor is identified at operation, resection is indicated because symptoms are likely to develop over time. At operation, a thorough search of the remainder of the small bowel is warranted because multiple tumors are not uncommon.

Stromal Tumors

GIST make up 20% of all soft tissue sarcomas occurring throughout the gastrointestinal tract, are most prevalent in the stomach (60%) and jejunum and ileum (30%), and rarely in duodenum (5%). Stromal tumors arise from the interstitial cell of Cajal, an intestinal pacemaker cell of mesodermal descent. Median age of diagnosis is 65 years of age, with similar rates in males and females. GISTs are often large, with a median size of 6 cm at diagnosis; some GISTs can even be larger than 20 cm.[30] GISTs can be malignant tumors and nearly 20% of patients are found to have metastatic disease, most commonly in the liver. Symptoms of GIST include abdominal pain, fullness, bowel obstruction, or tumor hemorrhage resulting in anemia, melena, or hematemesis. The workup of GIST is often initiated with a CT scan. MRI may provide more information for tumors in the rectum or duodenum. Next, an endoscopic core biopsy with immunohistochemical staining for KIT (95%) and anoctamin-1 (98%) confirms the diagnosis. More than 95% of stromal tumors express CD117, the KIT proto-oncogene protein that is a transmembrane receptor for the stem cell growth factor, and 70% to 90% express CD34, the human progenitor cell antigen. These tumors infrequently stain positive for actin (20%–30%), S100 (2%–4%), and desmin (2%–4%). In gross appearance, stromal tumors are firm, gray-white lesions with a whorled appearance noted on cut surface; microscopic examination demonstrates well-differentiated smooth muscle cells. These tumors may grow intramurally and cause obstruction. Alternatively, the tumors demonstrate intramural and extramural growth, sometimes achieving considerable size and eventually outgrowing their blood supply, resulting in bleeding manifestations.

Surgical resection is necessary for appropriate treatment. GIST malignancy risk and prognosis is stratified based on the number of mitoses per high-power field (hpf) and tumor size. The mitotic index is classified as low (<5 mitoses/50 hpf) or high (>5 mitoses/50 hpf). While benign tumors generally show a low mitotic index (<5 mitoses/50 hpf), the size of the tumor also must be considered. Tumors larger than 5 cm, regardless of mitotic index, have higher rates of metastasis and recurrence, while those with a high mitotic index have a higher risk of metastasis and recurrence regardless of size. Higher-risk GIST lesions may require adjuvant therapy after resection.

Adenomas. Adenomas account for approximately 15% of all benign small bowel tumors and are of three primary types: true adenomas, villous adenomas, and Brunner gland adenomas. Twenty percent of adenomas are found in the duodenum, 30% are found in the jejunum, and 50% are found in the ileum. Most of these lesions are asymptomatic; most occur singly and are found incidentally at autopsy. The most common presenting symptoms are bleeding and obstruction. Villous adenomas of the small bowel are rare, are most commonly found in the duodenum, and may be associated with the familial polyposis syndrome. Both true and villous adenomas are thought to proceed along a similar adenoma-carcinoma sequence as colorectal adenomas and should be considered premalignant. Villous adenomas have a particular propensity for malignant degeneration and may be relatively large (>5 cm) in diameter. They are usually noted secondary to abdominal pain or bleeding; obstruction may also occur. The malignant potential of these lesions is reportedly between 35% and 55%. Treatment is determined by location and adenoma type. The options for treatment are endoscopic and surgical. In the jejunum and ileum, the treatment of choice is segmental resection. Although only 5% of adenomas occur in the duodenum, they frequently cause symptoms, and decisions about surgical management must be carefully planned because of the potential morbidity (20%–30%) associated with duodenal resection by pancreaticoduodenectomy or pancreas-preserving duodenectomy. Endoscopic ultrasound has recently emerged as a useful modality in the preintervention evaluation and may help guide management planning. Endoscopic resection of these neoplasms is a safe alternative and may delay a more aggressive and potentially morbid surgical procedure; however, some series showed that the lifelong risk of recurrence is approximately 50% after endoscopic treatment (i.e., snare excision, thermal ablation, argon plasma coagulation, or photodynamic therapy). Endoscopic mucosal resection is gaining acceptance as a useful technique for the treatment of duodenal adenomas and Brunner gland tumors. A single-center study found that endoscopic mucosal resection, even in the setting of large (>2 cm) sessile duodenal adenomas, had a high success rate for complete removal; however, the risk of delayed bleeding is significant. Other studies have shown that endoscopic mucosal resection is associated with an approximate 17% risk of other complications, including perforation, hemorrhage, and pancreatitis. Invasive changes or a recurrence after polypectomy necessitates a more definitive approach (e.g., pancreaticoduodenectomy).

Familial adenomas typically occur in the presence of FAP syndrome and require a different algorithm. Extracolonic manifestations of FAP have significant consequences. Numerous studies have shown that adenomas in the duodenum can be found in 50% to 90% of cases, and increasing age was identified as an independent risk factor for adenoma development. Although these neoplasms grow slowly, FAP patients carry a 5% lifetime risk for development of duodenal adenocarcinoma, which represents the leading cause of cancer-related mortality in these patients; therefore, routine lifelong surveillance is a priority. To direct surveillance and treatment, patients are classified by the Spigelman classification (Table 50.8). Screening endoscopy with a forward- and side-viewing endoscope is performed at regular intervals with biopsy of all suspicious, villous, or large (>3 cm) adenomas in addition to random duodenal biopsy specimens. The frequency of endoscopic screening ranges from 1 to 5 years, depending on the Spigelman classification (Box 50.6).[31] Endoscopic mucosal resection or surgical polypectomy can be performed for large adenomas. Ablative therapy in the form of argon beam coagulation or photodynamic therapy has been attempted for these patients but with disappointing results. The presence of high-grade dysplasia, carcinoma in situ, or a Spigelman stage IV classification necessitates pancreaticoduodenectomy or pancreas-preserving duodenectomy. Adenomas of the remaining small bowel also occur more frequently in patients with FAP but are not as prevalent as duodenal disease in this population of patients.

Brunner gland adenomas represent benign hyperplastic lesions arising from the Brunner glands of the proximal duodenum. These adenomas may produce symptoms mimicking those of peptic ulcer disease. Diagnosis can usually be accomplished by endoscopy and biopsy, and symptomatic lesions in an accessible region can be resected by simple excision, either endoscopically or surgically. There is no malignant potential for Brunner gland adenomas, and a radical resection should not be used.

TABLE 50.8 Spigelman classification for duodenal adenomatosis.

PARAMETER	POINTS 1	2	3
No. of polyps	1–4	5–20	>20
Polyp size (mm)	1–4	5–10	>10
Histology	Tubular	Tubulovillous	Villous
Degree of dysplasia	Mild	Moderate	Severe

From Johnson MD, Mackey R, Brown N, et al. Outcome based on management for duodenal adenomas: sporadic versus familial disease. *J Gastrointest Surg*. 2010;14:229–235.

Stage 0, 0 points; stage I, 1–4 points; stage II, 5–6 points; stage III, 7–8 points; stage IV, 9–12 points.

BOX 50.6 Recommended surveillance interval for upper gastrointestinal endoscopic examination in relation to the Spigelman classification.

Spigelman Classification (Surveillance Interval in Years)

0 (4)
I (5)
II (2–3)
III (0.5–1)
IV (consider surgery)

Adapted from Campos FG, Sulbaran M, Safatle-Ribeiro AV, et al. Duodenal adenoma surveillance in patients with familial adenomatous polyposis. *World J Gastrointest Endosc*. 2015;7:950–959.

Lipomas. Lipomas, which are also included in the category of stromal tumors, are most common in the ileum and are manifested as single intramural lesions located in the submucosa. They usually occur in the sixth and seventh decades of life and are more frequent in men. Less than one third of these tumors are symptomatic, and of these, the most common manifestations are obstruction and bleeding from superficial ulcerations. The treatment of choice for symptomatic lesions is excision. Lipomas do not have malignant potential and, therefore, if found incidentally, should be removed only if the resection is simple.

Peutz-Jeghers syndrome. Hamartomas of the small bowel occur as part of the Peutz-Jeghers syndrome, an inherited syndrome of mucocutaneous melanotic pigmentation and gastrointestinal polyps. The pattern of inheritance is autosomal dominant, with a high degree of penetrance. The classic pigmented lesions are small, 1 to 2 mm, as brown or black spots located in the circumoral region of the face, buccal mucosa, forearms, palms, soles, digits, and perianal area. Hamartomas are most commonly found in the jejunum and ileum. However, 50% of patients may also have rectal and colonic lesions, and 25% of patients have gastric lesions. The most common symptom is recurrent colicky abdominal pain, usually the result of intermittent intussusception. Lower abdominal pain associated with a palpable mass has been reported in one third of patients. Hemorrhage as a result of autoamputation of the polyps occurs, but infrequently, and is most commonly manifested by anemia. Acute life-threatening hemorrhage is uncommon but may occur. Although once considered a purely benign disease, adenomatous changes have been reported in 3% to 6% of hamartomas. Extracolonic cancers are common, occurring in 50% to 90% of patients (small intestine, stomach, pancreas, ovary, lung, uterus, and breast). The small intestine represents the most frequent site for these cancers compared to other sites. The treatment for complications of Peutz-Jeghers syndrome is directed at bowel obstruction or persistent gastrointestinal bleeding. Resection should be limited to the segment of bowel that is producing complications. Because of the widespread nature of intestinal involvement, cure is not possible; therefore, extensive resection is not indicated.

Hemangiomas. Hemangiomas are developmental malformations consisting of submucosal proliferation of blood vessels. They can occur at any level of the gastrointestinal tract; the jejunum is the most commonly affected small bowel segment. Hemangiomas account for 3% to 4% of all benign tumors of the small bowel and are multifocal in 60% of patients. In addition, hemangiomas of the small bowel may occur as part of an inherited disorder known as *Osler-Weber-Rendu disease*. Hemangiomas may also occur in the lung, liver, and mucous membranes. Patients with Turner syndrome are likely also to have cavernous hemangiomas of the intestine. The most common symptom of small bowel hemangiomas is intestinal bleeding. Angiography and technetium Tc-99m red blood cell scanning are the most useful diagnostic studies. If a hemangioma is localized preoperatively, resection of the involved intestinal segment is warranted. Intraoperative transillumination and palpation may help to identify a nonlocalized hemangioma.

Malignant Neoplasms

Population-based analyses have shown that the incidence of malignant neoplasms of the small intestine has increased steadily during the past three decades. This increase has mirrored the increase in diagnosis of small bowel neuroendocrine neoplasms (NENs), which have increased more than fourfold (from 2.1–9.3 new cases per million population) during the past three decades, whereas changes in the frequency of adenocarcinomas, stromal tumors, and lymphomas were less pronounced. A large retrospective study evaluating the Surveillance, Epidemiology, and End Results (SEER) and Medicare database from 1992 to 2010 identified small bowel carcinoma 5-year survival rate of 34.9% compared to 51.5% survival rate for colorectal cancer over the same time period. Unlike colorectal cancer, chemotherapy for small bowel adenocarcinoma has not improved overall survival when matching for stage. In fact, chemotherapy with surgery has not resulted in an appreciable survival benefit compared to surgery alone, indicating, perhaps, an overuse of adjuvant chemotherapy in this population.[32] These findings highlight the need for more novel and effective treatment strategies.

In contrast to benign lesions, malignant neoplasms almost always produce symptoms, the most common of which are pain and weight loss. Obstruction develops in 15% to 35% of patients and, unlike the intussusception produced by benign lesions, is usually the result of tumor infiltration and adhesions. Diarrhea with tenesmus and passage of large amounts of mucus may occur.

Gastrointestinal bleeding, manifested by anemia and guaiac-positive stools or occasionally by melena or hematochezia, occurs to varying degrees with malignant lesions and is more common with GISTs. A palpable mass may be felt in 10% to 20% of patients, and perforations develop in approximately 10%, usually secondary to lymphomas and sarcomas. Although presentation may be similar, each tumor type has a distinct biology that dictates management and prognosis.

Neuroendocrine Neoplasms

Intestinal NENs arise from enterochromaffin cells (Kulchitsky cells), which are considered neural crest cells situated at the base of the crypts of Lieberkühn. These cells are also known as argentaffin cells because of their staining by silver compounds. These tumors were first described by Lubarsch in 1888; in 1907, Oberndorfer coined the term *Karzinoide* to indicate the carcinoma-like appearance and the presumed lack of malignant potential. However, the term "carcinoid" has become a misnomer, as all NENs have malignant potential. These tumors have been reported in a number of organs, including lungs, bronchi, and the gastrointestinal tract. Most patients with small bowel NENs are in their seventh decade of life, with a median age for gastroenteric NEN of 63 years. The classification of NENs is based predominately on tumor grade and differentiation. NENs are divided into NETs and neuroendocrine carcinomas. NETs may be benign or of the well-differentiated malignant type and are further subdivided into three groups, low-grade (grade 1, G1), intermediate-grade (grade 2, G2), or high-grade (grade 3, G3) tumors, based on the appearance, mitotic rates, behavior (invasion of other organs, angioinvasion), and Ki-67 proliferative index. On the other hand, neuroendocrine carcinomas are all G3, poorly differentiated malignant tumors. The distinction between a G3 well-differentiated NET and a G3 poorly differentiated NEC can be difficult and may require additional pathologic confirmation or immunohistochemical staining.[33]

NETs are also categorized based on the embryologic site of origin and secretory product. These tumors may derive from the foregut (respiratory tract, thymus), midgut (jejunum, ileum and right colon, stomach, proximal duodenum), and hindgut (distal colon, rectum). Foregut NETs characteristically produce low levels of serotonin (5-hydroxytryptamine) but may secrete 5-hydroxytryptophan or adrenocorticotropic hormone. Midgut NETs are characterized by having high serotonin production. Hindgut NETs rarely produce serotonin but may produce other hormones, such as somatostatin and peptide YY. The gastrointestinal tract is the most common site for NETs. After the appendix, the small intestine is the second most frequently affected site in the gastrointestinal tract. In the small intestine, NETs almost always occur within the last 2 feet of the ileum. NETs have a variable malignant potential and are composed of multipotential cells with the ability to secrete numerous humoral agents, the most prominent of which are serotonin and substance P (Table 50.9). In addition to these substances, NETs have been found to secrete corticotropin, histamine, dopamine, neurotensin, prostaglandins, kinins, gastrin, somatostatin, pancreatic polypeptide, calcitonin, and neuron-specific enolase.

The primary importance of NETs is the malignant potential of the tumors themselves. Additionally, carcinoid syndrome, secondary to serotonin or tachykinin production, is characterized by episodic attacks of cutaneous flushing, bronchospasm, diarrhea, and vasomotor collapse, is present mostly in those patients with hepatic metastases. Primary tumors that secrete directly into the venous system, bypassing the portal system (e.g., ovary, lung), give rise to carcinoid syndrome without metastasis.

Pathology. Seventy percent to 80% of NETs are asymptomatic and found incidentally at the time of surgery. In the gastrointestinal tract, more than 90% of NETs are found in five typical sites: small intestine (38%), rectum (34%), colon (16%), stomach (11%), and unknown sites (1%). The recent increase in incidence of NETs in the United States is due to improved diagnostic detection of both the rectal and gastric tumors. Interestingly, in Korea, the most common site for NETs is the rectum.[34] The malignant potential (ability to metastasize) is related to location, size, depth of invasion, and growth pattern. Only approximately 3% of appendiceal NETs metastasize, but about 35% of ileal NETs are associated with metastasis. Most (approximately 75%) gastrointestinal NETs are smaller than 1 cm in diameter, and about 2% of these are associated with metastasis. In contrast, NETs 1 to 2 cm in diameter and larger than 2 cm are associated with metastasis in 50% and 80% to 90% of cases, respectively.

In gross appearance, these tumors are small, firm, submucosal nodules that are usually yellow on the cut surface (Fig. 50.30A). They may be as subtle as a small whitish plaque seen on the antimesenteric border of the small intestine (Fig. 50.30B). Typically, they are associated with a larger mesenteric mass caused by nodal disease and desmoplastic invasion of the mesentery, which is often mistaken for the primary tumor. They tend to grow very slowly, but after invasion of the serosa, the intense desmoplastic reaction produces mesenteric fibrosis, intestinal kinking, and intermittent obstruction. Small bowel NETs are multicentric in 20% to 30% of patients. This tendency to multicentricity exceeds that of any other malignant neoplasm of the gastrointestinal tract. Another unusual observation is the frequent coexistence of a second primary malignant neoplasm of a different histologic type. This is usually a synchronous adenocarcinoma (most commonly in the large intestine) that can occur in 10% to 20% of patients with NETs.

TABLE 50.9 Secretory products of neuroendocrine tumors.*

AMINES	TACHYKININS	PEPTIDES	OTHER
5-HT	Kallikrein	Pancreatic polypeptide (40%)	Prostaglandins
5-HIAA (88%)	Substance P (32%)	Chromogranins (100%)	
5-HTP	Neuropeptide K (67%)	Neurotensin (19%)	
Histamine		HCG-α (28%)	
Dopamine		HCG-β	
		Motilin (14%)	

Compiled with the help of Zandee WT, Kamp K, van Adrichem RC, et al. Effect of hormone secretory syndromes on neuroendocrine tumor prognosis. *Endocr Relat Cancer*. 2017;24:R261–R274.

HCG, Human chorionic gonadotropin; *5-HIAA*, 5-hydroxyindoleacetic acid; *5-HT*, 5-hydroxytryptamine; *5-HTP*, 5-hydroxytryptophan.

*Values in parentheses represent percentage frequency.

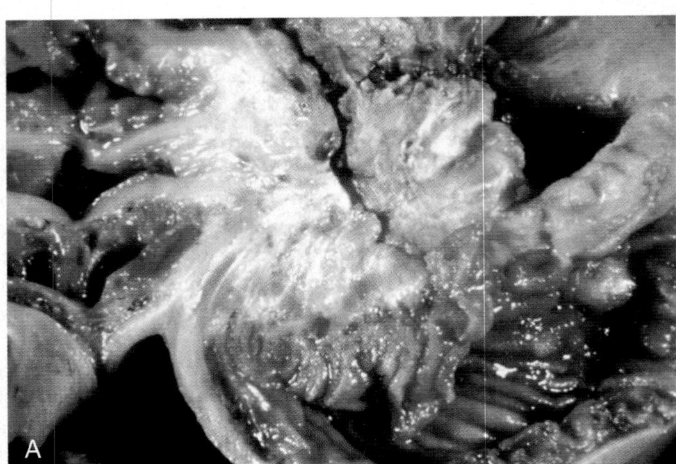

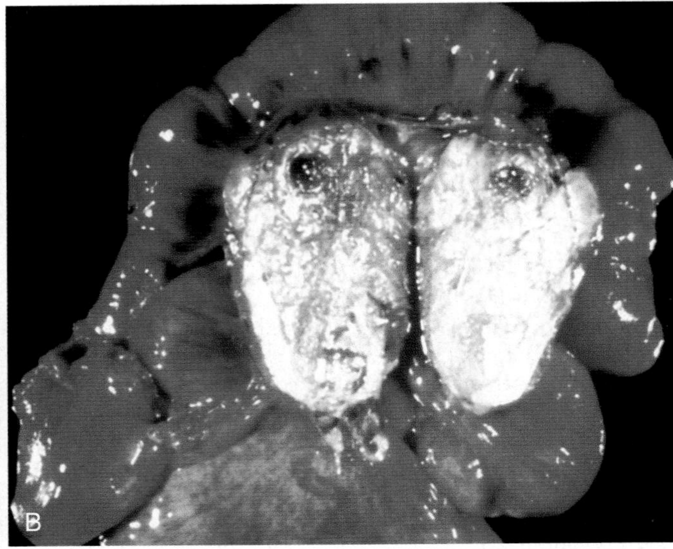

FIG. 50.30 Gross pathologic characteristics of neuroendocrine tumor (NET). (A) NET of the distal ileum demonstrates the intense desmoplastic reaction and fibrosis of the bowel wall. (B) Mesenteric metastases from a NET of the small bowel. (Adapted from Evers BM, Townsend CM Jr, Thompson JC. Small intestine. In: Schwartz SI, ed. *Principles of Surgery*. 7th ed. New York: McGraw-Hill; 1999:1245.)

Multiple endocrine neoplasia type 1 is associated with NETs in approximately 10% of cases.

Clinical manifestations. In the absence of carcinoid syndrome, symptoms of patients with NETs of the small bowel are similar to those of patients with small bowel tumors of other histologic types. The most common symptom is abdominal pain, which is variably associated with partial or complete small intestinal obstruction. Obstructive symptoms can be caused by intussusception but usually occur secondary to a local desmoplastic reaction, apparently produced by humoral agents elaborated by the tumor. Diarrhea and weight loss may also occur. The diarrhea is a result of a partial bowel obstruction rather than the secretory diarrhea noted in patients with the malignant carcinoid syndrome. As mesenteric and nodal extension progresses, local venous engorgement and, ultimately, ischemia of the affected segment of intestine contribute to most symptoms and complications related to the tumor.

Malignant carcinoid syndrome. Malignant carcinoid syndrome is a relatively rare disease, occurring in less than 10% of patients with NETs. The syndrome is usually associated with NETs of the gastrointestinal tract, particularly from the small bowel, but NETs in other locations, such as the bronchus, pancreas, ovary, and testes, have also been described in association with the syndrome. Because of the first-pass metabolism of the vasoactive peptides responsible for carcinoid syndrome, hepatic metastasis or extraabdominal disease is necessary to elicit the syndrome. The classic description of the carcinoid syndrome includes vasomotor, cardiac, and gastrointestinal manifestations. A number of humoral factors are produced by NETs, but those considered to contribute to the carcinoid syndrome include serotonin, 5-hydroxytryptophan (a precursor of serotonin synthesis), histamine, dopamine, tachykinin, kallikrein, substance P, prostaglandin, and neuropeptide K. Most patients who exhibit malignant carcinoid syndrome have massive hepatic replacement by metastatic disease. However, tumors that bypass the liver, specifically ovarian and retroperitoneal NETs, may produce the syndrome in the absence of liver metastasis.

Common symptoms and signs include cutaneous flushing (80%); diarrhea (76%); hepatomegaly (71%); cardiac lesions, most commonly right-sided heart valvular disease (41%–70%); and asthma (25%). Cutaneous flushing in the carcinoid syndrome may be of four varieties:

1. diffuse erythematous, which is short-lived and normally affects the face, neck, and upper chest;
2. violaceous, which is similar to a diffuse erythematous flush except that the attacks may be longer and patients may develop a permanent cyanotic flush, with watery eyes and injected conjunctivae;
3. prolonged flushes, which may last up to 2 or 3 days and involve the entire body and may be associated with profuse lacrimation, hypotension, and facial edema; and
4. bright-red patchy flushing, typically seen with gastric NETs.

The diarrhea associated with carcinoid syndrome is episodic (usually occurring after meals), watery, and often explosive. Increased circulating serotonin levels are thought to be the cause of the diarrhea because the serotonin antagonist, methysergide, effectively controls the symptom. Cardiac lesions usually involve the right side of the heart, but left-sided lesions are present in 15% of patients and can lead to congestive heart disease and symptomatic left-sided heart failure. The three most common cardiac lesions are pulmonary stenosis (90%), tricuspid insufficiency (47%), and tricuspid stenosis (42%). Asthmatic attacks are usually observed during the flushing symptom, and serotonin and bradykinin have been implicated in this symptom. Malabsorption and pellagra (dementia, dermatitis, and diarrhea) are occasionally present and are thought to be caused by excessive diversion of dietary tryptophan.

Diagnosis. The elevation of various humoral factors forms the basis for diagnostic tests in patients with NETs and the carcinoid syndrome. NETs produce serotonin, which is then metabolized in the liver and the lung to the pharmacologically inactive 5-hydroxyindoleacetic acid (5-HIAA). Elevated urinary levels of 5-HIAA measured during 24 hours with high-performance liquid chromatography are highly specific although not sensitive. For the last decade, chromogranin A (CgA) has been a well-established marker for carcinoid disease; it is elevated in more than 80% of patients with NETs. CgA alone may be used for the diagnosis of

NETs, given its specificity of 95%, but some investigators suggest that other tests should be used in conjunction with CgA for diagnostic purposes because its sensitivity is only 55%. A combination of serum CgA measurement with 24-hour urine 5-HIAA is an acceptable diagnostic combination with increased sensitivity. Studies suggest that serum CgA and N-terminal pro-brain natriuretic peptide may also be used in combination for both diagnosis and surveillance because patients with increased N-terminal pro-brain natriuretic peptide and CgA levels showed worse overall survival than patients with elevated CgA alone. In terms of surveillance after resection or as a prognostic marker to monitor response to therapy, CgA levels have proven efficacy over urine 5-HIAA levels.

Plasma serotonin, substance P, neurotensin, neurokinin A, and neuropeptide K levels can be measured, but these peptides may not be elevated in all patients. Provocative tests using pentagastrin, calcium, or epinephrine may be used to reproduce the symptoms of NETs. More recently, pentagastrin has been used to differentiate between NETs and chronic atrophic gastritis but is generally not used for the diagnosis of NETs, given the diagnostic reliability of 5-HIAA, CgA, and N-terminal pro-brain natriuretic peptide.

NETs of the small intestine are rarely diagnosed preoperatively. Barium radiographic studies of the small bowel may exhibit multiple filling defects as a result of kinking and fibrosis of the bowel (Fig. 50.31). A combination of anatomic and functional imaging techniques is routinely performed to optimize sensitivity and specificity.

Traditionally, CT scanning was the imaging modality of choice for identifying the site of disease and the presence of lymphatic or hematogenous metastases. CT scan findings depend on the size, the degree of mesenteric invasion and desmoplastic reaction, and the presence of regional lymph node invasion. If these entities are not well defined, CT has limited diagnostic capabilities in this disease. However, when CT scanning reveals a solid mass with spiculated borders and radiating surrounding strands that is associated with linear strands within the mesenteric fat and kinking of the bowel, a diagnosis of gastrointestinal NET can be made fairly confidently. CT angiography may be useful in cases associated with a large mesenteric process to identify encasement and pseudoaneurysm formation, typical of a malignant process in the mesentery. In general, MRI is not used in the diagnosis of gastrointestinal NETs but can be helpful in diagnosing metastatic disease, especially in the liver. Liver metastases are well demonstrated with MRI and usually have low signal intensity on T1-weighted images and high signal intensity on T2-weighted images. After the administration of a gadolinium-based contrast agent, liver metastases enhance peripherally in the hepatic arterial phase and appear as hypointense defects in the portal venous phase. Diffusion-weighted MRI and dynamic contrast-enhanced techniques represent promising advances in radiologic imaging, although these imaging techniques have not yet been validated for monitoring therapy of NETs.

Octreotide is a synthetic analogue of somatostatin, and indium (^{111}In)-labeled pentetreotide specifically binds to somatostatin receptor subtypes 2 and 5. Functional nuclear imaging studies capitalize on the concept of somatostatin receptor positivity and these techniques are used to image many NETs, including those with somatostatin-binding sites. Scintigraphic localization has a higher sensitivity than CT for delineating and localizing NETs and is particularly useful in the identification of extraabdominal metastatic disease or in cases in which the primary tumor cannot be identified by CT scan. An area of great interest is functional imaging by ^{18}F-fluorodeoxyglucose positron emission tomography

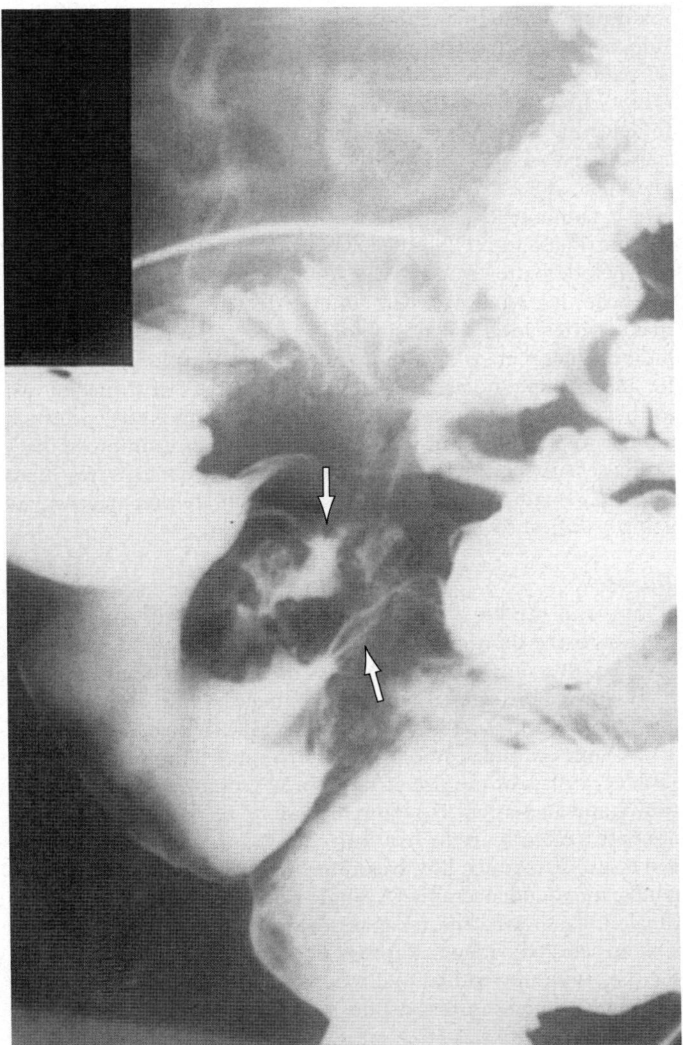

FIG. 50.31 Contrasted radiograph demonstrating a neuroendocrine tumor (NET). Barium radiograph of a NET of the terminal ileum demonstrates fibrosis with multiple filling defects and high-grade partial obstruction *(arrows)*. (Courtesy Dr. Melvyn H. Schreiber, The University of Texas Medical Branch, Galveston, TX.)

(^{18}FDG PET) scanning. However, this imaging modality alone has limited capabilities because ^{18}FDG is taken up only in high-grade NETs (e.g., high Ki-67 expression), whereas most NETs have low Ki-67 expression and are not apparent with this imaging modality. However, the addition of newer isotopes, such as ^{18}F-L-dihydroxyphenylalanine (^{18}F-DOPA), has dramatically improved the sensitivity of PET for the diagnosis and surveillance of neuroendocrine malignant neoplasms.

Somatostatin receptor imaging with gadolinium ^{68}Ga–DOTATATE PET/CT is increasingly used for the preoperative staging for patients with NETs. DOTATATE is an amide of 1,4,7,10-tetraazacyclododecane-1,4,7,10-tetraacetic acid (DOTA) and the octreotide derived radionuclide, tyrosine-3-octreotate (TATE). The latter binds to somatostatin receptors and thus directs the radioactivity into the tumor. ^{68}Ga-DOTATATE PET/CT is a clinically useful imaging technique to localize primary tumors in patients with neuroendocrine metastases of unknown origin as well as to define the existence and extent of metastatic disease. Combining the two modalities may be even more helpful in diagnosing and managing NETs. In a study designed to investigate the relationship between PET/CT results and histopathologic findings in 27 patients with NETs, the sensitivity of ^{68}Ga-DOTATATE and ^{18}FDG PET/CT was 95% and 37%, respectively. The sensitivity in detecting liver, lymph node, and bone metastases and the primary lesion was 95%, 95%, 90%, and 93% for ^{68}Ga-DOTATATE and 40%, 28%, 28%, and 75% for ^{18}FDG, respectively. Recently, a new radionuclide, ^{64}Cu-DOTATATE, was FDA approved for diagnostic use in NETs. The benefits of ^{64}Cu-DOTATATE imaging include better true positive lesion detection, longer shelf life and scanning window when compared with ^{68}Ga-DOTATATE, making it an ideal diagnostic tool.[35] Lastly, the peptide receptor radionuclide therapy agent lutetium-177 (^{177}Lu) is both diagnostic and therapeutic and belongs to a new class of drugs known as theranostics. The reason for developing compounds with high affinity for somatostatin receptors 2, 3, and 5 is to improve diagnostic sensitivity. Because resection is the only curative treatment in patients with small intestinal NETs, accurate preoperative imaging is critical to guide surgical management.

Treatment

Surgical therapy. The treatment of patients with small bowel NETs is based on tumor size, location, and presence of metastatic disease. For primary tumors smaller than 1 cm in diameter without evidence of regional lymph node metastasis, a segmental intestinal resection is adequate. For patients with lesions larger than 1 cm, with multiple tumors, or with regional lymph node metastasis, regardless of the size of the primary tumor, wide excision of bowel and mesentery is required. Lesions of the terminal ileum are best treated by right hemicolectomy. Small duodenal tumors can be excised locally; however, more extensive lesions may require pancreaticoduodenectomy. A single-center, prospective, longitudinal study showed that a laparoscopic approach is safe and feasible in selected patients. Laparoscopy was associated with similar R0 (i.e., without residual microscopic tumor) resection and morbidity rates but a shorter hospital stay compared with laparotomy. Median follow-up was 39 months, and progression-free survival at 1, 3, and 5 years was as follows: 95%, 83%, and 75%, respectively, for R0 patients without liver metastasis; 92%, 83%, and 57%, respectively, for R0 patients with resected liver metastasis; and 82%, 58%, and 30%, respectively, for patients with R2 resection (i.e., evidence of residual tumor on visual examination). Overall survival and progression-free survival did not show any difference in comparing the laparoscopic and open groups.[36]

Caution should be exerted in the anesthetic management of patients with NETs because anesthesia may precipitate a carcinoid crisis characterized by hypotension, bronchospasm, flushing, and tachyarrhythmias. Carcinoid crisis is treated with IV octreotide given as a bolus of 50 to 100 μg, which may be continued as an infusion at 50 μg/hr.

In addition to treatment of the primary tumor, it is important that the abdomen be thoroughly explored for multicentric lesions. There often is a large desmoplastic reaction causing shortening, folding and pleating of the small bowel mesentery resulting in intestinal angina and obstruction. In cases in which the mesenteric disease appears to involve a large portion of the mesentery, dissection of the tumor off the mesenteric vessels, with preservation of the blood supply to unaffected bowel, is appropriate, albeit technically demanding. Extensive mobilization of the small bowel mesentery is required to perform a difficult resection. Not only does removal of the mesenteric disease provide a significant survival advantage, but also mesenteric debulking ensures the most durable palliation for the patient. Aggressive surgical resection and debulking achieve relief of 93% of obstruction and 83% of mesenteric vessel encasement.[37]

In patients with NETs and widespread metastatic disease, surgery may still be indicated. In contrast to metastases from other tumors, there is a definite role for surgical debulking, which often provides beneficial symptomatic relief. In patients with limited hepatic involvement, metastasectomy provides the most durable survival benefit compared with other treatment modalities. For patients with liver metastases, surgical resection is an option as long as there are no extrahepatic metastases, liver function is not compromised, and there is no diffuse bilobar involvement. Unfortunately, most patients are not candidates for liver resection because of extensive disease at diagnosis. Even with liver metastasectomy, there is still a high recurrence rate of 75%. In these cases, transarterial chemoembolization or radioembolization has been shown to provide liver-directed control of disease. Furthermore, resection of the primary tumor, with or without mesenteric resection, has been shown to improve survival and to slow progression of hepatic metastases in patients with unresectable disease. Although there have been some small studies that evaluate hepatic transplantation for extensive liver metastases from NETs, unacceptably high recurrence rates limit this approach. Overall, due to the complexity of treatment regimens, all surgical resections should be performed at a high volume center.

Medical therapy. Medical therapy for patients with malignant carcinoid syndrome is primarily directed toward the relief of symptoms caused by the excess production of humoral factors. Table 50.10 summarizes medical therapies for NET treatment. Somatostatin analogs (SSAs) are the standard of care for controlling symptoms of patients with functional gastrointestinal NETs, and they control symptoms in more than 70% of patients with carcinoid syndrome.[38] SSAs such as octreotide (Sandostatin) and lanreotide and their depot formulations (Sandostatin LAR and Somatuline, respectively) relieve symptoms of the carcinoid syndrome (e.g., diarrhea, flushing, antisecretory effect) in most patients and delay cancer progression (antiproliferative effect). The antiproliferative effect was demonstrated in two randomized phase 3 trials. First, the PROMID trial of 85 patients confirmed that tumor burden is an important predictor of survival and octreotide LAR provided delayed tumor progression compared to placebo.[39] Octreotide LAR is recommended for Grade 1 and 2 NETs and not recommended in grade 3 disease. Second, the landmark controlled study of Lanreotide Antiproliferative Response In NeuroEndocrine Tumors (CLARINET) trial found that lanreotide, an SSA, was associated with prolonged progression-free survival among patients with metastatic grade 1 or 2 enteropancreatic NETs.[40] Currently, there is no guideline regarding the selection of Octreotide LAR versus lanreotide as a first-line therapy. The treatment of asymptomatic patients with low volume and unresectable disease requires a personalized decision on observation or initiation of SSAs. However, observation requires close monitoring with diagnostic imaging every 3 to 6 months.[41]

For patients who have disease progression on SSA therapy, several emerging treatment options remain. Everolimus, a mammalian target of rapamycin (mTOR) inhibitor, initially developed as immunosuppressant therapy, is approved for the treatment of nonfunctional gastrointestinal NETs with unresectable, locally advanced or metastatic disease. A randomized controlled trial (RADIANT-4) demonstrated that, with everolimus treatment, progression-free survival improved from 3.9 months to 11 months. Although everolimus can slow tumor progression, significant

TABLE 50.10 Medical therapies for neuroendocrine tumor treatment.

Approved Therapeutics	
Somatostatin analogs	Octreotide (Sandostatin; Sandostatin LAR)
	Lanreotide (Somatuline depot)
Cytotoxic therapies	Streptozotocin (pancreatic NET only)
mTOR inhibitor	Everolimus (Afinitor; gastrointestinal, pancreatic, lung NET)
Tyrosine kinase inhibitors	Sunitinib (Sutent; pancreatic NET only)
Peptide receptor radionuclide therapy	^{177}Lu isotopes conjugated with somatostatin analogs (Lutathera)
Serotonin synthesis inhibitors	Telotristat etiprate (Xermelo)
Used Off-Label	
Pan-receptor somatostatin agonists	Pasireotide (Signifor); approved indication for Cushing disease only
Interferons	Interferon alfa-2b (Intron A)
Cytotoxic therapies	5-Fluorouracil (5-FU)
	Capecitabine (Xeloda); oral 5-FU
	Temozolomide (Temodar)
Investigational	
Peptide receptor radiotherapy	^{177}Lu-OPS 201
	^{177}Lu-DOTA JR11
Dopamine agonists	Dopastatins
Checkpoint inhibitor	JS001
Somatostatin drug conjugate	PEN-221

Compiled with the assistance of Lowell B. Anthony, MD, University of Kentucky.

NET, Neuroendocrine tumor.

tumor reduction is rarely obtained. Targeting multiple signaling pathways is a treatment strategy that may provide better tumor control and overcome resistance mechanisms involved with simply targeting a single pathway. Results of ongoing and future studies will provide important information about the added benefit of combining mTOR inhibitors with other targeted agents, such as VEGF pathway inhibitors, and cytotoxic chemotherapy in the treatment of advanced NETs.[41]

Peptide receptor radionuclides are another class of therapy used in progressive disease. The NETTER-1 randomized control trial demonstrated that treatment with radionuclide ^{177}Lu-DOTATATE had a 79% improvement in progression-free survival when compared to high-dose octreotide. ^{177}Lu-DOTATATE can be used for PET imaging as well as to determine the distribution and the dosimetry of the tumor. There is also an interest in targeting incretin receptor family members, particularly glucagon-like peptide (GLP) 1, which are overexpressed in NETs. The GLP-1 inhibitor Lys^{40}(Ahx-DTPA/DOTA^{111}In) NH_2-exendin-4 is highly sensitive and can be detected up to 14 days after IV injection using a probe to facilitate surgical excision.

Second-generation SSAs have been developed to address the limitations of the current regimens. Studies are ongoing using pan-receptor agonists (e.g., pasireotide) as well as chimeric dimers, which possess features of somatostatin and dopamine agonists (dopastatins). These promising biologic therapies are thought to enhance symptom control by binding multiple receptors (somatostatin and dopamine receptors). Somatostatin receptor antagonists are also currently being developed for clinical use.

Other treatment options include interferon alpha, which was used as monotherapy for NET in 1983. Interferon binds to two different receptors to elicit effects that include cell cycle inhibition at G_1/S, antiangiogenesis effects through downregulation of VEGF, and upregulation of somatostatin receptors. Although some series showed tumor regression in 10% of patients and tumor stabilization in 65%, side effects, which included chronic fatigue, pancytopenia, thyroiditis, and systemic lupus erythematosus, were not tolerable, and thus, interferon alpha is no longer used. Pegylated interferon alpha-2b showed comparable survival rates to interferon alpha, but with more tolerable side effects. Some series showed that given the upregulation of somatostatin receptors by interferon alpha, its combination with SSAs may be efficacious. Prospective randomized controlled trials demonstrated variable findings, but one retrospective study determined that combined treatment resulted in a longer progression-free survival (58 vs. 55 months). Interferon is less expensive than the SSAs, but the increased incidence of side effects and variable outcomes preclude the widespread use of this drug.[41]

Patients with carcinoid syndrome that are resistant to SSAs have limited treatment options, which include increasing the dose of SSA or adding a short acting octreotide and starting antidiarrheals. An extensive workup is needed to rule out other causes of diarrhea, but few treatment options remain. Currently, the serotonin synthesis inhibitor, telotristat etiprate, is indicated for somatostatin refractory diarrhea in the setting of carcinoid syndrome. In the TELESTAR trial, telotristat treatment reduced daily bowel movements by 35%.[41] Serotonin receptor antagonists have been used with limited success. Methysergide is no longer used because of the increased incidence of retroperitoneal fibrosis. Ketanserin and cyproheptadine have been shown to provide some control of symptoms, and other antagonists, such as ondansetron, also have a role.

Historically, the only available treatment for metastatic NETs was cytotoxic chemotherapy, most frequently combinations that included streptozotocin, 5-fluorouracil (5-FU), and cyclophosphamide. These treatments resulted in a median survival of around 2 years. Currently, the role of chemotherapy is confined predominantly to patients with G2 metastatic disease who are symptomatic, are unresponsive to other therapies, or have high tumor proliferation rates. The duration of response, however, is short-lived. Temozolomide as monotherapy has acceptable toxicity and provides antitumoral effects in a small series of patients with advanced NETs, and in combination with capecitabine, it was shown to prolong survival in patients with well-differentiated, metastatic NETs who experienced progression with previous therapies. The use of cisplatin and etoposide has shown some promise, but only in patients with poorly differentiated neuroendocrine carcinomas.

The treatment of metastatic NENs requires a multidisciplinary approach; combined modalities may be the best option, including surgical debulking, hepatic artery embolization, chemoembolization, or radioembolization and medical therapy. In addition, newer and more targeted therapies are being developed that may be useful in the future. Sunitinib, which is a multitargeted or selective tyrosine kinase inhibitor that is active against alpha-type and beta-type platelet-derived growth factor receptor (PDGFR) and VEGF receptor (VEGFR), has been noted to decrease angiogenesis and to prolong progression-free survival in pancreatic NETs in multiple clinical trials, most notably those with mutations associated with exons 9 and 11.

Prognosis. NETs have the best prognosis of all small bowel tumors, whether the disease is localized or metastatic. Resection of a NET localized to its primary site approaches a 100% survival rate. Five-year survival rates are approximately 65% in patients with regional disease and 25% to 35% in those with distant metastasis. Metastatic disease at the time of diagnosis is approximately 20% to 50%, and tumors recur in 40% to 60% of patients. When widespread metastatic disease precludes cure, extensive resection for palliation may be indicated. In fact, long-term palliation often can be obtained because these tumors are relatively slow growing. A number of factors have been evaluated in an attempt to identify patients with NETs who have a poor prognosis. An elevated level of CgA, which is an independent predictor of an adverse prognosis, is probably the most useful factor identified.

Adenocarcinomas

Adenocarcinomas constitute approximately 40% of the malignant tumors of the small bowel. The median age at diagnosis is in the sixth decade of life, and most series show a slight male predominance. Most of these tumors are located in the duodenum and proximal jejunum (Fig. 50.32). Those arising in association with Crohn disease tend to occur at a somewhat younger age, and more than 70% arise in the ileum. Small bowel adenocarcinoma may have important gene mutations (*APC*, *β-CATENIN*, *EGFR*, *VEGF-A*, *KRAS*, *HER2*, *TP53*).[42] The most common familial causes include FAP, Lynch syndrome, and Peutz Jeghers syndrome. Tumors of the duodenum tend to manifest somewhat earlier than those in the jejunum and ileum because of the earlier presentation of symptoms, which are usually jaundice and chronic bleeding. Adenocarcinomas of the jejunum and ileum usually produce more nonspecific symptoms that include vague abdominal pain and weight loss. Intestinal obstruction and chronic bleeding may also occur. Perforation is uncommon. As with adenocarcinomas in other organs, survival of patients with small bowel adenocarcinomas is related to the stage of disease at the time of diagnosis. Unfortunately, diagnosis is often delayed, and the disease is advanced at the time of surgery secondary to a variety of factors (e.g., vagueness of symptoms, absence of physical findings, lack of clinical suspicion because of the rarity of these lesions). A variety of radiologic and endoscopic techniques such as CT of the abdomen and pelvis with enteroclysis, video capsule endoscopy, and double balloon enteroscopy (for biopsy and diagnosis) may be very useful in establishing the diagnosis prior to surgery.

Treatment of small bowel adenocarcinoma is determined by location and stage. An R0 resection of the primary tumor with locoregional lymph node resection is the only curative treatment. Neoadjuvant chemotherapy is appropriate to consider if there is tumor invasion into adjacent structures. Patients are then reevaluated for surgery after 2 to 3 months of treatment. Duodenal resection can be performed for a noninfiltrating tumor if it is located in the first, third, or fourth portion of the duodenum, but this is not recommended if an expected R0 resection (no microscopic tumor at margin) is not possible. Residual microscopic tumor (R1 status) or grossly visible tumor after resection (R2 status) are associated with poor prognosis. Resectable adenocarcinomas in the second portion of the duodenum are treated with pancreaticoduodenectomy. In addition, regional lymphadenectomy of the periduodenal, peripancreatic, and hepatic lymph nodes as well as involved vascular structures is necessary. Jejunal and ileal adenocarcinomas require surgical resection with regional lymphadenectomy and jejunojejunal or ileoileal anastomosis (Fig. 50.33). If the terminal ileum is involved, an ileocecectomy with right hemicolectomy should be performed with ligation of the ileocolic artery and subsequent regional lymphadenectomy.

There is currently no standard adjuvant protocol for small bowel adenocarcinoma. Despite this, most guidelines suggest that patients with poorly differentiated cancers or those who had incomplete lymph node resections (<10 nodes identified) should at least be considered for adjuvant chemotherapy. Adjuvant regimens are often dictated by location, although studies have suggested that fluoropyrimidine and oxaliplatin may increase overall survival in patients with advanced disease. A prospective international phase 3 trial (BALLAD study) comparing observation versus adjuvant chemotherapy in patients with an R0 resection is currently accruing subjects. This trial proposes that adjuvant chemotherapy will result in an improvement in disease-free survival and overall survival compared with observation alone after potentially curative surgery for patients with stage I, II, and III small bowel adenocarcinoma. In patients

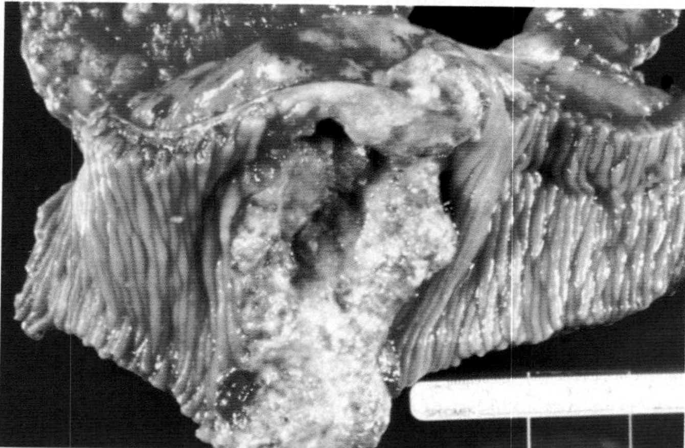

FIG. 50.32 Jejunal adenocarcinoma. Large circumferential mucinous adenocarcinoma of the jejunum. (Courtesy Dr. Mary R. Schwartz, Baylor College of Medicine, Houston, TX.)

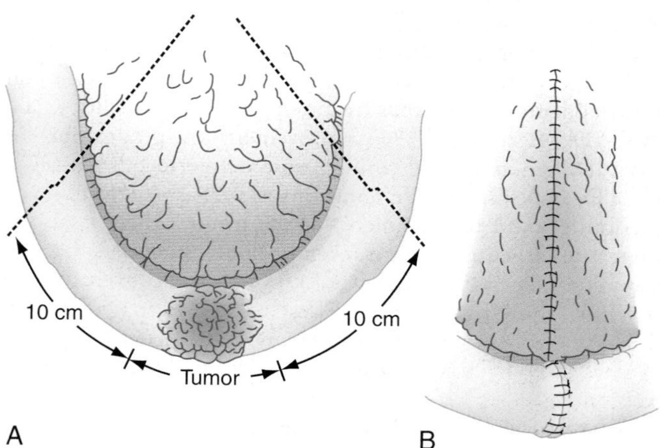

FIG. 50.33 Surgical management of carcinoma of the small bowel. (A) Malignant tumors should be resected with a wide margin of normal bowel and a wedge of mesentery to remove the immediate draining lymph nodes. (B) End-to-end anastomosis of the small bowel and repair of the mesentery. (Adapted from Thompson JC. *Atlas of Surgery of the Stomach, Duodenum, and Small Bowel.* St. Louis: Mosby-Year Book; 1992:299.)

with metastatic disease, studies have determined that using FOLFOX (oxaliplatin, 5-FU, and leucovorin) and FOLFIRI (irinotecan, 5-FU, and leucovorin) as first-line therapy significantly improves the performance status and progression-free survival. Unresectable metastatic disease may require surgical intervention for uncontrolled bleeding, bowel obstruction, or perforation.

The prognosis of small bowel adenocarcinoma is poor, probably because of the delayed presentation and presence of advanced disease at diagnosis. Five-year survival rates are typically in the 14% to 33% range, although duodenal adenocarcinoma has a 5-year survival rate of 50%, probably because of the earlier symptom presentation and diagnosis. Lymph node invasion is the main prognostic factor for local small bowel adenocarcinoma; moreover, the number of lymph nodes assessed and the number of positive lymph nodes are of prognostic value. In stage III patients, having more than three positive lymph nodes was associated with a worse 5-year disease-free survival rate than having one or two positive lymph nodes (37% vs. 57%, respectively). Multivariate analysis identified advanced age, advanced stage, ileal location, recovery of fewer than 10 lymph nodes, and number of positive nodes as significant predictors of poor overall survival. Notably, any attempts at curative resection should always include an extensive regional lymphadenectomy.[42]

Lymphoma

Malignant lymphomas involve the small bowel primarily or as a manifestation of systemic disease. Approximately one-third of gastrointestinal lymphomas occur in the small bowel, and these account for 5% of all lymphomas. Lymphomas constitute up to 25% of small bowel malignant tumors in the adult; in children younger than 10 years, they are the most common intestinal neoplasm. Lymphomas are most commonly found in the ileum, where there is the greatest concentration of gut-associated lymphoid tissue. An increased risk for development of primary small bowel lymphomas was reported in patients with celiac disease and immunodeficient states (e.g., AIDS). In gross appearance, small intestine lymphomas are usually large, with most greater than 5 cm and may extend beneath the mucosa (Fig. 50.34). On microscopic examination, there is often diffuse infiltration of the intestinal wall. Symptoms of small bowel lymphoma include pain, weight loss, nausea, vomiting, and change in bowel habits. Perforation may occur in up to 25% of patients (Fig. 50.35). Fever is uncommon and suggests systemic involvement.

The treatment of small bowel lymphoma remains controversial. Traditionally, a combination of surgery, chemotherapy, and radiation therapy was used for all small bowel tumors. However, in the absence of symptoms, small bowel lymphomas are often chemoresponsive and do not require surgery. This can typically be predicted by cell type because B-cell lymphomas are more chemosensitive than T-cell lymphomas and have high remission rates with or without surgery. T-cell lymphomas are traditionally more resistant to therapy and will progress to symptoms of obstruction or perforation if not resected. Regardless of cell type, resection is indicated at any onset of symptoms because progression to life-threatening hemorrhage or perforation portends a dismal prognosis. Five-year survival of 50% to 60% can be expected and is dictated by response to systemic therapy rather than by the success of surgical resection.

Gastrointestinal Stromal Tumors

Malignant GISTs arise from mesenchymal tissue and constitute about 20% of malignant neoplasms of the small bowel (Fig. 50.36).

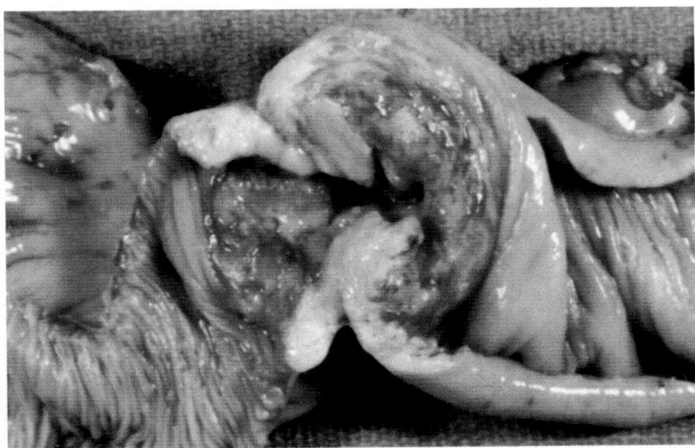

FIG. 50.34 Lymphoma of the small intestine. Gross photograph of primary lymphoma of the ileum shows replacement of all layers of the bowel wall with tumor. (Courtesy Dr. Mary R. Schwartz, Baylor College of Medicine, Houston, TX.)

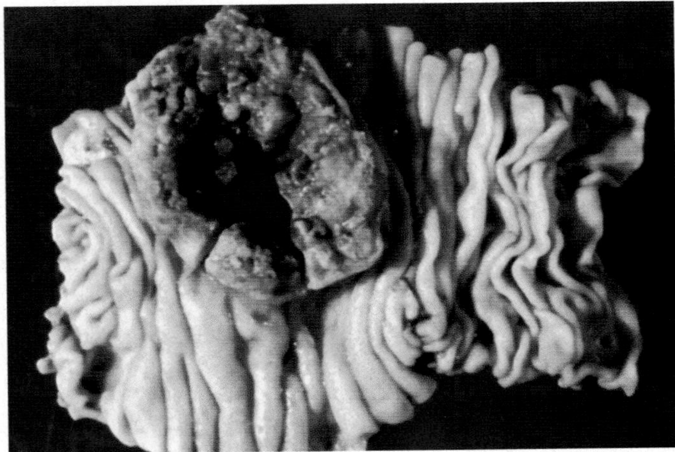

FIG. 50.35 Lymphoma of the small intestine. Small bowel lymphoma is manifested as perforation and peritonitis. (Courtesy Dr. Mary R. Schwartz, Baylor College of Medicine, Houston, TX.)

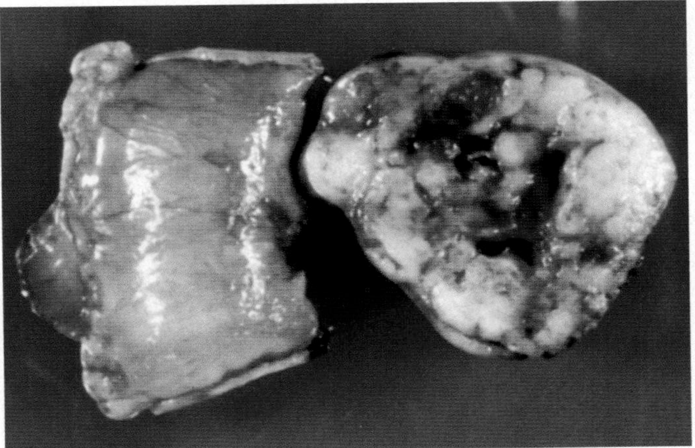

FIG. 50.36 Small intestine gastrointestinal stroma tumor (GIST). Small bowel GIST with hemorrhagic necrosis. (Courtesy Dr. Mary R. Schwartz, Baylor College of Medicine, Houston, TX.)

These tumors are more common in the jejunum and ileum, typically are diagnosed in the fifth and sixth decades of life, and occur with a slight male preponderance. Malignant GISTs are larger than 5 cm at the time of diagnosis in 80% of patients. GISTs mostly arise from the muscularis propria and generally grow extramurally. Most common indications for surgery include bleeding and obstruction, although free perforation may occur as a result of hemorrhagic necrosis in large tumor masses. Typically, GISTs tend to invade locally and to spread by direct extension into adjacent tissues and hematogenously to the liver, lungs, and bone; lymphatic metastases are unusual. The most useful indicators of survival and the risk for metastasis include the size of the tumor at presentation, mitotic index, and evidence of tumor invasion into the lamina propria.

Treatment of GISTs continues to evolve and represents one of the first breakthroughs in signal transduction manipulation. The treatment regimen is based on localized versus metastatic disease (Fig. 50.37). Surgical management includes complete resection for localized GISTs, with extreme care to avoid rupture of the tumor capsule, which results in relapse in 100% of these patients. If capsule rupture occurs, these patients should receive adjuvant therapy regardless of the extent of the tumor before surgery. It is advisable to perform an en bloc resection, to include adjacent organs, for prevention of tumor capsule rupture. A laparoscopic approach in patients with large tumors is strongly discouraged. Radiologic criteria for unresectability include infiltration of the celiac trunk, superior mesenteric artery, or portal vein. Lymphadenectomy is unnecessary, given the low frequency of lymph node metastasis.[30] Small GISTs (<2 cm) found incidentally in surgical specimens do not require further treatment. Before the development of tyrosine kinase inhibitors, adjuvant strategies for GISTs were lacking, and recurrence rates after resection were as high as 70%. However, the development of imatinib mesylate (Gleevec) has significantly altered previous treatment strategies. Imatinib mesylate is a tyrosine kinase inhibitor that blocks the unregulated mutant c-*kit* tyrosine kinase and inhibits the BCR-ABL and PDGF tyrosine kinases. Multiple randomized trials have confirmed its efficacy as a first-line agent in the treatment of GIST. Current guidelines suggest that patients with high-risk disease should receive 3 years of adjuvant treatment with imatinib, but it is not recommended for low-risk patients after an R0 resection. Neoadjuvant imatinib should be considered for patients requiring extensive surgery to allow for tumor shrinkage prior to resection.[30]

Relapse-risk assessment for a primary GIST is critical as it provides prognostic information as well as estimates the potential benefits of medical therapy. There are several available risk stratification systems, including the National Institute of Health GIST consensus criteria, the American Forces Institute of Pathology criteria, the Joensuu risk criteria, prognostic nomograms,

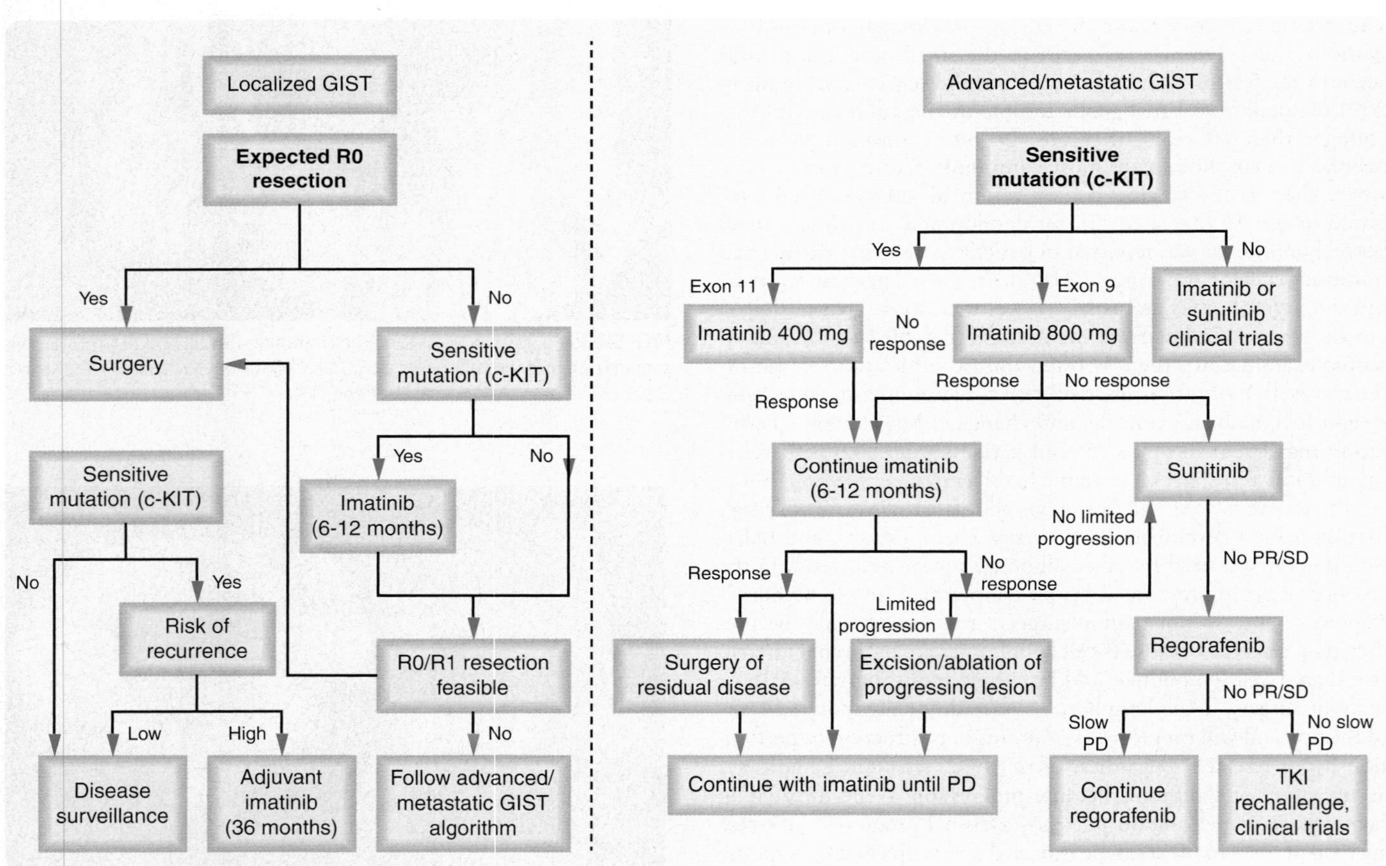

FIG. 50.37 Current algorithm for the management of GIST based on extent of disease. (Adapted from Casali PG, Abecassis N, Bauer S, et al. Gastrointestinal stromal tumours: ESMO-EURACAN clinical practice guidelines for diagnosis, treatment and follow-up. *Ann Oncol.* 2018;29:iv68–iv78.). *GIST*, Gastrointestinal stromal tumor; *PD*, progressive disease; *PR*, partial response; *R0*, no residual tumor; *R1*, microscopic residual tumor; *SD*, stable disease; *TKI*, tyrosine kinase inhibitor.

and mutational analysis. In addition to staging information, several mutations are found to have implications on prognosis. For example, deletions affecting exon 11, codon 557/558 of the c-*kit* gene, and D842V PDGFRα mutations have a higher risk of recurrence within the first 3 to 4 years after surgery. In fact, adjuvant imatinib therapy is not recommended in patients with D842V PDGFRα mutations, given its known resistance to this agent.

Imatinib is also a first-line treatment for unresectable and metastatic GISTs with characteristic tumor biology. Genotyping is standard of care for patients with advanced or metastatic GIST. Standard-dose therapy (400 mg daily) is recommended as no survival advantage is offered by increasing the dose unless the patient has an exon 9 mutation. A European trial determined that patients with exon 9 mutations exhibited a dose-dependent decrease in risk of progression. Therefore, in this select group of patients, imatinib 400 mg twice per day should be given.

New molecular targeted therapies may provide better treatments for patients with genetic mutations and GISTs. In phase 3 clinical trials evaluating imatinib dosing in patients with metastatic GIST, there was no objective response in patients who carry the D842V PDGFRα mutation. A recent phase 2 trial evaluated dasatinib, an oral tyrosine kinase inhibitor of c-*kit*, PDGFR, ABL (Abelson murine leukemia viral oncogene homologue), and the proto-oncogene *Src* with a distinct binding affinity for c-*kit* and PDGFR and showed that it has significant activity (as judged by CT response rates) in imatinib- and sunitinib-refractory GISTs; however, dasatinib did not meet the predefined 6-month progression-free survival rate of 30% in the patient population. Invitro studies suggest that dasatinib may provide the best response in patients with a D842V PDGFRα mutation and could prove to be useful in this particular subset of patients. Regorafenib is a second-generation tyrosine kinase inhibitor that targets c-*kit*, *RET*, *BRAF*, VEGFR, PDGFR, and fibroblast growth factor receptor. It is currently FDA approved and may be an effective treatment for advanced GISTs after failure of either imatinib or sunitinib. Nilotinib is a second-generation tyrosine kinase inhibitor active in chronic myeloid leukemia and has an inhibitory effect on c-*kit* and PDGF. Phase 3 trials have shown minimal differences between this drug and imatinib or sunitinib. Sorafenib is a VEGF, c-*kit*, PDGFR, and *BRAF* inhibitor and has been effective in imatinib- and sunitinib-resistant tumors. The combination of imatinib and doxorubicin has shown some benefit in patients with wild-type GISTs.[30]

Metastatic Neoplasms

Metastatic tumors involving the small bowel are much more common than primary neoplasms. Metastases to the small intestine usually arise from other intraabdominal organs, including the uterine cervix, ovaries, kidneys, stomach, colon, and pancreas. Small intestinal involvement is by direct extension or implantation of tumor cells. Metastases from extraabdominal tumors are rare but may be found in patients with adenocarcinoma of the breast and carcinoma of the lung. Cutaneous melanoma is the most common extraabdominal source to involve the small intestine, which is found in more than 50% of patients dying of malignant melanoma (Fig. 50.38). Common symptoms of metastatic disease include anorexia, weight loss, anemia, bleeding, and partial bowel obstruction. Treatment is often palliative to relieve symptoms or, occasionally, a bypass if the metastatic tumor is extensive and not amenable to resection. Nonoperative palliation of malignant bowel obstruction includes endoscopic or radiologic placement of self-expandable metal stents, especially in patients with very poor performance status who may not tolerate a surgical procedure. Gastrostomy and jejunostomy tubes also may be placed to provide decompression when other palliative methods are not possible.

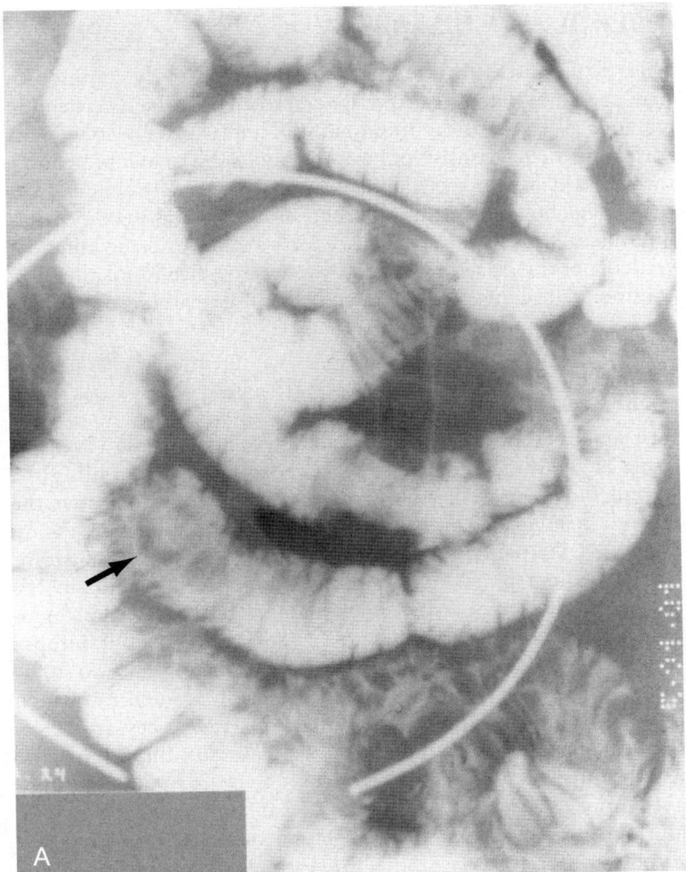

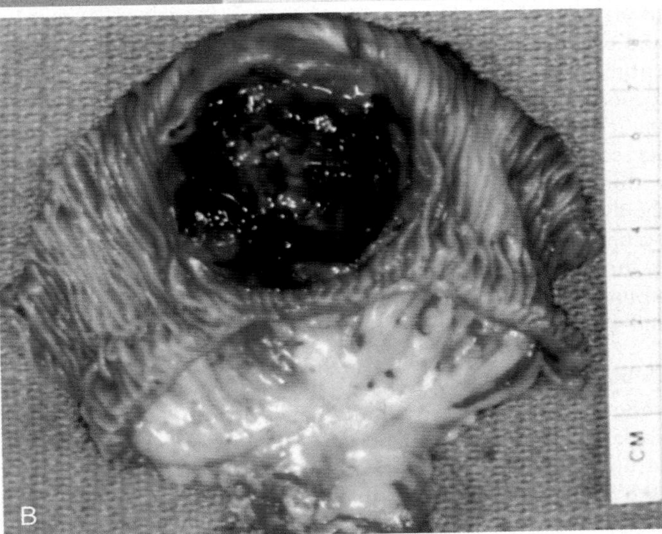

FIG. 50.38 Metastatic melanoma to the small intestine. (A) Barium radiograph shows target lesions consistent with metastatic melanoma of small bowel *(arrow)*. (B) Gross specimen demonstrating metastatic melanoma to the small bowel. (A, Courtesy Dr. Melvyn H. Schreiber, The University of Texas Medical Branch, Galveston, TX. B, Courtesy Dr. Mary R. Schwartz, Baylor College of Medicine, Houston, TX.)

DIVERTICULAR DISEASE

Diverticular disease of the small intestine is relatively common. It may be manifested as true or false diverticula. A true diverticulum contains all layers of the intestinal wall and is usually congenital. False diverticula consist of mucosa and submucosa protruding through a defect in the muscle coat and are usually acquired defects. Small bowel diverticula may occur in any portion of the small intestine. Duodenal diverticula are the most common acquired diverticula of the small bowel, and Meckel diverticulum is the most common true congenital diverticulum of the small bowel.

Duodenal Diverticula

Incidence and Cause

First described by Chomel, a French pathologist, in 1710, diverticula of the duodenum are relatively common, representing the second most common site for diverticulum formation after the colon. The incidence of duodenal diverticula varies, depending on the age of the patient and method of diagnosis. Upper gastrointestinal radiographic studies identify duodenal diverticula in 1% to 5% of all studies, whereas endoscopic retrograde cholangiopancreatography identifies 9% to 23% of cases. Previous autopsy series report the incidence as being approximately 15% to 20%. Duodenal diverticula occur twice as often in women as in men and are rare in patients younger than 40 years. They are classified as congenital or acquired, true or false, and intraluminal or extraluminal. Extraluminal duodenal diverticula are considerably more common than intraluminal diverticula, are acquired, and consist of mucosal or submucosal outpouchings herniated through a muscle defect in the bowel wall. Intraluminal duodenal diverticula (also known as windsock diverticula) are congenital and occur as a single saccular structure that is connected to the entire circumference or part of the wall of the duodenum to create a duodenal web. Incomplete recanalization of the duodenum during fetal development leads to intraluminal diverticula, which are exceedingly rare. In general, extraluminal diverticula usually occur within the second portion of the duodenum (62%) and less commonly in the third (30%) and fourth (8%) portions. They rarely occur in the first part of the duodenum (<1%). When they occur in the second portion, most (88%) are noted on the medial wall around the ampulla (i.e., periampullary), 8% are seen posteriorly, and 4% occur on the lateral wall.

Clinical Manifestations

Importantly, the overwhelming majority of duodenal diverticula are asymptomatic and are usually noted incidentally by an upper gastrointestinal series for an unrelated problem (Fig. 50.39). Upper gastrointestinal endoscopy identifies approximately 75% of duodenal diverticula, and the use of a side-viewing scope further increases the success rate. The diagnosis may be suggested by plain abdominal films showing an atypical gas bubble; CT can identify large diverticula by the presence of a mass-like structure interposed between the duodenum and pancreatic head containing air, air-fluid levels, fluid contrast material, or debris. Magnetic resonance cholangiopancreatography is particularly helpful to demonstrate the relationship of the diverticulum to the biliary and pancreatic ducts and associated pathologic changes in the biliary system and pancreas. Hemorrhage in diverticula is best diagnosed by a combination of angiography and ^{99m}Tc-labeled red blood cell scan; however, surgery should not be delayed to obtain imaging in the event of hemorrhage in a hemodynamically unstable patient. Less than 5% of duodenal diverticula will require surgery because of a complication from the diverticulum itself. Major complications of duodenal diverticula include obstruction of the biliary or pancreatic ducts that may contribute to cholangitis and pancreatitis, hemorrhage, perforation, and, rarely, blind loop syndrome. Iatrogenic injuries, most commonly acquired during endoscopic instrumentation of an asymptomatic diverticulum, can result in perforation or hemorrhage.

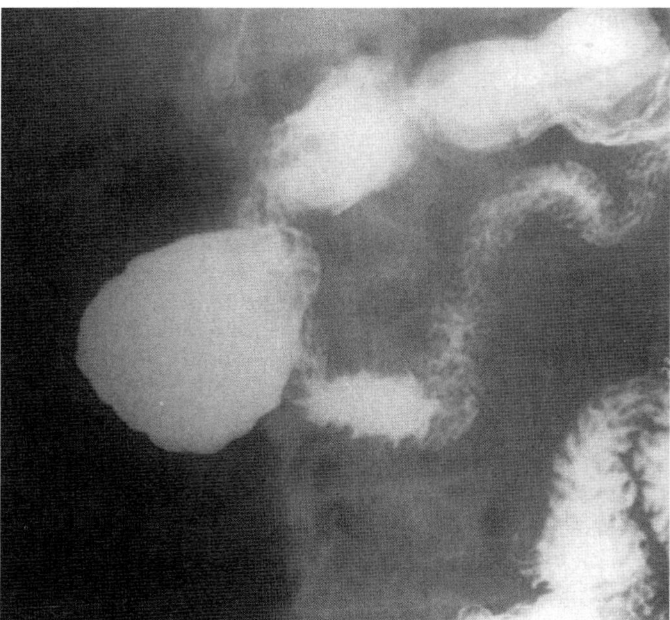

FIG. 50.39 Duodenal diverticulum. Large diverticulum arises from the second portion of the duodenum. (Courtesy Dr. Melvyn H. Schreiber, The University of Texas Medical Branch, Galveston, TX.)

Only those diverticula associated with the ampulla of Vater are significantly related to complications of cholangitis and pancreatitis. In these patients, the ampulla usually enters the duodenum at the superior margin of the diverticulum rather than through the diverticulum itself. A proposed etiology of biliary tract complications is the location of the perivaterian diverticulum, which may distort the common bile duct as it enters the duodenum, resulting in partial obstruction and stasis. In addition, hemorrhage can be caused by inflammation, leading to erosion of a branch of the superior mesenteric artery. Perforation of duodenal diverticula has been described but is rare. Finally, stasis of intestinal contents within a distended diverticulum can result in bacterial overgrowth, malabsorption, steatorrhea, and megaloblastic anemia, essentially producing a blind loop syndrome. Symptoms related to duodenal diverticula in the absence of any other demonstrable disease usually are nonspecific epigastric complaints that can be treated conservatively and may actually prove to be the result of another problem not related to the diverticulum itself.

Treatment

Most duodenal diverticula are asymptomatic and benign; when they are found incidentally, they should be left alone. For symptomatic duodenal diverticula, treatment consists of removal of the diverticulum, which can be accomplished endoscopically or surgically. Appropriate classification of these diverticula guides management. All intraluminal duodenal diverticula require treatment as recurrence of symptoms is certain. Curative treatment consists of removal of the intraluminal diverticulum by laparotomy and duodenotomy or by endoscopic resection. A large (>3 cm) or obstructing intraluminal duodenal diverticulum does not preclude endoscopic resection, but an endoscopic approach in the setting of massive hemorrhage or perforation with intraabdominal contamination secondary to intestinal contents is discouraged. These entities are relatively rare and often require a multidisciplinary approach to determine the best treatment strategy.

Extraluminal duodenal diverticula should be resected in the setting of symptomatic disease or need for urgent surgery, such as free perforation or hemorrhage. Several operative procedures have been described for the treatment of the symptomatic extraluminal duodenal diverticula. The most common and effective treatment is diverticulectomy, which is most easily accomplished by performing a wide Kocher maneuver that exposes the duodenum. The diverticulum is then excised, and the duodenum is closed in a transverse or longitudinal fashion, whichever produces the least amount of luminal obstruction. Careful identification of the ampulla is essential to prevent injury to the common bile duct and pancreatic duct. For diverticula embedded deep within the head of the pancreas, a duodenotomy is performed, with invagination of the diverticulum into the lumen, which is then excised, and the wall is closed (Fig. 50.40A–C). Alternative methods that have been described for duodenal diverticula associated with the ampulla of Vater include an extended sphincteroplasty through the common wall of the ampulla in the diverticulum (Fig. 50.40D–F). Laparoscopic duodenal diverticulectomy is safe and effective in patients with symptomatic and noncomplicated (i.e., not perforated or bleeding) diverticula. An endoscopic stapler is most commonly used to traverse and to resect the diverticulum at its base, and an omental patch reinforcement can be placed over the staple line.

The treatment of a perforated diverticulum may require procedures similar to those described for patients with massive trauma-related defects of the duodenal wall. The perforated diverticulum

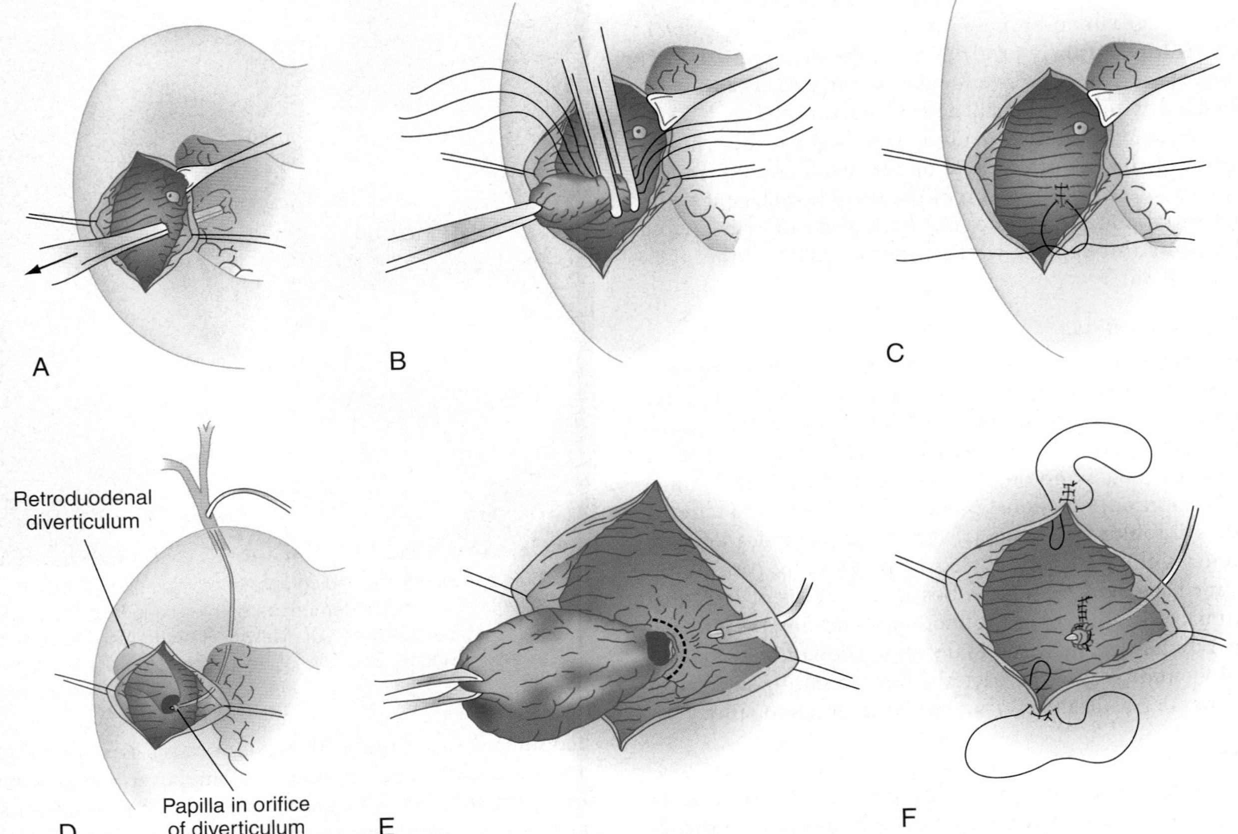

FIG. 50.40 (A–C) Treatment for diverticulum protruding into the head of the pancreas. The duodenum is opened vertically. A clamp is used to invert the diverticulum into the lumen, where it is excised, and the posterior wall defect is closed. (D–F) Management of the unusual duodenal diverticula that arise in the periampullary location. A tube stent should be placed into the common bile duct and passed distally into the duodenum to facilitate identification and later dissection of the sphincter of Oddi. The diverticulum is inverted into the lumen of the duodenum. The round opening in the wall of the base of the diverticulum is the site at which the ampullary structures were freed by a circumferential incision. (E) Line of division of the base of the diverticulum *(heavy broken line)*. which is accomplished by free-hand dissection. After the diverticulum has been removed, the stent and enveloping papilla are protruded into the defect left by the division of the base of the diverticulum. The mucosa and muscle wall of the papilla are then sewn circumferentially to the wall of the duodenum. (Adapted from Thompson JC. *Atlas of Surgery of the Stomach, Duodenum, and Small Bowel.* St. Louis: Mosby-Year Book; 1992:209–213.)

should be excised and the duodenum closed with a serosal patch from a jejunal loop. If the surrounding inflammation is severe, it may be necessary to divert the enteric flow away from the site of the perforation with a gastrojejunostomy or duodenojejunostomy. Interruption of duodenal continuity proximal to the perforated diverticulum may be accomplished by pyloric closure with suture or a row of staples. If the diverticulum is posterior and perforates into the substance of the pancreas, operative repair may be difficult and dangerous. Wide drainage with duodenal diversion may be all that is feasible in such cases. Great care should be taken if the perforation is adjacent to the papilla of Vater. Surgical jejunostomy should also be considered for all patients with acute perforation to ensure nutrition repletion.

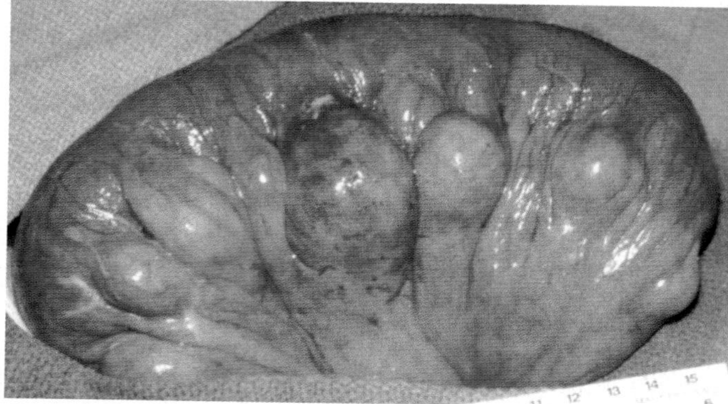

FIG. 50.41 Jejunal diveritculum. Multiple large jejunal diverticula located in the mesentery in an older patient presenting with obstruction secondary to an enterolith. (Adapted from Evers BM, Townsend CM Jr, Thompson JC. Small intestine. In: Schwartz SI, ed. *Principles of Surgery.* 7th ed. New York: McGraw-Hill; 1999:1248.)

Jejunal and Ileal Diverticula

Incidence and Cause

Diverticula of the small bowel are much less common than duodenal diverticula, with an incidence ranging from 0.1% to 1.4% in autopsy series and 0.1% to 1.5% in upper gastrointestinal studies. Jejunal diverticula are more common and are larger than those in the ileum. These are false diverticula, occurring mainly in an older age group (after the sixth decade of life). These diverticula are multiple, usually protrude from the mesenteric border of the bowel, and may be overlooked at surgery because they are embedded within the small bowel mesentery (Fig. 50.41). The cause of jejunoileal diverticulosis is thought to be a motor dysfunction of the smooth muscle or the myenteric plexus, resulting in disordered contractions of the small bowel, generating increased intraluminal pressure and herniation of the mucosa and submucosa through the weakest portion of the bowel (i.e., the mesenteric side).

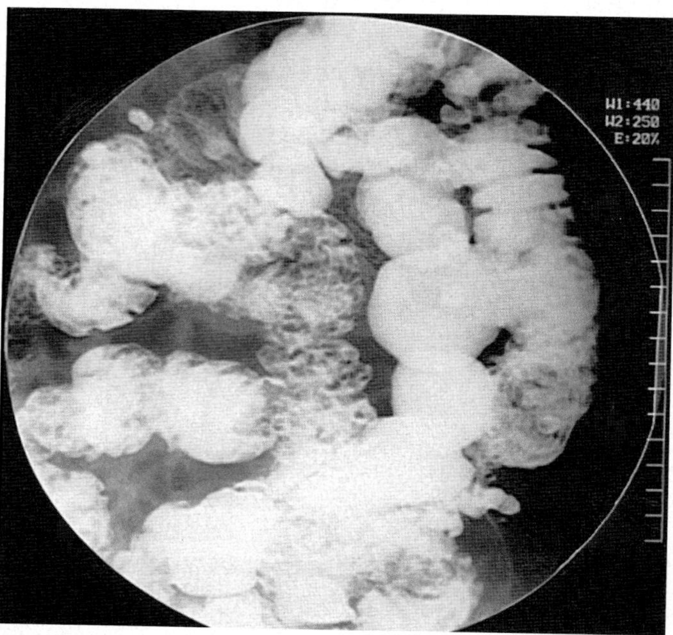

FIG. 50.42 Contrasted radiograph demonstrating jejunal diverticula. Multiple jejunal diverticula demonstrated by a barium contrast upper gastrointestinal study. (Courtesy Dr. Melvyn H. Schreiber, The University of Texas Medical Branch, Galveston, TX.)

Clinical Manifestations

Jejunoileal diverticula are usually found incidentally at laparotomy or during an upper gastrointestinal study (Fig. 50.42); the great majority remain asymptomatic. Acute complications, such as intestinal obstruction, hemorrhage, and perforation, can occur but are rare. Chronic symptoms include vague chronic abdominal pain, malabsorption, functional pseudo-obstruction, and chronic low-grade gastrointestinal hemorrhage. Acute complications are diverticulitis with or without abscess or perforation, gastrointestinal hemorrhage, and intestinal obstruction. Stasis of intestinal flow with bacterial overgrowth (blind loop syndrome), caused by the jejunal dyskinesia, may lead to deconjugation of bile salts and uptake of vitamin B_{12} by the bacterial flora, resulting in steatorrhea and megaloblastic anemia, with or without neuropathy.

Treatment

For incidentally noted, asymptomatic jejunoileal diverticula, no treatment is required. Treatment of complications of obstruction, bleeding, and perforation is usually by intestinal resection and end-to-end anastomosis. Patients presenting with malabsorption secondary to the blind loop syndrome and bacterial overgrowth in the diverticulum can usually be given antibiotics. Obstruction may be caused by enteroliths that form in a jejunal diverticulum and are subsequently dislodged and obstruct the distal intestine. This condition may be treated by enterotomy and removal of the enterolith, or sometimes the enterolith can be milked distally into the cecum. When the enterolith causes obstruction at the level of the diverticulum, bowel resection is necessary. When a perforation of a jejunoileal diverticulum is encountered, resection with reanastomosis is required because lesser procedures, such as simple closure, excision, and invagination, are associated with greater mortality and morbidity rates. Laparoscopic bowel resection with reanastomosis is a safe option in minimally contaminated surgical fields. In extreme cases, such as diffuse peritonitis, enterostomies may be required if judgment dictates that reanastomosis may be risky.

Meckel Diverticulum

Incidence and Cause

Meckel diverticulum is the most commonly encountered congenital anomaly of the small intestine, occurring in about 2% of the population. It was reported initially in 1598 by Hildanus and then described in detail by Johann Meckel in 1809. Meckel diverticulum is located on the antimesenteric border of the ileum 45 to

60 cm proximal to the ileocecal valve and results from incomplete closure of the omphalomesenteric, or vitelline, duct. An equal incidence is found in men and women. Meckel diverticulum may exist in different forms, ranging from a small bump that may be easily missed to a long projection that communicates with the umbilicus by a persistent fibrous cord (Fig. 50.43) or, much less commonly, a patent fistula. The usual manifestation is a relatively wide-mouthed diverticulum measuring about 5 cm in length, with a diameter of up to 2 cm (Fig. 50.44). Cells lining the vitelline duct are pluripotent; therefore, it is not uncommon to find heterotopic tissue within the Meckel diverticulum, the most common of which is gastric mucosa (present in 50% of all Meckel diverticula). Pancreatic mucosa is encountered in about 5% of diverticula; less commonly, these diverticula may harbor colonic mucosa.

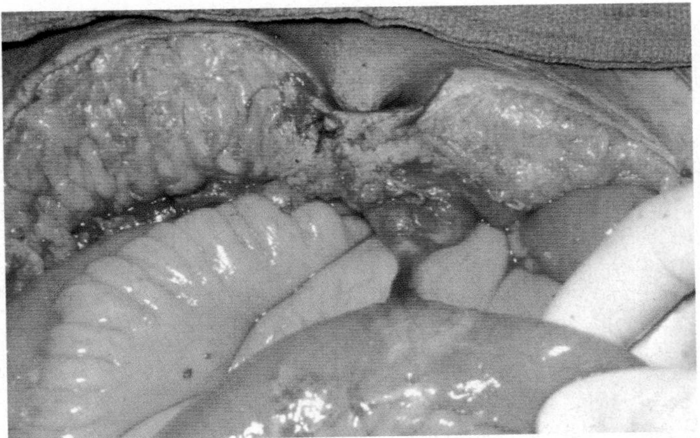

FIG. 50.43 Persistent omphalomesenteric remnant. Omphalomesenteric remnant persisting as a fibrous cord from the ileum to the umbilicus.

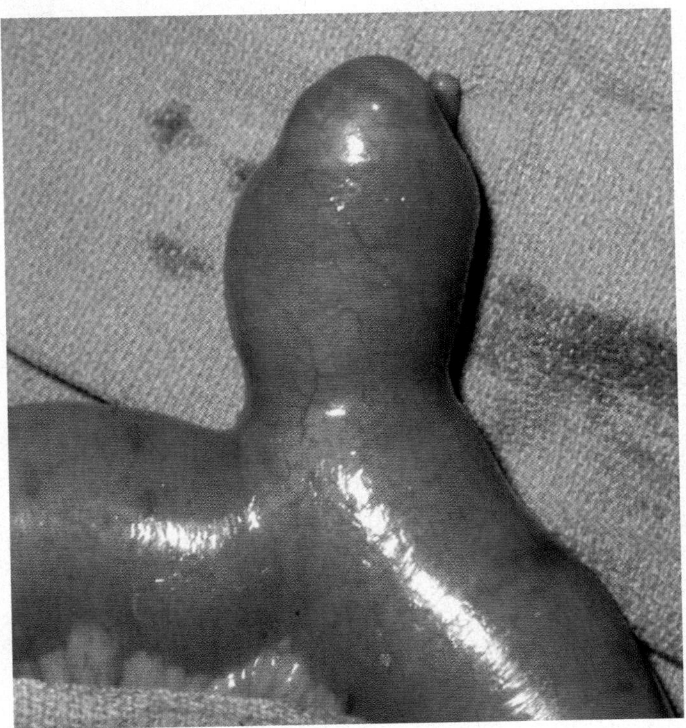

FIG. 50.44 Meckel diverticulum. Common presentation of a Meckel diverticulum projecting from the antimesenteric border of the ileum.

Clinical Manifestations

Most Meckel diverticula are benign and are incidentally discovered during autopsy, laparotomy, or barium studies (Fig. 50.45). The most common clinical presentation of Meckel diverticulum is gastrointestinal bleeding, which occurs in 25% to 50% of patients who present with complications; hemorrhage is the most common symptomatic presentation in children 2 years of age or younger. This complication may be manifested as acute massive hemorrhage, anemia secondary to chronic bleeding, or a self-limited recurrent episodic event. The usual source of the bleeding is a chronic acid-induced ulcer in the ileum adjacent to a Meckel diverticulum that contains gastric mucosa.

Another common presenting symptom of Meckel diverticulum is intestinal obstruction. Obstruction may result from a volvulus of the small bowel that surrounds the diverticulum and associated with a fibrotic band attached to the abdominal wall, intussusception, or, rarely, incarceration of the diverticulum in an inguinal hernia (Littre hernia). Volvulus is usually an acute event and, if allowed to progress, may result in strangulation of the involved bowel. In intussusception, a broad-based diverticulum invaginates and then is carried forward by peristalsis. This may be ileoileal or ileocolic and be manifested as acute obstruction associated with an urge to defecate, early vomiting, and occasionally passage of the classic currant jelly stool. A palpable mass may be present. Although reduction of an intussusception secondary to Meckel diverticulum can sometimes be performed by barium enema, the patient should still undergo resection of the diverticulum to negate subsequent recurrence of the condition.

Diverticulitis accounts for 10% to 20% of symptomatic presentations. This complication is more common in adult patients. Meckel diverticulitis, which is clinically indistinguishable from appendicitis, should be considered in the differential diagnosis of a patient with right lower quadrant pain. Progression of the diverticulitis may lead to perforation and peritonitis. When the appendix is found to be normal during exploration for suspected appendicitis, the distal ileum should be inspected for the presence of an inflamed Meckel diverticulum.

Neoplasms can also occur in a Meckel diverticulum, with NET as the most common malignant neoplasm (77%). Other histologic types include adenocarcinoma (11%), which generally originates from the gastric mucosa, GIST (10%), and lymphoma (1%).[43]

Diagnostic Studies

The diagnosis of Meckel diverticulum may be difficult. Plain abdominal radiography, CT, and ultrasonography are rarely helpful. In children, the single most accurate diagnostic test for Meckel diverticula is with sodium ^{99m}Tc-pertechnetate scintigraphy. The ^{99m}Tc-pertechnetate is preferentially taken up by the mucus-secreting cells of gastric mucosa and ectopic gastric tissue in the diverticulum (Fig. 50.46). The diagnostic sensitivity of this scan has been reported as high as 85%, with a specificity of 95% and an accuracy of 90% in the pediatric age group.

In adults, however, the sensitivity of ^{99m}Tc-pertechnetate scan falls to 63% because of the smaller presence of gastric mucosa in the diverticulum compared with that noted in the pediatric age group. The sensitivity and specificity can be improved by the use of pharmacologic agents. Cimetidine may be used to increase the sensitivity of scintigraphy by decreasing the peptic secretion, while not affecting radionuclide uptake, which may be caused by the release of pertechnetate from the diverticular lumen. Therefore, cimetidine treatment results in higher radionuclide concentrations in the wall of the diverticulum.

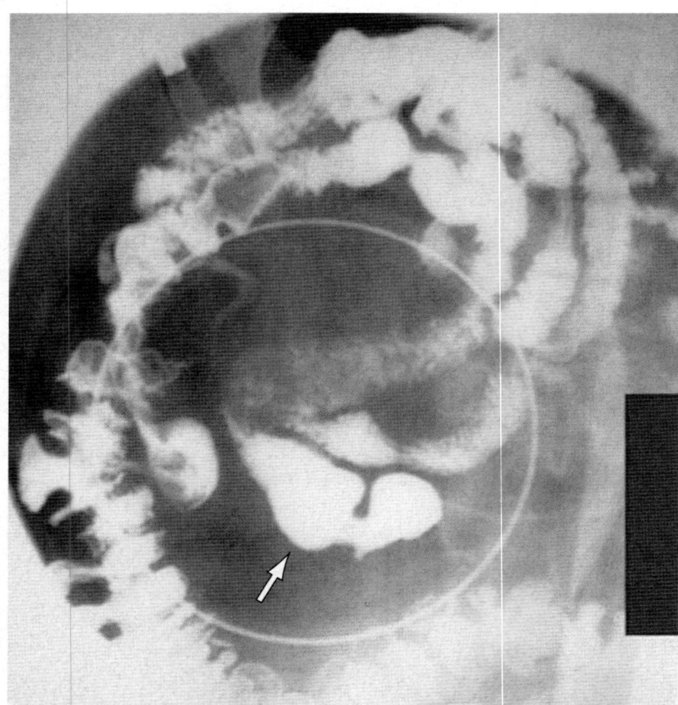

FIG. 50.45 Contrasted radiograph of Meckel diverticulum. Barium radiograph demonstrates an asymptomatic Meckel diverticulum *(arrow)*. (Courtesy Dr. Melvyn H. Schreiber, The University of Texas Medical Branch, Galveston, TX.)

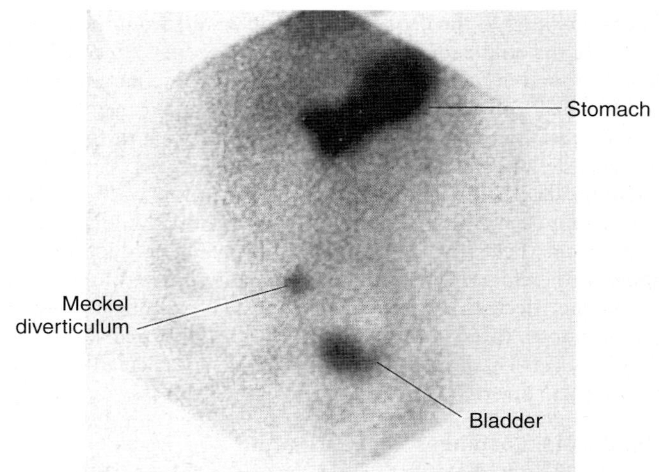

FIG. 50.46 Nuclear Imaging of Meckel diverticulum. A ^{99m}Tc-pertechnetate scintigram from a child demonstrates a Meckel diverticulum clearly differentiated from the stomach and bladder. (Courtesy Dr. Melvyn H. Schreiber, The University of Texas Medical Branch, Galveston, TX.)

False-negative results can occur because of absent gastric mucosal cells, inflammatory changes causing edema or necrosis, presence of outlet obstruction of the diverticulum, or anemia. In false-negative cases, barium contrast imaging, mesenteric arteriography, or double-balloon endoscopy can be helpful. In patients with acute hemorrhage, angiography is sometimes useful. Nevertheless, surgical intervention should not be delayed to obtain imaging for a patient with signs and symptoms of hemorrhage and hemodynamic instability.

Treatment

The treatment of a symptomatic Meckel diverticulum requires prompt surgical intervention with diverticulectomy or segmental resection of ileum containing the diverticulum. Segmental small bowel resection is required for treatment of patients with hemorrhage as the bleeding site is usually adjacent to the diverticulum. Diverticulectomy for nonbleeding Meckel diverticula can be performed with a hand-sewn technique or stapling across the base of the diverticulum in a diagonal or transverse line to minimize the risk for subsequent stenosis. Retrospective studies have demonstrated equivalent outcomes in laparoscopic resection as compared with open resection of Meckel diverticulum.

Although the treatment of a complicated or symptomatic Meckel diverticulum is straightforward, the optimal treatment of an asymptomatic diverticulum found incidentally is still debated. It is generally recommended that asymptomatic diverticula found in children during laparotomy should be resected. The treatment of Meckel diverticula encountered in the adult patient, however, remains controversial. A landmark paper by Soltero and Bill[44] formed the basis of the surgical management of asymptomatic Meckel's diverticula in adults for many years. In this study, the likelihood of a Meckel diverticulum becoming symptomatic in the adult patient was estimated to be 2% or less, and given that the morbidity rates from incidental removal were 12% at the time, the recommendation was to not remove the incidental Meckel diverticulum. This conservative approach was supported by a more recent systematic review by Zani etal.[45] identifying a clear increase in morbidity with resection and calculating that, to avoid one death related to the diverticulum, over 700 incidental diverticulum resections were required. However, other studies have challenged this more conservative approach to the adult patient with an incidental Meckel diverticulum. In a recent population-based study evaluating patients from 1973 to 2006, the mean annual incidence of malignancy in a Meckel diverticulum was noted to be approximately 1.44 per 10 million; therefore, the adjusted risk of cancer in the Meckel diverticulum was at least 70 times higher than in any other ileal site, thus identifying a Meckel diverticulum as a "hot spot" for malignant disease in the ileum.[43] Given the increased risk of malignant transformation over a lifetime, the authors also advocated for removal of an incidental Meckel diverticulum. A recent review suggested that the decision for resection of an incidentally found diverticulum should be based on the risk of future complications. The factors associated with a higher risk of complications, and warranting consideration of resection, include age younger than 50 years, male sex, diverticulum length >2 cm, and ectopic tissue or palpable abnormalities.[46] Taken together, the decision for surgical resection of Meckel diverticulum needs to be made on a personalized basis weighing the risk and benefits of malignancy, age, and complications. Future prospective trials are needed to clarify this controversy.

MISCELLANEOUS PROBLEMS

Small Bowel Ulcerations

Ulcerations of the small bowel are relatively uncommon and may be attributed to Crohn disease, typhoid fever, tuberculosis, lymphoma, and gastrinoma (Table 50.11). Drug-induced ulcerations can occur and were, in the past, attributed to enteric-coated potassium chloride tablets and corticosteroids. In addition, ulcerations of the small intestine in which no causative agent can be identified have been described. It is suggested that small bowel complications from NSAIDs may be more common than originally considered. NSAID-induced ulcers occur more commonly in the ileum, with single or multiple ulcerations

TABLE 50.11 Causes of small intestine ulceration.

CAUSE	EXAMPLES
Infections	Tuberculosis, syphilis, cytomegalovirus, typhoid, parasites, *Strongyloides* hyperinfection, *Campylobacter, Yersinia*
Inflammatory	Crohn disease, systemic lupus erythematosus, celiac disease, ulcerative enteritis
Ischemia	Mesenteric arterial insufficiency or venous thrombosis
Idiopathic	Primary ulcer, Behçet syndrome
Drug induced	Potassium, indomethacin, phenylbutazone, salicylates, antimetabolites
Radiation	Therapeutic, accidental
Vascular	Vasculitis, giant cell arteritis, amyloidosis (ischemic lesion), angiocentric lymphoma
Metabolic	Uremia
Hyperacidity	Zollinger-Ellison syndrome, Meckel diverticulum, stomal ulceration
Neoplastic	Lymphoma, adenocarcinoma, melanoma
Toxic	Acute jejunitis (β-toxin–producing *Clostridium perfringens*), arsenic
Mucosal lesions	Lymphocytic enterocolitis

Adapted from Rai R, Bayless TM. Isolated and diffuse ulcers of the small intestine. In: Feldman M, Scharschmidt BF, Sleisenger MH, eds. *Gastrointestinal and Liver Disease: Pathophysiology, Diagnosis, Management*. Philadelphia: WB Saunders; 1998:1771–1778.

noted. Complications necessitating operative intervention include bleeding, perforation, and obstruction. In addition to ulcerations, NSAIDs are known to induce an enteropathy characterized by increased intestinal permeability leading to protein loss and hypoalbuminemia, malabsorption, and anemia. Treatment of complications from small bowel ulcerations is segmental resection and intestinal reanastomosis.

Ingested Foreign Bodies

Ingested foreign bodies, which can lead to subsequent perforation or obstruction of the gastrointestinal tract, are swallowed, usually accidentally, by children or adults. These include glass and metal fragments, pins, needles, toothpicks, fish bones, coins, whistles, toys, and broken razor blades (Fig. 50.47). Intentional ingestion of foreign bodies is sometimes seen in the prison population and those who have a psychiatric illness. For most patients, treatment is observation, to permit safe passage of these objects through the intestinal tract. If the object is radiopaque, progress can be followed by serial abdominal films. Cathartic agents are contraindicated. Sharp pointed objects such as needles, razor blades, or fish bones may penetrate the bowel wall. If abdominal pain, tenderness, fever, or leukocytosis occurs, immediate laparotomy and surgical removal of the offending object(s) is indicated. Laparotomy is also required for intestinal obstruction.

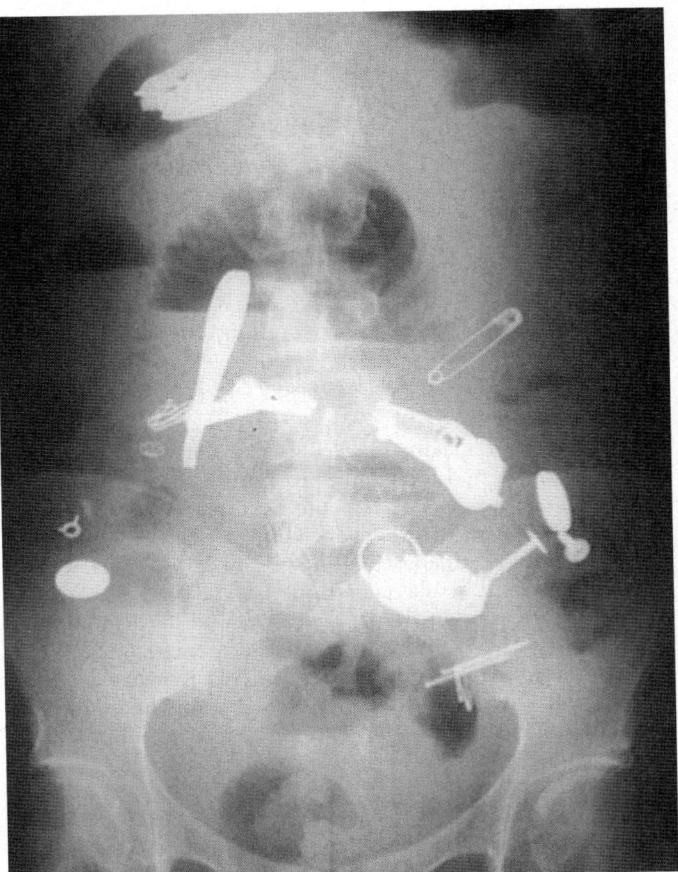

FIG. 50.47 Intestinal foreign bodies. Plain abdominal film demonstrates a number of ingested foreign bodies in a patient presenting with a small bowel obstruction. (Courtesy Dr. Melvyn H. Schreiber, The University of Texas Medical Branch, Galveston, TX.)

Small Bowel Fistulas

Despite improvements in surgical nutrition and critical care, mortality from enterocutaneous fistulas remains high, 10% in recent reports. Improvements in outcome focus on prevention and, when fistulas occur, prompt recognition and intervention. Multidisciplinary care is critical for improving fistula outcomes. Enterocutaneous fistulas are most commonly iatrogenic, as 75% to 85% occur during surgical intervention (e.g., anastomotic leakage, injury of the bowel or blood supply, erosion by suction catheters, laceration of the bowel by wire mesh or retention sutures). The remaining 15% to 25% of fistula occurrences are associated with predisposing conditions such as Crohn disease, malignant disease, radiation enteritis, diverticulitis, intraabdominal sepsis, or trauma.

Clinical Manifestations

Recognition of enterocutaneous fistulas is usually not difficult. The typical clinical presentation is that of a febrile postoperative patient with an erythematous wound. When a few skin sutures are removed, a purulent or bloody discharge is noted; leakage of enteric contents then occurs, sometimes immediately but often within 1 or 2 days. The diagnosis rarely eludes the surgeon for long. Small bowel fistulas can also be manifested with generalized peritonitis, although this is less common. Recently, the popularization of damage control laparotomy and staged management of the open abdomen has led to a more virulent form of small bowel fistula referred to as an *enteroatmospheric fistula*. These patients typically present with an open segment of intestine exposed through a large fascial defect, without a surrounding epidermal margin.

Enterocutaneous fistulas are classified according to their location and volume of daily output (Table 50.12). These factors dictate treatment and morbidity and mortality rates. Proximal fistulas are associated with higher output, greater fluid and electrolyte loss, and greater loss of digestive capacity. Distal fistulas tend to

TABLE 50.12 Factors predictive of nonoperative fistula closure.

FAVORABLE	UNFAVORABLE
Surgical etiology	Ileal, jejunal, nonsurgical etiology
Appendicitis or diverticulitis	Inflammatory bowel disease, cancer, radiation
Transferrin >200 mg/dL	Transferrin <200 mg/dL
No evidence of bowel obstruction, discontinuity, infection, inflammation	Distal small bowel obstruction, bowel is in discontinuity, adjacent infection, adjacent inflammation
Length >2 cm, end fistula	Length <2 cm, lateral or multiple fistulas
Output <200 mL/24 hours	Output >500 mL/24 hours
No sepsis, balanced electrolytes	Sepsis, electrolyte disturbances
Initial referral to tertiary care center and subspecialty care	Delay getting to tertiary care center and subspecialty care

Adapted from Gribovskaja-Rupp I, Melton GB. Enterocutaneous fistula: proven strategies and updates. *Clin Colon Rectal Surg.* 2016;29:130–137.

have lower output, making them easier to manage and more likely to close spontaneously. High-output fistulas are those that discharge 500 mL or more per 24 hours. Multiple factors prevent the spontaneous closure of fistulas including retained foreign body, radiation enteritis, inflammatory bowel disease or infection, epithelialization of the fistula tract, neoplasm, and distal obstruction. Once a fistula is identified, management should focus on prompt IV fluid resuscitation and consideration of potential factors that could prevent spontaneous closure. Successful management of patients with intestinal fistulas requires a coordinated staged approach that can be defined in three phases: (1) stabilization, (2) staging and supportive care, and (3) definitive management.

Treatment

Stabilization. Historically, malnutrition and fluid losses were the leading causes of death in patients with small bowel fistula. However, with better nutritional supplementation and critical care support, sepsis has become the most common cause of death in affected patients. Nevertheless, the fluid losses and volume depletion associated with small bowel fistula cannot be marginalized. Therefore, prompt fluid resuscitation and electrolyte replacement should occur on recognition of a fistula. Sepsis control is critical, and in the early period, CT scanning may be invaluable in identifying undrained abscesses, complete distal obstructions, or generalized intraabdominal sepsis with peritonitis. Numerous treatment options are available for enterocutaneous fistulas (Box 50.7). All infections should be adequately drained percutaneously or operatively, if necessary, along with appropriate antibiotic administration. Once sepsis is controlled and the patient is resuscitated, effluent control with skin protection and adequate nutrition are necessary. Fistula output is best controlled by intubation of the fistula tract with a drain. Protection of the skin around the fistulous opening is important to prevent excoriation and destruction of the skin. This is most easily accomplished by using a stomahesive product with applications of zinc oxide, aluminum paste, or karaya powder. The suction catheter can be brought out through the end of the stomahesive bag, which is cut to just fit the fistulous opening. This will allow collection and accurate measurement of the output. The use of TPN has been an important advance in the management of patients with high-output enterocutaneous fistulas and significantly decreases the incidence of malnutrition. TPN is particularly valuable in the stabilization period to help minimize high-output fistula losses and for immediate nutritional repletion while the fistula is being delineated. However, if the patient can meet calorie goals without the use of TPN, especially when a high-output fistula is not present, enteral feeding is preferable and recommended.

Staging and supportive care. When sepsis has been controlled and nutritional therapy has been instituted, the fistula must be adequately staged. The combined use of fluoroscopic contrast studies, fistulography if necessary, and CT, along with the patient's clinical behavior, will characterize the anatomy and underlying pathology of the fistula. Some have advocated conservative management for up to 3 months to allow spontaneous closure. However, others have shown that after sepsis is controlled, more than 90% of small intestinal fistulas that closed did so within 1 month. Less than 10% of the fistulas closed after 2 months, and none closed spontaneously after 3 months. In one large retrospective study, the majority of enterocutaneous fistulas closed spontaneously (54%), while 18% needed definitive surgery at a later time. Operative mortality was 9.8% while recurrence rate was 8%. Uncomplicated proximal fistulas have higher spontaneous closure rates, with duodenal fistulas closing within 2 to 4 weeks.[47] Therefore, a reasonable management plan would be to follow a 6-week period of convalescence, at which time, if closure has not been obtained, surgical management should be considered if the preoperative albumin level is above 25 g/L. However, knowledge that spontaneous closure is unlikely should not prompt immediate reexploration at 8 weeks. In general, a period of 3 to 6 months is beneficial to allow the profound inflammatory response associated with intraabdominal sepsis to subside completely and for the adhesion formation to stabilize. This period will provide a better opportunity for safe and successful operative intervention. Furthermore, as is the case with enteroatmospheric small bowel fistulas, it may take several months to stabilize the complex abdominal wound associated with the fistula.

Several adjuncts have been proposed to help assist in spontaneous fistula closure and management of the associated abdominal wound, although none are supported by vigorous level I data. Studies suggest that bowel rest with TPN therapy improves fistula closure rates and time to closure in patients with high-output fistulas. Low-output fistulas can successfully be managed with enteral therapy while avoiding the known complications of parenteral therapy. Dysmotility agents such as loperamide and codeine can also assist with attempts at enteral therapy. Furthermore, newer techniques, such as fistuloclysis, in which the distal limb of a proximal fistula is intubated and enteral therapy is delivered to the distal bowel, have proved effective. Several randomized trials have evaluated the role of octreotide in the management of fistulas. Although octreotide has been shown to decrease fistula output, which can be useful in the presence of a high-output fistula, octreotide has not convincingly provided an improvement in spontaneous closure rates. Vacuum devices are valuable in the setting of enteroatmospheric fistulas to help contract the open abdominal

BOX 50.7 Treatment strategy in patients with an enterocutaneous fistula.

Sepsis Control
Radiologic drainage of abscess
Relaparotomy on demand, minimally invasive if possible
Consider other infectious foci: intravenous line, urinary tract infection, pulmonary

Optimization of Nutritional Status
Rehydration and electrolyte supplementation
Enteral nutrition is preferred
Parenteral nutrition to meet calorie requirements, small bowel ECF
Allow 500 mL/day clear liquids orally

Wound Care
Gauzes for low-output ECF
Collect ECF fluids with bag (wound manager, fistula bag), paste to protect the skin
Drainage of excessive ECF fluid with sump suction
Proton pump inhibitors

Anatomy of ECF
Macroscopic
Biochemical analysis of ECF fluid (bilirubin/amylase)
Methylene blue
Preoperatively: fistulography or contrast computed tomography; length of intestine and localization of origin of ECF, stenosis, obstruction, and fluid collection

Timing of Surgery
Clinically stable (above)
Psychologically willing to undergo surgery
Albumin >25 g/L
Period of convalescence >6 weeks

Surgical Strategy
One-stage procedure
Careful adhesiolysis
Wedge excision of intestinal resection
Limit number of anastomoses to minimum
Cover sutures with healthy, viable tissue
Keep away from compromised area

Adapted from Visschers RG, van Gemert WG, Winkens B, et al. Guided treatment improves outcome of patients with enterocutaneous fistulas. *World J Surg*. 2012;36:2341–2348.
ECF, Enterocutaneous fistula.

wound around the associated fistula. Care should be given to avoid direct contact with visceral contents as this can cause new fistulas. Skin grafting up to the fistula has also been used in cases associated with an open abdomen, with a graft success rate of up to 80% in some series. Importantly, patients who could not be discharged before definitive repair also have higher mortality risk.

Definitive management. If the fistula persists despite adequately addressing the patient's nutritional, fluid, and wound care needs, reoperative intervention will ultimately be necessary for some patients. Surgery is most easily accomplished by entering the previous abdominal wound, with great care taken to avoid further damage to adherent bowel. The preferred operation is fistula tract excision and segmental resection of the involved segment of intestine and reanastomosis. Simple closure of the fistula after removal of the fistula tract almost always results in fistula recurrence. If an unexpected abscess is encountered or if the bowel wall is rigid and distended over a long distance, thus making primary anastomosis unsafe, exteriorization of both ends of the intestine should be accomplished. Various bypass procedures have also been described as part of a staged approach in which exclusion of the segment containing the fistula is accomplished in the first reoperation, and then another operation is required for resection of the involved segment and fistula tract. Although this may be necessary in extreme circumstances, this is certainly not the preferred surgical management. Basic surgical considerations include attempting a one-stage procedure, careful adhesiolysis, addressing compromised tissues with wedge excision or intestinal resection, covering sutures with viable tissues, and avoiding friable areas that are not directly involved with the fistula.

In summary, enterocutaneous fistulas occur most commonly as a result of a previous operative procedure. Once identified, a three-phase approach of stabilization, staging, and supportive care, and, in some cases, definitive surgical intervention is necessary. Most of these fistulas heal spontaneously within 6 weeks. If closure is not achieved after 6 weeks, surgery is indicated.

Pneumatosis Intestinalis

Pneumatosis intestinalis is an uncommon condition manifesting as multiple gas-filled cysts of the gastrointestinal tract. The cysts may be located in the subserosa, submucosa, and, rarely, muscularis layer and vary in size from microscopic to several centimeters in diameter. They can occur anywhere along the gastrointestinal tract, from the esophagus to the rectum; however, they are most common in the jejunum, followed by the ileocecal region and colon. Extraintestinal structures such as mesentery, peritoneum, and the falciform ligament may also be involved. There is an equal incidence in men and women, and the condition usually occurs in the fourth to seventh decades of life. Pneumatosis in neonates is usually associated with necrotizing enterocolitis. The cause of pneumatosis intestinalis has not been completely delineated. A number of theories have been proposed; mechanical, mucosal damage, bacterial, and pulmonary hypotheses seem to be most plausible.

There are two forms of pneumatosis intestinalis. Primary pneumatosis (15%) is a benign idiopathic condition that is not associated with any other conditions or symptoms and is found incidentally. The majority of pneumatosis intestinalis (85%) are associated with chronic obstructive pulmonary disease or an immunocompromised state (e.g., in AIDS; after transplantation; in association with leukemia, lymphoma, vasculitis, or collagen vascular disease; and in patients undergoing chemotherapy or taking corticosteroids). Other associated conditions include inflammatory, obstructive, or infectious conditions of the intestine; iatrogenic conditions, such as endoscopy and jejunostomy placement; small bowel ischemia; and extraintestinal diseases, such as diabetes.

Upon gross inspection, the cysts resemble cystic lymphangiomas or hydatid cysts. On histologic section, the involved portion has a honeycomb appearance. The cysts are thin walled and break easily. Spontaneous rupture gives rise to pneumoperitoneum. Symptoms are nonspecific, and in pneumatosis associated with other disorders, the symptoms may be those of the associated disease. Symptoms in primary pneumatosis intestinalis, when present, usually include diarrhea, abdominal pain, abdominal distention, nausea, vomiting, weight loss, and mucus in stools. Hematochezia and constipation have also been described. Complications associated with pneumatosis intestinalis occur in about 3% of cases and include volvulus, intestinal obstruction, hemorrhage, and intestinal perforation. Usually, pneumoperitoneum occurs in these patients, generally in association with small bowel rather than large bowel pneumatosis. Peritonitis is unusual. In fact, pneumatosis intestinalis represents one of the few cases of sterile pneumoperitoneum and should be considered in the patient with free abdominal air but no evidence of peritonitis. Pneumatosis intestinalis is an ominous sign when associated with peritonitis, mesenteric gas, or portovenous gas, as this is most concerning for life threatening small bowel ischemia.

The diagnosis is usually made radiographically by plain abdominal or barium studies. On plain films, pneumatosis intestinalis appears as radiolucent areas within the bowel wall, which must be differentiated from luminal intestinal gas (Fig. 50.48A). The radiolucency may be linear or curvilinear or appear as grape-like clusters or tiny bubbles. Alternatively, barium contrast or CT studies can be used to confirm the diagnosis (Fig. 50.48B). Visualization of intestinal cysts has also been described by ultrasound.

No treatment is necessary unless one of the very rare complications supervenes, such as small bowel ischemia, rectal bleeding, cyst-induced volvulus, or tension pneumoperitoneum. Prognosis in most patients is that of the underlying disease. The important point is to recognize that pneumatosis intestinalis is a radiographic finding and not a diagnosis. Treatment should be directed at the underlying cause of the pneumatosis, and surgical intervention should be predicated on the clinical course of the patient.

Blind Loop Syndrome

Blind loop syndrome is a rare condition manifested by diarrhea, steatorrhea, megaloblastic anemia, weight loss, abdominal pain, and deficiencies of the fat-soluble vitamins as well as neurologic disorders. The underlying cause of this syndrome is bacterial overgrowth in stagnant areas of the small bowel produced by stricture, stenosis, fistulas, or diverticula (e.g., jejunoileal or Meckel diverticulum). Under normal circumstances, the upper gastrointestinal tract contains fewer than 10^5 bacteria/mL, mostly gram-positive aerobes and facultative anaerobes. However, with stasis, the number of bacteria increases, with excessive proliferation of aerobic and anaerobic bacteria; bacteroides, anaerobic lactobacilli, coliforms, and enterococci are likely to be present in varying numbers. The bacteria compete for dietary vitamin B_{12}, producing a systemic deficiency of vitamin B_{12} and megaloblastic anemia.

The syndrome can be confirmed by a series of laboratory investigations. Bacterial overgrowth can be diagnosed with cultures obtained through an intestinal tube or by indirect tests such as the ^{14}C-xylose or ^{14}C-cholylglycine breath tests. Excessive bacterial use of ^{14}C substrate leads to an increase in ^{14}C-labeled CO_2. After bacterial overgrowth and steatorrhea are confirmed, the Schilling test (^{57}Co-labeled vitamin B_{12} absorption) may be performed, which should reveal a pattern of urinary excretion of vitamin B_{12} resembling that of pernicious anemia (a urinary loss of 0% to 6% of vitamin B_{12} compared with the normal of 7%–25%). In patients with blind loop syndrome, vitamin B_{12} excretion is not altered by the addition of intrinsic factor, but a course of a broad-spectrum antibiotic (e.g., tetracycline) should return vitamin B_{12} absorption to normal.

Treatment of patients with blind loop syndrome includes parenteral vitamin B_{12} therapy and broad-spectrum antibiotics. Tetracyclines have been the mainstay of treatment, but studies have shown that rifaximin and metronidazole demonstrate less resistance and are also effective. For most patients, a single course of therapy (7–10 days) is sufficient, and the patient may remain symptom free for months. Prokinetic agents have been used without real success. Surgical correction of the condition causing stagnation and blind loop syndrome produces a permanent cure and is indicated for patients who require multiple rounds of antibiotics or are receiving continuous therapy.

Radiation Enteritis

Radiation therapy is generally used as adjuvant therapy for various abdominal and pelvic cancers. In addition to tumor cells, however, other rapidly dividing cells in normal tissues may be affected by radiation. Surrounding normal tissue, such as the small

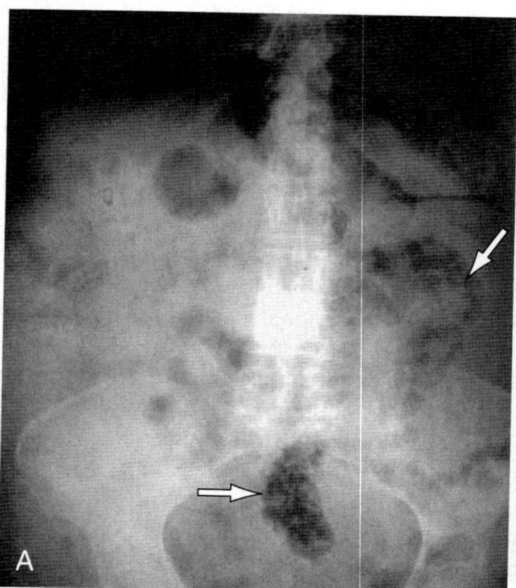

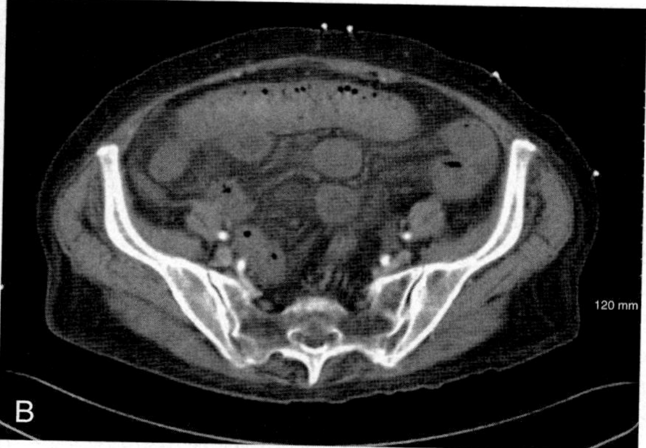

FIG. 50.48 Pneumatosis intestinalis. (A) Plain abdominal film demonstrates pneumatosis intestinalis *(arrows)*. (B) Computed tomography findings consistent with curvilinear radiolucency appearing as tiny bubbles in the antimesenteric border of the bowel consistent with pneumatosis intestinalis. (A, Courtesy Dr. Melvyn H. Schreiber, The University of Texas Medical Branch, Galveston, TX. B, Courtesy Dr. Kristin Long, University of Kentucky Medical Center, Lexington, KY.)

intestinal epithelium, may sustain severe, acute, and chronic deleterious effects. Radiation injury to the small bowel can be subdivided into acute and chronic forms. Acute radiation-induced small bowel disease usually is manifested with colicky abdominal pain, bloating, loss of appetite, nausea, diarrhea, and fecal urgency during or shortly after a course of radiotherapy. Most patients notice symptoms during the third week of treatment and these resolve 2 to 6 weeks after completion of radiation. Symptoms consistent with chronic radiation injury typically develop between 18 months and 6 years after a completed course of radiotherapy, but symptoms can be manifested up to 30 years after the treatment course.

The amount of radiation appears to correlate with the probability for the development of radiation enteritis. Serious late complications are unusual if the total radiation dosage is less than 4000 cGy; morbidity risk increases with dosages exceeding 5000 cGy. Other factors, including previous abdominal surgeries, preexisting vascular disease, hypertension, diabetes, and adjuvant treatment with certain chemotherapeutic agents (such as 5-FU, doxorubicin, dactinomycin, and MTX), contribute to the development of enteritis after radiation treatments. A previous history of laparotomy increases the risk for enteritis, presumably because of adhesions that fix portions of the small bowel into the irradiated field. Radiation damage leads to symptoms of diarrhea, abdominal pain, and malabsorption. The late effects of radiation injury are the result of damage to small submucosal blood vessels, with a progressive obliterative arteritis and submucosal fibrosis; these events eventually result in thrombosis and vascular insufficiency. This injury may produce necrosis and perforation of the involved intestine but, more commonly, leads to stricture formation with symptoms of obstruction or small bowel fistulas.

Multiple strategies are used to reduce radiation injury to the small bowel (Box 50.8). Radiation enteritis may be minimized by adjusting ports and dosages of radiation to deliver optimal treatment specifically to the tumor and not to surrounding tissues. Placement of radiopaque markers, such as titanium clips, at the time of the original operation facilitates better targeting of the radiation treatment. A reduction in field size, multiple field arrangements, conformal radiotherapy techniques, and intensity-modulated radiotherapy can reduce toxicity related to radiotherapy. Methods designed to exclude the small bowel from the irradiated field include reperitonealization, omental transposition, and placement of absorbable mesh slings.

A number of pharmacologic interventions have also been described to reduce the side effects of radiation enteritis. Angiotensin-converting enzyme inhibitors and statins significantly reduce acute gastrointestinal symptoms during radical pelvic radiotherapy. Sucralfate, a highly sulfated polyanionic disaccharide thought to stimulate epithelial healing and thereby form a protective barrier over damaged mucosal surfaces, may help in the treatment of bleeding from radiation proctitis, but no evidence exists supporting its use in the prevention of radiation-induced small bowel disease. Superoxide dismutase, a free radical scavenger, has been used successfully to reduce complications. Other compounds that have been evaluated include glutathione, antioxidants (e.g., vitamin A, vitamin E, beta-carotene), histamine antagonists, and the combination of pentoxifylline and tocopherols, a class of chemical compounds with vitamin E activity. In addition, early studies support the use of probiotics as having a radioprotective effect in the gut; however, further studies are required before a final assessment can be made. The most effective radioprotectant agent appears to be amifostine (WR-2721), a sulfhydryl compound that is converted intracellularly to an active metabolite, WR-1065, which in turn binds to free radicals and protects the cell from radiation injury.[48] A randomized controlled trial determined that glutamine offers little benefit, even when it is used before or during radiation therapy. Agents that may prove useful in the prevention of the acute symptoms of radiation enteritis include the hormones bombesin, growth hormone, GLP-2, and IGF-I, which, in experimental studies, demonstrated effectiveness in preventing or reducing symptoms associated with radiation enteritis.

The treatment of acute radiation enteritis is directed at controlling symptoms. Antispasmodics and analgesics may alleviate abdominal pain and cramping, and diarrhea usually responds to opiates or other antidiarrheal agents. The use of corticosteroids for acute radiation enteritis is of uncertain value. Dietary manipulation, including oral elemental diets, has also been advocated to ameliorate the acute effects of radiation enteritis; however, results are conflicting. Antibiotics are frequently used in the setting of bacterial overgrowth. Bile acid malabsorption, thought to be responsible for diarrheal symptoms in 35% to 72% of patients with radiation-induced small bowel disease, responds well to cholestyramine, but it is not well tolerated and many patients voluntarily discontinue use.

Operative intervention may be required for a subgroup of patients with the chronic effects of radiation enteritis. This is a small (1%–2%) subgroup of the total number of patients who received abdominal or pelvic irradiation. Indications for operation include obstruction, fistula formation, perforation, and bleeding, with obstruction being the most common presentation. Operative procedures include a bypass or resection with reanastomosis. Advocates for bypass procedures contend that this procedure is safer and controls the symptoms better than resection. Advocates of resection contend that the high morbidity and mortality rates previously reported with resection and reanastomosis reflect inadequate resection and anastomosis of diseased intestine. In patients presenting with obstruction, extensive lysis of adhesions should be avoided. Obstruction caused by rigid, fixed intestinal loops in the pelvis is best bypassed. If resection and reanastomosis are planned, at least one end of the anastomosis should be from intestine outside the irradiated field. Macroscopic inspection may not be accurate in evaluating the full extent of radiation damage. Frozen section and laser Doppler flowmetry techniques have been used to assist resection and

BOX 50.8 Prevention of radiation-induced small bowel disease.

Clinical Guidance

Use of modern imaging and radiotherapy techniques to minimize radiation exposure to normal tissues

Consideration of circadian rhythm effects and use of evening radiotherapy sessions

Continuation of angiotensin-converting enzyme inhibitors and statins and consideration of their introduction if appropriate

Consideration of the use of probiotics

Consideration of surgical techniques to minimize radiation exposure to the small bowel if appropriate and surgical team is experienced and competent at the procedure involved

Adapted from Stacey R, Green JT. Radiation-induced small bowel disease: latest developments and clinical guidance. *Ther Adv Chronic Dis.* 2014;5:15–29.

anastomosis. However, reports of their clinical usefulness are conflicting. Perforation of the intestine should be treated with resection and anastomosis. When reanastomosis is thought to be unsafe, the ends should be exteriorized.

Short Bowel Syndrome

The short bowel syndrome results from a total small bowel length that is inadequate to support nutrition. Of these cases of short bowel syndrome, 75% occur from massive intestinal resection. In the adult, mesenteric occlusion, midgut volvulus, and traumatic disruption of the superior mesenteric vessels are the most frequent causes. Multiple sequential resections, usually associated with recurrent Crohn disease, account for 25% of patients. In neonates, the most common cause of short bowel syndrome is bowel resection secondary to necrotizing enterocolitis. The clinical hallmarks of short bowel syndrome include diarrhea, fluid and electrolyte deficiency, and malnutrition. Other complications include an increased incidence of gallstones caused by disruption of the enterohepatic circulation and of nephrolithiasis from hyperoxaluria. Specific nutrient deficiencies must be prevented, and levels must be monitored closely; these nutrients include iron, magnesium, zinc, copper, and vitamins. The likelihood that a patient with short bowel syndrome will be permanently dependent on TPN is thought to be primarily influenced by the length, location, and health of the remaining intestine. In patients with short bowel syndrome, postabsorptive levels of plasma citrulline, a nonprotein amino acid produced by intestinal mucosa, may provide an indicator to differentiate transient from permanent intestinal failure.

The bowel has a remarkable capacity to adapt after small bowel resection; in many cases, this process of intestinal adaptation, termed *adaptive hyperplasia,* effectively prevents severe complications that result from the markedly decreased surface area available for absorption and digestion. However, any adaptive mechanism can be overwhelmed, and adaptation can be inadequate if too much small bowel is lost. Although there is considerable individual variation, resection of up to 70% of the small bowel usually can be tolerated if the terminal ileum and ileocecal valve are preserved. Length alone, however, is not the only determining factor of complications related to small bowel resection. For example, if the distal two thirds of the ileum, including the ileocecal valve, is resected, significant abnormalities of absorption of bile salts and vitamin B_{12} may occur, resulting in diarrhea and anemia, although only 25% of the total length of the small bowel has been removed. Proximal bowel resection is tolerated better than distal resection because the ileum can adapt and increase its absorptive capacity more efficiently than the jejunum.

Treatment

The most important issue to remember about short bowel syndrome is prevention. In patients with Crohn disease, limiting bowel resections to only segments with a particular complication should be performed. In addition, during surgery for problems related to intestinal ischemia, the smallest possible resection should be performed, and if necessary, second-look operations should be carried out to allow the ischemic bowel to demarcate, thus potentially preventing unnecessary extensive resection of the bowel.

After massive small bowel resection, the treatment course may be divided into early and late phases. In its early phase, treatment is primarily directed at the control of diarrhea, replacement of fluid and electrolytes, and prompt institution of TPN in patients who cannot safely tolerate enteral feedings. Volume losses may exceed 5 L/day, and vigorous monitoring of intake and output with adequate replacement must be carried out. Diarrhea in this early phase can be caused by a multitude of sources. For example, hypergastrinemia and gastric hypersecretion occur after massive small bowel resection and can significantly contribute to diarrhea after a massive small bowel resection. Acid hypersecretion can be managed by H_2 receptor antagonists or proton pump blockers, such as omeprazole. Diarrhea may also be caused by ileal resection, resulting in disruption of the enterohepatic circulation and excessive amounts of bile salts entering the colon. Cholestyramine may be beneficial when diarrhea is related to the cathartic effects of unabsorbed bile salts in the colon. In addition, the judicious use of agents that inhibit gut motility (e.g., codeine, diphenoxylate) may be helpful. The long-acting SSA octreotide also appears to reduce the amount of diarrhea during the early phase of short bowel syndrome. Some studies suggest that octreotide may inhibit gut adaptation; other studies, however, have not confirmed this deleterious effect of octreotide.

As soon as the patient has recovered from the acute phase, enteral nutrition should be started. The most common types of enteral diets are elemental (e.g., Vivonex, Flexical) and polymeric (e.g., Isocal, Ensure). Controversy exists about the optimal diet for these patients. Initially, a high-carbohydrate, high-protein diet is appropriate to maximize absorption. Milk products should be avoided, and the diet should begin at iso-osmolar concentrations and with small amounts. As the gut adapts, the osmolality, volume, and calorie content can be increased. The provision of nutrients in their simplest forms is an important part of the treatment. Simple sugars, dipeptides, and tripeptides are rapidly absorbed from the intestinal tract. Reduction in dietary fat has long been considered important in the treatment of patients with short bowel syndrome. Supplementation of the diet with 100 g or more of fat, however, should be carried out, often requiring the use of medium-chain triglycerides, which are absorbed in the proximal bowel. Vitamins, especially fat-soluble vitamins, as well as calcium, magnesium, and zinc supplementation should be provided. The roles of hormones administered systemically and glutamine administered enterally have been evaluated. The hormones neurotensin, growth hormone, bombesin, and GLP-2 have demonstrated marked mucosal growth in a variety of experimental studies and have been shown to prevent gut atrophy associated with TPN in experimental studies; combination therapy appears more efficacious than single-agent administration. Randomized controlled trials showed that teduglutide, a GLP-2 analogue that is resistant to degradation by the proteolytic enzyme dipeptidyl peptidase 4 and therefore has a longer half-life than natural GLP-2, is well tolerated and led to the restoration of intestinal functional and structural integrity through significant intestinotrophic and proabsorptive effects. It is the first targeted therapeutic agent to gain approval for use in pediatric and adult short bowel syndrome with intestinal failure.[49]

Two other hormones, not derived from the gut, that have been evaluated extensively in various experimental and limited clinical trials include growth hormone and IGF-I. A meta analysis of randomized controlled trials using growth hormone in short bowel syndrome suggests a possible short-term benefit in terms of body weight, lean body mass, and absorptive capacity; however, long-term efficacy was not noted. Somatropin, a recombinant human growth hormone that elicits anabolic and anticatabolic influence on various cells, either as a direct effect or indirectly through IGF-I, is currently indicated to treat short bowel syndrome in conjunction with nutritional support. The combination of various trophic hormones with glutamine and a modified diet may prove more efficacious in the treatment of this difficult group of patients.

The first step in terms of surgical intervention is to restore digestive continuity, which can be accomplished by the reversal of a proximal stoma to reduce rates of dehydration. A number of surgical strategies have been attempted in patients who are chronically TPN dependent, with limited success; these include procedures to delay intestinal transit time, methods to increase absorptive area, and small bowel transplantation. Methods to delay intestinal transit time include the construction of various valves and sphincters, with inconsistent results reported. Antiperistaltic segments of small intestine have been constructed to slow the transit, thus allowing additional contact time for nutrient and fluid absorption. Moderate successes have been described with this technique. Other procedures, including colonic interposition, recirculating loops of small bowel, and retrograde electrical pacing, have been tried but were found to be unsuccessful in humans and were largely abandoned. Surgical procedures to increase absorptive area include the intestinal tapering and lengthening procedure (e.g., Bianchi procedure), which improves intestinal function by correcting the dilation and ineffective peristalsis of the remaining intestine and by doubling the intestinal length while preserving the mucosal surface area. Serial transverse enteroplasty creates staple lines parallel to the mesenteric blood supply on alternating sides to create a channel of intestine that is both longer and smaller in diameter. This technique also increases the surface area of bowel for nutritional absorption.[50] Although beneficial in selected patients, potential complications can include necrosis of divided segments due to poor vasculature, stenosis from smaller caliber of bowel, and anastomotic leaks.

Intestinal transplantation remains the standard of care for patients for whom intestinal rehabilitation attempts have failed and who are at risk of life-threatening complications of TPN; these include impending liver failure, thrombosis of more than two major access veins, frequent severe line infections, and dehydration. Patient survival after intestinal transplantation has significantly improved with the use of the immunosuppressive agents alemtuzumab and tacrolimus and transplantation at a high volume center (≥10 grafts per year). The 1- and 5-year survival rates for isolated intestinal transplantation are 77% and 58%, respectively. Combined intestinal-liver transplants have comparable 1- and 5-year survival rates of approximately 66% and 54%, respectively. The challenges of small bowel transplantation continue to require better immunosuppression and earlier detection of rejection.[50]

Vascular Compression of the Duodenum

Vascular compression of the duodenum, also known as *superior mesenteric artery syndrome* or *Wilkie syndrome*, is a rare condition characterized by compression of the third portion of the duodenum by the superior mesenteric artery as it passes over this portion of the duodenum. Symptoms include profound nausea and vomiting, abdominal distention, weight loss, and postprandial epigastric pain, which varies from intermittent to constant, depending on the severity of the duodenal obstruction. Weight loss usually occurs before the onset of symptoms and contributes to the syndrome.

This syndrome is most commonly seen in young asthenic individuals, with women more commonly affected than men. Predisposing factors for vascular compression of the duodenum, aside from weight loss, include supine immobilization, scoliosis, and placement of a body cast, sometimes called the *cast syndrome*. An association between vascular compression of the duodenum and peptic ulcer has been observed. Vascular compression of the duodenum has been reported in association with anorexia nervosa and after proctocolectomy and J-pouch anal anastomosis, resection of an arteriovenous malformation of the cervical cord, abdominal aortic aneurysm repair, and orthopedic procedures, usually spinal surgery. One report in the literature described a family with a preponderance of vascular compression of the duodenum.

Diagnosis of this condition is made by a barium upper gastrointestinal series (Fig. 50.49) or hypotonic duodenography, which demonstrates abrupt or near-total cessation of flow of barium from the duodenum to the jejunum. CT is useful in certain cases. Treatment for this syndrome varies. Conservative measures should be tried initially and have been increasingly successful as definitive treatment. Operative management may include duodenojejunostomy, gastrojejunostomy to bypass the obstructing segment, or duodenal derotation (Strong procedure).

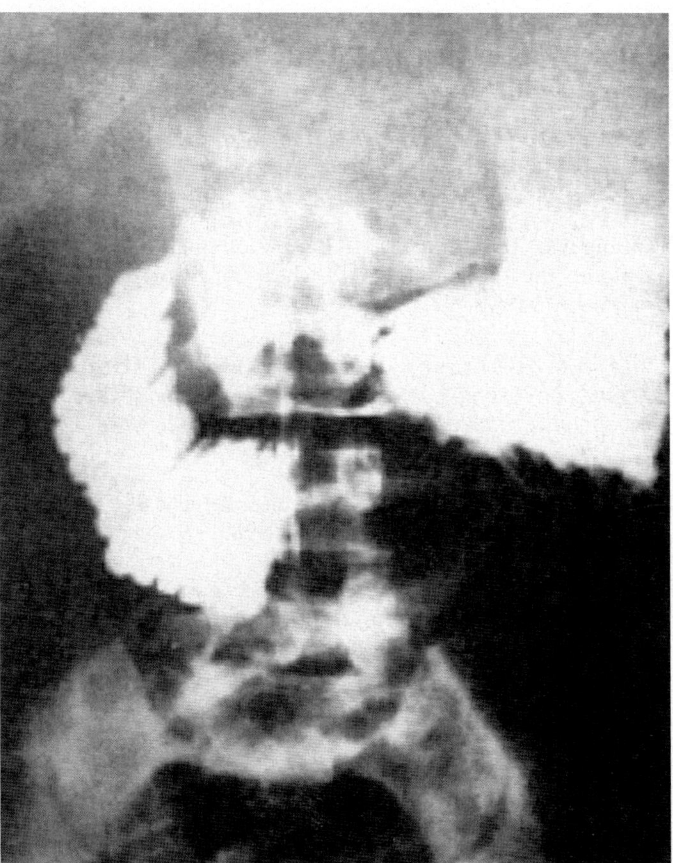

FIG. 50.49 Superior mesenteric artery (SMA) syndrome. Barium radiograph demonstrates obstruction of the third portion of the duodenum secondary to superior mesenteric artery compression as a consequence of burn injury. (Adapted from Reckler JM, Bruck HM, Munster AM, et al. Superior mesenteric artery syndrome as a consequence of burn injury. *J Trauma*. 1972;12:979–985.)

SELECTED REFERENCES

Caplin ME, Pavel M, Cwikla JB, et al. Lanreotide in metastatic enteropancreatic neuroendocrine tumors. *N Engl J Med*. 2014;371:224–233.

The landmark CLARINET trial (Lanreotide Antiproliferative Response in patients with GEP-NET) is the largest phase 3, randomized, double-blind, placebo-controlled, multinational study that evaluated the antiproliferative effect of the SSA lanreotide in patients with GEP-NETs. Lanreotide was associated with significantly prolonged progression-free survival among patients with grade 1 or 2 metastatic enteropancreatic NETs.

Crohn BB, Ginzburg L, Oppenheimer GD. Regional ileitis: a pathologic and clinical entity. *JAMA*. 1932;99:1323–1329.

This landmark paper succinctly crystallizes the clinical course, differential diagnosis, and pathologic findings of regional ileitis in young adults. Although other terms have been applied to this disease process, based on the descriptions in this classic paper, Crohn disease has been universally accepted as the name.

Feuerstein JD, Cheifetz AS. Crohn disease: epidemiology, diagnosis, and management. *Mayo Clin Proc*. 2017;92:1088–1103.

This paper provides an extensive review for current diagnostic and therapeutic options for Crohn disease, with a focus on medical and surgical management.

Paulson EK, Thompson WM. Review of small-bowel obstruction: the diagnosis and when to worry. *Radiology*. 2015;275:332–342.

This review identifies the important radiologic findings in bowel obstruction that are commonly used to make clinical decisions for operative intervention.

Shi HY, Ng SC. The state of the art on treatment of Crohn's disease. *J Gastroenterol*. 2018;53:989–998.

This represents a clear and concise review article highlighting critical issues in the medical management of Crohn disease, new evidence from clinical trials, and prospective studies.

Strosberg JR, Halfdanarson TR, Bellizzi AM, et al. The North American Neuroendocrine Tumor Society consensus guidelines for surveillance and medical management of midgut neuroendocrine tumors. *Pancreas*. 2017;46:707–714.

This paper provides an extensive review of current medical treatment guidelines for neuroendocrine tumors as agreed upon by the North American Neuroendocrine Tumor Society.

Thirunavukarasu P, Sathaiah M, Sukumar S, et al. Meckel's diverticulum—a high-risk region for malignancy in the ileum. Insights from a population-based epidemiological study and implications in surgical management. *Ann Surg*. 2011;253:223–230.

A national database study during 33 years that suggests Meckel diverticulum is a high-risk area for ileal cancer and supports the resection of incidental Meckel diverticulum.

Torres J, Mehandru S, Colombel JF, et al. Crohn's disease. *Lancet*. 2017;389:1741–1755.

A recent comprehensive review of Crohn disease from the etiology to diagnosis and medical/surgical treatment.

Young JI, Mongoue-Tchokote S, Wieghard N, et al. Treatment and survival of small-bowel adenocarcinoma in the United States: a comparison with colon cancer. *Dis Colon Rectum*. 2016;59:306–315.

This study represents a large, national database analysis of the outcomes of small intestine malignant neoplasms during the past two decades and its comparisons to colorectal cancer outcomes.

REFERENCES

1. Moore KL, Persaud TVN, Torchia MG. Alimentary system. In: Moore KL, Persaud TVN, eds. *The Developing Human: Clinically Oriented Embryology*. 10th ed. Philadelphia: Elsevier; 2016:209–240.
2. Bykov VL. [Paneth cells: history of discovery, structural and functional characteristics and the role in the maintenance of homeostasis in the small intestine]. *Morfologiia*. 2014;145:67–80.
3. Chung DH, Evers BM. The digestive system. In: O'Leary JP, ed. *The Physiologic Basis of Surgery*. 4th ed. Philadelphia: Lippincott Williams & Wilkins; 2007:475–507.
4. Li J, Song J, Zaytseva YY, et al. An obligatory role for neurotensin in high-fat-diet-induced obesity. *Nature*. 2016;533:411–415.
5. Allaire JM, Crowley SM, Law HT, et al. The intestinal epithelium: central coordinator of mucosal immunity. *Trends Immunol*. 2018;39:677–696.
6. Paulson EK, Thompson WM. Review of small-bowel obstruction: the diagnosis and when to worry. *Radiology*. 2015;275:332–342.
7. Aquina CT, Becerra AZ, Probst CP, et al. Patients with adhesive small bowel obstruction should be primarily managed by a surgical team. *Ann Surg*. 2016;264:437–447.
8. Quah GS, Eslick GD, Cox MR. Laparoscopic versus open surgery for adhesional small bowel obstruction: a systematic review and meta-analysis of case-control studies. *Surg Endosc*. 2019;33:3209–3217.
9. Tsuruta A, Itoh T, Hirai T, et al. Multi-layered intra-abdominal adhesion prophylaxis following laparoscopic colorectal surgery. *Surg Endosc*. 2015;29:1400–1405.

10. Crohn BB, Ginzburg L, Oppenheimer GD. Regional ileitis: a pathologic and clinical entity. *JAMA*. 1932;99: 1323–1329.
11. Feuerstein JD, Cheifetz AS. Crohn disease: epidemiology, diagnosis, and management. *Mayo Clin Proc*. 2017;92:1088–1103.
12. Wang MH, Picco MF. Crohn's disease: genetics update. *Gastroenterol Clin North Am*. 2017;46:449–461.
13. Lang BM, Biedermann L, van Haaften WT, et al. Genetic polymorphisms associated with smoking behaviour predict the risk of surgery in patients with Crohn's disease. *Aliment Pharmacol Ther*. 2018;47:55–66.
14. Torres J, Mehandru S, Colombel JF, et al. Crohn's disease. *Lancet*. 2017;389:1741–1755.
15. Cleynen I, Boucher G, Jostins L, et al. Inherited determinants of Crohn's disease and ulcerative colitis phenotypes: a genetic association study. *Lancet*. 2016;387:156–167.
16. Lichtenstein GR, Loftus EV, Isaacs KL, et al. ACG clinical guideline: management of Crohn's disease in adults. *Am J Gastroenterol*. 2018;113:481–517.
17. Adami HO, Bretthauer M, Emilsson L, et al. The continuing uncertainty about cancer risk in inflammatory bowel disease. *Gut*. 2016;65:889–893.
18. Kyriakidi KS, Tsianos VE, Karvounis E, et al. Neutrophil anti-neutrophil cytoplasmic autoantibody proteins: bactericidal increasing protein, lactoferrin, cathepsin, and elastase as serological markers of inflammatory bowel and other diseases. *Ann Gastroenterol*. 2016;29:258–267.
19. Shimoyama T, Yamamoto T, Umegae S, et al. Faecal biomarkers for screening small bowel inflammation in patients with Crohn's disease: a prospective study. *Therap Adv Gastroenterol*. 2017;10:577–587.
20. Deepak P, Park SH, Ehman EC, et al. Crohn's disease diagnosis, treatment approach, and management paradigm: what the radiologist needs to know. *Abdom Radiol (NY)*. 2017;42:1068–1086.
21. Niv Y, Gal E, Gabovitz V, et al. Capsule endoscopy Crohn's disease activity index (CECDAIic or Niv Score) for the small bowel and colon. *J Clin Gastroenterol*. 2018;52:45–49.
22. Shi HY, Ng SC. The state of the art on treatment of Crohn's disease. *J Gastroenterol*. 2018;53:989–998.
23. Rezaie A, Kuenzig ME, Benchimol EI, et al. Budesonide for induction of remission in Crohn's disease. *Cochrane Database Syst Rev*. 2015:CD000296.
24. Schlussel AT, Steele SR, Alavi K. Current challenges in the surgical management of Crohn's disease: a systematic review. *Am J Surg*. 2016;212:345–351.
25. Sevim Y, Akyol C, Aytac E, et al. Laparoscopic surgery for complex and recurrent Crohn's disease. *World J Gastrointest Endosc*. 2017;9:149–152.
26. Ponsioen CY, de Groof EJ, Eshuis EJ, et al. Laparoscopic ileocaecal resection versus infliximab for terminal ileitis in Crohn's disease: a randomised controlled, open-label, multicentre trial. *Lancet Gastroenterol Hepatol*. 2017;2:785–792.
27. Shimada N, Ohge H, Kono T, et al. Surgical recurrence at anastomotic site after bowel resection in Crohn's disease: comparison of Kono-S and end-to-end anastomosis. *J Gastrointest Surg*. 2019;23:312–319.
28. Schlussel AT, Cherng NB, Alavi K. Current trends and challenges in the postoperative medical management of Crohn's disease: a systematic review. *Am J Surg*. 2017;214:931–937.
29. Pavlinac PB, Tickell KD, Walson JL. Management of diarrhea in HIV-affected infants and children. *Expert Rev Anti Infect Ther*. 2015;13:5–8.
30. von Mehren M, Joensuu H. Gastrointestinal stromal tumors. *J Clin Oncol*. 2018;36:136–143.
31. Campos FG, Sulbaran M, Safatle-Ribeiro AV, et al. Duodenal adenoma surveillance in patients with familial adenomatous polyposis. *World J Gastrointest Endosc*. 2015;7:950–959.
32. Young JI, Mongoue-Tchokote S, Wieghard N, et al. Treatment and survival of small-bowel adenocarcinoma in the United States: a comparison with colon cancer. *Dis Colon Rectum*. 2016;59:306–315.
33. Tsoli M, Chatzellis E, Koumarianou A, et al. Current best practice in the management of neuroendocrine tumors. *Ther Adv Endocrinol Metab*. 2019;10:2042018818804698.
34. Kim JY, Hong SM. Recent updates on neuroendocrine tumors from the gastrointestinal and pancreatobiliary tracts. *Arch Pathol Lab Med*. 2016;140:437–448.
35. Johnbeck CB, Knigge U, Loft A, et al. Head-to-head comparison of (64)Cu-DOTATATE and (68)Ga-DOTATOC PET/CT: a prospective study of 59 patients with neuroendocrine tumors. *J Nucl Med*. 2017;58:451–457.
36. Figueiredo MN, Maggiori L, Gaujoux S, et al. Surgery for small-bowel neuroendocrine tumors: is there any benefit of the laparoscopic approach? *Surg Endosc*. 2014;28:1720–1726.
37. Farley HA, Pommier RF. Surgical treatment of small bowel neuroendocrine tumors. *Hematol Oncol Clin North Am*. 2016;30:49–61.
38. Paul D, Ostwal V, Bose S, et al. Personalized treatment approach to gastroenteropancreatic neuroendocrine tumors: a medical oncologist's perspective. *Eur J Gastroenterol Hepatol*. 2016;28:985–990.
39. Herrera-Martinez AD, Hofland J, Hofland LJ, et al. Targeted systemic treatment of neuroendocrine tumors: current options and future perspectives. *Drugs*. 2019;79:21–42.
40. Caplin ME, Pavel M, Cwikla JB, et al. Lanreotide in metastatic enteropancreatic neuroendocrine tumors. *N Engl J Med*. 2014;371:224–233.
41. Strosberg JR, Halfdanarson TR, Bellizzi AM, et al. The North American Neuroendocrine Tumor Society consensus guidelines for surveillance and medical management of midgut neuroendocrine tumors. *Pancreas*. 2017;46:707–714.
42. Aparicio T, Zaanan A, Mary F, et al. Small bowel adenocarcinoma. *Gastroenterol Clin North Am*. 2016;45:447–457.
43. Thirunavukarasu P, Sathaiah M, Sukumar S, et al. Meckel's diverticulum—a high-risk region for malignancy in the ileum. Insights from a population-based epidemiological study and implications in surgical management. *Ann Surg*. 2011;253:223–230.
44. Soltero MJ, Bill AH. The natural history of Meckel's diverticulum and its relation to incidental removal. A study of 202 cases of diseased Meckel's diverticulum found in King County, Washington, over a fifteen year period. *Am J Surg*. 1976;132:168–173.
45. Zani A, Eaton S, Rees CM, et al. Incidentally detected Meckel diverticulum: to resect or not to resect? *Ann Surg*. 2008;247:276–281.
46. Blouhos K, Boulas KA, Tsalis K, et al. Meckel's diverticulum in adults: surgical concerns. *Front Surg*. 2018;5:55.
47. Quinn M, Falconer S, McKee RF. Management of enterocutaneous fistula: outcomes in 276 patients. *World J Surg*. 2017;41:2502–2511.

48. Teo MT, Sebag-Montefiore D, Donnellan CF. Prevention and management of radiation-induced late gastrointestinal toxicity. *Clin Oncol (R Coll Radiol)*. 2015;27:656–667.
49. Kim ES, Keam SJ. Teduglutide: a review in short bowel syndrome. *Drugs*. 2017;77:345–352.
50. Billiauws L, Maggiori L, Joly F, et al. Medical and surgical management of short bowel syndrome. *J Visc Surg*. 2018;155:283–291.

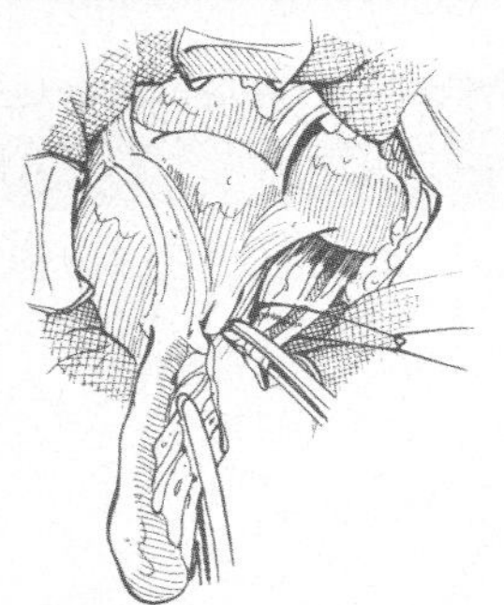

CHAPTER 51

The Appendix

Bryan Richmond

OUTLINE

Please access Elsevier eBooks for Practicing Clinicians to view the videos for this chapter https://expertconsult.inkling.com/.

Appendicitis remains one of the most common diseases faced by the surgeon in practice. It is the most common urgent or emergent general surgical operation performed in the United States and is responsible for as many as 300,000 hospitalizations annually.[1] Although appendectomy is frequently the first "major" case performed by the surgeon in training, the impact of a timely diagnosis and prompt treatment is as impressive as that of any other major surgical intervention. It is estimated that as much as 6% to 7% of the general population will develop appendicitis during their lifetime, with the incidence peaking in the second decade of life.[2] Despite its high prevalence in Western countries, the diagnosis of acute appendicitis can be challenging and requires a high index of suspicion on the part of the examining surgeon to facilitate prompt treatment of this condition, thereby avoiding the substantial morbidity (and even mortality) associated with delayed diagnosis and subsequent perforation. Appendicitis is much less common in underdeveloped countries, suggesting that elements of the Western diet, specifically a low-fiber, high-fat intake, may play a role in the development of the disease process.[3]

ANATOMY AND EMBRYOLOGY

The appendix is a midgut organ and is first identified at 8 weeks of gestation as a small outpouching of the cecum. As gestation progresses, the appendix becomes more elongated and tubular as the cecum rotates medially and becomes fixed in the right lower quadrant of the abdomen. The appendiceal mucosa is of the colonic type, with columnar epithelium, neuroendocrine cells, and mucin-producing goblet cells lining its tubular structure.[3] Lymphoid tissue is found in the submucosa of the appendix, leading some to hypothesize that the appendix may play a role in the immune system. In addition, evidence suggests that the appendix may serve as a reservoir of "good" intestinal bacteria and may aid in recolonization and maintenance of the normal colonic flora.[4] Although historically removal of the appendix was not felt to result in any adverse sequelae, this has recently been challenged. For example, patients who have had previous appendectomy have been demonstrated to have a more difficult clinical course and overall poorer outcomes in recurrent cases of *Clostridium difficile* infection when compared with patients who have not undergone appendectomy. The theory is that the microbiome of the appendix has a protective function and that the loss of this eliminates an element of beneficial immunologic redundancy.[5] In addition, a recently published epidemiological study found a significant link between appendectomy prior to age twenty and the development of prostate cancer, although a precise causative mechanism could not be elucidated.[6]

As a midgut organ, the blood supply of the appendix is derived from the superior mesenteric artery. The ileocolic artery, one of the major named branches of the superior mesenteric artery, gives rise to the appendiceal artery, which courses through the *mesoappendix*. The mesoappendix also contains lymphatics of the appendix, which drain to the ileocecal nodes, along with the blood supply from the superior mesenteric artery.[3,7]

The appendix is of variable size (5–35 cm in length) but averages 8 to 9 cm in length in adults. Its base can be reliably identified by defining the area of convergence of the taeniae at the tip of the cecum and then elevating the appendiceal base to define the course and position of the tip of the appendix, which is variable in location. The appendiceal tip may be found in a variety of locations, with the most common being retrocecal (but intraperitoneal) in approximately 60% of individuals, pelvic in 30%, and retroperitoneal in 7% to 10%. Agenesis of the appendix has been reported, as has duplication and even triplication.[3,7] Knowledge of these anatomic variations is important to the surgeon because the variable position of the appendiceal tip may account for differences in clinical presentation and in the location of the associated abdominal discomfort. For example, patients with a retroperitoneal appendix may present with back or flank pain, just as patients with the appendiceal tip in the midline pelvis may present with suprapubic pain. Both of these presentations may result in a delayed diagnosis, as the symptoms are distinctly different from the classically described anterior right lower quadrant abdominal pain associated with appendiceal disease.

APPENDICITIS

History

The first appendectomy was reported in 1735 by a French surgeon, Claudius Amyand, who identified and successfully removed the appendix of an 11-year-old boy that was found within an inguinal hernia sac and that had been perforated by a pin. Although autopsy findings consistent with perforated appendicitis appeared sporadically thereafter in the literature, the first formal description of the disease process, including the common clinical features and a recommendation for prompt surgical removal, was in 1886 by Reginald Heber Fitz of Harvard University.[3]

Notable advances in surgery for appendicitis include McBurney's description of his classic muscle-splitting incision and technique for removal of the appendix in 1894 and the description of the first laparoscopic appendectomy by Kurt Semm in 1982.[3] Laparoscopic appendectomy has become the preferred method for management of acute appendicitis among surgeons in the United States and may be accomplished using several (typically three) trocar sites or through single-incision laparoscopic surgical techniques. Finally, but of no less significance, was the development of broad-spectrum antibiotics, interventional radiologic techniques, and better surgical critical care strategies, all of which have resulted in substantial improvements in the care of patients with appendiceal perforation and its subsequent complications.

Pathophysiology and Bacteriology

Appendicitis is caused by luminal obstruction.[3] The appendix is vulnerable to this phenomenon because of its small luminal diameter in relation to its length. Obstruction of the proximal lumen of the appendix leads to elevated pressure in the distal portion because of ongoing mucus secretion and production of gas by bacteria within the lumen. With progressive distention of the appendix, the venous drainage becomes impaired, resulting in mucosal ischemia. With continued obstruction, full-thickness ischemia ensues, which ultimately leads to perforation. Bacterial overgrowth within the appendix results from bacterial stasis distal to the obstruction.[3] This is significant because this overgrowth results in the release of a larger bacterial inoculum in cases of perforated appendicitis. The time from onset of obstruction to perforation is variable and may range anywhere from a few hours to a few days. The presentation after perforation is also variable. The most common sequela is the formation of an abscess in the periappendiceal region or pelvis. On occasion, however, free perforation occurs that results in diffuse peritonitis.[3]

Because the appendix is an outpouching of the cecum, the flora within the appendix is similar to that found within the colon. Infections associated with appendicitis should be considered polymicrobial, and antibiotic coverage should include agents that address the presence of both gram-negative bacteria and anaerobes. Common isolates include *Escherichia coli*, *Bacteroides fragilis*, enterococci, *Pseudomonas aeruginosa*, *Klebsiella pneumoniae*, and others (Table 51.1).[8] The choice and duration of antibiotic coverage and the controversies surrounding the need for cultures are discussed later in the chapter.

TABLE 51.1 Bacteria commonly isolated in perforated appendicitis.

TYPE OF BACTERIA	ISOLATES (N = 694)
Gram-Negative Bacteria	
Escherichia coli	448 (64.6%)
Pseudomonas aeruginosa	114 (16.4%)
Klebsiella pneumoniae	37 (5.3%)
Citrobacter species	18 (2.6%)
Enterobacter species	10 (1.4%)
Serratia marcescens	3 (0.4%)
Raoultella planticola	3 (0.4%)
Comamomas testosteroni	2 (0.3%)
Aeromonas species	2 (0.3%)
Proteus species	2 (0.3%)
Acinetobacter species	1 (0.1%)
Yersinia species	1 (0.1%)
Morganella species	1 (0.1%)
Gram-Positive Bacteria	
Enterococcus species	27 (3.9%)
Streptococcus species	20 (2.9%)
Staphylococcus species	5 (0.7%)

Adapted from Song DW, Park BK, Suh SW, et al. Bacterial culture and antibiotic susceptibility in patients with acute appendicitis. *Int J Colorectal Dis*. 2018;33:441–447.

The causes of the luminal obstruction are many and varied. These most commonly include fecal stasis and fecaliths but may also include lymphoid hyperplasia, neoplasms, fruit and vegetable material, ingested barium, and parasites such as ascaris or pinworm infestation. Pain associated with appendicitis has both visceral and somatic components. Distention of the appendix is responsible for the initial vague abdominal pain (visceral) often experienced by the affected patient. The pain typically does not localize to the right lower quadrant until the tip becomes inflamed and irritates the adjacent parietal peritoneum (somatic) or perforation occurs, resulting in localized peritonitis.[3,9]

Differential Diagnosis

Appendicitis must be considered in every patient (who has not had an appendectomy) who presents with acute abdominal pain.[9] Knowledge of disease processes that may have similar presenting symptoms and signs is essential to avoid an unnecessary or incorrect operation. Consideration of the patient's age and gender may help narrow the list of possible diagnoses. In children, other considerations include but are not limited to mesenteric adenitis (often seen after a recent viral illness), acute gastroenteritis, intussusception, Meckel diverticulitis, inflammatory bowel disease, and (in males) testicular torsion. Nephrolithiasis and urinary tract infection may be manifested with right lower quadrant pain in either gender.[3,9]

In women of childbearing age, the differential diagnosis is expanded even further. Gynecologic pathology may be mistaken for appendicitis and result in a higher negative appendectomy rate than in male patients of comparable age. These processes include ruptured ovarian cysts, *mittelschmerz* (midcycle abdominal pain occurring with ovulation), endometriosis, ovarian torsion, ectopic pregnancy, and pelvic inflammatory disease.[3,9]

Two other patient populations deserve mention. In the elderly, consideration must be given to acute diverticulitis and malignant disease as possible causes of lower abdominal pain. In the neutropenic patient, *typhlitis* (also known as neutropenic enterocolitis) should also be considered within the differential diagnosis. Appendicitis in these special populations is discussed in greater detail later in the chapter.

Presentation

History

Patients presenting with acute appendicitis typically complain of vague abdominal pain that is most commonly periumbilical in origin and reflects the stimulation of visceral afferent pathways through the progressive distention of the appendix. Anorexia is often present, as is nausea with or without associated vomiting. Either diarrhea or constipation may be present as well. As the condition progresses and the appendiceal tip becomes inflamed, resulting in peritoneal irritation, the pain localizes to its classic location in the right lower quadrant. This phenomenon remains a reliable symptom of appendicitis[3,9] and should serve to further increase the clinician's index of suspicion for appendicitis (Fig. 51.1).

Whereas these symptoms represent the "classic" presentation of appendicitis, the clinician must be aware that the disease may be manifested in an atypical fashion. For example, patients with a retroperitoneal appendix may present in a more subacute manner, with flank or back pain, whereas patients with an appendiceal tip in the pelvis may have suprapubic pain suggestive of urinary tract infection.[3,9] Although cases such as these are less common than the typical presentation, knowledge of these variations is essential to maintain the necessary index of suspicion to permit a prompt and accurate diagnosis.

Physical Examination

Patients with appendicitis typically appear ill. They frequently lie still because of the presence of localized peritonitis, which makes any movement painful. Tachycardia and mild dehydration are often present to varying degrees. Fever is frequently present, ranging from low-grade temperature elevations (<38.5°C) to more impressive elevations of body temperature, depending on the status of the disease process and the severity of the patient's inflammatory response. Absence of fever does not exclude a diagnosis of appendicitis.[1,3,9]

Abdominal examination typically reveals a quiet abdomen with tenderness and guarding on palpation of the right lower quadrant. The location of the tenderness is classically over McBurney point, which is located one third the distance between the anterior superior iliac spine and the umbilicus. The pain and tenderness are typically accompanied by localized peritonitis as evidenced by the presence of rebound tenderness. Diffuse peritonitis or abdominal wall rigidity due to involuntary spasm of the overlying abdominal wall musculature is strongly suggestive of perforation.[1,3]

A number of signs have been described to aid in the diagnosis of appendicitis. These include the Rovsing sign (the presence of right lower quadrant pain on palpation of the left lower quadrant), the obturator sign (right lower quadrant pain on internal rotation of the hip), and the psoas sign (pain with extension of the ipsilateral hip), among others.[1] Although these are of historical interest, it is important to realize that they are simply indicators of localized peritonitis rather than a diagnostic of a specific disease process. Still, they are useful maneuvers to perform in examining a patient with suspected appendicitis and are supportive of the diagnosis if it is suspected clinically.

Rectal examination findings are typically normal. However, a palpable mass or tenderness may be present if the appendiceal tip is located within the pelvis or if a pelvic abscess is present. In female patients, pelvic examination is important to exclude pelvic disease. However, cervical motion tenderness, a finding typically associated with pelvic inflammatory disease, may be present in appendicitis because of irritation of the pelvic organs from the adjacent inflammatory process.[3,9]

Laboratory Studies

Laboratory studies should be interpreted with caution in cases of suspected appendicitis and should be used to support the clinical picture rather than definitively to prove or to exclude the diagnosis. A leukocytosis, often with a "left shift" (a predominance of neutrophils and sometimes an increase in bands), is present in 90% of cases. A normal white blood cell count is found in 10% of cases; however, and it should not be used as an isolated test to exclude the presence of appendicitis.[10–12] Urinalysis is typically normal as well, although the finding of trace leukocyte esterase or pyuria is not unusual and is presumably due to the proximity of the inflamed appendix to the bladder or ureter. If the presentation is strongly suggestive of appendicitis, a "positive" urinalysis should not be used as an isolated test to refute the diagnosis. Pregnancy testing is mandatory in women of childbearing age.

In addition to the white blood cell count, a number of biomarkers have been investigated as additional diagnostic clues to the diagnosis. These have included C-reactive protein, procalcitonin, interleukin 6, and others. Although C-reactive protein appears to provide the most sensitive of these, none provide sufficient specificity to definitively diagnose appendicitis.[10,12]

Ultimately, no symptom or sign has been demonstrated to be uniquely predictive of appendicitis.[1,10–12] The same may be said of laboratory tests, which are also weakly predictive when considered in isolation. Rather, it is the assessment of the collective body of information that allows more precise diagnosis.[1,10–12] For this reason, a number of clinical scoring systems have been developed to serve as predictive models for appendicitis. These have included the Alvarado score (which remains the most well known),[13] the pediatric appendicitis score, and the appendicitis inflammatory response score, and the adult appendicitis score—to name a few. Of these, the Alvarado score (Table 51.2), which includes eight clinical and laboratory variables used to assign a numerical score, remains the most widely used and was recently endorsed as the most clinically useful by two independent consensus statements.[11,12] Of note, however, both statements agreed that the sensitivity of an Alvarado score of <4 was most useful in excluding a diagnosis of appendicitis (96% sensitive) but that a higher score lacked specificity in diagnosing appendicitis as the cause of the patient's abdominal pain.[11,12]

Imaging Studies

Imaging studies in patients suspected to have acute appendicitis can reduce the negative appendectomy rate, which can be as high as 15%.[12] A variety of radiographic studies may be used to diagnose

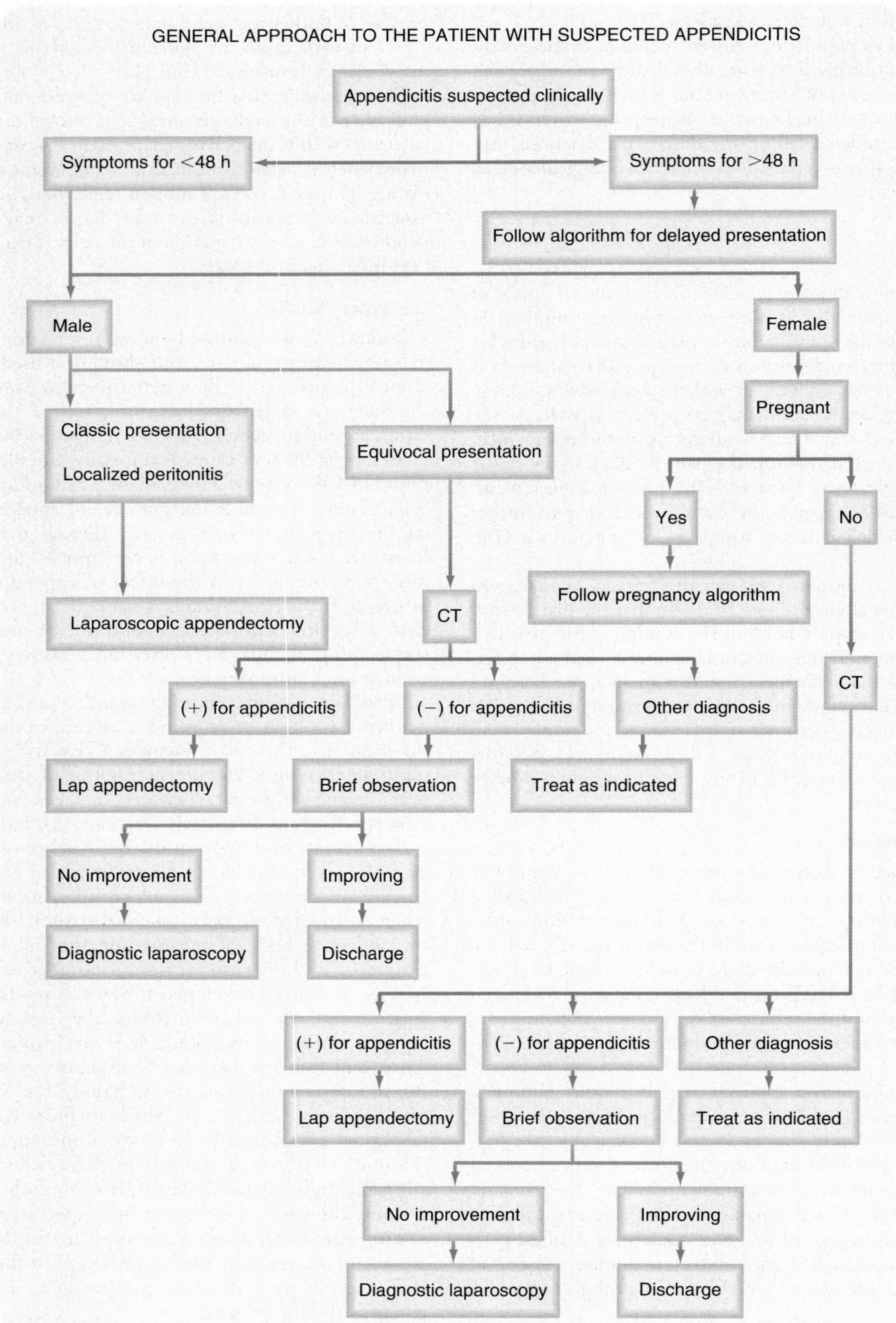

FIG. 51.1 Suggested algorithm for the approach to the patient with possible appendicitis. *CT*, Computed tomography ; Lap, laparoscopic.

appendicitis. These consist of plain radiographs, computed tomography (CT) scanning, ultrasound (US), and magnetic resonance imaging (MRI).

Plain radiographs are frequently obtained in the emergency department setting for the evaluation of acute abdominal pain but lack both sensitivity and specificity for the diagnosis of appendicitis and are rarely helpful. Findings that may support the diagnosis include the presence of a calcified fecalith in the right lower quadrant, although this finding must be placed into the appropriate clinical context and is typically present in only 5% of cases.[14] Pneumoperitoneum, if present, should alert the clinician to other causes of a perforated viscus (such as a perforated ulcer or diverticulitis), as this is not typically observed in cases of appendicitis, even with perforation.[14]

CT scanning is the most common imaging study used to diagnose appendicitis and is highly effective and accurate.[12,14] Modern helical CT scans have the advantage of being operator independent and easy to interpret. CT has been shown to have a sensitivity ranging from 76% to 100% and a specificity of 83% to 100%.[12] The recommended CT imaging technique involves the administration of intravenous contrast only. Enteral (oral and rectal) contrast is not recommended and is associated with lower sensitivity and specificity. In addition, techniques to reduce the radiation exposure to patients, a concern especially relevant to the pediatric population, have not resulted in lower sensitivity or specificity of diagnosis.[11,12]

The diagnosis of appendicitis on CT is based on the appearance of a thickened, inflamed appendix with surrounding "stranding" indicative of inflammation. The appendix is typically more than 7 mm in diameter with a thickened, inflamed wall and mural enhancement or "target sign" (Fig. 51.2). Periappendiceal fluid or air is also highly suggestive of appendicitis and suggests perforation. In cases in which the appendix is not visualized, the absence of inflammatory findings on CT suggests that appendicitis is not present.[11,14] Once again, although we do not recommend CT in cases in which appendicitis is strongly suspected on clinical grounds based on supportive history and physical and laboratory findings, published data do suggest that use of CT in equivocal cases does indeed reduce the negative appendectomy rate.[11,12,14]

US has been used for diagnosis of appendicitis since the 1980s. As US technology has become more advanced, so has its ability to visualize the appendix. The US probe is applied to the area of pain in the right lower quadrant, and graded compression is used to collapse normal surrounding bowel and to diminish the interference encountered with overlying bowel gas. The inflamed appendix is typically enlarged, immobile, and noncompressible (Fig. 51.3). If the appendix cannot be visualized, the study is inconclusive and cannot be relied on to guide treatment, although secondary signs such as free fluid, hyperemia of adjacent bowel loops, induration of mesenteric fat, and regional adenopathy may be considered in the overall picture and serve to increase the diagnostic accuracy of US.[15] Although US is time-efficient and provides the advantage of avoiding ionizing radiation, the success of the study depends greatly on the skill of the sonographer and is highly operator dependent. The sensitivity is reported to range from 71% to 94%, whereas the specificity ranges from 81% to 98%,[12] although once again, this varies greatly based on the skill and experience of the sonographer. Its greatest utility appears to be in the evaluation of the pediatric or pregnant patient, in whom the associated radiation exposure from CT is especially undesirable.[14] It has recently been suggested that a standardized reporting

TABLE 51.2 The Alvarado score.

		VALUE
Symptoms	Migration	1
	Anorexia	1
	Nausea	1
Signs	Tenderness in right lower quadrant	2
	Rebound	1
	Elevation of temperature	1
Laboratory	Leukocytosis	2
	Left shift	1
Total score		10

Adapted from Alvarado A. A practical score for the early diagnosis of acute appendicitis. *Ann Emerg Med.* 1986;15(5):557–564.
Interpretation:
<4 Appendicitis unlikely
5–6 Compatible with appendicitis
7–8 Probable appendicitis
9–10 Very probable appendicitis

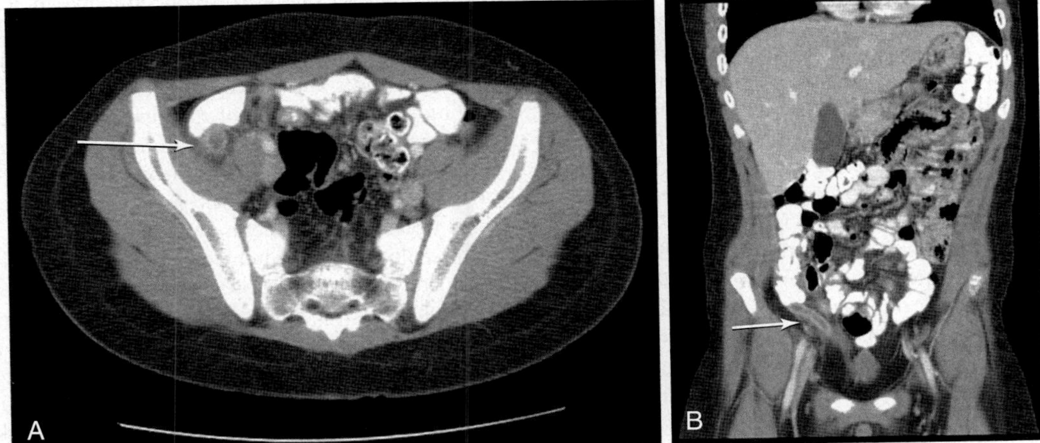

FIG. 51.2 Computed tomography scan of the abdomen demonstrating classic findings of acute appendicitis. (A) Sagittal view with *arrow* demonstrating a thickened, inflamed, and fluid-filled appendix (target sign). (B) Coronal view of same patient. The *arrow* points to the thickened, elongated appendix with periappendiceal fat stranding and fluid around the appendiceal tip.

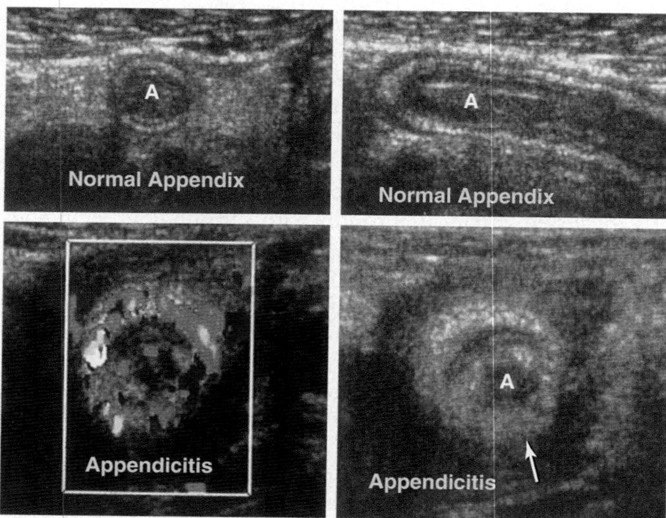

FIG. 51.3 Ultrasound image of a normal appendix (*top*) illustrating the thin wall in coronal (*left*) and longitudinal (*right*) planes. In appendicitis, there is distention and wall thickening (*bottom, right*), and blood flow is increased, leading to the so-called ring of fire appearance. *A*, Appendix.

method or "template" might improve the overall results of US in this clinical setting.[11,16]

MRI is typically reserved for use in the pregnant patient; the study is performed without contrast agents. If it is obtained in a pregnant woman, the study should be noncontrasted. MRI offers excellent resolution and is accurate in diagnosing appendicitis. Criteria for MRI diagnosis include appendiceal enlargement (>7 mm), thickening (>2 mm), and the presence of inflammation.[14] A recent meta analysis found the sensitivity of MRI to be 97% with a specificity of 95%.[12,17] MRI has the additional advantage of being operator independent and offers highly reproducible results. Drawbacks associated with the use of MRI include its higher cost, motion artifact, greater difficulty in interpretation by nonradiologists who may have limited experience with the technology, and limited availability (especially in the after-hours emergency setting).[12,14]

TREATMENT OF APPENDICITIS

Acute Uncomplicated Appendicitis

The gold standard and least controversial treatment of acute uncomplicated appendicitis remain prompt appendectomy. The patient should undergo fluid resuscitation as indicated, and the intravenous administration of broad-spectrum antibiotics directed against gram-negative and anaerobic organisms should be initiated immediately.[11,12] Operation should proceed without undue delay.

For open appendectomy, the patient is placed in the supine position. The choice of incision is a matter of the surgeon's preference, whether it is an oblique muscle-splitting incision (McArthur-McBurney; Fig. 51.4), a transverse incision (Rockey-Davis), or a conservative midline incision. The cecum is grasped by the taeniae and delivered into the wound, allowing visualization of the base of the appendix and delivery of the appendiceal tip. The mesoappendix is divided, and the appendix is crushed just above the base, ligated with an absorbable ligature, and divided. The stump is then either cauterized or, if desired, inverted by a purse-string or "Z" suture technique. Finally, the abdomen is irrigated and the wound closed in layers.

For laparoscopic appendectomy, the patient is placed in the supine position. The bladder is emptied by a straight catheter or by having the patient void immediately before the procedure. The abdomen is entered at the umbilicus, and the diagnosis is confirmed by inserting the laparoscope (Fig. 51.5). Two additional working ports are then placed, typically in the left lower quadrant and in either the suprapubic area or supraumbilical midline, based on the surgeon's preference. We have found it to be advantageous for both the surgeon and assistant to stand to the left side of the patient with the left arm tucked. This allows optimum triangulation of the camera and working instruments. Atraumatic graspers are used to elevate the appendix, and the mesoappendix is carefully divided using the harmonic scalpel. The base is then secured with endoloops and the appendix divided. Alternatively, the appendix and mesoappendix may be divided with an endoscopic stapling device. We prefer this technique in cases in which the entire appendix is friable because it allows the staple line to be placed slightly more proximally, on the edge of the healthy cecum, thereby theoretically reducing the risk of leakage from breakdown of a tenuous appendiceal stump. Retrieval of the appendix is accomplished by the use of a plastic retrieval bag. The pelvis is suctioned and irrigated, the trocars are removed, and the wounds are closed. Laparoscopic appendectomy may also be performed with single-site laparoscopic surgical techniques as well based on the experience and preferences of the surgeon. Laparoscopic appendectomy is demonstrated in Video 50.1.

Antibiotic administration is not continued beyond a single preoperative dose.[11,12] Oral alimentation is begun immediately and advanced as tolerated. Discharge is usually possible the day after operation.

Perforated Appendicitis

The operative strategy for perforated appendicitis is similar to that for uncomplicated appendicitis with a few notable exceptions. First of all, the patient may require more aggressive resuscitation before proceeding to the operating theater. As with uncomplicated appendicitis, antibiotic therapy should be initiated immediately on diagnosis.[11,12]

Both the open and laparoscopic approaches are acceptable for the treatment of perforated appendicitis. Although the technique of appendectomy for perforation is the same as for simple appendicitis, the level of difficulty encountered in removing a friable, gangrenous, perforated appendix can be a challenge to the most experienced surgeon and requires gentle meticulous handling of the friable appendix and inflamed periappendiceal tissues to avoid tissue injury. Cultures are not mandatory unless the patient has had exposure to a health care environment or has had recent exposure to antibiotic therapy because these factors increase the likelihood of encountering resistant bacteria.[18] However, we routinely obtain them because they sometimes yield resistant bacteria and are helpful in tailoring the switch to oral therapy on discharge. In addition, knowledge of regional and institutional bacterial resistance patterns should be considered when choosing empiric coverage to avoid "missing the mark" until culture results are available.[19] Once the appendix is successfully removed, careful attention should be given to the clearance of infectious material, including spilled fecal material or fecaliths from the abdomen. This task may be accomplished by suction and irrigation, with special attention given to the right lower quadrant and pelvis and manual removal of any obvious spilled solid fecal material. Although large volume irrigation has been traditionally advocated, recent data suggest that simple

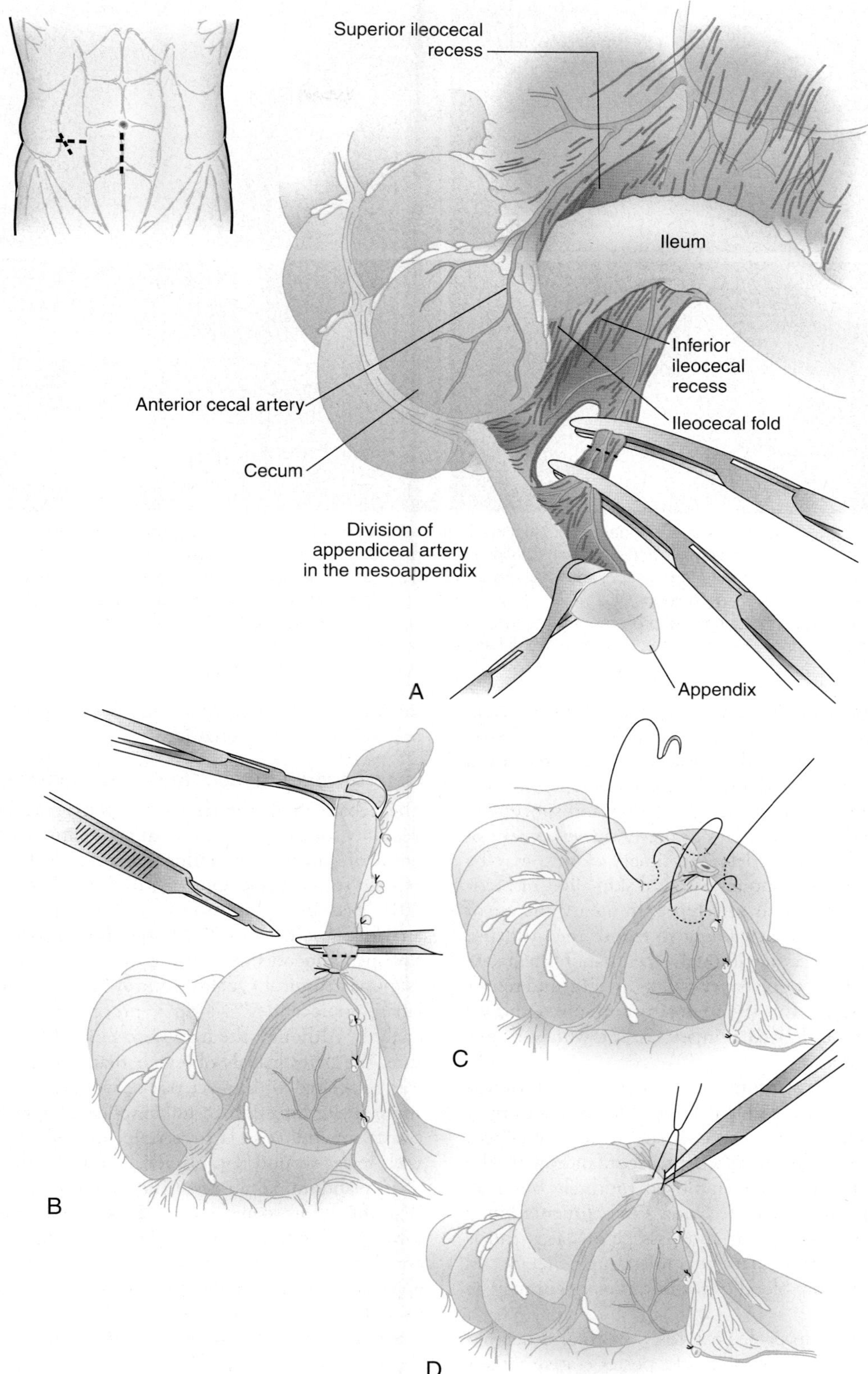

FIG. 51.4 (A) *Left,* Location of possible incisions for an open appendectomy. *Right,* Division of the mesoappendix. (B) Ligation of the base and division of the appendix. (C) Placement of purse-string suture or Z stitch. (D) Inversion of the appendiceal stump. (From Ortega JM, Ricardo AE. Surgery of the appendix and colon. In: Moody FG, ed. *Atlas of Ambulatory Surgery*. Philadelphia: WB Saunders: 1999.)

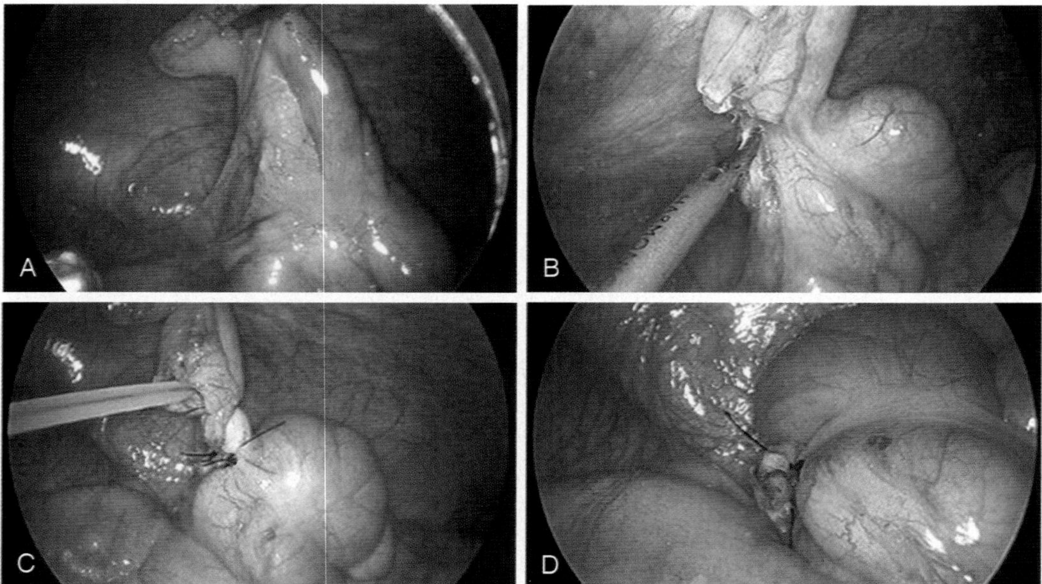

FIG. 51.5 Laparoscopic appendectomy. (A) Visualization and upward retraction of appendix. (B) Division of the mesoappendix using harmonic scalpel. (C) Application of endoloops to the appendix. Two loops are used to secure the base; a third loop is applied distally to avoid spillage of the luminal contents. The specimen is then divided between the endoloops. (D) View of completed appendectomy after removal of the specimen. (Note: Depending on the surgeon's preference, an endoscopic stapling device may be used to divide the mesoappendix and appendix instead of the harmonic scalpel and endoloops.)

suction aspiration of gross purulence may be just as effective in cases of appendiceal rupture.[11] Drains are not routinely placed unless a discrete abscess cavity is present. If an abscess cavity is present, a single closed suction drain is placed within its base and left for several days. If an open technique was used, the skin and subcutaneous tissues are left open for 3 or 4 days to prevent development of wound infection, at which time delayed primary closure may be performed at the bedside with sutures, surgical skin clips, or Steri-Strips, depending on the surgeon's preference. In theory, the use of delayed primary closure has been thought to reduce the incidence of postoperative wound infection, although recently published data suggest that it may actually not be beneficial in doing so and results in a longer length of stay.[11] This issue remains unresolved and we routinely perform bedside delayed primary closure with very few wound related complications.

Postoperatively, broad-spectrum antibiotics are continued for 4 to 7 days in accordance with Infectious Diseases Society of America (IDSA) guidelines.[19] If culture specimens were obtained, antibiotic therapy should be modified in accordance with the results. Nasogastric suction is not employed routinely but may be necessary if postoperative ileus develops. Oral alimentation is begun after return of bowel sounds and passage of flatus and is advanced as tolerated. Once the patient is tolerating a diet, is afebrile, and has a normal white blood cell count, the patient may be discharged home.

If the patient develops fever, leukocytosis, pain, and delayed return of bowel function, the possibility of a postoperative abscess must be entertained. Abscess complicates perforated appendicitis in 10% to 20% of cases and represents the major source of morbidity related to perforation.[1,3] A CT scan with intravenous administration of a contrast agent is diagnostic and also allows simultaneous placement of a percutaneous drain within the abscess cavity.[11,12] If CT drainage is not technically possible because of the location of the abscess, laparoscopic, transrectal, or transvaginal drainage is an alternative.

Laparoscopic Versus Open Appendectomy

The debate about the choice of open versus laparoscopic appendectomy for the treatment of appendicitis was historically a major point of controversy among surgeons. Although no level I data exist to support one approach over another, a study published in 2010 examined this issue in detail. Ingraham and colleagues[20] analyzed results from 222 hospitals comparing laparoscopic versus open appendectomy using the American College of Surgeons National Surgical Quality Improvement Program. In all, 24,969 laparoscopic and 7714 open procedures were included in the analysis. Although the data were limited by the retrospective nature, the investigators observed that laparoscopic appendectomy was associated with lower risk of wound complications and deep surgical site infection in uncomplicated appendicitis. In complicated appendicitis, laparoscopic appendectomy was associated with fewer wound complications but a slightly higher incidence of intraabdominal abscess. The overall conclusion, however, was that the laparoscopic approach was associated with an overall lower incidence of complications than the open procedure. The conclusions evident from a number of studies indicate that both approaches are acceptable and that the advantages with laparoscopy, although small, were a lower overall morbidity, reduced wound complications, reduced postoperative pain, and perhaps a slightly shorter recovery time. The slightly higher risk of intraabdominal abscess formation after laparoscopic appendectomy in cases of complicated appendicitis was a negative aspect of laparoscopic appendectomy, although the authors acknowledged that this has not been observed in all studies.[11] In fact, literature published since the Ingraham study suggest equal or even lower rates of intraabdominal abscess with the laparoscopic approach.[11]

We prefer the laparoscopic approach for several reasons. Laparoscopy allows examination of the entire peritoneal space, making it exceptionally useful to exclude other intraabdominal disease that may be manifested in a similar fashion, such as diverticulitis or tubo-ovarian abscess, whereas visualization of these structures would not be possible through a right lower quadrant incision. We find it to be technically simpler in most patients, particularly the obese, and have been impressed with our ability to discharge patients within several hours of the operation. Although the debate as to the least morbid and cost-effective approach to appendectomy may continue for some time, what remains crucial is that, regardless of the surgeon's preferred approach, the most important part of the technique of appendectomy is that it be done promptly and safely.

Delayed Presentation of Appendicitis

Patients may occasionally present several days to even weeks after the onset of appendicitis. In these cases, the treatment should be individualized on the basis of the nature of the presentation (Fig. 51.6). Although rare, a patient may present with diffuse peritonitis. More commonly, however, patients present with localized right lower quadrant pain and fever, with a history that is compatible with the onset appendicitis several days prior. A mass may be palpable in children or thin patients. Immediate exploration and attempted appendectomy in these patients may result in substantial morbidity, including failure to identify the appendix, postoperative abscess or fistula, and unnecessary extension of the operation to include ileocecectomy, all due to the extreme induration and friability of the involved tissues. For this reason, in general, treatment for these patients is initially accomplished nonoperatively.[11,12,21] Fluid resuscitation is initiated, and broad-spectrum antibiotic therapy is initiated. A CT scan is obtained, and perforated appendicitis with a localized abscess or phlegmon is confirmed (Fig. 51.7). If a localized abscess is identified, CT-guided percutaneous drainage is performed for source control. The drainage catheter is typically left in place for 4 to 7 days, during which the patient is treated with antibiotic therapy and after which time it is removed.[11,12,21] If CT-guided drainage is not technically feasible, operative drainage may be accomplished through transrectal or transvaginal approaches. Laparoscopic drainage is another option that we have found to be exceptionally useful. This technique is performed by visualizing the inflammatory mass with the laparoscope and then entering the abscess with a laparoscopic suction tip, evacuating the purulent material, and placing a drain within the residual abscess cavity. Postoperative management is identical to that of patients who are successfully drained percutaneously. If a periappendiceal phlegmon is present or if the amount of fluid present is not sufficient to drain, the patient may be treated with antibiotics alone, typically for 4 to 7 days also, as recommended by IDSA guidelines for treatment of intraabdominal infection.[20]

Traditionally, after successful nonoperative treatment of complicated appendicitis, patients were advised to undergo removal of the appendix, a procedure known as interval appendectomy, several weeks to months later. This practice has been reexamined. The rationale for interval appendectomy is based on the potential for development of recurrent appendicitis and the subsequent risks associated with emergent removal or reperforation of the appendix. However, the actual risk of recurrent appendicitis appears to be small, 8% at 8 years in one study of 6439 pediatric patients.[22] In addition, interval appendectomy can be challenging and consequently yield a higher risk of postoperative complications when performed.[23] The findings in these studies as well as similar results reported by others have led them to conclude that interval appendectomy should be reserved only for patients who present with symptoms of recurrent appendicitis.[11,22,23] In addition, the presence of an appendicolith on CT has also been shown to be predictive of a higher risk of recurrent appendicitis and has been used as a justification to proceed with interval appendectomy in that subgroup of patients. This selective approach to interval appendectomy has also been demonstrated to be more cost-effective than its routine performance in all affected patients.[24]

One argument favoring interval appendectomy in adults has been the observation by some investigators of a higher incidence of appendiceal neoplasms found in interval appendectomy specimens.[10,24–26] Also, perforated tumors of the cecum may be manifested in a similar fashion as perforated appendicitis.[26] For this reason, colonoscopy is recommended in all adult patients as routine follow-up after nonoperative management of complicated appendicitis.[23,25,26] In addition, no large-scale randomized controlled trials examining the outcomes of patients who do or do not undergo interval appendectomy after successful nonoperative treatment have been successful. For these reasons, this issue is likely to remain controversial for some time.

The Normal-Appearing Appendix at Operation

In cases of "negative appendectomy," in which a normal appendix is identified at operation, there is controversy as to whether the appendix should be removed.[27,28] Before that particular issue is examined, it is important to emphasize the need to thoroughly evaluate the abdomen for other causes of pain severe enough to warrant an operation. The abdominal and pelvic organs should be assessed for any abnormalities. In our experience, this is most easily done through the laparoscopic approach, which we believe to be a major advantage of laparoscopy over the open approach. Note should be made of any free fluid as such a finding may suggest perforation. The terminal 60 cm of ileum should be examined for a Meckel diverticulum and the serosa of the small bowel for any stigmata of Crohn disease, such as inflammation, stricture formation, or the characteristic "creeping fat" appearance of the mesentery. Inspection of the ileal mesentery may reveal enlarged lymph nodes suggestive of mesenteric adenitis. The uterine adnexa should be examined for any evidence of tubo-ovarian or salpingeal disease, such as ovarian torsion, tubo-ovarian abscess, endometriosis, or ruptured ovarian cysts. The sigmoid colon should be examined for evidence of acute diverticulitis, especially in cases in which a redundant sigmoid colon is found in the right lower quadrant. If these are all normal, attention should be turned to the upper abdomen for examination of the gallbladder and duodenum. Inability to perform an adequate evaluation of the intraabdominal organs or demonstration of disease of other organs requiring intervention may require conversion to a midline laparotomy if necessary.

We routinely remove the normal appendix for several reasons. First, many causes of right lower quadrant pain discussed before may be recurrent, such as pain from ruptured ovarian cysts or mesenteric adenitis. Appendectomy is also advisable in cases of Crohn disease when suggested by findings at operation, unless the base of the appendix and cecum are involved. In this scenario, appendectomy is deferred to avoid breakdown of the inflamed stump and subsequent fistula formation. In these clinical circumstances, appendectomy is advisable because it removes appendicitis from the differential diagnosis when the patient presents with recurrent right lower quadrant pain. In addition, abnormalities of the appendix not apparent on gross inspection at the time of operation are sometimes identified on pathologic examination.[27,28]

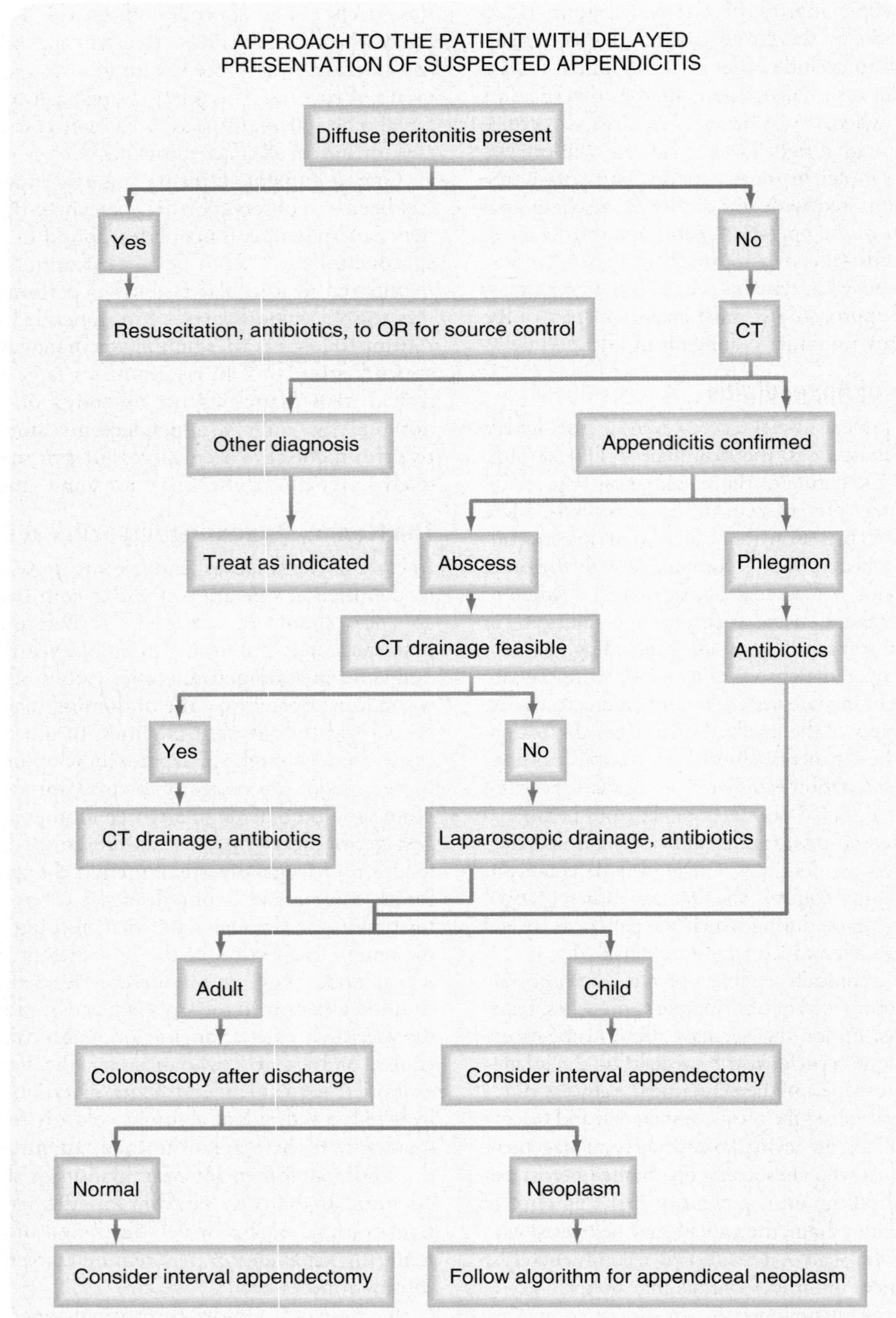

FIG. 51.6 Suggested algorithm for managing the patient with delayed presentation of appendicitis. *CT*, Computed tomography; *OR*, operating room.

NONOPERATIVE TREATMENT OF UNCOMPLICATED APPENDICITIS

Although prompt appendectomy is the current standard of care, few topics in surgery have been discussed as frequently in recent years as that of the nonoperative treatment of uncomplicated acute appendicitis. Two meta analyses analyzing the results of randomized controlled trials examining this issue concluded that nonoperative treatment was associated with a lower risk of complications (12% in the nonoperative group vs. 18% in the appendectomy group; $P = 0.001$).[29,30] In addition, the patients treated nonoperatively displayed no greater tendency to progress to complicated appendicitis.[29] Appendectomy, however, outperformed the nonoperative group in overall treatment failure rate (38% nonoperative vs. 9% in the appendectomy group; $P < 0.001$). The authors concluded that antibiotic therapy was safe as a treatment for uncomplicated appendicitis but was associated with a significantly, perhaps prohibitively high failure (recurrence) rate compared with appendectomy.[29,30] Criticism of both analyses included significant heterogeneity of the methodology of the examined studies.[12]

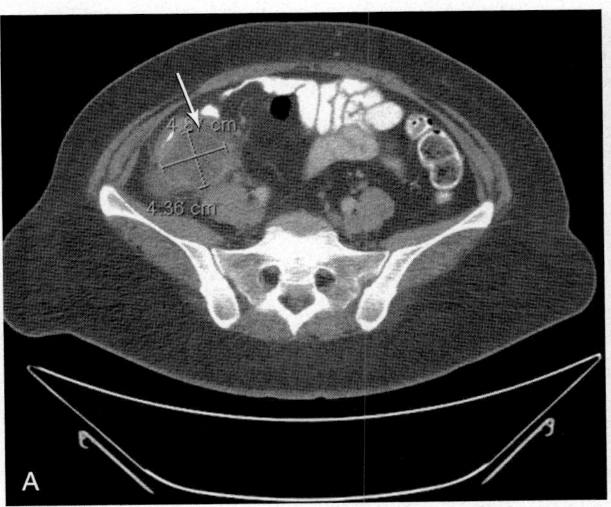

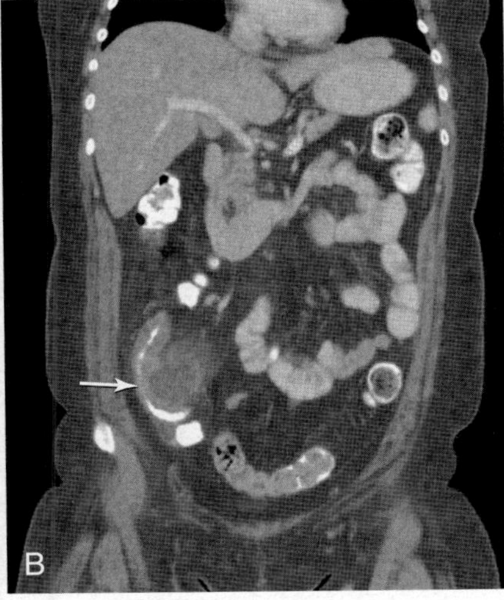

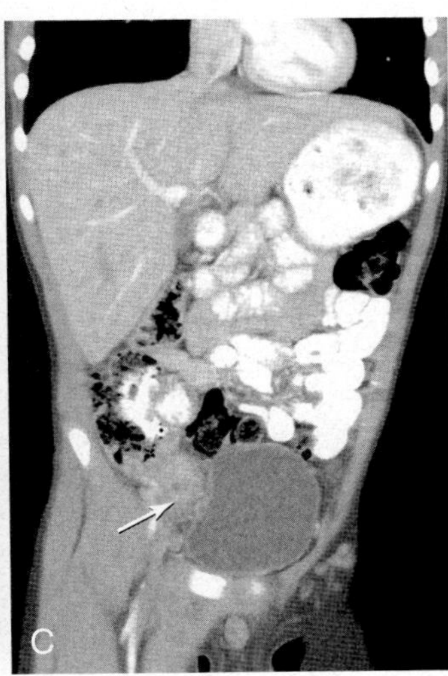

FIG. 51.7 Delayed diagnoses of appendicitis. Sagittal (A) and coronal (B) computed tomography images demonstrate an appendiceal abscess in a patient who presented with a 2-week history of abdominal pain and was found to have a palpable mass on examination. The *arrows* point to a periappendiceal abscess cavity. She was successfully managed with percutaneous drainage and antibiotic therapy. Image C is a similar case in which the patient presented with an appendiceal phlegmon and was successfully treated with antibiotics alone. The *arrow* points to the phlegmon. (Note the mass effect on the bladder.)

A number of studies have examined this controversy further. The Nonoperative Treatment for Acute Appendicitis (NOTA) study treated 159 patients with suspected appendicitis with antibiotics. The mean length of stay was 0.4 days and the mean sick leave period was 5.8 days. The 7-day failure rate was 11.9%. After 2 years of follow-up, 22 of the nonoperatively treated patients recurred (13.8%), 14 of which were once again treated nonoperatively.[31]

Svenssson and colleagues performed a randomized controlled trial in the pediatric population and reported similar results. Specifically, an initial success rate of 92% in patients treated nonoperatively and a 38% risk of recurrence at 1 year were shown.[32]

The Antibiotic Therapy vs. Appendectomy for Treatment of Uncomplicated Acute Appendicitis (APPAC) enrolled 530 patients with CT-confirmed appendicitis, of which 257 received antibiotics alone and 273 underwent appendectomy. The investigators reported a recurrence rate of 27% at the 1-year mark and an overall difference in treatment efficacy between the groups of −27%. They concluded that nonoperative therapy did not meet the specified criteria for noninferiority when compared with appendectomy.[33]

These more recent studies have also been analyzed via meta-analyses with similar conclusions. One such article by Findlay and colleagues examined six randomized controlled trials, all involving patients at least 16 years of age or older, with the primary endpoint being failure or recurrence. They reported an initial failure rate of 9.00% (95% confidence interval [CI], 4.00%–13.0%) and a 1-year recurrence rate of 25% (95% CI, 12.0%–35%).[34] Most significantly, however, they also noted a statistically significant increase in the likelihood of progressing to complicated appendicitis in the failed nonoperative group.[34] The authors also reported longer length of stay with antibiotic therapy but an overall lower cost of the initial treatment,[34] although the subsequent downstream cost of reintervention for recurrence was not considered.

For these reasons—specifically the low morbidity of prompt laparoscopic appendectomy, the reported high rates of recurrence, and the lack of high-quality data definitively supporting its routine practice—our approach is to reserve nonoperative therapy only for cases of acute uncomplicated appendicitis in those patients for whom the operative risk is prohibitive or when a patient is unable to undergo surgery immediately due to other reasons (e.g., patients receiving novel anticoagulants such as rivaroxaban for which no reversal agent is currently available). Failures of nonoperative therapy in these high-risk patients are then managed with adjunctive treatment measures, such as CT-guided drainage of periappendiceal abscesses. This approach has been supported in recent consensus papers; however, large, high-quality randomized controlled trials are required to definitively address this issue.[11,12] A simplified algorithm for this approach is provided (Fig. 51.8).

"Chronic" Appendicitis as a Cause of Abdominal Pain

On occasion, patients will present with a history of recurrent right lower quadrant pain, and a surgical opinion will be sought as to the benefit of elective appendectomy for treatment of this condition. Modest epidemiological data exist to suggest that appendicitis may spontaneously resolve, so it is conceivable that appendicitis may wax and wane in some patients.[1] In addition, some patients with pain are found to have a thickened appendix or an appendicolith on CT but have no evidence of a systemic illness or acute periappendiceal inflammation. In some cases, appendectomy will produce relief of symptoms, and in these cases, examination of the appendix will sometimes reveal findings consistent with chronic inflammation.[35] We will consider, on a case-by-case basis, elective appendectomy in cases in which the history is consistent with appendiceal disease and preferably is supported by radiographic (CT) evidence of appendiceal disease.

More troubling, however, is the patient with nonspecific lower abdominal pain in the absence of radiographic evidence of appendiceal disease. We typically pursue a multidisciplinary workup in these patients involving input from specialists in gastroenterology and gynecology as well as surgery. Appendectomy is typically not offered unless disease is demonstrated radiographically; however, if diagnostic laparoscopy is performed to investigate or to exclude other disease (typically by a gynecologist), we will usually perform appendectomy at that time, which is an approach advocated by

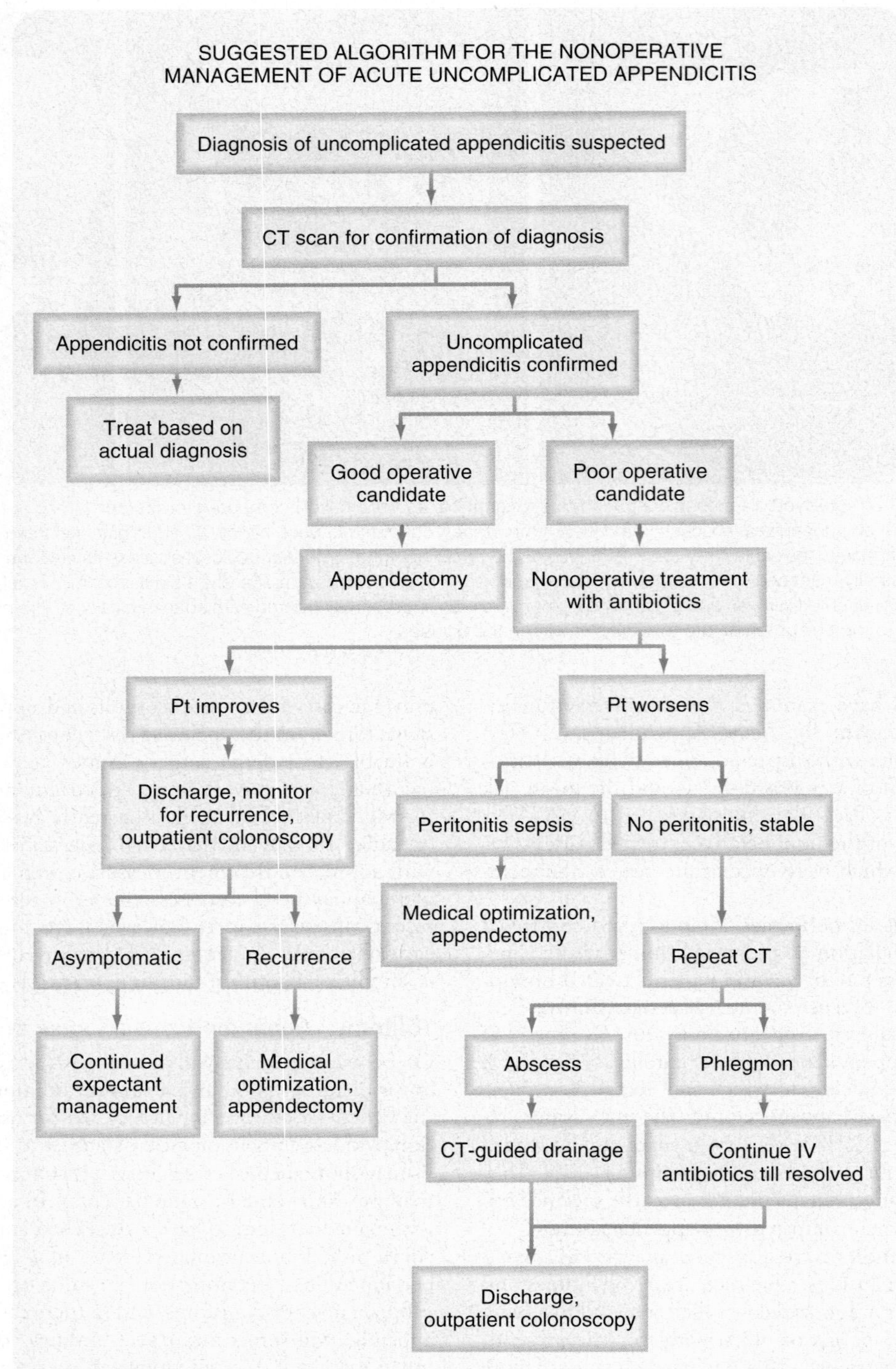

FIG. 51.8 Suggested algorithm for the nonoperative management of appendicitis. *CT,* Computed tomography; *IV,* intravenous; *Pt,* patient.

others.[36] This may result in resolution of the patient's symptoms if the appendix was the source. If not, it serves to remove the appendix from consideration and may save the patient from unnecessary imaging for what is likely to be recurring pain while also facilitating the search for other sources of pain. We have found that, as with the management of any chronic pain syndrome, management of the patients' expectations is critical in caring for this very difficult subgroup of patients.

Incidental Appendectomy

Incidental appendectomy is the term applied when a grossly normal appendix is removed at the time of an unrelated procedure, such as a hysterectomy, cholecystectomy, or sigmoid colectomy. Once commonly performed, incidental appendectomy has become a controversial procedure. The theoretical benefit is that of eliminating the patient's risk for development of appendicitis in the future, a concept that is thought to be most beneficial in patients

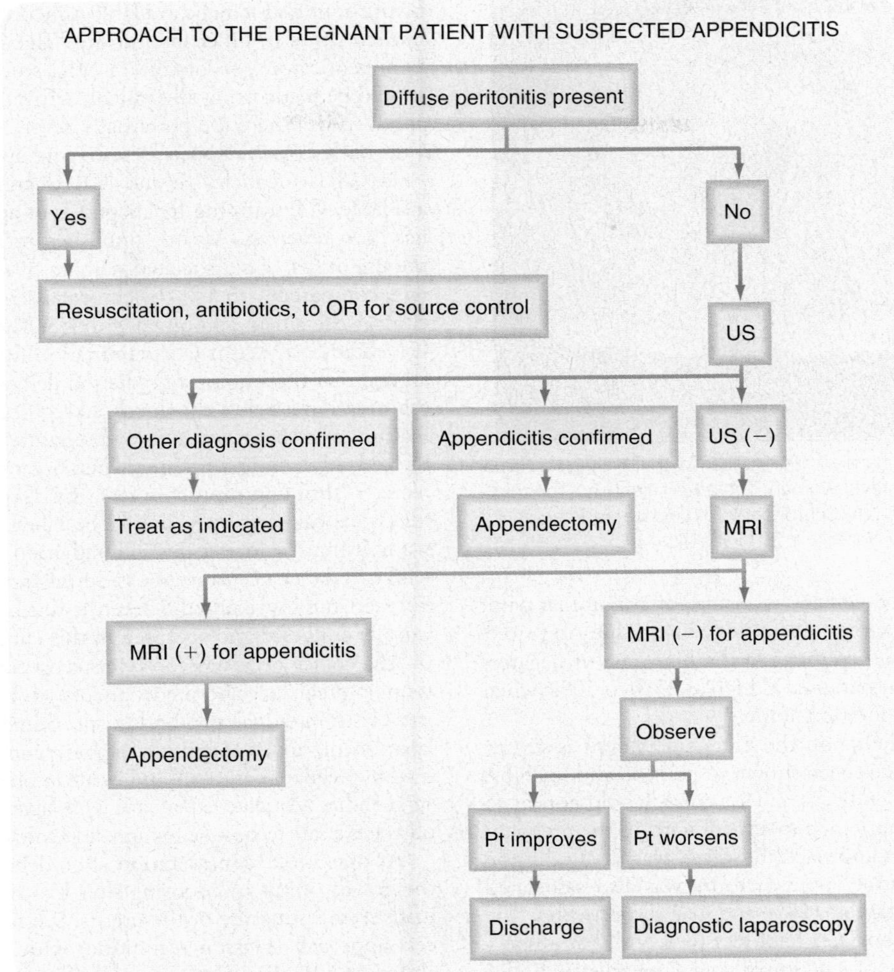

FIG. 51.9 Suggested algorithm for managing the pregnant patient with possible appendicitis. *MRI,* Magnetic resonance imaging; *OR,* operating room; *Pt,* patient; *US,* ultrasound.

younger than 35 years because of their greater lifetime risk for development of the disease when compared with older patients.[37] Data suggesting that incidental appendectomy may be performed with no additional morbidity have been criticized for not having been properly risk adjusted. When these data were scrutinized further, Wen and coworkers actually demonstrated that incidental appendectomy was associated with an increase in both morbidity and mortality.[38] Other investigators have demonstrated that incidental appendectomy does not appear to be cost-effective as a preventive measure.[39] Finally, the recent finding that the appendix may actually have a role in the maintenance of healthy colonic flora makes the practice of incidental appendectomy even more controversial.[4,5] For these reasons, we advocate careful inspection of the appendix for abnormalities during abdominal operations as part of a thorough exploration but do not advocate appendectomy unless an abnormality is detected.

APPENDICITIS IN SPECIAL POPULATIONS

Appendicitis in the Pregnant Patient

Appendicitis remains the most common nonobstetric emergency in pregnancy and is consequently the most frequent reason for general surgical intervention in this group of patients.[40] The diagnosis of appendicitis in pregnancy presents a special challenge to the surgeon. As with all conditions in pregnancy, the surgeon must consider the welfare of two patients, the mother and fetus, when considering possible diagnoses, workup, and treatment (Fig. 51.9).

In pregnancy, appendicitis has a typical clinical presentation in only 50% to 60% of cases.[40] The common symptoms of early appendicitis, such as nausea and vomiting, are nonspecific and are also often associated with normal pregnancy. The normal febrile response to illness may be blunted in pregnancy. Also, the physical examination of the pregnant patient is difficult and is altered because of the effect of the gravid uterus and its displacement of the appendix to a more cephalad location within the abdomen. Lower quadrant pain in the second trimester produced by traction on the suspensory ligaments of the uterus, a phenomenon known as round ligament pain, is a common occurrence and further complicates the clinical picture further because 50% of cases of appendicitis occur in the second trimester. Finally, biochemical and laboratory indicators used to support the diagnosis of appendicitis in the nonpregnant patient are unreliable in pregnancy. For example, a mild physiologic leukocytosis of pregnancy is a normal finding. C-reactive protein levels may also be physiologically elevated in pregnancy. In addition, the surgeon must be concerned about the

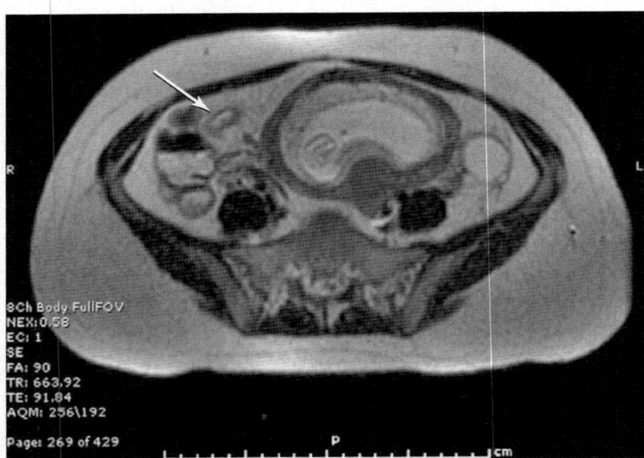

FIG. 51.10 Magnetic resonance imaging scan with T1-weighted axial image of the abdomen in a gravid woman. The *arrow* highlights the thickened appendix. (From Parks NA, Schroeppel TJ. Update on imaging for acute appendicitis. *Surg Clin North Am.* 2011;91:141–154.)

possibility of obstetric emergencies as a cause of abdominal pain, such as preterm labor, placental abruption, or uterine rupture.[40] All of these factors have contributed to the high rate of negative appendectomy in pregnant patients, as high as 25% to 50%, when it is based on clinical presentation alone.[40]

The impact of appendicitis on the pregnant patient is severe. The risk of preterm labor has been shown to be 11% and fetal loss 6% with complicated appendicitis.[41] These data would appear to favor an aggressive, early approach to appendicitis in the pregnant patient. Complicating this approach, however, was the finding in the same series that negative appendectomy was also associated with preterm labor and fetal loss (10% and 4%, respectively). The lowest rates of preterm labor and fetal loss (6% and 2%, respectively) were seen in cases of uncomplicated appendicitis.[41] For these reasons, preoperative accuracy of diagnosis is crucial in the pregnant patient with suspected appendicitis.

Routine imaging is recommended in pregnant patients. The initial study of choice is US with graded compression.[11] It has the advantage of being safe, inexpensive, and readily available. In addition, US may provide information as to fetal well-being and obstetric causes of abdominal pain, such as placental abruption. Scanning patients in a left posterior oblique or left lateral decubitus position rather than in the traditional supine position has been advocated to increase the chances of visualizing the appendix. The criteria for US diagnosis are the same as in the nonpregnant patient and have been discussed previously. Unfortunately, the sensitivity and specificity (83%) of US appear to be reduced in pregnancy because of the presence of the gravid uterus.[42]

If US examination findings are equivocal, MRI without gadolinium contrast, with its excellent soft tissue contrast resolution and lack of ionizing radiation, remains a safe alternative for confirmation or exclusion of appendicitis in the pregnant patient. In addition, the excellent sensitivity and specificity are preserved in the pregnant patient (Fig. 51.10).[11]A patient in whom MRI findings are normal likely does not require appendectomy. Routine use of MRI in pregnant patients has been demonstrated to reduce the negative appendectomy rate by 47% without a significant increase in the perforation rate, and it has been shown to be a cost-effective study.[42] For these reasons, we encourage liberal use of MRI in pregnant patients suspected to have acute appendicitis without frank peritonitis. However, MRI may not be available in some institutions and may be available only on a limited basis or during limited times in other institutions. The decision about any delay in appendectomy to obtain an MRI study is a complex one and should be made using all available clinical and imaging data available because there are potentially severe consequences associated with both negative appendectomy and appendiceal perforation.

If US is inconclusive and MRI scanning is not immediately available, CT scanning for diagnosis of appendicitis in pregnancy has been reported. A study published in 2008 demonstrated that the use of CT was associated with an 8% negative appendectomy rate, compared with 54% by clinical assessment alone and 32% by clinical assessment combined with US. The authors concluded that CT should be used if US examination findings are equivocal and argued that the amount of radiation delivered during a limited CT examination is below the threshold required to induce fetal malformations and that most cases of appendicitis in pregnancy occur in the second or third trimester, when organogenesis in already complete.[42] Although protocols vary, if CT is used during pregnancy for equivocal cases, care should be taken to perform as limited a study using the lowest possible radiation exposure technique and with avoidance of intravenous administration of contrast material. Further study is required before the routine use of CT can be universally endorsed and accepted in this clinical scenario.

The choice of laparoscopic versus open technique for appendectomy in pregnancy also merits discussion. Current Society of American Gastrointestinal and Endoscopic Surgeons guidelines state that laparoscopic appendectomy is the most common approach currently used in pregnant patients[43] and is safe in pregnancy provided that the surgeon has adequate experience with laparoscopy. Video 50.2 demonstrates a safe technique for appendectomy in a pregnant patient.

At operation, consideration should be given to the height of the gravid uterus in choosing sites for trocar placement to avoid inadvertent puncture of the uterus. We routinely use an open access approach (Hasson technique) with fingertip entry into the abdomen for initial trocar placement to avoid any chance of injury to the gravid uterus.

Our institutional experience with laparoscopic appendectomy in pregnancy has been positive, making it our preferred approach to the pregnant patient. In our hands, we believe it allows an easier identification of the highly variable location of the appendix in pregnancy, a more expeditious removal, and an opportunity for more thorough evaluation of the abdomen for any associated pathologic process.

Appendicitis in the Elderly

Although it is not the peak age for its occurrence, appendicitis is not infrequently seen in elderly patients and should remain in the differential diagnoses of any elderly patient presenting with acute abdominal pain who has not had an appendectomy. Data suggest that the reduced physiologic reserves and impaired immunologic and inflammatory responses result in a higher morbidity with a diagnosis of appendicitis.[12] The most important aspect when dealing with an elderly patient with abdominal pain is to realize the expanded differential diagnosis that must be considered. Other possible diagnoses include but are not limited to acute diverticulitis (uncomplicated or complicated), malignant disease, intestinal ischemia, ischemic colitis, complicated urinary tract infection, and perforated ulcer. Appendicitis may also be manifested in an atypical manner, so a high index of suspicion must be maintained. A careful history and physical examination may aid in diagnosis, but this may have little value in certain circumstances, such as in patients with dementia or an altered mental status. The higher perforation rate in the elderly population, as high as 40% to 70%, combined with the frequent coexistence of comorbidities resulting in higher morbidity, makes the diagnosis and treatment of appendicitis in the elderly a challenge, to say the least.[3,12]

When faced with an elderly patient with diffuse peritonitis, immediate laparotomy should be performed without delay. When the pain is localized and peritonitis is absent, CT scanning of the abdomen should be performed to confirm the diagnosis and to evaluate for other pathologic changes.

Laparoscopic appendectomy is safe in the elderly and is our procedure of choice in this group of patients,[12] provided the patient can safely undergo general anesthesia. Of note, we have successfully performed open appendectomy under spinal anesthesia in patients who are "pulmonary cripples" and in whom the risk of general anesthesia is prohibitive and likely to result in ventilator dependence. For patients too ill to undergo surgery, we have selectively utilized nonoperative therapy for appendicitis with success. Certainly, when dealing with the elderly and the infirm, the approach must be individually tailored to the specific challenges presented by the patient.

Appendicitis in the Immunocompromised Patient

Appendicitis in the immunocompromised patient is managed in the same manner as in the immunocompetent patient, with prompt appendectomy. The key in the evaluation of this population lies in maintenance of a high index of suspicion because the lack of the ability to mount an immune response may result in absence of fever, leukocytosis, and peritonitis. For this reason, early use of CT imaging is advisable. This allows confirmation of the diagnosis of appendicitis as well as the exclusion of diagnoses, such as neutropenic enterocolitis (typhlitis) that may be amenable to nonoperative treatment.[44] Video 50.3 demonstrates a single-incision laparoscopic approach (SILS) to a number of variants of appendiceal pathology.

NEOPLASMS OF THE APPENDIX

Neoplasms of the appendix, although rare, require appropriate treatment. An unanticipated appendiceal neoplasm may be encountered at any elective or emergency operation. It is estimated that as many as 50% of appendiceal neoplasms present as appendicitis and are diagnosed on pathologic examination of the surgical specimen, but variable presentations have been reported. It is further reported that appendiceal neoplasms are identified in 0.7% to 1.7% of pathology specimens. In addition, an appendiceal mass is sometimes noted as an incidental finding on abdominal CT (Fig. 51.11). The pathologic classification and biologic behavior of appendiceal neoplasms are diverse, which serves to make the classification, terminology, and treatment recommendations even more confusing.[1] Overall, appendiceal neoplasms are thought to account for 0.4% to 1% of all gastrointestinal malignant neoplasms.[1] After appendectomy for presumed appendicitis, the incidence of unexpected findings in the surgical specimen is low. Still, if identified, appropriate counseling and treatment are essential.

Appendiceal neuroendocrine neoplasms (ANENs)—once referred to in aggregate as carcinoids—are the most common primary tumor identified in the appendix, comprising approximately 65% of all appendiceal neoplasms. These neoplasms arise from neuroendocrine cells from within the appendix and are detected in 0.2% to 0.7% of appendectomy specimens.[45] These are typically small, well-circumscribed lesions that are located within the more distal aspect of the appendix. They are most commonly diagnosed in the second or third decade of life.[45]

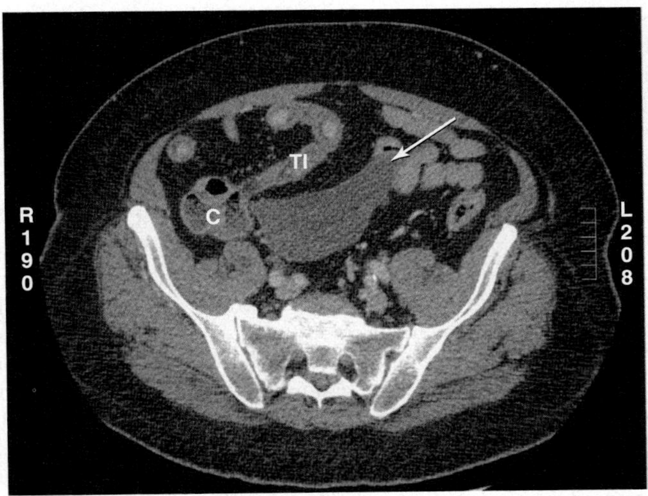

FIG. 51.11 Computed tomography scan of the abdomen in a patient with a benign 10-cm mucocele. The axial image shows a distended fluid-filled mass medial to the appendix *(arrow)*, without associated inflammation. *C*, Cecum; *TI*, terminal ileum.

The biologic behavior of ANENs is highly variable, and the prognosis subsequently depends greatly on the histologic type, malignant potential, grade, and stage at diagnosis. In 2010, the World Health Organization classified ANENs as follows: NET-G1 (well differentiated), NET-G2 (intermediately differentiated), NEC-G3 (poorly differentiated neuroendocrine carcinomas), and mixed neuroendocrine carcinomas (MANECs).[45] Size appears to be the best initial predictor of malignant behavior and metastatic potential, so recommendations regarding initial intraoperative decision making and extent of the initial surgical approach management are based on the size and location of the tumor. ANENs 1 cm or smaller are typically thought to behave in a benign manner and are most commonly treated with appendectomy with excision of the mesoappendix, as opposed to skeletonizing the appendix during removal, which should be explicitly avoided. ANENs larger than 2 cm are treated more aggressively, requiring right hemicolectomy and regional lymphadenectomy for adequate treatment. For lesions between 1 and 2 cm in size, recommendations should be made after careful consideration of the individual tumor characteristics, as metastases have been reported in this subgroup of patients.[1,45] Careful attention should be given to the Ki-67 index (>3%), as a high proliferative index portends a worse prognosis and also warrants right hemicolectomy for proper staging and treatment. The same is true for Grade 2 or greater tumors, or those showing lymphovascular or perineural invasion.[45] After definitive treatment, measurement of serum chromogranin A serves as a useful tumor marker.[45] Five-year survival rates based on Surveillance Epidemiology and End Results (SEER) data are 94% for confined disease, 84.6% for locoregional disease, and 33.7% when distant metastases are present.[45,46]

Adenocarcinoma of the appendix is rare and occurs at a frequency of 0.08% to 0.1% of all appendectomies.[1] Treatment is identical to that of cecal adenocarcinoma and consists of right hemicolectomy with regional lymphadenectomy. In addition, recently published literature utilizing SEER data suggests that, as in staging of adenocarcinoma of the colon, retrieval of more than 12 lymph nodes may be associated with improved staging and subsequently improved survival.[47]

Chemotherapy is also identical to that of adenocarcinoma of the colon with adjuvant administration of 5-fluorouracil, leucovorin, and oxaliplatin (FOLFOX) to selected patients. FOLFOX has also been used in the neoadjuvant setting in patients with mucinous adenocarcinoma before the implementation of cytoreductive (debulking) surgery.

Mucinous tumors of the appendix, which account for less than 0.4% to 1% of gastrointestinal malignancies overall, are a rare and heterogeneous disease for which clinical management is changing.[48] Low-grade appendiceal mucinous neoplasms (AMNs) are often diagnosed incidentally at appendectomy, where advanced-stage AMNs may present with advanced-stage disease and associated pseudomyxoma peritonei (PMP).[48,49] Early classification schemes considered AMN a benign disease, with different terminologies including appendiceal mucocele, cystadenoma, and cystadenocarcinoma.[48] Criteria for simple mucoceles were developed and distinguished from those of malignant histologies; however, intermediate-grade lesions were also identified that were more difficult to accurately characterize. Mucinous appendiceal tumors, if ruptured, can result in intraperitoneal spread and the development of PMP. Of note, it is now recommended that PMP be a term used to describe the existence of mucinous ascites and not be considered a histologic diagnosis itself.[48,49]

Classification and nomenclature of these lesions have been confusing and not universally agreed upon.[1,48] The most important distinction is between that of lesions that behave in a benign manner and those that have a more malignant course. Of note, it is thought that these tumors represent a spectrum of disease and that more aggressive malignant tumors likely evolved from lower grade tumors that were previously present (much like the polyp-cancer sequence seen in carcinoma of the colon), rather than arising de novo. It is also important to note that all AMNs may result in PMP regardless of their malignant potential.[48]

A number of changes in nomenclature and classification have emerged recently. First of all, the term "low-grade AMN" has replaced the term "benign mucocele." Also of note is the widely accepted Ronnet classification, which bases the nomenclature of AMNs primarily on cellularity, differentiation, and likelihood of malignant behavior.[48] The Ronnet scheme divides more clinically advanced AMNs into three major variants: disseminated peritoneal adenomucinosis (DPAM), peritoneal mucinous carcinomatosis (PMCA), and PMCA of indeterminant or discordant features.[48] The clinical course is highly variable among the three variants. Patients with DPAM have an indolent course without distant extraperitoneal spread, whereas patients with PMCA are far more likely to develop metastasis to lymph nodes and extraperitoneal organs, thus suffering a worse prognosis. The behavior of the intermediate category has a more unpredictable course, with authors reporting clinical courses similar to both DPAM and PMCA in individual patients, suggesting that other factors yet to be identified may be present which affect the prognosis and outcome.[47]

Treatment of AMNs varies according to histology and presentation. Low-grade AMNs less than 2 cm are treated adequately with appendectomy alone (with excision of the mesoappendix), with right hemicolectomy reserved for cases in which a positive margin is present, involvement of the appendiceal base, those exhibiting extra appendiceal extension, or those with invasive histology (adenocarcinoma) on final pathologic examination.[48] If PMP or peritoneal metastases are present or subsequently develop, additional therapeutic measures are warranted. First of all, because PMP results as a consequence of perforation and direct peritoneal seeding from the appendiceal contents, the surgeon should use great caution to avoid rupturing an intact appendix if a mucocele or mucinous neoplasm is suspected on preoperative imaging or diagnosed intraoperatively. If PMP or peritoneal metastases occur, treatment by extensive cytoreductive surgery combined with heated intraperitoneal chemotherapy (CRS-HIPEC) is typically employed and is associated with improved, often long-term survival.[48,49] Systemic chemotherapy may also be used in combination with HIPEC at the discretion of the treating oncologist, with 5-fluorouracil–based therapies as the mainstay of adjuvant treatment.[48]

Although the complexity of CRS-HIPEC precludes its complete discussion in this chapter, a brief description is provided for completeness. The goal of the operation is first to physically remove all tumor burden that can be possibly removed at operation, with the goal being to remove all macroscopic tumor via peritoneal stripping and excision of involved organs. This may involve omental excision, hysterectomy, colectomy, splenectomy, cholecystectomy, liver capsulectomy, and peritonectomy of the parietal, diaphragmatic, and pelvic surfaces. Heated chemotherapy (40.0°C) is then instilled into the peritoneal space and allowed to dwell. Mitomycin C is the most commonly used agent, although cisplatin and oxaliplatin are also sometimes administered.[48] The goal is to achieve maximum eradication of residual tumor burden while limiting systemic toxicity by administering the chemotherapy locally. These are extremely complex and difficult operations; operative times of 10 hours are not unusual.[49] Long-term survival with this approach is not unusual and is dependent on the presence of other metastases, histologic grade of the primary tumor, adequacy of cytoreduction, and response to chemotherapy.[48]

An excellent algorithm for the management of the incidentally identified appendiceal mass was proposed by Wray and colleagues, and a modified version is provided for review (Fig. 51.12).[1] This algorithm is useful both in cases of appendicitis and in cases in which an appendiceal tumor is identified incidentally. The availability of frozen-section diagnosis may provide additional help with intraoperative decision making.

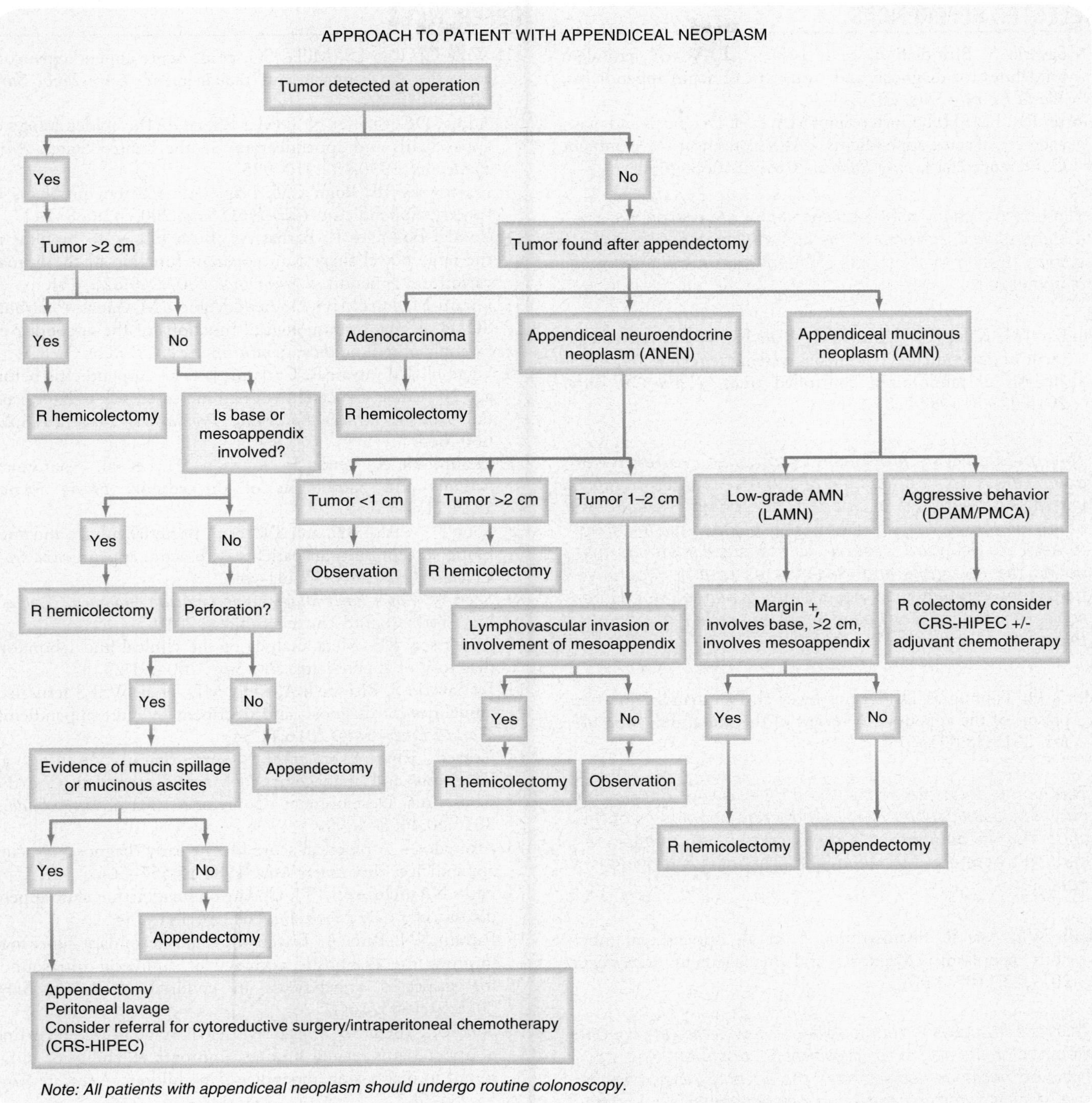

FIG. 51.12 Suggested algorithm for managing the patient with an appendiceal neoplasm. *DPAM,* Disseminated peritoneal adenomucinosis; *PMCA,* peritoneal mucinous carcinomatosis.

SELECTED REFERENCES

Di Saverio S, Birindelli A, Kelly MD, et al. WSES Jerusalem guidelines for diagnosis and treatment of acute appendicitis. *World J Emerg Surg*. 2016;11:34.

Gorter RR, Eker HH, Gorter-Stam MA, et al. Diagnosis and management of acute appendicitis. EAES Consensus Development Conference 2015. *Surg Endosc*. 2016;30:4668–4690.

These two recently published consensus statements provide a comprehensive review of the current literature and expert opinion relating to all aspects of the diagnosis and treatment of appendicitis.

Findlay JM, Kafsi JE, Hammer C, et al. Nonoperative management of appendicitis in adults: a systematic review and meta-analysis of randomized controlled trials. *J Am Coll Surg*. 2016;223:814–824 e812.

This meta analysis provides a comprehensive review of one of the most interesting and controversial topics relating to the treatment of appendicitis today: the concept of nonoperative management. The highest quality trials to date are analyzed in detail via statistical methods that define the strengths and weaknesses of a nonoperative treatment strategy and accentuate the need for large-scale randomized controlled trials to further investigate this evolving topic.

Moris D, Tsilimigras DI, Vagios S, et al. Neuroendocrine neoplasms of the appendix: A review of the literature. *Anticancer Res*. 2018;38:601–611.

This comprehensive and authoritative review details the newest classification of neuroendocrine neoplasms of the appendix. In addition, the most current information regarding treatment, follow-up, and prognosis is provided in detail.

Shaib WL, Assi R, Shamseddine A, et al. Appendiceal mucinous neoplasms: diagnosis and management. *Oncologist*. 2017;22:1107–1116.

This recently published authoritative review details the current literature on the diagnosis, classification, treatment, and prognosis of mucinous neoplasms of the appendix, including the role of initial surgical therapy and subsequent adjuvant strategies, and the role of adjuvant chemotherapy and heated intraperitoneal chemotherapy (HIPEC).

Silen W. *Cope's Early Diagnosis of the Acute Abdomen*. 22nd ed. New York: Oxford University Press; 2010.

This classic text, now in its 22nd edition, provides a masterful overview of the differential diagnoses and subtle historical findings of appendicitis and related disease. It is a timeless source of wisdom and is considered a "must read" by many surgeons.

REFERENCES

1. Wray CJ, Kao LS, Millas SG, et al. Acute appendicitis: controversies in diagnosis and management. *Curr Probl Surg*. 2013;50:54–86.
2. Addiss DG, Shaffer N, Fowler BS, et al. The epidemiology of appendicitis and appendectomy in the United States. *Am J Epidemiol*. 1990;132:910–925.
3. Prystowsky JB, Pugh CM, Nagle AP. Current problems in surgery. Appendicitis. *Curr Probl Surg*. 2005;42:688–742.
4. Randal Bollinger R, Barbas AS, Bush EL, et al. Biofilms in the large bowel suggest an apparent function of the human vermiform appendix. *J Theor Biol*. 2007;249:826–831.
5. Girard-Madoux MJH, Gomez de Aguero M, Ganal-Vonarburg SC, et al. The immunological functions of the appendix: an example of redundancy? *Semin Immunol*. 2018;36:31–44.
6. Ugge H, Udumyan R, Carlsson J, et al. Appendicitis before age 20 years is associated with an increased risk of later prostate cancer. *Cancer Epidemiol Biomarkers Prev*. 2018;27:660–664.
7. Deshmukh S, Verde F, Johnson PT, et al. Anatomical variants and pathologies of the vermix. *Emerg Radiol*. 2014;21:543–552.
8. Song DW, Park BK, Suh SW, et al. Bacterial culture and antibiotic susceptibility in patients with acute appendicitis. *Int J Colorectal Dis*. 2018;33:441–447.
9. Silen W. *Cope's Early Diagnosis of the Acute Abdomen*. 22nd ed. New York: Oxford University Press; 2010.
10. Andersson RE. Meta-analysis of the clinical and laboratory diagnosis of appendicitis. *Br J Surg*. 2004;91:28–37.
11. Di Saverio S, Birindelli A, Kelly MD, et al. WSES Jerusalem guidelines for diagnosis and treatment of acute appendicitis. *World J Emerg Surg*. 2016;11:34.
12. Gorter RR, Eker HH, Gorter-Stam MA, et al. Diagnosis and management of acute appendicitis. EAES Consensus Development Conference 2015. *Surg Endosc*. 2016;30:4668–4690.
13. Alvarado A. A practical score for the early diagnosis of acute appendicitis. *Ann Emerg Med*. 1986;15:557–564.
14. Parks NA, Schroeppel TJ. Update on imaging for acute appendicitis. *Surg Clin North Am*. 2011;91:141–154.
15. Partain KN, Patel A, Travers C, et al. Secondary signs may improve the diagnostic accuracy of equivocal ultrasounds for suspected appendicitis in children. *J Pediatr Surg*. 2016;51:1655–1660.
16. Sola R Jr, Theut SB, Sinclair KA, et al. Standardized reporting of appendicitis-related findings improves reliability of ultrasound in diagnosing appendicitis in children. *J Pediatr Surg*. 53:984–987.
17. Barger Jr RL, Nandalur KR. Diagnostic performance of magnetic resonance imaging in the detection of appendicitis in adults: a meta-analysis. *Acad Radiol*. 2010;17:1211–1216.
18. Solomkin JS, Mazuski JE, Bradley JS, et al. Diagnosis and management of complicated intra-abdominal infection in adults and children: guidelines by the Surgical Infection Society and the Infectious Diseases Society of America. *Clin Infect Dis*. 2010;50:133–164.
19. Sartelli M, Chichom-Mefire A, Labricciosa FM, et al. The management of intra-abdominal infections from a global perspective: 2017 WSES guidelines for management of intra-abdominal infections. *World J Emerg Surg*. 2017;12:29.

20. Ingraham AM, Cohen ME, Bilimoria KY, et al. Comparison of outcomes after laparoscopic versus open appendectomy for acute appendicitis at 222 ACS NSQIP hospitals. *Surgery.* 2010;148:625–635; discussion 635–627.
21. Deelder JD, Richir MC, Schoorl T, et al. How to treat an appendiceal inflammatory mass: operatively or nonoperatively? *J Gastrointest Surg.* 2014;18:641–645.
22. Puapong D, Lee SL, Haigh PI, et al. Routine interval appendectomy in children is not indicated. *J Pediatr Surg.* 2007;42:1500–1503.
23. Al-Kurd A, Mizrahi I, Siam B, et al. Outcomes of interval appendectomy in comparison with appendectomy for acute appendicitis. *J Surg Res.* 2018;225:90–94.
24. Raval MV, Lautz T, Reynolds M, et al. Dollars and sense of interval appendectomy in children: a cost analysis. *J Pediatr Surg.* 2010;45:1817–1825.
25. Schwartz JA, Forleiter C, Lee D, et al. Occult appendiceal neoplasms in acute and chronic appendicitis: a single-institution experience of 1793 appendectomies. *Am Surg.* 2017;83:1381–1385.
26. Furman MJ, Cahan M, Cohen P, et al. Increased risk of mucinous neoplasm of the appendix in adults undergoing interval appendectomy. *JAMA Surg.* 2013;148:703–706.
27. Garlipp B, Arlt G. Laparoscopy for suspected appendicitis. Should an appendix that appears normal be removed? *Chirurg.* 2009;80:615–621.
28. Lee M, Paavana T, Mazari F, et al. The morbidity of negative appendicectomy. *Ann R Coll Surg Engl.* 2014;96:517–520.
29. Varadhan KK, Neal KR, Lobo DN. Safety and efficacy of antibiotics compared with appendicectomy for treatment of uncomplicated acute appendicitis: meta-analysis of randomised controlled trials. *BMJ.* 2012;344:e2156.
30. Mason RJ, Moazzez A, Sohn H, et al. Meta-analysis of randomized trials comparing antibiotic therapy with appendectomy for acute uncomplicated (no abscess or phlegmon) appendicitis. *Surg Infect (Larchmt).* 2012;13:74–84.
31. Di Saverio S, Sibilio A, Giorgini E, et al. The NOTA Study (Non Operative Treatment for Acute Appendicitis): prospective study on the efficacy and safety of antibiotics (amoxicillin and clavulanic acid) for treating patients with right lower quadrant abdominal pain and long-term follow-up of conservatively treated suspected appendicitis. *Ann Surg.* 2014;260:109–117.
32. Svensson JF, Patkova B, Almstrom M, et al. Nonoperative treatment with antibiotics versus surgery for acute nonperforated appendicitis in children: a pilot randomized controlled trial. *Ann Surg.* 2015;261:67–71.
33. Salminen P, Paajanen H, Rautio T, et al. Antibiotic therapy vs appendectomy for treatment of uncomplicated acute appendicitis: the APPAC Randomized Clinical Trial. *JAMA.* 2015;313:2340–2348.
34. Findlay JM, Kafsi JE, Hammer C, et al. Nonoperative management of appendicitis in adults: a systematic review and meta-analysis of randomized controlled trials. *J Am Coll Surg.* 2016;223:814–824.e812.
35. Giuliano V, Giuliano C, Pinto F, et al. Chronic appendicitis "syndrome" manifested by an appendicolith and thickened appendix presenting as chronic right lower abdominal pain in adults. *Emerg Radiol.* 2006;12:96–98.
36. Teli B, Ravishankar N, Harish S, et al. Role of elective laparoscopic appendicectomy for chronic right lower quadrant pain. *Indian J Surg.* 2013;75:352–355.
37. Teixeira PG, Demetriades D. Appendicitis: changing perspectives. *Adv Surg.* 2013;47:119–140.
38. Wen SW, Hernandez R, Naylor CD. Pitfalls in nonrandomized outcomes studies. The case of incidental appendectomy with open cholecystectomy. *JAMA.* 1995;274:1687–1691.
39. Wang HT, Sax HC. Incidental appendectomy in the era of managed care and laparoscopy. *J Am Coll Surg.* 2001;192:182–188.
40. Brown JJ, Wilson C, Coleman S, et al. Appendicitis in pregnancy: an ongoing diagnostic dilemma. *Colorectal Dis.* 2009;11:116–122.
41. McGory ML, Zingmond DS, Tillou A, et al. Negative appendectomy in pregnant women is associated with a substantial risk of fetal loss. *J Am Coll Surg.* 2007;205:534–540.
42. Khandelwal A, Fasih N, Kielar A. Imaging of acute abdomen in pregnancy. *Radiol Clin North Am.* 2013;51:1005–1022.
43. Pearl JP, Price RR, Tonkin AE, et al. SAGES guidelines for the use of laparoscopy during pregnancy. *Surg Endosc.* 2017;31:3767–3782.
44. Rodrigues FG, Dasilva G, Wexner SD. Neutropenic enterocolitis. *World J Gastroenterol.* 2017;23:42–47.
45. Moris D, Tsilimigras DI, Vagios S, et al. Neuroendocrine neoplasms of the appendix: a review of the literature. *Anticancer Res.* 2018;38:601–611.
46. Modlin IM, Sandor A. An analysis of 8305 cases of carcinoid tumors. *Cancer.* 1997;79:813–829.
47. Fleischmann I, Warschkow R, Beutner U, et al. Improved survival after retrieval of 12 or more regional lymph nodes in appendiceal cancer. *Eur J Surg Oncol.* 2017;43:1876–1885.
48. Shaib WL, Assi R, Shamseddine A, et al. Appendiceal mucinous neoplasms: diagnosis and management. *Oncologist.* 2017;22:1107–1116.
49. Mittal R, Chandramohan A, Moran B. Pseudomyxoma peritonei: natural history and treatment. *Int J Hyperthermia.* 2017;33:511–519.

52 CHAPTER

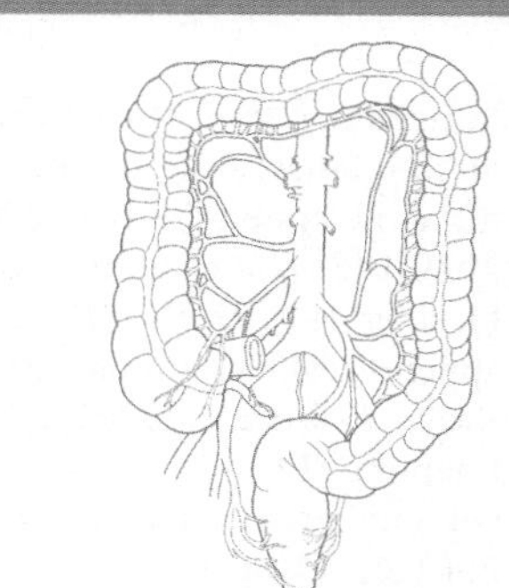

Colon and Rectum

Susan Galandiuk, Uri Netz, Emilio Morpurgo, Sara Maria Tosato, Naim Abu-Freha, C. Tyler Ellis

OUTLINE

Please access Elsevier eBooks for Practicing Clinicians to view the videos for this chapter https://expertconsult.inkling.com/.

Acknowledgments: Josè Adolfo Navarro, MD; Silvia Neri, MD; and Alberto Morabito, MD.

EMBRYOLOGY OF THE COLON AND RECTUM

A sound knowledge base of the gastrointestinal (GI) tract embryologic development is important in understanding colon and rectal anatomy and pathophysiology. The primitive gut tube is formed from the endodermal roof of the yolk sac. Early in the development process, beginning in the third week of gestation, the gut tube divides into three sections: the foregut, midgut, and hindgut (Fig. 52.1).

The foregut forms the oral (buccopharyngeal) membrane, esophagus, stomach, and proximal duodenum (to the duodenal ampulla) and is supplied by the celiac artery. The midgut, including the distal part of the duodenum, small intestine, right colon, and the proximal two thirds of the transverse colon, receives it blood supply from the superior mesenteric artery (SMA). The midgut temporarily herniates ventrally out of the abdomen, a key step in the physiologic development progress for acquiring length and correct positioning of its structures (Fig. 52.2). The hindgut develops into the distal third of the transverse colon, descending colon, sigmoid, and rectum all the way to the upper anal canal. It is supplied by the inferior mesenteric artery (IMA). The venous and lymphatic networks develop parallel to their corresponding sectional arteries.

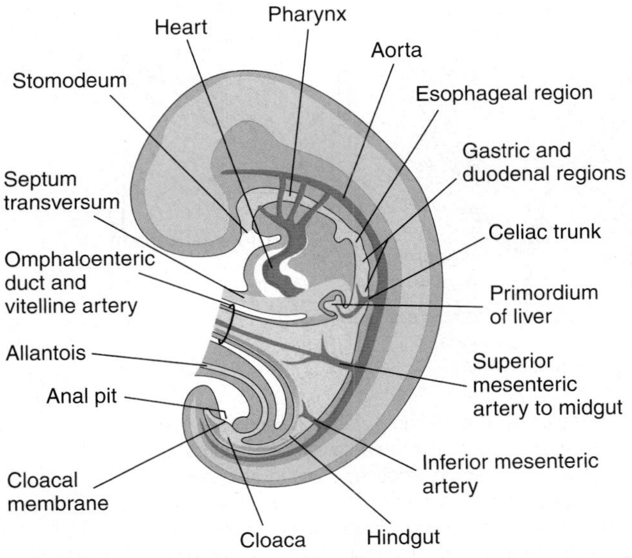

The embryologic development of the rectum is complex and prone to developmental complications (see Chapter 67, Pediatric Surgery). The proximal rectum develops similar to the colon. The distal regions develop from the terminal hindgut that enters into the cloaca (an endoderm-lined cavity in contact with the surface ectoderm at the cloacal membrane). Prior to 5 weeks, the intestinal and urogenital tracts terminate at a common cavity in the cloaca. During the next few weeks, the urorectal septum migrates caudally and divides the cloaca into an anterior urogenital sinus and posterior distal rectum and anal sinus (Fig. 52.3). The urorectal septum fusion with the cloacal membrane is represented in the adult by the perineal body. The external anal sphincter is formed by the posterior part of the cloacal sphincter, whereas the internal anal sphincter is formed from enlarging circular fibers of the rectum. The upper two thirds of the anal canal are derived from the hindgut and the lower third from the proctodeum. The dentate line marks the fusion of endodermal (hindgut) and ectodermal depression (proctodeum). The anal transition zone is formed from the cloacal part of the anal canal. The hindgut part of the anal canal is supplied by the IMA, while the lower third, by the internal pudendal artery.

Heart
Pharynx
Aorta
Stomodeum
Esophageal region
Gastric and duodenal regions
Septum transversum
Celiac trunk
Omphaloenteric duct and vitelline artery
Primordium of liver
Allantois
Superior mesenteric artery to midgut
Anal pit
Inferior mesenteric artery
Cloacal membrane
Cloaca
Hindgut

FIG. 52.1 Median section of the embryo showing the early alimentary system and its blood supply (week 4). (From Moore KL, Persaud TVN, Torchia MG. Alimentary system. In: *The Developing Human*. 11th ed. Philadelphia: Elsevier; 2020:193–221.)

ANATOMY OF THE COLON, RECTUM, AND PELVIC FLOOR

The large bowel including the colon and rectum is a tube of variable diameter, approximately 150 cm in length (Fig. 52.4).

Colon Anatomy

The cecum is the saccular beginning of the colon, with an average diameter of 7.5 cm and a length of 10 cm. It has no mesentery and is completely covered with peritoneum and is therefore considered an intraperitoneal structure. The cecum is variably connected to the posterior abdominal wall by a peritoneal reflection. Patients with an abnormally mobile cecum and ascending colon, found in a small proportion of patients, can be predisposed to volvulus (torsion) or cecal bascule (intermittent anterior and superior folding of the cecum associated with obstructive symptoms). The cecum has a thin wall compared to the rest of the colon, and considering its large diameter, in accordance with the law of Laplace, it is the site most likely to perforate in the presence of large bowel obstructions. Although it is distensible, acute dilation of the cecum to a diameter of more than 12 cm, which can be measured on a plain abdominal radiograph, is associated with risk of ischemic necrosis and perforation of the bowel wall and should be treated promptly, usually with surgery. The terminal ileum empties into the cecum along its medial border through the ileocecal valve, a thickened, nipple-shaped invagination containing circular muscle. In cases of large bowel obstruction, the ileocecal valve is clinically important. An ileocecal valve that does not allow reflux of colonic contents into the ileum (competent ileocecal valve) can result in a closed-loop obstruction, a surgical emergency, whereas a valve that allows retrograde flow into the ileum (incompetent ileocecal valve) will result in less colonic distension and a less acute clinical scenario.

The vermiform appendix extends from the cecum approximately 3 cm below the ileocecal valve as a blind-ending elongated tube, 8 to 10 cm in length (Fig. 52.5). It is most commonly found in a retrocecal position (65%), followed by pelvic (31%), subcecal (2.3%), preileal (1.0%), and retroileal (0.4%) locations. In the setting of inflammation and adhesions, locating the appendix can be difficult. One can reliably reach its base by following the anterior taenia of the cecum to the convergence with the other two taeniae. The bloodless fold of Treves extends from the antimesenteric border of the terminal ileum to the base of the appendix or the anterior surface of the mesoappendix, or to both areas. This fold contains no sizable blood vessels. Since it is the only part of the ileum that has a fold on the antimesenteric side of the bowel, it can help in the recognition of the ileocecal region and the base of the appendix.

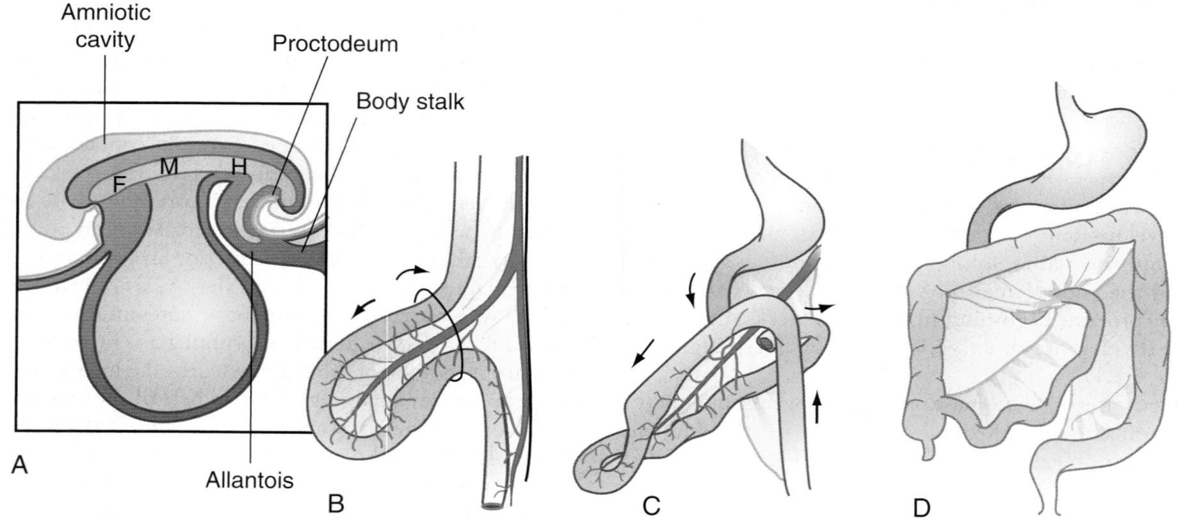

FIG. 52.2 At the third week of development, the primitive tube can be divided into three regions (A): the foregut *(F)* in the head fold, the hindgut *(H)* with its ventral allantoic outgrowth in the smaller tail fold, and the midgut *(M)* between these two portions. Stages of development of the midgut are physiologic herniation (B), return to the abdomen (C), and fixation (D). (From Corman ML, ed. *Colon and Rectal Surgery*. 4th ed. Philadelphia: Lippincott-Raven; 1998:2.)

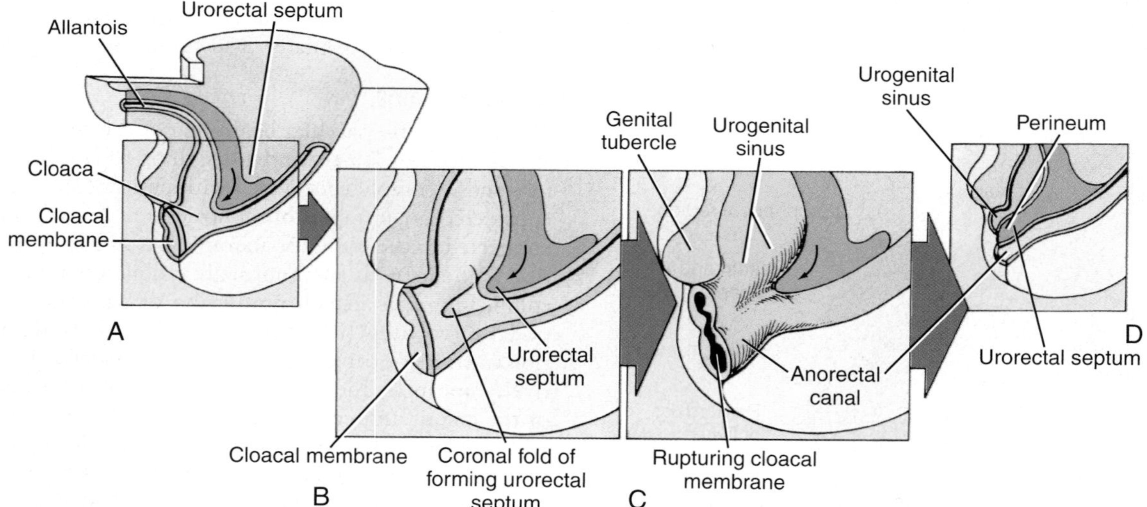

FIG. 52.3 Development of the distal rectum and anus. Progressive steps between 4 and 6 weeks in subdivision of the cloaca into a ventral primitive urogenital sinus and a dorsal anorectal canal (A–D). The urorectal septum is formed by the fusion of yolk sac extraembryonic mesoderm and allantois mesoderm, which produces a tissue wedge between the hindgut and urogenital sinus during craniocaudal folding of the embryo. As the tip of the urorectal septum approaches the cloacal membrane dividing the cloaca into the urogenital sinus and anorectal canal, the cloacal membrane ruptures, thereby opening the urogenital sinus and dorsal anorectal canal to the exterior. The tip of urorectal septum forms the perineum. A, B, and D, Sections through the cloacal and related endoderm-derived structures. C, Surface view of the caudal endoderm to better depict its three-dimensional shape. *Curved arrows* indicate the direction of growth of the developing urorectal septum. (From Schoenwolf GC, Bleyl SB, Brauer PR, et al. *Larsen's Human Embryology*. 5th ed. Philadelphia, PA: Churchill Livingstone, an imprint of Elsevier; 2015.)

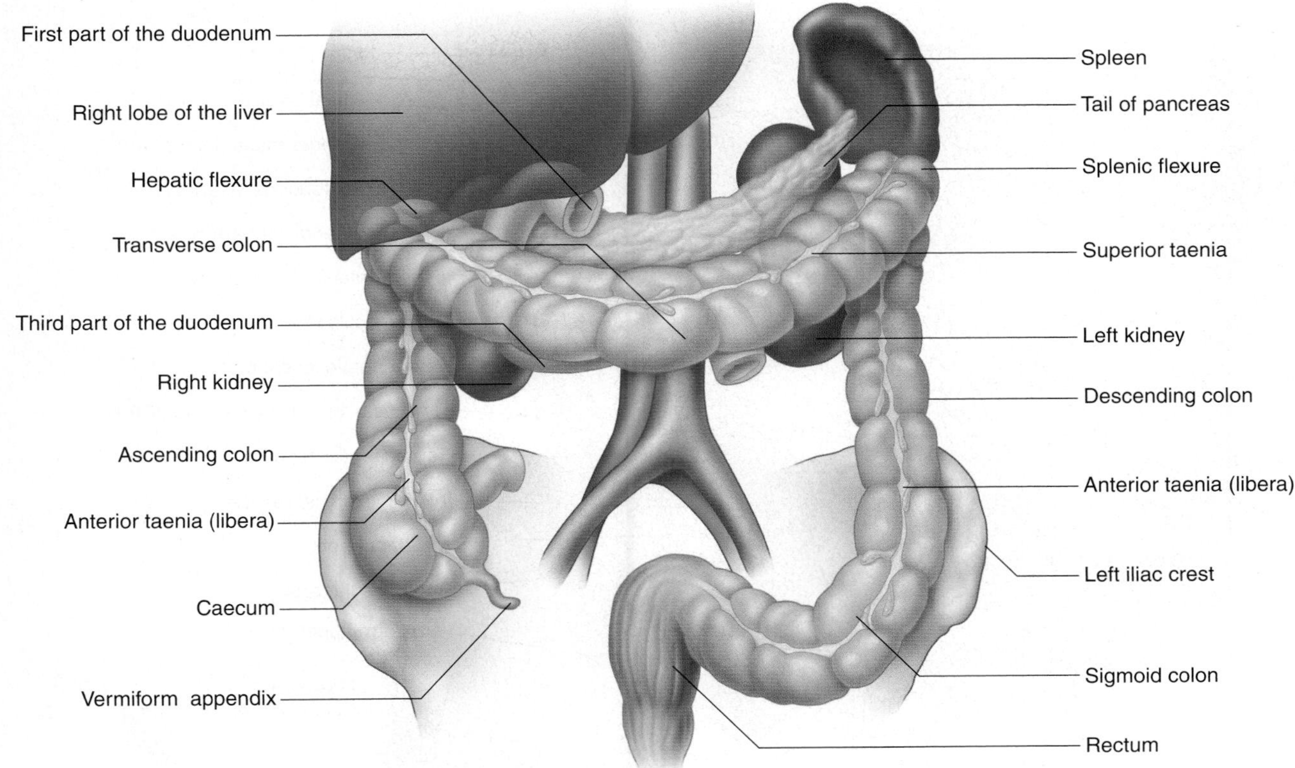

FIG. 52.4 The large bowel includes the colon, consisting of ascending, transverse, descending, and sigmoid colon and the rectum, shown here in relation to neighboring anatomic structures. (From Standring S, Anand N, Rolfe B, et al. *Gray's Anatomy*. 41st ed. Philadelphia: Elsevier; 2016.)

The ascending colon begins at the ileocecal junction and extends upward toward the hepatic flexure on the right side and is approximately 15 cm in length. The anterior and lateral surfaces are covered with peritoneum and are considered intraperitoneal, whereas the posterior surface is fixed against the retroperitoneum by the fascia of Toldt. The ascending colon is best mobilized along the lateral peritoneal reflection by incising the "white line of Toldt," which represents the fusion of the peritoneum with the posterior fascia of the same name. When releasing the hepatic flexure and lifting the colon medially, one must be aware of the proximity of the second part of the duodenum, which can be inadvertently injured.

The transverse colon, which is approximately 45 cm in length, is suspended between the hepatic and splenic flexures, which are fixed structures. It is completely covered by visceral peritoneum and connected to the posterior abdominal wall by the transverse mesocolon. It has a "U"-shaped curve, which can even reach down to the pelvis in some patients. Recognizing its variability in position is very important when attempting to exteriorize a loop of colon with a "target incision" for a transverse or sigmoid colostomy.

The greater omentum is attached to the superior aspect of the transverse colon. It has two parts, the superior gastrocolic ligament composed of two serous layers, and the inferior portion, which is composed of four serous layers draping over the anterior abdominal cavity like an apron. Its size and volume are highly variable, although in most cases correlated with body weight. Lifting the greater omentum upward with downward traction of the transverse colon will reveal an avascular plane adjacent to the colon most easily identified close to the midline. This plane is useful when separating these two structures. The greater omentum is commonly used to cover the intraperitoneal contents when closing abdominal incisions and also used to fill cavities after surgery helping to control infection. It also provides a good patch, or reinforcement, in cases when closure of inflamed and friable tissues is not possible or likely to fail, such as in the treatment of perforated duodenal ulcer. The omentum can be mobilized to create an omental pedicle that reaches the pelvis, by ligating and detaching either the right- or left-sided omental vessels, achieving extra omental length while the blood supply is adequately maintained by the distal arcade from the other side. Such an omental pedicle can be positioned between the rectum and vagina to buttress a colo- or rectovaginal fistula repair or used to fill the pelvic and perineal spaces after rectal excision.

The splenic flexure, where the transverse colon flexes downward, is found adjacent and inferior to the spleen. It is usually situated higher and deeper than the right colic or hepatic flexure. The splenic flexure is suspended by four mainly avascular ligaments: by the phrenicocolic ligament to the diaphragm, by the splenocolic ligament to the lower pole of the spleen, by the renocolic ligament to the Gerota fascia, which surrounds the left kidney, and by the pancreaticocolic ligament to the tail of the pancreas. The splenic flexure can be released or mobilized without dividing any major blood vessels if one is separating the correct plane (Fig. 52.6). Surgeons commonly dissect the descending colon along the line of Toldt from below and then enter the lesser sac by lifting the omentum above the transverse colon. This maneuver allows mobilization of the flexure to be achieved, with minimal traction. Bleeding is most commonly encountered from excessive downward traction resulting in avulsion of a portion of the splenic capsule.

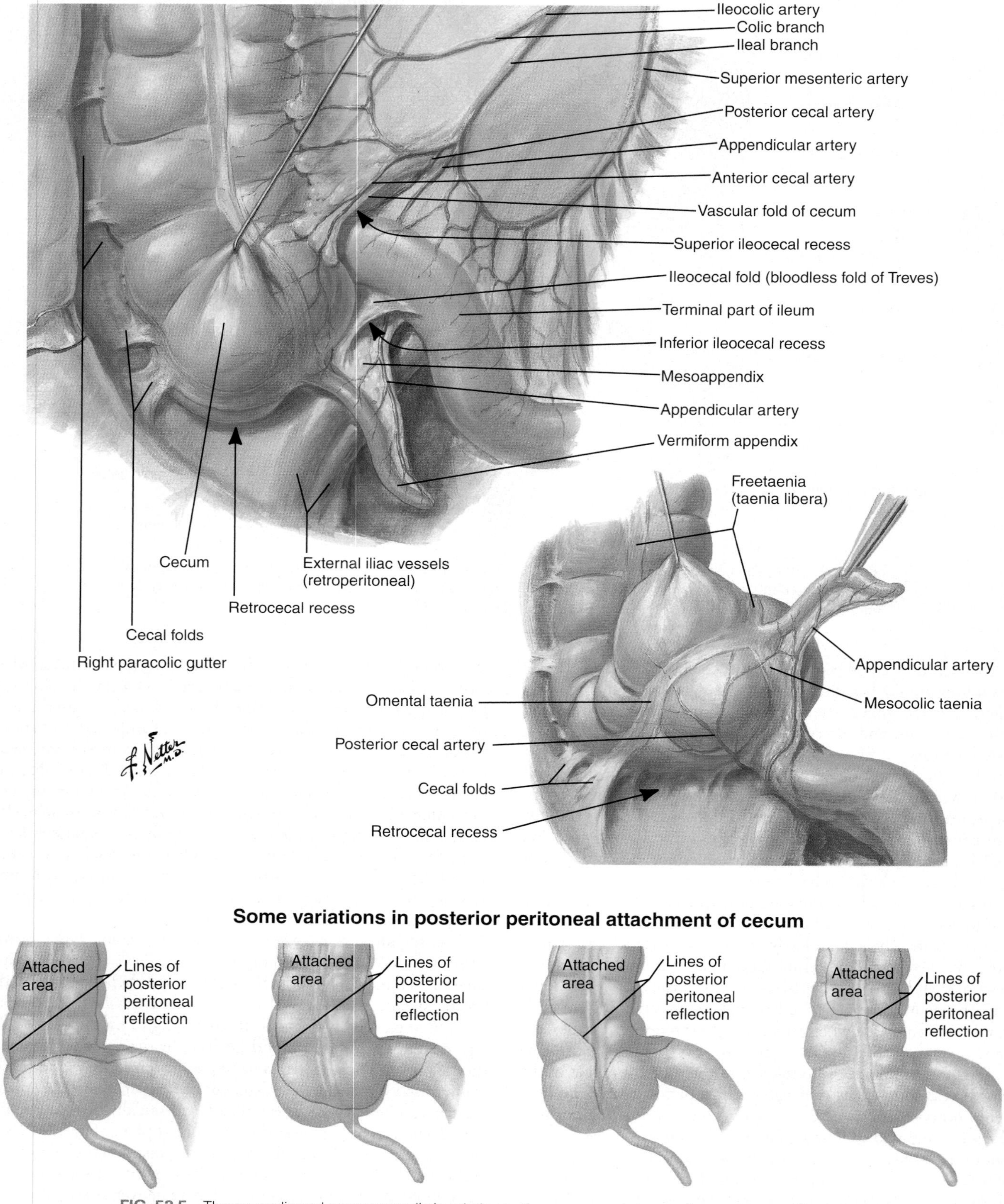

Ileocolic artery
Colic branch
Ileal branch
Superior mesenteric artery
Posterior cecal artery
Appendicular artery
Anterior cecal artery
Vascular fold of cecum
Superior ileocecal recess
Ileocecal fold (bloodless fold of Treves)
Terminal part of ileum
Inferior ileocecal recess
Mesoappendix
Appendicular artery
Vermiform appendix
Cecum
External iliac vessels (retroperitoneal)
Retrocecal recess
Cecal folds
Right paracolic gutter
Freetaenia (taenia libera)
Appendicular artery
Mesocolic taenia
Omental taenia
Posterior cecal artery
Cecal folds
Retrocecal recess
F. Netter M.D.
Some variations in posterior peritoneal attachment of cecum
Attached area
Lines of posterior peritoneal reflection
Attached area
Lines of posterior peritoneal reflection
Attached area
Lines of posterior peritoneal reflection
Attached area
Lines of posterior peritoneal reflection

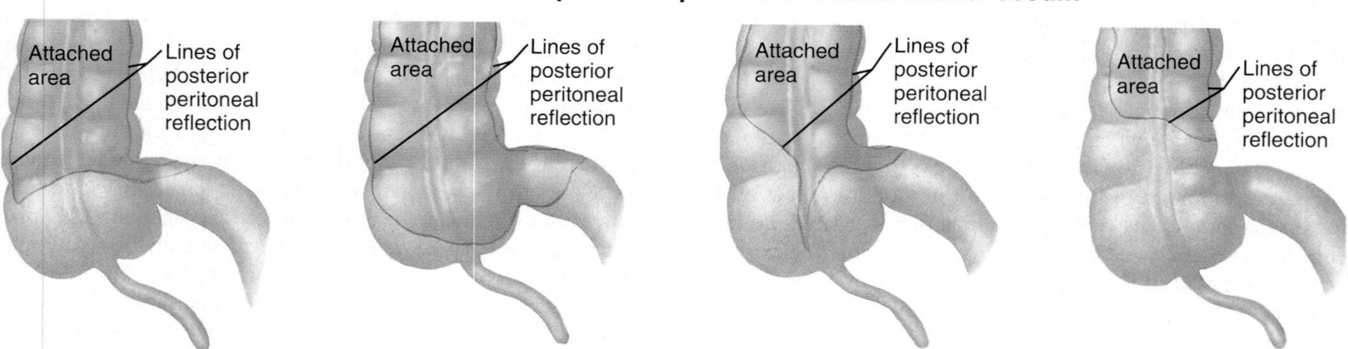

FIG. 52.5 The appendix and mesoappendix in relation to the cecum and surrounding structures. (From Netter FH. *Atlas of Human Anatomy*. Philadelphia: Elsevier; 2019.)

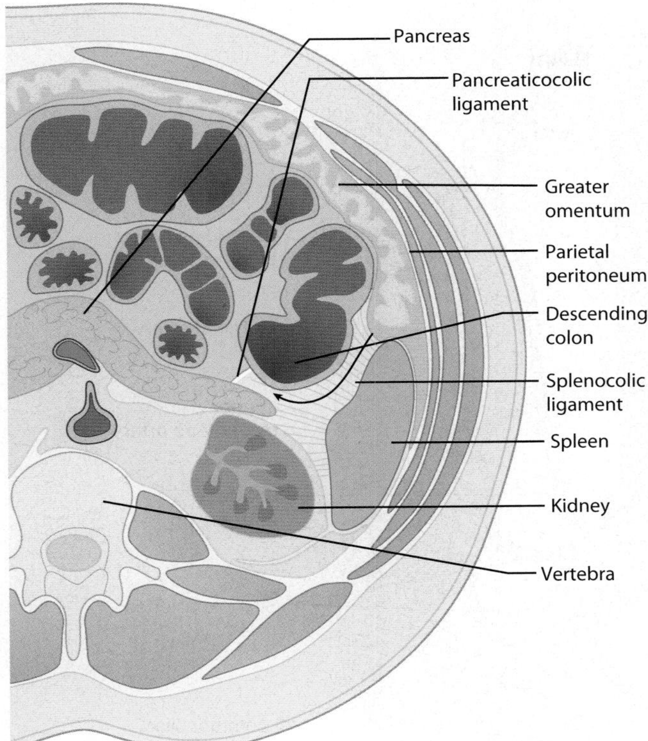

FIG. 52.6 Ligaments of the splenic flexure; the *arrow* indicates potential plane of dissection. (From Netz U, Galandiuk S. Clinical anatomy for procedures involving the small bowel, colon, rectum and anus. In: Fischer JE, Ellison EC, Upchurgh Jr. GR, et al., eds. *Fischer's Mastery of Surgery.* 7th ed. Philadelphia: Wolter Kluwer; 2019.)

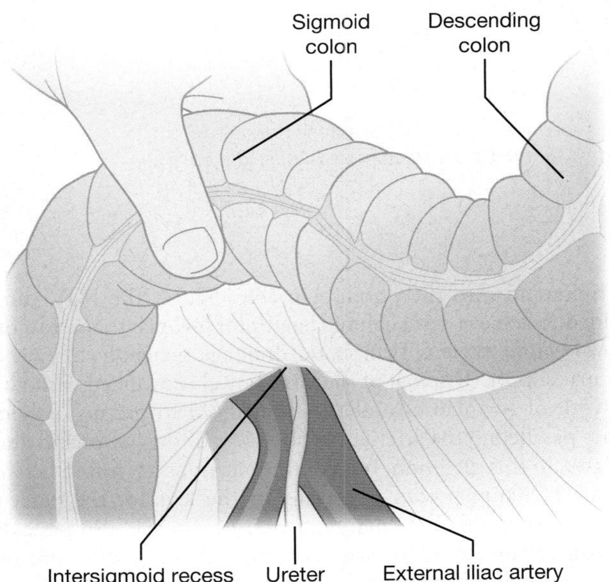

FIG. 52.7 The intersigmoid recess, the sigmoid colon being retracted upward and to the right. (From Hollinshead WH. *Anatomy for Surgeons.* Vol 2, 2nd ed. New York: Harper and Row; 1971.)

The descending colon begins at the splenic flexure where the intestine loses its mesentery and extends downward on the left side of the abdomen approximately 25 cm until it transitions into the sigmoid colon. It is smaller in diameter than the ascending colon. The descending colon is similar to the ascending colon with regard to its peritoneal coverage and approach to dissection.

The sigmoid colon begins at or below the level of the iliac crest, where the colon becomes completely intraperitoneal again, acquiring a mesentery covered on both sides with peritoneum. The sigmoid is thicker and more mobile compared to the descending colon varying in length from 15 to 50 cm (average, 38 cm). The mobile portion of the sigmoid colon is attached by the sigmoid mesocolon to the posterior abdominal wall and pelvis in the pattern of an inverted V creating the intersigmoid fossa (Fig. 52.7). When mobilizing the sigmoid colon, this mesenteric fold is a surgical landmark for the underlying left ureter. The sigmoid colon ends at the rectosigmoid junction, which is recognized as the point where the colonic taeniae confluence to form a complete longitudinal muscle layer, and the colon loses its mesentery, usually between the level of the sacral promontory and the S3 vertebra.

Blood Supply, Lymphatic Drainage, and Innervation of the Colon

Arterial blood supply. The anatomy of the blood supply is in accordance with the embryologic development of the GI tract. The celiac artery supplies the foregut, the SMA the midgut, and the IMA the hindgut. The colon receives its blood supply from the SMA and the IMA, both anterior branches of the abdominal aorta (Fig. 52.8).

The SMA is the second unpaired anterior branch of the aorta, arising at the level of the lower border of the L1 vertebra, it descends posterior to the pancreas and then crosses anteriorly to the uncinate process of the pancreas and the third part of the duodenum and enters the mesentery of the bowel. On the left side, it provides up to 20 branches to the small intestine. On the right, it gives off three major branches to the colon. The first branch is the middle colic artery, arising near the inferior border of the pancreas, followed by the right colic and ileocolic arteries. The ileocolic artery is the most constant of these arteries. It runs toward the ileocecal junction within the mesentery giving off the anterior and posterior cecal arteries and the appendicular artery, supplying the terminal ileum, cecum, and appendix. The avascular space between the SMA and the ileocolic artery is a safe region to begin vascular dissection in a minimally invasive right colectomy and can also be used as a space through which one can pull the transverse or right colon through in cases of "retroileal" colorectal anastomoses to gain bowel length. The right colic artery, absent in up to 20%, usually arises from the SMA but may be a branch of the ileocolic or left colic vessels. The middle colic artery enters the transverse mesocolon and divides into right and left branches, which supply the proximal and distal transverse colon, respectively. When lifting the transverse colon, the middle colic artery can be tracked to the base of the mesentery just to the right of the ligament of Treitz, and into the proximal SMA. The middle colic artery is the main blood supply to the splenic flexure in about a third of the cases.

The IMA is the third unpaired anterior artery arising from the aorta at the level of the L2–3 vertebrae approximately 3 cm above the aortic bifurcation. The IMA descends inferiorly and to the left giving off the left colic artery, followed by several sigmoid branches, and culminating in the superior rectal (hemorrhoidal) artery. The left colic artery divides into an ascending branch to the splenic flexure and a descending branch to the descending colon.

The marginal artery of Drummond runs along the mesenteric margin of the colon from the cecocolic junction to the

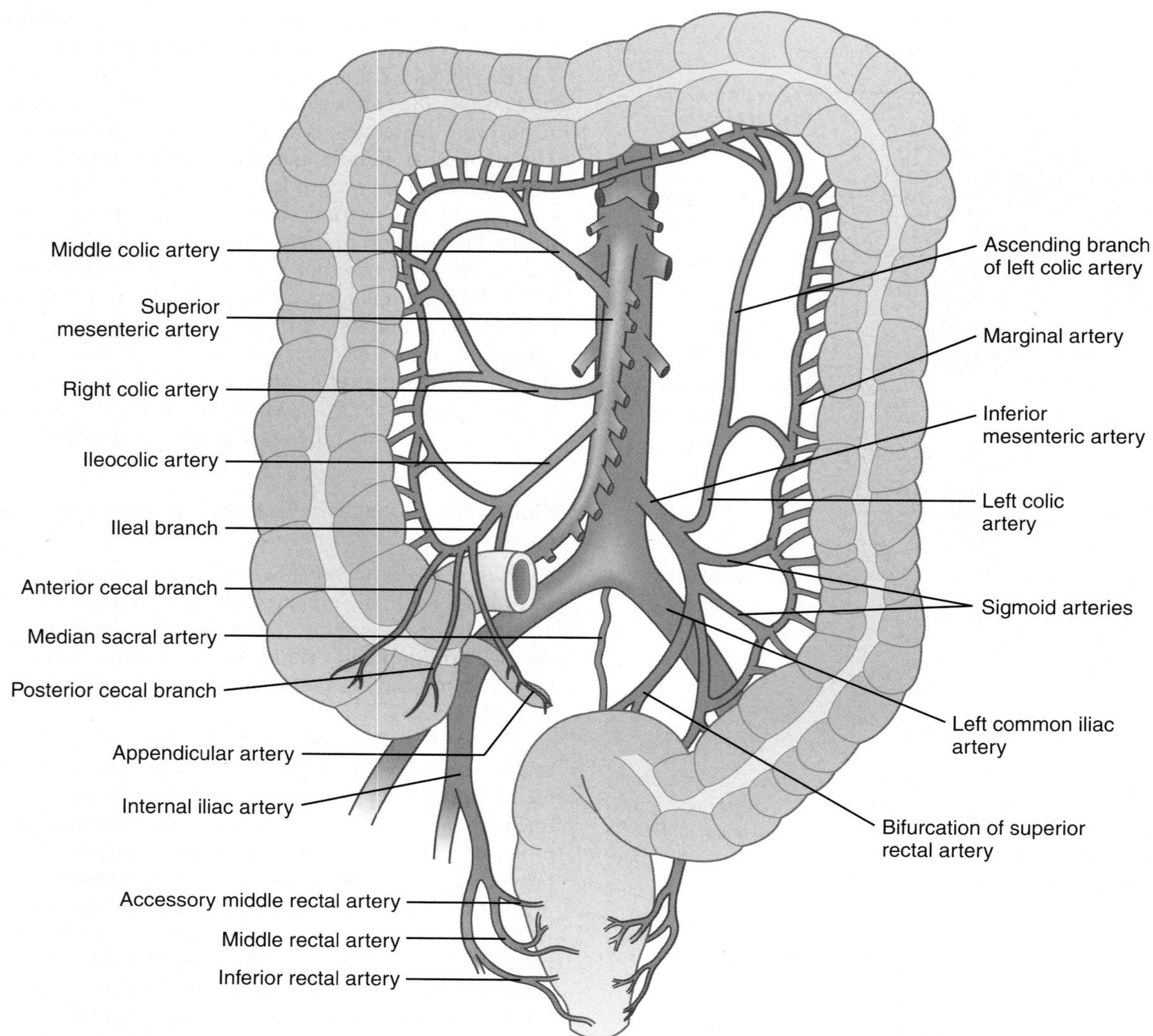

FIG. 52.8 The arterial blood supply to the colon is from the superior and inferior mesenteric arteries. (From Gordon PH, Nivatvongs S, eds. *Principles and Practice of Surgery for the Colon, Rectum and Anus.* 2nd ed. St. Louis: Quality Medical Publishing; 1999:23.)

rectosigmoid junction. Vasa recta from this artery branch off at short intervals and supply the bowel wall directly. The marginal artery is important clinically for when one of the larger arteries is obstructed (emboli, atherosclerosis, surgical ligation, etc.). The colon can receive collateral blood supply through this artery.

The meandering mesenteric artery, or "arc of Riolan," is an uncommon finding described as a thick tortuous collateral vessel that runs close to the base of the mesentery and connects the SMA or middle colic artery to the IMA or left colic artery. It can have an important role in blood delivery in cases of SMA or IMA occlusion. Flow can be forward (IMA stenosis) or retrograde (SMA stenosis), depending on the site of obstruction. The presence of a large arc of Riolan suggests occlusion of one of the major mesenteric arteries.

Venous drainage. Venous drainage somewhat follows the arterial supply through the superior mesenteric and inferior mesenteric veins (IMVs), which contribute to the formation of the portal vein. It is important to note that the IMV continues beyond the IMA along the base of the mesentery to the left of the ligament of Treitz and into the portal vein (Fig. 52.9). The IMV can be divided to achieve extra colonic length for low pelvic anastomoses.

Lymphatic system. Lymphatic drainage generally follows the vascular supply. The wall of the large bowel is supplied with a rich network of lymphatic capillaries that drain to groups of lymph nodes paralleling the arterial supply. Most of the lymphatic drainage goes in this direction, but communications are found between groups of lymph nodes, especially at the level of the paracolic groups at the level of the marginal arteries. There is also some dual drainage from the distal transverse and splenic flexure into both the superior and inferior mesenteric lymph nodes.

Innervation. The innervation of the large intestine has both sympathetic and parasympathetic components, which generally follow the blood supply.

Rectal Anatomy

The rectum begins at the rectosigmoid junction and ends at the level of the anus. Anatomists define the distal border as the dentate (pectinate) line based on the mucosal surface, whereas surgeons

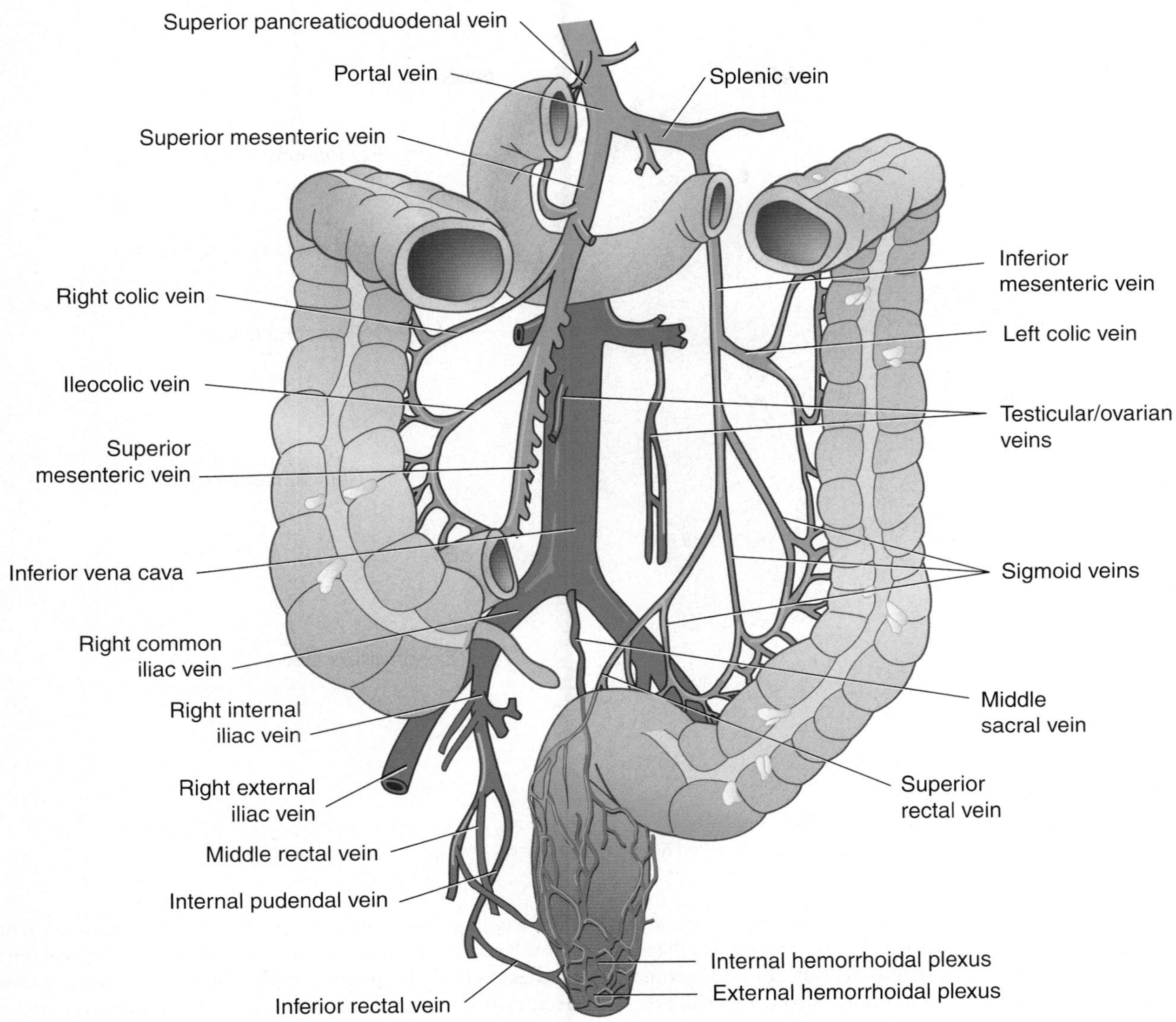

FIG. 52.9 Venous anatomy of the colon and rectum. (From Gordon PH, Nivatvongs S, ed. *Principles and Practice of Surgery for the Colon, Rectum and Anus.* 2nd ed. St. Louis: Quality Medical Publishing; 1999:30.)

define it as the proximal border of the anal sphincter complex at the level of the levator ani (about 2 cm above the dentate line). The rectum with a total length of around 15 to 20 cm is divided into thirds based on its peritoneal relationships. The upper rectum is covered by peritoneum anteriorly and laterally and its lower limit extends to approximately 10 cm above the dentate line. The middle third is covered by peritoneum only anteriorly and extends from 5 to 10 cm above the dentate line. The lower third of the rectum is totally extraperitoneal, extending from 1 to 5 cm above the dentate line. The rectum has three lateral curves or valves of Houston, the proximal and distal valves fold to the right and the middle to the left. They are lost after full surgical mobilization of the rectum, providing approximately 5 cm of additional length assisting the surgeon's ability to fashion an anastomosis deep in the pelvis. Structurally, the rectum lacks taeniae coli, epiploic appendices, and haustra. The anterior peritoneal reflection between the rectum and anterior structures, the rectovesicular pouch in males and rectouterine or Douglas pouch in females, is 7 to 9 cm from the anal verge in men and 5 to 7.5 cm in women (Fig. 52.10). The anterior peritoneal reflection is the lowest dependent part of the peritoneal cavity. It is clinically important as a common location of fluid and pus accumulation and may serve as a site of peritoneal metastases from visceral tumors. These "drop" metastases can form a mass in the cul-de-sac (Blumer shelf) that can be recognized on digital rectal examination. "Mesorectum" refers to the visceral mesentery of the rectum. Recognition of mesorectal planes during rectal surgery is extremely important as it allows for a relatively bloodless dissection with consistent excision of relevant lymphatic tissues, adhering to the basic surgical oncologic principle of removing the cancer in continuity with its blood and lymphatic supply. Total mesorectal excision (TME), based on a detailed understanding of anatomy, has been shown to reduce the incidence of local recurrence of rectal cancer and increase the preservation of urinary and sexual function. The mesorectum is relatively thick posteriorly, thinner along the sides, and very thin anteriorly.

Anatomic structures adjacent to the rectum are clinically important with regard to dissection planes and to direct extension of tumors and/or fistulas. In males, the rectum is adjacent anteriorly and extraperitoneally to the urinary bladder, ureters, vas deferens, seminal vesicles, and prostate. In women, intraperitoneally, it is

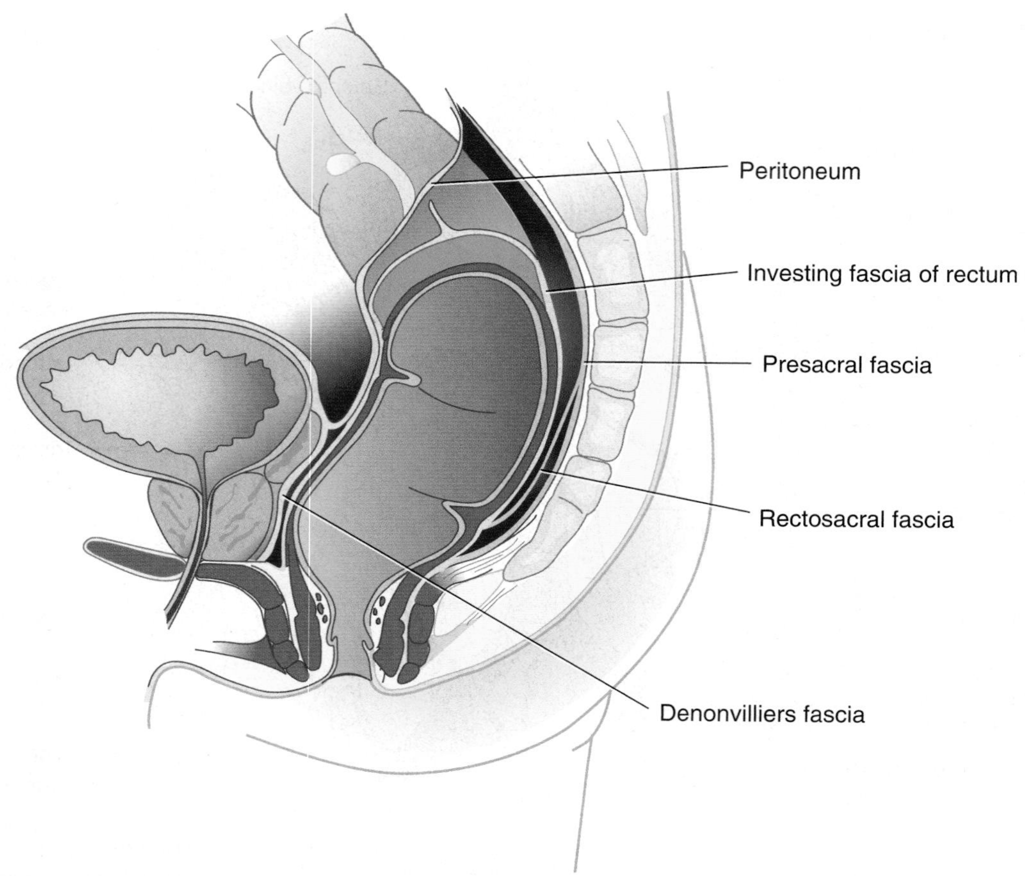

FIG. 52.10 Fascial relationships of the rectum. (From Gordon PH, Nivatvongs S, ed. *Principles and Practice of Surgery for the Colon, Rectum and Anus.* 2nd ed. St. Louis: Quality Medical Publishing; 1999:10.)

adjacent to the uterus, tubes, ovaries, and to the upper part of the posterior vaginal wall. Extraperitoneally, the rectum is adjacent to the uterine cervix and posterior vaginal wall. In both genders, the intraperitoneal cul-de-sac is commonly filled with small bowel and colon. The sacrum, sacral vessels, and sacral nerve roots are located posterior to the rectum.

The posterior aspect of the rectum is invested with a thick, closely applied mesorectum (Fig. 52.11). A thin layer of investing fascia (fascia propria) coats the mesorectum and represents a distinct layer from the presacral fascia against which it lies. During proctectomy for rectal cancer, mobilization and dissection of the rectum proceed between the presacral fascia and fascia propria. The presacral fascia covers the anterior sacrum and coccyx. A group of veins, on the presacral periosteum, the presacral veins, drain into the sacral foramina. Dissection deep to the presacral fascia can cause severe bleeding from the underlying presacral venous plexus. Such bleeding can be very difficult to control, as the torn vessels tend to withdraw into the sacral foramina. The rectosacral fascia, or Waldeyer fascia, is a thick condensation of endopelvic fascia connecting the presacral fascia to the fascia propria at the level of S4 that extends to the posterior-inferior rectum. Dividing Waldeyer fascia during dissection from an abdominal approach provides access to the deep retrorectal pelvis. Laterally, the rectum is connected to the pelvic sidewall by the "lateral stalks" or ligaments. These are found in the low pelvis at the level of the prostate or mid-vagina. It is important to remember that in about a quarter of the cases, a branch of the middle rectal artery traverses them and may cause bleeding when cutting through them. Denonvilliers fascia, located anterior to the rectum, is a membranous layer that is an extension of the inferior peritoneal reflection and extends to the perineal body. This fascial layer separates the rectum from the previously mentioned anterior structures and is considered as the anterior border of a TME.

Blood Supply, Lymphatic Drainage, and Innervation of the Rectum

The blood supply to the rectum is derived from the superior, middle, and inferior rectal (hemorrhoidal) arteries. All three rectal arteries are connected with a strong anastomotic network, which helps avoid rectal ischemia after dividing the superior rectal arteries during anterior resections (Fig. 52.12). The superior rectal artery is the end branch of the IMA. It usually divides into left and right branches that run posteriorly downward. The middle rectal arteries are paired vessels derived from the internal iliac arteries to the lower rectum through the lateral columns. They are not considered a major blood supply to the rectum and are found inconstantly. They can be inadvertently injured when dissecting the lateral ligaments. The inferior rectal arteries are branches of the internal pudendal arteries and generally supply the anus distal to the dentate line.

The superior rectal vein drains the upper two thirds of the rectum, draining into the IMV and portal system. The lower rectum and anus drain into the middle and inferior rectal veins, which are connected to the internal iliac and systemic circulation. This drainage pattern explains the higher rate of lung metastases observed with low rectal cancers as compared to mid and

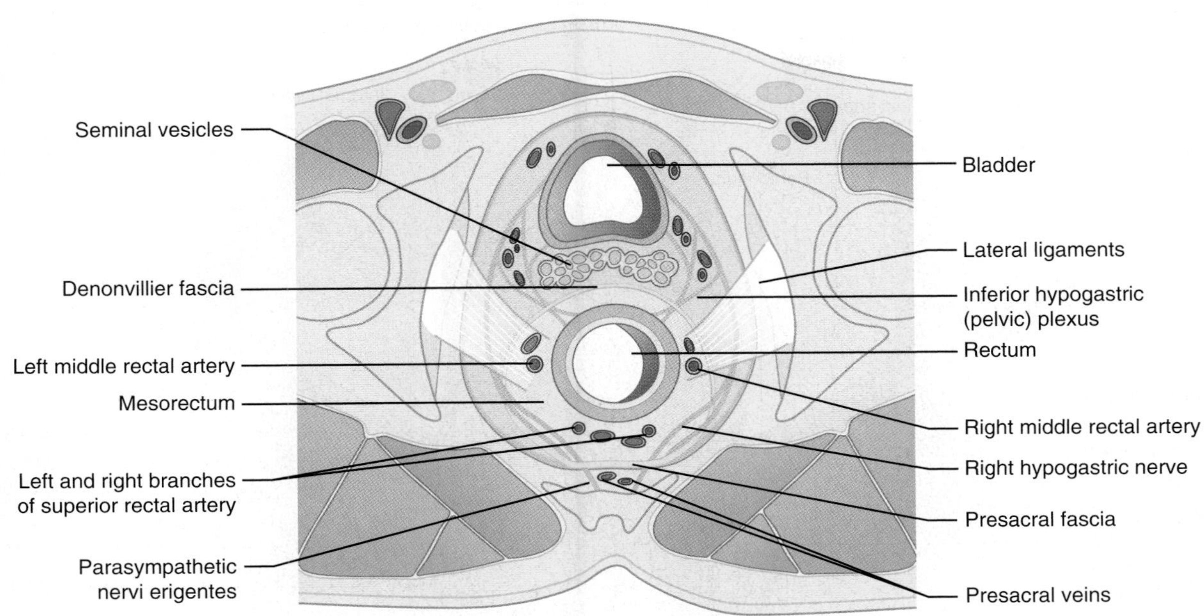

FIG. 52.11 Cross-section of mesorectum and surrounding structures. (From Netz U, Galandiuk S. Clinical anatomy for procedures involving the small bowel, colon, rectum and anus. In: Fischer JE, Ellison EC, Upchurgh Jr. GR, et al., eds. *Fischer's Mastery of Surgery*. 7th ed. Philadelphia: Wolter Kluwer; 2019.)

upper rectal cancers, which are much more likely to metastasize to the liver.

The lymph from the upper two thirds of the rectum drains upward toward the inferior mesenteric and paraaortic nodes. The lower part of the rectum drains in two directions, cephalad toward the inferior mesenteric nodes and laterally and inferiorly toward the internal iliac nodes. Below the dentate line, lymph drains toward the inguinal lymph nodes.

The sympathetic innervation of the rectum is derived from sympathetic nerves exiting at the level of L1–3, forming the superior hypogastric plexus (Fig. 52.13). At the level of the sacral promontory, they divide into left and right hypogastric nerves, traveling on both sides of the pelvis. These nerves supply the rectum and send branches to supply the genitourinary system anteriorly. When performing pelvic operations, it is important to be aware of these nerves and avoid injuring them if possible. A high IMA ligation injuring the superior hypogastric plexus or severing the hypogastric nerves near the sacral promontory may result in sympathetic dysfunction characterized by retrograde ejaculation in men. Division of the lateral stalks too close to the pelvic sidewall may injure the pelvic plexus and nervi erigentes and cause erectile dysfunction, impotence, and atonic bladder. Injury to the periprostatic plexus when dissecting anteriorly can also cause sexual and bladder dysfunction.

Pelvic Floor Anatomy

The pelvic floor or diaphragm supports the pelvic organs and, together with the anal sphincter, regulates defecation. The pelvic diaphragm resides between the sacrum, obturator fascia, ischial spines, and pubis. The levator ani muscle, which makes up the floor, consists of three subdivisions: the pubococcygeus, iliococcygeus, and the puborectalis (Fig. 52.14). The pubococcygeus forms the levator hiatus, which ellipses the top of the anal canal, urethra, and vagina in women and the dorsal vein in men. The puborectalis originates in the lower part of the symphysis pubis and courses parallel to the anorectal junction, forming a U-shaped sling of striated muscle posterior to the rectum. The puborectalis is in a state of constant contraction, increasing the anorectal angle, a factor critical to the maintenance of fecal continence. Relaxation of the puborectalis straightens the anorectal angle and permits defecation. Puborectalis dysfunction is an important cause of defecation disorders.

PHYSIOLOGY OF THE COLON

Absorption of Fluid and Electrolytes

The major functions of the colon are water absorption and electrolyte exchange. This process converts succus from the terminal ileus into formed stool that is stored in the rectal reservoir until it can be excreted at a convenient time. The body has the ability to adapt and sustain life without a colon, making it uniquely different to small bowel. The problems associated with colonic patients provide a simplistic view of colonic function—individuals with a diverting ileostomy are at particular risk for dehydration and electrolyte derangement.

By surface area, the colon is the most efficient site of absorption in the GI tract. It has the ability to absorb up to 5 L of fluid per day; however, only 1 to 2 L are generally excreted from the ileum. By the time succus reaches the terminal ileum, most of the nutrients have been absorbed, leaving a mix of electrolyte-rich fluid, bile salts, and some proteins and starches that have resisted digestion. Approximately 90% of the fluid in succus is reabsorbed in the colon, and the total volume of water in stool is only ~150 mL/day. The colon's ability to absorb sodium is equally impressive. Succus in the ileum has a sodium concentration of 200 mEq/L that is reduced to approximately 30 mEq/L in rectal stool.

Sodium and chloride are actively absorbed via Na^+/H^+, Na^+/K^+, and Cl^-/HCO_3^- exchange. Water is passively absorbed and follows sodium along an osmotic gradient. Potassium chloride and bicarbonate are actively secreted into the lumen.

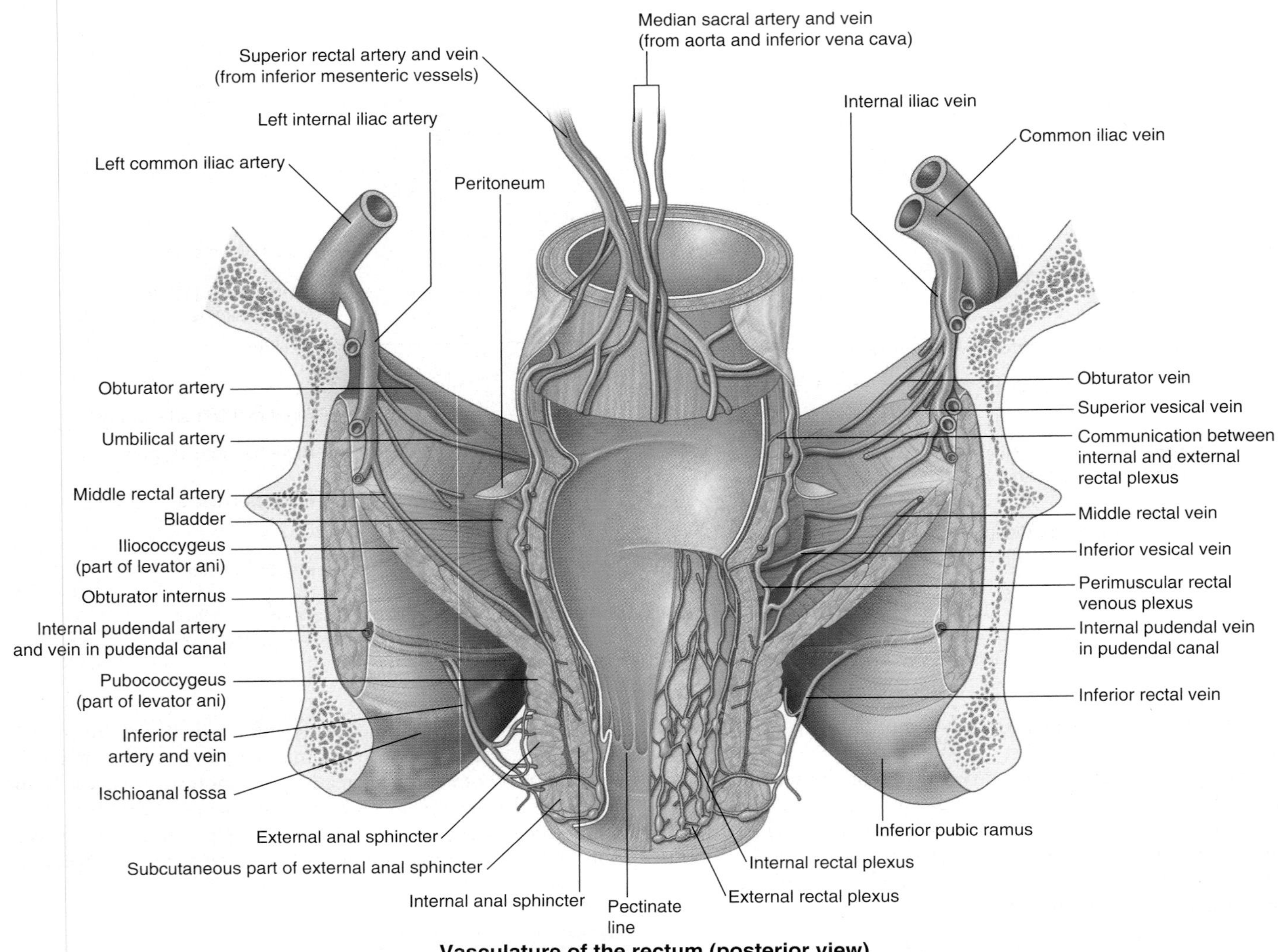

FIG. 52.12 Vasculature of the rectum, posterior view. (From Drake RL, Vogl AW, Mitchell AWM, et al. *Gray's Atlas of Anatomy*. 2nd ed. Philadelphia: Churchill Livingstone, an imprint of Elsevier; 2015.)

Secretion

The physiologic role of colon secretion is demonstrated in patients with chronic renal failure. Uremic patients can remain normokalemic while ingesting a normal amount of potassium before requiring dialysis. This phenomenon is associated with a compensatory increase in colonic secretion and fecal excretion of potassium. Aldosterone promotes colonic potassium secretion, and this effect is blocked by spironolactone.

Many forms of colitis are associated with increased potassium secretion, such as inflammatory bowel disease (IBD), cholera, and shigellosis. In addition, some forms of colitis impair colonic absorption or produce secretion of chloride, such as collagenous and microscopic colitis and congenital chloridorrhea. Chloride is secreted by colonic epithelium at a basal rate, which is increased in pathologic conditions such as cystic fibrosis and secretory diarrhea.

Colonic secretion of H^+ and bicarbonate is coupled to the absorption of Na^+ and Cl^-, respectively. It is through these exchangers that the colon is linked to systemic acid-base metabolism. The supply of H^+ and bicarbonate for these exchangers is catalyzed by colonic carbonic anhydrase. Changes in systemic pH induce changes in the activity of carbonic anhydrase, eliciting elimination of H^+ or bicarbonate as needed to bring the systemic pH back to normal.

Urea Recycling

Colonic bacteria are rich in urease, which is important for urea recycling. Since mammalian cells do not produce urease, this process relies on the symbiotic relationship found in a healthy colonic lumen. Ammonia is the by-product of urea metabolism, and its absorption depends on the concentration of bacteria present and the intraluminal pH. Antibiotics and lactulose decrease the amount of ammonia absorbed by lowering the concentration of bacteria and reducing the pH, respectively. Absorbed ammonia is transported to the liver.

Urea recycling is not beneficial in cases of liver failure. When the liver cannot reuse the urea nitrogen absorbed by the colon, ammonia crosses the blood-brain barrier and produces "false" neurotransmitters, which results in hepatic coma.

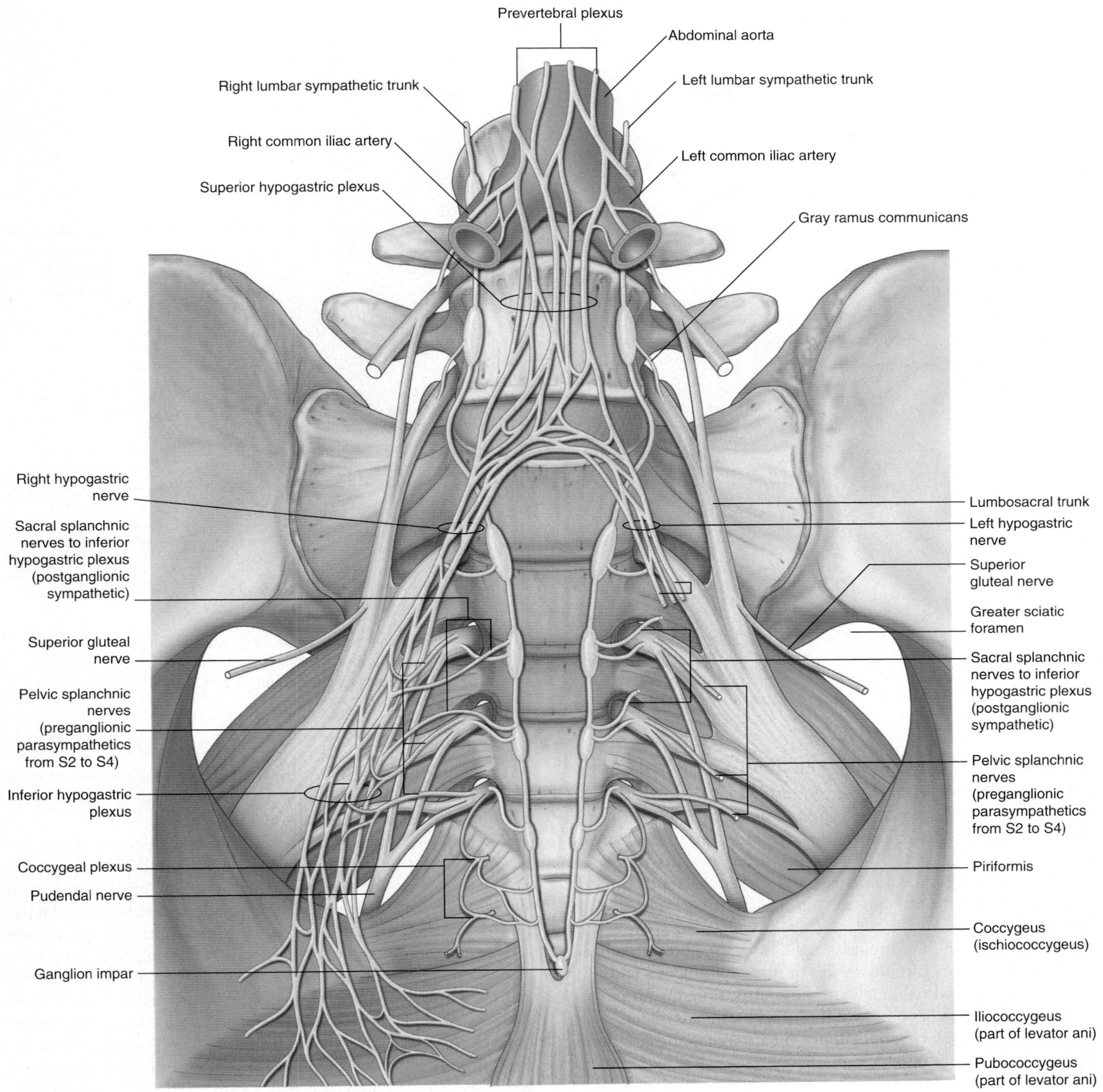

Pelvic extensions of the prevertebral nerve plexus (anterior view)

FIG. 52.13 Pelvic nerve plexus. (From Drake RL, Vogl AW, Mitchell AWM, et al. *Gray's Atlas of Anatomy*. 2nd ed. Philadelphia: Churchill Livingstone, an imprint of Elsevier; 2015.)

Recycling Bile Salts

The colon absorbs bile acids that escape absorption by the terminal ileum. Bile acids are passively transported across the colonic epithelium by nonionic diffusion. When the colonic absorptive capacity is exceeded, colonic bacteria deconjugate bile acids. Deconjugated bile acids can then interfere with sodium and water absorption, leading to secretory, or choleretic, diarrhea. Choleretic diarrhea is seen early after right hemicolectomy as a transient phenomenon and more permanently after extensive ileal resection. This diarrhea can often be effectively treated by administration of cholestyramine, which binds to bile acids.

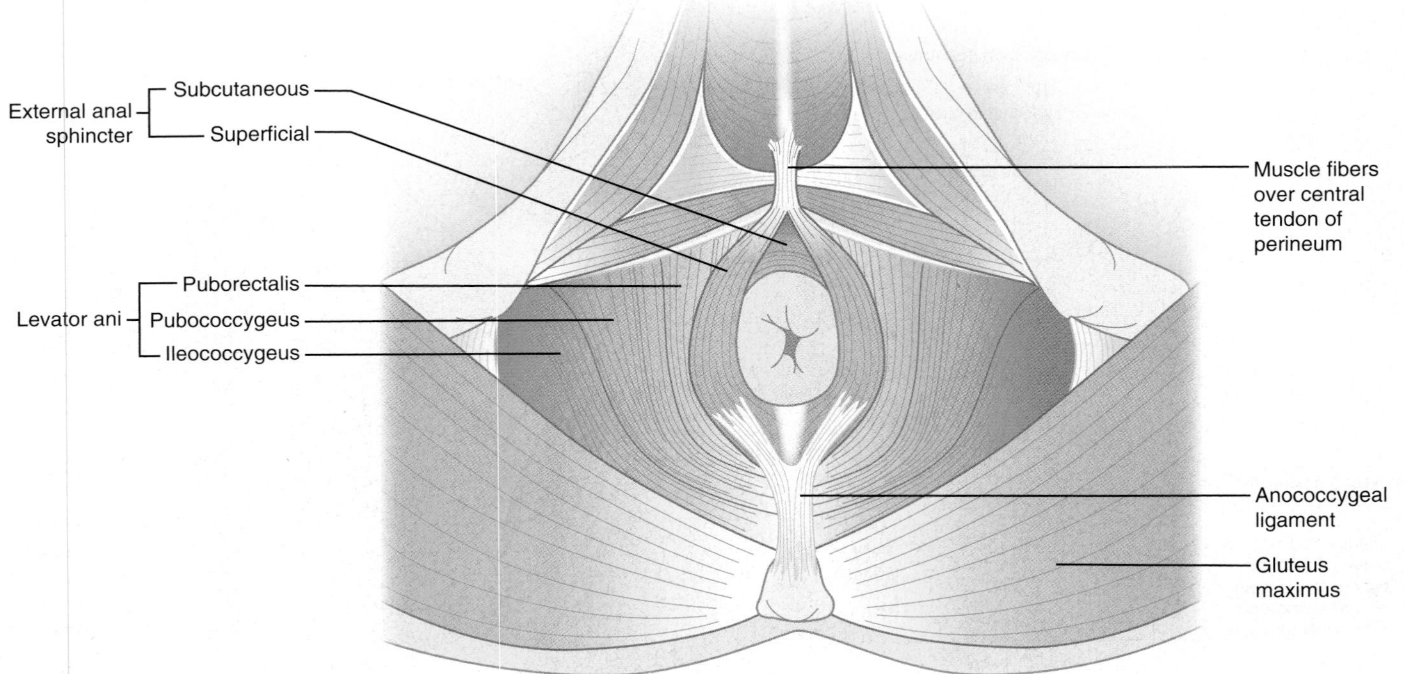

FIG. 52.14 The pelvic musculature and innervation from below. The deep anal sphincter muscles are hidden under the superficial part. (From Netz U, Galandiuk S. Clinical anatomy for procedures involving the small bowel, colon, rectum and anus. In: Fischer JE, Ellison EC, Upchurgh Jr. GR, et al., eds. *Fischer's Mastery of Surgery*. 7th ed. Philadelphia: Wolter Kluwer; 2019.)

Colonic Flora, Fermentation, and Short-Chain Fatty Acids

Large bowel contents have a concentration of 10^{11} to 10^{12} bacterial cells per gram, contributing approximately 50% of fecal mass. Over 400 bacterial species, mostly anaerobic, are present in the colon. Bacteroides species are obligate anaerobes that comprise two thirds of the total colonic bacteria. Other species commonly found in the colonic flora are the following facultative anaerobes: *Escherichia*, *Klebsiella*, *Proteus*, *Lactobacillus*, and *Enterococci*. These bacteria feed on proteins sloughed from the bowel wall and undigested complex carbohydrates. In turn, colonocytes and gut-associated lymphoid tissue rely on the colonic flora for nutrients.

The main source of energy for intestinal bacteria is dietary fiber, composed of complex carbohydrates (i.e., starches and nonstarch polysaccharides). However, not all complex carbohydrates are fermented in the same manner. Dietary recommendations (i.e., "adding fiber") generally refer to bulking agents, such as lignin and psyllium, which are nonabsorbable and nonfermentable by colonic bacteria. Bulking agents decrease intracolonic pressures and increase colonic transit time, which help prevent the formation of colonic diverticula and minimize colonic exposure to toxins.

For the fermentable complex carbohydrates available, colonic flora produce short-chain fatty acids (SCFAs). Butyrate, an SCFA, is the principal source of nutrition for the colonocyte. Because mammalian cells do not produce butyrate, the colonic epithelium and luminal bacteria form an essential and elegant symbiotic relationship. Antibiotics disrupt this cohabitation—decreased bacteria leads to less butyrate, which, in turn, negatively affects colonocyte function leading to diarrhea. Likewise, mucosal atrophy is seen after fecal diversion (i.e., diversion colitis). The other physiologic effects of SCFAs on the colon include stimulation of blood flow, mucosal cell renewal, and regulation of intraluminal pH for homeostasis of the bacterial flora.

The role of SCFAs on homeostasis extends beyond the colon. Besides butyrate, two other SCFAs, acetate and propionate, are produced in the colon, with acetate being the most common of all three. Over 90% of the SCFAs produced are absorbed. Hepatocytes metabolize SCFAs for use in gluconeogenesis, and muscle cells oxidize acetate to generate energy. Additionally, acetate is the primary substrate for cholesterol synthesis. The production of acetate is reduced by nonabsorbable, nonfermentable dietary fiber, such as psyllium, which in turn has a beneficial effect on cholesterol levels. Similarly, propionate, which has a glycolytic role in the liver, may also lower serum lipid levels by inhibiting cholesterol synthesis. Butyrate may also play an important role in maintaining cellular health by arresting the proliferation of neoplastic colonocytes while paradoxically being trophic for normal colonocytes.

The end products of fermentation are SCFAs and gas—carbon dioxide, methane, and hydrogen. In addition to nonstarch polysaccharides, colonic bacteria ferment poorly absorbed starches and proteins from the upper GI tract. Although highly variable from person to person, the gases produced by bacterial fermentation compose approximately 50% of flatus, with the remainder consisting of swallowed air.

Protein fermentation (i.e., putrefaction) results in the formation of potentially toxic metabolites, including phenols, indoles, and amines. The production of these toxins is inhibited in intestinal bacteria by the presence of carbohydrate energy sources. This process becomes accentuated more distally in the colon as carbohydrate sources become scarcer. These end products of bacterial metabolism can lead to mucosal injury and reactive hyperproliferation, which have been hypothesized to promote carcinogenesis.

Probiotics and Prebiotics

Probiotics can be defined as dietary supplements that contain live cultures of bacteria and/or yeast that are beneficial to colonic and host function. The two most widely used agents are *Lactobacillus* and *Bifidobacterium*. Studies have indicated that probiotics may have widespread health benefits, including stimulation of immune function, anti-inflammatory effects, and suppression of enteropathogenic colonization.[1] In addition, they may increase the digestibility of dietary proteins and enhance absorption of amino acids. Probiotics have been shown to prevent *Clostridium difficile*–associated diarrhea, but there are insufficient data to recommend probiotics for the primary prevention of *C. difficile* infection (CDI).[1] Indications for probiotics use are evolving. Currently, there are a small number of studies to support the role of probiotics for the following colorectal conditions: necrotizing enterocolitis in neonates, ulcerative colitis (UC), pouchitis, and constipation. Further research is needed, but the evidence for probiotic use in various settings is encouraging.

Prebiotics are nutrients that support the growth of probiotic bacteria. Prebiotics are nondigestible oligosaccharides (e.g., inulin) that help the host by stimulating the growth of certain species of beneficial intestinal bacteria. There is a growing body of data suggesting health benefits; however, there is currently little evidence to guide recommendations for their use.

Colonic Motility

In the colon, there is extrinsic and intrinsic innervation made up by the autonomic nervous system and enteric nervous system, respectively. The autonomic nervous system is comprised of parasympathetic and sympathetic innervation. Parasympathetic innervation is excitatory, and it reaches the colon via the vagus nerve and the rectum via the sacral nerves (S2–S4) through the pelvic plexus. Sympathetic innervation is, conversely, inhibitory. Sympathetic fibers originate from lumber ventral roots (L2–L5), postganglionic hypogastric nerves, and the splanchnic nerves (T5–T12), which reach the colon and rectum through perivascular plexuses (see also the section on Colon Anatomy).

The intrinsic colonic nervous system consists of the myenteric (Auerbach) plexus and the submucosal (Meissner) plexus. These plexus regulate colonic motility, as well as colonic blood flow, absorption, and secretion. The interstitial cells of Cajal are the primary pacemaker cells governing the function of the enteric nervous system and are important for colonic motility. Most motility is involuntary and is divided into two primary patterns: (1) low-amplitude propagated contractions (LAPCs) and (2) high-amplitude propagated contractions (HAPCs). LAPCs allow mixing, which promotes optimal absorption and are bursts of short-duration contractions. HAPCs propagate colonic contents distally in a coordinated fashion, and their role lies in shifting large quantities of contents through the colon one to three times per day. Other factors affecting motility are circadian rhythms and food ingestion.

Defecation

Normal defecation requires adequate colonic transit time, stool consistency, and fecal continence. The frequency of defecation is just as variable among individuals as is their perception of abnormal stool frequency. The definitions of diarrhea and constipation differ by individual patients and providers; therefore, reporting stool frequency and consistency provides a clearer understanding of defecation patterns.

Many factors influence colonic transit rate. Colonic transit is longer in women than in men and longer in premenopausal than in postmenopausal women. Supplementation with nonstarch polysaccharides shortens colonic transit time in individuals with idiopathic constipation.

PREOPERATIVE EVALUATION

Nutritional and Risk Assessment

Over the last 20 years since the original work on the National Veterans' Administration Surgical Risk Study, few parameters have been as reliable at predicting postoperative complications as the preoperative serum albumin level. Unfortunately, this laboratory value is seldom obtained preoperatively in elective surgery patients and therefore needs to be explicitly ordered. There are numerous preoperative indices such as POSSUM, CR-POSSUM, and the ACS-NSQIP calculators and others that have been used to predict operative risk. If operating on a patient with a condition such as diverticulitis, or IBD, the addition of an inflammatory marker such as C-reactive protein (CRP) may be beneficial. In general, patients with an albumin less than 3 are considered higher risk. Some studies suggest that preoperative correction of risk factors may result in improved postoperative outcomes. There is a growing field of immunonutrition suggesting that consumption of nutritional supplements rich in arginine may, in fact, boost the immune system and lead to a reduction in postoperative infectious complications, such as surgical site infection (SSI).[2]

Patients who are at particularly high risk are those who have chronic partial bowel obstruction and cancer and those who have lost a significant amount of weight (greater than 10% of body weight) in unintentional weight loss.

Preoperative Bowel Preparation

As human feces can have as much as 10^{12} bacteria/gram, colon surgery has been associated with a higher rate of SSI than small bowel and upper GI surgery. Issues of antibiotic prophylaxis have focused upon the choice of an antibiotic with an appropriate spectrum, administration prior to making the surgical incision, and discontinuation of the antibiotic postoperatively. Over the last 20 years, performing or omitting preoperative bowel preparation has been a cyclical phenomenon. The reader is referred to the American Society of Colon & Rectal Surgeons' Clinical Practice Guidelines for the Use of Bowel Preparation in Elective Colon and Rectal Surgery for a more in-depth coverage of this issue. Studies suggest that mechanical bowel preparation alone is not beneficial prior to *colon* resection. These recommendations were based upon findings that bowel preparation generally led to fluid and electrolyte abnormalities that, in turn, led to large volumes of fluid administration during surgery and subsequent bowel edema and ileus. In addition, bowel preparation is poorly tolerated in the elderly and in those with multiple medical comorbidities. Lower volume bowel preparations generally have higher patient compliance. Higher rates of spillage of liquid as opposed to more formed stool at the time of surgery following mechanical bowel preparation was thought to be the cause of the higher observed rates of SSI. However, for many surgeons performing rectal resection, either with minimally invasive or open techniques, particularly when inserting intraluminal staplers for the purpose of creating intestinal anastomoses, it was felt to be more convenient and safer to have the large bowel free of solid particulate matter. Recently, large administrative database studies have demonstrated that the combination of a mechanical and an oral antibiotic bowel preparation is associated with a very low rate of postoperative infectious complications in patients undergoing colorectal surgery. Generally, many surgeons believe that a formal mechanical bowel preparation is not required for patients undergoing surgery for IBD since these patients are already having numerous liquid bowel movements. Bowel preparation is also not used for patients with partial obstruction.

Planning Intestinal Stomas

When operating on a patient in whom there may be a need for a diverting stoma (e.g., patients with Crohn disease, diverticular disease, intestinal obstruction, and low rectal cancer), it is *always* wise to mark the patient for a preoperative stoma site. *Most* patients do not have an ideal abdomen. The area of the abdomen that usually is chosen for a stoma, the infraumbilical fat mound (Fig. 52.15), may not look the same in a patient who is sitting up as it does when they are recumbent. In many patients, there are skin folds that may prevent a stoma bag from sealing properly. It is essential to mark the patients in a sitting position and to avoid old scars and any skin folds that may interfere with adherence of a stoma appliance. Fig. 52.16 shows how important it is to avoid skin folds that would interfere with a normal adherence of a stoma appliance and how this can be underestimated if the patient is supine.

Stoma Types

Many different types of stoma configurations can be chosen at the time of surgery. Stomas can be differentiated by whether they:

- are small bowel stomas or colostomies
- drain stool or urine
- are temporary or permanent
- are end, loop, or end-loop stomas.

Temporary stomas are often chosen to aid in anastomotic healing or in the presence of sepsis or other conditions, when it is not considered not safe to perform an unprotected anastomosis. Loop ileostomies are often chosen for temporary diversion due to their lack of odor, ease of care, and ease of closing. Loop descending or sigmoid colostomies can similarly easily be closed. Transverse loop colostomies should seldom be used, as they are large, very prone to prolapse, and can be difficult to maintain pouch adherence, frequently being located in an area around the patient's belt line or mid-upper abdomen.

Temporary diversion can be performed for a number of situations. Most often, temporary diversion is used to aid in healing of distal anastomosis. Alternatively, diversion of the fecal stream is sometimes recommended in patients undergoing treatment of distal pathology, such as anal squamous cell carcinoma, in order to make the treatment (e.g., chemoradiation) more tolerable. In these scenarios, a diverting stoma is anticipated to be closed after healing of the anastomosis or after conclusion of treatment. Each of the three different types of stomas (end, loop, and end loop) has advantages and disadvantages. The **consistency** and **amount** of stoma effluent can differ significantly depending on:

- whether the small bowel or the colon is selected for stoma construction

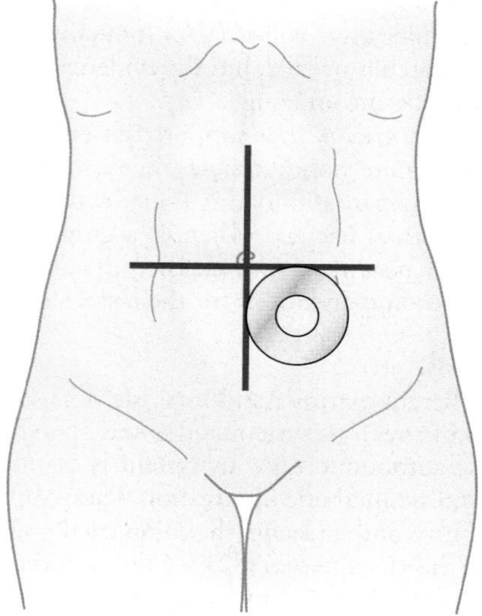

FIG. 52.15 Demonstration of the infraumbilical fat mound that is the ideal stoma site in many patients, here showing marking for a descending colostomy.

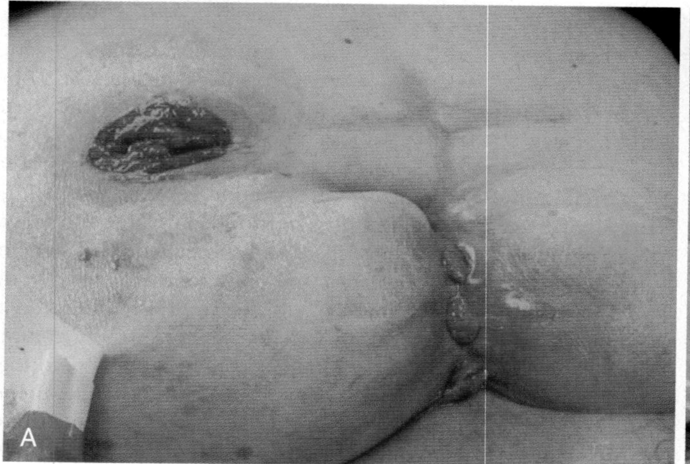

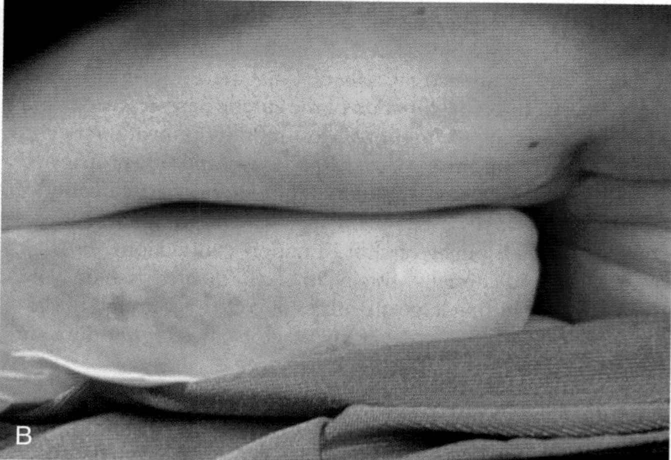

FIG. 52.16 Patient referred following surgery for ischemic colitis without preoperative stoma marking. (A) Patient in supine position. (B) Patient sitting up. Note the colostomy "disappears" within folds of her abdominal wall making pouching extremely difficult.

- if the colon is selected, upon which site of the colon is selected for stoma construction
- what types of treatment (radiation) the patient has undergone
- previous bowel resection(s) the patient may have had.

Colostomy

Ascending colostomies tend to have a higher amount of liquid effluent, while descending and left-sided colostomies are usually preferable, as most of the colon is in circuit, allowing for more colonic water absorption, with a more formed effluent, while still providing proximal diversion.

With the increasing body mass index of patients in the United States today, creating a well-functioning stoma can be a challenge. Both early and late complications can occur with stoma construction. Remember, **a stoma should look good at the end of an operation**! This is your best opportunity to address issues of stoma construction. One should not make the error of hoping that a suboptimal-appearing stoma will improve postoperatively. While edema secondary to obstruction may improve, ischemia does not and will only worsen over time. If there is doubt about stoma viability, construct the stoma *prior* to closing the abdomen, when revision is easy. A key aspect to creating a good stoma is to create a large enough aperture in the abdominal wall to allow the stoma to reach to the skin without tension, but not to create such a wide opening that the patient will develop a hernia at the site. Typically, creating an aperture that will admit two fingers is adequate (Fig. 52.17). In addition, one should ensure that the patient is marked for a stoma site preoperatively, as was discussed earlier. It is important to create a muscle-splitting stoma aperture within the rectus muscle and sharply divide the rectus sheath (Fig. 52.18). In creating a colostomy in an obese patient, especially with the left side of the colon, one frequently has to perform the same central vascular ligation as one does for a cancer resection merely to achieve the same degree of mobilization and mobility to enable the colon to reach to the abdominal wall in a tension-free manner. This can particularly be true with patients who have a very rigid abdominal wall and those with a very thick layer of subcutaneous tissue. In constructing an end colostomy, typically this does not need to protrude more than 0.5 to 1 cm above the level of the abdominal skin. However, there are some circumstances where the patient may be expected to have a more liquid effluent (e.g., due to receiving chemotherapy), and one may wish to have the stoma protrude more to permit easier pouch placement and adherence. In the presence of a liquid effluent, a protruding "spout-like" stoma is always easier to maintain pouch adherence compared with a flatter stoma. In the obese patient, it is sometimes easier to construct an end-loop colostomy than an end colostomy if complete fecal diversion is required. This is constructed in a similar fashion as a loop-end ileostomy (see later), whereby a loop of mesentery is brought up, rather than an end of mesentery. Remember, traditional loop colostomies are not always completely diverting. If one wishes total diversion, an end-loop stoma, with tacking of the distal limb in close proximity of the stoma site, may be a preferable option. Also remember that, in obese individuals, the thinnest part of the abdominal wall is often in the upper abdomen.

Ileostomy

As with colostomy, an ileostomy can be constructed as an end ileostomy, loop, or end-loop ileostomy (Fig. 52.19). Ileostomies are generally favored by colorectal surgeons for fecal diversion as they are easier to construct, especially in obese individuals, usually easier to close, and do not risk compromising the marginal vessels of the colon that are so important to the viability of low and ultralow colorectal and coloanal anastomoses. Ileostomy effluent usually has no odor, in contrast to colostomy effluent, which usually has odor associated with colonic flora. However, in contrast to a colostomy, an ileostomy will empty continuously and has a high rate of associated chemical dermatitis due to the more alkaline pH associated with small bowel effluent as opposed to the stool of the colon. There is also a much higher risk of dehydration with an ileostomy, which is a frequent reason for hospital readmission following elective colorectal surgery. Prior to hospital discharge, one should ensure that the 24-hour stoma output is less than 1000 mL.

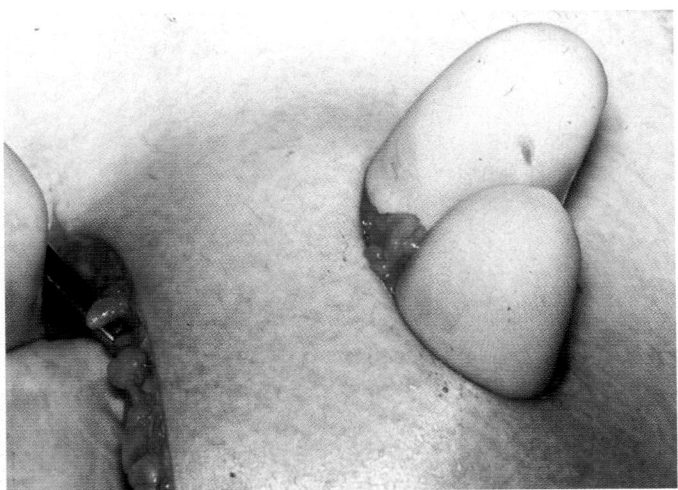

FIG. 52.17 A stoma aperture that admits two fingers is typically of adequate size to allow the bowel and mesentery to pass without tension. In cases of obstruction or an obese mesentery, a larger aperture will be needed.

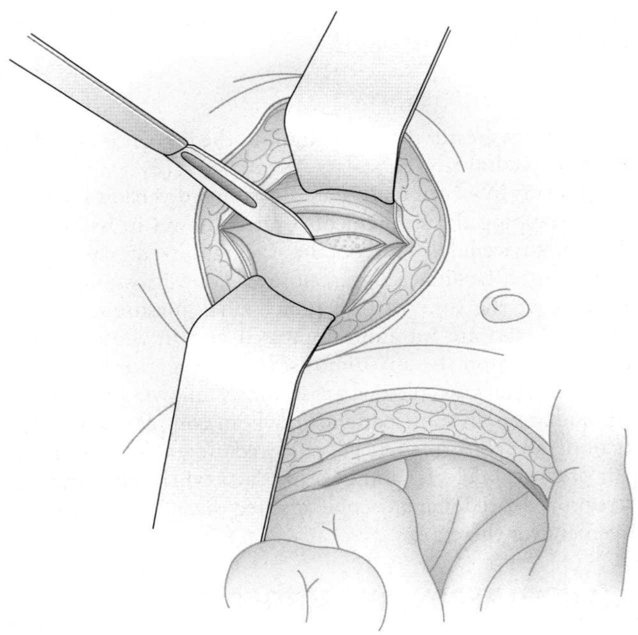

FIG. 52.18 In making the stoma aperture in the abdominal wall, the rectus muscle is split and the rectus sheath is divided sharply. In laparoscopic cases, one can cut down directly on the trocar inserted through this site.

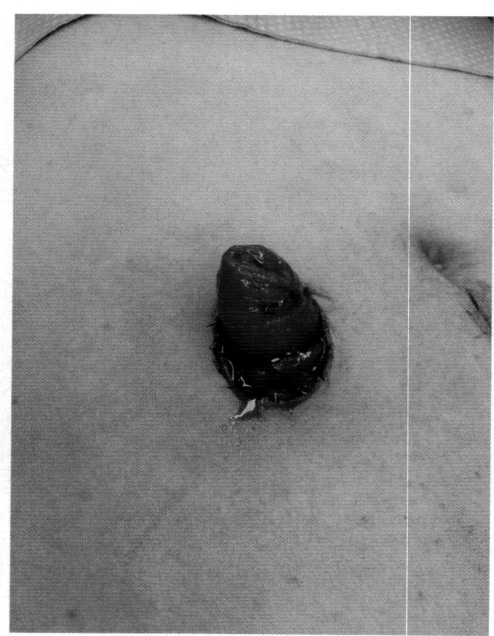

FIG. 52.19 The Intraoperative photo showing the "matured" loop ileostomy protruding 2 to 3 cm above the abdominal wall. The distal limb at skin level is located inferiorly.

If the output is greater than this amount, the patient is at high risk of hospital readmission.

In patients in whom temporary ileostomy diversion is contemplated, wrapping the segment of diverted bowel in hyaluronate-carboxymethylcellulose membrane (Seprafilm) at the time of stoma creation facilitates stoma closure. Loop ileostomy is often performed at the time of ileal pouch–anal anastomosis (IPAA) in patients who are immunosuppressed and in those in whom there is tension on the anastomosis. It is also performed in cases of low colorectal and coloanal anastomosis following neoadjuvant chemoradiation, in some patients in whom complex pelvic reconstructions are performed (e.g., redo rectovaginal fistula repairs, repair of cloacal defects) and in other cases when temporary fecal diversion is desired. Laparoscopic-assisted diversion is particularly convenient for these cases.

ENHANCED RECOVERY PROTOCOLS

The last edition of this textbook reported that protocols for enhanced recovery after surgery had not been widely implemented. Since that time, there has been much attention to enhanced recovery protocols (ERPs) in colorectal surgery with widespread dissemination and implementation in the community. These protocols, also called *fast-track* or *enhanced recovery after surgery protocols*, have been shown to reduce complications, length of stay, and cost of care without increasing readmission rates. Protocols include a bundle of components affecting the preoperative, intraoperative, and postoperative phases of care. The factors that comprise a single protocol are numerous and heterogeneous between centers, thus making it difficult to identify the most beneficial components in a bundled protocol. In 2017, the American Society of Colon and Rectal Surgeons (ASCRS) and the Society of American Gastrointestinal and Endoscopic Surgeons published evidence-based guidelines for the components of ERPs.[3]

Preoperative Interventions

Counseling before surgery to set expectations on milestones and discharge criteria is considered a cornerstone of successful ERPs. If an ostomy is a part of the planned operation, marking, education, and counseling on dehydration should be started in the preoperative period. Ostomy creation is an independent risk factor for increased postoperative length of stay, and structured education has been shown to mitigate this risk. Additionally, dehydration is the most common reason for readmission after an ileostomy creation.

Prehabilitation or increasing the patient's physical conditioning before elective surgery may be considered for patients with deconditioning or multiple comorbidities. The evidence to support prehabilitation is in evolution but appears promising.

Preadmission Nutrition and Bowel Preparation

There is strong evidence to support the recommendation of a clear liquid diet up until 2 hours before the induction of anesthesia. However, there is weaker evidence to support the use of per os carbohydrate loading prior to surgery.

Mechanical bowel preparation alone has not shown to be beneficial (strong recommendation based on high-quality evidence, 1A). In the United States, mechanical bowel preparation plus oral antibiotics preparation has become the preferred preparation to reduce complications, including SSIs, especially when left-sided and rectal resections are anticipated. In the American Society of Colon & Rectal Surgeons Clinical Practice Guidelines for the Use of Bowel Preparation in Elective Colon and Rectal Surgery, this practice was given a strong recommendation based on moderate-quality evidence, 1B. Interestingly, a recent randomized controlled trial found no evidence to support this practice for elective colon resection compared to no bowel preparation as a mechanism to reduce SSIs or postoperative morbidity.[4] It is important to note that the majority of reported studies, including this one, were performed in patients undergoing colon as opposed to rectal resections.

Perioperative Interventions

ERPs commonly involve preset orders for the preoperative, intraoperative, and postoperative care for all patients. Standardization requires collaborative buy-in from different stakeholders, which helps avoid confusion and promotes timely adherence to care.

Colorectal surgery patients have up to a 20% risk of developing a SSI postoperatively. Bundles of care aimed at SSI reduction have shown SSI rates to be significantly reduced. These bundles include some, if not all, of the following measures: preoperative chlorhexidine shower, mechanical bowel preparation with oral antibiotics, prophylactic antibiotic administration within 1 hour of incision, the use of wound protectors during surgery, changing gown, gloves, and instruments before fascial closure, euglycemia, and normothermia. The degree to which each element impacts the reduction of SSIs is unclear.

There is strong evidence to support the use of multimodal, opioid-sparing, pain management plans starting before the induction of anesthesia. Minimizing opioids is associated with earlier return of bowel function and shorter length of stay. Acetaminophen, nonsteroidal antiinflammatory drugs (NSAIDs), and gabapentin have all been incorporated into various ERPs. Transverse abdominis plane block with local anesthetic, including liposomal bupivacaine, have shown promising results. Epidural analgesia is generally recommended for open, but not laparoscopic, colorectal surgery.

The use of goal-directed fluid therapy in the intraoperative and postoperative phases of care is associated with a reduction in time to return of bowel function and length of stay. Lastly, minimally invasive surgical (MIS) approaches should be used, when possible, with avoidance of routine use of intraabdominal drains and nasogastric tubes.

Postoperative Interventions

Early patient mobilization with early feeding has good evidence to support its role in an ERP. Alvimopan use has been shown to hasten return of bowel function after open surgery, but not with MIS. In addition, intravenous (IV) fluids and urinary catheters should be discontinued early in the postoperative period.

In summary, ERPs are evidence-based protocols that benefit colorectal surgery patients. Local implementation involves buy-in for a range of stakeholders that may be in opposition to the preferences of individual healthcare professionals. Adherence to the constellation of ERP components and the outcomes of interest should be continually monitored and evaluated.

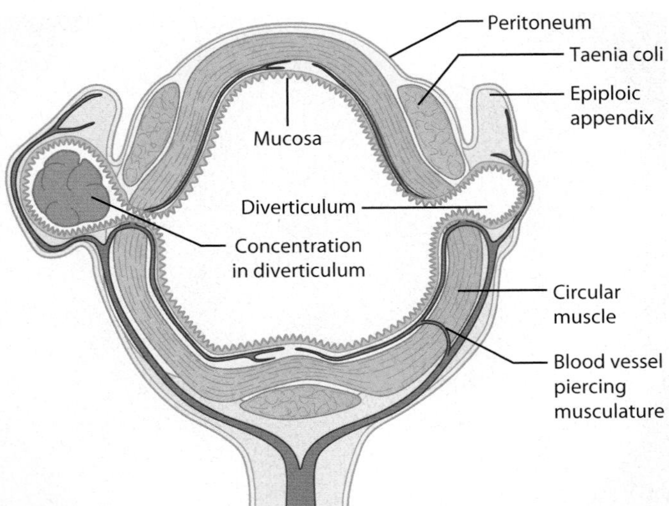

FIG. 52.20 Pathogenesis of diverticulosis. (From Netter FH. *Netter Collection of Medical Illustrations*. Vol 9. Philadelphia: Elsevier Saunders; 2016:145.)

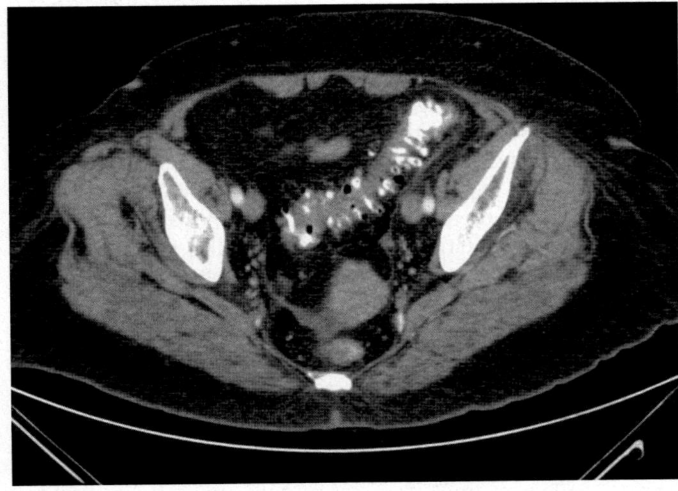

FIG. 52.21 Computed tomography scan of the pelvis showing extensive sigmoid diverticulosis.

DIVERTICULAR DISEASE

Background

Diverticular disease is used to describe a spectrum of manifestations associated with colonic diverticulosis. Diverticula are saccular outpouchings of the bowel wall. They are described as "true" diverticula when they contain all layers of the bowel wall; these are rare and usually congenital. The vast majority of diverticula in the colon are "false" diverticula (pulsion, pseudodiverticula), containing only the mucosa and muscularis mucosa. Diverticulitis is thought to be mainly a disease of the modern world, coinciding with dietary changes following the industrial revolution.

Pathophysiology and Epidemiology

Hypertrophy of the muscular layers of the colon wall, combined with a narrowed lumen and disordered colonic motility, causes localized high-pressure zones in which the mucosa herniates through areas of relative weakness. Diverticula are classically formed on the mesenteric side of the colonic wall in regions where vasa recta traverse through the muscular layer to provide blood to the mucosa (Fig. 52.20). The sigmoid and descending colon are typically affected, whereas the rectum, having an extra layer of muscle, is generally not affected (Fig. 52.21). This has implications for surgery and is why the distal anastomosis margin in operations for diverticulitis should always be within the rectum. Diverticulosis increases with age and is relatively rare in young adults. Colonic diverticula are noted in approximately 40% of individuals between the ages of 50 and 60 years and in over 60% of individuals over the age of 80 years (Fig. 52.22). The mechanism for developing diverticulitis is thought to be a result of obstruction of the orifice of a diverticulum, with stasis leading to bacterial overgrowth, inflammation, and increased pressure within the diverticulum, causing ischemia and microperforation. Interestingly, only a small proportion of patients with diverticulosis develop diverticulitis. Modern estimates indicate that fewer than 5% of patients with diverticulosis will develop diverticulitis; however, due to the high prevalence of diverticulosis, it has become a significant clinical and financial burden, accounting for more than 2.7 million outpatient visits in the United States annually and more than 200,000 inpatient admissions for diverticulitis at an estimated cost of more than $2 billion.

Diet and lifestyle factors play an important role in diverticular disease. Western dietary patterns high in red meat, fat, and refined grains are associated with an increased risk of the disease, whereas increased fiber intake, with abundant fruit, vegetables, and whole grains, reduces the risk of diverticulitis. Intake of nuts, seeds, and popcorn does not appear to increase the risk. Central obesity and smoking increase the risk, whereas physical activity such as running has been correlated with a decreased risk. A study examining the joint contribution of multiple lifestyle risk factors, defined as fewer than four servings of red meat per week, at least 23 g of fiber per day, 2 hours of vigorous activity per week, a body mass index 18.5 to 24.9 kg/m^2, and no history of smoking on the risk of incident diverticulitis, found that adherence to a low-risk lifestyle could prevent 50% of incident diverticulitis.[5]

Clinical Evaluation

Diverticular disease can manifest as diverticulitis, but it is also the most common reason for severe lower GI bleeding (discussed

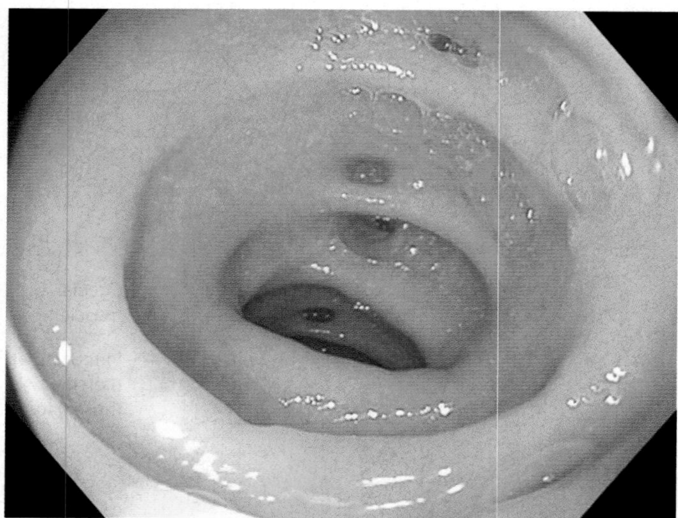

FIG. 52.22 Endoscopic view of diverticulosis.

TABLE 52.1 Modified Hinchey classification system.	
Stage 0	Mild clinical diverticulitis
Stage Ia	Confined pericolic inflammation—phlegmon
Stage Ib	Confined pericolic abscess (within sigmoid mesocolon)
Stage II	Pelvic, distant intraabdominal or intraperitoneal abscess
Stage III	Generalized purulent peritonitis
Stage IV	Fecal peritonitis

From Klarenbeek BR, de Korte N, van der Peet DL, et al. Review of current classifications for diverticular disease and a translation into clinical practice. *Int J Colorectal Dis*. 2012;27:207–214.

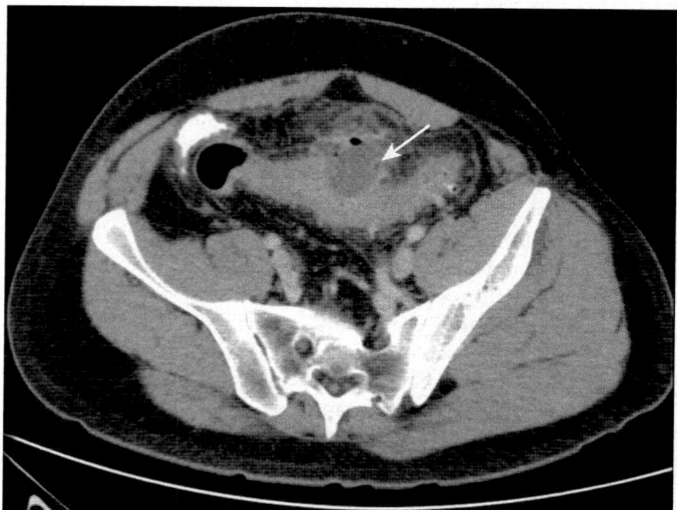

FIG. 52.23 Computed tomography of the pelvis demonstrating sigmoid diverticulitis with a thickened bowel wall, fat stranding a pericolonic abscess *(arrow)*, modified Hinchey grade 1b. 333

elsewhere). Since diverticulitis is caused by inflammation and perforation of a colonic diverticulum, signs and symptoms will generally result from the pericolonic inflammation. Patients will commonly present with abdominal pain localized to the left lower quadrant (following the location of the inflamed sigmoid colon). Additionally, fever, change in bowel habits, anorexia, and urinary urgency (in cases where the bladder is secondarily inflamed) are frequent. On physical examination, localized tenderness is noted, commonly with moderate abdominal distension. A tender mass can be palpable if there is a significant phlegmon. Rectal bleeding is rare in the presentation of acute diverticulitis and should raise suspicion of another diagnosis such as ischemic colitis or IBD. Leukocytosis is a common laboratory finding.

Several imaging modalities have been used to evaluate patients with suspected diverticular disease. Flat and upright plain films can be used to diagnose obstruction or free intraperitoneal air but are generally nonspecific. Contrast studies, ultrasound, and magnetic resonance imaging (MRI) have also been used, but currently, computed tomography (CT) has become the most useful examination to confirm the diagnosis, exclude other diagnoses, and classify the severity of the disease. Signs of diverticulitis on CT include the presence of diverticula, colonic wall thickening, pericolic fat stranding, and abscess formation. CT studies have the capacity to localize abscesses and fistulas and define the extent of the disease. The modified Hinchey classification[6] is the most commonly used tool to describe the severity of diverticulitis (Table 52.1).

Grade 0, not included in the original publication, is commonly used to describe mild clinical diverticulitis. If CT is performed, colonic wall thickening without pericolonic fat stranding can be seen. Grade 1a presents with a phlegmon with colonic wall thickening and pericolonic fat stranding, while grade 1b also includes a pericolonic or mesocolic abscess (Fig. 52.23). Patients with grade 2 disease have distant intraabdominal or pelvic abscesses. Patients with grade 3 disease have generalized purulent peritonitis, and grade 4 disease, fecal peritonitis. The ability of a CT scan to distinguish between grade 3 and grade 4 is limited, and in these cases, accurate diagnosis is usually made in the operating room.

Flexible endoscopy during the acute setting should be approached with caution because distention of the colon may result in worsening perforation.

Management

Complicated Diverticulitis

Patients with complicated diverticulitis are characterized by the presence of an abscess, fistula, obstruction, or free perforation.

Abscess. Signs and symptoms will depend on the size and location of the abscess, with diagnosis usually provided on imaging. Smaller abscesses can often be treated successfully with antibiotics alone. Larger abscesses will require drainage. Following recovery, elective surgery is generally recommended; however, some of these patients, especially those with smaller abscesses that were treated without drainage, can probably be managed nonoperatively. Patients with abscesses not amenable to percutaneous drainage and unresponsive to treatment require urgent surgery.

Fistula. Fistulas are abnormal connections to surrounding epithelial lined organs and are a relatively common complication of diverticulitis. They are a result of the local inflammation and development of an abscess that decompresses into a neighboring organ. The most common type, especially in men, is a colovesical fistula to the dome of the bladder. Patients will present with recurrent urinary tract infections, which are in many cases polymicrobial. Pneumaturia and fecaluria may also be present. CT can reveal air or contrast in the bladder in the absence of prior instrumentation. Cystoscopy will usually disclose inflammation at the site of the fistula. Colovaginal fistulas occur almost exclusively in women who have undergone previous hysterectomy and present with vaginal discharge and passing of air per vagina. Colocutaneous fistulas usually present at a previous drain site in patients who have undergone percutaneous drainage. Patients with fistulas usually do not need emergency surgery as the abscess has usually decompressed. Initial management includes broad spectrum antibiotics to decrease the inflammation. Patients are then investigated with colonoscopy and appropriate imaging (i.e., cystoscopy) to exclude malignancy and Crohn disease. Surgical principles then encompass resection of the involved colon and fistula tract with primary anastomosis. If possible, the fistula opening into the secondarily involved organ is primarily suture repaired; however, in many cases, the opening is small and difficult to recognize. In the case of the bladder, with small fistula openings, drainage of the bladder with a Foley catheter for 7 to 10 days will usually allow for healing. A cystogram can be done to confirm fistula healing prior to Foley removal. Fistulas to the small bowel will characteristically require resection and primary anastomosis.

Obstruction. Patients with recurrent and chronic diverticulitis can develop fibrosis of the colonic wall, leading to stricture formation. In most cases, these patients will present with insidious symptoms and a partial obstruction. Small bowel obstruction may also be seen as a result of a small bowel loop adhering to an area of inflamed colonic tissue or abscess. Management depends on the degree and type of obstruction. Patients with a partial obstruction can usually be initially treated with a nasogastric tube for decompression, antibiotics, fluids, and bowel rest. If the obstruction resolves, elective resection can be planned. It is usually important, prior to resection, to perform a colonoscopy to rule out malignancy. In cases where the stricture is impossible to pass using a colonoscope, virtual colonoscopy or a retrograde contrast study can be helpful to visualize the remainder of the bowel. Patients with a complete obstruction unresponsive to therapy will require emergency surgery.

Perforation. Patients with a free intraabdominal perforation with widespread contamination will present with diffuse peritonitis with rebound tenderness and guarding. Signs of sepsis including fever, tachycardia, and hemodynamic instability are frequently seen. Imaging can demonstrate free abdominal fluid, signs of peritonitis, and free intraabdominal air. The ability to distinguish between purulent and fecal diverticulitis prior to surgery is limited. Hinchey grades 3 and 4 are considered a surgical emergency. Following initial resuscitation, patients are taken to the operating room with a goal of controlling the source of infection by resection and washing out the abdominal contamination.

The mainstay of treatment in these cases has traditionally been the Hartmann procedure, which removes the involved colon and exteriorizes an end colostomy. Reversing the colostomy, however, requires a second major surgical procedure with its own significant morbidity and mortality. Practically, up to 50% of patients will never be reversed, with even higher rates in the elderly. Given these implications, several studies have investigated alternatives to the Hartmann procedure. One option has been laparoscopic lavage, which entails laparoscopic irrigation of the abdominal cavity to reduce the abdominal contamination and placement of drains without resection (mainly for Hinchey grade 3 diverticulitis). Although this approach results in lower stoma rates, it has been associated with significantly higher rates of ongoing and recurrent sepsis and emergency reoperations.[7] This approach is still controversial and should probably only be used in highly selected individuals. Another option is performing a resection with a primary anastomosis and diverting ileostomy. Although lengthening the initial surgery, this technique has been found to be safe and significantly simplifies and shortens the second operation. Overall morbidity and mortality are similar; however, a much higher proportion of patients will have their stomas reversed (94%–96% for primary anastomosis vs. 65%–72% for Hartmann).[8] This has become an attractive option for patients who are stable enough to withstand the additional time of the initial surgery.

Uncomplicated Diverticulitis

The treatment for uncomplicated diverticulitis depends on the severity of symptoms, and the approach is subsequently individualized. The majority of these patients can be managed as outpatients. The mainstay of treatment is based on pain medications, short-term alteration of diet, and antibiotics. Commonly, patients are initially prescribed clear liquids, followed by a low-residue diet until the inflammation subsides. Antibiotics have traditionally been prescribed to cover colonic bacteria. A systematic review and metaanalysis assessing the effect of antibiotic administration in patients with uncomplicated diverticulitis has not shown the usage of antibiotics to accelerate recovery or prevent complications or subsequent surgery.[9] As a result, some physicians have stopped prescribing antibiotics for uncomplicated diverticulitis.

A small proportion of patients diagnosed with diverticulitis will actually have a colonic neoplasm mimicking diverticulitis. Overall, this is currently estimated at around 1% to 3%, with significantly higher rates observed in complicated disease.[10] Upon recovery, it is recommended that patients undergo a colonoscopy after 4 to 8 weeks to exclude malignancy.

Following the initial episode of acute, uncomplicated diverticulitis, only 10% to 35% of individuals will have another episode.[11] After more episodes, the chances of recurrence increase significantly. In an attempt to avoid severe complicated diverticulitis, elective surgery was previously suggested following uncomplicated diverticulitis, depending on the number of episodes, with the thought that more episodes would lead to more chances of recurrence and a higher chance of severe complicated diverticulitis. However, recurrences in general tend to follow the severity of the initial episode. As a result, the number of attacks of uncomplicated diverticulitis has fallen out of favor as an indication for surgery. Currently, an individual assessment is performed on the frequency of attacks, ongoing symptoms, and their effect on quality of life versus the age and medical condition of the patient and their surgical risk.

The aim of elective surgery is to remove the affected segment of the colon (usually the sigmoid colon) and to perform a primary anastomosis of the healthy remaining bowel. When removing the sigmoid colon, the proximal margin should be in soft pliable bowel, but it is not necessary to include all proximal diverticula. The distal anastomosis, however, should be to the upper rectum, since leaving a section of distal sigmoid colon is associated with a higher risk of recurrent diverticulitis. Surgery can be performed by either an open, laparoscopic, hand-assisted, or robotic approach. MIS for diverticular disease has been shown to be safe, with advantages of more rapid recovery of bowel function, less pain, and shorter hospitalization.

Special Populations

Right-Sided Diverticulitis

This is common in Asian countries but rare in the west. This typically affects younger patients and may be challenging to diagnose as signs and symptoms are very similar to those of acute appendicitis. Other differential diagnoses to be considered include Meckel's diverticulitis, cholecystitis, ischemic colitis, mesenteric adenitis, pyelonephritis, and pelvic inflammatory disease. The recommended approach should generally be similar to that for diverticulitis in other sites. Patients who have recurrent episodes or complicated disease and patients with an uncertain diagnosis should be considered for resection with a right hemicolectomy.

Immunocompromised Patients

Immunocompromised patients include transplant patients; patients with diabetes mellitus, renal failure, or cirrhosis; and patients being treated with systemic steroids and/or chemotherapy. While the prevalence of diverticulitis in these patients is similar to the general population, they are more likely to present with free perforation and complicated disease because of their impaired ability to mount an inflammatory response. Because of this risk, there should be a lower threshold for resection after a single attack of diverticulitis. Immunocompromised patients who require emergency surgery and resection should probably not undergo primary anastomosis at the initial surgery because of their impaired immune system and healing.

Young Patients

Historically, patients younger than 50 were considered to have a more virulent form of diverticulitis and were recommended to undergo resection after one episode of uncomplicated disease. Although current evidence does demonstrate higher rates of recurrence, young patients do not have a higher rate of emergency surgical intervention. Current guidelines do not support treating young patients differently than others.

LARGE BOWEL OBSTRUCTION

Large bowel obstruction, defined as bowel obstruction distal to the ileocecal valve, can occur as a result of a variety of etiologies. Broadly, it is classified into mechanical (dynamic) obstruction and functional (adynamic or pseudoobstruction). Mechanical obstruction can be further characterized into endoluminal, mural, and extraluminal causes (Box 52.1).

The most common etiology of mechanical obstruction in the United States is colorectal cancer (CRC), whereas colonic volvulus is more common in Russia, Eastern Europe, Africa, the Middle East, and India. Presentation and symptoms depend on whether it is an acute obstruction or a more chronic progressive change, as well as partial, in which some gas/fecal contents are able to pass versus complete obstruction in which nothing passes distally. It is thought that worldwide, volvulus is responsible for roughly one third of the cases of large bowel obstruction. The most common site of volvulus is the sigmoid colon; however, cecal volvulus can also occur. Any portion of the colon that is not fixed to the retroperitoneum and that has an elongated mesentery has the potential for volvulus. In these cases, there is an axial twisting of the colon around the mesentery resulting in an obstruction.

BOX 52.1 Large bowel obstruction common etiologies.

Mechanical

Intraluminal

Intrinsic mass—neoplasm
Foreign body
Bezoar
Fecal impaction

Mural

Diverticular stricture
Crohn disease stricture
Ischemic stricture
Radiation stricture
Infectious (i.e., lymphogranuloma venereum, tuberculosis, schistosomiasis)
Hirschsprung disease

Extraluminal

Sigmoid volvulus
Cecal volvulus
Hernia (inguinal, ventral, internal)
Metastatic/intraabdominal tumor
Abdominal abscess
Retroperitoneal fibrosis
Adhesions (rare in large bowel)

Functional

Colonic pseudo-obstruction (Ogilvie)
Toxic megacolon
Paralytic ileus

Mechanical obstruction will generally present with increased peristalsis and low-grade colicky pain, but late, long-lasting obstruction may have decreased bowel sounds. In addition, patients will fail to pass stool and flatus and demonstrate increasing abdominal distention. Acute obstructions tend to present more dramatically with rapid onset of pain, distension, and abdominal tenderness, whereas patients with progressive obstruction may present with increasing constipation, pencil-thin stools, and intermittent abdominal pain. Functional obstruction usually presents with distension, vague abdominal pain, and weak or absent bowel sounds.

Patients with a closed-loop obstruction in which both the proximal and distal parts of a segment of bowel are blocked must be promptly recognized and treated, as they have the potential for ischemia and perforation with rapid deterioration. Closed-loop obstruction is commonly encountered in cases such as volvulus and strangulated hernias. Fig. 52.24 shows a plain film of a patient with a sigmoid volvulus. Note the bent, inner-tube appearance of the colon. The volvulus has resulted in a closed-loop obstruction. In these situations, the colon becomes progressively distended with pressure increasing to the point of ischemic necrosis and perforation. Fig. 52.25 shows a CT scan illustrating the characteristic mesenteric whorl seen in patients with a volvulus.

Another common circumstance of closed-loop obstruction is patients with obstructing colon cancers that have a competent ileocecal valve, which does not allow backflow of intestinal contents. Obstructing cancers with an incompetent ileocecal valve will usually present less acutely, with a much lower chance of

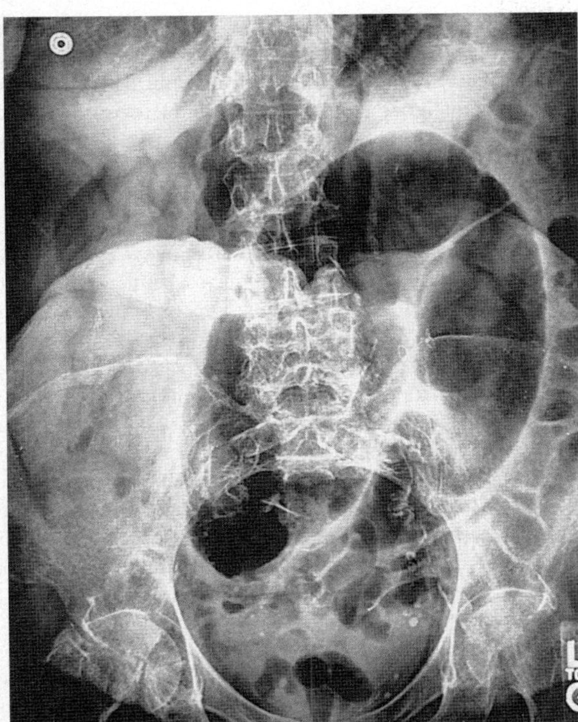

FIG. 52.24 Plain film of sigmoid volvulus. Note bent inner tube appearance.

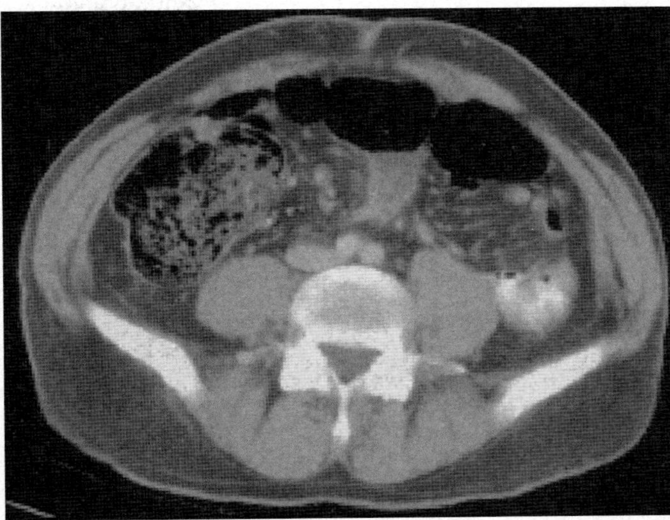

FIG. 52.25 Computed tomography scan of the abdomen in a patient with sigmoid volvulus. Note characteristic whorl in mesentery.

perforation as the valve allows backflow of intestinal contents into the small bowel, resulting in a progressively distended abdomen with nausea and vomiting of a feculent nature.

Distention of the colon occurs as a result of gas and stool that gather proximal to the obstruction. The gas originates both from swallowed air (around two thirds) and bacterial fermentation. In segments that undergo increasing distension, the pressure within the bowel wall can rise above the capillary pressure, diminishing adequate oxygenation, leading to ischemic necrosis and perforation. Although most malignant obstructions occur in the distal parts of the colon, the necrosis and perforation usually occur in the cecum as it has the largest diameter, and in accordance with the law of Laplace will distend more under lower pressures and develop higher wall stress.

In cases such as incarcerated hernias and volvulus, pressure on the mesentery can compromise the blood supply initially obstructing venous return, and with increasing edema and inflammation, eventually occluding the arterial blood supply. The resultant ischemia can also lead to early necrosis and perforation. In closed-loop obstructions, distention initially involves the trapped or incarcerated segment, but with time, the proximal bowel will also distend as a result of ongoing accumulation of gas and stool.

Diagnosis and Assessment

A good history and physical examination are critical in the diagnosis of large bowel obstruction. The onset and progression of symptoms, background illnesses, and medications can provide important clues. The abdomen should be palpated for masses, tenderness, and previous incisions; the groins should be examined for hernias; and a digital rectal examination should be performed to inspect for neoplasms and for the presence of fecal impaction (Fig. 52.26).

Plain films of the abdomen can help in localizing the obstruction, demonstrating the degree of distension as well as the status of the ileocecal valve (competent vs. incompetent), and, in some cases, provide the diagnosis. Water-soluble and IV contrast-enhanced CT scans provide significant information revealing the location and etiology of the obstruction such as diverticulitis, IBD, and extraluminal causes (e.g., abscesses and inflammation) (Fig. 52.27). CT can also provide clues regarding tissue ischemia and impending perforation. Flexible endoscopy can assist in the diagnosis of the obstruction and permit biopsies to be collected for further investigation. Endoscopy can also allow for treatment such as detorsion of a sigmoid volvulus and insertion of stents in cases of malignant or benign obstruction. Basic blood analyses are also important in the initial workup. Electrolyte abnormalities can be diagnosed, which are important both as a cause for adynamic nonfunction and being in the operative and perioperative care. Increased white blood cell counts and CRP, as well as increased lactate, base excess, and decreased pH, are all generally associated with a more severe state and can help guide the aggressiveness of treatment.

Treatment

The treatment of large bowel obstruction is tailored to the etiology of the obstruction, several of which are discussed in detail later in the chapter. Treatment options vary considerably depending on the cause of obstruction, suspicion of bowel ischemia, and impending perforation, as well as the patient's general condition and comorbidities. Patients who present with peritonitis, signs of perforation, or ischemic bowel should be taken immediately to surgery.

It is imperative to promptly relieve mechanical obstructions, particularly those with complete and closed-loop obstructions before compromise of the blood supply results in necrosis and perforation. Patients who do not present with immediate, ominous signs can be managed according to the cause of obstruction. In patients with sigmoid volvulus, endoscopic decompression is often successful using either a rigid or flexible sigmoidoscope with placement of a rectal tube proximal to the point of torsion. If this is unsuccessful, patients require surgery with resection, colostomy, and a Hartmann procedure. If decompression is successful, elective sigmoid resection with primary anastomosis should be performed due to the high rate of recurrence. With cecal volvulus, primary resection and anastomosis can typically be performed unless the patient is at increased risk of anastomotic leak (e.g., nonviable bowel, sepsis, hypotension, etc.). Patients with obstruction as a result of active IBD will commonly respond initially to steroids. Paracolic abscesses can be drained percutaneously. Foreign bodies can usually be removed endoscopically. Fecal impaction is commonly relieved with a combination of stool softeners and laxatives from above and manual disimpaction at the bedside or in the operating room under anesthesia. Hernias causing mechanical large bowel obstruction usually require surgery. Adult colonic intussusceptions, in contrast to pediatric intussusceptions, are almost always associated with a pathologic lead point, such as a polyp, cancer, Meckel, or colonic diverticulum. A recent meta-analysis found malignancy as the causative factor in 36.9% of ileocolonic and 46.5% of colonic intussusceptions.[12] Most authors recommend surgical resection adhering to oncologic principles without reduction.

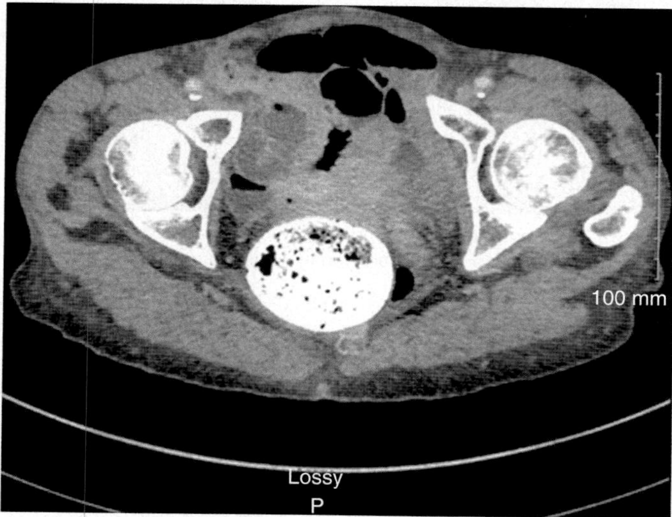

FIG. 52.26 Computed tomography scan of the pelvis showing a sizable barium impaction following a barium enema resulting in a large bowel obstruction. This patient required disimpaction in the operating room.

Patients with malignant obstruction of the low and mid rectum usually require an initial diverting stoma to allow for neoadjuvant chemoradiation prior to definitive surgery. Malignant obstructions of the sigmoid and left colon without signs of impending perforation can be treated with initial endoscopic stenting as a bridge to surgery, or initial surgery. Surgical options include segmental resection with Hartmann operation (end colostomy with internal closure of the rectal stump) or primary anastomosis with or without a diverting stoma. If the cecum is ischemic or nonviable, a subtotal colectomy is performed. In cases of right-sided obstruction, a right hemicolectomy is typically performed with primary anastomosis. Patients who are unstable with a high risk for anastomotic failure should undergo creation of a temporary diverting stoma or exteriorization of the anastomosis as a loop ileostomy.

COLONIC PSEUDO-OBSTRUCTION

Acute colonic pseudo-obstruction, also termed Ogilvie syndrome, was initially described by Sir William Heneage Ogilvie in 1948. It is characterized by acute colonic dilatation in the absence of a mechanical obstruction. Ogilvie syndrome is rare, with an estimated incidence of 100/100,000 admissions.[13] Dysregulation of the colonic autonomic innervation is hypothesized to play an important part. Several mechanisms have been implicated including autonomic imbalance with a relative excess of sympathetic over

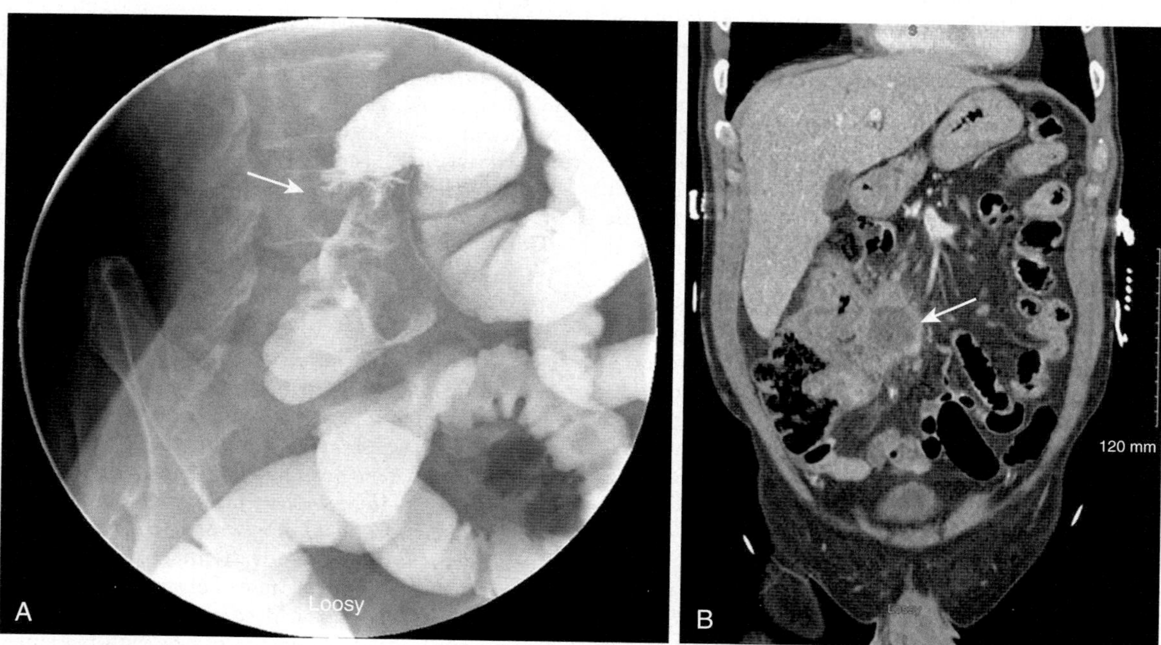

FIG. 52.27 (A) Gastrografin enema in a patient presenting with obstructing symptoms revealing an "apple-core" type lesion in the vicinity of the hepatic flexure *(arrow)*. (B) Computed tomography scan of the abdomen and pelvis in the same patient showing a large hepatic flexure carcinoma with perforation into the mesentery and associated mesenteric abscess *(arrow)*. Computed tomography–guided abscess drainage was not possible. This patient underwent extended right hemicolectomy with exteriorization of his ileocolic anastomosis as a loop ileostomy.

TABLE 52.2 Conditions associated with pseudo-obstruction.

CATEGORY	RISK FACTORS
Postsurgical	Following major orthopedic and/or spinal surgery, solid organ transplants, cardiac procedures
Neurologic disease	Parkinson disease, Alzheimer disease, stroke, spinal cord injury
Cardiac	Congestive heart failure, myocardial infarction
Pulmonary	Chronic obstructive pulmonary disease
Trauma	Major trauma, shock, burns
Metabolic	Diabetes mellitus, renal failure, electrolyte disturbances
Infectious	Cytomegalovirus, varicella-zoster virus
Obstetric/gynecologic	Caesarean section, normal and instrumental delivery
Miscellaneous	Lupus, scleroderma
Drugs	Opiates, chemotherapy, anti-Parkinson drugs, anticholinergics, antipsychotic drugs, clonidine

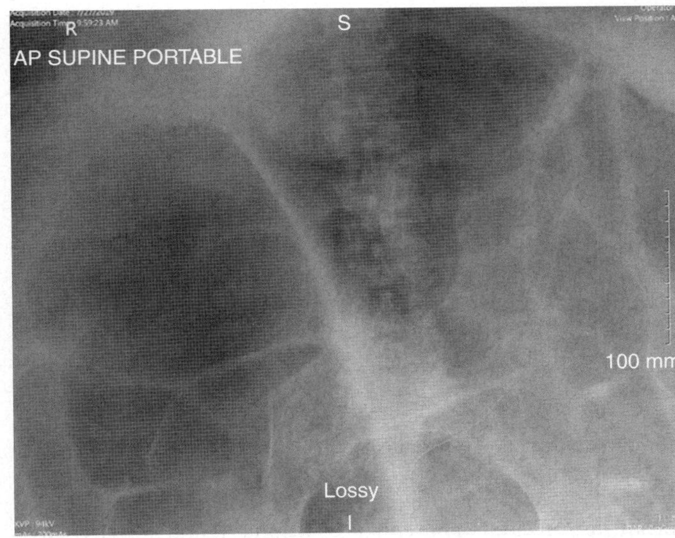

FIG. 52.28 Massive transverse colon distension due to Ogilvie syndrome in a woman with multiple comorbidities including a body mass index of 69, severe pulmonary hypertension, and cardiac disease.

parasympathetic activity, disrupted colonic reflex arcs, chronic disease, and medications.[13]

It is most commonly encountered among elderly and comorbid patients, classically following an acute illness on a background of neurologic, cardiac, or respiratory diseases. Common associated conditions are depicted in Table 52.2.

Diagnosis

The typical patient is elderly with multiple comorbidities who is hospitalized for an acute medical event or has undergone surgery (abdominal or nonabdominal). The presenting symptoms of the condition commonly include abdominal distension, pain, nausea, and vomiting. Obstipation is common, but some patients will have diarrhea due to hypersecretion of water. Lack of intestinal contractility is often associated with decreased or absent bowel sounds, but high-pitched, tinkling bowel sounds may also be encountered. Systemic toxicity and peritoneal signs are uncommon and should raise suspicion of ischemia and perforation. Initial evaluation should include a complete blood count, serum electrolytes, renal function assessment, and diagnostic imaging. Plain abdominal radiographs typically demonstrate a distended colon, with the largest diameter usually encountered in the cecum and right colon, which can reach 10 to 12 cm in diameter (Fig. 52.28). Dilation and gas continuing all the way down to the distal rectum support the suspicion of pseudo-obstruction in contrast to a mechanical obstruction in which a paucity of gas is commonly encountered distal to the obstruction. A water-soluble contrast enema can reliably distinguish between a mechanical obstruction and pseudo-obstruction. Currently, however, abdominal CT is typically utilized as the standard confirmatory test with the ability to commonly distinguish the type of obstruction as well as to assess for signs of ischemia and impending perforation (Fig. 52.29). Abdominal tenderness, leukocytosis, fever, and cecal dilation more than 12 cm are signs that may be indicative of colon ischemia, perforation, or impending perforation.

The differential diagnosis includes mechanical obstruction, toxic megacolon due to *C. difficile*, or toxic megacolon due to other causes.

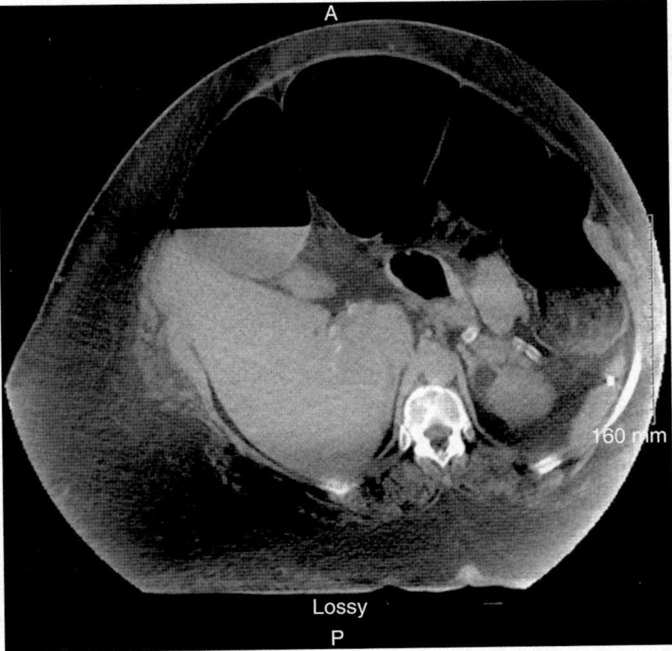

FIG. 52.29 Computed tomography scan showing massively distended colon without sign of ischemic change.

Management

The treatment of colonic pseudo-obstruction comprises a series of escalating interventions contingent on the degree of distension, risk for perforation, and the patient's response. Treatment options include supportive care, pharmacologic therapy (neostigmine), endoscopic decompression (colonoscopy), and surgery. Readers are referred to the American Society of Colon & Rectal Surgeons' Clinical Practice Guidelines.

Nonoperative, supportive care is initiated for patients with a cecal diameter that is less than 12 cm without evidence of ischemia or perforation. This includes nothing by mouth (NPO), correction of electrolyte disturbances, and discontinuation of medications that may be contributing such as opiates, anticholinergics, anti-Parkinson agents, antidepressants, neuroleptics, clonidine, atropines, and antihypertensives. Insertion of a nasogastric tube and rectal tube for decompression may be of help. Osmotic and stimulant laxatives should be avoided as they can worsen colonic dilation. Ambulation, prone positioning, and knee-chest position to encourage passage of flatus can assist. Patients should be monitored with serial physical exams and abdominal x-rays to assess for response or deterioration. Ischemia or perforation of the colon is the most feared complication and has been reported in the range of 3% to 15% of cases, leading to an associated mortality rate of close to 50%. In cases that do not improve with supportive care or with a cecal diameter of more than 12 cm, but without systemic toxicity and abdominal tenderness, colonic decompression is indicated.

Neostigmine is the keystone of pharmacologic decompression therapy. It is an acetylcholinesterase inhibitor that stimulates the muscarinic receptors and enhances colonic motor activity. Neostigmine is given as a 2 to 2.5 mg IV bolus injected over 3 to 5 minutes and results in significant parasympathetic stimulation causing strong colonic peristalsis that usually leads to subsequent flatus and bowel movements. It has been found to be a safe and effective option for patients with acute colonic pseudo-obstruction who have failed conservative management. Success rates for neostigmine treatment range from 60% to 94%, with recurrences observed in up to 31% of patients, with some patients requiring multiple drug administrations. Neostigmine is contraindicated in mechanical bowel obstruction and in patients with signs of ischemia or perforation. It should be used with caution among patients with asthma, chronic obstructive lung disease, bradycardia, and recent acute coronary syndrome and in those with renal failure. Neostigmine should be given in a monitored setting with atropine immediately available. Common side effects include vomiting, crampy abdominal pain, excessive salivation, and bradycardia. Colonoscopic decompression should be considered in patients with contraindications to neostigmine or for those who are unresponsive to it. The aim of endoscopic decompression is to advance the scope to the right colon with minimal insufflation and use of narcotics and place a colonic decompression tube while removing as much gas as possible from the colon. Endoscopic decompression has a high success rate of 61% to 95% for initial decompression and 70% to 90% for sustained decompression. Colonoscopic perforation rates following decompression for pseudo-obstruction are in the range of 1% to 3%.

Patients who do not respond to other lines of treatment or those who demonstrate signs of systemic toxicity, ischemia, or perforation require surgery. Surgical options are determined according to the condition of the colon and the patient. If the colon is viable, tube cecostomy or cecostomy can be performed, with high rates of success. For patients with signs of ischemia or perforation, a resection, usually with a diverting stoma, is recommended.

INFLAMMATORY BOWEL DISEASE

Epidemiology and Etiology

IBD, which includes both UC and Crohn disease, are largely diseases of the Western world. As Asian countries are adopting a more Western diet, the incidence of these disorders is increasing in these countries as well. The prevalence of IBD in Western countries is approximately 0.5% of the general population.[14] In the United States, over 1 million individuals are estimated to have IBD, with over 200,000 Canadians affected, and 2.5 to 3 million individuals in Europe having these disorders.[14] The highest incidence of UC has been reported in Europe, followed by the United States, whereas for Crohn disease, the highest incidence was observed in the United States, followed by Europe. Europe was noted to have the highest prevalence of IBD. Over time, the incidence of both disorders appears to be increasing. Both disorders appear to have a genetic predisposition with many contributing environmental factors. Over 10% of patients with IBD have a family history of IBD. To date, genome-wide association studies have linked to over 230 IBD susceptibility loci.[15] Cigarette smoking is the most studied environmental factor, having opposite effects in UC and Crohn disease. In UC, smoking tends to suppress symptoms, whereas in Crohn disease, smoking tends to exacerbate symptoms. Antibiotic use in early life has also been thought to predispose to IBD, as has NSAID use.

Disease Distribution and Classification

The extent of UC can also be graded with respect to the extent of inflammation within the colon. It can be limited only to the rectum and sigmoid colon (proctitis or proctosigmoiditis), restricted to the left side of the colon, or extended to involve the entire colon (pancolitis).

There are many classification schemes of Crohn disease. However, one of the most popular was initially the Vienna Classification, which was later updated to the Montreal Classification. With these classification schemes, patients are classified according to age of onset of disease, bowel location of their Crohn disease, as well as type of disease behavior. In addition to the different ages of onset, the Vienna Classification divided patients into whether or not they develop inflammatory Crohn disease at age of 40 or later. The Montreal Classification subdivides this into less than 20 or greater than 20 years old. In addition, the Montreal Classification adds a further subdivision of whether the patients have perianal Crohn disease. The three different types of behavior classifications for Crohn disease that are possible include inflammatory Crohn disease, fibrostenotic Crohn disease, and fistulizing Crohn disease. Many people feel that these three types of disease behaviors represent different time points in the progression of disease. In other words, a patient is initially diagnosed with inflammatory Crohn disease, which over time progresses to fibrostenotic Crohn disease. This, in turn, will frequently progress to an obstruction, with perforation proximal to the obstruction and abscess formation. When this abscess spontaneously drains into an adjacent structure or organ, fistula formation ensues. In this manner, there is a progression from inflammatory to fibrostenosing to fistulizing Crohn disease. It is with this thought in mind that the progression to "top-down" medical therapy has evolved (see later discussion on medical therapy). The goal is to interrupt this natural progression or cycle in the course of Crohn disease to prevent the progressive fibrosis that results in many of the complications leading to surgery.

Clinical Presentation and Disease Diagnosis

Clinical Presentation

Clinical presentation of both diseases can be similar. Diarrhea can be a presenting symptom in both diseases; however, this is typically more prevalent and severe in UC, where the diarrhea is characteristically bloody. Significant hemorrhage is much more common with UC than with Crohn disease. Typical UC symptoms also include tenesmus and urgency as well as associated anemia. In Crohn disease, symptoms of abdominal pain may predominate.

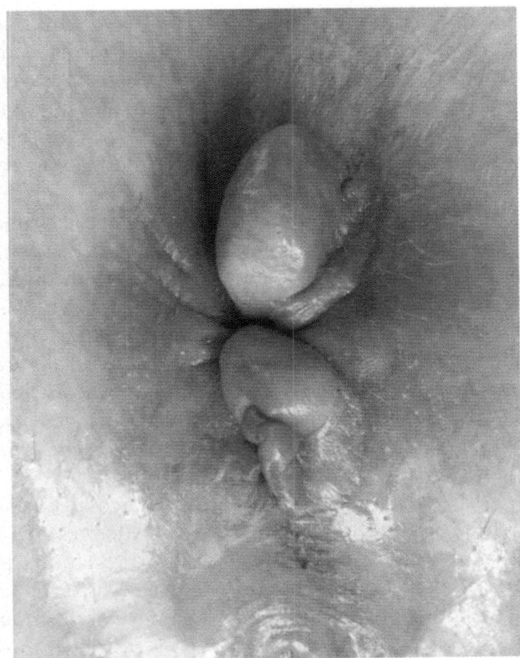

FIG. 52.30 Large anal Crohn tags. Note the bluish coloring and waxy appearance of the perianal skin

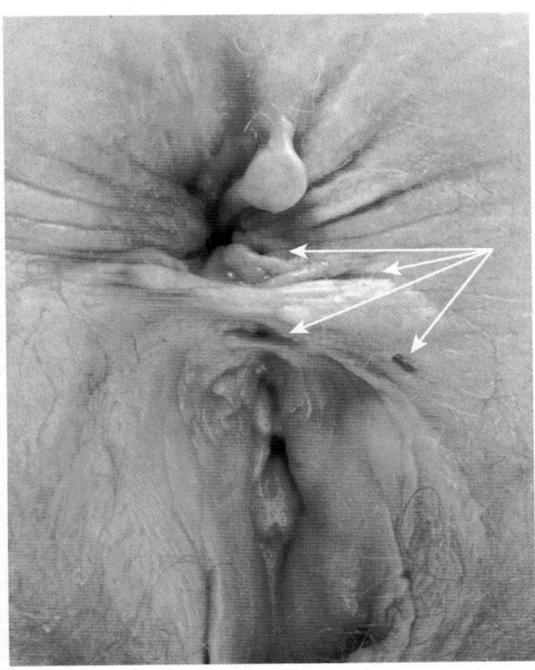

FIG. 52.31 A woman with significant fistulizing perianal Crohn disease. Note the multiple external fistula openings shown by the *white arrows*. These all had a common internal opening in the anterior midline, which was also associated with a rectovaginal fistula. This patient ultimately elected to undergo ileostomy diversion.

In any patient initially presenting with diarrhea, stool cultures should first be obtained to exclude the presence of infectious causes of diarrhea, such as *Salmonella*, *Giardia*, or community-acquired *C. difficile* that is now increasingly seen. Patients with Crohn disease may present with a palpable abdominal mass due to an intraabdominal abscess or have an external fistula. Roughly 25% of patients with Crohn disease will have associated perianal disease. This can include a variety of problems, including anal fissure, which in contrast to patients without Crohn, is often not painful and may be multiple. In addition, these patients can present with large anal skin tags (Fig. 52.30), which are not true external hemorrhoids. As a rule, these should not be excised, as they may lead to very delayed wound healing. These patients may also present with anorectal abscesses, fistula(s) (Fig. 52.31), and anal stenosis. Digital rectal examination should always be performed.

Extraintestinal manifestations. Extraintestinal manifestations can occur in many IBD patients, and it is estimated that up to half of IBD patients will have one or more extraintestinal manifestations. There is a slightly higher prevalence of extraintestinal manifestations in patients with Crohn disease as compared with those with UC and can be divided into those affecting the joints, eyes, and skin. Arthritis is by far the most common extraintestinal manifestation. One of the most common manifestations is sacroiliitis. One of the most serious joint manifestations is ankylosing spondylitis which runs a course independent of the bowel disease. These patients are HLA-B27 positive and may present in advanced cases with decreased cervical flexion, which has important anesthetic implications for intubation. These patients may require fiber optic intubation and will require specific preoperative anesthesia evaluation.

Cutaneous extraintestinal manifestations include erythema nodosum and pyoderma gangrenosum. From long experience of treating surgical patients with IBD, pyoderma is much more frequent than erythema nodosum. Erythema nodosum (Fig. 52.32) is characterized by red painful swollen nodules that can occur and

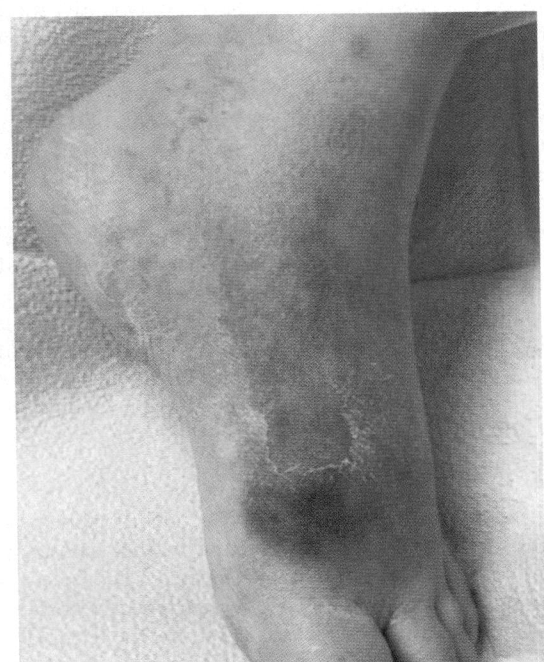

FIG. 52.32 A patient with a Crohn disease flare and active erythema nodosum. Note the red purplish nodule on the dorsum of the foot.

usually will respond to systemic steroid administration, whereas pyoderma gangrenosum is characterized by typically extremely painful ulcerating lesions that frequently occur at sites of repeated trauma such as in the vicinity of surgical incisions or more frequently around intestinal stomas (Fig. 52.33). There is a phenomenon called "pathergy," which refers to a worsening of the

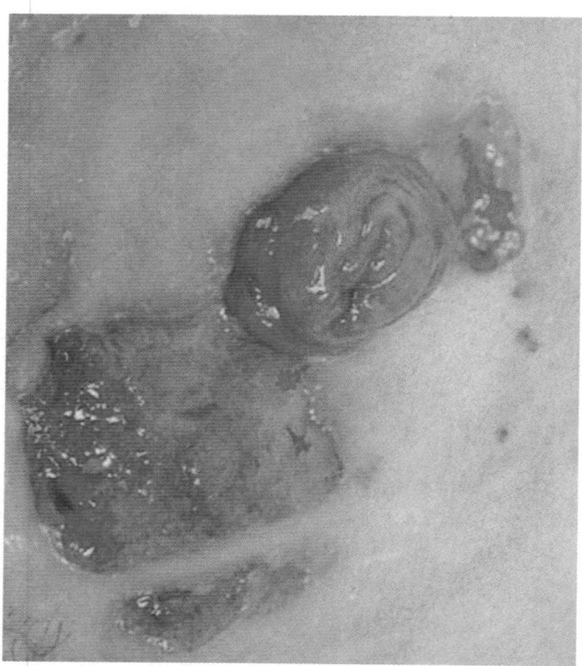

FIG. 52.33 Pyoderma gangrenosum adjacent to an end ileostomy in a patient with Crohn disease. Here, the lesions have started to heal with granulation tissue.

pyoderma with any type of surgical manipulation or debridement. These lesions are therefore best treated by nonoperative means and can include intralesional steroid injections (i.e., triamcinalone), topical (tacrolimus 0.1%), or systemic biologic therapy (antitumor necrosis factor [TNF] antibodies or similar agents). Such treatment will typically result in symptom resolution.

Ocular manifestations of UC can include uveitis, iritis, and episcleritis. Some of these can lead to significant irritation and require referral to an ophthalmologist.

Sclerosing cholangitis is estimated to affect approximately 5% of patients with IBD. It has a course that is curiously independent of the IBD. At its worst, it can progress to cirrhosis, result in liver failure, and require hepatic transplantation. Patients with sclerosing cholangitis are at higher risk for developing colorectal neoplasia, as will be discussed later, and are also at higher risk of developing pouchitis, as will be discussed in the section on IPAA and surgical treatment.

Disease Diagnosis

Endoscopy. The diagnosis of IBD is frequently made by endoscopy. This can be accomplished by either rigid proctoscopy, flexible sigmoidoscopy, or colonoscopy. Generally, a complete evaluation of the colon with colonoscopy is performed both to evaluate the extent of the disease as well as to examine the terminal ileum.

With UC, inflammation begins at the level of the dentate line and extends proximally, whereas in Crohn disease, in many cases, the inflammation is more patchy and there can be discontinuous inflammation (i.e., skip areas), with areas of intervening normal-appearing mucosa. In some cases, differentiation between the two diseases can be difficult, both endoscopically as well as histologically. A typical endoscopic view of UC is shown in Fig. 52.34. Note the more roughened or granular appearance of the colonic mucosa. One of the most common scoring systems for endoscopic assessment of UC is the Mayo Clinic Scoring System, which grades the endoscopic findings based upon the severity of the mucosal ulceration or the absence thereof. Grade 1 refers to a normal endoscopic appearance, grade 2 refers to slightly more erythematous, grade 3 refers to even more erythematous area with touch bleeding, and grade 4 refers to significant bleeding and friability. As the disease becomes more severe, there is an increasingly erythematous appearance of the mucosa with progressive mucosal ulceration.

With respect to endoscopy, Crohn disease is more characterized by deeper punched-out appearing ulcerations. In these cases, there are often longer serpiginous ulcerations covered with fibrin. These can oftentimes extend longitudinally along the lumen of the bowel, in which case they are sometimes referred to as "bear claw" ulcerations (Fig. 52.35). In many cases, Crohn disease ulcers are worse on the mesenteric side of the bowel. Regarding the distribution of Crohn disease, the most common site of involvement in nearly half of patients is ileocolic, followed by colonic involvement. Crohn disease can also affect the small bowel or upper GI tract.

Histologic evaluation. In UC, colonic mucosal biopsies will typically show significant inflammation with the presence of multiple polymorphonuclear leukocytes within the lamina propria. There may be depletion of mucin in goblet cells. One can also identify crypt abscesses, although this is somewhat of a nonspecific finding. As a rule, inflammation in UC is restricted to the surface epithelium (Fig. 52.36). The disease process is limited to the large intestine. Proximal colonic disease occurs in continuity with an involved rectum (i.e., no gross or histologic skip lesions). The inflammation is characterized by the absence of mural sinus tracts, deep fissural ulcers, and granulomas, as well as by the absence of transmural lymphoid aggregates in an area not deeply ulcerated.

In contrast, in patients with Crohn disease, there is often transmural inflammation, which is seen in histologic evaluation of resected specimens. In approximately one third of patients, there are noncaseating granulomas (Fig. 52.37). In biopsy specimens, the diagnosis of Crohn disease is made in the presence of non-necrotizing granulomas or the presence of transmural lymphoid aggregates in an area not deeply ulcerated. In patients with Crohn disease, just as one can macroscopically see "skip" disease with patchy inflammation, the same is true on microscopic evaluation. The term "focal active enteritis" is used. The differential diagnosis frequently includes infectious colitis or drug-induced colitis, and pathology reports often include this differential diagnosis when areas are biopsied during GI endoscopy. In patients who are suspected of having Crohn disease, it is important to make an effort to intubate the terminal ileum, as this is a common site of disease involvement.

IBD undetermined refers to a subset of patients who have overlapping characteristics of both Crohn disease as well as UC on endoscopic biopsy. It is thought that up to 10% to 15% of patients fall into this category. The diagnosis of **indeterminate colitis** is made in patients in whom there is uncertainty of the diagnosis on evaluation of the colectomy specimen, since histologic features of both Crohn and UC are seen. Overall, this diagnosis is more likely in patients with fulminant disease where the significant amount of inflammation interferes with precise disease diagnosis.

Medical Treatment

Changing medical treatment philosophy. The last two decades has seen a tremendous change in medical treatment for IBD. There has been a gradual evolution from a "bottom-up" approach to what is termed "top-down" approach. These terms refer to the

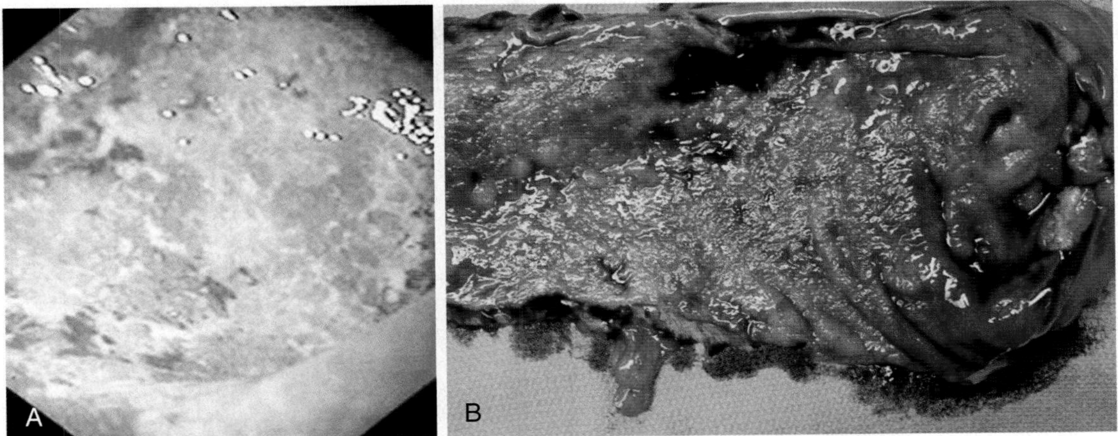

FIG. 52.34 (A) Endoscopic view of moderately severe ulcerative colitis. Note the bleeding and ulceration. (B) Macroscopic view of right colon following total proctocolectomy for fulminant ulcerative colitis.

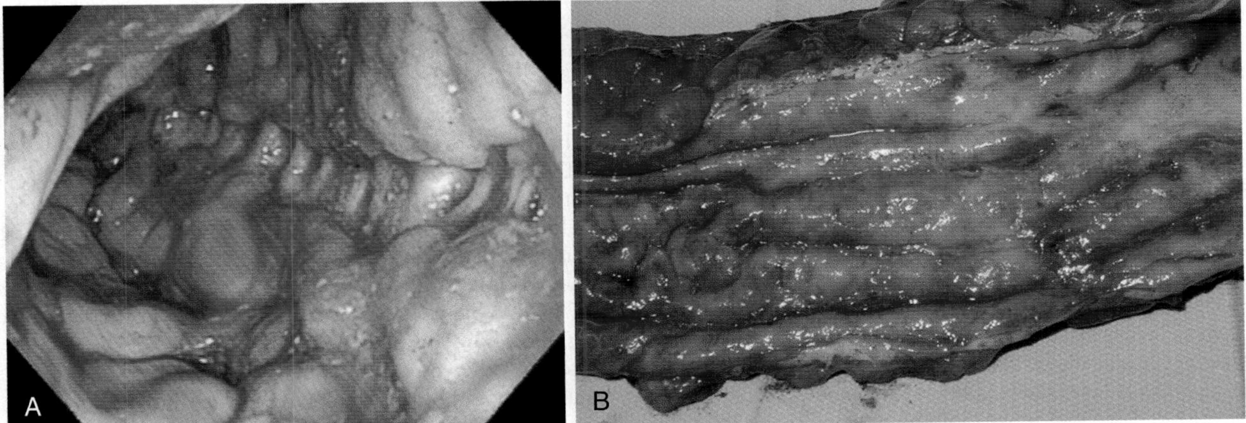

FIG. 52.35 Bear claw ulcers in Crohn colitis. (A) Endoscopic view. (B) Macroscopic view.

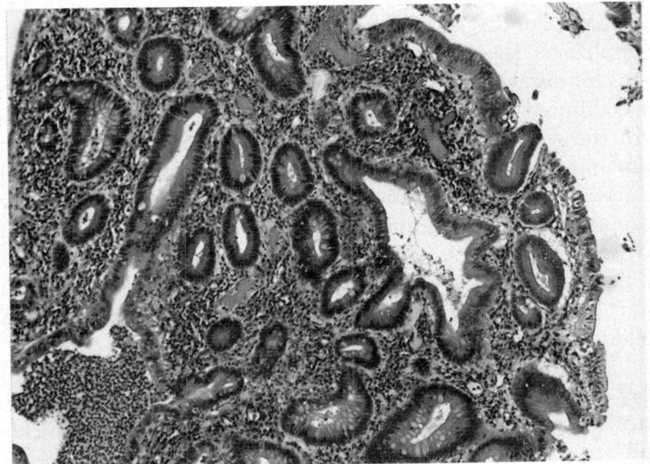

FIG. 52.36 Histologic section of active ulcerative colitis. There is glandular architectural distortion manifested by irregular branching and orientation of glands relative to the surface. The lamina propria is expanded with inflammatory cells, and intraepithelial neutrophils are present. A crypt abscess is noted *(lower left)*. (Courtesy Dr. Jeffrey P. Baliff, Thomas Jefferson University, Philadelphia.)

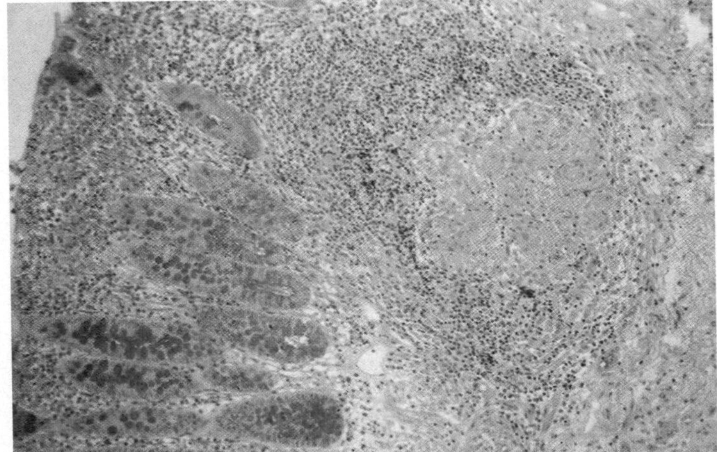

FIG. 52.37 Crohn colitis with noncaseating granuloma.

TABLE 52.3 Different types of medical treatment used for inflammatory bowel disease.

DRUG CLASS	EXAMPLES	INDICATION	ADMINISTRATION
Biologics	Infliximab	UC, CD	IV
	Adalimumab	UC, CD	SC
	Golimumab	UC	IV
	Natalizumab	CD	IV
	Vedolizumab	UC, CD	IV
	Ustekinumab	UC, CD	IV, SC
Antiinflammatory	Sulfasalazine	UC, CD	PO
	Mesalamine	UC, CD	PO, enema, suppository
Immunosuppressives	Conventional steroids	UC, CD	PO, IV, suppository
	Budesonide	UC, CD	PO, rectal foam
	Antimetabolites	UC, CD	PO
	Tofacitinib	UC	PO
Probiotics	*Lactobacillus*	UC, CD	Food, tablets, capsules, powders
	Bifidobacterium		
Antibiotics	Ciprofloxacin	UC, CD	PO, IV
	Metronidazole	UC, CD	PO, IV
	Rifaximin	Off-label	PO

CD, Crohn disease; *IV*, intravenous; *PO*, per os; *SC*, subcutaneous; *UC*, ulcerative colitis.

"bottom-up approach," beginning with the safest, least expensive medications first and only proceeding to the more potent, more expensive medications with a higher side effect profile once these have failed. This treatment approach has been largely replaced by the top-down approach, whereby patients are initially treated with the stronger, more potent medications which may, in turn, have a greater side effect profile and are associated with higher costs. Many of these drugs have been implicated with a higher rate of postoperative complications in patients undergoing surgery, and their use also has been associated with reactivation of certain remote infections. It is important for the surgeon to be aware of these medications and knowledgeable about their mechanism of action. Table 52.3 lists some of the more commonly utilized medications used in the treatment of IBD. The surgeon will find that these medications are being used increasingly not only in patients with IBD but also in patients with rheumatoid arthritis and psoriasis. Medical therapy formerly was based largely on medications such as sulfasalazine and steroids. However, the last 25 years has seen a revolution with the introduction of "biologic therapy," based largely on treatment with antibodies directed against TNF-α (anti-TNF-α). This began with the Food and Drug Administration (FDA) approval for infliximab (chimeric anti-TNF antibody) for Crohn disease in 1998, followed by adalimumab (humanized anti-TNF antibody) in 2007, certolizumab pegol (a PEGylated Fab' fragment of a humanized TNF antibody) and natalizumab (humanized monoclonal antibody to α4-integrin) both in 2008, golimumab (human monoclonal anti-TNF) approval for UC in 2013, vedolizumab (monoclonal antibody to integrin α4β7) in 2014, ustekinumab (human monoclonal antibody to p40 protein subunit used by interleukin [IL]-12 and IL-23) in 2016, and tofacitinib (janus kinase inhibitor) approval for UC in 2018. Currently, there is a wide assortment of drugs to choose from. There has also been a change in the philosophy of treatment with respect to IBD.

Medications for treatment of IBD

Aminosalicylates. Sulfasalazine has long been used for the treatment of colonic IBD. Originally used as a treatment for arthritis, it was noted that many arthritis patients with coexisting IBD noted an improvement in the latter when taking this medication. Use of this drug was limited by its sulfapyridine ring, which excludes use in patients with sulfa allergies. When this medication is used, patients require folic acid supplementation. Eventually, the sulfapyridine ring is cleaved, leaving the active 5-aminosalicylate (5-ASA) moiety. Pharmacologists rapidly realized that, depending upon how this drug was formulated, its delivery could be targeted to different portions of the GI tract. For example, mesalmine (Pentasa) begins to dissolve in the stomach and releases drug throughout the GI tract, whereas Asacol begins to be released in the terminal ileum by means of a pH-dependent mechanism and coats the entire colon. Drugs manufactured with an "MMX technology" are designed as once-a-day preparations and formulated so that they slowly dissolve, thus releasing medication throughout the colon. For this reason, they are thought to have greater patient compliance. There are also topical formulations of these medications for distal disease. Suppository formulations are administered at bedtime. While the patient sleeps, the suppositories melt and coat the rectum with mesalamine, which has a very potent antiinflammatory effect. The most popular brand of suppository is Canasa. The same medication in small-volume enema form (Rowasa enemas) can be administered also at bedtime. The patient is advised to lie on their left side, allowing the small volume of fluid to be delivered not only to the rectum but also sigmoid and, in some cases, the left colon. These medications are most effective for mild to moderate disease.

Corticosteroids. If the patient has severe disease, steroids still play a prominent role in the treatment of IBD. Although they have numerous side effects, they are inexpensive, act quickly, and are readily available, not requiring lengthy insurance preauthorizations as with the more expensive biologic medication alternatives. The recognized side effects of steroids include the following:

- Cushingoid appearance that is very unpopular, particularly among young patients
- Feared complication of aseptic necrosis of the hips

- Hypertension
- Mood changes that can escalate up to actual psychiatric conditions
- Hyperglycemia
- Increased risk of infectious complications after surgery
- Cataract formation
- Striae and others

Because of these complications, as well as the growth retardation seen when these drugs are used for prolonged periods in children, these medications should be used sparingly for as short a period as possible. Steroids are usually started at a high dose and then tapered quickly. Their main uses are either in the outpatient setting in the form of pulse therapy, as high doses that are tapered quickly, or intravenously in patients who are hospitalized with flares of their disease. In the outpatient setting, pulse therapy is usually given in the form of prednisone at doses starting at 40 to 60 mg/day, tapering by 5 to 10 mg at 2-week intervals until 10 mg/day is reached and then tapering by 5 mg every 2 weeks, at which time the drug is discontinued. In the hospital setting, 100 mg of hydrocortisone can be given intravenously every 6 to 8 hours depending on disease severity.

Immunomodulators

Thiopurines. Thiopurines are a "steroid-sparing" class of medication that are usually begun once patients are placed on steroids and perhaps have been unsuccessful in weaning off steroids after one or two attempts at pulse therapy. Thiopurines have been used for many decades in the treatment of Crohn disease and have long been used in the organ transplant population. Two drugs fall into this category: azathioprine and its metabolite 6-mercaptopurine. The side effects of this therapy include leukopenia and pancreatitis. These side effects are largely seen in individuals who are homozygous for a variant of the enzyme thiopurine methyltransferase responsible for metabolizing these drugs poorly. For this reason, many physicians now routinely perform thiopurine methyltransferase genotyping of patients to see whether they will be able to metabolize these drugs properly prior to initiating thiopurine treatment. These drugs have several advantages in that they are readily available and are an oral medication taken once a day, and dosing is based on body weight. On the downside, once a patient begins therapy, there is usually a 3- to 4-month lag time until these medications exert their therapeutic effect. For this reason, these medications cannot be used to treat a flare. Long-term thiopurine use is also associated with a higher risk of developing non-Hodgkin lymphoma than the general population.

Methotrexate. Methotrexate is another commonly used immunosuppressive for the treatment of IBD. This medication, which has long been used particularly in the treatment of patients with arthritis, can be dosed either orally or intramuscularly. Intramuscular dosing is particularly convenient in patients who have problems with significant diarrhea or absorption issues (e.g., short bowel syndrome). The side effects of methotrexate include elevations in liver function tests, as well as pulmonary fibrosis. When methotrexate is given, patients require folic acid supplementation.

Biologics in the Treatment of Inflammatory Bowel Disease

The term "biologics" as it pertains to drugs used for IBD initially referred to monoclonal antibodies directed against TNF-α. The first such agent, infliximab, was approved by the FDA for use in 1998. Since then, there has been a continued increase in both the number and type (based upon mechanism of action) of medications that have been approved (see Table 52.3). The side effects of these drugs include reactivation of infections including tuberculosis, histoplasmosis, actinomycosis, and hepatitis. For this reason, a careful patient history regarding these infections should be taken prior to consideration of treatment. In addition, before starting these drugs, the patient should have either a tuberculin skin test or undergo testing with QuantiFERON gold assay as well as obtain a hepatitis profile. There is currently no accurate test for past exposure for histoplasmosis. In addition, these types of agents, similar to the thiopurines, can be associated with a higher risk of developing non-Hodgkin lymphoma compared to the general population. In addition, anti-TNF-α antibody has been associated with a low risk of hepatosplenic T-cell lymphomas, particularly in young men who have been taking anti-TNF antibody therapy in combination with other immunosuppressive therapy such as a thiopurine.

Assessment of Symptom Severity

Truelove and Witts is a popular classification scheme that characterizes patients by the severity of their diarrhea, the presence of blood in stool, the presence of fever, tachycardia, anemia, or an elevated erythrocyte sedimentation rate. Many similar classification schemes are used, in addition to analyzing stool samples for either fecal calprotectin or lactoferrin that can be used as an inflammatory marker to assess disease activity. With Crohn disease, both the Crohn disease activity index (CDAI) and the Harvey Bradshaw index have been used to quantitate symptoms.[16] The CDAI is made up of eight clinical and laboratory variables, including the number of bowel movements/day, the presence of abdominal pain, hematocrit, and weight loss. A score of less than 150 indicates clinical remission, and a score of more than 450 denotes severe disease. Since the CDAI requires a 7-day patient symptom diary, the Harvey-Bradshaw Index was proposed as a modification of this scheme that only used clinical data.

Indications for Surgery for Ulcerative Colitis

There are several indications for surgery for UC, the foremost of which is failure to respond to maximum medical therapy. The frequency of surgery for UC has actually decreased over the last several decades with the improvement in efficacy and the number of new and more effective medical options such as the entire class of biologic therapies. However, despite these new therapies, patients still present with a failure to respond. Patients falling into this category range from those patients who have severe disease, namely, those patients with multiple bowel movements, poor nutritional status, "failure to thrive," and a need for surgery in order to regain their good physical health. These patients have a very poor quality of life with urgency, tenesmus, and low body weight; surgery represents a significant improvement in the quality of life. The second group of patients failing to respond to maximum medical therapy refers to patients with fulminant colitis. These patients have such severe disease that they need to be hospitalized and placed on IV steroids. In some cases, they have received in-hospital biologic therapy; in rare cases, these patients may be receiving intravenous cyclosporine as an attempt to avert colectomy. In these patients with fulminant colitis, toxic megacolon may be present (Fig. 52.38). This has arbitrarily been defined as having three or more of the following criteria present: tachycardia greater than 100, leukocytosis greater than 12,000/dL^3, hypoalbuminemia less than 3 g/dL^3, a temperature greater than 38°C, or a diameter of the transverse colon on a

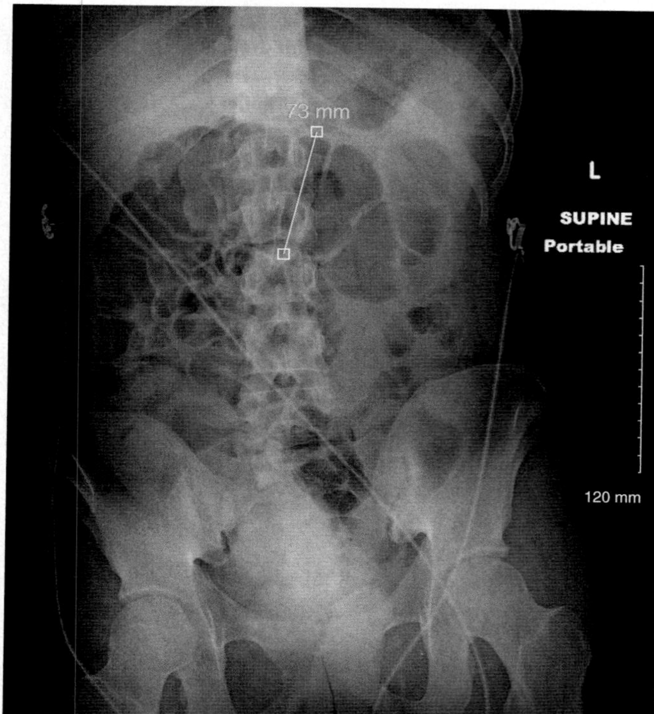

FIG. 52.38 Toxic megacolon. Abdominal film shows significant distension of the transverse colon in a 20-year-old man with toxic megacolon. (From Rojas-Khalil Y, Galandiuk S. Management of chronic ulcerative colitis. In: Cameron JL, Cameron A, eds. *Current Surgical Therapy*. 13th ed. Philadelphia: Elsevier; in press.)

plain abdominal radiograph greater than 5 cm. Three or more of these criteria meet the definition of toxic megacolon; note that a "megacolon" does not need to be present in order to meet this definition. Thus, the definition of toxic megacolon merely refers to a patient who is septic due to very severe colitis. Toxic megacolon can be present not only from severe UC but also due to severe Crohn colitis or severe infectious or ischemic colitis. When the colitis is severe enough, it is associated with a significant colonic ileus, and, in these cases, the colon becomes dilated and there is a significant risk of colonic perforation. The next category of indication for surgery occurs in patients in whom there is significant GI bleeding. Recalling basic anatomy, the vessels located underneath the colonic vessels are located underneath the mucosa. If the mucosa sloughs, this will, in effect, expose the underlying blood vessels of the colon and can result in massive GI hemorrhage if an ulcer erodes into these vessels. Significant hemorrhage can be one of the reasons for urgent surgery with UC, although the frequency of this complication has decreased over time. Another indication for surgery in children with UC is failure to grow, which is also an indication for surgery in patients with Crohn disease. The presence of a dysplasia or cancer is an indication for surgery, as well. Patients with longstanding UC (>8 years) have a high risk of developing dysplasia or cancer, as do those who have sclerosing cholangitis. Once the disease has been present longer than 8 years, patients are advised to undergo regular (yearly) colonoscopic surveillance with or without chromoendoscopy. If multiple areas of low-grade dysplasia or areas of high-grade dysplasia (Fig. 52.39) are found, a colectomy is recommended to prevent the development of invasive adenocarcinoma. The finding of colonic dysplasia in patients with longstanding UC is an indication for surgery that has undergone significant change over the last 20 years. There is currently somewhat of a controversy as to exactly who requires surgery and who requires continued observation with close surveillance. Much of this has arisen due to the development of high-definition colonoscopy, as well as the development of techniques of surveillance such as chromoendoscopy. Chromoendoscopy involves the performance of colonoscopy with the spraying of dyes such as methylene blue or indigo carmine onto the colonic mucosa at the time of colonoscopy to highlight areas suspicious for dysplasia to permit targeted biopsies rather than just performing the random biopsies that were previously standard of care. In addition to this, there has been recognition that there are different types of dysplasia. The flat dysplasia that is difficult to detect and blends in with the surrounding mucosa is very different from the "polypoid" dysplasia that is apparent and can be treated in many cases like a polyp and removed using techniques similar to that used for removal of a conventional polyp during colonoscopy. In some studies, patients with UC have undergone "polypectomy" removal of dysplastic lesions and have been followed long-term without interval development of cancer.[17] What is important to stress is that patients must have very close follow-up colonoscopy and that meticulous colonoscopy and pathology expertise are vital to this process, as is excellent patient compliance. If any one of these three factors is lacking, this is clearly not a viable treatment alternative. There is, however, still agreement that if there are multiple areas of flat dysplasia within the colon, colectomy is indicated. There is still much to be learned regarding the actual risk of cancer in patients with IBD. Overall, it is felt that approximately one fifth of the world's cancers arise in the setting of chronic inflammation. This mirrors t nhe problem with hepatitis, anal cancer, gastric cancer, and many others. With the advent of better medications and interruption in this chronic cycle of inflammation, it will be interesting to see whether the incidence of cancer and IBD begins to decline compared to historical data. The same is true regarding the indication for failure to grow in children. As more effective medications are identified and are able to be instituted at earlier ages, it is anticipated that there will be less of an indication to operate in these young patients.

Similarly, if an adenocarcinoma is identified, colectomy is indicated. In certain patients, the presence of severe extraintestinal disease is also an indication for surgery. In some cases, severe extraintestinal disease will respond to surgery; however, there are some cases in which the extraintestinal disease has a course relatively independent of the colon.

Indications for Surgery for Crohn Disease

Unlike indications for surgery for UC, indications for surgery for Crohn disease are generally reserved for complications of the disease. Similar to UC, surgery is also performed in children with Crohn disease when they show failure to grow. In addition, surgery is frequently performed for symptoms of obstruction secondary to fibrostenosing Crohn disease (Fig. 52.40). Also, if patients have a perforating Crohn disease associated with abscess or fistula, surgery may be indicated. The presence of many types of fistulas is also a relative indication for surgery. For example, the presence of a symptomatic ileal sigmoid fistula resulting in significant diarrhea bypassing the entire colon can be an indication for surgery. The occurrence of enterocutaneous fistulas is an indication for surgery. Enteroenteric fistulae are not an indication for surgery unless they are associated with significant symptoms of obstruction or discomfort. The

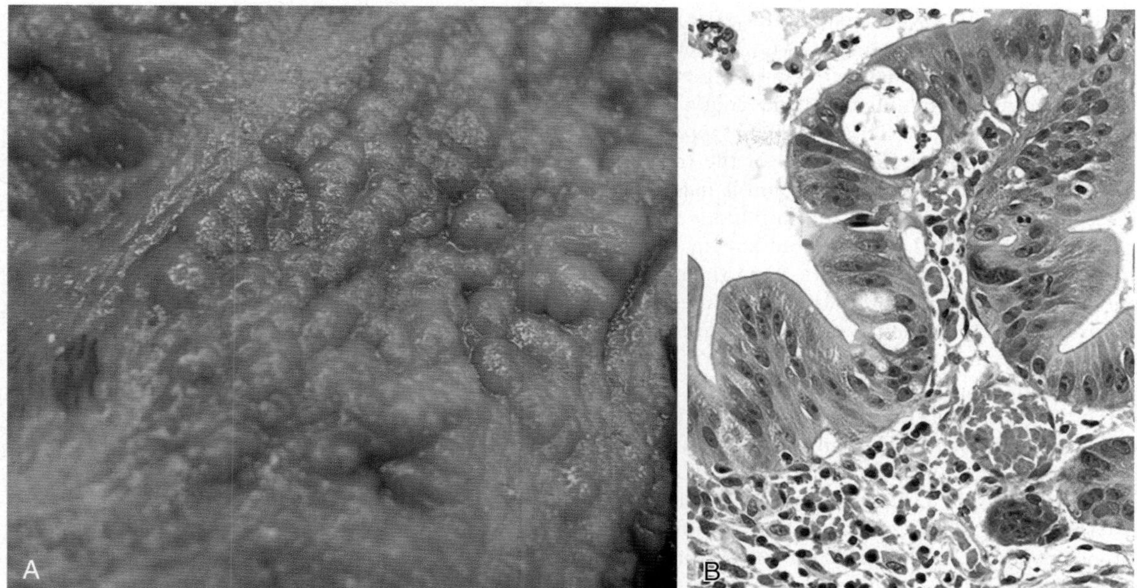

FIG. 52.39 (A) A dysplasia-associated lesion or mass (DALM) in a patient with long-standing ulcerative colitis and sclerosing cholangitis. (B) High-grade dysplasia within a DALM in a patient with long-standing ulcerative colitis and sclerosing cholangitis.

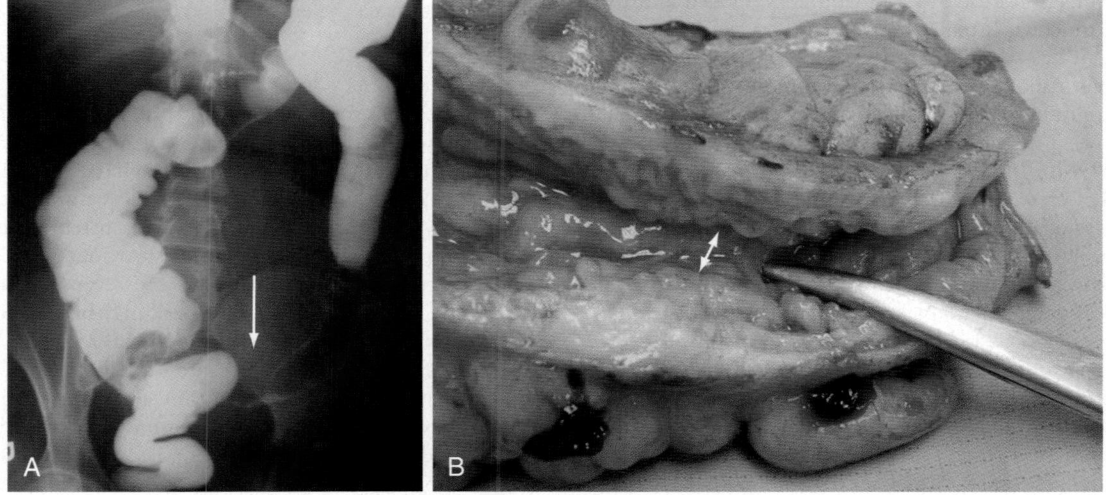

FIG. 52.40 (A) Gastrografin enema showing significant stricture *(arrow)* of sigmoid colon secondary to Crohn disease. (B) Segmental colonic resection for fibrostenotic disease. Note the significant wall thickening and narrowed lumen *(arrow)* and its size compared to the tip of the scissors.

presence of significant abdominal pain associated with obstruction is considered an indication for surgery. Patients with Crohn disease who have associated cancer or dysplasia, as with patients with UC, are an indication for surgery. In patients with Crohn disease, as with UC, areas of dysplasia in the colon can be multifocal, and for this reason, if this occurs in the colon, a total proctocolectomy is considered preferable to a segmental resection.

Surgical Options for Ulcerative Colitis

There are several operations that are currently performed for UC. These include subtotal colectomy, ileostomy, and Hartmann procedure, frequently performed for fulminant disease. Total proctocolectomy with end ileostomy and proctocolectomy with either stapled or hand-sewn IPAA are commonly performed in the elective setting. Subtotal colectomy and ileal rectal anastomosis and total proctocolectomy with continent ileostomy are less commonly performed procedures. We discuss these in order next.

Total Proctocolectomy With End Ileostomy

Subtotal colectomy and ileostomy and Hartmann procedure is the treatment for patients with fulminant colitis not responding to maximal medical therapy. The term "toxic megacolon" has long been used to refer to a condition arising when patients become toxic from colitis irrespective of its etiology (e.g., whether this be UC, Crohn colitis, infectious, or ischemic). In any of these conditions, as the mucosa sloughs, the endotoxins within the bowel lumen are absorbed leading to a septic state characterized by leukocytosis, tachycardia, fever, and in severe cases, hemodynamic instability. Many of these patients have protein-losing enteropathy and have associated hypoalbuminemia. If the colitis is severe enough to have an associated colonic ileus, this is apparent on an abdominal film with an increased diameter of the transverse colon (>5 cm). The definition of toxic megacolon is made when any three of these five factors are present. It is important to realize that a patient can have toxic megacolon without having a "megacolon" (i.e., they can just be "toxic" or septic from their colitis). When patients begin exhibiting symptoms of toxic megacolon, prompt surgery is indicated in order to prevent colonic perforation. With the improved medical therapy, this clinical scenario is becoming less common. In performing this operation, whether performed open or in a minimally invasive fashion, it is important to be gentle with the colon, as ordinary manipulation can result in perforation. If the colon is very dilated and there is loss of domain, the procedure may not be able to be safely performed in a minimally invasive fashion. One of the common complications of this procedure postoperatively is a "blow out" of the Hartmann stump, resulting in a pelvic abscess. This complication many times can be avoided simply by leaving a very long Hartmann stump and incorporating this into the fascial closure of the midline abdominal laparotomy wound or the specimen extraction site, depending on whether it is an open or minimally invasive procedure, and closing the incision over this. In this manner, if the stump dehisces and a wound infection develops, the wound is opened and there is a controlled mucous fistula rather than a deep pelvic infection. Once the patient has stabilized and weaned off immunosuppressant medications, usually after a period of 3 months, another procedure for restoration of intestinal continuity can be performed.

Subtotal Colectomy and Ileorectal Anastomosis

The option of ileal rectal anastomosis for the treatment of UC avoids complications of pelvic dissection such as disturbances of sexual function in men and reduced fertility seen in women, since there is no pelvic dissection. The key to good function following this operation is proper patient selection. Patients with limited rectal involvement do best, however, that is uncommon in UC, where the worst disease is usually located distally. In addition, since the patient retains the rectum with this procedure, these patients need to undergo continued surveillance for dysplasia because they are at in an increased risk of cancer in the retained rectum over time.

Ileal Pouch–Anal Anastomosis

IPAA has become the most popular procedure for UC not responding to medical therapy as well as for patients requiring colectomy for the presence of dysplasia. It has several advantages over ileal-rectal anastomosis in that it removes the entire colon as well as the majority of the at-risk mucosa, depending on how the operation is performed (i.e., stapled or hand-sewn anastomosis). IPAA was described in the mid to late 1970s and involves removing the entire colon and the majority of the rectum. It has two essential components: proctocolectomy and creation of a small bowel reservoir using the terminal ileum. This reservoir is then either sewn or sutured to the anal canal or lower rectum. There have been many different configurations of pouches or reservoirs that have been proposed in the past, including S Pouches, W Pouches, and H Pouches, all with relative advantages and disadvantages. However, by far, the simplest and easiest pouch and the one with the least complications is the J Pouch, which has withstood the test of time.

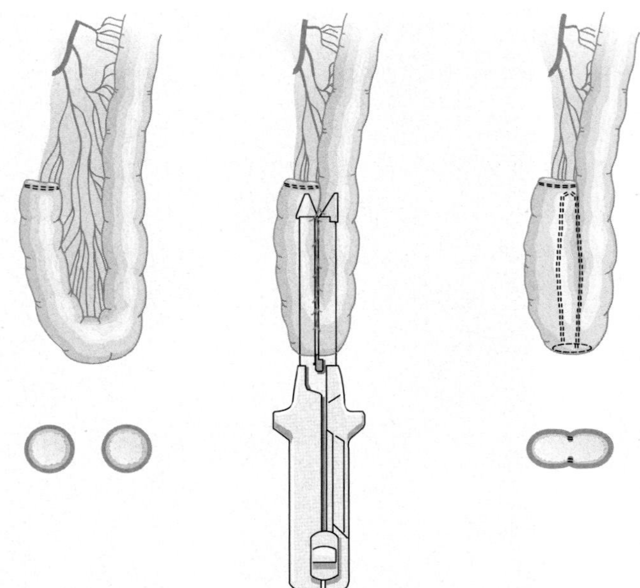

FIG. 52.41 Creation of an ileal J pouch using a cutting linear stapler. For replacement of the rectum, a reservoir is created from the distal ileum. The stapler joins two limbs of intestine with staples while dividing the intervening wall. The diameter of the pouch is created twice as large as the original diameter of the ileum. The limbs of the J pouch should be 15 cm in length. Two fires of a linear stapler are required; either a 75- or 100-mm stapler can be used.

This is created using 15-cm limbs of terminal ileum and two firings of a GIA stapler (Fig. 52.41). The apex of this J Pouch is then either stapled to the distal rectum, leaving a very short rectal cuff (Fig. 52.42), or hand-sewn to the distal rectum after a 2-cm mucosectomy is performed (Fig. 52.43). Currently, the stapled approach is preferred simply because it provides superior continence and it is much quicker to perform. However, in cases of dysplasia or cancer, hand-sewn approaches still may be warranted.

IPAA generally yields good functional results in patients with UC. Since many patients who are undergoing this operation are on immunosuppressives at the time of surgery or in poor nutritional state, this operation is commonly performed with temporary fecal diversion (temporary loop ileostomy). This is in place for 2 to 3 months, during which these immunosuppressant medications are weaned and the patient regains their normal nutritional state. The temporary ileostomy can then be closed, typically without requiring a laparotomy. In patients who are *not* on immune suppression and in good nutritional state (this usually refers to patients undergoing surgery for the findings of colonic dysplasia), the operation can safely be done in one stage *without* fecal diversion provided that there is no tension on the IPAA. Several technical maneuvers can be performed to lessen the tension on the IPAA. These include mobilization of the small bowel mesentery to the level of the pancreas (Fig. 52.44). When dividing the right colon mesentery, the ileocolic vessels should be preserved in their entirety. If distal traction is placed on the apex of the J pouch, it should easily reach just below the symphysis pubis (Fig. 52.45). When this maneuver is performed, one can either feel or visualize which small bowel mesenteric vessel is under more tension, the superior mesentery vessels or the ileocolic vessels. The vessel with the greater amount of tension can be divided, allowing greater length on the small bowel mesentery. "Peritoneal windowing" can

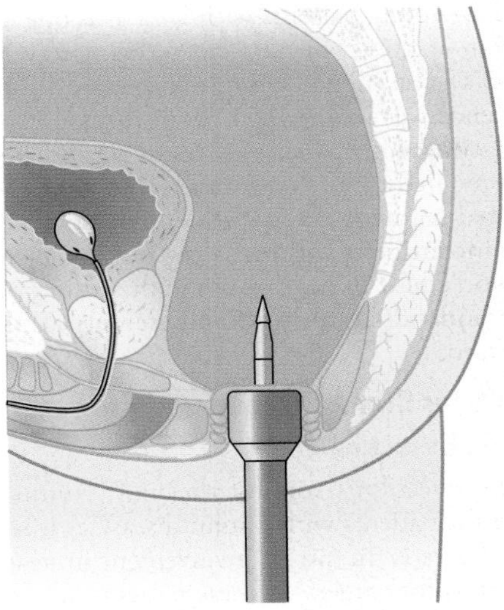

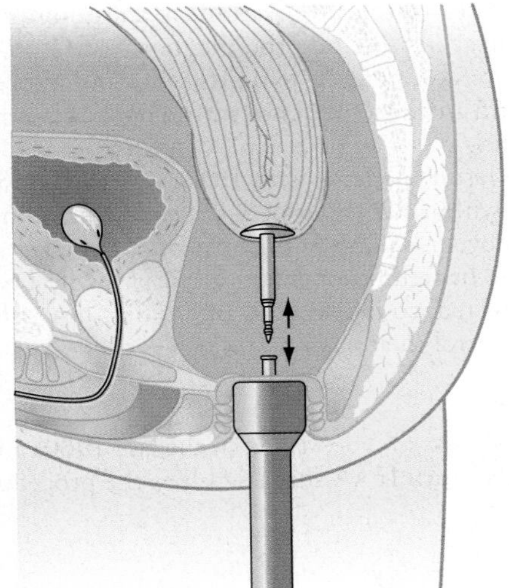

FIG. 52.42 Fashioning of stapled ileal pouch–anal anastomosis. A circular stapler is used; typically a 29-mm stapler is selected. A common error is to leave too long a segment of rectum, resulting in the persistent symptoms due to this retained segment of mucosa affected with inflammatory bowel disease (cuffitis).

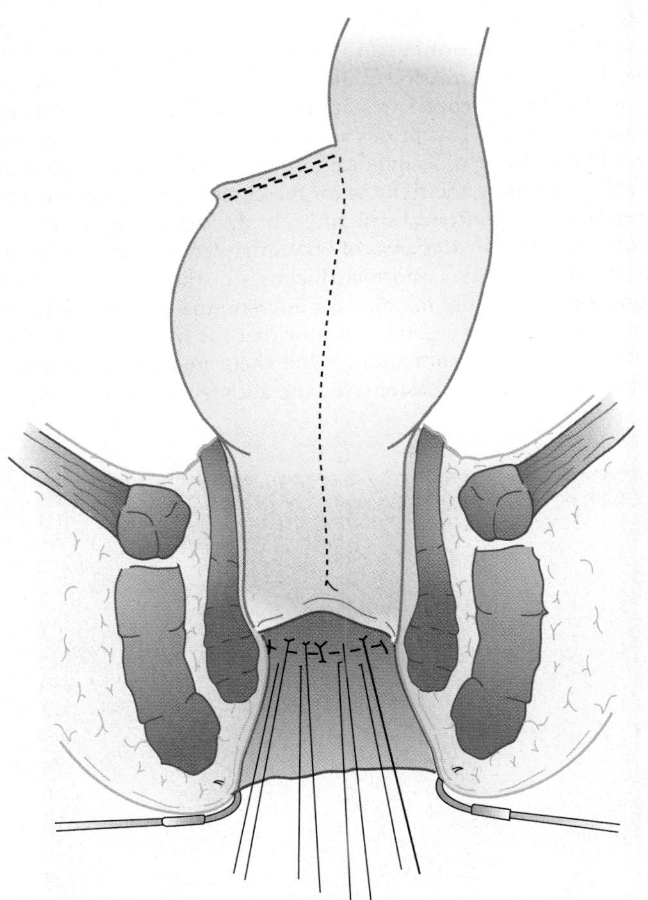

FIG. 52.43 Hand-sewn ileal pouch–anal anastomosis after anorectal mucosectomy.

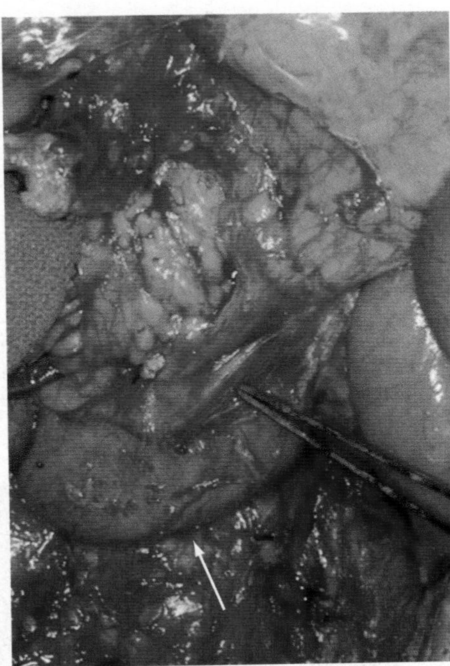

FIG. 52.44 Mobilization of the small bowel mesentery to the third portion of the duodenum. Here the small bowel mesentery has been retracted cephalad exposing the third portion of the duodenum *(arrow)*.

also provide mesenteric length. This is a maneuver whereby small slits are created in the anterior and posterior peritoneum covering the mesenteric vessels. These horizontal slits in the peritoneum, in most cases, provide for one or two extra centimeters of mesenteric length (Fig. 52.46). Needless to say, the more obese an individual is, the more difficult it can be to obtain sufficient mesenteric length for the small bowel to reach tension-free to the pelvis. In addition to this, with very tall individuals and those with a long torso, tension can be an issue as well.

Common early complications of IPAA include those associated with nonhealing of the IPAA: pelvic sepsis, ileal pouch–anal anastomotic fistulae, ileal pouch–vaginal fistulae, ileal pouch–anal anastomotic sinuses, and ileal pouch–anal anastomotic strictures (often a reflection of anastomotic tension). Late complications include the diagnosis of Crohn disease, which is more common in patients who undergo emergent colectomy and in those patients who have a diagnosis of indeterminate colitis.

With a "good" result, patients with IPAA will have up to six bowel movements within a 24-hour period, usually including one nocturnal bowel movement. In the majority of patients, at about 6 months, there will be significant enlargement of the ileal pouch, allowing patients to reduce the amount of antidiarrheal medication they take to control their output.

Continent Ileostomy

Continent ileostomy was first described in the late 1960s and remained very popular until IPAA surpassed it as the procedure of choice for young patients with UC. This operation involved construction of a reservoir, similar to that used with the IPAA. Here, instead of continence being maintained by the anal sphincter, continence was maintained by an intussuscepted segment of ileum positioned between this reservoir and the end ileostomy. A continent ileostomy is air and water tight; however, the intussuscepted segment is very prone to dessusception, rendering the stoma incontinent and requiring revisional surgery. This procedure works best in individuals with a thin body habitus as with heavier individuals the thicker mesentery also predisposes to dessusception.

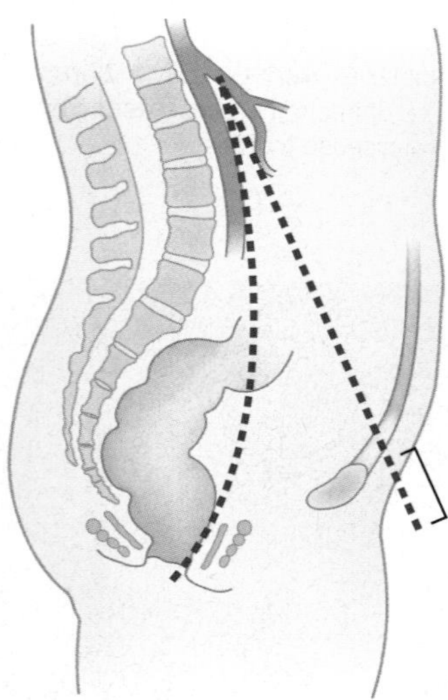

FIG. 52.45 Estimation of J-pouch length. The apex of the J pouch should be able to be brought down below the level of the symphysis pubis. This is a good estimate of a tension-free reach to the anal canal.

Surgery for Crohn Disease

Ileocolic Resection

Ileocolic resection is one of the most common operations performed for patients with Crohn disease as it is estimated that the ileocecal area is the site of involvement in nearly half of patients. Indications for surgery in these patients are usually either due to fibrostenosing disease with obstruction or associated fistulizing disease/mass/abscess or phlegmon. As the terminal ileum lies in the pelvis in close proximity to a number of pelvic structures, if there is a significant obstruction and a proximal perforation occurs, the resulting abscess can perforate into the sigmoid colon or bladder. The sigmoid colon is by far the more common, and the resulting ileosigmoid fistula fairly frequently occurs in these patients. When performing an ileocolic resection, one must always be alert to any "adhesions" and make sure these are not entero-enteric fistulas. Ileocolic resection lends itself well to the laparoscopic approach. Exceptions are cases in which there is extensive fistulizing disease or a significant phlegmon in which there is difficulty separating the right colon mesentery/terminal ileum away from the retroperitoneal structures. In deciding margins of resection, one should select areas of bowel that feel normal and are not thickened and have a normal thickness of the bowel-mesenteric junction. The ability to palpate a discrete small bowel-mesenteric junction is usually a good indicator that the lumen is free of significant Crohn inflammation. While there are many ways to construct the ileocolic anastomosis, the authors prefer a hand-sewn

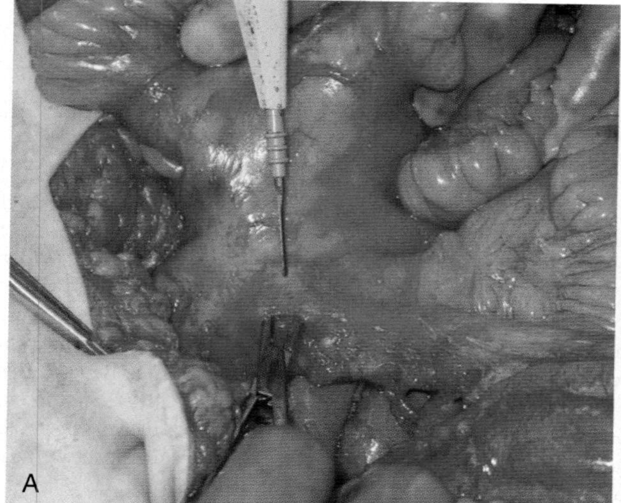

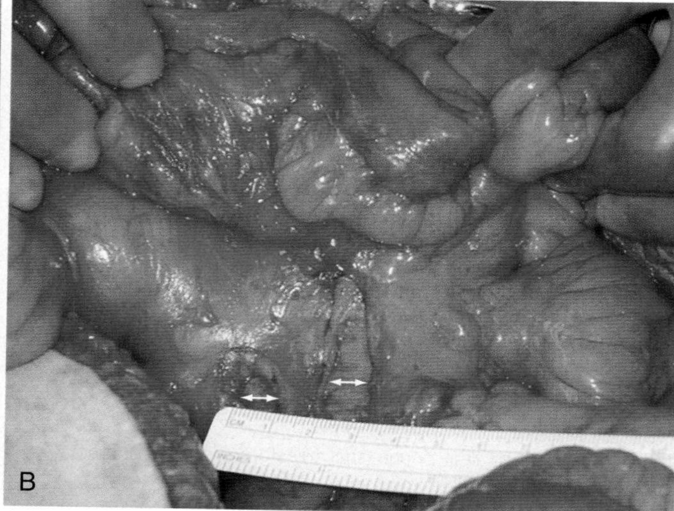

FIG. 52.46 Peritoneal windowing. (A) The mesenteric peritoneum is lifted away from the superior mesenteric artery by lifting it up with a hemostat and then divided using the electrocautery. (B) The mesenteric peritoneum has been divided perpendicular to the axis of the superior mesenteric artery. Note that at each area where the peritoneum has been divided, an additional 1 cm of mesenteric length has been obtained.

end-to-end anastomosis. Postoperatively, these anastomoses are very easy to evaluate endoscopically and to dilate in the event of recurrent disease, which is not true of side-to-side stapled anastomoses. It is paramount that however the anastomosis is constructed, it is made very wide.

Segmental Colon Resection

Segmental colonic resection has increasingly been used in the treatment of Crohn disease over the last two decades. This has been performed for two reasons: (1) recognition of the important role of water absorption (see section on colonic physiology) performed by the colon, and recognition that many of these patients will undergo repeated operations, and (2) availability of newer and more potent medications for Crohn disease allowing more effective suppression of recurrent disease. The idea of segmental resection for colonic Crohn disease can be performed in patients who have isolated areas of colonic stricture with relatively normal areas of "skipped" normal-appearing colon with normal colonic distensibility. In these patients, performing a segmental resection is associated with a much higher risk of recurrence, so this should always be accompanied by some type of postoperative chemoprophylaxis to reduce the risk of recurrence of the disease.

Subtotal Colectomy and Ileorectal Anastomosis

This is an operation that is well suited to patients with Crohn disease if they have a relative rectal-sparing and an otherwise diseased colon. Segmental resection is preferable if there are areas of normal intervening colon. However, this operation also, as with segmental colectomy, is associated with a much higher rate of recurrence. Options for this, if there is a smaller amount of retained rectum, are to perform an ileal pouch–rectal anastomosis in order to lessen the number of bowel movements that the patient has after surgery. Depending on the height of the anastomosis and the circumstances of the surgery (redo, associated immunosuppression, patients' nutritional state), this may require temporary fecal diversion (temporary loop ileostomy) to facilitate healing.

Proctocolectomy and Ileal-Pouch–Anal Anastomosis

In previous editions of the Sabiston textbook, there perhaps was only a passing mention of this procedure; however, every year, this is more frequently considered a possibility for patients with Crohn disease, providing that they do not have obvious perianal disease. With the advent of newer and more potent immunosuppressive drugs, this procedure is considered an option in an educated patient who is aware of the increased risk of morbidity and the less favorable functional results (i.e., greater number of bowel movements) as compared to when this operation is performed for patients with UC. In addition, there is, of course, a higher risk of fistulizing disease and the need to convert to an end ileostomy. However, in the motivated patient who recognizes and accepts these risks, this procedure can be performed. See the section on IPAA for UC for technical details regarding this procedure.

Cancer Risk

As with UC, there is an increased risk of colon cancer in patients with longstanding Crohn disease, although it is thought to be somewhat less than with UC. However, in patients in whom there has been a cancer identified, total colectomy should be performed, as there have been studies showing colonic procarcinogenic mutations tracking along the colon and the risk of a subsequent cancer in other areas of the colon is high.[18]

Postoperative Complications

Many patients with IBD who undergo surgery are on immunosuppressive medications, and in addition, many of these patients are hypoalbuminemic, since they have protein-losing enteropathy from their disease. Because of this, they are at increased risk for infectious postoperative complications. There are differing opinions as to the relative risk of complications with these different medications. However, overall, it is thought that steroids pose an increased risk for infectious complications, as do the administration of biologic medications, within several months before surgery.[19] Because of this, there should be a discussion with patients regarding the possibility of a temporary fecal diversion if an operation is undertaken in which an anastomosis is considered so that, if in the clinical judgment of the surgeon a temporary ileostomy is considered prudent, this can be performed.

Postoperative Recurrence

Recurrence rate following surgery for Crohn disease varies depending on the site of surgery as well as other factors such as environmental factors. It has been reported that Crohn patients who smoke are at higher risk of early disease recurrence, as are patients younger than 30 years old and those who have already had two or more operations for fistulizing disease.[20] There has been an increasing recognition that early intensive medical treatment beginning very soon postoperatively may successfully reduce the risk of recurrence. Regular endoscopic monitoring of the lower GI tract for signs of recurrent disease is important to allow therapeutic intervention prior to the development of therapy-resistant fibrosis.

INFECTIOUS COLITIS

Infectious colitis may be diagnosed among patients with acute diarrhea and colonic inflammation. Their importance for the surgeon arises in their capacity to mimic surgical conditions such as an acute abdomen or IBD and in some cases to deteriorate to the point where they require surgical treatment.

Clostridium difficile Infection

C. difficile is a common inhabitant of the GI tract that can manifest in a spectrum of symptoms ranging from that of an asymptomatic carrier to fulminant colitis.

Epidemiology

C. difficile is the most common cause of healthcare-associated diarrhea and is considered to be a major source of healthcare-associated morbidity occurring in 2% of all hospital discharges for all diseases. The prevalence of asymptomatic colonization of *C. difficile* among adult hospitalized patients ranges from 3% to 26% in different studies. Around 453,000 new cases of CDI are diagnosed annually in the United States, of which 83,000 are recurrent cases, with 29,300 attributed deaths.[21] Interestingly, after plateauing at historical high rates, some regions have begun to show a decline in incidence attributed to specific prevention and treatment programs. In participating Canadian hospitals, for example, the incidence of CDI has decreased from 7.9/10,000 patient-days in 2011 to 4.3/10,000 patient-days in 2015.[22]

Microbiology and Transmission

C. difficile is an anaerobic, spore-forming, gram-positive bacillus. Transmission routes include person-to-person spread through the fecal-oral route or through exposure to a contaminated environment by ingestion of spores from other patients and transmission via healthcare personnel's hands. Toxicogenic *C. difficile* pathogens can produce A and B toxins, both of which have been associated with colitis. Binding of toxin A or B to colonocyte glycoprotein receptors leads to colonocyte death and release of inflammatory mediators. The emergence of the *C. difficile* Ribotype 027 strain in the mid-2000s resulted in significant outbreaks across the Western world associated with more severe disease outcomes and deaths.

Risk Factors

The most important risk factor for the development of a clinical infection is recent exposure to antibiotics. Antibiotics affect the natural bowel flora, decreasing the natural ability to suppress the growth and spread of *C. difficile*. Virtually all antibiotics have been associated with *C. difficile*, but particularly third and fourth generation cephalosporins, fluoroquinolones, clindamycin, and carbapenems have been linked to a higher risk of CDI. Other risk factors include immunodeficiency (including human immunodeficiency virus infection), chemotherapy treatment, use of acid suppressing medications such as proton pump inhibitors, GI surgery or manipulation of GI tract including tube feeding, and prolonged hospitalization or lengthy stay in nursing homes or rehabilitation units. Patients with IBD have increased rates of CDI, along with worse outcomes [HIV] and higher rates of colectomy. These patients are more likely to receive immunosuppressants and antibiotics and have a different intestinal flora compared to healthy subjects. Differentiating between an IBD exacerbation and CDI can be difficult as the symptoms overlap, and a high index of suspicion must be maintained. Patients with an increased risk for death from CDI include those with advanced age, multiple comorbidities, hypoalbuminemia, leukocytosis, acute renal failure, and those infected with Ribotype 027.

Clinical Presentation

Symptoms of CDI commonly begin 4 to 9 days after initiation of antibiotics but can commence 10 weeks or more after antibiotic treatment. Patients presenting with new-onset, unexplained, watery diarrhea (with three or more unformed stools in 24 hours) should be suspected of having CDI. Patients may also have abdominal pain, fever, and an associated ileus. Patients with CDI can be categorized into asymptomatic colonization, nonsevere disease, severe disease, and fulminant disease. A variety of scores have been utilized to assess clinical severity and treatment response. Leukocytes of at least 15,000 cells/μL and/or serum creatinine of at least 1.5 cells/μL are predictors of severe disease according to the Infectious Disease Society of America. Fulminant or severe CDI is diagnosed in patients demonstrating hypotension or shock, ileus, or megacolon. The ATLAS criteria is a simple clinical bedside score, which includes age, temperature, leukocytosis, albumin, and systemic antibiotic treatment and has been used to assess response to treatment.[23]

Diagnosis

The diagnosis of CDI is based on typical symptoms in combination with stool testing. Laboratory testing is based on detection of *C. difficile* toxins, *C. difficile* antigen, or the bacteria itself. A variety of commercial tests are utilized, including enzyme-linked immunosorbent assay for toxin detection, glutamate dehydrogenase immunoassay for *C. difficile* antigen detection, nucleic acid amplification test, polymerase chain reaction testing, and stool cultures.

Flexible sigmoidoscopy may be helpful as a diagnostic modality for CDI. Although it is not a first-line modality for diagnosis, it can be helpful in cases of inconclusive stool testing or to help exclude other etiologies. Classically raised, yellowish-white small (2–10 mm) plaques (pseudomembranes) can be observed in approximately half of patients with CDI (Fig. 52.47). Nonspecific colitis can be found in an additional 25%. Histologic findings from the plaques reveal an inflammatory exudate with mucinous debris, fibrin, necrotic epithelial cells, and polymorphonuclear cells. In fulminant colitis, colonoscopy may increase the risk of perforation and should be considered only when the benefit is higher than the risk of complications.

Imaging is not very useful for diagnosis as it is not specific but can assist in assessing disease severity and response to treatment. Typical CT findings include significant colonic wall thickening, bowel dilation, pericolonic fat stranding, high attenuation oral contrast in the colonic lumen alternating with low-attenuation inflamed mucosa (accordion sign), and ascites. Ultrasound may also be useful, especially among critically ill patients who cannot be transported to the CT scanner in radiology. Ultrasonography may show bowel wall thickening, narrowing of the lumen, as well as pseudomembranes, which are seen as hyperechoic lines covering the mucosa.

Treatment

Initial treatment includes stopping or minimizing previous antibiotics, parenteral fluids, and correction of electrolytes. The use of antiperistaltic agents for the treatment of CDI should be avoided. Antibiotic treatment of CDI is determined according to the clinical setting and can be divided into the initial episode, recurrent episode, severe, and fulminant disease. Table 52.4 summarizes current antibiotic treatment recommendations for initial episodes and for severe and fulminant disease.

Treatment options for recurrent episodes generally include changing antibiotics (from metronidazole to vancomycin or fidaxomicin from vancomycin). In addition, tapered and pulsed regimens are used.

Fecal Microbiota Transplant

Fecal microbiota transplant (FMT) for patients with recurrent episodes of CDI is a relatively new treatment. Patients with CDI lack protective colonic microbiota to resist replication and colonization of *C. difficile*. Reimplantation of normal gut bacteria, particularly bacteria resistant to *C. difficile* from healthy donors can help restore normal gut biodiversity and correct the imbalance. Different routes of administration have been described in the literature including nasogastric, oral (frozen fecal microbial capsules), rectal enema, and colonic per colonoscopy. A recent comparison between upper and lower methods of delivery demonstrated the lower approaches being more effective.[24] The efficacy of FMT ranges from 77% to 100%, with multiple FMTs needed to achieve a good clinical response. Current guidelines recommend FMT for patients with multiple recurrences of CDI, in whom antibiotic treatment has failed.

Monoclonal Antibodies

Bezlotoxumab and actoxumab are monoclonal antibodies directed against *C. difficile* toxins B and A, respectively. These antibodies limit colonic damage by neutralization of the toxin and block the binding to host cells.[25] They can be used as coadjuvant treatment

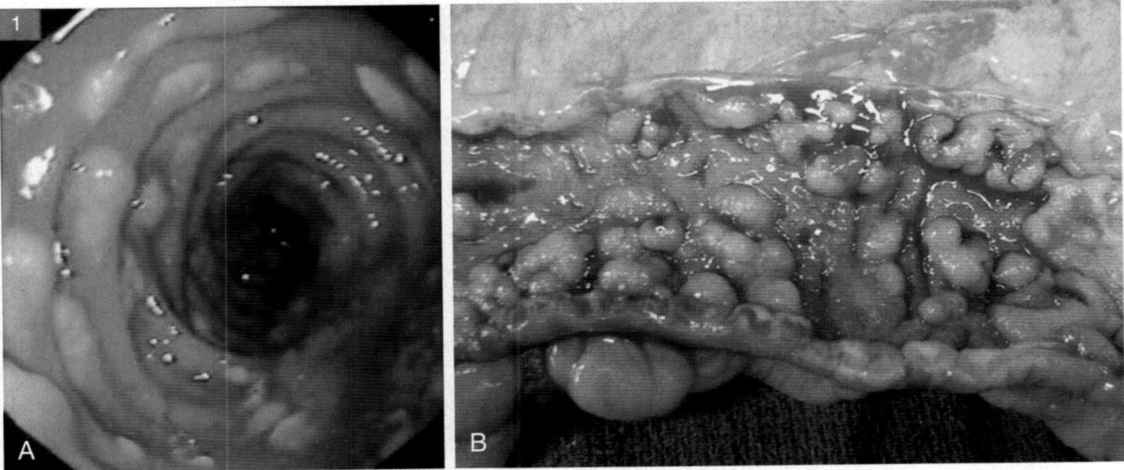

FIG. 52.47 (A) Endoscopic view of pseudomembranes associated with *Clostridium difficile*. (B) Pseudomembranes overlying the colon mucosa at the time of colectomy. The patient had active *Clostridium difficile* colitis with coexisting Crohn colitis.

TABLE 52.4 **Antibiotic treatment of *Clostridium difficile* infection.**

CLINICAL CONDITIONS	TREATMENT	TREATMENT DURATION
First episode	1. Oral vancomycin 125 mg 4 times daily OR 2. Fidaxomicin 200t mg twice Daily If vancomycin and fidaxomicin are not available: metronidazole 500 mg 3 times daily can be given for nonsevere disease.	10 days
First episode—fulminant (hypotension, shock, ileus, megacolon)	Vancomycin, 500 mg 4 times daily (oral or by nasogastric tube). In case of ileus: 1. Consider adding rectal instillation of vancomycin. 2. Intravenously administered metronidazole (500 mg every 8 hours) should be administered together with oral or rectal vancomycin.	At least 10 days, duration should be individualized

Adopted from McDonald LC, Gerding DN, Johnson S, et al, Clinical Practice Guidelines for *Clostridium difficile* infection in adults and children: 2017 update by the Infectious Diseases Society of America (IDSA) and Society for Healthcare Epidemiology of America (SHEA). *Clin Infect Dis.* 2018;66:987–994.

with antimicrobial therapy to help prevent recurrence, especially among patients infected by Ribotype 027, in severe CDI, and in immunocompromised patients.

Surgery

Patients with fulminant CDI who develop signs of systemic toxicity, toxic megacolon, or perforation should be operated upon emergently. Emergency colectomy for patients with fulminant colitis provides a survival advantage compared with continuing antibiotics. Among severely ill patients, a total or subtotal abdominal colectomy with preservation of the rectum has traditionally been performed. A newer option with similar results for patients without necrosis or perforation is exteriorization of a diverting loop ileostomy with on-table colonic lavage followed by antegrade vancomycin flushes.[26]

OTHER COLONIC INFECTIONS

Diarrhea and colitis can be caused by other pathogens. Most of these will not require surgery. A careful history can discover the source in many cases, such as polluted drinking or recreational water, consumption of contaminated fruits and vegetables, unpasteurized milk, undercooked meat and fish, shellfish, and eggs. International travel, as well as contact with animals and their feces should also be queried. Table 52.5 summarizes the important characteristics of common bacteria causing diarrhea and colitis.

The initial approach includes a careful history, evaluation for dehydration and electrolyte disturbances, and stool testing for ova and parasites and for culture and sensitivity. Patients with signs of sepsis or those who have traveled from enteric fever–endemic regions and immunocompromised patients should also have blood cultures obtained.

Initial treatment includes rehydration and correction of electrolyte disturbances. Oral rehydration solution is recommended for mild to moderate disease. Nasogastric administration of oral rehydration solution may be considered for patients who do not tolerate oral intake. Patients with signs of severe dehydration or ileus should be treated with isotonic IV fluids (normal saline or lactated Ringer's solution). The majority of patients who present with acute watery diarrhea and those without recent international travel *do not require* antimicrobial therapy. Immunocompromised

TABLE 52.5 Clinical characteristics of common enteric infections.

PATHOGEN	CHARACTERISTICS AND CLINCAL PRESENTATION
Campylobacter jejuni	Spiral, microaerophilic gram-positive rod. Exposure to improperly prepared chicken or beef. Fever, watery diarrhea, and abdominal pain. Commonly involves the cecum and terminal ileum. May mimic appendicitis or Crohn disease.
Yersinia enterocolitica	Gram-negative coccobacillus. Exposure to contaminated water or food. Abdominal pain and bloody diarrhea, may mimic appendicitis or Crohn disease.
Shigella	Gram-negative, facultative anaerobe. Common cause for dysentery in developing countries. Often affects rectum and sigmoid colon. Fever, abdominal pain, watery diarrhea that can progress to bloody diarrhea.
Salmonella typhi or *Salmonella enterica* serotypes Paratyphi	Gram-negative, facultatively anaerobic bacilli Recent travel to an endemic area, consumption of foods prepared by a traveler to an endemic area. Fever with or without diarrhea, abdominal pain, cramping and vomiting.

Adapted from Shane AL, Mody RK, Crump JA, et al. 2017 Infectious Diseases Society of America Clinical Practice Guidelines for the diagnosis and management of infectious diarrhea. *Clin Infect Dis*. 2017;65:1963–1973.

or septic patients, as well as those suspected of enteric fever, should be treated with empirical, broad-spectrum antimicrobial therapy, usually with fluoroquinolones, such as ciprofloxacin, or macrolides, such as azithromycin, depending on local susceptibility patterns. Surgical intervention is rarely required apart from those cases developing severe fulminant disease that lead to perforation or toxic megacolon.

Viruses can also cause acute diarrhea and colitis. Cytomegalovirus (CMV) is an important etiology to consider in immunocompromised hosts, particularly in advanced HIV infection, transplant patients, patients with IBD, and in those receiving chemotherapy. CMV colitis commonly presents with watery or bloody diarrhea, fever, and abdominal pain. Diagnosis is established by serology and by determining viral load in the blood. Endoscopy demonstrates patchy mucosal erythema in the colon. Inclusion bodies seen on biopsy are pathognomonic for CMV. CMV colitis can progress to sepsis, toxic megacolon and colon perforation. Treatment is usually supportive with the addition of ganciclovir. Patients with severe, complicated disease may require surgery.

ISCHEMIC COLITIS

Ischemic colitis is a common disorder that develops when the arterial blood supply to the colon is insufficient to support cellular metabolic demands. It is the most common form of GI ischemia, with rates of 7.1 to 22.9/100,000 person-years.[27] Severity varies within a wide spectrum, from mild self-limiting disease to severe life-threatening colonic ischemia. Considering the wide range of clinical findings with most patients presenting with mild nonspecific symptoms, the true incidence is likely much higher. It is important to differentiate ischemic colitis from situations of acute mesenteric ischemia, in which a major vessel of the bowel is obstructed, wherein patients commonly present with severe pain out of proportion to physical findings and require immediate vascular intervention. Ischemic colitis is considered a disease of small blood vessels and typically presents less dramatically, seldom requiring vascular intervention. Most cases, when recognized and managed promptly, do not require surgery. Delays in diagnosis and treatment, however, can result in the need for emergency colectomy with high morbidity and mortality.

Anatomic Considerations

The arterial blood supply to the colon is derived from the SMA and the IMA. The SMA gives off the ileocolic, right colic, and middle colic arteries. The IMA gives rise to the left colic and sigmoid arteries and ends as the superior rectal (hemorrhoidal) artery (Fig. 52.8). There are two well-described collateral networks that aid in preventing colonic ischemia by providing "backup" both within the territories of the two major arteries and between them. The main collateral vessel is the marginal artery of Drummond, which runs parallel and close to the mesenteric margin of the colon from the cecocolic junction to the rectosigmoid junction. The colon can receive collateral blood supply through this artery when one of the larger arteries is obstructed. It is important when resecting a section of colon to preserve this artery since only the vasa recta are located between it and the colon. When it is compromised, ischemia of that section of colon may result. The second collateral circulation can be found in the proximal region of the large arteries. The "arc of Riolan" (meandering mesenteric artery) is an infrequent finding, traversing close to the mesenteric root and connecting the SMA or middle colic artery to the IMA or left colic artery (Fig. 52.48). It can have a critical role in situations of SMA or IMA occlusion. The presence of a large arc of Riolan commonly indicates an obstruction of one of the major mesenteric arteries.

Watershed areas of the colon are potentially found at the edge of the region supplied by the two main arteries, the SMA and the IMA, zones that are frequently dependent upon collateral circulation (Fig. 52.49). There are two well-described watershed areas where the collateral circulation is classically inconsistent and vulnerable to ischemia. The first is the area of the splenic flexure (Griffiths point). In some studies, up to 50% of specimens were found to lack a marginal artery in the region where the SMA and IMA circulations meet. Commonly, surgeons avoid making anastomoses in this area for fear that the impaired blood supply will not be sufficient to permit anastomotic healing, leading to anastomotic leaks. A second potential watershed area is the

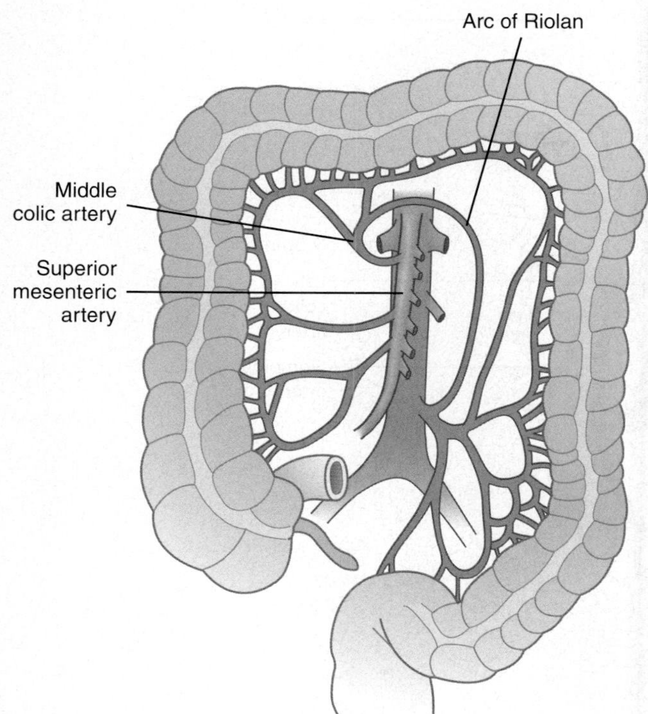

FIG. 52.48 The Arc of Riolan. (From Gordon PH, Nivatvongs S, ed. *Principles and Practice of Surgery for the Colon, Rectum and Anus.* 2nd ed. St. Louis: Quality Medical Publishing; 1999:27.)

rectosigmoid junction (Sudeck's point). This region receives it blood supply from the superior hemorrhoidal artery and distal sigmoid branches, both terminal branches of the IMA and prone to atherosclerotic changes. The right colon, although not classically considered a watershed area, it is also vulnerable to ischemia from embolic occlusion because the ileocolic artery is the terminal branch of the SMA. For this reason, the right colon is also particularly prone to low-flow conditions such as heart failure, hemorrhage, and sepsis. The rectum, which has a good blood supply from both the IMA and the iliac circulation, as well as a strong collateral network, is rarely the victim of ischemic injury.

Risk Factors

Ischemic colitis may occur in all ages but is significantly more common in elderly patients, in women, and in patients with multiple comorbidities. Several medical conditions and medications have been associated with ischemic colitis (Box 52.2)[28]

Patients with low-flow states, as a result of heart failure or sepsis, are especially prone to develop ischemic colitis. Diabetes mellitus, hypertension, chronic obstructive pulmonary disease, peripheral vascular disease, and renal disease have also been associated with this disorder. Patients undergoing aortic reconstructive surgery or abdominal surgery in which the IMA is ligated are also especially predisposed to colonic ischemia. In these patients, if the collateral circulation is not sufficient, acute occlusion of the IMA can result in sigmoid and left colon ischemia.

Several medications have been implicated in ischemic colitis. Constipation-inducing drugs can cause ischemic colitis, most likely as a result of reduced blood flow and increased intraluminal pressure. Immunomodulator drugs such as anti-TNF-α inhibitors can affect thrombogenesis, and illicit drugs such as cocaine and methamphetamines cause ischemia through vasoconstriction, hypercoagulation, and direct endothelial injury.

Presentation and Diagnosis

The majority of patients with partial-thickness ischemia of a localized section of colon present with relatively nonspecific signs and symptoms. A high index of suspicion is needed to make an early diagnosis. Presenting symptoms usually include sudden abdominal pain and cramping, tenesmus, and bloody diarrhea or hematochezia. The combination of these symptoms is present in close to 50% of the patients, with the pain usually beginning prior to the bleeding. Bleeding associated with ischemic colitis is usually minor and seldom requires blood transfusions. Patients may also experience nausea, vomiting, and a low-grade fever. On physical exam, abdominal distension may be noted, as well as tenderness overlying the involved region. A good medical history is important in establishing the diagnosis, with a focus on associated diseases and medications.

The most common affected region is the left colon (including the splenic flexure), followed by the sigmoid colon based on the affected blood supply. Pancolitis due to ischemia is associated with a worse prognosis. About a quarter of the patients present with isolated right-sided ischemic colitis. These patients are more likely to present with abdominal pain without bleeding and more commonly have atrial fibrillation, coronary artery disease, and/or chronic renal failure. Patients with isolated right-sided ischemic colitis have a higher chance of requiring surgery and have a poorer prognosis. A minority of patients will present with full-thickness ischemia. These patients are sicker and commonly present with high fever, leukocytosis, acidosis, and peritonitis.

Basic laboratory testing is nonspecific but can assist in predicting severity. Severe disease has been associated with an increased white blood cell count, blood urea nitrogen, lactate dehydrogenase, and decreased hemoglobin and albumin levels. Acidosis, decreased bicarbonate, and increased lactate levels are also associated with severe ischemic colitis. It is also recommended to test stool for *C. difficile* toxin, ova and parasites, and culture and sensitivity in order to exclude an infectious etiology.

Abdominal plain films may show bowel distension and "thumbprinting," which are rounded densities along the sides of a gas-filled colon indicative of submucosal edema. These are nonspecific to ischemic colitis since thumbprinting can be found with other situations of colonic inflammation. Free intraperitoneal air suggests bowel perforation and should lead to immediate operative management. Water-soluble contrast enemas have generally become obsolete in the diagnosis of ischemic colitis but may still be used for the evaluation of chronic ischemic strictures. CT scans of the abdomen have become the primary noninvasive modality for the initial diagnosis of colonic pathology. CT scans, performed using both IV and oral contrast, can assist in determining the location of involved areas, to assess the severity, identify complications, and exclude the presence of other diseases. Findings suggestive of ischemic colitis, although relatively nonspecific, include segmental bowel thickening, pericolonic fat stranding, and thumb printing. Pneumatosis intestinalis (the presence of gas in the colonic wall), portal venous gas, and the absence of large bowel enhancement on contrast-enhanced CT usually indicate severe transmural disease favoring immediate surgical intervention. Vascular imaging is usually not indicated in cases of ischemic colitis, as this is usually a disease of small vessels; however, in cases of pain of sudden onset

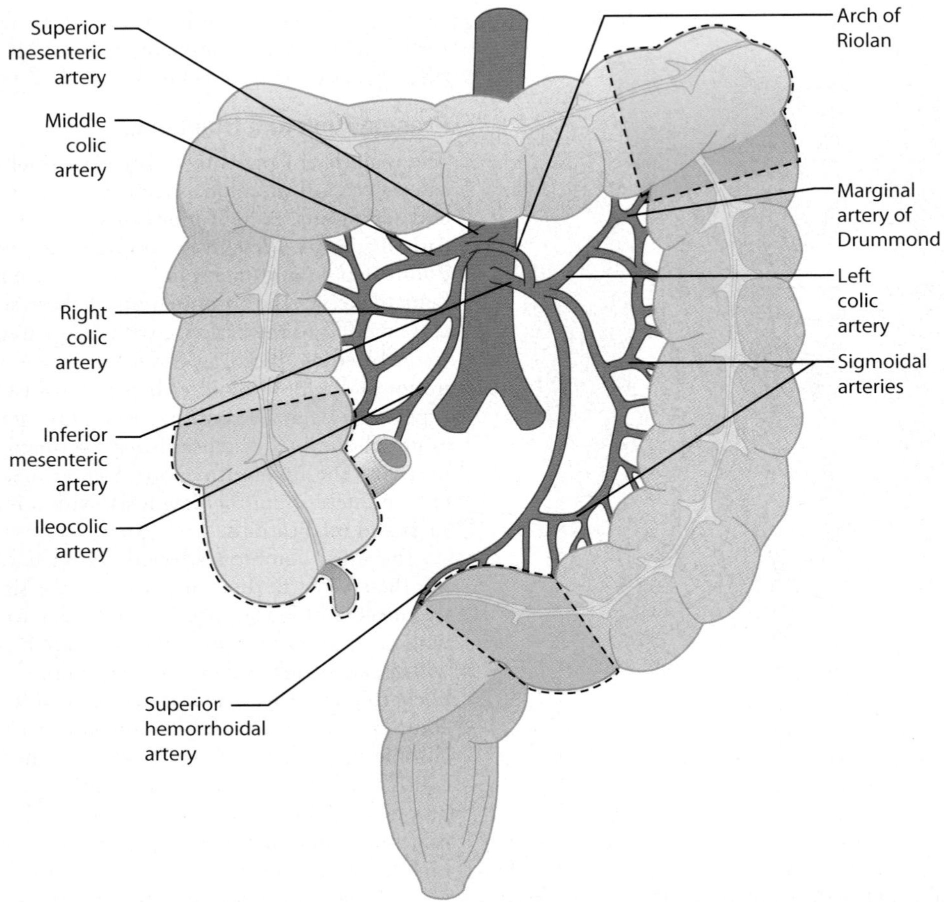

FIG. 52.49 Lightly shaded colonic regions especially vulnerable to ischemia. (From Netz U, Galandiuk S. Management of ischemic colitis. In: Cameron JL, Cameron A, eds. *Current Surgical Therapy*. 12th ed. Philadelphia: Elsevier; 2017:171–176.)

that is out of proportion to physical and laboratory findings and in isolated right colon ischemic colitis, multiphasic CT angiography should be performed to exclude acute proximal mesenteric ischemia.

The gold standard for the diagnosis of ischemic colitis is flexible endoscopy. Early colonoscopy should be performed (within 48 hours), except in cases of acute peritonitis or in cases of suspected severe transmural ischemia. In contrast to the expected increased risk of perforation due to endoscopy in the evaluation of ischemic colitis, current published literature does not demonstrate a higher rate of perforation compared to other patients. It is recommended, however, to refrain from overinsufflation and avoid advancing the scope beyond the most distal extent of disease. Common endoscopic findings characteristic of ischemic colitis include edematous and friable mucosa, erythema, petechial hemorrhage, and mucosal ulceration. The "single-stripe sign," a single linear ulcer running along the longitudinal axis of the colon is rare but considered specific for ischemic colitis. Segmental distribution, with abrupt transition between injured and noninjured mucosa, and sparing of the rectum support ischemia over IBD. It is important to note that diagnostic endoscopy usually cannot distinguish between partial-thickness and full-thickness ischemia. Fig. 52.50 depicts a recommended algorithm for diagnosis and treatment of ischemic colitis.

Treatment

The majority of patients, nearly 80%, will respond to conservative nonoperative treatment, with significant improvement within a few days. The mainstay of treatment includes bowel rest, IV fluids, and broad-spectrum antibiotics. A nasogastric tube should be inserted if ileus is present.

Efforts should be made to correct low-flow states and hypotension with aggressive fluid resuscitation and optimal treatment of associated conditions such as heart failure and sepsis. Colonic ischemia can result in failure of the intestinal epithelial barrier with bacterial translocation leading to overt sepsis. For this reason, empiric broad-spectrum antibiotics against both anaerobic and aerobic coliform bacteria are prescribed in ischemic colitis to cover the normal colonic bacterial flora. Cathartics are not recommended as they may lead to colon perforation. Glucocorticoids should be avoided unless treating a preexisting disorder such as lupus or rheumatoid arthritis.

Most episodes of ischemic colitis are mild and self-limiting. Patients who fail to improve or have worsening symptoms within a few days should raise the concern for the development of full-thickness ischemia and should have repeat imaging or endoscopy to help guide treatment.

A small proportion of patients with mild to moderate symptoms will develop a chronic colitis, with ongoing or recurrent bouts of

BOX 52.2 Conditions and drugs associated with ischemic colitis.

Low Flow State
- Septic shock
- Congestive heart failure
- Hemorrhagic shock
- Hypotension

Atherosclerosis
- Ischemic heart disease
- Cerebrovascular disease
- Peripheral vascular disease

Gastrointestinal
- Constipation
- Diarrhea
- Irritable bowel syndrome

Surgery and Invasive Interventions
- Abdominal surgery
- Aortic surgery (especially abdominal aortic aneurysm repair)
- Cardiovascular surgery
- Following endovascular abdominal manipulations (i.e., chemoembolization)
- Postcolonoscopy

Cardiovascular/Pulmonary
- Chronic obstructive pulmonary disease
- Atrial fibrillation
- Hypertension

Metabolic/Rheumatoid
- Diabetes mellitus
- Dyslipidemia
- Systemic lupus erythematosus
- Rheumatoid arthritis

Miscellaneous
- Hypercoagulable states
- Sickle cell disease
- Long-distance running

Drugs
- Constipation inducing drugs (opioids and nonopioids)
- Cocaine and methamphetamines
- Immunomodulatory drugs (anti-tumor necrosis factor-α, type 1 interferon-α, type 1 interferon-β)
- Chemotherapeutic drugs (i.e., taxanes)
- Female hormones and oral contraceptives
- Decongestants (pseudoephedrine)
- Serotoninergic (i.e., alosetron, sumatriptan)

symptoms of abdominal pain, bloody diarrhea, and sepsis. These patients have a higher rate of complications and commonly require surgical resection of the involved segment. Some patients who initially recover from partial-thickness ischemic colitis will eventually develop a chronic stricture at the involved segment. These patients may complain of constipation, narrowed stools, and abdominal pain. Diagnosis can be confirmed with a contrast enema, CT, or endoscopy. Symptomatic patients or those in which malignancy cannot be excluded should undergo elective resection.

Patients who present with, or develop signs of transmural ischemia and perforation, including peritonitis, hemodynamic instability, free peritoneal air, and ominous signs on CT as mentioned earlier, such as portal venous gas, require emergent surgical exploration. A recent large database study identified a 25% 30-day postoperative mortality rate for ischemic colitis[29] with other studies ranging up to 47% mortality following acute surgical intervention. Risk factors independently identified as associated with perioperative mortality after colectomy for ischemic colitis include the elderly, poor functional status, multiple comorbidities, preoperative septic shock, preoperative blood transfusions, preoperative acute renal failure, and delay from hospital admission to surgery.

During surgery, it is important to visualize and assess the entire small and large intestine for signs of ischemia and gangrene. Ischemia commonly affects a recognizable segment of the colon, frequently in watershed areas. In these cases, an anatomic resection should be performed to allow sufficient blood supply to the remaining colon with minimal reliance on stressed collaterals. Deciding how much to resect or whether a specific segment is likely to survive can be difficult. Visual examination tends to be inaccurate, especially when the bowel is ischemic but still viable. Intraoperative infrared angiography is a relatively new technique that has been gaining popularity as an adjunct for determining bowel viability and for determining the integrity of intestinal anastomoses. In this technique, indocyanine green is injected intravenously and distributes throughout the circulation. Then, using a variety of commercially available imaging systems, the indocyanine green undergoes laser excitation, demonstrating real-time tissue perfusion (Fig. 52.51). Creation of an anastomosis is usually not recommended in the acute setting, due to the concern for evolving ischemia and the existence of hemodynamic instability and sepsis commonly encountered in these situations. A temporary abdominal closure with a planned second-look after 24 hours may be prudent to determine the need for further resection. Staple the ends and leave them in the abdomen, avoiding complications of a stoma as in very obese patients. Pancolic ischemia is rare, but such cases require total colectomy with ileostomy. In contrast to mesenteric ischemia of the small intestine, there is usually no indication for revascularizing the large bowel in primary colonic ischemia, which is not generally related to large artery obstruction.

NEOPLASIA

Colorectal Cancer Genetics

As CRC is one of the most common cancers worldwide, much research has been directed into the genetics of CRC. It has long been appreciated that genetics play a role in the disorder and there has been an appreciation and recognition of specific inherited cancer syndromes that has greatly aided in our understanding of sporadic CRC. Before the reader passes on the next section, this section explains why some patients will develop a CRC very quickly and others, more slowly.

Chromosomal Instability Pathway

Much of our initial understanding of the genetic basis of CRC comes from the work of Vogelstein and colleagues, who evaluated nearly 200 samples of colorectal neoplasia ranging from polyps to invasive cancers. By checking for alterations in specific genes, they were able to propose a step-wise model of CRC carcinogenesis, involving the activation of an oncogene (a gene

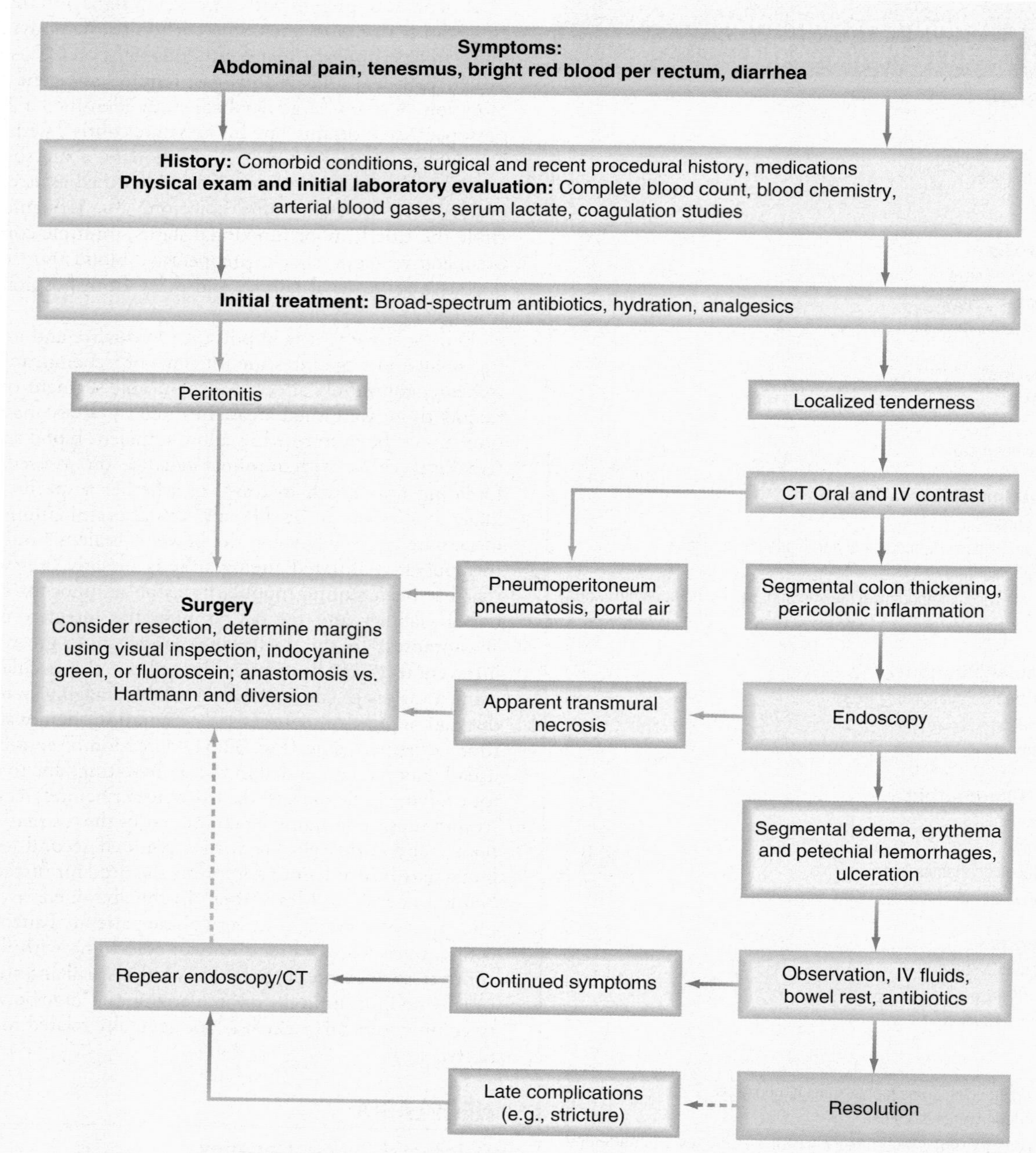

FIG. 52.50 Algorithm for investigation and treatment for ischemic colitis. (From Netz U, Galandiuk S. Management of ischemic colitis. In: Cameron JL, Cameron A, eds. *Current Surgical Therapy*. 12th ed. Philadelphia: Elsevier; 2017:171–176.) *CT*, Computed tomography; *IV*, intravenous.

that can induce cancer formation) and loss of several genes that act as tumor suppressors. Currently, it is thought that the majority of sporadic CRC arise in this fashion over the course of approximately 10 years from a precursor dysplastic adenoma. The molecular events involved include early *APC* (adenomatous polyposis coli) gene mutations, subsequent activating mutations in the oncogene *KRAS,* as well as mutations resulting in inactivation of the tumor suppressor gene *TP53*. Chromosomal instability refers to changes (gains or losses) in the numbers of chromosomes (aneuploidy) as well as subchromosomal genomic amplifications and loss of heterozygosity seen with this pathway of carcinogenesis. It is currently thought that this pathway accounts for approximately 60% of patients with CRC. The second major pathway accounting for approximately 35% of patients is the CpG island methylator phenotype cancer, and then the mutator phenotype associated with Lynch syndrome, accounting for 5%. Fig. 52.52 shows the different genetic pathways or mechanisms for development of CRC and their overlap. This is a complex topic, and a detailed discussion is beyond the scope of this chapter. The surgeon does, however, need to know the basics

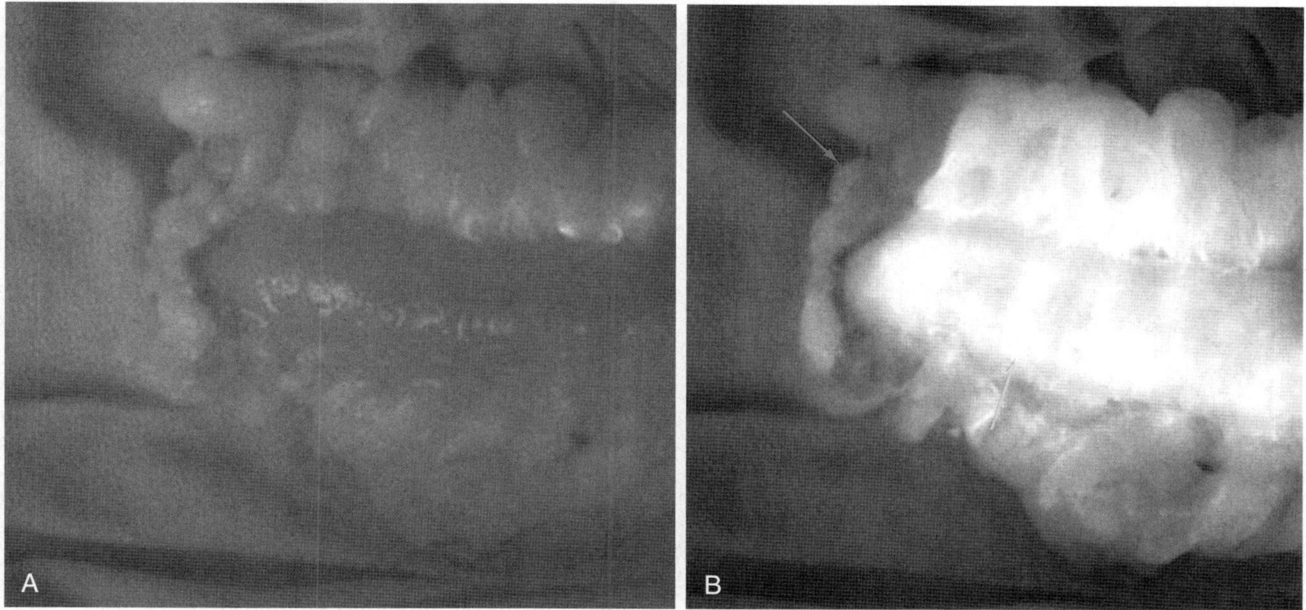

FIG. 52.51 Indocyanine green–based infrared angiography. (A) Colon before injection. (B) Colon after injection: ischemia of resection margin *(blue arrow)*; normal perfusion of colon *(yellow arrow)*. (From Netz U, Galandiuk S. Management of ischemic colitis. In: Cameron JL, Cameron A, eds. *Current Surgical Therapy*. 12th ed. Philadelphia: Elsevier; 2017:171–176.)

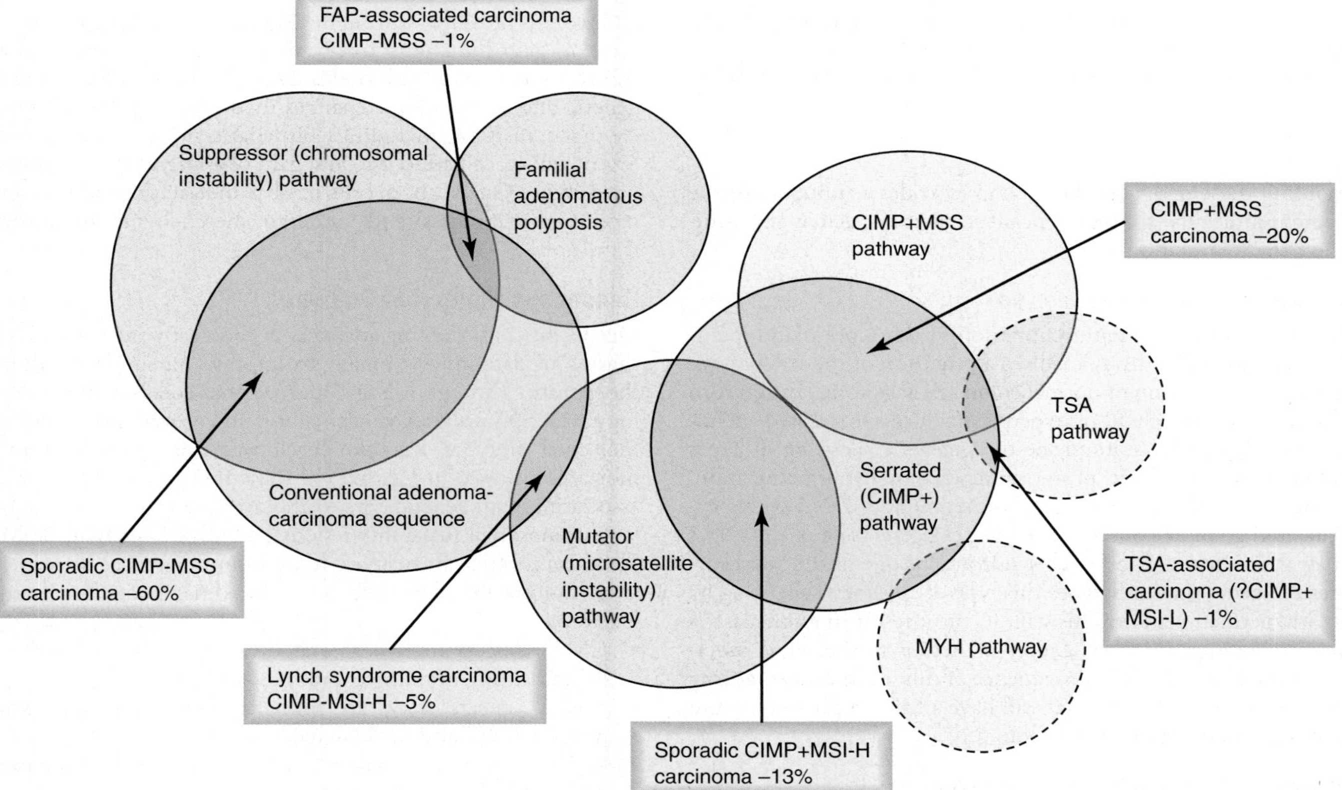

FIG. 52.52 Schematic represents several overlapping ways to describe the development of colorectal carcinoma. The *red circles* represent mechanisms based on suppressor and mutator pathways. The *blue circles* represent mechanisms based on the precursor lesion (the conventional adenoma-carcinoma sequence and serrated pathways). The *yellow circles* represent poorly characterized pathways. (From Snover DC. Update on the serrated pathway to colorectal carcinoma. *Hum Pathol.* 2011;42:1–10.) *CIMP-*, CpG island methylator phenotype negative; *CIMP+*, CpG island methylator phenotype positive; *FAP*, familial adenomatous polyposis; *MSI-H*, high degree of microsatellite instability; *MSI-L*, low degree of microsatellite instability; *MSS*, microsatellite stable; *TSA*, traditional serrated adenoma.

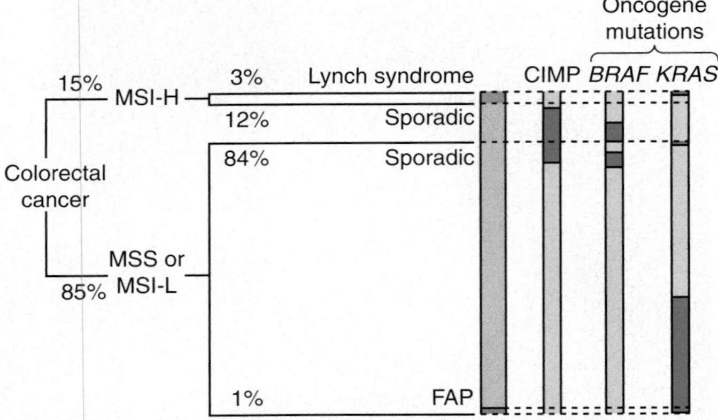

FIG. 52.53 Most colorectal cancers (85%, *light blue* and *dark blue*) show the MSS or MSI-L phenotype but are characterized by chromosomal changes. Most of these cancers develop through the classic adenoma-carcinoma pathway, but about 1% develop with an inherited syndrome FAP *(dark blue)*. About 15% of colorectal cancers (*red* and *pink*) have the MSI-H phenotype as a result of DNA mismatch repair deficiency. About 3% of colorectal cancers have MSI-H in context of the inherited Lynch syndrome (*red*), whereas 12% develop as sporadic tumors *(pink)*, with sessile serrated adenomas as a typical precursor lesion. The distribution of typical molecular changes including the CIMP and mutations of the BRAF or KRAS oncogenes are sketched in *green*. *Dark green* is the proportion of positive or mutant changes and *light green* is the proportion of negative or wild-type changes. (From Brenner H, Kloor M, Pox CP. Colorectal cancer. *Lancet*. 2014;383:1490–1502.) *CIMP*, CpG island methylator phenotype; *FAP*, familial adenomatous polyposis; *MSI-H*, high-level microsatellite instability in relation to the phenotypes in the first bar; *MSI-L*, low-level microsatellite instability; *MSS*, microsatellite-stable.

regarding these pathways. Fig. 52.53 provides a summary of the different molecular subtypes of cancer, their frequency, and common genetic mutations.

CpG Island Methylator Phenotype

The most common initiating mutation in this CpG island methylator phenotype pathway involves a mutation of the BRAF gene resulting in inhibition of normal colon cell apoptosis. This in turn leads to the development of hyperplastic or sessile serrated adenomas or polyps, which are prone to epigenetic silencing of genes within "CpG islands" in promoter regions by hypermethylation. A CpG island merely refers to a short segment of DNA with a cytosine and guanine content. The hMLH1 gene (one of the DNA repair genes involved in Lynch syndrome) is one of the best characterized genes that undergoes this type of epigenetic silencing by CpG hypermethylation. This will, in turn, result in a microsatellite instable-high (MSI-H) cancer if there is further gene mutation or methylation. As a consequence of this, most cancers arising from sessile serrated adenomas will have a MSI-H phenotype and are often located in the right colon.

Microsatellite Instability Mutator Pathway

The microsatellite instability (MSI) pathway is thought to be involved in up to 15% of early-stage CRCs. This is due to a mutation in genes that are responsible for repairing base mismatches in DNA. These genes include mutL homologue 1 (*MLH1*), *MLH3*, mutS homologue 2 (*MSH2*), *MSH3*, *MSH6*, or PMS1 homologue 2 (*PMS2*).[30] When mutations in these genes are present, mistakes that occur during DNA replication lead to mismatches between DNA base pairs that are not repaired and accumulate further, leading to a progressive accumulation of mutations (microsatellites). Microsatellites refer to normally occurring repeated sequences of one to six DNA base pairs. These associated cancers will be MSI-H and are often characterized by location in the proximal colon, large local tumor, typical absence of metastatic disease, and poor tumor differentiation. When this occurs in patients with sporadic cancer, they are often elderly; when this occurs in the hereditary form (i.e., Lynch syndrome), patients are often younger (<50 years old). These cancers can be associated with tumor-infiltrating lymphocytes. Testing for the presence of a BRAF mutation will aid in differentiating sporadic (BRAF mutation present) from inherited forms.

Hereditary CRCs are discussed later in this chapter; however, genetically, they account for approximately 5% of CRCs. In hereditary cancers, depending on the specific syndrome, either a tumor suppressor gene (e.g., *APC*) or DNA repair genes (e.g., Lynch syndrome) are inactivated by monoallelic expression in the germline and subsequent somatic event or second hit, which affects the function of the remaining allele, leading to cancer formation.

Epithelial-Mesenchymal Transition

CRC leads to death if it metastasizes. Epithelial-mesenchymal transition is the process whereby cells lose their epithelial functional and morphologic functional features and gain a "mesenchymal" phenotype. This process is not only important in cancer but is also a normal function during embryonic development and wound healing[31] Through this process, locally growing cancer cells gain the ability to invade through the bowel wall and spread to regional lymph nodes. Fig. 52.54 shows the numerous genetic and morphologic changes involved in epithelial mesenchymal transition, including epithelial cell loss of cell polarity, loss of cell-to-cell adhesion, and gain of a migratory and invasive phenotype. Once cancer cells reach a metastatic site, they must reverse this process and undergo mesenchymal-to-epithelial transition.

Consensus Molecular Subtypes

One of the most exciting advances in the treatment of CRC is the sharing of data internationally to improve our understanding of the disease. Through a large international collaboration evaluating transcription-based cancer subtyping, a system of "consensus molecular subtypes" has been developed. This system has four tumor types shown, in Fig. 52.55. These four tumor types have an association with genetic type, with CMS2–4 being more likely to be chromosomal instability lesions and CMS1 likely to be MSI-H cancers, which in turn are more immunogenic. Similarly, the latter cancers are more often in the proximal colon. Briefly summarized:

- CMS1 cancers are hypermutated, microsatellite unstable, and exhibit strong immune activation.
- CMS2 cancers show an epithelial phenotype and exhibit marked *WNT* and *MYC* signaling activation.
- CMS3 cancers are characterized by an epithelial phenotype and metabolic dysregulation; while
- CMS4 cancers show a mesenchymal phenotype, prominent transforming growth factor-β activation, stromal invasion, and angiogenesis.

The knowledge gained from such specific subtyping can be used for much more individualized and targeted, patient-specific treatment and gives hope for improved patient outcomes in years to come.

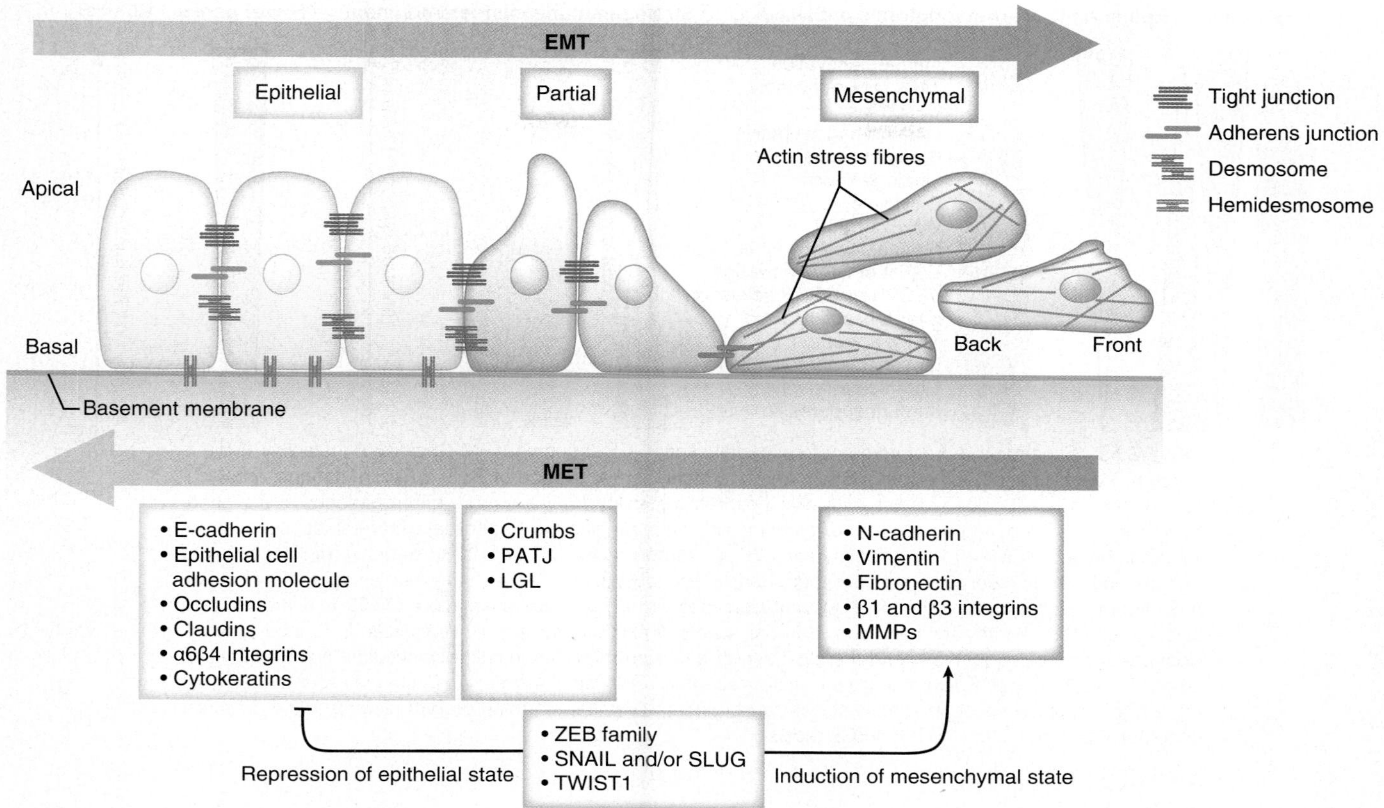

FIG. 52.54 Outline of a typical epithelial-mesenchymal transition *(EMT)* program. Epithelial cells displaying apical-basal polarity are held together by tight junctions, adherens junctions, and desmosomes and are tethered to the underlying basement membrane by hemidesmosomes. These cells express molecules that are associated with the epithelial state and help maintain cell polarity (listed in the *yellow* and *light orange boxes*, respectively). Induction of EMT leads to the expression of the EMT-inducing transcription factors (EMT-TFs) ZEB, SNAIL, and TWIST, which inhibit the expression of genes associated with the epithelial state (listed in the *yellow box*) and concomitantly activate the expression of genes associated with the mesenchymal state (listed in the *dark orange box*). These changes in gene expression result in cellular changes that include the disassembly of epithelial cell-cell junctions and the dissolution of apical-basal cell polarity via repression of crumbs, PALS1-associated tight junction protein *(PATJ)* and lethal giant larvae *(LGL)*, which are proteins that specifically regulate tight junction formation and apical-basal polarity. This progressive loss of epithelial features is accompanied by acquisition of a partial set of mesenchymal features with retention of certain epithelial features; in certain circumstances, a complete set of mesenchymal features may be acquired. Mesenchymal cells display front-to-back polarity and an extensively reorganized cytoskeleton and express a distinct set of molecules and EMT-TFs that promote and maintain the mesenchymal state. During EMT, cells become motile and acquire invasive capacities. EMT is a reversible process, and mesenchymal cells can revert to the epithelial state by undergoing mesenchymal-epithelial transition *(MET)*. EMT and MET occur during normal development and during cancer progression. It should be noted, however, that carcinoma cells in spontaneously arising tumors only very rarely advance into a completely mesenchymal state. (From Dongre A, Weinberg RA. New insights into the mechanisms of epithelial-mesenchymal transition and implications for cancer. *Nat Rev Mol Cell Biol*. 2019;20:69–84.) *E-cadherin*, Epithelial cadherin; *MMP*, matrix metalloproteinase; *N-cadherin*, neural cadherin.

COLORECTAL POLYPS

A colorectal polyp is a protrusion of tissue into the lumen above the surrounding intestinal mucosa. Polyps are usually asymptomatic, but may bleed or cause obstructive symptoms when large, and some are precursors for cancer. Polyps can be characterized according to their endoscopic appearance into pedunculated (with a stalk, Fig. 52.56) or sessile (flat, Fig. 52.57). Following excision or biopsy, they can be further classified according to their histologic appearance (adenomas, hamartomas, inflammatory, serrated, etc.). The main importance of polyps lies in their risk for the development of CRC. Neoplastic polyps that have the potential to develop into CRC should be removed in order to reduce cancer risk.

Nonneoplastic Polyps

Hyperplastic polyps are small sessile lesions, usually less than 5 mm, consisting of elongated colonic crypts with a papillary configuration of epithelial cells without atypia. They are common colonic polyps, frequently grossly indistinguishable from small adenomas. They have no malignant potential.

Inflammatory polyps (pseudopolyps) are found in regions of healing inflammation. They are usually formed in an area of regeneration after full-thickness epithelial ulceration in which the new mucosa forms in an irregular polypoid configuration. They do not have any intrinsic neoplastic potential but may be large, mimicking a neoplasm. Their significance is that they are

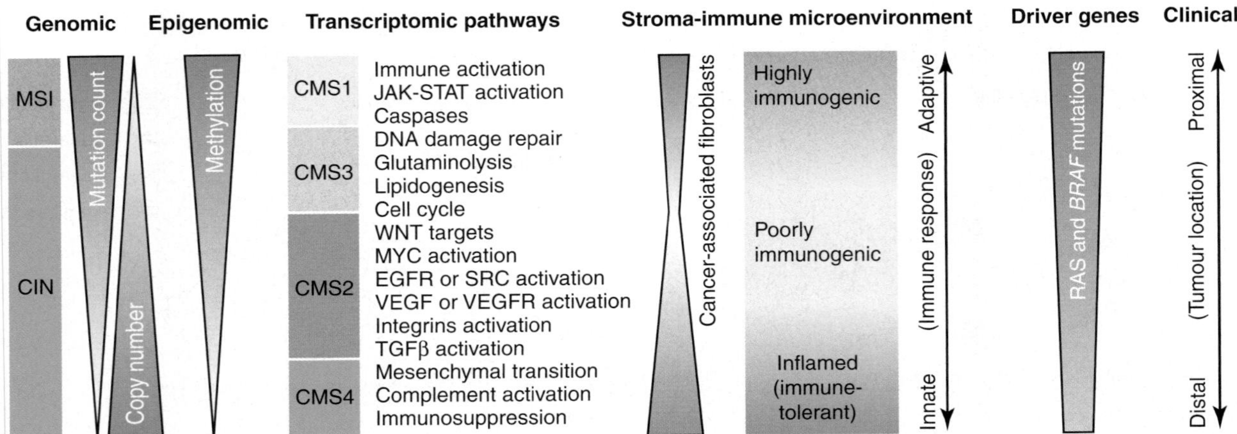

FIG. 52.55 Schematic representation of colorectal cancer (CRC) subtypes. Microsatellite instability *(MSI)* is linked to hypermutation, hypermethylation, immune infiltration, activation of RAS, *BRAF* mutations, and locations in the proximal colon. Tumors with chromosomal instability *(CIN)* are more heterogeneous at the gene-expression level, showing a spectrum of pathway activation ranging from epithelial canonical (consensus molecular subtype 2 *[CMS2]*) to mesenchymal *(CMS4)*. Tumors with CIN are mainly diagnosed in left colon or rectum, and their microenvironment is either poorly immunogenic or inflamed, with marked stromal infiltration. A subset of CRC tumors enriched for RAS mutations has strong metabolic adaptation *(CMS3)* and intermediate levels of mutation, methylation and copy number events. (From Dienstmann R, Vermeulen L, Guinney J, et al. Consensus molecular subtypes and the evolution of precision medicine in colorectal cancer. *Nat Rev Cancer.* 2017;17:79–92.) *EGFR*, Epidermal growth factor receptor; *JAK*, Janus kinase; *SRC*, steroid receptor coactivator; *STAT*, signal transducer and activator of transcription; *TGFβ*, transforming growth factor-β; *VEGF*, vascular endothelial growth factor; *VEGFR*, VEGF receptor.

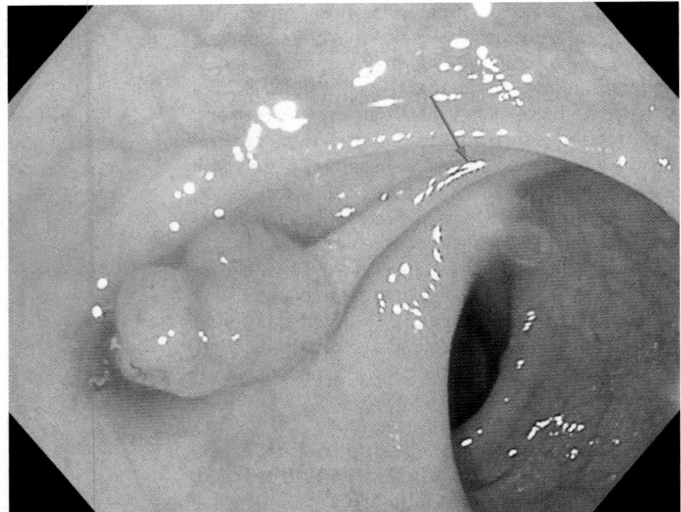

FIG. 52.56 Colonoscopic view of pedunculated polyp with a long narrow stalk (*arrow* showing stalk).

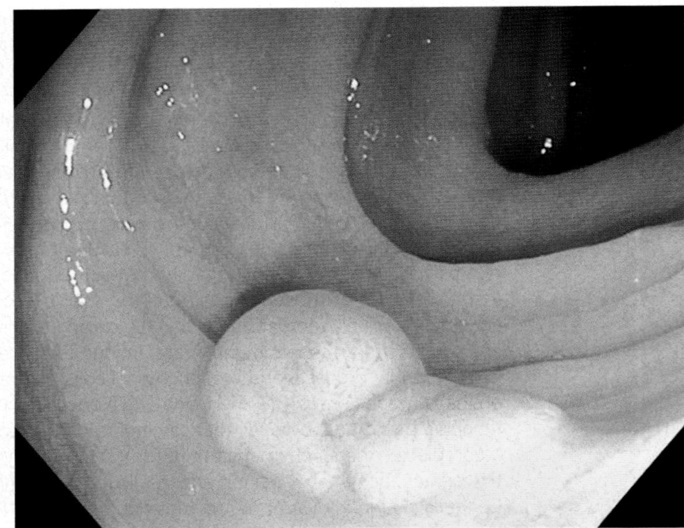

FIG. 52.57 Colonoscopic view of sessile polyp in colon.

found in diseased colons otherwise at risk for cancer (e.g., in IBD) and must be differentiated from neoplastic lesions.

Hamartomas are uncommon polyps found in the GI tract. They can be sporadic, but are commonly related to a genetic syndrome such as Peutz-Jeghers syndrome (PJS), juvenile polyposis syndrome, and PTEN hamartoma syndrome. They do not have an intrinsic malignant potential. Removal is indicated for obstructive symptoms or bleeding.

Serrated Polyps

Serrated polyps can be divided into three types: hyperplastic polyps (which are not considered precancerous), sessile serrated polyps, and traditional serrated adenomas. Sessile serrated polyps and traditional serrated adenomas are combinations of adenomatous and hyperplastic polyps, sharing features of both types including colonic crypts with a saw-tooth serrated configuration and nuclear atypia (Fig. 52.58). Patients with sessile serrated polyps and traditional serrated adenomas are recognized as having an increased

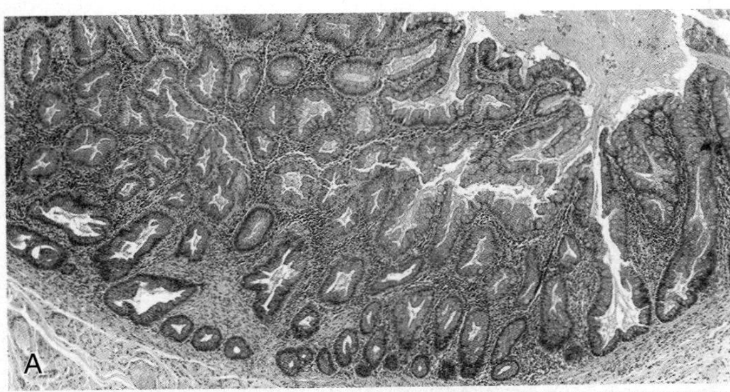

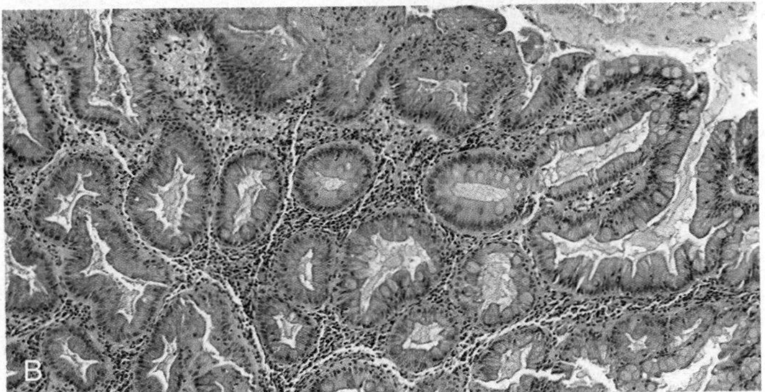

FIG. 52.58 (A) Histology of sessile serrated adenoma. (B) Histology of sessile serrated adenoma (high-power view). (Courtesy of Dr. Benzion Samueli, Department of Pathology, Soroka University Medical Center, Be'er Sheva, Israel.)

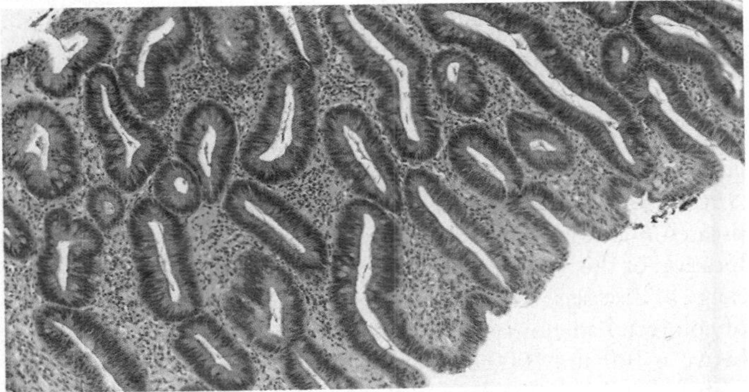

FIG. 52.59 Histology of tubular adenoma. (Courtesy of Dr. Benzion Samueli, Department of Pathology, Soroka University Medical Center, Be'er Sheva, Israel.)

risk of CRC.[32] The development of CRC in these patients usually follows the serrated neoplasia pathway in contrast to the classic adenoma–carcinoma pathway seen in adenomatous polyps. These polyps should be removed, and patients should be followed with serial endoscopy.

Neoplastic Polyps

All adenomas have a malignant potential. Tubular adenomas are characterized by branched tubular glands on histology (Fig. 52.59). Villous adenomas have long fingerlike projections of the surface epithelium (Fig. 52.60). Tubulovillous adenomas have elements of both types. The most common type are tubular adenomas, comprising 65% to 80% of polyps removed, and they are frequently pedunculated. Approximately 5% to 10% are villous

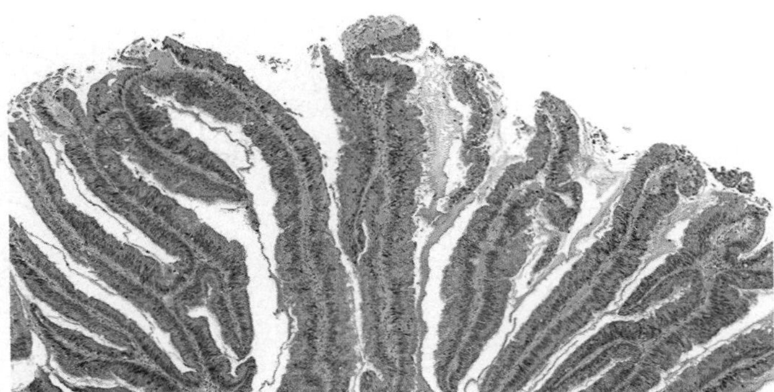

FIG. 52.60 Histology of a villous adenoma. (Courtesy of Dr. Benzion Samueli, Department of Pathology, Soroka University Medical Center, Be'er Sheva, Israel.)

adenomas and 10% to 25% are tubulovillous adenomas. Villous adenomas are commonly sessile. The risk of malignancy increases dependent on the size (large), gross shape (sessile), histologic type (villous), and grade of dysplasia. Patients with an advanced adenoma defined as size at least 1 cm, high-grade dysplasia, or tubulovillous or villous histology are at a significantly increased risk of developing CRC.[33] For example, there is less than a 5% incidence of carcinoma in a tubular adenoma smaller than 1 cm, whereas there is a 50% chance that a villous adenoma larger than 2 cm will contain a cancer.

Adenomatous polyps that are discovered during colonoscopy should be excised. A variety of techniques are employed for endoscopic removal of polyps, such as forceps and snares. Pedunculated polyps are commonly removed using cold or hot snare polypectomy. Sessile polyps are frequently elevated from the underlying muscularis by injection of saline and then excised using an assortment of techniques. Sessile polyps with a central depression that do not elevate adequately with saline injection (nonlifting sign) are at increased risk for perforation with endoscopic removal and at higher risk of harboring neoplasia and are commonly referred for surgical removal by segmental colectomy. Large polyps that cannot be removed endoscopically are also referred for surgery. Larger polyps can also be removed endoscopically using techniques such as endoscopic mucosal resection and endoscopic submucosal resection.

Malignant Polyps

Malignant polyps are those in which histologic examination following removal of a polyp reveals a focus of carcinoma that has invaded through the muscularis mucosa. The question that arises is whether complete endoscopic removal of these polyps is sufficient. Carcinomas that do not pass the muscularis mucosa are considered "carcinoma in situ" and do not carry metastatic risk. However, those that invade the muscularis mucosa harbor a significant risk of local recurrence and lymph node metastasis. One of the important risk factors is the depth of penetration. This can be defined by the Haggitt classification (Fig. 52.61):

Level 0: Carcinoma limited to the mucosa, carcinoma in situ.

Level 1: Carcinoma invading into the submucosa, limited to the head of the polyp.

Level 2: Carcinoma invading to the level of the neck (junction of the head and stalk).

Level 3: Carcinoma invading any part of the stalk.

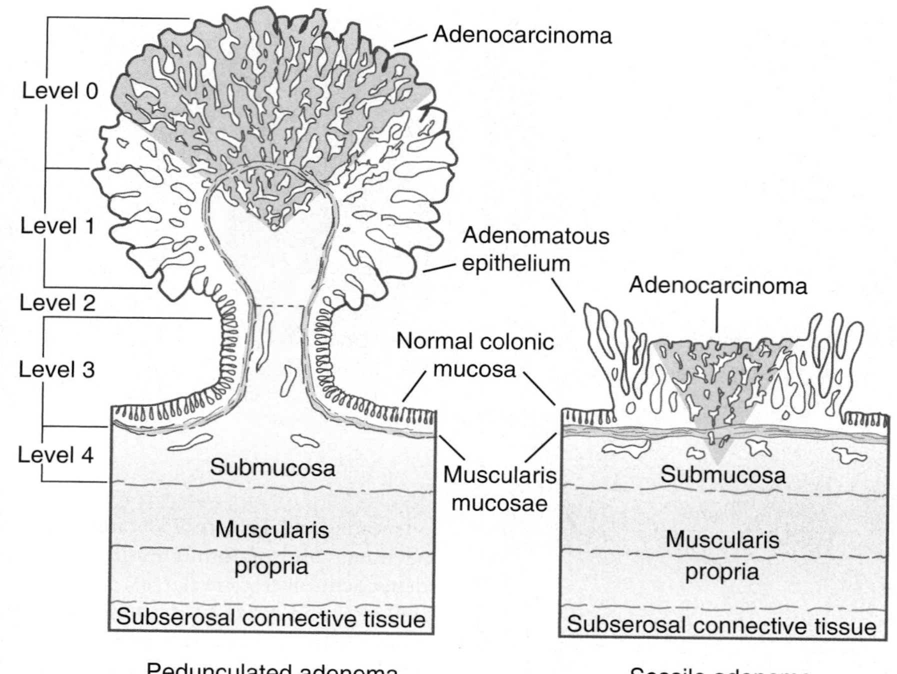

FIG. 52.61 Haggitt classification. Anatomic landmarks of pedunculated and sessile adenomas. (From Haggitt RC, Glotzbach RE, Soffer EE, et al. Prognostic factors in colorectal carcinoma arising in adenomas: implications for lesions removed by endoscopic polypectomy. *Gastroenterology.* 1985;89:328–336.)

Level 4: Carcinoma invading into the submucosa of the colon wall, below the level of the stalk, but above the muscularis propria.

Sessile polyps in which invasion of the muscularis mucosa is seen are by definition Haggit level 4. For these, the Kikuchi classification[34] can be used, in which Sm1 describes invasion into the upper third of the submucosa; Sm2, into the middle third; and Sm3, penetration into the lower third.

Malignant polyps are commonly referred for completion colectomy in cases of pedunculated Haggitt level 4, sessile Kikuchi level Sm2 and Sm3, histologic poor differentiation, lymphovascular invasion, and incomplete removal or close resection margins. In these cases, the risk of residual cancer and lymph node metastasis is higher than 10%.

Postpolypectomy Surveillance

The finding of adenomas in colonoscopy is considered a risk factor for future development of additional polyps. Table 52.6 depicts current recommendations for repeat colonoscopy following endoscopic removal of polyps.

Hereditary Cancer Syndromes

CRC is the third most common cancer in men and women in the United States. In approximately 20% to 30% of cases, these CRCs are associated with a family history of colorectal polyps or cancer, but only 3% to 5% of cases are associated with an identifiable inherited CRC syndrome such as Lynch syndrome, familial adenomatous polyposis (FAP), mutY Homolog (MUTYH)-associated polyposis (MAP), juvenile polyposis or PJS (Table 52.7). Timely identification of individuals at risk for hereditary CRC syndromes offers an opportunity to intervene to prevent the development of cancer. The reader is referred to the ASCRS Clinical Practice Guidelines for the Management of Inherited Polyposis Syndromes and for the Surgical Treatment of Patients with Lynch Syndrome.

Familial Adenomatous Polyposis

FAP is an autosomal dominant inherited disease that occurs in approximately 1:10,000 live births and affects genders and races equally. FAP is a syndrome caused by germline mutation in the *APC* tumor suppressor gene which is responsible for regulation of β-catenin and located on chromosome 5q21. Depending on the location of the APC mutation, the affected individuals can have a range of disease severity. Severe FAP is characterized by thousands of colorectal adenomas. Classical polyposis is described as having between 100 and 1000 colorectal adenomas (Fig. 52.62). Patients with fewer than 100 adenomas are considered to have attenuated FAP (AFAP). Germline mutations in the APC gene are found in 80% to 90% of patients with classic FAP and in 10% to 30% of patients with AFAP. About 25% of patients with FAP have a de novo mutation and thus have no family history. For individuals with the classic phenotype, the lifetime risk for CRC may exceed 90%, nearly 100% in the absence of treatment. If left untreated, patients with FAP develop CRC at an average age of 39 years (range 35–43 years).[35]

Clinically, FAP is characterized by early development of a wide range of colorectal adenomatous polyps after the second decade of life and many extracolonic manifestations. Patients with FAP may be asymptomatic or may present with bleeding, diarrhea, abdominal pain, or mucous discharge per rectum. Other symptoms such as anemia, obstruction, or weight loss usually occur as polyps grow larger in size or number and may foreshadow the presence of cancer. A variety of benign and malignant extracolonic manifestations have been described in FAP. These include gastroduodenal adenomas and carcinoma, desmoids, osteomas, epidermoid cysts, papillary thyroid

TABLE 52.6 Recommendations for repeat colonoscopy following endoscopic removal of polyps.

INDEX COLONOSCOPY FINDINGS	REPEAT COLONOSCOPY
Small (<10 mm) hyperplastic polyps in rectum or sigmoid	10 years
Low risk:	5–10 years (AGA guidelines)
One to two small tubular adenomas	10 years (ESGE guidelines)
<10 mm, with low-grade dysplasia	
High risk:	3 years
Villous histology or high-grade dysplasia or size ≥10 mm or ≥3 polyps	
Piecemeal removal of polyp	6 months
Sessile serrated polyp <10 mm	5 years
Sessile serrated polyp >10 mm or with dysplasia or traditional serrated adenoma	3 years

Adapted from Hassan C, Quintero E, Dumonceau JM, et al. Post-polypectomy colonoscopy surveillance: European Society of Gastrointestinal Endoscopy (ESGE) guideline. *Endoscopy.* 2013;45:842–851, and Lieberman DA, Rex DK, Winawer SJ, et al. Guidelines for colonoscopy surveillance after screening and polypectomy: a consensus update by the US Multi-Society Task Force on Colorectal Cancer. *Gastroenterology.* 2012;143:844–857.
AGA, American Gastroenterological Association; *ESGE*, European Society of Gastrointestinal Endoscopy.

TABLE 52.7 Inherited colorectal cancer syndromes.

SYNDROME	GENES	POLYP TYPE	INHERITANCE	CLINICAL FINDINGS	CRC RISK
Classical FAP	*APC*	Adenoma	AD	100–1000 adenomas; duodenal adenomas and carcinomas; gastric fundic gland polyps, desmoid tumors, epidermoid cysts, osteomas	100%
Severe FAP	*APC*	Adenoma	AD	>1000 adenomas	100%
Attenuated FAP	*APC*	Adenoma	AD	<100 adenomas	80%
MAP	*MUTYH (MYH)*	Adenoma	AR	0–1000 adenomas, CRC <50 years; gastric fundic gland polyps, duodenal adenomas, and carcinomas	80%
JPS	*SMAD4, BMPR1A*	Hamartoma	AD	≥5 juvenile polyps; any juvenile polyp and JPS family history	40%
PJP	*STK11*	Hamartoma	AD	Peutz-Jeghers polyps Orocutaneous pigmentation Family history of PJP; cancer of small bowel, colon, stomach, pancreas, breast, ovary, testis	40%
Lynch syndrome	*MLH1, MSH2, MSH6, PMS2, EpCAM*	Nonpolyposic adenoma	AD	Microsatellite-unstable CRC, advanced adenomas; gastric, duodenal, small bowel, transitional cell, gallbladder, pancreas, endometrial, ovarian	60%–80%

AD, Autosomal dominant; *AR*, autosomal recessive; *CRC*, colorectal cancer; *FAP*, familial adenomatous polyposis; *JPS*, juvenile polyposis syndrome; *MAP*, MUTYH-associated polyposis; *PJP*, Peutz-Jeghers polyposis.

carcinoma, small bowel polyps and carcinoma, congenital hyperplasia of the retinal pigment epithelium (CHRPE), and dental anomalies.

Nonneoplastic gastric fundic gland polyps are a common finding in about 50% of patients. Gastric adenomas are present in about 10% of patients with FAP, usually in the antrum. The risk of gastric cancer is low. Duodenal adenomas occur in 30% to 70% of patients with FAP, and there is a predilection for the ampullary and periampullary regions. The lifetime risk for duodenal cancer is 4% to 10%, constituting the second most common cause of death in FAP patients. The Spigelman classification is used to grade the severity of and guide the clinical management of duodenal polyposis (Table 52.8). Adenomas can occur rarely in the gallbladder, bile duct, and the small bowel, particularly the distal ileum. Most patients are eligible for chemoprevention for adenomas with NSAIDs (e.g., sulindac or celecoxib) after surgery, but this seems less effective than in the colorectum.[35]

Desmoid tumors are histologically benign but locally invasive monoclonal proliferations of fibroblasts. They are only occasionally seen in the general population but affect 10% to 15% of all patients with FAP. These tumors are associated with female gender and with a family history of desmoids. About half of FAP-associated desmoid tumors arise intraabdominally in the bowel mesentery and 40% develop in the abdominal wall. The remainder present in the back, neck, and limbs. Desmoids can manifest as flat, fibrous, sheet-like lesions or as defined discrete masses. This may result in pain, bowel or ureteral obstruction, vascular compromise, and perioperative complications. Desmoid tumors, together with duodenal polyposis and/or cancer, are the major causes of morbidity and mortality after proctocolectomy, leading to death in approximately 10% of patients. Surgery of intraabdominal desmoid tumors, in general, is not recommended and should typically be reserved for small, well-defined tumors when a clear margin can be obtained. Pharmacologic therapies with NSAIDs and antiestrogens showed similar outcomes to surgery. Combination chemotherapy, including doxorubicin, seems to be the best option for progressively growing intraabdominal desmoids.

The incidence of thyroid cancer in patients with FAP is 2%. Less frequently occurring extraintestinal malignancies in FAP include pancreatic adenocarcinomas, hepatoblastoma, and medulloblastoma.

CHRPE is a benign lesion characterized as well-delineated grayish-black or brown oval spots seen in 60% to 85% of FAP patients on fundoscopic scan. Normally, this does not require intervention but can be used to help make a diagnosis. Sebaceous or epidermoid cysts, lipomas, osteomas, fibromas, supernumerary teeth, juvenile nasopharyngeal angiofibromas, and adrenal adenomas have also been associated with FAP.

Two eponymous polyposis syndromes are recognized as belonging to the general disorder of FAP. These include Gardner syndrome (FAP with epidermal inclusion cysts, osteomas, desmoid tumors) and Turcot syndrome (FAP associated with malignant tumors of the central nervous system).

FAP may be diagnosed genetically or clinically. Genetic testing reveals an APC germline mutation in approximately 80% of cases. Indications for genetic counseling referral and testing include a family history of FAP, personal history of more than 10 adenomas, personal history of adenomas, and an extracolonic manifestation of FAP. For individuals suspected of AFAP, gene testing is recommended if 20 or more cumulative colorectal adenomas are found. Treatment should include thorough counseling about the nature of the syndrome, its natural history, its extracolonic manifestations, and the need for compliance with recommendations for management and surveillance.

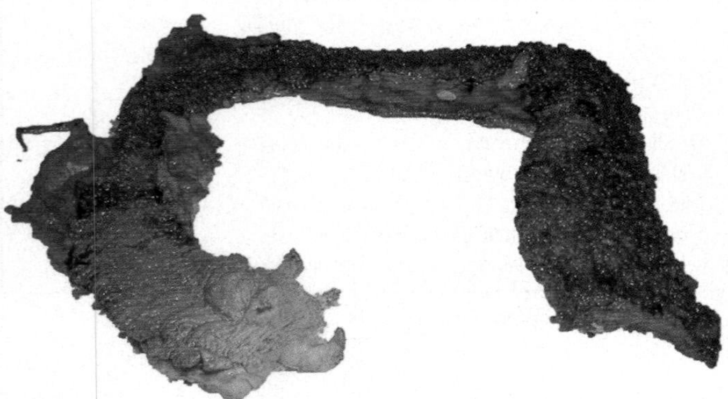

FIG. 52.62 Classical familial adenomatous polyposis in the resected specimen. Hundreds of polyps are well visible along the entire colon.

Colorectal screening in individuals of affected families begins at age 12 and can be initiated with flexible proctosigmoidoscopy. If polyps are seen, a full colonoscopy is warranted. If no polyps are identified on the initial flexible proctosigmoidoscopy, the exam should be repeated every 1 to 2 years until the age of 35 and every 3 to 5 years thereafter for at-risk first-degree relatives who have not undergone predictive testing or for those who have undergone DNA analysis that provides no information about whether they are affected. Patients at risk for AFAP should receive endoscopic screening with colonoscopy at ages 12, 15, 18, and 21 years, and then every 2 years. About one-third of patients with AFAP can be managed long-term endoscopically by polypectomy. For the upper GI tract, screening begins at 20 to 25 years of age. Screening intervals are based on the Spigelman staging system.

Annual thyroid screening by ultrasound should be recommended to FAP patients. Routine screening is not recommended for the other cancers.

The aims of treatment of the lower GI tract in patients with FAP are to prevent death from cancer and to maximize quality of life. The decisions that need to be made in affected patients to fulfill those aims center around the timing of surgery and the type of operation to be performed. Table 52.9 provides a list for timing of surgery. Decisions for surgery depend on the presence of symptoms, the age at diagnosis, and individual characteristics.

There are four surgical options in the treatment of FAP: restorative proctocolectomy with IPAA either with mucosectomy and a hand-sewn anastomosis or with a stapled anastomosis, colectomy with an ileorectal anastomosis (IRA), or proctocolectomy with a permanent end ileostomy. Each of these options has advantages and disadvantages.

- **Proctocolectomy and IPAA** greatly reduce the risk of rectal cancer, especially when performed with rectal mucosectomy and hand-sewn anastomosis. It is, however, a technically more demanding procedure and is associated with higher morbidity than IRA. IPAA also results in more frequent bowel movements compared to colectomy and IRA. Rectal dissection also poses a risk of nerve injury that can lead to sexual or urologic dysfunction. Pelvic dissection can cause infertility due to adhesions. Recently minimally invasive approaches reduce this risk significantly.

TABLE 52.8 Spigelman classification for duodenal polyps in familial adenomatous polyposis.

	POINTS		
CRITERIA	**1**	**2**	**3**
Polyp number	1	2	3
Polyp size (mm)	1–4	5–20	>20
Histology	Tubular	Tubulovillous	Villous
Dysplasia	Mild	Moderate	Severe

From Spigelman AD, Williams CB, Talbot IC, et al. Upper gastrointestinal cancer in patients with familial adenomatous polyposis. *Lancet.* 1989;2:783–785.

Stage 0 = 0 points; stage I = 1–4 points; stage II = 5–6 points; stage III = 7–8 points; stage IV= 9–12 points. Stage 0. Repeat endoscopy in 5 years. Stage I. Repeat endoscopy in 5 years. Stage II. Repeat endoscopy in 2–3 years. Stage III. Repeat endoscopy in 6–12 months and surgical evaluation. Stage IV. Repeat endoscopy in 6–12 months and surgical evaluation.

TABLE 52.9 **Timing of surgery in patients with familial polyposis.**

REASONS TO INDICATE OR POSTPONE SURGERY	TIMING FOR SURGERY
Presence of symptoms (> risk of CRC)	As soon as possible
Asymptomatic patient with mild disease	Discuss opportunity (before 20 years?) CRC before the age of 20 is rare
Patients diagnosed in their third decade or beyond	Immediately
Sized lesions or with high-grade dysplasia, not amenable to endoscopic resection	
Severe disease at colonoscopy or by family history/genotype	As soon as practicable
Attenuated polyposis at colonoscopy or by family history/genotype	Personal decision (16–20 years if mild or 21–25 years if attenuated polyposis)
Preoperative diagnosis, positive family history or genetically susceptible for desmoids	Delay surgery (after evaluating CRC risk)
Delaying surgery in women with a low polyp burden who wish to have children.	Reasonable to delay surgery as long as the patient remains in a strict surveillance program

From Campos FG: Surgical treatment of familial adenomatous polyposis: Dilemmas and current recommendations. *World J Gastroenterol.* 2014;20:16620–16629.
CRC, Colorectal cancer.

Patients with rectal cancer, a large polyp burden (>20 synchronous adenomas, adenoma with high-grade dysplasia, large (>30 mm) adenomas), or a severe familial phenotype (>1000 synchronous adenomas) should undergo IPAA. This operation is also the treatment of choice for patients with a large number of rectal adenomas, but the optimal timing of surgery should be individualized. IPAA should be performed with removal of the anal transitional zone by mucosectomy and a handsewn anastomosis or retaining some of the anal transitional zone with a stapled anastomosis. The choice of which is best to perform has been debated. The benefits of a stapled anastomosis include better function (less risk of incontinence) and fewer complications. A stapled IPAA is also easier to survey, and anal transitional zone adenomas may possibly be treated endoscopically or transanally. The benefit of a handsewn IPAA is a reduced incidence of anal transitional zone adenomas, but this is achieved at a potential cost of worse function. This procedure can be performed with or without a diverting ileostomy. A temporary diverting ileostomy proximal to the pouch has been classically performed in order to mitigate the effects of anastomotic leakage and to prevent pelvic sepsis (reported in as low as 6% and as high as 37%, respectively), fistulization, and thus compromised pouch function. Consequently, it should also prevent the need for relaparotomy. Ileostomy omission has been advocated in selected cases. The benefits of laparoscopy can be applied in this surgery, but in the literature, there is no evidence that this approach is better than the open approach. IPAA should be performed only in specialized centers and by skilled and experienced surgical teams.

- **Subtotal colectomy and IRA** provide good surgical and functional outcomes but require long-term follow-up of the retained rectum. The risk of metachronous rectal cancer is on the order of 30%. IRA is generally recommended for patients with few rectal polyps, AFAP, and a family history of a mild phenotype and for those young women with desire to become pregnant after recommendations of genetic counseling. IRA should not be performed in patients with a severely diseased rectum (adenomas >3 cm diameter, adenomas with severe dysplasia, cancer, sphincter dysfunction, or a rectum containing more than 20 rectal adenomas) or in the presence of colon cancer. IRA may provide good results in AFAP, MAP, and mild FAP patients who agree to undergo close follow-up, and proctocolectomy and IPAA should be reserved for those with profuse polyposis.
- **Proctocolectomy with end ileostomy** is currently rarely performed as a permanent stoma and is usually unacceptable to young patients. However, this option still has a role in the treatment of very low rectal cancer, when sphincter preservation is not possible, in cases of malignant transformation after IPAA or ileal pouch failure or in cases in which there is poor sphincter function.

Most patients are eligible for chemoprevention after surgery because proctocolectomy with IPAA or a colectomy with IRA can retain "at-risk" rectal mucosa, and the duodenal mucosa remains "at risk" in all these patients. Chemoprevention (i.e., taking medications that slow polyp growth such as sulindac or celecoxib) should *not* replace routine endoscopic surveillance.

Regular follow-up is mandatory after any procedure. Standard care includes perianal digital and flexible endoscopic examination at yearly intervals.

MUTYH-Associated Polyposis

MAP is an autosomal recessively inherited syndrome caused by germline mutation of both alleles of the *MUTYH* gene, located on chromosome 1. Because the autosomal recessive inheritance pattern requires that affected individuals have a biallelic mutation, both parents of affected individuals must be at least monoallelic carriers. If so, siblings of affected individuals have a 25% chance of biallelic mutations. Monoallelic MUTYH mutations are found in 0.7% to 1% of unselected individuals in population-based cohorts, with biallelic mutations identified in 1.7% of unselected individuals with CRC. CRC risk is increased twenty-eight fold for individuals with biallelic MUTYH mutations, while the risk for monoallelic carriers appears to be only moderately increased.[36]

The colonic phenotype mimics that of AFAP. The diagnosis of MAP should be considered in patients presenting with colorectal polyposis (>20 lifetime adenomas). Although most polyps in MAP are adenomas, patients can present with serrated polyps or a mixture of adenomas and serrated polyps. Bleeding or obstruction may occur, but the disease is suspected on findings from a screening colonoscopy. The syndrome is primarily characterized by multiple colorectal adenomas and an increased risk for CRC at a younger age (40–50 years of age). The colorectal polyp phenotype is highly variable usually with moderate polyposis (<100 adenomas). Approximately 20% of patients with MAP will have duodenal polyposis, and gastric fundic polyps are rare. Osteomas, desmoids, and CHRPE are not associated with MAP.

The following are indications for MUTYH gene testing: patients with 10 to 100 polyps, siblings of patients with biallelic MUTYH gene mutation, patients with early-onset CRC (<44–55 years), or children of monoallelic or biallelic MUTYH gene mutation carriers.

Patients with MAP should undergo colonoscopy every 1 to 2 years. Subtotal colectomy with IRA is recommended if endoscopic management fails or if CRC develops. Rectal cancer is uncommon in MAP. Patients with rectal cancer in MAP should be considered for proctocolectomy and IPAA.

Esophagogastroduodenoscopy with a side-viewing gastroscope to more accurately examine the ampulla should be performed to evaluate for duodenal adenomatous neoplasia. This screening should start at the age of 30 and be repeated every 3 to 5 years if the exam is normal. For patients with duodenal adenomas, management is similar to the recommendations for FAP patients with duodenal adenomas.

Peutz-Jeghers Syndrome

PJS is an autosomal-dominant hereditary cancer syndrome that carries a 39% lifetime risk of CRC characterized by benign hamartomatous, primarily GI, polyps, mucocutaneous pigmentation (dark blue or brown macules in the vermillion border of the lips, buccal mucosa, hands, and feet), and a high predisposition to many intestinal and extraintestinal cancers. Nearly 90% of PJS patients will develop hamartomatous polyps, most commonly in the small bowel, followed by the colon, stomach, and rectum in decreasing frequency. PJS patients have a 90% lifetime risk of cancer, including colorectal (most common), gastric, pancreatic, lung, breast, uterine, cervical, testicular, and ovarian.

PJS is caused by a mutation of the *STK11/LKB1* gene located on chromosome 19p. Approximately half of PJS cases are inherited from a parent; the remainder occur in patients with no family history and appear to result from a spontaneous mutation.

Polyps differ histologically from juvenile polyps in that they arise due to an overgrowth of the muscularis mucosa rather than the lamina propria.

PJS is a clinical diagnosis based on any one of the following World Health Organization criteria: (1) three or more histologically confirmed Peutz-Jeghers polyps; (2) any number of PJ polyps with a family history of PJS; (3) characteristic, prominent, mucocutaneous pigmentation with a family history of PJS; or (4) any number of Peutz-Jeghers polyps and characteristic prominent, mucocutaneous pigmentation.

PJS patients require special surveillance that includes multiple organs, as it is associated with an increased risk of cancer in many organs (small bowel, stomach, pancreas, colon, esophagus, ovary, lung, uterus, breast, testes, and others). Screening begins at 8 to 10 years of age with an evaluation of the small bowel. If initial exam is normal, a repeat evaluation is recommended at the age of 18 and then at 2- to 3-year intervals. Males should undergo annual testicular physical examination starting at age 10 years, and females should undergo an annual pelvic examination and Papanicolaou stain starting at age 18 to 20 years. Women should have breast physical examinations every 6 months and yearly mammogram and breast MRI starting at age 25 years. Colonoscopy and upper endoscopy should start in the late teens and be repeated every 2 to 3 years for both genders. Pancreatic cancer screening involves endoscopic ultrasound or magnetic resonance cholangiopancreatography along with serum CA19-9 every 1 to 2 years starting at age 25 to 30 years.

Polypectomy plays a key role in the management of PJS. Asymptomatic gastric or colonic polyps larger than 1 cm should be removed endoscopically. Small bowel polyps larger than 1 to 1.5 cm or those that are have grown rapidly should be removed to decrease future complications such as bleeding and intussusception.

Surgery is most commonly reserved for symptoms, the most common being obstruction (caused by intussusception) and bleeding in the small bowel. The goal of surgery is to remove the affected segment, preserving as much bowel as possible. Intervention may require push enteroscopy or combined laparoscopy/laparotomy with endoscopy in the operating room as these small bowel polyps may not be visualized by other means.[36]

Juvenile Polyposis Syndrome

Juvenile polyposis syndrome is an inherited autosomal-dominant pattern and is characterized by the development of hamartomatous intestinal polyps. Patients with JPS exhibit a 10% to 38% lifetime risk of colon cancer, and the average age at diagnosis is 34 years. JPS is clinically diagnosed when there are five or more juvenile polyps in the colorectum, multiple juvenile polyps throughout the GI tract, any number or juvenile polyps with a family history, or juvenile polyposis. Symptoms are related to the polyps and most commonly include acute or chronic GI bleeding, iron-deficiency anemia, prolapsed rectal polyps, abdominal pain, or diarrhea.

Two genes, *SMAD4* (chromosome 18q) and *BMPR1A* (chromosome 10q), have been linked to JPS. However, a pathogenic mutation in one of these two genes is detected in only 40%–50% of patients with JPS. There is an increased cancer risk in afflicted individuals, with a malignant potential of at least 10% in patients with multiple juvenile polyps.

Screening by colonoscopy should begin between the ages of 12 to 15 years. The interval between colonoscopies depends on exam findings. If there are no polyps, colonoscopy should be repeated in 2 to 3 years. When polyps are present and removed, colonoscopy should be done annually.

Surgical indications include the presence of high-grade dysplasia or cancer or if the polyp burden cannot be effectively managed endoscopically. Prophylactic colectomy may be considered for patients with poor surveillance compliance or in patients with family history of CRC. For colorectal disease, surgical options include subtotal colectomy and IRA, segmental colectomy or total colectomy, and IPAA.[36]

Lynch Syndrome

Lynch syndrome was previously used as a synonym for hereditary nonpolyposis CRC (HNPCC) but it was felt that the term "HNPCC" was a misnomer because patients can develop many non-CRCs, as well as one or more polyps or adenomas. This syndrome accounts for 3% to 5% of all CRCs and 10% to 19% of CRCs diagnosed before age 50. It is an autosomal dominantly inherited syndrome characterized by a mutation in one of the DNA mismatch repair (MMR) genes (*MLH1, MSH2, MSH6, PMS2, EpCAM*).These genes maintain fidelity of the DNA during replication by correction of nucleotide base mispairs and small insertions or deletions generated by misincorporations or slippage of DNA polymerase during DNA replication. Mutations in MLH1 and MSH2 account for up to 90% of patients with Lynch syndrome. Because of this genetic defect, Lynch syndrome tumors are characterized by MSI, in which ubiquitous mutations at simple

BOX 52.3 Amsterdam II citeria.

Three or more relatives with hereditary nonpolyposis colorectal cancer–associated cancer (colorectal cancer or cancer of the endometrium, small bowel, ureter, or renal pelvis) plus all of the following:

1. One affected patient is a first-degree relative of the other two.
2. Two or more successive generations are affected.
3. Cancer in one or more affected relatives is diagnosed before the age of 50 years.
4. Familial adenomatous polyposis is excluded.
5. Pathologic diagnosis of cancer is verified.

repetitive sequences (microsatellites) are found in the tumor DNA (but not in the DNA of adjacent normal colorectal mucosa) of individuals with MMR gene defects. Microsatellites are noncoding segments of DNA that contain repetitive sequences of one to six nucleotides. There are hundreds of thousands of microsatellites in the genome, and microsatellite patterns provide a unique DNA fingerprint. When these errors are not repaired due to MMR deficiency, the length of the microsatellite regions are altered and the fingerprint changes. MSI is found in most (>90%) colon malignancies in patients with Lynch syndrome. Immunohistochemistry test, using antibodies to the MMR gene proteins, evaluates for the loss of MMR protein expression and assists in the identification of patients with Lynch syndrome.

Somatic mutations in the BRAF gene are noted in 15% of sporadic CRCs but not in Lynch syndrome tumors. The presence of BRAF mutations in an MSI CRC is evidence against the presence of Lynch syndrome.

Lynch syndrome is characterized by an increased predisposition to the development of CRC and other tumors, which tend to develop at early ages. The estimated lifetime risk for CRC is 70% for men and 40% for women. The mean age of diagnosis for Lynch syndrome–related CRC is 44 to 61 years, compared with 69 years in patients with sporadic CRC. Lynch syndrome–associated CRCs show a predilection for the right colon as compared to sporadic CRC, but left-sided colon cancers, rectal cancers, and synchronous lesions at different sites of the colon and rectum are also common presentations. Among Lynch syndrome patients who have had an initial CRC treated by less than a total colectomy, the risk for a metachronous CRC is 16% at 10 years, 41% at 20 years, and 62% at 30 years. Compared with patients with AFAP or MAP, patients with Lynch syndrome develop few colorectal adenomas by the age of 50 years (usually fewer than three adenomas). Adenoma may progress to carcinoma within 2 to 3 years, compared with from 4 to 10 years in the general population. Histologic features showing poor differentiation, mucinous or signet-ring cell histology, tumor-infiltrating lymphocytes, and lymphoid host response are common.

Endometrial adenocarcinoma is the most common extracolonic cancer (lifetime risk of 32%–45%). Ovarian, gastric, small bowel, urinary tract, brain, and pancreas cancers are also frequently seen in these patients. Sebaceous adenomas and carcinomas of the skin, as well as keratoacanthomas, can be seen in the Muir-Torre variant of Lynch syndrome.[36]

Although germline sequencing of the MMR genes remains the "gold standard" for confirming the causative gene mutation for Lynch syndrome, patients with Lynch syndrome can be initially identified using Amsterdam (Box 52.3) or Bethesda (Box 52.4) criteria.

BOX 52.4 Bethesda criteria for testing colorectal tumors for microsatellite instability (MSI).

Tumors from individuals in the following situations should be tested for MSI:

1. Colorectal cancer diagnosed in a patient before age 50.
2. Presence of synchronous/metachronous colorectal or other hereditary nonpolyposis colorectal cancer (HNPCC)–related tumors (including endometrial, stomach, ovarian, pancreas, ureter and renal pelvis, biliary tract, brain (usually glioblastoma), sebaceous gland adenomas and keratoacanthomas, and carcinoma of the small bowel), regardless of age.
3. Colorectal cancer with the MSI histology (defined by the presence of tumor-infiltrating lymphocytes, Crohn-like lymphocytic reaction, mucinous/signet-ring differentiation, or medullary growth pattern) diagnosed in a patient before age 60.
4. Colorectal cancer diagnosed in at least one first-degree relative with an HNPCC-related tumor in which one cancer was diagnosed before age 50.
5. Colorectal cancer diagnosed in at least two first- or second-degree relatives with HNPCC-related tumors, regardless of age.

From Herzig DO, Buie WD, Weiser MR, et al. Clinical Practice Guidelines for the surgical treatment of patients with lynch syndrome. *Dis Colon Rectum*. 2017;60:137–143.

Screening for CRC by colonoscopy is recommended in persons at risk (first-degree relatives of known MMR gene mutation carriers who have not had genetic testing) or those affected with Lynch syndrome every 1 to 2 years, beginning at 20 to 25 years of age or 2 to 5 years before the youngest age of diagnosis of CRC in the family if diagnosed before age 25 years. This may not be covered by insurance in all cases. For MMR germline mutation–positive patients, consideration should be given to annual colonoscopy. For the endometrial cancer, the screening should be offered to women at risk for or affected with Lynch syndrome by pelvic examination and endometrial sampling annually starting at age 30 to 35 years. Similarly, screening of ovarian cancer should be offered beginning at the same age. Hysterectomy and bilateral salpingo-oophorectomy should be offered to women with Lynch syndrome undergoing colectomy, in all women over age 40 years or who have finished childbearing. Screening for gastric cancer should be considered in persons with Lynch syndrome by esophagogastroduodenoscopy with gastric biopsy of the antrum at 30 to 35 years, and subsequent surveillance every 2 to 3 years can be considered based on individual patient risk factors. Screening for cancer of the urinary tract should be considered for persons at risk for or affected with Lynch syndrome, with urinalysis annually starting at age 30 to 35 years.

In contrast to sporadic colon cancer, three issues must be evaluated when considering the appropriate surgical treatment for colon cancer in the setting of Lynch syndrome: (1) appropriate treatment of the primary tumor, (2) consideration of risk reduction with prophylactic removal of non-neoplastic colon, and (3) morbidity and quality of life after colectomy.

There is still no clear consensus on the surgical management of colon cancer. The options (partial or total colectomy) should be discussed with the patient, taking into account age, comorbidities, and cancer stage. There is no prospective randomized trial comparing extended resection with a limited resection. The cumulative risk of metachronous CRC in patients with segmental colectomy is 16% at 10 years, 41% at 20 years, and 62% at 30 years. However, based on currently available evidence, there is superior cancer risk reduction with total colectomy for the treatment of colon cancer in the setting of Lynch syndrome, and total abdominal colectomy with IRA is the preferred treatment for most patients. For patients with Lynch syndrome and rectal cancer, the rectal cancer should be treated based on standard oncologic principles, as in sporadic rectal cancer. The decision to remove the rest of the colon in patients with rectal cancer may be performed on an individual basis after discussion with the patient.

Consideration for less extensive surgery should be given in patients older than 60 to 65 years and those with underlying sphincter dysfunction. Annual colonoscopy should be performed after segmental resection of colon cancer.

STAGING

Following a diagnosis of CRC, the local and distant spread of the disease is defined and the tumor's stage is determined. Once an individual's stage has been designated, it can be used as a framework for information regarding survival with or without treatment, chance of cure, likelihood of residual disease, and recurrence as well as a support tool for planning treatment type. Staging is generally performed once the diagnosis has been established.

Rules for Classification

Historical staging systems for CRC include the Dukes classification and the modified Astler-Coller classification. Presently, the stage of the tumor is determined according to the tumor, node, metastasis (TNM) system, which assesses the depth of penetration of the tumor into the bowel wall (T stage), the extent of lymph node involvement (N stage), and the presence or absence of distant metastases (M stage). The TNM system was developed by the American Joint Committee on Cancer (AJCC) staging system and approved by the International Union Against Cancer. This classification combines clinical information obtained preoperatively with data obtained during surgery and after histologic examination of the specimen. There have been numerous and significant amendments in the classification system since its initial publication. The latest classification based on eighth edition of the AJCC Cancer Staging Manual is depicted in a table in Ref. 36a.

Clinical Staging

Clinical staging, given the prescript c (cTNM) is based on evidence obtained by medical history, physical examination, endoscopy, and imaging. Assessment for metastatic disease is usually completed with CT (including pelvis, abdomen, and chest). Other modalities such as MRI, positron emission tomography (PET), or fused PET/CT scans are usually not used for initial staging but may be used in patients with contrast allergy/renal failure or in equivocal cases. For rectal cancer, an accurate preoperative assessment of local spread is important in order to determine the need for preoperative neoadjuvant therapy. Modalities to assess the local spread of rectal cancer usually consist of pelvic MRI or endorectal ultrasound for superficial tumors and when MRI is contraindicated or unavailable.

Pathologic Staging

The pathologic examination of the resected specimen, given the prescript p (pTNM), provides additional information for prognosis and consideration of the need for additional (adjuvant) treatment. Patients who were given neoadjuvant therapy prior to resection based on their clinical staging will have a modified pathologic staging indicated by the y prescript (ypTNM). Once the three components of the TNM have been defined, they can be grouped together into overall stage as shown in a table in Ref. 36a

Additional Prognostic Factors

In addition to the classic TNM staging, the AJCC manual also recommends additional prognostic factors that should be determined and reported. Among these are the serum carcinoembryonic antigen (CEA) levels, the presence of tumor deposits within the lymph drainage area of a cancer, and their association with blood vessels and neural structures (lymphovascular and perineural invasion respectfully), all associated with a poorer prognosis. The histologic grade of the tumor (low grade vs. high grade) is determined by the pathologist, as well as specific histologic subtypes such as mucinous and signet ring adenocarcinomas, which are usually more aggressive and carry a worse prognosis. The circumferential resection margin should be reported by the pathologist, as well as the proximal and distal margin status and in rectal cancer, the completeness of the mesorectal excision. Pathologic response to neoadjuvant treatment is assessed on the primary tumor and reported as the tumor regression grade, a four-point regression grade scale from 0 (complete response) to 3 (poor or no response). In addition to the above, molecular markers for somatic and germline mutations are investigated, such as MSI, KRAS, BRAF, and NRAS mutations, which can help in both prognosis and treatment planning.

SURGICAL TREATMENT OF COLORECTAL CANCER

The goal of curative surgical treatment of CRC is the resection of the primary tumor with adequate free margins, en bloc with loco regional lymphadenectomy. Regional lymph nodes are located in the mesocolon along the main vascular pedicles. Therefore, an oncologically adequate resection implies the removal of the portion of colon where the primary cancer is located with its vascular pedicles, which must be ligated and divided at their origin. The aim of lymphadenectomy is to ensure an adequate pathologic staging and to remove any possible residual lymph node metastasis. No less than 12 lymph nodes are required for an oncologically adequate resection and for proper staging, but, in most cases, more than 20 nodes are retrieved from the specimen. The reader may wish to refer to the ASCRS Clinical Practice Guidelines for the Treatment of Colon Cancer and for the practice parameters for the management of rectal cancer.

There are some anatomic vascular landmarks when performing a colorectal resection.

- The ileocolic pedicle originates from the superior mesenteric vessels just caudal to the second portion of the duodenum (Fig. 52.63).
- The middle colic vessels originate from the superior mesenteric vessels at the level of the inferior margin of the pancreas.
- The inferior mesenteric vein can be easily identified at the level of the ligament of Treitz (Fig. 52.64).
- The IMA originates from the aorta, 2 to 3 cm caudal from the area where the IMV is identified; its origin is surrounded by the mesenteric and hypogastric nervous plexus (Fig. 52.65).
- The left colic artery originates about 2 cm distally to the origin of the IMA.

General Rules and Principles

- Surgery should be gentle, and manipulation of the tumor should be avoided as much as possible ("no touch" technique).

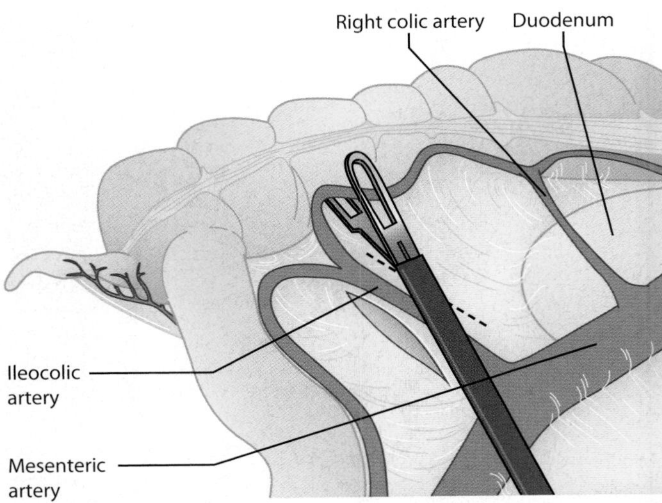

FIG. 52.63 Origin of the ileocolic pedicle from the mesenteric pedicle right below the duodenum.

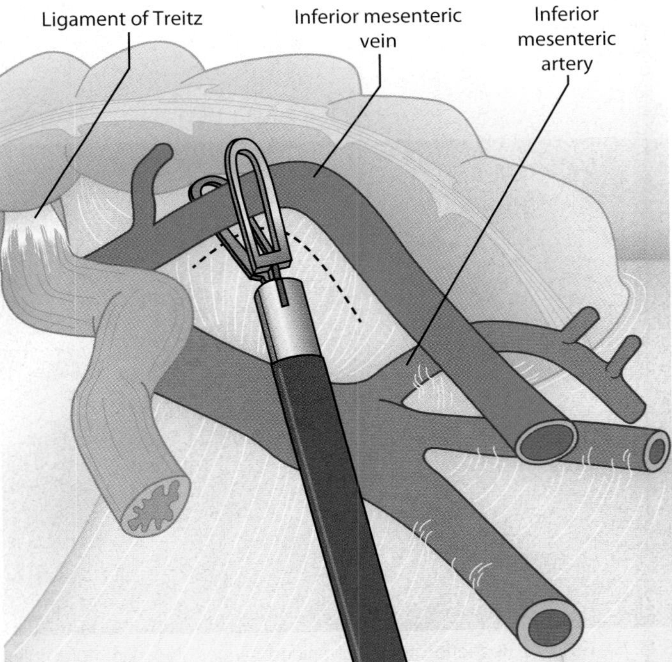

FIG. 52.64 In left-sided resections, the inferior mesenteric vein is identified at the ligament of Treitz and the mesocolon of the left colon is dissected away from the retroperitoneum along the fascia of Toldt. (From D'Annibale A, Morpurgo E, Menin N. Laparoscopic and robotic surgery in rectal cancer. In: Delaini GG, ed. *Rectal Cancer. New Frontiers in Diagnosis, Treatment and Rehabilitation*. New York: Springer; 2005:167–176.)

- "Free" margins must be adequate: for colon cancer, a 5-cm "free" margin is recommended in order to minimize the risk of recurrent cancer caused by distal spread and in order to avoid leaving behind perivisceral lymph nodes, which could be involved with metastatic disease.
- For rectal cancer, a 2-cm distal margin is sufficient: distal spread of the cancer occurs in 1% to 2% of cases when the distal margin is 2 cm. In ultradistal sphincter-sparing surgery

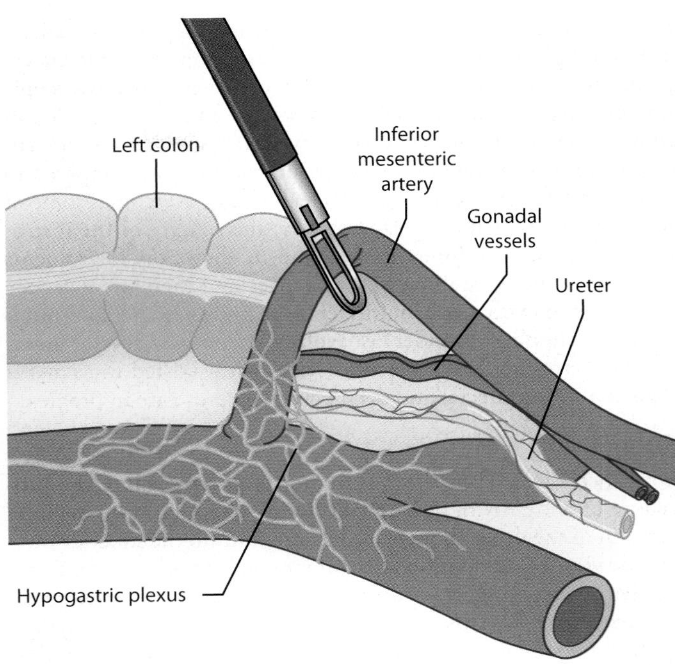

FIG. 52.65 The inferior mesenteric artery originates from the aorta, 2 to 3 cm caudal from the area where the inferior mesenteric vein is identified; its origin is surrounded by the mesenteric and hypogastric nervous plexus. (From D'Annibale A, Morpurgo E, Menin N. Laparoscopic and robotic surgery in rectal cancer. In: Delaini GG, ed. *Rectal Cancer. New Frontiers in Diagnosis, Treatment and Rehabilitation*. New York: Springer; 2005:167–176.)

resections, a cancer-free margin of 1 cm or, in selected cases, a free margin at frozen section examination can be accepted.

- In order to restore bowel continuity, the anastomosis must be constructed without any tension, utilizing well-vascularized segments of bowel.
- The vascular supply of the colon, which is mobilized and utilized for the anastomosis, relies on marginal vessels located in the mesocolon. Therefore, great care must be used during the manipulation of the mesocolon, as minimal injury of these vessels can result in irreversible ischemic damage of the transposed colon.

Surgical Technique

Colorectal resections can be approached by open access or with minimally invasive techniques. The latter have shown favorable short-term benefits when compared to standard open colectomies: less postoperative pain, shorter postoperative hospital stay, faster recovery of bowel function, and a lower wound infection rate. Surgical resection quality was proven to be noninferior in laparoscopy also for rectal cancer resections, and local recurrence rate and disease-free survival (DFS) are similar after open or laparoscopic resections.[37] Therefore, the laparoscopic approach should be preferred given the availability of expertise and proven experience. During the last decade, the use of laparoscopy for colorectal resections gradually increased to about 40%, with an overall conversion rate below 10%. The percentage varies greatly based on hospital setting (urban vs. rural, high volume vs. low volume) and the surgeon's expertise and may be as high as 80% in high-volume specialized institutions with a low conversion rate. Robotics is the evolution of MIS: the surgeon operates while sitting at a console and maneuvers the robotic instruments using joy sticks. The robot gives a deep three-dimensional vision and adds the capability of intracorporeal hand wristed movements to laparoscopic instruments. Randomized trials and results of metaanalysis do not show yet clear advantages in conversion rate and short-term oncologic results for robotic low anterior resections as compared to conventional laparoscopy, but this technology overcomes some of the intrinsic difficulties of laparoscopy: the rigidity of the instruments and the two-dimensional vision. It allows the instruments to move in the three dimensions of space and therefore gives the possibility to easily perform intracorporeal sutures and anastomosis. The technology is under fast evolution, and new developments of single arms and single access devices with wristed movements designed for intrarectal and deep pelvic space use are in progress.

Right-Sided Tumors

For cancers located in the cecum and ascending colon, the procedure of choice is right hemicolectomy. The procedure includes division of the ileocecal pedicle at its origin from the superior mesenteric vessels and division of the right colic vessels (Fig. 52.66A); the lymphatic tissue that surrounds the superior mesenteric vein can be removed en bloc in order to perform a complete lymph node dissection (Fig. 52.66B). The right branch of the middle colic vessels is divided. The terminal ileum is divided with a stapler 5 to 6 cm from the ileocecal valve and the transverse colon at the junction between its mid and proximal third. The omentum has to be removed en bloc, together with the gastrocolic ligament that is divided along the gastroepiploic arcade. Bowel continuity is restored with an ileotransverse anastomosis, in most cases laterolateral. When approached in laparotomy, the first maneuver is the detachment of the right abdominal side-wall attachment; the vascular pedicles are ligated once the right colon has been fully mobilized from the retroperitoneum and from the duodenum. In laparoscopy or robotics, the colectomy is usually performed with a medial to lateral approach with initial vascular control and then detachment from the abdominal side wall. If approached laparoscopically, the anastomosis can be extracorporeal (through an umbilical mini laparotomy, which is also utilized for specimen extraction) or intracorporeal. An intracorporeal anastomosis seems to bring advantages in terms of fewer anastomotic complications (leaks and twists) and faster recovery of bowel function and discharge when compared to extracorporeal anastomosis, but it is technically challenging in laparoscopy. The robot facilitates the anastomosis that can be done with the articulated robotic linear stapler and the enterotomies can be hand sewn with robotic instruments. Reported leak rates are about 1% and the specimen in these cases can be extracted through a Pfannenstiel incision that has fewer short- and long-term complications as compared to a midline mini-laparotomy.

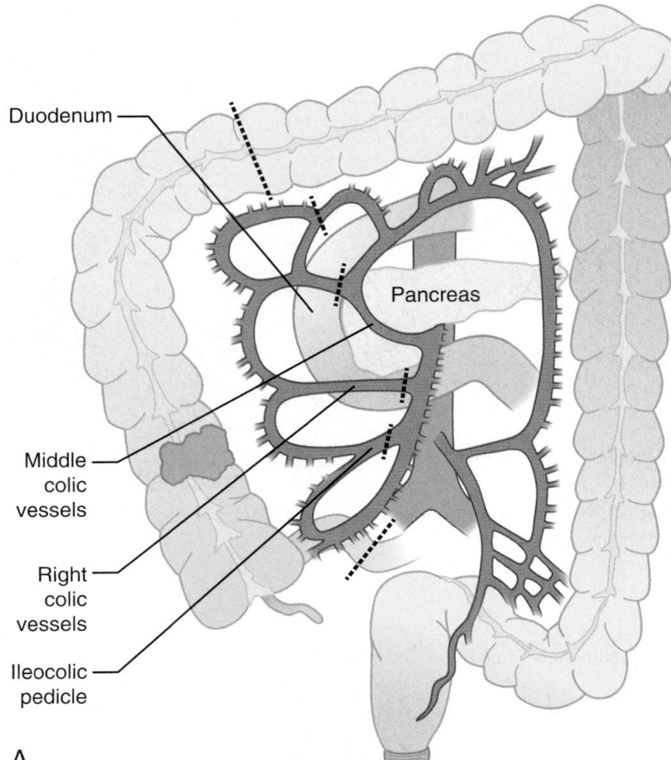

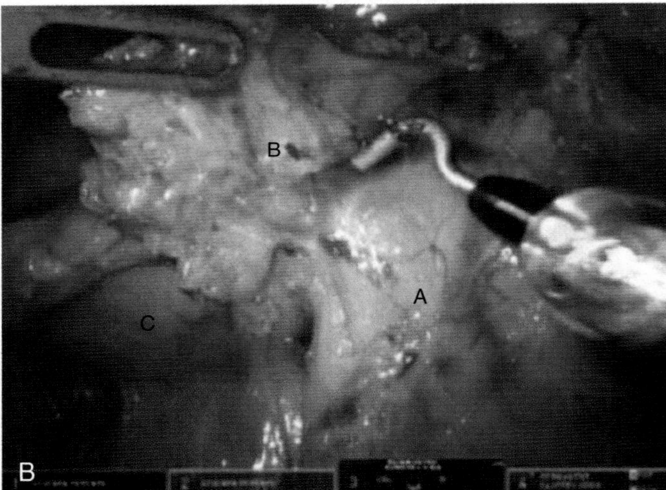

FIG. 52.66 (A) Resection for a right-sided cancer: ileocolic, right colic, and right branch of the middle colic vessels are ligated. The terminal ileum and the transverse colon are divided as shown. (B) Robotic dissection in right colectomy. The lymph nodes are peeled off the superior mesenteric vein, and the ileocolic vein is isolated at its origin. *A*, Superior mesenteric vein; *B*, ileocolic vein at its origin; *C*, duodenum.

Tumors of the Transverse Colon

The standard procedure for the majority of these cancers is right extended colectomy that differs from right colectomy because, here, the middle colic vessels are divided at their origin at the level of the inferior margin of the pancreatic neck (Fig. 52.67A). The ileocolic anastomosis is made at the distal third of the transverse colon. Indocyanine green angiography can allow one to assess the vascular supply of the residual colon and to identify the area of vascular demarcation. The transection with the stapler must be done in a well vascularized area (Fig. 52.67B). This test is crucial when multiple vascular pedicles are resected—as is the case in extended right hemicolectomy—or when the viability of the mobilized colon relies on small marginal vessels, especially in elderly atherosclerotic patients.

Tumors of the Splenic Flexure

This has been debated as to the ideal procedure for splenic flexure lesions—ranging from extended right-sided resection, to encompass the splenic flexure, to resection of the splenic flexure alone (Fig. 52.68). The inferior mesenteric vein is ligated at the level

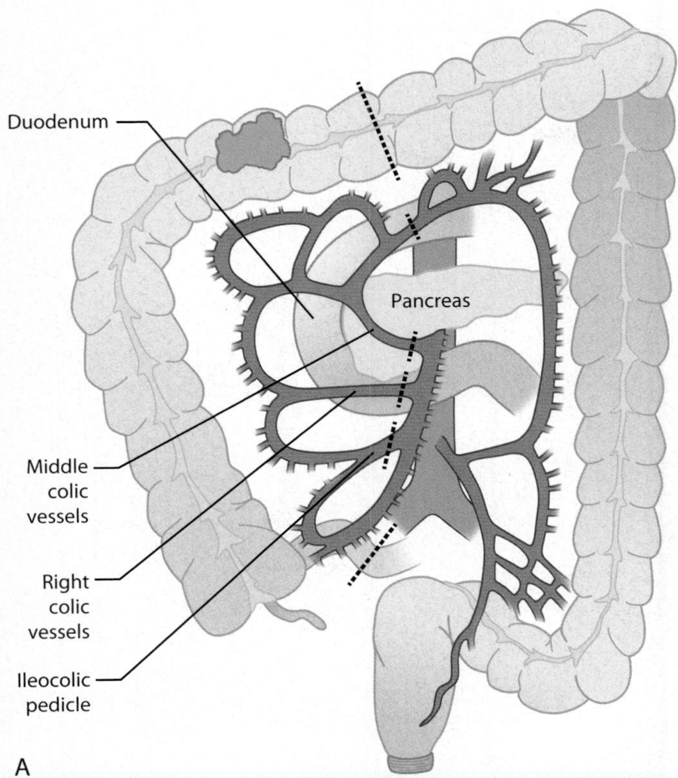

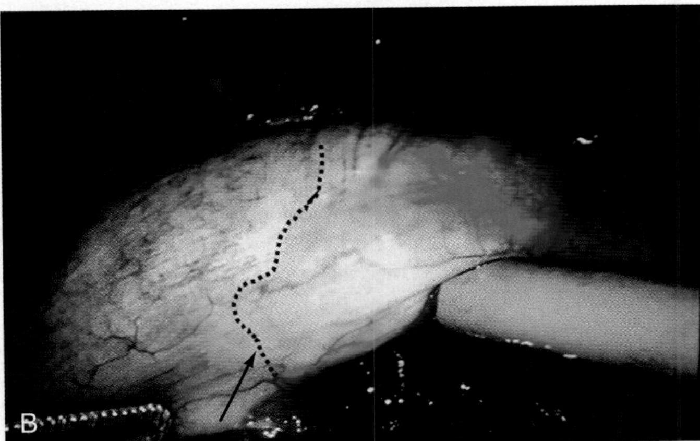

FIG. 52.67 (A) Resection for cancers of the transverse colon. The ileocolic, right, and middle colic vessels are ligated. The terminal ileum and the transverse colon are transected as shown. (B) Indocyanine green angiography. After transection of the middle colic vessels, the line of vascular demarcation is clearly visible *(arrow)*.

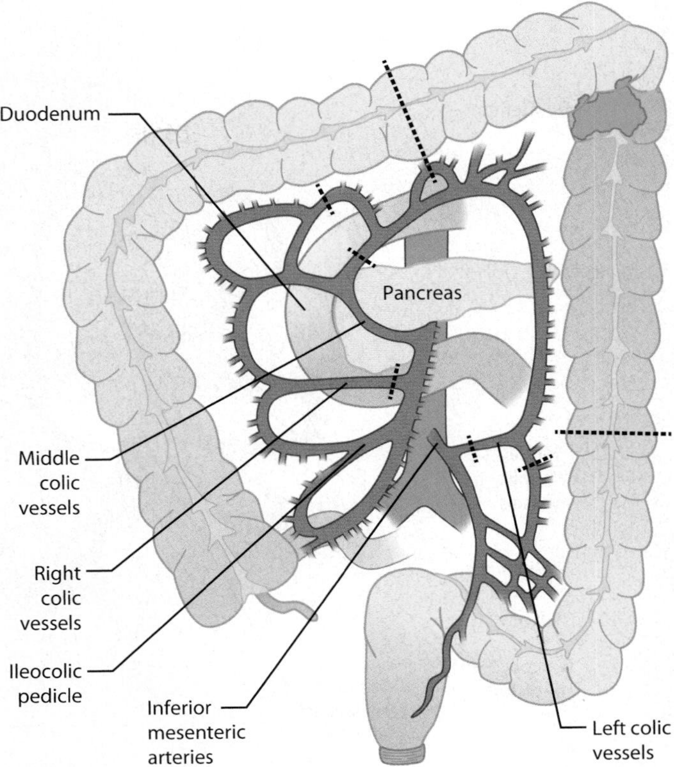

FIG. 52.68 Resection for cancers of the splenic flexure. The left colic artery and the left branch of the middle colic artery are ligated as shown.

of the ligament of Treitz and the left colic artery is divided at its origin from the IMA and the specimen is taken en bloc with the omentum. In the majority of cases, bowel continuity is restored with an anastomosis between the transverse and the descending colon. In selected cases, where the mesentery of the colon is thick and the colon is short, this colocolic anastomosis can compress and obstruct the duodenum at the ligament of Treitz. In these cases, extended right hemicolectomy with ileo-descending anastomosis is preferable.

Left-Sided Tumors

Left hemicolectomy includes the high ligation of the IMA at its origin (Fig. 52.69A). The IMA can also be ligated 2 to 3 cm more distally without compromising the oncologic outcome but lowering the risk of injuring the mesenteric and hypogastric nervous plexus. A damage of the nervous plexus carries the risk of genitourinary complications, including retrograde ejaculation in males, bladder dysfunction, and vaginal dryness in women. The inferior mesenteric vein is divided at the level of the ligament of Treitz. The splenic flexure must be fully mobilized with coloepiploic detachment, detachment of the mesocolon of the splenic flexure and distal transverse from the pancreas, and left abdominal gutter detachment. The detachment of the splenic flexure is necessary in order to guarantee an anastomosis without tension between the left colon and the proximal rectum below the rectosigmoid junction. Also, for left colectomies, in laparoscopy, the preferred approach is mediolateral with initial vascular control and then subsequent colon mobilization. Restoration of bowel continuity is made with a transanal circular stapler that should have a caliber of about 3 cm (Fig. 52.69B).

OBSTRUCTING COLON CANCERS

Patients with obstructing tumors of the colon may present indolently with pencil-thin stools, increasing constipation, and an increasingly distended abdomen, or acutely with obstipation, complete obstruction, abdominal pain, and vomiting, which may be feculent. Diagnosis is commonly confirmed with imaging such as plain films, contrast enemas, abdominal CT, and lower endoscopy. Treatment objectives entail relief of the obstruction, resection of ischemic or nonviable bowel, and resection of the tumor.

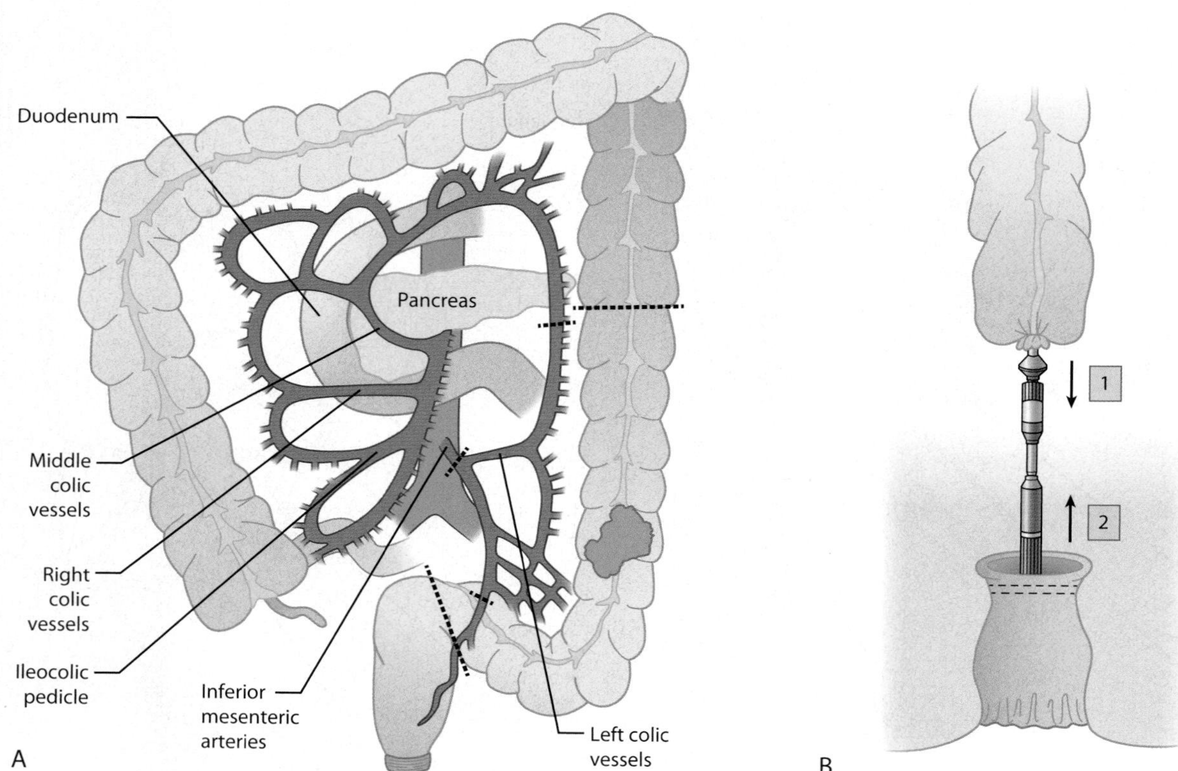

FIG. 52.69 (A) Left hemicolectomy. The inferior mesenteric artery is ligated and the marginal artery is ligated just distal to level of transection of the colon. The hemorrhoidal vessels are ligated within the proximal mesorectum. (B) Colorectal anastomosis with circular stapler. *1*, Anvil in the proximal colon; *2*, Shaft of the transanally placed circular stapler.

Management of Left-Sided Obstructions

The approach to left-sided obstructions is tailored according to the location of obstruction, viability of the proximal bowel, and general stability of the patient. In sigmoid and left colon obstructions, patients are commonly referred for urgent surgery. A segmental resection of the primary tumor is typically performed. If the proximal large bowel has perforated or is showing signs of ischemia, a subtotal colectomy is completed. Historically, primary anastomosis has been avoided, with the distal stump closed and a proximal stoma exteriorized (Hartmann operation). However, reestablishing intestinal continuity then entails a major operation, and a large proportion of patients will never be reversed. Current evidence supports the option of a primary anastomosis in appropriate patients who are hemodynamically stable, and a tension-free anastomosis with a good blood supply can be achieved, usually by specialized surgeons. In these cases, leak rates are in the range of 2% to 12%, which are almost comparable to the 2% to 8% leak rate in elective surgery.[38] Intraoperative colonic lavage or manual decompression prior to anastomosis can be performed with similar results between them, but evidence is lacking supporting either with regard to anastomotic leaks or infectious complications. A proximal diverting stoma may also be exteriorized combined with a primary anastomosis. This does not reduce the anastomotic leak rate but may decrease the quantity of leaks requiring reoperation.

Endoscopic stenting as a bridge for surgery has also emerged as an attractive technique to relieve obstructions and permit elective surgery under more favorable conditions. Stenting has been shown to permit higher rates of primary anastomosis, decreased wound infections, and a higher rate of completion of surgery laparoscopically. Stenting is contraindicated in suspected ischemic or perforated bowel. Clinical success is in the 70% to 80% range, with the main immediate risk being stent-related perforation. Concerns about inferior long-term oncologic outcomes have limited usage in patients with average risk curable disease. Although recent evidence has suggested that long-term oncologic outcomes may be acceptable,[39] current guidelines recommend stenting as a bridge for surgery on an individual basis, mainly in high-risk patients to allow optimization with interval colectomy.

Management of Right-Sided Obstructions

Treatment of right-sided obstructions generally includes an oncologic segmental resection. In most cases, a primary ileocolic anastomosis can be performed safely, but for patients with a high risk of anastomotic failure, a diverting stoma can be exteriorized.

RECTAL CANCER

Preoperative Evaluation of Patients With Rectal Cancer

Every year, there are approximately 44,000 new diagnoses of patients with rectal cancer in the United States. The main changing trend in the United States is the increasing number of young patients being diagnosed with rectal cancer. This is a significantly changing demographic that is projected to increase over the next 10 to 15 years. Similar to colon cancer, patients with rectal cancer are staged upon presentation to determine the extent of disease. Unlike colon cancers, rectal cancers have a much higher risk of

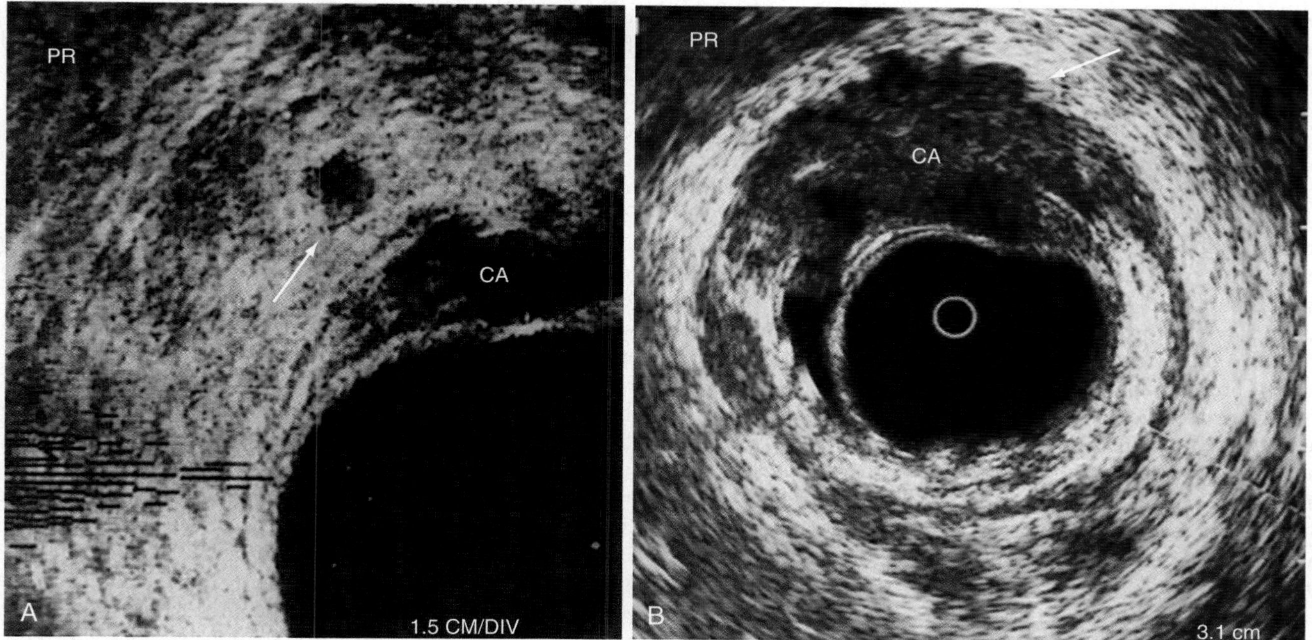

FIG. 52.70 (A) Endorectal ultrasound showing hypoechoic lymph node *(arrow)* between cancer and prostate. (B) Endorectal ultrasound showing irregular anterior border where cancer has grown through rectal wall *(arrow)* (T3). *CA*, Cancer; *PR*, prostate.

local recurrence; therefore, there has been an evolution in their treatment and preoperative assessment. Because of the boney confines of the pelvis, obtaining a clear "circumferential margin of resection" is less straightforward than within the true confines of the abdomen. As noted in the section on anatomy earlier in this chapter, the lower half of the rectum is either entirely or partly an extraperitoneal structure. Also, based on its blood supply, the lower half of the rectum drains into the systemic circulation and therefore can also metastasize through the systemic circulation to the lungs, whereas upper rectal cancers tend to metastasize, just as colon cancers do, to the liver. In assessing a patient with rectal cancer, the first thing would be to, on physical examination, assess if it is within reach of the examining finger of the surgeon. If it is palpable at the tip of the finger, one can ascertain whether there is good anal sphincter tone, in which case, in the majority of patients, the cancer will be amenable to treatment by a sphincter-sparing approach. Initial assessment of the patient with rectal cancer should include a physical examination, including digital exam. In evaluating patients with rectal cancer, one should always document any pathology as anterior, posterior, left, or right. Documentation of lesion location as at "six o'clock" or "twelve o'clock" is always confusing, as one does not know whether the patient is lying supine or prone. In women, it is always crucial to document whether or not there is invasion of the rectovaginal septum, as this will be a prime consideration of whether or not a vaginal resection will need to be performed at the time of surgery. In addition to this, assessment of sphincter involvement is critical.

A proctoscopic examination assessing for tumor height should be performed if possible as height assessments with flexible endoscopy are notoriously inaccurate. What is judged to be at 15 cm during a flexible endoscopic examination can be much closer or farther away on rigid endoscopy. Treating rectal cancers in men with a narrow pelvis, particularly obese males, is particularly challenging, as is the peritoneal reflection. Examining a patient on a tilt table in knee-chest position is particularly beneficial, especially in the extremely obese patients, as even in the very large patient this permits a fairly good digital examination and examination of the lower rectum.

Staging of the rectal cancer can be performed either with endorectal ultrasound or with MRI. The quality of MRI, as well as endorectal ultrasound, varies by center. Endorectal ultrasound is performed by a surgeon, gastroenterologist, or radiologist, whereas the MRI is performed by a radiologist. Both have advantages and disadvantages. Endorectal ultrasound is a much less expensive test, can be performed without sedation, and provides an accurate assessment of the T stage of a rectal cancer. Not all facilities have the equipment for performing endorectal ultrasonography. Some facilities may have endoscopic ultrasonography capability. Fig. 52.70 shows a representative endorectal ultrasound in a patient with rectal cancer. The rectal wall is indicated by three white lines and two hypoechoic lines. The innermost line represents the interface between the water-filled balloon and the transducer. The transducer rotates 360 degrees to give an image of the rectum. In most studies, the accuracy of lymph node detection is much less than the accuracy of detecting T stage.

With respect to MRI, in order to obtain a meaningful study for rectal cancer staging, the MRI has to be performed according to a specific rectal cancer protocol in which the MRI is accessed in the same axis as the rectum. In addition, it is very helpful to fill the rectum with ultrasound gel mixed with gadolinium. MRI interpretation is dependent upon the experience of the radiologist reading the MRI. A pelvic MRI will, however, permit assessment of lymph node involvement and circumferential resection margin status as well as assessment of extrarectal disease, which is not possible with endorectal ultrasound. Currently, clinically T3 and node positive rectal cancers and those with cancers in close proximity of the sphincter in whom sphincter sparing is desired are recommended to undergo preoperative neoadjuvant chemoradiation.

There has been an evolution in the overall treatment of rectal cancer with the recognition that patients' rectal cancers can be "downstaged," facilitating the surgery, increasing the chance of a sphincter-sparing operation, and also providing improved functional results (lesser number of bowel movements and improved control) as compared to when these treatments are given after surgery. These observations are derived from several studies. A major study was the German Rectal Cancer Study, whose results were published in 2004.[40] T3 and T4 rectal cancer patients were randomized to receive either preoperative or postoperative chemoradiation. There was no overall difference in morbidity or mortality; however, lower rates of local recurrence and both acute and long-term toxicity were seen with preoperative treatment. Importantly, significantly more patients in the preoperative treatment group were able to undergo sphincter-sparing procedures. Beginning in the 1980s, Richard Heald began to popularize a technique that many surgeons were already performing, namely, complete excision of the mesorectum. This involves removing the entire mesorectum intact using sharp dissection. This technique was associated with a much lower risk of local recurrence and improved survival rates. Publications from Quirke and colleagues emphasized the role of the circumferential margin in reducing recurrence. A combination of these techniques (i.e., performing preoperative chemoradiation) and TME and recognition of the importance of the circumferential margin have led to improved outcomes for rectal cancer surgery. In fact, much as has been done for anal squamous cell cancer; there have been variations in protocols, waiting different amounts of time from completion of chemoradiation until surgery. Professor Habr-Gama has been the lead of a new treatment philosophy entitled "watch and wait." The concept of "complete pathologic response" has been extensively studied. Initially reported in a small group of patients with rectal cancer undergoing preoperative neoadjuvant therapy, it was noted that 27% of patients had no clinically detectable evidence of cancer following this treatment.[41] When these patients were compared to those undergoing surgery with the finding of a complete response in their specimen, there was no difference in local or systemic recurrence between groups. Among rectal cancer patients undergoing neoadjuvant chemoradiation, approximately 20% will achieve a "complete response." Typically, a restaging is performed following treatment. In high-risk patients, or in select patients after an in-depth discussion, a watch and wait strategy may be chosen. This is currently not standard of care. The absence of luminal disease does not imply the absence of disease, and such patients must be followed longitudinally, not only with physical and endoscopic examination but also with cross-sectional imaging, preferably MRI. With respect to response to neoadjuvant therapy in patients undergoing resection for rectal cancer, there have been different staging systems proposed to grade the degree of tumor regression. One common scale ranges from 1 to 3, with respect to how many viable tumor cells remain, with 1 referring to a complete response and 3 referring to a minimal response.[42] As stated previously under Colon Cancer Staging, any staging that has a "y" prefix refers to an AJCC stage that is obtained following neoadjuvant treatment.

Local Excision

Local excision of rectal neoplasms can be accomplished through both endoscopic and transanal techniques. Endoscopic techniques include routine polypectomy, endoscopic mucosal resection, and endoscopic submucosal resection. Surgical excision can be performed via standard transanal excision, transanal MIS (TAMIS), as well as by transanal endoscopic microsurgery.

Endoscopy for the transanal removal of large rectal lesions has expanded with the availability of improved staging techniques, including endorectal and endoscopic ultrasound and MRI described elsewhere in this chapter. Careful digital examination is also accurate at staging lesions within reach of the examining finger, as a lesion that is soft to the touch typically is benign. This goes particularly for villous adenomas of the rectum. Villous adenomas of the lower rectum are commonly amenable to a transanal excision or endoscopic excision. The key here is, however, excision of a lesion with a free margin to reduce the risk of local recurrence.

Partial- or full-thickness (for cancers) excision of lesions can be performed. With partial-thickness excision, such as is done for benign lesions, these techniques are made easier by submucosal injection of a solution to elevate the lesion off of the underlying muscularis mucosa. Some of these solutions used for endoscopy are colored, making visualization even easier. Endoscopic submucosal dissection is used for lesions that are superficial. In doing this, a hollow cap is placed over the tip of the endoscope. After submucosal injection has been performed to lift the lesion away from the underlying muscularis, suction is applied to the colonoscope when the cap is positioned over the lesion. The lesion is drawn into the cap by suction, the snare that fits around the cap then is tightened, cutting off the area of mucosa that has been aspirated into the cap, much like a routine polypectomy. In using this technique, fairly large areas of mucosa can be safely removed. When lesions go somewhat deeper through the muscle wall, a technique called endoscopic submucosal resection can be performed. In this technique, submucosal injection is performed to facilitate dissection of a lesion off the underlying colon wall after the margin has been scored.

Surgical transanal resection of rectal lesions has long been popular as a form of sphincter-sparing surgery but has become less so with the advent of circular staplers and especially with minimally invasive techniques for resectional rectal surgery. Traditional criteria for performing a local excision for a rectal cancer have been small lesions (<2 cm in diameter), well-differentiated cancers within reach of the index finger, and lesions that are mobile (not fixed). T1 lesions are ideal, and patients with T2 or T3 lesions are not suitable, as the recurrence rate following local excision in this group of patients has been unacceptable. If a traditional local excision is performed, cautery is used to score a 1-cm margin around the lesion. Traction is used, and a full-thickness incision is performed down to perirectal fat (Fig. 52.71). Local excision is safe when performed for lesions that are located lateral to or posterior to the rectum due to the presence of the mesorectum. If these lesions are located in the anterior rectum in women, there is risk of iatrogenic rectovaginal fistula or, in the case of men, injury to the prostate. In addition, as one goes higher above 6 or 7 cm, there is concern that one may be intraperitoneal. These procedures are most safely performed in the lower rectum.

The development in the early 1990s of transanal endoscopic microsurgery made possible the excision of larger lesions and lesions higher than could be safely performed using conventional transanal surgery. This required a specialized set of instruments and demanded a very special set of skills working with rigid instruments with a high learning curve. This technique has now largely been supplanted with the technique of TAMIS, whereby standard laparoscopic instruments and an access port similar to that used for single-port laparoscopy is used in the anal canal to

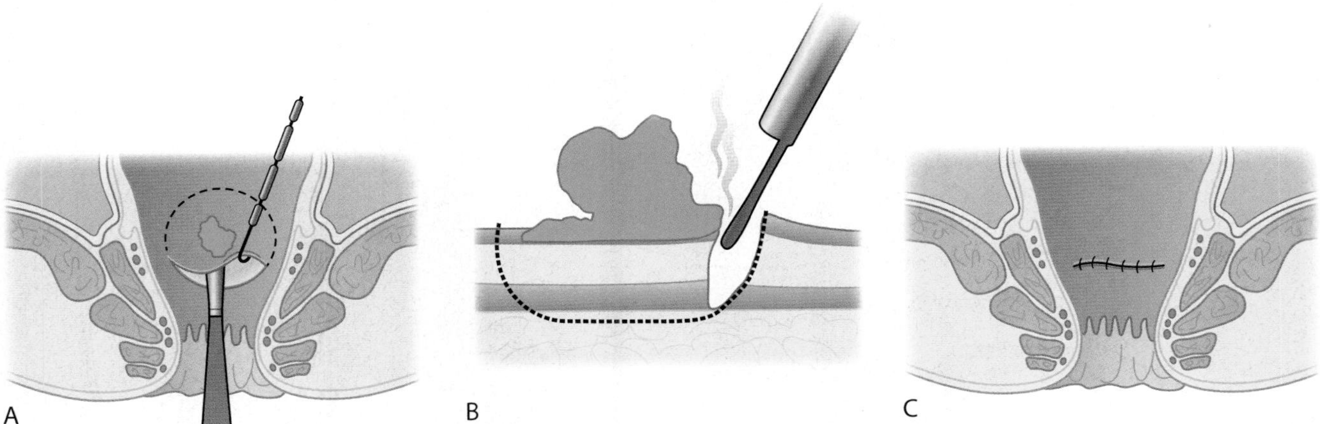

FIG. 52.71 (A) Transanal excision of a small rectal cancer. A 1-cm lesion has been scored around the lesion to be excised using electrocautery. Using careful traction, full-thickness excision is performed. (B) Transanal excision of a small rectal cancer. Electrocautery is used to perform a full-thickness excision extending into the mesorectum. (C) Transanal excision of a small rectal cancer. The defect can be sutured closed or left open to heal by secondary intention.

allow for safe excision of lesions above the level of the very distal rectum (Fig. 52.72, Video 52.1). Due to the anchoring of the laparoscopic access device itself, this technique is not suitable for lesions in the very lower rectum.

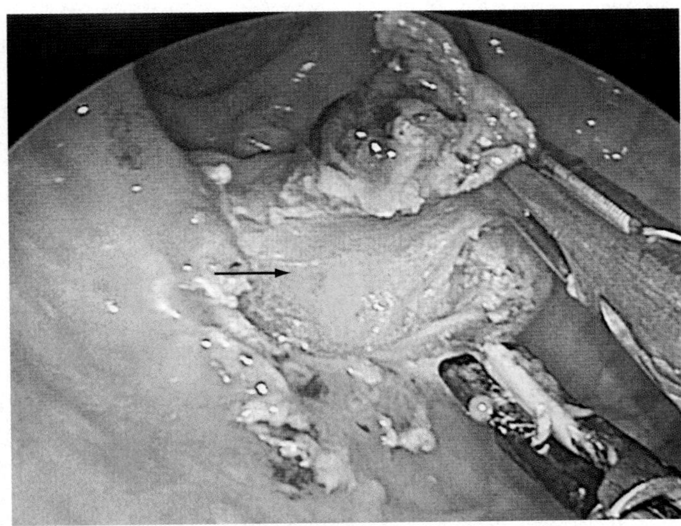

FIG. 52.72 Rectal cancer patient undergoing transanal minimally invasive surgical removal of residual scar following apparent complete clinical response following neoadjuvant chemoradiation. The *arrow* points to fat of rectal mesentery seen with full-thickness excision.

Resections for Rectal Cancers

The rectum is the distal portion of the large intestine. It is divided into three parts: proximal rectum (approximately from 15–10 cm from the anal verge), mid rectum (from 10–5 cm from anal verge), and distal rectum (5 cm and less). The upper portion of the mid rectum and distal rectum are extraperitoneal. The rectum is located in the narrow space of the pelvis. It has close anatomic relations with the genitourinary organs (bladder, seminal vesicles, prostate, vagina, uterus) and with the endopelvic nerves. It has an important role as a fecal reservoir. The rectum plays an active role in defecation and is in continuity with the sphincter apparatus. Its distal mucosa is fundamental to discriminate between stool and gas. An oncologically radical resection of the rectum must be performed along a very precise anatomic plane en bloc with its mesorectum where the lymphatics and the rectal lymph nodes are located. The mesorectum, in turn, is enveloped by the mesorectal fascia that has to be kept intact during the dissection because its integrity has been shown to be crucial to reduce the risk of local recurrence. For all these reasons, surgical resection of the rectum and the mesorectum—the so-called "total mesorectal excision" or TME—poses some specific challenges with respect to surgical technique.

Low Anterior Resection

After vascular division similar to left colectomies, the peritoneal reflection of the rectum is divided at the level of the sacral promontory and the rectum with its proximal mesorectum is gently pulled anteriorly entering the avascular "cotton candy" plane between the fascia of the mesorectum and the presacral fascia. Extra care must be taken in order to avoid any injury to the hypogastric nerves that must be visualized. Anteriorly, the cul-de-sac is divided, and the rectum is dissected from the anteriorly located seminal vesicles in males and the vagina in females. The dissection is continued distally and the rectum and the mesorectum are divided 5 cm below the cancer (Fig. 52.73), thus indicating a subtotal mesorectal excision. For cancers located in the distal two thirds of the rectum, the dissection must be continued more distally, dissecting the rectum away from the prostate along the fascia of Denonvilliers. Posteriorly, the rectum has to be dissected distally, up to the level of the levator muscles en bloc with the entire mesorectum, keeping the mesorectal fascia intact. The most distal part of the rectum is "naked" (i.e., not surrounded by the mesorectum that ends a few cm proximally) (Fig. 52.74). At this level, the rectum can be divided with a stapler. In laparoscopy, several reloads may be necessary to complete the transection of the rectum in the distal pelvis. This operation is called TME because it removes the rectum en bloc with its entire mesorectum. The integrity of the visceral

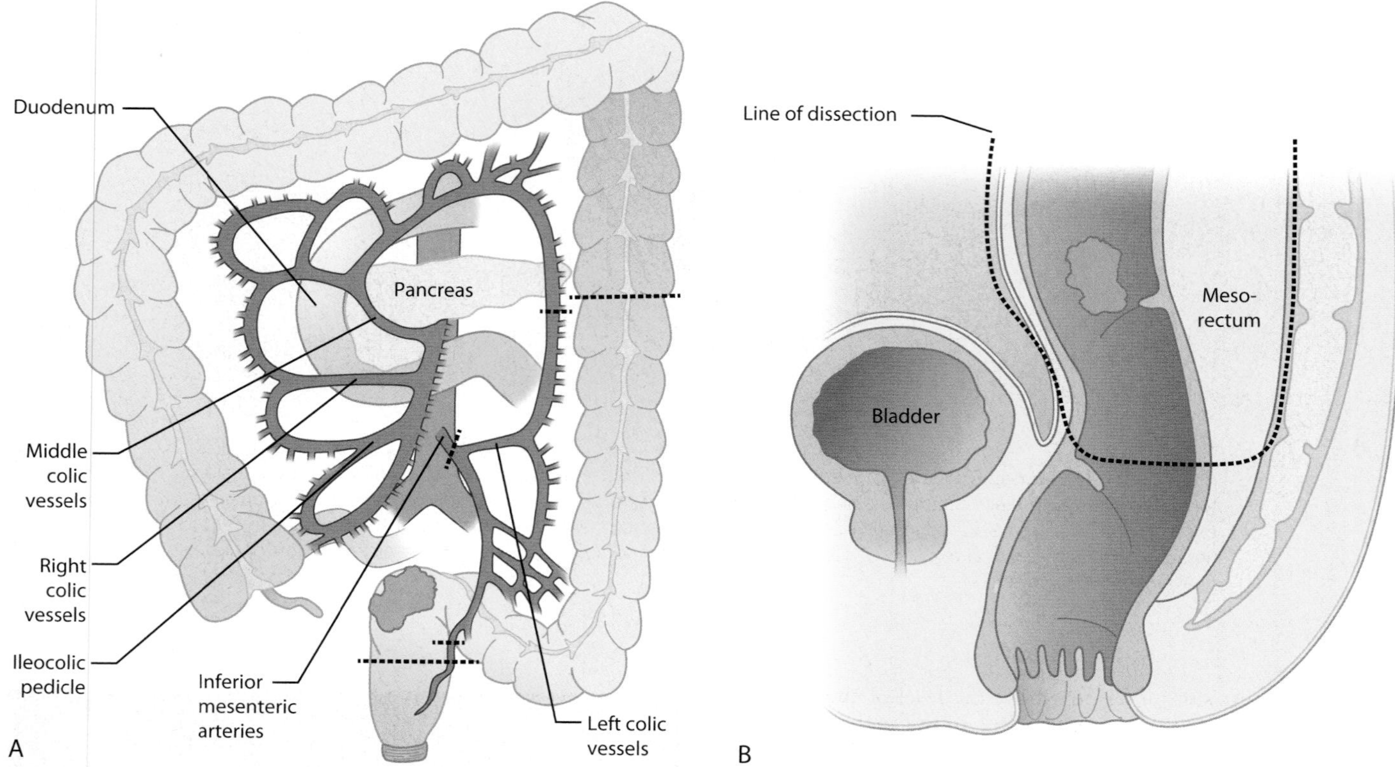

FIG. 52.73 (A) Low anterior resection for cancer of the upper rectum. The inferior mesenteric artery is ligated. The marginal artery is ligated just distal to level of colon transection; the hemorrhoidal vessels are ligated in the mesorectum. (B) Low anterior resection for cancer of the upper rectum. *(Dotted line)* A line of dissection of the rectum en bloc with the mesorectum.

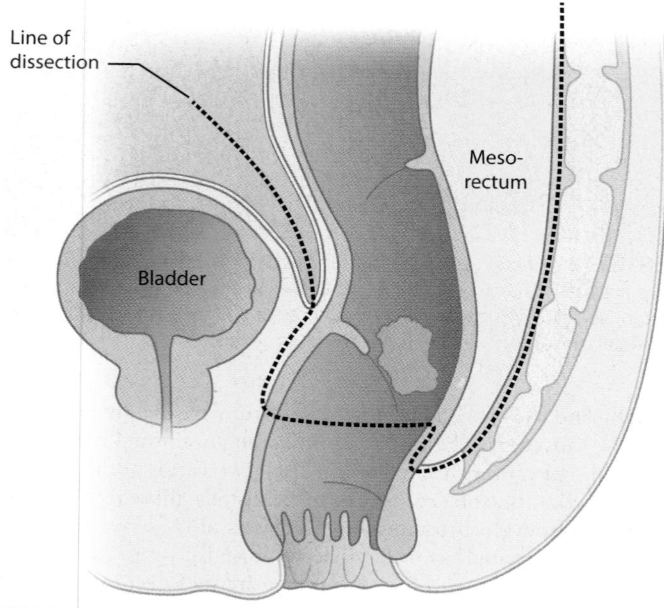

FIG. 52.74 Low anterior resection for cancer of the upper rectum. *Dotted line* of dissection of the rectum en bloc with the mesorectum.

fascia is a crucial point that defines the quality of a TME and is directly related to the DFS interval. The proper excision along the anatomic plane is essential in order to obtain free circumferential radial margins, thus reducing the local recurrence rate below 5%; it also results in a significant decrease in the frequency of urinary and sexual dysfunction (retrograde ejaculation and impotence). Recent evidence demonstrates that the laparoscopic approach has similar results with regard to the quality of resection, clear circumferential margins, and recurrence rate when compared to the open approach. The DFS for stages II–III cancer is about 75% regardless of the surgical approach utilized (i.e., laparoscopy or open surgery). The colorectal anastomosis is eventually made with a circular stapler inserted transanally. Air is then insufflated into the rectum through the anastomosis while the proximal colon is occluded, and the pelvis is filled with water in order to exclude the presence of leaks. In order to avoid the passage of stool through the anastomosis until complete healing, a loop diverting ileostomy is performed to protect the distal colorectal anastomosis, especially in patients who have received preoperative chemoradiation. The diverting stoma is usually maintained for at least 8 weeks after surgery and is closed only after the perfect healing of the anastomosis has been confirmed with a gastrografin enema or with endoscopy

Sphincter-Sparing Surgery Procedures for Low Rectal Cancers

Tumors located in the ultradistal portion of the rectum (i.e., at the level of the dentate line or just above it) are a specific entity due to their proximity to the anal sphincter and the implications that the resection may have upon sphincter function. In young and fit patients with good preoperative sphincter function, if the sphincters are not infiltrated with cancer and do not need to be sacrificed for oncologic reasons, an anastomosis between the colon and the anal

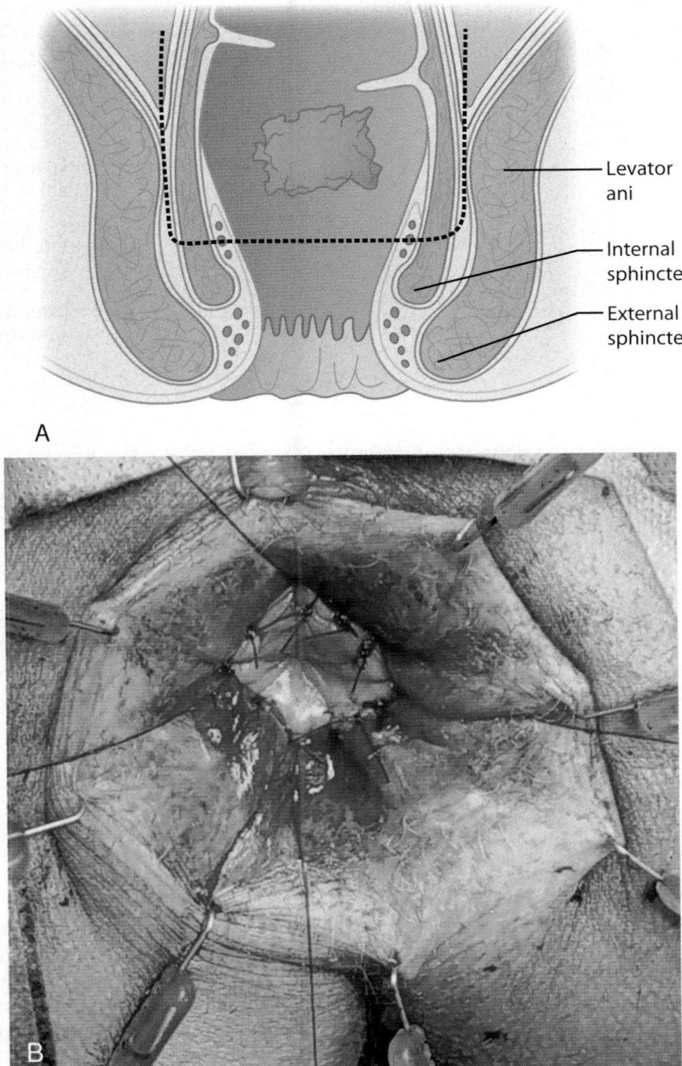

FIG. 52.75 Both external and internal sphincters and 1 to 2 cm of mucosa above the dentate line are left untouched. Sphincter-sparing surgery procedure. (B) Completed coloanal anastomosis. The anastomosis is handsewn with interrupted sutures between the colon and the distal rectum. About 1 cm of rectal mucosa is left intact above the dentate line.

canal is feasible. The ultradistal rectum cannot be stapled from the abdomen, and therefore, the dissection and reconstruction has to be performed transanally. Different instruments can be used: the sphincter is denuded starting just distally from the tumor with scissors or with a harmonic scalpel. Different types of dissection can be done and may have different functional results based on the structures that are excised with the dissection. With a standard mucosectomy, the distal mucosa is peeled off from the internal sphincter. Ideally, 1 to 2 cm of mucosa above the dentate line should be saved because this portion of distal mucosa has a critical importance in rectal sensibility and consequently for postoperative functional outcomes (Fig. 52.75). With this dissection, the internal sphincter that lies underneath the mucosa is spared. If the cancer is lower but small in size and involving only a small portion of the mucosa, an asymmetrical mucosectomy can be performed en bloc with the underlying internal sphincter on one side of the anal canal, sparing part of the distal mucosa and sphincter (Fig. 52.76). If the cancer involves a larger part of the anal canal, an intersphincteric dissection must be done (Fig. 52.77). With this dissection, the internal sphincter—responsible for resting pressure of the anal sphincter—is removed circumferentially: functional results are poor due to the loss of part of the sensation and the decrease of resting anal pressure.

Transanal Total Mesorectal Excision

Recently, a new emerging technique has been proposed when approaching sphincter-preserving procedures in order to facilitate the detachment of the rectum and to improve the vision in the narrow pelvic space.[43] This approach utilizes transanal platforms also used for TAMIS (Fig. 52.78). The distal rectum is closed with a purse string and is divided with a harmonic scalpel. At this point, the port platform for transanal surgery is positioned through the anus and the dissection of the rectum is continued from the bottom upward, thus gradually going from a narrow space to a wider space. Retropneumoperitoneum inflated through the port facilitates the blunt atraumatic dissection of the rectum with its

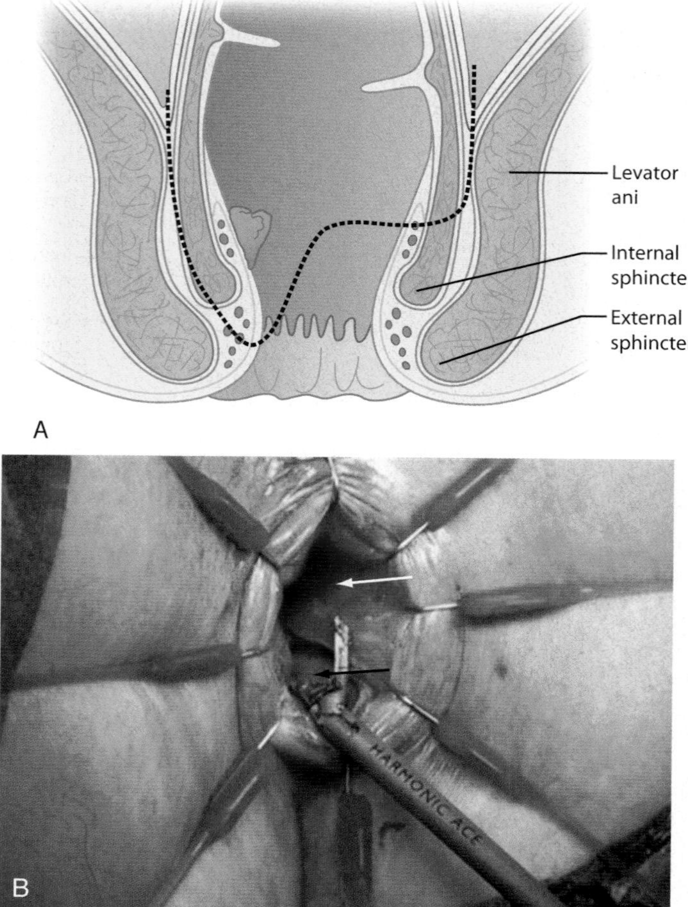

FIG. 52.76 (A) Sphincter-sparing surgery procedure. The cancer is ultradistal and located on the right side. In this case, the right side of the mucosa and the internal sphincter are dissected; on the patient's left side, 1 to 2 cm of mucosa are left untouched, together with part of the internal sphincter. (B) Resection of the distal mucosa of the rectum. A self-retaining retractor displays the dentate line; the mucosa of the distal rectum is indicated by the *white arrow*, while the *black arrow* indicates the underlying external anal sphincter in the area where the mucosa has already been dissected off using the harmonic scalpel.

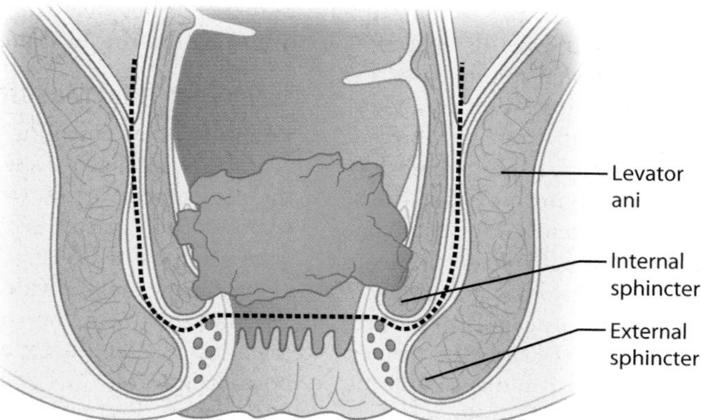

FIG. 52.77 Sphincter-sparing surgery procedure: intersphincteric dissection.

mesorectum along avascular planes under clear laparoscopic vision. The detachment of the rectum is first done posteriorly and then anteriorly from the prostate plane and can be continued until the cul-de-sac is entered. At this point, the procedure is continued within the abdomen with standard laparoscopic or robotic instruments. After the colon has been mobilized, when the pelvis is approached transabdominally, the distal rectum appears already fully detached and can be easily exteriorized (Video 52.2). The transanal TME technique has been shown to be oncologically safe with a low rate of involved circumferential margins and good quality of mesorectal excision. After the operation, all patients show a decrease of resting sphincter pressures, but the squeeze pressures are unchanged and functional results are acceptable.[44]

Abdominoperineal Resection

If the sphincters are infiltrated by tumor, complete excision of both the rectum and the anus, along with the sphincter apparatus, must be performed along with creation of a permanent colostomy. This procedure (abdominoperineal resection [APR], known as the Miles procedure) is also an option for elderly patients with distal

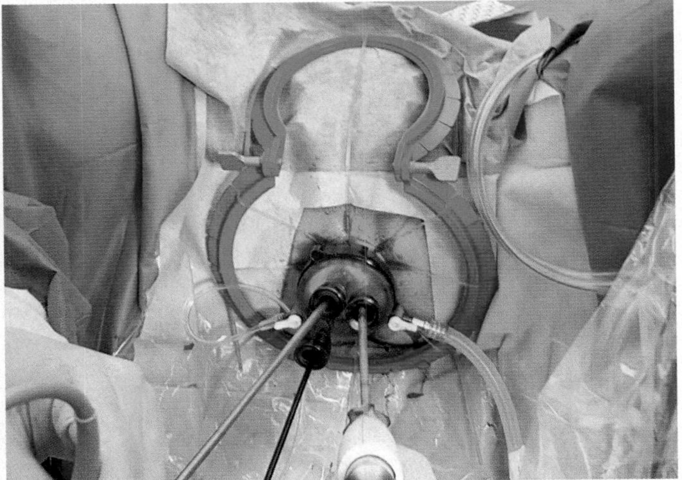

FIG. 52.78 Transanal total mesorectal excision (Ta TME). Transanal laparoscopy for the dissection of the rectum from below.

rectal cancer with poor sphincter function because an end colostomy offers a better quality of life if compared with an ultradistal coloanal anastomosis that could further compromise continence. The IMA is divided, the descending colon is mobilized and divided above the rectosigmoid junction, and the rectum is dissected according to the TME principles to the level of the levator ani. The colostomy aperture is created. At this point, the perineal part of the operation begins (Fig. 52.79A). A purse-string suture is placed around the anus, and an elliptical incision is made around the anus that is then excised en bloc with the sphincter. Dissection continues cephalad until the abdominal plane of dissection is reached. The specimen is removed through the pelvic incision and the perineum is closed in layers (Fig. 52.79BC). The empty space of the pelvis can often be filled with an omental pedicle. If wider perineal resections are needed, especially in irradiated pelvises that may have healing difficulties, the perineal defect can be closed using a rectus abdominis flap or gracilis muscle flap. The specimen includes the origin of the IMA, the mesorectum with hemorrhoidal vessels and the "naked" portion of the ultradistal rectum and the anal sphincters.

APR carries intrinsic risk of higher recurrence rates (up to 33%) compared to low anterior resection. This is in part explained by the fact that APR is done in more aggressive cancers, but another explanation is the fact that there is an intrinsic higher risk of specimen perforation and a higher rate of positive circumferential margins (up to 40%) in patients undergoing APR.

For this reason, a wider excision has been proposed that allows a more cylindrical resection avoiding the risk of "coning" toward the rectum (Fig. 52.80). After the abdominal part of the operation is completed, the patient is rotated in a prone jackknife position. A wider elliptical incision is made up to tip of the coccyx (that can be removed with the specimen) and the sphincter apparatus is removed en bloc with the levator ani in a cylindrical manner. The wide perineal defect, if needed, can be closed with a biologic mesh or with a muscle flap.

Special Circumstances

Synchronous Cancers

In patients with synchronous cancers, depending on the site of the tumors, more extended resections are indicated. For synchronous cancers of the right and left colon, an abdominal colectomy with

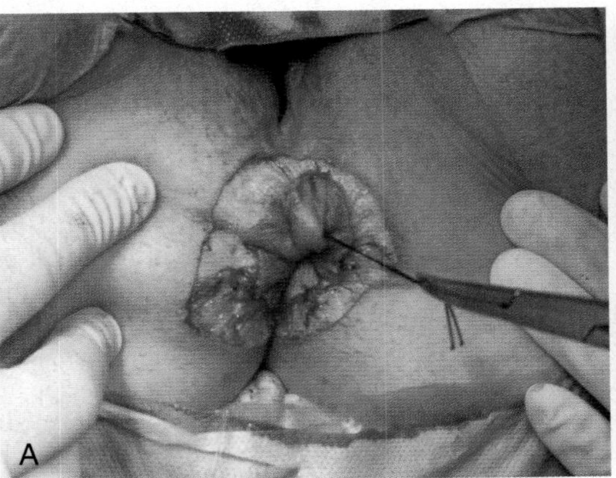

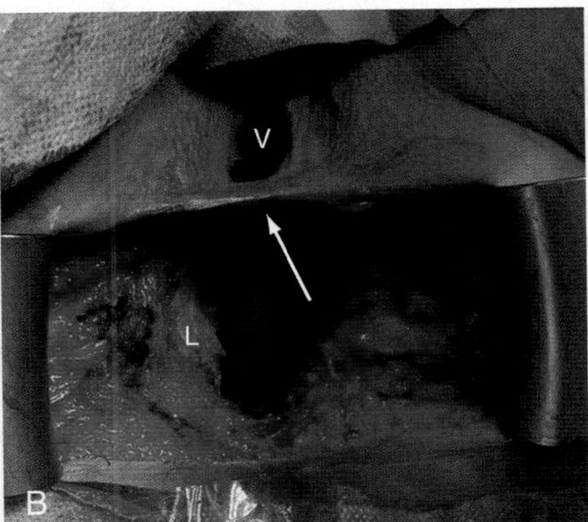

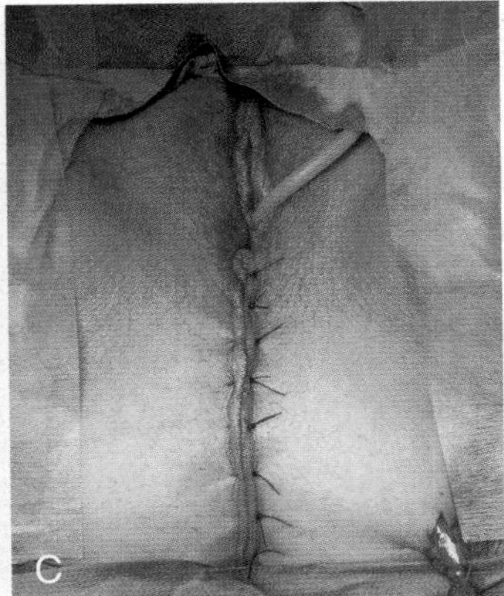

FIG. 52.79 (A) Perineal incision in Miles procedure. A purse-string suture is placed around the anal canal and the entire anal sphincter excised. (B) Photo of operative field after specimen has been removed. Perineal incision shows large defect in the pelvis (*white arrow* denotes posterior vaginal wall). *L*, Levator; *V*, vagina. (C) Perineal incision following skin closure following Miles procedure.

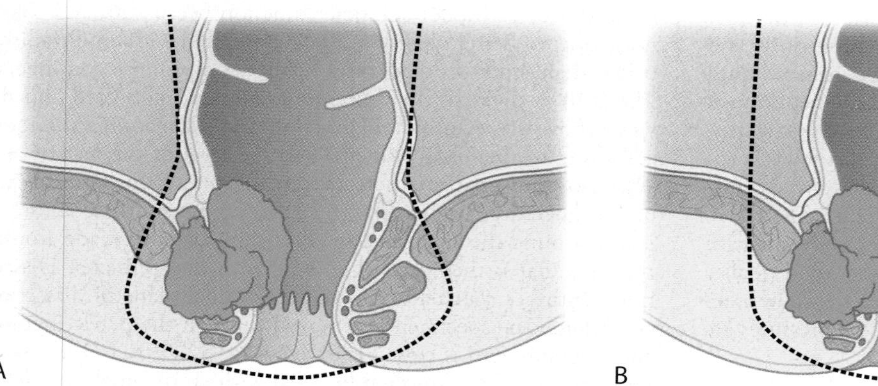

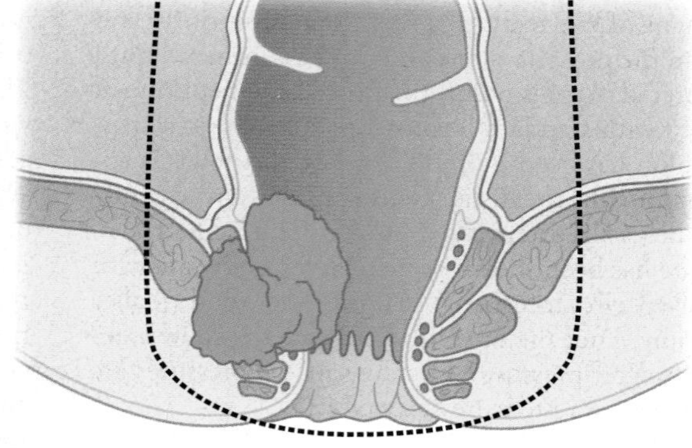

FIG. 52.80 (A) Conventional abdominoperineal resection. The line of the dissection tends to cone toward the rectum. (B) Cylindrical abdominoperineal resection with en bloc removal of the levator ani.

IRA is indicated. If the second cancer is located in the rectum, a total proctocolectomy with an IPAA may be necessary.

Short Residual Colon

In cases of re-resections for recurrent or metachronous cancers, the residual colon may be too short to reach the pelvis for a tension-free anastomosis, despite a complete mobilization of the splenic flexure. In such cases, the colon can be transposed through a "retroileal" transmesenteric route. Using this path, which is especially feasible in nonobese patients, the colon is pulled toward the pelvis more medially and led to the pelvis through the avascular space in the mesentery of the ileum just adjacent to the ileocolic resection. This gives the surgeon 4 to 5 cm of additional length that may be sufficient to reach for the tension-free anastomosis. If the colon is still under tension, another possibility is to rotate the right colon. In these cases, the middle colic and the right colic vessels, which are short and prevent the colon to be fully mobilized to the pelvis, are divided. The colon is transected at the site of ischemic demarcation (generally the hepatic flexure) and the residual right colon, whose blood supply now relies on the ileocolic pedicle, is rotated counterclockwise and mobilized to reach the rectal stump in the pelvis (Fig. 52.81)

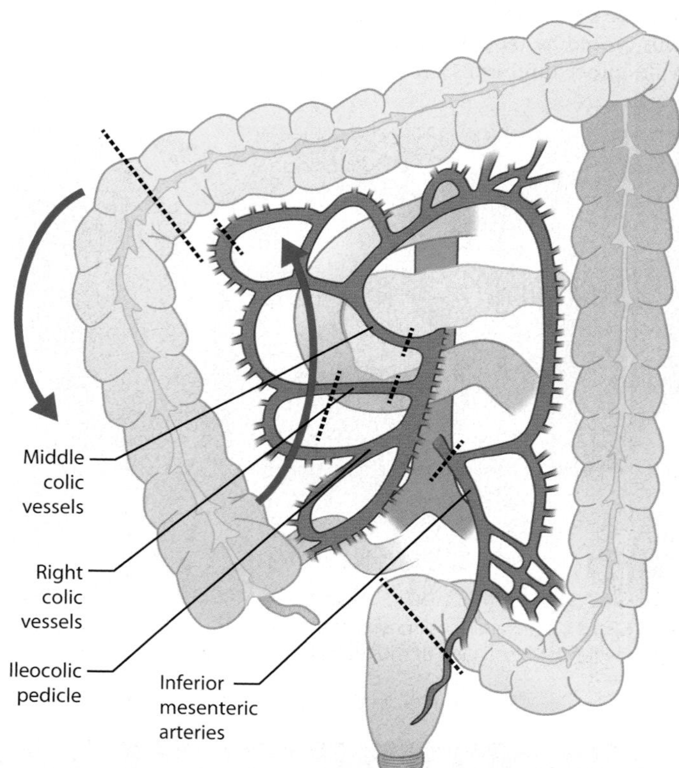

FIG. 52.81 Rotation of the right colon to reach the pelvis. The vascularization of the right colon is based on the ileocolic pedicle.

Complications

Patients undergoing colorectal resection can experience general complications just as those undergoing any major abdominal surgery, but complications related to the anastomosis are specific to these patients and include leaks, bleeding, twisting, strictures, and low anterior resection syndrome (LARS).

Anastomotic Leaks or Dehiscences

An anastomotic dehiscence is a leak of bowel content through an anastomosis. The incidence of anastomotic leaks varies widely from 1% to 3% in ileocolic anastomoses to up to 20% in coloanal anastomoses. Risk factors associated with postoperative dehiscence are male gender, obesity, low extraperitoneal anastomoses, ASA score III to V, emergency operations, intraoperative complications, use of oral anticoagulants, nutrition status, and hospital size and volume.[45] Anastomotic leak increases postoperative mortality and the length of postoperative hospital stay. The presence of a diverting stoma does not decrease the risk of a leak, but it reduces its severity and lowers the risk of reoperation. Diagnosis of a postoperative anastomotic leak is established when enteric, fecal, or purulent material, even if minimal, is detected in perianastomotic drains. Clinical signs of anastomotic leak are usually present including fever, signs of sepsis, abdominal pain, prolonged ileus, leukocytosis, increased CRP, and increased procalcitonin. The diagnosis can be confirmed by radiologic studies: CT scan demonstrates intraabdominal or perianastomotic fluid collections and gas (Fig. 52.82) or when gastrografin enema demonstrates leak of contrast. The majority of leaks become apparent between the second and seventh postoperative days with median time of 5.5 days, but up to 12% can appear 1 month after surgery, making the diagnosis more challenging.

Treatment. If the leak is subclinical with minimal discharge from the drains and no systemic signs, it can be managed conservatively with close clinical observation, broad spectrum antibiotics,

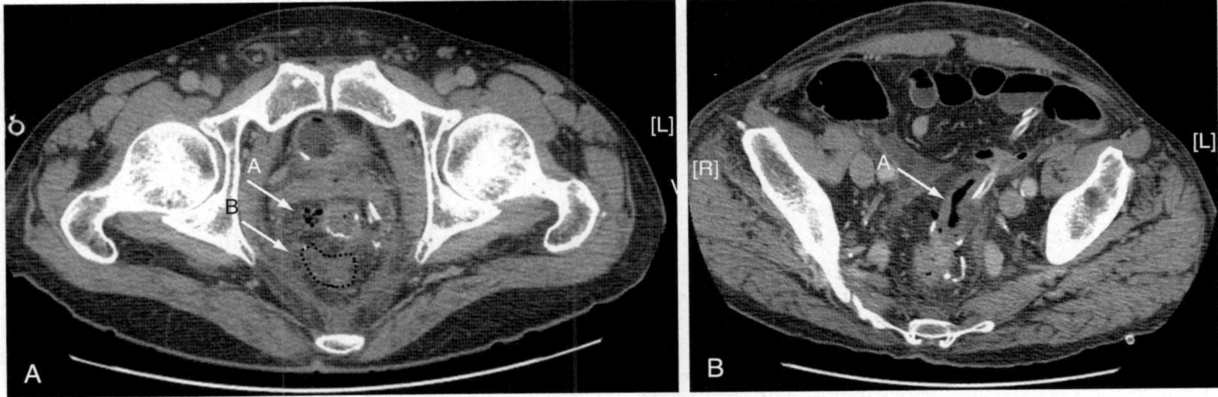

FIG. 52.82 (A) Leak at a colorectal anastomosis. *A*, Air around the anastomosis; *B*, a fluid collection behind the anastomosis. (B) Leak at a colorectal anastomosis. *A*, Air along the perianastomotic drains.

bowel rest, and parenteral nutrition. If a small perianastomotic abscess is demonstrated with no abdominal collections or free air and without systemic symptoms, an attempt of percutaneous drainage should be made with close clinical observation. In patients with signs of peritonitis or signs of sepsis, even if minimal, reoperation is required and should not be delayed. Abdominal exploration allows peritoneal lavage and reposition of new drains if needed. If possible, a laparoscopic approach may be preferred in order to minimize septic contamination of the abdominal wall. In left-sided colectomies, intraoperative endoscopic exploration of the anastomosis is helpful to determine the extent of the leak, and it also allows colonic lavage. If the leak involves less than one third of the anastomosis and the abdominal contamination is minimal, a diverting stoma may be sufficient. If the leak is larger or the anastomosis is disrupted, it has to be dismantled with the creation of a terminal stoma. An ileocolic anastomosis in right-sided resections can be managed ideally by redo of the anastomosis, but if the patient is unstable, the anastomosis has to be dismantled and an end ileostomy constructed.

Necrosis of the Transposed Colon

This is a rare and serious complication that has a subtle presentation characterized by malaise, early leukocytosis, and initially low-grade fever with foul-smelling material in the perianastomotic drains. It is a manifestation of ischemic injury of the transposed colon. Its presentation may mimic an anastomotic leak, but it must be immediately differentiated from a simple dehiscence because the treatment must be more aggressive. The diagnosis is often made with abdominal exploration or intraoperative endoscopy (Fig. 52.83) that shows a clear demarcation line. Its treatment requires immediate dismantling of the anastomosis with creation of a terminal stoma.

Bleeding

Minor bleeding—self-limited and not requiring blood transfusion or active treatment—is very common after colorectal resections and is observed with the first bowel movements. Major bleeding, with hemodynamic instability requiring active resuscitation, need of blood transfusion, and active treatment, can occur in up to 4% of cases. This may happen in the early postoperative period and in these cases is generally caused by small arterioles at the staple lining. Treatment is usually endoscopic with positioning of clips at the suture line, epinephrine injection, or electrocoagulation. If

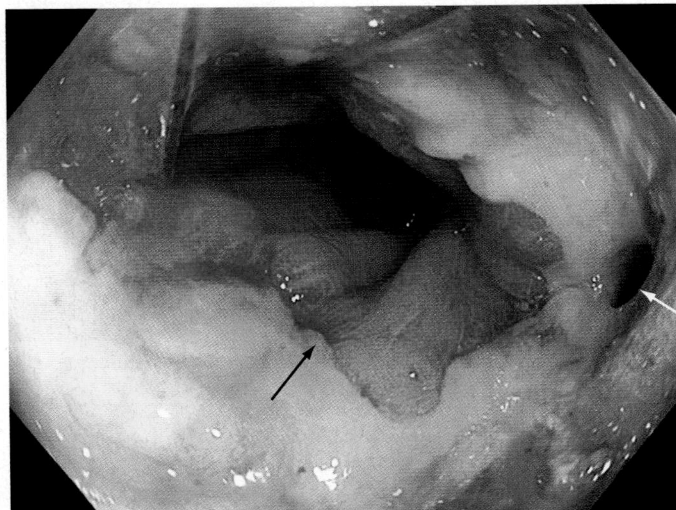

FIG. 52.83 A nonviable anastomosis with a visible leak *(white arrow)*. The necrotic appearance of one half of the anastomosed bowel is apparent with a clear line of demarcation *(black arrow)*.

endoscopy fails, angiographic treatment is possible, but it might lead to ischemia of the anastomotic rim and subsequent possible further leaks.

Twisting

Twist is another very rare but serious complication. It is described almost exclusively in extracorporeal ileocolic anastomosis after laparoscopic hybrid right colectomies, and it is caused by the lack of optimal visualization of the mesentery and mesocolon through the mini-laparotomy. When the anastomosis is twisted, there is an immediate swelling and edema of the small bowel that, if overlooked and if left untreated, can lead to ischemia and gangrene of the intestine. Immediate redo of the anastomosis is necessary.

Strictures

Clinically significant strictures are those that present with obstructive symptoms and occur in 4% to 10% of circular anastomoses (Fig. 52.84). Risk factors are the use of a small-diameter stapler (25-mm circular staplers should never be used in colorectal anastomosis in adults), anastomotic leaks, ischemia, and radiation.

Treatment is usually endoscopic with balloon dilation or placement of radial incisions or positioning of endoluminal stents. Redo of the anastomosis may be necessary in strictures not responding to the endoscopic treatment.

Low Anterior Resection Syndrome

Rather than a true complication, this is a consequence of low anterior resection and coloanal anastomosis and may be present in up to 80% of patients undergoing a low anterior resection. It is a syndrome characterized by a mixture of multiple symptoms that include frequency, multiple fragmented bowel movements, a sensation of incomplete emptying, incontinence, constipation, and diarrhea. Most of the symptoms improve 1 year or more after the resection, but long-term dysfunction is described in the majority of patients. The cause of LARS is multifactorial. It may be due to an injury of the internal sphincter, loss of sensitivity in the anorectal mucosa, loss or impairment of the rectoanal-inhibitory reflex, reduction of the capacity of the rectal reservoir, and/or loss of compliance of the transposed colon. The incidence is higher in patients undergoing TME, in those with coloanal anastomosis, in those who received neoadjuvant chemoradiation, and in those who had an anastomotic leak. Preventive technical mechanisms are currently used to improve LARS symptoms that aim to increase the capacity of the neorectum: anastomosis with a 5 to 6-cm colonic J-pouch or with a transverse coloplasty or side-to-end colorectal anastomosis (Fig. 52.85). The coloplasty is a possible alternative in obese patients in which the J pouch does not fit into the narrow pelvis. A longitudinal 10-cm colotomy is made about 5 cm from the distal end of the transposed colon and is then sutured transversely in order to widen the colon and increase it compliance. The treatment of LARS is often empirical, based on diet control, balanced use of loperamide associated with fiber products, physical therapy including biofeedback, and transanal irrigation. In a minority of highly symptomatic patients with low quality of life, after failure of conservative treatment, the construction of a stoma can be necessary as a definitive treatment.[46]

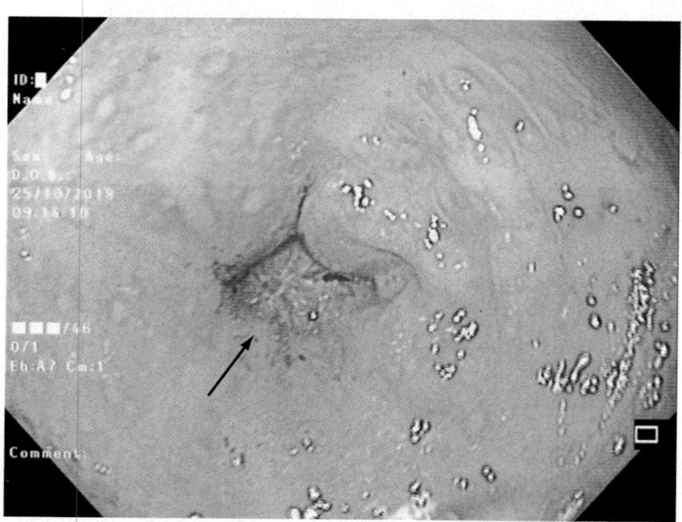

FIG. 52.84 Endoscopic view of a tight anastomotic stricture *(arrow)*.

Postoperative Treatment and Follow-up

Five-year survival rate for patients with stage I cancer is approximately 90%; for stage II, 75%; and for stage III (with positive lymph nodes), 50%. Patients with distant nonresectable metastases have a 5-year survival rate of about 5%. Patients with resectable liver metastases amenable to curative liver resection with

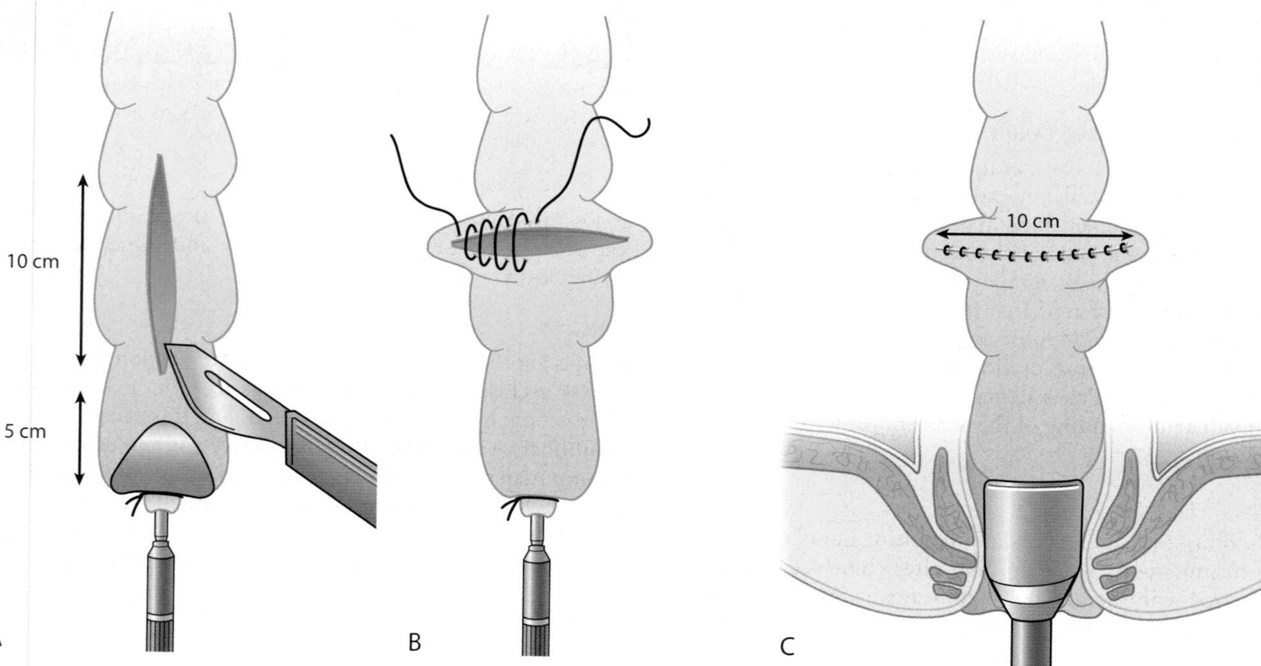

FIG. 52.85 Coloplasty. (A) A 10-cm longitudinal colotomy is made approximately 5 cm proximal to the end of the colon and the anvil of a circular stapler placed into the bowel lumen and pierced through adjacent to the distal staple line or secured using a purse-string suture (B). The colotomy is then closed transversely in one or two layers. (C) A circular stapled colorectal anastomosis is then performed.

free margins and favorable clinical risk factors may have a 5-year survival rate up to 60%. The majority of recurrences occur within the first 2 years after resection of the primary tumor. Close follow-up is therefore necessary especially within this interval in order to allow for early detection of any recurrence or metachronous tumor that could be amenable to curative treatment. The reader is referred to the ASCRS Practice Guideline for the Surveillance of Patients After Curative Treatment of Colon and Rectal Cancer.

Follow-up includes office visits with CEA levels obtained every 6 months for 5 years after surgery, then annually. Rising levels of CEA require additional tests in order to identify recurrent or metastatic disease. Colonoscopy should be scheduled 1 year after surgery (or 3–6 months after surgery if the entire colon was not completely investigated at the time of diagnosis); further colonoscopies should be repeated every 3 years if no adenomas were detected and every year if adenomatous polyps are found until the colon is found clean. Chest and abdominal CT scans are performed annually.

Postoperative Treatment

Adjuvant chemotherapy may be indicated in certain subsets of patients based on postoperative pathologic status.

Stage I: tumor invades muscularis propria, negative lymph nodes. Follow-up alone is the appropriate choice.

Stage II tumors: tumor penetrates into pericolic fat, negative lymph nodes. In general, in the absence of risk factors, there is limited evidence of any benefit from adjuvant chemotherapy: the absolute survival advantage with 5-fluorouracil (5-FU)/leucovorin (folinic acid [FA]) is about 3% to 4% (*P* borderline significant). In a recent metaanalysis by Bockelman et al., the 5-year DFS with or without chemotherapy is 81.4% versus 79.3%, respectively.

In stage II colon cancer patients, the following potential risk factors can be considered as relative indications for chemotherapy: poorly differentiated cancer (G3–4), vascular and perineural invasion, obstruction, perforation, adjacent organ invasion (pT4), and an inadequate number of examined number lymph nodes (<12). Even in these high-risk patients, no definite value for adjuvant chemotherapy has been demonstrated and the addition of oxaliplatin does not add any benefit. No difference in 10-year overall survival has been observed between low- and high-risk categories and no advantage has been derived from an oxaliplatin-based regimen.[47]

MSI is another relevant characteristic for oncologic postsurgical treatment in stage II disease. It is typical of Lynch syndrome (2%–4% of all colon cancers) but, in the majority of cases, somatic inactivation of MMR genes (*hMLH1, hMSH2, hMSH6, PMS2*) is due to the effect of other regulatory genes.

MSI-H condition (deficient expression of MMR genes) is more frequent in stage II disease (22%) than in stages III (12%) and IV (3%) and does appear to have a favorable prognostic significance in stage II. Moreover, adjuvant 5-FU treatment seems to have a detrimental effect on survival in stage II but not stage III colon cancer patients. All these elements are to be considered with respect to uncertain effectiveness.

Stage III disease: positive lymph nodes. Adjuvant chemotherapy is indicated in stage III patients. 5-FU and FA are combined with oxaliplatin in the FOLFOX protocol. In the CAPOX (or Xelox) regimen, oral capecitabine is used instead of 5-fluorouracil folinic acid (5-FUFA). Recently, a preplanned pooled analysis of data from six randomized phase III trials of adjuvant therapy in stage III colon cancer patients, was carried out[48]: a shorter treatment duration may reduce side effects, particularly neurotoxicity that is dose dependent and related to oxaliplatin. This analysis evaluated the noninferiority of 3 months versus 6 months of adjuvant FOLFOX/CAPOX therapy. The primary end point, the rate of DFS at 3 years, was not confirmed: 3 months is inferior to 6 months of adjuvant chemotherapy. However, in an analysis that had not been planned prior to starting the study, there was a difference between FOLFOX and CAPOX related to the risk class of patients. Low-risk patients were defined as pT3pN1, and high-risk patients, pT4 (any N) or N2.

In low-risk patients, 3 months (four cycles) of CAPOX was not inferior to 6 months of the same regimen (3 years DFS: 85.0% vs. 83.1%, 3 months vs. 6 months). In high-risk patients, 3 months of the CAPOX regimen was sufficient (3 years DFS: 64.1% vs. 64.0%, 3 months vs. 6 months).

With regard to the FOLFOX regimen, 6 months seems superior to 3 months, regardless of the risk group (3 years DFS in high-risk: 61.5% vs. 64.7%, 3 months vs. 6 months). One has to remember, however, that these are unexpected findings because a comparison between treatments was not preplanned: patients were not randomized to receive CAPOX or FOLFOX treatment.

Metastatic disease. There are several issues that have to be considered when choosing a treatment for metastatic disease: tumor burden, goal of the treatments chronicity, induction of resectability in borderline resectable disease, primary resection, age and comorbidities, patient's preferences, site of primary tumor, and molecular biology: N-Ras, K-Ras (i.e., pan-Ras), and BRAF mutation status.

Possible chemotherapy regimens are as follows:

1. Anti-EGFR antibodies (panitumumab, cetuximab) can be used in pan-Ras wild-type and BRAF wild-type neoplasia. The mutational analysis can be performed on the primary tumor but also preferably on the metastatic tumor
2. The standard treatment in BRAF-mutated metastatic disease is the administration of FOLFOXIRI (oxaliplatin + irinotecan + 5-FUFA) and bevacizumab. BRAF mutated patients have the worst prognosis.
3. If the primary tumor is right sided, anti-EGFR antibodies given in addition to chemotherapy (FOLFOX [oxaliplatin + 5-FUFA] or FOLFIRI [irinotecan + 5-FUFA]) are not superior to chemotherapy alone in first-line treatment: therefore, they are usually not administered in this phase. Doublets (FOLFOX or FOLFIRI) or the triplet FOLFOXIRI in fit patients, in combination with anti–vascular endothelial growth factor antibody (bevacizumab), could be the best choice.
4. In left-sided primary tumors, the addition of cetuximab or panitumumab to FOLFOX/FOLFIRI could be the first line of treatment. However, also in this case, the use of FOLFOXIRI can be considered.
5. In older or unfit patients, unable to tolerate doublets, capecitabine with bevacizumab is an appropriate treatment.

If the goal of treatment is the resection of hepatic disease, no more than six cycles of chemotherapy should be administered before surgery, in order to avoid hepatic toxicity (steatohepatitis with irinotecan and sinusoidal damage with oxaliplatin). In addition, bevacizumab needs to be stopped 6 weeks before hepatic resection because of its detrimental effects on wound healing. Bevacizumab can be started 4 weeks after surgery or once the wounds have healed.

PELVIC FLOOR DISORDERS AND CONSTIPATION

Disorders of the pelvic floor include multiple conditions, often involving colorectal, urologic, and gynecologic specialists.

Constipation is a dysfunction of colonic motility and of the defecation process. It can be present with several medical and colorectal conditions, including colon obstruction and pelvic floor diseases. Functional constipation is an entity that must be differentiated from distinct anatomic problems during patient evaluation and may be considered for surgical treatment if unresponsive to active medical therapy. The reader is again referred to the ASCRS Consensus Statement of Definitions for Anorectal Physiology Testing and Pelvic Floor Terminology, Clinical Practice Guidelines for the Treatment of Rectal Prolapse, and Clinical Practice Guideline for the Evaluation and Management of Constipation.

The pelvic floor disorders that present to the surgeon include:

- rectal prolapse or procidentia: a circumferential, full-thickness intussusception of the rectum
- rectocele: a bulging of the rectum into the posterior wall of the vagina
- cul-de-sac hernia: a protrusion of the peritoneum between the rectum and the vagina, referred to as "enterocele" if it contains the small bowel, and as "sigmoidocele" if it contains the sigmoid colon.
- anismus: the failure of the puborectalis and the external anal sphincter to relax during defecation (simple nonrelaxation or paradoxical contraction).

Even if functional disorders do not always require surgical operation, the surgeon is almost always involved in the evaluation of these patients and in establishing a treatment plan.

Diagnosis: Testing and Evaluation

Anorectal Physiology Laboratory Tests

Anorectal physiology tests are performed to evaluate anal canal pressures to determine the presence of anal reflexes, anal sensation, and electromyography recruitment.

Anorectal manometry evaluates the high-pressure zone (i.e., the length of the anal canal), the resting pressure, mostly due to the internal sphincter, the maximum voluntary pressure, and the squeeze pressure, due to the external anal sphincter (Fig. 52.86). The test is performed by placing a manometry catheter with a water-filled balloon at its tip in the anal canal, so that the balloon at the tip lies within the rectal lumen. Normal resting pressure values are 40 to 80 mm Hg. Anorectal manometry also provides information on intrarectal pressures, reflexes, rectal sensation, and rectal compliance. High-resolution manometry can provide greater physiologic resolution and minimizes motion artifacts.

The balloon expulsion test evaluates the ability of the patient to expel a balloon inflated with 50 to 60 cc of water/gas/air that simulates stool.

Pudendal nerve terminal motor latency measures the conduction of the pudendal nerve from its emergence at the level of the ischial spines to the internal anal sphincter, by the use of a transducer. Normal pudendal nerve terminal motor latency times are 2.0 ± 0.2 milliseconds. Prolonged values are seen in traumatic injuries (spinal cord) or with stretch injury from obstetric trauma due to prolonged labor, chronic stretch injury as seen in long-standing defecation disorders, sacral nerve root damage or chronic diseases as diabetes. This is typically measured with a special electrode taped to the index finger of the examiner, whereby the tip of the finger electrode stimulates the pudendal nerve and the recording electrode at the base of the finger measures anal sphincter contraction.

Electromyography records the change from basal electrical activity of motor units of the external sphincter and puborectalis muscle during activity. Patients with inappropriate or paradoxical puborectalis contraction fail to show a relaxation of the muscles when asked to push.

Imaging to Evaluate the Pelvic Floor and Colonic Transit

Endoanal ultrasound (Fig. 52.87) can be used to evaluate the integrity, thickness, and possible abnormalities (scars, fistulas) of the internal and external anal sphincter.

Defecography is a dynamic study of the anorectum and the pelvic floor during defecation. It provides information regarding anatomic abnormalities, such as rectocele, rectal prolapse, internal rectal intussusception, and cul-de-sac hernia, as well as about functional disorders, such as nonrelaxation or paradoxical puborectalis contraction, perineal descent, and the degree of rectal emptying. Dynamic images are captured with fluoroscopy, with the rectum and the vagina opacified with radiographic contrast and the patient in the sitting position on a radiolucent commode. If magnetic resonance defecography is performed, the rectum is opacified with a mixture of ultrasonography gel and gadolinium. The advantages of MRI are high-quality images of the pelvic soft tissues and viscera and avoiding use of ionizing radiation. It is, however, limited by the supine position of the patient that does not reproduce normal conditions of defecation (Fig. 52.88).

Colonic transit time is a test that studies colonic inertia. The patient is asked to ingest 24 radio-opaque markers contained in a capsule (Sitzmarks) and to refrain from using laxatives and any other mechanical measures that might interfere with colonic function. The progression of the markers through the three areas of the colon (right, left, and rectosigmoid) is studied with plain abdominal films that are taken every other day until day 7. In the healthy population, 80% of the markers should be expelled by day 5. Patients with slow transit constipation or colonic inertia retain a significant portion of the markers during the entire time of the study (Fig. 52.89).

Rectal Prolapse (Procidentia)

Anatomy and Pathophysiology

The rectal prolapse is a circumferential, full-thickness intussusception of the rectal wall. The degree of prolapse can vary from intrarectal or internal rectal prolapse (Fig. 52.90), to intra-anal prolapse, to external rectal prolapse (Fig. 52.91). Rectal prolapse is an uncommon condition that occurs in about 0.5% of the general population, with women older than 50 years 6 times more likely than men to develop rectal prolapse. The few men who present with rectal prolapse are usually younger than 40 years. Young patients (males and females) with prolapse often suffer from psychiatric diseases, such as autism or developmental delay, and take constipating medications. The cause of rectal prolapse is still unknown, but some anatomic defects are commonly found in patients with total rectal prolapse. These defects include a diastasis of the levator ani muscle, an abnormally deep cul-de-sac, a redundant sigmoid colon, a patulous anus, and a lack of fascial attachments of the rectum against the sacrum. Risk factors of rectal procidentia include: age over 40 years, female gender, prior pelvic surgery, chronic straining and constipation, chronic diarrhea, vaginal delivery, and multiparity (however, one third of the female rectal prolapse patients are nulliparous), pelvic floor dysfunction and/or anatomic defects, neurologic diseases/injuries, and psychiatric diseases that require constipating medications. Rectal prolapse usually has a progressive

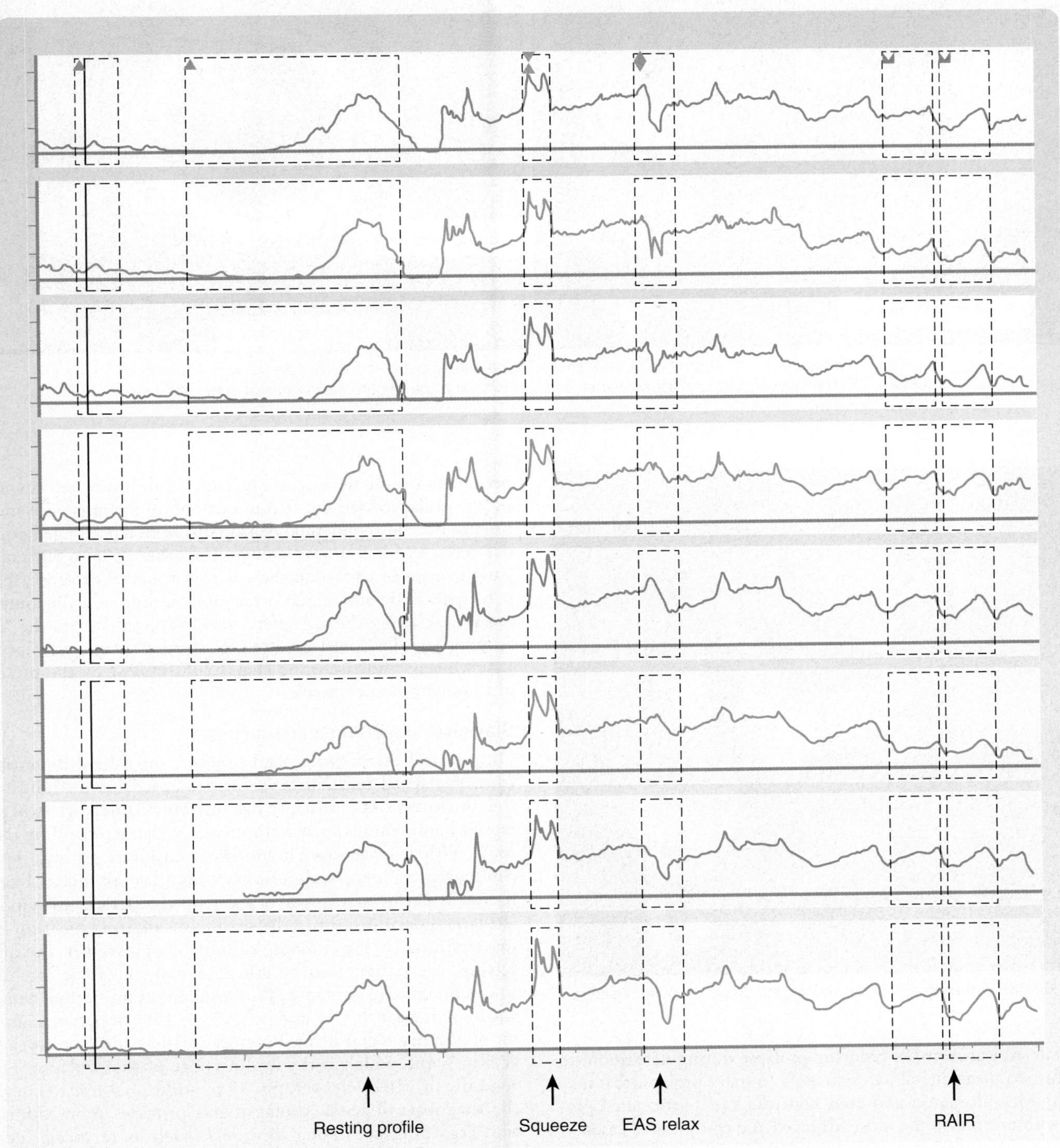

FIG. 52.86 A normal anorectal manometry: resting and squeeze pressure curves are evident, and the external anal sphincter relaxation when the patient is asked to push. The rectoanal inhibitory reflex is present. *EAS*, External anal sphincter.

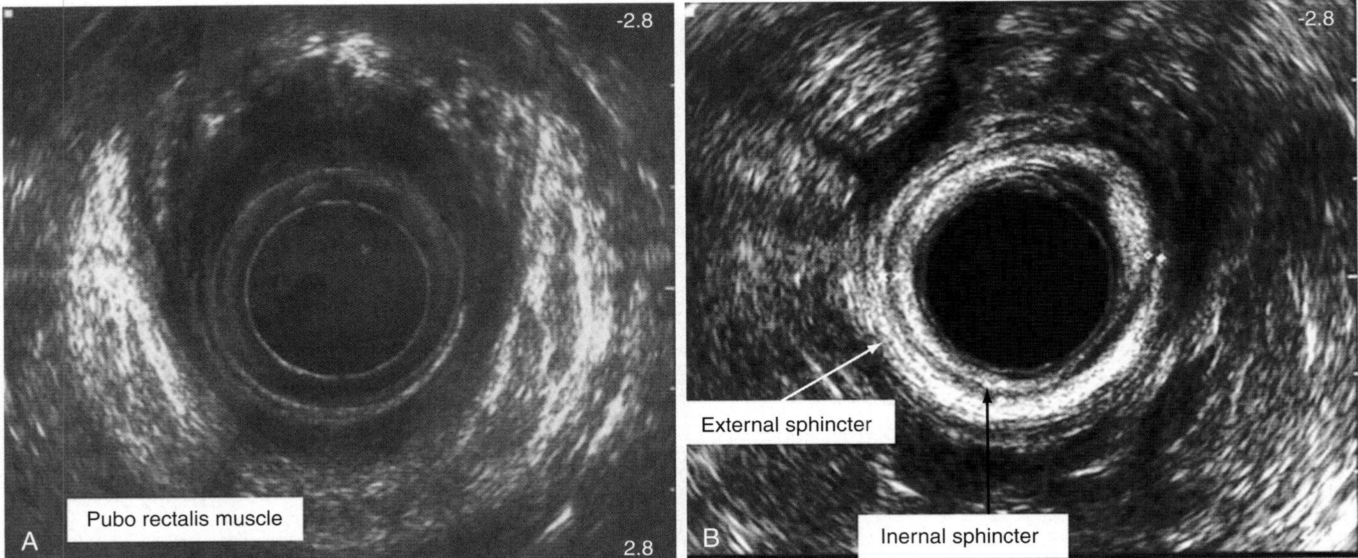

FIG. 52.87 Endoanal ultrasound. (A) The arch-shaped hyperechoic puborectalis muscle appears as a whitish structure. (B) The hypoechoic internal sphincter *(black arrow)* and the hyperechoic external sphincter *(white arrow)* are shown.

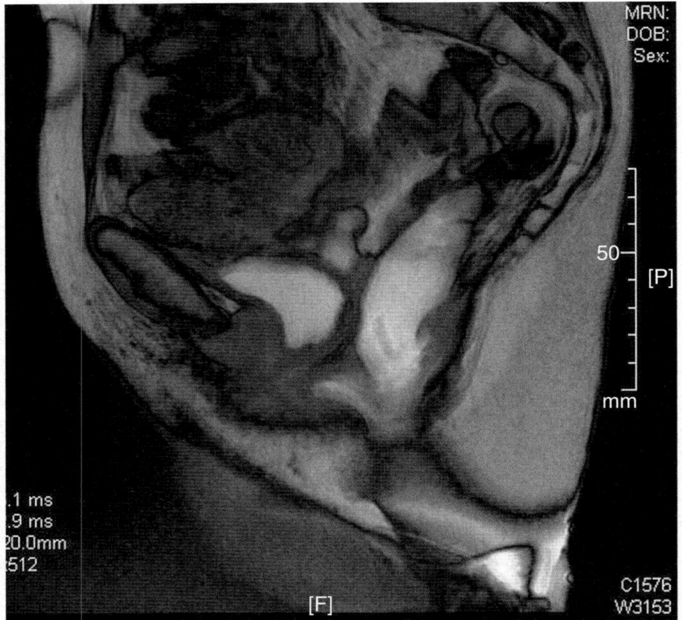

FIG. 52.88 A magnetic resonance imaging image of rectal prolapse.

course from transient self-reducing prolapse during defecation, to prolapse requiring digital self-reduction, to stable prolapse that may present with ulceration and even nonreducible, incarcerated prolapse with necrosis in the most advanced and complicated cases.

Symptoms

Symptoms include discomfort due to the prolapsed tissue, incontinence with drainage of mucous or blood, and constipation. The majority (50%–75%) of patients with evident rectal prolapse complain of fecal incontinence (passive or urge incontinence) that is caused by the presence of a direct conduit, by the chronic stretching of the sphincter due to the prolapse, and by persistent stimulation of the rectoanal inhibitory reflex caused by the prolapsed rectum. Up to one half of patients with incontinence have also pudendal neuropathy with a prolonged pudendal nerve terminal motor latency. The other 25% to 50% of the patients, and in particular those with intrarectal prolapse, report constipation or obstructed defecation (feeling of an incomplete rectal evacuation during defecation) that results from the "telescoping" of the bowel on itself creating a functional blockage that worsens with straining (Fig. 52.90B,C) or by the presence of a concomitant rectocele.

Diagnosis and Differential Diagnosis

On physical exam, true rectal prolapse must be differentiated from prolapsed rectal mucosa or prolapsed hemorrhoids: the full-thickness rectal prolapse has concentric folds, whereas prolapsed hemorrhoids or rectal mucosa is characterized by radial folds, with grooves along hemorrhoid cushions. At rest, typical findings include a patulous anus with a lax sphincter. Examination is performed in the office with the patient in standard left lateral decubitus or in the sitting or squatting position during straining. If the prolapse cannot be observed in the office setting, the patient can be asked to make a "selfie" at home to document the prolapse. Proctoscopic examination demonstrates redundant tissue and, in 10% to 15% of patients, an anterior solitary rectal ulcer. Proctoscopy may indicate erythema at 5 to 6 cm, which is the leading edge of the prolapse. Fluoroscopic or MRI defecography is an additional test to confirm the diagnosis of rectal prolapse and provides more information regarding coexisting disorders, such as rectocele, cystocele, vaginal vault prolapse, enterocele, and sigmoidocele (Fig. 52.92). Colonoscopy should be always performed to exclude the presence of CRC or other colonic pathology. A colonic transit study is performed in patients with a lifelong history of constipation in order to differentiate constipation due to obstructed defecation from constipation due to slow colonic transit. The two frequently coexist. Endoanal ultrasound usually shows a thickening of the internal anal sphincter.

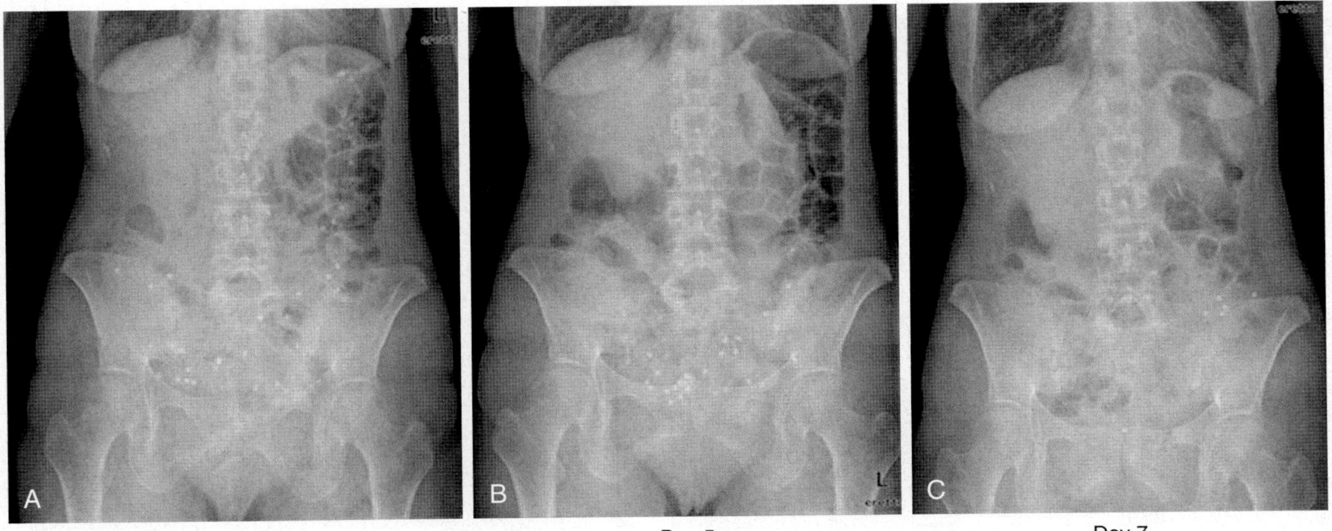

FIG. 52.89 Colonic transit study: plain abdominal films at 3, 5, and 7 days after ingestion of radiopaque markers. Note that at day 5, the majority of the radio-opaque markers are within the pelvis; however, by day 7, most markers have passed.

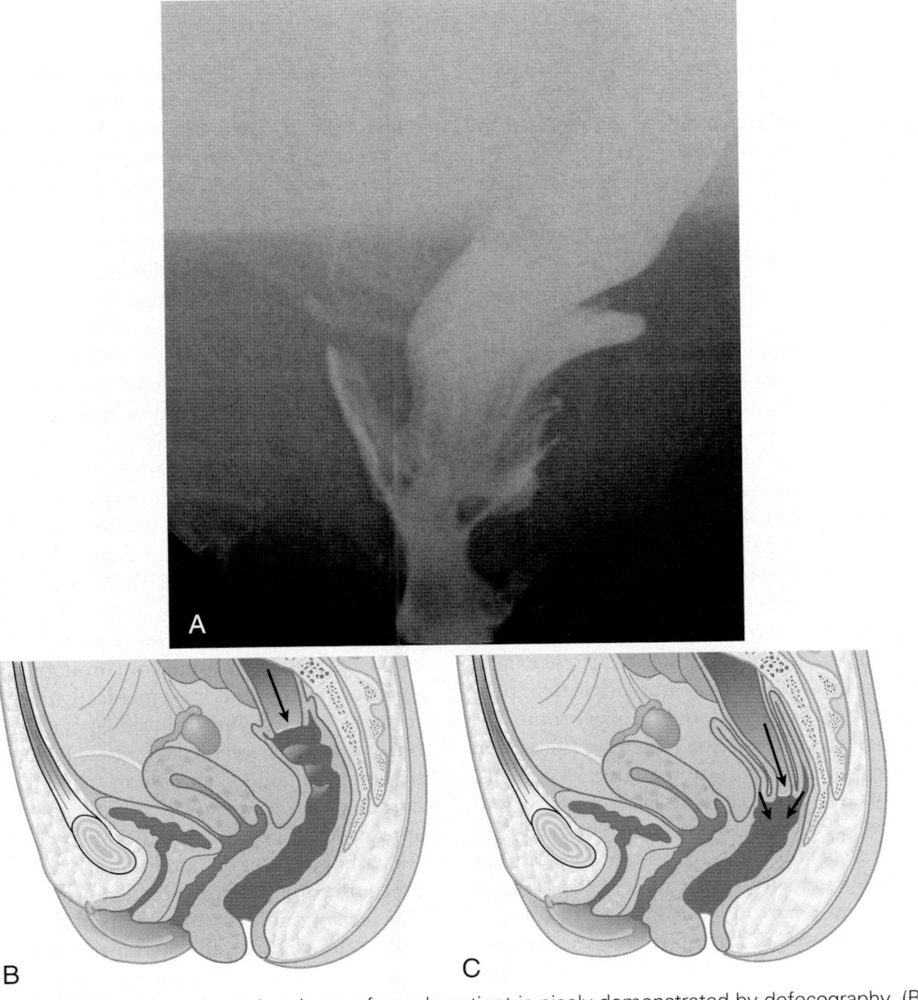

FIG. 52.90 (A) The internal rectal prolapse of a male patient is nicely demonstrated by defecography. (B and C) Progression of the internal rectal prolapse.

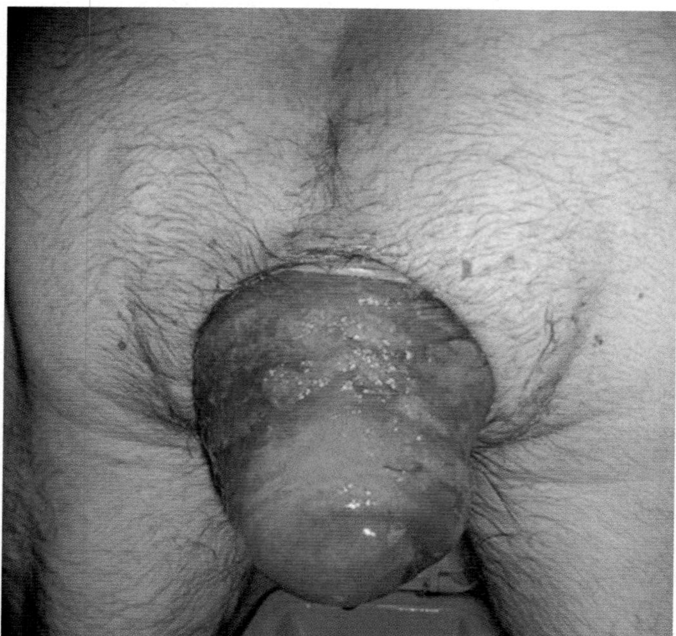

FIG. 52.91 A patient with a huge external rectal prolapse. (Courtesy of G. Sarzo, MD, Hospital Sant Antonio, Department of Surgery, Padova Italy.)

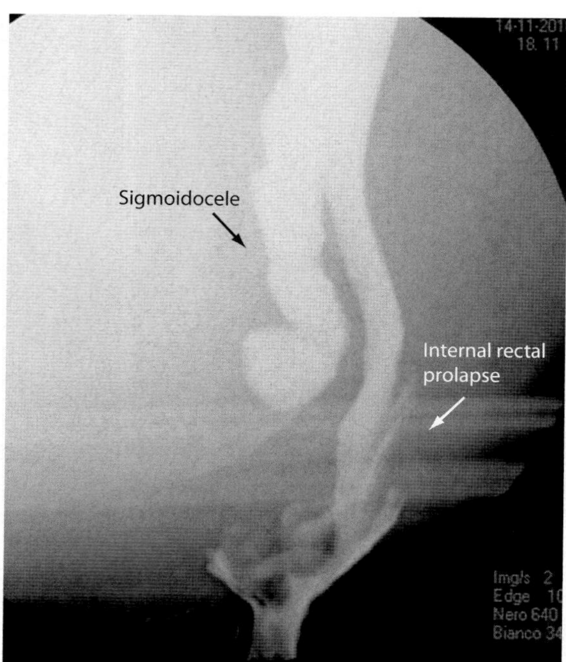

FIG. 52.92 Defecography of a young male patient who presents with internal rectal prolapse *(white arrow)* and sigmoidocele *(black arrow)*.

Nonoperative Management

Prolapse-associated symptoms of constipation and fecal incontinence can be palliated with medical treatment, in order to improve quality of life. Adequate fluid intake, fiber supplements, and stool softeners can treat constipation. Sugar or salt can be used topically to reduce rectal mucosal edema and facilitate reduction of the prolapsed tissue. Enemas and suppositories may be helpful to assist in defecation.

Operative Repair

The goals of surgery are to eliminate the prolapse and correct the anatomic and functional abnormalities. The approach can be transabdominal or transperineal. None have shown a clear superiority in terms of recurrence rates which vary between 13% and 31%. The choice of procedure is based upon the patient's comorbidities, the patient's age and bowel function, and the surgeon's preference.

Abdominal procedures. The rationale of the intraabdominal approach is to perform a fixation of the rectum with the goal of providing adequate upward tension to prevent a recurrence, but at the same time allowing appropriate evacuatory movements during defecation. The abdominal approach can be performed via open or minimally invasive approaches (laparoscopic or robotic). Both have equivalent clinical and functional results, recurrence rates (4%–8%), and morbidity (10%–33%). Laparoscopy offers benefits in terms of pain control, hospital stay, and recovery time. The advantages offered by robotic rectal prolapse repair are the ease in suturing and tying and improved visualization of the deep pelvis. The rectum must be dissected, retracted intraabdominally, and fixed to the presacral fascia with sutures (posterior rectopexy). In these cases, a simultaneous resection of the redundant sigmoid can be performed in selected patients with coexisting constipation. A mesh can be utilized to increase scarring and improve fixation of the rectum posteriorly or anteriorly. With the posterior mesh rectopexy, the rectum is mobilized posteriorly and laterally down to the levator ani muscles, and a mesh is fixed to the presacral fascia, below the sacral promontory, and to the rectum laterally (Fig. 52.93). This technique is associated with significant improvement in fecal incontinence in 20% to 60% of patients but has a 20% rate of postoperative complications and is associated with a 2% to 5% recurrence rate. The more recently described ventral mesh rectopexy is a technique that involves a limited anterior rectal mobilization and a mesh suspension to the sacral promontory. The mesh is fixed to the anterior wall of the rectum and suspended to the sacral promontory (Fig. 52.94). Advantages of this technique are the improvement in postoperative incontinence and constipation, with few cases of de novo postoperative constipation, and low complication and recurrence rates (3%–5%).[49] In published series, many different types of mesh and fixation devices are used: nonabsorbable or biologic grafts, tacks, sutures, or staples to fix the mesh. Mesh-related complications include erosion usually into the vagina, infection and pelvic sepsis, bowel obstruction, and mesh detachment and/or migration. In theory, with the use of biologic mesh, the risk of infection or erosion may be lower, and the risk of recurrence higher, but recent literature [49] shows no statistical improvement in recurrence and complication rates between biologic and nonabsorbable mesh. The follow-up for studies using biologic mesh is, however, short.

Perineal approach. Perineal procedures allow for the resection of the prolapse without concomitant fixation. They are recommended for the elderly or medically unfit patients and are thought to be associated with a lower operative morbidity and mortality but with higher recurrence rates. Recent reviews and trials have, however, concluded that there are no significant differences in recurrence and reoperation rates between perineal and abdominal approaches. Therefore, perineal procedures may have to be considered an option for all patients with rectal prolapse. The "Altemeier procedure" or perineal proctectomy or proctosigmoidectomy is a true rectosigmoidectomy. The prolapse is exteriorized, it is grasped with Allis clamps, and a full-thickness circumferential incision is made through the rectum 1 cm above the dentate line. The peritoneal cavity is entered anteriorly and the redundant sigmoid colon is extracted transanally (Fig. 52.95). The levator muscles are visualized and can be plicated posteriorly in order to reinforce

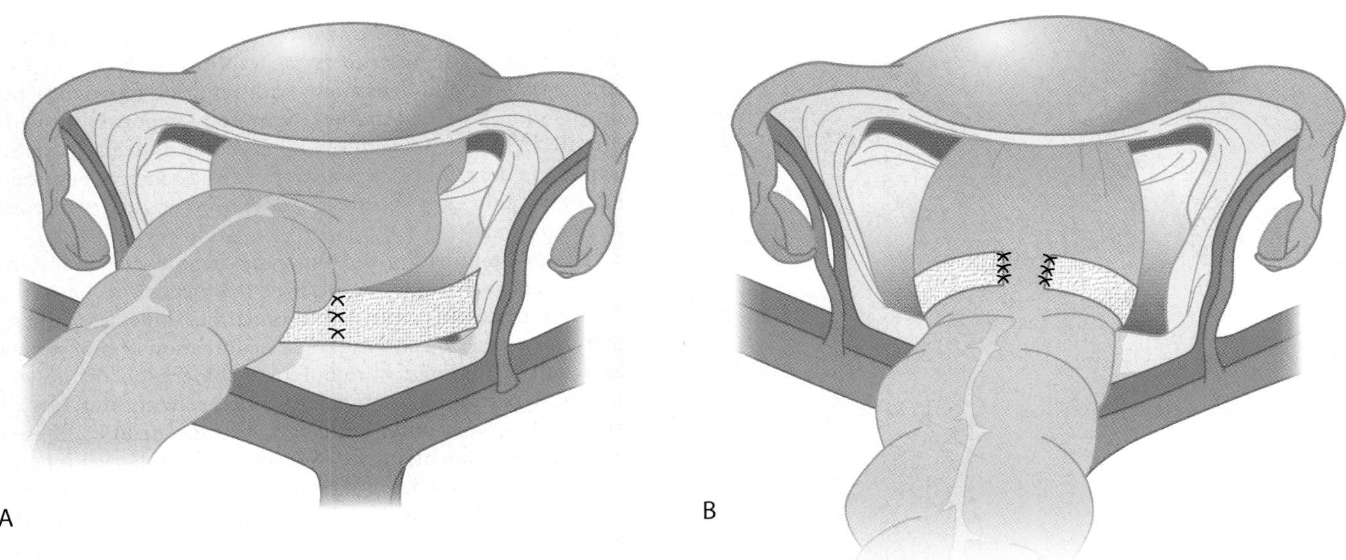

FIG. 52.93 The posterior mesh rectopexy (modified Ripstein operation). (A) The rectum is mobilized and the mesh is fixed to the presacral fascia. (B) The mesh is fixed to both sides of the rectum.

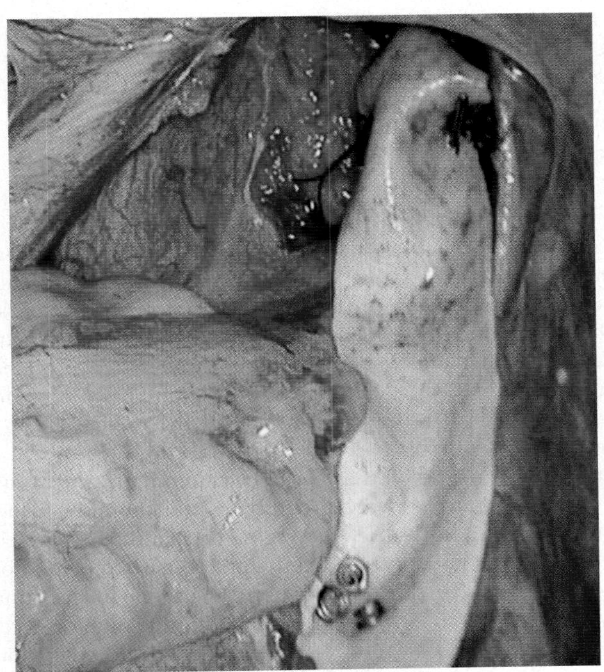

FIG. 52.94 Ventral mesh rectopexy. The mesh is attached to the anterior rectal wall and the sacral promontory. (Courtesy of G. Sarzo, MD, Hospital Sant Antonio, Department of Surgery, Padova Italy.)

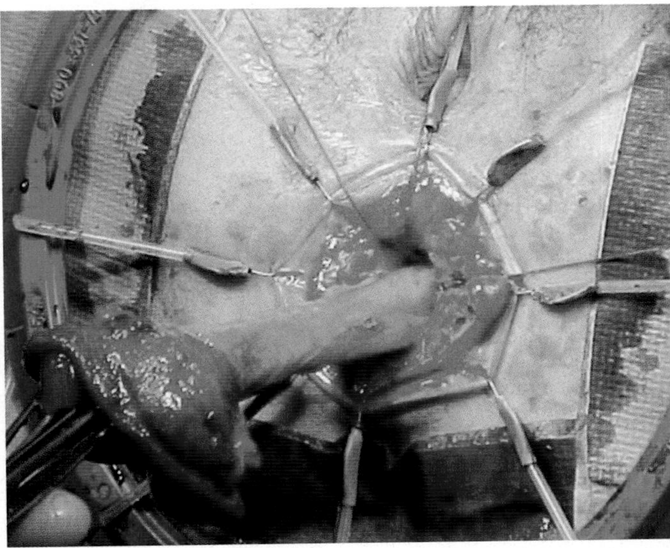

FIG. 52.95 The Altemeier procedure or perineal proctectomy. The redundant rectosigmoid colon is resected through a transperineal approach and a hand-sewn coloanal anastomosis is performed.

the pelvic floor and restore the anorectal angle (levatorplasty or Parks postanal repair). A handsewn or stapled coloanal anastomosis is then performed. The operation can be done under epidural anesthesia, with minimal postoperative pain. This technique allows for the resection of redundant bowel, it has low complication rates, and, especially when levator plication is done, it is associated with low recurrence rates (10%). For patients with a short (<5 cm) rectal prolapse, the Delorme procedure can be appropriate. A circumferential incision within the submucosal plane is made 1 cm proximal to the dentate line and the mucosa is stripped away from the muscularis propria of the rectum to the most proximal portion of prolapse. The stripped mucosa is then excised. A longitudinal suture plication of the muscularis propria is then performed. Finally, an anastomosis is performed between the proximal and distal mucosal edges (Fig. 52.96). This technique is very safe, entails a short hospital stay, and has lower complication rates than the abdominal approach. Incontinence and constipation are improved. Overall recurrence rates range from 7% to 27% and are comparable to the Altemeier or abdominal procedures. For symptomatic intrarectal prolapse, the stapled transanal rectal resection (STARR) has been proposed as an alternative possible technique. It consists of a full-thickness rectal resection including the internal prolapse with a circular stapler (STARR) or a specific curved-shape stapler (Transtar). These techniques have initially shown

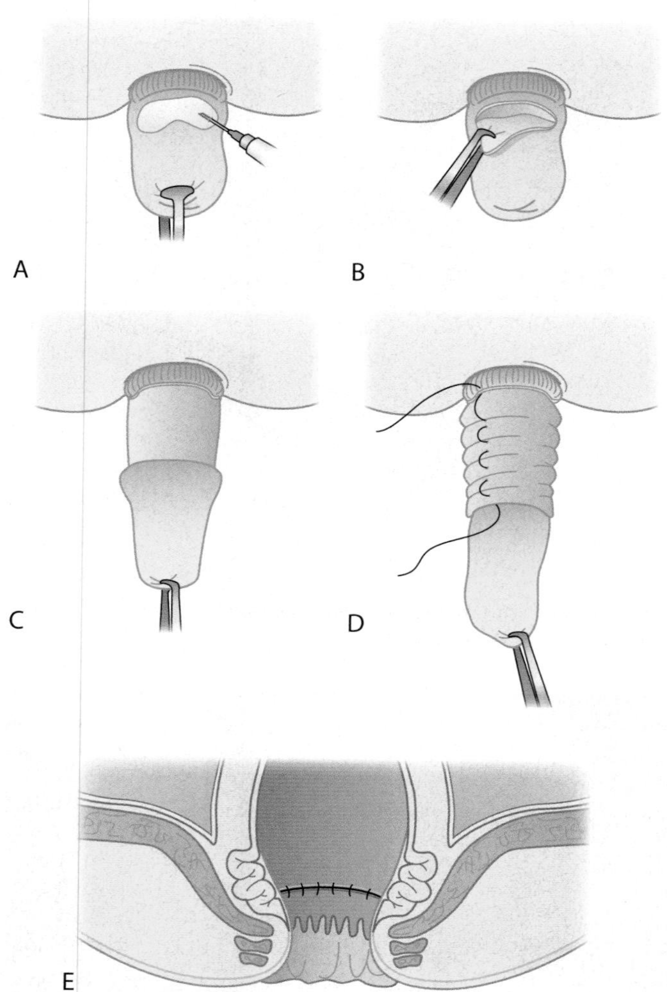

FIG. 52.96 The Delorme procedure. The mucosal layer is infiltrated with epinephrine containing solution (A), incised (B), and stripped off the underlying muscularis (C). Plication of the muscularis propria is performed (D).The operation concludes with an anastomosis between the proximal and distal mucosal edges (E).

good results in cases of obstructed constipation, but the onset of chronic proctalgia and stool urgency with postoperative incontinence have often been reported. Other complications of transrectal stapled repair are staple-line bleeding and, rarely, staple-line disruption and rectovaginal fistula (overall morbidity rate from 7%–21%). Because of the high rate of serious complications and poor functional outcome, this is not recommended by the ASCRS Clinical Practice Guidelines.

Solitary Rectal Ulcer

Solitary rectal ulcer syndrome (SRUS) is a rare chronic benign disorder characterized by a combination of symptoms, clinical findings, and histologic abnormalities. Twenty percent of patients have a single ulcer, while 40% of patients have multiple ulcers. The remainder have nonspecific lesions such as hyperemic mucosa or pseudopolyps.

SRUS is a disorder of young adults (30–40 years), with a slight female predominance. The cause is multifactorial and includes internal rectal prolapse and abnormal/paradoxical contraction of the puborectalis muscle. These two conditions result in trauma and compression of the anterior rectal wall on the upper anal canal during straining and defecation, with resulting mucosal ischemia and, in some cases, ulceration. Symptoms reported by patients with SRUS include rectal bleeding, prolonged excessive straining, incomplete defecation/tenesmus, mucous discharge, perineal and abdominal pain, and constipation. Up to one quarter of patients are asymptomatic.

Physical examination and anoscopy demonstrate an intrarectal prolapse and a 1 to 1.5-cm ulcer of the anterior rectal wall 3 to 10 cm from the anal verge that is sometimes difficult to differentiate from a rectal cancer. Histologic examination of biopsies shows characteristic findings: fibromuscular obliteration of the lamina propria, hypertrophied muscularis mucosae with muscular fibers between the crypts, and glandular crypt abnormalities. These specific findings differentiate SRUS from cancer and other inflammatory lesions such as IBD, ischemic colitis, and infectious proctitis.

For patients with mild to moderate symptoms and no significant mucosal prolapse, medical treatment is usually effective. It consists of patient education and behavioral modification: high-fiber diet, stool softeners and bulking laxatives, avoidance of straining and/or anal digitations, minimizing time on the toilet, and the use of sucralfate, corticosteroid, and/or mesalamine enemas. Surgery is rarely indicated and is reserved only for highly symptomatic patients absolutely unresponsive to medical treatment. Surgical options include local excision of the ulcer, treatment of the rectal prolapse, or a defunctioning stoma for patients who have failed other options. Unfortunately, many patients with SRUS continue to have symptoms of anorectal dysfunction regardless of the treatment.

Rectocele

A rectocele is a bulging of the anterior wall of the rectum into the posterior wall of the vagina. The most common risk factors are advanced age, history of pregnancy and vaginal childbirth, increasing body mass index, chronically elevated intraabdominal pressure, and a history of hysterectomy. The cause of rectocele is multifactorial and may be explained by a muscular and/or neurologic damage to the rectovaginal septum (usually due to obstetric trauma) and due to the effect of chronic straining on the endopelvic fascia and on the posterior wall of the vagina. It can be associated with other pelvic organ prolapses. Most rectoceles are asymptomatic, but when they become symptomatic, the cardinal symptom is difficulty in rectal emptying and the need to press against the posterior wall of the vagina or against the perineum in order to complete the rectal emptying (obstructed defecation). Other symptoms include the sensation of a vaginal bulge, urinary and/or sexual dysfunction, constipation, and in some cases fecal incontinence. The mechanism of incontinence is thought to be due to fecal trapping within the rectal pocket allowing for post-defecatory leakage, an associated mucosal prolapse that impairs anal closure or overflow incontinence. The diagnosis of rectocele is mainly clinical and based on physical examination. Digital vaginal and rectal examinations shows a bulging in the posterior vaginal wall and in the anterior rectal wall during straining that can be associated with the prolapse of other pelvic organs and with anterior cystocele. Associated stress urinary incontinence is assessed by making the patient cough or perform Valsalva maneuver with a full bladder.

On defecography, the rectocele appears as a bulging of the rectal wall toward the vagina. A rectocele is graded as small if it is less than 2 cm, moderate if it is between 2 and 4 cm, and large if it is larger than 4 cm in size (Fig. 52.97). This test also gives

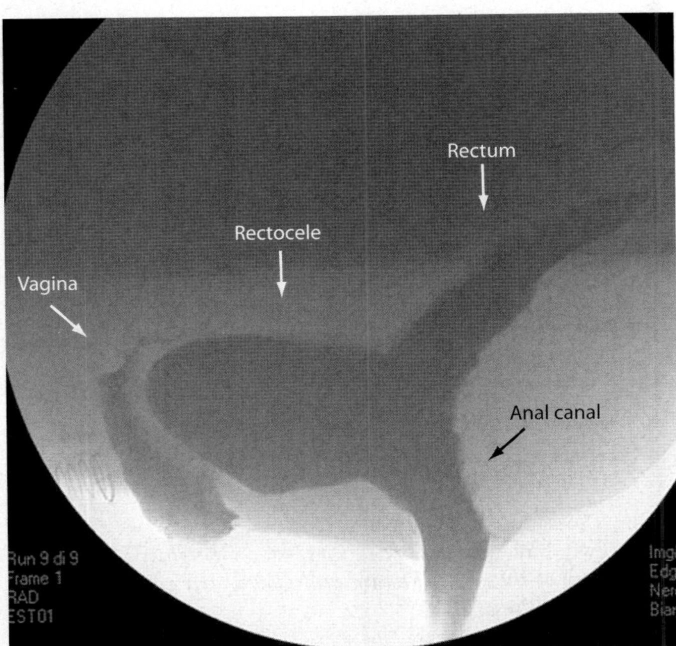

FIG. 52.97 A defecating proctogram. Both the vagina and the rectum are opacified. The rectocele is clearly evident.

information about the possible trapping of contrast within the rectocele during defecation and about the possible association with an enterocele or sigmoidocele. It is important to realize that the degree of anatomic distortion often does *not* correlate with the degree of functional impairment and symptoms. Dynamic MRI and MRI defecography are limited by the fact that they are performed with the patient in the supine position (i.e., not in the normal upright position for defecation). The balloon expulsion tests can identify the inability to expel an inflated balloon from the rectum after 4 minutes of sitting on a commode. Asymptomatic rectoceles do not need treatment, while patients with a symptomatic rectocele are initially managed with a bowel regimen and fiber products in order to improve defecation. Only selected patients with markedly symptomatic rectoceles unresponsive to medical treatment are candidates for surgery. The goal of surgery is to remove the redundant tissue of the rectocele and to strengthen the rectovaginal septum.

The transvaginal approach, preferred by gynecologists, allows for a better visualization and access to the levator muscles. A local anesthetic with epinephrine or vasopressin is injected below the vaginal mucosa to dissect the tissue and for hemostasis. The vaginal epithelium is opened in the posterior midline to the upper level of the defect; the fibromuscular layer is exposed and plicated in the midline with vertically or transversely placed sutures. The puborectalis can be reapproximated. The surplus vaginal epithelium is cut off if necessary and sutured with absorbable sutures.

An endorectal repair is performed by colorectal surgeons, with the patient in prone jackknife position. A local anesthetic plus epinephrine or vasopressin is injected in the submucosal plane to dissect the tissue and for hemostasis. A T-shaped or midline incision is made in the rectal mucosa just above the dentate line. Two lateral mucosal flaps are developed on either side of the midline to a level proximal to the rectocele. The excess rectal mucosa is excised. The underlying muscularis layer is exposed and plicated with transversely placed absorbable sutures and the mucosal edges are then approximated with absorbable sutures. The transperineal rectocele repair is performed by a transverse incision across the bulbocavernosus and transverse perineal muscles; the two limbs of the puborectalis muscle are reapproximated. A mesh can be placed in order to reinforce the plasty. This approach is indicated especially in patients with associated fecal incontinence, because a concomitant sphincteroplasty or levatorplasty can be performed.

Constipation

Constipation is a frequent condition that can affect more than 50% of population over 65, but in a small subset of patients, constipation may present at younger age. Several medical conditions can contribute to constipation, including metabolic, endocrine, neurologic, and psychiatric disorders. In adults, new-onset constipation is always a worrisome symptom and the primary cause must be excluded. Hypothyroidism and medication-induced constipation are common causes. The presence of colorectal malignancies and other cause of colonic obstruction must be excluded with colonoscopy. Patients should be counseled to increase fluid intake up to 1.5 to 2 L/day and to increase the fiber content in diet. Polyethylene-based solutions (e.g., MiraLAX), probiotics, and over-the-counter products may be helpful. Stimulant laxatives such as bisacodyl or senna should not be used long-term. A locally acting chloride channel activator (lubiprostone; Amitiza), a guanylate cyclase agonist (Linzess), and/or a serotonin 5-HT4 agonist (Motegrity) can all be used to treat symptoms of constipation. Long-term constipation, resistant to medical treatment and laxatives, should be further investigated. According to Rome IV criteria, functional constipation is diagnosed if (1) there are at least two of the following symptoms, during at least 25% of defecations, for at least 3 months[50]: straining, lumpy, or hard stools; a sensation of incomplete evacuation; sensation of anorectal obstruction/blockage; need for manual maneuvers to facilitate defecation (e.g., digital evacuation, support of the pelvic floor); or fewer than three spontaneous bowel movements per week; (2) loose stools rarely present without the use of laxatives; and (3) there are insufficient criteria for irritable bowel syndrome. In the presence of obstructed defecation symptoms, defecography, anorectal manometry, balloon expulsion testing, and electromyography can exclude the presence of pelvic floor disorders. Measuring the colonic transit time with the use of radiopaque markers (Sitzmark) can establish the diagnosis of slow transit constipation or colonic inertia. Slow transit constipation can have a neuropathic origin, even if a specific histologic change has not yet been demonstrated. The frequency of bowel movements varies in these patients from one to two per week to one per month. Some patients are unable to have a complete bowel movement in the absence of laxatives or colonic enemas. Severe constipation is associated with abdominal distension, abdominal pain, and nausea, and these symptoms can so affect the quality of a patient's life that they can be absolutely miserable. Chronic symptoms can be present from childhood or adolescence. Slow transit constipation can present with a megacolon on plain x-ray (Fig. 52.98); a water-soluble enema or colon CT can show a redundant, hypotonic colon, and colonoscopy similarly demonstrates a dilated hypotonic colon. In a subset of patients, the colon can be normal and not dilated at radiologic examination. In these patients, the diagnosis and the decision to initiate surgical treatment can be challenging. In highly symptomatic patients with slow transit constipation who failed aggressive medical therapy and whose quality of life is severely impaired, surgical treatment is indicated. Abdominal colectomy with IRA (total abdominal colectomy with ileorectal anastomosis [TAC-IRA] or colectomy with ileorectal

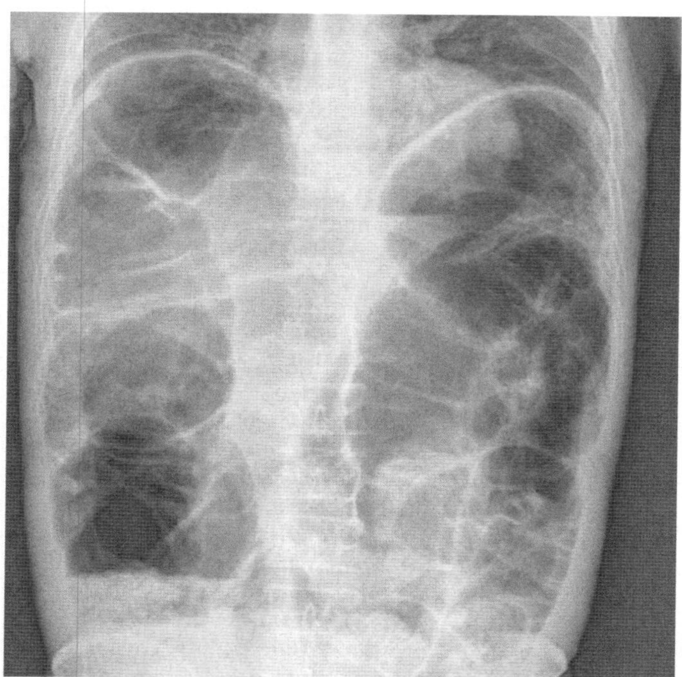

FIG. 52.98 Plain abdominal film of a patient with slow transit constipation and megacolon.

anastomosis [CIRA]) is an operation that has demonstrated good clinical improvement with acceptable morbidity. It can be performed with minimally invasive techniques. Despite postoperative diarrhea that occurs in 5% to 15%, abdominal pain (30%–50%), small bowel obstruction (10%–20%), fecal incontinence, and recurrence of constipation (10%–30%) that have been reported in long-term follow-up, most patients are satisfied with functional results following colectomy and IRA.

Segmental colon resections based on transit time measurements are no longer recommended. The extreme therapeutic solution proposed to patients with intractable constipation is a permanent ostomy, usually an ileostomy.

SELECTED REFERENCES

American Society of Colon & Rectal Surgeons Clinical Practice Guidelines published in Diseases of the Colon & Rectum. Available through a link to the Clinical Practice Guidelines on the journal website https://journals.lww.com/dcrjournal/pages/default.aspx.

Specifically referred to in this chapter are the Clinical Practice Guidelines for (1) Enhanced Recovery after Colon and Rectal Surgery, (2) the Use of Bowel Preparation in Elective Colon and Rectal Surgery, (3) Colon Volvulus and Acute Colonic Pseudo-obstruction, (4) the Management of Inherited Polyposis Syndromes, (5) the Surgical Treatment of Patients with Lynch Syndrome, (6) the Treatment of Colon Cancer, (7) the Management of Rectal Cancer, (8) the Surveillance of Patients after Curative Treatment of Colon and Rectal Cancer, (9) the Treatment of Rectal Prolapse, (10) the Evaluation and Management of Constipation, as well as (11) The Consensus Statement of Anorectal Physiology Testing and Pelvic Floor Terminology.

Beck DE, Wexner SD, Rafferty RF, eds. *Gordon and Nivatvongs Principles and Practice of Surgery for the Colon, Rectum, and Anus*. 4th ed. New York: Thieme Publishers; 2018.

This text provides excellent anatomic illustrations and detailed descriptions of all aspects of diseases of the colon, rectum, and anus.

Haggitt RC, Glotzbach RE, Soffer EE, et al. Prognostic factors in colorectal carcinomas arising in adenomas: implications for lesions removed by endoscopic polypectomy. *Gastroenterology*. 1985;89:328–336.

Description of Haggitt criteria, a classification for polyps with adenocarcinoma that assesses malignant potential according to the depth of invasion.

Sagar PM, Hill AG, Knowles CH, et al. *Keighley & Williams' Surgery of the Anus, Rectum and Colon*. 4th ed. Boca Raton, FL: CRC Press; 2019.

The most recently published two-volume textbook of colon and rectal surgery, with an international list of contributors.

Steele SR, Hull TL, Hyman N, et al. *The ASCRS Textbook of Colon and Rectal Surgery*. 3rd ed. New York: Springer; 2016.

This text is sponsored by the American Society of Colon and Rectal Surgeons (ASCRS), with chapters written by recognized authorities in their field, including an excellent chapter on the molecular basis of colorectal cancer and inherited syndromes written by Dr. Matthew Kalady.

REFERENCES

1. McDonald LC, Gerding DN, Johnson S, et al. Clinical Practice Guidelines for *Clostridium difficile* infection in adults and children: 2017 update by the Infectious Diseases Society of America (IDSA) and Society for Healthcare Epidemiology of America (SHEA). *Clin Infect Dis*. 2018;66:987–994.
2. Mazaki T, Ishii Y, Murai I. Immunoenhancing enteral and parenteral nutrition for gastrointestinal surgery: a multiple-treatments meta-analysis. *Ann Surg*. 2015;261:662–669.
3. Carmichael JC, Keller DS, Baldini G, et al. Clinical Practice Guidelines for enhanced recovery after colon and rectal surgery from the American Society of Colon and Rectal Surgeons and Society of American Gastrointestinal and Endoscopic Surgeons. *Dis Colon Rectum*. 2017;60:761–784.
4. Koskenvuo L, Lehtonen T, Koskensalo S, et al. Mechanical and oral antibiotic bowel preparation versus no bowel preparation for elective colectomy (MOBILE): a multicentre, randomised, parallel, single-blinded trial. *Lancet*. 2019;394:840–848.
5. Liu PH, Cao Y, Keeley BR, et al. Adherence to a healthy lifestyle is associated with a lower risk of diverticulitis among men. *Am J Gastroenterol*. 2017;112:1868–1876.
6. Wasvary H, Turfah F, Kadro O, et al. Same hospitalization resection for acute diverticulitis. *Am Surg*. 1999;65:632–635; discussion 636.

7. Penna M, Markar SR, Mackenzie H, et al. Laparoscopic lavage versus primary resection for acute perforated diverticulitis: review and meta-analysis. *Ann Surg*. 2018;267:252–258.
8. Lambrichts DPV, Vennix S, Musters GD, et al. Hartmann's procedure versus sigmoidectomy with primary anastomosis for perforated diverticulitis with purulent or faecal peritonitis (LADIES): a multicentre, parallel-group, randomised, open-label, superiority trial. *Lancet Gastroenterol Hepatol*. 2019;4:599–610.
9. Desai M, Fathallah J, Nutalapati V, et al. Antibiotics versus no antibiotics for acute uncomplicated diverticulitis: a systematic review and meta-analysis. *Dis Colon Rectum*. 2019;62:1005–1012.
10. Sharma PV, Eglinton T, Hider P, et al. Systematic review and meta-analysis of the role of routine colonic evaluation after radiologically confirmed acute diverticulitis. *Ann Surg*. 2014;259:263–272.
11. Bharucha AE, Parthasarathy G, Ditah I, et al. Temporal trends in the incidence and natural history of diverticulitis: a population-based study. *Am J Gastroenterol*. 2015;110:1589–1596.
12. Hong KD, Kim J, Ji W, et al. Adult intussusception: a systematic review and meta-analysis. *Tech Coloproctol*. 2019;23:315–324.
13. Wells CI, O'Grady G, Bissett IP. Acute colonic pseudo-obstruction: a systematic review of aetiology and mechanisms. *World J Gastroenterol*. 2017;23:5634–5644.
14. Kaplan GG. The global burden of IBD: from 2015 to 2025. *Nat Rev Gastroenterol Hepatol*. 2015;12:720–727.
15. Turpin W, Goethel A, Bedrani L, et al. Determinants of IBD heritability: genes, bugs, and more. *Inflamm Bowel Dis*. 2018;24:1133–1148.
16. Harvey RF, Bradshaw JM. A simple index of Crohn's-disease activity. *Lancet*. 1980;1:514.
17. Odze RD, Farraye FA, Hecht JL, et al. Long-term follow-up after polypectomy treatment for adenoma-like dysplastic lesions in ulcerative colitis. *Clin Gastroenterol Hepatol*. 2004;2:534–541.
18. Galandiuk S, Rodriguez-Justo M, Jeffery R, et al. Field cancerization in the intestinal epithelium of patients with Crohn's ileocolitis. *Gastroenterology*. 2012;142:855–864. e858.
19. Chang MI, Cohen BL, Greenstein AJ. A review of the impact of biologics on surgical complications in Crohn's disease. *Inflamm Bowel Dis*. 2015;21:1472–1477.
20. Nguyen GC, Loftus Jr EV, Hirano I, et al. American Gastroenterological Association Institute guideline on the management of Crohn's disease after surgical resection. *Gastroenterology*. 2017;152:271–275.
21. Lessa FC, Winston LG, McDonald LC, et al. Burden of *Clostridium difficile* infection in the United States. *N Engl J Med*. 2015;372:2369–2370.
22. Loo VG, Davis I, Embil J, et al. Association of Medical Microbiology and Infectious Disease Canada treatment practice guidelines for *Clostridium difficile* infection. *JAMMI*. 2018;3:71–92.
23. Miller MA, Louie T, Mullane K, et al. Derivation and validation of a simple clinical bedside score (ATLAS) for *Clostridium difficile* infection which predicts response to therapy. *BMC Infect Dis*. 2013;13:148.
24. Furuya-Kanamori L, Doi SA, Paterson DL, et al. Upper versus lower gastrointestinal delivery for transplantation of fecal microbiota in recurrent or refractory *Clostridium difficile* infection: a collaborative analysis of individual patient data from 14 studies. *J Clin Gastroenterol*. 2017;51:145–150.
25. Bartlett JG. Bezlotoxumab—a new agent for *Clostridium difficile* infection. *N Engl J Med*. 2017;376:381–382.
26. Ferrada P, Callcut R, Zielinski MD, et al. Loop ileostomy versus total colectomy as surgical treatment for *Clostridium difficile*–associated disease: an Eastern Association for the Surgery of Trauma multicenter trial. *J Trauma Acute Care Surg*. 2017;83:36–40.
27. Yngvadottir Y, Karlsdottir BR, Hreinsson JP, et al. The incidence and outcome of ischemic colitis in a population-based setting. *Scand J Gastroenterol*. 2017;52:704–710.
28. Brandt LJ, Feuerstadt P, Longstreth GF, et al. ACG clinical guideline: epidemiology, risk factors, patterns of presentation, diagnosis, and management of colon ischemia (CI). *Am J Gastroenterol*. 2015;110:18–44; quiz 45.
29. Tseng J, Loper B, Jain M, et al. Predictive factors of mortality after colectomy in ischemic colitis: an ACS-NSQIP database study. *Trauma Surg Acute Care Open*. 2017;2:e000126.
30. Dienstmann R, Vermeulen L, Guinney J, et al. Consensus molecular subtypes and the evolution of precision medicine in colorectal cancer. *Nat Rev Cancer*. 2017;17:79–92.
31. Dongre A, Weinberg RA. New insights into the mechanisms of epithelial-mesenchymal transition and implications for cancer. *Nat Rev Mol Cell Biol*. 2019;20:69–84.
32. He X, Hang D, Wu K, et al. Long-term risk of colorectal cancer after removal of conventional adenomas and serrated polyps. *Gastroenterology*. 2020;158:852–861.
33. Click B, Pinsky PF, Hickey T, et al. Association of colonoscopy adenoma findings with long-term colorectal cancer incidence. *JAMA*. 2018;319:2021–2031.
34. Kikuchi R, Takano M, Takagi K, et al. Management of early invasive colorectal cancer. Risk of recurrence and clinical guidelines. *Dis Colon Rectum*. 1995;38:1286–1295.
35. Brosens LA, Offerhaus GJ, Giardiello FM. Hereditary colorectal cancer: genetics and screening. *Surg Clin North Am*. 2015;95:1067–1080.
36. Stoffel EM, Mangu PB, Limburg PJ, et al. Hereditary colorectal cancer syndromes: American Society of Clinical Oncology clinical practice guideline endorsement of the familial risk-colorectal cancer: European Society for Medical Oncology clinical practice guidelines. *J Oncol Pract*. 2015;11:e437–e441.
36a. Amin MB, Edge SB, Greene, Fl et al: AJCC Cancer Staging Manual 8th edition, American College of Surgeons, NY: Springer, 2018.
37. Acuna SA, Chesney TR, Ramjist JK, et al. Laparoscopic versus open resection for rectal cancer: a noninferiority meta-analysis of quality of surgical resection outcomes. *Ann Surg*. 2019;269:849–855.
38. Pisano M, Zorcolo L, Merli C, et al. WSES guidelines on colon and rectal cancer emergencies: obstruction and perforation. *World J Emerg Surg*. 2017;13:36; 2018.
39. Amelung FJ, Borstlap WAA, Consten ECJ, et al. Propensity score-matched analysis of oncological outcome between stent as bridge to surgery and emergency resection in patients with malignant left-sided colonic obstruction. *Br J Surg*. 2019;106:1075–1086.
40. Sauer R, Becker H, Hohenberger W, et al. Preoperative versus postoperative chemoradiotherapy for rectal cancer. *N Engl J Med*. 2004;351:1731–1740.

41. Habr-Gama A, Perez RO, Nadalin W, et al. Operative versus nonoperative treatment for stage 0 distal rectal cancer following chemoradiation therapy: long-term results. *Ann Surg.* 2004;240:711–717.
42. Ryan R, Gibbons D, Hyland JM, et al. Pathological response following long-course neoadjuvant chemoradiotherapy for locally advanced rectal cancer. *Histopathology.* 2005;47:141–146.
43. Sylla P, Rattner DW, Delgado S, et al. NOTES transanal rectal cancer resection using transanal endoscopic microsurgery and laparoscopic assistance. *Surg Endosc.* 2010;24:1205–1210.
44. Penna M, Hompes R, Arnold S, et al. Transanal total mesorectal excision: international registry results of the first 720 cases. *Ann Surg.* 2017;266:111–117.
45. Frasson M, Flor-Lorente B, Rodriguez JL, et al. Risk factors for anastomotic leak after colon resection for cancer: multivariate analysis and nomogram from a multicentric, prospective, national study with 3193 patients. *Ann Surg.* 2015;262:321–330.
46. Martellucci J. Low anterior resection syndrome: a treatment algorithm. *Dis Colon Rectum.* 2016;59:79–82.
47. Andre T, de Gramont A, Vernerey D, et al. Adjuvant fluorouracil, leucovorin, and oxaliplatin in stage II to III colon cancer: updated 10-year survival and outcomes according to BRAF mutation and mismatch repair status of the MOSAIC Study. *J Clin Oncol.* 2015;33:4176–4187.
48. Grothey A, Sobrero AF, Shields AF, et al. Duration of adjuvant chemotherapy for stage III colon cancer. *N Engl J Med.* 2018;378:1177–1188.
49. Consten EC, van Iersel JJ, Verheijen PM, et al. Long-term outcome after laparoscopic ventral mesh rectopexy: an observational study of 919 consecutive patients. *Ann Surg.* 2015;262:742–747.
50. Mearin F, Lacy BE, Chang L, et al. *Bowel disorders.* Gastroenterology; 2016 18;S0016-5085(16)00222-5. doi: 10.1053/j.gastro.2016.02.031. Online ahead of print.

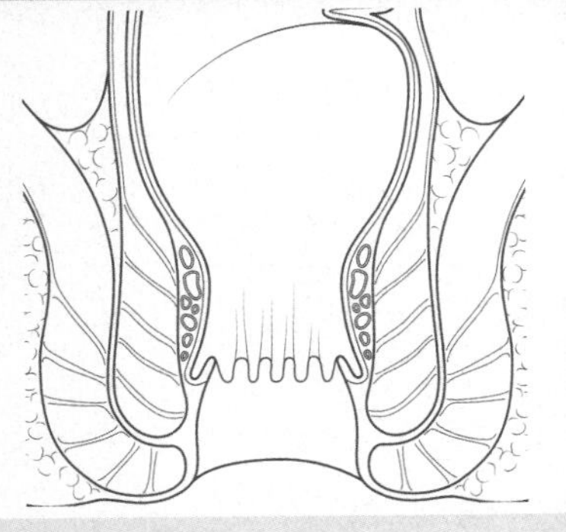

CHAPTER 53

Anus

Neil Hyman, Konstantin Umanskiy

OUTLINE

The anus comprises a relatively small anatomic region of the gastrointestinal tract, yet it plays a critical role in fecal continence and defecation. Because of its unique anatomy and physiology, the anus can present challenges to diagnosis and treatment. Although malignancy can occasionally develop, the anus is susceptible to a variety of common benign conditions that may cause considerable suffering and greatly impair a patient's quality of life. Understanding the applied anatomy and physiology of the anus is an invaluable asset to the surgeon and remains the cornerstone of accurate diagnosis and treatment.

ANATOMY

The anal canal, as defined by the surgeon/clinician, is approximately 4 cm in length, extending from the anal verge to the top of anorectal ring; the anatomist considers the anus to be the 2 cm from the anal verge to the dentate line (Fig. 53.1). The anus appears as an anteroposterior slit-like cutaneous opening, with its distal-most aspect referred to as the anal verge. The proximal anal canal is typically lined by columnar epithelium and the distal anus by squamous epithelium. The junction between the ectoderm and the endoderm, located at the midpoint of the anal canal, appears as an undulating demarcation referred to as the dentate line. Between the dentate line and the anal verge, the mucosa is lined by a modified squamous epithelium, similar to the epithelium of the skin, but devoid of hair follicles and glands.

The mucosa above the dentate line appears pleated with longitudinal folds, known as the columns of Morgagni. There is a small pocket or crypt at the base of most columns that communicate with the anal glands, which secrete lubricating fluid to assist with defecation. The glands number from 6 to 12 and are mostly concentrated in the posterior aspect of the anus. The anal gland duct traverses the submucosal plane and its branches terminate within the internal anal sphincter or extend into the intersphincteric plane. These glands are of substantial clinical importance; foreign debris may obstruct the ducts and result in the common perianal abscess, and its chronic counterpart, the fistula-in-ano.

The submucosa in the area of the distal anal canal is formed by a discontinuous layer of thickened tissue creating hemorrhoidal "cushions," typically found in the left lateral, right anterior, and right posterior positions. These cushions generally receive their blood supply from six hemorrhoidal arteries distributed along the circumference of the distal rectum and anus.[1] The venous drainage is provided by the superior, middle, and inferior hemorrhoidal vessels, allowing for communication between the portal and systemic circulations. These vessels form direct arteriovenous communications within the cushions, and for this reason, hemorrhoidal bleeding is arterial rather than venous in nature. Venous and lymphatic drainage above the dentate line flows into the internal iliac vessels; below the dentate line, blood supply and drainage are provided by the inferior hemorrhoidal system.

The anal opening and anal canal remain virtually closed at rest as a result of tonic circumferential contraction of both the internal and external sphincters, and compression of the anal cushions. The internal anal sphincter is composed of autonomically innervated smooth muscle and contributes between 50% to 85% of the resting tone of the anal canal. Anatomically, the internal anal sphincter is a thickened continuation of the circular layer of the muscularis propria of the distal rectum and occupies the distal 2 to 4 cm of the anal canal. The external anal sphincter is a funnel-shaped structure composed of the pelvic floor muscles enveloping the distal rectum and anus. The puborectalis muscle, often

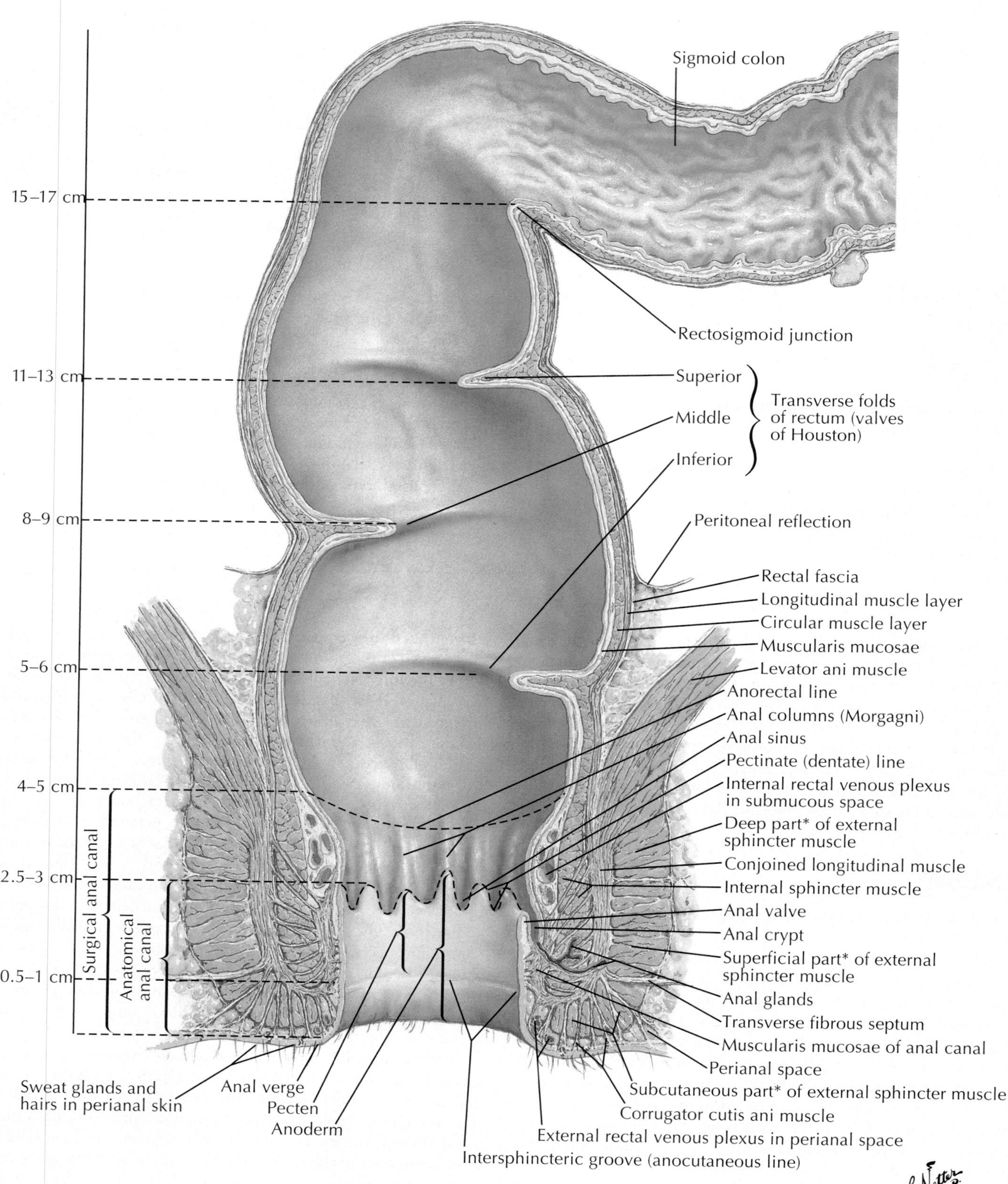

FIG. 53.1 Anatomy of the rectum and anus. (Netter image copyright by Elsevier.)

referred to as the rectal sling, is one of the main muscles contributing to the external anal sphincter. It originates at the pubis, passes around the rectum posteriorly, and returns to the pubis. The external anal sphincter is unique because it can be controlled both by the autonomic nervous system and by voluntary contraction. In response to increases in intraabdominal pressure or rectal distention, the external anal sphincter and puborectalis reflexively and voluntarily contract to prevent fecal leakage. Unlike the internal anal sphincter, the external anal sphincter can be subjected to muscular fatigue with maximal voluntary contraction sustained for only 30 to 60 seconds.

The internal anal sphincter is supplied by sympathetic (L5) and parasympathetic (S2, S3, and S4) nerves. The external anal sphincter is innervated on each side by the inferior rectal branch of the pudendal nerve (S2 and S3) and by the perineal branch of S4. Even though the puborectalis and external anal sphincter have somewhat different innervation, these muscles appear to act as a unit.[2] There is considerable redundancy in innervation of the anal sphincter— unilateral interruption of the pudendal nerve will not result in external anal sphincter dysfunction, but the loss of bilateral S3 nerve roots (e.g., by surgical transection) will typically result in fecal incontinence. If the S1 through S3 nerve roots remain intact only on one side, the patient is still expected to maintain control of the anal sphincters.

The rectal branch of the pudendal nerve transmits anal sensation, and it is thought to play a role in maintenance of anal continence. The anal canal contains a rich supply of free and organized sensory nerve endings, especially in the region of the anus. Organized nerve endings include Meissner corpuscles (touch), Krause bulbs (temperature sensation), Golgi-Mazzoni bodies (pressure), and genital corpuscules (friction).

Physiology

The process of defecation is a complex coordinated event involving increased intraabdominal pressure, rectal contraction, and synchronized relaxation of the anal sphincters. Distention of the rectum results in reflexive relaxation of the internal anal sphincter. This allows sensory epithelium of the anus to sample the fecal material in order to distinguish between solid stool, liquid stool, and gas. If defecation is deemed appropriate, the external anal sphincter relaxes together with the puborectalis muscle, which allows straightening of the rectoanal angle, opening of the anal canal, and evacuation of fecal material.

The physiology of continence is as complex as defecation. Continence requires rectal wall compliance to accommodate the fecal material, appropriate neurogenic control of the pelvic floor muscles, and properly functioning internal and external sphincter muscles. At rest, the puborectalis muscle creates a sling around the distal rectum, forming a relatively acute rectoanal angle that distributes intraabdominal forces onto the pelvic floor. With defecation, this angle straightens, allowing downward force to be applied along the axis of the rectum and anus. The internal anal and external sphincters, together with the hemorrhoidal cushions, provide a complete airtight and watertight seal.

Diagnosis

History

Most patients with clinically relevant diseases of the anus present with nonspecific complaints including rectal pain, bleeding, tissue prolapse, seepage, or anal itching. The skilled provider asks the focused questions that usually elucidate the nature of the problem. Patient history is the cornerstone of diagnosis and asking the right questions will almost always lead to a presumptive or even definitive diagnosis. It is pivotal that the provider has formed an impression of the likely problem before proceeding with the examination of the anus.

The history taking often includes detailed questioning about defecation. It is not sufficient to ask if the patient has "normal" bowel movements because most patients may believe/say that they do; rather, the number of daily bowel movements, straining with defecation, caliber of stool and consistency of bowel movements (soft, formed, liquid, or diarrhea), incontinence episodes, seepage, and soiling should be sought. A provider must inquire about the presence or absence of blood per anus, the character of the bleeding (bright vs. dark, amount of blood, presence or absence of blood clots), association with bowel movements, blood mixed within the fecal material or present as streaks of blood on stool, and whether blood is noted with wiping.

Anal pain or pressure is frequently a presenting complaint. Differentiating the type of pain can help accurately diagnose many conditions prior to examining the patient, as the common diagnoses typically present in distinct ways. Sharp, razor knife pain that occurs with bowel movements will almost always indicate an anal fissure. Pain occurring even without defecation, especially with bleeding, could indicate malignancy. Acute pain of relatively short duration may suggest a thrombosed hemorrhoid: when associated with fever and malaise, a perianal or ischiorectal abscess is a likely culprit.

Anal itching is a common and frustrating complaint, both for the patient and provider. The patient should be asked about the presence or absence of anal seepage or drainage, fecal soilage, or perianal moisture. Tactful questioning regarding sexual history, particularly anoreceptive intercourse, should be obtained from both men and women. Questions may include the number of partners, use of protection, sex without a partner, and a history of sexual trauma. If high-risk sexual behavior is reported, a focus on sexually transmitted diseases (STDs) and human immunodeficiency virus (HIV) status is suggested. Focused surgical history should include previous interventions for drainage of perirectal abscesses, fistula, hemorrhoid surgery, or sphincterotomy. Women should be asked about vaginal tears during delivery and a history of episiotomy.

Physical Examination

Anorectal examination in an outpatient setting should be tailored to the presenting complaints, as the patient may be very sensitive or uncomfortable with the examination. Again, the history will almost provide for at least a presumptive or differential diagnosis. Communication with the patient is the key. The provider should inform the patient of the proposed examination and ensure the patient is comfortable with proceeding. It is appropriate to have a chaperone present in the room throughout the examination.[3] The patient can be examined either in the knee-chest or Sims position; the latter being much more comfortable option for the patient, though perhaps more cumbersome for the provider.

The examination begins by observing the perianal skin and anal margin. Gentle spreading of the buttocks will reveal the anal verge and anoderm. The patient can be asked to squeeze and relax their sphincter muscle, which can reveal asymmetrical contraction or abnormal recruitment of the gluteus muscles to aid with anal squeeze. When asked to bear down, the patient is expected to reflexively relax their anal sphincter and may reveal rectal prolapse and/or abnormal pelvic floor descent.

TABLE 53.1 **Classification of internal hemorrhoids.**

GRADE OF INTERNAL HEMORRHOIDS	DESCRIPTION
Grade 1	No prolapse; hemorrhoidal bleeding
Grade 2	Hemorrhoids with bleeding and protrusion; reduce spontaneously
Grade 3	Hemorrhoids with bleeding and protrusion; manual reduction required
Grade 4	Prolapsed hemorrhoids that cannot be reduced

Digital rectal examination is performed next. Before inserting the examining finger into the anal canal, a gentle tap with a well-lubricated finger on the anoderm will allow the patient an opportunity to prepare for the exam. Digital rectal examination begins with evaluation of the length of the surgical anal canal to the top of puborectalis sling posteriorly, followed by a sweep around the sacrum with palpation of the tip of the coccyx and evaluation of the levator muscles on the posterolateral aspect of the rectal vault. In men, the prostate is palpated anteriorly; in women, the presence of a rectocele may be determined by gently flexing the examining finger anteriorly. If a mass is detected within the rectum or anal canal, its location, relationship to the anterior-posterior or lateral aspect of the rectum should be noted, size should be estimated, and the provider should observe if it is fixed or mobile and soft or firm.

Prior to concluding the digital rectal examination, the patient is asked to squeeze, which is followed by bearing down. With a Valsalva maneuver, the muscles of the internal and external sphincters should relax, indicating appropriate coordination of the anal sphincter complex. Particular attention should be paid to digital examination of the anus, which can be overlooked if the provider palpates only the rectal vault. Using the first phalanx of the examining finger, a sweep of the anal canal should be performed. The provider should feel for masses or other irregularities.

Anoscopy is a common adjunct to digital rectal examination. The objective of the anoscopic evaluation is to visually inspect the anus and distal rectal mucosa. It can be useful for evaluating suspected enlarged hemorrhoids, anal dysplasia, intraanal condyloma acuminata, or anal tags. If purulent drainage is noted, it may be swabbed for evaluation of an STD as applicable.

Imaging

Endoanal ultrasound may be used to evaluate the layers of the anal canal, internal anal sphincter, external sphincters, and puborectalis muscle. Ultrasound can be a used to accurately estimate the degree of anal sphincter disruption and to outline the anatomy of a complex anal fistula. Magnetic resonance imaging (MRI) is more sensitive than computed tomography (CT) for detecting pelvic lesions, and in defining the relationship to the pelvic muscular structures or pelvic sidewall. MRI can accurately determine the extent to which the distal rectal or anal cancer has spread into the adjacent mesorectum and pelvic organs, such as prostate or vagina, and it can reliably predict if the radial margin is threatened prior to surgical excision. MRI can be quite useful in detection and delineation of a complex fistula-in-ano.

Anorectal manometry provides a detailed physiologic assessment of anorectal function. This test measures the pressures generated by the anal sphincter muscles, sensation in the rectum, and the neural reflexes that are needed for normal bowel function. Using specially designed catheters and balloons, anorectal manometry and balloon expulsion testing provides important insights into the pathophysiology underlying incontinence and defecatory disorders and may serve as a guide to treatment.

COMMON BENIGN DISORDERS OF THE ANUS

Internal Hemorrhoids

Symptomatic hemorrhoids result from enlargement and/or protrusion of the anal hemorrhoidal cushions. The key etiologic factors contributing to the development of hemorrhoids include constipation and prolonged straining. Increased intraanal pressure leads to abnormal dilatation and engorgement of vascular channels, followed by chronic changes in the supporting connective tissue within the anal cushions.[4] An inflammatory reaction and vascular hyperplasia[5,6] may be evident in hemorrhoids. With time and aging, starting as early as the second or third decade of life, the tissue supporting hemorrhoids can deteriorate or weaken, leading to distal displacement of the cushions and venous distention, erosion, bleeding, thrombosis, and/or tissue prolapse.

Painless bleeding associated with bowel movements with or without intermittent tissue protrusion is the most common complaint of patients with symptomatic internal hemorrhoids. Focus should be on the extent, severity, and duration of symptoms such as bleeding and prolapse, issues of perineal hygiene, and the presence or absence of pain. A detailed review of fiber intake and bowel habits, including frequency, consistency, change in caliber of stool, and difficulty with evacuation, should also be sought. An assessment of fecal continence is helpful in guiding treatment decisions. Anorectal examination should include visual inspection of the anus, digital rectal examination, and anoscopy to evaluate the extent of hemorrhoidal disease and search for other abnormalities. Internal hemorrhoids can be assigned a grade based on the classification in Table 53.1.

The initial approach to a patient with symptomatic hemorrhoids usually includes the recommendation to increase fluid intake and start on fiber supplementation, along with counseling regarding defecation habits, such as avoidance of straining and limiting time on the toilet. The patient should be encouraged to drink at least 64 ounces of water per day and take fiber supplements with the goal of increasing the bulk of fecal material and caliber of stools. Even those patients who regularly consume dietary fiber and report having "normal" bowel movements will commonly benefit from additional fiber and water intake. Topical treatments for symptomatic hemorrhoids may include sitz baths 2 to 3 times per day and application of witch hazel topical pads as needed. A 6- to 8-week trial of medical management is usually indicated before considering more aggressive interventions.

Most patients with grade I and II (and select patients with grade III) internal hemorrhoidal disease who remain symptomatic despite medical management can be offered an office-based procedure, such as rubber band ligation (RBL), sclerotherapy, or infrared coagulation (IRC). Hemorrhoidal RBL is commonly the most effective option, and has been shown to be superior to sclerotherapy and IRC.[7] Band ligation strangulates hemorrhoidal tissue, which results in ischemia and necrosis of the prolapsing mucosa, followed by scar fixation to the rectal wall. This procedure alleviates symptoms by decreasing the size of the hemorrhoidal

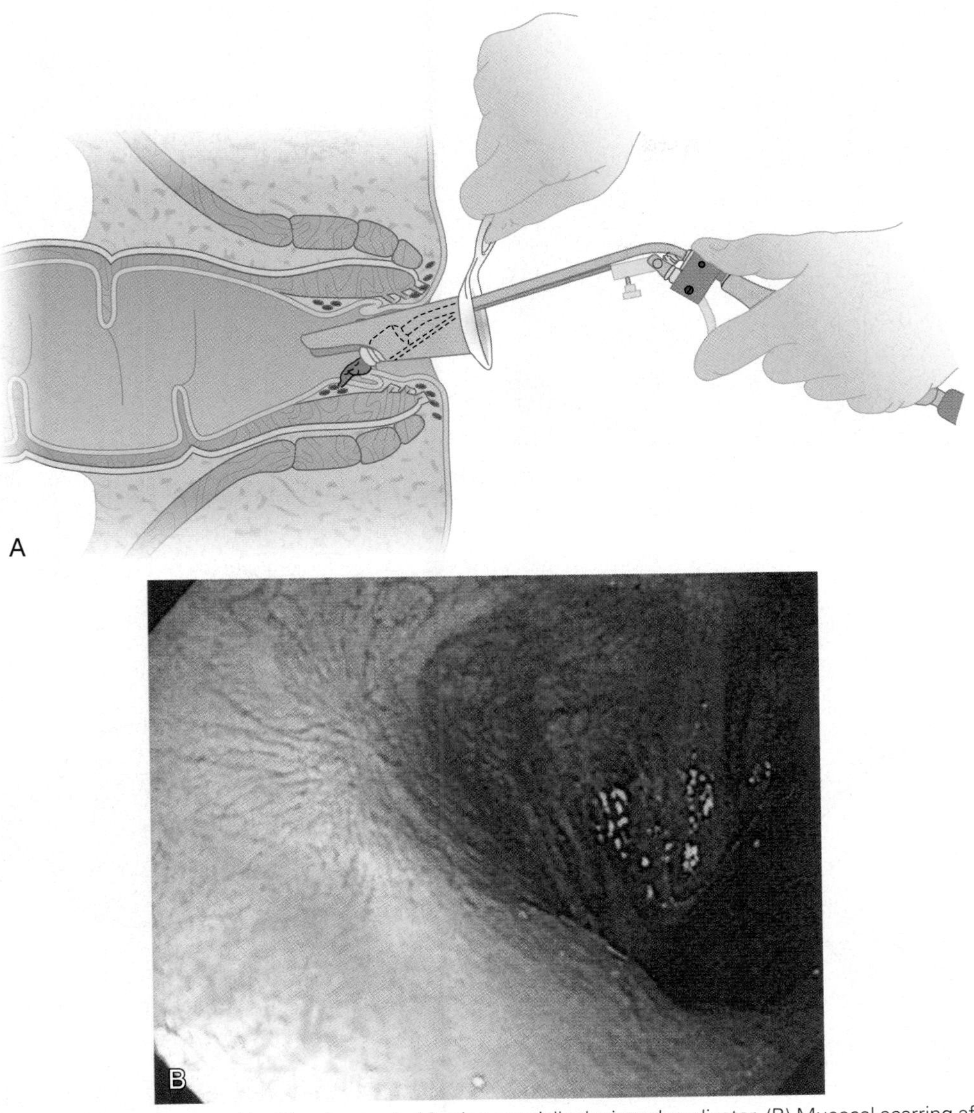

FIG. 53.2 (A) Placement of band on hemorrhoid using specially designed applicator. (B) Mucosal scarring after rubber band ligation, colonoscopic retroflexion.

cushion and increasing the fixation of the hemorrhoidal tissue to the rectal wall, thus minimizing hemorrhoidal prolapse (Fig. 53.2). RBL is generally well-tolerated because the rubber band is placed proximal to the dentate line, in the area of the anus devoid of somatic pain fibers. Sclerotherapy is accomplished by injection of a sclerosing agent directly into the hemorrhoid, which results in fibrosis of the submucosa with subsequent fixation of the hemorrhoidal tissue. The most commonly used sclerosing agents are 5% phenol in almond or vegetable oil and sodium tetradecyl sulfate. Injection is performed into the submucosa at the apex of a hemorrhoidal cushion, using approximately 1 ml of sclerosing agent. Sclerotherapy is appropriately offered to anticoagulated patients or those receiving antiplatelet therapy, who are often not optimal candidates for RBL or surgical excision. IRC utilizes direct application of infrared light resulting in protein coagulation within the hemorrhoid. This is most commonly used for grade I and II hemorrhoids.

External hemorrhoids are characterized by distended vascular tissue distal to the dentate line. Patients with thrombosed external hemorrhoids typically present with severe anal pain that may be exacerbated by sitting or defecation (Fig. 53.3). The thrombosed hemorrhoid is usually acute in onset and may be preceded by an episode of constipation or diarrhea. Most patients will experience resolution of their symptoms within 72 hours after the onset of symptoms with conservative measures, such as sitz baths, application of lidocaine ointment and stool softeners. Acutely tender, thrombosed external hemorrhoids are often surgically removed when pain is excessive and/or fails to respond to expectant management. Thrombectomy with evacuation of clot is often performed in the emergency department setting; however, excision of the hemorrhoid is usually a far better option, as it results in faster resolution of symptoms and a greatly decreased chance of recurrence. Both procedures may be readily accomplished with local anesthesia in an outpatient setting (Fig. 53.4).

Surgical excision of hemorrhoids is a very effective, albeit painful, approach for patients who did not improve or who are not candidates for an office-based treatment. Excisional hemorrhoidectomy can be offered to patients with symptomatic combined internal and external hemorrhoids with prolapse (grades III–IV) or patients with substantial associated skin tags. Either open or

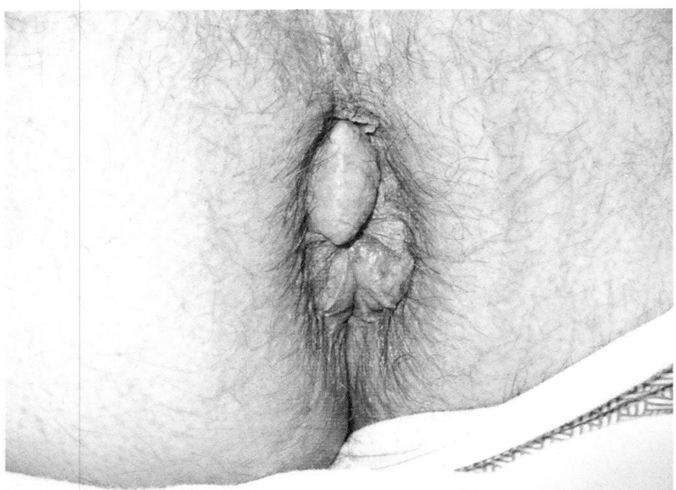

FIG. 53.3 Thrombosed external hemorrhoid.

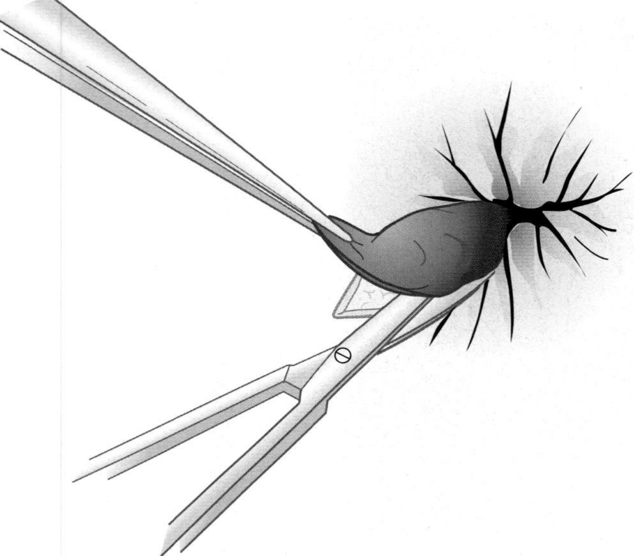

FIG. 53.4 Excision of thrombosed hemorrhoid.

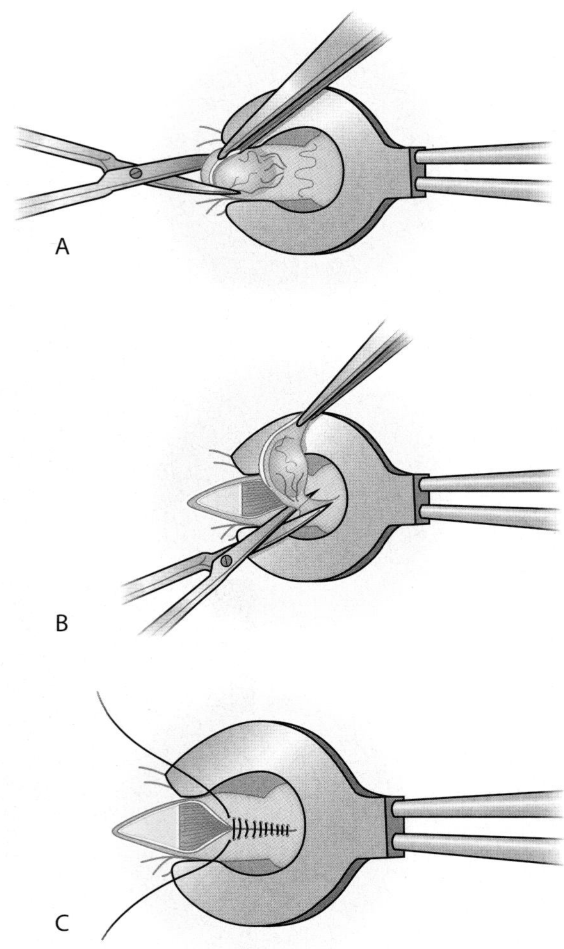

FIG. 53.5 Closed hemorrhoidectomy (Ferguson).

closed hemorrhoidectomy can be performed with a variety of surgical devices. The most commonly used technique is the closed (Ferguson) hemorrhoidectomy (Fig. 53.5). This approach is associated with decreased postoperative pain, faster wound healing, and a reduced risk of postoperative bleeding compared to an open (Milligan-Morgan) hemorrhoidectomy.

The principles of closed hemorrhoidectomy involve removal of only redundant hemorrhoidal tissue and pexy of hemorrhoidal mucosa to the rectal wall. In most instances, removal of the largest or most symptomatic hemorrhoid produces the desired symptomatic relief. Removal of all three hemorrhoidal columns can result in large mucosal defects and narrowing of the anal canal if not performed carefully. The procedure can be performed under general, local with monitored anesthesia, or spinal anesthesia. Prophylactic antibiotics are not indicated.[8] Either lithotomy or the prone jackknife position is acceptable. An anal block is induced with local anesthetic and exposure may be achieved with a Hill–Ferguson anoscope. The hemorrhoid is excised with a diamond-shaped excision extending onto the anoderm, using a scalpel, scissors, or energy device. Several bipolar or ultrasonic energy device-based techniques have been described. The use of a bipolar energy device was found to be faster and to cause less postoperative pain when compared with closed hemorrhoidectomy.

Regardless of the excision technique, the internal sphincter fibers should be identified and preserved. The base of the hemorrhoidal pedicle is oversewn with an absorbable braided suture to ligate the feeding arterial vessel. The edges of the hemorrhoidectomy wound are reapproximated with continuous locking braided absorbable suture. Complete hemostasis should be achieved with suture closure of the defect. If suture line bleeding is present, additional figure-of-eight sutures can be placed as needed. There is no benefit in packing the anal canal as it is unlikely to stop postoperative bleeding but can hide large quantities of blood accumulating above the packing.

Postoperative care should be aimed at maintaining regular bowel function with liberal use of milk of magnesia or polyethylene glycol laxatives to prevent constipation and impaction as needed. Pain is managed with sitz baths and judicious use of opioids. Complications after surgical hemorrhoidectomy are relatively low; the most common being postoperative hemorrhage, ranging in incidence between 1% and 2%.[9] Acute urinary retention occurs between 1% and 15% of cases. A rare, but feared complication of hemorrhoidectomy is pelvic sepsis. It can develop after excisional hemorrhoidectomy or office-based procedures. Early symptoms

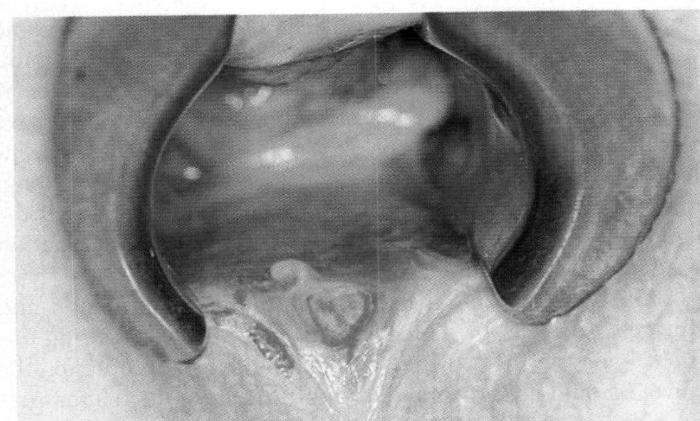

FIG. 53.6 Anal fissure. (From Tiernan JP, Brown SR. Benign anal conditions: Haemorrhoids, fissures, perianal abscess, fistula-in-ano and pilonidal sinus. *Surgery*. 2011;29:382–386.)

are often nonspecific, and may include urinary dysfunction, worsening anal pain, or fever; a high degree of suspicion is required to diagnose this potentially life-threatening complication.

Stapled hemorrhoidopexy utilizes a specially designed stapling device to create a mucosa-to-mucosa anastomosis, while removing redundant mucosa proximal to the dentate line; the procedure also disrupts the feeding hemorrhoidal arteries and displaces the hemorrhoidal cushions into the proximal anal canal. Unlike excisional hemorrhoidectomy, this technique does not address external hemorrhoids. Despite initial favorable reports, stapled hemorrhoidopexy has been associated with several concerning complications such as rectovaginal fistula, staple line bleeding, chronic pain, and stricture at the staple line. In one study, 35 patients were identified who required laparotomy with fecal diversion, and one patient was treated by low anterior resection. Despite surgical treatment and resuscitation, there were 4 deaths.[10]

Doppler-guided hemorrhoid artery ligation (HAL) utilizes a current understanding of the arterial blood supply of hemorrhoids to identify and ligate selected feeding vessels. There is no need for tissue excision, but mucosal pexy is required for patients with symptomatic hemorrhoidal prolapse. Several studies using HAL have demonstrated favorable short-term outcomes. This method, however, is expensive and was not found to be cost-effective compared with RBL in terms of incremental cost per quality-adjusted life-year.

Anal Fissure

An anal fissure is an elliptical or oval shaped tear in the anal canal starting at the anal verge and extending proximally for a varying length towards the dentate line (Fig. 53.6). Acute fissures appear as a shallow tear in the anoderm. The most common symptom is sharp anal pain with defecation, often described by patients as the feeling of "passing pieces of glass or razor blades." The sharp pain can be followed by throbbing and anal spasm. Anal bleeding can present as blood streaking on the stool or on the toilet paper. Anal fissures that are present for more than 6 to 8 weeks are considered to be chronic. Features of a chronic fissure include the presence of exposed internal sphincter fibers at the base, a hypertrophied anal papilla proximally, and a skin tag or sentinel pile distally. Pain with defecation tends to be less severe than with an acute fissure, but the symptoms are nonetheless unrelenting, and patients will often dread having bowel movements. Symptoms are commonly cyclical in nature, often making it challenging for patients to know whether any prescribed treatment is truly "helping."

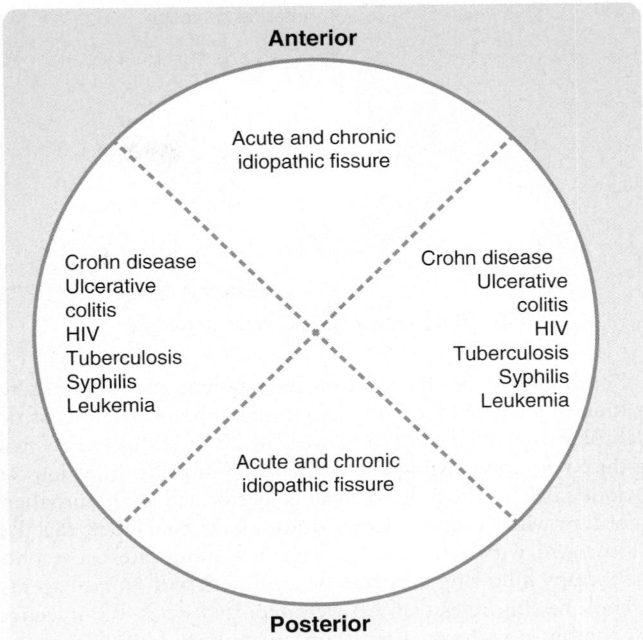

FIG. 53.7 Common and atypical locations of anal fissure. *HIV,* Human immunodeficiency virus.

Fissures may occur as a result of a tear caused by passage of a hard stool, explosive diarrhea, anal receptive intercourse or anal trauma. This, in turn, results in anal sphincter spasm, which further exacerbates constipation, ultimately decreasing blood flow to the anal mucosa and relative ischemia at the site of the tear. The most common location of an anal fissure is the posterior midline (75%). Another frequent location is the anterior midline, which is more common in women. Anal fissures found off the midline are considered atypical. The differential diagnosis of atypical fissures includes Crohn disease, anal cancer, tuberculosis, HIV, syphilis, herpes, and leukemia (Fig. 53.7).

The diagnosis of an anal fissure is usually straightforward and can often be made based on the patient's history alone. Gentle separation of the buttocks can reveal the fissure; however, just spreading the buttocks may cause intolerable pain and the examination may need to be stopped at this point. If the fissure is not clearly visible, gentle pressure with a cotton tip applicator on posterior and anterior aspect of the anal canal can reproduce the pain. Digital exam and anoscopic exam are often deferred to avoid exacerbating the patient's pain. If the diagnosis is unclear, an examination under anesthesia may be necessary.

The majority of acute anal fissures resolve with medical management alone. Chronic fissures, however, are less likely to heal with exclusively conservative measures. The goals of treatment are aimed at (1) addressing the inciting factors such as constipation or other causes of anal trauma, (2) relaxation and dilation of the internal anal sphincter to improve blood flow and allow healing, and (3) addressing the symptoms of pain and bleeding. The initial step in management should be to increase fluid and fiber ingestion as well as sitz baths and may include mineral oil or stool softeners to help with lubrication. Topical application of nitrates and calcium channel blockers are often used as an adjunct in nonoperative management. This results in internal anal sphincter relaxation and vasodilation, leading to improved blood flow to the anal mucosa and healing of the fissure.

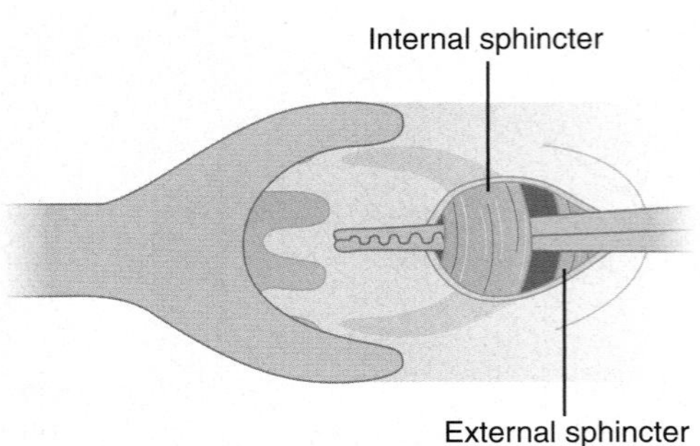

FIG. 53.8 Lateral internal sphincterotomy.

Botulinum toxin (BT) can produce potent and sustained relaxation of anal sphincter by inducing temporary paralysis of the anal sphincter muscle. A typical dose of 20 to 100 IU of BT will produce relaxation lasting approximately 3 months. Injection can be done safely in the office or may be performed as an outpatient procedure with sedation. Large studies have concluded that BT is associated with a modest increase in healing rates as second-line therapy following unsuccessful treatment with topical agents. Overall, healing rates of 65% were reported when BT injection was combined with concurrent topical application of diltiazem.[11] The most common side effects of BT injection are temporary incontinence to flatus. Other side effects include increased urinary residual volume, heart block, skin irritation, and allergic reactions.

Lateral internal sphincterotomy (LIS) induces sustained partial relaxation of the internal anal sphincter and reduces anal sphincter tone, enabling healing of the anal fissure. A radial incision in the anoderm exposes the internal sphincter muscle fibers (Fig. 53.8). The distal segment of the internal anal sphincter muscle is divided sharply for the length corresponding to that of the anal fissure. The wound can be left open or closed primarily. A closed LIS can be performed by inserting a narrow-bladed scalpel directly into the intersphincteric groove and dividing the internal sphincter laterally to medially toward the surgeon's finger within the anal canal. LIS has shown to be superior to topical nitrates, calcium channel blockers, or BT, with healing rates of 88% to 100%. Reported rates of fecal incontinence after LIS rates range from 8% to 30% but is usually limited to minor episodes of incontinence to flatus, most often in the first 30 days after the procedure.

Abscess/Fistula (Including Rectovaginal Fistula)

Perianal abscesses typically result from infection of the anal glands located at the level of dentate line and are attributed to obstruction of the draining duct from fecal debris; this is often referred to as a cryptoglandular abscess. Obstruction of the anal gland ducts leads to stasis, bacterial overgrowth, and ultimately abscesses that develop in the intersphincteric space.[12] These abscesses commonly expand by caudal extension to the anoderm (perianal abscess) or across the external sphincter into the ischiorectal fossa (ischiorectal abscess). Less common routes of spread are cephalad along the intersphincteric space and into supralevator space or within the submucosal plane (Fig. 53.9). Approximately 10% of perirectal abscesses occur due to other etiologies, such as Crohn disease, trauma, HIV, STDs, radiation therapy, or foreign body (Box 53.1).

Patients with anal abscess typically present with the indolent onset of a constant, throbbing anal pain associated with localized swelling, erythema, and fluctuance. Perianal abscess can be differentiated from other causes of acute anal pain such as anal fissure and thrombosed external hemorrhoid by history and gentle examination. Thorough digital rectal examination or anoscopic examination is often deferred in the acute setting owing to pain. A common error is diagnosing "cellulitis" when patients present with pain, erythema, and tenderness, but are not found to have fluctuance. The vast majority of these patients simply have a deeper abscess, making the need for drainage even more compelling; antibiotics alone in this situation are usually inappropriate. If the diagnosis is in question, imaging with a pelvic CT or examination under anesthesia should be considered.

Perianal abscess should be treated promptly by incision and drainage.[13] This can be done either in an ambulatory setting under local anesthesia or in the operating room as appropriate. The drainage should be performed starting at the most fluctuant aspect of the abscess, staying as close to the anus as possible to shorten the length of any subsequent fistula track. The size of the incision should be generous and tailored to the size of the abscess. This is accomplished by probing the cavity with the examining finger or an instrument to assess its extent. A cruciate incision with subsequent removal of the corners is a reliable way to assure adequate drainage. Loculations within the abscess cavity may be carefully broken up to achieve adequate drainage of the entire cavity. The practice of aggressive digital disruption of loculations, however, should be avoided as this maneuver may cause injury to the sphincter complex or pudendal nerve. If the abscess cavity is larger than 5 cm, one may consider placing counterincisions and bridge them with penrose drains. This technique avoids large gaping perineal wounds that may result in prolonged healing, scarring, and distortion of the perianal anatomy. An alternative to a wide incision and drainage is inserting a drainage catheter that can be left in place for several weeks until the abscess resolves, and then removed in the outpatient setting.

Packing of the abscess cavity is a common but usually unnecessary practice, as it often causes misery associated with the ongoing need to remove and replace gauze into a fresh, tender wound. However, packing may be necessary in selected patients at the time of abscess drainage to provide hemostasis of the inflamed, hypervascular abscess cavity. A well-drained abscess cavity typically does not require wet-to-dry dressing changes to achieve debridement and prevent premature closure of the skin. Further, patients can unwittingly retain the packing in the abscess cavity for days or weeks, despite being instructed to remove it.

A well-drained perirectal abscess does not typically require treatment with antibiotics, as they have not been shown to improve healing times or reduce the recurrence rate.[14] Antibiotics should be considered for patients with high-risk conditions such as immunosuppression, diabetes, extensive cellulitis, prosthetic devices, and high-risk cardiac, valvular, and related anatomical conditions.[13] Following successful drainage of the abscess, the patient may be instructed to use warm sitz baths, bulk-forming fiber supplements, and analgesics only for break-through pain. Oozing usually subsides within a few days, but drainage is to be expected to continue for 1 to 2 weeks as the cavity heals. The wound is typically expected to completely heal within 6 weeks. Surgical follow-up is recommended because the abscess may recur in about 10% of patients and development of a chronic fistula-in-ano occurs in up to 50% of patients.[15]

Fistula-in-ano results from persistent communication between the anal canal (internal opening) and perianal skin (external opening) following spontaneous or surgical drainage of a perianal abscess. Patients often report a cyclical pattern of pain and swelling, followed by drainage associated with relief of the symptoms. Physical examination usually identifies one or more external openings

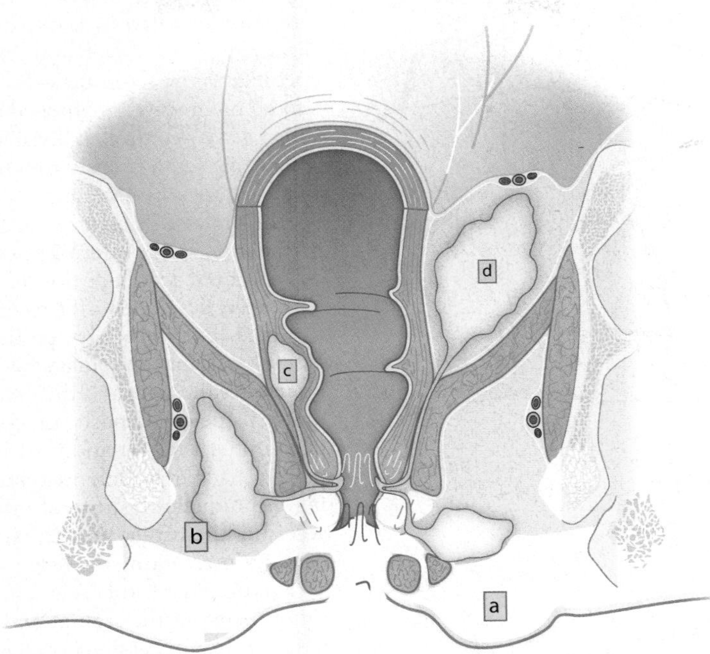

FIG. 53.9 Common extensions of anorectal abscesses: *(a)* superficial perianal, *(b)* ischiorectal, *(c)* intersphincteric, and *(d)* supralevator. (From McAneny D. Anorectal Disorders. In Noble J, ed: *Textbook of Primary Care Medicine*. 3rd ed. Philadelphia, PA: Mosby, 2001.)

BOX 53.1 Etiology of anorectal abscess.

- Nonspecific etiology
  - Cryptoglandular
- Specific etiology
  - Inflammatory condition
    - Crohn disease
    - Tuberculosis
    - Actinomycosis
    - Lymphogranuloma venereum
  - Traumatic etiology
    - Impalement
    - Foreign body
    - Anal fissure
    - Iatrogenic
    - Episiotomy
    - Hemorrhoidectomy
    - Prostatectomy
    - Radiation
  - Malignancy
    - Rectal or anal carcinoma
    - Leukemia
    - Lymphoma

with or without granulation tissue. Multiple external openings, or a so-called "watering can perineum," should trigger suspicion of perianal Crohn disease. Occasionally, the external opening may be subtle or located at a considerable distance from the anus. Careful inspection of the perianal region with gentle palpation searching for a cord-like subcutaneous structure can help to identify the course of the fistula track. The patient can often assist with identification of the fistula opening by pointing to the location of pain and drainage. If the course of the fistulous track remains unclear, a pelvic MRI can be useful in identifying the location of the primary and secondary openings and delineate the anatomy of the fistula tracks.

Fistula-in-ano can be classified as: intersphincteric, transsphincteric, suprasphincteric, and extrasphincteric based on the Parks classification (Fig. 53.10) The goals for treatment of an anal fistula are: (1) eliminate the septic focus, (2) remove or ablate epithelialized tracts, (3) avoid or minimize the risk of fecal incontinence, and (4) prevent recurrence. There is a progressive tradeoff between the extent of operative intervention and continence impairment stemming from sphincter division.[16] Preoperative planning should take into account preexisting incontinence, stool consistency, history of sphincter injury or surgery, the amount of sphincter that may need to be divided, anterior location in females, and the patient's attitude towards potential imperfections in continence.

Intraoperative evaluation begins with identification of the fistula tracks. Goodsall rule can be used as guide to predict the course of the fistula track and location of the internal opening (Fig. 53.11). Fistulas with an external opening anterior to the anus typically track in a radial fashion directly into the anal canal, except for those located at a distance greater than 3 cm from the anal verge; this usually indicates an anterior extension of a horseshoe

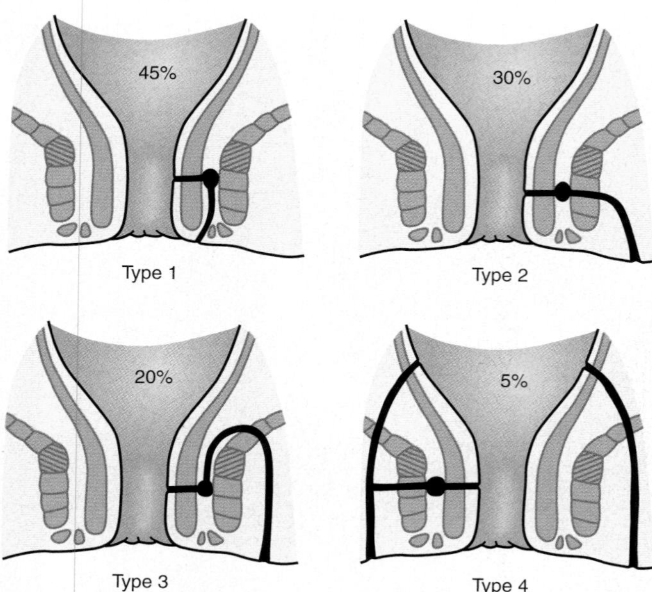

FIG. 53.10 Park classification of fistula-in ano: type 1, intersphincteric; type 2, transsphincteric; type 3, suprasphincteric; and type 4, extrasphincteric.

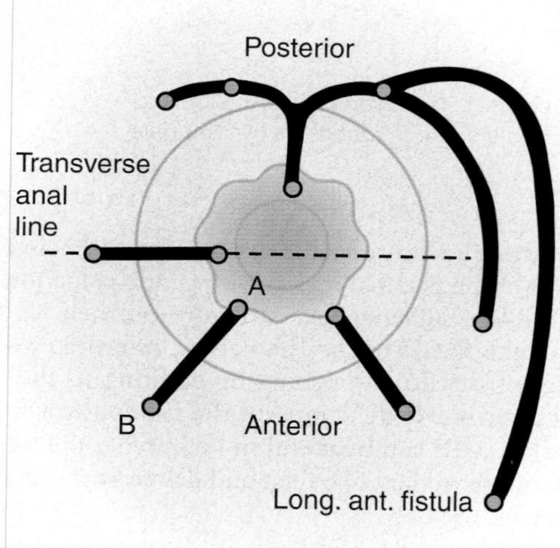

FIG. 53.11 Goodsall rule of fistula-in-ano tracks extension.

fistula originating posteriorly. Fistulas with an external opening posterior to the anus often track in a curvilinear fashion to a posterior midline internal opening.

Anoscopy allows direct inspection of the dentate line and may reveal an erythematous crypt or a visible internal opening. In the operating room, an anal fistula probe may be passed gently through the external opening into the fistula tract and through the internal opening to demonstrate the anatomy. The external opening can also be injected with dilute hydrogen peroxide, methylene blue, or milk when identification of the internal opening of the fistula in the anal canal is challenging. The anorectal mucosa should be evaluated to exclude a different origin of the perianal sepsis such as Crohn disease, atypical ulcers, or cancer.

Simple short fistulas may be treated by lay-open fistulotomy (Fig. 53.12). These incisions heal well, and derangements in fecal continence are uncommon. The recurrence rate for treatment of simple anal fistulas with fistulotomy is 2% to 8% with functional impairment generally between 0% and 17%.[16-18] In fistulas involving larger amounts of sphincter muscle, the initial treatment is often focused on controlling the fistula with a draining seton using a silastic vessel loop or a rubber band (Fig. 53.13). This allows formation of a narrow fistula track and prevents the recurrent cyclical symptoms of pain and drainage from closure of the external opening, as the seton provides continuous drainage. A seton can also be progressively tightened and used in a cutting manner, enabling a slow controlled division of the fistula track; alternatively, the cutting seton may shorten the tract over time and allowing for a safe lay open fistulotomy.

The preferred treatment of anal fistulas would ideally result in obliteration of the internal opening and all associated tracts without the need to divide any of the sphincter. Several techniques have been developed over recent years in the hopes of achieving this goal, but none have proven to provide a reliable cure. The fistula track may be plugged with a bioresorbable substance that obliterates the tract and theoretically provides a scaffold on which native tissue can deposit collagen and seal the fistula tract. Fibrin glue and several variations of fistula plugs have been developed but have achieved only marginal long-term success. The promising technique of ligation of intersphincteric fistula tract involves accessing the fistula tract through the intersphincteric plane and ligating/interrupting the fistula track (Fig. 53.14).[19]

Rectovaginal fistula is an abnormal epithelial-lined communication between the rectum and vagina. The spectrum of presentation is from occasional passage of flatus to continuous drainage of stool through the vagina, causing marked irritation and embarrassing symptoms. Rectovaginal fistulas may be caused by childbirth, as a result of prolonged labor with necrosis of the rectovaginal septum, obstetric injury with a third- or fourth-degree perineal tear, or episiotomy.[20,21] Breakdown of the repair of a third or fourth degree tear or infection can result in fistula development. Cryptoglandular anorectal abscesses and Bartholin gland infections may spontaneously drain through the rectovaginal septum, causing a low rectovaginal fistula.

Rectovaginal fistulas may be the result of iatrogenic injury such as a stapled colorectal anastomosis that incorporates vaginal wall or occur as a result of a colorectal anastomotic leak complicated by an abscess that drains into the vagina. Crohn disease may be associated with rectovaginal fistula as it may causes transmural inflammation of the anorectal wall with extension into the rectovaginal septum. Less common causes of rectovaginal fistulas include fecal impaction, viral and bacterial infections in patients with HIV, and trauma due to sexual assault. Diverticular disease is the most common infectious cause of a high colovaginal fistula and is discussed elsewhere. Malignancies, particularly anal cancer, may present as a rectovaginal fistula. In some patients, a fistula develops following radiation therapy. If suspicion for an undiagnosed malignancy is present, biopsy of the fistula should be performed.

Definitive surgical repair of a low rectovaginal fistula is typically recommended 3 to 6 months after onset to decrease the inflammation in surrounding tissues and enable a successful repair. A draining seton, antibiotics, or fecal diversion may be necessary depending on the size, location, and etiology of the fistula. Some fistulas may even close spontaneously during this time of expectant management. The most popular method of surgical repair is an endoanal sliding advancement flap. This repair involves excision of the fistula tract and closure of the rectal portion of the fistula with a vascularized mucosal flap (Fig. 53.15). A flap containing mucosa, submucosa, and circular muscle fibers is advanced to cover

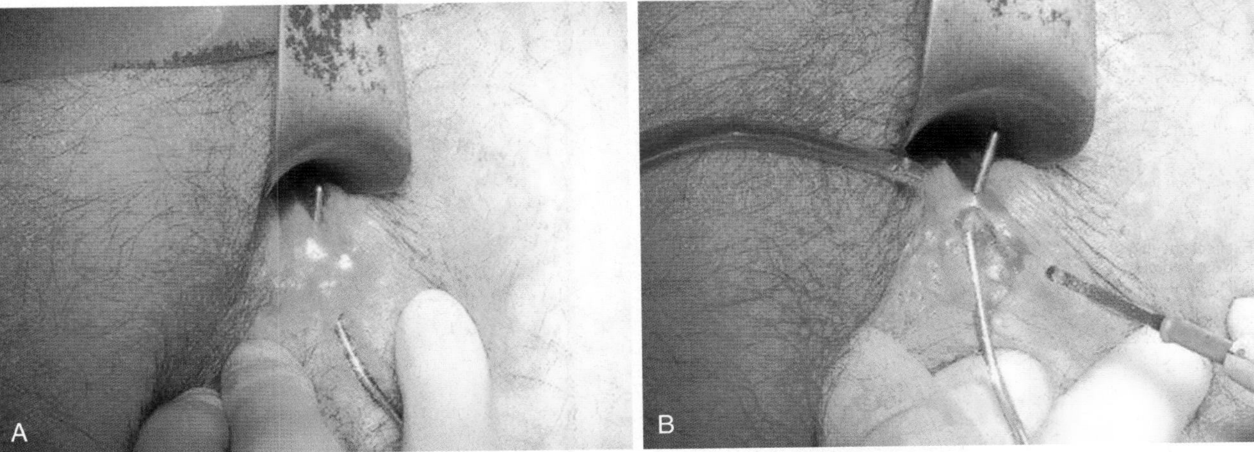

FIG. 53.12 (A) Lay-open fistulotomy. Fistula probe inserted through the fistula track. (B) Incision over the fistula probe to lay-open fistula track.

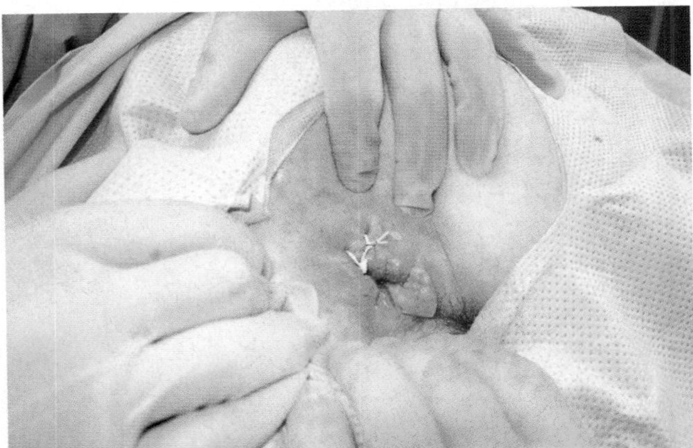

FIG. 53.13 Setons placed through fistula-in-ano tracks.

the anorectal side of the fistula (Fig 53.16). Success rates vary from 29% to 100%.[22] This procedure is well tolerated by patients and can be repeated if the initial repair is unsuccessful. Many other techniques have been used with success, depending on the etiology and anatomy of the fistula and the presence of a concomitant sphincter defect. These include labial fat pad interposition (Martius flap), episioproctotomy with sphincter interposition/reconstruction, and gracilis interposition. Other approaches for treatment of rectovaginal fistula have included the use of a bioprosthetic fistula plugs and the ligation of intersphincteric fistula tract procedure, but the outcomes of these techniques in patients with rectovaginal fistula have been disappointing.

Pilonidal Sinus

Pilonidal disease is a common anorectal problem affecting young people, typically in their middle to late 20s, with a reported incidence of 26 cases per 100,000 people. As the Latin origin of the name suggests—hair (pilus) and nest (nidus)—pilonidal disease is caused by shed hair drawn into the natal cleft by motion from the buttocks. This motion creates a vacuum effect forcing hair into the skin through the pits in the midline. The foreign body reaction produced by trapped hair may lead to a hair-filled abscess cavity (Fig. 53.17). The abscess can drain spontaneously through the skin or back through the sinus tracts. Men are at higher risk because they tend to be more hirsute. Other associations with pilonidal disease are obesity (37%), sedentary occupation (44%) and local irritation or trauma (34%).[23] While some patients are asymptomatic, the majority of patients will initially present with an acute abscess cephalad to the natal cleft. The location of the abscess is distinctly different from a perirectal abscess, which is typically found near the anus. The presence of sinus openings along the midline of the natal cleft 4 to 8 cm from the anus is the hallmark finding in pilonidal disease.

Treatment of pilonidal disease should be tailored to the severity of the disease. It may range from simple incision and drainage to wide excision with extensive reconstructive procedures. Simple pilonidal sinus in a patient with mild symptoms can be treated by laying open the tract. Acute pilonidal abscesses can be treated with incision and drainage. A lateral incision avoiding the midline should be made over the cavity whenever possible, to facilitate the healing of the wound. The cavity should also be thoroughly curetted, removing all of the embedded hair and devitalized tissue. The surrounding skin of the buttock, lower back and perianal region should meticulously depilated at the time of operation and maintained hair free. Trimming, shaving, waxing, or laser depilation have been shown to be effective in preventing recurrence.[24]

The importance of avoiding midline incisions was popularized by Bascom who advocated lateral incision over the sinus cavity, together with excision of the midline pits and sinus tracts.[25] The incision is left open with a light dressing to heal by secondary intention. In chronic or recurrent pilonidal sinuses, a more extensive excision of skin and subcutaneous tissue may be necessary for definitive treatment. These wounds may be left open with healing by secondary intention, closed off midline with a flap, or managed with negative pressure dressings. Complex or recurrent pilonidal disease my require transposition of healthy, well-vascularized tissue to close the defect. Several reconstructive techniques have been proposed to cover the defect including Z-plasty, rhomboid flap, V-to-Y advancement flap, and Limberg flap (Fig. 53.18). Antibiotics may be an important adjunct in surgical treatment of pilonidal disease as bacterial colonization was found to range from 50% to 70%, with typical isolates including *Staphylococcus aureus* and anaerobes such as *Bacteroides*.

Sexually Transmitted Diseases

Anorectal STDs are commonly the result of anoreceptive intercourse but may also be attributed to contiguous spread from a

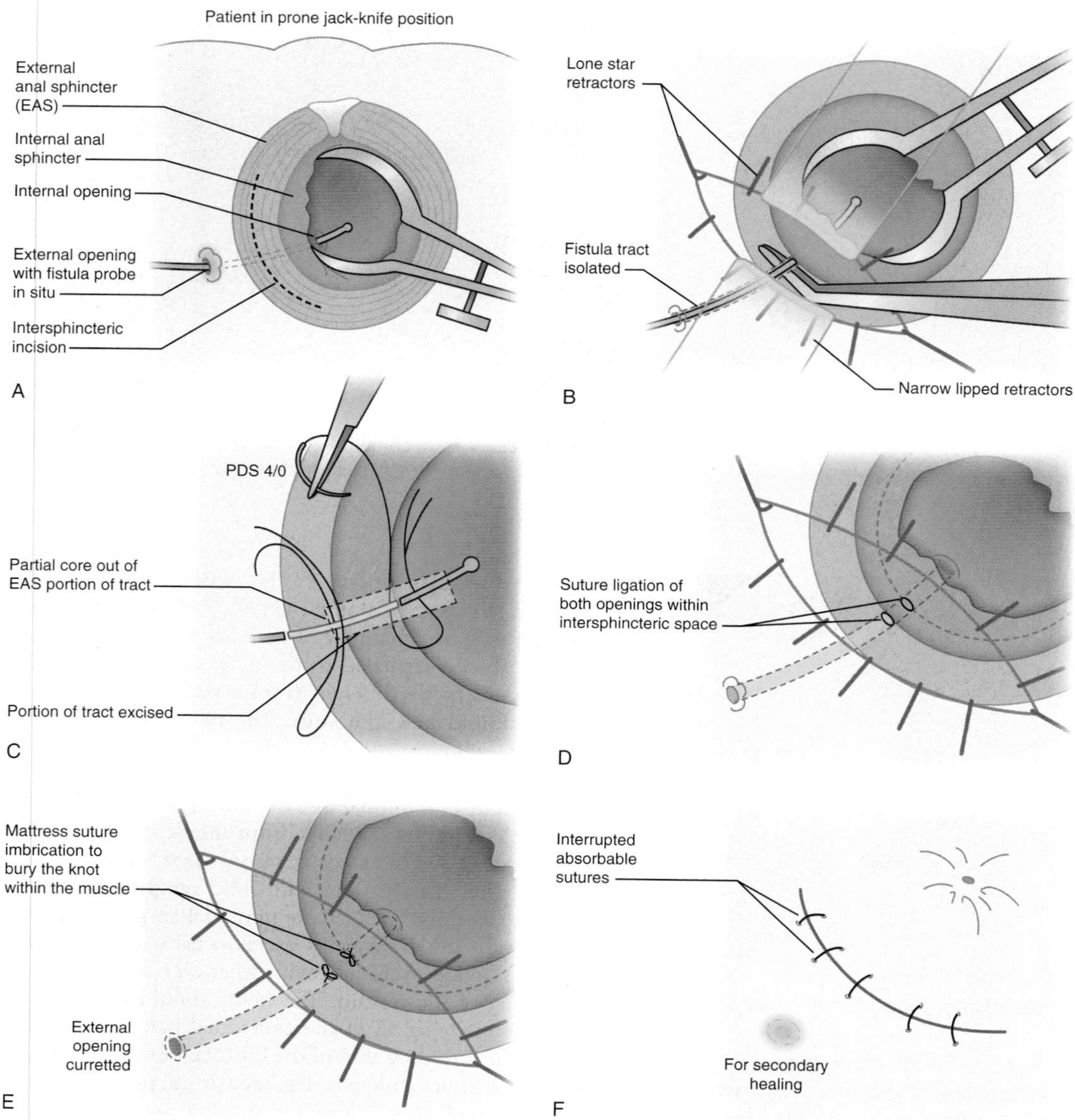

FIG. 53.14 Ligation of intersphincteric fistula tract (LIFT) procedure. (A) Fistula probe inserted into the fistula track: internal opening and external opening. (B) Intersphincteric plane is opened and fistula track identified within the intersphincteric space. (C) Fistula track is divided within intersphincteric space. (D) Both ends of divided track are suture-ligated. (E) Sphincter muscle fibers are approximated to obliterate the intersphincteric space. (F) Perianal skin is closed. (From Koh SZ, Tsang CB. The LIFT procedure. *Seminars in Colon and Rectal Surgery.* 2014;25:190–199.)

genital infection. The incidence of anorectal STDs has been increasing likely due to the increase in the practice of anal receptive intercourse. Both men who have sex with men (MSM) and heterosexual couples who engage in anal receptive intercourse are at increased risk. Transmission may occur through a variety of sexual practices, such as anoreceptive intercourse and oroanal sexual contact. Symptoms of STDs are often nonspecific and latent, with some infected individuals being completely asymptomatic. Complaints may include anal pain, tenesmus, urgency, purulent drainage, and bleeding. When evaluating a patient with an anorectal complaint, it is important to keep the diagnosis of STD in the differential when abnormalities such as ulcerations, vegetations, and proctitis are seen on examination (Table 53.2).

Human papillomavirus (HPV) is the most common STD in the United States, with 5.5 million new infections occurring every year. The classic lesion is the condyloma acuminatum or anal wart. Serotypes 6 and 11 are found in benign warts, while serotypes 16 and 18 are more commonly seen in dysplasia and malignancies.[26] Anal HPV is transmitted by anoreceptive intercourse and may be associated with immunosuppression caused by HIV infection or antirejection medications. The use of condoms lowers the risk of sexual transmission, although infection can be transmitted through the skin beyond the area covered by a condom. Symptoms include the presence of raised wart-like lesions, rectal bleeding or discharge, pain, and anal itching. Anoscopy may reveal extension of the disease into the anal canal. An aggressive variant of HPV infection, Buschke-Lowenstein disease, results in a giant condyloma. Anal condyloma can be treated by topical agents such as imiquimod, podophyllin, and 5-fluorouracil (5-FU) or surgical methods such as tangential excision, cryotherapy, and fulguration

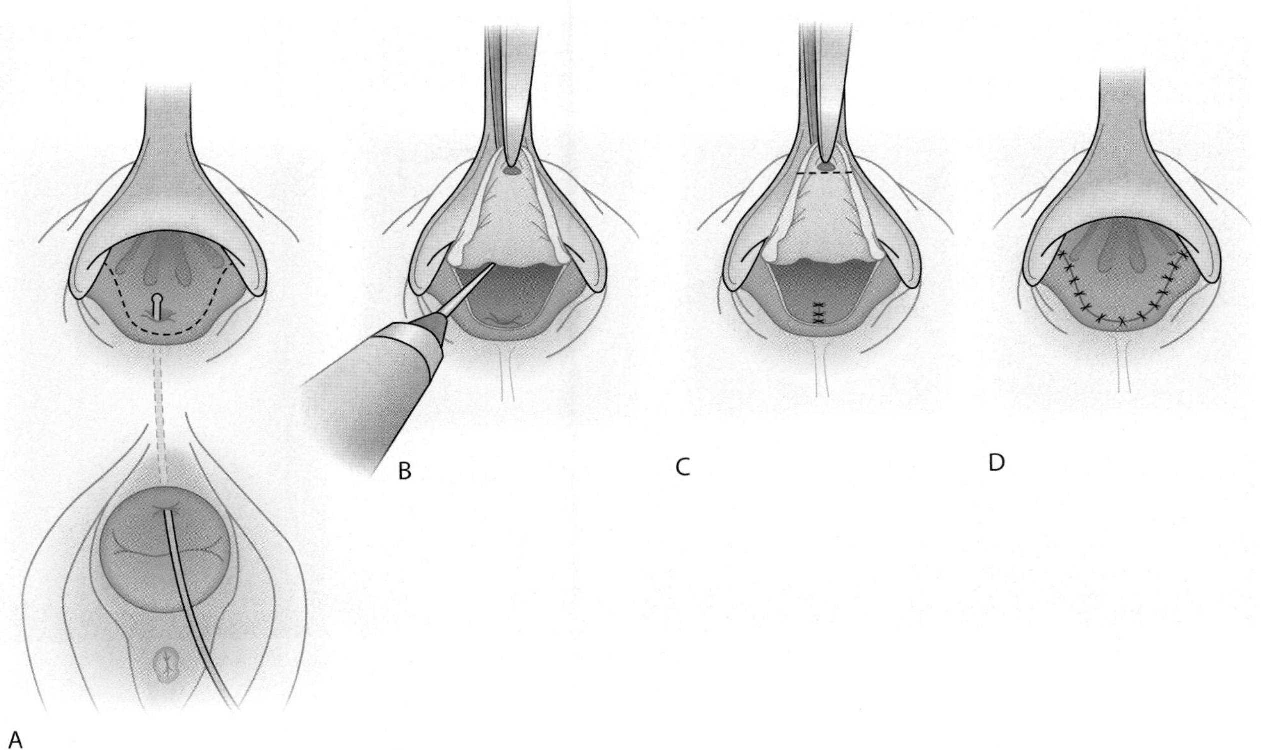

FIG. 53.15 Mucosal advancement flap for repair of a rectovaginal fistula. (A) Fistula probe inserted to identify fistula track. (B) Broad-based flap is raised. (C) Fistula opening is excised from the tip of the flap. (D) Flap is sutured in place.

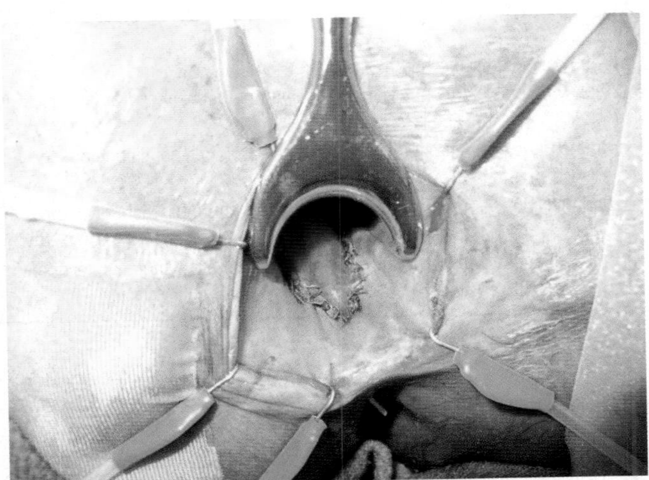

FIG. 53.16 Appearance of the mucosal advancement flap at the conclusion of the procedure.

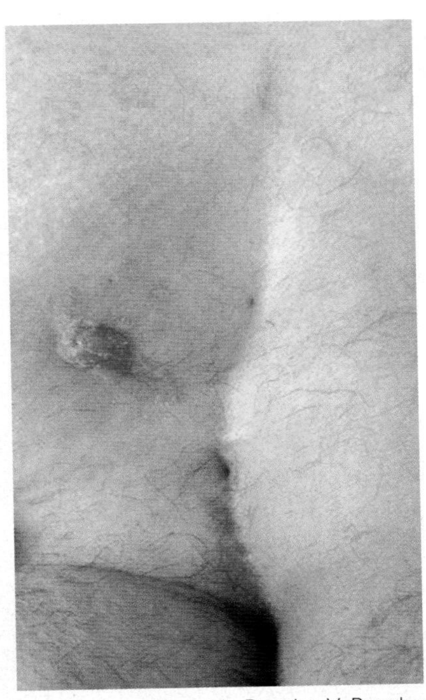

FIG. 53.17 Pilonidal sinus. (From de Parades V, Bouchard D, Janier M, et al: Pilonidal sinus disease. *J Visc Surg* 150:237-247, 2013.)

(Fig. 53.19). The clearance rate following surgical removal ranges from 60% to 90%, with recurrence rates of 20% to 30%.[27]

Herpes simplex virus is highly prevalent in the United States. Herpes simplex virus proctitis is commonly associated with the symptoms of anorectal pain, constipation, tenesmus, anal itching, difficulty with initiating urination, fever, and inguinal adenopathy.[28] Typical lesions are small vesicles that involve the perianal skin and anal canal but may also extend to the rectum. Treatment is with acyclovir, famciclovir, or valacyclovir for 7 to 10 days.

Gonorrhea is transmitted by anoreceptive intercourse with an infected partner. Rectal gonorrhea is often latent with 84% of MSM found to have rectal gonorrhea being asymptomatic.[29] Symptoms may include pruritus ani, constipation, mucopurulent or bloody anal discharge, pain, and tenesmus.[30] On anoscopic examination, the rectal mucosa can appear normal or erythematous

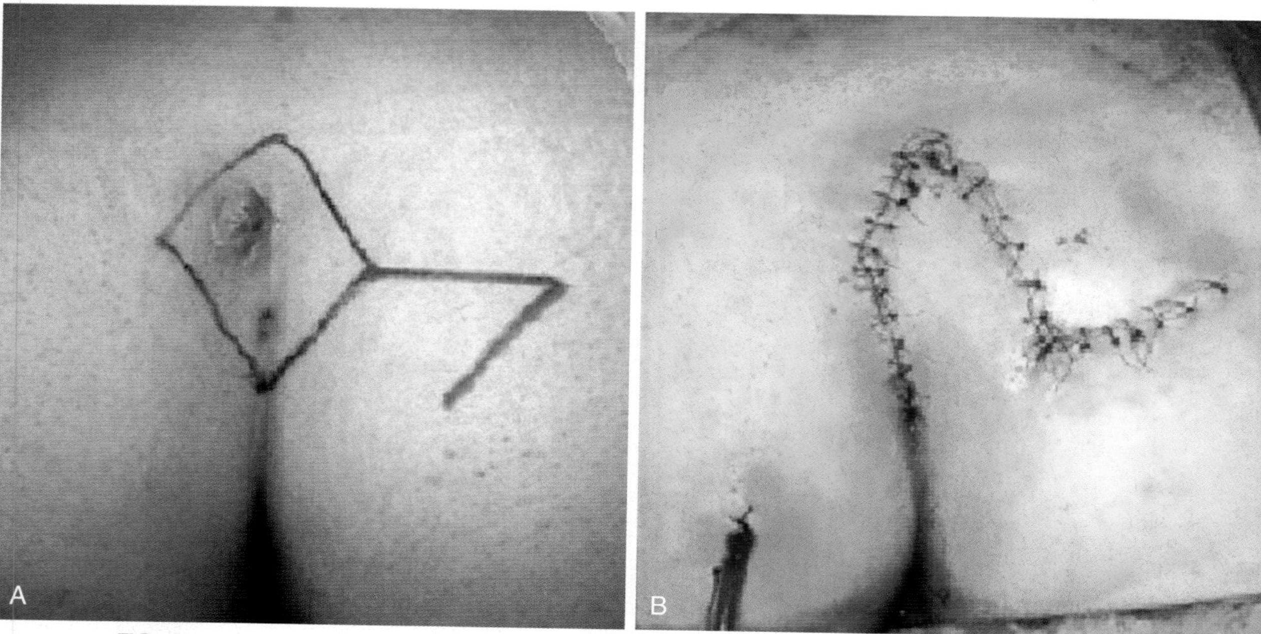

FIG. 53.18 Limberg flap. (A) Initial marking of a proposed incision. (B) Completed rotation of the flap.

TABLE 53.2 Etiology and symptoms of sexually transmitted proctitis.

ORGANISM	COMMON SIGNS AND SYMPTOMS
Gonorrhoea	Asymptomatic. If symptoms present: pruritus ani, constipation, mucopurulent anal discharge, rectal pain, and tenesmus
Chlamydia	Asymptomatic. If symptoms present: pruritus ani, mucous discharge, anal pain
Chlamydia (lymphogranuloma venereum)	Generalized illness: fever and malaise. Anal symptoms: purulent or bloody discharge. Anal pain and tenesmus. May mimic inflammatory bowel disease
Syphilis	Primary: anorectal chancre commonly asymptomatic. If symptomatic: pain or discomfort, itching, bleeding, and/or tenesmus.
	Secondary: ulcers and mucous patches. Perianal condylomata lata. Generalized manifestations: rash, fever, and lymphadenopathy
Herpes simplex virus	Vesicular lesions, severe pain, and tenesmus; difficulty with bowel movements. Generalized symptoms: fever and lymphadenopathy

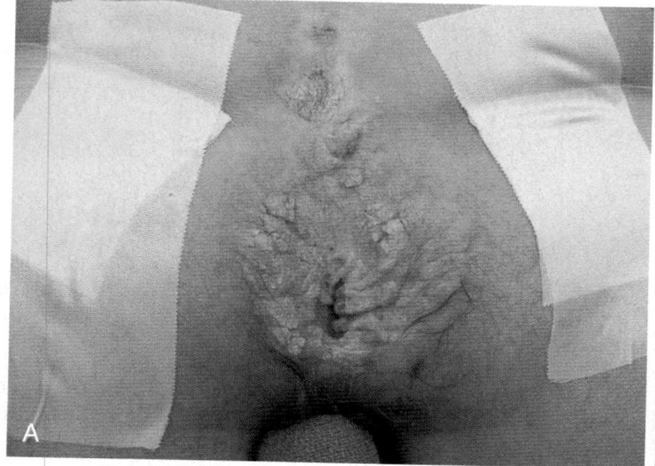

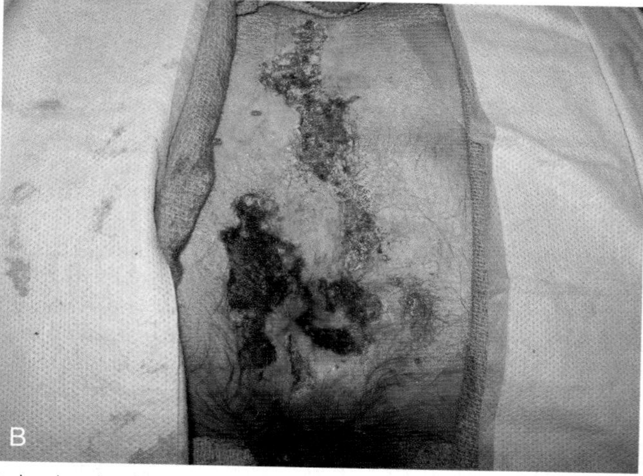

FIG. 53.19 (A) Extensive anal condyloma. (B) Perianal region following ablation of condyloma.

and friable with pus. Treatment is directed towards both gonorrhea and chlamydia, even if chlamydia testing is negative. The recommended regimen is ceftriaxone 250 mg in a single intramuscular dose plus azithromycin 1 g orally in a single dose, or doxycycline 100 mg orally twice daily for 7 days.

Chlamydial infection can cause a mild form of proctitis, but infections are commonly asymptomatic. On physical examination, the rectal mucosa can range from normal-appearing to erythematous and friable. Patients occasionally present with perirectal abscesses, anal fissures, and fistula formation mimicking Crohn disease. Recommended treatment is with azithromycin 1 g orally in a single dose or doxycycline 100 mg orally twice a day for 7 days.

Anorectal syphilis appears within 2 to 10 weeks of exposure following anal intercourse. Infections can be asymptomatic or manifest with proctitis, ulcers, and pseudotumors. Anal ulcers are frequently painful, in contrast to genital ulcers. Anal lesions usually heal within several weeks even if untreated. Secondary syphilis may present with a rectal mass, condylomata lata and mucous patches, generalized rash, fever, and lymphadenopathy. Tertiary syphilis presents many years later, commonly with debilitating ulcerating gummas. Primary or secondary syphilis is treated with benzathine penicillin G 2.4 million units intramuscularly in a single dose. Doxycyline, tetracycline, and possibly ceftriaxone can be used in patients with penicillin allergy.

HIV infection is a common contributing factor to STDs and may result in certain HIV-specific anorectal disorders. Idiopathic anal ulcers in HIV can be diagnosed after ruling out STDs and cancer. Clinical characteristics include a broad-based appearance, localization to the posterior midline, and more proximally in the anal canal erosion into the submucosa and sphincters with decreased anal sphincter tone. Treatment is with intralesional steroid injection and/or surgical debridement.

Anorectal Kaposi sarcoma presents with characteristic small, round, purple lesions and can be easily mistaken for hemorrhoids or other benign lesions. Diagnosis is confirmed with biopsy. Treatment with highly active antiretroviral therapy can induce rapid regression of the disease. Intralesional chemotherapy and radiation are associated with lesion regression, improved cosmesis, and palliation. Systemic chemotherapy is offered to patients with advanced or rapidly progressing disease.

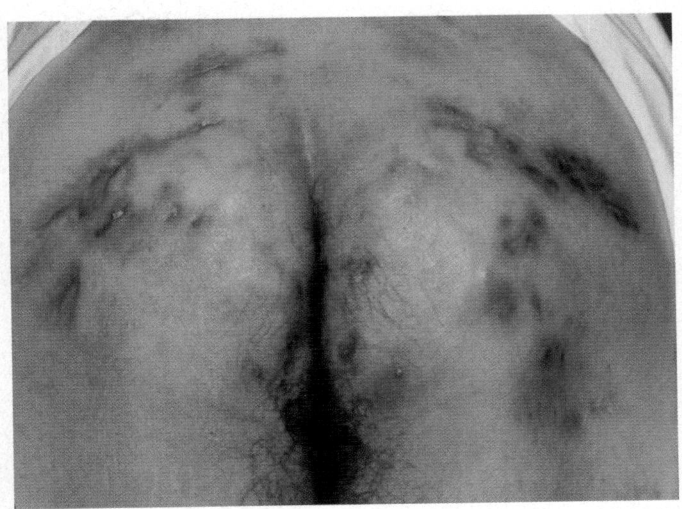

FIG. 53.20 Hidradenitis suppurativa.

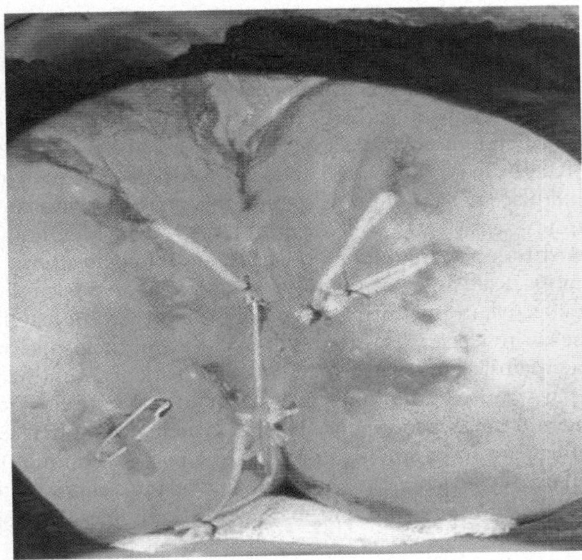

FIG. 53.21 Perianal Crohn disease with extensive fistulas.

Hidradenitis Suppurativa

Hidradenitis suppurativa (HS) is a chronic recurrent inflammatory skin disorder with chronically draining wounds and sinus tracks that can affect the hair and apocrine sweat glands bearing areas of the axillae, perineum, and inframammary regions.[31] Perineal disease is more commonly seen in men. HS typically occurs after puberty, with an incidence peaking between the second and fourth decades of life. The disease is thought to result from occlusion of the apocrine glands or the hair follicular duct. This results in stasis and dilatation of the apocrine gland followed by bacterial superinfection. When the glands rupture into the subcutaneous space, abscesses are formed that may lead to complex subcutaneous sinuses and draining tracks (Fig. 53.20). Longstanding inflammation may result in subcutaneous scarring, contractures, and chronic induration of the skin. Perianal HS may extend on to the buttocks, upper thighs and medially to the dentate line. While perianal HS should be differentiated from cryptoglandular abscess and fistula, HS may coexist with other inflammatory disorders such as Crohn disease.[32]

The differential diagnosis may be challenging, but the distribution of disease, characteristic subcutaneous "pitlike" scarring, distorting contractures, and induration of the skin should be considered pathognomonic for advanced HS. Treatment is based on the stage of disease at presentation and ranges from medical therapy (antibiotics, antiandrogens, and immunosuppression) to more invasive procedures where total excision of all effected apocrine sweat gland areas may be required.

Perianal Crohn Disease

Perianal Crohn disease typically manifests with fistula-in-ano, anal fissure, anal canal stricture, rectovaginal fistula, or abscess. It affects as many as 80% of patients with Crohn disease, depending on the criteria for diagnosis, as many patients have innocent findings such as simple skin tags that may or may not be true manifestations of the disease. Even though the majority of patients present with perianal disease after the diagnosis of Crohn disease has already been established, some patients may initially present with perianal disease. The diagnosis of Crohn disease should be considered in those patients who have complex fistulas, especially located bilaterally, large "elephant ear" type skin tags, or those with broad based anal fissures perhaps located off the midline (Fig. 53.21). A history of chronic diarrhea will also increase the level of suspicion in

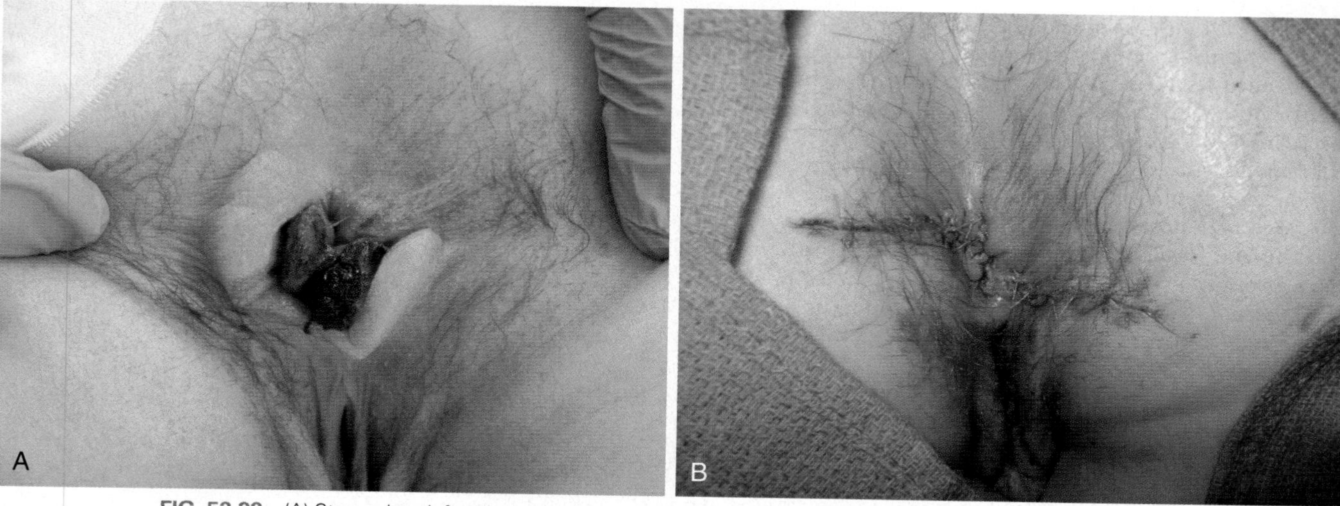

FIG. 53.22 (A) Strangulated, fourth-degree internal hemorrhoids. (B) Perianal region following urgent excision of strangulated internal hemorrhoids.

patients with atypical fissures/fistulas. Colonoscopy with ileal intubation will usually be sufficient to make the diagnosis.

The evaluation of patients with anorectal Crohn should include a careful anorectal examination and may be supplemented by MRI. The first priority is to drain any associated abscess with or without placement of draining setons. This should provide control of perineal sepsis and enable medical therapy, which typically includes antibiotics, immunomodulators, and biologic agents. The antitumor necrosis factor-α antibody, infliximab, has been shown to be effective in preventing the progression of Crohn fistulizing disease or, in select cases, may result in closure of the fistula track.

The mainstay of management in these patients is indwelling draining setons. Fistulotomy may result in a nonhealing rectal wound and cause incontinence in these patients who often suffer with frequent, loose stools. Asymptomatic tags are common and should usually be left alone. Anovaginal fistula presents a particularly challenging problem and may require early fecal diversion. An attempt at endoanal mucosal advancement flap repair is often appropriate when the rectal mucosa appears to be relatively healthy. Anal strictures are typically located at the top of anorectal ring and may be dilated if symptomatic. This can be done either by gentle dilation with an examining finger, self-dilation using anal dilators in an outpatient setting or dilation under anesthesia. In a long-standing perianal Crohn disease, malignancy may develop and requires a high index of suspicion in patients with long-standing disease and unusual appearing fistulas, strictures, or ulcerations.

Anorectal Emergencies

Even though the majority of anorectal maladies can be treated electively, there are several conditions that deserve special mention as they may require urgent attention and, if not treated in an expeditious fashion, may result in severe complications, permanent functional impairment, or worse.

Fourth-Degree Hemorrhoids

Patients with strangulated or acutely thrombosed internal hemorrhoids may present with severely painful and irreducible hemorrhoids. If the presentation is delayed, incarcerated hemorrhoids may become necrotic and drain bloody or malodorous material (Fig. 53.22). Patients who present with fourth degree hemorrhoids, but without compromised tissue, may be admitted for a trial of pain control, warm baths, and bowel management. The goal of this treatment is to allow resolution of the acute crisis so that a less invasive treatment modality such as hemorrhoid banding can be performed at a later time once swelling has subsided. However, patients who fail a limited trial of nonoperative management or those with strangulation and necrosis, require prompt operation. Manual reduction of the strangulated hemorrhoids should generally not be attempted in this setting. In patients suffering from circumferential fourth degree hemorrhoids with extensive thrombosis and inflammation, the anal canal is markedly distorted; special attention must be paid to anatomical planes, internal sphincter preservation, and meticulous hemostasis. Unless the tissue is necrotic, mucosa and anoderm should be preserved as much as possible to prevent postoperative anal stricture, which is a very real risk in this setting.

Fournier Gangrene

Fournier gangrene (FG) is a rare but life-threatening condition. It is a fulminant form of necrotizing fasciitis of the perineal, genital, or perianal regions, commonly affecting elderly men, but can also occur in women and children.[33] FG has been associated with diabetes, chronic alcohol abuse, and immunosuppression, although it can occur in healthy patients without significant comorbidities. The inciting focus is usually located in the genitourinary tract, or perianal region/skin. Bacterial infection results in microthrombosis of the small subcutaneous vessels leading to the development of gangrene of the overlying skin. FG is typically associated with a mixed flora, both aerobic and anaerobic. Cultures from the wounds commonly show Klebsiella, streptococci, staphylococci, clostridia, *Bacteroides*, and corynebacteria.

FG initially starts as an area of cellulitis at the initial focus of infection in the perineum or perianal region. The local signs and symptoms may include intense pain and swelling. Crepitus of the inflamed tissues is a common feature because of the presence of gas forming organisms. As the subcutaneous inflammation worsens, necrotic patches appear over the overlying skin and progress to more extensive necrosis (Fig. 53.23). The patient is likely to demonstrate signs of severe systemic illness, usually out of proportion to the local extent of the disease that may be appreciated on physical examination.

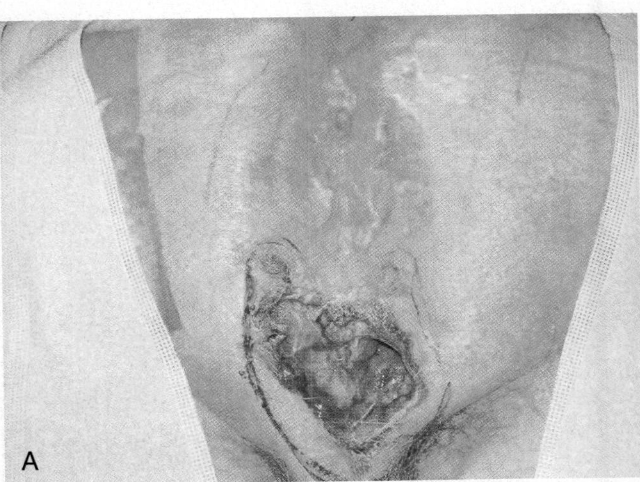

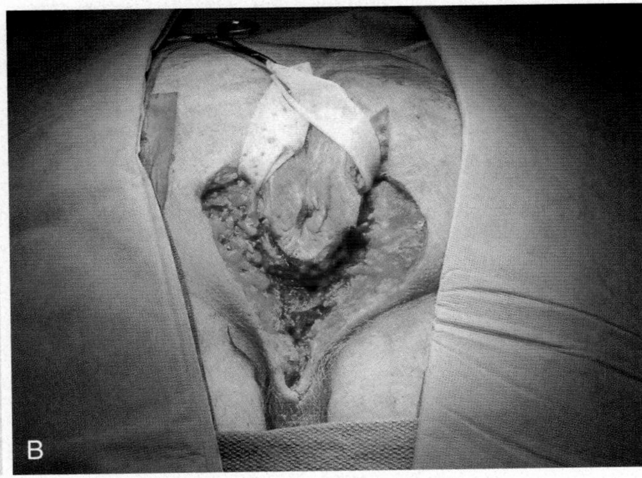

FIG. 53.23 (A) Fournier gangrene. (B) Perineum following excision of Fournier gangrene.

FG is a surgical emergency: it is usually rapidly progressive and quickly leads to sepsis, potentially with multiple organ failure and even death. Spread of infection occurs along the facial planes and is usually far more extensive than initially anticipated based on external appearance. Necrotizing fasciitis can extend to involve the scrotum and penis and can spread through the anterior abdominal wall, up to the clavicles.[34] Urogenital infections tend to extend posteriorly along Bucks and Dartos fascia up to the Colles fascia, but are limited from the anal margin by the attachment of the Colles fascia to the perineal body. In contrast, anorectal sources of infection usually involve the perianal skin. The location and the spread of infection can serve as a guide to identifying the initial focus of infection. Regardless of the cause of FG, the testes are usually spared as the blood supply originates intraabdominally.

Treatment of FG requires an aggressive multimodal approach, including hemodynamic stabilization and broad-spectrum antibiotics; however, early aggressive surgical debridement should be commenced without delay. It must be emphasized that early surgical debridement is the cornerstone of treatment and, if delayed, may have a negative impact on prognosis. All nonviable and necrotic tissue must be excised until well-perfused healthy tissue is reached. As noted earlier, the full extent of the disease may be far greater than estimated by the areas of cutaneous involvement. Urinary or fecal diversion may be necessary depending on the location and degree of tissue loss but is seldom necessary at the initial debridement. Multiple trips to the operating room are typically required, with an average of 3 to 4 procedures before complete debridement can be achieved. Although the testes are usually spared in FG, orchiectomy may be required in up to 21% of patients.[35] The use of vacuum-assisted closure system dressings have markedly improved wound care in these patients and accelerate wound healing. Split thickness skin grafts appear to be the treatment of choice in covering perineal and scrotal skin defects, but more extensive tissue coverage techniques may be necessary to enable reconstruction down the line.

Immunocompromised States

Perianal infection in immunocompromised patients often present a diagnostic and therapeutic challenge. Patients who are unable to mount an inflammatory response due to severe immunosuppression or neutropenia may present with serious perianal infection without "abscess" or localized soft tissue infection. Immunocompromised patients with perianal sepsis should be given broad-spectrum antibiotics and carefully watched. Cross sectional imaging modalities such as CT scanning may be helpful to assess the need for operative intervention; examination under anesthesia with drainage and/or debridement may be required.

Horseshoe Abscess

Horseshoe ischiorectal abscess can result from the lateral spread of infection originating in the deep postanal space. If untreated, the infection can spread to the lower abdominal wall, scrotum, and perineum. Deep postanal space abscesses are almost always associated with a posterior midline fistula-in-ano, but the external openings can be located anteriorly or anywhere along the course of the horseshoe extension. Drainage of the deep postanal space can be achieved by a midline incision between the coccyx and the anus. A fistula tract should be identified, and the lower half of the internal sphincter may be divided (Hanley procedure) or a seton placed through the fistula track. Counter incisions are made over the bilateral ischiorectal fossae to allow for drainage of the anterior extensions of the abscess (Fig. 53.24).

Incarcerated Rectal Prolapse

Incarcerated rectal prolapse typically results from obstruction of venous return from the prolapsed rectum, leading to a bulky edematous rectum that cannot be reduced back into the anal canal. Mucosal ischemia and ulcerations commonly occur and may progress to full thickness necrosis of the rectum. Initial conservative methods should be aimed at reducing the edema by the liberal application of sugar to allow manual reduction of the prolapse. If the rectal prolapse cannot be reduced or there is rectal necrosis, the patient needs to be taken to the operating room without delay for a perineal rectosigmoidectomy (Altemeier procedure) (Fig. 53.25).

Pelvic Floor

Fecal incontinence is defined as involuntary (accidental) leakage of fecal material in anyone over the age of four years. A prevalence up to 12% has been reported. Obstetric injury is the most common cause of fecal incontinence.[36] Changes in rectal sensation or rectal compliance can result in urgency, diminished capacity of the rectum, and loss of fecal control. Conditions causing inflammation of the anorectum such as inflammatory bowel disease can result in urgency and incontinence. Medical conditions such as diabetes, diarrhea, obesity, neurologic diseases, and urinary

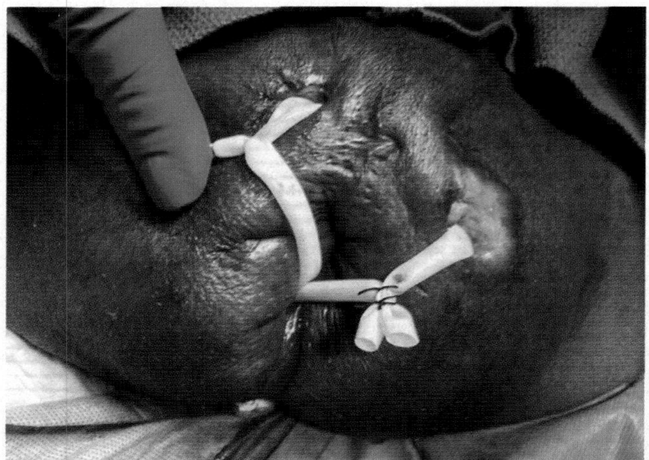

FIG. 53.24 Horseshoe abscess: incision and drainage.

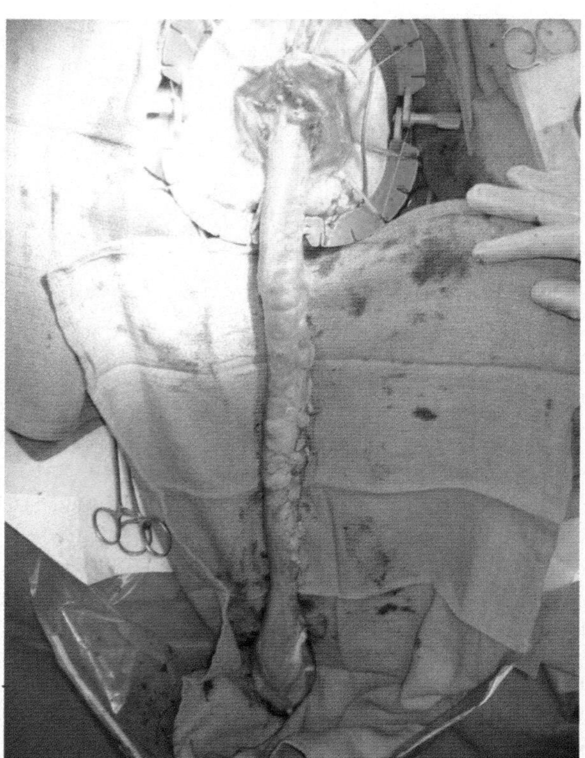

FIG. 53.25 Perineal proctosigmoidectomy (Altemeier procedure).

incontinence may result in, or contribute to, the symptoms of fecal incontinence.[37] A comprehensive evaluation of fecal incontinence includes a description of bowel habits including consistency of stools and frequency of bowel movements, type of incontinence (gas, liquid stool, solid stool, urge, passive, or postdefecation), associated urgency symptoms, awareness of incontinence versus complete lack of sensation, concomitant urinary incontinence, diet, and medications (Fig. 53.26). Colorectal cancer must be ruled out in those individuals with a recent change in bowel habits, particularly when blood per rectum is present. Patients should be asked about prior anal surgery, anal trauma or sexual instrumentation, prior radiation therapy, and systemic conditions such as diabetes and neurologic disease.

The physical examination should focus on the perineum and perianal region, evaluating for normal musculature, bulk of the perineal body, the perianal skin condition, and presence of any prolapsing tissue from the anus. Digital rectal examination evaluates resting tone of the anal canal and strength of the squeeze. Pelvic floor physiologic testing can be very helpful in patients when medical management has failed and in those being considered for surgical intervention. Initial management is typically focused on dietary modification; fiber supplementation is utilized to bulk and firm up stool consistency. Medical therapy may include antidiarrheal agents, such as loperamide, which can slow down transit time and decrease the frequency of loose stools.

Surgical intervention is usually reserved for highly selected patients in whom conservative management has failed. Anal sphincter repair can be beneficial in patients with anal sphincter disruption secondary to traumatic childbirth or prior anal surgery (Fig. 53.27). Although the majority of patients report improvement in continence shortly after surgery, long-term results and durability of the repair can be a problem. Sacral nerve stimulation (Medtronic, Minneapolis, MN, USA) has been successfully used in the treatment of fecal incontinence; although the mechanism of action is not entirely clear, patients report fewer episodes of incontinence and decreased urgency. Complications of sacral nerve stimulation include pain, infection, seroma formation, bleeding, and scarring.

Constipation is a common symptom accounting for 8 million annual visits to physicians in the United States. Constipation may occur because of a primary motor disorder involving the colon, rectum or anus, a defecation disorder, or as an adverse effect of medications. Initial management typically includes lifestyle changes, including increased intake of dietary fiber, fiber supplementation, increased fluid intake, and exercise (Fig. 53.28). Polyethylene glycol solutions are typically safe and effective when these measures are inadequate. Stimulant laxatives such as senna and bisacodyl may be used judiciously in those patients in whom lifestyle modification is inadequate. Prokinetics and secretagogues should be restricted to those not responding to simpler treatments.

Anorectal physiology testing and assessment of colorectal transit time are indicated if medical treatment fails and/or symptoms indicate severe slow transit or obstructed defecation. Barium or magnetic resonance evacuation proctography may be particularly helpful in the subset of patients with defecation disorders. Biofeedback therapy is often effective in patients with dyssynergic defecation, typically related to the failure of relaxation of the puborectalis muscle.

Surgery can be offered to some patients with severe constipation not responding to conservative treatment. Sacral nerve stimulation may alleviate symptoms of constipation in selected patients. The Malone antegrade colonic enema procedure with construction of a small stoma from the appendix can allow for colonic irrigations and cleansing.[38] Colectomy with ileorectal anastomosis is reserved for highly selected patients with severe colonic inertia and normal pelvic floor function, not responding to other methods of treatment. Ventral mesh rectopexy may address symptomatic rectocele and internal rectal intussusception. This technique involves mobilization of the rectum anteriorly without division of the lateral ligaments. The pelvic floor musculature and anterior aspect of rectum are suspended using a mesh sling sutured to the sacrum.

NEOPLASMS

Anal Intraepithelial Neoplasia

Anal intraepithelial neoplasia (AIN), previously known as Bowen disease, is characterized by dysplastic changes in the anal canal that are thought to be the precursor lesions to invasive anal carcinoma.

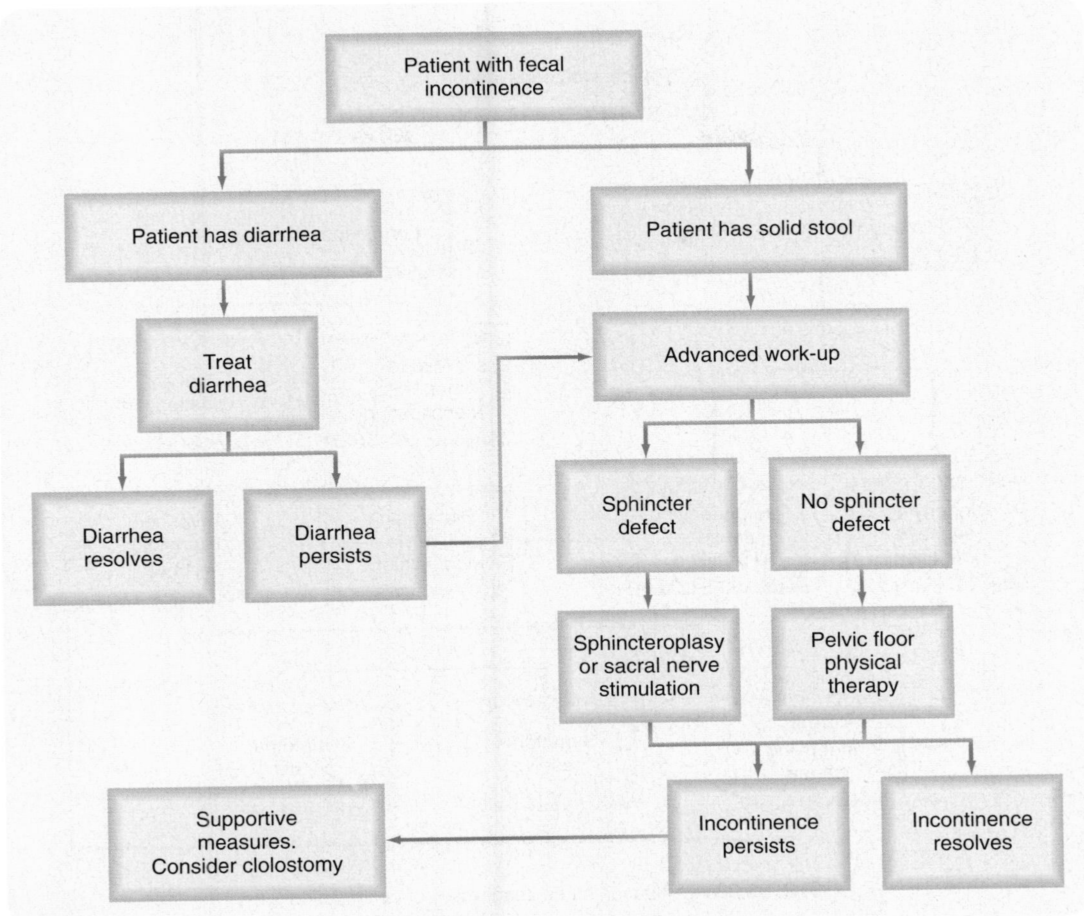

FIG. 53.26 Evaluation and management of fecal incontinence.

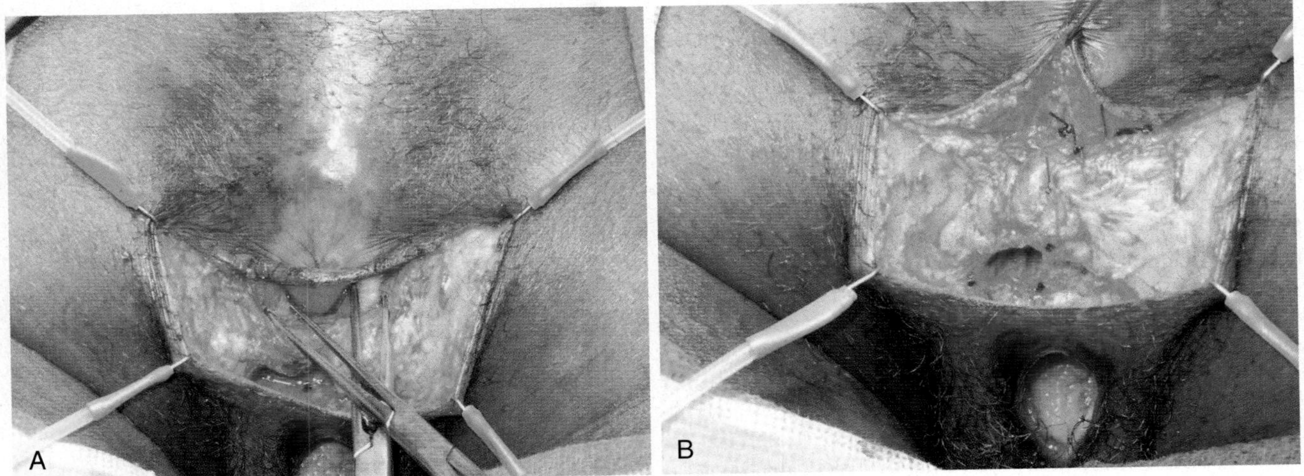

FIG. 53.27 (A) Surgical repair of anterior anal sphincter defect. Sphincter is dissected. (B) Completed overlapping sphincteroplasty.

There are three grades of AIN. Grade 1 is low-grade squamous intraepithelial lesion; grades 2 and 3 are often grouped together as high-grade squamous intraepithelial lesions and are associated with a higher risk of invasive cancer. These lesions are more frequently seen in HIV-positive MSMs and in immunosuppressed individuals such as transplant patients. Most cases of anal dysplasia are caused by the HPV, particularly the HPV-16 subtype. Other strains linked to anal cancer include HPV 18, 31, 33, and 45. The natural history of AIN is not entirely known; in particular, the rate of progression of untreated AIN to anal cancer is not well established, leading to considerable controversy surrounding just how aggressive efforts at the diagnosis and treatment of AIN should be. Current treatments for AIN include ablative and topical therapies. Topical therapies include immunomodulators such

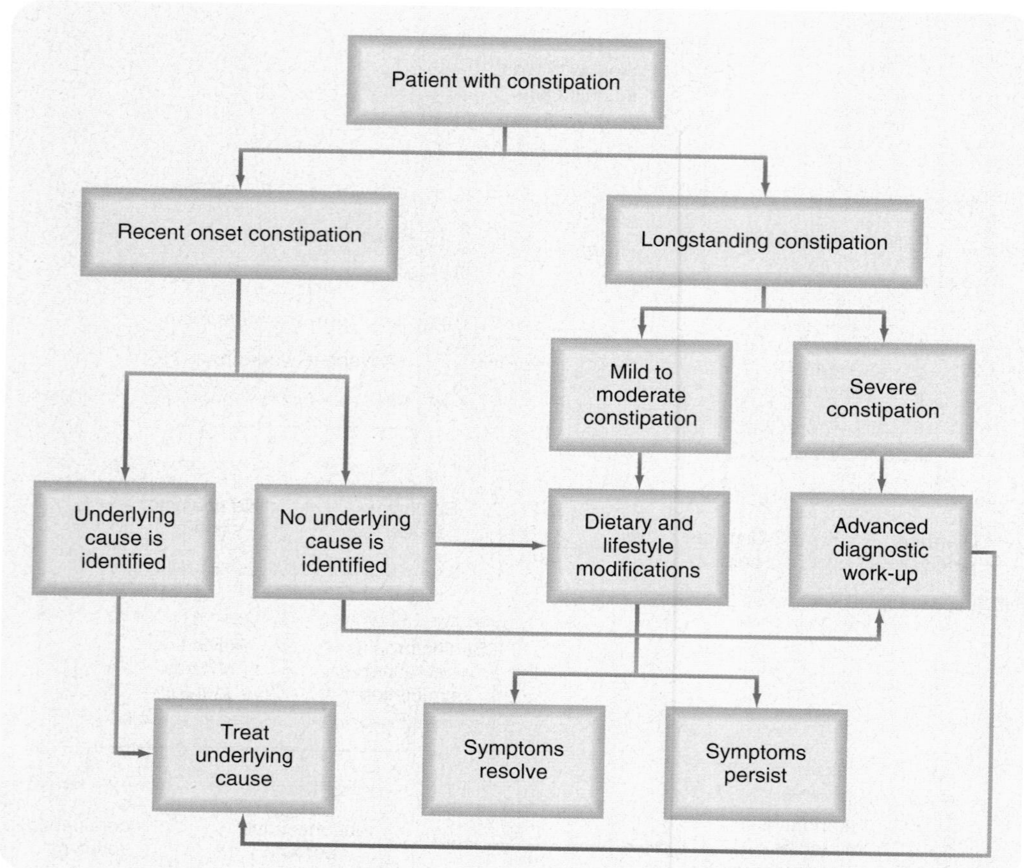

FIG. 53.28 Evaluation and management of constipation.

as imiquimod, podophyllin, or 5-FU. Ablative therapies include surgical excision, IRC, and thermal ablation.[39,40]

Screening of HIV-positive and HIV-negative MSM and bisexual men with Papanicolaou smear at 2- to 3-year intervals has been shown to be cost-effective with significant benefits on overall life-expectancy. Other groups that can benefit from screening include all HIV-positive individuals irrespective of their sexual practices, immunosuppressed organ transplant patients, and women with a past history of cervical dysplasia or cancer. Currently available quadrivalent HPV vaccines have the potential to reduce anal cancer incidence if administered before initiation of sexual activity.[41]

Squamous Cell Carcinoma

Squamous cell carcinoma (SCC) of the anal canal is most commonly associated with HPV infection; HIV is an additional independent risk factor for SCC of the anus. Sexual activity with multiple partners and anoreceptive intercourse increase the risk of HPV and HIV infection, thereby increasing the risk of anal cancer. People with reduced immunity such as immunosuppressed organ transplant patients also have higher rates of anal cancer. Women are more likely than men to suffer from anal cancer, presumably owing to the higher prevalence of HPV infection in women.[42]

Anal cancers tend to be locally aggressive with early invasion of the anal sphincters. Once the sphincter is invaded, the tumor can spread into the ischiorectal fossae, the prostatic urethra and bladder in men, and the vagina in women (Fig. 53.29). Anal canal cancer grows circumferentially and may result in narrowing and stenosis of the anal sphincter. Lymphatic spread occurs in 10% to 15% of patients, in the distribution of the perirectal and/or inguinal nodal basin. Hematogenous spread of anal canal cancer occurs in fewer than 10% of cases. Liver metastases are more common than lung or bone metastases and usually occur in the setting of a tumor arising at the anorectal junction. Metastases to distant organs such as the brain and iris have also been reported.[43,44]

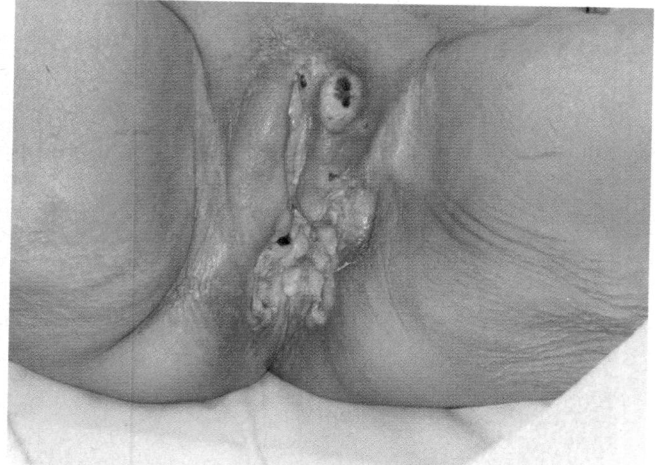

FIG. 53.29 Advanced anal squamous cell carcinoma.

Squamous cell cancer of the anus may manifest in different forms and is often confused with a wide range of benign anal disorders such as fissures, hemorrhoids, perianal dermatitis, and anorectal fistula.[45] The median age at diagnosis is 60 years. Patients typically present with a perianal mass, pain, anal discharge, and bleeding. A history of anal condyloma or dysplasia may be found in about 50% of MSM and 20% of women and heterosexual men. Physical examination may be limited due to discomfort, stricture, or induration of the perineal soft tissues. An examination under anesthesia may be required to evaluate and biopsy the lesion. Some patients with an anal cancer may present with isolated inguinal lymphadenopathy, which may be misdiagnosed as an inflammatory node or inguinal hernia.

Anal cancers are staged similarly to other tumors by the tumor, node, metastasis (TNM) staging system that has been developed by the American Joint Committee on Cancer (AJCC) 8th edition.[45a] Anal cancer may appear as a hypoattenuated necrotic mass on as CT scan; however, CT is primarily used to evaluate for distant metastatic disease. MRI is considered the modality of choice for assessment of locoregional disease. Tumors appear to be of high signal intensity relative to skeletal muscle on T2-weighted images and of low to intermediate signal intensity on T1-weighted images. Lymph node metastases tend to have similar signal intensity to the primary lesion. Positron emission tomography (PET)/CT with ^{18}F-fluorodeoxyglucose has been found to play an important role in the initial staging and posttreatment restaging of patients with anal cancer. PET/CT can help in differentiating residual viable anal cancer from post treatment necrosis and fibrosis.

Combined modality therapy (CMT) with mitomycin C, 5-FU, and radiotherapy (45–50.4 Gy) achieves a complete response in 64% to 86% of patients, and an overall 5-year survival rate of approximately 75% (66%–92%). Prophylactic bilateral inguinal radiation for patients with clinically negative nodes and the addition of a radiation boost for patients with clinically positive nodes is common practice. Evaluation of the response to therapy is important and entails careful examination of the anal canal. Since regression of anal canal cancers has been found to continue for up to three or more months after completion of CMT, it is recommended that a biopsy should be delayed for at least 3 months after treatment has been completed unless there is evidence of disease progression or other evidence to suggest inadequate response. Patients with anal cancer who have achieved complete remission at 12 weeks may be followed every 3 to 6 months for the first 2 years, and then every 6 to12 months up to 5 years. Clinical examination commonly includes digital rectal examination, anoscopy, and palpation of the inguinal lymph nodes. Locoregional relapse is more common than distant metastasis in anal cancer.

If pathologic evidence of recurrence is diagnosed, surgical management by an abdominoperineal resection is recommended. A salvage abdominoperineal resection is required in up to 30% of cases, either owing to primary nonresponse or subsequent recurrence of the tumor. In the majority of these cases, long-term survival is possible following these operations.[46] Patients with clear margins (R0) can achieve up to a 75% 5-year overall survival rate. Tumor size greater than 5 cm, adjacent organ involvement, male gender, and associated comorbidities are considered to be predictors of poor outcome following salvage surgery. Abdominoperineal resection in this setting is associated with substantial morbidity, with complications including delayed perineal wound healing, pelvic abscess, perineal wound hernia, urinary retention, and erectile dysfunction. Large perineal wound can be covered with tissue flaps including the pedicled omental flap, gracilis flap, gluteus maximus flap, and the vertical rectus abdominis myocutaneous flap. Inguinal lymph node dissection can also be offered for primary failure of chemoradiation and for recurrent disease.

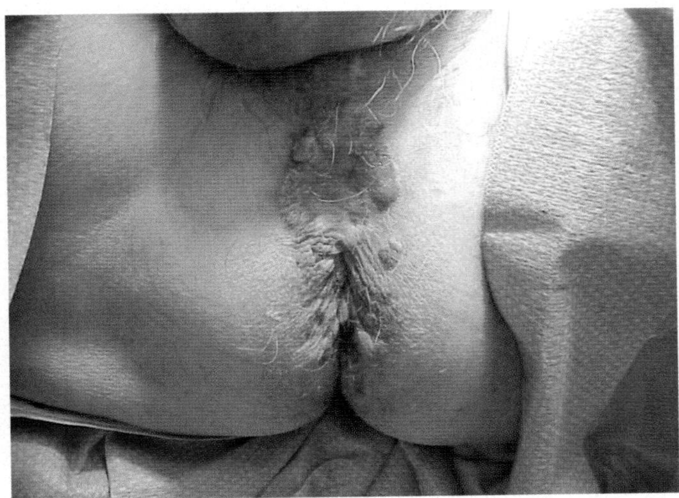

FIG. 53.30 Anal margin cancer.

Although CMT is the treatment of choice for most patients with SCC of the anal canal, wide local excision can be offered to selected patients with well-differentiated, early T1 tumors, especially those that arise on a hemorrhoidal cushion.

Anal margin cancers account for about 25% of all anal cancers; SCC is again the most common histologic subtype. As opposed to carcinomas in the anal canal, these cancers behave like skin lesions and are staged accordingly. Patients typically present between 65 and 75 years of age, with equal incidence in both genders. The presenting features are usually nonspecific and include pain, itching, burning, bleeding, palpable mass, and discharge. On examination, there is a typically an ulcerated lesion with rolled, everted edges (Fig. 53.30). Biopsy reveals well or moderately differentiated keratinizing SCC in the majority of cases.

Distant metastases occur rarely and may be ruled out with CT scan of the chest, abdomen, and pelvis. Lymph node involvement has been found to be an important adverse prognostic factor. Other predictive factors include the tumor size, differentiation, and invasion of extradermal structures. Bulky, advanced tumors of the anal margin extending into the anus are treated similarly to tumors of the anal canal with CMT. In contrast, tumors that are limited to the anal margin are treated like cutaneous SCC elsewhere on the body. Wide local excision is generally adequate treatment as it preserves continence and enables local control. If the margins are positive or close, radiotherapy can be administered with good results. If a large skin defect persists after excision, it can be reconstructed by a rotational skin flap or a split skin graft.

Perianal Paget Disease

Perianal Paget disease is thought to correspond to an intraepithelial adenocarcinoma arising from dermal apocrine sweat glands. Patients with this condition tend to present with nonspecific symptoms such as pruritus, discharge, or bleeding. The lesion appears as an erythematous plaque, which may be ulcerative and crusty or papillary (Fig. 53.31). Perianal Paget disease may represent primary (intraepidermal/intradermal) or secondary disease. Secondary disease is associated with anorectal adenocarcinomas. Approximately 50% of patients with anal margin Paget disease harbor a synchronous colorectal neoplasm, mandating full colonoscopy for complete evaluation. Patients with perianal Paget disease also

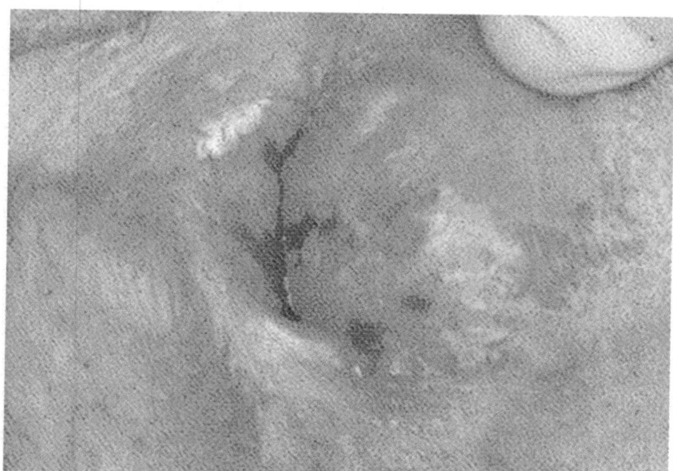

FIG. 53.31 Perianal Paget disease. (From St Peter SD, Pera M, Smith AA, et al. Wide local excision and split-thickness skin graft for circumferential Paget's disease of the anus. *Am J Surg*. 2004;187:413–416.)

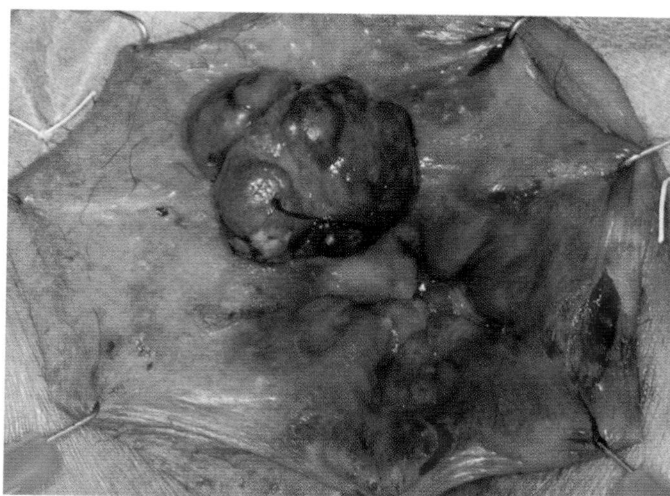

FIG. 53.32 Anal melanoma. (From Arakawa K, Kiyomatsu T, Ishihara S, et al. A case report of anorectal malignant melanoma with mucosal skipped lesion. *Int J Surg Case Rep*. 2016;24:206–210.)

frequently develop synchronous or metachronous malignancies of the adnexa and viscera.[47]

Wide local excision is recommended for most patients. The surgical defect created may require reconstruction with a cutaneous or myocutaneous flap. In the setting of a locally invasive lesion or a synchronous anorectal adenocarcinoma, abdominoperineal resection with neoadjuvant chemoradiotherapy is usually indicated. The recurrence rate can be as high as 30% to 60% at 5 years. The frequent association with synchronous and metachronous malignancies and high recurrence rate highlight the importance of long-term follow-up.

Basal Cell Carcinoma

Basal cell carcinoma (BCC) of the perianal region is a rare tumor. It comprises only 0.2% of BCCs diagnosed in the body and less than 1% of all cancers in the anorectal region. Men are predominantly affected (60%–80%) and the age of presentation is usually between 65 and 75 years. About 30% of patients have a past history of BCC at other sites. Lesions are generally small, with an average size of 1 to 2 cm. This cancer originates from the stratum basale of the epidermis and pilosebaceous follicle units. Radiation, immunodeficiency, trauma, burns or chronic irritation, or infection may also play role in development of perianal BCC.

Once perianal BCC is diagnosed, other cutaneous surfaces need to be thoroughly evaluated as there may be multiple associated lesions elsewhere. On local examination, BCC is a shallow, mobile, ulcerative lesion with raised edges and minimal potential for metastasis. Perianal BCC has not been shown to have any association with HPV infection. Management is dependent upon the dimension of the lesion and the extent of invasion into surrounding tissues. Tumors less than 2 cm are excised with at least a one cm margin. Larger lesions, without extension into the anal canal, are excised primarily but typically require coverage with skin grafts or flaps. Mohs microsurgery provides another viable option to excise the tumor with sacrifice of the least possible unaffected tissue. Large lesions with extension into the anal canal can be treated with radiation therapy and/or abdominoperineal resection. Five-year survival rates up to 100% have been reported after wide local excision, although the tumor can recur locally in up to 29% of cases.[48] Local recurrences with deep invasion of the anal canal are exceptionally rare.

Malignant Melanoma

Malignant melanoma of the anal margin accounts for 2% to 4% of all malignant anorectal neoplasms; the anus is the third most common site after skin and the eye, representing 0.2% to 0.3% of all melanomas. Symptoms are often nonspecific and include bleeding, pain, and mass. When a lesion is pigmented, melanoma can be confused with a thrombosed hemorrhoid (Fig. 53.32). Amelanotic lesions occur in 30% of cases. Overall prognosis is very poor irrespective of the surgical approach and efforts to improve survival with radical resection, including abdominoperineal resection, have not consistently shown benefit.[49] Wide local excision is usually recommended when feasible; patients with large lesions and/or extensive sphincter involvement generally require more aggressive surgery for local control. The response of anorectal melanoma to radiotherapy and chemotherapy is very limited. The reported five-year survival reported ranges from 10% to 26%.

Adenocarcinoma of the Anal Canal

Adenocarcinoma of anal canal accounts for 3% to 9% of all anal canal neoplasms. True anal canal adenocarcinoma needs to be differentiated from low rectal adenocarcinoma. Distinguishing features include prominent ductal structures, abundance of mucin with organized mucinous pools, and infiltration into the perirectal soft tissue. Anal canal adenocarcinoma usually originates from the anal glands but may develop in longstanding fistula-in-ano. Risk factors include infection with HPV and HIV, history of anoreceptive intercourse, smoking, and immunosuppression. Similar to colorectal adenocarcinoma, anal adenocarcinoma arises as a result of a multistep sequence of mutations that lead to the transformation of normal mucosa to adenoma and finally carcinoma. Because of the submucosal location of the anal glands, anal adenomas are not apparent until they undergo malignant transformation. Clinical features of anal adenocarcinoma include anal pain, induration of the anal canal, palpable mass, or abscess with mucous drainage.

Staging workup includes pelvic MRI and CT scanning. Adenocarcinoma arising in a fistula-in-ano has been reported to have three characteristic MRI findings: markedly hyperintense fluid on T2-weighted images, enhancing solid components, and a fistula between the mass and the anus.[50] Treatment is typically neoadjuvant chemoradiation followed by abdominoperineal resection for lesions larger than 2 cm. Wide local excision can be performed for smaller, well-differentiated tumors.

SELECTED REFERENCES

Davis BR, Lee-Kong SA, Migaly J, et al. the American Society of Colon and Rectal Surgeons Clinical Practice guidelines for the management of hemorrhoids. *Dis Colon Rectum.* 2018;61:284–292.

An authoritative, evidence-based guidelines for diagnosis and management of patients with symptomatic hemorrhoids.

Madoff RD, Mellgren A. One hundred years of rectal prolapse surgery. *Dis Colon Rectum.* 1999;42:441–450.

A historical perspective of surgery to repair rectal prolapse, summarizing much of the relevant data.

Nelson RL, Chattopadhyay A, Brooks W, et al. Operative procedures for fissure in ano. *Cochrane Database Syst Rev.* 2011;(11):CD002199.

An evidence-based review of the data on different surgical approaches to chronic anal fissure.

Parks AG, Gordon PH, Hardcastle JD. A classification of fistula-in-ano. *Br J Surg.* 1976;63:1–12.

A classic description of the anatomy, data, and classification of anorectal suppurative disease, including abscesses and fistulas.

Steele SR, Kumar R, Feingold DL, et al. Practice parameters for the management of perianal abscess and fistula-in-ano. *Dis Colon Rectum.* 2011;54:1465–1474.

A well-referenced summary of the current standards in the diagnosis and treatment of perianal suppurative disease.

Steele SR, Varma MG, Melton GB, et al. Practice parameters for anal squamous neoplasms. *Dis Colon Rectum.* 2012;55:735–749.

A comprehensive review of diagnostic and treatment issues pertinent to anal squamous neoplasms.

Tou S, Brown SR, Malik AI, et al. Surgery for complete rectal prolapse in adults. *Cochrane Database Syst Rev.* 2008;(4):CD001758.

A comprehensive review of the varying techniques for rectal prolapse repair.

REFERENCES

1. Aigner F, Bodner G, Conrad F, et al. The superior rectal artery and its branching pattern with regard to its clinical influence on ligation techniques for internal hemorrhoids. *Am J Surg.* 2004;187:102–108.
2. Shafik A. A new concept of the anatomy of the anal sphincter mechanism and the physiology of defecation. the external anal sphincter: a triple-loop system. *Invest Urol.* 1975;12:412–419.
3. Bignell CJ. Chaperones for genital examination. *BMJ.* 1999;319:137–138.
4. Loder PB, Kamm MA, Nicholls RJ, et al. Haemorrhoids: pathology, pathophysiology and aetiology. *Br J Surg.* 1994;81:946–954.
5. Aigner F, Gruber H, Conrad F, et al. Revised morphology and hemodynamics of the anorectal vascular plexus: impact on the course of hemorrhoidal disease. *Int J Colorectal Dis.* 2009;24:105–113.
6. Chung YC, Hou YC, Pan AC. Endoglin (CD105) expression in the development of haemorrhoids. *Eur J Clin Invest.* 2004;34:107–112.
7. MacRae HM, McLeod RS. Comparison of hemorrhoidal treatments: a meta-analysis. *Can J Surg.* 1997;40:14–17.
8. Nelson DW, Champagne BJ, Rivadeneira DE, et al. Prophylactic antibiotics for hemorrhoidectomy: are they really needed? *Dis Colon Rectum.* 2014;57:365–369.
9. Bhatti MI, Sajid MS, Baig MK. Milligan-Morgan (Open) versus ferguson haemorrhoidectomy (closed): a systematic review and meta-analysis of published randomized, controlled trials. *World J Surg.* 2016;40:1509–1519.
10. Faucheron JL, Voirin D, Abba J. Rectal perforation with life-threatening peritonitis following stapled haemorrhoidopexy. *Br J Surg.* 2012;99:746–753.
11. Minguez M, Herreros B, Espi A, et al. Long-term follow-up (42 months) of chronic anal fissure after healing with botulinum toxin. *Gastroenterology.* 2002;123:112–117.
12. Pares D. Pathogenesis and treatment of fistula in ano. *Br J Surg.* 2011;98:2–3.
13. Whiteford MH, Kilkenny 3rd J, Hyman N, et al. Practice parameters for the treatment of perianal abscess and fistula-in-ano (revised). *Dis Colon Rectum.* 2005;48:1337–1342.
14. Llera JL, Levy RC. Treatment of cutaneous abscess: a double-blind clinical study. *Ann Emerg Med.* 1985;14:15–19.
15. Vasilevsky CA, Gordon PH. The incidence of recurrent abscesses or fistula-in-ano following anorectal suppuration. *Dis Colon Rectum.* 1984;27:126–130.
16. Garcia-Aguilar J, Belmonte C, Wong WD, et al. Anal fistula surgery. factors associated with recurrence and incontinence. *Dis Colon Rectum.* 1996;39:723–729.
17. van Tets WF, Kuijpers HC. Continence disorders after anal fistulotomy. *Dis Colon Rectum.* 1994;37:1194–1197.
18. Vasilevsky CA, Gordon PH. Results of treatment of fistula-in-ano. *Dis Colon Rectum.* 1985;28:225–231.
19. Abcarian AM, Estrada JJ, Park J, et al. Ligation of intersphincteric fistula tract: early results of a pilot study. *Dis Colon Rectum.* 2012;55:778–782.
20. Homsi R, Daikoku NH, Littlejohn J, et al. Episiotomy: risks of dehiscence and rectovaginal fistula. *Obstet Gynecol Surv.* 1994;49:803–808.
21. Venkatesh KS, Ramanujam PS, Larson DM, et al. Anorectal complications of vaginal delivery. *Dis Colon Rectum.* 1989;32:1039–1041.

22. Stone JM, Goldberg SM. The endorectal advancement flap procedure. *Int J Colorectal Dis*. 1990;5:232–235.
23. Sondenaa K, Andersen E, Nesvik I, et al. Patient characteristics and symptoms in chronic pilonidal sinus disease. *Int J Colorectal Dis*. 1995;10:39–42.
24. Odili J, Gault D. Laser depilation of the natal cleft--an aid to healing the pilonidal sinus. *Ann R Coll Surg Engl*. 2002;84:29–32.
25. Bascom J. Pilonidal disease: origin from follicles of hairs and results of follicle removal as treatment. *Surgery*. 1980;87:567–572.
26. Lorincz AT, Temple GF, Kurman RJ, et al. Oncogenic association of specific human papillomavirus types with cervical neoplasia. *J Natl Cancer Inst*. 1987;79:671–677.
27. Silvera RJ, Smith CK, Swedish KA, et al. Anal condyloma treatment and recurrence in HIV-negative men who have sex with men. *Dis Colon Rectum*. 2014;57:752–761.
28. Goodell SE, Quinn TC, Mkrtichian E, et al. Herpes simplex virus proctitis in homosexual men. Clinical, sigmoidoscopic, and histopathological features. *N Engl J Med*. 1983;308:868–871.
29. 1993 revised classification system for HIV infection and expanded surveillance case definition for AIDS among adolescents and adults. *MMWR Recomm Rep (Morb Mortal Wkly Rep)*. 1992;41:1–19.
30. Hamlyn E, Taylor C. Sexually transmitted proctitis. *Postgrad Med J*. 2006;82:733–736.
31. Saunte DML, Jemec GBE. Hidradenitis suppurativa: advances in diagnosis and treatment. *J Am Med Assoc*. 2017;318:2019–2032.
32. Church JM, Fazio VW, Lavery IC, et al. The differential diagnosis and comorbidity of hidradenitis suppurativa and perianal crohn's disease. *Int J Colorectal Dis*. 1993;8:117–119.
33. Smith GL, Bunker CB, Dinneen MD. Fournier's gangrene. *Br J Urol*. 1998;81:347–355.
34. Saijo S, Kuramoto Y, Yoshinari M, et al. Extremely extended Fournier's gangrene. *Dermatol*. 1990;181:228–232.
35. Benizri E, Fabiani P, Migliori G, et al. Gangrene of the perineum. *Urology*. 1996;47:935–939.
36. Whitehead WE, Rao SS, Lowry A, et al. Treatment of fecal incontinence: state of the science summary for the national institute of diabetes and digestive and kidney diseases workshop. *Am J Gastroenterol*. 2015;110:138–146; quiz 147.
37. Markland A, Wang L, Jelovsek JE, et al. Symptom improvement in women after fecal incontinence treatments: a multicenter cohort study of the pelvic floor disorders network. *Female Pelvic Med Reconstr Surg*. 2015;21:46–52.
38. Malone PS, Ransley PG, Kiely EM. Preliminary report: the antegrade continence enema. *Lancet*. 1990;336:1217–1218.
39. Nagle D. Anal squamous cell carcinoma in the HIV-positive patient. *Clin Colon Rectal Surg*. 2009;22:102–106.
40. Goldstone SE, Hundert JS, Huyett JW. Infrared coagulator ablation of high-grade anal squamous intraepithelial lesions in HIV-negative males who have sex with males. *Dis Colon Rectum*. 2007;50:565–575.
41. Elbasha EH, Dasbach EJ. Impact of vaccinating boys and men against HPV in the United States. *Vaccine*. 2010;28:6858–6867.
42. Stanley M. Pathology and epidemiology of HPV infection in females. *Gynecol Oncol*. 2010;117:S5–S10.
43. Rughani AI, Lin C, Tranmer BI, et al. Anal cancer with cerebral metastasis: a case report. *J Neuro Oncol*. 2011;101:141–143.
44. Tougeron D, Tougeron-Brousseau B, Nasser Z, et al. Unusual iris metastasis from anal cancer: a case report. *Dig Liver Dis*. 2009;41:e1–3.
45. Crooms JW, Kovalcik PJ. Anal lesions. when to suspect carcinoma. *Postgrad Med*. 1985;77:85–88; 90.
45a. Gress DM, Edge SB, Greenwald JE, et al. Anus. In Amin MB, Edge SB, Green FL, et al., editors. AJCC Cancer Staging Manual, 8th edition, Chicago, IL: Springer. 2018, pp. 275–286.
46. Mullen JT, Rodriguez-Bigas MA, Chang GJ, et al. Results of surgical salvage after failed chemoradiation therapy for epidermoid carcinoma of the anal canal. *Ann Surg Oncol*. 2007;14:478–483.
47. Isik O, Aytac E, Brainard J, et al. Perianal Paget's disease: three decades experience of a single institution. *Int J Colorectal Dis*. 2016;31:29–34.
48. Paterson CA, Young-Fadok TM, Dozois RR. Basal cell carcinoma of the perianal region: 20-year experience. *Dis Colon Rectum*. 1999;42:1200–1202.
49. Matsuda A, Miyashita M, Matsumoto S, et al. Abdominoperineal resection provides better local control but equivalent overall survival to local excision of anorectal malignant melanoma: a systematic review. *Ann Surg*. 2015;261:670–677.
50. Fujimoto H, Ikeda M, Shimofusa R, et al. Mucinous adenocarcinoma arising from fistula-in-ano: findings on MRI. *Eur Radiol*. 2003;13:2053–2054.

CHAPTER 54

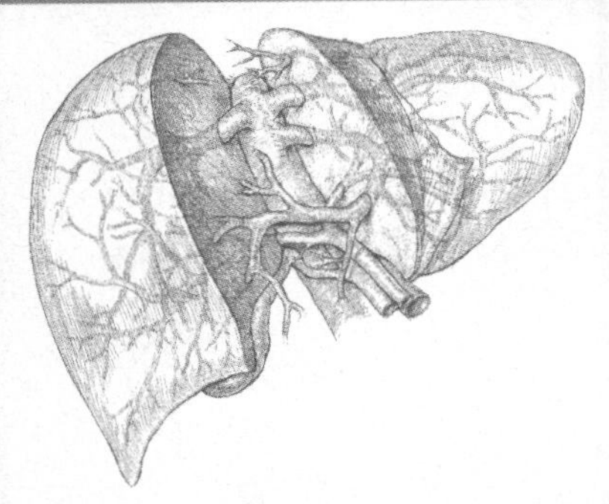

The Liver

Vikas Dudeja, Anthony Ferrantella, Yuman Fong

OUTLINE

HISTORICAL PERSPECTIVE

The surface anatomy of the liver was described as early as 2000 BC by the ancient Babylonians. Even Hippocrates understood and described the seriousness of liver injury. In 1654, Francis Glisson was the first physician to describe the essential anatomy of the blood vessels of the liver accurately. The beginnings of liver surgery are described as rudimentary excisions of eviscerated liver from penetrating trauma. The first documented case of a partial hepatectomy is credited to Berta, who amputated a portion of protruding liver in a patient with a self-inflicted stab wound in 1716.

In the late 1800s, the first gastrectomies and cholecystectomies were being performed in Europe. At that time, surgery on the liver was regarded as dangerous, if not impossible. In 1897, Elliot, in his report on liver surgery for trauma, said that the liver was so "friable, so full of gaping vessels and so evidently incapable of being sutured that it had always seemed impossible to successfully manage large wounds of its substance." European surgeons began to experiment with techniques of elective liver surgery on animals in the late 1800s. The credit for the first elective liver resection is a matter of debate and many surgeons have been given credit, but it certainly occurred during this period.

The early 1900s saw some small but significant advances in liver surgery. Techniques for suturing major hepatic vessels and the use of cautery for small vessels were applied and reported. The most significant advance of that time was probably that of J. Hogarth Pringle. In 1908, he described digital compression of the hilar vessels to control hepatic bleeding from traumatic injuries. The modern era of hepatic surgery was ushered in by the development of a better understanding of liver anatomy and formal anatomic liver resection. Credit for the first anatomic liver resection is usually given to Lortat-Jacob, who performed a right hepatectomy in 1952 in France. Pack from New York and Quattelbaum from Georgia performed similar operations within the next year and were unlikely to have had any knowledge of Lortat-Jacob's report. Descriptions of the segmental nature of liver anatomy by Couinaud, Goldsmith, and Woodburne in 1957 opened the door even wider and introduced the modern era of liver surgery.

Despite these improvements, hepatic surgery was plagued by tremendous operative morbidity and mortality from the 1950s into the 1980s. Operative mortality rates in excess of 20% were common and usually related to massive hemorrhage. Many surgeons were reluctant to perform hepatic surgery because of these results, and understandably, many physicians were reluctant to refer patients for hepatectomy. With the courage of patients and their families as well as the persistence of surgeons, safe hepatic surgery has now been realized. A complete list is not possible here, but courageous hepatic surgeons such as Blumgart, Bismuth, Longmire, Fortner, Schwartz, Starzl, and Ton deserve mention.

Advances in anesthesia, intensive care, antibiotics, and interventional radiologic techniques have also contributed tremendously to the safety of major hepatic surgery. Total hepatectomy with liver transplantation and live donor partial hepatectomy for transplantation are now performed routinely in specialized transplantation centers. Partial hepatectomy for a large number of indications is now performed throughout the world in specialized centers, with mortality rates of 5% or less. Partial hepatectomy on normal livers is now consistently performed, with mortality rates of 1% to 2%.

Safely performed open hepatic surgery with its liberal use in the management of a wide variety of diseases is now a reality. Moreover, minimally invasive approaches to liver surgery have been developed and are now being used in significant numbers. However, the learning curve remains steep, and the indications for this technique are still being carefully defined. Use of robotics in liver surgery may help in addressing the issues with learning curve with laparoscopy. The addition of robotics offers advanced suturing and articulation that closely approximate the open surgery. This allows a greater proportion of cases to be performed in total minimally invasive fashion. The role of robotics in liver surgery is rapidly evolving. Thermal ablative techniques to treat hepatic tumors, including radiofrequency and microwave ablation, have exploded in popularity. Finally, techniques to improve the safety of liver resection further, such as portal vein embolization to induce preoperative hypertrophy of the future liver remnant (FLR), have been developed and are now being used.

ANATOMY AND PHYSIOLOGY

Anatomy

Gross Anatomy

A precise knowledge of the anatomy of the liver is an absolute prerequisite to performing surgery on the liver or biliary tree. During the last several decades, a greater appreciation for the complex anatomy beyond the misleading minimal external markings has been realized. The anatomic contributions of Couinaud (see later) and the description of the segmental nature of the liver should be embraced and studied by students of hepatic surgery.

General description and topography. The liver is a solid gastrointestinal organ whose mass (1.2–1.6 kg) largely occupies the right upper quadrant of the abdomen. The costal margin coincides with the lower margin of the liver, and the diaphragm drapes over the superior surface of the liver. The large majority of the right liver and most of the left liver are covered by the thoracic cage. The posterior surface straddles the inferior vena cava (IVC). A wedge of liver extends to the left side of the abdomen. The liver is invested in peritoneum except for the gallbladder fossa, porta hepatis, and posterior aspect of the liver on either side of the IVC in two wedge-shaped areas. This region of liver to the right of the IVC, which is devoid of peritoneal coverage, is called the bare area of the liver. The peritoneal duplications on the liver surface are referred to as ligaments. The diaphragmatic peritoneal duplications are referred to as the coronary ligaments, whose lateral margins on either side are the right and left triangular ligaments. From the center of the coronary ligament emerges the falciform ligament, which extends anteriorly as a thin membrane connecting the liver surface to the diaphragm, abdominal wall, and umbilicus.

The ligamentum teres (the obliterated umbilical vein) runs along the inferior edge of the falciform ligament from the umbilicus to the umbilical fissure. The umbilical fissure is on the inferior surface of the left liver and contains the left portal pedicle. In early descriptions of hepatic anatomy, the falciform ligament, the most obvious surface marker of the liver, was used as the division of the right and left lobes of the liver. However, this description is

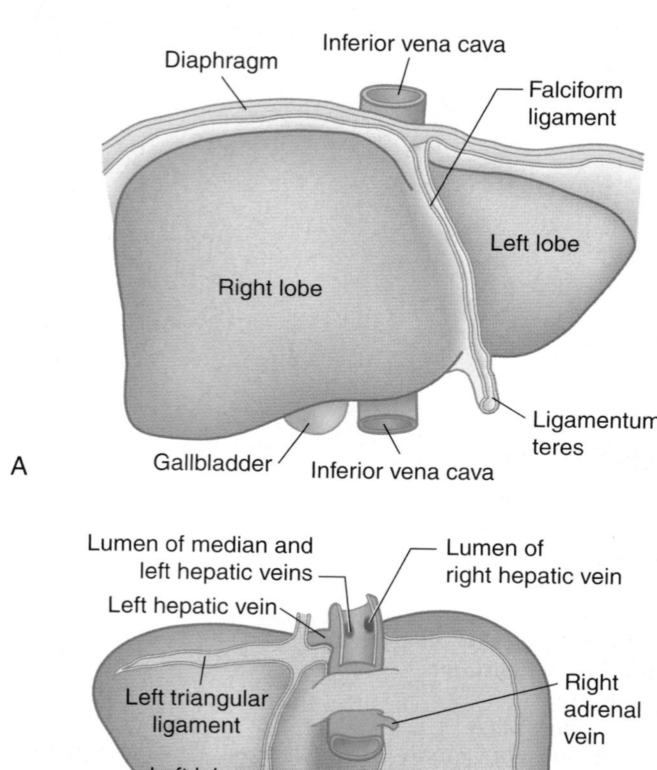

FIG. 54.1 (A) Historically, the liver was divided into right and left lobes by the external marking of the falciform ligament. On the inferior surface of the falciform ligament, the ligamentum teres can be seen entering the umbilical fissure. (B) The posterior and inferior surface of the liver is shown. The liver embraces the inferior vena cava (IVC) posteriorly in a groove. The lumens of the three major hepatic veins and right adrenal vein can be seen directly entering the IVC. The bare area, bounded by the right and left triangular ligaments, is illustrated. To the left of the IVC is the caudate lobe, which is bounded on its left side by a fissure containing the ligamentum venosum. The lesser omentum terminates along the edge of the ligamentum venosum, and thus the caudate lobe lies within the lesser sac and the rest of the liver lies in the supracolic compartment. A layer of fibrous tissue can be seen bridging the right lobe to the caudate lobe posterior to the IVC, thus encircling it. This ligament of tissue must be divided on the right side in mobilizing the right liver off the IVC. (From Blumgart LH, Hann LE. Surgical and radiologic anatomy of the liver and biliary tract. In: Blumgart LH, Fong Y, eds. *Surgery of the Liver and Biliary Tract*. London: WB Saunders; 2000:3–34.)

inaccurate and of minimal usefulness to the hepatobiliary surgeon (see later for detailed segmental anatomy). On the posterior surface of the left liver, running from the left portal vein in the porta hepatis toward the left hepatic vein and the IVC is the ligamentum venosum (obliterated sinus venosus) that also runs in a fissure (Fig. 54.1). Hepatic arterial blood and portal venous blood enter the liver at the hilum and branch throughout the liver as a single portal pedicle unit, which also includes a bile duct. These portal triads are invested in a peritoneal sheath that invaginates at the

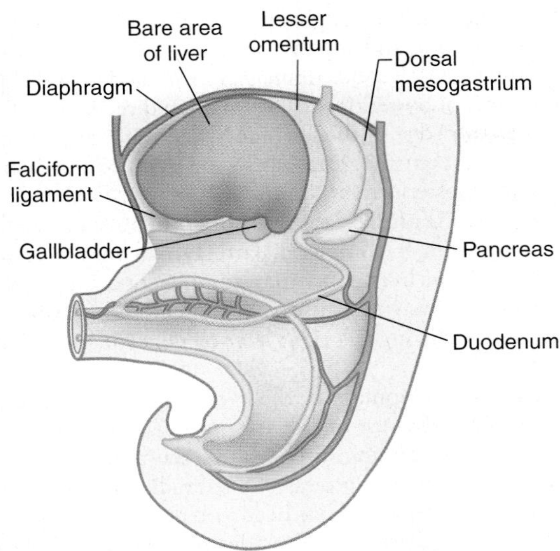

FIG. 54.2 An approximately 36-day-old embryo is shown. The extensions of the septum transversum can be seen developing as the liver protrudes into the abdominal cavity, stretching out and forming the lesser omentum and the falciform ligament. The liver is completely invested in visceral peritoneum, except for a portion next to the diaphragm known as the bare area. (From Sadler TW. *Langman's Medical Embryology*. 5th ed. Baltimore: Williams & Wilkins; 1985.)

hepatic hilum. Venous drainage is through the right, middle, and left hepatic veins that empty directly into the suprahepatic IVC.

Normal development and embryology. The developing liver shares a common progenitor with the biliary tree and pancreas. During embryogenesis, signals are transmitted from the cardiac mesenchyme and septum transversum. The molecules regulating this (e.g., fibroblast growth factor, bone morphogenetic protein, Wnt, tissue growth factor beta [TGF-β]) have begun to be elucidated. The liver primordium begins to form in the third week of development as an outgrowth of endodermal epithelium, known as the hepatic diverticulum or liver bud. The connection between the hepatic diverticulum and the future duodenum narrows to form the bile duct, and an outpouching of the bile duct forms into the gallbladder and cystic duct. Hepatic cells develop cords and intermingle with the vitelline and umbilical veins to form hepatic sinusoids. Simultaneously, hematopoietic cells, Kupffer cells, and connective tissue form from the mesoderm of the septum transversum. The mesoderm of the septum transversum connects the liver to the ventral abdominal wall and foregut. As the liver protrudes into the abdominal cavity, these structures are stretched into thin membranes, ultimately forming the falciform ligament and lesser omentum. The mesoderm on the surface of the developing liver differentiates into visceral peritoneum, except superiorly, where contact between the liver and mesoderm (future diaphragm) is maintained, forming a bare area devoid of visceral peritoneum (Fig. 54.2).

The primitive liver plays a central role in the fetal circulation. The vitelline veins carry blood from the yolk sac to the sinus venosus and ultimately form a network of veins around the foregut (future duodenum) that drain into the developing hepatic sinusoids. These vitelline veins eventually fuse to form the portal, superior mesenteric, and splenic veins. The sinus venosus, which empties into the fetal heart, becomes the hepatocardiac channel and then the hepatic veins and retrohepatic IVC. The umbilical veins, which are paired early on, carry oxygenated blood to the fetus. Initially, the umbilical veins drain into the sinus venosus, but at week 5 of development, they begin to drain into the hepatic sinusoids. The right umbilical vein ultimately disappears, and the left umbilical vein later drains directly into the hepatocardiac channel, bypassing the hepatic sinusoids through the ductus venosus. In the adult liver, the remnant of the left umbilical vein becomes the ligamentum teres, which runs in the falciform ligament into the umbilical fissure, and the remnant of the ductus venosus becomes the ligamentum venosum at the termination of the lesser omentum under the left liver (Fig. 54.3).

The adult liver is a complex system of numerous cell types, including hepatocytes, cholangiocytes, neuroendocrine cells, hepatic progenitors (known as oval cells), myofibroblastic mesenchymal cells (known as hepatic stellate cells and portal myofibroblasts), resident macrophages (known as Kupffer cells), and vascular endothelial cells.

Functional Anatomy

Historically, the liver was divided into left and right lobes by the obvious external landmark of the falciform ligament. Not only was this description oversimplified, but it was also anatomically incorrect in relation to the blood supply to the liver. Our understanding of functional liver anatomy has become more sophisticated.

The functional anatomy of the liver (Figs. 54.4 and 54.5) is composed of eight segments, each supplied by a single portal triad (also called a pedicle) composed of a portal vein, hepatic artery, and bile duct. These segments are further organized into four sectors, separated by scissurae containing the three main hepatic veins. The four sectors are even further organized into the right and left liver. The terms *right liver* and *left liver* are preferable to the terms *right lobe* and *left lobe* because there is no external mark that allows the identification of the right and left liver. This system was originally described in 1957 by Goldsmith and Woodburne and by Couinaud. It defines hepatic anatomy because it is most relevant to surgery of the liver. The functional anatomy is more often seen as cross-sectional imaging (Fig. 54.6).

The main scissura contains the middle hepatic vein, which runs in an anteroposterior direction from the gallbladder fossa to the left side of the vena cava. It divides the liver into right and left hemilivers. The line of the main scissura is also known as Cantlie line. The right liver is divided into anterior (segments V and VIII) and posterior (segments VI and VII) sectors by the right scissura, which contains the right hepatic vein. The right portal pedicle is composed of the right hepatic artery, portal vein, and bile duct. It splits into right anterior and right posterior pedicles, which supply the segments of the anterior and posterior sectors.

The left liver has a visible fissure along its inferior surface called the umbilical fissure. The ligamentum teres, containing the remnant of the umbilical vein, runs into this fissure. The falciform ligament is contiguous with the umbilical fissure and ligamentum teres. The umbilical fissure is not a scissura and does not contain a hepatic vein; it contains the left portal pedicle, which contains the left portal vein, hepatic artery, and bile duct. This pedicle runs in this fissure and branches to feed the left liver. The left liver is split into anterior (segments III and IV) and posterior (segment II, the only sector composed of a single segment) sectors by the left scissura. The left scissura runs posterior to the ligamentum teres and contains the left hepatic vein.

At the hilum of the liver, the right portal triad has a short extrahepatic course of approximately 1 to 1.5 cm before entering the substance of the liver and branching into anterior and posterior sectoral branches. The left portal triad, however, has a long extrahepatic course of up to 3 to 4 cm and runs transversely along the base of segment IV in a peritoneal sheath, which is the upper end of the lesser omentum. This connective tissue is known as the hilar plate (Fig. 54.7). The continuation of the left portal triad runs anteriorly and caudally in the umbilical fissure and gives branches to segments II and III on the left and recurrent branches to segment IV on the right side.

The caudate lobe (segment I) is the dorsal portion of the liver. It embraces the IVC on its ventral surface and lies posterior to the left portal triad inferiorly and the left and middle hepatic veins superiorly. The main bulk of the caudate lobe is to the left of the IVC, but inferiorly, it traverses between the IVC and left portal triad, where it fuses to the right liver (segments VI and VII). This part of the caudate lobe is known as the right portion or the caudate process. The left portion of the caudate lobe lies in the lesser omental bursa and is covered anteriorly by the gastrohepatic ligament (lesser omentum) that separates it from segments II and III anteriorly. The gastrohepatic ligament attaches to the ligamentum venosum (sinus venosus remnant) along the left side of the left portal triad (Fig. 54.8).

The vascular inflow and biliary drainage to the caudate lobe come from both the right and left pedicles. The right side of the caudate, the caudate process, largely derives its portal venous supply from the right portal vein or the bifurcation of the main portal vein. The left portion of the caudate derives its portal venous inflow from the left main portal vein. The arterial supply and biliary drainage are generally through the right posterior pedicle system for the right portion and through the left main pedicle for the left portion. The hepatic venous drainage of the caudate is unique because a number of posterior small veins drain directly into the IVC.

The posterior edge of the left side of the caudate terminates as a fibrous component that attaches to the crura of the diaphragm and also runs posteriorly, wrapping behind the IVC and attaching to segment VII of the right liver. In up to 50% of people, this fibrous component is composed partially or completely of liver parenchyma. Thus, liver tissue may completely encircle the IVC. This structure is known as the caval ligament and is important to recognize in mobilizing the right liver or the caudate lobe off the vena cava.

Anomalous development of the liver is uncommonly encountered. Complete absence of the left liver has been reported. A tongue of tissue extending inferiorly off the right liver has been described (Riedel lobe). Rare cases of supradiaphragmatic liver in the absence of a hernia sac have been noted.

Portal vein. The portal vein provides approximately 75% of the hepatic blood inflow. Despite being postcapillary and largely deoxygenated, its high flow rate provides 50% to 70% of the liver's oxygen requirement. The lack of valves in the portal venous system provides a system that can accommodate high flow at low pressure. This also allows the measurement of portal venous pressure at any point along the system.

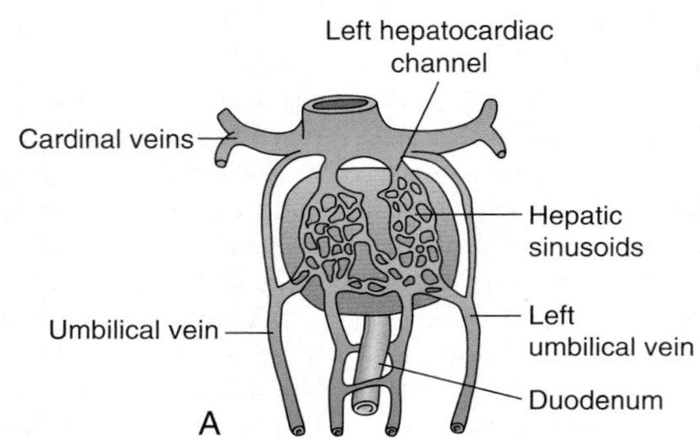

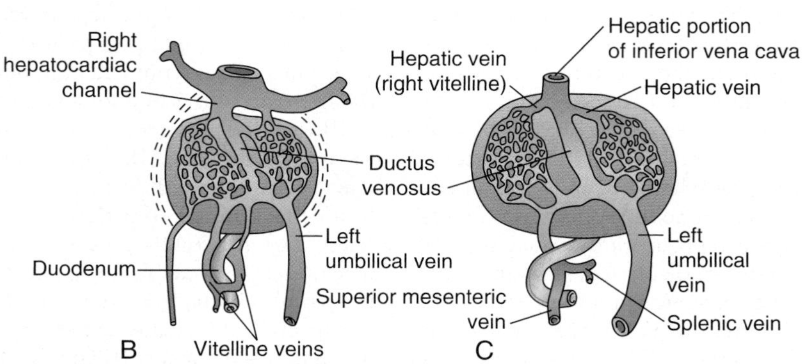

FIG. 54.3 (A) Umbilical and vitelline vein development of a 5-week-old embryo. The hepatic sinusoids have developed, and, although there are channels that bypass these sinusoids, the vitelline and umbilical veins are beginning to drain into them. (B) In the second month, the vitelline veins drain directly into the hepatic sinusoids. The ductus venosus has formed and accepts oxygenated blood from the left umbilical vein, bypasses the hepatic sinusoids, and directly enters the hepatocardiac channel. (C) By the third month, the vitelline veins have formed into the portal system (splenic, superior mesenteric, and portal veins). The right umbilical vein has disappeared, and the left umbilical vein (future ligamentum teres) drains into the sinus venosus, bypassing the hepatic sinusoids. Note the development of the inferior vena cava and hepatic veins. (From Sadler TW. *Langman's Medical Embryology*. 5th ed. Baltimore: Williams & Wilkins; 1985.)

The portal vein forms behind the neck of the pancreas at the confluence of the superior mesenteric vein and the splenic vein. The length of the main portal vein ranges from 5.5 to 8 cm, and its diameter is usually approximately 1 cm. Cephalad to its formation behind the neck of the pancreas, the portal vein runs behind the first portion of the duodenum and into the hepatoduodenal ligament, where it runs along the right border of the lesser omentum, usually posterior to the common bile duct and proper hepatic artery. The left gastric or coronary vein can variably drain into the portal vein, splenic vein, or the junction of the two.

The portal vein divides into main right and left branches at the hilum of the liver. The portal vein is the only vein with both tributaries and branches. The left branch of the portal vein runs transversely along the base of segment IV and into the umbilical fissure, where it gives off branches to segments II and III and feedback branches to segment IV. The left portal vein also gives off posterior branches to the left side of the caudate lobe. The right portal vein has a short extrahepatic course; it usually enters the substance of the liver, where it splits into anterior and posterior sectoral branches. These sectoral branches can occasionally be seen extrahepatically and can come off the main portal vein before its bifurcation. There is usually a small caudate process branch off the main right portal vein or at the right portal vein bifurcation that comes off posteriorly to supply this portion of liver (Fig. 54.9).

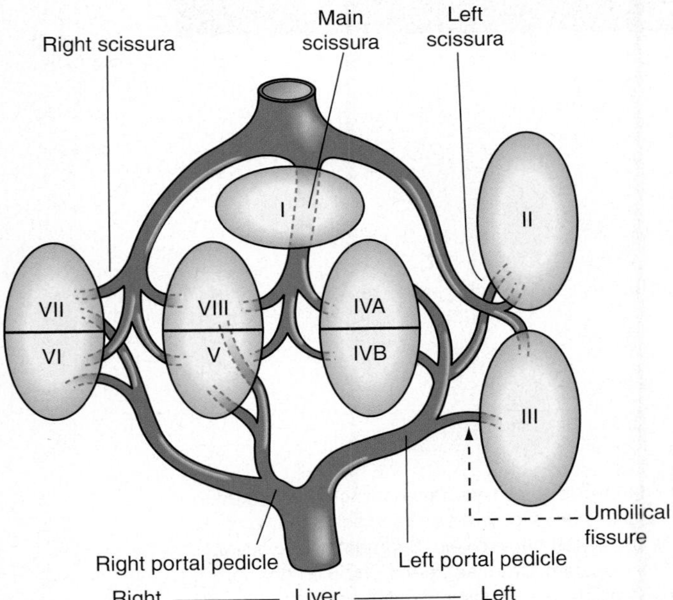

FIG. 54.4 Schematic depiction of the segmental anatomy of the liver. Each segment receives its own portal pedicle (triad of portal vein, hepatic artery, and bile duct). The eight segments are illustrated, and the four sectors, divided by the three main hepatic veins running in scissurae, are shown. The umbilical fissure (not a scissura) is shown to contain the left portal pedicle. (From Blumgart LH, Hann LE. Surgical and radiologic anatomy of the liver and biliary tract. In: Blumgart LH, Fong Y, eds. *Surgery of the Liver and Biliary Tract*. London: WB Saunders; 2000:3–34.)

There are a number of connections between the portal and systemic venous systems. Under conditions of high portal venous pressure, these portosystemic connections may enlarge secondarily to collateral flow. This concept is reviewed in more detail later in the chapter, but the most significant portosystemic collateral locations are the following: the submucosal veins of the proximal stomach and distal esophagus receive portal flow from the short gastric veins and the left gastric vein and can result in varices, with the potential for hemorrhage; the umbilical and abdominal wall veins recanalize from flow through the umbilical vein in the ligamentum teres, resulting in caput medusae; the superior hemorrhoidal plexus receives portal flow from inferior mesenteric vein tributaries and can form large hemorrhoids; and other retroperitoneal communications yield collaterals that can make abdominal surgery hazardous.

The anatomy of the portal vein and its branches is relatively constant and has much less variation than the biliary ductal and hepatic arterial systems. The standard configuration, where main portal vein divides into the left and right branches and the right portal vein then divides into right anterior and right posterior portal vein, is found in up to 70% of individuals. The most common variant from this configuration is the so-called "portal vein trifurcation," where the main portal vein divides into three branches: the left portal vein, the right anterior portal vein, and the right posterior portal vein. The second most common variant is the right posterior portal vein originating as the first branch of portal vein. This can also be envisioned as the right anterior portal vein arising from the left portal vein. These two variations account for the majority of the variations from the so-called normal anatomy. The portal vein is rarely found anterior to the neck of the pancreas and duodenum. Entrance of the portal vein directly into the vena

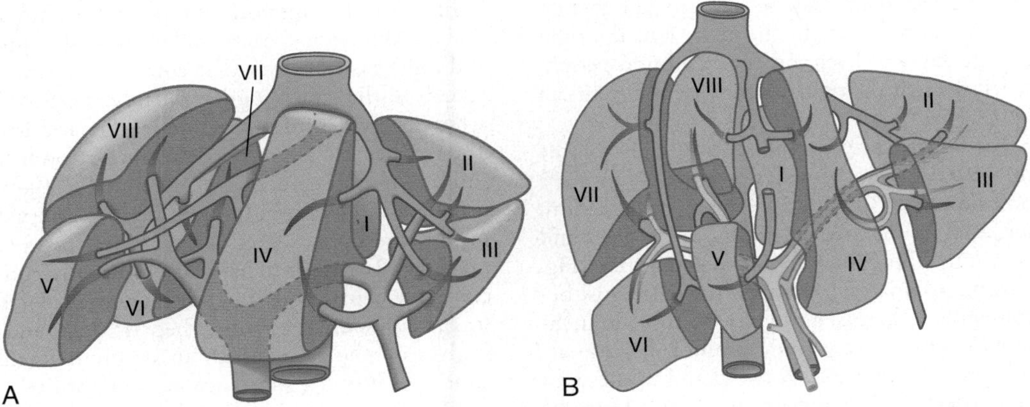

FIG. 54.5 Segmental anatomy of the liver. (A) As seen at laparotomy in the anatomic position. (B) In the ex vivo position. (From Blumgart LH, Hann LE. Surgical and radiologic anatomy of the liver and biliary tract. In: Blumgart LH, Fong Y, eds. *Surgery of the Liver and Biliary Tract*. London: WB Saunders; 2000:3–34.)

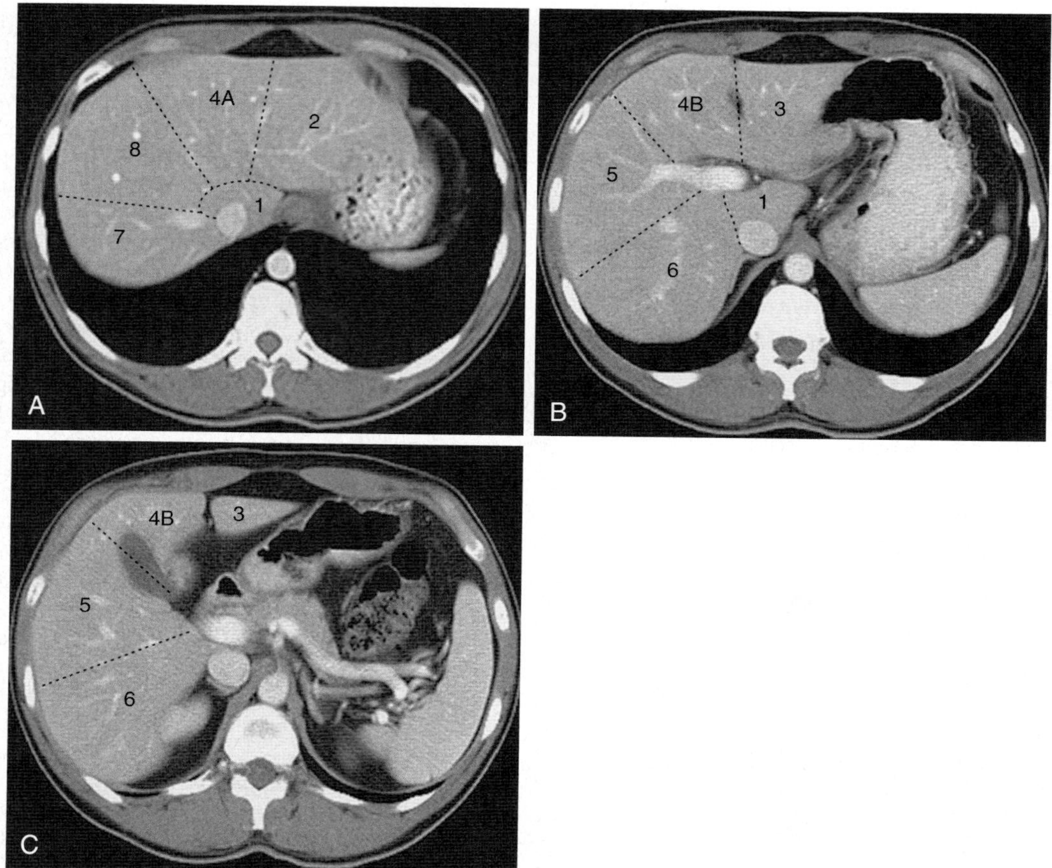

FIG. 54.6 Segmental anatomy of the liver is demonstrated at three levels on contrast-enhanced computed tomography images. (A) At the level of the hepatic veins, the caudate lobe (segment 1) is seen posteriorly embracing the vena cava. Segment 2 is separated from segment 4A by the left hepatic vein. Segment 4A is separated from segment 8 by the middle hepatic vein, and segment 8 is separated from segment 7 by the right hepatic vein. (B) At the level of the portal vein bifurcation, segment 3 is visible as it hangs inferiorly in its anatomic position and is separated from segment 4B by the umbilical fissure. Note that segment 2 is not visible at this level. Terminal branches of the middle hepatic vein separate segment 4B from segment 5, and terminal branches of the right hepatic vein separate segment 5 from segment 6. Note that segments 4A, 8, and 7 are not visible at this level. Segment 1 is seen posterior to the portal vein and embracing the vena cava. (C) Below the portal bifurcation, one can see the inferior tips of segments 3 and 4B. The terminal branches of the middle hepatic vein and the gallbladder mark the separation of segment 4B from segment 5. Segments 5 and 6 are separated by the distal branches of the right hepatic vein. Note how the right liver hangs well inferior to the left liver.

cava has also been described. Very rarely, a pulmonary vein may enter the portal vein. Finally, there may be a congenital absence of the left branch of the portal vein. In this situation, the right branch courses through the right liver and curves around peripherally to supply the left liver, or the right anterior sectoral vein can arise from the left portal vein.

Hepatic artery. The hepatic artery, representing high-volume oxygenated systemic arterial flow, provides approximately 25% of the hepatic blood flow and 30% to 50% of its oxygenation. The common description of the arterial supply to the liver and biliary tree is present only approximately 60% of the time (Fig. 54.10). The celiac trunk originates directly off the aorta, just below the aortic diaphragmatic hiatus, and gives off three branches—splenic artery, left gastric artery, and common hepatic artery. The common hepatic artery passes forward and to the right along the superior border of the pancreas and runs along the right side of the lesser omentum, where it ascends toward the hepatic hilum, lying anterior to the portal vein and to the left of the bile duct. At the point where the common hepatic artery begins to head superiorly toward the hepatic hilum, it gives off the gastroduodenal artery, followed by the supraduodenal artery and right gastric artery. The common hepatic artery beyond the takeoff of the gastroduodenal artery is called the proper hepatic artery; it divides into right and left hepatic arteries at the hilum. The left hepatic artery heads vertically toward the umbilical fissure to supply segments II, III, and IV. The left hepatic artery usually also gives off a middle hepatic artery branch that heads toward the right side of the umbilical fissure and supplies segment IV. The right hepatic artery usually runs posterior to the common hepatic bile duct and enters Calot triangle, bordered by the cystic duct, common hepatic duct, and liver edge, where it gives off the cystic artery to supply the gallbladder and then continues into the substance of the right liver.

Unlike portal vein anatomy, hepatic arterial anatomy is extraordinarily variable (Fig. 54.11). An accessory vessel is described as an aberrant origin of a branch that is in addition to the normal

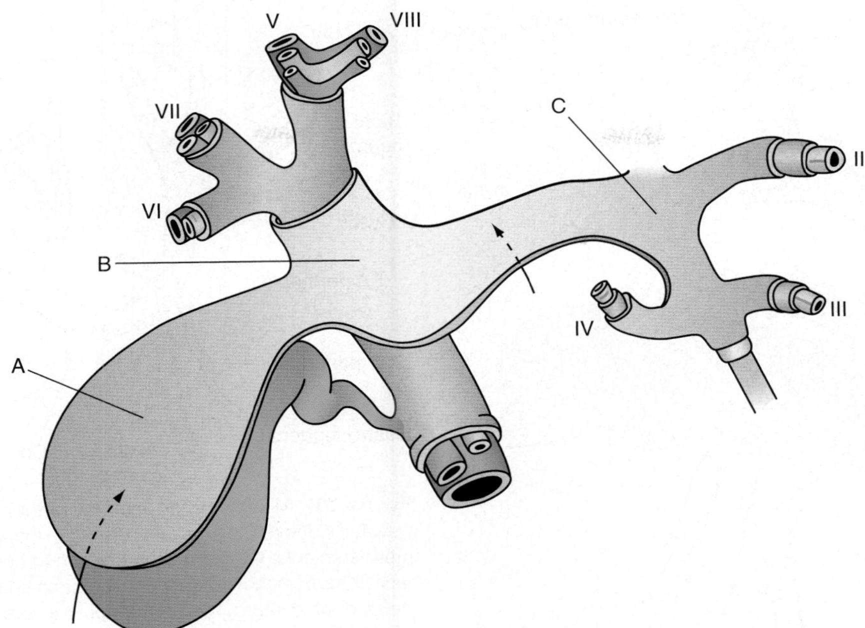

FIG. 54.7 The plate system: the cystic plate between the gallbladder and liver (A); the hilar plate at the biliary confluence at the base of segment IV (B); and the umbilical plate above the umbilical portion of the portal vein (C). Shown are the plane of dissection of the cystic plate for cholecystectomy and the hilar plate for exposure of the hepatic duct confluence and main left hepatic duct *(arrows)*. (From Blumgart LH, Hann LE. Surgical and radiologic anatomy of the liver and biliary tract. In: Blumgart LH, Fong Y, eds. *Surgery of the Liver and Biliary Tract*. London: WB Saunders; 2000:3–34.)

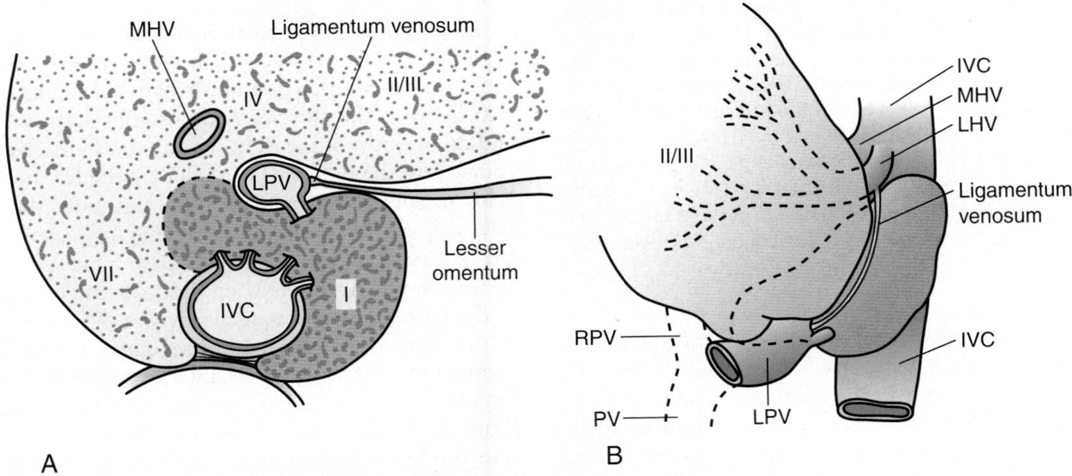

FIG. 54.8 Anatomy of the caudate lobe (segment I). (A) Seen in cross-section, most of the caudate is to the left of the inferior vena cava *(IVC)* and lies posterior to the lesser omentum, which separates the caudate from segments II and III. The termination of the lesser omentum at the ligamentum venosum is demonstrated. The caudate lobe traverses to the right, insinuating itself between the IVC and the left portal vein *(LPV)*, where it attaches to the right liver. Note the proximity of the middle hepatic vein *(MHV)* to these structures. (B) Segments II and III have been rotated to the patient's right, exposing the left side of the caudate. *LHV*, Left hepatic vein; *PV*, portal vein: *RPV*, right portal vein. (From Blumgart LH, Hann LE. Surgical and radiologic anatomy of the liver and biliary tract. In: Blumgart LH, Fong Y, eds. *Surgery of the Liver and Biliary Tract*. London: WB Saunders; 2000:3–34.)

branching pattern. A replaced vessel is described as an aberrant origin of a branch that substitutes for the lack of the normal branch. The hepatic artery usually originates off the celiac trunk. However, branches or the entire hepatic arterial system can originate off the superior mesenteric artery. The right and left hepatic arteries can also arise separately off the celiac axis. Replaced or accessory right hepatic arteries come off the superior mesenteric artery and are present approximately 11% to 21% of the time. Hepatic vessels replaced to the superior mesenteric artery run behind the head of the pancreas, posterior to the portal vein in the portacaval space. This is evident on cross-sectional imaging as well as during operative exploration by feeling hepatic artery pulsation in the

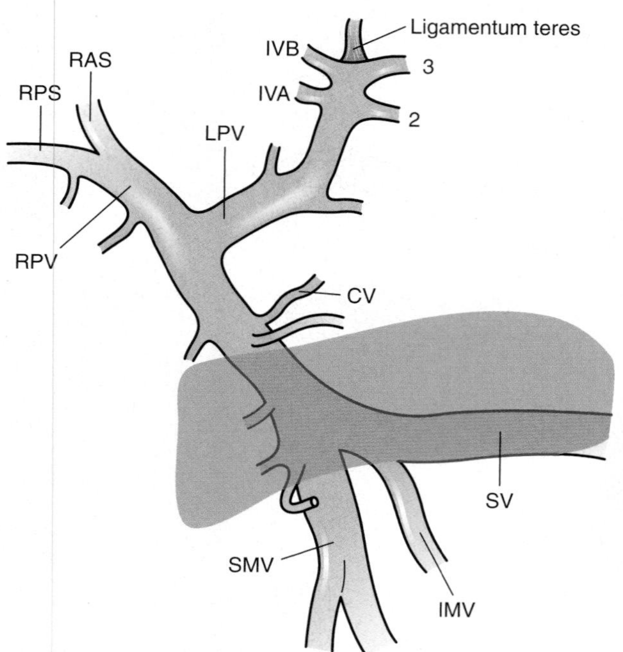

FIG. 54.9 Anatomy of the portal vein. The superior mesenteric vein *(SMV)* joins the splenic vein *(SV)* posterior to the neck of the pancreas *(shaded area)* to form the portal vein. Note the entrance of the inferior mesenteric vein *(IMV)* into the splenic vein, the most common anatomic arrangement. In its course superiorly in the edge of the lesser omentum posterior to the common bile duct and hepatic artery, the portal vein receives venous effluent from the coronary vein *(CV)*. At the hepatic hilum, the portal vein bifurcates into a larger right portal vein *(RPV)* and a smaller left portal vein *(LPV)*. The LPV runs transversely at the base of segment IV and enters the umbilical fissure to supply the segments of the left liver. Just before the umbilical fissure, the LPV usually gives off a sizable branch to the caudate lobe. The RPV enters the substance of the liver and splits into right anterior sectoral *(RAS)* and right posterior sectoral *(RPS)* branches. It also gives off a posterior branch to the right side of the caudate lobe–caudate process. (From Blumgart LH, Hann LE. Surgical and radiologic anatomy of the liver and biliary tract. In: Blumgart LH, Fong Y, eds. *Surgery of the Liver and Biliary Tract*. London: WB Saunders; 2000:3–34.)

lateral border of the hepatoduodenal ligament behind the portal vein and bile duct. The right hepatic artery, in its usual branching pattern, can also course anterior to the common hepatic duct. A replaced or accessory left hepatic artery is present approximately 3.8% to 10% of the time, originates from the left gastric artery, and courses within the lesser omentum, heading toward the umbilical fissure. Other important variations include the origin of the gastroduodenal artery, which has been found to originate from the right hepatic artery and is occasionally duplicated. The anatomy of the cystic artery is also variable; knowledge of these variations is of particular importance in the performance of cholecystectomy (Fig. 54.12). An accessory cystic artery can originate from the proper hepatic artery or gastroduodenal artery, where it runs anterior to the bile duct. A single cystic artery can originate anywhere off the proper hepatic artery or gastroduodenal artery or directly from the celiac axis. These variant cystic arteries can run anterior to the bile duct and are not necessarily present in the triangle of Calot. All these variations in hepatic arterial anatomy are of obvious importance during hepatic resection, hepatic arterial pump placement, cholecystectomy, and hepatic interventional radiologic procedures.

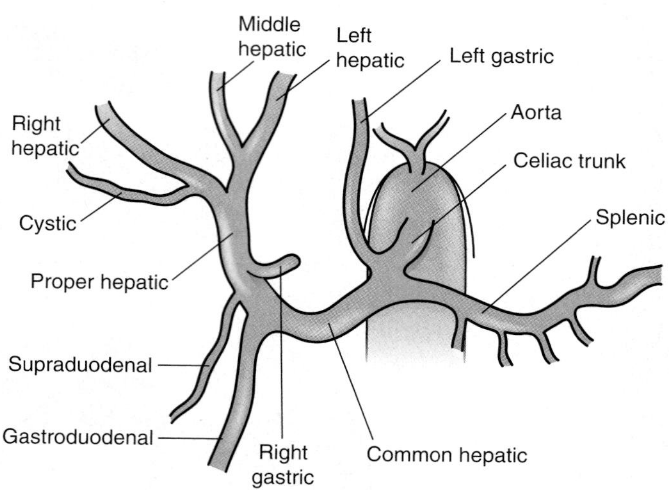

FIG. 54.10 Most common anatomy of the celiac axis and hepatic arterial system. The celiac axis, just below the diaphragmatic hiatus, trifurcates into the splenic, left gastric, and common hepatic arteries. The common hepatic artery heads to the right and turns superiorly toward the hilum. At the point of this turn, the gastroduodenal artery is given off, and the proper hepatic artery is formed. The common hepatic artery gives off right and left hepatic arteries in the hilum. Note the middle hepatic artery off the proximal left hepatic artery, which goes on to supply segment IV. The cystic artery usually comes off the right hepatic artery within the triangle of Calot. (From Blumgart LH, Hann LE. Surgical and radiologic anatomy of the liver and biliary tract. In: Blumgart LH, Fong Y, eds. *Surgery of the Liver and Biliary Tract*. London: WB Saunders; 2000:3–34.)

Hepatic veins. The three major hepatic veins drain from the superior-posterior surface of the liver directly into the IVC (see Figs. 54.4 to 54.6). The right hepatic vein runs in the right scissura between the anterior and posterior sectors of the right liver and drains most of the right liver after a short (1-cm) extrahepatic course into the right side of the IVC. The left and middle hepatic veins usually join intrahepatically and enter the left side of the IVC as a single vessel, although they may drain separately. The left hepatic vein runs in the left scissura between segments II and III and drains segments II and III; the middle hepatic vein runs in the portal scissura between segment IV and the anterior sector of the right liver, composed of segments V and VIII, and drains segment IV and some of the anterior sector of the right liver. The umbilical vein is an additional vein that runs under the falciform ligament, between the left and middle veins, and usually empties into the left hepatic vein. A number of small posterior venous branches from the right posterior sector and caudate lobe drain directly into the IVC. A substantial inferiorly located accessory right hepatic vein is commonly encountered. There is also often a venous tributary from the caudate lobe that drains superiorly into the left hepatic vein.

Biliary system. The intrahepatic bile ducts are the terminal branches of the right and left hepatic ductal branches that invaginate Glisson capsule at the hilum, along with their corresponding portal vein and hepatic artery branches, forming the peritoneal covered portal triads also known as portal pedicles. Along these intrahepatic portal pedicles, the bile duct branches are usually superior to the portal vein, whereas the hepatic artery branches run inferiorly. The left hepatic bile duct drains segments II, III, and IV, which constitute the left liver. The intrahepatic ductal branches of the left liver join to form the main left duct at the base of the umbilical fissure, where the left hepatic duct courses transversely

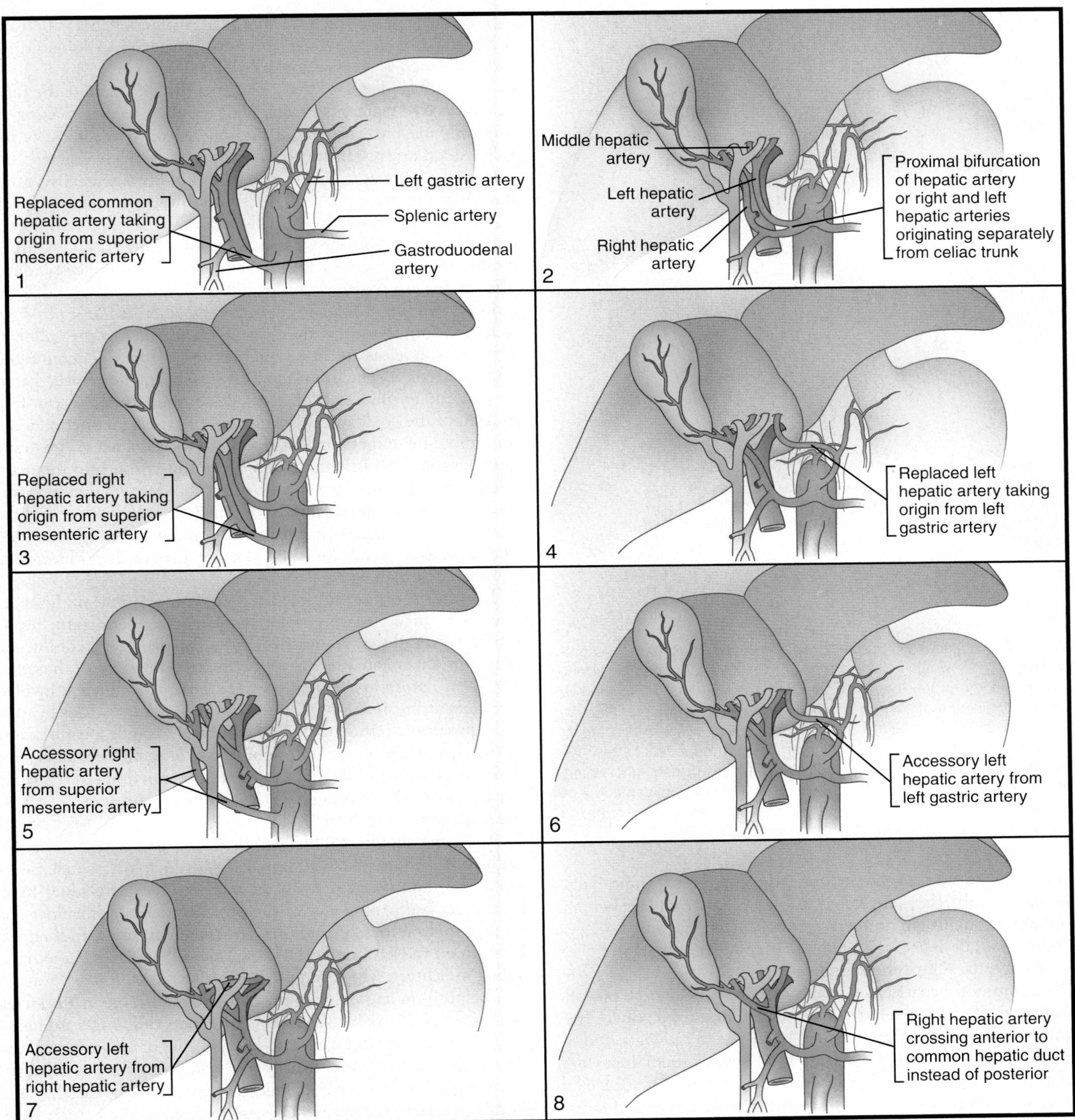

FIG. 54.11 Variable anatomy of the hepatic artery. The common hepatic artery can originate off the superior mesenteric artery instead of the celiac axis. A replaced or accessory right hepatic artery comes off the superior mesenteric artery and runs posterior to the head of the pancreas, to the right of the portal vein, and behind the common bile duct into the hilum. A replaced or accessory left hepatic artery originates off the left gastric artery and runs through the lesser omentum into the umbilical fissure. (From Netter FH. Netter anatomy collection. www.netterimages.com. ©Elsevier Inc. All rights reserved.)

across the base of segment IV to join the right hepatic duct at the hilum. In its transverse portion, the left hepatic duct drains one to three small branches from segment IV. The right hepatic duct drains the right liver and is formed by the joining of the anterior sectoral duct (draining segments V and VIII) and the posterior sectoral duct (draining segments VI and VII). The posterior sectoral duct runs in a horizontal and posterior direction; the anterior sectoral duct runs vertically. The main right hepatic duct bifurcates just above the right portal vein. The short right hepatic duct meets the longer left hepatic duct to form the confluence anterior

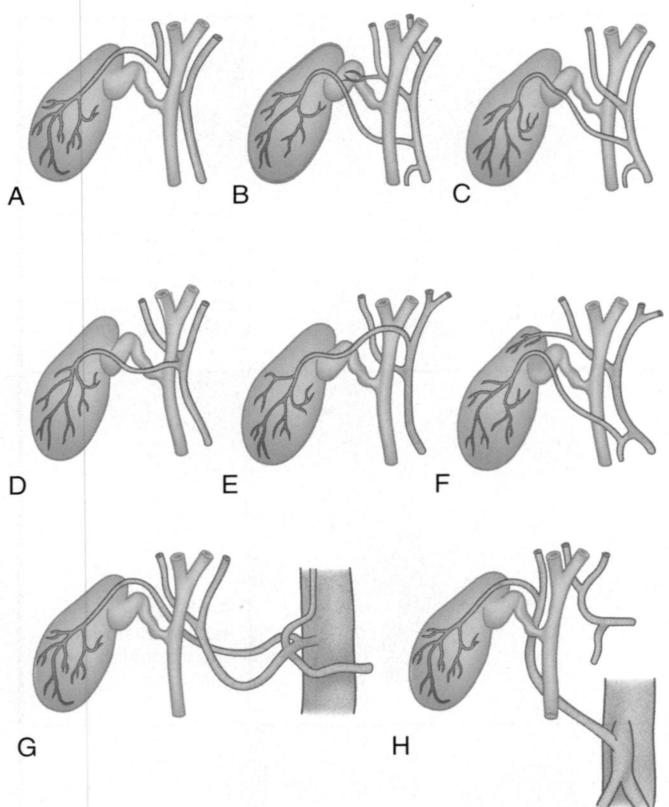

FIG. 54.12 Variations in the anatomy of the cystic artery. (A) Most common anatomy. (B) Double cystic artery, one off the proper hepatic artery. (C) Origin off the proper hepatic artery and coursing anterior to the bile duct. (D) Originating off the right hepatic artery and coursing anterior to the bile duct. (E) Originating from the left hepatic artery and coursing anterior to the bile duct. (F) Originating off the gastroduodenal artery. (G) Originating off the celiac axis. (H) Originating from a replaced right hepatic artery. (From Blumgart LH, Hann LE. Surgical and radiologic anatomy of the liver and biliary tract. In: Blumgart LH, Fong Y, eds. *Surgery of the Liver and Biliary Tract*. London: WB Saunders; 2000:3–34.)

to the right portal vein, constituting the common hepatic duct. The caudate lobe (segment I) has its own biliary drainage, which is usually through right and left systems. However, in up to 15% of individuals, drainage is through the left system only, and in 5%, it is through the right system only.

The common hepatic duct drains inferiorly. Below the takeoff of the cystic duct, it is referred to as the common bile duct. The common bile duct usually measures 10 to 15 cm in length and is typically 6 mm in diameter. The common hepatic (bile) duct runs along the right side of the hepatoduodenal ligament (free edge of the lesser omentum) to the right of the hepatic artery and anterior to the portal vein. The common bile duct continues inferiorly behind the first portion of the duodenum and into the head of the pancreas in an inferior and slightly rightward direction. The intrapancreatic distal common bile duct then joins with the main pancreatic duct (of Wirsung), with or without a common channel, and enters the second portion of the duodenum through the major papilla of Vater. At the choledochoduodenal junction, a complex muscular complex known as the sphincter of Oddi regulates bile flow and prevents reflux of duodenal contents into the biliary tree. There are three major parts to this sphincter: (1) the sphincter choledochus, which is a circular muscle that regulates bile flow and the filling of the gallbladder; (2) the pancreatic sphincter, present to variable degrees, which surrounds the intraduodenal pancreatic duct; and (3) the sphincter ampullae, made up of longitudinal muscle, which prevents duodenal reflux.

The gallbladder is a biliary reservoir that lies against the inferior surface of segments IV and V of the liver, usually making an impression against the liver. A peritoneal layer covers most of the gallbladder, except for the portion adherent to the liver. Here, the gallbladder adheres to the liver by a layer of fibroconnective tissue known as the cystic plate, an extension of the hilar plate (see Fig. 54.7). Variable in size but usually about 10 cm long and 3 to 5 cm wide, the gallbladder is composed of a fundus, body, infundibulum, and neck, which ultimately empty into the cystic duct. The fundus usually projects just slightly beyond the liver edge anteriorly; when it is folded on itself, it is described as a phrygian cap. Continuing toward the bile duct, the body of the gallbladder is usually close to the second portion of the duodenum and transverse colon. The infundibulum (or Hartmann pouch) hangs forward along the free edge of the lesser omentum and can fold in front of the cystic duct. The portion of gallbladder between the infundibulum and cystic duct is referred to as the neck. The cystic duct is variable in its length, course, and insertion into the main biliary tree. The first portion of the cystic duct is usually tortuous and contains mucosal duplications referred to as the folds of Heister, which regulate the filling and emptying of the gallbladder. The cystic duct usually joins the common hepatic duct to form the common bile duct.

Knowledge of the multiple and frequent variations in the anatomy of the biliary tree is absolutely essential for performing hepatobiliary procedures. Anomalies of the hepatic ductal confluence are common and are present approximately one third of the time. The most common anomalies of the biliary confluence involve variations in the insertion of the right sectoral ducts. Usually, this is the posterior sectoral duct. The confluence can be a trifurcation of the right anterior sectoral, right posterior sectoral, and left hepatic ducts. Either of the right sectoral ducts can drain into the left hepatic duct, the common hepatic duct, the cystic duct, or, rarely, the gallbladder (Fig. 54.13).

Anomalies of the gallbladder itself are rare. Agenesis of the gallbladder, bilobar gallbladder with two ducts or a single duct, septations, and congenital diverticulum of the gallbladder have been described. Anomalies of the position of the gallbladder are more common; these include an intrahepatic position and, rarely, location on the left side of the liver. The gallbladder can also have a long mesentery, which can predispose it to torsion.

The position and entry of the cystic duct into the main ductal system are also variable. Double cystic ducts draining a unilocular gallbladder and drainage into hepatic duct branches have been reported. The cystic duct usually joins the common hepatic duct at an angle; but it can run parallel and enter it more distally, and in this situation, the cystic duct can be fused to the hepatic duct along its parallel course by connective tissue. The cystic duct can also run a spiral course anteriorly or posteriorly and enter the left side of the common hepatic duct. Finally, the cystic duct can be very short or even absent (Fig. 54.14).

The supraduodenal and infrahilar bile ducts are predominantly supplied by two axial vessels that run at 3- and 9-o'clock positions. These vessels are derived from the superior pancreaticoduodenal, right hepatic, cystic, gastroduodenal, and retroduodenal arteries. It has been estimated that only 2% of the arterial supply to this portion of the bile duct is segmental, arising directly off the proper hepatic artery. The bile duct and its bifurcation in the hilum derive their arterial blood supply from a rich network of multiple small

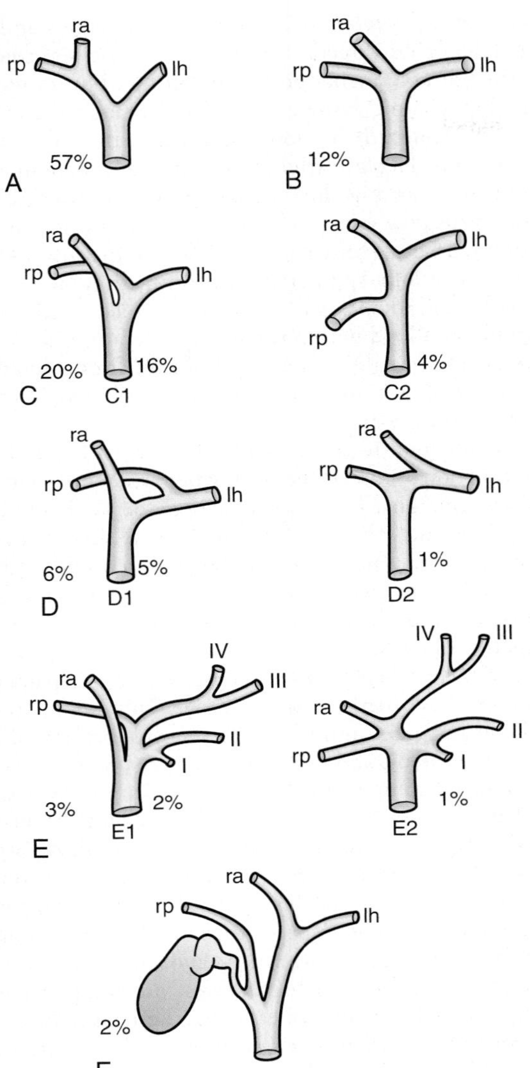

FIG. 54.13 Variations of the hepatic duct confluence. (A) Most common anatomy. (B) Trifurcation at the confluence. (C) Either of the right sectoral ducts drains into the common hepatic duct. (D) Either of the right sectoral ducts drains into the left hepatic duct. (E) Absence of a hepatic duct confluence. (F) Absence of right hepatic duct and drainage of right posterior sectoral duct into the cystic duct. (From Blumgart LH, Hann LE. Surgical and radiologic anatomy of the liver and biliary tract. In: Blumgart LH, Fong Y, eds. *Surgery of the Liver and Biliary Tract*. London: WB Saunders; 2000:3–34.)

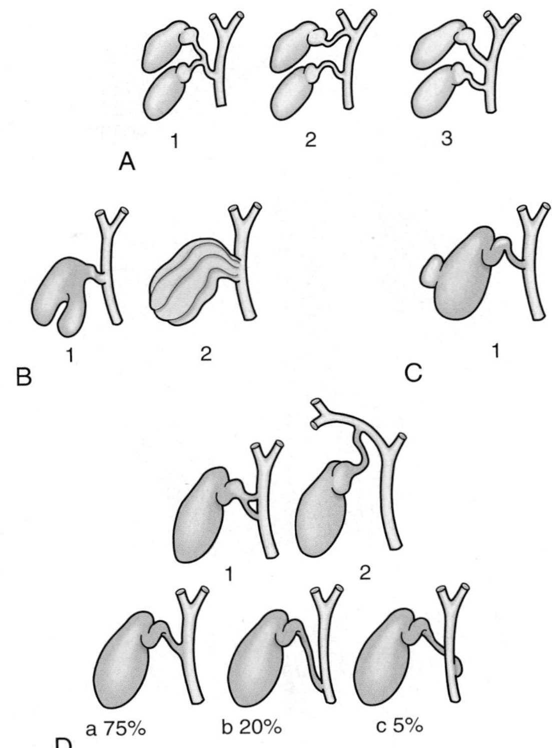

FIG. 54.14 Variations in the anatomy of the gallbladder and cystic duct. (A) Bilobar gallbladder. (B) Septations of the gallbladder. (C) Diverticulum of the gallbladder. (D) Variations in cystic duct anatomy. The three types of union of the cystic duct and common hepatic duct are illustrated. (From Blumgart LH, Hann LE. Surgical and radiologic anatomy of the liver and biliary tract. In: Blumgart LH, Fong Y, eds. *Surgery of the Liver and Biliary Tract*. London: WB Saunders; 2000:3–34.)

branches from surrounding vessels. Similarly, the retropancreatic bile duct derives its arterial supply from the retroduodenal artery, which provides a rich network of multiple small branches (Fig. 54.15). Venous drainage of the bile duct parallels the arterial supply and drains into the portal venous system. The venous drainage of the gallbladder empties into the veins that drain the bile duct and does not flow directly into the portal vein.

Nerves. The innervation of the liver and biliary tract is through sympathetic fibers originating from T7 through T10 as well as parasympathetic fibers from both vagal nerves. The sympathetic fibers pass through celiac ganglia before giving off postganglionic fibers to the liver and bile ducts. The right-sided celiac ganglia and right vagal nerve form an anterior hepatic plexus of nerves that runs along the hepatic artery. The left-sided celiac ganglia and left vagal nerve form a posterior hepatic plexus that runs posterior to the bile duct and portal vein. The hepatic arteries are supplied by sympathetic fibers, whereas the gallbladder and extrahepatic bile ducts receive innervation from sympathetic and parasympathetic fibers. The clinical significance of these nerves is still not well understood. Acute distention of the liver, and thus the liver capsule, can result in right upper quadrant pain, which may be referred to the right shoulder through phrenic nerve innervation of the diaphragmatic peritoneum.

Lymphatics. Most lymph node drainage from the liver is to the hepatoduodenal ligament. From here, lymphatic drainage usually continues along the hepatic artery to the celiac lymph nodes and then to the cisterna chyli. Lymphatic drainage can also follow the hepatic veins to lymph nodes in the area of the suprahepatic IVC and through the diaphragmatic hiatus. The lymphatic drainage of the gallbladder and most of the extrahepatic biliary tract is generally into the lymph nodes of the hepatoduodenal ligament. This drainage may follow along the hepatic artery to the celiac lymph nodes, but it can also flow into lymph nodes behind the head of the pancreas or within the aortocaval groove.

Microscopic Anatomy

Functional unit of the liver. The organization of hepatic parenchyma into microscopic functional units has been described in a number of ways, referred to as an acinus or a lobule (Fig. 54.16). This was originally described by Rappaport and then modified by Matsumoto and Kawakami. A lobule is made up of

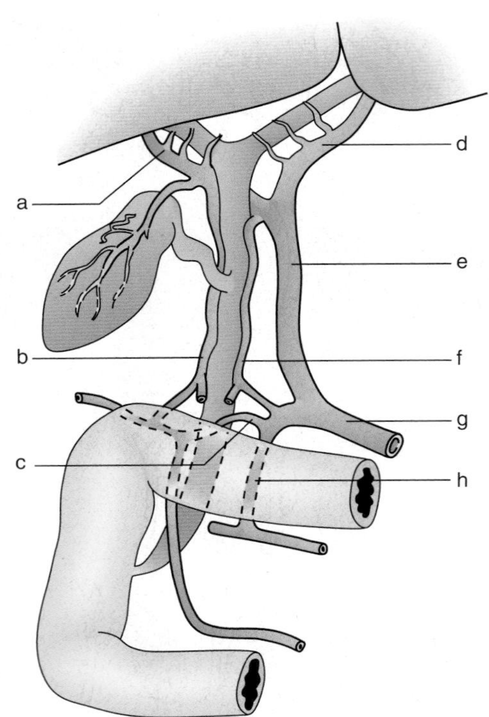

FIG. 54.15 Blood supply to the common bile duct and common hepatic duct: right hepatic artery *(a)*; 9:00 artery *(b)*; retroduodenal artery *(c)*; left hepatic artery *(d)*; proper hepatic artery *(e)*; 3:00 artery *(f)*; common hepatic artery *(g)*; gastroduodenal artery *(h)*. (From Blumgart LH, Hann LE. Surgical and radiologic anatomy of the liver and biliary tract. In: Blumgart LH, Fong Y, eds. *Surgery of the Liver and Biliary Tract*. London: WB Saunders; 2000:3–34.)

a central terminal hepatic venule surrounded by four to six terminal portal triads that form a polygonal unit. This unit is lined on its periphery between each terminal portal triad by terminal portal triad branches. In between the terminal portal triads and the central hepatic venule, hepatocytes are arranged in one-cell-thick plates, surrounded on each side by endothelium-lined and blood-filled sinusoids. Blood flows from the terminal portal triad through the sinusoids into the terminal hepatic venule. Bile is formed within the hepatocytes and empties into terminal canaliculi, which form on the lateral walls of the intercellular hepatocyte. These ultimately coalesce into bile ducts and flow toward the portal triads. This functional hepatic unit provides a structural basis for the many metabolic and secretory functions of the liver.

Between the terminal portal triad and central hepatic venule are three zones that differ in their enzymatic makeup as well as exposure to nutrients and oxygenated blood. There is debate about the shape of these zones and their relationship to the basic lobular unit, but in general, zones 1 through 3 splay out from the terminal portal triad toward the central hepatic venule. Zone 1 (periportal zone) is an environment rich in nutrients and oxygen. Zone 2 (intermediate zone) and zone 3 (perivenular zone) are exposed to environments that are poorer in oxygen and nutrients. The cells of the different zones differ enzymatically and respond differently to toxin exposure and hypoxia. This anatomic arrangement also explains the phenomenon of centrilobular necrosis from hypotension because zone 3 is the most susceptible to decreases in oxygen delivery.

Hepatic microcirculation. Terminal portal venous and hepatic arterial branches directly supply the hepatic sinusoids with blood. The portal branches provide a constant but minimal flow into this low-volume system; the arterial branches provide the sinusoids with pulsatile but low-volume flow that enhances flow in the sinusoids. Hepatic arterial branches terminate in a plexus around the terminal bile ductules and provide nutrients. Arterial and portal vein flow varies inversely in the sinusoids and can be compensatory. Local control of blood flow in the sinusoids likely depends on arteriolar sphincters and contraction of the sinusoidal lining by endothelial cells and hepatic stellate cells or portal myofibroblasts. Blood within the sinusoids empties directly into terminal hepatic venules at the center of a functional lobule. This process results in the unidirectional flow of blood in the liver from zone 1 to zone 3.

The endothelium-lined sinusoids of the hepatic lobule represent the functional unit of the liver, where afferent blood flow is exposed to functional hepatic parenchyma before being drained into hepatic venules (Fig. 54.17). The hepatic sinusoids are 7 to 15 μm wide but can increase in size by up to ten-fold. This yields a low-resistance and low-pressure (generally 2–3 mm Hg) system. The sinusoidal endothelial cells account for 15% to 20% of the total hepatic cell mass.

Sinusoidal endothelial cells are separated from hepatocytes by the space of Disse (perisinusoidal space). This is an extravascular fluid compartment into which hepatocytes project microvilli, which allows proteins and other plasma components from the sinusoids to be taken up by the hepatocytes. Within this space, the endothelial cells are specialized in that they lack intercellular junctions and a basement membrane but contain multiple large fenestrations. This arrangement provides for the maximal contact of hepatocyte membranes with this extravascular fluid compartment and blood in the sinusoidal space. Thus, this system permits bidirectional movement of solutes (high- and low-molecular-weight substances) into and out of hepatocytes, providing tremendous filtration potential. On the other hand, the fenestrations of the endothelial cells restrict movement of molecules between the sinusoids and hepatocytes and vary in response to exogenous and endogenous mediators.

Other cell types are found along the sinusoidal lining. Kupffer cells, derived from the macrophage-monocyte system, are irregularly shaped cells that also line the sinusoids insinuating between endothelial cells. Kupffer cells are phagocytic, can migrate along sinusoids to areas of injury, and play a major role in the trapping of foreign substances and initiating inflammatory responses. Major histocompatibility complex II antigens are expressed on Kupffer cells but do not confer efficient antigen presentation compared with macrophages elsewhere in the body. Other lymphoid cells also exist in hepatic parenchyma, such as natural killer, natural killer T, CD4 T, and CD8 T cells. These provide the liver with an innate immune system. Hepatic stellate cells, previously known as Ito cells, are cells high in retinoid content (accounting for their phenotypic identification) found in the space of Disse. They have dendritic processes that contact hepatocyte microvilli and also wrap around endothelial cells. The major functions of these stellate cells include vitamin A storage and the synthesis of extracellular collagen and other extracellular matrix proteins. In acute and chronic hepatic liver injuries, hepatic stellate cells are activated to a myofibroblastic state associated with morphologic changes, cellular contractility, decreases in intracellular vitamin A, and production of extracellular matrix. Ultimately, stellate cells play a central role in the development and progression of hepatic

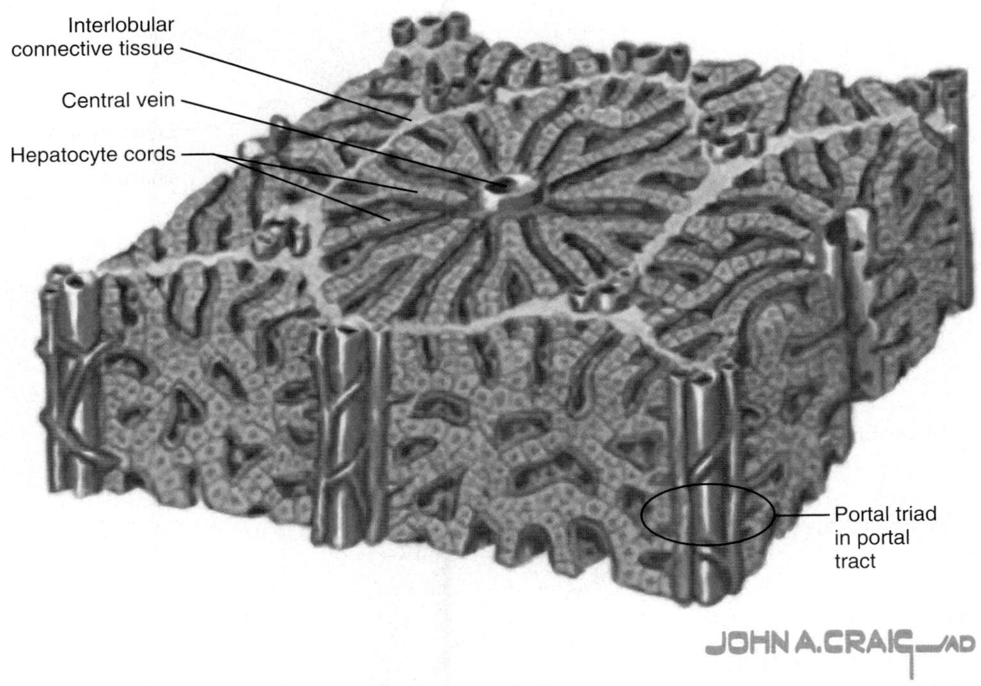

Hepatic lobule. Liver arranged as series of hexagonal lobules, each composed of series of hepatocyte cords (plates) interspersed with sinusoids. Each lobule surrounds a central vein and is bounded by 6 peripheral portal triads (low magnification).

FIG. 54.16 Schematic illustration of a hepatic lobule seen as a three-dimensional polyhedral unit. The terminal portal triads (hepatic artery, portal vein, and bile duct) are at each corner and give off branches along the sides of the lobule. Hepatocytes are in single-cell sheets with sinusoids on either end aligned radially toward a central hepatic venule. (From Netter FH. Netter anatomy collection. www.netterimages.com. ©Elsevier Inc. All rights reserved.)

fibrosis to cirrhosis and are the target for the development of antifibrotic treatments.

Hepatocytes. Hepatocytes are complex multifunctional cells that make up 60% of the hepatic cellular mass and 80% of the cytoplasmic mass of the liver (Fig. 54.17). The hepatocyte is a polyhedral cell with a central spherical nucleus. As noted, hepatocytes are arranged in single-cell-layer plates lined on either side by blood-filled sinusoids. Every hepatocyte has contact with adjacent hepatocytes, the biliary space (bile canaliculus), and the perisinusoidal space, enabling these cells to perform their broad range of functions. Among the many essential functions of the hepatocyte are the following: uptake, storage, and release of nutrients; synthesis of glucose, fatty acids, lipids, and numerous plasma proteins (including C-reactive protein and albumin); production and secretion of bile for digestion of dietary fats; and degradation and detoxification of toxins.

To carry out these functions, the plasma membrane of the hepatocyte is organized in a specific manner into three specific domains. The sinusoidal membrane is exposed to the space of Disse and has multiple microvilli that provide a surface specialized in the active transport of substances between the blood and hepatocytes. The lateral domain exists between neighboring hepatocytes and contains gap junctions that provide for intercellular communication. The canalicular membrane is a tube containing microvilli formed by two apposed hepatocytes. These bile canaliculi are sealed by zonula occludens (tight junctions), which prevent the escape of bile. The bile canaliculi form a ring around the hepatocyte that drains into small bile ducts known as canals of Hering, which empty into a bile duct at a portal triad. The canalicular membrane contains adenosine triphosphate (ATP)–dependent active transport systems that enable solutes to be secreted into the canalicular membrane against large concentration gradients.

The hepatocyte is one of the most diverse and metabolically active cells in the body, as reflected by its abundance of organelles. There are 1000 mitochondria/hepatocytes occupying approximately 20% of the cell volume. Mitochondria generate energy (ATP) through oxidative phosphorylation and provide the energy for the metabolic demands of the hepatocyte. The hepatocyte mitochondria are also essential for fatty acid oxidation. The monoclonal antibody HepPar1 (hepatocyte paraffin 1) identifies a unique antigen on hepatocyte mitochondria and is widely used to identify hepatocytes or hepatocellular neoplasms on immunohistochemical examination.

An extensive system of interconnected membrane complexes made up of smooth and rough endoplasmic reticulum and the Golgi apparatus compose what is known as the hepatocyte microsomal fraction. These complexes have a diverse range of functions, including the following: synthesis of structural and secreted proteins; metabolism of lipids and glucose; production and metabolism of cholesterol; glycosylation of secretory proteins; bile formation and secretion; and drug metabolism. Finally, hepatocytes also contain lysosomes, which are intracellular single-membrane vesicles that contain a number of enzymes. These vesicles store and degrade exogenous and endogenous substances. Coordination of these numerous organelles in the hepatocyte allows these cells to accomplish a large variety of functions.

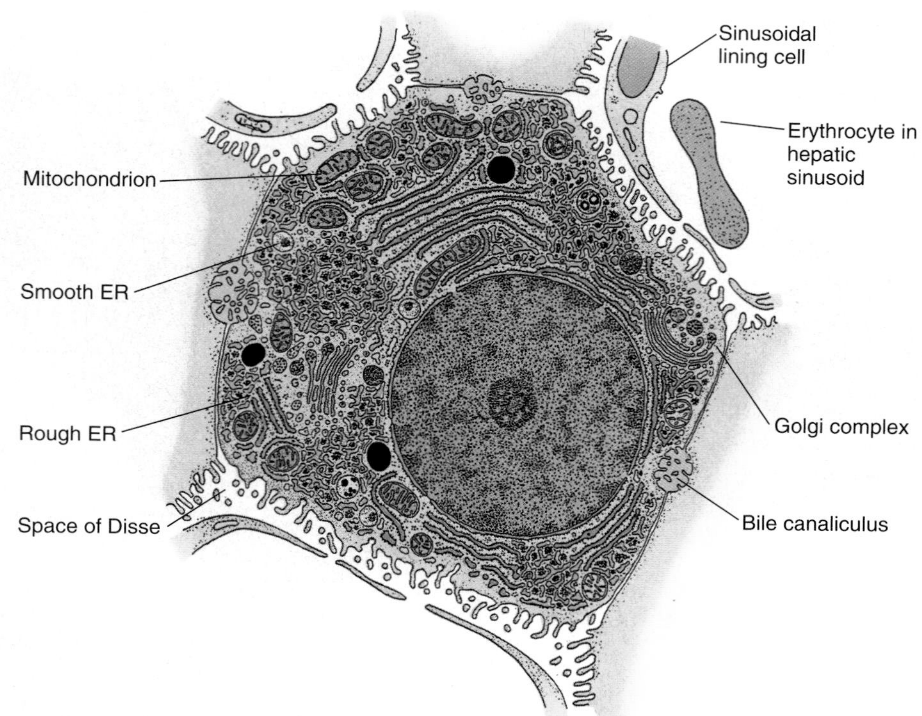

FIG. 54.17 A hepatocyte and its sinusoidal and lateral domains. (From Ross MH, Reith EJ, Romrell LJ. The liver. In: Ross RH, Reith EJ, Romrell LJ. *Histology: A Text and Atlas.* Baltimore: Williams & Wilkins; 1989:471–478.) *ER*, Endoplasmic reticulum.

Functions

The unique anatomic arrangement of the liver provides a remarkable landscape on which the multiple central and critical functions of this organ can be carried out. The liver is the center of metabolic homeostasis; it serves as the regulatory site for energy metabolism by coordinating the uptake, processing, and distribution of nutrients and their subsequent energy products. The liver also synthesizes a large number of proteins, enzymes, and vitamins that participate in a tremendously broad range of body functions. Finally, the liver detoxifies and eliminates many exogenous and endogenous substances, serving as the major filter of the human body. The following sections summarize this broad range of functions.

Energy

The liver is the critical intermediary between dietary sources of energy and the extrahepatic tissues that require this energy. The liver receives dietary byproducts through the portal circulation and sorts, metabolizes, and distributes them into the systemic circulation. The liver also plays a major role in regulating endogenous sources of energy, such as fatty acids and glycerol from adipose tissues and lactate, pyruvate, and certain amino acids from skeletal muscle. The two major sources of energy that the liver releases into the extrahepatic circulation are glucose and acetoacetate. Glucose is derived from the glycogenolysis of stored glycogen and from gluconeogenesis from lactate, pyruvate, glycerol, propionate, and alanine. Acetoacetate is derived from the β-oxidation of fatty acids. Also, storage lipids such as triacylglycerols and phospholipids are synthesized and stored as lipoproteins by the liver. These can be circulated systemically for uptake by peripheral tissues. These complex and essential functions are regulated by hormones, overall nutritional state of the organism, and requirements of obligate glucose-requiring tissues.

Functional Heterogeneity

To add to the metabolic complexity of the liver, hepatocytes vary in their function, depending on their location within the lobule. This functional heterogeneity of hepatocytes is anatomically related to their location in the three zones of the lobule and is specifically related to the distance from the incoming portal triad. For example, cells located in the periportal zone (zone 1) are exposed to a high concentration of substrates. Thus, uptake of oxygen and solutes is greater here. A critically important function of hepatocytes, however, is their ability to change their metabolic functionality and to be recruited to perform specific functions under varying physiologic conditions, regardless of anatomic location. Sinusoids in the periportal zone are narrower and more tortuous, facilitating increased uptake of substrate by the hepatocytes in this area. In contrast, sinusoids in zone 3 (perivenous) have larger fenestrations, allowing uptake of larger molecules. Thus, sinusoids are also variable in form and function.

Enzymatic makeup, plasma membrane proteins, and ultrastructure are also heterogeneous among the hepatocyte population. This cellular protein variability can also be distinguished on the basis of the hepatocyte location within the lobule. Glucose uptake and release, bile formation, and synthesis of albumin and fibrinogen take place in the periportal zone, whereas glucose catabolism, xenobiotic metabolism, and synthesis of α_1-antitrypsin and α-fetoprotein (AFP) occur in the perivenous zone. Another example of enzymatic heterogeneity according to lobular zones is the location of the urea cycle enzymes in zone 3, adjacent to the terminal hepatic veins. The functional hepatocyte heterogeneity and its anatomic relationship to the lobular unit account for patterns of damage from metabolic or physiologic insults to the liver.

Blood Flow

There is a dual blood supply to the liver that comes from the portal vein and hepatic artery. The portal vein provides approximately 75% of the blood flow to the liver, which is oxygen poor but rich in nutrients. The hepatic artery provides the other 25% of the blood flow, which is oxygen rich and represents systemic arterial blood flow. The large flow rate of the portal vein is still able to provide 50% to 70% of the afferent oxygenation to the liver. Overall, hepatic blood flow represents about 25% of the cardiac output, demonstrating its central role in whole body metabolism. Hepatic blood flow is decreased during exercise and increased after ingestion of food. Carbohydrates have the most profound effect on hepatic blood flow. Hepatic arterial pressure is representative of systemic arterial pressure. Portal pressure is generally 6 to 10 mm Hg, and sinusoidal pressure is usually 2 to 4 mm Hg.

Hepatic blood flow is regulated by various factors. Differences in afferent and efferent vessel pressures as well as muscular sphincters located at the inlet and outlet of the sinusoids play a major role. Muscular sphincter tone is regulated by the autonomic nervous system, circulating hormones, bile salts, and metabolites. Specific endogenous factors known to affect hepatic blood flow include glucagon, histamine, bradykinin, prostaglandins, nitric oxide, and many gut hormones, including gastrin, secretin, and cholecystokinin. The sinusoids are also the primary regulators of hepatic blood flow through contraction and expansion of their endothelial cells, Kupffer cells, and hepatic stellate cells.

A one-way reciprocal relationship between hepatic artery and portal vein flow has been demonstrated. Increases in hepatic arterial flow accompany decreases in portal vein flow, but the opposite does not occur. Hepatic arterial compensation, however, cannot provide complete compensation to support hepatic parenchyma in total portal vein occlusion, which is likely the cause of ipsilateral atrophy in this case. Experimental evidence has suggested that the buildup of adenosine in the liver plays an important role in this hepatic arterial compensatory response.

Bile Formation

One of the major functions of the liver is bile production and secretion. The physiologic role of bile is twofold. The first is to dispose of substances secreted into bile; the second is to provide enteric bile salts to aid in the digestion of fats. Bile is a substance containing organic and inorganic solutes produced by an active process of secretion and subsequent concentration of these solutes. The concentration of inorganic solutes in bile in the main biliary tree resembles that of plasma (Table 54.1). In the case of bile loss (e.g., from an external biliary fistula), the high concentrations of protein and electrolytes must be considered in replacing the losses. The osmolality of bile is approximately 300 mOsmol/kg and is accounted for by the inorganic solutes. The major organic solutes in bile are bile acids, bile pigments, cholesterol, and phospholipids.

The contents of bile are generally absorbed from the bloodstream through sinusoids into the hepatocyte through the sinusoidal membrane. Bile is initially secreted by hepatocytes into the canaliculi through specialized microvilli containing lateral membranes of the hepatocytes that form the canaliculi. Tight junctions along the canalicular membranes prevent leakage of bile in the normal state. This also provides a route for paracellular secretion of solutes and water into bile. The canaliculi coalesce into larger bile ductules containing biliary epithelium, which then form the intrahepatic and extrahepatic biliary tree. Thus, the liver, in part, serves as an epithelial structure that moves solutes from the blood to the bile and provides a route of secretion for bile into the intestines.

TABLE 54.1 Solute concentrations of hepatic bile.

SOLUTE	CONCENTRATION
Na^+	132–165 mEq/L
K^+	4.2–5.6 mEq/L
Ca^{2+}	1.2–4.8 mEq/L
Mg^{2+}	1.4–3.0 mEq/L
Cl^-	96–126 mEq/L
HCO_3^-	17–55 mEq/L
Bile acids	3–45 mM
Phospholipid	25–810 mg/dL
Cholesterol	60–320 mg/dL
Protein	300–3000 mg/L

Approximately 1500 mL of bile is secreted daily, and much of this (~80%) is secreted by hepatocytes into canaliculi. Such canalicular bile flow is largely the result of water flow in response to active solute transport. Bile acids are transported from the sinusoidal blood into the hepatocyte by ATP-requiring active transport. Intracellular transport to the canalicular membrane is through bile acid–binding proteins that are transported by a vesicular system derived from the Golgi apparatus. The bile acids are then actively pumped into the canaliculus through an ATP-requiring active transport system. It is well recognized that bile flow has a linear association with bile acid secretion, known as bile acid–dependent flow. Because bile acids form micelles in the bile and do not provide osmotic potential, it is likely that flow related to bile acid secretion is secondary to ions that accompany the bile acids (counterions). Bile flow can also occur in the near-absence of bile acid secretion, known as bile acid–independent flow. Experimental evidence has suggested that bile acid–independent flow is at least partially the result of biliary glutathione secretion.

Once bile has passed from the canaliculi to the biliary ductules and then to main bile ducts, bile undergoes further reabsorption and secretion. The epithelial cells of the biliary tract actively reabsorb and secrete water and electrolytes. Secretion is generally through a chloride channel activated by secretin, its most powerful activator, and its subsequent activation of cyclic adenosine monophosphate production. There is usually a net secretion of water and electrolytes, accounting for the other 20% of biliary secretion. Ultimately, bile becomes highly enriched in bicarbonate ions. Many organic substances, such as glutathione, are degraded in the biliary tree. Many drugs can be secreted into the biliary tree in a highly concentrated form (e.g., ceftriaxone). The gallbladder acts as the reservoir of the biliary tree; its function is to store bile in the fasting state. The gallbladder reabsorbs water, concentrating stored bile, and secretes mucin. Contraction of the gallbladder is mediated hormonally, largely through cholecystokinin, in response to a meal, with the simultaneous relaxation of the sphincter of Oddi and release of bile into the duodenum.

Enterohepatic Circulation

Bile salts are primarily produced in the liver and secreted to be used in the biliary tree and intestine. The primary bile salts cholic acid and chenodeoxycholic acid are produced in the liver from cholesterol and subsequently conjugated with glycine or taurine in the hepatocyte. Once secreted in the gut, the primary bile acids are modified by intestinal bacteria to form the secondary bile acids deoxycholic acid and lithocholic acid. Bile acids are reabsorbed passively into the jejunum and actively into the ileum. Thus, the bile acids reenter the portal venous system, and up to 90% of the bile acids are extracted by hepatocytes. Only a small fraction spills over into the systemic circulation because of efficient hepatic extraction, which accounts for low levels of plasma bile acids. After hepatic extraction, bile acids are recirculated into the canaliculi and back into the biliary tree, completing the circuit. A small amount of intestinal bile acids is not absorbed by the portal system and is excreted in the stool. Thus, the active secretion of bile salts from hepatocytes into bile and from ileal enterocytes into the portal vein is the engine behind the enterohepatic circulation.

The enterohepatic circulation is more than a unique mechanism for reusing physiologically valuable bile acids. This circulation of bile constitutes the major mechanism for eliminating excess cholesterol because cholesterol is consumed during the production of bile salts and is excreted in the feces by mixed micelles formed by organic biliary solutes. Bile salts also play a critical role in the absorption of dietary fats, fat-soluble vitamins (i.e., vitamins A, D, E, and K), and lipophilic drugs. Water movement from hepatocytes into bile and water absorption through the small bowel are also regulated by bile salts. The enterohepatic circulation is therefore central to a number of solubilization, transport, and regulatory functions.

Bilirubin Metabolism

Bilirubin is the result of heme breakdown. An early phase of heme breakdown, accounting for 20% of bilirubin, is from hemoproteins (heme-containing enzymes) and occurs within 3 days of labeling with radioactive heme. A late phase of heme breakdown, accounting for 80% of bilirubin, is from senescent red blood cells. This occurs approximately 110 days after administration of radioactive labeled heme and is consistent with the life span of red blood cells. Heme is initially broken down into a green biliverdin by heme oxygenase, which is then broken down into the orange bilirubin by biliverdin reductase.

Circulating bilirubin is bound to albumin, which protects many organs from the potentially toxic effects of this compound. The bilirubin-albumin complex enters hepatic sinusoidal blood, where it enters the space of Disse through the large sinusoidal fenestrations. The bilirubin-albumin complex is disassociated in this space. Free bilirubin is internalized into the hepatocyte, where it is conjugated to glucuronic acid. Conjugated bilirubin is then secreted in an energy-dependent fashion into canalicular bile against a large concentration gradient. Bilirubin is secreted with bile into the gastrointestinal tract. Within the gastrointestinal tract, bilirubin is deconjugated by intestinal bacteria to a group of compounds known as urobilinogens. These urobilinogens are further oxidized and reabsorbed into the enterohepatic circulation and secreted into bile. A small percentage of the reabsorbed urobilinogens is excreted into urine. These oxidized urobilinogens account for the colored compounds that contribute to the yellow color of urine and the brown color of stool.

Bilirubin has long been known to be a toxic compound and is the agent responsible for neonatal encephalopathy and cochlear damage secondary to severe unconjugated hyperbilirubinemia (kernicterus). The binding of serum bilirubin to albumin protects the tissues from exposure to bilirubin. However, binding sites can be overwhelmed by increasing amounts of bilirubin or displaced by other binding agents (e.g., various drugs). The mechanism of bilirubin toxicity appears to be related to a number of its effects. Free bilirubin can uncouple oxidative phosphorylation, inhibit ATPases, decrease glucose metabolism, and inhibit a broad spectrum of protein kinase activities.

Portosystemic shunts, such as those seen with cirrhosis and portal hypertension, decrease the first-pass hepatic clearance of bilirubin, resulting in a mildly increased serum unconjugated hyperbilirubinemia. A number of disorders can result in an unconjugated serum hyperbilirubinemia, including neonatal hyperbilirubinemia, an increased bilirubin load caused by hemolytic syndromes, and inherited enzymatic deficiencies such as Crigler-Najjar and Gilbert syndromes. Disorders presenting with serum conjugated hyperbilirubinemia include cholestasis, Dubin-Johnson, and Rotor syndromes.

Carbohydrate Metabolism

The liver is the center of carbohydrate metabolism because it is the major regulator of storage and distribution of glucose to the peripheral tissues and, in particular, to glucose-dependent tissues such as the brain and erythrocytes. Both liver and muscle are capable of storing glucose in the form of glycogen, but only the liver can break down glycogen to provide glucose for systemic circulation. Glycogen that is broken down can be used only in muscle and is therefore not a source of systemically circulated glucose.

In the fed state, carbohydrate absorbed through the intestines (mostly glucose) is circulated systemically. Carbohydrates reaching the liver are rapidly converted to glycogen for storage. The liver contains up to 65 g of glycogen per kilogram of liver tissue. Excess carbohydrate is mostly converted to fatty acids and stored in adipose tissue. In the postabsorptive state (between meals, nonfasting), there is no further systemic glucose coming directly from the gut, and the liver becomes the primary source of circulating glucose by the breakdown of glycogen. This is crucial for the brain and erythrocytes, which rely on glucose for their metabolism. In the postabsorptive state, most other tissues begin to rely on fatty acids derived from adipose tissue as their primary fuel. Highly active muscle may deplete its own glycogen and depend on liver-derived glucose for its substrate in the postabsorptive state. After 48 hours of fasting, hepatic glycogen is depleted and the liver shifts from glycogenolysis to gluconeogenesis. The substrate for hepatic gluconeogenesis is mostly from amino acids (mainly alanine) derived from muscle breakdown, but they also come from glycerol derived from adipose breakdown. During a prolonged fast, fatty acids from adipose breakdown are β-oxidized in the liver, which releases ketone bodies that then become the primary fuel for the brain.

Transition in and out of these various metabolic states and regulation of carbohydrate metabolism are mostly influenced by glucose concentration in sinusoidal blood and hormonal influences (e.g., insulin, catecholamines, glucagon). In the fasting state, during anaerobic metabolism, lactate is produced, largely from muscle. The liver uses this lactate, which is converted to pyruvate that enters into the gluconeogenic pathways, to produce glucose. This cycle is known as the Cori cycle.

Derangements of carbohydrate metabolism are common in liver disease. Cirrhotics often demonstrate abnormal glucose tolerance. Its mechanism is not completely clear but is probably related to associated insulin resistance. This phenomenon is not caused by shunting of glucose-containing blood away from the liver. Hypoglycemia is a distinctly uncommon entity in chronic liver disease because of the remarkable resilience of the liver and its metabolic function. Only with massive hepatocyte loss in fulminant hepatic failure does gluconeogenesis fail and hypoglycemia ensue.

Lipid Metabolism

Fatty acids are synthesized in the liver during states of glucose excess, when the liver's ability to store glycogen has been exceeded. Adipocytes have a limited ability to synthesize fatty acids. Therefore, the liver is the predominant source of synthesized fatty acids, although they are largely stored in adipose tissue. During lipolysis, free fatty acids are transported to the liver, where they are metabolized. Fatty acids in the liver undergo esterification with glycerol to form triglycerides for storage or transportation, or they undergo β-oxidation, yielding energy in the form of ATP and ketone bodies. In general, this process is regulated by the nutritional state; starvation favors oxidation, and the fed state favors esterification.

There is a constant cycling of fatty acids between the liver and adipose tissue that is under a delicate balance, which can easily be offset, resulting in fatty infiltration of the liver. A few factors influence this balance; for example, hepatic uptake of fatty acids is a function of plasma concentrations. Although there is no limit to the liver's ability to esterify fatty acids, its ability to dispose of or to break down fatty acids is limited, as is its ability to secrete triglycerides in the form of lipoproteins. Therefore, conditions of increased circulating fatty acids can easily override the liver's ability to handle them, resulting in fatty accumulation in the liver. This is known as steatosis or, when it is associated with chronic inflammation in more advanced cases, steatohepatitis. A number of conditions have been associated with hepatic steatosis, such as diabetes, steroid use, starvation, obesity, and extensive administration of cytotoxic chemotherapeutic agents. Fatty liver associated with alcohol intake has a number of causes; it is related to increased lipolysis, reduced oxygenation, and augmented esterification of hepatic fatty acids and may also be related to relative starvation in the chronic alcoholic.

Protein Metabolism

The liver is also a central site for the metabolism of proteins and is involved in the synthesis of protein, catabolism of proteins into energy or storage forms, and management of excess amino acids and nitrogen waste. Ingested protein is broken down into amino acids that are circulated throughout the body, where they are used as the building blocks for proteins, enzymes, and hormones. Excess amino acids not used in peripheral tissues are generally handled by the liver, in which they are oxidized for energy—providing 50% of the liver's energy needs—or converted into glucose, ketone bodies, or fats. When amino acids are catabolized for energy production throughout the body, ammonia, glutamine, glutamate, and aspartate are produced. These products are largely processed in the liver, where the waste nitrogen is converted to urea through the urea cycle, and the urea is generally excreted in the urine. Thus, the liver is central and critical to the body's nitrogen balance and amino acid metabolism.

Although the liver can catabolize most amino acids, yielding energy or other storable energy forms such as glucose and fats, notable exceptions are the branched-chain amino acids. Branched-chain amino acids cannot be catabolized in the liver and are mostly dealt with by muscle. It has been postulated that this may act as a so-called safety net that helps spare the liver some of the demands of protein and amino acid metabolism.

The liver also is the main site of synthesis for many proteins involved in such wide-ranging and critical functions as coagulation, transport, copper and iron binding, and protease inhibition. These proteins include ceruloplasmin, iron storage and binding proteins, and α_1-antitrypsin. Albumin is made exclusively in the liver and is the predominant serum binding protein. Hepatic insufficiency or specific genetic abnormalities can result in altered amounts and functions of these proteins, with wide-ranging pathologic effects.

The liver is also responsible for the so-called acute-phase response, a synthetic response by protein to trauma or infection. Its purpose is to restrict organ damage, to maintain vital hepatic function, and to control defense mechanisms. The response is incited by proinflammatory cytokines such as interleukin-1 (IL-1), IL-6, and tumor necrosis factor, which induce acute-phase protein gene expression in the liver. Some of the well-known hepatic acute-phase proteins are α_1-, α_2-, and β-globulin, as well as C-reactive protein and serum amyloid A. An equally important part of this response is its termination. Antiinflammatory cytokines such as IL-1 receptor antagonist, IL-4, and IL-10 appear to play important roles. The acute-phase response is usually completed in 24 to 48 hours but, in the context of ongoing injury, can be prolonged.

Vitamin Metabolism

Along with the intestine, the liver is responsible for the metabolism of the fat-soluble vitamins A, D, E, and K. These vitamins are obtained exogenously and absorbed in the intestine. Their adequate intestinal absorption is critically dependent on adequate fatty acid micellization, which requires bile acids.

Vitamin A is from the retinoid family and is involved in normal vision, embryonic development, and adult gene regulation. Storage of vitamin A is solely in the liver and occurs in the hepatic stellate cells. Overingestion of vitamin A can result in hepatic toxicity. Vitamin D is involved in calcium and phosphorus homeostasis. One of vitamin D's activation steps (25-hydroxylation) occurs in the liver. Vitamin E is a potent antioxidant and protects membranes from lipid peroxidation and free radical formation. Finally, vitamin K is a critical cofactor in the posttranslational γ-carboxylation of the hepatically synthesized coagulation factors II, VII, IX, and X, as well as of protein C and protein S, the so-called vitamin K–dependent cofactors. Cholestasis syndromes can result in the inadequate absorption of these vitamins secondary to poor micellization in the intestine. The associated vitamin deficiency syndromes, such as metabolic bone disease (vitamin D deficiency), neurologic disorders (vitamin E deficiency), and coagulopathy (vitamin K deficiency), can subsequently occur.

The liver is also involved in the uptake, storage, and metabolism of a number of water-soluble vitamins, including thiamine, riboflavin, vitamin B_6, vitamin B_{12}, folate, biotin, and pantothenic acid. The liver is responsible for converting some of these water-soluble vitamins to active coenzymes, transforming some to storage metabolites and using some for enterohepatic circulation (e.g., vitamin B_{12}).

Coagulation

The liver is responsible for synthesizing almost all the identified coagulation factors as well as many of the fibrinolytic system components and several plasma regulatory proteins of coagulation and fibrinolysis. As noted, the liver is critical for the absorption of vitamin K, synthesizes the vitamin K–dependent coagulation factors, and contains the enzyme that activates these factors. Also, the reticuloendothelial system of the liver clears activated clotting factors, activated complexes of the coagulation and fibrinolytic systems, and end products of fibrin degradation. Diseases of the liver are often associated with thrombocytopenia, qualitative platelet abnormalities, vitamin K deficiency with impaired modulation of vitamin K–dependent coagulation factors, and disseminated intravascular coagulation. It is no surprise that liver disease is firmly associated with coagulation disorders that are often challenging to deal with.

Warfarin, one of the most commonly dispensed anticoagulants, acts in the liver by blocking vitamin K–dependent activation of factors II, VII, IX, and X. Factor VII has the shortest half-life of the coagulation factors; its deficiency is manifested clinically as abnormalities of the measured prothrombin time (PT) or international normalized ratio (INR). Patients with hepatic synthetic dysfunction similarly have an abnormal PT.

Metabolism of Drugs and Toxins (Xenobiotics)

The human body is exposed to an inordinate amount of foreign chemicals during a lifetime. This poses a challenge to our ability to detoxify and to eliminate these potentially harmful chemicals. Many of these chemicals are not incorporated into cellular metabolism and are referred to as xenobiotics. The liver plays a central role in handling them through an enormously complex and numerous set of enzymes and reaction pathways, which are increasingly recognized as new chemicals are discovered.

Hepatic-based reactions to xenobiotics are broadly classified into phase I and phase II reactions. Phase I reactions, through oxidation, reduction, and hydrolysis, increase the polarity and, thus, water solubility of compounds. This in turn allows easier excretion. Phase I reactions do not necessarily detoxify chemicals and may, in fact, create toxic metabolites. Phase I reactions occur in the cytochrome P450 system. Phase II reactions generally act to create a less toxic or less active byproduct. This is generally accomplished through transferase reactions in which a compound is usually coupled to a conjugate, rendering the xenobiotic more innocuous.

Regeneration

The liver possesses the unique quality of adjusting its volume to the needs of the body. This is observed clinically in its regeneration after partial hepatectomy or after toxic liver injury. It is also seen in liver transplantation in that donor liver size mismatches adjust to the new host. This quality is highly conserved evolutionarily because of the critical functions of the liver and the fact that the liver is the first line of exposure to ingested toxic agents.

Liver regeneration is a hyperplastic response of all cell types of the liver, in which the microscopic anatomy of the functional liver is maintained. Much information that we have about the regenerative response of the liver is based on experimental evidence in rodents. Normally, quiescent hepatocytes rapidly enter the cell cycle after partial hepatectomy. Maximal hepatocyte DNA synthesis occurs 24 to 36 hours after partial hepatectomy, and maximal DNA synthesis occurs in the other cell types by 48 to 72 hours later. Most of the increase in hepatic mass in rodents is seen by 3 days after partial hepatectomy, and it is usually almost complete after 7 days.

In the late 1960s, it was recognized that circulating factors were responsible, in part, for the regenerative response, and much research has focused on the humoral and genetic control of hepatic regeneration. The major circulating factors that have been identified, largely from rodent studies, are hepatocyte growth factor, epidermal growth factor, transforming growth factors, insulin, and glucagon and the cytokines tumor necrosis factor-α, IL-1, and IL-6. These factors, when infused into a normal host, do not result in hepatic growth, indicating that hepatocytes must be primed in some way before responding to these growth factors. Remarkable progress in the understanding of liver regeneration has been made because of the development of improved genetic and molecular biologic techniques. Hundreds of genes involved at all stages of regeneration have been identified by RNA microarray techniques. Also, numerous cytokine-dependent and growth factor–independent pathways have been further defined. A complete description is beyond the scope of this chapter, however, and many questions still remain.

Future Developments

The study of the liver and its physiology continues to be a remarkable and exciting field. As the fields of molecular biology and genetic manipulation have exploded, so has the field of hepatology. Given the lack of alternative options to transplantation for patients with end-stage liver failure, tissue engineering and attempts to provide exogenous hepatic functional support continue to be studied. Liver repopulation with transplanted cells—hepatocytes or hepatic progenitor and stem cells—may also provide future options for patients with liver failure. Although the identification of specific and reliable markers for hepatic stem cells has been elusive, the concepts of liver progenitors and stem cells and their potential usefulness for hepatic repopulation have gained acceptance, making this an exciting area of research. Ongoing genetic comparisons of normal and diseased liver using new molecular biology and cell biology techniques will provide clues about the genetic regulation of liver diseases. Great strides have been made in the effectiveness of gene therapy, and many groups continue to study liver-directed gene therapy strategies to treat acquired and inherited disorders. Ongoing molecular biology studies are researching hepatic cell cycle regulation, with implications for hepatocarcinogenesis. Research studies about the pathogenesis of hepatic fibrosis and, perhaps more exciting, reversal of this process are ongoing and likely to result in significant advances in the future.

Assessment of Liver Function

A wide variety of tests are available to evaluate hepatic diseases. Screening for hepatic disease, assessing hepatic function, diagnosing specific disorders, and prognosticating are critical in the management of hepatic disease. For the surgeon, assessment of hepatic function and estimation of the ability of a hepatic remnant to be sufficient after liver resection are also of obvious importance. Unfortunately, most measures of hepatic disease are gross indicators and lack sensitivity, specificity, and accuracy. We have divided these hepatic function tests into three categories—routine screening, specific diagnostic, and quantitative tests.

Routine Screening Tests

Screening blood tests are often used to determine whether there is disease in the hepatobiliary system. Standard liver function tests (LFTs) are generally not tests of function and are not always specific to hepatic disease. Nonetheless, they are valuable as a general screening tool that can provide basic indications to recognize the presence of hepatic disease and to yield clues about the cause of that disease. Total bilirubin, direct bilirubin (conjugated), and indirect bilirubin (unconjugated) levels can be affected by a number of processes related to bilirubin metabolism. Unconjugated hyperbilirubinemia can be a reflection of increased bilirubin production (e.g., hemolysis), drug effects, inherited enzymatic disorders, or physiologic jaundice of the newborn. Conjugated hyperbilirubinemia is generally a result of cholestasis or mechanical biliary obstruction but can also be seen in some inherited disorders or hepatocellular disease.

The transaminases alanine aminotransferase (ALT) and aspartate aminotransferase (AST) are the most common serum markers of hepatocellular necrosis, with subsequent leak of these intracellular enzymes into the circulation. AST is found in other organs, such as the heart, muscle, and kidney, but ALT is liver specific. However, the degree of elevation of these enzyme levels has never been shown to be of prognostic value. Alkaline phosphatase (ALP) is expressed in liver, bile ducts, bone, intestine, placenta, kidney, and leukocytes. Isoenzyme determinations can sometimes be helpful for distinguishing the source of an elevated ALP level. Elevations of ALP levels in hepatobiliary diseases are generally secondary to cholestasis or biliary obstruction. Such elevations are caused by increased production of this enzyme. The ALP level can also be increased in malignant disease of the liver. Gamma-glutamyl transpeptidase (GGT) is an enzyme in many organs in addition to the liver, such as the kidneys, seminal vesicles, spleen, pancreas, heart, and brain. Its level can be elevated in diseases affecting any of these tissues. It is also induced by alcohol intake and is elevated in biliary obstruction. Thus, it is also a nonspecific marker of liver disease but can be helpful in determining whether an elevated ALP level is from hepatic disease. 5′-Nucleotidase is also found in a wide variety of organs in addition to the liver, but increased levels are fairly specific to hepatic disease. Like GGT, it can be helpful in determining whether an elevated ALP level is secondary to hepatic disease.

Albumin is synthesized exclusively in the liver and can be used as a general measure of hepatic synthetic function. Because chronic malnutrition and acute injury, infection, and/or inflammation can decrease albumin synthesis, these factors must be taken into account in evaluating a low serum albumin level. Because of the remarkable protein synthetic capacity of the liver, hypoalbuminemia is a marker of severe liver disease. However, it lacks sensitivity, and large decreases in hepatic function are required to be reflected in albumin levels. In general, it is most helpful in chronic liver disease.

Clotting factors are largely synthesized in the liver; abnormalities of coagulation can be a marker of hepatic synthetic dysfunction. Measurement of specific clotting factors, such as factors V and VII, has been used to evaluate hepatic function in the transplantation population. PT or INR is the best test to measure the effects of hepatic disease on clotting, and prolonged PT or elevated INR is usually a marker of advanced chronic liver disease. Hepatic disease can also affect clotting through intravascular coagulation and vitamin K malabsorption. Patients with liver disease have thrombocytopenia. While platelets are not incorporated in any measure of liver function and thrombocytopenia may be multifactorial, platelet levels provide insight into severity of portal hypertension in patients with liver disease.

Specific Diagnostic Tests

Once screening tests, along with clinical findings, have suggested liver disease, specific tests can be used to help elucidate the cause and to guide treatment, if necessary. Hepatitis serologies are important to determine the presence of viral hepatitis. Autoimmune antibodies are used to diagnose primary biliary cirrhosis (e.g., antimitochondrial), primary sclerosing cholangitis (e.g., antineutrophil), and autoimmune hepatitis. α_1-Antitrypsin and ceruloplasmin levels assist in the diagnosis of α_1-antitrypsin deficiency and Wilson disease, respectively. Tumor markers such as AFP and carcinoembryonic antigen (CEA) can be helpful in the diagnosis and management of primary and metastatic tumors of the liver.

In general, the LFTs discussed in this section are gross, nonspecific, and of little if any prognostic value. Many attempts have been made to formulate dynamic and quantitative tests of hepatic function based on the liver's ability to clear various exogenously administered substances. Despite many years of research, it still remains unclear whether these tests of hepatic function are any better than scoring systems derived from simple blood tests and clinical observations. For example, the aminopyrine breath test is based on cytochrome P450 clearance of radiolabeled aminopyrine. A breath test measuring radiolabeled CO_2 as a breakdown product of aminopyrine is performed after administration at a specified time. The results largely depend on the functional hepatic mass, which is generally not depleted until end-stage liver disease has developed. There are varying results of studies comparing the aminopyrine breath test with standard LFTs and scoring systems; its main value appears to be prognosis in chronic liver disease, but it is clearly not an effective test to detect subclinical hepatic dysfunction.

Substances such as antipyrine and caffeine can evaluate liver function in a similar way, with similar results. The lidocaine clearance test yields similar information to the aminopyrine test because it is based on its clearance by the hepatic cytochrome P450 test. Lidocaine clearance is dependent on blood flow and a complex distribution process, but measurement of one of its metabolites, monoethylglycinexylidide, has greatly simplified the test. It has been shown to have some prognostic value in the transplantation population. The galactose elimination test is based on the liver's role in phosphorylating galactose and converting it to glucose. The rate at which galactose is eliminated from the bloodstream can be used as a measure of hepatic function. Problems related to this test are that the enzymes involved are genetically heterogeneous, and considerable extrahepatic metabolism occurs. Also, multiple blood draws are necessary, which makes the test cumbersome. The value of this test is probably in assessing the prognosis of patients with chronic liver disease rather than in screening. Indocyanine green is a dye removed by the liver by a carrier-mediated process and excreted into bile. This dye is rapidly cleared from the bloodstream and is not metabolized. This is the only test that has been shown to have some prognostic ability in cirrhotic patients undergoing liver resection, although this is not universally demonstrated in studies, nor is it universally accepted.

Nuclear imaging studies overcome some of the limitations of the lidocaine and indocyanine green tests described above and have the advantage of providing simultaneous morphologic (visual) and physiologic (quantitative functional) information about the liver. This not only helps quantitate the liver function but also helps in determining the distribution of that function. Thus, regional (segmental) differentiation allows specific functional assessment of the future remnant liver. Technetium-99m (Tc 99m)-galactosyl human serum albumin scintigraphy and Tc 99m–mebrofenin hepatobiliary scintigraphy potentially identify patients at risk for postresectional liver failure who might benefit from liver-augmenting techniques.

Quantitative Tests

A large number of scoring systems based on clinical observation and standard blood tests have been proposed. The most commonly used system is Pugh modification of the Child score (Table 54.2). Although all these systems are less than perfect and not universally accepted, the Child-Pugh score is commonly used for cirrhotic patients who require liver surgery. Mortality and survival rates after hepatectomy have been shown to correlate with this

TABLE 54.2 Child-Pugh classification.

FACTOR	NO. OF POINTS 1	2	3
Bilirubin (mg/dL)	<2	2–3	>3
Albumin (g/dL)	>3.5	2.8–3.5	<2.8
Prothrombin time (increased seconds)	1–3	4–6	>6
Ascites	None	Slight	Moderate
Encephalopathy	None	Minimal	Advanced

Class A, 5–6 points; class B, 7–9 points; class C, 10–15 points.

score but are not always related to liver failure. Child-Pugh class B and C patients have higher perioperative mortality after any partial hepatectomy than Child-Pugh class A patients, who can generally withstand a major hepatectomy. The presence of portal hypertension has been shown to predict poor outcome after partial hepatectomy. Portal hypertension in cirrhotic patients is usually manifested as thrombocytopenia, splenomegaly, and presence of intraabdominal varices on imaging or at endoscopy. The best evidence for portal hypertension is a hepatic vein wedge pressure higher than 10 mm Hg, which has been shown to correlate strongly with postoperative liver failure.

PORTAL HYPERTENSION

Cirrhosis is the end result of a healing response initiated by chronic liver injury. Cirrhosis is characterized by the development of fibrous septa surrounding regenerating hepatocellular nodules. Besides development of synthetic deficiencies, cirrhosis is associated with development of portal hypertension. At present, effective treatments for cirrhosis are nonexistent. As a result, its treatment has largely been focused on the treatment of resultant portal hypertension and its complications. The major challenge for the hepatologist or surgeon who is treating patients with cirrhosis and end-stage liver disease is determining when definitive treatment (e.g., liver transplantation) rather than palliative treatment (e.g., interventions to prevent recurrent variceal hemorrhage) should be applied. Cirrhosis can be classified as compensated or decompensated based on the absence or presence of clinically evident decompensating events (variceal hemorrhage, encephalopathy, ascites). This classification provides important prognostic information, as patients with compensated cirrhosis have median survival exceeding 12 years whereas patients with decompensated cirrhosis have median survival of only 1.8 years.

Definition

Portal hypertension is defined by a portal pressure gradient (the difference in pressure between the portal vein and the hepatic veins) greater than 5 mm Hg. The best method to estimate this gradient is by transfemoral-hepatic vein catheterization with a balloon tip catheter. However, higher pressures (8–10 mm Hg) are typically required to begin stimulating the development of portosystemic collateralization. Collateral vessels usually develop where the portal and systemic venous circulations are in close apposition (Fig. 54.18). The collateral network through the coronary and short gastric veins to the azygos vein is clinically the most important because it results in the formation of esophagogastric varices. However, other sites include a recanalized umbilical vein from the left portal vein to the epigastric venous system (caput medusae), retroperitoneal collateral vessels, and the hemorrhoidal

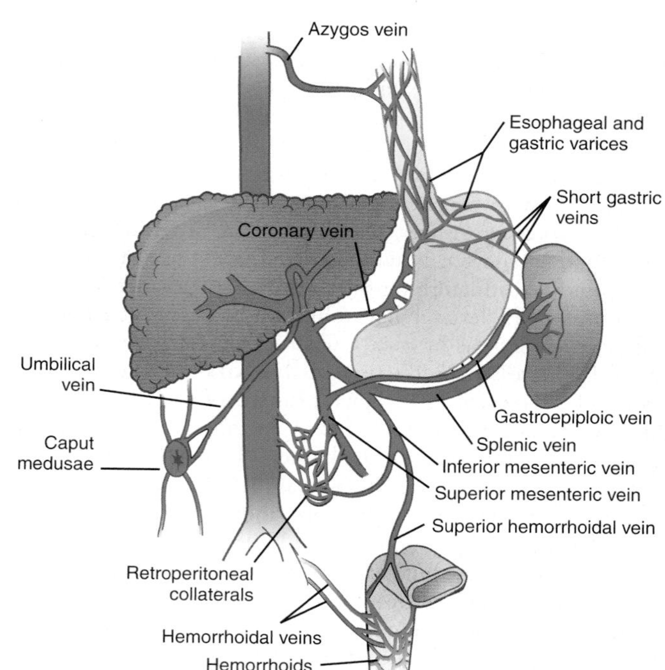

FIG. 54.18 Portosystemic collateral pathways develop where the portal venous and systemic venous systems are in close apposition. (From Rikkers LF. Portal hypertension. In: Miller TA, ed. *Physiologic Basis of Modern Surgical Care*. St Louis: Mosby; 1988:417–428.)

venous plexus. In addition to extrahepatic collateral vessels, a significant fraction of portal venous flow passes through anatomic and physiologic (e.g., capillarization of hepatic sinusoids) intrahepatic shunts. As hepatic portal perfusion decreases, hepatic arterial flow generally increases (buffer response).

Pathophysiology

Portal hypertension usually occurs because of increased portal venous resistance that is prehepatic, intrahepatic, or posthepatic in location. Several factors may contribute to this, including the following: increased passive resistance secondary to fibrosis and regenerative nodules; increased hepatic vascular resistance caused by active vasoconstriction by norepinephrine, endothelin, and other humoral vasoconstrictors; and increased portal venous inflow secondary to a hyperdynamic systemic circulation and splanchnic hyperemia. The last one is a major contributor to the maintenance of portal hypertension as portal systemic collaterals develop. Unfortunately, the exact causes remain unknown, but splanchnic hormones, decreased sensitivity of the splanchnic vasculature to catecholamines, and increased production of nitrous oxide and prostacyclin may be involved. Understanding the pathophysiology of portal hypertension may have therapeutic implications because these factors may represent targets for treatment.

The most common cause of prehepatic portal hypertension is portal vein thrombosis. This accounts for approximately 50% of cases of portal hypertension in children. When the portal vein is thrombosed in the absence of liver disease, hepatopetal (to the liver) portal collateral vessels develop to restore portal perfusion. This combination is termed cavernomatous transformation of the portal vein. Isolated splenic vein thrombosis (left-sided portal hypertension) is usually secondary to pancreatic inflammation or neoplasm. The result is gastrosplenic venous hypertension, with superior mesenteric and portal venous pressures remaining normal. The left gastroepiploic vein becomes a major collateral vessel, and gastric rather than esophageal varices develop. This variant of portal hypertension is important to recognize because it is easily reversed by splenectomy alone.

The site of increased resistance in intrahepatic portal hypertension may be at the presinusoidal, sinusoidal, or postsinusoidal level. Frequently, more than one level may be involved. The most common cause of intrahepatic presinusoidal hypertension is schistosomiasis. In addition, many causes of nonalcoholic cirrhosis result in presinusoidal portal hypertension. In contrast, alcoholic cirrhosis, the most common cause of portal hypertension in the United States, usually causes increased resistance to portal flow at the sinusoidal (secondary to deposition of collagen in the space of Disse) and postsinusoidal (secondary to regenerating nodules distorting small hepatic veins) levels.

Posthepatic or postsinusoidal causes of portal hypertension are rare; they include Budd-Chiari syndrome (hepatic vein thrombosis), constrictive pericarditis, and heart failure. Rarely, increased portal venous flow alone, secondary to massive splenomegaly (e.g., idiopathic portal hypertension) or a splanchnic arteriovenous fistula, causes portal hypertension.

Assessment of Chronic Liver Disease and Portal Hypertension

The key aspects of assessing a patient with suspected chronic liver disease or complications of portal hypertension are the following: diagnosis of the underlying liver disease; estimation of functional hepatic reserve; definition of portal venous anatomy and hepatic hemodynamic evaluation; and identification of the site of upper gastrointestinal hemorrhage, if present. These diagnostic categories take on varying degrees of importance, depending on the clinical situation. For example, estimation of functional hepatic reserve is useful in determining the risk associated with therapeutic intervention and whether definitive (e.g., hepatic transplantation) or palliative (e.g., endoscopic variceal ligation or a shunt procedure) treatment is indicated.

Variceal Hemorrhage

Bleeding from esophagogastric varices is the single most life-threatening complication of portal hypertension. It is responsible for approximately one third of all deaths in patients with cirrhosis. Approximately 50% of these deaths are caused by uncontrolled bleeding. The risk for death from bleeding is mainly related to the underlying hepatic functional reserve. Patients with extrahepatic portal venous obstruction and normal hepatic function rarely die of bleeding varices, whereas those with decompensated cirrhosis (e.g., Child-Pugh class C) may face a mortality rate in excess of 50%. Once bleeding is controlled, the greatest risk for rebleeding from varices is within the first few days after the onset of hemorrhage; the risk declines rapidly between that point and 6 weeks. Subsequently, the risk returns to the prehemorrhage rate.

Treatment

In a patient with upper gastrointestinal bleeding, general measures are instituted; these include securing the airway (especially in an encephalopathic patient), ensuring adequate access (two large-bore intravenous [IV] lines), fluid infusion, type and crossmatch of blood, and judicious blood and products transfusion. A randomized controlled trial comparing liberal transfusion (transfusion when the hemoglobin fell below 9 g/dL) to restrictive transfusion (transfusion when the hemoglobin levels fell below 7 g/dL) demonstrated that the restrictive strategy led to better survival at 6 weeks and reduced risk of rebleeding. Therapy for portal hypertension and variceal bleeding has evolved over time and now encompasses a spectrum of treatment modalities, in which sequential therapies are often necessary. For acutely bleeding patients with portal hypertension, nonoperative treatments are generally used as a first-line approach as these patients are high operative risks because of decompensated hepatic function. Endoscopic treatment (e.g., sclerosis or ligation) has become the mainstay of nonoperative treatment of acute hemorrhage because bleeding can be controlled in more than 85% of patients. This allows an interval of medical management for improvement of hepatic function, resolution of ascites and encephalopathy, and enhancement of nutrition before definitive treatment for prevention of recurrent bleeding is instituted. Pharmacotherapy can also be initiated, and trials have suggested that it may be as effective as endoscopic treatment. Balloon tamponade, which is infrequently used, can be lifesaving in patients with exsanguinating hemorrhage when other nonoperative methods are not successful. A transjugular intrahepatic portosystemic shunt (TIPS) is another treatment option whereby a percutaneous connection is created within the liver, between the portal and systemic circulations, to reduce portal pressure in patients with complications related to portal hypertension. TIPS has replaced operative shunts for managing acute variceal bleeding when pharmacotherapy and endoscopic treatment fail to control bleeding. As a result, emergency surgical intervention in most centers is reserved for select patients who are not TIPS candidates.

Endoscopy. About 80% to 90% of acute variceal bleeding episodes are successfully controlled by endoscopic measures. Sclerotherapy and band ligation of varices are the two main options available for control of acute variceal bleeding. Data suggest that band ligation is better than sclerotherapy in the initial control of bleeding and is associated with fewer complications. The literature also suggests that sclerotherapy, but not band ligation, may increase portal pressures. Thus, at this time, band ligation is the modality of choice for initial control of variceal bleeding. Endoscopic sclerotherapy may be used if technology for band ligation is not available. Early endoscopy, preferably within 12 hours of admission, with an attempt at control of bleeding is recommended. Patients should be started on vasoactive drugs early, and endoscopy with band ligation is performed after initial resuscitation.

Pharmacotherapy. Pharmacotherapy works by reducing variceal blood flow, which in turn reduces variceal pressure. Medical therapy should be initiated at the onset of variceal bleeding. Because infections are common in patients with variceal bleeding, antibiotic prophylaxis should be initiated. This has been shown to decrease the infection rate by more than 50%, to decrease rebleeding, and to improve survival. Randomized trials have also shown that somatostatin and its longer-acting analogue octreotide are as efficacious as endoscopic treatment for control of acute variceal bleeding. Because of the minimal adverse effects and ease of administration, octreotide is now commonly used as an adjunct to endoscopic therapy. In fact, the combination of octreotide and endoscopic therapy is more effective than octreotide alone in controlling bleeding and is the preferred treatment for most patients. In severe cases of hemorrhage, vasopressin can be used to diminish splanchnic blood flow. However, because of the adverse systemic effects of vasopressin, nitroglycerin should be simultaneously infused and then titrated to achieve blood pressure control.

Variceal tamponade. Controlled trials have demonstrated that balloon tamponade is as effective as pharmacotherapy and endoscopic therapy in controlling acute variceal bleeding. The major advantages of variceal tamponade using the Sengstaken-Blakemore tube are immediate cessation of bleeding in more than 85% of patients and the widespread availability of this device (Fig. 54.19). However, there are also significant disadvantages of balloon tamponade, including frequent recurrent hemorrhage in up to 50% of patients after balloon deflation, considerable discomfort for the patient, and a high incidence of serious complications when it is used incorrectly by an inexperienced healthcare provider.

Interventional approaches. In most institutions, TIPS has become the preferred treatment for acute variceal bleeding when pharmacotherapy and endoscopic treatment fail. With TIPS, a functional portacaval side-to-side shunt is established. TIPS is able to control bleeding in almost all patients. However, TIPS is associated with risk of encephalopathy. Furthermore, in the case of shunt dysfunction, there is risk of recurrent bleeding. Use of polytetrafluoroethylene (PTFE)-covered stents has been a major step forward. PTFE stents have higher patency rates over time and reduced mortality rates. Use of TIPS in patients with multiorgan failure or in patients with decompensated liver disease is associated with high 30-day mortality. In such patients, early use of TIPS, rather than after failure of other therapies, may be associated with better outcomes.

Operative approaches. Operative procedures are typically reserved for those situations in which TIPS is not indicated or is not available. Selection of the appropriate emergency operation should mainly be guided by the experience of the surgeon. Although nonoperative therapies are effective in most patients with acute variceal bleeding, an emergency operation should be promptly carried out when less invasive measures fail to control hemorrhage or are not indicated. The most common situations requiring urgent or emergency surgery are failure of acute endoscopic treatment, failure of long-term endoscopic therapy, hemorrhage from gastric varices or portal hypertensive gastropathy, and failure of TIPS placement.

Esophageal transection with a stapling device is rapid and relatively simple, but rebleeding rates after this procedure are high. Moreover, there is little evidence that operative mortality rates are lower than after surgical portal decompression.

A commonly performed shunt operation in the emergency setting is the portacaval shunt because it rapidly and effectively decompresses the portal venous circulation. Impressive results have been achieved by Orloff and colleagues, but not by others, when an emergency portacaval shunt is used as routine therapy for acute variceal bleeding. In patients who are not actively bleeding at the time of surgery and in those in whom bleeding is temporarily controlled by pharmacotherapy or balloon tamponade, a more complex operation, such as the distal splenorenal shunt, may be appropriate. The major disadvantage of emergency surgery is that operative mortality rates exceed 25% in most reported series. Early postoperative mortality is usually related to the status of hepatic functional reserve rather than to the type of emergency operation selected.

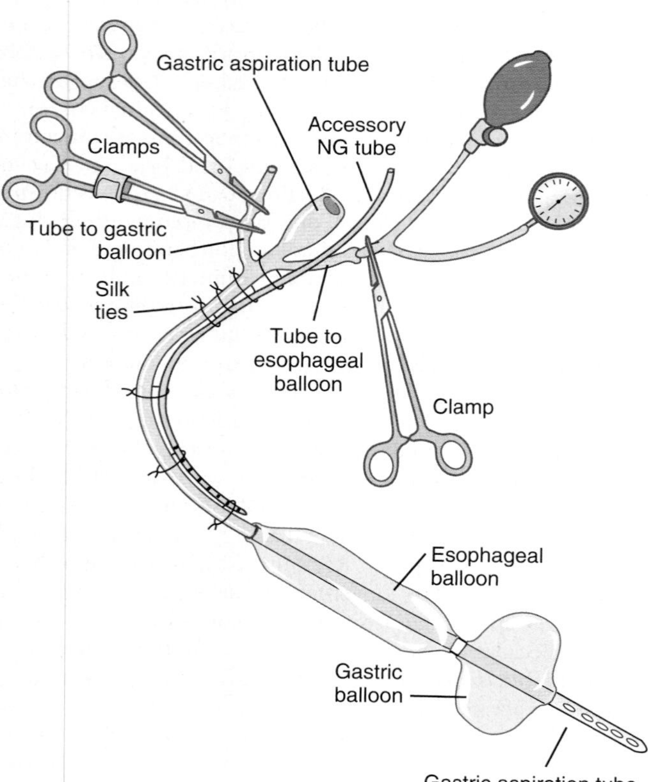

FIG. 54.19 Modified Sengstaken-Blakemore tube. Note the accessory nasogastric *(NG)* tube for suctioning of secretions above the esophageal balloon and the two clamps, one secured with tape, to prevent inadvertent decompression of the gastric balloon. (From Rikkers LF. Portal hypertension. In Goldsmith H, ed. *Practice of Surgery*. Philadelphia: Harper & Row; 1981:1–37.)

Prevention of Recurrent Variceal Hemorrhage

After a patient has bled from varices, the likelihood of a repeated episode exceeds 70%. Because most patients with variceal hemorrhage have chronic liver disease, the challenge of long-term management is prevention of recurrent bleeding and maintenance of satisfactory hepatic function. Options available for definitive treatment include pharmacotherapy, chronic endoscopic treatment, TIPS, shunt operations (e.g., nonselective, selective, partial), various nonshunt procedures, and liver transplantation. The most effective treatment regimen usually requires two or more of these therapies in sequence. In most centers, initial treatment consists of pharmacotherapy or endoscopic therapy, with portal decompression by means of TIPS or an operative shunt reserved for failures of first-line treatment. Hepatic transplantation is used for patients with end-stage liver disease.

Pharmacotherapy. A metaanalysis of controlled trials of nonselective β-adrenergic blockade has shown that this treatment significantly decreases the likelihood of recurrent hemorrhage and demonstrates a trend toward decreased mortality.[2] The combination of a beta blocker and long-acting nitrate (e.g., isosorbide 5-mononitrate) has been shown to be more effective than variceal ligation. Combination therapy is also more effective than beta blockade alone. Long-term pharmacotherapy should be used only in compliant patients who are observed closely by their physician.

Endoscopic therapy. Several controlled trials and a metaanalysis comparing endoscopic sclerotherapy with variceal ligation have shown a significant advantage to variceal ligation. Complications are less frequent after variceal ligation, and fewer treatment sessions are required to eradicate varices (Fig. 54.20). Rebleeding and mortality rates also appear to be lower after variceal ligation. The combination of variceal ligation and pharmacotherapy with nonselective beta blockade is more effective than variceal ligation alone. This result has been confirmed in a metaanalysis that included the data from 17 randomized controlled trials.[3] In this trial, combination of beta blocker and endoscopic treatment significantly reduced rebleeding rates at 6, 12, and 24 months. Furthermore, mortality at 24 months was significantly lower for the combined treatment group. Thus, at this time, combination therapy should be recommended as the first line of treatment for secondary prophylaxis of variceal bleeding.

Several controlled trials comparing chronic endoscopic therapy with conventional medical management have been completed. Although fewer patients receiving endoscopic treatment than medical treatment experienced rebleeding in all the investigations, recurrent bleeding still occurred in approximately 50% of endoscopic therapy patients. Rebleeding is most frequent during the initial year. Rebleeding rate decreases by about 15% annually thereafter. Although a single episode of recurrent hemorrhage does not signify failure of therapy, uncontrolled hemorrhage, multiple major episodes of rebleeding, and hemorrhage from gastric varices and hypertensive gastropathy all require that endoscopic therapy be abandoned, and another treatment modality substituted. Endoscopic treatment failure secondary to rebleeding occurs in as many as one third of patients. Thus, chronic endoscopic therapy is a rational initial treatment for many patients who bleed from esophageal varices, but subsequent treatment with TIPS, a shunt procedure, a nonshunt operation, or liver transplantation should be anticipated for a significant percentage of patients. Because of its relatively high failure rate, a course of chronic endoscopic therapy should not be undertaken for noncompliant patients and those living a long distance from advanced medical care.

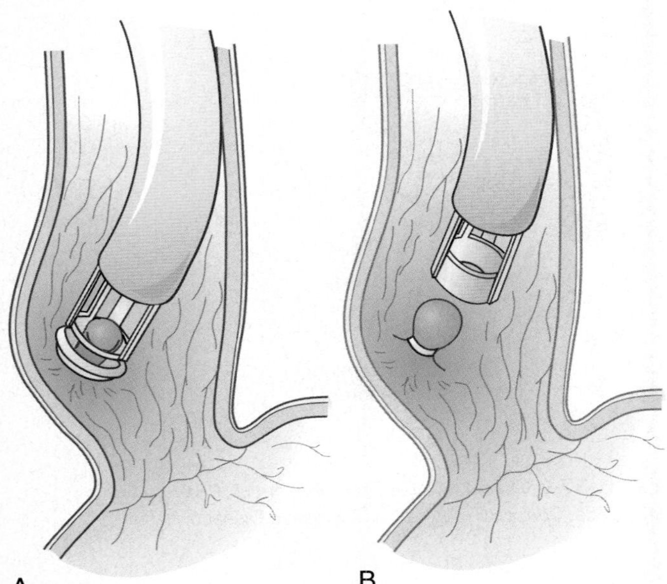

FIG. 54.20 Endoscopic ligation of esophageal varices. (A) The varix is drawn into the ligator by suction. (B) An O ring is applied. (From Turcotte JG, Roger SE, Eckhauser FE. Portal hypertension. In: Greenfield LJ, Mulholland MW, Oldham KT, eds. *Surgery: Scientific Principles and Practice.* Philadelphia: JB Lippincott; 1993:899.)

Interventional therapy. TIPS is being increasingly used for definitive treatment of patients who bleed from portal hypertension (Fig. 54.21). A major limitation of TIPS, however, is a high incidence (up to 50%) of shunt stenosis or shunt thrombosis within the first year. Shunt stenosis, which is usually secondary to neointimal hyperplasia, is more common than thrombosis and can often be resolved by balloon dilation of the TIPS or, in some cases, by placement of a second shunt. Total shunt occlusion occurs in 10% to 15% of patients. Shunt stenosis and shunt thrombosis are often followed by recurrent portal hypertensive bleeding. TIPS stenosis and occlusion have become less frequent with the use of PTFE-covered stents.

TIPS has been compared with chronic endoscopic therapy in 11 randomized controlled trials. Fewer patients rebled after TIPS (19%) than after endoscopic treatment (47%), but encephalopathy was significantly more common in TIPS patients (34%). TIPS dysfunction developed in 50% of patients. The major advantage of TIPS is that it is a nonoperative approach. Thus, it would appear to be the ideal therapy when only short-term portal decompression is required. Liver transplantation candidates who fail to respond to endoscopic therapy or pharmacotherapy are therefore well suited for TIPS followed by transplantation when a donor organ becomes available. As a result, the patient is protected from bleeding in the interim, and the transplantation procedure may

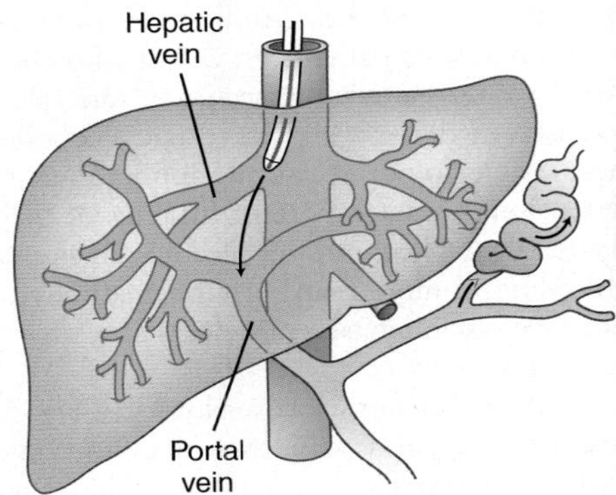

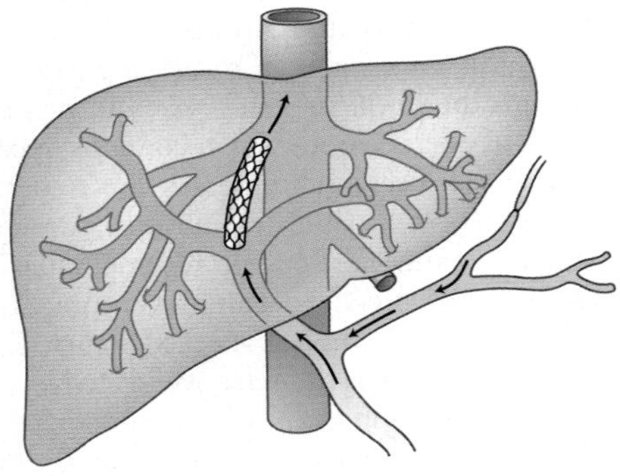

FIG. 54.21 Transjugular intrahepatic portosystemic shunt placement. The inferior vena cava is accessed through right internal jugular vein. If the right internal jugular vein is unsuitable, the left internal jugular vein may also be used. Through this access, a 5F catheter is placed into the right hepatic vein and wedged into a peripheral branch. Wedged hepatic venography is then performed with CO_2 gas to opacify the portal venous system. Using the wedged hepatic venogram image as a guide, a needle is advanced through the wall of the right hepatic vein and directed in an anteroinferior direction to access the right portal vein. Once the portal vein is cannulated, CO_2 is injected into the parenchymal tract to exclude transgression of the bile duct or hepatic artery. Once proper placement is confirmed, TIPS endoprosthesis is deployed, which creates a shunt between the portal vein and the hepatic vein, thus decreasing resistance and decompressing varices.

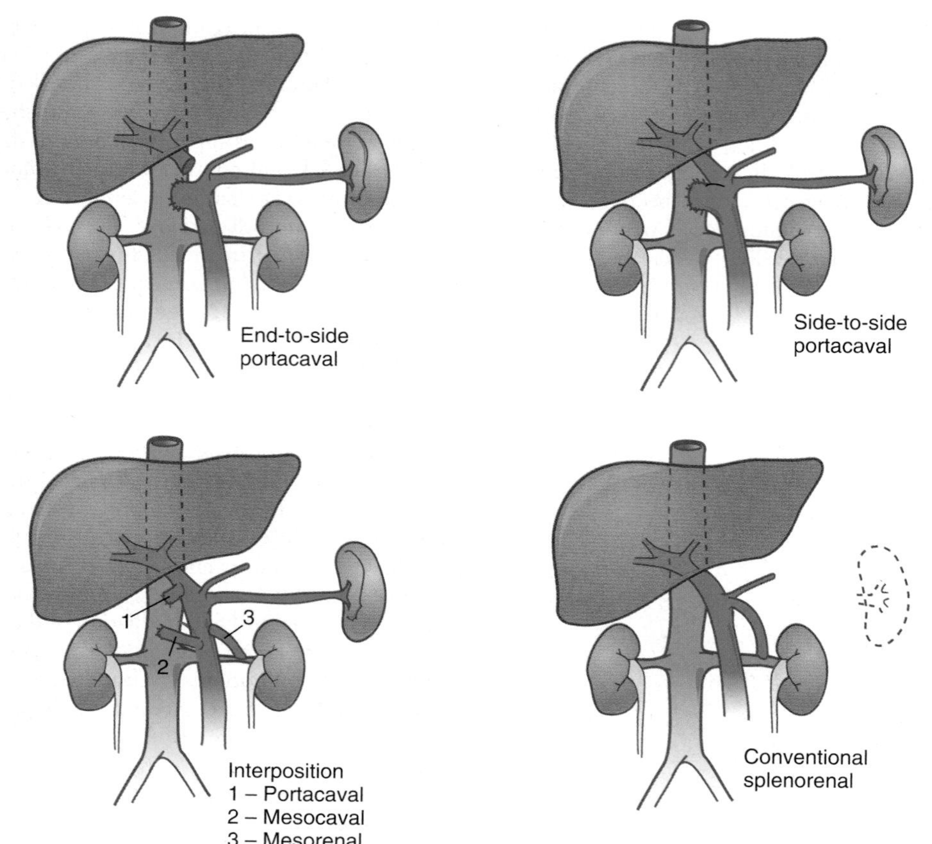

FIG. 54.22 Nonselective shunts completely divert portal blood flow away from the liver. (From Rikkers LF. Portal hypertension. In: Moody FG, Carey LC, Scott Jones RS, et al, eds. *Surgical Treatment of Digestive Disease.* Chicago: Year Book Medical; 1986:409–424.)

be facilitated by the lower portal pressure. Another group of patients in whom TIPS may be advantageous includes those with advanced hepatic functional decompensation who are unlikely to survive long enough for the TIPS to malfunction. Because it functions as a side-to-side portosystemic shunt, TIPS is also effective for the treatment of medically intractable ascites.

Surgical therapy. Portosystemic shunts are clearly the most effective means of preventing recurrent hemorrhage in patients with portal hypertension. These procedures are effective because they all decompress the portal venous system to varying degrees by shunting portal flow into the lower pressure systemic venous system. However, diversion of portal blood, which contains hepatotropic hormones, nutrients, and cerebral toxins, is also responsible for the adverse consequences of shunt operations, namely, portosystemic encephalopathy and accelerated hepatic failure. Depending on whether they completely decompress, compartmentalize, or partially decompress the portal venous circulation, portosystemic shunts can be classified as nonselective, selective, or partial. In addition to variceal decompression, selective and partial portosystemic shunts also aim to preserve hepatic portal perfusion and therefore to prevent or to minimize the adverse consequences of these procedures.

Nonselective shunts. Commonly used nonselective shunts, all of which completely divert portal flow, include the end-to-side portacaval shunt (Eck fistula), side-to-side portacaval shunt, large-diameter interposition shunts, and conventional splenorenal shunt (Fig. 54.22). The end-to-side portacaval shunt is the prototype of nonselective shunts and is the only shunt procedure that has been compared with conventional medical treatment in randomized controlled trials. Fig. 54.23 combines survival data from four controlled investigations of the therapeutic portacaval shunt, performed in patients with prior variceal hemorrhage. The most common causes of death in medically treated and shunted patients were rebleeding and accelerated hepatic failure, respectively. Although no survival advantage could be demonstrated for shunt patients, all these studies had a crossover bias in favor of medically treated patients, several of whom received a shunt when they developed intractable recurrent variceal hemorrhage. In addition, almost all the trial patients had alcoholic cirrhosis; therefore, these results do not necessarily apply to other causes of portal hypertension. Other important findings of these randomized trials included reliable control of bleeding in shunted patients, variceal rebleeding in more than 70% of medically treated patients, and spontaneous, often severe, encephalopathy in 20% to 40% of shunted patients.

All the other nonselective shunts in Fig. 54.22 maintain continuity of the portal vein, thereby connecting the portal and systemic venous systems in a side-to-side fashion. Therefore, these procedures decompress the splanchnic venous circulation and intrahepatic sinusoidal network. Because the liver and intestines are both important contributors to ascites formation, side-to-side portosystemic shunts are the most effective shunt procedures for relieving ascites as well as for preventing recurrent variceal bleeding. Because they completely divert portal flow, like the end-to-side portacaval shunt, however, side-to-side shunts also accelerate hepatic failure and lead to frequent postshunt encephalopathy.

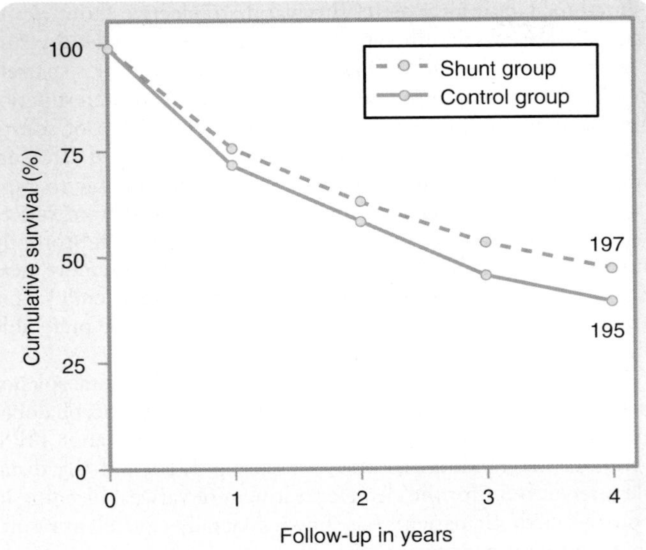

FIG. 54.23 Cumulative survival data from four controlled trials of the portacaval shunt versus conventional medical management. (From Boyer TD. Portal hypertension and its complications: bleeding esophageal varices, ascites, and spontaneous bacterial peritonitis. In Zakim D, Boyer TD, eds. *Hepatology: A Textbook of Liver Disease*. Philadelphia: WB Saunders; 1982:464–499.)

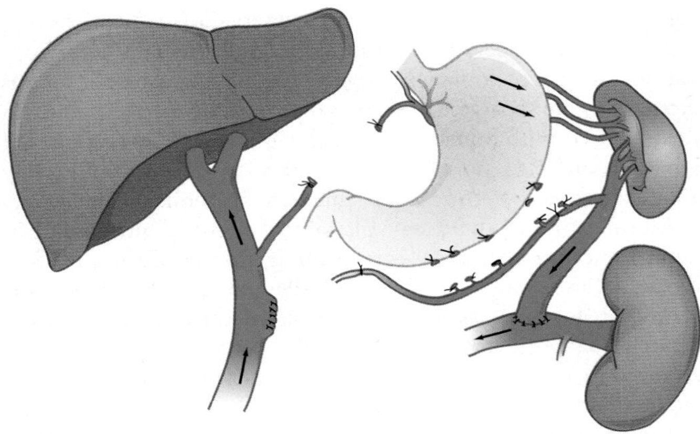

FIG. 54.24 The distal splenorenal shunt provides selective variceal decompression through the short gastric veins, spleen, and splenic vein to the left renal vein. Hepatic portal perfusion is maintained by interrupting the umbilical vein, coronary vein, gastroepiploic vein, and any other prominent collaterals. (From Salam AA. Distal splenorenal shunts: hemodynamics of total versus selective shunting. In: Baker RJ, Fischer JE, eds. *Mastery of Surgery*. 4th ed. Philadelphia: Lippincott Williams & Wilkins; 2001:1357–1366.)

The conventional splenorenal shunt consists of anastomosis of the proximal splenic vein to the renal vein. Splenectomy is also performed. Because the smaller proximal rather than the larger distal end of the splenic vein is used, shunt thrombosis is more common after this procedure than after the distal splenorenal shunt. Although early series noted that postshunt encephalopathy was less common after the conventional splenorenal shunt than after the portacaval shunt, subsequent analyses have suggested that this low frequency of encephalopathy was probably a result of restoration of hepatic portal perfusion after shunt thrombosis developed in many patients. A conventional splenorenal shunt that is of sufficient caliber to remain patent gradually dilates and eventually causes complete portal decompression and portal flow diversion. A purported advantage of the procedure is that hypersplenism is eliminated by splenectomy. The thrombocytopenia and leukopenia that accompany portal hypertension, however, are rarely of clinical significance, making splenectomy an unnecessary procedure in most patients.

In summary, nonselective shunts effectively decompress varices. Because of complete portal flow diversion, however, they are complicated by frequent postoperative encephalopathy and accelerated hepatic failure. Side-to-side nonselective shunts effectively relieve ascites and prevent variceal hemorrhage. Presently, nonselective shunts are only rarely indicated. TIPS, also a nonselective shunt, is the preferred therapy for most situations in which nonselective shunts were previously used (e.g., patients with both variceal bleeding and medically intractable ascites). In general, a nonselective shunt is constructed only when a TIPS cannot be performed or when a TIPS fails.

Selective shunts. The hemodynamic and clinical shortcomings of nonselective shunts stimulated development of the concept of selective variceal decompression. In 1967, Warren and colleagues introduced the distal splenorenal shunt. In the following year, Inokuchi and associates reported their initial results with the left gastric–vena cava shunt, which consists of interposition of a vein graft between the left gastric (coronary) vein and IVC. Therefore, it directly and selectively decompresses esophagogastric varices. However, only a minority of patients with portal hypertension have appropriate anatomy for this operation; experience with it has been limited to Japan, and no controlled trials have been conducted.

The distal splenorenal shunt consists of anastomosis of the distal end of the splenic vein to the left renal vein and interruption of all collateral vessels (e.g., coronary vein and gastroepiploic veins) that connect the superior mesenteric vein and gastrosplenic components of the splanchnic venous circulation (Fig. 54.24). This results in separation of the portal venous circulation into a decompressed gastrosplenic venous circuit and high-pressure superior mesenteric venous system that continues to perfuse the liver. Although the procedure is technically demanding, it can be mastered by most well-trained surgeons who are knowledgeable in the principles of vascular surgery.

Not all patients are candidates for the distal splenorenal shunt. Because sinusoidal and mesenteric hypertension is maintained and important lymphatic pathways are transected during dissection of the left renal vein, the distal splenorenal shunt tends to aggravate rather than to relieve ascites. Thus, patients with medically intractable ascites should not undergo this procedure. However, the larger population of patients who develop transient ascites after resuscitation from a variceal hemorrhage are candidates for a selective shunt. Another contraindication to a distal splenorenal shunt is prior splenectomy. A splenic vein diameter less than 7 mm is a relative contraindication to the procedure because the incidence of shunt thrombosis is high when a small-diameter vein is used. Although selective variceal decompression is a sound physiologic concept, the distal splenorenal shunt remains controversial after an extensive clinical experience spanning almost 40 years.

Although the distal splenorenal shunt results in portal flow preservation in more than 85% of patients during the early postoperative interval, the high-pressure mesenteric venous system gradually collateralizes to the low-pressure shunt, resulting in loss of portal flow in approximately 50% of patients by 1 year. The degree and duration of portal flow preservation depend on the cause of portal hypertension and the technical details of the operation (the extent to which mesenteric and gastrosplenic venous circulations are separated). Although portal flow is maintained in most patients with nonalcoholic cirrhosis and noncirrhotic portal hypertension (e.g., portal vein thrombosis), portal flow rapidly collateralizes to the shunt in patients with alcoholic cirrhosis.

Modification of the distal splenorenal shunt by purposeful or inadvertent omission of coronary vein ligation results in early loss of portal flow. Even when all major collateral vessels are interrupted, portal flow may be gradually diverted through a pancreatic collateral network (pancreatic siphon). This pathway can be discouraged by dissecting the full length of the splenic vein from the pancreas, splenopancreatic disconnection, which results in better preservation of hepatic portal perfusion, especially in patients with alcoholic cirrhosis. However, this extension of the procedure makes it technically more challenging and a significant disadvantage in an era when fewer shunts are being placed because of increased use of endoscopic therapy, TIPS, and liver transplantation.

Six of the seven controlled comparisons of the distal splenorenal shunt and nonselective shunts have included predominantly alcoholic cirrhotic patients. None of these trials has demonstrated an advantage to either procedure with respect to long-term survival. Three of the studies found a lower frequency of encephalopathy after the distal splenorenal shunt, whereas the other trials showed no difference in the incidence of this postoperative complication. In contrast to survival, encephalopathy is a subjective end point that was assessed with various methods in the trials. Another important end point in comparing treatments for variceal hemorrhage was the effectiveness with which recurrent bleeding was prevented. In almost all uncontrolled and controlled series of the distal splenorenal shunt, this procedure was equivalent to nonselective shunts in preventing recurrent hemorrhage. Mainly because of these inconsistent results of the controlled trials, there is no consensus as to which shunting procedure is superior in patients with alcoholic cirrhosis. Because the quality of life (e.g., lower encephalopathy rate) was significantly better in the distal splenorenal shunt group in three of the trials, there appears to be an advantage to selective variceal decompression, even in this population.

Considerably fewer data are available regarding selective shunting in nonalcoholic cirrhosis and noncirrhotic portal hypertension. Because hepatic portal perfusion after the distal splenorenal shunt is better preserved in these disease categories, one might expect improved results. A single controlled trial in patients with schistosomiasis (presinusoidal portal hypertension) has demonstrated a lower frequency of encephalopathy after the distal splenorenal shunt than after a conventional splenorenal shunt (nonselective). Another large series from Emory University has shown that distal splenorenal shunt is associated with better survival in patients with nonalcoholic cirrhosis than in those with alcoholic cirrhosis. However, this has not been a consistent finding in all centers in which the distal splenorenal shunts have been performed.

Several controlled trials have also compared the distal splenorenal shunt with chronic endoscopic therapy. In these investigations, recurrent hemorrhage was more effectively prevented by selective shunting than by sclerotherapy. However, hepatic portal perfusion was maintained in a significantly higher fraction of patients undergoing sclerotherapy. Despite this hemodynamic advantage, encephalopathy rates were similar after both therapies.

The two North American trials were dissimilar with respect to the effect of these treatments on long-term survival. Sclerotherapy with surgical rescue for the one third of sclerotherapy failures resulted in significantly better survival than selective shunt alone, whereas 85% of sclerotherapy failures could be salvaged by surgery. In contrast, a similar investigation conducted in a sparsely populated area (Intermountain West and Plains) showed superior survival after the distal splenorenal shunt. Only 31% of sclerotherapy failures could be salvaged by surgery in this trial. The survival results of these two studies suggest that endoscopic therapy is a rational initial treatment for patients who bleed from varices if sclerotherapy failure is recognized and these patients promptly undergo surgery or TIPS. However, patients living in remote areas are less likely to be salvaged by shunt surgery when endoscopic treatment fails, and therefore, a selective shunt may be preferable initial treatment for such patients.

In one nonrandomized comparison to TIPS, the distal splenorenal shunt had lower rates of recurrent bleeding, encephalopathy, and shunt thrombosis. Ascites was less prevalent after TIPS. A multicenter randomized trial comparing TIPS and the distal splenorenal shunt for the elective treatment of variceal bleeding in good-risk cirrhotic patients has shown generally equivalent results for these two procedures. Rebleeding rates were not significantly different between the distal splenorenal shunt (6%) and TIPS (11%), but this represents the lowest reported rate of rebleeding after TIPS. This was likely secondary to meticulous surveillance of TIPS patency by duplex ultrasound and angiography. Frequent reintervention in TIPS patients (82% compared with 11% for distal splenorenal shunt patients) was necessary to achieve these results. In this trial, postshunt encephalopathy and survival were similar after the two procedures.

Partial shunts. The objectives of partial and selective shunts are the same: effective decompression of varices, preservation of hepatic portal perfusion, and maintenance of some residual portal hypertension. Initial attempts at partial shunting consisted of small-diameter vein-to-vein anastomoses. In general, these thrombosed or dilated with time and thereby became nonselective shunts.

More recently, a small-diameter interposition portacaval shunt using a PTFE graft, combined with ligation of the coronary vein and other collateral vessels, was described (Fig. 54.25). When the prosthetic graft is 10 mm or less in diameter, hepatic portal perfusion is preserved in most patients, at least during the early postoperative interval. Early experience with this small-diameter prosthetic shunt is that less than 15% of shunts have thrombosed, and most of these have been successfully opened by interventional radiologic techniques. A small prospective randomized trial of partial (8 mm in diameter) and nonselective (16 mm in diameter) interposition portacaval shunts has shown a lower frequency of encephalopathy after the partial shunt but similar survival after both types of shunts. In another controlled trial, the small-diameter interposition shunt was discovered to have a lower overall failure rate than TIPS.

Hepatic transplantation. Liver transplantation is not a treatment for variceal bleeding but rather needs to be considered for all patients who present with end-stage hepatic failure, whether or not it is accompanied by bleeding. Transplantation in patients who have bled secondary to portal hypertension is the only therapy that addresses the underlying liver disease in addition to providing reliable portal decompression. Because of economic factors and a limited supply of donor organs, liver transplantation is not available to all patients. Also, transplantation is not indicated for some of the more common causes of variceal bleeding, such as schistosomiasis (normal liver function) and active alcoholism (noncompliance).

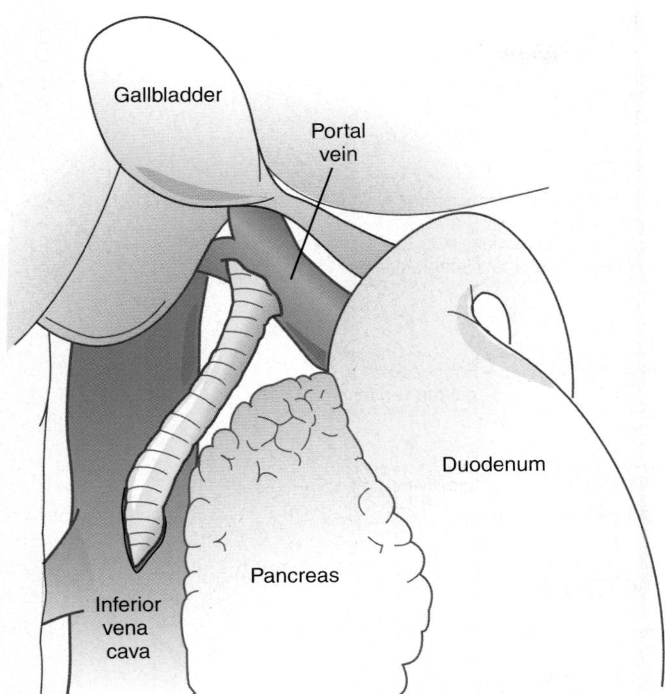

FIG. 54.25 A small-diameter (8- to 10- mm) interposition portacaval shunt partially decompresses the portal venous system and may preserve hepatic portal perfusion. (From Sarfeh IJ, Rypins EB, Mason GR. A systematic appraisal of portacaval H-graft diameters: clinical and hemodynamic perspectives. *Ann Surg.* 1986;204:356–363.)

There is accumulating evidence that variceal bleeders with well-compensated hepatic functional reserve (Child-Pugh class A and B+) are initially better served by nontransplantation strategies. The first-line treatment for such patients should be pharmacologic and endoscopic therapy. For those who fail to respond to first-line therapy, an operative shunt or TIPS can be performed. These can also be applied under circumstances in which pharmacologic or endoscopic treatment would be risky, such as patients with gastric varices and those geographically separated from tertiary medical care.

Patients with variceal bleeding who are transplantation candidates include nonalcoholic cirrhotic patients and abstinent alcoholic cirrhotic patients with limited hepatic functional reserve (Child-Pugh class B and C) or a poor quality of life secondary to the disease (e.g., encephalopathy, fatigue, bone pain). In these patients, the acute hemorrhage should be treated with endoscopic therapy and pharmacotherapy and the patient's transplantation candidacy immediately activated. If endoscopic treatment and pharmacotherapy are ineffective, a TIPS should be inserted as a short-term bridge to transplantation.

If a nontransplantation procedure (e.g., operative shunt or TIPS) is performed initially, these patients should be carefully assessed at regular intervals of 6 to 12 months. Hepatic transplantation should be considered when other complications of cirrhosis develop or hepatic functional decompensation is evident clinically or by careful assessment with quantitative LFTs.

Algorithm for Management of Variceal Hemorrhage

An algorithm for definitive management of variceal hemorrhage is shown in Fig. 54.26. Patients are first grouped according to their transplantation candidacy. This decision is based on a number of factors, including cause of portal hypertension, abstinence for alcoholic cirrhotic patients, presence or absence of other diseases, and physiologic rather than chronologic age. Transplantation candidates with decompensated hepatic function or a poor quality of life secondary to their liver disease should undergo transplantation as soon as possible.

Most future transplantation and nontransplantation candidates should undergo initial endoscopic treatment or pharmacotherapy unless they bleed from gastric varices or portal hypertensive gastropathy or live in a remote geographic location and have limited access to emergency tertiary care. Patients who live in remote locations and those who fail to respond to endoscopic and drug therapy should receive a selective shunt or TIPS. A controlled trial has shown that if careful surveillance of TIPS patency and frequent TIPS reinterventions are done, these procedures are equally efficacious.

Until improvements in TIPS technology are fully realized, the distal splenorenal shunt is likely to remain a more durable long-term solution and a reasonable alternative for TIPS failure. However, a TIPS is more commonly done, and few surgeons who are experienced in shunt surgery remain. Therefore, it is likely that operative shunts will play an even smaller role in the management of variceal bleeding in the future than they do now. Patients with medically intractable ascites in addition to variceal bleeding are best treated with TIPS when less invasive measures fail to control bleeding. If the TIPS eventually fails, an open side-to-side shunt can then be constructed if the patient has reasonable hepatic function and is not a transplantation candidate. On the other hand, TIPS is clearly indicated for patients with endoscopic treatment failure who may require transplantation in the near future and for nontransplantation candidates with advanced hepatic functional deterioration. Future transplantation candidates should be carefully monitored so that they undergo transplantation at the appropriate time before they become poor operative risks.

The treatment algorithm for variceal bleeding has changed considerably since the 1970s, during which time endoscopic therapy, liver transplantation, and TIPS have become available to these patients. Nontransplantation operations are now less frequently necessary, the survival results are better because patients at high operative risk are managed by other means, and emergency surgery has almost been eliminated.

INFECTIOUS DISEASES

Pyogenic Abscess

Epidemiology

Ochsner and DeBakey, in their classic paper on pyogenic liver abscess in 1938, described 47 cases and reviewed the world literature. This was the largest experience at that time and the first serious attempt to study this disease. In that era, pyogenic liver abscess was largely a disease of people in their 20s and 30s, mostly the result of acute appendicitis. With the marked changes in medical care since then, notably effective antibiotics and prompt effective treatments for acute inflammatory disorders, and an aging population, the spectrum of this disease has changed. Pyogenic liver abscess is now mostly seen in patients in their 50s or 60s and is more often related to biliary tract disease or is cryptogenic in nature.

However, the incidence of pyogenic liver abscess has remained similar. In 1938, Ochsner and DeBakey reported an incidence of 8/100,000 hospital admissions, whereas in 1975, Pitt and

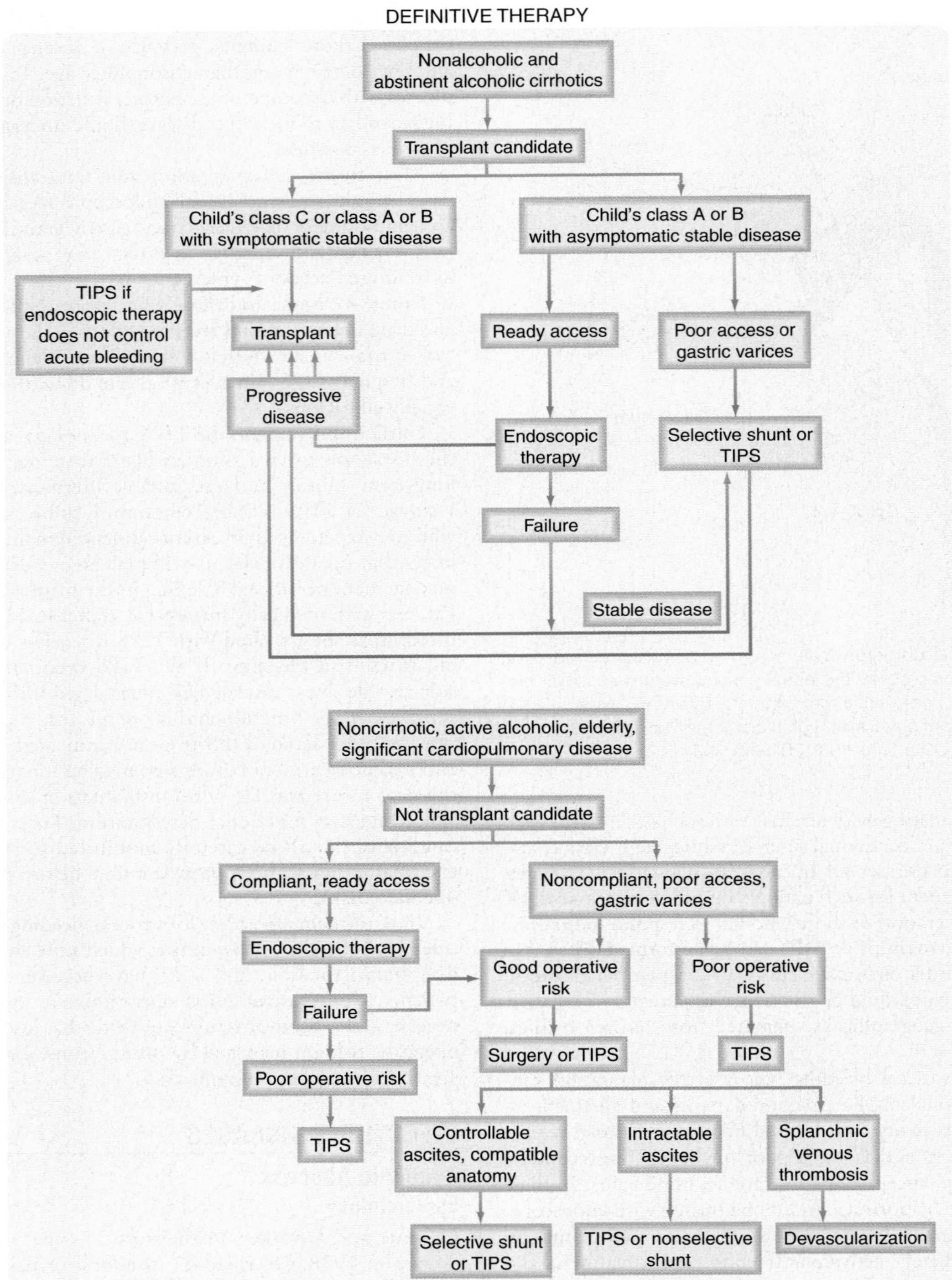

FIG. 54.26 Algorithm for definitive therapy of variceal hemorrhage (see text for details). (Adapted from Rikkers LF. Portal hypertension. In: Levine BA, Copeland E, Howard R, et al, eds. *Current Practice of Surgery*. Vol 3. New York: Churchill Livingstone; 1995.) *TIPS*, Transjugular intrahepatic portosystemic shunt.

Zuidema reported 13/100,000 hospital admissions. Two large autopsy studies, one from 1901 and another from 1960, have reported similar incidences of pyogenic liver abscess, 0.45% and 0.59%, respectively. More recent studies from the 1980s through the 2000s have suggested small but significant increases in the incidence of pyogenic liver abscess as high as 22/100,000 hospital admissions.[4] These figures may be declining on the basis of more recent data. This may reflect better, more available, and more frequently used high-quality imaging techniques. Hospital admission practices also affect these numbers. A recent population-based study from North America calculated an annual incidence of 3.6 cases/100,000 population.[5] There is no significant gender, ethnic, or geographic differences in disease frequency; the male-to-female ratio is approximately 1.5:1. Comorbid conditions associated with pyogenic abscess are cirrhosis, diabetes, chronic renal failure, and a history of malignant disease.

TABLE 54.3 Pyogenic abscesses attributable to specific cause.

YEAR OF REPORT	NO. OF PATIENTS	CAUSE (%)					
		PORTAL VEIN	HEPATIC ARTERY	BILIARY TREE	DIRECT EXTENSION	TRAUMA	CRYPTOGENIC
1927–1938 (one study*)	622	42	—	—	17	4	20
1945–1982 (eight studies)	521	17	9	38	10	4	16
1970–1999 (eight studies)	1264	5	3	38	1	2	43

*Ochsner A, DeBakey M, Murray S. Pyogenic abscess of the liver. *Am J Surg.* 1938;40:292–319. This is the classic study of Ochsner and DeBakey that reviewed 286 previously reported cases and 47 new cases.

Pathogenesis

The liver is probably exposed to portal venous bacterial loads on a regular basis and usually clears this bacterial load without problems. The development of a hepatic abscess occurs when an inoculum of bacteria, regardless of the route of exposure, exceeds the liver's ability to clear it. This results in tissue invasion, neutrophil infiltration, and formation of an organized abscess. The potential routes of hepatic exposure to bacteria are the biliary tree, portal vein, hepatic artery, direct extension of a nearby nidus of infection, and trauma. The relative contribution of these routes to the formation of hepatic abscess is summarized in Table 54.3.

Along with cryptogenic infections, infections from the biliary tree are the most common identifiable cause of hepatic abscess. Biliary obstruction results in bile stasis with the potential for subsequent bacterial colonization, infection, and ascension into the liver. This process is known as ascending suppurative cholangitis. The nature of biliary obstruction is mostly related to stone disease or malignant disease. In Asia, intrahepatic stones and cholangitis (recurrent pyogenic cholangitis [RPC]; see later) are common causes, whereas in the West, malignant obstruction has become a more predominant cause. Other factors associated with increased risk include Caroli disease, biliary ascariasis, and biliary tract surgery. The common link between all causes of hepatic abscesses from the biliary tree is obstruction and bacteria in the biliary tract. Prior biliary-enteric anastomosis has also been associated with hepatic abscess formation, likely because of unimpeded exposure of the biliary tree to enteric organisms.

The portal venous system drains the gastrointestinal tract; therefore, any infectious disorder of the gastrointestinal tract can result in an ascending portal vein infection (pyelophlebitis), with exposure of the liver to large amounts of bacteria. Historically, untreated appendicitis was considered the most common cause of hepatic abscess, but with the advent of antibiotics and the development of prompt and effective treatment of acute intra-abdominal infections, portal venous infections of the liver have become less frequent. The most common causes of pyelophlebitis are diverticulitis, appendicitis, pancreatitis, inflammatory bowel disease, pelvic inflammatory disease, perforated viscus, and omphalitis in the newborn. Hepatic abscess has also been associated with colorectal malignant disease. In a case-control study from Taiwan, the incidence of gastrointestinal cancers was increased fourfold among patients with pyogenic liver abscess compared with controls.[6]

Any systemic infection (e.g., endocarditis, pneumonia, osteomyelitis) can result in bacteremia and infection of the liver through the hepatic artery. Microabscess formation is a relatively common finding at autopsy in patients dying of sepsis, but these patients are generally not included in analyses of pyogenic liver abscess. Hepatic abscess from systemic infections may also reflect an altered immune response, such as in patients with malignant disease, acquired immunodeficiency syndrome (AIDS), or disorders of granulocyte function. Children with chronic granulomatous disease are particularly susceptible.

Hepatic abscess can be the result of direct extension of an infectious process. Common examples include suppurative cholecystitis, subphrenic abscess, perinephric abscess, and even perforation of the bowel directly into the liver.

Penetrating and blunt trauma can also result in an intrahepatic hematoma or an area of necrotic liver, which can subsequently develop into an abscess. Bacteria may have been introduced from the trauma, or the affected area may be seeded from systemic bacteremia. Hepatic abscesses associated with trauma can be manifested in a delayed fashion up to several weeks after injury. Other mechanisms of iatrogenic hepatic necrosis, such as hepatic artery embolization or, more recently, thermal ablative procedures, can be complicated by abscess. This is an uncommon complication of these procedures but is seen more often when there has been a previous biliary-enteric anastomosis.

Usually, no cause for a hepatic abscess is found. Cryptogenic abscesses predominate in many series and are more common in some case reports. Possible explanations for cryptogenic hepatic abscess are undiagnosed abdominal disease, resolved infectious process at the time of presentation, and host factors such as diabetes or malignant disease rendering the liver more susceptible to transient hepatic artery or portal vein bacteremia. In patients with cryptogenic hepatic abscess who have undergone computed tomography (CT) and ultrasonography, it has been argued whether a diligent search for a cause should ensue. In series evaluating colonoscopy and endoscopic retrograde cholangiopancreatography (ERCP) in patients with cryptogenic abscess, the yield has been low and often is only fruitful in patients with some objective finding that might have suggested a subclinical abnormality (e.g., mildly elevated bilirubin level). In general, these patients should undergo a thorough history, physical examination, and laboratory workup in search of abnormalities in the intestinal tract or biliary tree. Further invasive procedures or imaging studies should be based on clinical suspicions raised by this workup.

Pathology and Microbiology

Most hepatic abscesses involve the right hemiliver, accounting for about 75% of cases. The explanation for this is not known, but preferential laminar blood flow to the right side has been postulated. The left liver is involved in approximately 20% of the cases; the caudate lobe is rarely involved (5%). Bilobar involvement with

TABLE 54.4 **Pyogenic abscesses with noted symptoms.**

YEAR OF REPORT	NO. OF PATIENTS	SYMPTOM (%)								
		FEVER, CHILLS	NIGHT SWEATS	MALAISE	ANOREXIA, WEIGHT LOSS	NAUSEA, VOMITING	DIARRHEA	ABDOMINAL PAIN	CHEST PAIN	COUGH
1927–1938 (one study*)	333	94	—	—	—	33	—	92	—	—
1945–1982 (eight studies)	494	88	8	58	62	40	17	66	14	13
1970–1995 (ten studies)	1314	72	9	25	33	30	14	59	16	6

*Ochsner A, DeBakey M, Murray S. Pyogenic abscess of the liver. *Am J Surg.* 1938;40:292–319. This is the classic study of Ochsner and DeBakey that reviewed 286 previously reported cases and 47 new cases.

multiple abscesses is uncommon. Approximately 50% of hepatic abscesses are solitary. Hepatic abscesses can vary in size from less than 1 mm to 3 or 4 cm in diameter and can be multiloculated or a single cavity. At abdominal exploration, hepatic abscesses appear tan and are fluctuant to palpation, although deeper abscesses may not be visible and can be difficult to palpate. Surrounding inflammation can cause adhesions to local structures.

Studies of the microbiology of hepatic abscesses have had variable results for a number of reasons. In early series, sterile abscesses were commonly reported but probably reflected inadequate culture techniques, whereas in modern series, few abscesses are sampled before the administration of antibiotics. Also, the heterogeneity of the routes of infection makes the microbiology variable. Abscesses from pyelophlebitis or cholangitis tend to be polymicrobial with a high preponderance of gram-negative bacilli. Systemic infections, on the other hand, usually cause infection with a single organism.

Although the rate of sterility reported by Ochsner's review in 1938 was approximately 50%, series in the 1990s reported sterile abscess rates in approximately 10% to 20% of cases. Many hepatic abscesses are polymicrobial in nature and account for approximately 40% of cases. Some have suggested that solitary abscesses are more likely to be polymicrobial. Anaerobic organisms are involved approximately 40% to 60% of the time. The most common organisms cultured are *Escherichia coli* and *Klebsiella pneumoniae.* Other commonly encountered organisms are *Staphylococcus aureus, Enterococcus* sp., viridans streptococci, and *Bacteroides* spp. *Klebsiella* is frequently associated with gas-forming abscesses. Enterococci and viridans streptococci are generally found in polymicrobial abscesses, whereas staphylococcal infections are typically caused by a single organism. Uncommonly encountered organisms (<10% of cultures) include species of *Pseudomonas, Proteus, Enterobacter, Citrobacter, Serratia,* beta-hemolytic streptococci, microaerophilic streptococci, *Fusobacterium, Clostridium,* and other rare anaerobes. Blood cultures are positive in approximately 50% to 60% of cases. Of note, highly resistant organisms in patients with indwelling biliary catheters, multiple episodes of cholangitis, and repeated use of antibiotics are being encountered as the use of these catheters becomes more common. Fungal and mycobacterial hepatic abscesses are rare and are almost always associated with immunosuppression, usually from chemotherapy.

Clinical Features

The classic description of the presenting symptoms of hepatic abscess is fever, jaundice, and right upper quadrant pain, with tenderness to palpation. Unfortunately, this presentation is present in only 10% of cases. Fever, chills, and abdominal pain are the most common presenting symptoms, but a broad array of nonspecific symptoms can be present (Table 54.4). A study from Taiwan of 133 patients found fever in 96% of patients, chills in 80%, abdominal pain in 53%, and jaundice in 20%. Many of the symptoms, such as malaise and vomiting, were constitutional in nature. Involvement of the diaphragm may result in symptoms of cough or dyspnea. Rarely, patients can present with peritonitis secondary to rupture. Cases of rupture into the pleural space or pericardium have been reported but are distinctly uncommon. The duration of symptoms is variable, ranging from an acute presentation to a chronic illness lasting months. It has been suggested that acute presentation is associated with identifiable abdominal disease, whereas a chronic presentation is often associated with a cryptogenic abscess. A rare complication specific to *Klebsiella* hepatic abscesses is endogenous endophthalmitis, occurring in approximately 3% of cases. This serious complication is more common in diabetics. The best chance to preserve visual function is with early diagnosis and treatment.

On physical examination, fever and right upper quadrant tenderness are the most common findings. Tenderness is present in 40% to 70% of patients. Jaundice is also found in approximately 25% of cases and is often secondary to underlying biliary disease. Chest findings are often found in approximately 25% of patients, and hepatomegaly is also commonly noted in approximately 50%. Ascites, splenomegaly, and severe sepsis are uncommon signs of hepatic abscesses.

Nonspecific abnormalities of blood tests are common in pyogenic abscesses. Leukocytosis is present in 70% to 90% of patients, and anemia is commonly encountered. Abnormalities of LFT results are generally present. The ALP level is mildly elevated in 80% of patients, whereas total bilirubin concentration is elevated 20% to 50% of the time. Transaminases are mildly elevated in approximately 60% of patients. Severe abnormalities of liver function are almost always associated with underlying biliary disease. Hypoalbuminemia or mild elevations of the PT and INR can be present and reflect a degree of chronicity. None of these blood tests specifically help diagnose a hepatic abscess. However, together they may suggest a liver abnormality that often leads to imaging studies.

The most essential element to establishing the diagnosis of hepatic abscess is radiographic imaging. Chest radiographs are abnormal approximately 50% of the time, and findings generally reflect subdiaphragmatic disease, such as an elevated right

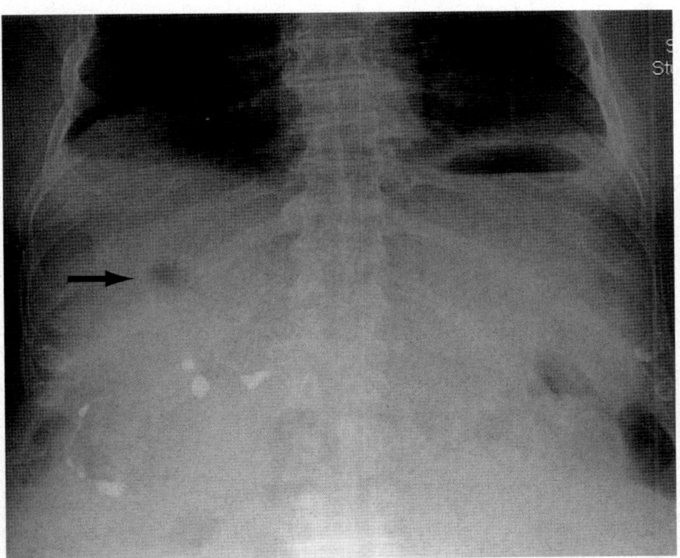

FIG. 54.27 Plain abdominal radiograph demonstrating an abnormal collection of air in the right upper quadrant consistent with a pyogenic hepatic abscess *(arrow)*.

hemidiaphragm, right pleural effusion, or atelectasis. On occasion, these can be left-sided findings in the case of an abscess involving the left liver. Plain abdominal radiographs, in rare cases, can be helpful. They can show air-fluid levels or portal venous gas (Fig. 54.27).

Ultrasound and CT are the mainstays of diagnostic modalities for hepatic abscess. Ultrasound usually demonstrates a round or oval area that is less echogenic than the surrounding liver. Ultrasound can reliably distinguish solid from cystic lesions. The limitations of ultrasound are in its ability to visualize lesions high up in the dome of the liver and that it is a user-dependent modality. The sensitivity of ultrasound in diagnosing hepatic abscess is 80% to 95%. CT demonstrates similar findings to ultrasound, and lesions are of lower attenuation than surrounding hepatic parenchyma. High-quality CT scans can demonstrate very small abscesses and can more easily identify multiple small abscesses. The abscess wall usually has an intense enhancement on contrast-enhanced CT. The sensitivity of CT in diagnosing hepatic abscess is 95% to 100%. Both CT and ultrasound are useful in diagnosing other intraabdominal pathologic processes, such as biliary disease (ultrasound) and inflammatory disorders such as appendicitis and diverticulitis (CT). Magnetic resonance imaging (MRI) can be helpful in distinguishing the cause of many hepatic masses and evaluating the biliary tree for pathologic changes, but it does not appear to have any distinct advantage over CT in diagnosing hepatic abscess.

Differential Diagnosis

Differentiating pyogenic abscess from other cystic infective diseases of the liver, such as amebic abscess or echinococcal cyst, is important because of differences in treatment. Pyogenic abscess (see later) is largely treated by antibiotics and drainage. Amebic abscess is mainly treated by antibiotics, whereas echinococcal cysts often require surgical management. Fortunately, echinococcal cysts can usually be diagnosed by history and characteristic radiologic findings (see later). The presentations of amebic and pyogenic abscess, however, are more similar, with some notable exceptions that are critical in distinguishing the two (Table 54.5). Amebic abscesses generally occur in young Hispanic men, whereas pyogenic abscess tends to occur in patients 50 to 60 years of age, with no predominant gender or race. Fever is common in both, but chills and symptoms of a severe acute bacteremia are more common in pyogenic abscess. On serologic testing, *Entamoeba histolytica* antibodies are almost always present in amebic abscesses but are uncommon in patients with pyogenic abscess. A study comparing 471 patients with amebic abscess to 106 patients with pyogenic abscess found age older than 50 years, pulmonary findings on physical examination, multiple abscesses, and low amebic serology titers to be independently predictive of pyogenic abscess. On occasion, differentiating the two is not possible, and diagnostic aspiration or a trial of antiamebic antibiotics may be necessary. Unfortunately, aspiration is diagnostic in amebic abscess only approximately 10% to 20% of the time.

TABLE 54.5 Features of amebic versus pyogenic liver abscess.

CLINICAL FEATURES	AMEBIC ABSCESS	PYOGENIC ABSCESS
Age	20–40 years	>50 years
Male-to-female ratio	≥10:1	1.5:1
Solitary versus multiple	Solitary 80%*	Solitary 50%
Location	Usually right liver	Usually right liver
Travel in endemic area	Yes	No
Diabetes	Uncommon (~2%)	More common (~27%)
Alcohol use	Common	Common
Jaundice	Uncommon	Common
Elevated bilirubin	Uncommon	Common
Elevated alkaline phosphatase	Common	Common
Positive blood culture	No	Common
Positive amebic serology	Yes	No

*In acute amebic abscess, 50% are solitary.

Treatment

Before the availability of antibiotics and the routine use of drainage procedures, untreated hepatic pyogenic abscess was almost uniformly fatal. It was not until the classic review by Ochsner and DeBakey in 1938 (see earlier) that routine surgical drainage was used and dramatic reductions in mortality were noted. Open surgical drainage of pyogenic abscesses was the sole treatment (with the addition of antibiotics eventually) for hepatic abscess until the 1980s. Since then, less invasive percutaneous drainage techniques and IV antibiotics have been used. Laparotomy is generally reserved for failures of percutaneous drainage.

Once the diagnosis of pyogenic hepatic abscess is suspected, broad-spectrum IV antibiotics should be started immediately to control ongoing bacteremia and its associated complications. Blood samples and specimens of the abscess from aspiration should be sent for aerobic and anaerobic cultures. In immunosuppressed patients, mycobacterial and fungal cultures of the aspirate should be considered. Patients who are at risk for amebic infections should have blood samples drawn for amebic serology. Until cultures have specifically identified the offending organisms, broad-spectrum antibiotics covering gram-negative, gram-positive, and anaerobic organisms should be used. Combinations such as ampicillin, an aminoglycoside, and metronidazole or a third-generation cephalosporin with metronidazole are appropriate. The optimal duration of antibiotic treatment is not well defined and

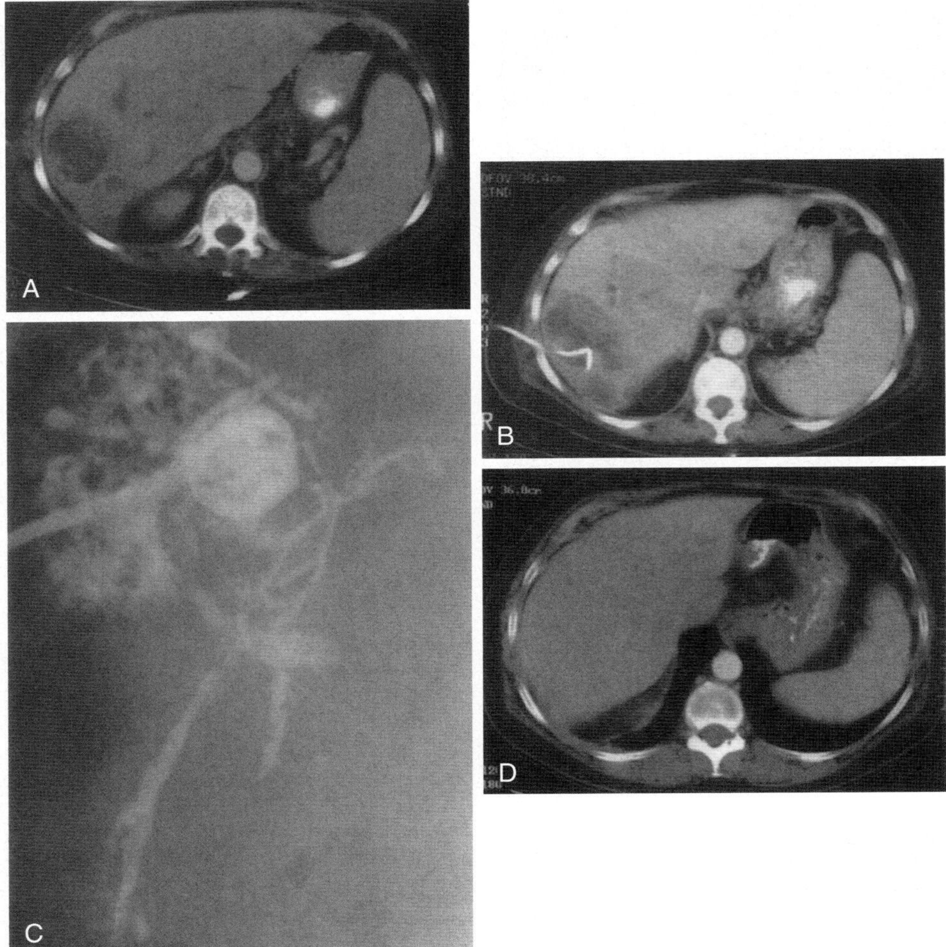

FIG. 54.28 (A) Computed tomography (CT) scan demonstrating multiloculated hepatic abscess in the right liver. (B) CT scan at the time of percutaneous drainage. (C) Contrast study through the drainage catheter demonstrating typical irregular loculated appearance as well as communication with biliary tree. (D) Follow-up CT scan 3 months after treatment demonstrating complete resolution of abscess. (From Brown KT, Getrajdman GI. Interventional radiologic techniques in the liver and biliary tract. In: Blumgart LH, Fong Y, eds. *Surgery of the Liver and Biliary Tract*. London: WB Saunders; 2000:575–594.)

must be individualized, depending on the success of the drainage procedure. Antibiotics should certainly be continued while there is evidence of ongoing infection, such as fever, chills, or leukocytosis. Beyond this, it is unclear how long to continue antibiotics, but recommendations are usually for 2 weeks or more.

Percutaneous drainage for pyogenic hepatic abscesses was first reported in 1953 but did not gain widespread acceptance until the 1980s with the development of high-quality imaging and expertise in interventional radiologic techniques. During the last 25 years, percutaneous catheter drainage has become the treatment of choice for most patients (Fig. 54.28). Success rates range from 66% to 90%. The obvious advantages are the simplicity of treatment (usually at the time of radiologic diagnosis) and avoidance of general anesthesia and a laparotomy. Relative contraindications to percutaneous catheter drainage include the presence of ascites, coagulopathy, and proximity to vital structures. Percutaneous drainage of multiple abscesses is usually met with a higher failure rate, but reports have demonstrated a high enough success rate that percutaneous approaches should be made first, reserving surgery for failures. A retrospective study comparing surgical with percutaneous drainage for large abscesses (>5 cm) has shown a better success rate with surgical drainage. Despite this, two thirds of percutaneous treatments were successful, and the overall morbidity and mortality rates were similar. There has never been a randomized prospective comparison between percutaneous and surgical therapy for hepatic abscess. However, case series have suggested that for most cases, there are similar success and mortality rates. Modern series attempting to compare these two techniques retrospectively must be read with caution because most patients treated surgically have failed to respond to other less invasive techniques. In general, surgery should be reserved for patients who require surgical treatment of the primary pathologic process (e.g., appendicitis) or for those who have failed to respond to percutaneous techniques. Laparoscopic drainage procedures have been reported with some success, and this can be considered a reasonable option to pursue in select cases.[4]

Percutaneous aspiration without the placement of an indwelling drain has been investigated by a number of groups. Success rates are generally 60% to 90% and are somewhat similar to those for percutaneous catheter drainage.[7] Most patients, however, require more than one aspiration, and 25% of patients require three or more aspirations. One randomized trial has evaluated percutaneous aspiration versus percutaneous catheter drainage. Success rates were 60% in the aspiration group and 100% in the catheter group. All but one patient in the aspiration group had a single aspiration. Another randomized trial of 64 patients has compared aspiration alone with catheter drainage. There were similar outcomes in terms of treatment success rate, hospital stay, antibiotic duration, and mortality. In the aspiration-only group, 40% required two aspirations and 20% required three aspirations. In general, catheter drainage remains the treatment of choice, although a trial of a single aspiration is reasonable to consider.

Some investigators have reported success with antibiotics alone. Most of these patients, however, have had a diagnostic aspiration and thus at least a partial drainage. Also, other series have reported that antibiotic treatment without drainage carries a prohibitively high mortality (59%–100%). In patients who are not surgical candidates or who refuse any invasive procedure, an attempt at antibiotic treatment is reasonable. However, this is not recommended in other situations.

Liver resection is occasionally required for hepatic abscess. This may be required for an infected hepatic malignant neoplasm, hepatolithiasis, or intrahepatic biliary stricture. If hepatic destruction from infection is severe, some patients may benefit from resection.

Outcomes

Mortality from pyogenic hepatic abscess has dramatically improved during the last 70 years. Before the routine use of surgical drainage, pyogenic abscess was uniformly fatal. With the routine use of surgical drainage and the use of IV antibiotics, mortality was reduced to approximately 50%, a figure that stayed relatively constant from 1945 until the early 1980s. Since then, the mortality has been reported from 10% to 20%, and series from the 1990s have demonstrated a mortality rate below 10%.[7] The most recent series from Memorial Sloan-Kettering Cancer Center (MSKCC) has reported a 3% mortality. A number of studies have analyzed factors predictive of a poor outcome in patients with hepatic pyogenic abscess. The presence of malignant disease, factors associated with malignant disease (e.g., jaundice, markedly elevated LFT results), and signs of sepsis appear to be consistent markers of poor prognosis. Signs of chronic disease, such as hypoalbuminemia, are also often associated with a poor outcome. Finally, signs of severe infection, such as marked leukocytosis, Acute Physiology and Chronic Health Evaluation II (APACHE II) scores, abscess rupture, bacteremia, and shock, are also associated with mortality.

Amebic Abscess

Epidemiology

Amebiasis is largely a disease of tropical and developing countries but is also a significant problem in developed countries because of immigration and travel between countries. *E. histolytica* is endemic in Mexico, India, Africa, and parts of Central and South America. In 1995, the World Health Organization estimated that 40 to 50 million people suffer from amebic colitis or amebic liver abscess worldwide, resulting in 40,000 to 100,000 deaths each year.[8] Before this, estimates of amebiasis were unreliable because *E. histolytica* (the pathogenic form) was not differentiated from *Entamoeba dispar* (the nonpathogenic form). Male homosexuals with diarrhea, previously thought to harbor *E. histolytica*, were actually found to be infected with *E. dispar*, which requires no treatment. Epidemiologic studies specifically addressing *E. histolytica* infections have estimated that as many as 55% of those in endemic regions are infected, although less than 50% are symptomatic.

In contrast to pyogenic hepatic abscesses, patients with amebic liver abscesses tend to be Hispanic men, 20 to 40 years of age, with a history of travel to (or origination from) an endemic area. Poverty and cramped living conditions are associated with higher rates of infection. A male preponderance of more than 10:1 has been reported in almost all studies. For unclear reasons, menstruating women have a low incidence of invasive amebiasis, and pregnancy appears to abrogate this resistance. Heavy alcohol consumption is commonly reported and may render the liver more susceptible to amebic infection. Patients with impaired host immunity also appear to be at higher risk of infection and have higher mortality rates. Patients with amebic liver abscess without a history of travel to an endemic area often have associated immunosuppression, such as human immunodeficiency virus (HIV) infection, malnutrition, chronic infection, or chronic steroid use.

Pathogenesis

E. histolytica is a protozoan and exists as a trophozoite or a cyst. All other species in the genus *Entamoeba* are considered nonpathogenic, and not all strains of *E. histolytica* are considered virulent. Ingestion of *E. histolytica* cysts through a fecal-oral route is the cause of amebiasis. Humans are the principal host, and the main source of infection is human contact with a cyst-passing carrier. Contaminated water and vegetables are also routes of human infection. Once ingested, the cysts are not degraded in the stomach and pass to the intestines, where the trophozoite is released and passed on to the colon. In the colon, the trophozoite can invade mucosa, resulting in disease.

It is thought that the trophozoites reach the liver through the portal venous system. There is no evidence for trophozoites passing through lymphatics. As implied by its name, *E. histolytica* trophozoites can lyse tissues through a complex set of events, including cell adherence, cell activation, and subsequent release of enzymes, resulting in necrosis. The principal mechanism is probably enzymatic cellular hydrolysis. Amebic liver abscesses are formed by progressing, localized hepatic necrosis producing a cavity containing acellular proteinaceous debris surrounded by a rim of invasive amebic trophozoites. Early development of an amebic liver abscess is associated with an accumulation of polymorphonuclear leukocytes, which are then lysed by the trophozoites.

Antiamebic antibodies develop rapidly in patients with invasive disease or an amebic hepatic abscess. Secretory immunoglobulin A (IgA) antibodies have been shown to inhibit adherence to colonic epithelium in vitro. However, the development of these antibodies does not halt the progression of disease. Interestingly, children who lack antiamebic IgG have innate resistance to invasive infection, suggesting an alternative immune-mediated response. There is now evidence that a cell-mediated helper T-cell response is probably the major mechanism of resistance.

Pathology

Hepatic amebic abscess is essentially the result of liquefaction necrosis of the liver producing a cavity full of blood and liquefied liver tissue. The appearance of this fluid is typically described as resembling anchovy sauce; the fluid is odorless unless secondary bacterial infection has taken place. The progressive hepatic necrosis continues until Glisson capsule is reached because the capsule is resistant to hydrolysis by the amebae. Thus, amebic abscesses tend to abut the liver capsule. Because of the resistance of Glisson capsule, the cavity is typically crisscrossed by portal triads protected by this peritoneal sheath. Early on, the formed cavity is ill-defined, with no real fibrous response around the edges. However,

TABLE 54.6 Signs, symptoms, and laboratory findings in amebic liver abscess.*

PARAMETER	AVERAGE	RANGE	NO. OF CASES REVIEWED
Symptoms and Signs			
Abdominal pain (%)	92	73–100	1701
Fever (%)	90	72–100	2192
Abdominal tenderness (%)	78	40–100	1424
Hepatomegaly (%)	62	20–100	1539
Anorexia (%)	47	28–89	499
Weight loss (%)	39	11–83	871
Diarrhea (%)	23	12–40	1426
Jaundice (%)	22	5–50	1630
Laboratory Tests			
Stool cysts, trophozoites (%)	12	4–30	4908
Amebae in cyst aspirate (%)	42	30–76	1402
Hemoglobin (g/dL)	12.1	10.2–12.8	229
Alkaline phosphatase (% >120 U/L)	76	65–91	589
Total bilirubin (g/dL)	1.4	0.8–2.4	509
Albumin (g/dL)	2.8	2.3–3.4	404
AST (× upper limit normal)	1.7	1.0–2.5	459

*In an extensive literature review.

a chronic abscess can ultimately develop a fibrous capsule and may even calcify. Like pyogenic abscesses, amebic abscesses tend to occur mainly in the right liver.

Clinical Features

Approximately 80% of patients with amebic liver abscess present with symptoms lasting from a few days to 4 weeks. The duration of symptoms has been found to be typically less than 10 days. The presenting clinical signs and symptoms are summarized in Table 54.6. The typical clinical picture is a patient 20 to 40 years of age who has recently traveled to an endemic area, with fever, chills, anorexia, right upper quadrant pain and tenderness, and hepatomegaly. The abdominal pain is typically constant, dull, and localized to the right upper quadrant. Although some studies report higher numbers, approximately 25% of patients have diarrhea despite an obligatory colonic infection. Synchronous hepatic abscess is found in one third of patients with active amebic colitis. Jaundice, as a result of a large abscess compressing the biliary tree, is not as rare as was once thought, with an average 22% of patients presenting with this feature worldwide. Weight loss and myalgias may occur when symptoms have been present for weeks. Pleuritic or right shoulder pain can occur if there is irritation of the right hemidiaphragm. Symptoms and tenderness may be epigastric or left sided if the abscess is located in the left liver. Rupture into the peritoneum with peritonitis occurs infrequently; when it does occur, it is more often with left-sided abscesses. Rare cases of rupture into the pleural space, pericardium, and other intra-abdominal organs have also been reported.

Patients presenting acutely (symptoms <10 days) versus those with a chronic presentation (>2 weeks) differ clinically. Acute presentations are typically more dramatic, with high fevers, chills, and significant abdominal tenderness. In the acute presentation, 50% of patients have multiple lesions, whereas with the chronic presentation, more than 80% of patients have a single right-sided

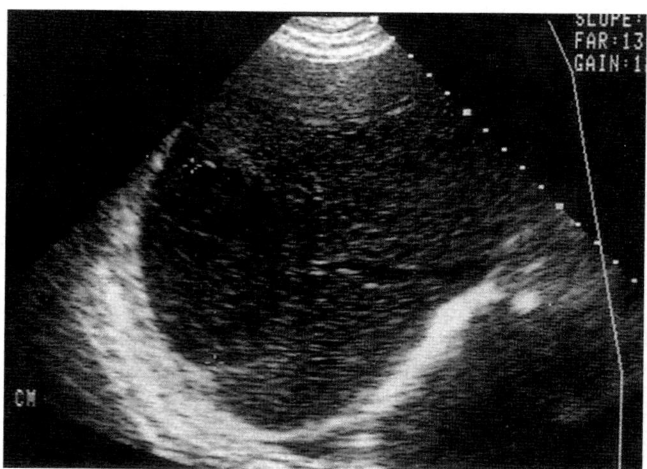

FIG. 54.29 Typical ultrasound image of an amebic hepatic abscess. Note the peripheral location, rounded shape with poor rim, and internal echoes. (From Thomas PG, Ravindra KV. Amebiasis and biliary infection. In: Blumgart LH, Fong Y, eds. *Surgery of the Liver and Biliary Tract*. London: WB Saunders; 2000:1147–1166.)

lesion. A more complicated course tends to ensue in the acute presentation, but response to therapy is similar in both groups.

Laboratory abnormalities are common in amebic abscess (Table 54.6). Patients typically have a mild to moderate leukocytosis, without eosinophilia. Anemia is common. Mild abnormalities of LFT results, including albumin, PT-INR, ALP, AST, and bilirubin levels, are typical. The most common LFT abnormality is an elevated PT-INR. Because more than 70% of patients with amebic liver abscess do not have detectable amebae in their stool, the most useful laboratory evaluation is the measurement of circulating antiamebic antibodies, which are present in 90% to 95% of patients. A number of serologic tests have been devised over the years. An indirect hemagglutinin test was used extensively in the past and has a sensitivity of 90%. This test has largely been replaced by enzyme immunoassays, which detect the presence of antibodies against the parasite and are simple, rapidly performed, and inexpensive. An enzyme immunoassay has a reported sensitivity of 99% and specificity higher than 90% in patients with hepatic abscess. Unfortunately, the presence of antibodies may reflect prior infection, and interpretation can be difficult in endemic areas. Ongoing studies are focusing on identifying specific *E. histolytica* antigens in an attempt to identify acute infection. Antigen detection kits have been evaluated in endemic areas. These kits can detect the *E. histolytica* lectin antigen in the serum and liver abscess pus and in small studies have been shown to have high sensitivity. However, the sensitivity may decrease if the test is performed after treatment with metronidazole.

Radiologic studies are a critical element in the diagnosis of amebic liver abscess. Plain chest radiographs are abnormal in approximately 50% of cases, usually demonstrating an elevated right diaphragm, pleural effusion, or atelectasis. Abdominal ultrasound has a reported accuracy of approximately 90% when it is combined with a typical history and clinical presentation. Typical findings on abdominal ultrasound are a rounded lesion abutting the liver capsule (see earlier) without significant rim echoes, interpreted as an abscess wall. The contents of the cavity are usually hypoechoic and nonhomogeneous (Fig. 54.29). These findings on ultrasound are found in 40% to 70% of cases. Abdominal CT scanning is probably more sensitive than

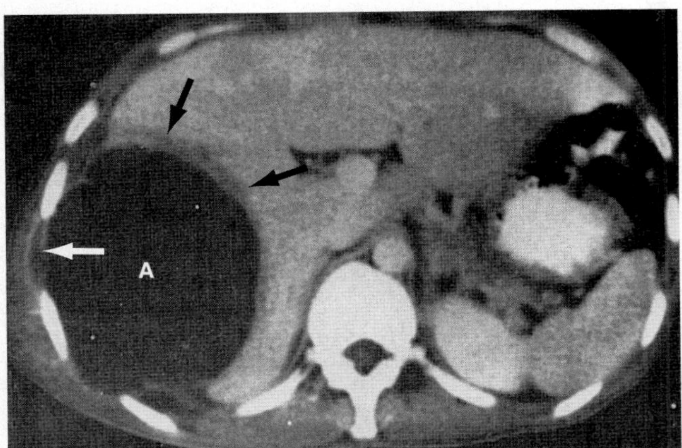

FIG. 54.30 Computed tomography scan of amebic abscess. The lesion is peripherally located and round. The rim is nonenhancing but shows peripheral edema *(black arrows)*. Note the extension into the intercostal space *(white arrow)*.

ultrasound and is helpful in differentiating amebic from pyogenic abscess, with rim enhancement noted in the pyogenic abscess (Fig. 54.30). CT can also be helpful in identifying simple cysts and necrotic tumors. MRI of the liver has no distinct advantages over CT or ultrasound in typical cases but may be helpful in differentiating atypical lesions. Nuclear medicine studies, such as gallium scanning or Tc 99m liver scans, can be helpful in differentiating pyogenic from amebic abscesses because the amebic abscesses typically do not contain leukocytes and therefore do not light up on these scans.

When this workup is still not definitive and diagnostic uncertainty persists, two options should be considered. First, a therapeutic trial of antiamebic drugs can be used. If a rapid improvement occurs, this supports the diagnosis. In situations in which amebic serology is inconclusive and a therapeutic trial of antibiotics is deemed inappropriate or has failed to improve symptoms, the second option, a diagnostic aspiration, should be considered. A pyogenic abscess would have bacteria and leukocytes, whereas an amebic abscess would contain the typical so-called anchovy sauce. Cultures of amebic abscess are usually negative and do not contain leukocytes. In patients for whom neoplasm or hydatid disease is in the differential diagnosis, aspiration should not be performed.

Differential Diagnosis

The differential diagnosis of an amebic liver abscess can be broad and include diseases such as viral hepatitis, echinococcal disease, cholangitis, cholecystitis, and even other inflammatory abdominal disorders, such as appendicitis. Malignant lesions of the liver can also have similar presentations in atypical situations. On occasion, primary pulmonary disorders must be considered. Usually, the most important distinction to be made is between pyogenic and amebic abscess. The essential elements of this distinction are summarized in Table 54.5 and in the earlier section on pyogenic abscess.

Treatment

The mainstay of treatment for amebic abscesses is metronidazole (750 mg orally, three times daily for 10 days), which is curative in more than 90% of patients. Clinical improvement is usually seen within 3 days. Other nitroimidazoles (e.g., secnidazole, tinidazole) are also as effective and are commonly used outside the United States. If response to metronidazole is poor or the drug is not tolerated, other agents can be used. Emetine hydrochloride is effective against invasive amebiasis, particularly in the liver, but requires intramuscular injections and has serious cardiac side effects. A more attractive option is chloroquine, but this is a less effective agent. After treatment of the liver abscess, it is recommended that luminal agents such as iodoquinol, paromomycin, and diloxanide furoate be administered to treat the carrier state.

Therapeutic needle aspiration of amebic abscesses has been proposed. However, a Cochrane systematic review did not support any benefit of therapeutic aspiration in addition to metronidazole treatment over metronidazole treatment alone to hasten clinical or radiologic resolution of amebic liver abscesses.[9] In general, aspiration is recommended for diagnostic uncertainty (see earlier), with failure to respond to metronidazole therapy in 3 to 5 days, or in abscesses thought to be at high risk for rupture. Abscesses larger than 5 cm in diameter and in the left liver are thought to carry a higher risk of rupture, and aspiration should be considered.

Outcomes

Although amebic liver abscesses usually respond rapidly to treatment, there are uncommon complications of which one must be aware. The most frequent complication of amebic abscess is rupture into the peritoneum, pleural cavity, or pericardium. The size of the abscess appears to be the most important risk factor for rupture, and the overall incidence of rupture ranges from 3% to 17%. Most peritoneal ruptures tend to be contained by the diaphragm, abdominal wall, or omentum, but rupture can fistulize into a hollow viscus. A peritoneal rupture usually is manifested as abdominal pain, peritonitis, and a mass or generalized distention. Laparotomy was advocated in the past for this complication, but now many patients are treated successfully with percutaneous drainage. Laparotomy is indicated in cases of doubtful diagnosis, hollow viscus perforation, fistulization resulting in hemorrhage or sepsis, and failure of conservative therapy. Rupture into the pleural space usually results in a large and rapidly accumulated effusion that collapses the involved lung. Treatment consists of thoracentesis, but if secondary bacterial infection ensues, more aggressive surgical approaches may be necessary. Rupture can occur into the bronchi and is usually self-limited with postural drainage and bronchodilators. Rarely, a left-sided abscess may rupture into the pericardium and can be manifested as an asymptomatic pericardial effusion or even tamponade. This must be treated with aspiration or drainage through a pericardial window. Other complications include compression of the biliary tree or IVC from a very large abscess and the development of a brain abscess.

The mortality for all patients with amebic liver abscess is approximately 5% and does not appear to be affected by the addition of aspiration to metronidazole therapy or by chronicity of symptoms. When an abscess ruptures, mortality ranges from 6% to as high as 50%. Factors independently associated with poor outcome are elevated serum bilirubin level (>3.5 mg/dL), encephalopathy, hypoalbuminemia (<2.0 g/dL), multiple abscess cavities, abscess volume larger than 500 mL, anemia, and diabetes. Although clinical improvement after adequate treatment with antiamebic agents is the rule, radiologic resolution of the abscess cavity is usually delayed. The average time to radiologic resolution is 3 to 9 months, and in some patients, it can take years. Studies have shown that more than 90% of the visible lesions disappear radiologically, but a small percentage of patients are left with a clinically irrelevant residual lesion.

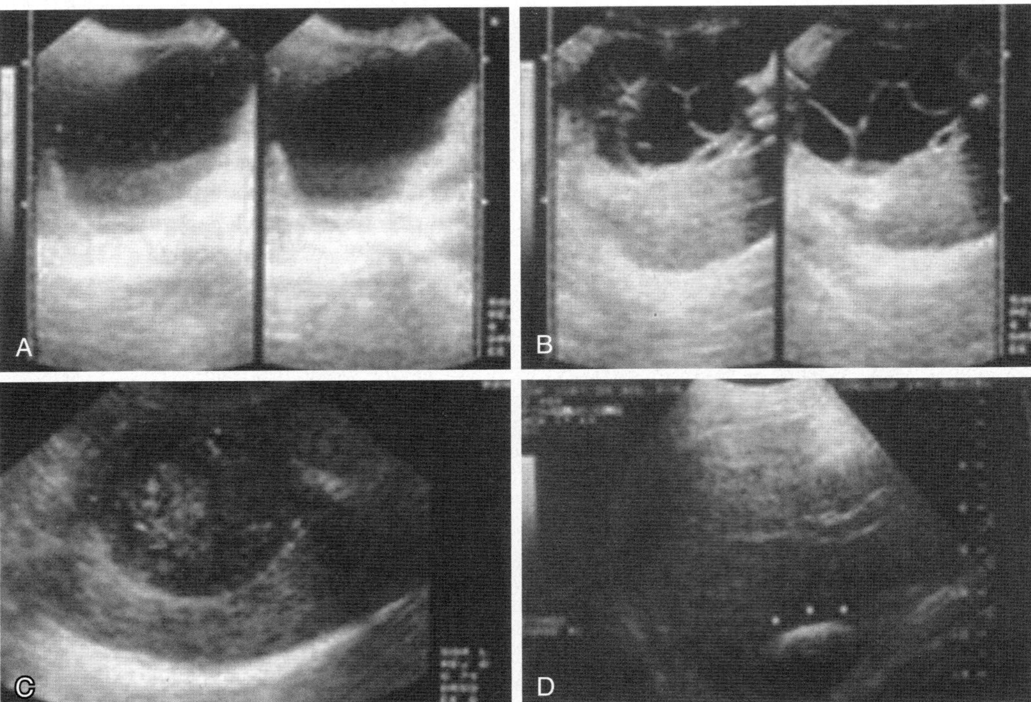

FIG. 54.31 Ultrasound image demonstrating typical characteristics of a hydatid cyst at varying stages. (A) Simple hydatid cyst with hydatid sand. (B) Daughter and granddaughter cysts and typical rosette appearance. (C) Hydatid cyst filled with amorphous mass, giving a solid or semisolid appearance. (D) Calcified cyst with egg-shell appearance. (From Thomas PG, Ravindra KV. Amebiasis and biliary infection. In: Blumgart LH, Fong Y, eds. *Surgery of the Liver and Biliary Tract.* London: WB Saunders; 2000:1147–1166.)

Hydatid Cyst

Hydatid disease or echinococcosis is a zoonosis that occurs primarily in sheep-grazing areas of the world but is common worldwide because the dog is a definitive host. Echinococcosis is endemic in Mediterranean countries, the Middle East, Far East, South America, Australia, New Zealand, and east Africa. Humans contract the disease from dogs, but there is no human-to-human transmission.

There are three species that cause hydatid disease. *Echinococcus granulosus* is the most common, and *Echinococcus multilocularis* and *Echinococcus ligartus* account for a small number of cases. Dogs are the definitive host of *E. granulosus*; the adult tapeworm is attached to the villi of the ileum. Up to thousands of ova are passed daily and deposited in the dog's feces. Sheep are the usual intermediate host, but humans are an accidental intermediate host. Humans are an end stage to the parasite. In the human duodenum, the parasitic embryo releases an oncosphere containing hooklets that penetrate the mucosa, allowing access to the bloodstream. In the blood, the oncosphere reaches the liver (most commonly) or lungs, where the parasite develops its larval stage—the hydatid cyst.

Three weeks after infection, a visible hydatid cyst develops, which then slowly grows in a spherical manner. A pericyst or fibrous capsule derived from host tissues develops around the hydatid cyst. The cyst wall itself has two layers, an outer gelatinous membrane (ectocyst) and an inner germinal membrane (endocyst). Brood capsules are small, intracystic cellular masses in which future worm heads develop into scoleces. In a definitive host, the scoleces develop into an adult tapeworm; but in the intermediate host, they can differentiate only into a new hydatid cyst. Freed brood capsules and scoleces are found in the hydatid fluid and form the so-called hydatid sand. Daughter cysts are true replicas of the mother cyst. Hydatid cysts can die with degeneration of the membranes, development of cystic vacuoles, and calcification of the wall. Calcification of a hydatid cyst, however, does not always imply that the cyst is dead.

Hydatid cysts are diagnosed in equal numbers of men and women at an average age of about 45 years. Approximately 75% of hydatid cysts are located in the right liver and are solitary. The clinical presentation of a hydatid cyst is largely asymptomatic until complications occur. The most common presenting symptoms are abdominal pain, dyspepsia, and vomiting. The most frequent sign is hepatomegaly. Jaundice and fever are each present in approximately 8% of patients. Bacterial superinfection of a hydatid cyst can occur and be manifested like a pyogenic abscess. Rupture of the cyst into the biliary tree or bronchial tree or free rupture into the peritoneal, pleural, or pericardial cavities can occur. Free ruptures can result in disseminated echinococcosis or a potentially fatal anaphylactic reaction. In cases of diagnostic uncertainty, a battery of serologic tests are available to evaluate antibody response, but all are plagued by low sensitivity and specificity.

Ultrasound is most commonly used worldwide for the diagnosis of echinococcosis because of its availability, affordability, and accuracy. A number of findings on ultrasound can be diagnostic but depend on the stage of the cyst at the time of the examination. A simple hydatid cyst is well circumscribed with budding signs on the cyst membrane and may contain free-floating hyperechogenic hydatid sand. A rosette appearance is seen when daughter cysts are present. The cyst can be filled with an amorphous mass, which can be diagnostically misleading. Calcifications in the wall of the cyst are highly suggestive of hydatid disease and can be helpful in the diagnosis (Fig. 54.31). Similar findings are seen on CT or

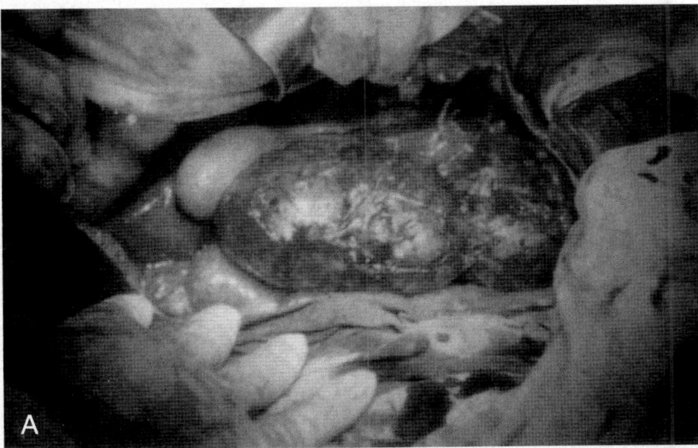

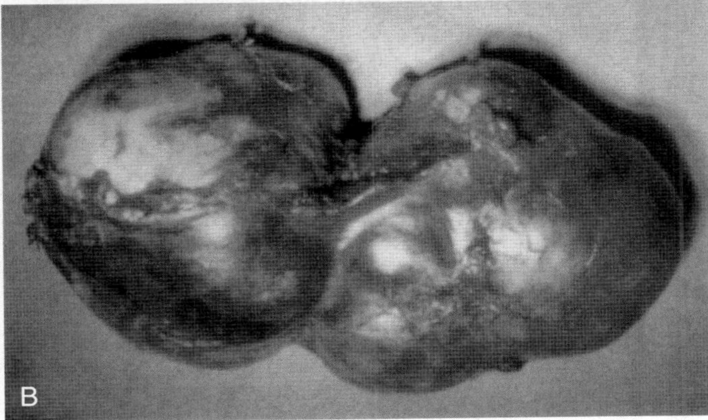

FIG. 54.32 (A) Peripheral hydatid cyst of the left liver. (B) Intact specimen after pericystectomy. Note that the entire pericyst has been removed. (From Milicevic MN. Hydatid disease. In: Blumgart LH, Fong Y, eds. *Surgery of the Liver and Biliary Tract*. London: WB Saunders; 2000:1167–1204.)

MRI scans. These cross-sectional imaging studies can also evaluate extrahepatic disease and demonstrate detailed hepatic anatomic relationships to the cyst. In patients with suspected biliary involvement, ERCP or percutaneous transhepatic cholangiography may be necessary.

Although the treatment of hepatic hydatid cysts is primarily surgical, alternative options are in evolution. In general, most cysts should be treated; but in older patients with small, asymptomatic, densely calcified cysts, conservative management is appropriate. In preparation for an operation, preoperative steroids have been recommended but are not universally used. The anesthesiologist should have epinephrine and steroids available in case of an anaphylactic reaction. A number of operations have been used, but in general, the abdomen is completely explored, the liver mobilized, and the cyst exposed. Packing off the abdomen is important because rupture can result in anaphylaxis and diffuse seeding. The cyst is usually then aspirated through a closed suction system and flushed with a scolicidal agent, such as hypertonic saline. The cyst is then unroofed, which can then be followed by a number of possibilities, including excision (or pericystectomy), marsupialization procedures, leaving the cyst open, drainage of the cyst, omentoplasty, and partial hepatectomy to encompass the cyst. Total pericystectomy or formal partial hepatectomy can also be performed without entering the cyst (Fig. 54.32). Both radical (resection) and conservative (drainage and evacuation) surgical approaches appear to be equally effective at controlling disease, although a prospective comparison has never been performed. When bile duct communication is diagnosed preoperatively or at operation, it must be meticulously sought after. Simple suture repair is often sufficient, but major biliary repairs, approaches through the common bile duct, or postoperative ERCP may be necessary. Laparoscopic techniques for drainage and unroofing of cysts have been reported in a number of series, with encouraging results. Recurrence rates after surgical treatment range from 1% to 20% but are generally 5% or less in experienced centers.

In the past, percutaneous aspiration of hydatid cysts was contraindicated because of the risk of rupture and uncontrolled spillage. However, percutaneous aspiration with injection of scolicidal agents has been reported with high success rates in highly selected patients. This technique is known as puncture, aspiration, injection, and reaspiration PAIR) and has become more accepted in some centers. Two randomized trials, one comparing PAIR with surgery ($N = 50$) and one comparing PAIR with medical therapy, have shown similar success rates. These trials were small and had significant methodologic problems, limiting the ability to draw firm conclusions.[10] Although surgery remains the treatment of choice, further prospective trials are clearly indicated to address this interesting and potentially useful technique. Treatment of echinococcosis with albendazole or mebendazole is effective at shrinking cysts in many patients with *E. granulosus* infection, but cyst disappearance occurs in well below 50% of patients. Preoperative treatment may decrease the risk of spillage and is a reasonable and safe practice.[7] Medical therapy without definitive resection or drainage should be considered only for widely disseminated disease or poor surgical candidates.

Recurrent Pyogenic Cholangitis

RPC is a syndrome of repeated attacks of cholangitis secondary to biliary stones and strictures that involve the extrahepatic and intrahepatic ducts. The condition has many names but is often referred to as Oriental cholangiohepatitis or hepatolithiasis. The disease is almost exclusively found in Asians and Asian medical centers. However, it is also seen in Asian immigrants throughout the world. Men and women are equally affected, and, historically, the disease strikes at an early age (20–40 years) in patients from lower socioeconomic classes.

The cause of RPC is unknown but is related to recurrent infection of biliary radicals with gut bacteria. Ultimately, stones and strictures develop in the biliary tree, but it is not known which occurs first. The stones are bilirubinate stones; in some patients, no stones are found and only biliary sludge is demonstrated. An association between RPC and *Clonorchis sinensis* and *Ascaris lumbricoides* infection has been noted, but a true causal relationship has never been proven.

Strictures can be found anywhere in the biliary tree but usually involve the intrahepatic main hepatic ducts, most often the left hepatic duct. The gallbladder is involved only in approximately 20% of cases. Cirrhosis and liver failure are seen only in long-standing disease, usually after multiple operations. Other complications include choledochoduodenal fistulas and acute pancreatitis from common bile duct stones. An increased incidence of cholangiocarcinoma has been noted, but a causal relationship is difficult to prove.

The typical patient with RPC is a young Asian of a lower socioeconomic background who presents with repeated bouts of cholangitis. The symptoms and presentation are those of cholangitis. These include fever, right upper quadrant abdominal pain, and jaundice. Biliary obstruction is usually incomplete, and

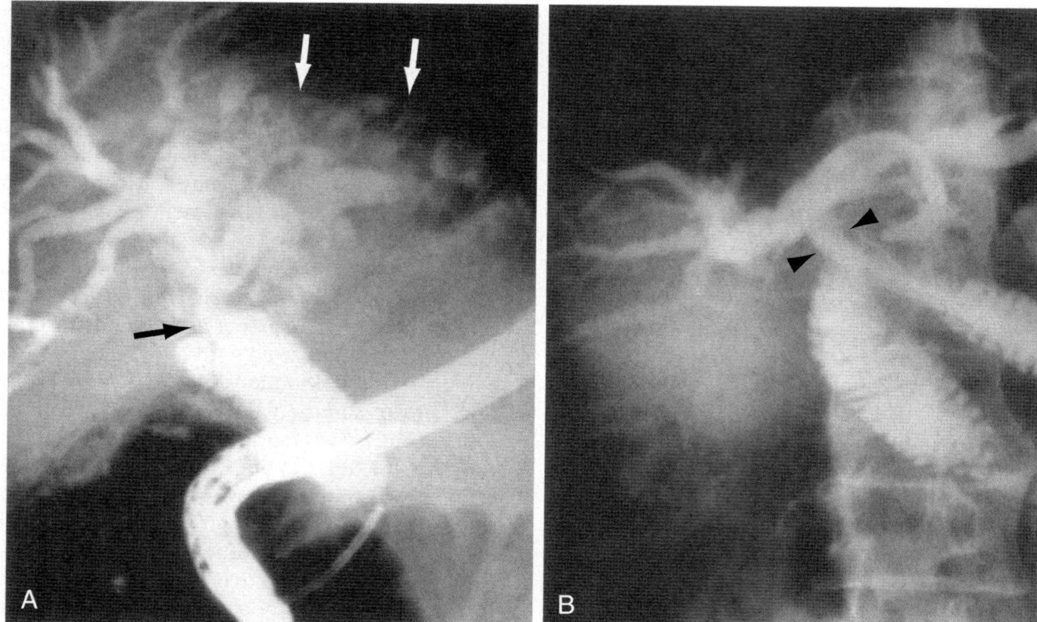

FIG. 54.33 (A) Cholangiogram of a patient with recurrent pyogenic cholangitis and a common hepatic duct stricture *(black arrow)*. There are numerous stones inside dilated left ducts *(white arrows)*. (B) A hepaticojejunostomy to the segment III duct *(arrowheads)* has been performed, and a flexible choledochoscope is shown passing through the anastomosis into the peripheral left ducts. All stones have been cleared. (From Fan ST, Wong J: Recurrent pyogenic cholangitis. In: Blumgart LH, Fong Y, eds. *Surgery of the Liver and Biliary Tract.* London: WB Saunders; 2000: 1205–1225.)

therefore, marked jaundice and pruritus are not common. There is usually leukocytosis and abnormal LFT results consistent with biliary obstruction. Evaluation of the anatomic distribution of disease is critical to formulation of a sound therapeutic plan. A combination of ultrasound, CT, and direct cholangiography is often necessary to evaluate these patients. Direct cholangiography is performed endoscopically or transhepatically and is considered an important study complementing the cross-sectional imaging. Magnetic resonance cholangiopancreatography can combine cross-sectional imaging and cholangiography in one noninvasive test and may ultimately replace direct cholangiography.

In an acute presentation, most patients improve with conservative management, allowing time for radiologic studies and planning of a definitive operation, which is the treatment of choice. If intervention is necessary during the acute phase, it must focus on adequate decompression of the biliary tree through open common bile duct exploration or endoscopic papillotomy with stenting. Although nonoperative approaches, such as percutaneous transhepatic cholangioscopic lithotomy, have been developed, surgical treatment remains the treatment of choice. Percutaneous transhepatic cholangioscopic lithotomy is generally used for poor-risk surgical patients and those who have failed to respond to surgical treatment. Stone clearance rates are high (>80%) and necessary for a successful long-term outcome. Unfortunately, stone recurrence is common and is mostly related to the presence of biliary strictures.

The goal of operative approaches is to clear the biliary tree of stones and to bypass, resect, or enlarge strictures. Many cases require only exploration of the common bile duct with or without hepaticojejunostomy. In complicated cases, providing permanent access to the biliary tree for interventional radiologic procedures by extending the end of the Roux-en-Y hepaticojejunostomy to the skin or subcutaneous space has been a successful approach (Fig. 54.33). Other potentially necessary procedures include strictureplasty and partial hepatectomy. Partial hepatectomy is advocated for patients with intrahepatic strictures, hepatic atrophy, liver abscess, or suspicion of cholangiocarcinoma.

In a large series from Asia, where surgery and hepatectomy are liberally applied, surgical mortality rates are 1%. Moreover, with aggressive treatment, there is almost a 100% stone clearance rate. Long-term outcome is excellent, with a less than 5% stone recurrence rate. Long-term survival is mostly related to the presence of cholangiocarcinoma, which is found in approximately 10% of patients. Particularly complicated cases can have a higher rate of recurrent symptoms.

NEOPLASMS

Solid Benign Neoplasms

It is estimated that benign focal liver masses are present in approximately 10% to 20% of the population in developed countries. With the increasing use of rapidly improving radiologic examinations, these entities have been encountered more frequently. Familiarity with the clinical characteristics, natural history, imaging characteristics, and indications for surgery in these tumors is essential. Many benign lesions can be adequately characterized by modern imaging studies, such as CT, ultrasound, and MRI. In unclear cases, serum tumor markers (e.g., AFP, CEA) and a search for a primary tumor in the case of suspected metastases should be carried out. A resection might be necessary to make a definitive diagnosis. Laparoscopy for assessment, biopsy, or resection has become an important diagnostic technique as well.

Liver Cell Adenoma

Liver cell adenoma (LCA) is a relatively rare benign proliferation of hepatocytes in the context of a normal liver. It is predominantly found in young women (aged 20–40 years) and is often associated with steroid hormone use, such as long-term oral contraceptive pill (OCP) use. Increased prevalence of LCA was observed in the 1970s, following the introduction of oral contraceptives. Male anabolic hormone use can also predispose to development of LCA. The female-to-male ratio is approximately 11:1. Other risk factors for LCA include vascular liver diseases, glycogenosis type 1A, and familial adenomatous polyposis. LCAs are usually singular, but multiple lesions have been reported in 12% to 30% of cases. Liver adenomatosis is defined by the presence of more than 10 LCAs in the liver. Interestingly, cases with multiple adenomas are not associated with OCP use and do not have as dramatic a female preponderance. On histologic evaluation, LCAs are composed of cords of benign hepatocytes containing increased glycogen and fat. Bile ductules are not observed histologically, and the normal architecture of the liver is absent in these lesions. Hemorrhage and necrosis are commonly seen. On the basis of detailed molecular pathology correlation studies, a French collaborative group has recently proposed a molecular-pathologic classification whereby the adenomas are classified as β-catenin mutated adenoma, *HNF1A* mutated adenoma, inflammatory adenoma, and not otherwise specified adenoma.[11] Molecular studies have also identified genetic signatures associated with a higher risk of malignant transformation. Specifically, highest risk of malignant transformation is observed in LCA with β-catenin activation.[11] With further research, new pathways driving the formation of adenomas are being identified and the "not otherwise specified adenoma" group is becoming smaller. For example, recently, sonic hedgehog activation has been observed in 5% of LCAs. Interestingly, these LCAs with sonic hedgehog activation are associated with obesity and bleeding. Furthermore, LCA with β-catenin mutations can be further classified by the nature of the mutation. For example, those with exon-3 mutation have increased risk of hepatocellular carcinoma (HCC) degeneration, whereas mutation in exon 7/8 leads to only weak activation of β-catenin and no risk of malignant transformation.

Patients with LCA present with symptoms approximately 50% to 75% of the time. Upper abdominal pain is common and may be related to hemorrhage into the tumor or local compressive symptoms. The physical examination is usually unrevealing, and tumor markers are normal. Dramatic presentations with free intraperitoneal rupture and bleeding can occur. Imaging tends to be characteristic and obviates the need for tissue diagnosis most of the time Because of intratumoral hemorrhage, the necrosis and fat component of LCA tends to be heterogeneous on CT. On contrast-enhanced CT, LCA tends to have peripheral enhancement with centripetal progression. MRI scans of LCA also have specific imaging characteristics, including a well-demarcated heterogeneous mass containing fat or hemorrhage. Despite high-quality imaging, resection may sometimes be necessary to secure a diagnosis in difficult cases. Intriguingly, studies are elucidating a correlation between the molecular subtypes described and imaging characteristics.

The two major risks of LCA are rupture, with potentially life-threatening intraperitoneal hemorrhage, and malignant transformation. Quantifying the risk of rupture is difficult, but it has been estimated to be as high as 30% to 50%, with all instances of spontaneous rupture occurring in lesions 5 cm and larger. Although there are numerous reports of transformation of LCA into HCC, the true risk of transformation is probably low. Hepatic adenomas with β-catenin activation should be considered for early surgical intervention as malignant transformation most commonly occurs in this subtype.

Patients who present with acute hemorrhage need emergent attention. If possible, hepatic artery embolization is a helpful and usually effective temporizing maneuver. Once the patient is stabilized and appropriately resuscitated, a laparotomy and resection of the mass are required. Symptomatic masses should be similarly resected. Patients with asymptomatic LCAs taking OCPs can be watched for regression after stopping of the OCPs, although progression and rupture have been observed in this setting. Behavior of LCAs during pregnancy has been unpredictable, and resection before a planned pregnancy is usually recommended. Overall, the surgeon must compare the risks of expectant management with serial imaging studies and AFP measurements against those of resection. Resection is usually recommended because of low mortality in experienced hands and the risks of observation. Margin status is not important in these resections, and limited resections can be performed. The management of adenomatosis is controversial, but large lesions should probably be resected because of the risk of rupture, whereas the risk of malignancy is low in lesions smaller than 5 cm. On occasion, liver transplantation is necessary for aggressive forms of adenomatosis.

Focal Nodular Hyperplasia

Focal nodular hyperplasia (FNH) is the second most common benign tumor of the liver after hemangioma and is predominantly discovered in young women.[12] FNH is characterized by a central fibrous scar with radiating septa, although no central scar is seen in approximately 15% of cases. On microscopic examination, FNH contains cords of benign-appearing hepatocytes divided by multiple fibrous septa originating from a central scar. Typical hepatic vascularity is not seen, but atypical biliary epithelium is found scattered throughout the lesion. The central scar often contains a large artery that branches out into multiple smaller arteries in a spoke wheel pattern. The cause of FNH is not known, but the most common theory is that FNH is related to a developmental vascular malformation. Female hormones and OCPs have been implicated in the development and growth of FNH, but the association is weak and difficult to prove.

In most patients, FNH is an incidental finding at laparotomy or, more commonly, on imaging studies. If symptoms are noted, vague abdominal pain is most often present, but a variety of nonspecific symptoms have been described. It is often difficult to ascribe these reported symptoms to the presence of FNH, and therefore, other possible causes must be sought. Physical examination is usually unrevealing, and mild abnormalities of liver function may be found. Serum AFP levels are normal.

With advances in hepatobiliary imaging, most cases of FNH can be diagnosed radiologically with reasonable certainty. Contrast-enhanced CT and MRI have become accurate methods of diagnosing FNH. FNH typically shows strong hypervascularity in the arterial phase of CT or MRI with central nonenhancing scar. The enhancement fades over time, and the lesion becomes isointense to the liver parenchyma in the portal and delayed phases. When no central scar is seen, however, radiologic diagnosis is difficult, and differentiation from LCA or a malignant mass, especially fibrolamellar HCC, can sometimes be impossible. On occasion, histologic confirmation is necessary, and resection is recommended for definitive diagnosis. Fine-needle aspiration for the diagnosis of FNH has been recommended but is often unrevealing.

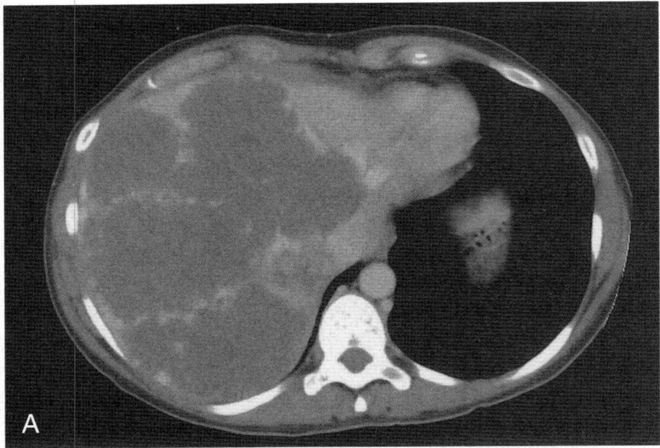

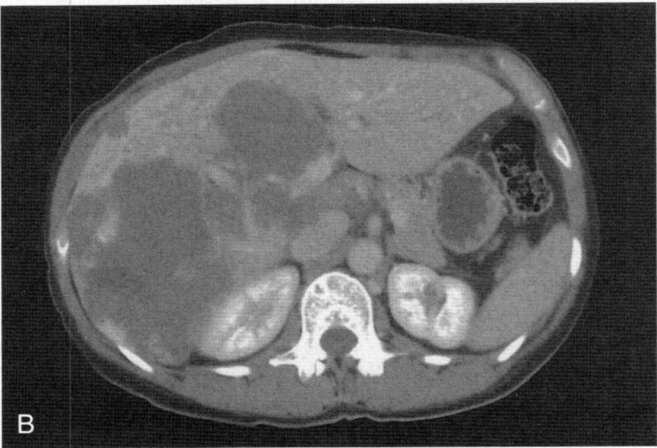

FIG. 54.34 (A and B) Computed tomography scans of a large cavernous hemangioma showing displacement of left and middle hepatic veins and abutment of the left portal vein. The mass was symptomatic and required an extended right hepatectomy for removal.

Most FNH tumors are benign and indolent. Rupture, bleeding, and infarction are exceedingly rare, and malignant degeneration of FNH has never been reported. The treatment of FNH therefore depends on diagnostic certainty and symptoms. Asymptomatic patients with typical radiologic features do not require treatment.[12] If diagnostic uncertainty exists, resection may be necessary for histologic confirmation. Symptomatic patients should be thoroughly investigated to look for other pathologic processes to explain the symptoms. Careful observation of symptomatic FNH with serial imaging is reasonable because symptoms may resolve in a significant number of cases. Patients with persistent symptomatic FNH or an enlarging mass should be considered for resection. Because FNH is a benign diagnosis, resection must be performed, with minimal morbidity and mortality.

Hemangioma

Hemangioma is the most common benign tumor of the liver.[12] It occurs in women more than in men (3:1 ratio) and at a mean age of approximately 45 years. Small capillary hemangiomas are of no clinical significance, whereas larger cavernous hemangiomas more often come to the attention of the liver surgeon (Fig. 54.34). Cavernous hemangiomas have been associated with FNH and are also theorized to be congenital vascular malformations. The enlargement of hemangiomas is by ectasia rather than by neoplasia. They are usually solitary and less than 5 cm in diameter, and they occur with equal incidence in the right and left hemilivers. Lesions larger than 5 cm are arbitrarily called giant hemangiomas. Involution or thrombosis of hemangiomas can result in dense fibrotic masses that may be difficult to differentiate from malignant tumors. On microscopic examination, they are endothelium-lined, blood-filled spaces separated by thin fibrous septa.

Hemangiomas are usually asymptomatic and found incidentally on imaging studies. Large compressive masses may cause vague upper abdominal symptoms. Symptoms ascribed to a liver hemangioma, however, mandate a search for other disease because an alternative cause of symptoms will be found in approximately 50% of cases. Rapid expansion or acute thrombosis can occasionally cause symptoms. Spontaneous rupture of liver hemangiomas is exceedingly rare. An associated syndrome of thrombocytopenia and consumptive coagulopathy known as Kasabach-Merritt syndrome is rare but well described.

LFT results and tumor markers are usually normal in liver hemangiomas. Radiologic investigation can make the diagnosis reliably in most cases. CT and MRI are usually sufficient if a typical peripheral nodular enhancement pattern is seen. Isotope-labeled red blood cell scans are an accurate test but are rarely necessary if high-quality CT and MRI are available. Percutaneous biopsy of a suspected hemangioma is potentially dangerous and inaccurate. Therefore, biopsy is not recommended.

The natural history of liver hemangioma is generally benign; it appears that most remain stable for a long time, with a low risk of rupture or hemorrhage.[12] Growth and development of symptoms do occur, however, occasionally requiring resection. There has never been a report of malignant degeneration of a liver hemangioma. An asymptomatic patient with a secure diagnosis can therefore be simply observed.[12] Symptomatic patients should undergo a thorough evaluation looking for alternative explanations for the symptoms but are candidates for resection if no other cause is found. Rupture, significant change in size, and development of the Kasabach-Merritt syndrome are indications for resection. In rare cases of diagnostic uncertainty, resection may be necessary for a definitive diagnosis to be made. Resection of liver hemangiomas should be performed, with minimal morbidity and mortality. The preferred approach to resection is enucleation with arterial inflow control, but anatomic resections may be necessary in some cases. Surgery on large central hemangiomas can be associated with significant morbidity.

Liver hemangiomas in children are common, accounting for approximately 12% of all childhood hepatic tumors. They are usually multifocal and can involve other organs. Large hemangiomas in children can result in congestive heart failure secondary to arteriovenous shunting. Untreated symptomatic childhood hemangiomas are associated with high mortality. On the other hand, almost all small capillary hemangiomas resolve. Symptomatic childhood hemangiomas may be treated with therapeutic embolization; medical therapy should be initiated for congestive heart failure. Radiation and chemotherapeutic agents have been used, but experience has been limited. Resection may be necessary for symptomatic lesions or rupture.

Other Benign Tumors

Most benign solid liver tumors are LCAs, FNHs, or hemangiomas, but there are other benign hepatic tumors. However, these are rare and can be difficult to differentiate from malignant neoplasms. Macroregenerative nodules, previously known as adenomatous hyperplasia, are single or multiple, well-circumscribed, bile-stained, bulging surface nodules that occur primarily in cirrhotics and result from the hyperplastic response to chronic liver injury. These lesions have malignant potential and can be difficult to distinguish from HCC. Nodular regenerative hyperplasia is a benign diffuse micronodular (usually <2 cm) process associated with lymphoproliferative disorders, collagen vascular diseases, and the use of steroids or chemotherapy. Nodular regenerative hyperplasia has no malignant potential and is not associated with cirrhosis. Biopsy may be necessary to distinguish these focal nodules from malignant neoplasms.

Mesenchymal hamartomas are rare solitary tumors of childhood that account for 5% of pediatric liver tumors. They are usually large cystic masses found in the right liver that present as progressive, painless, abdominal distention. Resection of mesenchymal hamartomas may be necessary in the case of large lesions causing a mass effect.

Fatty tumors of the liver are rarely encountered but can usually be distinguished by typical characteristics on CT or MRI scans. Fatty tumors of the liver include primary lipomas, myelolipomas (which contain hematopoietic tissue), angiolipomas (which contain blood vessels), and angiomyolipomas (which contain smooth muscle). Focal fatty change in the liver can be confused with a neoplastic process and is becoming more common with improved imaging and the increasing incidence of hepatic steatosis.

Benign fibrous tumors of the liver can become large and symptomatic, requiring resection. Inflammatory pseudotumors of the liver are localized masses of inflammatory cells that can mimic a neoplasm. The cause of these inflammatory lesions is unknown but may be related to thrombosed vessels or old abscesses. Other extremely rare benign hepatic tumors include leiomyomas, myxomas, schwannomas, lymphangiomas, and teratomas.

Intrahepatic biliary cystadenomas or bile duct adenomas are rare but can cause biliary symptoms. Biliary hamartomas and biliary hyperplasia are common and are often seen as small white surface lesions that can mimic small metastatic tumors at abdominal exploration. Adrenal and pancreatic rests have also been found in the liver.

Primary Solid Malignant Neoplasms

Hepatocellular Carcinoma

Epidemiology. Liver cancer is the fifth most common cancer and the second most frequent cause of cancer-related death globally. HCC is the most common primary malignant neoplasm of the liver and one of the most common malignant neoplasms worldwide. The epidemiology of HCC varies around the world, being affected by the varying etiologies in different parts of the world. Hepatitis B is the most common cause of HCC worldwide. Thus, the highest incidence of HCC occurs in geographical areas where hepatitis B is rampant, namely sub-Saharan Africa and Southeast Asia (>10–20 cases/100,000). The lowest incidence (1–3 cases/100,000) is found in Australia, North America, and Europe. Epidemiologic evidence strongly suggests that HCC is largely related to environmental factors; the incidence of HCC in immigrants eventually approaches that of the local population after several generations. An exception to this is that whites living in high-prevalence areas tend to have a low incidence of HCC. This is likely related to the continuation of the lifestyle and environment of their home country. It is probable that the variation in incidence rates among immigrants is related to hepatitis B virus (HBV) carrier rates. A significant rise in the incidence of HCC in the United States and other Western countries has been noted during the last 35 years. However, recent data suggest that at least in the United States, the epidemic may have peaked as the incidence rates have stabilized in the last few years. The explanation for the observed increase during the last few decades is not understood, but the emergence of hepatitis C virus (HCV) infection and immigration patterns have been suggested. In the United States, HCC incidence is highest in Asians, Pacific Islanders, and Native Americans and lowest among Caucasians. HCV is the most common cause of HCC, accounting for more than half of all cases in the United States and with HBV only present in up to 20% of cases. A third of HCC cases are not infected by either virus. Risk of HCC is further increased in obese patients and in those with nonalcoholic fatty liver disease and nonalcoholic steatohepatitis. Given that obesity and its ensuing complications are increasing at epidemic proportion in the Western world, obesity as the cause of HCC is becoming more important. Recent data also suggest that addressing the environmental factors can lead to reduction in incidence of HCC. In Taiwan, treatment of chronic hepatitis B and C under the auspices of a national viral hepatitis therapy program has met with a reduction in incidence and mortality due to HCC.

HCC is two to eight times more common in men than in women in low- and high-incidence areas. Although sex hormones may play a minor role in the development of HCC, the higher incidence in men is probably related to higher rates of associated risk factors, such as HBV infection, cirrhosis, smoking, alcohol abuse, and higher hepatic DNA synthesis in cirrhosis. In general, the incidence of HCC increases with age, but a tendency to development of HCC earlier in high-incidence areas has been noted. For example, in Mozambique, 50% of patients with HCC were found to be younger than 30 years. This may be related to differing ages at infection and the natural histories of hepatitis B and C.

Causative factors. A large number of associations between hepatic viral infections, environmental exposure, alcohol use, smoking, genetic metabolic diseases, cirrhosis, and OCP use and the development of HCC have been recognized. Overall, 75% to 80% of HCC cases are related to HBV (50%–55%) or HCV (25%–30%) infections. It is also clear from research that the development of HCC is a complex and multistep process that involves any number of these risk factors.

Many years of research have documented a clear association between persistent HBV infection and the development of HCC. Up to 5% of the world population is chronically infected with HBV. Chronic HBV infection accounts for up to 50% of the world's cases of HCC and most of the cases of childhood HCC. Studies have estimated relative risks of 5 to 100 for the development of HCC in HBV-infected individuals compared with noninfected individuals. The risk of developing HCC is also affected by the presence of other factors including, age, Asian or African ancestry, family history, viral factors (genotype, duration of infection, coinfection with HCV, HIV or hepatitis D), and environmental factors (exposure to aflatoxin, alcohol, and tobacco). Other evidence includes the following observations: geographic areas high in HBV infection have high rates of HCC; HBV infection precedes the development of HCC; the sequence of HBV infection to cirrhosis to HCC is well documented; and the HBV genome is found in the HCC genome. The HBV has no known oncogenes, but insertional mutagenesis into hepatocytes may be a contributing factor to the development of HCC. Another proposed mechanism is related to cirrhosis and chronic hepatic inflammation, which is present in 60% to 90% of patients with HBV infection and HCC. Cirrhosis, however, is not a prerequisite for the development of HBV-related HCC. The risk of HCC is not simply related to HBV exposure but requires chronic infection (i.e., chronically positive HBV surface antigen). There is a higher risk of persistent infection (carrier state) when the infection is acquired at birth or during early childhood. Familial clustering of HCC is probably related to early vertical transmission of the virus and establishment of the chronic carrier state. Individuals with greater HBV replication, evident from the presence of hepatitis B e antigen (HBeAg) and higher levels of HBV DNA, have higher risk of HCC development. HBV genotypes (A–H) also affect the clinical outcomes.

Hepatitis C has been discovered to be a major cause of chronic liver disease in Japan, Europe, and the United States, where there is a relatively low rate of HBV infection. 2% of the world's population is infected with HCV. Antibodies to the HCV are found in 76% of patients with HCC in Japan and Europe and in 36% of patients in the United States. HBV and HCV infections are both independent risk factors for the development of HCC but probably act synergistically when an individual is infected with both viruses. Although the natural history of HCV infection is not completely understood, it appears to be one of chronic infection, with a benign early course. However, the ultimate development of cirrhosis with increased risk of HCC may ensue. The rate of HCC among HCV-infected persons ranges from 1% to 3% over 30 years, and in individuals with HCV-related cirrhosis, HCC develops at an annual rate of 1%–4%. Studies on the rates of progression to cirrhosis estimate a median time of 30 years, but differing progression rates yield a range of less than 20 years to more than 50 years. Factors associated with a more rapid progression include male gender, chronic alcohol use, and older age at the time of infection. HCV is an RNA virus that does not integrate into the host genome, and therefore, the pathogenesis of HCV-related HCC may be related more to chronic inflammation and cirrhosis than to direct carcinogenesis. Data from era of interferon-based therapy suggests that the patients who achieved a sustained viral response had up to 75% reduction in their risk of HCC. This is exciting and has immense global health significance, especially now as there are many effective HCV treatments available. However, future studies will determine if these new treatments will change the incidence and course of HCC.

The true relationship of cirrhosis and HCC is difficult to ascertain, and suggestions of causation remain speculative. Cirrhosis is not required for the development of HCC, and hepatocarcinogenesis is not an inevitable result of cirrhosis. The relationship of cirrhosis and HCC is further complicated by the fact that they share common associations. Furthermore, some associations (e.g., HBV infection, hemochromatosis) are associated with higher risk of HCC, whereas others (e.g., alcohol, primary biliary cirrhosis) are associated with a lower risk of HCC. Research has demonstrated that cirrhotic livers with higher DNA replication rates are associated with the development of HCC.

Chronic alcohol abuse has been associated with an increased risk of HCC, and there may be a synergistic effect with HBV and HCV infection. Alcohol causes cirrhosis but has never been shown to be directly carcinogenic in hepatocytes. Thus, alcohol likely acts as a cocarcinogen. Cigarette smoking has been linked to the development of HCC, but the evidence is not consistent, and the contributing risk independent of viral hepatitis is likely to be small. Aflatoxin, produced by *Aspergillus* spp., is a powerful hepatotoxin. With chronic exposure, aflatoxin acts as a carcinogen and increases the risk of HCC. The offending fungi grow on grains, peanuts, and food products in tropical and subtropical regions. Ingestion of contaminated foods results in aflatoxin exposure. Levels of aflatoxin in these implicated foods are regulated in the United States.

Other chemicals have also been implicated as carcinogens related to HCC. These include nitrites, hydrocarbons, solvents, pesticide, and vinyl chloride. Thorotrast (colloidal thorium dioxide) is an angiographic medium that was used in the 1930s. It emits high levels of long-lasting radiation and has been associated with hepatic fibrosis, angiosarcoma, cholangiosarcoma, and HCC. Associations with inherited metabolic liver diseases, such as hereditary hemochromatosis, α_1-antitrypsin deficiency, and Wilson disease, have also been implicated as risk factors for HCC. Associations with hormonal manipulations, such as the use of OCPs and anabolic steroids, have been suggested but are weak and are probably better linked specifically to adenoma and well-differentiated HCC. Research has been focusing on relationships of HCC with diabetes, obesity, and metabolic syndrome.

Clinical presentation. Most commonly, patients presenting with HCC are men 50 to 60 years of age who complain of right upper quadrant abdominal pain and weight loss and have a palpable mass. In countries endemic for HBV, presentation at a younger age is common and probably related to childhood infection. Unfortunately, in unscreened populations, HCC tends to be manifested at a later stage because of the lack of symptoms in early stages. Presentation at an advanced stage is often with vague right upper quadrant abdominal pain that sometimes radiates to the right shoulder. Nonspecific symptoms of advanced malignant disease, such as anorexia, nausea, lethargy, and weight loss, are also common. Another common presentation of HCC is hepatic decompensation in a patient with known mild cirrhosis or even in patients with unrecognized cirrhosis.

HCC can rarely be manifested as a rupture, with the sudden onset of abdominal pain followed by hypovolemic shock secondary to intraperitoneal bleeding. Other rare presentations include hepatic vein occlusion (Budd-Chiari syndrome), obstructive jaundice, hemobilia, and fever of unknown origin. Less than 1% of cases of HCC are manifested with a paraneoplastic syndrome, usually hypercalcemia, hypoglycemia, and erythrocytosis. Small, incidentally noted tumors have become a more common presentation because of the knowledge of specific risk factors, screening programs for diagnosed HBV or HCV infection, and increasing use of high-quality abdominal imaging.

Diagnosis. Radiologic investigation is a critical part of the diagnosis of HCC. In the past, liver radioisotope scans and angiography were common methods of diagnosis, but ultrasound, CT, and MRI have replaced these studies. Ultrasound plays a significant role in screening and early detection of HCC, but definitive diagnosis and treatment planning rely on CT or MRI. Contrast-enhanced CT and MRI protocols aimed at diagnosing HCC take advantage of the hypervascularity of these tumors, and arterial-phase images are critical to assess the extent of disease adequately. Unlike many other cancers, the diagnosis of HCC can be established based on imaging findings alone. Typical imaging criteria for HCC include rapid arterial enhancement followed by washout in the delayed phase. An enhancing capsule supports the diagnosis of HCC. CT and MRI also evaluate the extent of disease in terms of peritoneal metastases, nodal metastases, and extent of vascular and biliary involvement. Detection of bland or tumor thrombus in the portal or hepatic venous system is also important and can be diagnosed with any of these modalities (Fig. 54.35).

AFP measurements can be helpful in the diagnosis of HCC. However, AFP measurement is associated with multiple problems. First, AFP measurements have low sensitivity and specificity. The

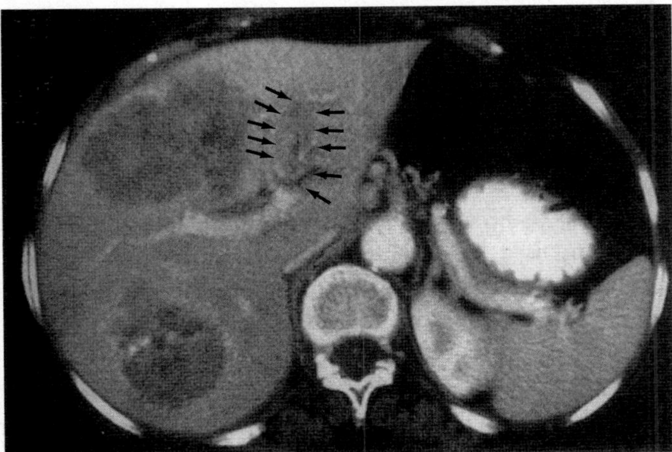

FIG. 54.35 Contrast-enhanced computed tomography scan demonstrating multifocal hepatocellular carcinoma. The left portal vein is invaded and expanded by tumor *(arrows)*. (From Roddie ME, Adam A. Computed tomography of the liver and biliary tree. In: Blumgart LH, Fong Y, eds. *Surgery of the Liver and Biliary Tract*. London: WB Saunders; 2000:309–340.)

specificity and positive predictive values of AFP improve with higher cutoff levels (e.g., 400 ng/mL) but at the cost of sensitivity. False-positive elevations of serum AFP levels can be seen in inflammatory disorders of the liver, such as chronic active viral hepatitis. Furthermore, AFP is not specific to HCC and can be elevated with intrahepatic cholangiocarcinoma (IHC) and colorectal metastases. With improvements in imaging technology and the ability to detect smaller tumors, AFP is largely used as an adjunctive test in patients with liver masses. AFP levels are particularly useful in monitoring treated patients for recurrence after normalization of levels.

Since the proposal of guidelines for the diagnosis of HCC by the Barcelona-2000 European Association for the Study of the Liver conference[13] and the American Association for the Study of Liver Disease,[14] new data have accumulated and the recommendations have evolved.[15,16] AFP used to play a major role in the diagnosis of HCC larger than 2 cm.[14] However, given the excellent performance of contrast-enhanced imaging modalities, AFP does not play a critical role in the diagnosis of HCC anymore.[15,16] For hepatic nodules 1 to 2 cm on a background of cirrhosis, a contrast-enhanced triple-phase CT and MRI scan is now recommended.[15,16] If typical features of HCC on imaging (arterially enhancing mass with washout of contrast material in delayed phases) are observed, diagnosis of HCC is presumed. For lesions larger than 2 cm, a single study may suffice. However, for lesions 1 to 2 cm, contrast-enhanced CT and MRI have a sensitivity of 53% to 62%, specificity of approximately 100%, positive predictive value of 95% to 100%, and negative predictive value of 80% to 84%. The performance of both MRI and CT in a sequential fashion can increase the sensitivity and may be required for difficult cases.

Patients with appropriate risk factors and suggestive radiologic features, with or without an elevated AFP level, who are candidates for potentially curative surgical therapy do not require preoperative biopsy unless the diagnosis is in question. Percutaneous fine-needle aspiration of HCC does run a small risk of tumor cell spillage (estimated to be ~1%) and rupture or bleeding, especially in cirrhotic livers and subcapsular tumors. Once the diagnosis of HCC has been made, the disease must be staged to develop an appropriate treatment plan. Most patients with HCC have two diseases, and survival is as much related to the tumor as it is to cirrhosis. Staging includes an extent of disease and extent of cirrhosis workup.

In assessing the extent of disease, the common sites of metastases must be considered. HCC largely metastasizes to the lung, bone, and peritoneum. Preoperative history should focus on symptoms referable to these areas. Extent of disease in the liver, including macrovascular invasion and the presence of multiple liver masses, must also be considered. Cross-sectional abdominal imaging, including arterial-phase images (see earlier), yields information on the extent of disease in the liver as well as peritoneal disease. Preoperative chest CT is mandatory because lung metastases are usually asymptomatic. Routine bone scans are not performed unless there are suggestive symptoms or signs.

Assessment of liver function is absolutely critical in considering treatment options for a patient with HCC. Liver resection is considered the treatment of choice for HCC, and the risk of postoperative liver failure and death must be considered. This risk is related to the degree of cirrhosis, portal hypertension, amount of liver resected (functional liver reserve), and regenerative potential response. Other successful treatments are available for HCC, such as ablative techniques, embolization techniques, and liver transplantation. Therefore, a complete assessment of tumor and liver function must be carried out. A number of tests of liver function are available, generally divided into clinical assessment and functional tests, and there are many clinical assessment schemes (see earlier). However, Child-Pugh status is used most often. Child-Pugh class C patients are not candidates for resectional therapy, whereas Child-Pugh class A patients can usually tolerate some extent of liver resection. Many consider Child-Pugh class B patients to be candidates for operation, but they are generally borderline, and therapy must be individualized.

Outside of scoring systems, it has been demonstrated that significant portal hypertension, regardless of biochemical assessments, is highly predictive of postoperative liver failure and death. Portal hypertension can be assessed directly through hepatic vein wedge pressures, but it is usually obvious on high-quality imaging in the form of splenomegaly, a cirrhotic-appearing liver, and intra-abdominal varices. Blood work usually demonstrates marked cytopenias. Most typically, patients have thrombocytopenia. Functional tests of liver function have been well described but are not routinely used in most Western centers because the results of studies evaluating their predictive value have been mixed.

Staging laparoscopy has been used as a staging tool in HCC and spares about one in five patients a nontherapeutic laparotomy. Laparoscopy yields additional information about the extent of disease in the liver, extrahepatic disease, and cirrhosis. The yield of laparoscopy is dictated by the extent of disease and is only selectively used. The presence of clinically apparent cirrhosis, radiologic evidence of vascular invasion, or bilobar tumors increases the yield to 30%, whereas without these factors, the yield is 5%.[17]

There are a number of staging systems for HCC, but none have been shown to be particularly superior; they probably depend on the specific population in which the disease is being staged as well as the cause of HCC in that particular population of patients. The tumor, node, metastasis (TNM) staging system is not routinely used for HCC because it does not accurately predict survival; it does not take liver function into account. Moreover, the TNM staging system relies on pathology that is frequently unavailable preoperatively. The Okuda staging system is an older but simple and effective system that takes liver function and tumor-related factors into account. It adds up a single point for the presence of

TABLE 54.7 Cancer of the Liver Italian Program score.*

CLINICAL PARAMETERS	CUTOFF VALUES	POINTS
Child-Pugh class	A	0
	B	1
	C	2
Tumor morphology	Uninodular, <50% extension	0
	Multinodular, <50% extension	1
	Massive or extension >50%	2
AFP level	<400 ng/dL	0
	>400 ng/dL	1
Portal vein thrombosis	No	0
	Yes	1

AFP, α-Fetoprotein.
*Score ranges from 0 to 6; a score of 4 to 6 is generally considered advanced disease, whereas a score of 0 to 3 has the potential for long-term survival.

tumor involving more than 50% of the liver, presence of ascites, albumin level less than 3 g/dL, and bilirubin level higher than 3 mg/dL. The Okuda staging system reliably distinguishes patients with a prohibitively poor prognosis from those with potential for long-term survival. The most well-validated staging system is the Cancer of the Liver Italian Program, which was rigorously developed and has been prospectively validated (Table 54.7). An example of a scoring system that is probably population specific is the Chinese University Prognostic Index, which takes into account TNM stage, symptoms, and ascites and the levels of AFP, bilirubin, and ALP; it appears to apply mainly to HBV-related HCC in China.

Pathology. On histologic evaluation, HCC is graded as well, moderately, or poorly differentiated. The grade of HCC, however, has never been shown to predict outcome accurately. In gross appearance, the growth patterns of HCC have been classified in a number of ways. The most useful scheme divides HCC into three distinct growth patterns that have distinct relationships to outcome. The hanging type of HCC is connected to the liver by a small vascular stalk and is easily resected without sacrifice of a significant amount of adjacent nonneoplastic liver tissue. This type can grow to substantial size without involving much normal liver tissue. The pushing type of HCC is well demarcated and often contains a fibrous capsule. It is characterized by growth that displaces vascular structures rather than invading them. This type is usually resectable. The last type is called the infiltrative type of HCC, which tends to invade vascular structures, even at a small size. Resection of the infiltrative type is often possible, but positive histologic margins are common. Small tumors (<5 cm) usually do not fall into any of these groups and are often discussed as a separate entity.

Finally, HCC can be manifested in a multifocal manner. Most HCC probably starts as a single tumor, but ultimately multiple satellite lesions can develop secondary to portal vein invasion and metastases. Multifocal tumors throughout the liver probably represent the end stage of HCC with multiple metastases and multiple primary tumors.

Treatment. There are a large number of treatment options for patients with HCC, reflecting the heterogeneity of this disease and the lack of a proven superior treatment, except complete resection (Box 54.1). Deciding on a treatment regimen for any one patient must take into consideration the stage of malignancy, the condition of the patient and of the liver, and the experience of the treating physician.

BOX 54.1 Treatment options for hepatocellular carcinoma.

Surgical
Resection
Orthotopic liver transplantation

Ablative
Ethanol injection
Acetic acid injection
Thermal ablation (cryotherapy, radiofrequency ablation, microwave)

Transarterial
Embolization
Chemoembolization

Radiotherapy
Combination transarterial and ablative: external beam radiation

Systemic
Chemotherapy
Hormonal
Immunotherapy

Surgical management

Resection. Complete excision of HCC by partial hepatectomy or by total hepatectomy and liver transplantation is the treatment of choice, when possible, because it has the highest chance of long-term survival. In general, however, only 10% to 20% of patients are considered to have resectable disease. Historically, mortality rates for partial hepatectomy have ranged from 1% to 20%, but if it is performed in healthy patients without advanced cirrhosis, most series have a mortality rate of less than 5%. Advances in surgical technique have also allowed the development of limited segmental resections when appropriate, which preserves liver function and improves early postoperative recovery. Selection of the appropriate patient for resection is critical and must take into account the condition of the liver and extent of disease. Hepatic resection is indicated as a potentially curative option in patients with adequate liver function (Child-Pugh Class A without portal hypertension) and solitary HCC without major vascular invasion. Patients with Child-Pugh class B or C cirrhosis or portal hypertension do not tolerate resection. The volume of the FLR is also an important consideration and is associated with postoperative complications and mortality. Preoperative portal vein embolization is an effective strategy to increase the volume and function of the FLR and should be used liberally in patients with Child-Pugh class A cirrhosis with a small FLR (i.e., <30%–40% of the total liver volume) who are being considered for a major resection. The overall postresection survival rates for HCC are 58% to 100% at 1 year, 28% to 88% at 3 years, 11% to 75% at 5 years, and 19% to 26% at 10 years. These results obviously depend on the stage of the tumor and degree of cirrhosis in each particular series. Together, they give a sense of the possibilities.

A variety of prognostic factors predictive of survival after resection have been identified, but none are universally agreed on. The most commonly cited negative prognostic factors are tumor size, cirrhosis, infiltrative growth pattern, vascular invasion, intrahepatic metastases, multifocal tumors, lymph node metastases, margin less than 1 cm, and lack of a capsule. The best outcomes are found in patients with single small tumors, but size alone should not contraindicate resection. Especially for patients with large tumors that are outside the criteria for transplantation, not many therapeutic options are available. In such patients with adequate liver function, adequate functional liver remnant, and resectable tumors, surgical resection may offer the best possible outcomes. Multifocal tumors and major vascular invasion are generally associated with a poor outcome, but some groups advocate resection in highly select patients. A randomized controlled trial corroborated these findings. In this study, patients with multifocal HCC outside Milan criteria were randomized to resection or transarterial chemoembolization.[18] In this study, resection provided better overall survival for patients with multifocal HCC compared with transarterial chemoembolization, suggesting that resection may be an option for these patients. For potentially resectable tumors that have high-risk features, various neoadjuvant strategies may help select patients for resection. For instance, a period of observation and tumor control with intraarterial therapies (e.g., transarterial chemoembolization/radioembolization) may help select patients who will benefit most from resection.

Transplantation. Theoretically, orthotopic liver transplantation is the ideal treatment for HCC because it addresses the liver dysfunction and cirrhosis and the HCC. The limitations of transplantation are the need for chronic immunosuppression and the lack of organ donors. There has been growing interest in the use of partial hepatectomy from live donors, which addresses the lack of organ donors but remains a somewhat controversial approach. Early series of transplantation for HCC had high recurrence rates and relatively poor long-term survival, largely attributed to the fact that most of these patients were undergoing transplantation for advanced disease. Refinements in patient selection—namely, patients with single tumors smaller than 5 cm or no more than three tumors 3 cm in size—have resulted in improved outcomes.[19] Long-term survival rates with more stringent selection criteria have ranged from 50% to 85%. Studies have begun to expand the indications for orthotopic liver transplantation without a major effect on long-term survival but likely an increase in overall recurrence rates. While the enlisted patient with HCC and cirrhosis awaits organ availability, the progression of HCC is typically controlled with locoregional therapy including ablation and transarterial therapies. Comparison of results of resection with transplantation is difficult as the patients considered for transplantation have a period of observation during which the patients with aggressive disease progress and dropout from the transplant list. As such, these two strategies should be viewed as complementary rather than competitive. Patients with advanced cirrhosis (Child class B and C) and early-stage HCC should be considered for transplantation, whereas those with Child class A cirrhosis have similar results with transplantation and resection and should probably be resected.

Locoregional therapies

Ablation. A number of other nonsurgical local ablative therapies are available for the treatment of small tumors. Percutaneous ethanol injection (PEI) is a useful technique for ablating small tumors. The tumor is killed by a combination of cellular dehydration, coagulative necrosis, and vascular thrombosis. Most tumors smaller than 2 cm can be ablated with a single application of PEI, but larger tumors may require multiple injections. Long-term survival after PEI for tumors smaller than 5 cm has been reported to range from 24% to 40%. Percutaneous injection of acetic acid is a technique similar to PEI but has stronger necrotizing abilities, making it more useful in septated tumors.

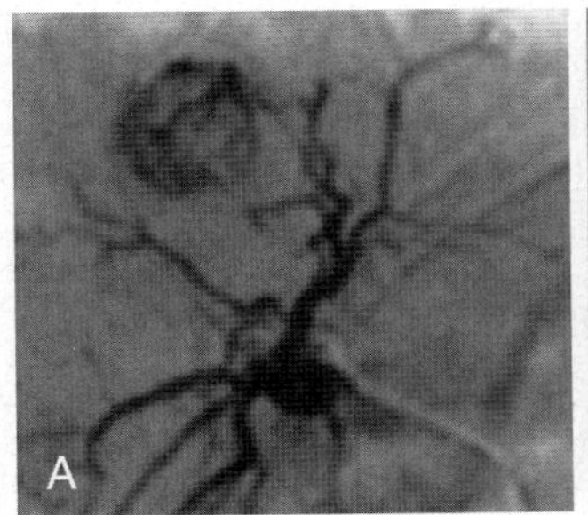

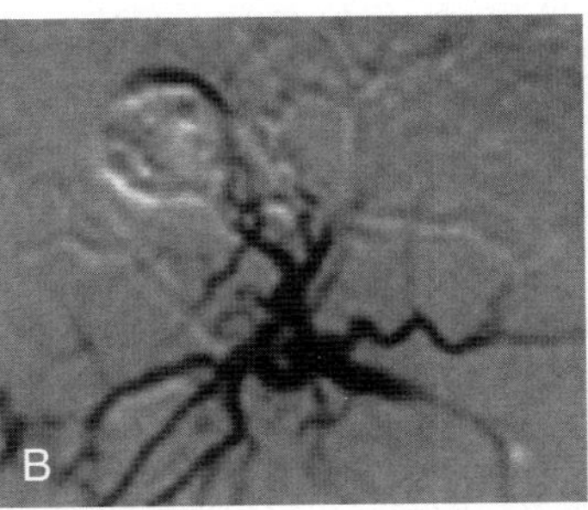

FIG. 54.36 Angiograms demonstrating hypervascular hepatocellular carcinoma before (A) and after (B) embolization.

Thermal ablative techniques that freeze or heat tumors to destroy them have become popular. Cryotherapy uses a specialized cryoprobe to freeze and thaw tumor and surrounding liver tissue, with resulting necrosis. Cryotherapy is usually performed at laparotomy or laparoscopically, but it has been performed with percutaneous techniques. One advantage is that the ice ball formed is easily monitored with ultrasound. Disadvantages include a heat sink effect, limiting the usefulness of freezing near major blood vessels and a relatively high complication rate of 8% to 41%. Reported 2-year survival rates for cryoablation of HCC range from 30% to 60%, but no comparative studies to resection have been carried out. Radiofrequency ablation (RFA) uses high-frequency alternating current to create heat around an inserted probe, resulting in temperatures higher than 60°C (140°F) and immediate cell death. Although initially limited to smaller tumors, improvements in technology have created RFA probes reportedly able to ablate tumors as large as 7 cm. Nonetheless, the efficacy of RFA for HCCs larger than 3 cm is limited because of increased local recurrence rates. RFA is also limited by the protective effect of blood vessels and does not ablate well in these areas. The procedure can easily be performed percutaneously, with low complication rates, and optimal guidance systems are being developed. Recent data suggest that resection may be superior to RFA for small HCCs in terms of both disease-free and overall survival. Microwave ablation has emerged as an alternative thermoablative procedure.

Arterially directed therapies. Transarterial therapy for HCC is based on the fact that most of the tumor's blood supply is from the hepatic artery. Today, the transarterial therapy is applied in a percutaneous fashion, thus avoiding morbidity and mortality of laparotomy. Percutaneous transarterial embolization can induce ischemic necrosis in HCC, resulting in response rates as high as 50% (Fig. 54.36). Attempts to improve the efficacy of arterial embolization have included adding chemotherapeutic agents (chemoembolization) to the bland embolization particles and oils, such as ethiodized oil (Ethiodol), that are selectively taken up by HCCs. Although chemoembolization has not been shown to be superior to bland embolization with regard to survival, a trial suggested an improvement in local control with chemoembolization.[20] Seven randomized trials have compared embolization or chemoembolization with conservative management. Two of these trials and a metaanalysis have confirmed an overall survival advantage from the embolization strategies.[21–23] The selection of appropriate candidates for embolization is important, and treatment should generally be limited to patients with preserved liver function and asymptomatic multinodular tumors without vascular invasion. Poor selection will result in a higher incidence of treatment-induced liver failure, offsetting the potential benefits. Intraarterial injections of iodine-131 with Ethiodol or yttrium-90 in glass microspheres have also been used to deliver localized radiation to HCCs, with reports of dramatic response rates. Transarterial radiotherapy is a potentially promising therapy for HCC as a primary or adjuvant therapy.

Radiation. External beam radiation therapy (EBRT) has a limited role in the treatment of HCC, although occasional dramatic responses are seen. EBRT is limited by damage to normal liver parenchyma and to surrounding organs, but newer methods of conformal radiotherapy and breath-gated techniques are improving the usefulness of this treatment modality.

Systemic therapies

Chemotherapy. Systemic chemotherapy with a variety of agents (e.g., cisplatin, doxorubicin, etoposide, 5-fluorouracil [5-FU], mitomycin C, amsacrine, mitoxantrone, picibanil, tamoxifen, uracil, VM-26) has been ineffective and has had a minimal role in the treatment of HCC. Response rates are generally below 20% and of short duration. Hormonal therapy has been used in small numbers of patients with HCC, with some early promising results, but have not yet demonstrated superiority to standard regimens.

Most recently, sorafenib, a molecular targeted therapy that inhibits the serine-threonine kinases Raf-1 and B-Raf and the receptor tyrosine kinase activity of vascular endothelial growth factor receptors 1, 2, and 3 and platelet-derived growth factor β, was evaluated. Llovet and colleagues[24] randomized 599 patients with advanced-stage HCC and Child-Pugh level A cirrhosis to oral sorafenib or placebo. The median overall survival was 10.7 months in the sorafenib group and 7.9 months in the placebo group ($P < 0.001$), a difference of 2.8 months. The median time to radiologic progression was 5.5 months in the sorafenib group and 2.8 months in the placebo group ($P < 0.001$), a difference of 2.7 months. Neither group demonstrated any complete responses by radiologic criteria. Although the adverse event profile of sorafenib was similar to the placebo group, this and earlier studies have shown that sorafenib is best tolerated in patients with Child-Pugh class A cirrhosis. With better understanding of the molecular pathogenesis, there is hope that novel therapeutics will be increasingly evaluated in this disease.[24]

Immunotherapy. Immunotherapy has shown some success against HCC. In a nonrandomized phase I/II multi-institution trial evaluating anti--program cell death protein-1 (anti-PD-1) antibody nivolumab objective response rate of ~20% was observed. A randomized controlled trial comparing efficacy of sorafenib to nivolumab as definitive treatment of advanced HCC is currently in process.

In summary, a plethora of treatment options are available for treatment of HCC. Selection of the appropriate treatment modality is based on disease extent, presence or absence of portal hypertension, and liver reserve. Patients with resectable disease with maintained liver reserve and absence of portal hypertension are best treated with resection. Patients with advanced underlying liver disease and with portal hypertension are best treated with liver transplantation. Liver transplantation is applicable only if the tumor is 5 cm or smaller or there are two or three tumors, the largest of which is 3 cm or smaller. Expanded criteria for transplantation are being increasingly used. In patients with very small tumors and with multiple comorbidities, percutaneous ablative techniques may be applied. The efficacy of ablation decreases with increasing size of the tumor. For multifocal disease in the absence of macrovascular invasion and extrahepatic disease, neither resection nor transplantation is applicable, and transarterial therapies offer the best results. For symptomatic patients with advanced disease, with macrovascular involvement, and in the presence of extrahepatic disease, sorafenib is an option. For patients with extensive disease who are symptomatic with deterioration of their performance status and who have severe deterioration of their liver function, any treatment modality is unlikely to provide significant benefit, and these patients should be offered supportive treatment only.

TABLE 54.8 Comparison of standard HCC and fibrolamellar HCC.

PARAMETER	HCC	FIBROLAMELLAR HCC
Male-to-female ratio	2:1–8:1	1:1
Median age	55 years	25 years
Tumor	Invasive	Well circumscribed
Resectability	<25%	50%–75%
Cirrhosis	90%	5%
AFP positive	80%	5%
Hepatitis B positive	65%	5%

AFP, α-Fetoprotein; *HCC,* hepatocellular carcinoma.

Postoperative adjuvant treatment. Currently, there is no recommended adjuvant treatment after HCC resection. This is largely due to lack of effective chemotherapy for HCC. In a phase III double-blind placebo-controlled study evaluating the efficacy of sorafenib in decreasing recurrence of HCC in patients who underwent complete radiologic response after resection or ablation, sorafenib treatment was not able to decrease recurrence.[25] However, antiviral treatment in patients with HBV infection has been shown to decrease the risk of HCC recurrence and HCC-related deaths. With availability of newer and effective antivirals for treatment of HCV, similar results are hoped for in patients infected with this virus. While lower level of evidence does suggest that sustained viral response is associated with improved OS and better recurrence-free survival following resection or locoregional therapy for HCV related HCC, this needs to be confirmed in better-designed trials.

Distinct variants of HCC. Fibrolamellar HCC[26] is a variant of HCC with remarkably different clinical features, summarized in Table 54.8. This tumor generally occurs in younger patients without a history of cirrhosis. The tumor is usually well demarcated and encapsulated and may have a central fibrotic area. The central scar can make distinguishing this tumor from FNH difficult. On histologic evaluation, fibrolamellar HCC is composed of large polygonal tumor cells embedded in a fibrous stroma, forming lamellar structures (Fig. 54.37). Fibrolamellar HCC does not produce AFP but is associated with elevated neurotensin levels. In general, fibrolamellar HCC has a better prognosis than HCC, probably related to high resectability rates, lack of chronic liver disease, and a more indolent course. Long-term survival can be expected in approximately 50% to 75% of patients after complete resection, but recurrence is common and occurs in at least 80% of patients. The presence of lymph node metastases predicts a worse outcome. Resection of lymph node metastases and recurrent disease has been advocated because of a lack of alternative therapy and the possibility of long-term survival. A study identified a chimeric transcript that is expressed in fibrolamellar HCC but not in the adjacent normal liver.[27] The study also suggested that this transcript codes

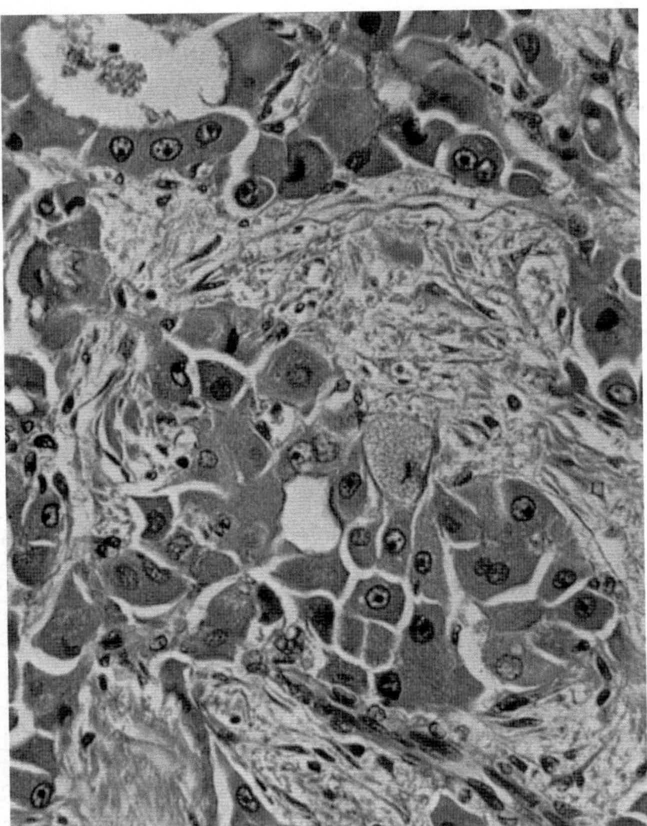

FIG. 54.37 Fibrolamellar hepatocellular carcinoma. Abundant collagen is evident interconnecting clusters of cells. The cells are often in single-layer sheets. An acinus is present in the left upper field.

for a chimeric protein containing the catalytic domain of protein kinase A, thus suggesting that this gain of kinase activity may have a role in the pathogenesis of fibrolamellar HCC. Elucidation of such novel processes can lead to the development of novel targeted therapies against this disease, which typically strikes young, healthy people.

Rarely, HCC can be manifested as a mixed hepatocellular-cholangiocellular tumor, with cellular differentiation of both types present. Whether this is two separate tumors growing into each other or mixed differentiation of the same tumor is not known. These mixed tumors tend to have a prognosis that is worse than for standard HCC but better than expected for intrahepatic cholangiocarcinoma.

A clear cell variant of HCC also exists, in which the cells contain a clear cytoplasm. These tumors can resemble renal cell neoplasms. The clear cell variant may have a better prognosis than standard HCC, but this is a subject of debate. A pleomorphic or giant cell variant of HCC has also been reported. Cells in this type are multinucleated, pleomorphic, and large and likely to originate from primary hepatic cells. Some HCCs show evidence of sarcomatoid differentiation and are referred to as a sarcomatoid variant or carcinosarcoma. These tumors tend not to produce AFP and have a higher incidence of metastases at presentation.

Childhood HCC is a distinct entity that represents almost 25% of pediatric liver tumors but rarely occurs in infancy. Viral hepatitis is associated with childhood HCC in Asia but less so in the United States. Other inherited metabolic liver diseases (see earlier) are often associated with childhood HCC. As in adult HCC, complete resection is the only potentially curative treatment. There is a high incidence of multifocality, vascular invasion, and extrahepatic metastases, resulting in relatively poor long-term survival rates of 10% to 20%.

Intrahepatic Cholangiocarcinoma

Cholangiocarcinoma is an uncommon neoplasm, with an incidence of 1 to 2/100,000 in the United States, and can develop anywhere along the biliary tree from the ampulla of Vater to the peripheral intrahepatic bile ducts. Most of these tumors (40% to 60%) involve the biliary confluence (Klatskin tumor), but approximately 10% emanate from intrahepatic ducts and are known as IHC. IHC is the second most common primary hepatic neoplasm. Studies on the incidence and natural history of IHC have been confused by the fact that, in the past, many of these tumors were mistaken for metastatic adenocarcinoma because biopsy is unable to differentiate the two.

IHC is associated with diseases that cause biliary inflammation and fibrosis. Historically, the most common risk factors for the development of cholangiocarcinoma (all types) were primary sclerosing cholangitis, choledochal cyst disease, hepatolithiasis, and RPC. Recent epidemiologic evidence has now linked IHC to HBV infection, HCV infection, cirrhosis, nonalcoholic steatohepatitis, and diabetes. Increases in the diagnosis of IHC in the United States are likely related to better recognition of the disease, changed classification, and perhaps the rise in HCV infections in the 1960s and 1970s.

The clinical presentation of IHC is similar to that of HCC. These tumors are asymptomatic in early stages. When present, the most common symptoms are right upper abdominal pain and weight loss. Jaundice occurs less commonly as these tumors tend to arise in the periphery of the liver. More commonly, patients present with incidentally found liver masses on cross-sectional imaging. Unlike in HCC, the AFP levels are normal, although CEA or CA 19-9 levels can be elevated in some cases. Because metastatic adenocarcinoma to liver is more common, IHC is a diagnosis of exclusion, and a search for a primary tumor with upper and lower gastrointestinal endoscopy and cross-sectional imaging of the chest, abdomen, and pelvis should be carried out. If a biopsy has been performed, it is often read as adenocarcinoma. Although special stains may suggest diagnosis of IHC, they are not conclusive. On CT and MRI, IHC is seen as a focal hepatic mass that may be associated with peripheral biliary dilation. The mass typically has peripheral or central enhancement on contrast-enhanced scans. Furthermore, unlike HCC there is persistent enhancement on delayed phases due to the fibrotic nature of cholangiocarcinoma, in contrast with the vascular nature of HCC. Hepatic capsular retraction is also frequently observed. Intrahepatic metastases, lymph node metastases, and growth along the biliary tree are often encountered.

Complete resection is the treatment of choice for IHC. The concept of optimal surgical margins in the treatment of IHC is evolving. However, surgeons should strive for R0 margins. Due to large tumor size and invasion into the surrounding structures, major hepatectomies with or without resection of surrounding organs may be required for achieving a margin negative resection. Resectability rates generally range up to 60%, and long-term survival in unresected patients is rare. If it is completely resected, 3-year survival rates range from 16% to 61%, and 5-year survival rates range from 24% to 44%. Factors associated with a poor outcome include multifocality, lymph node metastases, vascular invasion, and positive margins. These factors have now been included in the

American Joint Committee on Cancer (AJCC) staging system. A review of prospectively evaluated patients with IHC who underwent resection suggested that while patients with R0 resection did better when compared with R1 resection, width of margin did not influence outcomes.[28] Because of the rarity of IHC, little is known about the effectiveness of radiation therapy and chemotherapy for IHC in the adjuvant setting. Thus, their application is not routine. Use of chemotherapy as an adjuvant strategy is controversial. Due to the overall low incidence of biliary cancers, studies of adjuvant therapy have typically clubbed various disease sites to include both intrahepatic and extrahepatic cholangiocarcinoma as well as gallbladder cancer. In a recently reported clinical trial from the United Kingdom (phase III BILCAP study),[29] patients with completely resected gallbladder and cholangiocarcinoma were randomized to receive adjuvant capecitabine or observation. Although on intention-to-treat analysis, adjuvant capecitabine did not improve survival, when comparing patients who received adjuvant therapy per-protocol, adjuvant capecitabine was associated with 25% reduced risk of death. Retrospective studies have provided conflicting evidence regarding the benefits of adjuvant therapy. Regional hepatic artery chemotherapy is currently under study and may be a promising approach.

Other Primary Malignant Neoplasms

Hepatoblastoma is the most common primary hepatic tumor of childhood. There are approximately 50 to 70 new cases per year in the United States. Rare cases of adult hepatoblastoma have been reported, but overall, the median age at presentation is 18 months, and almost all cases occur before the age of 3 years. Hepatoblastoma has been associated with the familial polyposis syndrome. There are a number of histologic subtypes, but in general, the tumor is derived from fetal or embryonic hepatocytic progenitors, and mesenchymal elements are often present. This tumor generally is manifested as an asymptomatic mass. Mild anemia and thrombocytosis are commonly found at presentation. Serum AFP levels are elevated in 85% to 90% of patients and can serve as a useful marker for therapeutic response. Most studies have supported the use of chemotherapy followed by resection, and survival appears to be dependent on complete resection. Chemotherapy can serve to downstage tumors, which facilitates resection. In patients without metastatic disease or the anaplastic variant, long-term survival rates of 60% to 70% can be expected with complete resection. Interestingly, 50% of patients with pulmonary metastases can be cured with resection of the hepatic tumor and chemotherapy or resection of the pulmonary metastases.

A variety of sarcomas can rarely be manifested as primary liver tumors, but they must always be considered metastatic lesions until proven otherwise. Angiosarcoma is probably the best-described primary hepatic sarcoma because of its well-known association with vinyl chloride or Thorotrast exposure. Angiosarcoma typically is manifested as multiple hepatic masses and can appear in childhood. Long-term survival is uncommon with primary hepatic angiosarcoma. Other sarcomas, including leiomyosarcoma, malignant fibrous histiocytoma, embryonic sarcoma, and primary hepatic rhabdoid tumors, have been described but are rare. The last two lesions are typically seen in the pediatric population.

Non-Hodgkin lymphoma can be manifested primarily in the liver, with or without extrahepatic disease. Primary hepatic lymphoma should be treated in the same manner as lymphoma elsewhere in the body if the diagnosis can be made before a liver resection.

Primary hepatic neuroendocrine tumors or carcinoid tumors have been described but are probably extremely rare. Distinguishing the rare primary hepatic neuroendocrine tumor from a metastatic lesion can be difficult because the extrahepatic primary tumor can be radiologically occult for many years, and the liver is the most common site of metastases.

Malignant germ cell tumors of the liver including teratomas, choriocarcinomas, and yolk sac tumors are very rare and are principally described in the pediatric population.

Epithelioid hemangioendothelioma of the liver is a rare malignant vascular tumor that is manifested with multiple bilateral hepatic masses. Extrahepatic metastases occur in approximately 25% of patients and clinical behavior is unpredictable, with some patients having a prolonged indolent course. Most patients ultimately die of liver failure, but cases of successful transplantation have been reported.

Metastatic Tumors

The most common malignant tumors of the liver are metastatic lesions. The liver is a common site of metastases from gastrointestinal tumors, presumably because of dissemination through the portal venous system. The most relevant metastatic tumor of the liver to the surgeon is colorectal cancer because of the well-documented potential for long-term survival after complete resection. However, a large number of other tumors commonly metastasize to the liver, including cancers of the upper gastrointestinal system (stomach, pancreas, biliary), genitourinary system (renal, prostate), neuroendocrine system, breast, eye (melanoma), skin (melanoma), soft tissue (retroperitoneal sarcoma), and gynecologic system (ovarian, endometrial, cervical). The large majority of metastatic liver tumors that present with concomitant extrahepatic disease will have unresectable liver disease or are not curable with resection, limiting the role of the surgeon to highly select cases. Metastatic adenocarcinoma to the liver of unknown primary is often a primary IHC, and this diagnosis must always be kept in mind.

Traditionally, cancer spread to a distant site was considered a systemic disease in which locoregional therapies (i.e., surgery) were not effective. Some metastatic tumors to the liver, in particular, metastatic colorectal cancer, have been shown to be an exception to this rule. More than 35 years of clinical research has documented that metastatic colorectal cancer isolated in the liver can be resected with the potential for long-term survival and cure. Advances in systemic and regional chemotherapy have also broadened the number of patients eligible for surgical therapy and probably have improved long-term survival after resection. Selection of patients is the most important aspect of surgical therapy for metastatic disease in the liver, and clinical follow-up of resected patients has identified those most and least likely to benefit. Although long-term survival is common and occurs in up to 50% to 60% of patients in current series, recurrence and chronic multimodal therapy are common, occurring in approximately 75% of patients. Therefore, an important aspect of treatment is realistic expectations and honest patient education. Tumors other than colorectal cancer manifested as isolated or limited hepatic metastases can also be resected for potential long-term survival, but data on these other tumors are sparse and less compelling than for colorectal cancer.

Colorectal Metastases

Every year, there are more than 140,000 new cases of colorectal cancer in the United States. Up to 60% of these patients will develop metastases during the course of their disease. A large proportion of these patients will have metastases to the liver, which can be the only site of metastatic disease for some. In this regard, liver metastases can present synchronously (i.e., at the time of diagnosis of primary disease) or metachronously (arbitrarily defined as >1 year after the diagnosis of primary disease). Literature suggests that synchronous liver metastases portend to a worse prognosis than metachronous disease.[30] Most of these cases of liver metastases are associated with widespread metastatic disease or unresectable hepatic metastases. It is estimated that approximately 5% to 10% of these patients are candidates for a potentially curative liver resection. With improved response rates to modern chemotherapy and advances in hepatic surgery; however, more patients are now candidates for hepatectomy than in the past; at present, up to 20% of patients may be candidates.

Presentation. In the distant past, patients with hepatic colorectal metastases generally presented with symptoms and signs of advanced malignant disease, such as pain, ascites, jaundice, weight loss, and a palpable mass. Presentation with these symptoms is a poor prognostic sign; few of these patients are candidates for therapy aside from chemotherapy or supportive care. This has led most physicians to observe patients with resected primary colorectal cancer carefully who are potential candidates for aggressive therapy with serial physical examinations, cross-sectional imaging studies, LFTs, and determination of CEA levels. Although not supported by randomized trials, clinical observations have indicated that patients who are carefully observed with serial physical examinations, cross-sectional imaging studies, LFTs, and determination of CEA levels are those often found to have resectable metachronous disease and the greatest potential for long-term survival. In addition to these patients, some are found to have synchronous metastatic disease at the time of diagnosis of the primary colorectal cancer on preoperative imaging or at laparotomy.

Although an elevated CEA level is not specific for recurrent colorectal cancer, a rising CEA level on serial examinations and a new solid mass on imaging studies are diagnostic of metastatic disease. Mild elevations in LFT results are common in metastatic colorectal cancer to the liver but are not effective as a screening tool. The levels most commonly elevated are those of ALP, GGT, and lactate dehydrogenase. Imaging of hepatic metastases with high-quality CT or MRI is important for determining resectability and operative planning. Most physicians use thin-cut (5 mm), high-resolution, dynamic, contrast-enhanced helical scanning techniques. Timing with IV administration of a contrast agent should correspond to the portal venous phase to maximize hepatic parenchymal enhancement, which improves the disparity between parenchyma and tumor.

Workup. Once a patient with colorectal liver metastases is considered a candidate for surgical therapy, a complete extent of disease workup must be performed. Colonoscopy should be performed if it has been longer than 1 year since the last examination to rule out local recurrence or metachronous colorectal lesions. Complete abdominal and pelvic cross-sectional imaging must also be performed to rule out extrahepatic disease and aid with operative planning by identifying the number, location, and relationship of liver metastases to the hepatic vasculature. Chest CT is often performed but is of low yield. Many studies have evaluated the added benefit of positron emission tomography (PET) scans to detect occult extrahepatic disease. Approximately 25% of patients have a change in management based on PET scan

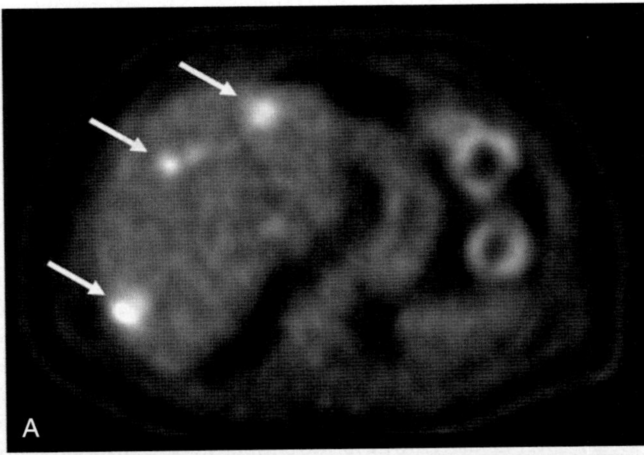

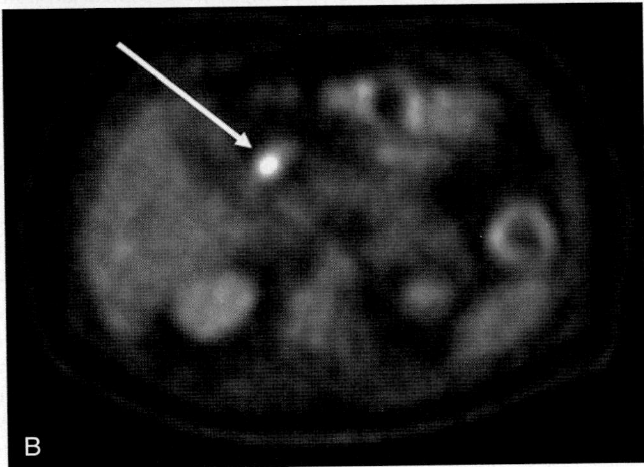

FIG. 54.38 Positron emission tomography (PET) from a patient with metastatic colorectal cancer to the liver. (A) shows three FDG-avid tumors in the liver identified by hypermetabolic activity seen on PET scan *(short arrows)*. (B) shows a positive porta-hepatis lymph node also seen on a PET scan *(long arrow)*.

findings, but this is highly variable, depending on the quality of cross-sectional imaging, radiologic interpretation, and patient selection (Fig. 54.38). A randomized trial of PET/CT versus CT in patients with potentially resectable colorectal liver metastases has been published.[31] In this trial, the use of PET/CT did not result in significant changes in surgical management, and there was no difference in resectability or long-term outcomes between the two groups. This trial provides definitive evidence that routine use of PET does not significantly affect outcomes among patients with potentially resectable colorectal cancer liver metastasis. With use of staging laparoscopy, 10% of patients are spared a nontherapeutic laparotomy, and the yield of laparoscopy correlates with the number of poor prognostic factors present, allowing it to be used on a selective basis.

Management

Surgical approach. To date, a prospective trial comparing surgery with no treatment or chemotherapy alone has not been performed, nor is this likely ever to be done. Therefore, the rationale for liver resection comes from retrospective comparisons of these treatment strategies. The surgeon must understand the natural history of colorectal liver metastases left untreated or treated with systemic chemotherapy to interpret survival data associated with hepatectomy appropriately. Before the 1980s, most hepatic metastases were left untreated. Two key studies retrospectively identified patients with isolated single hepatic metastases or multiple but resectable tumors who received no therapy. One study documented a 10% 3-year survival and the other a 2% 5-year survival for patients with limited and potentially resectable disease. It was clear from these studies that long-term survival is extremely rare without treatment and that survival is closely related to the extent of disease. In the past, 5-FU–based systemic chemotherapy was ineffective as sole therapy for hepatic colorectal metastases, with median survivals of approximately 12 months and response rates of 20% to 30%. Tremendous advances in systemic chemotherapy for metastatic colorectal cancer have now been achieved. Combination chemotherapy, including 5-FU with irinotecan or oxaliplatin combined with targeted antiangiogenic antibodies such as bevacizumab (antivascular endothelial growth factor antibody) or cetuximab (anti-epidermal growth factor antibody), has now resulted in response rates of more than 50% and median survivals of 20 months and longer for patients with advanced disease.[32] Although response rates and survival have improved, durable complete response and 5-year survival are rare with the administration of chemotherapy alone.

The sporadic partial hepatectomies performed for metastatic colorectal cancer before the 1980s were appropriately viewed with great skepticism. The high morbidity and mortality for liver surgery at that time and the questionable rationale of resecting blood-borne metastases were the major issues. During the last 30 years, however, large series have demonstrated that liver surgery can now be practiced with acceptable safety and that patients with isolated and resectable hepatic metastases have the potential for long-term survival. Five-year survival rates range from 25% to 58%. There is also a clear trend toward longer survival in more recent series (Table 54.9). Perioperative mortality in experienced centers is consistently less than 5% and in many series has been less than 2%. Almost all demonstrate that almost 50% of patients undergoing a liver resection for metastatic colorectal cancer will survive 3 years and 20% will survive 10 years. Despite the low operative mortality, liver surgery is still associated with significant morbidity rates of 30% to 50%. Complications are most commonly bleeding, bile leak, abscess, and other generalized cardiorespiratory complications. With improvements in chemotherapy, a higher proportion of patients undergoing hepatectomy have been treated preoperatively. However, some studies have shown that preoperative chemotherapy is associated with hepatic toxicity (steatohepatitis and sinusoidal obstructive syndrome) and higher rates of postoperative liver failure.

From these large series, we have learned much about prognostic factors as well as which patients are most likely to benefit from a liver resection for hepatic colorectal metastases. Although not all studies agree, it has been found that poor prognostic factors include extrahepatic metastases, involved lymph nodes with the primary colorectal tumor, synchronous presentation (or shorter disease-free interval), larger number of tumors, bilobar involvement, CEA level elevation more than 200 ng/mL, size of largest hepatic tumor more than 5 cm, and involved histologic margins. In a series of 1001 liver resections from MSKCC, a multivariate analysis[30] identified five preoperative factors as the most influential on outcome: size larger than 5 cm, disease-free interval less than 1 year, more than one tumor, lymph node–positive primary, and CEA level higher than 200 ng/mL. Using these five factors, we have developed a risk score predictive of recurrence after liver resection (Table 54.10).

Traditionally, the presence of extrahepatic disease, four or more hepatic metastases, close margins, and inability to resect all disease in the liver have been considered contraindications to hepatectomy. The only one of these historical contraindications that holds true today is the inability to resect all disease. Recent reports have shown that hepatectomy for four or more metastases is associated with an approximate 5-year survival of 33%, despite a high recurrence rate. Although the width of the closest margin has been shown to be associated with outcome, it is often confounded by its relationship to an overall poor prognostic tumor (i.e., multiple synchronous tumors). However, close or involved margins do not appear to preclude the possibility of long-term survival, but patients with positive margins tend to fare poorly. Nonetheless, attempts at wide margins more than 1 cm are appropriate, when possible. Resection of extrahepatic metastases that present simultaneously with liver metastases has been shown to be associated with long-term survival in highly select cases. The sites that appear to be associated with the best outcomes in this situation are limited lung metastases, locoregional recurrences of the primary tumor, and portal lymph nodes. These results have been further confirmed in a metaanalysis of 50 studies including 3481 patients with colorectal liver metastases with extrahepatic disease.[33] With availability of more effective chemotherapy, selected patients with extrahepatic disease should be considered for resectional therapy. Selection of patients is critical for this aggressive approach and generally requires preoperative chemotherapy to exclude progression and consideration of the overall bulk of metastatic disease.

Although long-term survival after liver resection for hepatic colorectal metastases is clearly possible, recurrence of disease is common. Overall, approximately 75% of patients have recurrence, but in high-risk situations (e.g., four or more tumors, extrahepatic disease), recurrence rates approach 100%. Approximately 50% of recurrences are isolated to the liver, and a small number of these patients (~5% of all patients undergoing liver resection) are candidates for a second liver resection. These highly select patients who undergo a second liver resection with complete removal of all disease can expect further 5-year survival rates of 30% to 40%. Limited and isolated lung recurrences can also be resected with the potential for further long-term survival. Furthermore, multiple lines of effective chemotherapy are now available, associated with prolongation of survival. Because of the potential for further effective therapeutic interventions after liver resection, patients eligible for such treatment should be observed with serial CEA level determinations and imaging studies to detect recurrences at an early, potentially treatable phase.

Adjuvant therapy. Adjuvant chemotherapy has been used in an attempt to reduce recurrence and to improve long-term survival. Prospective randomized clinical trials have shown a benefit to adjuvant hepatic intraarterial chemotherapy. However, results of randomized controlled trials on the benefit of adjuvant systemic chemotherapy after resection of hepatic metastases have been mixed. In a multicenter randomized trial, Portier and associates[34] randomized 173 patients to hepatic resection alone (87 patients) or to hepatic resection plus adjuvant chemotherapy (5-FU–folinic acid) for 6 months (86 patients). Even though this chemotherapy regimen is no longer standard, the 5-year disease-free survival rate was 26.7% for patients who had surgery alone and 33.5% for patients who had surgery plus chemotherapy ($P = 0.028$). A nonsignificant trend toward improved overall survival was also observed in the chemotherapy arm. The results of this trial were pooled with another phase 3 trial that failed to accrue. This pooled analysis failed to show a statistically significant improvement in progression-free survival or overall survival.[35] In this analysis, there were 278 patients (138 in the surgery with chemotherapy

TABLE 54.9 **Results of hepatic resection for hepatic colorectal metastases.***

STUDY	NO. OF PATIENTS	OPERATIVE MORTALITY RATE (%)	SURVIVAL RATE (%) 1 YEAR	5 YEARS	10 YEARS	MEDIAN SURVIVAL (MONTHS)
Adson, 1984	141	2	82	25	—	24
Hughes, 1986	607	—	—	33	—	—
Schlag, 1990	122	4	85	30	—	32
Doci, 1991	100	5	—	30	—	28
Gayowski, 1994	204	0	91	32	—	33
Scheele, 1995	469	4	83	33	20	40
Fong, 1995	577	4	85	35	—	40
Jenkins, 1997	131	4	81	25	—	33
Rees, 1997	150	1	94	37	—	
Jamison, 1997	280	4	84	27	20	33
Fong, 1999	1001	3	89	37	22	42
Minagawa, 2000	235	0	—	35	26	37
Scheele, 2000	597	—	—	36	—	35
Choti, 2002	226	1	—	40†	26	46
Abdalla, 2004	190	—	—	58	—	Not reached
Nicoli, 2004	228	0.9		16	9	
Andres, 2008	210	0.5	95	40	—	—
de Jong, 2009	243	—	—	47	—	36
House, 2010	1600					
1985–1998	1037	2.5	—	35	16	43
1999–2004	563	0.5	—	43	—	64
Faitot, 2014‡	272					
One stage	155	3	85	35		37.2
Two stage	117	4	82	49		34.5
Saxena, 2014	701	2	86	33	20	35
Marques, 2012§	676					
Preoperative chemotherapy‖	334	3.9	91	43		
No preoperative chemotherapy	342	3.4	93	55		
Matsumura, 2016 (major hepatectomy [MH] vs. parenchyma sparing hepatectomy [PSH])						
MH	32	0		29.4		
PSH	113	0		37		
Lordon, 2017 (major hepatectomy [MH] vs. parenchyma sparing hepatectomy [PSH])						
MH	238	3.8	82	34		
PSH	238	0.8	92	35		
Van Amerongen, 2016 (resection-only [ROG] vs. combination of resection and ablation [CG])						
ROG	534	1.3		62		
CG	98	1		42		

*In selected series with more than 100 patients.

†The 5-year survival rate in the patients operated on in the most current time period in this study was 58%.

‡Long-term results of two-stage hepatectomy versus one-stage hepatectomy used in combination with ablation approaches.

§Combined data from two hepatobiliary centers, data analyzed with respect to receipt of preoperative chemotherapy or not.

‖Number of tumors higher in the preoperative chemotherapy group (2.8 ± 2.2) compared with those with no preoperative therapy (1.8 ± 1.6).

arm and 140 in the surgery-alone arm). Median progression-free survival was 27.9 months in the chemotherapy arm compared with 18.8 months in the surgery arm (hazard ratio, 1.32; 95% CI, 1.00–1.76; $P = 0.058$). Median overall survival was 62.2 months in the chemotherapy arm compared with 47.3 months in the surgery arm (hazard ratio, 1.32; 95% CI, 0.95–1.82; $P = 0.095$).[35] Adjuvant chemotherapy was independently associated with both progression-free survival and overall survival in multivariable analysis.

In another multi-institutional randomized controlled trial (European Organization for Research and Treatment and Cancer, EORTC 40983 trial), Nordlinger and colleagues[36] randomized

TABLE 54.10 Clinical risk score and survival in 1001 patients undergoing liver resection for metastatic colorectal cancer.*

SCORE	SURVIVAL RATE (%) 1 YEAR	3 YEARS	5 YEARS	MEDIAN SURVIVAL (MONTHS)
0	93	72	60	74
1	91	66	44	51
2	89	60	40	47
3	86	42	20	33
4	70	38	25	20
5	71	27	14	22

Adapted from Fong Y, Fortner J, Sun RL, et al. Clinical score for predicting recurrence after hepatic resection for metastatic colorectal cancer: analysis of 1001 consecutive cases. *Ann Surg*. 1999;230:309–318.
*Each of the following five risk factors equals 1 point: node-positive primary, disease-free interval <12 months, >1 tumor, size >5 cm, carcinoembryonic antigen level >200 ng/mL. Score is total number of points in an individual patient.

364 patients into two groups; 182 patients were treated with surgery alone, and 182 patients had surgery plus systemic chemotherapy. Three cycles of systemic 5-FU–folinic acid plus oxaliplatin (FOLFOX4) were administered preoperatively and postoperatively in the chemotherapy group. Among eligible patients after randomization, the progression-free survival of patients at 3 years was 28.1% in the group with surgery alone and 36.2% in the group with surgery plus chemotherapy ($P = 0.041$). When analyzed by all patients, there was no significant difference in outcome. Long-term results of this trial have been released, and no difference in overall survival was observed with addition of chemotherapy.[37] Although this trial provides evidence that perioperative systemic chemotherapy can delay recurrence of disease, there is little difference in the recurrences at later time points. Also, the benefit of adjuvant chemotherapy may be related to better selection of patients. The role of adjuvant therapy in the treatment of colorectal liver metastases is further supported by a metaanalysis of 10 studies including 1896 patients.[38] In this metaanalysis, use of perioperative therapy significantly improved disease-free survival but did not affect the overall survival. In summary, there is level 1 clinical evidence that adjuvant systemic chemotherapy, when combined with liver resection, modestly improves progression-free survival in patients with colorectal liver metastases. At this time, the general consensus is that patients with liver metastases benefit from 6 months of perioperative adjuvant therapy.

Neoadjuvant chemotherapy for resectable metastases is also a common strategy to treat occult systemic disease and can be helpful in selecting the small group of patients (<10%) who progress while receiving chemotherapy and have a poor outcome after hepatectomy. A prospective randomized study by the National Surgical Adjuvant Breast and Bowel Project has begun accruing patients to study the role of adjuvant chemotherapy in these patients.

A convincing argument for adjuvant therapy with the use of hepatic arterial infusion (HAI) chemotherapy can be made.[39,40] The rationale for adjuvant hepatic artery chemotherapy is based on the fact that liver metastases derive most of their blood supply from the hepatic artery. Regional infusion of chemotherapeutic agents such as fluorodeoxyuridine has hepatic extraction rates of 90%, providing high local concentrations with minimal systemic toxicity. Furthermore, approximately 50% of all recurrences after hepatectomy involve the liver, so controlling the liver is likely to affect long-term outcome. There is clearly a higher response rate for liver tumors with HAI therapy compared with systemic therapy. A trial from MSKCC comparing HAI therapy with systemic chemotherapy to systemic chemotherapy alone has demonstrated significantly lower recurrence rates (9% and 36%) and a survival advantage at 2 years (86% vs. 72%).[41] Other trials have shown HAI therapy with fluorodeoxyuridine to be more effective than hepatectomy alone, with significantly improved disease-free survival. HAI has not been widely adopted due to the requirement of specific technical expertise and availability of effective systemic therapy. However, HAI is a useful strategy benefiting patients with liver-only colorectal metastases when applied in carefully selected patients.

Unresectable liver-only metastatic disease. For patients with unresectable liver-only metastatic disease, preoperative systemic and HAI chemotherapy has been shown to convert some patients to resection candidates. A critical observation in these patients is that outcome after complete resection appears to be as good as in those who were resectable at initial presentation. Strategies to extend the limits of liver resection have used parenchyma-preserving segmental resections, two-stage operations, and thermal ablative techniques, such as cryoablation or RFA. Most recently, microwave ablation is being studied as a treatment for these patients, and long-term results suggest that recurrence rates increase with the size of the tumor and when ablation is performed for the tumor close to the vessels. Recent results suggest that microwave ablation either alone or in combination with liver resection can provide good long-term results. Thus, multiple bilobar tumors can be extirpated by a combination of resection and ablation with preservation of sufficient hepatic parenchyma.

In summary, the treatment of hepatic colorectal metastases is evolving at a rapid pace, and improvements in hepatic surgery and chemotherapy have greatly improved prospects for patients. Chemotherapy has improved, but long-term survival with this modality alone is rare. Combinations of chemotherapy and complete resection of hepatic metastases are associated with long-term survival in up to 50% to 60% of patients. Long-term survival also appears to be possible in patients undergoing resection of extensive hepatic metastases and limited extrahepatic disease. Complete resection of hepatic metastases appears to be a critically important treatment modality that is necessary for long-term survival.

Neuroendocrine Metastases

Liver metastases from neuroendocrine tumors are common but vary according to the primary tumor type. Examples of primary tumors that commonly metastasize to the liver are gastrinomas, glucagonomas, somatostatinomas, and nonfunctional neuroendocrine tumors. Insulinomas and carcinoid tumors metastasize to the liver less commonly.

There are two issues to consider in determining the appropriate therapy for metastatic neuroendocrine tumors. First, these are slow-growing, indolent tumors in which long-term survival is possible even in the absence of treatment. Thus, assessing the effects of any treatment is difficult. Second, these tumors often secrete functional neuropeptides that can create debilitating syndromes of hormonal excess, so the goal of treatment is focused more often on quality of life rather than on prolongation of life.

A number of effective nonsurgical therapies exist for neuroendocrine liver metastases. Long-acting somatostatin analogues are useful for alleviating hormonal symptoms and may have a cytostatic role as well. Liver tumors can also be treated by hepatic arterial embolization or thermoablative approaches. Combinations of these therapies can be effective in cytoreducing tumor loads and alleviating symptoms of hormonal excess.

Liver resection can play a role in patients whose tumor can be completely encompassed. High-quality CT of the chest, abdomen, and pelvis with liver protocol should be obtained in all patients to define the extent of disease. Most well-differentiated neuroendocrine tumors express somatostatin receptors, and this has been leveraged previously by the ^{111}In-octreotide scan to diagnose and define the extent of disease. Now, where available, octreotide scan has been superseded by PET combined with CT (PET/CT) using ^{68}Ga-DOTA peptides. ^{68}Ga-DOTA PET/CT provides higher resolution than octreotide scan, thus allowing better localization and greater sensitivity (82%–100%) and specificity (67%–100%) for neuroendocrine metastases. Due to this increased sensitivity, preoperative use of ^{68}Ga-DOTA has been shown to influence the therapeutic strategy and/or extent of surgery for up to 60% of patients with neuroendocrine tumors. Whether that applies to patients with neuroendocrine liver metastases preparing for surgery remains to be seen.

Because these tumors are indolent, any therapy must be delivered with minimal morbidity. This has been the case in experienced hepatobiliary units. Five-year survival rates in excess of 50% to 75% can be expected if a complete resection is accomplished. Retrospective comparisons have suggested that this survival is better than that in untreated patients, but selection bias accounts for at least some of this difference. Because of the rarity of this diagnosis, no prospective data exist. The other role of surgery is for those patients who have failed to respond to medical therapy and have recalcitrant symptoms of hormonal excess. If preoperative staging suggests that at least 90% of tumor can be removed without prohibitive operative risk, surgical cytoreduction is reasonable. Symptom improvement can be expected in most patients if adequate cytoreduction is achieved. Formal resections with wide margins are not necessary for neuroendocrine tumors, and techniques such as enucleation and wedge resection are reasonable options. Thermoablative approaches, such as cryoablation and RFA, are also attractive alternatives in this type of cytoreductive surgery. Laparoscopic RFA has recently been used, although long-term follow-up is not available.

Noncolorectal, Nonneuroendocrine Metastases

Other tumors can be manifested as isolated liver metastases, but these are uncommon situations and therefore data for these situations are sparse.[42] There are many tumors that can be manifested in this way, including breast, lung, melanoma, soft tissue sarcoma, Wilms tumor, ocular melanoma, upper gastrointestinal (gastric, pancreas, esophagus, gallbladder), adrenocortical, urologic (bladder, renal cell, prostate, testicular), and gynecologic (uterine, cervical, ovarian) tumors. General principles that should be considered in dealing with these tumors as isolated liver metastases are similar to those for metastatic colorectal cancer. Prognosis tends to be dismal if there is extrahepatic disease, multiple tumors, large tumors, or a short disease-free interval, and patients should be carefully selected for surgery on the basis of these factors. Patients with liver-only metastatic disease should be treated with systemic chemotherapy before being considered for liver resection. This helps not only control the disease but also selects outpatients who have rapidly progressive disease and who will not benefit from liver resection.

Although there have been rare reports of long-term survival after resection of isolated liver metastases from upper gastrointestinal tumor, in general, these patients have a dismal prognosis and liver resection is not recommended. In most series, liver resection for genitourinary tumors has the best prognosis, and in well-selected patients, liver resection should be considered. Breast tumor, melanoma, and sarcoma patients rarely present with isolated liver metastases, and with a long disease-free interval or long-term stability on chemotherapy, liver resection should be considered. In general, liver resection for metastatic noncolorectal, nonneuroendocrine tumors has to be considered cytoreductive and should be used only in the most favorable situations (see earlier). Liver resection can also be an effective therapy for symptomatic tumors in patients who have a reasonable life expectancy and no other effective therapy.

Cystic Neoplasms

Simple Cyst

Simple cysts of the liver contain serous fluid, do not communicate with the biliary tree, and do not have septations. They are generally spherical or ovoid and can be as large as 20 cm. Large cysts can compress normal liver, inducing regional atrophy and sometimes compensatory contralateral hypertrophy. In 50% of cases, the cysts are singular. On histologic evaluation, a single layer of cuboidal or columnar cells without atypia lines these cysts. Simple cysts are generally regarded as congenital malformations.

Simple cysts are a relatively common finding in adults and are mostly asymptomatic incidental radiologic findings. On occasion, a large cyst will cause symptoms. Although CT demonstrates anatomic relationships, ultrasound is a helpful test of choice to confirm a single, thin-walled simple cyst. Hydatid disease, cystadenoma, and metastatic neuroendocrine tumor are the most important differential diagnoses to consider. A thick or nodular wall raises the suspicion of a cystadenoma but can also represent hemorrhage within the cyst. The most common complication is intracystic bleeding, but overall, complications are rare. The treatment of simple hepatic cysts is indicated only if they are symptomatic or there is diagnostic uncertainty. Because most cysts are asymptomatic, a thorough evaluation of the cause of the symptoms must be carried out before attributing them to the cyst. Nonsurgical treatment consists of aspiration and injection of a sclerosing agent. Few studies have documented long-term follow-up of sclerotherapy for hepatic cysts. Surgical therapy is achieved by fenestration or unroofing of the portion of the cyst that is extrahepatic. This can be performed at laparotomy with good long-term results or through laparoscopic approaches. The laparoscopic approach is favored, but long-term efficacy has not been well documented.[43] A metaanalysis including nine retrospective case-control studies involving 657 patients comparing laparoscopic fenestration with the open approach demonstrated that the laparoscopic approach was associated with shorter operative time, shorter hospital stay, and less operative blood loss with no difference in cyst recurrence rates.[44]

Cystadenoma and Cystadenocarcinoma

Cystadenoma of the liver is a rare neoplasm that generally is manifested as a large cystic mass, usually 10 to 20 cm. The cyst has a globular external surface with multiple protruding cysts and locules of various sizes. The fluid contained in these cysts is usually mucinous. On microscopic examination, atypical cuboidal or columnar cells resting on a basement membrane, with ovarian-like stroma, line the cysts. The epithelium often forms polypoid or papillary projections.

Cystadenoma of the liver mainly affects woman older than 40 years. Although many cystadenomas are asymptomatic, symptoms can include abdominal pain, anorexia, nausea, and abdominal distention. The diagnosis is usually suspected by a combination of cross-sectional imaging (CT or MRI) and ultrasound. Ultrasound usually demonstrates a cystic structure with varying wall thickness, nodularity, septations, and fluid-filled locules. Importantly, contrast-enhanced CT demonstrates enhancement of the cyst wall and septa. Hydatid disease must always be considered in the differential diagnosis. Cystadenomas tend to grow slowly but can eventually progress to their malignant counterpart, cystadenocarcinomas.

Cystadenocarcinoma is an extremely rare malignant neoplasm with little documentation of its natural history and outcome after resection. Malignant degeneration is typically suggested on imaging, with large projections and a markedly thickened wall. The treatment of cystadenoma or cystadenocarcinoma is complete excision, which can be done with an enucleation if there is no evidence of invasive malignant disease. Incomplete resection risks recurrence or the development of cystadenocarcinoma.

Polycystic Liver Disease

Liver cysts are commonly seen in patients with the autosomal dominant inherited adult polycystic kidney disease.[45] The cysts are histologically similar to simple cysts (see earlier). The main difference between the two entities is the number of cysts. When liver cysts are present in patients with adult polycystic kidney disease, they are always multiple in number. Also, there are usually numerous microscopic hepatic cysts as well as the grossly visible macrocysts. Despite the large number of liver cysts, hepatic parenchyma and function are usually preserved. Liver cysts are always preceded by kidney cysts, and their prevalence in adult polycystic kidney disease increases with age. In those younger than 20 years, the prevalence of liver cysts is 0%, whereas in those older than 60 years, it is 80%.

Liver cysts in patients with adult polycystic kidney disease are generally asymptomatic, but in a few patients, numerous large cysts may cause abdominal pain and distention. LFT results are almost always normal. Rare complications can occur; these include infection and intracystic bleeding. Ultrasound and CT reveal multiple simple cysts throughout the liver and kidneys. Treatment of polycystic liver disease is reserved for severe symptoms related to large cysts and complications. Treatment includes percutaneous aspiration with or without sclerotherapy, cyst fenestration (by laparotomy or laparoscopy), hepatic resection, and orthotopic liver transplantation. Liver transplantation is used only with progressive disease after fenestration or resection with liver or renal dysfunction. In the context of renal failure, a combined kidney and liver transplantation may be appropriate.

Bile Duct Cysts

Bile duct cysts or choledochal cysts are congenital dilations of the biliary tree that are usually diagnosed in childhood but can present in adulthood. Because of the risk of malignancy and recurrent cholangitis, treatment is excision with reestablishment of biliary-enteric continuity. Most bile duct cysts involve the extrahepatic biliary tree, but in type IV cysts, there is involvement of the extrahepatic bile duct and intrahepatic ducts. In contrast, Caroli disease (type V) is characterized by multiple intrahepatic cysts. Thus, bile duct cysts must be considered in the differential diagnosis of a patient with multiple hepatic cystic lesions. The intrahepatic lesions of type IV bile duct cysts and Caroli disease are multifocal dilations of the segmental bile ducts separated by portions of normal-caliber bile ducts. Approximately 50% of cases of Caroli disease are associated with congenital hepatic fibrosis; the cysts are diffusely located throughout the liver. In the other 50% of cases, the dilations may be confined to a portion of the liver, usually the left hemiliver. Recurrent bacterial cholangitis usually dominates the clinical course of these diseases, and death generally ensues within 5 to 10 years without adequate treatment. When intrahepatic bile duct cysts are localized, hepatic resection, with or without biliary reconstruction, is the treatment of choice. Treatment of diffuse hepatic involvement is poor; in complicated cases, the only probably effective treatment is transplantation.

Principles of Hepatic Resection

Although liver resections were performed in the late 1800s, it was not until 1952 that Lortat-Jacob was given credit for the first true anatomic right hepatectomy. This event ushered in the modern era of hepatic surgery. However, early series were plagued by high morbidity and mortality, which were largely related to massive intraoperative blood loss. Series from the 1970s and 1980s often reported mortality rates in excess of 10%, often as high as 20%, especially for major resections. This high mortality limited the use of liver resection, and there was reluctance to refer patients for such operations. During the last three decades, a number of advances have improved perioperative outcomes dramatically for patients undergoing major hepatic surgery. The understanding that most blood loss during a liver resection comes from the hepatic veins has prompted surgeons to perform these operations with a low central venous pressure. We perform partial hepatectomy with a central line in place, the patient in a mild Trendelenburg position, and fluid restriction and venodilators if necessary to maintain a central venous pressure lower than 5 mm Hg. The other major advance has been an improved understanding of the segmental anatomy of the liver, making intrahepatic dissection safer and more precise. There are numerous techniques to transect liver tissue and many methods to coagulate and to control vessels. The most important concept, however, is that dividing liver tissue is a dissection done by a surgeon with complete understanding of the liver's vascular anatomy.

In experienced centers, perioperative mortality is routinely 5% or less and depends on a number of factors. The three most critical factors related to perioperative morbidity are blood loss, the amount of normal liver resected, and the condition of the liver itself (e.g., cirrhosis). A partial hepatectomy must be performed with these factors in mind to minimize morbidity. In a review of more than 1800 liver resections during a 10-year period from MSKCC, the operative mortality was 3.1%.[46] The median blood loss was 600 mL, and two thirds of patients did not require a red blood cell transfusion. Overall, postoperative morbidity was 45%, but the median hospital stay was 8 days. Morbidity was mostly related to blood loss and the extent of resection. Minor resections were associated with a mortality of 1%. Most complications and deaths were seen in complex biliary tumors, cirrhotics with HCC, and extensive resections. Improving outcomes after partial hepatectomy continue, and experienced hepatobiliary centers have reported mortality rates that approach 1% to 2%, with fewer patients now requiring perioperative blood transfusions. As a result of the increasing safety of hepatic surgery, liver resection has become the treatment of choice for many malignant and benign hepatic conditions.

Bile leaks are a problem in cases requiring complex biliary reconstruction but can also occur in approximately 10% to 20%

TABLE 54.11 Nomenclature for most common major anatomic hepatic resections.*

SEGMENTS†	COUINAUD, 1957	GOLDSMITH AND WOODBURNE, 1957	BRISBANE, 2000
V–VIII	Right hepatectomy	Right hepatic lobectomy	Right hemihepatectomy
IV–VIII‡	Right lobectomy	Extended right hepatic lobectomy	Right trisectionectomy
II–IV	Left hepatectomy	Left hepatic lobectomy	Left hemihepatectomy
II, III	Left lobectomy	Left lateral segmentectomy	Left lateral sectionectomy
II, III, IV, V, VIII‡	Extended left hepatectomy	Extended left lobectomy	Left trisectionectomy

Adapted from the Terminology Committee of the International Hepato-Pancreatico-Biliary Association: The Brisbane 2000 terminology of liver anatomy and resections, 2000 <http://www.ahpba.org/assets/documents/Brisbane_Article.pdf>.
*The original terminology is based on the anatomic descriptions of Couinaud and of Goldsmith and Woodburne.
†See Fig. 54.40A–E.
‡Another common name for these operations is right or left trisegmentectomy.

of hepatectomies without biliary reconstruction. Careful ligation of biliary radicals is of obvious importance in minimizing this complication. Because of the regenerative capacity of the liver, resections of up to 80% of normal noncirrhotic livers can be performed, with functional compensation within a few weeks. Because many resections encompass tumors and normal liver, the concepts of functional liver parenchyma and FLR volume are important because there is often compensatory hypertrophy of normal liver when tumors occupy a significant amount of the liver volume. The risk of hepatic dysfunction is minimal if the reduction of functional liver parenchyma is less than 50% but begins to rise when this figure approaches 20% to 25%. Patients with cirrhosis have much higher rates of postoperative liver dysfunction because of impaired regenerative capacity and impaired primary liver function. Liver failure, extrahepatic multiorgan failure, and death are serious hazards to performance of major liver resections in cirrhotics. In general, patients with Child class B or C cirrhosis or portal hypertension do not tolerate liver resections, and selection of patients is therefore critical. Ascites and infectious complications are also common problems after major liver resection. One strategy to minimize postoperative liver dysfunction and morbidity after major hepatectomy is to embolize the portal vein percutaneously on the side of the liver to be resected. In approximately 4 weeks, this induces atrophy of the liver parenchyma to be resected and hypertrophy of the FLR. In turn, this increases the relative volume of the FLR.

Techniques of liver resection differ according to the disease being treated. In benign hepatic diseases requiring resection, the indications for operation are usually symptoms or infection. Removal of normal liver should be kept to a minimum in these cases, and techniques such as enucleation are appropriate, although a major resection is occasionally necessary. For malignant disease, a margin of normal tissue is important, and formal anatomic resections yield the best results. Techniques such as wedge resection often result in higher rates of margin involvement and disease recurrence and should therefore be used carefully and sparingly. It must be noted that for colorectal liver metastases, parenchymal sparing nonanatomic resection provides comparable oncologic outcomes with marked reduction in complications when compared to major hepatic resections.[47–49]

Detailed knowledge of liver anatomy is essential to the practice of safe hepatic surgery (see earlier). Unfortunately, detailed and complicated descriptions of liver anatomy and common liver resections can be confusing to the student. A 2000 consensus conference conducted in Brisbane, Australia, with the assistance of the Americas Hepato-Pancreato-Biliary Association has published guidelines for this terminology (Table 54.11 and Fig. 54.39). In general, the term *lobectomy* is not preferred because there are no external markings on the liver denoting a lobe. When in doubt, one should always revert to the numeric segments of the liver if there is any confusion about the description of a liver resection. Recall that the right liver is composed of segments V through VIII, and *right hepatectomy* and *right hemihepatectomy* are appropriate terms for resection of these segments. Segments II through IV compose the left liver, and *left hepatectomy* and *left hemihepatectomy* are appropriate terms for resection of these segments. A right hepatectomy can be extended farther to the left to include segment IV, and a left hepatectomy can be extended farther to the right to include segments V and VIII. Terms such as *extended right-left hepatectomy*, *right-left trisectionectomy*, and *trisegmentectomy* are appropriate to describe these resections. Resection of segments II and III is a commonly performed sublobar resection and is often referred to as a left lateral segmentectomy or left lateral sectionectomy. Other common sublobar resections, such as that of the right posterior sector (segments VI and VII) or the right anterior sector (segments V and VIII), are referred to as a right posterior sectorectomy-sectionectomy and right anterior sectorectomy-sectionectomy, respectively. Single or bisegmental resections can always be simply referred to by a numeric description of the segments to be resected.

A detailed discussion of the techniques of liver resection is beyond the scope of this chapter; in general, it requires specialty training, but general principles can be discussed. A liver resection must consider the disease to be treated and the goal of the operation, whether that is a margin-negative resection of a malignant neoplasm or the removal of benign tissue to alleviate symptoms. The most basic steps can be distilled down to inflow control (portal vein, hepatic artery, bile duct), outflow control (hepatic veins), and parenchymal transection, with preservation of a liver remnant of adequate size with intact inflow, biliary drainage, and venous outflow.

The most common approach to an anatomic resection, in the most common order, is mobilization of the liver to be resected, dissection of inflow and outflow structures, division of the inflow, division of the outflow, and parenchymal transection. Mobilization of the liver involves division of the right or left triangular ligaments, freeing up the liver from the diaphragm. Often, the liver must be mobilized completely off the vena cava, which it straddles, and this requires careful dissection and division of multiple retrohepatic caval venous branches. For major resections, the hepatic vein of the resected portion of liver is often encircled before the resection. There are various techniques to dissect, control, and divide inflow vessels. Classic inflow control is obtained by dissection of the liver hilum, with control of the portal vein and

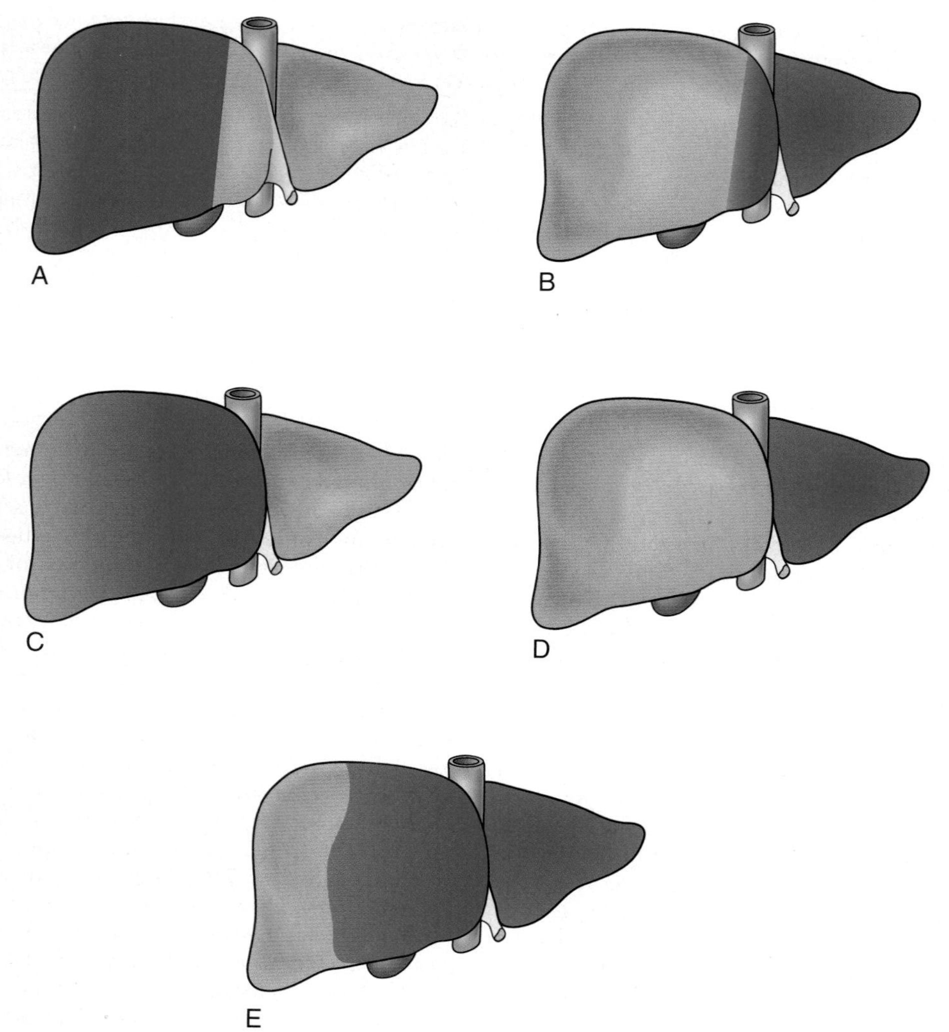

FIG. 54.39 Commonly performed major hepatic resections are indicated by the *shaded areas*. (A) Right hepatectomy, right hepatic lobectomy, or right hemihepatectomy (segments V to VIII). (B) Left hepatectomy, left hepatic lobectomy, or left hemihepatectomy (segments II to IV). (C) Right lobectomy, extended right hepatic lobectomy, or right trisectionectomy (trisegmentectomy; segments IV to VIII). (D) Left lobectomy, left lateral segmentectomy, or left lateral sectionectomy (segments II to III). (E) Extended left hepatectomy, extended left lobectomy, or left trisectionectomy (trisegmentectomy; segments II to V, VIII). See Table 54.11. (From Blumgart LH, Jarnagin W, Fong Y. Liver resection for benign disease and for liver and biliary tumors. In: Blumgart LH, Fong Y, eds. *Surgery of the Liver and Biliary Tract*. London: WB Saunders; 2000:1639–1714.)

hepatic artery to the hemiliver to be resected. These can be suture ligated or divided with vascular staplers. Unless tumor proximity mandates, we advocate dividing the bile duct within the liver substance to minimize absolutely contralateral biliary injuries related to anatomic anomalies. Inflow control can also be obtained by dissection of the intrahepatic inflow pedicle to the anatomic section of liver to be resected. Recall that the inflow structures invaginate peritoneum at the hepatic hilum and run intrahepatically as an invested pedicle of the three inflow structures. The inflow pedicles can be encircled by making flanking hepatotomies or by splitting parenchyma down to the pedicle of interest. The pedicle can usually be divided with a vascular stapler, but suture ligation is sometimes necessary. Typically, the hepatic vein is divided in its extrahepatic position, which can also usually be done with a vascular stapler.

The hepatic vein can also be divided within the substance of the liver during parenchymal transection. There are a number of methods of parenchymal transection, ranging from complex ultrasonic irrigators to radiofrequency energy coagulators to a simple clamp-crushing technique. In experienced hands, these can all be used effectively to minimize blood loss, and it is important to develop a specific technique that one is comfortable performing. Ultimately, parenchymal transection is about dissecting intrahepatic anatomy, controlling vascular and biliary structures, minimizing blood loss, and avoiding injury to the FLR.

HEMOBILIA

A case of lethal hemobilia secondary to penetrating abdominal trauma was first described by Glisson in 1654. It was not until 1948 that Sandblom coined the term *hemobilia* in his seminal paper on the subject. Hemobilia is defined as bleeding into the biliary tree from an abnormal communication between a blood vessel and bile duct. It is a rare condition that is often difficult to distinguish from common causes of gastrointestinal bleeding. The most common causes of hemobilia are iatrogenic trauma, accidental trauma, gallstones, tumors, inflammatory disorders, and vascular disorders. Major hemobilia is relatively uncommon, whereas minor inconsequential hemobilia is a common consequence of gallstone disease or interventional radiologic hepatic procedures.

Causes

The most common cause of hemobilia is iatrogenic trauma to the liver and biliary tree. Before the 1980s, the ratio of hemobilia attributed to accidental trauma compared with iatrogenic trauma was 2:1, but iatrogenic trauma is now regarded as the cause of hemobilia in 40% to 60% of cases. Percutaneous liver biopsy results in hemobilia in less than 1% of cases, but percutaneous transhepatic biliary drainage procedures have an incidence of 2% to 10%. Similarly, surgical exploration of the biliary tree can result in hemobilia from direct injury or arterial pseudoaneurysm. A number of cases of hemobilia after cholecystectomy have been reported. Hemobilia secondary to accidental trauma is more common with blunt than with penetrating abdominal trauma and occurs with a reported incidence of 0.2% to 3%. Risk factors for the development of hemobilia after accidental trauma are central hepatic rupture with a cavity, the use of packs, and inadequate drainage. The gallbladder can be a source of bleeding from trauma, gallstones, or acalculous cholecystitis. Primary vascular diseases, such as aneurysms, angiodysplasia, and hemangiomas, are rare causes of hemobilia. Malignant tumors of the liver, biliary tree, gallbladder, and pancreas as well as parasitic infections, hepatic abscesses, and cholangitis are uncommon causes of hemobilia.

Clinical Presentation

Portal venous bleeding into the biliary tree is rare and often self-limited unless the portal pressure is elevated. Minor hemobilia generally runs an uneventful asymptomatic clinical course. However, arterial hemobilia, the most common source, can be dramatic. Clinical sequelae of hemobilia are related to blood loss and the formation of potentially occlusive blood clots in the biliary tree. The classic triad of symptoms and signs of hemobilia is upper abdominal pain, upper gastrointestinal hemorrhage, and jaundice. In one report, all three were present in 22% of patients. The symptoms and signs of major hemobilia are melena (90% of cases), hematemesis (60% of cases), biliary colic (70% of cases), and jaundice (60% of cases). Upper gastrointestinal bleeding seen in conjunction with biliary symptoms must always raise the suspicion of hemobilia. One interesting aspect of hemobilia is the tendency for delayed presentations, up to weeks after the inciting causal event, as well as recurrent and brisk but limited bleeding during months and even years. Blood clots in the biliary tree can masquerade as stones if hemobilia goes unrecognized. These clots can cause cholangitis, pancreatitis, and cholecystitis.

Diagnostic Workup

Once hemobilia is suspected, the first evaluation should be upper gastrointestinal endoscopy, which rules out other sources of hemorrhage and may visualize bleeding from the ampulla of Vater. However, upper endoscopy is diagnostic of hemobilia in only approximately 10% of cases. If upper endoscopy is diagnostic and conservative management is planned, no further studies are necessary. Ultrasound or CT may be helpful in demonstrating intrahepatic tumor or hematoma. Evidence of active bleeding into the biliary tree may be seen on contrast-enhanced CT in the form of pooling contrast material, intraluminal clots, or biliary dilation. CT may also show risk factors associated with hemobilia, such as cavitating central lesions and aneurysms. Arterial angiography is now recognized as the test of choice when significant hemobilia is suspected and will reveal the source of bleeding in approximately 90% of cases. Cholangiography demonstrates blood clots in the biliary tree that may appear as stringy defects or smaller spherical defects that may be difficult to distinguish from stones.

Treatment and Outcomes

The treatment of hemobilia must be focused on stopping the bleeding and relieving biliary obstruction. Most cases of minor hemobilia can be managed conservatively with correction of coagulopathy, adequate biliary drainage (only if necessary), and close observation. In a review of 171 reported cases from 1996 to 1999, 43% of cases were successfully managed conservatively. The first line of therapy for major hemobilia was transarterial embolization, and success rates of 80% to 100% were reported. Angiography with transarterial embolization is indicated for major hemobilia requiring blood transfusion (Fig. 54.40).

Surgery is indicated when conservative therapy and transarterial embolization have failed. Surgical treatment of hemobilia is rarely necessary, and even in cases in which a laparotomy may be mandated for other reasons, transarterial embolization is still the therapy of choice for hemobilia because of its lower morbidity. Surgical approaches generally involve ligation of bleeding vessels, excision of aneurysms, or nonselective ligation of a main hepatic artery. Hepatic resection may be necessary for failed arterial ligation or for cases of severe trauma or tumor. Hemorrhage from the gallbladder or hemorrhagic cholecystitis mandates cholecystectomy. There have been isolated reports of successful management of hemobilia with endoscopic coagulation, somatostatin, and vasopressin. The management of hemobilia after percutaneous transhepatic biliary drainage usually consists of removal of the catheter or replacement with larger catheters but may require transarterial embolization.

At the time of Sandblom's report from the early 1970s, the mortality for hemobilia was at least 25%. A report from 1987 noted a mortality of 12%. In a review of cases from 1996 through 1999, only four deaths were reported. There has clearly been a reduction in mortality from hemobilia, which is probably related to two factors. First, the incidence of minor self-limited hemobilia has increased secondary to the rising number of percutaneous hepatic procedures. Second, improvements in selective angiography and transarterial embolization have greatly improved the treatment of major hemobilia.

Bilhemia

Bilhemia is an extremely rare condition in which bile flows into the bloodstream through the hepatic veins or portal vein branches. This flow occurs in the context of a high intrabiliary pressure exceeding that of the venous system. The cause can be gallstones eroding into the portal vein or accidental or iatrogenic trauma. The condition can be fatal secondary to embolization of large amounts of bile into the lungs. Usually, however, bile flow is low, and the fistulas close spontaneously. The clinical presentation is that of rapidly increasing jaundice, marked direct hyperbilirubinemia without elevation of hepatocellular enzyme levels (e.g., AST, ALT), and septicemia. This diagnosis is best determined by ERCP. Treatment is directed at lowering intrabiliary pressures through stents or sphincterotomy.

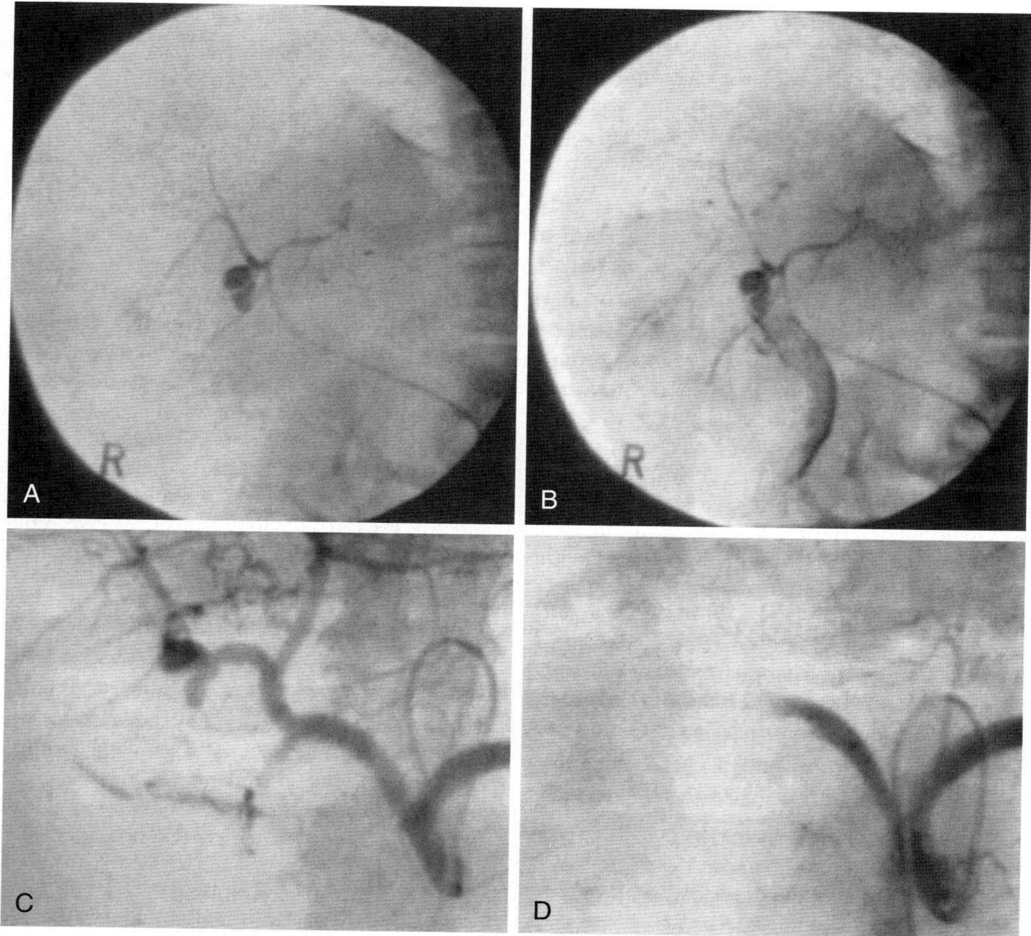

FIG. 54.40 Classic findings of hemobilia. After a complicated cholecystectomy, an iatrogenic pseudoaneurysm developed and ruptured into the biliary tree. Exsanguinating hemobilia ensued; the diagnosis was made by endoscopy and then treated by arterial embolization. (A) Arteriogram demonstrating a pseudoaneurysm of the hepatic artery at the hilum. (B) A few seconds later, the contrast material is seen flowing down the hepatic duct, with evidence of clot in the biliary tree. (C and D) The same aneurysm before (C) and after (D) successful embolization. (From Sandblom JP. Hemobilia and bilhemia. In: Blumgart LH, Fong Y, eds. *Surgery of the Liver and Biliary Tract.* London: WB Saunders; 2000:1319–1342.)

VIRAL HEPATITIS AND THE SURGEON

Epidemics of jaundice were noted in ancient civilizations and recorded by Hippocrates. During World War II, these epidemics were called catarrhal jaundice. More than 28,000 cases were documented at that time. Epidemiologic studies in the 1940s documented the difference between bloodborne hepatitis (hepatitis B) and enteric hepatitis (hepatitis A). The most important discovery was that of the Australia antigen by Blumberg and coworkers in 1965. This antigen proved to be the hepatitis B surface antigen (HBsAg) and provided a means for differentiating the two types of hepatitis and characterizing the epidemiology of this disease. This discovery also led to the development of HBV vaccines based on this antigen with obvious and profound effects worldwide. Further research led to the discovery of the delta virus (hepatitis D) and hepatitis C, explaining cases of non-A, non-B hepatitis. Hepatitis E has been found to be a unique enteral form of infectious hepatitis; the hepatitis G virus, discovered in 1995, is still being defined.

Viral hepatitis is a major health problem and is the most common cause of liver disease worldwide. Although fulminant acute hepatitis is uncommon, there are more than 5 million people who suffer from chronic hepatitis. It is estimated that more than 15,000 patients die each year of viral hepatitis in the United States alone. Viral hepatitis is not a surgical disease, but it has important consequences for surgeons and surgical patients. For any surgeon performing hepatic surgery, the functional state of the liver is extremely important, and patients with chronic viral hepatitis require special attention before any surgical intervention. Also, chronic viral hepatitis is a common cause of HCC. Finally, the risk of transmission from patient to surgeon and vice versa is an issue with which all surgeons should be familiar.

Definition

Viral hepatitis is an infection of the liver by one of six known viruses that have diverse genetic compositions and structures. Hepatitis A virus (HAV), HCV, hepatitis D virus (HDV), hepatitis E virus (HEV), and hepatitis G virus (HGV) have RNA genomes, whereas HBV has a DNA genome that replicates through RNA intermediates. HAV and HEV are both responsible for forms of epidemic hepatitis and are transmitted through the fecal-oral route. HBV is the only one with the potential to integrate into

TABLE 54.12 Serologic evaluation of the most common viral hepatitides.

VIRUS	ANTIGEN NAME	INTERPRETATION	ANTIBODY NAME	INTERPRETATION
HAV	HAV antigen	Acute infection	Anti-HAV IgM	Acute infection
			Anti-HAV IgG	Immunity
HBV	HBsAg	Acute or chronic infection	Anti-HBs	Immunity
	HBeAg	HBV replication, infectivity	Anti-HBc	All phases of infection
			Anti-HBe	Late convalescence
HCV	None	—	Anti-HCV	Late convalescence or chronic infection

HAV, Hepatitis A virus; *HBc*, hepatitis B core; *HBe*, hepatitis e-antigen; *HBs*, hepatitis surface antigen; *HBV*, hepatitis B virus; *HBeAg*, hepatitis B e antigen; *HBsAg*, hepatitis B surface antigen; *HCV*, hepatitis C virus; *IgG*, immunoglobulin G; *IgM*, immunoglobulin M.

host genomes, although this is not required for replication. HCV replicates in the cytoplasm of hepatocytes and has complex mechanisms of evading host immunity through hypervariable areas in its genome. HDV requires the presence of HBV coinfection for replication and infectivity and can alter the clinical course of HBV infection. HGV was discovered more recently and has similarities to HCV but has no definitive association with clinical hepatitis.

Diagnosis

Table 54.12 summarizes the serologic tests and their implications for HAV, HBV, and HCV. The diagnosis of HAV infection relies on the determination of antibodies to HAV. Both IgM and IgG antibodies are present early in the infection, but only IgG persists long term. HAV antigens and tests for HAV RNA have been developed but are generally restricted to research laboratories.

HBV infection has been characterized by a number of antigens and antibodies (Fig. 54.41). HBsAg is the hallmark of the diagnosis of HBV infection and appears in the serum 1 to 10 weeks after infection; it usually disappears in 4 to 6 months, but persistence in the serum beyond 6 months implies chronic infection. Anti-hepatitis B surface antigen (anti-HBs) antibodies usually appear during a window period after the disappearance of HBsAg and indicate recovery after HBV infection. Anti-HBs antibodies are also induced by the HBV vaccine. The hepatitis B core antigen (HBcAg) is an intracellular antigen that is not detectable in serum. On the other hand, anti-HBc antibodies are detectable early after infection and persist after recovery and in chronic infections. HBeAg is a secretory protein that is a marker of HBV replication and infectivity. It is usually present early and may persist for years in chronic infection but generally disappears within months in the absence of chronic infection. Seroconversion to anti-HBe antibodies is usually associated with resolution of infection. Determining the presence of HBeAg or anti-HBe antibodies helps decipher the phases of infection described below. It has also been shown that many patients who have seroconverted often have measurable HBV DNA, albeit at low levels. Quantification of HBV DNA in the serum has become the most accurate way of assessing HBV activity. Evidence has shown that many patients thought to have resolved acute HBV infection may have persistent viral infection and may be at risk for ongoing hepatitis or reactivation.

The diagnosis of HCV infection relies on the detection of antibodies to a number of HCV antigens. Current immunoassays are highly specific and sensitive. No specific HCV antigen tests exist, but there are a variety of quantitative and qualitative tests for HCV RNA, which have become important in confirming the diagnosis in unclear cases and assessing responses to therapy.

HDV coinfection of HBV-infected patients is best diagnosed by detection of HDV RNA, which can be measured in serum. The HDV antigen can be detected in liver specimens. HEV infection can

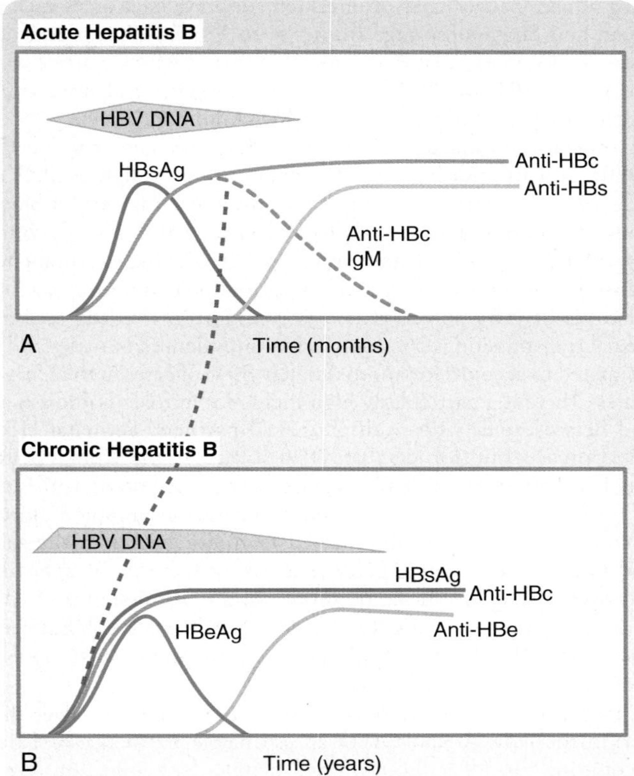

FIG. 54.41 Serologic makers in acute (A) and chronic (B) hepatitis B virus *(HBV)* infection. *Anti-HBc,* IgG antibodies against hepatitis B-core; *Anti-HBc IgM,* IgM antibodies against hepatitis B core; *Anti-HBe,* IgG antibodies against hepatitis e-antigen; *Anti-HBs,* IgG antibodies against hepatitis B surface antigen; *HBc,* hepatitis B core; *HBeAg,* hepatitis B e-antigen; *HBsAg,* hepatitis B surface antigen. (From Doo EC, Lian TJ. The hepatitis viruses. In Schiff ER, Sorrell MF, Maddrey WC, eds. *Schiff's Diseases of the Liver.* Philadelphia: Lippincott-Raven; 1999:725–744.)

be diagnosed by measurement of antibodies in serum or by detection of the virus or its components in feces, serum, or the liver itself.

Epidemiology and Transmission

The incidence of hepatitis A has fallen dramatically since the introduction of effective vaccines, but vaccination is not routine in all countries. Hepatitis A is common in third-world countries, with seropositivity rates approaching 100% in some populations. Infection occurs in childhood and is facilitated by poor hygiene and sanitation. Infection rates are much lower in developed countries. In the United States, approximately 10% of children and

35% of adults have been infected with HAV. Despite vaccination availability, 6000 cases were reported in the United States in 2004. The primary route of HAV infection is the fecal-oral route. Most cases of HAV occur because of ingestion of contaminated water or food and person-to-person contact. Parenteral transmission is possible but uncommon. Sexual transmission has been documented in homosexual men.

Hepatitis B is a major worldwide health problem. There are more than 300 million carriers and 250,000 associated deaths annually. The prevalence of HBV infection has considerable geographic variation. Low prevalence areas such as the United States and Western Europe have carrier rates of 0.1% to 2%. In these regions, transmission is generally through sexual intercourse or IV drug abuse. Carrier rates in intermediate-prevalence areas such as Japan and Singapore range from 3% to 5%. In high-prevalence areas such as Southeast Asia and sub-Saharan Africa, carrier rates range from 10% to 20%. Transmission in high-prevalence areas is largely perinatal and horizontal during childhood.

Transfusion-associated HBV infection was common in the 1960s, and the risk has been estimated to be as high as 50% at that time. Currently, screening programs and limitation of blood donation to voluntary donors have decreased the risk of acquiring HBV from a blood transfusion to 1 in 63,000. Percutaneous transmission through the use of any contaminated needle is a major route of HBV infection and is common in IV drug abusers. Sexual transmission is common in low-prevalence countries and is estimated to account for approximately 30% of cases in the United States. There is a particularly high incidence in male homosexuals and heterosexuals with multiple sexual partners. Perinatal HBV infection accounts for less than 10% of cases in the United States but is common in endemic regions, with rates of transmission of 90% in some areas. Horizontal transmission among children is common and is probably related to minor breaks in the skin and mucous membranes. HBV is the most commonly transmitted virus among healthcare personnel, and transmission is usually patient to patient or patient to worker. Needle-stick risk has been related to HBeAg positivity. Rare cases of physician-to-patient transmission have been reported.

Hepatitis C is the most common cause of chronic liver disease in the United States, with an estimated prevalence of 1.8% accounting for 3.9 million infected people. New infections typically occur at a younger age (20–39 years), and the most common risk factor is IV drug abuse. Healthcare workers have higher carrier rates than the general public. Transmission among healthcare workers is usually related to needle-stick incidents, and the risk of transmission is higher than that of HBV and HIV. In the past, blood transfusion was the major cause of HCV infection, accounting for at least 85% of cases. Currently, less than 2% of acute infections are caused by transfusions, and the risk of transfusion-associated transmission is estimated to be about 1 in 10,000. Although HCV has never been documented in semen, it is estimated that approximately 20% of HCV infections are caused by sexual transmission. Risk of sexual transmission appears to be related to the number of partners and presence of other sexually transmitted diseases. Monogamous sexual partners of HCV-infected people occasionally test positive for HCV in the absence of other risk factors, but this appears to be rare. Perinatal transmission has been documented but is also rare. No identifiable risk factors are found in 30% to 40% of HCV cases.

HDV infection occurs worldwide with a variable distribution that parallels that of HBV infection. Approximately 5% of HBsAg-positive patients also harbor HDV infection. Transmission of HDV is parenteral and can occur only in patients previously infected with HBV.

HEV is endemic in Southeast Asia and central Asia and occurs with low frequency in other areas of the world. HEV infection outbreaks are usually large, affecting hundreds to thousands of people at once, and often follow large rains and flooding. There is a particularly high incidence and mortality in pregnant women. Transmission is fecal-oral and usually related to contaminated drinking water or food. Person-to-person transmission and vertical transmission are rare.

Pathogenesis and Clinical Presentation

The pathogenesis of hepatic injury from these viral infections is not completely understood. For all the viruses discussed in this section, hepatic inflammation appears to be caused by direct cytotoxicity or immune-related phenomena. A combination of these two mechanisms probably underlies the cause of hepatic damage.

Humans are the only host for HAV, and no reservoir of infection has been identified. After oral intake, HAV can survive the acidic gastric pH, but the mechanism of hepatic uptake is not known. HAV infection results in acute inflammation of the liver and has no associated chronic sequelae. The most recent data suggest that hepatocyte damage is most likely an immunopathologic response rather than direct hepatotoxicity. Most children with HAV infection younger than 2 years are asymptomatic, whereas in pediatric patients older than 5 years, 80% will develop symptoms. Fulminant hepatitis develops in 1% to 5% of cases, and mortality is generally below 1%.

HBV is a member of the *Hepadnaviridae* family that is characterized by a genome consisting of partially double-stranded, circular DNA. After viral entry into the hepatocyte, the viral genome is delivered into the nucleus, where it is converted into fully double-stranded DNA and then covalently closed circular DNA. This stable form of HBV DNA is responsible for its persistence in infected hepatocytes. HBV also has the ability of integrating into the hepatocyte genome.

Approximately 70% of patients with acute HBV infection have subclinical or anicteric hepatitis; the other 30% have icteric hepatitis. The incubation period for HBV infection ranges from 1 to 4 months. A prodromal serum sickness–like syndrome may develop, followed by a multitude of constitutional symptoms, such as malaise, anorexia, and nausea. The constitutional symptoms last about 10 days and are followed by jaundice in 30% of patients. Clinical symptoms usually disappear within 3 months. Fulminant hepatic failure develops in 0.1% to 0.5% of patients. Almost 80% of patients with fulminant HBV-related hepatitis will die unless liver transplantation is performed.

Risk of chronic HBV infection is related to immunocompetence and age. Immunocompetent adults have a risk of less than 5%, whereas 30% of children and 90% of infants will develop chronic disease. The effect of age on HBV persistence is most likely due to difference in immune maturity between adults and young children. The natural history and disease course of chronic HBV infection are the result of complex interactions between the virus and host immune response. A substantial proportion of patients will develop liver injury, cirrhosis and its complications, and hepatocellular cancer, whereas others will harbor the virus with limited, if any, injury. Different phases of HBV infection, each with unique viral and biochemical profiles, have been described.[29] The first phase, **HBeAg-positive chronic infection** (previously known as immune tolerant phase), is characterized by high serum HBV DNA but normal liver enzymes. There is a high serum level of HBeAg, and patients in this phase are highly contagious due to the high level of HBV DNA. However, it must be noted that these phases are not necessarily sequential and can be reversed. The second phase, **HBeAg-positive chronic hepatitis B**, is characterized by all the features of phase I along with elevated ALT, suggesting liver damage. Liver biopsy at this stage will demonstrate moderate or severe liver necroinflammation. The third phase, **HBeAg-negative chronic HBV infection** (previously termed "inactive carrier" phase), is characterized by absence of HBeAg, presence of serum antibodies to HBeAg, undetectable or low levels of HBV DNA and normal liver enzymes. The fourth phase is termed **HBeAg-negative chronic hepatitis B** and is characterized by the lack of serum HBeAg, detectable anti-HBe levels, persistent moderate to high levels of serum HBV DNA, as well as fluctuating or persistently elevated ALT levels. Most patients with chronic HBV infection are asymptomatic, but some may experience exacerbations of symptoms. Progression to cirrhosis is marked by hepatic synthetic dysfunction and often cytopenias, related to hypersplenism. Extrahepatic manifestations of HBV infection, caused by circulating immune complexes, occur in approximately 10% to 20% of patients; these include polyarteritis nodosa, glomerulonephritis, essential mixed cryoglobulinemia, and papular acrodermatitis. The sequelae of chronic HBV infection range from none to cirrhosis, HCC, hepatic failure, and death. It has been noted that patients thought to have previously cleared the infection can have a reactivation, especially during a period of immunosuppression. In nonendemic areas, the long-term risk appears to be low, but in endemic areas, chronic HBV infection is a significant cause of morbidity and mortality.

HCV is an RNA virus with a single-stranded RNA genome. This genomic RNA encodes a single protein that can be cleaved by a protease enzyme into its components. HCV replicates in the hepatocyte cytoplasm. The components of viral replication are targeted by the recently successful direct-acting antivirals. For instance, protease inhibitors target the protease responsible for cleaving the initial protein into the various viral components. Acute HCV infection generally is manifested with mild elevation of hepatocellular enzyme levels. In general, 80% of cases occur 5 to 12 weeks after infection. Symptoms occur in less than 30% of patients and are usually so mild and nonspecific that they do not affect daily life. Jaundice occurs in less than 20% of patients, and fulminant hepatic failure caused by HCV is extremely uncommon. Chronic HCV infection develops in approximately two thirds of patients; the other third appear to clear the infection. Most patients with chronic HCV infection are asymptomatic without evidence of overt liver disease and present with only mildly elevated hepatocellular enzyme levels. Despite this quiet clinical course, patients with chronic HCV infection are at risk for development of cirrhosis and HCC. Estimates place the risk of cirrhosis at 2% to 20% at a 20- to 30-year interval. The risk for development of HCC from that point has been estimated at 1% to 4%/year. Progression of liver damage can be variable, and several factors appear to affect its rate. Factors associated with a more rapid progression include male gender, older age at infection, immunosuppression (e.g., HIV infection), coinfection with HBV, moderate alcohol intake, and obesity. Extrahepatic manifestations, such as autoimmune disorders and lymphoma, can occur with HCV infection and are likely related to circulating immune complexes.

The clinical presentation of HDV infection is related to a complex relationship between the degree of HBV and HDV infection. Simultaneous coinfection with high expression of HBV and HDV results in higher rates of acute fulminant hepatitis. Superinfection in a previous HBV carrier generally results in more rapidly progressive chronic liver damage. Some milder forms of acute HDV infection are associated with decreased expression of HDV and repression of HBV infection.

Hepatitis E has a histologic picture different from that of the other viral hepatitides in that a cholestatic type of hepatitis is seen in more than 50% of patients. HEV is introduced orally, and it is not known how the virus travels to the liver. The incubation period of HEV infection ranges from 2 to 9 weeks. The most common form of illness is acute icteric hepatitis; most series report jaundice in more than 90% of patients. Asymptomatic forms of the disease occur and are probably more common than the icteric form, but the actual frequency is unknown. The disease is usually self-limited, but fulminant hepatic failure can occur in a small percentage of patients. Overall, the mortality rate is probably significantly less than 1%. Pregnant women tend to have a more severe clinical course; mortality rates range from 5% to 25%.

Prevention

HAV infection prophylaxis relies on sanitary measures and administration of serum immunoglobulin. The development of safe and effective HAV vaccines, however, has made the use of preexposure immunoglobulin unnecessary. Serum immunoglobulin is still the therapy of choice for postexposure prophylaxis and may be safely given, along with active immunization. In the United States, the Centers for Disease Control and Prevention (CDC) has recommended universal vaccination of children on the basis of the safety and efficacy of the vaccine in high-risk populations. Public health researchers are investigating vaccination schemes to eradicate HAV infection in high-risk populations throughout the world. However, cost-benefit analyses have not supported universal vaccination worldwide. Similarly, HEV infection prophylaxis has focused on sanitary measures, particularly strategies aimed at drinking water. Unfortunately, HEV immunoglobulin has not been successful in preexposure or postexposure prevention of HEV infection, whereas anti-HEV antibodies appear to be effective at attenuating the clinical syndrome. Vaccines for HEV infection have been developed and evaluated in clinical trials.

Remarkable advances have been made in the prevention of HBV infection. In the past, prevention of HBV infection was limited to passive immunization with immunoglobulin containing high titers of antibody to HBsAg. Currently, immunoglobulin immunization is used only in postexposure prophylaxis. HBsAg-containing vaccines have been developed with good safety and efficacy profiles. These vaccines are used primarily for preexposure prophylaxis but can also be used in a postexposure setting along with immunoglobulin. Currently, CDC recommends a three-dose HBV vaccination for all children, with the first dose being administered preferably within 24 hours after birth followed by two subsequent booster doses. Although no vaccine is available for HDV infection, effective prevention of HBV infection prevents HDV infection.

The only effective preventive strategy for HCV infection relies on public health principles aimed at the major risk factors for transmission. Conventionally prepared anti-HCV immunoglobulin has been evaluated in a number of trials and has not been demonstrated to prevent transfusion-related non-A, non-B hepatitis. Screening of blood donors has rendered this issue irrelevant today. Unfortunately, because of various obstacles, a successful HCV vaccine has not been developed.

Treatment

Treatment of HAV or HEV infection is supportive in nature and is generally aimed at correcting dehydration and providing adequate calorie intake. Although fatigue may mandate significant periods of rest, hospitalization is usually not necessary, except in cases of fulminant liver failure.

The treatment of HBV infection is largely aimed at patients with chronic active disease. Interferon-alfa and the nucleoside analogue lamivudine used to be the only two approved therapies for the treatment of HBV. Now, many nucleoside analogues for the treatment of HBV infection have been developed and probably work through inhibition of DNA synthesis. Interferon-alfa is an immunomodulatory agent with some antiviral properties that can induce a virologic response in 35% to 40% of patients. However, long-term benefit with interferon therapy has not been proven. Oral nucleoside analogues are currently the main form of anti-HBV treatment, which include entecavir and two prodrugs of tenofovir. These three drugs are very effective in inducing virologic suppression in a high proportion of patients with favorable safety and tolerability profiles. Entecavir is not recommended in patients who have been previously treated with lamivudine or telbivudine. On the other hand, tenofovir derivatives are effective in patients with lamivudine and telbivudine resistance. Long-term viral suppression with nucleoside analog therapy leads to significant histologic improvement, including regression of cirrhosis, reduced complications of cirrhosis, and decreased risk of developing HCC. Indication for treatment of HBV infection is based on three parameters: serum HBV DNA, serum ALT levels, and severity of liver disease. All experts agree that patients with cirrhosis, with or without decompensation, should be treated when serum HBV DNA is detectable. Most experts will also suggest treatment with higher levels of HBV DNA with ALT elevations or with moderately elevated levels of HBV DNA with evidence of liver fibrosis.

During the last 20 years, tremendous advances in the treatment of HCV infection have occurred. Interferon-alpha and ribavirin were the recommended treatment for hepatitis C for the longest time. A benefit for interferon-alfa in the treatment of non-A, non-B hepatitis was originally demonstrated in 1986, before the discovery of HCV. With interferon-alfa treatment regimens, complete viral response, defined as sustained loss of serum viral RNA, occurs in 12% to 20% of patients. The addition of ribavirin to interferon-alfa resulted in response rates of 35% to 45%. In the most recent trials, treatment with pegylated interferon-alfa and ribavirin for 48 weeks resulted in viral clearance in 55% of patients. The specific genotype appears to be predictive of response, with some types resulting in response rates of 80% and others of 45%. Relapse can occur, but it usually occurs with monotherapy and shortened courses of therapy. Interferon-alfa regimens had significant side effects. During recent years, the treatment of chronic HCV infection has been revolutionized by the introduction of direct-acting antivirals (e.g., ledipasvir, sofosbuvir, glecaprevir, pibrentasvir, velpatasvir) that target specific nonstructural proteins of HCV and thus disrupt viral replication and infection. Combinations of these medications have now become the first-line treatment and have effectively replaced prior regimens of pegylated interferon-alpha and ribavirin as the standard of care where available. The current all-oral treatments are of shorter duration, have fewer side effects, and have higher cure rates. By tailoring the combination of direct-acting antiviral agents to patient factors and the specific HCV genotype, a sustained virologic response can be achieved in greater than 90% of patients.

SELECTED REFERENCES

Blumgart LH. *Video Atlas: Liver, Biliary and Pancreatic Surgery*. Philadelphia: Elsevier; 2011.

This video atlas includes an extensive library of narrated and captioned videos that present the history, radiologic evidence, and operative procedures for hepatic and biliary surgery. It also includes laparoscopic approaches to liver resections.

Blumgart LH. *Surgery of the Liver, Biliary Tract, and Pancreas*. 6th ed. Philadelphia: Elsevier; 2016.

A comprehensive and clinical review of hepatobiliary anatomy. The text is specifically oriented toward surgery of the liver and biliary tree. It covers anatomy, pathophysiology, immunology, molecular biology, genetics, diagnosis, and treatment. In addition, it is accompanied by a DVD with detailed video clips of laparoscopic procedures, effectively allowing one to use it as an operative atlas.

EASL. 2017 Clinical practice guidelines on the management of hepatitis B virus infection. *J Hepatol*. 2017;67:370–398.

These guidelines from "European Association for the Study of the Liver" provide a comprehensive update on the diagnosis, evaluation, and management of hepatitis B infection.

Fong Y, Fortner J, Sun RL, et al. Clinical score for predicting recurrence after hepatic resection for metastatic colorectal cancer: analysis of 1001 consecutive cases. *Ann Surg*. 1999;230:309–318.

At the time of publication, this was the largest single-institution series of liver resection for metastatic colorectal cancer. A very useful prognostic scoring system is presented and remains critically important in evaluating patients today.

Foster JH, Berman MM. *Solid Liver Tumors*. Philadelphia: WB Saunders; 1977.

A classic and comprehensive monograph that contains a complete history of liver surgery.

Herrera JL. Management of acute variceal bleeding. *Clin Liver Dis*. 2014;18:347–357.

This review article discusses the management of acute variceal bleeding with special emphasis on the appropriate role of various treatment modalities in the current era and when to escalate the therapy and move to the next stage.

Heimbach JK, Kulik LM, Finn RS, et al. AASLD guidelines for the treatment of hepatocellular carcinoma. *Hepatology*. 2018;67:358–380.

This is an update on the original AASLD guidelines on the management of hepatocellular carcinoma.

House MG, Ito H, Gonen M, et al. Survival after hepatic resection for metastatic colorectal cancer: trends in outcomes for 1,600 patients during two decades at a single institution. *J Am Coll Surg*. 2010;210:744–752.

This study analyzes factors associated with differences in long-term outcomes after hepatic resection for metastatic colorectal cancer. Despite worse clinical and pathologic features, survival rates after hepatic resection for colorectal metastases have improved, which might be attributable to improvements in patient selection, operative management, and chemotherapy.

Jang HJ, Yu H, Kim TK. Imaging of focal liver lesions. *Semin Roentgenol*. 2009;44:266–282.

Imaging modalities are key in diagnosing and differentiating various focal liver lesions. This monograph covers the critical elements of ultrasonography, computed tomography, and MRI of focal liver lesions.

Jarnagin WR, Gonen M, Fong Y, et al. Improvement in perioperative outcome after hepatic resection: analysis of 1,803 consecutive cases over the past decade. *Ann Surg*. 2002;236:397–406.

One of the largest series of hepatic resections that documents the remarkable improvement in perioperative outcomes.

Kelly K, Weber SM. Cystic diseases of the liver and bile ducts. *J Gastrointest Surg*. 2014;18:627–634, quiz 634.

This review article covers the diagnosis and management of cystic disease of the liver including hydatid disease.

Leung U, Fong Y. Robotic liver surgery. *Hepatobiliary Surg Nutr*. 2014;3:288–294.

This manuscript reviews the place and evolution of robotics in the current era of minimally invasive liver surgery.

Mayberry J, Lee WM. The revolution in treatment of hepatitis C. *Med Clin North Am*. 2019;103:43–55.

This review describes the epidemiology, risk factor, and natural history of hepatitis C infection. It also comprehensively, reviews the new developments which have revolutionized the treatment of hepatitis C.

Ochsner A, DeBakey M, Murray S. Pyogenic abscess of the liver. *Am J Surg*. 1938;40:292–319.

A classic landmark study on pyogenic abscesses of the liver. This was the first serious attempt to study hepatic abscesses and ushered in the modern era of treatment.

Sandhu BS, Sanyal AJ. Management of ascites in cirrhosis. *Clin Liver Dis*. 2005;9:715–732.

This is an excellent, comprehensive, and practical review of the treatment of ascites in patients with cirrhosis.

Stewart CL, Warner S, Ito K, et al. Cytoreduction for colorectal metastases: liver, lung, peritoneum, lymph nodes, bone, brain. When does it palliate, prolong survival, and potentially cure? *Curr Probl Surg*. 2018;55:330–379.

This excellent article analyzes the reasoning and the evidence underscoring the benefit of metastatectomy for colorectal liver and other metastases.

REFERENCES

1. Orloff MJ, Orloff MS, Orloff SL, et al. Three decades of experience with emergency portacaval shunt for acutely bleeding esophageal varices in 400 unselected patients with cirrhosis of the liver. *J Am Coll Surg*. 1995;180:257–272.
2. Bernard B, Lebrec D, Mathurin P, et al. Beta-adrenergic antagonists in the prevention of gastrointestinal rebleeding in patients with cirrhosis: a meta-analysis. *Hepatology*. 1997;25:63–70.
3. Funakoshi N, Segalas-Largey F, Duny Y, et al. Benefit of combination beta-blocker and endoscopic treatment to prevent variceal rebleeding: a meta-analysis. *World J Gastroenterol*. 2010;16:5982–5992.
4. Fong Y, Wong J. Evolution in surgery: influence of minimally invasive approaches on the hepatobiliary surgeon. *Surg Infect (Larchmt)*. 2009;10:399–406.
5. Meddings L, Myers RP, Hubbard J, et al. A population-based study of pyogenic liver abscesses in the United States: incidence, mortality, and temporal trends. *Am J Gastroenterol*. 2010;105:117–124.
6. Lai HC, Lin CC, Cheng KS, et al. Increased incidence of gastrointestinal cancers among patients with pyogenic liver abscess: a population-based cohort study. *Gastroenterology*. 2014;146:129–137.e121.
7. Mezhir J, Fong Y, Jacks L, et al. Current management of pyogenic liver abscess: surgery is now second-line treatment. *J Am Coll Surg*. 2010:975–983.
8. Salles JM, Salles MJ, Moraes LA, et al. Invasive amebiasis: an update on diagnosis and management. *Expert Rev Anti Infect Ther*. 2007;5:893–901.
9. Chavez-Tapia NC, Hernandez-Calleros J, Tellez-Avila FI, et al. Image-guided percutaneous procedure plus metronidazole versus metronidazole alone for uncomplicated amoebic liver abscess. *Cochrane Database Syst Rev*. 2009:CD004886.
10. Nasseri Moghaddam S, Abrishami A, Malekzadeh R. Percutaneous needle aspiration, injection, and reaspiration with or without benzimidazole coverage for uncomplicated hepatic hydatid cysts. *Cochrane Database Syst Rev*. 2006:CD003623.
11. Zucman-Rossi J, Jeannot E, Nhieu JT, et al. Genotype-phenotype correlation in hepatocellular adenoma: new classification and relationship with HCC. *Hepatology*. 2006;43:515–524.
12. Marrero JA, Ahn J, Rajender Reddy K. ACG clinical guideline: the diagnosis and management of focal liver lesions. *Am J Gastroenterol*. 2014;109:1328–1347; quiz 1348.
13. Bruix J, Sherman M, Llovet JM, et al. Clinical management of hepatocellular carcinoma. Conclusions of the Barcelona—2000 EASL Conference. European Association for the Study of the Liver. *J Hepatol*. 2001;35:421–430.
14. Bruix J, Sherman M. Management of hepatocellular carcinoma. *Hepatology*. 2005;42:1208–1236.

15. EASL-EORTC clinical practice guidelines: management of hepatocellular carcinoma. *J Hepatol.* 2012;56:908–943.
16. Bruix J, Sherman M. Management of hepatocellular carcinoma: an update. *Hepatology.* 2011;53:1020–1022.
17. Weitz J, D'Angelica M, Jarnagin W, et al. Selective use of diagnostic laparoscopy prior to planned hepatectomy for patients with hepatocellular carcinoma. *Surgery.* 2004;135:273–281.
18. Yin L, Li H, Li AJ, et al. Partial hepatectomy vs. transcatheter arterial chemoembolization for resectable multiple hepatocellular carcinoma beyond Milan Criteria: a RCT. *J Hepatol.* 2014;61:82–88.
19. Mazzaferro V, Regalia E, Doci R, et al. Liver transplantation for the treatment of small hepatocellular carcinomas in patients with cirrhosis. *N Engl J Med.* 1996;334:693–699.
20. Malagari K, Pomoni M, Kelekis A, et al. Prospective randomized comparison of chemoembolization with doxorubicin-eluting beads and bland embolization with BeadBlock for hepatocellular carcinoma. *Cardiovasc Intervent Radiol.* 2010;33:541–551.
21. Llovet JM, Bruix J. Systematic review of randomized trials for unresectable hepatocellular carcinoma: chemoembolization improves survival. *Hepatology.* 2003;37:429–442.
22. Llovet JM, Real MI, Montana X, et al. Arterial embolisation or chemoembolisation versus symptomatic treatment in patients with unresectable hepatocellular carcinoma: a randomised controlled trial. *Lancet.* 2002;359:1734–1739.
23. Lo CM, Ngan H, Tso WK, et al. Randomized controlled trial of transarterial lipiodol chemoembolization for unresectable hepatocellular carcinoma. *Hepatology.* 2002;35:1164–1171.
24. Llovet JM, Ricci S, Mazzaferro V, et al. Sorafenib in advanced hepatocellular carcinoma. *N Engl J Med.* 2008;359:378–390.
25. Bruix J, Takayama T, Mazzaferro V, et al. Adjuvant sorafenib for hepatocellular carcinoma after resection or ablation (STORM): a phase 3, randomised, double-blind, placebo-controlled trial. *Lancet Oncol.* 2015;16:1344–1354.
26. Lim II , Farber BA, LaQuaglia MP. Advances in fibrolamellar hepatocellular carcinoma: a review. *Eur J Pediatr Surg.* 2014;24:461–466.
27. Honeyman JN, Simon EP, Robine N, et al. Detection of a recurrent DNAJB1-PRKACA chimeric transcript in fibrolamellar hepatocellular carcinoma. *Science.* 2014;343:1010–1014.
28. Ribero D, Pinna AD, Guglielmi A, et al. Surgical approach for long-term survival of patients with intrahepatic cholangiocarcinoma: a multi-institutional analysis of 434 patients. *Arch Surg.* 2012;147:1107–1113.
29. EASL 2017 clinical practice guidelines on the management of hepatitis B virus infection. *J Hepatol.* 2017;67:370–398.
30. Fong Y, Fortner J, Sun RL, et al. Clinical score for predicting recurrence after hepatic resection for metastatic colorectal cancer: analysis of 1001 consecutive cases. *Ann Surg.* 1999;230:309–318; discussion 318–321.
31. Moulton CA, Gu CS, Law CH, et al. Effect of PET before liver resection on surgical management for colorectal adenocarcinoma metastases: a randomized clinical trial. *JAMA.* 2014;311:1863–1869.
32. Maithel SK, D'Angelica MI. An update on randomized clinical trials in advanced and metastatic colorectal carcinoma. *Surg Oncol Clin N Am.* 2010;19:163–181.
33. Hwang M, Jayakrishnan TT, Green DE, et al. Systematic review of outcomes of patients undergoing resection for colorectal liver metastases in the setting of extra hepatic disease. *Eur J Cancer.* 2014;50:1747–1757.
34. Portier G, Elias D, Bouche O, et al. Multicenter randomized trial of adjuvant fluorouracil and folinic acid compared with surgery alone after resection of colorectal liver metastases: FFCD ACHBTH AURC 9002 trial. *J Clin Oncol.* 2006;24:4976–4982.
35. Mitry E, Fields AL, Bleiberg H, et al. Adjuvant chemotherapy after potentially curative resection of metastases from colorectal cancer: a pooled analysis of two randomized trials. *J Clin Oncol.* 2008;26:4906–4911.
36. Nordlinger B, Sorbye H, Glimelius B, et al. Perioperative chemotherapy with FOLFOX4 and surgery versus surgery alone for resectable liver metastases from colorectal cancer (EORTC Intergroup trial 40983): a randomised controlled trial. *Lancet.* 2008;371:1007–1016.
37. Nordlinger B, Sorbye H, Glimelius B, et al. Perioperative FOLFOX4 chemotherapy and surgery versus surgery alone for resectable liver metastases from colorectal cancer (EORTC 40983): long-term results of a randomised, controlled, phase 3 trial. *Lancet Oncol.* 2013;14:1208–1215.
38. Wang ZM, Chen YY, Chen FF, et al. Peri-operative chemotherapy for patients with resectable colorectal hepatic metastasis: a meta-analysis. *Eur J Surg Oncol.* 2015;41:1197–1203.
39. Kemeny N, Capanu M, D'Angelica M, et al. Phase I trial of adjuvant hepatic arterial infusion (HAI) with floxuridine (FUDR) and dexamethasone plus systemic oxaliplatin, 5-fluorouracil and leucovorin in patients with resected liver metastases from colorectal cancer. *Ann Oncol.* 2009;20:1236–1241.
40. Kemeny N, Jarnagin W, Gonen M, et al. Phase I/II study of hepatic arterial therapy with floxuridine and dexamethasone in combination with intravenous irinotecan as adjuvant treatment after resection of hepatic metastases from colorectal cancer. *J Clin Oncol.* 2003;21:3303–3309.
41. Kemeny N, Huang Y, Cohen AM, et al. Hepatic arterial infusion of chemotherapy after resection of hepatic metastases from colorectal cancer. *N Engl J Med.* 1999;341:2039–2048.
42. D'Angelica M, Jarnagin W, Dematteo R, et al. Staging laparoscopy for potentially resectable noncolorectal, nonneuroendocrine liver metastases. *Ann Surg Oncol.* 2002;9:204–209.
43. Mimatsu K, Oida T, Kawasaki A, et al. Long-term outcome of laparoscopic deroofing for symptomatic nonparasitic liver cysts. *Hepatogastroenterology.* 2009;56:850–853.
44. Qiu JG, Wu H, Jiang H, et al. Laparoscopic fenestration vs open fenestration in patients with congenital hepatic cysts: a meta-analysis. *World J Gastroenterol.* 2011;17:3359–3365.
45. Gevers TJ, Drenth JP. Diagnosis and management of polycystic liver disease. *Nat Rev Gastroenterol Hepatol.* 2013;10:101–108.
46. Jarnagin WR, Gonen M, Fong Y, et al. Improvement in perioperative outcome after hepatic resection: analysis of 1,803 consecutive cases over the past decade. *Ann Surg.* 2002;236:397–406; discussion 406–397.
47. Matsumura M, Mise Y, Saiura A, et al. Parenchymal-sparing hepatectomy does not increase intrahepatic recurrence in patients with advanced colorectal liver metastases. *Ann Surg Oncol.* 2016;23:3718–3726.
48. Memeo R, de Blasi V, Adam R, et al. Parenchymal-sparing hepatectomies (PSH) for bilobar colorectal liver metastases are associated with a lower morbidity and similar oncological results: a propensity score matching analysis. *HPB (Oxford).* 2016;18:781–790.
49. Donadon M, Cescon M, Cucchetti A, et al. Parenchymal-sparing surgery for the surgical treatment of multiple colorectal liver metastases is a safer approach than major hepatectomy not impairing patients' prognosis: a bi-institutional propensity score-matched analysis. *Dig Surg.* 2018;35:342–349.

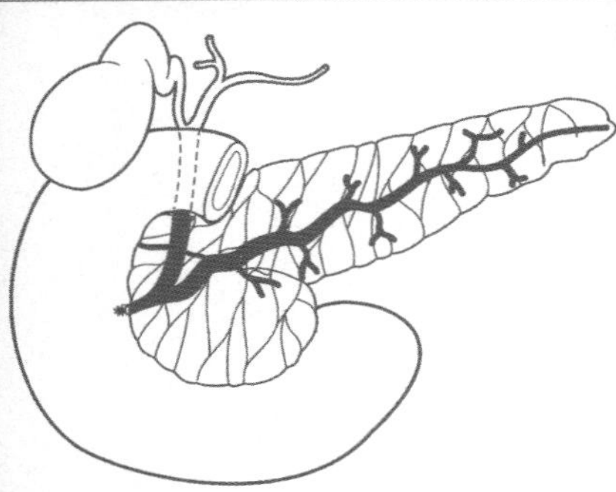

CHAPTER 55

Biliary System

Pejman Radkani, Jason Hawksworth, Thomas Fishbein

OUTLINE

ANATOMY AND PHYSIOLOGY

As anatomic variations in biliary anatomy are common, occurring in up to 30% of patients, understanding of both normal anatomy and the variations is important for the management of patients with biliary disease.

Bile ducts, either intrahepatic or extrahepatic, lie superior to the corresponding portal vein, which in turn are lateral and inferior to the arterial supply (Fig. 55.1). The left hepatic duct retains a longer transverse extrahepatic portion and travels under the edge of segment IV before diving before joining the bifurcation. It can receive a few subsegmental branches from segment IV in this transverse portion. The left duct drains segments I, II, III, and IV, with the most distal branch draining segment IVA. Further superolateral, the ducts draining segment IVB arise, and yet further up the left duct are the ducts for segments II and III. These ducts can generally be found just posterior and lateral to the umbilical recess. The caudate lobe drains through smaller ducts that enter the right and left hepatic duct systems. The drainage of the right duct system includes segments V, VI, VII, and VIII and is substantially shorter than the left duct, bifurcating almost immediately. The junction of two sectoral ducts, posterior and anterior, creates this short right hepatic duct. The anterior sectoral duct runs in a vertical direction to drain segments V and VIII, whereas the posterior sectoral duct follows a horizontal course to drain segments VI and VII.

The gallbladder is a partially intraperitoneal structure that lies attached to the undersurface of the liver on segments IVB and V. It is 7 to 10 cm in length, holds 30 to 60 mL of bile as a reservoir, and is divided into neck, infundibulum with Hartmann pouch, body, and fundus (Fig. 55.2). On the side of the gallbladder that is attached to the liver, there is no peritoneal covering; a fibrous lining known as the cystic plate occupies this space. Bile is drained via a cystic duct to the common bile duct (CBD). The cystic duct can range from 1 to 5 cm in length and drains at an acute angle into the CBD. There are numerous variations in this insertion, including into the right hepatic duct (Fig. 55.3). The valves of Heister, which are folds of mucosa oriented in spiral pattern within the neck of gallbladder, function to retain bile in the gallbladder until contraction in response to enteric stimulation.

The CBD is divided into three portions: supraduodenal, retroduodenal, and the pancreatic portion, which is the most inferior portion, encompassed by head of pancreas. The insertion of cystic duct marks the separation of the CBD (below) from the common hepatic duct (above). The CBD ends in the second portion of duodenum at the ampulla of Vater. The pancreatic duct also joins the ampulla, although in variants may have a separate orifice (Fig. 55.4).

As mentioned, the cystic duct divides the bile duct to common hepatic duct and CBD. The common hepatic duct drains the left and right hepatic ducts and their confluence at the hilar plate, which is an extension of Glisson's capsule. There are generally no vascular structures overlying bile ducts at this location, allowing exposure of the bifurcation by incision at the base of segment IV and lifting the liver off these structures. This technique, called lowering hilar plate, is used to expose the proximal extrahepatic biliary tree.

Vascular Anatomy

As described by Couinaud,[1] the hepatic parenchyma is divided into lobes, each of which is divided into lobar segments (Fig. 55.5) to define the basic hepatic anatomic resections.

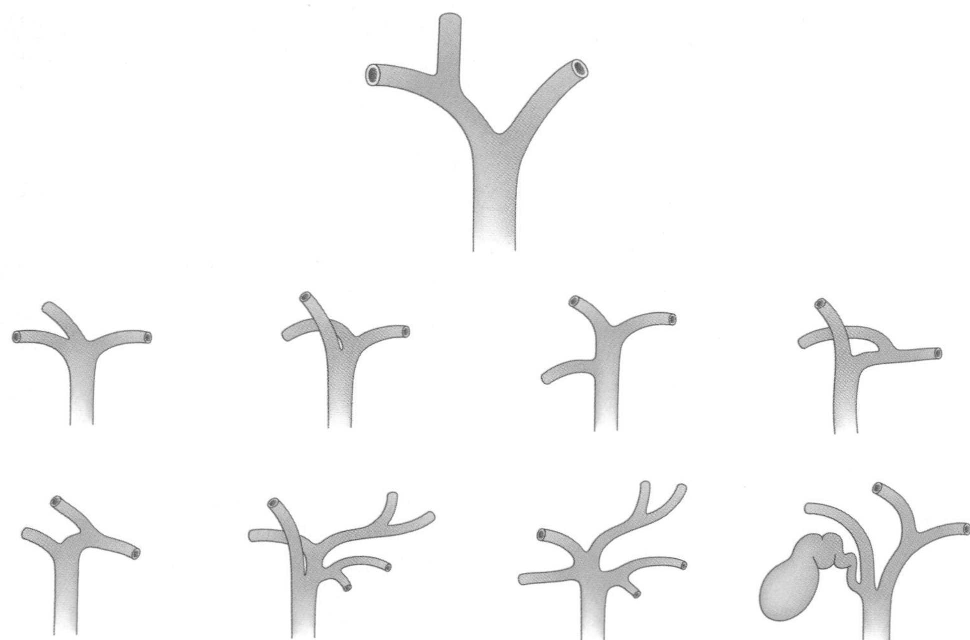

FIG. 55.1 Hepatic lobar segmental biliary anatomy.

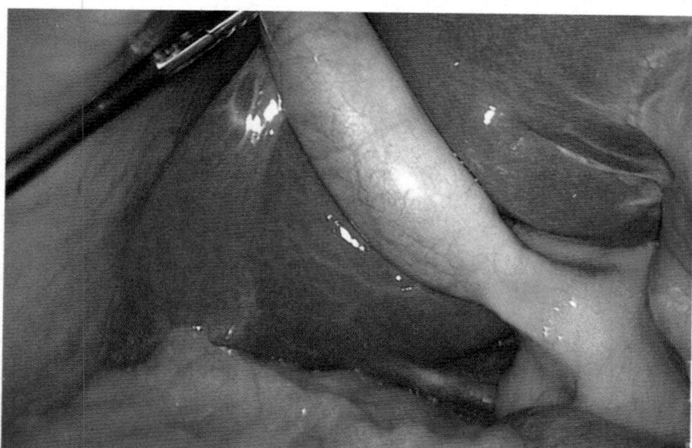

FIG. 55.2 Laparoscopic photograph of the gallbladder in situ. The gallbladder is being suspended by the fundus to expose the infundibulum and porta hepatis.

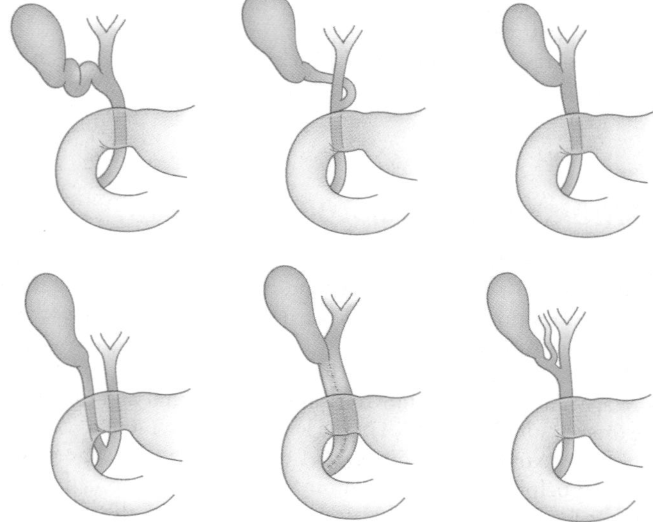

FIG. 55.3 Variability in cystic duct anatomy. Knowledge of these variations is important to try to avoid inadvertent injury to the biliary tree during cholecystectomy.

The blood supply to the entire biliary tree is solely arterial as contrasted with the hepatic parenchyma, where dual perfusion comes as well from the portal vein, which makes the biliary tree susceptible to ischemic injury.

The cystic artery normally arises from the right hepatic artery, and similar to the variability of the cystic duct, it may arise from the right hepatic, left hepatic, proper hepatic, common hepatic, gastroduodenal, or superior mesenteric artery. The cystic artery can pass posterior or anterior to the CBD to supply the gallbladder. Although variable, the cystic artery generally lies superior to the cystic duct and is usually associated with a lymph node, known as Calot node (Fig. 55.6). This node can be enlarged in the setting of gallbladder disease, whether inflammatory or neoplastic, due to the fact that it provides the lymphatic drainage of the gallbladder.

The blood supply of the common hepatic duct and CBD comes from the right hepatic and cystic artery. Typically, the right hepatic artery passes posterior to the common hepatic duct to supply the right lobe of the liver. It passes through the triangle of Calot (bordered by the cystic duct, common hepatic duct, and edge of the liver), after crossing the duct. The cystic artery takes off from the right hepatic artery in this triangle, which is at risk for injury during cholecystectomy. It is important to remember that in 20% of the population, there is an accessory or replaced right hepatic artery passing through the portacaval space and ascending to the right lobe along the lateral aspect of the CBD. A pulsatile structure palpated on the most lateral aspect of the porta during a Pringle maneuver identifies this anomaly. In addition, it can be noted on computed tomography (CT) as a vessel passing transversely between the portal vein and inferior vena cava behind the head of the pancreas.

The perfusion to the inferior bile duct, below the duodenal bulb, comes from tributaries of the posterosuperior pancreaticoduodenal and gastroduodenal arteries. The small branches coalesce to form the two vessels that run along the CBD at the 3- and 9-o'clock positions. These vessels can be damaged and leave the bile duct at risk for ischemic injury with close dissection of the areolar tissue surrounding the bile duct.

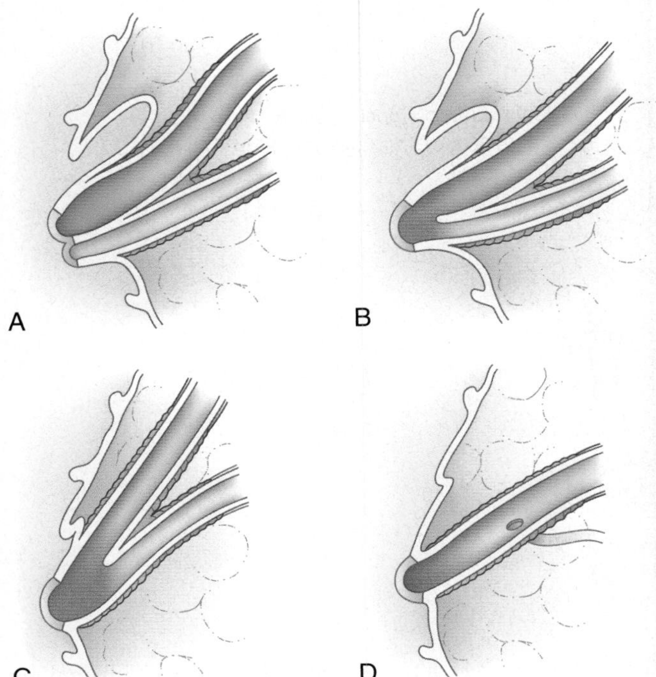

FIG. 55.4 Patterns of biliary duct–pancreatic duct junction and insertion into the duodenal wall. (A) Separate common bile duct (CBD) and pancreatic duct (PD) entry. (B) Joining ducts at the ampula. (C) Joining ducts before the ampula. (D) PD entering the CBD.

Physiology

The smallest functional unit of liver is the hepatic lobule. It is created by four to six portal triads and identified by its central terminal hepatic venule. Each hepatocyte is encircled by bile canaliculi, which coalesce to form small bile ducts, entering portal triad. Bile salts, such as cholic acid and deoxycholic acid, are originally created from cholesterol and secreted into bile canaliculi as cholic acid and its metabolite, deoxycholic acid. The liver actually makes only a small amount of the total bile salt pool used on a daily basis because most bile salts are recycled after use in the intestinal lumen, known as the enterohepatic circulation (Fig. 55.7). Bile is

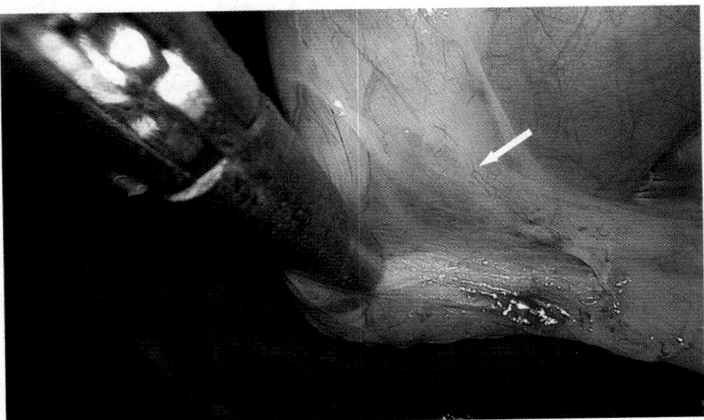

FIG. 55.6 Operative photograph of Calot node. This node *(arrow)* is useful for identification of the common location of the cystic artery.

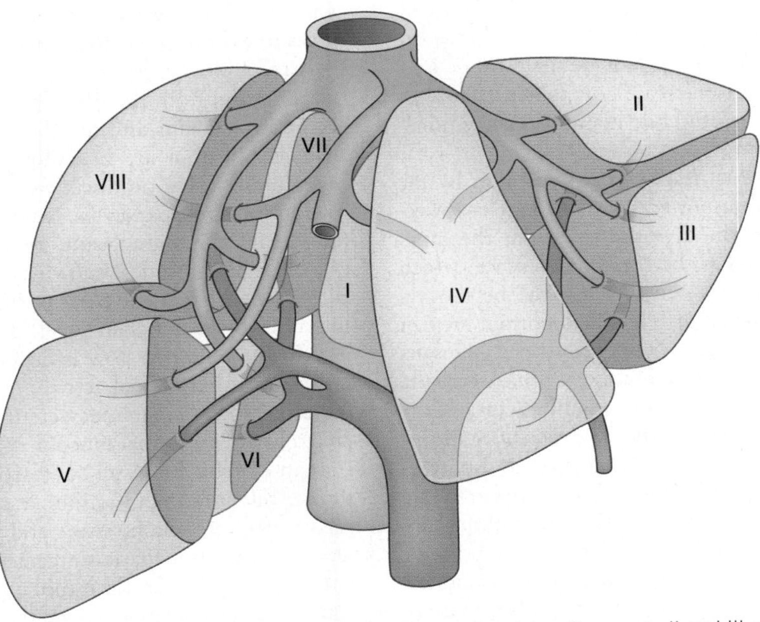

FIG. 55.5 Couinaud segmental anatomy. Segment I is the caudate lobe. Segments II and III are supplied by the lateral branch of the left portal vein, with segment II lying above the passage of the portal vein and segment III below it. Segment IV is supplied by the medial branch of the left portal vein and is further subdivided into IVA above and IVB below the segmental portal vein. Segment V is supplied by the inferior distribution of the anterior branch of the right portal vein, and segment VIII receives flow from the superior distribution of this branch. Similarly, with respect to the posterior branch of the right portal vein, segment VI lies inferior to the portal vein, whereas segment VII lies superior.

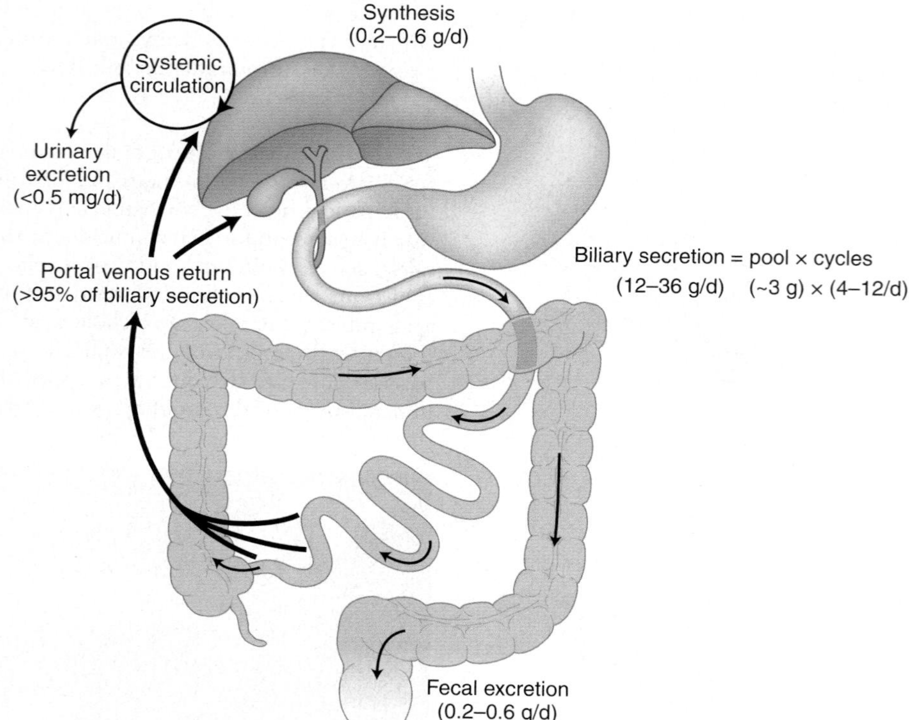

FIG. 55.7 Enterohepatic circulation.

secreted into canaliculi directly from hepatocytes. Once the bile components are secreted into the bile canaliculi, the tight junctions in the biliary tree keep these components within the bile secretory pathway. The secretion of bile components into the biliary tree is a major stimulus to bile flow, and the volume of bile flow is an osmotic process. Because bile salts combine to form spherical pockets, known as micelles, the salts themselves provide no osmotic activity. Instead, the cations that are secreted into the biliary tree along with the bile salt anion provide the osmotic load to draw water into the duct and to increase flow to keep bile electrochemically neutral. For this reason, bile maintains an osmolality approximately comparable to that of plasma.

After passage into the intestinal tract and reabsorption by the terminal ileum, bile acids are transported back to the liver for recycling bound to albumin. On the opposite side from the canalicular surface of the hepatocyte lies the sinusoidal surface, which contacts the space of Disse. In this contact area, the hepatocyte absorbs the circulating components of bile, an important step in the enterohepatic circulation. The passage of reabsorbed bile salts bound to albumin through the space of Disse allows uptake into the hepatocyte in an efficient process that involves sodium cotransport and sodium-independent pathways. In the less specific sodium-independent pathway, a number of organic anions are transported, including unconjugated and indirect bilirubin. The transport of bile salts across the canalicular membrane remains the rate-limiting step in bile salt excretion. Given the vast differences in concentration of bile salts, the transport of bile up an extreme concentration gradient is adenosine triphosphate dependent. Less than 5% of bile salts are lost each day in the stool. When sufficient quantities of bile salts reach the colonic lumen, the powerful detergent activity of the bile salts can cause inflammation and diarrhea. This can sometimes be seen after a cholecystectomy when the speed of the enterohepatic circulation of bile increases and may overwhelm the ability of the terminal ileum to absorb bile salts.

In addition to bile salts, bile contains proteins, lipids, and pigments. The major lipid components of bile are phospholipids and cholesterol. These lipids not only dispose of cholesterol from low- and high-density lipoproteins but also serve to protect hepatocytes and cholangiocytes from the toxic nature of bile. The sources of most biliary cholesterol are circulating lipoproteins and hepatic synthesis. Therefore, the biliary secretion of cholesterol actually serves to excrete cholesterol from the body.

Aside from absorption of nutrients from the intestinal tract, bile secretion from the liver serves an opposing function, namely, excretion of toxins and metabolites from the liver. Bile pigments such as bilirubin are breakdown products of hemoglobin and myoglobin. These products are transported in the blood, bound to albumin, to hepatocytes. Inside hepatocytes, they will be transferred into the endoplasmic reticulum and conjugated to form bilirubin glucuronides, known as conjugated or "direct" bilirubin. Bile pigment gives the color of bile and, when converted to urobilinogen by bacterial enzymes, gives stool its characteristic color.

Much of the bile flow is dependent on neural, humoral, and chemical stimuli. Vagal activity induces bile secretion as does the gastrointestinal hormone secretin. Cholecystokinin (CCK), secreted by the intestinal mucosa, serves to induce biliary tree secretion and gallbladder wall contraction, thereby augmenting excretion of bile into the intestines. Secreted bile will pass through the biliary tree into the intestine and be reabsorbed. The gallbladder serves as an extrahepatic storage site of bile, absorbing water and concentrating bile in an osmotic process performed through the active sodium transport. With the absorption of sodium and water across the gallbladder epithelium, the chemical composition of bile changes in the gallbladder lumen. Increases in cholesterol and calcium concentration calcium lead to decreased stability of phospholipid cholesterol vesicles. The reduced vesicle stability predisposes to nucleation of this stagnant pool of cholesterol and, thus, to cholesterol stone formation. The gallbladder neck and cystic

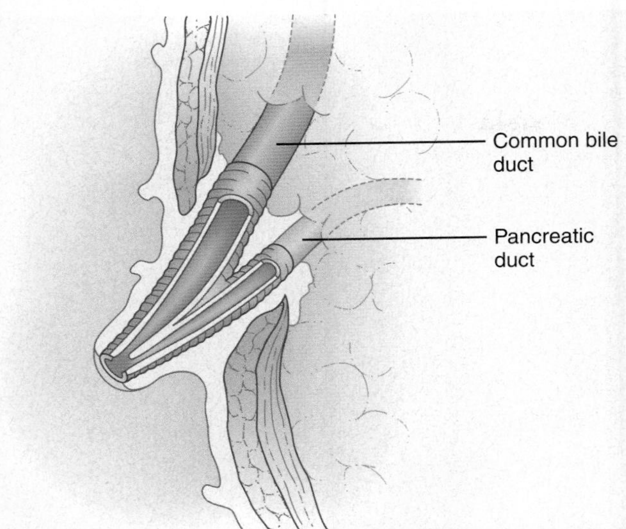

FIG. 55.8 Sphincter of Oddi. Because the sphincter is responsible for control of most bile flow, this sphincter maintains a high tonic contraction but is inhibited by cholecystokinin.

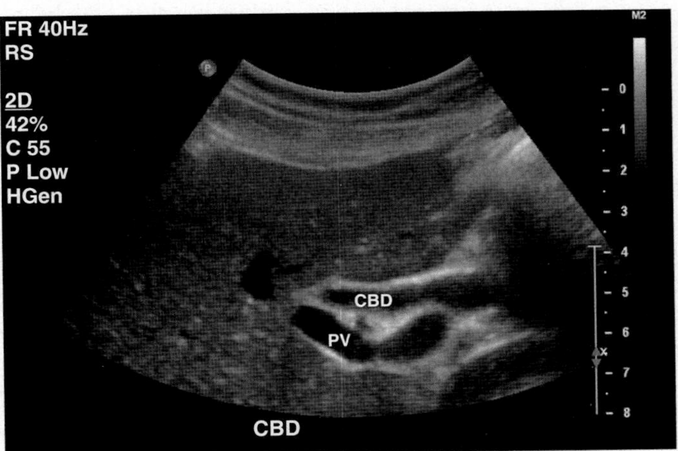

FIG. 55.9 Ultrasound image of dilated biliary tree. The common bile duct *(CBD)* is dilated. As it travels parallel to the portal vein *(PV)*, it is easy to identify. The depiction of the parallel stripes of duct and vein helps ensure that the common duct diameter is not overestimated by a tangential view, which would artificially increase the anteroposterior diameter.

duct also secrete glycoproteins to help protect the gallbladder from the detergent activity of bile. These glycoproteins also promote cholesterol crystallization.

An increase in the activity of the sphincter of Oddi in the fasting state (Fig. 55.8), whose musculature is independent from the duodenal intestinal wall, increases pressure in the CBD, filling the gallbladder, which is capable of storing up to 300 mL of daily bile production, through a retrograde mechanism. This muscular sphincter normally maintains high tonic and phasic activity, which is inhibited by CCK. The passage of fat, protein, and acid into the duodenum induces CCK secretion from duodenal epithelial cells. CCK, as its name suggests, then causes gallbladder contraction, with intraluminal pressures up to 300 mm Hg. Vagal activity also induces gallbladder emptying but is a less powerful stimulus to gallbladder contraction than CCK. At the same time, CCK induces relaxation of the sphincter, causing bile flow more readily from the biliary tree. Coordinated with gallbladder contraction, the relaxation of this sphincter allows evacuation of up to 70% of the gallbladder contents within 2 hours of CCK secretion. During the fasting state, the oblique passage of the bile duct through the duodenal wall and the tonic activity of the sphincter prevent duodenal contents from refluxing into the biliary tree.

BILIARY TREE PATHOPHYSIOLOGY

Laboratory Tests

A hepatic panel tests a number of metabolic and functional aspects of the liver and biliary system.

For example, increase in levels of bilirubin and alkaline phosphatase will be determinative in a cholestatic process, but serum transaminase level is suggestive of hepatocyte physiology.

Hyperbilirubinemia could be secondary to conjugated bilirubin, possibly due to obstruction, or to unconjugated hyperbilirubinemia caused by increased synthesis, impaired hepatocyte uptake of unconjugated bilirubin, and decreased intracellular conjugation. Although this is an oversimplification of a complex process, derangements up to and including conjugation will be manifested as elevated unconjugated bilirubin levels. Elevation in serum bilirubin caused by obstruction of the biliary system will be identifiable in the frenulum of the tongue, sclera, or skin. It is important to check the frenulum first, as the level of bilirubin must reach to 2.5 mg/dL to be seen in sclera and above 5 mg/dL to be manifested in skin.

Imaging Studies

Plain Films

As the simplest radiographic study, plain radiographs are of limited use in the overall evaluation of biliary tree disease. Gallstones are not regularly seen by plain films, and even when they are seen, it rarely changes therapy. Therefore, the role of plain radiographs in the evaluation of possible biliary disease is limited to exclusion of other diagnoses, such as a duodenal ulcer with free air, small bowel obstruction, or right lower lobe pneumonia causing right upper quadrant pain.

Ultrasound

Transabdominal ultrasound is a sensitive, inexpensive, reliable, and reproducible test to evaluate most of the biliary tree, being able to separate patients with medical jaundice, in which the source of hyperbilirubinemia is from hemoglobin breakdown through the process of conjugation, from those with surgical jaundice, in which the hyperbilirubinemia occurs from a blockage of excretion. Therefore, this modality is seen as the study of choice for the initial evaluation of jaundice or symptoms of biliary disease. The finding of a dilated CBD in the setting of jaundice suggests an obstruction of the duct from stones, usually associated with pain, or from a tumor, which is commonly painless (Fig. 55.9). Gallbladder diseases are regularly diagnosed by ultrasound because the superficial location of the gallbladder with no overlying bowel gas enables its evaluation by sound waves. Ultrasound has a high specificity and sensitivity for cholelithiasis, or gallstones. The density of gallstones allows crisp reverberation of the sound wave, showing an echogenic focus with a characteristic shadowing behind the stone (Fig. 55.10). Most gallstones, unless impacted, will move with positional changes in the patient. This feature allows their differentiation from gallbladder polyps, which are fixed, and from sludge, which will move more slowly and does not have the sharp echogenic pattern of gallstones. Pathologic changes seen in many gallbladder diseases can be identified by ultrasound. For example, the gallbladder wall

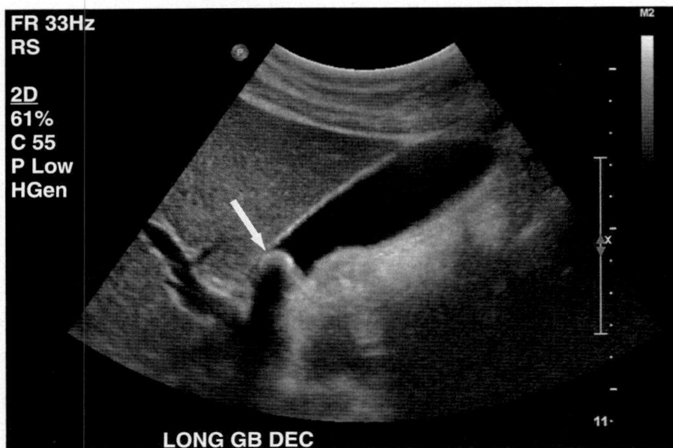

FIG. 55.10 Ultrasound image of a gallstone in the gallbladder neck. The sharp echogenic wall of the gallstone *(arrow)*, with the characteristic posterior shadowing stripe under the stone, helps differentiate it from other intraluminal findings.

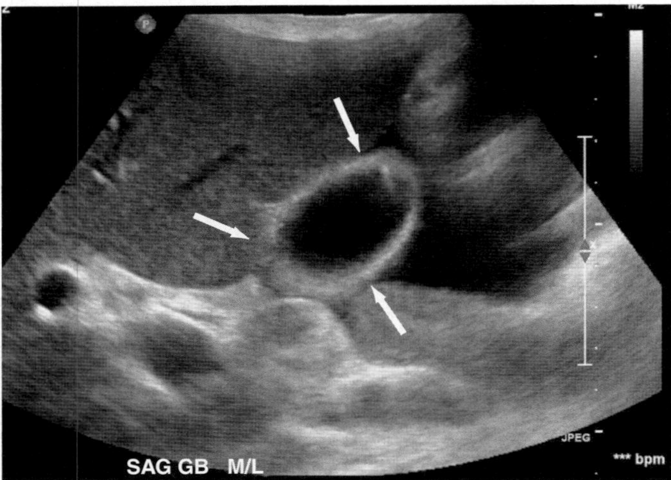

FIG. 55.11 Ultrasound image with acute cholecystitis and thickened gallbladder wall *(arrows)*.

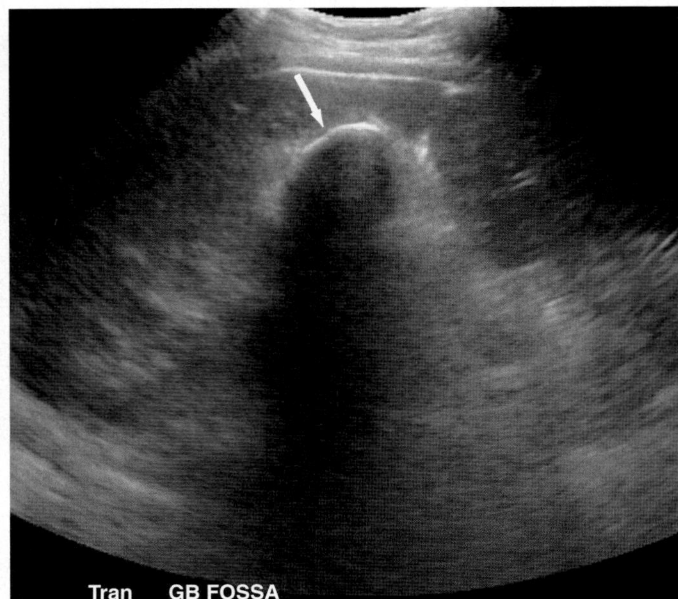

FIG. 55.12 Ultrasound image of porcelain gallbladder. The curvilinear sharp echogenic focus *(arrow)* combined with substantial posterior shadowing helps confirm this diagnosis.

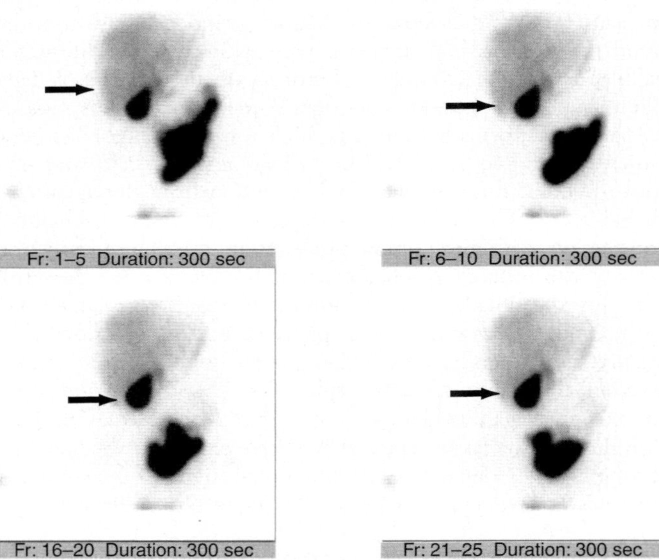

FIG. 55.13 Hepatic iminodiacetic acid scan showing filling of the gallbladder. With gallbladder filling *(arrows)*, the diagnosis of acute cholecystitis is effectively eliminated.

thickening and pericholecystic fluid seen in cholecystitis are visible by ultrasound (Fig. 55.11). Porcelain gallbladder, with its calcified wall, will appear as a curvilinear echogenic focus along the entire gallbladder wall, with posterior shadowing (Fig. 55.12). In addition to the division of medical versus surgical jaundice, ultrasound can sometimes identify the cause of obstructive jaundice, showing CBD stones or even cholangiocarcinoma.

Hepatic Iminodiacetic Acid Scan

Although incapable of providing any precise anatomic delineation, biliary scintigraphy, also known as a hepatic iminodiacetic acid (HIDA) scan, can be used to evaluate the physiologic secretion of bile. The injection of an iminodiacetic acid, which is processed in the liver and secreted with bile, allows identification of bile flow. Therefore, the failure to fill the gallbladder 2 hours after injection demonstrates obstruction of the cystic duct, as seen in acute cholecystitis (Figs. 55.13 and 55.14). In addition, the scan will identify obstruction of the biliary tree and bile leaks, which may be useful in the postoperative setting. HIDA scans can also be used to determine gallbladder function because the injection of CCK during a scan will document physiologic ejection of the gallbladder. This may be useful in patients with biliary tract pain but without stones because some patients have pain from impaired emptying, known as biliary dyskinesia. As a nuclear medicine test, the test demonstrates physiologic flow but does not provide fine anatomic detail, nor can it identify gallstones.

Computed Tomography

Although ultrasound is clearly the first test of choice for delineation of biliary disease, CT provides superior anatomic information and therefore is indicated when more anatomic delineation is required. Because most gallstones are radiographically isodense

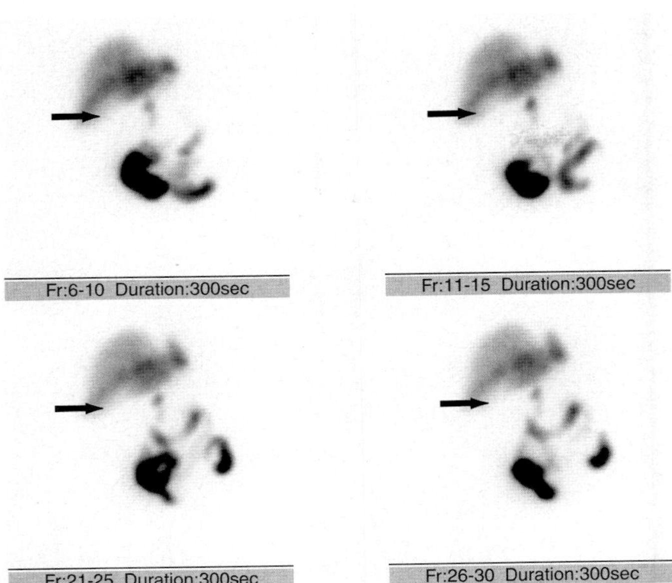

FIG. 55.14 Hepatic iminodiacetic acid (HIDA) scan showing nonfilling of the gallbladder. With no filling of the gallbladder *(arrows)* even on delayed images, HIDA confirms occlusion of the cystic duct, the characteristic feature of acute cholecystitis.

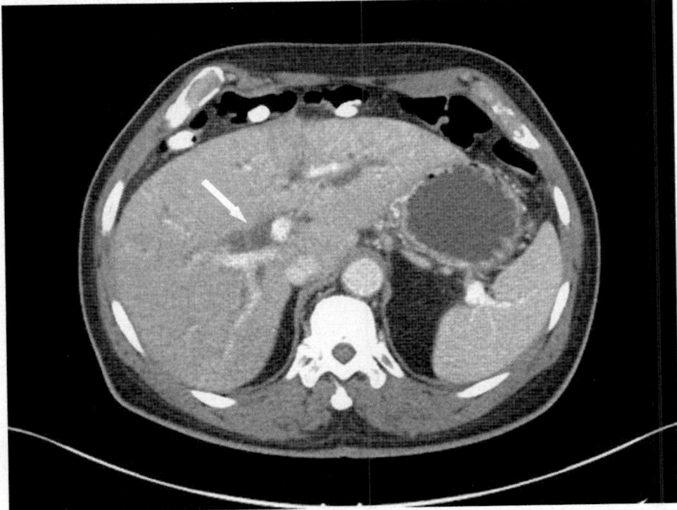

FIG. 55.15 Computed tomography scan showing dilated biliary tree *(arrow)* at the portal confluence. This dilation continued down to the head of the pancreas.

to bile, many will be indistinguishable from bile. However, because ultrasound is operator dependent and provides no anatomic reconstruction of the biliary tree, CT can be used to identify the cause and site of biliary obstruction (Fig. 55.15). When it is performed for the evaluation of hepatic or pancreatic parenchyma or possible neoplastic processes, CT is invaluable in preoperative planning, and the use of arterial phase, portal venous phase, and delayed phase imaging, known as a triple-phase CT, has essentially replaced diagnostic angiography of the liver.

Magnetic Resonance Imaging and Magnetic Resonance Cholangiopancreatography

Magnetic resonance imaging (MRI) uses the water in bile to delineate the biliary tree and thus provides superior anatomic definition

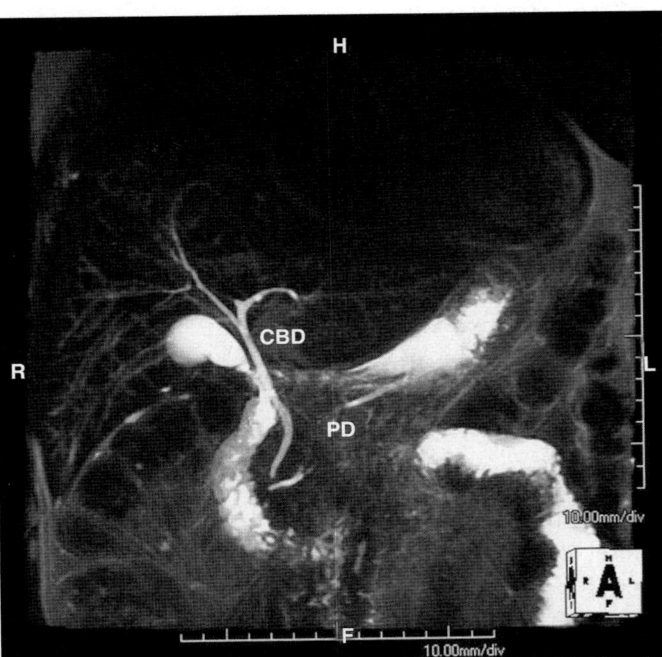

FIG. 55.16 Normal magnetic resonance cholangiopancreatography image. Note the normal common bile duct *(CBD)* and pancreatic duct *(PD)*.

of the intrahepatic and extrahepatic biliary tree and pancreas. Although management of most patients with biliary disease does not require the fine detail of anatomic evaluation shown by cross-sectional imaging, MRI is noninvasive, requires no radiation exposure, and can prove extremely useful in planning resection of biliary or pancreatic neoplasms or management of complex biliary disease. By use of the water content of bile, a cholangiopancreatogram can be created (Fig. 55.16), which makes it an excellent modality for cross-sectional imaging of the biliary tree.

Endoscopic Retrograde Cholangiopancreatography

Endoscopic retrograde cholangiopancreatography (ERCP) is an invasive test using endoscopy and fluoroscopy to inject contrast material through the ampulla to image the biliary tree (Fig. 55.17). Although it does carry a complication rate of up to 10%, its usefulness lies in its ability to diagnose and to treat many diseases of the biliary tree. For patients with malignant obstruction, ERCP can be used to provide tissue samples for diagnosis while also decompressing an obstruction, but it does not stage disease accurately. Many benign diseases, such as choledocholithiasis, can be easily treated by endoscopic means. ERCP has also proven extremely useful in the diagnosis and treatment of complications of biliary surgery.

Percutaneous Transhepatic Cholangiography

Interventional radiologic techniques can be used in the evaluation of biliary anatomy. Similar to ERCP, percutaneous transhepatic cholangiography (PTC) is an invasive procedure used to evaluate the biliary tree. A needle is passed directly into the liver to access one of the biliary radicals, and the tract is then used for contrast imaging and can serve to allow insertion of transhepatic catheters for drainage and sometimes biopsy. It can be useful for patients with intrahepatic biliary disease or in whom ERCP is not technically feasible; PTC can decompress biliary obstruction and stent obstructions nonoperatively and can provide anatomic information for biliary reconstruction (Fig. 55.18).

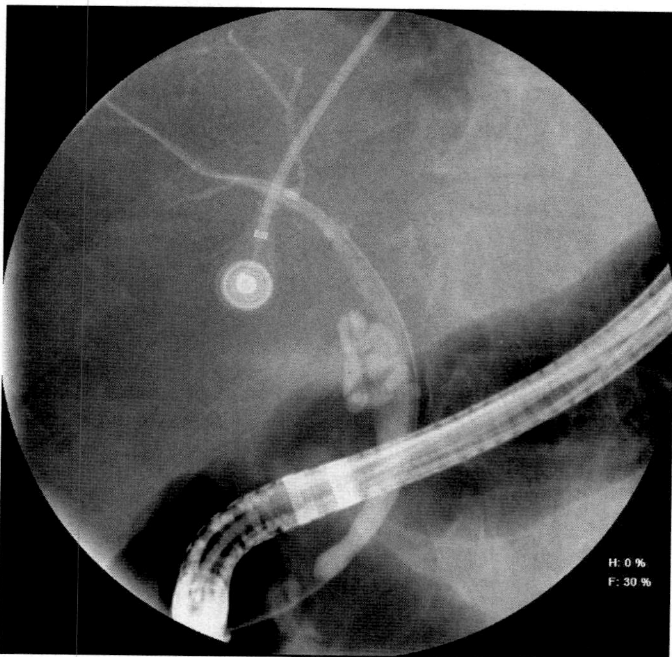

FIG. 55.17 Normal endoscopic retrograde cholangiopancreatography image.

Intraoperative Cholangiography

Another imaging tool for the diagnosis of biliary tract abnormalities is intraoperative cholangiography. With the injection catheter inserted through the cystic duct during a cholecystectomy or through another point in the biliary tree, intraoperative cholangiography can help delineate anomalous biliary anatomy, identify choledocholithiasis, or guide biliary reconstruction. Some surgeons advocate routine cholangiography during cholecystectomy. Advocates for routine cholangiography note that common duct injuries can be identified and managed immediately when cholangiography is used routinely. However, because it adds operative time and fluoroscopic exposure to the operation, many surgeons use intraoperative cholangiography selectively during the performance of a cholecystectomy. Although debated, the routine use of intraoperative cholangiography does not reduce significantly the incidence of injury to the biliary tree during laparoscopic cholecystectomy. Indications for the selective use of cholangiography include pain on the day of operation, abnormal hepatic function panel, anomalous or confusing biliary anatomy, and alteration in anatomy that precludes the ability to perform ERCP after cholecystectomy, such as Roux-en-Y gastric bypass, dilated biliary tree, or any preoperative suspicion of choledocholithiasis (Box 55.1).

Endoscopic Ultrasound

Although of limited use in the evaluation of gallbladder disease or intrahepatic disease of the biliary tree, endoscopic ultrasound is valuable in the assessment of distal CBD and ampulla. With the close apposition of the distal CBD and pancreas to the duodenum, sound waves generated by endoscopic ultrasound provide detailed evaluation of the bile duct and ampulla; this has proved most useful in assessing tumors for invasion into vascular structures. Echoendoscopes are subdivided into those that scan perpendicular to the long axis of the endoscope, known as radial echoendoscopes, and those that scan parallel, known as linear echoendoscopes. Radial echoendoscopes are most useful for providing a tomographic evaluation, whereas linear echoendoscopes

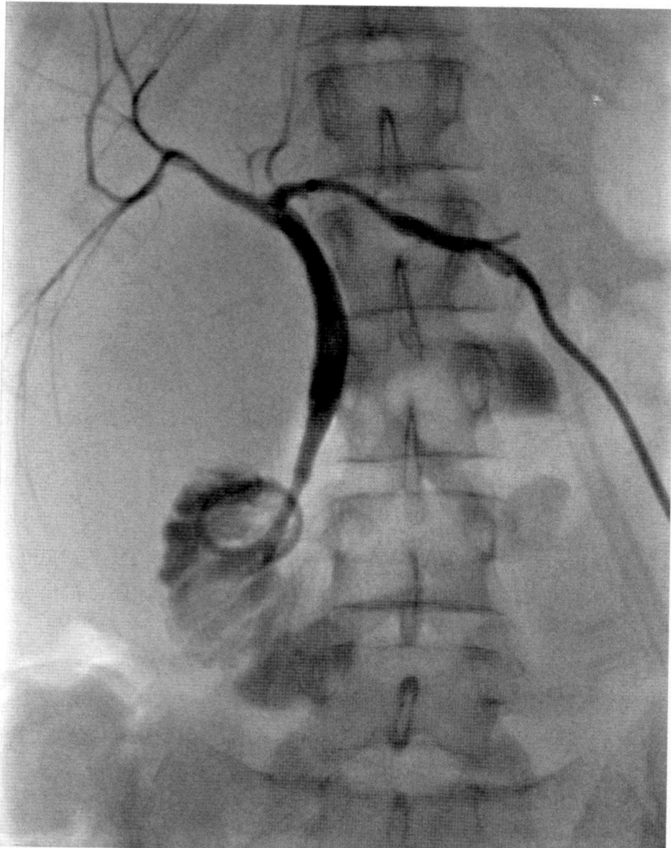

FIG. 55.18 Percutaneous transhepatic cholangiography image of hepatic biliary anatomy.

BOX 55.1 Indications for selective cholangiography.

- Pain at time of operation
- Abnormal hepatic function panel
- Anomalous or confusing biliary anatomy
- Inability to perform postoperative endoscopic retrograde cholangiopancreatography
- Dilated biliary tree
- Any suspicion of choledocholithiasis

can guide interventions such as needle biopsies under real-time ultrasound guidance (Fig. 55.19).

Fluorodeoxyglucose Positron Emission Tomography

Fluorodeoxyglucose positron emission tomography (FDG PET) exploits the metabolic difference between a highly metabolically active tissue, such as a neoplasm, and normal tissue. With the injection of a radiolabeled glucose molecule, FDG PET scans can differentiate benign and malignant lesions, detect recurrence, and identify metastatic disease. Unfortunately, FDG PET is incapable of demonstrating carcinomatosis and, given the high metabolism of the immune system, is of limited value in the setting of infection or inflammation.

Bacteriology

The biliary tree inserts into the duodenum and therefore cannot be considered truly sterile. Through a low bacterial load and with

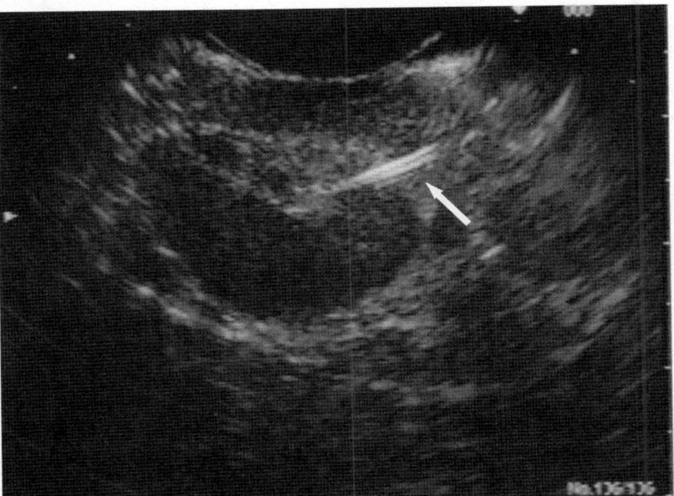

FIG. 55.19 Linear endoscopic ultrasound with needle *(arrow)* biopsy of a lymph node.

the flow of bile, infection in the absence of obstruction is rare. However, with the presence of stones or obstruction, the likelihood of bacterial infection increases. The most common types of bacteria found in biliary infections are Enterobacteriaceae, such as *Escherichia coli*, *Klebsiella*, and *Enterobacter*, followed by *Enterococcus* spp.

Prophylactic antibiotics should be used in most patients undergoing interventions in the biliary tree, such as ERCP or PTC. To cover the most common bacterial species, a first- or second-generation cephalosporin or fluoroquinolone should suffice. For those undergoing elective laparoscopic cholecystectomy for biliary colic, no antibiotic prophylaxis is necessary. However, antibiotics should be used for any patient with suspected or documented infection of the biliary tree, such as acute cholecystitis or ascending cholangitis, and should be chosen to cover gram-negative bacteria and anaerobes.

BENIGN BILIARY DISEASE

Calculous Biliary Disease

Cholelithiasis is the most common disease of gallbladder and biliary tree, affecting 10% to 15% of the population. Gallstones are generally classified into two major subtypes, cholesterol and pigment stones, depending on the principal solute that precipitates into a stone. More than 70% of gallstones in the United States are formed by precipitation of cholesterol and calcium, and pure cholesterol stones account for less than 10%. Pigment stones can be divided into black stones, as seen in hemolytic conditions and cirrhosis, and brown stones, which tend to be found in the bile ducts and are thought to be secondary to infection. The difference in color arises from incorporation of cholesterol into the brown stones. Because black pigment stones occur in hemolytic states from concentration of bilirubin, they are found almost exclusively in the gallbladder. Alternatively, brown stones can occur within the biliary tree and suggest a disorder of biliary motility and associated bacterial infection.

Four major factors explain most gallstone formation: supersaturation of secreted bile, concentration of bile in the gallbladder, crystal nucleation, and gallbladder dysmotility. High concentrations of cholesterol and lipid in bile secretion from the liver constitute one predisposing condition to cholesterol stone formation,

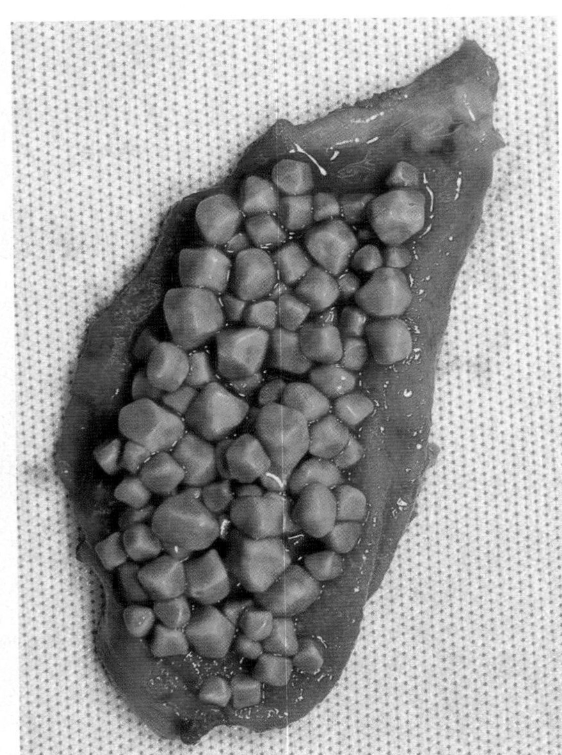

FIG. 55.20 Gallbladder with characteristic yellow cholesterol stones.

whereas increased hemoglobin processing is seen in most patients with pigment stones. Once in the gallbladder, bile is concentrated further through the absorption of water and sodium, increasing the concentrations of the bile solutes and calcium. Bile salts act to solubilize cholesterol. With respect to cholesterol stones (Fig. 55.20), cholesterol precipitates out into crystals when the concentration in the gallbladder vesicles exceeds the solubility of cholesterol (Fig. 55.21).[2] Crystal formation is further accelerated by pronucleating agents, including glycoproteins and immunoglobulins. Finally, abnormal gallbladder motility can increase stasis in the gallbladder, allowing more time for solutes to precipitate in the gallbladder. Therefore, increased stone formation can be seen in conditions associated with impaired gallbladder emptying, such as in prolonged fasting states, with use of total parenteral nutrition, after vagotomy, and with use of somatostatin analogues.

Natural History

Gallstones become symptomatic when they obstruct a visceral structure such as a cystic duct. However, gallstones often remain asymptomatic, only found incidentally on imaging. Biliary colic, caused by temporary blockage of the cystic duct, tends to occur after a meal in which the secretion of CCK leads to gallbladder contraction. Stones that do not obstruct the cystic duct or pass through the entire biliary tree into the intestines without impaction do not cause symptoms. Only 20% to 30% of patients with asymptomatic stones will develop symptoms within 20 years, and because approximately 1% of patients with asymptomatic stones develop complications of their stones before onset of symptoms, prophylactic cholecystectomy is not warranted in asymptomatic patients.

Certain subsets of patients, however, constitute a higher risk pool, so prophylactic cholecystectomy should be considered. Among these are patients with hemolytic anemias, such as sickle

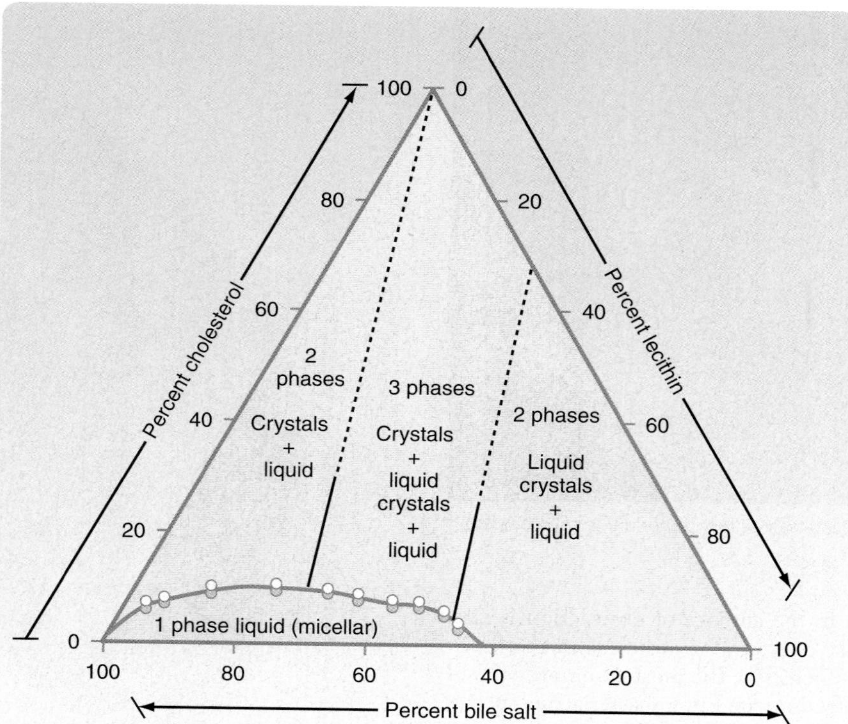

FIG. 55.21 Triangle of solubility. With the three major components of bile that determine cholesterol solubility and stability, each can be quantified by molar percentage to show a relative ratio to the other two. Cholesterol is completely soluble in only the small area in the left lower corner, where a clear micellar solution exists, below the *closed circles*. Just above this, in the area between the *open* and *closed circles*, cholesterol is supersaturated but stable and thus crystallized only with stasis. In the remainder of the triangle, cholesterol is significantly supersaturated and unstable. In this region, crystals form immediately. (From Admirand WH, Small DM. The physicochemical basis of cholesterol gallstone formation in man. *J Clin Invest*. 1968;47:1043–1052.)

cell anemia. These patients have an extremely high rate of pigment stone formation, and cholecystitis can precipitate a crisis. Patients with a calcified gallbladder wall (known as porcelain gallbladder), those with large (>2.5 cm) gallstones, and those with a long common channel of bile and pancreatic ducts all have a higher risk of gallbladder cancer and should consider cholecystectomy. In addition, patients with asymptomatic gallstones undergoing bariatric surgery may also benefit from cholecystectomy; however, it is still controversial. Not only does rapid weight loss favor stone formation, but also, after gastric bypass, ERCP to remove CBD stones in ascending cholangitis is extremely challenging and usually unsuccessful. Also, in diabetic patients with gallstones, one should have lower threshold for cholecystectomy, considering higher rate of gangrene.

Nonoperative Treatment of Cholelithiasis

Medical treatment of gallstones is generally unsuccessful and includes oral bile salt therapy, contact dissolution that requires cannulation of the gallbladder and infusion of organic solvent, and extracorporeal shock wave lithotripsy. With the dissolution strategies, unacceptable recurrence rates of up to 50% limit their application to the most select group of patients. Extracorporeal shock wave lithotripsy has a lower recurrence rate, approximately 20%, and can be used in patients with single stones 0.5 to 2 cm in size. The widespread use, safety, and efficacy of laparoscopic cholecystectomy have relegated nonoperative therapy to patients for whom general anesthesia presents a prohibitively high risk.

Chronic Cholecystitis

Recurrent attacks of biliary colic, with only temporary occlusion of the cystic duct, can cause inflammation and scarring of the neck of the gallbladder and cystic duct. This process causes fibrosis as histologic evidence of repeated self-limited episodes of inflammation and is called chronic cholecystitis. The diagnosis of chronic cholecystitis lies along a continuum with biliary colic because it results from recurrent attacks. Therefore, the presentation is that of symptomatic cholelithiasis, or biliary colic. Pain occurring after ingestion of a fatty meal, with the attendant increase in CCK secretion in response to duodenal intraluminal fat, is classic for biliary colic, although only 50% of patients will report an association with food. Pain from stones tends to locate in the epigastrium or right upper quadrant and may radiate around to the scapula. Biliary colic is a misnomer as the pain is typically constant rather than colicky. These attacks of pain generally last a few hours. Pain lasting longer than 24 hours or associated with fever suggests acute cholecystitis. The pain of biliary colic, even in the absence of cholecystitis, may also cause other gastrointestinal symptoms, such as bloating, nausea, or even vomiting.

Symptomatic stones constitute a risk profile different from that of asymptomatic stones, with a higher likelihood of complications. Therefore, symptomatic cholelithiasis is an indication for cholecystectomy. Documented stones and symptoms are the most common indications to perform a cholecystectomy.

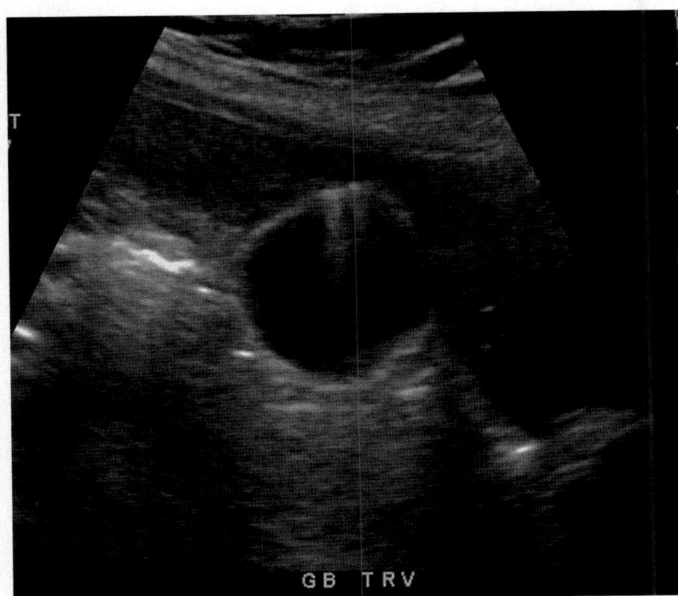

FIG. 55.22 Ultrasound image of cholesterolosis.

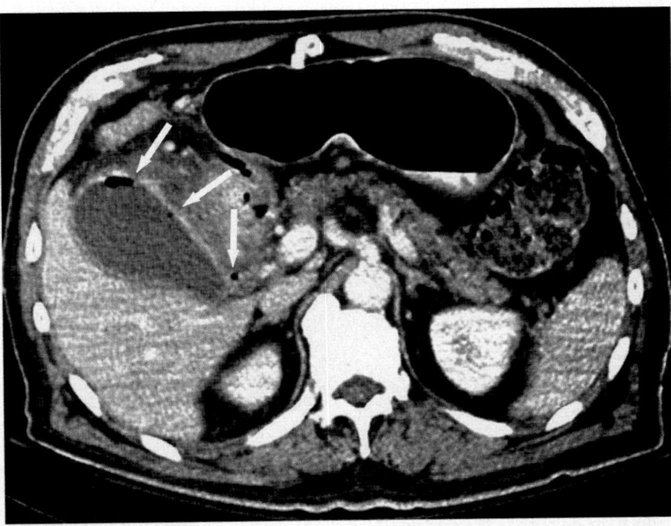

FIG. 55.23 Computed tomography scan of emphysematous cholecystitis. Significant pericholecystic inflammatory changes and air in the gallbladder wall *(arrows)* are signs of emphysematous cholecystitis.

Diagnosis

The diagnosis of chronic cholecystitis relies on a history consistent with biliary tract disease. Transabdominal ultrasonography reliably documents the presence of cholelithiasis. Ultrasound can provide other important information, such as CBD dilation, gallbladder polyps, porcelain gallbladder, or evidence of hepatic parenchymal processes. Cholesterolosis, or the accumulation of cholesterol found in gallbladder mucosal macrophages, can also be seen (Fig. 55.22). Even in the absence of frank stones, so-called sludge found in the gallbladder on ultrasonography, with appropriate symptoms, is consistent with biliary colic.

Treatment

Patients with sufficient symptoms from gallstones should undergo elective cholecystectomy. Cholecystectomy carries a low-risk profile but is not without complications, so an analysis of risks and benefits is important. Because patients with mild symptoms have a low rate of complications from gallstones (1%–3%/year), observation and dietary and lifestyle changes are appropriate in this population. Patients with more severe or recurrent symptoms have a higher rate of complications of the disease (7%/year), so elective laparoscopic cholecystectomy is warranted. In more than 90% of patients, cholecystectomy is curative, leaving them symptom free.

Acute Calculous Cholecystitis

Acute cholecystitis is the result of a blockage of the cystic duct and is called acute calculous cholecystitis when the blockage is by a stone. In chronic cholecystitis or biliary colic, the blockage is temporary and repetitive, while in acute cholecystitis, the blockage does not resolve, leading to inflammation with edema and subserosal hemorrhage. Obstruction is followed by infection of the stagnant pool of bile. Without resolution of the obstruction, the gallbladder will progress to ischemia and necrosis. Eventually, acute cholecystitis becomes acute gangrenous cholecystitis and, when complicated by infection with a gas-forming organism, acute emphysematous cholecystitis (Fig. 55.23).

Presentation

The inflammatory changes in the gallbladder wall are manifested as fever and right upper quadrant pain. On exam, patients will exhibit tenderness to palpation and guarding in the right upper quadrant. When the gallbladder lumen cannot fully empty because of a stone in the gallbladder neck, visceral pain fibers are activated, causing pain in the epigastrium or right upper quadrant. The same luminal obstruction of biliary colic but associated with sufficient stasis, pressure, and bacterial inoculum creates infection and, thereby, inflammation, therefore progressing to acute cholecystitis. With this infection and inflammation, the right upper quadrant pain of biliary colic will be accompanied by tenderness noted on palpation of the right upper quadrant. Specifically, the voluntary cessation of respiration when the examiner exerts constant pressure under the right costal margin, known as a Murphy sign, suggests inflammation of the visceral and parietal peritoneal surfaces and can be seen in diseases such as acute cholecystitis and hepatitis. Alternatively, biliary colic in the absence of infection and inflammation is not associated with any reproducible physical examination finding or systemic symptom.

There have been multiple grading systems evaluating severity of cholecystitis, most commonly the Tokyo Guidelines[3,4] and The American Association for the surgery of Trauma (AAST) Emergency General Surgery (EGS) guidelines.[5] AAST EGS categorizes acute cholecystitis into five grades, grade 1 being localized inflammation, to grade 5 with pericholecystic abscess, bilioenteric fistula, and peritonitis. The Tokyo Guidelines also grade the systemic effect of cholecystitis such as organ failure. Both classifications are helpful to categorize the management of these patients and consider treatment options relative to their severity of disease.

Mild elevations of alkaline phosphatase, bilirubin, and transaminase levels and leukocytosis support the diagnosis of acute cholecystitis. However, given that the CBD is not obstructed, profound jaundice in the setting of a picture of acute cholecystitis is rare and should raise the suspicion of cholangitis. Mirizzi syndrome should be suspected, in which inflammation or a stone in the gallbladder neck leads to inflammation of the adjoining biliary system, with obstruction of the common hepatic duct.

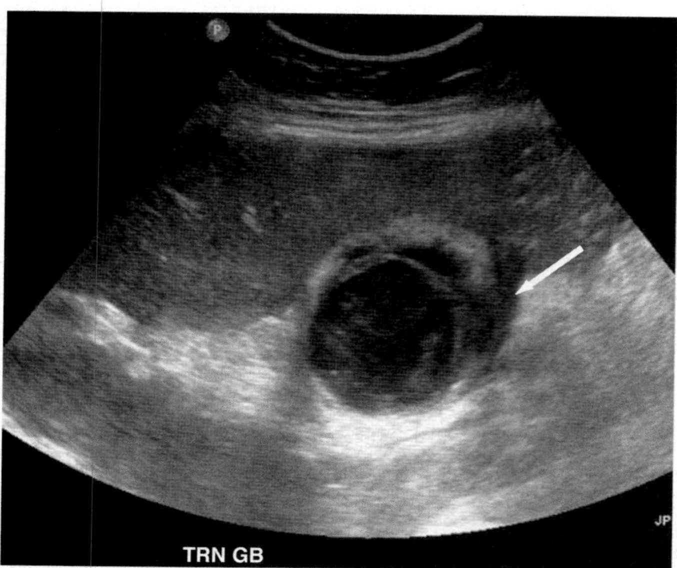

FIG. 55.24 Ultrasound image of pericholecystic fluid. The thickened gallbladder wall with pericholecystic fluid *(arrow)* indicates acute cholecystitis.

Diagnosis

Transabdominal ultrasonography is a sensitive, inexpensive, and reliable tool for the diagnosis of acute cholecystitis, with a sensitivity of 85% and specificity of 95%. In addition to identifying gallstones, ultrasound can demonstrate pericholecystic fluid (Fig. 55.24), gallbladder wall thickening, and even a sonographic Murphy sign, documenting tenderness specifically over the gallbladder. In most cases, an accurate history and physical examination, along with supporting laboratory studies and an ultrasound examination, make the diagnosis of acute cholecystitis. In atypical cases, a HIDA scan may be used to demonstrate obstruction of the cystic duct, which definitively diagnoses acute cholecystitis. Filling of the gallbladder during a HIDA scan essentially eliminates the diagnosis of cholecystitis. CT may show similar findings to ultrasound with pericholecystic fluid, gallbladder wall thickening, and emphysematous changes, but CT is less sensitive than ultrasound for the diagnosis of acute cholecystitis.

Treatment

Treatment of acute cholecystitis largely depends on the severity of disease and the physiologic status of the patient, and treatment can vary from immediate surgical intervention to conservative management. Although the primary pathophysiologic event in acute cholecystitis is the obstruction of the cystic duct and infection is a secondary event that follows stasis and inflammation, most cases of acute cholecystitis are complicated by superinfection of the inflamed gallbladder. Patients are given nothing by mouth, and intravenous (IV) fluids and parenteral antibiotics are started. Given that gram-negative aerobes are the most common organisms found in acute cholecystitis, followed by anaerobes and gram-positive aerobes, broad-spectrum antibiotics are warranted. Parenteral narcotics are usually required to control the pain.

Cholecystectomy, whether open or laparoscopic, is the treatment of choice for acute cholecystitis. The timing of operative intervention in acute cholecystitis has long been a source of debate. In the past, many surgeons advocated for delayed cholecystectomy with patients managed nonoperatively during their initial hospitalization and discharged home with resolution of symptoms. An interval cholecystectomy was then performed at approximately 6 weeks after the initial episode. More recent studies have shown that early in the disease process (within the first week), the operation can be performed laparoscopically with equivalent or improved morbidity, mortality, and length of stay as well as a similar conversion rate to open cholecystectomy.[6] In addition, approximately 20% of patients initially admitted for nonoperative management failed to respond to medical treatment before the planned interval cholecystectomy and required surgical intervention. Initial nonoperative therapy remains a viable option for patients who present in a delayed fashion and should be decided on an individual basis.

Given the inflammatory process occurring in the porta hepatis, early conversion to open cholecystectomy should be considered when delineation of anatomy is not clear or when progress cannot be made laparoscopically. With substantial inflammation, a partial cholecystectomy, transecting the gallbladder at the infundibulum with cauterization of the remaining mucosa, is acceptable to avoid injury to the CBD. Some patients present with acute cholecystitis but have a prohibitively high operative risk. For these patients, a percutaneously placed cholecystostomy tube should be considered. Frequently performed with ultrasound guidance under local anesthesia with some sedation, cholecystostomy can act as a temporizing measure by draining the infected bile. Percutaneous drainage results in improvement in symptoms and physiology, allowing a delayed cholecystectomy 3 to 6 months after medical optimization. In patients with cholecystostomy tubes, when fluoroscopy shows a patent cystic duct, the cholecystostomy tube can be removed and the decision for cholecystectomy determined by the patient's ability to tolerate surgical intervention.

Tokyo Guidelines, revised in 2018, predict the severity of gallbladder disorder, prognosis, and rate of conversion or bail-out procedure, can be used as a guideline to plan the management.[7]

Choledocholithiasis

CBD stones, or choledocholithiasis, are generally silent, and are seen in up to 10% of patients undergoing biliary imaging.[8,9] Primary common duct stones arise de novo in the bile duct, and secondary common duct stones pass from the gallbladder into the bile duct. Primary common duct stones are generally brown pigment stones, a combination of precipitated bile pigments and cholesterol. Brown pigment stones are associated with bacterial infections where free bilirubin is formed by hydrolyzing enzymes released by bacteria and then precipitates. Brown pigment stones are more common in Asian populations. Secondary stones are more common in the United States. Retained stones are secondary stones found in bile duct within 2 years of cholecystectomy and occur in 1% to 2% of patients (Fig. 55.25).

When symptomatic, common duct stones clinical manifestations range from biliary colic to obstructive jaundice, including darkening of the urine, scleral icterus, and lightening of the stools. Jaundice with choledocholithiasis is more likely to be painful because the onset of obstruction is acute, causing rapid distention of the bile duct and activation of pain fibers. Cholangitis, first described by Jean Martin Charcot in 1877, is ascending infection of CBD secondary to obstruction and increased intraluminal pressure. Cholangitis presents with right upper quadrant pain, fever, and jaundice, known as Charcot triad, and may progress to septic shock with mental status changes, and hypotension, known as Reynolds pentad, which is an ominous sign, and mortality approaches 100% without prompt treatment.

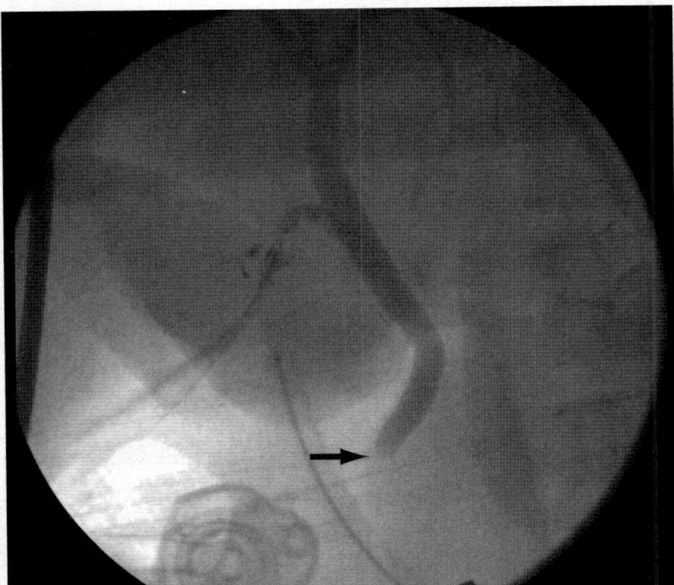

FIG. 55.25 Intraoperative cholangiogram showing choledocholithiasis in an asymptomatic patient with no filling of duodenum and outline of stone *(arrow)*.

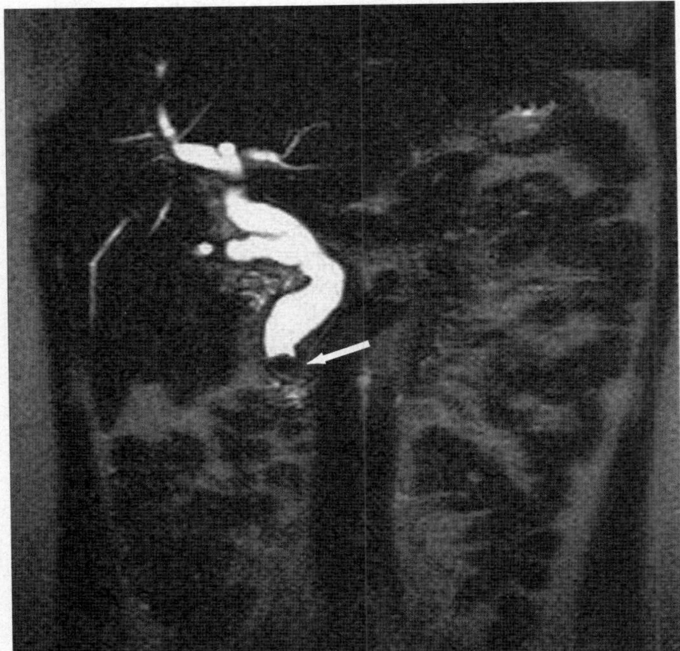

FIG. 55.26 Magnetic resonance cholangiopancreatography with choledocholithiasis. The dilated common bile duct ends abruptly with a convex intraluminal filling defect *(arrow)* consistent with choledocholithiasis.

Diagnosis

Asymptomatic choledocholithiasis is usually an incidental finding. Biliary type pain, jaundice, an abnormal liver function panel, and a dilated bile duct, usually more than 8 mm, are all highly suggestive of choledocholithiasis. Liver function panel abnormalities on their own are neither sensitive nor specific. Even without symptoms of biliary colic, a dilated bile duct in the presence of gallstones suggests choledocholithiasis.

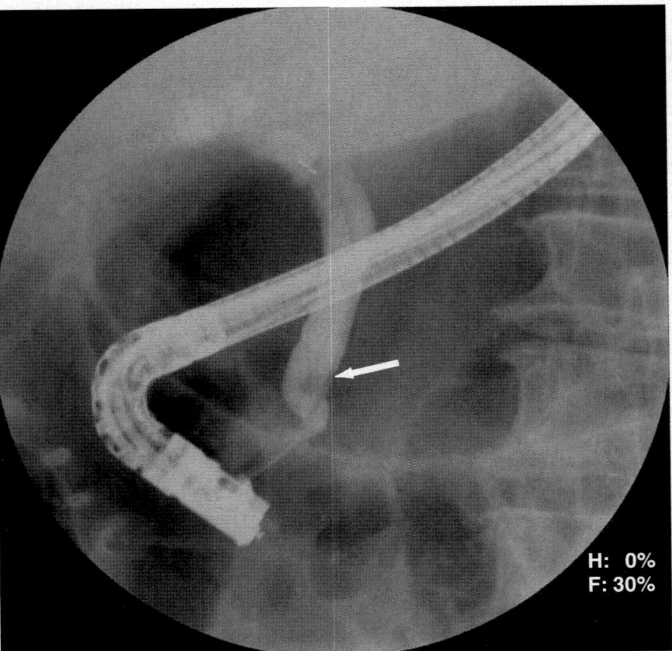

FIG. 55.27 Endoscopic retrograde cholangiopancreatography (ERCP) with choledocholithiasis. With retrograde injection of contrast material, a filling defect noted within the lumen of the common bile duct *(arrow)* identifies choledocholithiasis. ERCP can also be used to remove the stone through sphincterotomy and balloons or baskets.

Magnetic resonance cholangiopancreatography (MRCP), as mentioned earlier, is highly sensitive (>90%) and specific (>99%) in identifying CBD stones (Fig. 55.26). But as a noninvasive test, it will stay at diagnostic level, and a treatment procedure, such as ERCP or CBD exploration, still has to be done after diagnosis. Some surgeons resorted to preoperative MRCP to determine the need for preoperative ERCP.[10]

ERCP is also highly sensitive and specific for choledocholithiasis (Fig. 55.27) and often is the therapeutic procedure by clearing the duct in more than 75% of patients during first procedure and in 90% with repeated ERCP. A sphincterotomy with a balloon sweep is done and stones are extracted, with a less than 5% to 8% complication rate. Indications for preoperative ERCP include cholangitis, biliary pancreatitis, and patients with multiple comorbidities. However, some studies have suggested higher risk of surgical site infection in patients who receive preoperative ERCP before cholecystectomy.[11]

Finding of choledocholithiasis via intraoperative cholangiogram during cholecystectomy may be managed by either CBD exploration or postoperative ERCP. The experience of the surgeon with open biliary exploration may be a factor determining which route is chosen.

PTC can also be used to treat choledocholithiasis in case of unsuccessful ERCP, or anatomical difficulty for ERCP such as the patients' post-Roux-en-Y procedures. PTC is as effective as ERCP in patients with dilated biliary system with similar complication rate, but less effective in a nondilated biliary tree patient.

In short, in patients with likelihood of CBD stones, other modalities such as ERCP or MRCP must be considered on top of ultrasound. Choledocholithiasis identified but not removed during cholecystectomy mandates ERCP for stone extraction.

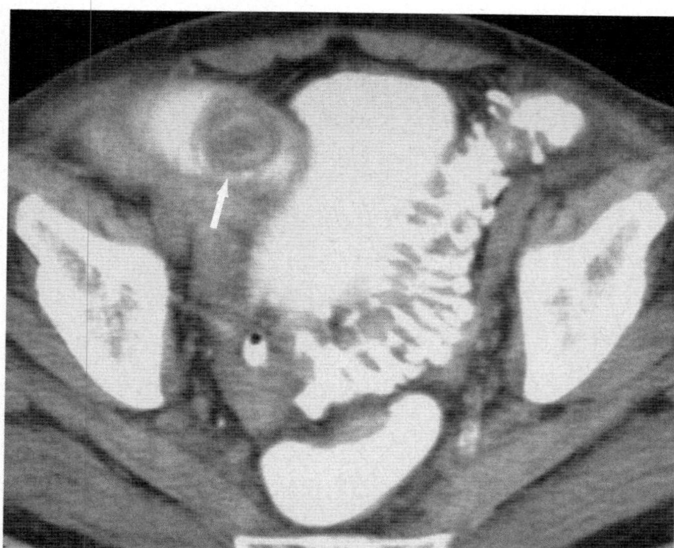

FIG. 55.28 Computed tomography scan of stone *(arrow)* obstructing the distal ileum.

Treatment

Treatment for choledocholithiasis is generally ERCP or CBD exploration, which can be performed via laparoscopic or open technique. Endoscopic sphincterotomy with stone extraction is effective for the treatment of choledocholithiasis. In the preoperative setting, it can clear the duct of stones, and when it is unsuccessful at removal of all stones, it will alter intraoperative decision-making. More than half of patients managed by ERCP without cholecystectomy will have recurrent symptoms of biliary tract disease.[12] Large stones (usually more than 2.5 cm), altered gastric or duodenal anatomy such as Roux-en-Y, impacted stones, intrahepatic stones, or multiple stones, are the most common causes of failure of ERCP.

Gallstone Pancreatitis

When a stone passes from the bile duct through the ampulla into the duodenum, this may cause secondary injury to the pancreas. Temporary elevation of the pancreatic duct pressure causes inflammation and may result in severe pancreatic injury. Symptoms usually persist even after passage of stone. Ultrasound usually shows gallstones, choledocholithiasis, or a dilated CBD. The offending stone usually passes spontaneously but the injury still can be severe. In most cases of gallstone pancreatitis, the pancreatitis is self-limited. Early ERCP to remove a stone that may not have passed is indicated and has been shown to reduce the morbidity of the episode of pancreatitis.[13] To prevent a future episode of gallstone pancreatitis, a cholecystectomy is warranted; this is generally recommended during the same hospitalization, just before discharge.[14] Given the suspicion of choledocholithiasis, intraoperative cholangiography should be performed if no other imaging has been performed to confirm the passage of the gallstone.

Gallstone Ileus

A misnomer, gallstone ileus is in fact a mechanical intestinal obstruction secondary to a gallstone. A large stone in the dependent portion of the gallbladder fistulizes into the adjacent duodenum, passing directly into the intestine. This usually happens in older patients and can be caused by inflammation or simply pressure necrosis. The most common site for obstruction is in the terminal ileum before entering the cecum (Fig. 55.28). The common presentation is an elderly patient with some history of biliary tree disorder, with no past surgical history or hernia, with a sudden mechanical small intestine obstruction.

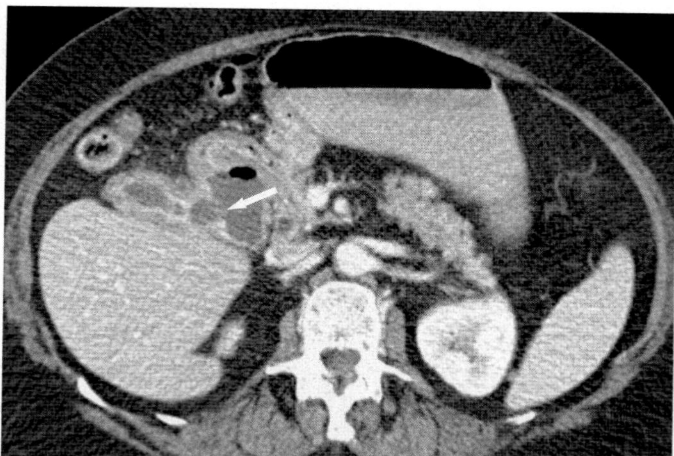

FIG. 55.29 Computed tomography scan of the cholecystoduodenal fistula *(arrow)*.

Although most patients will have constant pain from the obstruction, others can present with only episodic discomfort because the gallstone only intermittently obstructs the intestinal tract. Plain radiographs usually demonstrate air-fluid levels consistent with a small bowel obstruction, although the offending stone may or may not be identified. Pneumobilia, which may sometimes be identified only by CT scan, is a ubiquitous finding because the fistula that permitted a stone to pass into the duodenum allows air to enter the biliary tree (Fig. 55.29).

Treatment

Gallstone ileus is a surgical disorder. During an exploration, a longitudinal incision on the antimesenteric border of the ileum is made a few centimeters proximal to the stone. This site of impaction is at risk of perforation, so signs of ischemia may mandate resection. The stone is milked back through the enterotomy. Approximately 10% of patients have multiple large stones, so the remainder of the small intestine should be inspected.

Although some surgeons advocate surgical treatment of the biliary-enteric fistula at the same setting, the intense inflammatory process in the right upper quadrant may complicate the cholecystectomy and duodenal repair. In addition, because most of these patients are older, their overall physiologic status may not permit fistula repair in the emergent setting. One-stage repair should generally be performed in healthy patients without severe inflammatory changes in the right upper quadrant. Enterotomy with removal of the offending stone should suffice for patients with multiple comorbidities. Palpation of the remaining small intestine should be performed to exclude a second stone that could cause recurrent obstruction. A second operation for the cholecystectomy can be considered to avoid the possibility of future biliary complications.

Noncalculous Biliary Disease

Acute Acalculous Cholecystitis

Blockage of the cystic duct in the absence of stones is called acalculous cholecystitis. The exact mechanism and pathophysiology are poorly understood, but there is a role for bile stasis and gallbladder ischemia. Risk factors include old age, burns and trauma, prolonged

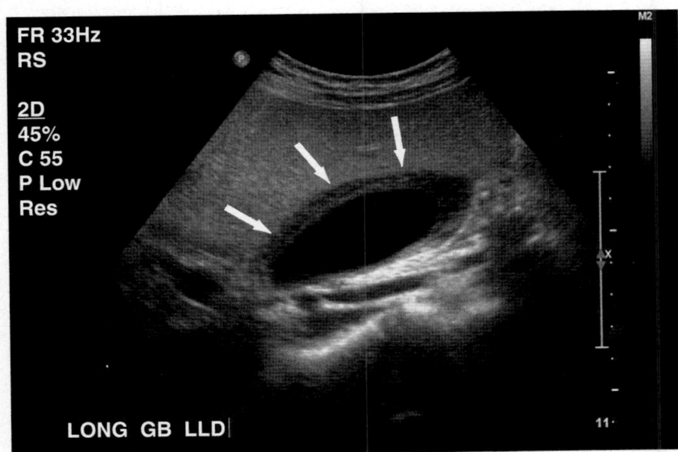

FIG. 55.30 Ultrasound image of a gallbladder with acute acalculous cholecystitis. The diffusely thickened gallbladder wall *(arrows)* is highly suggestive of cholecystitis.

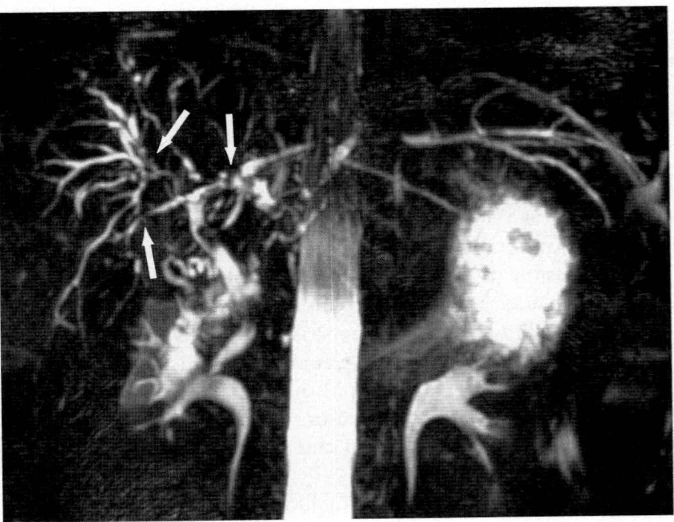

FIG. 55.31 Magnetic resonance cholangiopancreatography showing primary sclerosing cholangitis. Note the multilevel strictures *(arrows)*.

use of *total parenteral nutrition*, critical illness, immunosuppression, and diabetes, and the presentation can be similar or more fulminant than calculous cholecystitis and may progress to gangrenous gallbladder. Critically ill patients with acalculous cholecystitis may not have right upper quadrant pain and any fever with unknown origin in critically ill patients, especially with pericholecystic fluid and gallbladder wall thickening on imaging should raise suspicion for this disorder (Fig. 55.30). HIDA scan is diagnostic for acalculous cholecystitis but can have false-positive result. Treatment of acalculous cholecystitis is similar to that of calculous cholecystitis, with cholecystectomy being therapeutic. However, many of these patients are critically ill, raising the mortality and morbidity of this procedure. Therefore, percutaneous cholecystostomy tube placement under imaging to drain the gallbladder is a much more attractive and feasible treatment. More than 90% of these patients improve with a cholecystostomy tube, and interval cholecystectomy is necessary only if follow-up imaging continues to demonstrate the positive findings.

Biliary Dyskinesia

Biliary dyskinesia is a functional disorder of the biliary tree, generally defined by gallbladder dysmotility, and it is usually a diagnosis of exclusion. Patients may present with classic symptoms of calculous biliary disease but have no ultrasonographic evidence of stones or sludge. In some of these cases, the dysfunction of the gallbladder creates pain, even in the absence of stones. Rome criteria, which was defined in the late 1980s and has been updated multiple times,[15] helps in defining and diagnosing this functional disorder. Other diagnosis must be excluded first using different modalities such as CT and endoscopy. CCK-stimulated HIDA scan is helpful in confirming diagnosis. An ejection fraction of less than one third at 20 minutes after CCK administration in a patient without stone is considered diagnostic. More than 85% of patients show improvement in symptoms after cholecystectomy. In nonresponders, ERCP with sphincterotomy may prove useful.

Sphincter of Oddi Dysfunction

Similar to dyskinesia, sphincter of Oddi dysfunction is a functional disorder of the biliary tree; however, Rome IV criteria[15] recommends not using the term *functional*. It is caused by a structurally or physiologically abnormal sphincter with higher tone and failing to relax, manifested by pain, and recurrent pancreatitis with a usually normal liver function panel. Risk factors include chronic pancreatitis or calculous disease, which can cause fibrosis due to inflammation, and, subsequently, failure of the sphincter to relax. The diagnosis of sphincter of Oddi dysfunction should be suspected in patients with biliary pain and a common duct diameter of more than 12 mm. The bile duct in these patients tends to increase in diameter in response to CCK, as does the pancreatic duct after secretin administration. Sphincter manometry has also been used to make the diagnosis, with sphincter pressure higher than 40 mm Hg predicting good response to therapy. Therapy consists of endoscopic sphincterotomy or transduodenal sphincteroplasty with approximately equivalent results from the two approaches. In patients with objective evidence of sphincter of Oddi dysfunction, division of the sphincter will improve or resolve the pain in 60% to 80% of patients.

Primary Sclerosing Cholangitis

Primary sclerosing cholangitis (PSC) is an idiopathic disorder and considered an autoimmune process affecting the biliary tree. PSC is associated with other autoimmune disorders such as ulcerative colitis (in almost 70% of patients)[16] and Riedel thyroiditis.[17] PSC can be categorized into four anatomical subtypes depending on the level of biliary tree it involves, including intrahepatic, extrahepatic, combined, or small ducts disease. The course of PSC is characterized by progressive chronic cholestasis and advances at an unpredictable rate to biliary cirrhosis and eventually death from liver failure. With improved understanding of the disease and early diagnosis, PSC outcomes have improved.[17]

Clinical presentation. Most patients present with general symptoms such as fatigue and pruritus, but abnormal liver function studies are usually what prompts biliary imaging. Approximately 80% of patients have elevated perinuclear antineutrophil cytoplasmic antibodies, but the severity of disease does not correlate to titer levels. Abnormal liver function tests in a patient observed for inflammatory bowel disease should suggest PSC.

Imaging with cholangiography demonstrates a multifocal diffuse dilation and stricturing of the intrahepatic and/or extrahepatic biliary trees. This pattern is called "beading" or "chain of lakes" and is characteristic of PSC. MRCP is useful in the diagnosis and surveillance of PSC patients, while ERCP is reserved for the treatment of dominant strictures and to exclude malignancy, namely, cholangiocarcinoma (Fig. 55.31).

Liver biopsy tends to show an onionskin concentric periductal fibrosis. With disease progression, periportal fibrosis occurs, progressing to bridging necrosis and, eventually, biliary cirrhosis. Unfortunately, PSC is associated with cholangiocarcinoma, and distinguishing the strictures of PSC fibrosis from those of cholangiocarcinoma can be challenging.

Treatment. Ursodeoxycholic acid is commonly used as medical therapy for PSC and has demonstrated some improvement in liver function tests; however, it is controversial whether this alters the progression of disease. Ongoing trials in PSC include ursodeoxycholic acid homologs, antibiotics to alter the microbiome, and interruption of the enterohepatic bile circulation.[17] However, none of these agents has shown a consistent clinical benefit. In the symptomatic patient, endoscopic therapy, consisting of balloon dilation of the dominant strictures, has been shown to alleviate pruritus, to reduce likelihood of cholangitis, and even to prolong survival.

Surgical treatment options include biliary reconstruction in symptomatic patients with focal extrahepatic disease in some cases. Such patients are rare, and repeated operations for drainage have been shown to complicate definitive treatment by liver transplantation. Therefore, the use of biliary reconstructive procedures has decreased for this indication.

Although it is associated with ulcerative colitis, a proctocolectomy does not appear to affect biliary disease progression or survival in patients with both ulcerative colitis and PSC.

Orthotopic liver transplantation appears to be the only lifesaving option for patients with progressive hepatic dysfunction from PSC. The survival rate for patients undergoing liver transplantation for PSC is approximately equivalent to that of those undergoing transplantation for other causes of end-stage liver disease, with 5-year survival rates ranging from 75% to 85%.[18] Although the development of cholangiocarcinoma in a PSC liver is generally considered a contraindication to transplantation, some centers have shown excellent survival rates, up to 70% at 5 years, for patients with limited hilar disease who undergo a neoadjuvant protocol of chemotherapy and radiation followed by transplantation.[19] Because these results have not been reproduced universally, the use of liver transplantation for the treatment of cholangiocarcinoma occurring in the setting of PSC is limited to experimental protocols. After liver transplantation, 10% to 30% of PSC patients develop recurrent biliary strictures, suggestive of recurrence of disease in the donor liver. Even with the development of strictures, disease progression does not usually follow the aggressive course for which PSC is known. In cases where retransplantation is required, the morbidity and mortality are higher than for primary transplantation.

Biliary Strictures

Benign strictures can occur anywhere along the intrahepatic or extrahepatic portions of the biliary tree. Intrahepatic strictures are usually a result of cholangiohepatitis and/or ischemic events. Any inflammatory of ischemic process along the length of the CBD may cause an extrahepatic stricture. Chronic pancreatitis can cause strictures in the intrapancreatic portion of CBD and are usually long (2–4 cm) with gradually tapered narrowing. Stricturing at the middle portion of CBD is usually associated with a gallbladder process. The most common reason is iatrogenic and postcholecystectomy, reported in 0.1% to 1% of postcholecystectomy patients.[20] Alternatively, Mirizzi syndrome is a large stone in Hartmann pouch of the gallbladder, compressing the adjacent bile duct and leading to biliary obstruction (Fig. 55.32). These

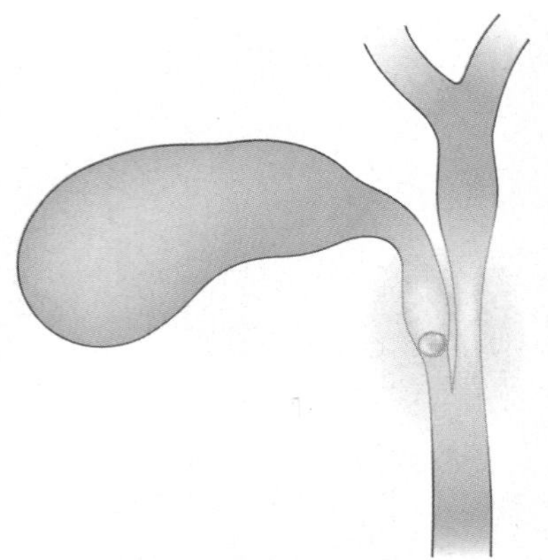

FIG. 55.32 Mirizzi syndrome. Obstruction of the bile duct from an inflammatory process is the hallmark of this syndrome; the cholecystocholedochal fistula may or may not be apparent.

patients often have a cystic duct parallel to common hepatic duct and an impacted gallstone in the neck or cystic duct. The resultant inflammation can cause a cholecystocholedochal fistula. The treatment of Mirizzi syndrome is cholecystectomy, which may require repair of the common duct; when a large fistula exists, a choledochojejunostomy may be necessary.

Long-standing choledocholithiasis also can cause fibrosis and stricture. ERCP with sphincterotomy, balloon dilation, and stent placement is generally regarded as primary treatment for benign bile duct strictures to make the diagnosis and potentially to treat the process. Endoscopic and percutaneous therapy can provide long-term success in more than 50% of patients. When this is unsuccessful, surgical management with anastomosis of the biliary tree to a Roux-en-Y jejunal limb has success rates of up to 90%.

Biliary Cysts

Choledochal cysts, or biliary cysts, are congenital intrahepatic and/or extrahepatic dilation anomalies. Due to new insights into epithelial markers, and different pathophysiology in different etiologic subtypes, now they are called biliary malformations rather than cysts. They are rare disorders, occurring in less than 1/100,000 patients. They occur more frequently in female patients and in Asian populations. These are considered premalignant conditions and are sometimes diagnosed in infancy; however, they can present in adulthood (Fig. 55.33).[21] Type I choledochal cyst is the most common form and involves only the extrahepatic biliary tree with a fusiform dilation. Type II cysts appear as a saccular diverticulum off the CBD and may be mistaken for an accessory gallbladder. Type III cysts appear as a cystic dilation of the intramural CBD, within the wall of the duodenum, and are also known as choledochoceles. Cysts involving the intrahepatic and extrahepatic biliary tree are known as type IVa, with type IVb being multiple cysts limited to the extrahepatic biliary tree. Type V cysts, also known as Caroli disease, involve the intrahepatic ducts only. Type V cysts may be solitary but usually occur diffusely in all segments. Although classified as a single disease, there are multiple theories for etiology, but mostly accepted, especially for types I and IV, is the anomalous pancreatobiliary junction (APBJ; Figs. 55.34 and 55.35).[22] With APBJ, the pancreatic duct and biliary tree fuse to form a common channel before passage through the duodenal wall; APBJ is seen in up to 90% of patients with choledochal cysts, but almost exclusively in types I and IV. The fused duct forms a long common channel, which allows pancreatic

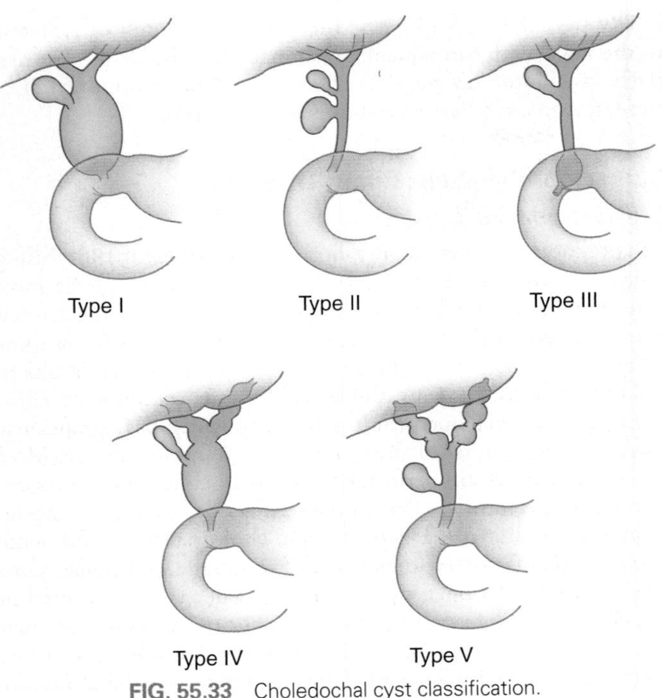

FIG. 55.33 Choledochal cyst classification.

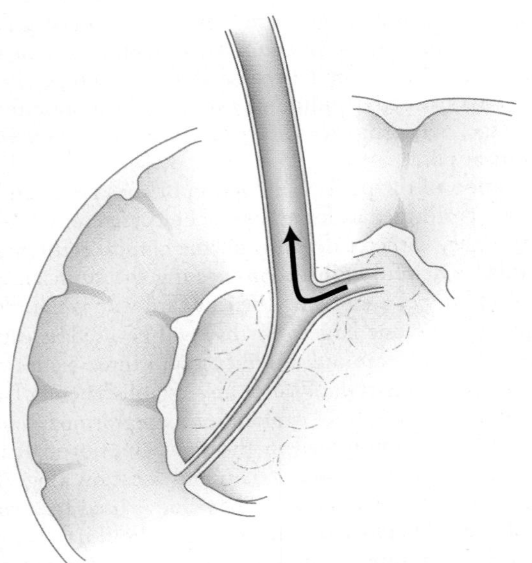

FIG. 55.34 Anomalous pancreaticobiliary junction. With fusion of the common bile duct and pancreatic duct long before they pass through the duodenal wall, the pancreatic secretions can reflux into the common bile duct and may cause damage to the common duct through pressure or chemical injury.

secretions to reflux into the biliary tree. Because the pancreatic duct has higher secretory pressures than the biliary tree, exocrine pancreatic secretions reflux up into the bile duct and can inflame and damage the biliary epithelium, leading to cystic degeneration. Types II and III almost never present with APBJ and are associated with minimal risk of malignancy.

Presentation. Jaundice is the most consistent symptom, sometimes accompanied with right upper quadrant pain and rarely a palpable mass. Patients may also suffer from nonspecific problems such as weight loss, nausea, and vomiting. Rarely, a long-standing malformation can cause liver injury and even cirrhosis. Diagnostic imaging is the only diagnostic confirmation test. With the current liberal use of CT, the diagnosis of a choledochal cyst is usually suspected in CT but it is further classified by MRCP or ERCP. Sometimes the distal bile duct is difficult to evaluate by MRCP, so ERCP is more useful for defining the distal biliary tree and pancreaticobiliary junction. Laboratory studies may identify cholestasis and jaundice. In late stages of disease, secondary hepatic injury and evidence of cirrhosis may be seen. Rarely, first presentation is cholangiocarcinoma. The incident of malignancy ranges between 5% and 30% over a lifetime, most commonly occurring in the seventh decade and almost exclusively occurring in types I and IV. Interestingly, malignancy has been seen in the nondilated intrahepatic biliary tree in type I choledochal cysts.[22]

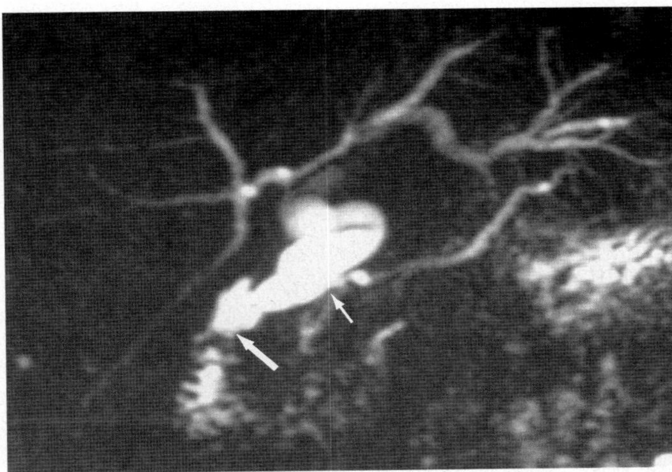

FIG. 55.35 Magnetic resonance cholangiopancreatography showing anomalous pancreaticobiliary junction with long common channel. The pancreatic duct fuses with the common bile duct *(slender arrow)*, and the common channel enters the duodenum *(bold arrow)*. Also noted in this illustration is the fusiform dilation of only the extrahepatic bile duct, as seen in a type I choledochal cyst.

Treatment. Historically, enteric drainage of the cyst was performed without resection, but this approach is complicated by the development of malignancy, recurrent biliary stasis, and infection.

Surgical management of choledochal cysts consists of resection of the entire cyst and appropriate surgical reconstruction. Type I cysts are treated by complete surgical excision, cholecystectomy, and Roux-en-Y hepaticojejunostomy. The proximal extent of resection should continue to the nondilated biliary tree and may require anastomosis to the left and right hepatic ducts.[22] The distal duct is oversewn, with care taken not to injure the pancreatic duct. Type II cysts should be excised entirely. Type III cysts are uncommon and may be approached transduodenally. Because the pathogenesis of type III cysts is not clear and almost always does not involve APBJ, endoscopic drainage may suffice. In the setting of duodenal or biliary obstruction, transduodenal excision or sphincteroplasty can be performed. Surgical treatment of type IV cysts must be carefully individualized to the affected anatomy. Type IV cysts affecting only the extrahepatic bile ducts are managed similarly to type I cysts, with excision and hepaticojejunostomy. Those with intrahepatic extension involving only one lobe can be treated with partial hepatectomy and reconstruction. Surgical treatment of Caroli disease ranges from resection if the disease is unilobar to liver transplantation when diffuse disease is detected.

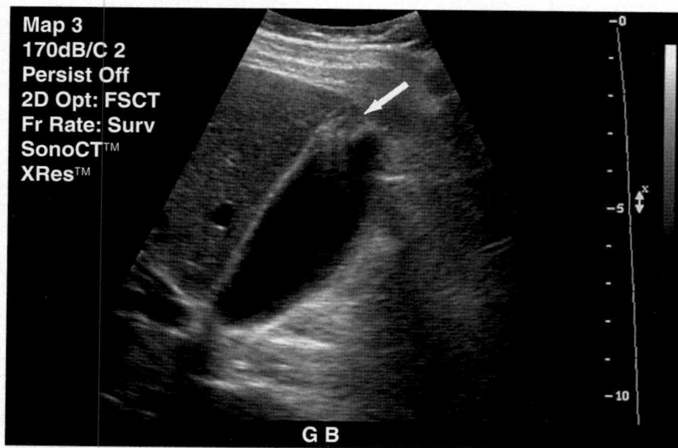

FIG. 55.36 Ultrasound image of adenomyomatosis. Seen in the fundus of the gallbladder is a sessile thickening *(arrow)* with smaller microcysts within it, consistent with adenomyomatosis.

Polypoid Lesions of the Gallbladder

Benign masses of the gallbladder are common. The estimated prevalence is between 3% and 12.3% of the population.[23] They can be divided into pseudopolyps and true polyps. Pseudopolyps are further divided into cholesterol polyps, focal adenomyomatosis, hyperplastic polyps, and inflammatory polyps. Cholesterol polyps appear as pedunculated echogenic lesions of the gallbladder, are usually smaller than 1 cm, and are frequently multiple. Alternatively, adenomyomatosis is seen as a sessile lesion, commonly in the fundus, with characteristic microcysts within the lesion, and is frequently larger than 1 cm (Fig. 55.36). True polyps are benign growths in the wall of the gallbladder and consist of only 5% of all polypoid disorders of gallbladder. True polyps may be difficult to differentiate from adenocarcinoma preoperatively due to imaging limitations in detecting mural invasion. This is discussed further in the malignancy section of this chapter. Asymptomatic lesions smaller than 10 mm with no other risk factors and no ultrasonographic features suggesting malignant disease can be observed with serial ultrasonography.

Benign Biliary Masses

Benign intraluminal lesions of the biliary tract have been a constant evolving field. The most accepted categorization of benign biliary lesions currently includes intraepithelial and intraductal types. Intraepithelial lesions are described in different grading system of "biliary intraepithelial neoplasms." These are considered precursors of epithelial malignancies of bile ducts. The intraductal lesions are described as "intraductal papillary neoplasms." These lesions include mucin producing neoplasms, adenomas, papillomas, and papillomatosis. Some of these lesions are premalignant, including mucin producing and papillomatosis.

The presentation is that of biliary obstruction with jaundice and sometimes right upper quadrant pain. Treatment consists of complete resection with a small rim of normal epithelium because incomplete excision of affected epithelium carries a high risk of recurrence. These lesions occur in the periampullary duct, so a transduodenal approach can be used. Rarely, intraductal papillary or mucin-producing lesions may be found in intrahepatic biliary radicles.

Inflammatory lesions of the biliary tree, known as pseudotumors or benign fibrosing disease, may be mistaken for cholangiocarcinoma. When this process follows surgical intervention on the biliary tree, the mass-like stricture may be the result of ischemia to the duct, with subsequent inflammation and fibrosis. Alternatively, pseudotumors may occur de novo; these commonly affect the extrahepatic biliary tree above the bifurcation.

Surgery for Calculous Biliary Disease

Laparoscopic Cholecystectomy

Laparoscopic cholecystectomy, first done by Muhe in 1985 (using a direct scope) and later in 1987 by Mouret, is one of the most commonly performed general surgery procedures in the United States. Laparoscopic cholecystectomy has a 0.1% to 0.5% mortality and 2% to 3% morbidity.[7] Laparoscopic surgery results in smaller incisions, less pain, and shorter hospitalization when compared to traditional open cholecystectomy, which has significantly increased the number of these procedures done worldwide. Most cholecystectomies are performed for biliary colic, but the operation can be performed safely in the setting of acute inflammation. Studies have shown that laparoscopic cholecystectomy for acute cholecystitis may carry longer operative times and a higher conversion rate to the open procedure than when it is performed in the elective setting, with possibly a higher risk of common duct injury.[24] General anesthesia with muscle relaxation is required when a laparoscopic cholecystectomy is performed. Therefore, one contraindication to the procedure is the inability to tolerate general anesthesia. Others include end-stage liver disease with portal hypertension, precluding safe portal dissection, and coagulopathy. Because most pneumoperitoneum laparoscopies are performed using CO_2 and has a number of adverse physiologic effects, severe chronic obstructive pulmonary disease, with poor ability for gas exchange, and congestive heart failure are considered relative contraindications.

Preparation of the patient, induction of anesthesia, and sterile draping are performed as for an open cholecystectomy. Although use of a urinary catheter depends on the clinical setting, an orogastric tube is helpful with decompressing the stomach and exposure of the upper abdomen. The standard way is the four-port technique, usually one large port that will be used as extraction site, typically placed around umbilicus, and three 5-mm or even smaller ports for dissection. After the establishment of a CO_2 pneumoperitoneum, a brief exploration is performed, and additional 5-mm ports are placed in the right anterior axillary line, right midclavicular line, and subxiphoid location (Fig. 55.37). The lateral port at the anterior axillary line is used to elevate the fundus of the gallbladder toward the right shoulder. This retraction provides exposure to the infundibulum and porta hepatis. The midclavicular trocar is used to grasp the gallbladder infundibulum, retracting it inferolaterally to open the triangle of Calot (Figs. 55.38 to 55.40). By distraction of Hartmann pouch laterally, the cystic duct no longer lies almost parallel to the common hepatic duct and is an extremely important maneuver to avoid injuring the CBD during this procedure.

The dissection is then carried along the infundibulum on the anterior and posterior surfaces to expose the base of the gallbladder to clear all fibrofatty tissue from the triangle of Calot. Then the cystic duct and artery are identified by inferolateral traction of the infundibulum. A useful landmark for the cystic artery is the overlying lymph node, known as Calot node. To minimize bile duct injury, a strategy known as the critical view of safety can be employed. Rotating the gallbladder infundibulum laterally and then medially, there should be only two structures entering the gallbladder, and the liver on the opposite side of the gallbladder

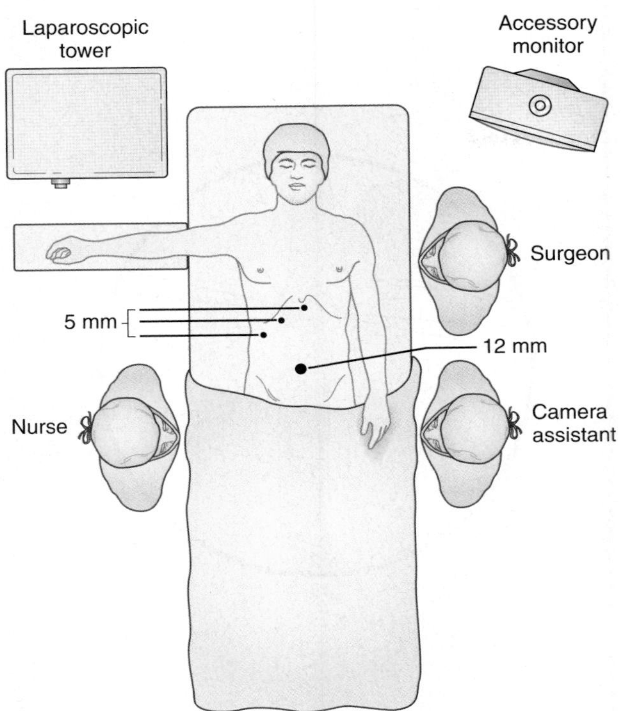

FIG. 55.37 Laparoscopic cholecystectomy ports. The assistant uses the periumbilical port to provide access for the camera and the most lateral port to elevate the fundus and to expose the neck. The surgeon can then provide inferolateral traction on the infundibulum and open the critical view of safety.

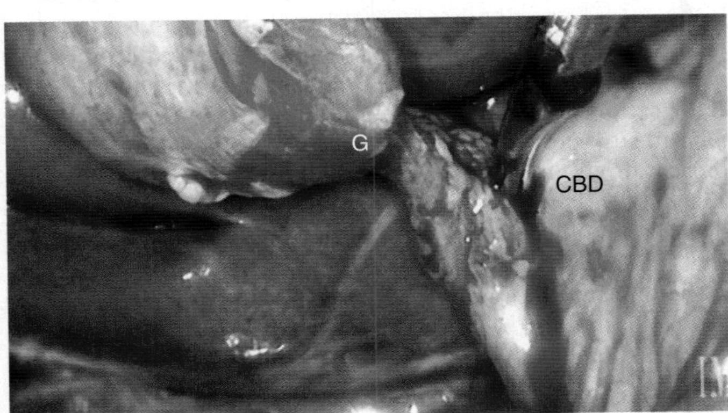

FIG. 55.38 Laparoscopic view of the porta and gallbladder infundibulum without inferolateral traction on the infundibulum. Note that the gallbladder infundibulum *(G)* lies immediately adjacent to the common bile duct *(CBD)*.

should be visible through the open spaces around each structure (Fig. 55.41).[24] Clips are then placed on the cystic artery and duct. If cholangiography is performed, the cystic duct is clipped only adjacent to the gallbladder, the cystic duct is incised but not transected so that the cholangiogram catheter can be passed into it, and fluoroscopic images are obtained (Fig. 55.42). On obtaining a normal cholangiogram or when cholangiography is not performed, the cystic duct is doubly clipped on the common duct side and transected. The previously clipped artery is also transected, and the gallbladder is dissected off the liver bed using electrocautery. Because the venous drainage of the gallbladder is directly into the liver bed through venules, excellent hemostasis must be achieved during

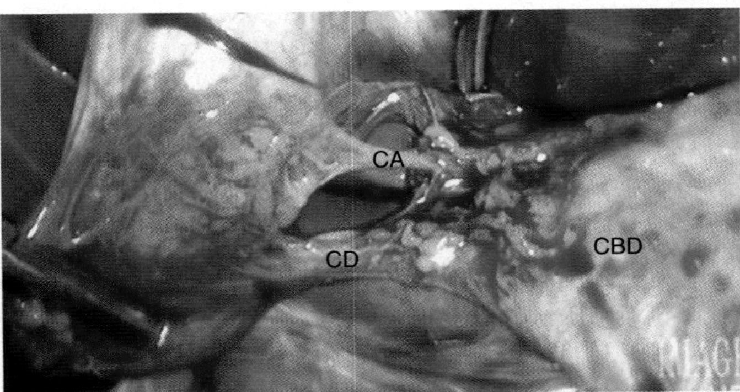

FIG. 55.39 Laparoscopic view of the same patient as in Fig. 55.38 but with inferolateral traction on the infundibulum. Note the angular change to the cystic duct *(CD)* compared with the common bile duct *(CBD)*. The dissecting tool indicates the location of the right hepatic artery. The key element to this view in minimizing CBD injury is the identification of the cystic artery *(CA)* and duct entering the gallbladder with the inferior aspect of segment V of the liver identified in the space on either side of the artery and duct.

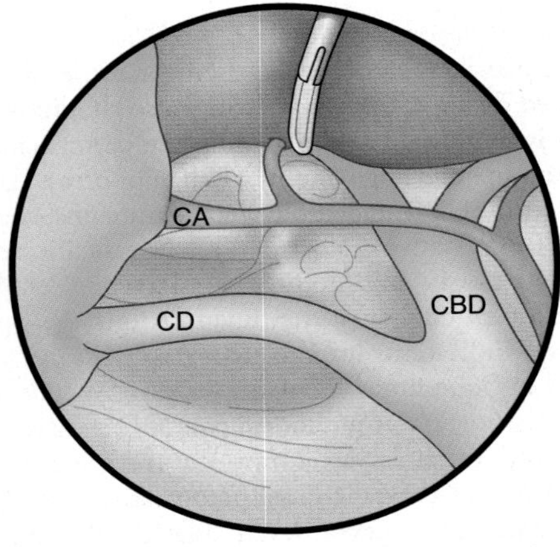

FIG. 55.40 An artist's representation of Fig. 55.39, showing hidden anatomy. *CA*, Cystic artery; *CBD*, common bile duct; *CD*, cystic duct.

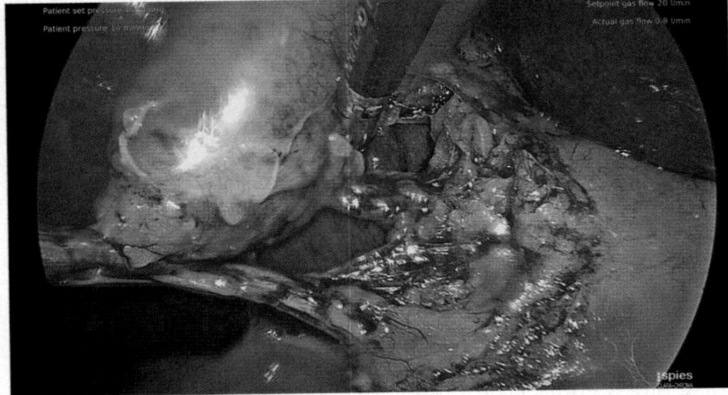

FIG. 55.41 Wide critical view.

this dissection. The cystic duct and cystic artery clips are inspected just before completion of the dissection of the fundic attachments because the superior traction of the fundus has provided exposure to the porta and triangle of Calot. The gallbladder is then brought out of the abdominal cavity through the umbilical port. In the setting of acute cholecystitis or if the gallbladder was entered during

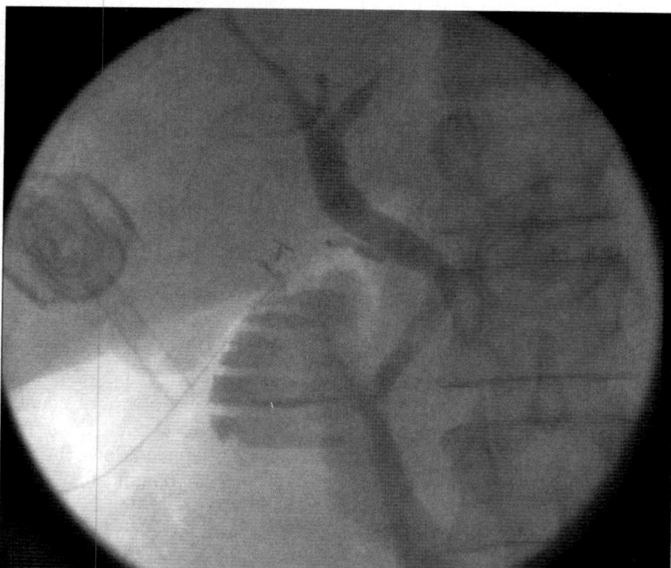

FIG. 55.42 Normal cholangiogram.

dissection, a plastic bag should be used for retrieval. Any stones that are spilled during a cholecystectomy also should be retrieved.

Opinion is sharply divided regarding the performance of selective versus routine cholangiography, with supportive data for each approach. Routine cholangiography will identify unsuspected stones in less than 10% of patients, does not decrease the incidence of biliary injury, and can be misinterpreted.[25] However, cholangiogram may capture a CBD injury at the time of surgery, as opposed to a later diagnosis. Indications for cholangiography in the selective setting include any questionable anatomy and difficulty identifying the structures, suspicion of intraoperative CBD injury, unexplained pain at the time of cholecystectomy, any suspicion of current or previous choledocholithiasis without preoperative duct clearance, elevated preoperative liver enzyme levels, dilated CBD in preoperative imaging, and suspicion of intraoperative biliary injury. The Tokyo Guidelines[7] does not encourage the routine use of cholangiography; however, many authors advocate its use in the academic setting to ensure that trainees are facile in its performance.[10] Although it is just as accurate as cholangiography for the identification of choledocholithiasis, laparoscopic ultrasonography is highly operator dependent, requires additional instrumentation, and is not widely available.

Bailout Procedures

As the grade of cholecystitis increases from I to II or III, a laparoscopic procedure becomes increasingly difficult to complete safely. The Tokyo Guidelines on recommendations for surgical management of cholecystitis recommend a few bailout options, and a surgeon must be prepared to perform these, especially with a higher-grade cholecystitis. The common bailout procedures include subtotal cholecystectomy, fundus first procedure (retrograde), and conversion to open.

Subtotal cholecystectomy is removing as much gallbladder as possible, from fundus to infundibulum, and is "reconstituting" (closed gallbladder remnant) or "fenestrated" (open gallbladder remnant, with or without closure of the internal opening of the cystic duct).[7]

Fundus first procedure refers to separation of the gallbladder from the liver surface starting from the fundus without visualizing the cystic duct and artery. This procedure can end with subtotal cholecystectomy or completion of cholecystectomy.[7]

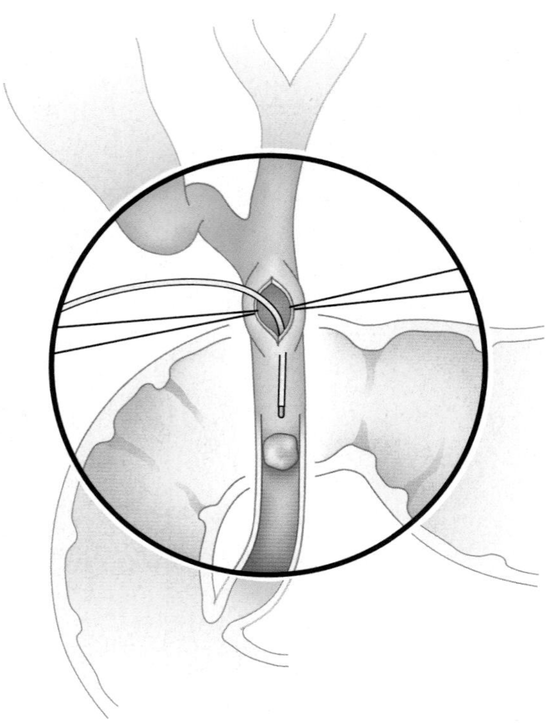

FIG. 55.43 Laparoscopic choledochotomy for common bile duct exploration.

Open Cholecystectomy

Although open cholecystectomy is considered a safe alternative or bailout procedure for the difficult laparoscopic cholecystectomy, experience with it has drastically declined, making this procedure not necessarily the safer technique.[7] Open cholecystectomy is generally performed after conversion from the laparoscopic approach, for patients who have a contraindication to the laparoscopic approach, or as a step during another operation, such as a pancreaticoduodenectomy. Open cholecystectomy can be performed through a midline or right subcostal incision. Early identification and ligation of the cystic artery limit the blood loss during the procedure but may prove difficult because of inflammation. This approach must be used with caution as the extension of the dissection continues inferiorly, putting portal vein and other portal structures at risk.[26] When it is performed for severe cholecystitis, the dissection of the gallbladder of the liver bed may be associated with substantial blood loss, but with removal of the infected gallbladder and packing of the area, the bleeding is usually well controlled.

Open CBD Exploration

Clearance of choledocholithiasis or any other reason for CBD exploration is typically performed by open technique. Most surgeons prefer right upper quadrant incision; however, an upper midline incision can be used as well. Gentle palpation of the distal bile duct will frequently find the offending stone, which may be milked backward. Stay sutures are then placed and a choledochotomy is performed in the supraduodenal bile duct. Flushing of the duct with a soft rubber catheter will frequently remove the offending stones. Balloon catheters and, with fluoroscopic guidance, wire baskets may be useful to withdraw the stone. Flexible choledochoscopes are used to visualize the distal bile duct (Fig. 55.43). With complete removal of stones, a T tube is placed, and a cholangiogram obtained before closure to document clearance.

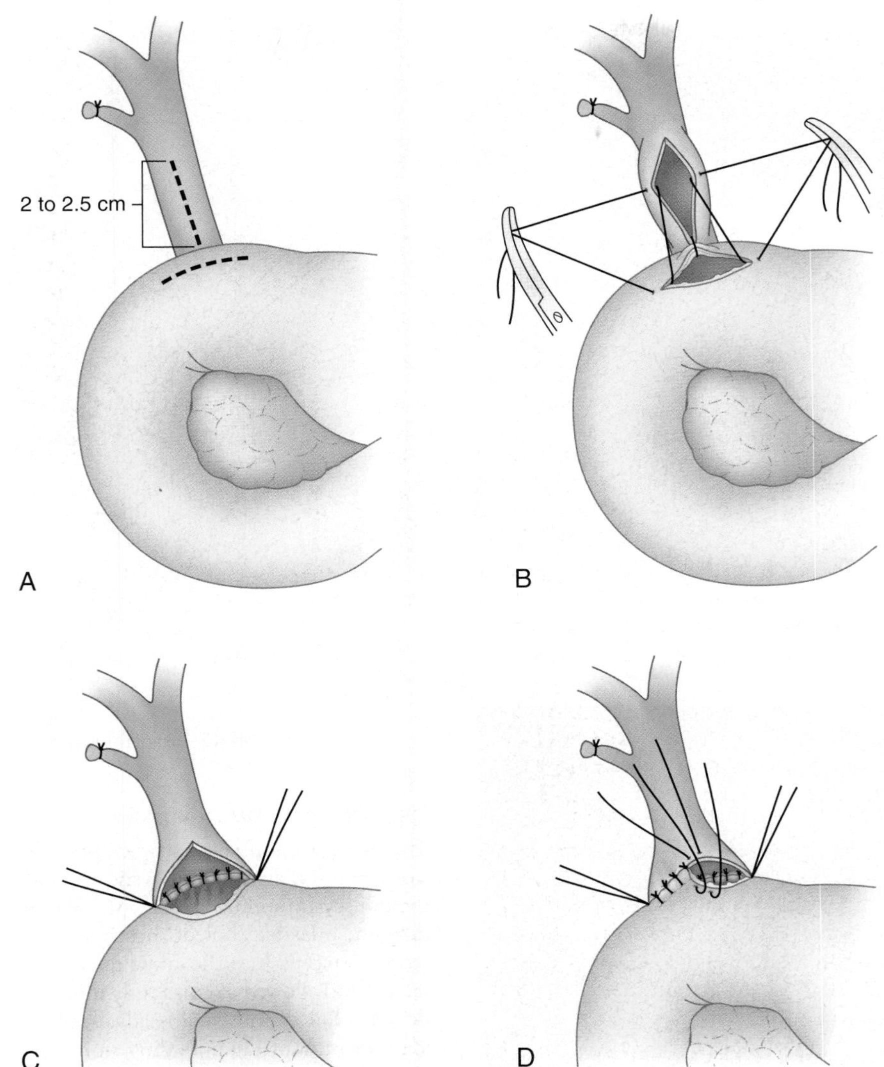

FIG. 55.44 Choledochoduodenostomy. In the setting of a dilated common bile duct *(CBD)* with inability to clear all the stones from the distal duct, an anastomosis can be performed between the CBD and adjacent duodenum. Although maintaining the possibility of future endoscopic therapy, this arrangement risks sump syndrome in the undrained distal duct. (A) Vertical incision on CBD and horizontal incision on duodenum. (B) Stay sutures on corners, creating open anastomosis. (C) Suturing posterior wall. (D) Suturing anterior wall.

With dilated bile ducts, multiple distal impacted stones, a distal duct stricture with stones, intrahepatic stones, or primary bile duct stones drainage procedures provide more successful long-term outcomes. Options in this setting include choledochoduodenostomy (Fig. 55.44), or Roux-en-Y hepaticojejunostomy (Fig. 55.45). A side-to-side or end-to-side choledochoduodenostomy allows future endoscopic intervention of the upper biliary tree, if necessary. An alternative to duodenostomy is a Roux-en-Y choledochojejunostomy.

Transduodenal sphincteroplasty must be the procedure of choice when impacted stones at the ampulla cannot be removed through choledochotomy or several stones are impacted in a *nondilated tree* (Figs. 55.46 and 55.47). After completion of the Kocher maneuver, a longitudinal duodenotomy is made on the lateral wall. Compression of the lateral wall against the medial wall will allow palpation of the ampulla to plan placement of the duodenotomy appropriately. With identification of the ampulla, an incision is made at the 11 o'clock position, and each wall is elevated with stay sutures. The pancreatic duct usually enters at the 5 o'clock position on the ampulla and must be avoided. It is also imperative to remember that the inferior pancreaticoduodenal arcade is adjacent to the distal part of the ampulla and can be injured during sphincterotomy. Sequential straight clamps are placed along the planned incision of the ampulla to guide visualization through hemostasis. With each step, the duodenal mucosa is sewn to the bile duct mucosa with absorbable 4-0 or 5-0 sutures. A 1.5-cm sphincterotomy is usually sufficient to allow stone removal and subsequent drainage. Closure of the longitudinal duodenotomy in transverse fashion avoids a future duodenal stricture.

Open exploration carries a low morbidity (8%–15%) and mortality (1%–2%), with a low rate of retained stones (<5%).

The downside of choledochoduodenostomy is that the bile duct distal to the anastomosis may drain poorly and may collect debris that obstructs the anastomosis or the pancreatic duct, a process known as *sump syndrome*. Anastomosis to the jejunum in a Roux-en-Y arrangement provides excellent drainage of the biliary tree without a risk of sump syndrome but does not allow future endoscopic evaluation of the biliary tree (Fig. 55.45).

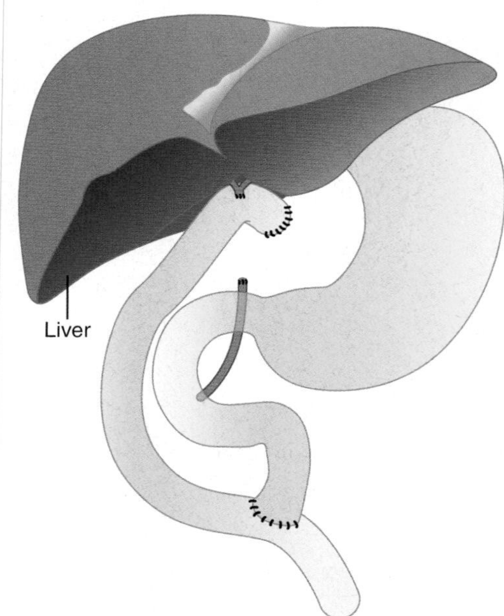

FIG. 55.45 Hepaticojejunostomy.

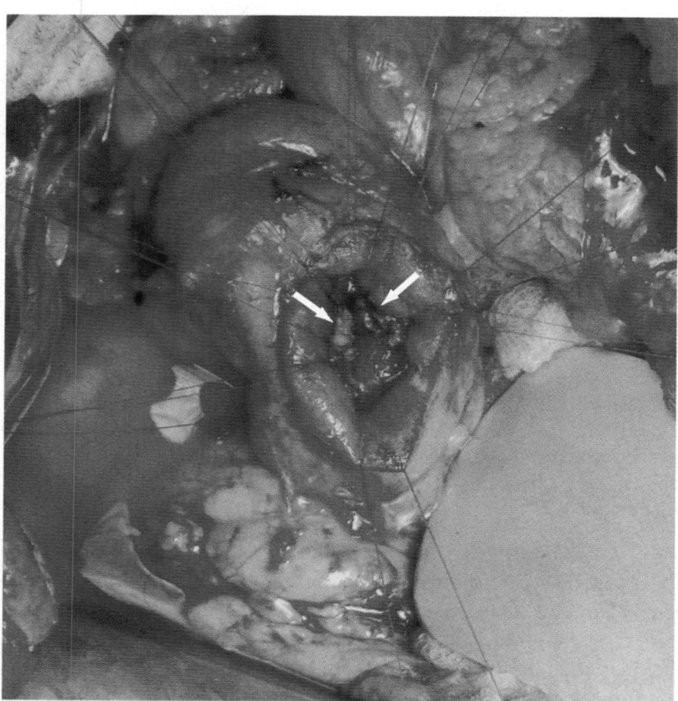

FIG. 55.46 Transduodenal sphincteroplasty. Note the generous opening of the distal common duct with sequential duct to mucosa approximation *(arrows)*.

With intrahepatic stones, the transhepatic approach to cholangiography is generally more successful. Percutaneous drainage catheters may be left in place and upsized to perform percutaneous stone extraction. Long-term management of intrahepatic stones must be carefully tailored to the disease but frequently requires hepaticojejunostomy for optimal biliary drainage. Liberal use of choledochoscopy at the time of a drainage procedure ensures removal of all current stones. This approach allows a stone clearance rate of more than 90%.

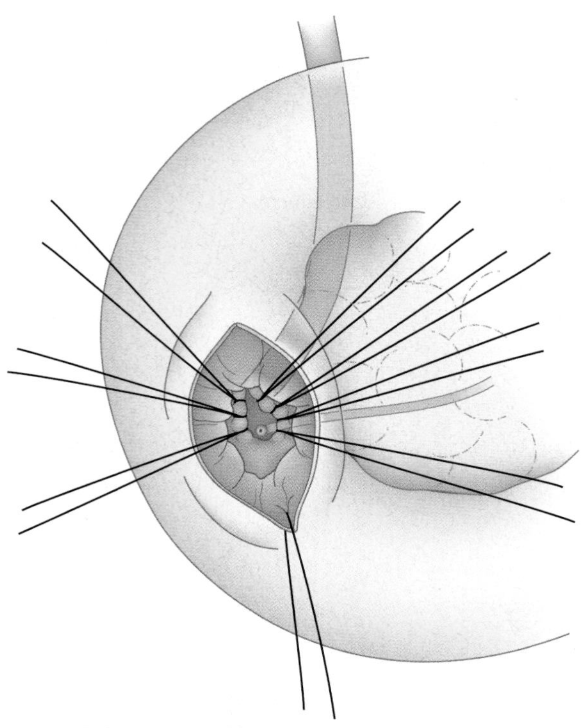

FIG. 55.47 Transduodenal sphincteroplasty.

Laparoscopic CBD Exploration

The two common laparoscopic approaches to explore the CBD for stone removal are the transcystic approach and choledochotomy. In the transcystic approach, using the Seldinger technique after balloon dilation, a flexible choledochoscope, or alternately a flexible ureteroscope, is passed into the cystic duct. A water irrigation system is attached and allowed to constantly infuse out the end of the scope. The flexible choledochoscope is advanced to the distal bile duct. With identification of the offending stone, a wire basket is passed to ensnare the stone, withdrawing it and the choledochoscope together.

In the laparoscopic choledochotomy approach, a longitudinal incision is made in the CBD (i.e., below the cystic duct). To expose the CBD, two stay sutures are placed on either side of the planned choledochotomy (Fig. 55.43). The size of the incision should be at least as large as the diameter of the largest stone. The choledochoscope can then be fed down into the distal bile duct and stone extraction performed as described earlier. At the completion of the exploration, a T tube should be placed through the choledochotomy and the bile duct closed with 4-0 absorbable sutures. Completion cholangiography through the T tube documents stone removal.

In addition to being technically easier, because it does not require fine laparoscopic suturing, the transcystic approach avoids a T tube. Contraindications to the transcystic approach include numerous (more than eight) stones, a stone larger than 1 cm, intrahepatic stones, and a cystic duct that does not allow dilation and choledochoscope passage. Both approaches are successful at stone removal, with most studies showing a 75% to 95% rate of stone clearance. This is comparable to that of laparoscopic cholecystectomy, followed by postoperative ERCP, with the only difference being a shorter hospitalization and lower physician fees for patients undergoing common duct exploration as the cholecystectomy and clearance of stones are performed in one setting by a single physician.[27]

Postcholecystectomy Syndromes

First described in 1947, postcholecystectomy syndrome, recurrence of heterogeneous symptoms similar to those experienced before a cholecystectomy, such as upper abdominal pain and dyspepsia, with or without jaundice, occurs in 10% to 15% of all cholecystectomies worldwide. These symptoms may manifest from 2 days up to 25 years postcholecystectomy and are more common in females.[28] The etiology ranges from surgical complications (in more severe forms) to primary unrelated etiology such as esophagitis, gastroesophageal reflux disease, etc. Biliary etiologies specifically include, but re not limited to, a retained stone, bile salt–induced diarrhea, biliary leak, long remnant cystic duct, or functional problems with biliary tree and/or sphincter of Oddi.

Bile Duct Injury

More than 80% of bile duct injuries occur during cholecystectomy. Variable anatomy, porta hepatis inflammation, inappropriate exposure, inadequate experience or skill, and aggressive hemostasis have been cited as risk factors. Studies have suggested that misperception of the anatomy is a much more common factor in iatrogenic injury than surgical skill.[10] With sufficient cephalad retraction of the gallbladder fundus, the cystic duct overlies the common hepatic duct, running in a parallel path. Without inferolateral traction of the gallbladder infundibulum to dissociate these structures, dissection of the apparent cystic duct may actually include the common hepatic duct, placing it in jeopardy. By retraction of Hartmann pouch inferolaterally and opening of the triangle of Calot, the cystic duct is displaced from the porta, no longer collinear with the hepatic duct. The use of a 30-degree laparoscope provides adequate visualization of the critical view of safety during laparoscopic cholecystectomy. Also, in many of these cases, a confirmation bias occurs in which surgeons tend to rely on evidence that supports their perception while simultaneously discounting visual cues that suggest an alternative explanation. Confirmation bias helps explain why most bile duct injuries are identified in the postoperative setting, not intraoperatively. Although the use of routine versus selective cholangiography is controversial, evidence has suggested that cholangiography does not completely avoid bile duct injury but may reduce the incidence and extent of injury and allow immediate recognition and management.[29] The original analysis of biliary reconstruction was based on the Bismuth classification and has been modified by Strasberg. Classification of bile duct injuries is determined by location and helps guide later surgical reconstruction (Fig. 55.48).[30] Injury to the bile duct that does not leak bile will usually be manifested with jaundice, with or without pain. Among postoperative bile duct strictures, occurring roughly in less than 1% of all cases,[28] types E1 and E2 involve the common hepatic duct but not the bifurcation, with type E1 maintaining more than 2 cm of common hepatic duct below the bifurcation and type E2 being within 2 cm of the confluence. Type E3 strictures occur at the confluence, preserving the extrahepatic ducts, and in type E4, the stricturing process includes the extrahepatic biliary tree. Type E5 strictures involve aberrant right hepatic duct anatomy, with injury to the aberrant duct and common hepatic duct.

Presentation. Bile duct injury can result in bile leakage or stricture. Leakage into peritoneal cavity followed by peritonitis tends to manifest earlier than stricture. Less than 10% of strictures are found in first week postoperation, and more than 70% are diagnosed within 6 months. In the setting of bile leakage, patients may present with fever, increasing abdominal pain, jaundice, or bile leakage from an incision. Regardless of timing or presentation, adequate repair and subsequent outcome depend on diagnosis, sufficient delineation of anatomy, creation of a tension-free anastomosis, and liberal use of transanastomotic stents.[31]

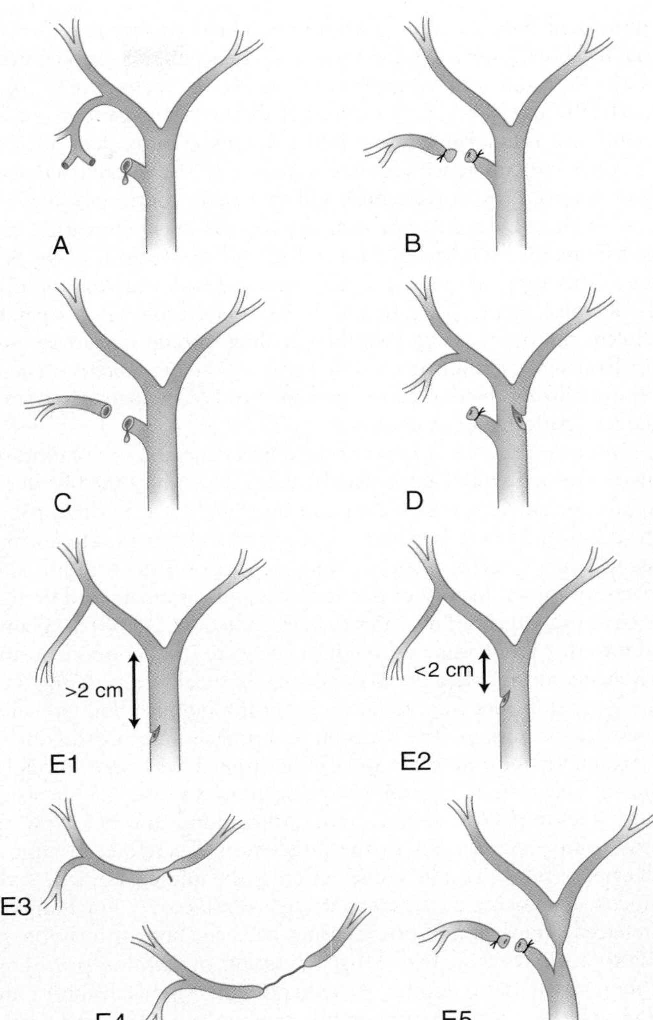

FIG. 55.48 Strasberg classification of postoperative bile duct strictures. (A) Injury to small ducts in continuity with the biliary system with a leak in the duct of Luschka or the cystic duct. (B) Injury to a sectoral duct, causing obstruction of portion of the biliary system. (C) Injury to a sectoral duct with bile leak; leak from a duct not continuous with the biliary system. (D) Lateral injury to the extrahepatic biliary ducts. (E1) Bismuth type 1: injury more than 2 cm from the confluence. (E2) Bismuth type 2: injury less than 2 cm from the confluence. (E3) Bismuth type 3: injury at the confluence; confluence intact. (E4) Bismuth type 4: destruction of the biliary confluence. (E5) Complete occlusion of all bile ducts, including sectoral ducts.

Treatment

Recognized at the time of cholecystectomy. When bile duct injury is suspected intraoperatively, conversion to an open operation and use of cholangiography help delineate management. Goals for the immediate treatment of bile duct injury include maintenance of ductal length, elimination of any bile leakage that would affect subsequent management, and creation of a tension-free repair. If the injury occurs to a larger than 3-mm duct but is not caused by electrocautery and involves less than 50% of the circumference of the wall, a T-tube placement through the injury, which is effectively a choledochotomy, usually will allow healing without the need for subsequent biliary-enteric anastomosis. Ducts smaller than 3 mm that by cholangiography drain only a single segment or subsegment of the liver and simple ligation may suffice for management. Any thermal injury in which the extent of thermal damage may not be manifested immediately or an injury involving more than 50% of the duct circumference requires resection of the injured segment with anastomosis to reestablish biliary-enteric continuity. Defects smaller than 1 cm and not near the hepatic duct bifurcation can be repaired by mobilization and end-to-end anastomosis of the bile duct. This approach should be accompanied with transanastomotic T-tube placement. The tube should be inserted through a separate choledochotomy and not exit the bile duct through the anastomosis. To ensure a tension-free anastomosis, a generous Kocher maneuver, mobilizing the duodenum and the head of the pancreas out of the retroperitoneum, is necessary.

More commonly, injuries occur adjacent to the bifurcation or involve more than a 1-cm defect between the ends of the bile duct, requiring reanastomosis to the gastrointestinal tract. In this setting, the distal end is oversewn and the proximal end debrided to normal tissue. The choice of reconstruction depends on the location and extent of injury, history of previous attempts at repair, and preference of the surgeon. Low injuries to the bile duct can be reimplanted into the duodenum, although the new choledochoduodenostomy anastomosis risks a duodenal fistula, especially considering that these anastomoses may require significant mobilization to avoid anastomotic tension. The Roux-en-Y approach to reconstruction is substantially more versatile and can be applied to injuries throughout the biliary tree. In addition, most injuries to the bile duct occur higher in the biliary tree, close to the hilum, thus not allowing tension-free anastomosis to the duodenum. Therefore, in almost all cases of bile duct injury, a resection of the injured segment with mucosa-to-mucosa anastomosis using a Roux-en-Y jejunal limb is preferred. Transanastomotic stenting has been shown to improve anastomotic patency, with longer duration of stenting providing a more favorable outcome. As concomitant vascular injuries are common, Doppler ultrasonography can confirm adequate hepatic arterial and portal venous flow to the hepatic parenchyma.

Recent data suggest that there is no significant difference in frequency of biliary injuries sustained at teaching hospitals compared with hospitals without residents.[32] Because most bile duct injuries and, therefore, most immediate repairs occur at centers where biliary reconstruction is performed infrequently, most immediate repairs go unreported in the literature. However, the importance of surgical judgment and experience in biliary reconstruction cannot be overemphasized. Although reports of previous failed attempts at reconstruction have not documented injuries successfully managed immediately, they do highlight the value of experience in the treatment of bile duct injuries.[33] Therefore, when one is confronted with a bile duct injury and no surgeon with experience in biliary reconstruction is available, the most appropriate management strategy is placement of a drain and immediate referral to an experienced center.

Identified after cholecystectomy. The diagnosis of iatrogenic bile duct injury should be suspected in any patient who presents with new or increasing symptoms after a laparoscopic cholecystectomy. Leakage may be manifested as bilious drainage into a subhepatic drain placed at the time of operation or bilious drainage from a surgical incision. Without a site for external drainage, bile leakage can be manifested as a biloma, whether sterile or infected, or with biliary ascites. Persistent or worsening postprandial pain, shoulder pain, malaise, and/or fever must raise the suspicion of a bile duct injury.

Patients suspected of having an iatrogenic bile duct injury should undergo imaging to assess for a fluid collection and to evaluate the biliary tree. Ultrasonography can achieve both these goals, but because percutaneous drainage may be required and anatomic delineation is valuable, cross-sectional imaging by CT will generally provide more useful data. Some surgeons advocate the use of radionuclide scanning to confirm bile leakage, but with any documentation of a leak, CT will be necessary to plan management. Also, ischemia is a common cause of bile duct stricture. In the setting of a bile duct injury, 20% or more of patients will have concomitant unrecognized vascular injuries.

BOX 55.2 Goals of therapy in iatrogenic bile duct injury.

1. Control of infection, limiting inflammation
   - Parenteral antibiotics
   - Percutaneous drainage of periportal fluid collections
2. Clear and thorough delineation of entire biliary anatomy
   - Magnetic resonance cholangiopancreatography or percutaneous transhepatic cholangiography
   - Endoscopic retrograde cholangiopancreatography (especially if cystic duct stump leak is suspected)
3. Reestablishment of biliary-enteric continuity
   - Tension-free, mucosa-to-mucosa anastomosis
   - Roux-en-Y hepaticojejunostomy
   - Long-term transanastomotic stents if bifurcation or higher is involved

In the delayed presentation of a bile duct injury, three major goals guide therapy (Box 55.2). *First, control of infection* with drainage of any fluid collections will minimize the inflammatory process. Inflammation in the porta hepatis leads to fibrosis, which acts only to increase stricture formation. Broad-spectrum antibiotics, decompression of the biliary tree, and drainage, whether percutaneous or operative, of any fluid collections will achieve this goal. With control of sepsis, there is no urgency for biliary reconstruction. In fact, with time, resolution of the periportal inflammation helps with the execution of a durable reconstruction. In addition, the retraction of an injured bile duct into the hilum of the liver, as well as inflammation in this region, makes successful repair in the immediate postoperative setting unlikely. Therefore, although immediate reexploration to manage the injury as expeditiously as possible is tempting, successful long-term management of bile duct injuries identified postoperatively depends on clear and deliberate preoperative planning of the reconstruction.

A second goal of management is clear and thorough delineation of the biliary anatomy with cholangiography. Without preoperative cholangiography, any attempts at repair are unlikely to be successful. The cholangiogram must indicate the intrahepatic anatomy and bile duct bifurcation. For patients with bile duct continuity, ERCP may be possible. However, PTC will demonstrate the intrahepatic biliary tree, identify the location of the injury, provide drainage of bile, and possibly even allow the leak to close (Fig. 55.49). Percutaneous biliary catheters can also be left in place during reconstruction to assist in dissection and to provide drainage perioperatively. PTC can be combined with ERCP as necessary, depending on the site and extent of injury. Small bile leaks with bile duct continuity and cystic duct stump leaks can be successfully managed by endoscopic stenting and sphincterotomy.

The third goal of management is to reestablish durable biliary-enteric drainage. Although a combination of percutaneous and endoscopic biliary dilations and stenting may establish continuity, surgical reconstruction has the highest patency rates. To achieve a successful and durable repair, the anastomosis must be performed between a minimally inflamed bile duct to intestines in a

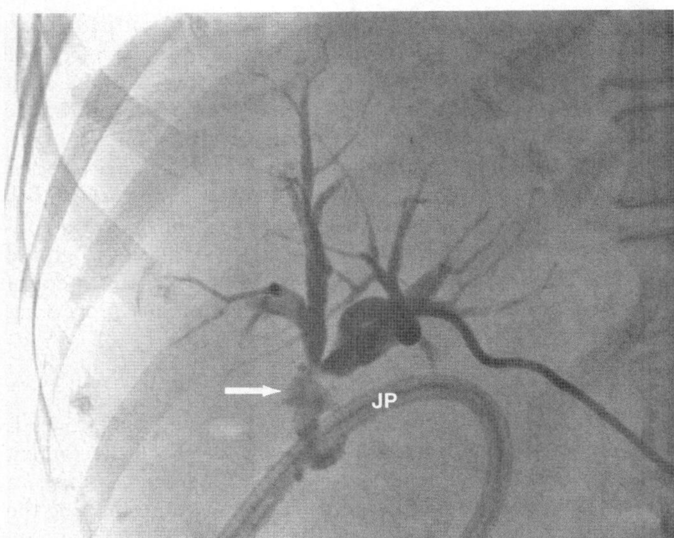

FIG. 55.49 Percutaneous transhepatic cholangiogram of bile duct injury. Note the extravasation of contrast material *(arrow)* and the Jackson-Pratt drain *(JP)* placed at the time of initial operation.

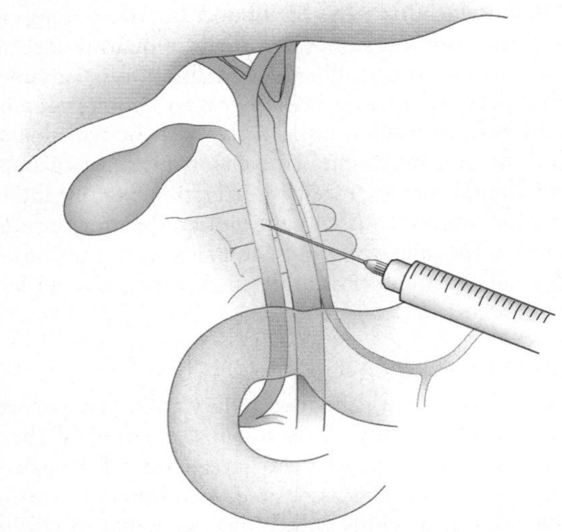

FIG. 55.50 Needle aspiration of porta used to identify the common bile duct in the setting of substantial inflammation.

tension-free, mucosa-to-mucosa fashion. When the anastomosis is within 2 cm of the hepatic duct bifurcation or involves intrahepatic ducts, some evidence suggests that long-term stenting may improve patency. If the bifurcation is involved, stenting of both right and left ducts should be performed. When the reconstruction involves the CBD or common hepatic duct more than 2 cm from the bifurcation, stenting is not necessary; therefore, a preoperatively placed transhepatic drain or intraoperatively placed T tube will provide adequate decompression in the immediate postoperative period.

At the time of operation, the adhesions of the duodenum and colon to the liver should be separated. The porta hepatis can be encircled with a Penrose drain. Although the bile duct should lie on the lateral border of the porta hepatis, preoperatively placed percutaneous biliary drainage catheters can assist in the dissection, as the marked fibrosis and inflammatory process may make its identification difficult. If necessary, a small-caliber needle attached to a syringe can be used to aspirate and to identify the bile duct while avoiding inadvertent injury to a vascular structure (Fig. 55.50).

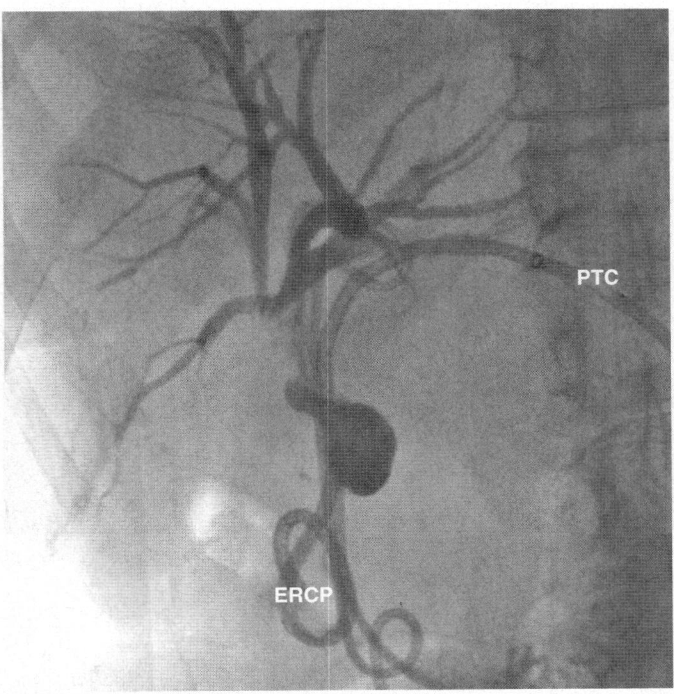

FIG. 55.51 Percutaneous transhepatic cholangiography catheter *(PTC)* traversing common bile duct iatrogenic injury. This catheter was used to guide endoscopic retrograde cholangiopancreatography stenting *(ERCP)* in a poor operative candidate with iatrogenic injury but common bile duct continuity.

Once identified, above the stricture, only a limited segment of bile duct (<5 mm) is dissected free. Any further dissection of normal duct risks vascular compromise of the segment to be used in the anastomosis. Preservation of as much normal biliary tree as possible remains a goal of the reconstruction. Next, the bile duct can be opened and the percutaneously placed catheters advanced through the incision. At this point, a wire can be used to exchange the catheters for long-term Silastic stents, if appropriate, or the catheters can be left in place for transanastomotic decompression. The mucosa-to-mucosa anastomosis can be created in an end-to-side fashion to the Roux-en-Y jejunal limb. In the setting of substantial inflammation at the bifurcation, another reconstruction option involves anastomosis of the Roux limb to the left hepatic duct. As noted, the left hepatic duct retains a substantial extraparenchymal length, allowing an anastomosis in this portion of normal duct. Before this section is used for drainage of the entire liver, cholangiography must confirm that the biliary bifurcation is widely patent, thus ensuring drainage of the right lobe across the bifurcation to the left duct system.

Interventional radiologic and endoscopic techniques. Fluoroscopic-guided management using percutaneous access to traverse the stricture can be used when the duct continuity of the duct is preserved. Balloon dilation can treat strictures and this (Fig. 55.51) approach is successful in up to 70% of patients.[34] Complications, although frequent, are generally limited and include cholangitis, hemobilia, and bile leaks requiring repeated intervention. Endoscopic balloon dilation of bile duct strictures is generally reserved for those with primary bile duct strictures or patients who have undergone choledochoduodenostomy for reconstruction because the Roux limb does not usually allow endoscopic strategies. Therefore, series are limited, but results are encouraging, with 88% of patients responding to therapy and a complication rate of 8% from pancreatitis and cholangitis.

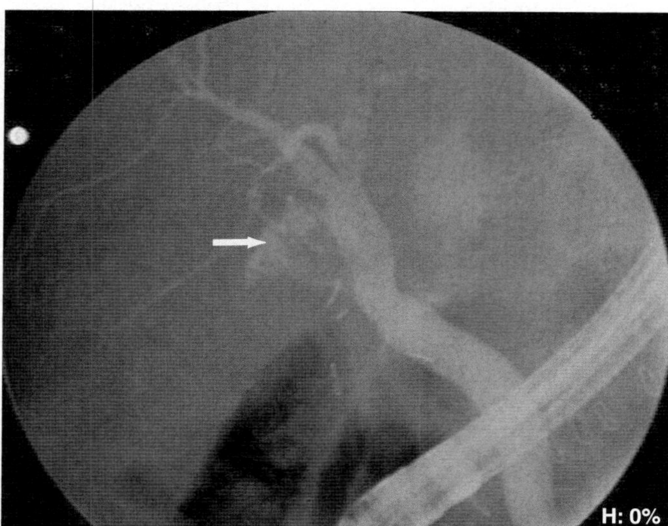

FIG. 55.52 Endoscopic retrograde cholangiopancreatography showing cystic duct stump leak *(arrow)*.

Outcomes. Successful outcomes can be achieved in patients undergoing biliary-enteric reconstruction after bile duct injury, with many series showing more than 90% of patients free of jaundice and cholangitis. High success rates are generally achieved when injuries are identified early, and patients are referred immediately to experienced centers. In several studies, referral to centers performing complex biliary surgery routinely was associated with better long-term success.[35] Surgical reconstruction provides a durable long-term management strategy.[36] Management of these injuries requires a multidisciplinary management and may need percutaneous techniques as well as surgical reconstruction. Sepsis at the time of reconstruction and biliary cirrhosis are predictors of stricture. In some studies, results were generally better if transanastomotic stents were used during reconstruction.[36] Chronic liver disease and hepatic fibrosis are associated with higher operative mortality and lower success rates. Although a devastating complication, management is highly successful and restores health-related quality of life scores to preinjury levels.[37]

Biliary Leak

After a cholecystectomy, patients may suffer a leak from the cystic duct or an unrecognized duct of Luschka. Fevers, chills, right upper quadrant pain, jaundice, leakage of bile from an incision or into a drain, or persistent anorexia or bloating are common signs and symptoms. Although it can be seen after any cholecystectomy, those performed for acute cholecystitis carry the greatest risk. With inflammation and fibrosis around an obstructed cystic duct, clips placed on the duct may not fully occlude it or may be dislodged as the inflammatory process resolves. Patients will generally present within 1 week of cholecystectomy as the bile collects and becomes clinically manifested. As discussed above in bile duct injury, CT should be performed and will show ascites or a right upper quadrant fluid collection consistent with a biloma. After drain placement and controlling the leak and infection, endoscopic cholangiography should be performed (Fig. 55.52). If the leak is from a cystic duct stump, sphincterotomy with stenting of the common duct will allow the leak to seal without need for surgical management.[36] Reexploration in this setting is rarely indicated, especially in patients with evidence of septic shock or those in whom the leakage is not percutaneously accessible. If percutaneous drainage is not feasible because of overlying bowel or the fluid is not localized and thus not amenable to percutaneous drainage, a laparoscopic washout of the abdomen and placement of subhepatic drains should be considered. No attempt should be made to fix the leak because any such intervention is almost always unsuccessful and carries a risk of further injury to the biliary tree. Persistence of a bile leak longer than 6 weeks should raise the suspicion of an unrecognized bile duct injury. Similar to CBD injuries, surgical treatment of a duct leak is most successful once the inflammatory process has resolved.

Lost Stones

Accidental opening of the gallbladder with spillage of stones is not infrequent, occurring in 20% to 40% of cholecystectomies, especially during a laparoscopic approach. Pigmented stones, a high number of stones, less experienced surgeons performing the surgery, and severe cholecystitis are all risk factors. Unfortunately, stones lost during a cholecystectomy can have significant and even substantially delayed consequences, such as chronic abscess, fistula, wound infection, and bowel obstruction. Most dropped stones settle into the Morison pouch or the retrohepatic space along the abdominal wall, which may develop into a chronic abscess in this location. The likelihood for the development of complications from lost stones is difficult to quantify because surgeon documentation of gallbladder perforation is variable and a substantial delay frequently exists between cholecystectomy and complication from lost stones. On the basis of available studies, lost stones do not necessitate conversion to an open operation; treatment should include extensive irrigation, significant attempt to retrieve lost stones, course of antibiotics, documentation of the perforation in the operative notes, and clear communication with the patient of the small possibility of delayed presentation from erosion or abscess.[38]

Postcholecystectomy Pain

Although unusual, pain similar to biliary colic may persist or recur after cholecystectomy. A thorough evaluation of the biliary tree should be undertaken after cholecystectomy if the pain recurs. Recurrence of pain, if it is associated with other system findings of jaundice, fever, or chills within days to weeks after cholecystectomy suggests a secondary choledocholithiasis or a bile leak. Other biliary tree phenomena may cause a similar picture, such as sphincter of Oddi dysfunction. Postoperative bile duct strictures, which usually are manifested with jaundice, are generally identified within the first year after cholecystectomy and may be manifested with pain or fever if only one lobar duct is obstructed. In the setting of normal liver chemistries, other causes of right upper quadrant pain should be investigated.

Retained Biliary Stones

Retained stones or secondary stones, originating in the gallbladder and passing into the common duct, are usually cholesterol stones and frequently become symptomatic within weeks of a cholecystectomy. They can be identified for up to 2 years after cholecystectomy. Hyperbilirubinemia and an elevated alkaline phosphatase level should raise the suspicion of a retained stone. Ultrasound may not show intrahepatic biliary ductal dilation if the stone does not fully occlude the duct or the obstruction is early. Endoscopic removal of these stones through a generous sphincterotomy is almost universally successful (Fig. 55.53).

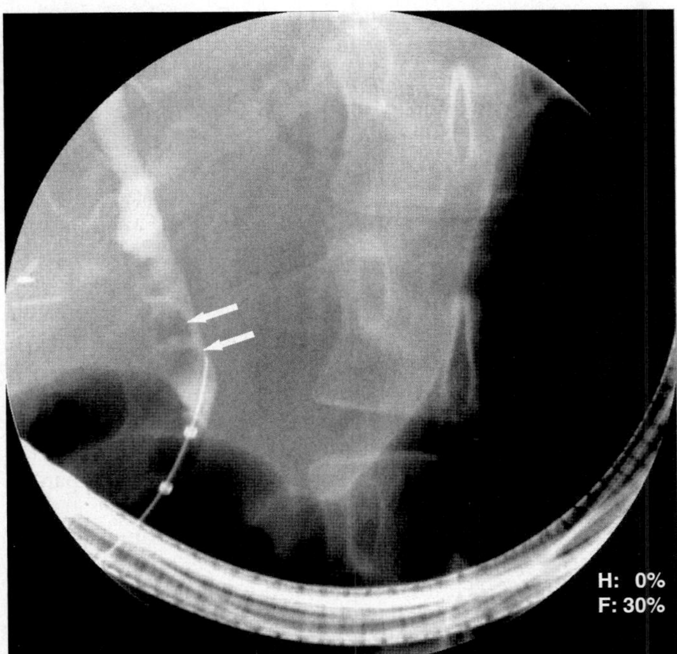

FIG. 55.53 Endoscopic retrograde cholangiopancreatography showing multiple retained common bile duct stones *(arrows)*.

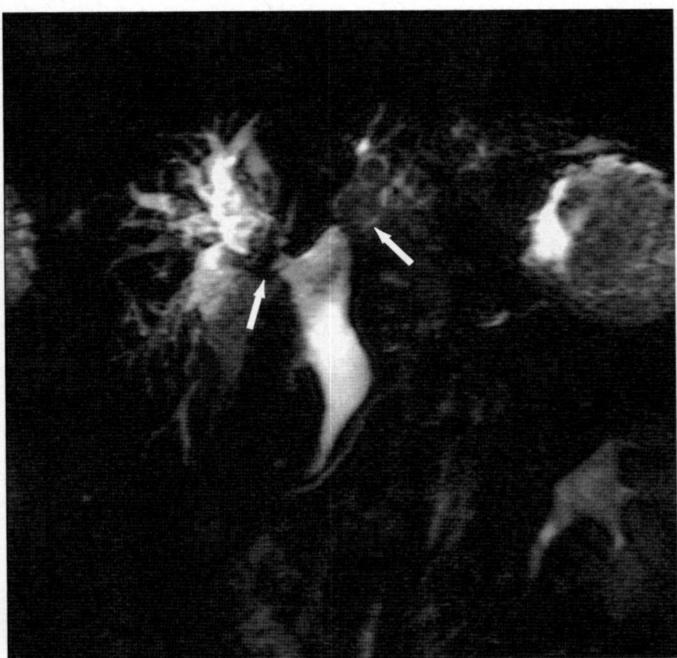

FIG. 55.54 Magnetic resonance cholangiopancreatography of recurrent pyogenic cholangitis. Intraluminal filling defects from stones are noted in both lobes *(arrows)*.

Acute Cholangitis

Any obstructing phenomenon, from biliary stones to neoplasms, can cause ascending bacterial infection of biliary tree, resulting in cholangitis. As cholecystitis, cholangitis requires obstruction and bacterial overgrowth. With obstruction from a stone, bactibilia can be identified in up to 90% of patients. The most common pathogens include *Klebsiella*, *E. coli*, *Enterobacter*, *Pseudomonas*, and *Citrobacter* spp.

The classic Charcot triad of fever, jaundice, and right upper quadrant pain can be seen in less than 50% of all patients, the least common finding being jaundice. Leukocytosis with an abnormal liver panel is common. Hepatocellular injury from the infection and inflammation elevate serum transaminase and alkaline phosphatase levels. Ultrasound should be the first screening test and will commonly show dilation of the biliary tree. HIDA scans should be interpreted with caution because infection of the biliary tree reduces the secretion of these agents into the biliary tree. CT can be helpful in identifying the site of obstruction although not always the case. The most valuable modalities are cholangiography through ERCP or PTC as they are not only diagnostic but also therapeutic.

Adequate hydration and IV antibiotics should be started immediately. Many patients will improve with medical therapy; however, these patients require emergent decompression of the biliary tree for definitive therapy. Endoscopic or percutaneous drainage achieves this goal with less morbidity than surgical intervention. If endoscopic and percutaneous means are unavailable or unsuccessful, surgical drainage consists of common duct exploration with placement of a T tube. Given the unstable nature of the patient, definitive surgical treatment of the cause is deferred until the patient is stabilized, the cholangitis is treated, and the diagnosis is confirmed.

Recurrent Pyogenic Cholangitis

More common in East Asian populations, recurrent pyogenic cholangitis is caused by cholangiohepatitis or intrahepatic stones. Biliary pathogens such as *Clonorchis sinensis* and *Ascaris lumbricoides* populate the biliary tree. These and other pathogens secrete an enzyme that hydrolyzes water-soluble bilirubin glucuronides to form free bilirubin, which then precipitates to form brown pigment stones. These stones may partially or fully obstruct the biliary tree, causing recurrent episodes of cholangitis and, eventually, abscesses or even cirrhosis. The chronicity of the infection and inflammation places these patients at risk for the development of cholangiocarcinoma. It is unclear whether the primary inciting event is infection causing inflammatory stricture or inflammatory stricture with subsequent infection of stagnant bile.

Recurrent pyogenic cholangitis tends to occur in the third to fourth decade of life, affecting men and women equally. The clinical presentation is that of cholangitis with fever, right upper quadrant pain, and jaundice. Because the infection, inflammation, and stones commonly present in a segmental or lobar pattern, the jaundice tends to be mild. Serum studies are similar to other causes of cholangitis, with a leukocytosis and elevated bilirubin and high alkaline phosphatase levels. Diagnosis is usually made by a combination of CT or MRCP with ERCP (Fig. 55.54). Lobar or segmental atrophy or hypertrophy may be seen in chronic cases.

In the setting of an acute attack, conservative treatment with parenteral antibiotics, IV fluids, and analgesics will usually suffice. Failure of this approach, with clinical deterioration, mandates biliary drainage by ERCP or percutaneous methods. Once the attack has subsided, a thorough investigation of biliary tree anatomy will help direct treatment. Definitive operative treatment is almost always required. The goals of surgical therapy are threefold: (1) remove all stones; (2) bypass, enlarge, or resect the strictures; and (3) provide adequate biliary drainage. The variability of presentation and location of disease have spurred the development of a number of operations to achieve these goals. The presence of intrahepatic strictures connotes a complicated case and may warrant resection, stricturoplasty, or hepaticojejunostomy. When clearance of all stones is not possible or future need for endoscopic therapy is anticipated, the terminal end of the Roux limb for a hepaticojejunostomy can be brought out as a stoma to provide easy access for choledochoscopy. Given the risk of cholangiocarcinoma, disease affecting predominantly one lobe should be resected in patients with adequate hepatic reserve. In the absence of the development of cholangiocarcinoma, surgical management is highly successful.[39]

MALIGNANT BILIARY DISEASE

Gallbladder Cancer

Gallbladder cancer is an aggressive malignant disease and carries an extremely poor prognosis. Patients have no specific presenting symptoms, and, therefore, presentation with late-stage disease is common. The poor prognosis corresponds to the high proportion of patients presenting with advanced disease. For patients with earlier stage disease, a more aggressive surgical approach is warranted.

Incidence

Gallbladder cancer generally occurs in the sixth and seventh decades of life and is two to three times more common in women than in men. Ethnicity plays an important role in the development of gallbladder cancer, with the highest incidence in women from India and Pakistan. Among North American populations, Native Americans and immigrants from Latin America have the highest rates. In the United States overall, gallbladder cancer is the most common cancer of the biliary tract and the fifth most common gastrointestinal cancer.[40]

Cause

Although not proven scientifically, the prevailing theory of gallbladder cancer focuses on chronic inflammation with subsequent development of neoplasia. Therefore, the presence of gallstones is considered to be the primary risk factor, and larger stones (>3 cm) carry an increased risk of cancer development. More than 80% of patients with gallbladder cancer have cholelithiasis, and gallbladder cancer is approximately seven times more common in patients with gallstones than in those without stones. The type of stone does not correlate with incidence of gallbladder cancer. Other risk factors include entities that may also cause inflammation in the gallbladder wall, such as APBJ, choledochal cysts, and PSC.

Extensive calcification of the wall of the gallbladder, termed porcelain gallbladder, carries a risk of cancer development. The calcification is probably the result of long-standing inflammation. Whereas the risk of gallbladder cancer is higher in patients with gallbladder wall calcification, malignant disease in this setting is unusual, occurring in less than 10% of patients with porcelain gallbladder.[41]

There is some suggestion of an adenoma-carcinoma progression in the development of gallbladder cancer as severe dysplasia and carcinoma in situ are often adjacent to gallbladder carcinomas.[42] However, there is no evidence that patients with gallbladder polyposis carry an increased risk of gallbladder malignancy. Conversely, several studies have demonstrated that the presence of a single gallbladder polyp larger than 10 mm carries an increased malignancy risk and cholecystectomy is generally recommended.[43]

Pathology and Staging

Gallbladder cancer is generally adenocarcinoma. It is staged by the standard tumor node metastasis (TNM) staging system (Table 55.1). Gallbladder cancer spreads via lymphatics, hematogenously, and notoriously into the peritoneal cavity or along biopsy or surgical wound tracts.

Gross descriptions of gallbladder cancer have been grouped into infiltrative, nodular, papillary, and combined forms. Most tumors have an infiltrative pattern and spread in a subserosal plane and can invade the entire gallbladder wall and even into the porta hepatis. Nodular types tend to grow as a more circumscribed mass and can invade the liver. A small subset of gallbladder cancers are of the papillary subtype and carry a better prognosis as they tend to have an indolent course and are commonly limited to the gallbladder wall at the time of diagnosis (Fig. 55.55).

The first draining nodal basin for gallbladder cancer includes the cystic and pericholedochal nodes. From these, the primary drainage areas are the retroportal and pancreaticoduodenal notes. Progressing from these lower portal areas, the lymphatics course to the celiac, superior mesenteric, and finally to aortocaval notes. Thereby, it is important to explore the retropancreatic area with a full Kocher maneuver at time of surgery to properly stage a patient with gallbladder cancer.[44]

The gallbladder wall is thin, contains a narrow lamina propria, and is only a single muscular layer with no serosal covering between it and the liver. Thereby, gallbladder malignancies can invade the liver early in their progression. In addition, because the venous drainage of the gallbladder includes direct venous tributaries into the liver parenchyma, these tumors may spread directly into segment IV of the liver. Transperitoneal spread is also common and can progress to carcinomatosis.

Clinical Presentation

Because 90% of gallbladder cancers originate in the fundus or body of the gallbladder, most do not produce symptoms until the disease is advanced (Fig. 55.56). Most gallbladder carcinomas have systemic disease at the time of presentation, with nodal disease in 35% and distant metastases in 40%. Symptoms of acute cholecystitis, with obstruction of the neck of the gallbladder, may portend a better prognosis because patients with these symptoms may present with earlier stages of disease. This presentation is often indistinguishable from hilar cholangiocarcinoma. Weight loss, jaundice, or an abdominal mass is associated with later stages of disease. Some patients describe symptoms of chronic cholecystitis in which the pain has recently changed in quality or frequency. Other common symptoms include chronic epigastric pain, early satiety, and a sense of fullness.[45]

Diagnosis

Laboratory examination generally is not helpful except to identify signs of advanced disease, such as anemia, hypoalbuminemia, leukocytosis, and elevated alkaline phosphate or bilirubin levels. Carcinoembryonic antigen and carbohydrate antigen 19-9 may be elevated in gallbladder cancer.

Ultrasonography is generally the first examination used in the evaluation of right upper quadrant pain. Ultrasonographic findings of gallbladder cancer include an irregularly shaped lesion in the subhepatic space, heterogeneous mass in the gallbladder lumen, and asymmetrically thickened gallbladder wall (Fig. 55.57). The finding of a polyp larger than 10 mm should raise the suspicion of gallbladder cancer.

Cross-sectional imaging with CT or MRI is an important part of the preoperative assessment of gallbladder cancer and can provide critical information on the local extent of disease and whether distant metastases are present. CT and MRI may demonstrate peritoneal metastases, hepatic parenchymal metastases,

TABLE 55.1 Staging for gallbladder cancer.

Definition of Primary Tumor (T)

T Category	T Criteria
TX	Primary tumor cannot be assessed
T0	No evidence of primary tumor
Tis	Carcinoma in situ
T1	Tumor invades the lamina propria or muscular layer
T1a	Tumor invades the lamina propria
T1b	Tumor invades the muscular layer
T2	Tumor invades the perimuscular connective tissue on the peritoneal side without involvement of the serosa (visceral peritoneum) or tumor invades the perimuscular connective tissue on the hepatic side, with no extension into the liver
T2a	Tumor invades the perimuscular connective tissue on the peritoneal side without involvement of the serosa (visceral peritoneum)
T2b	Tumor invades the perimuscular connective tissue on the hepatic side with no extension into the liver
T3	Tumor perforates the serosa (visceral peritoneum) and/or directly invades the liver and/or one other adjacent organ or structure, such as the stomach, duodenum, colon, pancreas, omentum, or extrahepatic bile ducts
T4	Tumor invades the main portal vein or hepatic artery or invades two or more extrahepatic organs or structures

Definition of Regional lymph Node (N)

N Category	N Criteria
NX	Regional lymph nodes cannot be assessed
N0	No regional lymph node metastasis
N1	Metastases to one to three regional lymph nodes
N2	Metastases to four or more regional lymph nodes

Definition of Distant Metastasis (M)

M Category	M Criteria
M0	No distant metastasis
M1	Distant metastasis

AJCC Prognostic Stage Groups

When T is...	And N is...	And M is...	Then the stage group is...
Tis	N0	M0	0
T1	N0	M0	I
T2a	N0	M0	IIA
T2b	N0	M0	IIB
T3	N0	M0	IIIA
T1–3	N1	M0	IIIB
T4	N0–1	M0	IVA
Any T	N2	M0	IVB
Any T	Any N	M1	IVB

Histologic Grade (G)

G	G definition
GX	Grade cannot be assessed
G1	Well differentiated
G2	Moderately differentiated
G3	Poorly differentiated

From Amin MB,[1] Greene FL,[2] Edge SB,[3,4] Compton CC,[5,6] Gershenwald JE,[7] Brookland RK,[8] Meyer L,[9] Gress DM,[10] Byrd DR,[11] Winchester DP.[12] *AJCC Cancer Staging Manual*. 8th ed. New York: Springer; 2017:303–310.

AJCC, American Joint Committee on Cancer.

[1]Professor and Chairman, UTHSC Gerwin Chair for Cancer Research, Department of Pathology and Laboratory Medicine, University of Tennessee Health Science Center, Memphis, TN.
[2]Medical Director, Cancer Data Services, Levine Cancer Institute, Charlotte, NC.
[3]Vice President, Healthcare Outcomes and Policy, Department of Cancer Prevention and Control, Roswell Park Cancer Institute, Buffalo, NY.
[4]Professor of Oncology, Department of Surgical Oncology, Roswell Park Cancer Institute, Buffalo, NY.
[5]Chief Medical Officer, Complex Adaptive Systems Initiative, Arizona State University, Scottsdale, AZ.
[6]Professor of Laboratory Medicine and Pathology, Mayo Clinic, Rochester, MN.
[7]Professor of Surgery and Cancer Biology, The University of Texas MD Anderson Cancer Center, Houston, TX.
[8]Radiation Oncologist, Greater Baltimore Medical Center, Baltimore, MD.
[9]Eighth Edition Project Manager and Managing Editor, American Joint Committee on Cancer, Chicago, IL.
[10]Technical Specialist and Technical Editor, American Joint Committee on Cancer, Chicago, IL.
[11]Section Chief of Surgical Oncology and Professor of Surgery, University of Washington, Seattle, WA.
[12]Medical Director, American Joint Committee on Cancer, Chicago, IL.

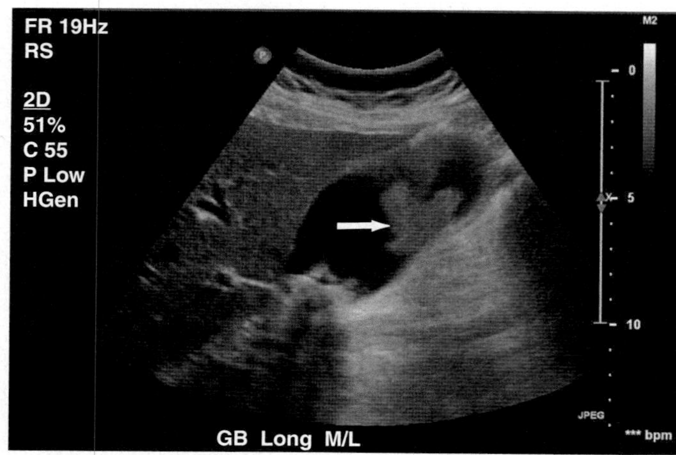

FIG. 55.55 Ultrasound image showing intraluminal polypoid gallbladder wall mass *(arrow)* but without extraluminal extension.

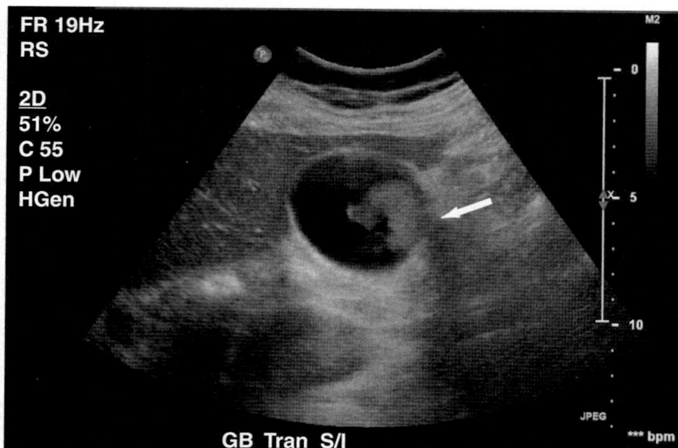

FIG. 55.57 Ultrasound image of gallbladder mass with loss of continuity of gallbladder wall *(arrow)*, suggesting extraluminal growth.

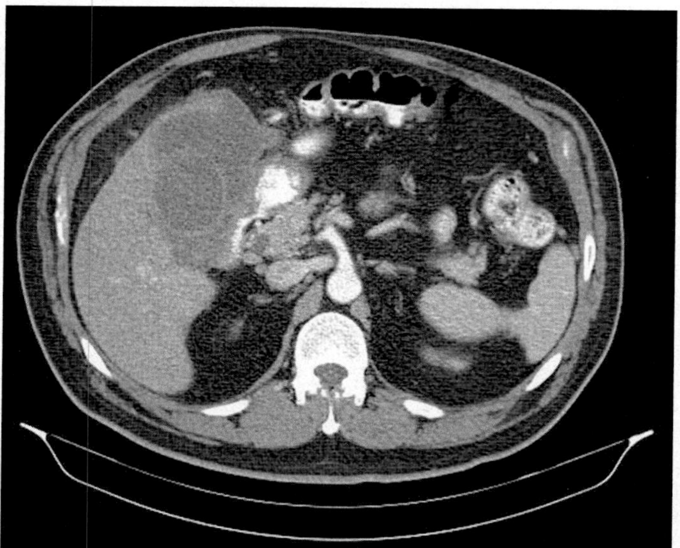

FIG. 55.56 Computed tomography scan showing gallbladder cancer with invasion into the duodenum and liver parenchyma.

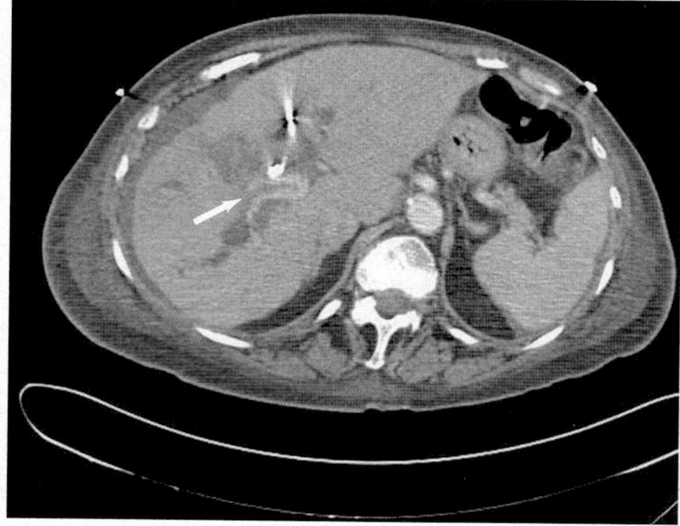

FIG. 55.58 Computed tomography scan showing gallbladder mass with local invasion into portal vein *(arrow)*.

lymphadenopathy, and adjacent vascular involvement (Fig. 55.58). Invasive diagnostic cholangiography has largely been replaced by MRI cholangiography in most high-volume centers.[46] PET can also be a valuable adjunct in searching for metastatic disease or when CT or MRI provides limited information about the primary tumor.

Gallbladder cancer has a tendency to seed biopsy tracts and unnecessary biopsies simply increase this risk. If the diagnosis is suspected, the surgeon and patient must be prepared for a definitive operation. In the setting of unresectability (vascular encasement or extensive hepatic involvement) or incurability (hepatic or peritoneal metastases), a biopsy for confirmatory tissue diagnosis should be used.

Treatment

Resection of gallbladder cancer remains the only potential for cure. Patients with gallbladder cancer can be divided into four specific subgroups of presentation: patients with a gallbladder polyp, patients with an incidental finding of gallbladder cancer at the time of or after cholecystectomy, patients suspected of having gallbladder cancer preoperatively, and patients with advanced disease at presentation.

Gallbladder polyp. The only polypoid lesions that have malignant potential and are associated with a significant rate of harboring malignancy are adenomatous polyps. The most consistent predictors of malignancy in gallbladder polyps are single polyp, size greater than 1 cm, and age older than 50 years.[47] Cholecystectomy is generally recommended for polyps larger than 1 cm and can safely be performed laparoscopically. Polyps smaller than 1 cm can undergo surveillance to demonstrate stability, with the exception in the setting of PSC, where the threshold for cholecystectomy should be lower in the population.

Gallbladder cancer after cholecystectomy. With the finding of carcinoma after cholecystectomy, subsequent treatment depends on depth of penetration of the gallbladder wall and surgical margins. With T1a lesions, in which the carcinoma penetrates the lamina propria but does not invade the muscle layer, cholecystectomy suffices for therapy. The likelihood of nodal disease in this setting is less than 3% and cholecystectomy cures 85% to 100%

of patients. The cystic duct margin should be reviewed to ensure a negative margin, and sometimes, it is necessary to resect the CBD to obtain a negative margin. For those penetrating the muscularis but not the deeper connective tissue or serosa, classified as T1b lesions, cholecystectomy may be sufficient as long as the margins are negative, although this remains controversial. With T1b lesions and perineural, lymphatic, or vascular invasion, the likelihood of nodal disease increases significantly. Therefore, extended cholecystectomy is generally recommended for all patients who are medically fit with T1b or greater level of invasion.

The extended cholecystectomy is directed at obtaining an R0 resection of the disease, including the draining lymph node basins. Therefore, removal of the hepatoduodenal, gastrohepatic, and retroduodenal lymph nodes should be included. Resection of the cystic duct margin to uninvolved mucosa may require resection of the CBD with Roux-en-Y reconstruction. Because local extension into the hepatic parenchyma is common, 2 cm of apparently normal hepatic parenchyma from the gallbladder fossa is resected. As port site recurrences have been reported for patients with even in situ disease, some surgeons recommend port site excision, although this remains controversial as port site recurrences rarely occur in isolation and may represent aggressive disease. In patients with T2 lesions, in which the cancer extends past the muscularis but not beyond the serosa, a similar approach with radical cholecystectomy is indicated because more than 40% of these patients have lymph node metastases and up to 25% have positive margins when treated with standard cholecystectomy alone. Because gallbladder cancer is generally unresponsive to other therapies, the presence of any residual disease after operative intervention predicts poor outcome.[48]

Patients suspected of having gallbladder cancer preoperatively. Patients in whom preoperative evaluation suggests possibly resectable gallbladder cancer without metastatic disease should be offered an attempt at resection, even though survival is poor compared with those found incidentally. These patients tend to present with advanced locoregional disease and may require an extended liver resection. Because surgical intervention provides the only potential for cure or prolongation of life, radical resection should be considered for adequate operative candidates. The operation begins with a diagnostic laparoscopy to identify small-volume peritoneal or hepatic metastases that would preclude a resection, thereby avoiding an unnecessary operation. In the setting of metastatic disease, nonoperative strategies should be used to palliate symptoms. Radical resection in the setting of T3 and T4 lesions includes at least segments IVB and V but more often requires a central hepatectomy, including all of segments IV, V, and VIII. To achieve R0 margin status in large tumors, a right trisegmentectomy may be required. Direct extension of tumor into adjacent structures such as the hepatic flexure is not a contraindication to resection as long as negative margins can be obtained and all disease resected. Debulking without the possibility of complete resection has no role in the management of gallbladder cancer.

Patients with advanced disease at presentation. Many patients with gallbladder cancer will present with advanced disease, and therefore, the goal of therapy is palliation of symptoms. Common symptoms requiring palliation include jaundice, pain, and intestinal obstruction. Jaundice can be managed by endoscopic biliary stenting, and self-expanding endobiliary metal stents can provide a durable solution, with less need for repeated interventions than with plastic stents. Pain is generally treated with oral narcotics but may progress to require parenteral opioids in the hospice setting. Percutaneous neurolysis of the celiac ganglion can help with the palliation of pain. Intestinal obstruction is usually gastric outlet obstruction from local extension of tumor and is generally managed by an endoscopic duodenal wall stent. Unfortunately, neither chemotherapy nor radiation therapy has shown a survival benefit in the management of gallbladder cancer.

Adjuvant Therapy

The majority of gallbladder cancer recurrences include distant sites as part of the recurrence pattern, highlighting the importance of systemic therapies.[49] Much of the data for the adjuvant setting has been extrapolated from the metastatic setting. Gemcitabine-based regimens, often combined with a platinum agent, are typically used for treating gallbladder cancer. Patients with high-risk lesions (T4 tumors, positive lymph nodes, R1 resection) should be considered for adjuvant therapy in consultation with an oncologist.

Survival

Survival of patients diagnosed with gallbladder cancer is dependent on the stage of disease at presentation and whether surgical resection is performed. Independent factors affecting survival include T status, N status, histologic differentiation, CBD involvement, and R0 resection. Advances in surgical management and extent of resection have led to improvements in survival in surgical patients, although most patients present with late-stage disease and are not candidates for resection. Patients with T1a lesions, limited to the mucosa and lamina propria, have an excellent prognosis. Complete resection of T1b lesions to negative margins also affords an excellent prognosis. Survival of patients with T2 lesions depends on nodal status, and radical resection in this setting improves 5-year survival from approximately 20% to more than 60%. The 5-year survival of patients with T3 tumors is less than 20%, and patients with T4 lesions have a survival measured in months. Patients with metastatic disease at presentation have a median survival of 13 months. Because most patients with gallbladder cancer present with advanced disease, the overall survival of gallbladder cancer is less than 15%.

Bile Duct Cancer

Cholangiocarcinoma is a rare disease entity that carries a dismal prognosis. The incidence of cholangiocarcinoma is rising worldwide and is now the second most common primary cancer of the liver behind hepatocellular carcinoma. Historically, evaluation and management of cholangiocarcinoma required arbitrary division of the bile duct into thirds based on the location of obstruction. Lesions of the middle third, however, are decidedly rare, so investigations have recently focused on perihilar and intrahepatic lesions, known as proximal lesions, versus those involving the periampullary region, known as distal disease. More than two thirds of all cholangiocarcinomas involve the proximal biliary tree near the bifurcation, known as a Klatskin tumor.

Risk Factors

Although most patients with cholangiocarcinoma have no identifiable cause, the risk of development of cholangiocarcinoma appears to correlate with chronic inflammation in the biliary tree and compensatory cellular proliferation. Therefore, many predisposing disease states carry an increased risk for development of cholangiocarcinoma. Congenital lesions, such as choledochal cysts, predispose to the development of cholangiocarcinoma from exposure of the biliary epithelium to toxic pancreatic secretions. The incidence of cholangiocarcinoma is estimated between 10% and 20% if the cyst is not resected by age 20 years old. Cholangiocarcinoma is more prevalent in Southeast Asia, where infection with the liver flukes *Clonorchis sinensis* and *Opisthorchis viverrini* creates chronic biliary inflammation, with obstructions and strictures. Recurrent pyogenic cholangitis is characterized by primary bile duct stone formation with infections and carries a risk of cholangiocarcinoma development. PSC, with its autoimmune multifocal strictures of the intrahepatic and extrahepatic biliary trees, carries an increased risk of cholangiocarcinoma. PSC is the most common risk factor for cholangiocarcinoma in the West. PSC carries a cumulative annual risk for cholangiocarcinoma of 1.5% per year, and this risk is increased in those with associated inflammatory bowel disease. Although sporadic cases of cholangiocarcinoma tend to occur at the bifurcation, patients with PSC may have multifocal disease not amenable to resection. Medications and chemical carcinogens have been associated with the development of cholangiocarcinoma, including Thorotrast, oral contraceptives, asbestos, and cigarette smoke. Finally, cirrhosis is an important risk factor for cholangiocarcinoma with a risk of 10.7% versus 0.7% in the general population.

Staging and Classification

The three distinct pathologic subtypes include sclerosing, nodular, and papillary cholangiocarcinoma. Sclerosing cholangiocarcinoma tends to occur in the proximal bile ducts, causing periductal fibrosis in a concentric pattern and a circumferential duct occlusion. The papillary and nodular subtypes tend to occur in distal cholangiocarcinomas and are manifested with intraluminal growths. In the nodular subtype, a firm mass based in the duct wall can be seen growing into the duct lumen, whereas the more common papillary subtype appears as a polypoid lesion that is soft with less periductal fibrosis and a better prognosis.

The staging of cholangiocarcinoma relies on the TNM staging system but is slightly different on the basis of anatomic location. The three staging subdivisions include intrahepatic (Table 55.2), perihilar (Table 55.3), and distal bile duct (Table 55.4).[50] Similar to many adenocarcinomas, direct local invasion and local lymph node spread are common and portend a worse prognosis. Tumors confined to the bile duct (T1) and those extending outside the bile duct but not invading adjacent structures such as the hepatic artery or portal vein (T2) carry a significantly better prognosis than those invading any nearby structure. The two pathologic factors most influencing prognosis after resection are complete (R0) resection to negative margins and absence of lymph node metastases.

Clinical Presentation

The presentation of cholangiocarcinoma depends on the site of origin and manifestations of biliary obstruction at that site. Painless jaundice is a common symptom, but patients with unilobar obstruction of a bile duct may present with unilateral lobar atrophy and subsequent contralateral lobar hypertrophy (Fig. 55.59). The resultant hepatic compensation can delay presentation until the later stages of disease. Therefore, cholangiocarcinoma causing obstruction at or below the hepatic bifurcation tends to be manifested at earlier stages than intrahepatic cholangiocarcinoma. With obstruction of the biliary tree, the common manifestations of direct hyperbilirubinemia, such as pruritus, dark urine, and steatorrhea, can be seen. Cholangiocarcinoma tends to extend in a submucosal route, with associated perineural invasion, but constant pain on presentation suggests more advanced disease.

Diagnosis and Assessment of Resectability

At the time of presentation, most patients will have manifestations of obstructive jaundice with hyperbilirubinemia and an elevated alkaline phosphatase level. Other markers of hepatic synthetic function, such as prothrombin time and albumin level, are generally unaffected until later in the disease or when the biliary obstruction is long-standing. Tumor markers, including carcinoembryonic antigen and carbohydrate antigen 19-9, are unreliable for diagnosis of cholangiocarcinoma but, if elevated, may be useful postoperatively in the surveillance of recurrence.

The radiologic evaluation of jaundice includes a right upper quadrant ultrasound examination, which may show intrahepatic biliary ductal dilation but does not usually identify the actual site of obstruction. With hilar cholangiocarcinomas, the gallbladder and visualized extrahepatic biliary tree are usually decompressed, whereas distal lesions will have extrahepatic biliary ductal dilation and gallbladder distention. Cross-sectional imaging by triphasic CT allows not only assessment of metastatic disease but also evaluation of resectability. The location of the tumor can be identified, and its relationship to vascular structures also can be assessed. Identification of aberrant anatomy and determination of segmental or lobar involvement by CT are helpful for preoperative planning.

Typically, CT alone is insufficient for the assessment of feasibility and appropriateness of resection. Cholangiography by MRCP, PTC, or ERCP helps determine the proximal extent of resection. Endoscopic cholangiography carries the additional risk of cholangitis by the introduction of enteric bacteria into an undrained portion of the biliary tree. Bilobar intrahepatic metastases and any extrahepatic disease are contraindications to resection, as is the involvement of bilateral secondary biliary radicals. Because complete (R0) resection is the only strategy that affords the possibility of cure, other contraindications to resection include encasement of the main portal vein (Fig. 55.60), bilateral hepatic lobar artery involvement, and lobar atrophy with involvement of the contralateral portal vein or biliary radicals. Involvement of unilobar vascular structures is managed with resection of the primary and affected lobe in continuity, and therefore, it is not a contraindication.

Tissue diagnosis before resection in operative patients is unnecessary. With obstructive jaundice, bile cytology and brushings are unreliable, and thus, a negative cytology report does not exclude malignant disease. Therefore, invasive attempts to establish a diagnosis before resection carry risk but do not alter subsequent management. Establishment of a tissue diagnosis is important only when the patient is not a surgical candidate. However, preoperative biliary drainage may be useful in select cases. In patients with distal cholangiocarcinoma, preoperative biliary drainage increases the rate of infectious complications of resection but is generally useful for those with preoperative hyperbilirubinemia (bilirubin level >10 mg/dL) and those with a prolonged time interval between presentation and resection. For patients with hilar cholangiocarcinoma, hepatic resection remains an important feature of the operative strategy. In the setting of complete biliary obstruction, hepatic resection carries an additional risk of bleeding, sepsis, and hepatic failure. Drainage of the obstructed but unaffected segments can enhance the postresection hypertrophy of the remaining liver but may increase perioperative infectious complications.

Treatment

Operative management. With the clinical suspicion of cholangiocarcinoma in adequate operative candidates without contraindications to resection, exploration should proceed, even in the absence of a confirmed tissue diagnosis. Between 7% and 15%

TABLE 55.2 Staging for intrahepatic bile duct cancer.

Definition of Primary Tumor (T)

T Category	T Criteria
TX	Primary tumor cannot be assessed
T0	No evidence of primary tumor
Tis	Carcinoma in situ (intraductal tumor)
T1	Solitary tumor without vascular invasion, ≤5 cm or >5 cm
T1a	Solitary tumor ≤5 cm without vascular invasion
T1b	Solitary tumor >5 cm without vascular invasion
T2	Solitary tumor with intrahepatic vascular invasion or multiple tumors, with or without vascular invasion
T3	Tumor perforating the visceral peritoneum
T4	Tumor involving local extrahepatic structures by direct invasion

Definition of Regional Lymph Node (N)

N Category	N Criteria
NX	Regional lymph nodes cannot be assessed
N0	No regional lymph node metastasis
N1	Regional lymph node metastasis present

Definition of Distant Metastasis (M)

M Category	M Criteria
M0	No distant metastasis
M1	Distant metastasis

AJCC Prognostic Stage Groups

When T is...	And N is...	And M is...	Then the stage group is...
Tis	N0	M0	0
T1a	N0	M0	IA
T1b	N0	M0	IB
T2	N0	M0	II
T3	N0	M0	IIIA
T4	N0	M0	IIIB
Any T	N1	M0	IIIB
Any T	Any N	M1	IV

From Amin MB,[1] Greene FL,[2] Edge SB,[3,4] Compton CC,[5,6] Gershenwald JE,[7] Brookland RK,[8] Meyer L,[9] Gress DM,[10] Byrd DR,[11] Winchester DP.[12] *AJCC Cancer Staging Manual.* 8th ed. New York: Springer; 2017:295–302.

AJCC, American Joint Committee on Cancer.

[1]Professor and Chairman, UTHSC Gerwin Chair for Cancer Research, Department of Pathology and Laboratory Medicine, University of Tennessee Health Science Center, Memphis, TN.

[2]Medical Director, Cancer Data Services, Levine Cancer Institute, Charlotte, NC.

[3]Vice President, Healthcare Outcomes and Policy, Department of Cancer Prevention and Control, Roswell Park Cancer Institute, Buffalo, NY.

[4]Professor of Oncology, Department of Surgical Oncology, Roswell Park Cancer Institute, Buffalo, NY.

[5]Chief Medical Officer, Complex Adaptive Systems Initiative, Arizona State University, Scottsdale, AZ.

[6]Professor of Laboratory Medicine and Pathology, Mayo Clinic, Rochester, MN.

[7]Professor of Surgery and Cancer Biology, The University of Texas MD Anderson Cancer Center, Houston, TX.

[8]Radiation Oncologist, Greater Baltimore Medical Center, Baltimore, MD.

[9]Eighth Edition Project Manager and Managing Editor, American Joint Committee on Cancer, Chicago, IL.

[10]Technical Specialist and Technical Editor, American Joint Committee on Cancer, Chicago, IL.

[11]Section Chief of Surgical Oncology and Professor of Surgery, University of Washington, Seattle, WA.

[12]Medical Director, American Joint Committee on Cancer, Chicago, IL.

of patients undergoing resection for suspected biliary malignant disease will prove to have benign disease. Alternatively, more than 50% of patients undergoing exploration have historically had findings precluding resection, such as peritoneal metastases, hepatic metastases, or locally advanced lesions. With experienced judgment and advances in the quality of preoperative imaging, this rate is decreasing. Staging laparoscopy can also be an important initial step at the time of resection to reduce the incidence of nontherapeutic laparotomy.

Distal cholangiocarcinoma. Distal cholangiocarcinoma is managed by pancreaticoduodenectomy. Because these lesions tend to grow in a submucosal plane, a frozen section of the proximal bile duct margin helps ensure an R0 resection. An R0 resection remains one of the most important prognostic factors for this disease, with 5-year survival rates of up to 50% in node-negative patients with an R0 resection.

Proximal cholangiocarcinoma. Surgical management of proximal cholangiocarcinoma involves resection of regional nodal tissue and en bloc resection of the CBD with hepatic parenchyma as necessary to achieve negative margins. The Bismuth-Corlette classification of the tumor by assessment of the involvement of biliary radicals helps with operative planning (Fig. 55.61).[51]

TABLE 55.3 Staging for perihilar bile duct cancer.

Definition of Primary Tumor (T)

T Category	T Criteria
TX	Primary tumor cannot be assessed
T0	No evidence of primary tumor
Tis	Carcinoma in situ/high-grade dysplasia
T1	Tumor confined to the bile duct, with extension up to the muscle layer or fibrous tissue
T2	Tumor invades beyond the wall of the bile duct to surrounding adipose tissue, or tumor invades adjacent hepatic parenchyma
T2a	Tumor invades beyond the wall of the bile duct to surrounding adipose tissue
T2b	Tumor invades adjacent hepatic parenchyma
T3	Tumor invades unilateral branches of the portal vein or hepatic artery
T4	Tumor invades the main portal vein or its branches bilaterally, or the common hepatic artery; or unilateral second-order biliary radicals with contralateral portal vein or hepatic artery involvement

Definition of Regional Lymph Node (N)

N Category	N Criteria
NX	Regional lymph nodes cannot be assessed
N0	No regional lymph node metastasis
N1	One to three positive lymph nodes typically involving the hilar, cystic duct, common bile duct, hepatic artery, posterior pancreatoduodenal, and portal vein lymph nodes
N2	Four or more positive lymph nodes from the sites described for N1

Definition of Distant Metastasis (M)

M Category	M Criteria
M0	No distant metastasis
M1	Distant metastasis

AJCC Prognostic Stage Groups

When T is...	And N is...	And M is...	Then the stage group is...
Tis	N0	M0	0
T1	N0	M0	I
T2a–b	N0	M0	II
T3	N0	M0	IIIA
T4	N0	M0	IIIB
Any T	N1	M0	IIIC
Any T	N2	M0	IVA
Any T	Any N	M1	IVB

From Amin MB,[1] Greene FL,[2] Edge SB,[3,4] Compton CC,[5,6] Gershenwald JE,[7] Brookland RK,[8] Meyer L,[9] Gress DM,[10] Byrd DR,[11] Winchester DP.[12] *AJCC Cancer Staging Manual*. 8th ed. New York: Springer; 2017:311–316.

AJCC, American Joint Committee on Cancer.

[1]Professor and Chairman, UTHSC Gerwin Chair for Cancer Research, Department of Pathology and Laboratory Medicine, University of Tennessee Health Science Center, Memphis, TN.

[2]Medical Director, Cancer Data Services, Levine Cancer Institute, Charlotte, NC.

[3]Vice President, Healthcare Outcomes and Policy, Department of Cancer Prevention and Control, Roswell Park Cancer Institute, Buffalo, NY.

[4]Professor of Oncology, Department of Surgical Oncology, Roswell Park Cancer Institute, Buffalo, NY.

[5]Chief Medical Officer, Complex Adaptive Systems Initiative, Arizona State University, Scottsdale, AZ.

[6]Professor of Laboratory Medicine and Pathology, Mayo Clinic, Rochester, MN.

[7]Professor of Surgery and Cancer Biology, The University of Texas MD Anderson Cancer Center, Houston, TX.

[8]Radiation Oncologist, Greater Baltimore Medical Center, Baltimore, MD.

[9]Eighth Edition Project Manager and Managing Editor, American Joint Committee on Cancer, Chicago, IL.

[10]Technical Specialist and Technical Editor, American Joint Committee on Cancer, Chicago, IL.

[11]Section Chief of Surgical Oncology and Professor of Surgery, University of Washington, Seattle, WA.

[12]Medical Director, American Joint Committee on Cancer, Chicago, IL.

Types I and II lesions are treated with common duct resection, cholecystectomy, and a 5- to 10-mm margin of resection. Type II lesions may also require partial hepatic resection, which commonly includes resection of the caudate lobe. Resection of the bile duct and nodal tissue requires skeletonization of the hepatic artery and portal vein. Reconstruction is performed using a Roux limb of jejunum. Types III and IV lesions may involve complex resection and reconstruction of the portal vein, hepatic artery, or both. With resection to secondary biliary radicals, transanastomotic stenting is used liberally to allow healing and even confirmation of anastomotic integrity. A substantial improvement in long-term survival has correlated with the increasing use of hepatic resection to achieve negative margins. Negative margin status is the most important variable associated with outcome.[52]

TABLE 55.4 **Staging for distal bile duct cancer.**

Definition of Primary Tumor (T)

T Category	T Criteria
TX	Primary tumor cannot be assessed
Tis	Carcinoma in situ/high-grade dysplasia
T1	Tumor invades the bile duct wall with a depth less than 5 mm
T2	Tumor invades the bile duct wall with a depth of 5–12 mm
T3	Tumor invades the bile duct wall with a depth greater than 12 mm
T4	Tumor involves the celiac axis, superior mesenteric artery, and/or common hepatic artery

Definition of Regional Lymph Node (N)

N Category	N Criteria
NX	Regional lymph nodes cannot be assessed
N0	No regional lymph node metastasis
N1	Metastasis in one to three regional lymph nodes
N2	Metastasis in four or more regional lymph nodes

Definition of Distant Metastasis (M)

M Category	M Criteria
M0	No distant metastasis
M1	Distant metastasis

AJCC Prognostic Stage Groups

When T is...	And N is...	And M is...	Then the stage group is...
Tis	N0	M0	0
T1	N0	M0	I
T1	N1	M0	IIA
T1	N2	M0	IIIA
T2	N0	M0	IIA
T2	N1	M0	IIB
T2	N2	M0	IIIA
T3	N0	M0	IIB
T3	N1	M0	IIB
T3	N2	M0	IIIA
T4	N0	M0	IIIB
T4	N1	M0	IIIB
T4	N2	M0	IIIB
Any T	Any N	M1	IV

From Amin MB,[1] Greene FL,[2] Edge SB,[3,4] Compton CC,[5,6] Gershenwald JE,[7] Brookland RK,[8] Meyer L,[9] Gress DM,[10] Byrd DR,[11] Winchester DP.[12] *AJCC Cancer Staging Manual*. 8th ed. New York: Springer; 2017:317–326.

AJCC, American Joint Committee on Cancer.

[1]Professor and Chairman, UTHSC Gerwin Chair for Cancer Research, Department of Pathology and Laboratory Medicine, University of Tennessee Health Science Center, Memphis, TN.

[2]Medical Director, Cancer Data Services, Levine Cancer Institute, Charlotte, NC.

[3]Vice President, Healthcare Outcomes and Policy, Department of Cancer Prevention and Control, Roswell Park Cancer Institute, Buffalo, NY.

[4]Professor of Oncology, Department of Surgical Oncology, Roswell Park Cancer Institute, Buffalo, NY.

[5]Chief Medical Officer, Complex Adaptive Systems Initiative, Arizona State University, Scottsdale, AZ.

[6]Professor of Laboratory Medicine and Pathology, Mayo Clinic, Rochester, MN.

[7]Professor of Surgery and Cancer Biology, The University of Texas MD Anderson Cancer Center, Houston, TX.

[8]Radiation Oncologist, Greater Baltimore Medical Center, Baltimore, MD.

[9]Eighth Edition Project Manager and Managing Editor, American Joint Committee on Cancer, Chicago, IL.

[10]Technical Specialist and Technical Editor, American Joint Committee on Cancer, Chicago, IL.

[11]Section Chief of Surgical Oncology and Professor of Surgery, University of Washington, Seattle, WA.

[12]Medical Director, American Joint Committee on Cancer, Chicago, IL.

Five-year survival rates as high as 59% have been reported in selected series, and with vascular resection and reconstruction techniques, resectability rates have also increased. Increases in the magnitude of the operation have also correlated with an expected increase in surgical mortality, from 2% to 4% in limited resection up to 3% to 11% when more complex.

Although the importance of achieving an R0 resection is clear, the role of routine lymph node dissection is debated. There has been no demonstrable benefit of routine lymph node dissection; however, lymph nodes are one of the most important prognostic factors in cholangiocarcinoma and may help direct adjuvant therapy.

As noted previously, an extensive neoadjuvant therapy protocol followed by transplantation has shown promising results in tightly controlled trials where hilar cholangiocarcinoma occurs in the setting of underlying liver disease. In spite of these findings, the role of transplantation in the management of cholangiocarcinoma remains experimental, and substantial debate remains about the routine use of an extremely limited resource in this disease process. Many patients entering such a protocol develop disseminated disease prior to achieving transplantation.

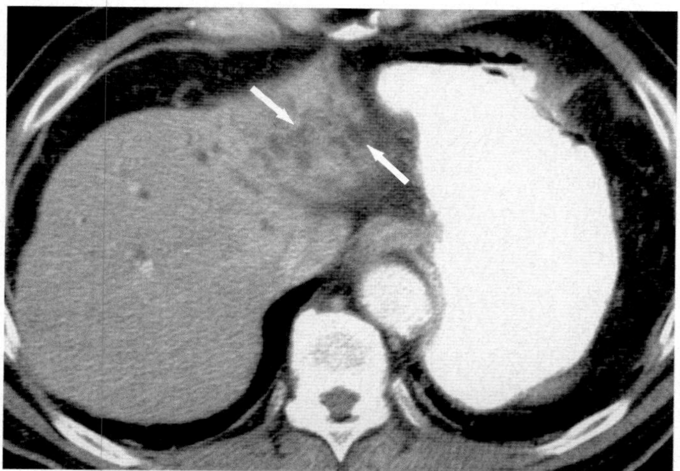

FIG. 55.59 Computed tomography scan of cholangiocarcinoma with left lobar atrophy caused by obstruction of the left duct. Noted in the atrophied left lobe are dilated biliary radicals *(arrows)*.

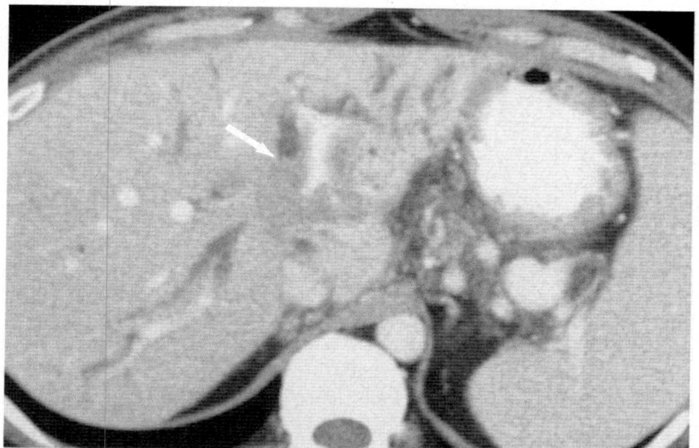

FIG. 55.60 Computed tomography scan of Klatskin tumor *(arrow)* encasing the main portal vein, consistent with unresectable disease.

Palliation. In patients found to have unresectable or incurable disease preoperatively, all attempts to palliate their symptoms nonoperatively should be used. The goals of palliation should include relief of jaundice, alleviation of pain, and relief of duodenal obstruction, if necessary. Surgical palliation has not been shown to prolong survival or to reduce complication rates and thus should be reserved for candidates found to be unresectable or metastatic at time of operation. Depending on the location of the biliary obstruction, endoscopic or percutaneous routes of drainage can be used, and placement of a self-expandable metallic stent provides a durable solution. When plastic stents are used, additional manipulation or placement of subsequent stents may be required. For distal cholangiocarcinomas, ERCP is the preferred route of nonoperative biliary drainage, whereas PTC is more useful for proximal lesions. Drainage of atrophic lobes with stents does not improve palliation of disease. Pain can be treated with oral narcotics. IV narcotics and even percutaneous destruction of the celiac plexus have demonstrated some benefit. For distal cholangiocarcinomas, in which duodenal obstruction may occur, endoscopic duodenal stenting can relieve obstruction in this preterminal condition.

Medical treatment. Chemotherapy has not been shown to improve survival in patients with cholangiocarcinoma. In addition, radiation therapy has not been proven in a prospective fashion to affect survival. Therefore, neither chemotherapy nor radiation therapy is used routinely in the adjuvant or neoadjuvant setting. Although some retrospective studies have shown a small survival advantage with adjuvant radiation, prospective studies of adjuvant radiotherapy have shown no benefit in completely resected patients. Radiation therapy may provide a small survival advantage as an adjunct to resection when microscopic residual disease remains. Most studies have reported a clinical response rate of less than 10%. Even in the absence of supportive data, adjuvant chemoradiation is used routinely at many centers but should be limited to patients with nodal disease, those with R1 resections, and those undergoing a clinical trial.

Outcomes

Long-term survival is highly dependent on stage at presentation and complete surgical resection to negative margins. With the use of common duct resection with partial hepatectomy, negative margin rates have increased to more than 75%. This has resulted in 5-year survival rates of 20% to 45% in most series. The principal reason for the variability in survival appears to be the presence of lymph node metastases. Although

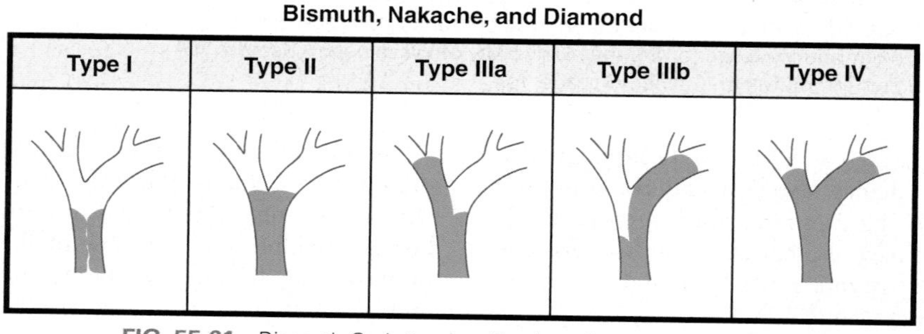

FIG. 55.61 Bismuth-Corlette classification of tumor involvement.

morbidity rates of 35% to 50% are common, mortality rates are generally low (<10%). In the setting of distal bile duct cancers, resection rates are generally higher, with approximately similar 5-year survival among patients undergoing R0 resections. Alternatively, because there is no reliable therapeutic alternative, the median survival of unresected patients ranges from 5 to 8 months.

Because negative margin status is easier to obtain by explanting the liver, some have advocated total hepatectomy with liver transplantation for treatment. Unfortunately, initial experience with therapeutic transplantation was plagued by early mortality and high recurrence rates. Recently, some centers have attempted neoadjuvant chemoradiation followed by exploration for the evaluation of resectability and metastases, and finally transplantation, with improved survival over resection alone.[19] At present, the role of transplantation in the management of cholangiocarcinoma is at best controversial, and it should be limited to research protocols.

METASTATIC AND OTHER TUMORS

Any primary or secondary tumor affecting the liver can cause biliary obstruction. The most common examples include portal nodal disease from adenocarcinomas, such as hepatocellular carcinoma, pancreatic adenocarcinoma, and colorectal carcinoma. The metastatic nodes can compress the CBD at any point along its length. Lymphoma may affect the portal lymph node chain and, when isolated to periportal nodes, is notoriously difficult to differentiate from cholangiocarcinoma. Placement of temporary plastic stents to relieve the obstruction is usually the only therapeutic biliary intervention required because these lymphomas will generally respond to chemotherapy and the obstruction will usually resolve.

Primary lesions of the liver or metastatic disease may obstruct the biliary tree from direct compression or extension, as seen in hepatocellular carcinoma, but this phenomenon does not create an intraluminal biliary growth. Rarely, tumor cells may actually pass into the biliary tree and embolize distally. As the exfoliated cellular mass grows, it may be manifested with intraluminal biliary obstruction. Intrahepatic biliary cystadenomas and cystadenocarcinoma may obstruct the bile duct directly or by passage of the mucin that they produce.

SELECTED REFERENCES

Butte JM, Kingham TP, Gonen M, et al. Residual disease predicts outcomes after definitive resection for incidental gallbladder cancer. *J Am Coll Surg.* 2014;219:416–429.

This article evaluated the survival of gallbladder cancer after attempted surgical resection, noting the import of R0 resection status on survival.

Darwish Murad S, Kim WR, Harnois DM, et al. Efficacy of neoadjuvant chemoradiation, followed by liver transplantation, for perihilar cholangiocarcinoma at 12 US centers. *Gastroenterol.* 2012;143:88–98.e3.

This article evaluated the results of transplantation for cholangiocarcinoma after a rigorous neoadjuvant therapy protocol.

Drossman DA. Functional gastrointestinal disorders: history, pathophysiology, clinical features and rome IV. *Gastroenterol.* 2016;150:1262–1279.

This article is a review article on functional disorders of gastrointestinal tract, with updated guidelines and recommendations for these functional disorders, their diagnosis, and their management.

Fogel EL, Sherman S. ERCP for gallstone pancreatitis. *N Engl J Med.* 2014;370:150–157.

This article reviews the current status of the role of endoscopic retrograde cholangiopancreatography in the diagnosis and management of biliary pancreatitis, depending on severity.

Horwood J, Akbar F, Davis K, et al. Prospective evaluation of a selective approach to cholangiography for suspected CBD stones. *Ann R Coll Surg Engl.* 2010;92:206–210.

This article evaluates the criteria for selective cholangiography during routine cholecystectomy.

Pitt HA, Sherman S, Johnson MS, et al. Improved outcomes of bile duct injuries in the 21st century. *Ann Surg.* 2013;258:490–499.

This article reviewed a large series of iatrogenic bile duct injuries, highlighting the success of surgical intervention and the multidisciplinary approach to management.

Sirinek KR, Schwesinger WH. Has intraoperative cholangiography during laparoscopic cholecystectomy become obsolete in the era of preoperative endoscopic retrograde and magnetic resonance cholangiopancreatography? *J Am Coll Surg.* 2015;220:522–528.

This article highlights current practice patterns of imaging in the management of suspected choledocholithiasis, noting the application of magnetic resonance cholangiopancreatography as a screening tool for referral for endoscopic retrograde cholangiopancreatography before laparoscopic cholecystectomy.

Strasberg SM, Gouma DJ. 'Extreme' vasculobiliary injuries: association with fundus-down cholecystectomy in severely inflamed gallbladders. *HPB.* 2012;14:1–8.

This article discusses the surgical pitfalls of a "dome down" approach to the inflamed gallbladder.

Strasberg SM, Hertl M, Soper NJ. An analysis of the problem of biliary injury during laparoscopic cholecystectomy. *J Am Coll Surg.* 1995;180:101–125.

This is the most cited article for classification of iatrogenic bile duct injuries and is considered the seminal comprehensive article on the topic.

Wakabayashi G, Iwashita Y, Hibi T, et al. Tokyo Guidelines 2018: surgical management of acute cholecystitis: safe steps in laparoscopic cholecystectomy for acute cholecystitis (with videos). *J Hepatobiliary Pancreat Sci*. 2018;25:73–86.

This article is a new guideline called "Tokyo Guidelines" for surgical steps and techniques of cholecystectomy, after international multicenter expert reviews.

REFERENCES

1. Couinaud C. Les envelopes vasculobiliares de foie ou capsule de glisson: leur interet dans la chirurgie vesiculaire, les resections hepatique et l'abord du hile du foie. *Lyon Chir*. 1954;49:589–615.
2. Admirand WH, Small DM. The physicochemical basis of cholesterol gallstone formation in man. *J Clin Invest*. 1968;47:1043–1052.
3. Hirota M, Takada T, Kawarada Y, et al. Diagnostic criteria and severity assessment of acute cholecystitis: Tokyo Guidelines. *J Hepatobiliary Pancreat Surg*. 2007;14:78–82.
4. Kimura Y, Takada T, Kawarada Y, et al. Definitions, pathophysiology, and epidemiology of acute cholangitis and cholecystitis: Tokyo Guidelines. *J Hepatobiliary Pancreat Surg*. 2007;14:15–26.
5. Shafi S, Priest EL, Crandall ML, et al. Multicenter validation of American Association For The Surgery Of Trauma grading system for acute colonic diverticulitis and its use for emergency general surgery quality improvement program. *J Trauma Acute Care Surg*. 2016;80:405–410; discussion 410–401.
6. de Mestral C, Rotstein OD, Laupacis A, et al. Comparative operative outcomes of early and delayed cholecystectomy for acute cholecystitis: a population-based propensity score analysis. *Ann Surg*. 2014;259:10–15.
7. Wakabayashi G, Iwashita Y, Hibi T, et al. Tokyo Guidelines 2018: surgical management of acute cholecystitis: safe steps in laparoscopic cholecystectomy for acute cholecystitis (with videos). *J Hepatobiliary Pancreat Sci*. 2018;25:73–86.
8. Verbesey JE, Birkett DH. Common bile duct exploration for choledocholithiasis. *Surg Clin North Am*. 2008;88:1315–1328, ix.
9. Horwood J, Akbar F, Davis K, et al. Prospective evaluation of a selective approach to cholangiography for suspected common bile duct stones. *Ann R Coll Surg Engl*. 2010;92:206–210.
10. Sirinek KR, Schwesinger WH. Has intraoperative cholangiography during laparoscopic cholecystectomy become obsolete in the era of preoperative endoscopic retrograde and magnetic resonance cholangiopancreatography? *J Am Coll Surg*. 2015;220:522–528.
11. Peponis T, Panda N, Eskesen TG, et al. Preoperative endoscopic retrograde cholangio-pancreatography (ERCP) is a risk factor for surgical site infections after laparoscopic cholecystectomy. *Am J Surg*. 2019;218:140–144.
12. Lee JK, Ryu JK, Park JK, et al. Roles of endoscopic sphincterotomy and cholecystectomy in acute biliary pancreatitis. *Hepato-Gastroenterology*. 2008;55:1981–1985.
13. Fogel EL, Sherman S. ERCP for gallstone pancreatitis. *N Engl J Med*. 2014;370:150–157.
14. Lyu YX, Cheng YX, Jin HF, et al. Same-admission versus delayed cholecystectomy for mild acute biliary pancreatitis: a systematic review and meta-analysis. *BMC Surg*. 2018;18:111.
15. Drossman DA. Functional gastrointestinal disorders: history, pathophysiology, clinical features and rome IV. *Gastroenterol*. 2016;150:1262–1279.
16. Weismuller TJ, Trivedi PJ, Bergquist A, et al. Patient age, sex, and inflammatory bowel disease phenotype associate with course of primary sclerosing cholangitis. *Gastroenterol*. 2017;152:1975–1984.e1978.
17. Tabibian JH, Ali AH, Lindor KD. Primary sclerosing cholangitis, part 1: epidemiology, etiopathogenesis, clinical features, and treatment. *Gastroenterol Hepatol*. 2018;14:293–304.
18. Carbone M, Neuberger JM. Autoimmune liver disease, autoimmunity and liver transplantation. *J Hepatol*. 2014;60:210–223.
19. Darwish Murad S, Kim WR, Harnois DM, et al. Efficacy of neoadjuvant chemoradiation, followed by liver transplantation, for perihilar cholangiocarcinoma at 12 US centers. *Gastroenterol*. 2012;143:88–98.e83; quiz e14.
20. Zhang X, Wang X, Wang L, et al. Effect of covered self-expanding metal stents compared with multiple plastic stents on benign biliary stricture: a meta-analysis. *Medicine (Baltimore)*. 2018;7:e12039.
21. Todani T, Watanabe Y, Narusue M, et al. Congenital bile duct cysts: classification, operative procedures, and review of thirty-seven cases including cancer arising from choledochal cyst. *Am J Surg*. 1977;134:263–269.
22. Ten Hove A, de Meijer VE, Hulscher JBF, et al. Meta-analysis of risk of developing malignancy in congenital choledochal malformation. *Br J Surg*. 2018;105:482–490.
23. McCain RS, Diamond A, Jones C, et al. Current practices and future prospects for the management of gallbladder polyps: a topical review. *World J Gastroenterol*. 2018;24:2844–2852.
24. Strasberg SM, Hertl M, Soper NJ. An analysis of the problem of biliary injury during laparoscopic cholecystectomy. *J Am Coll Surg*. 1995;180:101–125.
25. Way LW, Stewart L, Gantert W, et al. Causes and prevention of laparoscopic bile duct injuries: analysis of 252 cases from a human factors and cognitive psychology perspective. *Ann Surg*. 2003;237:460–469.
26. Strasberg SM, Gouma DJ. 'Extreme' vasculobiliary injuries: association with fundus-down cholecystectomy in severely inflamed gallbladders. *HPB*. 2012;14:1–8.
27. Rogers SJ, Cello JP, Horn JK, et al. Prospective randomized trial of LC+LCBDE vs ERCP/S+LC for common bile duct stone disease. *Arch Surg*. 2010;145:28–33.
28. Schofer JM. Biliary causes of postcholecystectomy syndrome. *J Emerg Med*. 2010;39:406–410.
29. Nieuwenhuijs VB. Impact of routine intraoperative cholangiography during laparoscopic cholecystectomy on bile duct injury (*Br J Surg* 2014; 101: 677–684). *Br J Surg*. 2014;101:685.
30. Bismuth H, Majno PE. Biliary strictures: classification based on the principles of surgical treatment. *World J Surg*. 2001;25:1241–1244.
31. Lillemoe KD. Current management of bile duct injury. *Br J Surg*. 2008;95:403–405.
32. Harrison VL, Dolan JP, Pham TH, et al. Bile duct injury after laparoscopic cholecystectomy in hospitals with and without surgical residency programs: is there a difference? *Surg Endosc*. 2011;25:1969–1974.
33. Sicklick JK, Camp MS, Lillemoe KD, et al. Surgical management of bile duct injuries sustained during laparoscopic cholecystectomy: perioperative results in 200 patients. *Ann Surg*. 2005;241:786–792; discussion 793–785.

34. Eum YO, Park JK, Chun J, et al. Non-surgical treatment of post-surgical bile duct injury: clinical implications and outcomes. *World J Gastroenterol.* 2014;20:6924–6931.
35. Pottakkat B, Vijayahari R, Prakash A, et al. Factors predicting failure following high bilio-enteric anastomosis for post-cholecystectomy benign biliary strictures. *J Gastrointest Surg.* 2010;14:1389–1394.
36. Pitt HA, Sherman S, Johnson MS, et al. Improved outcomes of bile duct injuries in the 21st century. *Ann Surg.* 2013;258:490–499.
37. Ejaz A, Spolverato G, Kim Y, et al. Long-term health-related quality of life after iatrogenic bile duct injury repair. *J Am Coll Surg.* 2014;219:923–932.e910.
38. Pazouki A, Abdollahi A, Mehrabi Bahar M, et al. Evaluation of the incidence of complications of lost gallstones during laparoscopic cholecystectomy. *Surg Laparosc Endosc Percutan Tech.* 2014;24:213–215.
39. Co M, Pang SY, Wong KY, et al. Surgical management of recurrent pyogenic cholangitis: 10 years of experience in a tertiary referral centre in Hong Kong. *HPB.* 2014;16:776–780.
40. Carriaga MT, Henson DE. Liver, gallbladder, extrahepatic bile ducts, and pancreas. *Cancer.* 1995;75:171–190.
41. Kim JH, Kim WH, Yoo BM, et al. Should we perform surgical management in all patients with suspected porcelain gallbladder? *Hepato-Gastroenterology.* 2009;56:943–945.
42. Lazcano-Ponce EC, Miquel JF, Munoz N, et al. Epidemiology and molecular pathology of gallbladder cancer. *CA Cancer J Clin.* 2001;51:349–364.
43. Yang HL, Sun YG, Wang Z. Polypoid lesions of the gallbladder: diagnosis and indications for surgery. *Br J Surg.* 1992;79:227–229.
44. Shukla VK, Tiwari SC, Roy SK. Biliary bile acids in cholelithiasis and carcinoma of the gall bladder. *Eur J Cancer Prev.* 1993;2:155–160.
45. Duffy A, Capanu M, Abou-Alfa GK, et al. Gallbladder cancer (GBC): 10-year experience at Memorial Sloan-Kettering Cancer Centre (MSKCC). *J Surg Oncol.* 2008;98:485–489.
46. Schwartz LH, Black J, Fong Y, et al. Gallbladder carcinoma: findings at MR imaging with MR cholangiopancreatography. *J Comput Assist Tomogr.* 2002;26:405–410.
47. Shinkai H, Kimura W, Muto T. Surgical indications for small polypoid lesions of the gallbladder. *Am J Surg.* 1998;175:114–117.
48. D'Angelica M, Dalal KM, DeMatteo RP, et al. Analysis of the extent of resection for adenocarcinoma of the gallbladder. *Ann Surg Oncol.* 2009;16:806–816.
49. Jarnagin WR, Ruo L, Little SA, et al. Patterns of initial disease recurrence after resection of gallbladder carcinoma and hilar cholangiocarcinoma: implications for adjuvant therapeutic strategies. *Cancer.* 2003;98:1689–1700.
50. Amin MB, Greene FL, Stephen BE, et al., eds. Gallbladder. *AJCC Cancer Staging Manual.* 8th ed. New York: Springer; 2017:303–310.
51. Bismuth H, Nakache R, Diamond T. Management strategies in resection for hilar cholangiocarcinoma. *Ann Surg.* 1992;215:31–38.
52. Maithel SK, Gamblin TC, Kamel I, et al. Multidisciplinary approaches to intrahepatic cholangiocarcinoma. *Cancer.* 2013;119:3929–3942.

56 CHAPTER

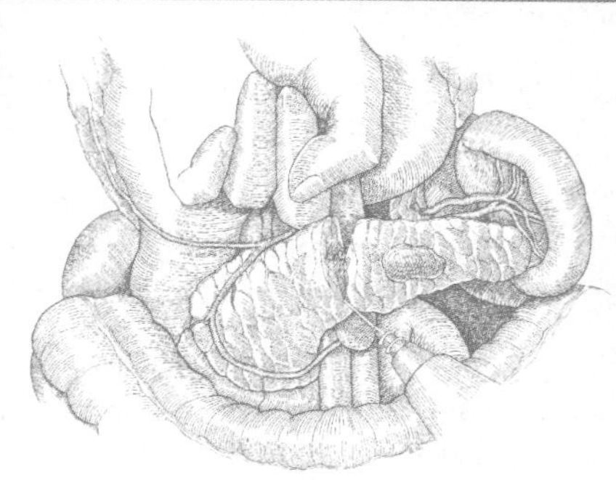

Exocrine Pancreas

Vikas Dudeja, J. Bart Rose, Eric H. Jensen, Selwyn M. Vickers

OUTLINE

Please access Elsevier eBooks for Practicing Clinicians to view the videos for this chapter https://expertconsult.inkling.com/.

ANATOMY

The average pancreas weighs between 75 g and 125 g and measures 10 cm to 20 cm. It lies in the retroperitoneum just anterior to the first lumbar vertebra and is anatomically divided into five sections, the head, uncinate, neck, body, and tail. The head lies to the right of midline within the C loop of the duodenum, immediately anterior to the vena cava at the confluence of the renal veins. The uncinate process extends from the head of the pancreas behind the superior mesenteric vein (SMV) and terminates adjacent to the superior mesenteric artery (SMA). The neck is the short segment of pancreas that immediately overlies the SMV. The body and tail of the pancreas then extend across the midline, anterior to Gerota fascia and slightly cephalad, terminating within the splenic hilum. The transition point between body and tail is nebulous. (Fig. 56.1).

Arterial Blood Supply

The pancreas is supplied by a complex arterial network arising from the celiac trunk and SMA. The head and uncinate process are supplied by the pancreaticoduodenal arteries (superior and inferior). The superior pancreaticoduodenal artery arises from the gastroduodenal artery and divides into anterior and posterior branches as it runs inferiorly within the pancreaticoduodenal groove. The inferior pancreaticoduodenal artery arises from SMA and also divides into anterior and posterior branches as it runs superiorly within pancreaticoduodenal groove. Terminal branches of superior and inferior pancreaticoduodenal arteries join each other to form the arcade, which supplies the head and uncinate process of the pancreas and the duodenum. The neck, body, and tail receive arterial supply from the splenic arterial system. Several small branches originate from the length of the splenic artery, including the dorsal pancreatic artery and greater pancreatic artery. The dorsal pancreatic courses posterior to the body of the gland to become the inferior pancreatic artery (also known as the transverse pancreatic artery). The inferior pancreatic artery then runs along the inferior border of the pancreas, terminating at its tail.

Venous Drainage

The venous drainage mimics the arterial supply, with blood flow from the head of the pancreas draining into the anterior and posterior pancreaticoduodenal veins. The posterior superior

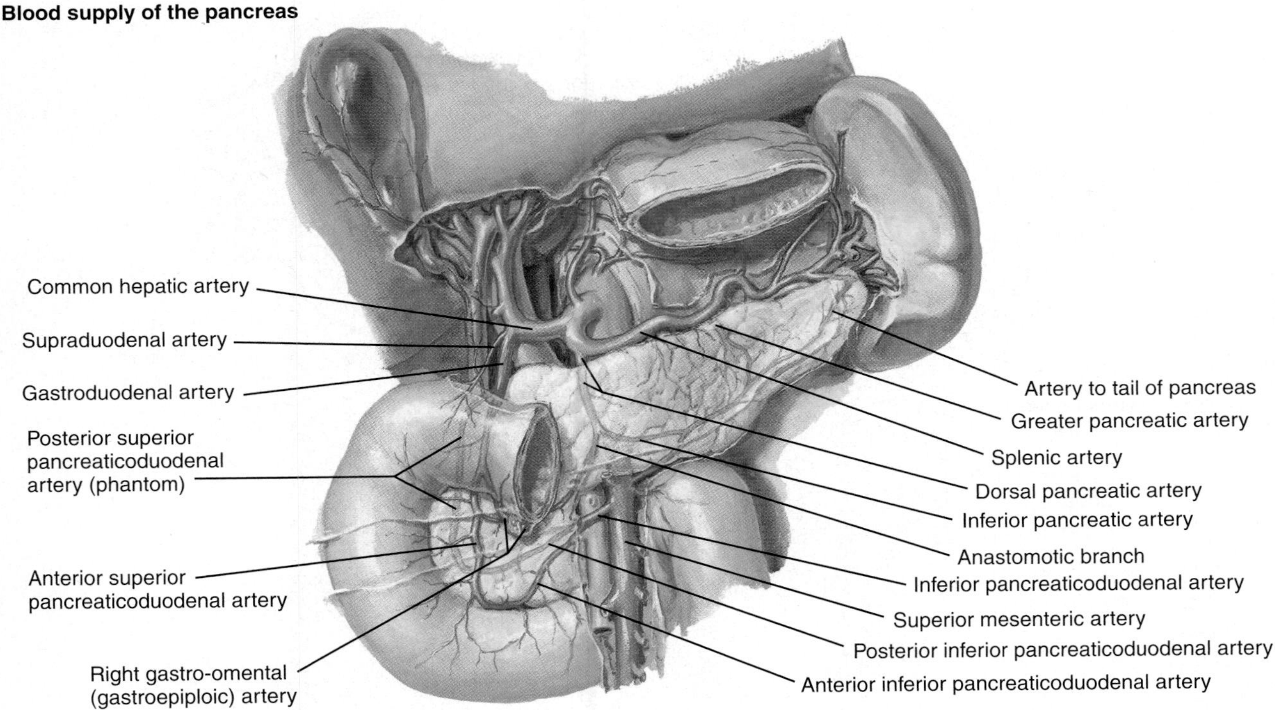

FIG. 56.1 Anatomy. (Netter illustration from www.netterimages.com. © Elsevier Inc. All rights reserved.)

pancreaticoduodenal vein enters the SMV laterally at the superior border of the neck of the pancreas. The anterior superior pancreaticoduodenal vein enters the right gastroepiploic vein just before its confluence with the SMV at the inferior border of the pancreas. The anterior and posterior inferior pancreaticoduodenal veins enter the SMV along the inferior border of the uncinate process. The remaining body and tail are drained through the splenic venous system.

Lymphatic Drainage

Understanding the lymphatic drainage of the pancreas is paramount to performing an appropriate oncologic resection. The pancreas can be thought of as having four quadrants of primary drainage. The tissue in the left side of the gland drains to lymph nodes in the splenic hilum or gastrosplenic omentum via lymphatics along the superior and inferior border of the pancreas. Small lymph nodes are present along this drainage pathway. Tissue in the right side of the gland drains superiorly to gastroduodenal lymph nodes and inferiorly to infrapancreatic lymph nodes. Again, small lymph nodes are present along these lymphatic channels. These four pathways form a "ring" around the border of the pancreas. A secondary drainage pathway occurs via retropancreatic lymph nodes located anterior to the aorta between the celiac and SMAs. These lymph nodes can receive drainage either directly from the pancreatic tissue (first order lymph nodes) or from the "ring" (second order).[1] A schematic of this drainage is shown in Fig. 56.2.

EMBRYOLOGY

The exocrine pancreas begins development during the fourth week of gestation. Pluripotent pancreatic epithelial stem cells give rise to exocrine and endocrine cell lines as well as the intricate pancreatic ductal network. Initially, dorsal and ventral buds appear from the primitive duodenal endoderm (Fig. 56.3A). The dorsal bud typically appears first and ultimately develops into the superior head, neck, body, and tail of the mature pancreas. The ventral bud develops as part of the hepatic diverticulum and maintains communication with the biliary tree throughout development. The ventral bud will become the inferior part of the head and uncinate process of the gland. Between the fourth and eighth weeks of gestation, the ventral bud rotates posteriorly in a clockwise fashion to fuse with the dorsal bud (Fig. 56.3B). At approximately eight weeks of gestation, the dorsal and ventral buds are fused (Fig. 56.3C).

The initiation of pancreas bud formation and differentiation of the ventral bud from the hepatic-biliary fates is dependent on the expression of pancreatic duodenal homeobox 1 (PDX1) protein and pancreas-specific transcription factor 1 (PTF1). In the absence of PDX1 expression in mice, pancreatic agenesis occurs, indicating its importance in the early phases of organogenesis. PTF1 expression is first detectable shortly after PDX1 in cells of the early endoderm, which will become the dorsal and ventral pancreas. By lineage analysis, 95% of acinar cells express PTF1. In PTF1 null mice, acini do not form. The notch signaling pathway is also critical to duct and acinar differentiation. In the absence of notch signaling, embryonic cells commit to endocrine lineage, suggesting that notch signaling is vital to exocrine differentiation. In addition to PDX1, PTF1, and notch signaling, complex interactions between mesenchymal growth factors such as transforming growth factor-β (TGF-β) and other signaling pathways, including hedgehog and Wnt, seem to play critical roles in pancreas development.[2] The precise interactions that lead to normal organogenesis continue to be defined. Table 56.1 summarizes the factors and pathways that affect pancreas development.[2]

Pancreas Divisum

During normal organogenesis, the primitive ducts of both the dorsal and ventral anlage contribute to the mature ductal system

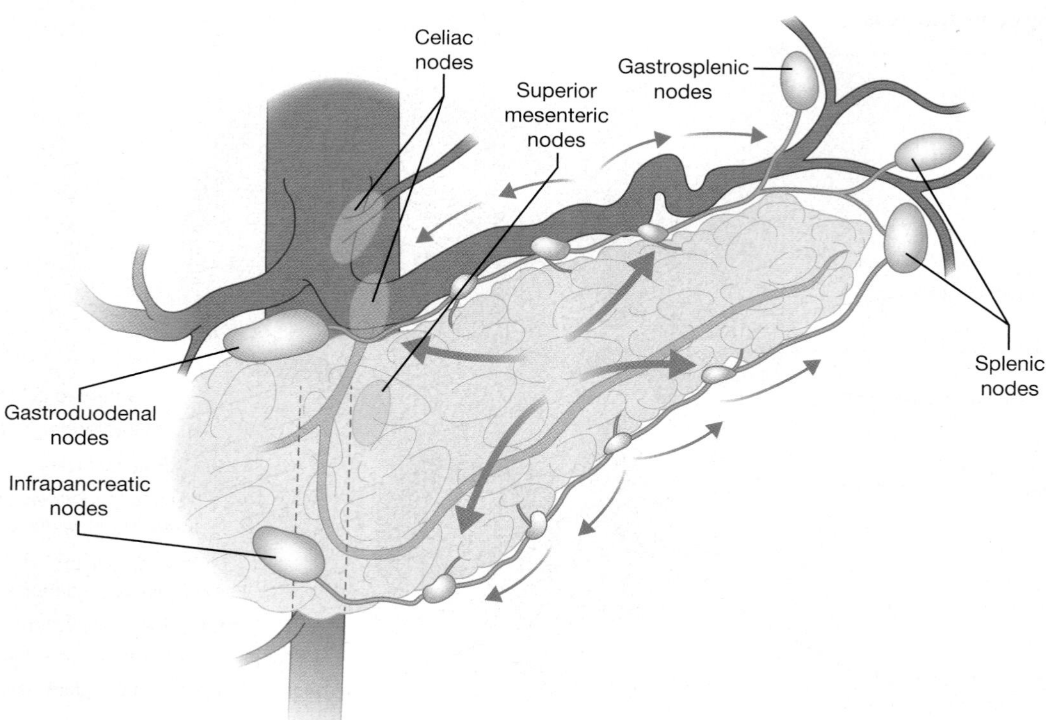

FIG. 56.2 Lymphatic drainage of the pancreas. (Adapted from Strasberg SM, Drebin JA, Linehan D: Radical antegrade modular pancreatosplenectomy. *Surgery* 133:521-527, 2003.)

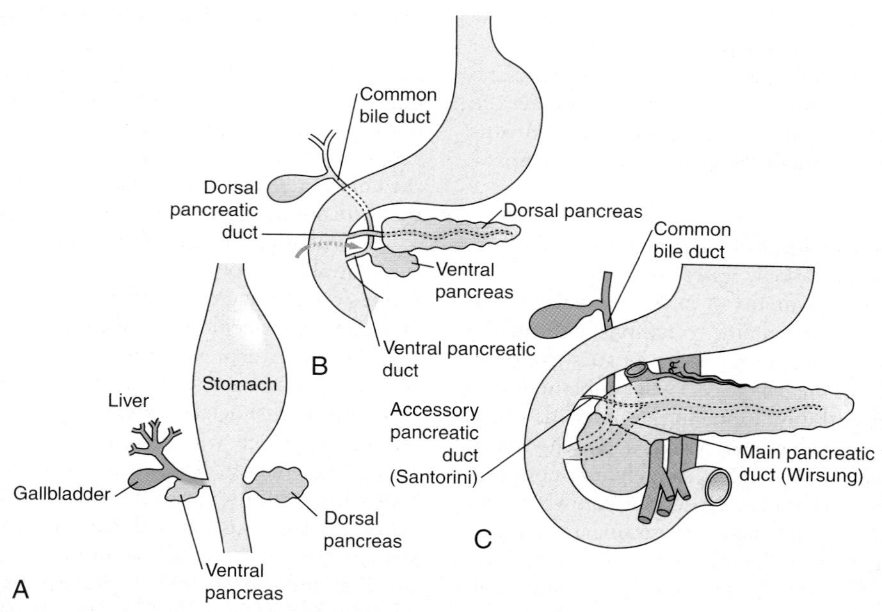

FIG. 56.3 Embryologic development of the pancreas.

of the pancreas. These ducts fuse together such that the proximal aspect of the dorsal anlage duct forms the duct of Santorini, while the distal aspect combines with the duct of the ventral bud to form the duct of Wirsung. The duct of Wirsung is generally the major exocrine drainage pathway of the pancreas, joins the common bile duct at the ampulla of Vater, and enters the duodenum through the major papilla. The duct of Santorini may drain through a minor papilla that is more proximal in the duodenum. Failure of the dorsal and ventral ducts to fuse during embryogenesis leads to pancreas divisum, a condition identified by a ventral pancreatic duct and common bile duct that enter the duodenum through a major papilla, whereas a dorsal pancreatic duct enters through a minor papilla that is slightly proximal (Fig. 56.4). Because most pancreatic exocrine secretions exit through the dorsal duct, pancreas divisum can lead to a condition of partial obstruction caused by a small minor papilla, leading to chronic backpressure in the

TABLE 56.1 Molecular factors and pathways associated with pancreatic organogenesis.

GENE	RELEVANCE
PDX1	Critical role in exocrine differentiation; knockout mice develop primitive pancreatic buds but agenesis of the organ
PTF1	Coexpression with *PDX1* determines progenitor cells to pancreatic fate
Notch signaling pathway	Suppresses endocrine differentiation, promoting exocrine development via induction of *Hes1* transcription factor. Prolonged notch expression prevents acinar formation via *RBP-Jκ* binding of *Ptf1a*
Hedgehog	Inhibition of hedgehog in *PDX1*-positive cells leads to initiation of endoderm differentiation into pancreas lineage
Wnt	Complex Wnt signaling is important in all aspects of pancreas development; lack of Wnt signaling results in varying levels of pancreatic agenesis
Neurogenin 3	Repressed by notch signaling, drives endocrine lineage differentiation.
Arx and *Pax-4*	*Arx* expression favors α/PP cell differentiation, while *Pax-4* expression favors β vs δ cell differentiation depending on length of exposure.

Arx, Aristaless related homeobox; *Pax-4*, paired box gene 4; *PDX1*, insulin promoter factor 1; *PTF1*, pancreas-specific transcription factor 1.

duct. This relative outflow obstruction has been implicated in the development of relapsing acute or chronic pancreatitis. Although 10% of the population is affected by pancreas divisum, only rarely do affected individuals develop pancreatitis.

Annular Pancreas

Annular pancreas results from aberrant migration of the ventral pancreas bud, which leads to circumferential or near-circumferential pancreas tissue surrounding the second portion of the duodenum. This abnormality may be associated with other congenital defects, including Down syndrome, malrotation, intestinal atresia, and cardiac malformations. If symptoms of obstruction occur, surgical bypass through duodenojejunostomy is performed instead of dividing the pancreatic tissue, as this annular pancreas has a pancreatic duct and its division will likely lead to pancreatic fistula formation.

Ectopic Pancreas

Ectopic pancreas may arise anywhere along the primitive foregut but is most common in the stomach, duodenum, and Meckel's diverticulum. Clinically, ectopic nodules may result in bowel obstruction caused by intussusception, bleeding, or ulceration. They can sometimes be found incidentally as firm yellow nodules that arise from the submucosa. Although there have been rare case reports of adenocarcinoma arising in ectopic pancreas tissue, resection is not necessary unless symptoms occur.

PHYSIOLOGY

The human pancreas is a complex gland with endocrine and exocrine functions. It is mainly composed of acinar cells (85% of the gland) and islet cells (2%) embedded in a complex extracellular matrix, which composes 10% of the gland. The remaining 3% to 4% of the gland is composed of the epithelial duct system and blood vessels.

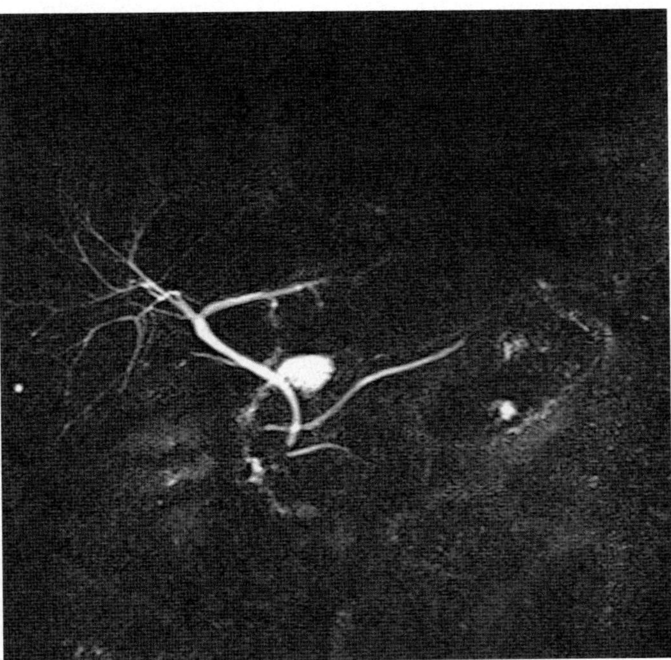

FIG. 56.4 MRCP showing pancreas divisum, with the dorsal pancreatic duct draining through the minor papilla and the ventral pancreatic duct joining the biliary tree draining through the major papilla. *MRCP*, Magnetic resonance cholangiopancreatography.

Major Components of Pancreatic Juice

The main function of the exocrine pancreas is to provide most of the enzymes needed for alimentary digestion. Acinar cells synthesize many enzymes that digest food proteins, such as trypsin, chymotrypsin, carboxypeptidase, and elastase. Under physiologic conditions, acinar cells synthesize these proteases as inactive proenzymes that are stored as intracellular zymogen granules. With stimulation of the pancreas, these proenzymes are secreted into the pancreatic duct and eventually the duodenal lumen. The duodenal mucosa expresses enterokinase on its brush boarder, which catalyzes the enzymatic activation of trypsin from trypsinogen.[3] Trypsin also plays an important role in protein digestion by propagating pancreatic enzyme activation through autoactivation of trypsinogen and other proenzymes, such as chymotrypsinogen, procarboxypeptidase, and proelastase. Fig. 56.5 summarizes the mechanisms of pancreatic exocrine secretion.

In addition to protease production, acinar cells also produce pancreatic amylase and lipase, also known as glycerol ester hydrolase, as active enzymes. With the exception of cellulose, pancreatic amylase hydrolyzes major polysaccharides into small oligosaccharides, which can be further digested by the oligosaccharidases present in the duodenal and jejunal epithelium. Pancreatic lipase hydrolyzes ingested fats into free fatty acids and 2-monoglycerides. In addition to pancreatic lipase, acinar cells produce other enzymes that digest fat, but they are secreted as proenzymes, like the proteases previously mentioned. These include colipase, cholesterol ester hydrolase, and phospholipase A2. The main function of colipase is to stabilize the activity of pancreatic lipase in the presence of bile salts. Pancreatic acinar cells also secrete deoxyribonuclease and ribonuclease, enzymes required for the hydrolysis of DNA and RNA, respectively.

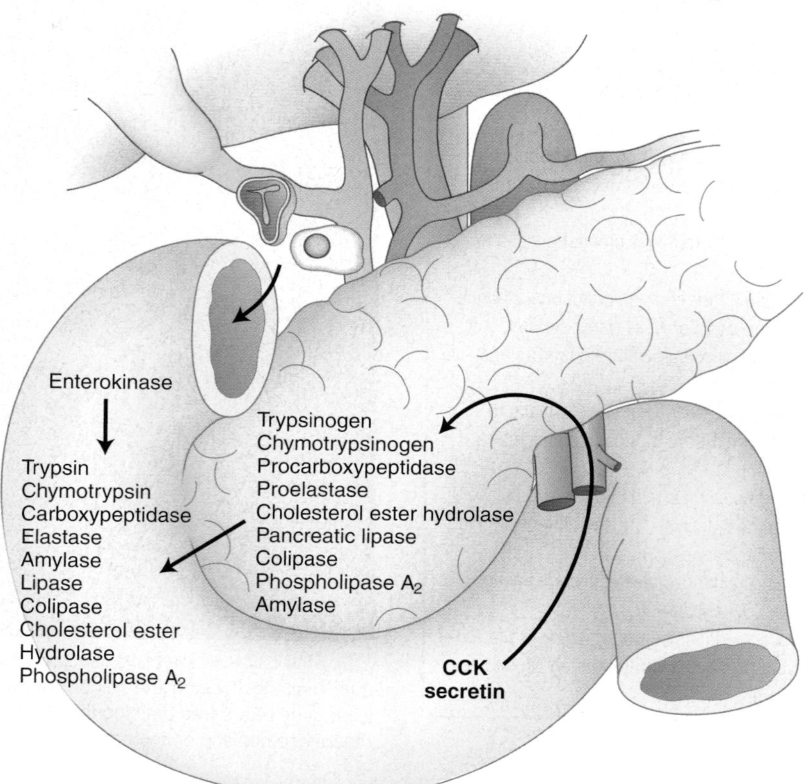

FIG. 56.5 Physiology of the secretion of pancreatic enzymes. The presence of peptides and fatty acids from food triggers the release of cholecystokinin *(CCK)*. CCK induces the release of pancreatic enzymes into the duodenal lumen. Conversely, S cells located in the duodenum release secretin in response to the acidification of the duodenum. Secretin induces the secretion of HCO_3^- from pancreatic cells into the duodenum.

Pancreatic enzymes are inactive inside acinar cells because they are synthesized and stored as inactive enzymes. In addition to this autoprotective mechanism, acinar cells synthesize pancreatic secretory trypsin inhibitor, which also protects acinar cells from autodigestion because it counteracts premature activation of trypsinogen inside acinar cells. Pancreatic secretory trypsin inhibitor is encoded by serine protease inhibitor Kazal type 1 *(SPINK1)* gene. *SPINK1* gene mutations are associated with the development of chronic pancreatitis, especially in childhood.

The primary function of pancreatic duct cells is to provide the water and electrolytes required to dilute and to deliver the enzymes synthesized by acinar cells. Although the concentrations of sodium and potassium are similar to their respective concentrations in plasma, the concentrations of bicarbonate and chloride vary significantly according to the secretion phase.

The mechanism responsible for the secretion of bicarbonate was first described in 1988 on the basis of in vitro studies. According to this model, extracellular CO_2 diffuses across the basolateral membrane of ductal cells. Once CO_2 is inside pancreatic duct cells, it is hydrated by intracellular carbonic anhydrase; as a result of this reaction, HCO_3^- and H^+ are generated. The apical membrane of pancreatic duct cells contains an anion exchanger that secretes intracellular HCO_3^- into the lumen of the cell and favors the exchange of luminal Cl^- inside the ductal epithelium. Studies have shown that this exchanger interacts with the cystic fibrosis transmembrane conductance regulator (CFTR); mutations in the *CFTR* gene have been linked to chronic pancreatitis. This may correlate with the inability of patients with cystic fibrosis to secrete water and bicarbonate. Although the nature of this exchanger has not been completely elucidated, it is possible that this anion exchanger is an SLC26 family member. This family contains different anion exchangers that transport monovalent and divalent anions, such as Cl^- and HCO_3^-. Some of these exchangers are known to interact with CFTR. Thus, HCO_3^- level in the pancreatic juice varies inversely to the Cl^- level. Secretin hormone is the major stimulator of the HCO_3^- secretion. Cholecystokinin (CCK) weakly stimulates HCO_3^- secretion and also synergizes with the effect of secretin.

In addition to HCO_3^- CO_2 hydration also generates H^+ ions, which are secreted by Na^+ and H^+ exchangers present in the basolateral membrane of ductal cells. These exchangers belong to the *SLC9* gene family. The main function of these exchangers is to maintain the intracellular pH within a physiologic range. In addition, the basolateral membrane of duct cells contains multiple Na^+,K^+-ATPases that provide the primary force that drives HCO_3^- secretion; the Na^+,K^+-ATPase maintains the Na^+ gradient used to extrude H^+ as well. Finally, K^+ channels present in the basolateral membrane of acinar cells maintain the membrane potential to allow recirculation of K^+ ions brought by the Na^+,K^+ pump inside the cell. Fig. 56.6 illustrates HCO_3^- secretion inside pancreatic duct cells. The level of Na^+ and K^+ in pancreatic juice remains relatively constant without much variation with the secretory rate.

Once the HCO_3^- secreted by pancreatic duct cells reaches the duodenal lumen, it neutralizes the hydrochloric acid secreted by gastric parietal cells. Pancreatic enzymes are inactivated at a low

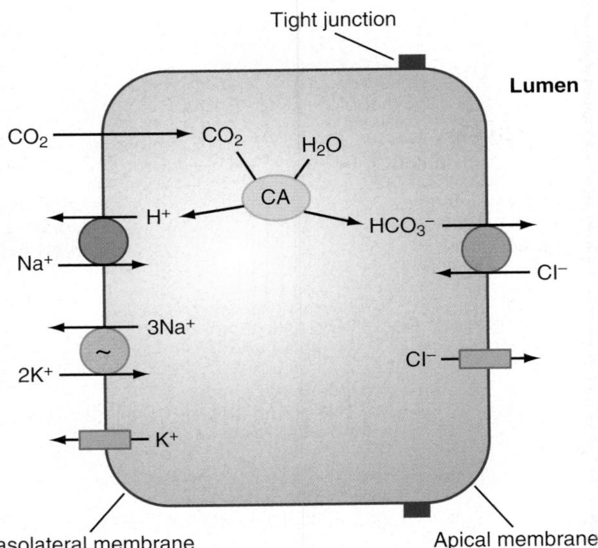

FIG. 56.6 Cellular mechanism proposed for HCO_3^- secretion by pancreatic duct epithelium. (From Steward MC, Ishiguro H, Case RM. Mechanisms of bicarbonate secretion in the pancreatic duct. *Annu Rev Physiol.* 2005;67:377–409.)

pH; therefore, pancreatic bicarbonate provides an optimal pH for pancreatic enzyme function. The optimal pH for the function of chymotrypsin and trypsin is 8.0 to 9.0; for amylase, the optimal pH is 7.0; and for lipase, it is 7.0 to 9.0.

Phases and Regulation of Pancreatic Secretion

Pancreatic exocrine secretion occurs during the interdigestive state and after the ingestion of food, which is also known as the digestive state. The same phases of secretion that have been identified in the stomach during the digestive state have also been described in pancreatic secretion. The first phase is the cephalic phase, in which the pancreas is stimulated by the vagus nerve in response to the sight, smell, or taste of food. This phase is generally mediated by the release of acetylcholine at the terminal endings of postganglionic fibers. The main effect of acetylcholine is to induce acinar cell secretion of enzymes. This phase accounts for 20% to 25% of the daily secretion of pancreatic juice.

The second phase of pancreatic secretion is known as the gastric phase. It is mediated by vagovagal reflexes triggered by gastric distention after the ingestion of food. These reflexes induce acinar cell secretion. It accounts for 10% of the pancreatic juice produced daily.

The most important phase of pancreatic secretion is the intestinal phase, which accounts for 65% to 70% of the total secretion of pancreatic juice. It is mediated by secretin and CCK. Acidification of the duodenal lumen induces the release of secretin by S cells. Secretin was the first polypeptide hormone identified more than 100 years ago. It is the most important mediator of the secretion of water, bicarbonate, and other electrolytes into the duodenum. Secretin receptors are located in the basolateral membrane of all pancreatic duct cells but cannot be identified in other pancreatic components, such as islet cells, blood vessels, or extracellular matrix. Secretin receptors are members of the G protein–coupled receptor superfamily. The most important effect of secretin stimulation is an increase of intracellular cyclic adenosine monophosphate, which activates the HCO_3^--Cl^- anion exchanger in the apical membrane of pancreatic duct cells. It also increases the activity of the enzyme carbonic anhydrase, the excretion of H^+ outside the duct cell, and the activity of the CFTR.

The presence of lipid, protein, and carbohydrates inside the duodenum induces the secretion of CCK-releasing factor and monitor peptide. Both peptides induce release of CCK by I cells present in the duodenal mucosa. Whereas secretin is the main mediator of the secretion of water and bicarbonate in the intestinal phase, CCK is the main mediator of the secretion of pancreatic enzymes. CCK exerts a number of effects:

1. CCK travels through the bloodstream and induces the release of pancreatic enzymes by acinar cells.
2. CCK induces local duodenal vagovagal reflexes that cause the release of acetylcholine, vasoactive intestinal peptide, and gastrin-releasing peptide, which promotes the release of pancreatic enzymes.
3. CCK induces the relaxation of the sphincter of Oddi. Also, CCK potentiates the effects of secretin, and vice versa.

ACUTE PANCREATITIS

The incidence of acute pancreatitis (AP) has increased during the past 20 years. AP is responsible for more than 300,000 hospital admissions annually in the United States. Most patients develop a mild and self-limited course; however, 10% to 20% of patients have a rapidly progressive inflammatory response associated with prolonged length of hospital stay and significant morbidity and mortality. Patients with mild pancreatitis have a mortality rate of less than 1%, but in severe pancreatitis, this increases up to 10% to 50%. The highest mortality rates in this group of patients are those who present with multiple organ dysfunction syndrome. Mortality in pancreatitis has a bimodal distribution. In the first two weeks (early phase), it is a result of multiple organ dysfunction caused by the intense inflammatory cascade triggered by pancreatic inflammation. Mortality after two weeks (late phase) is often caused by septic complications.[3]

Pathophysiology

The exact mechanism whereby predisposing factors such as ethanol and gallstones produce pancreatitis is not completely known. Most researchers believe that AP is the final result of abnormal pancreatic enzyme activation inside acinar cells. Immunolocalization studies have shown that after 15 minutes of pancreatic injury, both zymogen granules and lysosomes colocalize inside the acinar cells. The fact that zymogen and lysosome colocalization occurs before amylase level elevation, pancreatic edema, and other markers of pancreatitis are evident suggests that colocalization is an early step in the pathophysiologic process and not a consequence of pancreatitis. Studies also suggest that lysosomal enzyme cathepsin B activates trypsin in these colocalization organelles. In vitro and in vivo studies have elucidated an intricate model of acinar cell death induced by premature activation of trypsin. In this model, once cathepsin B in lysosomes and trypsinogen in zymogen granules are brought in contact by colocalization induced by pancreatitis-inciting stimuli, activated trypsin then induces leak of colocalized organelles, releasing cathepsin B into the cytosol. It is the cytosolic cathepsin B that then induces apoptosis or necrosis, leading to acinar cell death. Thus, acinar cell death and to a degree the inflammatory response seen in AP can be prevented if acinar cells are pretreated with cathepsin B inhibitors. In vivo studies have also shown that cathepsin B knockout mice have a significant decrease in the severity of pancreatitis.[4]

Intraacinar pancreatic enzyme activation induces autodigestion of normal pancreatic parenchyma. In response to this initial insult, acinar cells release proinflammatory cytokines, such as tumor necrosis factor-α (TNF-α) and interleukin (IL)-1, IL-2, and IL-6, and antiinflammatory mediators, such as IL-10 and IL-1 receptor antagonist. These mediators do not initiate pancreatic injury but propagate the response locally and systemically. As a result, TNF-α, IL-1 and IL-6, neutrophils, and macrophages are recruited into the pancreatic parenchyma and cause the release of more TNF-α, IL-1 and IL-6, reactive oxygen metabolites, prostaglandins, platelet-activating factor, and leukotrienes. The local inflammatory response further aggravates the pancreatitis because it increases the permeability and damages the microcirculation of the pancreas. In severe cases, the inflammatory response causes local hemorrhage and pancreatic necrosis. In addition, some of the inflammatory mediators released by neutrophils aggravate the pancreatic injury because they cause pancreatic enzyme activation.

The inflammatory cascade is self-limited in approximately 80% to 90% of patients. However, in the remaining patients, a vicious circle of recurring pancreatic injury and local and systemic inflammatory reaction persists. In a small number of patients, there is a massive release of inflammatory mediators to the systemic circulation. Active neutrophils mediate acute lung injury and induce the adult respiratory distress syndrome frequently seen in patients with severe pancreatitis. The mortality seen in the early phase of pancreatitis is the result of this persistent inflammatory response. A summary of the inflammatory cascade seen in AP is shown in Fig. 56.7.

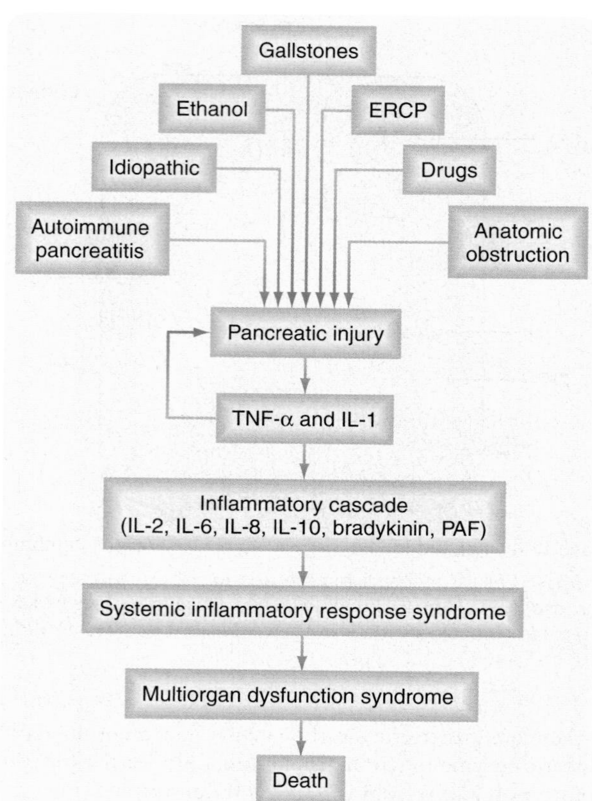

FIG. 56.7 Pathophysiology of severe acute pancreatitis. The local injury induces the release of tumor necrosis factor-alpha (TNF-α) and interleukin-1 (IL-1). Both cytokines produce further pancreatic injury and amplify the inflammatory response by inducing the release of other inflammatory mediators, which cause distant organ injury. This abnormal inflammatory response is responsible for the mortality seen during the early phase of acute pancreatitis. *ERCP,* Endoscopic retrograde cholangiopancreatography; *PAF,* XXX.

Risk Factors

Gallstones and ethanol abuse account for 70% to 80% of AP cases. In pediatric patients, abdominal blunt trauma and systemic diseases are the two most common conditions that lead to pancreatitis. Autoimmune and drug-induced pancreatitis should be a differential diagnosis in patients with rheumatologic conditions such as systemic lupus erythematosus and Sjögren syndrome.

Biliary or Gallstone Pancreatitis

Gallstone pancreatitis is the most common cause of AP in the West. It accounts for 40% of U.S. cases. The overall incidence of AP in patients with symptomatic gallstone disease is 3% to 8%. It is seen more frequently in women between 50 and 70 years of age. The exact mechanism that triggers pancreatic injury has not been completely understood, but two theories have been proposed.[5] In the obstructive theory, pancreatic injury is the result of excessive pressure inside the pancreatic duct. This increased intraductal pressure is the result of continuous secretion of pancreatic juice in the presence of pancreatic duct obstruction. Animal studies suggest that high intraductal pressure initiates pancreatitis through a mechanism dependent on calcineurin signaling.[6] The second, or reflux, theory proposes that stones become impacted in the ampulla of Vater and form a common channel that allows bile salt reflux into the pancreas. Animal models have shown that bile salts cause direct acinar cell necrosis because they increase the concentration of calcium in the cytoplasm; however, this has never been proven in humans.[3]

Alcohol-Induced Injury

Excessive ethanol consumption is the second most common cause of AP worldwide. It accounts for 35% of cases and is more prevalent in young men (30–45 years of age) than in women. However, only 5% to 10% of patients who drink alcohol develop AP. Factors that contribute to ethanol-induced pancreatitis include heavy ethanol abuse (>100 g/day for at least 5 years), smoking, and genetic predisposition. Compared with nonsmokers, the relative risk of alcohol-induced pancreatitis in smokers is 4.9.[7]

Alcohol has a number of deleterious effects in the pancreas and its mechanism of injury is likely multifaceted. It has been shown to: 1) trigger proinflammatory pathways via upregulation of nuclear factor κB (NF-κB), TNF-α, and IL-1, 2) cause inappropriate basolateral exocytosis of pancreatic zymogens, 3) increased autophagy possibly due to dysregulation of cathepsin L and B, 4) increased oxidative stress leading to mitochondrial dysfunction, 5) activation of pancreatic stellate cells (PSCs) leading to increased secretion of matrix metalloproteases, 6) impaired pancreatic cell repair due to dysregulation in developmental factors PDX1, PTF1a, and Notch, and 7) a shift in cell death caused by apoptosis to necrosis by decreasing caspase 3/8 activity and loss of adenosine triphosphate (ATP) production via mitochondrial depolarization.

Anatomic Obstruction

Abnormal flow of pancreatic juice into the duodenum can result in pancreatic injury. AP has been described in patients with pancreatic tumors, parasites, and congenital defects.

Pancreas divisum is an anatomic variation present in 10% of the population. Its association with AP is controversial. Patients with this variation have a 5% to 10% lifetime risk for development of AP caused by relative outflow obstruction through the minor papilla. Endoscopic retrograde cholangiopancreatography (ERCP) with minor papillotomy and stenting may be beneficial for such patients.

Infrequent anatomic obstructions that have been associated with AP include *Ascaris lumbricoides* infection and annular pancreas. Although pancreatic cancer is not uncommon, patients with pancreatic cancer usually do not develop AP.

Endoscopic Retrograde Cholangiopancreatography–Induced Pancreatitis

AP is the most common complication after ERCP, occurring in up to 5% of patients. However, the incidence of this complication after ERCP could be as high as 15% in high-risk patients. PostERCP pancreatitis is more common in female patients, young individuals, and in patients with prior history of ERCP induced pancreatitis. AP occurs more frequently in patients who have undergone therapeutic procedures compared with diagnostic procedures. It is also more common in patients who have had multiple attempts of cannulation, sphincter of Oddi dysfunction, and abnormal visualization of the secondary pancreatic ducts after injection of contrast material. The clinical course is mild in 90% to 95% of patients. ERCP-induced pancreatitis is one of the rare opportunities where primary prevention of development of AP may be possible. First, ERCP should only be performed when absolutely necessary. With improvement in other diagnostic modalities including magnetic resonance cholangiopancreatography (MRCP), the use of diagnostic ERCP with its associated complications including ERCP-induced pancreatitis has decreased. Among pharmacologic agents to prevent ERCP-induced pancreatitis, use of indomethacin has gained the most traction. Technique related and interventional strategies, which have been shown to reduce the risk of postERCP pancreatitis, include use of pancreatic stents and using minimal pressure while performing ERCP.

Drug-Induced Pancreatitis

Up to 2% of AP cases are caused by medications. The most common agents include sulfonamides, metronidazole, erythromycin, tetracyclines, didanosine, thiazides, furosemide, 3-hydroxy-3-methylglutaryl-coenzyme A (HMG-CoA) reductase inhibitors (statins), azathioprine, 6-mercaptopurine, 5-aminosalicylic acid, sulfasalazine, valproic acid, and human immunodeficiency virus antiretroviral agents.

Metabolic Factors

Hypertriglyceridemia and hypercalcemia can also lead to pancreatic damage. Direct pancreatic injury can be induced by triglyceride metabolites. It is more common in patients with type I, II, or V hyperlipidemia. It should be suspected in patients with a triglyceride level higher than 1000 mg/dL. A triglyceride level higher than 2000 mg/dL confirms the diagnosis. Hypertriglyceridemia secondary to hypothyroidism, diabetes mellitus, and alcohol does not typically induce AP.

Hypercalcemia is postulated to induce pancreatic injury through the activation of trypsinogen to trypsin and intraductal precipitation of calcium, leading to ductal obstruction and subsequent attacks of pancreatitis. Approximately 1.5% to 13% of patients with primary hyperparathyroidism develop AP.

Miscellaneous Conditions

Blunt and penetrating abdominal trauma can be associated with AP in 0.2% and 1% of cases, respectively. Prolonged intraoperative hypotension and excessive pancreatic manipulation during abdominal surgery can also result in AP. Pancreatic ischemia in association with acute pancreatic inflammation can develop after splenic artery embolization. Other rare causes include scorpion venom stings and perforated duodenal ulcers.

Clinical Manifestations

The cardinal symptom of AP is epigastric or periumbilical pain that radiates to the back. Up to 90% of patients have nausea or vomiting that typically does not relieve the pain. The nature of the pain is constant; therefore, if the pain disappears or decreases, another diagnosis should be considered.

Dehydration, poor skin turgor, tachycardia, hypotension, and dry mucous membranes are commonly seen in patients with AP. Severely dehydrated and older patients may also develop mental status changes.

The physical examination findings of the abdomen vary according to the severity of the disease. With mild pancreatitis, the physical examination findings of the abdomen may be normal or reveal only mild epigastric tenderness. Significant abdominal distention associated with generalized rebound and abdominal rigidity is present in severe pancreatitis. The nature of the pain described by the patient may not correlate with the physical examination findings or the degree of pancreatic inflammation.

Rare findings include flank and periumbilical ecchymosis (Grey Turner and Cullen signs, respectively). Both are indicative of retroperitoneal bleeding associated with severe pancreatitis. Patients with concomitant choledocholithiasis or significant edema in the head of the pancreas that compresses the intrapancreatic portion of the common bile duct can present with jaundice. Dullness to percussion and decreased breathing sounds in the left or, less commonly, in the right hemithorax suggest pleural effusion secondary to AP.

Diagnosis

The diagnosis of AP requires two of the following three features to be present according to international consensus: 1) abdominal pain consistent with AP (acute onset of a persistent, severe, epigastric pain often radiating to the back), 2) a threefold or higher elevation of serum amylase or lipase levels above the upper laboratory limit of normal, or 3) characteristics findings of pancreatitis by imaging. The serum half-life of amylase (10 hours) is shorter than that of lipase (6.9–13.7 hours) and therefore normalizes faster (3–5 vs. 8–14 days, respectively). In patients who do not present to the emergency department within the first 24 to 48 hours after the onset of symptoms, determination of lipase levels is a more sensitive indicator to establish the diagnosis. Lipase is also a more specific marker of AP because serum amylase levels can be elevated in a number of conditions, such as peptic ulcer disease, mesenteric ischemia, salpingitis, and macroamylasemia.

Patients with AP are typically hyperglycemic; they can also have leukocytosis and abnormal elevation of liver enzyme levels. The elevation of alanine aminotransferase levels in the serum in the context of AP confirmed by high pancreatic enzyme levels has a positive predictive value of 95% in the diagnosis of acute biliary pancreatitis.[5]

Imaging Studies

Imaging studies are not required for diagnosis, but may be helpful in determining need for intervention in severe AP or elucidating an elusive etiology. Although simple abdominal radiographs are not useful for diagnosis of pancreatitis, they can help rule out other conditions, such as perforated ulcer disease. Nonspecific findings in patients with AP include air-fluid levels suggestive of ileus, cutoff colon sign as a result of colonic spasm at the splenic flexure and widening of the duodenal C loop caused by severe pancreatic head edema.

The usefulness of ultrasound for diagnosis of pancreatitis is limited by intraabdominal fat and increased intestinal gas as a result of the ileus. Nevertheless, this test should always be ordered in patients with AP because of its high sensitivity (95%) in diagnosing gallstones. Combined elevations of liver transaminase and pancreatic enzyme levels and the presence of gallstones on ultrasound have an even higher sensitivity (97%) and specificity (100%) for diagnosing acute biliary pancreatitis.

Contrast-enhanced computed tomography (CT) is currently the best modality for evaluation of the pancreas, especially if the study is performed with a multidetector CT scanner. Indications for CT include diagnostic uncertainty, confirmation of severity based on clinical predictors, failure to respond to conservative treatment, or clinical deterioration. The most valuable contrast phase in which to evaluate the pancreatic parenchyma is the portal venous phase (65–70 seconds after injection of contrast material), which allows evaluation of the viability of the pancreatic parenchyma, amount of peripancreatic inflammation, and presence of intraabdominal free air or fluid collections. Noncontrast CT scanning may also be of value in the setting of renal failure by identifying fluid collections or extraluminal air.

Abdominal magnetic resonance imaging (MRI) is also useful to evaluate the extent of necrosis, inflammation, and presence of free fluid. However, its cost and availability and the fact that patients requiring imaging are critically ill and need to be in intensive care units limit its applicability in the acute phase. Although MRCP is not indicated in the acute setting of AP, it has an important role in the evaluation of patients with unexplained or recurrent pancreatitis because it allows noninvasive complete visualization of the biliary and pancreatic duct anatomy. For difficult to view pancreatic ducts, intravenous (IV) administration of secretin can be injected prior to imaging to stimulate pancreatic juice secretion, thereby causing a transient distention of the pancreatic duct. Any pain associated with the timing of secretin stimulation should be noted as it may help in confirming an uncertain etiology of epigastric pain. For example, secretin stimulated MRCP is useful in patients with AP and no evidence of a predisposing condition to rule out pancreas divisum, intraductal papillary mucinous neoplasm (IPMN), or a small tumor in the pancreatic duct.

In the setting of gallstone pancreatitis, endoscopic ultrasound (EUS) may play an important role in the evaluation of persistent choledocholithiasis. Several studies have shown that routine ERCP for suspected gallstone pancreatitis reveals no evidence of persistent obstruction in most cases and may actually worsen symptoms because of manipulation of the gland. EUS has been proven to be sensitive for identifying choledocholithiasis; it allows examination of the biliary tree and pancreas with no risk of worsening of the pancreatitis. In patients in whom persistent choledocholithiasis is confirmed by EUS, ERCP can be used selectively as a therapeutic measure.

Assessment of Severity of Disease

The earliest scoring system designed to evaluate the severity of AP was introduced by Ranson and colleagues in 1974. It predicts the severity of the disease on the basis of 11 parameters obtained at the time of admission or 48 hours later. The mortality rate of AP directly correlates with the number of parameters that are positive. Severe pancreatitis is diagnosed if three or more of the Ranson criteria are fulfilled. The main disadvantage is that it does not predict the severity of disease at the time of the admission because six parameters are assessed only after 48 hours of admission. The Ranson score has a low positive predictive value (50%) and high negative predictive value (90%). Therefore, it is mainly used to rule out severe pancreatitis or to predict the risk of mortality. The original scoring symptom designed to predict the severity of the disease and its modification for acute biliary pancreatitis are shown in Boxes 56.1 and 56.2.

AP severity can also be addressed by the Acute Physiology and Chronic Health Evaluation (APACHE II) score. Based on the patient's age, previous health status, and 12 routine physiologic measurements, APACHE II provides a general measure of the severity of disease. An APACHE II score of eight or higher defines severe pancreatitis. The main advantage is that it can be used on admission and repeated at any time. However, it is complex, not specific for AP, and based on the patient's age, which easily upgrades the AP severity score. APACHE II has a positive predictive value of 43% and a negative predictive value of 89%.

Using imaging characteristics, Balthazar and associates have established the CT severity index. This index correlates CT findings

BOX 56.1 Ranson Prognostic Criteria for Nongallstone Pancreatitis

At presentation

- Age >55 years
- Blood glucose level >200 mg/dL
- White blood cell count >16,000 cells/mm^3
- Lactate dehydrogenase level >350 IU/L
- Aspartate aminotransferase level >250 IU/L

After 48 hours of admission

- Hematocrit*: decrease >10%
- Serum calcium level <8 mg/dL
- Base deficit >4 mEq/L
- Blood urea nitrogen level: increase >5 mg/dL
- Fluid requirement >6 L
- Pa_{O_2} <60 mm Hg

Ranson score ≥3 defines severe pancreatitis.

*Compared with admission value.

BOX 56.2 Ranson prognostic criteria for gallstone pancreatitis.

At presentation

- Age >70 years
- Blood glucose level >220 mg/dL
- White blood cell count >18,000 cells/mm^3
- Lactate dehydrogenase level >400 IU/L
- Aspartate aminotransferase level >250 IU/L

After 48 hours of admission

- Hematocrit*: decrease >10%
- Serum calcium level <8 mg/dL
- Base deficit >5 mEq/L
- Blood urea nitrogen level: increase >2 mg/dL
- Fluid requirement >4 L
- Pa_{O_2}: Not available

Ranson score ≥3 defines severe pancreatitis.

*Compared with admission value.

TABLE 56.2 Computed Tomography Severity Index (CTSI) for acute pancreatitis.

FEATURE	POINTS
Pancreatic Inflammation	
Normal pancreas	0
Focal or diffuse pancreatic enlargement	1
Intrinsic pancreatic alterations with peripancreatic fat inflammatory changes	2
Single fluid collection or phlegmon	3
Two or more fluid collections or gas, in or adjacent to the pancreas	4
Pancreatic Necrosis	
None	0
≤30%	2
30%–50%	4
>50%	6

CTSI 0–3, mortality 3%, morbidity 8%; CTSI 4–6, mortality 6%, morbidity 35%; CTSI 7–10, mortality 17%, morbidity 92%.

BOX 56.3 Definition of systemic inflammatory response syndrome (SIRS).

Two or more of the following conditions must be met:

- Temperature >38.3°C or <36.0°C
- Heart rate of >90 beats/minute
- Respiratory rate of >20 breaths/minute or $PaCO_2$ of <32 mm Hg
- WBC count of >12,000 cells/mL, <4000 cells/mL, or >10% immature (band) forms

From Annane D, Bellissant E, Cavaillon JM. Septic shock. *Lancet.* 2005;365:63–78.

BOX 56.4 Atlanta criteria for acute pancreatitis.

Organ Failure, as Defined by

Shock (systolic blood pressure <90 mm Hg)
Pulmonary insufficiency (Pao_2 <60 mm Hg)
Renal failure (creatinine level >2 mg/dL after fluid resuscitation)
Gastrointestinal bleeding (>500 mL/24 hour)

Systemic Complications

Disseminated intravascular coagulation (platelet count ≤100,000)
Fibrinogen <1 g/L
Fibrin split products >80 μg/dL
Metabolic disturbance (calcium level ≤7.5 mg/dL)

Local Complications

Necrosis
Abscess
Pseudocyst
Severe pancreatitis is defined by the presence of any evidence of organ failure or a local complication.

with the patient's outcome. The CT severity index is shown in Table 56.2.

While many prognostic indices have been developed to predict severity of disease, most are hindered by complexity, need for imaging, or inability to be calculated at admission. This has led to multiple professional societies recommending the use of the systemic inflammatory response syndrome (SIRS) scoring system (Box 56.3) as a fast, inexpensive, and reliable replacement.[8,9] Having a persistent SIRS throughout hospital admission, having a transient SIRS, or never meeting SIRS criteria has been associated with mortality rates of 25%, 8%, and 0%, respectively.

In 1992, the International Symposium on Acute Pancreatitis defined severe pancreatitis as the presence of local pancreatic complications (necrosis, abscess, or pseudocyst) or any evidence of organ failure. Severe pancreatitis is diagnosed if there is any evidence of organ failure or a local pancreatic complication (Box 56.4). In 2012, the International Symposium on Acute Pancreatitis updated their three-tiered grading schema of pancreatitis severity. Mild pancreatitis has no organ dysfunction or local/systemic complications, moderate pancreatitis can have organ failure lasting less than 48 hours and/or local/systemic complications, while severe pancreatitis is characterized by organ failure lasting beyond 48 hours. With increasing severity comes increased rates of morbidity and mortality.

C-reactive protein (CRP) is an inflammatory marker that peaks 48 to 72 hours after the onset of pancreatitis and correlates with the severity of the disease. A CRP level of 150 mg/mL or higher defines severe pancreatitis. The major limitation is that it cannot be used on admission; the sensitivity of the assay decreases if CRP levels are measured within 48 hours after the onset of symptoms. In addition to CRP, a number of studies have shown other biochemical markers (e.g., serum levels of procalcitonin, IL-6, IL-1, elastase) that correlate with the severity of the disease. However, their main limitation is their cost, and they are not widely available.

Treatment

Regardless of the cause or the severity of the disease, the cornerstones of treating AP are aggressive fluid resuscitation with isotonic crystalloid solution, pain control, and early nutrition. The rate of fluid administration should be individualized and adjusted on the basis of age, comorbidities, vital signs, mental status, skin turgor, and urine output. Patients who do not respond to initial fluid resuscitation or have significant renal, cardiac, or respiratory comorbidities often require invasive monitoring with central venous access and a Foley catheter. While the nature of fluid which should be used for initial resuscitation is still being debated, some evidence suggest that Ringer's lactate may be the best fluid for initial resuscitation.[10]

In addition to fluid resuscitation, patients with AP require continuous pulse oximetry because one of the most common systemic complications of AP is hypoxemia caused by the acute lung injury associated with this disease. Patients should receive supplementary oxygen to maintain arterial saturation above 95%.

It is also essential to provide effective analgesia. Narcotics are usually preferred, especially morphine. One of the physiologic effects described after systemic administration of morphine is an increase in tone in the sphincter of Oddi; however, there is no evidence that narcotics exert a negative impact on the outcome of patients with AP.

Nutritional support is vital in the treatment of AP. Oral feeding may be impossible because of persistent ileus, pain, or intubation. In addition, 20% of patients with severe AP develop recurrent pain shortly after the oral route has been restarted.

The main options to provide this nutritional support are enteral feeding and total parenteral nutrition (TPN). Although there is no difference in the mortality rate between both types of nutrition, enteral nutrition is associated with fewer infectious complications and reduces the need for pancreatic surgery. Although TPN provides most nutritional requirements, it is associated with mucosal atrophy, decreased intestinal blood flow, increased risk of bacterial overgrowth in the small bowel, antegrade colonization with colonic bacteria, and increased bacterial translocation. In addition, patients with TPN have more central line infections and metabolic complications (e.g., hyperglycemia, electrolyte imbalance). Whenever possible, enteral nutrition should be used rather than TPN and TPN should be used only if there is intolerance to enteral feeding. Nasojejunal feeding tube placement is currently favored, but there is some low-level evidence suggesting that nasogastric feeding can safely be considered as an alternative if significant gastric outlet obstruction is not present.

Given the significant increase in mortality associated with septic complications in severe pancreatitis, a number of physicians advocated the use of prophylactic antibiotics in the 1970s. Recent meta-analyses and systematic reviews that have evaluated multiple randomized controlled trials have proved that prophylactic antibiotics do not decrease the frequency of surgical intervention, infected necrosis, or mortality in patients with severe pancreatitis. In addition, they are associated with gram-positive cocci infection, such as by *Staphylococcus aureus*, and *Candida* infection, which is seen in 5% to 15% of patients. Current recommendations are to only administer antibiotics if a preexisting infection is present on presentation or radiographic imaging suggests infected peripancreatic fluid collections (e.g., air within collection or rim enhancement).

Special Considerations

Endoscopic retrograde cholangiopancreatography. Early ERCP, with or without sphincterotomy, was initially advocated to reduce the severity of pancreatitis because the obstructive theory of AP states that pancreatic injury is the result of pancreatic duct obstruction. However, multiple randomized trials have evaluated the use and efficacy of early ERCP in the management of acute biliary pancreatitis. The results of these trials do not support the use of ERCP in the management of acute biliary pancreatitis regardless of the severity. Routine use of ERCP is not indicated for patients with mild pancreatitis because the bile duct obstruction is usually transient and resolves within 48 hours after the onset of symptoms. Based on a meta-analysis of these clinical trials[11] as well as two major society guidelines based on these clinical trials,[8] ERCP is only indicated for patients who develop cholangitis and those with persistent bile duct obstruction demonstrated by other imaging modalities, such as EUS. Finally, in older patients with poor performance status or severe comorbidities that preclude surgery, ERCP with sphincterotomy is a safe alternative to prevent recurrent biliary pancreatitis.

Laparoscopic cholecystectomy. In the absence of definitive treatment, 30% of patients with acute biliary pancreatitis will have recurrent disease. With the exception of older patients and those with poor performance status, laparoscopic cholecystectomy is indicated for all patients with mild acute biliary pancreatitis. Studies have shown that early laparoscopic cholecystectomy, defined as laparoscopic cholecystectomy during the initial admission to the hospital, is a safe procedure that decreases recurrence of the disease.[5] Choledocholithiasis can be excluded by intraoperative cholangiography, EUS, or MRCP. For patients with severe pancreatitis, early surgery may increase the morbidity and length of stay. Current recommendations suggest conservative treatment for at least 6 weeks before laparoscopic cholecystectomy is attempted in this setting. This approach has significantly decreased morbidity.[5]

Complications

Sterile and Infected Peripancreatic Fluid Collections

Discussion regarding appropriate management of pancreatic and peripancreatic fluid collections requires an understanding of the current classification of these entities as defined in Table 56.3. Fluid collections are divided into acute (present for less than four weeks) and chronic (lasting past four weeks) and either being simple or complex in nature. Acute peripancreatic fluids collections are simple in nature and after four weeks are referred to as a pseudocyst. Fluid collections associated with necrotizing pancreatitis are referred to as an acute necrotic collection (ANC) before four weeks and as walled off necrosis after that period. The presence of acute peripancreatic fluids collection during an episode of AP has been described in 30% to 57% of patients. In contrast to pseudocysts and cystic neoplasias of the pancreas, fluid collections are not surrounded or encased by epithelium or fibrotic capsule. Treatment is supportive because most fluid collections will be spontaneously reabsorbed by the peritoneum. All of these fluid collections may become infected. The usual signs and symptoms of infection (e.g., fever, elevated white blood cell count, and abdominal pain) may also be present without an infection in AP due to a robust SIRS response in many of these patients, making diagnosis of infection difficult. Evidence of gas within a fluid collection on imaging is highly suggestive. Acute decompensation or failure to improve after 10 to 14 days may suggest infection and consideration should be given to CT-guided fluid sampling. Drainage (percutaneous or endoscopic) and IV administration of antibiotics should be instituted if infection is present. Antibiotics known to penetrate pancreatic necrosis include carbapenems, quinolones, metronidazole, and high-dose cephalosporins.

Pancreatic Necrosis and Infected Necrosis

Necrosis is the presence of nonviable pancreatic parenchyma or peripancreatic fat and can manifest as a focal area or diffuse involvement of the gland. Contrast-enhanced CT is the most reliable technique to diagnose ANC and are typically seen as areas of low attenuation (<40–50 HU) after the IV injection of contrast material. Normal parenchyma usually has a density of 100 to 150 HU. Up to 20% of patients with AP develop ANCs. It is important to identify and to provide proper treatment of these complications because most patients who develop multiorgan failure have necrotizing pancreatitis; pancreatic necrosis has been documented in up to 80% of the autopsies of patients who died after an episode of AP.[4]

The main complication of ANC is infection. The risk is directly related to the amount of necrosis; in patients with pancreatic necrosis involving less than 30% of the gland, the risk of infection is 22%. The risk is 37% for patients with pancreatic necrosis that involves 30% to 50% of the gland and up to 46% if more than 70% of the gland is affected.[4] This complication is associated with bacterial translocation usually involving enteric flora, such as gram-negative rods (e.g., *Escherichia coli, Klebsiella,* and *Pseudomonas* spp.) and *Enterococcus* spp.

Infected necrotic collection should be suspected in patients with prolonged fever, elevated white blood cell count, or progressive clinical deterioration. It should also be suspected if the patient

TABLE 56.3 **Revised definitions of morphological features of acute pancreatitis.**

TIME FROM ONSET	SUBTYPE OF PANCREATITIS	FLUID COLLECTION NOMENCLATURE	COMPUTED TOMOGRAPHY FINDINGS
4 Weeks			
	Interstitial edematous*	Acute peripancreatic fluid collection	• Homogeneous collection with fluid density • Confined by normal peripancreatic fascial planes • No definable wall encapsulating the collection • Adjacent to pancreas (no intrapancreatic extension)
	Necrotizing†	Acute necrotic collection	• Heterogeneous and nonliquid density of varying degrees in different locations (some appear homogeneous early in their course) • No definable wall encapsulating the collection • Location—intrapancreatic and/or extrapancreatic
>4 Weeks			
	Interstitial edematous*	Pseudocyst	• Well circumscribed, usually round or oval • Homogeneous fluid density • No nonliquid component • Well-defined wall; that is, completely encapsulated
	Necrotizing†	Walled-off necrosis	• Heterogeneous with liquid and nonliquid density with varying degrees of loculations (some may appear homogeneous) • Well-defined wall; that is, completely encapsulated • Location—intrapancreatic and/or extrapancreatic

Adapted from: Banks,P, Bollen, T, Dervenis C. Classification of acute pancreatitis—2012: revision of the Atlanta classification and definitions by internationa1. Banks PA, Bollen TL, Dervenis C, et al: Classification of acute pancreatitis–2012: revision of the Atlanta classification and definitions by international consensus. *Gut.* 2013;62:102–111.
*Acute inflammation of the pancreatic parenchyma and peripancreatic tissues but without recognizable tissue necrosis.
†Inflammation associated with pancreatic parenchymal necrosis and/or peripancreatic necrosis.

develops sepsis, SIRS, and/or organ failure later in the course of the disease (>7 days after the onset of the AP). Evidence of air within the pancreatic necrosis seen on a CT scan confirms the diagnosis but is a rare finding. If infected necrosis is suspected, fine-needle aspiration (FNA) may be performed if the diagnosis is equivocal; from the aspirate, a positive Gram stain or culture establishes the diagnosis. Although positive cultures are confirmatory, a review has demonstrated that despite negative preoperative cultures, 42% of patients with so-called persistent unwellness will have infected necrosis.[12] Fig. 56.8 illustrates the pathophysiologic process of pancreatic necrosis infection.

With decades of experience with treatment of pancreatic necrosis, few general concepts have emerged. First, all sterile necrotic collections do not need to be intervened upon. Indications for intervening in sterile necrotizing pancreatitis include: persistent pain, failure to improve clinically with conservative management, and/or symptomatic biliary or enteric obstruction. Intervention for these indications should be delayed as much as possible to allow development of walled off necrosis. Second, clinical suspicion of or documented infected necrotic collection with clinical deterioration is a clear indication for intervention. Even in this situation, the intervention should be delayed as much as possible to allow the collection to become walled off.

Once infection has been demonstrated, IV antibiotics should be given. Because of their penetration into the pancreas and spectrum coverage, carbapenems are the first option of treatment. Alternative therapy includes quinolones, metronidazole, third-generation cephalosporins, and piperacillin. Historically, the definitive treatment of infected pancreatic necrosis is surgical

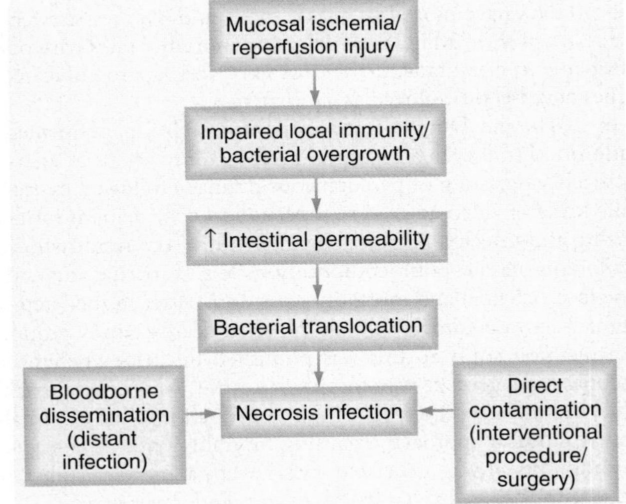

FIG. 56.8 Pathophysiology of pancreatic necrosis infection. The acute inflammatory injury that occurs during the first 48 to 72 hours causes mucosal ischemia and reperfusion injury. Both effects favor bacterial overgrowth because they alter local immunity. Mucosal ischemia also produces an increase in the permeability of intestinal cells, which is initiated 72 hours after the acute episode but typically peaks one week later. These transient episodes of bacteremia are associated with pancreatic necrosis infection. Less frequently, distant sources of infection, such as pneumonia and vascular or urinary tract infection associated with central lines and catheters, are associated with bacteremia and pancreatic necrosis. Finally, local contamination after surgery or interventional procedures such as endoscopic retrograde cholangiopancreatography is responsible for necrosis infection.

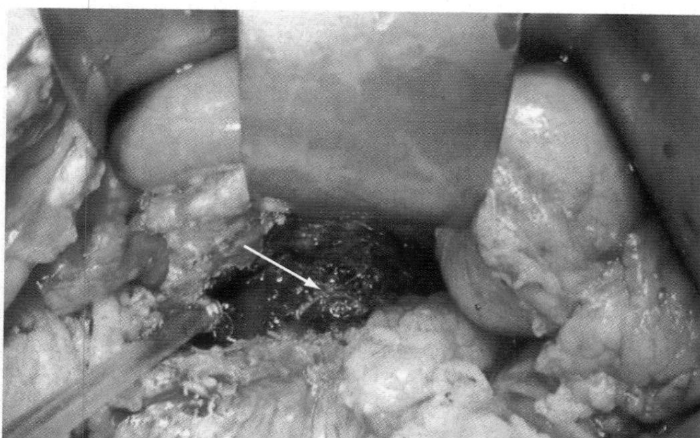

FIG. 56.9 Infected pancreatic necrosis. This 45-year-old man had severe ethanol-induced pancreatitis. Four weeks after the initial episode, the patient developed fever (39.5°C [103°F]), hypotension, and leukocytosis (19,000 cells/mm^3). The computed tomography (CT) scan documented pancreatic necrosis involving 35% of the gland. After fine-needle aspiration (FNA), Gram staining documented the presence of gram-negative rods. The exploratory laparotomy indicated pancreatic necrosis involving mainly the body of the gland *(arrow)*. The patient was treated with necrosectomy, closed drainage, and intravenous meropenem. Final culture documented the presence of *Escherichia coli*. The patient was discharged home 56 days after the initial episode.

debridement with necrosectomy, closed continuous irrigation, or open packaging (Fig. 56.9). The overall mortality rate after open necrosectomy has been as high as 25% to 30%[12] because of the severe nature of the disease as well as the high complication rate of an open debridement. Outcomes are time dependent; patients who undergo surgery in the first 14 days have a mortality rate of 75%, and those who undergo surgery between 15 and 29 days and after 30 days have mortality rates of 45% and 8%, respectively.[13] As a result of the elevated morbidity and mortality rates with open debridement, percutaneous, endoscopic, and laparoscopic techniques have been employed as alternatives.

In 2010, the Dutch Pancreatitis Study Group performed a randomized trial evaluating open necrosectomy versus a "step-up approach" consisting of percutaneous drainage followed by minimally invasive video-assisted retroperitoneal debridement for necrotizing and infected necrotizing pancreatitis. The results showed that long-term end-point complications (e.g., exocrine and endocrine insufficiency) and mortality rates were better in the "step-up approach" group compared with the open necrosectomy group.[14] A companion study to this was published in 2018 wherein endoscopic management was compared to the "step-up approach". While the endoscopic approach was nonsuperior to the minimally invasive surgical approach regarding mortality and most secondary endpoints, it was associated with fewer pancreatic fistulae, reduced cumulative hospital length of stay, and lower cost.[15]

Currently, an endoscopic drainage with a large-bore stent and possible endoscopic debridement with or without percutaneous drainage can avoid an operation in most patients. If the endoscopic and/or percutaneous management fails, a minimally invasive operation will usually be more straightforward and the results improved. Regardless of which route is taken, physiologic and nutritional support of the patient will have a large impact on outcome.

Pancreatic Pseudocysts

Pancreatic pseudocysts occur in 5% to 15% of patients who have peripancreatic fluid collections after AP. By definition, the capsule of a pseudocyst is composed of collagen and granulation tissue, and it is not lined by epithelium. The fibrotic reaction typically requires at least four to eight weeks to develop. Fig. 56.10 shows CT scans of a large pseudocyst arising in the tail of the pancreas.

Up to 50% of patients with pancreatic pseudocysts will develop symptoms. Persistent pain, early satiety, nausea, weight loss, and elevated pancreatic enzyme levels in plasma suggest this diagnosis. The diagnosis is corroborated by CT or MRI. EUS with FNA is indicated for patients in whom the diagnosis of pancreatic pseudocyst is not clear. Characteristic features of pancreatic pseudocysts include high amylase levels associated with the absence of mucin and low carcinoembryonic antigen (CEA) levels.

Observation is indicated for asymptomatic patients because spontaneous regression has been documented in up to 70% of cases; this is particularly true for patients with pseudocysts smaller than 4 cm in diameter, located in the tail, and no evidence of pancreatic duct obstruction or communication with the main pancreatic duct. Invasive therapies are indicated for symptomatic patients or when the differentiation between a cystic neoplasm and pseudocyst is not possible. Because most patients are treated with decompressive procedures and not with resection, it is imperative to have a pathologic diagnosis. Surgical drainage had been the traditional approach for pancreatic pseudocysts. However, modern evidence suggests that transgastric and transduodenal endoscopic drainage are safe and effective approaches for patients with pancreatic pseudocysts in close contact (defined as <1 cm) with the stomach and duodenum, respectively. In addition, transpapillary drainage can be attempted in pancreatic pseudocysts communicating with the main pancreatic duct. For patients in whom a pancreatic duct stricture is associated with a pancreatic pseudocyst, endoscopic dilation and stent placement are indicated.

Surgical drainage is generally reserved for patients with pancreatic pseudocysts that cannot be treated with endoscopic techniques for anatomic reasons and for patients who fail to respond to endoscopic treatment. Definitive treatment depends on the location of the cyst. Pancreatic pseudocysts closely attached to the stomach should be treated with a cystogastrostomy. In this procedure, an anterior gastrostomy is performed (see Video 56.1). Once the pseudocyst is located, it is drained through the posterior wall of the stomach using a linear stapler. The defect in the anterior wall of the stomach is closed in two layers. Pancreatic pseudocysts located in the head of the pancreas that are in close contact with the duodenum are treated with a cystoduodenostomy. Finally, some pseudocysts are not in contact with the stomach or duodenum. The surgical treatment for these patients is a Roux-en-Y cystojejunostomy. Surgical cyst enterostomy is successful in achieving immediate cyst drainage in more than 90% of cases. After initial resolution, pseudocyst formation may recur in up to 12% of cases during long-term follow-up, depending on the location of the cyst and underlying cause of the disease.

Complications of pancreatic pseudocysts include bleeding and pancreaticopleural fistula secondary to vascular and pleural erosion, respectively; bile duct and duodenal obstruction; rupture into the abdominal cavity; and infection. Percutaneous drainage is indicated only for septic patients secondary to pseudocyst infection because it has a high incidence of external fistula.

Pancreatic Ascites and Pancreaticopleural Fistulas

Although very rare, complete disruption of the pancreatic duct can lead to significant accumulation of fluid. This condition should be suspected in patients who have an episode of AP, develop significant abdominal distention, and have free intraabdominal

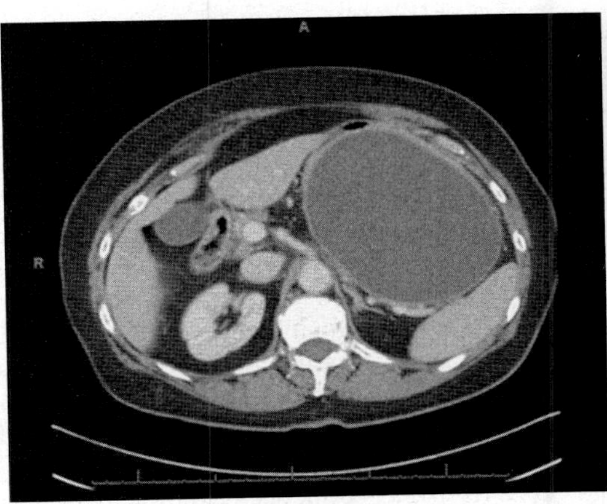

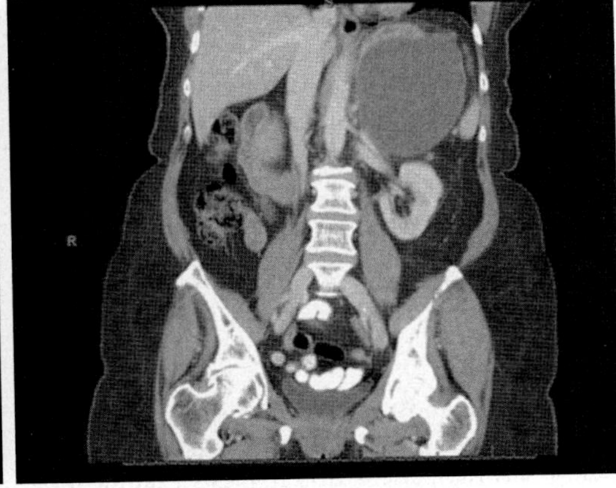

FIG. 56.10 Computed tomography (CT) scans showing a large pseudocyst arising in the tail of the pancreas.

fluid. Diagnostic paracentesis typically demonstrates elevated amylase and lipase levels. Treatment consists of abdominal drainage combined with endoscopic placement of a pancreatic stent across the disruption. Failure of this therapy requires surgical treatment; it consists of distal resection and closure of the proximal stump.

Posterior pancreatic duct disruption into the pleural space has been described rarely. Symptoms that suggest this condition include dyspnea, abdominal pain, cough, and chest pain. The diagnosis is confirmed with chest radiography, thoracentesis, and CT scan. Fig. 56.11 demonstrates a large, left-sided pleural effusion caused by a pancreatic-pleural fistula. Amylase levels above 50,000 IU in the pleural fluid confirm the diagnosis. It is more common after alcoholic pancreatitis and in 70% of patients is associated with pancreatic pseudocysts. Iatrogenic pancreaticopleural fistulas may also be seen after placement of percutaneous drainage catheters that traverse the diaphragm. Initial treatment requires chest drainage, parenteral nutritional support, and administration of octreotide. Up to 60% of patients respond to this therapy. Persistent drainage should also be treated with endoscopic sphincterotomy and stent placement. Patients who do not respond to these measures require surgical treatment, similar to that described for pancreatic ascites.

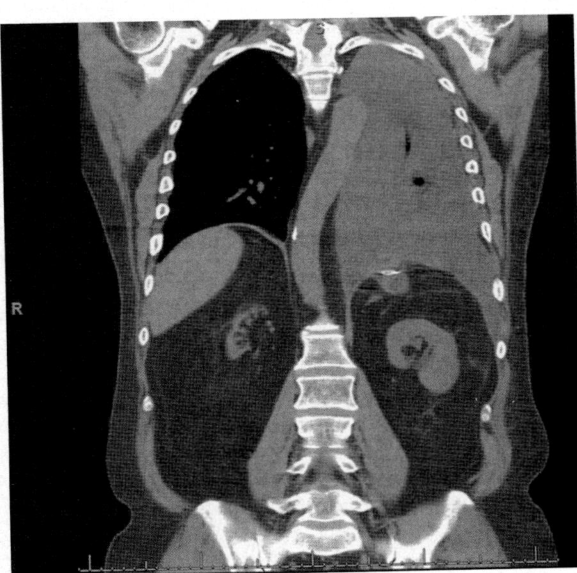

FIG. 56.11 Massive left-sided pleural effusion secondary to a pancreaticopleural fistula.

Vascular Complications

AP is rarely associated with arterial vascular complications. The most common vessel affected is the splenic artery, but the SMA, cystic artery, and gastroduodenal artery (GDA) have also been found to be affected. It has been proposed that pancreatic elastase damages the vessels, leading to pseudoaneurysm formation. Spontaneous rupture results in massive bleeding. Clinical manifestations include sudden onset of abdominal pain, tachycardia, and hypotension. If possible, arterial embolization should be attempted to control the bleeding. Refractory cases require ligation of the vessel affected. The mortality ranges from 28% to 56%.

Pancreatic inflammation can also produce vascular thrombosis; the vessel usually affected is the splenic vein, but in severe cases, it can extend into the portal venous system. Imaging demonstrates splenomegaly, gastric varices, and splenic vein occlusion. Thrombolytics have been described in the acute early phase; however, most patients can be managed with conservative treatment. Anticoagulation for splanchnic vein thrombosis related to pancreatitis has not been shown to improve recanalization rates compared to expectant management.[16] Recurrent episodes of upper gastrointestinal bleeding caused by venous hypertension should be treated with splenectomy.

Pancreatocutaneous Fistula

The frequency of pancreatic fistulas is low. Only 0.4% of patients have this complication after an acute episode. However, the incidence of this complication increases in patients with other complications after AP: 4.5% in patients with pancreatic pseudocysts (4.5%) and 40% in patients with infected necrosis after surgical debridement.[12] Treatment is conservative for most patients.

CHRONIC PANCREATITIS

In contrast to AP, the histologic hallmark of chronic pancreatitis is the persistent inflammation and irreversible fibrosis associated with atrophy of the pancreatic parenchyma. These histologic features are associated with chronic pain and endocrine and exocrine insufficiency that significantly decrease the quality of life of these patients. Chronic pancreatitis affects between 3 and 10/100,000 persons.

Risk Factors

The specific cause and frequency of each condition vary among countries, hospital populations, and referral practices. In general, heavy alcohol consumption is the most common cause of chronic pancreatitis (70%–80% of cases), especially in urban hospitals. Conditions such as chronic duct obstruction, trauma, pancreas divisum, cystic dystrophy of the duodenal wall, hyperparathyroidism, hypertriglyceridemia, autoimmune pancreatitis, tropical pancreatitis, and hereditary pancreatitis are rare and account for less than 10% of all cases. However, hereditary, chronic, and autoimmune pancreatitis are more common in referral centers. In up to 20% of patients, a clear cause cannot be documented and cases are considered to be idiopathic.

Alcohol Abuse

Prolonged alcohol abuse is the most important risk factor associated with chronic pancreatitis. The fact that only 3% to 7% of heavy drinkers develop chronic pancreatitis suggests that alcohol is only a cofactor and that other factors are required for development of this complication. Alcohol exerts multiple noxious effects in the pancreas: it increases the total protein concentration in the pancreatic juice, it promotes the synthesis and secretion of lithostathine by acinar cells, and it increases glycoprotein 2 secretion in pancreatic juice. These factors lead to protein precipitation and subsequent formation of protein plugs and eventually stones inside the pancreatic duct. As a result of the obstruction, acinar cells are no longer able to secrete pancreatic enzymes and are predisposed to autodigestion. In addition, several products of alcohol metabolism, such as fatty acid ethyl esters and reactive oxygen species, cause fragility of intraacinar organelles, such as zymogen granules and lysosomes, which leads to abnormal pancreatic enzyme activation inside acinar cells. Acetaldehyde, another alcohol metabolite, causes direct acinar injury. Chronic alcohol consumption is associated with enhanced NF-κB activity, decreased perfusion in the microcirculation of the pancreas, and increased intracellular calcium levels.

The identification of PSCs in the late 1990s is one of the most important discoveries in the pathophysiology of chronic pancreatitis.[17] PSCs are specialized quiescent fibroblasts found at the base of acinar cells. Once stimulated, PSCs differentiate into activated myofibroblasts, which synthesize proteins that form the extracellular matrix. Examples of these proteins include collagen I and III, fibronectin, laminin, and matrix metalloproteinases. PSCs have responses similar to hepatic stellate cells; chronic necrosis and inflammation (necroinflammation) induce the release of inflammatory mediators, such as platelet-derived growth factor, TGF-β, TNF-α, IL-1, and IL-6, which are known to activate PSCs. Consequently, the synthesis of collagen and other components of pancreatic fibrosis is increased. It has been postulated that the chronic necroinflammation induced by ethanol activates PSCs and induces pancreatic fibrosis. Interestingly, it has also been shown that alcohol and some of its metabolites (e.g., acetaldehyde) cause activation of PSCs.

Although they have been evaluated only in preclinical studies, novel therapies that target the activation of PSCs are being investigated. It has been reported that antioxidants, angiotensin-converting enzyme inhibitors, peroxisome proliferator-activated receptor gamma ligands, and vitamin A inhibit the activity of PSCs.

Smoking

Epidemiologic studies have shown that smoking increases the risk of alcohol-induced chronic pancreatitis. Active smokers develop chronic pancreatitis at a younger age compared with nonsmokers. In addition, the risk of pancreatic calcifications and diabetes mellitus is increased in patients who smoke compared with nonsmokers.

Gene Mutations

Under physiologic conditions, pancreatic enzyme activation is strictly controlled. Mutations in proteins that regulate this activation increase the risk of chronic pancreatitis. Mutations in the cationic trypsinogen gene, also known as protease serine 1 *(PRSS1)* gene, are common in hereditary chronic pancreatitis. *PRSS1* is located on chromosome 7 and regulates trypsinogen production; mutations in this gene are associated with intraacinar trypsinogen activation. *PRSS1* mutations have been documented in hereditary pancreatitis but are uncommon in other forms of chronic pancreatitis.

SPINK-1 is a peptide secreted by acinar cells that regulates the premature activation of trypsinogen. Because *SPINK1* mutations are present in 1% to 2% of healthy patients but the prevalence of chronic pancreatitis is much lower, it has been hypothesized that *SPINK1* mutations are not enough to trigger pancreatic inflammation. However, they lower the threshold for its development and influence the severity of the disease. *SPINK1* mutations are more prevalent in alcoholic, hereditary, and idiopathic pancreatitis.

The secretion of bicarbonate and chloride in respiratory and pancreatic secretions is regulated by the *CFTR* gene. *CFTR* mutations affect the normal secretion of bicarbonate, decrease pancreatic juice volume, and augment the concentration of pancreatic enzymes inside the pancreatic duct. Homozygous *CFTR* mutations result in cystic fibrosis; heterozygous mild mutations predispose to pancreatic exocrine insufficiency and chronic pancreatitis. The prevalence of *CFTR* gene mutations is higher in patients with alcoholic, idiopathic, and hereditary pancreatitis compared with the general population. Similarly, mutation in human chymotrypsin C gene has been found to be associated with development of chronic pancreatitis. It seems that chymotrypsin C protects against pancreatitis by degrading trypsinogen and thereby curtailing harmful intrapancreatic trypsinogen activation.[18]

While our understanding of pathogenesis of chronic pancreatitis has evolved in a largely trypsin centric fashion, animal studies in trypsin knockout mice suggest that even in the absence of trypsin, chronic noxious stimuli can induce chronic pancreatitis.[19] These results suggest that alternative pathways independent of trypsin may exist that can lead to chronic injury in pancreatitis, and elucidation of these pathways may lead to development of novel therapeutics.

Types of Chronic Pancreatitis

Autoimmune Pancreatitis

Autoimmune pancreatitis is a chronic inflammatory disorder that involves the pancreas. At least two different histologic variants have been defined: 1) Type 1, which is the pancreatic manifestation of an immunoglobulin G4-related disease; and 2) Type 2, a pancreatic specific disorder, not associated with immunoglobulin G4. Type 1 is the most common; it is characterized by dense, periductal lymphoplasmacytic infiltrates, storiform fibrosis, and obliterative venulitis. Plasmatic cells typically stain positive for immunoglobulin G4. In type 2, the pancreas is infiltrated by neutrophils, lymphocytes, and plasma cells that destroy and obliterate the epithelium in the pancreatic duct. Autoimmune pancreatitis is more common in men than in women. Up to 80% of patients are older than 50 years. Patients with autoimmune pancreatitis can

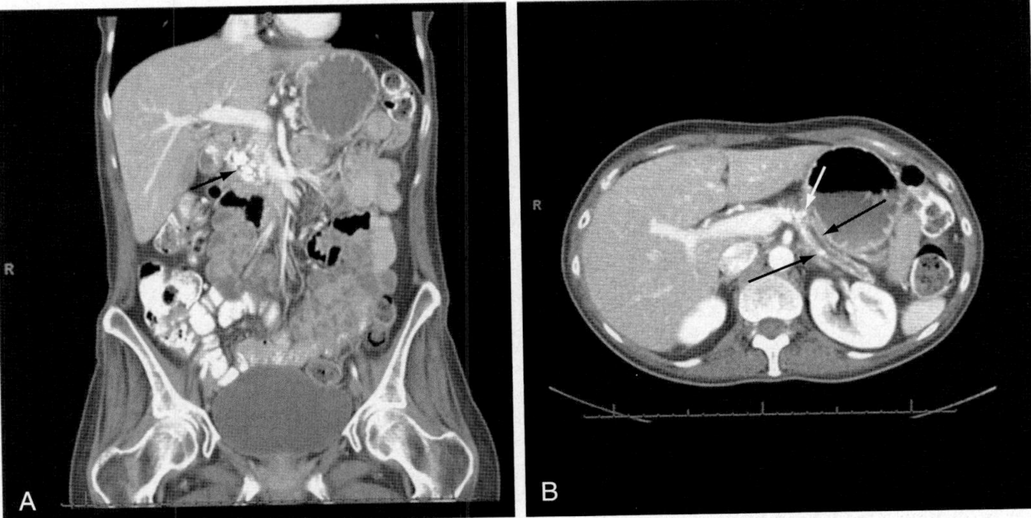

FIG. 56.12 Typical computed tomography (CT) findings associated with chronic pancreatitis. Shown are pancreatic duct dilation *(long arrow)* and intrapancreatic calcifications, which are also typical of chronic pancreatitis *(small arrow)*.

develop acute symptoms such as jaundice or AP, closely mimicking patients with pancreatic adenocarcinoma. However, most patients with chronic pancreatitis develop chronic abdominal discomfort associated with abnormal elevation of amylase and lipase levels.

Tropical Pancreatitis

Tropical pancreatitis is not common in the United States; it is more common in tropical areas within 30 degrees of the equator, particularly in India. Its pathophysiology has not been completely delineated, but it has been associated with cassava ingestion and *SPINK1* mutations. Up to 45% to 50% of patients with tropical pancreatitis have *SPINK1* mutations.

Idiopathic Pancreatitis

In up to 10% to 20% of patients with chronic pancreatitis, a clear cause that predisposed to the disease is not evident. Future identification of genetic defects associated with chronic pancreatitis may allow the identification of individuals at highest risk for development of this disease.

Clinical Manifestations

Pain is the primary manifestation of chronic pancreatitis. Initially precipitated by oral intake, the intensity, frequency, and duration of pain gradually increase with worsening disease. Quality of life of these patients is significantly affected because of decreased oral intake, interference with daily activities, and dependence on narcotic pain medications. Nausea and vomiting are not common early on; however, they may appear as the disease progresses.

Pancreatic inflammation and fibrosis not only affect the pancreatic ducts but also decrease the number and function of acinar cells. At least 90% of the gland needs to be dysfunctional before steatorrhea, diarrhea, and other symptoms of malabsorption develop. In severe cases, diseases associated with fat-soluble vitamin deficiency, such as bleeding, osteopenia, and osteoporosis, develop. Exocrine insufficiency occurs in 80% to 90% of patients with long-standing chronic pancreatitis.

Chronic pancreatitis also affects islet cell populations. As a result, 40% to 80% of patients will have clinical manifestations of diabetes mellitus, typically occurring years after the onset of abdominal pain and pancreatic exocrine insufficiency.

Jaundice or cholangitis occurs in 5% to 10% of patients because of fibrosis of the distal common bile duct. Extensive scarring in the head of the pancreas can also obstruct the duodenum, leading to severe nausea, vomiting, and abdominal pain. Upper gastrointestinal bleeding secondary to portal or splenic vein thrombosis is a rare manifestation of chronic pancreatitis.

Diagnosis

Imaging Studies

Cross-sectional imaging plays an important role in the diagnosis of chronic pancreatitis; however, a standardized approach to the diagnosis and assessment of disease is lacking. The most common CT findings in chronic pancreatitis include dilated pancreatic duct (68%), parenchymal atrophy (54%), and pancreatic calcifications (50%; Fig. 56.12). Other findings include peripancreatic fluid, focal pancreatic enlargement, biliary duct dilation, and irregular pancreatic parenchyma contour. CT has a sensitivity of 56% to 95% and a specificity of 85% to 100% for the diagnosis of chronic pancreatitis. In addition to establishing the diagnosis, CT is particularly useful to assess complications, such as pancreatic duct disruption, pseudocysts, portal and splenic vein thrombosis, and splenic and pancreaticoduodenal artery pseudoaneurysms.

MRI is a reliable alternative to evaluate patients with chronic pancreatitis. The sensitivity for the diagnosis of pancreatic calcifications is lower, but MRI is useful to detect changes in the pancreatic parenchyma suggestive of chronic inflammation, such as changes in intensity, pancreatic atrophy, and irregularities in the contour. In addition, MRCP with secretin injection is particularly useful to evaluate intraductal strictures and pancreatic duct disruption. Efforts to standardize imaging evaluation of chronic pancreatitis patients are underway.

Although ERCP was historically considered the "gold standard" for the diagnosis of chronic pancreatitis, current indications include patients for whom other diagnostic tests, including CT and MRCP, are contraindicated or have failed to corroborate the diagnosis. ERCP should be considered a therapeutic modality in patients who develop pancreatic duct complications amenable to endoscopic therapy, such as stricture, stone, pseudocysts, and biliary stenosis.

EUS has emerged as the most accurate technique to diagnose chronic pancreatitis in patients with minimal change disease or in the early stages. The criteria required for diagnosis of chronic pancreatitis based on EUS are known as the Rosemont criteria (Box 56.5). Histologic evidence of inflammation, atrophy, and fibrosis is the gold standard for the diagnosis of chronic pancreatitis; however, current evidence does not support the use of EUS-guided FNA or Tru-Cut biopsies to diagnose this disease. While positive Rosemont criteria are predictive of histologic pancreatitis, a finding of Rosemont "normal" has a poor negative predictive value, with as many as 55% of cases ultimately found to have chronic pancreatitis on histopathologic exam.

Functional Tests

Measurement of the fecal elastase 1 level is the preferred noninvasive study to diagnose pancreatic exocrine insufficiency. It quantifies the amount of fecal elastase 1 using monoclonal or polyclonal anti–human elastase 1 antibodies. A fecal elastase 1 concentration above 200 μg/g feces is normal; a fecal elastase 1 concentration between 100 and 200 μg/g defines mild to moderate pancreatic insufficiency; and a fecal elastase 1 concentration below 100 μg/g establishes the diagnosis of severe pancreatic exocrine insufficiency.

The fecal fat and weight estimation test measures the stool content of fat after a nutritional fat intake of 100 g/day for 3 days. If the stool fat content exceeds 7 g/day, the diagnosis of steatorrhea is established.

Treatment

Medical Treatment

The main goal in the treatment of chronic pancreatitis is palliation of symptoms, and removal of predisposing factors. Optimal treatment requires that a multidisciplinary team follow a systematized and well-structured therapeutic plan. Patient counseling is an important component because current evidence suggests that this disease is irreversible, but disease progression can be delayed if the predisposing condition is eradicated. Patients should be strongly encouraged to stop drinking and smoking. Furthermore, other risk factors, such as hypertriglyceridemia, should be treated, and diet modification (i.e., low-fat diet) may benefit some patients.

Pain Management

Because most patients develop pain during the natural history of the disease, analgesic selection is a cornerstone of treatment. Nonsteroidal antiinflammatory drugs are the first line of treatment. Moderate to severe pain that does not respond to nonsteroidal antiinflammatory drugs should be treated with tramadol. Patients with severe pain that does not respond to these recommendations should be treated with potent long-acting narcotics. It cannot be overemphasized that adjuvant measures to prevent addiction, depression, and poor quality of life should be considered for patients with severe pain who require narcotics. Alternative drugs useful in the treatment of other conditions associated with chronic pain, such as tricyclic antidepressants, selective serotonin reuptake inhibitors, combined serotonin and norepinephrine reuptake inhibitors, gabapentin, and $\alpha 2\delta$ inhibitors, may also be considered. Randomized controlled trials have shown that nonnarcotic medications can reduce pain and reduce the need for opioids in chronic pancreatitis patients, highlighting the need for a multidisciplinary team including pain management experts. For patients with unrelenting pain, celiac neurolysis has been attempted but without sustained success in those with chronic pancreatitis.

BOX 56.5 Rosemont consensus-based endoscopic ultrasound features for diagnosis of chronic pancreatitis.

Parenchymal Features

Major A Criteria

- Hyperechoic foci with postacoustic shadowing

Major B Criteria

- Honeycombing lobularity*

Minor Criteria

- Hyperechoic, nonshadowing foci ≥3 mm in length and width
- Lobularity including three or more noncontiguous lobules in the body or tail
- Pancreatic cysts ≥2 mm in short axis
- At least three strands†

Ductal Features

Major A Criteria

- Main pancreatic duct calculi‡

Minor Criteria

- Irregular main pancreatic duct contour
- Dilated side branches§
- Main pancreatic duct dilation (≥3.5 mm in the body or ≥1.5 mm in the tail)
- Hyperechoic main pancreatic duct margin >50% of the main pancreatic duct in the body and tail*

Diagnosis of Chronic Pancreatitis

Consistent With Chronic Pancreatitis

- 1 major A criterion + ≥3 or more minor criteria
- 1 major A criterion + major B criterion
- 2 major A criteria

Suggestive of Chronic Pancreatitis¶

- 1 major A criterion + <3 minor criteria
- 1 major B criterion + ≥3 minor criteria
- ≥5 minor criteria

Indeterminate for Chronic Pancreatitis¶

- 3–4 minor criteria in the absence of major criteria
- Major B criterion + <3 minor criteria

Normal

- <3 minor criteria

Adapted from Catalano MF, Sahai A, Levy M, et al. EUS-based criteria for the diagnosis of chronic pancreatitis: The Rosemont classification. *Gastrointest Endosc*. 2009;69:1251–1261.

*Defined as lobularity that includes at least three contiguous lobules in the body or tail. It should be assessed in the body and tail.

†Strands are defined as hyperechoic lines ≥3 mm in length seen in at least two different directions in the body or tail of the pancreas.

‡The presence of calculi in the main pancreatic duct, regardless of location, is the most predictive finding of chronic pancreatitis.

§Defined as at least three tubular anechoic structures, each one ≥1 mm in width, budding from the main pancreatic duct.

¶With suggestive and indeterminate chronic pancreatitis, the diagnosis needs to be confirmed with another imaging modality.

Pancreatic Exocrine Insufficiency

There is no question about the digestive benefits of pancreatic enzyme replacement in patients with pancreatic exocrine insufficiency. In the absence of pancreatic enzyme replacement therapy, patients with chronic pancreatitis may suffer from steatorrhea or diarrhea, leading to malabsorption, malnutrition, and vitamin and mineral deficiencies. A thorough nutritional evaluation should be performed prior to initiation of therapy; however generally, 90,000 USP of lipase is required to avoid malabsorption. Therapeutic trials with pancreatic enzymes should last at least six weeks and should be given along with proton pump inhibitors because acid suppression improves the effects of uncoated pancreatic enzymes.

Endocrine Insufficiency

Endocrine insufficiency and resulting diabetes is not always present early on, but may develop in patients with chronic pancreatitis. Unlike more common type 1 or type 2 diabetes, patients with chronic pancreatitis may develop diabetes, which includes deficiency of insulin and other regulatory hormones such as glucagon. These patients are at higher risk of suboptimal glucose control; particularly severe hypoglycemia related to insulin use and should be managed by an endocrinologist with experience in managing these complex patients.

Interventional Therapy: Endoscopic Treatment

ERCP is the primary modality for treating symptomatic pancreatic duct obstruction with dilation and polyethylene stent placement. Note that the differential diagnosis of pancreatic duct strictures includes pancreatic cancer. Only after a thorough evaluation, which includes CT, MRCP, or EUS, has completely ruled out the possibility of malignant disease should endoscopic treatment be considered. Surgical resection is indicated if any concern of malignant disease exists.

Endoscopic stone extraction should be considered for patients with pain and pancreatic duct dilation secondary to stones. Extracorporeal shock wave lithotripsy followed by therapeutic ERCP may be required for the treatment of large impacted stones. The success rate varies from 44% to 77% for this technique. In conjunction with stone extraction, pancreatic duct stenting may benefit patients by relieving obstruction. Although this relief may be temporary, during this interim a patient may be able to improve nutritional and functional status before further, perhaps more invasive therapy.

Biliary obstruction caused by chronic pancreatitis occurs in 10% of patients and is best treated with surgical bypass. Temporary relief of the obstruction with plastic stents is indicated for patients with cholangitis or for those who are severely malnourished.

Surgical Treatment

Several factors, including intractable pain, biliary or pancreatic duct obstruction, duodenal obstruction, pseudocyst or pseudoaneurysm formation, and the inability to rule out malignant disease, may prompt surgical intervention. The choice of surgical procedure depends on the symptoms requiring palliation and the presence or absence of pancreatic ductal dilation. In general, patients with a dilated pancreatic duct (defined as diameter >7 mm), or large duct disease, require a decompressing procedure; patients with a nondilated pancreatic duct, or small duct disease, require a resectional procedure. Several clinical scenarios that require surgical intervention are described here.

Pancreatic duct dilation secondary to duct stones or strictures. Pancreatic duct dilation is defined as a main pancreatic duct measuring at least 7 mm in diameter. Pancreatic duct dilation can be secondary to a single stone or stricture; however, it is often caused by multiple strictures and stones in the pancreatic duct. The pancreatic duct dilation observed on pancreatography for chronic pancreatitis is classically described as a chain of lakes, which reflects the presence of multiple dilations and stenoses. When it is accompanied by intractable pain, this condition is best treated with side-to-side Roux-en-Y pancreaticojejunostomy, also known as the modified Puestow procedure or lateral pancreaticojejunostomy.

The anterior surface of the pancreatic duct is opened, and the anterior surface of the duct is completely unroofed. This tissue may be sent for frozen section analysis to rule out underlying malignant disease. The proximal extent of tissue resection is within 1 cm of the duodenum, and the distal limit is within 1 cm to 2 cm of the end of the pancreas. Failure to cross the GDA into the neck and head of the pancreas may leave undrained pancreatic head or uncinate process ducts obstructed by stones or strictures, which may give incomplete relief or early recurrence of symptoms. After all stones are extracted, a standard Roux-en-Y is used to create a lateral pancreaticojejunostomy. The main advantage offered by this procedure is parenchymal conservation, which preserves endocrine and exocrine function. The modified Puestow procedure provides palliation of pain in 80% of cases; however, 30% of cases will recur, usually 3 to 5 years after surgery. Decompressive procedures temporarily relieve the ductal obstruction, but in most cases, they do not modify the natural history of the disease, and chronic pancreatitis progresses. Other factors associated with recurrence include smoking and alcohol ingestion after surgery, failure to decompress the head and uncinate process properly, and length of the pancreaticojejunostomy.

In 1987, Andersen and Frey described the local resection of the pancreatic head with longitudinal pancreaticojejunostomy as an alternative procedure. The surgical approach is similar to the Puestow procedure; however, once the anterior surface of the pancreatic duct has been completely exposed, the anterior portion of the head of the pancreas is also resected, leaving a 1-cm rim of pancreatic tissue along the duodenal margin. Fig. 56.13 shows intraoperative images of a Frey procedure. This procedure is also an alternative for patients with a dilated pancreatic duct secondary to a benign stricture in the head of the pancreas associated with severe inflammation, scarring, or portal hypertension surrounding the head of the pancreas that precludes a safe pancreaticoduodenectomy. The main disadvantage is the removal of pancreatic parenchyma. A study has demonstrated that 62% of patients are completely free of pain and 95% of patients have satisfactory pain control after this procedure. In the same series, 34% of patients developed endocrine or exocrine pancreatic insufficiency.[20]

Pancreatic duct dilation secondary to a single stricture or stone. On occasion, a single stricture that is proximal to the papilla produces pancreatic duct dilation. As an alternative to a Puestow or Frey procedure, a pancreaticoduodenectomy (or pancreatoduodenectomy) can be performed to relieve the obstruction. This procedure is described later in the surgical treatment of pancreatic adenocarcinoma. It must be emphasized that this procedure is absolutely contraindicated if more than one obstruction is present in the duct. Single distal obstructions can occasionally be treated with a distal pancreatectomy. The main disadvantage of both procedures is that they can be associated with pancreatic insufficiency because normal parenchyma is removed. This issue may be ameliorated with autotransplantation of islet cells derived from the resected parenchyma, further discussed below.

Focal inflammatory mass without significant dilation of the pancreatic duct. In a small percentage of patients with chronic pancreatitis, a predominant mass in the head or, less commonly, in the tail of the pancreas without any evidence of pancreatic duct dilation is seen. Long-standing chronic pancreatitis is also a risk

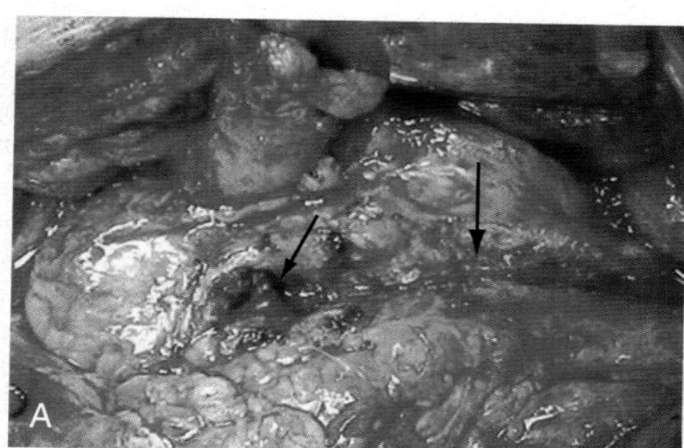

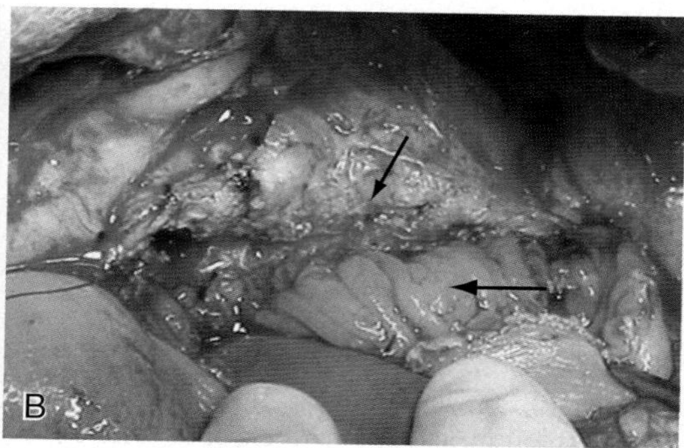

FIG. 56.13 Frey procedure, intraoperative photographs. (A) Significant dilation of the main pancreatic duct at the level of the head *(short arrow)* and body of the pancreas *(long arrow)* after the anterior surface of the pancreas has been opened. (B) Side-to-side anastomosis between the pancreatic duct *(short arrow)* and jejunum *(long arrow)*.

factor for development of pancreatic cancer; therefore, even in patients with a known history of chronic pancreatitis, finding a focal mass is concerning because it may represent an area of pancreatic adenocarcinoma that has developed in the setting of chronic pancreatitis. Resection is recommended for surgical candidates to avoid any error in diagnosis.

Once malignant disease is ruled out with percutaneous or EUS biopsy, resection of the pancreatic head may be done with either of two operations: pancreaticoduodenectomy or duodenum-preserving pancreatic head resection, otherwise known as the Beger procedure. The Beger procedure was designed to remove the pancreatic head while preserving the remainder of the foregut anatomy and therefore function. Once the pancreatic head is removed, a Roux-en-Y is created and anastomosed to the rim of pancreas or duodenum, pancreatic duct, and body and perhaps the bile duct if it was entered. Randomized controlled trials have demonstrated that the Beger procedure offers symptomatic relief that is equivalent to the pancreaticoduodenectomy and Frey procedure in appropriately selected patients.

Diffuse glandular involvement without dilation of the pancreatic duct. The most effective treatment to eliminate pain in patients without dilation of the pancreatic duct is total pancreatectomy. However, this procedure is invariably associated with diabetes mellitus. In contrast to type 1 diabetes mellitus, the severity and risk of hypoglycemia are increased in these patients. In 1977, researchers at the University of Minnesota described islet autotransplantation after total pancreatectomy to prevent the effects of surgically induced diabetes. In the largest experience there, one third of patients who underwent this procedure were insulin independent, an additional one-third required insulin intermittently, and the other third was fully dependent. According to this study, 90% had pain relief or reduction and 50% were able to discontinue narcotics. Similar results were demonstrated at the University of Cincinnati; up to two thirds of patients had complete or partial islet function, and 40% were insulin independent. Narcotics were discontinued in 66% of patients.[21] Although preliminary results have been encouraging, routine implementation of this operative intervention has been controversial. Major limitations associated with this procedure include the cost and lack of islet processing facilities.

As several other centers have established islet autotransplantation programs and laboratories, it has become clear that the treatment of patients with severe diffuse chronic pancreatitis should be coordinated by a multidisciplinary team. This should include a pancreatic surgeon, pancreatologist, interventional endoscopist, radiologist, anesthesia pain specialist, endocrinologist, nutritional expert, and perhaps a neuropsychologist or psychiatrist. The multifaceted approach to the decision and the type of treatment is crucial to long-term success. The groups at the Medical University of South Carolina and at the University of Alabama at Birmingham have shown that patients with depression or substance abuse, such as alcoholism, have a poor outcome compared with those patients without depression or alcoholism.

In pediatric patients with genetic predisposition to pancreatitis, early pancreatectomy and islet autotransplantation is highly effective at improving quality of life.

Biliary strictures. Chronic scarring and fibrosis of the head of the pancreas result in external compression of the intrapancreatic portion of the common bile duct. Up to one third of patients with chronic pancreatitis develop radiologic evidence of bile duct dilation; however, significant biliary obstruction occurs in 6% of patients. Biliary strictures typically appear as a long symmetrical narrowing that involves the intrapancreatic portion of the common bile duct in MRCP or ERCP (Fig. 56.14). IV fluid and antibiotic therapy and temporary bile duct decompression with plastic stents is indicated for patients who present with cholangitis. Pancreaticoduodenectomy is indicated for patients in whom malignant disease cannot be excluded before surgery. A Roux-en-Y hepaticojejunostomy is an alternative treatment for patients without evidence of malignant disease or significant scarring that precludes resection of the head of the pancreas.

Duodenal stenosis. Up to 1.2% of patients with chronic pancreatitis develop duodenal strictures. Clinical manifestations include abdominal pain, nausea, vomiting, and significant weight loss. Differential diagnoses include other causes of gastric outlet obstruction secondary to upper gastrointestinal malignant neoplasms and gastroparesis. Severely malnourished patients require IV hydration, nutritional support, and gastric decompression with a nasogastric tube. Permanent treatment requires a gastrojejunostomy.

Pancreatic pseudocyst. Pancreatic pseudocysts develop more frequently in patients with chronic pancreatitis compared with AP. Up to 30% to 40% of patients develop pseudocysts during the course of their disease. Only 10% of patients have spontaneous pancreatic pseudocyst regression. Spontaneous regression is less likely to occur in these patients because pancreatic pseudocysts arise more frequently in the setting of pancreatic duct obstruction. Indications for treatment include symptoms secondary to gastric, duodenal, or biliary compression or associated complications, such as bleeding, pancreaticopleural fistulas, rupture, or spontaneous bleeding. Alternative modalities in the treatment include endoscopic and surgical drainage (see earlier).

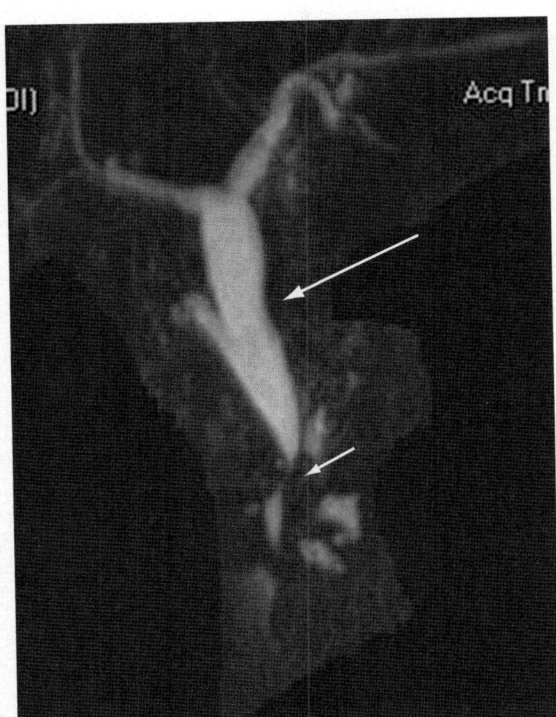

FIG. 56.14 Bile duct stricture secondary to chronic pancreatitis. Magnetic resonance cholangiopancreatography (MRCP) indicates common bile duct dilation *(large arrow)* secondary to a stricture at the level of the intrapancreatic portion of the common bile duct *(small arrow)*.

Traditionally, management of a symptomatic or persistent pseudocyst has been open operation and, depending on location, drainage through either cystogastrostomy or Roux-en-Y cystojejunostomy. With advancements in interventional endoscopy, drainage has proven successful with ERCP. More recently, drainage with EUS has been shown to be more successful because of improved visualization of vasculature as well as fluid collections and necrosis. Small-caliber plastic stents may be used for simple pancreatic fluid collections or larger metal stents for complex collections or those with infection or necrosis. At the University of Alabama at Birmingham, a prospective randomized trial of endoscopic versus operative cystogastrostomy showed equal efficacy but quicker improvement in quality of life and less hospital expenditure from the endoscopic approach for simple pancreatic pseudocysts.[22]

CYSTIC NEOPLASMS OF THE PANCREAS

Second only to adenocarcinoma, cystic neoplasms of the pancreas have become an increasingly recognized entity, with sometimes complex treatment decision algorithms. Over the last two decades, significant effort has been placed on standardizing the diagnosis and on characterization of these lesions in an effort to create universally accepted guidelines for management. Initially created in 2006 at a consensus meeting of the International Association of Pancreatology in Sendai, Japan, the international guidelines for the management of cystic lesions of the pancreas continue to evolve.

Types of Cystic Neoplasms

Serous Cystic Neoplasm

Serous cystic neoplasms (SCNs) have a predilection for the head of the pancreas and occur in patients with a higher median age. Patients commonly present with vague abdominal pain and less

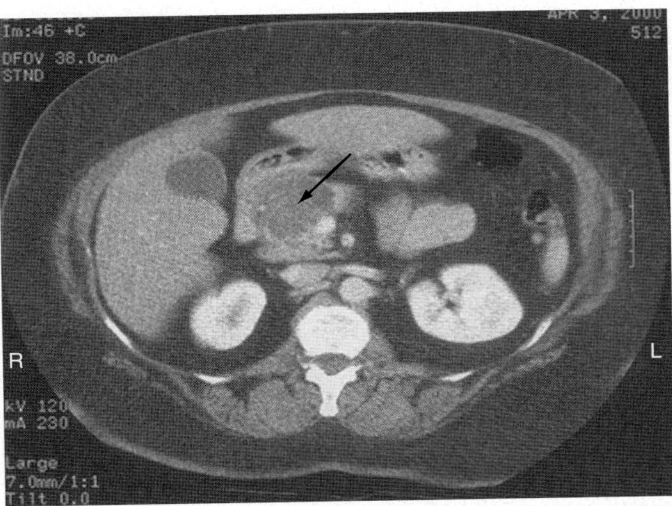

FIG. 56.15 Computed tomography (CT) scan of serous cyst neoplasm. The *arrow* depicts the sunburst appearance and central calcification.

frequently with weight loss and obstructive jaundice. On gross inspection, SCNs are large, well-circumscribed masses. Microscopic examination reveals multiloculated, glycogen-rich small cysts. Central calcification, with radiating septa giving the sunburst appearance, is a radiographic sign on CT in 10% to 20% of patients (Fig. 56.15). With the advent of EUS, these features can now be better delineated. Recently, differential cyst fluid protein expression was observed between SCNs and IPMNs, with accurate discrimination in 92% of patients.[23] Although serous cystic tumors are generally considered benign, pancreatectomy is suggested when the diagnosis of malignant disease is uncertain or in symptomatic serous cystadenomas. Patients with a tumor larger than 4 cm are more likely to be symptomatic and to display a more rapid median growth rate than patients with tumors smaller than 4 cm. Thus, in select patients with large (>4 cm) or rapidly growing lesions, resection of an SCN is appropriate.

Mucinous Cystic Neoplasm

Mucinous cystic neoplasms (MCNs) are the mucin producing cyst tumors which, unlike IPMNs (described below), lack communication with the pancreatic duct. These tumors span the histologic spectrum from benign to invasive carcinomas. MCNs contain mucin-producing epithelium and are identified histologically by the presence of mucin-rich cells and ovarian-like stroma surrounding the cyst (Fig. 56.16). Staining for estrogen and progesterone is positive in most cases. Frequently seen in young women, the mean age at presentation is in the fifth decade. Men are rarely affected. MCNs are typically found in the body and tail of the pancreas but infrequently can occur elsewhere. Although incidental MCN is becoming increasingly common, up to 50% of patients present with vague abdominal pain. A history of pancreatitis may be found in up to 20% of patients, which explains the common misdiagnosis of pseudocyst.

The radiologic characteristic of an MCN on a CT scan is the presence of a solitary cyst, which may have fine septations and be surrounded by a rim of calcification (Fig. 56.17). Cross-sectional imaging may not be able to distinguish between benign and malignant MCNs; however, the presence of eggshell calcification, larger tumor size, or a mural nodule on cross-sectional imaging is suggestive of malignancy.

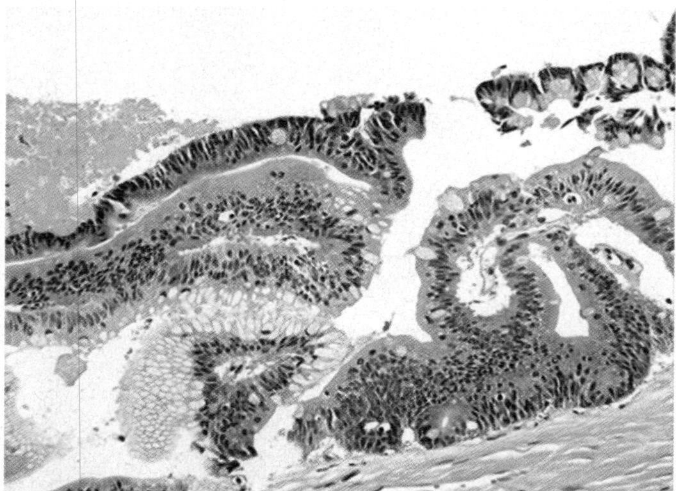

FIG. 56.16 Ovarian-like stroma is a histologic feature often seen in mucinous cystic neoplasms (MCNs).

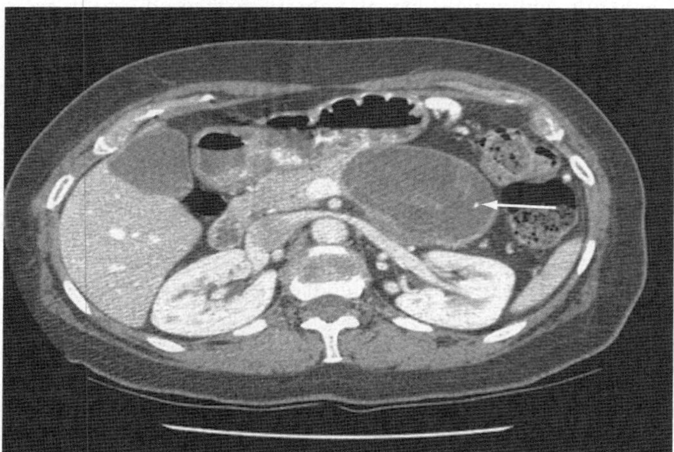

FIG. 56.17 Computed tomography (CT) scan of the tail of the pancreas mucinous cystic neoplasm (MCN) showing a large multiloculated cyst arrow in the absence of pancreatic ductal communication.

EUS and cyst fluid analyses play an important role in the diagnosis of MCN and other cystic neoplasms. FNA with cyst fluid analysis of MCNs demonstrates mucin-rich aspirate, high CEA levels (>192 ng/mL; log scale), and low amylase. Fig. 56.18 illustrates the sensitivity and specificity of CEA in identifying mucinous neoplasms on the basis of fine-needle fluid aspiration. These fluid analyses provide accurate diagnosis in up to 80% of cases.[24] Table 56.4 summarizes the distinguishing features of cystic neoplasms of the pancreas.

Pancreatic resection is the standard treatment for MCNs, given the potential for malignant transformation. In the absence of invasive malignant disease, resection is curative and no further surveillance is required. The prognosis of patients who undergo pancreatectomy for invasive MCNs is poor although more favorable than that of patients with ductal adenocarcinoma of the pancreas. Invasive MCNs exhibit slower growth, less frequent nodal involvement, and less aggressive clinical behavior compared with ductal adenocarcinoma; a 5-year survival of 50% to 60% can be expected after resection. Despite limited experience with invasive MCNs, most centers offer adjuvant systemic chemotherapy after surgical resection, especially when node-positive disease is present.

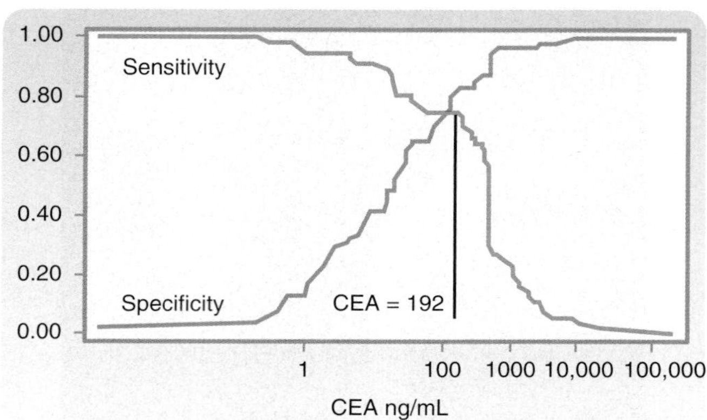

FIG. 56.18 Sensitivity and specificity curves of cyst fluid carcinoembryonic antigen *(CEA)* concentrations (ng/mL; log scale) for differentiating between mucinous and nonmucinous cystic lesions. An optimal cutoff value of 192 ng/mL correlated with the crossover of the sensitivity and specificity curves. (From Brugge WR, Lewandrowski K, Lee-Lewandrowski E, et al. Diagnosis of pancreatic cystic neoplasms: A report of the cooperative pancreatic cyst study. *Gastroenterology. 2004*;126:1330–1336.)

Intraductal Papillary Mucinous Neoplasm

IPMNs of the pancreas are mucinous epithelial neoplasms, which arise from the main pancreatic ducts or branch ducts or both. IPMNs were first described by Ohashi and typically manifest in the sixth to seventh decade of life. Due to increasing use of cross-sectional imaging (CT and MRI), this entity is being increasingly diagnosed. IPMNs encompass a wide spectrum of epithelial changes. Recent efforts to standardize nomenclature for IPMN has been critical to allow for better study of diagnosis, management, and outcomes for IPMN. The terms "adenoma" and "carcinoma in situ" have been abandoned in order to standardize reporting. Current histopathologic grading includes low, moderate, or high-grade dysplasia, and presence or absence of invasive malignancy.

There are three subtypes of IPMN which are defined by the pattern of ductal involvement that is present. IPMNs are further characterized by the extent to which they involve the pancreatic ducts. Neoplasia that affects only the small side branches is termed side branch or branch duct IPMN (BD-IPMN), whereas involvement of the main pancreatic duct is termed main duct IPMN (MD-IPMN). Side branch IPMNs that extend into the main duct, often leading to upstream dilation, are termed mixed-type IPMNs.

Management Strategies for Intraductal Papillary Mucinous Neoplasm

Risk of malignant transformation has been described in IPMN and is related to multiple factors that have been stratified as worrisome and high risk. These factors have been identified through international consensus and are reported in the international consensus guidelines for the management of IPMN of the pancreas, most recently updated in 2017.[25]

Worrisome features of IPMN based on imaging include BD-IPMN cyst size larger than 3 cm, enhancing mural nodule smaller than mm, thickened enhancing cyst wall, main pancreatic duct size of 5 to 9 mm, abrupt change in caliber of main pancreatic duct with distal pancreatic atrophy, and lymphadenopathy. In addition, patients who present with clinical signs of pancreatitis, an elevated CA19-9 level or cyst growth of more than 5 mm over two years should be considered to have worrisome features. These features are summarized in Table 56.5.

TABLE 56.4 Defining characteristics of pseudocysts and pancreatic cystic neoplasms.

CHARACTERISTICS	PSEUDOCYST	SCN	MCN	IPMN
Epidemiology				
Gender	F = M	F ≫ M (4:1)	F ⋙ M (10:1)	F = M
Age (years)	40–60	60–70	50–60	60–70
Imaging Findings				
Location	Evenly distributed	Evenly distributed	Head ≪ body/tail	Head > diffuse > body/tail
Appearance	Round, thick-walled large cyst; gland atrophy ± calcification	Multiple small cysts separated by internal septations with central starburst calcifications	Thick-walled, septated macrocyst with smooth contour; ± solid component, eggshell calcifications	Poorly demarcated, lobulated, polycystic mass with dilation of main or branch ducts
Communication with ducts	Yes	No	Very rare	Yes
Cyst Fluid Analysis				
Cytology	Inflammatory cells	Scant glycogen-rich cells, with positive periodic acid–Schiff stain	Sheets and clusters of columnar, mucin-containing cells	Tall, columnar, mucin-containing cells
Mucin stain	Negative	Negative	Positive	Positive
Amylase	Very high	Low	Low	High
CEA	Low	Low	High	High

CEA, Carcinoembryonic antigen; *F*, female; *M*, male; *IPMN*, intraductal papillary mucinous neoplasm; *MCN*, mucinous cystic neoplasm; *SCN*, serous cystic neoplasm.
From Tran Cao HS, Kellogg B, Lowy AM, et al. Cystic neoplasms of the pancreas. *Surg Oncol Clin N Am*. 2010;19:267–295.

High-risk features of IPMN include the presence of an enhancing nodule larger than 5 mm within the cyst and main pancreatic duct dilation of more than 1 cm. Patients who present with clinical signs of jaundice should also be considered at high risk.

Numerous genetic mutations which may lead to malignant transformation of IPMN have been evaluated, including *KRAS*, *p53*, *MUC* and others. To date, genetic analysis of cyst fluid has failed to improve our ability to predict malignancy or select patients for surgical resection over existing clinical guidelines.

Branch duct intraductal papillary mucinous neoplasm. As the name implies, BD-IPMN involves dilation of the pancreatic duct side branches that communicate with but do not involve the main pancreatic duct. BD-IPMNs may be focal, involving a single side branch, or multifocal, with multiple cystic lesions throughout the length of the pancreas. Multiplicity of cysts favors a diagnosis of BD-IPMN.

All cysts with worrisome features on CT or MRI should undergo EUS; all cysts with high-risk features should be resected. Recommendations for management of suspected BD-IPMN are summarized in Fig. 56.19. [25] For asymptomatic patients with BD-IPMN who have no worrisome or high-risk features, surveillance may be a reasonable initial strategy; however, multiple variables including patient age and comorbidities also play a role in decision making.[25] Based on size alone, asymptomatic patients with cysts larger than 3 cm (worrisome feature) should be strongly considered for surgical resection, while those with 2- to 3-cm cysts may be considered for resection or observation depending on age and physical condition. Cysts smaller than 2 cm generally have a low risk for malignancy and therefor are most appropriate for surveillance.

Any patient with symptoms or high-risk features related to BD-IPMNs (e.g., jaundice, enhancing mural nodule, and dilated main pancreatic duct) should undergo surgical resection because the risk of malignant disease in symptomatic patients is heightened. Overall, the risk of invasive malignant disease in the setting of BD-IPMN is approximately 10% to 15%; however, it is increasingly clear that not all patients with IPMNs require surgery. Overall, for BD-IPMN, the risk of invasive malignant disease is approximately 2% to 3% per year. A plan for watchful surveillance with delayed intervention in these patients is reasonable because the risk for malignant transformation with small, asymptomatic branch duct tumors is low, most patients are older, and the time required for development of invasive malignant disease may be longer than the patient's life expectancy.

TABLE 56.5 A summary of worrisome and high-risk features of intraductal papillary mucinous neoplasm.

WORRISOME FEATURES	HIGH-RISK FEATURES
Main duct 5–9 mm	Main duct >1 cm
Enhancing mural nodule <5 mm	Enhancing mural nodule >5 mm
Thickened, enhancing cyst wall	Jaundice
BD-IPMN >3 cm	
Abrupt caliber change in main duct with upstream atrophy	
Lymphadenopathy	
Pancreatitis	
Increased serum 19–9	
Cyst growth >5 mm over 2 years	

BD-IPMN; Branch-duct intraductal papillary mucinous neoplasm.

Main duct intraductal papillary mucinous neoplasm. In contrast to BD-IPMN, MD-IPMN indicates abnormal cystic dilation of the main pancreatic duct with columnar metaplasia and thick mucinous secretions, which can be seen oozing from a patulous papilla on endoscopic evaluation (Fig. 56.20). Involvement of the main pancreatic duct may be focal or diffuse; it is most relevant because of the significantly increased risk of malignant degeneration. Individuals with MD-IPMN have a 30% to 50% risk of harboring invasive pancreatic cancer at the time of presentation.

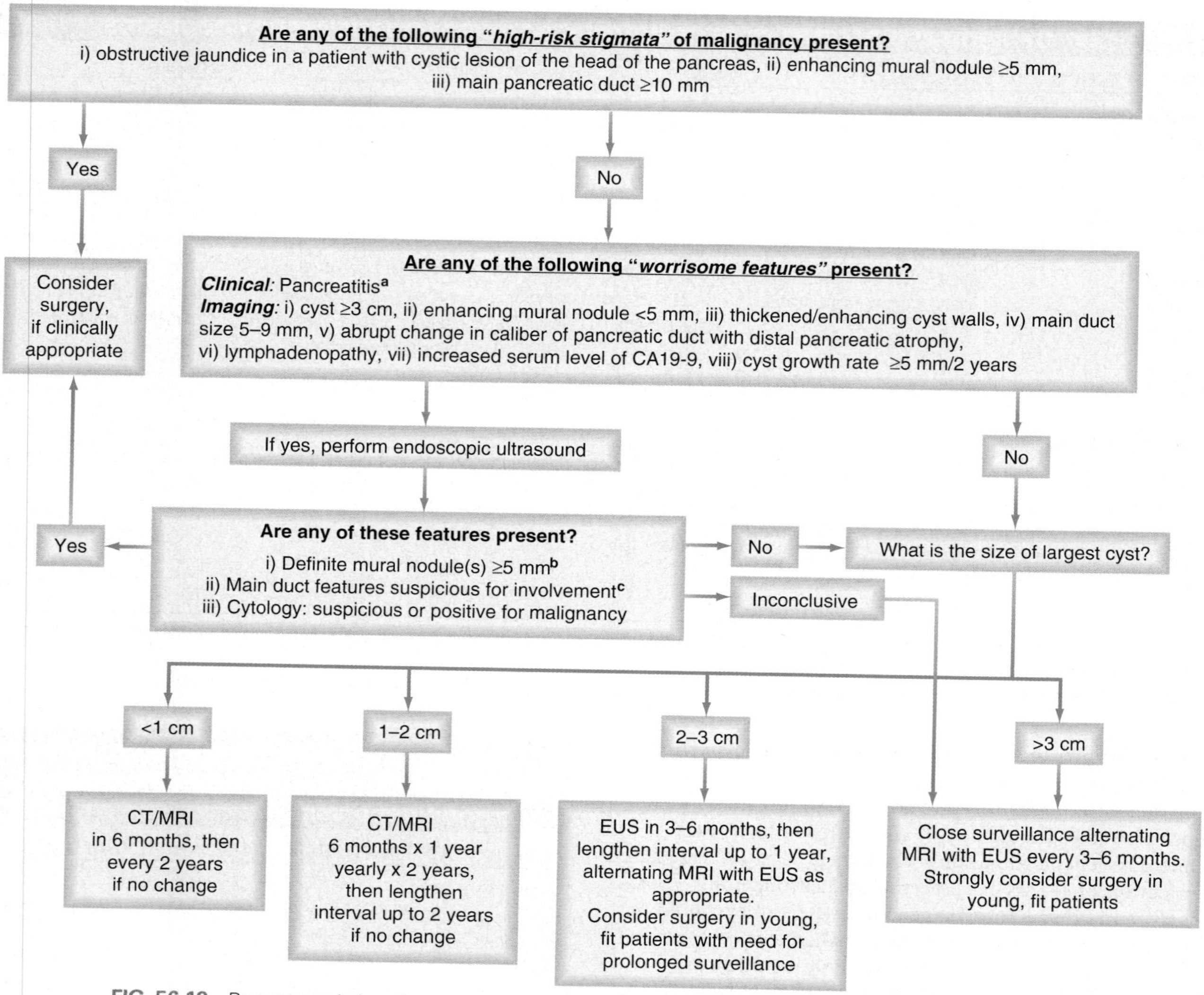

Are any of the following *"high-risk stigmata"* of malignancy present?
i) obstructive jaundice in a patient with cystic lesion of the head of the pancreas, ii) enhancing mural nodule ≥5 mm, iii) main pancreatic duct ≥10 mm

Yes → Consider surgery, if clinically appropriate

No ↓

Are any of the following *"worrisome features"* present?
Clinical: Pancreatitis[a]
Imaging: i) cyst ≥3 cm, ii) enhancing mural nodule <5 mm, iii) thickened/enhancing cyst walls, iv) main duct size 5–9 mm, v) abrupt change in caliber of pancreatic duct with distal pancreatic atrophy, vi) lymphadenopathy, vii) increased serum level of CA19-9, viii) cyst growth rate ≥5 mm/2 years

If yes, perform endoscopic ultrasound

Are any of these features present?
i) Definite mural nodule(s) ≥5 mm[b]
ii) Main duct features suspicious for involvement[c]
iii) Cytology: suspicious or positive for malignancy

Yes → Consider surgery, if clinically appropriate

No → What is the size of largest cyst?

Inconclusive → Close surveillance alternating MRI with EUS every 3–6 months. Strongly consider surgery in young, fit patients

No (worrisome features) → What is the size of largest cyst?

<1 cm → CT/MRI in 6 months, then every 2 years if no change

1–2 cm → CT/MRI 6 months x 1 year yearly x 2 years, then lengthen interval up to 2 years if no change

2–3 cm → EUS in 3–6 months, then lengthen interval up to 1 year, alternating MRI with EUS as appropriate. Consider surgery in young, fit patients with need for prolonged surveillance

>3 cm → Close surveillance alternating MRI with EUS every 3–6 months. Strongly consider surgery in young, fit patients

FIG. 56.19 Recommendations for management of suspected branch-duct intraductal papillary mucinous neoplasm (BD-IPMN). (From Tanaka M, Fernandez-del Castillo C, Adsay V, et al. International consensus guidelines 2012 for the management of IPMN and MCN of the pancreas. *Pancreatology.* 2012;12:183–197)

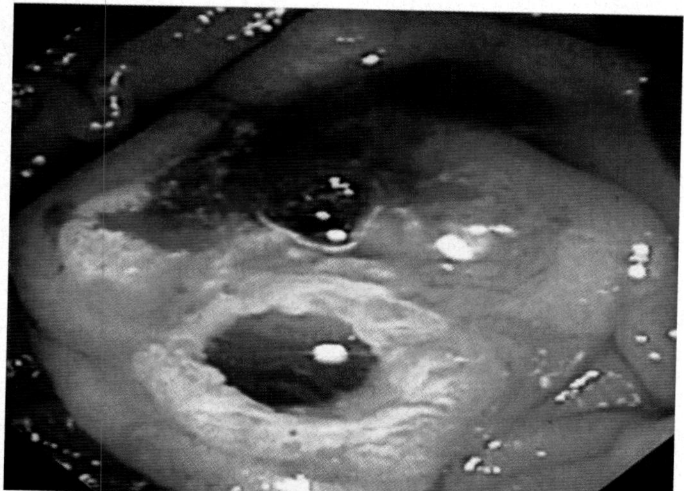

FIG. 56.20 Classic endoscopic view of intraductal papillary mucinous neoplasm (IPMN) showing viscous fluid oozing from a patulous ampulla of Vater.

Thus, surgical resection is the cornerstone of treatment. Fig. 56.21 demonstrates MD-IPMN with dilation of the entire pancreatic duct.

Unlike patients with pancreatic ductal adenocarcinomas (PDACs), 50% of patients with IPMNs of the pancreas present with abdominal pain and up to 25% present with AP, which, not surprisingly, has led to the diagnosis of chronic pancreatitis in many series. Several investigators have studied clinical and pathologic markers as predictors of malignancy and found that jaundice, elevated serum alkaline phosphatase level, mural nodules, diabetes, and main pancreatic duct diameter of 7 mm or larger are strongly associated with invasive IPMNs. Current guidelines suggest that main duct dilation of more than 5 mm is consistent with a diagnosis of MD-IPMN and a worrisome feature, while more than 1 cm is considered high risk. Given the overall high risk of malignant transformation, all patients with evidence of MD-IPMN should be considered for surgical resection if they are surgically fit.

The radiographic features of IPMNs on pancreatic CT scans may include a dilated main pancreatic duct, cysts of varying sizes,

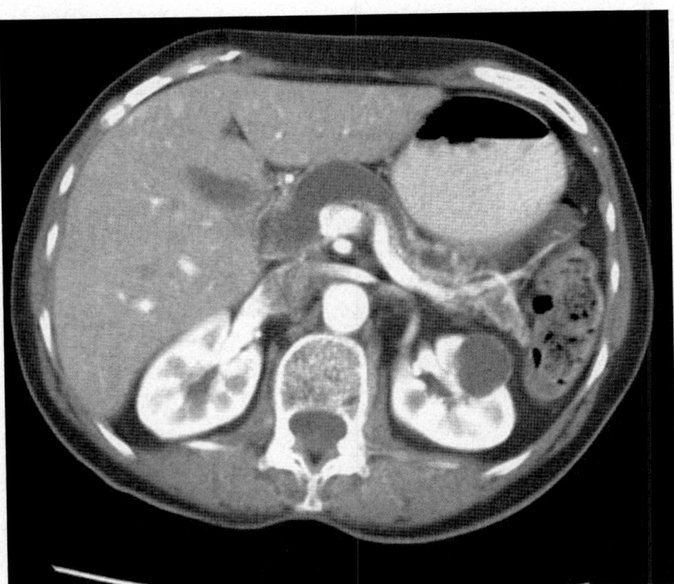

FIG. 56.21 Cross-sectional imaging of main-duct intraductal papillary mucinous neoplasm (MD-IPMN) throughout the entire pancreatic gland and a prominent ampulla of Vater.

and possibly mural nodules (Fig. 56.21). MRCP and EUS are important secondary diagnostic studies for the evaluation of patients with suspected IPMN. MRCP may allow localization of mural nodules and pretreatment classification of suspected side branch or main duct types of IPMN. EUS can evaluate the pancreatic duct and assess the fluid and solid components of the neoplasm. Aspirated fluid is typically viscous and clear and contains mucin. Cytology studies demonstrate mucin-rich fluid with variable cellularity; columnar mucinous cells with variable atypia may also be seen. As in MCNs and BD-IPMNs, fluid aspirates characteristically reveal an elevated CEA level (>192 ng/mL; log scale). This elevation of the CEA level is not predictive of invasive malignant disease, only the presence of mucinous metaplasia.

Mixed-type intraductal papillary mucinous neoplasm. Mixed-type IPMN denotes a side branch IPMN that has extended to involve the main pancreatic duct to a varying degree. Concern for mixed-type IPMNs should be raised in individuals with side branch cysts who exhibit upstream dilation of the pancreatic duct because this is an indication of main duct involvement. The biologic behavior of mixed-type IPMNs most closely resembles that of MD-IPMNs, with a significant risk of invasive malignant disease at the time of presentation (30% to 50%). As for MD-IPMN, surgical resection is indicated for the treatment of mixed-type IPMN.

Treatment: Surgical Resection for Intraductal Papillary Mucinous Neoplasm

Partial pancreatectomy is the primary treatment for high-risk lesions; however, the optimal extent of pancreatic resection for some patients remains unknown. For BD-IPMN, resection should target the lesion of concern, and therefore surgical decision making is usually straightforward. For MD-IPMN, however, it is not always possible to determine the extent of microscopic abnormality within the duct. In the absence of diffuse polyps or enhancing nodules in the main duct, a right-sided pancreatectomy is preferred. Intraoperative frozen section of the pancreas neck margin is obtained, and total pancreatectomy is reserved for those cases with high-grade dysplasia or invasive carcinoma identified at the margin. Although some investigators continue to advocate total pancreatectomy for the treatment of any IPMN, the evidence supporting this approach is decreasing with longer follow-up of patients treated by R0 and R1 partial pancreatectomy. It is appropriate to recommend partial pancreatectomy and to discuss management of the pancreatic margin preoperatively, advising the patient that approximately 15% of patients will require conversion to total pancreatectomy to achieve negative parenchymal resection margins.

Survival outcomes are significantly better in patients with IPMNs than in patients with PDACs. Sohn and associates[26] have analyzed a series of 136 patients with IPMNs; survival rates for patients with noninvasive IPMNs are 97% at 1 year, 94% at 2 years, and 77% at 5 years. When the group of patients with noninvasive IPMNs was analyzed further, no survival differences were found between patients with IPMNs and those with borderline IPMNs. On the contrary, there was a significant difference in survival rate between patients with noninvasive IPMNs and those with invasive IPMNs. The 1-, 3-, and 5-year survival rates for patients with invasive IPMNs were 72%, 58%, and 43%, respectively. Therefore, survival is clearly dependent on the invasive component of the lesion.

Following resection, surveillance of the remnant pancreas is advocated due to risk of recurrence of IPMN or invasive malignancy, which has been reported to range between 5% and 22%. The decision to terminate surveillance should depend on the age and condition of the patient. Reoperation should be considered for patients who present with recurrence or progression of disease in the pancreas remnant.

ADENOCARCINOMA OF THE EXOCRINE PANCREAS

Epidemiology

In 2018, it is estimated that PDAC will affect approximately 55,440 individuals in the United States and 44, 330 will die of the disease. In comparison, two decades ago in 1995, there were 24,000 new cases of pancreatic cancer. While the increasing and aging population is the most likely cause of this increase, whether factors other than population size and age have contributed to this increase is not known. Although it is the ninth most common cancer diagnosis, pancreatic cancer has recently out ranked breast cancer and has become the third most common cause of cancer deaths in United States. Despite significant advances in the treatment of other cancers, the prognosis of pancreatic cancer remains dismal. Overall, less than 8% of individuals will survive 5 years beyond their diagnosis. One of the reasons for these dismal outcomes is that most patients with pancreatic cancer have locally advanced or distant metastatic disease at presentation. Efforts at early detection of pancreatic cancer may change these outcomes by detecting pancreatic cancer at an early and curable stage. In a recent study, the authors performed a quantitative analysis of the timing of evolution of metastatic clones in pancreatic cancer. This elegant study suggested that on average, 5 years are required for the acquisition of metastatic ability in pancreatic cancer, thus suggesting that a window of opportunity does exist when the cancer is a locoregional disease and potentially curable.[27] Men are affected slightly more commonly than women, with a 1.3 : 1 incidence ratio. African Americans have a slightly higher risk for development of pancreatic cancer and dying of their disease compared with whites. The risk of pancreatic cancer increases with age beyond the sixth decade; the mean age at diagnosis is 72 years.

TABLE 56.6 Hereditary risk factors associated with development of pancreatic cancer.

GENE	ASSOCIATED SYNDROME	CLINICAL SIGNIFICANCE
PRSS1	Familial pancreatitis	Mutation results in chronic pancreatitis and 40% lifetime risk of PDAC
STK11	Peutz-Jeghers syndrome	Mutation results in >100-fold increase in risk of PDAC
CDKN2A	Familial atypical mole and multiple melanoma syndrome	Mutation leads to increased risk of melanoma and >40-fold increase in risk of PDAC
CFTR	Cystic fibrosis	Thick secretions result in chronic pancreatitis and 30-fold increase in risk of PDAC
BRCA2	Hereditary breast and ovarian cancer	Mutation results in elevated risk of breast and ovarian cancer and 10-fold increase in risk of PDAC
MLH1	Lynch syndrome	Mismatch repair gene mutation leads to increased risk of colon cancer and eightfold increase in risk of PDAC
APC	Familial adenomatous polyposis	Mutation results in polyposis coli and colon cancer with fourfold increase in risk of PDAC

PDAC; Pancreatic ductal adenocarcinoma.

Risk Factors

Environmental Risk Factors and Causes

Although the cause of pancreatic cancer remains unclear, several environmental risks have been associated with its increased incidence. The most notable risk factor is related to smoking. Several epidemiologic studies have shown an association of the amount and duration of smoking history with an elevated risk of pancreatic cancer. On average, smokers face a onefold to threefold increase in risk for development of pancreatic cancer compared with nonsmokers. This risk seems to be a linear association, with pancreatic cancer incidence directly related to the number of pack-years smoked (packs per day × number of years smoking). As with other cancers, the risk of pancreatic cancer persists many years beyond smoking cessation. Over the years, there have been several other factors, including chronic pancreatitis and occupational exposure, that were thought to contribute to an elevated risk of pancreatic cancer; however, population data have been somewhat controversial. It is likely that these factors are associated with an elevated risk, but the magnitude of the risk is uncertain. Obesity has recently become the focus of investigation; several authors have found that obese patients may be up to three times more likely to develop pancreatic cancer than nonobese individuals. It remains unclear whether obesity itself or one of the comorbidities related to obesity is associated with the higher incidence of pancreatic cancer seen in this population.

The relationship between diabetes and pancreatic cancer is a complicated one. Studies suggest that patients with new-onset diabetes have higher incidence of pancreatic cancer.[28] The association with pancreatic cancer is especially strong if the new diagnosis of diabetes is made in those who are elderly, have a lower body mass index, or have weight loss and in those who do not have family history of diabetes. In these patients with new-onset diabetes, diabetes may be caused by pancreatic cancer. The diagnosis of diabetes may precede the diagnosis of pancreatic cancer by up to 36 months, suggesting that there may be a window of opportunity for early diagnosis. Thus, patients with new onset diabetes constitute a high-risk group at which the pancreatic cancer early diagnosis effort may be focused. The mechanism of pancreatic cancer–induced diabetes is unclear at this time. Other studies have suggested that long-term diabetes may increase the risk of pancreatic cancer. However, these observations may be confounded by the fact that factors like obesity are associated with both diabetes and pancreatic cancer. It is clear, though, that in elderly patients with new-onset diabetes in the presence of unusual symptoms like weight loss and abdominal symptoms, diagnosis of pancreatic cancer should be considered and may lead to early diagnosis of pancreatic cancer.

Hereditary Risk Factors

An inherited predisposition to pancreatic cancer is seen in a range of clinical settings. Several hereditary cancer syndromes (e.g., Peutz-Jeghers syndrome, familial atypical mole and multiple melanoma syndrome, hereditary breast and ovarian cancer syndrome) are known to be associated with increased risk of pancreatic cancer. Increased risk of pancreatic cancer is present in patients with inheritable inflammatory disease of the pancreas, namely, hereditary pancreatitis and cystic fibrosis. These patients with known genetic syndromes are responsible for about 20% of hereditary cases of pancreatic cancer. The term *familial pancreatic cancer* (FPC) applies to the remaining 80% of patients with an inherited predisposition but who do not have an identifiable genetic syndrome. Table 56.6 summarizes several known gene mutations and their clinical significance.

Hereditary pancreatitis (PRSS1 and SPINK1 gene mutation). It has long been noted that individuals with familial pancreatitis have an elevated risk of pancreatic cancer. Mutations in the cationic trypsinogen gene *(PRSS1)* are responsible for 80% of the cases of hereditary pancreatitis and lead to increased trypsin activity and chronic inflammation in the pancreas. The *SPINK1* gene codes for a serine protease inhibitor that inhibits active protein, and mutations in this gene have been associated with hereditary pancreatitis. Individuals with hereditary pancreatitis have a greater than 50-fold increase in their risk for development of pancreatic cancer compared with unaffected individuals.[29]

Peutz-Jeghers syndrome (STK11 gene mutation). Individuals with Peutz-Jeghers syndrome are distinguished by the development of gastrointestinal hamartomatous polyps and pigmented mucocutaneous lesions. The specific role of *STK11* is not defined, although it is thought to act as a tumor suppressor gene, with loss of heterozygosity leading to the development of gastrointestinal tumors. In addition to gastrointestinal cancers, individuals with Peutz-Jeghers syndrome are at a higher risk of lung, ovarian, breast, uterine, and testicular cancers. The risk of pancreatic cancer in the setting of Peutz-Jeghers syndrome is more than 100 times greater than that in unaffected individuals.[29]

Cystic fibrosis (CFTR gene mutation). Although the cause remains unclear, those with cystic fibrosis (*CFTR* gene mutation) are up to 30 times more likely to develop pancreatic cancer than the general population. It is postulated that this elevated risk is caused by the chronic inflammatory condition of the pancreas resulting from a lifetime of thickened secretions and partial ductal obstruction.[29]

Familial atypical mole and multiple melanoma syndrome (CDKN2A gene mutation). *CDKN2A* encodes protein p16, which normally inhibits cell proliferation by binding to cyclin-dependent kinases (CDKs). Mutations of *CDKN2A* lead to uninhibited cell cycle activation and proliferation. Although *CDKN2A* is most noted for its associated increased risk of melanoma, individuals with *CDKN2A* mutations have up to a 20-fold increase in risk for the development of pancreas cancer.[29]

Hereditary breast and ovarian cancer (BRCA2 gene mutation). Although germline *BRCA* mutations are most recognized because of their association with breast cancer, 10% of individuals from high-risk pancreatic cancer families (at least two first-degree relatives with pancreas cancer) have been found to have *BRCA2* mutations. Germline mutations of the *BRCA2* gene lead to an elevated risk for pancreatic cancer, which is up to 10 times that of the general population.[29]

Lynch syndrome (mismatch repair gene mutations). Although most strongly associated with colon cancers caused by mutations in mismatch repair genes *(MLH1, MSH2, MSH6),* Lynch syndrome also leads to an increased risk of pancreatic cancer. The microsatellite instability noted in colon cancer cells has also been seen in pancreatic cancer cells from individuals with Lynch syndrome, indicative of a common genetic cause. It is estimated that the risk of pancreatic cancer is increased eightfold in individuals with Lynch syndrome.[29]

Familial adenomatous polyposis (APC gene mutation). Familial adenomatous polyposis results from mutation of the adenomatous polyposis coli *(APC)* gene, leading to the development of thousands of colonic polyps. It has been found that individuals affected by familial adenomatous polyposis are also significantly more likely to develop pancreas cancer, with a fourfold increase above that in the general population. These data remain observational because the cause of pancreatic cancer in this setting has not been defined.[29]

Familial pancreatic cancer (unknown gene). FPC is defined by families with two or more first-degree relatives with pancreatic adenocarcinoma that do not fulfill the criteria of other inherited tumor syndromes with an increased risk for the development of pancreatic adenocarcinoma. Compared with relatives of patients with sporadic pancreatic cancer, the risk for development of pancreatic cancer is markedly elevated in FPC kindreds. Family members of FPC kindreds are at an 18-fold increased risk for development of pancreatic cancer compared with the general population. Furthermore, this risk increases with increasing numbers of first-degree relatives with pancreatic cancer in FPC kindreds and if one of the affected individuals is diagnosed before 50 years of age. Segregation analysis suggests that the aggregation of pancreatic cancer in these families is due to unidentified, autosomal dominantly inherited genes with reduced penetrance. This entity is being increasingly appreciated, and guidelines for pancreatic cancer screening and management of identified suspicious lesions in this population are under evolution.

Pathogenesis of Sporadic Pancreatic Cancer

Although there are several inherited forms of PDAC, most cases are sporadic. As for many other cancers, a sequential pathway has been observed in the development of PDAC from pancreatic intraepithelial neoplasia (PanIN) to invasive cancer. A number of tumor suppressor genes and oncogenes have been identified that play a significant role in the pathogenesis of PDAC, including *PDX1, KRAS2, CDKN2A/p16, P53,* and *SMAD4.* Novel techniques like sleeping beauty transposon-mediated insertional mutagenesis has helped identify tumor suppressor genes like deubiquitinase USP9X which is mutated in as many as 50% of the tumors. It must be noted that up to 5% of patients who, due to lack of any family history, are believed to have sporadic pancreatic cancer, harbor germline mutation in pancreatic cancer susceptibility genes. This has led to *National Comprehensive Cancer Network* (NCCN) recommendation to consider offering germline gene testing in all patients with a personal history of pancreatic cancer, regardless of family history or age at diagnosis

Genetic Progression of Pancreatic Intraepithelial Neoplasia to Invasive Pancreatic Ductal Adenocarcinoma

PanIN is defined histologically by progressive abnormality of the ductal epithelium from columnar metaplasia (PanIN-1A) through carcinoma in situ (PanIN-3). PanIN-1A is histologically characterized by the presence of columnar, mucin-producing ductal epithelium that maintains basally located homogeneous nuclei without atypia. The development of papillary architecture defines PanIN-1B, but it is otherwise identical to PanIN-1A. PanIN-2 denotes the progression from simple papillary growth to evidence of nuclear atypia not seen in PanIN-1B. Enlarged nuclei with nuclear crowding and loss of polarity are present. Prominent nuclear abnormalities with complete loss of polarity and marked cytologic atypia are characteristic of PanIN-3 (carcinoma in situ). Clusters of abnormal cells can usually be seen within the duct lumen.

The *KRAS2* oncogene is activated in more than 95% of pancreatic cancers and is thought to be the initiating event in tumorigenesis. *KRAS2* is activated by point mutation (codon 12, 13, or 61), which causes constitutive activation and loss of regulation of mitogen-activated protein kinase cell signal transduction. Mutation of the *KRAS2* oncogene is one of the earliest genetic abnormalities identified in the progression of PanIN to PDAC and has been noted in 36% of PanIN-1 cases, 44% of PanIN-2 cases, and 87% of PanIN-3 cases.

CDKN2A/p16, P53, and *SMAD4* are tumor suppressor genes that also appear to play critical roles in the development of PDAC. *CDKN2A* encodes a protein, p16, that binds to CDK4 and CDK6, resulting in cell cycle arrest. Mutation of *CDKN2A* and loss of p16 lead to a loss of cell cycle regulation. Like mutation of *KRAS,* mutation of *CDKN2A* (loss of p16 expression) has been identified in 30% of PanIN-1 cases, 55% of PanIN-2 cases, and 71% of PanIN-3 cases. Approximately 90% of PDACs demonstrate loss of p16 function. Also, *P53* encodes the protein p53, which regulates cell proliferation through cell cycle arrest and proapoptotic mechanisms. Although it is rare in PanIN, 79% of invasive PDACs demonstrate *P53* mutations, indicating its potential importance in the transition from noninvasive to invasive tumors. Similarly, *SMAD4* mutations occur late in the pathway from PanIN to PDAC. Loss of *SMAD4,* which normally functions as a downstream mediator related to TGF-β, leads to decreased inhibition of cell growth and proliferation. Loss of *SMAD4* function has been observed in 20% to 30% of PanIN-3 and localized cancers, whereas 78% of widely metastatic tumors show loss of *SMAD4.* Fig. 56.22 demonstrates the molecular genetic alterations involved in the PanIN-PDAC pathway.

Clinical Presentation

The defining presenting symptom of patients with PDACs in the periampullary region is jaundice. Although painless jaundice has

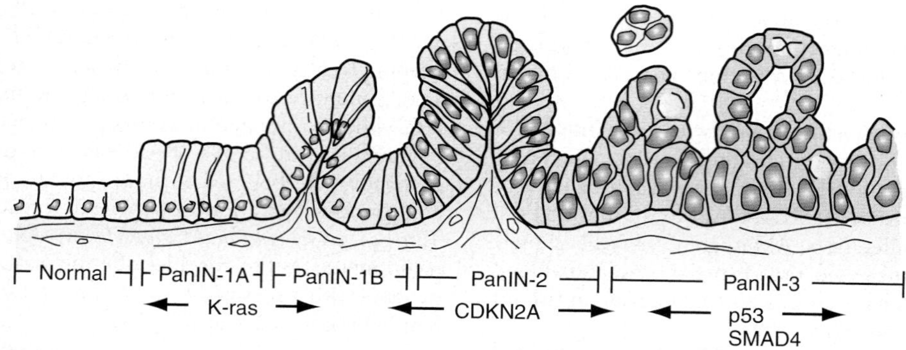

FIG. 56.22 Molecular genetic progression from pancreatic intraepithelial neuroplasia *(PanIN)* to invasive ductal adenocarcinoma. (Adapted from Wilentz RE, Iacobuzio-Donahoe CA, Argani P, et al. Loss of expression of SMAD4 in pancreatic intraepithelial neoplasia: Evidence that SMAD4 inactivation occurs late in neoplastic progression. *Cancer Res.* 2000;60:2002–2006.)

frequently been described, a significant number of patients present with pain in addition to jaundice, typically arising in the epigastrium and radiating to the back. Weight loss is also common at the time of presentation, affecting more than 50% of individuals. For tumors of the body and tail of the pancreas, pain and weight loss become more common at presentation. Table 56.7 lists the most common presenting symptoms and their frequency. As mentioned before, new-onset diabetes in an elderly patient with weight loss may be an early presenting symptom of pancreatic cancer. Except for jaundice, the physical examination findings are otherwise unremarkable for most patients with PDAC. A palpable distended gallbladder can be identified in approximately one third of patients with periampullary PDAC, an association first described by Courvoisier, a Swiss surgeon, in 1890. He noted that choledocholithiasis was commonly associated with a shrunken fibrotic gallbladder, whereas the slow progressive occlusion by other causes, including tumors, was more likely to result in ectasia of the organ. Although not diagnostic in itself, Courvoisier sign is familiar to medical students as a defining characteristic of PDACs. With widespread disease, a left supraclavicular node (Virchow node) may be palpable. Similarly, periumbilical lymphadenopathy may be palpable (Sister Mary Joseph node). In cases of peritoneal dissemination, perirectal tumor involvement may be palpable through digital rectal examination, referred to as Blumer shelf.

Diagnosis

Laboratory Evaluation

Laboratory evaluation of patients presenting with suspected PDAC should include hepatic function evaluation, including a coagulation profile and nutritional assessment. An elevated bilirubin level is expected, but careful attention should be paid to nutritional values, including prealbumin and albumin levels if surgical intervention is to be considered. Individuals with malnutrition should be given preoperative nutritional supplementation. Several tumor markers may be appropriate at the initial evaluation, including CEA, carbohydrate antigen 19-9 (CA 19-9), and α-fetoprotein. Of these, CA 19-9 is most sensitive for pancreatic adenocarcinoma, with a sensitivity of approximately 79% and a specificity of 82%. A notable limitation of CA 19-9 testing in the setting of periampullary tumors is the false elevation caused by biliary obstruction, which can be misleading. In addition, 10% to 15% of individuals do not have elevation of the CA 19-9 level, a finding that has been associated with blood Lewis antigen–negative status and is caused by a lack of the fucosyltransferase gene. Accepting these limitations, CA 19-9 continues to be the most

TABLE 56.7 Presenting symptoms for periampullary tumors of the pancreas.

PRESENTING SYMPTOM	FREQUENCY (%)
Jaundice	75
Weight loss	51
Abdominal pain	39
Nausea/vomiting	13
Pruritus	11
Fever	3
Gastrointestinal bleeding	1

reliable tumor marker for pretreatment evaluation and posttreatment surveillance for pancreatic adenocarcinoma. Besides being used in the diagnosis of pancreatic cancer, CA 19-9 is also used as a predictive and prognostic marker. For instance, some studies have suggested its use for identifying patients who will benefit from staging laparoscopy.[30] Similarly, normalization of CA 19-9 after neoadjuvant therapy has been suggested as an important prognostic factor.[31]

Imaging Studies

Multidetector CT is the imaging study of choice for the evaluation of lesions arising in the pancreas. CT allows an accurate determination of the level of biliary obstruction, the relationship of the tumor to critical vascular anatomy, and the presence of regional or metastatic disease. For suspected periampullary disease, a three-phase (noncontrast, arterial, and portal venous) CT scan with 3-mm slices and coronal and three-dimensional reconstruction should be routine. Because of its widespread availability and excellent sensitivity (85%), CT has become the imaging modality of choice for the evaluation of suspected pancreatic cancer. Pancreatic adenocarcinoma is typically seen as a hypoattenuating lesion during the portal venous phase of the imaging.

ERCP is frequently used in the assessment of the jaundiced patient because of its ability to perform a biopsy and to palliate jaundice, if necessary. Although palliative biliary stenting remains routine for PDAC tumors resulting in jaundice, its usefulness is questionable for patients who are candidates for surgical resection. Preoperative biliary decompression may increase the rate of wound infection caused by bactibilia, although overall morbidity and mortality are unchanged. In modern medical practice, ERCP should be reserved for cases requiring therapeutic or palliative intervention because other imaging modalities provide superior diagnostic abilities without the invasiveness of ERCP. The use of ERCP for biliary decompression is bound to increase, given the increased use of neoadjuvant chemotherapy approach. In such cases, use of short metal stent rather than plastic stents is recommended, given the propensity of plastic stents to get blocked thus requiring repeat procedures.

EUS is becoming widely used for the evaluation of suspected pancreatic disease. Perhaps its most important ability is to provide tissue diagnosis of suspected tumors through the use of FNA before initiation of systemic therapy. FNA has a sensitivity and specificity that are far superior to those of brush cytology, with a diagnostic accuracy of 92% to 95%. It may also play a crucial role in the molecular evaluation of tumor samples from patients undergoing neoadjuvant therapy. Although the use of EUS is increasing for the evaluation of peritumoral vasculature and regional lymph nodes, it has not been shown to provide any significant benefit over CT alone in the absence of a need for tissue diagnosis. EUS may be beneficial for the identification of small tumors that do not appear on CT scans and for the delineation of more clearly suspicious lesions smaller than 2 cm; it therefore plays an important complementary role.

For cases that require detailed assessment of luminal pancreatobiliary anatomy, MRCP should be considered. MRCP has become useful for the investigation of cystic lesions of the pancreas, with sensitivity and specificity slightly superior to CT alone. MRCP also provides several advantages over ERCP; it is noninvasive, has no risk of inciting pancreatitis, and provides three-dimensional reconstruction of the ductal system.

Biologic imaging. ^{18}F-fluorodeoxyglucose positron emission tomography (FDG PET) in combination with CT scanning has been increasingly used in the evaluation of pancreatic cancer. The ability of FDG PET to detect cancers is based on the principle that cells that are actively metabolizing will preferentially take up ^{18}F-labeled glucose compared with surrounding normal tissues. Several studies have noted the potential benefits of FDG PET with CT, including the ability to differentiate between benign and malignant pancreas tumors (autoimmune pancreatitis vs. adenocarcinoma) and also to identify unsuspected disease, which alters clinical planning in more than 10% of cases. False-positive findings are also possible, most notably because of inflammatory conditions, and the risk-benefit ratio of FDG PET with CT has not yet been determined. Further studies will be necessary to clarify the role of FDG PET with CT in the evaluation of pancreatic cancer before its routine use should be advocated.

Staging

Pancreatic cancer staging is based on the American Joint Committee on Cancer (AGCC) tumor, node, metastasis (TNM) system.[31a] After biopsy confirmation, typically by EUS-FNA, accurate staging is accomplished by multidetector CT scanning of the abdomen and pelvis with three-phase administration of contrast material and three-dimensional reconstruction. Chest radiography is sufficient for the evaluation of potential pulmonary metastasis and should be followed by CT of the chest if any suspicious lesions are noted. In the 8th edition of AJCC staging, the T category is revised from descriptive to size-based definitions, as tumor size is the best surrogate of pancreatic cancer biology.

After CT imaging, tumors are classified into resectable, borderline resectable, or unresectable. Resectable tumors are defined as localized to the pancreas, with no evidence of SMV or portal vein involvement (i.e., no abutment, distortion, thrombus, or encasement) and a preserved fat plane surrounding the SMA and celiac artery branches, including the hepatic artery. Traditionally patients with imaging consistent with resectable disease used to proceed with operative resection. Currently, given the success of neoadjuvant strategy in the treatment of borderline resectable pancreatic cancer, there is increased use of preoperative chemotherapy for the treatment of even resectable disease. However, use of neoadjuvant therapy for the treatment of resectable pancreatic cancer is highly variable amongst various institutes.

The appropriate definition of borderline resectable tumors continues to evolve. The NCCN defines borderline resectable as tumors that exhibit one or more of the following characteristics:

1. Venous involvement: solid tumor contact with SMV or portal vein of more than 180 degrees or contact of less than or equal to 180 degrees with contour irregularity of the vein or thrombosis of the vein but with suitable vessel proximal and distal to the site of involvement allowing for safe and complete resection and vein reconstruction.
2. Arterial involvement:
   a. Hepatic artery involvement: solid tumor contact with common hepatic artery (abutment or encasement) without extension to the celiac axis or hepatic artery bifurcation allowing for safe and complete resection and reconstruction.
   b. SMA involvement: solid tumor contact with the SMA of less than or equal to 180 degrees.

Currently, these patients are started for surgical resection only after neoadjuvant therapy. There is limited evidence with respect to the type and duration of neoadjuvant therapy and this varies widely at various institutions (see below).

Unresectable tumors are those that exhibit metastasis (including lymph node metastasis outside the field of resection), ascites, or vascular involvement beyond what has been detailed here.

Laparoscopy

Staging laparoscopy has been advocated by several authors as a means to reduce the frequency of nontherapeutic laparotomy for patients with unsuspected metastatic or locally advanced unresectable disease identified at the time of surgery. For patients who appear to have resectable disease on imaging studies alone, laparoscopy identifies additional unresectable disease in up to 30% of cases. Others have argued that with current imaging used properly, the benefit of additional laparoscopy only rarely alters surgical planning. Recently, there has been some consensus on a more selective use of laparoscopy for those at particularly high risk for occult disease, including those with large tumors (>3 cm), significantly elevated CA 19-9 level (>100 U/mL), uncertain findings on CT, or body or tail tumors. It may be clinically prudent also to consider laparoscopy for patients with clinical indicators of widespread disease, including significant weight loss, malnutrition, and pain. There are no level I data available to define the role of staging laparoscopy, and therefore its use remains at the discretion of the surgeon. Furthermore, the role and place of peritoneal cytology are unclear at this time. However, patients with positive findings on peritoneal cytology have very poor prognosis and behave like patients with metastatic disease.

Treatment

Surgical resection remains the only potentially curative treatment of pancreas cancer.

Surgery for Tumors of the Head of the Pancreas

For tumors involving the head of the pancreas, pancreaticoduodenectomy is the procedure of choice. Although first described in 1909 by Kausch, the technique became widely known after the first successful surgical resection was performed by Whipple and Parsons and presented to the American Surgical Association by Parsons in 1935. The first two attempts, in 1934, resulted in operative mortality; but in 1935, a two-stage procedure, which included biliary decompression followed by pancreaticoduodenectomy, was successful. The initial operative description included ligation of the pancreas remnant without reanastomosis.

The first one-stage Whipple procedure was reported by Trimble and colleagues at Johns Hopkins University in 1941.[32] The modern Whipple procedure maintained a perioperative mortality of 25% and morbidity of well above 50% up until the late 1970s. The advent of improved outcomes for this complex procedure can be attributed to many surgeons and institutions. Most notable on this list of early and seminal leaders in regard to improved mortality and outcome are Cameron (Johns Hopkins Hospital, Baltimore), Tredi (Mannheim Clinic, Mannheim, Germany), Warshaw (Massachusetts General Hospital, Boston), and Brennan (Memorial Sloan Kettering Cancer Center, New York). Each surgeon and center performed more than 100 procedures without any deaths in the 1980s and 1990s.

Surgical technique. The modern pancreaticoduodenectomy begins with exploration of the peritoneal surfaces for evidence of metastatic disease, which would deem the patient inoperable. A Kocher maneuver is performed to the level of the left lateral border of the aorta. The transverse mesocolon is separated off the head of the pancreas, exposing the infrapancreatic SMV. Fig. 56.23 shows complete mobilization of the head of the pancreas and gallbladder. The lesser sac is entered through the gastrocolic ligament, sparing the gastroepiploic vessels. The right gastroepiploic vein is ligated at its confluence with the SMV, allowing the SMV to be dissected from the inferior border and posterior neck of the pancreas. The middle colic vein may also be sacrificed, if necessary, to allow adequate dissection at this level.

Once the infrapancreatic SMV is dissected and the head of the pancreas is fully mobilized, the gallbladder is removed and the common hepatic duct is circumferentially dissected. Division of the common hepatic duct allows visualization of the suprapancreatic portal vein. In pylorus preserving pancreaticoduodenectomy, the duodenum is divided at least 2 cm distal to the pylorus. The hepatic artery is exposed proximally and distally and assessed for replacement or aberrant anatomy. The GDA and right gastric artery are visualized. Before division of the GDA, the vessel is temporarily occluded, and blood flow through the distal common hepatic artery is ensured using a Doppler device. This maneuver is vital in patients with atherosclerosis of celiac origin to ensure that the hepatic blood supply is not dependent on collateral retrograde arterial flow from the SMA through the GDA. Once hepatic arterial flow is confirmed, the right gastric artery and GDA are ligated and divided. If flow in the hepatic artery is interrupted by occlusion of the GDA, resection may proceed only with preservation of the GDA or arterial resection and bypass, typically as an aortohepatic conduit.

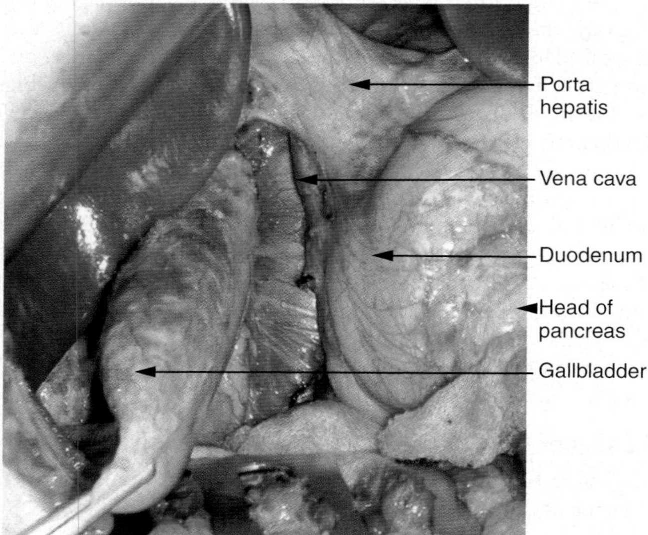

FIG. 56.23 Complete mobilization of the head of the pancreas is shown. The vena cava is visible posteriorly. The gallbladder has been freed from the gallbladder fossa.

The pancreas is then divided after four-point ligation of the inferior and superior pancreaticoduodenal arteries. The jejunum is divided approximately 10 cm distal to the ligament of Treitz, and the short mesenteric vessels are divided to allow retromesenteric rotation of the jejunum and third and fourth portions of the duodenum. The head of the pancreas and attached small bowel are then retracted to the patient's right, and the remaining portal vein and uncinate dissection is completed.

With the portal vein completely free, the gland is retracted farther to the right to allow complete visualization of the uncinate process and SMA. The retroperitoneal tissue is dissected from the SMA, allowing complete removal of the periarterial lymphatic tissue. Fig. 56.24A shows the anatomy after removal of the head of the pancreas, and Fig. 56.24B highlights complete clearance of periarterial tissue from the SMA. If portal venous or SMV tumor involvement is encountered, as shown in Fig. 56.25A and B, venous resection should be performed. Resections that compromise less than 50% of the venous diameter can be closed primarily (Fig. 56.25C); otherwise, segmental resection with primary anastomosis or interposition graft using internal jugular or femoral vein should be performed.

Reconstruction. Before reconstruction, some surgeons will obtain a frozen section evaluation of the pancreatic neck margin. Once negative margins are ensured, the proximal jejunum is brought through the transverse mesocolon or the retromesenteric defect in preparation for pancreaticojejunostomy and hepaticojejunostomy. The pancreaticojejunostomy is created in two layers, anterior and posterior, with a duct-to-mucosa anastomosis (Fig. 56.26). An internal or external[33,34] pancreatic stent can be left in place for ducts smaller than 5 mm. The hepaticojejunostomy anastomosis is then created downstream from the pancreaticojejunostomy in an end-to-side fashion. If the duct is smaller than 5 mm, it can be spatulated to improve patency. After this, a duodeno- or gastrojejunostomy is completed. External drains are selectively placed adjacent to the pancreaticojejunostomy and hepaticojejunostomy. A feeding jejunostomy can be considered in selected patients with significant preoperative malnutrition (albumin level <3.5 g/dL).

Surgery for Tumors of the Body and Tail of the Pancreas

Tumors arising in the body and tail of the pancreas are rarely resectable at the time of presentation, given the lack of symptoms with small tumors. Only 5% to 7% of individuals with body or tail PDACs will ultimately undergo surgery, and median survival is significantly shorter than with PDACs of the pancreatic head because of the more advanced nature of resected tumors.

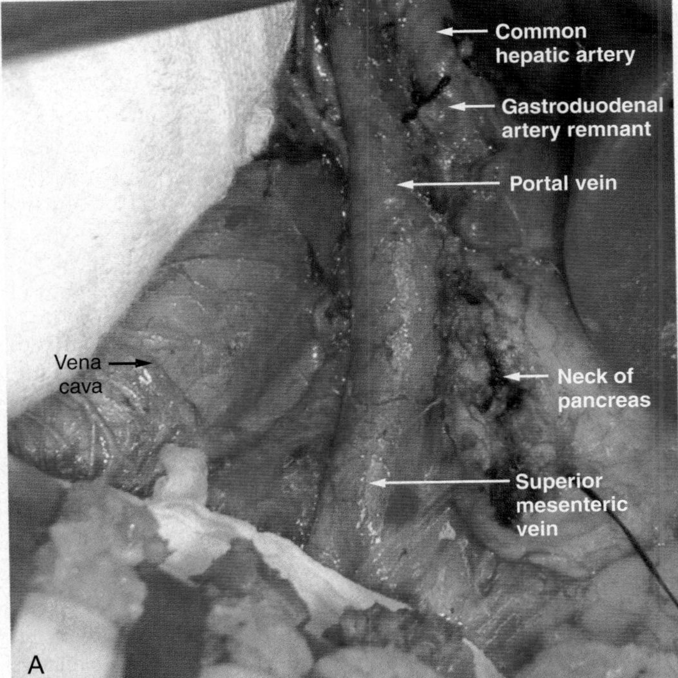

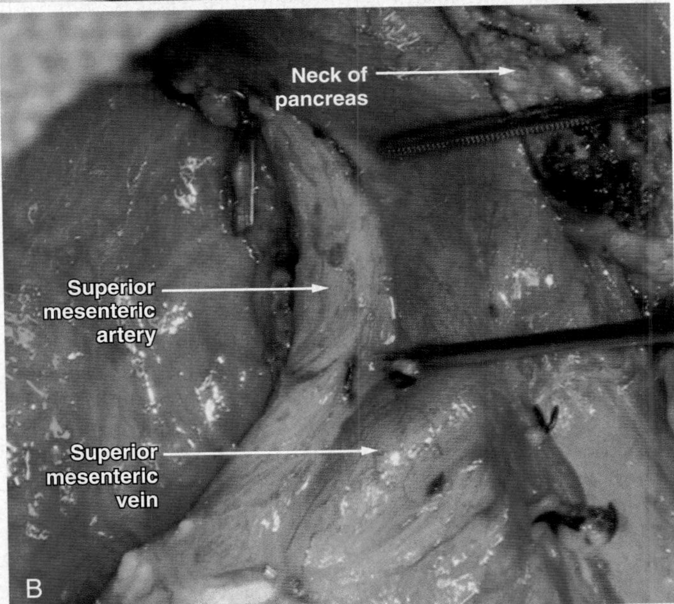

FIG. 56.24 (A) Surgical anatomy after pancreaticoduodenectomy. The SMV, portal vein, hepatic artery, and vena cava are visualized. Complete lymphatic clearance is noted. (B) SMA dissection illustrating complete clearance of periarterial lymphatic tissue.

Although tumor involvement of the splenic artery or vein does not preclude surgery, involvement of the celiac axis is a contraindication to resection. For resectable tumors, distal pancreatectomy and en bloc splenectomy should be performed. Distal pancreatectomy and splenectomy can be performed in a retrograde fashion whereby the spleen and pancreas are mobilized lateral to medial en bloc, thus providing access to splenic vasculature located superior and behind the pancreas. Alternatively, the dissection can proceed antegrade in a medial to lateral fashion. In this approach, the pancreatic neck is encircled and divided away from the tumor early in the procedure. This medial-to-lateral approach in combination with extensive lymph node dissection has been termed radical antegrade modular pancreatosplenectomy.[35] The medial-to -lateral or antegrade approach is described here, but depending on the situation, a combination of these two approaches can be used.

After inspection of the peritoneal surfaces, the gastrocolic and splenocolic ligaments and short gastric vessels are divided to expose the pancreas and spleen. The inferior border of the pancreas is dissected, exposing the retroperitoneal plane behind the gland. This anatomic plane can be used to mobilize the body and tail of the pancreas anterior to Gerota fascia completely. At the superior border of the pancreas, the splenic artery is circumferentially dissected and divided at its origin from the celiac trunk. The splenic vein is carefully dissected from the posterior wall of the pancreas at its confluence with the SMV and divided. At this point, the distal pancreas and spleen are devascularized and the neck of the pancreas is divided. A medial to lateral dissection is completed, and the spleen is detached from its posterior peritoneal attachments to allow en bloc removal of the specimen and surrounding lymph node basin. Several techniques may be used to close the pancreatic duct remnant, with the most common being direct suture ligation or use of a linear stapling device. Either technique is appropriate, with similar risk for the development of pancreatic fistula.

Laparoscopic Distal Pancreatectomy

There has been growing interest in the use of minimally invasive surgery for the resection of tumors of the distal pancreas. Laparoscopic distal pancreatectomy (LDP) may offer advantages over open resection for select patients, with smaller incisions and shorter hospital stay. In a review of more than 800 LDPs, Borja-Cacho and colleagues[36] described an overall morbidity rate of 38% and hospital length of stay of 5 days, which compare favorably with large series after open pancreatectomy. Although LDP is increasingly used for benign conditions, its usefulness for the treatment of PDAC remains to be fully validated. For benign conditions, a spleen preserving LDP can be considered. This can be done by either preserving the splenic vessels (see Video 56.2) or by sacrificing them proximally and relying on the short gastric vessels for perfusion (see Video 56.3).

The DIPLOMA trial recently reported outcomes for a matched cohort of over 1200 patients, comparing open to minimally invasive approaches (robotic or laparoscopic), and did not identify any inferiority of minimally invasive techniques.[37] To date, there have been no randomized trials to assess minimally invasive versus open surgical approaches.

Minimally invasive pancreaticoduodenectomy has similarly seen a rise in popularity despite a lack of evidence as to its proposed benefits. Several authors have reported favorable results in single institution series; however, broader population analysis has raised concern about the risk of increased morbidity and mortality seen with minimally invasive procedures. In an effort to evaluate the efficacy of minimally invasive pancreaticoduodenectomy, a multicenter, randomized controlled trial known as LEOPARD-2 was initiated, however, was recently closed early by the data safety monitoring board due to significantly increased mortality seen in the minimally invasive group. After enrolling 99 patients, the risk of mortality after minimally invasive surgery was 10% (five patients) versus 2% (one patient) for open surgery.[38] Debate continues as to the appropriateness of minimally invasive pancreaticoduodenectomy.

Outcomes

Perioperative Mortality: Long-Term Survival

Perioperative mortality has become a rare event after the Whipple procedure, occurring in less than 2% of cases at high-volume

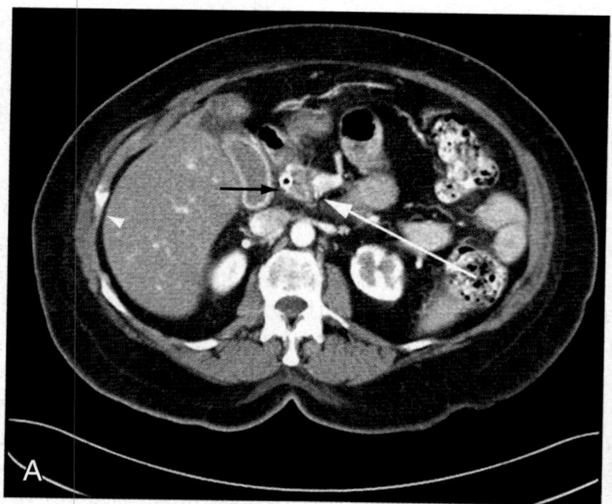

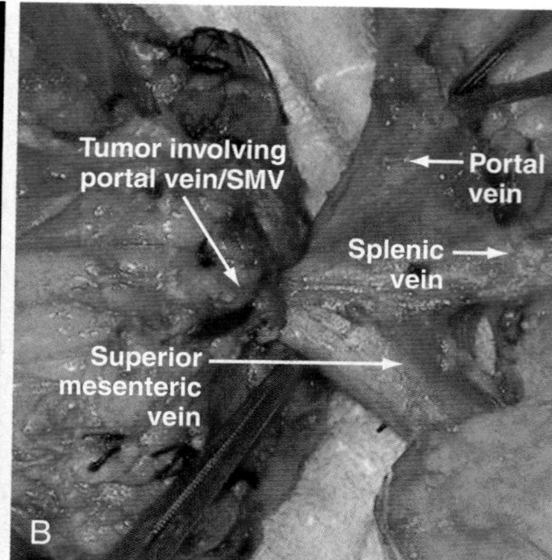

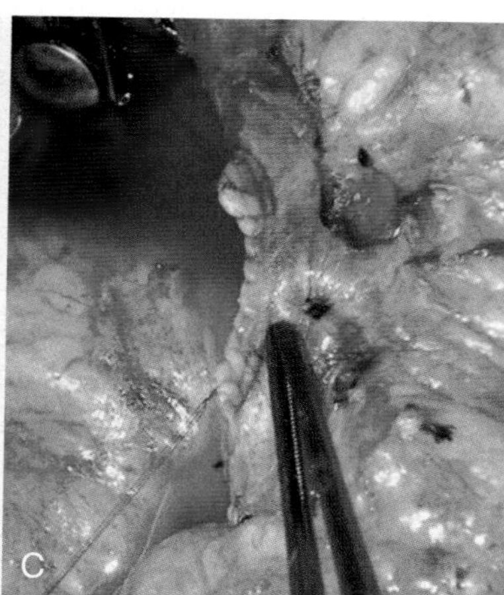

FIG. 56.25 (A) Computed tomography (CT) scan showing pancreatic ductal adenocarcinoma (PDAC) of the pancreatic head with involvement of portal vein–superior mesenteric vein *(SMV)* confluence *(large arrow)*. A metal biliary stent is in place *(small arrow)*. (B) Operative image demonstrating tumor involvement of the lateral aspect of the portal vein–SMV confluence. (C) Primary closure of portal vein–SMV confluence after tumor removal with lateral vein resection.

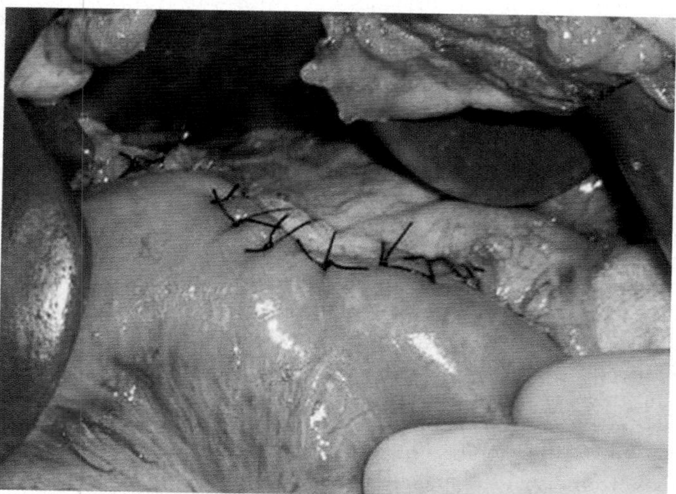

FIG. 56.26 Completed pancreaticojejunostomy.

TABLE 56.8 Morbidity after pancreaticoduodenectomy.

COMPLICATION	FREQUENCY (%)
Delayed gastric emptying	18
Pancreas fistula	12
Wound infection	7
Intraabdominal abscess	6
Cardiac events	3
Bile leak	2
Overall reoperation	3

centers. Despite significant reduction in mortality, however, morbidity remains common, occurring after 30% to 50% of procedures. Table 56.8 lists several of the most common postoperative morbidities and their frequencies.

After surgical resection and adjuvant therapy for pancreatic cancer, the median survival is approximately 22 months, with 5-year survival of 15% to 20%. Most patients experience relapse of disease in the form of metastatic disease (85%) and, less commonly, local recurrence (40%). In the absence of surgical resection, those with locally advanced disease who receive palliative chemotherapy may survive 10 to 12 months, whereas those with metastases rarely survive beyond 6 months. The role of adjuvant chemotherapy and radiation is described later in this chapter.

Morbidity

Delayed gastric emptying characterized by the need for prolonged nasogastric decompression or inability to tolerate oral intake is a frequent complication after pancreaticoduodenectomy, occurring 5% to 15% of the time. Few studies have demonstrated an association of delayed gastric emptying with pylorus preservation, but this finding has not been confirmed by all. When patients have the inability to tolerate solid foods or a prolonged nasogastric tube requirement, it is critical to perform cross-sectional imaging to rule out a secondary cause, such as pancreatic leak or intraabdominal abscess. An underlying structural abnormality, like stricture or other anastomotic complications, is ruled out with imaging and endoscopy. Enteral feeding with a feeding tube placed during surgery or percutaneously through endoscopy is used to maintain nutrition while waiting for stomach function to return.

Pancreatic leak or pancreatic fistula, which has been defined by the International Study Group on Pancreatic Fistula[39] as "output via an intraoperatively placed drain (or percutaneous drain) of any measurable volume on or after postoperative day 3, with amylase >3 times normal serum value," is a frequent complication after pancreaticoduodenectomy, occurring after 5% to 22% of surgeries. Perhaps the most predictive factor is the texture of the gland, with soft fatty glands at significantly higher risk of leak. Most fistulas are controlled by drainage catheters placed at the time of surgery and require no additional intervention. Rarely, uncontrolled fistulas require additional drain placement or operative exploration, sometimes mandating completion pancreatectomy to eliminate further abdominal contamination. The classification of pancreatic fistulas is given in Table 56.9.

Anastomotic leaks from the hepaticojejunostomy and duodenojejunostomy are rare and occur after less than 5% of procedures. Infectious complications (e.g., intraabdominal abscess, wound infection) are slightly more common and may require intervention with percutaneous drainage or open wound dressing changes.

TABLE 56.9 International Study Group on Pancreatic Fistula Classification of Pancreatic Fistulas.

	GRADE		
PARAMETER	A	B	C
Clinical conditions	Well	Often well	Ill-appearing, bad
Specific treatment	No	Yes/no	Yes
US/CT (if obtained)	Negative	Negative/ positive	Positive
Persistent drainage (after 3 weeks)	No	Usually yes	Yes
Reoperation	No	No	Yes
Death related to POPF	No	No	Possibly yes
Signs of infections	No	Yes	Yes
Sepsis	No	No	Yes
Readmission	No	Yes/no	Yes/no

From Bassi C, Dervenis C, Butturini G, et al: Postoperative pancreatic fistula: An international study group (ISGPF) definition. *Surgery* 138:8–13, 2005.
CT, Computed tomography; *POPF*, postoperative pancreatic fistula; *US*, ultrasound.

Pancreatic endocrine and exocrine insufficiency can occur after pancreaticoduodenectomy, but the risk of these events is unpredictable. For individuals with a normal gland, pancreatic insufficiency is rare. However, for those with preexisting chronic pancreatitis, fibrosis of the gland, or insulin resistance, exogenous enzyme and insulin replacement is usually needed.

Controversies

Palliative Bypass in the Case of Unresectable/Metastatic Disease

Despite availability of high quality thin cut cross-sectional imaging, up to 10% of patients are still found to have locally advanced or metastatic disease at the time of operation. Metastatic disease may be observed during laparoscopy. Given that palliation of gastrointestinal obstruction as well as biliary obstruction can be achieved by endoscopic (duodenal stents, ERCP with metallic stents for biliary system) means, proceeding with laparotomy and palliative bypass when metastatic disease is observed on staging laparoscopy is usually not indicated. If metastases or unresectable disease is observed once laparotomy has been performed, decision to proceed with biliary and/or gastrointestinal bypass needs to be individualized. Options include proceeding with operative palliation or closing the abdomen and pursuing endoscopic interventions if the patient did not already undergo preoperative biliary drainage. Unfortunately, there are no definitive data describing survival and quality of life of patients undergoing surgical bypass versus closure and rapid placement of endoscopic stents. To make this decision, the surgeon needs to assimilate data on patient's symptoms, performance status, and projected survival. In the setting of carcinomatosis or multifocal metastatic disease, regardless of performance status, endoscopic intervention should be favored due to the short median survival. However, these should be obvious on staging laparoscopy. If patient has had obstructive gastrointestinal symptoms or a need for placement of duodenal stent previously, it may be prudent to do gastrointestinal bypass. Similarly, in those patients with good functional status and low-volume metastatic disease or locally advanced disease, operative biliary bypass is a reasonable option.

Pylorus-Preserving versus Non–Pylorus-Preserving Whipple Procedure

We have described the pylorus-preserving Whipple procedure, which is the operation of choice for a growing number of pancreatobiliary surgeons. It was initially proposed as a means to reduce postpancreatectomy dumping and bile reflux, which is common after a non–pylorus-preserving Whipple procedure. Although initial results were encouraging, none of the randomized controlled trials have suggested superiority of a pylorus-preserving over a non–pylorus-preserving Whipple procedure.

Pancreaticojejunostomy Versus Pancreatogastrostomy

The pancreaticojejunostomy remains the Achilles heel of the Whipple procedure because of the frequency of pancreatic fistula. Several studies have reported successful outcomes with pancreatogastrostomy and reduced leak rates compared with pancreaticojejunostomy, but this finding has not been reproducible in several randomized trials, and most surgeons continue to prefer pancreaticojejunostomy.[40] In cases in which the pancreatic duct is not identified, invagination of the gland into the jejunal stump or pancreatogastrostomy may be performed.

Use of Somatostatin Analogues to Reduce Pancreatic Fistula

Although the mortality of pancreaticoduodenectomy has gone down, postoperative morbidity continues to be a significant problem. Pancreatic fistula is the major source of morbidity after the Whipple operation. Because pancreatic exocrine secretion is the proposed mechanism by which postoperative fistula occurs, inhibition of this secretion by means of somatostatin and its analogues has been evaluated in multiple trials with mixed results. Whereas European studies have shown that use of octreotide perioperatively leads to a decreased incidence of postoperative pancreatic fistula, North American trials have not confirmed these results. A recent trial from Memorial Sloan Kettering Cancer Center evaluated the efficacy of pasireotide, a somatostatin analogue with a longer half-life (11 hours for pasireotide vs. 2 hours for octreotide) and a broader binding profile (pasireotide binds to somatostatin-receptor subtypes 1, 2, 3, and 5, whereas octreotide binds only to receptor subtypes 2 and 5), in reducing pancreatic fistula, leak, or abscess of grade 3 or higher after pancreatic surgery (both pancreaticoduodenectomy and distal pancreatectomy). In this trial, pasireotide treatment significantly lowered the rate of grade 3 or higher postoperative pancreatic fistula, leak, or abscess (9% vs. 21%; relative risk, 0.44; 95% confidence interval, 0.24–0.78; $P = 0.006$). This finding was seen consistently in patients who underwent pancreaticoduodenectomy or distal pancreatectomy as well as in patients with dilated duct versus nondilated pancreatic duct.[41] A follow-up prospective observational study from Memorial Sloan Kettering Cancer Center confirmed the findings of the clinical trial.[42] Unfortunately, these results have not been reproduced outside this institute.[43]

Extent of Lymphadenectomy

Given the fact that 75% to 80% of patients are found to have lymph node involvement at the time of the Whipple procedure and, overall, 80% to 85% of patients will experience tumor recurrence and cancer-related death, some have proposed that radical lymphadenectomy may improve outcomes. Regional pancreatectomy was first proposed by Fortner in 1973 and has been used widely in Japan, where significant improvements in survival of patients undergoing extended lymphadenectomy have been reported. In addition to peripancreatic, portal, and pyloric lymph nodes, extended lymphadenectomy includes retrieval of hilar and retroperitoneal lymph nodes, extending from the celiac origin to the level of the inferior mesenteric artery and including all tissue between the renal hilum laterally. Several randomized controlled trials have since been completed, with no evidence to suggest improved survival after extended lymphadenectomy. In fact, more than one trial has shown increased morbidity associated with extended lymphadenectomy, including delayed gastric emptying, pancreatic fistula, and dumping. In view of the current evidence, standard pancreaticoduodenectomy is the operation of choice for localized pancreatic adenocarcinoma.

Laparoscopic and Robotic Pancreaticoduodenectomy

The first laparoscopic pancreaticoduodenectomy was performed in 1994 by Gagner and Pomp. Since then, several case reports and small series have demonstrated the feasibility of the minimally invasive approach. In the largest U.S. series to date, Kendrick and Cusati[44] have reported outcomes of 65 laparoscopic pancreaticoduodenectomies, with an overall morbidity rate of 42%: pancreatic fistula, 18%; delayed gastric emptying, 15%; bleeding, 8%; wound infection, 6%; reoperation, 5%; and mortality, 1.5%. These results indicate that laparoscopic pancreaticoduodenectomy has similar short-term outcomes to the open approach. Recently, the authors have presented the updated experience with 108 laparoscopic pancreaticoduodenectomies. Their data suggested that the median length of hospital stay was shorter with the laparoscopic approach. Furthermore, the authors observed that compared with the laparoscopic approach, a significantly higher proportion of patients had delay in delivery of adjuvant therapy with the open approach.[45] Pancreaticoduodenectomy is one of the most complex intraabdominal operations, and to perform it laparoscopically, the operator needs advanced training in both hepatopancreatobiliary and laparoscopic approaches, not to mention years of high-volume experience. Given the complexity of the procedure and the fact that the major morbidities that follow pancreaticoduodenectomy are not related to the size of the incision, the laparoscopic Whipple procedure has not become widely adopted.

Robotics has emerged as both an alternative and an adjunct to laparoscopy. Given the limitations of current laparoscopic technology and the need for meticulous vascular control and complex reconstruction in pancreatic surgery, robotic pancreaticoduodenectomy has been proposed as an alternative to laparoscopic pancreaticoduodenectomy. There are only a few centers in the United States that are pursuing robotics as an approach to pancreaticoduodenectomy. The largest series on robotic pancreaticoduodenectomy is from the University of Pittsburgh. Zureikat and colleagues published their experience with 132 robotic pancreaticoduodenectomies.[46] However, as mentioned before, the major morbidity of pancreaticoduodenectomy does not emanate from the incision, and it is too early to predict whether robotic pancreaticoduodenectomy will ever be widely adopted. At this time, open pancreaticoduodenectomy remains the standard of care.

Antecolic versus Retrocolic Duodenojejunostomy

Delayed gastric emptying is a common occurrence after pancreaticoduodenectomy with an elusive cause. Emerging data suggest that creation of an antecolic duodenojejunostomy may improve gastric emptying compared with the retrocolic technique.

Drain Versus No Drain

Given the high frequency of pancreatic fistula after pancreatic resection and morbidity associated with uncontrolled pancreatic leak, drains are routinely used after pancreatic resections. However, surgical drains are not without untoward effects, and their use has been associated with increased rates of intraabdominal and wound infection, increased pain, and prolonged hospital stay. Use of surgical drains after pancreatic resection has been evaluated in randomized controlled trials. In a randomized controlled trial from Memorial Sloan Kettering Cancer Center comparing outcomes in patients undergoing pancreatic resection with and without placement of surgical drains, no difference in complication rate was observed between the two groups. Furthermore, presence of a drain failed to reduce the need for radiologic intervention or surgical exploration. However, a multiinstitution randomized controlled trial comparing drain versus no drain in patients undergoing pancreaticoduodenectomy had to be terminated early as a result of increased morbidity as well as a fourfold increase in mortality in the no-drain group. In this trial, the use of a drain decreased the adverse clinical impact of pancreatic fistula. Good results without use of surgical drains have been achieved only at high-volume specialized centers that have vast experience in dealing with intraabdominal complications after pancreaticoduodenectomy. These centers have access to advanced interventional radiology techniques as well as experienced endoscopists who can drain many of the intraabdominal collections internally through the stomach. At this time, use of a surgical drain should be considered standard of care.

Irreversible Electroporation

The use of irreversible electroporation for treatment of locally advanced nonresectable pancreas cancers, or as "margin accentuation" to treat grossly positive margins is being investigated at many specialty centers. Irreversible electroporation preserves collagen rich structures such as blood vessels and ducts, while killing tumor cells, and therefore is proposed to provide improved local control or overall survival for patients with pancreas cancer. Currently, however, its utility in the management of locally advanced pancreas cancer remains to be determined.

Adjuvant Therapy for Pancreatic Cancer

Chemotherapy and Radiation Therapy

During the last 30 years, there have been conflicting reports about the survival benefit of adjuvant therapy after surgical resection of localized pancreatic cancer, particularly with regard to radiation therapy. Although the use of chemotherapy is widely accepted, the usefulness of radiation therapy has been increasingly questioned. In the United States, chemotherapy and radiation therapy are still widely used, whereas European centers have stopped using radiation therapy as part of standard adjuvant therapy because of lack of evidence to support a survival benefit.

Several randomized trials have attempted to clarify the roles of chemotherapy and radiation therapy for adjuvant treatment of pancreatic cancer after surgical resection. Table 56.10 summarizes the findings of several important trials. In 1974, the Gastrointestinal Tumor Study Group (GITSG) began a prospective randomized trial comparing adjuvant 5-fluorouracil (5-FU) and 40-Gy radiation with observation after curative resection.[47] The trial was terminated prematurely because of low accrual and the observation that the chemoradiation arm had a significant survival advantage. During an 8-year period, only 49 patients were accrued and randomized (43 patients were included in the final analysis because of withdrawal of 5 individuals and misdiagnosis of 1). Median survival was 20 months for the chemoradiation group compared

TABLE 56.10 Summary of Clinical Trials Defining Role of Adjuvant Therapy After Resection of Pancreatic Cancer.

TRIAL	CONCLUSIONS
GITSG	Adjuvant chemoradiation with 5-FU and 40-Gy radiation therapy improves survival compared with observation alone.
ESPAC-1	Adjuvant chemotherapy improves survival; chemoradiation is deleterious.
CONKO-001	Adjuvant gemcitabine improves disease-free survival compared with observation.
RTOG 97-04	Gemcitabine before and after 5-FU–based chemoradiation provides similar overall survival compared with 5-FU but with significantly less toxicity.
ESPAC-3	Adjuvant chemotherapy alone with gemcitabine provides similar overall survival compared with 5-FU but with significantly less toxicity.
ESPAC-4	Adjuvant combination of gemcitabine and capecitabine is superior to gemcitabine alone.

with 11 months for the observation group. Despite its limitations, this was the first randomized controlled trial that demonstrated an overall survival benefit after chemoradiation.

The European Study Group for Pancreatic Cancer-1 (ESPAC-1) trial was a 2 × 2 factorial design that compared chemoradiotherapy alone (5-FU, 20 Gy during 2 weeks) versus chemotherapy alone (5-FU) versus chemoradiotherapy and chemotherapy versus observation.[48] At a median follow-up of 47 months, it was noted that the estimated 5-year survival for those who underwent chemoradiotherapy was significantly less than that for those who did not (10% vs. 20%; $P = 0.05$). At the same time, those who received chemotherapy had a 5-year survival of 21% versus 8% for those who did not ($P < 0.009$). These findings led to the conclusion that although chemotherapy provided significant improvement in overall survival, the routine use of chemoradiation may be detrimental.

In 2007, the Charité Onkologie (CONKO-001) trial of 368 individuals enrolled during a 6-year period evaluated whether chemotherapy with gemcitabine (without radiation) could extend disease-free survival compared with observation.[49] Trial patients received six cycles of gemcitabine (days 1, 8, and 15 every 4 weeks for 6 months), and outcomes were compared with observation alone. Median disease-free survival was significantly improved in the gemcitabine group compared with the observation group (13.4 vs. 6.9 months). There was a trend toward improved overall survival, but this did not meet statistical significance (median, 22.1 vs. 20.2 months). This trial established the use of adjuvant gemcitabine for the treatment of pancreatic cancer.

The Radiation Therapy Oncology Group (RTOG 97-04) trial compared 5-FU versus gemcitabine chemotherapy before and after 5-FU–based chemoradiation.[50] The purpose of the study was to determine whether gemcitabine provided a survival benefit over 5-FU in combination with 5-FU–based chemoradiation. It was noted that although overall survival was similar (20.5 months for gemcitabine vs. 16.9 months for 5-FU; P = NS), the treatment-related toxicity was significantly higher in the 5-FU group. These data have led to the use of gemcitabine as the first-line agent for adjuvant chemotherapy, with or without radiation therapy.

ESPAC-3 trial was designed to evaluate overall survival comparing 5-FU (425 mg/m^2 IV bolus injection, given on days 1–5 every 28 days) versus gemcitabine (1000 mg/m^2 IV infusion, days 1, 8, and 15 every 4 weeks) after curative surgery. No observation arm was included because it was thought to be unethical, given the existing data suggesting a survival benefit of chemotherapy over observation alone. More than 1000 participants from 16 countries were randomized. Overall survival was similar between the groups (23.0 months for 5-FU, 23.6 months for gemcitabine), but gemcitabine was found to have less treatment-related toxicity, with fewer severe adverse events and better compliance. The current NCCN guidelines recommend gemcitabine or 5-FU alone or in combination with 5-FU–based chemoradiation as adjuvant treatment after resection for PDAC. Given the overall poor prognosis, enrollment into clinical trials is encouraged.

ESPAC-4 trial is the most recent international randomized controlled trial to finish.[51] ESPAC-4 was aimed to determine the efficacy and safety of gemcitabine and capecitabine compared with gemcitabine monotherapy for resected pancreatic cancer. In this two-group, open-label, multicenter randomized clinical trial, patients who had undergone complete macroscopic resection for ductal adenocarcinoma of the pancreas (R0 or R1 resection) were randomly assigned patients (1:1) within 12 weeks of surgery to receive six cycles of either 1000 mg/m^2 gemcitabine alone administered once a week for three of every 4 weeks (one cycle) or with 1660 mg/m^2 oral capecitabine administered for 21 days followed by 7 days rest (one cycle). The median overall survival for patients in the gemcitabine plus capecitabine group was 28.0 months (95% CI, 23.5–31.5) compared with 25.5 months (22.7–27.9) in the gemcitabine group (hazard ratio 0.82 [95% CI, 0.68–0.98], $P = 0.032$). This trial has established gemcitabine and capecitabine as the new standard for adjuvant therapy following resection for PDAC.

In the America Society of Clinical Oncology (ASCO) 2018 results of a randomized, multicenter phase III PRODIGE 24 trial was reported. In this trial, patients with surgical resected pancreatic cancer were randomized to receive either modified regimen of 5-FU, leucovorin, irinotecan, and oxaliplatin (mFOLFIRINOX) or gemcitabine for 6 months. The median disease-free survival was nearly 9 months longer in the mFOLFIRINOX arm compared to the gemcitabine arm. Median overall survival was 54 months for the mFOLFIRNOX arm and 35 months for gemcitabine arm. While promising, FOLFIRINOX is associated with higher rate of toxicity and may be difficult to administer in a community setting, especially in postoperative setting.

Role of Neoadjuvant Therapy

It is clear that for the optimal outcome, patients with pancreatic cancer require multimodal treatment that includes a combination of surgery and chemotherapy with or without radiation treatment. The administration of chemotherapy, with or without radiation therapy, before planned surgical resection for pancreatic cancer is becoming increasingly common. The rationale for the neoadjuvant approach is multifaceted. After surgical resection, approximately 25% of patients do not receive adjuvant therapy because of refusal, surgical complications, or an inability to recover physiologically. Giving therapy before surgery ensures that all patients will receive multimodality therapy, and by delivery of therapy to an intact gland with an established blood supply, the efficacy of therapy may be maximized. In addition, by treatment of patients with measurable disease, response to therapy can be assessed more readily. Progression of disease during neoadjuvant treatment is indicative of aggressive tumor biology and may prevent these patients from undergoing extensive surgery, which is unlikely to provide any survival benefit. Finally, the administration of chemotherapy and radiation therapy before surgery has been viewed as a physiologic stress test and helps select patients who would be unlikely to tolerate the major stress of surgical resection. Neoadjuvant therapy may provide improved selection of patients, avoiding surgery for those who progress, but also improved negative margin rates and reduced lymph node metastasis.

Both retrospective data and recently emerging level 1 data support use of neoadjuvant approaches. In a study from MD Anderson Cancer Center, the authors retrospectively reviewed and compared the outcomes of patients with resectable pancreatic adenocarcinoma who underwent neoadjuvant therapy followed by surgery with the outcomes of patients who were treated with the surgery first approach. In this study, 83% of patients with neoadjuvant therapy completed all components of therapy, including surgery with chemotherapy or radiotherapy, compared with 58% of patients treated with the surgery first approach. In this study, patients who completed all components of multimodal therapy had better outcomes compared with those who received only one component, whether surgery or chemotherapy. Although the rate of complications in both groups was similar, patients who received neoadjuvant therapy and suffered postoperative major complication had longer survival compared with patients with the surgery first approach who had a major postoperative complication. This may suggest that neoadjuvant therapy protects patients with pancreatic cancer who undergo pancreatectomy for pancreatic cancer from early recurrence and death. Alternatively, these results may just be a reflection of the fact that the patients who underwent surgery first and developed a complication were unable to receive adjuvant therapy, which is an equally critical component of treatment.

In select patients, the role of neoadjuvant therapy is clearer, particularly for those with significant venous or limited arterial involvement whose disease is classified as borderline resectable. In these patients, for whom upfront surgical exploration has a significant risk of exposing them to nontherapeutic laparotomy, the argument for neoadjuvant therapy is strengthened and is now supported by level 1 evidence. The results of PREOPANC-1 randomized controlled multicenter trial, which randomized patients with borderline resectable pancreatic cancer into immediate surgery versus preoperative chemoradiotherapy, were recently released.[52] Both groups received adjuvant therapy. The study demonstrated that the patients undergoing neoadjuvant approach had significantly better overall survival (median 17.1 months vs. 13.5 months in surgery first approach), better disease-free survival (median 11.2 months vs. 7.9 months in surgery first approach). No significant difference was observed in grade ≥3 adverse events between both groups. Another small-randomized controlled trial from South Korea[53] demonstrated that neoadjuvant treatment of borderline resectable pancreatic cancer patients led to improvement in overall survival and R0 resection rate when compared with upfront surgery. Furthermore, for individuals with significant SMV–portal vein involvement (>180 degrees or short-segment encasement) or hepatic arterial or SMA abutment (<180 degrees), neoadjuvant therapy may play an important role in identifying the subset of patients most likely to derive benefit from aggressive multimodality therapy, including surgical resection with vascular reconstruction. This type of aggressive treatment should be undertaken only by an experienced multidisciplinary team in the setting of a clinical trial.

Chemotherapy for Metastatic Pancreatic Adenocarcinoma

More than 80% of patients with pancreatic cancer present with locally advanced or metastatic disease and are primarily managed with chemotherapy. There has been some progress in the chemotherapy treatment of locally advanced or metastatic pancreatic adenocarcinoma. It is vital for the surgeons taking care of patients with pancreatic cancer to know these studies as regimens used to treat locally advanced and metastatic pancreatic adenocarcinoma slowly find their way into the treatment of patients with resectable pancreatic cancer in both adjuvant and neoadjuvant settings. Gemcitabine has been the standard of care for the treatment of metastatic pancreatic cancer since the late 1990s. Few chemotherapy regimens have shown greater efficacy than gemcitabine. Compared with gemcitabine alone, FOLFIRINOX (combination of 5-FU, oxaliplatin, irinotecan, and leucovorin) improves the median overall survival (gemcitabine, 6.8 months; FOLFIRINOX, 11.1 months) and progression-free survival (gemcitabine, 3.3 months; FOLFIRINOX, 6.4 months).[54] FOLFIRINOX is being used as the neoadjuvant regimen of choice in patients with borderline resectable pancreatic cancer and good performance status who can tolerate this aggressive regimen.

In a similar vein, the combination of gemcitabine with nab-paclitaxel improves overall and progression-free survival of patients with metastatic pancreatic cancer compared with gemcitabine alone.[55] The results with targeted therapies in pancreatic cancer have not been very promising as yet. The addition of erlotinib, which targets epidermal growth factor receptor–dependent growth pathways to gemcitabine, leads to statistically significant but marginal improvement in overall survival and progression-free survival in patients with metastatic pancreatic cancer.[56] Evaluation of gemcitabine-erlotinib combination as adjuvant therapy is currently ongoing. Randomized controlled trials evaluating addition of the vascular endothelial growth factor inhibitor bevacizumab or epidermal growth factor receptor inhibitor cetuximab to gemcitabine have not demonstrated improvement in outcomes of patients with metastatic pancreatic cancer compared with gemcitabine alone.

Palliative Therapy for Pancreatic Cancer

Given that 80% to 85% of those with pancreatic cancer have locally advanced or metastatic disease at the time of presentation and are therefore not candidates for surgical resection, it is imperative that all surgeons be familiar with nonoperative and operative palliative options. In general, nonoperative management should be pursued whenever possible to expedite systemic therapy and to optimize quality of life for these patients.

Biliary Obstruction

Palliation of biliary obstruction is commonly required for patients who are not candidates for surgical resection. ERCP with metal stent placement provides excellent palliation of jaundice, and at high-volume university centers, successful biliary drainage is possible in more than 90% of cases. In patients for whom endoscopic palliation is impossible, percutaneous biliary drainage with subsequent internalization may be required. For patients who are found at laparotomy to have unresectable disease or those for whom nonsurgical measures have failed, a surgical biliary-enteric bypass may be performed by Roux-en-Y hepaticojejunostomy, with excellent long-term patency.

Gastric Outlet Obstruction

Approximately 20% of patients with locally advanced pancreatic cancer will develop gastric outlet obstruction. For those with metastatic disease or disease found to be unresectable on the basis of imaging findings who have symptoms of gastric outlet obstruction, endoscopic luminal stenting should be carried out. Palliative endoscopic stenting has excellent short-term results, with almost immediate improvement in oral intake, but is limited in its ability to provide long-term patency. For this reason, patients who are found to have unresectable cancer at the time of laparotomy may benefit from preventive gastrojejunostomy, with no increase in perioperative morbidity. For patients who require surgical intervention, a double bypass consisting of a Roux-en-Y hepaticojejunostomy and gastrojejunostomy may be performed.

Pain Relief

Pain is a common component in the natural history of pancreatic cancer, affecting most patients with advanced disease. Palliation of pain is paramount for optimizing the quality of life for patients and should be a primary goal for physicians. The initial management of pain may include antiinflammatories or long-acting opioids, taken orally or through a cutaneous patch. For patients with pain that is not well controlled or who suffer side effects of narcotic use, celiac nerve block should be considered. The procedure involves injecting a combination of 3 mL of 0.25% bupivacaine and 10 mL of absolute alcohol into each celiac plexus. For cases that are found at exploration to be unresectable, this can be performed intraoperatively, as described by Lillemoe and coworkers.[57] For those with unresectable disease based on staging evaluation who do not undergo surgical exploration, neurolysis can be achieved through EUS guidance, with pain relief expected in 80% of patients. CT-guided percutaneous neurolysis may also be performed.

PANCREATIC TRAUMA

Pancreatic injuries are uncommon. The mechanism of injury varies according to the age of the patient. The most common mechanism in pediatric patients is abdominal blunt trauma. Direct compression of the epigastrium against the vertebral column and a blunt object (handlebar) is typically seen after bicycle injuries. The most common segment of the pancreas affected is the body. Penetrating injuries into the abdomen are the most common injuries seen in adults.

Isolated pancreatic injuries are not common. Up to 90% of patients present with associated hepatic, gastric, splenic, renal, colonic, or vascular lesions. The diagnosis and therapy in unstable patients with severe retroperitoneal injuries, gunshot wounds, or penetrating injury into the abdomen are usually straightforward, and they do not require further evaluation. Hemodynamically stable patients represent a challenge because isolated pancreatic injuries are normally associated with subtle or absent physical symptoms and signs. Undiagnosed pancreatic injuries are associated with significant complications, such as intraabdominal abscess, fistula, and fluid collections, in 60% of patients. Pancreatic injuries should always be considered after epigastric compression during a car or bicycle accident.

The modality of choice to evaluate patients with abdominal trauma is CT scanning of the abdomen. Findings such as peripancreatic hematomas, free fluid in the lesser sac, and abnormal thickening of Gerota fascia suggest pancreatic injury. Studies have shown that MRCP provides excellent visualization of the pancreatic duct, peripancreatic fluid contiguous to fractured segments of the pancreas, and hemorrhage after nonpenetrating trauma. Its main limitations include high cost, availability, and amount of time required to perform the study. Isolated pancreatic amylase measurement is not recommended because up to 40% of patients with transected pancreatic duct have normal serum amylase levels.

TABLE 56.11 American Association for the Surgery of Trauma pancreatic injury grading.

GRADE		INJURY DESCRIPTION
I	Hematoma	Minor contusion without ductal injury
	Laceration	Superficial laceration without ductal injury
II	Hematoma	Major contusion without ductal injury or tissue loss
	Laceration	Major laceration without ductal injury or tissue loss
III	Laceration	Distal transection or pancreatic parenchymal injury with ductal injury
IV	Laceration	Proximal transection or pancreatic parenchymal injury involving the ampulla
V	Laceration	Massive disruption of the pancreatic head

From Subramanian A, Dente CJ, Feliciano DV. The management of pancreatic trauma in the modern era. *Surg Clin North Am.* 2007;87:1515–1532.

Serial quantification levels increase the sensitivity of the assay. Abnormal amylase level elevations require further imaging.

The most reliable test to demonstrate pancreatic duct integrity is ERCP. However, its applicability is frequently limited by the risk of inducing pancreatitis, availability, and severity of the trauma.

Pancreatic injuries are classified according to the system described by the American Association for the Surgery of Trauma (Table 56.11). Definitive treatment is based on surgical findings. Major pancreatic resections have been described in stable patients with isolated pancreatic injury. However, pancreatic resections in unstable patients are associated with significant morbidity and mortality. Therefore, damage control surgery is indicated for complex injuries or unstable patients. Most pancreatic lesions can be temporarily controlled with drains. Once the physiologic insult has been controlled, definitive treatment should be considered, if indicated. Up to 75% of deaths occur within the 48 to 72 hours after trauma, and most are related to hypovolemic shock.

SELECTED REFERENCES

Abrams RA, Lowy AM, O'Reilly EM, et al. Combined modality treatment of resectable and borderline resectable pancreas cancer: expert consensus statement. *Ann Surg Oncol.* 2009;16:1751–1756.

A consensus statement about recommending multimodality therapy to optimize outcomes for patients with resectable and borderline resectable pancreatic cancer.

Andersen DK, Frey CF. The evolution of the surgical treatment of chronic pancreatitis. *Ann Surg.* 2010;251:18–32.

A review of the pathophysiology of acute pancreatitis and clinical management strategies.

Gittes GK. Developmental biology of the pancreas: A comprehensive review. *Dev Biol.* 2009;326:4–35.

A comprehensive review of pancreatic embryology and development.

IAP/APA evidence-based guidelines for the management of acute pancreatitis. *Pancreatology*. 2013;4:e1–e16.

This manuscript provides evidence-based guidelines addressing multiple issues in the management of acute pancreatitis, including the role and timing of endoscopic retrograde cholangiopancreatography and use of antibiotics.

Tanaka M, Fernandez-Del Castillo C, Kamisawa T, et al. Revisions of international consensus Fukuoka guidelines for the management of IPMN of the pancreas. *Pancreatology*. 2017;17:738–753.

The latest version of the consensus guidelines (2017) for diagnosis and management of cystic neoplasms of the pancreas points out the issues and provides guidelines and the evidence behind the guidelines.

van Santvoort HC, Besselink MG, Bakker OJ, et al. A step-up approach or open necrosectomy for necrotizing pancreatitis. *N Engl J Med*. 2010;362:1491–1502.

Clinical trial showing minimally invasive step-up approach for infected necrotizing pancreatitis had fewer major complications and mortalities than open necrosectomy.

REFERENCES

1. O'Morchoe CC. Lymphatic system of the pancreas. *Microsc Res Tech*. 1997;37:456–477.
2. Gittes GK. Developmental biology of the pancreas: a comprehensive review. *Dev Biol*. 2009;326:4–35.
3. Beger HG, Rau BM. Severe acute pancreatitis: clinical course and management. *World J Gastroenterol*. 2007;13:5043–5051.
4. Saluja AK, Lerch MM, Phillips PA, et al. Why does pancreatic overstimulation cause pancreatitis? *Annu Rev Physiol*. 2007;69:249–269.
5. Larson SD, Nealon WH, Evers BM. Management of gallstone pancreatitis. *Adv Surg*. 2006;40:265–284.
6. Wen L, Javed TA, Yimlamai D, et al. Transient high pressure in pancreatic ducts promotes inflammation and alters tight junctions via calcineurin signaling in mice. *Gastroenterology*. 2018;155:1250–1263 e1255.
7. Frossard JL, Steer ML, Pastor CM. Acute pancreatitis. *Lancet*. 2008;371:143–152.
8. Tenner S, Baillie J, DeWitt J, et al. American College of Gastroenterology guideline: management of acute pancreatitis. *Am J Gastroenterol*. 2013;108:1400–1415; 1416.
9. IAP/APA evidence-based guidelines for the management of acute pancreatitis. *Pancreatology*. 2013;13:e1–e15.
10. Wu BU, Hwang JQ, Gardner TH, et al. Lactated Ringer's solution reduces systemic inflammation compared with saline in patients with acute pancreatitis. *Clin Gastroenterol Hepatol*. 2011;9:710–717.e711.
11. Tse F, Yuan Y. Early routine endoscopic retrograde cholangiopancreatography strategy versus early conservative management strategy in acute gallstone pancreatitis. *Cochrane Database Syst Rev*. 2012:CD009779.
12. Rodriguez JR, Razo AO, Targarona J, et al. Debridement and closed packing for sterile or infected necrotizing pancreatitis: insights into indications and outcomes in 167 patients. *Ann Surg*. 2008;247:294–299.
13. Besselink MG, Verwer TJ, Schoenmaeckers EJ, et al. Timing of surgical intervention in necrotizing pancreatitis. *Arch Surg*. 2007;142:1194–1201.
14. van Santvoort HC, Besselink MG, Bakker OJ, et al. A step-up approach or open necrosectomy for necrotizing pancreatitis. *N Engl J Med*. 2010;362:1491–1502.
15. van Brunschot S, van Grinsven J, van Santvoort HC, et al. Endoscopic or surgical step-up approach for infected necrotising pancreatitis: a multicentre randomised trial. *Lancet*. 2018;391:51–58.
16. Harris S, Nadkarni NA, Naina HV, et al. Splanchnic vein thrombosis in acute pancreatitis: a single-center experience. *Pancreas*. 2013;42:1251–1254.
17. Apte MV, Haber PS, Applegate TL, et al. Periacinar stellate shaped cells in rat pancreas: identification, isolation, and culture. *Gut*. 1998;43:128–133.
18. Szabo A, Ludwig M, Hegyi E, et al. Mesotrypsin Signature Mutation in a Chymotrypsin C (CTRC) Variant Associated with Chronic Pancreatitis. *J Biol Chem*. 2015;290:17282–17292.
19. Sah RP, Dudeja V, Dawra RK, et al. Cerulein-induced chronic pancreatitis does not require intra-acinar activation of trypsinogen in mice. *Gastroenterology*. 2013;144:1076–1085. e1072.
20. Keck T, Wellner UF, Riediger H, et al. Long-term outcome after 92 duodenum-preserving pancreatic head resections for chronic pancreatitis: comparison of Beger and Frey procedures. *J Gastrointest Surg*. 2010;14:549–556.
21. Blondet JJ, Carlson AM, Kobayashi T, et al. The role of total pancreatectomy and islet autotransplantation for chronic pancreatitis. *Surg Clin North Am*. 2007;87:1477–1501; x.
22. Varadarajulu S, Bang JY, Sutton BS, et al. Equal efficacy of endoscopic and surgical cystogastrostomy for pancreatic pseudocyst drainage in a randomized trial. *Gastroenterology*. 2013;145:583–590. e581.
23. Allen PJ, Qin LX, Tang L, et al. Pancreatic cyst fluid protein expression profiling for discriminating between serous cystadenoma and intraductal papillary mucinous neoplasm. *Ann Surg*. 2009;250:754–760.
24. Brugge WR, Lewandrowski K, Lee-Lewandrowski E, et al. Diagnosis of pancreatic cystic neoplasms: a report of the cooperative pancreatic cyst study. *Gastroenterology*. 2004;126:1330–1336.
25. Tanaka M, Fernandez-Del Castillo C, Kamisawa T, et al. Revisions of international consensus Fukuoka guidelines for the management of IPMN of the pancreas. *Pancreatology*. 2017;17:738–753.
26. Sohn TA, Yeo CJ, Cameron JL, et al. Intraductal papillary mucinous neoplasms of the pancreas: an updated experience. *Ann Surg*. 2004;239:788–797; discussion 797-789.
27. Yachida S, Jones S, Bozic I, et al. Distant metastasis occurs late during the genetic evolution of pancreatic cancer. *Nature*. 2010;467:1114–1117.
28. Chari ST, Leibson CL, Rabe KG, et al. Probability of pancreatic cancer following diabetes: a population-based study. *Gastroenterology*. 2005;129:504–511.
29. Klein AP, Hruban RH, Brune KA, et al. Familial pancreatic cancer. *Cancer J*. 2001;7:266–273.
30. Maithel SK, Maloney S, Winston C, et al. Preoperative CA 19-9 and the yield of staging laparoscopy in patients with radiographically resectable pancreatic adenocarcinoma. *Ann Surg Oncol*. 2008;15:3512–3520.

31. Tsai S, George B, Wittmann D, et al. Importance of normalization of CA19-9 levels following neoadjuvant therapy in patients with localized pancreatic cancer. *Ann Surg*. 2018.

31a. Amin MB, Edge SB, Greene FL, et al. AJCC Cancer Staging Manual 8th edition, American College of Surgeons, NY: Springer, 2018.

32. Trimble IR, Parsons JW, Sherman CP. One-stage operation for the cure of carcinoma of the ampulla of Vater and the head of the pancreas. *Surg Gynecol Obstet*. 1941;73:711–722.

33. Jang JY, Chang YR, Kim SW, et al. Randomized multicentre trial comparing external and internal pancreatic stenting during pancreaticoduodenectomy. *Br J Surg*. 2016;103:668–675.

34. Ecker BL, McMillan MT, Allegrini V, et al. Risk Factors and mitigation strategies for pancreatic fistula after distal pancreatectomy: analysis of 2026 resections from the international, multi-institutional distal pancreatectomy study group. *Ann Surg*. 2019;269:143–149.

35. Strasberg SM, Drebin JA, Linehan D. Radical antegrade modular pancreatosplenectomy. *Surgery*. 2003;133:521–527.

36. Borja-Cacho D, Al-Refaie WB, Vickers SM, et al. Laparoscopic distal pancreatectomy. *J Am Coll Surg*. 2009;209:758–765; quiz 800.

37. van Hilst J, de Rooij T, Klompmaker S, et al. Minimally invasive versus open distal pancreatectomy for ductal adenocarcinoma (DIPLOMA): a pan-european propensity score matched study. *Ann Surg*. 2019;269:10–17.

38. van Hilst J, de Rooij T, Bosscha K, et al. Laparoscopic versus open pancreatoduodenectomy for pancreatic or periampullary tumours (LEOPARD-2): a multicentre, patient-blinded, randomised controlled phase 2/3 trial. *Lancet Gastroenterol Hepatol*. 2019;4:199–207.

39. Bassi C, Dervenis C, Butturini G, et al. Postoperative pancreatic fistula: an international study group (ISGPF) definition. *Surgery*. 2005;138:8–13.

40. Wente MN, Shrikhande SV, Muller MW, et al. Pancreaticojejunostomy versus pancreaticogastrostomy: systematic review and meta-analysis. *Am J Surg*. 2007;193:171–183.

41. Allen PJ, Gonen M, Brennan MF, et al. Pasireotide for postoperative pancreatic fistula. *N Engl J Med*. 2014;370:2014–2022.

42. Kunstman JW, Goldman DA, Gonen M, et al. Outcomes after pancreatectomy with routine pasireotide use. *J Am Coll Surg*. 2019;228:161–170. e162.

43. Dominguez-Rosado I, Fields RC, Woolsey CA, et al. Prospective evaluation of pasireotide in patients undergoing pancreaticoduodenectomy: The Washington University Experience. *J Am Coll Surg*. 2018;226:147–154 e141.

44. Kendrick ML, Cusati D. Total laparoscopic pancreaticoduodenectomy: feasibility and outcome in an early experience. *Arch Surg*. 2010;145:19–23.

45. Croome KP, Farnell MB, Que FG, et al. Total laparoscopic pancreaticoduodenectomy for pancreatic ductal adenocarcinoma: oncologic advantages over open approaches?. *Ann Surg*. 2014;260:633–638; discussion 638-640.

46. Zureikat AH, Moser AJ, Boone BA, et al. 250 robotic pancreatic resections: safety and feasibility. *Ann Surg*. 2013;258:554–559; discussion 559-562.

47. Kalser MH, Ellenberg SS. Pancreatic cancer. Adjuvant combined radiation and chemotherapy following curative resection. *Arch Surg*. 1985;120:899–903.

48. Neoptolemos JP, Stocken DD, Friess H, et al. A randomized trial of chemoradiotherapy and chemotherapy after resection of pancreatic cancer. *N Engl J Med*. 2004;350:1200–1210.

49. Oettle H, Post S, Neuhaus P, et al. Adjuvant chemotherapy with gemcitabine vs observation in patients undergoing curative-intent resection of pancreatic cancer: a randomized controlled trial. *JAMA*. 2007;297:267–277.

50. Regine WF, Winter KA, Abrams RA, et al. Fluorouracil vs gemcitabine chemotherapy before and after fluorouracil-based chemoradiation following resection of pancreatic adenocarcinoma: a randomized controlled trial. *JAMA*. 2008; 299:1019–1026.

51. Neoptolemos JP, Palmer DH, Ghaneh P, et al. Comparison of adjuvant gemcitabine and capecitabine with gemcitabine monotherapy in patients with resected pancreatic cancer (ESPAC-4): a multicentre, open-label, randomised, phase 3 trial. *Lancet*. 2017;389:1011–1024.

52. Tienhoven GV, Versteijne E, Suker M, et al. Preoperative chemoradiotherapy versus immediate surgery for resectable and borderline resectable pancreatic cancer (PREOPANC-1): a randomized, controlled, multicenter phase III trial. *J Clinl Oncolo*. 2018;36:LBA4002.

53. Jang JY, Han Y, Lee H, et al. Oncological benefits of neoadjuvant chemoradiation with gemcitabine versus upfront surgery in patients with borderline resectable pancreatic cancer: a prospective, randomized, open-label, multicenter phase 2/3 trial. *Ann Surg*. 2018;268:215–222.

54. Conroy T, Desseigne F, Ychou M, et al. FOLFIRINOX versus gemcitabine for metastatic pancreatic cancer. *N Engl J Med*. 2011;364:1817–1825.

55. Von Hoff DD, Ervin T, Arena FP, et al. Increased survival in pancreatic cancer with nab-paclitaxel plus gemcitabine. *N Engl J Med*. 2013;369:1691–1703.

56. Moore MJ, Goldstein D, Hamm J, et al. Erlotinib plus gemcitabine compared with gemcitabine alone in patients with advanced pancreatic cancer: a phase III trial of the National Cancer Institute of Canada Clinical Trials Group. *J Clin Oncol*. 2007;25:1960–1966.

57. Lillemoe KD, Cameron JL, Kaufman HS, et al. Chemical splanchnicectomy in patients with unresectable pancreatic cancer. A prospective randomized trial. *Ann Surg*. 1993;217:447–455; discussion 456.447.

57 CHAPTER

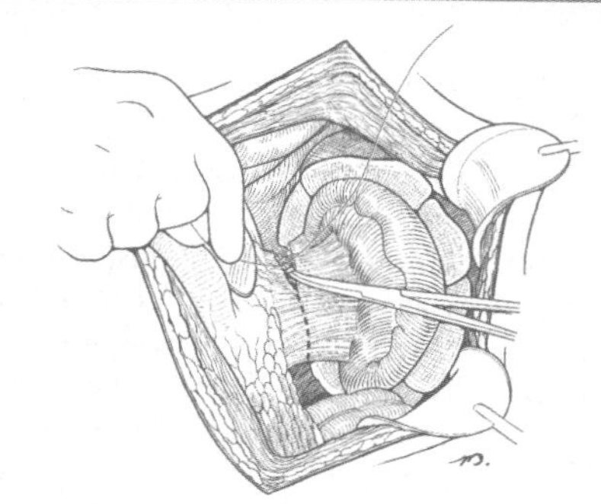

The Spleen

Aussama K. Nassar, Mary Hawn

OUTLINE

SPLENIC ANATOMY

The spleen is the largest lymphoid tissue mass in the body; it measures 7 to 13 cm in length and weighs up to 250 g. The spleen develops from mesenchymal cells in the dorsal mesogastrium during week 5 of embryogenesis. It is initially adherent to dorsal pancreatic bud and ultimately separates from the pancreatic bud and settles into the left uppermost aspect of the abdomen in the intraperitoneal cavity. Anatomically, it comprises of two surfaces: the diaphragmatic surface and visceral surface. The diaphragmatic surface is roofed by the diaphragm, separating it from the pleura. However, the costodiaphragmatic recess extends to the inferior-most aspect of a normal-sized spleen. The spleen's visceral surface is in close proximity to the greater curvature of the stomach, splenic flexure of the colon, apex of the left kidney, and tail of the pancreas (Fig. 57.1). On topographic anatomy, it lies in the left lower thorax and it is normally protected by ribs 9, 10, and 11. In healthy adult individuals, it is not palpated below the costal margin. However, in infants it is palpated below the costal margin at the midaxillary line. This relationship is crucially important in trauma patients who present with fractured left lower ribs as risk of splenic injury is high. Spleen is an intraperitoneal organ and is suspended in the peritoneal cavity by multiple peritoneal reflections misreferred to as "ligaments" (Fig. 57.2); at the diaphragmatic surface is the splenophrenic ligament, the visceral surface, and the gastrosplenic, splenorenal, and splenocolic ligaments. In patients without portal hypertension, the splenophrenic and splenocolic ligaments are relatively avascular. The gastrosplenic ligament carries the short gastric vessels in its superior aspect and the left gastroepiploic in its inferior aspect. The splenorenal ligament houses the splenic artery and vein as well as the tail of the pancreas. The tail of the pancreas abuts the splenic hilum in 30% of individuals and is within 1 cm of the hilum in 70% of cases, thus it is important to ligate the splenic vessels within 1 cm from the splenic hilum to avoid injury to the tail of the pancreas.

Vascular Anatomy

The splenic artery, a branch of the celiac trunk together with its branches of the short gastric arteries provide the arterial blood supply of the spleen. The splenic artery is a tortuous vessel that gives off multiple branches (16–18 branches) to the pancreas as it travels along its posterior aspect (Fig. 57.3). Understanding the variant anatomy of the splenic artery helps surgical planning to avoid potential intraoperative bleeding. There are two common variations of the splenic artery with regards to the relation between the splenic artery branches and the hilum. The magistral type, which branches into terminal and polar arteries near the hilum of the spleen; and the distributed type, which, as the name implies, gives off its branches early and distant from the hilum. The magistral type of splenic arterial anatomy occurs in 30% of individuals compared with the distributed type (70%). The splenic artery branches to approximately five to six polar arteries and six short gastric arteries. The superior polar artery which sometimes communicates with the short gastric arteries, the superior, middle, and inferior terminal arteries, and an inferior polar artery. Knowing these variable distributions are necessary in performing resections, especially a spleen-preserving distal pancreatectomy, in an effort to preserve splenic function.

The splenic vein created by the union of several splenic veins and the left gastroepiploic vein then travels posteriorly to the pancreas, joining with pancreatic branches and often the inferior mesenteric vein to join the superior mesenteric vein to form the portal vein.

The spleen is encased within a fibroelastic capsule. From the capsule trabeculae extend and compartmentalize the spleen. The spleen is also segmented by the divisions of the splenic vessels as they branch within the organ and merge with these trabeculae (Figs. 57.4 and 57.5). The arterioles branch into even smaller vessels and leave these trabeculae to merge with the splenic pulp, where their adventitia is replaced by a covering of lymphatic tissue that continues until the vessels thin to capillaries. These lymphatic

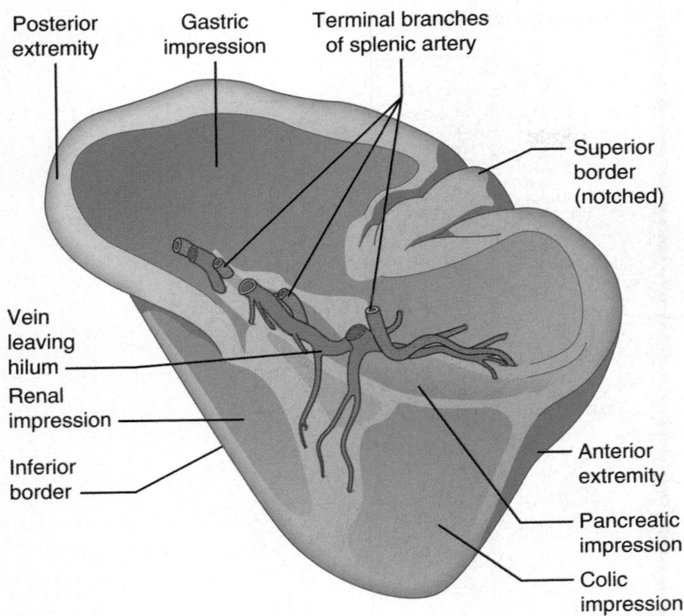

FIG. 57.1 The spleen and its visceral surface relationships. (From Ellis H. Anatomy of splenectomy for ruptured spleen. *Surgery (Oxford)*. 2010;28:226–228.)

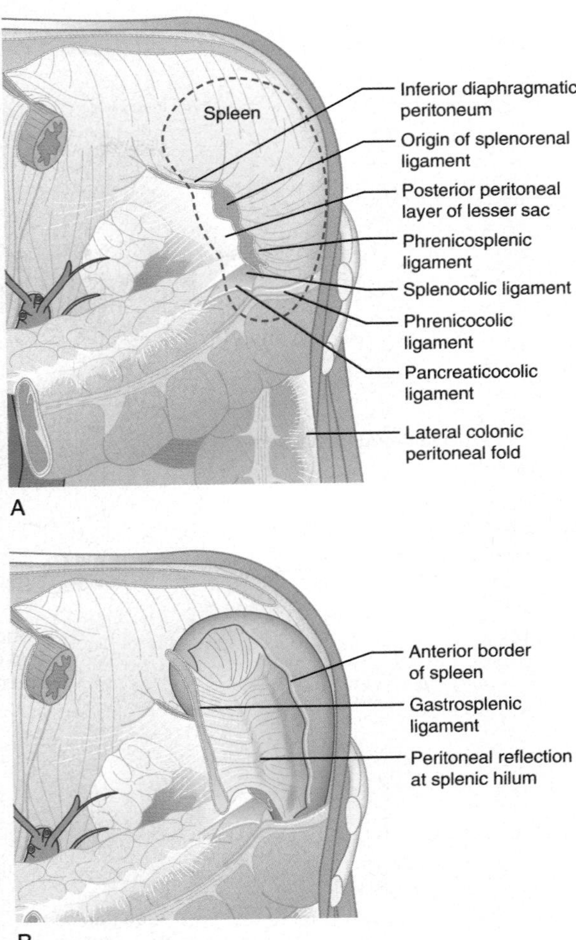

FIG. 57.2 (A) Posterior peritoneal attachments. (B) Anterior peritoneal attachments. (From Ellis H. Anatomy of splenectomy for ruptured spleen. *Surgery (Oxford)*. 2010;28:226–228.)

sheaths make up the white pulp of the spleen and are interspersed among the arteriolar branches as lymphatic follicles. The white pulp then interfaces with the red pulp at the marginal zone. It is in this marginal zone that the arterioles lose their lymphatic tissue and the vessels evolve into thin-walled splenic sinuses and sinusoids. The sinusoids then merge into venules, draining into veins that travel along the trabeculae to form splenic veins that mirror their arterial counterparts.

SPLENIC FUNCTION

Splenic function can be summarized into hematopoietic, reservoir, filtration, and immunity.

Hematopoietic

During fetal development between 3 to 5 weeks of fetal life, the spleen has important hematopoietic functions, which include white and red blood cell (RBC) production. This production is assumed by the bone marrow during the fifth month of gestation, and under normal conditions, the spleen has no significant hematopoietic function beyond this point. However, in certain pathologic conditions such as myelodysplastic syndrome, the spleen is one of the main organs involved in extramedullary erythropoiesis.

Reservoir

The spleen functions as a reservoir, where it pools in platelets. Normally one third of the platelets are pooled within the spleen. Thus, patients with splenomegaly are able to sequestrate large volume of platelets (up to 80%) with resultant thrombocytopenia. Due to that, after splenectomy, patients usually present with thrombocytosis which could be one of the factors that play a role in increasing thrombotic complications after splenectomy.

Filtration

The splenic filtration process consists of two methods of blood flow, the closed and open systems. In the closed system, blood flows directly from arteries to veins. In the open system, the blood flows through the arterioles and then trickles through a sieve-like parenchyma made up of reticuloendothelial cells into the splenic sinuses before draining into the venous system (Figs. 57.4 and 57.5). The cellular elements are directed toward these reticuloendothelial cells, in which cellular cleansing processes take place. These include removal of senescent cells, cellular inclusions (e.g., RBC nucleoli), and parasites and the sequestration of RBCs (for maturation) and platelets (reservoir). The plasma is directed to the lymphoid tissue, where soluble antigens stimulate the production of antibodies. RBC morphology, and thus RBC function, is maintained by splenic filtration. Normal RBCs are biconcave and deform easily. This plasticity allows passage through the microvasculature and optimizes the exchange of oxygen and carbon dioxide. Imperfect RBCs with inclusions such as nucleoli, Howell-Jolly bodies (nuclear remnant), Heinz bodies (denatured hemoglobin), Pappenheimer bodies (iron granules), acanthocytes (spur cells), codocytes (target cells), and stippling cause these RBCs to undergo cleansing in the spleen. The presence of Howell-Jolly bodies on a peripheral blood smear is one of the most characteristic finding for asplenia; surgical or medical (hemoglobinopathies) (Fig. 57.6). Howell-Jolly bodies are strongly basophilic inclusion bodies found in the cytoplasm of RBCs and represent nuclei remnants that were

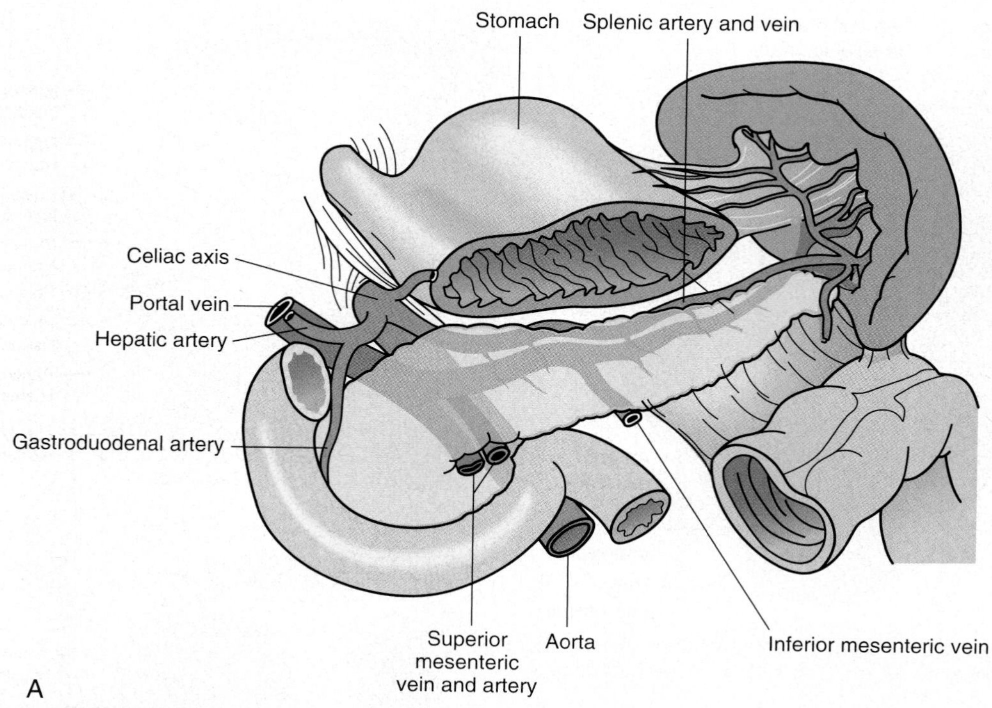

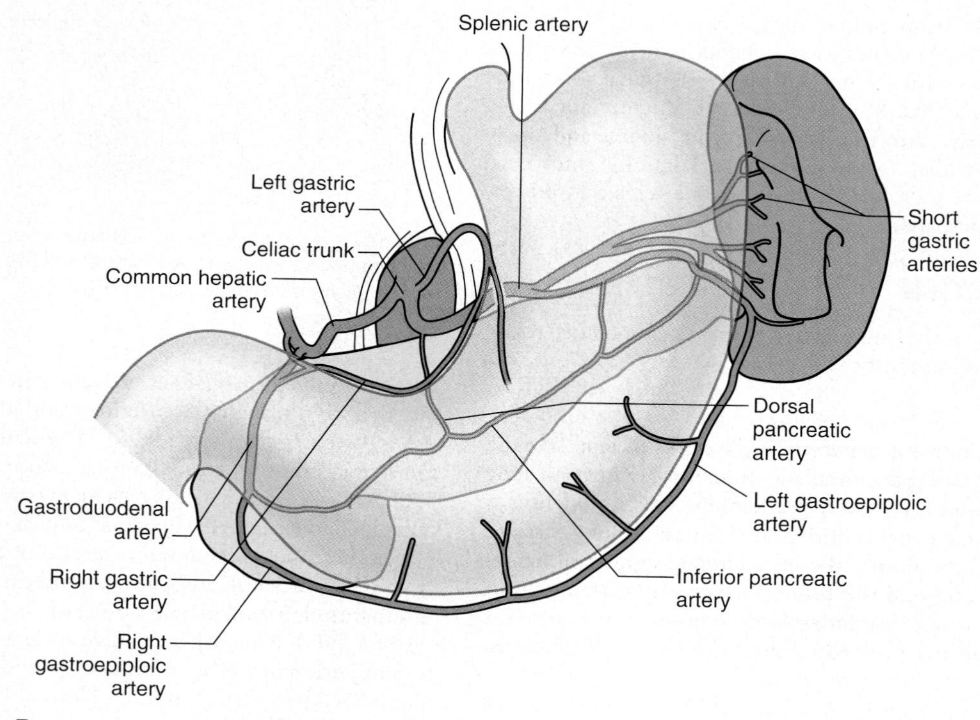

FIG. 57.3 Anatomic relationships of the splenic vasculature. The magistral type of splenic artery anatomy (A) occurs in 30% of individuals. The more common distributed type of anatomy (B) occurs in 70% of individuals. (From Economou SG, Economou TS. *Atlas of surgical techniques.* Philadelphia, PA: WB Saunders; 1966:562.)

unable to be cleared by a functioning spleen. Aged RBCs with decreased plasticity (>120 days) become trapped and destroyed in the spleen. Abnormal erythrocytes that result from hemoglobinopathies such as sickle cell anemia, hereditary spherocytosis, thalassemia, or pyruvate kinase deficiency (PKD) are also trapped and destroyed by the spleen. The overall effect is worsening anemia, splenomegaly, and sometimes autoinfarction of the spleen. Similarly, the spleen is involved in platelet destruction in immune thrombocytopenia (ITP), formerly known as idiopathic thrombocytopenia purpura.

Immunity

It functions by antibody synthesis and phagocytosis. Asplenic patients have been found to express subnormal immunoglobulin M

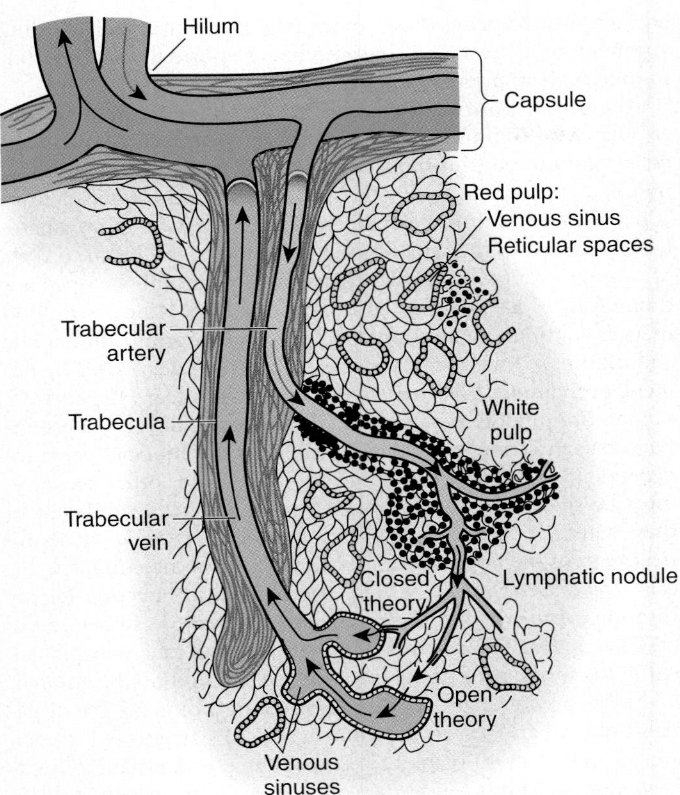

FIG. 57.4 Structure of the sinusoidal spleen showing the open and closed blood flow routes. (From Bellanti JA. *Immunology: Basic processes*. Philadelphia, PA: WB Saunders ,1979.)

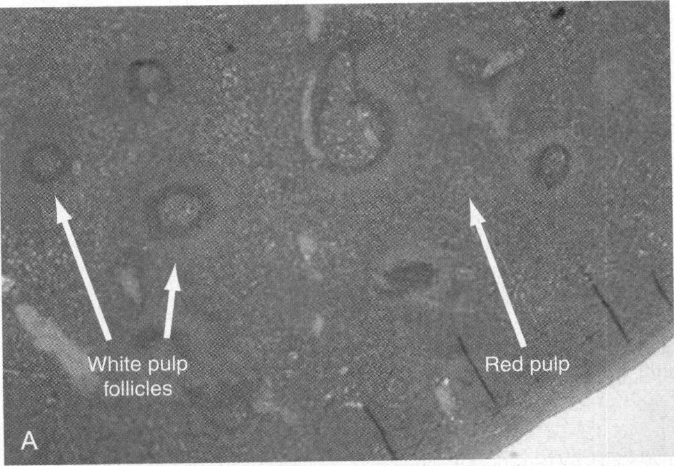

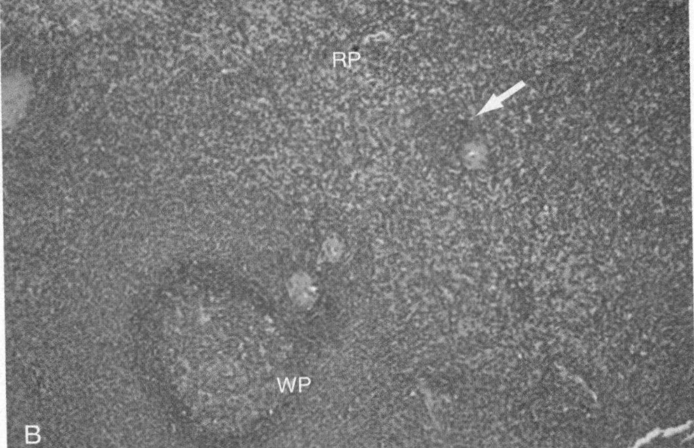

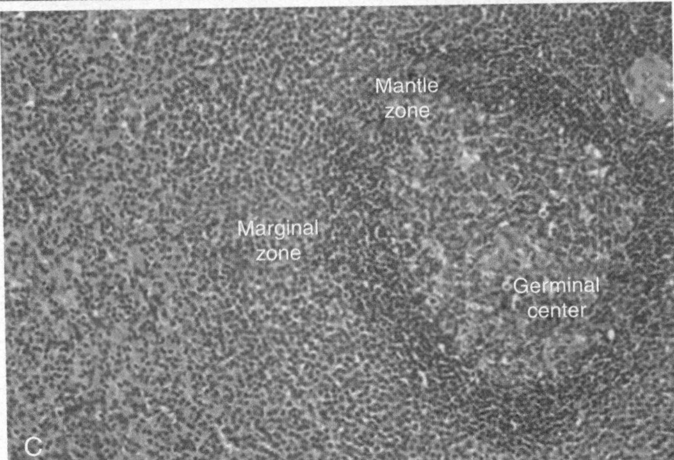

FIG. 57.5 Normal human spleen on hematoxylin-eosin staining. (A) Low-power photomicrograph showing relationship and relative proportions of red and white pulp. (B) Medium-power photomicrograph (*arrow* indicates periarterial lymphoid sheath). (C) High-power photomicrograph showing detailed secondary follicle architecture. (From Pernar LIM, Tavakkoli A. Anatomy and physiology of the spleen. In: Yeo CJ, eds. *Shackelford's surgery of the alimentary tract*. 8th ed. Philadelphia, PA: Elsevier; 2019:1595.). *RP*, Red pulp; *WP*, white pulp (secondary follicle).

levels, and their peripheral blood mononuclear cells exhibit a suppressed immunoglobulin response. Other factors involved in the immune response are opsonins, such as properdin and tuftsin. Opsonins, produced in the spleen, exhibit reduced serum levels after splenectomy. Properdin, a globulin protein also known as factor P, initiates the alternate pathway of complement activation; this increases the destruction of bacteria and abnormal cells. Tuftsin, a tetrapeptide, enhances the phagocytic activity of mononuclear phagocytes and polymorphonuclear leukocytes. Absence of a circulating mediator appears to result in suppressed neutrophil function. The spleen also plays a key role in cleaving tuftsin from the heavy chain of immunoglobulin G; thus, circulating levels of tuftsin are subnormal in asplenic patients. Additionally, splenic filtration may be particularly important for removal of microorganisms for which the host does not have a specific antibody (Box 57.1).

The immune functions of the spleen become evident after splenectomy, when patients are noted to be at risk for specific infections related to encapsulated bacteria *Streptococcus pneumoniae*, *Haemophilus influenza,* and *Neisseria meningitidis*. Asplenia and hyposplenism could be a result of surgical absence of spleen or lack of functioning of an anatomically present spleen. The most serious sequela is overwhelming postsplenectomy infection (OPSI). OPSI is discussed in detail at the end of this chapter.

SPLENECTOMY

Splenectomy may be indicated for conditions other than trauma. These indications encompass mainly hematologic disorders in addition to other mass lesions and splenic vascular lesions that are discussed elsewhere in this textbook.

Benign Hematologic Conditions

Immune Thrombocytopenia

ITP is the most common hematologic indication for splenectomy and is discussed here in detail. ITP was previously known as

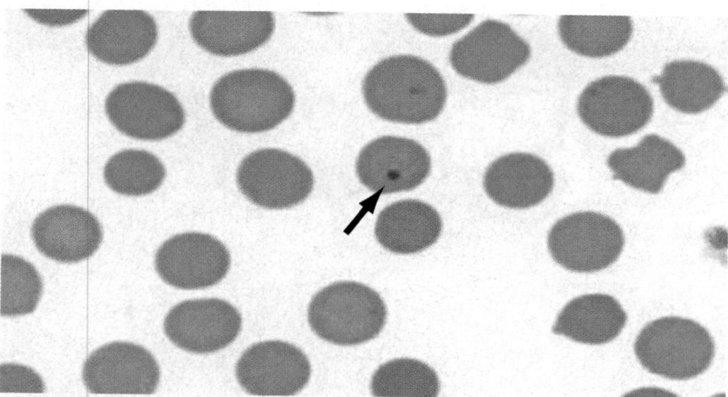

FIG. 57.6 The presence of Howell-Jolly bodies (arrow) on the peripheral blood smear is suggestive of asplenia or hyposplenism. (From Hashimoto N. Management of overwhelming postsplenectomy infection syndrome. *Clin Surg.* 2016;1:1148.)

BOX 57.1 Biologic substances removed by the spleen.

Normal Subjects

- Red blood cell membrane
- Red blood cell surface pits and craters
- Howell-Jolly bodies
- Heinz bodies
- Pappenheimer bodies
- Acanthocytes
- Senescent red blood cells
- Particulate antigen

Patients With Disease

- Spherocytes (hereditary spherocytosis)
- Sickle cells, hemoglobin C cells
- Antibody-coated red blood cells
- Antibody-coated platelets
- Antibody-coated white blood cells

Adapted from Eichner ER. Splenic function: Normal, too much and too little. *Am J Med.* 1979;66:311–320.

idiopathic thrombocytopenic purpura. In 2009, the ITP workgroup (IWG) published guidelines and defined the abbreviation to be ITP and dropped idiopathic and purpura as pathophysiology is better understood and the majority do not present with purpura.[1] ITP is characterized by a low platelet count below 100 × 10^9/L despite normal bone marrow and the absence of other causes of thrombocytopenia that could be responsible for the finding.[2] The pathogenesis is not fully understood. However, immunoglobulin G autoantibodies directed towards the platelet membranes are believed to be responsible for platelet destruction within the reticuloendothelial system by macrophages and cytotoxic T cells. In addition to the destruction, there is dysfunction of megakaryocytes with low level of thrombopoietin. It is classified as primary ITP when there is no clear etiology.[1] Primary ITP is further classified into three subtypes based on disease chronicity: newly diagnosed (within 3 months), persistent (3–12 months), and chronic (greater than 12 months). Secondary ITP is due to a known cause such as medication-induced, infectious, or rheumatologic conditions (i.e., systemic lupus erythromatosis). The typical presentation of ITP is characterized by purpura, epistaxis, and gingival bleeding. Less commonly, gastrointestinal bleeding and hematuria are noted. Intracerebral hemorrhage is a rare but sometimes fatal presentation.

The diagnosis of primary ITP involves the exclusion of other relatively common causes of thrombocytopenia—pregnancy, drug-induced thrombocytopenia (e.g., heparin, quinidine, quinine, sulfonamides), viral infections, and hypersplenism (Box 57.2). Mild thrombocytopenia may be seen in approximately 6% to 8% of otherwise normal pregnancies and in up to 25% of women with preeclampsia. Drug-induced thrombocytopenia is thought to occur rarely, in approximately 20 to 40 cases/million users of common medications, such as trimethoprim-sulfonamide and quinine. Other medications, such as gold salts, have a higher incidence, almost 1% of users. Viral infection (e.g., hepatitis C, human immunodeficiency virus (HIV) infection, rarely Epstein-Barr virus infection) can be responsible for thrombocytopenia independent of splenic sequestration. Once again, other processes must be ruled out, but healthcare providers can be confident of these causative factors if platelet counts improve with successful treatment of the responsible infection. Bacterial infection, specifically *Helicobacter pylori,* has also been linked to infection-related thrombocytopenia that improves with eradication. Other causes are listed in Box 57.2; spurious laboratory values caused by platelet clumping or the presence of giant platelets should not be ignored.

ITP is predominantly a disease of young women; 72% of patients older than 10 years are women, and 70% of affected women are younger than 40 years. ITP is manifested somewhat differently in children; both genders are affected equally, onset is sudden, thrombocytopenia is severe, and complete spontaneous remissions are seen in approximately 80% of affected children. Girls older than 10 years with more chronic purpura are those in whom the disease seems to persist.

Management of ITP depends primarily on the severity of the thrombocytopenia. Asymptomatic patients with platelet counts higher than 50,000/mm^3 may be observed without further intervention. Platelet counts of 50,000/mm^3 and higher are rarely associated with clinical sequelae, even with invasive procedures. Patients with slightly lower platelet counts, between 30,000 and 50,000/mm^3, may be observed but with more routine follow-up because they are at increased risk for progressing to severe thrombocytopenia. Initial medical treatment of patients with platelet counts below 50,000/mm^3 and symptoms such as mucous membrane bleeding, high-risk conditions (e.g., active lifestyle, hypertension, peptic ulcer disease), or platelet counts below 20,000 to 30,000/mm^3, even without symptoms, is glucocorticoid administration (typically, prednisone, 1 mg/kg body weight per day). Clinical response with increases in platelet levels to higher than 50,000/mm^3 is seen in up to two thirds of patients within 1 to 3 weeks of initiating treatment. Of patients treated with steroids, 25% will experience a complete response. Patients with platelet counts higher than 20,000/mm^3 who remain symptom free or who experience minor purpura as their only symptom do not require hospitalization. Hospitalization may be required for patients whose platelets counts remain below 20,000/mm^3 with significant mucous membrane bleeding and is required for those who have life-threatening hemorrhage. Platelet transfusion is indicated only for those who experience severe hemorrhage. Intravenous immune globulin is important for the treatment of acute bleeding, in pregnancy, or for patients being prepared for operation, including splenectomy. The usual dose is 1 g/kg body weight per day for 2 days. This dose usually increases the platelet count within 3 days; it also increases the efficacy of platelet transfusions.

BOX 57.2 Differential diagnosis of immune thrombocyopenia (ITP).

Falsely Low Platelet Count

In vitro platelet clumping caused by ethylenediaminetetraacetic acid (EDTA)–dependent or cold-dependent agglutinins, insufficiently anticoagulated specimen, glycoprotein IIb/IIIa inhibitors (e.g., abciximab)

Giant platelets that are miscounted as WBC by automated counters rather than platelets

Common Causes of Thrombocytopenia

Pregnancy (gestational thrombocytopenia, preeclampsia, HELLP syndrome)

Drug-induced thrombocytopenia (common drugs include heparin, quinidine, quinine, sulfonamides, acetaminophen, cimetidine, ibuprofen, naproxen, ampicillin, piperacillin, vancomycin, linezolid, glycoprotein IIb/IIIa inhibitors

Viral infections, such as HIV, HCV, EBV (infectious mononucleosis), rubella

Helicobacter pylori

Malaria

Hypersplenism caused by chronic liver disease

Alcohol

Nutrient deficiencies (e.g., vitamin B_{12}, folate, copper)

Rheumatologic/autoimmune disorders (e.g., systemic lupus erythematosus, rheumatoid arthritis)

Other Causes of Thrombocytopenia Mistaken for Immune Thrombocytopenia (ITP)

Myelodysplasia

Congenital thrombocytopenias

Thrombotic thrombocytopenic purpura and hemolytic-uremic syndrome

Chronic disseminated intravascular coagulation

Thrombocytopenia Associated With Other Disorders

Autoimmune diseases, such as systemic lupus erythematosus

Lymphoproliferative disorders (chronic lymphocytic leukemia, non-Hodgkin lymphoma)

Adapted from George JN, El-Harake MA, Raskob GE. Chronic idiopathic thrombocytopenic purpura. *N Engl J Med.* 1994;331:1207–1211.

HELLP, Hemolysis, elevated liver enzymes, and a low platelet count; *EBV*, Epstein-Barr virus; *HCV*, hepatitis C virus; *HIV*, human immunodeficiency virus.

Should initial therapy for ITP fail, medical options for refractory ITP include oral prednisone, oral dexamethasone (40 mg/day for 4 days), rituximab (375 mg/m^2/week intravenously for 4 weeks), and thrombopoietin receptor antagonists (eltrombopag, romiplostim). Successful response for months is observed in 28% to 44% of patients using rituximab; more transient responses are observed from thrombopoietin receptor antagonists.[3]

Before the establishment of glucocorticoids for treatment of ITP in 1950, splenectomy was the treatment of choice. For those two thirds of patients in whom glucocorticoids result in the normalization of platelet counts, no further treatment is necessary. For patients with severe thrombocytopenia with counts below 10,000/mm^3 for 6 weeks or longer, with thrombocytopenia refractory to glucocorticoid treatment, and who require toxic doses of steroid to achieve remission, the treatment of choice is to proceed to splenectomy. Splenectomy is also the treatment of choice for patients with incomplete response to glucocorticoid treatment and for pregnant women in the second trimester of pregnancy who have also failed to respond to steroid treatment or intravenous immune globulin therapy with platelet counts below 10,000/mm^3 without symptoms or below 30,000/mm^3 with bleeding problems. It is not necessary to proceed to splenectomy for patients who have platelet counts higher than 50,000/mm^3, who have had ITP for longer than six months, who are not experiencing bleeding symptoms, and who are not engaged in high-risk activities. A review of short-term and long-term failure of laparoscopic splenectomy has reported an overall approximate failure rate of 28% at five years after splenectomy.[4]

A systematic review of 436 published articles from 1966 to 2004 has reported that 72% of patients with ITP had a complete response to splenectomy. Relapse occurred in a median of 15% of patients (range, 1%–51%), with a median follow-up of 33 months.[5]

In addition to relapse rates, predictors of successful splenectomy were examined. Of the variables in the multivariate model, age at the time of splenectomy was an independent variable that was most correlated with response.[5]

Most patients will exhibit improved platelet counts within 10 days postoperatively, and durable platelet responses are associated with patients who have platelet counts of 150,000/mm^3 by postoperative day 3 or more than 500,000/mm^3 by postoperative day 10. Even with splenectomy, however, some patients may relapse (12%, range 4%–25%). A review of 1223 ITP patients has estimated the long-term failure rate of laparoscopic splenectomy at approximately 8% and approximately 44/1000 patient-years of follow-up.[4] Another study has estimated the complete response of ITP patients after splenectomy to be 66%.[5]

Although a thorough search for accessory spleens is completed during the initial surgery, evaluation for a missed accessory spleen must be undertaken in patients who experience a relapse. In their evaluation of 394 patients treated with laparoscopic splenectomy, Katkhouda and colleagues noted 15% of patients with accessory spleens. In those with accessory spleens, examination of a peripheral blood smear will lack the characteristic RBC morphology resulting from excision of the spleen. Radionuclide imaging may also be helpful in locating the presence and location of any accessory splenic tissue. Patients with chronic ITP in whom an accessory spleen is identified should have this removed, as long as the patient can withstand the surgical risk.

Other treatment options for these patients include observation of stable nonbleeding patients with platelet counts higher than 30,000/mm^3, long-term glucocorticoid therapy, and treatment with azathioprine or cyclophosphamide. Recent evidence indicates that thrombopoietin receptor agonists can be used as a novel medical therapy for patients with chronic ITP with no response to steroids, intravenous immune globulin therapy, or splenectomy.[6]

Approximately 10% to 20% of otherwise asymptomatic patients with HIV infection will develop ITP. Splenectomy is a safe treatment option for this cohort of patients and may actually delay HIV disease progression.[7]

Hereditary Anemia

This is usually classified into: 1) defects of the RBC membrane (e.g., hereditary spherocytosis); 2) defect in erythrocyte enzyme (e.g., glucose-6-phosphate dehydrogenase deficiency [G6PD]); and 3) defect in hemoglobin synthesis (e.g., thalassemia, sickle cell anemias [hemoglobin S]).

Hereditary Spherocytosis

Hereditary spherocytosis is the most common anemia and results from a defect in the erythrocyte cell membrane. Hereditary spherocytosis is usually transmitted as an autosomal dominant disease;

however, albeit rare autosomal recessive transmission also occurs. Hereditary spherocytosis is thought to be most commonly caused by mutation of genes affecting the production of the RBC cytoskeleton proteins such as spectrin, ankryin, band 3 (anion exchanger AE1), and band 4.2. Mutations of spectrin and band 3 proteins are the most frequently associated with hereditary spherocytosis.[8] Loss of function of those proteins causes RBCs to lack their characteristic biconcave shape. This affects the deformability of RBCs because lack of this protein results in rigid erythrocytes that are small and sphere shaped. Also, these cells have increased osmotic fragility and are more susceptible to trapping and destruction by the spleen. The most common resulting clinical features are moderate hemolytic anemia, occasionally with jaundice, folate deficiency, and splenomegaly. Diagnosis is made by hematologic workup: complete blood count with indices, increased reticulocyte count on peripheral blood smear with spherocytes, elevated lactate dehydrogenase, increased indirect bilirubin, absence of decreased haptoglobin, increased osmotic fragility, and negative Coombs test result.

The resultant anemia can be successfully treated with splenectomy, but normalization of the erythrocyte morphology does not occur. Splenectomy should be delayed until the age of five years to preserve immunologic function of the spleen and to reduce the risk of OPSI. If patient requires splenectomy before that age, partial splenectomy is an option. Just as with other hemolytic anemias, the presence of pigmented gallstones is common. The preoperative workup should include ultrasound evaluation; if gallstones are present, cholecystectomy may be performed at the same time as splenectomy.

Hereditary elliptocytosis, hereditary pyropoikilocytosis, hereditary xerocytosis, and hereditary hydrocytosis also result in anemia secondary to RBC membrane abnormalities. Splenectomy is indicated in cases of severe anemia with these conditions, except hereditary xerocytosis, which results in only mild anemia of limited clinical significance.

Hemolytic Anemia Caused by Erythrocyte Enzyme Deficiency

PKD and G6PD deficiency are the predominant hereditary conditions associated with hemolytic anemia. Although PKD is the second most common enzymopathy after G6PD deficiency, it is the most common cause for hemolytic anemia compared to G6PD deficiency. PKD is an autosomal recessive disease caused by a mutation to the pyruvate kinase L/R (*PKLR* gene). The gene is expressed as liver (L) and RBC (R) isoforms of pyruvate kinase. Mature RBC lack mitochondria and rely on anaerobic glycolysis as their sole source of energy. Pyruvate kinase is involved in glycolysis and adenosine triphosphate (ATP) production, therefore a *PKLR* mutation causes reduced pyruvate kinase production leading to reduced levels of ATP in red cells and increased production of other byproducts of glycolysis. This results in the rapid depletion of ATP and the inability of the RBC to maintain its membrane integrity. They are subsequently destroyed by the spleen via phagocytosis.

In G6PD deficiency, however, splenectomy is rarely indicated. This X-linked condition is typically seen in people of African, Middle Eastern, or Mediterranean ancestry. G6PD catalyzes the first step in the oxidative part of the pentose phosphate pathway leading to the production of NDPH. NDPH is a crucial enzyme in combatting oxidative stress in cells. Therefore, cells with G6PD deficiency are especially susceptible to oxidative stress. RBCs with G6PD deficiency are unable to protect themselves from reactive oxygen species, which is precipitated by infection or exposure to certain foods, medications, or chemicals. Primary treatment, therefore, is avoidance of exacerbation of the condition.

Thus, PKD causes chronic hemolysis compared to G6PD deficiency, which is more episodic. As a result, there is a role for splenectomy in PKD.[9] Splenectomy has been shown to eliminate or decrease transfusion requirements through elevating the hemoglobin and reticulocyte count.[9]

Hemoglobinopathies

In addition to cellular membranes or enzyme gene mutation, hereditary anemias may also result from globin chain of the hemoglobin molecule mutations. Almost 1000 different globin mutations have been discovered. Out of all these hemoglobin mutations, sickle cell disease and thalassemia are the two most clinically important disorders. Sickle cell disease is a point mutation in the beta globin gene resulting a single amino acid substitution (valine for glutamic acid) in the sixth position of the β chain of hemoglobin A). Sickle cell disease results from homozygous inheritance of the defective hemoglobin (hemoglobin S), although sickling can also be seen when hemoglobin S is inherited along with other hemoglobin variants, such as hemoglobin C or sickle cell β-thalassemia. In African Americans, 8% are heterozygous for hemoglobin S (sickle cell trait), and approximately 0.5% are homozygous for hemoglobin S. The affected hemoglobin chains become rigid, sickle shaped, and unable to deform under reduced oxygen conditions. These misshapen cells are unable to pass through the microvasculature, which results in capillary occlusion, thrombosis, and ultimately microinfarction. This cascade of events frequently occurs in the spleen. These episodes of vasoocclusion and progressive infarction result in autosplenectomy. The spleen, which is usually hypertrophied early in life, typically atrophies by adulthood, although splenomegaly may occasionally persist.

Other causes of hemolytic anemia are the thalassemias. The thalassemias are a group of disorders with disproportional alpha to beta chain ratio, this results in precipitation of the unpaired chain and subsequent RBC destruction.[10] These abnormal cells are destroyed either in the bone marrow (ineffective erythropoiesis) or in the blood stream (hemolysis). Thalassemia is classified into two main types depending on which globin chain is defective: alpha thalassemia and beta thalassemia. The mode of inheritance is autosomal recessive. Splenomegaly, hypersplenism, and splenic infarction, common in sickle cell disease, are also commonly seen in patients with thalassemia.

Acute splenic sequestration crises are life-threatening disorders in children with sickle cell disease or sickle-Beta thalassemia. In this condition, there is rapid drop in hemoglobin level due to vasoocclusion and RBC sequestration in the spleen. This could lead to life-threatening hypovolemic shock and require multiple blood transfusions. Patients with acute splenic sequestration crisis present with severe anemia, splenomegaly, and an acute bone marrow response, with reticulocytosis. There may be a concurrent decrease in hemoglobin levels, abdominal pain, and circulatory collapse. Resuscitation with hydration and transfusion may be followed by splenectomy in these patients. Splenectomy is usually indicated after the first attack to prevent subsequent attacks. Hypersplenism related to sickle cell disease is characterized by anemia, leukopenia, and thrombocytopenia requiring transfusions; transfusions may be reduced by performing splenectomy. Symptomatic massive splenomegaly that interferes with daily activities may also be improved by splenectomy. Finally, in children with sickle cell disease who exhibit growth delay or even weight loss because of increased metabolic rate and whole body total protein turnover, splenectomy may relieve these symptoms.

Splenic abscesses may also be seen in patients with sickle cell anemia. These patients present with fever, abdominal pain, and a tender enlarged spleen. Most patients with splenic abscesses will have a leukocytosis as well as thrombocytosis and Howell-Jolly bodies, indicating a functional asplenia. *Salmonella* and *Enterobacter* spp. and other enteric organisms are common pathogens. These patients require resuscitation, antibiotics, and may require urgent splenectomy after stabilization.

Malignant Disease

Hematopoietic Neoplasm

Lymphomas

Hodgkin lymphoma. Hodgkin lymphoma, formerly known as Hodgkin disease, is a group of malignant conditions that are characterized by the presence of Reed-Sternberg cells on histology. Hodgkin lymphoma usually affects young adults in their 20s and 30s with a second peak in adults over the age of 50. Rarely, patients present with constitutional symptoms such as night sweats, weight loss, and pruritus; but more typically, asymptomatic lymphadenopathy usually involves the cervical nodes. Hodgkin lymphoma histologic subtypes are lymphocyte predominant, nodular sclerosing, mixed cellularity, or lymphocyte depleted. The disease staging is based on the Ann Arbor staging with Cotswold modifications.[11]

Stage I is disease in a single lymphatic site. Stage II is disease in two or more lymphatic sites on the same side of the diaphragm. Stage III indicates disease on both sides of the diaphragm and includes splenic involvement. Stage IV disease is disease with additional noncontiguous extralymphatic implication with or without associated lymphatic involvement. The addition of a subscript E to stage I, II, or III indicates single or contiguous extralymphatic spread; subscript S indicates splenic involvement. Patients who exhibit constitutional symptoms are denoted with a B (presence), and those without symptoms are denoted with an A (absence).

Historically, patients with Hodgkin lymphoma underwent a staging laparotomy that included splenectomy to provide pathologic staging information required to determine appropriate therapy. Staging methods have evolved to include imaging techniques. The recommended imaging modality is computed tomography (CT) and ^{18}F-fluorodeoxyglucose positron emission tomography (PET). Hodgkin lymphoma is a fluorodeoxyglucose-avid lymphoma. In the absence of a PET scan, CT with intravenous contrast is recommended.

Early-stage Hodgkin lymphoma is now often treated with the combination of radiation and chemotherapy. Advanced stage is usually managed with chemotherapy with or without radiation. Splenectomy for Hodgkin lymphoma is currently rarely indicated. However, it may be performed for symptomatic splenomegaly.[12]

Non-Hodgkin lymphoma. Non-Hodgkin lymphoma is a group of malignant neoplasms derived from progenerates of B cell, T cell, mature B cells, and mature T cells. Staging relies mostly on integrated PET/CT, this also helps with targeting fluorodeoxyglucose-avid lymph nodes with biopsy. Surgeons are frequently involved with obtaining a lymph node or tissue biopsy. Ideally, biopsy is obtained before initiation of steroid therapy as steroids would lyse lymphoid tissue and might obscure the diagnosis.

Splenomegaly or hypersplenism is a common occurrence during the course of non-Hodgkin lymphoma. Splenectomy is indicated for non-Hodgkin lymphoma patients with massive splenomegaly leading to abdominal pain, early satiety, and fullness. It may also be indicated for patients who develop anemia, neutropenia, and thrombocytopenia associated with hypersplenism.

Splenectomy may also be instrumental in the diagnosis and treatment of a rare subtype of non-Hodgkin lymphoma currently known as splenic marginal zone lymphoma (previously termed splenic lymphoma).[13] Most of these patients present with splenomegaly, lymphocytosis with anemia, and thrombocytopenia. Diagnosis of splenic marginal zone lymphoma is based on clinical feature of unexplained lymphocytosis and splenomegaly, triggering splenectomy and/or immunophenotypic findings on bone marrow biopsy. PET/CT is also indicated as part of the workup. Splenectomy is indicated for symptomatic splenomegaly and with those suspected large cell transformations on PET/CT scan. In patients with spleen-predominant features, survival is significantly improved after splenectomy and could be considered as a mainstay therapy for those that are surgical candidates.

Leukemia

Hairy cell leukemia. Hairy cell leukemia, a rare disease that accounts for approximately 2% of adult leukemias, is characterized by splenomegaly, pancytopenia, and neoplastic mononuclear cells in the peripheral blood and bone marrow. The cells that give the disease its name are B lymphocytes that have a ruffling of the cell membrane. This ruffling causes the cells to appear to have cytoplasmic projections under the light microscope. The male-to-female ratio is approximately 4:5. They usually present with palpable splenomegaly. Approximately 10% of patients require no treatment because of the indolent course of the disease. Treatment for cytopenias or splenomegaly typically begins with first line therapy with purine analogue chemotherapy.[14] For more refractory cancers, a second-line immunotherapy may be instituted. In others, however, the extent of splenomegaly or symptoms from hypersplenism can lead to splenectomy. Most patients show improvement after the procedure, with a response lasting approximately 10 years after splenectomy, and some patients (~40%–60%) show normalization of blood counts after splenectomy. Patients with diffusely involved bone marrow without massive splenomegaly are less responsive to splenectomy. Patients with hairy cell leukemia are also at a twofold to threefold risk for development of other malignant neoplasms after their diagnosis of hairy cell leukemia. Most of these second malignant neoplasms are solid tumors, such as skin cancers, lung cancer, prostate cancer, and gastrointestinal adenocarcinomas. Hairy cell leukemia behaves like a chronic leukemia; many patients can achieve a clinical remission, with a normal or near-normal life span.[15]

Chronic lymphocytic leukemia. Chronic lymphocytic leukemia (CLL) is the most common leukemia in the western world. It is a clinically heterogeneous disease of B lymphocytes characterized by the progressive accumulation of relatively morphologically normal, mature but functionally incompetent lymphocytes. CLL is seen with a slight predominance in men, mainly after the age of 50 years. CLL is staged according to the Rai system and correlates fairly well with survival. Low-risk CLL (formerly stage 0) involves bone marrow and blood lymphocytosis only; intermediate-risk CLL (formerly stages I and II) involves lymphocytosis and lymphadenopathy in any site or splenomegaly, hepatomegaly, or hepatosplenomegaly; and high-risk CLL (formerly stages III and IV) involves lymphocytosis and anemia or thrombocytopenia. The Rai system helps clinicians determine when therapy should be started. Other genetic and biologic markers are also used for prognostication. An International prognostication score (CLL-IPI) integrates clinical, genetic, and biologic variables. Medical treatment is reserved for fit patients with symptomatic disease and advanced Rai stages.[16] Treatment involves chemotherapy with fludarabine, rituximab, and cyclophosphamide. Conversely, unfit patients have two options: anti-CD20 antibody combined with chlorambucil or ibrutinib. The indication for splenectomy in CLL has declined dramatically in the past decade and is rarely performed.

Chronic myelogenous leukemia. Chronic myelogenous leukemia (CML) is a myeloproliferative disorder that develops as a result of a neoplastic transformation of myeloid elements. CML is characterized by the progressive replacement of normal diploid elements of the bone marrow with mature-appearing neoplastic myeloid cells. Although CML can be asymptomatic at presentation, patients commonly present with fever, fatigue, malaise, effects of pancytopenia (e.g., infections, anemia, easy bruising), and occasionally splenomegaly. Peripheral blood smear analysis shows leukocytosis of white blood cell count up to 100,000/μL with white blood cell count from myeloblasts to mature neutrophils. The gold standard for the diagnosis of CML is a chromosomal marker, the Philadelphia chromosome, is caused by the fusion of fragments of chromosomes Abelson gene (*ABL1*) 9q34 and breakpoint cluster region gene (*BCR*) on chromosome 22q11.2. This fusion results in expression of the BCR-ABL1 fusion oncogene and trannslates to BCR-ABL1 oncoprotein which then accelerates cell division and inhibits DNA repair.[17]

CML may occur in patients from childhood to old age. It usually is manifested with an asymptomatic chronic phase but may progress to an accelerated phase associated with fever, night sweats, and progressive splenomegaly. The accelerated phase may be asymptomatic and may be detectable only by changes in peripheral blood or bone marrow. The accelerated phase may then progress to the blastic phase. This phase is also characterized by fever, night sweats, and splenomegaly but is also associated with anemia, infections, and bleeding.

The BCR-ABL gene product is the target for therapy with tyrosine kinase inhibitors (imatinib, dasatinib, and nilotinib) and other chemotherapeutic modalities. Bone marrow transplantation is an option, but prognosis has improved dramatically with the advent of recent therapies, making transplantation less common. Studies evaluating the efficacy of newer therapies and combination therapies are ongoing. Symptomatic splenomegaly and hypersplenism in CML can be effectively treated with splenectomy, but there does not appear to be a survival benefit when it is performed during the early chronic phase. Surgery is therefore reserved for patients with significant symptoms attributable to splenomegaly or hypersplenism.

Nonhematologic Tumors of the Spleen

Lymphoma is the most common tumor involving the spleen. Other primary and secondary neoplasms are rare.

Primary tumors of the spleen are commonly vascular neoplasms and include benign and malignant variants. Splenic hamartomas are rare and are usually composed of malformed disorganized red pulp elements. Hemangiomas are frequent findings in spleens removed for other reasons. Angiosarcomas (or hemangiosarcomas) of the spleen usually occur spontaneously but have been linked to environmental exposures, such as to thorium dioxide and monomeric vinyl chloride. Patients with angiosarcomas may present with splenomegaly, hemolytic anemia, ascites, pleural effusions, or even spontaneous splenic rupture. These tumors are aggressive and have a poor prognosis. Lymphangiomas, by contrast, are endothelium-lined cysts that come to attention because of splenomegaly secondary to cyst enlargement. These are usually benign tumors; however, lymphangiosarcoma has been found within lymphangiomas. Splenectomy is appropriate for the diagnosis, treatment, and palliation of these conditions.

Secondary metastatic splenic neoplasms are rare and thought to be due to lack of afferent lymphatics.[18] They are seen in up to 7% of autopsies of cancer patients. The solid tumors that most frequently spread to the spleen are carcinomas of the breast, lung, and melanoma. Any primary malignant neoplasm, however, can metastasize to the spleen. Metastases are often asymptomatic but may be associated with splenomegaly and even splenic rupture; thus, splenectomy may provide palliation for carefully chosen patients with symptomatic splenic metastases.

Miscellaneous Benign Conditions

Splenic Cysts

Splenic cysts have been seen with increasing frequency since the advent of CT and ultrasound scanning. They are classified as parasitic and nonparasitic cysts. The nonparastic cysts are further divided into true cysts and pseudocysts. True cysts are lined with epithelium and may be considered congenital. They account for 10% of all splenic cysts. Tumors of the spleen may also appear to be cystic; these include lymphangiomas and cavernous hemangiomas (see earlier).

Parasitic cysts occur in areas of endemic hydatid disease (*Echinococcus* spp.). Radiographic imaging, usually with ultrasound, reveals cyst wall calcifications or daughter cysts, and although hydatid disease is uncommon in North America, this diagnosis must be excluded before invasive procedures are undertaken that might result in spillage of the cyst contents. Rupture of the cyst and expulsion of contents into the abdomen may precipitate anaphylactic shock and can also lead to intraperitoneal dissemination of the infection. Serologic testing is helpful for verifying the presence of these parasites. Splenectomy is the treatment of choice. As with hydatid cysts of the liver, the cysts may be sterilized by injection of a 3% sodium chloride solution, alcohol, or 0.5% silver nitrate. Even so, great care should be taken to avoid intraoperative rupture of the cyst.

Nonparasitic true cysts of the spleen account for approximately 10% of all splenic cysts. These epithelial cells are often positive for carbohydrate antigen 19-9 and carcinoembryonic antigen by immunohistochemistry. Patients with splenic epidermoid cysts may have elevated serum levels of one or both of these tumor markers. These cysts, however, are benign and apparently do not have malignant potential beyond that of the surrounding native tissue.

True splenic cysts are often asymptomatic and discovered incidentally. Patients may complain of abdominal fullness, early satiety, pleuritic chest pain, shortness of breath, and left shoulder or back pain. They may also experience renal symptoms from compression of the left kidney. On physical examination, an abdominal mass may be palpable. Rarely, splenic cysts are manifested with acute symptoms related to rupture, hemorrhage, or infection. Diagnosis is best made by CT, and operative intervention is indicated for those with symptomatic or large cysts. Total or partial splenectomy may provide appropriate treatment. Partial splenectomy has the advantage of preserving splenic function; 25% of the spleen appears to be sufficient to protect against pneumococcal pneumonia. Open and laparoscopic procedures allow total or partial splenectomy, cyst wall resection, or partial decapsulation.[19]

Nonparasitic pseudocysts represent the remaining 70% to 80% of nonparasitic splenic cysts. A history of prior trauma can typically be elicited. Pseudocysts of the spleen are not lined with epithelium.

Radiologic imaging usually reveals a smooth, unilocular, thick-walled lesion, sometimes with focal calcifications. Asymptomatic, small (<4 cm) pseudocysts do not require treatment and may involute with time. Symptomatic pseudocysts are manifested in a fashion similar to true splenic cysts; these are treated surgically with total or partial splenectomy, again remembering that partial splenectomy preserves splenic function. Percutaneous drainage has also been reported for splenic pseudocysts, although, in a case series, recurrence was common and subsequent complications were deemed too high.[20]

Splenic Abscess

Splenic abscess is an unusual but potentially life-threatening illness if not promptly identified and treated, with a 0.2% to 0.007% incidence in autopsy series. The mortality rate for splenic abscess ranges from 15% to 20% in previously healthy patients with single unilocular lesions up to 80% for multiple abscesses in immunocompromised patients. Illnesses and other factors that predispose to splenic abscess include malignant neoplasms, polycythemia vera, endocarditis, prior trauma, hemoglobinopathies, urinary tract infections, intravenous drug use, and acquired immune deficiency syndrome.

Approximately 70% of splenic abscesses result from hematogenous spread of the infective organism from another location, as in endocarditis, osteomyelitis, and intravenous drug use. Spread may also occur in a contiguous fashion from local infections of the colon, kidney, or pancreas. Gram-positive cocci (commonly *Staphylococcus, Streptococcus,* or *Enterococcus* spp.) and gram-negative enteric organisms are typically involved. *Mycobacterium tuberculosis, Mycobacterium avium,* and *Actinomyces* spp. have also been found. Fungal abscesses (e.g., *Candida* spp.) also occur, typically in immunosuppressed patients.

Splenic abscesses are manifested with nonspecific symptoms—vague abdominal pain, fever, peritonitis, and pleuritic chest pain. Splenomegaly is not typical. CT is the preferred method for diagnosis; however, the diagnosis can also be made with ultrasound.

Treatment of splenic abscesses depends on whether the abscess is unilocular or multilocular. In one third of adult patients, the abscess is multilocular. In one third of children, the abscess is unilocular. Unilocular abscesses are often amenable to percutaneous drainage, along with antibiotics, with high success rates for unilocular lesions. Multilocular lesions, however, are usually treated with splenectomy, drainage of the left upper quadrant, and antibiotics.[21] Laparoscopic splenectomy for abscess has been reported.[22]

Wandering Spleen

Wandering spleen is a rare finding seen in children and in women between the ages of 20 and 40 years. There are two potential theories. The first theory is a failure to form normal splenic peritoneal attachments that suspend the organ securely within its usual anatomic position. Failure to form these attachments is thought to arise from lack of fusion of the dorsal mesogastrium to the posterior abdominal wall during embryogenesis. The second theory surmises that in multiparous women, hormonal changes and abdominal laxity lead to an acquired defect in splenic attachments. In either case, without these attachments, the splenic pedicle is unusually long and prone to torsion.

Intermittent abdominal pain, splenomegaly resulting from venous congestion, and severe persistent pain are suggestive of wandering spleen and tension or intermittent torsion of the splenic pedicle. A mobile mass may be palpable on physical examination. CT of the abdomen with intravenous administration of contrast material provides confirmation of the diagnosis, with the spleen located outside its usual position. A noncontrasted spleen or whorled appearance of the vascular pedicle provides additional evidence for the condition and may be helpful in choosing splenopexy or splenectomy.[23]

Other Considerations

Splenic Trauma (See Chapter 17)

Vascular conditions. Splenectomy could be indicated for vascular conditions these will be discussed elsewhere in this textbook. These vascular disorders are; portal hypertension (Chapter 54), splenic artery aneurysm (Chapter 63) and splenic vein thrombosis (Chapter 65).

Elective Laparoscopic Splenectomy

Laparoscopic splenectomy is now the preferred method for resecting the spleen. This technique was first described in 1991,[24] and many studies have supported its use in terms of outcomes and patient safety. Disadvantages of the laparoscopic technique are longer operating times and difficulty in removing large spleens; however, reduced hospital stay and more rapid postoperative recovery alleviate these limitations. Complications are typically linked to the patient's comorbidities.

Laparoscopic splenectomy has been reported for most splenic diseases and is the preferred method for most situations, barring trauma or cases of massive splenomegaly. In deciding whether to pursue laparoscopic methods for splenectomy, certain considerations should be taken into account, such as operative indication (e.g., benign or malignant disease), splenic size, and any potential contraindications to laparoscopy. Preoperative planning is essential and is aided by CT imaging, however, CT scan is unreliable in detecting accessory splenic tissue and surgical exploration at the time of surgery is essential to avoid disease recurrence in ITP. In addition, maintaining communication with the hematologist in the preoperative period is essential to determine the need for steroids, platelets transfusion and immunoglobulins. Preoperative planning with CT imaging is especially crucial in determining splenomegaly. Melman and Matthews[25] have noted that spleens measuring more than 22 cm in craniocaudal dimension or more than 19 cm in width and with an estimated weight of more than 1600 g will require hand-assisted laparoscopic procedures, if not open splenectomy. A more recent study, although from a single institution, doubted the benefit of laparoscopic splenectomy versus open for moderate and massive splenomegaly defined by weight over 500 g and 1000 g, respectively, showing no advantage of laparoscopic splenectomy over open with longer operative time in laparoscopic splenectomy.[26] Laparoscopic splenectomy can be completed in approximately 90% of patients. The reported conversion to open splenectomy is between 0% and 20%. Most conversions are caused by intraoperative bleeding, lack of surgical experience, prohibitive adhesions, massive splenomegaly, and obesity.[26] As with other laparoscopic procedures, there is a learning curve, and with increasing experience, conversion to open splenectomy declines. Published guidelines regarding laparoscopic splenectomy reiterate the importance of indications for the procedure, preoperative imaging for determining size and volume and presence of accessory splenic tissue, choices regarding hand-assisted techniques (early in cases of splenomegaly), contraindications (e.g., portal hypertension, major medical comorbidities), and splenic vaccinations.[27] Vaccinations for *N. meningitidis, S. pneumoniae,* and *Haemophilus influenzae* should be given at least 14 days before elective splenectomy or 14 days after or upon discharge of an emergent splenectomy to reduce the risk of OPSI (see later).

Less blood loss and shorter hospital stays are a major advantage of laparoscopic procedures.[28] A prospective randomized controlled trial comparing open and laparoscopic approaches was performed in patients with β-thalassemia major. This study reported a shorter median hospital stay in the laparoscopic patients but longer operative times and an increase in blood transfusions.[29] It is not known whether these results can be generalized to all patients with splenic disease. Several case series have also compared the laparoscopic with the open approach and consistently favored the laparoscopic approach, particularly in regard to earlier resumption of diet, decreased postoperative pain, and shorter hospital stay.[30]

Treatment outcomes are the primary concern in comparing these approaches. In published results to date, laparoscopic outcomes are equivalent to those of open splenectomy. In a review of laparoscopic splenectomy for malignant disease, Burch and associates[31] have reported that this population of patients benefits from laparoscopic splenectomy, similar to those with benign disease. Katkhouda and coworkers have reported that in the treatment of ITP, laparoscopic and open splenectomy results appear to be similar.

Laparoscopic splenectomy needs careful consideration for special populations. Portal hypertension and its risk of uncontrollable operative hemorrhage is a relative contraindication for laparoscopic splenectomy. However, with advancement in laparoscopic techniques and the advent of laparoscopic energy devices and staplers, laparoscopic splenectomy can be safely carried out in patients with portal hypertension.[32] Splenectomy is sometimes indicated during pregnancy for refractory ITP. Case studies have shown that laparoscopic approach during pregnancy is generally safe and is preferably conducted during the second trimester of pregnancy. Operating during the first trimester is associated with fetal loss and the third trimester is technically difficult due to loss of operative domain.[33,34]

Patient positioning. The laparoscopic technique may be performed with the patient in the lateral or supine position. This depends on the surgeon's preference, concomitant surgery, and patient's body habitus. The lateral technique is the most widely used position. For all positions, the patient is placed on the table so that the kidney rest can be raised to maximize the space between the iliac crest and costal margin. Finally, the patient is tilted in a reverse Trendelenburg position to facilitate retraction of the viscera caudally away from the left upper quadrant.

In the right lateral decubitus position (Fig. 57.7), the patient is placed in a 60-degree right lateral decubitus position using a beanbag and axillary roll. In this case, the patient's left arm is placed on an arm board or supported by a splint with protection of all pressure points with gel pads or foams. With this approach, the surgeon and scrub nurse stand to the patient's right and the assistants stand to the patient's left.[35] The spleen will thus be suspended from its diaphragmatic attachments; gravity retracts the stomach, omentum, and colon; and the splenic hilum will be under some degree of tension. Alternatively, in the supine position, the surgeon stands to the patient's left, and the first assistant and camera assistant stand to the patient's right. It may be easier for a right-handed surgeon to work from a position between the patient's legs, with the patient in a modified lithotomy position. The scrub nurse stands to the patient's left side, near the foot of the table.

Trocar placement. Trocar access to the abdomen is gained with an open (Hasson) or Veress needle technique, medial to the left

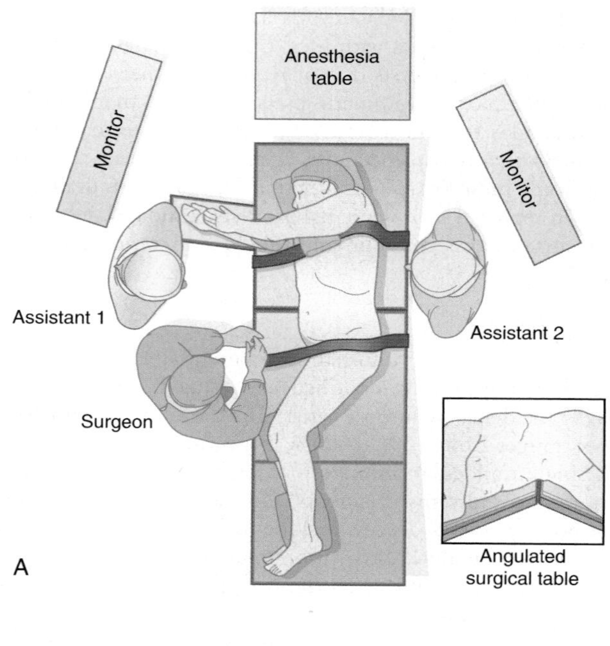

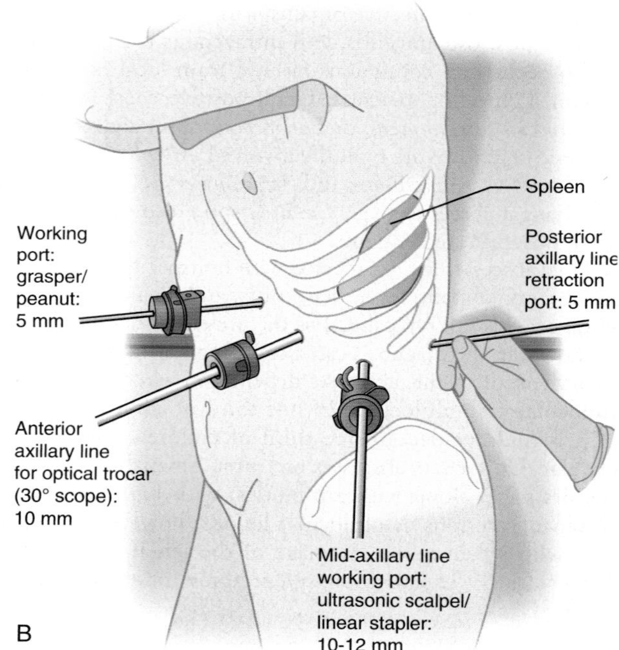

FIG. 57.7 (A) Patient positioning and (B) trocar placement-lateral decubitus position. (Copyright Lianne Krueger Sullivan, From Jenkins M, Parikh M, Pachter HL: Technique of Splenectomy. In Yeo CJ (editors): *Shackelford's surgery of the alimentary tract,* ed 8. Philadelphia: Elsevier, 2019.)

anterior axillary line 2 to 3 cm below the costal margin, and pneumoperitoneum is established to a pressure of 12 to 15 mm Hg. Three to four additional ports are used.

Surgical technique. The operation is begun with a thorough search of the abdominal cavity for the presence of accessory splenic tissue (Fig. 57.8); the stomach is retracted to the right side to facilitate examination of the gastrosplenic ligament. The splenocolic ligament, greater omentum, and phrenosplenic ligament are

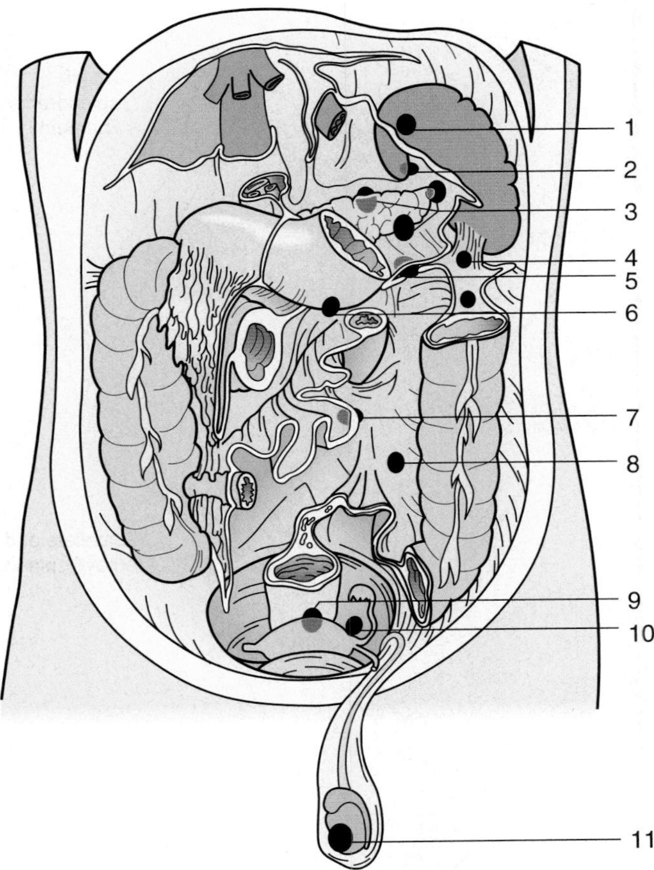

FIG. 57.8 Usual location of accessory spleens: (1) gastrosplenic ligament, (2) splenic hilum, (3) tail of the pancreas, (4) splenocolic ligament, (5) left transverse mesocolon, (6) greater omentum along the greater curvature of the stomach, (7) mesentery, (8) left mesocolon, (9) left ovary, (10) Douglas pouch, and (11) left testis. (From Gigot JF, Lengele B, Gianello P, et al. Present status of laparoscopic splenectomy for hematologic diseases: certitudes and unresolved issues. *Semin Laparosc Surg.* 1998;5:147–167.)

inspected next. The small and large bowel mesenteries, pelvis, and adnexal tissues are examined. Finally, the gastrosplenic ligament is opened, and the tail of the pancreas is confirmed to be free of splenic tissue (Fig. 57.8).

Our preference has been to use the right lateral decubitus approach, with the operating room table flexed 45 degrees from horizontal and the kidney rest elevated. The initial dissection is begun by mobilizing the splenic flexure of the colon. By use of sharp dissection, the splenocolic ligament is divided. The spleen can then be retracted cephalad; care should be taken not to rupture the splenic capsule during retraction. The lateral peritoneal attachments of the spleen are incised next, with use of scissors or ultrasonic shears. A 1-cm cuff of peritoneum is left along the lateral aspect of the spleen, which can then be grasped to facilitate medial retraction (Fig. 57.9). The lesser sac is entered along the medial border of the spleen. Continuing the cephalad retraction, the short gastric vessels and main vascular pedicle can be identified. The tail of the pancreas is also visualized, and care is taken to avoid it as it nears the splenic hilum. The short gastric vessels are divided. A number of options are currently available for this, including ultrasonic dissectors, hemoclips, bipolar devices, LigaSure (Covidien, Boulder, CO), and endovascular stapling devices. Hemoclips are used minimally around the area of the splenic hilum to prevent interference with future use of a stapling device, which could lead to significant bleeding from improperly ligated hilar vessels.

After the short gastric vessels are divided, the splenic pedicle is carefully dissected from the medial and lateral aspects. After the artery and vein are dissected, the vessels are divided by application of endovascular staplers or suture ligatures. In the more prevalent distributed mode, there are multiple vascular branches entering the spleen close to the hilum, so the dissection is carried out approximately 2 cm from the splenic capsule. Several branches may still be encountered, but these may be individually controlled more easily. A pedicle formed by the artery and vein that enters the hilum is known as the magistral type of arterial anatomy. If this is seen, the pedicle is transected en bloc using a linear vascular stapler. The tail of the pancreas, which is within 1 cm of the splenic hilum in 75% of patients and touches the hilum in 30%, should be well visualized as the stapler is applied to avoid injury.

The now-devascularized spleen is suspended only from a small cuff of avascular splenophrenic tissue at the superior pole. This tissue facilitates transfer of the spleen into a retrieval bag. To remove the detached spleen, the puncture-resistant nylon bag is grasped by its drawstring, which can be drawn through a port, usually the epigastric or supraumbilical site. The bag is opened slightly, providing access to the still intra-abdominal spleen. The spleen is then morcellated with ring forceps or finger fracture and removed piecemeal (Fig. 57.9). In the rare cases requiring pathologic examination of an intact spleen, an incision large enough to allow extraction of the spleen must be made. Care must be taken to avoid spillage of any splenic fragments into the abdominal cavity or wound. The laparoscope is then reinserted and the splenic bed assessed for hemostasis. Drains may be placed, if necessary. Pneumoperitoneum is then released, and the fasciae of all trocar ports larger than 5 mm are closed.

Robotic Splenectomy

Laparoscopic splenectomy is considered the gold standard for normal size spleen. The role of robotic splenectomy is still controversial. There have been a few studies specifically comparing laparoscopic with robotic splenectomy. In a recent retrospective cohort study by Cavaliere and colleagues,[36] they concluded that robotic splenectomy for splenomegaly is associated with less blood loss and longer operative times with comparable outcomes. In another study, Bodner and colleagues[37] compared operative times, hospital stay, and cost. They concluded that although the robotic procedure is feasible and safe for the patient, cost and operative times are both higher in the robotic group. In another study, Corcione and associates[38] evaluated the use of a robotic system in common general surgical procedures. Although they noted some benefits (e.g., availability of three-dimensional vision, greater dexterity with instruments), they reported concerns about the ability to control bleeding with only two instruments available; in these cases, they were required to convert to a traditional laparoscopic procedure. Overall, the addition of the robot to a straightforward procedure such as laparoscopic splenectomy is currently deemed unnecessary.

Short-Term Complications After Splenectomy

Splenectomy just like any other technique is associated with postoperative complications regardless of the technique; open, laparoscopic, or robotic. Predictors of technical difficulties and postoperative complications with a minimally invasive approach are splenic size over 19 cm, surgeons experience, and older

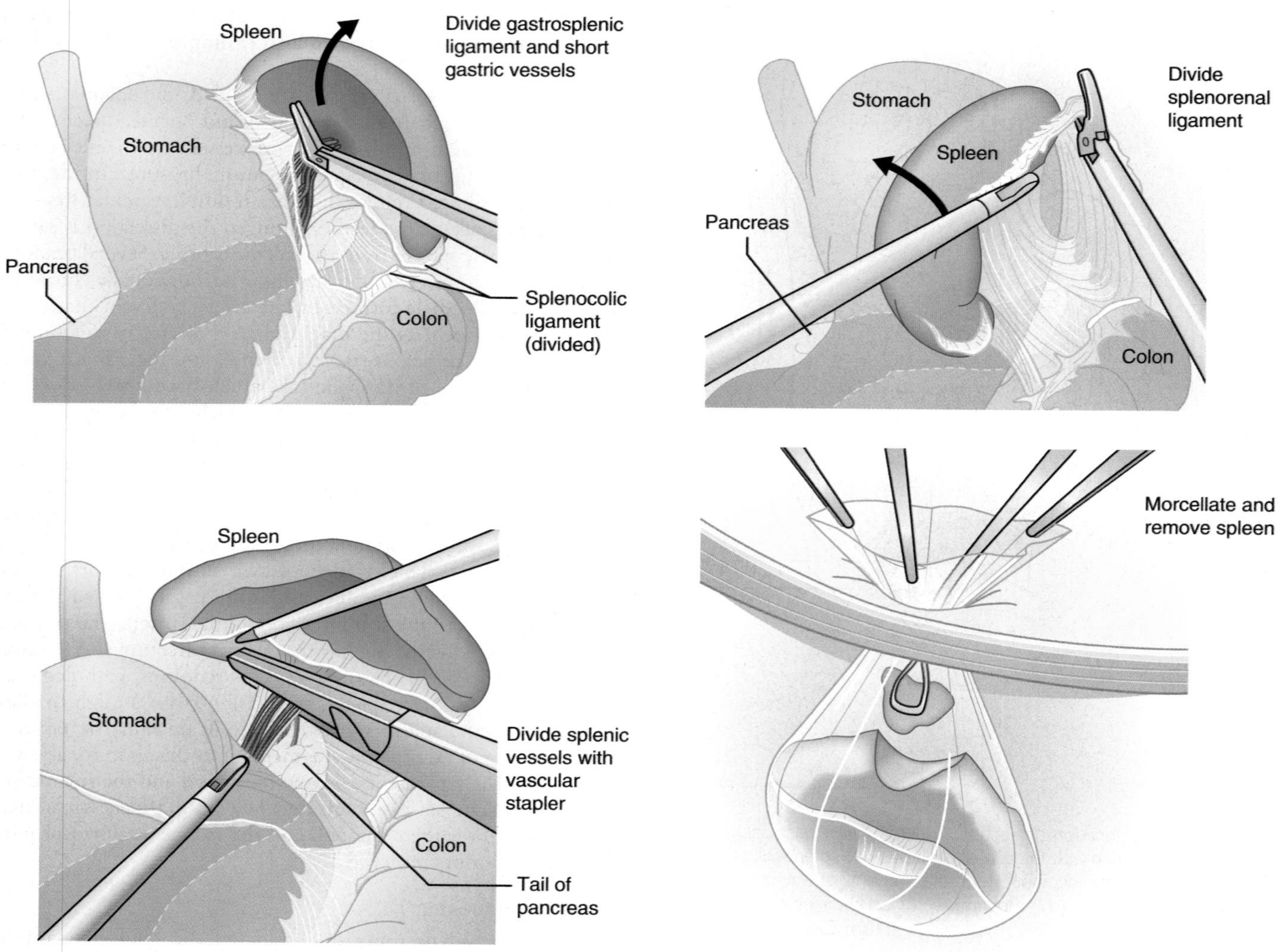

FIG. 57.9 Surgical technique. (Copyright Jennifer N. Gentry, From: Jenkins M, Parikh M, Pachter HL. Technique of Splenectomy. In: Yeo CJ, eds. *Shackelford's surgery of the alimentary tract.* 8th ed. Philadelphia, PA: Elsevier; 2019:1600.)

patients.[39] Complications in the immediate postoperative period are usually related to postoperative bleeding due to slipped ligature from the hilar vessels or other small vascular tributaries or branches not recognized. Other short-term complications include pneumonia, left-sided pleural effusion, and pancreatic leak and fistula. Pancreatic leak is related to unrecognized pancreatic tail injury during splenic hilum dissection. Pancreatic leak usually manifest with upper abdominal pain, leukocytosis, and feeling unwell.[40] Pancreatic leak is typically managed with percutaneous drainage with or without endoscopic retrograde cholangiopancreatography and sphincterotomy to reduce resistance forward flow of pancreatic secretions. Another important, yet rare, complication is gastric perforation at the greater curvature of the stomach, caused by inadvertent injury to the greater curvature during dissection of the short gastric arteries. This commonly necessities reoperation and could lead to chronic fistula if associated with concomitant pancreatic injury. Thromboembolism is one of the most serious complications after splenectomy. It is thought that it is related to the reactive thrombocytosis after splenectomy; however, the correlation is not linear. Abdominal venous thrombosis referred as postsplenectomy thrombosis of the splenic, mesenteric, and portal veins (PST-SMPv) has an incidence of 8% to 10%, splenic size and myeloproliferative disorder are the main risk factors.[41,42] Presentation is usually with nonspecific postoperative gastrointestinal symptoms of abdominal pain and ascites. Management is usually medical with systemic anticoagulation. Currently there is an increasing role for interventional radiology with catheter-based thrombolysis, stents, and/or thrombectomy.[43] Management of this condition is described in detail in Chapter 64.

Late Morbidity After Splenectomy

Postsplenectomy thrombocytosis occurs particularly in patients with myeloproliferative disorders (e.g., CML, polycythemia vera, essential thrombocytosis), which can result in thrombosis of the mesenteric, portal, and renal veins and can be life-threatening because it can lead to hemorrhage and thromboembolism. The lifelong risk for deep venous thrombosis and pulmonary embolism has not been established but may be significant. Also, there have

BOX 57.3 Overwhelming postsplenectomy infection–associated risk factors.

- Young age
- Thalassemia major (8.2%)
- Sick cell anemia (7.3%)
- Idiopathic thrombocytopenia (2.1%)
- Lymphoma
- Immunosuppression

Hashimoto N. Management of overwhelming postsplenectomy infection syndrome. *Clin Surg.* 2016;1:1148.

been case reports of acute myocardial infarction in postsplenectomy patients with thrombocytosis.

OPSI is the most common fatal late complication of splenectomy. Infection may occur at any time after splenectomy. In one series, most infections occurred more than two years after splenectomy and 42% occurred more than five years after splenectomy, with the overall incidence reported to be 3.2% to 3.5%. For those who acquire OPSI, the mortality is between 40% and 50%.[44] The risk is greatest in patients with thalassemia major and sickle cell disease (Box 57.3). OPSI is typically caused by polysaccharide-encapsulated organisms, such as *S. pneumoniae, N. meningitidis,* and *H. influenzae with S. pneumoniae* estimated to be responsible for between 50% and 90% of cases. The risk for fatal OPSI is estimated to be 1/300 to 350 patient-years of follow-up for children and 1/800 to 1000 patient-years of follow-up for adults. A review of selected reported splenectomy series of 7872 total cases, including children and adults, has revealed 270 episodes of sepsis (3.5%) with 169 septic fatalities (2.1%).[7] The incidence of nonfatal infection and sepsis is therefore likely to be significantly greater.

Clinical presentation usually begins with flue-like symptoms characterized by fever, rigors, chills, and other nonspecific symptoms, including sore throat, malaise, myalgias, diarrhea, and vomiting. These symptoms quickly progress to fulminant infection with multiorgan system failure with the development of hypotension, disseminated intravascular coagulation, respiratory distress, coma, and death within hours of presentation or within 24 to 48 hrs.[44] Survivors also often have a long and complicated hospital course with multiple sequelae, such as peripheral gangrene requiring amputation, deafness from meningitis, mastoid osteomyelitis, bacterial endocarditis, and cardiac valvular destruction.

Immunization

The immunization recommendations and formulations differ depending on patient's age and region. Currently, the standard of care for asplenic and hyposplenism patients includes immunization with the 13-valent pneumococcal conjugate vaccine (PCV13) followed by the 23-valent pneumococcal polysaccharide vaccine (PPSV23) at least 8 weeks later, *H. influenzae* type b conjugate, the quadrivalent meningococcal conjugate ACWY vaccine series (MenACWY) and the monovalent meningococcal serogroup B vaccine series (MenB-4C or MenB-FHbp). In addition, all asplenic or hyposplenic patients should receive seasonal influenza vaccination, measles, mumps, and rubella, varicella, and tetanus diphtheria pertussis. Visit the U.S. Centers for Disease Control and Prevention (CDC) website for details (https://www.cdc.gov/vaccines/schedules/hcp/imz/adult-conditions.html#f11). These vaccines should be ideally given 10 to 12 weeks prior to elective splenectomy and at least 14 days prior to surgery. If the patient did not receive these vaccines before surgery such as in emergency surgery, vaccine should be given 14 days after splenectomy or upon discharge (to improve compliance) whichever comes first. In patients with functional asplenia or hyposplenism they should be given as soon it is recognized (Table 57.1).[45,46]

The CDC has concluded that despite physician and patient education, pamphlets, and MedicAlert bracelets, the patient's retention regarding the risks of the postsplenectomy sepsis is poor. The CDC recommended that all splenectomy patients, including those with hereditary spherocytosis, be revaccinated and reeducated between two and six years after splenectomy. Recommendations include determination of pneumococcal antibody titers after immunization of every splenectomized patient because nonresponders to vaccination may be at high risk for OPSI. Subsequent follow-up of antibody titers is recommended at three to five years to evaluate for possible need for revaccination.

In an effort to improve host immunocompetence, partial splenic salvage or splenic autotransplantation has been considered because this may improve the humoral immune response to PPV23.[47] The difficulty with splenic salvage techniques is the lack of objective functional immune testing in humans. This is also true for patients who have undergone angiographic embolization for cessation of splenic hemorrhage in trauma. No studies are available regarding the risk of these patients for OPSI. Preclinical studies have examined the optimal site and amount of splenic tissue for autotransplantation. The most effective site of splenic autotransplantation was found to be the omental pouch, and approximately 50% of the spleen would be necessary for the prevention of pneumococcal sepsis. Although all efforts need to be made to preserve the spleen in trauma victims, the strategy of splenic autotransplantation seems to have limited applicability in humans.

Currently, it is suggested that educational intervention for patients who have undergone splenectomy is necessary; patients may require a number of instructional sessions. Communication with and educational efforts for primary care providers who assume medical care for asplenic patients are also extremely important because OPSI is preventable if appropriate precautions are taken. CDC immunization guidelines for 2020 (https://www.cdc.gov/vaccines/schedules/hcp/imz/adult-conditions.html) have recommended the following vaccines in addition to what has been discused above, for asplenic patients: tetanus (Tdap or Td), human papillomavirus (HPV), measles, mumps, and rubella (MMR), varicella, zoster, influenza, hepatitis A (hep A) and hepatitis B (hep B), and meningococcal.

Antibiotics

Significant controversy still exists about antibiotic prophylaxis in postsplenectomy patients. The primary goal of this prophylaxis is to prevent OPSI, particularly that secondary to pneumococcal infection, which is reported to be the cause of OPSI in 50% to 90% of patients. However, OPSI secondary to penicillin-sensitive pneumococcal infection has been reported in children and adults receiving penicillin prophylaxis.

There are two general approaches for antibiotic prophylaxis in asplenic or hyposplenic patients. One is daily and the other is having an emergency supply. There is variability of practice among different societies. The published Australian spleen society recommends daily antibiotic prophylaxis for children preferably up to age 16 or a minimum up to age five or three years after splenectomy. In addition, they recommend lifelong prophylaxis for immunocompromised states and an emergency supply of oral antibiotics (standby antibiotics) for postsplenectomy adults, with instructions to begin taking the medication at the onset of a febrile illness or rigors if there is no access to immediate medical evaluation.[48]

TABLE 57.1 Centers for Disease Control and Prevention vaccine recommendations for asplenic patients*†

	PNEUMOCOCCAL VACCINATION	MENINGOCOCCAL VACCINATION	HAEMOPHILUS INFLUENZAE TYPE B VACCINATION
Children	Immunologically naïve 2–6 years‡: PCV13 followed by PVC13 8 weeks later; PPSV23 8 weeks later; repeat PPSV23 at 5 years Immunologically naïve 6–18 years‡: PCV13 followed by PPSV23 8 weeks later; repeat PPSV23 at 5 years	MenACWY series AND MenB series§	Hib once if 15 months or older and previously not vaccinated
Adults (age 19 and older)	Immunologically naïve‡: PCV13 followed by PPSV23 8 weeks later; repeat PPSV23 every 5 years	MenACWY or MPSV4 2 months apart; repeat MenACWY every 5 years AND MenB series§ once	Hib once

From Pernar LIM, Tavakkoli A. Anatomy and physiology of the spleen. In: Yeo CJ, eds. *Shackelford's surgery of the alimentary tract.* 8th ed. Philadelphia, PA: Elsevier; 2019:1595.
Hib, H. influenzae type b; *MenACWY,* meningococcal 4-valent conjugate; *MPSV4,* meningococcal 4-valent polysaccharide; *PCV13,* 13-valent pneumococcal conjugate vaccine; *PPSV23,* pneumococcal 23-valent polysaccharide.
*First vaccination should be administered at least 2 weeks before splenectomy if elective.
†Even with vaccination, oral antibiotic prophylaxis with penicillin V or amoxicillin should be considered for children under 2 years of age or high-risk postsplenectomy patients.
‡For patients who have previously received any PCV or PPSV23 or a combination of these vaccinations, the recommendations vary and are outlined in the CDC Guidelines accessible online.
§MenB-4C 2 doses 1 month apart or MenB-FHbp 3 doses, 1 each at 0, 2, and 6 months.

The oral antibiotic of choice is amoxycillin or oral penicillin; for those who have confirmed hypersensitivity, the second choice would be a macrolide. For the emergency supply, we recommend the use of amoxycillin plus clavulanate and in penicillin-allergic patients, macrolides or quinolones are a second-choice agent.

The length of the above prophylactic treatment may be unacceptable to patients, and there is evidence that there is no difference in the incidence of sepsis in postsplenectomy sickle cell patients when the antibiotic prophylaxis is ceased after five years. OPSI has been reported in patients taking prophylactic medications, and patients should be made aware that even with daily antibiotics, not all infections may be preventable.

There is evidence that the risk of OPSI is lowest in patients who exhibit the greatest understanding of the infectious risks of asplenia.[49] This highlights the importance of education of the patient, particularly at follow-up visits, to ensure compliance with antibiotic and vaccine prophylaxis.

Whether the patient elects to take antibiotic prophylaxis, and because of the risk of OPSI and the extreme level of associated mortality, any asplenic or hyposplenic patient who presents with rigors or fever must be started immediately on aggressive empirical antibiotic coverage, even without culture data.

SELECTED REFERENCES

Feldman LS. Laparoscopic splenectomy: standardized approach. *World J Surg.* 2011;35:1487–1495.

This article provides a useful overview of indications and technique for laparoscopic splenectomy. It also provides useful tips on minimally invasive approaches to specific scenarios in splenic disease (e.g., splenomegaly, accessory spleens).

Gigot JF, Jamar F, Ferrant A, et al. Inadequate detection of accessory spleens and splenosis with laparoscopic splenectomy. A shortcoming of the laparoscopic approach in hematologic diseases. *Surg Endosc.* 1998;12:101–106.

Despite being more than 10 years old, this article provides good technical tips for the surgeon. The article discusses numerous hematologic indications for splenectomy and their surgical outcome.

Habermalz B, Sauerland S, Decker G, et al. Laparoscopic splenectomy: the clinical practice guidelines of the European Association for Endoscopic Surgery (EAES). *Surg Endosc.* 2008;22:821–848.

Publication of an expert panel using a Delphi process to develop practice guidelines for laparoscopic splenectomy; covers indications, preoperative evaluation, management, and operative and postoperative issues.

Kanhutu K, Jones P, Cheng AC, et al. Spleen Australia guidelines for the prevention of sepsis in patients with asplenia and hyposplenism in Australia and new zealand. *Intern Med J.* 2017;47:848–855.

Well-written and comprehensive guidelines for the prevention of sepsis in asplenia and hyposplenism with illustrations.

Lambert MP, Gernsheimer TB. Clinical updates in adult immune thrombocytopenia. *Blood.* 2017;129:2829–2835.

This study provides the latest clinical guidelines for the management of immune thrombocytopenia.

Musallam KM, Khalife M, Sfeir PM, et al. Postoperative outcomes after laparoscopic splenectomy compared with open splenectomy. *Ann Surg.* 2013;257:1116–1123.

This study provides one of the few reliable comparative evaluations assessing the differences between open and laparoscopic splenectomy.

REFERENCES

1. Lambert MP, Gernsheimer TB. Clinical updates in adult immune thrombocytopenia. *Blood*. 2017;129:2829–2835.
2. Provan D, Stasi R, Newland AC, et al. International consensus report on the investigation and management of primary immune thrombocytopenia. *Blood*. 2010;115:168–186.
3. Abrams CS. Thrombocytopenia. In: Goldman L, Schafer AI, eds. *Goldman's Cecil Medicine*. 24th ed. Philadelphia, PA: Saunders/Elsevier; 2012:1124–1130.
4. Mikhael J, Northridge K, Lindquist K, et al. Short-term and long-term failure of laparoscopic splenectomy in adult immune thrombocytopenic purpura patients: a systematic review. *Am J Hematol*. 2009;84:743–748.
5. Kojouri K, Vesely SK, Terrell DR, et al. Splenectomy for adult patients with idiopathic thrombocytopenic purpura: a systematic review to assess long-term platelet count responses, prediction of response, and surgical complications. *Blood*. 2004;104:2623–2634.
6. Arai Y, Matsui H, Jo T, et al. Comparison of treatments for persistent/chronic immune thrombocytopenia: a systematic review and network meta-analysis. *Platelets*. 2018:1–11.
7. Hansen K, Singer DB. Asplenic-hyposplenic overwhelming sepsis: postsplenectomy sepsis revisited. *Pediatr Dev Pathol*. 2001;4:105–121.
8. Narla J, Mohandas N. Red cell membrane disorders. *Int J Lab Hematol*. 2017;39(suppl 1):47–52.
9. Grace RF, Zanella A, Neufeld EJ, et al. Erythrocyte pyruvate kinase deficiency: 2015 status report. *Am J Hematol*. 2015;90:825–830.
10. Benz EJ, Ebert BL. Hemoglobin variants associated with hemolytic anemia, altered oxygen affinity, and methemoglobinemias. In: Hoffman R, Benz EJ, Silberstein LE, et al., eds. *Hematology Basic Principles and Practice*. 7th ed. Philadephia, PA: Elsevier; 2018:608–615.
11. Cheson BD, Ansell S, Schwartz L, et al. Refinement of the Lugano classification lymphoma response criteria in the era of immunomodulatory therapy. *Blood*. 2016;128:2489–2496.
12. Taner T, Nagorney DM, Tefferi A, et al. Splenectomy for massive splenomegaly: long-term results and risks for mortality. *Ann Surg*. 2013;258:1034–1039.
13. Xing KH, Kahlon A, Skinnider BF, et al. Outcomes in splenic marginal zone lymphoma: analysis of 107 patients treated in British Columbia. *Br J Haematol*. 2015;169:520–527.
14. Kreitman RJ, Arons E. Update on hairy cell leukemia. *Clin Adv Hematol Oncol*. 2018;16:205–215.
15. Goodman GR, Bethel KJ, Saven A. Hairy cell leukemia: an update. *Curr Opin Hematol*. 2003;10:258–266.
16. Hallek M. Chronic lymphocytic leukemia: 2017 update on diagnosis, risk stratification, and treatment. *Am J Hematol*. 2017;92:946–965.
17. Jabbour E, Kantarjian H. Chronic myeloid leukemia: 2018 update on diagnosis, therapy and monitoring. *Am J Hematol*. 2018;93:442–459.
18. Lam KY, Tang V. Metastatic tumors to the spleen: a 25-year clinicopathologic study. *Arch Pathol Lab Med*. 2000;124:526–530.
19. Breitenstein S, Scholz T, Schafer M, et al. Laparoscopic partial splenectomy. *J Am Coll Surg*. 2007;204:179–181.
20. Wu HM, Kortbeek JB. Management of splenic pseudocysts following trauma: a retrospective case series. *Am J Surg*. 2006;191:631–634.
21. Green BT. Splenic abscess: report of six cases and review of the literature. *Am Surg*. 2001;67:80–85.
22. Carbonell AM, Kercher KW, Matthews BD, et al. Laparoscopic splenectomy for splenic abscess. *Surg Laparosc Endosc Percutan Tech*. 2004;14:289–291.
23. Sayeed S, Koniaris LG, Kovach SJ, et al. Torsion of a wandering spleen. *Surgery*. 2002;132:535–536.
24. Delaitre B, Maignien B. Splenectomy by the laparoscopic approach. Report of a case. *Presse Med*. 1991;20:2263.
25. Melman L, Matthews BD. Current trends in laparoscopic solid organ surgery: spleen, adrenal, pancreas, and liver. *Surg Clin North Am*. 2008;88:1033–1046, vii.
26. Shin RD, Lis R, Levergood NR, et al. Laparoscopic versus open splenectomy for splenomegaly: the verdict is unclear. *Surg Endosc*. 2019;33:1298–1303.
27. Habermalz B, Sauerland S, Decker G, et al. Laparoscopic splenectomy: the clinical practice guidelines of the European Association for Endoscopic Surgery (EAES). *Surg Endosc*. 2008;22:821–848.
28. Feng S, Qiu Y, Li X, et al. Laparoscopic versus open splenectomy in children: a systematic review and meta-analysis. *Pediatr Surg Int*. 2016;32:253–259.
29. Konstadoulakis MM, Lagoudianakis E, Antonakis PT, et al. Laparoscopic versus open splenectomy in patients with beta thalassemia major. *J Laparoendosc Adv Surg Tech*. 2006;16:5–8.
30. Gigot JF, Jamar F, Ferrant A, et al. Inadequate detection of accessory spleens and splenosis with laparoscopic splenectomy. A shortcoming of the laparoscopic approach in hematologic diseases. *Surg Endosc*. 1998;12:101–106.
31. Burch M, Misra M, Phillips EH. Splenic malignancy: a minimally invasive approach. *Cancer J*. 2005;11:36–42.
32. Zhan XL, Ji Y, Wang YD. Laparoscopic splenectomy for hypersplenism secondary to liver cirrhosis and portal hypertension. *World J Gastroenterol*. 2014;20:5794–5800.
33. Gernsheimer T, McCrae KR. Immune thrombocytopenic purpura in pregnancy. *Curr Opin Hematol*. 2007;14:574–580.
34. Stavrou E, McCrae KR. Immune thrombocytopenia in pregnancy. *Hematol Oncol Clin North Am*. 2009;23:1299–1316.
35. Flowers JL, Lefor AT, Steers J, et al. Laparoscopic splenectomy in patients with hematologic diseases. *Ann Surg*. 1996;224:19–28.
36. Cavaliere D, Solaini L, Di Pietrantonio D, et al. Robotic vs laparoscopic splenectomy for splenomegaly: a retrospective comparative cohort study. *Int J Surg*. 2018;55:1–4.
37. Bodner J, Kafka-Ritsch R, Lucciarini P, et al. A critical comparison of robotic versus conventional laparoscopic splenectomies. *World J Surg*. 2005;29:982–985; discussion 985-986.
38. Corcione F, Esposito C, Cuccurullo D, et al. Advantages and limits of robot-assisted laparoscopic surgery: preliminary experience. *Surg Endosc*. 2005;19:117–119.
39. Wysocki M, Radkowiak D, Zychowicz A, et al. Prediction of technical difficulties in laparoscopic splenectomy and analysis of risk factors for postoperative complications in 468 cases. *J Clin Med*. 2018;7:547.
40. Buzele R, Barbier L, Sauvanet A, et al. Medical complications following splenectomy. *J Visc Surg*. 2016;153:277–286.
41. Tsamalaidze L, Stauffer JA, Brigham T, et al. Postsplenectomy thrombosis of splenic, mesenteric, and portal vein (PST-SMPv): a single institutional series, comprehensive systematic review of a literature and suggested classification. *Am J Surg*. 2018;216:1192–1204.
42. Tsamalaidze L, Stauffer JA, Vishnu P, et al. Incidence of postsplenectomy thrombosis of splenic, mesenteric and portal vein

(PST-SMPv) in 953 patients at a multi-site single-institution and validation of PST-SMPv classification. *J Ame Col Surg.* 2018;227:S102.
43. Wichman HJ, Cwikiel W, Keussen I. Interventional treatment of mesenteric venous occlusion. *Pol J Radiol.* 2014;79:233–238.
44. Spelman D, Buttery J, Daley A, et al. Guidelines for the prevention of sepsis in asplenic and hyposplenic patients. *Intern Med J.* 2008;38:349–356.
45. Bonanni P, Grazzini M, Niccolai G, et al. Recommended vaccinations for asplenic and hyposplenic adult patients. *Hum Vaccin Immunother.* 2017;13:359–368.
46. Rubin LG, Schaffner W. Clinical practice. Care of the asplenic patient. *N Engl J Med.* 2014;371:349–356.
47. Leemans R, Harms G, Rijkers GT, et al. Spleen autotransplantation provides restoration of functional splenic lymphoid compartments and improves the humoral immune response to pneumococcal polysaccharide vaccine. *Clin Exp Immunol.* 1999;117:596–604.
48. Kanhutu K, Jones P, Cheng AC, et al. Spleen Australia guidelines for the prevention of sepsis in patients with asplenia and hyposplenism in Australia and New Zealand. *Intern Med J.* 2017;47:848–855.
49. El-Alfy MS, El-Sayed MH. Overwhelming postsplenectomy infection: is quality of patient knowledge enough for prevention? *Hematol J.* 2004;5:77–80.

SECTION XI

Chest

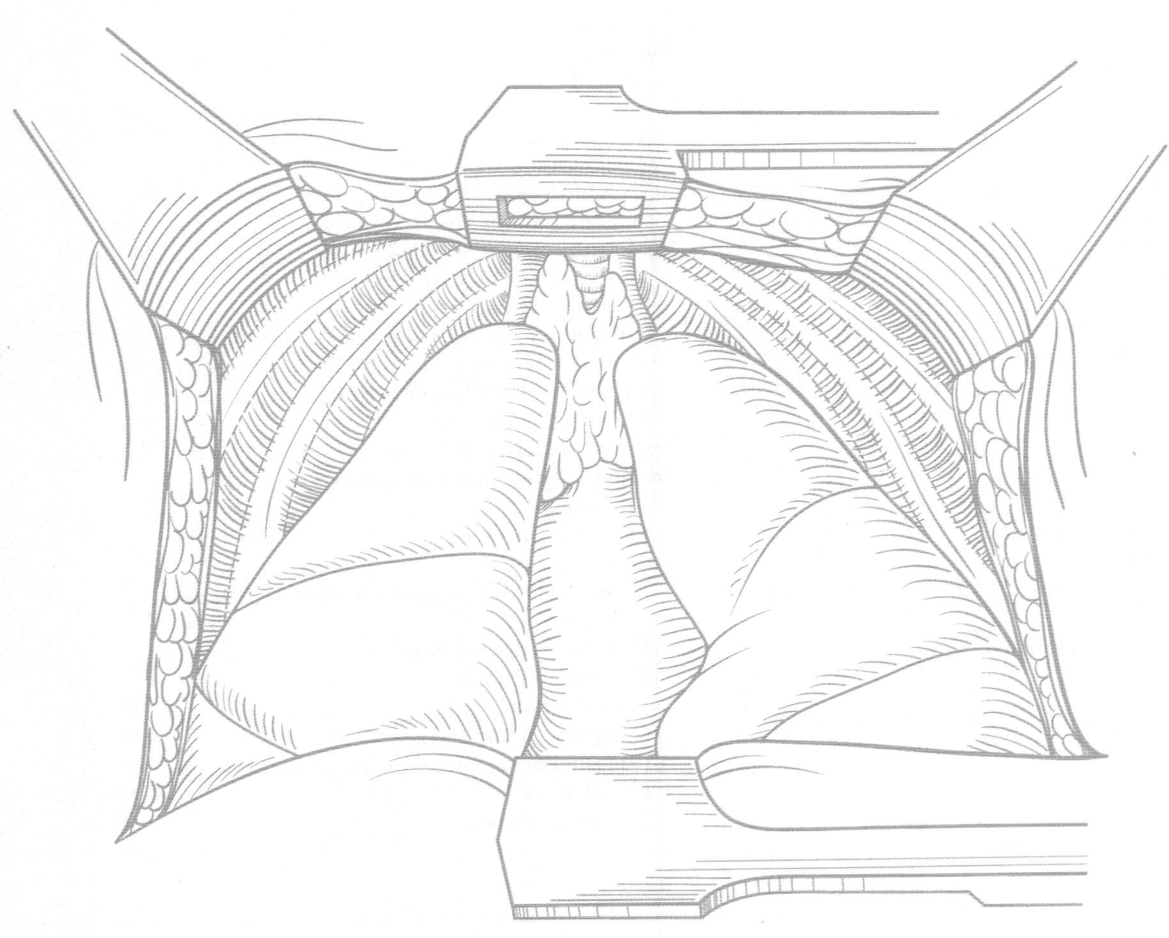

58 CHAPTER

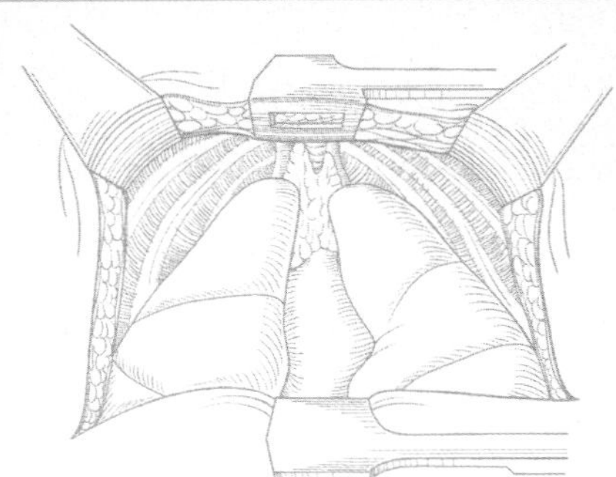

Lung, Chest Wall, Pleura and Mediastinum

Ori Wald, Uzi Izhar, David J. Sugarbaker

OUTLINE

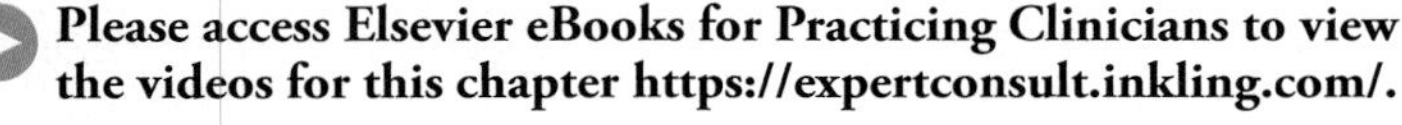

Please access Elsevier eBooks for Practicing Clinicians to view the videos for this chapter https://expertconsult.inkling.com/.

The term *thorax* refers to the area between the neck and abdomen enclosed by the ribs, sternum, and vertebrae radially, the thoracic inlet superiorly, and the diaphragm inferiorly. The chest or thorax supports and protects the internal thoracic organs, provides for the negative inspiratory force that initiates ventilation and the positive expiratory force needed for vocalization, and creates a frame for the neck, upper extremities, thoracic structures, and abdomen.

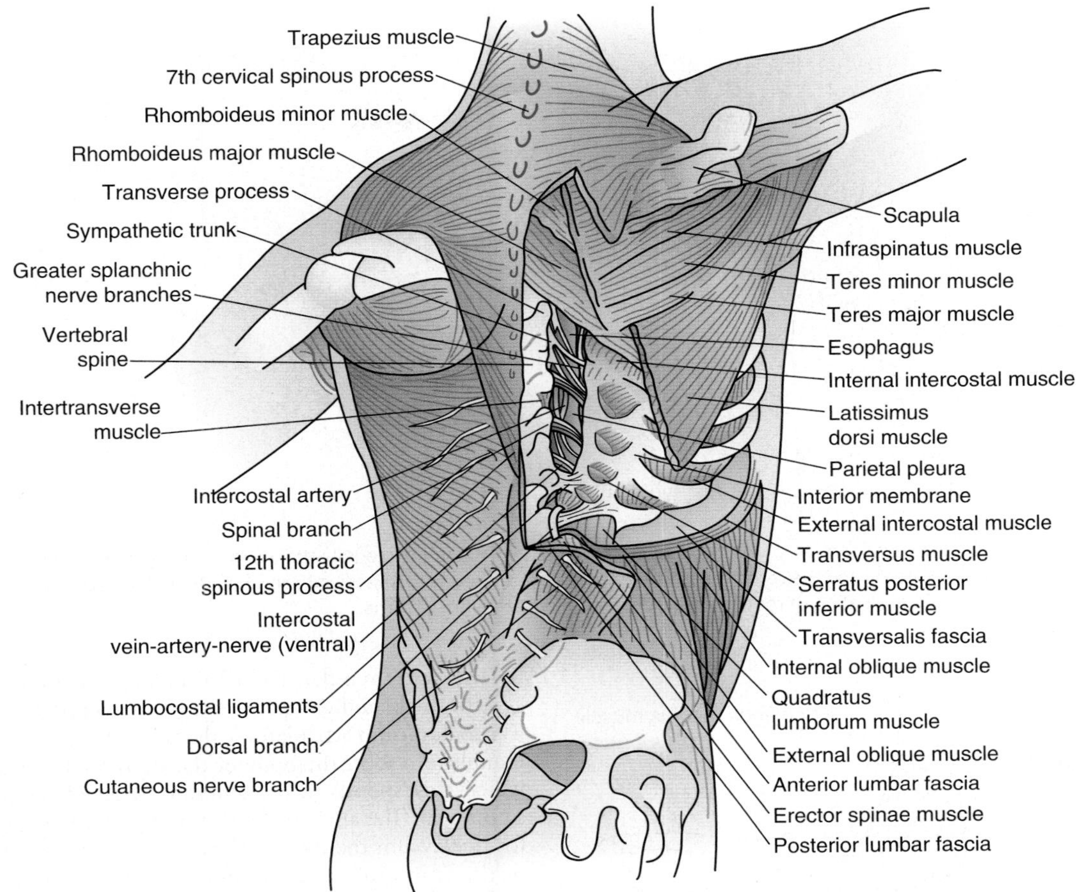

FIG. 58.1 Musculature of the chest wall. (From Ravitch MM, Steichen FM. *Atlas of general thoracic surgery.* Philadelphia, PA: Saunders;1988.)

The major thoracic structures include the heart and lungs, chest wall—including the overlying musculature, ribs, sternum, and vertebrae—diaphragm, trachea, esophagus, and great vessels.

ANATOMY

The thoracic organs are protected by the bony thorax and overlying chest musculature. The parietal pleura, the internal lining of the chest wall, is separated from the visceral pleura, the outer lining of the lung, by a small amount of pleural fluid. The parietal pleura covers the chest wall, mediastinum, diaphragm, and pericardium. The visceral pleura covers the lung and separates the lobes from one another. The pleural space is a potential space that may compress the lungs or heart with fluid, tumor, or infection. The right and left pleural spaces are separated from one another by the mediastinum.

The bony thorax is covered by three groups of muscles: the primary and secondary muscles for respiration and the muscles attaching the upper extremity to the body (Fig. 58.1). The primary muscles include the diaphragm and intercostal muscles. The intercostal muscles of the intercostal spaces include the external, internal, and transverse or innermost muscles. The 11 intercostal spaces, each associated numerically with the rib *superior* to it, contain the intercostal bundles (vein, artery, and nerve) that travel along the lower edge of each rib. All intercostal spaces are wider anteriorly, and each intercostal bundle falls away from the rib posteriorly to become more centrally located within each space. The intercostal muscle layers assist with respiration and protect the thoracic structures. The extrinsic muscles of the chest, latissimus dorsi muscle, serratus anterior muscle, pectoralis major and minor muscles, and cervical muscles (sternocleidomastoid, scalene muscles) attach to the bony thorax, protect the chest wall itself, and may assist with ventilatory efforts in patients with chronic obstructive pulmonary disease (COPD).

The secondary muscles consist of the sternocleidomastoid, serratus posterior, and levatores costarum. The third muscle group attaches the upper extremity to the body. The pectoralis major and minor muscles lie anteriorly and superficially. Posterior superficial musculature includes the trapezius and latissimus dorsi. Deep muscles include the serratus anterior and posterior, the levatores, and the major and minor rhomboids. These superficial and deep muscles help to hold the scapulae to the chest wall. In respiratory distress, the deltoid, pectoralis, and latissimus dorsi muscles form a tertiary system for ventilatory assistance through fixation of the upper extremities.

The bony thorax consists of 12 ribs peripherally extending from the vertebrae posteromedially to the sternum or costal arch anteriorly (Fig. 58.2). The 11th and 12th ribs are "floating ribs" and are not attached directly to the sternum. Ribs 1 to 5 are directly attached to the sternum by costal cartilages. The lower ribs (6–10) coalesce into the costal arch. The first rib is relatively flat and dense and travels from the first thoracic vertebra to the manubrium to create the thoracic inlet (Fig. 58.3). Through this relatively small area pass the great vessels, trachea, esophagus, and innervation to the upper extremity, diaphragm, and larynx.

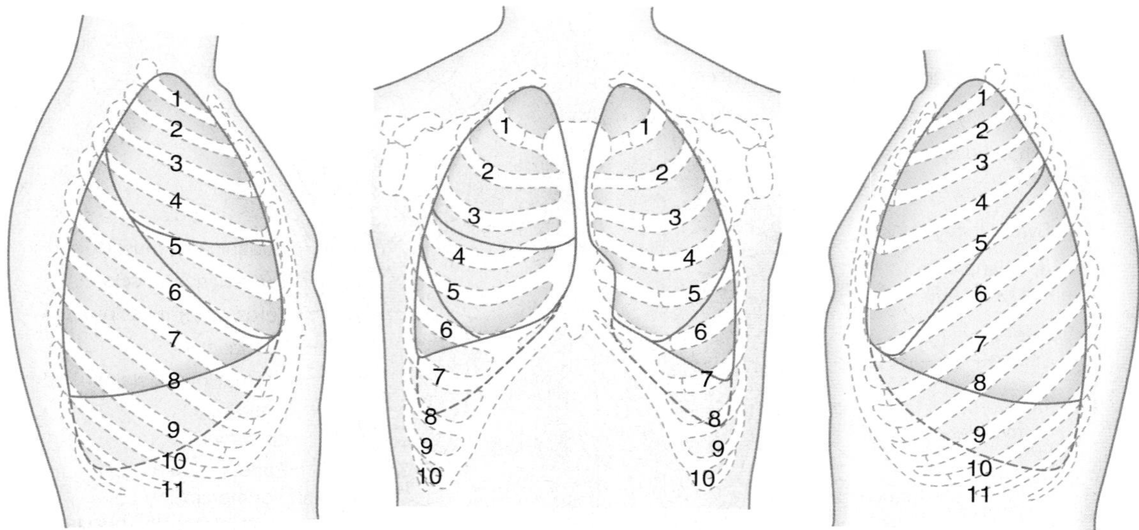

FIG. 58.2 The relationships of the lobes of the lung to the ribs and the pleural reflections with respiration. The topographic anatomy and the relationship of the fissures of the lobes to specific ribs in inspiration and expiration are important in evaluation of routine posteroanterior and lateral chest films.

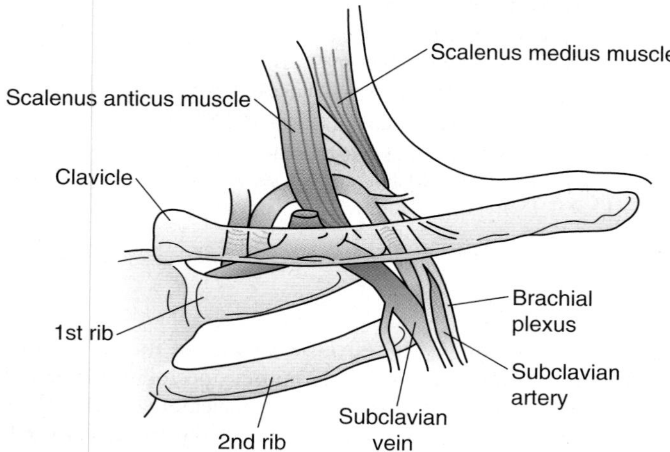

FIG. 58.3 Relationship of the neurovascular bundle to the scalenus muscles, clavicle, and first rib. (From Urschel HC. Thoracic outlet syndromes. In Baue AE, Geha AS, Hammond GL, et al, ed. *Glenn's thoracic and cardiovascular surgery*. 6th ed. Stamford, CT: Appleton & Lange;1996: 567.)

Trauma to this area, manifested by a first rib fracture, is the consequence of a significant mechanical force with likelihood of injury to one or more of these structures. Other structures within the thoracic inlet include the phrenic nerve, the recurrent laryngeal nerve in the tracheoesophageal groove (which recurs around the aorta at the ligamentum arteriosum on the left and around the innominate artery on the right), and the insertion of the thoracic duct posteriorly at the junction of the left subclavian with the left internal jugular veins. The remaining ribs gradually slope downward. Each rib is composed of a head, neck, and shaft. Each head has an upper facet, which articulates with the vertebral body above it, and a lower facet, which articulates with the corresponding thoracic vertebra to that rib, establishing the costovertebral joint. The neck of the rib has a tubercle with an articular facet; this articulates with the transverse process, creating the costotransverse joint and imparting strength to the posterior rib cage.

The sternum is flat, 15 to 20 cm long and approximately 1.0 to 1.5 cm thick, and comprises the manubrium, body, and xiphoid. The manubrium articulates with each clavicle and the first rib. The manubrium joins the body of the sternum at the angle of Louis, which corresponds to the anterior aspect of the junction of the second rib. The angle of Louis is a superficial anatomic landmark for the level of the carina. The anterior cartilaginous attachments of the true ribs to the sternum, along with intercostal muscles and the hemidiaphragms, allow for movement of the ribs with respiration.

The trachea in adults is approximately 12 cm long with 18 to 22 cartilaginous rings. The internal diameter is 2.3 cm laterally and 1.8 cm anteroposteriorly. The larynx ends with the inferior edge of cricoid cartilage. The cricoid is the only complete cartilaginous ring in the trachea. The trachea begins approximately 1.5 cm below the vocal cords and is not rigidly fixed to surrounding tissues. Vertical movement is easily possible. The most rigid point of fixation is where the aortic arch forms a sling over the left mainstem bronchus. The innominate artery crosses over the anterior trachea in a left inferolateral to high right anterolateral direction. The azygos vein arches over the proximal right mainstem bronchus as it travels from posterior to anterior to empty into the superior vena cava. The esophagus is closely applied to the membranous trachea and lies to the left of the midline of the trachea. The recurrent laryngeal nerves run in the tracheoesophageal groove on both the right and the left. The blood supply to the trachea is lateral and segmental from the inferior thyroid, the internal thoracic, the supreme intercostal, and the bronchial arteries. During trachea reconstruction, circumferential dissection greater than 1 to 2 cm may lead to vascular insufficiency with necrosis or anastomotic dehiscence.

Lung development begins at approximately 21 to 28 days' gestation. The true alveolar stage, with air sacs surrounded on all sides by capillaries, occurs from approximately 7 months to term. Alveolar proliferation continues after birth. There are approximately 20 million alveoli at birth, which increase to approximately 300 million by age 10 years, with no more increase after that time. There are 23 generations of bronchi between the trachea and terminal alveoli. Air accounts for 80% of the lung volume, blood accounts for 10%, and solid tissue accounts for

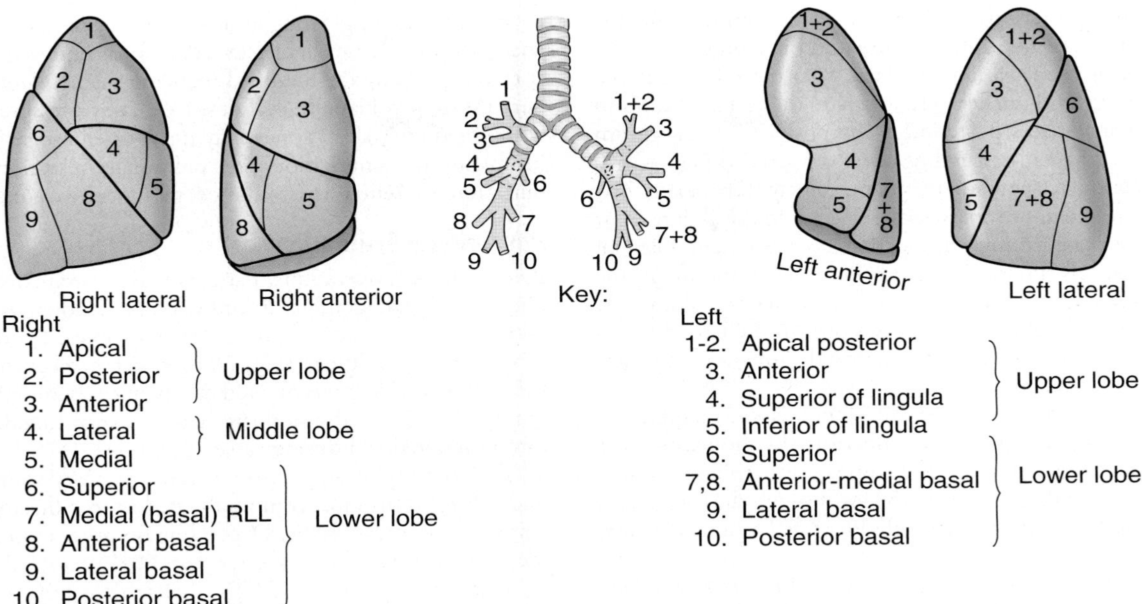

FIG. 58.4 Segments of the pulmonary lobes. (Adapted from Jackson CL, Huber JF. Correlated applied anatomy of the bronchial tree and lungs with a system of nomenclature. *Dis Chest.* 1943;9:319.) *RLL,* Right lower lobe.

approximately 10%. Alveoli make up approximately half of the entire lung volume.

The lungs are broadly divided into five lobes and multiple segments within each lobe (Fig. 58.4). The right lung is composed of three lobes: upper, middle, and lower. Two fissures separate these lobes. The major, or oblique, fissure separates the lower lobe from the upper and middle lobes. The minor or horizontal fissure separates the upper lobe from the middle lobe. The left lung has two lobes—the upper lobe and the lower lobe; the lingula corresponds embryologically to the right middle lobe. A single oblique fissure separates the lobes.

The bronchopulmonary segments are divisions of each lobe that contain anatomically separate arterial, venous, and bronchial supply. There are 10 bronchopulmonary segments on the right and 8 bronchopulmonary segments on the left.

The blood supply of the lung is twofold. Unoxygenated blood circulates from the right ventricle through the pulmonary artery to each lung. After oxygenation in the lung, the blood is returned to the left atrium through the pulmonary veins. Blood supply to the bronchi is from the systemic circulation by bronchial arteries arising from the superior thoracic aorta or the aortic arch, either as discrete branches or in combination with the intercostal arteries.

Lymphatic vessels are present throughout the lung parenchyma and pleura and gradually coalesce toward the hilar areas of the lungs. Generally, lymphatic drainage from the lung affects the ipsilateral lymph nodes; however, flow of lymph from the left lower lobe may drain to the right mediastinal (paratracheal) lymph nodes. Lymphatic drainage within the mediastinum moves cephalad. The pulmonary parenchyma does not contain a nerve supply.

The visceral pleura is separated from the parietal pleura by a small amount of pleural fluid, which allows nearly frictionless movement during respiration. The blood supply of the parietal pleura comes from the systemic arteries and veins, including the posterior intercostal, internal mammary, anterior mediastinal, and superior phrenic arteries and corresponding systemic veins. The blood supply of the visceral pleura is both systemic and pulmonary. The lymphatic drainage of the parietal pleura is into regional lymph nodes, including intercostal, mediastinal, and phrenic nodes. Visceral pleural lymphatics follow the superficial lung lymphatics and drain into the mediastinal lymph nodes. The parietal pleura underlying the ribs has rich nerve endings from the intercostal nerves. Generous local anesthesia is necessary for chest tube insertion. The visceral pleura is innervated by vagal branches and the sympathetic system.

The anatomic boundaries of the mediastinum include the thoracic inlet superiorly, the diaphragm inferiorly, the sternum anteriorly, the vertebral column posteriorly, and medially to the parietal pleura. Thoracic tumors that penetrate through the pleura (by definition) invade the mediastinum. Traditionally, the mediastinum can be divided into anterosuperior, middle, and posterior compartments. No specific anatomic planes define these areas. Fat and lymph nodes are found throughout the mediastinum.

The anterosuperior compartment includes the thymus gland. The right and left lobes of the thymus extend into the cervical areas, and these portions of the thymus must be resected to provide for complete extirpation of the gland.

The middle mediastinum contains the heart; pericardium; great vessels, including the ascending, transverse, and descending aorta; superior and inferior vena cava; pulmonary artery and veins; trachea and bronchi; and phrenic, vagus, and recurrent laryngeal nerves. The phrenic nerve enters the thorax through the thoracic inlet on the anterior aspect of the anterior scalene muscle.

The vagus nerve enters the thoracic inlet through the carotid sheath. It lies anterior to the subclavian and posterior to the innominate artery on the right. The right recurrent laryngeal nerve loops or "recurs" around the innominate artery to innervate the right vocal cord. The vagus nerve then continues posteriorly in the tracheoesophageal groove to innervate the trachea and continues down to innervate the esophagus. On the left side, the vagus nerve enters the thorax through the thoracic inlet, and as it exits the carotid sheath, it moves along the anterior aspect of the aortic arch. The recurrent laryngeal nerve arises from the vagus nerve and loops around under the ligamentum arteriosum and continues superiorly under the aorta and lies in the tracheoesophageal groove as it innervates the left recurrent laryngeal nerve. The left vagus continues posteriorly within the mediastinum along the esophagus to innervate both the trachea and the esophagus.

The posterior mediastinum contains structures between the heart/pericardium and trachea anteriorly and the vertebral column and paravertebral spaces posteriorly. The posterior mediastinum contains the esophagus, descending aorta, azygos and hemiazygos veins, thoracic duct, sympathetic chain, and lymph nodes. The thoracic duct originates from the cisterna chyli in the abdomen. It enters into the chest through the aortic hiatus in an anterolateral position and travels superiorly just to the right of midline in the chest along the anterolateral surface of the vertebral column. At approximately the level of T5, it crosses over to the left and continues superiorly to empty, posteriorly, into the junction of the left jugular and subclavian veins.

The inferior border of the mediastinum is the diaphragm, which separates the abdominal contents from the thorax. Hernias through the esophageal hiatus (paraesophageal hernias), through the foramen of Bochdalek (posteriorly), or through the foramen of Morgagni (anteriorly) may be initially identified as a mediastinal mass.

Each spinal root exits the neural foramina of the vertebral body and bifurcates to form a branch to the intercostal nerve to innervate the skin and intercostal musculature and a branch to the sympathetic ganglion. Intercostal nerves innervate the skin and musculature of the intercostal muscles. The spinal root divides as it exits the neural foramina. One branch goes to the intercostal nerve, and one lies in the posterior vertebral gutter to form the sympathetic ganglion. The thoracic sympathetic trunk comprises several ganglia that lie along the ribs. The most superior ganglion is the stellate ganglion.

SELECTION OF PATIENTS FOR THORACIC OPERATIONS

The physiologic evaluation of the thoracic surgical patient must be individualized for each patient but generally emphasizes the pulmonary and cardiac function. The assessment of a patient's ability to tolerate lung resection from a cardiopulmonary standpoint is fundamental to patient selection for surgery. Patients with advanced pulmonary disease and severe pulmonary dysfunction may have prohibitive risk, which may exist in greater than one third of patients with otherwise resectable lung disease.[1]

Cigarette smoking is associated with increased postoperative pulmonary complications. If the patient is a smoker, he or she must stop smoking immediately. The physician must clearly communicate this message. Although there are few studies specific to pulmonary resection, there is evidence that smoking abstinence of 4 to 8 weeks' duration preoperatively is necessary to reduce the incidence of complications. Ideally, patients are smoke-free for a minimum of 2 weeks and preferably for 4 to 8 weeks before surgery, although smoking cessation at any time is valuable. Smoking cessation programs may be helpful for these patients, and patients may need pharmacologic assistance. This combination may have increased efficacy in smoking cessation efforts over counseling alone.

Before the operation and in the perioperative period, deep venous thrombosis prophylaxis is provided by subcutaneous heparin or low-molecular–weight heparin and by sequential compression stockings. Perioperative antibiotics are used to minimize complications from infections. Postoperative morbidity may also be minimized by adequate pain control to facilitate early ambulation. Routine use of a thoracic epidural catheter, or intercostal rib blocks with long-acting local anesthetics, or patient-controlled analgesia provide excellent pain control. Incentive spirometry assists in expanding the lung and reducing the incidence of pulmonary morbidity. Nasal bilevel positive airway pressure for patients with obstructive sleep apnea may delay or eliminate the need for intubation or reintubation after pulmonary resection. Early mobilization is essential to avoid most perioperative complications.

Physiologic Evaluation

Before thoracic operations, patients may be evaluated by a combination of radiographic and physiologic studies. A plain chest x-ray (CXR) is commonly obtained (Fig. 58.5). Spirometry measures the lung volumes (Fig. 58.6) and the mechanical properties of lung elasticity, recoil, and compliance. Pulmonary function testing (Fig. 58.7) also evaluates gas exchange functions, such as carbon monoxide diffusing capacity (DLCO).

The predicted postoperative forced expiratory volume in 1 second (FEV_1) is the most commonly used as an indicator of postoperative pulmonary reserve. Depending on other evaluable factors, most patients with FEV_1 greater than 60% predicted can tolerate an anatomic lobectomy. If FEV_1 is less than 60% of predicted, further testing in an attempt to estimate postoperative FEV_1 (predicted postoperative FEV_1 [ppo-FEV_1]) could be considered. The quantitative ventilation-perfusion lung scan is used to assist in the calculation of postoperative residual pulmonary function after resection. Patients with a ppo-FEV_1 of 35% to 40% should functionally tolerate the operation.

Quantitative radionucleotide lung perfusion (Fig. 58.8) provides a measurement of the relative function of each lobe and lung and allows an estimation of pulmonary function after lung resection:

$$ppo - FEV_1 = preopFEV_1 \times (1 - \textit{fraction of perfusion to region of planned resection})$$

A ppo-FEV_1 of 30% or less carries a greater risk for supplemental oxygen and ventilator dependence, but a decision to deny surgical resection to this group of patients must be considered on an individual basis because some will do better than expected with careful selection at experienced centers. Finally, in the immediate postoperative period, the ppo-FEV_1 is not likely to be realized secondary to limited ambulation, pain, or other emotional or physical factors.

DLCO can be measured by several methods, although the single-breath test is most commonly performed. DLCO measures the rate at which test molecules such as carbon monoxide move from the alveolar space to combine with hemoglobin in the red blood cells. DLCO is determined by calculating the difference between inspired and expired samples of gas. DLCO levels less than 40% to 50% are associated with increased perioperative risk.

The ratio of FEV_1 to forced vital capacity (FEV_1/FVC) describes the relationship between the FEV_1 and the functional lung volume. In obstructive disease, the ratio is low (FEV_1 is low, and FVC is high); in restrictive disease, the ratio is about normal because both FEV_1 and FVC are reduced.

Flow-volume loops derived from spirometry describe the relationship between lung volume and air flow as the lung volume changes during a forced expiration and inspiration. The typical test consists of tidal breathing at rest, followed by maximal inspiratory effort to total lung capacity, then maximal expiratory effort to residual volume, concluding with maximal inspiratory effort to total lung capacity.

Cardiopulmonary exercise testing (CPET) can be extremely useful in the evaluation of marginal candidates (ppo-FEV_1 or

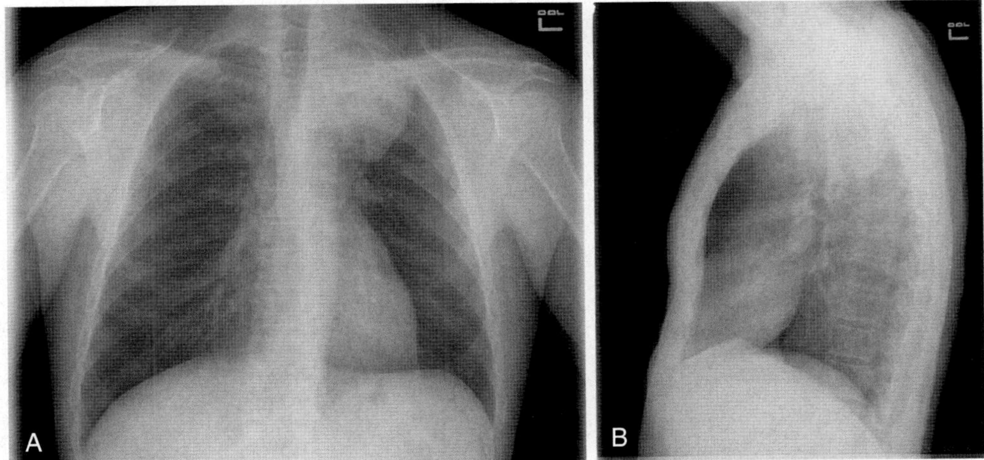

FIG. 58.5 Initial chest x-rays. This patient is a 67-year-old man with a weight loss of 10 pounds in 4 weeks and a 35–pack-year history of cigarette smoking. He quit smoking 10 years ago. He had left shoulder pain for 4 months with no dyspnea, cough, hemoptysis, or other symptoms. Massage and other musculoskeletal manipulation did not improve his symptoms. A chest x-ray with posteroanterior (A) and lateral (B) views demonstrates an 8.4-cm left upper lung mass. Some deviation of the distal trachea is noted.

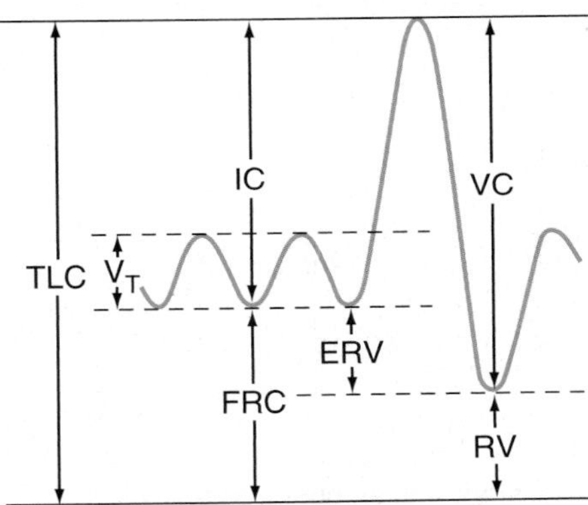

FIG. 58.6 Spirometry with subdivisions of lung volumes. *ERV*, Expiratory reserve volume; *FRC*, functional residual capacity (i.e., lung volume at end expiration); *IC*, inspiratory capacity; *RV*, residual volume (i.e., lung volume after forced expiration from FRC); *TLC*, total lung capacity; *VC*, vital capacity (i.e., maximal volume of gas inspired from RV); V_T, tidal volume.

predicted postoperative DLCO <50% predicted) or patients who appear more disabled than expected from simple spirometry measurements. CPET includes exercise electrocardiography, heart rate response to exercise, and measurements of minute ventilation and oxygen uptake per minute. CPET allows a calculation of maximal oxygen consumption (VO_2 max) and provides insight into overall cardiopulmonary function (the "cardiopulmonary axis") that cannot be ascertained from other objective studies. CPET may identify clinically occult cardiac disease and provide a more accurate assessment of pulmonary function than spirometry and DLCO, which tend to overestimate functional loss after resection.

A patient's risk of perioperative morbidity and mortality may be stratified by VO_2 max. A level less than 11 to 15 mL/kg/min is associated with an increased risk, and VO_2 max less than 10 mL/kg/min indicates high risk.[2]

In patients undergoing evaluation for lung volume reduction surgery or for lung transplantation, a 6-minute walk test is used for a measure of the cardiac and pulmonary reserve. Patients are told to walk as far and as fast as they can during this time period. Distances of more than 1000 feet suggest an uncomplicated course.

Measurement of diaphragm function by fluoroscopy, the "sniff test," or by ultrasonography is needed to determine symmetry of effort and to exclude paradoxical movement of the diaphragm. Paradoxical movement (elevation of one hemidiaphragm with active contraction/retraction of the other diaphragm) suggests paresis or paralysis. This finding may suggest a specific reason for breathlessness. Diaphragm plication may be therapeutic.

No single test result should be viewed as an absolute contraindication to surgical resection. Although the physiologic assessment for patients undergoing normal spirometry and minimal comorbidity is straightforward, patients with marginal preoperative indices must be considered on an individual basis.

Thoracic Incisions

The choice of incision depends on the operation, the patient's underlying physiologic condition, and the anticipated benefits and limitations of the planned approach. Video-assisted thoracoscopic surgery (VATS), robotic surgery, and other minimally invasive surgical techniques have been developed to treat most thoracic problems, including lung cancer, mediastinal tumors, pleural diseases, and parenchymal diseases, and to diagnose and stage thoracic malignancies. Various small incisions are made for the camera and other instruments depending on the location of the tumor. The ribs are not spread. Improved lighting and optics create excellent exposure and visualization. Advantages of minimally invasive surgical techniques include minimizing pain and surgical trauma from the incisions, decreasing hospitalization, and improving convalescence.

A thoracotomy requires spreading the ribs with a retractor and is used for operations on a single thorax. The patient is placed in a lateral decubitus position. The location of the incision may be posterior, axillary, or anterior. Posteriorly, an oblique incision is used with or without sparing the latissimus dorsi muscle. The chest is typically entered through the fifth interspace for pulmonary resection. A vertical axillary incision is made anterior to the latissimus dorsi muscle, and the chest is entered through the fourth interspace. This approach provides excellent hilar visualization. The anterior or anterolateral thoracotomy is created by a curvilinear incision underneath the inferior border of the pectoralis

Section of Pulmonary Medicine
Pulmonary Function Report

Last Name:		First Name:	
Identification:			
Age:	56 years	Room:	Out-patient
Sex:	Male	Race:	Caucasian
Height:	65 inches	Physician:	
Weight:	177 lbs	Operator:	
Date			
Time			

Spirometry	Pred	Pre BD	%Pred	Post BD	%Pred	%Chg
FVC....[l]	3.48	3.07	88	3.07	88	0
FEV_1....[l]	2.83	2.23	79	2.26	80	1
FEV_1/VC....[%]	80.81	72.26	89	69.78	86	–3
FEF 25–75....[l/s]	3.01	1.37	45	1.46	49	7
PEF....[l/s]	7.57	6.43	85	7.10	94	10
FIVC....[l]	3.48	3.09	89	3.24	93	5
FIV_1....[l]		3.09		3.24		5
FIV_1/FVC.... [%]		100.00		100.00		0

Lung Volumes	Pred	Measured	%Pred
SVC....[l]	3.48	3.04	87
TLC....[l]	5.51	5.54	101
RV....[l]	1.96	2.49	127
RV/TLC....[%]	35.9	45.0	125
FRC-Box....[l]	2.24	3.01	134

Diffusion SB	Pred	Measured	%Pred
DLCO SB....[ml/min/mm Hg]	22.59	23.81	105
DLCO Hb Corr[ml/min/mm Hg]	22.6	24.2	107
VA....[l]		5.27	
DLCO/VA....[ml/min/mm Hg/l]	3.93	4.52	115
Hb....[g/100ml]		14.1	

Interpretation

Spirometry reveals an isolated reduction in mid-expiratory flows consistent with an obstructive small airways defect. Increased residual volume (RV) is consistent with air trapping. Following the inhalation of a bronchodilator, there is no improvement of the obstructive airway defect. The diffusing capacity is normal.

FIG. 58.7 The pulmonary function report provides complete spirometry data based on predicted values for height and weight. In this patient, the forced expiratory volume in one second (FEV_1) is 2.26 L after bronchodilators, which is 80% of predicted. The carbon monoxide diffusing capacity (DLCO) is measured as 23.81 mL/min/mm Hg, which is 105% of predicted. *FEF*, Forced expiratory flow; *FIV_1*, forced inspiratory volume in one second; *FIVC*, forced inspiratory vital capacity; *FRC*, functional reserve capacity; *FVC*, forced vital capacity; *Hb*, hemoglobin; *PEF*, peak expiratory flow; *SB*, single breath; *SVC*, slow vital capacity; *TLC*, total lung capacity; *VA*, alveolar volume; *VC*, vital capacity.

major muscle at the inframammary fold. A median sternotomy is performed using a vertical incision from the sternal notch to the xiphoid. A sternal saw is then used to divide the sternum in the midline. With gentle retraction, the sternum can be spread approximately 8 to 10 cm to allow access to the mediastinum, heart, great vessels, and right and left thorax. The pleura can be opened on either side to explore the hemithorax. The sternum is usually closed with stainless steel wire.

The transverse sternotomy or "clamshell" incision is larger than a median sternotomy and more uncomfortable for the patient. This incision combines two anterior thoracotomy incisions in the inframammary fold with transverse division of the sternum at the fourth intercostal space. Both internal mammary arteries are ligated. This approach is ideal for accessing both the right and the left hilum and providing additional exposure for large mediastinal tumors, bilateral hilar dissections, bilateral lung transplantation, or posterior-based metastases in both lungs.

LUNG

Congenital Lesions of the Lung

Various congenital lung abnormalities can occur as a consequence of disturbed embryogenesis. Bilateral agenesis of the lungs is fatal. Unilateral agenesis may occur more frequently on the left (~70%) than on the right (~30%), with more than a 2:1 male-to-female ratio.

Hypoplasia of the lungs may occur as a result of interference with the development of the alveolar system during the last 2 months of gestation. Bochdalek hernia is the most frequent cause

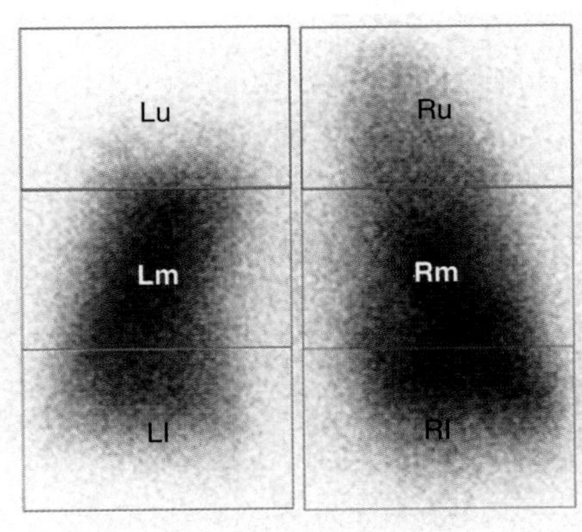

	Left lung		Right lung	
	%	Kct	%	Kct
Upper zone:	4.7	22.66	9.5	46.27
Middle zone:	24.0	116.91	28.3	138.05
Lower zone:	13.2	64.20	20.3	99.02
Total lung:	41.8	203.77	58.2	283.34

FIG. 58.8 The quantitative perfusion lung scan report provides the lung volume and the perfusion to each lung. In a patient with a large left hilar tumor, perfusion may be reduced in the involved left lung compared with the uninvolved right lung. The predicted post–left pneumonectomy right lung function can be obtained by multiplying the right lung percent perfusion (58.2%) by the observed best FEV_1 (2.26 L). The resulting value, 1.31 L, 46.5% predicted, is the predicted postoperative FEV_1 (after left pneumonectomy). This value suggests that a left pneumonectomy would be functionally tolerated. *Ll,* Left lower zone; *Lm,* left middle zone; *Lu,* left upper zone; *Rl,* right lower zone; *Rm,* right middle zone; *Ru,* right upper.

of hypoplasia. Conditions associated with hypoplasia of the lungs include oligohydramnios, prune-belly syndrome (deficiency in the abdominal musculature, genitourinary abnormalities), scimitar syndrome (abnormal pulmonary vein draining into the inferior vena cava, demonstrated as a crescent along the right heart border on cardiac angiography), and dextrocardia. Isolated pulmonary hypoplasia is rare.

Hyaline membrane disease (or infant respiratory distress syndrome) is frequent in premature infants (24–28 weeks' gestation) and infants of diabetic mothers. At a gestational age of 24–28 weeks, infants have an immature surfactant system. Hyaline membrane disease develops in the alveoli, causing congestion and a lung with a deep purple gross appearance. Respiratory distress frequently ensues, requiring high concentrations of oxygen. CXRs demonstrate a reticulogranular ground-glass appearance from the interstitial edema. As needs for oxygen and ventilator pressure increase to counteract this interstitial edema, pneumothorax frequently occurs.

Congenital Cystic Lesions

Congenital cystic lesions present in 1 in 10,000 to 35,000 births and present as a spectrum of anomalies. Majority of these cystic lesions comprise congenital pulmonary airway malformations (CPAM)/congenital cystic adenomatoid malformations, pulmonary sequestrations, congenital lobar emphysema, and bronchogenic cysts. They generally occur as a result of separation of the pulmonary remnants from airway branchings. Clinically, approximately one third of patients do not have symptoms; one third have cough; and one third have infection or, rarely, hemoptysis. Treatment may be with antibiotics or, for more severe localized cases, with resection. Any cystic lesion that enlarges on serial radiographs needs to be considered for resection.[3]

Bronchogenic cysts arises from a tracheal or bronchial diverticulum (see also "Primary Mediastinal Cysts"). This diverticulum becomes completely separated from the trachea and is frequently found as an asymptomatic mass on routine CXRs. Symptoms may arise from compression of adjacent airways and from infection. On computed tomography (CT) of the chest, a homogeneous, well-circumscribed mass adjacent to the trachea may be seen (Fig. 58.9). Infected cysts are characterized by an air fluid level. Bronchogenic cysts accounts for 10% of mediastinal masses in children, they are located in the midmediastinum. Treatment consists of excision in symptomatic cases while controversy exists regarding resection in asymptomatic patients.

Lobar emphysema is the most commonly resected congenital cystic lesion (50%). Its pathogenesis is related to intrinsic or extrinsic airway obstruction leading to the creation of a "ball-valve" mechanism and consequently to air trapping. The onset of rapidly progressive respiratory distress usually occurs 4 to 5 days to several weeks after birth. It rarely occurs after 6 months of age. It affects the upper lobes predominately. Treatment is lobectomy.

CPAMs, previously termed *congenital cystic adenomatoid malformations,* are the second most commonly resected congenital cystic lesion.[4] They result from abnormalities in branching morphogenesis of the lung. There are five types of CPAM according to the Stocker classification (types 0-4), with type 1 being the most common one (60%–70%). In this type of malformation, single or multiple cysts larger than 2 cm that are covered by pseudostratified columnar epithelium are formed yielding an "adenomatoid" malformation. The lung has the appearance of Swiss cheese and feels like a large rubbery mass. With air trapping and overdistention, respiratory distress may occur, which is optimally relieved by lobectomy. Type 4 CPAM is strongly associated with malignancy in particular pleuropulmonary blastoma.

Bronchopulmonary sequestration (BPS) is an area of embryonic lung tissue, separate from the tracheobronchial tree, which receives blood supply from an anomalous systemic artery from the aorta, not the pulmonary artery. This condition occurs secondary to an accessory lung bud caudal to the normal lung, but with a lack of absorption of primitive surrounding splanchnic vessels. During lung development, interlobar sequestration (75%) occurs early. Later, after the pleura forms, extralobar sequestration occurs (25%), primarily on the left side (66%), and is completely enclosed by its own pleura. The extralobar sequestration blood supply is usually from the thoracic or upper abdominal aorta to systemic (azygos or hemiazygos veins). Extralobar sequestration is more common in male patients. Intralobar sequestration occurs within the lower lobes predominately (>95%) and is equally distributed between the right and left lower lobes. Intralobar sequestration blood supply is from the descending thoracic aorta that usually traverses the pulmonary ligament. Venous drainage is via the pulmonary veins. The thoracic aorta provides 95% of the systemic blood supply to the pulmonary sequestration. Infants with respiratory symptoms or with large BPS are treated by surgical excision. Asymptomatic small BPS can either be treated by embolization of the feeding artery or may be conservatively managed by observation (Fig. 58.10). Hybrid BPS/CPAM lesions have been reported in a substantial proportion of cases of BPS. These hybrid

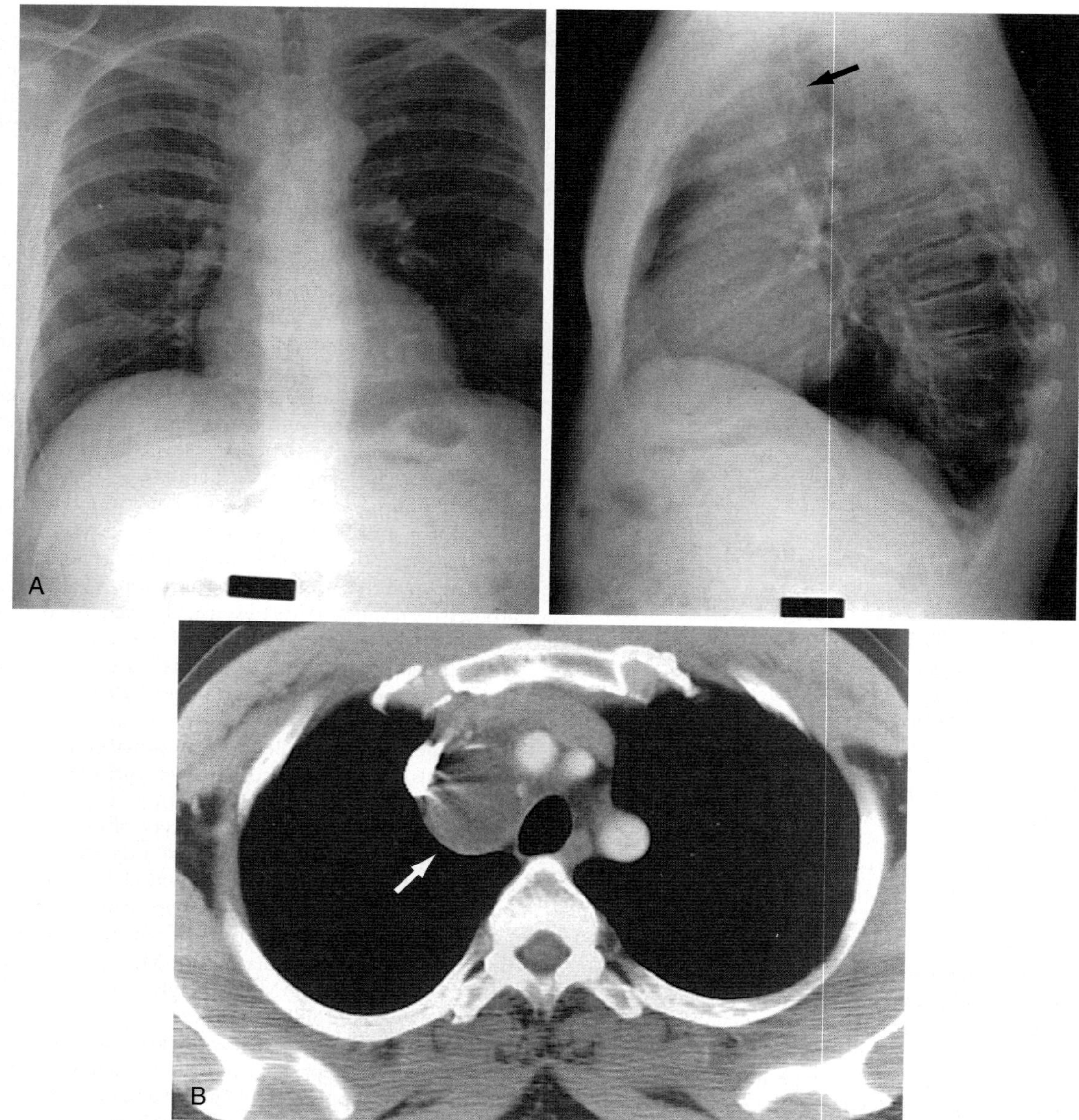

FIG. 58.9 Two chest x-rays (A) and a computed tomography scan (B) of the chest of a patient with a bronchogenic cyst *(arrow)*.

lesions have histologic features of CPAM and a blood supply from a systemic artery.

Cystic fibrosis is an autosomal recessive disorder that is found more commonly in whites. Excessively thick mucus leads to recurrent infections, bronchitis, and bronchiectasis. Fibrosis and cystic changes on pathologic examinations are identified. Pneumothorax may occur secondary to air trapping. Lung failure is the most frequent cause of death. Bilateral lung transplantation should be considered when the disease rapidly progresses and the remaining pulmonary reserve is low.

Congenital Abnormalities of the Trachea and Bronchi

Esophageal atresia with tracheoesophageal fistula is the most frequent abnormality of the trachea in infants (see Chapter 67). Bronchial atresia is the second most frequent congenital pulmonary lesion after tracheoesophageal fistula.[5] The lung tissue distal to the atresia expands and becomes emphysematous as a result of air entry through collateral airways/pores. With no exit for air or mucus because of this blind bronchial stump, emphysema from air trapping or development of a mucocele may occur. CXRs may demonstrate hyperinflation of a lobe or a segment. The oval density may be identified between the hyperinflated lung and the hilum. The left upper lobe is the most frequently involved of all lobes within the lung. Diagnosis may be confirmed with bronchography or CT. The surgeon must rule out a mucous plug, adenoma, vascular compression, or sequestration.

Tracheal agenesis is a rare phenomenon and is fatal. The trachea is absent from the larynx to the carina, and bronchi communicate with the esophagus.

Tracheal stenosis is also rare and consists of generalized hypoplasia, a funnel-like trachea, and bronchial and segmental malformations. The right upper lobe bronchus may come from the trachea directly and may be associated with an aberrant left pulmonary artery (so-called pulmonary artery sling). Completely

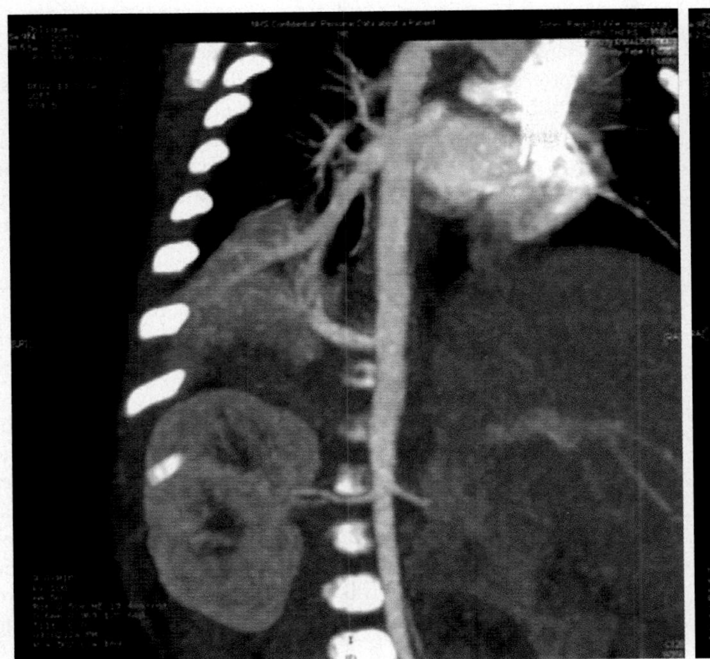
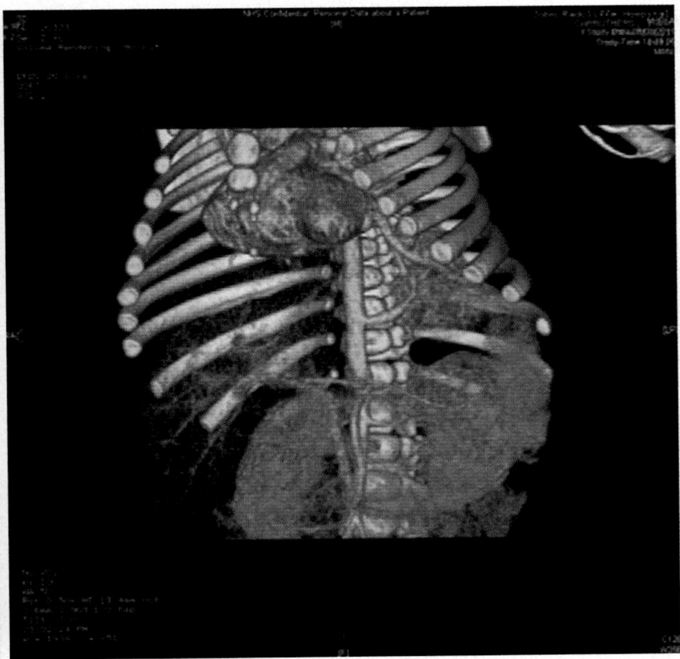

FIG. 58.10 Contrast-enhanced computed tomography and a 3D-reconstruction image showing bronchopulmonary sequestration in the right lower lung field. Note the feeding vessel arising from the aorta. (From Durell J, Lakhoo K. Congenital cystic lesions of the lung. *Early Hum Dev.*2014; 90:935–939.)

circular tracheal rings are commonly associated with a pulmonary sling. Repair of the trachea is by vertical incision and widening of the tracheal lumen.

Tracheomalacia can be identified by diagnostic imaging (dynamic expiratory CT) or bronchoscopy. The surgeon should notice marked variation of the tracheal lumen with inspiration and expiration. Collapse of greater than 70% of the lumen during expiration is consistent with this condition. Respiratory difficulty ensues from the intermittently collapsing trachea. Relief of the extrinsic compression is needed. Stent placement in adults or posterior splinting or primary tracheobronchoplasty may be required. This condition may have a congenital predisposition but is most often seen in adults with COPD.

Congenital Vascular Disorders

Congenital vascular disorders of the lungs may occur.[6] In Swyer-James and Macleod syndrome, there is idiopathic hyperlucent lung. This problem develops from chronic pulmonary infections such as bronchiectasis. As the consolidation persists, decreased pulmonary artery blood supply may cause an "autopneumonectomy" and a hyperlucent lung.

Scimitar syndrome is associated with hypoplastic right lung with drainage of the pulmonary vein to the inferior vena cava. The anomaly is usually corrected using extracorporeal cardiopulmonary support. A patch from the pulmonary vein to the left atrium via an atrial septal defect corrects this problem.

Pulmonary arteriovenous malformations may exist as one or more pulmonary artery-to-pulmonary vein connections, bypassing the pulmonary capillary bed. This connection results in a right-to-left shunt. Approximately one third of these patients have hereditary hemorrhagic telangiectasia (Osler-Weber-Rendu syndrome). Approximately half of the malformations are small (<1 cm) and tend to be multiple. Half are greater than 1 cm and usually less than 5 cm and tend to be subpleural. These lesions need to be considered in the differential diagnosis of any patient with hemoptysis that is unexplained on the basis of bronchoscopy or routine imaging. Either local resection or catheter embolization of these lesions can be curative.

A pulmonary vascular sling consists of an anomalous or aberrant left pulmonary artery, which causes airway obstruction, and is associated with other anomalies. The aberrant left pulmonary artery arises from the right (main) pulmonary artery and courses between the trachea and the esophagus to supply the left lung. More than 90% of patients have wheezing and stridor. Esophagoscopy shows the anomalous vessel anterior to the esophagus; bronchoscopy demonstrates the vessel posterior to the trachea. Surgical correction requires relocation of the left pulmonary artery from its right-sided origin to the main pulmonary artery. If tracheal stenosis with complete tracheal rings are identified segmental resection of the trachea or tracheoplasty should be performed.

Vascular rings[7] constitute 7% of all congenital heart problems. The most common vascular ring is a double aortic arch, which occurs in 60% of these patients. The right, or posterior, arch is the larger arch and gives rise to the right carotid and right subclavian arteries. The ring wraps around both the trachea and the esophagus. A posterior indentation is noted in the esophagus on barium swallow. Simple division corrects the anomaly. A right aortic arch with a retroesophageal left subclavian artery and left ligamentum arteriosum occurs in approximately 25% to 30% of patients with vascular rings. Intracardiac defects occur with a double aortic arch. Most of these infants require operation within the first weeks or months of life. Patients with vascular rings require a careful history and barium swallow for diagnosis. Bronchoscopy or esophagoscopy are not routinely ordered because they may be harmful. Echocardiography is a complementary test. CT scan and magnetic resonance imaging (MRI) may be used to further delineate the anatomy. Repair is performed through the left chest. Division of the smaller arch, usually the left one, is undertaken. The ligamentum is divided, and the trachea and the esophagus are freed from the surrounding tissues. When a retroesophageal right subclavian artery with left ligament occurs, the patient may complain of dysphagia, which is referred to as *dysphagia lusoria.* The differential diagnosis includes neuromotor diseases of the esophagus or stricture.

LUNG CANCER

Lung cancer is a significant global health problem. In the United States in 2018, there were estimated to be 234,030 new cases of lung cancer. Lung cancer is the most frequent cause of death from cancer in men and women and accounts for 13.0% of all cancer diagnoses and 26% of all cancer deaths in the United States. Lung cancer deaths exceed the combined total deaths from breast, prostate, and colorectal cancer. Since 1987, more women have died of lung cancer than breast cancer. Lung cancer deaths have decreased by approximately 3% per year in men and by approximately 2% per year in women. Smoking cessation in women has lagged behind smoking cessation in men, and thus the incidence of lung cancer in women has not declined as much as the incidence in men (Fig. 58.11). The decline in lung cancer incidence and mortality rate likely reflects decreasing cigarette smoking and potentially earlier detection of smaller, asymptomatic lung cancers. African American men have both the highest incidence and the highest death rate from cancer of the lung and bronchus.[8]

Lung cancer survival is stage specific. The overall 1-year and 5-year survival rates are 44% and 17%, respectively. Patients presenting with localized (early-stage) lung cancer have a 5-year survival rate of 54%. However, greater than 50% of patients present with locally advanced or metastatic disease and their 1-year and 5-year survival rates do not exceed 26% and 4%, respectively.[9]

Cigarette smoking is unequivocally the most important risk factor in the development of lung cancer. Other environmental factors may predispose to lung cancer. Environmental radon gas exposure is estimated to be the second most important risk factor. Other factors include asbestos, arsenic, chromium, nickel, organic chemicals, iatrogenic radiation exposure, air pollution, and secondary smoke from nonsmokers.

Radon is associated with approximately 18,000 lung cancer deaths a year. Radon is a natural radioactive gas released from the normal decay of uranium in the soil. Inhalation is associated with health risk. Inexpensive test kits are available to determine the amount of radon present in homes.

Optimal treatment of lung cancer requires accurate diagnosis and clinical staging before treatment begins. The anatomic basis for staging (tumor, lymph nodes, and metastases) includes the physical properties of the tumor and the presence of regional or systemic metastases. The biologic and immunologic basis for staging/disease characterization (molecular and immunologic markers prognostic for survival and indicative of the potential to respond to specific treatments) may be incorporated into staging systems of the future.

Pathology

In 2015 the World Health Organization (WHO) issued a revised classification of tumors of the lung. By expanding the use

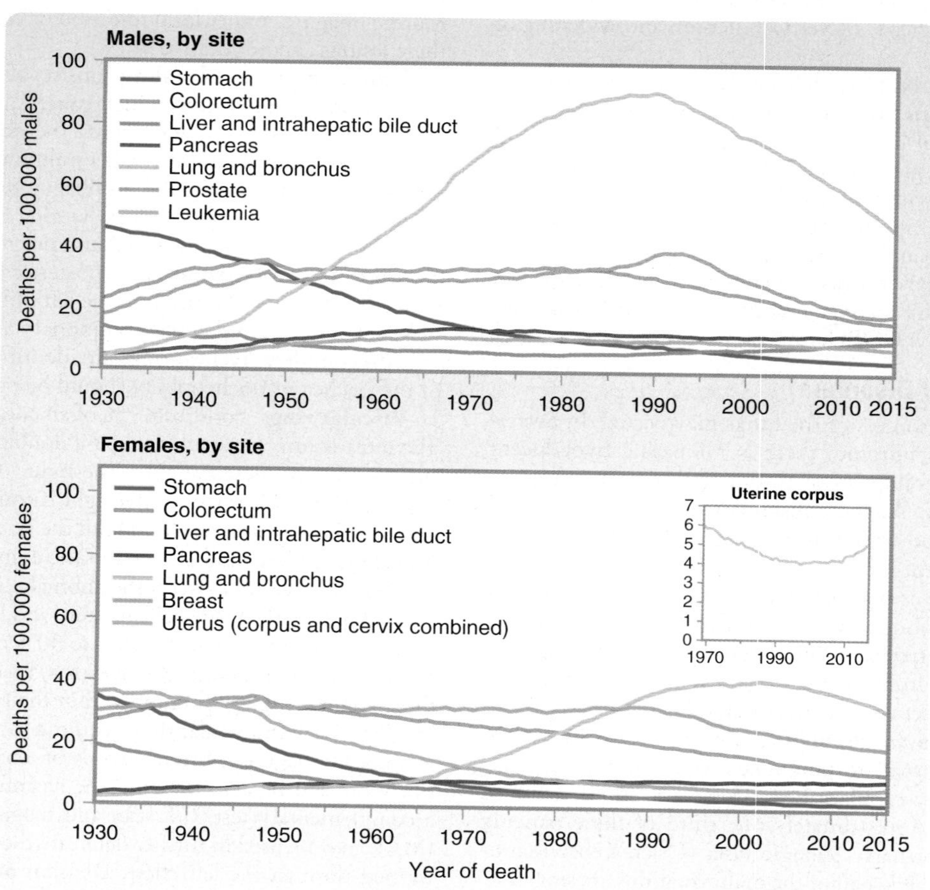

FIG. 58.11 Trends in cancer death rates by sex for selected cancers, United States 1930 to 2015. Rates are age adjusted to the 2000 United States standard population. (From Siegel RL, Miller KD, Jemal A. Cancer statistics, 2018. *CA Cancer J Clin.* 2018;68:7–30.)

of immunohistochemistry and by providing recommendations for genetic characterization of the tumors more accurate and clinically relevant subtyping of the tumors was established. The major types of malignant tumors of the lung are adenocarcinomas, squamous cell carcinomas (SCCs), large cell carcinomas, and neuroendocrine tumors of the lung; each of these groups has multiple subtypes that differ by their morphologic, genetic, and biologic properties. Key characteristics of these tumors are described below.

Adenocarcinomas are malignant epithelial tumors with glandular differentiation or mucin production, showing acinar, papillary, lepidic (bronchioloalveolar), or solid with mucin growth patterns or a mixture of these patterns. Adenocarcinoma of the lung is the most frequent histologic type of lung cancer accounting for approximately 45% of all lung cancers. Microscopic features consist of cuboidal to columnar cells with adequate to abundant pink or vacuolated cytoplasm and some evidence of gland formation. Most of these tumors (75%) are peripherally located. Adenocarcinoma of the lung tends to metastasize earlier than SCC of the lung and more frequently to the central nervous system.

The pathology of adenocarcinoma has been revised.[10] Bronchoalveolar or bronchioloalveolar carcinoma and mixed type adenocarcinoma have been eliminated, and adenocarcinoma in situ (pure lepidic growth, tumor cells proliferating along the surface of intact alveolar walls without stromal or vascular invasion) and minimally invasive adenocarcinoma (predominantly lepidic growth with <5 mm invasion) have been created. A solitary tumor focus of adenocarcinoma in situ or minimally invasive adenocarcinoma is treated in a manner similar to invasive adenocarcinoma (in the majority of cases anatomic resection of the affected segment/lobe of the lung). The management of multifocal adenocarcinoma in situ disease is generally more complex. In this scenario, surgical resection, ablation, and radiation of the most active lesions is performed while following up on the progression of the additional lesions. The aim is to eliminate the lesion that progress while preserving as much lung tissue as possible.

SCC is a malignant epithelial tumor showing keratinization and/or intercellular bridges that arises from bronchial epithelium. Over 90% of SCC occur in cigarette smokers, these tumors occur in approximately 30% of patients with lung cancer. Approximately two thirds of these tumors are centrally located and tend to expand against the bronchus, causing extrinsic compression. SCC are prone to undergo central necrosis and cavitation. SCC tends to metastasize later than adenocarcinoma. Microscopically, keratinization, stratification, and intercellular bridge formation are exhibited. SCC may be more readily detected on sputum cytology than adenocarcinoma.

A diagnosis of large cell undifferentiated carcinoma may be made when specific cytologic features of SCC or adenocarcinoma or neuroendocrine differentiation are lacking. These tumors tend to occur peripherally and may metastasize relatively early. Microscopically, these tumors show sheets of round to polygonal cells with prominent nucleoli and abundant pale-staining cytoplasm without differentiating features.

Neuroendocrine tumors of the lung share specific morphologic, ultrastructural, immunohistochemical, and molecular features; they arise from cells derived from the embryologic neural crest. This group of tumors includes small cell carcinomas, large cell neuroendocrine carcinomas, and typical and atypical carcinoids. Typical carcinoids show a relatively indolent growth pattern while small cell carcinoma and large cell neuroendocrine carcinomas are highly aggressive. Small cell lung cancer represents approximately 20% of all lung cancers. In the majority of cases (80%), these tumors are centrally located and tend to spread early to mediastinal lymph nodes and distant sites, especially the bone marrow and brain. Microscopically, the tumors appear as sheets or clusters of cells with dark nuclei and little cytoplasm. Neurosecretory granules are evident on electron microscopy. Small cell lung cancer is staged according to the lung cancer TNM staging system; however, from a clinical perspective, the disease may also be addressed as *limited stage* (disease restricted to an ipsilateral hemithorax within a single radiation port) and *extensive stage* (obvious metastatic disease). These tumors are often advanced at presentation with an aggressive tendency to metastasize. Chemoradiotherapy is generally used for treatment. Prophylactic cranial irradiation is considered in a patient with limited or extensive disease that responds well to first-line therapy. Complete responses may occur in approximately 30%, of patients; however, the 5-year survival rate is only 5%. Patients with early-stage disease (e.g., <3 cm in size, no nodal metastases, and no extrathoracic metastases) may be considered for surgical resection, followed by adjuvant systemic therapy. Staging before resection includes ^{18}F-fluorodeoxyglucose positron emission tomography (FDG-PET), brain CT or MRI, and mediastinoscopy. Mediastinal metastases on clinical staging suggest advanced disease, which is best treated with chemoradiotherapy.[10,11]

Lung cancers commonly metastasize to the pulmonary and mediastinal lymph nodes (lymphatic spread). Hematogenous spread of lung cancer commonly results in metastases to the adrenal glands, brain, lung, and bone. Adenocarcinoma is more likely to metastasize to the central nervous system. Bone metastases are osteolytic. Extrathoracic metastases may occur without hilar nodes or mediastinal metastases.

Screening

Patients with lung cancer often present with advanced disease stage and symptoms. The pulmonary parenchyma does not contain nerve endings, and tumors may grow undetected until symptoms of pain, hemoptysis, or obstructive pneumonia arise. With the increased use of CT in the United States, smaller asymptomatic lung cancers are being identified.

Screening for lung cancer has been evaluated by the National Lung Screening Trial (NLST). The NLST is a prospective randomized multicenter study evaluating annual low-dose helical CT with annual chest radiography. The 53,454 enrolled patients were randomly assigned between the two arms. The men and women screened were asymptomatic and older (age range: 55 to 74 years), with 30 pack-years or more of cigarette smoking at the beginning of the trial, and were either current smokers or had recently quit (within 15 years). The NLST found that patients randomly assigned to low-dose helical CT screening for 3 years (compared with CXR) had a reduced lung cancer-specific mortality and all-cause mortality. The death rate from lung cancer in this high-risk population was reduced by 20%, and all-cause mortality was reduced by 7%. The study showed the benefit is statistically significant, as 354 lung cancer deaths occurred in the CT group compared with 442 lung cancer deaths in the CXR group (P = 0.0041), leading to early study closure.[12]

More recently, the results of the European Nelson lung cancer screening trial have been reported. In this population-based controlled trial, 15,792 individuals were randomized 1:1 to either the study arm or control arm. Study arm participants were offered CT screenings at baseline, one, three, and five and one-half years after randomization. No screenings were offered to control arm participants. The follow-up period comprised a minimum of 10 years, unless deceased, for 93.7% of enrolled participants. Detection rates across the rounds varied between 0.8% and 1.1%, and 69% of screen-detected lung cancers were detected at Stage IA or IB. A total of 261 lung cancers (52 interval cancers) were detected before the fourth round of follow-ups. In a subset of analyzed patients, surgical treatment was three times significantly more prevalent in the study lung cancer patients than in control arm patients (67.7% vs. 24.5%, $P < 0.001$). Overall the study has shown that the use of CT screening among asymptomatic men at high risk for lung cancer led to a 26% (9-41%, 95% confidence interval [CI]) reduction in lung cancer deaths at 10 years of study follow-up (at 86% compliance). In the smaller subset of women, the rate-ratio of dying from lung cancer varied between 0.39 and 0.61 in different years of follow-up, indicating an even larger reduction in lung cancer mortality than in men.

Screening for early lung cancer detection using low-dose helical CT is recommended by the National Comprehensive Cancer Network (NCCN) for 1) individuals aged 55 to 74 years with a 30 or more pack-year history of smoking tobacco who currently smoke or, if a former smoker, have quit within 15 years and 2) individuals aged 50 years or older with a 20 or more pack-year history of smoking tobacco who are either current or former smokers and whose risk for lung cancer is greater than 1.3%[13,14] (key risk factors include personal history of cancer or lung disease, family history of lung cancer, radon exposure, and occupational exposure to carcinogens). The U.S. Preventive Services Task Force is currently revising its recommendations for lung cancer screening.

Physicians may discuss testing for early-stage lung cancer with their patients on an individual basis. This discussion with the patient should include the risks, benefits, and limitations associated with lung cancer screening with low-dose helical CT and should occur before a decision is made to start any lung cancer screening. Screening is not an alternative to smoking cessation. A clear and unambiguous statement is needed from the physician that smoking cessation is essential. Pharmacologic or other strategies need to be tailored to the individual patient. Screening of asymptomatic patients may identify nonspecific findings, such as over diagnosis of benign nodules, which could result in patient anxiety as well as additional radiation exposure.

Diagnosis

The diagnosis of lung cancer can be challenging. Many benign conditions mimic lung cancer. Physical examination should focus on the cardiorespiratory system. In addition, the presence of cancer in supraclavicular lymph nodes, identified by a careful examination of the cervical and supraclavicular lymph nodes, suggests advanced disease (N3 lymph node descriptor), and therapy other than resection is recommended. Paraneoplastic syndromes are distant manifestations of lung cancer (not metastases) as revealed in extrathoracic nonmetastatic symptoms. The lung cancer causes an effect on these extrathoracic sites by producing one or more biologic or biochemical substances. Small cell lung cancer frequently causes neurologic paraneoplastic syndromes. Other lung cancers may cause hypertrophic osteoarthropathy.

Non–small cell lung cancer (NSCLC) typically occurs in patients who are 50 to 70 years old with a history of cigarette smoking. Patients develop symptoms based on the physical impact of tumor growth within the lung parenchyma. Symptoms such as cough, dyspnea, chest wall pain, and hemoptysis are related to the physical presence of the tumor and its interactions with the structures of the lung and chest wall.[15]

Once a clinical suspicion for NSCLC arises the clinician should aim to achieve a timely diagnosis and accurate staging so that appropriate therapy can be administered. The workup of a primary solitary pulmonary nodule (SPN) involves the combination of imaging modalities including CXR, CT, and often also a PET-CT. In addition, a tissue biopsy is often performed based on the suspicion level for malignancy. Guidelines for management of a SPNs are available. Under certain circumstances, a SPN may be deemed benign with adequate confidence in the absence of a pathologic diagnosis. SPNs that are entirely calcified, or radiologically stable on CT of the chest over a minimum of 2 years, are very likely to be benign. Review of old radiographs or other prior imaging studies can assist in evaluation of changes in the mass.[16]

In patients with a clinically suspicious SPN, histologic information may be needed to assess risk and benefit of the various available treatment options. The least invasive strategy compatible with obtaining a diagnosis would be recommended. Diagnostic bronchoscopy, transthoracic needle aspiration, or navigational bronchoscopy can be selected based on the size, location, and condition of the patient. In a physiologically fit patient with a suspicious yet undiagnosed SPN, nonanatomic wedge or sublobar resection provides a diagnosis. Confirmation of NSCLC by the pathologist should be followed by definitive (anatomic) resection in the same setting. For a SPN in the absence of a cancer diagnosis (that cannot be removed by wedge resection), a lobectomy can be considered for diagnosis (and treatment). A pneumonectomy is not performed without a cancer diagnosis.

One third of patients with NSCLC may have a pleural effusion at the time of presentation. Pleural fluid sampling with thoracentesis is required for cytologic examination. Malignant pleural effusion (MPE) is a contraindication to resection, but many pleural effusions in this setting may be reactive in origin.[17]

Bronchoscopy is recommended before any planned pulmonary resection. The surgeon independently assesses (via bronchoscopy) the endobronchial anatomy to exclude secondary endobronchial primary tumors and to ensure that all known cancer will be encompassed by the planned pulmonary resection. Secretions can be cleared with suctioning and gentle irrigation. When pneumonectomy or bronchoplastic resection is contemplated for a central tumor, the surgeon's assessment at bronchoscopy is critical to the determination of whether complete (R0) resection can be achieved.

If the patient has hard palpable lymph nodes in the cervical or supraclavicular area, fine-needle aspiration or biopsy may provide an accurate diagnosis of N3 disease.

Staging

Staging is a description of the extent of the cancer based on similarities in survival for the group of patients with those characteristics. The staging system creates a shorthand description of the tumor, lymph nodes, and metastatic characteristics of the patient to facilitate the choice of optimal therapy and to evaluate outcomes based on the clinical and pathologic stage. The American Joint Committee on Cancer (AJCC) and the Union for International Cancer Control work to establish and promulgate staging system guidelines. The 2018 eighth edition TNM stage classification for lung cancer provides the basis for specific patient stage groupings and is used for initial treatment recommendations based on the clinical stage and on the pathologic stage after pulmonary resection.

The clinician's responsibility is to ensure the highest possible degree of certainty of the extent of the disease and to recommend the therapy or therapeutic combination of greatest efficacy based on the disease stage. Optimal staging assists the clinician in providing the best recommendations for therapeutic interventions for the patient. The clinical stage is the physician's best and final estimate of the extent of disease based on all available information from invasive and noninvasive studies before the initiation of definitive therapy. Key imaging modalities used in clinical staging of NSCLC patients are CT, PET-CT, and MRI of the brain. Invasive staging of the mediastinum, pleural taps and biopsies from suspected metastatic sites are also often performed to complement and more accurately determine disease stage. The pathologic stage is the determination of the physical extent of the disease based on histologic examination of the resected tissues, including the hilar and mediastinal lymph nodes.

Evaluation of Tumor (T) Stage

As the tumor size increases, survival decreases. Diagnostic imaging commonly includes a CXR and CT scan of the chest and upper abdomen, including the liver and adrenals (Fig. 58.12). The CXR provides information on the size, shape, density, and location of the primary tumor and its relationship to the mediastinal structures. CT scan of the chest provides more detail on tumor characteristics and provides information on the relationship of the tumor to the mediastinum, chest wall, and diaphragm as well as invasion into the vertebrae or mediastinal structures. MRI of the chest may complement CT in better delineating tumor invasion in such patients. MRI of the brain is reserved for patients with stage I or II cancer with new neurologic symptoms (vertigo, headache) and for all patients with stage III and IV cancer, as well as patients with small cell carcinoma or superior sulcus tumors (Pancoast tumor) because these patients have a higher incidence of occult brain metastases.

Evaluation of Nodal (N) Stage

Determination of metastases to mediastinal lymph nodes constitutes a critical point in staging and treatment recommendations. Mediastinal lymph node metastases are present in 26% to 32% of patients at the time of diagnosis and initially assessed with chest CT. Lymph nodes may be enlarged normally from infection (e.g., histoplasmosis, previous bronchitis, or pneumonia) or other inflammatory processes, such as granulomatous disease. Mediastinal adenopathy is most often defined as lymph nodes with a maximal transverse diameter greater than 1 cm on axial tomographic images. In the absence of mediastinal nodes greater than 1 cm in diameter, the likelihood of N2 or N3 disease is low. If mediastinal nodes greater than 1 cm are identified, nodal tissue must be examined (e.g., with endoscopic bronchial ultrasound (EBUS), cervical mediastinoscopy, endoscopic ultrasound, VATS) for histologic evidence of metastases before definitive resection can be considered.

CT has a reported sensitivity of 57% to 79% for mediastinal lymph node assessment in NSCLC, with a positive predictive value of 56%. No CT size criteria are entirely reliable for the determination of mediastinal lymph node involvement. Larger

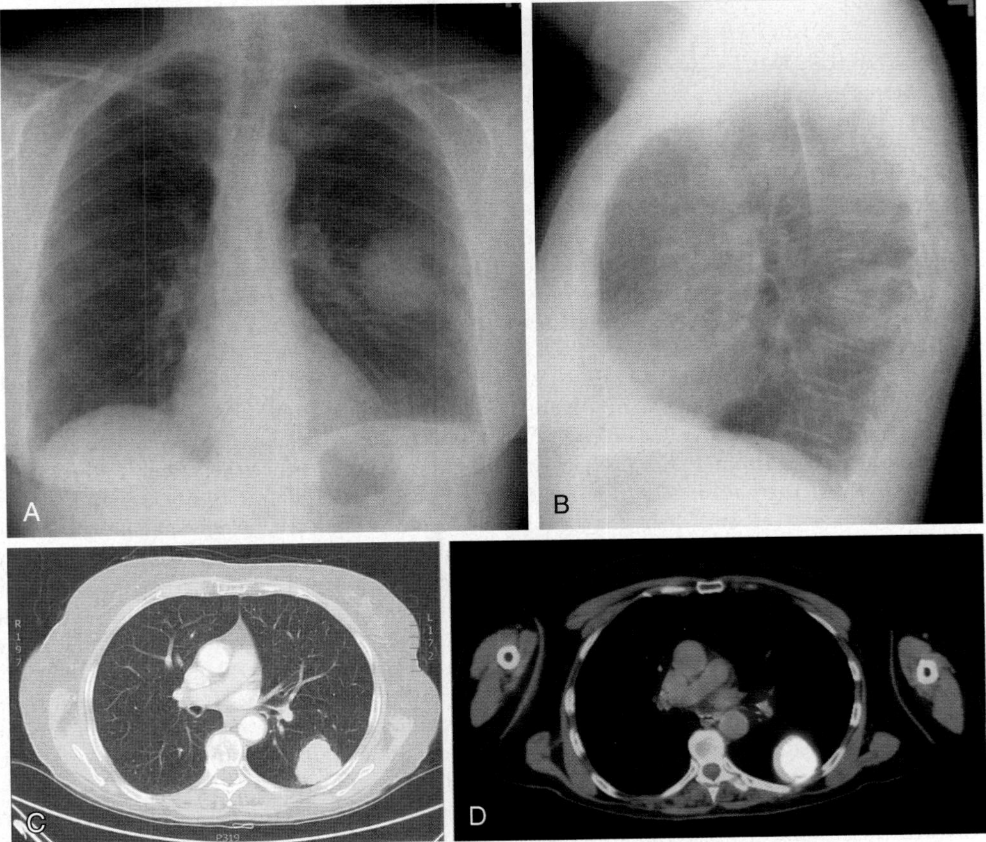

FIG. 58.12 Radiographic evaluation for any patient with known or suspected lung cancer includes a plain chest x-ray, posteroanterior (A) and lateral (B) views. Evaluation of the plain films and computed tomography (CT) (C) guides subsequent evaluations. ^{18}F-Fluorodeoxyglucose positron emission tomography (FDG-PET) with fused CT (D) provides the ability to correlate metabolic activity with physical findings. Although FDG-PET uses the increased metabolism in most neoplasms to create the FDG-PET image, other processes, such as infection, inflammation, or sequelae of trauma or fractures, can be identified as well. Sites of increased metabolism should be carefully evaluated for metastases.

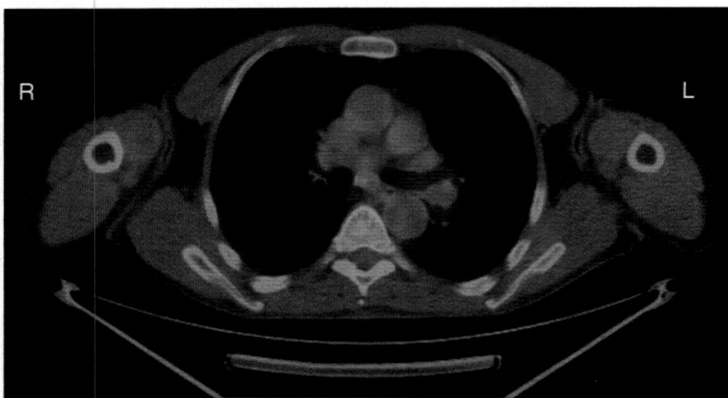

FIG. 58.13 A subcarinal lymph node has mild ^{18}F-fluorodeoxyglucose (FDG) uptake. Based on these findings, additional invasive staging is warranted, including bronchoscopy and invasive staging of mediastinal lymph nodes. Endobronchial ultrasound with transtracheal needle aspiration can be performed with real-time ultrasound guidance to facilitate transtracheal needle placement. Biopsies of other stations can be performed as well. If needed, cervical mediastinoscopy is performed with biopsy of high paratracheal (2R and 2L), low paratracheal (4R and 4L), pretracheal (3A), and subcarinal (7) lymph nodes. If left-sided aortopulmonary lymph nodes were FDG avid, a Chamberlain procedure (anterior mediastinotomy) or video-assisted thoracic surgery with biopsy of aortopulmonary window lymph nodes or hilar lymph nodes could also be performed. Additional evaluation of the patient would be warranted if the patient would be considered a surgical candidate.

mediastinal lymph nodes are more likely to be associated with metastasis (>70%); however, normal-sized lymph nodes (<1 cm) have a 7% to 15% chance of containing metastases.[18]

PET may assist in evaluating the local extent and presence of known or occult metastases based on the differential increased metabolism of glucose by cancer cells compared with normal tissues (Fig. 58.13). A PET scan is not a cancer-specific study or a "cancer scan," as high cellular glucose metabolism is seen in inflammatory processes in addition to malignancy. Histologic confirmation of FDG avid mediastinal lymph node involvement is indicated to complete clinical staging before final treatment decisions. FDG-PET coupled with CT may yield increased sensitivity and specificity in determining the stage of patients with lung cancer before treatment interventions. The negative predictive value of PET-CT for mediastinal lymph node metastases from NSCLC is in the range of 85% to 95% being more accurate in smaller (T1) rather than larger (T2) tumors and in larger (>1 cm) than smaller (<1 cm) lymph nodes.

Invasive staging includes cervical mediastinoscopy or mediastinotomy (Chamberlain procedure), EBUS, or endoscopic ultrasound. Cervical mediastinoscopy is traditionally indicated in patients with otherwise operable NSCLC with enlarged paratracheal or subcarinal lymph nodes, particularly if the cancer is proximal, if pneumonectomy is planned, or if the patient is at increased risk for the planned resection. Cervical mediastinoscopy is commonly performed for biopsy of bilateral paratracheal (levels 2 and 4) and subcarinal (level 7) lymph nodes. A left anterior mediastinotomy is used to gain access to the mediastinum after resection of the second costosternal cartilage to evaluate the aortopulmonary window (level 5) or anterior mediastinum (level 6) lymph nodes. Cervical mediastinoscopy has a negative predictive value greater than 90%, it may be performed as an outpatient procedure, and is associated with a low rate of significant complications. When pathologic "frozen section" evaluation fails to demonstrate malignant nodal involvement, mediastinoscopy may be followed by resection under the same anesthetic. The use of cervical mediastinoscopy regardless of radiographic evidence of nodal involvement ("routine mediastinoscopy") is not a cost-effective approach and adds little to the accuracy of staging in patients with an adequate noninvasive preoperative evaluation.[19] Additional sampling techniques may be helpful. In particular, EBUS, which provides access to nodal stations 2, 4, 7, 10, 11, and endoscopic ultrasound via the esophagus, which provides access to nodal stations 2, 4, 7, 8, and 9, may be as sensitive as and less invasive than mediastinoscopy. VATS techniques can evaluate enlarged level 4, 7, 8, 9, and 10 lymph nodes bilaterally and levels 5 or 6 lymph nodes on the left.

Evaluation of Metastasis (M) Stage

Endothoracic (M1a) and extrathoracic metastases (single extrathoracic metastasis M1b or multiple extrathoracic metastasis [M1c]) are common in lung cancer. Beyond a thorough history, physical examination, and standard imaging based staging techniques (CT, PET-CT, and MRI of the brain), additional evaluation for metastatic disease is indicated only in selected cases. In particular, a tissue diagnosis should be obtained if confirmation of metastasis is anticipated to alter the treatment plan. When pleural effusion is present a diagnostic tap is usually performed to confirm tumor spread to the pleural space. Up to 7% of patients have metastatic adrenal involvement at presentation. The standard CT evaluation of the chest should also include evaluation of the upper abdomen including the liver and the adrenal glands. Indeterminate adrenal lesions on CT may be further evaluated with MRI or with CT-guided percutaneous biopsy.

Current Lung Cancer Eighth Edition Staging System

The International Association for the Study of Lung Cancer (IASLC), together with the AJCC, has recently issued the eighth edition of lung cancer staging system.[20] For this project the IASLC has collected data on a total of 94,708 patients diagnosed with lung cancer from 1999 to 2010. The data has originated from 35 different databases in 16 countries on 5 continents. The information was provided by credible centers, which facilitated data collection and analysis of a large patient population. After exclusions, 77,156 patients remained evaluable, including 70,967 with NSCLC and 6189 with small cell lung cancer. Nearly 85% of the patients included in the database underwent surgical treatment, either alone (57.7%) or together with chemotherapy (21.1%), radiotherapy (1.5%), or both (4.4%). Survival was analyzed using Kaplan-Meier methods, and survival estimates were compared using the likelihood ratio test from Cox proportional hazards regression. Extensive analysis allowed definition of TNM categories and stage groupings that demonstrated consistent discrimination overall and within multiple different patient cohorts (e.g., clinical or pathologic stage, R0 or R-any resection status, geographic region). Additional analyses provided evidence of applicability over time, across a spectrum of geographic regions, histologic types, evaluative approaches, and follow-up intervals.[21,22]

The TNM definitions, nodal characteristics, and stage groupings of the TNM subsets are shown in Tables 58.1 to 58.3. Other schematics have been created for the lymph node map and T characteristics. The mediastinal and regional lymph node classification schema is presented in Fig. 58.14. This map presents a graphic representation of mediastinal and pulmonary lymph nodes in relation to other thoracic structures for optimal dissection and anatomic labeling by the surgeon.[23]

TABLE 58.1 **Tumor, node, metastasis (TNM) descriptors for the eighth edition of TNM Classification for Lung Cancer**

T: Primary Tumor

TX Primary tumor cannot be assessed, or tumor proven by the presence of malignant cells in sputum or bronchial washings but not visualized by imaging or bronchoscopy

T0 No evidence of primary tumor

Tis Carcinoma in situ

T1 Tumor ≤3 cm in greatest dimension, surrounded by lung or visceral pleura, without bronchoscopic evidence of invasion more proximal than the lobar bronchus (i.e., not in the main bronchus)[a]

T1a(mi) Minimally invasive adenocarcinoma[b]

- **T1a** Tumor ≤1 cm in greatest dimension[a]
- **T1b** Tumor >1 cm but ≤2 cm in greatest dimension[a]
- **T1c** Tumor >2 cm but ≤3 cm in greatest dimension[a]

T2 Tumor >3 cm **but ≤5 cm** or tumor with any of the following features[c]:

- **Involves main bronchus regardless of distance from the carina but without involvement of the carina**
- Invades visceral pleura
- **Associated with atelectasis or obstructive pneumonitis that extends to the hilar region, involving part or all of the lung**

T2a **Tumor >3 cm but ≤4 cm in greatest dimension**

T2b **Tumor >4 cm but ≤5 cm in greatest dimension**

T3 **Tumor >5 cm but ≤7 cm in greatest dimension** or associated with separate tumor nodule(s) in the same lobe as the primary tumor or directly invades any of the following structures:
chest wall (including the parietal pleura and superior sulcus tumors), phrenic nerve, parietal pericardium

T4 **Tumor >7 cm in greatest dimension** or associated with separate tumor nodule(s) in a different ipsilateral lobe than that of the primary tumor or invades any of the following structures: **diaphragm**, mediastinum, heart, great vessels, trachea, recurrent laryngeal nerve, esophagus, vertebral body, and carina

N: Regional Lymph Nodes Involvement

NX Regional lymph nodes cannot be assessed

N0 No regional lymph node metastases

N1 Metastasis in ipsilateral peribronchial and/or ipsilateral hilar lymph nodes and intrapulmonary nodes, including involvement by direct extension

N2 Metastasis in ipsilateral mediastinal and/or subcarinal lymph node(s)

N3 Metastasis in contralateral mediastinal, contralateral hilar, ipsilateral or contralateral scalene, or supraclavicular lymph node(s)

M (Distant Metastasis)

M0 No distant metastasis

M1 Distant metastasis present

- **M1a** Separate tumor nodule(s) in a contralateral lobe; tumor with pleural or pericardial nodule(s) or malignant pleural or pericardial effusion[d]
- **M1b** Single extrathoracic metastasis[e]
- **M1c** Multiple extrathoracic metastases in one or more organs

From Goldstraw P, Chansky K, Crowley J, et al. The IASLC Lung Cancer Staging Project: Proposals for Revision of the TNM Stage Groupings in the Forthcoming (Eighth) Edition of the TNM Classification for Lung Cancer. *J Thorac Oncol.* 2016;11:39–51.

Note: Changes to the seventh edition are in bold.

[a]The uncommon superficial spreading tumor of any size with its invasive component limited to the bronchial wall, which may extend proximal to the main bronchus, is also classified as T1a.

[b]Solitary adenocarcinoma, ≤3cm with a predominately lepidic pattern and ≤5mm invasion in any one focus.

[c]T2 tumors with these features are classified as T2a if ≤4 cm in greatest dimension or if size cannot be determined, and T2b if >4 cm but ≤5 cm in greatest dimension.

[d]Most pleural (pericardial) effusions with lung cancer are due to tumor. In a few patients, however, multiple microscopic examinations of pleural (pericardial) fluid are negative for tumor and the fluid is nonbloody and not an exudate. When these elements and clinical judgment dictate that the effusion is not related to the tumor, the effusion should be excluded as a staging descriptor.

[e]This includes involvement of a single distant (nonregional) lymph node.

Tumor (T)

In the eighth edition of the IASLC/AJCC, lung cancer staging project significant innovations were introduced into the definitions of the T descriptor. In particular, the eighth edition includes for the first time special definitions for carcinoma in situ (Tis) and for minimally invasive carcinomas (T1mi). Tis are less than 3-cm noninvasive tumors that histologically display a pure lepidic growth pattern. T1mi are less than 3-cm tumors that histologically display a predominant lepidic growth pattern; however, they also have a small (<0.5-cm) invasive component. In addition, the definitions of the four classic lung cancer T categories (T1–T4) have also been refined. In the current edition, T1 tumors (<3 cm) are subcategorized as T1a <1 cm, T1b >1 to 2 cm, T1c >2 to 3 cm. T2 tumors (>3 to 5 cm) are subcategorized as T2a >3 to 4 cm, T2b >4 to 5 cm. T3 tumors are defined as >5 up to 7 cm and T4 tumors are defined as >7 cm. Other important tumor characteristics that

TABLE 58.2 Proposed stage grouping for the Eighth Edition of the TNM Classification for Lung Cancer

OCCULT CARCINOMA	TX	N0	M0
Stage 0	Tis	N0	M0
Stage IA1	**T1a(mi)**	**N0**	**M0**
	T1a	**N0**	**M0**
Stage IA2	**T1b**	**N0**	**M0**
Stage IA3	**T1c**	**N0**	**M0**
Stage IB	T2a	N0	M0
Stage IIA	T2b	N0	M0
Stage IIB	**T1a-c**	**N1**	**M0**
	T2a	**N1**	**M0**
	T2b	N1	M0
	T3	N0	M0
Stage IIIA	**T1a-c**	**N2**	**M0**
	T2a–b	N2	M0
	T3	N1	M0
	T4	N0	M0
	T4	N1	M0
Stage IIIB	**T1a-c**	**N3**	**M0**
	T2a–b	N3	M0
	T3	**N3**	**M0**
	T4	N2	M0
Stage IIIC	**T3**	**N3**	**M0**
	T4	**N3**	**M0**
Stage IVA	**Any T**	**Any N**	**M1a**
	Any T	**Any N**	**M1b**
Stage IVB	**Any T**	**Any N**	**M1c**

From Goldstraw P, Chansky K, Crowley J, et al. The IASLC Lung Cancer Staging Project: Proposals for Revision of the TNM Stage Groupings in the Forthcoming (Eighth) Edition of the TNM Classification for Lung Cancer. *J Thorac Oncol.* 2016;11:39-51.
TNM, tumor, node, metastasis; *Tis*, carcinoma in situ; *T1a(mi)*, minimally invasive adenocarcinoma.
Note: Changes to the seventh edition are highlighted in bold and underlined.

dictate the T stage are involvement of the main bronchus/invasion of the visceral pleural/associated lobar or lung atelectasis in the T2 descriptor, invasion of the parietal pleura/chest wall/phrenic nerve/parietal pericardium or associated separate tumor nodule(s) in the same lobe as the primary tumor in the T3 descriptor, and invasion of the diaphragm/mediastinum/heart/great vessels/trachea/recurrent laryngeal nerve/esophagus/vertebral body/carina or separate tumor nodule(s) in a different ipsilateral lobe to that of the primary tumor in the T4 descriptor. Contrast-enhanced CT of the chest is the main imaging modality used to determine the T stage. MRI of the chest wall may assist in identifying chest wall involvement and in staging of superior sulcus tumors.

Lymph Nodes (N)

The node descriptor (N0–N3) is defined according to the extent of lymph node metastasis along a predefined lymph node map. There are 14 lymph node stations: stations 10 to 14 are confined to the lung, and metastasis to these nodes indicates N1 disease if ipsilateral to the tumor and N3 disease if contralateral to the tumor; stations 9 to 2 are confined to the mediastinum, and metastasis to these nodes indicates N2 disease if ipsilateral to the tumor and N3 disease if contralateral to the tumor; station 1 are supraclavicular or suprasternal or low cervical nodes, and metastasis to these nodes indicates N3 disease. The nodal characteristics and designations did not change in the eighth edition of the IASLC lung cancer staging project. However, a recommendation is made to define nodal involvement not only by the N0 to N3 descriptors, but also by quantifying the number of involved lymph nodes. In particular, nodal quantification by the number of involved nodal stations is defined as follows: N1a: involvement of a single N1 nodal station; N1b: involvement of multiple N1 nodal stations; N2a1: involvement of a single N2 nodal station without N1 involvement (skip metastasis); N2a2: involvement of a single N2 nodal station with N1 involvement; and N2b: involvement of multiple N2 nodal stations. Prognosis worsens as the number of involved nodal stations increases, but N1b and N2a1 have the same prognosis. Asamura and colleagues[24] have shown that the five-year survival rates in the population of patients who underwent complete resection for the different N subcategories were: N1a, 59%; N1b, 50%; N2a1, 54%; N2a2, 43%; and N2b, 38%. FDG-PET combined with contrast-enhanced CT is the main imaging modality used to determine the N stage. Hilar and mediastinal nodes that are suspected to be involved by cancer (>1 cm) or have positive FDG uptake are in the majority of cases sampled to confirm tumor metastasis.

Metastases (M)

The eighth edition of lung cancer stating system has refined the categorization of the M descriptor. It defines two M descriptors, M0 and M1, with M1 being subcategorized to M1a, M1b, and M1c. M1a indicates endothoracic metastasis (malignant pleural/pericardial effusion or malignant pleural/pericardial nodules or separate tumor nodule in a contralateral lobe). M1b indicates the presence of a single extrathoracic metastasis in a single organ. M1c indicates the presence of a multiple extrathoracic metastases in a single organ or in multiple organs. Remarkably, M1a and M1b tumors have similar prognosis; however, since they represent different forms of metastatic involvement and require different diagnostics and therapeutics, they were separately categorized. FDG-PET combined with contrast-enhanced CT is the main imaging modality used to determine the M stage. Brain MRI is used to identify brain metastasis. Suspected metastatic lesions may be samples in order to confirm NSCLC diagnosis or if biopsy results will alter the treatment plan. Otherwise routine sampling of metastatic lesions in not performed.

Stages. The eighth edition of lung cancer stating system has refined and expanded the lung cancer stage definitions to produce a more precise tool to predict prognosis and guide treatment plan (Fig. 58.15).

Results of Treatment for Lung Cancer

The choice of initial therapy (whether single-modality or multimodality therapy) depends on the patient's clinical stage at presentation and on his or her functional class and comorbidities. Treatment options may vary, even among different subsets of patients within the same clinical stage. Pretreatment staging is the critical step before initiating therapy. With current efforts, 5-year survival rates by pathologic stage are 90% for stage IA1, 85% for stage IA2, 80% for stage IA3, 73% for stage IB, 65% for stage IIA, 56% for stage IIB, 41% for stage IIIA, 24% for stage IIIB, and 12% for stage IIIB. The 5-year survival rates by clinical stage are 13% for

TABLE 58.3 Anatomic limits of the nodal stations of the International Association for the Study of Lung Cancer Lymph Node Map and their grouping in nodal zones.

LYMPH NODE STATION NO.	ANATOMIC LIMITS
Supraclavicular Zone	
1: Low cervical, supraclavicular, and sternal notch nodes	• Upper border: Lower margin of cricoid cartilage • Lower border: Clavicles bilaterally and, in the midline, the upper border of the manubrium; 1R designates right-sided nodes, and 1L designates left-sided nodes in this region • For lymph node station 1, the midline of the trachea serves as the border between 1R and 1L
Upper Zone	
2: Upper paratracheal nodes	• 2R: Upper border: Apex of the right lung and pleural space and, in the midline, the upper border of the manubrium • Lower border: Intersection of caudal margin of innominate vein with the trachea • Similar to lymph node station 4R, 2R includes nodes extending to the left lateral border of the trachea • 2L: Upper border: Apex of the lung and pleural space and, in the midline, the upper border of the manubrium • Lower border: Superior border of the aortic arch
3: Prevascular and retrotracheal nodes	• 3a: Prevascular • On the right: Upper border, apex of chest; lower border, level of carina; anterior border, posterior aspect of sternum; posterior border, anterior border of superior vena cava • On the left: Upper border, apex of chest; lower border, level of carina; anterior border, posterior aspect of sternum; posterior border, left carotid artery • 3p: Retrotracheal • Upper border, apex of chest; lower border, carina
4: Lower paratracheal nodes	• 4R: Includes right paratracheal nodes and pretracheal nodes extending to the left lateral border of the trachea • Upper border: Intersection of caudal margin of innominate vein with the trachea • Lower border: Lower border of the azygos vein • 4L: Includes nodes to the left of the left lateral border of the trachea, medial to the ligamentum arteriosum • Upper border: Upper margin of the aortic arch • Lower border: Upper rim of the left main pulmonary artery
Aortopulmonary Zone	
5: Subaortic (aortopulmonary window)	• Subaortic lymph nodes lateral to the ligamentum arteriosum • Upper border: The lower border of the aortic arch • Lower border: Upper rim of the left main pulmonary artery
6: Para-aortic nodes (ascending aorta or phrenic)	• Lymph nodes anterior and lateral to the ascending aorta and aortic arch • Upper border: A line tangential to the upper border of the aortic arch • Lower border: The lower border of the aortic arch
Subcarinal Zone	
7: Subcarinal nodes	• Upper border: The carina of the trachea • Lower border: The upper border of the lower lobe bronchus on the left; the lower border of the bronchus intermedius on the right
Lower Zone	
8: Paraesophageal nodes (below carina)	• Nodes lying adjacent to the wall of the esophagus and to the right or the left of the midline, excluding subcarinal nodes • Upper border: The upper border of the lower lobe bronchus on the left; the lower border of the bronchus intermedius on the right • Lower border: The diaphragm
9: Pulmonary ligament nodes	• Nodes lying within the pulmonary ligament • Upper border: The inferior pulmonary vein • Lower border: The diaphragm
Hilar/Interlobar Zone	
10: Hilar nodes	• Includes nodes immediately adjacent to the mainstem bronchus and hilar vessels, including the proximal portions of the pulmonary veins and main pulmonary artery • Upper border: The lower rim of the azygos vein in the right, upper rim of the pulmonary artery on the left • Lower border: Interlobar region bilaterally

Continued

TABLE 58.3 Anatomic limits of the nodal stations of the International Association for the Study of Lung Cancer Lymph Node Map and their grouping in nodal zones.—cont'd

LYMPH NODE STATION NO.	ANATOMIC LIMITS

11: Interlobar nodes	• Between the origins of the lobar bronchi
	• Optional notations for subcategories of station:
	  • 11s: Between the upper lobe bronchus and bronchus intermedius on the right
	  • 11i: Between the middle and lower bronchi on the right

Peripheral Zone	
12: Lobar nodes	Adjacent to the lobar bronchi
13: Segmental nodes	Adjacent to the segmental bronchi
14: Subsegmental nodes	Adjacent to the subsegmental bronchi

Adapted from: Rusch VW, Asamura H, Watanabe H, et al. The IASLC lung cancer staging project: a proposal for a new international lymph node map in the forthcoming seventh edition of the TNM classification for lung cancer. *J Thorac Oncol.* 2009;4:568–577.

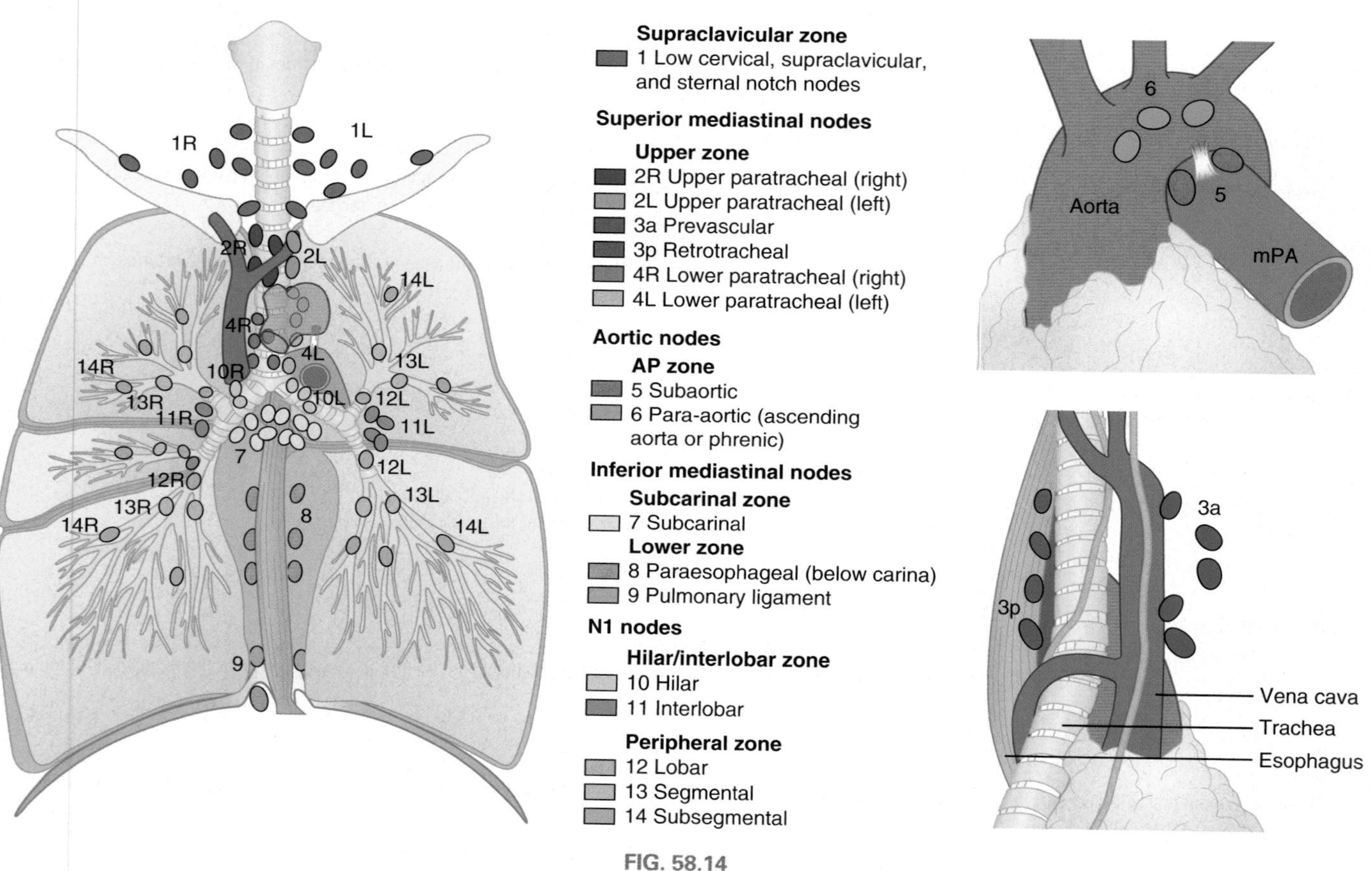

FIG. 58.14

stage IVA and 0% for stage IVB. Treatment for lung cancer can broadly be grouped into three major categories, as follows:

1. *Stage I* disease and *stage II* disease indicate the presence of tumor that is contained within the lung and that may be completely resected with surgery. Anatomic resection of the lobe where the tumor resides with complete sampling of mediastinal lymph nodes is the treatment of choice. The key aim of this treatment approach is to achieve complete resection of the tumor and its intralobar draining lymph nodes. In certain cases, sublobar anatomic resections may be considered for small and peripheral tumors. Nonanatomic resections (wedge resection) are considered inferior to anatomic resection and should be performed only when more extensive surgery cannot be tolerated by the patient (due to reduced pulmonary reserve for example). Stereotactic body radiation therapy (SBRT) has had good early results (local control rates of 90% at 3 years) in selected patients that cannot withstand surgical resection.[25]
2. *Stage IV* disease (metastatic disease) and *stage IIIB* disease (advanced disease presenting either as a relatively small tumor with N3 nodes or as a large tumors with N2 nodes) are not typically treated by surgery except in patients requiring surgical palliation. Systemic therapies for metastatic disease are common. Chemoradiation is often used in stage IIIB disease. Targeted therapies and immunotherapy are providing encouraging results in properly screened and selected patient groups.

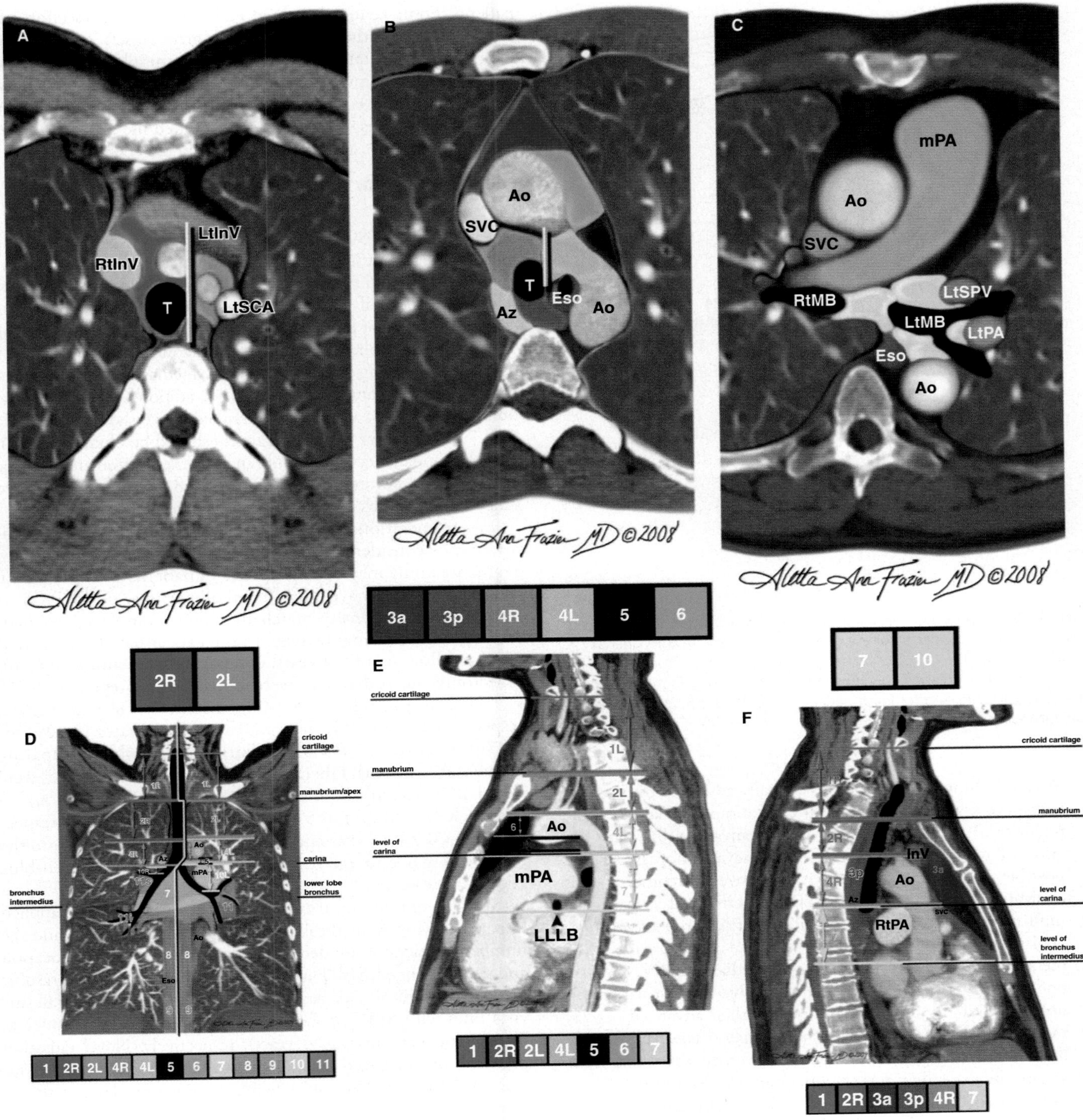

B

FIG. 58.14—cont'd (A) The International Association for the Study of Lung Cancer (IASLC) lymph node map, including the proposed grouping of lymph node stations into "zones" for the purposes of prognostic analyses. (B) *A–F*: Illustrations of how the IASLC lymph node map can be applied to clinical staging by computed tomography scan in axial *(A–C)*, coronal *(D)*, and sagittal *(E, F)* views. The border between the right and left paratracheal region is shown in *A* and *B*. (From Rusch VW, Asamura H, Watanabe H, et al. The IASLC lung cancer staging project: A proposal for a new international lymph node map in the forthcoming seventh edition of the TNM classification for lung cancer. *J Thorac Oncol*. 2009;4:568–577.) *Ao*, Aorta; *AV*, azygos vein; *Br*, bronchus; *IA*, innominate artery; *IV*, innominate vein; *LA*, ligamentum arteriosum; *LIV*, left innominate vein; *LSA*, left subclavian artery; *PA*, pulmonary artery; *PV*, pulmonary vein; *RIV*, right innominate vein; *SVC*, superior vena cava.

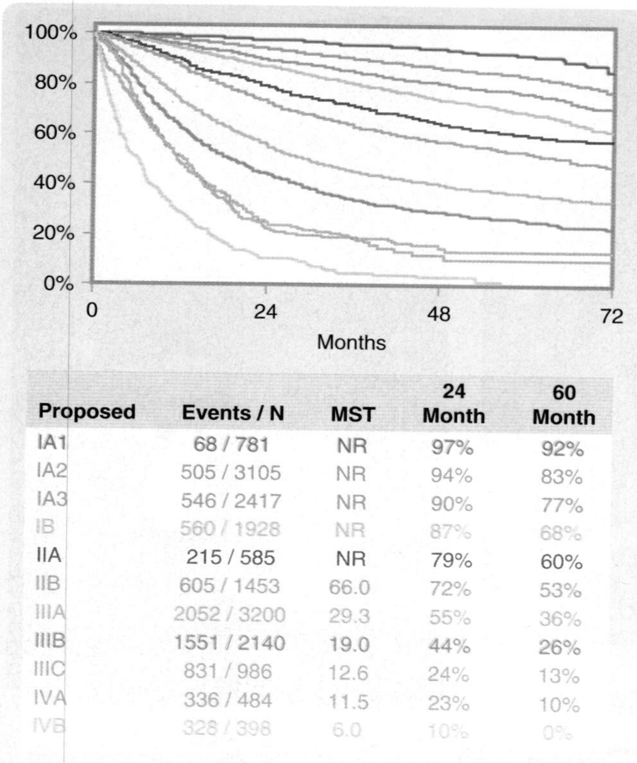

Proposed	Events / N	MST	24 Month	60 Month
IA1	68 / 781	NR	97%	92%
IA2	505 / 3105	NR	94%	83%
IA3	546 / 2417	NR	90%	77%
IB	560 / 1928	NR	87%	68%
IIA	215 / 585	NR	79%	60%
IIB	605 / 1453	66.0	72%	53%
IIIA	2052 / 3200	29.3	55%	36%
IIIB	1551 / 2140	19.0	44%	26%
IIIC	831 / 986	12.6	24%	13%
IVA	336 / 484	11.5	23%	10%
IVB	328 / 398	6.0	10%	0%

FIG. 58.15 Overall survival by clinical stage according to the eighth edition of the lung cancer staging project. (From Goldstraw P, Chansky K, Crowley J, et al. The IASLC Lung Cancer Staging Project: Proposals for Revision of the TNM Stage Groupings in the Forthcoming (Eighth) Edition of the TNM Classification for Lung Cancer. *J Thorac Oncol.* 2016;11:39–51.) *MST*, Median survival time.

3. *Stage IIIA* lung cancer indicates a locally advanced disease that may have a wide spectrum of presentations. Remarkably, the majority of stage IIIA tumors are too advanced for consideration of resection; however, if complete resection is deemed possible, it may be associated with improved outcomes. In this clinical scenario, surgical resection is performed as part of a multimodality treatment protocol. In particular, *resectable stage IIIA* tumors are either small tumors that present with a low metastatic burden to the ipsilateral mediastinal (N2) lymph nodes or larger tumors that do not involve mediastinal lymph nodes (T4N0/1M0). These tumors, by their advanced nature, may be mechanically removed with surgery; however, surgery does not consistently control the micrometastases that exist within the general area of the operation or systemically. Combinations of chemotherapy and radiotherapy, and in recent years also immunotherapy, are used for locally advanced disease either in the adjuvant or neoadjuvant settings. A multidisciplinary team of experts usually predefines the desired treatment plan in each case.[26]

More broadly, lung carcinoma should be resected when the local disease can be controlled, the patient's physical condition can tolerate the planned resection and reconstruction, and the anticipated operative morbidity and mortality are reasonable. Conditions such as superior vena cava syndrome, tumor invasion across the mediastinum into the main pulmonary artery, N3 nodal metastases, malignant pleural or pericardial disease, or extrathoracic metastases carry greater risk than benefit for resection in most patients. Some centers have had good results with resection and reconstruction of the trachea, atrium, great vessels, or other mediastinal or vertebral structures. These are complex operations requiring dedicated multidisciplinary teams during the preoperative phase and multispecialty teams in the operating room. Patients with tracheoesophageal fistula have a limited life expectancy, and palliative care with stent placement would be recommended.

Local Therapy for Early-Stage Non–Small Cell Lung Cancer

Stages I and II NSCLC can be treated safely with surgery and mediastinal lymph node dissection alone, and most patients have long-term survival. Anatomic resection with lobectomy, with systematic mediastinal lymph node dissection/sampling, is the procedure of choice for lung cancer confined to one lobe (Fig. 58.16). The American College of Surgeons Oncology Group defined a systematic sampling strategy for specific mediastinal lymph nodes. At a minimum, samples of nodal (not adipose) tissue from stations 2R, 4R, 7, 8, and 9 for right-sided cancers and stations 4L, 5, 6, 7, 8, and 9 for left-sided cancers should be obtained. Mediastinal lymphadenectomy should include exploration and removal of lymph nodes from stations 2R, 4R, 7, 8, and 9 for right-sided cancers and stations 4L, 5, 6, 7, 8, and 9 for left-sided cancers.

Lesser operations, such as wedge resection or segmentectomy, may be considered for patients at greater risk for lobectomy. Segmentectomy may be appropriate in patients with peripheral small tumors that have a low metabolic activity on PET-CT. A retrospective propensity matched analysis comparing segmentectomy to lobectomy in stage I lung cancer has shown that at a mean follow-up of 5.4 years, comparing segmentectomy with lobectomy, no differences were noted in locoregional (5.5% vs. 5.1%, respectively; $P = 1.00$), distant (14.8% vs. 11.6%, respectively; $P = 0.29$), or overall recurrence rates (20.2% vs. 16.7%, respectively; $P = 0.30$). Furthermore, when comparing segmentectomy with lobectomy, no significant differences were noted in 5-year freedom from recurrence (70% vs. 71%, respectively; $P = 0.467$) or 5-year survival (54% vs. 60%, respectively; $P = 0.258$).[27] Patients with NSCLC that invades into the chest wall may undergo resection with lobectomy with en-bloc chest wall resection.

SBRT is another local control modality that may be applied in patients who are medically inoperable. Radiation dose and the number of fractions are determined according to tumor location and size. In general, SBRT is well tolerated with good early results. Prospective clinical trials have shown local control and overall survival rates with SBRT to be more than 85% and about 60% at 3 years (median survival, 4 years), respectively. Novel radiation protocols use advanced technologies to better plan and direct radiation delivery to the tumor while minimizing damage to the surrounding tissues.

Neoadjuvant and Adjuvant Therapy

Advanced stage lung cancer, particularly with extensive nodal spread, cannot typically be considered a disease effectively treated with a single modality. Survival after resection may be improved in selected patients with adjuvant chemotherapy. The International Adjuvant Lung Trial enrolled 1,867 patients with completely resected stage I to III NSCLC. These patients were randomly assigned to observation or chemotherapy. Radiation therapy was at the discretion of the institution. The treatment group received one of four cisplatin-based doublet adjuvant regimens. Survival was increased 5% in the adjuvant chemotherapy group. Consequently,

SURGICAL PATHOLOGY REPORT

DIAGNOSIS:
1) LYMPH NODE, 4R, EXCISION: FRAGMENTS OF LYMPH NODE, NEGATIVE FOR MALIGNANCY.
2) LYMPH NODE, 2R, EXCISION: FRAGMENTS OF LYMPH NODE, NEGATIVE FOR MALIGNANCY.
3) LYMPH NODE, PRE-CARINAL, EXCISION: FRAGMENTS OF LYMPH NODE, NEGATIVE FOR MALIGNANCY.
4) LYMPH NODE, LEVEL 4, EXCISION: FRAGMENTS OF LYMPH NODE, NEGATIVE FOR MALIGNANCY.
5) LYMPHNODE, LEVEL 2L, EXCISION: FRAGMENTS OF LYMPH NODE, NEGATIVE FOR MALIGNANCY.
6) LYMPH NODE, LEVEL 7, EXCISION: FRAGMENTS OF LYMPH NODE, NEGATIVE FOR MALIGNANCY.
7) LYMPH NODE, LEVEL 8, EXCISION: INVOLVED BY METASTATIC ADENOCARCINOMA.
8) LYMPH NODE, LEVEL 11, EXCISION: 1 LYMPH NODE, NEGATIVE FOR MALIGNANCY (0/1).
9) LYMPH NODE, LEVEL 10, EXCISION: FRAGMENTS OF LYMPH NODE, NEGATIVE FOR MALIGNANCY.
10) LUNG, LEFT LOWER LOBE, LOBECTOMY: POORLY- DIFFERENTIATED ADENOCARCINOMA, SIMILAR TO PREVIOUS (SEE S10-37167), PREDOMINANTLY SOLID TYPE, 4.9 CM IN GREATEST EXTENT, INVADING INTO VISCERAL PLEURA; RESECTION MARGINS NEGATIVE FOR MALIGNANCY; LARGE VESSEL INVASION PRESENT; CENTRIACINAR EMPHYSEMA.
11) LYMPH NODE, LEVEL 5, EXCISION: FRAGMENTS OF LYMPH NODE, NEGATIVE FOR MALIGNANCY.

COMMENT: These findings correspond to AJCC 7th Edition pathologic Stage IIIA (pT2a, pN2, pM n/a).

Lung Carcinoma Summary Findings

Specimen type: lobectomy
Laterality: left
Tumor site: lower lobe
Tumor size: 4.9 x 4.1 x 3.8 cm
Tumor focality: unifocal
Histologic type: adenocarcinoma
Histologic grade: poorly-differentiated
Visceral pleural invasion: present (confirmed with elastin stain)
Direct extension of tumor: limited to lung and visceral pleura
Venous (large vessel invasion): present
Arterial (large vessel invasion): negative
Lymphatic (small vessel invasion): negative
Treatment effect: n/a

Margins: 1.1 cm from parenchymal margin

Ancillary testing:
EGFR mutational analysis: yes
KRAS mutational analysis: yes
Other (specify): ALK
Pathologic staging (pTNM): IIIA
Primary tumor: pT2a
Regional lymph nodes: pN2
Distant metastasis: pM n/a

FIG. 58.16 Structured pathology report after left lower lobectomy. Lung carcinoma summary findings are helpful in identifying factors critical for pathologic staging and factors that may influence subsequent survival. Ancillary testing for mutational analysis of epidermal growth factor receptor (EGFR), KRAS, and ALK is done routinely.

all patients staged IB and IIB should be considered for adjuvant chemotherapy after resection.

Surgery alone for stage IIIA (N2), IIIB, or IV lung cancer is infrequently performed; however, selected patients may benefit from a multidisciplinary approach to treatment. Resection for isolated brain metastasis is warranted for improvement in symptoms, quality of life, and survival rate. The primary lung tumor can be treated according to T and N stage. Additional treatment beyond resection is needed.[28]

Even with complete resection, patients with resectable NSCLC have poor survival. Preoperative therapy (induction/neoadjuvant) has been evaluated: preoperative paclitaxel and carboplatin followed by surgery was compared with surgery alone in patients with stage IB to IIIA NSCLC without N2 involvement. Overall survival (62 months vs. 41 months) and progression-free (33 months vs. 20 months) survival were higher with preoperative chemotherapy, although the differences did not reach statistical significance.[29] Further, a metaanalysis of randomized clinical trials evaluating preoperative chemotherapy in resectable NSCLCs has indicated that the overall survival of NSCLC patients receiving neoadjuvant chemotherapy was significantly improved compared to those in who had surgery alone (hazard ratio [HR] 0.84; 95% CI, 0.77–0.92; $P = 0.0001$).[30] Other studies have shown that the benefit from preoperative chemotherapy is similar to that attained with postoperative chemotherapy. These results further confirm the recognition that operable NSCLC patients with disease stage IB or higher should be considered for preoperative chemotherapy. Induction chemoradiotherapy has been evaluated for treatment of clinical stage IIIA (N2) NSCLC. In one phase III trial, concurrent chemotherapy and radiotherapy followed by resection was compared with standard concurrent chemotherapy and definitive radiotherapy without resection. The median overall survival was similar in both groups (~23 months). Progression-free survival was better in the surgery group (12.8 months median vs. 10.5 months; $P = 0.017$). The authors reported pneumonectomy was associated with poor outcomes. In an exploratory analysis, overall survival was improved for patients who were found to have undergone induction chemoradiotherapy and lobectomy.[31] In selected patients with resectable stage IIIA NSCLC, induction chemoradiotherapy followed by resection is an alternative treatment to chemoradiotherapy alone. Patients with local extension of lung cancer at the apex of the lung into the thoracic inlet may have characteristics of shoulder and arm pain, Horner syndrome, and occasionally paresthesia in the ulnar nerve distribution of the hand (fourth and fifth fingers) (Fig. 58.17). Patients with all these characteristics may be classified as having Pancoast syndrome. Pain comes from the C8 and T1 nerve roots. Sympathetic nerve involvement may result in Horner syndrome (miosis, ptosis, anhidrosis, and enophthalmos). Typically, the first, second, and third ribs are involved and require resection, but the bony spine and intraforaminal spaces can also be involved. MRI is necessary, in addition to CT, to plan the surgical procedure. Preoperative therapy includes chemoradiotherapy.

Treatment of Metastatic Disease

Metastatic disease (stage IV NSCLC) is usually incurable. Performance and quality of life decline. Patients and families should be informed of the diagnosis and potential outcomes of treatment. Treatment decisions should take into consideration the wishes of the patient and family, and realistic expectations should be set and monitored during therapy. Nevertheless, in recent years, a growing number of biologic and immunologic therapies have been approved for the treatment of advanced NSCLC. Utilization of such therapeutics and their incorporation into conventional anti NSCLC protocols (chemotherapy and radiation) has significantly expanded the therapeutic options for patients with advanced inoperable NSCLC (stages IV and IIIB). Modern NSCLC therapeutics is based on genetic and immunologic phenotyping of the tumor. Treatment is often tailored according to disease characteristics and according to the patients' functional status. NSCLC tumors may be categorized as oncogene addicted, as highly sensitive to immunotherapy, and as tumors that are less likely to respond to either targeted or immunologic therapies (Figs. 58.18 and 58.19).[32] Oncogene addicted tumors are treated with specific small molecules and antibodies that target key NSCLC driving mutations (epidermal growth factor receptor [EGFR], BRAF, ALK, ROS, and MET). Resistance to such therapies eventually develops; however, newer and more efficient second line agents are continuously being developed. To illustrate, osimertinib a novel EGFR tyrosine kinase inhibitor (TKI) had significantly greater efficacy than platinum therapy plus pemetrexed in patients with T790M-positive (a mutation conferring resistance to first line EGFR TKI) advanced NSCLC (including

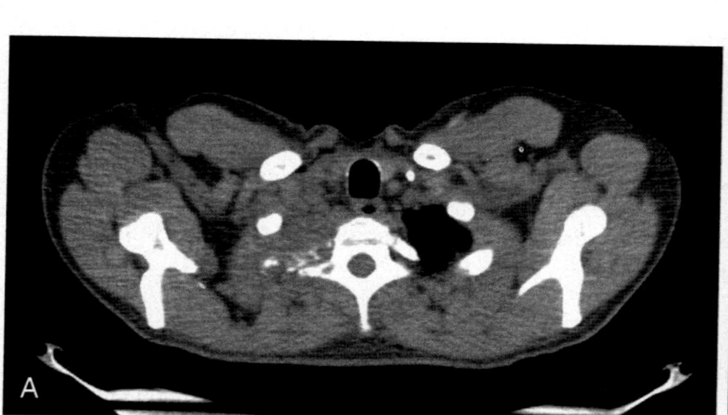

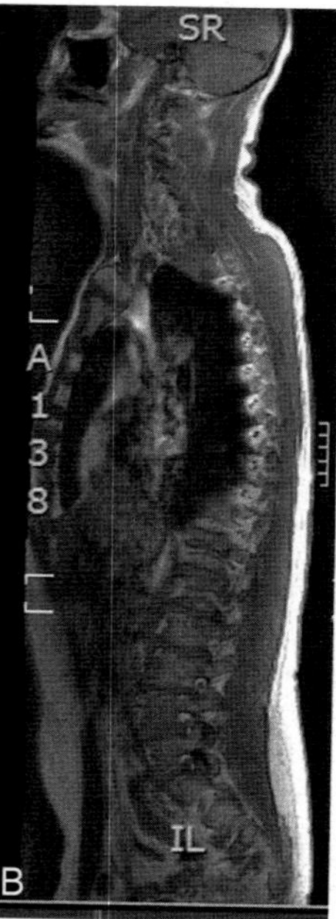

FIG. 58.17 The patient is a 50-year-old man with a right superior sulcus tumor. Diagnostic imaging revealed a right apical mass and destruction of the posterior aspect of the second rib. Transthoracic biopsy was positive for poorly differentiated adenocarcinoma (non–small cell lung carcinoma). Endobronchial ultrasound for mediastinal staging was negative; cervical mediastinoscopy was also negative. Induction chemoradiotherapy was given with 48 Gy in 24 fractions over 1 month with chemotherapy (carboplatin AUC of 5 + pemetrexed 500 mg/m^2). (A) Computed tomography (CT) scan of the chest demonstrates the mass is present in the apex of the chest with complete destruction of the posterior aspect of the right second rib and cortical erosion of the right T2 vertebral body secondary to the mass. The patient is left hand–dominant. (B) Magnetic resonance imaging of the thoracic spine demonstrates a medial right apical lung mass consistent with a Pancoast tumor involving the right lateral aspect of the T2 vertebral body, articular facet, and transverse process. There was also extension into the neural foramen and involvement of the nerve roots on the right at T1-2 and T2-3. There was no extension into the central canal or involvement of the spinal cord. CT scan of the head demonstrated no acute findings involving the brain. Complete resection was performed with a two-surgeon team, a thoracic surgeon and neurosurgeon. The patient required a right upper lobectomy with en-bloc chest wall and vertebral body resection and mediastinal lymph node dissection. Spine stabilization was required.

those with CNS metastases) in whom disease had progressed during first-line EGFR-TKI therapy (progression-free survival of (10.1 months vs. 4.4 months; HR 0.30; 95% CI, 0.23–0.41; $P < 0.001$). Tumors that are considered to be highly sensitive to immunotherapy are treated with immune checkpoint inhibitors that block the PD-1/PD-L1 and CTLA4/CD80/CD86 pathways. In particular, immunotherapy is effective against tumors that express high levels of the immune inhibitory molecule PD-L1, against tumors that have a high mutational burden (as seen in smoke induced NSCLC), and against tumors that have defective DNA repair mechanisms. To illustrate, in patients with advanced NSCLC and PD-L1 expression on at least 50% of tumor cells, pembrolizumab (an anti PD-1 antibody) was associated with significantly longer progression-free and overall survival and with

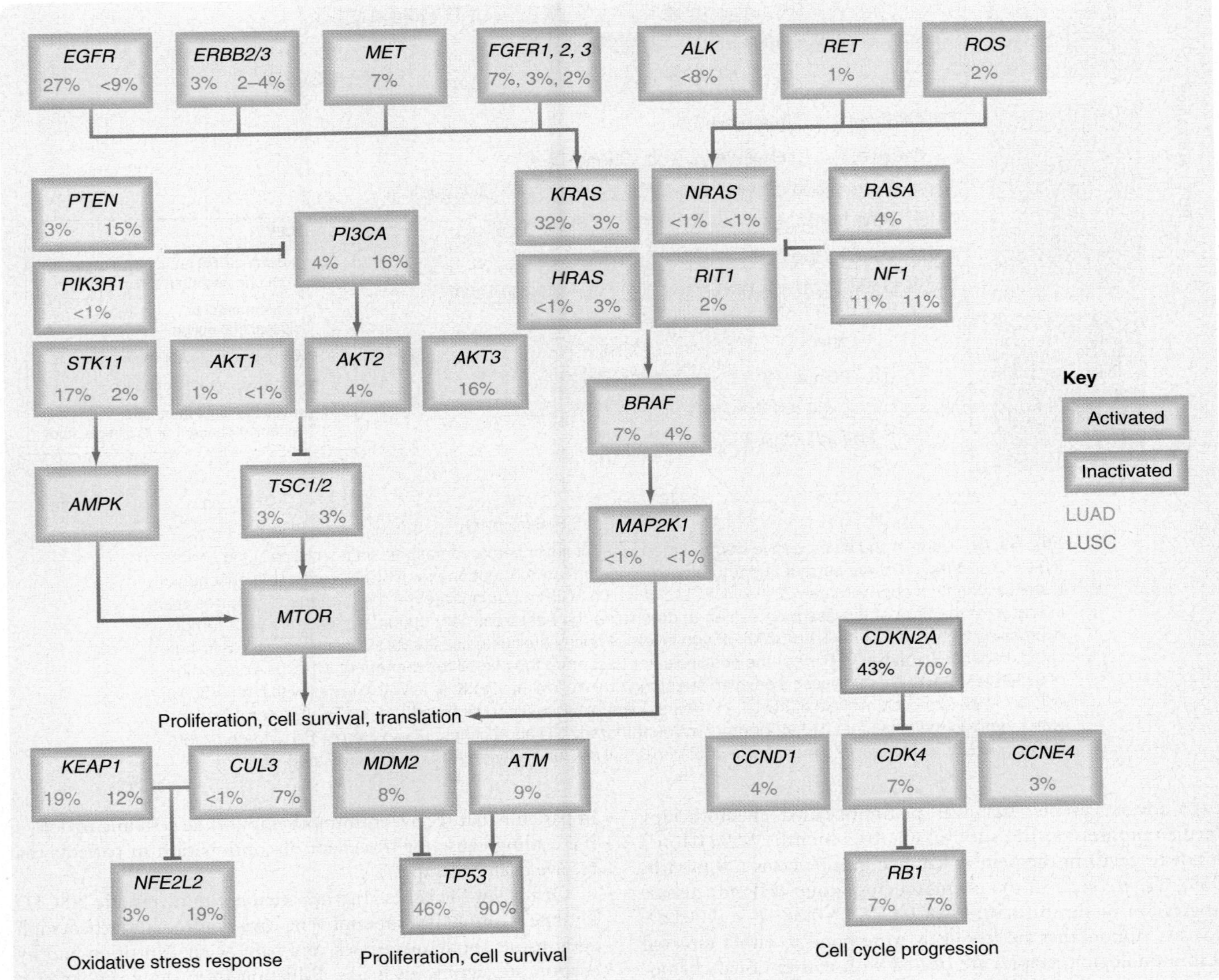

FIG. 58.18 Alterations in targetable oncogenic pathways in LUAD and LUSC. Pathway diagram showing the percentage of non–small cell lung cancer with alterations involving key pathway components for receptor tyrosine kinase signaling, mTOR signaling, oxidative stress response, proliferation, and cell cycle progression. The frequency of alterations is based on the sum of somatic mutations, homozygous deletions, focal amplifications, and by significant up- or downregulation of gene expression (for example, *AKT3, FGFR1, PTEN*). The most commonly mutated genes in LUAD include *KRAS* and *EGFR*, and the tumor suppressor genes *TP53, KEAP1, STK11*, and *NF1*. The frequency of EGFR-activating mutations varies greatly by region and ethnicity. *KEAP1* inactivation in the presence of *KRAS* mutations confers sensitivity to inhibition of glutaminase in preclinical lung cancer models, providing a potential therapeutic strategy in dual *KEAP1*- and *KRAS*-mutant LUAD139. Common mutated genes in LUSC include the tumor suppressors *TP53*, which is present in more than 90% of tumors, and *CDKN2A*. The latter, which encodes the p16INK4A and p14ARF proteins, is inactivated in over 70% of LUSC through epigenetic silencing by methylation (21%), inactivating mutation (18%), exon 1β skipping (4%), or homozygous deletion (29%). Although EGFR amplification occurs, unlike LUAD, actionable mutations in receptor tyrosine kinases are rarely observed in LUSC. (From Herbst RS, Morgensztern D, Boshoff C. The biology and management of non-small cell lung cancer. *Nature*. 2018 ;553:446–454.)

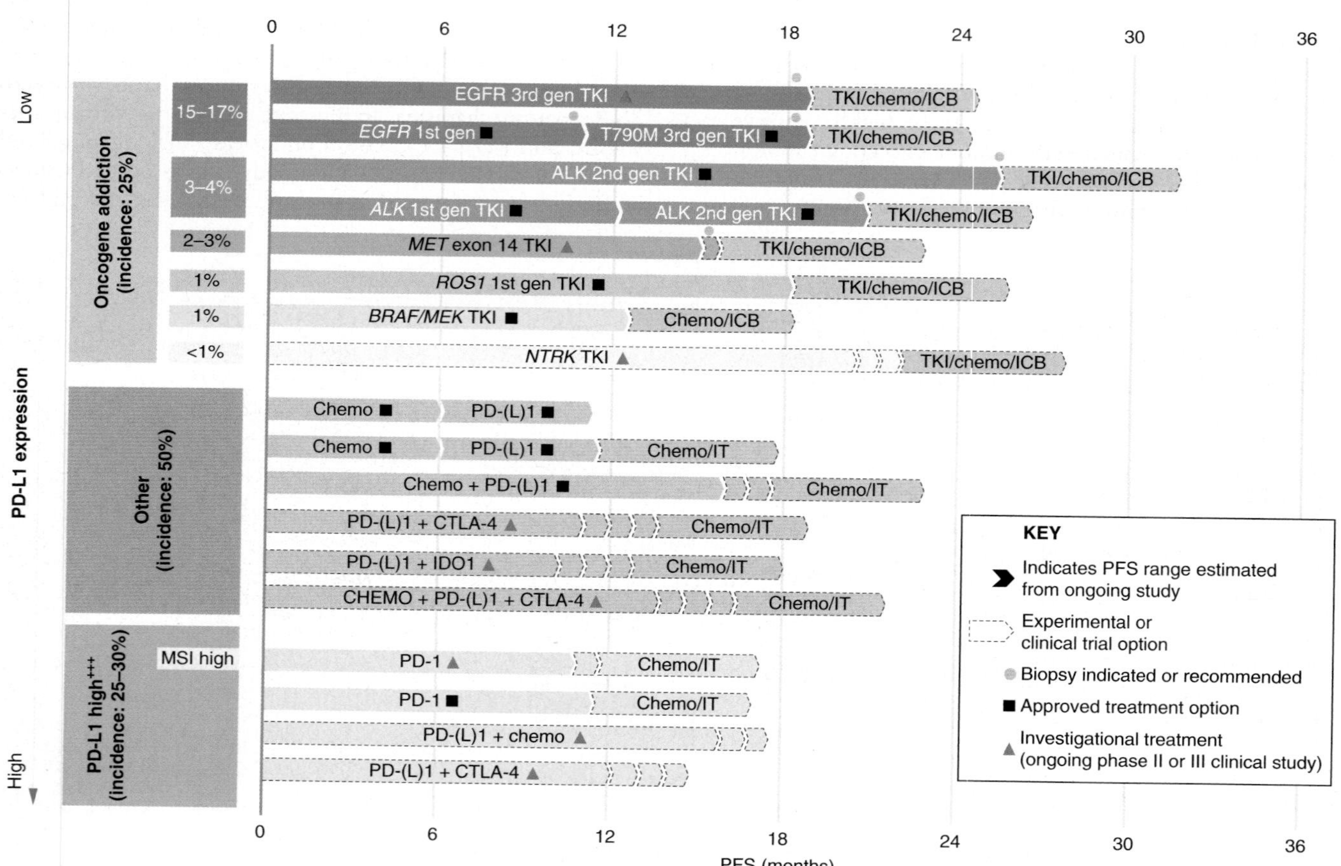

FIG. 58.19 Current and investigative treatment options for advanced or metastatic non–small cell lung cancer (NSCLC). Illustration of the current and future personalized treatment options for NSCLC. Targetable oncogenic drivers account for approximately 25% of NSCLC, of which EGFR mutations are the most frequent. Biopsies are indicated at the time of disease progression to determine the best treatment option. For patients with tumors expressing high levels of PD-L1 (>50%) or high levels of microsatellite instability (MSI), single-agent ICB is indicated. In general, median PFS is not the best indicator to capture the overall true benefit of ICBs, as a proportion of patients remain alive or disease-free even after long-term follow-up. In patients with tumors with high (>50%) or low (>1%) expression levels of PD-L1, current studies are assessing the benefit of anti-PD-(L)1 combinations with cytotoxic therapy, anti-CTLA-4, or other immunotherapy (IT) approaches. (From Herbst RS, Morgensztern D, Boshoff C. The biology and management of non-small cell lung cancer. *Nature*. 2018;553:446–454.)

fewer adverse events than was platinum-based chemotherapy (median progression-free survival was 10.3 months; 95% CI, 6.7 to not reached) in the pembrolizumab group versus 6.0 months (95% CI, 4.2–6.2) in the chemotherapy group (HR for disease progression or death, 0.50; 95% CI, 0.37–0.68; $P < 0.001$).[33] NSCLC tumors that are less likely to respond to either targeted or immunologic therapies are treated with conventional chemotherapy (therapeutics for squamous and nonsquamous NSCLC slightly differ). Platinum-based combinations produce 1-year survival rates of 30% to 40% and are more efficacious than single agents. In the United States, for patients with good functional status, frequently used initial cytotoxic regimens for nonsquamous NSCLC include: 1) cisplatin (or carboplatin)/pemetrexed or 2) carboplatin/paclitaxel with (or without) bevacizumab. Gemcitabine/cisplatin is recommended for patients with either SCC or nonsquamous NSCLC. More recently combination of immunotherapy with chemotherapy have shown promising anti-NSCLC effects even in subgroups of patients whose tumors where less likely to respond to immunotherapy.[34] The side-effect profile of chemotherapy and immunotherapy significantly differs. Autoimmunity it the leading cause for treatment discontinuation in patients that receive immunotherapy while systemic toxicity is the leading cause for treatment discontinuation in patients that receive chemotherapy.

Quality-of-life issues arise in patients with metastatic NSCLC. Dyspnea from MPE, superior vena cava syndrome, tracheoesophageal fistula, bone metastases, and pain occur. Nutrition and hydration are significant issues. Palliation from symptoms may be accomplished with good results. For MPE associated dyspnea, insertion of a tunneled indwelling pleural catheter such as the pleurX drainage systems is indicated.

TRACHEA

The trachea is a semi-flexible tube of 1.5 to 2 cm in width and 10 to 13 cm in length, reaching from the lower portion of the larynx at the level of the sixth to seventh cervical vertebra to the fourth to fifth thoracic vertebra, where it bifurcates to form the two bronchi for the lungs.

The location of the carina is at the level of the angle of Louis anteriorly and the T4 vertebra posteriorly. The tracheal wall consists of up to 20 incomplete rings of hyaline cartilage forming the anterior and lateral circumference, and smooth muscle at the posterior side, which are both embedded into a fibrous membrane of elastic connective tissue.

Its major physiologic role is to conduct air between the larynx and the bronchi, exchange heat and moisture and remove particles. The transport of air is critically dependent on the inner diameter of the trachea. Mucosal swelling, constriction of airway muscles, or tumors that reduce the airway space, but also endotracheal tubes, considerably increase the resistance to airflow: a 50% reduction of the inner diameter increases the resistance sixteenfold, and during turbulent flow up to thirty-twofold. During inspiration, the upper airways warm and humidify the inspired air. This process is very efficient. During quiet breathing at room temperature, air is completely warmed up to 37°C and humidified to 100% saturation shortly distal of the bifurcation; this is called the isothermal saturation point. Tracheobronchial glands produce a mucin-rich secretion that forms a protective barrier between the epithelium and the environment. This secretion is largely controlled by the autonomic nervous system. The mucus collects debris and microorganisms and is transported orally by the mechanical forces of coordinated ciliary beating and the airflow during expiration.[35]

Benign Stenosis of the Trachea

Stenosis of the trachea implies significant functional impairment. A normal 2 cm trachea has a 100% peak expiratory flow rate. A 10 mm opening provides an 80% peak expiratory flow rate. At 5 to 6 mm, only a 30% expiratory flow rate is obtained. Benign stenosis of trachea results mainly from tracheotomy, ventilation, or trauma. Tracheotomy leads to a transmural defect of the ventral part of the cervical trachea. The tracheotomy wound is colonized by bacteria with local necrosis by mechanical alteration. After removal of the tracheostomy tube, the defect is closed by the secondary scar tissue healing, which tends to contract. This process of healing results in an A-shaped stenosis of the trachea (Fig. 58.20). The severity of shrinkage depends on the extension of the defect, necrosis, and infection. Low-volume, high-pressure cuffs of ventilation tubes induce circular necrosis of the tracheal mucosa. Depending on the pressure, the duration of ischemia, and local infection, the underlying cartilages may be bare, necrotic, and destroyed. Mucosal defects without infection can be recovered from surrounding epithelium without relevant morbidity. Deeper destruction and infection of the tracheal wall leads to a ring of granulation tissue forming a sand-glass stenosis. Cuff-induced stenosis appears in the middle part of the trachea. The introduction of low-pressure, high-volume cuffs make this kind of tracheal stenosis a rare disease.[36]

Symptoms of tracheal obstruction can occur immediately after extubation or slowly over several years. Clinical signs like stridor and dyspnea appear when the lumen is obliterated by more than 50%; however, clinical signs and lung function testing are not very sensitive or specific for tracheal stenosis. Standard of treatment for symptomatic patients consists of resection of the pathologic segment of the trachea with end-to-end anastomosis. In case of involvement of the larynx, partial resections of the anterior cricoid cartilage or division of the larynx with tracheolaryngeal silicone stents is used. Short-term and long-term results are satisfying.

Primary Neoplasm of the Trachea

Most tumors of the trachea in adult patients are malignant, with approximately one half to two thirds being SCCs; adenoid cystic carcinomas (ACCs) were the second most common, accounting for approximately 10% to 15% of cases. Less common primary tracheal tumors include mucoepidermoid carcinoma,

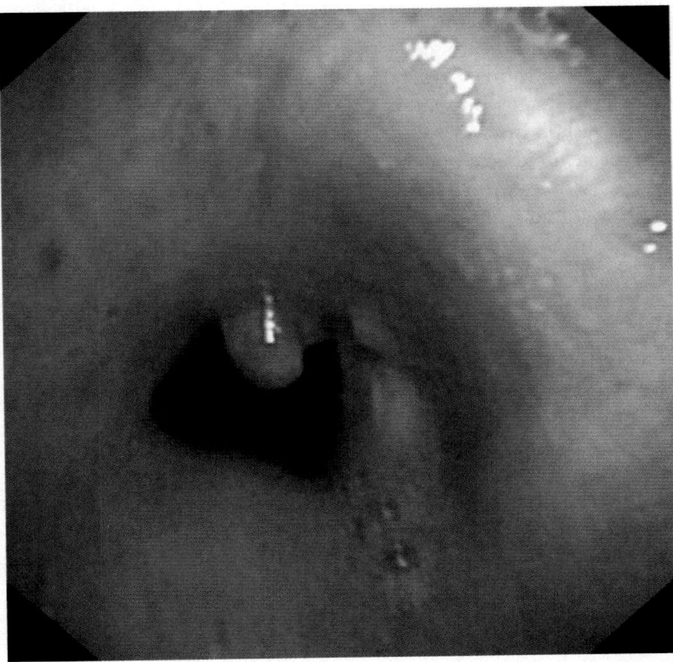

FIG. 58.20 Tracheoscopy three months after decannulation with stenosis of the trachea by shrinkage and granulation tissue. (From Stoelben E, Koryllos A, Beckers F, et al. Benign stenosis of the trachea. *Thorac Surg Clin.* 2014;24:59–65.)

nonsquamous cell bronchogenic carcinomas, sarcomas, carcinoid tumors, and pleomorphic adenoma. Benign tracheal lesions include hemangioma, hamartoma, neurogenic tumors, granular cell tumor, and squamous papillomas. Rather than being primary tracheal tumors, the majority of tracheal tumors occur via direct invasion of the trachea from carcinoma of the lung, esophagus, larynx, or thyroid gland. Hematogenous tracheal metastases have been described in patients with carcinoma of the breast, colon, and kidney, as well as those with melanoma.[37]

SCCs are the most common histopathologic type of tracheal malignancy. Up to 10% can be multifocal. Tumors may arise as an intraluminal nodule and progress to include mediastinal extension or lymph node metastases and may lead to stenosis or tracheoesophageal fistula. They are histologically identical to SCCs of the lung.

ACCs, previously called cylindroma, of the tracheobronchial tree are well-differentiated, slow-growing neoplasms. ACCs typically form polypoid lesions in the trachea or main stem bronchi, but they may form infiltrative plaques with longitudinal or circumferential extension and often breach the cartilaginous plate. Perineural invasion and extension along vascular structures is very common and accounts for the high rate of positive surgical margins, well beyond the gross limits of the tumor. ACCs can have multiple recurrences with late metastases. They are histologically identical to ACCs of the salivary glands.

The most common presenting symptoms of tracheal tumors are due to the presence of a mass within the trachea. These symptoms frequently do not arise until the tumor is large enough to obstruct at least 50% of the diameter of the lumen. Symptoms vary based on the location of the tumor as well as the histologic subtype.

SCCs often present with hemoptysis, given mucosal irritation and ulceration, and are typically diagnosed within four to six months of symptom onset. Dysphagia and hoarseness may also be present. The peak incidence is in the sixth to seventh decade of life. These tumors are seen primarily in smokers.

ACC commonly presents with wheezing or exertional dyspnea, with hemoptysis present in only a minority of cases. Diagnosis is established on average 18 months after symptom presentation. The peak incidence occurs in the fourth and fifth decade of life. It affects men and women equally and usually affects nonsmokers. Low-grade tumors, such as mucoepidermoid carcinomas or benign tumors, may be asymptomatic for years before diagnosis.[38]

The diagnosis of tracheal tumors is often delayed due to similar presenting symptoms with other etiologies, including asthma, COPD, and pneumonia. Chest CT is typically ordered for patients in whom a tracheal pathology is suspected. This study may reveal polypoid lesions, focal stenosis, eccentric narrowing, or circumferential wall thickening. Bronchoscopy is mandatory to obtain a tissue diagnosis and to differentiate between benign and malignant tumors. PET/CT may be useful for staging the cancer, but data on tracheal tumors are limited. Preoperative PET/CT scans may help to assess extent of disease and resectability, particularly for SCC.

The primary treatment modalities for tracheal tumors are surgery and radiation therapy; there are no randomized trials directing the most efficacious treatment approach. The outcome of treatment depends on the stage, as well as the histology of the tracheal tumor. Complete surgical resection is the treatment of choice for malignant tracheal tumors whenever possible, given retrospective data suggesting improved disease outcomes and acceptable postoperative morbidity. Because of the lack of suitable replacement material, the suggested maximum resected length of trachea is 5 cm. Available data suggest that postoperative radiotherapy improves survival for patients with incompletely resected squamous SCC and ACC, but not for those with completely resected tumors. For patients with unresectable, nonmetastatic SCC or ACC, concurrent chemoradiotherapy with a platinum-based regimen may be attempted, though data are limited.[39]

Involvement of the trachea because of local extension from bronchogenic carcinoma may contraindicate resection. Involvement of the trachea because of local extension of esophageal carcinoma may require palliative therapy or stent placement.

Tracheal Trauma

Blunt or penetrating injuries of the tracheobronchial tree are most often accompanied by a variety of different and sometimes life-threatening injuries. Almost 75% to 80% of penetrating injuries involve the cervical trachea, whereas 75% to 80% of blunt injuries occur within 2.5 cm of the carina and 40% occur within the first 2 cm of the right main bronchus.

Blunt or penetrating trauma to the neck or trachea can produce lacerations, transections, or shattering injuries of both the cervical and the mediastinal trachea. Blunt trachea-bronchial injuries are associated with major accompanying injuries in 40% to 100% of cases, primarily involving orthopedic, facial, pulmonary, and intraabdominal injuries. Major associated injuries, mainly of the esophagus and great vessels, were reported in 50% to 80% of penetrating injuries.[40]

Tachypnea and subcutaneous emphysema are the most common clinical signs. Other signs include air escaping from the neck wound, massive air leak after placement of a tube thoracostomy, hemoptysis, stridor, and dysphagia. Chest roentgenogram and chest CT scan are the first step in diagnosis. Paratracheal air, deep cervical emphysema, and pneumomediastinum are common findings. Associated injuries include pneumothorax/hemothorax, ribs fractures, pulmonary contusion, laryngeal fracture, esophageal injury, cervical spine, and great vessels injuries. Bronchoscopy is the most important procedure to exactly locate and assess trachea-bronchial injuries. Early airway assessment followed by definitive airway protection is the key to neck trauma management and trachea-bronchial injuries. Concurrent esophageal injury needs to be excluded by barium esophagography or esophagoscopy. Anesthetic management with laryngeal mask airway may be helpful for initial examination for full visualization of the airway before endotracheal intubation.

Patients with blunt trauma and small injuries or no appreciable air leaks, who do not require positive pressure ventilation and are nonprogressive, may be treated nonoperatively with close monitoring. For all other cases, immediate exploration of neck wounds is crucial for survival because vascular and esophageal injuries are frequent and the tracheal injury often includes cartilages as well as ligamentous portions. Primary surgical repair represents the treatment of choice to reestablish airway continuity. Bronchial disruption may require thoracotomy for repair. Right thoracotomy provides excellent visualization of the carina and proximal left mainstem bronchus.

Acquired tracheoesophageal fistula can occur from cancer or from prolonged intubation with erosion posteriorly. Repair is with separation of the trachea and esophagus, repair of the fistulous tract, and interposition of normal tissue, such as muscle between the two structures.

Tracheoinnominate fistula may result from prolonged cuff erosion inferiorly and anteriorly in the trachea. Inappropriate low stoma may further increase the likelihood of a direct erosion of the trachea by the innominate artery. The tip of the endotracheal tube may predispose to erosions or granulomas within the trachea. Tracheoinnominate fistula may manifest with a sentinel hemorrhage before sudden exsanguinating hemorrhage. Investigation of these sentinel hemorrhage episodes is critical. Evaluation in the operating room may provide for optimal situational control should additional interventions be required.

Principles of Tracheal Surgery

Elective or emergent tracheal surgical procedures are typically performed to improve tracheal patency or repair loss of tracheal integrity. Anesthetic challenges include abnormal airway anatomy and physiology, likely requirements for specialized endotracheal tubes for initial airway management and additional airway devices to meet evolving intraoperative needs, and changes to alternative modes of ventilation if the trachea is open or obstructed.

General inhalational anesthesia is used, and induction may take a long time if the stenosis is tight. The patient should be maintained spontaneously breathing if possible. If the stenosis is less than 5 to 6 mm, dilation may be required before passing the endotracheal tube; the dilation may be performed with rigid bronchoscopy. If the stenosis is greater than 5 to 6 mm, the endotracheal tube may be positioned to a point above the stricture for induction. Stenoses that are subglottic must be dilated for intubation. The endotracheal tube often goes alongside tumors.

The cervical approach for tracheal resection is usually used for tumors of the upper half of the trachea plus all benign tracheal stenoses (because these usually occur as a result of endotracheal tube placement). Occasionally, an upper sternal split may be needed (Fig. 58.21). The posterolateral thoracotomy (fourth interspace) is used for tumors of the lower half of the trachea plus carinal reconstruction. Rigid bronchoscopy for diagnosis, biopsy, dilation,

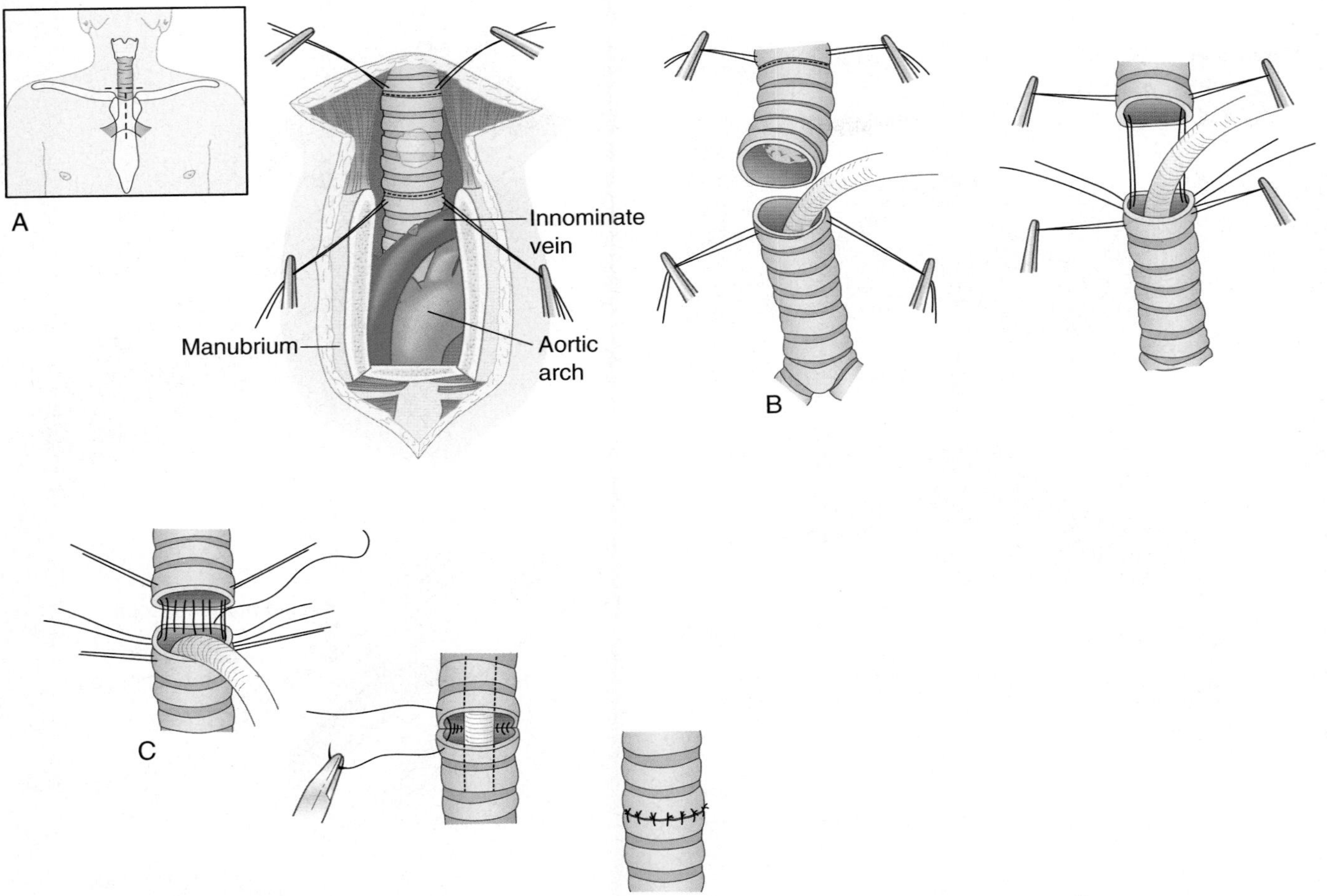

FIG. 58.21 (A) Exposure of the midtrachea through a cervical and partial sternal-splitting incision. The extent of the resection has been marked by sutures. (B) After distal division, a sterile, armored endotracheal tube is placed. After proximal resection, two mattress sutures are placed in the edges of the cartilaginous rings. A simple running suture completes the membranous anastomosis. (C) At this point, the original endotracheal tube is positioned in the distal trachea so that the anastomosis can be completed with interrupted simple sutures between cartilaginous rings.

or morcellation of tumor or other treatment may be required if the tumor cannot be immediately resected (Fig. 58.22).

In general, the maximal amount of trachea that can be resected is approximately 5 cm, but this varies from person to person. Various techniques are used to mobilize the trachea to create a repair without undue tension on the anastomosis. The anterior cervical approach plus mobilization of the trachea and neck flexion can allow for 4 to 5 cm of trachea resection. A suprahyoid release may achieve 1 cm of additional length. Mobilization of the right hilum, together with division of the pericardium around the right hilum, may achieve an additional length.[41]

Procedures to repair subglottic larynx or cricoid stenosis are technically challenging. The recurrent nerves innervate the larynx just superior to the posterolateral cricoid on each side. If the tracheal lesions involve only the anterior surface, the anterior cricoid can be removed and the distal trachea beveled to match the defect. This maneuver spares the recurrent laryngeal nerves. With circumferential involvement, it may be necessary to perform a laryngectomy.

Reconstruction of the lower trachea is performed in the right fourth intercostal space. Intubation of the distal trachea or the left main stem bronchus is performed. Carinal reconstruction is usually performed for tumor and is the most feasible of alternative reconstructions chosen.

Contraindications to trachea repair include (1) inadequately treated laryngeal problem (which does not include single vocal cord paralysis); (2) need for ventilatory support or permanent tracheostomy for patients with amyotrophic lateral sclerosis, myasthenia gravis, or quadriplegia; (3) use of high-dose steroids; and (4) inflamed or recent tracheostomy. Poor pulmonary reserve is not a contraindication for repair in patients who have been weaned from the ventilator.

PULMONARY INFECTIONS

Pulmonary infections requiring surgical interventions are infrequent compared with pleural space infections. Clinical features are similar to pneumonia, including fever, cough, leukocytosis, pleuritic pain, and sputum production. The patient is specifically questioned about aspiration of a foreign body. Evaluation includes CXR and CT scan of the chest and upper abdomen. Bronchoscopy can be performed to clear secretions and, when the diagnosis is suspected, to rule out cancer, foreign body, bronchial stenosis, or stricture. Cultures may be obtained to facilitate antibiotic treatment. Medical treatment is optimized; this includes

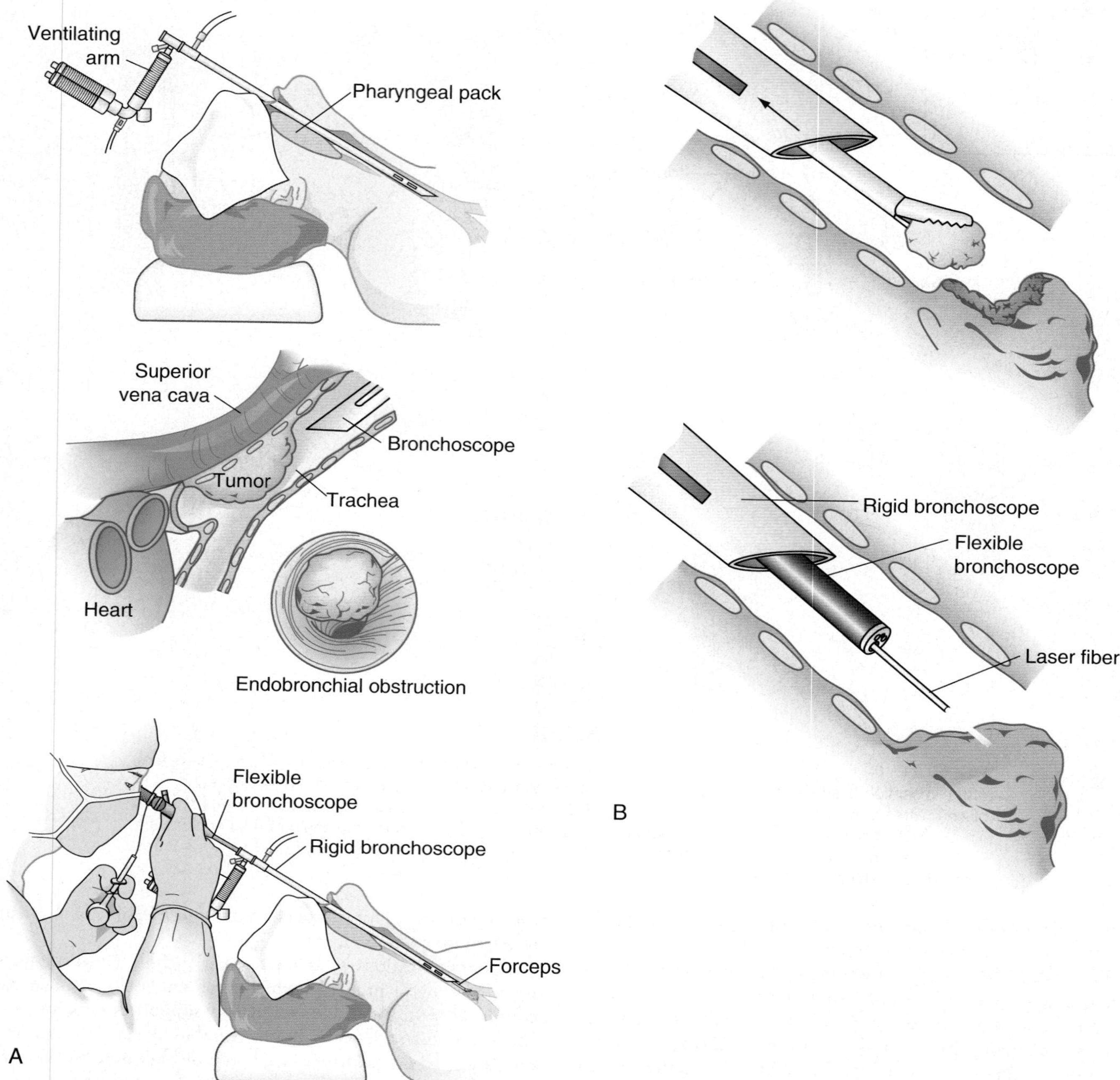

FIG. 58.22 (A) Proper technique for rigid bronchoscopy in a patient with a tracheal mass. *Top,* Pharyngeal packing used to protect the esophagus is shown. The surgeon should be cautious because this packing can move and may obstruct the larynx. Complete removal of the packing is done at the end of the operation. *Middle,* A nearly obstructing tumor is shown. *Bottom,* A flexible bronchoscope is placed into the rigid scope for the biopsy. This protects the airway. (B) Technique for endoscopic resection of a tracheal mass with a rigid bronchoscope without *(top)* and with *(bottom)* use of the laser. (From Sugarbaker DJ, Mentzer SJ, Strauss G, et al. Laser resection of endobronchial lesions: Use of the rigid and flexible bronchoscopes. *Oper Tech Otolaryngol Head Neck Surg.* 1992;3:93.)

discontinuation of smoking and institution of postural drainage, bronchodilator medications, and oral antibiotics.

Bronchiectasis

Bronchiectasis is a chronic respiratory disease characterized by a clinical syndrome of cough, sputum production, and bronchial infection and radiologically by abnormal and permanent dilation of the bronchi.

There are numerous predisposing factors, including cystic fibrosis; α_1-antitrypsin deficiency, primary ciliary syndrome (Kartagener syndrome), bronchial obstruction from foreign body, extrinsic lymph nodes that compress the bronchus, neoplasm, or mucous plug (Fig. 58.23).

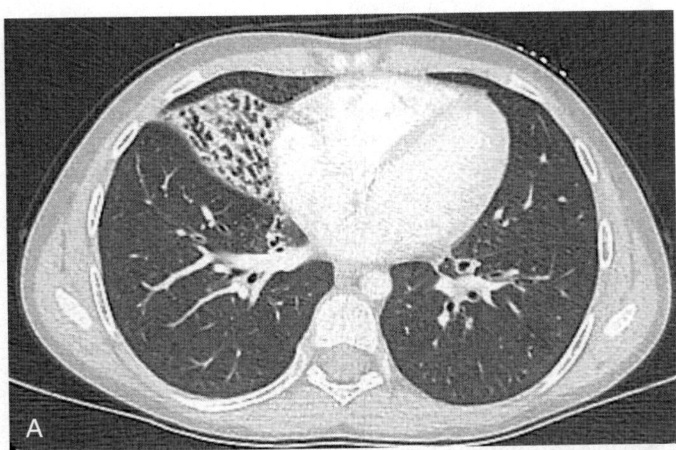

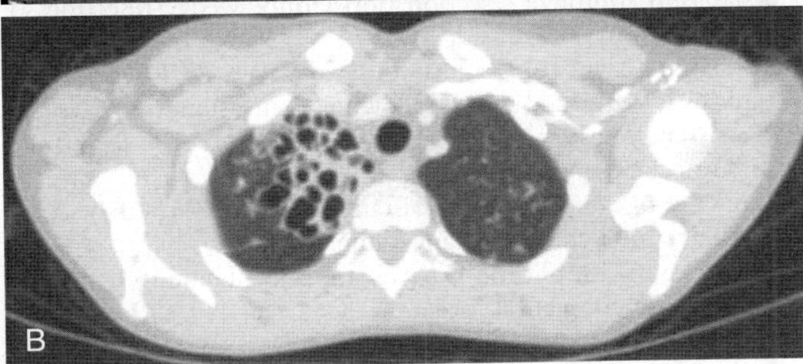

FIG. 58.23 (A) A chest computed tomography (CT) scan of an 8-year-old girl with primary ciliary dyskinesia shows sever bronchiectasis of the right middle lobe *(arrow)*. (B) A chest CT scan of a 6-year-old boy with cystic fibrosis shows severe bronchiectasis of the right upper lobe *(arrow)*.

Exacerbations of bronchiectasis are associated with increased airways and systemic inflammation and progressive lung damage, lung function decline, and mortality. Chronic airways infection, most frequently with *Haemophilus influenzae* and *Pseudomonas aeruginosa* and less frequently with Moraxella catarrhalis, *Staphylococcus aureus*, and Enterobacteriaceae, stimulate and sustain lung inflammation. Persistent isolation of these organisms in sputum or bronchoalveolar lavage is associated with an increased frequency of exacerbations, worse quality of life, and increased mortality.

Inflammation in bronchiectasis is primarily neutrophilic and closely linked to persistent bacterial infection. Excessive neutrophilic inflammation is linked to an increased frequency of exacerbations and rapid lung function decline through degradation of airway elastin, among other mechanisms. Mucociliary clearance is impaired by the impact of structural bronchiectasis, airway dehydration, excess mucus volume and viscosity.

Structural changes in the lung associated with the disease include bronchial dilation, bronchial wall thickening, and mucus plugging as well as small airways disease and emphysema. More than 50% of patients have airflow obstruction, but restrictive, mixed ventilatory pattern and preserved lung function are also frequently observed.

Therapies may aim to treat airflow obstruction (e.g., bronchodilators), to improve exercise capacity (pulmonary rehabilitation), or to remove poorly functioning or diseased lung (surgical resection). Treatment is primarily based on the principles of preventing or suppressing acute and chronic bronchial infection, improving mucociliary clearance, and reducing the impact of structural lung disease.

Patients with localized disease and a high exacerbation frequency despite optimization of all other aspects of their bronchiectasis management are candidates for surgical resection. The rationale for surgical treatment of bronchiectasis is to break the vicious circle of bronchiectasis by removing the lung segments that are no longer functional and preventing the contamination of adjacent lung zones. Surgery is also the procedure of choice for massive haemoptysis refractory to bronchial artery embolization, but emergency surgery in unstable patients is associated with higher morbidity and mortality. Lobectomy is the most frequently performed operation. VATS is often preferred to better preserve lung function and reduce morbidity. In comparison with open surgery, VATS has been reported to produce comparable symptomatic improvement, but with shorter hospital stay, fewer complications, and less pain.[42]

Although bilateral bronchiectasis (reported in 5.8%–30% of surgical series) is not an absolute contraindication for surgery, other options such as prolonged conservative treatment or bronchial artery embolization are frequently used as an alternative.

Lung Abscess

Lung abscess is defined as necrosis of the pulmonary parenchyma caused by microbial infection. Most lung abscesses arise as a complication of aspiration pneumonia and are caused by species of anaerobes that are normally present in the gingival crevices. The most common organisms are *Peptostreptococcus*, *Prevotella*, *Bacteroides* (usually not *B. fragilis*), and *Fusobacterium* spp. Many other bacteria can also cause lung abscesses, including Streptococcus anginosus, *S. aureus*, *K. pneumoniae*, *Streptococcus pyogenes*, *Burkholderia pseudomallei*, *Haemophilus influenzae* type b, *Legionella*, *Nocardia*, and *Actinomyces*. In the immunocompromised host, the most common causes of lung abscess are *Pseudomonas aeruginosa* and other aerobic gram-negative bacilli, *Nocardia* spp, and fungi (*Aspergillus* and *Cryptococcus* spp).

Most patients with lung abscesses, and nearly all patients with lung abscesses due to anaerobic bacteria, present with indolent symptoms that evolve over a period of weeks or months. The characteristic features suggest pulmonary infection, including fever, cough, and sputum production. Evidence of chronic systemic disease is usually present, with night sweats, weight loss, and anemia.

A chest radiograph will often demonstrate infiltrates with a cavity, frequently in a segment of the lung that is dependent in the recumbent position (e.g., the superior segment of a lower lobe or a posterior segment of the upper lobes). A better anatomic definition can be achieved with CT. It can be particularly helpful if there is a question of cavitation that cannot be clearly delineated on the chest radiograph or if an associated mass lesion is suspected. A CT will also distinguish between a parenchymal lesion and a pleural collection, which are managed very differently (Fig. 58.24).

The antibiotic treatment of lung abscess is almost always empiric. Empiric regimens should penetrate the lung parenchyma and target both strict anaerobes and facultatively anaerobic streptococci. Drugs that are reasonable to use are any combination of a beta-lactam–beta-lactamase inhibitor or a carbapenem. The duration of therapy is controversial. Some treat for three weeks as a standard and others treat based upon the response.

Bronchoscopy may be used for treatment to assist in drainage of the cavity either directly or via transbronchial catheterization of the cavity. Most patients (85%–95%) respond to medical management with rapid decrease in fluid, collapse of the walls, and complete healing in 3 to 4 months. Patients with symptoms for longer than 3 months before treatment or cavities larger than 4 to 6 cm are less likely to respond.

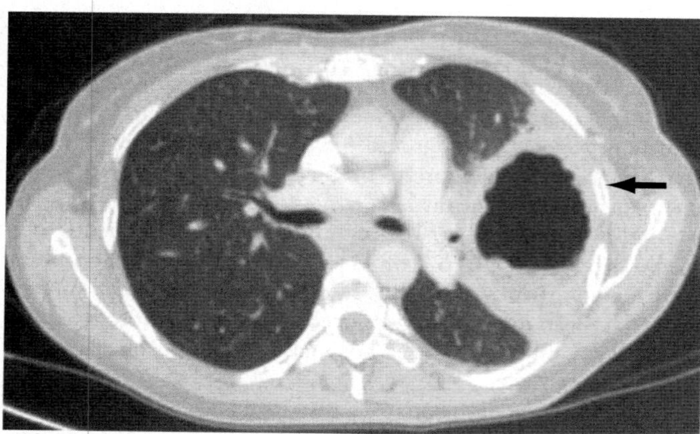

FIG. 58.24 A chest computed tomography scan of a 43-year-old woman shows a left upper lobe abscess *(arrow)*, a complication of pulmonary infection with *Streptococcus milleri.*

Surgery is rarely required for patients with uncomplicated lung abscess. Surgical therapy is indicated for persistent cavity (≥2 cm and thick-walled), failure to clear sepsis after 8 weeks of medical therapy, hemoptysis, and exclusion of cancer. If a lung abscess ruptures into the pleural cavity, simple drainage may suffice, and the patient is managed for empyema or bronchopleural fistula. Lobectomy is typically required; the mortality rate is 1% to 5%. Occasionally, external drainage may be required in critically ill patients if pleural symphysis has occurred.

Other Bronchopulmonary Disorders

Bronchopulmonary disorders caused by inflammatory lymph node disease are usually caused by tuberculosis or histoplasmosis. Lobar atelectasis, hemoptysis, or broncholithiasis can occur. Bronchial compressive disease typically occurs most commonly in the middle lobe. More than 20% of disorders are caused by cancer. This condition results in repeated infection in the same area of the lung, which usually responds to antibiotics. Bronchoscopy is essential to rule out cancer and foreign body and to evaluate for stricture. Medical management is required to treat infection. Surgery is indicated to treat bronchostenosis, irreversible bronchiectasis, or severe recurrent infection.

Broncholithiasis is a calcified node tightly adherent to a bronchus. An innocent hemoptysis may occur even with a negative CXR. Sudden bleeding caused by erosion of a small bronchial artery and mucosa by a spicule in the calcified node causes this hemoptysis. Bright red blood occurs and usually stops with sedation and antitussive therapy. This type of hemoptysis is almost never massive (≥600 mL in 24 hours). Bronchoscopy is possible during a bleeding episode to localize the site of the bleeding. Nasal or pharyngeal lesions or hematemesis from a gastrointestinal source should be excluded.

Organizing pneumonia may replace lung parenchyma with scar tissue or persistent atelectasis or consolidation. If the shadow or mass persists over 6 to 8 weeks, resection is performed to exclude carcinoma. The differential diagnosis includes pneumonia, congenital abnormality, and aneurysm of the aorta.

Mycobacterial Infections

Mycobacterium tuberculosis infects approximately 7% of patients exposed, and tuberculosis develops in 5% to 10% of patients who are infected. A primary infection develops. The exudative response progresses to caseous necrosis. Postprimary tuberculosis tends to occur in apical and posterior segments of the upper lobes and superior segments of the lower lobes. Healing occurs with fibrosis and contracture. Extensive caseation with cavitation may occur early. Coalescing areas of caseous necrosis may form cavities. There are frequently incomplete septations and lobulations. Erosions of septations supplied by bronchial arteries cause hemoptysis and may be secondarily infected.

Medical management is with isoniazid, rifampin, ethambutol, streptomycin, and pyrazinamide. Bronchoscopy may be required for patients who do not respond to medical management. Cancer should be excluded for a newly identified mass on CXR even with a positive tuberculosis skin test and acid-fast bacillus-positive sputum. In general, surgery for treatment of tuberculosis is most effective for patients with poor clinical response or intolerance to supervised medical therapy who have pulmonary disease that is amenable to complete resection (lobectomy, wedge resection, or pneumonectomy).[43] Consideration of surgery for management of multidrug-resistant tuberculosis and extensively drug-resistant tuberculosis is warranted in the following circumstances:

- Persistently positive sputum cultures beyond four to six months of antituberculous therapy.
- Presence of extensive drug resistance that is unlikely to be cured with antituberculous therapy alone.
- Presence of complications such as massive hemoptysis or persistent bronchopleural fistula.

In general, surgery should be performed only after several months of antituberculous therapy has been administered, after smear conversion (if possible) and ideally after culture conversion. A full course of antituberculous therapy should be administered following surgical resection. Surgical therapy may be considered when medical therapy fails and persistent tuberculosis-positive sputum remains and when surgically correctable residua of tuberculosis may be of potential danger to the patient. This is not the same management as for atypical mycobacteria; many of these patients remain clinically well even with positive sputum.

Surgical complications are doubled if the sputum is positive for *M. tuberculosis* and decreased if remaining lung tissue is fully expanded within the chest. Infectious complications include empyema, bronchopleural fistula, and endobronchial spread of the disease and are associated with a higher mortality rate. Tuberculosis infection of the pleural space without lung destruction is primarily treated medically.

Thoracoplasty or muscle flap interposition may be used to control postresection empyema space. Collapse therapy, with thoracoplasty or plombage, is rarely used to manage parenchymal disease alone.

Fungal and Parasitic Infections

The surgical management of fungal infections includes diagnosis and management of complications of fungal disease. Frequently, cancer has to be excluded or other infectious or benign conditions have to be confirmed. Medical management may be considered as initial treatment of fungal diseases in the lung and as part of the patient's overall management.

Immunocompromised patients experience *Aspergillus* spp. infection as the most frequent opportunistic infection, followed by *Candida* and *Nocardia* spp. and mucormycosis. Normal, or immunocompetent, patients may be affected by histoplasmosis, coccidioidomycosis, or blastomycosis. Immunocompromised and immunocompetent patients may be affected by actinomycosis and cryptococcosis. Although *Nocardia* and *Actinomyces* spp. are bacteria, they are usually discussed with fungal infections. Diagnosis

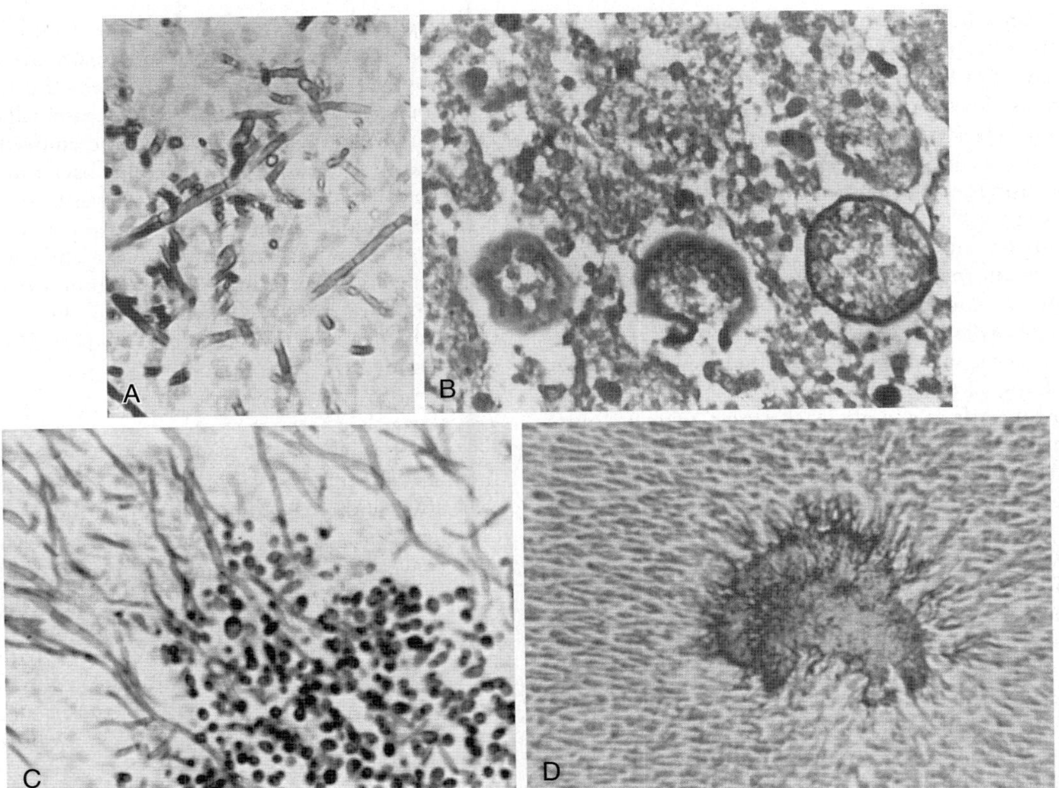

FIG. 58.25 (A) The coarse fragmented, septate mycelia of *Aspergillus fumigatus*. (B) Microscopic section of a coccidioidal granuloma (×400) shows spherules packed with endospores. (C) *Candida albicans* with both the mycelial and the yeast forms. (D) Actinomycotic granule shows branching filaments of a microscopic colony of *Actinomyces israelii*. (Gomori stain, ×250.) (A and C, From Takaro T. Thoracic mycotic infections. In: *Lewis' practice of surgery*. New York, NY.: Hoeber Medical Division, Harper & Row;1968. (B) from Scott S, Takaro T. Thoracic mycotic and actinomycotic infections. In: Shields TW, ed. *General thoracic surgery*. 4th ed. Baltimore; Williams & Wilkins:1994.)

is most often made by sputum examination using potassium hydroxide preparations (Fig. 58.25). Cultures may take some time for results to be obtained; Papanicolaou test cytology may be best. Silver methenamine stain is used for microscopic evaluation. Most infections are self-limited and do not require treatment. Intravenous or oral antifungal agents may be used for treatment of the diseases.

Aspergillosis is an opportunistic infection, characterized by coarse fragmented septa and hyphae (see Fig. 58.25A). There are three types of aspergillosis: aspergilloma, invasive pulmonary aspergillosis, and allergic bronchopulmonary aspergillosis. Aspergilloma is the most common form of aspergillosis. The fungus colonizes an existing lung cavity, commonly a tuberculosis cavity. CXR may demonstrate a crescent radiolucency next to a rounded mass. Cavities may form because of destruction of the underlying pulmonary parenchyma, and debris and hyphae may coalesce and form a fungus ball, which lies free in the cavity and can move with the patient's change in position. Invasion and destruction of parenchymal blood vessels occur within this cavity. Patients with aspergilloma fungus balls are at high risk for fatal hemorrhage; they are treated aggressively and undergo resection when possible. Involvement and destruction of parenchymal blood vessels occur. Prophylactic resection is controversial, although some physicians recommend resection if isolated disease is present in low-risk patients. Surgery is indicated for treatment, for massive or recurrent hemoptysis, or to rule out neoplasm. The procedure of choice is lobectomy. The operation can be complex with a significant inflammatory response within the hilum. Invasive aspergillosis occurs in immunocompromised patients and manifests with chest pain, cough, and hemoptysis. The treatment is primarily medical, although lung biopsy may be necessary for diagnosis. Allergic aspergillosis is diagnosed by bronchoscopy and represents the allergic reaction to chronic colonization with the fungus. It is usually treated medically. Rarely, resection is performed for localized bronchiectasis.

Histoplasmosis is the most common of all fungal infections in the United States and is most frequently a serious systemic fungal disease. *Histoplasma capsulatum* is endemic to the Mississippi and Ohio River valleys as well as portions of the southwestern United States. A high percentage of patients are affected usually with a subclinical form of this disease. An inoculum (from the mycelial form found in soil, decaying materials, and bat or bird guano) can produce an acute pneumonic illness in immunocompetent hosts, which usually resolves without specific treatment. The yeast form exists in macrophages or within the cytoplasm of the alveoli. Pathologic examination demonstrates granulomas (e.g., tuberculosis) or caseating epithelioid granulomas. The lymphogenous reaction to *Histoplasma* causes mediastinal lymph node enlargement, middle lobe syndrome, bronchiectasis, esophageal traction diverticulum, broncholithiasis with hemoptysis, tracheoesophageal fistula, constrictive pericarditis, or fibrosing mediastinitis with superior vena cava syndrome or other problems relating to compression of mediastinal structures. In addition to the compressive symptoms, the lymphadenopathy caused by histoplasmosis may confound radiographic evaluation of the mediastinal lymph nodes in patients with lung cancer and may complicate lung resection.

Coccidioidomycosis is endemic to the Southwest and is localized in the soil. It is second only to histoplasmosis in frequency. Inhaling the organism results in a primary lung disease that is usually self-limited (see Fig. 58.25B). In endemic areas, coccidioidomycosis is a frequent cause of lung nodules, and resection may be required to rule out malignancy. Medical management is preferred. Surgery may be considered for treatment of cavitary disease or complications of cavitary disease.

Cryptococcosis is the second most common lethal fungus after histoplasmosis. Lungs are frequently involved. Central nervous system involvement with meningitis is the most frequent cause of death. Any patient diagnosed with pulmonary cryptococcosis undergoes lumbar puncture to rule out central nervous system involvement. Surgery may be required for open lung biopsy for diagnosis or to exclude lung cancer.

Mucormycosis is a rare, opportunistic, rapidly progressive infection; it occurs in immunocompromised patients, including patients with diabetes. The appearance is that of a black mold; it has wide nonseptate branching hyphae. The infection causes blood vessels to thrombose and lung tissue to infarct. Clinically, the rhinocerebral form occurs much more frequently than the pulmonary form of consolidation and cavities. Medical management involves cessation of steroids and antineoplastic drugs and initiation of amphotericin and control of diabetes. The disease is often too advanced for effective treatment. Aggressive surgical and medical treatment may improve what is usually a grave prognosis.

Candida is a small, thin-walled budding yeast that occurs in immunocompromised patients (see Fig. 58.25C). Lung involvement alone is rare. Surgery may be needed to confirm the diagnosis.

Pneumocystis carinii is an opportunistic infection that is positive on silver methenamine stain. Bronchoalveolar lavage is diagnostic in more than 90% of patients. However, lung biopsy may be required to confirm the diagnosis.

Surgery may also be used to manage the sequelae and complications of parasitic infections. Infections with *Entamoeba histolytica* are usually confined to the right lower thorax and are related to extension from a liver abscess below the diaphragm via direct extension or lymphatics to the right thorax. Metronidazole (Flagyl) is usually effective, although Flagyl and tube drainage may be required for treatment of empyema. Open resection is infrequently required. Similarly, infection with *Echinococcus* spp. may occur. The hydatid cyst may rupture, flooding the lung or producing a severe hypersensitivity reaction. A lung abscess could occur with compression of the airway, great vessels, or esophagus. Surgery, if feasible, may include simple enucleation via cleavage of planes between the cyst and the normal tissue. Aspiration and hypertonic saline 10% may be performed before enucleation. Positive pressure on the lung needs to be maintained until the cyst is out to prevent contamination, soilage, or hypersensitivity reaction. Nonoperative therapy for small asymptomatic calcified cysts may be considered. Paragonimiasis is another common infection and cause of hemoptysis in Asia. In endemic areas, prevalence may be 5%, and hemoptysis from paragonimiasis must be differentiated from tuberculosis or lung cancer.

Actinomycosis is a bacterium that is not found free in nature. It produces a chronic anaerobic endogenous infection deep within a wound. "Sulfur granules" draining from infected sinuses are microcolonies (see Fig. 58.25D). The cervicofacial form is the most common. The thoracic form usually occurs as pulmonary parenchymal disease resembling cancer. The treatment is most commonly penicillin. Surgery may occasionally be required for radical excision of chest wall disease and empyema.

Nocardiosis is caused by an aerobic bacterium widely disseminated in soil and domestic animals; it was formerly rare, although it is increasing in immunocompromised patients. Nocardiosis resembles actinomycosis in invading the chest wall and produces subcutaneous abscesses and sinuses draining sulfur granules. Surgery is performed to exclude cancer, to obtain a diagnosis, or to treat complications of the disease. Medical therapy may include sulfonamides.

MASSIVE HEMOPTYSIS

In clinical practice, massive hemoptysis may be defined as greater than 500 to 600 mL of blood loss from the lungs in 24 hours, or bleeding at a rate of more than 100 mL/hr, regardless of whether abnormal gas exchange or hemodynamic instability exists. The proximal airways may be occluded with only 150 mL of clotted blood, and even lower volume hemoptysis may be life-threatening. The physiologic impact and threat to the patient who presents with massive hemoptysis are greatly affected by the degree of underlying lung and heart disease. The current mortality rate is approximately 13% and is related to drowning or suffocation rather than exsanguination.

There are numerous causes of massive hemoptysis that originate in the lower respiratory tract. Bronchiectasis, tuberculosis, bronchogenic carcinoma, and various lung infections are still believed to be the most common causes of massive hemoptysis.

The principles of the initial management of a patient with massive hemoptysis include establishing a patent airway, ensure adequate gas exchange and cardiovascular function, and control the bleeding. Flexible bronchoscopy is usually the preferred initial diagnostic study. It can be performed in the intensive care unit, is readily available, and provides a view of the more distal airways. Rigid bronchoscopy is an acceptable alternative if flexible bronchoscopy is either inadequate or seems likely to be insufficient in light of the amount of bleeding. If bronchoscopy fails to identify the cause of the massive hemoptysis and the patient continues to bleed, arteriography should next be performed because it may be useful for therapy (embolization) as well as diagnosis. If bronchoscopy fails to identify the cause of the massive hemoptysis, but the bleeding has ceased, CT of the chest with high-resolution cuts should be performed. Definitive therapy for massive hemoptysis is treatment of the underlying cause.

Conservative management may consist of maintaining a functional and patent airway, bronchoscopy, clearing the airway of blood, cough suppression (with codeine), and monitoring until stabilized. Angiographic catheterization for massive hemoptysis may be considered in patients with hemoptysis. Risks include spinal cord ischemia and paralysis. Small particles of polyvinyl alcohol or other synthetic materials used for embolization occlude vessels at a peripheral level. Embolization may be repeated. Patients who continue to bleed despite both a flexible bronchoscopic intervention and arteriographic embolization may benefit from another attempt at bronchoscopic bleeding control via rigid bronchoscopy. If the bleeding cannot be controlled via rigid bronchoscopy, surgery may be the best option. The morbidity and mortality of emergent surgery for persistent massive bleeding are high. Common complications of surgery for massive hemoptysis include

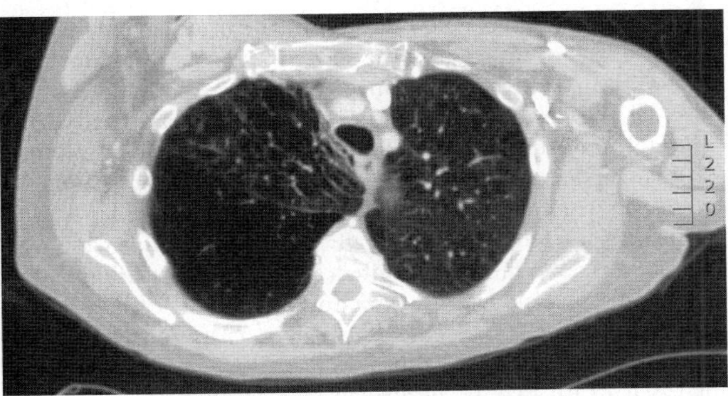

FIG. 58.26 Bullous emphysema. The patient is a chronic smoker (>100 pack-years) and developed emphysema, which is progressing. The superior segment of the right lower lobe is completely destroyed, and the resultant bullae are compressing functioning lung parenchyma in the right and the left lung.

empyema, bronchopleural fistula, postoperative pulmonary hemorrhage, lung infarction, respiratory insufficiency, wound infection, and hemothorax. Empyema and bronchopleural fistula are especially frequent after emergent surgery.

EMPHYSEMA AND DIFFUSE LUNG DISEASE

Emphysema

Emphysema is defined as dilation and destruction of the terminal air spaces. These air cavities are blebs (subpleural air space separated from the lung by a thin pleural covering with only minor alveolar communications) or bullae (larger than a bleb with some destruction of the underlying lung parenchyma). Bullous emphysema (Fig. 58.26) is either congenital without general lung disease or a complication of COPD with more or less generalized lung disease. The challenge is to separate the disability related to the bullae from that caused by the chronic emphysema or chronic bronchitis. DLCO is a good index of the state of severity of the generalized lung disease. On pulmonary angiography, bullae are vacant and do not contain vessels. The bullae may compress normal lung with crowding of the relatively normal pulmonary vasculature. COPD may show abrupt narrowing and tapering of vessels. Surgical therapy includes resection of the bullae to leave functioning lung tissue. Simple removal of the bullae alone is required. Lobectomy is seldom indicated because good lung tissue is removed, which is frequently needed for independent function by these patients, who have significant lung impairment.

Treatment of emphysema is primarily medical, but there are surgical therapies. Although emphysema usually diffusely involves the lung, it may have a heterogeneous distribution within the lung. These areas may be identified by CT and perfusion scan. Often the disease predominates in the upper lobes and the superior segment of the lower lobes. Lung volume reduction surgery removes areas of greatest emphysematous involvement. The remaining lung tissue expands with improved elastic recoil, improved aeration and perfusion of the remaining lung, and improved chest wall mechanics. The National Emphysema Treatment Trial compared lung volume reduction surgery with the best medical therapy. Patients with predominantly upper lobe emphysema and low exercise capacity had lower mortality with lung volume reduction surgery than medical therapy.[44] In patients with nonupper lobe emphysema and high exercise capacity, mortality was higher in the operative group. Long-term results have been favorable. Endoscopic therapies have been developed, including airway bypass and one-way valves.

Lung transplantation is performed for COPD (including α_1-antitrypsin deficiency), pulmonary fibrosis, primary pulmonary hypertension, cystic fibrosis, and bronchiectasis. The survival rates after lung transplantation are approximately 80% at 1 year, 65% at 3 years, 54% at 5 years, and 32% at 10 years.[45] Long-term immunosuppression is required. Unilateral lung transplantation is more readily tolerated than bilateral lung transplantation; however, bilateral lung transplantation is more frequently performed and has a survival advantage after 1 year.

Diffuse Lung Disease

The surgeon's role in diffuse lung disease is to obtain a diagnosis, typically by open lung biopsy after other methods (e.g., transthoracic needle aspiration; bronchoscopy with transbronchial biopsy) have failed. The CXR may demonstrate an alveolar pattern (fluffy with air bronchograms) or an interstitial pattern (ground-glass or granular appearance, indicating a diffuse increase in interstitial tissue) (Box 58.1). Patients may be mildly symptomatic, and biopsy may be needed to confirm or exclude a specific diagnosis before embarking on aggressive medical therapy, such as cyclophosphamide for Wegener granulomatosis, or patients may be critically ill and in the intensive care unit, requiring mechanical ventilation.

Sarcoidosis affects the lungs in 90% of patients with this diagnosis, causing symptoms of dyspnea and dry cough. Foci of noncaseating epithelioid granulomas may be found in any part of the body. In 40% to 50% of cases, patients have insidious respiratory complaints without constitutional symptoms. Severe progressive pulmonary fibrosis may develop in 10% to 20% of patients. Bilateral hilar mediastinal lymph nodes are involved in 60% to 80% of patients. Bronchoscopic lung biopsy is the initial diagnostic procedure. If required, biopsy of mediastinal lymph nodes may be performed. Steroids may be used for treatment.

Lung biopsy may be required for progressive interstitial parenchymal changes for which no diagnosis can be obtained. Lung biopsies can be performed using minimally invasive techniques. Biopsy specimens are sent for routine, fungal, and acid-fast bacillus culture. In immunocompromised patients, *Nocardia* cultures are considered. If possible, the surgeon should sample more than one area of the lung. One method is to resect the worst-appearing region on radiography and the most normal-appearing area. The normal-appearing lung may exhibit early-stage disease and may aid the pathologist in making the diagnosis. Frozen section is used only to confirm that adequate samples of the pathologic process were obtained. In the acute setting of a critically ill patient, an open lung biopsy is performed only when the results would significantly modify subsequent treatment, such as the initiation of protocol-based treatment for experimental antibiotics, or to withdraw futile care.

Adult Respiratory Distress Syndrome

Adult respiratory distress syndrome is a complex biologic and clinical process. Acute deterioration of pulmonary function occurs exclusive of pulmonary edema, pneumonia, or exacerbation of COPD. Approximately 50,000 cases occur each year in the United States, with a mortality rate of 30% to 40%.

The initial clinical presentation of dyspnea, tachypnea, hypoxemia, and mild hypocapnia is nonspecific. CXR may show diffuse bilateral infiltrates secondary to increased interstitial fluid. Pathologically, vascular congestion occurs with alveolar collapse, edema, and inflammatory cell infiltration. The underlying mechanism is

BOX 58.1 Classification of diffuse lung diseases.

Infections (more commonly cause focal disease, granuloma formation)
- Viruses—especially influenza, cytomegalovirus
- Bacteria—tuberculosis, all types of regular bacteria, Rocky Mountain spotted fever
- Fungi—all types can cause diffuse disease
- Parasites—Pneumocystis species infection, toxoplasmosis, paragonimiasis, among others

Occupational causes
- Mineral dusts
- Chemical fumes—NO_2 (silo filler disease), Cl, NH_3, SO_2, CCl_4, Br, HF, HCl, HNO_3, kerosene, acetylene

Neoplastic disease
- Lymphangitic spread
- Hematogenous metastases
- Leukemia, lymphoma, bronchioloalveolar cell cancer

Congenital—familial
- Niemann-Pick disease, Gaucher disease, neurofibromatosis, and tuberous fibrosis

Metabolic and unknown
- Liver disease, uremia, inflammatory bowel disease

Physical agents
- Radiation, O_2 toxicity, thermal injury, blast injury

Heart failure and multiple pulmonary emboli

Immunologic causes

Hypersensitivity pneumonia
- Inhaled antigens
- Farmer lung (actinomycosis)
- Bagassosis (sugar cane)
- Malt workers (Aspergillus spp.)
- Byssinosis (cotton)

Drug reactions
- Hydralazine, busulfan, nitrofurantoin (Macrodantin), hexamethonium, methysergide, bleomycin

Collagen diseases
- Scleroderma, rheumatoid disease, systemic lupus erythematosus, dermatomyositis, Wegener granulomatosis, Goodpasture syndrome

Other
- Sarcoidosis
- Histiocytosis
- Idiopathic hemosiderosis
- Pulmonary alveolar proteinosis
- Diffuse interstitial fibrosis, idiopathic pulmonary fibrosis
- Desquamative interstitial pneumonia
- Eosinophilic pneumonia (Note: some are caused by drugs, actinomycosis, and parasites)
- Lymphangioleiomyomatosis

increased pulmonary capillary permeability with extravasation of intravascular fluid and protein into the interstitium and alveoli. The leukocyte is the most prominent mediator of this injury. Stimuli, such as sepsis, activate the complement pathway, causing recruitment of leukocytes to the site of the infection. The lung releases potent mediators, such as oxygen free radicals, arachidonic acid metabolites, and proteases. If the underlying disease is not controlled, these changes progress to vascular thrombosis and interstitial fibrosis and hyaline membrane deposition in the alveoli. This process causes hypoxemia; pulmonary hypertension; carbon dioxide retention; secondary infections; and eventually right heart failure, hypoxia, and death. The severity of acute respiratory distress syndrome (ARDS) is defined according to the degree of hypoxemia as follows: mild ARDS (200 mm Hg > PaO_2/FiO_2 ≤300 mm Hg), moderate ARDS (100 mm Hg > PaO_2/FiO_2 ≤200 mm Hg), and severe ARDS (PaO_2/FiO_2 ≤100 mm Hg), mortality increases with more severe ARDS.[46]

Treatment is supportive and directed toward improving oxygenation. Maintaining an inspired oxygen concentration as low as possible and positive end-expiratory pressure (PEEP) as low as possible to maintain adequate oxygenation and carbon dioxide exchange is helpful. Tidal volumes and PEEP are kept low; however, increased PEEP may be needed in selected patients to facilitate oxygenation. A conservative fluid management protocol is used in order to avoid volume overload. Based on a more recent meta-analysis, prone or rotational therapy may improve outcomes of ARDS patients. In patients that do not improve with aggressive supportive care measures, mechanical support with extracorporeal membrane oxygenation (ECMO) should be considered.

PULMONARY METASTASES

Isolated pulmonary metastases represent a unique manifestation of systemic spread of a primary neoplasm. Patients with metastases located only within the lungs may be more amenable to local or local and systemic treatment options than other patients with multiorgan metastases. Although primary tumors can be locally controlled with surgery or radiation, extraregional metastases are usually treated with systemic chemotherapy. Radiation therapy may be used to treat or palliate the local manifestations of metastatic disease, particularly when metastases occur within the bony skeleton and cause pain. Resection of solitary and multiple pulmonary metastases from sarcomas and various other primary neoplasms has been performed, with improved long-term survival rates in 40% of patients. Therefore, isolated pulmonary metastases are treatable.

Certain clinical characteristics (prognostic indicators) may be used to select patients with more favorable disease-free and overall survival expectations. Patients who have complete resection of all metastases have associated longer survival than patients whose metastases are unresectable. Long-term survival (>5 years) may be expected in approximately 20% to 30% of all patients with resectable pulmonary metastases. Optimal (and more consistent) survival statistics await improvements in local control, systemic therapy, or regional drug delivery to the lungs.

Surgical Treatment

Predictors for improved survival rate have been studied retrospectively for various tumor types. These predictors may allow the clinician to identify selected patients who would optimally benefit from pulmonary metastasectomy. Patients should have pulmonary parenchymal nodules consistent with metastasis, absence of uncontrolled or untreated extrathoracic metastases, control of the primary tumor, sufficient physiologic and pulmonary reserve to tolerate the operation, and the probability of complete resection. Regardless of histology, patients with pulmonary metastases isolated to the lungs that are completely resected have improved survival rates compared with patients with unresectable metastases. Resectability consistently correlates with improved post-thoracotomy survival rates for patients with pulmonary metastases. In one series of more than 5000 patients with metastases treated with resection, overall actuarial 5-year survival rate was 36%. Favorable clinical indicators included a disease-free interval of greater than

3 years, a SPN, and germ cell histology. Soft tissue sarcomas of all types predominantly metastasize to the lungs. CT usually underestimates the number of metastases by 50% to 100%.

Resection can be accomplished safely. Open or minimally invasive procedures may be used. These procedures have minimal mortality and morbidity. Patients with pulmonary metastases may also undergo multiple procedures for reresection of metastases with prolonged survival expectations after complete resection. VATS procedures limit the ability of the surgeon to palpate the lung to identify occult metastases. Follow-up with radiographic screening at regular intervals is recommended to exclude recurrence.

MISCELLANEOUS LUNG TUMORS

Slow-growing lung tumors may arise from the epithelium, ducts, and glands of the bronchial tree and account for 1% to 2% of all lung neoplasms. Most are of low-grade malignant potential.

Neuroendocrine Tumors of the Lung

Carcinoid tumors (1% of lung neoplasms) arise from Kulchitsky (amine precursor uptake and decarboxylation [APUD]) cells in bronchial epithelium. They have positive histologic reactions to silver staining and to chromogranin. Special stains and examination can identify neurosecretory granules by electron microscopy. Typical carcinoid tumors are the most indolent of the spectrum of pulmonary neuroendocrine tumors (typical carcinoid, atypical carcinoid, large cell neuroendocrine carcinoma, and small cell carcinoma—most malignant). Histologic findings include less than 2 to 10 mitoses per 10 high-power fields. With complete surgical resection, 5-year survival rates are in the range of 85% to 90%. Peripheral carcinoid tumors are usually symptom-free, although central tumors may cause endobronchial obstruction with cough, hemoptysis, recurrent infection or pneumonia, bronchiectasis, lung abscess, pain, or wheezing. Symptoms may persist for many years without diagnosis, particularly if only an endobronchial component partially obstructs the airway. Carcinoid syndrome (flushing, tachycardia, wheezing, and diarrhea) is uncommon and occurs with large tumors or extensive metastatic disease. Atypical carcinoid may have lymph node or vascular invasion with metastasis. The location is in the mainstem bronchi (20%), lobar bronchi (70%–75%), or peripheral bronchi (5%–10%). They rarely occur in the trachea. Local invasion with involvement of peribronchial tissue occurs. Atypical carcinoids have more mitoses (>2–10 mitoses per 10 high-power fields) than typical carcinoid. These tumors are more aggressive, they tend to metastasize to the liver, bone, or adrenal, and their 5-year survival rate is in the range of 50% to 75%. Diagnosis of a carcinoid tumor can often be achieved by bronchoscopy, unless the nodule or mass is peripheral. Although these tumors tend to bleed, biopsy can usually be performed safely. Morphologically at bronchoscopy, most carcinoids are sessile, although a few are polypoid.

Surgical resection is standard, using the same surgical principles as applied for NSCLC. The aim of surgery is achieve anatomic complete resection of the tumor. Lobectomy is the most common procedure; endoscopic removal is performed only for rare polypoid tumors if surgery is contraindicated. Survival rate is typically 85% at 5 to 10 years. Large cell neuroendocrine tumors and small cell cancer are not typically treated with surgery and may be best treated with combinations of chemotherapy and radiation; survival of these patients is poor.

ACC is a slow-growing malignancy involving the trachea and mainstem bronchi that is similar to salivary gland tumors. ACC is more malignant than carcinoid tumors and has a slight female

BOX 58.2 Miscellaneous lung tumors.

Hamartoma
Epithelial origin tumors
- Papilloma—single or multiple, squamous epithelium, occurs in childhood, probably viral, may require bronchial resection but frequently recur
- Polyp—inflammatory-squamous metaplasia on a stalk; bronchial resection may be needed; these do not usually recur

Mesodermal origin tumors
- Fibroma—most frequent mesodermal tumor
- Chondroma
- Lipoma
- Leiomyoma—intrabronchial or peripheral; conservative resection

Granular cell tumors
- Rhabdomyoma
- Neuroma
- Hemangioma—subglottic larynx or upper trachea of infants; radiation therapy
- Lymphangioma—similar to cystic hygroma; upper airway obstruction in neonates
- Hemangioendothelioma—newborn lungs, often progressive and lethal
- Lymphangiomyomatosis—rare, slowly progressive; death from pulmonary insufficiency; fine, multinodular lesions, loss of parenchyma and honeycombing; usually women in their reproductive years
- Arteriovenous fistula—congenital, right-to-left shunt; cyanosis, dyspnea on exertion, clubbing, brain abscess; associated with hereditary hemorrhagic telangiectasia of lower lobes

Inflammatory tumors and pseudotumors
- Plasma cell granuloma
- Pseudolymphoma
- Xanthoma

Teratoma

preponderance. The tumor typically involves the lower trachea, carina, and take-off of the mainstem bronchi. Stridor is often the presenting symptom of adenoid cystic tumors because these tumors are most often found in the trachea and mainstem bronchi. One third of patients have tumors that have metastasized at the time of treatment. These patients typically have involvement of the perineural lymphatics, regional nodes, or liver, bone, or kidneys. The tumor arises from ducts in the submucosa and extends proximally and distally in that plane. Microscopic examination demonstrates cells with large nuclei and a small cytoplasm and surrounding cystic spaces (pseudoacinar type); the medullary type has a Swiss cheese appearance. Treatment is wide en-bloc resection with conservation of as much lung tissue as possible. Radiation treatment alone may be effective in patients not amenable to surgical resection.

Benign tumors of the lung account for less than 1% of all lung neoplasms and arise from mesodermal origins (Box 58.2). Hamartomas are the most frequent benign lung tumor; they consist of normal tissue elements found in an abnormal location. Hamartomas are manifested by overgrowth of cartilage. Hamartomas are typically identified in patients 40 to 60 years old and have a 2:1 male-to-female predominance. They are usually peripheral and slow-growing. CXR demonstrates a 2- to 3-cm mass that is sharply demarcated and frequently lobulated. It is usually not calcified, but the "popcorn" appearance on CXR may provide the diagnosis of hamartoma. Cystic adenomatoid malformation may represent adenomatous hamartomas, which occur in infants as cysts or immature elements in the lung.

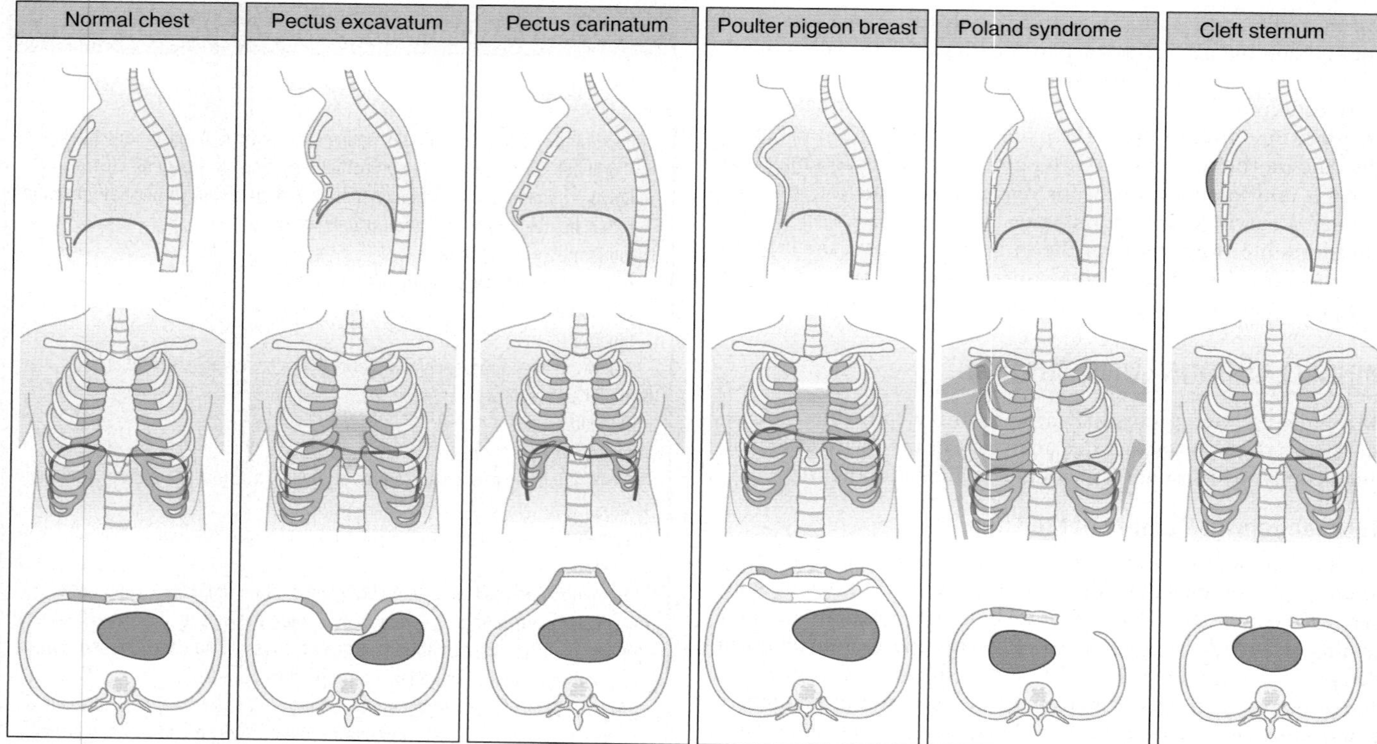

FIG. 58.27 Classification of chest wall deformities. (From Fokin AA, Steuerwald NM, Ahrens WA, et al. Anatomical, histologic, and genetic characteristics of congenital chest wall deformities. *Semin Thorac Cardiovasc Surg.* 2009;21:44–57.)

Very low-grade malignancies include hemangiopericytoma and pulmonary blastoma that arises from embryonic lung tissue. Treatment is resection. Tumorlets are epithelial proliferative lesions that may resemble oat cell carcinoma or carcinoid. These are typically incidental findings noted on examination of resected lung specimens. They rarely metastasize.

Primary sarcomas of the lung occur rarely. Resection, similar to lung carcinoma, is feasible in 50% to 60% of patients. Prognosis of patients with leiomyosarcoma is excellent, with approximately a 50% survival rate at 5 years; all other sarcomas have poor survival expectations.

Lymphoma of the lung most commonly occurs as disseminated lymphoma involving the lung. Disseminated lymphoma occurs in 40% of patients with Hodgkin disease and in 7% of patients with non-Hodgkin disease. Primary lymphoma of the lung is rare. The diagnosis is usually made at surgery. A thorough evaluation for other primary sites of lymphoma is done if primary pulmonary lymphoma is suspected preoperatively.

CHEST WALL

Congenital Deformities

There is a large group of congenital abnormalities of the thoracic cage that manifest as deformities and/or defect of the anterior chest wall. This diverse group includes pectus excavatum, pectus carinatum, pouter pigeon breast, Poland syndrome, and cleft sternum (Fig. 58.27).[47]

Pectus Excavatum

Pectus excavatum is the most common chest wall deformity, occurring in 1 of 400 children with a male predominance (4:1). It comprises approximately 90% of all chest wall deformities and is usually sporadic, although a definitive group of familial cases has been well documented.

Pectus excavatum refers to the sternal depression (depressed dorsally) caused by unequal growth rates or development of the lower ribs and costal cartilages (usually after the third rib). Pectus excavatum could be symmetric or asymmetric with a right-side predominance of the depression. The asymmetry is defined by rotation of the sternum, uneven height of the sides of the concavity, or both and is caused primarily by uneven elongation of costal cartilages. The severity of the depression is one of the most important characteristics of pectus excavatum and is defined by the amount of reduction in sternovertebral distance. The main assessment of pectus excavatum includes the measurement of the relative depth of the concavity by comparing it to the estimated normal anteroposterior diameter of the thorax or to the width of the chest (Fig. 58.28).

This syndrome may be associated with other musculoskeletal abnormalities. Most patients are asymptomatic, but some have decreased exercise capacity or pulmonary reserve. Patients are evaluated with plain CXRs, CT scans, pulmonary function studies, ventilation-perfusion lung scans, and other physiologic studies.

Indications for surgery for patients with pectus excavatum would include a significant history of compromise, which may be with exercise or daily activities and endurance issues, significant anterior chest wall pain, or significant body image issues. Patients also should have a caliper measurement depth of greater than 2.5 cm or a Haller index on CT scan of greater than 3. The timing for surgery is problematic in the very young child and younger school-age child. Currently, it is recommended to wait for patients to reach the middle teenage years to perform a pectus excavatum repair.[48]

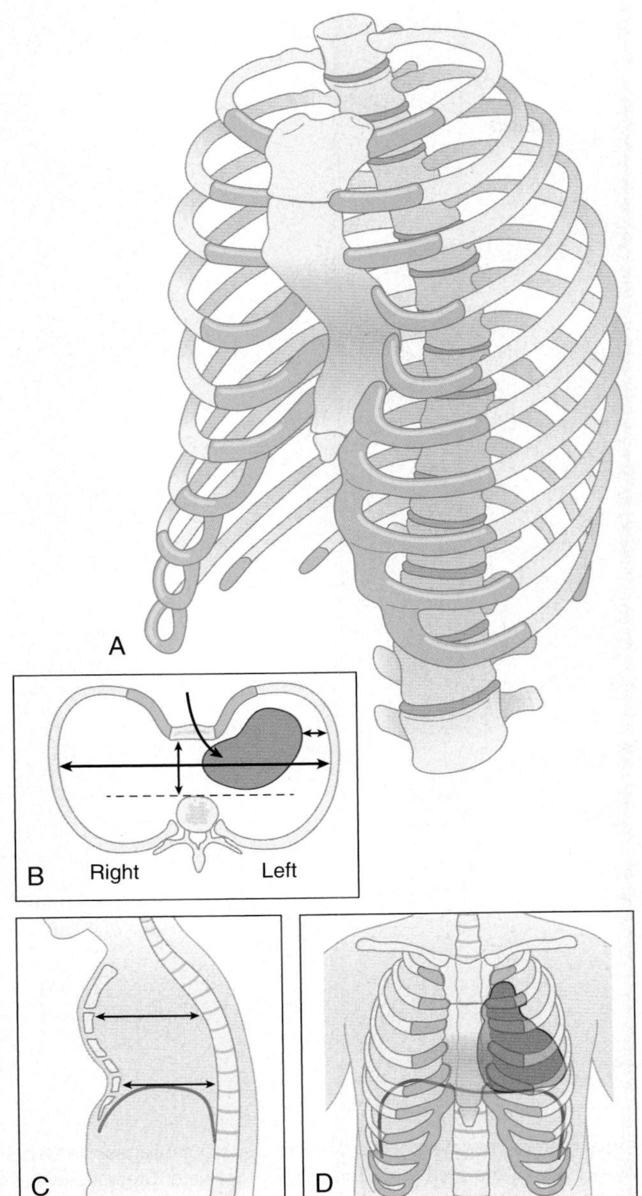

FIG. 58.28 Anatomic representation of pectus excavatum (PE). (A) Three-dimensional view. Classic, cup-shaped PE. (B) Cross-sectional view. Symmetric depression of the anterior chest wall. Cup-shaped concavity. Heart shifted to the left and rotated. (C) Lateral view. Depression of the lower third of mesosternum with a reduction in the anteroposterior thorax diameter. (D) Frontal view. Heart shifted to the left. (From Fokin AA, Steuerwald NM, Ahrens WA, et al. Anatomical, histologic, and genetic characteristics of congenital chest wall deformities. *Semin Thorac Cardiovasc Surg.* 2009;21:44–57.)

Repair of pectus excavatum can be accomplished by various techniques including open surgical repair and minimally invasive technique. Most methods of open surgical correction of pectus excavatum include the basic steps described by Ravitch in 1949. These include bilateral parasternal and subperichondrial resection of the deformed costal cartilages, detachment of the xiphoid process, transverse wedge osteotomy at the upper edge of the sternal depression, and bending the sternum anteriorly to straighten its course, and securing the corrected position of the sternum (Fig. 58.29).[49]

In 1987, during the early stages of laparoscopic and minimally invasive surgery, a pediatric surgeon from Virginia, Donald Nuss, performed the first minimally invasive operation for the correction of pectus excavatum (The Nuss technique). A convex stainless steel bar is placed under the sternum through 2 small lateral thoracic incisions, allowing anterior displacement of sternum and ribs, without the need for any type of bone or cartilage resection. The bar is removed after 3 years. The apparent simplicity of this technique, combined with the early good results reported, contributed to the enthusiastic widespread use of this operation by many pediatric and thoracic surgeons since its introduction.[50]

Pectus Carinatum

Pectus carinatum is the second most common deformity of the anterior chest wall. It is defined by the outward displacement of the sternum and/or abnormal protrusion of the ribs. Most cases of pectus carinatum are sporadic; however, familial incidence has been reported in as many as one-third of cases. Pectus carinatum can also be a part of a syndrome or connective tissue disorder. *Carinatum* deformities may be divided into 3 main types: keel chest, lateral precuts carinatum, and pouter pigeon chest. The classic one, is represented by *keel chest* or chondrosternal prominence, is the most frequent variety of pectus carinatum. This condition is characterized by protrusion of the lower third of the elongated sternum with maximum prominence at the sternoxiphoidal junction, which can be very noticeable ("pyramidal chest") (Fig. 58.30). This type of pectus carinatum could be associated with lateral depressions of the ribs. Keel chest may be symmetric or asymmetric, depending on the uneven elongation of the ribs and sternal rotation. Pouter pigeon chest, the most intriguing deformity, is characterized by a protrusion of the manubriosternal junction and the adjacent ribs with premature ossification of the sternum. Symptoms of pain and significant body image impairment are the main indications for surgical repair. The timing for repair of should be when patients have finished their teenage growth spurt. Patients that are still in their growth years are placed in a corrective constricting brace. Corrective bracing is successful in more than 80% of patients to eliminate the pectus carinatum defect. Patients who fail bracing can undergo surgical repair. Surgical repair includes bilateral parasternal and subperichondrial resection of the deformed costal cartilages and linear transverse osteotomy. The xiphoid process is detached and a 3- to 4-cm portion is resected from the caudal end of the sternum and then is reattached to the distal sternum (Fig. 58.31). This way, the shortened sternum is held straight and "in-line" by the pulling force of the rectus abdominis muscles. Results of this repair are excellent.[49]

Poland syndrome is a unilateral pectoral aplasia/dysdactylia syndrome characterized by unilateral absence of the costosternal portion of the pectoralis major muscle, absence of the pectoralis minor muscle, aplasia or deformity of the costal cartilages of the second through the fifth ribs, hypoplasia or absence of the breast and nipple, hypoplasia of the subcutaneous tissue of the region, alopecia of the axillary and mammary region, and brachysyndactyly, all on the same side. The pathogenesis of Poland syndrome remains unclear with the prevailing theory being "subclavian artery blood supply disruption sequence," which implies that hypoplasia of the internal thoracic artery or a reduction in blood flow at crucial periods leads to the absence of the pectoralis major muscle, whereas hypoplasia of branches of the brachial artery causes the hand abnormalities.

Characteristics of this syndrome include absence of the pectoralis major muscle, absence or hypoplasia of the pectoralis minor

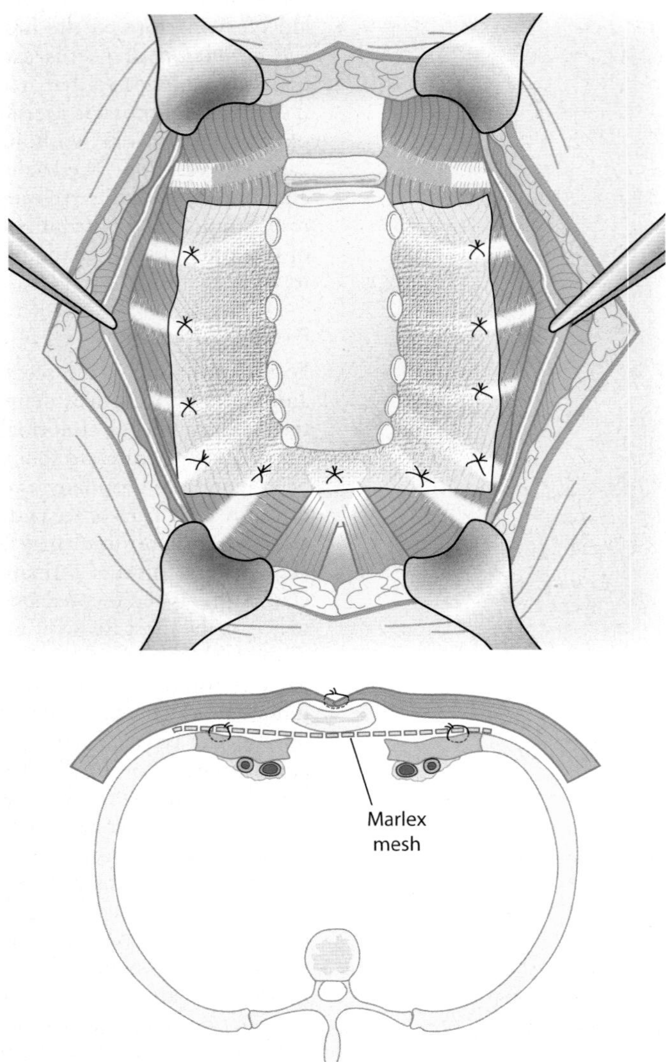

FIG. 58.29 Surgical repair of pectus excavatum: Robicsek method. Subperichondrial bilateral resection of the deformed costal cartilages. Transverse wedge sternotomy. Detachment of xiphoid process and perichondrial and intercostal strips of the sternum. Sternum bent forward. Sternal support is achieved with Marlex mesh sutured taut to the resected costal cartilages. Xiphoid process reattached to the mesh. Insert: Cross-sectional view. Intact internal thoracic vessels. Sternum in corrected position rests on the mesh hammock. (From Robicsek F, Watts LT, Fokin AA. Surgical repair of pectus excavatum and carinatum. *Semin Thorac Cardiovasc Surg.* 2009;21:64–75.)

muscle, absence of costal cartilages, hypoplasia of breast and subcutaneous tissue (including the nipple complex), and various hand anomalies.

Cleft sternum (CS) is a rare abnormality in which failed fusion of the two sternal halves results in defects of different lengths in the breast bone. It is also known by the term "sternum bifidum."[47]

Chest Wall Tumors

General

Chest wall tumors are rare. These tumors are more commonly either metastases or local invasion of an underlying adjacent tumor. Primary chest wall tumors account for only 0.04% of all new cancers diagnosed and 5% of all thoracic neoplasms. Primary chest wall tumors are best classified according to their tissue of origin, bone, or soft tissue and further subclassified according to whether or not they are benign or malignant (Table 58.4). Approximately 60% of primary chest wall tumors are malignant. Although primary chest wall tumors are diagnosed in every age group, they are more likely malignant in the extremes of age: in the young and the elderly.

Patients with primary chest wall tumors often present with a palpable enlarging mass. Less commonly, asymptomatic patients are diagnosed due to an incidental finding on imaging study. Soft tissue masses are often painless, whereas bony lesions, both benign and malignant, are typically painful due to growth and periosteal damage. Symptoms develop as the tumor grows and can be associated with local invasion of adjacent structures. There are no specific signs or symptoms that distinguish between benign and malignant lesions. Local tumor extension onto the lung or mediastinum can create associated symptoms. Due to the rarity of chest wall tumors, the time between onset of symptoms and diagnosis is often long.[51]

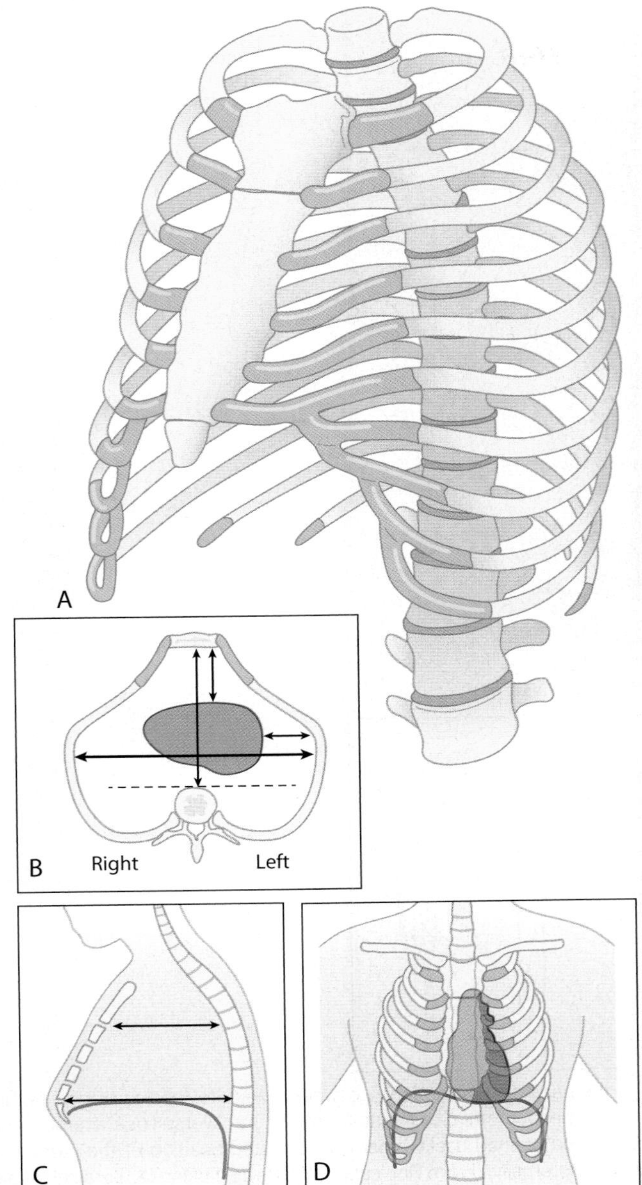

FIG. 58.30 Anatomic representation of keel chest deformity with lateral rib depressions. (A) Three-dimensional view. Protruding sternum accentuated by lateral rib depressions. (B) Cross-sectional view. Pyramidal chest with severe lateral rib depressions. (C) Lateral view. Sharp protrusion at the sternoxiphoidal junction. Abnormal posture. (D) Frontal view. Central position of the heart. (From Fokin AA, Steuerwald NM, Ahrens WA, et al. Anatomical, histologic, and genetic characteristics of congenital chest wall deformities. *Semin Thorac Cardiovasc Surg*. 2009;21:44–57.)

Evaluation requires diagnostic imaging, such as CXR, CT, MRI, and FDG-PET. A chest CT assesses the extent of bone, soft tissue, pleural and mediastinal involvement, and pulmonary metastases. MRI further delineates soft tissue, vascular and nerve involvement, and the presence of spinal cord or epidural extension. Benign soft tissue tumors are often small and superficial. Some tumors have classic appearances on imaging. Malignant tumors are often deep to the fascia and appear dark on T1-weighted MRI images and bright on T2-weighted MRI images.

Tissue biopsy is usually mandatory to confirm the diagnosis and for therapy strategies. Biopsy methods include core needle as well as open incisional and excisional biopsy techniques.

Consideration for future resection may dictate size and location of the incisional biopsy.

The indication for surgery is based on evaluation of the tumor histology, location, degree of local invasion, and presence of metastases. Complete resection and reconstruction of the chest wall defect is the principle surgical approach for most of the chest wall tumors. Exceptions include patients with the diagnosis of Ewing tumors or solitary plasmacytomas. Ewing sarcoma is first treated with chemotherapy or sequential with radiation, followed by possible surgical resection. Solitary plasmacytoma is treated solely with radiation. Surgical resection of all tumors must ensure negative margins to prevent local recurrence. There are no clear guidelines for the exact margins size, and it is mainly depending on the specific tumor type and its size. The excision of tumors that involve the ribs should generally incorporate resection of all or most of the rib involved, a portion of any adjacent ribs, and en-bloc resection of any attached structures, including portions of pleura, lung, pericardium, thymus, or diaphragm. Malignant tumors of the manubrium, sternum, clavicle, and scapula generally require excision of the entire bone and surrounding soft tissue to ensure negative margins.[51] Chest wall closure of small defect for small lesions can usually be done primarily. Large tumors in which a considerable defect is anticipated, both skeletal reconstruction and soft tissue coverage are often necessary. Local thoracic pedicle or myocutaneous flaps are generally used for reconstruction of large defects, and include pectoralis major, latissimus dorsi, serratus anterior, rectus abdominis, and external oblique muscles. Synthetic materials used included polypropylene (Marlex), polytetrafluorethylene patch, methyl methacrylate and osteosynthesis system with titanium implantable material.[52] These reconstructive techniques are mainly used to provide a chest wall stability to prevent flail segments and postoperative respiratory compromise (Fig. 58.32).

Bone Tumors

Benign bone tumors include fibrous dysplasia of the bone, which accounts for approximately 30% of these tumors. Chondromas account for 15% to 20% of benign chest wall lesions and arise from the anterior costochondral junction. Osteochondroma occurs commonly in young men as an asymptomatic tumor originating from the cortex of the rib. Eosinophilic granuloma is a benign component of malignant fibrous histiocytosis and primarily affects men. Skull and rib involvement are common and appear as expansile lesions on radiographic evaluation. Excisional biopsy is indicated for solitary lesions, and radiotherapy is indicated for multiple lesions. Aneurysmal bone cysts occur in the ribs and may be associated with previous trauma. Radiographic characteristics include a blow-out lytic lesion (Fig. 58.33). Resection is recommended for diagnosis and for relief of pain.

Malignant bone tumors include chondrosarcoma, which is the most common malignant tumor of the chest wall, accounting for 20% of all bone tumors. Chondrosarcomas arise in the third and fourth decades of life. Radiographic characteristics include a poorly defined tumor mass that is destroying cortical bone. Resection with wide margins (3–5 cm) is the treatment of choice. The 5-year survival after complete resection is approximately 70%. Osteosarcoma (osteogenic sarcoma) most frequently arises in the long bones of adolescents and young adults. Primary osteosarcomas in the chest account for 10% to 15% of malignant tumors. The tumor grows rapidly, and radiographic characteristics include

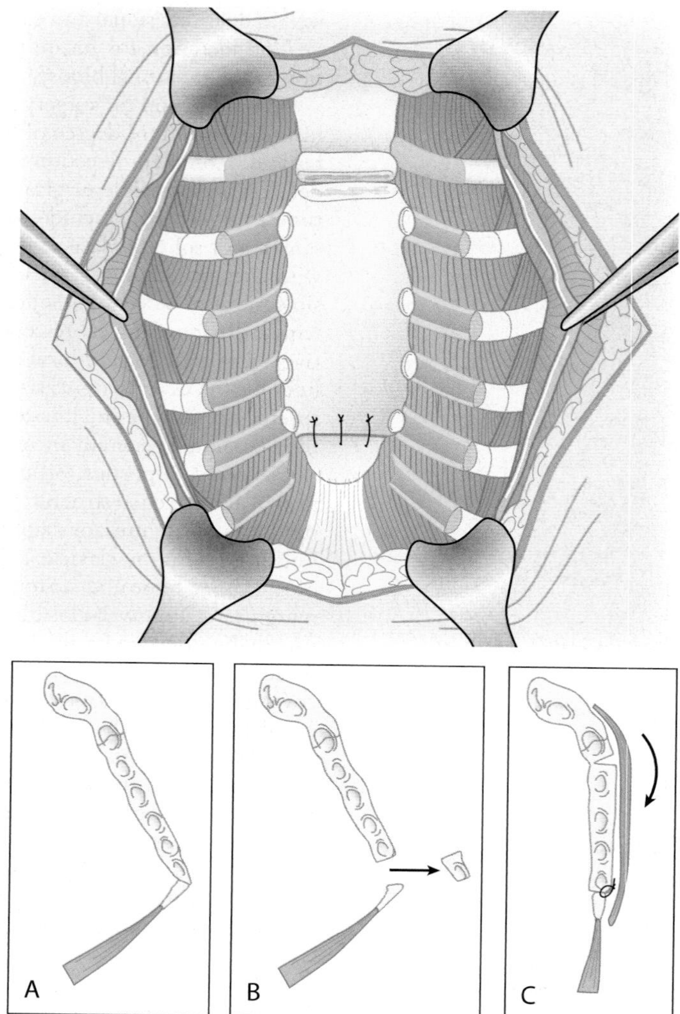

FIG. 58.31 Keel chest repair. Upper: Frontal view. Transverse linear sternotomy at the beginning of the forward curve. The deformed cartilages are bilaterally resected subperichondrially. Lower: lateral cross-section view. (A) Protrusion of the lower third of the sternum. (B) Transverse linear sternotomy at the beginning of the forward curve; sternum is shortened using a distal resection and pushed backwards. (C) Corrected position of the sternum. Xiphoid process is reattached to the shortened sternum. Pectoralis muscles reunited presternally. (From Robicsek F, Watts LT, Fokin AA. Surgical repair of pectus excavatum and carinatum. *Semin Thorac Cardiovasc Surg.* 2009;21:64–75.)

a sunburst pattern on CXR. Ewing sarcoma commonly arises in bones of the pelvis, humerus, or femur of young men. It is the third most common malignant chest wall tumor (5%–10%). The radiographic characteristics include an onion-peel appearance with periosteal elevation and bony remodeling. With multimodality therapy, 5-year survival is 50%. Solitary plasmacytoma is a rare tumor that occurs in older men as a painful solitary tumor arising from plasma cells. Multiple myeloma is the same tumor arising in more than one location. Radiographic characteristics include a diffuse, moth-eaten, or punched-out appearance of the bone. Systemic disease can be confirmed using serum protein electrophoresis, urinalysis (Bence-Jones protein), and bone marrow aspiration. Local radiotherapy for solitary plasmacytoma is recommended.

Soft Tissue Tumors

Soft tissue sarcomas are the most common malignant primary chest wall tumors. Core needle or incisional biopsy is performed to establish the diagnosis (Fig. 58.34). Resection with wide local excision (3–5 cm) is required. These tumors should not be shelled out despite the presence of a pseudocapsule. Complete resection is associated with excellent local control and prolonged survival. Combinations of chemotherapy and radiation therapy may be used as components of the multidisciplinary treatment plan.

Metastatic Tumors

Metastatic neoplasms may involve the chest wall by direct extension, by lymphatic metastasis, or by hematogenous metastasis. Lung cancer and breast cancer can involve the chest wall by direct extension, and if identified, chest wall resection should be performed concurrently with resection of the primary neoplasm.

Chest Wall Infections

Infections of the chest wall are relatively uncommon. Soft tissue necrosis secondary to infection and radiation injury account for the majority of chest wall resections performed today that are unrelated to malignancy. The risk for chest wall infection is significantly

TABLE 58.4 Classification of tumors of the chest wall.

	BENIGN (40%)	MALIGNANT (60%)
Bone Tumors		
Bone	Osteoblastoma	Ewing sarcoma
	Osteoid osteoma	Osteosarcoma
Cartilage	Chondroma (enchondroma)	Chondrosarcoma
	Osteochondroma	
Fibrous tissue	Fibrous dysplasia	
Bone marrow	Eosinophilic granuloma	Solitary plasmacytoma
Osteoclast	Aneurysmal bone cyst	
	Giant cell tumor (osteoclastoma)	
Vascular	Hemangioma	Hemangiosarcoma
	Cystic angiomatosis	
Other	Mesenchymal hamartoma	
Soft Tissue Tumors		
Adipose tissue	Lipoma	Liposarcoma
	Ossifying lipoma	
Fibrous tissue	Fibroma (desmoid tumor)	Fibrosarcoma
	Ossifying fibroma	MFH
Muscle	Leiomyoma	Leiomyosarcoma
	Rhabdomyoma	Rhabdomyosarcoma
		Tendon sheath sarcoma
Nerve	Neurofibroma	Askin tumor (PNET)
	Schwannoma (neurilemoma or neurinoma)	Malignant schwannoma
		Neurofibrosarcoma
		Neuroblastoma
Vascular	Hemangioma	Hemangiosarcoma
	Vascular leiomyoma	
Other		Hodgkin disease
		Leukemia
		Lymphoma
		Lymphosarcoma
		Mixed sarcoma
		Reticulosarcoma

From Smith SE, Keshavjee S. Primary chest wall tumors. *Thorac Surg Clin.* 2010;20:495–507.
MFH, Malignant fibrous histiocytoma; *PNET*, primitive neuroectodermal tumor.

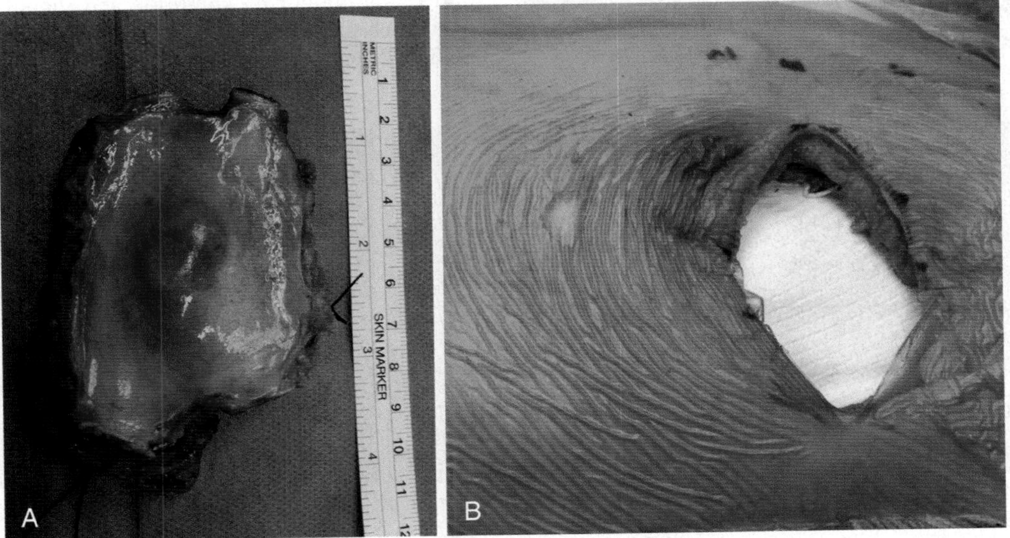

FIG. 58.32 Chest wall synovial sarcoma in a 9-year-old child. (A) Shown is a segment of the left chest wall (ribs 3 and 4). Complete resection was performed. The macroscopic clear margins are verified in final pathology. (B) Reconstruction of chest wall defect with a synthetic polytetrafluoroethylene Gore-Tex patch.

increased by immune compromised states and a history of surgery or trauma to the region. In addition, patients with a history of intravenous drug use are at increased risk for developing septic arthritis of the sternoclavicular, sternochondral, and manubriosternal joints.[53] Clinical findings and laboratory tests can be unreliable or nonspecific in the diagnosis of chest infection. A chest CT is accurate in detecting bone destruction and MRI visualizes a soft tissue involvement. Both CT and ultrasound may also be useful adjuncts, guiding percutaneous biopsies and drainage procedures.

Inflammatory breast carcinoma is not an infection but may mimic a chest wall infection. Biopsy may be needed to confirm the diagnosis. Mondor disease, thrombophlebitis of the superficial veins of the breast and anterior chest wall, is also not an infection. Ultrasound or biopsy may be necessary to confirm the diagnosis. Tietze syndrome or costochondritis is usually self-limited and can be treated with nonsteroidal antiinflammatory drugs and rest. Because of the limited blood supply to the cartilage, infection in this area may be difficult to diagnose. Debridement and reconstruction may be necessary. Sternal wound infections are complications following median sternotomy or cardiac surgery. Spontaneous primary chest wall infections can arise from various sources as a consequence of immunosuppression, drug-resistant organisms, including tuberculosis, or HIV infection.

Chest Wall Trauma

Thoracic trauma comprises 10% to 15% of all traumas, and 30% to 55% of polytraumas involve the chest wall. Reportedly, 10% to 15% of blunt chest trauma will result in a flail chest with an overall mortality around 20%. In spite of the common nature of chest injuries, most do not require any surgical intervention. Blunt trauma results from significant compression of the thorax, yielding rib fractures, soft tissue injuries, and intrathoracic damage of different degree, due to a stretch-and-shear strain effect. Open chest wall injuries are usually penetrating thoracic wounds.[54]

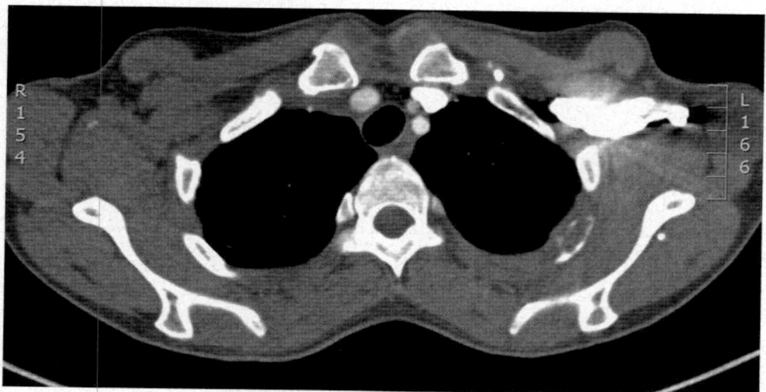

FIG. 58.33 Aneurysmal bone cyst.

CXR and chest CT scan are obtained often as part of the secondary survey in chest wall trauma. CT can identify rib, parenchymal, or other abnormalities. Blunt chest wall trauma commonly results in contusion of the chest wall tissues and the underlying lung parenchyma. Supportive care is warranted.

Rib fractures are perhaps the most common traumatic injury sustained after blunt chest wall trauma. Four percent to 10% of all hospitalized trauma patients usually have associated rib fractures. Pneumothorax, hemothorax, or hemopneumothorax are common associated findings with rib fracture requiring tube thoracostomy.

Symptoms include pain on inspiration and localized point tenderness. Plain films can confirm the diagnosis. Optimal therapy includes proper pain relief, aggressive physiotherapy, incentive spirometry, and a semi-sitting position.

Some locations where rib fractures are encountered require special considerations. In fractures of the uppermost three ribs, the possibility of brachial plexus and thoracic outlet vascular injuries, including aortic disruption, should be considered. Middle-zone fractures (ribs from third to eighth) should be diagnosed carefully, since 6% to 8% of rib fractures are bilateral and can easily compromise lung function on a longer run if pain relief or tracheobronchial toilette is insufficient. Advanced age, smoking, underlying lung disease, and low patient compliance are poor prognostic factors for severe morbidity. Potential liver, spleen, and kidney injuries should be ruled out in case of fracture of the lower-most ribs (ninth and below). Diaphragmatic tears may coexist as well. Contusion or injury to underlying structures should be suspected with any rib fracture.

Flail chest may occur with multiple rib fractures, when a segment of at least four ribs fractures in two different places on the same side. Flail chest results in an unstable chest wall that develops paradoxical motion during respiration (e.g., depression during the negative inspiratory phase and extrusion during the positive expiratory phase). Flail chest is often associated with an underlying pulmonary contusion and should be supported with pain relief, stabilization of the chest wall, or even mechanical ventilation. There are no clear guidelines to define indications for

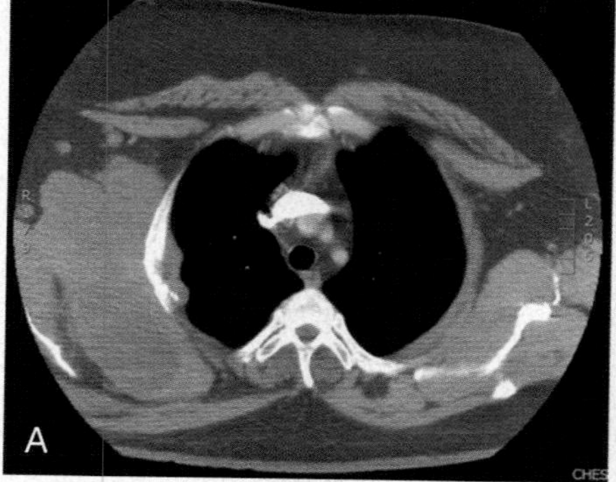

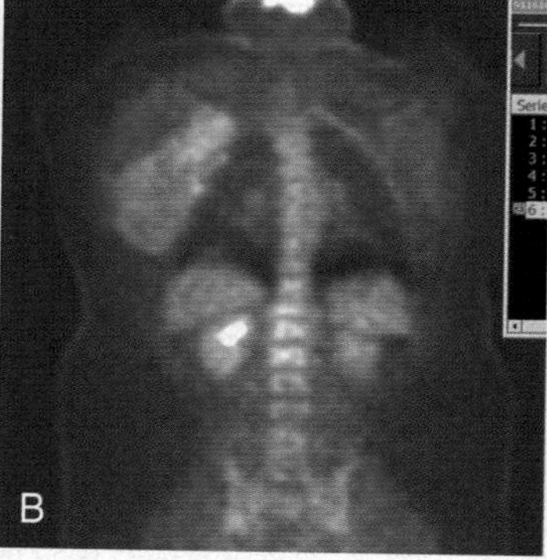

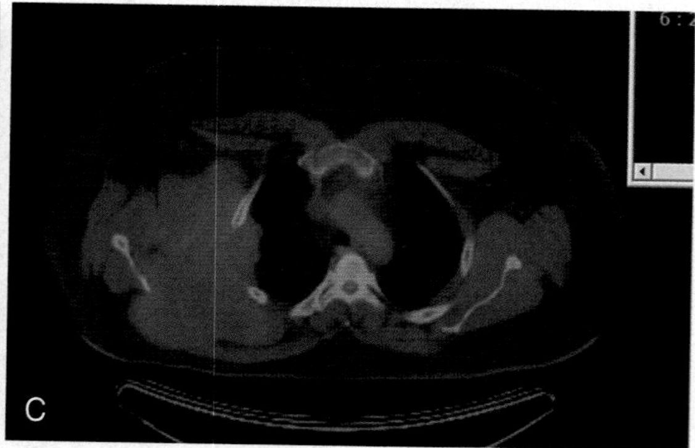

FIG. 58.34 (A) Primary chest wall tumor, desmoid tumor of the right lateral and posterior chest wall, is shown on computed tomography (CT) image. (B) ^{18}F-Fluorodeoxyglucose positron emission tomography (FDG-PET) demonstrates mild FDG avidity. No sites of metastases were identified. (C) A fused image of CT and FDG-PET is shown. Resection of the tumor included chest wall musculature and chest wall. Reconstruction was performed with prosthetic material, and a muscle flap was required.

osteosynthesis in order to restore chest wall stability. It is justified for flail chest which causes severe deformity, and exceptionally for intractable pain.

Sternal injuries are uncommon and may result from blunt trauma to the anterior chest, typically from a steering wheel injury during a motor vehicle accident. An underlying cardiac injury, such as aortic disruption, cardiac contusion, pericardial effusion, or arrhythmia, must be considered. Heart rhythm monitoring, serial cardiac observations with electrocardiography and cardiac enzymes, and echocardiography are used to exclude these injuries. Clavicular fractures may be associated with injury to the great vessels or the brachial plexus. Supportive care and stabilization are recommended.

THORACIC OUTLET SYNDROME

Thoracic outlet syndrome (TOS) refers to compression of the subclavian vessels and nerves of the brachial plexus in the region of the thoracic inlet. Symptoms most commonly develop secondary to neural compromise; however, vascular and neurovascular symptoms are reported. Middle-aged women are most commonly affected by TOS. The subclavian vessels and the brachial plexus can be compressed at various locations as they pass between the thoracic inlet and the upper extremity (Fig. 58.35). From medial to lateral, these anatomic regions are as follows:

1. Interscalene triangle (artery and nerves)
2. Costoclavicular space (vein)
3. Subcoracoid area (artery, vein, nerves)

Diagnosis

The symptoms associated with TOS vary depending on the anatomic structure that is compressed. Neurogenic manifestations are reported in more than 90% of cases. Symptoms of subclavian artery compression include fatigue, weakness, coldness, upper extremity claudication, thrombosis, and paresthesia. Thrombosis with distal embolization rarely can occur, producing vasomotor symptoms (Raynaud phenomenon) in the hand or ischemic changes. Venous compression results in edema, venous distention, collateral formation, and cyanosis of the affected limb. Venous TOS may be characterized by upper extremity edema, venous distention, or effort thrombosis, also known as *Paget-Schroetter syndrome.*

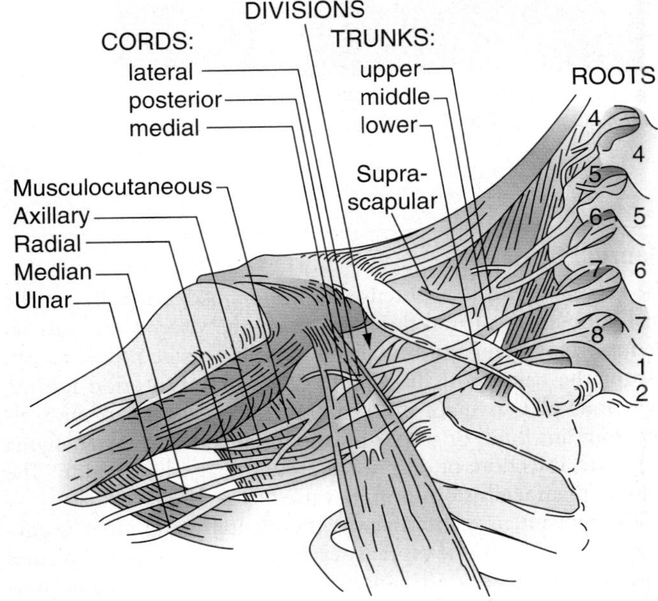

FIG. 58.35 Detailed view of brachial plexus. (From Urschel HC, Razzuk M. Upper plexus thoracic outlet syndrome: Optimal therapy. *Ann Thorac Surg.* 1997;63:935–939.)

The diagnosis of neurogenic TOS is initially made clinically. Objective evaluation for TOS includes chest and cervical spine films. A cervical rib or bony degenerative cervical spine changes may be present. CT and MRI are helpful to rule out narrowing of the intervertebral foramina or cervical disc pathology. Doppler studies and/or vascular imaging (using either CT or conventional angiography/venography) may be indicated to evaluate the extent of vascular impairment and to assess for aneurysm formation or venous thrombosis. Neurogenic TOS needs to be confirmed with nerve conduction studies to localize the area of slowing of nerve conduction and to rule out other compression syndromes, such as carpal tunnel syndrome. Nonsurgical management is indicated first in most patients with neurogenic TOS. Surgery is warranted in patients with neurogenic TOS who have persistent symptoms, muscle atrophy, or a progressive deficit. Vascular TOS must be confirmed with objective studies.

Clinical maneuvers to evaluate a patient suspected to have TOS are performed to identify the loss or decrease of radial pulse or to reproduce neurologic symptoms. A clear, objective, validated definition for TOS is needed. Evocative tests to illicit symptoms include the following (Fig. 58.36):

- Adson (scalene) test. The patient inspires maximally and holds his or her breath while the neck is fully extended and the head is turned toward the affected side. This maneuver narrows the space between the scalenus anticus and medius, resulting in compression of the subclavian artery and the brachial plexus. Decrease or loss of ipsilateral radial pulse suggests compression.
- Halsted (costoclavicular) test. The patient is instructed to place his or her shoulders in a military position (drawn backward and downward) to narrow the costoclavicular space between the first rib and the clavicle, causing neurovascular compression. Reproduction of neurologic symptoms or decrease or loss of ipsilateral radial pulse suggests compression.
- Wright (hyperabduction) test. The patient's arm is hyperabducted 180 degrees, which causes the neurovascular structures to be compressed in the subcoracoid region by the pectoralis tendon, the head of the humerus, or the coracoid process. Decrease or loss of ipsilateral radial pulse suggests compression.
- Roos test. The patient abducts the involved arm 90 degrees with external rotation of the shoulder. Maintaining this body position, the modified Roos test is performed by opening and closing the hand rapidly for 3 minutes in an attempt to reproduce symptoms. Additionally, neurogenic compromise may be detected using provocative tests, such as percussion of the nerve (Tinel sign) or flexion of the elbow or wrist (Phalen sign).

Management

Results of treatment of TOS are variable because there are inconsistent objective criteria for the diagnosis of TOS other than clinical diagnosis. Initial management of TOS is nonoperative. Physical therapy is needed. Repetitive upper extremity mechanical work and muscular trauma are eliminated. Indications for operation include failure of conservative management, progressive neurologic symptoms, prolonged ulnar or median nerve conduction velocities, narrowing or occlusion of the subclavian artery, and thrombosis of the axillary or subclavian vein. The key aim of surgery is to release the narrowing/pressure point at the thoracic

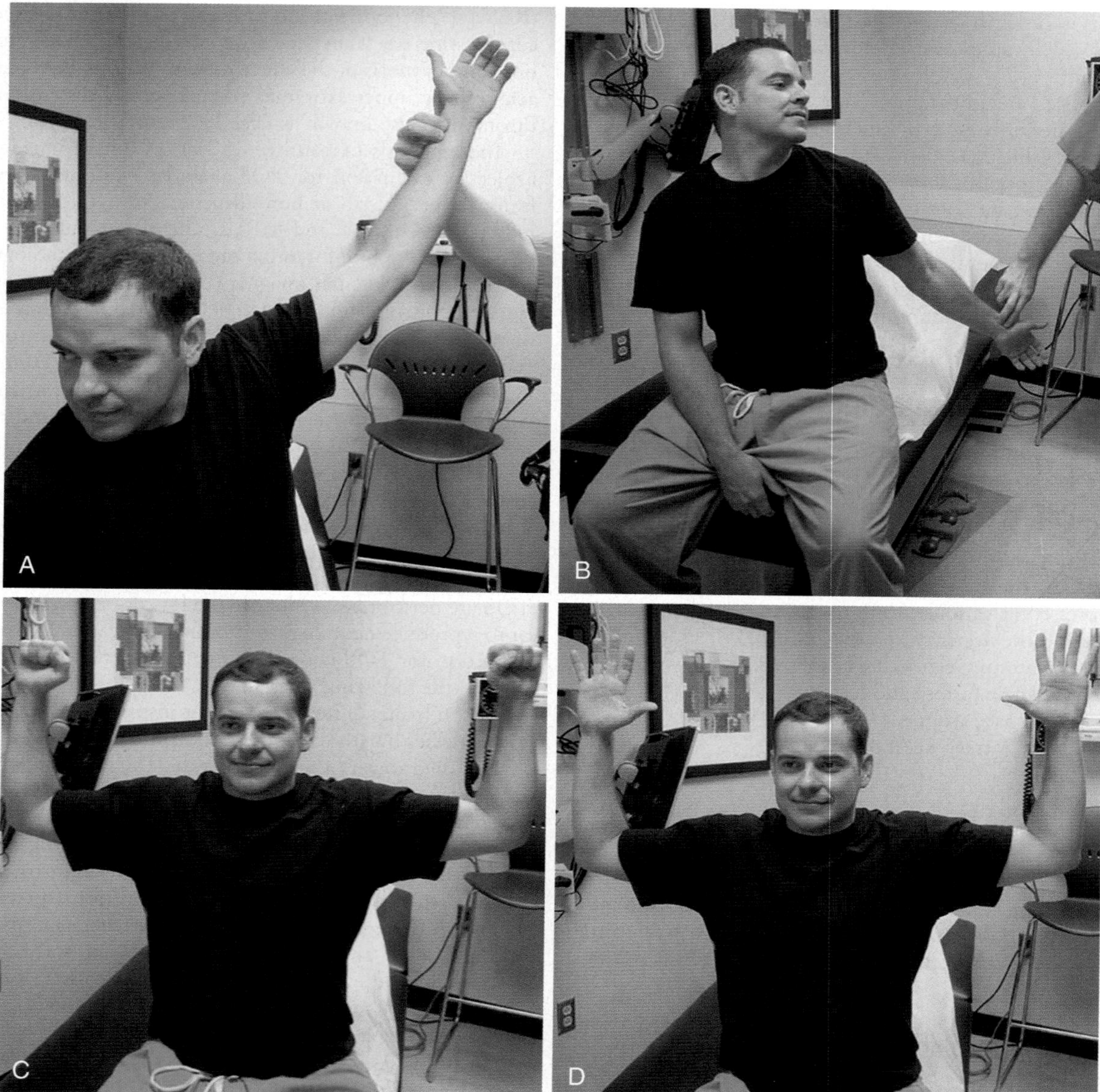

FIG. 58.36 Clinical photographs demonstrating provocative physical tests for thoracic outlet syndrome. (A) Wright test. (B) Adson test. (C and D) Roos test. (From Kuhn JE, Lebus VG, Bible JE. Thoracic outlet syndrome. *J Am Acad Orthop Surg*. 2015;23:222–232.)

outlet. This is achieved in the majority of cases by detachment of the anterior and middle scalene muscle from the first rib and by resection of the rib (in the presence of an accessory rib, it is resected). Additional interventions may include release of the pectorals minor muscle from its insertion on the coracoid process and neurolysis of dense fibrosis along the brachial plexus. Supraclavicular, axially, posterior, and thoracoscopic/robotic approaches have been applied for first rib resection. Regardless of the approach, identification and preservation of the brachial plexus, the phrenic nerve, the lung thoracic nerve, and the subclavian vein and artery is a key component of surgery. Operative management can provide excellent results in properly selected patients. Objective agreed-upon outcome measures and clinical trials are needed to compare outcomes of surgery for TOS compared with no surgery. Success rates with surgery approach 70% at 5 years. Recurrent symptoms may prompt reoperation in up to one third of patients.[55]

PLEURA

Pleural Effusions

The pleural space is a potential space defined normally by the small amount of pleural fluid separating the visceral and parietal pleura. Many benign and malignant pleural space problems can disrupt the balance of fluid production and absorption leading to various pleural space problems, including increased mass effect from air, fluid, or tumor on the ipsilateral lung parenchyma and heart, infection, or dyspnea and pulmonary dysfunction. The cause of pleural effusions is quite varied (Box 58.3).

The movement of fluid across the pleural membranes is governed by Starling law of capillary exchange. The amount of pleural fluid is controlled by a balance of oncotic and hydrostatic pressure within the pleural space and the pleural capillaries. Under normal circumstances, the net pressure moves fluid from the parietal pleura into the pleural space. It is estimated that the pleural

BOX 58.3 Pleural effusions.

Cause of Transudative Effusions
Congestive heart failure
Cirrhosis
Nephrotic syndrome
Hypoalbuminemia
Fluid retention/overload
Pulmonary embolism
Lobar collapse
Meigs syndrome

Cause of Exudative Effusions
Malignant
- Primary lung or metastatic carcinoma
- Lymphoma
- Mesothelioma

Infectious
- Bacterial (parapneumonic)/empyema
- Tuberculosis
- Fungal
- Viral
- Parasitic

Collagen vascular disease related
- Rheumatoid arthritis
- Wegener granulomatosis
- Systemic lupus erythematosus
- Churg-Strauss syndrome

Abdominal/gastrointestinal disease related
- Esophageal perforation
- Subphrenic abscess
- Pancreatitis/pancreatic pseudocyst
- Meigs syndrome

Others
- Chylothorax
- Uremia
- Sarcoidosis
- After coronary artery bypass grafting
- Radiation/trauma
- Dressler syndrome
- Pulmonary embolism with infarction
- Asbestosis related

space contains a tiny amount (≈0.3 mL·kg^{-1}) of fluid and that in homeostasis the fluid turnover is about ≈0.15 mL·kg^{-1}·h^{-1}. Under physiologic conditions, most pleural fluid is also reabsorbed through lymphatics of the parietal pleura because protein that enters the pleural space cannot enter the relatively impermeable visceral pleura. The parietal pleura and its lymphatics have significant capacity for protein and fluid removal. A small imbalance of accumulation and absorption can lead to the development of a pleural effusion. The causative factors include increased hydrostatic pressure, increased negative intrapleural pressure, increased capillary permeability, decreased plasma oncotic pressure, and decreased or interrupted lymphatic drainage.

Pleural fluid is characterized as a transudate or an exudate. Transudative effusions are protein-poor and result in change in fluid balance in the pleural space. Exudative effusions are protein-rich and may be related to disruption of pleural or lymphatic reabsorption. After drainage, the fluid is evaluated according to Light's criteria. An exudate is defined as (1) pleural fluid protein-to-serum protein ratio greater than 0.5, (2) pleural fluid lactate dehydrogenase (LDH)-to-serum LDH ratio greater than 0.6, or (3) pleural fluid LDH 1.67 times the normal serum level or higher. In addition, the pleural fluid should also be assessed for its visual characteristics (serous, bloody, milky, turbid, or frankly purulent). Pleural fluid should be analyzed for cytology; cell counts; Gram stain; culture for aerobic, anaerobic, and fungal organisms; tuberculosis testing; and chemistry with simultaneous pleural and serum protein, glucose, LDH, and pH. The treatment goals for patients with pleural effusion include obtaining a diagnosis, relieving or eliminating symptoms such as dyspnea, optimizing lung expansion, and minimizing or eliminating hospitalization.[18,56]

Benign Pleural Effusions

Most benign pleural effusions are transudates, free-flowing, without loculation, and treatment should be directed toward the underlying cause, such as congestive heart failure, ascites, or malnutrition. Symptoms are typically dyspnea or cough. Pleural fluid can be identified on CXR; the presence of 300 mL of fluid causes blunting of the costophrenic angle on upright CXR. Clinical examination can detect 500 mL of fluid or greater. Initial thoracentesis should achieve complete drainage for diagnosis and treatment. In addition, radiographic evidence of complete reexpansion of the lung should be sought. Failure of the lung to expand completely suggests a "trapped" lung, which may require decortication, particularly if symptoms, such as dyspnea, persist. Relief of symptoms with thoracentesis usually indicates the pleural effusion as the cause. Occasionally, symptoms are not relieved by thoracentesis, and an alternative diagnosis is required.

Recurrent effusions can occur, and repeat thoracenteses may be required. Alternative therapies, such as chest tube insertion (tube thoracostomy) or thoracoscopic drainage with or without mechanical and chemical pleurodesis, can be considered. Visceral and parietal pleural apposition is required to achieve pleurodesis. Drainage of the effusion can be diagnostic and therapeutic. Sclerosing agents can be placed to facilitate pleural symphysis. This pleurodesis is most effectively accomplished with slurry of 5 g of talc in 100 mL of saline placed through the chest tube. Video-assisted thoracoscopic drainage of effusions can also be diagnostic and therapeutic. Pleural biopsy or wedge resection of the lung can be easily performed to facilitate diagnosis. During surgery, mechanical pleural abrasion or chemical pleurodesis with talc is typically used. The talc is insufflated within the hemithorax to cover all visceral pleural surfaces (e.g., talc poudrage). Pleurectomy is not commonly needed; however, persistent pleural effusions and trapped lung may not be amenable to more conservative measures. Decortication may be required.

Malignant Pleural Effusion

Patients with known or previous malignancy can develop MPE. In 25% of MPEs, a histologic diagnosis of cancer is not made within the fluid after two thoracenteses. Drainage is required for relief of dyspnea (Fig. 58.37).

MPE is an effusion with positive cytopathology. Not all pleural effusions associated with malignancy are caused by direct or metastatic pleural involvement. Other mechanisms for their development (bronchial or lymphatic obstruction, hypoproteinemia, and accumulation from infradiaphragmatic involvement) exist. Although repeated cytologic evaluation of a pleural effusion achieves high positive and negative predictive values, this diagnostic procedure has important limitations. A cancer diagnosis is obtained

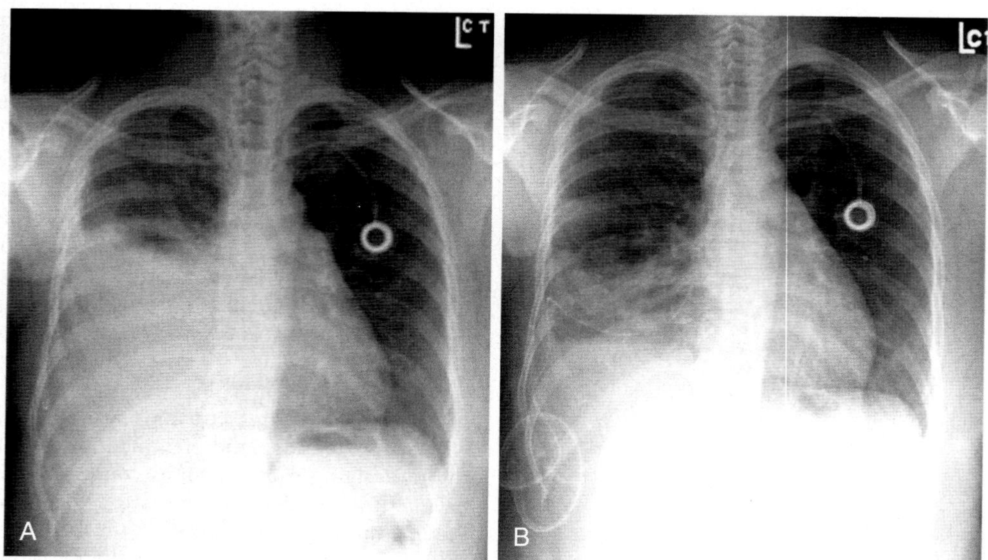

FIG. 58.37 (A) Malignant pleural effusion causing dyspnea. A long-term indwelling pleural catheter was placed as an outpatient procedure to facilitate drainage at home to prevent dyspnea. Hospitalization was not required. (B) Following drainage. A long-term indwelling pleural catheter is effective in patients with trapped lung. Every-other-day drainage reduces impairment of the contralateral lung and prevents mediastinal shift.

after three thoracenteses in 70% to 80% of patients. Thoracoscopy is diagnostic in 92% of patients.

A patient with MPE has a median survival of 90 days. Patients with breast cancer and MPE have a median survival of approximately 5 months. Patients with lymphoma typically have a longer median survival. Local treatment of MPE does not affect the systemic disease process but may provide significant symptomatic relief. Repeated pleural taps as indicated by symptoms may help relief dyspnea. Alternatively insertion of a long-term indwelling pleural catheter should be considered as these devices not only permit for repeated drainage of the MPE, but they may also induce pleurodesis in up to 70% of cases. Insertion of a pigtail catheter or a chest tube with attempt to perform talc pleurodesis is an additional treatment option. Complications of treatments include hemothorax, loculation of fluid, empyema, failure of pleurodesis with recurrence of effusion, and lung entrapment caused by tumor growth and fibrin deposition on the lung. Open surgical pleurectomy and pleurodesis are reserved for patients who fail other therapies and who have a reasonably long life expectancy. Talc slurry following chest tube insertion and drainage of the effusion is as effective as VATS with talc pleurodesis.

Empyema

Empyema is an infection of the pleural space and commonly an exudate. Empyemas progress from an acute phase with fluid that is thin and can be drained completely with a chest tube or small bore catheter. This process typically worsens as the fluid becomes more turbid and thick and begins to loculate. Mucopurulent debris occurs within the pleural space and compresses the underlying lung parenchyma. The organizing or chronic phase is reflected in more lung entrapment with capillary ingrowth and creation of a pleural rind, which traps the lung.

An empyema typically occurs after a reactive pleural effusion as a consequence of a lung infection. These infections historically were due to streptococcal or pneumococcal pneumonia. At the present time, gram-negative and anaerobic organisms are common causes of empyema. Tuberculous empyema can also be identified. Empyema can follow trauma or thoracic surgery (from residual pleural space or bronchopleural fistula), hematologic spread, rupture of a pulmonary or mediastinal abscess, or esophageal perforation.

Symptoms typically include constitutional symptoms of general malaise, fever, loss of appetite, and weight loss. Cough and dyspnea are common if lung infection is present. Evaluation includes CXR and CT scan of the chest and upper abdomen.

Treatment of empyema depends on the extent of the disease and its location. Complete drainage is required. Antibiotics and supportive care (e.g., fluids, nutrition, skin care) are commonly initiated. In an uncomplicated pleural space complete drainage can be achieved by ultrasound-guided insertion of a pleural drain (pigtail catheter). In loculated effusion more than one catheter may be necessary. Larger chest tubes may assist in drainage of turbid effusions. Use of fibrinolytic agents can be effective. Intrapleural tissue plasminogen activator and DNase when used may improve drainage of the pleural space and reduce the need for surgical drainage. VATS decortication and thoracotomy with debridement or formal decortication in later stage empyema is reserved for treatment failures with persistent symptoms of dyspnea, loculations, or continued sepsis.

Bronchopleural fistula after lobectomy or pneumonectomy predisposes to empyema. Management of bronchopleural fistula requires evaluation of the underlying cause of the fistula, drainage of the infection, and obliteration of the residual pleural space along with general supportive care. Chronic empyema with a residual pleural space can be treated with drainage, gauze packing, or skin flap (Eloesser flap) with eventual muscle transposition and skin closure. Lung resection or pleuropneumonectomy is rarely required.

Chylothorax

Chylothorax occurs when chyle from the thoracic duct empties into the pleural space. Chyle is a milky white fluid with a high concentration of triglycerides and chylomicrons and white blood cells. It is nutritionally rich and depends on the nutritional and

BOX 58.4 Chylothorax.

Traumatic (chest and neck)
- Blunt
- Penetrating

Iatrogenic
- Catheterization, particularly subclavian vein
- Postsurgical
- Excision of cervical/supraclavicular lymph nodes
- Radical lymph node dissections of the neck or chest
- Lung, esophageal, or mediastinal resection
- Thoracic aneurysm repair
- Sympathectomy
- Congenital cardiovascular surgery

Neoplasms
- Lymphoma, lung, esophageal, or mediastinal neoplasms
- Metastatic carcinoma

Infectious
- Tuberculous lymphadenosis
- Mediastinitis
- Ascending lymphangitis

Other
- Lymphangioleiomyomatosis
- Venous thrombosis
- Congenital

dietary status of the patient. It may be clear. Chylothorax has multiple causes Box 58.4.

Symptoms from chylothorax include dyspnea or cough. In addition, because of the nutritional consequences of chronic chyle leak (e.g., loss of fat, protein) and the volume of the leak (0.5–3.0 L/day), fluid and nutritional replacement and correction of the underlying problem are necessary. The diagnosis may be made with thoracentesis or drainage of the fluid with a chest tube. Analysis of pleural fluid with chylomicrons confirms the diagnosis. Conservative measures such as medium-chain triglyceride diet or total parenteral nutrition and administration of octreotide are used initially. If conservative measures fail, operative intervention may be considered between days 7 and 14. Commonly ligation of thoracic duct where it enters the chest through the diaphragmatic hiatus is achieved via a right thoracotomy or thoracoscopy. Placement of olive oil or ice cream by nasogastric tube at the time of the operation may increase chyle drainage into the operative field and help to identify the area of thoracic duct disruption. Percutaneous techniques with needle cannulation and duct occlusion are emerging in recent years as efficient and less invasive methods for the treatment of chyle leak.

Pneumothorax

Pneumothorax is the accumulation of air within the pleural space. It may occur as a result of trauma, surgery, needle aspiration, central line insertion, increased pressure from mechanical ventilation, or lung diseases (e.g., COPD, cystic or pulmonary fibrosis) or other conditions (e.g., catamenial pneumothorax) (Box 58.5). A primary spontaneous pneumothorax occurs as a consequence of subpleural blebs or other pulmonary disease. Tension pneumothorax occurs when air continues to enter the pleural space without decompression. This problem results in positive intrathoracic pressure causing compression of the lung and mediastinum, shift of the mediastinum into the contralateral chest, and decrease in ventilation and venous return. Cardiopulmonary collapse and death ensue. Immediate decompression with needle or chest tube insertion is lifesaving.

BOX 58.5 Pneumothorax.

Spontaneous
- Primary
- Secondary
  - COPD
  - Bullous disease
  - Cystic fibrosis
  - Pneumocystis related
  - Congenital cysts
  - IPF
  - Pulmonary embolism
- Catamenial
- Neonatal

Traumatic
- Penetrating
- Blunt

Iatrogenic
- Mechanical ventilation
- Needle puncture: thoracentesis, FNA lung nodule, central line insertion
- Postsurgical

COPD, Chronic obstructive pulmonary disease; *FNA*, fine-needle aspiration; *IPF*, idiopathic pulmonary fibrosis.

Symptoms of pneumothorax include pain and dyspnea. Patients with spontaneous pneumothorax are usually tall and thin young men. Diagnostic imaging includes CXR and occasionally CT. Apical blebs and bullae are common. CT scan can be performed to assess for the cause of spontaneous pneumothorax or the presence of other occult lung disease. Subcutaneous emphysema may or may not be present.

Treatment depends on size and symptoms. Smaller pneumothorax may be followed and may resolve spontaneously, particularly pneumothorax that occurs after needle aspiration for lung biopsy. Progression in the size of pneumothorax requires intervention with drainage. Initial spontaneous pneumothorax may be treated with small bore catheter drainage or chest tube and drainage with resolution of the air space and cessation of air leak. Persistent air leak (>5 days) or failure of the lung to expand fully suggests additional intervention may be needed.

Operative intervention is recommended for patients who have a persistence or recurrence of spontaneous pneumothorax or who develop a contralateral pneumothorax. Patients that had experienced an event of spontaneous pneumothorax and have not had surgery should avoid high-risk professions (e.g., scuba diver, airplane pilot) since the risk for recurrence is not negligible. Operative repair typically includes thoracoscopy to identify apical blebs, which are resected with endoscopic staplers. Mechanical abrasion of the parietal pleura is performed. Pleurodesis with talc in patients with malignancy or in older patients may be considered.

Mesothelioma

Diffuse malignant pleural mesothelioma (MPM) is a highly aggressive malignancy that arises from the mesothelial cells lining the parietal and visceral pleura. MPM pathogenesis is tightly linked to asbestos exposure and a long latency period (15–40 years) exists between primary exposure and disease development. Histologic subtypes include epithelial, sarcomatoid, or mixed histology. Pure epithelial histology has a more favorable prognosis. Symptoms include shortness of breath, cough, pleural effusion, weight loss, chest pain, and fever. Diagnostic imaging includes CXR, CT, MRI, and FDG-PET scan to determine the extent of tumor invasion and to evaluate for occult metastases, including mediastinal metastases. Echocardiography is performed to determine cardiac involvement and function. The diagnosis is made with pleural biopsy, which may include thoracentesis or pleural biopsy alone or incisional biopsies via thoracoscopy or open techniques. Disease stage is dictated by the extent and invasiveness of the tumor in the thorax (T descriptor), the spread of tumor to intra- and extrathoracic lymph nodes (N descriptor) and the presence of metastasis (M descriptor). Due to the insidious onset of clinical symptoms, majority of MPM patient are diagnosed with advanced disease. In this scenario, survival is extremely poor, ranging from 4 to 12 months. Advanced chemotherapeutic protocols may somewhat extend survival (median survival of 19 months) however they do not offer cure (5-year survival rates <5%). Selected patient that are diagnosed with early stage disease, with pure epithelial histology and are in good functional status may be considered for a multimodality surgery based therapeutic approach. Various cisplatin-based neoadjuvant and adjuvant chemotherapy and radiotherapy protocols are available and these are sequentially administered in conjunction with surgery in order to achieve extend survival. The surgical aim in MPM is to perform complete macroscopic resection (CMR) of the tumor. This can be achieved either by extrapleural pneumonectomy (EPP – resection of the entire lung, including the visceral and parietal pleura and the diaphragm +/- pericardium through a large posterolateral thoracotomy) or by extended pleurectomy and decortication (EPD – resection of the parietal and visceral pleura and the diaphragm +/- pericardium while preserving the lung parenchyma through a large posterolateral thoracotomy). EPP is the most extensive surgery for MPM, it is considered to offer the most extensive CMR, however it is associated with high mortality (5%–20%) and morbidity (40%–60%) rates. EPD is a lung preserving surgery that offers somewhat less extensive CMR; however, it is much safer than EPP. Consequently, in many centers EPD has replaced EPP as the procedure of choice to achieve CMR in MPM. The median survival period of patients that had completed a multimodality treatment for MPM is in the range of 24 to 36 months. Palliative care for MPM patients may include insertion of pleural indwelling catheters and pleurodesis.[57]

Solitary Fibrous Tumor of the Pleura

Solitary fibrous tumors are rare fibroblastic mesenchymal tumors that arise either from the visceral or the parietal pleura. They rarely metastasize; however, local recurrence and malignant transformation to a sarcomatous type of tumor may occur. The tumors often attach to the pleura with a thin pedicle and they may grow quite large. Symptoms are related in the majority of cases to a mass effect in the thorax and up to 20% are associated with digital clubbing and hypertrophic pulmonary osteoarthropathy. Treatment is based on surgical resection of the tumor, its pedicle and the pleura/lung at the base of the pedicle. Wedge resection of lung tissue is sufficient in the vast majority of cases to remove the pedicle and other adhesions of the tumors to the lung. Long-term follow-up of these patients is indicated.

MEDIASTINUM

Mediastinal abnormalities may manifest as an asymptomatic mass identified on screening CXR or with significant symptoms, including hypoxia, facial swelling, and acute respiratory distress. Symptoms are related to the involvement of the specific mediastinal structures. Thoracic imaging with contrast-enhanced CT and MRI play critical role in the characterization of mediastinal masses. Cytology from fine-needle aspiration or core biopsy or surgical biopsy may be needed to make the diagnosis and to determine optimal therapy. Mediastinal masses differ between adults and children. The most common mediastinal masses (Box 58.6) in adults are thymomas and thymic cysts, neurogenic tumors, other cysts, germ cell tumors, and

BOX 58.6 Mediastinum: classificaton of primary mediastinal tumors and cysts.

- Thymoma
  - Thymic carcinoma
- Lymphoma
  - Hodgkin disease
  - Lymphoblastic lymphoma
  - Large cell lymphoma
- Germ cell tumors
  - Teratodermoid (benign/malignant)
  - Seminoma
  - Nonseminoma
    - Embryonal
    - Choriocarcinoma
    - Endodermal
- Primary carcinomas
  - Mesenchymal tumors
    - Fibroma/fibrosarcoma
    - Lipoma/liposarcoma
    - Leiomyoma/leiomyosarcoma
    - Rhabdosarcoma
    - Xanthogranuloma
    - Myxoma
    - Mesothelioma
    - Hemangioma
    - Hemangioendothelioma
    - Hemangiopericytoma
    - Lymphangioma
    - Lymphangiomyoma
    - Lymphangiopericytoma
  - Endocrine tumors
    - Intrathoracic thyroid
    - Parathyroid adenoma/carcinoma
    - Carcinoid
- Cysts
  - Bronchogenic
  - Pericardial
  - Enteric
  - Thymic
  - Thoracic duct
  - Nonspecific
- Giant lymph node hyperplasia
  - Castleman disease
- Chondroma
- Extramedullary hematopoiesis
- Neurogenic tumors
  - Neurofibroma
  - Neurilemoma
  - Paraganglioma
  - Ganglioneuroma
  - Neuroblastoma
  - Chemodectoma
  - Neurosarcoma

lymphomas. In children, the most common pathologies are neurogenic tumors, germ cell tumors, primary cysts, and lymphomas. Pericardial cysts and thymomas are uncommon in children. Malignant mediastinal neoplasms account for 25% to 50% of mediastinal masses in adults. Lymphomas, thymomas, germ cell tumors, primary carcinomas, and neurogenic tumors are the most common.

Many mediastinal lesions occur in characteristic sites within the mediastinum (Fig. 58.38). They may cause specific symptoms due to compression or invasion of adjacent structures. Approximately half of all mediastinal masses are located in the anterosuperior mediastinum, with the remainder divided between the posterior and middle mediastinum.

Anterosuperior Compartment

The anterosuperior compartment of the mediastinum borders the undersurface of the sternum ventrally, the pericardium dorsally, and the visceral pleura laterally (at the apposition of the pleura and pericardium). Among adults older than 40 years old, thymomas are the most frequently occurring neoplasm of the anterior mediastinum, and the second most common pathology is retrosternal goiter. Other pathologies are lymphomas, seminomas, nonseminoma germ cell tumors, and teratomas. Between the ages of 10 and 40 years old, lymphomas and teratomas in women and lymphomas, seminomas, nonseminoma germ cell tumors, and teratomas in men are the most frequently occurring neoplasms of the anterior mediastinum. In children younger than 10 years of age, lymphomas and teratomas are the most frequently occurring neoplasms of the anterior mediastinum. In this age group, benign thymic pathologies, such as thymic cysts or hyperplasia, are also encountered. Additional pathologies of the anterior mediastinum include carcinoid tumors, which may be found within the thymus, and primary carcinomas of the mediastinum, which are often unresectable and respond poorly to treatment (Fig. 58.39).[58]

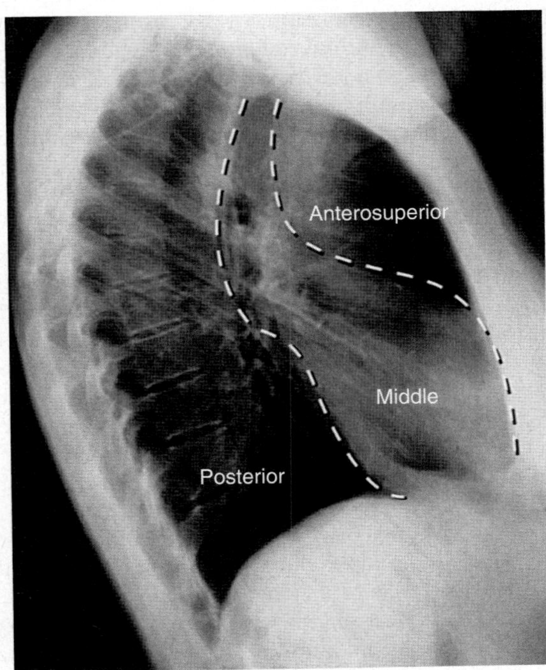

FIG. 58.38 Lateral chest radiograph demonstrating the mediastinum divided into three anatomic subdivisions.

Middle Compartment

The middle (or visceral) compartment extends from (and contains) the structures of the thoracic inlet (superiorly), the pericardium anteriorly, to the anterior surface of the vertebrae posteriorly. Lymphomas can occur in the middle mediastinum. Tumors of the heart and great vessels as well as tumors of the trachea, mainstem bronchi, and esophagus may be considered tumors of the middle compartment. Benign diseases, such as pericardial cysts and bronchogenic cysts, also occur here. Vascular masses and enlargement may represent aortic pathologies such as aortic aneurism, abscess, or dissection.

Posterior or Paravertebral Sulci Compartment

The posterior compartment is bounded by the middle compartment anteriorly and the costophrenic angle laterally. Neurogenic tumors are usually the most common primary tumors of the mediastinum, and approximately 25% of these tumors are malignant. These tumors are located within the paravertebral sulcus and may erode the adjacent vertebra or rib. Schwannomas and neurilemomas are the most common neurogenic tumors. Neurofibromas arise from the nerve sheath and fibers and occur in middle-aged patients. In children, ganglioneuroma is the most common neurogenic tumor. Posterior mediastinal tumors frequently attain a large size before presentation of symptoms. Surgical resection of these neurogenic tumors is usually the procedure of choice.

Embryologic development of the neural crest cells forms the basis of neuroendocrine tumors in the mediastinum. Of pheochromocytomas, 1% occurs within the mediastinum. Chemodectomas or paragangliomas may arise from chemoreceptor tissues around the aorta and great vessels, including the carotid. Symptoms may result from catecholamine production and are alleviated by surgical resection.

Clinical Manifestations and Diagnosis

Approximately one third of adult patients may develop symptoms from a mediastinal mass. Symptoms include chest pain, dyspnea, and cough. The symptoms may vary widely and relate to size (fatigue, weight loss), location, extent of compression or invasion of mediastinal structures (superior vena cava syndrome), and production of hormones, markers, or other biochemical materials (e.g., myasthenia gravis, fatigue, night sweats). Larger mediastinal tumors are more likely to produce symptoms. Benign lesions are more often asymptomatic. Superior vena cava syndrome (obstruction of the superior vena cava with head and neck and

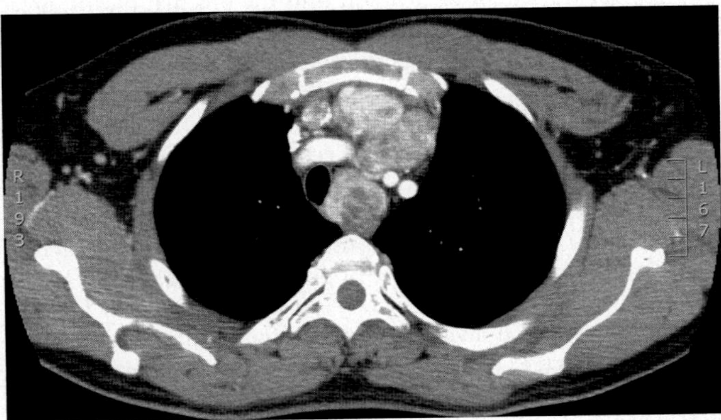

FIG. 58.39 Thyroid carcinoma within the mediastinum. The tumor was resected via median sternotomy. No invasion was identified. A complete resection was accomplished.

upper extremity swelling), cough, hoarseness (from involvement of the recurrent laryngeal nerve), dyspnea from tumor volume or phrenic nerve paralysis, and dysphagia occur with compression or invasion of mediastinal structures. Other manifestations include Horner syndrome and Pancoast syndrome.

Infections within the mediastinum are devastating. Because of the extensive thin areolar planes between major structures, infections within a limited portion of the mediastinum may spread vertically or horizontally to create an extensive infection. Synergistic aerobic and anaerobic infections from the perforated esophagus are particularly life-threatening. Treatment consists of surgical drainage and antibiotics.

Specific clinical syndromes may occur as a result of mediastinal tumors. Physical examination may reveal swelling of the head, neck, or upper extremities. Dyspnea may result from compression of the trachea, bronchus, or a portion of the lung parenchyma. Recurrent respiratory symptoms may occur for some time until a CXR is obtained and the abnormality is identified. Postobstructive pneumonitis or infection of benign pericardial or enteric duplication cysts may produce fever or sepsis. Myasthenia gravis may result from thymomas. In addition, thymomas may result in autoimmune problems, such as hypogammaglobulinemia, red cell aplasia, and smooth muscle degeneration. Mediastinal Hodgkin disease may produce an intermittent fever. Patients with hypertension from pheochromocytoma, thyrotoxicosis from goiter, hypercalcemia from ectopic mediastinal parathyroid adenoma or carcinoma, or hypogammaglobulinemia should be evaluated carefully; mediastinal findings may affect subsequent therapeutic recommendations.

Evaluation and Diagnostic Imaging

Diagnostic imaging typically includes a plain CXR taken in two planes (posteroanterior and left lateral), which provides basic information about the location of the mass within the mediastinum. Given the known propensity of specific lesions to occur in the anterior, visceral (middle), or paravertebral (posterior) sulcus based on the anatomy and embryologic development of cervicothoracic organs, a differential diagnosis may be obtained.

CT scan of the chest has replaced plain CXRs as the diagnostic procedure of choice for mediastinal masses. MRI is used if invasion to specific anatomic structures/location in the mediastinum is in doubt. To illustrate, an anterior mediastinal mass, such as a thymoma, can be evaluated for the extent of compression or possible invasion into the pulmonary artery, innominate vein, or superior vena cava. Similarly, posterior mediastinal masses can be evaluated by MRI for the extent of invasion into the brachial plexus, great vessels, vertebral body, neural foramina, and spinal column. Echocardiography may identify pericardial and cardiac involvement. When malignancy is suspected PET-CT is used to evaluate the extent of systemic disease. Additional scans may be used in specific scenarios (technetium scan for ectopic thyroid tissue or a substernal goiter and 131-I metaiodobenzylguanidine for mediastinal pheochromocytoma). If the CXR shows an elevated diaphragm, fluoroscopy or ultrasonography is used to evaluate paradoxical motion of the diaphragm indicative of phrenic nerve paralysis.

Mediastinal tumors may secrete specific hormones or biologic markers. Parathyroid adenomas or functioning parathyroid carcinomas may secrete parathormone. Pheochromocytomas may secrete various catecholamines (in serum and urine), which may cause hypertension. Carcinomas may secrete carcinoembryonic antigen. Nonseminomatous germ cell neoplasms may secrete α-fetoprotein (AFP) or β-human chorionic gonadotropin (β-HCG). Lymphomas may be associated with elevated levels of LDH and alkaline phosphatase. Thymomas may be associated with production of antiacetylcholine receptor (AChR) antibodies. Skin tests for tuberculosis, histoplasmosis, and coccidioidomycosis may also yield positive results. Other diagnostic tests for mediastinal tuberculosis include sputum cytology, CXR, and urine cytology.

Histologic Diagnosis

Radiographic diagnosis may be sufficient for the design of a treatment plan for mediastinal cysts and for other solid lesions that are clearly resectable (early stage thymoma). However, tissue for definitive diagnosis is required for the workup of more complex solid masses. Fine-needle aspiration or needle biopsy with CT guidance of a mediastinal mass may provide sufficient tissue for diagnosis for thymic carcinoma or other defined neoplasms. For lymphomas in particular, as well as thymomas and neural tumors, larger amounts of tissue may be required for cellular analysis. In these patients, core needle biopsy, mediastinoscopy, or intrathoracic biopsy (via thoracoscopy or open thoracotomy) may be considered. For recurrent lymphomas, after chemotherapy, open techniques for incisional biopsy are often required.

When upfront resection is considered for diagnosis and treatment, median sternotomy provides a direct visual approach to the anterior and middle mediastinum. Thoracotomy provides direct visual approach to the posterior mediastinum. VATS techniques and robotic techniques of resection are increasingly used for treatment of noninvasive tumors. More extensive approaches include the transverse sternotomy or "clam-shell" incision. Anesthetic considerations should include avoidance of airway obstruction, awake intubation, and use of muscle paralytics in patients with myasthenia gravis.

PRIMARY MEDIASTINAL CYSTS

Primary cysts of the mediastinum account for approximately 20% of mediastinal masses in most collected series. Cysts are characterized from the organ of origin and may be bronchogenic, pericardial, enteric, or thymic, or may be of an unspecified nature. More than 75% of cases are asymptomatic, and these tumors rarely cause morbidity; however, with proximity to vital structures within the mediastinum and increasing size, the cyst may cause significant problems. Benign cysts may be resected with minimally invasive techniques.

Bronchogenic cysts account for most primary cysts of the mediastinum (see Fig. 58.9). They originate as sequestrations from the ventral foregut, the antecedent of the tracheobronchial tree, and can be situated within the lung parenchyma or the mediastinum. Bronchogenic cysts are usually located proximal to the trachea or bronchi and may be just posterior to the carina. A connection to the bronchus rarely exists; however, when it occurs, these cysts may become infected. Diagnostic imaging may reveal an air-fluid level within the mediastinum. Two thirds of bronchogenic cysts are asymptomatic. In infants, cysts cause severe respiratory compromise by compressing the trachea or the bronchus. Resection is recommended.

Pericardial cysts are second in frequency to bronchogenic cysts and occur in the cardiophrenic angle mostly on the right side (70%). These cysts may or may not communicate with the pericardium. Typically, clear fluid is encountered. The characteristics of pericardial cysts include location in the cardiophrenic angle, characteristic appearance, smooth borders, and attenuation approximating water for the cyst fluid. Needle aspiration and routine surveillance may be all that is needed. Resection may be used for diagnosis and to exclude malignant tumors.

Enteric cysts or duplication cysts arise from the primitive foregut, which develops into the upper division of the gastrointestinal tract. These cysts are usually attached to the esophagus. Symptoms occur as size increases with compression of the esophagus and dysphagia. Neuroenteric cysts are associated with anomalies of the vertebral column. Excision is recommended.

PRIMARY MEDIASTINAL NEOPLASMS

Thymoma

Thymomas are the most common neoplasm of the anterosuperior compartment of the mediastinum. They are considered as malignant tumors with varying degrees of aggressiveness. The major histologic subtypes are A, AB, and B1–B3 thymomas, with type A being the most indolent subtype and type B3 being the most aggressive subtype. Thymic carcinomas are more aggressive than thymomas and are separately classified. Thymoma peak incidence is in the third through fifth decades, but they may occur throughout adulthood. Thymoma is rare in the first two decades of life. A thymoma may appear on a radiograph as a small, well-circumscribed mass or as a bulky, lobulated mass confluent with adjacent mediastinal structures (Fig. 58.40). Symptoms at presentation are related to local mass effects causing chest pain, dyspnea, hemoptysis, cough, and superior vena cava syndrome or systemic syndromes caused by immunologic mechanisms. The most common syndrome is myasthenia gravis (in up to 50% of cases); other syndromes include pure red blood cell aplasia, hypogammaglobulinemia, and thymoma-associated multiorgan autoimmunity. Staging of thymomas and thymic carcinomas is based on the extent of the primary tumor and the presence of invasion into adjacent structures and/or dissemination. Until recently, thymomas were staged according to the modified Masaoka-Koga system; however, a formal TNM-based staging system for thymic tumors has recently been issued by the AJCC as part of its eighth edition cancer staging manual (Table 58.5).

From a surgical perspective, thymomas may be viewed as those that can be completely resected, those that are potentially resectable, and those that cannot be completely resected. Patients presenting with small fully encapsulated thymomas should undergo surgery. Patients that present with invasive but potentially resectable tumors are managed by a multidisciplinary team of expert. Neoadjuvant and adjuvant chemotherapy, radiation, and immunotherapy are applied in conjunction with extensive surgery to achieve complete or at least macroscopic complete resection of the tumor with the aim of preventing or deferring disease recurrence. Resection and reconstruction of involved mediastinal structures, including the superior vena cava and innominate vein, as well as resection of droplet metastatic lesions, may in selected patient achieve significant prolongation of survival. As a rule of thumb, survival is dictated by the histologic subtype, by disease stage, and by the extent of resection.

For patients with myasthenia gravis and thymoma, surgery is advocated as soon as the patient's degree of weakness is sufficiently controlled to permit surgery. Attentive perioperative management in these patients is crucial to prevent complications. Anticholinesterase inhibitors, plasmapheresis, and/or intravenous immunoglobulin are used pre- and postoperatively to control generalized weakness. Intensive pulmonary toilet, early extubation if possible, chest physiotherapy, and avoidance of paralyzing agents and narcotics are central in assuring proper recovery from surgery. During surgery, complete resection of the entire thymus and all accessible mediastinal fatty areolar tissue is performed to ensure removal of all ectopic thymic tissue and to reduce the incidence of tumor recurrences. Protection and preservation of the phrenic nerves is an important integral component of thymectomy. Improvement in myasthenia gravis symptoms and reduction in the dosages of drugs required to control the disease is anticipated to a certain extent in the months following surgery.[59]

Germ Cell Tumors

Germ cell tumors arise from primordial germ cells that fail to complete the migration from the urogenital ridge and rest in the mediastinum. Treatment depends on histology. The anterosuperior mediastinum is the most common extragonadal primary site of these tumors. Although these lesions are identical histologically to germ cell tumors originating in the gonads, they are not considered metastatic from primary gonadal tumors. The current recommendations for evaluating the testes of a patient with mediastinal germ cell tumor are careful physical examination and ultrasonography of the testes. Biopsy is reserved for positive findings. Blind biopsy or orchiectomy is contraindicated.

Teratomas

Teratomas are the most common mediastinal germ cell neoplasms and are located most commonly in the anterosuperior

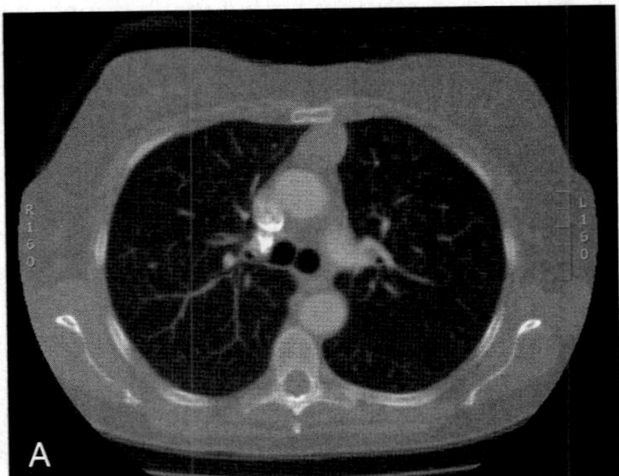

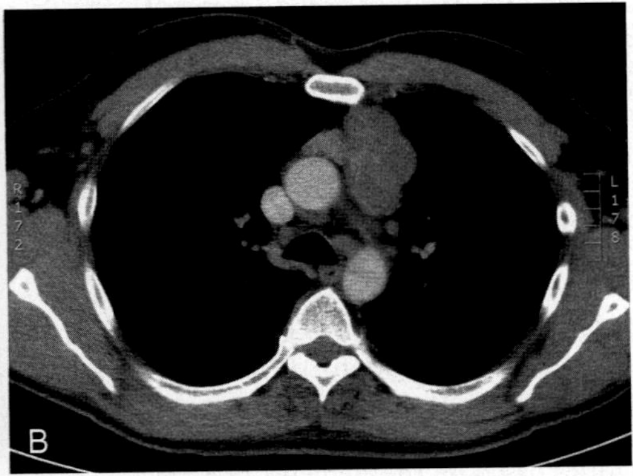

FIG. 58.40 (A) Computed tomography (CT) scan of the chest in a patient with myasthenia gravis and thymoma. The thymoma is small with a plane of separation between the tumor and the pericardium. (B) Chest CT scan in a patient with a larger mediastinal mass. The location, character, and size are noted. Transthoracic core needle biopsy was performed. Germ cell tumor markers were normal. Pathology demonstrated thymoma. A 6.5-cm thymoma was subsequently resected. There was no invasion of the pericardium. A complete resection (R0) was accomplished.

TABLE 58.5 Thymoma staging.

T Descriptors

CATEGORY	DEFINITION (INVOLVEMENT OF)[a,b]
T1	
a	Encapsulated or unencapsulated, with or without extension into mediastinal fat
b	Extension into mediastinal pleura
T2	Pericardium
T3	Lung, brachiocephalic vein, superior vena cava, chest wall, phrenic nerve, hilar (extrapericardial) pulmonary vessels
T4	Aorta, arch vessels, main pulmonary artery, myocardium, trachea, or esophagus

N and M Descriptors

CATEGORY	DEFINITION (INVOLVEMENT OF)[a]
N0	No nodal involvement
N1	Anterior (perithymic) nodes
N2	Deep intrathoracic or cervical nodes
M0	No metastatic pleural, pericardial, or distant sites
M1	
A	Separate pleural or pericardial nodule(s)
B	Pulmonary intraparenchymal nodule or distant organ metastasis

Stage Grouping

STAGE	T	N	M
I	T1	N0	M0
II	T2	N0	M0
IIIa	T3	N0	M0
IIIb	T4	N0	M0
IVa	T any	N1	M0
	T any	N0,1	M1a
IVb	T any	N2	M0,1a
	T any	N any	M1b

From Detterbeck FC, Stratton K, Giroux D, et al. The IASLC/ITMIG Thymic Epithelial Tumors Staging Project: proposal for an evidence-based stage classification system for the forthcoming (8th) edition of the TNM classification of malignant tumors. *J Thorac Oncol.* 2014;9:S65–72.

[a]Involvement must be pathologically proven in pathologic staging.

[b]A tumor is classified according to the highest T level of involvement that is present with or without any invasion of structures of lower T levels.

mediastinum. They are composed of multiple tissue elements that are derived from the three primitive embryonic layers foreign to the area in which they occur. The peak incidence is in the second and third decades of life. There is no gender predisposition. Radiographic evidence of normal tissue (e.g., well-formed teeth or globular calcifications, a fatty mass) in an abnormal location can be considered specific. The teratodermoid (dermoid) cyst is the simplest form of a teratoma and is composed of derivatives of the epidermal layer, including dermal and epidermal glands, hair, and sebaceous material. Teratomas are histologically more complex. The solid component of the tumor often contains well-differentiated elements of bone, cartilage, teeth, muscle, connective tissue, fibrous and lymphoid tissue, nerve, thymus, mucous and salivary glands, lung, liver, or pancreas. Malignant tumors are differentiated from benign tumors by the presence of primitive (embryonic) tissue or by the presence of malignant components. Immature teratomas contain combinations of mature epithelial and connective tissues with immature areas of mesenchymal and neuroectodermal tissues. Teratomas with malignant components are divided into categories based on the elements present.

Diagnosis and therapy rely on surgical excision. For benign tumors of large size or with involvement of adjacent mediastinal structures such that complete resection is impossible, partial resection has led to resolution of symptoms, frequently without relapse. For malignant teratomas, chemotherapy, and radiation therapy, combined with surgical excision, are individualized for the type of malignant components contained in the tumors. The overall prognosis is poor for malignant teratomas.

Malignant Nonteratomatous Germ Cell Tumors

Malignant germ cell tumors occur predominantly in the anterosuperior mediastinum with a marked male decades of life.[60] Most patients have symptoms of chest pain, cough, dyspnea, and hemoptysis; the superior vena cava syndrome occurs commonly. A large anterior mediastinal mass is identified on diagnostic imaging. There is evidence of intrathoracic spread of disease. CT and MRI are helpful to define the extent of the disease and involvement of mediastinal structures. Serologic measurements of AFP and β-HCG are useful for differentiating seminomas from nonseminomatous tumors, assessing response to therapy, and diagnosing relapse or failure of therapy. Seminomas rarely produce β-HCG and never produce AFP; in contrast, more than 90% of nonseminomatous tumors secrete one or both of these hormones. This differentiation is important, as seminomas are radiosensitive, and nonseminomatous tumors are relatively radioinsensitive.

Seminomas

Seminomas constitute 50% of malignant germ cell tumors. Seminomas usually remain intrathoracic. Symptoms are related to the mechanical effects of the tumor on adjacent mediastinal and pulmonary structures. The superior vena cava syndrome occurs in 10% to 20% of patients. These tumors are sensitive to irradiation and chemotherapy. Therapy is determined by the stage of the disease. Cytoreductive resection before chemotherapy or radiation therapy is unnecessary. Treatment consists of systemic and local therapy—chemotherapy with salvage surgery or combined chemoradiotherapy. Radiation therapy may be considered for early-stage disease but is not recommended for regional disease. Platinum-based chemotherapy is common. Occasionally, excision is possible without injury to vital structures and can be recommended. When complete resection is possible, the use of adjuvant therapy is unnecessary. When excision is impossible, a biopsy sample of sufficient size to establish the diagnosis is obtained.

Nonseminomatous Tumors

Malignant nonseminomatous germ cell tumors include choriocarcinomas, embryonal cell carcinomas, immature teratomas, teratomas with malignant components, and endodermal cell (yolk sac) tumors and occur mostly in men in their third or fourth decades. Diagnostic imaging reveals a large anterior mediastinal mass with frequent extension to the lung, chest wall, and mediastinal structures. Nonseminomatous germ cell neoplasms are more aggressive tumors and more frequently disseminated at the time of diagnosis, they are rarely radiosensitive, and more than 90% produce either β-HCG or AFP. All patients with choriocarcinoma and some patients with embryonal cell tumors have elevated levels of β-HCG. AFP is most commonly elevated in patients with embryonal cell carcinomas and yolk sac tumors. Mediastinal nonseminomatous germ cell tumors, but not testicular germ cell tumors, are associated with the development of rare hematologic malignancies, such as acute megakaryocytic leukemia, systemic mast cell disease, and malignant histiocytosis, as well as other hematologic abnormalities, including myelodysplastic syndrome and idiopathic thrombocytopenia refractory to treatment.

Treatment of these nonseminomatous tumors currently is with cisplatin and etoposide-based regimens. Advanced disease, invasion into thoracic structures, and metastasis preclude surgical resection. Serum markers, AFP or β-HCG, are followed to assess response to systemic treatment. If a complete serologic and radiologic response is achieved, patients are closely observed. If the disease progresses during therapy, salvage chemotherapy is initiated. Operative intervention may be required to establish a histologic diagnosis in patients without elevations in serum AFP or β-HCG or for salvage resection after tissue or serologic response to therapy. The pathology of the resected postchemotherapy specimen appears to be the most significant predictor of survival. The presence of residual disease after chemotherapy portends a poor prognosis and the need for additional chemotherapy. When tumor necrosis or a benign teratoma is found during surgical exploration after chemotherapy, an excellent or intermediate prognosis is conferred, respectively.

Neurogenic Tumors

Neurogenic tumors are usually located in the posterior mediastinum and originate from the sympathetic ganglia (ganglioma, ganglioneuroblastoma, and neuroblastoma), the intercostal nerves (neurofibroma, neurilemoma, and neurosarcoma), and the paraganglia cells (paraganglioma). Although the peak incidence occurs in adults, neurogenic tumors make up a proportionally greater percentage of mediastinal masses in children. Although most neurogenic tumors in adults are benign, a greater percentage of neurogenic tumors are malignant in children.

The most common neurogenic tumor is neurilemoma or schwannoma, which originates from perineural Schwann cells. They are benign, slow-growing neoplasms that frequently arise from a spinal nerve root but can involve any thoracic nerve. These tumors are well circumscribed and have a defined capsule. They arise from the nerve sheath and extrinsically compress the nerve fibers. The peak incidence of these tumors is in the third through fifth decades of life; men and women are equally affected.

Many of these tumors are asymptomatic. Symptoms such as pain occur from compression or invasion of intercostal nerve, bone, and chest wall; cough and dyspnea resulting from compression of the tracheobronchial tree; Pancoast syndrome; and Horner syndrome resulting from involvement of the brachial and the cervical sympathetic chain. Approximately 10% of neurogenic tumors have extensions into the spinal column and are termed *dumbbell tumors* because of their characteristic shape with relatively large paraspinal and intraspinal portions connected by a narrow isthmus of tissue traversing the intervertebral foramen. Patients with paraspinal tumors should undergo MRI to evaluate the presence and extent of the tumor and its relationship to the neural foramen and the intraspinal space. During resection, the intraspinal component should be removed first via a posterior laminectomy. This approach minimizes the potential for spinal column hematoma, cord ischemia, and paralysis. A separate transthoracic approach is needed for resection of the intrathoracic component.

Neuroblastoma

Neuroblastomas originate from the sympathetic nervous system. The most common location for a neuroblastoma is in the retroperitoneum; however, 10% to 20% occur primarily in the mediastinum. These are highly invasive neoplasms that have frequently metastasized before diagnosis. Most of these tumors occur in children 4 years old or younger. A 24-hour urine collection to measure catecholamines is obtained in children with a posterior mediastinal mass. Therapy is determined by the stage of the disease: stage I, surgical excision; stage II, excision and radiation therapy; stages III and IV, multimodality therapy using surgical debulking, radiation therapy, and multiagent chemotherapy and a second-look exploration to resect residual disease when necessary. The usual chemotherapeutic agents are cisplatin, vincristine, doxorubicin, cyclophosphamide, and etoposide.

Ganglion Tumors

Ganglioneuroblastomas are composed of mature and immature ganglion cells. Treatment of ganglioneuroblastoma ranges from surgical excision alone to various chemotherapeutic strategies depending on histologic characteristics, age at diagnosis, and stage of disease. Ganglioneuromas are benign tumors that originate from the sympathetic chain and are composed of ganglion cells and nerve fibers. These tumors typically manifest at an early age and are the most common neurogenic tumors occurring during childhood. The usual location is the paravertebral region. These tumors are well encapsulated and, when cross-sectioned, frequently exhibit areas of cystic degeneration. Surgical excision provides cure.

Paraganglioma (Pheochromocytoma)

Mediastinal paragangliomas are rare tumors, representing less than 1% of all mediastinal tumors and less than 2% of all pheochromocytomas. Although most are found in the paravertebral sulcus, an increasing number occur in the branchial arch structures, coronary and aortopulmonary paraganglia, atria, and islands of tissue in the pericardium. Although adrenal pheochromocytomas often produce both epinephrine and norepinephrine, extra-adrenal paragangliomas rarely secrete epinephrine. Multiple paragangliomas occur in 10% of patients. These tumors are more common in patients with multiple endocrine neoplasia syndromes, a family history of disease, and Carney syndrome (pulmonary chondroma, gastric leiomyosarcoma, and functioning extra-adrenal paraganglioma). In patients who have had excision of an adrenal pheochromocytoma and continue to have symptoms, a search for an extra-adrenal lesion is undertaken with careful attention to the mediastinum. Tumor localization has improved through the use of CT and iodine-131 metaiodobenzylguanidine scintigraphy, particularly when the tumors are hormonally active. When appropriate, surgical resection is the optimal therapy. In patients with tumors involving the middle mediastinum, cardiopulmonary bypass may be necessary to enable resection. Preoperative embolization to reduce perioperative bleeding may be considered. Although half of tumors appear malignant morphologically, metastatic disease rarely develops.

Lymphomas

Although the mediastinum is frequently involved in patients with lymphoma at some time during the course of their disease, it is infrequently the sole site of disease at the time of presentation. Hodgkin and non-Hodgkin lymphoma are distinct clinical entities with overlapping features. Patients usually have symptoms, with chest pain, cough, dyspnea, hoarseness, and superior vena cava syndrome being the most common clinical manifestations. Nonspecific systemic symptoms of fever and chills, weight loss, and anorexia are frequently noted.

Surgical excision of all disease is rarely possible; the surgeon's primary role is to provide sufficient tissue for diagnosis and to assist in pathologic staging. A needle biopsy is often unsuccessful because larger tissue samples are needed to make a histologic diagnosis, particularly with nodular sclerosing lesions. Thoracoscopy, mediastinoscopy, or mediastinotomy and, rarely, thoracotomy or median sternotomy may be necessary to obtain sufficient tissue.

Patients with non-Hodgkin lymphoma usually have symptoms because of involvement of adjacent mediastinal structures. Superior vena cava syndrome is relatively common. Lymphoblastic lymphoma occurs predominantly in children, adolescents, and young adults and represents 60% of cases of mediastinal non-Hodgkin lymphoma.

After treatment of lymphomas, residual radiographic abnormalities within the mediastinum are commonly noted (64% to 88%). CT cannot differentiate fibrosis or necrosis from residual tumor. FDG-PET has shown promise as a noninvasive way to detect active mediastinal disease and predict relapse in patients with lymphoma, but tissue confirmation is required. Needle biopsy does not provide significant diagnostic material. Transthoracic incisional biopsy under general anesthesia is often needed given the significant fibrosis that remains after therapy.

Endocrine Tumors

Thyroid Tumors

Although substernal extension of a cervical goiter is common, totally intrathoracic thyroid tumors are rare and make up only 1% of all mediastinal masses in collected series. These tumors arise from heterotopic thyroid tissue, which occurs most commonly in the anterosuperior mediastinum but may also occur in the middle mediastinum between the trachea and the esophagus as well as in the posterior mediastinum. Although there may be a demonstrable connection with the cervical gland (usually a fibrous connective tissue band), a true intrathoracic thyroid gland derives its blood supply from thoracic vessels. Substernal extensions of a cervical goiter can usually be excised using a cervical approach.

Parathyroid Tumors

Although parathyroid glands may occur in the mediastinum in 10% of patients, they are usually accessible through the cervical incision. Most often, these adenomas are found in the anterosuperior mediastinum (80%) embedded in or near the superior pole of the thymus. This anatomic relationship is the result of the common embryogenesis of the inferior parathyroid glands from the third branchial cleft. The superior parathyroid glands and the lateral lobes of the thyroid gland are derived from the fourth branchial pouch. Because they migrate with the lateral lobes of the thyroid gland to a paraesophageal position, parathyroid adenomas can also be found in the posterior mediastinum.

Most frequently, the mediastinal parathyroid adenoma may be excised after a negative exploration of the cervical region through the existing cervical incision. Usually the vascular supply extends from cervical blood vessels. In patients with persistent hyperparathyroidism after cervical exploration, if localization studies show residual parathyroid in the mediastinum, mediastinal exploration using a median sternotomy or thoracoscopy is indicated.

Parathyroid carcinomas have been reported and are usually hormonally active. Patients differ in clinical presentation in that they often have higher serum calcium levels and manifest more severe symptoms of hyperparathyroidism. When possible, resection is the optimal therapy.

Neuroendocrine Tumors

Mediastinal neuroendocrine tumors and carcinoid tumors, arise from cells of Kulchitsky located in the thymus and commonly occur in men in their 40s and 50s. They are usually located in the anterosuperior mediastinum. These tumors are aggressive and 20% have metastatic spread to mediastinal and cervical lymph nodes, liver, bone, skin, and lungs. More than 50% of thymic neuroendocrine tumors are hormonally active, often associated with Cushing syndrome because of production of adrenocorticotropic hormone, less frequently associated with multiple endocrine neoplasia syndromes, and only rarely associated with carcinoid syndrome (0.6%). If possible, resection is recommended; however, local invasion and metastasis often preclude complete excision. Adjuvant therapy is controversial, but irradiation should probably be added, particularly in patients with capsular invasion.

SELECTED REFERENCES

Carter BW, Marom EM, Detterbeck FC. Approaching the patient with an anterior mediastinal mass: a guide for clinicians. *J Thorac Oncol.* 2014;9:S102–109.

Anterior mediastinal masses are relatively uncommon, include a wide variety of entities, and often pose a diagnostic challenge for clinicians. In this article, available data is assembled in a clinically oriented manner to develop a structured approach to evaluation of these patients. Attention to age and gender, combined with identification of certain radiographic and clinical characteristics, allows a presumptive diagnosis to be established in most patients. This structure efficiently guides what additional workup is needed.

Feller-Kopman D, Light R. Pleural disease. *N Engl J Med.* 2018;378:740–751.

This review nicely summarizes the approach and guidelines to evaluation and management of pleural space problems including benign and malignant pleural effusion and pneumothorax.

NCCN Clinical Practice Guidelines in Oncology. Non-small cell lung cancer. National Comprehensive Cancer Network. Retrieved November 20, 2019, from http://www.nccn.org/professionals/physician_gls/f_guidelines.asp.

Guidelines for diagnosis, treatment, and surveillance are published by various organizations based on evidence and consensus of experts. Two sets of guidelines for the management of non–small cell lung cancer were published by the American College of Chest Physicians and the National Comprehensive Cancer Network.

Rami-Porta R, Asamura H, Travis WD, et al. Lung cancer - major changes in the american joint committee on cancer eighth edition cancer staging manual. *CA Cancer J Clin.* 2017;67:138–155.

This manuscript and website provide valuable information regarding the 8th edition of staging of lung cancer and other thoracic malignancies.

REFERENCES

1. Brunelli A, Kim AW, Berger KI, et al. Physiologic evaluation of the patient with lung cancer being considered for resectional surgery: diagnosis and management of lung cancer, 3rd ed: american college of chest physicians evidence-based clinical practice guidelines. *Chest.* 2013;143:e166S–e190S.
2. Beckles MA, Spiro SG, Colice GL, et al. The physiologic evaluation of patients with lung cancer being considered for resectional surgery. *Chest.* 2003;123:105S–114S.
3. Durell J, Lakhoo K. Congenital cystic lesions of the lung. *Early Hum Dev.* 2014;90:935–939.
4. Fowler DJ, Gould SJ. The pathology of congenital lung lesions. *Semin Pediatr Surg.* 2015;24:176–182.
5. Jaquiss RD. Management of pediatric tracheal stenosis and tracheomalacia. *Semin Thorac Cardiovasc Surg.* 2004;16:220–224.
6. Berrocal T, Madrid C, Novo S, et al. Congenital anomalies of the tracheobronchial tree, lung, and mediastinum: embryology, radiology, and pathology. *Radiographics.* 2004;24:e17.
7. Maldonado JA, Henry T, Gutierrez FR. Congenital thoracic vascular anomalies. *Radiol Clin North Am.* 2010;48:85–115.
8. Siegel RL, Miller KD, Jemal A. Cancer statistics, 2018. *CA Cancer J Clin.* 2018;68:7–30.
9. Rami-Porta R, Asamura H, Travis WD, et al. Lung cancer - major changes in the american joint committee on cancer eighth edition cancer staging manual. *CA Cancer J Clin.* 2017;67:138–155.
10. Travis WD, Brambilla E, Noguchi M, et al. International association for the study of lung cancer/american thoracic society/european respiratory society: international multidisciplinary classification of lung adenocarcinoma: executive summary. *Proc Am Thorac Soc.* 2011;8:381–385.
11. Travis WD, Brambilla E, Nicholson AG, et al. The 2015 World health organization classification of lung tumors: impact of genetic, clinical and radiologic advances since the 2004 classification. *J Thorac Oncol.* 2015;10:1243–1260.
12. Aberle DR, Adams AM, Berg CD, et al. Reduced lung-cancer mortality with low-dose computed tomographic screening. *N Engl J Med.* 2011;365:395–409.
13. Tammemagi MC, Katki HA, Hocking WG, et al. Selection criteria for lung-cancer screening. *N Engl J Med.* 2013;368:728–736.
14. National Comprehensive Cancer Network. Retrieved January 2, 2019, from https://www.nccn.org/default.aspx.
15. Simoff MJ, Lally B, Slade MG, et al. Symptom management in patients with lung cancer: diagnosis and management of lung cancer, 3rd ed: american college of chest physicians evidence-based clinical practice guidelines. *Chest.* 2013;143:e455S–e497S.
16. MacMahon H, Naidich DP, Goo JM, et al. Guidelines for management of incidental pulmonary nodules detected on CT images: from the fleischner society 2017. *Radiology.* 2017;284:228–243.
17. Feller-Kopman D, Light R. Pleural disease. *N Engl J Med.* 2018;378:740–751.
18. Silvestri GA, Gonzalez AV, Jantz MA, et al. Methods for staging non-small cell lung cancer: diagnosis and management of lung cancer, 3rd ed: american college of chest physicians evidence-based clinical practice guidelines. *Chest.* 143:e211S–e250S.
19. Fernandez FG, Kozower BD, Crabtree TD, et al. Utility of mediastinoscopy in clinical stage I lung cancers at risk for occult mediastinal nodal metastases. *J Thorac Cardiovasc Surg.* 2015;149:35–41, 42 e31.
20. IASLC 8th Edition Staging Educational Materials. Retrieved January 2, 2020, from https://www.iaslc.org/Research-Education/IASLC-Staging-Project/Staging-Educational-Materials.
21. Goldstraw P, Chansky K, Crowley J, et al. The IASLC lung cancer staging project: proposals for revision of the TNM stage groupings in the forthcoming (eighth) edition of the TNM classification for lung cancer. *J Thorac Oncol.* 2016;11:39–51.
22. Detterbeck FC, Chansky K, Groome P, et al. The IASLC lung cancer staging project: methodology and validation used in the development of proposals for revision of the stage classification of NSCLC in the forthcoming (eighth) edition of the TNM classification of lung cancer. *J Thorac Oncol.* 2016;11:1433–1446.
23. Rusch VW, Asamura H, Watanabe H, et al. The IASLC lung cancer staging project: a proposal for a new international lymph node map in the forthcoming seventh edition of the TNM classification for lung cancer. *J Thorac Oncol.* 2009;4:568–577.
24. Asamura H, Chansky K, Crowley J, et al. The international association for the study of lung cancer lung cancer staging project: proposals for the revision of the N descriptors in the forthcoming 8th edition of the TNM classification for lung cancer. *J Thorac Oncol.* 2015;10:1675–1684.
25. Timmerman R, Paulus R, Galvin J, et al. Stereotactic body radiation therapy for inoperable early stage lung cancer. *J Am Med Assoc.* 2010;303:1070–1076.
26. Forde PM, Chaft JE, Smith KN, et al. Neoadjuvant PD-1 blockade in resectable lung cancer. *N Engl J Med.* 2018;378:1976–1986.
27. Landreneau RJ, Normolle DP, Christie NA, et al. Recurrence and survival outcomes after anatomic segmentectomy versus lobectomy for clinical stage I non-small-cell

lung cancer: a propensity-matched analysis. *J Clin Oncol.* 2014;32:2449–2455.
28. Ramnath N, Dilling TJ, Harris LJ, et al. Treatment of stage III non-small cell lung cancer: diagnosis and management of lung cancer, 3rd ed: american college of chest physicians evidence-based clinical practice guidelines. *Chest.* 2013;143:e314S–e340S.
29. Pisters KM, Vallieres E, Crowley JJ, et al. Surgery with or without preoperative paclitaxel and carboplatin in early-stage non-small-cell lung cancer: southwest oncology group trial S9900, an intergroup, randomized, phase III trial. *J Clin Oncol.* 2010;28:1843–1849.
30. Song WA, Zhou NK, Wang W, et al. Survival benefit of neoadjuvant chemotherapy in non-small cell lung cancer: an updated meta-analysis of 13 randomized control trials. *J Thorac Oncol.* 2010;5:510–516.
31. Albain KS, Swann RS, Rusch VW, et al. Radiotherapy plus chemotherapy with or without surgical resection for stage III non-small-cell lung cancer: a phase III randomised controlled trial. *Lancet.* 2009;374:379–386.
32. Ferrara R, Mezquita L, Besse B. Progress in the management of advanced thoracic malignancies in 2017. *J Thorac Oncol.* 2018;13:301–322.
33. Reck M, Rodriguez-Abreu D, Robinson AG, et al. Pembrolizumab versus chemotherapy for PD-L1-positive non-small-cell lung cancer. *N Engl J Med.* 2016;375:1823–1833.
34. Gandhi L, Rodriguez-Abreu D, Gadgeel S, et al. Pembrolizumab plus chemotherapy in metastatic non-small-cell lung cancer. *N Engl J Med.* 2018;378:2078–2092.
35. Brand-Saberi BEM, Schafer T. Trachea: anatomy and physiology. *Thorac Surg Clin.* 2014;24:1–5.
36. Stoelben E, Koryllos A, Beckers F, et al. Benign stenosis of the trachea. *Thorac Surg Clin.* 2014;24:59–65.
37. Junker K. Pathology of tracheal tumors. *Thorac Surg Clin.* 2014;24:7–11.
38. Sherani K, Vakil A, Dodhia C, et al. Malignant tracheal tumors: a review of current diagnostic and management strategies. *Curr Opin Pulm Med.* 2015;21:322–326.
39. Behringer D, Konemann S, Hecker E. Treatment approaches to primary tracheal cancer. *Thorac Surg Clin.* 2014;24:73–76.
40. Welter S. Repair of tracheobronchial injuries. *Thorac Surg Clin.* 2014;24:41–50.
41. Hecker E, Volmerig J. Extended tracheal resections. *Thorac Surg Clin.* 2014;24:85–95.
42. Polverino E, Goeminne PC, McDonnell MJ, et al. European respiratory society guidelines for the management of adult bronchiectasis. *Eur Respir J.* 2017;50:1700629. https://doi.org/10.1183/13993003.00629-2017.
43. Fox GJ, Mitnick CD, Benedetti A, et al. Surgery as an adjunctive treatment for multidrug-resistant tuberculosis: an individual patient data metaanalysis. *Clin Infect Dis.* 2016;62:887–895.
44. Fishman A, Martinez F, Naunheim K, et al. A randomized trial comparing lung-volume-reduction surgery with medical therapy for severe emphysema. *N Engl J Med.* 2003;348:2059–2073.
45. Yusen RD, Edwards LB, Dipchand AI, et al. The registry of the international society for heart and lung transplantation: thirty-third adult lung and heart-lung transplant report-2016; focus theme: primary diagnostic indications for transplant. *J Heart Lung Transplant.* 2016;35:1170–1184.
46. Ranieri VM, Rubenfeld GD, Thompson BT, et al. Acute respiratory distress syndrome: the berlin definition. *J Am Med Assoc.* 2012;307:2526–2533.
47. Fokin AA, Steuerwald NM, Ahrens WA, et al. Anatomical, histologic, and genetic characteristics of congenital chest wall deformities. *Semin Thorac Cardiovasc Surg.* 2009;21:44–57.
48. Colombani PM. Preoperative assessment of chest wall deformities. *Semin Thorac Cardiovasc Surg.* 2009;21:58–63.
49. Robicsek F, Watts LT, Fokin AA. Surgical repair of pectus excavatum and carinatum. *Semin Thorac Cardiovasc Surg.* 2009;21:64–75.
50. Hebra A. Minimally invasive repair of pectus excavatum. *Semin Thorac Cardiovasc Surg.* 2009;21:76–84.
51. Smith SE, Keshavjee S. Primary chest wall tumors. *Thorac Surg Clin.* 2010;20:495–507.
52. Thomas PA, Brouchet L. Prosthetic reconstruction of the chest wall. *Thorac Surg Clin.* 2010;20:551–558.
53. Blasberg JD, Donington JS. Infections and radiation injuries involving the chest wall. *Thorac Surg Clin.* 2010;20:487–494.
54. Molnar TF. Surgical management of chest wall trauma. *Thorac Surg Clin.* 2010;20:475–485.
55. Burt BM. Thoracic outlet syndrome for thoracic surgeons. *J Thorac Cardiovasc Surg.* 2018;156:1318–1323 e1311.
56. Havelock T, Teoh R, Laws D, et al. Pleural procedures and thoracic ultrasound: british thoracic society pleural disease guideline 2010. *Thorax.* 2010;65(suppl 2):ii61–76.
57. Wald O, Sugarbaker DJ. New concepts in the treatment of malignant pleural mesothelioma. *Annu Rev Med.* 2018;69:365–377.
58. Carter BW, Marom EM, Detterbeck FC. Approaching the patient with an anterior mediastinal mass: a guide for clinicians. *J Thorac Oncol.* 2014;9:S102–S109.
59. Wolfe GI, Kaminski HJ, Aban IB, et al. Randomized trial of thymectomy in myasthenia gravis. *N Engl J Med.* 2016;375:511–522.
60. Kesler KA, Einhorn LH. Multimodality treatment of germ cell tumors of the mediastinum. *Thorac Surg Clin.* 2009;19:63–69.

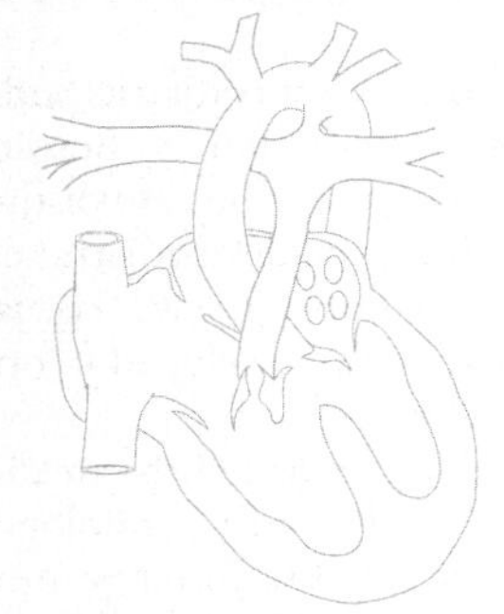

CHAPTER 59

Congenital Heart Disease

Andrew Well, Chuck D. Fraser Jr.

OUTLINE

This chapter is designed to provide medical students, general surgery residents, and practicing general surgeons with a working tool to aid in their understanding of the features of anatomy and physiology in patients presenting for general surgical procedures in the setting of repaired or unrepaired congenital cardiac lesions. The large scope and breadth of the evolving field of congenital heart surgery precludes an exhaustive treatise on all aspects of this specialty. Several excellent and thorough textbooks of congenital heart surgery are referenced in this chapter, and the reader is encouraged to use them for additional in-depth understanding of the lesions to be reviewed. A general surgeon practicing today needs to be well versed in the basics of cardiac anatomy, physiology, and specific derangements associated with the various known congenital cardiac lesions. Furthermore, few patients with complex congenital cardiac lesions may be considered cured of their cardiac problem, even after successful reconstructive surgery. Thus, it is imperative that a general surgeon who needs to perform a noncardiac operation on such a patient be familiar with the specific issues of ongoing concern in patients with congenital cardiac disease.

HISTORY AND OTHER CONSIDERATIONS

The era of surgical treatment for congenital cardiac anomalies was initiated in November 1944, when Alfred Blalock and associates Vivien Thomas and Helen Taussig combined their unique talents and vision to treat a young child dying of cyanotic congenital heart disease (CHD).[1] This palliative operation involved the surgical creation of a systemic–pulmonary artery connection in the patient, who had inadequate pulmonary blood flow. The procedure has since been recalled as miraculous and now more than 60 years later is known by the eponym Blalock-Taussig (BT) shunt. The striking success of this simple concept and the reproducible nature of the operation in children with otherwise fatal cardiac conditions have emboldened subsequent surgical innovators to venture inside the congenitally malformed heart. At first, the parent was asked to serve as a biologic oxygenator using the technique of controlled cross-circulation; soon thereafter, the mechanical, extracorporeal, heart-lung bypass pump was developed.[2,3] With the aid of this ability to support the patient's circulation during intracardiac exploration, surgeons have sequentially attacked almost every described congenital cardiac anomaly. The prospect of meaningful survival for patients born with otherwise devastating congenital cardiac lesions is now expected in most, if not all, cases.

As a result of this success story, there is now a large and growing population of adults with repaired or unrepaired CHD; estimates in the United States for 2010 placed the number of adult patients surviving with repaired or palliated congenital cardiac lesions at more than one million.[4] There has been an increase of greater than 50% in CHD prevalence since 2000, and by 2010, adults accounted for two thirds of patients with CHD in the general population.[5] This reality has been associated with new challenges in the ongoing medical maintenance of such patients, with particular focus on the care of patients with congenital cardiac lesions presenting for surgery for noncardiac illnesses. The evolving subspecialty of adult CHD points to the unique needs of this population of patients.

PATHWAYS FOR PRACTICING CONGENITAL HEART SURGERY

Before embarking on a review of the field, it is worthwhile to describe the setting in which patients with CHD seek and receive care in today's medical environment. With the development of sophisticated methods of fetal ultrasound, a large percentage of children requiring surgery for CHD are diagnosed during gestation (Fig. 59.1). A fetal diagnosis of complex CHD is extremely helpful to parents and the medical management team. Fetal diagnosis is particularly important in the setting of lesions dependent on persistent patency of the ductus arteriosus for postnatal survival. In these individuals, survival after delivery is predicated on the maintenance of ductal patency through the intravenous infusion of prostaglandin E1 (PGE1) initiated in the delivery suite, often through an umbilical vein catheter. Several studies have shown a decrease in morbidity, but there is inconclusive evidence that mortality rates are decreased.[6,7]

A growing number of congenital cardiac lesions are known to be associated with specific genetic mutations, many clearly inherited and some presumed to be sporadic. A chromosomal analysis is frequently performed in individuals found to have major structural cardiac abnormalities; this analysis may be performed during gestation through amniocentesis or after delivery. The chromosomal evaluation is beneficial to the family when planning the risk of such an occurrence in future offspring. For the clinician, knowledge of chromosomal abnormalities, such as DiGeorge sequence, velocardiofacial syndrome, and Marfan syndrome, aids in the delivery of acute medical management.

In general terms, the timing of surgery for various congenital cardiac conditions depends on the presenting symptoms and expectations for further associated complications. Neonates presenting with limited pulmonary blood flow or atretic pulmonary connections typically require surgery during the first few days of life and occasionally within hours of delivery. Lesions associated with excessive pulmonary blood flow result in early heart failure, which may manifest as poor feeding, tachypnea, or respiratory failure. These patients are operated on during early infancy to ameliorate their symptoms and prevent the development of pulmonary vascular disease.

Preterm and low-birth-weight infants with CHD have been presenting for surgical consideration with more frequency. This treatment strategy requires thoughtful planning and coordination among the surgery, anesthesia, cardiology, intensive care, and neonatology teams. We have successfully operated on an 800-g infant with transposition of the great arteries (TGA).

The specialty of congenital heart surgery is now recognized as a subspecialty of cardiothoracic surgery. Congenital heart surgeons were previously certified in cardiothoracic surgery by the American Board of Thoracic Surgery and received additional fellowship training in the United States or abroad in congenital heart surgery. As of 2009, the American Board of Thoracic Surgery offers a formal certification process for subspecialty training in congenital heart surgery. At the present time, there are 12 congenital cardiac surgery residency programs approved by the Accreditation Council for Graduate Medical Education.[8] Most pediatric cardiac surgery is performed in large, multispecialty children's hospitals in association with formal programs focused on the care of these complex patients. The management team includes pediatric cardiac anesthesiologists, perfusionists, and nursing staff. Focused pediatric cardiac intensive care units have been developed to optimize the patients' opportunity for recovery.

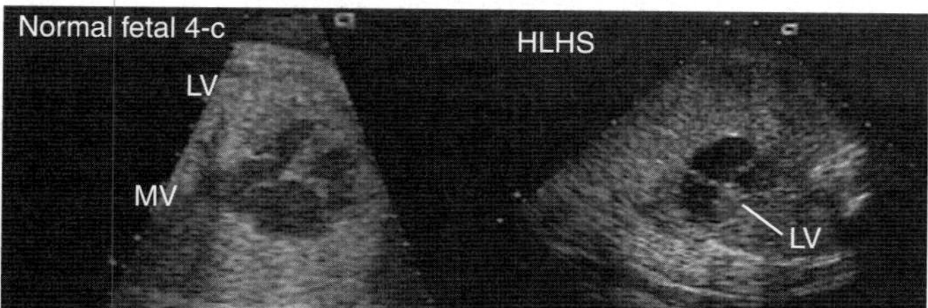

FIG. 59.1 Normal fetal ultrasound (four chamber; *left*) and fetal ultrasound of a child with hypoplastic left heart syndrome *HLHS; (right)*. *LV*, Left ventricle; *MV*, mitral valve.

Historically, pediatric cardiologists have provided the medical management of patients born with CHD. Pediatric cardiology is also evolving. With advances in catheter-based technology, interventional pediatric cardiologists are now addressing lesions previously treated with surgery. Examples include device closure of atrial septal defects (ASDs) and ventricular septal defects (VSDs), occlusion of patent ductus arteriosus (PDA), and dilation and stenting of stenotic vessels in the systemic and pulmonary circulation. For a more in-depth review of this specialty, see the excellent technical text by Mullins.[9]

The care for adults with CHD is in evolution. This issue is of particular relevance to the general surgeon faced with operating on an adult patient with significant CHD. One overriding message needs to be clear to the general surgeon in this setting: It must be assumed that in patients with previously repaired congenital cardiac lesions, even without overt cardiac symptoms, the potential for significant perioperative cardiorespiratory derangement exists. More simply stated, the presence of a surgical scar on the chest of a patient with known CHD does not suggest that the lesion has been cured. With this message firmly in mind, the general surgeon may find it challenging to determine the best source for a qualified consultation for such a patient. At the present time, many adult cardiologists are not adequately trained in CHD to provide competent consultation on adult patients with CHD.

Pediatric cardiologists are not educated in adult medicine and cardiology, and many feel uncomfortable providing consultation on adult patients with CHD. The subspecialty of adult CHD is currently becoming more formalized, but the number of physicians who have been educated specifically to care for these patients is still few. In 2015, the American Board of Internal Medicine offered the first certification examination in Adult Congenital Heart Disease. The Accreditation Council for Graduate Medical Education–accredited fellowship became available in 2019 with 21 accredited programs.[10,11] The practicing general surgeon needs to become familiar with the specific issues of concern for patients with CHD to ascertain that the patient's unique anatomic and physiologic issues have been evaluated properly. A pediatric cardiologist, in coordination with an adult cardiologist, must evaluate adult patients with CHD who present for care in a center without a designated qualified specialist. Of equal importance, the anesthesiologists and intensivists caring for an adult patient with CHD must have a working understanding of the complexities and nuances of the patient's cardiac condition. The anesthetic management of patients with CHD undergoing general surgical procedures is complicated and can become disastrous if managed improperly.

ANATOMY, TERMINOLOGY, AND DIAGNOSIS

Anatomy and Terminology

One of the most intimidating aspects for the student of CHD is developing a level of comfort with the terminology used for describing specific lesions. A thorough and sound understanding of normal cardiac anatomy is mandatory. There are several excellent texts on this subject; in particular, the text edited by Wilcox and coworkers[12] is especially concise and clear. One difficulty that challenges proper understanding of anatomy is the frequent use of abbreviations and eponyms for various congenital lesions—for example, congenitally corrected TGA (ccTGA), ventricular inversion, and L-transposition all describe the same heart, but none provides a complete anatomic description. Unless otherwise clear to all clinicians involved in the care of these complicated patients, the anatomic description needs to be segmental and complete to avoid mistakes and misinterpretations of structure.

In describing congenital cardiac lesions, a segmental approach is used to determine the relationship of the various structural elements. The situs describes the relationship of sidedness—situs solitus (normal), situs inversus (reversed), or situs ambiguus (indeterminate). The cardiac elements described include (in sequence) the atria, ventricles, and great vessels. The relationship of the connections must be understood; connections are concordant (e.g., the right atrium connecting to the right ventricle) or discordant (e.g., the right ventricle connecting to the aorta). The chamber sidedness must be clarified (e.g., a morphologic right atrium may be on the left side of the patient). The relationship and connections of the cardiac valves must then be assessed; connections may be normal, stenotic, atretic, or straddling. Of note to the general surgeon, abnormal sidedness of the cardiac structures is frequently associated with abnormal relationships of the thoracic and abdominal organs. A thorough assessment of the patient's anatomy is recommended before surgery. Commonly used tools in evaluation of anatomy include echocardiogram, computed tomography (CT), magnetic resonance imaging (MRI), and cardiac catheterization.

There are two widely accepted and applied schools of cardiac morphologic description. The Van Praagh nomenclature uses abbreviations to describe the relationship of the atria, ventricular looping, and position of the aorta sequentially. The first letter describes the situs of the atrial chambers (and usually the abdominal organs): "S" for situs solitus (normal), "I" for situs inversus (reversed), or "A" for situs ambiguus (indeterminate). The second letter describes the relationship of the embryologic looping of the ventricles: "D" for dextro looping or right-handed topology (normal), or "L" (levo) for left-handed topology. The third and last letter describes the relationship of the aortic valve to the pulmonary valve: "D" for right-sided and "L" for left-sided as well as "S" for solitus and "I" for inversus (Fig. 59.2).

The Anderson nomenclature is more wordy and longer but is perhaps simpler to understand. The descriptions are again of the sequential relationship of the structures. Starting with the atria, the connections and relationships are sequentially described. Thus, the atrial sidedness is described, followed by the sequence of connections to the ventricles and then great vessels. For example, "atrial situs solitus (normal) with atrioventricular discordance (reversed) and ventriculoarterial (A-V) discordance (reversed)" describes the heart mentioned earlier as corrected transposition, or S,L,L by the Van Praagh classification (Fig. 59.3).

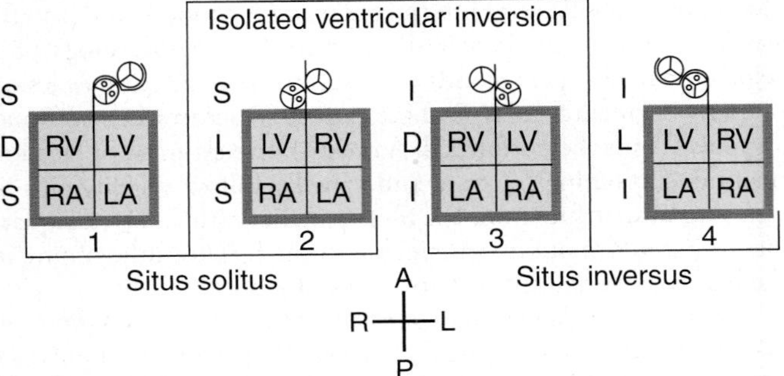

FIG. 59.2 Model depicting cardiac morphology for normal hearts—that is, hearts with atrioventricular concordance and ventriculoarterial concordance—using Van Praagh nomenclature. The *vertical line* above the box denotes the position of the ventricular septum. (From Kirklin JW, Barratt-Boyes BG. General considerations: Anatomy, dimensions, and terminology. In *Cardiac surgery*. 2nd ed. New York, 1993, Churchill Livingstone.)

Diagnosis

As with all aspects of surgery, a wide variety of highly sophisticated diagnostic tools are available to examine cardiac structure and function. Despite the widespread availability and application of these tools, none has replaced or eliminated the necessity of a thorough history and physical examination. Most patients who have a history of CHD become very well informed about the specifics of their cardiac conditions, as do their parents. A detailed review of the patient's past medical history is mandatory. This review includes, when possible, securing records from all previous diagnostic and procedural reports. An incorrect assumption often is made about a patient's previous surgical history and anatomy, frequently in a setting in which a patient's old operative report or clinical summary could easily clarify the misunderstanding.

In adults with CHD, in particular, there are specific points of medical history that must be elucidated. A history of palpitations, syncope, and neurologic deficit must be investigated further. The incidence of significant dysrhythmias in certain categories of adults with CHD is high and, in many cases, warrants further investigation, including continuous monitoring (Holter), electrophysiologic study, or provocative testing.

Physical Examination

A complete physical examination in a patient with previously repaired CHD often yields critical information for the proper planning of a general surgical procedure. Patients need to be completely undressed and thoroughly examined. In many cyanotic patients, color changes may be prominent, particularly in the nail beds, lips, and mucous membranes. Clubbing of fingers may be noted. In other patients, cyanosis may be more subtle, giving the patient a gray or even pale appearance. Previous surgical incisions need to be noted and reconciled with the known medical history. Thoracotomy incisions on either side may indicate a previous BT shunt using the turned-down, divided subclavian artery or with a prosthetic interposition graft—the so-called modified BT shunt.

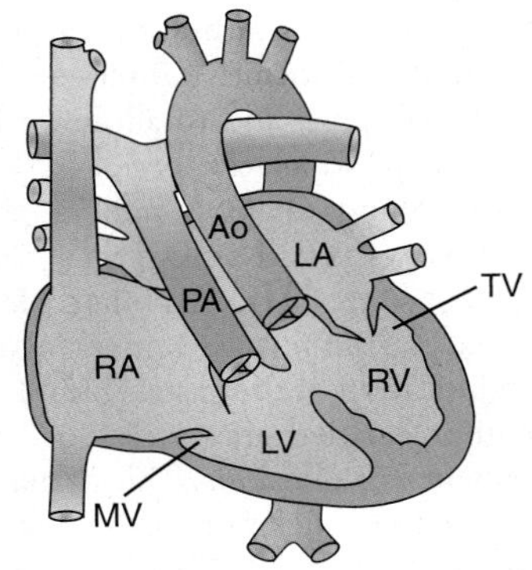

FIG. 59.3 Congenitally corrected transposition of the great arteries. Atrial situs solitus (normal) with atrioventricular discordance and ventriculoarterial discordance using Anderson nomenclature, S,L,L by Van Praagh classification. *Ao*, Aorta; *LA*, left atrium; *LV*, left ventricle; *MV*, mitral valve; *PA*, pulmonary artery; *RA*, right atrium; *RV*, right ventricle; *TV*, tricuspid valve.

In patients with a left aortic arch, a left thoracotomy incision is present if a previous coarctation repair has been carried out. Median sternotomy incisions or anterior thoracotomy incisions may indicate previous intracardiac or extracardiac surgery.

A complete vascular examination is often overlooked in patients with CHD. It is important to assess pulses and obtain blood pressure measurements in all four extremities. Patients who have an existing or have previously had a BT shunt often have diminished or absent pulses in the upper extremity corresponding to the previous shunt. Also, patients with previous coarctation repairs may have diminished or absent pulses in the left upper extremity, especially if a subclavian flap angioplasty was performed (Waldhausen procedure). Furthermore, a history of previous coarctation repair does not guarantee that the lower extremity pulses and blood pressures will be normal. Moreover, patients who have undergone previous cardiac catheterization may have chronically stenosed or occluded femoral vessels. All these issues may be of significance for monitoring and vascular access in a patient undergoing a general surgical procedure.

Later in this chapter, the Fontan procedure for single-ventricle palliation is reviewed. Briefly, this operation results in significant systemic venous hypertension, often measuring 12 to 15 mm Hg (normal 0 to 8 mm Hg). In patients with a Fontan circulation, physical examination may reveal hepatic congestion, ascites, pedal edema, venous varicosities, and jugular venous distention. In some patients, macronodular hepatic cirrhosis may be suspected on the basis of a firm, fibrotic liver edge on palpation.

Entire textbooks have been dedicated to the physical examination of patients with cardiac disease, and a thorough discussion of this issue, particularly the specifics of cardiac auscultation, is beyond the scope of this chapter. In general, the cardiac examination includes an assessment of the patient's rhythm, point of maximal impulse, and character of any auscultated murmurs. Importantly, the absence of a significant cardiac murmur does not rule out significant cardiac pathology.

Diagnostic Tests

Pulse oximetry. Four-extremity pulse oximetry is an essential part of the clinical assessment of a patient with suspected CHD. Patients with ductal-dependent circulation to the lower body (severe aortic coarctation or aortic arch interruption) may present with differential cyanosis. This presentation indicates the ejection of desaturated pulmonary arterial blood through the patent ductus to the descending aorta contrasted with fully saturated pulmonary venous blood ejected to the ascending aorta and the upper extremities. Baseline (room air) saturation must be documented in all patients for whom an operative intervention is anticipated to establish their normal range and to allow for identification of changes throughout the perioperative period.

Plain radiography. Standard chest radiography with anteroposterior and lateral views is still an essential component of the assessment of a patient with CHD. Standard elements to be examined include a skeletal survey, assessment of the diaphragms, hepatic shadow, and location of the gastric bubble. The lung fields are assessed for pulmonary plethora (arterial or venous), air space disease, and the presence of effusions. The cardiac silhouette may reveal essential information, such as a cardiothoracic ratio indicative of cardiomegaly or pericardial effusion, the presence of atrial enlargement, the presence or absence of the pulmonary artery shadow, and arch sidedness (Fig. 59.4).

Electrocardiography. The electrocardiogram (ECG) is important in assessing patients with CHD. The rate and rhythm must be noted, including the presence or absence of P wave activity and axis. Many patients with CHD, especially patients with complex conditions such as heterotaxy syndrome, may exhibit deranged or absent sinus node activity, giving rise to a predominant junctional rhythm, which may significantly compromise cardiac output. The QRS duration and axis reveal information concerning conduction delay and abnormal ventricular forces. For example, patients with A-V canal defects are known to have left axis deviation. Furthermore, in patients undergoing repair of certain forms of CHD, there may be an early or late predisposition to malignant dysrhythmias. It is particularly important to elucidate a history of palpitations from a patient with repaired or unrepaired CHD; such a history may warrant further investigation with 24-hour continuous ECG monitoring (Holter).

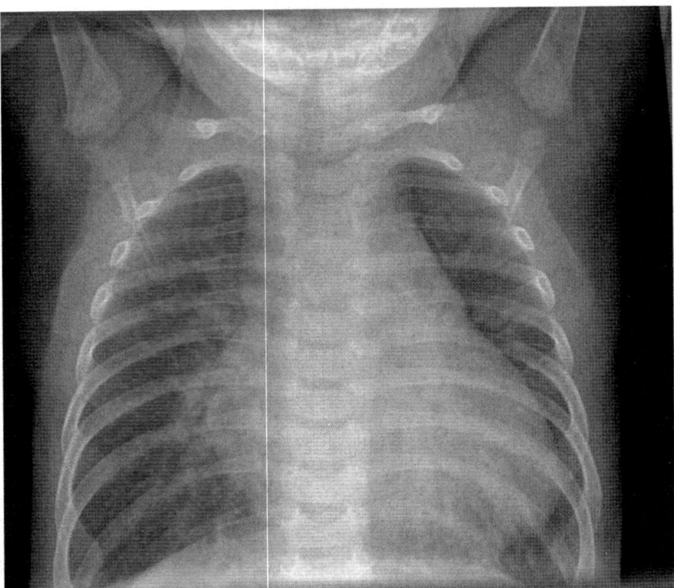

FIG. 59.4 Cardiomegaly and increased pulmonary vascular markings in a patient with complete atrioventricular canal defect.

Echocardiography. Noninvasive imaging is well established as the primary diagnostic modality for structural cardiac disease. For most patients, excellent anatomic detail may be obtained using two-dimensional transthoracic imaging. Standard images include subcostal, suprasternal, parasternal, and subxiphoid views and are oriented in long and short axis directions. Furthermore, significant hemodynamic information may be inferred using echo Doppler blood flow velocities and interpreted using the modified Bernoulli formula (pressure gradient = $4V^2$, where V is echocardiographic velocity in meters per second). To assess the patient's cardiac lesion properly, segmental analysis of the cardiac structures, connections, and valves must be performed. A quantitative estimate of ejection fraction, shortening fraction, and valvular inflow velocity aids in assessing cardiac function. For most patients with CHD, adequate diagnostic information is attainable through echocardiography in the hands of a qualified pediatric cardiologist.

Magnetic resonance imaging and computed tomography. Cardiac MRI and CT are adjuncts to echocardiography for noninvasive structural and functional assessment of the heart. MRI has been used with increasing frequency to provide anatomic detail in congenitally malformed hearts in which echocardiographic detail is lacking or unattainable. Cardiac MRI has proved particularly useful for imaging the extracardiac great vessels, systemic and pulmonary venous connections, and for providing accurate estimates of cardiac

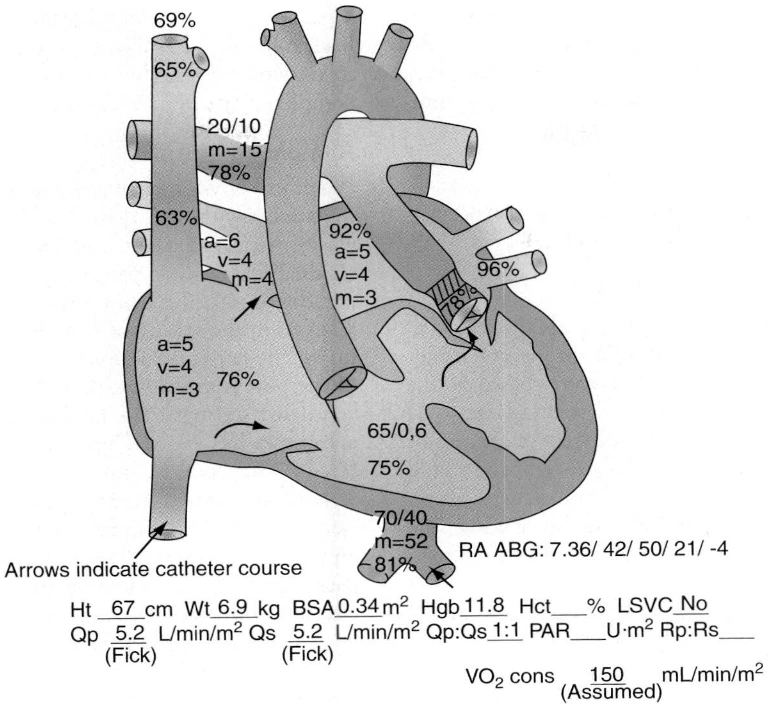

FIG. 59.5 Hemodynamic information obtained after cardiac catheterization.

function, especially right ventricular ejection fraction. MRI has the added benefit of using nonionizing electromagnetic fields. CT may also be used for such imaging detail but has the potential detrimental association with significant radiation exposure. A CT scan of the chest averages 5 to 7 mSv, and CT coronary angiography averages 9 to 11 mSv (chest x-ray: 0.1 mSv).[13]

Cardiac catheterization. Cardiac catheterization was long considered the gold standard for diagnostic imaging of congenitally malformed hearts. With the current sophistication of echocardiography, CT, and MRI, this is no longer the case for most patients. Nonetheless, there are still circumstances in which diagnostic cardiac catheterization is necessary to obtain accurate anatomic detail. One such circumstance may be patients who have poor echocardiographic windows, although even this issue may be overcome using transesophageal echocardiography. More often, there are specifics of anatomic detail that neither echocardiography nor MRI can delineate, such as branch pulmonary artery (or segmental) stenosis, origin and course of aortopulmonary collateral vessels, fistulous connections, and intracardiac communications (septal defects) not clarified by other imaging modalities.

Usually, diagnostic cardiac catheterization is performed to obtain precise hemodynamic information needed to make an informed assessment of the consequences of the patient's cardiac lesions. Using oximetric measurements, pressure data, and thermodilution cardiac output determination, accurate assessment of the patient's hemodynamic profile is obtained. Measured or derived data include central venous pressure, atrial pressure, ventricular pressures (including end-diastolic pressure), shunt fraction (in the case of ASDs or VSDs), pulmonary artery pressures, pulmonary capillary wedge pressure, systemic arterial pressure, and segmental oximetry of cardiac structures, including systemic and pulmonary venous return (Fig. 59.5). Thus, critical information is obtained about the presence and degree of shunting, systemic and pulmonary vascular resistance (PVR), and cardiopulmonary function. In certain clinical settings, these data are mandatory to a successful clinical management strategy. This may be particularly true for an adult patient with CHD requiring noncardiac surgery.

A thorough understanding of normal cardiorespiratory physiology is critical in interpreting data obtained by cardiac catheterization in a patient with CHD. Specifically, the normal pressure range, pulse waveforms, and oxygen saturations for the various cardiac chambers must be compared against data obtained in a deranged circulation. In the atria, there are characteristic waveforms— the *a* wave corresponding to atrial contraction, the *c* wave corresponding to A-V valve closure, and the *v* wave corresponding to atrial filling from venous return against the closed A-V valve. Typical normal right atrial mean pressures range from 1 to 5 mm Hg, and left atrial mean pressures range from 2 to 10 mm Hg. Right ventricular pressure tracings in normal hearts demonstrate a more gradual upstroke when compared with the left ventricle. Filling or end-diastolic pressures in both ventricles are between 2 and 10 mm Hg in normal hearts. The normal right ventricular systolic pressure (and thus pulmonary artery systolic pressure) is 15 to 30 mm Hg, and the left ventricular systolic pressure is 90 to 110 mm Hg.

In normal hearts, there is a small, physiologically insignificant right-to-left shunt, which results from ventilation-perfusion (VQ) mismatch in the lungs and coronary venous return directly to the left ventricle (thebesian venous return). This physiologic shunt represents less than 5% of the cardiac output and, in normal circumstances, does not produce detectable systemic arterial desaturation. Thus, significant systemic arterial desaturation represents a pathologic finding, consistent with pulmonary disease, intracardiac shunting, or both. As noted, the origin and degree of intracardiac shunting may be assessed by echocardiography. However, in certain circumstances, cardiac catheterization is necessary to measure cardiac oximetry, calculate shunt fraction, and derive systemic and PVR. Using a derivation of the Fick principle, the ratio of pulmonary blood flow (Qp) to systemic blood flow (Qs) can be determined as follows: where Sao_2 is systemic arterial oxygen saturation, $\bar{M}O_2$ sat is mixed venous oxygen saturation, $\bar{P}O_2$ sat is pulmonary venous oxygen saturation, and Pao_2 is pulmonary arterial oxygen saturation.

$$Qp/Qs = (Sa_{O2} - \bar{M}O_2 \text{ sat}) / (\bar{P}O_2 \text{ sat} - Pa_{O2})$$

Thus, in a patient with $\bar{M}O_2$ sat of 60%, $\bar{P}O_2$ sat of 100%, Sao_2 of 100%, and Pao_2 of 80%, the equation is as follows:

$$Qp/Qs = (100 - 60) / (100 - 80) = 40/20 = 2:1$$

Calculating pulmonary vascular resistances may also be crucial in determining operability in a patient with CHD. In many settings, a precise measure of vascular resistance is unnecessary based on the clinical evidence. For example, in a small child with a large VSD seen on echocardiogram, the clinical findings of tachypnea, cardiomegaly, and failure to thrive confirm a large left-to-right shunt and infer acceptable PVR. However, in less clear circumstances, a precise calculation may be important in clinical decision-making. The PVR may be calculated from cardiac catheterization data as follows:

$$PVR = \frac{(\text{Mean PA pressure [mm Hg]} - \text{Mean LA pressure [mm Hg]})}{\textit{Pulmonary Blood Flow } (Qp)\ [L/min/m^2]}$$

In general, patients with an elevated PVR are further evaluated with pulmonary vasodilation—hyperventilation, hyperoxygenation, and inhaled nitric oxide—to determine whether the PVR is responsive. This information may be critical for patients who are otherwise marginal candidates.

Finally, cardiac catheterization has been evolving as the primary therapeutic method for many important structural cardiac defects. In many children's hospitals, most catheterizations now performed are for interventional procedures rather than diagnostic procedures. This fact may be particularly pertinent to a general surgeon faced with treating a patient with a previous catheter-based correction of a cardiac defect. For example, the patient may have had an ASD or VSD closed with an occluder device in the past. This information may have important ramifications for infectious exposure and vascular access.

PERIOPERATIVE CARE

Perioperative management of a patient with unrepaired or palliated CHD can be extremely challenging. Standard hemodynamic, respiratory, and pharmacologic manipulations appropriate for structurally normal hearts may be entirely inappropriate in settings of complex CHD. This is especially true in the operating room and intensive care settings. General rules include a thorough knowledge of the patient's intracardiac anatomy and expected physiology. It is possible to make significant management errors based on incorrect physiologic expectations in the setting of incomplete understanding of the patient's anatomy. For example, in a patient with unrepaired tetralogy of Fallot (TOF) and associated significant right ventricular outflow tract obstruction (RVOTO), it is expected that the patient will exhibit some degree of systemic arterial desaturation. However, a patient with repaired TOF with no residual intracardiac shunts is expected to be fully saturated, and a finding of desaturation likely represents a complication that warrants expedient investigation. This clinical scenario is a frequent one; a patient with a specific cardiac diagnosis, despite having undergone a successful correction, continues to be incorrectly presumed to have ongoing physiologic perturbation. Further, it is important to understand whether previous cardiac intervention resulted in complete correction of the lesion or only palliation.

Anesthesia Pitfalls

Providing physiologic anesthetic management can be challenging in patients with CHD, especially in situations such as chronic single-ventricle palliation, unrepaired CHD, chronic cyanosis, and residual intracardiac pathology. Standard anesthetic management paradigms may be completely inappropriate and potentially disastrous in the setting of complex CHD. A thorough understanding of the patient's anatomy is mandatory, along with knowledge of the potential for unexpected response to anesthetic agents and ventilator settings. The field of pediatric and congenital cardiac anesthesia has evolved relative to this specific clinical need; the text by Andropoulos and colleagues[14] is an excellent resource.

Several points concerning anesthesia management warrant discussion. The first is vascular access for intraoperative and postoperative management. In patients with complex CHD, especially patients who have undergone previous complex surgical and catheterization procedures, obtaining appropriate vascular access may be challenging. Typically, a large-bore, multilumen central venous line is necessary for appropriate resuscitation and monitoring of right-sided filling pressures. In some patients, the placement of a thermodilution pulmonary artery catheter (oximetric) must be considered because one cannot presume that right-sided filling pressures correlate well with left heart volume or functional status (e.g., after a Fontan operation). Options for central access mirror those of non-CHD patients and include percutaneous internal jugular or subclavian routes with a secondary option of common femoral access to the inferior vena cava (IVC). However, access may be difficult in the setting of previous catheterization or venous reconstruction; this situation may be addressed with the aid of ultrasound-guided catheter placement, which has become a standard in many cardiac operating rooms. Arterial access for continuous blood pressure monitoring and sampling is important for many patients. Percutaneous radial arterial cannulation can be readily achieved in most patients; however, upper extremity blood pressure values may be factitiously altered by previous systemic-to-pulmonary artery shunts, previous aortic arch surgery (especially coarctation), and abnormalities of vascular origin (e.g., aberrant subclavian origin from the descending aorta).

Ventilator management in the perioperative setting of CHD requires special understanding. In settings of large potential left-to-right shunts (e.g., unrepaired VSDs), hyperventilation and hyperoxygenation promote excessive pulmonary blood flow and potentially diminish systemic cardiac output. Positive pressure ventilation, particularly positive end-expiratory pressure, negatively influences hemodynamics in many patients, especially in palliated patients with a single ventricle and passive cavopulmonary flow after the Fontan procedure. Early extubation in these patients can be done to limit the deleterious effects of positive end-expiratory pressure on the Fontan circulation. Data has shown that early extubation is feasible, safe, improves outcomes, and reduces overall hospital costs for these patients.[15] Finally, pharmacologic manipulation of systemic and PVR and cardiac performance are important adjuncts in the perioperative management of patients with CHD. In general, a low-dose infusion of epinephrine 0.05 mcg/kg/min (0.02–0.05 mcg/kg/min) with the addition of a phosphodiesterase inhibitor is an effective pharmacologic cocktail to promote a cardiac inotropic state, lower systemic and PVR, and limit tachycardia. Dopamine, vasopressin, sodium nitroprusside, and nitroglycerin are other frequently used agents. Appropriate perioperative analgesia and sedation are also important aspects of the patient's management.

Neurologic Outcomes

With expectations of almost 100% survival after surgery for CHD, emphasis has been placed on the long-term neurologic outcomes and quality of life of these patients. The potential for neurologic insult in children after CHD arises from the nature of their disease (e.g., cyanotic defects, low cardiac output state, genetic syndromes, effects of cardiopulmonary bypass, circulatory arrest). Evidence also suggests that patients with CHD may be genetically predisposed to neurologic insult. Gestational age has been found to be an important factor to consider in the optimization of neurologic outcomes.[16]

LESION OVERVIEW

Defects Associated With Increased Pulmonary Blood Flow

Persistent Arterial Duct (Patent Ductus Arteriosus)

A persistent arterial duct, or PDA, is a frequently encountered congenital cardiac condition. PDA is found in 1 in 2000 term neonates but has significantly increased incidence in preterm neonates with incidence of 40% in infants with birth weights less than 2000 g and 80% for less than 1200 g. The arterial duct is necessary during gestation to shunt right ventricular blood away from the unventilated pulmonary vasculature; ductal flow is from the pulmonary artery to the aorta during gestation. At delivery, after the first breath of the neonate, ductal flow reverses and becomes left to right in most individuals. Over the first several hours to days of postnatal life, the PDA closes spontaneously and is completely closed in most infants by 2 to 3 weeks of age.

In the absence of other congenital cardiac lesions, a PDA becomes pathologic related to its presence and the degree of left-to-right shunting. A PDA may be present in association with other structural cardiac conditions and may sometimes be necessary for systemic or pulmonary blood flow. The amount of shunting produced relates to the size and geometry of the duct and the PVR. A PDA may be responsible for a large Qp/Qs ratio and result in pulmonary overcirculation, left heart volume overload, and congestive heart failure (CHF). A large unrestricted PDA is associated with pulmonary hypertension; if left untreated, this proceeds to irreversible pulmonary vascular disease (Eisenmenger syndrome), which ultimately proceeds to pulmonary and right heart failure, treatable only by pulmonary transplantation. Even with a small, pressure-restrictive PDA, there is an ongoing risk for pulmonary congestion and left heart volume overloading; endocarditis is always of concern even for small PDAs. Closure is recommended for all PDAs.

The gold standard of therapy for closure of PDA is surgery, usually accomplished through a left posterolateral thoracotomy using ductal division, ligation, or clipping (Fig. 59.6). Surgery needs to be a low-risk procedure associated with minimal potential for persistence of the PDA. Nonetheless, the invasive nature of this proven method has led to the development of alternative strategies for ductal occlusion. From a surgical perspective, many PDAs are amenable to thoracoscopic clipping through very small port incisions; robot-assisted PDA occlusion has been performed in many patients with good results.[12] Medical treatment with indomethacin (0.1 mg/kg for <1 kg, 0.2 mg/kg ≥ 1 kg on day 1, then 0.1 mg/kg daily for days 2–7 oral or IV over 1 hour) can be attempted in a neonate but carries risk of necrotizing enterocolitis, intracranial hemorrhage, and renal toxicity. However, at the present time, most PDAs are occluded in the cardiac catheterization laboratory using occlusive devices. Even the repair of large defects

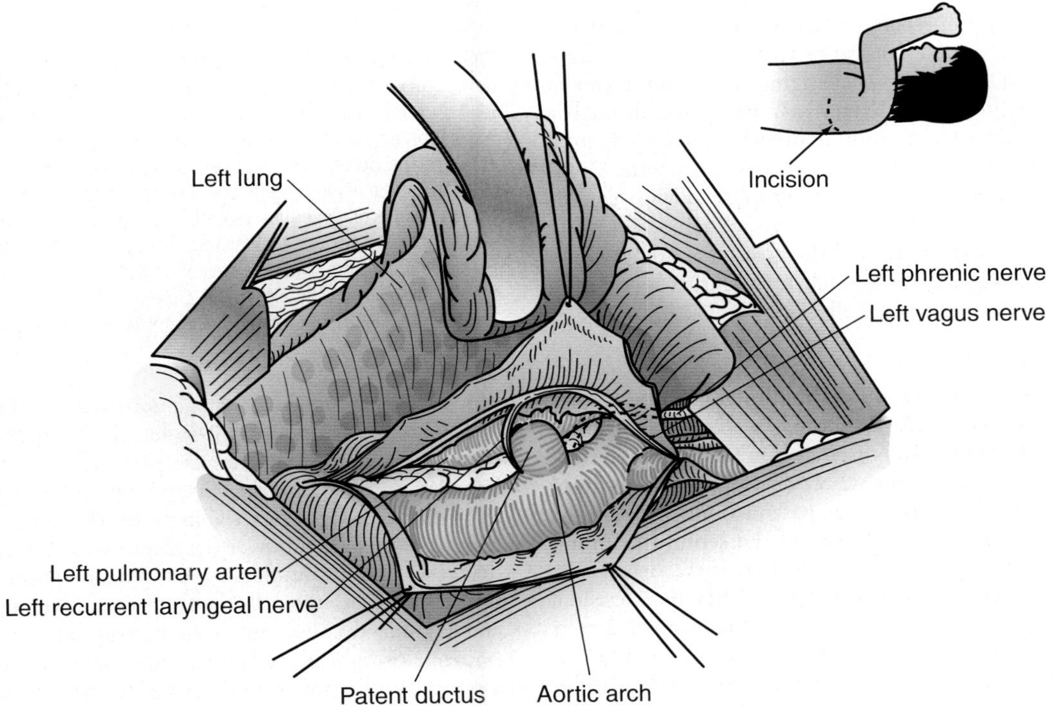

FIG. 59.6 Anatomic relationships of a patent ductus arteriosus exposed from a left thoracotomy. (From Castaneda AR, Jones RA, Mayer JE, Jr, et al. Patent ductus arteriosus. In: *Cardiac surgery of the neonate and infant.* Philadelphia, PA: Saunders;1994.)

in small infants has been successfully addressed. The long-term effects of the devices remaining in the vascular tree are not fully understood yet; however, successful device closure appears to be an extremely effective, safe, and durable therapy. Recently, catheter-based devices have been approved for PDA occlusion on preterm infants as small as 700 g.

A PDA in an adult patient can be challenging. As noted, a long-standing large PDA may be associated with pulmonary vascular disease. A right-to-left shunt in a PDA is cause for significant concern and warrants further investigation with concern for significantly elevated PVR. In adults with PDAs, the arterial wall may calcify, making an attempt at ligation or division hazardous. In these patients, ductal occlusion may require resection of the adjacent descending aorta with patch grafting or short-segment graft replacement (e.g., Dacron).

Aortopulmonary Septal Defect (Aortopulmonary Window)

An aortopulmonary septal defect is a communication between the ascending aorta and, usually, the main pulmonary artery. This is a rare defect comprising 0.1% to 0.6% of CHD. This lesion results from the failure of complete separation of the embryologic common arterial trunk into the aorta and pulmonary artery. Defects are classified by their location: Type I is proximal, just above the aortic sinuses; type II is more distal on the ascending aorta and often involves the origin of the right pulmonary artery; and type III is more distal and associated with a separate origin of the right pulmonary artery from the aorta (Fig. 59.7). An aortopulmonary septal defect may occur in isolation or in association with other conditions, including interrupted aortic arch (IAA) and anomalous origin of a coronary artery. Defects are typically large and responsible for a large left-to-right shunt with systemic pulmonary artery pressures. Children with this defect typically present with CHF, failure to thrive, and frequent respiratory infections. Echocardiography, MRI, or cardiac catheterization may be used to make the diagnosis.

The gold standard for repair of aortopulmonary septal defects is surgical closure. Case reports of transcatheter closure exist; however, this is a technically challenging feat without known long-term durability.[17] A small defect may be ligated through a thoracotomy or median sternotomy approach, but this method is not recommended because of significant risk for rupture or incomplete closure. Surgical closure is accomplished with cardiopulmonary bypass support. Options for closure include complete division and separate patch repairs of the great vessel defects or a sandwich type of closure, using a patch to construct a common intervening wall; both methods are effective (Fig. 59.8).

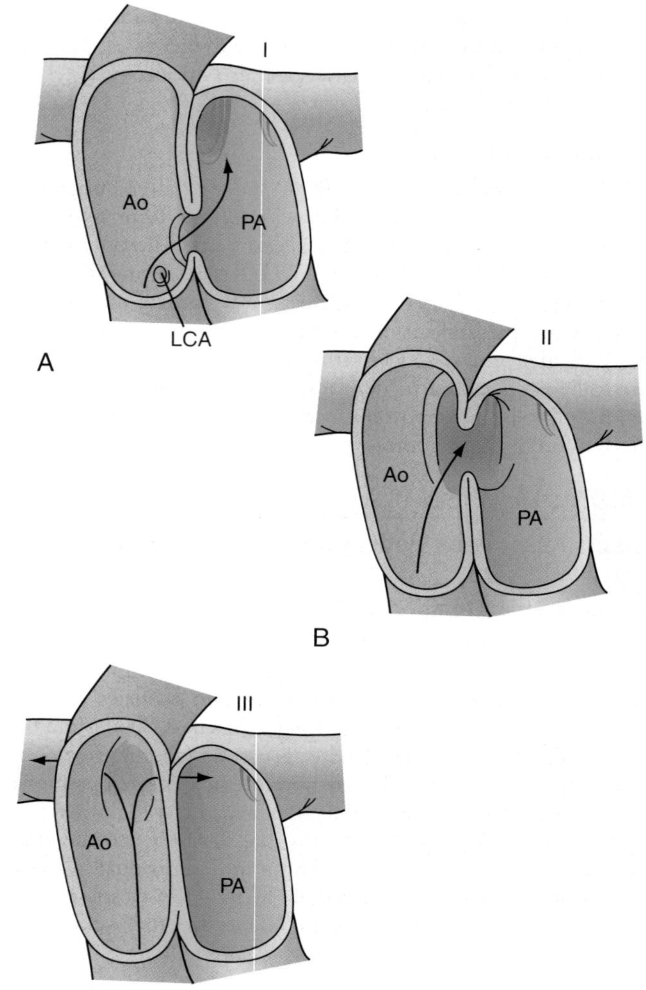

FIG. 59.7 Native anatomy and classification of aortopulmonary septal defect. (A) In type I, the communication is between the ascending aorta *(Ao)* and the main pulmonary artery *(PA)* on the posterior medial wall of the ascending aorta. The left main coronary artery *(LCA)* orifice may be close to the defect. (B) In type II, the defect is more cephalic on the ascending aorta. (C) In type III, the defect is more posterior and lateral in the aorta. The communication is with the right pulmonary artery, which may be completely separate from the main pulmonary artery. (Adapted from Fraser CD. Aortopulmonary septal defects and patent ductus arteriosus. In: Nichols DG, Ungerleider RM, Spevak PJ, et al, eds. *Critical heart disease in infants and children.* Philadelphia, PA: Mosby; 2006:664–666.)

Atrial Septal Defect

An isolated ASD is one of the most common congenital cardiac lesions occurring in 13 of every 10,000 live births. The most frequently encountered ASD relates to a defect in the interatrial wall, as defined by the fossa ovalis. The defect develops as the result of incomplete closure of the embryologic patent foramen ovale; the defect is a result of incomplete closure of the septum primum. Although the terminology can be confusing, these defects are typically termed *secundum atrial septal defects.* They manifest in a wide variety of configurations, ranging from single small defects to multiple fenestrations to complete absence of the septum primum. The confines of the defect may extend from the IVC orifice up to the superior atrial wall adjacent to the aortic root (Fig. 59.9).

The primary pathophysiologic derangement in ASDs relates to a significant left-to-right shunt in the setting of normal PVR. However, even in the setting of a normal PVR, patients with ASDs are capable of transient right-to-left shunting, particularly during times of increased intrathoracic pressure. The effects of chronic, large left-to-right shunting (in some patients producing a Qp/Qs >3:1) include right heart volume overloading and enlargement. Most children are not overtly symptomatic but may exhibit some degree of exercise intolerance or frequent respiratory tract infection. Symptoms typically become more prevalent in adulthood and include dyspnea on exertion, palpitations, and, ultimately, evidence of right heart failure. Pulmonary vascular disease is not a typical finding in secundum ASDs, but one may demonstrate an ASD in a patient with primary pulmonary hypertension. A rare form of presentation relates to the potential of right-to-left shunting at the atrial level; the ever-present risk for paradoxical

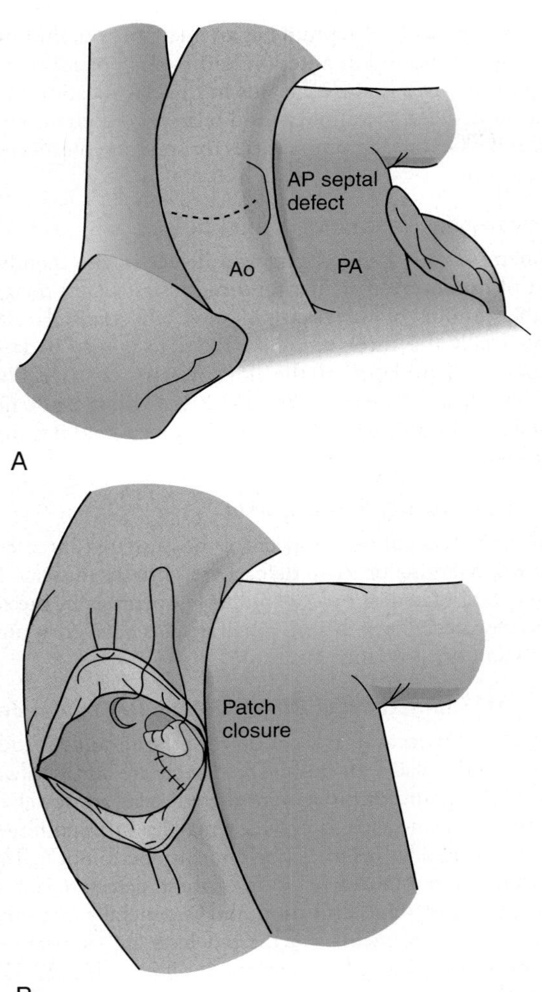

FIG. 59.8 (A) Surgical exposure of aortopulmonary *(AP)* septal defect includes a transverse incision in the ascending aorta *(Ao)*. (B) The aortopulmonary septal defect is closed by suturing a patch over the aortic side of the defect. (Adapted from Fraser CD. Aortopulmonary septal defects and patent ductus arteriosus. In: Nichols DG, Ungerleider RM, Spevak PJ, et al, eds. *Critical heart disease in infants and children.* Philadelphia, PA: Mosby; 2006:664–666.) *PA,* Pulmonary artery.

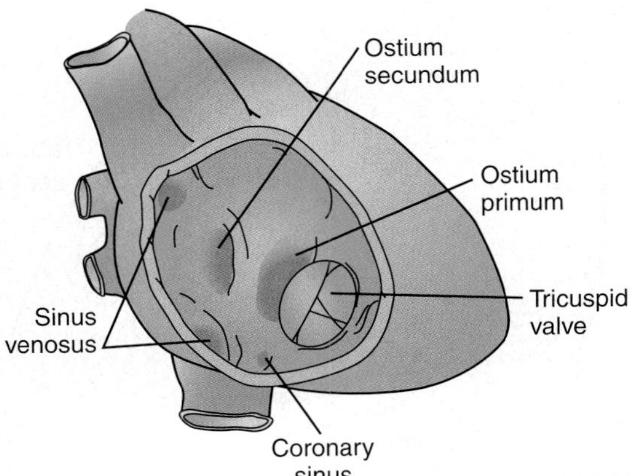

FIG. 59.9 Types of atrial septal defects as viewed through the right atrium, ostium secundum, ostium primum, and sinus venosus. (Adapted from Redmond JM, Lodge AJ. Atrial septal defects and ventricular septal defects. In Nichols DG, Ungerleider RM, Spevak PJ, et al, eds. *Critical heart disease in infants and children.* Philadelphia, PA: Mosby; 2006:580.)

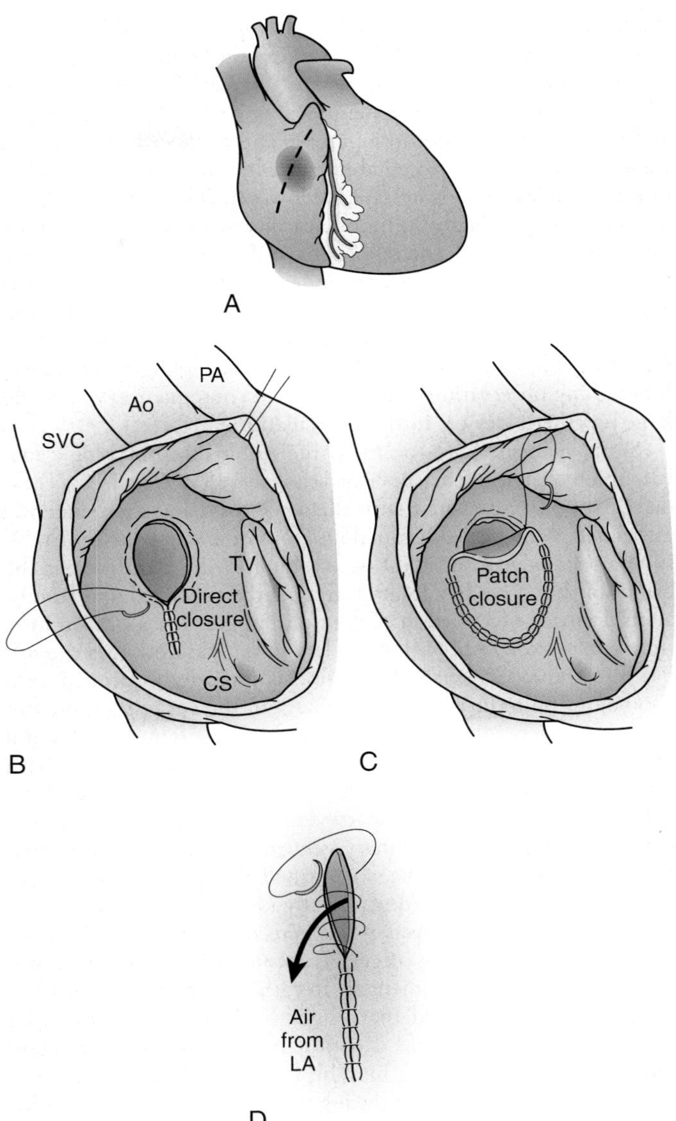

FIG. 59.10 Surgical closure for atrial septal defect. (A) Right atriotomy. (B) Direct suture closure. (C) Patch closure. (D) Deairing the left atrium *(LA)*. (Adapted from Redmond JM, Lodge AJ. Atrial septal defects and ventricular septal defects. In: Nichols DG, Ungerleider RM, Spevak PJ, et al, eds. *Critical heart disease in infants and children.* Philadelphia, PA: Mosby; 2006:583.) *Ao,* Aorta; *CS,* coronary sinus; *PA,* pulmonary artery; SVC, superior vena cava; *TV,* tricuspid valve.

embolus and cerebrovascular accident must be considered when recommending ASD closure.

Most centers recommend ASD closure in patients before school age. Since the late 1950s, the standard therapy for ASDs has been surgical closure using cardiopulmonary bypass support. The defect is closed using direct suture closure, autologous pericardium, or prosthetic patch material (Fig. 59.10). This is an effective method with a low associated perioperative risk including the virtual absence of residual or recurrent defects.[18] Minimally invasive techniques for ASD closure have also gained popularity with good safety profiles and outcomes.[19]

The potential for closing defects using nonsurgical methods has led to the development of catheter-based therapies, which are now being widely applied to large numbers of patients worldwide for the treatment of ASD. Currently upwards of 60% of ASD interventions are catheter based.[20] The most commonly used device is the Amplatzer septal occluder device (St. Jude Medical, St. Paul, MN), made of nitinol metal mesh, which is placed percutaneously and delivered with echocardiographic and fluoroscopic guidance. Reports indicated an acceptable procedure-related complication rate and successful closure rate.[21] However, the long-term effects of having such a device in mobile cardiac structures are not fully understood. More recent reports have documented an alarming incidence of device erosion through the atrial wall and into the adjacent ascending aorta as well as disruption of the conduction system.[22,23] A case report showing severe endocarditis involving a previously placed Amplatzer ASD device has highlighted the need for ongoing observation of the long-term consequences of placing large prosthetic devices into the circulation.[24]

Sinus venosus ASDs occur as the result of embryologic malalignment between the superior vena cava (SVC) or IVC. These defects are not associated with the ovale fossa and are frequently associated with partial anomalous pulmonary venous return. A superior sinus venosus ASD occurs high in the atrium, near the orifice of the SVC. This lesion is frequently associated with anomalous drainage of a portion of the right lung to the SVC. An inferior sinus venosus ASD is located low in the atrium, often extending into the IVC orifice. This lesion is typically associated with anomalous pulmonary venous drainage of the entire right lung to the IVC (potentially intrahepatic); pulmonary sequestration and an abnormal systemic artery perfusing the right lower lobe, with origin from the abdominal aorta, may also be present. In patients with total anomalous pulmonary venous return (TAPVR) to the IVC, the anomalous pulmonary vein may be obvious on a plain chest radiograph and has been described as appearing like a saber (scimitar syndrome), first described by Neill and colleagues.[25]

Surgery for sinus venosus ASDs is recommended for the same pathophysiologic reasons surgery is recommended for secundum ASDs. The repair is not amenable to catheter techniques, and surgery is more complicated than for an isolated secundum ASD. Superior sinus venosus defects with partial anomalous pulmonary venous return to the SVC may be treated with an intracardiac patch baffle; however, in the setting of high drainage of the anomalous pulmonary veins, an SVC translocation operation (Warden procedure) may be necessary. Surgery for an inferior sinus venosus ASD with a scimitar vein can be more complicated, potentially involving the need for a patch baffle within the intrahepatic IVC, which may require periods of hypothermic circulatory arrest.

Ventricular Septal Defect

A VSD is a pathologic communication involving a defect in the interventricular septum. Isolated VSD is present in 0.3% of newborns. Defects are classified in terms of their location and surrounding structures. Patients may be entirely asymptomatic, depending on the size and location of the VSD, along with associated lesions and PVR. In the setting of otherwise normal cardiac morphology and appropriate PVR, the net shunt in patients with VSD is left to right; the Qp/Qs depends on the size of the defect and pulmonary resistance. Large defects result in large shunts, high right ventricular and pulmonary artery pressures, significant pulmonary overcirculation, CHF, and left heart volume overload. In these settings, unrestrictive pulmonary blood flow exposes the patient to the risk for pulmonary vascular disease and Eisenmenger syndrome.

The ventricular septum can be best thought of in terms of the pathway of blood and associated cardiac anatomy. Thus, the right ventricular aspect of the septum has an inlet portion; midmuscular portion; apical, posterior, anterior, and outlet portions; and subaortic portion. This knowledge aids in the classification of VSDs. Furthermore, defects are understood relative to their embryologic origins and have varying propensities for spontaneous decreases in size or closure.

Perimembranous Ventricular Septal Defect

A perimembranous VSD occurs as a defect in the membranous portion of the interventricular septum; its associated margins include the annulus of the tricuspid valve, the muscular septum, and potentially the aortic annulus. The defects may be large and have associated prolapse of the noncoronary or right coronary aortic valve cusps. Perimembranous VSDs exhibit a potential for spontaneous closure, particularly small defects manifesting early in childhood.

Muscular Ventricular Septal Defect

Muscular VSDs occur in all aspects of the muscular interventricular septum. Margins of these defects are entirely muscle. The lesions may be isolated or involve multiple openings in the septum (so-called Swiss cheese septum). Small defects have great potential for regression or spontaneous closure.

Subarterial (Supracristal or Outlet) Ventricular Septal Defect

Subarterial VSDs occur in association with the annulus of the aortic valve, pulmonary valve, or both. The defects are almost always associated with significant prolapse of the adjacent aortic valve cusp, usually the right coronary cusp, which may lead to significant cusp distortion, aortic valve insufficiency, and cusp perforation. The only mechanism for spontaneous closure of these defects relates to the cusp prolapse and valve distortion and is generally not complete or a favorable arrangement. All these defects are surgically closed because of the ongoing risk for aortic valve injury (Fig. 59.11).

The indications for surgery to close VSDs relate to the size of the VSD, degree of shunting, and associated lesions. Small infants presenting with large VSDs, refractory heart failure, and large shunts undergo surgical closure of the defects in the newborn

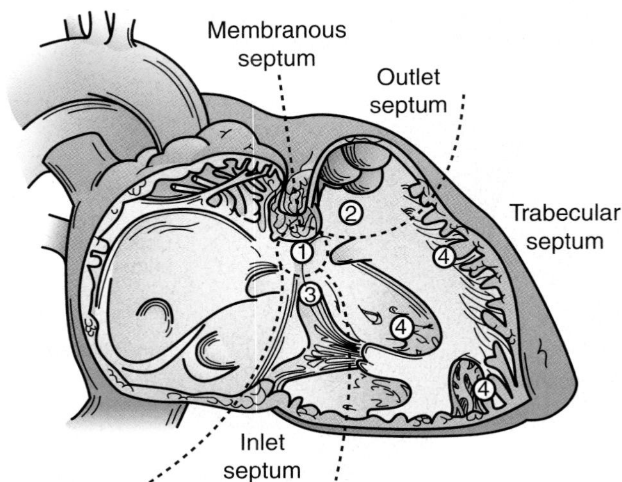

FIG. 59.11 Location of ventricular septal defects (VSDs) in the ventricular septum (view of the ventricular septum from the right side). (From Tchervenkov CI, Shum-Tim D. Ventricular septal defect. In: Baue AE, Geha AS, Hammond GL, eds. Glenn's thoracic and cardiovascular surgery, 6th ed. Stamford, CT: Appleton & Lange; 1996.) *1*, Perimembranous VSD; *2*, subarterial VSD; *3*, atrioventricular canal–type VSD; *4*, muscular VSD.

period, regardless of age or size. Other defects are addressed based on the ongoing concerns of left-to-right shunting, aortic valve cusp distortion, and risk for endocarditis. Asymptomatic patients with evidence of significant shunts and cardiomegaly are proposed for surgical therapy. Prophylactic closure of small defects in asymptomatic patients with normal cardiac size and function is advocated by some surgeons because of the lifelong risk for endocarditis and comparatively low risk for surgery.

Percutaneous VSD closure is an acceptable alternative to surgical closure of VSDs with very high procedural success.[26] The complex relationship of many defects, including close association with the aortic valve and cardiac conduction tissue, makes the existing technology less than ideal. At the present time, surgery remains the primary mode of therapy for VSD closure. Defects are approached with the aid of cardiopulmonary bypass support and may be closed with various materials, including autologous pericardium (our preference), Dacron, polytetrafluoroethylene, and homograft material. Surgical closure of VSDs is a low-risk procedure with a high expectation of complete closure. Challenging anatomic situations, such as Swiss cheese septum or multiple apical muscular VSDs, may be initially palliated by limiting pulmonary blood flow with a pulmonary artery band and deferring corrective surgery to later in life.

Atrioventricular Septal Defect (Atrioventricular Canal Defect)

Atrioventricular septal defects (AVSDs) are a complex constellation of cardiac lesions involving deficiency of the atrial septum, ventricular septum, and A-V valves and occur in approximately 1 in every 2100 live births. This lesion results from an embryologic maldevelopment involving the endocardial cushions; thus, the term *endocardial cushion defect* is often applied. AVSDs may be partial, involving no ventricular level component; intermediate or transitional, involving a small restrictive VSD; or complete, involving a large nonrestrictive VSD. The A-V valve tissue is always abnormal in AVSD, although there is great individual variability in terms of the severity of the valvular malformation and valve function. Complete AVSDs are frequently seen in patients with trisomy 21 but also occur in patients with normal chromosomes. The morphology of the septal defects in this condition is different from that previously discussed. The ASD in this defect is termed a *primum ASD* and is distinctly separate from the ovale fossa. There is displacement of the A-V node and bundle of His to the inferior aspect of the primum defect and A-V junction, a feature of critical importance during surgical repair. Patients with AVSD have an *inlet VSD*, which may extend into the subaortic region and have a component of septal malalignment. The chordal support of the A-V valves has a variable relationship to the interventricular septum. The relationship of the chordal support and superior bridging component of the left A-V valve has been used to classify complete AVSD, as described by Rastelli and associates:[27] type A, with superior leaflet and chordal support committed to the left side of the ventricular septum; type B, with straddling and shared chordal support; and type C, with a floating left superior leaflet component and chordal support on the right side of the ventricular septum (Fig. 59.12).

Patients with complete AVSD typically present in infancy with large left-to-right shunts, cardiomegaly, and CHF. Without surgical treatment, patients exhibit severe failure to thrive, a susceptibility to severe respiratory infections, and potential for early development of pulmonary vascular disease. Surgical repair is recommended in infancy (usually before 6 months of age) but may be necessary in the newborn period for neonates with refractory heart failure, especially in association with aortic arch anomalies. Patients with partial or intermediate defects may have the surgery deferred until later in childhood, depending on the degree of atrial level shunting and the presence of A-V valve regurgitation. AVSD may also manifest in unbalanced forms with dominance of right-sided or left-sided components. In severely affected individuals, biventricular repair is not feasible, and patients are managed along a single-ventricle pathway. AVSD may also be found in association with TOF; this combination is associated with cyanosis, and repair is more challenging than for either condition considered in isolation.

Surgery is the primary mode of therapy for patients with AVSD. Operative goals include complete closure of ASDs and VSDs and effective use of available A-V valve tissue to achieve valve competence. As noted, the inferiorly displaced conduction tissue must be protected to avoid the complication of surgically induced A-V block (Fig. 59.13). Surgical intervention is performed with the use of the cardiopulmonary bypass machine. The atrial and ventricular septal components are closed with a common patch (single-patch method) or separate patches (two-patch technique). We believe the two-patch method to be superior in preserving A-V valve tissue (Fig. 59.14).[28] The critical component of the repair lies in the valve repair; typically, after suspending the valve tissue to the reconstructed septum, the line of coaptation between the superior and inferior leaflet components (cleft) is closed; however, care must be exercised to avoid valvular stenosis.

Perioperative care is predicated on an accurate and hemodynamically favorable repair. Patients with long-standing pulmonary overcirculation may have a potential for early perioperative pulmonary hypertensive crisis. This condition may require therapy,

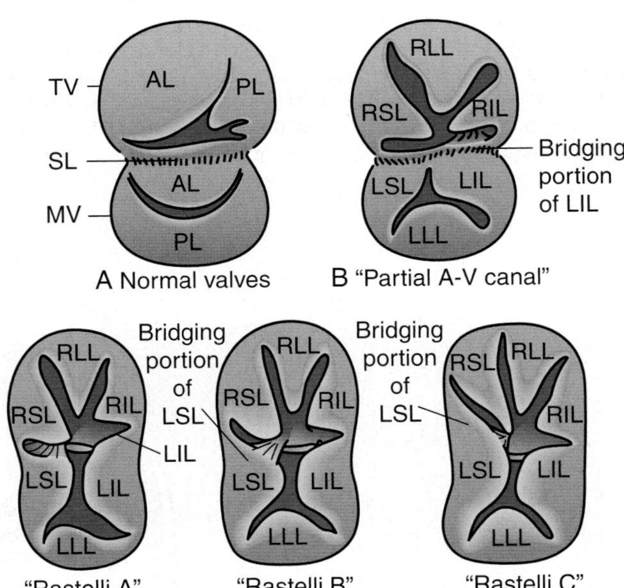

FIG. 59.12 Rastelli classification type A, B, or C. The difference in valve morphology in a normal (A), partial (B), and complete (C) canal defect is illustrated. (From Kirklin JW, Pacifico AD, Kirklin JK. The surgical treatment of atrioventricular canal defects. In: Arciniegas E, ed. *Pediatric cardiac surgery*. Chicago, IL: Year Book Medical Publishers: 1985.) *AL*, Anterior leaflet; *A-V*, atrioventricular; *LIL*, left inferior leaflet; *LLL*, left lateral leaflet; *LSL*, left superior leaflet; *MV*, mitral valve; *PL*, posterior leaflet; *RIL*, right inferior leaflet; *RLL*, right lateral leaflet; *RSL*, right superior leaflet; SL, superior leaflet; *TV*, tricuspid valve.

including oxygen, optimization of fluid balance, continuous sedation, hyperventilation, and, possibly, inhaled nitric oxide.

Adult Patients With Atrioventricular Septal Defect

Numerous patients with partial or transitional AVSD survive well into adulthood without surgery. These patients have variable presentations but may exhibit severe exercise intolerance; evidence of right heart dysfunction; some elevation of PVR; and, possibly, atrial dysrhythmias, including atrial fibrillation. In patients with late presentation of AVSD, cardiac catheterization is often recommended to rule out occult coronary artery lesions and to evaluate PVR. Nonetheless, in the absence of obvious surgical contraindication, surgery is recommended for adults with unrepaired AVSD to eliminate the chronic left-to-right shunt and repair the typically insufficient A-V valves.

Other patients present well into adulthood with previously repaired AVSDs. These patients may have a widely disparate constellation of findings, including atrial and ventricular dysrhythmias, valvular insufficiency or stenosis, and right heart dysfunction. In many of them, secondary reparative surgery may become necessary. Furthermore, in the setting of a patient with remotely repaired AVSD requiring noncardiac surgery, potential ongoing hemodynamic concerns that would affect the perioperative course must be expected.

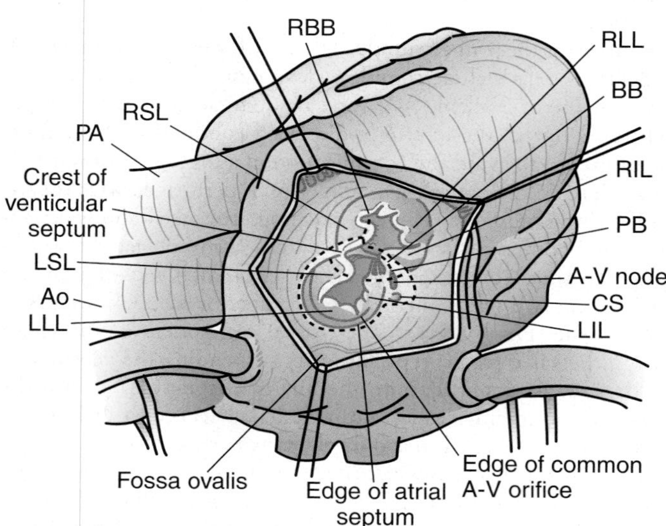

FIG. 59.13 Position of the conducting system in complete atrioventricular canal defect. The anatomic relationships and morphology of the common atrioventricular *(A-V)* valve are shown. The view is through a right atriotomy. (From Bharati S, Lev M, Kirklin JW. *Cardiac surgery and the conducting system.* New York, NY: Churchill Livingstone: 1983.) *Ao,* Aorta; *BB,* left bundle branch; *CS,* coronary sinus; *LIL,* left inferior leaflet; *LLL,* left lateral leaflet; *LSL,* left superior leaflet; *PA,* pulmonary artery; *PB,* penetrating bundle; *RBB,* right bundle branch; *RIL,* right inferior leaflet; *RLL,* right lateral leaflet; *RSL,* right superior leaflet.

Persistent Arterial Trunk (Truncus Arteriosus)

Truncus arteriosus or persistent arterial trunk results from failure of separation of the embryonic arterial trunk and semilunar valves and occurs in approximately 1 in 10,000 live births. It is almost always associated with a large nonrestrictive perimembranous VSD, and is associated with varying degrees of truncal override of the interventricular septum, including 100% association of the trunk with the right ventricle. The condition is classified by the relationship of the origins of the pulmonary arteries. In type I truncus arteriosus, there is a demonstrable common main pulmonary artery with subsequent origins of the branch pulmonary arteries; in type II truncus arteriosus, the branch pulmonary arteries arise closely, but separately, from the trunk; in type III truncus arteriosus, the branch pulmonary arteries are widely separated in origin on the ascending aorta; and in type IV truncus arteriosus, no pulmonary arterial branch arises from the common trunk. Type IV truncus arteriosus is now recognized as a form of pulmonary atresia with VSD (Fig. 59.15).

In contrast to patients with aortopulmonary septal defects, patients with truncus arteriosus have a single outlet valve of highly variable morphology. The valve may have a normal appearance, with three well-formed and distinct cusps similar to those of a

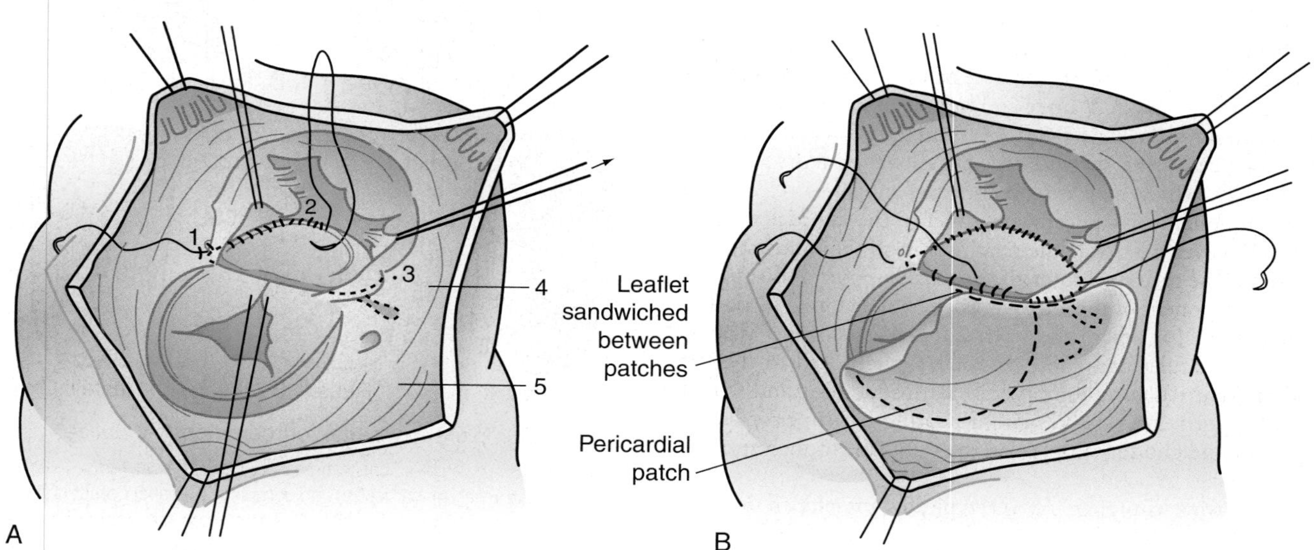

FIG. 59.14 Two-patch closure of complete atrioventricular canal defect. (A) A ventricular septal patch is placed first, and a separate patch is used to close the atrial septal defect (ASD) component. (B) Note the position of the coronary sinus and conducting system relative to the ASD patch suture line to avoid injury to the atrioventricular node. (From Kirklin JW, Barratt-Boyes BG. *Cardiac surgery.* New York, NY: Churchill Livingstone; 1986.)

normal aortic valve. In other patients, the truncal valve may be severely malformed, with multiple cusps, dysmorphic leaflets, and abnormal commissural relationships. The truncal valve morphology and function have significant bearing on patient symptoms and the difficulty of surgery. Patients with truncus arteriosus frequently have coronary ostial abnormalities, including juxta-commissural origin and intramural course. There is an associated interruption of the aortic arch in 25% of newborns presenting with truncus arteriosus. Abnormalities of thymic genesis, T cell function, and calcium homeostasis may frequently be seen in this group of patients in association with a chromosome 22 deletion (DiGeorge syndrome).

Patients with truncus arteriosus present in the newborn period with unrestricted pulmonary blood flow and systemic pulmonary artery pressure. With the expected postnatal decrease in PVR, massive pulmonary overcirculation, and CHF, patients may exhibit a wide pulse pressure because of diastolic runoff of blood into the pulmonary vasculature. This situation is further exacerbated in the setting of significant truncal valve insufficiency, resulting in poor systemic perfusion and cardiovascular collapse. Some infants can be initially managed with medical decongestive therapy (e.g., diuretics, angiotensin-converting enzyme inhibitors, and digoxin) and fortified nutritional support (through gastric intubation); however, this is a precarious arrangement. In the few individuals who survive infancy, irreversible pulmonary vascular disease develops rapidly, and patients become inoperable. In other patients, refractory CHF results in poor weight gain, respiratory insufficiency, and susceptibility to infection. The profound hemodynamic compromise places many newborns with unrepaired truncus arteriosus at high risk for necrotizing enterocolitis. Patients with truncus arteriosus and IAA have ductal-dependent systemic blood flow and are dependent on intravenous PGE1 to maintain ductal patency until they undergo repair. Given these considerations, it is recommended that most newborn patients undergo repair in the first several weeks of life.

The surgical repair is performed on cardiopulmonary bypass support. Components of the repair include division of the common trunk and reconstruction of confluent central branch pulmonary arteries. The large VSD is closed with a patch, typically through a right ventriculotomy. In patients with an abnormal, insufficient truncal valve, a valve repair may be necessary. It is unusual to have to replace the truncal valve at the initial operation; most valves can be at least partially repaired to provide the patient with an adequate aortic valve. Right ventricle–pulmonary artery continuity then must be established. Most surgeons prefer to interpose a valved conduit between the right ventriculotomy and pulmonary artery bifurcation (Fig. 59.16).

Conduits are limited and include homografts (pulmonary artery or aorta, valved) or heterografts (bovine or porcine). Experience with a commercially available, glutaraldehyde-preserved, bovine jugular vein valved conduit (Contegra; Medtronic, Minneapolis, MN) had been encouraging. However, there is a concerning increased incidence of endocarditis with Contegra valved conduits compared with other conduits, including homografts and heterografts.[29] Successful repair of truncus arteriosus in infants using a direct hooded anastomosis between the pulmonary artery bifurcation and right ventriculotomy has also been reported.[30] No option available at the present time offers patients the lifetime solution of a connection capable of somatic growth along with a competent, durable pulmonary valve. Thus, it is expected that all infants undergoing successful truncus repair will require multiple subsequent cardiac surgeries as they outgrow their current right ventricle–pulmonary artery conduit. Experience with a percutaneously delivered, catheter-mounted pulmonary valve has been encouraging as an interim solution for these patients in an effort to limit the number of required cardiac reoperations.

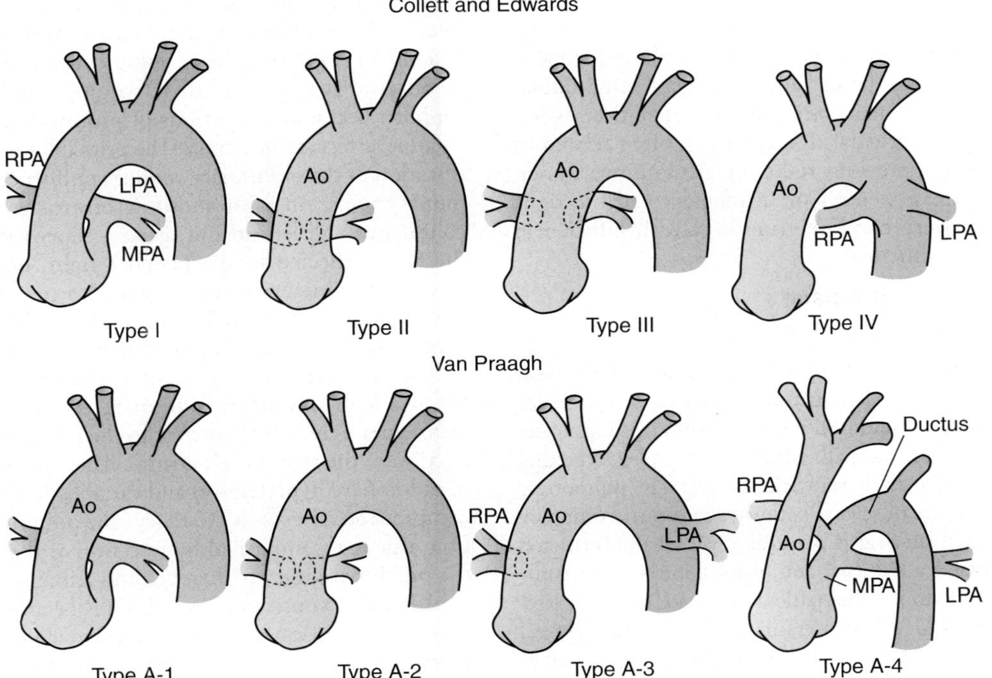

FIG. 59.15 Collett-Edwards and Van Praagh classification systems for persistent truncus arteriosus (see text for details). (Adapted from St Louis JD. Persistent truncus arteriosus. In: Nichols DG, Ungerleider RM, Spevak PJ, et al, eds. *Critical heart disease in infants and children*. Philadelphia, PA: Mosby; 2006:690.) *Ao,* Aorta; *LPA,* left pulmonary artery; *MPA,* main pulmonary artery; *RPA,* right pulmonary artery.

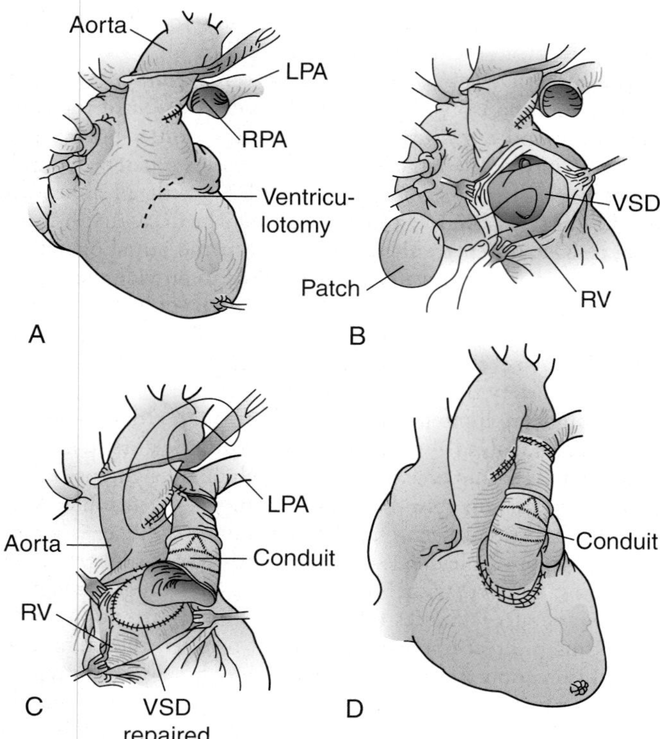

FIG. 59.16 Surgical repair of truncus arteriosus. (A) The origin of the truncus arteriosus is excised, and the truncal defect is closed with a direct suture. The incision is made high in the right ventricle *(RV)*. (B) The ventricular septal defect *(VSD)* is closed with a prosthetic patch. (C) Placement of a valved conduit into the pulmonary arteries. (D) Proximal end of conduit is anastomosed to the RV. (From Wallace RB. Truncus arteriosus. In: Sabiston DC, Jr, Spencer FC, eds. *Gibbons surgery of the chest.* 3rd ed. Philadelphia, PA: Saunders; 1976.) *LPA,* Left pulmonary artery; *RPA,* right pulmonary artery.

A growing number of adults have survived childhood truncus arteriosus repair. All these patients require diligent longitudinal cardiology surveillance, and many will require reoperation. Issues of concern include late ventricular dysrhythmias, often related to surgical scarring from the previous right ventriculotomy; branch pulmonary artery stenosis; stenosis or insufficiency of the right ventricle–pulmonary artery conduit; truncal valve insufficiency; and right ventricular dysfunction.

Abnormalities of Venous Drainage

Total Anomalous Pulmonary Venous Return

TAPVR results from embryonic failure of connection of the fetal pulmonary venous sinus to the left atrium and occurs in 1 in every 10,000 live births. This fatal condition has a spectrum of clinical presentations and may be associated with additional complex structural cardiac disease, including a single ventricle. In TAPVR, pulmonary venous return may take one of several pathways to return eventually to the right heart. Initial survival is predicated on an unobstructed pathway and unrestricted atrial-level communication so that sufficient intracardiac mixing affords the patient adequate systemic oxygenation. Patients with TAPVR are desaturated to varying degrees, depending on the adequacy of the anomalous pathway, atrial mixing, and pulmonary function. The abnormal venous connection drains in several typical patterns.

In supracardiac TAPVR, the pulmonary veins drain to a vertical vein, which courses cephalad to join a systemic vein. In the most common variation, the vertical vein courses anterior to the left pulmonary artery to join the left innominate vein. This vein may course posterior to the left pulmonary artery, resulting in compression of the pulmonary venous pathway between the left pulmonary artery and left mainstem bronchus (so-called pulmonary artery vise). The vertical vein may also join the SVC or azygos vein. In intracardiac TAPVR, the pulmonary veins drain into the coronary sinus and, in most cases in which the coronary sinus is intact, into the right atrium. This variant is rarely obstructed and may not be diagnosed until later in life in some patients. In infracardiac TAPVR, the vertical veins descend in a caudal direction through the diaphragm to join the embryologic ductus venosus and then through the liver to join the IVC. This variation is almost always obstructed at some level (Fig. 59.17). In mixed TAPVR, the pulmonary venous pathway drains in several pathways to reach the heart. Frequently, in mixed TAPVR, one or several pulmonary veins connect to the SVC, with others draining to an infracardiac or supracardiac connection.

Obstructed total anomalous pulmonary venous return. Obstructed TAPVR is one of the few true surgical emergencies in congenital heart surgery. When the condition is suspected, it is diagnosed with transthoracic echocardiography. Obstructed TAPVR occurs when one of the drainage patterns noted earlier is obstructed, resulting in severe pulmonary venous hypertension. Secondary effects include pulmonary edema, pulmonary artery hypertension, and profound hypoxemia. Interstitial pulmonary emphysema and frank pneumothorax may develop while attempting vigorous ventilatory support in profoundly desaturated children. Patients with obstructed TAPVR may present within hours of birth in extremis and do not respond to resuscitative efforts. The only useful therapy is rapid surgical repair, regardless of the severity of the patient's preoperative status.

For other forms of TAPVR, elective surgical repair is recommended after the condition is diagnosed. Occasionally, the diagnosis is not made until later in childhood in patients with an unobstructed vertical vein and widely patent atrial communication. These patients undergo elective repair to relieve cyanosis, intracardiac mixing, and right heart volume overload.

Surgical repair of TAPVR requires cardiopulmonary bypass support; occasionally, periods of profound hypothermia and circulatory arrest are necessary. The principles of repair include identification of the pulmonary venous confluence and individual pulmonary veins. An anastomosis is constructed between the venous confluence and left atrium using a superolateral approach, with the heart reflected to the patient's right, or an incision directly through the interatrial septum and corresponding region of the posterior right atrial wall. The ASD and PDA that are typically present are closed as well (Fig. 59.18).

Cor triatriatum. Cor triatriatum is a rare condition accounting for ~0.1% of all congenital heart defects in which the pulmonary veins enter a chamber posterior to the left atrium with a small connection to the right or left atrium. These patients exhibit evidence of pulmonary hypertension and variable desaturation. Surgical decompression is necessary to relieve the pulmonary venous obstruction; this is accomplished by resection of the membrane between the pulmonary venous chamber and left atrium.

A dreaded consequence of TAPVR occurs when there is a progressive, malignant sclerosing process involving the individual pulmonary veins. This process may be initiated by inaccurate surgery resulting in obstruction of the venous confluence and individual veins, or it may progress independently of surgical manipulation. It may progress to intrapulmonary pulmonary venous stenoses. A technique to deal with individual pulmonary venous stenoses

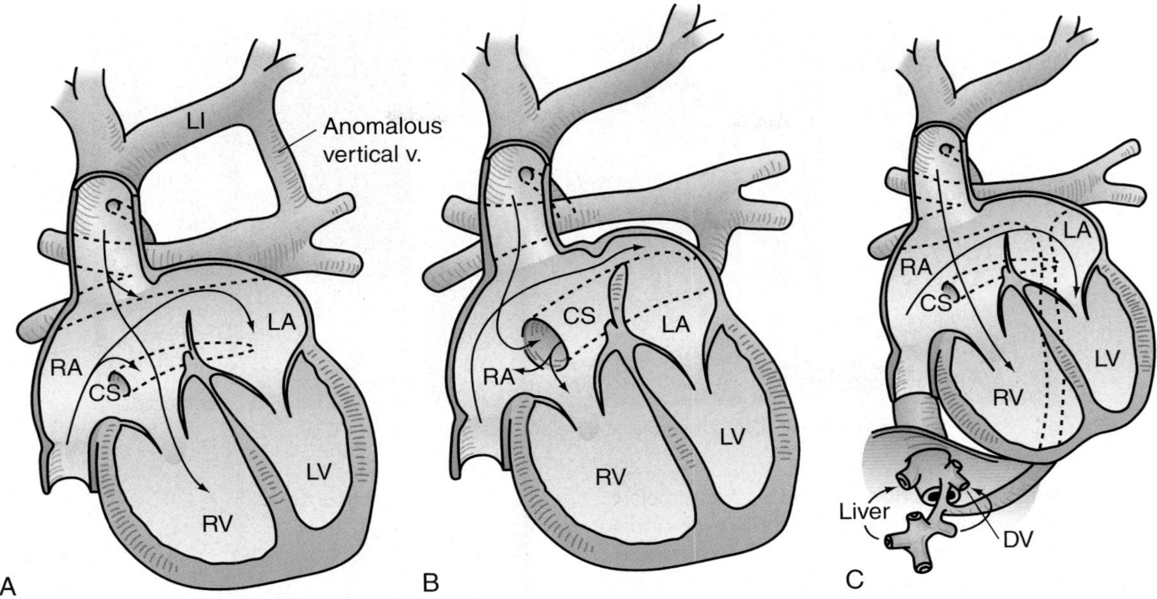

FIG. 59.17 Types of total anomalous pulmonary venous connection. (A) Supracardiac type with a vertical vein joining the left innominate *(LI)* vein. (B) Intracardiac type with connection to the coronary sinus *(CS)*. (C) Infracardiac type with drainage through the diaphragm via an inferior connecting vein. (From Hammon JW, Jr, Bender HW, Jr. Anomalous venous connections: Pulmonary and systemic. In: Baue AE, ed. *Glenn's thoracic and cardiac surgery*. 5th ed. Norwalk, CT; Appleton & Lange; 1991.) *DV,* Ductus venosus; *LA,* left atrium; *LV,* left ventricle; *RA,* right atrium; *RV,* right ventricle; *v,* vein.

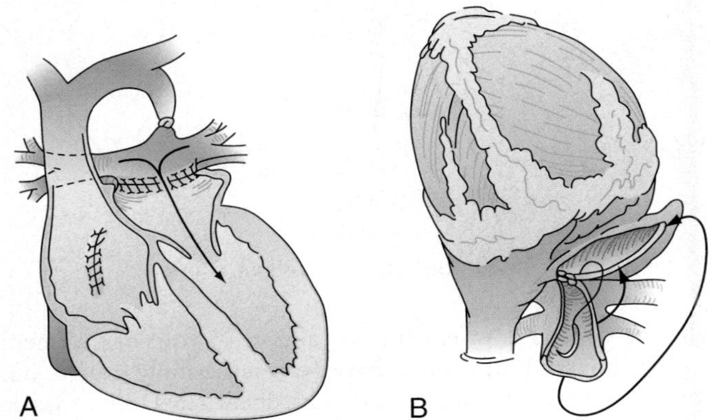

FIG. 59.18 (A) Repair of supracardiac total anomalous pulmonary venous connection (TAPVC) through a superior approach. (B) Repair of infracardiac TAPVC. Elevating the apex of the heart to the right side exposes the left atrium and pulmonary confluence. Anastomosis is created as shown. (From Lupinetti FM, Kulik TJ, Beekman RH, et al. Correction of total anomalous pulmonary venous connection in infancy. *J Thorac Cardiovasc Surg*. 1993;106:880–885.)

uses a pedicled flap of adjacent pericardium to augment the pulmonary venous orifices (sutureless technique), but this method is not applicable to all patients with pulmonary venous obstruction. Catheter-based dilation and stenting have been attempted in this setting with good acute relief of obstruction but have a high rate of reintervention and unknown long-term success, with 50% survival at 5 years.[31] In the most severe cases, the only meaningful surgical option is lung transplantation.

Anomalous Systemic Venous Drainage

Congenital abnormalities of systemic venous drainage may occur in isolation or in association with other significant structural cardiac defects. In the setting of an otherwise normal heart, the anomaly is frequently not of physiologic significance. The most common example is a persistent left SVC draining to the coronary sinus. In the absence of an intracardiac communication or unroofing of the coronary sinus, this is of anatomic significance only. In many cases, a persistent left SVC occurs, with absence of a communicating innominate vein. This condition becomes important in situations of mechanical occlusion, which may be seen with trauma or chronic venous intubation with thrombosis. A persistent left SVC frequently is incidentally discovered after placement of a left internal jugular central line, which is apparently found to track into the heart on plain chest radiography. A persistent left SVC becomes more significant in patients requiring intracardiac or extracardiac surgery. If the left SVC drains to an unroofed coronary sinus in a patient undergoing atrial septation, the patient will be profoundly desaturated after surgery. This situation requires reconstruction of the coronary sinus or some other method to reroute the left SVC to the right atrium.

An interrupted IVC usually occurs in association with other structural cardiac disease. The IVC drainage in these settings is to the azygos (azygos continuation) or hemiazygos vein and ultimately the SVC. In these patients, the hepatic veins drain into the atrium as a common confluence or as individual veins. The physiologic significance of the interrupted IVC relates to the coexisting cardiac lesion and the necessity of appreciating the abnormality of systemic venous drainage in performing corrective surgery. In patients requiring noncardiac surgery or catheter intervention, the presence of an interrupted IVC is noted when an attempt is being made to pass a venous catheter from the groin into the heart.

Cyanotic Congenital Heart Disease

Tetralogy of Fallot

TOF is a common form of cyanotic CHD occurring in approximately 1 in 2500 live births and is probably the most studied

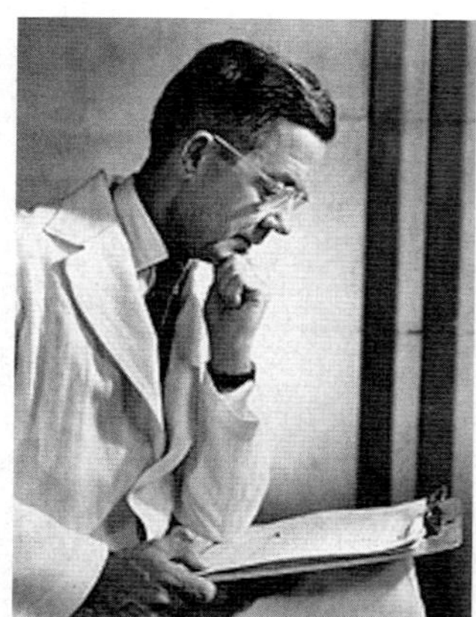
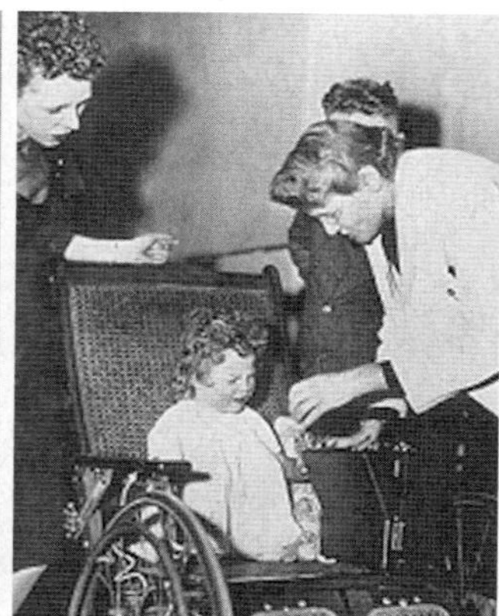
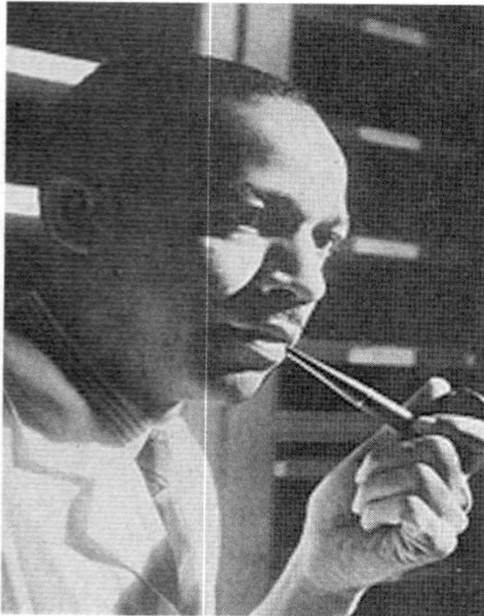

FIG. 59.19 Drs. Alfred Blalock, Helen Taussig, and Vivien Thomas.

lesion in the era of surgical correction for CHD. Many believe that The Johns Hopkins Hospital was the birthplace of cardiac surgery. Blalock performed the first successful palliative operation for TOF in November 1944, assisted by his laboratory technician, Vivian Thomas.[1] Blalock was encouraged by Taussig, the matriarch of pediatric cardiology (Fig. 59.19). Until more recently, some degree of controversy has surrounded the relative degree of contribution by these three individuals in bringing this historical event to fruition. In actuality, all three were significant participants in this momentous medical advance. While working at Vanderbilt Medical School, Blalock had charged his young and capable laboratory technician, Vivien Thomas, with the development of a surgical model of pulmonary hypertension. Thomas and Blalock developed a method of anastomosing the left subclavian artery to the divided left pulmonary artery in a canine model. Specifically, Thomas worked out the technical details, including crafting the necessary surgical instruments, and mastered the operation. This work did not produce the desired effect; canine PVR is almost infinitely low, and the animals did not develop a hypertensive pulmonary vasculature. Nonetheless, the technique was developed and published approximately 10 years in advance of the clinical application in 1944.

Blalock subsequently became the Chair of Surgery at Johns Hopkins. Taussig had by that time established a reputation as a meticulous diagnostician of complex congenital heart lesions. She had a large clinic of critically ill children with disabling cyanosis—"blue babies." At her suggestion (and probably her insistence), Blalock was convinced to attempt a surgical palliation for TOF by constructing in a human the subclavian-to-pulmonary artery anastomosis that had been perfected in the research laboratory (Fig. 59.20). Blalock performed the operation in conditions and with instruments that would be considered extremely crude by today's standards. Thomas stood immediately behind Blalock during that operation and many subsequent cases, providing instruction and encouragement. The clinical success was an earth-shattering event; hundreds of patients subsequently traveled to Johns Hopkins for surgical treatment, and the era of cardiac surgery was ushered in. (These historic accounts are factual, the result of personal interviews with many of those in attendance at that event, including Thomas, Taussig, J. Alex Haller, and Denton Cooley.)

The historic account of the development of the BT shunt has relevance to the practice of congenital heart surgery today. First, it is important that the facts surrounding this achievement are acknowledged. Second, this remarkably simple concept still remains a frequently applied technique for children with inadequate pulmonary blood flow. Finally, over almost 75 years of treatment of TOF, thousands of patients have been successfully treated, but most are not cured; many require subsequent reoperative cardiac surgery, even after complete repair.

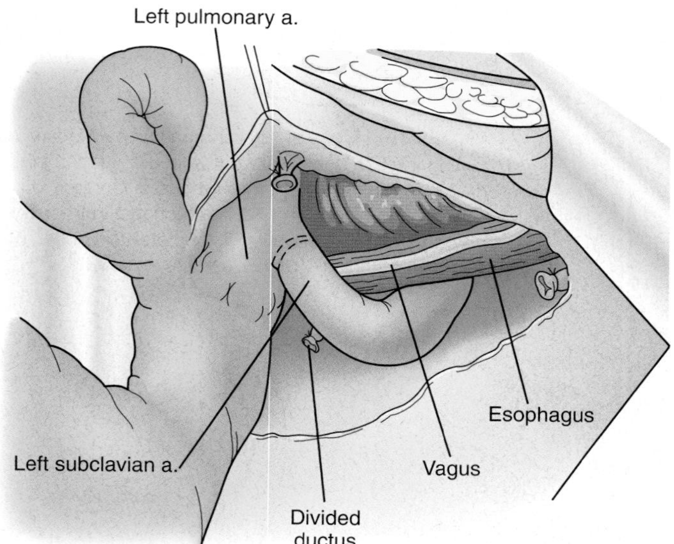

FIG. 59.20 Blalock-Taussig shunt. *a,* Artery.

The anatomic hallmark of TOF is anterior malalignment of the infundibular septum, which leaves a deficiency in the subaortic region—a malalignment VSD. This VSD is usually perimembranous, large, and pressure-nonrestrictive. The relative degree of malalignment influences the relationship of the aorta to the interventricular septum, producing varying degrees of aortic override. The deviated infundibular septum produces varying degrees of RVOTO. The path of pulmonary blood flow may be impeded at numerous levels, including the infundibulum, pulmonary valve and annulus, and main and branch pulmonary arteries. Secondary right ventricular hypertrophy occurs relative to the degree and duration of the obstruction and is progressive, contributing to the propensity for the lesion to worsen over time (Fig. 59.21).

The pathophysiology of TOF relates to shunting of desaturated, systemic venous blood through the VSD to mix with the systemic cardiac output. The greater the degree of obstruction to pulmonary blood flow, the larger the right-to-left shunt and the worse the desaturation. There are several modes of presentation. Newborns with TOF and severe RVOTO may present soon after

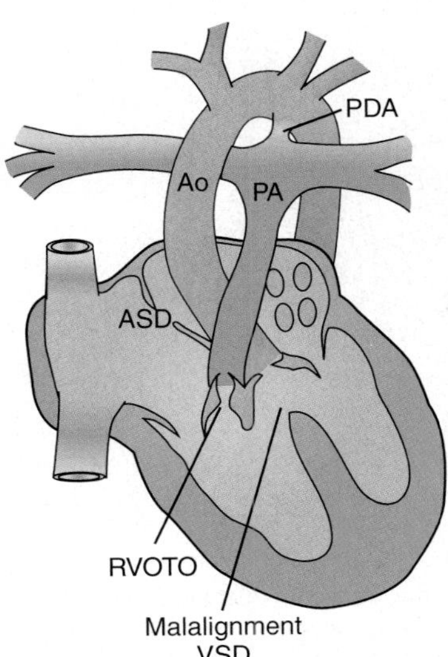

FIG. 59.21 Anatomy of tetralogy of Fallot. A malalignment ventricular septal defect *(VSD)*, aortic override, right ventricular outflow tract obstruction *(RVOTO)*, and subsequent right ventricular hypertrophy. (Adapted from Davis S. Tetralogy of Fallot with and without pulmonary atresia. In: Nichols DG, Ungerleider RM, Spevak PJ, et al, eds. *Critical heart disease in infants and children*. Philadelphia, PA: Mosby; 2006:756.) *Ao,* Aorta; *ASD,* atrial septal defect; *PA,* pulmonary artery; *PDA,* patent ductus arteriosus.

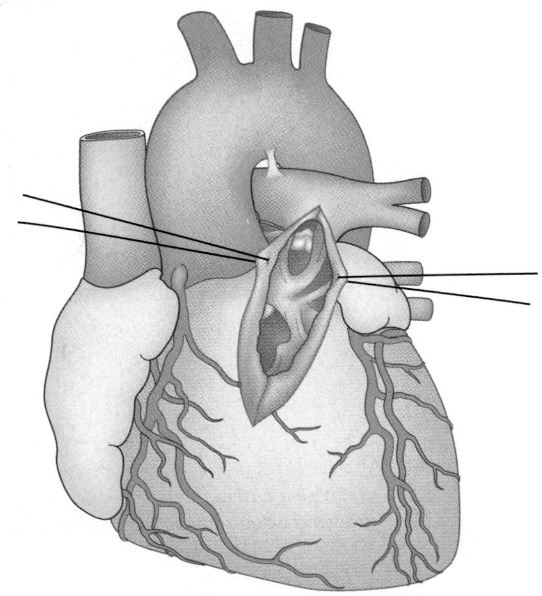

FIG. 59.22 Long right ventriculotomy in a classic transventricular approach. (From Morales DL, Zafar F, Heinle JS. Right ventricular infundibulum sparing [RVIs] tetralogy of Fallot repair: A review of over 300 patients. *Ann Surg*. 2009;250:611–617.)

birth with profound cyanosis; some require PGE1 to maintain ductal patency for adequate oxygenation. At the other end of the spectrum are children with little infundibular obstruction and normal pulmonary valve and branch pulmonary arteries. These patients may have net left-to-right flow through the VSD, occasionally to the extent that they experience pulmonary overcirculation and CHF (so-called pink TOF). Most children present between these extremes; an initially mild to moderate degree of infundibular stenosis progresses over time to become severe with worsening desaturation. A TOF spell occurs when there is an acute change in the cardiac inotropic state, often in the setting of agitation and dehydration. The infundibular stenosis acutely worsens, and patients become profoundly desaturated; this may be an extremely serious event, leading to brain damage or death. Acute treatment modalities include sedation, hydration, systemic afterload augmentation (α-adrenergic agonists), beta blockade to reduce the inotropic state, and endotracheal intubation with supplemental inspired oxygen.

The natural history of untreated TOF is dismal, with most children dying of progressive cyanosis before 10 years of age. Surgery is the mainstay of therapy. Medical and catheter-based therapy may be used to temporize, but TOF is a surgical disease. The principles of surgical correction include patch closure of the VSD and relief of all levels of the RVOTO and pulmonary artery stenosis. The classic method of TOF repair uses a longitudinal incision through the right ventricular outflow tract (RVOT); this provides an excellent transventricular view of the VSD, which is closed with a patch. The pulmonary artery, pulmonary valve, and annulus are incised if stenotic, and then the RVOT is patched. This method was used for many years but has the complicating feature of the long ventriculotomy, with attendant right ventricular dysfunction and often severe pulmonic insufficiency (Fig. 59.22). An alternative method, the transatrial or transpulmonary approach, first proposed by Imai, has gained popularity. In this method, the VSD closure and RVOT resection are accomplished through a right atriotomy via the tricuspid valve. The main pulmonary artery and pulmonary annulus are incised only if stenotic, but there is no transmural infundibular incision. This method is technically more demanding than the classic method but may offer the patient improved long-term right ventricular function (Figs. 59.23 to 59.25). The approach has been further developed as a right ventricular infundibulum-sparing strategy that focuses on minimizing the right ventricular incision and preserving the pulmonary valve. The right ventricular infundibulum-sparing strategy includes an algorithm for optimal timing of the repair that considers the individual patient's weight, age, and overall clinical picture (Fig. 59.26). Midterm results with this approach have demonstrated preserved right ventricular function.[32]

The long-term sequelae of TOF repair have been unfolding. For most patients, successful childhood repair of TOF does not translate into a cure. As patients age after TOF repair, long-term complications may develop. Patients with long RVOT incisions (transannular) by necessity have severe pulmonary insufficiency and a noncontractile infundibulum. Over time, the effects of chronic right heart volume overload include right ventricular dilation and decreased function, often with progressive tricuspid insufficiency and elevated central venous pressure. These patients may present with hepatomegaly, peripheral edema, and severe exercise intolerance. Dysrhythmias may frequently occur; patients with large right ventriculotomies develop endocardial scarring, which may be the substrate for ventricular tachycardia. Chronic right atrial dilation may ultimately lead to atrial dysrhythmias, including atrial tachycardia and fibrillation. Relative to these and other potential issues after TOF repair, patients require careful and lifelong medical follow-up. Many need reintervention; this is frequently the case in patients with chronic, severe pulmonary insufficiency, which is indicated when right ventricular dilation and dysfunction become significant. In these patients, placing a competent pulmonary valve is necessary to relieve chronic right ventricular overload. These issues are of particular importance to a patient with repaired TOF presenting for noncardiac surgery. A

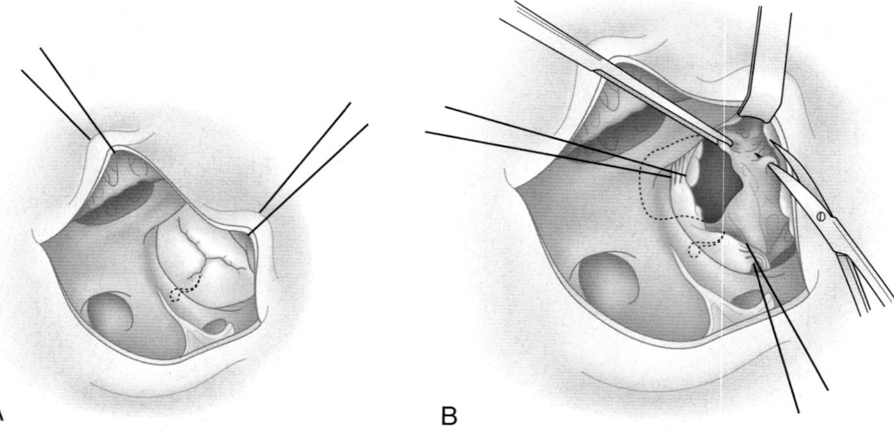

FIG. 59.23 (A) Surgeon's view through a transatrial incision in the transatrial/transpulmonary approach. (B) Right ventricular outflow tract muscle resection through the right atriotomy. (From Morales DL, Zafar F, Heinle JS. Right ventricular infundibulum sparing [RVIs] tetralogy of Fallot repair: A review of over 300 patients. *Ann Surg*. 2009;250:611–617.)

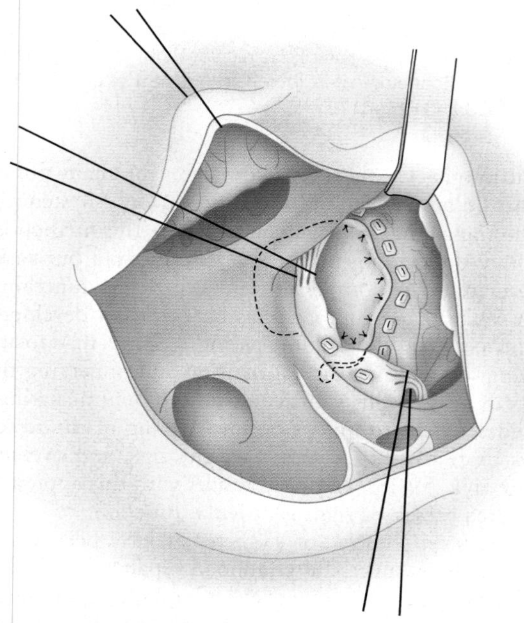

FIG. 59.24 Ventricular septal defect patch closure with pledgets around the defect and onto the tricuspid valve annulus to avoid the conduction system. (From Morales DL, Zafar F, Heinle JS. Right ventricular infundibulum sparing [RVIs] tetralogy of Fallot repair: A review of over 300 patients. *Ann Surg*. 2009;250:611–617.)

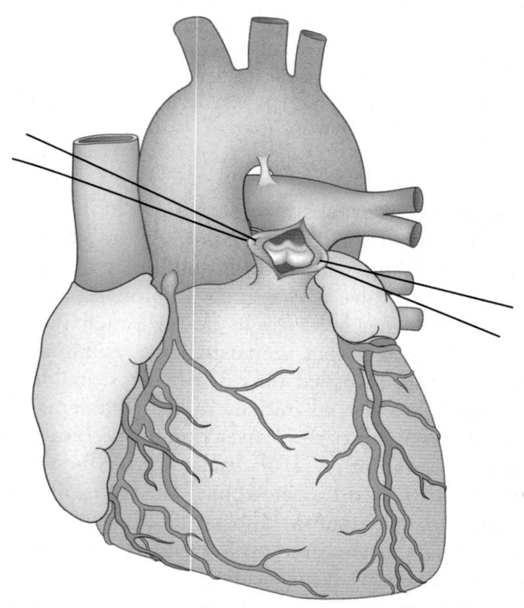

FIG. 59.25 Mini–transannular incision in the transatrial-transpulmonary approach. (From Morales DL, Zafar F, Heinle JS. Right ventricular infundibulum sparing [RVIs] tetralogy of Fallot repair: A review of over 300 patients. *Ann Surg*. 2009;250:611–617.)

careful assessment of the patient's cardiac anatomy and function is performed, including echocardiography, Holter monitoring, and occasionally cardiac catheterization.

Pulmonary Atresia and Intact Ventricular Septum

Pulmonary atresia with an intact ventricular septum (IVS) manifests with profound desaturation and ductal-dependent pulmonary blood flow in newborns. The cardiac morphology in this condition varies widely. On the most severe end of the spectrum, patients have very small right ventricles, tiny tricuspid inlets, and often a right ventricle–dependent coronary circulation. In these cases, the right ventricle must remain hypertensive to provide flow to these segments of the coronary circulation. At the other end of the anatomic spectrum, patients have a relatively normal tricuspid valve and right ventricle. Most patients fall in between these extreme with some degree of tricuspid valve and right ventricle underdevelopment.

Because patients are ductal-dependent at birth, an assessment must be made as to whether the right heart will be capable of ultimately supporting a biventricular circulation. If the coronary circulation is truly right ventricle–dependent, decompressing the right ventricle would result in coronary insufficiency. In these situations, a palliative BT shunt is created in anticipation of promoting the patient down a single-ventricle pathway. In other patients, the atretic pulmonary valve must be opened with percutaneous balloon dilation or open surgical valvotomy. Over time, the hypertensive, often apparently underdeveloped right ventricle will improve in size and function and become capable of supporting all or a significant proportion of the cardiac output. At initial presentation, many patients have a large patent foramen ovale or ASD; in

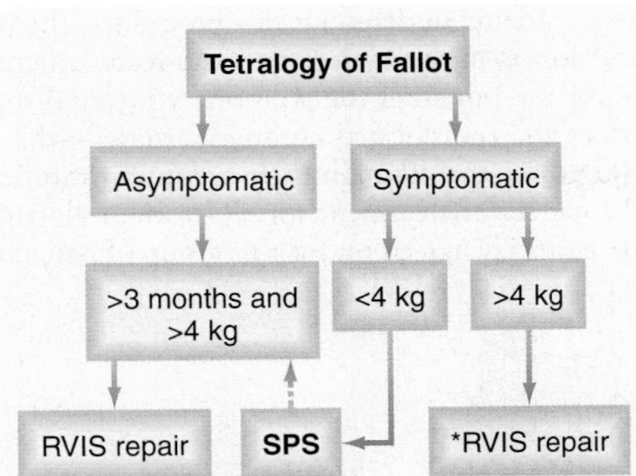

FIG. 59.26 Algorithm for the right ventricular infundibulum-sparing (*RVIS*) strategy. The goal of this strategy is to minimize the right ventricular incision and preserve the pulmonary valve. It is an individualized approach that considers the patient's weight, age, and overall clinical picture. (From Morales DL, Zafar F, Heinle JS. Right ventricular infundibulum sparing [RVIs] tetralogy of Fallot repair: A review of over 300 patients. *Ann Surg.* 2009;250:611–617.) *SPS,* Systemic-to-pulmonary artery shunt.

patients with a restrictive ASD and marginal right heart, an atrial septostomy (balloon) allows for atrial-level right-to-left shunting until the right ventricle improves. Ultimately, if the right ventricle is adequate, the ASD can be closed.

Pulmonary Atresia With Ventricular Septal Defect

Pulmonary atresia with VSD is morphologically similar to TOF, with the exception of an atretic pulmonary valve. Patients may have confluent, normal-sized pulmonary arteries perfused by a PDA. In severe cases, the pulmonary arteries are discontinuous, and the lungs are variably perfused by diminutive native branch pulmonary arteries and muscularized, collateral vessels originating from the descending aorta and brachiocephalic vessels. These major aortopulmonary collateral arteries (MAPCAs) have a propensity to develop severe stenoses as they are exposed to systemic arterial pressure. Many of these MAPCAs eventually occlude at an unpredictable rate during childhood. Because they may provide the only blood supply to some lung segments, patients become progressively desaturated.

The goal of surgical therapy for pulmonary atresia with VSD is biventricular repair to achieve normal cardiac workload and systemic arterial saturations. In patients with confluent native pulmonary arteries of adequate caliber, the VSD is surgically closed, and a valved conduit (homograft or heterograft) is interposed between the right ventricle and pulmonary bifurcation. In patients with pulmonary atresia with VSD and MAPCAs, the pulmonary arteries must be repaired by connecting the various lung segments into a common trunk through a process termed *pulmonary artery unifocalization*. Depending on the source and size of the MAPCAs and native pulmonary arteries, this may be a challenging surgical procedure, but the goal is constructing a pulmonary tree as close to normal as possible so that biventricular repair is feasible (see earlier).

The long-term issues of repair of pulmonary atresia with VSD are similar to concerns described earlier for TOF. The addition of a right ventricle–pulmonary artery conduit guarantees the need for reoperation because no currently available conduit choice offers the potential for somatic growth or an indefinitely durable valve.

Valvular Pulmonic Stenosis

Patients with isolated valvular pulmonary stenosis are almost always treated in infancy with a percutaneous balloon pulmonary valvotomy. The intermediate-term results of this treatment are good; however, all patients are left with significant pulmonary valve insufficiency and eventually require pulmonary valve replacement.

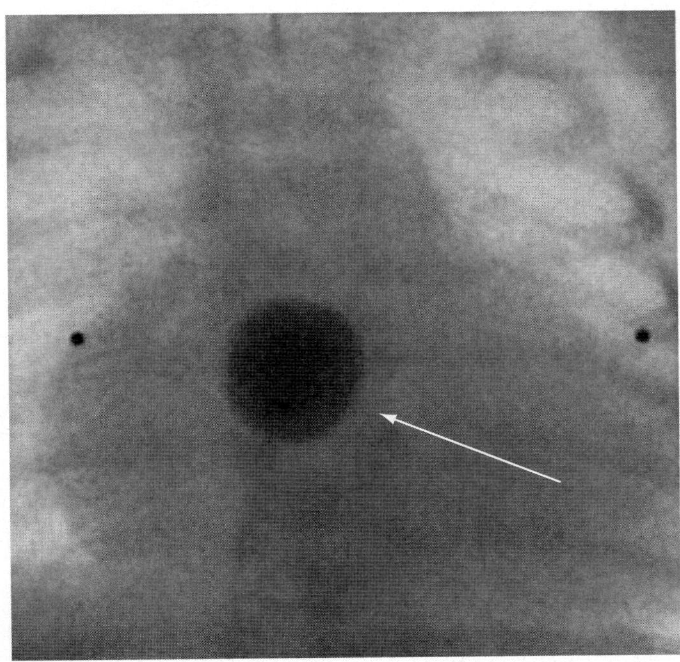

FIG. 59.27 Angiogram during balloon atrial septostomy. The *arrow* points to the inflated balloon catheter at the atrial septum. The interventional cardiologist forcefully pulls the balloon across the patent foramen ovale to create an open, unobstructed secundum atrial septal defect.

Conotruncal Anomalies

Transposition of the Great Arteries

Transposition of TGA is a common cyanotic congenital cardiac lesion occurring in 2 to 3 per 10,000 live births. In this section, our discussion relates only to TGA in which there are two good ventricles identified as being capable of independent function as the right and left ventricle. TGA is commonly referred to as D-TGA, in relationship to the typically normal D (dextro) ventricular looping that occurs in association with the discordant ventriculoarterial connection and normal A-V connection. TGA occurs in the setting of an IVS (TGA-IVS) or with associated VSD (TGA-VSD). In TGA-VSD, there may be associated aortic arch hypoplasia and coarctation. On the other extreme, there may be severe pulmonic and subpulmonic stenosis (left ventricular outflow tract obstruction [LVOTO]) or even pulmonary atresia (TGA-VSD with pulmonary atresia).

Patients with TGA-IVS typically present in the early newborn period with profound cyanosis associated with normal perinatal PDA closure. In the absence of a significant ASD, the cyanosis is severe and progresses to death if left untreated. Administration of intravenous PGE1 is almost uniformly successful in reestablishing ductal patency to improve the patient's arterial saturation by providing left-to-right shunting and improved pulmonary blood flow.

In most patients, a balloon atrial septostomy is performed (percutaneous through the umbilical vein or femoral vein) to allow atrial-level mixing (Fig. 59.27). This procedure is usually effective in allowing sufficient atrial-level mixing so that the patient is adequately saturated (70%–80%).

After the procedure, the prostaglandin infusion can be discontinued. In TGA-VSD, there is often sufficient shunting at the level of the VSD to promote adequate systemic saturation; in patients with large VSDs, the predominant presenting symptom may be pulmonary overcirculation and CHF. Patients with TGA with pulmonary atresia have ductal-dependent pulmonary blood flow. In patients with TGA-VSD and aortic arch hypoplasia or coarctation, PGE1 may be necessary to maintain ductal patency and systemic perfusion. Echocardiography is the primary diagnostic modality for TGA.

The treatment of TGA has evolved significantly during the past 60 years of surgical therapy for CHD. Initial success was achieved by surgical reconstruction to create a physiologic repair. The atrial switch operation involves a series of intraatrial baffles using a patch channel (Mustard procedure)[33] or infolding of the native atrial wall and interatrial septum (Senning procedure).[34] Both procedures achieve the same physiologic result: The systemic venous blood is redirected to the left ventricle (and the pulmonary circulation), and the pulmonary venous blood is redirected to the right ventricle. After a successful atrial switch, patients are fully saturated but are left with their morphologic right ventricle supporting the entire systemic cardiac output. In many (perhaps ultimately all) patients undergoing the atrial switch procedure, the right ventricle becomes dysfunctional over time, which is manifested by dilation, decreased ejection fraction, tricuspid insufficiency, and dysrhythmias. The observation of problems with the systemic right ventricle in patients after the atrial switch operation was the primary impetus behind the development and application of the arterial switch operation (ASO), which is now established as the surgical treatment of choice for patients with TGA. At the present time, operative survival rates for the ASO approach 100%.[35]

The ASO provides physiologic and anatomic correction of TGA by establishing ventriculoarterial concordance. The procedure involves transection and translocation of the malposed great vessels. The technically challenging requirement of the ASO relates to the translocation of the coronary arteries to the pulmonary root (the neoaorta). As noted, there are numerous possible branching patterns for the coronary arteries in TGA—some are easily transferred in the ASO, whereas others are more challenging (including single coronary ostium and intramural course) (Fig. 59.28).[36] Nonetheless, precise surgical techniques have been described and successfully applied to all coronary branching patterns. Given this as well as the known benefit of aligning the morphologic left ventricle with the systemic circulation, the ASO is offered to all patients with TGA regardless of the coronary branching pattern. There is no need for precise anatomic definition before surgery; all patients undergo the

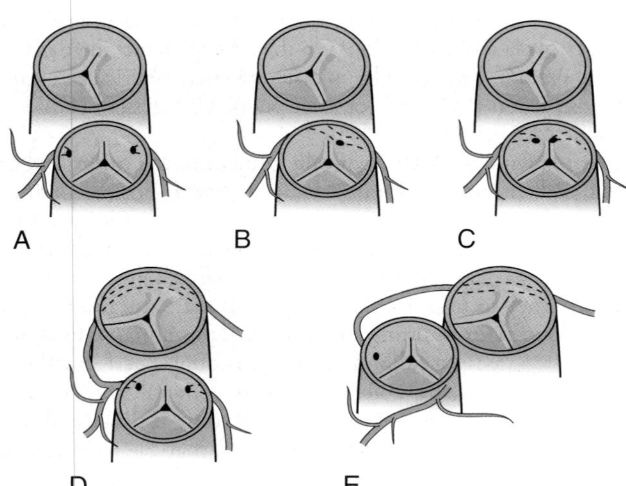

FIG. 59.28 (A-E) Five basic coronary artery configurations, as described by Yacoub and Radley-Smith. (Adapted from Mee R. The arterial switch operation. In: Stark J, de Leval M, eds. *Surgery for congenital heart defects.* 2nd ed. Philadelphia, PA: Saunders; 1994:484.)

ASO. In most patients undergoing this procedure, the pulmonary artery bifurcation is moved anterior to the reconstructed neoaorta to minimize the potential for pulmonary artery distortion and compression of the translocated coronary arteries—the Lecompte maneuver (Fig. 59.29). Although there are interinstitutional biases in terms of nuances of treatment for TGA, the following surgical strategies are generally agreed on for this group of patients.

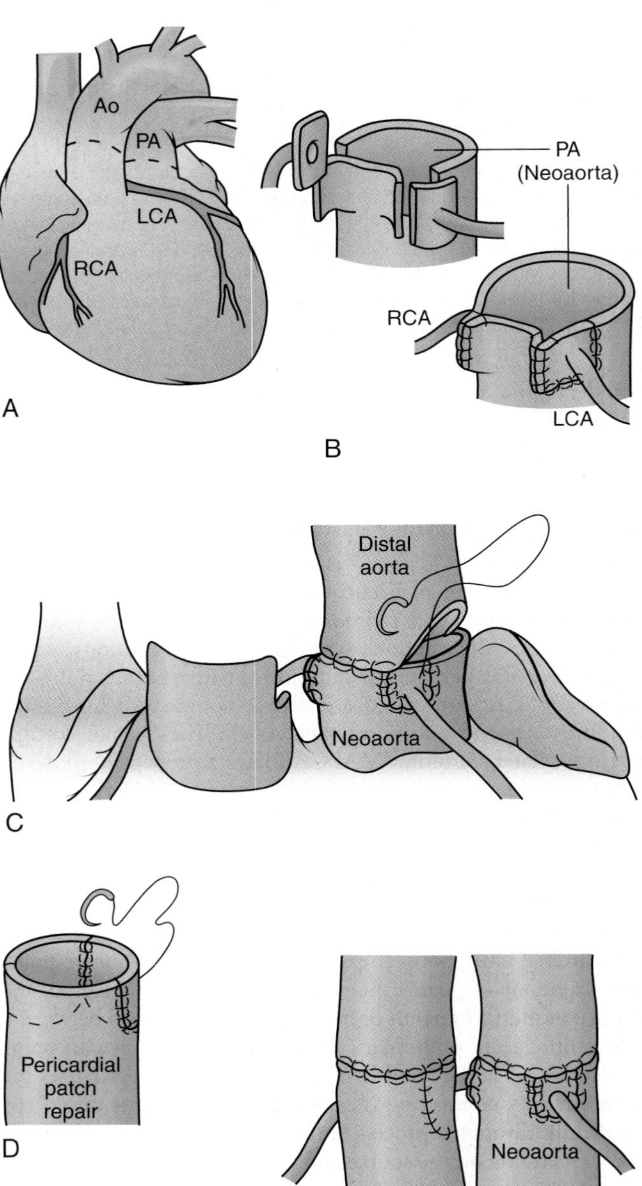

FIG. 59.29 Arterial switch operation. (A) The aorta *(Ao)* and pulmonary artery *(PA)* are transected above the sinuses of Valsalva. (B) The coronary arteries are excised from the aorta and anastomosed to the pulmonary artery using a trapdoor technique. (C) The distal aorta is brought behind the pulmonary artery (Lecompte maneuver) and anastomosed to the neoaorta. (D) Separate pericardial patches are sutured to replace the excised coronary artery tissue from the aorta. (E) Completed repair. (Adapted from Karl TR, Kirshbom PM. Transposition of the great arteries and the arterial switch operation. In: Nichols DG, Ungerleider RM, Spevak PJ, et al, eds. *Critical heart disease in infants and children.* Philadelphia, PA: Mosby; 2006:721.) *LCA,* Left coronary artery; *RCA,* right coronary artery.

Transposition of the great arteries–intact ventricular septum. After balloon atrial septostomy and weaning from PGE1, if possible, newborns with TGA-IVS undergo semielective ASO in the first few days to weeks of life. Rarely, patients present with profound desaturation refractory to balloon atrial septostomy and PGE1; in this setting, an emergent ASO is indicated. We have found this to be necessary in one patient during the past decade in an experience involving more than 200 ASOs performed in newborns. For other patients, the ASO needs to be performed in a timely but nonemergent setting. Even in the presence of adequate systemic saturation, the patient's morphologic left ventricle is functioning in a low-pressure work environment—supporting the pulmonary circulation. Thus, left ventricle mass and function involute rapidly in the first few weeks of life. By 6 weeks of life, the left ventricle may be incapable of supporting the normal systemic workload after the ASO. As such, the preferred timing for the operation is in the first 1 to 2 weeks of life.

Transposition of the great arteries–ventricular septal defect with or without arch hypoplasia. There are several modes of presentation for patients with TGA-VSD. In patients with small, pressure-restrictive VSD, the presenting symptoms are similar to those of TGA-IVS. These patients require the ASO early in life, along with VSD closure before left ventricle involution. In patients with TGA and nonrestrictive VSD, there may be adequate mixing to allow reasonable systemic arterial saturation. In this setting, the left ventricle remains pressure-loaded and does not involute; thus, the necessity of early promotion to the ASO is less time-compressed. Many newborns with TGA and a large VSD are relatively asymptomatic soon after birth; they go on to develop CHF in the first 1 to 2 months of life as the normal decrease in newborn pulmonary resistance occurs. Our preference for these patients is to follow them closely for evidence of CHF and perform semielective ASO and VSD closure in the first 4 to 6 weeks of life. Some centers prefer to proceed with this surgery sooner; this appears to be a matter of surgeon preference and has not been shown to affect long-term outcome. In patients with TGA-VSD with arch hypoplasia or coarctation, early surgery is required. In this setting, the preferred treatment involves one-stage, complete correction, including ASO, VSD closure, and aortic arch repair.

Transposition of the great arteries–ventricular septal defect with pulmonary stenosis–left ventricular outflow tract obstruction or pulmonary atresia. The issue of concern in this group of patients is the degree of LVOTO. In patients with TGA-VSD and organic LVOTO, with a relatively normal pulmonary valve, the treatment strategy is as described earlier, with ASO, VSD closure, and left ventricular outflow tract (LVOT) resection. The situation becomes more complex in the setting of severe pulmonary stenosis or pulmonary atresia. These patients may be ductal-dependent as newborns (pulmonary atresia) and require newborn complete correction or a palliative modified BT shunt in the newborn period, followed by biventricular repair later in infancy (our preference). The goal in these patients is to achieve biventricular repair to create an unobstructed connection between the morphologic left ventricle and systemic circulation. Several operations have been described and successfully used in this setting.

The Rastelli procedure involves an interventricular patch baffle, which commits the left ventricle to the aorta through the VSD. Typically, a right ventricle–pulmonary artery conduit is then placed to achieve pulmonary blood flow. Issues of concern include the potential for LVOTO (at or below the level of the VSD) and the certain need for future right ventricle–pulmonary artery conduit revision. The REV procedure is designed to minimize the potential of LVOT obstruction and to use all possible native tissue-tissue connections to limit the potential need for future surgery. This procedure involves resection of the muscular conus between the aorta and pulmonary roots, interventricular baffle of the left ventricle to the aorta, and translocation of the native main pulmonary artery to the right ventricle (by a Lecompte maneuver) without the use of an intervening conduit. The final option involves aortic root translocation, which includes resection of the entire native aortic root and coronary origins, resection of the intervening muscular conus, and posterior translocation of the aortic root to the surgically enlarged pulmonary root to achieve a direct connection between the left ventricle and aorta. The VSD is then closed, and a conduit is placed or a direct connection is created between the right ventricle and pulmonary arteries.

Transposition of the great arteries in adults. The long-term prognosis of adult patients who have undergone childhood repair of TGA is still incompletely understood; however, all these patients require lifelong surveillance and have the potential of developing significant anatomic and functional cardiac problems. Patients who were treated with the atrial switch operation have a morphologic right ventricle supporting their systemic circulation, which will predictably fail in many patients. Although fully saturated, these patients may present later in life with signs and symptoms of CHF and dysrhythmia. For severely affected individuals, the only realistic treatment option ultimately may be cardiac transplantation.

The long-term issues related to the ASO are less well understood. Despite technical advances in reconstructive methods, there is still a troubling incidence of postoperative supravalvular and branch pulmonic stenosis. The neoaortic root may dilate in some patients undergoing the ASO, leading to neoaortic insufficiency and coronary artery distortion. The fate of the surgically translocated coronary ostia is unclear; there is clearly a risk for late sudden cardiac death related to unsuspected coronary insufficiency noted elsewhere in this chapter. For an adult patient undergoing noncardiac surgery after previous surgery for complex congenital cardiac disease, including TGA, a high index of suspicion is warranted.

Double-Outlet Right Ventricle

Double-outlet right ventricle occurs when both great vessels are anatomically committed to the right ventricle. Double-outlet right ventricle occurs in 3 to 9 per 100,000 live births. This condition may occur in association with a subaortic VSD, a noncommitted (remote) VSD, or a subpulmonary VSD (Taussig-Bing anomaly). As with other complex cardiac conditions, the goal of treatment relates to the presenting hemodynamic conditions and patient symptoms. The ultimate goal is to achieve a biventricular circulation when possible. Patients may present with severe cyanosis and require corrective or palliative therapy in the newborn period. Conversely, they may present with unrestricted pulmonary blood flow and develop CHF. The challenging issue of constructing a biventricular repair relates to achieving unobstructed outlets from the right and left ventricles. In patients with double-outlet right ventricle with subaortic VSD and RVOTO, reconstruction is similar to that for TOF. More remote VSDs may require enlargement with interventricular tunnel repair. For the Taussig-Bing anomaly, the relationship of the VSD to the pulmonary artery makes the ASO the procedure of choice. These patients often have RVOTO and aortic arch hypoplasia, which require attention at the time of complete correction. For rare individuals, the relationship of the great vessels and complexity of the VSD preclude a biventricular repair, and the patient must be treated as if he or she has a functional single ventricle.

Congenitally Corrected Transposition of the Great Arteries (L-Transposition)

Congenitally corrected TGA (ccTGA, or L-TGA), describes a constellation of conditions with the common feature of A-V and ventriculoarterial discordance and occurs in approximately 1 in 33,000 live births. ccTGA may occur in association with VSD, pulmonic and subpulmonic stenosis, and displaced left A-V valve (Ebsteinoid left A-V valve). In ccTGA, the morphologic mitral valve is right-sided and associated with the morphologic left ventricle; the morphologic tricuspid valve is associated with the morphologic right ventricle. Patients with this condition are physiologically corrected in that in the absence of ventricular-level shunting, they are fully saturated—hence, the term *corrected transposition.* The age and mode of patient presentation in this condition depend on the contribution of associated defects and the function of the morphologic right ventricle, which acts as the systemic ventricle. Controversy exists regarding the timing and mode of surgical treatment for patients presenting with various manifestations of ccTGA.

Congenitally corrected transposition of the great arteries with intact ventricular septum. Patients with ccTGA-IVS may be entirely asymptomatic throughout childhood and early adulthood. Frequently, the diagnosis is made incidentally. In other patients, the disease manifests with symptoms of CHF in association with right ventricular dysfunction or left A-V valve insufficiency. There is also a high incidence of complete heart block in patients with ccTGA, and the first manifestation may be this dysrhythmia with associated symptoms.

Treatment for patients presenting with CHF is a challenging management scenario. For patients with ccTGA and preserved right ventricular function, left A-V valve repair or replacement may be considered. In many of these patients, the valvular insufficiency may be more a manifestation of declining systemic RV function, with septal shift and annular dilation, rather than intrinsic valve pathology. In this setting, valve replacement would not correct the progression of right ventricular dysfunction. For patients with systemic right ventricular dysfunction, one option for treatment is a complex reconstruction known as a *double switch* (Fig. 59.30). This procedure includes an atrial switch in combination with an arterial switch to align the morphologic left ventricle with the systemic circulation. In almost all patients with ccTGA-IVS and right ventricular dysfunction (and in the absence of structural LVOTO), a period of left ventricle retraining is required before the double-switch procedure. This requirement relates to the fact that the left ventricle will have been functioning

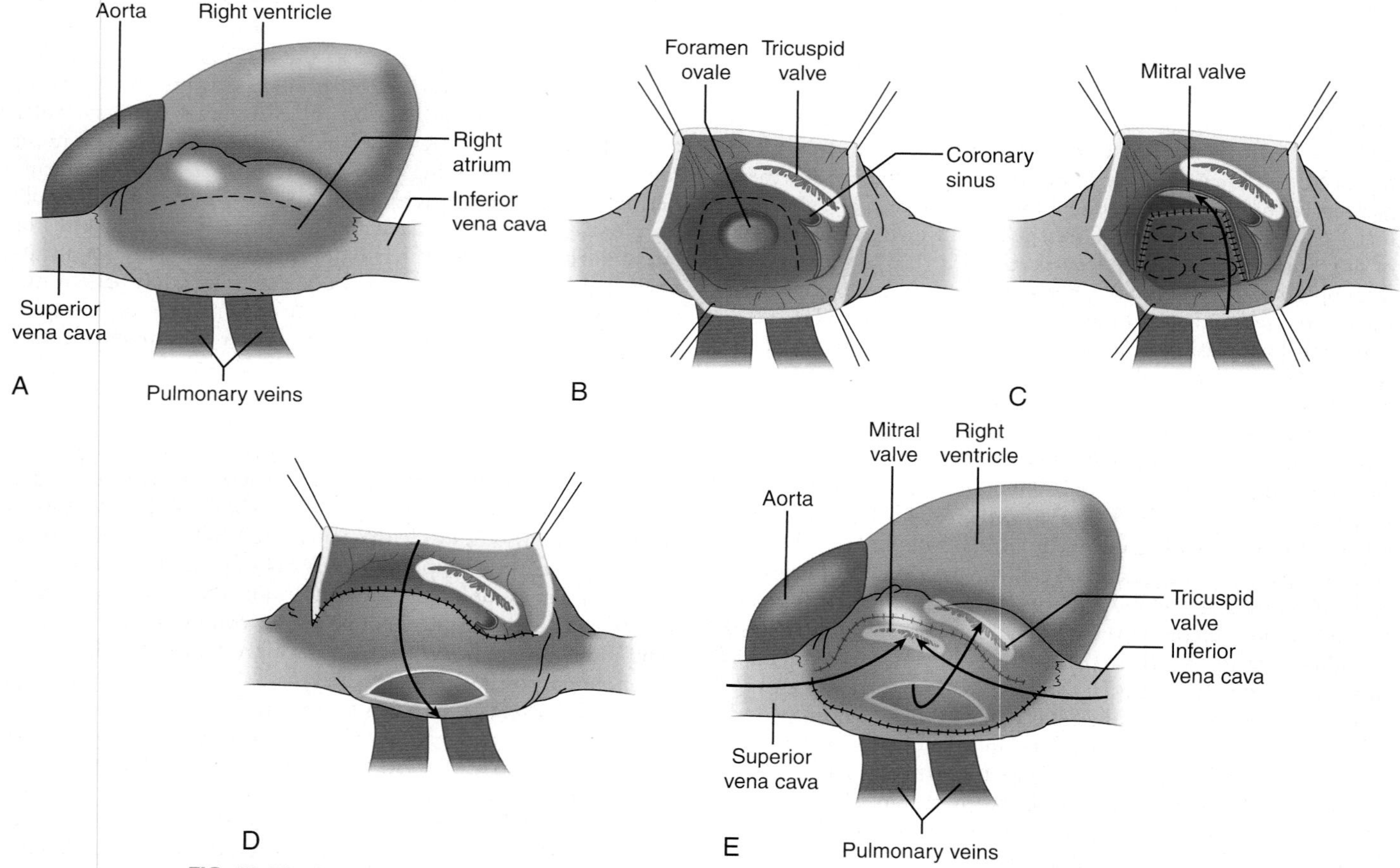

FIG. 59.30 Schematic representation of the Senning procedure for transposition of the great arteries. (A) Two separate incisions, one in the right atrium and the other in the left atrium near the insertion of the pulmonary veins. (B) Location of the incision in the atrial septum. (C) The atrial septum sewn down to the pulmonary veins preparing for oxygenated blood to be directed to the tricuspid valve. The inferior free wall of the right atrium is sewn along the cut edge of the atrial septum redirecting the deoxygenated blood to the mitral valve. (D) The superior free wall of the right atrium is now sewn to the cut edge of the left atrium, redirecting the oxygenated blood from the pulmonary veins to the tricuspid valve. (E) Schematic representation of the oxygenated blood and deoxygenated blood pathways. (Reprinted with permission from Texas Children's Hospital, 2016.)

in the low-pressure pulmonary circulation and will be incapable of performing systemic work. Retraining or conditioning the left ventricle requires the surgical creation of pulmonary stenosis by the placement of a pulmonary artery band. Most surgeons agree that the left ventricle must work at or very near systemic blood pressure for many months (we favor a minimum of 6 months) before the double-switch operation. The double switch is a technically challenging operation, with significant perioperative risk. Because of the small numbers of patients treated worldwide with this complicated surgical strategy, there are only limited data of the acute and midterm results.[37] An issue of concern centers on the long-term ability of the retrained left ventricle to function as the systemic ventricle. Nonetheless, patients with ccTGA and depressed right ventricular function have a poor prognosis otherwise, and, as such, the complexity and risk of the double-switch operation appear justified. The only other surgical option for these patients is cardiac transplantation.

Congenitally corrected transposition of the great arteries with ventricular septal defect and pulmonic stenosis. Patients in this category are often well balanced and have mild cyanosis, with minimal symptoms in childhood, whereas others with more severe pulmonary stenosis or pulmonary atresia present early in life with symptomatic cyanosis. Treatment for an overtly cyanotic infant with ccTGA with pulmonary stenosis is initially palliative in the form of a modified BT shunt. The ultimate goal for all patients is a biventricular circulation, with normal arterial oxygen saturation. One option for these patients is to close the VSD surgically and place a conduit between the morphologic left ventricle and pulmonary arteries to relieve the pulmonary obstruction. This classic repair benefits the patient by separating the systemic and pulmonary circulations and allowing normal oxygen tension. The issue of concern in patients undergoing this repair is that the morphologic right ventricle must act independently as the systemic ventricle after repair. As noted, the ability of the right ventricle to support the systemic circulation may be questionable over the long-term in some patients. As such, an alternative strategy in these patients is to baffle the left ventricular outflow to the aorta through the VSD, then to perform an atrial switch to reroute the systemic and pulmonary venous return, and finally to place a conduit from the morphologic right ventricle to the pulmonary arteries. This option is a modification of the double-switch arrangement, affording the patient the benefit of a systemic left ventricle. Because the left ventricle has been working at systemic pressure before correction, a period of retraining is unnecessary.

Adult patients with ccTGA, with or without previous surgery, warrant careful attention before any noncardiac operation. These patients may have various complex ongoing cardiac issues, including rhythm disturbance, ventricular dysfunction, and valvular insufficiency.

Left Ventricular Outflow Tract Obstruction

Left ventricular outflow tract obstruction (LVOTO) may manifest in isolation or in combination with other complex cardiac lesions. The physiologic consequences of severe LVOTO may be catastrophic, including diminished systemic cardiac output and tremendous left ventricular pressure overload. Newborns with severe LVOTO may present in shock with diminished peripheral perfusion, cardiomegaly, and pulmonary congestion. There is a significant risk for necrotizing enterocolitis in these infants. In older patients, gradual onset of LVOTO may be initially asymptomatic, only to manifest over time as decreasing exercise tolerance and declining left ventricular function. Patients with severe LVOTO and cardiomegaly are at high risk for myocardial ischemia and sudden cardiac death. The resting ECG often demonstrates left ventricular hypertrophy, with a strain pattern. If an exercise stress test is performed, it may demonstrate worrisome ST segment depression and ventricular dysrhythmias. Echocardiography is the primary diagnostic tool for patients with LVOTO. In rare cases, diagnostic cardiac catheterization may be considered to delineate the level of obstruction.

Valvular Aortic Stenosis

Congenital valvular aortic stenosis (AS) is a common cause of LVOTO and represents approximately 5% of all CHD. The degree of obstruction may range from mild in patients with a congenitally bicuspid aortic valve to severe in patients with critical AS with unidentifiable valve commissures and annular hypoplasia. Infants presenting with critical AS are often symptomatic early in the newborn period, presenting with shock and profoundly depressed ventricular function. At the present time, almost all patients are taken to the cardiac catheterization laboratory for balloon aortic valvotomy. This procedure may be lifesaving in relieving AS and allowing for recovery of ventricular function. However, for most patients, the procedure is palliative, with a significant incidence of recurrence of AS or development of significant aortic insufficiency after the procedure. In patients with AS refractory to balloon dilation, an open aortic valvotomy may be necessary (Fig. 59.31). A surgical valvotomy, especially in small infants with adequate annular dimension, can be accomplished by an accurate incision down a rudimentary commissure or raphe to improve cusp mobility.

Recurrent AS after previous ballooning may be amenable to repeat dilation; however, when associated with significant aortic insufficiency, the patient requires surgery. Severe aortic insufficiency after previous balloon dilation is usually related to an avulsed cusp. In these cases, valve repair may be possible, but replacement may become necessary. Published series have confirmed the usefulness of aortic valve repair procedures, which is a particularly attractive option for growing children.[38]

The decision to replace the aortic valve in growing children is clouded by the lack of an ideal aortic valve substitute—a valve

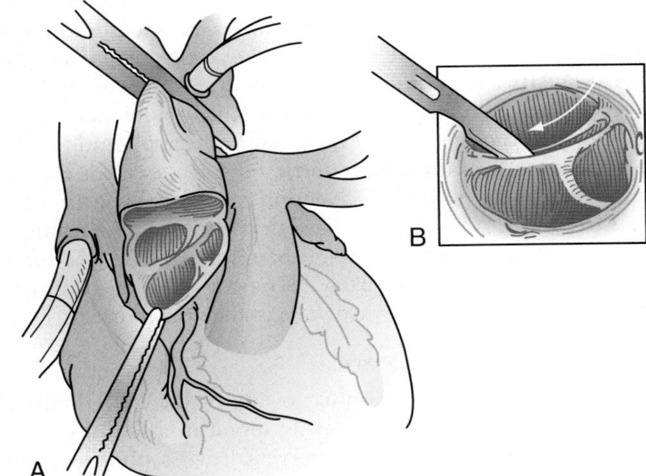

FIG. 59.31 Close-up view of the aortic valve demonstrating a surgical valvectomy. (A) The valve is bicuspid, with a prominent raphe in the anterior valve leaflet. (B) The orifice is enlarged by incising the fused commissure between the two leaflets. (From Chang AC, Burke RP. Left ventricular outflow tract obstruction. In: Chang AC, Hanley FL, Wernovsky G, et al, eds. *Pediatric cardiac intensive care*. Baltimore, MD: Williams & Wilkins; 1998.)

capable of lifelong durability, appropriate somatic growth, easily implantable, and not requiring anticoagulation. Criteria for aortic valve replacement are beyond the scope of this chapter; however, severe valvular AS not amenable to catheter or open valvotomy is an appropriate indication. Options for aortic valve replacement in children include a mechanical prosthesis, heterograft, homograft, and pulmonary autograft. A mechanical prosthesis may be considered in childhood; however, the valve size must be sufficient to provide adequate function as the patient grows. Most surgeons and cardiologists recommend therapeutic anticoagulation in children with a mechanical valve prosthesis, but this can be challenging and potentially dangerous in growing children and adolescents. Many surgeons believe the risk for such medical treatment outweighs the potential benefit of a theoretically durable valve.

Heterograft aortic valve prostheses historically have been associated with limited durability in children and are not capable of somatic growth. A recent analysis in children has confirmed a significantly reduced long-term durability of heterografts when compared to mechanical valves and the Ross Operation.[39] Human cadaver aortic valves (aortic homograft) have been used extensively in children and young adults. These valves are usually implanted as a complete aortic root replacement, which requires coronary ostial implantation. Thus, surgery to place an aortic homograft is considerably more complex and with potentially higher risk. The positive features of an aortic homograft include improved durability compared with heterograft and avoidance of anticoagulation. Nonetheless, these valves eventually fail, necessitating a complicated reoperative aortic root replacement.

Pulmonary autograft aortic root replacement (Ross operation) involves translocation of the pulmonary valve to the aortic position with subsequent replacement of the pulmonary valve with a homograft or heterograft valved conduit (Fig. 59.32). The theoretical advantages of the Ross procedure include the potential for somatic growth, avoidance of anticoagulation, and possibility of extended durability. Enthusiasm for this procedure has been tempered by the recognition that the need for extensive cardiac dissection to harvest the autograft, along with a more complex implantation, is associated with increased operative risk. Furthermore, the unsupported pulmonary root may dilate in the presence of systemic arterial pressure, leading to progressive autograft aortic insufficiency. This observation has led to various modifications of the implantation technique to support the aortic annulus and the sinus segment. Given these considerations and the certain need for reoperation to replace the right ventricular–pulmonary artery conduit, great caution must be exercised in the application of the Ross operation.[40] Transcatheter aortic valve replacement has become a frequently utilized intervention for acquired aortic valve disease in adults. With the continued development of increasingly sophisticated and smaller means to perform transcatheter aortic valve replacement, this will likely become a potential treatment algorithm for congenital aortic disease in the near future.

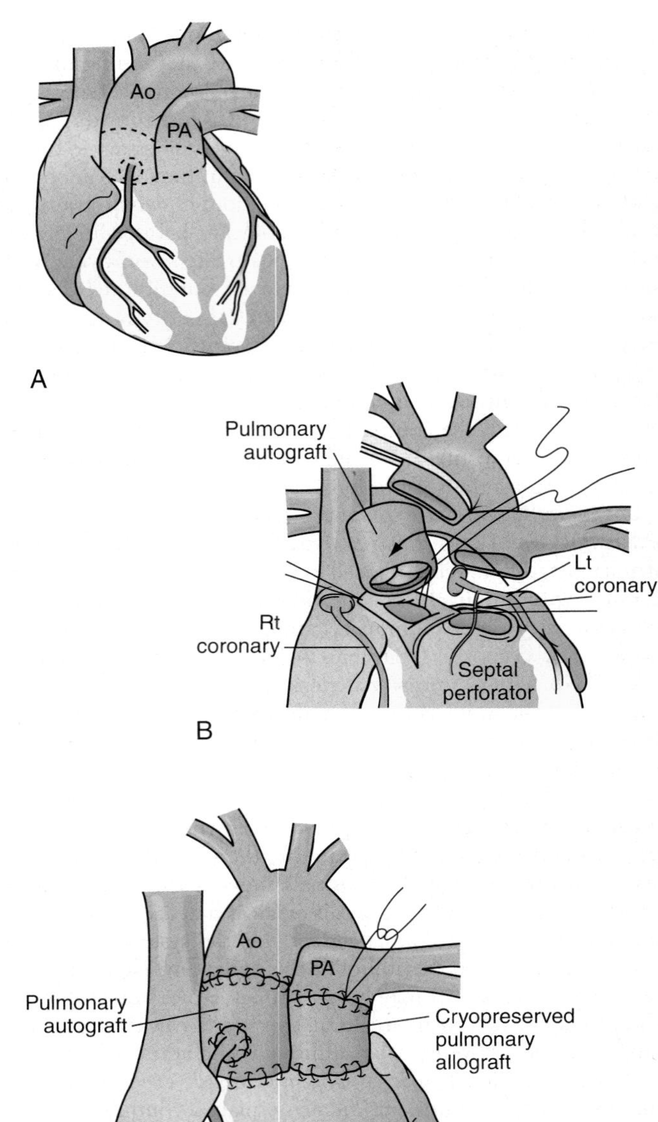

FIG. 59.32 Ross procedure. (A) The great arteries are transected above the sinotubular ridge. The coronary arteries are excised using coronary artery buttons. (B) The pulmonary autograft is excised from the right *(Rt)* ventricular outflow tract, and the proximal end of the autograft is anastomosed to the annulus. (C) The coronary artery buttons are anastomosed to the pulmonary autograft. (Adapted from St Louis JD, Jaggers J. Left ventricular outflow tract obstruction. In: Nichols DG, Ungerleider RM, Spevak PJ, et al, eds. *Critical heart disease in infants and children.* Philadelphia, PA; Mosby; 2006:615.) *Ao,* Aorta; *Lt,* left; *PA,* pulmonary artery.

Fibromuscular Subaortic Stenosis

This condition is a progressive narrowing of the LVOT related to a dense fibrous membrane usually found in association with asymmetrical protrusion of the interventricular septum into the outflow tract. Fibromuscular subaortic stenosis accounts for approximately 6% of all CHD. The membrane is often concentric and becomes densely adherent to the septum and mitral valve. The membrane progresses toward and eventually onto the undersurface of the aortic valve cusps, which leads to progressive LVOTO, aortic valve cusp retraction, and aortic insufficiency.

Echocardiography is the primary diagnostic tool when assessing the degree of obstruction and progression of subaortic stenosis. However, it is not accurate for assessing subtle degrees of cusp extension.[41] Cardiac catheterization is rarely needed to diagnose this condition; balloon dilation is of no use in treating the LVOTO.

Surgery is the mainstay of treatment for subaortic stenosis, but there is disagreement about surgical indications. Most surgeons believe that new onset of any degree of aortic insufficiency in association with a subaortic membrane, regardless of the pressure gradient, is an indication for surgery. In other patients, an escalating LVOT gradient, associated left ventricular hypertrophy, and

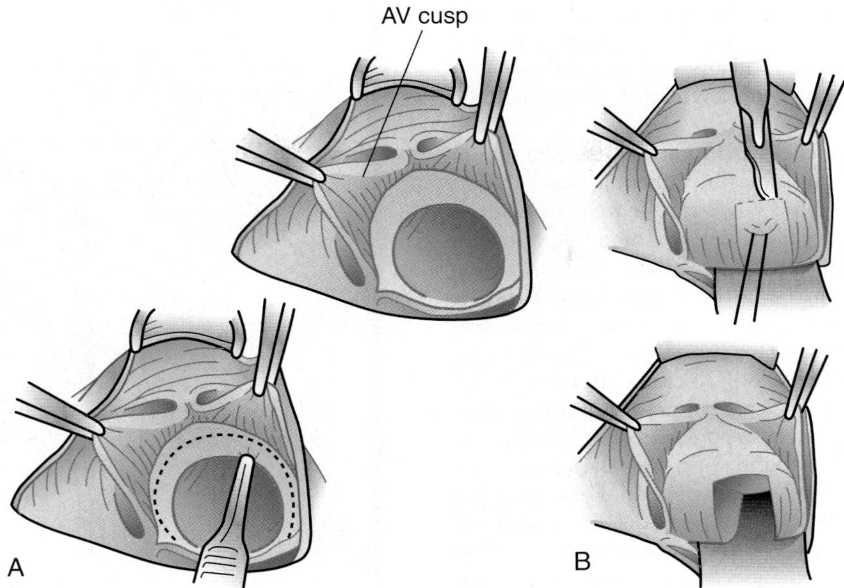

FIG. 59.33 (A) Excision of discrete subaortic stenosis. The aorta is opened obliquely, and the aortic valve *(AV)* leaflets are retracted to expose the subaortic membrane. The membrane is excised circumferentially *(dotted line)*. (B) This is usually combined with a muscle resection. (From de Leval M. Surgery of the left ventricular outflow tract. In: Stark J, de Leval M, eds. *Surgery for congenital heart defects*. 2nd ed. Philadelphia, PA: Saunders; 1994.)

appropriate anatomic substrate are acceptable indications for operation.

The surgical procedure for subaortic stenosis involves a transaortic resection of the subaortic membrane, including all attachments to the mitral valve, septum, and aortic valve cusps. A septal myectomy is performed, along with membrane resection, in most patients (Fig. 59.33). Complications include membrane recurrence, injury to the bundle of His, and iatrogenic VSD creation. Nonetheless, with careful technique, the risk for these complications is minimized. Despite surgical intervention, a significant proportion of patients will have recurrence which requires reintervention and upwards of 40% will develop some degree of aortic insufficiency.[42]

Tunnel Subaortic Stenosis

Tunnel subaortic stenosis is a more severe form of LVOTO that is often associated with aortic annular hypoplasia and valvular AS. In severe cases, the LVOTO is not amenable to subaortic resection alone. In this situation, an aortic root–enlarging procedure may be necessary to relieve the obstruction (aortoventriculoplasty, or Konno procedure). This complex reconstruction generally is associated with the necessity of aortic valve replacement using one of the aforementioned options. Moreover, all degrees of LVOTO may be seen in association with numerous left heart obstructive lesions (Shone syndrome) that may require extensive reconstruction.

Aortic Arch Anomalies

Aortic Coarctation

Coarctation of the aorta is one of the most frequently encountered congenital cardiac lesions occurring in 3 of every 10,000 live births. This condition has a wide range of presentations, from a severely symptomatic newborn with CHF and depressed ventricular function to an adult with proximal hypertension and minimal symptoms. Coarctation is classified relative to its association with the ligamentum arteriosus and aortic arch. An infantile or preductal aortic coarctation is seen in combination with a large PDA,

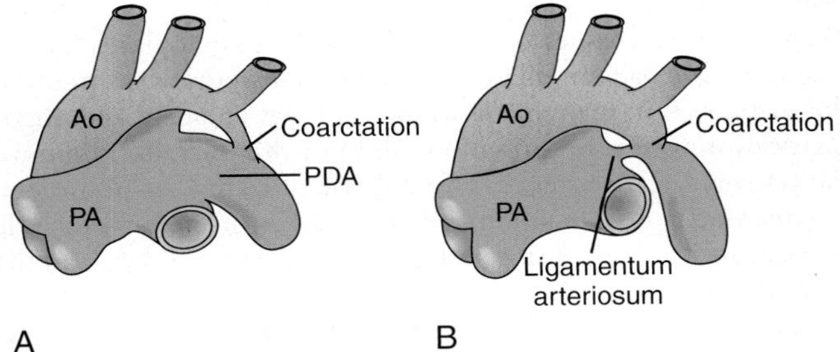

FIG. 59.34 Coarctation of the aorta *(Ao)*. (A) Infantile or preductal coarctation. (B) Adult coarctation. (From Backer CL, Mavroudis C. Coarctation of the aorta. In: Mavroudis C, Backer CL, eds. *Pediatric heart surgery*. Philadelphia, PA: Mosby; 2003:252.) *PA,* Pulmonary artery; *PDA,* patent ductus arteriosus.

which may have predominantly right-to-left flow to the lower descending aorta. In this setting, the patient is ductal-dependent for systemic blood flow until the coarctation is repaired, and a PGE1 infusion must be maintained to prevent ductal closure. A periductal or juxtaductal coarctation occurs in the region of the ductal insertion and is distal to the aortic isthmus, which may be normal or hypoplastic (Fig. 59.34).

Aortic coarctation with or without aortic arch hypoplasia is frequently associated with intracardiac anomalies, including multiple left heart obstructive lesions (e.g., mitral stenosis, left ventricular hypoplasia or endocardial fibroelastosis, subaortic stenosis or AS) known as Shone syndrome. Patients with large VSDs may present in infancy with severe aortic coarctation, with or without subaortic stenosis.

Aortic coarctation may be suspected on clinical examination by a significant upper extremity–lower extremity blood pressure gradient and diminished or absent femoral and pedal pulses. In older patients with well-developed intercostal collateral arteries, a continuous murmur may be auscultated over the posterior thorax. Echocardiography is now the primary diagnostic modality for aortic coarctation. MRI and CT angiography may also be useful in some patients. In rare cases, cardiac catheterization is required to define the anatomy, but this modality is now used more frequently for treatment, including balloon dilation with or without stenting.

Treatment strategies for aortic coarctation have evolved significantly since the first successful surgical treatment almost 70 years ago. Newborns presenting with severe aortic coarctation with or without associated ductal-dependent systemic blood flow are best treated by surgery. Initial enthusiasm regarding balloon dilation in these patients has diminished as it has become clear that there is a high incidence of recurrent coarctation after neonatal dilation.[43] Most congenital cardiac surgeons perform isolated coarctation repair through a left thoracotomy incision (third or fourth interspace) using resection of the coarctation and primary anastomosis. For patients with relative hypoplasia of the distal aortic arch, the anastomosis can be brought along the lesser curve of the aortic arch using an extended end-to-end method. For coarctation with a hypoplastic transverse arch, we favor the aortic arch advancement procedure, which uses all native tissue repair to allow for growth.[44] Other methods include subclavian artery flap aortoplasty (Waldhausen method) and prosthetic patch aortoplasty. These latter methods are used less frequently than primary repair (Fig. 59.35). Catheter therapy as a primary treatment for aortic coarctation is a controversial therapy in the opinion of most surgeons. Although this methodology has been widely applied, its true comparability to surgery requires further prospective study. There are several issues of concern regarding angioplasty for coarctation. The balloon dilation results in transmural disruption of the aortic wall in many patients, and there is an acute and ongoing risk for aneurysm formation. To limit this risk and minimize the potential of recurrence, off-label use of stents has been done for treatment of coarctation. Obvious issues of concern include somatic growth and lifetime risk potential of a metal device in the descending aorta.

Another controversial issue surrounds the concomitant treatment of coarctation and significant intracardiac pathology. Several series have demonstrated superior outcomes for simultaneous therapy in selected groups of patients, including neonates with large VSDs and coarctation with arch hypoplasia. Our approach to this condition has included one-stage complete repair of intracardiac defects along with aortic arch advancement through median sternotomy on cardiopulmonary bypass.

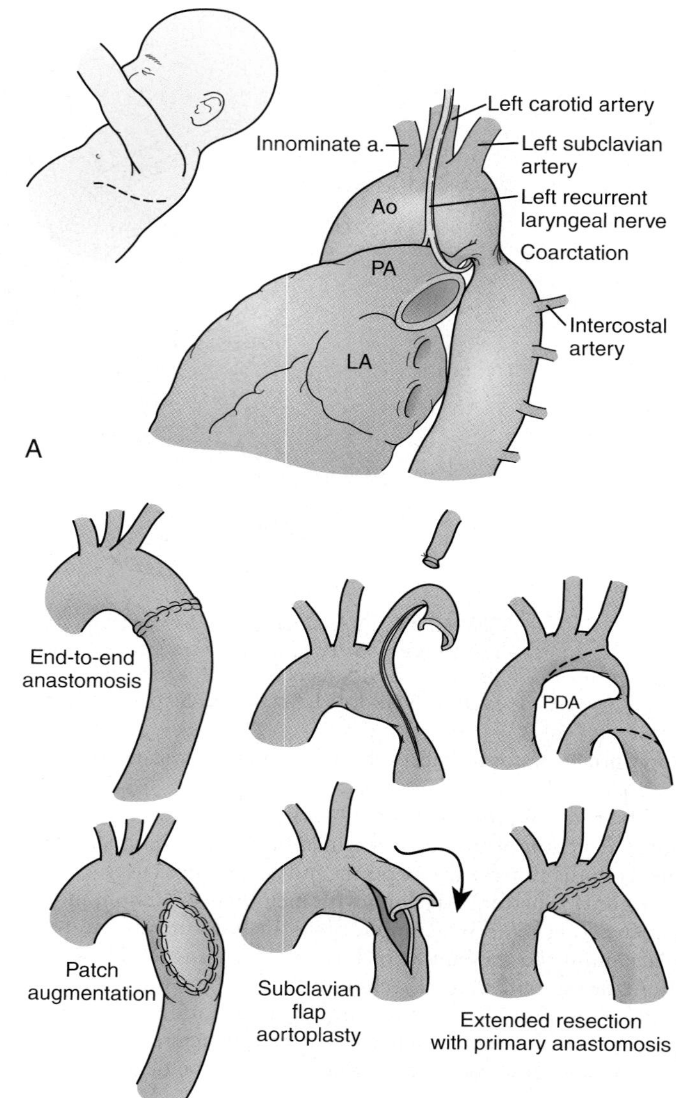

FIG. 59.35 Surgical repair for aortic coarctation. (A) Surgical incision and anatomic orientation. (B) Four different methods are shown: end-to-end anastomosis, patch augmentation, subclavian flap aortoplasty, and extended resection with primary anastomosis. (Adapted from Hastings LA, Nichols DG. Coarctation of the aorta and interrupted aortic arch. In: Nichols DG, Ungerleider RM, Spevak PJ, et al, eds. *Critical heart disease in infants and children*. Philadelphia, PA: Mosby; 2006:635.) *Ao*, Aorta; *LA*, left atrium; *PA*, pulmonary artery; *PDA*, patent ductus arteriosus.

Interrupted Aortic Arch

IAA results from lack of proper fusion and involution of the fetal aortic arches and represents 1.3% of all CHD. This is a fatal condition without treatment, and IAA is frequently associated with serious intracardiac pathology. IAA is classified based on the level of the interruption. Type A is distal to the left subclavian artery, type B occurs between left subclavian and common carotid arteries, and type C occurs proximal to the left subclavian artery (Fig. 59.36). There is a frequent finding of an aberrant right subclavian artery (retroesophageal) from the descending aorta. Survival for patients with IAA is initially predicated on ductal patency; thus, a PGE1 infusion is required to stabilize the patient. Diagnosis is confirmed by echocardiography; other methods, including cardiac catheterization, are needed infrequently.

IAA requires surgical treatment in the newborn period, which typically involves simultaneous repair of intracardiac lesions (Fig. 59.37). Repair may be accomplished with the aid of an aortic arch augmentation patch, although researchers at Texas Children's Hospital reported a series confirming that a primary tissue-tissue repair can be performed in most patients and minimizes the potential for recurrent aortic arch obstruction.[45]

SINGLE VENTRICLE

Single-ventricle physiology is a frequently encountered form of CHD. Patients may present as newborns with inadequate pulmonary blood flow, excessive pulmonary blood flow, or balanced circulations. The single ventricle may be of right, left, or indeterminate morphology. Surgical treatment is required to provide adequate systemic oxygen delivery, while protecting the pulmonary

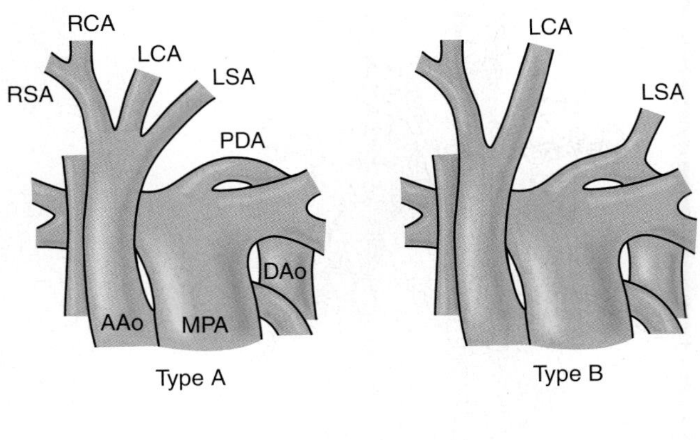

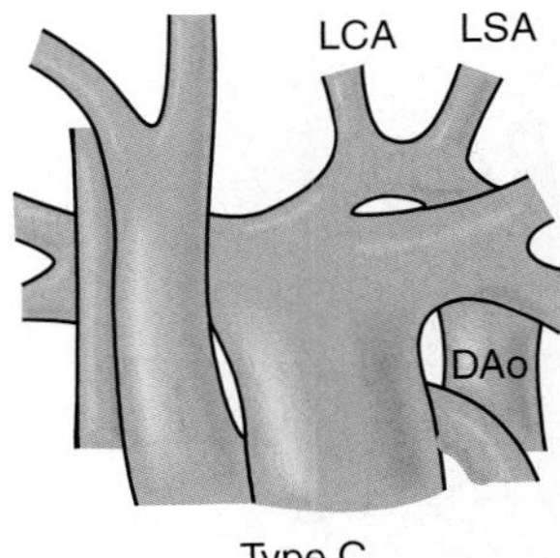

FIG. 59.36 Classification of interrupted aortic arch. (Adapted from Monro JL. Interruption of aortic arch. In: Stark J, de Leval M, eds. *Surgery for congenital heart defects.* 2nd ed. Philadelphia, PA: Saunders; 1994:299.) *AAo,* Ascending aorta; *DAo,* descending aorta; *LCA,* left common carotid artery; *LSA,* left subclavian artery; *MPA,* main pulmonary artery; *PDA,* patent ductus arteriosus; *RCA,* right common carotid artery; *RSA,* right subclavian artery.

vasculature. The function of the single ventricle must be preserved to afford the patient the best possible long-term outcome.

The rapid evolution of successful palliation for patients with various forms of single-ventricle physiology since the late 1970s has led to a large and growing population of adults with a single ventricle. For most of these patients, lifelong cardiac attention is needed, and the potential for subsequent cardiac reoperation is high. Patients in this category who present for noncardiac surgery may be especially difficult to manage because of their challenging physiology.

An exhaustive discussion of the various forms of single ventricles is well beyond the scope of this chapter. This discussion is limited to common forms of single right and left ventricles to provide examples of the surgical management strategies for a single ventricle.

Tricuspid Atresia

Tricuspid atresia is the template of a single-ventricle lesion for which most current palliative strategies were developed. Tricuspid atresia occurs in 1 of every 10,000 live births. Patients with tricuspid atresia have a single morphologic left ventricle and may have normally related or transposed great vessels (Fig. 59.38). They may present with excessive pulmonary blood flow and require pulmonary artery banding early in infancy to relieve pulmonary overcirculation and CHF. Conversely, patients may have pulmonary stenosis or pulmonary atresia and require creation of a Blalock shunt to provide adequate pulmonary blood flow and systemic oxygenation.

As noted, the initial palliative goals in patients with tricuspid atresia include adequate systemic oxygenation, protection of ventricular function, and adequate pulmonary arterial growth. Patients with ductal-dependent pulmonary blood flow require a Blalock shunt in the newborn period. We prefer to construct the shunt to the morphologic right pulmonary artery through a right thoracotomy. This construction allows shunt flow to be governed by the size of the subclavian artery. Furthermore, the right pulmonary artery is typically longer and runs in a more horizontal plane compared with the left pulmonary artery; this facilitates avoiding distortion of a lobar branch. The goal of the shunt is to protect the pulmonary arteries, promote adequate pulmonary artery development, and support systemic arterial oxygenation for the first 4 to 6 months of life until the next planned stage of palliation (see later discussion of Glenn and Fontan operations). The shunt is not designed for long-term use; thus, in most patients, a small interposition graft (expanded polytetrafluoroethylene, 3.0 to 4.0 mm) is selected. In the early era of single-ventricle palliation, less well-controlled shunts were constructed, including classic Blalock (divided native subclavian artery-to-branch pulmonary artery), Pott's (side-to-side left pulmonary artery to descending aorta), and Waterston (side-to-side right pulmonary artery to ascending aorta) shunts (Fig. 59.39). These native tissue-tissue connections are capable of somatic growth but have the confounding risks for pulmonary overcirculation, pulmonary artery hypertension (potentially irreversible), and branch pulmonary artery distortion with hypoplasia. During the early stages of development of single-ventricle palliation, many patients were treated with these poorly controlled shunts. Thus, significant numbers of adult patients present with complications of these palliations, including chronic cardiac volume overload and decreased ventricular function, severe pulmonary artery distortion or isolation, pulmonary vascular disease, and profound cyanosis. These patients may present for surgery for noncardiac illness and are extremely difficult to manage.

Hypoplastic Left Heart Syndrome

Hypoplastic left heart syndrome (HLHS) is the prototypical single right ventricle. HLHS occurs in 8 to 25 per 100,000 live births. Patients with this condition present with inadequate left heart structures ranging from mitral stenosis and AS with left ventricular hypoplasia to almost complete absence of the left heart structures with aortic and mitral atresia. In the case of aortic and mitral atresia, the ascending aorta is typically small (1–2 mm) and is perfused through retrograde aortic arch flow provided by the PDA. In HLHS, ductal closure results in rapid cardiovascular collapse, with profound systemic hypoperfusion and hypoxia, followed quickly by death. Therefore, in cases of prenatal diagnosis, patients must be born in a facility qualified to institute appropriate medical management immediately, including the establishment of suitable vascular access (umbilical artery catheter) and institution of intravenous PGE1 to maintain ductal patency. Patients with HLHS undiagnosed at birth typically have an early grace period of a few hours, but with the initiation of ductal closure, these children become critically ill and require aggressive resuscitation for survival. Although most children with HLHS are otherwise normal, without treatment, HLHS is a uniformly fatal condition (Fig. 59.40).

After delivery, medical treatment is directed at maintaining ductal patency and balancing systemic and pulmonary blood flow. Balancing the circulations becomes increasingly challenging with the normal decline in neonatal PVR, resulting in massive pulmonary overcirculation. As the overcirculation progresses, infants become tachypneic and may exhibit decreased systemic perfusion.

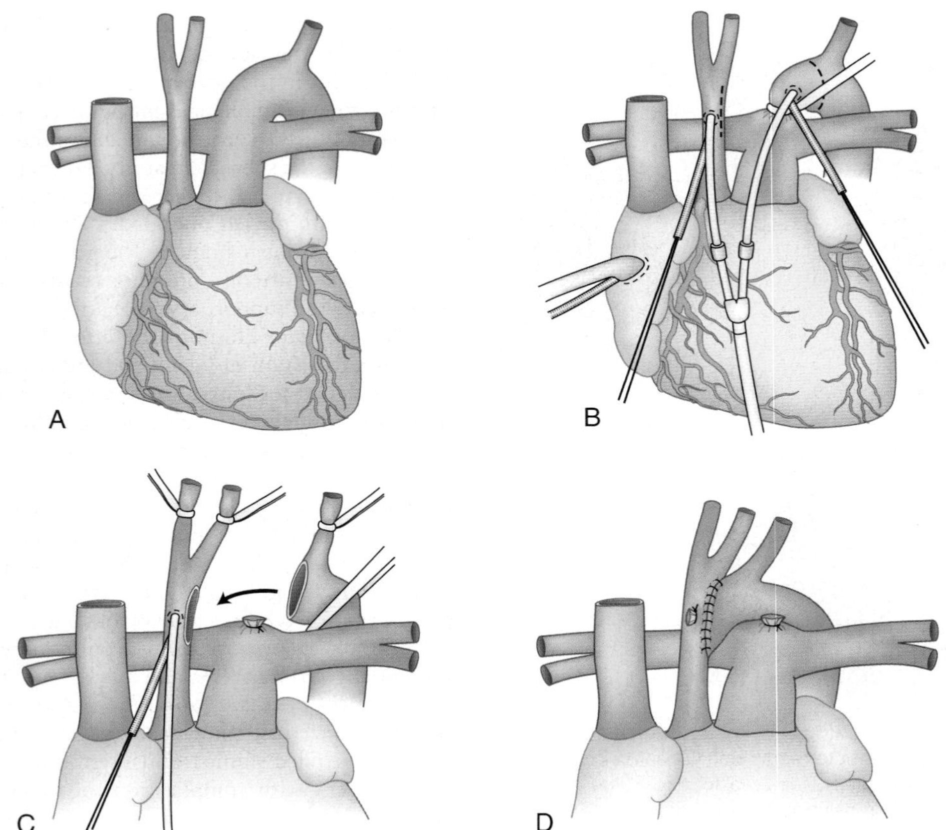

FIG. 59.37 (A) Type B interrupted aortic arch. (B) Cannulation and site of incision for repair. The descending thoracic aorta is brought upward into the mediastinum (C) and then anastomosed to the ascending aorta in an end-to-side fashion (D). (From Hirooka K, Fraser CD. One-stage neonatal repair of complex aortic arch obstruction or interruption. *Tex Heart Inst J.* 1997;24:317–321.)

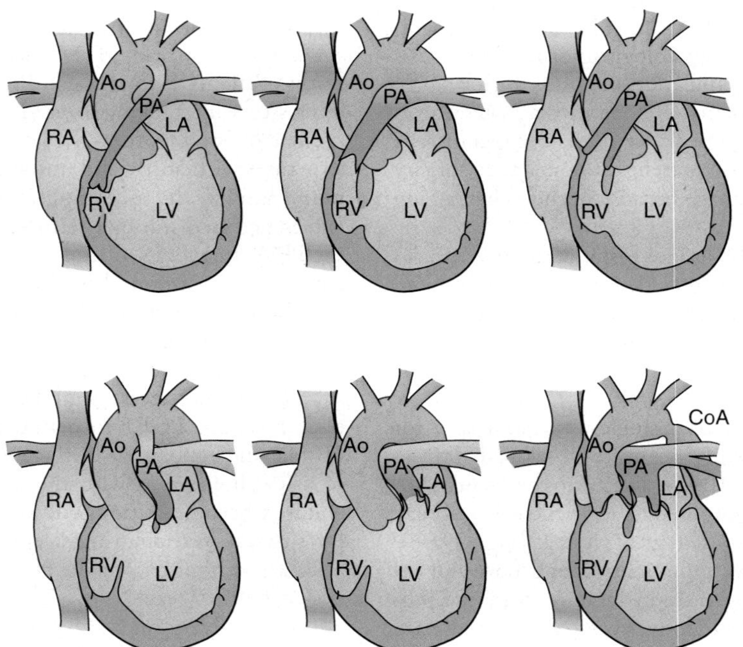

FIG. 59.38 Anatomy of the various types of tricuspid atresia. *Top,* Normally related great vessels. *Bottom,* D-Transposition of the great vessels. (Adapted from Lok JM, Spevak PJ, Nichols DG. Tricuspid atresia. In: Nichols DG, Ungerleider RM, Spevak PJ, et al, eds. *Critical heart disease in infants and children.* Philadelphia, PA: Mosby; 2006:800–801.) *Ao,* Aorta; *CoA,* coarctation of the aorta; *LA,* left atrium; *LV,* left ventricle; *PA,* pulmonary artery; *RA,* right atrium; *RV,* right ventricle.

CLASSIC RIGHT BLALOCK-TAUSSIG

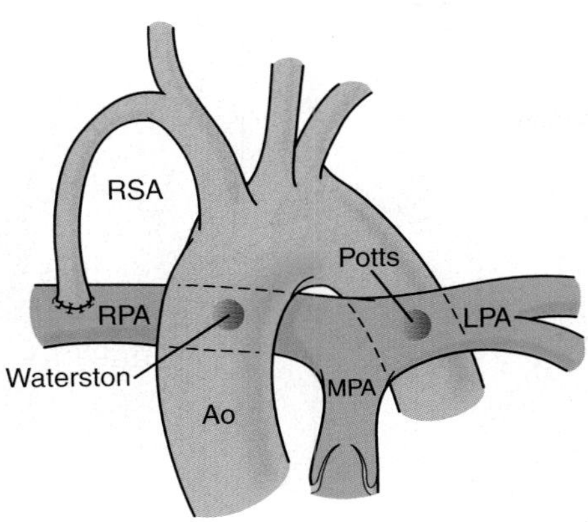

RIGHT MODIFIED BLALOCK-TAUSSIG

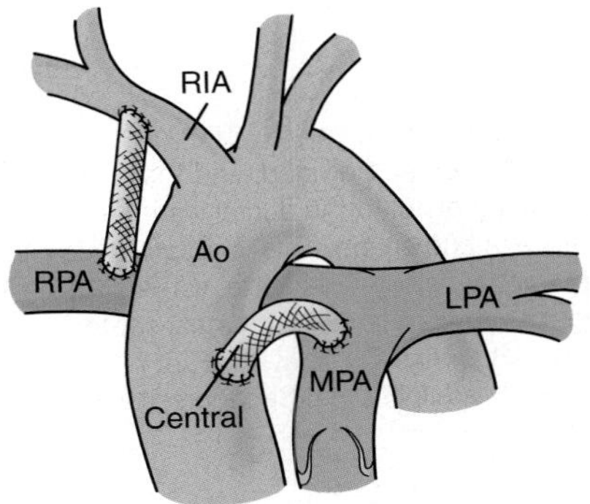

FIG. 59.39 Systemic-to-pulmonary artery shunts. (Adapted from Marino BS, Wernovsky G, Greeley WJ. Single-ventricle lesions. In: Nichols DG, Ungerleider RM, Spevak PJ, et al, eds. *Critical heart disease in infants and children.* Philadelphia, PA: Mosby; 2006:793.) *Ao,* Aorta; *LPA,* left pulmonary artery; *MPA,* main pulmonary artery; *RIA,* right innominate artery; *RPA,* right pulmonary artery; *RSA,* right subclavian artery.

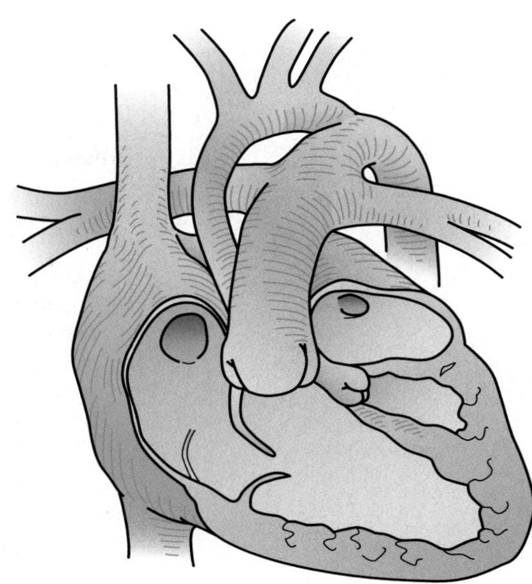

FIG. 59.40 Anatomy of hypoplastic left heart syndrome. The tiny ascending aorta is seen arising from a markedly hypoplastic left ventricle. The ductus arteriosus is large, providing forward flow to the systemic circuit. The right ventricle is hypertrophied, and the pulmonary artery is enlarged. (From Wernovsky G, Bove EL. Single ventricle lesions. In: Chang AC, Hanley FL, Wernovsky G, et al, eds. *Pediatric cardiac intensive care.* Baltimore, MD: Williams & Wilkins; 1998.)

Necrotizing enterocolitis is a significant risk in these children, and if there is any question of visceral malperfusion, many centers avoid enteral nutrition in an effort to minimize this potential. Other medical maneuvers include deliberate hypoventilation, low inspired oxygen concentration, and additional carbon dioxide in an attempt to increase PVR and limit pulmonary flow. These options are of limited use in newborns with HLHS; over days to weeks, the infants become progressively ill with pulmonary congestion and marginal systemic cardiac output. Patients who are maintained have the potential of developing increased PVR as they age, and there is a known association with advanced age (>30 days) and increased operative mortality.

Surgery in the newborn period is the only realistic option for long-term survival in infants born with HLHS. Outcomes for surgical palliation of HLHS have come to be synonymous with the reputation of the treating center and surgeons. As with tricuspid atresia, patients with HLHS require a staged palliative approach. In the experiences of all centers, the first stage is the most challenging and risk-laden. The various first-stage options are described in the following sections.

Neonatal Cardiac Transplantation

Transplantation is a theoretically attractive option in infants with HLHS that replaces the malformed heart with a structurally normal one. Leonard Bailey was an influential champion of this approach and was the first to report exciting results with transplantation in newborns with HLHS.[46] Furthermore, although there is an ever-present risk for rejection and infection in children with heart transplants, long-term meaningful survival is possible, and the quality of life of the recipients is good. The option of cardiac transplantation is limited by the small numbers of suitable donor hearts, and most children with HLHS are unable to survive the wait time for a donor graft. This situation has led most centers to abandon cardiac transplantation as the primary mode of therapy for most neonates with HLHS.

Norwood Reconstruction

After initial work and success at Boston Children's Hospital, Norwood and colleagues[47] gained international attention at the Children's Hospital of Philadelphia for developing and implementing a reconstructive technique to palliate newborns with HLHS; this methodology now carries the widely used eponym of the Norwood procedure. This procedure was gradually refined as experience accrued. The most common method involves surgical connection of the divided main pulmonary artery to the reconstructed aortic arch. In almost all children with HLHS, there is associated aortic arch hypoplasia with coarctation. A critical feature of the operation is to reconstruct the aortic arch to provide unrestricted systemic blood flow. Most surgeons use some form of prosthetic material, usually pulmonary artery homograft patching. Some surgeons have reported accomplishing the arch reconstruction without the necessity of additional material. After reconstructing the aortic arch, the divided main pulmonary artery is anastomosed to the arch and small ascending aorta to create a neoaortic confluence providing systemic output from the right ventricle. The challenging feature of the reconstruction involves the accurate connection of this often-miniscule ascending aorta to the confluence of the arch and main pulmonary artery stump.

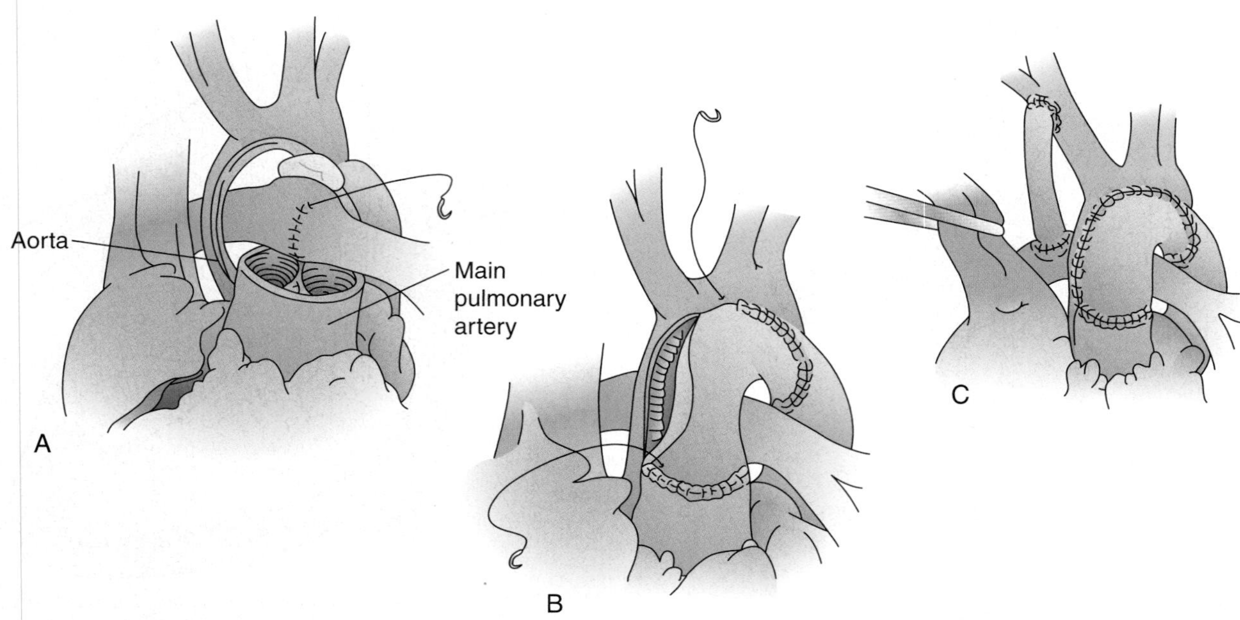

FIG. 59.41 Norwood procedure for first-stage palliation of hypoplastic left heart syndrome. (A), The main pulmonary artery is divided proximal to the bifurcation, the ductus arteriosus is ligated and divided, and the aortic arch is opened from the level of the transected main pulmonary artery to a point distal to the ductal insertion in the descending aorta. (B) A segment of homograft is cut to an appropriate size and shape. This is sutured into place, creating an unobstructed outflow from the right ventricle to the pulmonary artery and aorta. (C) Polytetrafluoroethylene tube graft is placed from the innominate artery to the right pulmonary artery. The atrial septectomy is done while the patient is under circulatory arrest. (From Castaneda AR, Jonas RA, Mayer JE, et al. Hypoplastic left heart syndrome. In: *Cardiac surgery of the neonate and infant*. Philadelphia, PA: Saunders; 1994.)

The risk for torsion and coronary insufficiency is high. The final element of the classic Norwood reconstruction is the creation of a controlled source of pulmonary blood flow in the form of a modified BT shunt (Fig. 59.41).

Sano Modification of the Norwood Operation

Achieving survival after the Norwood operation is challenging, involving innumerable technical and medical details. At best, after a Norwood procedure, the patient is fragile, with a delicate balance between systemic and pulmonary blood flow. This fact and the observation of widely disparate outcomes for the procedure have led to many important advances in the treatment of these children. One issue relates to the difficulty of balancing the systemic to pulmonary artery shunt, which lowers diastolic blood pressure (and coronary perfusion pressure) and volume loads the heart. Sano and associates[48] from Okayama University in Japan were the first to report a series of infants undergoing a successful Norwood procedure with the modification of a right ventricle–pulmonary artery conduit rather than a Blalock shunt. The theoretical advantage of this approach is the increase in diastolic pressure, creating a physiology more similar to a banded circulation rather than shunted circulation. Early reports with this method were encouraging, although patients appeared to become more rapidly desaturated as they aged compared with the shunted patients. The long-term effects of the right ventriculotomy on cardiac function are unknown. In one report, patients undergoing the Norwood operation were randomly assigned to receive a right ventricle-to-pulmonary artery shunt or modified BT shunt. Transplantation-free survival was higher 12 months after randomization in the right ventricle-to-pulmonary artery shunt group, as was the rate of unplanned reinterventions and complications.[49] More recent updates on the same cohort revealed no difference in transplant-free survival at 6 years after randomization between the right ventricle to pulmonary artery shunt group and the modified BT shunt group. However, the right ventricle to pulmonary artery group did have a greater number of catheter-based interventions.[50]

Hybrid Procedure

The notion of a combined therapy between interventional cardiology and surgery for the first-stage palliation of HLHS has achieved significant attention. The idea is to minimize the risk of the first operation by banding the branch pulmonary arteries and delivering a stent into the ductus to maintain patency. This hybrid arrangement is designed to allow newborn survival so that a more complete reconstruction may be performed later in infancy in a larger child. There appears to be a significant learning curve with this approach, as with any new procedure, and the incidence of complications warrants further study. Data have shown that the prevalence of necrotizing enterocolitis after the hybrid procedure is significant and comparable to reports after the Norwood procedure.[51] A recent meta analysis revealed increased early mortality and worse 1-year transplant-free survival in patients undergoing the hybrid procedure compared to the Norwood. However, it is noted that the hybrid procedure was preferentially utilized in higher risk patients thus making it difficult to draw firm conclusions.[52] In addition, concerning features include the effect of the banding on long-term pulmonary artery growth, the fact that cardiac perfusion is still retrograde through the aortic arch, and the risk profile of the more extensive reconstruction later in life. The true place for this mode of therapy is unclear at the present time, but it represents an important direction of advancement to optimize the opportunity of survival for these children.

Fontan Operation

The long-term goal of single-ventricle palliation is to optimize ventricular function and promote systemic oxygen delivery. As noted earlier, patients with a single ventricle who are shunted or banded have ongoing concerns, including systemic desaturation, continued intracardiac mixing, and chronic cardiac volume overload. The current strategy for addressing these concerns uses a direct connection between the branch pulmonary arteries and systemic venous return, as initially proposed by Fontan in the early 1970s. The Fontan operation is now the treatment of choice for children born with all varieties of single ventricle and provides acceptable long-term palliation in suitable patients. However, the Fontan circulation is not normal and even in the best of circumstances results in significant alteration in normal cardiorespiratory physiology.

The Fontan circulation is established by connecting the systemic venous return directly into isolated branch pulmonary arteries without an intervening power source. Thus, blood flow in the Fontan circuit is passive, being promoted only by the pressure differential between the systemic venous system and pulmonary venous atrium. An impediment to flow in the systemic-to-pulmonary pathway results in a poor Fontan outcome. Established criteria for creating an effective Fontan circulation include the ability to connect the systemic venous return surgically to the pulmonary arteries in an unobstructed manner, normal pulmonary artery architecture and resistance, normal pulmonary venous drainage and low left atrial pressure, absence of significant A-V valve regurgitation, good ventricular function (and low ventricular end-diastolic pressure), an unobstructed systemic arterial outlet, and good aortic valve function. Compromise of any of these elements may compromise the quality of the Fontan circulation.

The Fontan operation has undergone several technical modifications in the almost 40 years of successful application to patients with single-ventricle physiology. Many patients underwent an atriopulmonary connection in which the open right atrial appendage was directly anastomosed to the pulmonary artery bifurcation with surgical closure of the ASD. Many of these patients present as adults with extreme dilation of the right atrium, with resulting sluggish flow, hepatic congestion, and atrial dysrhythmias (Fig. 59.42). Today, the most widely practiced modification of the Fontan operation is the total cavopulmonary connection. First described by DeLeval, this operation involves connection of the divided SVC to the superior and inferior aspects of the right pulmonary artery (typically offset), along with the creation of a channel to direct the IVC flow into the pulmonary arteries. The channel may be created using a surgically created lateral tunnel in the right atrium (Fig. 59.43) or interposing a conduit between the IVC and pulmonary arteries (extracardiac Fontan) (Fig. 59.44).

The change from a volume-loaded circulation in patients with a single ventricle who are shunted or banded to a Fontan circulation results in acute volume unloading of the systemic ventricle. In the chronic overloaded heart, this acute change may be poorly tolerated, with resultant diastolic dysfunction and decreased ventricular compliance. To deal with this problem, patients with a single ventricle typically undergo an intervening stage of palliation in the form of a bidirectional, superior cavopulmonary anastomosis (Glenn shunt). The bidirectional Glenn shunt is constructed by anastomosing the cephalad end of the divided SVC to the superior aspect of the right pulmonary artery (Fig. 59.45). Other sources of pulmonary blood flow are typically eliminated, and the heart is volume-unloaded; however, systemic cardiac output is maintained because the IVC return is preserved. After the Glenn shunt, the patients are not fully saturated; typically, patients have saturations of approximately 80%. Over time, the unloaded ventricle remodels, and the patient is promoted to reoperation and completion of the Fontan circulation.

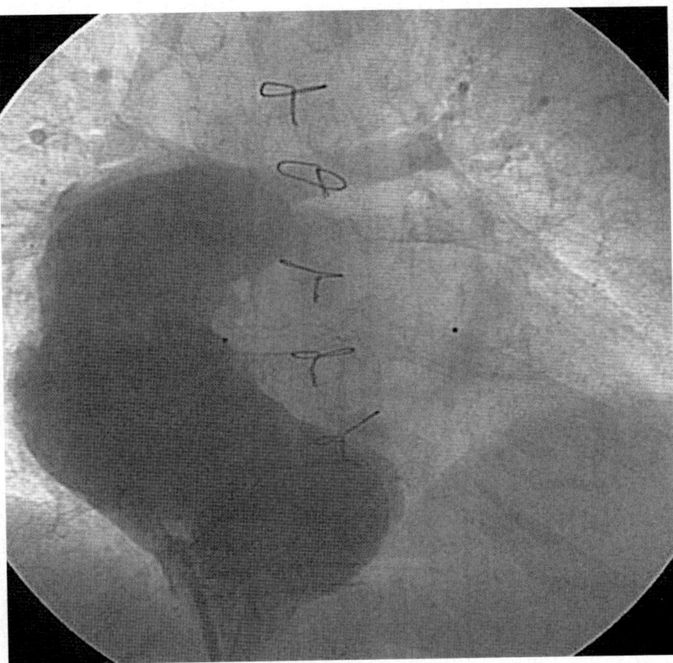

FIG. 59.42 Angiogram of a dilated right atrium in a patient with an atriopulmonary Fontan connection.

Perioperative care of a patient after a Fontan procedure can be challenging. The acute changes in cardiac volume loading may negatively affect cardiac output. Even in patients with supposedly ideal Fontan connections, the central venous pressure acutely increases to 12 to 15 mm Hg. Consequences of this increased venous pressure include pleural effusions, hepatic congestion, and ascites. In marginal Fontan candidates, some surgeons routinely place an intentional leak, or fenestration; the goal here is to preserve systemic ventricular volume loading and decrease systemic venous congestion at the expense of some degree of desaturation caused by the right-to-left shunting. The practice of routine fenestration after the Fontan operation has been examined, and some early data have shown that excellent outcomes can be achieved with highly selective application of a fenestration, which mitigates the risks associated with such a procedure, including hypoxia and systemic embolism.[53] Any impediment to passive pulmonary blood flow will inhibit Fontan flow and result in right heart failure. Positive pressure ventilation, especially elevated levels of positive end-expiratory pressure, impedes pulmonary blood flow in the Fontan patient. Conversely, early extubation and effective spontaneous ventilation will improve pulmonary blood flow in the Fontan patient. Data have suggested that early extubation in the operating room for patients after the Fontan procedure improves hemodynamics, decreases the length of stay for patients, and decreases hospital costs.

The chronic complications of living with a Fontan circulation are still unfolding and include chronic hepatic congestion and cirrhosis, protein-losing enteropathy, atrial dysrhythmias, and venous stasis disease. Management of patients with failing Fontan circulations is especially challenging. These patients are at high risk for severe cardiac compromise while undergoing general anesthesia with positive pressure ventilation or any procedure

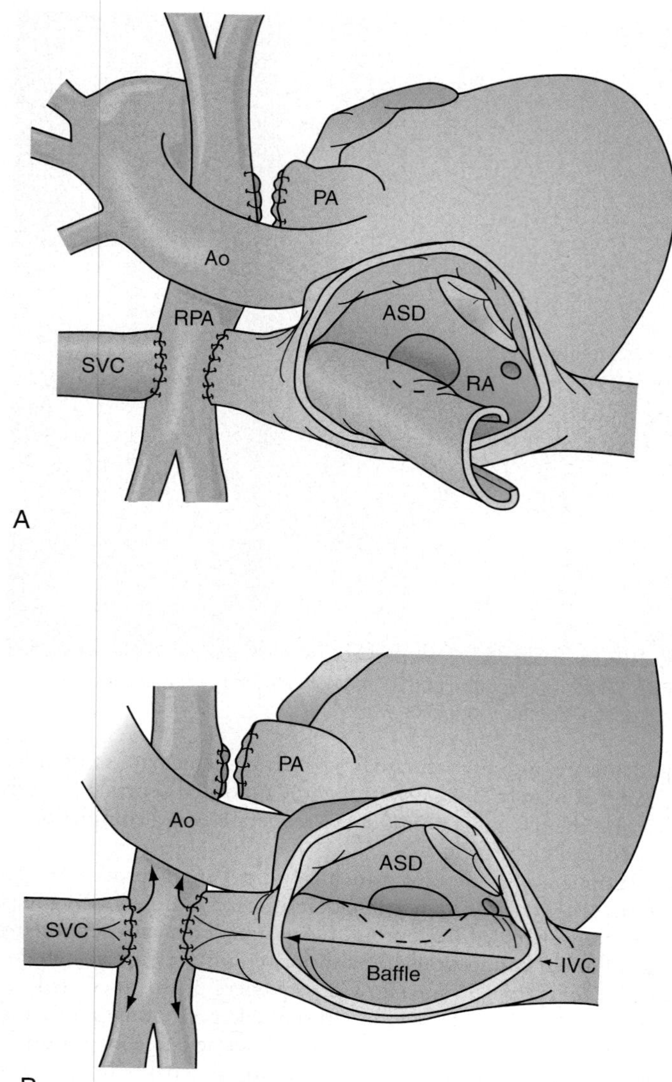

FIG. 59.43 (A) and (B), Lateral tunnel Fontan procedure. (Adapted from Lok JM, Spevak PJ, Nichols DG. Tricuspid atresia. In: Nichols DG, Ungerleider RM, Spevak PJ, et al, eds. *Critical heart disease in infants and children.* Philadelphia, PA: Mosby; 2006:813.) *Ao,* Aorta; *ASD,* atrial septal defect; *IVC,* inferior vena cava; *PA,* pulmonary artery; *RA,* right atrium; *RPA,* right pulmonary artery; *SVC,* superior vena cava.

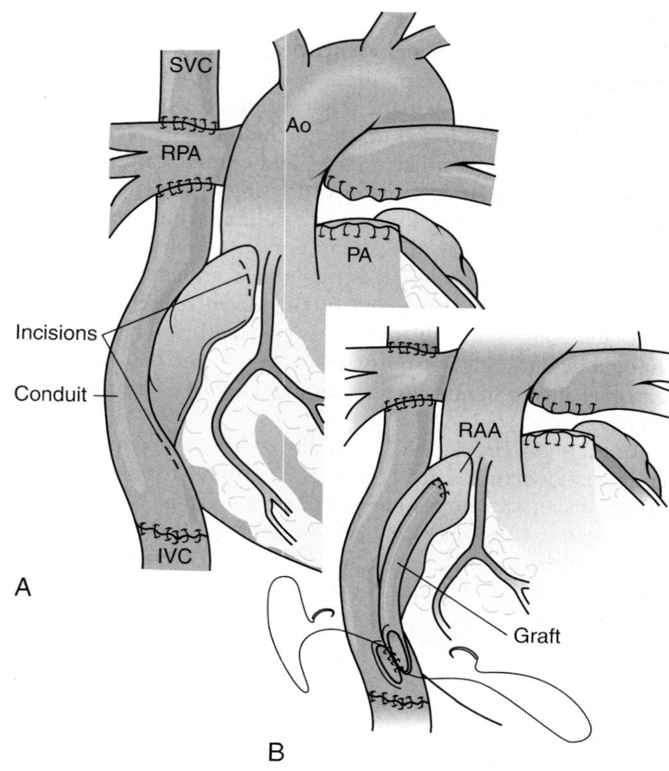

FIG. 59.44 (A) Extracardiac Fontan procedure. (B) Creation of a fenestration in an extracardiac Fontan procedure using a graft between the extracardiac conduit and right atrial appendage *(RAA).* (Adapted from Lok JM, Spevak PJ, Nichols DG. Tricuspid atresia. In: Nichols DG, Ungerleider RM, Spevak PJ, et al, eds. *Critical heart disease in infants and children.* Philadelphia, PA: Mosby; 2006:814.) *Ao,* Aorta; *IVC,* inferior vena cava; *PA,* pulmonary artery; *RPA,* right pulmonary artery; *SVC,* superior vena cava.

involving large fluid shifts, including abdominal surgery. Patients with chronic hepatic congestion may develop a coagulopathy related to a decrease in factor production.

MISCELLANEOUS ANOMALIES

Vascular Rings and Pulmonary Artery Slings

Vascular Rings

Vascular rings are abnormalities of the aortic arch and its branches, compressing the trachea, esophagus, or both. The ring may be complete or partial. Categorization of the defects is useful for description:

- Complete vascular rings
- Double arch: Equal arches or left or right arch dominant (Fig. 59.46)
- Right arch: Left ligamentum arteriosus from anomalous left subclavian artery
- Right arch: Mirror image branching, with left ligamentum from descending aorta
- Partial vascular rings
- Left arch: Aberrant right subclavian artery
- Left arch: Innominate artery compression

The double aortic arch is the most common form of complete ring. Two arches arise from the ascending aorta, forming a true ring. The left arch is usually smaller. The right arch–left ligamentum complex is formed from persistence of the right fourth arch and regression of the left fourth arch. The anomalously arising left subclavian artery is often associated with a diverticulum at its base (Kommerell diverticulum). In partial rings, the most common form is an aberrant right subclavian artery arising distal to the left subclavian artery with a left arch. The right subclavian artery passes behind the esophagus from left to right. Innominate artery compression arises from a more posterior and leftward origin of the innominate artery from a left arch, leading to anterior compression of the trachea.

Pulmonary Artery Slings

A pulmonary artery sling occurs when the left pulmonary artery arises from the right pulmonary artery, passing leftward between the trachea and the esophagus. The ligamentum arteriosum attachment from the main pulmonary artery to the undersurface of the aorta forms a vascular ring around the trachea but not the esophagus. The trachea may be compressed, the cartilage may be soft, or there may be intrinsic stenosis of the trachea in the form of complete cartilage rings.

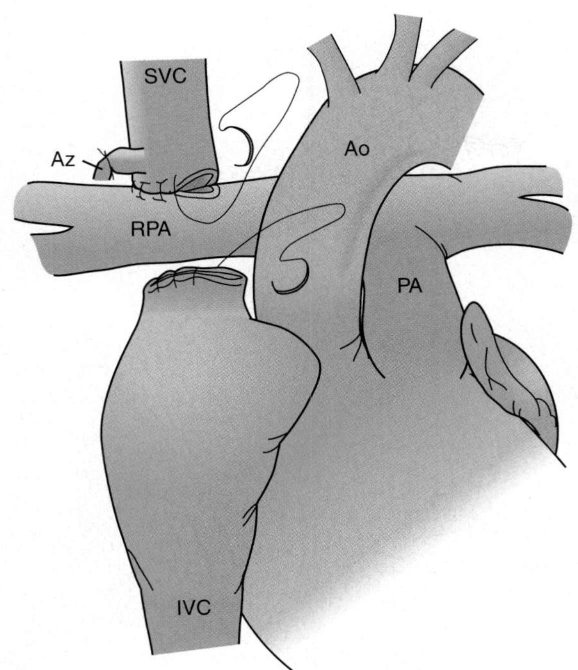

FIG. 59.45 Bidirectional Glenn shunt. (Adapted from Lok JM, Spevak PJ, Nichols DG. Tricuspid atresia. In: Nichols DG, Ungerleider RM, Spevak PJ, et al, eds. *Critical heart disease in infants and children.* Philadelphia, PA: Mosby; 2006:809.) *Ao,* Aorta; *Az,* azygos vein; *IVC,* inferior vena cava; *PA,* pulmonary artery; *RPA,* right pulmonary artery; *SVC,* superior vena cava.

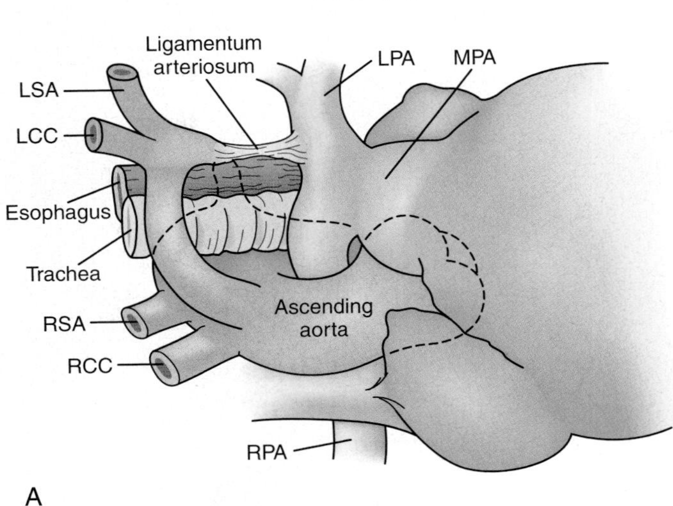

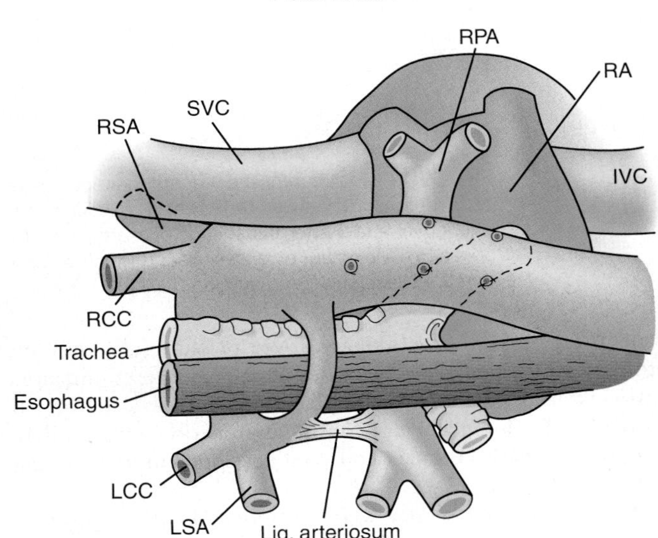

FIG. 59.46 Double aortic arch, anterior (A) and posterior (B) views. (Adapted from Jonas RA. *Comprehensive surgical management of congenital heart disease.* New York, NY: Oxford University Press; 2004:499.) *IVC,* Inferior vena cava; *LCC,* left common carotid artery; *Lig.,* ligamentum; *LPA,* left pulmonary artery; *LSA,* left subclavian artery; *MPA,* main pulmonary artery; *RA,* right atrium; *RCC,* right common carotid artery; *RPA,* right pulmonary artery; *RSA,* right subclavian artery; *SVC,* superior vena cava.

Diagnosis and Indications for Intervention

Symptoms reflect the degree of tracheal and esophageal compression from complete rings as well as the presence of coexistent tracheomalacia or stenosis. Upper respiratory symptoms predominate, with a characteristic brassy cough, recurrent respiratory infections, failure to thrive, and sometimes esophageal motility problems. In children, documentation of a ring is an indication for surgery. Older patients are often asymptomatic. Initially, the diagnosis is based on a high index of suspicion, and barium swallow is the first investigation. Echocardiography can document an abnormal head and neck vessel branching pattern, excluding intracardiac abnormalities. MRI provides complete anatomic detail.

Surgery

Most vascular rings are accessible through a left posterolateral thoracotomy; the exception is a left arch with right-sided ligamentum. Division of the ring and, in the case of double arch, preservation of the dominant arch is performed. Preservation of the recurrent laryngeal nerve is important. Initial experience with endoscopic robotically assisted repair of vascular rings has also been reported. Pulmonary artery slings are approached through the midline; the use of cardiopulmonary bypass facilitates tracheal reconstruction and relocation of the right pulmonary artery (Fig. 59.47). Repair can be achieved with low risk. Symptoms may take months to resolve, with slow resolution of the underlying tracheomalacia.

Coronary Artery Anomalies

Anomalies occur as a result of anomalous origin, termination, courses, and aneurysm formation. Of these variables, only an anomalous left coronary artery rising from the pulmonary artery (ALCAPA) and coronary artery fistulas are discussed here.

Anomalous Left Coronary Artery Rising From the Pulmonary Artery

An ALCAPA is a rare, often lethal lesion in early infancy. Untreated, the mortality rate approaches 90%.

Anatomy and pathophysiology. Developmentally, failure of the normal connection of the left coronary artery bud to the aorta results in an abnormal connection to the pulmonary artery. The abnormal origin can be situated in the main pulmonary artery or proximal branches. Associated abnormalities are rare but important to recognize because lowering of the pulmonary artery pressure by PDA ligation or closure of a VSD can be fatal if the ALCAPA is not noted. In utero, with equal pulmonary arterial and aortic pressures, satisfactory perfusion of the ALCAPA can

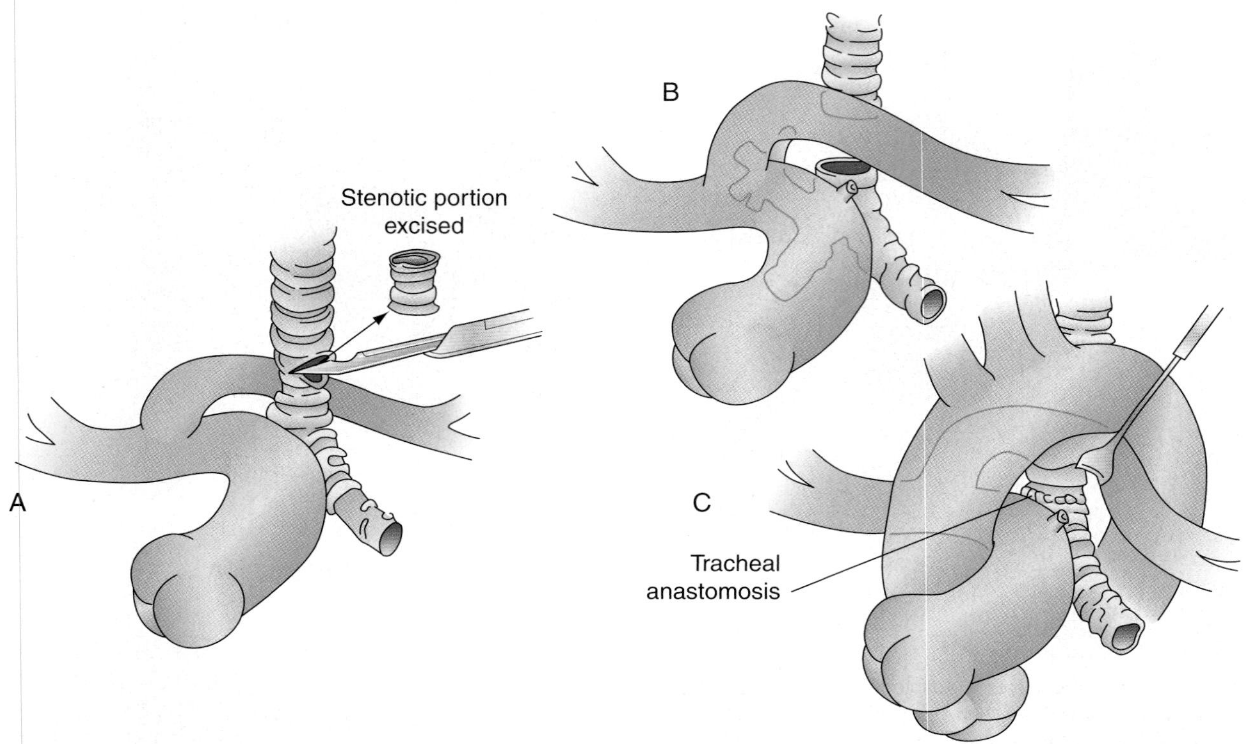

FIG. 59.47 Method for the management of a pulmonary artery sling with associated tracheal stenosis, using cardiopulmonary bypass. (A) Tracheal resection of the involved segment. (B) Anterior translocation of the left pulmonary artery after transection of the trachea. (C) Direct anastomosis of the trachea. (From Castaneda AR, Jonas RA, Mayer JE, et al. Vascular rings, slings, and tracheal anomalies. In: *Cardiac surgery of the neonate and infant.* Philadelphia, PA: Saunders; 1994.)

occur. After birth, the pulmonary artery pressure falls, and left coronary artery perfusion decreases. Ischemia causes impaired ventricular function and myocardial infarcts and leads to left ventricular dilation. Papillary muscle dysfunction causes mitral regurgitation. Early coronary collateral development may prevent ongoing infarction.

Diagnosis and indications for intervention. ALCAPA is suspected in any infant with mitral regurgitation, ventricular dysfunction, or dilated cardiomyopathy. Infants present with low cardiac output and systemic heart failure. Feeding may also precipitate sudden death and angina in infants. Sudden death has been described in older children. The ECG may reflect ischemic changes. The echocardiogram is usually diagnostic. However, because this diagnosis is often confused with dilated cardiomyopathy, there is an argument in favor of catheterizing all patients with dilated cardiomyopathy in whom the coronary artery anatomy cannot be clearly defined on echocardiography. Secondary findings of dilated cardiac chambers and segmental wall motion abnormalities together with mitral regurgitation prompt a search for an ALCAPA. Diagnosis of an ALCAPA is an indication for intervention.

Surgery. A degree of ventricular dysfunction is usually present. Preoperative inotropic support and optimization of hemodynamics may be required before surgical intervention. Severe cardiomyopathy rarely may necessitate cardiac transplantation. Current experience indicates that creation of a dual coronary system is safe and reproducible and offers the best opportunity for recovery of function. Operative considerations include optimal myocardial protection and prevention of left heart distention. Direct reimplantation of the ALCAPA into the ascending aorta is the procedure of choice (Fig. 59.48). Sometimes, limited mobility of the

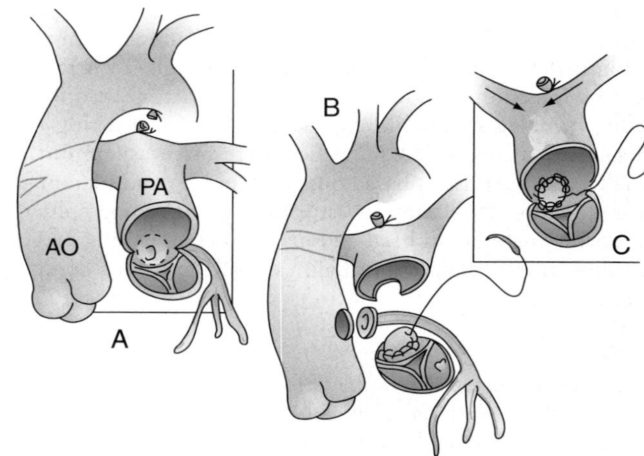

FIG. 59.48 Direct reimplantation of anomalous left coronary artery rising from the pulmonary artery (ALCAPA). (A) Excision of ALCAPA from the pulmonary artery *(PA).* (B) Aortic reimplantation of the coronary ostium into the aorta. (C) Reconstruction of the PA with autologous pericardium. (From Vouhe PR, Tamisier D, Sidi D, et al. Anomalous left coronary artery from the pulmonary artery: Results of isolated aortic reimplantation. *Ann Thorac Surg.* 1992;54:621–626.) *AO,* Aorta.

coronary artery precludes reimplantation, and a surgically created aorta–pulmonary artery–coronary artery tunnel is created; this is known as the *Takeuchi procedure.* Ligation of the ALCAPA is not recommended.

Postoperative management is directed toward maintaining adequate coronary perfusion and cardiac output. Mechanical support of the heart may be temporarily required. Mitral regurgitation usually improves, and valve replacement is rarely necessary. Current intervention has a low operative mortality. Risks for nonsurvival relate to preoperative ventricular dysfunction and cardiogenic shock. The Takeuchi repair is associated with tunnel complications such as obstruction, leak, aortic valve damage, and RVOTO in the long-term.

Coronary Arteriovenous Fistula and Aneurysms

Isolated coronary artery fistula is more rare than ALCAPA. Drainage of coronary artery fistula is reported to terminate more commonly in the right side of the heart or pulmonary artery than in the left side of the heart. A shunt from the high-pressure coronary artery system into a low-pressure cardiac chamber may result in coronary steal and some degree of cardiac volume overload. Coronary artery aneurysms are associated with Kawasaki disease.

Diagnosis and indications for intervention. Presentation depends on the amount of functional compromise produced by the ischemia and volume overload. Echocardiography may be able to delineate the anomaly, but coronary angiography is diagnostic. Details of coronary anatomy are essential for determining intervention. Interventional catheterization is useful for the obliteration of fistulas and terminal aneurysms.

Surgery. If the lesion is not amenable to transcatheter intervention, surgery is indicated. Options include suture ligation without bypass, cardiopulmonary bypass, and aneurysmectomy with closure of the fistula. Early and late mortality rates are low. Risk factors for death and ventricular dysfunction relate to coronary artery insufficiency and infarction after fistula ligation or aneurysmectomy.[54]

Ebstein Anomaly of the Tricuspid Valve

Ebstein anomaly of the tricuspid valve is a rare defect in which the tricuspid valve attachments are displaced into the right ventricle to varying degrees. Ebstein anomaly includes a spectrum of abnormalities involving a degree of displacement of the tricuspid valve, variable right ventricular size, and variable pulmonary outflow obstruction. Associated abnormalities are ASD, pulmonary atresia, and ccTGA. The posterior and septal leaflets of the tricuspid valve are variably displaced to the apex of the right ventricle, which results in an atrialized portion of the right ventricle. The anterior leaflet remains large and sail-like. The major hemodynamic issue is tricuspid incompetence with decreased pulmonary blood flow and, if an ASD is present, right-to-left shunting causing cyanosis. Long-standing tricuspid incompetence leads to volume overload of an abnormal right ventricle. Variable pulmonary outflow tract obstruction limits effective pulmonary blood flow. If adequate pulmonary blood flow requires continued ductal patency, the need for neonatal intervention is almost certain.

Diagnosis and Intervention

The more severe forms of Ebstein anomaly manifest with cyanosis in infancy. Critically ill neonates tend to have a severe form of the disease, with a grossly inefficient right ventricle compounded by the high pulmonary resistance of the neonate or by pulmonary valve atresia. The mortality rate in this group is high. Older patients present in heart failure and may have cyanosis. Supraventricular dysrhythmias and the preexcitation syndrome (Wolff-Parkinson-White syndrome) are associated with Ebstein anomaly. Echocardiography is diagnostic. Critically ill neonates have poor survival rates, and surgery is indicated only after stabilization with PGE1 and controlled ventilation. In older patients, cyanosis and heart failure are indications to intervene, although earlier intervention in asymptomatic patients, before excessive right ventricular dilation, is being more actively pursued.

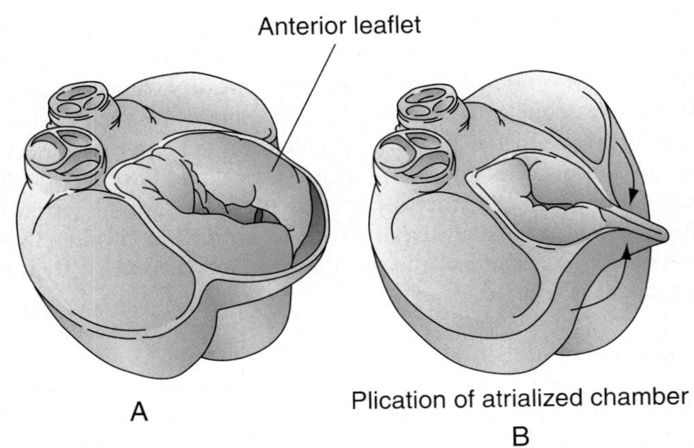

FIG. 59.49 Repair of Ebstein malformation using the Carpentier method. (A) The anterior and posterior leaflets of the tricuspid valve are detached from the annulus. (B) The atrium is plicated, reducing the annular diameter. The detached leaflets are reattached to the annulus. (From Castaneda AR, Jonas RA, Mayer JE, et al. Ebstein's anomaly. In: *Cardiac surgery of the neonate and infant*. Philadelphia, PA: Saunders; 1994.)

Surgery

In critically ill neonates, after stabilization, palliation with a systemic-to-pulmonary artery shunt may be required. The Starnes operation has allowed salvage in previously hopeless cases. This operation consists of patch closure of the tricuspid orifice, atrial septectomy, and a systemic-to-pulmonary artery shunt.[55] In patients with less severe forms of this disease, tricuspid valve repair or replacement is also an option. Surgical techniques for the treatment of Ebstein anomaly have been evolving, and outcomes are improving for this challenging group of patients (Fig. 59.49).[56]

Mitral Valve Anomalies

Most abnormalities of the mitral valve are associated with other complex lesions (e.g., Shone complex). More commonly, mitral disease in children is inflammatory in nature—that is, rheumatic disease or infective endocarditis. It may also be associated with collagen vascular disease and Marfan syndrome.

Mitral Stenosis

Mitral stenosis is caused by obstruction at a supravalvular, valvular, or subvalvular level, singly or in combination. Supravalvular stenosis is caused by a ring of fibrous tissue above the annulus of the mitral valve or attached to the proximal leaflets. Valvular stenosis involves the leaflets, with commissural fusion occurring with or without hypoplasia of the valve ring. Hypoplasia of the mitral valve is often associated with left ventricular hypoplasia. Frequently, the leaflets and subvalvular apparatus are also dysplastic. Fusion of the leaflets can lead to an accessory orifice and produce mitral stenosis at a purely valvular level (so-called double-orifice mitral valve). Three types of subvalvular stenosis have been recognized—parachute mitral valve, hammock valve, and absence of one or both papillary muscles. Mitral regurgitation is a result of secondary annular dilation, congenital isolated clefts of the valve, and prolapse of the leaflets from abnormal chordae or papillary muscle insertion.

Echocardiography is diagnostic. Intervention includes balloon valvuloplasty, particularly for selected forms of rheumatic mitral stenosis, and surgical intervention. Intervention is timed to avoid irreversible sequelae related to chronic volume overload or pulmonary hypertension. Surgical intervention is aimed at preserving the mitral valve, and valvuloplasty techniques have a valuable place in children. Prosthetic valves are the least desirable option. Bioprosthetic or tissue valves need to be avoided in children. Supraannular placement of the prosthesis may be necessary. Repeat placement is ensured.

SUMMARY

This chapter provides a basic overview of the major congenital cardiac lesions and a framework for the diagnosis and treatment of these conditions. For most patients, the diagnosis of CHD, whether surgically treated or not, carries lifelong implications. For patients with CHD presenting for noncardiac surgery, a thorough understanding of the patient's unique anatomy and physiology is mandatory when planning a rational management strategy. The reader is directed to several excellent texts on CHD for a more thorough review of each of the lesions reviewed in this chapter.

SELECTED REFERENCES

Bailey LL, Nehlsen-Cannarella SL, Doroshow RW, et al. Cardiac allotransplantation in newborns as therapy for hypoplastic left heart syndrome. *N Engl J Med.* 1986;315:949–951.

This classic reference describes the first report of cardiac transplantation in newborns with hypoplastic left heart syndrome (HLHS). Although limited in its applicability because of limited donor organs, neonatal cardiac transplantation has provided children born with HLHS a new option for survival.

Blalock A, Taussig HB. The surgical treatment of malformations of the heart in which there is pulmonary stenosis or pulmonary atresia. *JAMA.* 1945;128:189–202.

This landmark article describes the surgical procedure that initiated the era of elective cardiac surgery. The study reported the initial experience with palliative surgical treatment of patients with pulmonary stenosis or pulmonary atresia using the Blalock-Taussig shunt.

Fontan F, Baudet E. Surgical repair of tricuspid atresia. *Thorax.* 1971;26:240–248.

This article represents a milestone in the evolution of surgical management of patients with single-ventricle physiology. It described the first corrective operation for patients with tricuspid atresia. Although previous palliative procedures, provided by various systemic-to-pulmonary artery shunts, improved the clinical condition of patients, systemic blood was still a mixture of oxygenated and deoxygenated blood. The Fontan operation redirected superior and inferior vena cava blood flow to the lungs so that only oxygenated blood returned to the heart and subsequently to the systemic circulation.

Kirklin JW, Dushane JW, Patrick RT, et al. Intracardiac surgery with the aid of a mechanical pump-oxygenator system (gibbon type): report of eight cases. *Mayo Clin Proc.* 1955;30:201–206.

This landmark article demonstrated that open repairs of congenital cardiac defects using mechanical pump oxygenator systems could be performed with minimal risk to patients.

Mustard W. Successful two-stage correction of transposition of the great vessels. *Surgery.* 1964;55:469–472.

This classic reference describes one of the initial surgical approaches to the treatment of transposition of the great arteries (D-TGA). Although the arterial switch operation is now the surgical treatment of choice for D-TGA, there are many adult patients with congenital heart disease who have been palliated with the Mustard operation. Understanding the operation and resulting physiology is critical to general surgery management strategies for noncardiac operations.

Norwood WI, Lang P, Casteneda AR, et al. Experience with operations for hypoplastic left heart syndrome. *J Thorac Cardiovasc Surg.* 1981;82:511–519.

In this landmark article, Norwood and colleagues reported the outcomes of what was then a new reconstructive surgical technique to palliate newborns with hypoplastic left heart syndrome (HLHS). Until the Norwood operation, the only option for survival of patients with HLHS was cardiac transplantation. At most centers today, the Norwood operation is the primary mode of therapy for most neonates with HLHS.

Sano S, Ishino K, Kawada M, et al. Right ventricle-pulmonary artery shunt in first-stage palliation of hypoplastic left heart syndrome. *J Thorac Cardiovasc Surg.* 2003;126:504–509.

This classic reference describes the right ventricle–to–pulmonary artery conduit used in the Norwood procedure. This novel procedure, named after the author, Sano, allowed for more hemodynamic stability postoperatively from the Norwood procedure and improved intrastage survival.

Senning A. Surgical correction of transposition of the great vessels. *Surgery.* 1959;45:966–980.

This classic reference describes the initial surgical approach to management of transposition of the great arteries (D-TGA). Although the arterial switch operation is currently the surgical treatment of choice for D-TGA, there are many adult patients with congenital heart disease in the community who have had the Senning operation. Understanding the operation and resulting physiology is critical to general surgery management strategies for noncardiac operations.

Starnes VA, Pitlick PT, Bernstein D, et al. Ebstein's anomaly appearing in the neonate. A new surgical approach. *J Thorac Cardiovasc Surg.* 1991;101:1082–1087.

This classic reference describes the first report of a new surgical approach to Ebstein anomaly in neonates. The procedure was named after the surgeon, Starnes. This approach has provided children born with severe Ebstein anomaly a new option for survival.

Ungerleider RM, Meliones JN, McMillian KN, et al. *Critical Heart Disease in Infants and Children*. 3rd ed. Philadelphia, PA: Elsevier; 2019.

This text provides a comprehensive and current review of heart disease in infants and children. It contains numerous surgical drawings and diagnostic images to supplement the didactic material.

Warden HE, Cohen M, Read RC, et al. Controlled cross circulation for open intracardiac surgery: physiologic studies and results of creation and closure of ventricular septal defects. *J Thorac Surg*. 1954;28:331–341.

This landmark article described the technique of cross-circulation to facilitate cardiopulmonary bypass and intracardiac repair of congenital heart lesions. Warden and colleagues documented the successful use of cross-circulation to correct defects such as ventricular septal defect.

Wilcox B, Cook A, Anderson R. *Surgical Anatomy of the Heart*. 3rd ed. Cambridge, UK: Cambridge University Press; 2004.

This text provides an excellent reference manual for understanding the complex anatomy of the heart. It contains color photographs and diagrams and is an invaluable resource for any student of cardiac surgery.

REFERENCES

1. Blalock A, Taussig HB. The surgical treatment of malformations of the heart in which there is pulmonary stenosis or pulmonary atresia. *J Am Med Assoc*. 1945;128:189–202.
2. Warden HE, Cohen M, Read RC, et al. Controlled cross circulation for open intracardiac surgery: physiologic studies and results of creation and closure of ventricular septal defects. *J Thorac Surg*. 1954;28:331–341; discussion, 341–333.
3. Kirklin JW, Dushane JW, Patrick RT, et al. Intracardiac surgery with the aid of a mechanical pump-oxygenator system (gibbon type): report of eight cases. *Proc Staff Meet Mayo Clin*. 1955;30:201–206.
4. Marelli A, Gilboa S, Devine O, et al. Estimating the congenital heart disease population in the United States in 2010—what are the numbers? *J Am Coll Cardiol*. 2012;59; E787–E787.
5. Marelli AJ, Ionescu-Ittu R, Mackie AS, et al. Lifetime prevalence of congenital heart disease in the general population from 2000 to 2010. *Circulation*. 2014;130:749–756.
6. Levey A, Glickstein JS, Kleinman CS, et al. The impact of prenatal diagnosis of complex congenital heart disease on neonatal outcomes. *Pediatr Cardiol*. 2010;31:587–597.
7. Morris SA, Ethen MK, Penny DJ, et al. Prenatal diagnosis, birth location, surgical center, and neonatal mortality in infants with hypoplastic left heart syndrome. *Circulation*. 2014;129:285–292.
8. American Board of Thoracic Surgery. *American Board of Thoracic Surgery*. https://www.abts.org. Retrieved September 26, 2019.
9. Mullins CE. *Cardiac Catheterization in Congenital Heart Disease: Pediatric and Adult*. Malden, MA: Blackwell Futura; 2006.
10. American Board of Internal Medicine www.abim.org. *American Board of Internal Medicine*. Retrieved September 26, 2019.
11. Accreditation Council for Graduate Medical Education (ACGME). *Congenital Cardiac Surgery Programs*. https://apps.acgme.org/ads/Public/Reports/ReportRun. Retrieved September 24, 2019.
12. Wilcox BR, Cook AC, Anderson RH. *Surgical Anatomy of the Heart*. 3rd ed. Cambridge, MA: Cambridge University Press; 2004.
13. Morin RL, Gerber TC, McCollough CH. Radiation dose in computed tomography of the heart. *Circulation*. 2003;107:917–922.
14. Andropoulos DB, Stayer SA, Russell IA, et al. *Anesthesia for Congenital Heart Disease*. 2nd ed. Hoboken, NJ: Wiley-Blackwell; 2010.
15. Kintrup S, Malec E, Kiski D, et al. Extubation in the operating room after fontan procedure: does it make a difference? *Pediatr Cardiol*. 2019;40:468–476.
16. Licht DJ, Shera DM, Clancy RR, et al. Brain maturation is delayed in infants with complex congenital heart defects. *J Thorac Cardiovasc Surg*. 2009;137:529–536; discussion 536–527.
17. Noonan PM, Desai T, Degiovanni JV. Closure of an aortopulmonary window using the amplatzer duct occluder II. *Pediatr Cardiol*. 2013;34:712–714.
18. Hopkins RA, Bert AA, Buchholz B, et al. Surgical patch closure of atrial septal defects. *Ann Thorac Surg*. 2004;77:2144–2149; author reply 2149–2150.
19. Vida VL, Zanotto L, Tessari C, et al. Minimally invasive surgery for atrial septal defects: a 20-year experience at a single centre. *Interact Cardiovasc Thorac Surg*. 2019;28:961–967.
20. Farooqi M, Stickley J, Dhillon R, et al. Trends in surgical and catheter interventions for isolated congenital shunt lesions in the UK and Ireland. *Heart*. 2019;105:1103–1108.
21. Knepp MD, Rocchini AP, Lloyd TR, et al. Long-term follow up of secundum atrial septal defect closure with the amplatzer septal occluder. *Congenit Heart Dis*. 2010;5:32–37.
22. Clark JB, Chowdhury D, Pauliks LB, et al. Resolution of heart block after surgical removal of an amplatzer device. *Ann Thorac Surg*. 2010;89:1631–1633.
23. Piatkowski R, Kochanowski J, Scislo P, et al. Dislocation of amplatzer septal occluder device after closure of secundum atrial septal defect. *J Am Soc Echocardiogr*. 2010;23:1007.e1001–e1002.
24. Slesnick TC, Nugent AW, Fraser Jr CD, et al. Images in cardiovascular medicine. incomplete endothelialization and late development of acute bacterial endocarditis after implantation of an amplatzer septal occluder device. *Circulation*. 2008;117:e326–e327.
25. Neill CA, Ferencz C, Sabiston DC, et al. The familial occurrence of hypoplastic right lung with systemic arterial supply and venous drainage "scimitar syndrome". *Bull Johns Hopkins Hosp*. 1960;107:1–21.
26. Balzer D. Current status of percutaneous closure of ventricular septal defects. pediatr therapeut. *Pediatr Therapeut*. 2012;2:1000112.

27. Rastelli GC, Weidman WH, Kirklin JW. Surgical repair of the partial form of persistent common atrioventricular canal, with special reference to the problem of mitral valve incompetence. *Circulation*. 1965;31:31–35.
28. Bakhtiary F, Takacs J, Cho MY, et al. Long-term results after repair of complete atrioventricular septal defect with two-patch technique. *Ann Thorac Surg*. 2010;89:1239–1243.
29. Beckerman Z, De Leon LE, Zea-Vera R, et al. High incidence of late infective endocarditis in bovine jugular vein valved conduits. *J Thorac Cardiovasc Surg*. 2018;156:728–734. e722.
30. Chen JM, Glickstein JS, Davies RR, et al. The effect of repair technique on postoperative right-sided obstruction in patients with truncus arteriosus. *J Thorac Cardiovasc Surg*. 2005;129:559–568.
31. Balasubramanian S, Marshall AC, Gauvreau K, et al. Outcomes after stent implantation for the treatment of congenital and postoperative pulmonary vein stenosis in children. *Circ Cardiovasc Interv*. 2012;5:109–117.
32. Morales DL, Zafar F, Heinle JS, et al. Right ventricular infundibulum sparing (RVIS) tetralogy of fallot repair: a review of over 300 patients. *Ann Surg*. 2009;250:611–617.
33. Mustard WT. Successful two-stage correction of transposition of the great vessels. *Surgery*. 1964;55:469–472.
34. Senning A. Surgical correction of transposition of the great vessels. *Surgery*. 1959;45:966–980.
35. Dibardino DJ, Allison AE, Vaughn WK, et al. Current expectations for newborns undergoing the arterial switch operation. *Ann Surg*. 2004;239:588–596; discussion 596–588.
36. Yacoub MH, Radley-Smith R. Anatomy of the coronary arteries in transposition of the great arteries and methods for their transfer in anatomical correction. *Thorax*. 1978;33:418–424.
37. Ly M, Belli E, Leobon B, et al. Results of the double switch operation for congenitally corrected transposition of the great arteries. *Eur J Cardio Thorac Surg*. 2009;35:879–883; discussion 883–874.
38. Bacha EA, McElhinney DB, Guleserian KJ, et al. Surgical aortic valvuloplasty in children and adolescents with aortic regurgitation: acute and intermediate effects on aortic valve function and left ventricular dimensions. *J Thorac Cardiovasc Surg*. 2008;135:552–559, 559 e551–e553.
39. Sharabiani MT, Dorobantu DM, Mahani AS, et al. Aortic valve replacement and the ross operation in children and young adults. *J Am Coll Cardiol*. 2016;67:2858–2870.
40. Shinkawa T, Bove EL, Hirsch JC, et al. Intermediate-term results of the ross procedure in neonates and infants. *Ann Thorac Surg*. 2010;89:1827–1832; discussion 1832.
41. Booth JH, Bryant R, Powers SC, et al. Transthoracic echocardiography does not reliably predict involvement of the aortic valve in patients with a discrete subaortic shelf. *Cardiol Young*. 2010;20:284–289.
42. Donald JS, Naimo PS, d'Udekem Y, et al. Outcomes of subaortic obstruction resection in children. *Heart Lung Circ*. 2017;26:179–186.
43. Cowley CG, Orsmond GS, Feola P, et al. Long-term, randomized comparison of balloon angioplasty and surgery for native coarctation of the aorta in childhood. *Circulation*. 2005;111:3453–3456.
44. Mery CM, Guzman-Pruneda FA, Carberry KE, et al. Aortic arch advancement for aortic coarctation and hypoplastic aortic arch in neonates and infants. *Ann Thorac Surg*. 2014;98:625–633; discussion 633.
45. Morales DL, Scully PT, Braud BE, et al. Interrupted aortic arch repair: aortic arch advancement without a patch minimizes arch reinterventions. *Ann Thorac Surg*. 2006;82:1577–1583; discussion 1583–1574.
46. Bailey LL, Nehlsen-Cannarella SL, Doroshow RW, et al. Cardiac allotransplantation in newborns as therapy for hypoplastic left heart syndrome. *N Engl J Med*. 1986;315:949–951.
47. Norwood WI, Lang P, Casteneda AR, et al. Experience with operations for hypoplastic left heart syndrome. *J Thorac Cardiovasc Surg*. 1981;82:511–519.
48. Sano S, Ishino K, Kado H, et al. Outcome of right ventricle-to-pulmonary artery shunt in first-stage palliation of hypoplastic left heart syndrome: a multi-institutional study. *Ann Thorac Surg*. 2004;78:1951–1957; discussion 1957–1958.
49. Ohye RG, Sleeper LA, Mahony L, et al. Comparison of shunt types in the norwood procedure for single-ventricle lesions. *N Engl J Med*. 2010;362:1980–1992.
50. Newburger JW, Sleeper LA, Gaynor JW, et al. Transplant-free survival and interventions at 6 years in the SVR trial. *Circulation*. 2018;137:2246–2253.
51. Luce WA, Schwartz RM, Beauseau W, et al. Necrotizing enterocolitis in neonates undergoing the hybrid approach to complex congenital heart disease. *Pediatr Crit Care Med*. 2011;12:46–51.
52. Cao JY, Lee SY, Phan K, et al. Early outcomes of hypoplastic left heart syndrome infants: meta-analysis of studies comparing the hybrid and norwood procedures. *World J Pediatr Congenit Heart Surg*. 2018;9:224–233.
53. Salazar JD, Zafar F, Siddiqui K, et al. Fenestration during Fontan palliation: now the exception instead of the rule. *J Thorac Cardiovasc Surg*. 2010;140:129–136.
54. Valente AM, Lock JE, Gauvreau K, et al. Predictors of long-term adverse outcomes in patients with congenital coronary artery fistulae. *Circ Cardiovasc Interv*. 2010;3:134–139.
55. Starnes VA, Pitlick PT, Bernstein D, et al. Ebstein's anomaly appearing in the neonate. a new surgical approach. *J Thorac Cardiovasc Surg*. 1991;101:1082–1087.
56. Brown ML, Dearani JA, Danielson GK, et al. The outcomes of operations for 539 patients with ebstein anomaly. *J Thorac Cardiovasc Surg*. 2008;135:1120–1136, 1136 e1121–e1127.

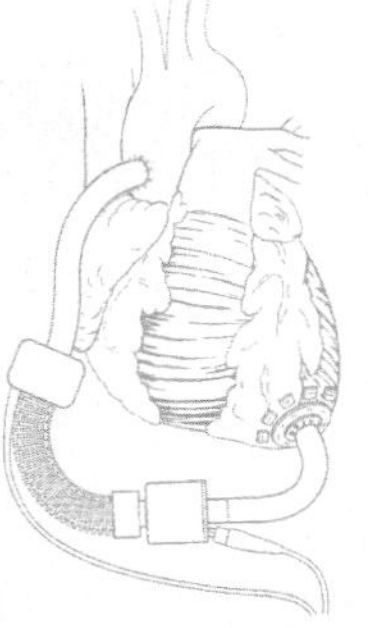

CHAPTER 60

Acquired Heart Disease: Coronary Insufficiency

Shuab Omer, Faisel G. Bakaeen

OUTLINE

Ischemic heart disease (IHD) is the predominant public health problem worldwide. Coronary heart disease (43.8%) is the leading cause of death attributable to cardiovascular disease (CVD) in the United States, followed by stroke (16.8%), high blood pressure (9.4%), heart failure (9.0%), diseases of the arteries (3.1%), and other CVDs (17.9%).

It is estimated that by 2035, more than 130 million adults in the U.S. population (45.1%) are projected to have some form of CVD, and total costs of CVD are expected to reach $1.1 trillion in 2035, with direct medical costs projected to reach $748.7 billion and indirect costs estimated to reach $368 billion.[1–3]

Despite recent advances in percutaneous intervention, coronary artery bypass grafting (CABG) still remains the most effective treatment for coronary artery disease (CAD) and is the most commonly performed open cardiac procedure in the United States.

CORONARY ARTERY ANATOMY AND PHYSIOLOGY

Anatomic Considerations

The coronary arteries, the predominant blood supply to the heart, arise from the sinuses of Valsalva. They are the first arterial branches of the aorta, and two are usually present. The coronary arteries are

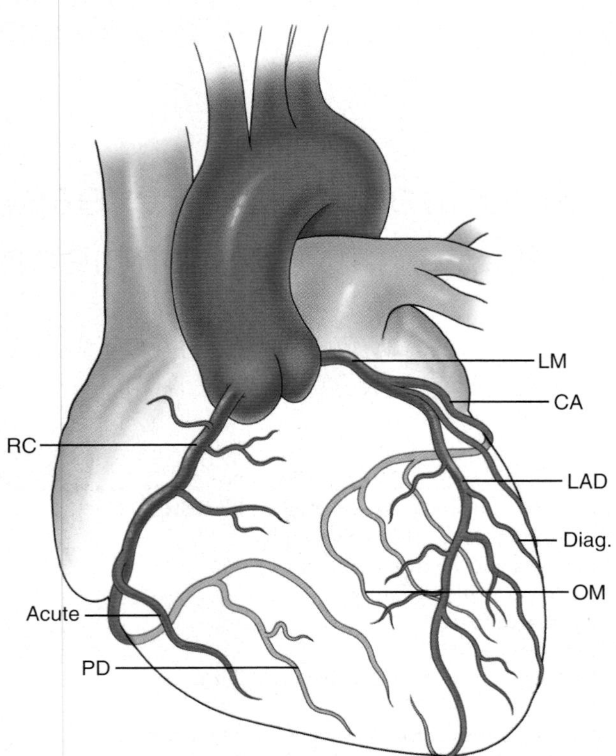

FIG. 60.1 Anatomy of normal coronary artery vasculature. *CA*, Circumflex artery; *LAD*, left anterior descending; *LM*, left main; *OM*, obtuse marginal; *PD*, posterior descending; *RC*, right coronary.

designated right and left according to the embryologic chamber that they predominantly supply. The left coronary artery (LCA) arises from the left coronary sinus, which is located posterior; the right coronary artery (RCA) arises from the right coronary sinus, which is located anterior. The LCA, also called the left main coronary artery, averages approximately 2 to 3 cm in length and courses in a left posterolateral direction, winding behind the main pulmonary artery trunk and then splitting into the left anterior descending (LAD) and left circumflex arteries. The LAD courses in an anterolateral direction to the left of the pulmonary trunk and runs anteriorly over the interventricular septum. The diagonal branches of the LAD supply the anterolateral wall of the left ventricle (LV). The LAD is considered the most important surgical vessel because it supplies more than 50% of the LV mass and most of the interventricular septum. The LAD has several septal perforating branches that supply the interventricular septum from its anterior aspect. The LAD extends over the interventricular septum up to the apex of the heart, where it may form an anastomosis with the posterior descending artery (PDA), which is typically a branch of the right coronary system (Fig. 60.1).

The circumflex artery passes in the atrioventricular (AV) groove and gives off the obtuse marginal branches that extend toward but do not quite reach the apex of the heart. The obtuse marginal branches are designated numerically from proximal to distal. The circumflex coronary artery usually terminates as the left posterolateral branch after taking a perpendicular turn toward the apex.

The term *ramus intermedius* is used to designate a dominant coronary vessel that arises from the occasional trifurcation of the LCA. This branch can be intramyocardial and difficult to locate at times.

The RCA supplies most of the right ventricle as well as the posterior part of the LV. The RCA emerges from its ostium in the right coronary sinus and passes deep in the right AV groove. At the superior end of the acute margin of the heart, the RCA turns posteriorly toward the crux and usually bifurcates into the PDA over the posterior interventricular sulcus and right posterolateral artery. The RCA also supplies multiple right ventricular branches (i.e., the acute marginal branches). On occasion, the PDA arises from both the RCA and LCA, and the circulation is considered to be codominant. The AV node artery arises from the RCA in approximately 90% of patients. The sinoatrial node artery arises from the proximal RCA in 50% of patients. Although the source of the PDA is often used clinically to define dominance of circulation in the heart, anatomists define it according to where the sinoatrial node artery arises. Table 60.1 summarizes the hierarchy of the coronary artery anatomy.

TABLE 60.1 Anatomic architecture of coronary arteries.

NAMED VESSELS	BRANCHES
Left main coronary artery	Left anterior descending Circumflex coronary Ramus intermedius
Left anterior descending	Diagonal arteries Septal perforators
Circumflex coronary artery	Obtuse marginal branches Left posterolateral artery
Right coronary artery	Acute marginal artery Posterior descending artery Right posterolateral artery

All the epicardial conductance vessels and septal perforators from the LAD give rise to a multitude of branches, termed resistance vessels, that penetrate into the ventricular wall. These vessels play a crucial role in oxygen and nutrient exchange with the myocardium by forming a rich capillary plexus. This plexus offers a low-resistance sink that allows arterial blood flow to increase unimpeded when oxygen demand rises. This is important because the myocardial vascular bed extracts oxygen at its full capacity, even in low-demand circumstances, thereby allowing no margin for further oxygen extraction when demand is high.

An intricate network of veins drains the coronary circulation, and the venous circulation can be divided into three systems: the coronary sinus and its tributaries, the anterior right ventricular veins, and the thebesian veins. The coronary sinus predominantly drains the LV and receives 85% of coronary venous blood. It lies within the posterior AV groove and empties into the right atrium. The anterior right ventricular veins travel across the right ventricular surface to the right AV groove, where they enter directly into the right atrium or form the small cardiac vein, which enters into the right atrium directly or joins the coronary sinus just proximal to its orifice. The thebesian veins are small venous tributaries that drain directly into the cardiac chambers and exit primarily into the right atrium and right ventricle. Understanding of the anatomy of the coronary sinus is essential for placement of the retrograde cardioplegia cannula during cardiopulmonary bypass (CPB).

Physiology and Regulation of Coronary Blood Flow

Aortic pressure is a driving force in the maintenance of myocardial perfusion. During resting conditions, coronary blood flow is maintained at a fairly constant level over a wide range of aortic perfusion pressures (70–180 mm Hg) through the process of autoregulation.

Because the myocardium has a high rate of energy use, normal coronary blood flow averages 225 mL/min (0.7–0.9 mL per gram of myocardium per minute) and delivers 0.1 mL/g/min of oxygen

BOX 60.1 Unique features of coronary blood flow.

- Autoregulated over wide pressure ranges
- Blood flow: 0.7–0.9 mL per gram of myocardium per minute
- 75% oxygen extraction
- Coronary sinus blood is the most deoxygenated blood in the body
- 4- to 7-fold increase in flow with increased demand
- 60% blood flow occurs during diastole
- Flow-limited oxygen supply

to the myocardium. Under normal conditions, more than 75% of the delivered oxygen is extracted in the coronary capillary bed, so any additional oxygen demand can be met only by increasing the flow rate. This highlights the importance of unobstructed coronary blood flow for proper myocardial function. Box 60.1 summarizes the unique features of coronary blood flow.

In response to increased load, such as that caused by strenuous exercise, the healthy heart can increase myocardial blood flow four- to sevenfold. Blood flow is increased through several mechanisms. Local metabolic neurohumoral factors cause coronary vasodilation when stress and metabolic demand increase, thereby lowering the coronary vascular resistance. This results in increased delivery of oxygen-rich blood, mimicking the phenomenon of reactive hyperemia. When a transient occlusion to the coronary artery is released (e.g., during the performance of a beating-heart operation), blood flow immediately rises to exceed the normal baseline flow and then gradually returns to its baseline level. The autoregulatory mechanism responsible is guided by several metabolic factors, including carbon dioxide, oxygen tension, hydrogen ions, lactate, potassium ions, and adenosine. Adenosine, a potent vasodilator and a degradation product of adenosine triphosphate, accumulates in the interstitial space and relaxes vascular smooth muscle. This results in vasomotor relaxation, coronary vasodilation, and increased blood flow. Another substance that plays an important role is nitric oxide, which is produced by the endothelium. Without the endothelium, coronary arteries do not autoregulate, suggesting that the mechanism for vasodilation and reactive hyperemia is endothelium dependent.

Extravascular compression of the coronaries during systole also plays an important role in the regulation of blood flow. During systole, the intracavitary pressures generated in the LV wall exceed intracoronary pressure, and blood flow is impeded. Hence, approximately 60% of coronary blood flow occurs during diastole. During exercise, increased heart rate and reduced diastolic time can compromise flow time, but this can be offset by vasodilatory mechanisms of the coronary vessels. Buildup of atherosclerotic plaques and fixed coronary occlusion significantly impair coronary arterial compensatory mechanisms while heart rate is elevated. This forms the basis for exercise-induced stress tests, in which abnormal physiologic responses to increased physical activity unmask underlying CAD.

HISTORY OF CORONARY ARTERY BYPASS SURGERY

One of the first attempts at myocardial revascularization was made by Arthur Vineberg from Canada.[4] He operated on a series of patients who presented with symptoms of myocardial ischemia and implanted the left internal mammary artery (LIMA) into the myocardium by creating a pocket. The operation did not entail a direct anastomosis to any coronary vessel and was performed on a beating heart through a left anterolateral thoracotomy. Dr. David Sabiston, Jr., performed the first CABG with venous grafting on April 4, 1962, in a patient with an occluded RCA. A saphenous vein graft (SVG) was taken from the leg and anastomosed from the ascending aorta to the RCA. Unfortunately, the patient had a stroke and died shortly thereafter. Michael DeBakey performed a successful aortocoronary SVG in 1964. At the Cleveland Clinic, Mason Sones, who is credited with inventing cardiac catheterization, and cardiac surgeon, Rene Favaloro, helped establish CABG surgery as a planned and consistent therapy in patients with angiographically documented CAD.

TABLE 60.2 Evolution of surgical coronary artery interventions: timeline.

1950	A. Vineberg	Direct implantation of mammary artery into myocardium
1953	J. H. Gibbon	First successful use of cardiopulmonary bypass machine
1962	F. M. Sones	Successful cineangiography
1964	M. E. DeBakey	First successful coronary artery bypass grafting
1964	T. Sondergaard	Introduced routine use of cardioplegia for myocardial protection
1964	D. A. Cooley	Routine use of normothermic arrest for all cardiac cases
1968	R. Favoloro	First large series showing success of coronary artery bypass grafting
1973	V. Subramanian	Beating-heart coronary artery bypass grafting
1979	G. Buckberg	First use of blood cardioplegia as preferred method for arrested myocardial protection

The development of the heart-lung machine and its successful clinical use by John Heysham Gibbon in the 1950s, along with the advancement of cardioplegia techniques in later years by Gerald Buckberg, allowed surgeons to perform coronary anastomosis on an arrested (nonbeating) heart with a relatively bloodless field, thus increasing the safety and accuracy of the coronary bypass. In the 1990s, the advent of devices that could atraumatically stabilize the heart provided another pathway for the development of off-pump techniques of myocardial revascularization. Today, an armamentarium of techniques ranging from conventional on-pump CABG to minimally invasive robotic and percutaneous approaches is available to manage CAD. Table 60.2 summarizes the timeline of major historical events in the development of surgery for myocardial revascularization.

ATHEROSCLEROTIC CORONARY ARTERY DISEASE

Coronary atherosclerosis is a process that begins early in the patient's life. Epicardial conductance vessels are the most susceptible and intramyocardial arteries, the least. Risk factors for atherosclerosis include elevated plasma levels of total cholesterol and low-density lipoprotein cholesterol, cigarette smoking, hypertension, diabetes mellitus, advanced age, low plasma levels of high-density lipoprotein cholesterol, and family history of premature CAD.

Epidemiologic evidence suggests that coronary artery atherosclerosis is closely linked to the metabolism of lipids, specifically low-density lipoprotein cholesterol. The development of lipid-lowering drugs has resulted in a significant reduction in mortality. In one observational study of patients who received statin therapy and were known to have CAD, statin treatment was associated with improved survival in all age groups. The greatest survival benefit was found in those patients in the highest quartile of plasma levels of high-sensitivity C-reactive protein, a biomarker of inflammation

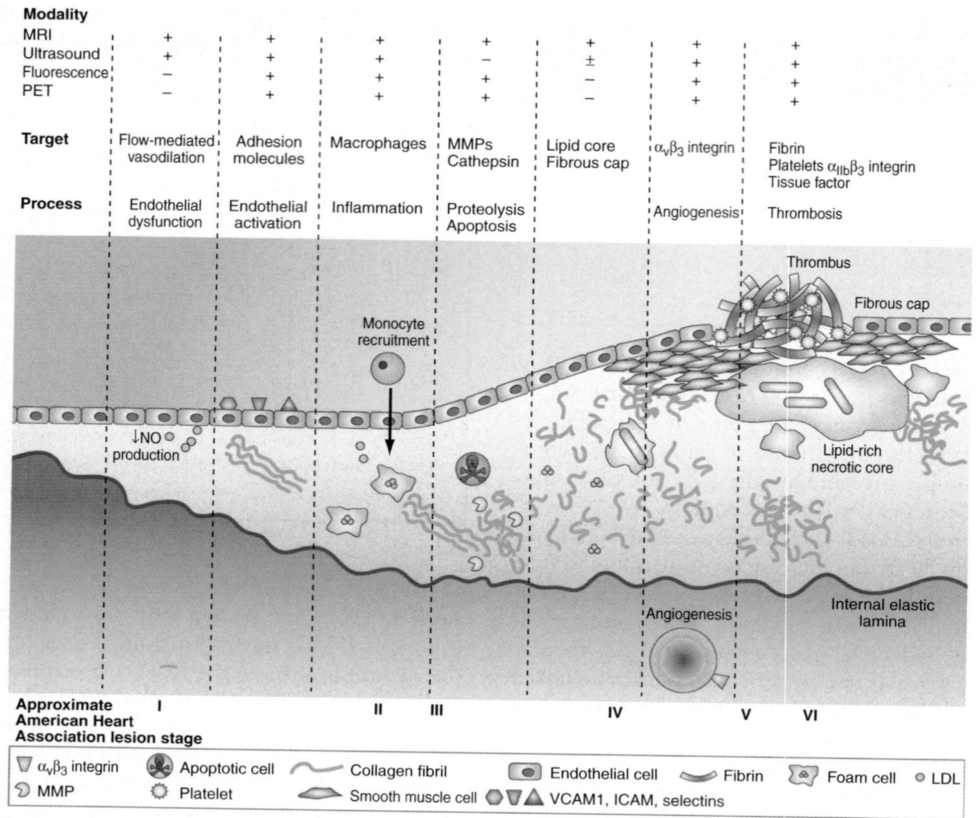

FIG. 60.2 Components of atherosclerotic plaque. Thinning of the fibrous cap eventually results in plaque rupture and extrusion of highly thrombogenic lipid-laden material into the coronary artery. This causes an acute occlusion of the coronary artery, resulting in myocardial infarction. (Adapted from Choudhury RP, Fuster V, Fayad ZA. Molecular, cellular and functional imaging of atherothrombosis. *Nat Rev Drug Discov.* 2004;3:913–925.) *ICAM,* Intercellular adhesion molecule; *LDL,* low-density lipoprotein; *MMP,* matrix metallopeptidases; *MRI,* magnetic resonance imaging; *PET,* positron emission tomography; *VCAM1,* vascular cell adhesion molecule 1.

and CAD. Animal and human studies have demonstrated that statin therapy also modifies the lipid composition within plaques by lowering the amount of low-density lipoprotein cholesterol and stabilizing the plaque through various mechanisms, including reduced macrophage accumulation, collagen degradation, reduced smooth muscle cell protease expression, and decreased tissue factor expression.

Pathogenesis

The primary cause of CAD is endothelial injury induced by an inflammatory wall response and lipid deposition. There is evidence that an inflammatory response is involved in all stages of the disease, from early lipid deposition to plaque formation, plaque rupture, and coronary artery thrombosis. Vulnerable or high-risk plaques that are prone to rupture have the following characteristics: a large, eccentric, soft lipid core; a thin fibrous cap; inflammation within the cap and adventitia; increased plaque neovascularity; and evidence of outward or positive vessel remodeling.

Thinner fibrous caps are at a higher risk for rupture, probably because of an imbalance between the synthesis and the degradation of the extracellular matrix in the fibrous cap that results in an overall decrease in the collagen and matrix components (Fig. 60.2). Increased matrix breakdown caused by matrix degradation by an inflammatory cell-mediated metalloproteinase or reduced production of extracellular matrix results in thinner fibrous caps. Not all plaque ruptures are symptomatic; whether they are depends on the thrombogenicity of the plaque's components. Tissue factor within the lipid core of the plaque, secreted by activated macrophages, is one of the most potent thrombogenic stimuli. Rupture of a vulnerable plaque may be spontaneous or caused by extreme physical activity, severe emotional distress, exposure to drugs, cold exposure, or acute infection.

Fixed Coronary Obstructions

More than 90% of patients with stable IHD (SIHD) have advanced coronary atherosclerosis caused by a fixed obstruction. Atherosclerotic plaques of the coronary arteries are concentric (25%) or eccentric (75%). Eccentric lesions compromise only a portion of the lumen; through vascular remodeling, the arterial lumen may remain patent until late in the disease process. The impact of an arterial stenosis on coronary blood flow can be appreciated in the context of the Poiseuille law. Reductions in luminal diameter up to 60% have minimal impact on flow, but when the cross-sectional area of the vessel has decreased by 75% or more, coronary blood flow is significantly compromised. Clinically, this loss of flow often coincides with the onset of exertional angina. A 90% reduction in luminal diameter results in resting angina.

CLINICAL MANIFESTATIONS AND DIAGNOSIS OF CORONARY ARTERY DISEASE

Clinical Presentation

Clinically, IHD has two predominant modes of presentation:

- Stable angina

- Acute coronary syndrome: ST-segment elevation myocardial infarction (STEMI) and its complications, non-STEMI (NSTEMI), and unstable angina (UA)

Anginal pain is the main presenting symptom of IHD. It typically lasts minutes. The location is usually substernal, and pain can radiate to the neck, jaw, epigastrium, or arms. Anginal pain is precipitated by exertion or emotional stress and relieved by rest. Sublingual nitroglycerin also usually relieves angina within 30 seconds to several minutes.

On presentation, angina must be classified as stable or unstable. Patients are said to be having UA if the pain is increasing (in frequency, intensity, or duration) or occurring at rest. Such patients should be transferred promptly to an emergency department.

Patients, especially female and elderly patients, sometimes present with atypical symptoms, such as nausea, vomiting, midepigastric discomfort, or sharp (atypical) chest pain. In the Women's Ischemic Syndrome Evaluation (WISE) study, 65% of women with ischemia presented with atypical symptoms.[5]

The term *acute coronary syndrome* has evolved to refer to a constellation of clinical symptoms that represent myocardial ischemia. It encompasses both STEMI and NSTEMI. Myocardial infarction (MI) often is manifested as crushing chest pain that may be associated with nausea, diaphoresis, anxiety, and dyspnea. Symptoms of the hypoperfusion that follows MI may include dizziness, fatigue, and vomiting. Heart rate and blood pressure may be initially normal, but both increase in response to the duration and severity of pain. Loss of blood pressure is indicative of cardiogenic shock and indicates a poorer prognosis. At least 40% of the ventricular mass must be involved for cardiogenic shock to occur.

Mechanical complications of MI include acute ventricular septal defect (VSD), papillary muscle rupture, and free ventricular rupture. They usually occur approximately 7 to 10 days after the initial MI.

Physical Examination

Some clinical findings are generic and are related to the systemic manifestations of atherosclerosis. Eye examination may reveal a copper wire sign, retinal hematoma or thrombosis secondary to vascular occlusive disease, and hypertension. Corneal arcus and xanthelasma are features noticed in cases of hypercholesterolemia. Other clinical manifestations are caused by sequelae of CAD (Box 60.2).

A thorough vascular evaluation is essential for any patient who presents with CAD because atherosclerosis is a systemic process. In addition, if surgery is being planned, the extremities should be evaluated for any previous surgical scars or fractures that could potentially preclude conduit harvest.

Diagnostic Testing

Biochemical Studies

Patients suspected of having an acute coronary syndrome should undergo appropriate blood testing. Levels of creatine kinase muscle and brain subunits (CK-MB) and troponin T or I should be assessed at least 6 to 12 hours apart. Additional laboratory tests include a complete blood count, comprehensive metabolic panel, and lipid profile (total cholesterol, triglycerides, low-density lipoprotein cholesterol, high-density lipoprotein cholesterol). Elevated brain natriuretic peptide and C-reactive protein levels suggest a worse outcome.

Chest Radiography

The chest radiograph is helpful in identifying causes of chest discomfort or pain other than CAD. Chest radiography does not detect CAD directly; it only identifies sequelae, such as cardiomegaly, pulmonary edema, and pleural effusions, that are indicative of heart failure. From a surgical standpoint, preoperative chest radiography is important because it can identify obvious abnormalities, such as porcelain aorta, lung masses, effusion, and pneumonias, that may affect further workup or prompt a change in operative strategy.

BOX 60.2 Sequelae of coronary artery disease.

Clinical Manifestations

- Abnormal neck vein pulsations, which may be seen in patients with second- or third-degree heart block or CHF
- Bradycardia—a subtle presentation of ischemia involving the right coronary territories and a possible sign of heart block
- Weak or thready pulse suggestive of ectopic or premature ventricular beats
- Third heart sound that is noted with elevated left ventricular filling pressures/CHF
- Fourth heart sound, which is commonly heard in patients with acute and chronic CAD
- Mitral regurgitant heart murmurs caused by ischemic papillary muscles
- Ejection systolic murmur indicative of aortic stenosis, which can contribute to coronary ischemia
- Holosystolic murmurs caused by ventricular septal rupture
- Manifestations of CHF, such as rales, hepatomegaly, right upper abdominal quadrant tenderness, ascites, and marked peripheral and presacral edema

CAD, Coronary artery disease; *CHF*, congestive heart failure.

Resting Electrocardiography

A 12-lead resting electrocardiogram (ECG) should be obtained in all patients with suspected IHD or sequelae thereof. The ECG is evaluated for evidence of LV hypertrophy, ST-segment depression or elevation, ectopic beats, or Q waves. In addition, arrhythmias (atrial fibrillation or ventricular tachycardia) and conduction defects (left anterior fascicular block, right bundle branch block, left bundle branch block) are suggestive of CAD and MI. Persistent ST-segment elevation or an evolving Q wave is consistent with myocardial injury and ongoing ischemia. Fifty percent of patients with significant CAD nonetheless have normal electrocardiographic results, and 50% of ECG recordings obtained during chest pain at rest will be normal, indicating the inaccuracy of the test. Patients with SIHD tend to have a worse prognosis if they have the following abnormalities on a resting ECG: evidence of prior MI, especially Q waves in multiple leads or an R wave in V_1 indicating a posterior infarction; persistent ST-T wave inversions, particularly in leads V_1 to V_3; left bundle branch block, bifascicular block, second- or third-degree AV block, or ventricular tachyarrhythmia; or LV hypertrophy.[6]

Functional (Stress) Tests

In patients with suspected stable ischemic CAD, functional or stress testing is used to detect inducible ischemia. These are the most common noninvasive tests used to diagnose SIHD (Box 60.3). All functional tests rely on the principle of inducing cardiac ischemia by using exercise or pharmacologic stress agents, which increase myocardial work and oxygen demand, or by causing vasodilation-elicited heterogeneity in induced coronary flow. Whether ischemia is induced, however, depends on the severity of both the stress imposed (e.g., submaximal exercise can fail to produce ischemia) and the flow disturbance. Approximately 70% of

BOX 60.3 Stress tests to identify coronary artery disease.

Exercise Stress ECG

- Bruce protocol
- Five 3-minute bouts of treadmill exercise
- Determines the ischemia threshold
- 12 metabolic equivalents of energy expenditure needed for complete test
- Low cost and short duration
- Highly sensitive in multivessel disease

Limitations

- Suboptimal sensitivity
- Low detection rate of one-vessel disease
- Nondiagnostic with abnormal baseline ECG
- Poor specificity in premenopausal women
- Many cannot accomplish the 12 metabolic equivalents for a complete test or an appropriate heart rate response

Exercise and Pharmacologic Stress SPECT Perfusion Imaging

- Simultaneous evaluation of perfusion and function
- Higher sensitivity and specificity than exercise ECG
- Quantitative image analysis

Limitations

- Long procedure time with Technetium-99m
- Higher cost
- Radiation exposure
- Poor-quality images in obese patients

Exercise and Pharmacologic Stress Echocardiography

- Higher sensitivity and specificity than exercise ECG
- Comparable value with dobutamine stress
- Short examination time
- Identification of structural cardiac abnormalities
- Simultaneous evaluation of perfusion with contrast agents
- No radiation

Limitations

- Decreased sensitivity for detection of one-vessel disease or mild stenosis
- Highly operator dependent
- No quantitative image analysis
- Poor imaging in some patients
- Infarct zone poorly defined

ECG, Electrocardiogram; *SPECT*, single-photon emission computed tomography.

coronary stenoses are not detected by functional testing. Because abnormalities of regional or global ventricular function occur later in the ischemic cascade, they are more likely to indicate severe stenosis; thus, such abnormalities have a higher diagnostic specificity for SIHD than do perfusion defects, such as those seen on nuclear myocardial perfusion imaging (MPI).

Exercise versus pharmacologic testing. In patients capable of performing routine activities of daily living without difficulty, exercise testing is preferred to pharmacologic testing because it induces greater physiologic stress than drugs can. This may make exercise testing the better means of detecting ischemia as well as providing a correlation to a patient's daily symptom burden and physical work capacity not offered by pharmacologic stress testing.

The treadmill protocols initiate exercise at 3.2 to 4.7 metabolic equivalents of the task (METs) and increase by several METs every 2 to 3 minutes of exercise (e.g., modified or standard Bruce protocol). Performance of most activities of daily living requires approximately 4 to 5 METs of physical work. Patients unable to perform moderate physical activity and those with disabling comorbidities should undergo pharmacologic stress imaging instead.

Diagnostic accuracy of stress testing for SIHD

Exercise electrocardiography (Bruce protocol). The criterion for diagnosis of ischemia is an ECG showing 1-mm horizontal or downsloping (at 80 milliseconds after the J point) ST-segment depression at peak exercise. The diagnostic sensitivity and specificity of this sign is 61%. It is lower in women than in men[7,8] and lower than that of stress imaging modalities.

Exercise and pharmacologic stress echocardiography. These tests rely on detecting new or worsening wall motion abnormalities and changes in global LV function during or immediately after stress. In addition to the detection of inducible wall motion abnormalities, most stress echocardiography includes screening images to evaluate resting ventricular function and valvular abnormalities.

Pharmacologic stress echocardiography is usually performed using dobutamine with an end point of producing wall motion abnormalities. Vasodilator agents such as adenosine can be used to the same effect.

The diagnostic sensitivity is 70% to 85% for exercise and 85% to 90% for pharmacologic stress echocardiography. The use of intravenous ultrasound contrast agents, by improving endocardial border delineation, can result in improved diagnostic accuracy.

Exercise and pharmacologic stress nuclear myocardial perfusion imaging. Myocardial perfusion single-photon emission computed tomography (SPECT) generally is performed with rest and with stress. Technetium-99m agents are generally used; one of these, thallium Tl 201, has limited applications (e.g., viability) because of its higher radiation exposure. Pharmacologic stress is generally induced with vasodilator agents administered by continuous infusion (adenosine, dipyridamole) or bolus injection (regadenoson).

The diagnostic end point of nuclear MPI is a reduction in myocardial perfusion after stress. The diagnostic accuracy for detection of obstructive CAD of exercise and pharmacologic stress nuclear MPI has been studied in detail.[9,10] Studies suggest that nuclear MPI's sensitivity ranges from 82% to 88% for exercise and 88% to 91% for pharmacologic stress, and its diagnostic specificity ranges from 70% to 88% and 75% to 90% for exercise and pharmacologic stress nuclear MPI, respectively.

For myocardial perfusion SPECT, global reductions in myocardial perfusion, such as in the patients with left main or three-vessel CAD, can result in balanced reduction and an underestimation of ischemic burden.

Echocardiography

From a surgical standpoint, most patients with SIHD should undergo preoperative echocardiography. Echocardiography provides information not only for surgical planning but also regarding prognosis. A resting left ventricular ejection fraction (LVEF) of 35% is associated with an annual mortality rate of 3% per year. Resting two-dimensional Doppler echocardiography provides information on cardiac structure and function, including identifying the mechanism of heart failure and differentiating systolic from diastolic LV dysfunction. Echocardiography can identify LV or left atrial dilation, identify aortic stenosis (a potential non-CAD cause of angina-like chest pain), measure pulmonary artery pressure, quantify mitral regurgitation, identify LV aneurysm, identify LV thrombus (which increases the risk of death), and measure LV mass and the ratio of wall thickness to chamber radius—all of which predict cardiac events and mortality.[11,12]

Multidetector Computed Tomography

From a surgical standpoint, multidetector computed tomography (CT) has two pertinent applications in the management of CAD: to detect CAD and to inform the planning of grafting sites for CABG by providing additional information about coronary lesions, especially calcification and the course of coronary arteries. It also gives additional pertinent information about aortic disease and calcification, which might profoundly influence surgical decision making. However, the timing of cardiac CT should be carefully weighed against the risk of renal injury as a result of contrast nephropathy. Although revascularization decisions are currently made on the basis of coronary angiography, there have been tremendous improvements in temporal and spatial resolution of cardiac CT that make it useful for this purpose as well. Coronary CT angiography (CCTA) can now provide high-quality images of the coronary arteries.[13] When it is performed with 64-slice CT, CCTA has a sensitivity of 93% to 97% and a specificity of 80% to 90% for detecting obstructive CAD.[14–17]

The potential advantages of CCTA over standard functional testing for CAD screening include the high negative predictive value of CCTA for obstructive CAD. This can reassure caregivers that it is a sensible strategy to provide guideline-directed medical therapy (GDMT) and to defer consideration of revascularization. Among the greatest potential advantages of CCTA over conventional angiography, in addition to documentation of stenotic lesions, is that CCTA can assess remodeling and identify nonobstructive plaque, including calcified, noncalcified, and mixed plaque.[18]

Magnetic Resonance Imaging

Myocardial first-pass perfusion magnetic resonance imaging has been considered a good alternative to nuclear cardiac ischemia and viability testing. However, the procedure has not gained widespread popularity because special training and expertise are required to perform this type of imaging and to interpret the results.

Cardiac Catheterization and Intervention

Coronary catheterization is the "gold standard" for diagnosis of CAD. Coronary angiography defines coronary anatomy, including the location, length, diameter, and contour of the epicardial coronary arteries; the presence and severity of coronary luminal obstructions; the nature of the obstruction; the presence and extent of angiographically visible collateral flow; and coronary blood flow.

The classification for defining coronary anatomy that is still used today was developed for the Coronary Artery Surgery Study (CASS)[19] and further modified by the Balloon Angioplasty Revascularization Investigation (BARI) study group.[20] This scheme assumes that there are three major coronary arteries: the LAD, the circumflex, and the RCA, with a right-dominant, left-dominant, or codominant circulation. The extent of disease is defined as one-vessel, two-vessel, three-vessel, or left main disease; a luminal diameter reduction of at least 70% is considered to be significant stenosis (Figs. 60.3 and 60.4). Left main disease, however, is defined as stenosis of at least 50% (Fig. 60.5). Despite being recognized as the traditional gold standard for clinical assessment of coronary atherosclerosis, this test is not without limitations. There is marked variation in interobserver reliability, and investigators have found only 70% overall agreement among readers with regard to the severity of stenosis; this was reduced to 51% when restricted to coronary vessels rated as having some stenosis by any reader. Also, angiography provides only anatomic data and is not a reliable indicator of the functional significance of a given

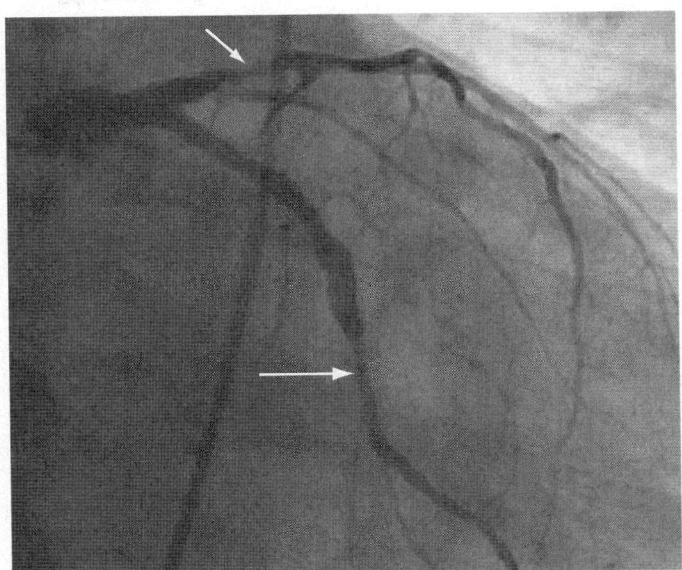

FIG. 60.3 Left coronary angiogram showing hemodynamically severe lesions in the left anterior descending artery *(small arrow)* and the circumflex artery *(large arrow)*.

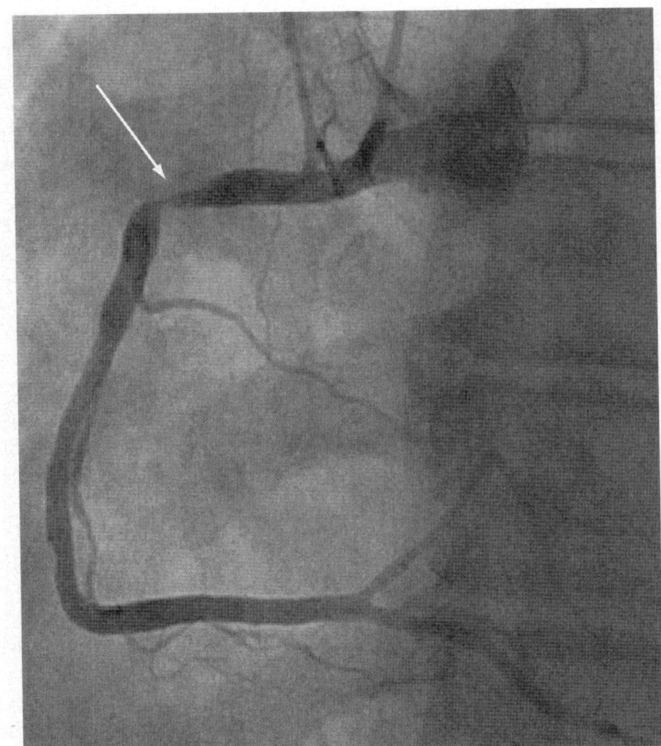

FIG. 60.4 Right coronary angiogram showing hemodynamically significant lesion *(arrow)*. The right coronary artery terminates as a posterior descending artery in the right dominant system.

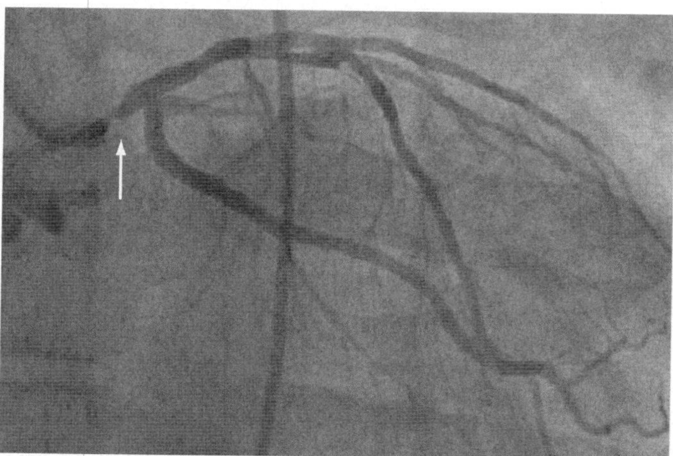

FIG. 60.5 Coronary angiogram showing critical left main coronary artery stenosis *(arrow)*.

coronary stenosis unless a technique such as fractional flow reserve (FFR) is used to provide information about the physiologic effects of the stenosis. FFR is measured by passing a sensor guidewire into the LAD or circumflex vessels for LCA lesions. Thereafter, the flow reserve in the artery is checked by using adenosine to induce hyperemia in the coronary system, which is discussed in the next section on FFR. In addition, angiography cannot distinguish between vulnerable and stable plaques. In angiographic studies performed before and after acute events and early after MI, plaques causing UA and MI commonly were found to be 50% obstructive before the acute event and were therefore angiographically "silent."[19,20] Diagnostic testing methods to identify vulnerable plaque and, therefore, the patient's risk of MI are being intensely studied, but no gold standard has yet emerged. Despite these limitations of coronary angiography, the extent and severity of CAD as revealed angiographically remain important predictors of long-term patient outcomes.[21,22]

In the CASS registry[23] of medically treated patients, the 12-year survival rate of patients with normal coronary arteries was 91% compared with 74% for those with one-vessel disease, 59% for those with two-vessel disease, and 40% for those with three-vessel disease.

Importantly, besides informing the decision whether to intervene surgically or with percutaneous coronary intervention (PCI), the salient characteristics of coronary lesions (e.g., stenosis severity, length, and complexity and presence of thrombus), the number of lesions threatening regions of contracting myocardium, the effect of collaterals, and the volume of jeopardized viable myocardium also can afford some insight into the potential consequences of subsequent vessel occlusion and therefore the haste with which surgery should be scheduled.

PCI techniques in current use include balloon dilation, stent-supported dilation, atherectomy and plaque ablation with a variety of devices, thrombectomy with aspiration devices, specialized imaging, and physiologic assessment with intracoronary devices.

Coronary artery stents were the first substantial breakthrough in the prevention of restenosis after angioplasty. Although stent recoil and compression are not completely insignificant problems, the greatest cause of lumen loss in stented coronary arteries is neointimal hyperplasia. This is the principal mechanism of in-stent stenosis and results from inappropriate cell proliferation—hence, the advent of cytotoxic drug-eluting stents (DESs).

Fractional Flow Reserve

Angiography can underestimate the severity of CAD, especially LCA disease.[24,25] This underestimation may be due to the lack of a reference segment or to very ostial or distal disease. Therefore, in cases with intermediate lesions, FFR has emerged as a helpful modality.

FFR is measured by passing a sensor guidewire into the LAD or circumflex vessels for LCA lesions. Thereafter, the flow reserve in the artery is checked by using adenosine to induce hyperemia in the coronary system. An FFR below 0.75 is considered to signify ischemia-producing lesions. Some studies have used a threshold of 0.8.

Intravascular Ultrasonography

Intravascular ultrasonography (IVUS) provides high-quality cross-sectional images of the coronary system. It is done by inserting an IVUS wire into the LAD or circumflex artery and gradually pulling it out while obtaining real-time images of the coronary system. In indeterminate lesions of the LCA, an IVUS minimum luminal diameter of 2.8 or a minimum luminal area of 6 mm^2 suggests a physiologically significant lesion.

Hybrid Imaging

Hybrid imaging has the potential of taking coronary artery assessment one step further by combining the advantages of two different modalities to give both anatomic and physiologic information in one snapshot. Hybrid imaging can combine positron emission tomography (PET) and CT or SPECT and CT, thus allowing combined anatomic and functional testing. In addition, novel scanning techniques make it possible to use CCTA alone to assess perfusion and FFR, in addition to coronary anatomy. Interestingly, these combined assessments can produce a fused image in which physiologic information about flow is combined with information about the anatomic extent and severity of CAD, plaque composition, and arterial remodeling. Robust evidence to support the use of hybrid imaging is lacking at this point, despite its reported accuracy in predicting cardiac events with both ischemic and anatomic markers. The strength of combined imaging is that it provides anatomic information to guide the interpretation of ischemic and scarred myocardium as well as information to guide therapeutic decision-making. Hybrid imaging also can overcome technical limitations of myocardial perfusion SPECT or myocardial perfusion PET by providing anatomic correlates to guide interpretative accuracy, and it can provide the functional information that an anatomic technique like CCTA or magnetic resonance angiography lacks; however, use of hybrid techniques requires increasing the radiation dose.

INDICATIONS FOR CORONARY ARTERY REVASCULARIZATION

Per the most current American College of Cardiology/American Heart Association guidelines, the only class Ia indication for PCI is acute STEMI. In all other indications, CABG has superior class based on current evidence (Table 60.3). These guidelines are based on the existing literature, which spans four decades. Many of the studies on which current recommendations are based were conducted in the 1970s and 1980s.

Coronary Artery Bypass Grafting Versus Contemporaneous Medical Therapy

In the 1970s and 1980s, three landmark randomized controlled trials (RCTs) established the survival benefit of CABG compared

TABLE 60.3 Guidelines for coronary revascularization.

CORONARY ARTERY LESIONS	RECOMMENDATIONS
Unprotected Left Main	
CABG	I
PCI	IIa—For SIHD when both of the following are present: • Cardiac catheterization reveals a low risk of PCI procedural complications with a high likelihood of good long-term outcome (low SYNTAX score 22, ostial or trunk left main). • Significantly increased risk of adverse surgical outcomes (STS-predicted risk of operative mortality 5%) IIa—For UA/NSTEMI if not a CABG candidate IIa—For STEMI when distal coronary flow is TIMI flow grade 3 and PCI can be performed more rapidly and safely than CABG IIb—For SIHD when both of the following are present: • Cardiac catheterization reveals a low to intermediate risk of PCI procedural complications and an intermediate to high likelihood of good long-term outcome (low–intermediate SYNTAX score of 33, bifurcation left main) • Increased risk of adverse surgical outcomes (moderate–severe COPD, disability from prior stroke, or prior cardiac surgery; STS-predicted operative mortality 2%) III: Harm—For SIHD in patients (versus performing CABG) with unfavorable anatomy for PCI and who are good candidates for CABG
Three-Vessel Disease With or Without Proximal LAD Artery Disease	
CABG	I IIa—It is reasonable to choose CABG over PCI in patients with complex three-vessel CAD (SYNTAX score 22) who are good candidates for surgery
PCI	IIb—Of uncertain benefit
Two-Vessel Disease With Proximal LAD Artery Disease	
CABG	I
PCI	IIb—Of uncertain benefit
Two-Vessel Disease Without Proximal LAD Artery Disease	
CABG	IIa—With extensive ischemia IIb—Of uncertain benefit without extensive ischemia
PCI	IIb—Of uncertain benefit
One-Vessel Proximal LAD Artery Disease	
CABG	IIa—With LIMA for long-term benefit
PCI	IIb—Of uncertain benefit
One-Vessel Disease Without Proximal LAD Artery Involvement	
CABG	III: Harm
PCI	III: Harm
LV Dysfunction	
CABG	IIa—LVEF 35% to 50% IIb—LVEF 35% without significant left main CAD
PCI	Insufficient data
Survivors of Sudden Cardiac Death With Presumed Ischemia-Mediated VT	
CABG	I
PCI	I
No Anatomic or Physiologic Criteria for Revascularization	
CABG	III: Harm
PCI	III: Harm

Class I: benefit ⋙ risk. Procedure should be performed.
Class IIa: benefit ≫ risk. Additional studies with focused objectives needed. It is reasonable to perform procedure.
Class IIb: benefit ≥ risk. Additional studies with broader objectives and additional registry data may be needed. Procedure treatment may be considered.
Class III: no benefit or
Class III: harm
From Reference 28.
CABG, Coronary artery bypass grafting (major adverse events occurred less frequently with CABG); *CAD*, coronary artery disease; *COPD*, chronic obstructive pulmonary disease; *LAD*, left anterior descending; *LIMA*, left internal mammary artery; *LV*, left ventricle; *LVEF*, left ventricular ejection fraction; *PCI*, percutaneous coronary intervention; *SIHD*, stable ischemic heart disease; *STEMI*, ST-elevation myocardial infarction; *STS*, Society of Thoracic Surgeons; *SYNTAX*, Synergy between Percutaneous Coronary Intervention with Taxus and Cardiac Surgery; *TIMI*, thrombolysis in myocardial infarction; *UA/NSTEMI*, unstable angina/non–ST-elevation myocardial infarction; *VT*, ventricular tachycardia.

with medical therapy without revascularization in certain patients with SIHD: the Veterans Affairs Cooperative Study,[26] European Coronary Surgery Study,[27] and CASS.[22] Subsequently, a 1994 metaanalysis of seven studies in which 2649 patients were randomly assigned to medical therapy or CABG[24] showed that CABG offered a survival advantage over medical therapy for patients with LCA or three-vessel CAD. The studies also established that CABG is more effective than medical therapy for relieving anginal symptoms. These studies have been replicated only once during the past decade. In Medicine, Angioplasty, or Surgery Study II (MASS II), patients with multivessel CAD who were treated with CABG were less likely than those treated with medical therapy to have a subsequent MI, to need additional revascularization, or to experience cardiac death in the 10 years after randomization.[25] Surgical techniques and medical therapy have improved substantially during the intervening years. Some critics state that if CABG were compared with GDMT in RCTs today, the relative benefits in terms of survival and angina relief observed several decades ago might no longer be observed. However, it should also be understood that the concurrent administration of GDMT, which most post–cardiac surgery patients now receive, may also substantially improve long-term outcomes in patients treated with CABG in comparison with those receiving medical therapy alone. Thus, the survival difference might still favor CABG over GDMT.

Percutaneous Coronary Intervention Versus Medical Therapy

Although contemporary interventional treatments have lowered the risk of restenosis compared with earlier techniques, metaanalyses have not shown that the use of bare-metal stents (BMS) confers a survival advantage over balloon angioplasty[26,27] or that the use of DES confers a survival advantage over BMS.[28] Evaluation of trials of PCI conducted during the last 30 years show that, despite improvements in PCI technology and pharmacotherapy, PCI has not reduced the risk of death or MI in patients without recent acute coronary syndrome. The findings from individual studies and systematic reviews of PCI versus medical therapy can be summarized as follows:

- PCI reduces the incidence of angina
- PCI has not been demonstrated to improve survival in stable patients
- PCI may increase the short-term risk of MI
- PCI does not lower the long-term risk of MI

Coronary Artery Bypass Grafting Versus Balloon Angioplasty or Bare-Metal Stents

From a review of multiple RCTs comparing CABG with balloon angioplasty or BMS, the following conclusions can be drawn[28]:

- Survival was similar for CABG and PCI (with balloon angioplasty or BMS) at 1 year and 5 years. Survival was similar for CABG and PCI in patients with one-vessel CAD (including those with disease of the proximal portion of the LAD artery) or with multivessel CAD
- Incidence of MI was similar at 5 years
- Procedural stroke occurred more commonly with CABG than with PCI (1.2% vs. 0.6%)
- Relief of angina was more effective with CABG than with PCI at 1 year and 5 years
- At 1 year after the index procedure, repeated coronary revascularization was performed less often after CABG than after PCI (3.8% vs. 26.5%). This was also found after 5 years of follow-up (9.8% vs. 46.1%). This difference was more pronounced with balloon angioplasty than with BMS.

Coronary Artery Bypass Grafting Versus Drug-Eluting Stents

Multiple observational studies comparing CABG and DES implantation have been published, but most of them had short (12–24 months) follow-up periods. A large RCT comparing CABG and DES implantation in patients with three-vessel or left main disease has been published, called the Synergy between Percutaneous Coronary Intervention with Taxus and Cardiac Surgery (SYNTAX) trial, in which 1800 patients (of a total of 4337 who were screened) were randomly assigned to undergo DES implantation or CABG. Major adverse cardiac events (a composite of death, stroke, MI, or repeated revascularization during the 3 years after randomization) occurred less frequently in CABG patients (20.2%) than in DES patients (28.0%; $P = 0.001$). The rates of death and stroke were similar; however, MI (3.6% for CABG, 7.1% for DES) and repeated revascularization (10.7% for CABG, 19.7% for DES) were more likely to occur with DES implantation. In SYNTAX, the extent of CAD was assessed by using the SYNTAX score, which is based on the location, severity, and extent of coronary stenoses, with a low score indicating less complicated anatomic CAD. In post hoc analyses, a low score was defined as 22 or lower; intermediate, 23 to 32; and high, 33 or higher. The occurrence of major adverse cardiac events correlated with the SYNTAX score for DES patients but not for those undergoing CABG. At 12-month follow-up, the primary end point was similar for CABG and DES in those with a low SYNTAX score. In contrast, major adverse cardiac events occurred more often after DES implantation than after CABG in those with an intermediate or high SYNTAX score. At 3 years of follow-up, the mortality rate was greater in patients with three-vessel CAD treated with PCI than in those treated with CABG (6.2% vs. 2.9%). The differences in major adverse cardiac events of those treated with PCI or CABG increased with an increasing SYNTAX score. Although the utility of using a SYNTAX score in everyday clinical practice remains uncertain, it seems reasonable to conclude from SYNTAX and other data that the outcomes of patients undergoing PCI or CABG in those with relatively uncomplicated and lesser degrees of CAD are comparable, whereas in those with complex and diffuse CAD, CABG appears to be preferable. At 5-year follow-up, a similar trend was seen, with CABG superior to PCI for intermediate or high SYNTAX scores.[29]

Left Main Coronary Artery Disease

CABG or PCI Versus Medical Therapy for Left Main CAD

CABG confers a survival benefit over medical therapy in patients with LCA CAD. Subgroup analyses from RCTs performed three decades ago demonstrated a 66% reduction in relative risk of death with CABG, with the benefit extending to 10 years.[23,24]

Studies Comparing PCI Versus CABG for Left Main CAD

Of all patients undergoing coronary angiography, approximately 4% are found to have LCA CAD, 80% of whom have significant (70% diameter) stenoses in other epicardial coronary arteries. Published cohort studies have found that major clinical outcomes for ostial LCA are similar with PCI or CABG 1 year after revascularization and that mortality rates are similar at 1 year, 2 years, and 5 years of follow-up; however, the risk of needing target vessel revascularization is significantly higher with stenting than with CABG.

Multiple RCTs have looked at this topic: the SYNTAX trial,[29] the Study of Unprotected Left Main Stenting versus Bypass Surgery (LE MANS) trial, the Premier of Randomized Comparison of Bypass Surgery versus Angioplasty Using Sirolimus-Eluting Stent in Patients with Left Main Coronary Artery Disease (PRECOMBAT) trial, the Percutaneous Coronary Angioplasty Versus CABG in Treatment of Unprotected Left Main Stenosis (NOBLE) trial,[30] and the Everolimus-Eluting Stents or Bypass Surgery for Left Main Coronary Artery Disease (EXCEL) trial.[31] The results from these RCTs suggest (but do not definitively prove) that major clinical outcomes in *selected* patients with LCA CAD are similar with CABG and PCI at 1- to 2-year follow-up, but repeated revascularization rates are higher after PCI than after CABG. RCTs with extended follow-up of 5 years are required to provide definitive conclusions about the optimal treatment of LCA CAD.

In the NOBLE trial comparing PCI versus CABG, Kaplan-Meier 5-year estimates of major adverse cardiac event (MACE) were 28% for PCI (121 events) and 18% for CABG (80 events) (hazard ratio, 1.51; 95% confidence interval, 1.13–2.00), exceeding the limit for noninferiority, and CABG was significantly better than PCI ($P = 0.0044$). As-treated estimates were 28% versus 18% (1.48, 1.11–1.98; $P = 0.0069$). Comparing PCI with CABG, 5-year estimates were 11% versus 9% (1.08, 0.67–1.74; $P = 0.84$) for all-cause mortality, 6% versus 2% (2.87, 1.40–5.89; $P = 0.0040$) for nonprocedural MI, 15% versus 10% (1.50, 1.04–2.17; $P = 0.0304$) for any revascularization, and 5% versus 2% (2.20, 0.91–5.36; $P = 0.08$) for stroke.[30]

Revascularization Options for LCA CAD

Although CABG has been considered the gold standard for unprotected LCA CAD revascularization, PCI has more recently emerged as a possible alternative mode of revascularization in carefully selected patients. Lesion location is an important determinant when PCI is considered for unprotected LCA CAD. Stenting of the LCA ostium or trunk is more straightforward than treatment of distal bifurcation or trifurcation stenoses, which generally requires a greater degree of operator experience and expertise. In addition, PCI of bifurcation disease is associated with higher restenosis rates than PCI of disease confined to the ostium or trunk. Although lesion location influences technical success and long-term outcomes after PCI, location exerts a negligible influence on the success of CABG. In subgroup analyses, patients with LCA CAD and a SYNTAX score of 33 with more complex or extensive CAD had a higher mortality rate with PCI than with CABG. Physicians can estimate operative risk for all CABG candidates by using a standard instrument, such as the risk calculator from the Society of Thoracic Surgeons (STS) database. These considerations are important factors when one is choosing among revascularization strategies for unprotected LCA CAD and have been factored into revascularization recommendations. Use of a Heart Team approach has been recommended in cases in which the choice of revascularization is not straightforward. The patient's ability to tolerate and to comply with dual antiplatelet therapy is also an important consideration in revascularization decisions.

Experts have recommended immediate PCI for unprotected LCA CAD in the setting of STEMI. The impetus for such a strategy is greatest when LCA CAD is the site of the culprit lesion, antegrade coronary flow is diminished (e.g., thrombolysis in MI flow grade 0, 1, or 2), the patient is hemodynamically unstable, and it is believed that PCI can be performed more quickly than CABG. When possible, the interventional cardiologist and cardiac surgeon should decide together on the optimal form of revascularization for these patients, although it is recognized that they are usually critically ill and therefore not amenable to a prolonged deliberation or discussion of treatment options.

Proximal LAD Artery Disease

Multiple studies have suggested that CABG confers a survival advantage over contemporaneous medical therapy for patients with disease in the proximal segment of the LAD artery. Cohort studies and RCTs, as well as collaborative analyses and metaanalyses, have shown that PCI and CABG result in similar survival rates in these patients.

Completeness of Revascularization

Most patients undergoing CABG receive complete or nearly complete revascularization, which seems to influence long-term prognosis positively.[32,33] In contrast, complete revascularization is accomplished less often in patients receiving PCI (e.g., in 70% of patients), and the extent to which the incomplete initial revascularization influences outcome is less clear. Rates of late survival and survival free of MI appear to be similar in patients with and without complete revascularization after PCI. Nevertheless, the need for subsequent CABG is usually higher in those whose initial revascularization procedure was incomplete (compared with those with complete revascularization) after PCI.

Left Ventricular Systolic Dysfunction

Several older studies and a metaanalysis of the data from these studies reported that patients with LV systolic dysfunction (predominantly mild to moderate in severity) had better survival with CABG than with medical therapy alone. In the Surgical Treatment for Ischemic Heart Failure (STICH) trial of CABG and GDMT in patients with an LVEF of 35% with or without viability testing, both treatments resulted in similar rates of survival (i.e., freedom from death from any cause, the study's primary outcome) after 5 years of follow-up. In the same study at 10 years, the rates of death from any cause, death from cardiovascular causes, and death from any cause or hospitalization for cardiovascular causes were significantly lower among patients who underwent CABG in addition to receiving medical therapy than among those who received medical therapy.[34,35]

Only limited data are available comparing PCI with medical therapy in patients with LV systolic dysfunction. The data that exist at present on revascularization in patients with CAD and LV systolic dysfunction are more robust for CABG than for PCI, although data from contemporary RCTs in this population of patients are lacking.

The choice of revascularization method in patients with CAD and LV systolic dysfunction is best based on clinical variables (e.g., coronary anatomy, presence of diabetes mellitus, presence of chronic kidney disease), magnitude of LV systolic dysfunction, preferences of the patient, clinical judgment, and consultation between the interventional cardiologist and the cardiac surgeon.

Revascularization Options for Previous CABG

In patients with recurrent angina after CABG, repeated revascularization is most likely to improve survival in patients at highest risk, such as those with obstruction of the proximal LAD artery and extensive anterior ischemia. Patients with ischemia in other locations and those with a patent LIMA to the LAD artery are unlikely to experience a survival benefit from repeated revascularization.[36] Cohort studies comparing PCI and CABG among post-CABG patients report similar rates of midterm and long-term survival after the two procedures. In patients with previous CABG who are referred for revascularization for medically refractory ischemia, factors that may support the choice of repeated CABG include vessels unsuitable for PCI, multiple diseased bypass grafts, availability of the internal mammary artery (IMA) for grafting of chronically occluded coronary arteries, and good distal targets for bypass graft placement. Factors favoring PCI over CABG include limited areas of ischemia causing symptoms, suitable PCI targets, patent graft to the LAD artery, poor CABG targets, and comorbid conditions.

Unstable Angina/Non–ST-Segment Elevation Myocardial Infarction

The main difference between treating a patient with SIHD and a patient with UA/NSTEMI is that the impetus for revascularization is stronger in the treatment of UA/NSTEMI because myocardial ischemia occurring as part of an acute coronary syndrome is potentially life-threatening, and associated angina symptoms are more likely to be reduced with a revascularization procedure than with GDMT.[37] Thus, the indications for revascularization are strengthened by the acuity of presentation, the extent of ischemia, and the likelihood of achieving full revascularization. The choice of revascularization method is generally dictated by the same considerations used to decide between PCI or CABG for patients with SIHD.

ST-Segment Elevation Myocardial Infarction–Acute Myocardial Infarction

Percutaneous Coronary Intervention Versus Medical Management for Acute Myocardial Infarction

In general, PCI confers a greater survival advantage than thrombolytics as an initial treatment for STEMI–acute MI (AMI), and the use of delayed PCI as an adjunct to therapy, including therapy with thrombolytics, does not affect survival. In the Global Use of Strategies to Open Occluded Coronary Arteries in Acute Coronary Syndromes (GUSTO) IIb trial,[38] the 30-day rate of the composite end point of death, nonfatal MI, and nonfatal disabling stroke was 9.6% for PCI patients and 13.7% for recipients of thrombolytics.

Prospective observational data collected from the Second National Registry of Myocardial Infarction between June 1994 and March 1998 included data from a cohort of 27,080 consecutive patients with AMI associated with ST-segment elevation or left bundle branch block. These patients were all treated with primary angioplasty. The study revealed that the adjusted odds of mortality were significantly higher (62% vs. 41%) for patients with door-to-balloon times longer than 2 hours. The longer the door-to-balloon time, the higher the mortality risk, emphasizing that door-to-balloon time has a significant impact on outcomes for patients with AMI.[39]

On the basis of this evidence, PCI facilities have been required to establish a target door-to-balloon time of no longer than 90 minutes. Depending on the available facilities in a particular region, it is the responsibility of emergency medical services personnel to determine whether that goal can be achieved by transferring the patient to a PCI-capable facility. If this cannot be accomplished, a medical management strategy should be considered, with the goal being a door-to-needle time of 30 minutes or less.[40]

Role of Coronary Artery Bypass Grafting

Although an increasing number of patients undergo catheterization early after AMI, the initial treatment is directed by the interventionalist, which has significantly diminished the role of emergency CABG. In general, patients who undergo CABG early after AMI are sicker, and efforts to improve myocardial function are typically refractory to medical therapy. These patients typically have a higher incidence of comorbidities and are more likely to require intraaortic balloon pump (IABP) insertion. The optimal timing of CABG after AMI is not well established. A review of California discharge data identified 9476 patients who were hospitalized for AMI and subsequently underwent CABG. Of these, 4676 (49%) were in the early CABG group and 4800 (51%) were in the late CABG group. The mortality rate was highest (8.2%) among patients who underwent CABG on day 0 and declined to a nadir of 3.0% among patients who underwent CABG on day 3. The mean time to CABG was 3.2 days. Early CABG was an independent predictor of mortality, suggesting that CABG may best be deferred for 3 days or more after admission for AMI in nonurgent cases.[41]

The Should We Emergently Revascularize Occluded Coronaries for Cardiogenic Shock (SHOCK) trial has shown the survival advantage of emergency revascularization versus initial medical stabilization in patients in whom cardiogenic shock developed after AMI. A subanalysis that compared the effects of PCI and CABG on 30-day and 1-year survival showed that survival rates were similar at both time points. Among SHOCK trial patients randomly assigned to undergo emergency revascularization, those treated with CABG had a greater prevalence of diabetes and worse CAD than those treated with PCI. However, survival rates were similar.

In patients with AMI, CABG is usually performed in conjunction with an operation to treat a specific complication, such as refractory postinfarction angina, papillary muscle rupture with mitral regurgitation, and infarction VSD. The rationale for urgent or emergent surgery is often based on high early mortality risk from mechanical complications.

Preoperative Evaluation

The success of coronary artery revascularization depends on proper workup and patient selection. Currently, a multidisciplinary approach with cardiologists and cardiac surgeons is needed to give the patient the most appropriate form of revascularization based on guidelines (Fig. 60.6). Comorbidities that affect CABG outcomes and that are typically incorporated into risk models include age, gender, urgency of the procedure, ejection fraction, need for mechanical circulatory support, MI, smoking status, use of immunosuppressive drugs, prior coronary interventions, hypertension, diabetes, peripheral vascular disease (PVD), and cerebrovascular disease. In addition, the severity of angina, as designated by the Canadian Cardiovascular Society classification of angina, and the New York Heart Association classification of congestive heart failure (CHF) are important risk variables.

The following are essential components of a preoperative workup for CABG patients:

- Detailed history and physical examination, including conduit evaluation
- Review of medications, including angiotensin-converting enzyme inhibitors, beta blockers, antiplatelet agents, and anticoagulants
- Carotid duplex ultrasonography in patients who have clinical bruit or are at high risk for cerebrovascular disease
- Cardiac echocardiography to evaluate ventricular function and the structural integrity of valves and chambers
- Cardiac viability study in patients with depressed LVEF, chronic total occlusions, frailty, and high-risk operations to decide between PCI and CABG

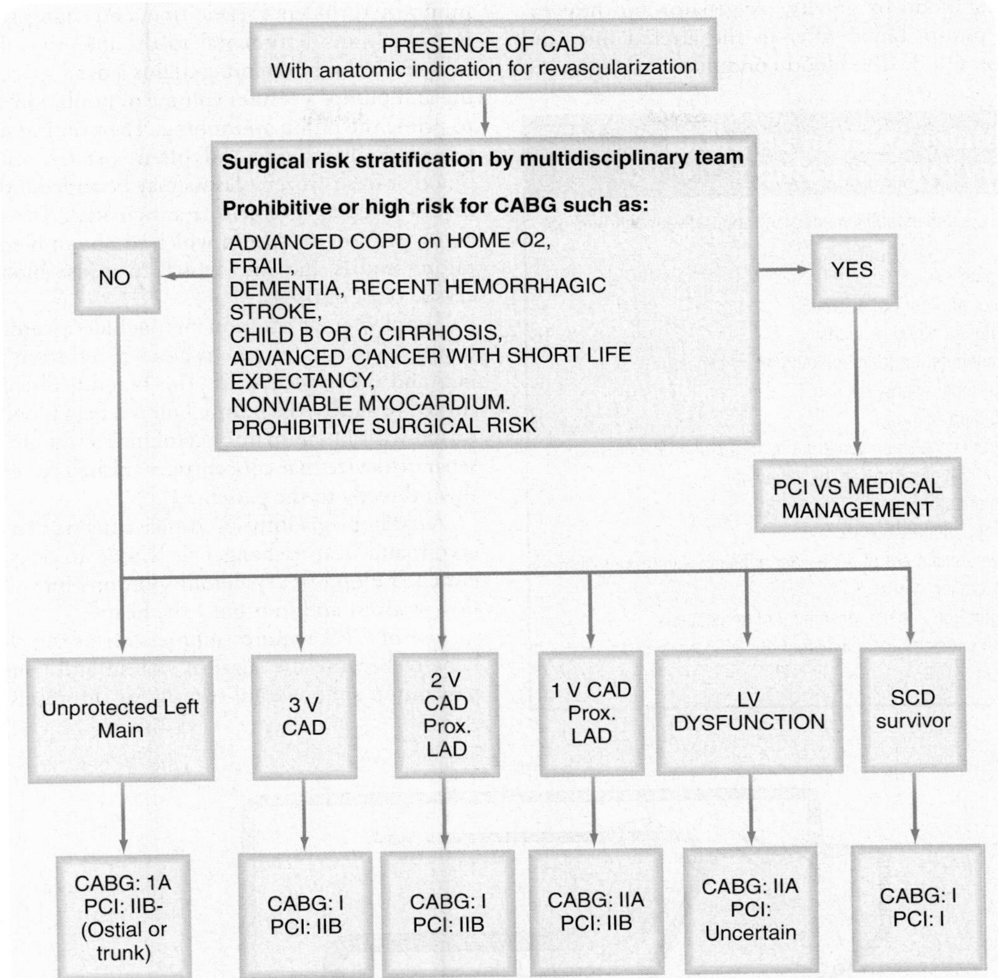

FIG. 60.6 Surgical decision-making tree for coronary revascularization. *CABG*, Coronary artery bypass grafting; *CAD*, coronary artery disease; *COPD*, chronic obstructive pulmonary disease; *LAD*, left anterior descending; *LV*, left ventricle; *PCI*, percutaneous coronary intervention; *SCD*, sudden cardiac death (sudden cardiac arrest).

- Cardiac catheterization to delineate the coronary anatomy
- Chest radiography
- Coagulation and platelet profile, comprehensive metabolic panel, and complete blood count

Depending on the findings of these tests, patients may need additional workup. In emergency circumstances, several of these tests may be skipped so that immediate revascularization can be performed.

Technique of Myocardial Revascularization: Conventional On-Pump Cardiopulmonary Bypass

Box 60.4 outlines all the major steps of an on-pump CABG operation.

Positioning and Draping

General anesthesia with a single-lumen endotracheal tube is the anesthetic technique of choice. After anesthetic induction and placement of necessary access and monitoring lines, the patient is positioned supine, with or without a roll underneath the shoulder blades according to the surgeon's preference. The arms are tucked beside the patient with appropriate padding to minimize the chance of any nerve injury. A warming blanket is typically placed underneath the patient to assist in rewarming after controlled hypothermia during CPB. The entire chest, abdomen, and lower extremities are prepared. Circumferential preparation of the lower extremities is important because the leg may have to be maneuvered during harvesting of the saphenous vein conduit. If radial artery harvesting is being contemplated, the arm also has to be circumferentially prepared and positioned 90 degrees from the bedside on an arm board because most patients have a multilumen central line in the internal jugular vein or a Swan-Ganz catheter. Anchor points on the drapes are designated appropriately to allow CPB circuit lines to be secured without compromising sterility.

Cardiopulmonary Bypass

CPB is the establishment of extracorporeal oxygenation and perfusion of the human body by diverting all returning venous blood from the body to the heart-lung machine and returning the oxygenated blood in a controlled, pressurized manner. In essence, most blood flow to the heart and lungs is bypassed. Establishment of CPB is a critical step for any major cardiac procedure and allows complete control of the operation.

The basic components of an extracorporeal heart pump circuit are venous cannulas to drain the returning venous blood, venous reservoir that collects blood by gravity, oxygenator and heat exchanger, perfusion pump, blood filter in the arterial line, and arterial cannula (Fig. 60.7). The blood conduits are designed to minimize turbulence, cavitation, and changes in blood flow velocity, which are detrimental to the integrity of component blood cells. Because the circuit contains a dead space created by the tubing and pump, a certain volume of nonblood solution is necessary to prime the pump and tubing. The priming solution consists of a balanced salt solution and, often, a starch solution. Homologous blood or fresh-frozen plasma may be added if the patient is anemic or if a bleeding problem is anticipated. The circuit has multiple access ports or sites from which to obtain blood samples for laboratory studies and into which to infuse blood, blood products, crystalloids, or drugs.

Supplemental components include a cardiotomy suction system to collect undiluted or clean blood from open cardiac chambers and the surgical field. This blood is filtered, de-aired, and returned to the bypass pump. Diluted field blood and blood that has mixed with inflammatory cytokines or fat are collected through a separate device that concentrates washed red cells before returning them directly to the patient.

A cardioplegia infusion device consists of a separate pump, reservoir, and heat exchanger. It is used to deliver cold, potassium-enriched blood or crystalloid solutions into the coronary circulation to arrest and to protect the heart.

Use of CPB requires suppression of the clotting cascade with heparin because the surgical wound and components of the bypass pump are powerful stimuli for thrombus formation. A strict

BOX 60.4 Major steps in on-pump coronary artery bypass grafting.

- Induction of anesthesia and establishment of intraoperative monitoring adjuncts
- Positioning and draping
- Median sternotomy or appropriate approach
- Harvest and evaluation of blood conduits
- Heparinization and cannulation for cardiopulmonary bypass
- Establishment of cardiopulmonary bypass
- Myocardial arrest and protection
- Identification of target vessels and construction of distal anastomoses
- Restoration of myocardial electromechanical activity
- Creation of proximal anastomoses
- Weaning from cardiopulmonary bypass
- Evaluation for and establishment of necessary adjuncts—inotropes, intra-aortic balloon pump, pacing wires
- Reversal of anticoagulation and establishment of hemostasis
- Evaluation of surgical sites and establishment of surgical drainage
- Closure of sternotomy

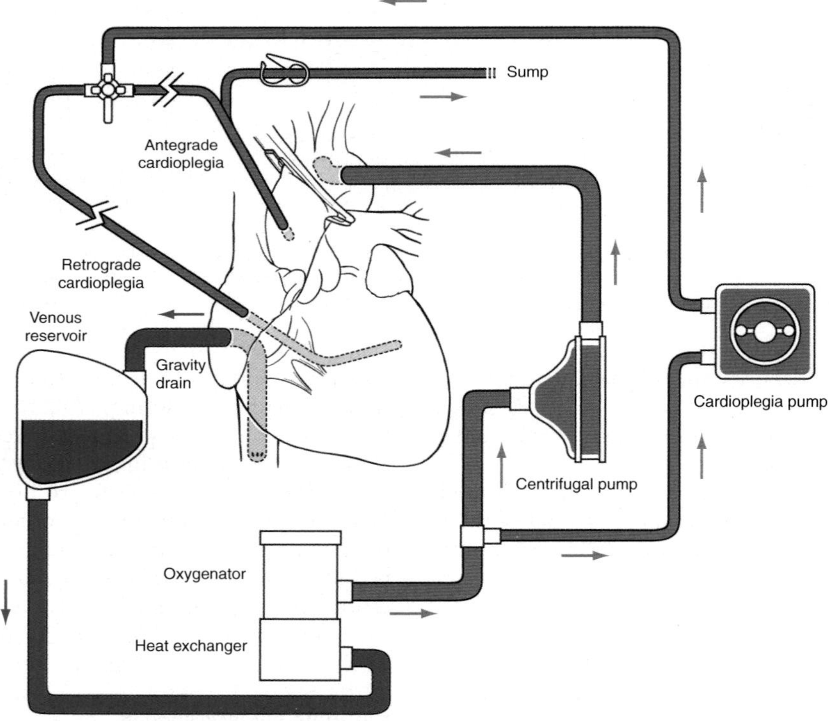

FIG. 60.7 Schematic of total cardiopulmonary bypass circuit. All returning venous blood is siphoned into a venous reservoir and is oxygenated, and temperature is regulated before being pumped back through a centrifugal pump into the arterial circulation. The most common site for inflow cannulation is the ascending aorta; alternative sites include the femoral arteries and the right axillary artery in special circumstances. A parallel circuit derives oxygenated blood that is mixed with cold (4°C) cardioplegia solution in a 4:1 ratio and administered in antegrade or retrograde fashion to induce cardiac arrest. Cardioplegia solution is administered antegrade into the aortic root and retrograde through the coronary sinus. During the retrograde administration of cardioplegia solution, the efflux of blood from the coronary ostium is siphoned off through the sump drain, a return parallel circuit connected to the venous reservoir (not shown) that also helps to keep the heart decompressed during the arrest phase.

anticoagulation protocol should be enforced before CPB is initiated. The pump prime is premixed with 4 U/mL heparin, and the patient is systemically heparinized with 300 U/kg before cannulation. An activated clotting time obtained approximately 3 minutes after heparin administration should be more than 400 seconds before cannulation is begun and should be maintained for more than 450 seconds throughout CPB, with intermittent doses given as needed during the operation.

The usual pumps are roller head pumps, which consist of circumferential tubing that is compressed by a roller on the outside, thereby forcing blood in one direction. This pump mechanism is associated with higher rates of hemolysis compared with centrifugal pumps, so roller head pumps are used only in cardiotomy suction and cardioplegia pumps. The main systemic pump is a centrifugal pump that consists of a vortex polyurethane-embedded magnetic cone housed in a conical chamber. The vortex spins at approximately 2000 to 5000 rpm, thereby generating enough centrifugal force to pump blood. Because the flow is entirely caused by a nonturbulent vortex generated by a finless cone, this mechanism is almost atraumatic to the blood cells and is therefore associated with less hemolysis than the roller head pump mechanism (Fig. 60.8).

Neurologic Protection During Cardiopulmonary Bypass

The incidence of stroke after CPB is approximately 1.5%, but neurocognitive deficits are more frequent. Thus, several steps should be taken during CPB to minimize the risk of neurologic insult, including maintaining adequate cerebral perfusion, minimizing fat microemboli by eliminating the unnecessary use of cardiotomy suction, minimizing aortic manipulation by using single-clamp techniques when feasible, and instituting moderate hypothermia.

The oxygen consumption of a patient on CPB at normal temperatures averages 80 to 125 mL/min/m^2, similar to that of an anesthetized adult not on bypass. However, with the use of hypothermia, the oxygen consumption is markedly lower, and the flow rate can be reduced to less than 2.2 L/min/m^2. This is because the mean oxygen consumption of the body decreases by 50% for every 10°C decrease in body temperature. Below 28°C, a flow rate of 1.6 L/min/m^2 may be safe for as long as 2 hours. Significant

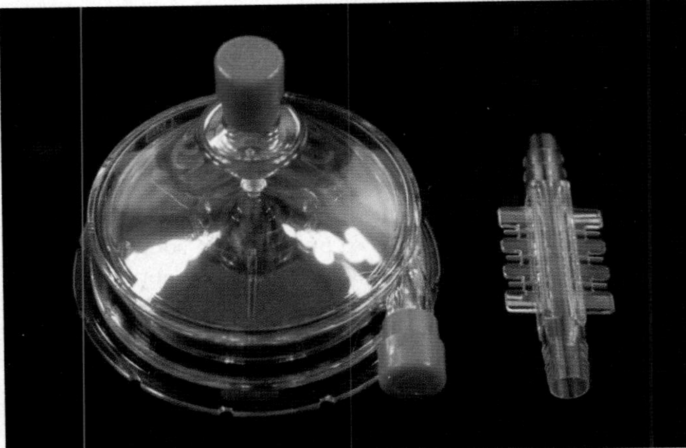

FIG. 60.8 Main centrifugal pump used in most cardiopulmonary bypass circuits. The entire unit is sterile molded and contains a finless cone that spins at 2000 to 5000 rpm, generating a powerful yet nonturbulent vortex. A flow meter (shown) must be used with these pumps because the ultimate volume of flow depends on outflow resistance rather than on pump speed. The conventional roller head pumps are still used for the auxiliary circuits, such as cardiotomy suction and cardioplegia circuits.

disadvantages of using systemic hypothermia to accommodate lower flow rates include the extra time required to rewarm the patient and associated changes in the reactivity of blood elements, particularly platelets. These changes may increase the rewarmed patient's propensity for bleeding.

Median Sternotomy

The most common approach for performing CABG is a median sternotomy, although anterolateral thoracotomy is used in certain circumstances. A traditional sternotomy incision commences at the midpoint of the manubrium and is carried down to the xiphoid. The sternum is split through the middle with a sternal saw. It is essential that gentle upward force and a backward tilt be applied to the saw to prevent it from engaging the lung or soft tissues in the anterior mediastinum. Once the sternotomy is completed, the periosteum of the posterior table is cauterized, and a passive hemostatic agent such as bone wax or a reconstituted mixture of vancomycin may be used to prevent bleeding from the marrow. The most important consideration during the sternotomy is staying in the midline because the most common cause of sternal dehiscence is an off-midline sternotomy and the consequent technically suboptimal closure. Other potential problems associated with the sternotomy include indirect injury to the liver and direct injury to the heart, innominate vein, and lungs.

Conduit Choice and Harvesting

Left internal mammary artery. In a seminal study from the Cleveland Clinic, Loop and colleagues[42] have shown improved 10-year survival in patients who received a LIMA graft; patients who received an SVG had 1.6 times the risk of death that LIMA graft recipients had. The long-term patency rate of the LIMA graft has been shown to be approximately 95% and 90% at 10 and 20 years, respectively. The best patency rates are achieved when the LIMA is used as an in situ pedicled graft and is anastomosed to the LAD.

Bilateral internal mammary artery. Observational studies from major CABG centers suggested that the use of bilateral IMA (BIMA) grafts improves survival and significantly reduces the need for reoperation without increasing mortality. However, early results from a randomized trial demonstrated that compared with SVGs, BIMA grafts are associated with a higher (twofold) incidence of deep sternal wound infection. BIMA grafts are best used by experienced surgeons in younger, nondiabetic, nonobese patients. Four major studies that tilted the balance in favor of BIMA grafts were the two Cleveland Clinic studies (1999 and 2004), in which propensity scores were used to match single and BIMA graft recipients; the Oxford metaanalysis (2001); and a retrospective study from Japan (2001). Skeletonization of the IMA grafts may reduce the wound complication rate.

The ART trial has revealed no significant difference in mortality and cardiovascular events with the use if BIMA at 5 years. At 10-year follow-up of the ART trial among patients who were scheduled for CABG and had been randomly assigned to undergo bilateral or single internal-thoracic-artery grafting, there was no significant difference between-group difference in the rate of death from any cause at 10 years in the intention-to-treat analysis.[43]

The IMA is harvested after the sternotomy is completed. A specially designed mammary retractor is used to elevate the appropriate hemithorax, typically the left for harvesting the LIMA. Adequately exposing the undersurface of the sternum is essential for successful harvest of the IMA (Fig. 60.9). The artery may be harvested as a pedicle that includes the two venae comitantes and surrounding soft

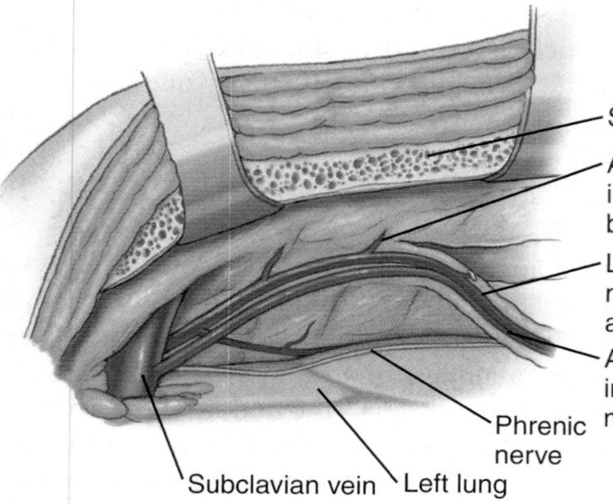

FIG. 60.9 Surgeon's view of the left internal mammary artery (LIMA) as it is being harvested. A mammary retractor is used to elevate the left hemithorax to provide adequate visualization. The LIMA is dissected away from the chest wall as a pedicle with its accompanying venae comitantes. Low-voltage electrocautery with no-touch technique is crucial for the atraumatic harvest of this important conduit. Understanding of its relation to the phrenic nerve and subclavian veins is important to avoid injury to these structures during LIMA harvest.

tissue from the level of the subclavian vein to the level of the bifurcation of the artery into the superior epigastric and musculophrenic branches. The alternative method of harvesting is the skeletonized harvest, in which only the IMA is dissected away from the chest wall.

The basic principle of harvesting the IMA relies exclusively on the no-touch technique, use of low-voltage electrocautery, and clipping of the anterior intercostal branches. Care must be taken during the harvest to identify the course of the phrenic nerves and to avoid injury to them. This is particularly important while harvesting the right IMA because the phrenic nerve is more closely related to it at the level of the second or third intercostal space. The IMA is a fragile vessel, and direct handling or undue traction should be avoided because it may cause traumatic dissection of the vessel. The distal end of the IMA should be divided only after the patient is fully heparinized to avoid thrombosis of the conduit. Once the IMA is divided, the distal end is spatulated appropriately to fashion the anastomosis.

Greater saphenous vein. Vein grafts have a patency rate of 90% at 1 year.[44] Beyond 5 years after surgery, graft atherosclerosis develops in a substantial number of SVGs. Historically, by 10 years, only 60% to 70% of SVGs are patent, and 50% of those have angiographic evidence of atherosclerosis.

While the sternotomy is being done, a separate team begins harvesting saphenous or radial artery conduits. Saphenous vein harvesting can be performed by open or endoscopic techniques. The conventional method of open vein harvesting involves making a long incision along the entire length of the harvested vein. Alternatively, a bridging technique can be used in which multiple 1- to 2-inch incisions are made, with intact bridges of skin between them. The most common complications associated with long open incisions are pain, slow wound healing, and dehiscence, which is compounded by the fact that a significant number of CABG patients have diabetes or PVD. The use of endoscopic or bridging techniques significantly alleviates but does not entirely eliminate these problems. There are some centers that avoid endoscopic vein harvesting entirely on the assumption that the technique is too traumatic to the vein itself, may be associated with intimal trauma, and may impair the long-term patency of the conduit. However, a recent randomized trial (REGROUP)

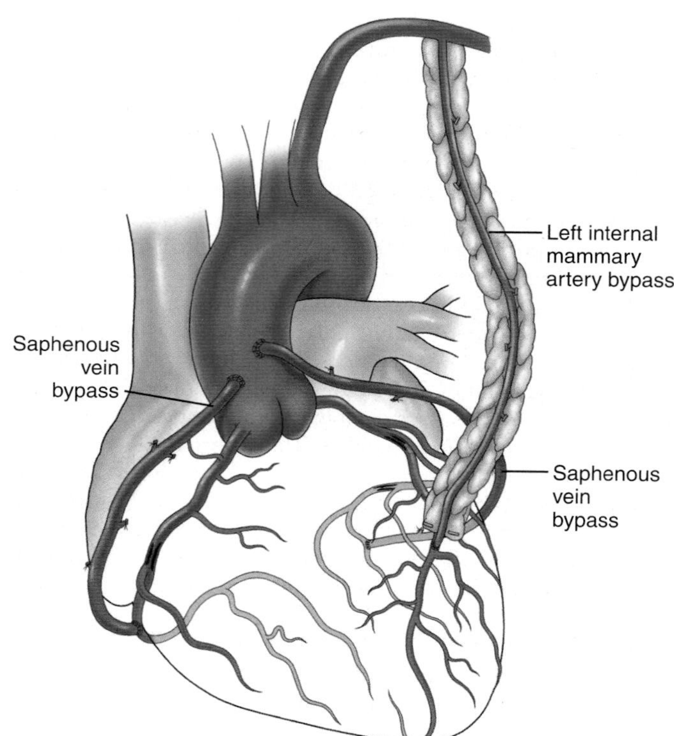

FIG. 60.10 Typical configuration for a three-vessel coronary artery bypass. The left internal mammary artery is anastomosed to the left anterior descending artery. Aortocoronary bypasses are created with reversed saphenous vein to the distal right coronary artery and an obtuse marginal branch of the circumflex coronary artery. The circumflex coronary artery is usually avoided as a target for bypass because its location well inside the atrioventricular groove makes it difficult to visualize.

demonstrated the safety and efficacy of endoscopic vein harvesting.[45] These reports were based on post hoc analyses of data from trials designed to address other aspects of coronary revascularization. Once the vein is extracted and the branches are ligated, the graft is soaked in a heparin solution while awaiting implantation. The veins are typically used in a reversed fashion and hence may not require valvotomy. A typical configuration of a three-vessel coronary artery bypass graft is shown in Fig. 60.10.

Alternative conduits may be needed in patients who have had previous coronary bypass, peripheral vascular surgery with the use of vein conduits, or lower extremity amputations and in those who have unusable saphenous vein conduits because of severe varicosities of the saphenous vein. Other manifestations of venous insufficiency or disease may also pose problems. In addition, patients who have severely calcified ascending aortas may not be amenable to a vein-based aortocoronary bypass because anastomosis to the ascending aorta is complicated. In these cases, alternative bypass strategies include total arterial revascularization with BIMA pedicles (Fig. 60.11). In addition, the IMA may be used as the main conduit from which further arterial conduits may be Christmas-treed in an off-pump setup so that any aortic manipulation is avoided.

Other conduits

Radial artery. The radial artery graft is easily harvested and can reach all coronary territories, making it an attractive option for an arterial conduit. Both the Radial Artery Patency Study and the Radial Artery versus Saphenous Vein Patency study showed

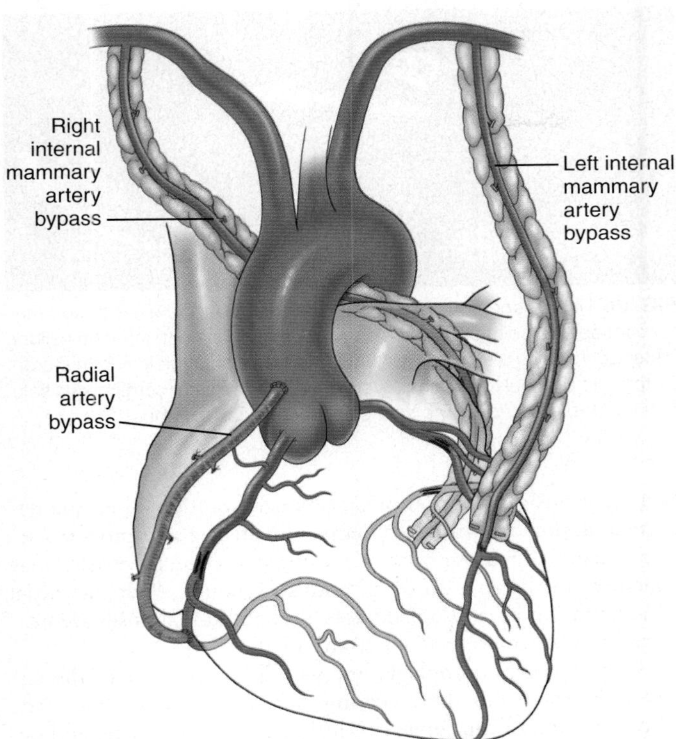

FIG. 60.11 Total arterial revascularization by use of bilateral mammary artery and radial artery conduits. The right internal mammary artery, bypassed to an obtuse marginal branch, is routed behind the aorta, and the pulmonary artery is routed through the transverse sinus.

radial artery grafts to have better patency than SVGs on 5-year angiographic follow-up. However, the radial artery is associated with a significantly higher incidence of conduit spasm and string sign. In addition, to date, no study has shown a survival advantage of radial artery over SVG grafting. Also, patency is much worse if the radial grafts are not placed on critically stenotic vessels.

Gastroepiploic artery. The gastroepiploic artery is rarely used today, although some centers in Asia still use gastroepiploic grafts and continue to report acceptable outcomes associated with them. Evidence from RCTs and a recent metaanalysis suggests that the saphenous vein has better early (6-month) and midterm (3-year) graft patency than the right gastroepiploic artery when it is used for RCA revascularization.

Total Arterial Revascularization

More than 90% of all CABG operations performed in the United States, United Kingdom, and Australia involve only one arterial graft.[46,47] The LIMA and SVG remain the standard CABG grafts; SVGs account for most of the conduits used. In an effort to ameliorate the shortcomings of SVGs, which are vulnerable to atherosclerosis and stenosis over time, some centers have been heavily emphasizing total arterial revascularization in which the LIMA, right IMA, and radial arteries are used.

Results from retrospective series have shown some survival benefit with total arterial revascularization, as would be expected. However, there are certain pragmatic reasons that total arterial revascularization has not totally replaced the use of SVGs:

- Concern about arterial spasm: Arterial grafts, particularly radial grafts, are prone to spasm, and their use necessitates vasodilator administration
- Use of arterial grafts appropriate only for severely stenotic arteries as they are more vulnerable to competitive flow compared to veins: Most experts would not use a radial graft unless there is at least 70% stenosis and probably 90% or more for larger vessels such as the main right coronary
- Inadequate length: As an in situ graft, the right IMA is typically not long enough to reach the PDA, mid or distal circumflex, or distal LAD and cannot be used easily as a sequential graft. It can, however, be used as a free graft
- Concern about sternal nonunion and mediastinitis: There is a higher risk of sternal nonunion and mediastinitis with the use of BIMA grafts versus SVGs. Most experts will not use BIMA grafts in patients with poorly controlled diabetes, severe PVD, use of steroids, severe chronic obstructive pulmonary disease, or morbid obesity. Also, in the event that BIMA is used, most would recommend the skeletonized technique of BIMA harvest with preservation of the intercostal blood supply
- Longer operative times: Using BIMA grafts obviously prolongs operative times

Because of all these practical considerations, multiarterial revascularization has not become as popular as would be expected, and most surgeons would offer total arterial revascularization only to younger patients because of their longer life expectancy.

Cannulation for Cardiopulmonary Bypass

Cannulation for the establishment of CPB commences after conduit harvest and preparation are completed, the pericardium is opened, and the thymus is divided along the embryologic fusion plane. The patient is fully heparinized at a dose of 3 mg/kg. A purse-string is created on the anterior surface of the distal ascending aorta at the cannulation site. The aortic purse-string should involve only a partial thickness of the aorta, incorporating the adventitia and media but entirely avoiding the intimal layer. It is essential that the cannulation site be free of calcified plaques or atheroma to minimize the chance of embolization and cannulation site bleeding. Manual palpation, the commonly practiced method of assessment, is unreliable. Doppler transesophageal or epiaortic ultrasonographic guidance should be used whenever aortic disease is suspected. Also, the presence of calcium elsewhere in the ascending aorta may preclude safe clamp application. Although cannulation of the aorta may be a simple task, loss of control of the aortic cannulation site or inadvertent dissection could lead to a disastrous situation.

With a sharp scalpel, the adventitia is teased, and a full-thickness stab incision is made. The aortic cannula is inserted with the outflow bevel aimed toward the aortic arch. Tourniquet snares are used to secure the cannula in position and are tied. After the cannula is de-aired, it is connected to the arterial line of the CPB circuit. Alternative sites of arterial cannulation include the femoral artery and right axillary artery, which are used in reoperations or cases in which concomitant complex aortic and arch reconstruction may be required. Axillary artery cannulation is usually achieved with an 8-mm graft anastomosed end to side to the axillary artery.

For venous cannulation, a purse-string is then placed around the right atrial appendage. The tip of this appendage is amputated, and a dual-stage venous cannula is inserted and positioned with the tip at the level of the diaphragm. The basket of the dual-stage cannula should rest in the main chamber of the right atrium to capture drainage from the superior vena cava into the right atrium (Figs. 60.12 and 60.13).

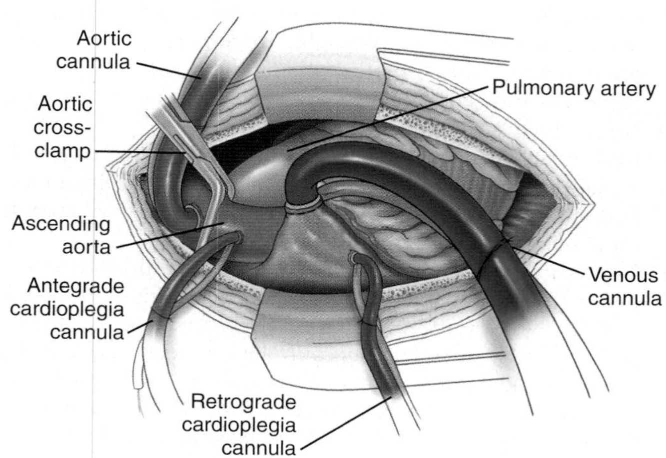

FIG. 60.12 Surgeon's view of the heart after cannulation. The cross-clamp isolates the aortic root and coronary vessels from the rest of the systemic circulation. This allows administration of cardioplegia solution in a closed circuit and prevents the systemic blood from washing the cardioplegia solution out of the coronary system during the arrest phase. Applying the cross-clamp prevents active blood flow through the coronary arteries and thus allows the surgeon to perform the distal anastomoses in a bloodless field.

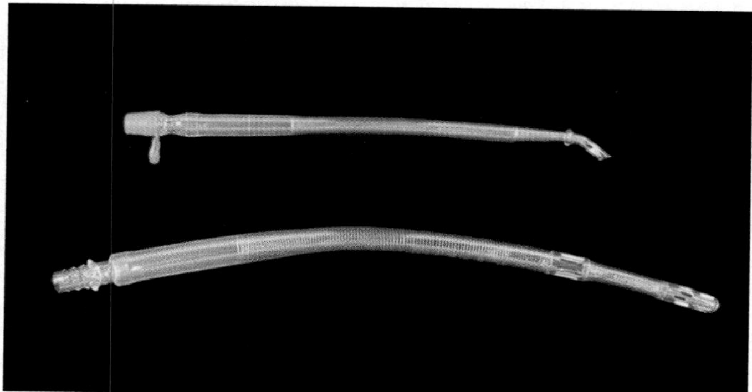

FIG. 60.13 Aortic cannula *(top):* The specially designed tip is angulated to allow laminar flow of blood into the aortic arch. Dual-stage venous cannula *(bottom):* The first stage is the fenestrated basket that usually rests at the level of the hepatic veins and captures all venous return from the inferior vena cava. The second-stage basket is located such that it remains within the right atrium and captures venous return from the superior vena cava, azygos vein, coronary sinus, and direct collateral drainage into the right atrium. The venous drainage is a passive siphon aided by gravity.

Cardiac Arrest and Myocardial Protection

The initiation of CPB allows the heart to be stopped. To achieve cardiac arrest, a large dose of potassium solution (cardioplegia) is injected into the coronary vessels. This requires the coronary blood flow to be completely isolated from the systemic circulation, which is done by applying a cross-clamp to the ascending aorta proximal to the aortic cannula.

There are several different delivery options for cardioplegia solutions. One involves taking a balanced approach; the cardioplegia solution is administered antegrade through the ascending aorta proximal to the cross-clamp and then retrograde through a coronary sinus catheter inserted through a purse-string suture placed in the right atrium by use of special cannulas (Fig. 60.14). The extensive collateralization among the coronary veins and arteries and the paucity of valves in the coronary vein system ensure a relatively

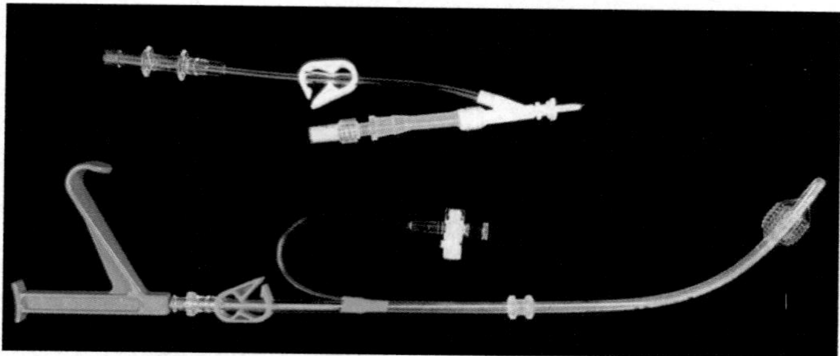

FIG. 60.14 Retrograde cardioplegia cannula *(bottom)* used to administer cardioplegia solution into the coronary sinus. The self-inflating balloon distends, forming a seal only when cardioplegia solution is administered. Antegrade cardioplegia cannula *(top)* used to administer cardioplegia solution into the aortic root. The side port functions as a sump.

homogeneous distribution of cardioplegia solution when the retrograde approach is used. Patients with high-grade proximal lesions, especially those with suboptimal collateral vessels, may benefit from the application of both techniques. After the initial administration of cardioplegia solution, additional doses are usually administered every 15 to 20 minutes.

An antegrade cardioplegia line with a Y-connector to the circuit is inserted into the ascending aorta. This allows antegrade administration of cardioplegia solution and also sumping and decompression of the ascending aorta while cardioplegia solution is administered retrogradely into the coronary sinus. The sump drain also functions to keep the coronary arteries free of any blood, thus providing the surgeon with a bloodless field in which to fashion the distal anastomoses. In addition, the sump drain performs the important function of decompressing the LV while the heart is arrested (see Figs. 60.7 and 60.12).

The most important task for ensuring myocardial protection is establishing complete diastolic arrest with an unloaded heart. In this state, the myocardial consumption of adenosine triphosphate is extremely low and allows maximal preservation of myocytes. In conventional CABG with total CPB, the decompression of the ventricle by off-loading, systemic cooling, topical cooling, and diastolic arrest of the heart with potassium cardioplegia solution serves to decrease myocardial oxygen consumption. Approximately 40% of the myocardial metabolic demand is eliminated when total CPB is established before diastolic arrest and cooling are instituted.

Target Identification and Distal Anastomosis

Once successful diastolic arrest of the heart is accomplished, the target coronary arteries to be bypassed are identified. Some of the epicardial conductance vessels are intramyocardial and therefore may not be directly visible. Once a target vessel is identified, it is opened with a sharp blade. Typically, the arteriotomy is approximately 5 mm long. The conduit, which is prepared and spatulated, is then grafted in an end-to-side fashion with running 7-0 or 8-0 Prolene suture. This component of the operation is technically the most challenging and requires precision. The flow and integrity of each vein conduit are tested by flushing it with cold blood or cardioplegia solution mix. The LIMA to left descending artery anastomosis is usually the last one to be performed (Fig. 60.15) because it is best to avoid manipulating the heart once this anastomosis is completed in case avulsion of the LIMA conduit occurs. Bypassing the PDA and obtuse marginal targets requires lifting the apex of the heart out of the pericardium.

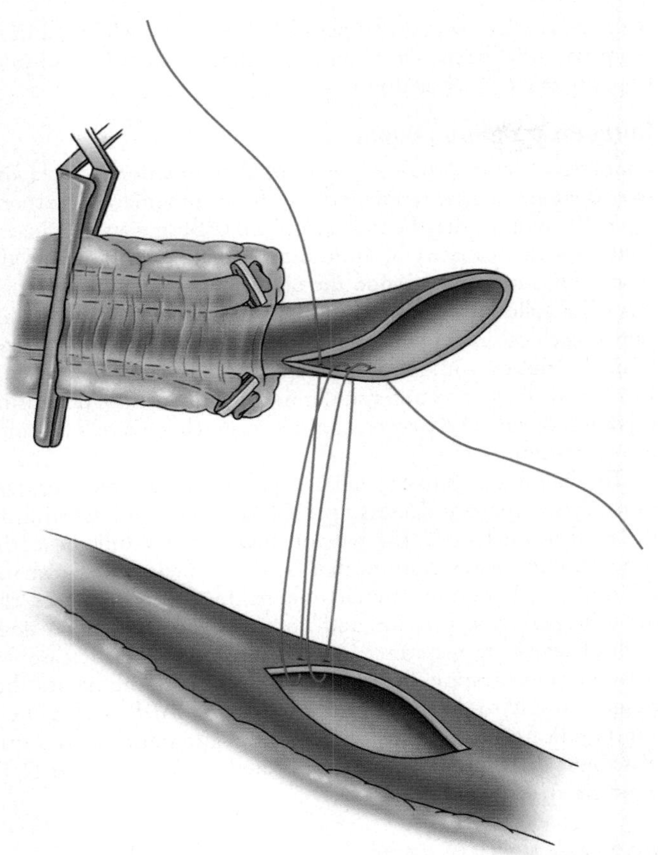

FIG. 60.15 Technique of constructing the distal anastomoses: left internal mammary artery to left anterior descending artery, magnified surgeon's view. A 5-mm longitudinal arteriotomy is made on the coronary artery to be bypassed. The distal end of the left internal mammary artery is spatulated to an appropriate size match. A 7-0 Prolene suture is used to create the anastomosis with a parachuting technique.

Typically, a single segment of conduit is anastomosed to each planned distal target. On occasion, a single conduit can be used to supply blood to two targets, which is known as a sequential anastomosis. This is a good technique to use when there is a shortage of available vein conduits or when the target vessels are small; in these cases, use of this technique ensures a higher rate of blood flow through the vein conduit, reducing the risk of graft thrombosis (Fig. 60.16).

As the last distal anastomosis is being completed, the patient is warmed back to physiologic temperature. The cross-clamp is released after the final dose of warm cardioplegia solution is administered, which helps in scavenging the accumulated free radicals in the myocardium. A partial clamp is then applied to the ascending aorta, and the proximal anastomoses are constructed in an end-to-side fashion with running 5-0 Prolene suture. If there are concerns about the quality of the aorta, use of a partial clamp is typically avoided in favor of a single-clamp technique, which involves constructing the proximal anastomoses on an arrested heart, as for the distal anastomoses.

In patients in whom the ascending aorta is calcified or a free IMA pedicle needs to be used, a branching pattern of proximal anastomoses is made. This conserves vein length to a certain extent but also minimizes the number of aortotomies, especially if the ascending aorta is short or a concomitant aortic procedure has been performed. The ascending aorta is allowed to de-air as the aortic clamp is released, after which the vein grafts are de-aired.

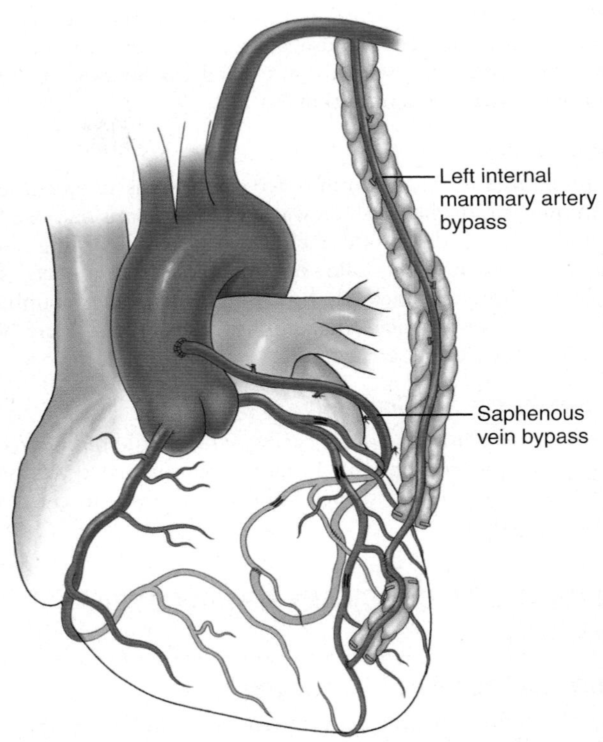

FIG. 60.16 Alternative configuration for a three-vessel coronary artery bypass. The left internal mammary artery is anastomosed sequentially to a diagonal branch and to the distal left anterior descending artery. Aortocoronary bypasses are constructed with reversed saphenous vein in sequential configuration to the left posterolateral artery and an obtuse marginal branch of the circumflex coronary artery. The ideal configuration depends on the extent and distribution of the coronary blockages.

Separation from Cardiopulmonary Bypass

Separation from CPB commences once the following physiologic criteria have been met:

- Resumption of rhythmic electromechanical activity
- Attainment of physiologic temperature above 36.5°C
- Availability of adequate reserve blood volume
- Restoration of normal systemic potassium levels
- Resumption of ventilation with an acceptable arterial blood gas level

A few other actions that may be considered at this point are placement of temporary pacing wires and insertion of an IABP, if needed. Typically, the CPB flows are progressively decreased as the following parameters are closely observed:

- Data from the Swan-Ganz catheter
- Direct visual observations of cardiac function and chamber volume
- The transesophageal echocardiogram

Most patients have a transient systemic inflammatory response, causing vasodilation that becomes more pronounced as they are warmed. Thus, restoration of volume with intravascular fluids or administration of vasopressors may be necessary to maintain systemic blood pressure. Inotropic agents may be used if ventricular function is not adequate. Separating patients from CPB is primarily the surgeon's responsibility but requires dynamic communication with the perfusionist and anesthesiologist.

After CPB is discontinued, the venous cannula is removed and the purse-string is tied down. Once it is confirmed that the heart is providing satisfactory perfusion, protamine is administered. Close monitoring is needed because adverse reactions to protamine range from transient hypotension to fatal anaphylaxis. Such reactions necessitate the resumption of CPB.

Hemostasis

As protamine is being administered, hemostasis is expeditiously accomplished. As the patient rewarms, blood vessels that had been hemostatic may dilate and rebleed. Persistent bleeding should alert the surgeon to the following possible causes: aspects of the surgical technique, platelet dysfunction, inadequate protamine reversal, and hypothermia. The administration of blood and blood products may be necessary.

Sternal Closure and Completion of Surgery

The chest tube and temporary pacing wires should be checked for appropriate positioning. The sternum is approximated with stainless steel wires. The soft tissues and skin are closed in layers with absorbable sutures.

ADJUNCTS TO CORONARY ARTERY BYPASS GRAFTING

Transesophageal Echocardiography

Use of transesophageal echocardiography (TEE) enables the assessment of ventricular wall motion abnormalities and the detection of any chamber or valve anomalies that may change the strategy of the operation. Examples of TEE findings that may affect the conduct of the operation include an incidentally discovered large patent foramen ovale or fibroelastoma of the valves. New-onset or worsening mitral regurgitation after CABG suggests inferior wall ischemia and may indicate reevaluation of the bypass grafts or valve repair or replacement. Also, TEE helps in assessing ejection fraction and the volume status of the heart after surgery.

Inotropes and Pharmacotherapy

Cardioplegic arrest causes transient myocardial ischemia and lactic acid accumulation. After perfusion is reestablished, the ventricles are stiffer and require higher filling pressures to maintain adequate stroke volume. Also, CPB may cause significant third spacing and vasodilation. Thus, epinephrine as an inotropic agent is ideal to maintain adequate contractility in the initial recovery phase and during separation from CPB. Alpha agonists such as norepinephrine, phenylephrine, and vasopressin may be used to counteract the effects of inflammatory vasodilation. In patients with depressed myocardial function, such as left- or right-sided heart failure, dobutamine or a phosphodiesterase inhibitor such as milrinone may be required to enhance myocardial contractility and to decrease afterload or pulmonary vascular resistance. Because hypotension is a common side effect of these drugs, the systemic volume must be adequate, and an alpha agonist may be required. Calcium channel blockers or nitroglycerin may be needed in patients with preexisting hypertension.

It is essential to maintain a mean arterial pressure higher than 60 mm Hg in the initial postoperative period, but hypertension should be avoided because it puts stress on a myocardium that is trying to recover and increases the risk of bleeding from anastomotic suture lines. Blood pressure management requires a thorough understanding of physiologic and pharmacologic principles. It is a balancing act geared toward maintaining adequate systemic pressure, cardiac output, and peripheral perfusion while minimizing myocardial stress. Urine output is the most reliable indicator of peripheral organ perfusion.

Intraaortic Balloon Pump

For patients whose profound myocardial dysfunction is unresponsive to volume resuscitation and significant pharmacologic therapy, IABP support may be indicated. The IABP is a special Silastic balloon with a capacity of 40 to 60 mL that is positioned in the descending aorta just beyond the origin of the left subclavian artery. The balloon is designed to be actively inflated and deflated during each cardiac cycle; its timing is controlled by a specially designed computer with input from an arterial line tracing or ECG. Intra-aortic balloon counterpulsation has the benefit of decreasing myocardial work and oxygen consumption while increasing coronary perfusion.

The balloon is actively deflated just before systolic contraction begins, thereby decreasing LV impedance and assisting in the ejection of blood. The balloon then actively inflates at the time of aortic valve closure; that is, it is timed to occur at the dicrotic notch of the arterial line tracing. This increases the diastolic perfusion pressure and improves coronary blood flow, both of which decrease the time-tension index and increase the diastolic pressure-time index, thereby increasing the myocardial oxygen supply-to-demand ratio. The use of IABP is absolutely contraindicated in patients with aortic regurgitation and aortic dissection. It is relatively contraindicated in patients with PVD or aortic aneurysm.

POSTOPERATIVE CARE

Postoperative care in the intensive care unit (ICU) begins with a thorough physical and hemodynamic assessment. Mediastinal chest tube drainage should be recorded and assessed hourly. Initial ventilator settings should be set to match those in the operating room. Further adjustments in ventilator settings are made according to the postoperative blood gases. High positive end-expiratory pressure should be avoided in patients with hemodynamic instability. The ideal mode of ventilation is that with which the surgical or intensive care team is comfortable. A portable chest radiograph is obtained to confirm the position of the endotracheal tube, central lines, Swan-Ganz catheter, and IABP and to identify any pneumothorax, atelectasis, pulmonary edema, or pleural effusions. Initial laboratory studies should include hemoglobin, hematocrit, electrolyte, blood urea nitrogen, creatinine, and arterial blood gas levels and platelet count, prothrombin time, and partial thromboplastin time.

The patient should have an ECG monitor that can assess ST-T wave abnormalities; an arterial line to measure arterial blood pressure; and a line to measure central venous pressure, pulse oximetry, and core temperature. In select patients, pulmonary artery pressures and cardiac output are monitored continuously with a Swan-Ganz catheter. Neurologic assessment should be completed as soon as the patient wakes up to ensure that no cerebrovascular accident has occurred.

The primary considerations during the first 12 hours after the operation should be maintaining adequate blood pressure and cardiac output, correcting coagulation defects and electrolyte levels, stabilizing intravascular volume, and normalizing the peripheral vascular resistance. This often involves administration of crystalloid solutions, blood or blood products, inotropic agents, calcium, and vasodilators or vasoconstrictors.

Some of the goals in the postoperative period are as follows:

- Avoiding marked elevations in blood pressure
- Maintaining adequate perfusion pressure (60–80 mm Hg)
- Maintaining core body temperature higher than 36.5°C by warming the patient with forced hot air blankets
- Maintaining adequate cardiac output and a cardiac index of 2.2 L/min/m^2
- Keeping mixed venous oxygenation at 60%
- Reducing afterload, as appropriate, to minimize myocardial work
- Volume resuscitation with crystalloid or blood products, as necessary
- Maintaining hemoglobin level higher than 8 g/dL, or higher than 10 g/dL in older patients or those with severe cerebrovascular disease
- Maintaining homeostatic pH. Metabolic acidosis may be caused by hypoperfusion from low cardiac output, poor resuscitation, hypovolemia, or end-organ ischemia from embolism.
- Monitoring neurologic and peripheral vascular status
- Maintaining a sinus or perfusing rhythm at a rate of 70 to 100 beats/min
- Monitoring for and treating postoperative cardiac arrhythmias
- Ensuring adequate pain control to minimize fluctuations in blood pressure and myocardial stress
- Keeping blood glucose levels below 180 mg/dL. Standardized insulin-infusion regimens should be initiated, if needed

Pulmonary Care

It is desirable to separate patients from the ventilator as soon as they awaken, are hemodynamically stable with minimal chest tube drainage, and can maintain a satisfactory spontaneous tidal volume and respiratory rate. Coughing and deep breathing exercises with appropriate sternal precautions are essential for postoperative recovery. Suboptimal postoperative pulmonary function may indicate additional therapy, including the use of bronchodilators, mucolytics, and chest physical therapy. Although β-adrenergic bronchodilators and *N*-acetylcysteine are useful adjuncts, they also can induce atrial fibrillation.

After extubation, it is important to provide the patient with sufficient pain relief to minimize emotional distress, poor coughing, and reluctance to begin ambulation. Unrelieved pain can also be a source of tachycardia, hypertension, myocardial ischemia, atelectasis, hypoxia, and pneumonia.

Discharge From the Intensive Care Unit

Before the patient leaves the ICU, unnecessary lines and catheters should be removed. Chest tubes are removed approximately 48 hours postoperatively, when the combined drainage is less than 200 mL per shift and chest radiography reveals no effusion. Removal of temporary atrial and ventricular pacing wires is often deferred to the third postoperative day.

Outcomes

Hospital Mortality

Seven core variables—emergency of operation, age, prior heart surgery, gender, LVEF, percentage stenosis of LCA, and number of major coronary arteries with more than 70% stenosis—have the greatest impact on CABG mortality. Other variables are important but have minimal impact when added to these core variables; these include recent MI (<1 week), angina severity, ventricular arrhythmia, CHF, mitral regurgitation, diabetes, PVD, renal insufficiency, and creatinine level.

In cardiac surgery, operative mortality has traditionally included 30-day and in-hospital mortality. The mortality figure for CABG is 1% to 3% in most modern series. Risk-adjusted outcomes have become the gold standard for reporting and comparing cardiac surgery outcomes. The STS database is the largest and most authoritative voluntary national database to date. The STS has developed a risk calculator that estimates morbidity and mortality for a given patient's risk profile. The observed-to-expected mortality ratio for a given surgeon or institution can then be determined.

Long-Term Survival

Survival after CABG is related to cardiac and noncardiac comorbidities. Risk factors for atherosclerosis, particularly cigarette smoking, hypercholesterolemia, hypertension, and diabetes, are associated with decreased survival.

In no longitudinal study has CABG obliterated the negative impact of abnormal LV function on late survival. Incomplete revascularization is associated with decreased survival, whereas complete revascularization, the use of the LIMA, and, in some studies, the use of BIMA are associated with improved survival.

The CASS documented overall survival of 96%, 90%, 74%, 56%, and 45% at 1, 5, 10, 15, and 18 postoperative years, respectively. These figures are inferior to those for the age-matched U.S. population and for modern series of patients who receive single or bilateral mammary grafts.

Morbidity

Tamponade. Pericardial tamponade is caused by the formation of pericardial clot and compression of the heart. The condition should be suspected if there is evidence of low cardiac output, hypotension coincident with tachycardia, and elevated central venous pressure. The quantity of mediastinal drainage is an unreliable predictor of tamponade, although an abrupt decline in mediastinal chest tube drainage should raise suspicion of tamponade caused by absence of an exit path for the blood. Widening of the mediastinum on chest radiography and echocardiographic evidence of a pericardial effusion should confirm the diagnosis.

If a Swan-Ganz catheter is in place and right- and left-sided heart pressures are monitored, the central venous pressure and pulmonary capillary wedge pressure are usually elevated and equal. The earliest manifestation of tamponade is an acute drop in mixed venous oxygen saturation. After the diagnosis is made, the patient should be returned to the operating room for evacuation of the clot and relief of the compression. If the patient's condition is rapidly deteriorating, the sternotomy incision may have to be reopened at the bedside.

Postoperative bleeding. The combination of heparinization, hypothermia, CPB, and protamine reversal is associated with increased risk for bleeding after CABG. Post-CABG bleeding that requires transfusion or reoperation is associated with a significant increase in morbidity and mortality risk. A minority of patients having cardiac procedures (15%–20%) consume more than 80% of all blood products transfused at operation. Blood must be viewed as a scarce resource that carries significant risks and unproven benefits. There is a high-risk subset of patients who require multiple preventive measures to reduce the chance of postoperative bleeding. Nine variables stand out as important indicators of risk (Box 60.5).

Available evidence-based blood conservation techniques include the following:

- Administration of drugs that increase preoperative blood volume (e.g., erythropoietin) or decrease postoperative bleeding

BOX 60.5 Risk factors for postoperative bleeding.

- Advanced age
- Low preoperative red blood cell volume (preoperative anemia or small body size)
- Preoperative antiplatelet or antithrombotic drugs
- Reoperative or complex procedures
- Emergency operations
- Noncardiac patient comorbidities
- Renal failure
- Chronic obstructive pulmonary disease
- Congestive heart failure

BOX 60.6 Causes of immediate postoperative bleeding.

Surgical
- Conduit
- Anastomoses
- Cannulation sites
- Mammary bed
- Thymic veins
- Pericardial edge
- Sternal wire sites

Platelet dysfunction
Inadequate protamine reversal
Hypothermia

(e.g., ε-aminocaproic acid). Aprotinin is currently banned in the United States because some studies have associated it with increased mortality, stroke, and renal failure when it is administered to cardiac surgery patients
- Intraoperative blood salvage and blood-sparing interventions
- Interventions that protect the patient's own blood from the stress of operation (e.g., autologous predonation, normovolemic hemodilution)
- Institution-specific blood transfusion algorithms supplemented with point-of-care testing

Despite efforts at blood conservation to limit perioperative bleeding and blood transfusions, 2% to 3% of patients will require reexploration for bleeding, and as many as 20% will have excessive bleeding and blood transfusion postoperatively. Bleeding of more than 500 mL in the first hour or persistent bleeding of more than 200 mL/hr for 4 hours is an indication for mediastinal exploration. Exploration is also indicated if a large hemothorax is identified on chest radiography or pericardial tamponade occurs. Usually, a specific bleeding site is not identified. Box 60.6 summarizes the common causes of immediate postoperative bleeding.

Neurologic complications. There are two types of neurologic deficits after CABG: type I deficit, which is a focal neurologic deficit; and type II deficit, which is manifested as nonspecific encephalopathy. In a 1996 multi-institutional prospective study, 6% of patients had these adverse outcomes, which were evenly distributed between the two types of deficit. Associated mortality was 20% for type I, which was twice the mortality for type II deficit. Age (especially >70 years) and hypertension are consistent risk factors for both types. History of previous neurologic abnormality, diabetes, and atherosclerosis of the aorta are risk factors for type I. Significant atherosclerosis of the ascending aorta mandates a surgical approach that will minimize the possibility of atherosclerotic emboli. Patients with concomitant carotid stenosis are at an elevated risk for neurologic complications. One approach used in such patients involves a staged procedure in which the more symptomatic and more critical vascular bed is addressed first. Otherwise, a combined approach may be used, but this poses a greater overall risk.

Mediastinitis. The incidence of deep sternal wound infection is 1% to 2% in modern-era CABG. Risk factors include obesity, reoperation, diabetes, and duration and complexity of operation. Using a BIMA graft can increase the risk of sternal wound complications in high-risk patients. The use of perioperative antibiotics and a strict protocol aimed at controlling the blood glucose level to less than 180 mg/dL by continuous intravenous infusion of insulin has been shown to reduce the incidence of mediastinitis significantly. Early debridement and muscle flap closure improve outcome. More recently, good outcomes have also been reported with the use of wound vacuum-assisted closures after adequate debridement.

Renal dysfunction. Mangano and coworkers have reported a 7.7% incidence of postoperative renal dysfunction in CABG patients and mortality rates of 0.9%, 19%, and 63% in patients without postoperative renal dysfunction, patients with postoperative renal dysfunction but without need for dialysis, and patients who required dialysis, respectively. The 63% figure was confirmed in a large Veterans Administration study.

Medical Adjuncts for Postoperative Management

The following drugs are considered essential components of the postoperative management of CABG patients:
- Aspirin administration, 81 to 325 mg orally or rectally, is begun on the same day after CABG, unless the patient is bleeding because of platelet dysfunction. This is a quality-of-care index and has been shown to improve long-term graft patency
- Beta blocker administration should begin after all inotropes have been discontinued. The goal is to maintain a heart rate of 60 to 80 beats/min and adequate mean perfusion pressures
- Afterload reduction is important in all patients with a low LVEF. Afterload reduction is commenced after all inotropes are discontinued and adequate beta blockade is achieved. The angiotensin-converting enzyme inhibitors are first-line drugs for afterload reduction. Creatinine levels should be monitored
- For antiarrhythmic treatment, amiodarone is used in many cardiac centers as prophylaxis against or treatment of atrial fibrillation. This drug should be used with caution in patients with preexisting interstitial lung disease and those taking warfarin. A prolonged Q-T interval is a contraindication
- Administration of furosemide, a diuretic, is begun on the first postoperative day; the goal is to maintain a negative fluid balance. Chest radiography, creatinine levels, physical examination, and input-output charts help guide the dose of furosemide

ALTERNATIVE METHODS FOR MYOCARDIAL REVASCULARIZATION

Cardiopulmonary Bypass With Hypothermic Fibrillatory Arrest

Hypothermic fibrillatory arrest is a good on-pump alternative to conventional cardioplegic arrest and avoids the use of the aortic cross-clamp. Although cardioplegic arrest offers maximal myocardial protection while providing a stable, immobile target for the distal anastomoses, not all patients are amenable to cardioplegia-based arrest. In patients with an extensively calcified aorta, cross-clamp application may be precarious and associated with an elevated incidence of stroke.

In these cases, a hypothermic fibrillatory arrest strategy may be used in which aortic manipulation is minimized. Once CPB is initiated, the patient is cooled to 28°C. The heart typically begins fibrillating at approximately 32°C. An LV sump is usually introduced through the right superior pulmonary vein to ensure LV decompression. Handling of the distal and proximal targets is similar to off-pump CABG (OPCAB) techniques because the coronary arteries are still fully perfused while the anastomoses are being performed. Vessel loops or occluders may be needed. In patients with extensive aortic calcification, there may not be any room to place an aortic cannula in or a proximal vein graft on the ascending aorta. In these cases, the right axillary artery may be used for arterial perfusion, and the saphenous vein can be anastomosed to the innominate artery if it is free of disease, or a total arterial vascularization approach should be considered with the use of one or both mammary arteries.

Once the anastomoses are completed, the patient is rewarmed to physiologic temperature and the heart is defibrillated into sinus rhythm. The use of hypothermic fibrillatory arrest is contraindicated in patients with significant aortic valve incompetence because the ventricle would distend with the regurgitant blood once fibrillation sets in, and no stroke volume is generated. Increased ventricular wall tension and energy consumption could lead to myocardial ischemia.

On-Pump Beating-Heart Bypass

On-pump beating-heart bypass is a selective strategy used for patients who have a very low LVEF and have suffered a recent MI. The logic behind this approach is that the myocardium is severely compromised and would poorly tolerate further ischemic compromise. Despite currently available techniques for myocardial protection, cardioplegic arrest is always associated with a certain degree of ischemia. This is especially true in patients with severe CAD and a stunned myocardium, in whom uniform protection of the ventricle with cardioplegia may be difficult to achieve, and an on-pump beating-heart strategy can be considered. The coronary arteries continue to be perfused, and exposure and handling of the anastomoses are similar to those for OPCAB. The use of CPB offloads the ventricle and offers a safety margin to manipulate the heart and to visualize all the targets that need to be bypassed. Use of IABP should be considered for most of these patients because their hemodynamic state is precarious to begin with.

Off-Pump Coronary Artery Bypass Grafting

The main rationale for using OPCAB was to avoid the adverse effects of CPB related to the systemic inflammatory response caused by contact of blood components with the surface of the bypass circuit. This hypothesis, although not supported by much sound scientific clinical data, spawned the belief that CPB contributed to various adverse outcomes, including postoperative bleeding, neurocognitive dysfunction, thromboembolism, fluid retention, and reversible organ dysfunction. Because OPCAB eliminated the use of a CPB circuit and could potentially reduce some of these pump-associated complications, there was a great enthusiasm for OPCAB. In fact, throughout Asia and particularly in India, 95% of CABG operations are still performed off-pump.

In a nationwide review of the STS database by Bakaeen and colleagues, the use of off-pump procedures peaked in 2002 (23%) and again in 2008 (21%), followed by a progressive decline in off-pump frequency to 17% by 2012. Interestingly, after 2008, off-pump rates declined among both high-volume and intermediate-volume centers and surgeons, and currently in the United States, this technique is used in fewer than one in five patients who undergo surgical coronary revascularization. A minority of surgeons and centers, however, continue to perform OPCAB in most of their patients.

This decline in OPCAB is presumably due not only to the procedure's technical complexity and steep learning curve but also, and more important, to the decreased long-term patency, higher rate of incomplete revascularization, and inferior long-term survival associated with OPCAB.

Data from multiple studies have not supported the belief that OPCAB decreases inflammatory mediator release. Some investigators have shown that even though complement activation may be reduced, there is no difference in production of cytokines and chemokines that modulate neutrophils and platelets.[43,48] In addition, myocardial ischemia by itself activates complement such as C5b-9. Thus, great caution should be used in interpreting studies regarding activation of the inflammatory cascade.

The Randomized On/Off Bypass (ROOBY) trial was a prospective RCT of CABG and OPCAB that involved 2203 patients at 18 Veterans Affairs medical centers. There was no difference in 30-day mortality or short-term major adverse cardiovascular events. The OPCAB patients received significantly fewer grafts per patient. One-year rates of cardiac-related death (8.8% vs. 5.9%; $P = 0.01$) and major adverse events (9.9% vs. 7.4%; $P = 0.04$) were significantly higher in the OPCAB group. Furthermore, graft patency was significantly lower in the OPCAB group (82.6% vs. 87.8%; $P < 0.001$). The results did not differ when the operation was performed by a resident or attending physician or by a high- or low-volume surgeon.

The Surgical Management of Arterial Revascularization Therapy (SMART) trial examined long-term survival and graft patency in a prospective RCT involving 297 patients who underwent isolated elective CABG or OPCAB. After 7.5 years of follow-up, there was no difference in mortality or late graft patency between OPCAB and on-pump CABG. Although recurrent angina was more common in the OPCAB group, this difference did not reach statistical significance. Hence, this study, performed by one of the world's experts in OPCAB surgery, could not demonstrate any superiority of OPCAB over on-pump CABG.

Another prospective study, the Coronary Artery Bypass Surgery Off or On Pump Revascularization Study (CORONARY) trial, involved 4752 patients randomly assigned to either CABG or OPCAB at 79 centers in 19 countries. There were no significant differences in the incidence of recurrent angina between the OPCAB (0.9%) and CABG (1.0%) groups, but the need for repeated revascularization was higher in the OPCAB group, and the difference approached statistical significance (1.4% OPCAB vs. 0.8% CABG; $P = 0.07$).

The CORONARY trial included twice as many participants as the ROOBY trial. Each off-pump procedure was performed by an experienced surgeon who had more than 2 years of experience and had performed more than 100 OPCAB cases. Trainees were not allowed to be the primary surgeon. The rate of crossover from the off-pump to the on-pump group was lower in the CORONARY trial (7.9% versus 12.4%), suggesting a higher level of surgical expertise. Despite the improved technical experience of highly qualified off-pump surgeons, the need for revascularization remained higher in the off-pump group.

In the German Off-Pump Coronary Artery Bypass Grafts in Elderly Patients (GOPCADE) trial, patients aged 75 years and older scheduled for isolated bypass surgery were randomly assigned to on-pump or off-pump surgery. The trial was undertaken to attempt to define the potential benefits of OPCAB in an elderly group of high-risk patients with multiple comorbidities. The study involved 2539 patients from 12 centers. The primary end point was the composite of death or major adverse events (MI, cerebrovascular accident, acute renal failure requiring renal replacement therapy, or need for repeated revascularization) within 30 days and within 12 months after surgery. The secondary end points included operating room time, duration of mechanical ventilation, transfusion requirements, and ICU and hospital length of stay.

There was no difference in the primary composite end point (7.0% off-pump vs. 8.0% on-pump; $P = 0.40$). However, additional revascularization procedures within 30 days were more frequent in the off-pump group (1.3% vs. 0.3%; $P = 0.03$). Patients in the off-pump group were less likely to receive blood products; however, the study had no protocols to determine when transfusions should be given. There was no difference in any of the other secondary end points. The mean number of grafts was significantly lower in the off-pump group (2.7 vs. 2.8; $P < 0.001$). The investigators concluded that OPCAB did not improve outcomes in these elderly high-risk patients. Furthermore, concerns were raised that the increased need for early repeated revascularization and the decreased number of grafts in the off-pump group would lead to an increased incidence of future cardiovascular events, thus exposing these elderly patients to increased morbidity and mortality.

These findings have dampened the enthusiasm for OPCAB at most centers. However, it is our practice to offer OPCAB to patients with single-vessel CAD in the LAD system.

The technique and operative strategy of OPCAB differ significantly from those of on-pump CABG. Certain adjuncts are needed to provide adequate exposure of the coronary vessels. Because the heart is fully contractile and maintaining systemic perfusion, the manipulation should proceed in a planned and systematic manner. Both the pleural spaces are opened to allow the heart to rotate into either side to allow the surgeon to visualize the targets, especially the lateral and inferior wall. The more critical areas of the myocardium are revascularized first, which minimizes ischemia time, improves myocardial reserve, and permits more complex manipulation of the heart for the other targets. Mammary artery–based pedicles are typically approached first because these do not require a proximal anastomosis, thus providing immediate coronary blood flow to the bypassed vessel.

Once the target vessel is selected, a small area of the coronary artery is exposed proximal and distal to the planned area of anastomosis to allow placement of vessel loops or bulldog clamps for proximal and distal control. A coronary occluder may also be used. Two stabilizers are used to stabilize the myocardium (Fig. 60.17). The fork-octopus has a suction padded tip and is attached to a multifunctional arm. The fork is positioned so that the limbs straddle the coronary target, and suction is applied, which attaches the device to the myocardium while the arm is secured in position. The other device consists of a suction cup that is applied to the apex of the heart and is used to lift it out of the chest to expose its posterior aspect. A sling attached to the posterior pericardium allows the heart to be elevated out and enhances visualization of the posterior targets.

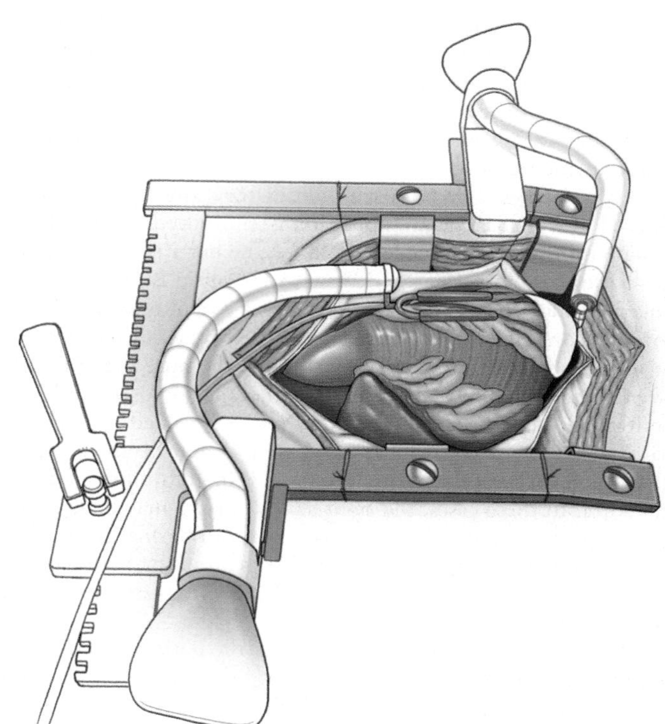

FIG. 60.17 Off-pump coronary artery bypass with vacuum-assisted multiarticulating arms to position and to stabilize the myocardium. This minimizes the movement of the heart, allowing the surgeon to feasibly perform the distal anastomoses. Here, the stabilizer is positioned in preparation for creating a bypass to the left anterior descending artery.

Full heparinization is not needed; in general, 50% of the usual dose is used. Success of the operation requires coordinated efforts between the surgeon and anesthesiologist so that adequate systemic perfusion is maintained throughout the operation while allowing a comfortable milieu in which the surgeon can operate. Short-acting beta blockers to slow the heart rate and alpha constrictors to maintain systemic perfusion pressures are important adjuncts for this procedure.

The postoperative management of OPCAB patients is significantly different from that of patients who undergo conventional CABG, primarily because of the reduced inflammatory effects, which are more prominent in patients who have undergone CPB. The OPCAB patients do not manifest the vasodilatory response or massive fluid shifts seen with CPB. Rather, these patients are more like those who have undergone major general surgery and require early deep venous thrombosis and balanced postoperative fluid management. In our practice, all patients who undergo OPCAB are given aspirin and clopidogrel (Plavix) on the day of surgery.

Minimally Invasive Direct Coronary Artery Bypass

Minimally invasive direct coronary artery bypass (MIDCAB) describes any technique of coronary artery bypass that uses a minimally invasive approach, such as an anterolateral thoracotomy (Fig. 60.18), ministernotomy, or subxiphoid approach, without the use of a robot. Most MIDCABs are performed on the beating heart and involve vascularization of the anterior wall. A metaanalysis of all published outcome studies of MIDCAB grafting performed from January 1995 through October 2007 has revealed early and late (>30 days) death rates of 1.3% and 3.2%, respectively. Of the grafts that were studied angiographically immediately after

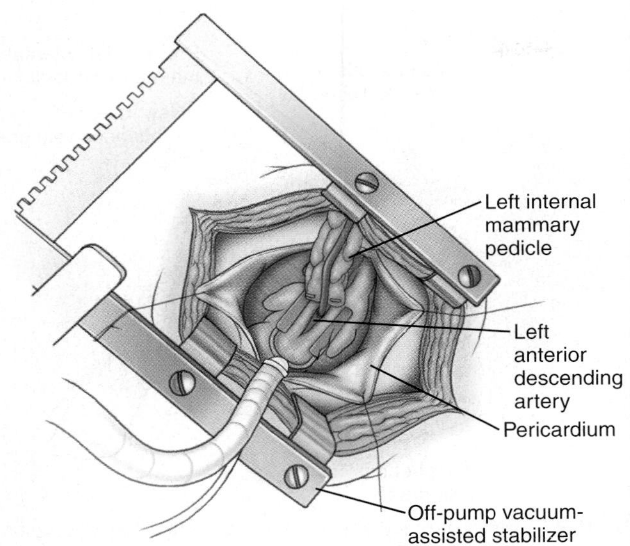

FIG. 60.18 Left thoracotomy approach for performing off-pump left internal mammary to left anterior descending bypass. This is commonly used in the minimally invasive direct coronary artery bypass approach. Multiarticulating stabilizers are essential for this technique.

surgery, 4.2% were occluded and 6.6% had a significant stenosis (50%–99%). At 6-month follow-up, 3.6% were occluded and 7.2% had significant stenosis. Long-term follow-up results and further prospective RCTs comparing MIDCABs with standard revascularization procedures in large patient cohorts are needed. Although MIDCAB offers several advantages, such as the avoidance of sternotomy and CPB, it is subject to the same limitations as OPCAB in addition to its own technical challenges and limited revascularization territory.

Robotics: Totally Endoscopic Coronary Artery Bypass

With the popularity of robotic technology in other surgical specialties, robotic totally endoscopic coronary artery bypass (TECAB) has been in use at select centers. Robotically assisted microsurgical systems have the theoretical advantage of enhancing surgical dexterity and minimizing the invasiveness of otherwise conventional coronary artery surgery. The da Vinci system (Intuitive Surgical, Mountain View, CA) is the most commonly used system. It consists of three major components: surgeon-device interface module, computer controller, and specific patient interface instrumentation. It allows real-time surgical manipulation of tissue, advanced dexterity in multiple degrees of freedom, and optical magnification of the operative field, all through minimal access ports. The technology has seen significant use in valve repair operations and other surgical specialties as well.

With regard to coronary artery bypass, TECAB can be performed on-pump or totally off-pump, and multivessel TECAB is currently a reality. However, operating times and conversion rates are much higher with this technology. More important, it is technically more difficult and expensive, and it has a steep learning curve. Long-term data regarding its durability and safety are unavailable at this point.

In the largest TECAB series to date (about 500 cases), success and safety rates were 80% (n = 400) and 95% (n = 474), respectively. Intraoperative conversion to larger thoracic incisions was required in 49 (10%) patients. The median operative time was 305 minutes (range, 112–1050 minutes), and the mean lengths of stay in the ICU and in the hospital were 23 hours (range, 11–1048 hours) and 6 days (range, 2–4 days), respectively. Independent predictors of success were single-vessel TECAB (P = 0.004), arrested-heart TECAB (P = 0.027), non–learning curve case (P = 0.049), and transthoracic assistance (P = 0.035). The only independent predictor of safety was EuroSCORE (P = 0.002). Interestingly, the mean time per anastomosis was 27 minutes (range, 10–100 minutes), which is significantly longer than an average surgeon would take to accomplish an open anastomosis (i.e., well below 10 minutes per anastomosis). Also, the LIMA injury rate was high (n = 24; 5%).[49] All these data point to less than perfect procedures and technology that require further development before they can replace open CABG, which has an excellent track record and is a proven and reproducible procedure.

The current limitations of robotic TECAB include its lack of applicability to all patients, prolonged operating room time, limited access to all vessels, difficulty in achieving multiarterial coronary grafting, cost, and limited training opportunities. However, over time, robotic surgery is likely to become a niche specialty for a subset of surgeons who treat a specific population of patients.

Transmyocardial Laser Revascularization

Patients with chronic, severe angina refractory to medical therapy who cannot be completely revascularized with percutaneous catheter intervention or CABG present clinical challenges. Transmyocardial laser revascularization (TMLR), either as sole therapy or as an adjunct to CABG surgery, may be appropriate for some of these patients. The STS Evidence-Based Workforce has reviewed available evidence and recommends the use of TMLR for patients with an LVEF greater than 0.30 and Canadian Cardiovascular Society class III or class IV angina that is refractory to maximal medical therapy. These patients should have reversible ischemia of the LV free wall and CAD corresponding to the regions of myocardial ischemia. In all regions of the myocardium, the CAD must not be amenable to CABG or PCI.

The TMLR procedure uses a high-energy laser beam to create myocardial transmural channels that were originally thought to provide direct access to oxygenated blood in the LV cavity. This is no longer considered to be the mechanism whereby TMLR reduces the symptoms of IHD. Although some local neovascularization has been documented, the magnitude of changes does not account for any substantive increases in myocardial perfusion. One mechanism that has been proposed relates to a local effect on cardiac neuronal signaling. It has been hypothesized that local tissue injury by TMLR damages ventricular sensory neurons and autonomic efferent axons, which leads to local cardiac denervation and anginal relief. Regardless of the mechanism, TMLR therapy is associated with a reproducible improvement in symptoms. Patients who undergo TMLR show a persistent improvement in Canadian Cardiovascular Society angina class. This improvement is observed in 60% to 80% of patients within 6 months after the operation.

Hybrid Procedures

It is generally accepted that the LIMA to LAD anastomosis is the single most important component of CABG and confers long-term benefits unmatched by those of any other intervention. State-of-the-art PCIs with DES have produced outcomes competitive with those of vein grafts to non-LAD targets. This has led to an integrated approach to coronary revascularization, termed the hybrid procedure. The hybrid procedure consists of a minimally invasive LIMA to LAD anastomosis in conjunction with PCI of non–LAD-obstructed coronary arteries.

This approach has met with initial success, but many potential pitfalls exist. The procedural costs may be greater than those of either CABG or DES implantation alone. The timing and staging of the procedures are uncertain, and limited data are available on long-term outcomes.

Technical Aspects of Reoperative Coronary Artery Bypass Grafting

Within 5 years, 15% of CABG patients experience a recurrence of symptoms, typically angina. This increases to approximately 40% within 10 years. Recurrent symptoms almost always indicate either progression of disease in the native coronary circulation or graft disease. In most cases, the indications for coronary angiography, PCI with or without stenting, or repeated CABG are the same as for the first operation. Patients who are considered candidates for reoperative CABG are usually older, have more diffuse CAD, and have diminished ventricular function. Factors that increase the risk for reoperation include the absence of an IMA graft, younger age at the time of the index operation, prior incomplete revascularization, CHF, and New York Heart Association class III or class IV angina.

The technical aspects of reoperative CABG differ significantly from those of the index procedure. Reentry into the chest and dissection of the old grafts are sometimes challenging. Preparation for femoral cannulation for femorofemoral bypass or axillary cannulation should be considered with preemptive availability of blood products. Redo sternotomy is typically completed with an oscillating saw or after the heart is dissected away from the sternum through a subxiphoid approach. Injury to the right ventricle or to the aorta or vein grafts is of potential concern. A poorly placed LIMA graft from the prior operation is also at risk during the sternotomy. If a cardiac or vascular injury is identified, an assistant holds the sternum together to prevent further bleeding, and expeditious cannulation of alternative sites is begun with the institution of CPB. Preoperative CT scans are helpful in planning the operation.

Once the sternotomy is completed, the rest of the adherent cardiac structures are dissected away from the underside of the sternum to allow placement of a sternal retractor. No retractor should be placed unless the heart is adequately dissected away; this will result in disruption of the aorta or right ventricle, which may be difficult to control.

The next steps are geared toward establishing sites for cannulation. The right atrium and aorta are dissected first; then, the rest of the heart is dissected away from the pericardium, which may be performed on CPB. The areas of previous cannulation and vein grafts are the most adherent regions, whereas the diaphragmatic aspect is least adherent and provides a good starting point to gain entry into the correct plane.

Manipulation of the old grafts should be kept to a minimum to avoid distal coronary bed microembolization. Isolation of the LIMA pedicle is often necessary and should be carefully performed with the ability to start bypass rapidly if an inadvertent injury occurs (Fig. 60.19). The rest of the operation proceeds in a similar fashion to primary CABG and can be performed on-pump or off-pump. In some cases, the procedure can be performed through a left anterolateral thoracotomy approach. Typically, this approach is used in patients with previous mediastinitis or multiple sternotomies or when an extensive area of the heart is adherent to the sternum, precluding a safe entry. The vein conduit is anastomosed to the descending aorta in these cases (Fig. 60.20).

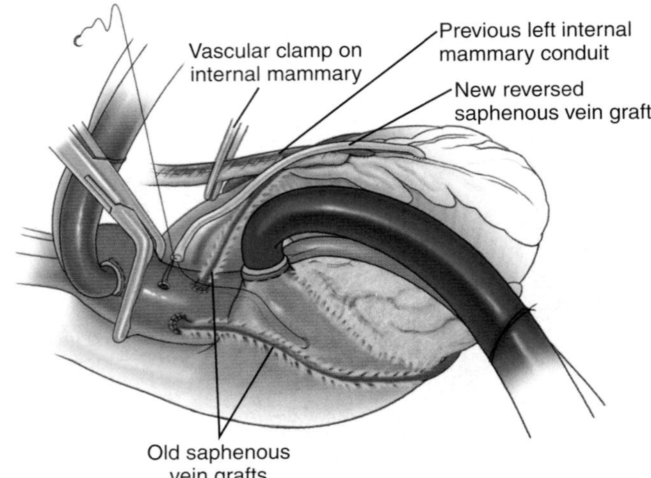

FIG. 60.19 Redo coronary artery bypass grafting. The cannulation is similar to that used in a first-time coronary artery bypass operation in most cases. However, identification of coronary targets is much more difficult because of scarring. The course of the prior grafts is useful in identifying the targets. In addition to clamping of the aorta above the previous vein grafts, the left internal mammary pedicle should be dissected and clamped separately, if feasible. A single-clamp technique is preferred because it avoids the tedious and potentially dangerous dissection around the proximal aorta that may be needed to place a partial side-biting clamp.

To summarize, some of the unique difficulties that can be encountered in redo CABG are as follows:

- Injury to heart during sternotomy
- Injury to mammary pedicle
- Limited space on ascending aorta for placement of new grafts
- Inability to identify distal targets because of scars and adhesions
- Limited availability of conduits
- Increased risk of perioperative MI because atheroembolic embolization from diseased vein grafts and diffuse CAD preclude optimal cardioplegia
- Increased bleeding because of higher inflammatory response and a more raw surface
- Injury to pulmonary artery during cross-clamping of the aorta

In most published series, the mortality rate of reoperative CABG patients exceeds that of primary CABG patients.

MECHANICAL COMPLICATIONS OF CORONARY ARTERY DISEASE

Left Ventricular Aneurysm

The incidence of ventricular aneurysm after AMI has been declining because of early interventional therapies. Of LV aneurysms, 90% are the result of a transmural MI secondary to an acute occlusion of the LAD. Patients may develop an aneurysm (pseudoaneurysm) as early as 48 hours after infarction, but most patients develop one within weeks. Approximately two thirds of patients who develop ventricular aneurysms remain asymptomatic.

The 10-year survival rate is 90% for asymptomatic patients and 50% for symptomatic patients. The most common causes of death are arrhythmias (>40%), CHF (>30%), and recurrent MI (>10%). The risk of thromboembolism is low, so long-term anticoagulation is not recommended unless there is a mural thrombus. The

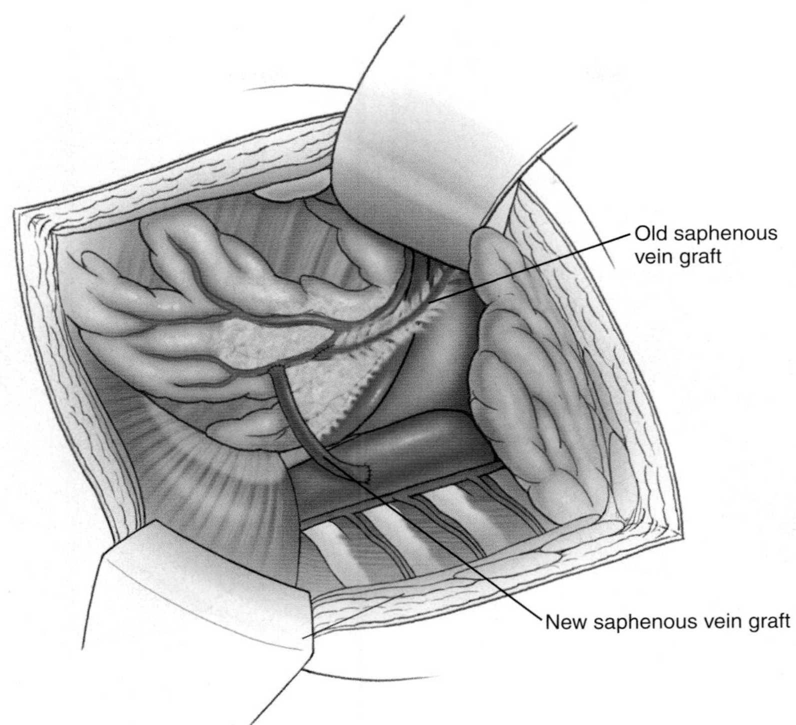

FIG. 60.20 Left thoracotomy approach for recurrent coronary artery disease. This approach avoids the hazards of a difficult redo sternotomy and is used as an alternative in some cases. New saphenous vein graft: descending thoracic aorta to obtuse marginal bypass.

diagnosis is usually made by echocardiography. Thallium imaging or PET is useful for determining the extent of the aneurysm and viability of adjacent regions.

Surgery for LV aneurysm is indicated if the patient is scheduled to undergo CABG for symptomatic CAD, there is contained rupture or evidence of a false aneurysm, or the patient has a thromboembolic event despite anticoagulation. The 5-year postoperative survival rate has been reported to range between 60% and 80%. In general, surgical repair or resection in conjunction with CABG results in angina relief and resolution of heart failure symptoms for most patients.

Surgical ventricular restoration is a technical term that describes the surgical resection of the aneurysm and reconstruction of the native ventricular geometric shape. This is ideally performed with CPB and without cardioplegic arrest as long as the aortic valve is competent. The aneurysm is usually recognized by the paradoxical movement of the walls compared with the rest of the viable LV myocardium. The aneurysm is opened, and a purse-string Fontan stitch is placed at the junction of the viable and nonviable myocardium, which can be manually palpated on the beating heart. A Dacron or bovine pericardial patch is used to exclude the aneurysm, and the aneurysm is closed over the patch. Two potentially acute complications that require surgical intervention are postinfarction VSD and postinfarction mitral regurgitation caused by papillary muscle rupture.

Ventricular Septal Defect

This occurs in less than 1% of patients and is associated with acute LAD occlusion. The defect is more common in men than in women (3:2) and typically is manifested within 2 to 4 days of the infarction. However, a VSD that occurs in the first 6 weeks after an infarct is still considered acute. The VSD is usually located in the anterior or apical aspect of the ventricular septum. Approximately 25% of affected patients have a posterior VSD caused by an inferior wall MI due to occlusion of the RCA system or a distal branch LCA. A full-thickness infarct is a prerequisite for VSD formation. A new, loud, systolic cardiac murmur after an MI suggests the diagnosis; echocardiography is effective for determining the size and character of the VSD as well as the degree of left-to-right shunting. Right-sided heart catheterization typically shows an increase in oxygen saturation levels in the right ventricle and pulmonary artery. The defect is usually approximately 1 to 2 cm in size.

After the diagnosis is established, patients should undergo immediate left-sided heart catheterization to characterize the degree of CAD and the magnitude of LV dysfunction and to detect any mitral valve insufficiency. Approximately 60% of patients with an infarction VSD have significant CAD in an unrelated vessel. The mortality rate in untreated patients is high; 25% of patients die within 24 hours of refractory heart failure. Survival rates of patients at 1 week, 1 month, and longer than 1 year are 50%, 20%, and less than 3%, respectively.

Patients who are considered candidates for surgery should be treated early with closure of the defect and concomitant CABG. In the absence of refractory heart failure and hemodynamic instability, the survival rate may be as high as 75%. The infarct exclusion technique is used to repair the VSD and is one of the most technically challenging procedures. The LV is opened longitudinally on the infarct, and the defect is evaluated. Multiple VSDs may be present, and necrotic myocardium is debrided to viable tissue. A prosthetic Dacron patch or bovine pericardium is then sutured to the LV side of the septal defect and brought out through the ventriculotomy, where it is incorporated into the closure (Fig. 60.21).

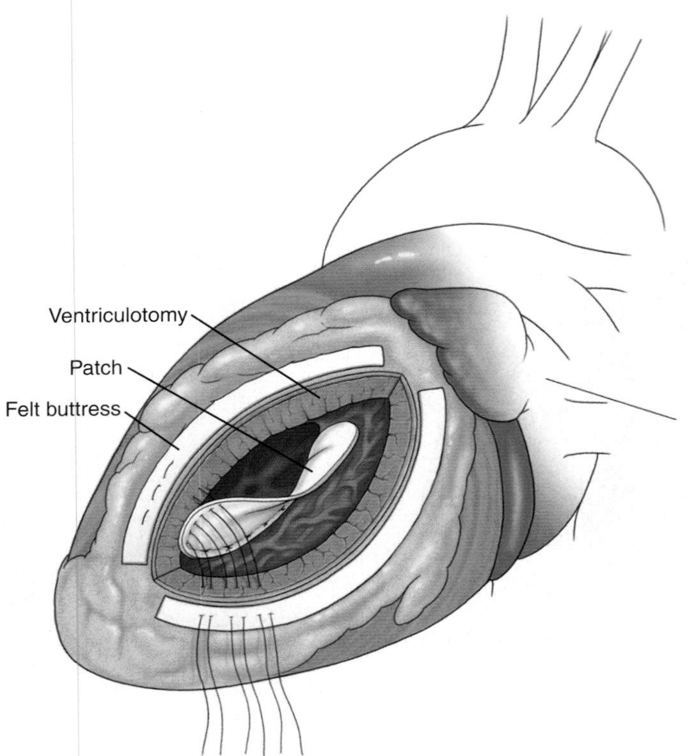

FIG. 60.21 Infarct exclusion technique for repair of acute ventricular septal defect secondary to acute myocardial infarction. A ventriculotomy is made through the zone of infarct, and all necrotic muscle is debrided. The repair is accomplished with a patch placed on the left ventricular aspect of the septum. Felt buttresses are used to reinforce the closure of the ventriculotomy, and it is essential that all sutures be incorporated into healthy myocardium to ensure durability of the repair.

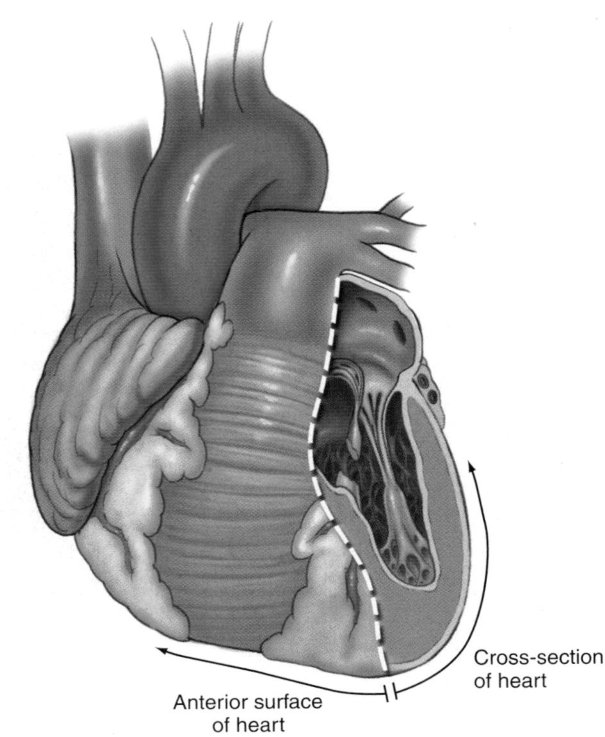

FIG. 60.22 Mechanical complication of acute myocardial infarction. Acute papillary muscle rupture (shown here) and acute ventricular septal defect are two sequelae in a patient with extensive zones of infarct. Acute papillary muscle rupture results in acute mitral regurgitation that is manifested as cardiogenic shock and immediate pulmonary decompensation. If the patient is a surgical candidate, mitral valve replacement is the only option.

In this method, the posterior aspect of the patch is thus anchored to the remnant viable septum, and the anterior aspect is incorporated with the free ventricular wall, forming the neo–interventricular septum. Felt strips are used to buttress the closure.

In addition to the traditional repair of postinfarction VSD, there has been recent enthusiasm about transcatheter closure of postinfarction VSD. This obviates a pump run in an otherwise tenuous patient. In both patients treated surgically and with transcatheter closure, temporary circulatory support in the form of extracorporeal membrane oxygenation or ventricular assist device can be lifesaving.

Mitral Regurgitation

Approximately 40% of patients who sustain an AMI develop chronic ischemic mitral regurgitation (IMR) detectable by color flow Doppler echocardiography. In 3% to 4% of cases, the degree of mitral regurgitation is moderate or severe.

The cause of chronic IMR is ischemic papillary muscle dysfunction and LV dilation associated with mitral annular dilation and restriction of the posterior leaflet. The operation for chronic IMR is usually performed on an elective basis. It consists of complete myocardial revascularization and mitral valve repair with the use of an annuloplasty ring.

Acute IMR may result from papillary muscle necrosis and rupture caused by occlusion of the overlying epicardial arteries that give rise to the penetrating vessels that supply the papillary muscles. The posterior papillary muscle is involved three to six times more often than the anterior muscle (Fig. 60.22), and either the entire trunk of the muscle or one of the heads to which chordae attach may rupture partially or totally.

In most cases, prompt surgical intervention provides the best chance for survival. Predictors of in-hospital death include CHF, renal insufficiency, and multivessel CAD. Emergent surgical treatment usually involves mitral valve replacement and concomitant CABG. The hospital mortality rate may be as high as 50% in acute cases. Mitral repair should not be attempted in such cases because it may not be feasible in papillary muscle rupture; it requires prolonging the cross-clamp time (compared with replacement), which is not ideal in acute cases. Operations on patients with acute mechanical complications from MI are challenging; the surgeon has to anticipate and be prepared for placement of an LV assist device if the patient cannot be separated from CPB (Fig. 60.23).

CORONARY ARTERY BYPASS GRAFTING AND SPECIAL POPULATIONS OF PATIENTS

Patients With Diabetes

Mortality and morbidity rates after CABG are higher in diabetic patients than in the general population. The BARI trial showed that diabetic patients with multivessel disease benefit more from CABG than from any other treatment. Similarly, the FREEDOM trial also demonstrated superiority of CABG over PCI.

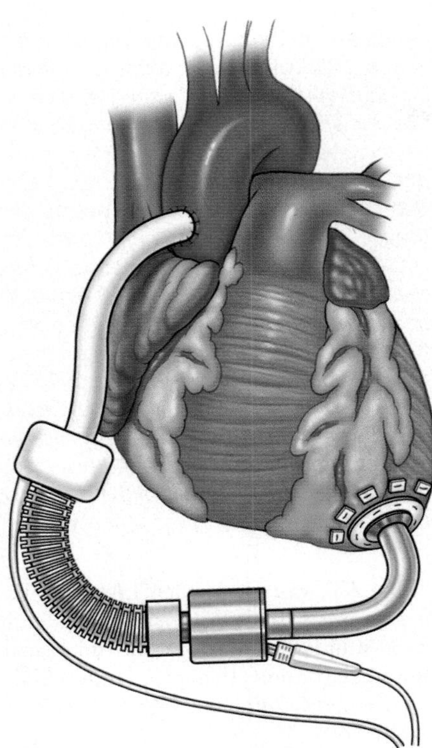

FIG. 60.23 An axial flow left ventricular assist device, which can be used as temporary mechanical support or a bridge to transplantation for a patient in end-stage cardiomyopathy due to coronary artery disease not amenable to bypass surgery. The inflow of blood into the pump is from the apex of the left ventricle. The blood is then pumped into the ascending aorta through specially designed grafts that are incorporated into the pump. The axial flow pumps are less bulky and relatively easy to implant. They have only a single moving part, which is the axial impeller.

Older Patients

Approximately 10% of patients who undergo CABG are older than 80 years. Older age is an independent predictor of surgical morbidity and mortality and a nonroutine discharge status. Although CABG should not be denied to patients on the basis of age alone, it should be considered during risk assessment. Appropriate arrangements should be made beforehand with the expectation that only one in five postoperative patients will be able to go home without additional support.

Women

Although women in every age group have a lower incidence of CAD than men, CAD is still the leading cause of death in women in the United States. Historically, serious manifestations and associated complications of CAD in women were considered uncommon. Examination of the STS database in two separate studies has revealed that the operative mortality rate is higher in women, 3.2% versus 2.6% in men.

With evolving strategies, studies have been designed to evaluate specific aspects of coronary artery bypass that would benefit women. For example, OPCAB has produced favorable outcomes in women. A review of 42,477 patients in the STS National Cardiac Database revealed that women have a significantly greater adjusted risk of death and prolonged ventilation and longer length of stay than do men who undergo on-pump CABG. In contrast, among OPCAB cases, women had a lower risk of reexploration than men did and a similar risk of death, MI, and prolonged ventilation and hospital stay.

Patients With Renal Disease

Renal insufficiency is also an independent risk factor for mortality after CABG. A preoperative serum creatinine level higher than 1.4 to 2.5 mg/dL is independently associated with a twofold increase in mortality. In a retrospective study of 59,576 patients who underwent CABG or PCI, CABG had a survival benefit in patients with a serum creatinine level higher than 2.5 mg/dL. The 1-, 2-, and 3-year survival rates were 84.1%, 77.4%, and 65.9%, respectively, for CABG compared with 70.8%, 51.9%, and 46.1%, respectively, for PCI. This effect was more dramatic in diabetic patients.

Obese Patients

The incidence of postoperative renal failure, prolonged ventilation, and sternal wound infection is significantly higher in obese patients than in normal-weight patients. Both extremes of weight are risk factors for CABG-related mortality.

ACKNOWLEDGMENTS

We would like to acknowledge Scott Weldon and Michael DeLaflor for graphic services, and Johnny Airheart for photographic support.

SELECTED REFERENCES

Chu D, Bakaeen FG, Dao TK, et al. On-pump versus off-pump coronary artery bypass grafting in a cohort of 63,000 patients. *Ann Thorac Surg*. 2009;87:1820–1826.

This study was a nationwide comparison of on-pump versus off-pump coronary artery bypass surgery in the United States. The study highlighted the fact that off-pump coronary artery bypass does not produce lower postoperative mortality or stroke rates than conventional on-pump coronary artery bypass. Furthermore, off-pump coronary artery bypass was associated with longer hospital stays and higher hospital costs.

Edwards FH, Carey JS, Grover FL, et al. Impact of gender on coronary bypass operative mortality. *Ann Thorac Surg*. 1998;66:125–131.

This study analyzed the outcomes of more than 300,000 patients from the Society of Thoracic Surgeons database and used multivariate analysis and risk model stratification to examine the outcomes of female patients. Female gender was shown to be an independent predictor of higher mortality in low- to moderate-risk patients but not in high-risk patients.

Influence of diabetes on 5-year mortality and morbidity in a randomized trial comparing CABG and PTCA in patients with multivessel disease: the Bypass Angioplasty Revascularization Investigation (BARI). *Circulation*. 1997;96:1761–1769.

Follow-up results from the initial randomized controlled trial established that patients with treated diabetes mellitus who were assigned to undergo coronary artery bypass grafting (CABG) had a striking reduction in mortality compared with patients who underwent percutaneous transluminal coronary angioplasty. This benefit was attributed predominantly to the use of the left internal mammary artery conduit in CABG.

Loop FD, Lytle BW, Cosgrove DM, et al. Influence of the internal-mammary-artery graft on 10-year survival and other cardiac events. *N Engl J Med.* 1986;314:1–6.

This retrospective study of 5931 coronary artery bypass grafting patients operated on at a single institution compared the outcomes of patients who had an internal mammary artery (IMA) graft with those of patients who had only vein grafts. The findings of this landmark study established the superiority of the IMA over any other conduit. During a 10-year period, patients who had only vein grafts had a 1.6 times higher risk of mortality than those who had mammary grafts.

Lopes RD, Hafley GE, Allen KB, et al. Endoscopic versus open vein-graft harvesting in coronary-artery bypass surgery. *N Engl J Med.* 2009;361:235–244.

This retrospective study evaluated the effects of endoscopic vein harvesting on the rate of vein graft failure and on clinical outcomes. Endoscopic vein harvesting was shown to be independently associated with vein graft failure and adverse clinical outcomes compared with open vein harvesting.

Parisi AF, Khuri S, Deupree RH, et al. Medical compared with surgical management of unstable angina: 5-year mortality and morbidity in the Veterans Administration Study. *Circulation.* 1989;80:1176–1189.

This prospective, multicenter Veterans Administration randomized controlled trial compared surgical and medical management and established that, for patients with triple-vessel coronary disease, surgical intervention better promotes survival than medical management.

Peduzzi P, Kamina A, Detre K. Twenty-two-year follow-up in the VA Cooperative Study of Coronary Artery Bypass Surgery for Stable Angina. *Am J Cardiol.* 1998;81:1393–1399.

This study compared the 22-year results of initial coronary artery bypass grafting surgery with saphenous vein grafts with those of initial medical therapy with regard to survival, the incidences of myocardial infarction (MI) and reoperation, and symptomatic status in 686 patients with stable angina who participated in the Veterans Affairs Cooperative Study of Coronary Artery Bypass Surgery. This trial provided strong evidence that initial bypass surgery did not improve survival for low-risk patients and did not reduce the overall risk of MI. The early survival benefit with surgery in high-risk patients did not translate to comparable long-term survival rates for both treatment groups.

Serruys PW, Morice MC, Kappetein AP, et al. Percutaneous coronary intervention versus coronary-artery bypass grafting for severe. *N Engl J Med.* 2009;360:961–972.

This was a landmark contemporary study of percutaneous coronary intervention (PCI) with drug-eluting stents versus coronary artery bypass grafting (CABG). The primary end point was a major adverse cardiac or cerebrovascular event (i.e., death from any cause, stroke, myocardial infarction (MI), or repeated revascularization) during the 12-month period after randomization. Rates of major adverse cardiac or cerebrovascular events at 12 months were significantly higher in the PCI group (17.8% vs. 12.4% for CABG; P = 0.002), in large part because of an increased rate of repeated revascularization (13.5% vs. 5.9%; P < 0.001); as a result, the criterion for noninferiority was not met. At 12 months, the rates of death and MI were similar between the two groups; stroke was significantly more likely to occur with CABG (2.2% vs. 0.6% with PCI; P = 0.003). The investigators concluded that CABG remains the standard of care for patients with three-vessel or left coronary artery disease because the use of CABG, compared with PCI, resulted in lower rates of the combined end point of major adverse cardiac or cerebrovascular events at 1 year.

Serruys PW, Ong AT, van Herwerden LA, et al. Five-year outcomes after coronary stenting versus bypass surgery for the treatment of multivessel disease: the final analysis of the Arterial Revascularization Therapies Study (ARTS) randomized trial. *J Am Coll Cardiol.* 2005;46:575–581.

The final results of the Arterial Revasularization Therapies Study were summarized and showed that the overall rate of major adverse cardiac and cerebrovascular events was higher in patients who underwent coronary artery stenting than in those who underwent coronary artery bypass grafting. This difference was driven by the increased need for repeated revascularization in the stent group.

Shroyer AL, Grover FL, Hattler B, et al. On-pump versus off-pump coronary-artery bypass surgery. *N Engl J Med.* 2009;361:1827–1837.

This study was a randomized, multicenter Veterans Affairs trial that compared conventional coronary artery bypass grafting with off-pump coronary artery bypass (OPCAB) in 2203 patients. The primary end point was a composite of death from any cause, repeated revascularization, or nonfatal myocardial infarction within 1 year after surgery. At 1-year follow-up, the OPCAB patients had worse composite outcomes and poorer graft patency. The presumed benefit of fewer neuropsychological adverse outcomes was not found in OPCAB patients.

Taggart DP, Altman DG, Gray AM, et al. Randomized trial of bilateral versus single internal-thoracic-artery grafts. *N Engl J Med.* 2016;375:2540–2549.

The use of bilateral internal thoracic (mammary) arteries for coronary artery bypass grafting (CABG) may improve long-term outcomes as compared with the use of a single internal thoracic artery plus vein grafts. Patients undergoing CABG were randomized to undergo single or bilateral internal thoracic artery grafting in 28 cardiac surgical centers in 7 countries. Among patients undergoing CABG, there was no significant difference between those receiving single internal thoracic artery grafts and those receiving bilateral internal thoracic artery grafts regarding mortality or the rates of cardiovascular events at 5 years of follow-up. There were more sternal wound complications with bilateral internal thoracic artery grafting than with single internal thoracic artery grafting. Ten-year follow-up is ongoing.

Velazquez EJ, Lee KL, Jones RH, et al. Coronary-artery bypass surgery in patients with ischemic cardiomyopathy. *N Engl J Med.* 2016;374:1511–1520.

The survival benefit of a strategy of coronary artery bypass grafting (CABG) added to guideline-directed medical therapy, as compared with medical therapy alone, in patients with coronary artery disease, heart failure, and severe left ventricular systolic dysfunction remains unclear. This study randomized patients with very low ejection fraction (<35%) to GDMT vs. CABG. At 10 years in a cohort of patients with ischemic cardiomyopathy, the rates of death from any cause, death from cardiovascular causes, and death from any cause or hospitalization for cardiovascular causes were significantly lower over 10 years among patients who underwent CABG in addition to receiving medical therapy than among those who received medical therapy alone.

White HD, Assmann SF, Sanborn TA, et al. Comparison of percutaneous coronary intervention and coronary artery bypass grafting after acute myocardial infarction complicated by cardiogenic shock: results from the Should We Emergently Revascularize Occluded Coronaries for Cardiogenic Shock (SHOCK) trial. *Circulation.* 2005;112:1992–2001.

This randomized controlled trial was designed to compare coronary artery bypass grafting (CABG) surgery with percutaneous coronary intervention in patients who presented with cardiogenic shock. The trial evaluated 30-day and 1-year mortality and found comparable results between the two groups, even though the CABG patients had a higher prevalence of diabetes and worse coronary artery disease preoperatively.

REFERENCES

1. Benjamin EJ, Virani SS, Callaway CW, et al. Heart disease and stroke statistics—2018 update: a report from the American Heart Association. *Circulation.* 2018;137:e67–e492.
2. Ford ES, Capewell S. Coronary heart disease mortality among young adults in the U.S. from 1980 through 2002: concealed leveling of mortality rates. *J Am Coll Cardiol.* 2007;50:2128–2132.
3. Murphy SL, Xu J, Kochanek KD. Deaths: preliminary data for 2010. *Natl Vital Stat Rep.* 2012;60:1–52.
4. Bakaeen FG, Blackstone EH, Pettersson GB, et al. The father of coronary artery bypass grafting: Rene Favaloro and the 50th anniversary of coronary artery bypass grafting. *J Thorac Cardiovasc Surg.* 2018;155:2324–2328.
5. Pepine CJ, Balaban RS, Bonow RO, et al. Women's Ischemic Syndrome Evaluation: current status and future research directions: report of the National Heart, Lung and Blood Institute Workshop: October 2–4, 2002: section 1: diagnosis of stable ischemia and ischemic heart disease. *Circulation.* 2004;109:e44–46.
6. Hammermeister KE, DeRouen TA, Dodge HT. Variables predictive of survival in patients with coronary disease. Selection by univariate and multivariate analyses from the clinical, electrocardiographic, exercise, arteriographic, and quantitative angiographic evaluations. *Circulation.* 1979;59:421–430.
7. Kwok Y, Kim C, Grady D, et al. Meta-analysis of exercise testing to detect coronary artery disease in women. *Am J Cardiol.* 1999;83:660–666.
8. Shaw LJ, Mieres JH, Hendel RH, et al. Comparative effectiveness of exercise electrocardiography with or without myocardial perfusion single photon emission computed tomography in women with suspected coronary artery disease: results from the What Is the Optimal Method for Ischemia Evaluation in Women (WOMEN) trial. *Circulation.* 2011;124:1239–1249.
9. Fleischmann KE, Hunink MG, Kuntz KM, et al. Exercise echocardiography or exercise SPECT imaging? A meta-analysis of diagnostic test performance. *JAMA.* 1998;280:913–920.
10. Underwood SR, Anagnostopoulos C, Cerqueira M, et al. Myocardial perfusion scintigraphy: the evidence. *Eur J Nucl Med Mol Imaging.* 2004;31:261–291.
11. Badran HM, Elnoamany MF, Seteha M. Tissue velocity imaging with dobutamine stress echocardiography—a quantitative technique for identification of coronary artery disease in patients with left bundle branch block. *J Am Soc Echocardiogr.* 2007;20:820–831.
12. Levy D, Garrison RJ, Savage DD, et al. Prognostic implications of echocardiographically determined left ventricular mass in the Framingham Heart Study. *N Engl J Med.* 1990;322:1561–1566.
13. Mark DB, Berman DS, Budoff MJ, et al. ACCF/ACR/AHA/NASCI/SAIP/SCAI/SCCT 2010 expert consensus document on coronary computed tomographic angiography: a report of the American College of Cardiology Foundation Task Force on Expert Consensus Documents. *Catheter Cardiovasc Interv.* 2010;76:E1–42.
14. Hamon M, Biondi-Zoccai GG, Malagutti P, et al. Diagnostic performance of multislice spiral computed tomography of coronary arteries as compared with conventional invasive coronary angiography: a meta-analysis. *J Am Coll Cardiol.* 2006;48:1896–1910.
15. Janne d'Othee B, Siebert U, Cury R, et al. A systematic review on diagnostic accuracy of CT-based detection of significant coronary artery disease. *Eur J Radiol.* 2008;65:449–461.
16. Miller JM, Rochitte CE, Dewey M, et al. Diagnostic performance of coronary angiography by 64-row CT. *N Engl J Med.* 2008;359:2324–2336.
17. Schuijf JD, Bax JJ, Shaw LJ, et al. Meta-analysis of comparative diagnostic performance of magnetic resonance imaging and multislice computed tomography for noninvasive coronary angiography. *Am Heart J.* 2006;151:404–411.
18. Shmilovich H, Cheng VY, Tamarappoo BK, et al. Vulnerable plaque features on coronary CT angiography as markers of inducible regional myocardial hypoperfusion from severe coronary artery stenoses. *Atherosclerosis.* 2011;219:588–595.

19. Ambrose JA, Tannenbaum MA, Alexopoulos D, et al. Angiographic progression of coronary artery disease and the development of myocardial infarction. *J Am Coll Cardiol.* 1988;12:56–62.
20. Little WC, Constantinescu M, Applegate RJ, et al. Can coronary angiography predict the site of a subsequent myocardial infarction in patients with mild-to-moderate coronary artery disease? *Circulation.* 1988;78:1157–1166.
21. Eleven-year survival in the Veterans Administration randomized trial of coronary bypass surgery for stable angina. *N Engl J Med.* 1984;311:1333–1339.
22. Ringqvist I, Fisher LD, Mock M, et al. Prognostic value of angiographic indices of coronary artery disease from the Coronary Artery Surgery Study (CASS). *J Clin Invest.* 1983;71:1854–1866.
23. Passamani E, Davis KB, Gillespie MJ, et al. A randomized trial of coronary artery bypass surgery. Survival of patients with a low ejection fraction. *N Engl J Med.* 1985;312:1665–1671.
24. Yusuf S, Zucker D, Peduzzi P, et al. Effect of coronary artery bypass graft surgery on survival: overview of 10-year results from randomised trials by the Coronary Artery Bypass Graft Surgery Trialists Collaboration. *Lancet.* 1994;344:563–570.
25. Hueb W, Lopes N, Gersh BJ, et al. Ten-year follow-up survival of the Medicine, Angioplasty, or Surgery Study (MASS II): a randomized controlled clinical trial of 3 therapeutic strategies for multivessel coronary artery disease. *Circulation.* 2010;122:949–957.
26. Eighteen-year follow-up in the Veterans Affairs Cooperative Study of coronary artery bypass surgery for stable angina. *Circulation.* 1992;86:121–130.
27. Varnauskas E. Twelve-year follow-up of survival in the randomized European Coronary Surgery Study. *N Engl J Med.* 1988;319:332–337.
28. Fihn SD, Gardin JM, Abrams J, et al. 2012 ACCF/AHA/ACP/AATS/PCNA/SCAI/STS guideline for the diagnosis and management of patients with stable ischemic heart disease: a report of the American College of Cardiology Foundation/American Heart Association Task Force on Practice Guidelines, and the American College of Physicians, American Association for Thoracic Surgery, Preventive Cardiovascular Nurses Association, Society for Cardiovascular Angiography and Interventions, and Society of Thoracic Surgeons. *Circulation.* 2012;126:e354–471.
29. Mohr FW, Morice MC, Kappetein AP, et al. Coronary artery bypass graft surgery versus percutaneous coronary intervention in patients with three-vessel disease and left main coronary disease: 5-year follow-up of the randomised, clinical SYNTAX trial. *Lancet.* 2013;381:629–638.
30. Makikallio T, Holm NR, Lindsay M, et al. Percutaneous coronary angioplasty versus coronary artery bypass grafting in treatment of unprotected left main stenosis (NOBLE): a prospective, randomised, open-label, non-inferiority trial. *Lancet.* 2016;388:2743–2752.
31. Stone GW, Sabik JF, Serruys PW, et al. Everolimus-eluting stents or bypass surgery for left main coronary artery disease. *N Engl J Med.* 2016;375:2223–2235.
32. Jones EL, Craver JM, Guyton RA, et al. Importance of complete revascularization in performance of the coronary bypass operation. *Am J Cardiol.* 1983;51:7–12.
33. Omer S, Cornwell LD, Rosengart TK, et al. Completeness of coronary revascularization and survival: impact of age and off-pump surgery. *J Thorac Cardiovasc Surg.* 2014;148:1307–1315:e1301.
34. Velazquez EJ, Lee KL, Jones RH, et al. Coronary-artery bypass surgery in patients with ischemic cardiomyopathy. *N Engl J Med.* 2016;374:1511–1520.
35. Velazquez EJ, Lee KL, Deja MA, et al. Coronary-artery bypass surgery in patients with left ventricular dysfunction. *N Engl J Med.* 2011;364:1607–1616.
36. Subramanian S, Sabik 3rd JF, Houghtaling PL, et al. Decision-making for patients with patent left internal thoracic artery grafts to left anterior descending. *Ann Thorac Surg.* 2009;87:1392–1398: discussion 1400.
37. Choudhry NK, Singh JM, Barolet A, et al. How should patients with unstable angina and non–ST-segment elevation myocardial infarction be managed? A meta-analysis of randomized trials. *Am J Med.* 2005;118:465–474.
38. Berger PB, Ellis SG, Holmes Jr DR, et al. Relationship between delay in performing direct coronary angioplasty and early clinical outcome in patients with acute myocardial infarction: results from the global use of strategies to open occluded arteries in Acute Coronary Syndromes (GUSTO-IIb) trial. *Circulation.* 1999;100:14–20.
39. Cannon CP, Gibson CM, Lambrew CT, et al. Relationship of symptom-onset-to-balloon time and door-to-balloon time with mortality in patients undergoing angioplasty for acute myocardial infarction. *JAMA.* 2000;283:2941–2947.
40. Weiss ES, Chang DD, Joyce DL, et al. Optimal timing of coronary artery bypass after acute myocardial infarction: a review of California discharge data. *J Thorac Cardiovasc Surg.* 2008;135:503–511, 511:e501–503.
41. White HD, Assmann SF, Sanborn TA, et al. Comparison of percutaneous coronary intervention and coronary artery bypass grafting after acute myocardial infarction complicated by cardiogenic shock: results from the Should We Emergently Revascularize Occluded Coronaries for Cardiogenic Shock (SHOCK) trial. *Circulation.* 2005;112:1992–2001.
42. Loop FD, Lytle BW, Cosgrove DM, et al. Influence of the internal-mammary-artery graft on 10-year survival and other cardiac events. *N Engl J Med.* 1986;314:1–6.
43. Castellheim A, Hoel TN, Videm V, et al. Biomarker profile in off-pump and on-pump coronary artery bypass grafting surgery in low-risk patients. *Ann Thorac Surg.* 2008;85:1994–2002.
44. Comparison of coronary bypass surgery with angioplasty in patients with multivessel disease. *N Engl J Med.* 1996;335:217–225.
45. Zenati MA, Bhatt DL, Bakaeen FG, et al. Randomized trial of endoscopic or open vein-graft harvesting for coronary-artery bypass. *N Engl J Med.* 2019;380:132–141.
46. Tabata M, Grab JD, Khalpey Z, et al. Prevalence and variability of internal mammary artery graft use in contemporary multivessel coronary artery bypass graft surgery: analysis of the Society of Thoracic Surgeons National Cardiac Database. *Circulation.* 2009;120:935–940.
47. Tatoulis J, Buxton BF, Fuller JA. The right internal thoracic artery: is it underutilized? *Curr Opin Cardiol.* 2011;26:528–535.
48. Hoel TN, Videm V, Mollnes TE, et al. Off-pump cardiac surgery abolishes complement activation. *Perfusion.* 2007;22:251–256.
49. Bonaros N, Schachner T, Lehr E, et al. Five hundred cases of robotic totally endoscopic coronary artery bypass grafting: predictors of success and safety. *Ann Thorac Surg.* 2013;95:803–812.

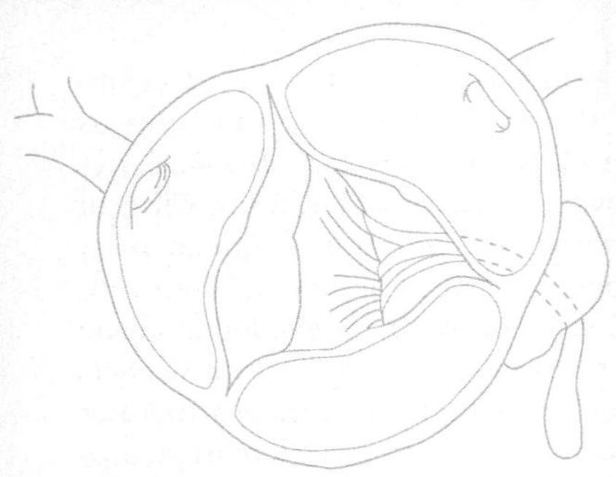

CHAPTER 61

Acquired Heart Disease: Valvular

Todd K. Rosengart, Corinne M. Aberle, Christopher Ryan

OUTLINE

The heart contains four one-way valves that regulate the directional flow of blood through its chambers. Effective cardiac pumping activity is dependent on the proper functioning of these valves. The atrioventricular (mitral and tricuspid) valves close during systole to allow for stepwise pressure gradients to be maintained between the atria and ventricles, while the semilunar (aortic and pulmonic) valves likewise close during diastole to maintain pressure gradients between the ventricles and great arteries.

The heart on average beats 100,000 times per day and more than 2.5 billion times over an average lifespan. Given the great number of open-close cycles the heart valves are subjected to and the relative infrequency of cardiac valvular heart disease - with a reported prevalence of less than 2% of the population,[1] it must be concluded that the valvular structures are exceedingly well adapted to meet these physical demands.

The cardiac valves may, nevertheless, succumb to injury or degeneration due to a variety of pathophysiologic processes, and valvular dysfunction can result in significant morbidity and mortality. The advent in the past century of open surgical valve repair and replacement procedures have delivered extended life and improved health to millions of individuals with cardiac valve disease. Today, for example, approximately 90,000 patients in the United States and 280,000 worldwide undergo valve replacement each year. More recently, percutaneous interventions to repair or replace damaged valves are increasingly utilized to deliver these benefits without requiring open-heart surgery or cardiopulmonary bypass.

HISTORY OF HEART VALVE SURGERY

Notwithstanding investigations in the nineteenth century into the treatment of rheumatic heart disease, the modern history of heart valve surgery can be traced back to Sir Thomas Lauder Brunton, a Scottish physician, who in 1902 proposed a technique for closed repair of stenotic rheumatic mitral valve disease, with access to the valve gained by passing a dilator through the left ventricular (LV) wall. Unfortunately, this idea was shunned by Brunton's colleagues as reckless and was never attempted clinically. Fortunately, however, Elliot Cutler and Peter Levine further developed Brunton's early theory, and successfully performed the first surgical correction of the mitral valve in 1923 after their extensive experimentation in the research laboratories of the Peter Bent Brigham Hospital in Boston.

Henry Souttar of England adapted the Cutler and Levine technique and in 1925 reported the first successful case of closed digital commissurotomy, inserting the surgeon's index finger through the left atrial (LA) appendage to accomplish mechanical mitral valve (MV) dilatation. This procedure was not widely adopted until 1948, following reports by Charles Bailey of Philadelphia and Dwight Harken of Boston of clinically successful closed digital mitral commissurotomies (Fig. 61.1).

Blinded aortic valvular surgery followed a similar course. In 1912, Theodore Tuffier of Paris reported the first clinical attempt to dilate a stenotic aortic valve, pushing his finger against the aorta and invaginating the aortic wall through the valve to approach the valve. Mechanical dilation using an instrument passed retrograde through

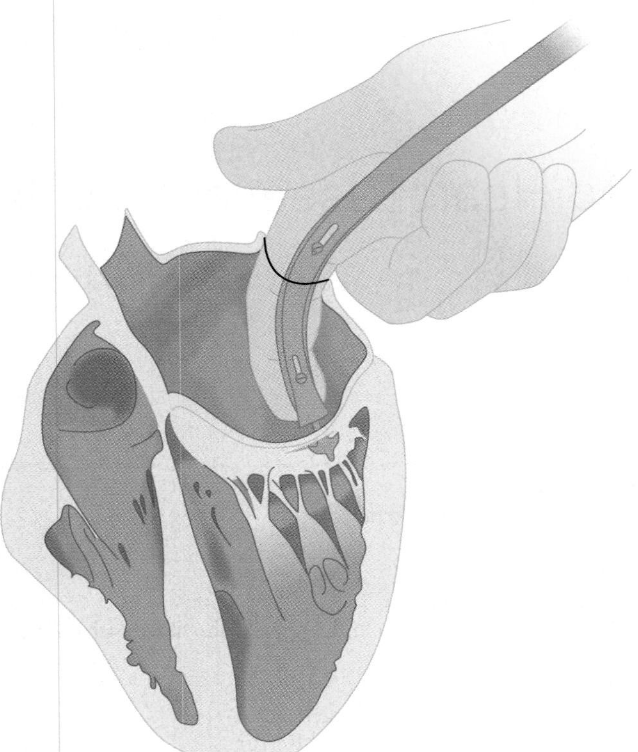

FIG. 61.1 Closed mitral commissurotomy. Dwight Harken developed a closed mitral commissurotomy procedure to correct rheumatic mitral stenosis that became the first widespread approach to treating valvular heart disease. (From Muller WH, Jr. The surgical treatment of mitral stenosis. *Calif Med.* 1951;75:285–289.)

the innominate artery was reported by Russell Brock of London in 1940. Neither of these efforts gained acceptance, but paved the way for Horace Smithy of Charleston, South Carolina, who in 1948 performed the first successful aortic valvotomy. Three years later, Charles Bailey of Philadelphia reported the first successful aortic valvotomy using a transventricular expanding dilator.

Two major landmarks occurring in the twentieth century marked the beginning of the modern era of "open" heart valve surgery: the development of a prosthetic valve, and the advent of cardiopulmonary bypass. The first successful implantation of a prosthetic valve was performed without bypass and was reported by Charles Hufnagel of Georgetown University in 1952. Given the inability to access the aortic valve in situ, Hufnagel implanted a caged-ball valve into the *descending aorta* in patients with aortic insufficiency. Following the first successful clinical use of cardiopulmonary bypass by Gibbon in 1953, Harken in 1960 completed the first successful in situ aortic valve replacement using a caged-ball device inserted in place of an excised aortic valve. That same year, Albert Starr and Lowell Edwards in Oregon replaced the mitral valve using a similar caged-ball prosthesis of their own design. What followed was an explosion of improvements in prosthetic valve design and surgical implantation techniques allowing for progressive improvement in outcome after valve replacement, and more recently, valve repair.

VALVE ANATOMY

The four human heart valves follow similar early embryologic development, beginning at four weeks of gestation with formation of the valve primordia in the primitive heart tube. This development is closely linked to the division of the heart tube into its chambers, including septation of the outflow tract (truncus arteriosus) and fusion of the atrioventricular canal cushions. Most of the cells, which migrate to form the valve primordia originate from the endocardial cushion, although epicardial and neural crest cells also appear to contribute. The valve primordia grow and elongate between 20 and 39 weeks of gestation, thinning to form leaflets and cusps. In late gestation and early after birth, these structures become stratified into highly organized layers to differentiate into formal valve leaflets. Valve maturation and remodeling continues into the juvenile stages of life.

All four cardiac valves are supported by internal plates of dense collagen-, proteoglycan- and elastin-rich connective tissue that are continuous with the fibrous skeleton at the base of the heart (Fig. 61.2). The extracellular matrix of each valve is organized into three layers: the fibrosa, made of fibrillar collagen; the spongiosa, made of proteoglycans; and an elastin layer termed the ventricularis on the semilunar valves or the atrialis on the atrioventricular valves, in reference to the heart chamber, the layer faces (Fig. 61.3). Covered in a thin layer of epithelium, the atrialis or ventricularis form the surface over which blood flows through the valve, with the underlying spongiosa and fibrosa contributing structural support.

The aortic and pulmonic semilunar valves are freestanding structures seated atop the outflow tracts of their respective ventricles. They do not have discrete annuli but are instead attached in a curvilinear fashion to the wall of the aorta or pulmonary artery at their junction with the left or right ventricular (RV) outflow tracts, respectively. These valves have three *cusps* with a semilunar shape from which they derive their name (Fig. 61.4). Each cusp is in turn made up of four components: the hinge region where the cusp connects to the annulus; the belly, which make up the majority of the cusp; the coapting surface at the cusp periphery; and the lannulae, which are thin, crescent shaped segments of the cusp surrounding a central fibrous nodule at the midpoint of its free edge (termed the nodes of Aranti in the aortic valve).

In contrast to the freestanding semilunar valves, the mitral and tricuspid valves exist within a functional valve complex composed of discrete, fibrous annular rings (the annuli fibrosis), the valve leaflets, fibrous chordae tendinae, and papillary muscles. The fibrous chordae tendinae arise from the leaflet free edges (marginal or primary chordae) or undersurface (intermediate or secondary chordae), with basal (tertiary) chordae also arising from the posterior leaflet base and annulus. These chordae attach to intraventricular papillary muscles, which in turn arise from the ventricular myocardium. These additional support structures allow the atrioventricular (AV) valves to maintain the high transvalvular pressures to which they are exposed during systole.

The mitral valve proper has two *leaflets* possessing approximately equal surface area (Fig. 61.5). The square-shaped anterior leaflet originates from approximately the anterior one third of the valve annulus. The posterior mitral leaflet is less wide ("tall") but is longer than the anterior leaflet, attaching to approximately two thirds of the annulus. The anterior and posterior leaflets each have three scallops (e.g., A1, P1, etc.), based upon indentations found in the posterior leaflet (Fig. 61.5). In comparison, the tricuspid valve is comprised of anterior, posterior, and septal leaflets, of which the anterior leaflet is the largest and the septal leaflet the smallest.

The mitral valve is supported by an anterior and posterior papillary muscle that each sends chordae to the anterior and posterior leaflets. In comparison, the tricuspid valve is supported by a large anterior papillary muscle that sends chordae to the anterior

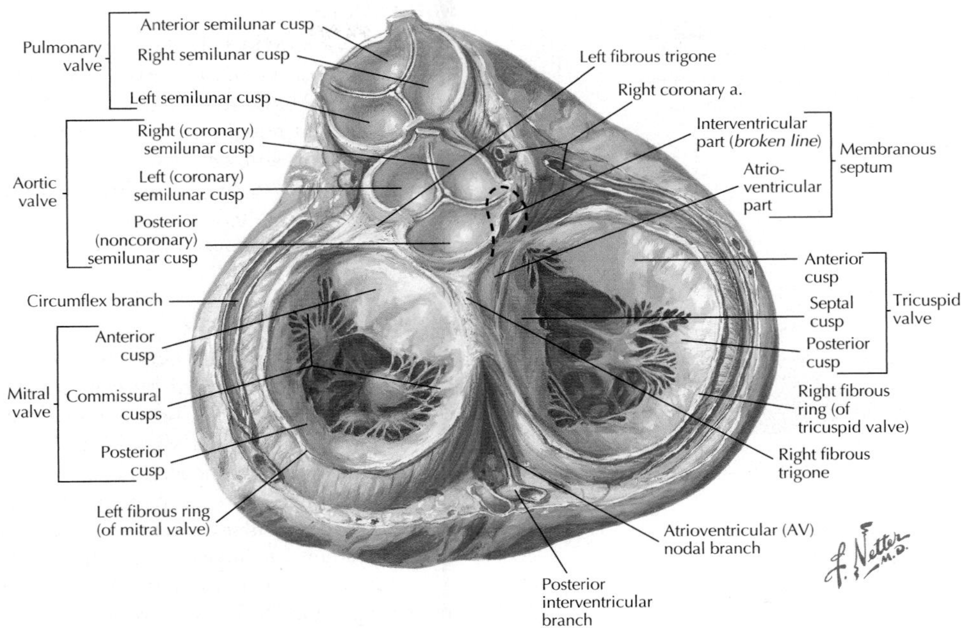

FIG. 61.2 Fibrous cardiac skeleton. The base of the heart contains an integrated 'skeleton' of connective tissue which invests the tricuspid, mitral, and aortic valves. Note the close anatomic relationship of these valves to each other, the coronary circulation, and the electrical conduction system of the heart. (Adapted from Conti CR. *Netter collection of medical illustrations: Cardiovascular system*. 2nd ed. Philadelphia, PA: Elsevier Saunders; 2014.)

and posterior leaflets, and a variable medial or posterior papillary muscle that provides chordae to the posterior and septal leaflets. The RV septal wall also provides chordae to the anterior and septal tricuspid leaflets, but there is no formal septal papillary muscle.

As suggested by their anatomy, the semilunar and AV valves differ in the mechanisms employed to maintain coaptation. The semilunar valve cusps depend largely upon mechanisms intrinsic to the cusps themselves. During diastole, the cusps falling passively to the center and seal the orifice by coapting with the corresponding midpoint nodules on adjoining cusps. The AV valves, on the other hand, are tethered in their closed position by their chordal attachments to the papillary muscles, which contract during systole to maintain leaflet coaptation and prevent leaflet prolapse into the atria (Fig. 61.6).

Surgical Anatomic Relationships

While the pulmonary valve is relatively easily accessed and isolated at the anterior of the heart, the aortic and atrioventricular valves are closely invested with each other at the base of the heart, with both the electrical conduction and coronary arterial systems in close proximity and at risk during cardiac valve procedures (Fig. 61.7). The central location of the aortic valve at the base of the heart in particular imparts complex anatomic relationships to the other cardiac chambers and valves. The aortic valve cusps, for example, are named for their intimate relationship with the coronary arteries (i.e., the right coronary, left coronary, and noncoronary [posterior] cusps), which arise from the coronary ostia in the sinuses of Valsalva, gentle dilatations of the aorta just distal to the valve which direct flow into the ostia (Fig. 61.7).

In direct continuity with the left and noncoronary cusps of the aortic valve, from about the 5 to the 8 o'clock position in the traditional surgical perspective, is the anterior leaflet of the mitral valve (Fig. 61.8). The noncoronary cusp of the aortic valve and the anterior leaflet of the mitral valve are therefore at risk of injury during mitral and aortic valve surgery, respectively. Likewise, the atrioventricular node lies embedded in the top of the ventricular membranous septum, just beneath the commissure between the noncoronary and right coronary aortic leaflets, from the 3 to the 5 o'clock position in the surgical perspective. Only the remaining circumference of the aortic annulus is relatively free anatomically from surgical injury during aortic valve surgery.

The mitral valve bears two important surgical anatomic relationships. The posterior (mural or lateral) leaflet is in continuity with the posterior LV wall. Deep (posterior) to the posterior leaflet lies the AV groove, within which lies the circumflex coronary artery and the coronary sinus, which are thereby at risk of surgical injury. The atrioventricular node and bundle of His likewise lie deep to the posteromedial commissure of the mitral valve, with errant sutures having potential to cause complete atrioventricular conduction block (Fig. 61.9).

Tricuspid valve surgery also entails risk to the atrioventricular node, as the tricuspid annulus is positioned on the opposite side of the membranous septum from the mitral valve. The atrioventricular node lies in the apex of "Koch triangle," which is bounded by the septal leaflet of the tricuspid valve anteriorly, the tendon of Todaro posteriorly, and the central fibrous body containing the bundle of His superiorly, leading to the coronary sinus inferiorly (Fig. 61.10). Additionally, the coronary sinus ostium lies adjacent

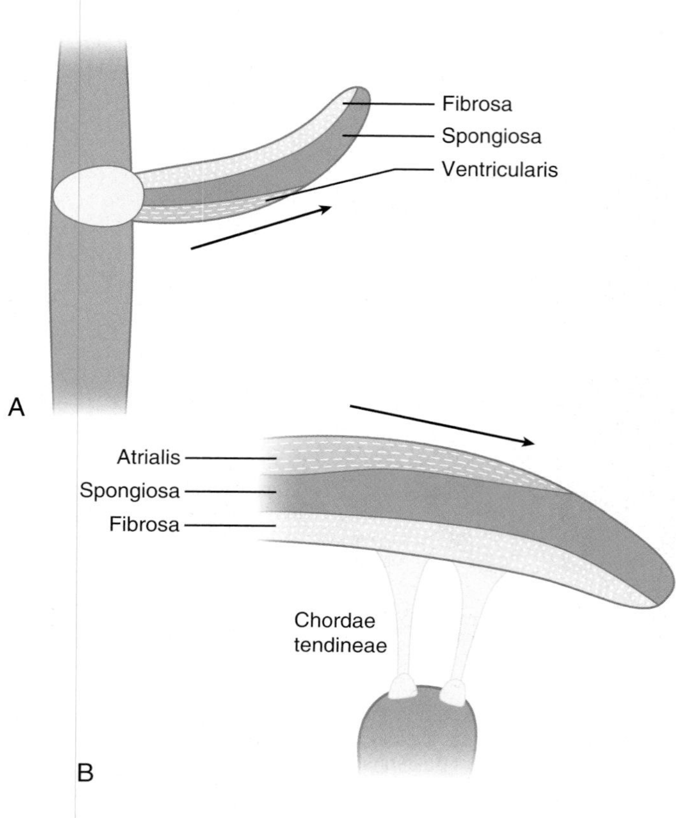

FIG. 61.3 Valve histology. The mature valve is composed of a highly organized extracellular matrix, which is compartmentalized into three layers: the fibrosa (F), made of fibrillar collagen; the spongiosa (S), made of proteoglycans; and either the ventricularis (V) of the semilunar valves or the atrialis (A) of the atrioventricular valves, made of elastin fiber. (From Combs MD, Yutzey KE. Heart valve development: regulatory networks in development and disease. *Circ Res.* 2009;105:408–421.)

to the commissure of the septal and posterior leaflets of the valve and can be inadvertently oversewn if it is not carefully identified.

ETIOLOGY AND PATHOLOGY OF VALVULAR HEART DISEASE

The cardiac valves may become impaired through two fundamental forms of dysfunction, stenosis and insufficiency. Valvular stenosis is an obstruction to forward flow due to incomplete opening of the valve. Valvular insufficiency, also referred to as regurgitation or incompetence, describes backward flow through a valve when its cusps or leaflets are unable to obtain or maintain coaptation. Both stenosis and insufficiency may exist simultaneously in any one valve.

Valvular stenosis is almost always caused by a primary abnormality of the cusp or leaflet from a chronic disease process. Regurgitation may be caused by an acute or chronic disease process affecting the valve itself or may be secondary to a structural abnormality of associated supporting structures, such as the great arteries, annuli fibrosi, chordae tendinae, papillary muscles, or ventricular myocardium (Table 61.1).

Although degenerative disease is a more common cause of valve disease in the developed world, rheumatic fever and ensuing rheumatic heart disease (RHD) likely remains the most common (albeit decreasing) cause of valvular dysfunction worldwide.

Mitral Stenosis

Mitral stenosis (MS) is by far most commonly caused by RHD and RHD most commonly involves the mitral valve. It is highly uncommon to have valvular RHD without mitral involvement. For reasons that remain incompletely understood, the prevalence of RHD is approximately twice as great in women as men. Other less common causes of MS include endocarditis, mitral annular calcification, and congenital anomalies such as parachute mitral valve and as a component of Shone complex, which is associated with supramitral rings.

Rheumatic Heart Disease

Acute rheumatic fever develops because of a cross-reactive host immune response exhibited by genetically susceptible individuals in response to group A beta-hemolytic streptococcal infection acquired during the first decade of life, driven by molecular mimicry between streptococcal proteins and host cardiac proteins such as laminin.[2] In some patients, this initial response causes clinically evident inflammation in the cardiac valves and/or conduction system several weeks after the streptococcal infection.

Rarely, acute rheumatic valvulitis can result in severe acute mitral regurgitation (MR) and may be associated with other manifestations of carditis such as atrioventricular conduction abnormalities or pericarditis. More typically, chronic RHD silently develops as ongoing valvular damage occurs due to repeated exposures to streptococcal infection and ongoing hemodynamic damage to a deformed valve in adolescence and adulthood.

Chronic RHD most commonly presents as either mitral valve stenosis or mixed valve lesions (stenotic and regurgitant). Mixed stenotic/regurgitant pathology takes the form of a pathognomonic "fish mouth" funnel valve lesion with associated fusion and shortening of the leaflets and chordae tendinae (Fig. 61.11). Sclerosis induced from chronic inflammation reducing leaflet mobility and prevents both complete opening of the valve during diastole and adequate coaptation during systole. Clinically apparent heart failure typically develops from these RHD lesions in the third or fourth decade of life due to progressive valve dysfunction and/or exhaustion of compensatory mechanisms.[3]

RHD next most frequently leads to aortic valve stenosis through a similar pattern of chronic inflammation with resultant sclerosis impairing valve opening leading to a narrowed orifice. Tricuspid regurgitation (TR) is a common secondary valvular abnormality in RHD due to upstream hemodynamic stresses caused by MS, with resultant pulmonary hypertension and dilation of the pulmonary artery compromising valvular coaptation.

Aortic Stenosis

In the developed world, aortic valvular stenosis (AS) is the most common form of valvular heart disease requiring surgical intervention. AS is almost always acquired, resulting from degenerative changes to the aortic valve, but unicuspid aortic valves or other congenital anomalies of the LV outflow tract may also present as early in life. Because of the aging population, the prevalence of AS continues to rise, and is now found in 4% of the population over 85-years old.[4]

Stenotic disease of the aortic valve is relatively equally divided between that affecting initially normal trileaflet valves and that arising in congenitally bicuspid valves. Bicuspid aortic valves are

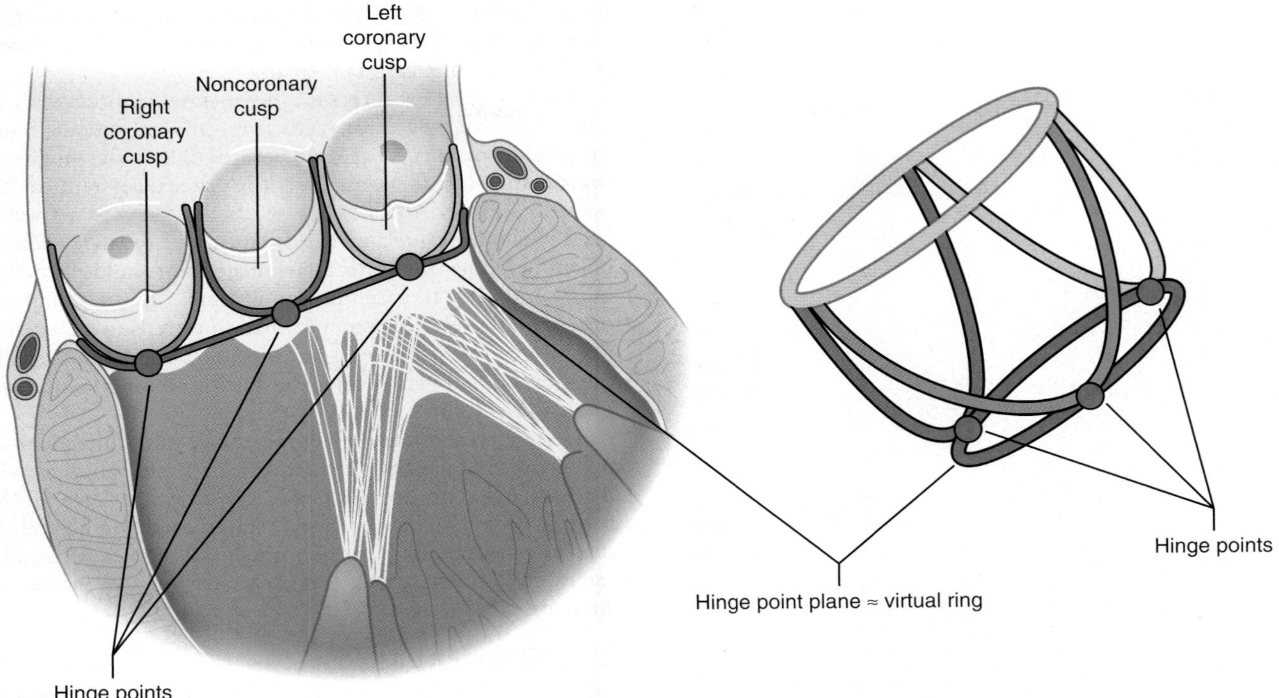

FIG. 61.4 Anatomy of the semilunar valves. Each valve is comprised of three cusps arising directly from the juncture of the great vessel and ventricular outflow tract walls. (From Kasel AM, Cassese S, Bleiziffer S, et al. Standardized imaging for aortic annular sizing: implications for transcatheter valve selection. *JACC Cardiovasc Imaging.* 2013;6:249–262.)

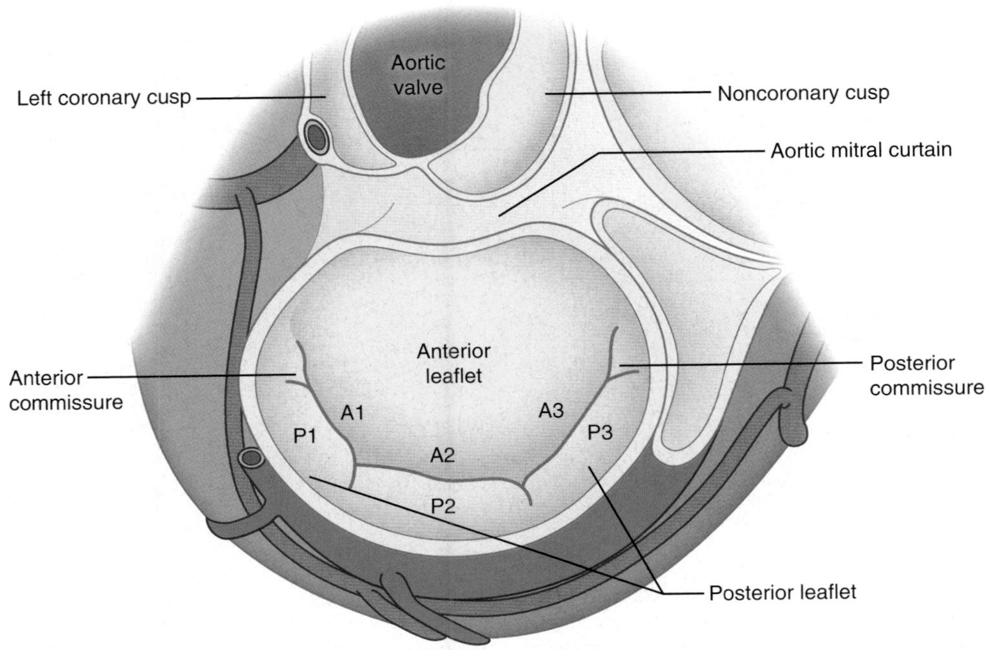

FIG. 61.5 Anatomy of the atrioventricular valves. The atrioventricular valves are comprised of leaflets arising from a distinct fibrous annulus. The depicted mitral valve is comprised of an anterior and posterior leaflet, each subdivided into three scallops. (With permission, Decker Medicine LLC)

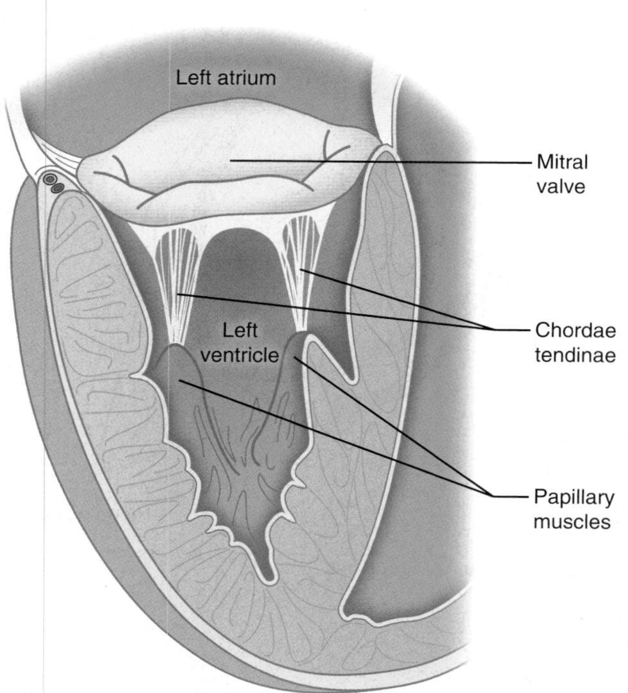

FIG. 61.6 Subvalvular apparatus of the atrioventricular valves. The mitral and tricuspid valves are supported by a robust subvalvular apparatus featuring the chordae tendinae that tether the leaflets and annuli to the papillary muscles which contract during systole to maintain leaflet coaptation and prevent leaflet prolapse into the atria. (From Filsoufi F, Carpentier A. http://www.themitralvalve.org/mitralvalve/anatomy-subvalvular-apparatus. Accessed August 11, 2020.)

present in 1% to 2% of the population, making this anomaly the most prevalent of the congenital valve lesions, and are more commonly found in males than females.

Stenosis develops through a degenerative process with prevalence increasing with age, with over 80% of patients requiring surgery for trileaflet AS aged 60 years or older.[5] The progression of degenerative (calcific) aortic stenosis (previously termed "senile" or "wear and tear" disease) is now thought to be an actively regulated phenomenon related to atherosclerotic disease, wherein turbulent blood flow at leaflet attachment points induces endothelial injury and leads to accumulation of lipids, infiltration of macrophages and T-cells, and transformation of cells to an osteoblastic phenotype.[4,6] It is believed that this process leads to aortic leaflet calcification and may involve the aortic and mitral annuli as well as the mitral leaflets.

Degenerative disease of bicuspid aortic valves presents as about two decades earlier than it does with tricuspid valves, peaking in the fifth and sixth decades of life. AS occurs in 20% to 30% of patients born with bicuspid aortic valves. Increased hemodynamic stresses associated with the abnormally configured bicuspid valve leaflets are thought to accelerate degenerative valve changes in this anomaly.

Mitral Regurgitation

MR is the most frequent form of valve dysfunction overall, with at least trivial MR present in most healthy adults, and is the second most common form of valvular heart disease requiring surgical intervention. The diagnosis and treatment of MR was greatly facilitated by the work of Carpentier, who in innovating surgical approaches to repair the mitral valve also described a functional classification of MR based on abnormal patterns of leaflet motion (Table 61.2).[7] Degenerative changes to the mitral valve apparatus

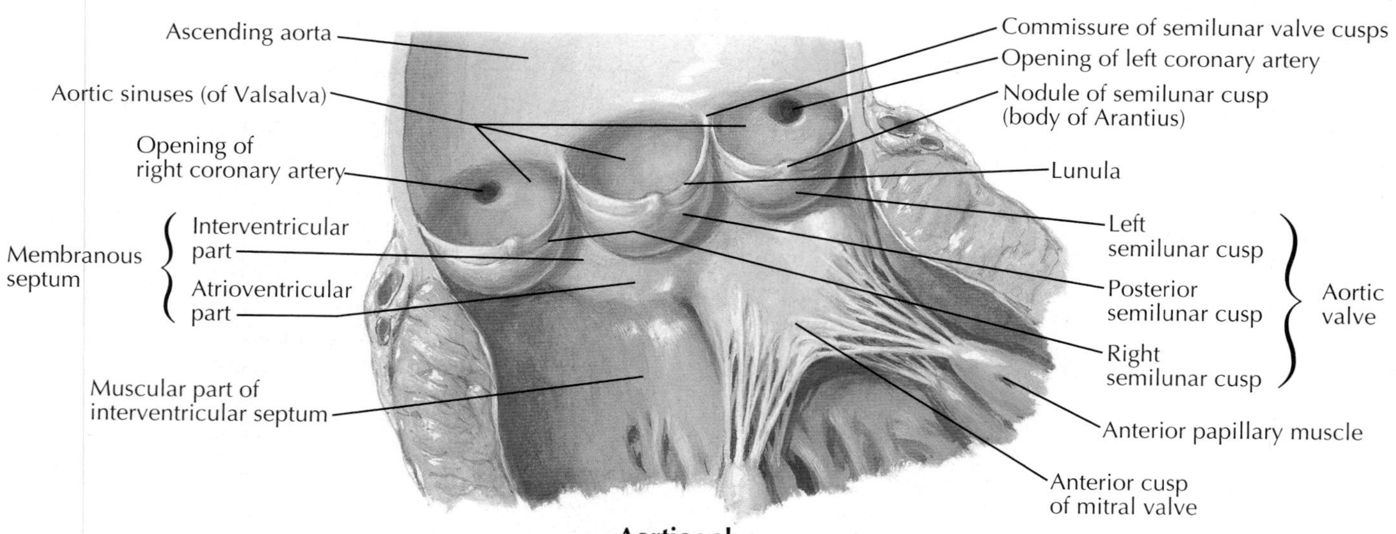

FIG. 61.7 Sinuses of Valsalva. The coronary arterial circulation originates at the Sinuses of Valsalva, gentle dilatations of the aorta just distal to the valve proper which impart important facilitation to valve closure and coronary and blood flow. (From http://cdn.agilitycms.com/applied-radiology/MediaGroupings/124/Fiss_figure04.jpg. https://www.appliedradiology.com/articles/normal-coronary-anatomy-and-anatomic-variations. Accessed August 11, 2020.)

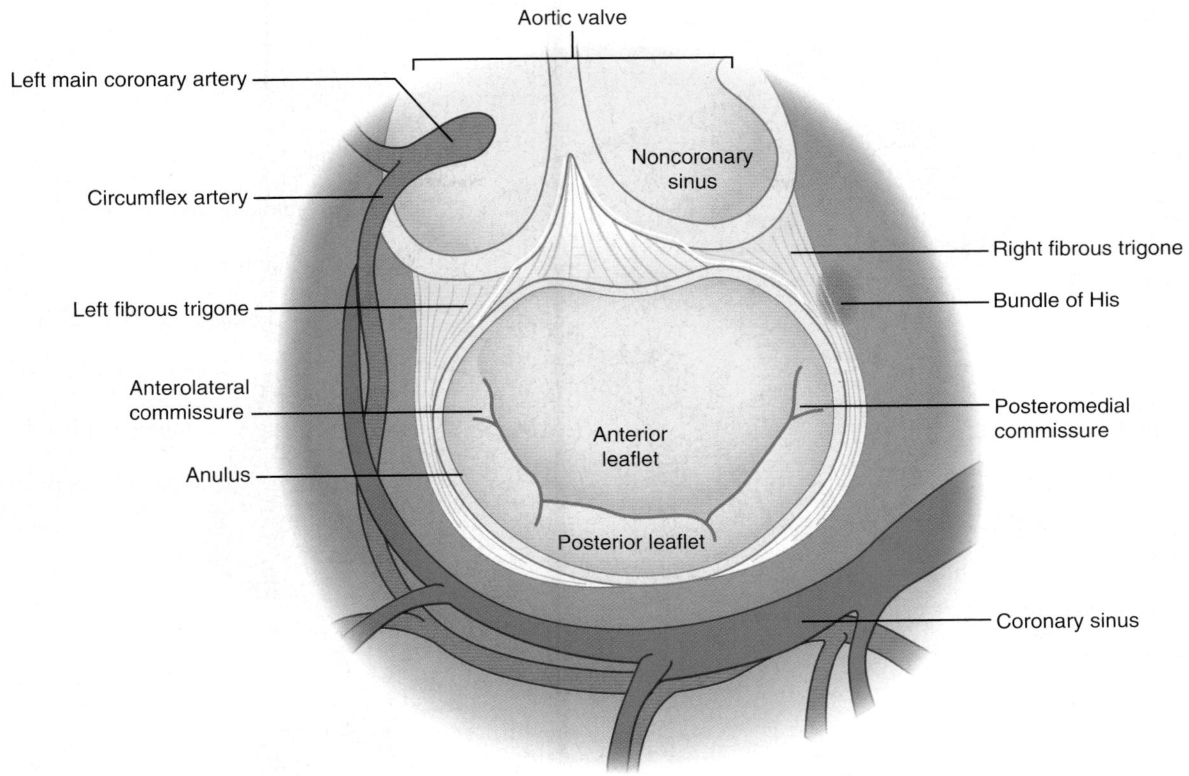

FIG. 61.8 Surgical anatomy of the aortic and mitral valves. The anterior leaflet of the mitral valve is in direct continuity with the left and noncoronary cusps of the aortic valve from about the 5 to the 8 o'clock position in the traditional surgical perspective. (From Sellke FW, del Nido PJ, Swanson SJ. *Sabiston and Spencer's Surgery of the Chest*. 9th ed. Philadelphia, PA: Saunders Elsevier; 2015, p. 1384.)

are the most common cause of MR and are typically found in young patients (Table 61.1). Surgical intervention for MR is related to degenerative disease in 60% to 70% of cases, to ischemic disease in 20% of cases, and to endocarditis or rheumatic disease in 2% to 5%.

A wide variety of connective tissue diseases may lead to degenerative disease of the mitral valve, typically causing annular dilation (Carpentier Type I lesion) and/or leaflet or subvalvular deformations resulting in excessive leaflet motion (Carpentier Type II lesion). The most prevalent of these diseases is Marfan syndrome. "Myxomatous disease" describes a common pathologic end point of these degenerative diseases, which typically presents as MR in the third or fourth decade of life. This process is characterized by glycosaminoglycan infiltration of the valve leaflets, thickening of the spongiosa, and separation of collagen bundles in the fibrosa.

Myxomatous disease of the mitral valve typically leads to redundant, "billowing" valve leaflets, annular dilatation, and/or chordae enlargement or elongation with consequent abnormal systolic leaflet prolapse into the atrium. This syndrome typically occurs in young women and is also known as Barlow disease after the clear identification in 1963 of the etiology of this "click-murmur syndrome."[8] Mitral disease is the most common manifestation of myxomatous disease, but it may also present as aortic and tricuspid valve disease.

Myxomatous disease should be differentiated from fibroelastic deficiency syndrome, which is typically characterized by thinned leaflets and chordal rupture and presents in older patients. Prolapse or flail of the middle posterior leaflet cusp (P2) due to chordae rupture is a common manifestation of fibroelastic deficiency syndrome.[9]

Mitral annular calcification is an extremely common degenerative change found in older patients that is typically without functional sequelae. It may be associated with similar changes involving the aortic or mitral valves. Mitral annular calcification can, however, on occasion produce MR by reducing annulus pliability and systolic contraction, which prevent appropriate leaflet coaptation. Less frequently, mitral annular calcification disorders manifest through a more widespread degenerative pathology.

Coronary ischemia causing rupture of a papillary muscle or acute myocardial infarction, particularly in the inferior distribution, can also lead to significant MR. This typically involves the posterior papillary muscle leading to prolapse or flail of the posterior leaflet, because the blood supply to the posterior papillary muscle is from a single (terminal) branch of the posterior descending coronary artery, compared to dual blood supply to the anterolateral papillary muscle from the left anterior descending and circumflex arteries.

In contrast to the causes of primary MR noted above, secondary or "functional" MR, is not caused by abnormalities of the valve itself, but rather by distortion of the subvalvular apparatus and ventricle. Typically, functional MR is a result of myocardial ischemic events and/or cardiomyopathy-induced ventricular dilatation. Dilation of the ventricle results in outward (lateral) and apical (inferior) displacement of the posteromedial papillary muscle, causing tethering of the valve leaflets and loss of central coaptation (Carpentier Type IIIb lesion).

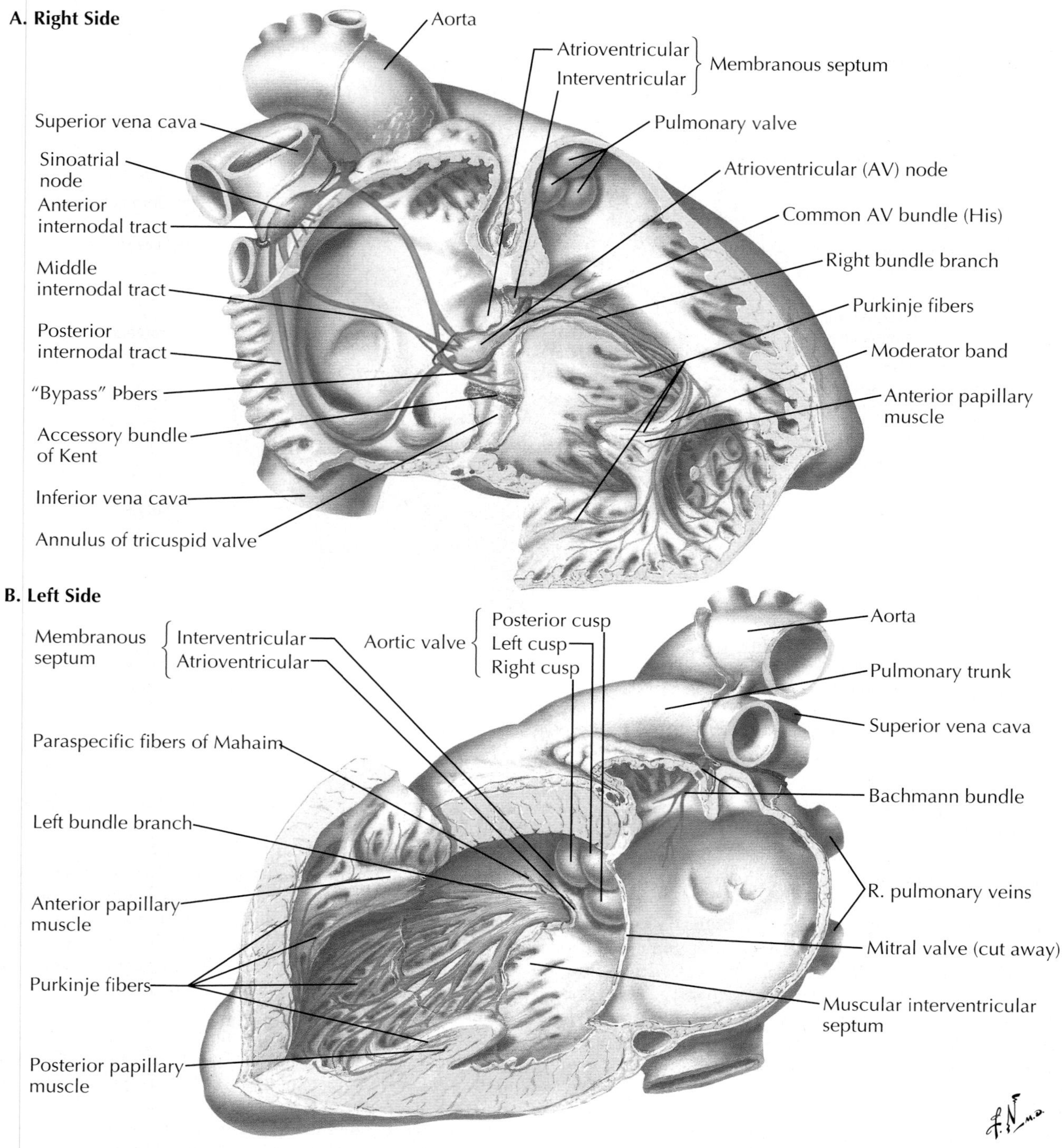

FIG. 61.9 Anatomic relations of cardiac valves and conduction system. The fibrous skeleton, which provides structure to the atrioventricular and aortic valves also contains the electrical conduction system, placing this system at risk for injury during cardiotomy for valve exposure and/or valve interventions by open or percutaneous techniques. (From Conti CR. *Netter Collection of Medical Illustrations: Cardiovascular System*. 2nd ed. Philadelphia, PA: Elsevier Saunders; 2014, Plate 1-12.)

In addition to these and other acquired forms of MR, including those that limit systolic motion of the mitral leaflets (Carpentier IIIa lesion), congenital anomalies such as cleft leaflets and atrioventricular canal/endocardial cushion defects may lead to MR as well.

Aortic Insufficiency

Aortic valve insufficiency (AI) may be caused by myxomatous disease leading to thinning, enlargement, perforation and/or prolapse of the aortic valve cusps themselves. AI may also be caused by chronic or acute dilatation of the aortic root, which prevents proper aortic valve coaptation by increasing intravalvular closing distances. Root enlargement is typically caused by hypertension and/or connective tissue disorders such as cystic medial necrosis, Marfan syndrome, Ehlers-Danlos syndrome, or Loeys Dietz syndrome, either directly or as a result of acute or chronic aortic dissection.

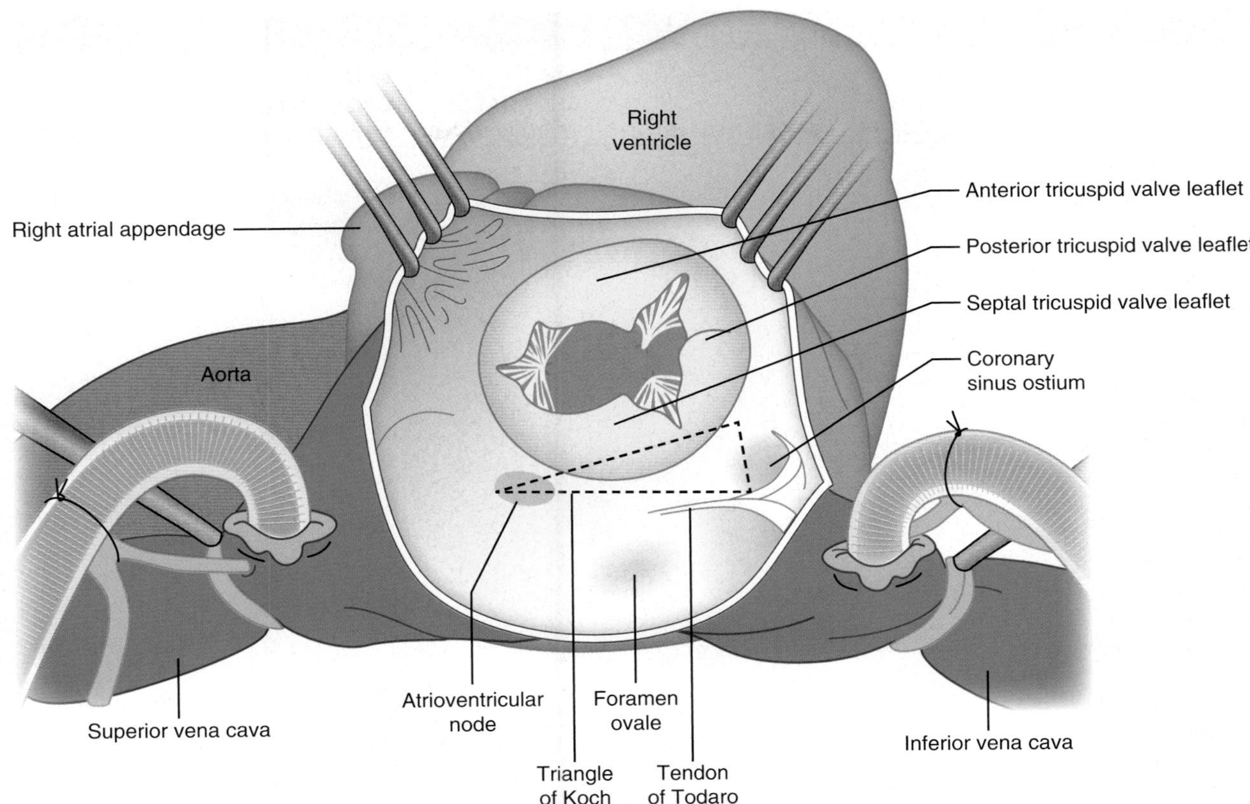

FIG. 61.10 Surgical anatomy of the tricuspid valve. The atrioventricular node lies in the apex of a triangular area first described by Koch, which is bounded by the septal annulus of the tricuspid valve anteriorly, the tendon of Todaro posteriorly, and the central fibrous body containing the bundle of His superiorly, leading to the coronary sinus inferiorly. (From Rogers JH, Bolling SF. The tricuspid valve: current perspective and evolving management of tricuspid regurgitation. *Circulation*. 2009;119:2718–2725.) *A*, Anterior tricuspid valve leaflet; *AVN*, atrioventricular node; *CS*, coronary sinus ostium; *FO*, foramen ovale; *IVC*, inferior vena cava; *P*, posterior tricuspid valve leaflet; *RAA*, right atrial appendage; *RV*, right ventricle; *S*, septal tricuspid valve leaflet; *SVC*, superior vena cava.

Importantly, (Mendelian) inheritance of a bicuspid aortic valve anomaly is also associated with dilation of the proximal ascending aorta in up to 50% of patients, which can lead to bicuspid-related AI. This association is hypothesized to be due to a currently unidentified common genetic defect causing abnormalities in aortic wall elasticity, or through hemodynamic "blast" effects of abnormal flow through the bicuspid valve orifice. AI due to bicuspid valve-related root enlargement typically develops at a much younger age than AS that develops from accelerated degeneration, and with a lower rate of progression requiring surgical intervention.

Less common causes of aortic root enlargement and/or aortic dissection include trauma, syphilitic aortitis, rheumatoid arthritis, lupus erythematosus, or other systemic vasculopathies such as Takayasu and giant cell aortitis, and osteogenesis imperfecta.

Endocarditis

Endocarditis is a relatively common cause of AI, and a frequent cause of valve pathology overall. The incidence of endocarditis varies from 3 to 10 episodes per 100,000 person-years. Endocarditis typically causes valvular insufficiency by progressive inflammatory destruction of the affected valve. Less frequently, endocarditis can cause functional valve stenosis, with valve orifice obstruction developing from endocarditic vegetations–masses of platelets, fibrin, microcolonies of microorganisms, and inflammatory cells.

Although endocarditis is typically relatively indolent, it is the most common cause of death secondary to acute AI in the adult population and carries a relatively high mortality compared to other valve lesions. Endocarditis may affect previously normal valves, but it typically affects valves deformed by congenital or rheumatic disease, degenerative processes such as calcification, or previously replaced prosthetic valves. Infectious endocarditis is usually left-sided, reflecting the normal distribution of such preexisting valvular disease.

The pathophysiology of endocarditis is typically initiated by platelets and fibrin deposition on normal or deformed valves occurring as part of a normal healing process following normal disruptions of the valvular endothelium, which are in turn caused by hemodynamic or metabolic injuries. Endocarditis results from subsequent seeding onto thus damaged valves of microbiologic organisms after bacteremia or fungemia episodes; most commonly staphylococci, streptococci, or enterococci.

Acute endocarditis, increasingly affecting normal valves, may follow an aggressive course with valvular perforation or more extensive destruction of the leaflet and/or surrounding support structures, resulting in acute valvular regurgitation. With subacute or chronic presentations of endocarditis, valve insufficiency may result from residual leaflet deformities caused by fibrotic healing of endocarditic lesions. The growth of large vegetations may also uncommonly lead to improper leaflet coaptation and AI as well.

Right-Sided Valvular Disease

Nearly all the pathophysiologic mechanisms causing left-sided valve disease may analogously lead to primary right-sided valve disease;

TABLE 61.1 **Etiology of valve pathology.**

	LEAFLETS	ANNULUS	CHORDAE TENDINAE	VENTRICULAR WALL/ PAPILLARY MUSCLE (PM)	AORTIC ROOT
Mitral Stenosis					
Rheumatic valve disease	++	++	++	+/- (PM fusion/ shortening)	NA
Endocarditis (vegetation)	+/-	-	-	-	NA
Congenital*	++	-	-	+/-	NA
Supravalvular (thrombus, myxoma)	++	-	-	-	NA
Mitral Regurgitation					
Mitral valve prolapse (myxomatous/connective tissue disorder)	++	++	++	-	NA
Rheumatic fever	++	-	+/-	-	NA
Endocarditis	++	+/-	++	+	NA
Congenital anomaly**	++	-	+/-	-	NA
Systemic lupus erythematosus***	++	+/-	+/-	+/- (PM)	NA
Mitral annular calcification (MAC)	=/-	++	-	-	NA
Myocardial ischemia/ infarction	-	+/-	-	++	NA
Hypertrophic cardiomyopathy				++	NA
Aortic Stenosis					
Degenerative disease (trileaflet)	++	+	NA	-	-
Bicuspid valve disease	++	+	NA	-	-
Rheumatic valve disease	++	+	NA	-	-
Endocarditis (vegetation)	++	+	NA	-	-
Other congenital anomaly^	++	+	NA	++	+
Hypertrophic cardiomyopathy	-	-	-	++	-
Aortic Insufficiency					
Degenerative/connective tissue disease^^	++	++	NA	-	++
Rheumatic disease	++	-	NA	-	-
Inflammatory disease^^^	+	-	NA	-	++
Endocarditis	++	+	NA	-	+
Congenital (bicuspid, unicuspid)	++	-	NA	-	+
Aortic dissection/ aortic aneurysm#	-	++	NA	-	++

(++) Common; (+) fairly common; (+/-) possibly involved; (-) rarely involved.
NA, Not applicable; *PM*, papillary muscle.
*Parachute mitral valve, supramitral ring.
**Cleft leaflet, endocardial cushion defect, parachute mitral valve.
***Liebman-Sacks lesion.
^Unicuspid/unicommisural valve, hypoplastic annulus/root, subaortic membrane/stenosis.
^^Marfan syndrome, myxomatous degeneration, osteogenesis imperfecta, Ehlers-Danlos syndrome.
^^^Ankylosing spondylitis, Reiter syndrome, Takayasu disease, giant cell aortitis.

however, the most common presentation of right-sided valvular disease is functional TR caused by RV failure (which itself is typically secondary to left sided dysfunction and pulmonary hypertension). Less commonly, functional TR may also be caused by RV infarction or ischemia. Transvalvular pacemaker or cardioverter-defibrillator leads can also uncommonly cause mild or even higher-grade TR.

Tricuspid stenosis (TS) occurs infrequently in developed countries since rheumatic disease accounts for over 90% of such lesions.

Carcinoid syndrome is the most common of a group of unusual disorders that lead to the deposition of pathologic materials in the tricuspid and/or pulmonic leaflets as a far less frequent cause of primary TR, TS, or pulmonic valve disease.

Congenital anomalies causing pulmonic valve stenosis, often associated with tetralogy of Fallot; tricuspid atresia; and TR occurring as part of the Ebstein anomaly are three of the most common of the congenital disorders leading to right-sided valve disease.

PATHOPHYSIOLOGY OF VALVULAR HEART DISEASE

Two fundamental pathophysiologic derangements may affect the heart valves: stenosis and insufficiency. The hemodynamic hallmark of cardiac valve stenosis is the occurrence of an increased pressure gradient between an upstream pumping chamber and downstream receiving chamber or great artery. This increased gradient is necessary to maintain the baseline flow rate through the valve due to the increased resistance to laminar flow introduced by the smaller effective cross-sectional area of the stenotic valve orifice, as described by Poiseuille law (flow α Δp/resistance, where Δp signifies pressure gradient). The hemodynamic hallmark of regurgitant valvular disease is the retrograde flow of blood from downstream structures (ventricle or great vessel) into an upstream chamber during the diastolic interval during which the malfunctioning valve should normally be closed. Uncompensated, both stenotic and regurgitant lesions cause an increase in upstream chamber afterload and consequent wall stress – predominating either during ventricular systolic ejection against the resistance of stenotic valves, or with increased chamber filling by regurgitant volumes peaking at the end of diastole, respectively.

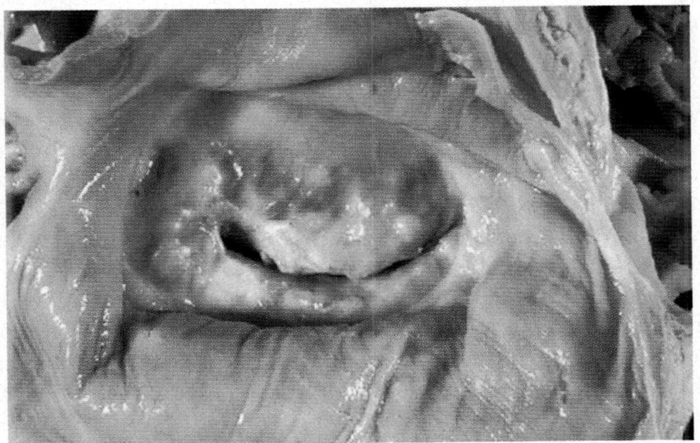

FIG. 61.11 Mitral valve pathology in rheumatic heart disease. Typical pathology of rheumatic mitral valve disease presenting as a pathognomonic, mixed stenotic/regurgitant "fish mouth" funnel valve lesion, often associated with fusion and shortening of the leaflets and chordae tendinae. (From http://library.med.utah.edu/WebPath/CVHTML/CV061.html. Accessed August 11, 2020.)

Two compensatory mechanisms provide robust reserves in cardiac function before the volume and pressure overload stresses of valve disease translate into significant cardiac physiologic derangements. The first, described by the Frank-Starling law (Fig. 61.12), produces increases in ventricular contractile force as a function of end-diastolic volume (EDV), or preload, which enhances stroke volume and ventricular emptying. The second involves stress-induced ventricular hypertrophy, which leads to increased wall thickness. By decreasing chamber radius (volume) or increasing wall thickness, respectively, each of these processes can improve wall stress, as described by Laplace law: (wall stress α (pressure $\times$ radius)/(2 $\times$ wall thickness). Decreased wall stress in turn translates into decreased myocardial work and oxygen demand and improved cardiac function.

The microanatomic basis of the Frank-Starling relationship is the orientation between actin and myosin fibers of the cardiomyocyte sarcomere, which become ideally aligned to generate contractile force as cardiac muscle is stretched from a "zero-load" status. Ideal actin-myosin alignment occurs at a sarcomere length of 2.2 micrometers, at which point contractile proteins become optimally sensitized to calcium fluxes, resulting in maximized sarcomere contractility as well as rates of contraction and relaxation. As cardiomyopathy progress, contractile function diminishes at a given level of cellular stretch, and eventually heart failure ensues.

TABLE 61.2 Carpentier classification of mitral valve regurgitation.

CARPENTIER CLASSIFICATION	DYSFUNCTION	LESIONS	ETIOLOGY
Type I	Normal leaflet motion	Annular dilatation Leaflet perforation/tear	Dilated cardiomyopathy Endocarditis
Type II	Excessive leaflet motion (prolapse)	Elongation/rupture of chordae Elogation/rupture of papillary muscle	Degenerative valve disease Fibroelastic deficiency Barlow disease Marfan disease Rheumatic (acute) Endocarditis Trauma Ischemic cardiomyopathy
Type IIIa	Restricted leaflet motion (diastole and systole)	Leaflet thickening/retraction Leaflet calcification Chordal thickening/retraction/fusion Commissural fusion	Rheumatic (chronic) Carcinoid heart disease
Type IIIb	Restricted leaflet motion (systole)	Left ventricular dilatation/aneurysm Papillary muscle displacement Chordae tethering	Ischemic/dilated cardiomyopathy

From Carpentier A. Cardiac valve surgery–the "French correction". *J Thorac Cardiovasc Surg.* 1983;86:323–337.

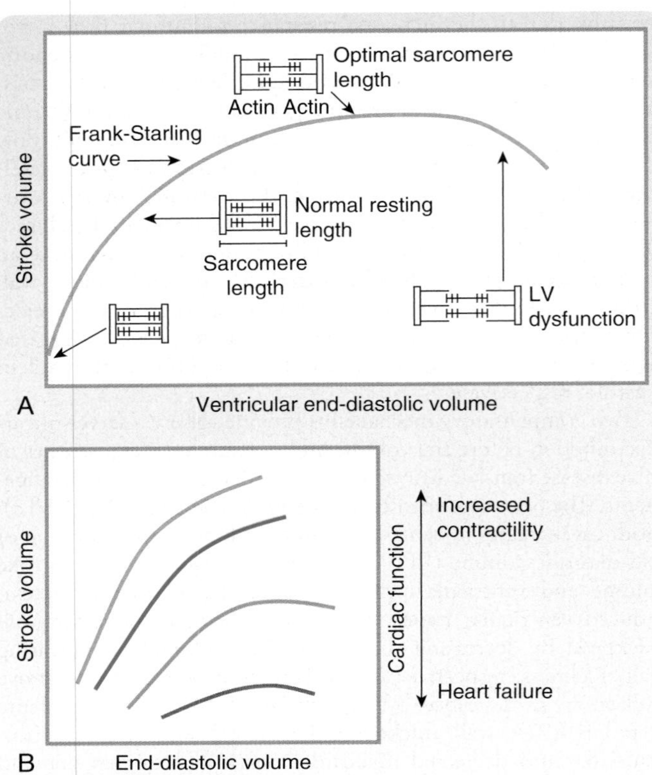

FIG. 61.12 Frank Starling curve. The Frank-Starling law describes a generally linear relationship between increasing end-diastolic volume (EDV), or preload, and generated ventricular pressure. (A) Shifts in volume change generated pressure/stroke volume along a given pressure-volume curve. (B) Cardiomyopathy shifts curve downward. (From http://cardiovascres.oxfordjournals.org/content/cardiovascres/77/4/627/336033. Accessed August 11, 2020.)

VALVE DISEASE SYNDROMES

Patients with valvular heart disease typically progress through a series of disease stages, from Stage A ("at risk") to Stage D ("symptomatic severe").[10,11] Asymptomatic patients demonstrating mild to moderate valve pathology are classified as Stage B and asymptomatic patients with severe valve pathology are classified as Stage C, either with compensated (C1) or decompensated (C2) left or RV function. Regular assessment is recommended for patients with valvular heart disease (i.e., echocardiograms every 3–5 years for Stage B patients, increasing to every 6–12 months for Stage C patients). This surveillance should allow appropriately timed intervention to minimize valve-related symptomatology, sequelae (e.g., atrial fibrillation, stroke, pulmonary dysfunction) and mortality risk, while balancing the risks of intervention with the natural history of advanced disease.

Mitral Stenosis

There is typically no pressure gradient across a normally-sized mitral valve (4–6 cm^2 cross-sectional area) and "upstream" LA pressure is typically less than 10 to 15 mm Hg. As the mitral valve orifice narrows to a cross sectional area of 2 to 2.5 cm^2 (mild MS), resistance to flow leads to increased LA blood volume "pooling." Increased LA pressure generated by Frank Starling mechanics maintains adequate diastolic flow across the resistive valve orifice.

When progressive MS leads to a transvalvular gradient of greater than 5 to 10 mm Hg, typically corresponding to a valve orifice of less than 1.5 cm^2, MS is classified as "severe". The resultant increase in LA pressure is transmitted upstream to the pulmonary veins, capillaries, and arteries. At an LA pressure of 25 mm Hg, pulmonary edema typically develops, with prolonged arterial vasoconstriction and vascular remodeling eventually leading to fixed pulmonary hypertension with chronically increased pulmonary pressure. Elevated pulmonary arterial systolic pressure greater than 60 mm Hg imparts significant RV afterload may also ultimately lead to RV dilatation, TR, and RV failure. MS spares left ventricle function in two-thirds of cases, with normal or less than normal LV chamber hemodynamics in 85% of cases and impaired output primarily due to restricted LV inflow.

Any increase in cardiac output, as with exercise, will lead to an increase in mitral transvalvular pressure gradients according to the law of Poiseuille: flow α Δp/resistance, where Δp signifies pressure gradient. At a given cardiac output, decreased diastolic filling time caused by increased heart rates, such as with exercise or the onset of atrial fibrillation, will also cause increased transvalvular gradient as more flow must occur per unit time.

Chronically increased transmitral pressure gradients caused by MS typically lead to atrial hypertrophy and dilatation. Associated LA fibrosis and disorganization of the atrial muscle fibers cause abnormal atrial conduction velocities and refractory times. Increased automaticity, ectopic foci, and reentry circuits eventually lead to supraventricular tachyarrhythmias in nearly 40% of patients. Loss of the "kick" generated by normal atrial contraction, responsible for 30% of ventricular filling, results in a 20% decrease in cardiac output and necessitates increased atrial pressure to allow ventricular loading. Atrial fibrillation consequently causes increased diastolic pressures and volume overload, potentially leading to worsening congestion.

Diagnosis of Mitral Stenosis

Symptoms and signs. MS patients may remain asymptomatic for many years. As valvular stenosis gradually worsens, however, symptoms characteristic of low cardiac output and pulmonary venous congestion eventually develop, including fatigue, dyspnea, and orthopnea. Ultimately, peripheral edema and other congestive symptoms caused by volume overload and right heart failure ensue. Increased heart rate caused by atrial fibrillation or supraventricular tachycardia, exercise or other factors may exacerbate symptomatology.

Patients with MS who develop atrial fibrillation may complain of palpitations and symptomatic tachycardia. More ominously, thromboembolization will occur in 20% of patients with MS and may be its first symptom in 10% of cases, presenting as stroke, myocardial ischemia or infarction, renal infarction, and gut or limb ischemia. Half of all thromboembolic events will involve the cerebral circulation. Rarely, a large, pedunculated atrial thrombus may form and obstruct the valve inlet, resulting in hemodynamic collapse and sudden death. With advanced disease, LA enlargement may cause hoarseness from left recurrent laryngeal nerve compression onto the pulmonary artery, dysphagia from esophageal compression, or persistent cough from bronchial compression. Pulmonary venous congestion may induce hemoptysis from sudden rupture of a dilated bronchial vein. RV failure and TR can cause abdominal pain and swelling from hepatomegaly and ascites, or even florid peripheral edema.

Physical exam. The characteristic physical finding of MS is a low-pitched, rumbling diastolic murmur which is best heard at the apex with the patient in the left lateral decubitus position. In patients who are in sinus rhythm, the murmur increases in intensity during late diastole (known as presystolic accentuation) due to the increased flow across the stenotic valve with atrial contraction. A high-pitched "opening snap" or an accentuated first heart sound caused by forceful opening or closing, respectively, of an inflexible but still mobile mitral leaflet may be heard with early MS. The Graham Steell diastolic murmur of MS can result from pulmonary regurgitation caused by pulmonary hypertension and right-sided overload.

Advanced MS is typically associated with rales developing with the onset of pulmonary edema. As RV failure develops, an RV heave, jugular venous distension, hepatomegaly, ascites, and lower extremity edema may be found.

Diagnostic testing. The earliest appreciable changes of MS discernable by routine chest radiography include evidence of an enlarged LA seen as a straightening of the left cardiac border, a double shadow in the cardiac silhouette, or an elevated left main stem bronchus. Prominent pulmonary vessels may also be appreciated. If stenosis is severe, congested pulmonary lymphatics in the lower lung fields may be present as horizontal linear opacities, known Kerley B lines. Mitral valve calcification may also be visible. Stigmata of heart failure, such as opacification of the lung fields and pleural effusions, may follow.

The electrocardiogram of MS patients is often grossly normal, although 90% of patients will demonstrate evidence of LA enlargement as a widened, notched P wave (p mitrale). Atrial arrhythmias may also be appreciated if present. With advanced MS, RV hypertrophy may be associated with right-axis deviation.

Echocardiography, as with other valve lesions, is the primary diagnostic method to determine the presence and severity of MS and associated abnormalities. Commissural fusion, leaflet immobility and leaflet as well as annular/subvalvular thickening and calcification can be well assessed by transthoracic and especially by transesophageal echo. Three-dimensional (3D) echocardiography provides further definition of valve morphology and function.

Doppler echocardiography has largely replaced cardiac catheterization in accurately assessing the hemodynamic parameters of MS as well as other valve lesions. Doppler blood velocity measurement allows mean and peak transvalvular mitral pressure gradient determination as a function of the simplified Bernoulli equation: $p = 4v^2$, where v equals the velocity of blood crossing the valve orifice. Orifice area can be measured by planimetry (tracing the valve-opening orifice on a still echocardiographic image) or as a derivative of velocity measurements, based on continuity equations. Mitral valve area can also be determined based upon the pressure half-time, the time in which the transvalvular velocity decreases by half. Pressure half-time will become prolonged with increasing severity of stenosis.

Natural History

Ten-year patient survival is greater than 80% in the asymptomatic patient with MS, and interventional treatment is consequently not recommended in this setting. In comparison, 10-year survival for symptomatic patients with severe MS who forgo intervention is less than 15%, and mean survival is less than three years in patients with MS and severe pulmonary hypertension.

Treatment

Medical management. Medical management of patients with symptomatic MS includes the use of diuretics to reduce LA pressure and vascular congestion. Beta-blockers and calcium channel-blocking agents are recommended to provide heart rate control and help maintain sinus rhythm. Anticoagulation therapy is recommended via $CHADS_2$ and the updated $CHADS_2$-VASc (modification to better assess low-risk patients) scoring systems in patients developing atrial fibrillation (Table 61.3), and in patients without atrial fibrillation but who have suffered a prior embolic event or have a documented LA thrombus.[11] Use of anticoagulation therapy must be tempered against the risk of major bleeding, which can now be calculated using the Hypertension, Abnormal renal/liver function, Stroke, Bleeding history or predisposition, Labile international normalized ratio, Elderly [>65 years], Drugs/alcohol concomitantly (HAS-BLED) scoring system developed in 2010 from data in the Euro Heart Survey to assess 1-year risk of major bleeding in patients taking anticoagulants with atrial fibrillation.[12]

Interventional Management

Early intervention is associated with improved long-term survival for patients with MS compared to patients in whom intervention is delayed until the development of symptomatology. Five-year survival is 62% for NHYA Class III patients, and 15% for Class IV patients.[13] The current American Heart Association/

TABLE 61.3 $CHADS_2$ and $CHADS_2$-VASc score for atrial fibrillation stroke risk and recommended anticoagulation.

	$CHADS_2$ SCORE	POINTS*	$CHADS_2$ - VASc SCORE	POINTS*
C	Congestive heart failure	1	Congestive heart failure	1
H	Hypertension	1	Hypertension	1
A	Age ≥ 75 years	1	Age ≥ 75 years	2
D	Diabetes mellitus	1	Diabetes mellitus	1
S	Prior stroke, TIA or thromboembolism	2	Prior stroke, TIA, or thromboembolism	2
V			Vascular disease	1
A			Age 65–74 years	1
Sc			Sex category (female)	1

$CHADS_2$: Score of 0, low risk; 1, moderate risk; 2–6, high risk.

$CHADS_2$-VASc: Score of 0 (male) or 1 (female), low risk; 1, moderate risk (male); 2–9, high risk.

TIA, Transient ischemic attack.

Recommended therapy for moderate or high risk is typically oral anticoagulant, with well-controlled vitamin K antagonist (VKA, e.g., warfarin with time in therapeutic range >70%), or a Non-VKA Oral Anticoagulant (NOAC, e.g., dabigatran, rivaroxaban, edoxaban, or apixaban).

*Points for each risk factor are additive.

American College of Cardiology (AHA/ACC) guidelines accordingly recommend intervention for MS in patients with symptomatic severe or asymptomatic very severe MS (valve orifice area <1.5 cm^2 or <1 cm^2, respectively).[10,11] Additionally, surgery is recommended for patients with moderate or severe MS undergoing cardiac surgery for other reasons, and for patients with severe MS who have recurrent embolic events while on anticoagulation (with LA excision recommended). Options for mechanical intervention include percutaneous mitral balloon commissurotomy, open mitral commissurotomy and surgical repair, or replacement of the mitral valve.

Percutaneous Balloon Mitral Commissurotomy

This endovascular procedure, first reported by Inoue and colleagues in 1984, uses a balloon catheter advanced into the left atrium via transseptal puncture or retrograde transaortic delivery to dilate the stenotic mitral valve. Based upon compelling safety and efficacy data, percutaneous balloon mitral commissurotomy (PBMC) has largely replaced surgical interventions in appropriately selected patients based upon (Wilkins) echocardiographic criteria (Table 61.4). In general, PBMC is indicated by the presence of mobile, noncalcified, thin valves with minimal fusion, scarring or calcification of the subvalvular apparatus, and the absence of moderate-to-severe MR or a LA thrombus.[10,11]

PBMC is associated with a mortality risk of 0.5%, and a less than 10% risk of cardiac or vascular complications, embolization, or creation of severe MR.[14] Successful PBMC, defined as a postdilation valve area of more than 1.5 cm^2 with MR less than 2/4, is achieved in over 80% of patients. Although reintervention is often required, over half of patients can expect to remain free from surgery at 20 years.[15]

Open Mitral Commissurotomy

Open mitral commissurotomy is the primary form of surgical repair of MS, and is limited to use for patients in whom intervention is needed but PBMC is contraindicated, or have failed previous percutaneous intervention. Open mitral commissurotomy requires use of cardiopulmonary bypass, and involves division of fused commissures, mobilization of scarred chordae, and ligation of the LA appendage. The mortality rate for open commissurotomy is less than 2%, and the 10-year freedom from reoperation rate after open mitral commissurotomy is approximately 90%.[16,17]

Mitral Valve Replacement

Mitral valve replacement is the most commonly employed surgical management of MS and is considered a very safe procedure, providing excellent long-term results. Regardless of whether a mechanical or tissue valve is employed, there is well-documented evidence that preservation of the subvalvular apparatus is critical for the maintenance of optimal LV geometry and function and improving 30-day and long-term survival.[10,11,14,18]

Mitral Regurgitation

Pathologic changes to any portion of the mitral valve apparatus or its function may cause improper systolic coaptation between the anterior and posterior mitral leaflets with subsequent valvular regurgitation. MR is subdivided into primary and secondary MR, which are distinct in their pathophysiology, natural history, and treatment approach. Primary MR, classified as Type I or II in the Carpentier system (Table 61.2), is secondary to pathologies affecting the structure of the mitral valve apparatus, specifically the leaflets, chordae, and annulus.[7] In contrast, secondary or functional MR, classified as Carpentier Type IIIb, is secondary to LV dysfunction and dilation, primarily due to ischemic cardiomyopathy. The severity of MR is dependent upon the size of the mitral orifice, the pressure gradient between the LV and LA, and the systemic afterload. Because LV pressure exceeds LA pressure well before it exceeds systemic pressure, mitral valve incompetency may allow a significant amount of regurgitant volume (up to one half of the ventricular preload) into the LA well before the opening of the aortic valve and forward flow into the aorta.

In the acute phase of MR, retrograde flow into the small, low-compliance LA receiving chamber may be poorly tolerated, and high atrial pressures may be transmitted into the pulmonary vasculature. Pulmonary hypertension with fulminant heart failure can ensue, and even prove to be fatal. When the onset of MR is more insidious, the LA can dilate and hypertrophy, and a chronic compensated state without pulmonary hypertension may be sustained for many years. On the other hand, LA dilatation may be accompanied by atrial fibrillation with the potential for thrombosis and episodic embolization.

Critical compensatory changes in LV hemodynamics are characteristic of chronic MR. Regurgitant volumes returning to the LV during diastole result in increased left ventricular end-diastolic volume (LVEDV) and supranormal ejection fractions, based both

TABLE 61.4 Wilkins score for assessing appropriateness of percutaneous balloon mitral commissurotomy.

GRADE	MOBILITY	THICKENING	CALCIFICATION	SUBVALVULAR THICKENING
1	Highly mobile valve with only leaflet tips restricted	Leaflets near normal in thickness (4–5 mm)	A single area of increased echocardiographic brightness	Minimal thickening just below the mitral leaflets
2	Leaflet mid and base portions have normal mobility	Midleaflets normal, considerable thickening of margins (5–8 mm)	Scattered areas of brightness confined to leaflet margins	Thickening of chordal structures extending to one-third of the chordal length
3	Valve continues to move forward in diastole, mainly from the base	Thickening extending through the entire leaflet (5–8 mm)	Brightness extending into the midportions of the leaflets	Thickening extended to distal third of the chords
4	No or minimal forward movement of the leaflets in diastole	Considerable thickening of all leaflet tissue (>8–10 mm)	Extensive brightness throughout much of the leaflet tissue	Extensive thickening and shortening of all chordal structures extending down to the papillary muscles

Sum of the four items ranges between 4 and 16. With a score of 8 or less, percutaneous balloon mitral valvuloplasty is likely to be successful. If the score is more than 8, surgery is recommended.

upon standard Frank-Starling mechanics as well the presence of LV ejection into the relatively low resistance/low afterload left atrium. Although net forward blood flow is reduced, this supranormal ejection serves to marginally unload the LV and normalize LVEDV. Wall stress resulting from increased LVEDV also leads to compensatory myocardial hypertrophy and restoration of normal wall tension, as per Laplace law.

While a hypertrophied and/or hyperdynamic LV is typical of acute or compensated chronic MR, the finding of diminished ejection fraction despite the afterload reduction associated with MR is suggestive of a decompensated state with rightward or downward shifts in Frank-Starling curve pressure-volume relationships (Fig. 61.12). In this setting, net forward flows continue to decrease and LVEDV increases. Consequent LA and LV dilatation lead to an increase in mitral orifice size. A self-perpetuating cycle of worsening heart failure with worsened MR eventually takes hold. LV failure may then lead to pulmonary hypertension and right-sided heart failure.

Diagnosis of Mitral Regurgitation

Symptoms and signs. Acute decompensated MR may cause the sudden onset of dyspnea secondary to pulmonary venous hypertension and congestion. An associated decrease in forward cardiac output may cause hypotension or even hemodynamic collapse. More typically, patients with chronic, mild MR may be asymptomatic for most of their lives. When MR more gradually becomes moderate to severe, typical symptoms of left heart failure, atrial fibrillation, or even right heart failure may become manifested.

Physical exam. Palpation of patients with MR may reveal a hyperdynamic, laterally displaced cardiac impulse. Auscultation typically reveals a holosystolic, high-pitched, blowing apical murmur that radiates to the axilla. Isolated posterior leaflet dysfunction may cause the murmur to radiate to the sternum or aortic area, while isolated anterior leaflet dysfunction may cause the murmur to radiate to the back or head. Other findings may include a diminished first heart sound, wide splitting of the second heart sound due to early aortic valve closure, or a third heart sound due to increased blood flow across the mitral valve.

Diagnostic Testing

Echocardiography is the mainstay of diagnosing and monitoring MR, although cardiac magnetic resonance imaging (MRI) can also provide useful regurgitant volume and cardiac function data. Routine chest radiography may demonstrate an enlarged cardiac silhouette and LA enlargement, or signs of pulmonary congestion associated with heart failure. Echocardiography may reveal atrial fibrillation and/or signs of LA enlargement (p mitrale), and QRS or ST-T interval changes reflective of ventricular hypertrophy and/or bundle branch conduction abnormalities.

Transthoracic and especially transesophageal echo studies allow precise visualization of the mechanisms responsible for inducing MR, including single or bileaflet prolapse and/or flail, enlarged or "billowing" leaflets, annular dilatation, chordal rupture, papillary muscle rupture, or restricted leaflet motion and tethering caused by an enlarged or infarcted ventricle. Leaflet disruption or perforation, valvular vegetations or annular abscesses secondary to infective endocarditis may also be visualized.

Doppler analysis provides important prognostic data on regurgitant jet localization and quantification, typically based upon flow dynamics related to the proximal isovolumetric surface area, which is seen on echo as a hemispheric area of flow convergence proximal to a regurgitant orifice (i.e., ventricular side of MR valves [Fig. 61.13]). Analysis of the radius and the MR flow velocity in this flow convergence area allows calculation of the regurgitant fraction, effective regurgitant orifice area, and regurgitant volume based on the equation: flow = velocity x area. The flow convergence area narrows just downstream to the orifice of a regurgitant valve into a waist of highest blood flow velocity as the regurgitant volume passes through the valve orifice, called the vena contracta, the width of which is also a marker of MR severity. Severe MR is thus now defined as an effective regurgitant orifice of at least 40 cm^2, a regurgitant volume of at least 60 mL, or a regurgitant fraction of at least 50% or a vena contracta larger than 7 mm or a central MR jet larger than 40% of the LA area or a holosystolic eccentric jet.[11]

Natural History

Acute MR is typically caused by chordal rupture due to degenerative disease, papillary muscle rupture due to myocardial infarction, or infective endocarditis causing leaflet perforation or chordal rupture. It is typically poorly tolerated and often requires urgent intervention. In the absence of intervention, severe pulmonary edema, cardiac decompensation, and/or the development of pulmonary hypertension often lead to rapid deterioration and poor outcomes.

The subacute/chronic asymptomatic MR patient was long thought to not pose an increased mortality risk, but a rich body of data developed over the past two decades now clearly demonstrate that even in the asymptomatic patient, the presence of severe MR with ventricular dysfunction, pulmonary hypertension, or atrial fibrillation carries a diminished prognosis.[10,19] Moderate primary MR has likewise now been shown to be associated with an annual

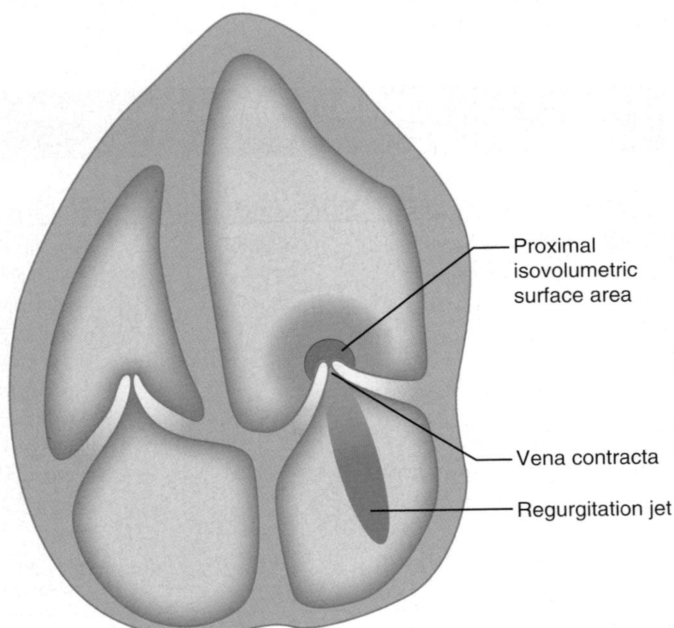

FIG. 61.13 Echocardiographic assessment of severity of mitral regurgitation. The proximal isovolumetric surface area (PISA) is seen on echo as a hemispheric area of flow convergence proximal to a regurgitant orifice; i.e., ventricular side of MR valves. Analysis of the radius and the MR flow velocity in this flow convergence area allows calculation of the regurgitant fraction, effective regurgitant orifice (ERO) area, and regurgitant volume based on the equation: flow = velocity x area. The flow convergence area narrows just downstream to the orifice of a regurgitant valve into a waist of highest blood flow velocity as the regurgitant volume passes through the valve orifice, called the vena contracta, the width of which is also a marker of MR severity.

mortality risk of 3%, representing excessive risk compared to results now achievable with mitral repair.[19]

Patients with functional ("secondary") MR, typically occurring on the basis of ischemic disease, carry a far worse prognosis than patients with primary MR.[19] Data from the STICH trial examining patients with ischemic heart disease and diminished ejection fraction (≤35%) demonstrated that mortality over approximately 4.5 years was about two-fold greater in patients with moderate to severe MR compared to those with mild or no MR.[20]

Treatment

Medical treatment. The medical management of acute MR involves afterload reduction with vasodilators. The resultant decrease in aortic pressure and afterload enhances forward cardiac output and decreases regurgitant flow into the LA. When vasodilator use is ineffective, or is limited by systemic hypotension, intraaortic balloon pump counterpulsation effectively lowers systolic afterload and increases forward flow. Prompt mitral valve surgery is typically needed in acute MR, particularly in the symptomatic or hemodynamically compromised patient, but intraaortic balloon pump can be used to temporize surgery and stabilize the patient.

In symptomatic patients with chronic MR, standard vasodilator and diuretic medical therapy can be useful in improving ventricular hemodynamics and reducing pulmonary congestion. Diuretics may be particularly effective in reducing volume overload and ventricular distension and thus annular orifice size and regurgitant MR fractions. Contrary to popular practice, however, there is no evidence to support the use of vasodilator or other afterload-reducing medications in order to attempt to delay the need for surgery in asymptomatic patients with chronic MR and normal LV systolic function.[11]

For patients with functional, secondary MR, medical therapy should specifically address underlying ventricular dysfunction. Treatment should include carefully titrated use of nitrates, diuretics, ACE inhibitors or angiotensin receptor antagonists, beta-blockers, and aldosterone antagonists in the presence of heart failure.[10,11,14]

Surgical treatment. Surgical indications for MR have broadened considerably as morbidity and mortality associated with surgery have decreased and the pathophysiology of this syndrome is better understood. Specifically, current understanding that the onset of ventricular dysfunction is associated with diminished prognosis and expectation for postoperative ventricular functional recovery has expanded indications to asymptomatic patients with severe MR regardless of LV function.

Surgery now carries a Class I indication for asymptomatic patients with chronic severe primary MR and evidence of LV dysfunction (LV ejection fraction [LVEF] 30%–60% or LV end-systolic diameter [LVESD] ≥40 mm) as well as symptomatic patients and an LVEF greater than 30% (Class IIb indication for LVEF <30%).[10,11] Further, because of the above considerations, Class IIa indications have now been added for asymptomatic patients with chronic primary severe MR *without* LV dysfunction LVEF (LVEF >60% and LVESD <40 mm) who exhibit a progressive increase in LV size or decrease in EF on serial imaging studies.[10]

Mitral repair now also carries a specific Class IIa indication for asymptomatic patients with preserved LV function (LVEF >60% and LVESD <40 mm) in whom a 95% chance of successful repair with <1% mortality is predicted, or in those with new onset atrial fibrillation or resting pulmonary hypertension (pulmonary artery systolic pressure >50 mm Hg).[10] Patients with chronic moderate or severe primary MR undergoing cardiac surgery for other indications also carry Class I and IIa indications, respectively (Table 61.5).[10,11]

TABLE 61.5 Indications for intervention for the treatment of valvular heart disease (excerpted).

VALVE LESION	PRESENTATION	PROCEDURE	INDICATION	CLASS OF INDICATION	LEVEL OF EVIDENCE
Mitral stenosis	Symptomatic	PBMC†	Severe MS (MVA ≤1.5 cm²)	I	A*
			Evidence of hemodynamically significant MS during exercise (despite MVA >1.5 cm²)	IIb	C
			Severe MS with suboptimal valve anatomy, but with NYHA Class II/IV symptoms and high risk for surgery	IIb*	C
		MVR‡	Severe MS (MVA 1.5 cm²) with NYHA class III/IV symptoms	I	B**
	Asymptomatic	PBMC*	Very severe MS (MVA ≤1.0 cm²)	IIa*	C
			Severe MS (MVA ≤1.5 cm²) and new onset of AF	IIb*	C
		MVR**	Severe MS with recurrent embolic events despite adequate anticoagulation^	IIb	C

MS, Mitral stenosis; *MVA*, mitral valve area; *MVR*, mitral valve surgery (repair or replacement); *NYHA*, New York Heart Association classification for heart failure symptom severity; *PBMC*, Percutaneous balloon mitral commissurotomy.

*In the ESC/EACTS guidelines,[14] PBMC is: Indicated for symptomatic patients without unfavorable characteristics – **Class I**, level of evidence **B**; Indicated in *any* symptomatic patients with contraindication or high risk for surgery – **Class I**, Level C; Considered in asymptomatic patients without unfavorable characteristics and with high thromboembolic risk (previous history of embolism, dense spontaneous contrast in the left atrium, recent or paroxysmal atrial fibrillation) or risk of hemodynamic decompensation (pulmonary hypertension, need for major noncardiac surgery, desire for pregnancy)– **Class IIa,** Level C

*In the ESC/EACTS guidelines, [14] MVR is indicated in symptomatic patients who are not suitable for PBMC (symptoms do not have to be severe) – **Class I**, Level C

†PBMC indicated if favorable valve morphology based on Wilkins score (Table 61.4) in the absence of contraindications

‡If appropriate risk and not candidates for PMBC due to valve morphology or clinical criteria (e.g., left atrial thrombus present)

^With excision of the left atrial appendage.

TABLE 61.5 Indications for intervention for the treatment of valvular heart disease (excerpted). (cont'd)

VALVE LESION	PRESENTATION	PROCEDURE	INDICATION	CLASS OF INDICATION	LEVEL OF EVIDENCE
Mitral regurgitation (primary)	Symptomatic	MV Surgery§	Severe MR and LVEF >30%	I	B
			Consider for severe MR and LVEF ≤30%	IIb	B
	Asymptomatic	MV Surgery	Severe primary MR and LV dysfunction (LVEF 30%–60% and/or LVESD ≥40 mm)**	v	B*
			Reasonable for severe MR and preserved LV function (LVEF ≥60% and LVESD <40 mm) but progressive increase in LV size or decrease in EF on serial imaging	IIa	C
		MV Repair	Severe primary MR which is: Limited to the posterior leaflet OR Involving the anterior leaflet or both leaflets, when a successful and durable repair can be accomplished	I	B
			Reasonable for severe primary MR with preserved LV function (LVEF ≥60% and LVESD <40 mm), in patients with a >95% likelihood of durable repair without residual MR and either: - An expected mortality rate of <1% when performed at a Heart Valve Center of Excellence OR - Nonrheumatic disease and 1) new onset of AF or 2) resting pulmonary hypertension (systolic pulmonary arterial pressure >50 mm Hg)	IIa	B
	+/- Symptoms	MV Surgery	Reasonable for moderate primary MR when undergoing cardiac surgery for other indication(s)	IIa	C
Mitral regurgitation (secondary)	Symptomatic	MV Surgery	Consider for severe secondary MR with NYHA class III/IV symptoms despite medical therapy	IIb	B
		MV Replacement	Reasonable to choose chordal-sparing valve replacement over downsized annuloplasty repair in severely symptomatic patients (NYHA class II/IV) with chronic ischemic MR and persistent symptoms despite medical therapy	IIa	B
	+/- Symptoms	MV Surgery	Reasonable for severe secondary MR when undergoing CABG or AVR	IIa**	C
		MV Repair	Uncertain benefit for patients with chronic, moderate secondary MR who are undergoing CABG	IIb***	B

AVR, Aortic valve replacement; *CABG*, coronary artery bypass grafting; *LVEF*, left ventricular ejection fraction; *LVESD*, left ventricular end-systolic diameter; *MR*, mitral regurgitation; *MV*, mitral valve; *NYHA*, New York Heart Association classification for heart failure symptom severity.
§Mitral valve repair is preferred over replacement for primary MR, when possible.
*In the ESC/EACTS guidelines,[14] surgery indicated in asymptomatic patients with left ventricular dysfunction (LVESD ≥45 mm and/or LVEF ≤60%). – **Class I** Level C.
In the ESC/EACTS guidelines,[14] surgery indicated in patients with severe MR undergoing CABG, and LVEF >30%. – **Class I, Level C.
***In the ESC/EACTS guidelines,[14] surgery considered in symptomatic patients with severe MR, LVEF <30%, option for revascularization, and evidence of viability. – **Class IIa,** Level C.

It has been traditional to defer surgical treatment of functional MR, especially in the setting of coronary artery bypass surgery (CABG), under the presumption that improvements in the ischemic milieu after CABG would lead to the resolution of functional MR. Data from recent studies suggest, however, that deferring intervention for moderate to severe MR leads to worse outcomes in the setting of concomitant CABG.[20] As such, surgery carries a Class IIa indication for patients with chronic severe secondary MR undergoing aortic valve replacement or CABG and a IIb indication for severely symptomatic (New York Heart Association [NYHA] class III/IV) patients with chronic severe secondary MR.[10,11]

Repair of the mitral valve is preferred over mitral valve replacement for patients with primary MR when technically feasible and indicated.[7,10,11] Successful mitral valve repair provides an improved quality of life, with less morbidity and improved long-term event-free survival when compared to mitral valve replacement in appropriately selected patients. Mitral repair is considered very durable, with reoperations rates less than 10% at 10 years when postoperative echocardiography demonstrates mild or absent MR.[21,22]

Repair can today be accomplished through a variety of techniques including anterior or posterior leaflet resection, chordae transfer, leaflet folding plasty, edge-to-edge leaflet sutures, creation of neochordae, and ring annuloplasty. Ring annuloplasty is now generally indicated with all mitral valve repairs as it has been clearly shown to improve the durability of repair.[22] Some debate continues, however, whether rings should be flexible or rigid, contoured or uniplanar, and completely or partially circumferential (open or closed).

TABLE 61.5 **Indications for intervention for the treatment of valvular heart disease (excerpted). (cont'd)**

VALVE LESION	PRESENTATION	PROCEDURE	INDICATION	CLASS OF INDICATION	LEVEL OF EVIDENCE
Aortic stenosis	Symptomatic	AVR (surgical or transcatheter)	Severe, high-gradient AS (symptoms by history or on exercise testing)	I	B
			Reasonable for severe, low-gradient AS, reduced LVEF (<50%), and dobutamine study with aortic velocity ≥4.0 m/s (or mean pressure gradient ≥40 mm Hg) and valve area ≤1.0 cm² at any dobutamine dose	IIa*	B*
			Reasonable for severe, low-gradient AS, preserved LVEF (≥50%), but valve obstruction the most likely cause of symptoms	IIa*	B*
	Asymptomatic	AVR	Severe AS and reduced LVEF (<50%)	I	B
			Reasonable for very severe AS (aortic velocity ≥5.0 m/s) with preserved LVEF (≥50%), but low surgical risk	IIa	B*
			Reasonable for severe AS with preserved LVEF (>50%), but decreased exercise tolerance or fall in blood pressure during exercise	IIa*	B*
			May be considered for severe AS with preserved LVEF (≥50%), but rapid disease progression and low surgical risk	IIb*	C
	+/- Symptoms	AVR	- Severe AS (with or without symptoms) and undergoing cardiac surgery for another indication	I	B*
			Reasonable for moderate AS and undergoing cardiac surgery for other indication(s)	IIa	B
Aortic insufficiency	Symptomatic	AVR	Symptomatic AI^ (regardless of LVEF)	I	B
	Asymptomatic	AVR	Severe chronic AI and reduced LVEF (<50%)	I	B
			Reasonable for severe AI with preserved LVEF (≥50%), but systolic dysfunction suggested by severe end-systolic LV dilation (LVESD >50 mm)	IIa	B**
			Consider for severe AI and preserved LVEF (≥50%), but progressive severe LV dilation (LVEDD >65 mm) and low surgical risk	IIb	C**
	+/- Symptoms	AVR	Severe AR while undergoing cardiac surgery for other indication(s)	I	C
			Reasonable for moderate AR while undergoing cardiac surgery for other indication(s)	IIa	C

From Nishimura RA, Otto CM, Bonow RO, et al. 2017 AHA/ACC Focused Update of the 2014 AHA/ACC Guideline for the Management of Patients With Valvular Heart Disease: A Report of the American College of Cardiology/American Heart Association Task Force on Clinical Practice Guidelines. *J Am Coll Cardiol*. 2017;70:252–289, and Nishimura RA, Otto CM, Bonow RO, et al. 2014 AHA/ACC Guideline for the Management of Patients With Valvular Heart Disease: executive summary: a report of the American College of Cardiology/American Heart Association Task Force on Practice Guidelines. *Circulation*. 2014;129:2440–2492.

AI, Aortic insufficiency; *AS*, aortic stenosis; *AVR*, aortic valve replacement (denotes surgical replacement unless specified); *LVEF*, left ventricular ejection fraction; *MV*, mitral valve.

*In the ESC/EACTS guidelines,[14] AVR is indicated for severe AS if undergoing CABG, surgery of the ascending aorta, or another valve. **Class I,** Level C; indicated in asymptomatic patients with severe AS and exercise testing with symptoms clearly related to aortic stenosis **Class I**, Level C; considered in abnormal exercise test showing fall in blood pressure below baseline. **Class IIa,** Level C; considered in symptomatic patients with severe AS and LV dysfunction without flow reserve. **Class IIb,** Level C.

In the ESC/EACTS guidelines,[14] AVR is considered for asymptomatic, severe AR with resting EF >50% but severe LV dilatation (LVESD >50 mm or LVEDD >70 mm) **Class IIa, Level B.

^By definition, symptomatic AI is categorized as severe.

The appropriate surgical intervention for patients with secondary MR is less clearly defined than for primary MR, with a growing understanding of the role of ventricular pathology in perpetuating ischemic MR undermining previous recommendations for using (exaggerated or undersized ring annuloplasty) mitral repair to correct this pathophysiology. Specifically, randomized controlled trial data from the Cardiothoracic Surgical Trials Network showed no difference in overall LV remodeling or survival for patients undergoing repair versus replacement, but a higher 2-year rate recurrence rate for moderate or severe MR with repair versus replacement (59% vs. 4%, $P < 0.001$).[23] Likewise, while the addition of MV repair to patients undergoing CABG with moderate ischemic MR did significantly decrease the incidence of residual moderate or severe residual MR versus the CABG-alone group (11% vs. 32%, $P < 0.001$), MV repair failed to improve mortality.[24] In the 2017 ACC/

AHA guidelines, chordal sparing mitral valve replacement was consequently given a IIa indication over downsized annuloplasty repair for severely symptomatic patients with chronic secondary MR, and the usefulness of repair downgraded to "uncertain" with a IIb recommendation for patients with moderate ischemic MR undergoing CABG.[10] A variety of new techniques, including papillary muscle "sling" procedures, are also consequently being tested to address primary subvalvular and ventricular pathology as the primary focus of secondary MR repair.[25]

AORTIC STENOSIS

The normal aortic valve orifice measures 3 to 5 cm^2. Aortic valve stenosis to less than half this size causes hemodynamic obstruction and a transvalvular pressure gradient as the primary pathophysiology of AS. This gradient induces compensatorily increased ventricular pressure generated through Frank Starling mechanisms and concentric LV hypertrophy via parallel replication of sarcomeres as a response to increased myocardial wall tension. Wall tension thereby normalizes according to the law of Laplace, and a compensated state preserving the systolic function of a hypertrophied but nondilated LV may persist for many years.

Two-thirds of patients who progress to severe AS develop myocardial ischemia as a result of the increased work and consequently elevated myocardial oxygen demands of the hypertrophied ventricle, which must generate increased ejection pressures over prolonged systolic intervals against the increased afterload of the narrowed aortic valve. Myocardial ischemia, particularly in the subendocardial region, is accentuated by the reduction of perfusion gradients during diastolic coronary flow intervals across the hypertrophied, hyperpressurized myocardial wall. Resultant cell death and myocardial fibrosis leading to cardiomyopathy may then exacerbate heart failure.

Myocardial hypertrophy can also precipitate ventricular diastolic dysfunction, which typically occurs prior to the onset of systolic dysfunction. Decreased ventricular compliance leads to increased left ventricular end-diastolic pressure (LVEDP), prolonged LV relaxation time, and shortened diastolic filling time. These increased pressures are transmitted back through the LA and pulmonary circulation, leading to pulmonary congestion. Pulmonary hypertension and right heart failure may develop in severe cases. Eventually, maximal ventricular hypertrophy is reached, and an adequate pressure gradient can no longer be achieved, resulting in inadequate cardiac outputs and overt, self-reinforcing systolic LV failure.

Increased LA pressure and consequent LA dilatation also increase the risk for atrial arrhythmias in patients with AS, albeit less commonly than in patients with mitral valve disease. The loss of normal atrial contraction severely compromises filling of the noncompliant ventricle, leading to a sometimes precipitous decrease in cardiac output. Reduced forward flow can further increase LVEDP and aggravate the symptoms of heart failure.

Presyncope and syncope are unusual sequelae of AS related to inadequate (cerebral) organ perfusion, typically caused by inadequate forward flow through the restrictive aortic valve. Symptoms are typically associated with periods of peripheral vasodilatation such as occurring during exercise or in changing from recumbent to standing positioning when increased cardiac output is required to maintain peripheral vascular filling.

Diagnosis of Aortic Stenosis

Symptoms and Signs

Patients with AS will typically remain asymptomatic for an extended time. The onset of symptoms occurs when the valve orifice area decreases to approximately 1 cm^2, which marks a critical point in the natural history of the disease. The classic symptoms of AS typically progress from the appearance of angina and (pre-) syncope to the occurrence of dyspnea associated with heart failure (pneumonic: "ASD"). Whereas angina is the presenting symptom of AS in 35% of patients, syncope is a relatively sporadic event that is the presenting symptom in 15% of patients. Although heart failure typically appears late in the course of AS, dyspnea or other heart failure symptoms are presenting signs in 50% of patients.

Physical Exam

The diagnosis of AS based upon physical findings is frequently made prior to the onset of symptoms. The typical finding of AS is a crescendo-decrescendo ejection murmur best heard along the left sternal border and that radiates to the upper right sternal border and carotid arteries. The apical impulse in AS is forceful and slightly enlarged. If heart failure develops, the apical impulse may become laterally displaced. The characteristic carotid upstroke of AS has a slow rate of rise and a reduced peak (*pulsus parvus et tardus*) and may have an associated thrill.

Diagnostic Testing

Nonspecific findings of AS on chest radiography include a boot-shaped heart typical of concentric hypertrophy of the left ventricle, calcification of the valvular cusps, and poststenotic dilatation of the aorta. Roentgenographic signs of heart failure may ensue. Electrocardiographic changes are similar to that seen for MR.

Echocardiography allows the precise assessment of aortic valve anatomy, calcification, and effective orifice size, measured by planimetry. Ventricular hypertrophy and function can also be assessed. As with MS, Doppler echo allows measurement of transvalvular pressure gradients and valve area as a derived function (e.g., severe AS: Doppler velocity >4 m/sec = mean aortic valve gradient >40 mm Hg = valve area <1.0 cm^2). Pressure gradients may be decreased in AS patients with low cardiac output, leading to miscalculated (falsely increased) aortic valve areas. Low-dose dobutamine may be used during echo to increase cardiac output and assess the true severity of the AS lesion in these patients.

Cardiac catheterization may occasionally be needed to measure pressure gradients in ambiguous cases. Simultaneous pressure readings can be obtained in such instances with one pressure measuring port in the body of the left ventricle and a second device in the proximal aorta. Valvular area may then be determined using the Gorlin formula. Catheterization may be needed to assess the presence of coronary artery disease, coexistent in up to 50% of AS patients.

Natural History

Calcific AS is a progressive disease marked by a long, asymptomatic latent period that may vary greatly between individuals. Patients with moderate AS can, however, be expected to undergo a 7-mm Hg increase in mean pressure gradient or a 0.1-cm^2 decrease in valve area annually. Conversely, only about 10% of patients with mild aortic valve sclerosis (aortic velocity <2.5 m/sec), progress to severe AS within 5 years.

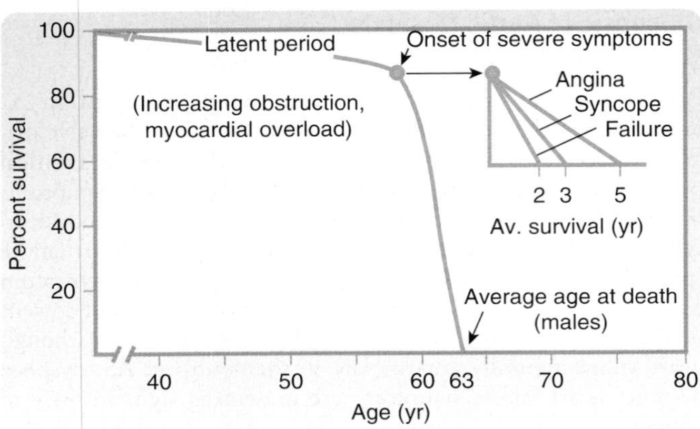

FIG. 61.14 Symptoms and survival in aortic valvular stenosis. Ross and Braunwald's classic 1968 report first described the onset of symptoms of heart failure, syncope, or angina in patients with aortic valvular stenosis as a marker of impending death. (From Ross J, Jr., Braunwald E. Aortic stenosis. *Circulation.* 1968;38:61–67.)

Ross and Braunwald's classic 1968 report first described the onset of symptoms as survival indicators in patients with AS (Fig. 61.14).[26] As reported in this study, and subsequently confirmed by others, mean survival after the appearance of angina is about five years, less than three years after the onset of syncope, and only one to two years once heart failure symptoms develop. Sudden death may also occur in symptomatic patients at a rate of 2% per month but appears to be rare (<1%/yr) in asymptomatic patients.[27]

Treatment

Medical management. Medical therapy is important in the treatment of early signs and symptoms of heart failure and other common comorbidities, such as hypertension. Treatment of hypertension may also serve to unload the AS ventricle, helping to relieve adverse ventricular remodeling. Although there are no medical therapies currently proven to alter the natural history of calcific AS, ongoing investigations are seeking to slow disease progression via an apparent endothelial injury/atherosclerosis AS pathway.

Surgical treatment

Because the natural history of untreated symptomatic AS is grave, mechanical relief of AS is recommended as a Class I indication in all symptomatic patients with evidence of severe AS (aortic velocity ≥4.0 m/sec or greater or mean pressure gradient ≥40 mm Hg; Table 61.5).[10,11] In addition to history-taking, exercise or dobutamine stress echo has now also been shown to be useful in eliciting symptoms and/or abnormal physiology (e.g., fall in systolic blood pressure or decreased exercise tolerance) as a Class IIa indicator for surgical intervention.[10,11]

Surgical intervention now also carries a Class I indication in the asymptomatic patient with severe AS and evidence of LV dysfunction (LVEF <50%). A Class IIa indication exists also for asymptomatic patients with very severe AS (aortic velocity ≥5.0 m/sec or greater or mean pressure gradient ≥60 mm Hg) who present low (≥4%) predicted surgical mortality risk, given that symptoms are expected to present in 50% of these patients within two years and evidence suggesting that overall mortality risk is reduced in these patients with early surgery.[10,11] Patients with at least moderate AS who are undergoing cardiac surgery for other reasons can be considered for aortic valve replacement as well. Likewise, because smaller patients, for example, may have relatively low transvalvular flows, symptomatic patients with aortic velocities less than 4 m/sec and an EF greater than 50% are Class IIa candidates when their indexed valve area is no more than 0.6 cm^2.[10,11]

Surgery for AS almost always requires valve replacement, either with a mechanical or tissue valve (see below) and is associated with excellent immediate and long-term outcomes (Table 61.6), especially when conducted before the onset of ventricular dysfunction. Aortic valve surgery improves symptoms, increases life expectancy, and often improves or normalizes systolic function, depending upon pathophysiologic status of the LV prior to surgery.[10,11,14]

Repair options for the treatment of AS are limited, and earlier efforts at valve debridement met with disastrous intermediate term outcomes with delayed onset of regurgitation, which led to the general abandonment of this technique. In comparison, percutaneous, catheter-based "transcatheter aortic valve replacement" (TAVR) is an increasingly prevalent alternative to surgical aortic valve replacement (SAVR), as discussed below.

Aortic Insufficiency

The aortic valve like the mitral valve is dependent on the coordinated function of a complex and dynamic anatomy to preserve its competency. This apparatus includes the aortic valve cusps, annulus, sinuses of Valsalva, and the sinotubular junction above the sinuses. AI may be induced by pathologic processes that may alter any one or more of these components and/or their anatomic relationships with each other.

Acute AI, usually the consequence of endocarditis or aortic dissection, produces sudden increases in LVEDV caused by acute regurgitant flow into a relatively small, nonadapted, noncompliant ventricle. Even greater increases in LVEDP result, and equalization of systemic and ventricular pressure may occur, which may temporarily curtail increased regurgitation. Transmission of increased LVEDP into the pulmonary circuit may, however, produce fulminant pulmonary edema, particularly in the setting of coexisting MR induced or exacerbated by sudden increases in LV dimensions. Consequent increased LV wall tension typically leads to myocardial ischemia, exacerbated if aortic dissection extends to the coronary ostia, and hemodynamic collapse and/or early, sudden death.

Chronic AI, like chronic MR, is an insidiously progressive process that triggers compensatory mechanisms including LV enlargement and hypertrophy that help maintain net forward stroke volume and decrease wall tension. At first, increases in LV filling caused by mild or moderate regurgitant flow lead to increases in LVEDV and improvement in LV contractility along the Frank Starling curve. Increases in afterload and wall stress caused by increases in LVEDV likewise lead to eccentric ventricular hypertrophy characterized by sarcomere replication in series and elongation of myofibers. This hypertrophy tends to preserve ventricular compliance and minimize increases in LVEDP, while still decreasing wall tension. Increases in heart rate and decreases in peripheral vascular resistance that reduce diastolic filling time and decrease afterload also act to decrease regurgitant flow. Because of these mechanisms, patients with chronic AI often consequently remain well compensated for many years.

Ultimately, the sum effect of myocardial hypertrophy and LV enlargement in AI patients is a dramatically enlarged heart known as *cor bovinum*, characterized by the largest EDV and mass of any form of heart disease. AI ventricles can ultimately weigh as much as three times normal and have a capacitance of over 200 mL (≈ 4X normal) to accommodate massive regurgitant volumes.

TABLE 61.6 Indications for surgical and transcatheter interventions for symptomatic aortic stenosis (excerpted).

PROCEDURE	INDICATIONS^	CLASS OF INDICATION	LEVEL OF EVIDENCE
SAVR	Symptomatic, severe AS with *low or intermediate* surgical risk	I*	B
TAVR	Indicated in symptomatic, severe AS and *prohibitive* surgical risk with a predicted post-TAVR survival >12 months	I	A
	Not indicated in patients with predicted survival <12 months or in whom comorbidities would preclude the expected benefit from correction of AS	III	B
	Reasonable alternative to surgical AVR for symptomatic, severe AS and *high* surgical risk	I	A
	Reasonable alternative to surgical AVR for symptomatic, severe AS and *intermediate* surgical risk, depending on patient-specific procedural risks, values, and preferences - Preferred in elderly patients suitable for transfemoral access°	IIa**	B
PBAV	Consider as a bridge to surgical AVR or TAVR for patients with severe AS who are severely symptomatic, require urgent noncardiac major surgery, or with hemodynamic instability	IIb	C

From Nishimura RA, Otto CM, Bonow RO, et al. 2017 AHA/ACC Focused Update of the 2014 AHA/ACC Guideline for the Management of Patients With Valvular Heart Disease: A Report of the American College of Cardiology/American Heart Association Task Force on Clinical Practice Guidelines. *J Am Coll Cardiol*. 2017;70:252–289 and Nishimura RA, Otto CM, Bonow RO, et al. 2014 AHA/ACC Guideline for the Management of Patients With Valvular Heart Disease: executive summary: a report of the American College of Cardiology/American Heart Association Task Force on Practice Guidelines. *Circulation*. 2014;129:2440–2492.

PBAV, Percutaneous balloon aortic valvuloplasty; *SAVR*, surgical aortic valve replacement; *TAVR*; transcatheter aortic valve replacement;

*In the ESC/EACTS Guidelines,[14] SAVR is recommended in patients at low surgical risk (STS or EuroSCORE II <4% and/or logistic EuroSCORE I <10% and no other risk factors not included in these scores, such as frailty, porcelain aorta, or sequelae of chest radiation).

**In the ESC/EACTS Guidelines,[14] patients with increased surgical risk (STS or EuroSCORE II ≥4% or logistic EuroSCORE I ≥10% and/or with other risk factors such as frailty, porcelain aorta, sequelae of chest radiation), the decision between SAVR and TAVR whould be made by a multidisciplinary Heart Team according to patient characteristics; with TAVR.

^TAVR is not indicated for asymptomatic aortic stenosis based on currently available evidence.

°Per the ESC/EACTS Guidelines.[14] Specific characteristics favoring either modality in intermediate risk patients are not delineated in AHA/ACC Guidelines.

Progressive changes in LV dynamics eventually exhaust preload reserve and overwhelm compensation mechanisms, and increased LVEDV and LVEDP lead to ventricular dilatation, increased wall tension, and increased myocardial oxygen demand. Decreased systemic diastolic pressure and increased intramyocardial wall tension decrease coronary perfusion gradients and further exacerbate myocardial ischemia. Ultimately, ischemia may lead to myocardial fibrosis and cardiomyopathy. When the ventricle can no longer maintain adequate forward flow, overt heart failure ensues.

Diagnosis and Treatment of Aortic Insufficiency

Symptoms and signs. Severe acute AI may be difficult to recognize clinically, although acute AI patients may present with dyspnea, hemodynamic instability or shock. Frequently, symptoms reflecting the underlying cause of the AI, such as fever from endocarditis or chest pain from aortic dissection, may mask AI symptoms and obscure a correct diagnosis. Chronic AI typically presents with heart failure symptomatology when decompensation develops, although severe chronic AI patients may also present with angina or palpitations during stress or exertion.

Physical exam. Acute AI may yield few if any diagnostic signs other than those of fulminant heart failure and/or hemodynamic collapse. In comparison, chronic AI typically offers many physical findings, primarily related to the increases in stroke volume and pulse pressure due to regurgitant flow back into the ventricle in AI patients. These signs include peripheral pulses that rise abruptly and rapid collapse (water-hammer pulse), a bounding carotid pulse (Corrigan pulse), head bobbing with each heartbeat (de Musset sign), pulsation of the uvula (Müller sign), a "pistol shot" auscultated with compression of the femoral artery (Traube sign), and capillary pulsations seen with fingernail compression using a glass slide (Quincke sign).

Cardiac exam typically reveals an apical impulse that is diffuse, hyperdynamic and displaced inferiorly and laterally. It may be associated with a systolic thrill at the base of the heart, suprasternal notch, and carotid arteries due to high stroke volume. Auscultation reveals a high frequency blowing, decrescendo diastolic murmur best heard with the diaphragm at the left sternal border with the patient sitting up, leaning forward and at end-exhalation. The murmur is increased by maneuvers such as squatting or hand-grip, which increase diastolic pressure. The examiner may appreciate a mid- and late-diastolic apical rumble (Austin-Flint murmur), which is thought to be secondary to vibration of the anterior mitral leaflet caused by a posteriorly directed AI jet. The second heart sound may be soft or absent, and a third heart sound may be present.

Diagnostic Testing

Chest radiography in patients with acute AI may reveal only pulmonary edema, and electrocardiography may reveal evidence of LV strain, but echo may be the only test useful in diagnosing this condition. With chronic AI, chest radiography typically shows a significantly enlarged cardiac silhouette. The ascending aorta may be enlarged if AI is due to an aortic aneurysm. Electrocardiography will typically show signs of increased LV mass, with left axis deviation and increased QRS amplitude with strain patterns and conduction abnormalities.

Echocardiography allows the comprehensive evaluation of aortic apparatus abnormalities, LV size and compliance, and the character and magnitude of the regurgitant jet. Severe AI, for example, may be diagnosed by a jet width ≥65% of the LV outflow tract) >0.6 cm vena contracta, regurgitant fraction ≥50% or an effective regurgitant orifice area ≥0.3 cm^2.[10,11]

Natural History

While acute AI may lead to the sudden onset of heart failure and/or hemodynamic collapse, patients with chronic AI typically enjoy years of asymptomatic, compensated LV function. The combined likelihood of onset of adverse events for such patients (LV dysfunction, onset of symptoms, or death) is less than 5% per year. Overall, the freedom from ventricular dysfunction or death in asymptomatic patients is about 75% at five years, but this incidence decreases to 60% at 10 years.[28,29] Further, once the end-systolic diameter of the left ventricle is greater than 50 mm, adverse event rates increase to about 20% per year.[11,14,29] Once symptoms develop in AI patients, mortality rates rise to over 10% per year.[10,11,29]

Treatment

Medical management. Medical therapy should be considered only as a temporizing measure for patients with acute severe AI and acute volume overload, hypotension, and/or pulmonary edema who will require emergent surgery. In this scenario, vasodilators and inotropes may be valuable in augmenting forward flow and reducing LVEDP. Beta blockers used for aortic dissection should be employed with great caution in other causes of acute AI because they block compensatory tachycardia and could cause a significant drop in blood pressure. Importantly, intraaortic balloon pump is contraindicated in AI because it will worsen regurgitation and forward output.

Patients with chronic severe AI may benefit from medical management with the primary goal of reducing systolic hypertension, therefore reducing wall stress and improving ventricular function. Vasodilating drugs may improve hemodynamic abnormalities and forward flow, but their effect in favorably prolonging the asymptomatic period in patients with chronic severe AI and normal ventricular function is uncertain.[10,11,14] Medical treatment of symptomatic patients with AI is appropriate only until surgical intervention can be undertaken.

Surgical Treatment

Urgent or emergent surgical intervention to repair or replace the aortic valve and address underlying pathologic mechanisms is nearly always indicated in patients with acute severe AI (e.g., for endocarditis, aortic dissection). Surgery is also indicated (Class I) for symptomatic patients with severe chronic AI (Table 61.5).[10,11] Importantly, based on improved current understandings of the natural history of chronic AI, aortic valve surgery is now also a Class I indication for asymptomatic chronic severe AI patients with LV systolic dysfunction (LVEF <50%), and a Class IIa and Class IIb indication, respectively, for asymptomatic severe AI with normal LV systolic function (LVEF ≥50%) but with severe LV dilation (LVESD >50 mm [indexed LVESD >25 mm/m^2]) or progressive severe LV dilation (LV end-diastolic diameter >65 mm).[10,11]

Valve replacement with mechanical or biologic prostheses has yielded excellent results in correcting isolated AI (Table 61.7); however, over the past two decades, increasing numbers of centers are employing repair strategies in selected patients, as described below.[30] For patients with aortic root disease, these procedures are typically combined with root repair or replacement and coronary reimplantation, as discussed elsewhere in this text.

In selected patients, the aortic valve may alternatively be replaced with a pulmonary autograft, with heterograft substitution of the native pulmonic valve (Ross procedure). Excellent results with this technically demanding procedure have been demonstrated in highly experienced centers, especially for younger (<30 year-old) patients in whom traditional valve replacement procedures carry high risks of valve-related complications over time.[11,14,30]

Tricuspid Regurgitation and Other Right-Sided Valve Disease

TR accounts for most right-sided valvular disease, of which secondary or functional TR is the most prevalent. Secondary TR is most often the result of left-sided valve disease and/or heart failure. Primary causes of TR include endocarditis, rheumatic valvular disease, carcinoid disease, and iatrogenic injuries including injuries resulting from pacemaker/defibrillator implantation. Unlike left-sided disease, altered RV mechanics and geometry associated with RV failure may cause irreversible dilatation of the saddle-shaped ellipsoid of a healthy tricuspid annulus into a more planar circular shape, leading to persistence of TR despite the correction of inciting hemodynamics. Increased central venous pressure resulting from tricuspid valve disease can lead to venous congestion, hepatic enlargement, ascites, and peripheral edema as well as right atrial enlargement and arrhythmias. Decreased RV output can lead to LV underfilling and inadequate left-sided output.

Diagnosis of Tricuspid Valve Disease

Symptoms and signs. Because patients with tricuspid disease almost invariably have coexisting left-sided valve disease, it is difficult to separate symptoms of tricuspid pathology from that of multivalvular disease, and tricuspid valve disease itself may frequently be asymptomatic. Dyspnea, fatigue, and exercise intolerance may; however, result as heart failure develops.

Physical exam. A holosystolic murmur that increases with inspiration (Carvallo sign) and that may be heard along the sternal border is typical of TR. With TS, an opening snap followed by a diastolic rumble may be heard at the right sternal border. The physical exam of patients with tricuspid valve disease may otherwise reveal only jugular venous distension with a prominent systolic "v" wave. With progressive central venous congestion, physical findings are often out of proportion to symptoms and may include pleural effusions, hepatic enlargement (pulsatile liver typical of TR), abdominal tenderness, ascites, and peripheral edema.

Diagnostic testing. Because of the overlay of concomitant left-sided disease, echocardiography is the sole reliable testing modality useful in assessing tricuspid disease, similar in application to that for assessing mitral disease. Estimation of pulmonary arterial systolic pressure based on the velocity of the TR jet measured by continuous-wave Doppler is a useful prognostic criterion. An annular diameter of greater than 40 mm defines significant tricuspid annular dilation, and is also an important consideration when selecting appropriate treatment of TR.[31]

Natural History

Decreased survival is associated with increasing TR severity, regardless of other indices of cardiac function.[31] Although patients who undergo surgical treatment of left-sided valve disease may experience improved or resolved functional TR, such improvement is highly unpredictable, and survival for patients with uncorrected

TABLE 61.7 Outcomes of surgery for valvular heart disease.

VALVE SURGERY	VALVE LESION	OPERATIVE MORTALITY	SURVIVAL AFTER SURGERY	FREEDOM FROM REOPERATION
Aortic valve replacement	Aortic stenosis	1%–3%[1]	85% at 10 years[2]	75% (lifetime; biologic) 97% (lifetime; mechanical)[3]
	Aortic insufficiency	1%–4%[1]	63% at 10 years[4]	75% (lifetime; biologic) 97% (lifetime; mechanical)[3]
Aortic valve repair	Aortic insufficiency	1%–4%[1]	95% at 13 years[4]	83%–93% at 8 years[5]
Mitral valve replacement	Mitral stenosis	3%–10%[1]	15%–62% at 5 years[15]	92% at 10 years[8]
	Primary MR	4%[7]	60% at 10 years[8]	92% at 10 years[8]
	Functional MR	3%–5%[10,13]	66% at 5 years[11]	70%–85% at 4 years[10]
Mitral valve repair	Primary MR	0%–1%[6]	87% at 10 years[8]	94% at 10 years[8]
	Functional MR	~5%[9]	50%–75% at 5 years[11,12]	63% at 10 years[13]
Percutaneous balloon mitral commissurotomy	Mitral stenosis	0.5%–2%[1]	80% at 9 years[14]	50% at 20 years*[15]
Open mitral commissurotomy	Mitral stenosis	<2%[14]	96% at 10 years[16]	98% at 9 years[13]

[1]Vahanian A, Alfieri O, Andreotti F, et al. Guidelines on the management of valvular heart disease (version 2012): the Joint Task Force on the Management of Valvular Heart Disease of the European Society of Cardiology (ESC) and the European Association for Cardio-Thoracic Surgery (EACTS). *Eur J Cardiothorac Surg.* 2012;42:S1–44.
[2]Kvidal P, Bergstrom R, Horte LG, et al. Observed and relative survival after aortic valve replacement. *J Am Coll Cardiol.* 2000;35:747–756.
[3]van Geldorp MW, Eric Jamieson WR, Kappetein AP, et al. Patient outcome after aortic valve replacement with a mechanical or biological prosthesis: weighing lifetime anticoagulant-related event risk against reoperation risk. *J Thorac Cardiovasc Surg.* 2009;137:881–886, 886e881–885.
[4]Chaliki HP, Mohty D, Avierinos JF, et al. Outcomes after aortic valve replacement in patients with severe aortic regurgitation and markedly reduced left ventricular function. *Circulation.* 2002;106:2687–2693.
[5]Talwar S, Saikrishna C, Saxena A, et al: Aortic valve repair for rheumatic aortic valve disease. *Ann Thorac Surg.* 2005;79:1921–1925.
[6]Donndorf P, Park H, Vollmar B, et al. Impact of closed minimal extracorporeal circulation on microvascular tissue perfusion during surgical aortic valve replacement: intravital imaging in a prospective randomized study. *Interact Cardiovasc Thorac Surg.* 2014;19:211–217.
[7]Gammie JS, Sheng S, Griffith BP, et al. Trends in mitral valve surgery in the United States: results from the Society of Thoracic Surgeons Adult Cardiac Surgery Database. *Ann Thorac Surg.* 2009;87:1431–1437; discussion 1437–1439.
[8]Gillinov AM, Blackstone EH, Nowicki ER, et al. Valve repair versus valve replacement for degenerative mitral valve disease. *J Thorac Cardiovasc Surg.* 2008;135:885–893, 893 e881–882.
[9]Braunberger E, Deloche A, Berrebi A, et al. Very long-term results (more than 20 years) of valve repair with carpentier's techniques in nonrheumatic mitral valve insufficiency. *Circulation.* 2001;104:I8–11.
[10]Lorusso R, Gelsomino S, Vizzardi E, et al. Mitral valve repair or replacement for ischemic mitral regurgitation? The Italian Study on the Treatment of Ischemic Mitral Regurgitation (ISTIMIR). *J Thorac Cardiovasc Surg.* 2013;145:128–139; discussion 137–128.
[11]Calafiore AM, Di Mauro M, Gallina S, et al. Mitral valve surgery for chronic ischemic mitral regurgitation. *Ann Thorac Surg.* 2004;77:1989–1997.
[12]Oliveira JM, Antunes MJ. Mitral valve repair: better than replacement. *Heart.* 2006;92:275–281.
[13]DiBardino DJ, ElBardissi AW, McClure RS, et al. Four decades of experience with mitral valve repair: analysis of differential indications, technical evolution, and long-term outcome. *J Thorac Cardiovasc Surg.* 2010;139:76–83; discussion 83–74.
[14]Song JK, Kim MJ, Yun SC, et al. Long-term outcomes of percutaneous mitral balloon valvuloplasty versus open cardiac surgery. *J Thorac Cardiovasc Surg.* 2010;139:103–110.
[15]Bouleti C, Iung B, Himbert D, et al. Reinterventions after percutaneous mitral commissurotomy during long-term follow-up, up to 20 years: the role of repeat percutaneous mitral commissurotomy. *Eur Heart J.* 2013;34:1923–1930.
[16]Antunes MJ, Vieira H, Ferrao de Oliveira J. Open mitral commissurotomy: the 'golden standard'. *J Heart Valve Dis.* 2000;9:472–477.

moderate to severe TR has been reported to be less than 50% at four years.[32] The natural history of other right-sided valve lesions is poorly documented since such lesions are uncommon in adulthood and typically require surgical correction as congenital anomalies, or are associated with rheumatic disease of the mitral and aortic valves.

Treatment

Medical management. The medical treatment of tricuspid valve disease involves optimization of RV preload and afterload, using diuretics and ACE inhibitors, respectively. If atrial fibrillation is present, rate control may optimize diastolic filling. With functional TR, medical treatment to reduce pulmonary hypertension may also improve cardiac output.

Surgical treatment. The timing and method of surgical treatment for functional TR are controversial. Until recent years, the notion that functional TR would improve after primary left-sided valve treatment led to recommendations of avoiding tricuspid surgery. This has, however, proven not to be a reliable strategy. Left uncorrected, secondary TR may worsen in about 25% of patients, which has functional and survival implications due to irreversible progression of RV damage and organ failure.[32] Further, while adding tricuspid repair during left-sided heart surgery does not significantly increase operative risk, reoperation due to persistent TR after left-sided heart surgery carries a perioperative mortality of 10% to 25%.

On the basis of these considerations, severe TR has emerged as a Class I indication for concomitant tricuspid valve surgery in patients who are undergoing left-heart surgery.[11,14] Concomitant repair is also probably indicated in those with mild or greater TR and either tricuspid annular dilation (>40 mm diameter) or evidence of right heart failure (Class IIa).[10,11,33] Additionally, patients with symptomatic severe primary TR unresponsive to medical therapy are candidates for tricuspid valve surgery (Class IIa), as are patients with moderate TR and pulmonary hypertension

(Class IIb), and asymptomatic or minimally symptomatic patients with evidence of progressive RV dysfunction (Class IIb).

Tricuspid valve repair is generally preferred to replacement whenever possible. For severe TR due to isolated annular dilation, annuloplasty using a prosthetic ring has been shown in several studies to have better long-term results than traditional suture annuloplasty.[10,11] Valve replacement should be considered for functional TR due to leaflet tethering and RV remodeling.

Symptomatic patients with isolated TS do not benefit from medical management and are best treated with valve replacement. Those with TS and left-sided valve disease should likewise undergo concomitant correction during the same operation.[10,11,14] Percutaneous tricuspid valvulotomy may be considered, but outcomes are less optimistic than those seen with MS and may induce significant TR.[34]

Mixed Valve Disease

Patients with mixed valve disease typically present with a predominant lesion that dictate symptoms and pathophysiology. There is very limited data on the natural history of mixed valve disease and therefore the optimal timing of serial evaluation is not clear. Patients with multivalvular disease likewise present even more complex diagnostic and therapeutic challenges than patients with single valve disease. The coexistence of aortic valve disease and MR, for example, will mitigate LV changes induced by aortic valve pathology, but worsen pulmonary and right sided complications.

Limited data are available to guide treatment in cases of multivalvular disease, and indications for interventions should be based on symptoms and objective analysis of surgical outcome rather than severity indices for the individual lesions.[14] In general, therapy should be targeted to the predominant lesion while considering the severity of concomitant valve disease.

OPERATIVE APPROACHES

Surgery for valvular heart disease is today associated with excellent short- and long-term outcomes, with some evidence suggesting even better outcomes for surgery performed at high volume centers.[35] Operative mortality, which in the modern era is generally <5% for all types of valve pathology, can now be predicted using several widely available multivariable risk calculation scoring systems, such as those provided by the Society of Thoracic Surgeons (STS) and the European Association for Cardiothoracic Surgery (EACTS).[10,11,14]

In general, operative mortality is predicted by risk factors such as age, female gender, emergency surgery, symptomology, concomitant procedures, decreased ejection fraction, and comorbidities such as diabetes mellitus, renal dysfunction, pulmonary disease, peripheral vascular disease, and prior operation (Table 61.8). Typically,

TABLE 61.8 European system for valvular surgery operative risk evaluation (EuroSCORE).

PATIENT-RELATED FACTORS	DEFINITION	SCORE
Age	Per 5 years or part thereof over 60 years	1
Sex	Female	1
Chronic pulmonary disease	Long-term bronchodilators/steroids	1
Extracardiac arteriopathy	Claudication, carotid occlusion or >50% stenosis, intervention on abdominal aorta, limb arteries, carotids	2
Neurologic dysfunction	Severely affecting ambulation or day-to-day functioning	2
Previous cardiac surgery	Requiring opening of the pericardium	3
Serum creatinine	>200 mmol/L preoperatively	2
Active endocarditis	Antibiotic treatment for endocarditis at the time of surgery	3
Critical preoperative state	Ventricular tachycardia, fibrillation, aborted sudden death; preoperative cardiac massage, ventilation, inotropic support, IABP, or acute renal failure (anuria or oliguria <10 mL/h)	3
Cardiac-Related Factors		
Unstable angina	Rest angina requiring intravenous nitrates preoperatively	2
LV dysfunction	Moderate or LVEF 30%–50%	1
	Poor or LVEF <30	3
Recent myocardial infarct	Within 90 days	2
Pulmonary hypertension	Systolic PA pressure >60 mm Hg	2
Operation-Related Factors		
Emergency	Carried out on referral prior to next working day	2
Other than isolated CABG	Major cardiac procedure other than or in addition to CABG	2
Surgery on thoracic aorta	For disorder of ascending, arch or descending aorta	3
Postinfarct septal rupture		4

Adapted from Roques F, Nashef SA, Michel P, et al. Risk factors and outcome in European cardiac surgery: analysis of the EuroSCORE multinational database of 19030 patients. *Eur J Cardiothorac Surg*. 1999;15:816–822.

isolated tricuspid surgery is associated with the highest operative mortality risk (primarily related to coexistent cardiac pathophysiology), followed by MR, and AI. Surgery for AS and MS offers the best operative mortality outcomes. Complications most frequently associated with surgery for valvular heart disease include infection, bleeding, stroke, conduction block (potentially requiring permanent pacemaker placement), and heart failure (Table 61.9).

Long-term outcomes and resolution of ventricular hemodynamic pathophysiology can generally be predicted by the duration and/or severity of symptoms associated with valvular disease, as well as the extent of ventricular dysfunction and/or the presence and severity of pulmonary hypertension.[11,14] Complete hemodynamic recovery from valvular disease, including resolution of ventricular hypertrophy and enlargement, may be seen as early as the first several weeks postop, but may progress for up to a year after surgery. Long-term complications frequently associated with valve surgery include thromboembolic events including stroke, reoperation for valve deterioration or perivalvular leaks, bleeding associated with anticoagulation, and endocarditis (Table 61.9).

Conduct of Heart Valve Surgery

The use of cardiopulmonary bypass and cardioplegic arrest of the heart are standard to performing open-heart procedures on the cardiac valves (although are not used for percutaneous interventions, as described below). A full midline median sternotomy has traditionally been the predominant means to obtain wide exposure for heart valve surgery. However, a variety of minimally invasive approaches are now also used and proven to be equally safe and effective to traditional open approaches. Specific minimally invasive approaches include partial upper or lower sternotomies, as well as small right third or fourth interspace thoracotomies, using either direct visualization with specialized instruments or indirect, robotic surgical techniques (Fig. 61.15). These approaches have been associated with decreased transfusion, wound infection, hospital stay, atrial fibrillation, and quicker recovery and improved cosmesis.

Mitral Valve Replacement and Repair

The mitral valve is typically exposed through a left atriotomy, made anterior to the pulmonary veins (Fig. 61.16). A right atriotomy and incision through the atrial septum also provides excellent exposure to the mitral valve. Even greater exposure can be provided by a "superior septal" approach joining the right atrial and septostomy incisions onto the dome of the left atrium, but this approach requires more extensive closure.

Mitral Valve Replacement

Minimal valve leaflet resection (typically of a portion of the anterior leaflet) is currently preferred for mitral valve replacement, making best efforts to preserve the chordae and subvalvular apparatus in continuity with the valve annulus. If the chordae or leaflets are severely calcified or fibrotic, resection may be required to facilitate implantation of an adequately sided valve prosthesis without perivalvular leak. After the resected valve orifice is sized (using a plastic avatar), the selected valve prosthesis is typically secured to the valve annulus using circumferentially-placed, nonabsorbable, braided pledgeted horizontal mattress sutures (Fig. 61.16B). The sutures are tied securely so there is no perivalvular defect, which would allow a regurgitant leak, and the atriotomy is closed after de-airing of the heart (Fig. 61.16C).

Mitral Valve Repair

A wide variety of surgical techniques may be employed to repair primary MR lesions. Most commonly, flail or prolapsing segments of the valve can be excised via limited triangular or more extensive quadrangular resections, and leaflet continuity restored by suturing the resected leaflet edges back together (Fig 61.17A). Relaxing incisions along the posterior leaflet base facilitate a sliding annuloplasty, which may be used to reduce tension on the repair and to decrease the height of the posterior leaflet. This helps prevent postresection MR resulting from systolic anterior motion (SAM) of the anterior mitral leaflet, which may become displaced towards the aortic outflow tract after inadequate resections.

Another option for mitral repair is the creation of neochordae, which can be created or preselected using Gore-Tex suture and should be sized to the height of the annulus. The neochordae are attached to the papillary muscle and the free edge of the leaflet to provide appropriate leaflet support and prevent leaflet prolapse.

A ring annuloplasty should be performed with all mitral valve leaflet repairs as this maneuver has been shown to significantly improve the durability of repair and can be used as a stand-alone procedure to address MR arising from a dilated annulus (Fig. 61.17B). Insertion of an annuloplasty ring helps restore normal annular geometry and ensure an appropriate coaptation zone of 6 to 8 mm between anterior and posterior leaflets. Numerous device options are available for annuloplasty, including rigid or flexible and partial or complete rings, and specially configured "3D" rings have also been developed to correct the apical and lateral displacement of the posterior valve leaflet associated with functional MR, as have subvalvular procedures seeking to realign the papillary muscles.[25] Data is indefinite on which of these ring types provides the best outcomes.

TABLE 61.9 Complications associated with valvular heart surgery.

OUTCOME	AVR	MVR
Prolonged ventilation	7%	10.8%
Renal failure	3.7%	5.2%
Reoperation for bleeding	4.1%	4.7%
Permanent stroke	1.6%	2.2%
Deep sternal infection	0.5%	0.3%
Postoperative hospital stay*	8.5 ± 8.4	9.9 ± 10.3
Overall hospital stay*	10.6 ± 9.6	12.8 ± 12.6

Adapted from Edwards FH, Peterson ED, Coombs LP, et al. Prediction of operative mortality after valve replacement surgery. *J Am Coll Cardiol.* 2001;37:885–892.

AVR, aortic valve replacement; *MVR,* mitral valve replacement.

Interpretation: Low risk 0–2; Medium risk 3–5; High risk 6 or more. *CABG,* coronary artery bypass graft surgery; *IV,* intravenous; *IABP,* intraaortic balloon counterpulsation; *LV,* left ventricular; *LVEF,* left ventricular ejection fraction; *PA,* pulmonary artery.

*Mean days ± standard deviation.

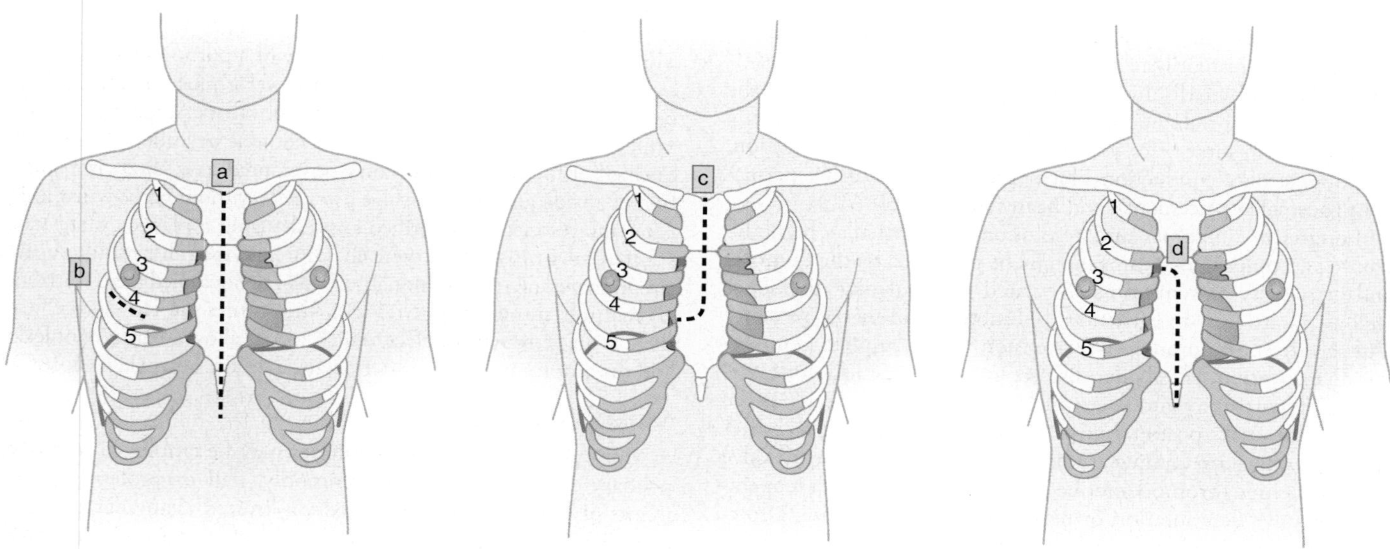

FIG. 61.15 Surgical access for valvular heart surgery. Median sternotomy *(a)* versus minimally invasive access via minithoracotomy *(b)*, partial upper *(c)* or lower *(d)* sternotomy. (From Byrne JG, Leacche M, Vaughan DE, et al. Hybrid cardiovascular procedures. *JACC Cardiovasc Interv.* 2008;1:459–468.)

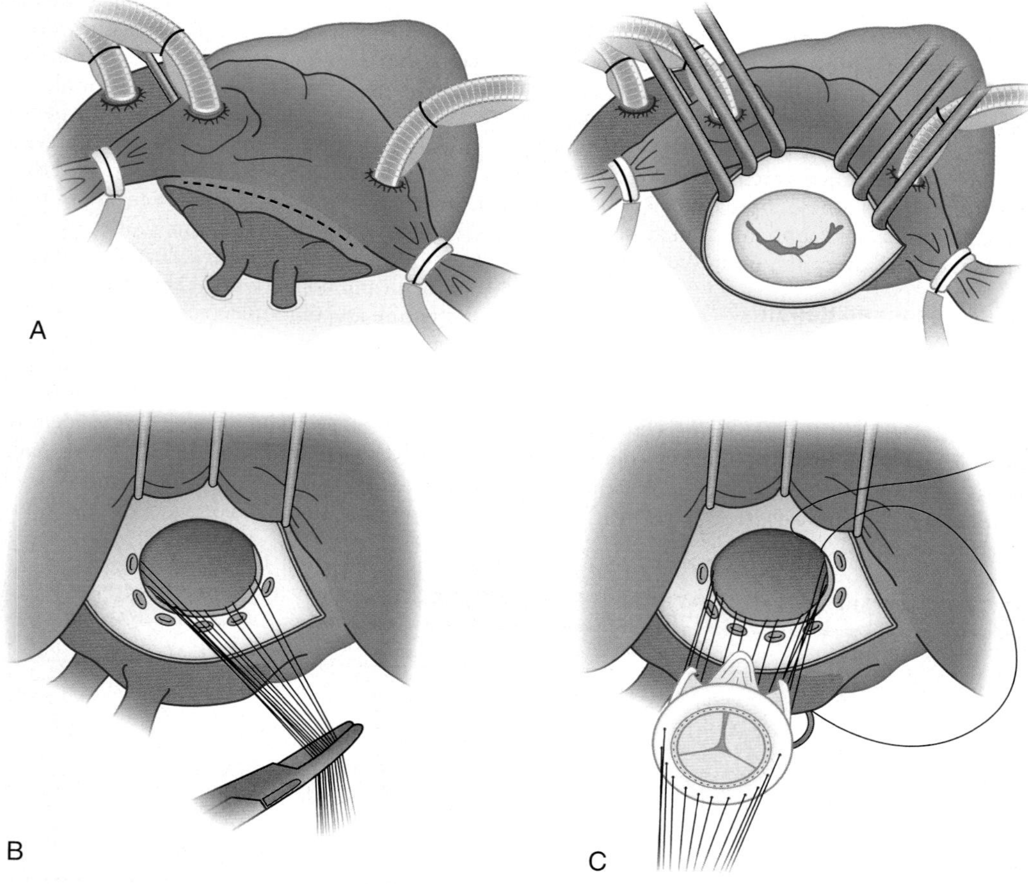

FIG. 61.16 Mitral valve replacement surgery. (A) The mitral valve is typically exposed through a left lateral atriotomy made just anterior to the pulmonary veins. (B) After partial excision of the native valve, pledgeted horizontal mattress sutures are placed circumferentially into the valve annulus and then into the cloth sewing ring of the prosthesis. (C) Valve lowered into position and sutures securely tied. (From Glower DD. Surgical approaches to mitral regurgitation. *J Am Coll Cardiol.* 2012;60:1315–1322.)

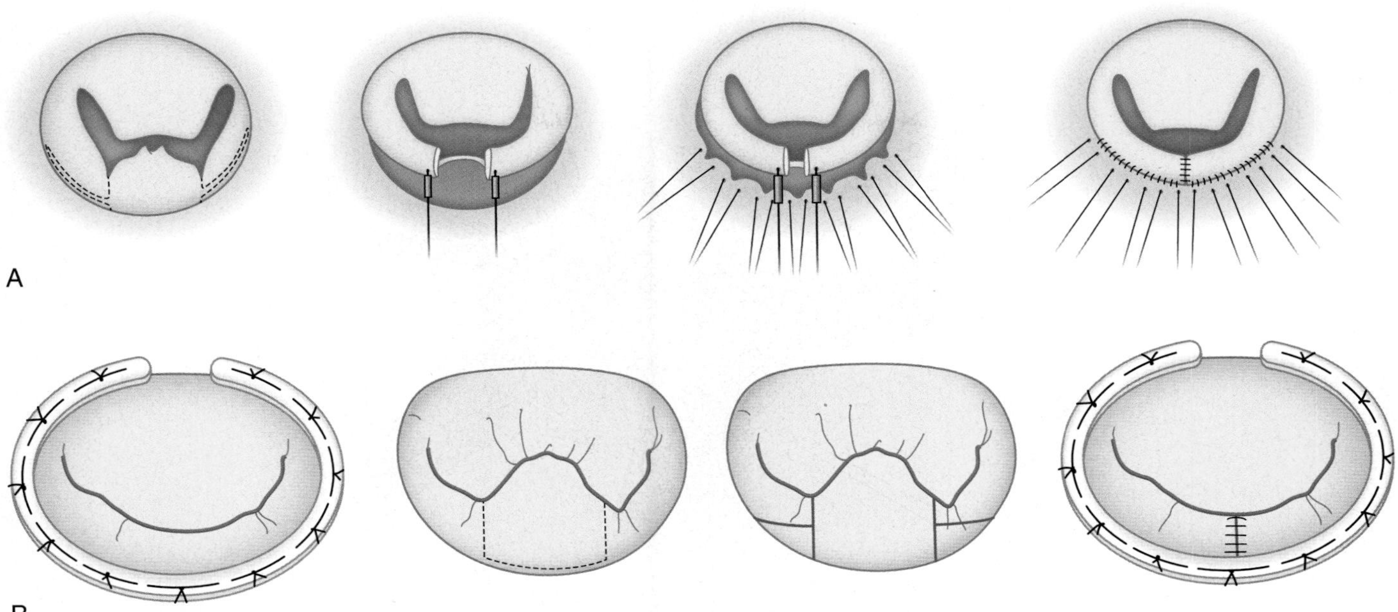

FIG. 61.17 Mitral valve repair surgery. (A) Resection of leaflet tissue incorporating triangular or quadrangluar resection, most commonly, flail or prolapsing (typically posterior [P2]) segments of the valve. Leaflet continuity is restored simply by suturing the resected leaflet edges back together. (B) Annuloplasty ring. An annuloplasty ring is almost always implanted to supplement resectional repairs or may be used alone to address MR arising from a dilated annulus. Circumferentially placed simple, nonpledgeted sutures are typically used to implant annuloplasty rings in a manner similar to valve implantation.

Surgical Aortic Valve Replacement and Aortic Valve Repair

Exposure of the aortic valve is typically obtained via a transverse or "hockey stick" incision of the proximal ascending aorta (Fig. 61.18A). For valve replacement, the native aortic valve cusps are carefully excised to avoid perforation of the aortic wall and a thorough decalcification of residual annular tissue is performed to improve prosthetic valve fit. Implantation of mechanical or bioprosthetic valves is similar to that described for the mitral valve (Fig. 61.18B). Homografts or "free style" stentless aortic valve homografts may sometimes be used, if aortic root replacement is concomitantly required.[36]

Aortic valve repair may be an option for selected patients with aortic insufficiency or a normally functioning aortic valve associated with an aortic root or ascending aortic aneurysm. When aortic insufficiency is secondary to dilation of the aortic root or ascending aorta, valve sparing operations which remodel the sinotubular junction can be very effective. Valve-sparing root replacement, commonly known as the "David" procedure after Dr. Tirone David, the pioneer of this operation, is a complex but highly successful procedure involving reimplantation of the native valve inside a Dacron graft.[30,37,38]

Prosthetic valves

Prosthetic heart valves used currently are typically made from a synthetic material (mechanical valves; Fig. 61.19A), allogeneic biologic tissue (bioprosthetic valves; Fig. 61.19B), or (cadaveric) homografts. Each have distinct advantages and disadvantages. Anticoagulation with a vitamin-K antagonist (warfarin) and monitoring of the international normalized ratio (INR) is recommended in nearly all patients with mechanical prosthetic valves, and typically for the first three months following bioprosthetic mitral implants (Table 61.10).[10,11] Aspirin may be added to warfarin therapy to reduce rates of major embolism, stroke, and overall mortality.

The current generation of mechanical valves, nearly all bileaflet pyrolitic carbon in design, can be expected to provide an extremely low incidence of structural deterioration, but a 0.6% to 2.3% per patient-year incidence of thromboembolic complications, even utilizing warfarin anticoagulation.[10,11,39] The need for anticoagulation with warfarin in turn is associated with approximately a 1% annual risk of bleeding complications. Both bleeding and thromboembolic complications may be reduced through more frequent (e.g., weekly) INR surveillance and/or home testing.[40]

Bioprosthetic valves are almost universally fabricated from preserved (bovine) pericardium or from porcine valves specially harvested for this use. Modern antimineralization and tissue preservation techniques involving treatment of valves with alpha-oleic acid (AOA) reduces cusp calcification and typically provide ~ 90% freedom from structural valve deterioration and reoperation at 10 years in patients over 65 years of age.[41] Failure rates may be higher in younger patients as a result of greater hemodynamic stresses and/or metabolic (calcium turnover) rates.

Based upon the above considerations, some surgeons now recommend implantation of bioprosthetic valves in patients less than the recommended Class IIa cutoff recommendation of 50 to 70 years of age, accepting the risk of reintervention by open or percutaneous technique as being less than the lifelong risk of anticoagulation/mechanical valve thromboembolism. The decision for a mechanical versus a bioprosthetic valve is complex; however, and must take into account many variables, including patient age, likelihood for pregnancy, and indications or contraindications to anticoagulation. In contrast to more the complex xenograft stentless aortic bioprosthetic roots and homografts implants, technical considerations in prosthetic valve implantation are generally considered similar between valve types.

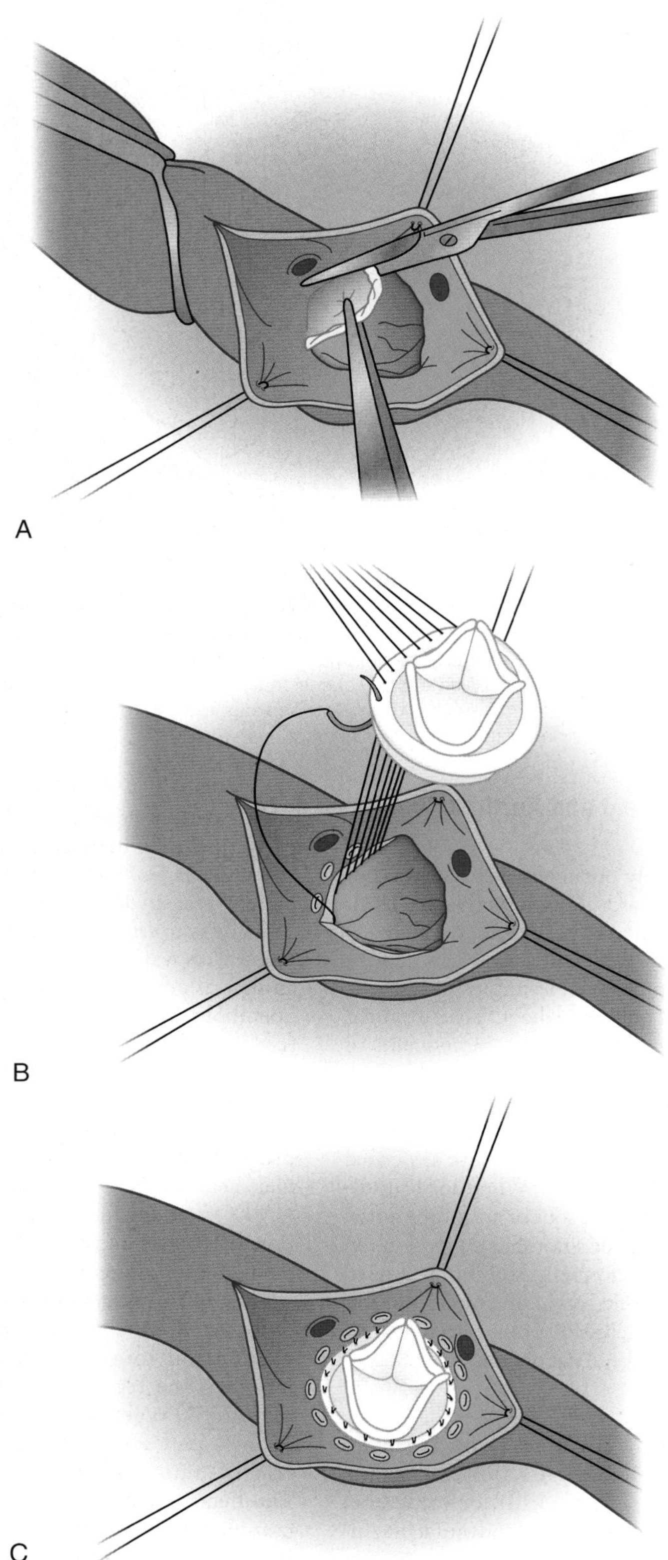

FIG. 61.18 Aortic valve replacement surgery. Exposure of the aortic valve is typically obtained via a transverse or "hockey stick" incision of the proximal ascending aorta. After aortic valve excision (A), implantation is conducted as for mitral valve replacement (B,C).

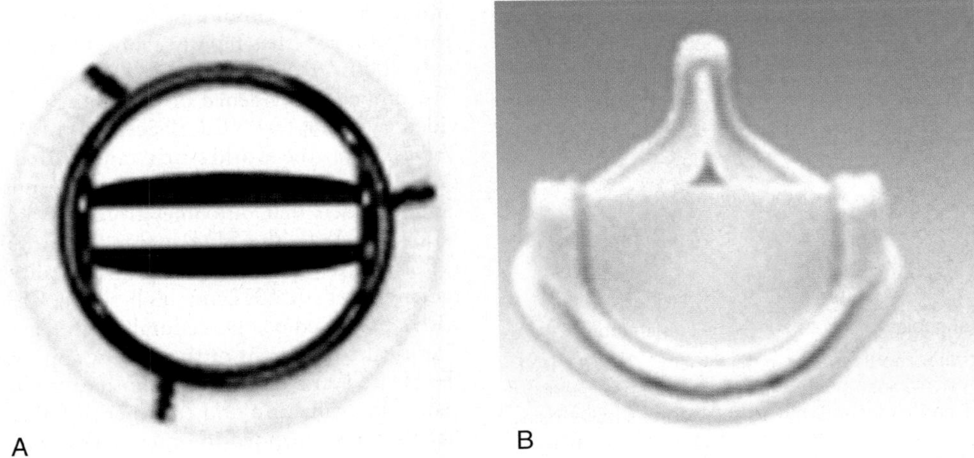

FIG. 61.19 Prosthetic valves. Prosthetic heart valves most often implanted are made from (A) synthetic material such as pyrolitic carbon (mechanical valve) or (B) allogeneic biologic tissue such as bovine pericardium (bioprosthetic valve). (From Pibarot P, Dumesnil JG. Prosthetic heart valves: selection of the optimal prosthesis and long-term management. *Circulation.* 2009;119:1034–1048.)

TABLE 61.10 Anticoagulation recommendation with prosthetic valves.

VALVE TYPE	ANTICOAGULATION RECOMMENDATION		DURATION	INDICATION CLASS
Mechanical	Aspirin*	Warfarin (INR goal)		
MVR	+	(3.0)	Long-term	I
AVR (+ risk factors)†	+	(3.0)	Long-term	I
AVR (- risk factors)†	+	(2.5)	Long-term	I
Bioprosthetic				
AVR/MVR		(2.5)	3–6 Months	IIa
AVR/MVR	+	-	Long-term	IIa
TAVR		2.5	3 Months	IIb
TAVR	+‡		6 Months	IIb

From Nishimura RA, Otto CM, Bonow RO, et al. 2017 AHA/ACC Focused Update of the 2014 AHA/ACC Guideline for the Management of Patients With Valvular Heart Disease: A Report of the American College of Cardiology/American Heart Association Task Force on Clinical Practice Guidelines. *J Am Coll Cardiol.* 2017;70:252–289 and Nishimura RA, Otto CM, Bonow RO, et al. 2014 AHA/ACC Guideline for the Management of Patients With Valvular Heart Disease: executive summary: a report of the American College of Cardiology/American Heart Association Task Force on Practice Guidelines. *Circulation.* 2014;129:2440–2492.

AVR, Aortic valve replacement; *MVR,* mitral valve replacement; *TAVR,* transcatheter aortic valve replacement.

*Risk factors: atrial fibrillation, previous thromboembolism, LV dysfunction, hypercoagulable condition, older-generation valve.

†Recommended aspirin dose 75–100 mg daily.

‡For TAVR, aspirin plus clopidogrel 75 mg daily.

Excellent early and long-term survival outcomes can be expected following valve implantation (Tables 61.7 and 61.9).[10,11] One of the most frequent and dangerous complications of valve implantation is prosthetic valve endocarditis (PVE), which is 50 times more likely to occur compared in implant patients than in the general population. PVE typically requires prosthetic valve excision and rereplacement, especially when PVE is caused by virulent organisms such as *Staph Aureus* or fungi, although antibiotic therapy alone may occasionally be used to sterilize lesions in high risk individuals.[10,11] Even with appropriate antibiotic therapy and surgical intervention, PVE carries a mortality rate up to 40% at 1-year. Accordingly, practitioners and patients with prosthetic valves like individuals at increased risk for native valve endocarditis should be well versed and strictly adhere to recommendations for antibiotic prophylaxis against endocarditis.[10,11]

Another potential complication of valve implantation is patient-prosthesis mismatch, arising from an undersized (aortic) prosthetic effective orifice area compared to patient body surface area. Inadequate prosthetic valve effective orifice area can lead to residual transvalvular gradients, resulting in persistent ventricular hypertrophy, impaired ventricular remodeling, and excessive late cardiac events. Patient-prosthesis mismatch is unusual with the excellent hemodynamic performance of current valves, and root enlargement can be performed to accommodate a sufficiently sized prosthesis.

Transcatheter Aortic Valve Replacement and Other Emerging Technologies

TAVR describes a procedure coupling balloon aortic valvuloplasty, which of itself does not provide long-term relief of AS, with implantation of an expandable bioprosthesis delivered and expanded

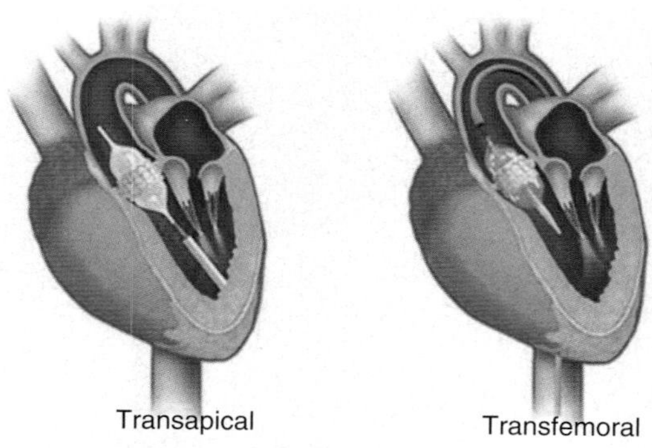

FIG. 61.20 Transcatheter aortic valve replacement *(TAVR)*. TAVR couples balloon aortic valvuloplasty with implantation of an expandable bioprosthesis delivered and expanded into to the aortic annulus using catheter technology. (From http://www.heart-valve-surgery.com/heart-surgery-blog/2013/09/18/tavr-transfemoral-transapical-approaches/ Accessed August 11, 2020.)

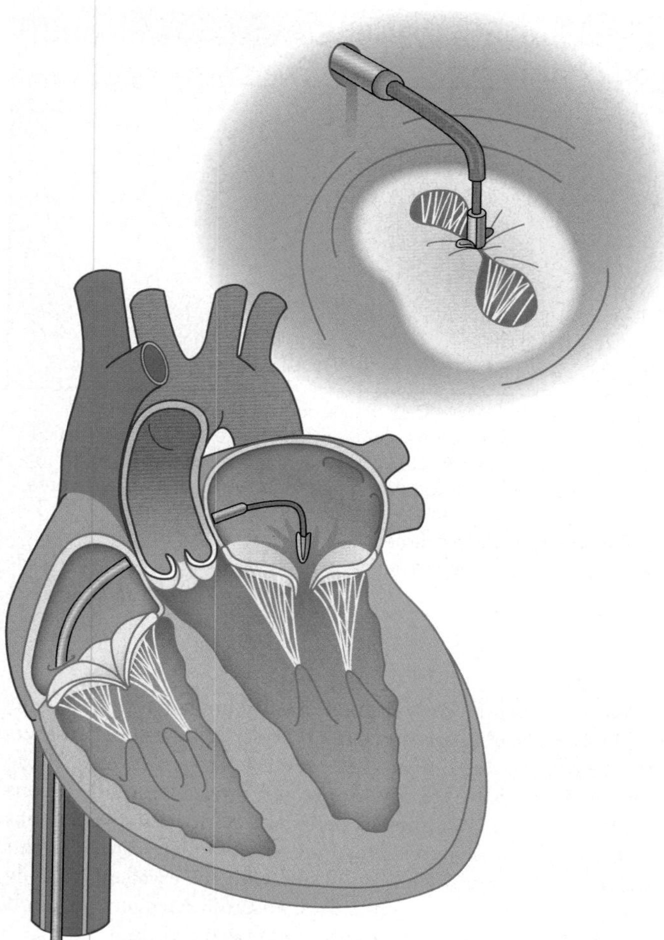

FIG. 61.21 Percutaneous mitral valve repair. Using a catheter-based clip delivery system, the operator grasps the mitral valve leaflet edges and places a clip that emulates the edge-to-edge leaflet repair. (MitraClip is a trademark of Abbott or its related companies. Reproduced with permission of Abbott, © 2020. All rights reserved.)

into to the aortic annulus using catheter technology (Fig. 61.20). This technology has rapidly evolved since its introduction in the early 2000s.[42,43]

Compelling evidence of the efficacy of TAVR was first provided by the PARTNER (Placement of AoRtic TraNscathetER Valves) trial, the world's first randomized study of this procedure.[44–46] Based on PARTNER and subsequent trials which demonstrated that outcomes from TAVR were at least noninferior to SAVR, the FDA granted approval for TAVR in 2011 for prohibitive risk (>50% 1-year mortality or major morbidity) patients, and in 2012 for high-risk (>10% mortality) patients with a predicted postprocedural survival greater than 12 months. A critical component of these FDA approvals was the advent of the Heart Team, consisting of both cardiologists and cardiac surgeons, in evaluation and treatment of TAVR patients – a practice that has expanded to other cardiac surgery decision-making processes.[10,11]

Expansion of indication to lower risk patients is expected given results of the more recently completed PARTNER IIA and other trials using self-expanding balloons (SurTAVI), in which TAVR was noninferior to SAVR for intermediate risk (STS score ≥4%) symptomatic patients with severe AS.[47,48] Improved overall outcomes, stroke rates, and vascular complication rates in these second-generation trials have been generated through innovation of smaller caliber valves and catheters, and improved patient selection and deployment strategies (including rapid placing during deployment to minimize prosthesis displacement).[47,48]

Despite these encouraging data, surgical aortic valve replacement still remains the gold standard for low- and intermediate-risk patients, especially since long-term (>5 year) durability data are not yet available. Complications such as complete heart block and paravalvular regurgitation still also remain higher after TAVR than SAVR, and these complications have been linked to higher long-term mortality.[44–48] Other unanticipated complications also remain a concern, including the recent finding of increased valve thrombosis rates in TAVR versus SAVR valves, with up to 18% of patients with a thrombus formation developed clinically overt obstructive valve thrombosis.[49]

Percutaneous Mitral Interventions

Percutaneous therapies for mitral valve disease lag behind TAVR, in part because of the greater difficulty in accessing the mitral valve as opposed to the aortic annulus, as well as the lack of a secure landing zone for a transcatheter mitral valve.

The MitraClip System, clinically introduced in 2003, has seen the greatest advancement of all percutaneous mitral valve therapies, receiving FDA approval for high risk patients in 2013.[50] Using a catheter-based clip delivery system, this device emulates the edge-to-edge "Alfieri" leaflet repair (Fig. 61.21). Although the reduction of severe MR is less effective than surgical therapy, this technology is potentially attractive for nonsurgical candidates.[50]

Other experimental mitral valve therapies include "indirect annuloplasty" strategies using compression devices placed inside the coronary sinus designed to apply radial forces as an annuloplasty strategy, although results have been inconsistent. Sutureless valves developed based upon TAVR technology that are placed under direct vision surgically or more recently via experimental percutaneous approaches are also being tested.[51–53]

SELECTED REFERENCES

Carpentier A. Cardiac valve surgery--the "French correction". *J Thorac Cardiovasc Surg.* 1983;86:323–337.

This work by Alain Carpentier for the first time described a comprehensive strategy for repairing regurgitant lesions of the mitral valve. It remains a relevant classic today.

David TE, Feindel CM. An aortic valve-sparing operation for patients with aortic incompetence and aneurysm of the ascending aorta. *J Thorac Cardiovasc Surg.* 1992;103:617–621.

David and Feindel report their initial cohort of patients treated with a novel technique for aortic valve-sparing root replacement. This technique is used around the world today to preserve the native aortic valve.

Leon MB, Smith CR, Mack M, et al. Transcatheter aortic-valve implantation for aortic stenosis in patients who cannot undergo surgery. *N Engl J Med.* 2010;363:1597–1607.

This is the original prospective randomized study report from the PARTNER investigators demonstrating the feasibility of percutaneous aortic valve replacement.

Nishimura RA, Otto CM, Bonow RO, et al. 2014 AHA/ACC Guideline for the Management of Patients With Valvular Heart Disease: executive summary: a report of the American College of Cardiology/American Heart Association Task Force on Practice Guidelines. *Circulation.* 2014;129:2440–2492.

These are the most recent comprehensive American College of Cardiology/American Heart Association Task Force guidelines for diagnosis and treatment of valvular heart disease (The 2017 update provides some revision of these recommendations).

Ross Jr J, Braunwald E. Aortic stenosis. *Circulation.* 1968;38:61–67.

This article first describes the onset of symptoms of heart failure, syncope, or angina in patients with aortic stenosis as survival indicators.

REFERENCES

1. Nkomo VT, Gardin JM, Skelton TN, et al. Burden of valvular heart diseases: a population-based study. *Lancet.* 2006;368:1005–1011.
2. Marijon E, Mirabel M, Celermajer DS, et al. Rheumatic heart disease. *Lancet.* 2012;379:953–964.
3. Seckeler MD, Hoke TR. The worldwide epidemiology of acute rheumatic fever and rheumatic heart disease. *Clin Epidemiol.* 2011;3:67–84.
4. Stewart BF, Siscovick D, Lind BK, et al. Clinical factors associated with calcific aortic valve disease. Cardiovascular Health Study. *J Am Coll Cardiol.* 1997;29:630–634.
5. Roberts WC, Ko JM. Frequency by decades of unicuspid, bicuspid, and tricuspid aortic valves in adults having isolated aortic valve replacement for aortic stenosis, with or without associated aortic regurgitation. *Circulation.* 2005;111:920–925.
6. Rajamannan NM, Evans FJ, Aikawa E, et al. Calcific aortic valve disease: not simply a degenerative process: a review and agenda for research from the National Heart and Lung and Blood Institute Aortic Stenosis Working Group. Executive summary: Calcific aortic valve disease-2011 update. *Circulation.* 2011;124:1783–1791.
7. Carpentier A. Cardiac valve surgery--the "French correction". *J Thorac Cardiovasc Surg.* 1983;86:323–337.
8. Barlow JB, Pocock WA, Marchand P, et al. The significance of late systolic murmurs. *Am Heart J.* 1963;66:443–452.
9. Anyanwu AC, Adams DH. Etiologic classification of degenerative mitral valve disease: Barlow's disease and fibroelastic deficiency. *Semin Thorac Cardiovasc Surg.* 2007;19:90–96.
10. Nishimura RA, Otto CM, Bonow RO, et al. 2017 AHA/ACC Focused Update of the 2014 AHA/ACC Guideline for the Management of Patients With Valvular Heart Disease: A Report of the American College of Cardiology/American Heart Association Task Force on Clinical Practice Guidelines. *J Am Coll Cardiol.* 2017;70:252–289.
11. Nishimura RA, Otto CM, Bonow RO, et al. 2014 AHA/ACC Guideline for the Management of Patients With Valvular Heart Disease: executive summary: a report of the American College of Cardiology/American Heart Association Task Force on Practice Guidelines. *Circulation.* 2014;129:2440–2492.
12. Pisters R, Lane DA, Nieuwlaat R, et al. A novel user-friendly score (HAS-BLED) to assess 1-year risk of major bleeding in patients with atrial fibrillation: the Euro Heart Survey. *Chest.* 2010;138:1093–1100.
13. Olesen KH. The natural history of 271 patients with mitral stenosis under medical treatment. *Br Heart J.* 1962;24:349–357.
14. Baumgartner H, Falk V, Bax JJ, et al. 2017 ESC/EACTS Guidelines for the management of valvular heart disease. *Eur Heart J.* 2017;38:2739–2791.
15. Bouleti C, Iung B, Himbert D, et al. Reinterventions after percutaneous mitral commissurotomy during long-term follow-up, up to 20 years: the role of repeat percutaneous mitral commissurotomy. *Eur Heart J.* 2013;34:1923–1930.
16. Song JK, Kim MJ, Yun SC, et al. Long-term outcomes of percutaneous mitral balloon valvuloplasty versus open cardiac surgery. *J Thorac Cardiovasc Surg.* 2010;139:103–110.
17. Antunes MJ, Vieira H, Ferrao de Oliveira J. Open mitral commissurotomy: the 'golden standard'. *J Heart Valve Dis.* 2000;9:472–477.
18. Sa MP, Ferraz PE, Escobar RR, et al. Preservation versus non-preservation of mitral valve apparatus during mitral valve replacement: a meta-analysis of 3835 patients. *Interact Cardiovasc Thorac Surg.* 2012;15:1033–1039.
19. Enriquez-Sarano M, Avierinos JF, Messika-Zeitoun D, et al. Quantitative determinants of the outcome of asymptomatic mitral regurgitation. *N Engl J Med.* 2005;352:875–883.
20. Deja MA, Grayburn PA, Sun B, et al. Influence of mitral regurgitation repair on survival in the surgical treatment for ischemic heart failure trial. *Circulation.* 2012;125:2639–2648.
21. Gillinov AM, Blackstone EH, Nowicki ER, et al. Valve repair versus valve replacement for degenerative mitral valve disease. *J Thorac Cardiovasc Surg.* 2008;135:885–893, 893.e881–e882.

22. Gillinov AM, Cosgrove DM, Blackstone EH, et al. Durability of mitral valve repair for degenerative disease. *J Thorac Cardiovasc Surg*. 1998;116:734–743.
23. Goldstein D, Moskowitz AJ, Gelijns AC, et al. Two-year outcomes of surgical treatment of severe ischemic mitral regurgitation. *N Engl J Med*. 2016;374:344–353.
24. Michler RE, Smith PK, Parides MK, et al. Two-year outcomes of surgical treatment of moderate ischemic mitral regurgitation. *N Engl J Med*. 2016;374:1932–1941.
25. Pantoja JL, Ge L, Zhang Z, et al. Posterior papillary muscle anchoring affects remote myofiber stress and pump function: finite element analysis. *Ann Thorac Surg*. 2014;98:1355–1362.
26. Ross Jr J, Braunwald E. Aortic stenosis. *Circulation*. 1968;38:61–67.
27. Bach DS, Cimino N, Deeb GM. Unoperated patients with severe aortic stenosis. *J Am Coll Cardiol*. 2007;50:2018–2019.
28. Gillam LD, Marcoff L, Shames S. Timing of surgery in valvular heart disease: prophylactic surgery vs watchful waiting in the asymptomatic patient. *Can J Cardiol*. 2014;30:1035–1045.
29. Bekeredjian R, Grayburn PA. Valvular heart disease: aortic regurgitation. *Circulation*. 2005;112:125–134.
30. David TE. Surgical treatment of aortic valve disease. *Nat Rev Cardiol*. 2013;10:375–386.
31. Van de Veire NR, Braun J, Delgado V, et al. Tricuspid annuloplasty prevents right ventricular dilatation and progression of tricuspid regurgitation in patients with tricuspid annular dilatation undergoing mitral valve repair. *J Thorac Cardiovasc Surg*. 2011;141:1431–1439.
32. Benedetto U, Melina G, Angeloni E, et al. Prophylactic tricuspid annuloplasty in patients with dilated tricuspid annulus undergoing mitral valve surgery. *J Thorac Cardiovasc Surg*. 2012;143:632–638.
33. Nath J, Foster E, Heidenreich PA. Impact of tricuspid regurgitation on long-term survival. *J Am Coll Cardiol*. 2004;43:405–409.
34. Yeter E, Ozlem K, Kilic H, et al. Tricuspid balloon valvuloplasty to treat tricuspid stenosis. *J Heart Valve Dis*. 2010;19:159–160.
35. Goodney PP, O'Connor GT, Wennberg DE, et al. Do hospitals with low mortality rates in coronary artery bypass also perform well in valve replacement? *Ann Thorac Surg*. 2003;76:1131–1136; discussion 1136–1137.
36. El-Hamamsy I, Clark L, Stevens LM, et al. Late outcomes following freestyle versus homograft aortic root replacement: results from a prospective randomized trial. *J Am Coll Cardiol*. 2010;55:368–376.
37. David TE, Feindel CM. An aortic valve-sparing operation for patients with aortic incompetence and aneurysm of the ascending aorta. *J Thorac Cardiovasc Surg*. 1992;103:617–621; discussion 622.
38. David TE. Aortic valve sparing operations: outcomes at 20 years. *Ann Cardiothorac Surg*. 2013;2:24–29.
39. Pibarot P, Dumesnil JG. Prosthetic heart valves: selection of the optimal prosthesis and long-term management. *Circulation*. 2009;119:1034–1048.
40. Garcia-Alamino JM, Ward AM, Alonso-Coello P, et al. Self-monitoring and self-management of oral anticoagulation. *Cochrane Database Syst Rev*. 2010:CD003839.
41. Flameng W, Rega F, Vercalsteren M, et al. Antimineralization treatment and patient-prosthesis mismatch are major determinants of the onset and incidence of structural valve degeneration in bioprosthetic heart valves. *J Thorac Cardiovasc Surg*. 2014;147:1219–1224.
42. Cribier A, Eltchaninoff H, Bash A, et al. Percutaneous transcatheter implantation of an aortic valve prosthesis for calcific aortic stenosis: first human case description. *Circulation*. 2002;106:3006–3008.
43. Bonhoeffer P, Boudjemline Y, Saliba Z, et al. Percutaneous replacement of pulmonary valve in a right-ventricle to pulmonary-artery prosthetic conduit with valve dysfunction. *Lancet*. 2000;356:1403–1405.
44. Leon MB, Smith CR, Mack M, et al. Transcatheter aortic-valve implantation for aortic stenosis in patients who cannot undergo surgery. *N Engl J Med*. 2010;363:1597–1607.
45. Smith CR, Leon MB, Mack MJ, et al. Transcatheter versus surgical aortic-valve replacement in high-risk patients. *N Engl J Med*. 2011;364:2187–2198.
46. Kodali SK, Williams MR, Smith CR, et al. Two-year outcomes after transcatheter or surgical aortic-valve replacement. *N Engl J Med*. 2012;366:1686–1695.
47. Leon MB, Smith CR, Mack MJ, et al. Transcatheter or surgical aortic-valve replacement in intermediate-risk patients. *N Engl J Med*. 2016;374:1609–1620.
48. Reardon MJ, Van Mieghem NM, Popma JJ, et al. Surgical or transcatheter aortic-valve replacement in intermediate-risk patients. *N Engl J Med*. 2017;376:1321–1331.
49. Hansson NC, Grove EL, Andersen HR, et al. Transcatheter aortic valve thrombosis: incidence, predisposing factors, and clinical implications. *J Am Coll Cardiol*. 2016;68:2059–2069.
50. Munkholm-Larsen S, Wan B, Tian DH, et al. A systematic review on the safety and efficacy of percutaneous edge-to-edge mitral valve repair with the MitraClip system for high surgical risk candidates. *Heart*. 2014;100:473–478.
51. Shrestha M, Folliguet TA, Pfeiffer S, et al. Aortic valve replacement and concomitant procedures with the perceval valve: results of European trials. *Ann Thorac Surg*. 2014;98:1294–1300.
52. Englberger L, Carrel TP, Doss M, et al. Clinical performance of a sutureless aortic bioprosthesis: five-year results of the 3f Enable long-term follow-up study. *J Thorac Cardiovasc Surg*. 2014;148:1681–1687.
53. Pollari F, Santarpino G, Dell'Aquila AM, et al. Better short-term outcome by using sutureless valves: a propensity-matched score analysis. *Ann Thorac Surg*. 2014;98:611–616; discussion 616–617.

SECTION XII

Vascular

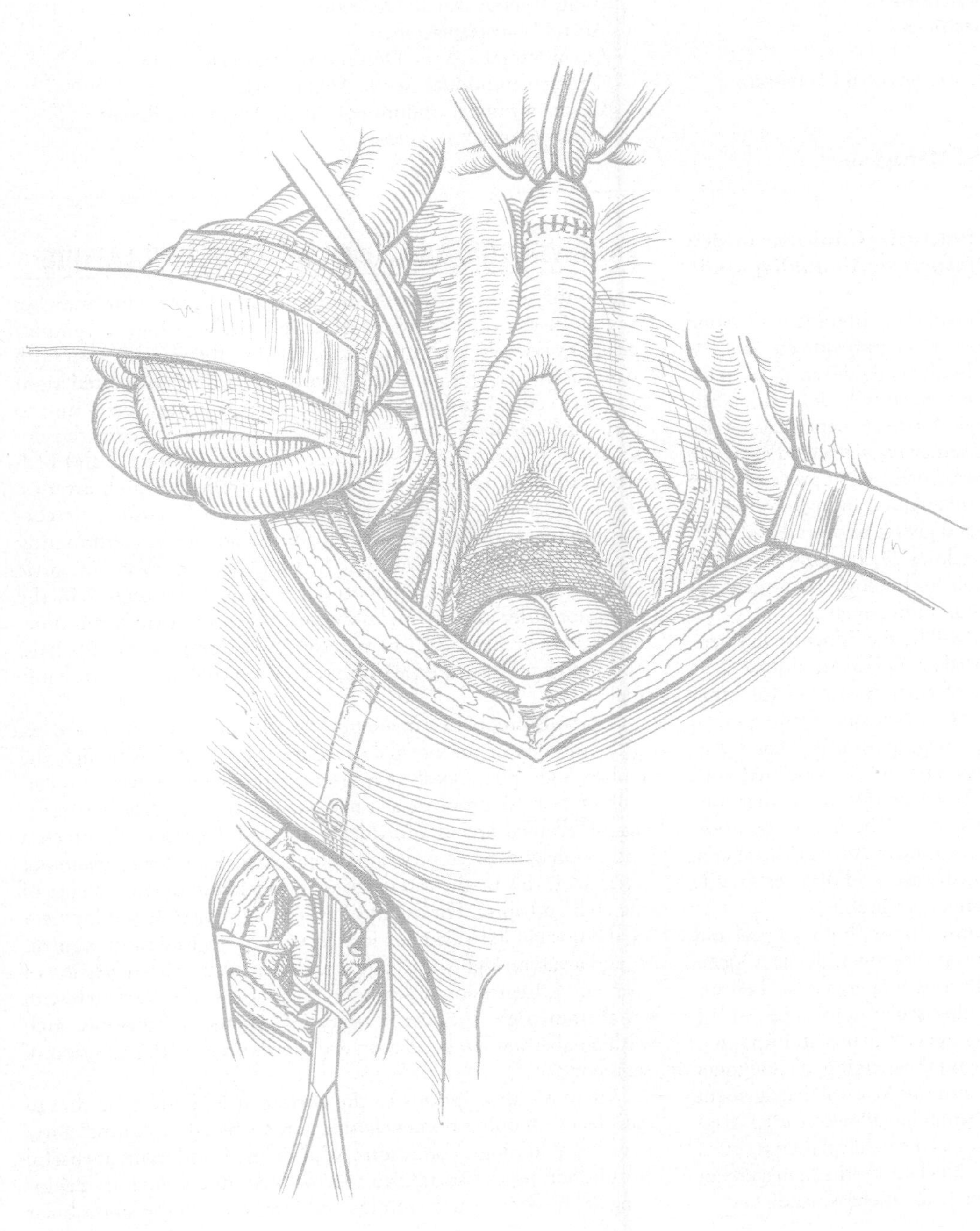

62 CHAPTER

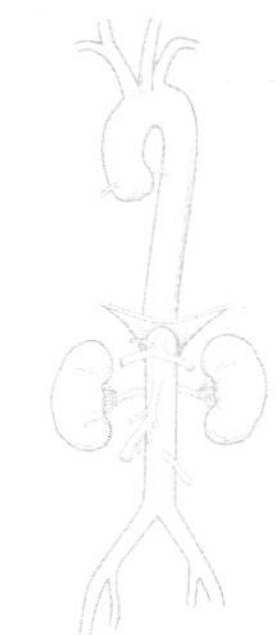

The Aorta

Abe DeAnda Jr., Jennifer Worsham, Matthew Mell

OUTLINE

Please access Elsevier eBooks for Practicing Clinicians to view the videos for this chapter https://expertconsult.inkling.com/.

Diseases of the aorta encompasses a broad range of topics far beyond the scope of a book chapter. However, we can provide an overview of common diseases and surgical issues involving the aorta, with the caveat that both our understanding of the pathophysiology of aortic disease as well as the medical and surgical management of aortic disease is constantly evolving. With the somewhat simplified acknowledgement that surgeons are either disease-oriented or procedure-oriented, this chapter aims to provide residents-in-training information regarding common disease processes and giving an overview of technical considerations. Systematic procedural descriptions are mostly avoided and information on available technology minimized, as both will change as part of the evolution in treatment.

A common theme in this chapter will be the difficulty in documenting the true incidence and prevalence of aortic disease. The reasons are many, patients may die of aortic processes (or other diseases) prior to diagnosis, and pathology involving the aorta is often only found incidentally during imaging for other issues. Aneurysmal disease is typically asymptomatic unless associated with rapid growth, aortitis, or rupture. The very definition of what constitutes an aneurysm may be up for debate. The first recognition of aortic dissection (AD) may occur at autopsy. Aortic disease may present as only one part of a systemic disease, and diagnosis made after preventative measures are no longer applicable.

Despite the late presentation of aortic disease, both surgical and medical therapeutic and management options are available. Operative therapy for patients previously deemed inoperable has become available with the introduction of endovascular approaches to the thoracic and abdominal aorta. Open surgery remains an important part of the surgeon's armamentarium, and the merging of techniques with hybrid approaches has become common. Medical management also retains a role, the use of genetic testing has allowed earlier diagnosis and in some cases treatment with specific medical therapy, such as in the case of angiotensin II receptor blockers for the management of Loey-Dietz syndrome or beta-blockade for aneurysmal disease.

EMBRYOLOGY, ANATOMY, AND NOMENCLATURE

The embryologic formation of the aorta and its major branches begins in the third week of gestation and is a highly complex process of development that lends itself to the variants seen both structurally as well as histologically. Starting with paired right and left ventral and dorsal aortae, the two ventral pairs fuse to form the aortic sac and the dorsal pairs fuse to form the descending thoracoabdominal aorta. During the fourth and fifth weeks of development, the pharyngeal arches, or arch arteries, form, and as they develop in a cephalocaudal manner, six corresponding aortic arches form from the aortic sac, terminating on the dorsal aortae (Fig. 62.1). While the embryologic aortic arches develop in a cephalocaudal fashion, they regress in the opposite order and are not necessarily present at the same time. The aortic arches begin to regress day 27 and by day 29 have completely disappeared with remnants contributing to the normal aorta.

Edwards proposed a theoretical double aortic arch system to explain variants of the normal anatomy (Fig. 62.2).[1] Although the embryologic pharyngeal arch arteries appear and regress sequentially, Edwards's proposal pictured the developing aorta as consisting of bilateral arches and ductus arteriosi encircling the trachea and esophagus. By considering the persistence and/or regression of a segment, this model can describe most variants and anomalies of the arch and aorta. For example, as seen in Fig. 62.2, development of the normal left-sided aortic arch requires regression of segment 1, and a variant right-sided aortic arch will occur with regression of segment 4. Regression of segment 2 results in a left-sided arch with an aberrant right subclavian artery (SCA), and a right-sided arch with an aberrant left subclavian artery will occur with regression of segment 3.

Anatomic descriptions of the aorta can be perplexing due to various overlapping nomenclature systems based on normal aorta as well as pathologic conditions. Well-defined landmarks are useful in subdividing the aorta into specific anatomic segments. Beginning at the aortic valve annulus and extending to the sinotubular junction is the aortic root, which traditionally includes the aortic valve. Embryologically, the root derives from the truncus arteriosus, the fused portion of the ventral aorta. Continuing from the sinotubular junction to either the take-off of the innominate artery or the pericardial reflection is the ascending aorta. Like the root, the ascending aorta originates embryologically from the ventral aorta. Distally, the ventral aorta during development bifurcates into two horns, the right becoming the brachiocephalic artery and the left the proximal portion of the aortic arch. The aortic arch starts at the terminal end of the ascending aorta and ends immediately distal to the left SCA. The remnant of the fourth embryologic aortic arch forms the portion of the aortic arch between the left common carotid and the left SCA. The descending thoracic aorta begins at the left SCA and extends to the aortic hiatus and transitions to the abdominal aorta, which then becomes the supra- and, subsequently, infrarenal aorta (the juxtarenal or pararenal tag is usually reserved for diseased segment terminology).

Aortic pathologic conditions have their own unique nomenclature. Aneurysmal disease is perhaps the easiest to describe since typically the label is simply the location (e.g., root aneurysm, arch aneurysm, etc.) with some exceptions. For example, Estrera and colleagues[2] subdivide the descending thoracic aorta into three subtypes (A: proximal to the sixth rib, B: distal to the sixth rib, C: entire descending thoracic aorta) as this has implications on the risk of postoperative paraplegia (Fig. 62.3). The Society for Vascular Surgery (SVS) divides the aorta into "zones" as it pertains to endograft attachment sites rather than to disease extent (Fig. 62.4).[3]

In the case of thoracoabdominal aortic aneurysms (TAAA), first catalogued and subsequently refined by Crawford and colleagues,[4,5] the original groupings attempted to describe the aneurysm in relationship to the extent of thoracic and abdominal involvement. The label "group" later evolved into "extent" or "type." Extent I involved the descending thoracic aorta and abdominal aorta to the level of the celiac artery. Extent II involved the entire thoracic and abdominal aorta, and Extent III had "... lesser involvement of the thoracic aorta" and most of the abdominal aorta. Extent IV involved the entire abdominal aorta. In the original classification scheme there was also an Extent V, which involved the lower abdominal aorta and renal arteries. This classification scheme was refined to four groups, or extents, and later modified to five extents to account for aneurysms involving only a portion of the thoracic aorta with sparing of the infrarenal aorta (Fig. 62.5).[6] The Crawford classification system remains as an important tool in comparing procedural outcomes for TAAAs.

There are two major classification schemes for ADs (Fig. 62.6). The DeBakey classification was the first attempt of distinguishing two clinically different scenarios (i.e., dissections limited to the descending aorta as compared to those involving the ascending aorta).[7] When the ascending is involved, the dissection is either a Type I (involving the entire ascending, arch, and to some extent descending aorta) or a Type II (limited to the ascending aorta only). Dissection of the descending aorta alone is a DeBakey Type III with the further subdivisions of IIIa (tear only in the descending thoracic aorta) and IIIb (tear extending below the diaphragm). The Stanford classification scheme is limited to Type A, which encompasses

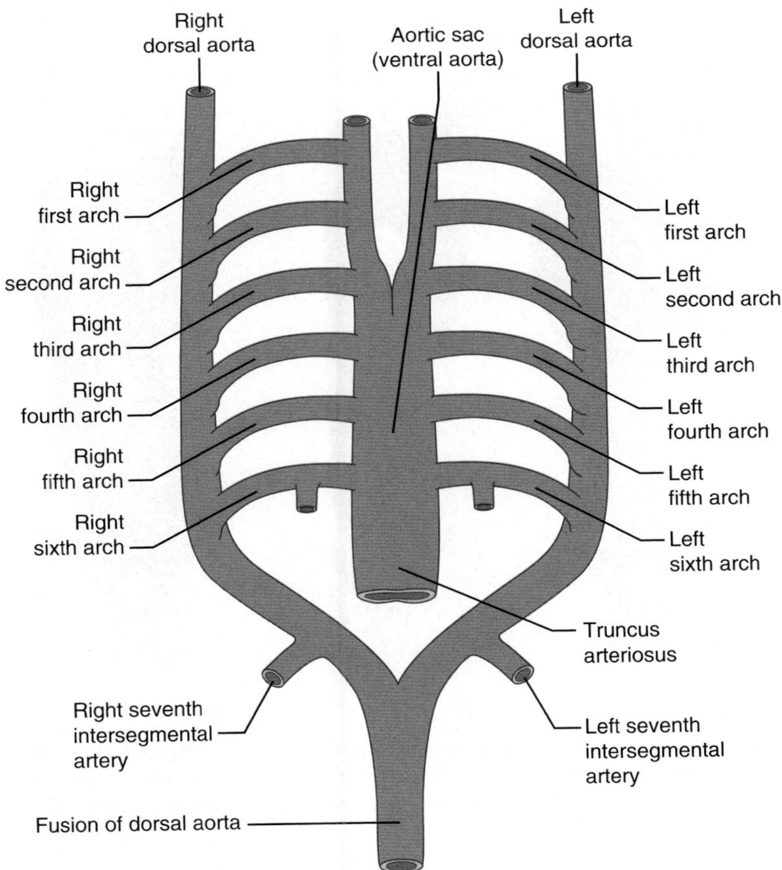

FIG. 62.1 Embryologic development of the aortic arch and branches.

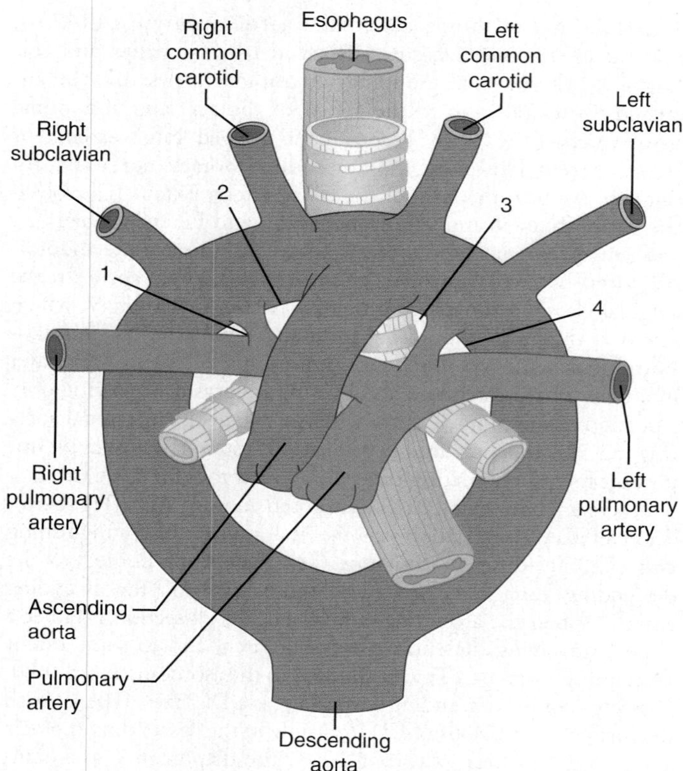

FIG. 62.2 Edwards theoretical arch.

dissections with *any* involvement of the ascending aorta, and Type B, which is for dissections distal to the left SCA.[8] The Stanford scheme thus could, in a broad sense, distinguish between surgical management (Type A) and medical management (Type B), although there are exceptions, and with the ability for endovascular therapy of the descending aorta there is a shift of Type B's away from medical management towards surgical intervention. The DeBakey scheme can also be separated into surgical (Types I and II) and nonsurgical (Type III), but in contrast to the Stanford classification, it also provides information on the extent of the disease process. By convention, the classical separation between an acute and chronic dissection occurs at the two-week mark, but a recent modification includes four time domains: hyperacute (<24 hours), acute (2–7 days), subacute (8–30 days) and chronic (>30 days).[9]

Both the DeBakey and Stanford classifications conveniently ignore dissections beginning or limited to the arch. Lansman and colleagues expanded on the Stanford classification to specify the site of intimal tear, and in this case, included arch dissections.[10] In their series of 168 acute dissections, 139 patients had a Type A dissection (TAAD), and 30% of these had arch tears. There was a nonstatistically significant decrease in 10-year survival when an arch tear was present, although this did not affect hospital mortality. The Task Force on Aortic Dissection of the European Society of Cardiology proposed an entirely different classification based on anatomic presentation.[11] The five classes are 1) classic AD with a distinct intimal flap separating the true and false lumen, 2) intramural hematoma (IMH), 3) subtle or discrete AD, 4) penetrating atherosclerotic aortic ulcer (PAU), and 5) iatrogenic or traumatic dissection. In this chapter, we consider traumatic dissection/transection, IMH, and PAU as separate, nondissection processes.

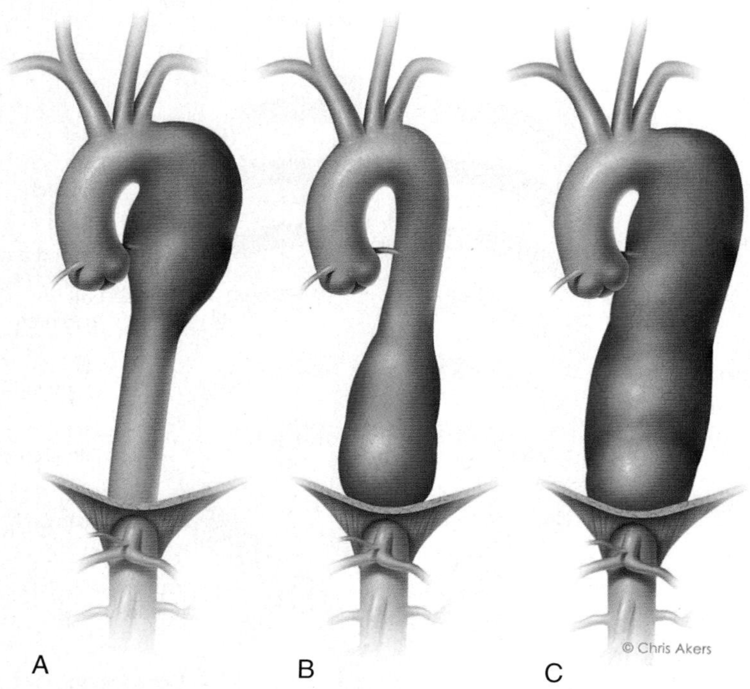

FIG. 62.3 Classification, descending thoracic aortic aneurysm. (A) Type A, distal to the left subclavian artery to the sixth intercostal space. (B) Type B, sixth intercostal space to above the diaphragm (twelfth intercostal space). (C) Type C, entire descending thoracic aorta, distal to the left subclavian artery to above the diaphragm (twelfth intercostal space). (Courtesy Chris Akers, 2006.)

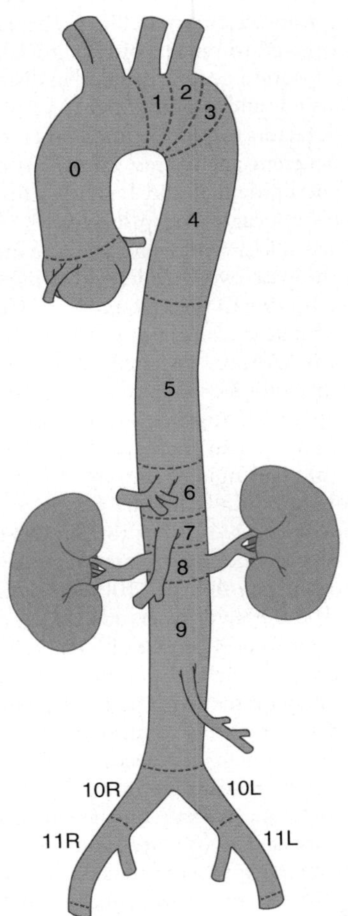

FIG. 62.4 Aortic endograft attachment zones. (Adapted from Fillinger MF, Greenberg RK, McKinsey JF, et al. Reporting standards for thoracic endovascular aortic repair (TEVAR). *J Vasc Surg.* 2010;52:1022–1033.)

More recently, the Penn classification scheme has been introduced which combines the Stanford classification with the DeBakey dissection extent and a further distinction focused on clinical presentation and distal malperfusion.[12,13] The Penn classification was initially for TAAD. The four subgroups in the Penn classification are absence of branch vessel malperfusion or circulatory collapse (Penn class Aa), branch vessel malperfusion with ischemia (Penn class Ab), circulatory collapse with or without cardiac involvement (Penn class Ac), and finally both branch vessel malperfusion and circulatory collapse (Penn class Aabc). The rationale for this approach was an appreciation of the consequences of malperfusion in patient interventions, prognosis, and outcomes.[13] Subsequently the classification was modified for Type B dissection to better differentiate complicated and uncomplicated Type B dissection. Similar to the TAAD classification, the four subgroups are absence of branch vessel malperfusion or circulatory collapse (Class A), branch vessel malperfusion with ischemia (Class B), circulatory collapse with or without cardiac involvement (Class C), and finally both branch vessel malperfusion and circulatory collapse (Class BC). Class A is subdivided into Type I (high risk for future aortic complications) and Type II (low risk), and Class C is subdivided into Type I (aortic rupture with hemorrhage outside the aortic wall) and Type II (threatened aortic rupture).[14]

PATHOLOGY, MANAGEMENT, AND OUTCOMES

Acute Aortic Syndromes

Aneurysm

Aneurysms, typically defined as an increase in size of more than 50% above the normal arterial diameter,[15] may occur anywhere along the aorta, from the aortic root to the bifurcation. As the mean aortic diameter differs between the ascending, descending, and infrarenal aorta, the absolute size criteria for aneurysm changes. Normal values will also vary due to methods of measurement, patient's age, sex, and other factors.[15] As an example based on a population-based magnetic resonance imaging (MRI) study

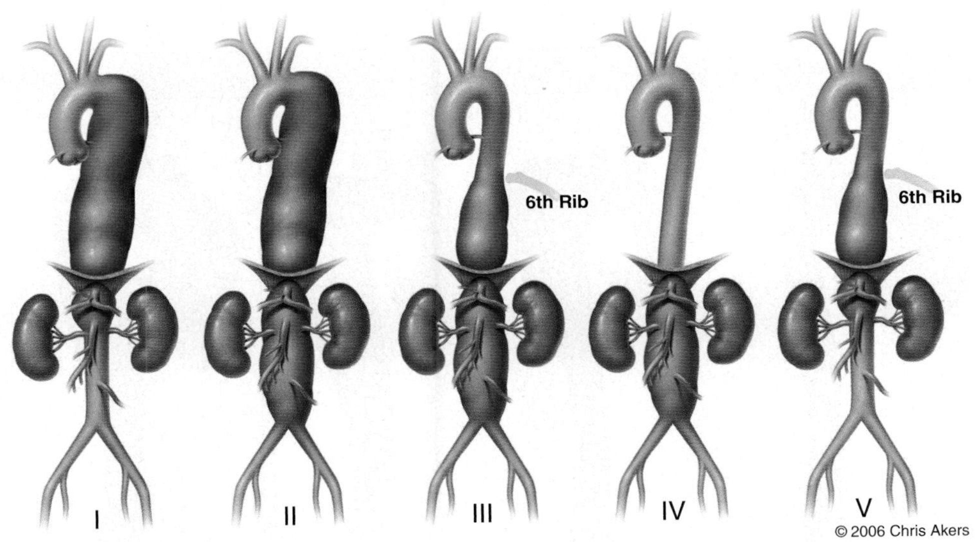

FIG. 62.5 Normal thoracoabdominal aorta aneurysm classification. Extent I, distal to the left subclavian artery to above the renal arteries; Extent II, distal to the left subclavian artery to below the renal arteries; Extent III, from the sixth intercostal space to below the renal arteries; Extent IV, from the twelfth intercostal space to the iliac bifurcation (total abdominal aortic aneurysm); Extent V, below the sixth intercostal space to just above the renal arteries (modified Crawford classification). (Courtesy Chris Akers, 2006.)

of 70-year-olds, Wanhainnen and colleagues defined aneurysms of the ascending aorta as 4.7 cm in men and 4.2 cm in women, descending aorta as 3.7 cm in men and 3.3 cm in women, and infrarenal aorta as 3.0 cm in men and 2.7 cm in women.[16] Anatomy or etiology may also be the basis for characterization of aneurysms. Anatomically, fusiform aneurysms exhibit smooth, circumferential dilatation across the entire vessel as opposed to saccular aneurysms, which appear as a focal outpouching of the arterial wall. Whereas true aneurysms involve all three layers of the vessel wall, false aneurysm or pseudoaneurysm describes a focal defect in the artery with an associated collection of blood contained by surrounding connective tissue. Pseudoaneurysms may be degenerative, infectious, or traumatic in etiology. These pseudoaneurysms may occur at sites of prior surgical anastomosis and represent anastomotic disruption. The majority of aneurysms addressed in this chapter are degenerative in nature. Less frequently, aneurysms may be associated with infection (mycotic aneurysms), inflammation, or autoimmune or connective tissue disease. These cases merit special consideration in their evaluation and management.

Aneurysmal enlargement of the aorta is associated with factors that result in weakening of the arterial wall and increased local hemodynamic forces. These may include heritable conditions, such as Marfan syndrome, familial thoracic aortic aneurysm and dissection, and vascular-type Ehlers-Danlos, as well as less well-defined entities that contribute to the significantly elevated incidence of aneurysm in patients with a family history of aneurysm. Factors that contribute to the degradation of extracellular matrix and reduction of elastin concentration are also associated with aneurysmal disease, and research in this area has focused on the role of matrix metalloproteinases, both their presence in the aneurysm specimens and for deficits of antiproteolytic enzymes that normally inhibit metalloproteinases.[17] Ongoing avenues of investigation in this area also include the role of the immune response and hormone milieu.[18] Finally, aneurysmal dilatation may also occur as a degenerative complication after AD.

As alluded to earlier, determining the incidence and prevalence of aneurysmal disease is difficult, in part because of the tendency for aneurysms to be asymptomatic and found incidentally during imaging for unrelated medical problems or symptoms. The incidence of abdominal aortic aneurysm (AAA), based on large screening studies, is estimated to range from 3% to 10%. A number of risk factors, in addition to genetic or familial disorders, for the development, expansion, and rupture of AAAs have been identified (Table 62.1). Risk factors for development of an AAA include age, male gender, concurrent aneurysms, family history, tobacco use, hypertension, hyperlipidemia, and height. Female gender, black race, and diabetes appear to be protective.[19–21] Recent studies have suggested that in first-world countries the incidence has been decreasing over the past two decades, most likely related to the decreased tobacco burden in those countries.[22] Gender differences extend to the presentation, associations, and natural history of aneurysms. Men with AAA, for instance, are more likely to present with concurrent iliac or femoropopliteal aneurysms.[23] Women are more likely to experience rupture and consistently demonstrate poorer outcomes after repair, perhaps because of a significantly higher incidence of challenging anatomy.[24] With screening of an at-risk population, specifically for the 65- to 89-year-old demographic, the incidence of AAA is 5% to 7% with a male to female ratio of roughly four to one.[25] Estimates of the prevalence of thoracic aortic aneurysms are 400 per 100,000 patients in 65-year-olds and 670 per 100,000 in 80-year olds, and in contrast to AAA, there does not appear to be a gender difference.[26]

While aneurysms may be asymptomatic, an acutely enlarging or inflamed aorta may present with pain. Depending on the location of the aneurysm, other less common signs or symptoms may occur. For example, an enlarged ascending aorta or proximal arch may result in superior vena cava syndrome.[27] An expanding proximal descending aorta can impinge on the left recurrent laryngeal nerve, leading to hoarseness (Ortner syndrome)[28] or pulmonary embarrassment from extrinsic compression of the left main stem bronchus.[29] Large AAAs may give a feeling of fullness or early satiety after small meals.

Chest x-ray (CXR) studies may detect incidentally thoracic aneurysm due to abnormalities in aortic contour, size, or calcifications, but CXR is not a good screening tool.[30] A number of other noninvasive and invasive modalities are available for screening,

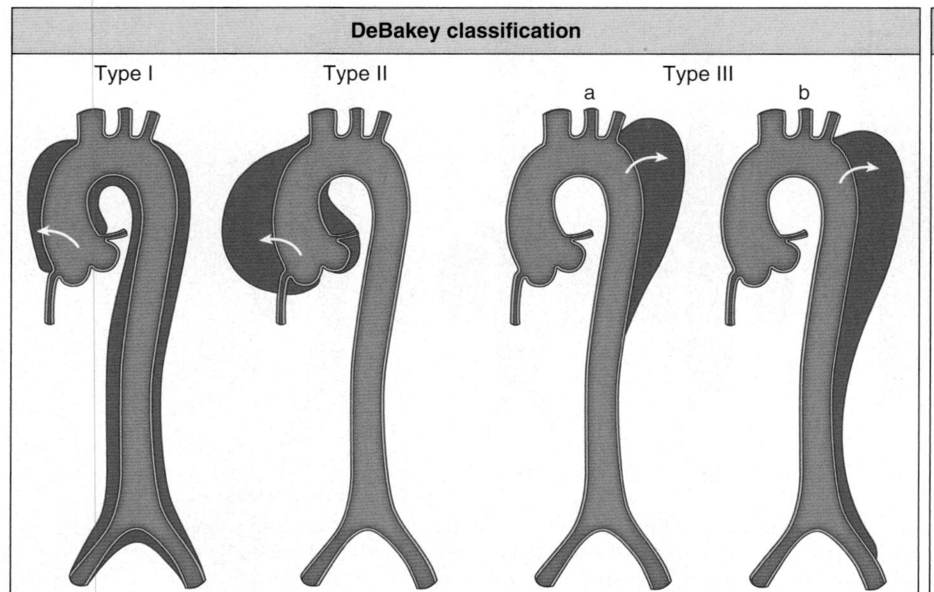

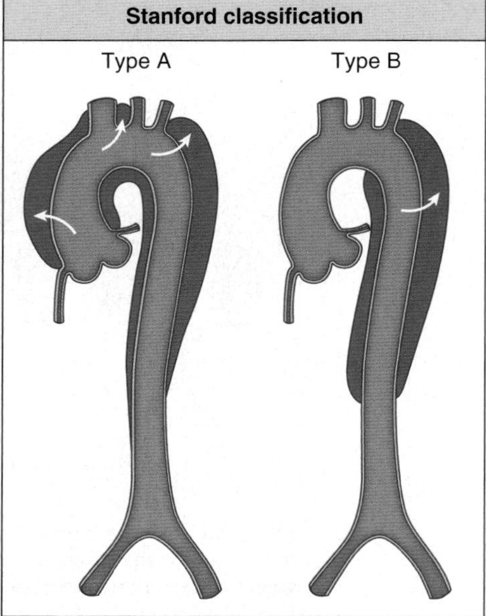

FIG. 62.6 DeBakey *(left)* and Stanford *(right)* aortic dissection classifications.

TABLE 62.1 Risk factors for aneurysm development, expansion, and rupture.

SYMPTOM	RISK FACTORS
AAA development	Tobacco use Hypercholesterolemia Hypertension Male gender Family history (male predominance)
AAA expansion	Advanced age Severe cardiac disease Previous stroke Tobacco use Cardiac or renal transplantation
AAA rupture	Female gender ↓ FEV_1 Larger initial abdominal aortic diameter Higher mean blood pressure Current tobacco use (length of time smoking ≫ amount) Cardiac or renal transplantation Critical wall stress–wall strength relationship

Adapted from Chaikof EL, Brewster DC, Dalman RL, et al. The care of patients with an abdominal aortic aneurysm: the Society for Vascular Surgery practice guidelines. *J Vasc Surg*. 2009;50:S2–49.
AAA, Abdominal aortic aneurysm; *FEV_1*, forced expiratory volume.

case management, and surveillance. Ultrasound is an important tool in AAA management, as it is accurate, noninvasive, and cost-effective.[19] Contrast-enhanced ultrasound is particularly useful in patients after endovascular aneurysm repair (EVAR) in detecting, localizing, and quantifying endoleaks.[31] Echocardiography is ultrasonography when performed on the chest and its contents, and the noninvasive technique is transthoracic echocardiography (TTE). TTE is useful for measuring certain segments of the ascending aorta as well as assessing the degree of aortic valve insufficiency, if present.[32] The invasive transesophageal echocardiogram (TEE) is capable of seeing the thoracic aorta from the aortic annulus to the celiac axis, with the exception of a short segment of the ascending aorta proximal to the innominate artery.[33] This technique usually requires at least a modest level of sedation. Intravascular ultrasound (IVUS) is an additional modality for imaging of the aorta, and while it not typically utilized for diagnostic purposes, it is invaluable as an adjunct in endovascular procedures.

Computed tomography (CT) provides excellent imaging of the aorta, with greater reproducibility of diameter measurements than by ultrasound,[19] and remains an important tool in the diagnosis, management, and surveillance of aortic disease. CT, particularly with the adjunctive use of iodinated contrast agents to perform CT angiography (CTA), provides a wealth of anatomic information; it detects vessel calcification, thrombus, and concurrent arterial occlusive disease and permits multiplanar and three-dimensional reconstruction and analysis for operative planning. Drawbacks include substantial radiation exposure, particularly in the setting of serial examinations, and the use of iodinated contrast media in a population with a high incidence of comorbid kidney disease.

MRI provides a reasonable alternative to CT for imaging of the aorta, with the benefits being the elimination of ionizing radiation and iodinated contrast. Spin-echo black blood and gradient echo sequences provide an intrinsic contrast between the blood flow and aortic wall to provide dimensional and geometric information.[34] With the addition of intravenous gadolinium as a contrast agent, magnetic resonance angiography (MRA) provides rapid 3D imaging of the aorta without the need for electrocardiogram (ECG)-gating. The ability to acquire dynamic images throughout the cardiac cycle allows physiologic parameters such as estimates of wall shear stress to be determined, which may lead to clinical applications.[35] Unlike CT, MRI does not demonstrate aortic wall calcification, which may be important in operative planning especially for endovascular approaches. MRI does not necessarily use iodinated contrast material but instead can utilize gadolinium, which has been associated with the development of nephrogenic systemic fibrosis in patients with low glomerular filtration rate. Additionally, a contraindication for MRI is the presence of incompatible metallic implants or foreign bodies. Mechanical valves, pacemakers, and implantable cardioversion devices currently marketed in the United States are MRI compatible. Newer ferrous-based contrast agents coupled with MRA may provide a viable alternative to vascular imaging when iodinated contrast or gadolinium is contraindicated.[36]

Size and symptoms play a large role in determining the management of aortic aneurysms (Table 62.2). For aneurysms that do not meet criteria or appropriateness for surgical intervention, medical management is a mainstay. Lifestyle modifications may be necessary, such as tobacco use cessation. Current smoking has been associated with significantly increasing the expansion rate of AAA (~ 0.4 mm/yr).[37] While moderate levels of exercise have a beneficial impact on patient's cardiopulmonary health and progression of atherosclerosis, patients should avoid vigorous levels of activity and contact sports. Activities that cause a sudden spike in blood pressure may lead to aortic rupture or dissection in the presence of underlying aortic pathology.[38] Blood pressure management, both in the reduction of systolic pressure as well as the pulse pressure (an indirect measure of dP/dt and wall stress), may require multiple medications. β-blockers, both selective and nonselective, are useful in accomplishing both goals.

Prevention of aneurysmal dilatation or even regression would be an ideal consequence of medical therapy. This has been shown to be the case in the specific clinical scenario of the patient with Marfan syndrome treated with β-blockers, angiotensin II receptor blockers, and angiotensin-converting enzyme inhibitors.[37,39] None of these drugs has been shown to be effective in patients who do not have Marfan syndrome. HMG–coenzyme A reductase inhibitor (statin) therapy has been associated with reduced rates of AAA enlargement[40] and is otherwise appropriate in a population with a high prevalence of concurrent atherosclerotic disease. Statin therapy improves survival following open and endovascular repair of AAAs and has been shown to decrease the incidence of major cardiovascular events (stroke, myocardial infarction, and death) for patients with the diagnosis of AAA.[41] Finally, antiplatelet therapy using aspirin offers a secondary preventive benefit in this population.

Screening recommendations of aneurysms are informed by the sensitivity and specificity of ultrasound screening (or other imaging modality), the detection yield of screening based on various risk factor selection criteria, and cost. Screening for thoracic aneurysms is generally not done without a pretest high probability (e.g., suspicion of an aortic syndrome). The caveat is when an AAA is diagnosed it is a general recommendation that the thoracic aorta be screen to rule out metasynchronous disease.[42] Current consensus guidelines recommend one-time screening of all men aged 65 years and older or men 55 years and older with a family history of AAA.[19] In 2014, the U.S. Preventive Services Task Force

TABLE 62.2 Recommended size for intervention of asymptomatic aortic aneurysm.

LOCATION	SIZE CRITERIA	COMMENT
Ascending/root	≥55 mm	All patients, including BAV
	≥50 mm	Patients with Marfan syndrome
		BAV with risk factors for dissection
	≥45 mm	Selected patients with Marfan syndrome
	>45 mm	When aortic valve is being intervened on
	>27.5 mm/m^2	For patients with a small body size
Arch	≥55 mm	All patients
	Any size	Signs or symptoms of local compression
Descending	≥55 mm	When TEVAR possible
	≥60 mm	Open repair (less for Marfan syndrome)
Abdominal	≥55 mm	All patients

Adapted from Erbel R, Aboyans V, Boileau C, et al. 2014 ESC Guidelines on the diagnosis and treatment of aortic diseases: Document covering acute and chronic aortic diseases of the thoracic and abdominal aorta of the adult. The Task Force for the Diagnosis and Treatment of Aortic Diseases of the European Society of Cardiology (ESC). *Eur Heart J.* 2014;35:2873–2926.
BAV, bicuspid aortic valve; *TEVAR*, thoracic endovascular aortic repair.

(USPSTF) issued a more limited recommendation for one-time screening for AAA using ultrasonography of men between 65 and 75 years of age who have a personal smoking history and selective screening for nonsmokers.[43] For women the recommendations remain controversial. The USPSTF concluded that there was insufficient evidence to recommend routine screening in women who smoke and recommended against routine screening in nonsmoking women. One issue that may have biased these results is the paucity of women in large screening trials. In one metaanalysis that looked at a combination of four studies with over 125,000 patients enrolled, less than 10,000 subjects were women.[44] Payer policies regarding reimbursement may not track either of these recommendations. Medicare, for instance, because of the Screening Abdominal Aortic Aneurysms Very Efficiently (SAAAVE) Act, reflects an intermediate approach in offering a screening benefit for men with a personal smoking history and men or women with a family history of AAA, although only as a part of the initial Welcome to Medicare physical examination. In a single-institution study of ruptured AAAs, only 17% of patients would have been eligible for screening.[45]

Following the initial detection of a nonsurgical aneurysm, surveillance is necessary in addition to optimal medical management. Ideally, surveillance should be low-cost, high-sensitivity, and pose minimal harm to the patient. For the abdominal aorta, ultrasound follow-up is advisable. Those patients with a known AAA who do not have appropriate surveillance may have up to a sixfold increase in rate of rupture.[46] The Society for Vascular Surgery Clinical Practice Council recommends the following screening intervals based on aneurysm size (maximum external aortic diameter) and associated risk of rupture:[19]

- <2.6 cm: no further screening recommended
- 2.6–2.9 cm: reexamination at 5 years
- 3–3.4 cm: reexamination at 3 years
- 3.5–4.4 cm: reexamination at 12 months
- 4.5–5.4 cm: reexamination at 6 months

These recommendations, as is the case for thoracic aortic aneurysms, stem from our understanding of growth rates of normal and abnormal aortas as well as published rates of rupture at given sizes. No large, prospective studies that compare surveillance intervals exist. For the abdominal aorta, while the SVS recommends no further screening for aneurysms less than 2.6 cm, others have suggested 3 cm as the cutoff.[47] Countering this is the findings that a significant proportion of 65-year-old men (13.8%) with an initial aortic diameter of 2.6 to 2.9 cm developed aneurysms exceeding 5.5 cm at 10 years.[48] Given current life expectancy projections, it is evident that a subset of patients deem "normal" at screening will go on to develop clinically significant aneurysms.

Surveillance of thoracic aortic aneurysms is more an art than science. With the exception of the aortic root, visible with TTE, the thoracic aorta generally requires CT or MRI contrast imaging. For the ascending, arch, and descending aortas, after the initial diagnosis a second study at 6 months should suffice to determine if there is measurable growth in the aortic diameter. This is followed with yearly scans until there is reasonable certainty of stability in size, at which time extending surveillance to a 2- to 3-year interval is tolerable. Conversion to MRI for surveillance avoids exposure of the patient to ionizing radiation.

Prevention of rupture of the growing aorta is the rationale for surveillance imaging, and risk models for rupture do exist. Juvonen and colleagues developed a model that included risk factors of age, presence of pain, chronic obstructive pulmonary disease, and maximal diameters of the thoracic and abdominal aorta. Based on this model, surgery was recommended when the calculated risk of rupture within one year exceeded the anticipated mortality risk of an elective procedure, even if the recommended aortic diameter for intervention was not reached.[49]

Outcomes for surgical intervention of aneurysmal disease are dependent on location of the lesion, extent of disease, and technique of repair. Endovascular technology has had a dramatic impact on treatment options and outcomes, but open repair or hybrid approaches remain an important part of the armamentarium of the surgeon. For aneurysms involving the aortic root and ascending aorta, repaired electively, the mortality rate is approximately 5%[50] for all patients and likely less when performed in high-volume centers. When aneurysms involve the arch, the mortality outcomes are similar to the ascending aorta, but there is an increase in morbidity, specifically with cerebrovascular injury.

With the descending thoracic aorta, the thoracic endovascular aorta repair (TEVAR) approach has become the standard of care for most aneurysmal disease. Since the first reported series by Dake and colleagues in 1994, the indications for TEVAR have expanded[51] with a paucity of randomized controlled studies comparing TEVAR to open repair of descending thoracic aortic aneurysms. A metaanalysis of forty two nonrandomized studies with

5888 patients demonstrated a reduction of all-cause mortality and paraplegia, as well as a decrease in complications and length of stay. Beyond one year, there was no difference in mortality or surgical reintervention.[52]

For treatment of TAAAs, no endovascular devices are currently approved for use in the United States, and open surgery is the mainstay of treatment. Recently reported surgical mortality has ranged from 2.3% to 7.5% in specialized centers[53] and over 20% in "real-world" practice.[54] A metaanalysis demonstrated a pooled mortality rate of 11.26% with Crawford Extent II having the highest risk of death.[55] Pooled spinal cord ischemic rates (paraparesis and paraplegia) were estimated at 8.26%.[55] Successful repair is reliant on a cohesive team approach, including cardiothoracic and/or vascular surgeons, cardiac anesthesiologists, trained nursing staff, and intensivists knowledgeable of the nuances and subtleties for caring for this patient population.

For infrarenal AAA, reported outcomes for open abdominal aortic repair vary from 1% to 4% for infrarenal repair performed in centers of excellence[56] to 4% to 8% noted in statewide or nationwide databases.[56,57] Complications associated with open repair occur in 15% to 30% of patients.[57] Both early mortality and complication rates are better with an endovascular approach to AAAs, although this may represent a selection bias. The United Kingdom EVAR trial investigators randomized 1252 patients with AAAs larger than 5.5 cm for elective open repair versus EVAR, and while the 30-day mortality rate was favorable for EVAR (1.8% vs. 4.3%, $P = 0.02$), this benefit was lost by the end of the study.[58] Additionally, EVAR was more costly in part due to increased rates of graft-related complications and need for reintervention.[58] A similar study by the Dutch Randomized Endovascular Aneurysm Management (DREAM) trial group found early advantages of EVAR to have disappeared by the two-year follow-up mark.[59]

With currently approved and available technology, roughly 80% of nonemergent AAAs can be repaired with an endovascular approach. When considering an endovascular approach, accurate evaluation of anatomy is essential. This includes the neck of the aneurysm, which should be of sufficient length and without severe angulation, extensive mural thrombus, or calcification. The diameter of the proximal seal zone must not be too large to prevent a proximal seal. Access vessels (iliac and femoral arteries) should be of sufficient diameter to allow passage of appropriately sized sheaths.

As newer generation devices have become available, anatomic indications have expanded. AAAs with necks as short as 4 mm long can be treated with custom-made fenestrated stent-grafts or with suprarenal fixation and endoanchors. Many aortoiliac aneurysms can be treated with iliac-branched devices. Arteriotomy closure devices have allowed many aneurysms to be safely repaired with a totally percutaneous approach, and while postprocedure pseudoaneurysms are more common with arteriotomy closure devices, there are fewer seromas, wound dehiscences, and surgical site infections associated with the use of arteriotomy closure devices.[60] On the horizon may include branched endografts to treat pararenal or TAAAs. As of yet, these devices are not available in the United States.

Postoperative evaluation of a successful EVAR includes serial CT scans and/or color duplex ultrasonography,[61] looking for aortic sac diameter or volume, graft migration, and endoleaks. Surveillance imaging is generally recommended at 1 month, 6 months, 12 months, and yearly thereafter provided a stable exam. Because of the need for ongoing surveillance, patients who may be unwilling or unable to undergo postoperative imaging may not be appropriate candidates for EVAR.[61]

When identified, endoleaks are classified as:

- Type 1A (proximal seal zone)
- Type 1B (distal seal zone)
- Type 2 (retrograde flow from lumbar and/or inferior mesenteric arteries [IMAs])
- Type 3 (component separation)
- Type 4 (fabric porosity)
- Type 5 (expanding aneurysm without demonstrable blood flow)

Type 1 and 3 endoleaks require repair. Type 2 endoleaks are common early after EVAR, with most resolving by 1 to 6 months.[62] Management of persistent type 2 endoleaks is controversial, with most favoring observational management in the absence of sac growth.[62] If sac growth occurs after EVAR with an otherwise stable type 2 endoleak, delayed type 1 or 3 endoleak may be the underlying culprit.[63]

When anatomic considerations fall outside the "Instructions for Use" for endovascular devices, open repair remains the most acceptable treatment option. Additional potential considerations for open repair include younger patients, patients with connective tissue disorders, and, as discussed above, those who are unable or unwilling to participate in postoperative surveillance. For such patients whose comorbidity excludes open repair, novel approaches to endovascular repair have been described. These options may include snorkel/chimney EVAR,[64] physician modified endografts,[65] and use of investigational devices not currently available for clinical use in the United States.[66] These options necessitate local expertise and may require federally approved Individual Device Exemption (IDE) prior to proceeding with these alternatives.

Ruptured AAAs deserve special attention. Approximately 15,000 annual deaths from ruptured AAAs occur in the United States.[67] In ruptured AAAs where it would be ideal to treat with an endovascular approach, there has not been any statistical evidence of a short-term benefit of one approach versus another. In one European trial, comparison between open and EVAR showed no difference in operative mortality (39% vs. 35%, respectively) or 90-day mortality (42% vs. 40%).[68] In the IMPROVE trial (The Immediate Management of the Patient with Ruptured Aneurysm: Open Versus Endovascular repair) there was no difference in 30- or 90-day mortality, but there was an advantage for EVAR at three years (42% vs. 54%); but once again this advantage was gone by 7 years.[69] Interpreting these trials is challenging, as intention-to-treat and treatment received may not align, thereby biasing the conclusions. Post hoc analysis of these data suggest that those who were able to receive an endovascular repair enjoyed better outcomes,[69] and therefore it is the recommendation of many to consider an "endovascular-first approach."

Rapidly and effectively treating ruptured AAA requires trained personnel, access to endovascular inventory, and standard standardized protocols.[70] Examples of such may include systems for rapid transport to an operating room with both open surgical and endovascular capability, minimal preoperative testing and imaging, and placement of an aortic occlusion balloon.[71,72] The latter should be placed prior to induction of anesthesia, as it may support blood pressure regardless of the type of repair offered. For patients amenable to EVAR for ruptured AAA, outcomes may be improved if general anesthesia is avoided altogether and the procedure performed under local anesthesia.[71,72]

Of note, many patients with ruptured AAA present with significant comorbidities or severe acutely deteriorating clinical condition. For this reason over the past two to three decades, many scoring systems have been proposed to predict nonsurvivability and therefore consider comfort care instead of attempts at definitive repair. These scoring systems either were developed before the advent of EVAR or have not been validated with contemporary care. The University of Washington scoring system[73] is one of the few that predicts futility rather than increased mortality risk and therefore may be more useful. A recent institutional study demonstrated that only a very small proportion of patients met futility criteria with this scoring system. Additionally, outcomes out-performed all predictive models, thereby raising concerns of the clinical usefulness of such scoring systems.[74] As such, each patient should be judged individually to determine suitability for intervention and definitive repair.

With increasing specialization of vascular surgery and expansion of EVAR for ruptured AAA, many hospitals are no longer equipped to provide care, thereby necessitating the need for transfer of these critically ill patients. Utilization of transfer appears to be increasing,[70] creating additional challenges for timely intervention. When available, local care may represent the best treatment; for although operative mortality is better for transferred patients, overall mortality is worse.[70] This paradox is most likely explained by selection bias of those who are clinically stable to receive treatment once they arrive at the receiving hospital. In fact, approximately one in seven patients who are transferred do not receive treatment,[70] which may be due to clinical deterioration, severe comorbidities that may not have been recognized at the sending hospital, or patient refusal. To address this, current guidelines[19] as well as regional societies[75] provide recommendations for transferring patients with ruptured AAA to optimize the transfer process and provide the greatest opportunity for definitive repair in transferred patients.

Aortic Dissection, Intramural Hematoma, and Penetrating Aortic Ulcers

We consider AD, IMH, and PAU together because of the interplay between these three disease states, and each may be representative of the same disease within a spectrum and in fact may occur together. What separates the three, in part, is the level of involvement of the aortic wall. While aneurysmal disease involves all three layers of the aorta, PAU is a disease of the intima and media, and AD and IMH a disease of the media, with significant overlap between the three.

Aortic Dissection

Acute AD is the most common clinical emergency involving the aorta, but the incidence is only an estimate due to a number of factors, including difficulties in making the diagnosis antemortem. Various prospective population studies and retrospective registries give estimates of the incidence range from 3.5 to 16.3 cases per 100,000 patient-years.[76,77] Men are more frequently diagnosed with an AD compared to women (16 per 100,000 compared to 7.9 per 100,000), and women present later, are older, and have worse in-hospital and surgical mortalities.[78] TAADs occur more commonly than Type B AD by a 2:1 ratio for the population as a whole, although Type B AD is more common than TAAD amongst black patients (52.4% vs. 47.6%).[79] Compared to aneurysmal disease, dissections occur in all age groups, although there is a bimodal pattern with older patients having associated risk factors of hypertension and atherosclerosis and younger patients having connective tissue and genetic disorders as well as bicuspid aortic valve disease.

Predisposing risk factors of hypertension,[80] connective tissue disorders, vascular inflammation, and disruption of the intima and media (e.g., PAU and IMH) may play a role in the mechanisms leading to the initiation of an AD. Syndromes associated with AD include those with well-known genetic markers and mutations such as Marfan syndrome (mutation of FBN1) and Loey-Dietz (mutation of TGF-β1, TGF-βR2, TGF-β), as well as less common affected genes such as MYH11, ACTA2, and SMAD3. Some of these mechanisms also may be responsible in the development of aneurysmal dissection as well as IMHs. When illicit drug use, including cocaine and methamphetamines, is present or suspected, patients tend to be younger and have Type B dissections.[81] It may not be the acute use of cocaine but rather the long-term atherogenic effects of cocaine that predisposes to AD.[82] Finally, there are potential environmental and social factors that may transcend genetic factors alone. The Registry of Aortic Dissection in China (Sino-RAD), in comparison to the International Registry of Acute Aortic Dissection (IRAD) describes acute TAADs in the Chinese population to occur at an earlier age (mean age 50.5 vs. 61.1 years), less hypertension (51.4% vs. 67%), and greater predominance of men (76.3% vs. 66.9%).[83]

As noted by Elefteriades and colleagues, a dissection can mimic a variety of other medical problems, including an acute coronary syndrome, stroke, paraplegia, lower extremity ischemia, acute renal failure, and an abdominal catastrophe;[84] each of these problems are due to malperfusion. In a review of 526 patients who were ultimately diagnosed with an acute TAAD, 90% had pain as a presenting symptom while slightly over 20% had pain localized in the abdomen.[85] In the same study, the so-called pathognomonic sign of absent or differential pulses was present in only 139 of the 526 patients, and only 31% of patients had normal ECGs with more than 25% of patients having ECG findings of myocardial ischemia, infarction, new Q waves, or ST segment deviations. Such ECG findings could lead to the misdiagnosis of an acute coronary syndrome. Putting the difficulty in diagnosis in perspective, while the incidence of AD is up to 16 per 100,000, this pales in comparison to acute coronary syndromes (440 per 100,000) and pulmonary embolism (69 per 100,000), both conditions which can present similar to AD.[80]

Prior to the widespread introduction and implementation of CT scan, the diagnosis of an AD was made at autopsy in more than 25% of patients with the disease.[86] Both CT and MRI are useful in the diagnostic confirmation of a dissection, with sensitivities and specificities reported to be as high as 100%.[87] CT imaging has the added benefit of providing the "triple-rule-out" (i.e., specific protocols regarding the timing of contrast to rule out [or in] dissection, pulmonary embolism, or coronary artery calcification).[88] TTE is of limited utility for TAAD and no utility in Type B. For TAAD, TTE has a sensitivity range of 35% to 80% and a specificity range of 35% to 96% depending on the location of the tear,[87] and a normal TTE cannot exclude the possibility of a dissection. TEE is more specific (63%–96%) and sensitive (98%) in diagnosing TAAD and will also detect a flap in the descending thoracic aorta.[87] Shiga and colleagues[89] demonstrated that pooled sensitivities (98%–100%) and specificities (95%–98%) were comparable between TEE, contrast CT, and MRI.

TAADs are surgical emergencies requiring, with rare exceptions, open surgical repair. Medical management with impulse control therapy can be used either as a temporizing measure or for palliation in patients not deemed to be surgical candidates.

There are reports of endovascular repairs of TAAD, but this is not the standard of care;[90] although hybrid approaches are becoming more common.[91] An example is the frozen elephant trunk technique that addresses the proximal descending aorta with a covered stent at the time of open therapy of the ascending aorta and arch.[92]

A frequently quoted risk of mortality is 1% to 2%/hr in the first 24 hours.[80] While this is likely true for untreated TAAD, medical management with blood pressure and antiimpulse therapy will reduce the 24-hour mortality rate. Subsequently with surgical intervention, hospital and operative mortality becomes more of a function of patient characteristics than time to diagnosis and treatment. Large clinical databases such as IRAD provide fodder for univariate and multivariate analyses to develop risk models. Mehta and colleagues identified age older than 70 years, abrupt onset of chest pain, shock/tamponade, kidney failure, pulse deficit, and abnormal ECG to be factors in postoperative mortality.[93] A subsequent refinement divided the model into preoperative factors as well as intraoperative findings, with the need for coronary artery bypass grafting and the observation of right ventricular dysfunction boding poorly.[94] Interestingly, right hemiarch replacement was a favorable factor. More recently, an observation that patients without evidence of malperfusion had a lower mortality rate than those who presented with malperfusion has led to the development of a risk-score that considers three variables: creatinine, lactic acid, and evidence of liver malperfusion.[95] The gamut of symptoms described by Elefteriades and colleagues[84] is primarily due to different degrees and distributions of malperfusion raising the issue of whether to address the malperfusion prior to surgical repair of the dissection. This appears to have some benefit for operative mortality but may increase the risk for early and late mortality,[96] and the challenge is to develop an algorithm to identify patients who will benefit from revascularization prior to central repair.[97] Overall operative mortality rates for acute TAAD are typically reported in the range of 15% to 25%[85,98] and are in single digits in specialized, multidisciplinary aortic surgery programs.[99]

Medical management of Type B dissections is favored initially unless there is evidence of rupture or malperfusion (complicated Type B AD). Selective β-blockade remains the preferred first line treatment with the dual ability to lower blood pressure and reduce aortic tension from the pressure impulse (dP/dt). The ultimate goal is a reduction of pulse pressure while maintaining end-organ perfusion with an appreciation that some antihypertensive medications may increase pulse pressure while reducing mean arterial pressure secondary to their preferential impact on lowering diastolic pressure. This conservative approach preendovascular era comes from the finding that in the acute phase for stable Type B dissections, the risk of intervention exceeds the risk of waiting.[100] With the development of endovascular techniques, TEVAR has emerged as the treatment of choice for complicated dissections (i.e., with rupture or malperfusion)[101,102] and as an option for noncomplicated dissections;[103] although medical management remains the recommended standard of care for noncomplicated AD.[104] The primary goals of endovascular therapy include coverage of the primary intimal tear and obliteration and/or thrombosis of the false lumen. Fattori and colleagues showed that in-hospital mortality for open surgical repair of acute Type B AD was almost 34%, compared to TEVAR and medical management, which were both in the range of 10%.[105] The majority of patients (68.3%) in this study were medically managed, and open surgical repair and TEVAR reserved for complicated dissections.

The mortality rate for open surgically managed patients seen in Fattori and colleagues[105] was substantially higher than other studies, as noted in a subsequent metaanalysis[106] in which the pooled mortality rate was 17.5%. The disparity in results may reflect the paucity of studies that directly and randomly compare TEVAR with open surgery or medical management, as well as clear distinctions of complicated versus uncomplicated designations and acuity.

The first prospective trial to investigate TEVAR for uncomplicated acute Type B AD was the INSTEAD (Investigation of Stent Grafts in Aortic Dissection) trial.[102] At two years, there was no difference in all-cause deaths or aortic-related deaths, but remodeling was favorable in the TEVAR group compared to the medical management cohort.[107] These results were attributed to an underpowered study. The ADSORB trial (Acute Dissection: Stent Graft OR Best Medical Therapy)[103] was a small trial prospectively comparing best medical therapy (BMT, n = 31) with BMT and TEVAR (n = 30) in patients with uncomplicated Type B acute AD. The end-point was a composite of completeness of false lumen thrombosis, continued aortic growth more than 5 mm or a maximum aortic diameter larger than 55 mm, or descending or abdominal aortic rupture at one year. At one year, the results favored BMT and TEVAR, chiefly due to completeness of false lumen thrombosis in the BMT and TEVAR group (57% vs. 3%, $P < 0.001$).[108] The clinical significance of the findings from ADSORB, which was not powered to detect differences in aortic-related and all-cause mortality, remains unclear. An extension of the INSTEAD trial (INSTEAD-XL) did find a benefit in aortic-related mortality in the TEVAR cohort at 5 years.[109]

The PETTICOAT (Provisional Extension to Induce Complete Attachment) technique was initially described as an adjunct to TEVAR for complicated acute Type B dissection.[110] The original report noted that in 12 of 100 patients treated with TEVAR, there was persistent flow in the distal false lumen with true lumen collapse. With the subsequent deployment of an uncovered stent distal to the previously implanted stent-graft, there was reperfusion of the true lumen and abolishment of malperfusion. These results persisted at one year and there was evidence of improved aortic remodeling.[110] This technique has been modified further to address the distal aorta in open repair of acute TAAD (DeBakey type 1) as part of a frozen elephant trunk technique.[111] An "extended" technique (e-PETTICOAT) has been proposed to preemptively address the entire descending thoracic and abdominal aorta with the anticipated benefits being complete aortic remodeling and prevention of aneurysmal progression.[112]

Intramural Hematoma

IMH is a subadventitial lesion usually involving the outer third of the media. The nomenclature of IMH follows the Stanford dissection classification, so IMH involving the ascending aorta is Type A IMH, and that confined to the descending aorta is Type B IMH. One common hypothesis for the development of IMH is the rupture of a vaso vasorum with subsequent intramural bleeding and hematoma formation,[113] but others have suggested that IMH may reflect an unrecognized AD subsequently seen on pathologic examination[114] or demonstrated using submillimeter spatial resolution contrast-enhanced multidetector computer tomography.[115]

IMH accounts for approximately 10% of acute aortic syndromes in Western countries[116] and may be higher in Asian countries.[117] The incidence may be underestimated either due to misclassification of IMH as a discrete dissection or the evolution of IMH into an AD during transfer to a tertiary center for treatment.[116] In contrast to AD, there is a slight predominance of IMH seen in women compared to men,[118] Type B IMH occurs more frequently than Type A IMH,[116] and patients with IMH tend to be older and more likely hypertensive.[98] Marfan's syndrome or other connective tissue disorders do not appear to play a role in the development of IMH.[119] Similar to AD and PAU, patients present with chest or back pain, but in contrast, the pain in IMH does not often radiate.[98] The clinical presentation of IMH may be suggestive in differentiating from AD before diagnostic imaging confirms the diagnosis; in Type A IMH aortic valve insufficiency, distal malperfusion, and ECG abnormalities are not as frequent as in AD, but the presence of a pericardial effusion is increased in incidence.[116,120]

The *sine qua non* for diagnostic noninvasive imaging requires the presence of a thickened aortic wall (localized or circumferential) greater than 5 mm with no detectable blood flow on CT imaging, and the combination of CT imaging with and without contrast has reported sensitivities greater than 95%.[42] TEE has been shown to have both a high sensitivity (100%) and specificity (91%) for IMH.[121]

Management of IMH is similar to that of AD, with medical management generally limited to Type B IMH, and antiimpulse therapy with a selective β-blocker as the therapy of choice. As in the case of AD, medical management failure includes persistent pain and uncontrollable hypertension, as well as progressively enlarging wall thickness more than 11 mm and recurrent pleural effusions.[42] Interestingly, in contrast to AD, Falconi and colleagues demonstrated that medical and surgical management of Type B IMH had similar mortality rates (19% vs. 17%, respectively),[122] and because of this Type B IMH is more likely to be managed medically than Type B AD.[116]

Emergent or urgent management of Type A IMH is typically recommended, especially in the setting of a pericardial effusion and ongoing pain;[42] although in a selected group of patients, initial medical management and optimization has been reported.[123] Open surgical repair of Type A IMH proceeds similar to that of TAAD with two caveats. First, "normal" aorta may not be identified distally, so surgical judgement as to the extent of resection is important, and second, clamping of the aorta may convert the IMH into a dissection upon release of the cross clamp, presumably due to the creation of intimal tears with the placement of the clamp.

Similar to Type B AD, endovascular repairs have emerged as a treatment option for Type B IMH. For an uncomplicated Type B IMH, the European Consensus Guidelines recommend initial medical management and surveillance with noninvasive imaging (Class I recommendation). With expansion of the hematoma, development of a periaortic hematoma, recurrent pain, or conversion to a frank dissection, the recommendations switch to TEVAR (Class IIa) or open repair (Class IIb).[42] Li and colleagues compared TEVAR with optimal medical management and in their small series showed no progression of IMH or mortality with the endovascular approach.[124] Bischoff and colleagues also compared TEVAR with medical management, and in support of the equipoise seen by Falconi and colleagues,[122] showed no difference in early or late mortality, incidence of complete remodeling, or regression between the two groups.[125] The results suggested that TEVAR might be reserved for specific cases of Type B IMH. The difficulty with TEVAR in Type B IMH is determining the extent of coverage, similar to determining the extent of open repair. Since there (by definition) is no primary intimal tear, coverage territory becomes either presumptive of where the process started or targeted in the case of a periaortic hematoma or associated PAU.[126]

Penetrating Aortic Ulcer

As noted, PAU involves both the intima and media, arising from an ulceration of an atherosclerotic plaque that has penetrated the elastic lamina. PAU can be associated with IMH, serve as a nidus for AD, or lead to the development of a saccular pseudoaneurysm. Coady and colleagues found that in 7.6% of their patients treated for either Type A or B AD had an associated PAU.[127] Isolated PAU accounts for 2% to 7% of AAS,[128] and while there is an overall slight predominance in men,[127] PAU occurs more frequently in the thoracic aorta in women and more frequently in the abdominal aorta in men.[129] When considering only the thoracic aorta in PAU, for both men and women the descending aorta is the predominant site of occurrence 90% of the time.[130]

In contrast to AD and IMH, pain may not be a component of PAU. In a Mayo Center study, 87% of patients with PAU were asymptomatic at the time of diagnosis,[129] and often the ulcer is detected incidentally. PAU is defined by a distinct, focal outpouching through an area of intimal calcification or in an area with associated diffuse atherosclerosis when contrast-enhanced CT scanning is performed.

Asymptomatic PAU may be managed medically with antiimpulse therapy and routine surveillance noninvasive imaging, but early intervention has been suggested for large PAUs, specifically when the greatest diameter is larger than 20 mm or the neck is larger than 10 mm.[131] This approach has not been validated longitudinally.[128] With open surgical repair, the involved segment is resected and replaced with a prosthetic graft or homograft. However, since PAU is associated with, and defined by the presence of, severe atherosclerosis and calcification, finding normal aorta proximally and/or distally to sew to may be difficult. While studies on the efficacy of endovascular repair for PAU are lacking, limited data have shown good results for TEVAR in the setting of PAU and pseudoaneurysm formation or rupture.[128] The same challenges for open repair of PAU, namely extensive atherosclerosis, may pose problems if the atherosclerotic disease extends into the peripheral (and therefore, access) vessels or if the presence of laminated thrombus associated with PAU makes achieving a safe landing zone difficult.[126]

Blunt Thoracic Aortic Injury

The overall incidence of blunt thoracic aortic injury (BTAI) as a component of trauma admissions is 0.3%, based on an analysis of the National Trauma Databank over a 5-year period.[132] Of the 3114 patients with BTAI, 4% were dead on arrival and 19% died during triage. Excluding these patients, 31% also had a major head injury and 29% had a major abdominal injury.[132] Motor vehicle crashes remain the most common mechanism of aortic injury (>70%),[133] and BTAI may have been involved in 33% of the motor vehicle deaths in 2010.[134]

Although the entire aorta is susceptible to BTAI, the most common site of injury is at the isthmus (approximately 54%–66%) based on autopsy studies[135] and is typically a transverse tear. There are different proposed mechanisms for the pathogenesis of BTAI based on the variety of mechanical forces potentially being applied to the aorta. One proposed mechanism is "stretching" of the aortic wall secondary to intrinsic weakness at the isthmus and rather immobile distal descending aorta relative to the arch and ascending aorta.[136] Another hypothesis includes bending, torsion, and shearing stresses over the spine in high impact injuries.[137] A third is the Archimedes Lever Hypothesis that proposes a lever system where the long arm is the proximal aorta and aortic arch, the short arm is the aortic isthmus, and the great vessels serve as

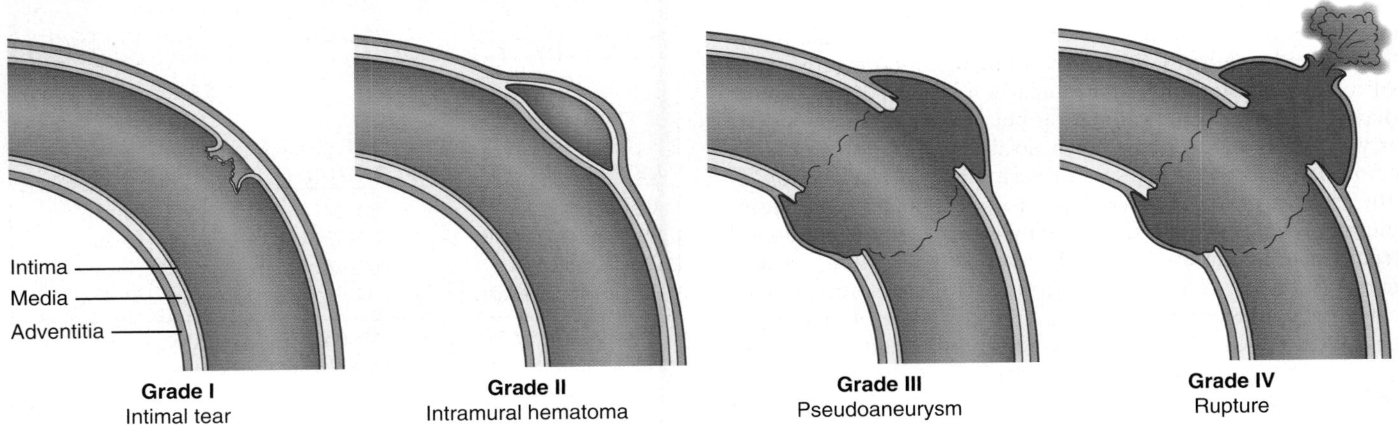

FIG. 62.7 Classification of blunt thoracic aortic injury.

a fulcrum.[138] Simulations of lateral impact motor vehicle crashes have shown that the magnified forces mediated by the "long arm" provide sufficient strain on the "short arm" to result in rupture.[138] It is likely that a combination of all of mechanisms play a role in BTAI etiology.

The classification of BTAI is based on the extent of the damage to the aortic wall layers. There are four different grades ranging from intimal tear (grade I) to rupture (grade IV), each with different management strategies (Fig. 62.7). Grade I injuries do not cause any changes to the external aortic contour and is best visualized with either CTA or IVUS as angiogram may be interpreted as normal. Grade II injury causes an abnormal aortic contour that can be visualized on CTA, IVUS, or angiography. Grade III and IV injuries can be visualized with any imaging modality. At the time of the American Association for the Surgery of Trauma multicenter trial of BAI (AAST I trial), aortography was the most common diagnostic modality and the standard treatment was open operative repair if the patient was stable.[139]

The most common finding on plain film chest radiograph is a widened mediastinum, but it may also show apical pleural cap, loss of the aortopulmonary window, rightward deviation of the mediastinal structures or endotracheal tube (if present), or depression of the left mainstem bronchus. Multidetector CTA is now the gold standard diagnostic modality for BTAI in the updated AAST.[139] Modern treatment has changed dramatically with treatment options of aggressive blood pressure control and increasing indications for endovascular repair. Current guidelines by the SVS recommend expectant management with strict blood pressure control and serial imaging (repeat CTA in six weeks) for grade I injuries—as most heal spontaneously[140]—and repair of grades II to IV injuries. In Arthurs and colleagues' review, 68% of patients with BTAI surviving to treatment were treated medically, but aortic repair independently improved survival after controlling for associated injuries.[132]

For medical management of grade I BTAI, Fabian and colleagues recommended maintenance systolic blood pressure less than 100 mm Hg or mean arterial pressure less than 80 mm Hg along with heart rate control less than 100 beats per minute.[139] These parameters were achieved using intravenous β-blockade (esmolol or labetalol).[139] Nitroprusside was added if satisfactory blood pressure not achieved with β-blockers alone.

Since the first report of endovascular repair of a traumatic injury to the thoracic aorta in 1997 by Kato and colleagues,[141] data have increased substantially to support use of endovascular stent graft over traditional open repair. Earlier experience did not show a difference in mortality rates between open and endovascular repair (19% vs. 18%, respectively).[132] Improvements in techniques and technology have led to consistently reduced rates of mortality (8%–9% vs. 19%), paraplegia (0.5%–3% vs. 3%–9%), and end-stage renal disease (5% vs. 8%) as well as a comparable stroke rate (2.5% vs. 1%).[142] The Society of Vascular Surgery recommends that for those undergoing repair that the timing is within 24 hours in the absence of other serious injuries, repaired immediately after other injuries have been treated, or at the latest before the patient is discharged from the hospital.[140] They also advocate endovascular repair in anatomically suitable candidates with selective revascularization of the left SCA, routine heparin administration (at a lower dose than elective TEVAR), general anesthesia, and open femoral exposure.[140] The presence of an adequate 2-cm proximal seal zone in many cases requires partial or complete coverage of the left SCA, as the aortic isthmus is the most common site of injury. According to the SVS practice guidelines, the decision to perform revascularization of the left SCA is individualized and must consider the status of the right vertebral anatomy and posterior circulation, availability of surgical expertise, condition of the patient, and presence of other injuries.[140] Revascularization is accomplished with a carotid subclavian bypass. Patients with ascending aorta or aortic arch injuries should undergo open repair if feasible, as they are not candidates for endovascular repair.

SPECIFIC CONSIDERATIONS IN SURGICAL MANAGEMENT

The surgical management of aortic disease, whether open, endovascular, or a hybrid approach, is continuously being refined as new techniques, devices, and understanding of disease processes evolve. What follows is not meant to be a "how I do it" synopsis but rather a brief summary of special considerations for specific pathologies with an appreciation that every patient presents a unique set of challenges.

Acute Type A Aortic Dissection

Open surgical repair of an acute TAAD remains the standard of care when the patient is a surgical candidate. As reported by IRAD, in tertiary medical centers with expertise in the treatment of acute TAAD in the years from 1995 to 2013, the proportion of patients relegated to medical management declined from 21% to 10% with a corresponding decline in surgical mortality rate from 25%

to 18%.[143] Relative contraindications to surgery would include advanced age,[144] multiple comorbidities, and neurologic status. Stamou and colleagues did not see a difference in operative mortality or major morbidity in a comparison between patients older than 70 years and those younger,[145] but octogenarians do not fare as well.[146] IRAD data has shown no difference in outcomes for octogenarians treated with surgical versus medical intervention.[147] The presence of cerebrovascular accident or coma has a significant impact on hospital survival, but for patients who undergo surgical repair there is improved survival compared to medical management. In 84.3% of patients presenting with cerebrovascular accident who underwent surgical repair, there was resolution of the neurologic deficit.[148] Softer contraindications include concern for the risk of bleeding secondary to antithrombotic medication,[83] and the patient's refusal for blood transfusions (i.e., in the case of a Jehovah Witness).

Once the decision is made to proceed with surgery, the primary goal of surgery is the elimination of the entry tear and obliteration of the false lumen in the aortic root and ascending aorta. Successful completion of these goals will often address secondary issues, such as aortic valve insufficiency and distal visceral malperfusion. Specific considerations are the cannulation strategy, cerebral protection, conduct of cardiopulmonary bypass, and the proximal and distal extent of resection and repair.

Traditionally, femoral cannulation was the primary access for establishing arterial inflow for cardiopulmonary bypass due in part to the ability to rapidly establish access via surgical cut-down or percutaneously. The decision as to which vessel to approach is paradoxical in the sense that the femoral artery most likely to be in continuity with the true lumen is the one without the pulse (due to true lumen collapse). The clinical situation in which true lumen collapse was occurring and the wrong vessel cannulated would result in high circuit line pressures. Malperfusion from femoral cannulation is uncommon. Axillary artery access grew popular in part by the ability to use this approach as part of a selective cerebral perfusion technique during periods of circulatory arrest.[149] Additional benefits include the avoidance of atheroembolization and false lumen perfusion.[150] Other approaches include arterial access via the apex of the left ventricle with the cannula traversing the aortic valve,[151] direct cannulation of the true lumen after transection of the ascending aorta ("Samurai" technique[152]), and echo-guided cannulation of ascending aorta/arch using a Seldinger technique.[153]

With some exceptions, acute TAAD repair is performed with a period of hypothermic circulatory arrest. The initial approach to the arch reported by DeBakey and colleagues[154] included a multicatheter approach to the great vessels and one of the femoral arteries to provide arterial inflow without circulatory arrest. Hypothermic circulatory arrest (Table 62.3) allows the establishment of a bloodless field allowing for the evaluation of the distal ascending aorta and arch to confirm intimal integrity, ensures graft continuity to the true lumen, and assists in obliteration of the false lumen.[155] Profound hypothermic circulatory arrest provides 30 to 40 minutes of protective cerebral time; deep hypothermia alone should be sufficient for open-distal and hemi-arch repairs. The use of unilateral selective antegrade (SACP) or bilateral antegrade cerebral circulatory perfusion extends this protective time. With the adjunct of SACP, moderate hypothermia has been shown to be safe and effective.[156] Cerebral perfusion during SACP (with right axillary cannulation) is via the right carotid and assumes the absence of right carotid stenosis and an intact Circle of Willis. Concern for coagulopathy secondary to hypothermia has been raised,[157] but adequate rewarming should be sufficient to address this concern.[158]

TABLE 62.3 Level of hypothermia and duration of circulatory arrest.

LEVEL	NASOPHARYNGEAL TEMPERATURE (ºC)	ESTIMATED SAFE DURATION OF CIRCULATORY ARREST (MIN)
Mild hypothermia	28.1–34	<10
Moderate hypothermia	20.1–28	10–20
Deep hypothermia	14.1–20	20–30
Profound hypothermia	≤14	30–40

Adapted from Yan TD, Bannon PG, Bavaria J, et al. Consensus on hypothermia in aortic arch surgery. *Ann Cardiothorac Surg.* 2013;2:163–168.

Once the patient is successfully cannulated and cardiopulmonary bypass initiated, systemic cooling is started with the target temperature based on surgeon preference, experience, and patient characteristics. Topical ice on the patient's head is typically included, although evidence of its efficacy is limited.[159] There is currently no consensus regarding the rate of cooling or the acid-based management strategy (alpha stat vs. pH stat) during cooling, and the surgeon should discuss with the anesthesia and perfusion team the target temperature as part of the operative plan. Routine clamping of the ascending aorta during cooling is not necessary. Distention of the left ventricle may occur because of the presence of aortic valve insufficiency. If the distention is significant, the ventricle can be vented a number of ways, including catheters inserted via the right superior pulmonary vein, the pulmonary artery, or directly via the apex of the ventricle. If unsuccessful in reducing the distention, the ascending aorta can be clamped and transected proximally with concomitant myocardial protection via retrograde or direct antegrade cardioplegia. The suggestion is made for routine clamping of the ascending aorta during the cooling phase, with the proximal portion of the repair completed during this phase to lessen the length of cardiopulmonary bypass period.[160] However, the length of the surgery is more impacted by the rewarming than the cooling phase. Additionally, when the distal anastomosis is completed first, the anastomosis can be tested with direct vision of the entire suture line, and rewarming then initiated while the proximal aorta is dealt with.[42]

If selective cerebral perfusion and circulatory arrest is used, when the target temperature is achieved, the patient is placed in a Trendelenburg position and the surgical field can be flooded with CO_2 to minimize cerebral microbubbles when the arch is opened. The ascending aorta is then opened and the arch examined. Once the extent of repair has been decided, the base of the innominate artery is clamped and SACP started with a typical rate of 10 to 15 cc/kg and perfusion pressure of 40 to 50 mm Hg. The extent of repair, both proximally and distally, has also been a subject of debate. The aortic root is not infrequently involved, and oftentimes resuspension of the aortic valve commissures in addition to reapproximating the walls of the sinuses is sufficient to provide integrity to the aorta as well as correcting aortic valve insufficiency. Barring this, the root should be addressed at the time of repair. As in the case of elective root replacement (see below) there are a number of ways of accomplishing this, but the goal should be to pick the procedure that can be most efficiently and successfully accomplished.

Aortic Root Replacement

Aortic root replacement is primarily for aneurysmal disease or TAAD but is also performed in certain cases of aortic valve endocarditis as well as reoperative aortic valve replacement. There are three standard approaches to replacement of the aortic root: composite valve grafts (CVGs; mechanical or biologic), complete tissue replacement (either cadaveric homograft or autograft [Ross Procedure]), and valve-sparing root replacement (remodeling, reattachment, and Florida sleeve).

As noted earlier, the boundaries of the aortic root are the aortic annulus proximally and the sinotubular junction distally; components of the root include the aortic valve and ostia of the coronary arteries. Thus, when the aortic root is repaired or replaced, with few specific exceptions, the coronaries are always reimplanted or bypassed, the valve is addressed (replaced or spared), and circulatory arrest is not needed unless the ascending aorta is also impacted and needs to be replaced.

Modifications to the procedure, as originally described by Bentall and colleagues,[161] have made the term Bentall procedure an anachronism. The original description was a CVG with an inclusion technique to deal with the coronaries (i.e., sewing the coronaries onto the graft not as Carrel buttons but rather in a side-to-side fashion). Wheat preceded Bentall in an earlier publication describing a technique where the valve and graft were separate and the coronaries reimplanted on "tongues of aortic wall" extending from the annulus.[162] Subsequent work by Kouchoukos and colleagues[163] incorporated the now familiar coronary button technique. The composite valve graft concept evolved into preconstructed composites, initially with a mechanical valve followed with biologic valves as an option. With a mechanical and tissue option, the indications for the type of CVG used is the same as for a valve-replacement (e.g., mechanical valves favored in younger patients due to durability, tissue valves in older patients, or when life-long anticoagulation is not a reasonable option).

Balancing the desire for a durable valve or root replacement with avoidance of life-long anticoagulation led to a number of innovated techniques. Work by Lower and Shumway[164,165] and promoted by Ross resulted in the eponymous Ross procedure.[166] This technique is an autotransplantation of the pulmonary valve into the aortic position and subsequent replacement of the pulmonary artery root with a cadaveric homograft. While the procedure never gained popularity in adult patients, it remains a viable alternative, especially when performed in high-volume environments.[167] An alternative to the Ross procedure is replacement of the aortic root with a cadaveric homograft, notably in the setting of aortic valve endocarditis with destruction of the aorta annulus. Both of these procedures have the theoretical advantage of the lack of need for anticoagulation as well as an increase in durability compared to a tissue valve. However, both procedures are technically challenging and the outcomes dependent on the experience of the surgeon.

Dilatation of the aortic root or of the sinotubular junction because of an ascending aortic aneurysm may result in valve insufficiency in the face of normal valve leaflets. In this setting, the replacement of the normal valve while addressing the aortic root or ascending aorta seems like overkill. With sinotubular junction dilatation alone, replacement of the ascending aorta with a downsized graft may be sufficient to restore the aortic valve competency.[168] With root dilatation and an anatomically normal valve, two valve-sparing approaches have been popularized: the remodeling technique and the reimplantation technique, championed respectively by Yacoub and David. Miller has summarized the techniques referenced as David I through V (Table 62.4).[169] While expansion on each of the valve-sparing techniques is beyond the scope of this chapter, Miller summarizes the differences between the Yacoub remodeling and David reimplantation technique by the number of suture lines; remodeling employs two aortic suture lines, and reimplantation three. Both techniques use a Dacron graft as the neoaorta and both, as previously mentioned for root replacements, require reimplantation of the coronary ostia. There is an exception to the comment that the coronaries are always reimplanted (i.e., the Florida Sleeve technique[170] where "slots" are made on the Dacron graft to accommodate the coronaries).

TABLE 62.4 Miller classification of David valve-sparing root replacement.

NAME	CLASSIFICATION	DESCRIPTION
David I	Reimplantation	Implantation in cylindric tube graft
David II	Remodeling	Classic Yacoub
David III	Remodeling	David II combined with aortic annuloplasty
David IV	Reimplantation	David I with 4-mm larger graft and plication at the sinotubular junction
David V	Reimplantation	David I with 6–8 mm larger graft and plication at sinotubular junction and annulus to create pseudosinuses

Adapted from Miller DC. Valve-sparing aortic root replacement in patients with the Marfan syndrome. *J Thorac Cardiovasc Surg*. 2003;125:773–778.

Open Surgery of the Descending Thoracic Aorta

Open surgical repair of thoracic aortic pathology has changed dramatically since the introduction of endovascular techniques.[51] While TEVAR has a predominant role in the management of thoracic aortic disease, there remain clinical scenarios in which knowledge of open approaches to the thoracic aorta are an important part of the surgeon's armamentarium. As mentioned previously, TEVAR may not always be appropriate or doable for some Type B ADs and, with a few exceptions, not applicable to patients with Marfan disease or other connective tissue disorders. Issues regarding spinal cord protection and intraoperative monitoring are pertinent to open and endovascular techniques. Considerations specific to open surgery include the need and approach to distal perfusion ("clamp-and-sew," left heart bypass, cardiopulmonary bypass) as well as access. Many of the issues and considerations with open thoracic aortic surgery also pertain to TAAAs (see below).

Hemodynamic monitoring, specifically invasive arterial lines, during open repair of thoracic aneurysms and dissections is required and may necessitate transducing from both upper and lower body sites depending on the surgical plan. Pulmonary artery catheterization is not typically helpful during the intraoperative period but can be useful in postoperative management. Use of TEE is reasonable in open surgery (as well as TEVAR) and carries a Class IIa recommendation in a 2010 consensus statement.[171] A second Class IIa monitoring recommendation relates to spinal cord perfusion, acknowledging the potential for the devastation of spinal cord ischemia following surgery on the thoracic aorta. While not a therapeutic modality, motor or somatosensory evoked potential monitoring can help guide therapy and alterations in intraoperative management.[171]

Avoidance of spinal cord injury secondary to ischemia is paramount in surgery of the thoracic and thoracoabdominal aorta for both open and endovascular approaches. Adjuncts used include cerebrospinal fluid (CSF) drainage, distal perfusion (either left-heart bypass or cardiopulmonary bypass with femorofemoral cannulation), hypothermia, and pharmacotherapeutics. The rationale for CSF drainage is to increase spinal cord perfusion pressure (SCPP) by lowering CSF pressure. By definition, SCPP is:

$$\text{SCPP} = \text{Mean distal aortic pressure} - (\text{CSF pressure} + \text{Central venous pressure})$$

Thus, SCPP can be favorably increased with increases in distal aortic pressure, decreasing CSF pressure (by drainage) and decreasing central venous pressure. Management of the CSF drain varies between setting a limit of CSF pressure (e.g., 10–15 mm Hg) to draining at a constant rate (e.g., 10–20 cc/h). Whichever approach is used, two things must be remembered. First, in instances of acute changes in neurologic status, an immediate drainage of 10 to 20 ccs of CSF may salvage the spinal cord. Second, the two other variables related to SCPP—namely, mean aortic pressure and central venous pressure—can also be manipulated to maximize SCPP. CSF drainage is not innocuous with almost 10% of patients developing a postdural puncture headache and 2.8% reported risk of intracranial hemorrhage, the majority being subdural hematomas.[172]

Maintenance of distal aortic pressure and perfusion of visceral branches (including collaterals to the spinal cord) can be supplemented with circulatory support. For procedures of the thoracic aorta associated with dissection, cardiopulmonary bypass may be preferable since it provides not only circulatory support but also a mechanism for temperature regulation and rapid volume infusion. For both thoracic and thoracoabdominal procedures, the use of hypothermic circulatory arrest has been championed because of the elimination of the need for proximal and sequential aortic clamping (and the periaortic dissection required), easy proximal access to the arch, a bloodless field, and the ability to return all shed blood back to the perfusion circuit.[173] Interestingly, Coselli and colleagues found no difference in paraplegia rates for descending thoracic aortic aneurysms with left heart bypass compared to the "clamp-and-sew" technique (4% vs. 2.3%, respectively, $P = 0.3$).[174]

Thoracoabdominal Aortic Aneurysms

For TAAA repair, an incision entering both the thoracic and abdominal compartments is required and represents a significant physiologic stress. For this reason, preoperative work-up may be more extensive, including pulmonary function tests and more intense evaluation of cardiac function. Although repair can be performed with a clamp-and-sew technique, most high-volume centers perform repair with either left heart bypass or full cardiopulmonary bypass with hypothermic arrest.[173,175] This approach is specifically advantageous for Extent II TAAA that do not have a safe location for clamping the most proximal aorta.

As in descending thoracic aortic procedures, paraplegia is an uncommon but feared complication of TAAA repair. Mortality after TAAA repair is significantly increased should paraplegia develop.[176] The risk of paraplegia is increased with Extent II TAAA, TAAA associated with AD, acute presentations, or previous infrarenal aortic surgery.[177] Increase in SCPP as previously discussed may be protective. Other approaches to maximize spinal cord perfusion include intercostal artery reimplantation[178] and maintenance of central perfusion. Strategies to decrease the metabolic rate of the spinal cord may include preoperative steroids,[179] the use of a naloxone drip,[180] moderate hypothermia (to 34°C),[181] and injection of propofol just prior to clamping.[182]

Construction of the visceral component of the graft may depend on the underlying cause for repair. For patients with degenerative TAAA, a Carrel patch may be considered for the reimplantation of the visceral vessels. This approach many simplify the operation and decrease the visceral ischemia time but may run the risk of future degeneration of the residual aorta and subsequent pseudoaneurysm formation.[183] For those with connective tissue disorders or aneurysmal degeneration of a previous dissection, most would consider individual branch grafts to each visceral artery, thereby eliminating any suspect aortic tissue in the repair.

Open Infrarenal Abdominal Aortic Aneurysm Repair

Open repair can be performed through a transabdominal or retroperitoneal approach. Advantages of the transabdominal approach include the ability to inspect the abdominal contents, supraceliac control without entering the thorax, and better exposure of the right iliac bifurcation and external iliac arteries. Potential disadvantages may include hernia formation, increased risk of bowel obstruction, and perhaps an increased risk of late aortoenteric fistula. With this approach, after the abdominal contents are inspected, the omentum and transverse colon is retracted cephalad and the small intestines are retracted to the patient's right to expose the retroperitoneum and the ligament of Treitz. The ligament is taken down and the duodenum is retracted to the right. A slip of tissue should be left attached to the duodenum for closure of this space after the repair. A self-retaining retractor can be helpful to maintain optimal exposure.

The posterior parietal peritoneum is incised to expose the aorta and the dissection carried proximally to expose the neck. The inferior mesenteric vein is generally encountered and should be identified, retracted, or ligated. As the dissection is carried cephalad the left renal vein is encountered. This vein can be duplicated or travel behind the aorta; its course can and should be identified on preoperative imaging. The left renal vein can be retracted and, if needed, the adrenal and gonadal veins can be divided to provide more mobility of the left renal vein. Some have advocated for division of the left renal vein;[184] if this is considered, the adrenal and gonadal veins must be left intact, as they will subsequently provide the venous drainage of the left kidney. Proximal aortic control should be obtained at healthy aorta and with enough room to safely place sutures. Control can be either circumferential, which may allow a transversely oriented aortic occlusion clamp, or anterior and on either side of the aorta with the dissection carried down to the spine.

The dissection is then carried distally. If a tube graft is considered, it is safer to control the bilateral proximal iliac arteries to avoid injury to the iliac veins that travel directly behind the arteries and may be more densely adherent at the aortic bifurcation. If dissection and arterial control is required at or past the iliac bifurcation, care should be taken to avoid the ureters as they traverse anteriorly at this level.

Once the dissection is complete, the patient should be given heparin at 10 units/kg prior to clamping with a goal activated clotting time (ACT) of 250 to 300 seconds. Once clamped, the aneurysm is opened and thrombus is removed. Back-bleeding from lumbar vessels should be controlled with suture ligatures. The origin of the IMA should be inspected. If back-bleeding is absent or brisk it can also be suture-ligated; however, if back bleeding is scant the IMA should be preserved for possible reimplantation.

Appropriately sized polyester or polytetrafluoroethylene graft is then sewn into place, first proximally and then distally. The vessels are flushed to remove all debris and then flow is slowly reestablished, making certain that the blood pressure remains stable. If a bifurcated graft is required, flow should be reestablished to one limb at a time. Heparin is then reversed if needed, hemostasis is secured, and then the sigmoid colon is interrogated for ischemia visually and with a Doppler probe; if present, the IMA should be reimplanted with either a Carrel patch or interposition graft.

The wound is closed in layers, starting with the aneurysm sac and then posterior parietal peritoneum to protect the repair from the intestines. The remainder of the incision is then closed in a standard fashion.

Retroperitoneal exposure is generally performed with the patient in a semilateral position and through an oblique incision to the tip of the eleventh rib. The incision can be extended into the chest for more proximal control if needed. With this approach the left kidney is usually left down for infrarenal exposure but can be retracted upward with the peritoneum for more proximal exposure.

Endovascular Principles

For all endovascular procedures, certain principles apply beginning with careful planning and correct sizing based on device-specific manufacturer's instructions for use. Evaluation of access vessels (typically the common femoral or external iliac arteries) ensures adequate diameter as well as noting the presence of tortuosity and calcification. Verifying healthy arteries will allow for percutaneous access, performed by accessing the anterior noncalcified surface of the common femoral artery with a 5F micropuncture sheath under ultrasound guidance with angiographic confirmation of successful puncture. Deployment of closure devices (if used) occurs after exchanging the micropuncture sheath over a wire to a 7-French sheath. Subsequently after removal of the 7-French sheath, a series of wire and catheter exchanges occurs resulting in the appropriately sized sheath for the chosen endograft device.

Questionable access vessels may require open femoral exposure, with or without a conduit to the more proximal iliac artery. If a conduit is used, generally a 10 mm diameter will assure passage of the delivery device. Once open access is obtained, stiff wires should be place and used for endograft delivery. The patient is anticoagulated with heparin to achieve ACT goal of 250 to 300 seconds, maintained for the remainder of the case. Limiting radiation exposure is paramount, and the recent implementation of image fusion (projection of preoperative CTA scan onto two-dimensional intraoperative fluoroscopic images [2D-3D fusion imaging]) demonstrates a reduction in exposure.[185] When the endograft placement is complete and balloon molding performed, a final angiogram is obtained to investigate the presence of endoleaks. Types 1 and 3 endoleaks are addressed, if present, prior to completion of the case. If a fenestrated endograft is used, perfusion of the kidneys and absence of renal artery kinking, dissection, or renal injury should be confirmed.

Closure of open incisions is standard after reversal of heparin. For percutaneous access, sheaths are removed over a wire as the sutures are secured. Maintaining wire access at this point is important should there be either an iliac artery injury requiring vascular control and/or endovascular repair or the need for placement of an additional closure device. Wires can then be removed after satisfactory hemostasis.

Endovascular Approaches to the Thoracic Aorta

There have not been any randomized controlled trials to compare endovascular to open repair of the thoracic aorta, but nonrandomized studies, metaanalyses, and comparisons to historical data have suggested a decreased incidence of perioperative mortality and morbidity, including paraplegia. In the FDA phase II trial of the GORE TAG device (TAG; W.L. Gore, Flagstaff, AZ), Makaroun and colleagues documented mortality rates of 1.5%, 1.5%, and 0% at 30 days, 1 year, and 2 years, respectively.[186] Early major adverse events included stroke (4%) and paraplegia (3%), which compared favorably with historical numbers. At five years the aneurysm-related mortality was 2.8% in the endovascular patients versus 11.7% in the open controls, although there was no difference when considering all-cause related mortality (68% survival in the endovascular group vs. 67% in the open group).[187] As noted previously, a metaanalysis by Cheng and colleagues of TEVAR versus open surgical repair showed a reduction in 30-day and one-year all-cause mortality (odds ratio of 0.44 and 0.73, respectively) with this reduction in all-cause mortality lost beyond one year.[52] The overall stroke rate was similar between the two groups. This metaanalysis revealed the primary benefit of TEVAR over open surgery to be a significant reduction in the risk of paraplegia and paraparesis.[52] Thus, at least in the early follow-up period, reductions in all-cause mortality and complications favor TEVAR, especially in high surgical risk patients with suitable anatomy.

Considerations for suitable anatomy include appropriate landing zones with possible coverage of the left SCA, vertebral artery anatomy, angulation and tortuosity of the aorta, size and amount of disease in the planned access arteries, and concurrent AAA. For landing zones, it is usually adequate to obtain a 2- to 3-cm seal zone proximally with extension if the aorta is particularly tortuous or angulated. As seen in Figure 62.4, there are five potential landing zones for the ascending aorta, arch, and proximal descending thoracic aorta.

- Zone 0: proximal to the innominate artery
- Zone 1: proximal to the left common carotid artery
- Zone 2: proximal to the origin of the left SCA
- Zone 3: proximal descending thoracic aorta less than 2 cm from the left SCA
- Zone 4: greater than 2 cm from the left SCA and extends to the proximal portion of the descending aorta (level of T6 vertebral body)

Proximal lesions of the thoracic aorta may require coverage of the left SCA, (i.e., Zone 2 landing). In patients with previous coronary revascularization where an *in situ* left internal mammary was used as a conduit, it is essential to perform left SCA revascularization prior to Zone 2 coverage to prevent myocardial ischemia. The overall reported incidence of left SCA coverage in single-center studies ranges from 23% to over 40% incidence with or without left SCA revascularization.[188,189] In a multicenter study, the European Collaborators on Stent/Graft Techniques for Aortic Aneurysm Repair (EUROSTAR) reported 26% of 606 requiring left SCA coverage.[190] In the EUROSTAR study, there was a 2.5% incidence of paraplegia or paraparesis and a 3.1% incidence of stroke. Multivariate regression analysis demonstrated a correlation of spinal cord ischemia and SCA coverage without revascularization (odds ratio 3.9, $P = 0.027$). Paraplegia or stroke occurred in 8.4% of patients with left SCA coverage when prophylactic revascularization was not performed, compared with 0% when it was performed.[190] Freezor and colleagues found that in their TEVAR patients that had strokes, 78% of strokes were in the posterior circulation territory, highlighting the importance in evaluating the vertebral artery anatomy preoperatively to determine those who might be at a higher risk for posterior circulation strokes with acute coverage of the left SCA. All of the patients in Freezor and colleagues[191] had coverage of Zones 0–2 and only one of the six patients had preemptive carotid-subclavian bypass.

Buth and colleagues also found that, in addition to SCA coverage, the use of three or more stents had a significant impact on the development of spinal cord ischemia (odds ratio 3.5, $P = 0.43$). A metaanalysis by Cooper and colleagues reported an incidence of spinal cord ischemia of 2.3% without SCA coverage versus 2.8% with SCA coverage (pooled odds ratio 2.39).[192] As the thyrocervical trunk branches and vertebral artery contribute to the anterior spinal artery, revascularization may be important for prevention of spinal cord ischemia. Woo and colleagues reported their indications for left subclavian revascularization included a dominant left vertebral artery, a stenotic, atretic, hypoplastic (or absent right vertebral artery), an incomplete vertebrobasilar system, a history of arm ischemia, and a patent LIMA-LAD bypass.[189] In a single-center comparison, the reported incidence of spinal cord ischemia with TEVAR was less compared to open repair (6.7% vs. 8.6%, respectively), although it did not reach statistical significance.[193]

Other proposals to reduce the risk of spinal cord ischemia, other than selective left SCA revascularization as mentioned above, include avoiding intraoperative and postoperative hypotension, spinal fluid drainage, and naloxone infusion.[194] It is important to have both preoperative and postoperative protocols in conjunction with your anesthesia team to achieve this. If the patient needs both treatment of abdominal and thoracic aortic pathology, staging the procedures should allow adequate collateralization to develop. The EUROSTAR study found that concomitant open abdominal aorta surgery had a significant impact on the development of spinal cord ischemia (odds ratio 5.5) presumably from interruption of the IMA and/or intercostal and lumbar artery branches.[190]

Finally, another consideration to determine the feasibility of TEVAR is adequacy of access vessels. Ideally, an access vessel measuring at least 8 mm in diameter will be adequate for most device delivery systems. The size of the thoracic aorta generally requires larger endograft devices when compared to EVAR and will therefore require larger sheath access. It is important to have imaging of the abdominal aorta and iliac arteries to determine the best access vessel based on size, disease, and tortuosity. If the femoral and/or external iliac arteries are not adequate, then a common iliac conduit graft can be considered. In rare cases, if neither iliac system is adequate, then an aortic conduit may be feasible. A dreaded complication of TEVAR is disruption of the iliac vessel upon removal of the access sheath, requiring either endovascular or open repair usually with temporary endovascular balloon inflation for control of hemorrhage.

REFERENCES

1. Edwards JE. Anomalies of the derivatives of the aortic arch system. *Med Clin North Am.* 1948;32:925–949.
2. Charlton-Ouw KM, Estrera AL. Thoracic endovascular aortic repair for aneurysm: how I Teach it. *Ann Thorac Surg.* 2018;106:646–650.
3. Fillinger MF, Greenberg RK, McKinsey JF, et al. Reporting standards for thoracic endovascular aortic repair (TEVAR). *J Vasc Surg.* 2010;52:1022–1033.
4. Crawford ES, Snyder DM, Cho GC, et al. Progress in treatment of thoracoabdominal and abdominal aortic aneurysms involving celiac, superior mesenteric, and renal arteries. *Ann Surg.* 1978;188:404–422.
5. Crawford ES, Crawford JL, Safi HJ, et al. Thoracoabdominal aortic aneurysms: preoperative and intraoperative factors determining immediate and long-term results of operations in 605 patients. *J Vasc Surg.* 1986;3:389–404.
6. Estrera AL, Miller 3rd CC, Huynh TT, et al. Neurologic outcome after thoracic and thoracoabdominal aortic aneurysm repair. *Ann Thorac Surg.* 2001;72:1225–1230; discussion 1230–1221.
7. DeBakey ME, Henly WS, Cooley DA, et al. Surgical treatment of dissecting aneurysm of the aorta analysis of seventy-two cases. *Circulation.* 1961;24:290–303.
8. Daily PO, Trueblood HW, Stinson EB, et al. Management of acute aortic dissections. *Ann Thorac Surg.* 1970;10:237–247.
9. Booher AM, Isselbacher EM, Nienaber CA, et al. The IRAD classification system for characterizing survival after aortic dissection. *Am J Med.* 2013;126;730 e719–724.
10. Lansman SL, McCullough JN, Nguyen KH, et al. Subtypes of acute aortic dissection. *Ann Thorac Surg.* 1999;67:1975–1978; discussion 1979–1980.
11. Erbel R, Alfonso F, Boileau C, et al. Diagnosis and management of aortic dissection. *Eur Heart J.* 2001;22:1642–1681.
12. Augoustides JG, Geirsson A, Szeto WY, et al. Observational study of mortality risk stratification by ischemic presentation in patients with acute type A aortic dissection: the Penn classification. *Nat Clin Pract Cardiovasc Med.* 2009;6:140–146.
13. Augoustides JG, Szeto WY, Desai ND, et al. Classification of acute type A dissection: focus on clinical presentation and extent. *Eur J Cardio Thorac Surg.* 2011;39:519–522.
14. Augoustides JG, Szeto WY, Woo EY, et al. The complications of uncomplicated acute type-B dissection: the introduction of the Penn classification. *J Cardiothorac Vasc Anesth.* 2012;26:1139–1144.
15. Johnston KW, Rutherford RB, Tilson MD, et al. Suggested standards for reporting on arterial aneurysms. Subcommittee on reporting standards for arterial aneurysms, Ad hoc Committee on reporting standards, society for vascular surgery and North American chapter, international society for cardiovascular surgery. *J Vasc Surg.* 1991;13:452–458.
16. Wanhainen A, Themudo R, Ahlstrom H, et al. Thoracic and abdominal aortic dimension in 70-year-old men and women--a population-based whole-body magnetic resonance imaging (MRI) study. *J Vasc Surg.* 2008;47:504–512.
17. Lijnen HR. Metalloproteinases in development and progression of vascular disease. *Pathophysiol Haemost Thromb.* 2003;33:275–281.
18. Wassef M, Upchurch Jr GR, Kuivaniemi H, et al. Challenges and opportunities in abdominal aortic aneurysm research. *J Vasc Surg.* 2007;45:192–198.
19. Chaikof EL, Brewster DC, Dalman RL, et al. The care of patients with an abdominal aortic aneurysm: the Society for Vascular Surgery practice guidelines. *J Vasc Surg.* 2009;50:S2–S49.
20. Bengtsson H, Sonesson B, Lanne T, et al. Prevalence of abdominal aortic aneurysm in the offspring of patients dying from aneurysm rupture. *Br J Surg.* 1992;79:1142–1143.
21. Lederle FA, Johnson GR, Wilson SE, et al. Prevalence and associations of abdominal aortic aneurysm detected through screening. Aneurysm detection and management (ADAM) veterans affairs cooperative study group. *Ann Intern Med.* 1997;126:441–449.

22. Sidloff D, Stather P, Dattani N, et al. Aneurysm global epidemiology study: public health measures can further reduce abdominal aortic aneurysm mortality. *Circulation*. 2014;129:747–753.
23. Lawrence PF, Lorenzo-Rivero S, Lyon JL. The incidence of iliac, femoral, and popliteal artery aneurysms in hospitalized patients. *J Vasc Surg*. 1995;22:409–415; discussion 415-406.
24. Velazquez OC, Larson RA, Baum RA, et al. Gender-related differences in infrarenal aortic aneurysm morphologic features: issues relevant to Ancure and Talent endografts. *J Vasc Surg*. 2001;33:S77–S84.
25. Golledge J, Muller J, Daugherty A, et al. Abdominal aortic aneurysm: pathogenesis and implications for management. *Arterioscler Thromb Vasc Biol*. 2006;26:2605–2613.
26. Svensjo S, Bengtsson H, Bergqvist D. Thoracic and thoracoabdominal aortic aneurysm and dissection: an investigation based on autopsy. *Br J Surg*. 1996;83:68–71.
27. Dayan V, Michelis V, Lorenzo A. Giant aortic aneurysm as a rare cause of superior vena cava syndrome. *Ann Thorac Surg*. 2008;86:1383.
28. Van Melle JP, Meyns B, Budts W. Ortner's syndrome, presentation of two cases with cardiovocal hoarseness. *Acta Cardiol*. 2010;65:703–705.
29. Singh SM, Safi HJ, Estrera AL. Aortobronchial syndrome: extrinsic compression of the left main bronchus secondary to a descending thoracic aortic aneurysm. *Ann Thorac Surg*. 2011;91:1292.
30. von Kodolitsch Y, Nienaber CA, Dieckmann C, et al. Chest radiography for the diagnosis of acute aortic syndrome. *Am J Med*. 2004;116:73–77.
31. Karthikesalingam A, Al-Jundi W, Jackson D, et al. Systematic review and meta-analysis of duplex ultrasonography, contrast-enhanced ultrasonography or computed tomography for surveillance after endovascular aneurysm repair. *Br J Surg*. 2012;99:1514–1523.
32. Evangelista A, Flachskampf FA, Erbel R, et al. Echocardiography in aortic diseases: EAE recommendations for clinical practice. *Eur J Echocardiogr*. 2010;11:645–658.
33. Flachskampf FA, Badano L, Daniel WG, et al. Recommendations for transoesophageal echocardiography: update 2010. *Eur J Echocardiogr*. 2010;11:557–576.
34. Holloway BJ, D, Jones RG. Imaging of thoracic aortic disease. *Br J Radiol*. 2011;84 Spec No 3:S338–S354.
35. Barker AJ, Markl M, Burk J, et al. Bicuspid aortic valve is associated with altered wall shear stress in the ascending aorta. *Circ Cardiovasc Imaging*. 2012;5:457–466.
36. Finn JP, Nguyen KL, Hu P. Ferumoxytol vs. Gadolinium agents for contrast-enhanced MRI: Thoughts on evolving indications, risks, and benefits. *J Magn Reson Imaging*. 2017;46:919–923.
37. Brady AR, Thompson SG, Fowkes FG, et al. Abdominal aortic aneurysm expansion: risk factors and time intervals for surveillance. *Circulation*. 2004;110:16–21.
38. Hatzaras I, Tranquilli M, Coady M, et al. Weight lifting and aortic dissection: more evidence for a connection. *Cardiology*. 2007;107:103–106.
39. Groenink M, den Hartog AW, Franken R, et al. Losartan reduces aortic dilatation rate in adults with Marfan syndrome: a randomized controlled trial. *Eur Heart J*. 2013;34:3491–3500.
40. Stein LH, Berger J, Tranquilli M, et al. Effect of statin drugs on thoracic aortic aneurysms. *Am J Cardiol*. 2013;112:1240–1245.
41. de Bruin JL, Baas AF, Heymans MW, et al. Statin therapy is associated with improved survival after endovascular and open aneurysm repair. *J Vasc Surg*. 2014;59:39–44 e31.
42. Erbel R, Aboyans V, Boileau C, et al. 2014 ESC Guidelines on the diagnosis and treatment of aortic diseases: document covering acute and chronic aortic diseases of the thoracic and abdominal aorta of the adult. The Task Force for the Diagnosis and Treatment of Aortic Diseases of the European Society of Cardiology (ESC). *Eur Heart J*. 2014;35:2873–2926.
43. Abdominal aortic aneurysm: Screening. U.S. Preventive Services Task Force Web Site https://www.uspreventiveservicestaskforce.org/Page/Document/UpdateSummaryFinal/abdominal-aortic-aneurysm-screening Published June 23, 2014. Accessed January 1, 2019.
44. Takagi H, Goto SN, Matsui M, et al. A further meta-analysis of population-based screening for abdominal aortic aneurysm. *J Vasc Surg*. 2010;52:1103–1108.
45. Eckroth-Bernard K, Garvin RP, Ryer E, et al. The SAAAVE Act and routine ambulatory medical care fail to diagnose patients with abdominal aortic aneurysms prior to rupture: a single-institution experience. *ISRN Vascular Medicine*. 2013;2013:134019.
46. Mell MW, Baker LC, Dalman RL, et al. Gaps in preoperative surveillance and rupture of abdominal aortic aneurysms among Medicare beneficiaries. *J Vasc Surg*. 2014;59:583–588.
47. Scott RA, Vardulaki KA, Walker NM, et al. The long-term benefits of a single scan for abdominal aortic aneurysm (AAA) at age 65. *Eur J Vasc Endovasc Surg*. 2001;21:535–540.
48. McCarthy RJ, Shaw E, Whyman MR, et al. Recommendations for screening intervals for small aortic aneurysms. *Br J Surg*. 2003;90:821–826.
49. Juvonen T, Ergin MA, Galla JD, et al. Prospective study of the natural history of thoracic aortic aneurysms. *Ann Thorac Surg*. 1997;63:1533–1545.
50. Pan E, Kyto V, Savunen T, et al. Early and late outcomes after open ascending aortic surgery: 47-year experience in a single centre. *Heart Ves*. 2018;33:427–433.
51. Dake MD, Miller DC, Semba CP, et al. Transluminal placement of endovascular stent-grafts for the treatment of descending thoracic aortic aneurysms. *N Engl J Med*. 1994;331:1729–1734.
52. Cheng D, Martin J, Shennib H, et al. Endovascular aortic repair versus open surgical repair for descending thoracic aortic disease a systematic review and meta-analysis of comparative studies. *J Am Coll Cardiol*. 2010;55:986–1001.
53. Coselli JS, de la Cruz KI, Preventza O, et al. Extent II thoracoabdominal aortic aneurysm repair: how I do it. *Semin Thorac Cardiovasc Surg*. 2016;28:221–237.
54. Cowan Jr JA, Dimick JB, Henke PK, et al. Surgical treatment of intact thoracoabdominal aortic aneurysms in the United States: hospital and surgeon volume-related outcomes. *J Vasc Surg*. 2003;37:1169–1174.
55. Moulakakis KG, Karaolanis G, Antonopoulos CN, et al. Open repair of thoracoabdominal aortic aneurysms in experienced centers. *J Vasc Surg*. 2018;68; 634–645 e612.

56. Brewster DC, Cronenwett JL, Hallett Jr JW, et al. Guidelines for the treatment of abdominal aortic aneurysms. Report of a subcommittee of the Joint Council of the American association for vascular surgery and society for vascular surgery. *J Vasc Surg*. 2003;37:1106–1117.
57. Lee WA, Carter JW, Upchurch G, et al. Perioperative outcomes after open and endovascular repair of intact abdominal aortic aneurysms in the United States during 2001. *J Vasc Surg*. 2004;39:491–496.
58. Greenhalgh RM, Brown LC, Powell JT, et al. Endovascular versus open repair of abdominal aortic aneurysm. *N Engl J Med*. 2010;362:1863–1871.
59. Blankensteijn JD, de Jong SE, Prinssen M, et al. Two-year outcomes after conventional or endovascular repair of abdominal aortic aneurysms. *N Engl J Med*. 2005;352:2398–2405.
60. Vierhout BP, Pol RA, El Moumni M, et al. Editor's choice - arteriotomy closure devices in EVAR, TEVAR, and TAVR: a systematic review and meta-analysis of randomised clinical trials and cohort studies. *Eur J Vasc Endovasc Surg*. 2017;54:104–115.
61. Rooke TW, Hirsch AT, Misra S, et al. 2011 ACCF/AHA focused update of the guideline for the management of patients with peripheral artery disease (updating the 2005 guideline): a report of the American College of Cardiology Foundation/American heart association Task force on practice guidelines: developed in collaboration with the society for cardiovascular angiography and interventions, society of interventional Radiology, society for vascular medicine, and society for vascular surgery. *Catheter Cardiovasc Interv*. 2012;79:501–531.
62. Sidloff DA, Gokani V, Stather PW, et al. Type II endoleak: conservative management is a safe strategy. *Eur J Vasc Endovasc Surg*. 2014;48:391–399.
63. Higashiura W, Greenberg RK, Katz E, et al. Predictive factors, morphologic effects, and proposed treatment paradigm for type II endoleaks after repair of infrarenal abdominal aortic aneurysms. *J Vasc Interv Radiol*. 2007;18:975–981.
64. Donas KP, Lee JT, Lachat M, et al. Collected world experience about the performance of the snorkel/chimney endovascular technique in the treatment of complex aortic pathologies: the PERICLES registry. *Ann Surg*. 2015;262:546–553; discussion 552-543.
65. Tsilimparis N, Heidemann F, Rohlffs F, et al. Outcome of surgeon-modified fenestrated/branched stent-grafts for Symptomatic complex aortic pathologies or contained rupture. *J Endovasc Ther*. 2017;24:825–832.
66. Oderich GS, Ribeiro MS, Sandri GA, et al. Evolution from physician-modified to company-manufactured fenestrated-branched endografts to treat pararenal and thoracoabdominal aortic aneurysms. *J Vasc Surg*. 2019;70:31–42 e37.
67. Murphy SL, Xu J, Kochanek KD, et al. Centers for disease control and prevention. National vital statistics reports. *Deaths: Final date for 2015*. 2017;66:6.
68. Peppelenbosch N, Geelkerken RH, Soong C, et al. Endograft treatment of ruptured abdominal aortic aneurysms using the Talent aortouniiliac system: an international multicenter study. *J Vasc Surg*. 2006;43:1111–1123; discussion 1123.
69. Improve Trial Investigators. Comparative clinical effectiveness and cost effectiveness of endovascular strategy v open repair for ruptured abdominal aortic aneurysm: three year results of the IMPROVE randomised trial. *BMJ*. 2017;359:j4859.
70. Mell MW, Wang NE, Morrison DE, et al. Interfacility transfer and mortality for patients with ruptured abdominal aortic aneurysm. *J Vasc Surg*. 2014;60:553–557.
71. Malina M, Veith F, Ivancev K, et al. Balloon occlusion of the aorta during endovascular repair of ruptured abdominal aortic aneurysm. *J Endovasc Ther*. 2005;12:556–559.
72. Powell JT, Hinchliffe RJ, Thompson MM, et al. Observations from the IMPROVE trial concerning the clinical care of patients with ruptured abdominal aortic aneurysm. *Br J Surg*. 2014;101:216–224; discussion 224.
73. Hansen SK, Danaher PJ, Starnes BW, et al. Accuracy evaluations of three ruptured abdominal aortic aneurysm mortality risk scores using an independent dataset. *J Vasc Surg*. 2019;70:67–73.
74. Thompson PC, Dalman RL, Harris EJ, et al. Predictive models for mortality after ruptured aortic aneurysm repair do not predict futility and are not useful for clinical decision making. *J Vasc Surg*. 2016;64:1617–1622.
75. Mell MW, Starnes BW, Kraiss LW, et al. Western Vascular Society guidelines for transfer of patients with ruptured abdominal aortic aneurysm. *J Vasc Surg*. 2017;65:603–608.
76. Olsson C, Thelin S, Stahle E, et al. Thoracic aortic aneurysm and dissection: increasing prevalence and improved outcomes reported in a nationwide population-based study of more than 14,000 cases from 1987 to 2002. *Circulation*. 2006;114:2611–2618.
77. Clouse WD, Hallett Jr JW, Schaff HV, et al. Acute aortic dissection: population-based incidence compared with degenerative aortic aneurysm rupture. *Mayo Clin Proc*. 2004;79:176–180.
78. Nienaber CA, Fattori R, Mehta RH, et al. Gender-related differences in acute aortic dissection. *Circulation*. 2004;109:3014–3021.
79. Bossone E, Pyeritz RE, O'Gara P, et al. Acute aortic dissection in blacks: insights from the international registry of acute aortic dissection. *Am J Med*. 2013;126:909–915.
80. Hagan PG, Nienaber CA, Isselbacher EM, et al. The international registry of acute aortic dissection (IRAD): new insights into an old disease. *J Am Med Assoc*. 2000;283:897–903.
81. Dean JH, Woznicki EM, O'Gara P, et al. Cocaine-related aortic dissection: lessons from the international registry of acute aortic dissection. *Am J Med*. 2014;127:878–885.
82. Lange RA, Hillis LD. Cardiovascular complications of cocaine use. *N Engl J Med*. 2001;345:351–358.
83. Wang W, Duan W, Xue Y, et al. Clinical features of acute aortic dissection from the Registry of Aortic Dissection in China. *J Thorac Cardiovasc Surg*. 2014;148:2995–3000.
84. Elefteriades JA, Ziganshin BA. Examining the face of aortic dissection outside the Western world. *J Thorac Cardiovasc Surg*. 2014;148:3001–3002.
85. Trimarchi S, Nienaber CA, Rampoldi V, et al. Contemporary results of surgery in acute type A aortic dissection: the International Registry of Acute Aortic Dissection experience. *J Thorac Cardiovasc Surg*. 2005;129:112–122.
86. Spittell PC, Spittell Jr JA, Joyce JW, et al. Clinical features and differential diagnosis of aortic dissection: experience with 236 cases (1980 through 1990). *Mayo Clin Proc*. 1993;68:642–651.
87. Khan IA, Nair CK. Clinical, diagnostic, and management perspectives of aortic dissection. *Chest*. 2002;122:311–328.
88. Rogers IS, Banerji D, Siegel EL, et al. Usefulness of comprehensive cardiothoracic computed tomography in the evaluation of acute undifferentiated chest discomfort in the emergency department (CAPTURE). *Am J Cardiol*. 2011;107:643–650.

89. Shiga T, Wajima Z, Apfel CC, et al. Diagnostic accuracy of transesophageal echocardiography, helical computed tomography, and magnetic resonance imaging for suspected thoracic aortic dissection: systematic review and meta-analysis. *Arch Intern Med*. 2006;166:1350–1356.
90. Nordon IM, Hinchliffe RJ, Morgan R, et al. Progress in endovascular management of type A dissection. *Eur J Vasc Endovasc Surg*. 2012;44:406–410.
91. Liu JC, Zhang JZ, Yang J, et al. Combined interventional and surgical treatment for acute aortic type a dissection. *Int J Surg*. 2008;6:151–156.
92. Sun LZ, Qi RD, Chang Q, et al. Surgery for acute type A dissection using total arch replacement combined with stented elephant trunk implantation: experience with 107 patients. *J Thorac Cardiovasc Surg*. 2009;138:1358–1362.
93. Mehta RH, Suzuki T, Hagan PG, et al. Predicting death in patients with acute type a aortic dissection. *Circulation*. 2002;105:200–206.
94. Rampoldi V, Trimarchi S, Eagle KA, et al. Simple risk models to predict surgical mortality in acute type A aortic dissection: the International Registry of Acute Aortic Dissection score. *Ann Thorac Surg*. 2007;83:55–61.
95. Ghoreishi M, Wise ES, Croal-Abrahams L, et al. A novel risk score predicts operative mortality after acute type A aortic dissection repair. *Ann Thorac Surg*. 2018;106:1759–1766.
96. Patel HJ, Williams DM, Dasika NL, et al. Operative delay for peripheral malperfusion syndrome in acute type A aortic dissection: a long-term analysis. *J Thorac Cardiovasc Surg*. 2008;135:1288–1295; discussion 1295-1286.
97. Goldberg JB, Lansman SL, Kai M, et al. Malperfusion in type A dissection: consider reperfusion first. *Semin Thorac Cardiovasc Surg*. 2017;29:181–185.
98. Mussa FF, Horton JD, Moridzadeh R, et al. Acute aortic dissection and intramural hematoma: a systematic review. *J Am Med Assoc*. 2016;316:754–763.
99. Beller JP, Scheinerman JA, Balsam LB, et al. Operative strategies and outcomes in type A aortic dissection after the Enactment of a multidisciplinary aortic surgery team. *Innovations*. 2015;10:410–415.
100. Marui A, Mochizuki T, Mitsui N, et al. Toward the best treatment for uncomplicated patients with type B acute aortic dissection: a consideration for sound surgical indication. *Circulation*. 1999;100:II275–280.
101. Wilkinson DA, Patel HJ, Williams DM, et al. Early open and endovascular thoracic aortic repair for complicated type B aortic dissection. *Ann Thorac Surg*. 2013;96:23–30; discussion 230.
102. Nienaber CA, Zannetti S, Barbieri B, et al. INvestigation of STEnt grafts in patients with type B Aortic Dissection: design of the INSTEAD trial--a prospective, multicenter, European randomized trial. *Am Heart J*. 2005;149:592–599.
103. Nienaber CA, Kische S, Akin I, et al. Strategies for subacute/chronic type B aortic dissection: the investigation of stent grafts in patients with type B aortic dissection (INSTEAD) trial 1-year outcome. *J Thorac Cardiovasc Surg*. 2010;140:S101–S108; discussion S142-S146.
104. Hughes GC, Andersen ND, McCann RL. Management of acute type B aortic dissection. *J Thorac Cardiovasc Surg*. 2013;145:S202–S207.
105. Fattori R, Tsai TT, Myrmel T, et al. Complicated acute type B dissection: is surgery still the best option?: a report from the International Registry of Acute Aortic Dissection. *JACC Cardiovasc Interv*. 2008;1:395–402.
106. Fattori R, Cao P, De Rango P, et al. Interdisciplinary expert consensus document on management of type B aortic dissection. *J Am Coll Cardiol*. 2013;61:1661–1678.
107. Nienaber CA, Rousseau H, Eggebrecht H, et al. Randomized comparison of strategies for type B aortic dissection: the INvestigation of STEnt Grafts in Aortic Dissection (INSTEAD) trial. *Circulation*. 2009;120:2519–2528.
108. Brunkwall J, Kasprzak P, Verhoeven E, et al. Endovascular repair of acute uncomplicated aortic type B dissection promotes aortic remodelling: 1 year results of the ADSORB trial. *Eur J Vasc Endovasc Surg*. 2014;48:285–291.
109. Nienaber CA, Kische S, Rousseau H, et al. Endovascular repair of type B aortic dissection: long-term results of the randomized investigation of stent grafts in aortic dissection trial. *Circ Cardiovasc Interv*. 2013;6:407–416.
110. Nienaber CA, Kische S, Zeller T, et al. Provisional extension to induce complete attachment after stent-graft placement in type B aortic dissection: the PETTICOAT concept. *J Endovasc Ther*. 2006;13:738–746.
111. Hsu HL, Chen YY, Huang CY, et al. The Provisional Extension to Induce Complete Attachment (PETTICOAT) technique to promote distal aortic remodelling in repair of acute DeBakey type I aortic dissection: preliminary results. *Eur J Cardio Thorac Surg*. 2016;50:146–152.
112. Kazimierczak A, Jedrzejczak T, Rynio P, et al. Favorable remodeling after hybrid arch debranching and modified provisional extension to induce complete attachment technique in type a aortic dissection: a case report. *Medicine (Baltim)*. 2018;97:e12409.
113. Gore I. Pathogenesis of dissecting aneurysm of the aorta. *AMA Arch Pathol*. 1952;53:142–153.
114. Park KH, Lim C, Choi JH, et al. Prevalence of aortic intimal defect in surgically treated acute type A intramural hematoma. *Ann Thorac Surg*. 2008;86:1494–1500.
115. Kitai T, Kaji S, Yamamuro A, et al. Detection of intimal defect by 64-row multidetector computed tomography in patients with acute aortic intramural hematoma. *Circulation*. 2011;124:S174–S178.
116. Harris KM, Braverman AC, Eagle KA, et al. Acute aortic intramural hematoma: an analysis from the international registry of acute aortic dissection. *Circulation*. 2012;126:S91–S96.
117. Song JK, Yim JH, Ahn JM, et al. Outcomes of patients with acute type a aortic intramural hematoma. *Circulation*. 2009;120:2046–2052.
118. Tittle SL, Lynch RJ, Cole PE, et al. Midterm follow-up of penetrating ulcer and intramural hematoma of the aorta. *J Thorac Cardiovasc Surg*. 2002;123:1051–1059.
119. Song JK. Update in acute aortic syndrome: intramural hematoma and incomplete dissection as new disease entities. *J Cardiol*. 2014;64:153–161.
120. Matsushita A, Fukui T, Tabata M, et al. Preoperative characteristics and surgical outcomes of acute intramural hematoma involving the ascending aorta: a propensity score-matched analysis. *J Thorac Cardiovasc Surg*. 2016;151:351–358.
121. Di Cesare E, Giordano AV, Cerone G, et al. Comparative evaluation of TEE, conventional MRI and contrast-enhanced 3D breath-hold MRA in the post-operative follow-up of dissecting aneurysms. *Int J Card Imaging*. 2000;16:135–147.

122. Falconi M, Oberti P, Krauss J, et al. Different clinical features of aortic intramural hematoma versus dissection involving the descending thoracic aorta. *Echocardiography*. 2005;22:629–635.
123. Kitai T, Kaji S, Yamamuro A, et al. Clinical outcomes of medical therapy and timely operation in initially diagnosed type a aortic intramural hematoma: a 20-year experience. *Circulation*. 2009;120:S292–S298.
124. Li DL, Zhang HK, Cai YY, et al. Acute type B aortic intramural hematoma: treatment strategy and the role of endovascular repair. *J Endovasc Ther*. 2010;17:617–621.
125. Bischoff MS, Meisenbacher K, Wehrmeister M, et al. Treatment indications for and outcome of endovascular repair of type B intramural aortic hematoma. *J Vasc Surg*. 2016;64:1569–1579 e1562.
126. Svensson LG, Kouchoukos NT, Miller DC, et al. Expert consensus document on the treatment of descending thoracic aortic disease using endovascular stent-grafts. *Ann Thorac Surg*. 2008;85:S1–S41.
127. Coady MA, Rizzo JA, Hammond GL, et al. Penetrating ulcer of the thoracic aorta: what is it? How do we recognize it? How do we manage it?. *J Vasc Surg*. 1998;27:1006–1015; discussion 1015-1006.
128. Eggebrecht H, Plicht B, Kahlert P, et al. Intramural hematoma and penetrating ulcers: indications to endovascular treatment. *Eur J Vasc Endovasc Surg*. 2009;38:659–665.
129. Gifford SM, Duncan AA, Greiten LE, et al. The natural history and outcomes for thoracic and abdominal penetrating aortic ulcers. *J Vasc Surg*. 2016;63:1182–1188.
130. Cho KR, Stanson AW, Potter DD, et al. Penetrating atherosclerotic ulcer of the descending thoracic aorta and arch. *J Thorac Cardiovasc Surg*. 2004;127:1393–1399; discussion 1399-1401.
131. Ganaha F, Miller DC, Sugimoto K, et al. Prognosis of aortic intramural hematoma with and without penetrating atherosclerotic ulcer: a clinical and radiological analysis. *Circulation*. 2002;106:342–348.
132. Arthurs ZM, Starnes BW, Sohn VY, et al. Functional and survival outcomes in traumatic blunt thoracic aortic injuries: an analysis of the National Trauma Databank. *J Vasc Surg*. 2009;49:988–994.
133. Fabian TC, Richardson JD, Croce MA, et al. Prospective study of blunt aortic injury: multicenter trial of the American association for the surgery of trauma. *J Trauma*. 1997;42:374–380; discussion 380-373.
134. Estrera AL, Miller 3rd CC, Guajardo-Salinas G, et al. Update on blunt thoracic aortic injury: fifteen-year single-institution experience. *J Thorac Cardiovasc Surg*. 2013;145:S154–S158.
135. Teixeira PG, Inaba K, Barmparas G, et al. Blunt thoracic aortic injuries: an autopsy study. *J Trauma*. 2011;70:197–202.
136. Mohan D, Melvin JW. Failure properties of passive human aortic tissue. I--uniaxial tension tests. *J Biomech*. 1982;15:887–902.
137. Symbas PN. Great vessels injury. *Am Heart J*. 1977;93:518–522.
138. Siegel JH, Yang KH, Smith JA, et al. Computer simulation and validation of the Archimedes Lever hypothesis as a mechanism for aortic isthmus disruption in a case of lateral impact motor vehicle crash: a Crash Injury Research Engineering Network (CIREN) study. *J Trauma*. 2006;60:1072–1082.
139. Fabian TC, Davis KA, Gavant ML, et al. Prospective study of blunt aortic injury: helical CT is diagnostic and antihypertensive therapy reduces rupture. *Ann Surg*. 1998;227:666–676; discussion 676-667.
140. Lee WA, Matsumura JS, Mitchell RS, et al. Endovascular repair of traumatic thoracic aortic injury: clinical practice guidelines of the Society for Vascular Surgery. *J Vasc Surg*. 2011;53:187–192.
141. Kato N, Dake MD, Miller DC, et al. Traumatic thoracic aortic aneurysm: treatment with endovascular stent-grafts. *Radiology*. 1997;205:657–662.
142. Fox N, Schwartz D, Salazar JH, et al. Evaluation and management of blunt traumatic aortic injury: a practice management guideline from the Eastern Association for the Surgery of Trauma. *J Trauma Acute Care Surg*. 2015;78:136–146.
143. Pape LA, Awais M, Woznicki EM, et al. Presentation, diagnosis, and outcomes of acute aortic dissection: 17-year Trends from the international registry of acute aortic dissection. *J Am Coll Cardiol*. 2015;66:350–358.
144. Rylski B, Hoffmann I, Beyersdorf F, et al. Acute aortic dissection type A: age-related management and outcomes reported in the German Registry for Acute Aortic Dissection Type A (GERAADA) of over 2000 patients. *Ann Surg*. 2014;259:598–604.
145. Stamou SC, Hagberg RC, Khabbaz KR, et al. Is advanced age a contraindication for emergent repair of acute type A aortic dissection? *Interact Cardiovasc Thorac Surg*. 2010;10:539–544.
146. Hata M, Sezai A, Niino T, et al. Should emergency surgical intervention be performed for an octogenarian with type A acute aortic dissection? *J Thorac Cardiovasc Surg*. 2008;135:1042–1046.
147. Trimarchi S, Eagle KA, Nienaber CA, et al. Role of age in acute type A aortic dissection outcome: report from the International Registry of Acute Aortic Dissection (IRAD). *J Thorac Cardiovasc Surg*. 2010;140:784–789.
148. Di Eusanio M, Patel HJ, Nienaber CA, et al. Patients with type A acute aortic dissection presenting with major brain injury: should we operate on them? *J Thorac Cardiovasc Surg*. 2013;145:S213–S221 e211.
149. Sabik JF, Lytle BW, McCarthy PM, et al. Axillary artery: an alternative site of arterial cannulation for patients with extensive aortic and peripheral vascular disease. *J Thorac Cardiovasc Surg*. 1995;109:885–890; discussion 890-881.
150. Strauch JT, Spielvogel D, Lauten A, et al. Axillary artery cannulation: routine use in ascending aorta and aortic arch replacement. *Ann Thorac Surg*. 2004;78:103–108; discussion 103-108.
151. Wada S, Yamamoto S, Honda J, et al. Transapical aortic cannulation for cardiopulmonary bypass in type A aortic dissection operations. *J Thorac Cardiovasc Surg*. 2006;132:369–372.
152. Kitamura T, Nie M, Horai T, et al. Direct true lumen cannulation ("Samurai" cannulation) for acute Stanford type A aortic dissection. *Ann Thorac Surg*. 2017;104:e459–e461.
153. Ma H, Xiao Z, Shi J, et al. Aortic arch cannulation with the guidance of transesophageal echocardiography for Stanford type A aortic dissection. *J Cardiothorac Surg*. 2018;13:106.
154. De Bakey ME, Crawford ES, Cooley DA, et al. Successful resection of fusiform aneurysm of aortic arch with replacement by homograft. *Surg Gynecol Obstet*. 1957;105:657–664.
155. Ott DA, Frazier OH, Cooley DA. Resection of the aortic arch using deep hypothermia and temporary circulatory arrest. *Circulation*. 1978;58:I227–I231.

156. Keeling WB, Leshnower BG, Hunting JC, et al. Hypothermia and selective antegrade cerebral perfusion is safe for arch repair in type A dissection. *Ann Thorac Surg.* 2017;104:767–772.
157. Westaby S. Coagulation disturbance in profound hypothermia: the influence of anti-fibrinolytic therapy. *Semin Thorac Cardiovasc Surg.* 1997;9:246–256.
158. Stein LH, Rubinfeld G, Balsam LB, et al. Too cold to clot? Does intraoperative hypothermia contribute to bleeding after aortic surgery? *Aorta (Stamford).* 2017;5:106–116.
159. O'Neill B, Bilal H, Mahmood S, et al. Is it worth packing the head with ice in patients undergoing deep hypothermic circulatory arrest? *Interact Cardiovasc Thorac Surg.* 2012;15:696–701.
160. Shemin RJ. Acute type A aortic dissection: to crossclamp or not to crossclamp? That is the question. *J Thorac Cardiovasc Surg.* 2015;150:302–303.
161. Bentall H, De Bono A. A technique for complete replacement of the ascending aorta. *Thorax.* 1968;23:338–339.
162. Wheat Jr MW, Wilson JR, Bartley TD. Successful replacement of the entire ascending aorta and aortic valve. *J Am Med Assoc.* 1964;188:717–719.
163. Kouchoukos NT, Wareing TH, Murphy SF, et al. Sixteen-year experience with aortic root replacement. Results of 172 operations. *Ann Surg.* 1991;214:308–318; discussion 318-320.
164. Lower RR, Stofer RC, Shumway NE. Autotransplantation of the pulmonic valve into the aorta. *J Thorac Cardiovasc Surg.* 1960;39:680–687.
165. Pillsbury RC, Shumway NE. Replacement of the aortic valve with the autologous pulmonic valve. *Surg Forum.* 1966;17:176–177.
166. Ross DN. Replacement of aortic and mitral valves with a pulmonary autograft. *Lancet.* 1967;2:956–958.
167. Ouzounian M, Mazine A, David TE. The Ross procedure is the best operation to treat aortic stenosis in young and middle-aged adults. *J Thorac Cardiovasc Surg.* 2017;154:778–782.
168. David TE, Feindel CM, Bos J. Repair of the aortic valve in patients with aortic insufficiency and aortic root aneurysm. *J Thorac Cardiovasc Surg.* 1995;109:345–351; discussion 351-342.
169. Miller DC. Valve-sparing aortic root replacement in patients with the Marfan syndrome. *J Thorac Cardiovasc Surg.* 2003;125:773–778.
170. Hess Jr PJ, Klodell CT, Beaver TM, et al. The Florida sleeve: a new technique for aortic root remodeling with preservation of the aortic valve and sinuses. *Ann Thorac Surg.* 2005;80:748–750.
171. Hiratzka LF, Bakris GL, Beckman JA, et al. 2010 ACCF/AHA/AATS, guidelines for the diagnosis and management of patients with thoracic aortic disease. A report of the American College of Cardiology Foundation/American heart association Task force on practice guidelines, American association for thoracic surgery, American College of Radiology,American stroke association, society of cardiovascular anesthesiologists, society for cardiovascular angiography and interventions, society of interventional Radiology, society of thoracic Surgeons,and society for vascular medicine. *J Am Coll Cardiol.* 2010;55:e27–e129.
172. Youngblood SC, Tolpin DA, LeMaire SA, et al. Complications of cerebrospinal fluid drainage after thoracic aortic surgery: a review of 504 patients over 5 years. *J Thorac Cardiovasc Surg.* 2013;146:166–171.
173. Kouchoukos NT. Thoracoabdominal aortic aneurysm repair using hypothermic cardiopulmonary bypass and circulatory arrest. *Ann Cardiothorac Surg.* 2012;1:409–411.
174. Coselli JS, LeMaire SA, Conklin LD, et al. Left heart bypass during descending thoracic aortic aneurysm repair does not reduce the incidence of paraplegia. *Ann Thorac Surg.* 2004;77:1298–1303; discussion 1303.
175. Coselli JS, LeMaire SA, Preventza O, et al. Outcomes of 3309 thoracoabdominal aortic aneurysm repairs. *J Thorac Cardiovasc Surg.* 2016;151:1323–1337.
176. Coselli JS, LeMaire SA, Miller 3rd CC, et al. Mortality and paraplegia after thoracoabdominal aortic aneurysm repair: a risk factor analysis. *Ann Thorac Surg.* 2000;69:409–414.
177. Acher CW, Wynn MM, Mell MW, et al. A quantitative assessment of the impact of intercostal artery reimplantation on paralysis risk in thoracoabdominal aortic aneurysm repair. *Ann Surg.* 2008;248:529–540.
178. Safi HJ, Miller 3rd CC, Carr C, et al. Importance of intercostal artery reattachment during thoracoabdominal aortic aneurysm repair. *J Vasc Surg.* 1998;27:58–66; discussion 66-58.
179. Acher CW, Wynn MM, Hoch JR, et al. Combined use of cerebral spinal fluid drainage and naloxone reduces the risk of paraplegia in thoracoabdominal aneurysm repair. *J Vasc Surg.* 1994;19:236–246; discussion 247-238.
180. Laschinger JC, Cunningham Jr JN, Cooper MM, et al. Prevention of ischemic spinal cord injury following aortic cross-clamping: use of corticosteroids. *Ann Thorac Surg.* 1984;38:500–507.
181. Sinha AC, Cheung AT. Spinal cord protection and thoracic aortic surgery. *Curr Opin Anaesthesiol.* 2010;23:95–102.
182. Baars JH, Dangel C, Herold KF, et al. Suppression of the human spinal H-reflex by propofol: a quantitative analysis. *Acta Anaesthesiol Scand.* 2006;50:193–200.
183. Murana G, Castrovinci S, Kloppenburg G, et al. Open thoracoabdominal aortic aneurysm repair in the modern era: results from a 20-year single-centre experience. *Eur J Cardio Thorac Surg.* 2016;49:1374–1381.
184. Mehta T, Wade RG, Clarke JM. Is it safe to ligate the left renal vein during open abdominal aortic aneurysm repair? *Ann Vasc Surg.* 2010;24:758–761.
185. Hertault A, Maurel B, Sobocinski J, et al. Impact of hybrid rooms with image fusion on radiation exposure during endovascular aortic repair. *Eur J Vasc Endovasc Surg.* 2014;48:382–390.
186. Makaroun MS, Dillavou ED, Kee ST, et al. Endovascular treatment of thoracic aortic aneurysms: results of the phase II multicenter trial of the GORE TAG thoracic endoprosthesis. *J Vasc Surg.* 2005;41:1–9.
187. Makaroun MS, Dillavou ED, Wheatley GH, et al. Five-year results of endovascular treatment with the Gore TAG device compared with open repair of thoracic aortic aneurysms. *J Vasc Surg.* 2008;47:912–918.
188. Feezor RJ, Lee WA. Management of the left subclavian artery during TEVAR. *Semin Vasc Surg.* 2009;22:159–164.

189. Woo EY, Carpenter JP, Jackson BM, et al. Left subclavian artery coverage during thoracic endovascular aortic repair: a single-center experience. *J Vasc Surg*. 2008;48:555–560.
190. Buth J, Harris PL, Hobo R, et al. Neurologic complications associated with endovascular repair of thoracic aortic pathology: incidence and risk factors. a study from the European Collaborators on Stent/Graft Techniques for Aortic Aneurysm Repair (EUROSTAR) registry. *J Vasc Surg*. 2007;46:1103–1110; discussion 1110-1101.
191. Feezor RJ, Martin TD, Hess PJ, et al. Risk factors for perioperative stroke during thoracic endovascular aortic repairs (TEVAR). *J Endovasc Ther*. 2007;14:568–573.
192. Cooper DG, Walsh SR, Sadat U, et al. Neurological complications after left subclavian artery coverage during thoracic endovascular aortic repair: a systematic review and meta-analysis. *J Vasc Surg*. 2009;49:1594–1601.
193. Stone DH, Brewster DC, Kwolek CJ, et al. Stent-graft versus open-surgical repair of the thoracic aorta: mid-term results. *J Vasc Surg*. 2006;44:1188–1197.
194. Acher C, Acher CW, Marks E, et al. Intraoperative neuroprotective interventions prevent spinal cord ischemia and injury in thoracic endovascular aortic repair. *J Vasc Surg*. 2016;63:1458–1465.

63

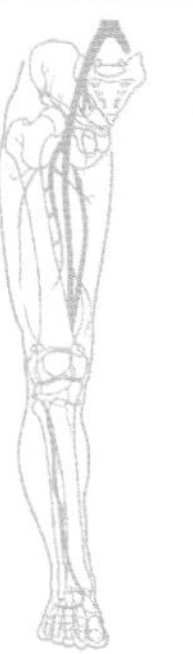

Peripheral Arterial Disease

Joseph L. Mills Sr., Zachary S. Pallister

OUTLINE

Peripheral artery disease (PAD) is the most common condition requiring treatment by vascular surgeons and vascular specialists. Over the last decade, the global prevalence of PAD has continued to rise, and it is a major contributor to rising healthcare resource consumption.[1,2] An estimated 8 to 12 million individuals in the United States are afflicted with PAD, and at least 202 million people suffer from PAD across the globe.[3] A recent metaanalysis of more than 34 studies showed a 23.5% increase in the prevalence of PAD during the first decade of the twenty-first century.[4] The primary drivers of this dramatic rise in PAD prevalence are the underlying increases in the major risk factors for the development of PAD around the world. These risk factors include population aging (i.e., increased longevity); the global epidemic of diabetes, hypertension, and obesity; and the persistence of tobacco smoking in many parts of the world (Fig. 63.1). An increased PAD prevalence has been noted in both high- and low-income countries (Fig. 63.2), although the rise has been more dramatic in low- and middle-income countries (28.7% increase) than in high-income countries (13.1% increase).[3]

The economic impact of PAD has been growing in parallel with its increased prevalence, especially in the United States and in many industrialized countries. In 2001, PAD-related treatments comprised approximately 13% of all Medicare Part A and B expenditures and contributed to an estimated economic burden of over $4.3 billion. By 2004, according to a detailed analysis of the Reduction of Atherothrombosis for Continued Health (REACH) Registry, the total estimated costs of vascular-related hospitalizations in the United States was $21 billion.[3,5] The main contributor to these costs was revascularization procedures, particularly rises in the use of endovascular therapy (EVT).

The chapter which follows will review the pathophysiology, anatomy, patient presentations, natural history, diagnosis, and management of lower extremity PAD. While there have been many advances in therapy over the last decade, there is still a striking relative lack of high-level evidence for many of the treatments in common use. The condition is underdiagnosed, medical management is underutilized and often not maximized, and there are wide regional differences and disparities in the application of revascularization procedures and strategies.

EPIDEMIOLOGY AND DEMOGRAPHICS

Aging is a major risk factor for the development of PAD. Lower extremity PAD most commonly presents in patients more than 50 years of age and increases markedly with each decade beginning at 60 years of age. The prevalence of PAD has been estimated at 14.5% in patients more than 69 years of age and as high as 20% in patients 80 years of age and older.[3] Cigarette smoking and its intensity is also strongly associated with PAD with one study estimating its population attributable fraction at 44%.[6] In the last 20 years, it has become evident that diabetes has become one of the most prominent risk factors for the development of PAD.[7] There is an ongoing global epidemic of diabetes and currently over 383 million people are affected; this number is expected to almost double in the next 15 to 20 years. Diabetes is strongly associated with PAD; population-based studies have reported odds ratios of 1.9 to 4 (Fig. 63.1).[3] Patients with diabetes are more likely to develop a foot ulcer and to present with chronic limb-threatening ischemia (CLTI). Hypertension and hyperlipidemia are the other major risk factors associated with the development of PAD.

PATIENT PRESENTATIONS AND NATURAL HISTORY

Patients may have detectable PAD and yet be completely asymptomatic; this situation is not uncommon in the aging population as other factors may limit activity levels while PAD lurks in the background. Individuals may also present with atypical leg symptoms that result from other conditions such as lumbar spine disease, neuropathy, degenerative joint disease, and myopathy. Typical symptoms of PAD include vasculogenic claudication and CLTI. The latter category includes ischemic rest pain, ischemic ulcer, and gangrene.

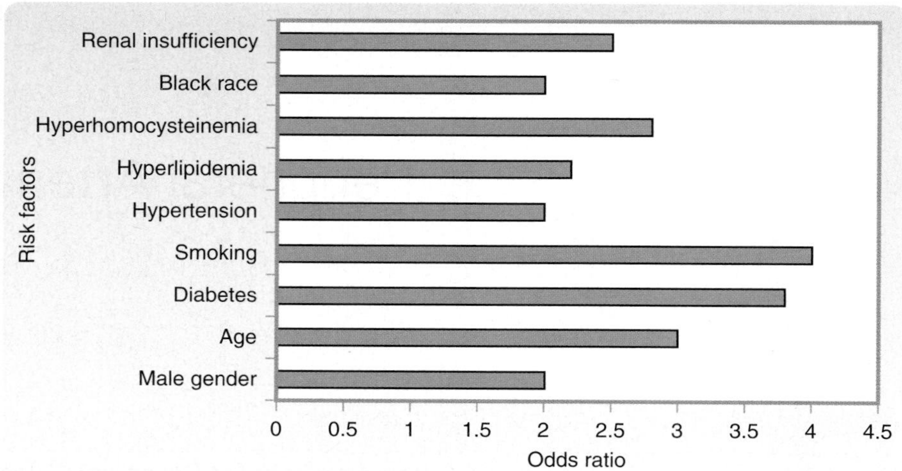

FIG. 63.1 The approximate odds ratios (ORs) for risk factors associated with the development of peripheral arterial disease (PAD). (Adapted from Norgren L, Hiatt WR, Dormandy JA, et al. Inter-Society Consensus for the Management of Peripheral Arterial Disease (TASC II). *J Vasc Surg.* 2007;45 Suppl S:S5–67.)

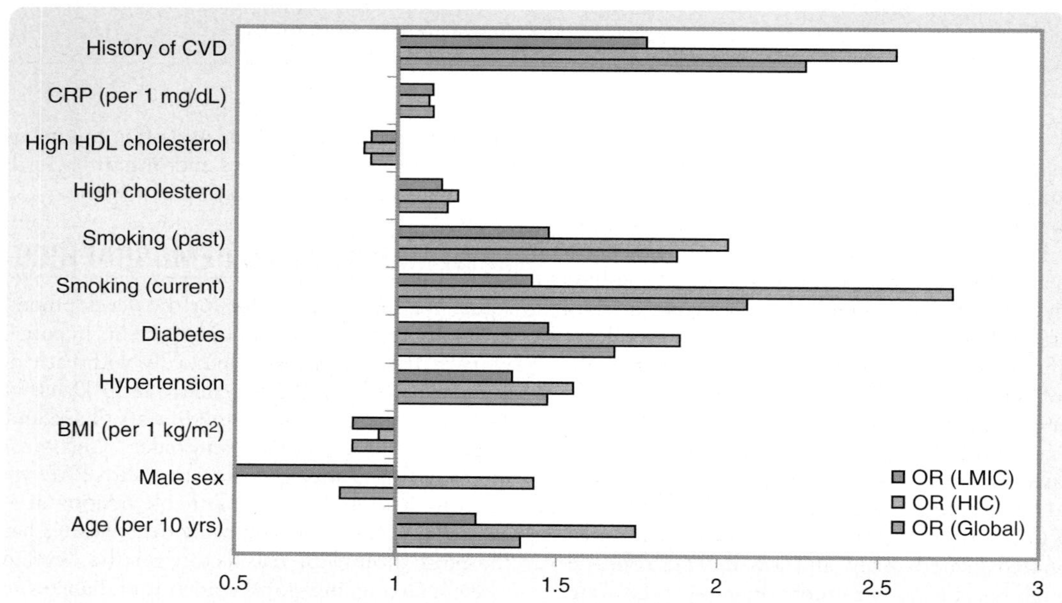

FIG. 63.2 Odds ratios *(ORs)* for peripheral artery disease (PAD) in high-income countries *(HICs)* and low- and middle-income countries *(LMICs)*. (From Criqui MH, Aboyans V. Epidemiology of peripheral artery disease. *Circ Res.* 2015; 116:1509–1526.) *BMI*, Body mass index; *CRP*, C-reactive protein; *CVD*, cardiovascular disease; *HDL*, high-density lipoprotein.

Symptoms typical of vasculogenic claudication are characterized by cramping or aching discomfort in the buttock, thigh, or calf muscles that is induced by walking and relieved by rest. The location of muscular symptoms often correlates with the anatomic site of disease, such that aortoiliac disease produces buttock and thigh claudication, while femoropopliteal occlusive disease results in calf claudication. Such complaints are usually reproducible in onset but may arise sooner by walking at a faster pace or uphill. Vasculogenic claudication typically resolves with a short period of rest (which reduces the muscular metabolic requirement), and in contrast to neurogenic claudication, is neither variable in onset nor does it require a change in position for symptom resolution. Symptoms related to nerve root compression are often variable in onset, can take a long time for recovery, may arise from standing alone (without walking), and are often relieved by changes in spine position (such as spine flexion or sitting down). These two conditions may coexist, and a good history and physical examination will often help the clinician differentiate them.

Complementing the history, qualitative components of a physical examination form the cornerstone of PAD diagnosis. These components include pulse examination (brachial, radial, femoral, popliteal, posterior tibial, and dorsalis pedis), observation for lack of distal hair growth on the involved extremity and dry skin which may result from apocrine gland dysfunction. The measurement of ankle-brachial index (ABI) forms the objective, quantitative basis of PAD assessment. An ABI of less than 0.9 has a sensitivity of 79%

to 95% and a specificity exceeding 95% to establish the diagnosis of PAD in patients in whom it is suspected.[2,3] In some individuals, particularly those with diabetes or the aged, medial calcinosis will result in falsely elevated ABIs. Because the toe arteries are often spared calcification, a toe-brachial index may be measured to quantitate PAD in individuals found to have noncompressible ankle arteries. A toe-brachial index less than or equal to 0.7 is abnormal and indicates hemodynamically significant PAD.[3] If the diagnosis of PAD is still in doubt, particularly when compelling symptoms are present in the setting of palpable pulses, an ABI test with exercise can be helpful. This test and other useful studies will be subsequently discussed in more detail under "Evaluation of the Patient with PAD."

Ischemic rest pain has long been recognized as a classic symptom of advanced PAD and is one manifestation of CLTI. It is more common in smokers than patients with diabetes mellitus, likely masked in the latter by peripheral sensory neuropathy related to underlying diabetes. It occurs in the forefoot and is typically described as having its onset with leg elevation or recumbency (i.e., when going to bed at night) and is relieved by dependency (i.e., dangling the foot off the bed at night). The increase in pedal blood pressure related to gravity is sufficient to relieve the pain. Affected patients lack pedal pulses and usually suffer from distal hair loss in the affected extremity. Pallor on elevation and dependent rubor are common physical findings. The diagnosis is confirmed by one or more of several hemodynamic parameters, including an ABI less than 0.4, an ankle systolic pressure less than 50 mm Hg, a systolic toe pressure less than 30 mm Hg, a transcutaneous partial pressure of oxygen ($TcPO_2$) less than 30 mm Hg, and flat or minimally pulsatile pulse volume recording waveforms in the forefoot.[8] It is simple and important to objectively confirm the diagnosis with hemodynamic testing, as other conditions such as diabetic neuropathy, night cramps, degenerative joint disease, and gout may be confused with rest pain.

Tissue loss (lower leg or foot ulcer) and gangrene can be obvious manifestations of CLTI. The strict definition of CLTI-related tissue loss requires that it be present for at least two weeks (to exclude minor traumatic lesions that heal spontaneously) and that it be accompanied by objective evidence of PAD of sufficient severity to impede wound healing. This topic will be addressed in more detail below when the wound, ischemia, and foot infection (WIfI) classification[9] of CLTI is reviewed as one of the key management concepts recently recommended by the Global Guidelines Committee on CLTI.[8]

PATHOPHYSIOLOGY AND ANATOMY

This chapter focuses on PAD due to atherosclerotic occlusive disease. Other uncommon arteriopathies and vasculitides that may produce peripheral ischemia are beyond its scope. These nonatherosclerotic conditions include giant cell arteritis, Takayasu arteritis, polyarteritis nodosa, Wegener granulomatosis, thromboangiitis obliterans (Buerger disease), Behcet disease, pseudoxanthoma elasticum, iliac artery endofibrosis, popliteal entrapment syndrome, and cystic adventitial disease.

Arteries are generally grouped into three types: elastic, muscular, and arterioles. The elastic arteries are the aorta and the pulmonary arteries. They need to be elastic because they receive blood directly from the heart and are relatively thin compared to their diameters. With each contraction of the heart, blood is forcibly ejected into the elastic arteries, whose walls must stretch to accommodate this systolic force. During diastole, their elastic walls recoil, thus continuing to propel blood forward while the heart refills. The muscular arteries are distributive in nature and include the coronary and peripheral arteries. These arteries are thicker relative to their diameters than the elastic arteries, with reduced sheets of elastin and characteristically well-defined longitudinal and circular smooth muscle layers. Contraction and relaxation of the muscular arteries alter the amount of blood flow delivered depending on local requirements (e.g., increased peripheral arterial flow is induced by exercise). Arterioles are the vessels of blood delivery to the capillary bed. Arterioles are characterized by concentric rings of smooth muscle whose contraction and dilation control blood flow into the capillary bed; they are generally less than 300 microns in diameter.

Arteries consist of three layers: the endothelium, media, and adventitia (with vasa vasorum). These layers vary in composition and thickness depending on location and health/disease state. The endothelium is considered an organ. As such, it has autocrine, paracrine, and endocrine functions that regulate blood flow and thrombogenicity. The endothelium is remarkable in that it synthesizes multiple compounds that regulate vascular tone and provide vascular homeostasis. Dysfunction of the endothelium is the earliest hallmark of vessel injury (Ross hypothesis of atherosclerosis) and it can be detected before histologic changes associated with atherosclerosis are evident. The injury response is currently thought to be similar in many ways to a chronic inflammatory response. After initial epithelial dysfunction, changes in the arterial wall permeability occur and in response to a multitude of growth factors, stimulatory factors, and interactions between smooth muscle cells (SMCs), monocytes, lymphocytes and platelets, a fibroproliferative response takes place that results in plaque deposition. There are three stages of plaque, with the earliest stage termed the fatty streak. Fatty streaks are focal, yellow, usually linear streaks that can be seen on the luminal surface of arteries and are evident in most individuals after three years of age. These streaks are microscopically macrophages (foam cells) full of lipid that accumulate in the intima. They often occur at branch points. Atherosclerotic plaque also tends to develop at branch points. The intermediate stage is a fibrofatty lesion characterized by increased deposition of layers of matrix around layered macrophages, T lymphocytes, and SMCs. The most advanced stage is the complicated or fibrous plaque. Such plaques have begun to compromise the arterial lumen and protrude into it. On their surface is a fibrous cap beneath which lie dense layers of connective tissue and SMCs with a core containing lipid and necrotic debris. Rupture of the cap characterizes an unstable plaque, which exposes the vessel lumen to lipid and cellular debris, leading to the thrombotic complications associated with atherosclerotic plaque (Fig. 63.3).

Atherosclerotic disease is a chronic, degenerative, inflammatory process to which the body attempts to adapt to maintain both the structure and underlying function of the arterial circulation. Although systemic in nature, atherosclerosis tends to develop at specific, anatomic locations within the arterial tree. Adaptive responses include compensatory changes in wall thickness and luminal diameter, which are thought to result from changes in shear stress. Glagov and associates were among the first to note that as atherosclerotic plaques enlarge, the lumen enlarges to compensate and maintain similar flow rates.[10] This process has been shown to occur in the coronary, carotid, and superficial femoral arteries as well as the aorta. Such compensatory enlargement may serve to prevent flow-limiting luminal stenosis until the plaque area reaches approximately 40% of the cross-sectional area of the affected lumen. While coronary, carotid, and aortoiliac lesions tend to occur at branch points, obstructive superficial femoral artery plaque tends to develop in the distal portion of the vessel, which is generally

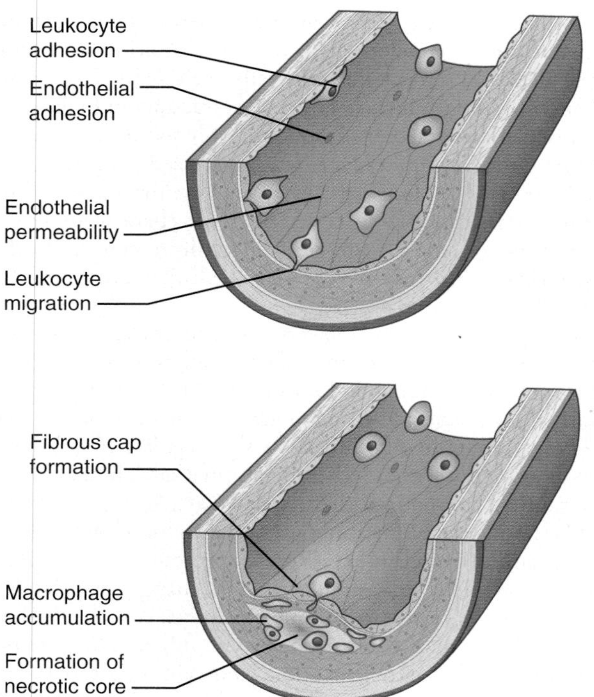

FIG. 63.3 Initiation and progression of atherosclerotic plaque. Cardiovascular risk factors, hemodynamic forces, toxins, and infectious agents interact with the vessel at the level of the endothelium to produce injury, resulting in decreased nitric oxide production and increased permeability. Once injured, the endothelium increases the expression of leukocyte adhesion molecules such as vascular cell adhesion molecule-1, intracellular adhesion molecule-1, and P- and E-selectin, which increases the adherence of macrophages and other leukocytes. Permeability of the endothelium also increases and permits entry of leukocytes and lipoproteins into the subendothelial space. Chemokines and cytokines such as monocyte chemotactic protein-1 and interleukin-8 further enhance the recruitment of leukocytes and smooth muscle cells (SMCs) into the subendothelial space. Lipoproteins retained in the subendothelial space are biochemically modified such that they can be taken up by macrophages and SMCs to form foam cells. Foam cells at the central-most position of the developing atheroma become necrotic and form the central lipid core, whereas the shoulder regions contain SMCs, macrophages, and other leukocytes. Platelet-derived growth factor and transforming growth factor-β stimulate SMC migration and collagen formation in the subendothelial space, as well as formation of the fibrous cap. (From Owens CD, Ho KJ. Atherosclerosis. In: Sidawy AN, Perler BA, eds. *Rutherford's vascular surgery and endovascular therapy*. 9th ed. Philadelphia, PA: Elsevier; 2019:44–53.)

straight, with few branches. This predilection for PAD to occur in the superficial femoral artery at the adductor hiatus has been attributed to the anatomic compression by the adductor tendons, which limits compensatory arterial dilation to growing plaque.

In general, patients with claudication will be found to have single level disease, frequently involving either the aortoiliac segment or the femoropopliteal segment, with relative sparing of the distal extremity arteries. These patterns of disease are common in cigarette smokers. Patients with CLTI more often have multilevel disease. Patients with PAD associated with diabetes tend to have patterns of more distal occlusive disease and more frequently have involvement of the deep femoral (profunda) artery and the infrapopliteal arteries.[11] CLTI patients often have femoropopliteal artery stenosis or occlusion along with tibial occlusive disease, but especially in diabetes, they may be found to have isolated infrapopliteal occlusive disease. The pedal arteries are often spared, with more than 85% of patients having a patent pedal vessel,[12] although severe pedal occlusive disease seems to be increasing in frequency, especially among patients with end-stage renal disease. For reasons that remain yet unexplained, the anterior tibial and posterior tibial arteries are most frequently involved, with relative sparing of the peroneal artery. These patterns of disease are important to recognize as they have significant implications for management (Fig. 63.4).

EVALUATION OF THE PATIENT WITH PERIPHERAL ARTERY DISEASE

A detailed history and thorough physical examination should be performed in every patient suspected of having PAD. It should include elucidation of pertinent symptoms and the degree of disability associated with them; past medical history (particularly prior surgical operations or revascularization procedures); assessment of all major cardiovascular risk factors (smoking, diabetes, hypertension, hyperlipidemia, obesity, and sedentary lifestyle); palpation of all accessible peripheral pulses (carotid, brachial, radial, ulnar, femoral popliteal, posterior tibial, and dorsal pedal); auscultation of the neck, abdomen and groin for bruits; auscultation of the heart and lungs; and palpation of the abdomen, femoral, and popliteal regions for aneurysm. The extremities should be inspected for temperature changes, color (elevation pallor or dependent rubor), signs of muscle atrophy, distal hair loss, and ulcers of the leg and foot, especially examining all surfaces of the foot and between the toes in patients with diabetes. An adequate extremity examination requires removal of the socks and shoes bilaterally, even if there are only complaints in one limb. The shoes themselves should also be closely examined for signs of uneven wear and foreign bodies within them or stuck in the soles (nails, tacks, screws, etc.). Patients with diabetic neuropathy will not feel these items. All patients with foot ulcers should be tested for neuropathy to detect loss of protective sensation (the Semmes-Weinstein monofilament test is the simplest) and probe-to-bone test should be performed in any patient with a foot ulcer.[7]

MEDICAL MANAGEMENT

PAD is a localized manifestation of systemic atherosclerosis. PAD is associated with high cardiovascular morbidity and mortality from myocardial infarction and stroke. These risks are particularly high among CLTI patients. Major risk factors for the development of PAD include age, sex, hypertension, hyperlipidemia, diabetes mellitus, smoking status, and sedentary lifestyle. Major cardiovascular risk factors should be evaluated in all patients with PAD. Medical management of patients with PAD includes modification of these medical comorbidities when feasible to reduce lower cardiac morbidity and mortality. The Society for Vascular Surgery Global Vascular Guidelines were used as a framework on which the following recommendations were based.[3,8]

Antithrombotic therapy is strongly recommended for all patients with PAD to reduce major adverse cardiac events (MACEs), defined as a composite of nonfatal stroke, nonfatal myocardial infarction, and cardiovascular death. The mainstay of this therapy is low-dose aspirin. Recent data suggests that further benefit might result from the use of alternative antiplatelets agents such as clopidogrel or ticlopidine. The benefit achieved in these patients is a lowering of MACEs. A metaanalysis performed comparing single-agent antithrombotic use in PAD patients suggested that clopidogrel monotherapy was

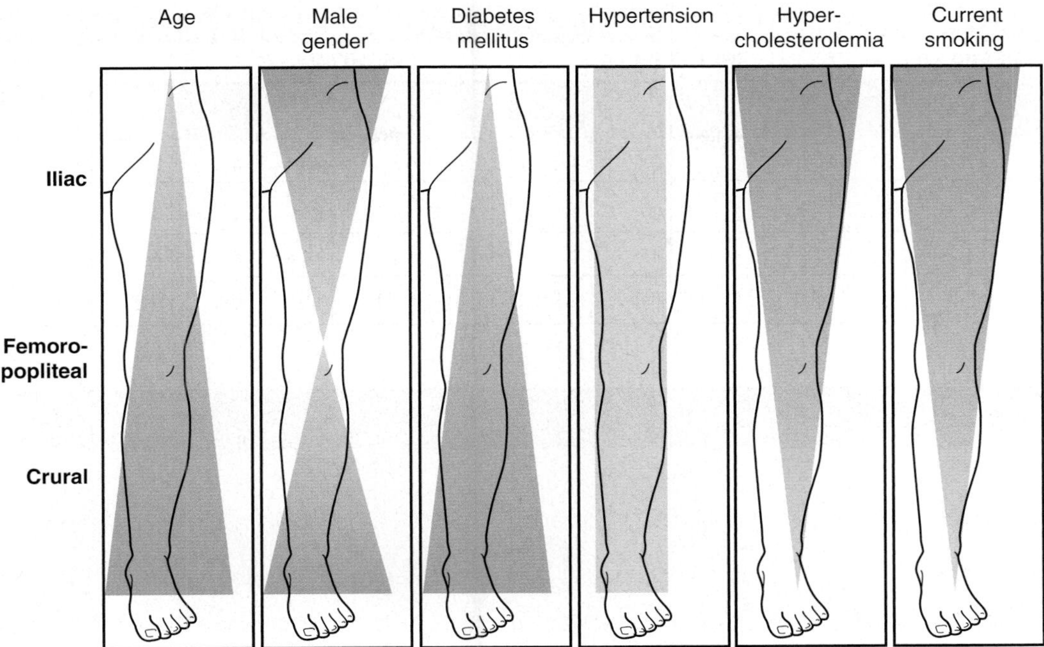

FIG. 63.4 Association of risk factors with the level of atherosclerotic target lesions. The red overlay on the anatomic cartoon illustrates the association of risk factor with patterns of atherosclerotic disease. (From Diehm N, Shang A, Silvestro A, et al. Association of cardiovascular risk factors with pattern of lower limb atherosclerosis in 2659 patients undergoing angioplasty. *Eur J Vasc Endovasc Surg.* 2006;31:59–63.)

most effective for lowering MACEs. Currently, there is no clear benefit for dual antiplatelet therapy (DAPT) or systemic anticoagulation in patients with PAD to lower MACEs, though there are several ongoing clinical trials to evaluate this issue further.

Lipid-lowering therapy is essential in patients with PAD and has been demonstrated to decrease MACEs. Additionally, there appears to be a direct antiinflammatory effect in PAD patients, which has been postulated to lead to atherosclerotic plaque stability and reduce vascular events. It has been well established that high-intensity statin therapy decreases MACEs in patients with PAD. Specifically, this includes high intensity rosuvastatin (20–40 mg/day) or simvastatin (40–80 mg/day).

Control of hypertension has been shown to decrease MACEs in patients with PAD. Data suggests that targeting systolic blood pressure (SBP) less than 140 mm Hg and diastolic blood pressure (DBP) less than 90 mm achieves optimal reduction in MACEs in patients with PAD. Specific categories of antihypertensives have not clearly been demonstrated to be optimal in PAD patients, with angiotensin-converting enzyme (ACE) inhibitors, calcium channel blockers, beta blockers, and diuretics all being effective to lower MACEs.

Diabetes mellitus is a significant risk factor and contributor to the development of atherosclerosis and PAD. The extent and severity of disease correlates with blood glucose control. Therefore, glycemic control should be a focus of care in patients with PAD. The specific goal is for patients is to maintain a Hemoglobin A1c level of less than 7%. There has been a noted advantage for using metformin as the primary hypoglycemic agent for patients with Type II diabetes and CLTI. Adjunctive medications as well as insulin should be considered to achieve this A1c target.

Tobacco abuse is a frequent comorbid condition for patients with PAD and specifically those with CLTI. The extent of cigarette smoking has been shown to correlate with PAD severity. Tobacco abuse leads to higher MACEs in patients with PAD and also contributes to PAD disease progression. Patients should be asked about the status of their tobacco use at every visit. Clinical support, adjunctive medications, and counseling should be offered to all active smokers with PAD.

Exercise has been shown to have clear benefits for patients with PAD and intermittent claudication and should be the attempted prior to revascularization in these patients. This is especially true for patients with stable symptoms that are not lifestyle limiting. Specifically, patients should be referred for a supervised exercise therapy program with an exercise physiologist if possible. There is greater established benefit for supervised compared to nonsupervised programs, but home-based plans have also shown benefit. Exercise has been shown to improve walking distances in claudicants by increasing calf blood flow, improving endothelial function, reducing local inflammation, and inducing angiogenesis. The general recommendations are for these patients to perform a minimum of 45 to 60 minutes of exercise, 3 times per week for 12 weeks, typically walking on a treadmill. The exercise should be sufficiently intense to elicit claudication. No specific randomized controlled trial has been used to evaluate this benefit in CLTI patient symptoms, although the benefit from reduced MACEs associated with cardiac rehabilitation regimens has been demonstrated.

KEY MANAGEMENT CONCEPTS: WIfI, GLASS, TAP AND PLAN

Perhaps the most significant recent change in the diagnosis and management of PAD relates to concepts concerning CLTI. These changes were driven in large part by the global epidemic of diabetes. Diabetes currently affects nearly 400 million people around the world and its prevalence is increasing in virtually every country for which data are available. Due to neuropathy and PAD, about one in four patients with diabetes will develop a foot ulcer during their lifetime; 80% of diabetes-related amputations are preceded

TABLE 63.1 SVS WIfI clinical limb stage based on estimated risk of amputation at one year.

	ISCHEMIA - 0				ISCHEMIA - 1				ISCHEMIA - 2				ISCHEMIA - 3			
W-0	1	1	2	3	1	2	3	4	2	2	3	4	2	3	3	4
W-1	1	1	2	3	1	2	3	4	2	3	4	4	3	3	4	4
W-2	2	2	3	4	3	3	4	4	3	4	4	4	4	4	4	4
W-3	3	3	4	4	4	4	4	4	4	4	4	4	4	4	4	4
	fI-0	fI-1	fI-2	fI-3	fI-0	fI-1	fI-2	fI-3	fI-0	fI-1	fI-2	fI-3	fI-0	fI-1	fI-2	fI-3

Key: *fI*, foot infection; *W*, wound.

Clinical Stage 1 or very low risk

Clinical Stage 2 or low risk

Clinical Stage 3 or moderate risk

Clinical Stage 4 or high risk

Clinical Stage 5 = unsalvageable limb

Adapted from Mills JL, Sr., Conte MS, Armstrong DG, et al. The Society for Vascular Surgery Lower Extremity Threatened Limb Classification System: Risk stratification based on wound, ischemia, and foot infection (WIfI). *J Vasc Surg.* 2014;59:220–234 e221–222.

IDSA, Infectious Diseases Society of America; *PAD,* peripheral artery disease; *PEDIS,* perfusion, extent/size, depth/tissue loss, infection, sensation; *WIfI,* wound, ischemia, and foot infection.

Premises:

a. Increase in wound class increases risk of amputation (based on WIfI, PEDIS, University of Texas, and other wound classifications systems).
b. PAD and infection are synergistic (Eurodiale); infected wound + Pad increases likelihood revascularization will be needed to heal wound.
c. Infection 3 category (systemic/metabolic instability): moderate to high-risk of amputation regardless of other factors (validated IDSA infection guidelines).

by a diabetic foot ulcer (DFU).[7,9] A significant fraction (49%–66%) of people with DFUs have detectable underlying PAD.[9,13] Even in many, modern, complex healthcare systems, patients with DFU are not routinely evaluated for PAD and the opportunity for diagnosis and revascularization is missed. All too often, DFUs are managed with wound care alone or even amputation (both major and minor) without any evaluation for correctable PAD, despite the well-known association of PAD with delayed wound healing and amputation in such patients.[13] It became apparent that the dated concept of "critical limb ischemia"[14] first proposed in 1982, as well as the most common classification systems used for decades by vascular surgeons (Fontaine[15] and Rutherford[16]), failed to address numerous issues related to management of DFU. In fact, the authors of the original consensus statement on critical limb ischemia specifically stated that patients with diabetes were to be excluded from the definition as wounds in such patients were often complicated by neuropathy and infection, and the perfusion requirements to achieve healing in patients with diabetes were likely greater than in patients with foot ulcers and gangrene occurring in the setting of pure chronic ischemia from PAD seen in cigarette smokers without diabetes.[14] The hemodynamic parameters for "critical" limb ischemia proposed in the existing classifications were likely too rigid, and both the Fontaine and Rutherford systems lacked sufficient detail about wound characteristics and failed to consider the presence and severity of infection. Both of these factors influence care and outcomes of care, especially in patients with DFU. With these considerations in mind, the Society for Vascular Surgery created and published a new classification system intended to stratify amputation risk and impact clinical management. This classification is applicable to patients with and without diabetes and is based on three major factors: wound, ischemia, and foot infection (WIfI).[9] Since its publication in 2014, the WIfI concept has achieved broad acceptance and has been adopted and recommended by many societies across the globe including, among others, the Society for Vascular Surgery, the European Society of Vascular and Endovascular Surgery, the European Society of Cardiology, the International Working Group on the Diabetic Foot (IWGDF), the American Podiatric Medical Association, and the very recently published Global Vascular Guidelines Committee.[8]

WIfI is a limb staging system. The underlying principle of WIfI is that the limb must be staged at presentation, prior to planning treatment, and in that way, it is analogous to the tumor, node, metastasis (TNM) system for cancer staging. Each of the three factors is graded on an objective scale from 0 to 4, a process which therefore yields 64 potential combinations of WIfI. By Delphi consensus, these combinations were grouped into one of four clinical stages (I–IV), each associated with progressively increasing risk of amputation at one year (Tables 63.1 and 63.2). Although initially based on a consensus approach, when subsequently applied in clinical practice, WIfI has been shown to have considerable prognostic value in predicting amputation risk. A recent metaanalysis[17] of 12 studies comprising 2669 patients with CLTI demonstrated that the likelihood of amputation at 1 year increased progressively with increasing WIfI stage, 0%, 8% (95% confidence interval [CI] 3%–21%), 11% (95% CI 6%–18%) and 38% (95% CI 21%–58%), for WIfI stages I–IV, respectively. Other analyses have yielded similar findings.[18] WIfI may also be used to predict the likelihood of benefit of revascularization, although the data supporting this particular utility of WIfI are less robust.[19,20]

TABLE 63.2 Society for Vascular Surgery Lower Extremity Threatened Limb (SVS WIfI) classification system.

I. **W**ound
II. **I**schemia
III. **F**oot **I**nfection
W I fI score

W: Wound/clinical category

SVS grades for rest pain and wounds/tissue loss (ulcers and gangrene):
0 (ischemic rest pain, ischemia grade 3; no ulcer), 1 (mild), 2 (moderate), 3 (severe).

GRADE	ULCER	GANGRENE
0	No ulcer	No gangrene
Clinical description: ischemic rest pain (requires typical symptoms + ischemia grade 3); no wound.		
1	Small, shallow ulcer(s) on distal leg or foot; no exposed bone, unless limited to distal phalanx	No gangrene
Clinical description: minor tissue loss. Salvageable with simple digital amputation (1 or 2 digits) or skin coverage.		
2	Deeper ulcer with exposed bone, joint, or tendon; generally not involving the heel; shallow heel ulcer, without calcaneal involvement	Gangrenous changes limited to digits
Clinical description: major tissue loss salvageable with multiple (≥3) digital amputations or standard TMA ± skin coverage.		
3	Extensive, deep ulcer involving forefoot and/or midfoot; deep, full thickness heel ulcer ± calcaneal involvement	Extensive gangrene involving forefoot and/or midfoot; full thickness heel necrosis ± calcaneal involvement
Clinical description: extensive tissue loss salvageable only with a complex foot reconstruction or nontraditional TMA (Chopart or Lisfranc); flap coverage or complex wound management needed for large soft tissue defect.		

TMA, Transmetatarsal amputation.

I: Ischemia

Hemodynamics/perfusion: Measure TP or $TcPO_2$ if ABI incompressible (>1.3)
SVS grades 0 (none), 1 (mild), 2 (moderate), and 3 (severe).

GRADE	ABI	ANKLE SYSTOLIC PRESSURE	TP, $TcPO_2$
0	≥0.80	>100 mm Hg	≥60 mm Hg
1	0.6–0.79	70–100 mm Hg	40–59 mm Hg
2	0.4–0.59	50–70 mm Hg	30–39 mm Hg
3	≤0.39	<50 mm Hg	<30 mm Hg

ABI, Ankle-brachial index; *PVR,* pulse volume recording; *SPP,* skin perfusion pressure; *TP,* toe pressure; *$TcPO_2$,* transcutaneous oximetry.

Patients with diabetes should have TP measurements. If arterial calcification precludes reliable ABI or TP measurements, ischemia should be documented by $TcPO_2$, SPP, or PVR. If TP and ABI measurements result in different grades, TP will be the primary determinant of ischemia grade.

Flat or minimally pulsatile forefoot PVR = grade 3.

fI: foot Infection:

SVS grades 0 (none), 1 (mild), 2 (moderate), and 3 (severe: limb and/or life-threatening)

SVS adaptation of Infectious Diseases Society of America (IDSA) and International Working Group on the Diabetic Foot (IWGDF) perfusion, extent/size, depth/tissue loss, infection, sensation (PEDIS) classifications of diabetic foot infection.

CLINICAL MANIFESTATION OF INFECTION	SVS	IDSA/PEDIS INFECTION SEVERITY
No symptoms or signs of infection	0	Uninfected
Infection present, as defined by the presence of at least two of the following items: • Local swelling or induration • Erythema >0.5 to ≤2 cm around the ulcer • Local tenderness or pain • Local warmth • Purulent discharge (thick, opaque to white, or sanguineous secretion) Local infection involving only the skin and the subcutaneous tissue (without involvement of deeper tissues and without systemic signs as described below). Exclude other causes of an inflammatory response of the skin (e.g., trauma, gout, acute Charcot neuroosteoarthropathy, fracture, thrombosis, venous stasis)	1	Mild
Local infection (as described above) with erythema >2 cm, or involving structures deeper than skin and subcutaneous tissues (e.g., abscess, osteomyelitis, septic arthritis, fasciitis), and No systemic inflammatory response signs (as described below)	2	Moderate
Local infection (as described above) with the signs of SIRS, as manifested by two or more of the following: • Temperature >38°C or <36°C • Heart rate >90 beats/min • Respiratory rate >20 breaths/min or $PaCO_2$ <32 mm Hg • White blood cell count >12,000 or <4000 cu/mm or 10% immature (band) forms	3	Severe*

From Lipsky BA, Berendt AR, Cornia PB, et al. 2012 Infectious Diseases Society of America clinical practice guideline for the diagnosis and treatment of diabetic foot infections. *Clin Infect Dis.* 2012;54:e132–173.

$PACO_2$, Partial pressure of arterial carbon dioxide; *SIRS,* systemic inflammatory response syndrome.

*Ischemia may complicate and increase the severity of any infection. Systemic infection may sometimes manifest with other clinical findings, such as hypotension, confusion, vomiting, or evidence of metabolic disturbances, such as acidosis, severe hyperglycemia, new-onset azotemia.

The limb itself, however, is only one issue to be considered in the treatment of patients with CLTI. Patient risk factors, life expectancy, and the underlying vascular anatomy in patients felt to benefit from revascularization also constitute integral components of the decision-making process. The Global Vascular Guidelines on CLTI were recently published in an effort to initiate evidence-based guidelines for the diagnosis, evaluation, and management of such patients. The guidelines include an expanded and more modern definition of CLTI, are based upon a three-step process that includes limb staging with WIfI, and introduce three other new concepts: patient, limb, anatomy (PLAN), target artery path (TAP), and Global Limb Anatomic Staging System (GLASS).[8] These guidelines are succinctly summarized below as they represent an important advance in CLTI care.

The Global Vascular Guideline begins by establishing important definitions and nomenclature. The Global Vascular Guidelines suggest abandoning the outdated term "critical limb ischemia"[14] as it fails to encompass the complete spectrum of patients in modern day practice who are evaluated and treated to prevent limb amputation. Instead, the term CLTI is now proposed so as to include a much broader spectrum of patients with varying degrees of ischemia sufficient to contribute to the development of foot and leg ulcers, delay healing, and increase amputation risk. CLTI includes only patients with chronic atherosclerotic disease and is not intended to be applied to patients with acute thrombotic or embolic leg ischemia, trauma, pure venous disease, or nonatherosclerotic conditions such as the vasculitides and Buerger disease. The target population therefore includes any adult with CLTI, defined as a patient with objectively documented PAD and any of the following clinical presentations: ischemic rest pain with confirmatory hemodynamic measurements; DFU or any lower limb ulcer present for at least two weeks; and gangrene involving any part of the lower limb or foot. CLTI is thus a more inclusive and well-defined term that can be more appropriately applied to the spectrum of patients presenting with limb threat than the dated or imprecise terms, critical limb ischemia or severe limb ischemia.

Given a patient presenting with any of the above manifestations of CLTI, the next step is to stage the limb with the WIfI classification system, which provides an evidence-based estimation of the degree of limb threat and helps focus limb salvage efforts.

PLAN includes a focus on the patient and his/her estimated risk for intervention, in particular estimates of short- and long-term mortality. In contrast to patients with CLTI, patients with claudication are generally at lower risk, with a predicted 75% to 80% 5-year life expectancy and a 5-year risk of amputation of only 5%.[3] Interventions should only be undertaken in claudicants after failure of exercise and medical therapy, when anatomic factors are favorable for intervention, and prolonged patency and symptom relief is likely. In contrast, CLTI patients overall have a 50% 5-year mortality,[21] but also a much higher amputation risk, based primarily on the limb stage at presentation. Simons and associates[22] suggested that CLTI patients could be grouped into three risk groups for mortality based on a combination of factors including age older than 80 years, oxygen-dependent chronic obstructive lung disease, stage 5 chronic kidney disease, and bedbound status. Using a predictive model based on these factors from a large cohort of over 38,000 patients derived from the Vascular Quality Initiative, patients were defined as low-risk (30-day survival >97% and 2-year survival >70%), medium-risk (30-day survival 95%–97% or 2-year survival 50%–70%), or high-risk (30-day survival <95% or 2-year survival <50%).[22] These data and those from the BASIL trial[23] were considered in the Global Guidelines and it was recommended that CLTI patients be grouped into average (anticipated periprocedural mortality <5% and estimated 2-year survival >50%) and high-risk groups (anticipated periprocedural mortality ≥5% and estimated 2-year survival ≤50%). One of the reasons for this adjustment was because the BASIL trial had shown that EVT for severe limb ischemia patients had similar outcomes compared to open surgical bypass for patients living less than two years from their initial revascularization attempt, whereas patients living longer than two years appeared to benefit from bypass surgery.[24,25] Other factors have also been examined including functional status and frailty,[26–33] but the data in CLTI patients in predicting perioperative and long-term survival is not yet well defined. The final component of PLAN, after assessing individual patient risk and WIfI limb stage, is to evaluate the arterial anatomy in those patients in need of revascularization and who would be candidates for revascularization. These three pieces are then considered to formulate a revascularization strategy (Fig. 63.5).

To define the arterial anatomy, many groups start with duplex imaging because it can be done in the office, is relatively inexpensive, and requires neither an intravenous catheter nor contrast administration. Computed tomography angiography and magnetic resonance angiography can be considered, especially when inflow disease (aortoiliac disease) is suspected. Most commonly, patients are evaluated with catheter-based digital subtraction angiography because it is the most direct method and offers the best views of the foot (Fig. 63.6). Studies which do not include the foot in CLTI patients are inadequate.[7,8] Contrast can be diluted in patients with kidney disease and CO_2 arteriography offers excellent views of the proximal vessels down the popliteal level and is therefore often used to limit contrast in patients with significant baseline renal impairment.

Any inflow disease, if present, must be corrected, most commonly with angioplasty with or without stenting. The entire affected limb is evaluated angiographically and classified using the GLASS. GLASS classifies the limb disease burden from the groin to the foot, with the underlying assumption that inflow disease is not present or has already been corrected. GLASS was designed to address inconsistencies and the overall lack of utility of the older, TransAtlantic Inter-Society Consensus (TASC) I and II anatomic classification systems, which were lesion and arterial segment based and did not correlate with expected patency rates and outcomes of therapy.[8] There are several underlying key assumptions and principles defined by GLASS. The first is that in-line flow to the ankle and the foot is a primary goal of therapy, and to accomplish that, one must select a TAP. The TAP is selected by the operator and is a continuous route of in-line flow from groin to foot. Assessment of patency is limb based, not lesion or segment based. The femoropopliteal and infrapopliteal segments are each graded in severity on a scale from 0 to 4 based on length and other important characteristics of the stenosis or occlusion, such as whether or not the origin of the vessel is involved and whether or not significant calcification is present (Figs. 63.7 and 63.8). Pedal anatomy is used as a modifier/descriptor (Fig. 63.9). CLTI is most often a multilevel disease, so GLASS combines the grades of the infrainguinal segments to create an arterial anatomic stage, analogous to the way in which the WIfI system is used to stage the limb itself. Stages range in progressive severity from I to III, based on consensus estimates of the estimated technical failure rates and 1-year limb-based patency (Table 63.3). The system is geared toward an endovascular approach but should allow meaningful comparison with open bypass surgery for comparable WIfI limb stage and GLASS arterial anatomic stages. Although based on current best evidence and expert consensus, the GLASS classification has not yet been validated. However, neither were the TASC systems it is intended to replace and GLASS makes more clinical sense because the entire limb is staged from an arterial anatomic standpoint and it

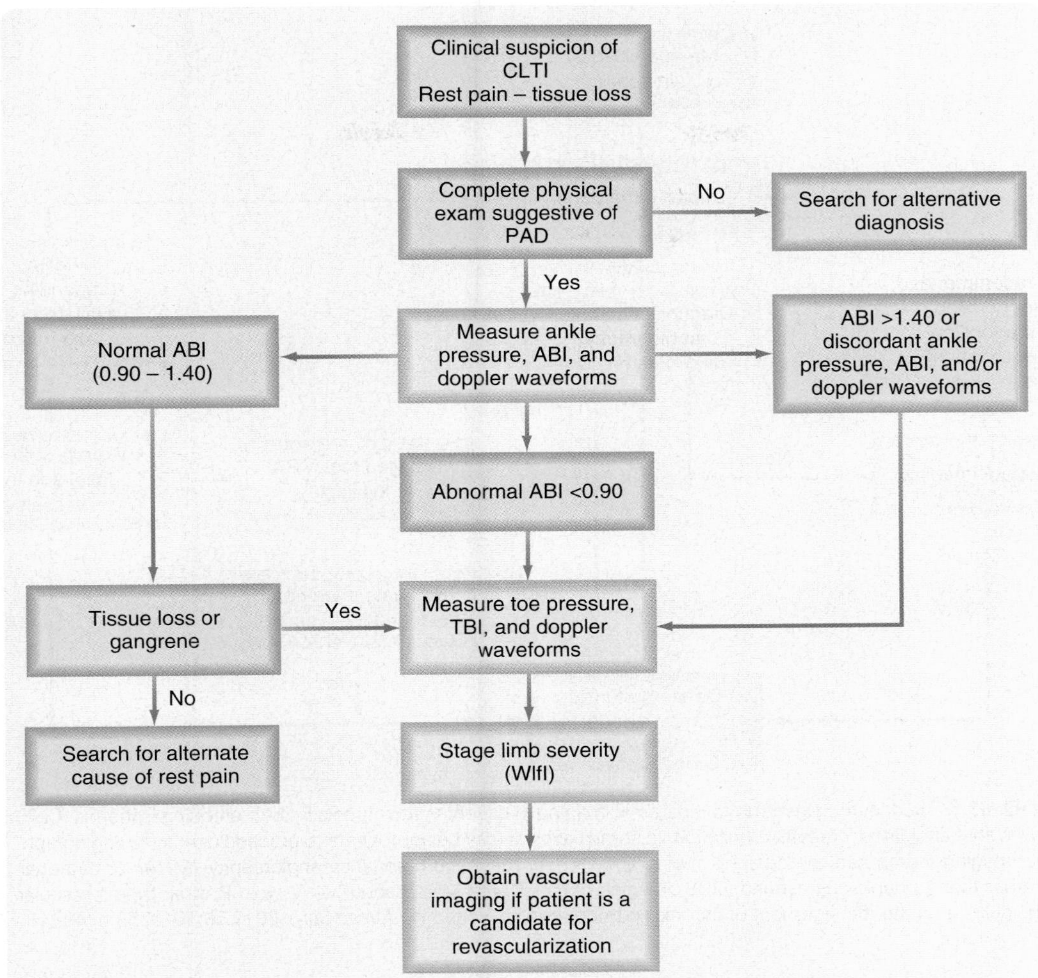

FIG. 63.5 Flow diagram for the investigation of patients presenting with suspected chronic limb-threatening ischemia *(CLTI)*. (From Conte MS, Bradbury AW, Kolh P, et al. Global vascular guidelines on the management of chronic limb-threatening ischemia. *J Vasc Surg*. 2019;69:3S–125S e140.) *ABI*, Ankle-brachial index; *PAD*, peripheral artery disease; *TBI*, toe-brachial index; *WIfI*, wound, ischemia, and foot infection.

considers that more than one level of disease may have to be treated to obtain in-line flow to heal the foot (Fig. 63.10). Going forward, it is anticipated that the combination of patient risk, WIfI limb stage, and GLASS anatomic stage can be put together to predict the benefit of revascularization and the best means of accomplishing it (i.e., EVT vs. bypass, see Figs. 63.11 and 63.12)

ENDOVASCULAR VERSUS OPEN SURGICAL THERAPY

The emergence of EVT for the treatment of PAD has created the dilemma of which revascularization option to select for any given patient. Once the determination has been made that an indication for revascularization exists, vascular surgeons are charged with determining the appropriate avenue of intervention. EVT has advanced to such an extent that it is often the first option selected for patients undergoing infrainguinal revascularization in contemporary practice.

A paucity of Level 1 data exists to direct the decision-making for choosing endovascular versus open surgical intervention. In fact, the sole completed randomized, controlled, prospective, multicenter trial comparing angioplasty to open surgery therapy is the BASIL Study from the United Kingdom.[24,25] While this trial demonstrated no significant differences between the open bypass first group versus the balloon angioplasty group at six months, a trend toward improved amputation-free survival was noted at two years in the group initially undergoing open surgical bypass.

Anatomic considerations previously deemed to necessitate open surgical therapy have become less stringent in parallel with these endovascular advancements. The now dated TASC 2007 guidelines suggest that bypass is still preferable in TASC D (long segment, extensive) aortoiliac and femoropopliteal lesions. Additionally, extensive literature suggests that patients with limited tibial runoff should be considered for open revascularization to avoid further damage to the remaining runoff vessels.[34] It is important to note that despite these recommendations, all lesions are considered by some to be appropriate for either open or EVT based solely on anatomic considerations.

The underlying indication is important to consider at the time of operative planning. Expected long-term patency rates should be considered prior to selecting a treatment plan. Patients with claudication or ischemic rest pain treated with EVT will often have

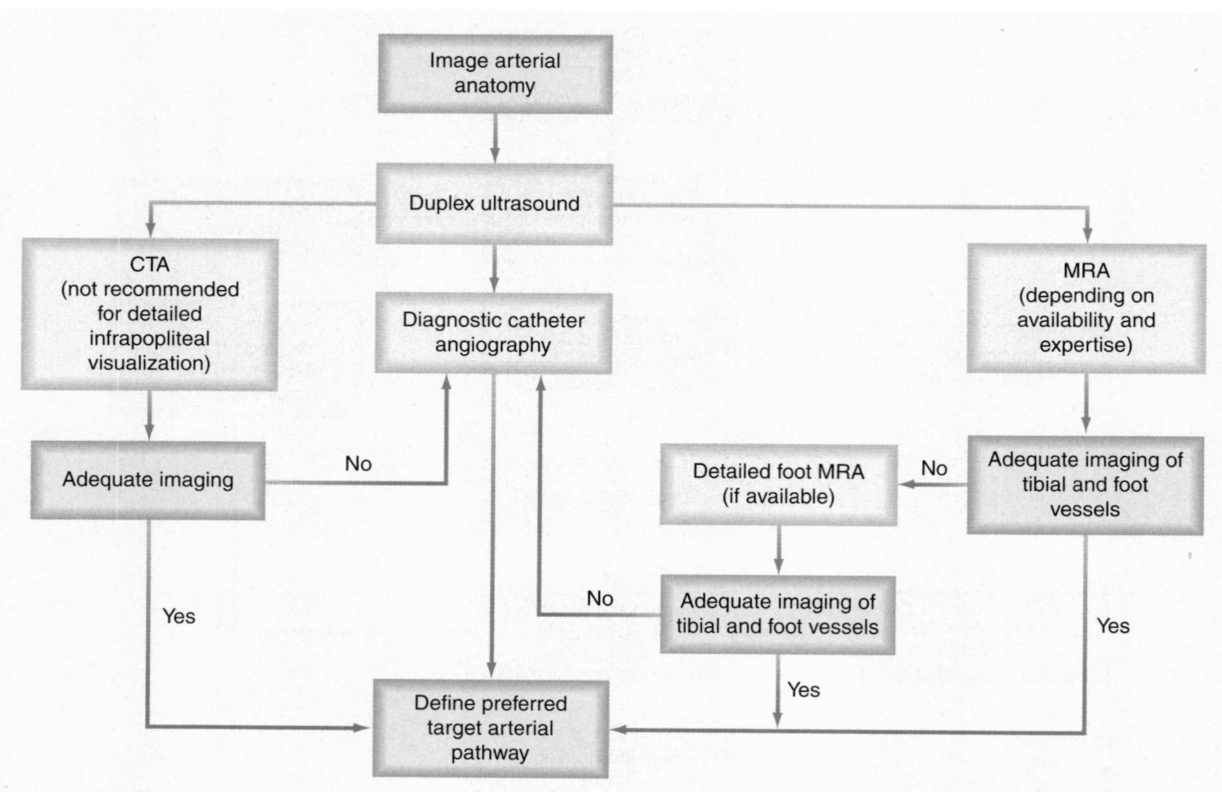

FIG. 63.6 Suggested algorithm for anatomic imaging in patients with chronic limb-threatening ischemia (CLTI) who are candidates for revascularization. In some cases, it may be appropriate to proceed directly to angiographic imaging (computed tomography angiography *[CTA]*, magnetic resonance angiography *[MRA]*, or catheter) rather than to duplex ultrasound (DUS) imaging. (From Conte MS, Bradbury AW, Kolh P, et al. Global vascular guidelines on the management of chronic limb-threatening ischemia. *J Vasc Surg*. 2019;69:3S–125S e140.)

recurrence of symptoms when the intervention fails. Conversely, patients with tissue loss can often heal their wounds or amputation incisions in the period of EVT patency and may not require further intervention if the index wound(s) have healed, despite recurrence of the underlying arterial lesions. Restenosis is extremely common after EVT, especially for complex and more calcified lesions. Patients with CLTI often have long segment and multilevel disease which has inferior patency rates after endovascular intervention.[35]

Medical comorbidities should also be considered when determining the type of intervention. EVT can often be performed under local anesthesia with monitored conscious sedation (avoiding general anesthesia), with minimal blood loss and reduced physiologic stress to the patient. These considerations may lead to the selection of an EVT approach in patients with severe medical comorbidities, including advanced coronary artery disease or chronic obstructive pulmonary disease. However, some patients with severe medical comorbidities can be medically optimized and may then tolerate open intervention. Finally, as demonstrated in the BASIL trial, one must consider patient life expectancy. A significant benefit for open surgical bypass over angioplasty was not evident until two years following intervention. Therefore, angioplasty should be strongly considered as the primary therapy for patients with shorter life expectancies to avoid prolonged hospitalization or morbidity, as these considerations likely outweigh issues of patency and durability of the revascularization.

The BASIL trial also demonstrated a very high level of treatment crossover. Specifically, patients undergoing EVT first had a high rate of subsequent open bypass and those treated first with open bypass frequently required subsequent endovascular intervention to maintain patency. This finding suggests that the two forms of intervention are complementary and reinforces the need to have both options available when treating patients with PAD.[35]

Of note, due to the lack of level 1 data to guide this decision-making process, two additional randomized controlled trials are currently ongoing. The BASIL 2 trial (United Kingdom) and the BEST-CLI (primarily United States and Canada) trial seek to further inform surgeons and patients determining appropriate treatment courses.

Endovascular Therapy

EVT has exploded due to rapid evolution of devices and techniques over the last two decades such that it has now become the first option for intervention in many patients with clinical manifestations of PAD. While initially limited to focal lesions in larger diameter vessels, it currently is used even to treat long segment lesions in the tibial and pedal vessels. Historically, this same evolution of treatment from proximal to distal vessel occurred with open surgical therapy. Although in many cases EVT patency rates remain inferior to those of open surgical bypass, with appropriate patient and lesion selection and with the use of advanced, meticulous techniques, favorable patient-centered outcomes can be achieved.

General Considerations

There are certain aspects of technique applicable to all forms of EVT and these include gaining arterial access and sheath, catheter,

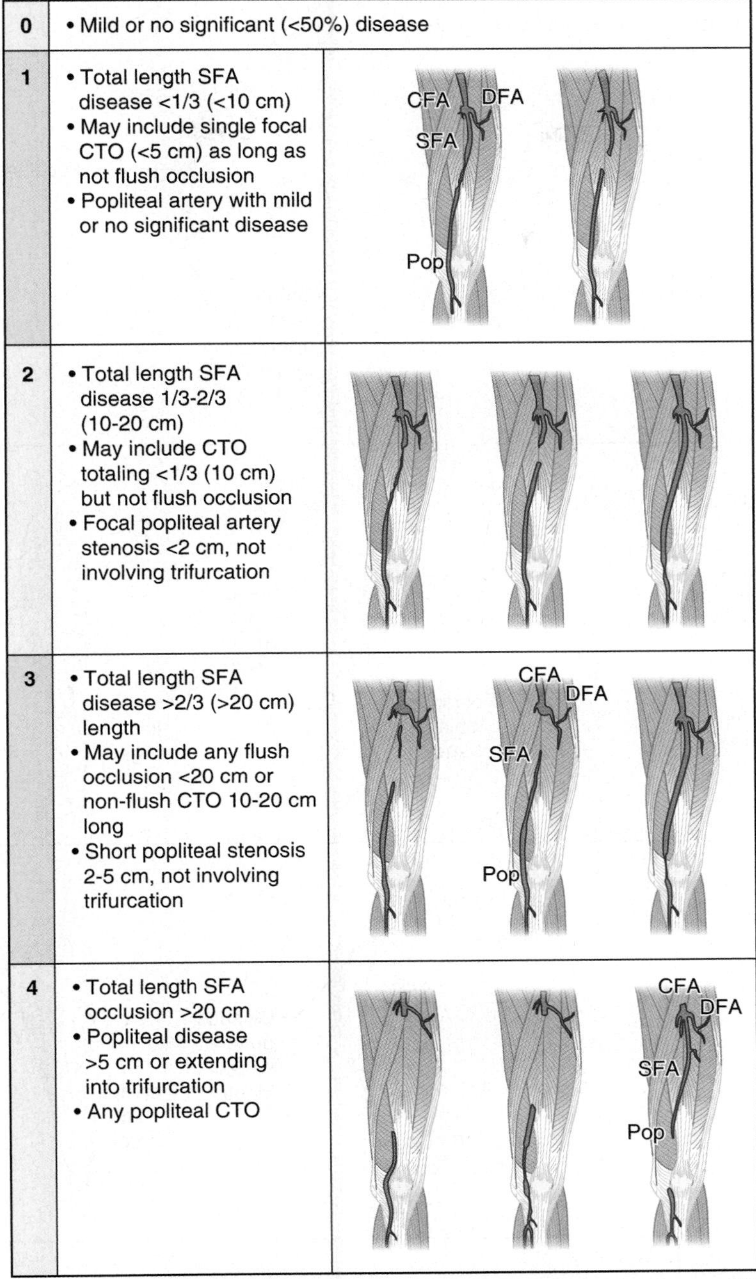

FIG. 63.7 Femoropopliteal (FP) disease grading in Global Limb Anatomic Staging System (GLASS). Trifurcation is defined as the termination of the popliteal artery at the confluence of the anterior tibial (AT) artery and tibioperoneal trunk. (From Conte MS, Bradbury AW, Kolh P, et al. Global vascular guidelines on the management of chronic limb-threatening ischemia. *J Vasc Surg.* 2019;69:3S–125S e140.) *CFA*, Common femoral artery; *CTO*, chronic total occlusion; *DFA*, deep femoral artery; *Pop*, popliteal; *SFA*, superficial femoral artery.

and wire selection. Choice and technique of arterial access are of fundamental importance to the success of endovascular therapies and careful attention to access reduces complications. Access should be obtained in every case using a combination of anatomic landmarks (based on palpable bony or fluoroscopic landmarks), pulse palpation (if present), and ultrasound guidance. Most operators routinely employ ultrasound guidance to optimize vessel access and subsequent access site closure. The most common complications of EVT are related to the access site; they can be minimized by careful site selection and meticulous technique. In general, retrograde common femoral artery access is most commonly used for aortic and common iliac artery interventions, with up and over retrograde common femoral artery access for contralateral external iliac and superficial femoral/above-knee popliteal interventions. Antegrade common or proximal superficial femoral artery accesses are preferred by many when treating infrageniculate disease, and because of the characteristics of proximal and distal caps for longer or calcified occlusive lesions, retrograde access of a tibial or pedal vessel is often used either alone or in combination with antegrade access in treating more complex CLTI cases. All

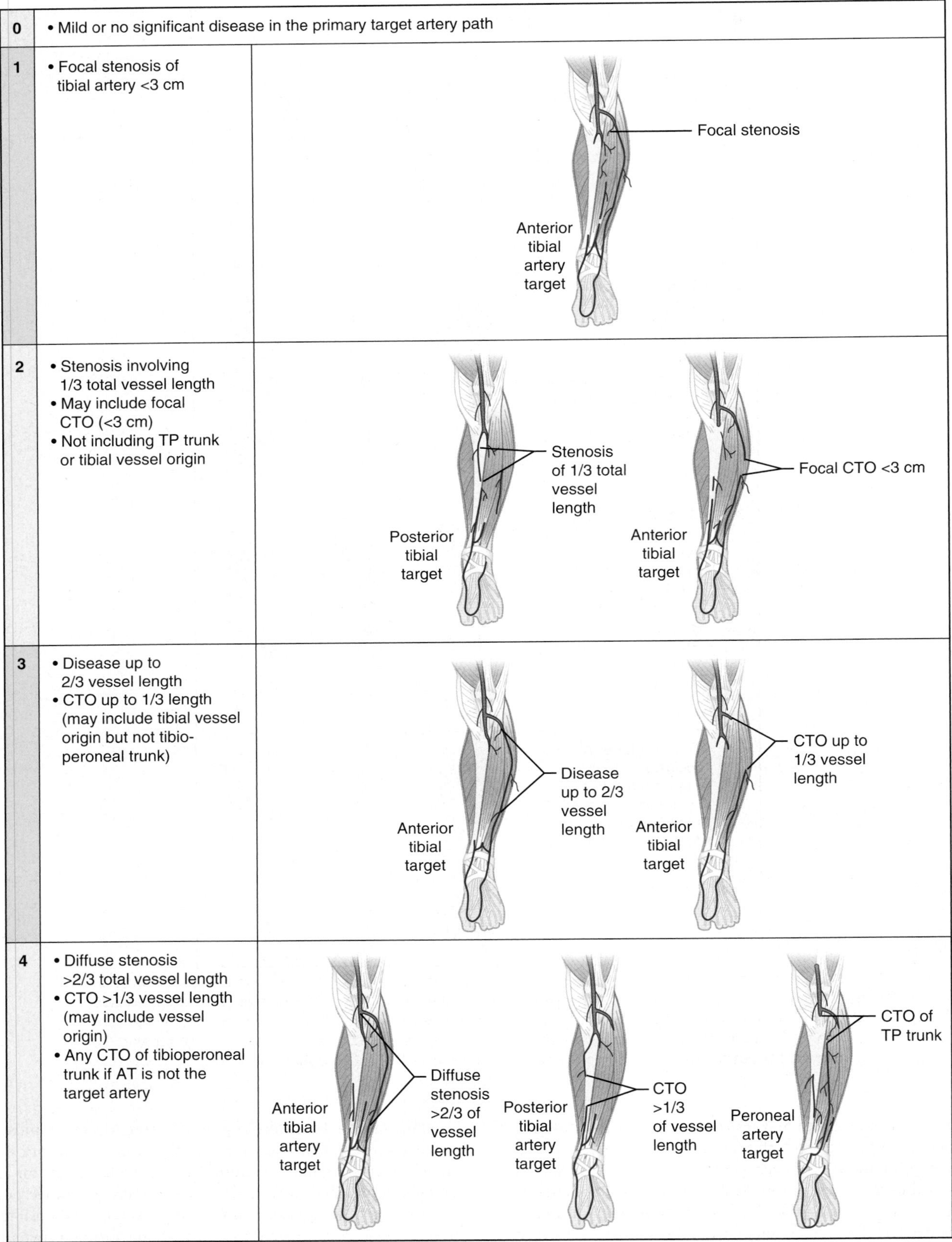

FIG. 63.8 Infrapopliteal (IP) disease grading in Global Limb Anatomic Staging System (GLASS). (From Conte MS, Bradbury AW, Kolh P, et al. Global vascular guidelines on the management of chronic limb-threatening ischemia. *J Vasc Surg.* 2019;69:3S–125S e140.) *AT*, Anterior tibial; *CTO*, chronic total occlusion; *TP*, tibioperoneal.

Inframalleolar/pedal descriptor	
P0	Target artery crosses ankle into foot, with intact pedal arch
P1	Target artery crosses ankle into foot; absent or severely diseased pedal arch
P2	No target artery crossing ankle into foot

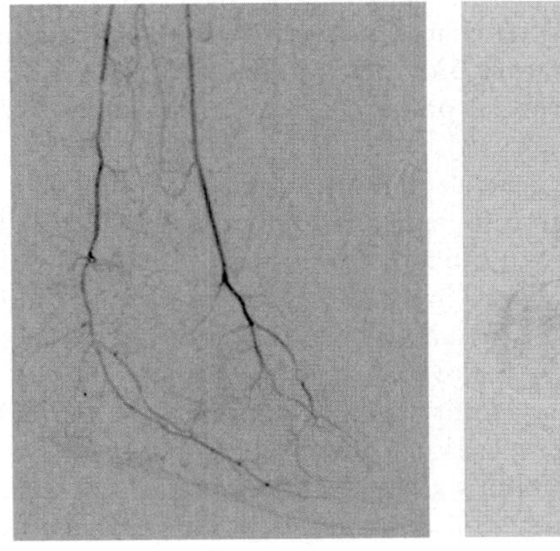
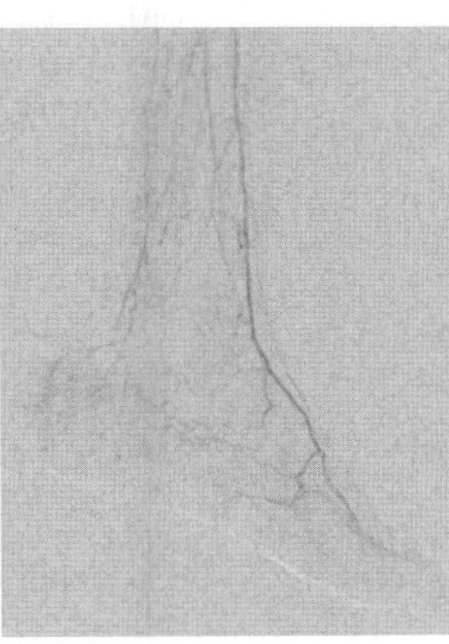
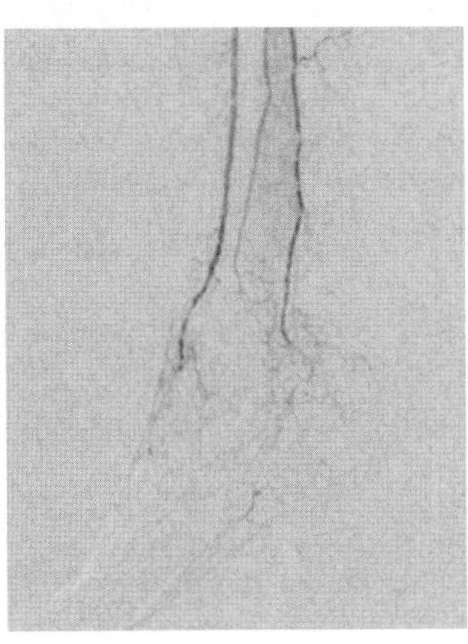

P0 P1 P2

FIG. 63.9 Inframalleolar (IM)/pedal disease descriptor in Global Limb Anatomic Staging System (GLASS). Representative angiograms of *P0* (left), *P1* (middle), and *P2* (right) patterns of disease. (From Conte MS, Bradbury AW, Kolh P, et al. Global vascular guidelines on the management of chronic limb-threatening ischemia. *J Vasc Surg.* 2019;69:3S–125S e140.)

TABLE 63.3 Assignment of Global Limb Anatomic Staging System (GLASS) stage.

		INFRAINGUINAL GLASS STAGE (I–III)				
FP Grade	4	III	III	III	III	III
	3	II	II	II	III	III
	2	I	II	II	II	III
	1	I	I	II	II	III
	0	NA	I	I	II	III
		0	1	2	3	4
		IP Grade				

From Conte MS, Bradbury AW, Kolh P, et al. Global vascular guidelines on the management of chronic limb-threatening ischemia. *J Vasc Surg.* 2019;69:3S–125S e140.

After selection of the target arterial path (TAP), the segmental femoropopliteal (FP) and infrapopliteal (IP) grades are determined from high-quality angiographic images. Using the table, the combination of FP and IP grades is assigned to GLASS stages I to III, which correlate with technical complexity (low, intermediate, and high) of revascularization. *NA*, Not applicable.

of these approaches are facilitated by a thorough understanding of bony, skin, and fluoroscopic landmarks as well as facility with ultrasound guidance. After access is obtained, diagnostic angiography is usually performed to confirm lesions suspected on preoperative assessment. Once the lesion(s) are identified, they must be crossed with a suitable wire to allow treatment.

Wires come in a variety of lengths, diameters, weights and relative stiffnesses. Wires 0.035 inch in diameter are used for most aortoiliac and femoral interventions, while 0.014 and 0.018 are most often used for tibial interventions (and renal and carotid arteries). Wire tips vary but are generally floppier than the rest of the wire and may be preshaped or be shaped by the operator depending on preference. Some wires are hydrophilic and must be kept moistened/wet or they will become sticky and not function properly. A torque device may be attached to the wire to make it more steerable. For nearly all stenoses, and many occlusions, the goal is to maintain the wire in the true lumen of the artery, cross the lesion, and then treat it with either angioplasty, atherectomy, or primary stenting depending upon the type and length of the lesion. If difficulty crossing a particular lesion occurs, the use of additional catheters for support, which can be telescoped through a long access sheath, may help, as well as using a stiffer or heavier wire. More recently, several devices have become available to facilitate crossing of difficult/resistant lesions and true lumen reentry, including plaque microdissection (Frontrunner XP CTO Catheter; Cordis, Bridgewater, NJ), fast and bidirectional catheter spinning (CrossBoss CTO Catheter; BridgePoint Medical, Plymouth, MN), and catheter tip deflection capability with spiral wedges to facilitate advancement (Wildcat Catheter; Avinger, Redwood City, CA).[36]

A useful alternative to difficult transluminal lesion crossing is intentional subintimal angioplasty, a technique initially

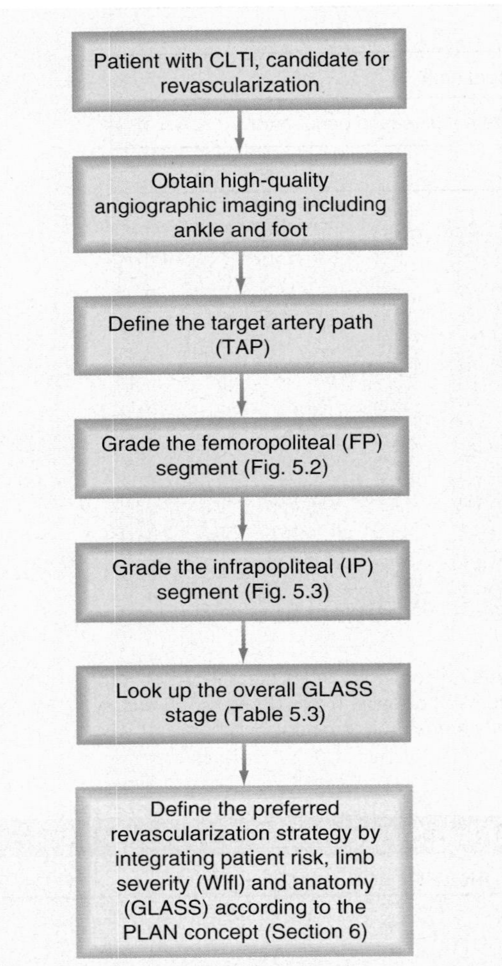

FIG. 63.10 Flow chart illustrating application of Global Limb Anatomic Staging System *(GLASS)* to stage infrainguinal disease pattern in chronic limb-threatening ischemia *(CLTI)*. (From Conte MS, Bradbury AW, Kolh P, et al. Global vascular guidelines on the management of chronic limb-threatening ischemia. *J Vasc Surg*. 2019;69:3S–125S e140.) *FP*, Femoropopliteal; *IP*, infrapopliteal; *PLAN*, patient risk estimation, limb staging, anatomic pattern of disease; *TAP*, target arterial path; *WIfI*, wound, ischemia, and foot infection.

described 30 years ago by Bolia and colleagues.[37] A wire, typically with a short J-shaped tip is formed and directed via the catheter against the arterial wall just proximal to the occlusion and used to initiate a subintimal dissection plane. The wire formed in this fashion is then intentionally advanced in this subintimal plane until the lesion is crossed, and then attempts are made to reenter the true lumen with catheter support. True lumen reentry is confirmed by return of blood through the catheter and easy advancement of the wire without resistance. If there is minimal disease in the reentry zone, this step is not difficult and often occurs spontaneously. If true lumen reentry is difficult, there are reentry devices available or, in complex cases, one may combine with retrograde access.[36]

Once the culprit arterial lesion has been successfully crossed, balloon angioplasty can be performed. Balloon angioplasty fractures the plaque and may cause focal dissection, so appropriate sizing is important. Many operators use IVUS (intravascular ultrasound) to size balloons and stents and to assess results after angioplasty or stent deployment. Balloons come in a wide variety of lengths and sizes and may be compliant or noncompliant. There are also scoring and cutting balloons, which are used to treat fibrotic and resistant lesions such as those due to intimal hyperplasia. Cutting balloons have three or four microtomes oriented longitudinally around the balloon that create controlled cuts in the fibrotic lesion and then allow standard angioplasty with a larger balloon to enlarge the stenotic lumen. There are also drug-coated balloons available analogous to the coronary circulation but their use has become controversial due to concerns about potential increased mortality risk when used in the periphery.[38]

In general, angioplasty results with respect to primary patency are better in larger, more proximal arteries and for shorter lesions. However, the rapid evolution of smaller profile systems with longer balloons has facilitated the treatment of disease in the smaller arteries, including tibial and even pedal arteries. Although not comparable to the results of open bypass with vein conduit, distal lower extremity angioplasty results are improving and with careful patient selection, patency of distal angioplasty may be sufficient to heal wounds and prevent amputation. Recently compiled results for infrapopliteal angioplasty are presented in Table 63.4. Endovascular techniques have improved such that even long segment disease in CLTI patients can successfully be treated endoluminally, an important option to have available for higher risk patients or those with no suitable autogenous conduit (Fig. 63.13).

Stents are reserved by some for residual stenosis, dissection or other complications of plain balloon angioplasty. However, for iliac lesions, data would suggest that primary stenting is superior to angioplasty (percutaneous transluminal angioplasty) alone (Table 63.5) with primary patency rates at four years better in both in claudicants (77% stenting vs. 68% percutaneous transluminal angioplasty) and those presenting with CLTI (67% vs. 55%).[39] Stents may be balloon expandable or self-expanding, covered or uncovered, drug-coated, or bare. Balloon expandable stents are often used when precise deployment and landing are critical. Covered stents may be used for a variety of indications, such as to treat embolic lesions or to prevent or treat vessel rupture (e.g., "pave and crack" technique for iliac lesions). Stenting in the femoral-popliteal segment is widely used. Stent selection is beyond the scope of this book, but good discussions are available elsewhere.[36,39]

Atherectomy devices (orbital and laser) are widely used, but high-level data supporting their use compared to numerous alternatives are still lacking. One possible advantage is that debulking the lesion may allow treatment with angioplasty alone, avoiding the expense and potential long-term sequelae of long-term stent implantation.

The results of EVT depend on a multitude of factors, especially the following: procedure indication (claudication vs. CLTI); lesion length; vessel calcification; poor runoff status; and specific comorbidities such as diabetes and end-stage renal disease.[36,39] Despite current limitations, EVT is widely used; short-term results have improved over the last decade and EVT would currently appear to be the better choice in older, higher risk patients with shorter life expectancies who would not benefit from the long-term patency afforded by bypass surgery and would be at increased risk for open surgery. Application of the WIfI, PLAN and GLASS approach to therapy of CLTI should help define the role of EVT versus bypass in the future, as well as the awaited publication of trial results from BEST-CLI and BASIL 2 and 3.

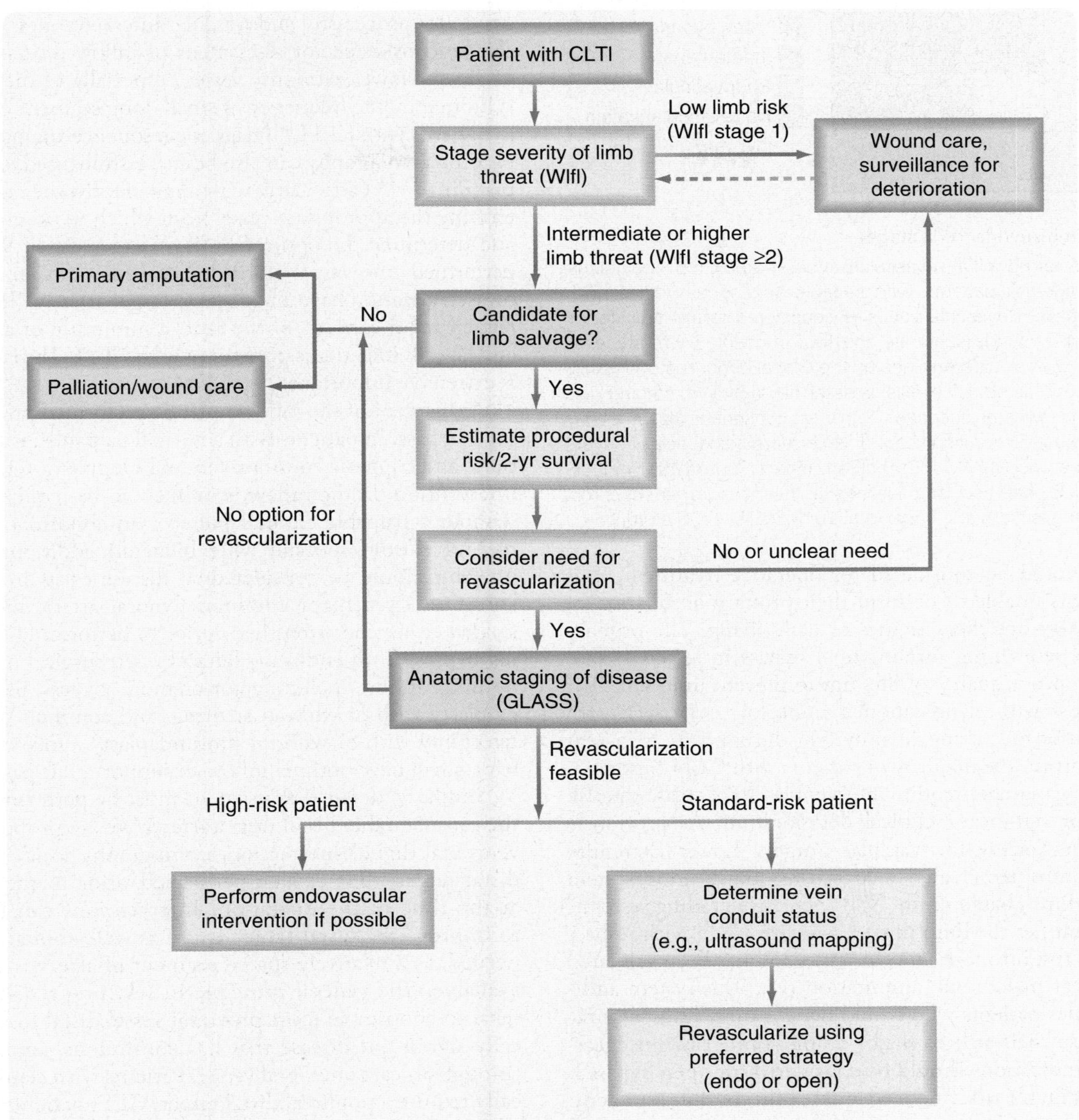

FIG. 63.11 The patient, limb, anatomy (PLAN) framework of clinical decision-making in chronic limb-threatening ischemia *(CLTI);* infrainguinal disease. Refer to Fig. 63.12 for preferred revascularization strategy in standard-risk patients with available vein conduit, based on limb stage at presentation and anatomic complexity. Approaches for patients lacking suitable vein are reviewed in the text. (From Conte MS, Bradbury AW, Kolh P, et al. Global vascular guidelines on the management of chronic limb-threatening ischemia. *J Vasc Surg.* 2019;69:3S–125S e140.) *GLASS,* Global Limb Anatomic Staging System; *WIfI,* Wound, ischemia, and foot infection.

Open Surgical Therapy

Despite the rapid evolution and utilization of EVT in the treatment of patients with lower extremity PAD, open surgical therapy is still a viable and often preferable option for these patients. The hallmark of open lower extremity revascularization remains arterial bypass, including aortofemoral bypass and infrainguinal bypass. There are extraanatomic reconstructions available to bypass to the lower extremity in the presence of aortoiliac occlusive disease, including axillofemoral bypass, femoral-femoral bypass, and thoracofemoral bypass. However, a discussion of these is beyond the scope of this chapter, as these procedures are typically only performed to address complications of previous aortofemoral revascularization or other endovascular aortoiliac reconstructions. Aortofemoral bypass most often utilizes prosthetic bifurcated conduits to bypass from the aorta to the common femoral, profunda femoris, or superficial femoral arteries. Infrainguinal bypass is defined as any major arterial reconstruction using a bypass conduit, either autogenous or prosthetic, that originates below the inguinal ligament.

Indications

The two primary indications for infrainguinal bypass are claudication and CLTI. Nonoperative management is appropriate, and initially preferable, for most patients presenting with claudication. However, following an exercise program, smoking cessation, and optimization of medical therapy, patients significantly disabled by

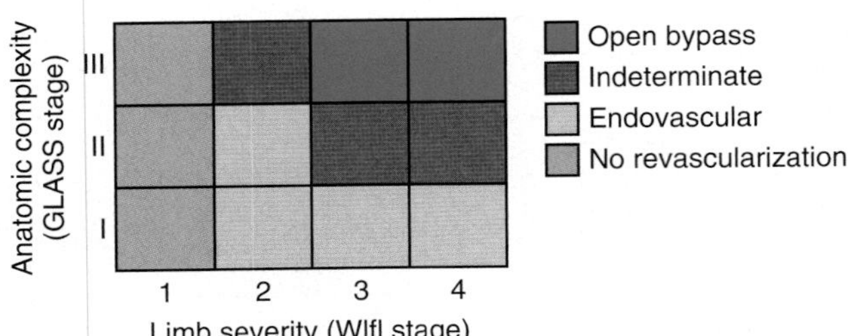

FIG. 63.12 Preferred initial revascularization strategy for infrainguinal disease in average-risk patients with suitable autologous vein conduit available for bypass. Revascularization is considered rarely indicated in limbs at low risk (wound, ischemia, and foot infection *[WIfI]* stage 1). Anatomic stage (y-axis) is determined by the Global Limb Anatomic Staging System *(GLASS)*; limb risk (x-axis) is determined by WIfI staging. The dark gray shading indicates scenarios with least consensus (assumptions inflow disease either is not significant or is corrected; absence of severe pedal disease (i.e., no GLASS P2 modifier). (From Conte MS, Bradbury AW, Kolh P, et al. Global vascular guidelines on the management of chronic limb-threatening ischemia. *J Vasc Surg.* 2019;69:3S–125S e140.)

claudication should be considered for operative treatment. This includes patients unable to perform their primary occupation or who cannot carry out the activities of daily living. The primary indication for performing infrainguinal bypass in selected claudicants is to improve quality of life, not to prevent limb loss. The risk of limb loss with claudication is quite low (<1%/yr), with major amputation occurring in only 5% during a 3- to 5-year period.[3] In contrast, the majority of patients with CLTI (rest pain, ischemic ulcer, gangrene) require intervention to decrease the risk of limb loss or significant clinical deterioration. As previously mentioned, the Society for Vascular Surgery Lower Extremity Guidelines Committee created a consensus stratification system for threatened limbs based on the WIfI objective grading system.[9] This system stratifies the limb in patients with CLTI with respect to amputation risk into four clinical stages and has been validated to predict 1-year major limb amputation risk. This system additionally identifies patients who would benefit from revascularization to decrease their risk of major amputation. Patients meeting these two indications should be considered for open bypass if functional, of suitable risk, and if adequate vein conduit is present.

Prior to intervention, it is imperative to assess the medical comorbidities of potential open surgical candidates. There is a high rate of concordant chronic obstructive pulmonary disease, diabetes mellitus, renal insufficiency, and coronary artery disease. The patients should have optimized control of blood pressure, diabetes, congestive heart failure, and angina prior to intervention. Postponement of intervention should only routinely occur for patients with unstable angina, recent myocardial infarction or uncontrolled congestive heart failure.

Preoperative Planning

A successful bypass has several prerequisites to support long-term patency. Adequate inflow and outflow must exist. Additionally, the conduit used must be optimized to ensure long-term patency. In the case of lower extremity revascularization in patients with CLTI, it is also important to determine the best outflow target vessel to provide "in-line flow" to the foot.

As with all surgical bypasses, it is imperative to obtain adequate preoperative imaging to evaluate for each of these criteria. The traditional route to obtain this necessary anatomic information is by performing standard angiography of the lower extremity. This will often be available at the time of planning if the patient underwent previous unsuccessful endovascular intervention. CT angiography can be considered for assessment of inflow disease, although its use in the lower extremity vessels, especially in the CLTI cohort, is limited by the frequency of small, long segment calcified vessels in patients with CLTI.[40] Magnetic resonance angiography and duplex ultrasonography can also be successfully used for preoperative planning.[41,42] Particularly with angiography, the operator can determine the appropriate vessel from which to originate the bypass and determine the optimal outflow target vessel. When properly performed, the vast majority of patients with an indication for revascularization have an adequate target artery.[43] Target artery selection requires views of the foot (a minimum of anteroposterior and lateral) in patients presenting with CLTI. The lateral foot view is extremely important (Fig. 63.14).

Assessment of the inflow must be performed prior to performing a bypass. In patients with a normal palpable ipsilateral femoral pulse and triphasic common femoral Doppler arterial waveforms, intervention on the inflow is unlikely to be required. In patients without a palpable femoral pulse or an abnormal femoral Doppler waveform (especially when bilateral), additional preoperative imaging should be considered. If disease exists in the ipsilateral aortoiliac segment or common femoral artery, these should be treated either concurrently or prior to performing the infrainguinal bypass. Both endovascular and open surgical options exist to optimize inflow, including aortofemoral bypass, iliac balloon angioplasty with or without stenting, and common femoral endarterectomy with or without profundaplasty. Once completed, the bypass will have optimal inflow to support graft patency.

Similarly, detailed assessment must be performed to identify the most suitable distal target artery. We are proponents of conventional digital subtraction arteriography to identify the ideal distal target. This can be performed prior to the operation or at the time of the operation. Interventions can be performed to improve the distal target artery as well, though this is rarely needed, as a relatively spared segment of artery is almost always available. The general principle in selecting a distal target vessel is to choose the most proximal vessel distal to hemodynamically significant disease that has continuous runoff to the foot through at least one tibial vessel. Patients with claudication typically require a popliteal distal target. CLTI patients often require a more distal target to a tibial, peroneal, dorsalis pedis or plantar artery (Fig. 63.15).

Conduit selection is perhaps the most critical factor underlying successful infrainguinal bypass. Autologous vein conduits include ipsilateral and contralateral great saphenous vein (GSV), short saphenous vein (SSV), femoral vein, arm (basilic and cephalic) vein, endarterectomized superficial femoral artery, cryopreserved vein, and radial artery. Preoperative imaging, typically with duplex ultrasound, is adequate to determine the presence, caliber, and quality of adequate autologous veins. Prosthetic conduits include Dacron, heparin-bonded Dacron, human umbilical vein, polytetrafluoroethylene (PTFE) with and without covalently bonded heparin, and expanded PTFE bonded with heparin.

Autologous vein outperforms all other conduits for infrainguinal bypass, including above knee popliteal bypasses. A single segment of autologous vein is superior to spliced segments. GSV and SSV are superior to arm veins. Autologous vein should be used for infrainguinal bypass whenever feasible. Prosthetic conduits for infrainguinal bypass should only be considered when autologous conduits are truly not available. Dacron has recently been shown to outperform expanded PTFE in above knee popliteal bypasses.[44]

TABLE 63.4 Results of infrapopliteal angioplasty, stenting, and atherectomy.

AUTHOR	YEAR	NUMBER TREATED	CLI	MEAN LESION LENGTH	TECHNICAL FAILURES	PRIMARY PATENCY	LIMB SALVAGE RATE
Angioplasty							
Giles and colleagues	2008	176	100%	NR	7%	53%, 1 year 51%, 2 years	84%, 3 years
Conrad and colleagues	2009	155	86%	NR	5%	71%, 2 years 62%, 3.3 years	86%, 3.3 years
Sadek and colleagues (single vs. multilevel PTA)	2009	89	77%	NR	9%	34%, 1 year Single level 58%, 1 year Multilevel NR	67% 1.5 years Single level 63%, 1.5 years Multilevel 76%, 1 year
Peregrin and colleagues	2010	1445	100%	NR	11%		
Schmidt and colleagues	2010	62	100%	18.3 cm	5%	50%, 3 months	100%, 15 months
Subintimal Angioplasty							
Ingle and colleagues	2002	70	91%	NR	14%	NR	94%, 3 years
Vraux and Bertoncello	2006	50	100%	78% >10 cm	18%	46%, 1 year 42%, 2 years	87%, 1 year 87%, 2 years
Tartari and colleagues (SFA only in 27 limbs)	2007	109	100%	59% ≥10 cm	17%	NR	87%, 1 year 85%, 2 years
Cutting-Balloon Angioplasty							
Engelike and colleagues	2002	16	31%	NR	6%	67%, 1 year	93%, 10 months
Ansel and colleagues	2004	73	71%	2.7 cm	0%	NR	89%, 1 year
Vikram and colleagues	2007	11	NR	NR	18%	50%, 1 year	NR
Drug-Coated Balloon[a]							
Tepe and colleagues	2008	48	15%	7.5 cm	2% all cases	80%, 6 months	96%, 6 months
Stenting							
Feiring and colleagues	2004	92	68%	NR	7%	NR	87%, 1 year
Bosiers and colleagues	2006	300	100%	NR	NR	76%, 1 year	99%, 1 year
Donas and colleagues	2009	34	100%	6.5 cm stenosis; 7.5 cm occlusion	3%	91%, 10 months	100%, 10 months
Randon and colleagues	2010	16	100%	38% ≥10 cm	13%	56%, 1 year	92%, 1 year
Drug-Eluting Stent							
Scheinert and colleagues	2006	30	63%	NR	0%	100%, 6 months	100%, 9 months
Fering and colleagues	2010	130	100%	NR	9%	NR	88%, 3 years
Karnabatidis and colleagues	2011	51	100%	7.7 cm	0%	30%, 3 years	NR
Rastan and colleagues	2011	82	51%	3.0 cm	0%	81%, 1 year	98%, 1 year
Atherectomy							
Zeller and colleagues	2007	36	53%	4.6 cm	2%	67%, 1 year 60%, 2 years	100%, 2 years
Safian and colleagues	2009	124	32%	3.0 cm	2.5%	NR	100%, 6 months

From Montero-Baker M, Mills JL. Endovascular repair of infrapopliteal arterial occlusive disease. In: Moore WS, Lawrence PF, Oderich GS, eds. *Moore's Vascular and endovascular surgery: A comprehensive review.* 9th ed. Philadelphia, PA: Elsevier; 2019:460–468.
CLI, Critical limb ischemia; *NR*, not reported; *PTA*, percutaneous transluminal angioplasty; *SFA*, superficial femoral artery.

Our group generally does not perform infrainguinal bypass with prosthetic conduit solely for the indication of claudication, since graft failure frequently converts a patient with stable claudication to one with acute limb-threatening ischemia, and may thus actually increase amputation risk.

Aortofemoral Bypass Techniques

Aortofemoral bypass should be considered when hemodynamically significant aortic and iliac stenosis leads to the aforementioned indications. The typical reconstruction performed is an aortobifemoral bypass with the outflow target either the common femoral arteries

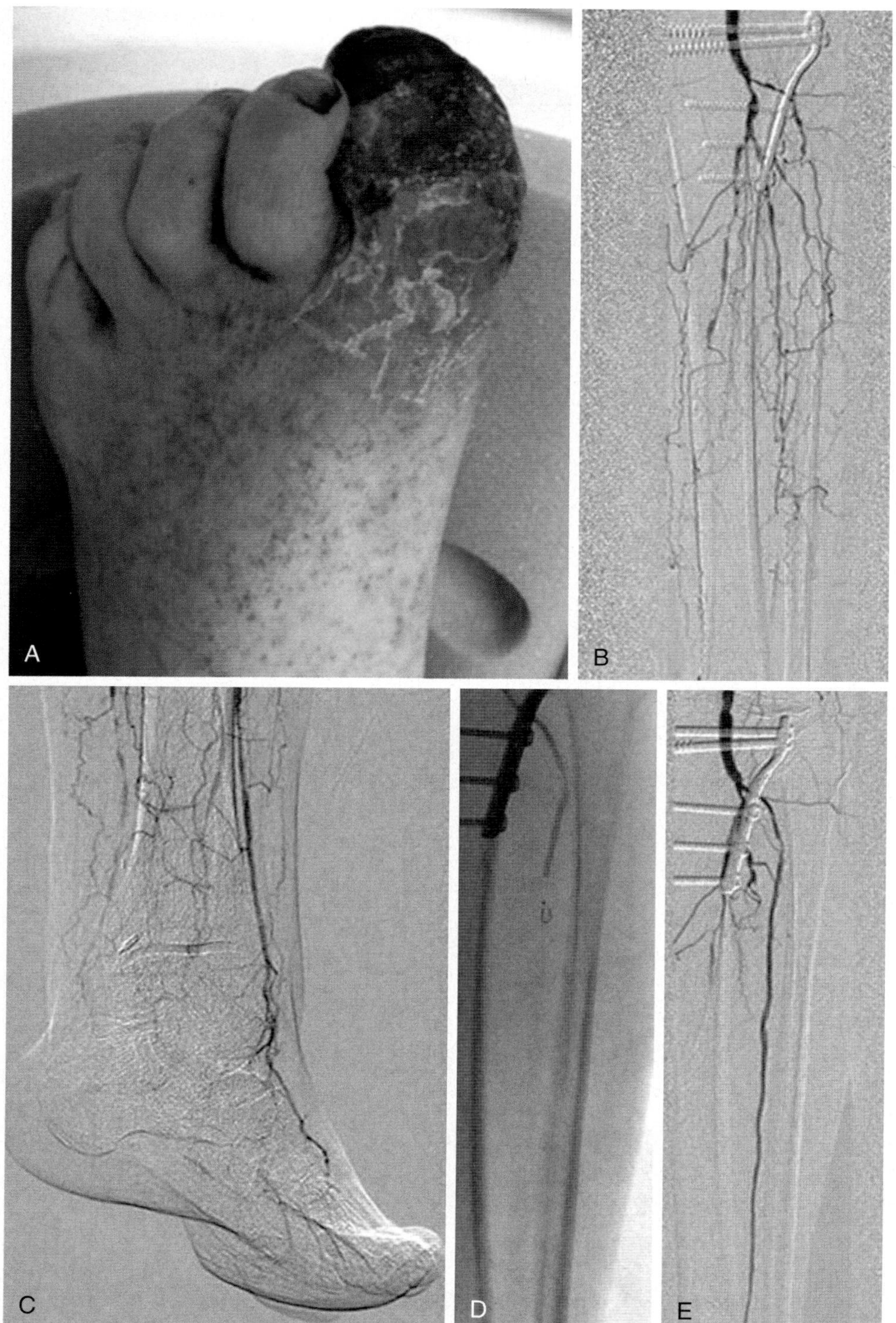

FIG. 63.13 A 77-year-old high-risk patient with diabetes and great toe gangrene. (A) Critical limb ischemia with ankle-brachial index (ABI) of 0.39. (B) Three-vessel long-segment (>25 cm) tibial artery occlusions with (C) distal anterior tibial artery reconstitution. (D) Subintimal angioplasty of long-segment occlusion. (E) Anterior tibial artery after long-segment subintimal angioplasty with ABI improved to 0.81. Toe amputation healed and the vessel remains patent 6 months after intervention. (From Montero-Baker M, Mills JL. Endovascular repair of infrapopliteal arterial occlusive disease. In: Moore WS, Lawrence PF, Oderich GS, ed. *Moore's Vascular and endovascular surgery: A comprehensive review*. 9th ed. Philadelphia, PA: Elsevier; 2019:460–468.)

or the profunda femoris arteries bilaterally. With respect to the surgical reconstruction of aortoiliac occlusive disease, the optimal inflow site is almost always just inferior to the renal arteries. Prosthetic conduits (Dacron or expanded PTFE) are generally used except when the indication is infection of a previously placed prosthetic conduit, in which case, after excision of the infected prosthetic, the choice of replacement conduit may be the femoral vein(s) to create a neo-aortoiliac system (NAIS) or cryopreserved arteries and veins.

TABLE 63.5 Review of outcomes in interventional treatment of aortoiliac occlusive disease.

SERIES	YEAR	NUMBER OF PATIENTS	INDICATION	TYPE OF INTERVENTION	PRIMARY PATENCY (%)
Parsons et al	1998	45		PTA	74 (5 year)
Klein	2006	279		Primary stenting versus selective stenting	83 (5 year)
Bosch and Hunink	1997	1300	Claudication vs. CLI	Selective stenting versus primary stenting	70 (5 year)
(metaanalysis)	1997	1300		Primary stenting	77 (4 year)
					67 (4 year)
Murphy (metaanalysis)	1998	2058		Primary stenting	73 (5 year)
Schurmann et al	2002	110	93% claudication	Primary stenting	66 (5 year)
Galaria and Davies	2005	276	TASC A and B	Primary stenting	71 (10 year)
Leville et al	2006	92	TASC C and D	Primary stenting	76 (3 year)
Rzucidlo et al	2005	34	TASC B, C, and D	Stent grafting	80 (5 year)
Chang et al	2008	171	TASC B, C, and D	Stent graft 41%, bare metal sent 59%	60 (5 year)
Mwipatayi	2011	40	TASC C and D	Stent graft	95 (18 month)
		24		Bare metal sent	50 (18 month)
Psacharopulo	2015	11	TASC D	Stent graft	91 (2 year)

From Powell RJ, Rzucidlo EM. Aortoiliac disease: Endovascular treatment. In: Sidawy AN, Perler BA, eds. *Rutherford's vascular surgery and endovascular therapy*. 9th ed. Philadelphia, PA: Elsevier; 2019:1423–1437.
CLI, Critical limb ischemia; *PTA*, percutaneous transluminal angioplasty; *TASC*, TransAtlantic Inter-Society Consensus.

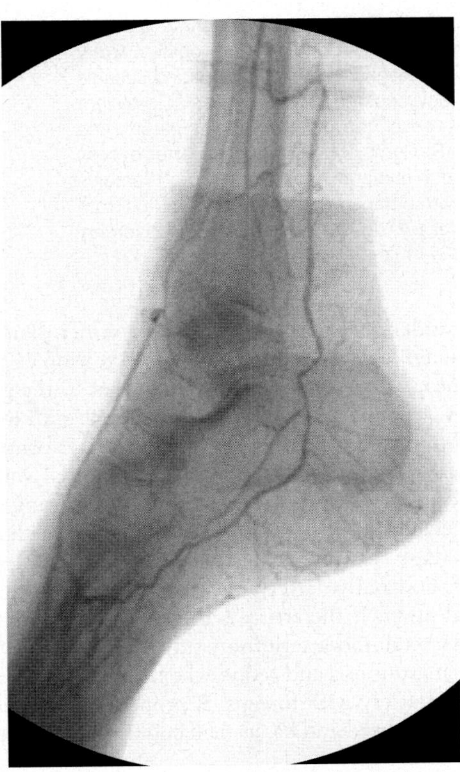

FIG. 63.14 Lateral foot view obtained by distal selective superficial femoral arterial catheter injection identifies excellent collaterals from the distal peroneal artery to both the dorsal pedal and posterior tibial circulations. (From Mills JL. Infrainguinal disease: Surgical treatment. In: Sidawy AN, Perler BA, ed. *Rutherford's vascular surgery and endovascular therapy*. 9th ed. Philadelphia, PA: Elsevier; 2019:1438–1462.)

Rifampin-bonded Dacron grafts are also occasionally used, both for primary reconstructions, as well as in the replacement of infected grafts in the setting of low virulence organisms. The preferred proximal aortic anastomosis by many vascular surgeons is end-to-end, as it is thus easier to cover/protect the prosthetic from the adjacent duodenum and although unproven, it has been felt by some to be hemodynamically superior. There are certain settings, however, in which an end-to-side proximal anastomosis may be considered or even be mandatory. These circumstances include the presence of a large, patent inferior mesenteric artery and in anatomic situations in which an end-to-end aortic anastomosis would eliminate flow, even retrograde, to the hypogastric arteries. For example, if the common iliac and external iliac arteries are both occluded on one side, and the common iliac and internal iliac arteries are patent on the contralateral side with contralateral external iliac artery occlusion, creation of a proximal aortic end-to-side anastomosis would preserve perfusion to one hypogastric artery. In contrast, an end-to-end aortic anastomosis would eliminate pulsatile flow to the pelvis, increasing the risk of colonic and pelvic ischemia (including buttock necrosis or so called "trash can," a disastrous complication). If the surgeon elects to perform the proximal anastomosis end-to-end in the former circumstance, the inferior mesenteric artery should be reimplanted into the body of the aortofemoral graft (Fig. 63.16). When faced with anatomy such as that described in the second circumstance, the distal limb on the ipsilateral side is brought down to the common femoral artery while the contralateral limb is sewn to the distal common iliac artery or proximal patent hypogastric artery An additional graft limb is then sewn to the hood of the contralateral limb and brought down to that common femoral artery (Fig. 63.17). This approach preserves hypogastric flow and simplifies the pelvic anastomoses, as the deeper anastomosis to the iliac artery is performed first, and the more superficial anastomosis to the limb that will be extended to the common femoral artery is relatively easily performed.

Clamp application and release are important maneuvers. The clamp should be applied to a normal arterial segment whenever possible. This can be assured by thorough preoperative preparation and review of all pertinent images (duplex ultrasound, CT or conventional angiography, depending on which are available). Intraoperative arterial palpation with a right angle behind the artery can also be used to identify significant posterior plaque. If clamp application to normal or near normal artery is not possible, particularly when posterior plaque is present, one should consider a clamp that compresses the artery from front to back rather than from side to side. If anastomosis to a very diseased vessel is needed,

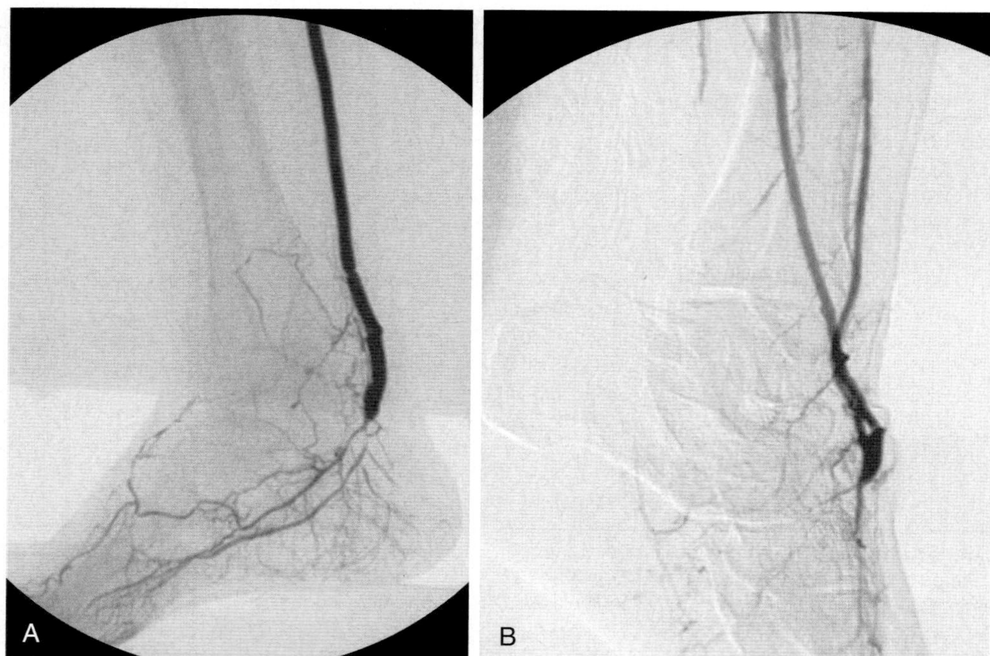

FIG. 63.15 Detailed diagnostic arteriography with fixed imaging, proper timing, and appropriate catheter placement almost always identifies suitable target arteries. Each of the patients depicted had popliteal artery occlusion and extensive trifurcation and long-segment tibial disease, but diagnostic studies identified suitable target arteries in the foot. (A) Completion arteriogram after inframalleolar posterior tibial bypass in a patient with diabetes and forefoot gangrene. Despite a small-caliber outflow vessel, the bypass remains patent, and the ischemic foot ulcers healed and have not recurred at two years. (B) Completion arteriogram after bypass to a diseased dorsal pedal artery. Despite poor outflow and diseased arch and pedal vessels, the graft remains patent at one year. This patient with diabetes healed and ambulates with a transmetatarsal amputation. (From Mills JL. Infrainguinal disease: Surgical treatment. In: Sidawy AN, Perler BA, ed. *Rutherford's vascular surgery and endovascular therapy*. 9th ed. Philadelphia, PA: Elsevier; 2019:1438–1462.)

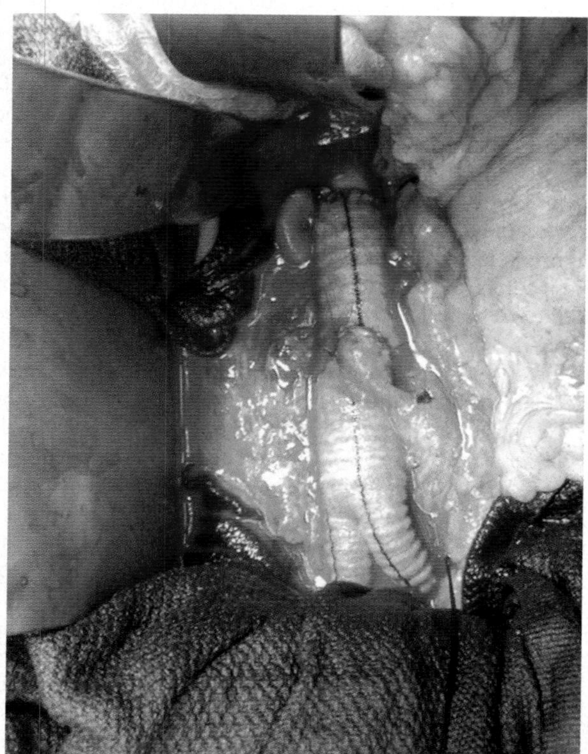

FIG. 63.16 Inferior mesenteric artery reimplantation into body of bifurcated aortic graft sewn end-to-end proximally.

one can consider proximal balloon control rather than ill-advised clamping of a diseased segment. Following creation of an arteriotomy of appropriate length, and matching that to the graftotomy, the needle is generally directed from outside the graft to inside the graft and from inside the artery to out when performing arterial anastomoses, especially in the presence of arterial wall thickening from occlusive disease. These clamping and sewing techniques reduce the chance of lifting up native arterial intima and creating an intimal flap. This sewing technique also encourages eversion of the graft and native artery, making the anastomosis creation simpler and faster. If the artery is thickened and resists eversion, medial and lateral mid-arteriotomy stay sutures can be used to facilitate the anastomosis and reduce the need for repeatedly grasping a diseased artery with forceps. A properly created end-to-side anastomosis is everted and has a small cobra-head appearance (Fig. 63.15).

Aortofemoral bypass is an operation of considerable physiologic magnitude and is associated with several major complications. Immediate complications include hemorrhage, intestinal ischemia, buttock and pelvic necrosis, acute renal failure, myocardial infarction, pulmonary complications, and death. Late complications include limb thrombosis, aortoenteric fistula, graft infection, and anastomotic pseudoaneurysm.

Infrainguinal Bypass Techniques

There are multiple variations available for performing infrainguinal bypass, including reversed vein, nonreversed vein, in-situ vein, spliced veins, and prosthetic bypass. When available, in-situ

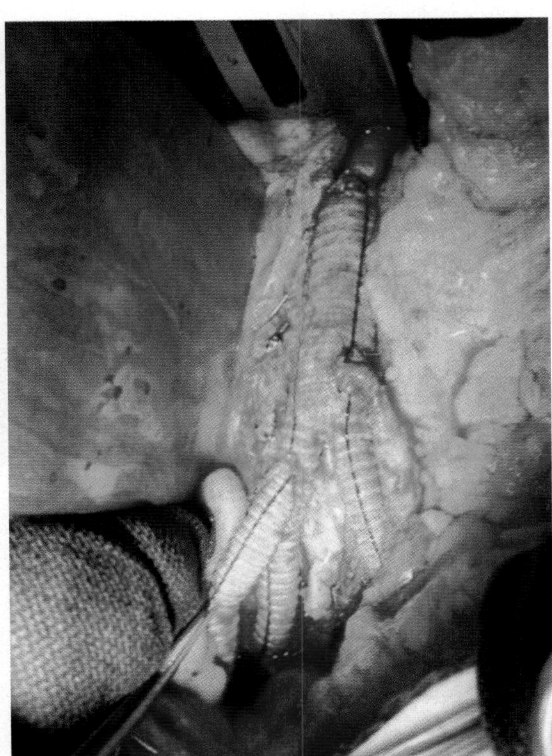

FIG. 63.17 Inferior mesenteric artery reimplantation into aortic graft body, right limb sewn to sole patent hypogastric artery with jump graft to the right common femoral artery to preserve pelvic and colonic flow.

GSV can be used by mobilizing the proximal GSV to the inflow artery, performing valve lysis and subsequently mobilizing the distal segment of the GSV and anastomosing it to the target artery. This technique has the advantage of avoiding full length GSV harvesting and matches vein conduit vein to native artery diameter for both the inflow artery and the target vessel. Nonreversed vein bypass also allows for easier matching of vein to artery diameters. However, using the nonreversed vein requires full vein harvesting, tunneling of the graft and valve lysis. Reversing the vein avoids the need for valve lysis but does require full harvest and potentially creates the issue of vein bypass to artery size mismatch. Despite the theoretical size mismatch with reversed vein, no data suggest that reversed vein conduits are inferior to techniques requiring valve lysis, and reversing the vein obviates problems with incomplete valve lysis and allows significant latitude in tunnelling the bypass. All grafts can be tunnelled either anatomically along the vessel which is being bypassed or subcutaneously. Subcutaneous bypasses require a longer vein conduit than anatomic bypasses but are often very useful in reoperative cases to avoid scarring from previous operations. Many of these issues are avoided with the use of prosthetic bypass, especially harvest time, conduit length issues, and dealing with vein valves. Avoiding vein harvest also decreases the operative time and decreases the incisional lengths, potentially avoiding morbidity. However, the inferior patency rates and increased risk of infection associated with prosthetic bypasses greatly outweigh these potential benefits for most patients.

Inflow for infrainguinal bypasses can arise from the common femoral artery, the profunda femoris artery, the superficial femoral artery and the popliteal artery, and less commonly, even a tibial artery. The profunda femoris artery is often an excellent option when previous common femoral artery procedures have been performed, as this artery can be exposed from a lateral approach, thereby avoiding dense scarring from previous operative site in the femoral triangle. Additionally, when an adjunctive inflow procedure has been performed, the bypass can originate from the hood of the proximal bypass, from an arterial patch, or even from the native artery beneath the inflow graft-artery anastomosis. Bypass graft origins distal to the common femoral artery are especially useful in reoperative cases and when available vein length is limited. Distal origin grafts do not compromise long-term graft patency when vein conduit is utilized and if there are no hemodynamically significant lesions proximal to the graft origin. A metaanalysis of popliteal origin grafts, which are especially applicable to patients with CLTI and diabetes, reported nearly 80% 2-year patency with this configuration.[8]

Completion studies following bypass should be considered to avoid potentially early graft thrombosis or hemorrhage and subsequent “take back” operations. Options include distal pulse palpation and Doppler flow assessment with and without graft compression, completion arteriography, intraoperative duplex scanning and angioscopy. Not all bypasses require completion imaging and unfortunately clear consensus on when to use these adjuncts currently does not exist. However, one should note that the best opportunity to salvage a potential problem is at the time of the original operation. We therefore remain advocates of completion angiography, especially in an era when open surgical bypass operations are being performed with diminishing frequency.

Complications. Major complications following infrainguinal bypass include wound problems, graft occlusion, graft infection, bleeding, and death. The PREVENT III trial demonstrated the following complication rates associated with infrainguinal vein bypass procedures: death (2.7%), myocardial infraction (4.7%), major amputation (1.8%), graft occlusion (5.2%), major wound complication (4.8%), and graft hemorrhage (0.4%).[26] Late complications include lymphedema, infection, graft aneurysm, and graft stenosis or occlusion. Early graft occlusion is typically associated with technical or judgment error and should be remedied as soon as possible. If an underlying cause for graft failure is not identified, long-term patency is poor. Intermediate and late graft occlusion occurs due to a number of underlying causes, including intimal hyperplasia (with a peak incidence in the first 18 postoperative months), anastomotic aneurysm, and recurrent atherosclerotic disease. These should generally only be treated for high-grade restenosis or whenever the patient has return of symptoms or a nonhealing wound. For vein grafts, structured serial duplex graft surveillance has been shown to reduce intermediate and late bypass graft occlusion.

SURVEILLANCE

Surveillance is a fundamental aspect of longitudinal PAD management and is an important component of providing comprehensive care to maximize patient outcomes. The mode and frequency of surveillance depend on the patient, the specific intervention, and the anticipated time frame and modes of failure of the intervention performed. Structured follow-up is intended to identify threatened interventions prior to actual failure and to guide appropriate and timely reintervention. Concurrent clinical evaluation is paramount to add adjunctive information with respect to recurrent symptoms and wound status. The Society for Vascular Surgery published a guideline in 2018 regarding surveillance following lower extremity arterial procedures, which will serve as a reference for our recommendations.[45]

Endovascular Therapy Surveillance

There has not been an established interval or optimal algorithm for following lower extremity endovascular interventions. However, it is clear that longitudinal follow-up to ensure adequate medical management of comorbid conditions is essential and may improve patency as well as amputation-free survival after endovascular intervention.[46] Follow-up requires full history and physical examination to assess new medical conditions, wounds, symptoms, and measurement of ankle-brachial indices. Additionally, a baseline duplex ultrasound surveillance (DUS) within the first month after EVT is recommended. Following EVT, arterial restenosis frequently occurs through several mechanisms including neointimal hyperplasia, constrictive arterial remodeling, and recurrent atherosclerotic disease. Routine imaging with DUS or contrast imaging beyond the first month following the procedure has not produced clear benefit with respect to limb salvage. Part of the reason for this lack of benefit is difficulty establishing velocity thresholds and criteria predictive of progression that are sufficiently accurate to recommend reintervention following angioplasty, atherectomy, and stenting. Further imaging and subsequent reintervention are generally only required if the patient has developed recurrent symptoms or has failed to heal existing wounds. The Society for Vascular Surgery guideline suggests continued clinical follow up at 3 months and then subsequently at 6-month intervals. However, routine DUS is currently not recommended beyond 1 month in the absence of recurrent symptoms or without the presence of nonhealing or recurrent wounds. For patients with recurrent symptoms or unresolved CLTI, duplex imaging may help identify an area of restenosis (peak systolic velocity [PSV] greater than 300 cm/sec, velocity ratio [Vr] greater than 3.5).[45] Such restenosis merit reintervention in patients with unresolved or recurrent symptoms and in very selected patients who are asymptomatic after catheter-based intervention.

Open Surgical Bypass Graft Surveillance

As opposed to the unestablished surveillance recommendations after lower extremity EVT, open surgical therapy has clearer guidelines for clinical and imaging surveillance. These surveillance mechanisms include clinical monitoring, ABI assessment, and DUS. A general guideline following open surgical revascularization includes early postoperative assessment within 4 weeks of intervention and then at 3-, 6, and 12-month intervals following the operation. Thereafter, surveillance can be continued every 6 to 12 months.[45,47] DUS criteria have been established to define recurrent stenosis and vein bypass graft-threatening stenoses. These criteria are based on duplex-derived PSV and Vr at the site of the stenosis.

Surveillance has been especially well established for autologous vein grafts, for which identification and treatment of restenosis has clear benefit to prolonging graft patency and avoiding thrombosis of valuable vein conduit.[45,47–50] DUS has added utility over ABI assessment alone. A full evaluation of the bypass is performed, including the native inflow and outflow, proximal and distal anastomoses, and at multiple intervals along the entire length of the graft. Criteria have been established based on PSV, Vr, low flow velocity, and changes in ABI to stratify the risk of thrombosis of infrainguinal vein grafts. Grafts are at high risk for thrombosis when any of the following are identified: PSV greater than 300 cm/s and/or the Vr greater than 3.5 at the site of a stenosis; globally low peak systolic graft flow velocity less than 45 cm/s; or a drop in ABI greater than 0.15.[49,50] Any of these findings should prompt consideration for diagnostic angiography and reintervention on

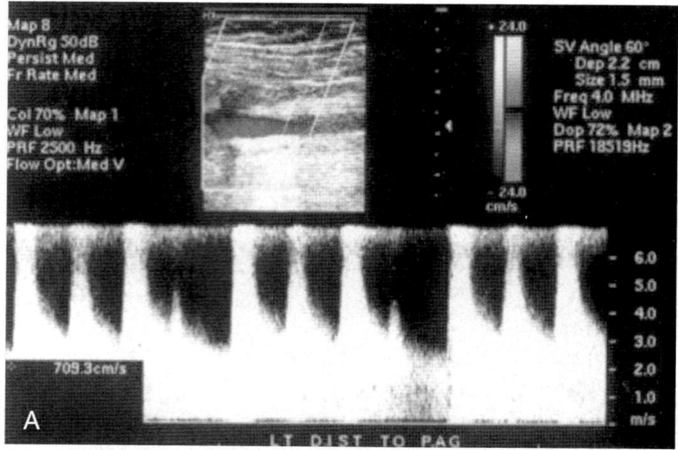

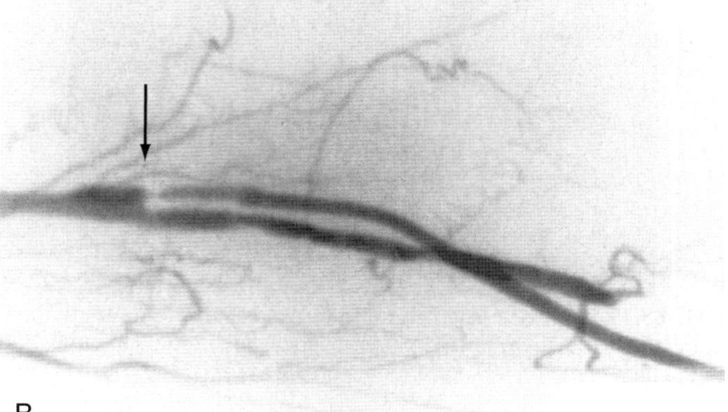

FIG. 63.18 Duplex surveillance identified a critical vein graft stenosis in the proximal aspect of a femoropopliteal vein graft. (A) Marked spectral broadening and pronounced elevation of both the peak systolic and end-diastolic velocities are diagnostic of a high-grade vein graft stenosis. (B) A focal, severe proximal graft stenosis *(arrow)* was confirmed by arteriography and treated with a short interposition vein graft harvested from the upper extremity. (From Mills JL. Infrainguinal disease: Surgical treatment. In: Sidawy AN, Perler BA, ed. *Rutherford's vascular surgery and endovascular therapy*. 9th ed. Philadelphia, PA: Elsevier; 2019:1438–1462.)

the culprit lesion to prevent graft thrombosis (Fig. 63.18). Primary patency is the term applied to a bypass graft when patency is maintained over a specified time interval without reintervention on the graft itself or its anastomoses. Successful reintervention on a patent, but restenotic graft, is termed assisted-primary patency. Resurrection of an occluded bypass results in loss of primary patency, but if successful, is termed secondary patency. The purpose of vein graft surveillance is to prevent loss of primary patency, as reintervention for "failed (occluded) vein grafts is not as durable as reintervention for patent, but "failing" grafts. Vein graft surveillance is generally recommended every 3 to 6 months for the first 2 years, and then annually thereafter. The most common cause of vein graft failure (75%–80%) in the first 3 to 8 postoperative months is an intrinsic vein graft stenosis due to intimal hyperplasia. Such lesions are readily detectable and can be monitored for progression by serial duplex surveillance. After 18 to 24 months, the de-novo vein graft stenosis rate falls off markedly, so in the absence of recurrent symptoms, annual surveillance is sufficient.[50]

Following prosthetic lower extremity bypass, surveillance does not clearly predict graft failure, and specific DUS criteria have not been established to accurately identify threatened prosthetic grafts. Early baseline ABI should be established and repeated at 6 and 12 months. Subsequently, clinical evaluation and ABI assessment should occur at yearly intervals or with changes in patient clinical condition. If the ABIs are suprasystolic due to medial calcinosis, as is common in patients with CLTI, diabetes or renal failure, toe systolic pressure, and waveforms can be very useful to monitor hemodynamics.

ASSESSMENT OF OUTCOMES

Longitudinal assessment of vascular interventions, particularly those performed for lower extremity PAD, have long focused on endpoints such as patency (primary, assisted primary, and secondary), hemodynamic success (based on ABI or toe pressure), limb salvage (lack of major amputation), and mortality. However, quality evidence to support indications and type of revascularization is generally of poor quality and quite weak when compared to that available for pharmacologic risk reduction and interventions for coronary artery disease and stroke. Many device trials have used anatomic or surrogate markers such as the presence or absence of restenosis, target lesion revascularization, and target vessel revascularization to define treatment success. None of these markers, however, are highly meaningful limb or patient outcome measurements. In an effort to address this issue, suggested objective performance goals were published in 2009 for evaluating catheter-based treatment of CLTI and to permit suitable comparison with surgical bypass.[51] This document suggested the following endpoints as safety and efficacy measures: major adverse limb event; MACE; major limb (proximal to ankle) amputation; amputation-free survival; and DEATH. Reinterventions were grouped into major and minor categories. Major reinterventions include the creation of a new bypass graft, graft thrombectomy or thrombolysis for graft occlusion, or a major surgical revision such as a jump or interposition graft. Minor reinterventions include primarily simpler reinterventions for patent reconstructions with restenosis, both endovascular (angioplasty, atherectomy, or stenting) and minor open procedures such as focal patch angioplasty. The objective performance goals set targets for EVT for CLTI based on the datasets from three large trials, which had a surgical control group.

Important patient outcomes of revascularization for CLTI include freedom from death, relief of ischemic pain, complete healing of any index wounds, freedom from major amputation, relative freedom from reinterventions, resumption or maintenance of ambulation; and independent living status. Numerous studies have shown more sanguine results of lower extremity bypass when all of the latter endpoints are evaluated in the CLTI subpopulation. As one example, a study from the Oregon group evaluated 112 consecutive patients 5 to 7 years after infrainguinal bypass. While only 26% of these patients lost their limb during this extended follow-up period, the authors reported that less than 20% of patients had an ideal outcome as defined by the presence of all of the following criteria: patent graft, healed wound, no need for reoperation, continued ambulation, and independent living status.[27] This report and other studies clearly demonstrate that longitudinal follow-up and care are clearly necessary for PAD patients, particularly those with CLTI, and that ongoing efforts are required to maintain limb salvage and preserve ambulatory and functional status.[31-33] From this longitudinal perspective, while timely and appropriate revascularization for CLTI can undoubtedly offer clinically important and often prolonged palliation, it does not cure and rarely yields what would be viewed by most patients and objective surgeons as ideal patient-centered, functional outcomes.

SELECTED REFERENCES:

Bradbury AW, Adam DJ, Bell J, et al. Bypass versus angioplasty in severe ischaemia of the leg (BASIL) trial: Analysis of amputation free and overall survival by treatment received. *J Vasc Surg*. 2010;51:18S–31S.

Remains the only randomized prospective trial of angioplasty versus bypass for severe limb ischemia. Patients surviving more than two years are likely to benefit from bypass first.

Conte MS, Bradbury AW, Kolh P, et al. Global vascular guidelines on the management of chronic limb-threatening ischemia. *J Vasc Surg*. 2019;69; 3S–125S e140.

Multidisciplinary, global collaborative effort to redefine diagnosis, management, and treatment of chronic limb-threatening ischemia (CLTI). Important new concepts include wound, ischemia, and foot infection (WIfI) threatened limb classification, patient, limb, and anatomy (PLAN), target artery path (TAP) and Global Limb Anatomic Staging System (GLASS)). While the concepts need to be validated, these systems will finally allow comparison of alternative methods of treatments for comparably risk stratified patients, limbs, and anatomic lesions.

Fowkes FG, Rudan D, Rudan I, et al. Comparison of global estimates of prevalence and risk factors for peripheral artery disease in 2000 and 2010. A systematic review and analysis. *Lancet*. 2013;382:1329–1340.

Important systematic review on prevalence and risk factors for the development of peripheral artery disease.

Mills JL Sr, Conte MS, Armstrong DG, et al. The Society for vascular surgery lower extremity threatened limb classification system: risk stratification based on wound, ischemia, and foot infection (WIfI). *J Vasc Surg*. 2014;59:220–234 e221– e222.

Key change in perspective to classify threatened limb at baseline based on the combination of three factors (wound, ischemia, and foot infection) that correlate with likelihood of healing, risk of amputation, and potential benefit of revascularization.

Prompers L, Schaper N, Apelqvist J, et al. Prediction of outcome in individuals with diabetic foot ulcers: focus on the differences between individuals with and without peripheral arterial disease. The EURODIALE Study. *Diabetologia*. 2008;51:747–755.

Important data on frequent association of diabetic foot ulcer (DFU) and peripheral artery disease (PAD), and critical impact of PAD + infection on risk of amputation in patients with DFU.

REFERENCES

1. Selvin E, Erlinger TP. Prevalence of and risk factors for peripheral arterial disease in the United States: results from the national health and nutrition examination survey, 1999-2000. *Circulation*. 2004;110:738–743.
2. Hirsch AT, Criqui MH, Treat-Jacobson D, et al. Peripheral arterial disease detection, awareness, and treatment in primary care. *JAMA*. 2001;286:1317–1324.
3. Conte MS, Pomposelli FB, Clair DG, et al. Society for vascular surgery practice guidelines for atherosclerotic occlusive disease of the lower extremities: management of asymptomatic disease and claudication. *J Vasc Surg*. 2015;61:2S–41S.
4. Fowkes FG, Rudan D, Rudan I, et al. Comparison of global estimates of prevalence and risk factors for peripheral artery disease in 2000 and 2010: a systematic review and analysis. *Lancet*. 2013;382:1329–1340.
5. Mahoney EM, Wang K, Keo HH, et al. Vascular hospitalization rates and costs in patients with peripheral artery disease in the United States. *Circ Cardiovasc Qual Outcomes*. 2010;3:642–651.
6. Joosten MM, Pai JK, Bertoia ML, et al. Associations between conventional cardiovascular risk factors and risk of peripheral artery disease in men. *JAMA*. 2012;308:1660–1667.
7. Hingorani A, LaMuraglia GM, Henke P, et al. The management of diabetic foot: a clinical practice guideline by the society for vascular surgery in collaboration with the American Podiatric Medical Association and the Society for Vascular Medicine. *J Vasc Surg*. 2016;63:3S–21S.
8. Conte MS, Bradbury AW, Kolh P, et al. Global vascular guidelines on the management of chronic limb-threatening ischemia. *J Vasc Surg*. 2019;69; 3S–125S.e140.
9. Mills JL Sr, Conte MS, Armstrong DG, et al. The society for vascular surgery lower extremity threatened limb classification system: risk stratification based on wound, ischemia, and foot infection (WIfI). *J Vasc Surg*. 2014;59:220–234; e221–222.
10. Glagov S, Weisenberg E, Zarins CK, et al. Compensatory enlargement of human atherosclerotic coronary arteries. *N Engl J Med*. 1987;316:1371–1375.
11. Faglia E, Favales F, Quarantiello A, et al. Angiographic evaluation of peripheral arterial occlusive disease and its role as a prognostic determinant for major amputation in diabetic subjects with foot ulcers. *Diabetes Care*. 1998;21:625–630.
12. Graziani L, Silvestro A, Bertone V, et al. Vascular involvement in diabetic subjects with ischemic foot ulcer: A new morphologic categorization of disease severity. *Eur J Vasc Endovasc Surg*. 2007;33:453–460.
13. Prompers L, Schaper N, Apelqvist J, et al. Prediction of outcome in individuals with diabetic foot ulcers: focus on the differences between individuals with and without peripheral arterial disease. The EURODIALE Study. *Diabetologia*. 2008;51:747–755.
14. Bell PRF, Charlesworth D, DePalma RG, et al. The definition of critical ischemia of a limb. Working Party of the International Vascular Symposium. *Br J Surg*. 1982;69:S2.
15. Fontaine R, Kim M, Kieny R. Surgical treatment of peripheral circulation disorders. *Helv Chir Acta*. 1954;21:499–533.
16. Rutherford RB, Baker JD, Ernst C, et al. Recommended standards for reports dealing with lower extremity ischemia: revised version. *J Vasc Surg*. 1997;26:517–538.
17. van Reijen NS, Ponchant K, Ubbink DT, et al. Editor's Choice - The prognostic value of the WIfI classification in patients with chronic limb threatening ischaemia: A systematic review and meta-analysis. *Eur J Vasc Endovasc Surg*. 2019;58:362–371.
18. Mayor JM, Mills JL. The correlation of the society for vascular surgery wound, ischemia, and foot infection threatened limb classification with amputation risk and major clinical outcomes. *Indian J Vasc Endovasc Surg*. 2018;5:83–86.
19. Leithead C, Novak Z, Spangler E, et al. Importance of post-procedural wound, ischemia, and foot infection (WIfI) restaging in predicting limb salvage. *J Vasc Surg*. 2018;67:498–505.
20. Mayor J, Chung J, Zhang Q, et al. Using the society for vascular surgery wound, ischemia, and foot infection classification to identify patients most likely to benefit from revascularization. *J Vasc Surg*. 2019;70:776–785; e771.
21. Biancari F. Meta-analysis of the prevalence, incidence and natural history of critical limb ischemia. *J Cardiovasc Surg (Torino)*. 2013;54:663–669.
22. Simons JP, Schanzer A, Flahive JM, et al. Survival prediction in patients with chronic limb-threatening ischemia who undergo infrainguinal revascularization. *J Vasc Surg*. 2019;69:137S–151S. e133.
23. Bradbury AW, Adam DJ, Bell J, et al. Bypass versus Angioplasty in Severe Ischaemia of the Leg (BASIL) trial: a survival prediction model to facilitate clinical decision making. *J Vasc Surg*. 2010;51:52S–68S.
24. Adam DJ, Beard JD, Cleveland T, et al. Bypass versus angioplasty in severe ischaemia of the leg (BASIL): multicentre, randomised controlled trial. *Lancet*. 2005;366:1925–1934.
25. Bradbury AW, Adam DJ, Bell J, et al. Bypass versus Angioplasty in Severe Ischaemia of the Leg (BASIL) trial: analysis of amputation free and overall survival by treatment received. *J Vasc Surg*. 2010;51:18S–31S.
26. Conte MS, Bandyk DF, Clowes AW, et al. Results of PREVENT III: a multicenter, randomized trial of edifoligide for the prevention of vein graft failure in lower extremity bypass surgery. *J Vasc Surg*. 2006;43:742–751; discussion 751.
27. Nicoloff AD, Taylor Jr LM, McLafferty RB, et al. Patient recovery after infrainguinal bypass grafting for limb salvage. *J Vasc Surg*. 1998;27:256–263; discussion 264–256.
28. Taylor SM, York JW, Cull DL, et al. Clinical success using patient-oriented outcome measures after lower extremity bypass and endovascular intervention for ischemic tissue loss. *J Vasc Surg*. 2009;50:534–541; discussion 541.
29. Kraiss LW, Beckstrom JL, Brooke BS. Frailty assessment in vascular surgery and its utility in preoperative decision making. *Semin Vasc Surg*. 2015;28:141–147.
30. Kraiss LW, Al-Dulaimi R, Presson AP, et al. A vascular quality initiative-based frailty instrument predicts 9-month postoperative mortality. *J Vasc Surg*. 2016;64:551–552.
31. Goshima KR, Mills Sr JL, Hughes JD. A new look at outcomes after infrainguinal bypass surgery: Traditional reporting standards systematically underestimate the expenditure of effort required to attain limb salvage. *J Vasc Surg*. 2004;39:330–335.
32. Morgan MB, Crayford T, Murrin B, et al. Developing the vascular quality of life questionnaire: a new disease-specific quality of life measure for use in lower limb ischemia. *J Vasc Surg*. 2001;33:679–687.
33. Nguyen LL, Moneta GL, Conte MS, et al. Prospective multicenter study of quality of life before and after lower extremity

vein bypass in 1404 patients with critical limb ischemia. *J Vasc Surg*. 2006;44:977–983; discussion 983–974.
34. Johnston KW, Rae M, Hogg-Johnston SA, et al. 5-year results of a prospective study of percutaneous transluminal angioplasty. *Ann Surg*. 1987;206:403–413.
35. Mills Sr JL. Open bypass and endoluminal therapy: complementary techniques for revascularization in diabetic patients with critical limb ischaemia. *Diabetes Metab Res Rev*. 2008;24(suppl 1):S34–39.
36. Montero-Baker M, Mills JL. Endovascular repair of infrapopliteal arterial occlusive disease. In: Moore WS, Lawrence PF, Oderich GS, eds. *Moore's Vascular And Endovascular Surgery: A Comprehensive Review*. 9th edition. Philadelphia, PA: Elsevier; 2019:460–468.
37. Bolia A, Brennan J, Bell PR. Recanalisation of femoro-popliteal occlusions: Improving success rate by subintimal recanalisation. *Clin Radiol*. 1989;40:325.
38. Katsanos K, Spiliopoulos S, Kitrou P, et al. Risk of death following application of paclitaxel-coated balloons and stents in the femoropopliteal artery of the leg: a systematic review and meta-analysis of randomized controlled trials. *J Am Heart Assoc*. 2018;7:e011245.
39. Powell R.J., Rzucidlo E.M.. Aortoiliac disease: endovascular treatment. In: Sidawy A.N., Perler B.A., eds. Rutherford's vascular surgery and endovascular therapy. 9th edition. Philadelphia, PA: Elsevier; 2019:1423–1437.
40. Ouwendijk R, Kock MC, van Dijk LC, et al. Vessel wall calcifications at multi-detector row CT angiography in patients with peripheral arterial disease: effect on clinical utility and clinical predictors. *Radiology*. 2006;241:603–608.
41. Dorweiler B, Neufang A, Kreitner KF, et al. Magnetic resonance angiography unmasks reliable target vessels for pedal bypass grafting in patients with diabetes mellitus. *J Vasc Surg*. 2002;35:766–772.
42. Mazzariol F, Ascher E, Hingorani A, et al. Lower-extremity revascularisation without preoperative contrast arteriography in 185 cases: lessons learned with duplex ultrasound arterial mapping. *Eur J Vasc Endovasc Surg*. 2000;19:509–515.
43. Kozak BE, Bedell JE, Rosch J. Small vessel leg angiography for distal vessel bypass grafts. *J Vasc Surg*. 1988;8:711–715.
44. Rychlik IJ, Davey P, Murphy J, et al. A meta-analysis to compare Dacron versus polytetrafluroethylene grafts for above-knee femoropopliteal artery bypass. *J Vasc Surg*. 2014;60:506–515.
45. Zierler RE, Jordan WD, Lal BK, et al. The society for vascular surgery practice guidelines on follow-up after vascular surgery arterial procedures. *J Vasc Surg*. 2018;68:256–284.
46. Chung J, Timaran DA, Modrall JG, et al. Optimal medical therapy predicts amputation-free survival in chronic critical limb ischemia. *J Vasc Surg*. 2013;58:972–980.
47. Hodgkiss-Harlow K, Bandyk DF. Ultrasound assessment during and after carotid and peripheral intervention. In: Pellerito JS, Polak JF, eds. *Introduction To Vascular Ultrasonography*. 6th ed. Philadelphia, PA: Elsevier Saunders; 2012:307–323.
48. Lundell A, Lindblad B, Bergqvist D, et al. Femoropopliteal-crural graft patency is improved by an intensive surveillance program: a prospective randomized study. *J Vasc Surg*. 1995;21:26–33; discussion 33-24.
49. Mills JL, Bandyk DF, Gahtan V, et al. The origin of infrainguinal vein graft stenosis: a prospective study based on duplex surveillance. *J Vasc Surg*. 1995;21:16–22; discussion 22–23.
50. Mills JL Sr, Wixon CL, James DC, et al. The natural history of intermediate and critical vein graft stenosis: recommendations for continued surveillance or repair. *J Vasc Surg*. 2001;33:273–278; discussion 278–280.
51. Conte MS, Geraghty PJ, Bradbury AW, et al. Suggested objective performance goals and clinical trial design for evaluating catheter-based treatment of critical limb ischemia. *J Vasc Surg*. 2009;50:1462–1473; e1461–1463.

64 CHAPTER

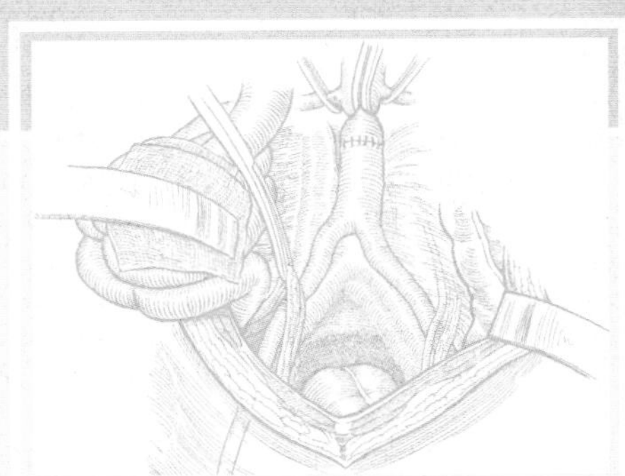

Vascular Trauma

Michael J. Sise, Carlos V.R. Brown, Howard C. Champion

OUTLINE

The prompt recognition and rapid and effective surgical management of vascular trauma remain challenging despite major advances in access to care produced by trauma systems development. The risk to life and limb remains significant, and the margin for error in both diagnosis and treatment of these injuries is very thin. Either delay in recognition of or failure to adequately manage vascular injuries remains alarmingly common in trauma centers. An organized approach with well-planned and implemented practice guidelines is essential to convert an error-prone process into one of timely diagnosis and safe and effective treatment.

The widespread preference for endovascular techniques for elective vascular surgery, coupled with fewer and fewer open vascular surgery cases, has produced a shortage of surgeons who feel capable of and comfortable in performing open vascular repairs for vascular trauma. The steadily decreasing volume of open vascular procedures in both general surgery residencies and vascular fellowships has significantly eroded the skill level of both trauma surgeons and the vascular surgeons who support them in managing vascular injuries. The need for innovative solutions to restore the skill level among trauma and vascular surgeons is compelling.

This chapter reviews the pathophysiology, clinical presentation, diagnostic workup, management, and outcome of vascular injuries. Education and training solutions to restore the skills required to manage vascular injuries are also presented. The educational objectives of this review are the following: to elucidate the mechanisms of vessel injury and the resulting clinical manifestations; to provide an organized approach to rapid assessment of injured patients for the presence of vascular injuries in the neck, torso, and extremities; to present management guidelines to assist in the decision of which treatment options best apply and how to effectively implement them; to identify the clinically important sequelae of vascular injuries and the appropriate measures required to maximize functional recovery; and to review the available education and training opportunities to maintain the open surgical skills that are essential to effective management of vascular trauma.

MECHANISM OF INJURY AND PATHOPHYSIOLOGY

Vascular injury can be produced by either a blunt or a penetrating mechanism. Penetrating injury tends to be more discrete and to produce focal injuries; blunt trauma is more diffuse, producing injuries not only to the vascular structures but also to the bone, muscle, and nerves. Blunt injury not only affects major arteries, it also disrupts smaller vessels that would normally provide collateral flow. As a result, ischemia may be worsened. Knife wounds produce focal injury along their track. Gunshot wounds produce injury of varying degrees dependent on the characteristics of both the weapon and the projectile.

Penetrating gunshot wound injury is generally classified as low velocity (<2500 ft/sec, typically a handgun wound) or high velocity (>2500 ft/sec, such as a military rifle wound).[1] High-velocity military-style weapons produce significantly more tissue damage than low-velocity weapons because of the high amount of kinetic energy (energy = mass × velocity^2). The bullet creates a cavity by the rapidly expanding and rapidly contracting tissue surrounding the bullet's course that can reach a size equal to 30 times the diameter of the projectile at right angles to the missile track. Tearing of the adjacent tissue can be devastating. Impact with bone can lead to further damage from secondary bullet and bone fragment impact on the adjacent tissue. Civilian gunshot injuries involve predominantly low-velocity projectiles and create more focal injuries with little cavitation.[2]

Shotgun wounds, depending on the proximity to the gun barrel, the gunpowder load, and the size of the shot, cause highly variable injury patterns. The spread and force of the shot determine the extent of injury. Close-range gunshot wounds are defined as within 6 feet; intermediate, 6 to 18 feet; and long range, beyond 18 feet.[3] Close-range injures are devastating and often lethal. Intermediate-range injuries are often severe, and longer range injuries may be mild.

Vascular trauma produces a spectrum of findings from life-threatening hemorrhage from major vessel laceration to no overtly detectable findings in minimal injuries. Hemorrhage is produced when all of the vessel layers (intima, media, and adventitia) are disrupted or lacerated. If the bleeding is controlled locally, a hematoma is produced, which may or may not be pulsatile. If bleeding is not contained, exsanguination can occur. Completely transected extremity vessels often retract and constrict secondary to spasm of the muscular middle layer of the vessel wall. The surrounding adventitia is highly thrombogenic. Subsequently, hemorrhage may cease secondary to thrombosis. Paradoxically, partially transected arteries and veins cannot retract and thrombose and may cause much more extensive hemorrhage.

Arterial thrombosis occurs if there is damage to the intima, exposing the underlying media and causing local thrombus formation, which may propagate and either occlude the lumen or embolize distally. In addition, the injured intima can prolapse into the lumen as a result of blood flow dissecting this layer into the lumen, producing partial or complete obstruction. Trauma to the surrounding bone structures may cause external compression of the vessel, interrupting flow and producing thrombosis. Spasm occurs if there is external trauma to the vessel, such as stretching or contusion, which can stimulate the release of mediators (such as hemoglobin) that cause constriction of the vascular smooth muscle. Spasm, by reducing the cross-sectional area of the vessel, reduces flow.

Vascular trauma can produce subacute, chronic, or occult injuries. The most common of these are arteriovenous fistula and pseudoaneurysm. An arteriovenous fistula typically occurs after penetrating trauma that causes injury to both an artery and a vein in proximity. The high-pressure flow from the artery will follow the path of least vascular resistance into the vein, producing local, regional, and systemic signs and symptoms. These include local tenderness and edema, regional ischemia from "steal," and congestive heart failure if the fistula enlarges.[4] A pseudoaneurysm is a result of a puncture or laceration of an artery that bleeds into and is controlled by the surrounding tissue. Pseudoaneurysms can enlarge and produce local compressive symptoms, erode adjacent structures, or, rarely, be a source of distal emboli.[4] They can initially be clinically occult but with time become symptomatic.[4]

CLINICAL PRESENTATION

Vascular injuries have a broad spectrum of clinical manifestations varying from profound hemorrhagic shock to subtle findings, such as an asymptomatic bruit. Patients who present in hemorrhagic shock must be assumed to have a major vascular injury until proven otherwise.[5] There are five anatomic areas to consider, each with specific considerations. In the head and neck, external hemorrhage is required for vascular injuries to result in shock. Relatively small and tightly organized tissue planes preclude significant internal hemorrhage. In the chest, each hemithorax can accommodate lethal amounts of hemorrhage from cardiac, pulmonary, or great vessel arterial and venous injuries. Abdominal and pelvic vascular injuries can also result in lethal hemorrhage, particularly from the aorta and iliac arteries. As in the head and neck, extremity vascular injuries generally cause hemorrhagic shock only if there is significant external hemorrhage. The patient with hypotension and a lack of chest, abdomen, and pelvic findings may have what appears to be a trivial neck or extremity laceration that initially communicated with a major vessel injury. A hemorrhage sufficient to produce hypotension can be followed by thrombosis. It is therefore necessary to obtain a history from the prehospital personnel about the amount of blood at the scene or the initial presence of severe wound hemorrhage. It is also necessary to thoroughly examine the patient for additional wounds and to carefully assess each of them.[5]

Extremity vascular trauma may be immediately apparent on presentation because of external hemorrhage, hematoma, or obvious limb ischemia. A history of penetrating trauma associated with hypotension, pulsatile bleeding, or a large quantity of blood at the scene suggests vascular injury. Blunt trauma is also capable of causing significant vascular injury that can be overlooked when serious head, chest, or abdominal injuries are present. Extremity fractures may result in vascular injury. Supracondylar humerus fracture can be associated with brachial artery injury, and knee dislocation carries a significant risk of popliteal artery injury.[6] Crush injuries of the extremity without fracture may also result in vascular injury.

A relatively small number of vascular injuries are manifested in a delayed fashion without initial findings. These are limited to thrombosis of a previously partially disrupted but initially patent vessel, distal emboli from an intimal tear of the arterial wall with formation of platelet debris, and, least commonly, rupture or expansion of a pseudoaneurysm that was initially small and contained by the outer arterial wall and local tissue.[4] Local signs of hematoma, diminished pulses, and patterns of associated injuries should point to the presence of these vascular injuries. A thorough history and physical examination and appropriate adjunctive imaging studies will result in effective initial diagnosis and a decrease in the frequency of these delayed presentations.

Because such a broad spectrum of clinical findings are associated with vascular trauma, it is best to assume that vascular injury is present until proven otherwise in all patients with hemorrhagic shock and all patients with extremity fractures.[5]

DIAGNOSIS

Physical Examination

Vascular injury can produce systemic symptoms of hypotension, tachycardia, and altered mental status by hypovolemic

TABLE 64.1 History and physical examination findings of vascular injury.

Hard Findings

Indicate need for immediate intervention for vascular injury

- Pulsatile bleeding
- Expanding hematoma
- Palpable thrill or audible bruit
- Evidence of extremity ischemia
  - Pallor
  - Paresthesia
  - Paralysis
  - Pain
  - Pulselessness
  - Poikilothermia

Soft Findings

- Consider further imaging and evaluation for vascular injury
- History of moderate hemorrhage
- Proximity fracture, dislocation, or penetrating wound
- Diminished but palpable pulse
- Level of peripheral nerve deficit in proximity to major vessel
- Wounds in proximity to extremity or neck vessels in patients with unexplained hemorrhagic shock

shock caused by hemorrhage. As a result, vascular injury can be life-threatening, and attention must initially be directed to the primary survey using the principles of advanced trauma life support.[5] The airway must be assessed, adequate oxygenation and ventilation ensured, and intravenous access achieved. Once this is completed and resuscitation is under way, the secondary survey is undertaken. A thorough history and careful physical examination are then performed. This examination must include a careful inspection of the injured sites and wounds, a complete sensory and motor assessment, and a pulse examination of each extremity. The presence of a hematoma, bruit, or thrill must be noted. If distal pulses are diminished or absent, ankle or wrist systolic blood pressure should be determined with a continuous-wave Doppler device and compared with the uninjured side. A significant difference in systolic blood pressure (>10 mm Hg) between extremities may be an indication of vascular injury. Patients with "hard" findings of vascular injury (Table 64.1) should be taken directly to the operating room.

In patients with "soft" findings (Table 64.1), vascular imaging can be used to rule out the need for operation. In addition, patients with hard findings but with multilevel injuries in the same extremity may also need imaging. Catheter arteriography is both sensitive and specific in the diagnosis of extremity vascular injuries (Fig. 64.1). However, computed tomography (CT) angiography with the latest generation scanners is readily available and highly accurate and obviates the delay caused by mobilizing the angiography suite for catheter angiography (Fig. 64.2).[7–9] Although this imaging technique requires an infusion of contrast material, it does not require arterial catheterization, is easily performed, and is less costly and less time-consuming than conventional angiography.[7] The important distinction, however, is the ability to perform endovascular techniques with catheter access in the angiography suite or properly equipped operating room. Therefore, an orchestration of CT imaging and catheter imaging to meet the patient's needs and to manage vascular injuries in a timely and effective manner is essential.

Severely injured patients who must be taken to the operating room for treatment of life-threatening associated injuries, such as penetrating thoracic injury or ruptured spleen, may not be able to undergo CT angiography. In such cases, it is not prudent to delay operative therapy to obtain formal vascular imaging. An arteriogram can be obtained in the operating room by cannulating the artery proximal to the suspected vascular injury, injecting 20 to 25 mL of a full-strength radiographic contrast agent, and taking a radiograph or using fluoroscopy (Fig. 64.3).[10] If doubt remains about the presence of a vascular injury and the imaging studies and other diagnostic tests are inconclusive, there is a role for operative exploration and direct assessment of the artery. Routine operative exploration in the stable patient with soft signs, however, has a 5% to 30% incidence of morbidity, occasional mortality, and low diagnostic yield.[11] These patients are better served with formal vascular imaging.

Duplex color flow imaging is not used for the acute assessment of vascular injury. Wounds, swelling, air in the tissue, and dressings or splints impair the ability to obtain satisfactory images. Duplex imaging does have a role in the follow-up of treated lesions (i.e., to assess patency of bypass grafts or to detect luminal stenosis at an anastomosis) or in the follow-up of nonoperative management of minimal vascular injury, such as small pseudoaneurysms or arteriovenous fistulas.

MINIMAL VASCULAR INJURY AND NONOPERATIVE MANAGEMENT

The widespread application of CT angiography in the evaluation of injured extremities results in the detection of clinically insignificant lesions.[12] There is now an extensive body of experience with lesions that are not limb-threatening. These minimal vascular injuries include intimal irregularity, small nonocclusive intimal flaps, focal spasm with minimal narrowing, and small pseudoaneurysms. They are often asymptomatic and usually do not progress.[6,12]

A small, nonocclusive intimal flap is the most commonly encountered clinically insignificant minimal vascular injury. The likelihood that it will progress to cause either occlusion or distal embolization is approximately 10% or less.[6,12] This progression, if

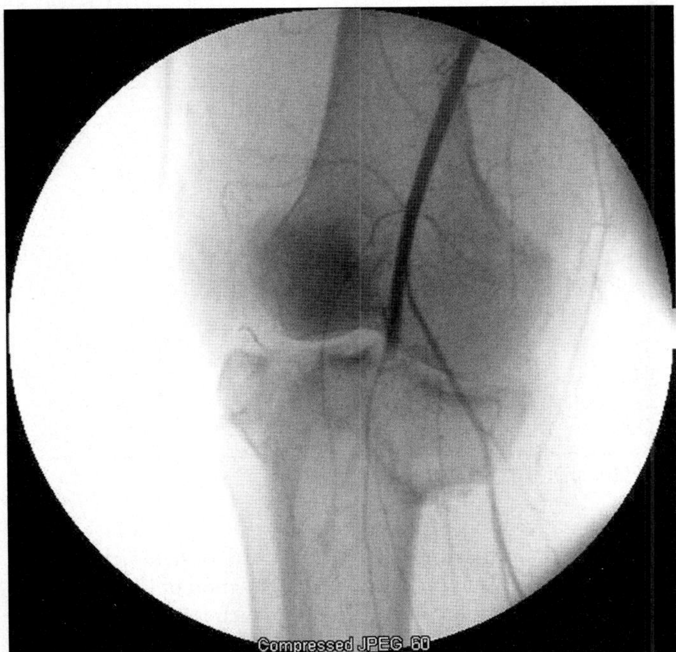

FIG. 64.1 Catheter arteriogram demonstrating an acute occlusion of right popliteal artery secondary to blunt injury with associated tibial plateau fracture.

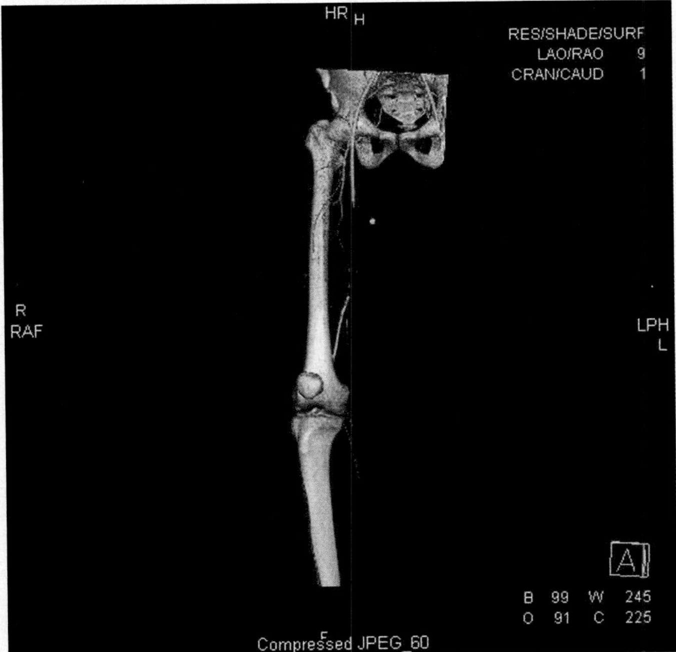

FIG. 64.2 Computed tomography angiogram with VTR view of a gunshot wound to the right superficial femoral artery resulting in segmental thrombosis.

it occurs, will be early in the postinjury course. Spasm is another common minimal vascular injury. This finding should resolve promptly after initial discovery. Failure of the return of normal extremity perfusion pressure indicates that a more serious vascular injury is present and intervention is needed. Small pseudoaneurysms are more likely to progress to the point of needing repair

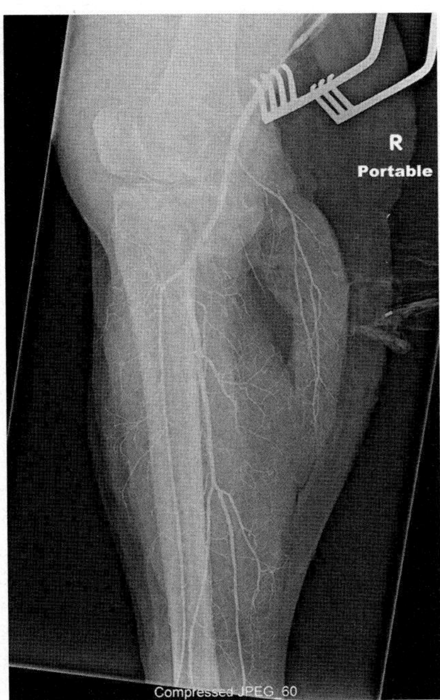

FIG. 64.3 Intraoperative plain film (direct injection arteriogram) in the patient described in Fig. 64.2 with blunt injury of the knee. Exploration of the popliteal artery with fasciotomy of the posterior compartments released compression of the artery with return of flow. This intraoperative arteriogram confirms a normal popliteal artery.

and must be actively observed with Duplex color flow imaging. Arteriovenous fistulas always enlarge over time and should be promptly repaired.

There is extensive evidence supporting nonoperative therapy for many asymptomatic lesions. However, successful nonoperative therapy requires continuous surveillance for subsequent progression, occlusion, or hemorrhage. Operative therapy is required for thrombosis, symptoms of chronic ischemia, and failure of small pseudoaneurysms to resolve.[12]

ENDOVASCULAR MANAGEMENT

Endovascular repair of vascular injuries is increasingly common.[13,14] This approach has become particularly effective in stable large-vessel injuries and in areas difficult to expose for direct repair. However, despite advances in endovascular techniques and devices, this approach has not supplanted open surgery in the management of most peripheral vascular injuries. Endovascular therapy for atherosclerotic arterial disease has become the first choice in management. Endoluminal stent deployment for occlusive lesions and stent graft for aortic aneurysms have become widely accepted. However, there is a strong tendency to generalize from this elective experience in elderly patients with atherosclerosis to the treatment of younger patients with acute vascular injuries. The evidence to support these approaches in preference to traditional open techniques in peripheral arterial injuries is yet to be demonstrated and there have been problems.[6,15] The striking decrease in open vascular surgical experience among general surgeons and vascular surgeons trained in the twenty-first century creates a lack of comfort and competence in performing open vascular repairs.[16,17] A balanced approach using each of these techniques where they best apply supported by clinical evidence is essential to good outcomes in patients with vascular trauma.

TABLE 64.2 **Comparison of endovascular and open blunt thoracic aortic injury repairs.**

	RELATIVE DEGREE OF RISK		
TECHNIQUE	**CLAMP AND SEW**	**PARTIAL BYPASS**	**ENDOVASCULAR**
Complications			
Physiology impact	High	Medium	Low
Blood loss	Medium	Medium	Low
Operative time	Medium	High	Low
Paraplegia	High	Medium	Low
Clinical Variables			
High surgical risk	High	Medium	Low
Severe lung injury	High	Medium	Low
Severe head injury	High	High	Low
Challenging aortic anatomy	Medium	Low	High

From Neschis DG, Scalea TM, Flinn WR, et al. Blunt aortic injury. *N Engl J Med.* 2008;359:1708–1716.

Endovascular Operating Rooms

There is a widespread proliferation of "hybrid" operating rooms. These high-technology suites have both advanced imaging capability and traditional operating room properties. They require a major commitment of resources and personnel to be effective. They are ideal for complex elective endovascular cases. Not all trauma centers have hybrid operating rooms, or, if they do, they cannot staff them on an emergency basis for the often after-hours management of vascular trauma.

Many centers create "hybrid operating rooms of opportunity" with high-resolution digital subtraction C-arm fluoroscopy equipment, mobile cabinets with the appropriate catheters and stent grafts, and on-call technical staff. They can create hybrid suite capabilities in an operating room large enough for the C-arm and the rolling cabinets with a standard orthopedic surgery operating table that accommodates fluoroscopy. An unstable trauma patient taken directly to the operating room with a major vascular injury or solid organ hemorrhage can be placed on an orthopedic surgery table and then be managed with all the functionality of a dedicated hybrid operating room. Many trauma centers already provide these mobile capabilities to their vascular surgeons performing elective endovascular abdominal aortic aneurysm repair. All trauma centers need to develop this capacity for their trauma patients.

Endovascular Management of Torso Vascular Injuries

Endovascular techniques offer a variety of options for hemorrhage control in the torso. Intra arterial catheter-directed embolization has become a mainstay of the management of solid organ hemorrhage in the abdomen.[18,19] Whether it is used as the sole treatment or in combination with open procedures, this approach has been effective in liver, spleen, and kidney injuries. Less commonly used intra arterial balloon occlusion for proximal control is a promising adjunct to open repair.[20,21] The availability of retrograde endovascular balloon occlusion of the aorta is growing and will soon be common practice in the same clinical setting of exsanguinating abdominal hemorrhage in which an aortic cross-clamp in the chest is needed. In trauma centers with the appropriately trained surgeons and proper equipment, these techniques are quick, accurate, and easily performed. The reluctance to adopt new and promising technology must be avoided, and trauma surgeons need either to add surgeons or radiologists with endovascular capabilities to their specialty physician call panels or to obtain the training themselves.

The early use of catheter-directed control of hemorrhage associated with pelvic fracture is an effective method of limiting blood loss and improving outcome.[22] This approach is well tolerated and has proved superior to open attempts at hemorrhage control by packing in most patients. Unstable patients benefit from an immediate trip to the operating room. If intraoperative endovascular capability is present, a combined approach may offer the best results.

Endovascular stent graft placement for the management of great vessel injuries has become the procedure of choice.[23,24] New devices with better proximal fixation seems to be preventing many of the early catastrophic graft failures of older devices. The comparison of the relative degree of risk of endovascular techniques to open repair reveals why this newer approach has gained widespread application (Table 64.2).[24,25] Lifelong CT imaging is necessary because of the possibility of delayed endoleak and the possible loss of device fixation as the aorta enlarges over time. There is a definite role for covered stents in proximal branches of the aorta in both the thorax and abdomen. In stable injuries at risk for delayed hemorrhage or thrombosis, carefully placed stents have the potential to lower morbidity compared with open procedures that require extensive operative dissection for exposure and control. Endoluminal management with stent grafts appears most effective in those torso injuries that are surgically inaccessible with the potential for significant hemorrhage in stable patients (Fig. 64.4). These techniques should be used only in centers with an active elective endovascular practice that has experience in treating trauma patients.

Endovascular Management of Cerebrovascular Vascular Injuries

Endovascular techniques offer advantages in anatomic regions where direct operative control is difficult or impossible. For example, hemorrhage from a penetrating injury at the base of the skull is extremely difficult to control (Fig. 64.5). Catheter-directed placement of coils, balloons, or hemostatic agents in the injured carotid or vertebral artery could be lifesaving. Stent placement initially appeared less effective than anticoagulation in partially occluded injuries without associated hemorrhage.[26] However, the role of stents in cerebrovascular trauma has yet to be defined and may prove safe.[27,28] This use of endoluminal cerebrovascular interventions requires significant expertise and experience. If such experience does not exist at the receiving hospital, consideration

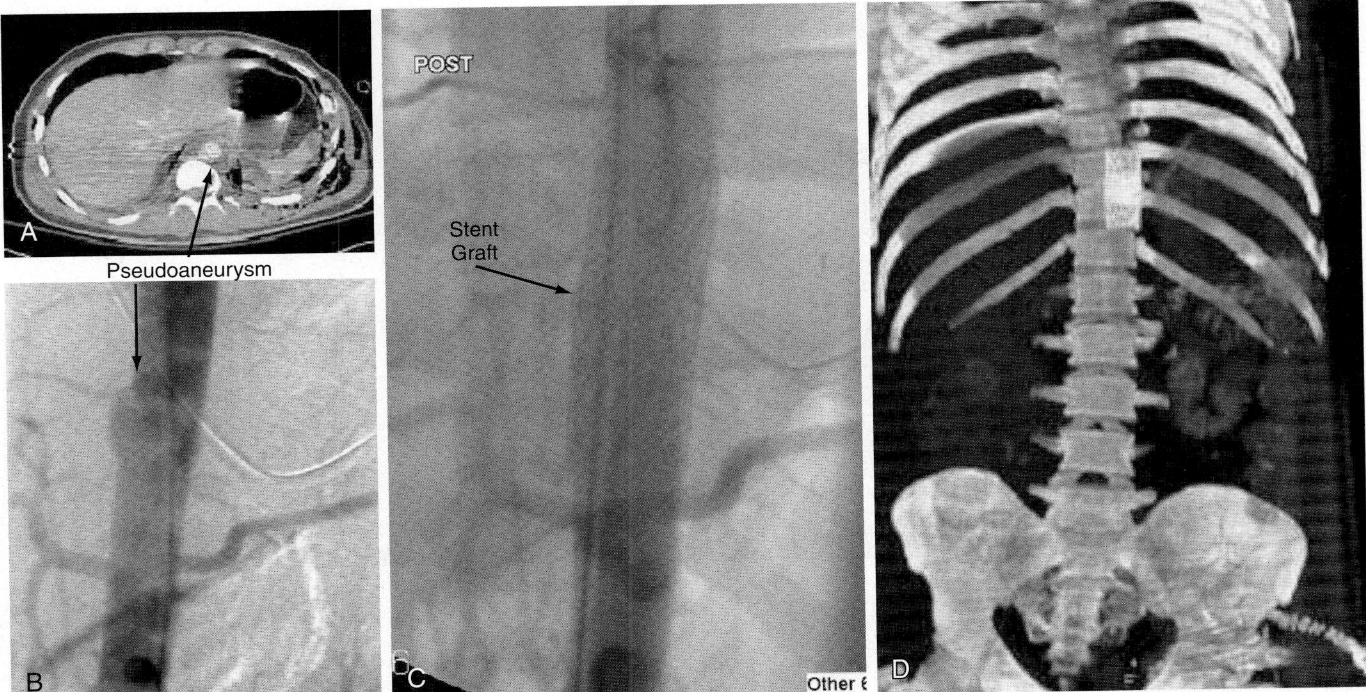

FIG. 64.4 Endovascular repair of a difficult-to-expose aortic injury with pseudoaneurysm at the diaphragm from blunt-force trauma. (A) Computed tomography (CT) angiogram showing the cross-sectional view of the pseudoaneurysm and associated thoracic spine fracture. (B) Catheter arteriogram demonstrating the pseudoaneurysm. (C) Deployed stent graft. (D) CT scan of level of aortic stent graft in mid-torso (VTR view).

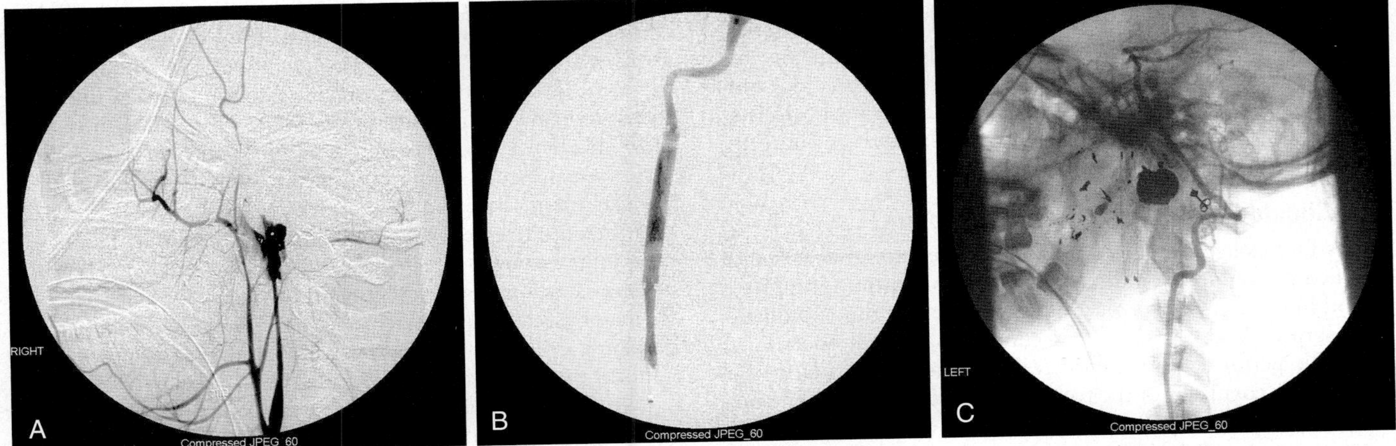

FIG. 64.5 (A) Gunshot wound with laceration and hemorrhage of internal carotid artery at the base of the skull. (B) Covered stent placed at the site of internal carotid artery injury. (C) After placement of a covered stent in the internal carotid artery at base of the skull.

should be given to transferring the patient to a medical center with experience in this mode of therapy.

Endovascular Management of Extremity Vascular Injuries

The use of stent grafts in extremity vascular injuries is becoming more common.[13,14] The long-term results, however, have not been documented, and caution should be used in considering this type of treatment. In hemodynamically stable patients with contained hemorrhage, difficult-to-access proximal subclavian or iliac arterial injuries may be effectively treated with covered stents. In the extremities distal to these areas, autologous vein interposition grafts have excellent long-term patency rates and remain the "gold standard" for vascular repairs.

The loss of open vascular surgery experience in general surgery residencies and vascular fellowship has resulted in many trauma and vascular surgeons resorting to endovascular repair in the extremities. This trend is particularly dangerous in the popliteal artery, where there is a high risk of stent or endograft thrombosis and subsequent limb threatening ischemia. Early patency of endovascular repairs can be, unfortunately followed by delayed thrombosis with extremely high rate of severe distal ischemia.

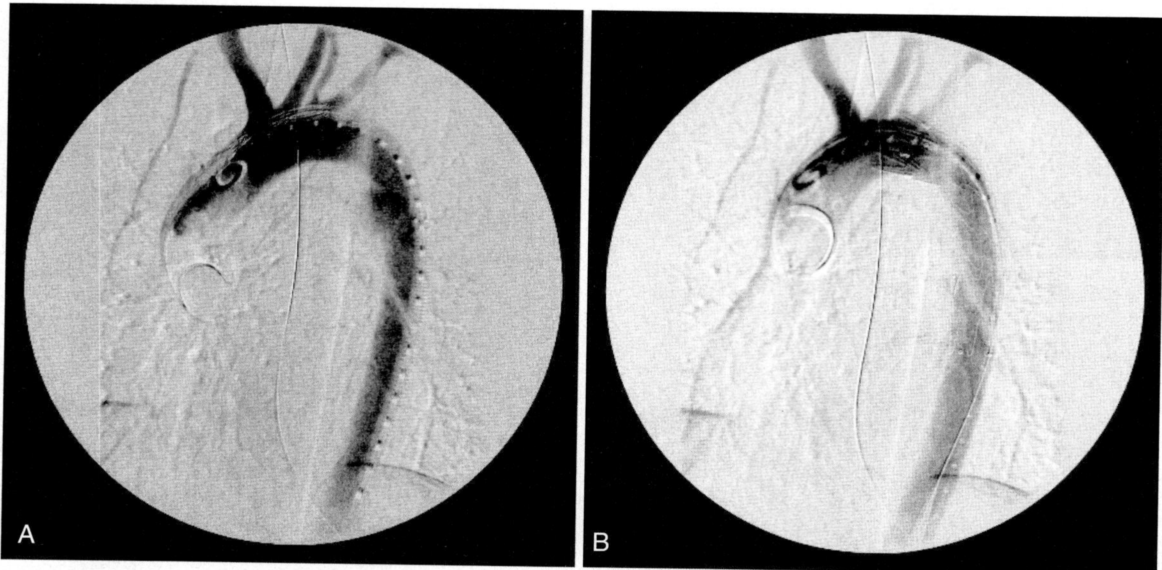

FIG. 64.6 (A) Aortogram of acute traumatic pseudoaneurysm of the thoracic aorta. (B) Image after stent graft deployment.

Open repair with suitable saphenous vein interposition graft placement is the best approach, and the results of all other techniques need to be compared to this traditional standard treatment.

Catheter-directed therapies for controlling hemorrhage from large branch vessels in the extremities are often effective and sufficient to manage these injuries. Endoluminal treatment is used sparingly for pseudoaneurysms of extremity arteries. Small pseudoaneurysms are likely to resolve without any intervention, and large pseudoaneurysms are best treated with open techniques because the risk of arterial thrombosis or distal embolization is high with this endovascular intervention (Fig. 64.6).

Who Should Perform Endovascular Repairs?

Successful management of vascular injuries requires that the most qualified person do the indicated intervention in the appropriate patient in the appropriate place at the appropriate time. Endovascular surgery is an operative procedure and, like all operations, should be performed by readily available trained clinicians who not only are cognizant of the technical aspects of a procedure but are also knowledgeable about the disease for which the procedure is being performed. In many centers, this person is the interventional radiologist. Other centers have catheter-trained vascular surgeons, and a few others have trauma surgeons who are capable of performing endovascular procedures. Catheter skills training is being integrated in many surgical critical care fellowships and may subsequently become more available in the near future at many trauma centers. (See later section on training and preparation.)

Endoluminal management of vascular trauma does not require a full endovascular hybrid operating room, as explained before. Planning and preparation, however, are essential for the endovascular capability, which more often than not is needed in the middle of the night. Preparing a team who can perform these techniques and who can organize the appropriate equipment with brief notice requires commitment, dedication, collaboration, and training.

OPEN SURGICAL MANAGEMENT

Preparation for Operative Management

Operative procedures to manage vascular injuries should be limited to those surgeons who are capable, experienced, and qualified. Board certification in vascular surgery is not enough to qualify a surgeon as capable to handle these injuries, just as the lack of certification does not necessarily disqualify a surgeon. Many surgeons who perform elective vascular surgery are not sufficiently experienced in the management of vascular trauma. Conversely, there are many trauma surgeons who are very skilled in vascular technique by virtue of their interest and experience. The results of major open vascular repairs are dependent on the skill level of the vascular trauma–capable surgeon independent of board preparation. In a multicenter review of close to 700 major extremity vascular injuries, board-certified general surgeons and board-certified vascular surgeons had nearly identically high limb salvage rates for major vascular surgical repairs.[29] Every trauma center needs to develop a call panel of surgeons with the skill and knowledge to perform the full spectrum of vascular trauma repairs.

Successful operative management of vascular injuries requires a systematic approach with careful preparation. This begins with airway control, adequate intravenous access, and availability of blood products. The administration of these blood products, however, should not begin before obtaining control of hemorrhage unless the patient is profoundly hypotensive.[5] If the blood pressure is below 80 to 90 mm Hg, the goal should be to provide adequate volume restoration with type O-negative packed cells and type AB fresh-frozen plasma infusion to support transport to the operating room for definitive hemorrhage control without delay. Volume infusion that raises the blood pressure above a systolic pressure of 90 to 100 mm Hg may increase bleeding and have a negative impact on outcome, particularly if the infusion delays transport to the operating room.[5]

Broad-spectrum preoperative antibiotics (and tetanus toxoid, if it is a penetrating wound) should be administered, and if there is an isolated extremity injury without significant hemorrhage, a bolus of 5000 units of heparin should also be given intravenously.

Systemic heparinization should be avoided in patients with torso injuries, head injuries, or multiple extremity injuries. The most commonly omitted step in preparation is a failure to document preoperative extremity neurologic status. The presence of a neurologic deficit after operative vascular repair without knowing the preoperative status presents a difficult management challenge. A new neurologic deficit after vascular repair merits investigation and, possibly, reoperation. Therefore, a thorough preoperative neurologic examination and careful documentation are essential to effective management.

The operative management of extremity vascular injuries must be carefully orchestrated with the overall care of the patient. The choice between definitive repair and damage control should be made as soon as possible in patients with life-threatening torso injuries or severe head injuries. This includes coordinating two surgical teams to work simultaneously to care for the torso injury and the extremity vascular injury at the same time. Associated injuries to the soft tissue and bone require a coordinated assessment and treatment with orthopedic and plastic surgery consultants. These specialists should be involved as early as possible to facilitate any additional imaging or diagnostic procedures before proceeding to the operating room. The conduct of the operation should also be discussed with these colleagues. For example, the use of damage control procedures with shunt placement, followed by orthopedic stabilization, can remove the sense of urgency to restore blood flow. Extensive soft tissue injuries may compromise the proper coverage of vascular repairs and fracture fixation. The advice and assistance of a plastic and reconstructive surgeon can be helpful in obtaining coverage of exposed grafts and fractures.

Vascular Exposure and Control

Always place the patient with major hemorrhage or suspected vascular injury on a fluoroscopy-capable operating room table to allow the endovascular therapy option for hemorrhage control or vascular repair. A generous sterile field should be prepared to allow adequate exposure of vessels to obtain proximal and distal control. In torso injuries, this includes preparing the chest and abdomen to the table laterally on both sides and both legs in case distal access or an autologous conduit is needed. For proximal vascular injuries of the extremities (at the groin crease or axilla), the chest or abdomen should be prepared to obtain proximal control out of the zone of injury. An uninjured leg should also be prepared for harvesting of autologous venous conduit.

Proximal control is the first priority in the exposure of vascular injuries. In the torso, chest injuries with life-threatening hemorrhage are best approached through a fourth intercostal space anterolateral thoracotomy that can be extended across the sternum into the third intercostal space of the right side of the chest to create a "clamshell" incision.[30] Thoracic outlet and proximal neck vascular injuries may require median sternotomy with extension above the clavicle up along the ipsilateral sternocleidomastoid muscle.

Retrograde endovascular balloon occlusion of the aorta with the 7 Fr catheter via common femoral access should be considered for patients with suspected abdominal vascular injury.[21] In unstable patients, it can be advanced to the descending aorta in the chest and inflated. In stable patients in whom difficulty with proximal control is anticipated, it can be similarly positioned but left uninflated. For abdominal vascular injury, a generous xiphoid to pubis incision is needed for adequate exposure.[31] Proximal control for abdominal aortic injuries should be obtained just below the aortic hiatus of the diaphragm or may require a left anterolateral thoracotomy to clamp the distal thoracic aorta. If retrograde endovascular balloon occlusion of the aorta or intrathoracic aortic clamping is used, it should be converted to a clamp low on the aorta while providing proximal control as possible to allow visceral artery perfusion to prevent ischemic injury.

In the proximal extremity injuries with active hemorrhage, the first incision site is chosen to give the fastest exposure of inflow vessels for clamping. For proximal upper extremity injuries, this may include incisions over the infraclavicular region of the chest to expose the axillary artery. For injuries in the groin, prepare to enter the lower quadrant of the abdomen for access to the external iliac vessels. In mid and distal extremity vascular injuries associated with active hemorrhage, tourniquets can rapidly obtain control in the trauma resuscitation room. In the operating room, have one team member precisely compress the bleeding site with a gloved hand and a sponge, remove the tourniquet, and prepare the extremity. A 5000-unit heparin bolus is then given, if appropriate, and the extremity is prepared and draped and a sterile tourniquet is placed proximal to the wound and inflated. The injury site can then be explored in a controlled fashion and clamps or vessel loops placed above and below the vascular injury. In certain injuries, distal arterial occlusion and retrograde intraluminal insertion of a Fogarty catheter with a stopcock to maintain balloon inflation will provide rapid hemorrhage control.[6]

Incisions used to manage vascular injuries are often the same as those used to manage elective cases but are generally more generous. The use of smaller incisions may lead to error in identifying the extent of vascular injury, adequately controlling branch vessel hemorrhage, and identifying associated venous lacerations. This is particularly true for popliteal artery and vein injuries. A limited approach with separate medial above- and below-knee incisions will not adequately expose the site of injury. Similarly, the posterior approach with the patient prone is not recommended because of the difficulty in obtaining adequate proximal and distal exposure for both vascular repair and bleeding control of associated venous injuries. A medial incision from the proximal popliteal space to the distal popliteal space with division of the medial head of the gastrocnemius muscle and the semimembranosus and semitendinosus muscles with full exposure of the popliteal artery and vein and the tibial nerve provides adequate exposure. This ensures adequate vascular control and the opportunity for successful repair. Closure of the wound to include approximation of the divided muscles yields an excellent functional result. Dividing the inguinal ligament in the groin, dividing the pectoralis major in the axilla, and removing the mid clavicle may rarely be necessary. In each of these areas, rapid endovascular balloon occlusion offers an excellent adjunct to proximal control. In the presence of life-threatening hemorrhage that cannot be controlled by any other approach, these structures should not stand in the way of adequate exposure and control.

Vascular Damage Control

Damage control has gained wide acceptance in trauma surgery and is directed at rapid control of hemorrhage and closure of enteric wounds so that the patient can be warmed and resuscitated. The choice between definitive time-consuming vascular repair and temporary measures that achieve control must be made early in care of patients with vascular injury and hypovolemic shock. This is particularly important when an extremity vascular injury is associated with major torso injuries. Ligation and placement of intraluminal shunts are the mainstays of vascular damage control.[32,33]

Ligation should be reserved for vessels with adequate distal collateral flow in patients who are too unstable for definitive repair. In the torso, this includes the subclavian and innominate arteries, the celiac artery, and the inferior mesenteric artery. In the upper extremity, proximal injuries of the axillary artery and distal injuries to either the radial or ulnar artery may be ligated, provided there is evidence of adequate distal collateral flow assessed by either physical examination or continuous-wave Doppler interrogation. In the groin, profunda femoris artery injuries can be ligated if the common and superficial femoral arteries (SFAs) are intact. Similarly, in the lower extremity, ligation of a single tibial artery or the peroneal artery can be performed after a similar assessment. If distal perfusion is compromised, an intraluminal shunt should be inserted, rather than ligating the vessel. Superior mesenteric artery (SMA) ligation is associated with a high risk of bowel necrosis, and damage control is best accomplished with placement of an intraluminal shunt. In the extremities, ligation of the brachial, external iliac, superficial femoral, or popliteal artery has a high likelihood of producing limb-threatening ischemia and should be avoided, if possible.

A variety of commercially available shunts can be used for damage control. If these are not available, sterile intravenous tubing is of adequate size to "shunt" both the artery and the vein, if necessary. Venous shunt placement (instead of ligation) may improve extremity perfusion and lower the risk of compartment syndrome. Damage control shunt placement begins with obtaining adequate proximal and distal control. Thrombus should be cleared with a Fogarty embolectomy catheter, followed by the instillation of regional heparinized saline (5000 units heparin/500 mL saline). The shunt should be placed in a straight line and be long enough to remain safely held in place in the proximal and distal vessel with a tied umbilical tape or 2-0 silk tie at each end. Long, looped shunts run the risk of becoming dislodged during subsequent dressing changes and should be avoided. The ties securing the shunt cause intimal damage, and those portions of the artery must be resected at the time of definitive vascular repair.

The condition of the patient determines the timing of definitive vascular repair after damage control. Hemorrhage must be controlled, coagulopathy and acidosis corrected, and temperature normalized.

Choice of Repair and Graft Material

Vessel injuries that cannot be repaired by primary end-to-end technique will require an interposition graft. The most desirable graft is autologous great saphenous vein harvested from an uninjured leg.[6] Native vein graft is preferable because it has elastic properties that make it compliant with the normal pulsatile flow of an artery; it has a diameter that approximates that of an extremity artery, producing an adequate size match for grafting in the arm and leg; it is not thrombogenic; and it has superior long-term patency in elective vascular surgery compared with prosthetic material when it is used with smaller vessels (popliteal and tibial). Cephalic vein and lesser saphenous vein have been suggested as suitable second choices, but cephalic vein is less muscular than the greater saphenous and, like the lesser saphenous, may present problems with harvesting in a trauma patient.[6] Also, upper extremity venous access becomes compromised when the cephalic vein is used.

Saphenous vein may not be suitable in all instances because of inadequate size or because it has been traumatized or harvested previously. In such cases, a prosthetic conduit may be needed. Initial experiences with the use of prosthetic material (Dacron) in traumatic vascular injuries were not good. Rich and Hughes reported a complication rate of 77% (infection and thrombosis were the most common) in 26 patients.[34] However, more recent experience with newer graft material (polytetrafluoroethylene [PTFE]) has shown improved patency (70%–90% short term) and rare infection (even in contaminated wounds).[35] Early rates of patency with PTFE grafts are equivalent to those with vein for injuries proximal to the popliteal artery and in the brachial artery. Distal to these levels, PTFE is inferior to vein for popliteal and more distal vessels and in the arm and leg. PTFE grafts of less than 6 mm should not be used.[35] PTFE and vein grafts must be covered or there is a significant risk of hemorrhage from desiccation of the vein with subsequent autolysis or breakdown of the anastomosis.[21,35]

Intraoperative Imaging and Noninvasive Evaluation

The successful management of vascular injury requires knowing precisely the status of blood flow in the area of the vessel injury. Preoperative imaging with catheter angiography or CT angiography is not always possible. In addition, when a vascular repair has been completed, the presence of thrombus, kinking, or unexpected technical problems may cause early failure. Intraoperative imaging is therefore an important part of assessing the injured vessels and the repair site.[6] Either single-injection radiography or fluoroscopy is effective in providing images in the operating room (see Fig. 64.6). Intraoperative duplex scanning is also effective but requires significant training and experience for it to be performed adequately. Hand-held continuous-wave Doppler interrogation can be helpful but requires considerable experience to be used effectively. Ankle or wrist pressure measurements may be misleading because of regional vasospasm in the proximal injured extremity, resulting in a reduced distal pressure compared with the uninjured leg. Intraoperative radiographic imaging remains the most accurate and useful method to detect technical problems with a vascular repair or to determine the presence of thrombus in the runoff vessels distal to a repair. Routine completion arteriography after vascular repairs will yield findings of clinical importance in approximately 10% of patients.[6]

Role of Tissue Coverage

All vascular repairs must be covered to prevent desiccation and disruption. In crushed or badly mangled extremities, this can be a difficult challenge. Rotation of regional muscle or skin flaps may be required. The early involvement of a plastic and reconstructive surgeon is essential to obtain tissue coverage when there is extensive soft tissue injury or loss. Local muscle can be advanced into the wound at the initial operation. If there is a large contaminated wound and local muscle viability is questionable, early reexploration and preparation for a free flap should be considered. On occasion, tissue loss may be so extensive that an extra-anatomic course for an interposition graft may be required. Attention to coverage is also essential in damage control procedures to avoid shunt dislodgment during dressing changes.

Role of Fasciotomy

Failure to perform an adequate fasciotomy after revascularization of an acutely ischemic limb is the most common cause of preventable limb loss.[6] Calf compartment syndrome is the most common indication for fasciotomy. Forearm and thigh compartment syndromes are less common. Any muscle group can develop compartment syndrome, including those in the hands and feet.

Compartment syndrome may be manifested immediately or delayed to 12 to 24 hours after reperfusion. If it is not promptly diagnosed and treated, the risk of limb loss or limb dysfunction is high. Calf compartment syndrome most commonly results from prolonged ischemia or a crush injury. Frequent physical examinations augmented with compartment pressure measurements are necessary to detect this complication in its early stage. The first clinical findings are pain and loss of light touch sensation in the distribution of the nerve in the compartment. The diagnosis of compartment syndrome should be suspected in any patient complaining of increasing pain after injury. Other physical findings include a tense compartment, pain on passive range of motion, progressive loss of sensation, and weakness. The loss of arterial pulses is a late finding, which usually indicates a poor prognosis. Neurologic signs and symptoms, although helpful, are neither sensitive nor specific in the upper extremity after arterial injury because associated peripheral nerve injury often exists. Early diagnosis must be predicated on measurement of compartment pressures. The normal tissue compartment pressure ranges from 0 to 9 mm Hg. Much controversy exists about what constitutes a pathologic elevation. However, the safest approach is to perform fasciotomy when compartment pressure exceeds 25 mm Hg.[6,36,37]

A compartment syndrome can also develop in either the upper arm (triceps, deltoid, or along the axillary sheath) or the forearm. The forearm compartment syndrome is more common. Increased tissue pressure can follow either blunt or penetrating trauma because of hematoma, posttraumatic transudation of serum into the interstitial space, venous thrombosis, or reperfusion after ischemia.[36] The possibility of a compartment syndrome must always be a consideration in a patient who has been injured, particularly one with prolonged ischemia before reperfusion.

Role of Immediate Amputation

A very limited role for primary amputation exists in the management of complex extremity vascular injuries. Patients with extensive soft tissue loss, neurologic deficit, extensive fractures, and vascular injuries should be evaluated collaboratively with orthopedic, neurosurgical, and plastic and reconstructive surgery colleagues to determine if primary amputation is the best initial management. Scoring systems to predict the need for amputation have not been useful.[38,39] Because of the emotional impact of amputation and because marginally viable tissue often takes hours to demarcate or declare, it may be best to proceed with initial intraoperative evaluation and documentation (pictures, radiographs, and consultation), damage control using intravascular shunts for the vascular injuries, and a second look in 24 hours. The interval of time allows communication with the patient and the family and a more planned approach. Immediate amputation should also be considered in patients with extensive soft tissue, bone, and neurovascular disruption who have life-threatening torso injuries as mentioned earlier in the discussion of damage control techniques. If immediate amputation is required, extensive documentation of the extremity injury with photographs placed in the chart will be helpful in later explaining the decision to the patient and family and will help with their acceptance of this drastic surgical procedure.

Common Errors and Pitfalls

The management of vascular injuries is challenging. An organized approach is necessary to avoid the common errors and pitfalls. One of the most common errors is the lack of recognition of an extremity vascular injury in a patient with multiple torso injuries. Failure to recognize and adequately treat compartment syndrome is another error that is all too common and has devastating consequences. In torso injuries to the great vessels, failure to adequately expose and control the injured site can lead to a rapid death from exsanguination. Finally, failure to recognize the need for damage control techniques and a rapid completion of the operation in an unstable patient can also be deadly. The three most common factors in generating errors in caring for the injured are fatigue, distraction, and familiarity.[40] Each of these factors is inherent to the process of care at busy trauma centers. An organized approach mitigates these factors and intercepts errors in progress before they are completed and the patients suffer.

SPECIFIC INJURIES

Head, Neck, and Thoracic Outlet

Vascular injuries of the head, neck, and thoracic outlet are often challenging to manage. Penetrating trauma can injure large vessels, such as the innominate and subclavian arteries, which can lead to exsanguination. Blunt trauma to the carotid and vertebral arteries, collectively known as blunt cerebrovascular injuries, is often occult and, if not diagnosed and treated rapidly, can lead to cerebral ischemia, infarction, and possibly death.

The principles of management of penetrating trauma to this region are based on the location of the injury relative to the three zones of the neck: zone 1, inferior to the cricoid cartilage; zone 2, cricoid cartilage to the angle of the mandible; and zone III, cephalad from the angle of the mandible. In a stable patient with a suspected vascular injury in either zone 1 or zone 3, vascular imaging is mandatory to confirm the suspicion of vascular injury and to plan proximal and distal control.[41] Vascular imaging is also recommended for stable patients with penetrating trauma in zone 2, but exploration should be undertaken expeditiously for patients with an expanding hematoma or impending airway compromise (manifested by hoarseness and tracheal deviation).[41] In the unstable patient, a Foley urinary catheter with the balloon inflated can be inserted into the wound to achieve temporary tamponade of injuries in these regions. Conventional angiography can have a dual role for injuries in zone 1 or zone 3. It not only can provide the diagnosis but also may provide a venue for endoluminal management—coiling of bleeding vessels or pseudoaneurysms in zone 3 or placement of covered stents in zone 1.

Blunt cerebrovascular injuries are often occult and asymptomatic. Therefore, rapid diagnostic screening is essential and provides the underpinning of successful management. Initially, blunt cerebrovascular injuries were thought to be rare, occurring in about 0.1% of patients; but with use of the screening criteria developed by the group at Denver General Hospital, the incidence is actually 10 to 20 times that.[27] Factors associated with these injuries include displaced midface fractures, basilar skull fracture with carotid canal involvement, cervical spine fracture, closed head injury consistent with diffuse axonal injury and Glasgow Coma Scale score below 6, and blunt neck trauma from hanging or seat belt injuries. Both carotid and vertebral artery injuries occur from stretching or tearing of the intima of the vessels produced by rapid extreme extension or flexion of the neck or by direct blunt-force injury. The carotid artery is particularly vulnerable where it lies close to the second and sixth cervical transverse processes. The vertebral artery is also vulnerable to stretch injuries and fractures of the transverse process of the cervical vertebrae that involve the foramen transversarium. Cerebrovascular injuries vary from minor intimal irregularities to arterial rupture and severe hemorrhage (Table 64.3).[27]

Patients who fulfill the Denver criteria should undergo CT angiography of the neck.[26,27] The treatment of blunt carotid and

TABLE 64.3 **Spectrum of severity of blunt cerebrovascular arterial injury.**

Grade I	Luminal irregularity with <25% luminal narrowing
Grade II	Dissection of hematoma with >25% luminal narrowing
Grade III	Pseudoaneurysm
Grade IV	Occlusion
Grade V	Transection with extravasation

vertebral artery injuries is anticoagulation in patients who do not have a contraindication.[26] Aspirin is the only alternative in patients who cannot be safely anticoagulated. The use of endovascular techniques has a very limited role as discussed before. However, in patients with carotid injuries at the base of the skull or injuries of the vertebral artery, covered stents or embolization offers the best results (see Fig. 64.5).

Vascular injuries of the thoracic outlet are challenging because they involve large-caliber vessels that can be difficult to expose and to control. Unstable patients with vascular injury in the region of the thoracic outlet must be expeditiously taken to the operating room. Stable patients should have preoperative imaging with catheter or CT angiography to locate the injury and to determine its extent. This will allow planning for endoluminal treatment or open exposure.[42,43] Operative control may require a simple supraclavicular incision, a sternotomy, or a combination of the two incisions, depending on the location and extent of the injury. Clamp application on the proximal subclavian and carotid arteries must be precise to avoid injury to the vagus, phrenic, or recurrent laryngeal nerves, all of which reside in this anatomic region. Sternotomy is frequently used for proximal innominate, proximal right subclavian, and proximal right carotid arterial injuries. Left subclavian artery proximal control is best obtained through a posterolateral thoracotomy for definitive repair. However, for supraclavicular injuries, a third intercostal space anterolateral thoracotomy provides exposure for proximal control. Distal control of the carotid arteries is obtained by extending the median sternotomy superiorly along the border of the ipsilateral sternocleidomastoid muscle. Distal subclavian arterial control is obtained through a supraclavicular incision. Resection of the clavicle results in little or no morbidity and can be performed quickly to control hemorrhage if needed. Suturing of the subclavian and axillary arteries must be done with extreme caution. Undue tension or traction will result in a tear of these vessels.[44] Endovascular balloon occlusion, when it is rapidly available, is an excellent adjunctive measure for proximal control.

Intrathoracic Great Vessels

Penetrating injuries of the intrathoracic great vessels (aorta, superior and inferior venae cavae, pulmonary arteries and veins) usually cause death at the time of injury from exsanguination. The small number of patients with penetrating injuries of the intrathoracic great vessels who arrive to the trauma center alive often present hemodynamically unstable and require emergent operative intervention. Repair of intrathoracic great vessel injuries may be achieved through sternotomy, left or right anterolateral thoracotomy, or, in many cases, bilateral (or clamshell) anterolateral thoracotomy.[30] Although many of these structures are exposed through a posterolateral thoracotomy in the elective setting, patients who present in hemorrhagic shock and without a distinct diagnosis should be managed with more versatile incisions, such as median sternotomy and anterolateral thoracotomy.

Injuries to the ascending aorta and the superior or inferior vena cava are best exposed and treated through a median sternotomy.[30] These injuries should be controlled with digital pressure and then placement of a side-biting clamp to allow suture repair of the injury and may require cardiopulmonary bypass to achieve repair. Injuries of the descending aorta are ideally approached through a left posterolateral thoracotomy. However, most of these injuries will be discovered during emergent left anterolateral thoracotomy and will need to be quickly repaired. Injuries of the pulmonary arteries and veins can be approached through a sternotomy or anterolateral thoracotomy, depending on their proximity to the heart.[30] If possible, these injuries should be repaired primarily. However, destructive injuries to the pulmonary arteries and veins may necessitate pneumonectomy for definitive control.

Blunt injuries to the intrathoracic great vessels consist primarily of blunt thoracic aortic injury (BTAI). BTAI occurs as a result of high-energy blunt trauma. The most common mechanisms of injury resulting in BTAI are high-speed motor vehicle crashes and falls from a height. The aorta is typically injured in a location where it is relatively fixed (root of the aorta, ligamentum arteriosum, diaphragmatic hiatus), and the majority (85%–90%) of patients die at the scene. Patients with BTAI who arrive at the hospital alive have typically sustained multisystem associated injuries. BTAI must be ruled out when there is a high-energy mechanism injury or a chest radiograph shows a widened mediastinum. However, definitive diagnosis of BTAI is established with a high-resolution CT scan of the chest. Injuries vary from an intimal injury to pseudoaneurysm or a contained periaortic hematoma just distal to the left subclavian artery.[7,9]

Once the diagnosis of BTAI is confirmed, the initial management is focused on blood pressure control and addressing associated immediately life-threatening injuries. Blood pressure is best controlled with a short-acting intravenous beta blocker (e.g., esmolol) that can be titrated to a systolic blood pressure of less than 110 mm Hg while also keeping heart rate below 100 beats/min.[30] If beta blockade does not achieve blood pressure goals, other intravenous agents, such as calcium channel blockers, nitroglycerin, and nitroprusside, may be used. Whereas some stable minimal BTAIs may be managed nonoperatively, most will require definitive repair through the endovascular or open approach. Regardless of the approach, most BTAIs in stable patients with a stable aortic pseudoaneurysm may be repaired in a delayed fashion after the patient's concomitant injures are dealt with. Early repair of these injuries has been associated with increased mortality.[30]

Open repair of BTAI was once the mainstay of treatment for decades. Open repair is achieved through a left posterolateral thoracotomy, cardiopulmonary bypass, and placement of a synthetic aortic interposition graft. Endovascular repair of BTAI has become increasingly more common during the past decade (Fig. 64.7). The advent of new and improved stent graft and the widespread adoption of endovascular techniques have made this approach the first choice at most centers. Although there are no prospective, randomized trials comparing open versus endovascular

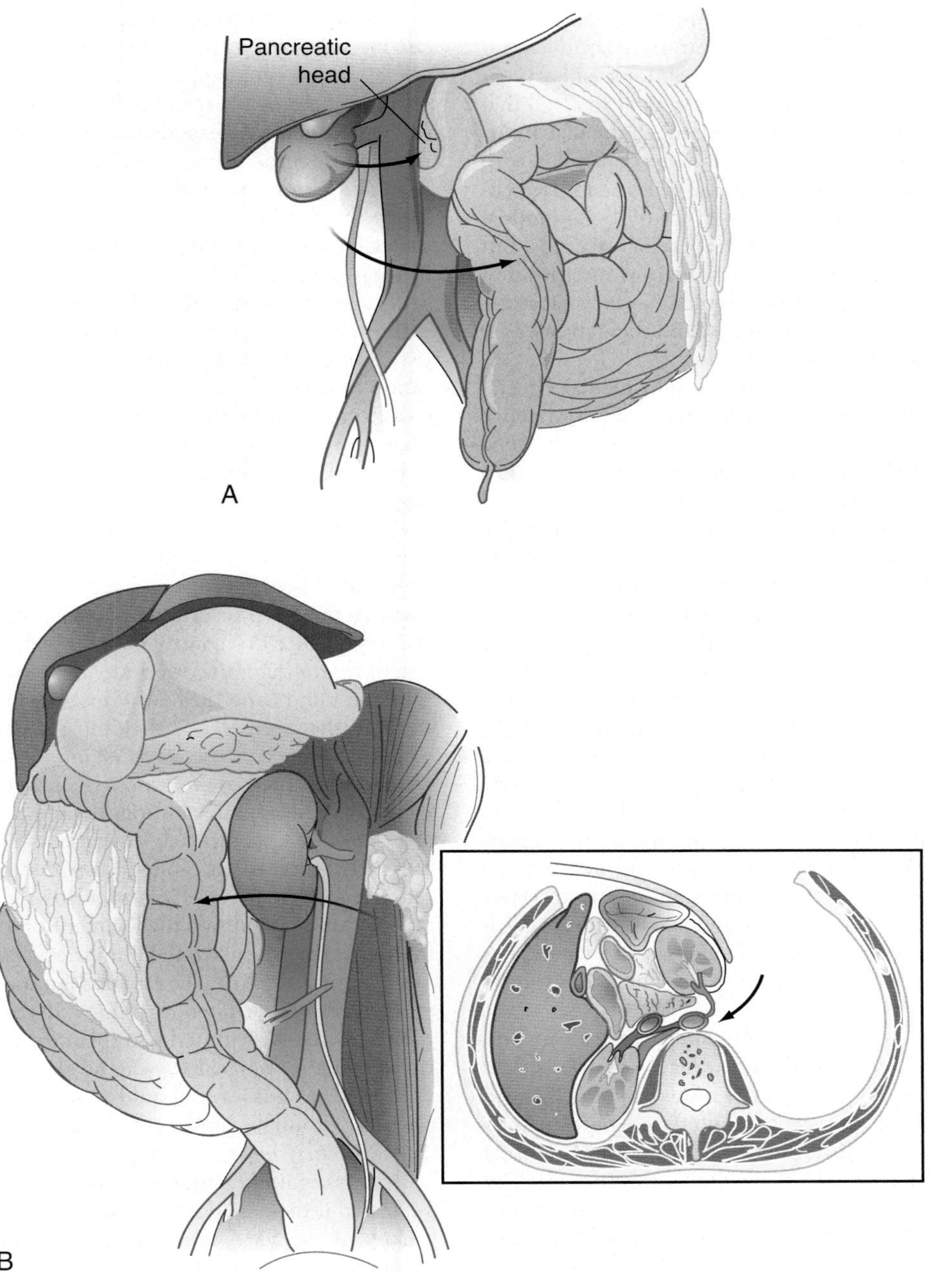

FIG. 64.7 (A) Left-sided medial visceral rotation for exposure of great vessels in the retroperitoneum. (B) Right-sided medial visceral rotation for exposure of vena cava and renal veins in the retroperitoneum.

management of BTAI, there have been two multicenter American Association for the Surgery of Trauma trials showing lower morbidity (spinal cord ischemia, stroke) and mortality with the endovascular approach.[24,25] However, patients who undergo endovascular repair require lifelong surveillance because there is no information about long-term sequelae of endovascular grafts in the aortic position in young patients. In addition, many young patients do not have favorable anatomy for endovascular repair and still require the open approach. More recent series of open repair with spinal cord protection from partial cardiopulmonary bypass have a competitively low rate of paraplegia.[25] The widespread preference for thoracic endovascular aortic repair may suffer from the famous British thoracic surgeon Ronald Belsey's observation that "the follow-up clinics are the shoals upon which founder many attractive theories in surgery."[45] Late graft failure due to endoleak and possible collapse within aortas susceptible to the elongation and widening that occur with age may be a future source of major morbidity and mortality. Despite this lack of conclusive evidence, in 2011, the Society of Vascular Surgery endorsed endovascular aortic repair as the preferable approach in BTAI.[46] As of 2019, the time of writing this chapter, there is not conclusive evidence that early and late results with thoracic endovascular aortic repair in young patients are superior to well-performed open repairs with partial bypass for spinal cord protection.[25]

Abdominal Vascular Injury

Abdominal vascular injury most often results from penetrating trauma, and all are treated through a generous midline laparotomy.[31] Many of these injuries will require supraceliac control of the aorta to achieve adequate visualization to complete exposure and repair. Penetrating injuries to the abdominal aorta are best exposed and repaired with a left medial visceral rotation that exposes the aorta from the diaphragmatic hiatus to the iliac bifurcation (see Fig. 64.7). The injury can typically be controlled with direct digital pressure, which allows time for placement of vascular clamps proximal and distal to the site of injury.[31] Abdominal aortic injuries may be repaired primarily after stab wounds, but gunshot wounds will often require a patch repair or interposition graft. Uncommonly, patients will sustain a blunt abdominal aortic injury without life-threatening hemorrhage, and these injuries are best repaired by endovascular techniques.

The inferior vena cava is exposed with a right medial visceral rotation that exposes the vena cava from iliac vein confluence to inferior edge of the liver (see Fig. 64.7).[31] Injury to the vena cava is best controlled with direct digital pressure, with subsequent proximal and distal control using sponge sticks or vessel loops. Lumbar tributaries and renal veins may also need to be controlled to clearly visualize and repair the injury. Injuries to the anterior or lateral surfaces of the vena cava can most often be repaired primarily as long as the repair does not narrow the lumen more than 50%. Penetrating injuries to the vena cava may be through-and-through and require repair of a posterior injury as well. Injuries to the posterior vena cava may be repaired through the anterior injury, or the vena cava may be mobilized after ligating and dividing lumbar veins. Complex injuries may require patch repair, interposition graft, shunting with delayed reconstruction, or ligation.[31] Complexity of repair will depend on the physiologic status of the patient and the location of the injury. Hemodynamically unstable patients with ongoing hemorrhage are not candidates for complex repairs and should have the vena cava ligated or shunted. Hemodynamically stable patients with injuries at or above the level of the renal veins may be candidates for complex reconstruction, but ligation is still an option for the exsanguinating patient.[31]

The right common, external, and internal iliac arteries are best exposed by widely mobilizing the cecum, whereas injuries to the left iliac arteries are exposed by completely mobilizing the sigmoid colon.[31] Keep in mind the course of the ureter on both sides as it crosses the iliac vessels. Injuries to the common and external iliac arteries are initially controlled with digital pressure to allow proximal and distal control with vascular clamps or vessel loops. Injuries to the common and external iliac arteries may be repaired primarily but will often require a synthetic interposition graft. The common and external iliac arteries should never be ligated; if a patient is hemodynamically unstable, these injuries should be shunted and repaired in a delayed fashion. However, injuries to the internal iliac artery can be routinely ligated.[31]

Iliac veins are exposed in the same manner as for iliac arteries. Exposure is made more challenging by the location of the confluence of the iliac veins with the inferior vena cava directly posterior to the right common iliac artery. It will need to be widely mobilized to allow access to the confluence of the iliac veins. However, we do not advocate division of the right iliac artery to achieve exposure of the iliac vein confluence. Once the common, external, and internal iliac veins are exposed, the injury is best controlled with direct digital pressure, then proximal and distal control may be achieved with vessel loops. If possible, simple injuries to the iliac veins should be repaired with primary venorrhaphy. However, complex repairs of destructive injuries to the iliac veins should not be attempted, and these injuries should be ligated.[31]

Injuries to the mesenteric vessels are some of the most challenging injuries to expose and to repair. In the elective setting, the celiac trunk is often approached through the lesser sac; but in the setting of trauma, this may prove difficult because of a large lesser sac hematoma that obscures the usual landmarks. In the setting of trauma, the celiac trunk is best exposed through a wide left medial visceral rotation that mobilizes the spleen and tail of pancreas but leaves the left kidney in situ.[31] Once exposed, most injuries to the celiac trunk should be ligated because repair is difficult and ligation is well tolerated in the majority of patients. Although the SMA and celiac trunk take off from the aorta within 1 to 2 cm of each other, the exposure and treatment algorithm for SMA injuries is different. Management of SMA injuries will depend on location based on the Fullen classification: zone I, beneath the pancreas; zone II, between the pancreaticoduodenal and middle colic branches; zone III, beyond the middle colic branch; zone IV, enteric branches. Injuries that present with a large contained central hematoma at the root of the mesentery are best approached with a left medial visceral rotation. Active hemorrhage is controlled by manual compression, followed by left medial visceral rotation.[31] This will allow exposure and control of the aorta proximal and distal to the SMA or direct clamping of the SMA as it comes off the aorta. Once this control has been achieved, attention is turned anteriorly for definitive exposure and repair of the SMA injury.

Zone I and zone II SMA injuries can be exposed and repaired through the lesser sac by dividing the gastrocolic ligament. The pancreas will need to be retracted inferiorly to expose the origin of the SMA or superiorly to expose the proximal SMA. Uncommonly, in active bleed SMA injuries behind the pancreas, it may need to be divided to completely visualize and control that segment of the SMA. Zone III and zone IV injuries should be approached by reflecting the transverse colon and its mesentery superiorly with or without taking down the ligament of Treitz. All zones of SMA injuries (except distal zone IV injuries) should always be repaired, with a primary repair, end-to-end anastomosis, or interposition graft of reversed saphenous vein.[31] If the patient is in extremis, the SMA may be shunted with plan for delayed repair. The superior mesenteric vein (SMV) can be exposed in the same fashion as the SMA. SMV injuries should be repaired or reconstructed when possible, although shunting with delayed repair is also an option. The SMV may be ligated for patients in extremis who would otherwise exsanguinate. Injuries to the inferior mesenteric artery may be ligated if there is adequate collateral flow from the middle colic branch of the SMA and the inferior and middle hemorrhoidal branches of the internal iliac arteries. The inferior mesenteric vein may be safely ligated if required.

The portal vein runs close to the inferior vena cava and is the most posterior structure within the portal triad, closely associated with the common bile duct and hepatic artery. Portal vein injuries are initially controlled with direct manual pressure. A right medial visceral rotation, including a generous Kocher maneuver, is performed to expose and to visualize the lateral and inferior portal vein. The common bile duct and hepatic artery will need to be mobilized to expose the anterior surface of the portal vein. Similar to SMA and SMV exposure, the neck of the pancreas may need to be divided to visualize the entirety of the portal vein.[31] These injuries should be managed in the same fashion as SMV injuries, with repair or reconstruction in the majority of cases, shunting and delayed repair if necessary, and ligation only for patients in extremis who would otherwise exsanguinate.

Penetrating renal vascular injuries are easily exposed on either side after medial visceral rotation. Gerota fascia is opened, and the kidney is bluntly mobilized into the wound. Once the kidney is mobilized, the vascular injury can be controlled with direct manual pressure while proximal and distal control is obtained with vessel loops. Renal artery injuries can be managed with primary repair, end-to-end anastomosis, vein patch, interposition graft, or nephrectomy (after confirming a normal contralateral kidney by palpation). Treatment of renal artery injuries is based on complexity of the injury and physiologic status of the patient. Renal vein injuries can be repaired with primary venorrhaphy or ligation. On the right, ligation of the renal vein will require a nephrectomy, and patch angioplasty or interposition graft should be considered in stable patients. The left renal vein may be safely ligated near the inferior vena cava because of collateral flow through the adrenal, gonadal, and lumbar veins.[31] Combined injuries to the renal artery and vein should be treated with nephrectomy in unstable patients. Renal artery injuries rarely occur after blunt trauma. These injuries may be managed nonoperatively with expected involution of the affected kidney or nephrectomy. It is uncommon to successfully salvage renal function with vascular reconstruction of complete blunt renal artery occlusion. Management must consider several factors, including overall status of the patient, warm ischemia time, and need for laparotomy for associated intra abdominal injuries.

Upper Extremity

Penetrating injury often presents with a history of either arterial hemorrhage or ongoing bleeding. Blunt injury usually causes thrombosis and the signs of acute arterial occlusion with resultant ischemia. Significant neurologic injury, usually involving the median nerve, is present in 60% of patients with upper extremity arterial injury.[6,47] Concomitant venous injury is common. In the setting of multisystem injury, arterial occlusion in the upper extremity is easily missed. Delay in diagnosis resulting in prolonged ischemia is an important contributing factor to preventable limb loss or long-term disability from irreversible ischemic nerve injury. All significant vascular injuries of the upper extremity result in clinical findings that are apparent on thorough physical examination. Unfortunately, associated severe torso or lower extremity injuries distract the trauma team from the injured and ischemic upper extremity. Delays in diagnosis and treatment are common in collected series of patients with upper extremity arterial injury and are more common after blunt-force trauma.[6,47]

The diagnosis of upper extremity arterial injury is often made on physical examination alone, particularly in penetrating injuries. Noninvasive evaluation of the injured upper extremity adds little to a thorough history and physical examination. Patients with obvious arterial or venous laceration from penetrating trauma or those with blunt trauma and hard findings (see Table 64.1) should be taken directly to the operating room. The arterial bed of the upper extremity is extremely reactive to vasoconstriction produced by hypovolemic shock, pain, and drugs, including cocaine and methamphetamine. Absent pulses in the presence of complex fractures or crush injuries of the upper extremity need to be assessed with imaging (either multidetector CT or conventional angiography) if normal perfusion does not return after resuscitation and the administration of adequate pain medications.

There is currently not a role for endovascular therapy in the brachial artery and forearm vessels. Traditional operative exposure, catheter thrombectomy, and repair remain the best approach to optimize results.[6,47] In patients unstable from associated torso injuries, damage control with arterial shunt placement followed by repair when the patient is hemodynamically stable is the best management option. Vascular injuries in the upper extremity are often associated with significant musculoskeletal, neurologic, and soft tissue injuries. When this occurs, a multidisciplinary approach is often required with orthopedics, neurosurgery, and plastic surgery. Venous injuries of the upper extremity can be ligated unless there is extensive soft tissue injury and loss of venous collaterals. In that setting, some form of venous reconstruction should be considered.

On occasion, bleeding from a partially transected arm or forearm vessel can be significant. The senior surgeon should make certain that adequate control is obtained and maintained during resuscitation, transportation to the operating room, and surgical preparation and draping. Tourniquets have proved lifesaving in the field for management of hemorrhage from extremities and they have a role in the trauma bay for obtaining hemorrhage control during resuscitation and a timely thorough evaluation for other injuries. Tourniquets from the field or applied in the trauma bay should carefully monitored for both adequacy of compression and duration of application by the senior surgeon present.

The patient should be widely prepared and draped with generous inclusion of the entire upper extremity, the shoulder, and the anterior-superior aspect of the chest to allow incisions for proximal control.[6] An uninjured leg should also be prepared and draped from inguinal region to toes to allow saphenous vein harvest. Adjunctive measures, such as bolus intravenous systemic heparinization, administration of a continuous infusion of low-molecular-weight dextran, and administration of intravenous antibiotics, should be considered and used where appropriate. In patients with multisystem injuries, especially head injury, local or regional infusion of heparin should be used in place of systemic administration. Loupe magnification and coaxial lighting ("headlight") are technical adjuncts that may be useful in suturing small blood vessel with fine suture.

Surgical exposure requires generous incisions placed to maximize exposure and to provide appropriate options for further exploration and repair. The brachial artery is best exposed through a longitudinal incision along the medial aspect of the upper arm over the groove between the triceps and biceps muscles. The incision can be extended distally with an S-shaped extension across the antecubital fossa from ulnar to radial aspect and onto the forearm to expose the origins of the forearm vessels.[6,47] Proximal brachial artery injuries may require control of the infraclavicular axillary artery. Vascular repair requires attention to detail in all phases. Balloon catheter thrombectomy and flushing with heparinized saline followed by debridement of damaged arterial wall are essential to successful repair. Lacerated veins should be ligated. However, if there is extensive soft tissue injury and collateral venous flow is compromised, the vein should be repaired. In repairing both venous and arterial injuries, the vein should be repaired first. If the duration of arterial occlusion and ischemia is a concern, temporary intraluminal shunts may be placed in the artery. Primary arterial repair of undamaged ends of vessel (end-to-end anastomosis) should be performed only if the repair is tension free. Saphenous vein interposition should be chosen whenever vessel injury is extensive or if primary tension-free repair is not possible. PTFE needs to remain a second choice to autologous vein in the management of injuries of the brachial artery and forearm vessels.[2,6,47]

Forearm fasciotomy, particularly in the setting of prolonged ischemia, must always be considered before completion of the operation, and compartment pressures should be measured at the completion of the operation. If normal pressures are obtained, fasciotomy is not necessary, but pressure measurements should be repeated frequently because compartment syndrome can occur in the postoperative period as a consequence of reperfusion.[37,47]

There is a limited but important role for "primary" or early amputation in the management of upper extremity vascular injuries. Patients with extensive soft tissue loss or with scapulothoracic dissociation who have severe neurologic deficits, extensive fractures, and vascular injuries should be evaluated collaboratively with orthopedic, neurosurgery, and plastic surgery colleagues to determine if early amputation is appropriate. The best approach is intraoperative, multidisciplinary assessment, damage control, and plan for reoperative assessment in 24 to 48 hours. This will allow discussions with the patient and family and a second look.

Combined ulnar and radial artery injury in the forearm requires repair of at least one vessel. The ulnar artery is usually larger in the proximal forearm and is a better target for direct repair or saphenous vein bypass. Distally, the vessel repair should be performed in whichever vessel is largest or amenable to simple repair.[6,47]

Isolated ulnar or radial artery injuries can be managed with simple ligation only if there is absolute certainty that flow through the remaining vessel is adequate. Close inspection of the forearm and hand with palpation of pulses augmented by continuous-wave (hand-held) Doppler interrogation is essential.[6]

Lower Extremity

Vascular injuries in the legs are more common in military settings (30%–40%) than in civilian practice (20%).[2,48] Although penetrating injuries are more common, blunt vascular trauma in the lower extremity remains a significant challenge. In the thigh and the leg, fractures and dislocations can be associated with vascular injuries. The popliteal artery is at particularly high risk of injury after dislocation of the knee.[2,48]

Findings at presentation vary from significant hemorrhage from a wound (i.e., open fracture, stab, or gunshot) to occult arterial occlusion from blunt injury. A systematic approach with a thorough extremity vascular examination is essential to avoid errors in recognition and delays in treatment.

Exposure is obtained with incisions used for elective surgical procedures. The common femoral artery is best exposed through a longitudinal incision overlying its course from the inguinal ligament inferiorly for 8 to 12 cm. Proximal control may require exposure of the external iliac artery, best accomplished through an oblique muscle-splitting lower quadrant abdominal incision carried into retroperitoneum, where the artery and vein can be controlled. SFA injuries are best exposed through a longitudinal groin incision similar to that used for femoral bifurcation exposure for the proximal portion. The mid-SFA is approached through an oblique incision over the sartorius muscle. The junction of the SFA and popliteal can be exposed by extending this incision, dividing the adductor tendon.

Popliteal injuries are exposed through a generous medial incision. Exposure of the artery in the area at the knee joint requires division of the medial head of the gastrocnemius muscle and the semimembranosus and semitendinosus muscles. The distal popliteal artery is exposed with an incision along the posterior margin of the tibia.

Repair of lower extremity vascular injuries usually requires an interposition graft. This is particularly true in the popliteal artery. Reverse saphenous vein from the contralateral extremity is the first choice for interposition grafts. In the common femoral artery, PTFE is an acceptable choice for interposition if the saphenous vein is not of sufficient size. However, saphenous vein remains the best graft for repair of the superficial femoral, popliteal, and tibial vessels.[35]

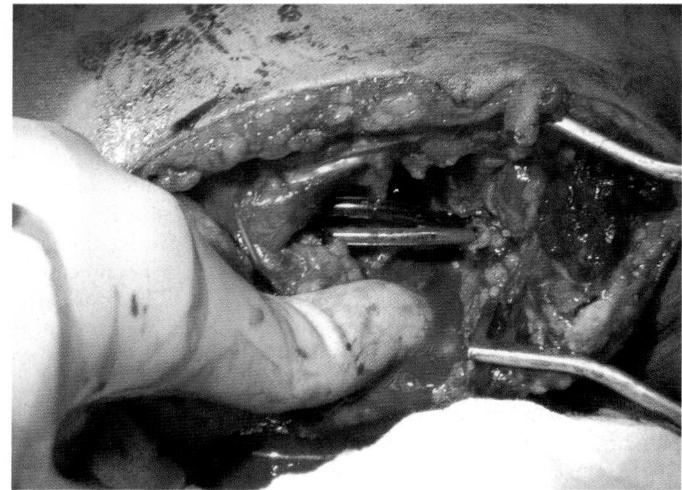

FIG. 64.8 Damage control for multiple gunshot wounds with shunt placement in the popliteal artery and vein in a patient with associated major torso hemorrhage.

Injuries below the popliteal artery at the level of the tibial vessels are best managed by ligation if two of the three calf vessels are patent and there is adequate collateral flow. In the presence of both anterior and posterior tibial vessel occlusion, the peroneal artery is usually not sufficiently connected to the distal arterial bed by collaterals, and repair of one of the injured vessels should be performed. The choice of which vessel to repair is based on both the extent of associated soft tissue injury and the patency of the distal segments of those vessels.

Damage control techniques with arterial and venous shunt placement with delayed definitive repair are an important part of managing lower extremity vascular injury associated with major torso injuries and hemodynamic instability (Fig. 64.8). All efforts should be made early postoperatively to achieve adequate stability as rapidly as possible to allow a timely return to the operating room for definitive vascular repair before shunt thrombosis and prolonged ischemia.

Operative Techniques for Extremity Fasciotomy

Fasciotomy of the forearm compartments requires release of individual muscle bundles. Generous incisions are required to release the dorsal and volar compartments and the mobile wad. Fasciotomy in the leg requires release of the anterior and lateral compartments on the anterior lateral aspect of the calf and the deep and superficial posterior compartments through incisions on the lateral and medial aspects of the calf (Fig. 64.9). These incisions should be generous in their length to accommodate subsequent muscle swelling and to avoid further compression.[6]

Thigh compartment syndrome is uncommon. The most common cause is thigh crush injury associated with femur fracture. Fasciotomy should release the three compartments: lateral, medial, and posterior. Two incisions, one lateral for the lateral compartment and one medial for the other two compartments, are sufficient. These need to be generous in their length. Compartment syndromes occur in the hands and feet, and these are best managed by orthopedic surgeons or hand surgeons.[6]

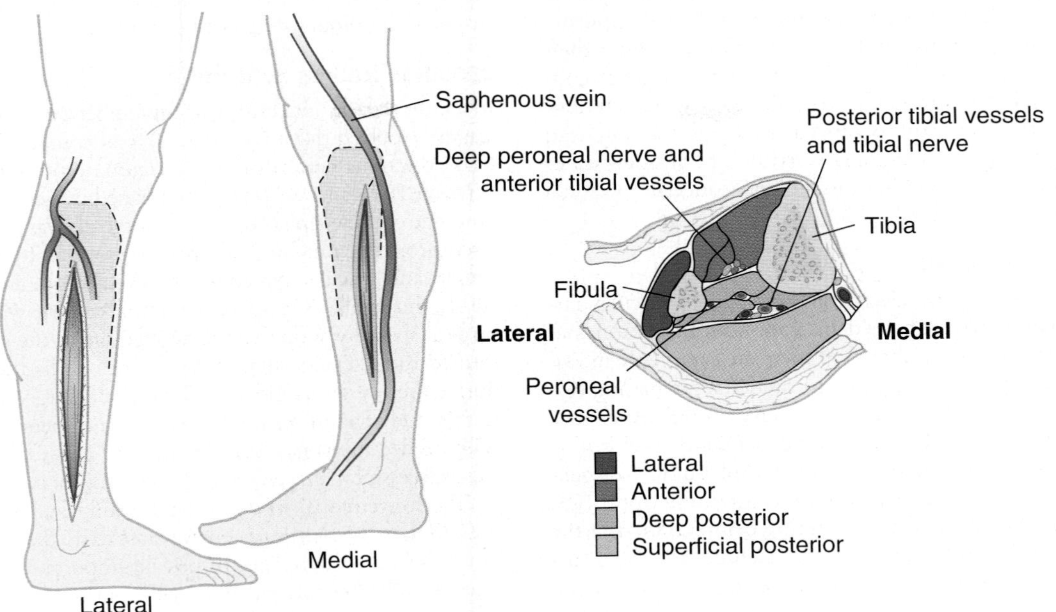

FIG. 64.9 Calf muscle compartments and incisions for fasciotomy.

POSTOPERATIVE MANAGEMENT

The cornerstone of postoperative management is close follow-up to detect a change in the vascular examination findings. This includes frequent assessment of the vital signs, the distal extremity pulse, the continuous-wave Doppler signal, the capillary refill, and the neurologic examination findings of the injured extremity. If there is concern about any portion of the examination, an immediate return to the operating room may avert a potentially limb-threatening problem. Because failure of a vascular repair due to thrombosis can occur during the first 48 hours after the repair, careful follow-up with frequent examinations should continue for at least that length of time.

Reperfusion edema or intracompartmental hemorrhage can lead to a delayed onset of a compartment syndrome.[37] Physical examination alone may not detect the presence of compartment syndrome. Frequent postoperative compartment pressure measurements are the only way to accurately assess the injured extremity in patients who are not conscious and cooperative. The presence of a new postoperative extremity neurologic deficit is an important indicator of ongoing ischemia and should prompt assessment of both the patency of the vascular repair and the pressure within muscle compartments.

OUTCOMES AND FOLLOW-UP

The most common cause of amputation after vascular injury is the neurologic insult from either direct trauma to the nerve or ischemia. This should be remembered as one contemplates repair of a vascular injury in a "flail extremity" (permanently denervated secondary to irreversible neurologic injury).[38,39] Functional outcome after vascular repair is related to the severity of the associated injuries of muscle, bone, and nerve. Regular follow-up of patients with vascular repairs should continue to assess patency of the repair and to determine the presence of late complications. These include aneurysmal dilation or segmental stenosis of vein grafts, venous insufficiency from venous ligation, thrombosis of a pseudoaneurysm, and arteriovenous fistula. Ideally, these patients should be seen in yearly follow-up. Pulse examination and, if indicated, noninvasive imaging should be performed on a regular basis. Imaging with CT angiography or catheter angiography should be used if there is a suspicion of a complication.

Torso vascular injuries have relatively few late complications. Venous interposition grafts, when used, should be observed with periodic noninvasive imaging and, if indicated, CT angiography. Aortic and iliac arterial repairs should be observed similarly, and surveillance should ascertain signs and symptoms of arterial occlusive disease, such as upper or lower extremity claudication. Patients with synthetic interposition grafts should be counseled on the need for antibiotic prophylaxis during subsequent dental work or invasive procedures. Although late infections are uncommon, patients should be made aware of this possibility and counseled to notify all of their healthcare providers of the presence of a vascular prosthesis.

TRAINING AND PREPARATION FOR SUCCESSFUL MANAGEMENT

Vascular surgery carries a high risk of technical surgical error compared with many other areas of surgery. The optimal treatment of vascular trauma remains challenging and is rapidly evolving. Establishing goals for training in vascular trauma cannot be discussed without understanding the trends of increasing endovascular approaches and declining numbers of open repairs. Although one can acquire the didactic knowledge base from reading chapters such as this, the acquisition of decision-making abilities and surgical skills is based on experience that is becoming more and more difficult to obtain during surgical training. The average general surgical resident completes surgical residency having managed less than one vascular trauma case.[49,50] The average high-volume major trauma center in the United States manages approximately 10 to 15 vascular training cases a year. Fellowship-trained vascular surgeons receive vastly more exposure to chronic vascular disease and endovascular techniques than training in the rapid exposure of major vessels for proximal and distal control, let alone their open surgical management. The number of trauma surgeons contemporarily trained in endovascular techniques is extremely low. Many military general surgeons deployed to Afghanistan and Iraq for combat surgical care of wounded warriors site deficiencies in open vascular surgeries as their number one concern (personal communication to the authors).

General Surgery Training

The shrinking volume of open elective and emergency vascular surgery operations combined with resident work hour limitations has created significant obstacles to obtaining adequate experience in vascular surgical technique.[49] As opposed to residents graduating two decades ago, today's general surgeons rarely have enough experience to make them competent and capable of independently performing vascular surgery. Currently, there are a significant number of general surgeons who include vascular surgical cases in their practices. However, almost all completed their training before 2000 and the advent of the extensive use of endovascular techniques. These surgeons honed skills on open aortic aneurysm repairs, aortobifemoral bypass, and femoral popliteal bypass procedures.

The numbers of vascular surgery cases done by residents appears to be rising according to the Residency Review Committee. However, a closer look reveals the harsh reality that the case logs include a growing number of endovascular and venous procedures and an alarming decrease in open arterial procedures.[49–51] There has been as much as a 65% decrease in open arterial reconstruction case volume for graduate general surgery residents.[49,50] Open aortic surgery experience is much more uncommon, with many residents participating in five or fewer open aortic cases. Most surgery residents, however, claim endovascular aortic aneurysm repair (EVAR) among their vascular surgery numbers. Dialysis access cases have ironically become one of the last bastions of giving residents training in vascular techniques. The above-knee elective femoral popliteal bypass on mildly or moderately diseased vessels has all but disappeared. Most lower extremity bypasses are performed to very small distal vessels, and residents are often not able to perform these anastomoses.

Vascular Fellowship Training

The shrinking volume of open cases has also had an impact on vascular fellowship training. EVAR has become the treatment of choice for elective aneurysm repair, and emergency EVAR capabilities for ruptured abdominal aortic aneurysm have become a widespread practice. Consequently, there is real concern about the lack of open aortic cases available for training vascular surgery fellows. A conservative estimate of the number of cases required to give a surgeon adequate experience to competently handle the difficult ruptured aorta is well above 20 to 30 cases. The old saying that it takes up to 50 to 100 aortic repairs before the surgeon's fear transforms to profound respect for the aorta is probably accurate. Very few training programs come close to that volume. In reality, with widespread use of EVAR as the first-line therapy for elective abdominal aortic aneurysm repair, most graduating fellows will not see 100 open cases in the first 10 to 15 years of practice. The "fear factor" remains a considerable issue for these surgeons to contend with.

The decrease in open case volume during training and the significant rise in endovascular experience have produced a generation of vascular fellowship graduates who are more comfortable with closed techniques versus open techniques in many areas. This translates to a reluctance to convert to open technique and a discomfort with situations such as vascular trauma in which endovascular techniques may not be an option.

Vascular Trauma Realities

In a multi-institutional study in September 2012, Shackford and colleagues reported that more than 60% of complex extremity vascular reconstructions performed at 12 trauma centers across the country between 1995 and 2010 were performed by general surgeons.[29] The outcome of these repairs by general surgeons was not significantly different from the outcome of repairs performed by fellowship-trained cardiac and vascular surgeons. The overall amputation rate was low. All 12 hospitals were mature trauma centers with well-organized surgical specialty support. The average age of the surgeons who performed these repairs suggested that they all had adequate exposure during their surgical residency. What all the surgeons from the centers in this study had in common was a commitment to maintaining the skills needed to manage vascular injuries. The results of this approach were successful management of these complex injuries.

The conventional wisdom at successful trauma centers has always been to have the right surgeon available to do the right operation in a timely fashion. This has been especially important in repair of vascular injuries. Whether this capability will continue to be widely available remains to be seen. Few recent graduates of general surgery residencies feel confident in managing vascular injuries or other vascular emergencies. The alarming lack of open abdominal vascular procedures in most fellowship training programs has similarly eroded the confidence and competence of recently trained vascular surgeons. The paucity of capable vascular surgical emergency backup represents a threat to most of our trauma and emergency centers.

Need for Remedial Training and Review

We cannot expect the current general surgery and vascular surgery training programs to mitigate this lack of technical and cognitive competence without adding additional educational content focusing on areas of limited experience. The alternatives to hands-on operative experience remain limited. Simulation, although promising, has yet to accomplish the vision that it can replace actual experience as an adequate teaching opportunity. Maximizing open experience by resident participation in abdominal organ harvest by the transplantation team has been somewhat helpful.

There are two approaches in residency and fellowship training programs that hold promise. One is to actively audit general surgery and vascular fellowship trainee case logs to detect which resident should be the next participant in a major abdominal vascular procedure. These cases are precious training opportunities and should be shared evenly with all trainees. At this operation, the resident must be taught by actually performing the procedure, not simply watching. Attending surgeons must have the patience and forbearance to actually allow the trainee to perform the operation. Preparation with thoughtful didactic material focusing on these key operations should occur early in the trainee's rotation so that the operative experience has maximum educational impact. Postprocedure debriefing with a thorough discussion of decision points, troubleshooting, and management of different versions of the anatomy and pathologic findings needs to be rigorously performed.

The second important educational opportunity is participation in courses such as the American College of Surgeons–sponsored Advanced Surgical Skills for Exposure in Trauma and Advanced Trauma Operative Management. These courses combine appropriate focused didactic material with either cadaver or live animal dissection. They are highly successful in improving both the knowledge and skill set of the participants. Equally important is the increase in confidence all participants report.

Additional courses developed through international cooperation are extremely promising. The Definitive Surgical Trauma Care course was developed by the International Association for Trauma and Surgical Intensive Care. The Definitive Surgical Trauma Skills course was developed by the Royal College of Surgeons of England with the Royal Defence Medical College and the Uniformed Services University of the Health Sciences in the United States. Completing either of these two courses provides excellent surgical training in trauma surgery decision making, vascular exposures, and vascular repairs.

Many centers are developing perfused cadaver labs for simulation training for general surgery residents. This method of training is particularly relevant to vascular exposures. Residents and fellows have the opportunity to dissect along pressurized cadaver vessels and learn the techniques for proper exposure and proximal and distal control. Their performance is recorded and critiques with the identification of opportunities for improvement. The trainee then repeats the procedure and demonstrates improved performance. This approach has had demonstrable results in improving operative skills in the trauma centers where it has been implemented.

The Need for Action

The rapidly disappearing knowledge and experience base of major open vascular surgical technique threaten all trauma centers' ability to provide effective care for patients with major vascular injury and other vascular emergencies. Not taking action ensures a crisis in the near future that will result in poor outcomes. New education strategies are called for. Combining the maximal education value of a decreasing number of key open cases with appropriate courses that use cadaver and live animal operative experience will partially mitigate this looming deficit of open operative cases. Simulation is a cornerstone of training and maintenance of competence in commercial aviation. Simulation in surgery has yet to achieve its promise to augment real operative experience. However, in the future, it may become an important method for both acquiring and maintaining skills.

The over 100-year history of major advances in the management of vascular injuries lead by surgeons with an interest in trauma needs to be sustained.[52] New and innovative ways of training and preparation will insure that the art and the science of the surgical management of these challenging injuries will endure. The coming generations of surgeons can and will carry on in the finest traditions of our profession.

SELECTED REFERENCES

Biffl WL, Cothren CC, Moore EE, et al. Western Trauma Association critical decisions in trauma: screening for and treatment of blunt cerebrovascular injuries. *J Trauma.* 2009;67:1150–1153.

This practice recommendation from the Western Trauma Association offers an evidence-based approach to the diagnosis of blunt cerebrovascular injuries.

Chang R, Fox EE, Greene TJ, et al. Multicenter retrospective study of noncompressible torso hemorrhage: anatomic locations of bleeding and comparison of endovascular versus open approach. *J Trauma Acute Care Surg.* 2017;83:11–18.

This multicenter study frames the current practice of open versus endovascular techniques to control torso hemorrhage. It is valuable report of the state of the practice in managing these challenging and often life-threatening injuries.

Feliciano DV. For the patient—evolution in the management of vascular trauma. *J Trauma Acute Care Surg.* 2017;83:1205–1212.

This excellent review traces the evolution of the surgical management for the last 100 years. The advances in surgical science, imaging, antibiotics, anticoagulation, and graft materials are thoughtfully discussed. This is a unique and valuable contribution to the literature.

Feliciano DV, Mattox KL, Graham JM, et al. Five-year experience with PTFE grafts in vascular wounds. *J Trauma.* 1985;25:71–82.

This is a landmark report establishing the acceptability of polytetrafluoroethylene in vascular trauma repairs. It remains the best work in this area.

Mattox KL, Feliciano DV, Burch J, et al. Five thousand seven hundred sixty cardiovascular injuries in 4459 patients. Epidemiologic evolution 1958 to 1987. *Ann Surg.* 1989;209:698–705.

This is the largest epidemiological study in the literature on civilian vascular injuries, and it remains the best work on the subject.

Neschis DG, Scalea TM, Flinn WR, et al. Blunt aortic injury. *N Engl J Med.* 2008;359:1708–1716.

This review of series of both open and endovascular repairs of blunt thoracic injury provides a valuable overview of the risks versus benefits of each technique.

Patel MB, Guillamondegui OD, May AK, et al. Twenty-year analysis of surgical resident operative trauma experiences. *J Surg Res.* 2013;180:191–195.

This report gives a sobering perspective on the dwindling open surgical experience for surgical residents and highlights the need for alternative training modalities.

Patterson BO, Holt PJ, Cleanthis M, et al. Imaging vascular trauma. *Br J Surg.* 2012;99:494–505.

This systematic review was performed of literature relating to radiologic diagnosis of vascular trauma from 2000 to 2010. This excellent review conclusively established the superiority of computed tomography angiography for the diagnosis of vascular injuries.

Reuben BC, Whitten MG, Sarfati M, et al. Increasing use of endovascular therapy in acute arterial injuries: analysis of the National Trauma Data Bank. *J Vasc Surg*. 2007;46:1222–1226.

This report was a harbinger of the shift away from open vascular repairs and, from the perspective of 2016, was a predictor of the loss of open surgical experience and skills in the management of vascular injuries.

Sirinek KR, Levine BA, Gaskill 3rd HV, et al. Reassessment of the role of routine operative exploration in vascular trauma. *J Trauma*. 1981;21:339–344.

This report was the basis for the cessation of operative exploration in stable patients in favor of angiography. In its time, it was a landmark paper and vastly improved the workup of patients with suspected vascular injury.

REFERENCES

1. Amato JJ, Rich NM, Billy LJ, et al. High-velocity arterial injury: a study of the mechanism of injury. *J Trauma*. 1971;11:412–416.
2. Mattox KL, Feliciano DV, Burch J, et al. Five thousand seven hundred sixty cardiovascular injuries in 4459 patients. Epidemiologic evolution 1958 to 1987. *Ann Surg*. 1989;209:698–705; discussion 706–697.
3. National Association of Emergency Medical Technicians and the Committee on Trauma of the American College of Surgeons. *PHTLS Prehospital Trauma Life Support*. 8th ed. Burlington, MA: Jones & Bartlett Learning; 2016.
4. Rich NM. Historic review of arteriovenous fistulas and traumatic false aneurysms. In: Rich NM, Mattox KL, Hirshberg A, eds. *Vascular Trauma*. Philadelphia: Elsevier Saunders; 2004:457–524.
5. Henry S. *ATLS Advanced Trauma Life Support for Doctors: Student Course Manual*. 10th ed. Chicago: American College of Surgeons; 2018.
6. Shackford SR, Sise MJ. Peripheral vascular injury. In: Moore EE, Feliciano DV, Mattox KL, eds. *Trauma*. 8th ed. New York: McGraw-Hill; 2017:817–847.
7. Patterson BO, Holt PJ, Cleanthis M, et al. Imaging vascular trauma. *Br J Surg*. 2012;99:494–505.
8. Seamon MJ, Smoger D, Torres DM, et al. A prospective validation of a current practice: the detection of extremity vascular injury with CT angiography. *J Trauma*. 2009;67:238–243.
9. White PW, Gillespie DL, Feurstein I, et al. Sixty-four slice multidetector computed tomographic angiography in the evaluation of vascular trauma. *J Trauma*. 2010;68:96–102.
10. O'Gorman RB, Feliciano DV, Bitondo CG, et al. Emergency center arteriography in the evaluation of suspected peripheral vascular injuries. *Arch Surg*. 1984;119:568–573.
11. Sirinek KR, Levine BA, Gaskill 3rd HV, et al. Reassessment of the role of routine operative exploration in vascular trauma. *J Trauma*. 1981;21:339–344.
12. Dennis JW. Minimal vascular injury. In: Rich NM, Mattox KL, Hirshberg A, eds. *Vascular Trauma*. 2nd ed. Philadelphia: Elsevier Saunders; 2004:85–96.
13. DuBose JJ, Savage SA, Fabian TC, et al. The American Association for the Surgery of Trauma Prospective Observational Vascular Injury Treatment (PROOVIT) registry: multicenter data on modern vascular injury diagnosis, management, and outcomes. *J Trauma Acute Care Surg*. 2015;78:215–222; discussion 222–213.
14. Faulconer ER, Branco BC, Loja MN, et al. Use of open and endovascular surgical techniques to manage vascular injuries in the trauma setting: a review of the American Association for the Surgery of Trauma Prospective Observational Vascular Injury Trial registry. *J Trauma Acute Care Surg*. 2018;84:411–417.
15. Cothren CC, Moore EE, Ray Jr CE, et al. Carotid artery stents for blunt cerebrovascular injury: risks exceed benefits. *Arch Surg*. 2005;140:480–485; discussion 485–486.
16. Patel MB, Guillamondegui OD, May AK, et al. Twenty-year analysis of surgical resident operative trauma experiences. *J Surg Res*. 2013;180:191–195.
17. Schanzer A, Steppacher R, Eslami M, et al. Vascular surgery training trends from 2001–2007: a substantial increase in total procedure volume is driven by escalating endovascular procedure volume and stable open procedure volume. *J Vasc Surg*. 2009;49:1339–1344.
18. David Richardson J, Franklin GA, Lukan JK, et al. Evolution in the management of hepatic trauma: a 25-year perspective. *Ann Surg*. 2000;232:324–330.
19. Dent D, Alsabrook G, Erickson BA, et al. Blunt splenic injuries: high nonoperative management rate can be achieved with selective embolization. *J Trauma*. 2004;56:1063–1067.
20. Martinelli T, Thony F, Declety P, et al. Intra-aortic balloon occlusion to salvage patients with life-threatening hemorrhagic shocks from pelvic fractures. *J Trauma*. 2010;68:942–948.
21. Chang R, Fox EE, Greene TJ, et al. Multicenter retrospective study of noncompressible torso hemorrhage: anatomic locations of bleeding and comparison of endovascular versus open approach. *J Trauma Acute Care Surg*. 2017;83:11–18.
22. Velmahos GC. Pelvis. In: Moore EE, Feliciano DV, Mattox KL, eds. *Trauma*. 8th ed. New York: McGraw-Hill; 2017:655–668.
23. Mattox KL, Whigham C, Fisher RG, et al. Blunt trauma to the thoracic aorta: current challenges. In: Lumsden AB, Lin PH, Chen C, et al., eds. *Advanced Endovascular Therapy of Aortic Disease*. London: Blackwell Publishing; 2007: 127–133.
24. Demetriades D, Velmahos GC, Scalea TM, et al. Operative repair or endovascular stent graft in blunt traumatic thoracic aortic injuries: results of an American Association for the Surgery of Trauma Multicenter Study. *J Trauma*. 2008;64:561–570; discussion 570–561.
25. Neschis DG, Scalea TM, Flinn WR, et al. Blunt aortic injury. *N Engl J Med*. 2008;359:1708–1716.
26. Cothren CC, Biffl WL, Moore EE, et al. Treatment for blunt cerebrovascular injuries: equivalence of anticoagulation and antiplatelet agents. *Arch Surg*. 2009;144:685–690.
27. Biffl WL, Cothren CC, Moore EE, et al. Western Trauma Association critical decisions in trauma: screening for and treatment of blunt cerebrovascular injuries. *J Trauma*. 2009;67:1150–1153.
28. DuBose J, Recinos G, Teixeira PG, et al. Endovascular stenting for the treatment of traumatic internal carotid injuries: expanding experience. *J Trauma*. 2008;65:1561–1566.
29. Shackford SR, Kahl JE, Calvo RY, et al. Limb salvage after complex repairs of extremity arterial injuries is independent of surgical specialty training. *J Trauma Acute Care Surg*. 2013;74:716–723; discussion 723–714.
30. Wall MJ, Tsai P, Mattox KL. Heart and thoracic vascular injuries. In: Moore EE, Feliciano DV, Mattox KL, eds. *Trauma*. 8th ed. New York: McGraw-Hill; 2017:485–511.

31. Dente CJ, Feliciano DV. Abdominal vascular injury. In: Mattox KL, Moore EE, Feliciano DV, eds. *Trauma*. 7th ed. New York: McGraw-Hill; 2013:633–654.
32. Ding W, Wu X, Li J. Temporary intravascular shunts used as a damage control surgery adjunct in complex vascular injury: collective review. *Injury*. 2008;39:970–977.
33. Inaba K, Aksoy H, Seamon MJ, et al. Multicenter evaluation of temporary intravascular shunt use in vascular trauma. *J Trauma Acute Care Surg*. 2016;80:359–364; discussion 364–355.
34. Rich NM, Hughes CW. The fate of prosthetic material used to repair vascular injuries in contaminated wounds. *J Trauma*. 1972;12:459–467.
35. Feliciano DV, Mattox KL, Graham JM, et al. Five-year experience with PTFE grafts in vascular wounds. *J Trauma*. 1985;25:71–82.
36. Kim JY, Buck 2nd DW, Forte AJ, et al. Risk factors for compartment syndrome in traumatic brachial artery injuries: an institutional experience in 139 patients. *J Trauma*. 2009;67:1339–1344.
37. Branco BC, Inaba K, Barmparas G, et al. Incidence and predictors for the need for fasciotomy after extremity trauma: a 10-year review in a mature level I trauma centre. *Injury*. 2011;42:1157–1163.
38. Ly TV, Travison TG, Castillo RC, et al. Ability of lower-extremity injury severity scores to predict functional outcome after limb salvage. *J Bone Joint Surg Am*. 2008;90:1738–1743.
39. Loja MN, Sammann A, DuBose J, et al. The mangled extremity score and amputation: time for a revision. *J Trauma Acute Care Surg*. 2017;82:518–523.
40. Dekker S. *The Field Guide to Understanding Human Error*. Hampshire, UK: Ashgate Publishing Ltd; 2006.
41. Feliciano DV, Vercruysse GA. Neck. In: Moore EE, Feliciano DV, Mattox KL, eds. *Trauma*. 7th ed. New York: McGraw-Hill; 2013:414–442.
42. Du Toit DF, Lambrechts AV, Stark H, et al. Long-term results of stent graft treatment of subclavian artery injuries: management of choice for stable patients? *J Vasc Surg*. 2008;47:739–743.
43. Gilani R, Tsai PI, Wall Jr MJ, et al. Overcoming challenges of endovascular treatment of complex subclavian and axillary artery injuries in hypotensive patients. *J Trauma Acute Care Surg*. 2012;73:771–773.
44. Carrick MM, Morrison CA, Pham HQ, et al. Modern management of traumatic subclavian artery injuries: a single institution's experience in the evolution of endovascular repair. *Am J Surg*. 2010;199:28–34.
45. Lee WA, Matsumura JS, Mitchell RS, et al. Endovascular repair of traumatic thoracic aortic injury: clinical practice guidelines of the Society for Vascular Surgery. *J Vasc Surg*. 2011;53:187–192.
46. Cooper JD. The history of surgical procedures for emphysema. *Ann Thorac Surg*. 1997;63:312–319.
47. Franz RW, Goodwin RB, Hartman JF, et al. Management of upper extremity arterial injuries at an urban level I trauma center. *Ann Vasc Surg*. 2009;23:8–16.
48. Franz RW, Shah KJ, Halaharvi D, et al. A 5-year review of management of lower extremity arterial injuries at an urban level I trauma center. *J Vasc Surg*. 2011;53:1604–1610.
49. Varley I, Keir J, Fagg P. Changes in caseload and the potential impact on surgical training: a retrospective review of one hospital's experience. *BMC Med Educ*. 2006;6:6.
50. Kairys JC, McGuire K, Crawford AG, et al. Cumulative operative experience is decreasing during general surgery residency: a worrisome trend for surgical trainees?. *J Am Coll Surg*. 2008;206:804–811; discussion 811–803.
51. Grabo DJ, DiMuzio PJ, Kairys JC, et al. Have endovascular procedures negatively impacted general surgery training?. *Ann Surg*. 2007;246:472–477; discussion 477–480.
52. Feliciano DV. For the patient-Evolution in the management of vascular trauma. *J Trauma Acute Care Surg*. 2017;83:1205–1212.

65 CHAPTER

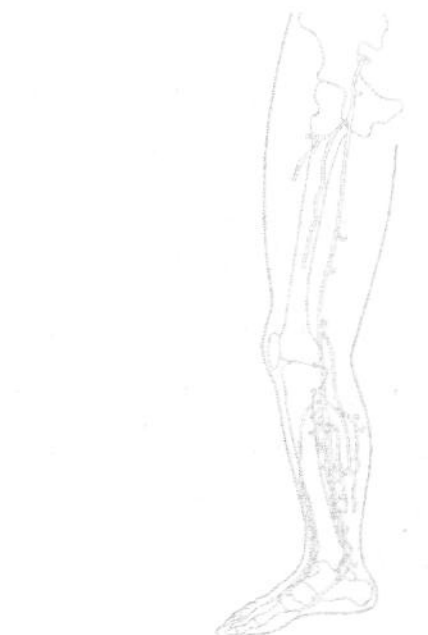

Venous Disease

Luigi Pascarella, William Marston

OUTLINE

Please access Elsevier eBooks for Practicing Clinicians to view the videos for this chapter https://expertconsult.inkling.com/.

An understanding of venous physiology provides the surgeon with valuable information with which to formulate a diagnostic and treatment plan. Technologic advances have broadened the therapeutic armamentarium. This chapter provides the reader with a thorough overview of the physiology and pathophysiology of the venous system. Pathognomonic features of superficial and deep venous disorders are described with discussion of appropriate diagnostic modalities and therapeutic interventions.

VIDEOS

VIDEO 65.1 TriVex 1
VIDEO 65.2 TriVex 2

ANATOMY

To determine whether a pathophysiologic process is present, knowledge of venous anatomy is essential. Venous drainage of the legs is the function of two parallel systems: the superficial and the deep venous system, in anatomic continuity through connecting veins, called perforating veins. The nomenclature of the venous system of the lower limb was revised in 2002, and the most relevant changes are addressed here.[1] The revised nomenclature is delineated in Tables 65.1 and 65.2.

Superficial Venous System

The superficial veins of the lower extremity form a network that connects the superficial dorsal veins of the foot and deep plantar veins. The dorsal venous arch, into which empty the dorsal metatarsal veins, is continuous with the great saphenous vein medially and the small saphenous vein laterally (Fig. 65.1).

The great saphenous vein arises from dorsal veins of the foot. The great saphenous vein extends cephalad and travels over the medial aspect of the tibia and in parallel to the saphenous nerve. As the great saphenous vein ascends through the thigh, multiple accessory branches are demonstrated, and variability of the number and location of these branches is the norm. The great saphenous vein travels within its own fascia, called the saphenous sheath (Fig. 65.2). This structure is superior to the deep fascia of the leg. Although a classic feature, the great saphenous vein can be contained completely within the saphenous sheath or exit the fascia and reenter at another point in its course along the extremity. In some cases, patients exhibit an incomplete saphenous sheath, which makes identification of the great saphenous vein difficult. The great saphenous vein terminates into the saphenofemoral junction, where it is joined by the confluence of the superficial circumflex iliac veins, the external pudendal veins, and the superficial epigastric veins. It then ascends in the superficial compartment and empties into the common femoral vein after entering the fossa ovalis (Fig. 65.2). The saphenofemoral junction is a complex anatomic entity composed of one or several external pudendal veins, the superficial epigastric vein, the superficial circumflex vein, and one or several accessory saphenous veins, whose course in the leg can be anterior and posterior to the great saphenous vein. At the saphenofemoral junction and a few millimeters distal in thigh, the terminal valve and the preterminal, are located.

The small saphenous vein arises from the dorsal venous arch at the lateral aspect of the foot and ascends posterior to the lateral

TABLE 65.1 Superficial veins.

ANATOMIC TERMINOLOGY	NEW TERMINOLOGY
Greater or long saphenous vein	Great saphenous vein
	Superficial inguinal veins
External pudendal vein	External pudendal vein
Superficial circumflex vein	Superficial circumflex iliac vein
Superficial epigastric vein	Superficial epigastric vein
Superficial dorsal vein of clitoris or penis	Superficial dorsal vein of clitoris or penis
Anterior labial veins	Anterior labial veins
Anterior scrotal veins	Anterior scrotal veins
Accessory saphenous vein	Anterior accessory great saphenous vein
	Posterior accessory great saphenous vein
	Superficial accessory great saphenous vein
Smaller or short saphenous vein	Small saphenous vein
	Cranial extension of small saphenous vein
	Superficial accessory small saphenous vein
	Anterior thigh circumflex vein
	Posterior thigh circumflex vein
	Intersaphenous veins
	Lateral venous system
Dorsal venous network of the foot	Dorsal venous network of the foot
Dorsal venous arch of the foot	Dorsal venous arch of the foot
Dorsal metatarsal veins	Superficial metatarsal veins (dorsal and plantar)
Plantar venous network	Plantar venous subcutaneous network
Plantar venous arch	
Plantar metatarsal veins	Superficial digital veins (dorsal and plantar)
Lateral marginal vein	Lateral marginal vein
Medial marginal vein	Medial marginal vein

TABLE 65.2 Deep veins.

ANATOMIC TERMINOLOGY	NEW TERMINOLOGY
Femoral vein	Common femoral vein
	Femoral vein
Profunda femoris vein or deep vein of thigh	Profunda femoris vein or deep femoral vein
Medial circumflex femoral vein	Medial circumflex femoral vein
Lateral circumflex femoral vein	Lateral circumflex femoral vein
Perforating veins	Deep femoral communicating veins (accompanying veins of perforating arteries)
	Sciatic vein
Popliteal vein	Popliteal vein
	Sural veins
	Soleal veins
	Gastrocnemius veins
	Medial gastrocnemius veins
	Lateral gastrocnemius veins
	Intergemellar vein
Genicular veins	Genicular venous plexus
Anterior tibial veins	Anterior tibial veins
Posterior tibial veins	Posterior tibial veins
Fibular or peroneal veins	Fibular or peroneal veins
	Medial plantar veins
	Lateral plantar veins
	Deep plantar venous arch
	Deep metatarsal veins (plantar and dorsal)
	Deep digital veins (plantar and dorsal)
	Pedal vein

malleolus, rising cephalad in the midposterior calf. The small saphenous vein continues to ascend, penetrates the superficial fascia of the calf, and then terminates into the popliteal vein. However, this anatomy is extremely variable. Most commonly, the small saphenous vein terminates within a lateral branch of the thigh, bypassing the classic saphenopopliteal junction. The sural nerve lies parallel to the small saphenous vein. This relationship becomes more intimate at the distal calf. A common vein branch, the vein of Giacomini, connects the small saphenous vein with the great saphenous vein.

Deep Venous System

The plantar digital veins in the foot empty into a network of metatarsal veins that compose the deep plantar venous arch. This continues into the medial and lateral plantar veins, which then drain into the posterior tibial veins. The dorsalis pedis veins on the dorsum of the foot form the paired anterior tibial veins at the ankle.

The paired posterior tibial veins, adjacent to and flanking the posterior tibial artery, run under the fascia of the deep posterior compartment. These veins enter the soleus and join the popliteal vein, after joining with the paired peroneal and anterior tibial veins. There are large venous sinuses within the soleus

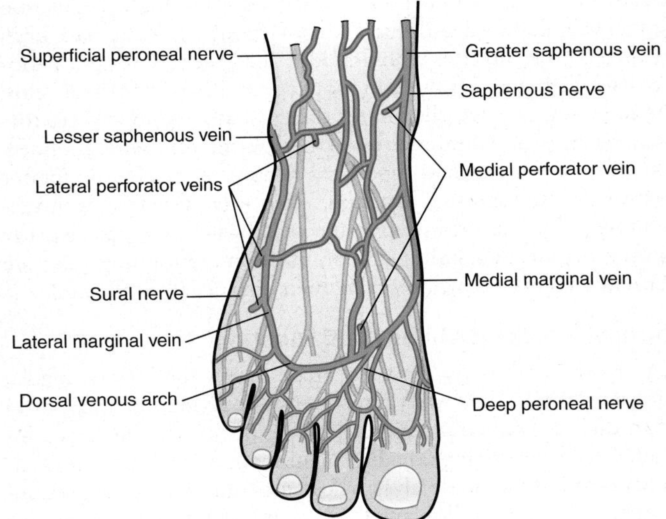

FIG. 65.1 Venous drainage of the foot.

muscle—soleal sinuses—that empty into the posterior tibial and peroneal veins. Bilateral gastrocnemius veins empty into the popliteal vein distal to the point of entry of the small saphenous vein into the popliteal vein.

The popliteal vein enters a window in the adductor magnus, at which point it is termed the femoral vein, previously known as the superficial femoral vein. The femoral vein ascends and receives venous drainage from the profunda femoris vein, or deep femoral vein, and after this confluence, it is the common femoral vein.

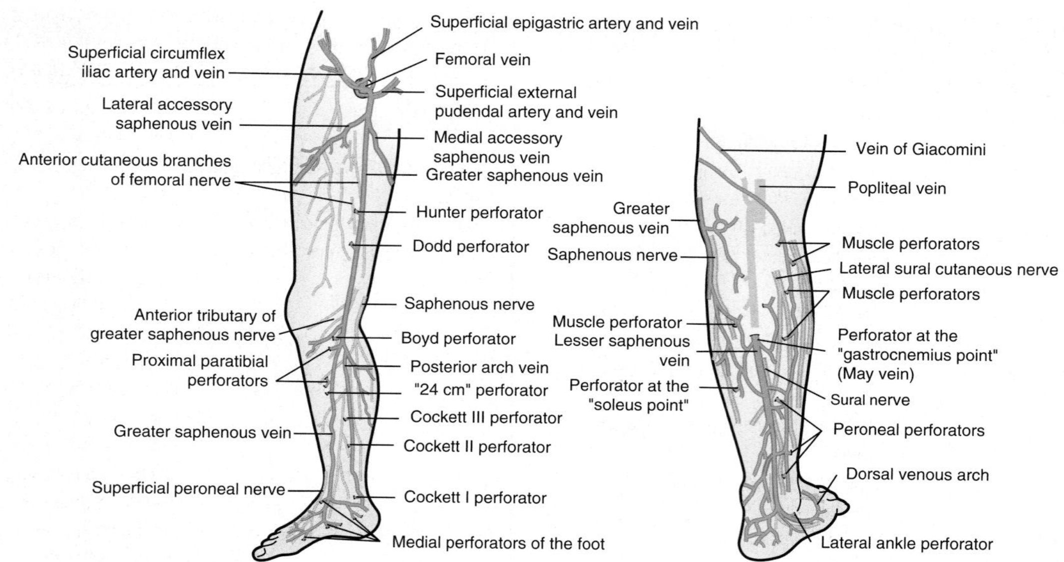

FIG. 65.2 Venous drainage of the lower limb.

As the common femoral vein crosses the inguinal ligament, it becomes the external iliac vein.

Venous System Perforators

Perforating veins connect the superficial venous system to the deep venous system by penetrating the fascial layers of the lower extremity. These perforators run in a perpendicular fashion to the axial veins previously described. Although the total number of perforator veins is variable, up to 100 have been documented. The perforators enter at various points in the leg—the foot, medial and lateral calf, and mid and distal thigh (Fig. 65.3). Some have been named by the surgeons who first identified them: Crockett perforators, which connect the posterior arch and posterior tibial veins; Boyd perforators, which connect the great saphenous and gastrocnemius veins; and hunterian and Dodd perforators, which connect the great saphenous and superficial femoral veins. The perforator veins have an important function. Their valve system aids in preventing reflux from the deep to the superficial system, particularly during periods of standing and ambulation. Perforating veins are currently identified by measuring their distance from the heel.

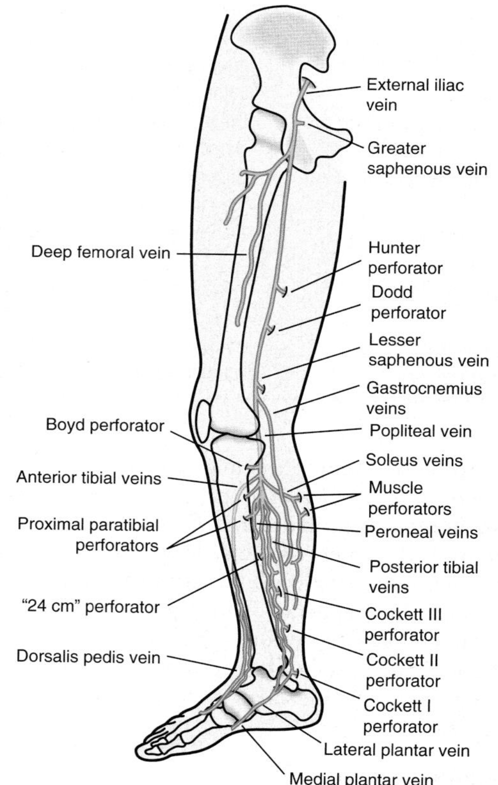

FIG. 65.3 Perforating veins of the lower limb.

Normal Venous Histology and Function

The venous wall is composed of three layers, the intima, media, and adventitia. Vein walls have less smooth muscle and elastin than their arterial counterparts. The venous intima has an endothelial cell layer resting on a basement membrane. The intima enfolds forming bicuspid valves whose function is to assure venous return to the heart. The media is composed of smooth muscle cells and elastin connective tissue. The adventitia of the venous wall contains adrenergic fibers, particularly in the cutaneous veins. Central sympathetic discharge and brainstem thermoregulatory centers can alter venous tone, as can other stimuli, such as temperature changes, pain, emotional stimuli, and volume changes.

The histologic features of veins vary, depending on the caliber of the veins. The venules, the smallest veins, range from 0.1 to 1 mm and contain mostly smooth muscle cells, whereas the larger extremity veins contain relatively few smooth muscle cells. These larger caliber veins have limited contractile capacity in comparison to the thicker walled great saphenous vein. The venous valves prevent retrograde flow; it is their failure or valvular incompetence that leads to reflux and its associated symptoms. Venous valves are most prevalent in the distal lower extremity, whereas as one proceeds proximally, the number of valves decreases to the point that no valves are present in the superior vena cava and inferior vena cava (IVC).

Most of the capacitance of the vascular tree is in the venous system. Because veins do not have significant amounts of elastin, veins can withstand large volume shifts with comparatively small changes in pressure. A vein has a normal elliptical configuration until the limit of its capacitance is reached, at which point the vein assumes a round configuration.

The calf muscles augment venous return by functioning as a pump. In the supine state, the resting venous pressure in the foot is the sum of the residual kinetic energy minus the resistance in the arterioles and precapillary sphincters. Thus, a pressure gradient is generated to the right atrium of approximately 10 to 12 mm Hg. In the upright position, the resting venous pressure of the foot reflects the hydrostatic pressure from the upright column of blood extending from the right atrium to the foot.

The return of the blood to the heart from the lower extremity is facilitated by the muscle pump function of the calf, a mechanism whereby the calf muscle, functioning as a bellows during exercise, compresses the gastrocnemius and soleal sinuses and propels the blood toward the heart. The normally functioning valves in the venous system prevent retrograde flow; when one or more of these valves become incompetent, symptoms of venous insufficiency can develop. During calf muscle contraction, the venous pressure of the foot and ankle drops dramatically. The pressures developing in the muscle compartments during exercise range from 150 to 200 mm Hg, and when there is failure of perforating veins, these high pressures are transmitted to the superficial system.

VENOUS INSUFFICIENCY

Chronic venous insufficiency (CVI) is dominated by venous reflux through incompetent venous valves.

There are three categories of venous insufficiency—congenital, primary, and secondary. Congenital venous insufficiency comprises predominantly anatomic variants that are present at birth. Examples of congenital venous anomalies include venous ectasias, absence of venous valves, and syndromes such as Klippel-Trénaunay syndrome. While the secondary venous insufficiency can be considered a sequela of a previous acute thrombotic disorder (postthrombotic syndrome [PTS]), the etiology of primary CVI cannot be clearly identified.

Risk Factors

Risk factors for the development of varicose veins include advancing age, female gender, multiparity, heredity, history of trauma to the extremity, and prolonged standing. Additional risk factors include obesity and a positive family history. Advancing age appears to be an important significant risk factor. Venous function is undoubtedly influenced by hormonal changes. In particular, progesterone liberated by the corpus luteum stabilizes the uterus by causing the relaxation of smooth muscle fibers.[2] This directly influences venous function. The result is passive venous dilation, which in many cases causes valvular dysfunction. Although progesterone is implicated in the first appearance of varicosities in pregnancy, estrogen also has profound effects. It produces the relaxation of smooth muscle and a softening of collagen fibers. Furthermore, the estrogen-to-progesterone ratio influences venous distensibility. This ratio may explain the predominance of venous insufficiency symptoms on the first day of a menstrual period, when a profound shift occurs from the progesterone phase of the menstrual cycle to the estrogen phase. Autosomal dominant penetrance has been identified as the underlying genetic risk factor for subsequent development of varicose veins.

Pathology

Venous reflux through incompetent venous valves has been described as the main pathogenetic factor underlying CVI. However, obstruction of venous channels, due to either intrinsic narrowing, postthrombotic thickening and scarring, or external compression, may also result in venous hypertension leading to CVI. In many cases, particularly after venous thrombosis, obstruction, and reflux coexist resulting in severe CVI.

Mechanical Abnormalities

Anatomic differences in the location of the superficial veins of the lower extremities may contribute to the pathogenesis. Primary venous insufficiency may involve both the axial veins (great and small saphenous), either vein, or neither vein. Perforating veins may be the sole source of venous pathophysiologic changes, perhaps because the great saphenous vein is supported by a well-developed medial fibromuscular layer and fibrous connective tissue that bind it to the deep fascia. In contrast, tributaries to the small saphenous vein are less supported in the subcutaneous fat and are superficial to the membranous layer of superficial fascia (Fig. 65.4). These tributaries also contain less muscle mass in their walls. Thus, these veins, and not the main trunk, may become selectively varicose.

When these fundamental anatomic peculiarities are recognized, the intrinsic competence or incompetence of the valve system becomes important. For example, failure of a valve protecting a tributary vein from the pressures of the small saphenous vein allows a cluster of varicosities to develop. Furthermore, communicating veins connecting the deep with the superficial compartment may have valve failure. Pressure studies have shown that there are two sources of venous hypertension. The first is gravitational and is a result of venous blood coursing in a distal direction down linear axial venous segments. This is referred to as hydrostatic pressure and is the weight of the blood column from the right atrium. The highest pressure generated by this mechanism is evident at the ankle and foot, where measurements are expressed in centimeters of water or millimeters of mercury.

The second source of venous hypertension is dynamic. It is the force of muscle contraction, usually contained within the compartments of the leg. If a perforating vein fails, high pressures (range, 150–200 mm Hg) developed within the muscular compartments during exercise are transmitted directly to the superficial venous system. Here, the sudden pressure transmitted causes dilation and lengthening of the superficial veins. Progressive distal valvular incompetence may occur. If proximal valves such as the saphenofemoral valve become incompetent, systolic muscular contraction is supplemented by the weight of the static column of blood from the heart. Furthermore, this static column becomes a barrier. Blood flowing proximally through the femoral vein spills into the saphenous vein and flows distally. As it refluxes distally through progressively incompetent valves, it is returned through perforating veins to the deep veins. Here, it is conveyed once again to the femoral veins, only to be recycled distally.

Regardless of the precise source of the elevated hydrostatic pressure, the ultimate end result is increased ambulatory venous hypertension.

A number of authors have demonstrated that the development of all the clinical manifestations of CVI can be ascribed to a blood flow driven inflammatory process. Leukocytes are activated and marginalize. Adhesion to the endothelium is prompted by the expression of adhesion molecules, such as Intracellular Adhesion Molecule 1 (ICAM-1), Vascular Cell Adhesion Molecule 1(VCAM-1), L and P-selectins. Ultimately, they infiltrate the venous wall, lyse, and release activated extracellular matrix enzymes (Matrix Metallopeptidase 1, 2, and 9 [MMP1, MMP2, and MMP9]).[3] The extracellular matrix is degraded and the venous

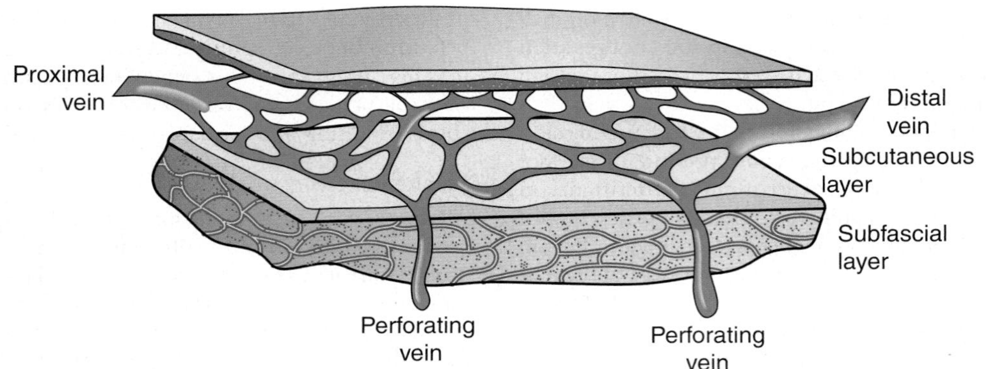

FIG. 65.4 Dilation of superficial venous tributaries caused by increased transmission of pressure by the perforating veins.

wall, including the valves, undergoes remodeling. Decreased amounts of elastin and an imbalance between collagen I and III have been identified in surgical specimens, suggesting that the loss of the venous wall intimal architecture leads to dilation, tortuosity, and the formation of varicose veins.[2,4]

Symptoms

The patient with symptomatic varicose veins commonly reports heaviness, discomfort, and extremity fatigue. The pain is characteristically dull, does not usually occur during recumbency or early in the morning, and is exacerbated in the afternoon, especially after periods of prolonged standing. Swelling is commonly described. The discomforts of aching, heaviness, and fatigue are usually relieved by leg elevation or elastic support. Cutaneous burning, termed venous neuropathy, can also occur in patients with advanced venous insufficiency. Pruritus occurs from excess hemosiderin deposition and tends to be located at the distal calf or in areas of phlebitic varicose branch segments. Patients may report cramping pain that occurs during or after exercise and is relieved with rest and leg elevation. This syndrome is termed venous claudication and is a clinical manifestation of venous outflow obstruction, secondary venous insufficiency. Predominant causes of venous claudication include a prior deep venous thrombosis (DVT) and May-Thurner syndrome.

Multiparous female patients in their childbearing years may report a constellation of symptoms that involve varicosities of the leg in conjunction with chronic pelvic pain. The lower extremity symptoms may or may not be present. Additional symptoms include a feeling of bladder fullness with standing, dyspareunia, and chronic pelvic pain. This clinical picture suggests pelvic congestion syndrome. As the differential diagnosis for pelvic pain is extensive, the diagnosis of pelvic venous congestion tends to be one of exclusion; diagnostic modalities to confirm its presence include magnetic resonance venous imaging (MRVI) of the pelvis and conventional pelvic venography, which can be both diagnostic and therapeutic.

Physical Examination

A comprehensive examination includes assessment of the arterial circulation. Briefly, palpation of the femoral, popliteal, dorsalis pedis, and posterior tibialis pulses is performed. Nonpalpable pulses necessitate further evaluation. Auscultation of pulse flow is indicated when a thrill or widened pulse is appreciated. Decreased hair, dependent rubor, pallor on elevation, and tissue loss are all indicative of advanced arterial ischemia.

The venous examination includes assessment of the patient in the standing and supine positions. The examination room must be well lighted and warm so that vasospasm does not occur, limiting a comprehensive evaluation. Standing increases venous hypertension and dilates veins, thereby facilitating examination. Patients with superficial axial incompetence commonly exhibit palpable great saphenous veins (Fig. 65.5).

Visual inspection is critical. There are three main anatomic categories of primary venous insufficiency—telangiectasias, reticular veins, and varicose veins. Telangiectasias, reticular varicosities, and varicose veins are similar but exhibit distinct variations in caliber. Telangiectasias are very small intradermal venules. These structures measure less than 3 mm. Without associated symptoms and stigmata of other venous disease, they are idiopathic in nature and are not medically necessary to treat.

Leg telangiectasias of multiple causes may be a manifestation of a systemic disease. Some of these disorders include autoimmune diseases (such as lupus erythematosus and dermatomyositis), exogenous causes, and xeroderma pigmentosum. Reticular veins are vein branches that enter the tributaries of the main axial, perforating, or deep veins. The axial veins, the great and small saphenous veins, represent the largest caliber veins of the superficial venous system.

Location of varicosities can commonly identify an incompetent valve or the axial vein from which the varicosities developed. For example, medial thigh varicose veins are likely to develop from an incompetent great saphenous vein, whereas posterior calf or lateral calf varicose veins tend to originate from the small saphenous vein. In addition, the location of varicose veins can be a diagnostic predictor of a larger process. Varicosities of the scrotum can be associated with gonadal vein incompetence, otherwise termed the nutcracker syndrome (compression of the left renal vein between the aorta and the superior mesenteric artery). Perineal or vulvar varicosities can be a sign of ovarian or pelvic venous insufficiency, or iliac vein obstruction.

The physical examination can provide the physician with important information on the history of the venous disease that the patient might have neglected or forgotten to mention during the history. For example, signs of a chronic or resolved thrombophlebitis may include a partially thrombosed varicosity; a brownish discoloration around a varicosity or along a palpable segment of the axial veins, consistent with hemosiderin deposition; and palpable segments of axial vein, suggesting partially or completely occluded axial vein segments.

Signs of advanced venous insufficiency include hyperpigmentation in the distal calf or gaiter distribution, secondary to

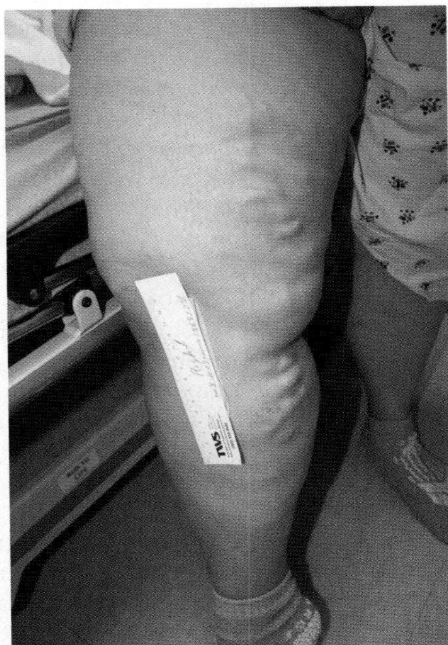
FIG. 65.5 Varicose veins.

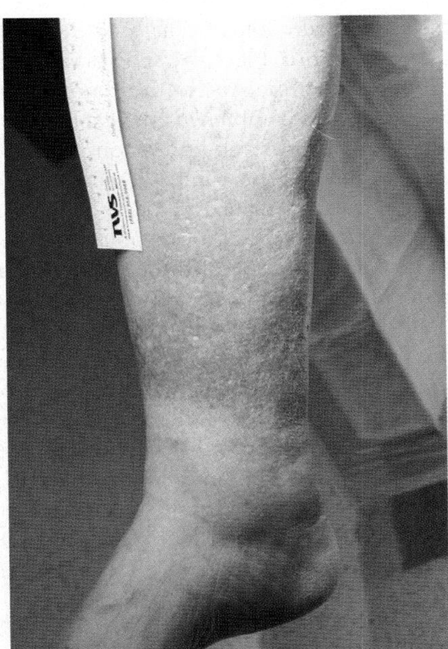
FIG. 65.6 Lipodermatosclerosis, atrophie blanche, and brawny edema.

hemosiderin deposition, and lipodermatosclerosis. Lipodermatosclerosis develops over time because of prolonged ambulatory venous hypertension and chronic inflammation. Physical examination findings that reflect lipodermatosclerosis are brawny edema of the distal calf, "champagne bottle leg," fibrotic and hypertrophic skin, and hyperpigmentation. Advanced lipodermatosclerosis may involve fibrosis of the Achilles tendon, impairing motor function of the extremity. Therefore, examination should include motor function at the ankle. Atrophie blanche is an area of pale hue, visualized around the medial malleolus; it is commonly mistaken for a healed ulcer because of its lighter pigmentation (Fig. 65.6). Corona phlebectatica is a term used to describe an accumulation of tiny telangiectasias or venous flare, usually located at the medial malleolus or the dorsum of the foot. Skin changes from CVI can mimic other dermatologic phenomena; both dermatitis and eczematous changes can be seen from venous disease.

Venous stasis ulcers exhibit pathognomonic features that distinguish them from their arterial or neuropathic counterparts. Venous ulcers are not generally painful and appear at the medial malleolus, not in the mid to distal foot. Lack of arterial pulses in patients with a venous ulcer is unusual.

Venous stasis dermatitis is visualized at the distal ankle and can mimic eczema or dermatitis of another cause. It is this important attention to supporting features of the physical examination and history as well as confirmation with duplex reflux examination that will distinguish advanced venous stasis disease from dermatologic conditions.

Diagnostic Evaluation of Venous Dysfunction

The Perthes test for deep venous occlusion and the Brodie-Trendelenburg test of axial reflux have been replaced by in-office use of the continuous-wave, hand-held Doppler instrument supplemented by duplex ultrasound evaluation. The hand-held Doppler instrument can confirm an impression of saphenous reflux, which in turn dictates the operative procedure to be performed in a given patient. A common misconception is the belief that the Doppler instrument is used to locate perforating veins. Instead, it is used in specific locations to determine incompetent valves, for example, the hand-held, continuous-wave, 8-MHz flow detector placed over the great and small saphenous veins near their terminations. With distal augmentation of flow and release, normal deep breathing, and performance of a Valsalva maneuver, valve reflux is accurately identified. Formerly, the Doppler examination was supplemented by other objective studies, including photoplethysmography, mercury strain-gauge plethysmography, and photorheography. These are no longer in common use.

Another instrument reintroduced to assess physiologic function of the muscle pump and venous valves is air displacement plethysmography.[5] Its use was discontinued after the 1960s because of its cumbersome nature. Computer technology has now allowed its reintroduction, as championed by Christopoulos and colleagues.[6] It consists of an air chamber that surrounds the leg from knee to ankle. During calibration, leg veins are emptied by leg elevation, and the patient is then asked to stand so that leg venous volume can be quantitated and the time for filling recorded. The filling rate is then expressed in milliliters per second, thus giving readings similar to those obtained with the mercury strain-gauge technique.

Today, duplex imaging is the first and best modality to assess for the normal function and presence of venous insufficiency of the lower extremities. Duplex technology more precisely defines which veins are refluxing by imaging the superficial and deep veins. The duplex examination is commonly done with the patient supine, but this yields an erroneous evaluation of reflux. In the supine position, even when no flow is present, the valves remain open. Valve closure requires a reversal of flow with a pressure gradient that is higher proximally than distally. Thus, the duplex examination needs to be done with the patient standing or in the markedly trunk-elevated position.[7]

There are many advantages of ultrasound imaging. The ultrasound examination is noninvasive, requires no contrast material, and can be performed in the office as well as in the hospital. Drawbacks to the modality include interobserver variability and limitations in imaging in patients with an elevated body mass index and extensive dressings. Imaging is obtained with a 7.5- or 10-MHz probe; the pulsed Doppler consists of a 3.0-MHz probe. The examination begins with the probe placed longitudinally on the groin. First, all of the deep veins are examined. Next, the superficial veins are evaluated. There are four basic components of the examination that should be included to complete a comprehensive venous evaluation of the lower extremity veins: compressibility, venous flow, augmentation after reflux, and visibility. Reflux can be demonstrated with the patient performing a Valsalva maneuver or by manual compression and release of the extremity distal to the point of the examination. A Valsalva maneuver is performed for the proximal extremity, that is, the thigh and groin, whereas compression is used for the calf. Reflux times of 500 milliseconds or longer are considered significant. Perforator veins can be visualized well with the duplex examination. Significant perforator reflux is defined as a diameter of more than 3.5 mm and a reflux time of 500 milliseconds or longer. Demonstration on duplex images of to-and-fro flow, with the presence of dilated segments, constitutes findings compatible with a refluxing perforator. In addition, Doppler studies can provide the clinician with information about the deep system. Widespread use of duplex scanning has allowed a comparison of findings between standard clinical examinations and duplex Doppler studies.[8,9]

Phlebography and Venography

In general, phlebography is unnecessary in the diagnosis and treatment of primary venous insufficiency. In cases of secondary CVI, phlebography has specific usefulness. Ascending phlebography is performed by injection of contrast material into a superficial pedal vein after a tourniquet is applied at the ankle to prevent flow into the superficial venous system. Observation of flow defines anatomy and regions of thrombus or obstruction. Therefore, ascending phlebology differentiates primary from secondary venous insufficiency. Descending phlebography is performed with retrograde injection of contrast material into the deep venous system at the groin or popliteal fossa (femoral vein or popliteal vein). This diagnostic modality identifies specific valvular incompetence suspected on B-mode scanning and clinical examination. These studies are performed only as preoperative adjuncts when deep venous reconstruction is being planned.

Magnetic Resonance and Computed Tomography Venous Imaging

Advancements in technology have led to a paradigm change in the imaging of the venous system. MRVI is a diagnostic imaging modality reserved for evaluation of the abdominal and pelvic venous vasculature. MRVI, unlike venography, is noninvasive and does not require intravenous (IV) administration of contrast material. Studies have documented similar rates of specificity and sensitivity compared with venography. MRVI is used to evaluate pelvic venous outflow obstruction, providing information from the IVC through the iliac venous system. Furthermore, it is an excellent test to evaluate for pelvic congestion syndrome. Computed tomography (CT) venography has similar applications to MRVI. A recent metaanalysis showed that CT venography has sensitivity from 71% to 100% and specificity ranging 93% to 100% for the diagnosis of proximal DVT. Anatomy of the abdominal and pelvic venous system can be well characterized by CT venography. Limitations may include artifacts from orthopedic implants and/or adjacent pathology, administration of contrast, and pelvic radiation in young patients.

Classification Systems

In 1994, the American Venous Forum devised the Clinical-Etiological-Anatomical-Pathophysiological (CEAP) classification system, which is a scoring system that stratifies venous disease on the basis of clinical presentation, etiology, anatomy, and pathophysiology (Table 65.3). It is useful in helping the physician assess a limb afflicted with venous insufficiency and then arrive at an appropriate treatment plan. A revised CEAP classification was introduced in 2004 that included a Venous Disability Score to document a patient's ability to perform activities of daily living.[10] Although the CEAP classification is a valuable tool to grade venous disease, assessment of outcomes after intervention cannot be realized. As a result, two additional scoring systems, the Venous Clinical Severity Score and the Venous Segmental Disease Score, enhance the CEAP score with the increased ability to plot outcome. These three classification modalities now provide clinical researchers with invaluable tools to study treatment outcomes.[11]

Treatment of Superficial Venous Insufficiency

Nonoperative Management

Nonoperative management of patients with CVI includes lifestyle modifications, compression, and pharmacologic therapies.[12] Initial recommendations for lifestyle changes are avoidance of vigorous exercise and leg elevation in order to improve symptoms caused by venous hypertension. While vigorous exercise has shown to increase the risk of developing venous ulcerations, however, increased mobility and moderate physical activity may be beneficial for ulcer healing and may be a useful adjunct to compression therapy. Leg elevation 30 cm above the heart, aids venous drainage, venous return, thus reducing lower extremity venous edema. Leg elevation has also shown to enhance cutaneous microcirculation in patients with lipodermatosclerosis (45% Doppler flux increase).[12] A retrospective study of 122 patients with healed venous ulcer over a period of 12 to 40 months documented statistically significant lower rates of ulcer recurrence with a combination of compression therapy and longer leg elevation times (median 33 min/day). Increased recurrence was observed with a median period of leg elevation of 14 min/day.[12]

Compression therapy is an integral component of the care with patients with CVI. The rationale of compression therapy is to oppose the reflux induced venous hypertension. Considering 60 to 80 mm Hg to be within normal limits standing venous pressure, hemodynamic effects can be expected with an interface compression of 30 to 40 mm Hg. External compression of greater than 60 mm Hg has been shown to occlude lower extremity veins in standing individuals. Investigations conducted via dermal blood flow assessment have demonstrated that 30 to 40 mm Hg compression rates are beneficial also in patients with combined chronic venous disease and peripheral arterial disease with ankle brachial indexes greater than 0.5. The biomolecular mechanisms by which compression therapy functions are unclear. Animal and clinical studies have described an overall improvement of the cutaneous microcirculation, increased capillary density and decreased capillary diameter, and pericapillary halo at video capillary microscopy, increased transcutaneous oxygen saturation levels, and decreased levels of cytokines, such as tumor necrosis factor α and vascular endothelial growth factors.[12]

Compression therapy can be achieved via gradient compression stockings and bandages,

Gradient elastic stockings are considered the most initial intervention in patients with clinical stigma of venous disease. They are currently available in four tensions: 10 to 15 mm Hg (class 1; over-the-counter); 20 to 30 mm Hg (class 2; prescription); 30 to 40 mm Hg (class 3; prescription); and 40 to 50 mm Hg (class 4 high compression; prescription). They are also

TABLE 65.3 Classification of chronic lower extremity venous disease.

C	Clinical signs (grade$_{0\text{-}6}$), supplemented by A for asymptomatic and S for symptomatic presentation
E	Classification by cause (etiology)—*c*ongenital, *p*rimary, *s*econdary
A	Anatomic distribution—*s*uperficial, *d*eep, or *p*erforator, alone or in combination
P	Pathophysiologic dysfunction—*r*eflux or *o*bstruction, alone or in combination

Clinical Classification ($C_{0\text{-}6}$)

Any limb with possible chronic venous disease is first placed into one of seven clinical classes ($C_{0\text{-}6}$), according to the objective signs of disease.

Clinical Classification of Chronic Lower Extremity Venous Disease*

Class	***Features***
0	No visible or palpable signs of venous disease
1	Telangiectasia, reticular veins, malleolar flare
2	Varicose veins
3	Edema without skin changes
4	Skin changes ascribed to venous disease (e.g., pigmentation, venous eczema, lipodermatosclerosis)
5	Skin changes as defined above with healed ulceration
6	Skin changes as defined above with active ulceration

*Limbs in higher categories have more severe signs of chronic venous disease and may have some or all of the findings defining a less severe clinical category. Each limb is further characterized as asymptomatic (A)—for example, $C_{0\text{-}6,A}$—or symptomatic (S)—for example, $C_{0\text{-}6,S}$. Symptoms that may be associated with telangiectatic, reticular, or varicose veins include lower extremity aching, pain, and skin irritation. Therapy may alter the clinical category of chronic venous disease. Limbs should therefore be reclassified after any form of medical or surgical treatment.

Classification by Cause (E_c, E_p, or E_s)

Venous dysfunction may be congenital, primary, or secondary. These categories are mutually exclusive. Congenital venous disorders are present at birth but may not be recognized until later. The method of diagnosis of congenital abnormalities must be described. Primary venous dysfunction is defined as venous dysfunction of unknown cause but not of congenital origin. Secondary venous dysfunction denotes an acquired condition resulting in chronic venous disease—for example, deep venous thrombosis.

Classification by Cause of Chronic Lower Extremity Venous Disease

Congenital (E_c)	Cause of the chronic venous disease present since birth
Primary (E_p)	Chronic venous disease of undetermined cause
Secondary (E_s)	Chronic venous disease with an associated known cause (e.g., postthrombotic, posttraumatic, other)

Anatomic Classification (A_s, A_d, or A_p)

The anatomic site(s) of the venous disease should be described as superficial (A_s), deep (A_d), or perforating (A_p) vein(s). One, two, or three systems may be involved in any combination. For reports requiring greater detail, the involvement of the superficial, deep, and perforating veins may be localized by use of the anatomic segments.

Segmental Localization of Chronic Lower Extremity Venous Disease

Segment no.	***Veins***
Superficial Veins ($A_{s1\text{-}5}$)	
1	Telangiectasia/reticular veins
	Greater (long) saphenous vein
2	Above knee
3	Below knee
4	Lesser (short) saphenous vein
5	Nonsaphenous
Deep Veins ($A_{d6\text{-}16}$)	
6	Inferior vena cava
	Iliac
7	Common
8	Internal
9	External
10	Pelvic: gonadal, broad ligament
	Femoral

(Continued)

TABLE 65.3 Classification of chronic lower extremity venous disease.—cont'd

11	Common
12	Deep
13	Superficial
14	Popliteal
15	Tibial (anterior, posterior, or peroneal)
16	Muscular (gastrointestinal, soleal, other)
17	Thigh
18	Calf

Pathophysiologic Classification ($P_{r,o}$)

Clinical signs or symptoms of chronic venous disease result from reflux (P_r), obstruction (P_o), or both ($P_{r,o}$).

Pathophysiologic Classification of Chronic Lower Extremity Venous Disease

Reflux (P_r)

Obstruction (P_o)

Reflux and obstruction ($P_{r,o}$)

available in different sizes and length. Gradient compression stockings have shown to be beneficial in symptom control in patients with moderate CVI.[12]

Patients who exhibit venous stasis ulceration will require local wound care (Fig. 65.7). A triple-layer compression dressing with a zinc oxide paste gauze wrap in contact with the skin is used most commonly from the base of the toes to the anterior tibial tubercle with snug graded compression. This is an example of what is generally known as an Unna boot. A 15-year review of 998 patients with one or more venous ulcers treated with a similar compression bandage demonstrated that 73% of the ulcers healed in patients who returned for care (Fig. 65.8). The median time to healing for individual ulcers was 9 weeks. In general, snug, graded-pressure, triple-layer compression dressings result in more rapid healing than compression stockings alone.

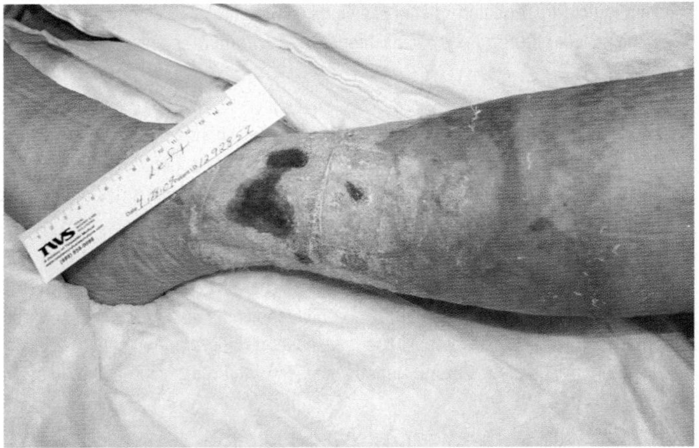

FIG. 65.7 Venous stasis ulcer.

For most patients, well-applied, sustained compression therapy offers the most cost-effective and efficacious therapy in the healing of venous ulcers. After healing, most cases of CVI are controlled with elastic compression stockings to be worn during waking hours. On occasion, older patients and those with arthritic conditions cannot apply the compression stocking required, and control must be maintained by triple-layer zinc oxide compression dressings, which can usually be left in place and changed once a week. In addition to compression, wound care, and surgery, large chronic venous ulcers may benefit from venoactive medications, in particular, pentoxifylline and micronized purified flavonoid fraction.

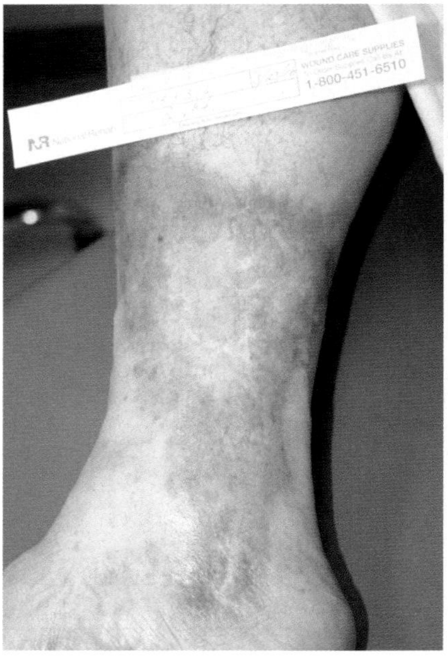

FIG. 65.8 Healed venous stasis ulcer.

Indications for interventional treatment are symptoms refractory to conservative therapy, recurrent superficial thrombophlebitis, variceal bleeding, and venous stasis ulceration. After clinical and objective criteria have established the presence of symptomatic varicose veins, the next step is to plan a course of therapy. The Eschar Trial randomized 500 patients with saphenous insufficiency and venous leg ulcers to conservative management with compression therapy to saphenous stripping and compression therapy. At 4 years of follow-up, there was no evidence of a significant difference in ulcer healing rates but the incidence of ulcer recurrence after healing was significantly lower in patients who underwent saphenous stripping. [12,13]

The efficacy of conservative versus surgical treatment for varicose veins was studied in the Randomised Clinical Trial, Observational Study and Assessment of Cost-Effectiveness of the Treatment of Varicose veins (REACTIV) trial. The authors concluded that

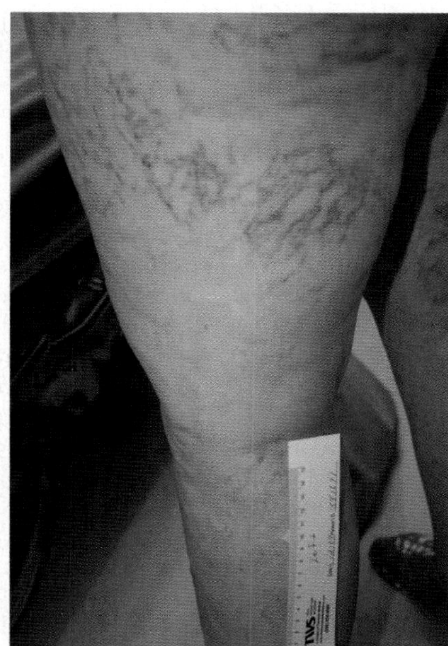

FIG. 65.9 Spider telangiectasias.

surgical treatment was more cost-effective and patients had a higher quality of life benefit than the group who had maintained conservative management alone with compression therapy.[12,13]

Treatment Options for Telangiectasias

By definition, telangiectasias, as they are structures with diameters smaller than 3 mm, are not appropriate for surgical treatment. Asymptomatic telangiectasias are of cosmetic concern only. In these asymptomatic patients with only C_1 disease, a reflux examination is not indicated. However, if the patient describes symptoms consistent with possible venous insufficiency or has concomitant varicosities or more advanced disease on physical examination, a reflux examination is indicated. Treatment options for telangiectasias (spider veins and reticular veins) include injection sclerotherapy and transdermal laser treatment (Fig. 65.9).

Injection sclerotherapy is a technique that involves direct injection of a sclerosant agent into the feeding vein (reticular vein) or spider vein. This procedure is performed in the office setting. There is no preprocedural preparation of the patient. However, patients are asked not to shave or to apply lotions to the extremity before the treatment. Patients leave the office and are able to perform regular activities immediately. Direct sunlight exposure to the treatment area is avoided for a few weeks after the injection. Although it is a safe technique, injection sclerotherapy is contraindicated in the following situations: pregnancy, patients receiving anticoagulation, patients with acute superficial thrombophlebitis, patients with acute DVT, and patients with a history of severe allergy or severe asthma.

Sclerosants act to disrupt the venous endothelium, causing a periphlebitic reaction, which acts to obliterate the vein segment. There are many sclerosants available, and there are particular categories of sclerosants. They include osmotic, detergent, chemical, and corrosive. Hypertonic saline, in various concentrations, was long considered the agent of choice; however, it can be painful with injection (despite the addition of lidocaine) and appears to exhibit a higher incidence of hyperpigmentation after treatment. Therefore, varying concentrations of sodium tetradecyl sulfate (Sotradecol) and polidocanol (Aethoxysklerol) are now the preferred agents.

The procedure should be performed in a well-lit room. Dilute solutions of sclerosant (e.g., 1% to 3% sodium tetradecyl sulfate; polidocanol 0.5%, 1%, 1.5%) can be injected directly into the venules. Care must be taken to ensure that no single injection dose exceeds 0.1 mL but that multiple injections completely fill all feeding vessels. Larger spider veins should be injected first. Injection should begin proximally and proceed distally. When the session is complete, a pressure dressing is applied, consisting of cotton balls at each injection site, and then covered with compression stockings. Patients are advised to ambulate frequently during the first 24 hours and to abstain from direct sun exposure and airline travel for 2 weeks. On occasion, entrapped blood may form, and patients report significant discomfort. Needle drainage is performed at the site, which facilitates healing and cosmesis and rapidly improves discomfort. This liberation of entrapped blood is as important to success as the primary injection. This therapy is remarkably successful in achieving an excellent cosmetic result. C_1 larger than 1 mm and smaller than 3 mm can also be injected with a sclerosant of slightly greater concentration, but the amount injected at one site needs to be limited to less than 0.5 mL. A total volume of sclerosant should not exceed 4 mL during a treatment session. If one is using hypertonic saline, maximum treatment volume can be 10 mL. Although injection sclerotherapy has met with significant success, complications do occur. They include hyperpigmentation, venous matting, postsclerotherapy necrosis, and an allergic reaction to the sclerosant. In addition, telangiectasia formation after injection sclerotherapy treatment tends to occur. Patients will commonly observe return of spider veins 8 to 12 months after treatment. Although patients may report localized discomfort, sclerotherapy of telangiectasias is considered cosmetic and does not influence the venous circulation of the extremity.[14]

Laser treatment of spider telangiectasias has been performed with a variety of wavelengths and varying techniques, such as high-intensity pulsed light, fiber-guided laser coagulation, and neodymium:yttrium-aluminium-garnet laser with a wavelength of 1064 nm. Evaluation of all existing laser modalities has suggested that the neodymium:yttrium-aluminium-garnet laser has the most success. However, to date, there have not been any prospective randomized trials to support this presumption. Laser treatment does tend to be more painful. Laser treatment in most centers will be used in conjunction with injection sclerotherapy, that is, injection treats the feeding venules; laser treatment will be used to treat the extremely small branches not adequately addressed with the injection technique. Most patients are satisfied with the injection-only method.

Surgery for Axial Venous Incompetence

Vein stripping. It has been more than a century since surgeons began to develop techniques to treat superficial axial venous reflux. Keller introduced saphenous vein invagination and stripping, and Mayo pioneered use of an external stripper to remove the saphenous vein. Babcock described stripping the saphenous vein intraluminally from the ankle to groin. High ligation of the great saphenous vein briefly gained popularity as a method for treating venous reflux without removing the great saphenous vein. Enthusiasm for high ligation of the great saphenous vein quickly faded as it proved to be ineffective because the reflux in the axial vein was not eliminated. Today, traditional surgical treatment of superficial venous reflux involves high ligation as well as stripping of the great saphenous vein from the knee to the groin. Stripping at the ankle has been largely abandoned because of a high incidence of saphenous nerve injury.

High ligation and vein stripping usually require general or spinal anesthesia. A transverse or oblique groin incision is made just medial to the femoral artery pulse and inferior to the inguinal crease. Sharp dissection allows identification of the proximal great saphenous vein and other venous tributaries that can be ligated and divided. A brief exploration to identify the presence of a duplicate saphenous system should be performed. The great saphenous vein can then be brought up into the surgical field with gentle traction on the saphenofemoral junction. This maneuver affords further visualization of any missed tributaries that require ligation. The great saphenous vein should be ligated with a nonabsorbable suture and transected near its confluence with the femoral vein.

Attention is then directed to the below-knee segment of the great saphenous vein by making a small transverse incision on the proximal, medial calf. The great saphenous vein is identified, ligated distally, and transected. The Codman stripper is then advanced proximally through the great saphenous vein to exit the transected vein in the groin incision. The bulb is attached to the end of the Codman stripper that exits the groin incision, and a handle is attached to the other end (exiting the calf incision). The saphenous vein should be secured to the bulb of the stripper and inverted onto itself. Forcefully pulling on the handle of the Codman stripper removes the great saphenous vein from the groin to the knee. Before stripping, the lower extremity should be wrapped circumferentially to aid in hemostasis and to prevent postoperative edema and permanent hyperpigmentation due to blood extravasation.

Small saphenous vein stripping requires placing the patient in the prone position to optimize surgical exposure. The procedure starts with a proximal dissection involving the saphenopopliteal junction and follows the same techniques used in stripping of the great saphenous vein. Stripping of the small saphenous should be done only to the level of the midcalf to avoid injury to the closely aligned sural nerve.

Complications. Neovascularization refers to the development of new venous tributaries and varicose veins around the previously ligated and divided saphenofemoral junction. The incidence of neovascularization after high ligation and stripping of the great saphenous vein exceeds 30% according to some reports. Interestingly, neovascularization does not occur after endovenous ablation procedures, which obviate the need for a groin dissection or venous tributary ligation. This observation challenges the long-held tenet of varicose vein surgery that stressed the importance of a thorough groin dissection with ligation of all visible venous tributaries. Rather than being beneficial, surgical dissection and tributary ligation may actually trigger neovascularization and varicose vein recurrence. Monitoring for this complication usually involves periodic duplex ultrasound examination.

Saphenous nerve injury is a well-documented complication that occurs more frequently when the great saphenous vein is stripped from the ankle to the groin. The saphenous nerve runs close to the great saphenous vein in the calf compared with the thigh, where the nerve and vein have more separation. This anatomic detail may explain why stripping from the knee to the thigh only reduces the risk of nerve injury (Fig. 65.10).[15]

Although axial venous stripping was considered the "gold standard" of therapy for several decades, several disadvantages to the technique have been realized. Patients required general anesthesia and a hospitalization. In addition, once discharged, patients experienced a prolonged convalescence before resuming baseline activity. Also, the problems of nerve injury and neovascularization were frustrating to surgeons and patients.

In an effort to address and to correct these limitations, endovenous techniques have been developed. They are discussed in the next section. As a result of their efficacy, stripping is now considered only in select cases.

Endovenous Thermal Ablation

Percutaneous vein ablation. Percutaneous endovenous ablation of the superficial axial veins revolutionized the treatment of superficial venous insufficiency. As a minimally invasive alternative to surgical vein stripping, percutaneous endovenous ablation can be performed on an outpatient basis with local anesthesia. Advantages of this technique include less discomfort of the patient and a more rapid recovery. Patients now actively seek treatment for varicose veins, prompting the proliferation of outpatient vein treatment centers. There are three types of endovenous thermal therapy for the superficial axial veins: radiofrequency ablation, laser ablation, and ultrasound-guided sclerotherapy (UGS).

Endovenous thermal ablation requires minimal preprocedure preparation. Healthy patients with no medical history do not require laboratory work, whereas standard laboratory evaluation is usually obtained for patients with significant medical comorbidities. Patients who are receiving anticoagulation should remain on their standard regimen. The risk of bridging therapy is greater than the risk of keeping patients on their baseline anticoagulation as long as the international normalized ratio (INR) is 3 or less. Guidelines for periprocedural DVT prophylaxis remain unclear. The author gives a single preprocedure dose of low–molecular-weight heparin (LMWH) to patients with two or more risk factors for DVT. All antiplatelet medications can be continued throughout the procedural course. The author does not routinely administer prophylactic antibiotics. Patients with advanced CVI and skin changes usually receive a preprocedure dose of cefazolin.

Anesthesia for endovenous thermal ablation procedures can range from local injections to conscious sedation. Many patients tolerate the procedure with minimal anesthesia consisting only of tumescent infusion of dilute lidocaine around the great saphenous vein. Ideally, these patients can be treated in an office setting. Moderate sedation requires hemodynamic monitoring equipment and is more suited for an outpatient surgical center. The choice of anesthesia ultimately depends on the preferences of the patient and physician as well as the available resources and practice environments.

The venous duplex ultrasound examination plays an essential role in planning of endovenous thermal ablation procedures. The ultrasound examination should provide the treating physician with the following information: patency of the deep venous system, location of normal and refluxing axial veins, areas of communication between the varicosities and the axial vein, and presence of duplicate or accessory refluxing vein segments.

An acute occlusive DVT is an absolute contraindication to endovenous thermal ablation, whereas a chronically recanalized deep venous system in the extremity to be treated is a relative contraindication. In patients who harbor secondary venous insufficiency, the superficial veins play a more important role in venous drainage compared with patients with a pristine deep venous system and primary venous insufficiency. Care must be taken to ensure that superficial venous ablation will not compromise the venous outflow of the postthrombotic limb.

The site of percutaneous access depends on the patient's symptoms and the location of the varicose vein tributaries. If endovenous thermal ablation of the great saphenous vein is planned in a patient with painful varicosities on the proximal calf, it is helpful

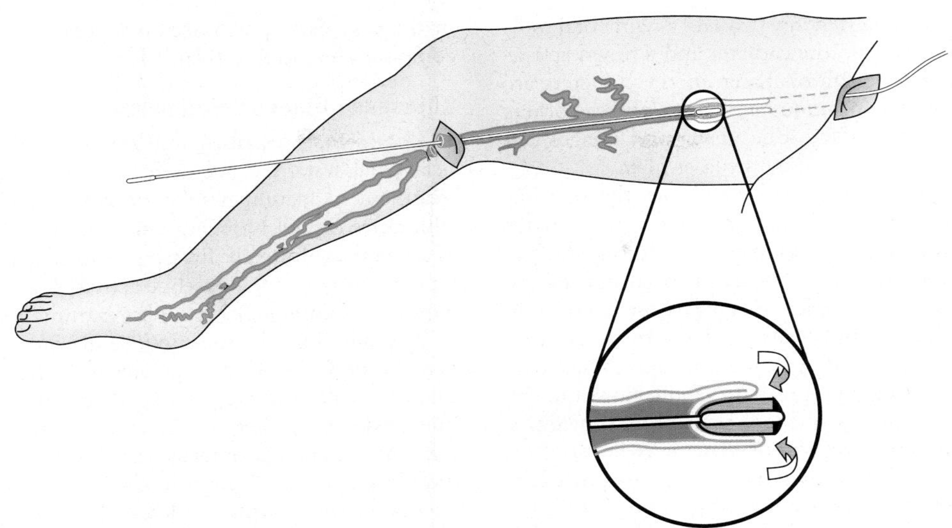

FIG. 65.10 Inversion stripping of the saphenous vein for superficial venous reflux caused by an incompetent saphenofemoral junction.

to evaluate these branches with ultrasound. Percutaneous access on the distal calf just inferior to the varicose veins will ensure that maximum resolution of the tributary branches is achieved with endovenous thermal treatment.

Radiofrequency ablation and laser energy deliver two different types of energy to the vein lumen. Radiofrequency heat is delivered at a temperature of 120°C. The radiofrequency directly injures the vein wall endothelium, resulting in collagen contraction and thrombosis of the treated vein. Laser energy delivers energy to the blood itself. Steam bubbles are generated with the laser energy, and coagulation occurs after completion of laser energy delivery. Radiofrequency catheters vary in length but not in temperature delivered. In contrast, laser energy generators come in different wavelengths ranging from 810 nm to 1470 nm and laser catheters continues to evolve, and as such, updated laser therapy strategies are frequently introduced into the evolving therapeutic armamentarium. Investigators have demonstrated that the higher wavelength fibers appear to be associated with less postprocedural discomfort.

Technique. In most cases, the extremity should be placed in a position of external rotation with the knee slightly flexed. A sheet "bump" may help the patient maintain this position. Placing the patient in reverse Trendelenburg can help dilate the vein to be accessed. After the standard sterile preparation and draping, the ultrasound probe is brought onto the field in a sterile transducer cover. The author reexamines the vein to be treated along its entire course, noting areas of aneurysmal dilation or tortuosity that may affect catheter placement. Ideally, the puncture site should be distal to the lowest level of truncal reflux and provide unobstructed access to the refluxing vein segment.

At the chosen site of percutaneous access, the ultrasound probe is positioned to obtain a stable gray-scale image of the vein in either the transverse or sagittal plane. After puncture of the skin, limited, small movements of the 21-gauge needle help identify its tip on the ultrasound image. On real-time imaging, the needle is guided into the vein lumen and exchanged over a wire for a 6 Fr or 7 Fr sheath using the modified Seldinger technique. With ultrasound guidance, the radiofrequency catheter or laser catheter is then advanced through the sheath, and the ultrasound probe is positioned in the groin to visualize the catheter tip, the saphenofemoral junction, and the deep system. Using ultrasound guidance, the tip of the ablation catheter is placed 2 to 3 cm distal to the saphenofemoral junction to minimize the chance of heat transmission into the femoral vein. Definitive positioning of the therapeutic catheter must be completed at this point, before the administration of local anesthesia during the next stage of the procedure. Imaging artifacts from the tumescent anesthesia tend to impede visualization of the catheter tip, making it difficult to adjust its position.

Before tumescent anesthesia is begun, the patient should be placed in the Trendelenburg position to help empty the vein. Tumescent anesthesia is the infusion of a large volume of dilute local anesthetic. Although there are many recipes for tumescent solution, the main components are lidocaine, epinephrine, and sodium bicarbonate diluted with lactated Ringer solution or normal saline. During laser treatment and radiofrequency ablation procedures, tumescent anesthesia performs three functions: it provides anesthesia over a large area; it compresses the vein around the therapeutic catheter; and it acts as a protective barrier to prevent heating of nontarget tissues, including skin, nerves, arteries, and the deep veins.

For great saphenous vein procedures, the target of tumescent anesthesia is the saphenous sheath. When it is viewed in the transverse plane, the saphenous canal resembles an eye, and the ultrasound image is often referred to as the "saphenous eye." Administration of tumescent anesthesia starts distally on the lower extremity and progresses proximally. Real-time ultrasound imaging guides a 21- to 25-gauge needle into the saphenous canal to deliver the tumescent anesthesia. When it is injected into the proper perivenous tissue plane, the tumescent anesthesia will track up and around the target vein. A long-axis ultrasound view gives the best image of fluid spreading up the saphenous canal. Multiple skin punctures and injections are performed until the vein has a 10-mm halo of tumescent anesthesia along its entire course. The targeted vein segment is then reinspected by ultrasound to ensure that the vein is compressed around the therapeutic catheter and adequately separated from the overlying skin.

Radiofrequency energy or laser energy is then applied to the vein segment by activating and slowly withdrawing the therapeutic catheter. The specifics of retrograde pullback depend on the type of catheter. Radiofrequency energy involves a segmental pullback governed by hash marks on the catheter and a timed activation on the accompanying generator. Laser energy catheters are variable; some have a slow continuous pullback, whereas others require a segmental pullback. Gray-scale ultrasound images can often detect steam bubbles generated by the laser fiber.

Regardless of the type of energy delivered, once the vein has been completely treated, the sheath and accompanying catheter are removed. Ultrasound imaging resumes, confirming the patency of the femoral vein as well as successful occlusion of the great saphenous vein. Color Doppler imaging is often the only way to assess patency at this point because of the distortion caused by the ablation and the surrounding tumescent anesthesia. It is also important to verify retrograde epigastric venous flow into the proximal segment of the great saphenous vein. This provides a "protective flush" of the great saphenous vein. It is believed by many venous experts that this flow pattern prevents postprocedural development of endovenous heat-induced thrombus (EHIT).

Postprocedural instructions vary by practitioner. The patient's extremity is usually wrapped in a layered compression dressing, or a 20 to 30 mm Hg compression stocking is applied. The patient is instructed to walk every hour until bed. Regular activity except for vigorous cardiovascular exercise can be resumed the following day. After a satisfactory postprocedural duplex examination, all activity restrictions are lifted.

Most venous specialists recommend a physical examination or duplex ultrasound examination 2 to 5 days after the procedure. The duplex ultrasound examination ensures that the deep venous system remains patent and confirms the ablation of the great saphenous vein. Reported rates of DVT after endovenous ablation range from 0% to 16% after radiofrequency ablation and 0% to 7.7% after laser ablation. Although the incidence of postablation DVT is extremely low, duplex ultrasound examination can detect thrombus in the proximal great saphenous vein that can extend into the common femoral vein. Lowell Kabnick coined the term *endovenous heat-induced thrombus* to describe this ultrasound finding. He classified EHIT into four different levels based on of the size of the thrombus and its extension into the deep venous system.

The mechanism of EHIT formation remains unclear. General consensus assumes that heat-triggered thrombus in the great saphenous vein propagates into the saphenofemoral junction and encroaches on the deep venous system. EHIT and acute DVT differ in their sonographic characteristics and natural history. EHIT becomes sonographically echogenic quickly (<24 hours), whereas acute DVT usually remains hypoechoic for several days after its initial detection. Although EHIT appears to have a low propensity to propagate or to embolize, pulmonary embolism has been reported after venous ablation procedures. Follow-up ultrasound examinations usually demonstrate retraction or complete resolution of EHIT within 7 to 10 days. Given this benign natural history, most practitioners do not treat class 1 and class 2 EHIT. Class 3 EHIT, which involves partial, nonocclusive extension into the deep venous system, usually warrants anticoagulation therapy, the duration of which can vary on the basis of the physician's discretion. Because class 4 EHIT represents occlusive DVT, it requires a 3-month course of anticoagulation.

The choice of whether to use radiofrequency ablation or laser as the energy source for venous ablation procedures remains a matter of the physician's preference. Randomized prospective studies comparing the two techniques have detected few differences. Patients treated with laser ablation tended to have more discomfort in the very early postprocedural period; however, all other outcome variables were similar.[16,17]

Ultrasound-Guided Sclerotherapy

UGS was first described in 1989 as a treatment for the superficial axial system. Since then, the use of UGS has expanded to treatment of incompetent perforator branches and large venous tributaries caused by neovascularization. UGS gained popularity as a simple, minimally invasive technique that allows patients to rapidly return to their baseline activity level. Preparation for UGS requires a comprehensive duplex examination.

The closed needle technique is the most common method for performing UGS. A 25-gauge needle is used as this is the smallest caliber needle that can be visualized with gray-scale ultrasound. The needle is attached to a syringe containing the sclerosant. The vein can be sonographically visualized in a transverse or longitudinal plane, depending on the operator's preference. The frequency of the transducer depends on the depth of the vein to be treated. High-frequency transducers visualize superficial veins better, whereas deeper veins require lower frequency transducers. The needle tip must be visualized immediately as it penetrates the dermis. After entering the vein, the needle should be aspirated to confirm its position within the vein lumen. Injecting a small test dose of sclerosant provides further confirmation of the needle's position. An alternative method of UGS uses a butterfly needle instead of the needle attached to a syringe.

Volumes and concentrations of sclerosant are dependent on the size and length of vein to be treated. In general, UGS requires high concentrations of sclerosant because of the large caliber of the targeted veins. Specific details about sclerosant preparation are outside the scope of this chapter. Early investigational studies reported promising results. Further study using randomized prospective trials with all modalities is necessary before true standards of practice can be formalized.

Nontumescent Ablation and Future Modalities for Axial Vein Incompetence

In addition to the ultrasound-guided foam sclerotherapy, many other newer techniques have been recently introduced into the therapeutic armamentarium. One device is mechanical chemical ablation. The catheter device is composed of two components. A mechanical portion rotates inside the vein lumen and denudes the venous endothelium. The second component is the chemical portion, which involves concomitant injection of a liquid sclerosant as the mechanical rotation inside the vein is taking place. Potential advantages over the endothermal devices are the lack of tumescence because no heat is required and the small profile of the catheter. Access of the vein is similar. The glue and foam injectable category comprises another group of devices that are also "tumescent free." Time will tell as further data are obtained to determine the role of each therapy in superficial axial insufficiency.

Treatment of Branch Varicosities

There are three techniques to treat secondary branch varicosities: conventional stab phlebectomy, powered phlebectomy (TriVex; InaVein, Lexington, MA), and foam sclerotherapy. Ambulatory phlebectomy is performed by the stab avulsion technique (Fig. 65.11). The patient's varicosities are marked after standing to allow optimal dilation and visualization of affected veins. A variety of anesthetic methods are used successfully, including local anesthesia with tumescence and IV sedation. First, 1-mm incisions are made along Langer skin lines, and the vein is retrieved with a

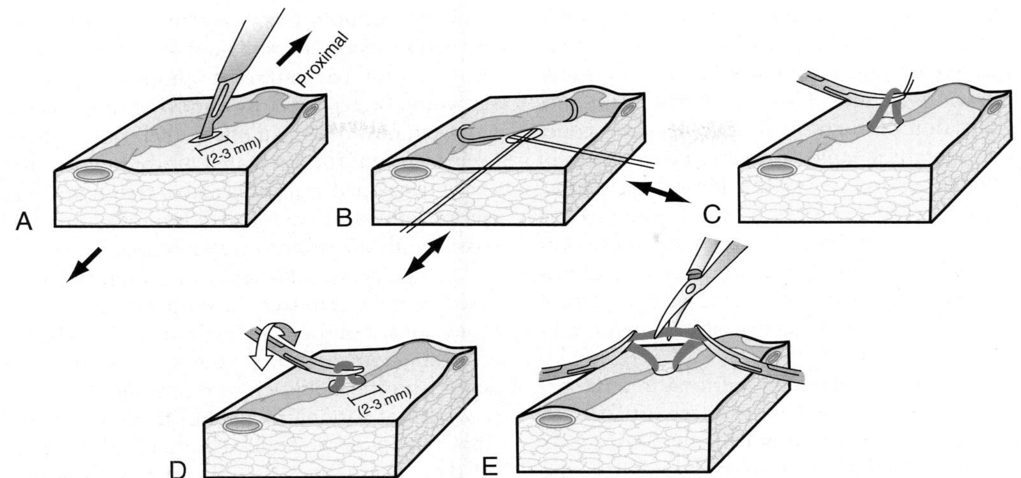

FIG. 65.11 (A–E) Technique of ambulatory phlebectomy (otherwise known as stab avulsions of varicosities).

hook. Continuous retraction of the vein segment affords maximal removal of the vein, and direct pressure is applied over the site. Incisions are made at approximately 2-cm intervals. The extremity is wrapped with a layered compression dressing, and patients are instructed to ambulate on the day of surgery. The postoperative course is brief, and rarely do patients require more than acetaminophen or nonsteroidal antiinflammatory drugs for discomfort. Compression stockings are worn for 2 weeks after the procedure. Complications are unusual but include bleeding, infection, temporary or permanent paresthesias, and phlebitis from retained vein segments. There can be recurrence.

Powered phlebectomy (TriVex) is a modality that can be used to treat extensive secondary branch varicosities. The patient's varicosities are circumferentially marked preoperatively; in the operating room, 2-mm incisions are made at these boundary sites. These incisions permit placement of a transilluminator and resection device. The instruments are inserted through a subcutaneous plane, just deep to the varicosities. The transilluminator not only provides visualization of the veins but also administers tumescent anesthesia. The resector is a rotating blade that transects the veins and then removes them through a high-suction tubing system. The extremity is wrapped with a multilayer compression dressing, and the patient is discharged with instructions to ambulate hourly. The patient returns to the office for a dressing change within 48 hours and usually is changed to standard compression hose. Discomfort is minimal, and over-the-counter analgesia is sufficient. A second-generation TriVex device has been developed; technical issues with the first-generation instrument were revised, and studies now focus on methods to use the TriVex system in an outpatient setting. A steep learning curve occurs with this device, but once it is achieved, experienced physicians can perform most TriVex procedures within 30 minutes. Complications are unusual but can include contained hematoma, bleeding, temporary or permanent paresthesias, and phlebitis.[18]

Secondary Venous Insufficiency

Secondary venous insufficiency is usually caused by a deep venous thrombus. Clinical manifestations of secondary venous insufficiency usually present in a more advanced stage than their primary counterparts. In addition, patients may describe venous claudication, or a bursting pain in the calf, that is classic for secondary venous insufficiency. Conservative treatment regimens are similar to those described in the preceding section for primary insufficiency; however, these patients require a higher grade of compression for efficacy (30–40 mm Hg). Interventional treatment focuses on the superficial and deep systems. Diagnostic interrogation of the deep venous system must be more comprehensive in these patients to determine whether they are candidates for deep surgical or endovenous reconstruction.

Treatment

Surgery for deep venous insufficiency. While conservative therapy is being pursued or ulcer healing is achieved, appropriate diagnostic studies generally reveal patterns of venous reflux or segments of venous occlusion so that specific therapy can be prescribed for the individual limb being evaluated. Imaging by duplex ultrasound suffices for the detection of reflux if the examination is carried out while the patient is standing. Such noninvasive imaging may prove the only testing necessary beyond the hand-held, continuous-wave Doppler instrument if superficial venous ablation is contemplated. If direct venous reconstruction by bypass or valvuloplasty techniques is planned, ascending and descending phlebography is required.[19]

Surprisingly, superficial reflux may be the only abnormality present in advanced chronic venous stasis. Correction goes a long way toward permanent relief of the chronic venous dysfunction and its cutaneous effects. Using duplex technology, Hanrahan and associates[20] found that in 95 extremities with current venous ulceration, 16.8% had only superficial incompetence and another 19% showed superficial incompetence combined with perforator incompetence. Another study has demonstrated ulcer healing and decreased ulcer recurrence with perforator reconstruction.[21]

A significant proportion of patients with venous ulceration have normal function in the deep veins, and surgical treatment is a useful option that can definitively address the hemodynamic derangements. Maintaining that all venous ulcers are surgically incurable is not reasonable when data suggest that superficial vein surgery holds the potential for ameliorating the venous hypertension. A randomized controlled trial comparing compression therapy and surgery for superficial reflux versus conservative management alone has revealed significant improvement in patients who had been treated by the surgical component.[21] Early success in patients with CVI, superficial valvular incompetence, and venous ulceration has been obtained with endovenous radiofrequency and laser therapies.

In the 1938, Linton[22] emphasized the importance of perforating veins, and their direct surgical interruption was advocated. This has fallen into disfavor because of a high incidence of postoperative wound healing complications. However, video techniques that allow direct visualization through small-diameter endoscopes have made endoscopic subfascial exploration and perforator vein interruption the desirable alternative to the Linton technique, minimizing morbidity and wound complications. The connective tissue between the fascia cruris and underlying flexor muscles is so loose that this potential space can be opened up easily and dissected with the endoscope. This operation, done with a vertical proximal incision, accomplishes the objective of perforator vein interruption on an outpatient basis.

The availability of subfascial endoscopic perforator vein surgery has had an impact on the care of venous ulcers in Western countries, albeit not as dramatic as its proponents had hoped. As the limbs of patients with severe CVI were studied accurately, the term *postthrombotic syndrome* (PTS) had to give way to the term *CVI;* a link to platelet and monocyte aggregates in the circulation reflected the leukocytic infiltrate of the ankle skin, with its lipodermatosclerosis and healed and open ulcerations.[23]

Data regarding leukocytes in CVI accumulated and were consistent, showing that the activation of leukocytes sequestered in the cutaneous microcirculation during venous stasis was important to the development of the skin changes of CVI. This is reflected in the finding of adhesion markers between leukocytes and endothelial cells and increased production of leukocyte degranulation enzymes and oxygen free radicals. Nevertheless, experimental evidence was still required for decisive proof of the leukocyte hypothesis.

In the United States, several groups have performed perforating vein division using laparoscopic instrumentation. Initial data have suggested that perforator-interruption produces rapid ulcer healing and a low rate of recurrence. The North American Registry, which voluntarily recorded the results of perforating venous surgery, has confirmed a low 2-year recurrence rate of ulcers and more rapid ulcer healing.[24]

A comparison of the three methods of perforator vein interruption, including the classic Linton procedure, laparoscopic instrumentation procedure, and single open-endoscope procedure, has revealed that the endoscopic technique produces results comparable to those of the open Linton operation, with much less scarring and a greater tendency toward a fast recovery. More perforating veins were identified with the open technique. However, the mean hospital stay and period of convalescence were more favorable with the endoscope procedures.[25]

In general, registry reports and individual institution clinical experience have shown that patients with true postthrombotic limbs are disadvantaged by the procedure, enough so that at Leicester (England), the students of the procedure said, "We conclude that perforating vein surgery is not indicated for the treatment of venous ulceration in limbs with primary deep venous incompetence."[25] Nevertheless, studies were reported in which previous superficial reflux was corrected with failures of such treatment. Rescue of these limbs with perforating vein division produced satisfactory results and verified that perforating veins are important in the genesis of venous ulceration and that their division accelerates healing and may reduce recurrence of ulceration.

Part of the difficulty in understanding the need for perforating vein division is the disparity between venous hemodynamics and the severity of cutaneous changes. This is not surprising because the cutaneous changes of CVI are dependent on leukocyte-endothelium interactions, which may not be directly related to venous hemodynamics. However, endoscopic perforator vein division has improved venous hemodynamics in some limbs, as would be expected, by removing superficial reflux and perforating vein outflow. In an effort to eliminate incompetent perforator veins without the associated morbidity described earlier, UGS has been developed as an alternative technique. Early study results are promising and have revealed improved wound healing rates compared with the subfascial endoscopic perforator surgery.[26]

Percutaneous endovenous techniques are also now commonly used modalities to treat incompetent perforator veins. These therapies consist of the same treatments described in the percutaneous vein ablation section. Further study is required to determine the safest and most efficacious technique. For now, the physician has a wealth of varying modalities from which to treat. Interestingly, this may serve the field well; there may be a unique role for each of these techniques. Radiofrequency ablation, laser ablation, and UGS are all commonly used modalities.

Direct venous reconstruction. Historically, the first successful procedures done to reconstruct major veins were the femorofemoral crossover graft of Eduardo Palma and the saphenopopliteal bypass he described, also used by Richard Warren of Boston. These operations were elegant in their simplicity, use of autogenous tissue, and reconstruction by a single venovenous anastomosis.

With regard to femorofemoral crossover grafts, the only group to provide long-term physiologic data on a large number of patients has been Halliday and coworkers from Sydney, Australia. Although phlebography was used in selecting patients for surgery, no other details of preoperative indications were given. These investigators documented that 34 of 50 grafts remained patent in the long term, as assessed by postoperative phlebography. They believed that the best clinical results were achieved in relief of postexercise calf pain but thought that a patent graft also slowed the progression of distal liposclerosis and controlled recurrent ulceration. No proof of this was given in their report. The history of application of bypass procedures for venous obstruction is a fascinating one. Nevertheless, the advent of endovascular techniques has made those operations almost obsolete.[27] However, as a small subset of patients who have had endovascular stenting of the iliac vein develop stent narrowing and recurrent obstruction, the need for bypass procedures may reemerge. If a Palma vein crossover is considered, it appears that saphenous vein provides more durable results than prosthetic graft, but a large saphenous vein of at least 6 mm is required to provide meaningful outflow volume for the obstructed limb.

Perforator interruption, combined with superficial venous ablation, has been effective in controlling venous ulceration in 75% to 85% of patients. However, emphasis on failures of this technique led to Masuda and Kistner's[28] significant breakthrough in direct venous reconstruction with valvuloplasty in 1968 and the general recognition of this procedure after 1975. Late evaluations of direct valve reconstruction have indicated good to excellent long-term results in more than 80% of patients.[29] One cannot overestimate Kistner's contributions. The technique of directing the incompetent venous stream through a competent proximal valve by venous segment transfer was his next achievement. After Kistner's studies, surgeons were provided with an armamentarium that included Palma's venous bypass, direct valvuloplasty (of Kistner), and venous segment transfer (of Kistner). Moreover, external valvular reconstruction, as performed by various techniques, including monitoring by endoscopy, has led to renewed interest in this form of treatment of venous insufficiency. Axillary to popliteal autotransplantation of valve-containing venous segments has been considered since the early observations of Taheri and colleagues.[30] However, long-term verification of the preliminary excellent results has not been accomplished.

DEEP VENOUS THROMBOSIS

Lower Extremity Deep Venous Thrombosis

Acute DVT is a major cause of morbidity and mortality in the hospitalized patient, particularly in the surgical patient. The triad of venous stasis, endothelial injury, and hypercoagulable state, first posited by Virchow in 1856, has held true more than a century and a half later.

Acute DVT poses several risks and has significant morbid consequences. The thrombotic process initiated in a venous segment, in the absence of anticoagulation or in the presence of inadequate anticoagulation, can propagate to involve more proximal segments of the deep venous system, thus resulting in edema, pain, and immobility. The most dreaded sequel to acute DVT is that of pulmonary embolism, a condition of potentially lethal consequence. The late consequence of DVT, particularly of the iliofemoral veins, can be CVI and ultimately PTS as a result of valvular dysfunction in the presence of luminal obstruction.

Thus, understanding the pathophysiology, standardizing protocols to prevent or to reduce DVT, and instituting optimal treatment promptly are critical to reducing the incidence and morbidity of this unfortunately common condition.

Causes

The triad of stasis, hypercoagulable state, and vessel injury is present in most surgical patients. It is also clear that increasing age places a patient at a greater risk, with those older than 65 years representing a higher risk population. In addition, many epidemiological studies have reviewed additional factors that place patients at risk for the development of deep venous thrombus, including malignant disease, increased body mass index, increasing age (especially >60 years), pregnancy, prolonged immobilization, tobacco use, and prior deep vein thrombus.[31]

Stasis

Labeled fibrinogen studies in patients as well as in autopsy studies have demonstrated convincingly that the soleal sinuses are the most common sites of initiation of venous thrombosis. The stasis may contribute to the endothelial cellular layer contacting activated platelets and procoagulant factors, thereby leading to DVT. Stasis, in and of itself, has never been shown to be a causative factor for DVT.

Hypercoagulable State

Our knowledge of hypercoagulable conditions continues to improve, but it is still in its early stages. The standard array of conditions screened for in searching for a hypercoagulable state is listed in Box 65.1. If any of these conditions is identified, a treatment regimen of anticoagulation is instituted for life, unless specific contraindications exist. It is generally appreciated that the postoperative patient, after major surgery, is predisposed to the formation of DVT. After major operations, large amounts of tissue factor may be released into the bloodstream from damaged tissues. Tissue factor is a potent procoagulant expressed on the leukocyte cell surface as well as in a soluble form in the bloodstream. Increases in platelet count, adhesiveness, changes in coagulation cascade, and endogenous fibrinolytic activity result from physiologic stress, such as major operation or trauma, and have been associated with an increased risk for thrombosis.

BOX 65.1 Hypercoagulable states.

- Factor V Leiden mutation
- Prothrombin gene mutation
- Protein C deficiency
- Protein S deficiency
- Antithrombin III deficiency
- Homocysteinemia
- Antiphospholipid syndrome
- Lupus antibody
- Anticardiolipin antibody

Venous Injury

It has been clearly established that venous thrombosis occurs in veins that are distant from the site of operation; for example, it is well known that patients undergoing total hip replacement frequently develop contralateral lower extremity DVT.

In a series of experiments, animal models of abdominal and total hip operations were used to study the possibility of venous endothelial damage distant from the operative site. In these studies, jugular veins were excised after the animals were perfusion fixed. These experiments demonstrated that endothelial damage occurred after abdominal operations and was more severe after hip operations. There were multiple microtears noted within the valve cusps that resulted in exposure of the subendothelial matrix. The exact mechanisms whereby this injury at a distant site occurs and which mediators, cellular or humoral, are responsible are not clearly understood, but that the injury occurs is evident from these and other studies.

Diagnostic Considerations

Incidence

Venous thromboembolism occurs for the first time in approximately 100 persons/100,000 each year in the United States. This incidence increases with increasing age, with an incidence of 0.5%/100,000 at 80 years of age. More than two thirds of these patients have DVT alone, and the rest have evidence of pulmonary embolism. The recurrence rate with anticoagulation has been noted to be 6% to 7% in the ensuing 6 months.

In the United States, pulmonary embolism causes 50,000 to 200,000 deaths annually. A 28-day case-fatality rate of 9.4% after first-time DVT and of 15.1% after first-time pulmonary thromboembolism has been observed. Aside from pulmonary embolism, secondary CVI (resulting from DVT) is significant in terms of cost, morbidity, and lifestyle limitations.

If the consequences of DVT in terms of pulmonary embolism and CVI are to be prevented, the prevention, diagnosis, and treatment of DVT must be optimized.

Clinical Diagnosis

The diagnosis of DVT requires a high index of suspicion. Most are familiar with Homan sign, which refers to pain in the calf on dorsiflexion of the foot. Although the absence of this sign is not a reliable indicator of the absence of venous thrombus, the presence of Homan sign should prompt one to attempt to confirm the diagnosis. The extent of venous thrombosis in the lower extremity is an important factor in the manifestation of

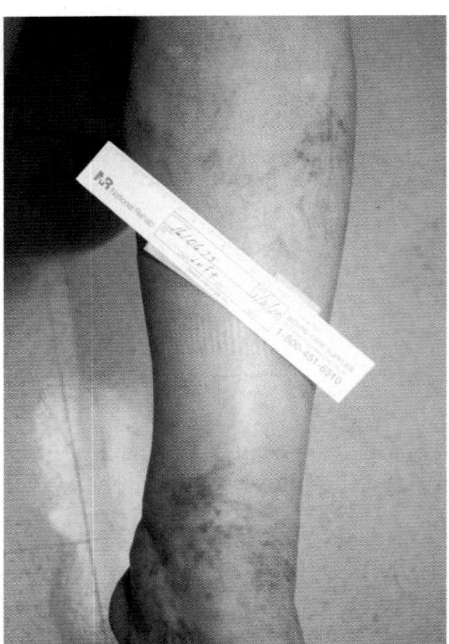

FIG. 65.12 Edema. Note the loss of ankle definition.

symptoms. For example, most calf thrombi may be asymptomatic unless there is proximal propagation. This is one reason that radiolabeled fibrinogen testing demonstrates a higher incidence of DVT than studies using imaging modalities. Only 40% of patients with venous thrombosis have any clinical manifestations of the condition.

Major venous thrombosis involving the iliofemoral venous system results in a massively swollen leg, with pitting edema (Fig. 65.12), pain, and blanching, a condition known as phlegmasia alba dolens. With further progression of disease, there may be such massive edema that arterial inflow can be compromised. This condition results in a painful blue leg, a condition called phlegmasia cerulea dolens. With this evolution of the condition, venous gangrene can develop unless flow is restored.

PTS is a common and unfortunate manifestation of deep venous thrombus. It occurs in 20% to 50% of patients after a documented episode of DVT. The clinical presentation includes chronic edema, pain, and venous claudication. Venous ulcerations occur. Risk factors for the development of PTS include persistent leg symptoms for months after the acute episode of DVT, an anatomically extensive DVT involving the iliofemoral system, recurrent ipsilateral DVTs, and a prolonged state of subtherapeutic anticoagulation for DVT. Unfortunately, treatment of PTS remains supportive, and compression therapy remains the mainstay of treatment for PTS. Some investigators have advocated the early use of thrombolysis to prevent PTS, but its use remains controversial.

Imaging Studies and Laboratory Tests

Venography

Injection of contrast material into the venous system has been long considered the most accurate method of confirming DVT and its location. The superficial venous system has to be occluded with a tourniquet, and the veins in the foot are injected for visualization of the deep venous system. Although this is a good test for finding occlusive and nonocclusive thrombus, it is also invasive, subject to risks of IV administration of contrast material. As a result, this technique has been replaced by less invasive modalities.

Impedance Plethysmography

Impedance plethysmography measures the change in venous capacitance and rate of emptying of the venous volume on temporary occlusion and release of the occlusion of the venous system. A cuff is inflated around the upper thigh until the electrical signal has plateaued. When the cuff is deflated, there is usually rapid outflow and reduction of volume. With a venous thrombosis, one notes a prolongation of the outflow wave. It is not useful clinically for the detection of calf venous thrombosis and of patients with prior venous thrombosis.

Fibrin and Fibrinogen Assays

Fibrin and fibrinogen levels can be determined by measuring the degradation of intravascular fibrin. The D-dimer test measures cross-linked degradation products, which is a surrogate of plasmin's activity on fibrin. In combination with clinical evaluation and assessment, the sensitivity exceeds 90% to 95%. The negative predictive value is 99.3% for proximal evaluation and 98.6% for distal evaluation. In the postoperative patient, D-dimer is causally elevated because of surgery, and as such, a positive result of the D-dimer assay for evaluating for DVT is not useful. However, a negative D-dimer test result in patients with suspected DVT has a high negative predictive value, ranging from 97% to 99%.[32]

Duplex Ultrasound

The current test of choice for the diagnosis of DVT is duplex ultrasound, a modality that combines Doppler ultrasound and color flow imaging. The advantage of this test is that it is noninvasive, comprehensive, and without any risk of reaction to contrast angiography. This test is also highly operator dependent, which is one of its potential drawbacks.

Doppler ultrasound is based on the principle of the impairment of an accelerated flow signal caused by an intraluminal thrombus. A detailed interrogation begins at the calf with imaging of the tibial veins and then proximally over the popliteal and femoral veins. A properly done examination evaluates flow with distal compression, which results in augmentation of flow, and with proximal compression, which should interrupt flow. If any segment of the venous system being examined fails to demonstrate augmentation on compression, venous thrombosis is suspected.

Real-time B-mode ultrasonography with color flow imaging has improved the sensitivity and specificity of ultrasound scanning. With color flow duplex imaging, blood flow can be imaged in the presence of a partially occluding thrombus. The probe is also used to compress the vein. A normal vein is easily compressed, whereas in the presence of a thrombus, there is resistance to compression. In addition, the chronicity of the thrombus can be evaluated on the basis of its imaging characteristics, namely, increased echogenicity and heterogeneity. Duplex imaging is significantly more sensitive than indirect physiologic testing. There are many advantages associated with duplex ultrasound: noninvasiveness, portability, and no need for a contrast agent. However, there are significant disadvantages as well; these include interuser variability and skill, body habitus, and suboptimal visualization in regions such as the lower pelvis.

Magnetic Resonance Venous Imaging

With major advances in imaging technology, MRVI has come to the forefront of imaging for proximal venous disease. The cost and the issue of patient tolerance because of claustrophobia limit its widespread application, but this has been changing. It is a useful test for imaging the iliac veins and IVC, an area where the use of duplex ultrasound is limited. MRVI is less invasive than conventional venography and is able to directly visualize the thrombus.

Prophylaxis

The patient who has undergone major abdominal or orthopedic surgery, has sustained major trauma, or has prolonged immobility (>3 days) represents an elevated risk for the development of venous thromboembolism. The specific risk factor analysis and epidemiological studies detailing the causes of venous thromboembolism are beyond the scope of this chapter. The reader is referred to a more extensive analysis of this problem.[31]

The methods of prophylaxis can be mechanical or pharmacologic. The simplest method is for the patient to walk. Activation of the calf pump mechanism is an effective means of prophylaxis, as evidenced by the fact that few active people without underlying risk factors develop venous thrombosis. A patient who is expected to be up and walking within 24 to 48 hours is at low risk for development of venous thrombosis. The practice of having a patient out of bed into a chair is one of the most thrombogenic positions that could be ordered for a patient. Sitting in a chair, with the legs in a dependent position, causes venous pooling, which in the postoperative milieu could easily be a predisposing factor for the development of thromboembolism.

The most common method of surgical prophylaxis has traditionally revolved around sequential compression devices, which periodically compress the calves and essentially replicate the calf bellows mechanism. This has clearly reduced the incidence of venous thromboembolism in the surgical patient. The most likely mechanism for the efficacy of this device is prevention of venous stasis. Some studies have suggested that fibrinolytic activity systemically is enhanced by a sequential compression device. However, this has not been definitively established because a considerable number of studies have demonstrated no enhancement of fibrinolytic activity.[33]

Another traditional method of thromboprophylaxis has been the use of low-dose unfractionated heparin. The dosage traditionally used was 5000 units of unfractionated heparin every 12 hours. However, analyses of trials comparing placebo versus fixed-dose heparin have shown that the stated dose of 5000 units subcutaneously every 12 hours is no more effective than placebo. When subcutaneous heparin is used on a dosing regimen of every 8 hours rather than every 12 hours, there is a reduction in the development of venous thromboembolism.

More recently, a number of studies have revealed the efficacy of fractionated LMWH for the prophylaxis and treatment of venous thromboembolism. LMWH inhibits factor Xa and IIa activity, with the ratio of antifactor Xa to antifactor IIa activity ranging from 1:1 to 4:1. LMWH has a longer plasma half-life and significantly higher bioavailability. The consistent bioavailability and clearance of LMWH do not require monitoring of factor Xa levels, which facilitates use by the patient. Dosing is merely based on the patient's weight. There is a more predictable anticoagulant response than with unfractionated heparin. No laboratory monitoring is necessary because the partial thromboplastin time (PTT) is unaffected. Various analyses, including a major metaanalysis, have shown that LMWH results in equivalent if not better efficacy, with significantly fewer bleeding complications. It was first thought that LMWH results in less bleeding than unfractionated heparin, but no clinical observations have confirmed this. This property may be more a function of dose than an intrinsic drug action.

Comparison of LMWH with mechanical prophylaxis has demonstrated the superiority of LMWH for reduction of the development of venous thromboembolic disease.[34–36] Prospective trials evaluating LMWH in head-injured and trauma patients have also proved the safety of LMWH with no increase in intracranial bleeding or major bleeding at other sites.[37] In addition, LMWH shows a significant reduction in the development of venous thromboembolism compared with other methods.

Thus, LMWH is considered the optimal method of prophylaxis for moderate- and high-risk patients. Even the traditional reluctance to use heparin in high-risk groups, such as the multiple injured trauma patient and head-injured patient, must be reexamined, given the efficacy and safety profile of LMWH in multiple prospective trials.

Treatment

After a diagnosis of venous thrombosis has been made, a treatment plan must be instituted. Complications of calf DVT include proximal propagation of thrombus in up to one third of hospitalized patients and PTS. In addition, untreated lower extremity DVT carries a 30% recurrence rate.

Any venous thrombosis involving the femoropopliteal system is treated with full anticoagulation. Traditionally, the treatment of DVT has centered around heparin treatment to maintain the PTT at 60 to 80 seconds, followed by warfarin therapy to obtain an INR of 2.5 to 3.0. If unfractionated heparin is used, it is important to use a nomogram-based dosing therapy. The incidence of recurrent venous thromboembolism increases if the time to therapeutic anticoagulation is prolonged. Therefore, it is important to reach therapeutic levels within 24 hours. An initial bolus of 80 units/kg or 5000 units IV bolus is administered, followed by 18 units/kg/hr. The rate is dependent on a target PTT corresponding to an antifactor Xa level of 0.3 to 0.7 unit/mL.[38] The PTT needs to be checked six hours after any change in heparin dosing. Warfarin is started on the same day. If warfarin is initiated without heparin, the risk for a transient hypercoagulable state exists because protein C and protein S levels fall before the other vitamin K–dependent factors are depleted. With the advent of LMWH, it is no longer necessary to admit the patient for IV heparin therapy. It is now accepted practice to administer LMWH on an outpatient basis, as a bridge to warfarin therapy, which is also monitored on an outpatient basis.

The recommended duration of anticoagulant therapy continues to evolve. A minimum treatment time of three months is advocated in most cases. The recurrence rate is the same with three months versus six months of warfarin therapy. If the patient has a known hypercoagulable state or has experienced episodes of venous thrombosis, however, lifetime anticoagulation is required in the absence of contraindications. The accepted INR range is 2.0 to 3.0; a randomized double-blind study has confirmed that a goal INR of 2.0 to 3.0 is more effective in preventing recurrent venous thromboembolism than a low-intensity regimen with a goal INR of 1.0 to 1.9.[39] In addition, the low-intensity regimen did not reduce the risk for clinically important bleeding.

Oral anticoagulants are teratogenic and thus cannot be used during pregnancy. In the case of the pregnant patient with venous thrombosis, LMWH is the treatment of choice; this is continued through delivery and can be continued postpartum, as indicated.

Catheter directed thrombolysis. The advent of thrombolysis has resulted in increased interest in thrombolysis for DVT. The purported benefit is preservation of valve function, with a subsequently lesser chance for development of PTS. In the

ATTRACT (Acute Venous Thrombosis: Thrombus Removal with Adjunctive Catheter-Directed Thrombolysis) Trial, 692 patients with acute proximal deep vein thrombosis were randomized to receive anticoagulation therapy alone or anticoagulation plus pharmacomechanical thrombolysis (catheter mediated, thrombus aspiration, and/or maceration with or without stenting) with the primary outcome of development of PTS between 6- to 24-months follow-up. Overall, there was no significant difference in PTS occurrence between the groups (47% in the thrombolysis group vs. 48% in the anticoagulation group; risk ratio 0.96; 95% confidence interval [CI]). Pharmacomechanical thrombolysis was associated with an increased rate of major bleeding events within 10 days (1.7% vs. 0.3% of patients, P = 0.049). Moderate to severe PTS occurred in 18% of patients in the pharmacomechanical thrombolysis group versus 24% of the anticoagulation alone group (risk ratio 0.73; 95% CI 0.54–0.98; P = 0.04). Severity scores for PTS were lower in the pharmacomechanical thrombolysis group than in the control group at 6-, 12-, 18- and 24-month follow-ups. Quality of life improvement from baseline did not differ between the groups at 24 months. Based on the result of the ATTRACT trial, catheter directed thrombolysis may be recommended in patients with a more proximal, iliofemoral involvement and moderate to severe symptoms.[27]

In patients with phlegmasia, thrombolysis is advocated for relief of significant venous obstruction. In this condition, thrombolytic therapy probably results in better relief of symptoms and fewer long-term sequelae than heparin anticoagulation alone. The alternative for this condition is surgical venous thrombectomy. No matter which treatment is chosen, long-term anticoagulation is indicated.

Endovascular reconstruction. Chronic proximal venous occlusion of the iliofemoral system is a challenging clinical problem. The presentation is variable, and there is no reliable diagnostic modality to measure proximal iliofemoral venous stenosis and to assess outflow obstruction accurately. The pathophysiologic mechanism is often a combination of primary and secondary venous insufficiency. Therefore, evaluation and treatment can be challenging. Endovascular reconstruction removes the need for surgical bypass and has been used successfully. Recanalization of the occluded iliac vein is performed endovascularly. Balloon dilation of the lesion is then performed, and a stent is placed across the dilated segment. Excellent results have been achieved, thereby obviating an open surgical procedure. Endovascular iliac therapy has evolved to become first-line therapy for iliac occlusions. A prospective multicenter randomized trial has recently been initiated known as the C-TRACT study that will randomize 375 patients with PTS and proximal venous obstruction to compression therapy compared to interventional therapy with stenting of the obstructed segments. It is hoped that this trial will provide evidence to identify whether intervention is warranted and which patients with PTS benefit most from venous stenting.

Upper Extremity Deep Venous Thrombosis

Upper extremity DVT is much less common than its lower extremity counterpart, constituting only approximately 5% of all documented DVTs. Although not as common, it is a serious problem; pulmonary embolism occurs in up to one third of all patients with an upper extremity DVT. Upper extremity DVT usually refers to thrombosis of the axillary or subclavian veins. The syndrome can be divided into two categories, primary idiopathic and secondary.

Primary causes include Paget-Schroetter syndrome and idiopathic upper extremity DVT. Patients with Paget-Schroetter syndrome develop effort thrombosis of the extremity caused by compression of the subclavian vein, the venous component of thoracic outlet syndrome. A classic presentation involves a young athlete who uses the upper extremity in a repetitive motion, such as swimming, which causes repetitive extrinsic compression of the subclavian vein. In these patients, anatomic anomalies such as a cervical rib or myofascial bands cause the venous compression. Plain films are one of the first diagnostic tests used to confirm thoracic outlet syndrome. Treatment with initial thrombolysis followed by thoracic outlet decompression (anterior and middle scalene resection, first rib resection) with possible balloon angioplasty or surgical reconstruction of the axillary and subclavian veins is the standard of care. In our institution, thoracic outlet decompression is performed within four weeks from the initial thrombotic episode and thrombolysis. We favor a combined supraclavicular and infraclavicular approach, that allows adequate exposure for surgical reconstruction of the vein (patch angioplasty or interposition graft). After surgery, we recommend anticoagulation for a 6- to 12-month period.

Idiopathic upper extremity DVT is sometimes eventually attributed to an occult malignant neoplasm, and therefore a diagnosis of idiopathic upper extremity DVT warrants evaluation for an undetected malignant neoplasm.

Secondary causes of upper extremity DVT are more common. These include an indwelling central venous catheter, pacemaker, thrombophilia, and malignant disease.

Classic findings on physical examination include unilateral swelling, pain, extremity discomfort, erythema, and a palpable cord. Diagnosis is confirmed by duplex ultrasonography. Because the clavicle obscures the midportion of the subclavian vein, venography or magnetic resonance venography may be required; these are second-line imaging modalities.

Treatment

Treatment of upper extremity DVT involves anticoagulation therapy. Therapeutic dosing parameters are the same as for lower extremity DVT. Treatment should be for 3 months and consist of heparin or LMWH plus warfarin for at least 3 months. Long-term complications of upper extremity DVT include recurrence and PTS. Thrombolysis has not been shown to decrease long-term manifestations from upper extremity DVT and thus PTS. PTS is treated with extremity elevation and graduated elastic compression.[40,41]

Vena cava filter. The most worrisome and potentially lethal complication of DVT is pulmonary embolism. The symptoms of pulmonary embolism, ranging from dyspnea, chest pain, and hypoxia to acute cor pulmonale, are nonspecific and require a high index of suspicion. The gold standard remains pulmonary angiography, but increasingly, this has been displaced by CT angiography.

Adequate anticoagulation is usually effective for stabilizing venous thrombosis, but if a patient develops a pulmonary embolism in the presence of adequate anticoagulation, a vena cava filter is indicated. The general indications for a vena cava filter are listed in Box 65.2. Modern filters are placed percutaneously over a guidewire. The Greenfield filter, most extensively used and studied, has a 95% patency rate and a 4% recurrent embolism rate. This high patency rate allows safe suprarenal placement if there is involvement of the IVC up to the renal veins or if it is placed in a woman in her childbearing years.

BOX 65.2 Indications for a vena cava filter.

- Recurrent thromboembolism despite adequate anticoagulation
- Deep venous thrombosis in a patient with contraindications to anticoagulation
- Chronic pulmonary embolism and resultant pulmonary hypertension
- Complications of anticoagulation
- Propagating iliofemoral venous thrombus in anticoagulation

BOX 65.3 Indications for placement of a retrievable inferior vena cava filter.

- Prophylactic placement in a high-risk trauma patient (orthopedic, spinal cord patients)
- Short-term duration, contraindication to anticoagulation therapy
- Protection during venous thrombolytic therapy
- Extensive iliocaval thrombosis

Device-related complications are wound hematoma, migration of the device into the pulmonary artery, and caval occlusion caused by trapping of a large embolus. In the last situation, the dramatic hypotension that accompanies acute caval occlusion can be mistaken for a massive pulmonary embolism. The distinction between the hypovolemia of caval occlusion and the right-sided heart failure from pulmonary embolism can be made by measuring filling pressures of the right side of the heart. The treatment of caval occlusion is volume resuscitation.

Retrievable vena cava filters. Although they are generally safe, IVC filters are not without risk and significant morbidity. Therefore, permanent placement of a caval filter, particularly in a young patient who may require only short-term caval protection, is not generally recommended. Retrievable filters entered the field as a potential solution for the patient with temporary indications for pulmonary embolus prophylaxis. Currently there are numerous options for retrievable IVC filtration, allowing insertion via the femoral vein or internal jugular vein using smaller caliber (6- to 8-Fr) insertion catheter systems. Before retrieval, venography is performed to ensure that there is no nidus of IVC thrombus in the filter. These filters can be placed in an angiography suite or at the bedside using intravascular ultrasound. A major advantage to retrievable filters is that they may be removed when the patient no longer requires pulmonary embolism protection or can undergo anticoagulation. Insertion complications are rare but include vena cava perforation, filter migration, and venous thrombosis at the insertion site. Retrieval complications include failure to retrieve the filter, thrombus embolization from the filter, vein retrieval site thrombus, and groin hematoma.

Recently, increased attention has focused on the importance of removing retrievable IVC filters that are no longer required for PE prophylaxis. A number of studies indicated that a very low rate of filter retrieval actually is achieved. Complications with retained filters have been reported including migration, penetration of legs into structures around the IVC including the small intestine, aorta, and spine, and infection. For these reasons, recent authors recommend informing all patients with IVC filters that they must return for evaluation of the need for ongoing filtration and removal of filters when no contraindication to removal is present.

Further investigation is required before definitive practice guidelines can be established (Box 65.3).[42,43]

SUPERFICIAL THROMBOPHLEBITIS

Superficial thrombophlebitis is a common disorder, diagnosed in the hospital and outpatient setting. Cardinal signs of a superficial thrombophlebitis are rubor, calor, dolor, and, tumor describing a linear, erythematous, tender, and swollen lesion along the course of a superficial vein. The condition is self-limiting in the majority of patients and as result of the inflammatory reaction; the superficial vein becomes a palpable fibrotic cord. In hospitalized patients, superficial thrombophlebitis is usually caused by an indwelling catheter. In the clinic, patients with thrombophlebitis report common predisposing risk factors, such as recent surgery, recent childbirth, venous stasis, varicose veins, or IV drug use. Patients who deny any of these factors may be classified with idiopathic thrombophlebitis. In these cases, care must be taken to ensure that the patient does not harbor an occult hypercoagulable state or occult malignant disease. In 1876, Trousseau identified the phenomenon of migratory thrombophlebitis and malignant disease, particularly involving the tail of the pancreas. Mondor disease involves superficial thrombophlebitis of the superficial veins of the breast. Diagnosis of superficial thrombophlebitis can be easily made by physical examination of an erythematous palpable cord coursing along a superficial vein, usually located along the lower extremities. Duplex ultrasonography is recommended to confirm diagnosis and if there is suspicion of possible proximal propagation into the deep venous system. With this diagnosis of DVT, anticoagulation is indicated. If, however, thrombus abuts the saphenofemoral junction, treatment of this more elusive condition is controversial. Some authors recommend serial ultrasound examinations and others anticoagulation; another alternative is operative ligation at the junction.

The initial treatment of localized noncomplicated thrombophlebitis involves conservative therapy, which consists of antiinflammatory medication and compression stockings. The recommended treatment of a superficial thrombophlebitis, involving a ≥5 cm great saphenous vein segment is a midtreatment dose of LMWH (enoxaparin 60 mg daily subcutaneously) or fondaparinux (2.5 mg daily subcutaneously) for a 6-week period. A similar treatment is recommended if the thrombophlebitis ascends the great saphenous vein with 3 cm from the saphenofemoral junction. Results from the SURPRISE (superficial vein thrombosis treated for 45 days with rivaroxaban vs. fondaparinux) have shown noninferiority of rivaroxaban at the dosage of 10 mg daily compared to fondaparinux (2.5 mg daily subcutaneously) for 45 days in the treatment of superficial thrombophlebitis. When the thrombophlebitis involves clusters of varicosities, particularly in the lower extremities, excision may be indicated. Selective removal of the entire vein along its course is indicated only in the rare case of suppurative septic thrombophlebitis after all other sources of sepsis have been excluded.

CONCLUSION

The spectrum of venous disease is widespread and diverse, providing surgeons who fully understand the unique physiology of veins a rewarding and rich arena for future investigation.

SELECTED REFERENCES

Bergan JJ, Pascarella L, Schmid-Schönbein GW. Pathogenesis of primary chronic venous disease: insights from animal models of venous hypertension. *J Vasc Surg*. 2008;47:183–192.

This article provides a comprehensive review of the known aspects of venous hypertension pathophysiology.

Caggiati A, Bergan JJ, Gloviczki P, et al. Nomenclature of the veins of the lower limbs: an international interdisciplinary consensus statement. *J Vasc Surg*. 2002;36:416–422.

Revised terminology for the venous anatomy of the lower extremity is outlined.

Eklöf B, Rutherford RB, Bergan JJ, et al. American Venous Forum International Ad Hoc Committee for Revision of the CEAP Classification: revision of the CEAP classification for chronic venous disorders: consensus statement. *J Vasc Surg*. 2004;40:1248–1252.

Essential adjunct to the original Clinical-Etiological-Anatomical-Pathophysiological document.

Leopardi D, Hoggan BL, Fitridge RA, et al. Systematic review of treatments for varicose veins. *Ann Vasc Surg*. 2009;23:264–276.

Systematic overview of current treatment modalities for superficial venous disease.

Meissner MH, Eklof B, Smith PC, et al. Secondary chronic venous disorders. *J Vasc Surg*. 2007;46(suppl):68S–83S.

Meissner MH, Gloviczki P, Bergan J, et al. Primary chronic venous disorders. *J Vasc Surg*. 2007;46(suppl):54S–67S.

These two supplements provide an extremely comprehensive evaluation of venous insufficiency, including pathophysiology, medical and surgical management, and outstanding references.

Wakefield TW, Caprini J, Comerota AJ. Thromboembolic diseases. *Curr Probl Surg*. 2008;45:844–899.

Excellent review of secondary venous disorders.

REFERENCES

1. Caggiati A, Bergan JJ, Gloviczki P, et al. Nomenclature of the veins of the lower limbs: an international interdisciplinary consensus statement. *J Vasc Surg*. 2002;36:416–422.
2. Pascarella L, Schonbein GW, Bergan JJ. Microcirculation and venous ulcers: a review. *Ann Vasc Surg*. 2005;19:921–927.
3. Raffetto JD. Inflammation in chronic venous ulcers. *Phlebology*. 2013;28(suppl 1):61–67.
4. Kowalewski R, Malkowski A, Sobolewski K, et al. Evaluation of transforming growth factor-beta signaling pathway in the wall of normal and varicose veins. *Pathobiology*. 2010;77:1–6.
5. Neglen P, Raju S. A rational approach to detection of significant reflux with duplex Doppler scanning and air plethysmography. *J Vasc Surg*. 1993;17:590–595.
6. Christopoulos D, Nicolaides AN, Szendro G. Venous reflux: quantification and correlation with the clinical severity of chronic venous disease. *Br J Surg*. 1988;75:352–356.
7. van Bemmelen PS, Bedford G, Beach K, et al. Quantitative segmental evaluation of venous valvular reflux with duplex ultrasound scanning. *J Vasc Surg*. 1989;10:425–431.
8. Gloviczki P, Comerota AJ, Dalsing MC, et al. The care of patients with varicose veins and associated chronic venous diseases: clinical practice guidelines of the Society for Vascular Surgery and the American Venous Forum. *J Vasc Surg*. 2011;53:2S–48S.
9. Singh S, Lees TA, Donlon M, et al. Improving the preoperative assessment of varicose veins. *Br J Surg*. 1997;84:801–802.
10. Eklof B, Rutherford RB, Bergan JJ, et al. Revision of the CEAP classification for chronic venous disorders: Consensus statement. *J Vasc Surg*. 2004;40:1248–1252.
11. Rutherford RB, Padberg Jr FT, Comerota AJ, et al. Venous severity scoring: an adjunct to venous outcome assessment. *J Vasc Surg*. 2000;31:1307–1312.
12. Pascarella L, Shortell CK. Nonoperative management of chronic venous insufficiency. In: Sidawy AN, Perler B, ed. Rutherford's vascular surgery and endovascular therapy. 9th ed. Philadelphia: Elsevier; 2019:2055–2066.
13. Barwell JR, Davies CE, Deacon J, et al. Comparison of surgery and compression with compression alone in chronic venous ulceration (ESCHAR study): Randomised controlled trial. *Lancet*. 2004;363:1854–1859.
14. Franz RW, Knapp ED. Transilluminated powered phlebectomy surgery for varicose veins: a review of 339 consecutive patients. *Ann Vasc Surg*. 2009;23:303–309.
15. Dwerryhouse S, Davies B, Harradine K, et al. Stripping the long saphenous vein reduces the rate of reoperation for recurrent varicose veins: Five-year results of a randomized trial. *J Vasc Surg*. 1999;29:589–592.
16. Raju S, Hollis K, Neglen P. Use of compression stockings in chronic venous disease: patient compliance and efficacy. *Ann Vasc Surg*. 2007;21:790–795.
17. van den Bos R, Arends L, Kockaert M, et al. Endovenous therapies of lower extremity varicosities: a meta-analysis. *J Vasc Surg*. 2009;49:230–239.
18. Marston WA, Owens LV, Davies S, et al. Endovenous saphenous ablation corrects the hemodynamic abnormality in patients with CEAP clinical class 3-6 CVI due to superficial reflux. *Vasc Endovascular Surg*. 2006;40:125–130.
19. Neglen P, Hollis KC, Olivier J, et al. Stenting of the venous outflow in chronic venous disease: Long-term stent-related outcome, clinical, and hemodynamic result. *J Vasc Surg*. 2007;46:979–990.
20. Hanrahan LM, Araki CT, Rodriguez AA, et al. Distribution of valvular incompetence in patients with venous stasis ulceration. *J Vasc Surg*. 1991;13:805–811; discussion 811–802.
21. O'Donnell Jr TF. The present status of surgery of the superficial venous system in the management of venous ulcer and the evidence for the role of perforator interruption. *J Vasc Surg*. 2008;48:1044–1052.
22. Linton RR. The communicating veins of the lower leg and the operative technic for their ligation. *Ann Surg*. 1938;107:582–593.

23. Powell CC, Rohrer MJ, Barnard MR, et al. Chronic venous insufficiency is associated with increased platelet and monocyte activation and aggregation. *J Vasc Surg*. 1999;30:844–851.
24. Gloviczki P, Bergan JJ, Rhodes JM, et al. Mid-term results of endoscopic perforator vein interruption for chronic venous insufficiency: Lessons learned from the North American subfascial endoscopic perforator surgery registry. The North American Study Group. *J Vasc Surg*. 1999;29:489–502.
25. Murray JD, Bergan JJ, Riffenburgh RH. Development of open-scope subfascial perforating vein surgery: lessons learned from the first 67 cases. *Ann Vasc Surg*. 1999;13:372–377.
26. Masuda EM, Kessler DM, Lurie F, et al. The effect of ultrasound-guided sclerotherapy of incompetent perforator veins on venous clinical severity and disability scores. *J Vasc Surg*. 2006;43:551–556; discussion 556–557.
27. Vedantham S, Goldhaber SZ, Julian JA, et al. Pharmacomechanical catheter-directed thrombolysis for deep-vein thrombosis. *N Engl J Med*. 2017;377:2240–2252.
28. Kistner RL. Surgical repair of the incompetent femoral vein valve. *Arch Surg*. 1975;110:1336–1342.
29. Masuda EM, Kistner RL. Long-term results of venous valve reconstruction: a four- to twenty-one-year follow-up. *J Vasc Surg*. 1994;19:391–403.
30. Taheri SA, Lazar L, Elias S, et al. Surgical treatment of postphlebitic syndrome with vein valve transplant. *Am J Surg*. 1982;144:221–224.
31. Anderson Jr FA, Spencer FA. Risk factors for venous thromboembolism. *Circulation*. 2003;107:I9–16.
32. Kovacs MJ, MacKinnon KM, Anderson D, et al. A comparison of three rapid D-dimer methods for the diagnosis of venous thromboembolism. *Br J Haematol*. 2001;115:140–144.
33. Killewich LA, Cahan MA, Hanna DJ, et al. The effect of external pneumatic compression on regional fibrinolysis in a prospective randomized trial. *J Vasc Surg*. 2002;36:953–958.
34. Bernardi E, Prandoni P. Safety of low molecular weight heparins in the treatment of venous thromboembolism. *Expert Opin Drug Saf*. 2003;2:87–94.
35. Couturaud F, Julian JA, Kearon C. Low molecular weight heparin administered once versus twice daily in patients with venous thromboembolism: a meta-analysis. *Thromb Haemost*. 2001;86:980–984.
36. Offner PJ, Hawkes A, Madayag R, et al. The role of temporary inferior vena cava filters in critically ill surgical patients. *Arch Surg*. 2003;138:591–594; discussion 594–595.
37. Mismetti P, Laporte S, Darmon JY, et al. Meta-analysis of low molecular weight heparin in the prevention of venous thromboembolism in general surgery. *Br J Surg*. 2001;88:913–930.
38. Norwood SH, McAuley CE, Berne JD, et al. Prospective evaluation of the safety of enoxaparin prophylaxis for venous thromboembolism in patients with intracranial hemorrhagic injuries. *Arch Surg*. 2002;137:696–701; discussion 701–692.
39. Kearon C, Ginsberg JS, Kovacs MJ, et al. Comparison of low-intensity warfarin therapy with conventional-intensity warfarin therapy for long-term prevention of recurrent venous thromboembolism. *N Engl J Med*. 2003;349:631–639.
40. Joffe HV, Goldhaber SZ. Upper-extremity deep vein thrombosis. *Circulation*. 2002;106:1874–1880.
41. Martinelli I, Battaglioli T, Bucciarelli P, et al. Risk factors and recurrence rate of primary deep vein thrombosis of the upper extremities. *Circulation*. 2004;110:566–570.
42. Rosenthal D, Wellons ED, Lai KM, et al. Retrievable inferior vena cava filters: initial clinical results. *Ann Vasc Surg*. 2006;20:157–165.
43. Kearon C, Akl EA, Comerota AJ, et al. Antithrombotic therapy for VTE disease: Antithrombotic Therapy and Prevention of Thrombosis, 9th ed: American College of Chest Physicians Evidence-Based Clinical Practice Guidelines. *Chest*. 2012;141:e419S–e496S.

66 CHAPTER

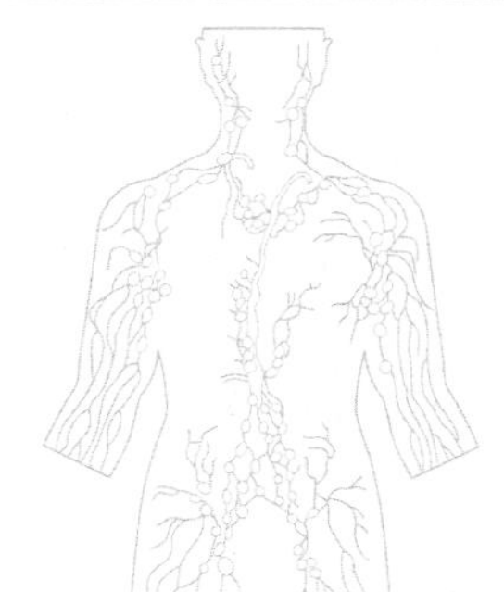

The Lymhatics

Jonathan R. Thompson, Iraklis I. Pipinos

OUTLINE

EMBRYOLOGY AND ANATOMY

The primordial lymphatic system is first seen during the sixth week of development in the form of lymph sacs located next to the jugular veins. During the eighth week, the cisterna chyli forms just dorsal to the aorta, and, at the same time, two additional lymphatic sacs corresponding to the iliofemoral vascular pedicles begin forming. Communicating channels connecting the lymph sacs, which will become the thoracic duct, develop during the ninth week.

From this primordial lymphatic system sprout endothelial buds that grow with the venous system to form the peripheral lymphatic plexus (Fig. 66.1). Failure of one of the initial jugular lymphatic sacs to develop proper connections and drainage with the lymphatic system and, subsequently, the venous system may produce focal lymph cysts (cavernous lymphangiomas), also known as cystic hygromas.[1] Similarly, failure of embryologic remnants of lymphatic tissues to connect to efferent channels leads to the development of cystic lymphatic formations (simple capillary lymphangiomas) that, depending on their location, are classified as truncal, mesenteric, intestinal, and retroperitoneal lymphangiomas. Hypoplasia or failure of development of drainage channels connecting the lymphatic systems of extremities to the main primordial lymphatic system of the torso may result in primary lymphedema of the extremities.

Lymphangiogenesis appears to be regulated by the vascular endothelial growth factors C and D (VEGF-C, VEGF-D); their receptor, VEGFR-3; and their binding protein, neuropilin 2 (Nrp2). Consistent with these findings, Nrp2-deficient mice have lymphatic hypoplasia, and heterozygous inactivating mutation of VEGFR-3 is found in Chy mice, an animal model of primary lymphedema, which appears to be the underlying problem in patients with Milroy disease (congenital familial lymphedema).[2] A number of additional genes have recently been found to be related to lymphatic disorders.[3] The best studied at this point are the gene for the forkhead family transcription factor FOXC2 (responsible for the hereditary lymphedema-distichiasis syndrome) and the gene for the transcription factor SOX18 (related to recessive and dominant forms of hypotrichosis-lymphedema-telangiectasia). As more causal genes are identified, the possibility arises for a classification built on patient phenotypes for which the gene is known.[4] Receptor activity-modifying protein 1 (RAMP1) has also been identified as an important factor for lymphangiogenesis. RAMP1 knockout mice have greater amounts of surgery-associated lymphedema compared to controls. This is thought to occur from a lack of attenuation of proinflammatory macrophage recruitment in the RAMP1 knockout mice.[5]

FUNCTION AND STRUCTURE

The lymphatic system is composed of three elements: (1) the initial or terminal lymphatic capillaries, which absorb lymph; (2) the collecting vessels, which serve primarily as conduits for lymph transport; and (3) the lymph nodes, which are interposed in the pathway of the conducting vessels, filtering the lymph and serving a primary immunologic role.

The terminal lymphatics have special structural characteristics that allow entry not only of large macromolecules but even of cells and microbes. Their most important structural feature is a high porosity resulting from a very small number of tight junctions between endothelial cells, a limited and incomplete basement membrane, and anchoring filaments (4–10 nm) tethering the interstitial matrix to the endothelial cells. These filaments, once the turgor of the tissue increases, are able to

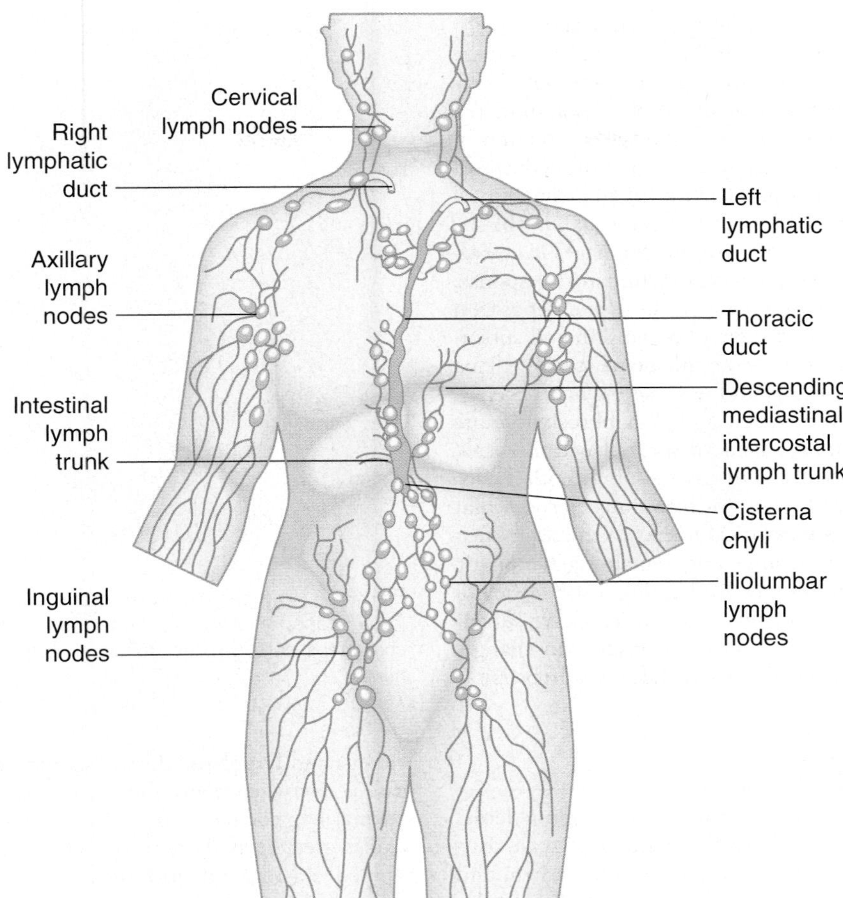

FIG. 66.1 Major anatomic pathways and lymph node groups of the lymphatic system.

pull on the endothelial cells and essentially introduce large gaps between them, which then allow very low resistance influx of interstitial fluid and macromolecules in the lymphatic channels. The collecting vessels ascend alongside the primary blood vessels of the organ or limb, pass through the regional lymph nodes, and drain into the main lymph channels of the torso. These channels eventually empty into the venous system through the thoracic duct. There are additional communications between the lymphatic and the venous systems. These smaller lymphovenous shunts mostly occur at the level of lymph nodes and around major venous structures, such as the jugular, subclavian, and iliac veins. Several structures in the body contain no lymphatics. Specifically, lymphatics have not been found in the epidermis, cornea, central nervous system, cartilage, tendon, and muscle.

The lymphatic system has three main functions. First, tissue fluid and macromolecules that undergo ultrafiltration at the level of the arterial capillaries are reabsorbed and returned to the circulation through the lymphatic system. Every day, 50% to 100% of the intravascular proteins are filtered this way in the interstitial space. Normally, they then enter the terminal lymphatics and are transported through the collecting lymphatics back into the venous circulation. Second, antigens, immune cells, microbes, and mutant cells arriving in the interstitial space enter the lymphatic system and are presented to the lymph nodes, which represent the first line of the immune system. Last, at the level of the gastrointestinal tract, lymph vessels are responsible for the uptake and transport of most of the fat absorbed from the bowel. Recent data suggest that a relationship between fat and lymphatics may exist well beyond the gut alone. It appears that peripheral tissue lipid transport and homeostasis may be, in part, determined by lymphatic function, hence the increased fat deposition seen in lymphedema.[3,6]

In contrast to what happens with venous forward flow, lymph's centripetal transport occurs mainly through intrinsic contractility of the individual lymphatic vessels, which in concert with competent valvular mechanisms is effective in establishing constant forward flow of lymph. In addition to the intrinsic contractility, other factors, such as surrounding muscle activity, negative pressure secondary to breathing, and transmitted arterial pulsations, have a lesser role in the forward lymph flow. These secondary factors appear to become more important under conditions of lymph stasis and congestion of the lymphatic vessels.

PATHOPHYSIOLOGY AND STAGING

Lymphedema is the result of an inability of the existing lymphatic system to accommodate the protein and fluid entering the interstitial compartment at the tissue level.[7] Impaired lymphatic vasculature can be either aplastic, hypoplastic, or hyperplastic. All of these patterns can lead to clinical lymphedema. In aplasia and hypoplasia an absent or diminished number of lymphatics are seen. In hyperplasia, the vessels are incompetent and tortuous. Hyperplasia is only a cause in 8% of patients with lymphedema.[8]

An international working group developed a clinical staging for lymphedema.[9] In the latent phase, excess fluid accumulates and the lymphatics become fibrosed. In the latent phase, there is no clinical evidence of edema. In the first stage of lymphedema, impaired lymphatic drainage results in protein-rich fluid accumulation in the interstitial compartment. Clinically, this is manifested as soft pitting edema. In the second stage of lymphedema, the clinical condition is further exacerbated by accumulation of fibroblasts, adipocytes, and, perhaps most important, macrophages in the affected tissues, which culminates in a local inflammatory response. This results in important structural changes from the deposition of connective tissue and adipose elements at the skin and subcutaneous level. In the second stage of lymphedema, tissue edema is more pronounced, is nonpitting, and has a spongy consistency. Elevation does not reduce the edema and skin fibrosis is more apparent. In the third and most advanced stage of lymphedema, the affected tissues sustain further injury as a result of both the local inflammatory response and recurrent infectious episodes that typically result from minimal subclinical breaks in the skin. Such repeated episodes injure the incompetent, remaining lymphatic channels, progressively worsening the underlying insufficiency of the lymphatic system. This eventually results in excessive subcutaneous fibrosis and scarring with associated severe skin changes characteristic of lymphostatic elephantiasis. Edema is irreversible at this stage.

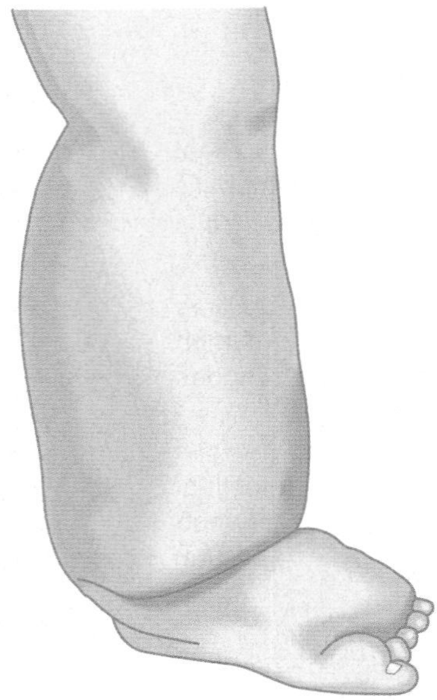

FIG. 66.2 Lymphedema with characteristic loss of the normal perimalleolar shape, resulting in a "tree trunk" pattern. Dorsum of the foot is characteristically swollen, resulting in the appearance of the "buffalo hump."

DIFFERENTIAL DIAGNOSIS

In most patients with second- or third-stage lymphedema, the characteristic findings on physical examination can usually establish the diagnosis. The edematous limb has a firm and hardened consistency. There is loss of the normal perimalleolar shape, resulting in a "tree trunk" pattern. The dorsum of the foot is characteristically swollen, resulting in the appearance of the "buffalo hump," and the toes become thick and squared known as Stemmer sign (Fig. 66.2). In advanced lymphedema, the skin undergoes characteristic changes, such as lichenification, development of peau d'orange, and hyperkeratosis.[7] In addition, the patients give a history of recurrent episodes of cellulitis and lymphangitis after trivial trauma and frequently present with fungal infections affecting the forefoot and toes. Patients with isolated lymphedema usually do not have the hyperpigmentation or ulceration one typically sees in patients with chronic venous insufficiency. Lymphedema does not respond significantly to overnight elevation, whereas edema secondary to central organ failure or venous insufficiency does.

The evaluation of a swollen extremity should start with a detailed history and physical examination. The most common causes of bilateral extremity edema are of systemic origin. The most common cause is cardiac failure followed by renal failure.[10] Hypoproteinemia secondary to cirrhosis, nephrotic syndrome, and malnutrition can also produce bilateral lower extremity edema. Another important cause to consider with bilateral leg enlargement is lipedema. Lipedema is not true edema but rather excessive subcutaneous fat typically found in obese women. It is bilateral, nonpitting, and greatest at the ankle and legs, with characteristic sparing of the feet. There are no skin changes, and the enlargement is not affected by elevation. The history usually indicates that this has been a lifelong problem that "runs in the family."

Once the systemic causes of edema are excluded in the patient with unilateral extremity involvement, edema secondary to venous and lymphatic disease should be entertained. Venous disease is overwhelmingly the most common cause of unilateral leg edema. Leg edema secondary to venous disease is usually pitting and is greatest at the legs and ankles with a sparing of the feet. The edema responds promptly to overnight leg elevation and is controlled with regular compression. In the later stages, the skin is atrophic with brawny pigmentation from hemosiderin deposition. Ulceration associated with venous insufficiency occurs above or posterior to and beneath the malleoli.

CLASSIFICATION

Lymphedema is generally classified as primary when there is no known cause and secondary when its cause is a known disease or disorder.[11] Primary lymphedema has generally been classified on the basis of the age at onset and presence of familial clustering. Primary lymphedema with onset before the first year of life is called congenital lymphedema. The familial version of congenital lymphedema is known as Milroy disease and is inherited as a dominant trait. Primary lymphedema with onset between the ages of 1 and 35 years is called lymphedema praecox. The familial version of lymphedema praecox is known as Meige disease with an onset around puberty. Finally, primary lymphedema with onset after the age of 35 years is called lymphedema tarda. The primary lymphedemas are relatively uncommon, occurring in one out of every 10,000 individuals. The most common form of primary lymphedema is praecox, which accounts for approximately 80% of the patients. Congenital and tarda lymphedemas each account for 10%. Worldwide, the most common cause of secondary lymphedema is infestation of the lymph nodes by the parasite *Wuchereria bancrofti* in the disease state called filariasis. In the developed countries, the most common causes of secondary lymphedema involve resection or ablation of regional lymph nodes by surgery, radiation therapy, tumor invasion, direct trauma, or, less commonly, an infectious process.

DIAGNOSTIC TESTS

The diagnosis of lymphedema is relatively easy in the patient who presents in the second and third stages of the disease. It can, however, be a difficult diagnosis to make in the first stage, particularly when the edema is mild, pitting, and relieved with simple maneuvers such as elevation.[11,12] For patients with suspected secondary forms of lymphedema, computed tomography and magnetic resonance imaging are valuable and indeed essential for exclusion of underlying oncologic disease states.[13] In patients with known lymph node excision and radiation treatment as the underlying problem of their lymphedema, additional diagnostic studies are rarely needed except as these studies relate to follow-up of an underlying malignant disease. For patients with edema of unknown cause and a suspicion for lymphedema, lymphoscintigraphy is the diagnostic test of choice. When lymphoscintigraphy confirms that lymphatic drainage is delayed, the diagnosis of primary lymphedema should never be made until neoplasia involving the regional and central lymphatic drainage of the limb has been excluded through computed tomography or magnetic resonance imaging. If a more detailed diagnostic interpretation of lymphatic channels is needed for operative planning, contrast lymphangiography may be considered.

Lymphoscintigraphy (or isotope lymphography) has emerged as the test of choice in patients with suspected lymphedema.[13,14] It cannot differentiate between primary and secondary lymphedemas; however, it has a sensitivity of 70% to 90% and a specificity of nearly 100% in differentiating lymphedema from other causes of limb swelling. The test assesses lymphatic function by quantitating the rate of clearance of a radiolabeled macromolecular tracer (Fig. 66.3). The advantages of the technique are that it is simple, safe, and reproducible, with small exposure to radioactivity (approximately 5 mCi). It involves the injection of a small amount of radioiodinated human albumin or technetium-99m–labeled sulfur colloid into the first interdigital space of the foot or hand. Migration of the radiotracer within the skin and subcutaneous lymphatics is easily monitored with a whole body gamma camera, thus producing clear images of the major lymphatic channels in the leg as well as measuring the amount of radioactivity at the inguinal nodes 30 and 60 minutes after injection of the radiolabeled substance in the feet. An uptake value that is less than 0.3% of the total injected dose at 30 minutes is diagnostic of lymphedema. The normal range of uptake is between 0.6% and 1.6%. In patients with edema secondary to venous disease, isotope clearance is usually abnormally rapid, resulting in more than 2% ilioinguinal uptake. Importantly, variation in the degree of edema involving the lower extremity does not appear to significantly change the rate of clearance of the isotope.

Direct contrast lymphangiography provides the finest details of the lymphatic anatomy.[15] However, it is an invasive study that involves exposure and cannulation of lymphatics at the dorsum of the forefoot, followed by slow injection of contrast medium (ethiodized oil). The procedure is tedious, the cannulation often necessitates aid of magnification optics (frequently an operating microscope is needed), and the dissection requires some form of anesthetic. After cannulation of a superficial lymph vessel, contrast material is slowly injected into the lymphatic system. A total of 7 to 10 mL of contrast material is ideal for lower extremity evaluation and 4 to 5 mL for upper extremity evaluation. Potential complications include damage of the visualized lymphatics, allergic reactions, and pulmonary embolism if the oil-based contrast agent enters the venous system through lymphovenous anastomoses. Lymphangiography in present surgical practice is used infrequently and solely reserved for the preoperative evaluation of selected patients who are candidates for direct operations on their lymphatic vessels.

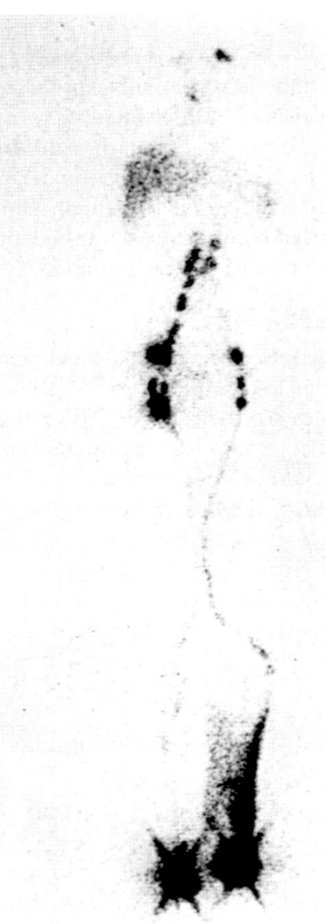

FIG. 66.3 Lymphoscintigraphic pattern in primary lymphedema. Note area of dermal backflow on the left and diminished number of lymph nodes in the groin. (From Cambria RA, Gloviczki P, Naessens JM, et al. Noninvasive evaluation of the lymphatic system with lymphoscintigraphy: A prospective, semiquantitative analysis in 386 extremities. *J Vasc Surg*. 1993;18:773–782.)

New Diagnostic Tests

The field of lymphatic imaging is ever evolving, and we can expect that technologic advances, combined with the development of new contrast agents, will continue to improve diagnostic accuracy.[13] The most promising new test appears to be contrast magnetic resonance lymphangiography.[13,16] The test is performed after intracutaneous injection of gadobenate dimeglumine into the interdigital webs of the dorsal foot. Reported data suggest that the new test is capable of visualizing the anatomy and functional status of lymph flow transport of lymphatic vessels and lymph nodes of lymphedematous limbs in both primary and secondary lymphedema. Another new test which holds promise to detect early disease is bioimpedance spectroscopy. Flow of electrical current in a particular region of the body is inversely related to the amount of fluid in the tissue. With early lymphedema and increased interstitial fluid, impedance decreases. While tested in small samples, sensitivity and specificity has been found to be 100%.[17]

THERAPY

The majority of lymphedema patients can be treated with a combination of limb elevation, a high-quality compression garment, complex decongestive physical therapy, and compression pump therapy. We currently have no effective medications for the treatment of lymphedema. Operative treatment may be considered for patients with advanced complicated lymphedema for whom management with nonoperative means has failed.

General Therapeutic Measures

All patients with lymphedema should be educated in meticulous skin care and avoidance of injuries.[12,18,19] The patients should always be instructed to see their physicians early for signs of infections because these may progress rapidly to serious systemic infections. Infections should be aggressively and promptly treated with appropriate antibiotics directed at gram-positive cocci. Eczema at the level of the forefoot and toes requires treatment, and hydrocortisone-based creams may be considered. In addition, basic range of motion exercises for the extremities have been shown to be of value in the management of lymphedema in the long term. Finally, the patients should make every effort to maintain ideal body weight.

Elevation and Compression Garments

For lymphedema patients in all stages of disease, management with high-quality elastic garments is necessary at all times except when the legs are elevated above the heart.[20,21] The ideal compression garment is custom fitted and delivers pressures in the range of 30 to 60 mm Hg. Such garments may have the additional benefit of protecting the extremity from injuries, such as burns, lacerations, and insect bites. The patients should avoid standing for prolonged periods and should elevate their legs at night by supporting the foot of the bed on 15-cm blocks.

Complex Decongestive Physical Therapy

This specialized massage technique for patients with lymphedema is designed to stimulate the still functioning lymph vessels, to evacuate stagnant protein-rich fluid by breaking up subcutaneous deposits of fibrous tissue, and to redirect lymph fluid to areas of the body where lymph flow is normal.[22] The technique is initiated on the normal contralateral side of the body, evacuating excessive fluid and preparing first the lymphatic zones of the nonaffected extremity, followed by the zones in the trunk quadrant adjacent to the affected limb, before attention is turned to the swollen extremity. The affected extremity is massaged in a segmental fashion, with the proximal zones being massaged first, proceeding to the distal limb. The technique is time-consuming but effective in reducing the volume of the lymphedematous limbs.[22] After the massage session is complete, the extremity is wrapped with a low-stretch wrap, and then the limb is placed in the custom-fitted garment to maintain the decreased girth obtained with the massage therapy. This kind of therapy is appropriate for patients with all stages of lymphedema.

When the patient is first referred for complex decongestive physical therapy, the patient undergoes daily to weekly massage sessions for up to 8 to 12 weeks (initial or reductive stage). Limb elevation and elastic stockings are a necessary adjunct in this phase. After maximal volume reduction is achieved, the patient returns for maintenance massage treatments every 2 to 3 months while continuing to wear compression garments (maintenance phase). Without adherence to therapy, lymphatic fluid will reaccumulate. Lifelong maintenance is imperative to maintain reduction. Volume reduction is generally 60% to 70% and compliant patients retain 90% of this reduction.[23]

Compression Pump Therapy

Pneumatic compression pump therapy is another effective method of reducing the volume of the lymphedematous limb by a similar principle to massage therapy. The device consists of a sleeve containing several compartments. The lymphedematous limb is positioned inside the sleeve, and the compartments are serially inflated to milk the stagnant fluid out of the extremity.[24]

When a patient with advanced lymphedema is first referred for therapy, an initial approach with hospitalization for 3 or 4 days involving strict limb elevation, daily complex decongestive physical therapy, and compression pump treatments may be necessary to achieve optimal control of the lymphedema. It is particularly important that patients with cardiac or renal dysfunction be monitored for fluid overload. After this initial period of intensive therapy, the patients are fitted with high-quality compression garments to maintain the limb volume. Maintenance sessions are then prescribed for the patients on an as-needed basis.

Drug Therapy

Benzopyrones have attracted interest as potentially effective agents in the treatment of lymphedema. This class of medications including coumarin (1,2-benzopyrone) is thought to reduce lymphedema through stimulation of proteolysis by tissue macrophages and stimulation of the peristalsis and pumping action of the collecting lymphatics. Benzopyrones have no anticoagulant activity. The first randomized, crossover trial of coumarin in patients with lymphedema of the arms and legs was reported in 1993.[25] The study concluded that coumarin was more effective than placebo in reducing not only volume but other important parameters, including skin temperature, attacks of secondary acute inflammation, and discomfort of the lymphedematous extremities; skin turgor and suppleness were improved with coumarin. A second randomized, crossover trial was reported in 1999.[26] This study focused on effects of coumarin in women with secondary lymphedema after treatment of breast cancer. The trial investigators found that coumarin was not effective therapy for the specific group of women. Because of the disagreement between these two major trials, coumarins are not recommended for lymphedema treatment.

Diuretics may temporarily improve the appearance of the lymphedematous extremity with stage I disease, leading patients to request continuous therapy. However, other than producing temporary intravascular volume depletion, there is no long-term benefit as lymphedema fluid is not in the vascular space. Thus, diuretics have no role in the treatment of lymphedema at any stage.

Molecular Lymphangiogenesis

Fundamental discoveries in lymphatic development have pointed to the potential of exciting new treatments for lymphedema. These molecular treatments are based on the activation of the VEGFR-3 pathway by administration of cognate ligands VEGF-C and VEGF-D using a variety of methods.[27] At this point, these treatments have been tested only in animal models, with promising results. Formal clinical trials are now needed to evaluate the therapeutic potential and possible untoward effects (including the possibility of stimulation of dormant tumor cells as a consequence of increased angiogenesis) of therapeutic lymphangiogenesis.[28]

Operative Treatment

Ninety-five percent of patients with lymphedema can be managed nonoperatively. Surgical intervention may be considered for patients with stage II or stage III lymphedema who have severe functional impairment, recurrent episodes of lymphangitis, and severe pain despite optimal medical therapy. Two main categories of operations are available for the care of patients with lymphedema: reconstructive and excisional.

Reconstructive operations[29,30] should be considered for those patients with proximal (either primary or secondary) obstruction of the extremity lymphatic circulation with preserved, dilated lymphatics peripheral to the obstruction. In these patients, the residual dilated lymphatics can be anastomosed either to nearby veins or to transposed healthy lymphatic channels (usually mobilized or harvested from the healthy lower extremity) in an attempt to restore effective drainage of the lymphedematous extremity (Fig. 66.4). Some of the most common candidates for reconstructive procedures are patients with upper extremity lymphedema secondary to axillary lymphadenectomy or patients with leg lymphedema secondary to inguinal or pelvic lymphadenectomy. Treatment of selected lymphedema patients with lymphovenous anastomoses or lymphovenous bypass or lymphaticolymphatic bypass has resulted in objective improvement in 30% to 80% of the patients, with an average initial reduction in the excess limb volume of 30% to 84%.[31–34]

Excisional operations are essentially the only viable option for patients without residual lymphatics of adequate size for reconstructive procedures. For patients with recalcitrant stage II and early stage III lymphedema in whom the edema is moderate and the skin is relatively healthy, an excisional procedure that removes a large segment of the lymphedematous subcutaneous tissues and overlying skin is the procedure of choice. This palliative procedure was introduced by Kontoleon in 1918 and was later popularized by Homan as "staged subcutaneous excision underneath flaps" (Fig. 66.5). The operative approach starts with a medial incision extending from the level of the medial malleolus through the calf into the midthigh.[35,36] Flaps about 1 to 2 cm thick are elevated anteriorly and posteriorly, and all subcutaneous tissue beneath the flaps along with the underlying medial calf deep fascia is removed with the redundant skin. The sural nerve is preserved. After the first-stage procedure is completed and if additional lymphedematous tissue removal is necessary, a second operation is performed usually 3 to 6 months later. The second-stage operation is performed by similar techniques through an incision on the lateral aspect of the limb. In a recent long-term follow-up study, 80% of patients undergoing staged subcutaneous excision underneath flaps had significant and long-lasting reduction in extremity size associated with improved function and extremity contour. Wound complications were encountered in 10% of the patients.[35]

A minimally invasive version of the Kontoleon procedure is gaining increasing support among lymphedema experts.[37,38] A number of reports have demonstrated that use of liposuction through small incisions is safe and is able to achieve control, at least on a short-term basis, of clinically disabling conditions associated with advanced stages of lymphedema. Surgeons with experience in this technique recommend initial conservative treatment of pitting lymphedema to remove excess fluid, followed by liposuction to remove remaining excess volume bothersome to the patient.[38]

When the lymphedema is extremely pronounced and the skin is unhealthy and infected, the simple reducing operation of Kontoleon is not adequate. In this case, the classic excisional operation originally described by Charles in 1912 is performed (Fig. 66.6). The procedure involves complete and circumferential excision of the skin, subcutaneous tissue, and deep fascia of the involved leg and dorsum of the foot.[39] The excision is usually performed in one stage, and coverage is provided preferably by full-thickness grafting from the excised skin. In a follow-up report, patients subjected to the Charles operation had immediate volume and circumference reduction. Skin graft take was 88%, and complications of the operation consisted primarily of wound infections, hematomas, and necrosis of skin flaps. The hospital stay was 21 to 36 days.[40] Although this is a successful and radically reducing operation, the behavior in the healing skin graft is unpredictable. Between 10% and 15% of the grafted segments do not take and can be difficult to manage because of frequent localized sloughing, excessive scarring, focal recurrent infections, and hyperkeratosis or dermatitis. These complications seem to be worse in patients in whom leg resurfacing is performed with split-thickness grafts from the opposite extremity. In advanced cases, the exophytic changes within the grafted skin, chronic cellulitis, and skin breakdown may eventually lead to leg amputation.[41]

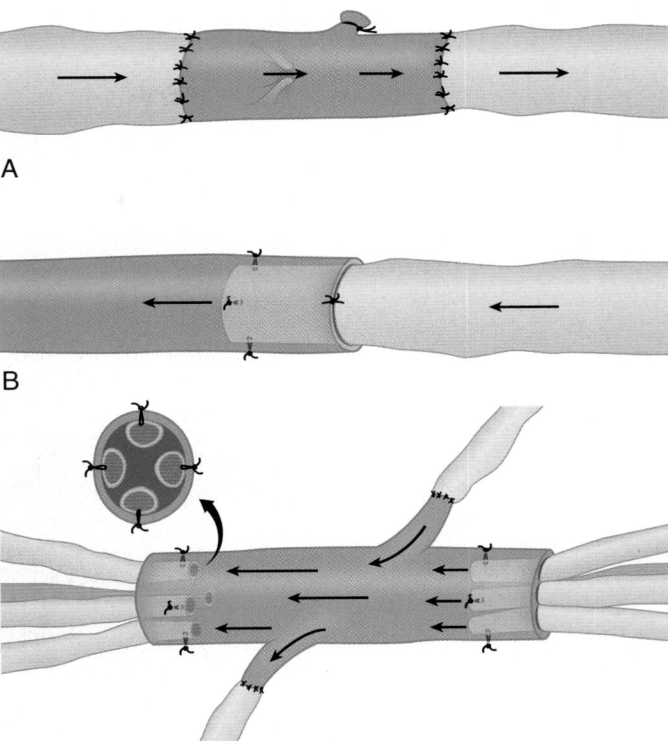

FIG. 66.4 Lymphatic reconstruction techniques with a venous interposition graft (A), a lymphovenous anastomosis (B), and invagination of multiple lymphatics into a vein graft (C). (From Campisi C, Boccardo F, Tacchella M. Reconstructive microsurgery of lymph vessels: The personal method of lymphatic-venous-lymphatic (LVL) interpositioned grafted shunt. *Microsurgery*. 1995;16:161–166.)

CHYLOTHORAX

Chylous pleural effusion is usually secondary to thoracic duct trauma (usually iatrogenic after chest surgery) and rarely a manifestation of advanced malignant disease with lymphatic metastasis.[42] Presence of chylomicrons on lipoprotein analysis and a triglyceride level of more than 110 mg/dL in the pleural fluid are diagnostic. Initially, patients can be treated nonoperatively with tube thoracostomy, medium-chain triglyceride diet or total

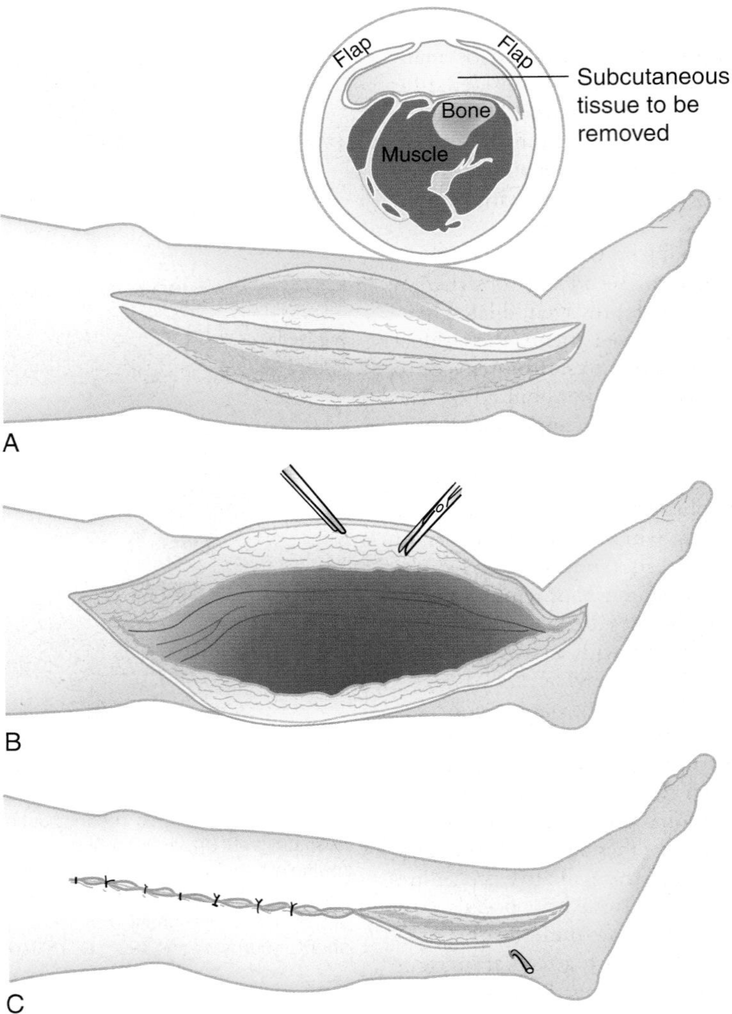

FIG. 66.5 (A–C) Schematic representation of the Kontoleon or Homan procedure. Relatively thick skin flaps are raised anteriorly and posteriorly, and all subcutaneous tissue beneath the flaps and the underlying medial calf deep fascia are removed along with the necessary redundant skin.

parenteral nutrition, and octreotide/somatostatin therapy.[43] For patients with thoracic duct injury and an effusion that persists after 1 week of treatment with appropriate diet, octreotide, and thoracostomy drainage, an intervention should be considered to identify and to occlude the thoracic duct above and below the leak. The operative approach of choice has been video-assisted thoracoscopy or thoracotomy to identify and to ligate the thoracic duct above and below the leak (the site of the leak can be identified if heavy cream is given to the patient a few hours before operation). However, a new endoluminal technique has been introduced and is becoming the optimal first approach for the management of persistent postoperative chylothorax. The approach starts with lymphangiography, usually through a groin lymph node access, to identify the location and anatomy of the cisterna chyli and the location of the divided thoracic duct. Once the cisterna chyli is opacified, it is percutaneously accessed with a spinal needle, using radiographic guidance, and is catheterized. The location of the divided thoracic duct is then identified with repeated lymphangiography, and the duct is embolized. In expert hands, this technique has a more than 50% success rate.[44,45] For patients with cancer-related chylothorax and persistent drainage despite optimal chemotherapy and radiation therapy, pleurodesis is highly successful in preventing recurrences.

CHYLOPERITONEUM

In contrast to chylothorax, the most common cause of chylous ascites is congenital lymphatic abnormalities in children and malignant disease involving the abdominal lymph nodes in adults. Postoperative injury to abdominal lymphatics resulting in chylous ascites is rare.[46] Presence of chylomicrons on lipoprotein analysis and a triglyceride level of more than 110 mg/dL are diagnostic. Initial treatment includes paracentesis followed by medium-chain triglyceride diet or total parenteral nutrition. In patients with postoperative chyloperitoneum, if ascites does not respond after 1 to 2 weeks of nonoperative management, percutaneous embolization[44,45] or surgical exploration should be employed to identify and to occlude or ligate the leaking lymphatic duct. Congenital and malignant causes should be given longer periods (up to 4–6 weeks) of nonoperative management. If ascites persists in patients with congenital ascites, lymphoscintigraphy or lymphangiography is performed before an attempt is made to control the leak with laparotomy or laparoscopy. At the time of exploration, control of the leak can be achieved by ligation of leaking lymphatic vessels or resection of the bowel associated with the leak. Patients with malignant neoplasms should receive aggressive management for their underlying disease, which generally is effective at controlling the chyloperitoneum.

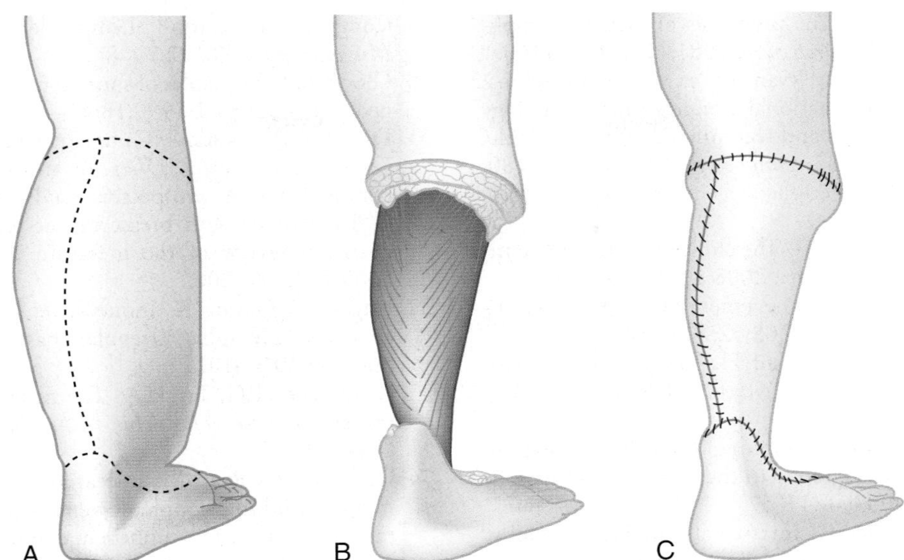

FIG. 66.6 (A–C) Schematic representation of the Charles procedure. It involves complete and circumferential excision of the skin, subcutaneous tissue, and deep fascia of the involved leg and dorsum of the foot. Coverage is provided preferably by full-thickness grafting from the excised skin.

TUMORS OF THE LYMPHATICS

Lymphangiomas are the lymphatic analogue of the hemangiomas of blood vessels. They are generally divided into two types, (1) simple or capillary lymphangioma and (2) cavernous lymphangioma or cystic hygroma.[47] They are thought to represent isolated and sequestered segments of the lymphatic system that retain the ability to produce lymph. As the volume of lymph inside the cystic tumor increases, it grows larger within the surrounding tissues. The majority of these benign tumors are present at birth, and 90% of them can be identified by the end of the first year of life. The cavernous lymphangiomas almost invariably occur in the neck or the axilla and very rarely in the retroperitoneum. The simple capillary lymphangiomas also tend to occur subcutaneously in the head and neck region as well as in the axilla. Rarely, however, they can be found in the trunk within the internal organs or the connective tissue in and about the abdominal or thoracic cavities. The treatment of lymphangiomas should be surgical excision, with care taken to preserve all normal surrounding infiltrated structures.

Lymphangiosarcoma, or Stewart Treves syndrome, is a rare tumor that develops as a complication of long-standing (usually more than 10 years) lymphedema.[48] Clinically, the patients present with acute worsening of the edema and appearance of subcutaneous nodules that have a propensity toward hemorrhage and ulceration. The tumor can be treated, like other sarcomas, with preoperative chemotherapy and radiation followed by surgical excision, which usually may take the form of radical amputation. Overall, the tumor has a very poor prognosis.[49]

SELECTED REFERENCES

Campisi CC, Ryan M, Boccardo F, et al. A single-site technique of multiple lymphatic-venous anastomoses for the treatment of peripheral lymphedema: long-term clinical outcome. *J Reconstr Microsurg*. 2016;32:42–49.

Granzow JW, Soderberg JM, Kaji AH, et al. Review of current surgical treatments for lymphedema. *Ann Surg Oncol.* 2014;21:1195–1201.

These comprehensive reviews summarize the important elements in the surgical management of patients with lymphedema.

Rockson SG. Diagnosis and management of lymphatic vascular disease. *J Am Coll Cardiol.* 2008;52:799–806.

Rockson SG. Update on the biology and treatment of lymphedema. *Curr Treat Options Cardiovasc Med.* 2012;14:184–192.

These two reviews focus on the current knowledge and controversies in the pathophysiology, classification, natural history, differential diagnosis, and treatment of primary and secondary lymphedema.

Rockson SG. Lymphedema: evaluation and decision making. In: Sidawy AN, Perler BA, eds. *Rutherford's Vascular Surgery and Endovascular Therapy*. 9th ed. Philadelphia, PA: Elsevier; 2019:2193–2205.

This authoritative text provides a succinct summary of the evaluation of lymphatic disorders.

REFERENCES

1. Levine C. Primary disorders of the lymphatic vessels--a unified concept. *J Pediatr Surg*. 1989;24:233–240.
2. Alitalo K, Tammela T, Petrova TV. Lymphangiogenesis in development and human disease. *Nature*. 2005;438:946–953.
3. Mortimer PS, Rockson SG. New developments in clinical aspects of lymphatic disease. *J Clin Invest*. 2014;124:915–921.
4. Connell FC, Gordon K, Brice G, et al. The classification and diagnostic algorithm for primary lymphatic dysplasia: an update from 2010 to include molecular findings. *Clin Genet*. 2013;84:303–314.
5. Mishima T, Ito Y, Nishizawa N, et al. RAMP1 signaling improves lymphedema and promotes lymphangiogenesis in mice. *J Surg Res*. 2017;219:50–60.
6. Dixon JB. Lymphatic lipid transport: sewer or subway. *Trends Endocrinol Metab*. 2010;21:480–487.
7. Browse NL, Stewart G. Lymphoedema: pathophysiology and classification. *J Cardiovasc Surg (Torino)*. 1985;26:91–106.

8. Wolfe JH, Kinmonth JB. The prognosis of primary lymphedema of the lower limbs. *Arch Surg*. 1981;116:1157–1160.
9. Casley-Smith JR, Foldi M, Ryan TJ, et al. Lymphedema: summary of the 10th International Congress of Lymphology Working Group discussions and recommendations, Adelaide, Australia, August 10-17:1985. *Lymphology*. 1985;18:175–180.
10. Cho S, Atwood JE. Peripheral edema. *Am J Med*. 2002;113:580–586.
11. Radhakrishnan K, Rockson SG. The clinical spectrum of lymphatic disease. *Ann N Y Acad Sci*. 2008;1131:155–184.
12. Rockson SG. Diagnosis and management of lymphatic vascular disease. *J Am Coll Cardiol*. 2008;52:799–806.
13. Barrett T, Choyke PL, Kobayashi H. Imaging of the lymphatic system: New horizons. *Contrast Media Mol Imaging*. 2006;1:230–245.
14. Szuba A, Shin WS, Strauss HW, et al. The third circulation: radionuclide lymphoscintigraphy in the evaluation of lymphedema. *J Nucl Med*. 2003;44:43–57.
15. Weissleder H, Weissleder R. Interstitial lymphangiography: initial clinical experience with a dimeric nonionic contrast agent. *Radiology*. 1989;170:371–374.
16. Liu NF, Lu Q, Jiang ZH, et al. Anatomic and functional evaluation of the lymphatics and lymph nodes in diagnosis of lymphatic circulation disorders with contrast magnetic resonance lymphangiography. *J Vasc Surg*. 2009;49:980–987.
17. Rockson SG. Current concepts and future directions in the diagnosis and management of lymphatic vascular disease. *Vasc Med*. 2010;15:223–231.
18. The diagnosis and treatment of peripheral lymphedema. 2009 Concensus Document of the International Society of Lymphology. *Lymphology*. 2009;42:51–60.
19. Kerchner K, Fleischer A, Yosipovitch G. Lower extremity lymphedema update: pathophysiology, diagnosis, and treatment guidelines. *J Am Acad Dermatol*. 2008;59:324–331.
20. Yasuhara H, Shigematsu H, Muto T. A study of the advantages of elastic stockings for leg lymphedema. *Int Angiol*. 1996;15:272–277.
21. Badger CM, Peacock JL, Mortimer PS. A randomized, controlled, parallel-group clinical trial comparing multilayer bandaging followed by hosiery versus hosiery alone in the treatment of patients with lymphedema of the limb. *Cancer*. 2000;88:2832–2837.
22. Franzeck UK, Spiegel I, Fischer M, et al. Combined physical therapy for lymphedema evaluated by fluorescence microlymphography and lymph capillary pressure measurements. *J Vasc Res*. 1997;34:306–311.
23. Ko DS, Lerner R, Klose G, et al. Effective treatment of lymphedema of the extremities. *Arch Surg*. 1998;133:452–458.
24. Richmand DM, O'Donnell Jr TF, Zelikovski A. Sequential pneumatic compression for lymphedema. A controlled trial. *Arch Surg*. 1985;120:1116–1119.
25. Casley-Smith JR, Morgan RG, Piller NB. Treatment of lymphedema of the arms and legs with 5,6-benzo-[alpha]-pyrone. *N Engl J Med*. 1993;329:1158–1163.
26. Loprinzi CL, Kugler JW, Sloan JA, et al. Lack of effect of coumarin in women with lymphedema after treatment for breast cancer. *N Engl J Med*. 1999;340:346–350.
27. Nakamura K, Rockson SG. Molecular targets for therapeutic lymphangiogenesis in lymphatic dysfunction and disease. *Lymphat Res Biol*. 2008;6:181–189.
28. Tervala T, Suominen E, Saaristo A. Targeted treatment for lymphedema and lymphatic metastasis. *Ann N Y Acad Sci*. 2008;1131:215–224.
29. Campisi C, Boccardo F. Lymphedema and microsurgery. *Microsurgery*. 2002;22:74–80.
30. Gloviczki P. Principles of surgical treatment of chronic lymphoedema. *Int Angiol*. 1999;18:42–46.
31. Damstra RJ, Voesten HG, van Schelven WD, et al. Lymphatic venous anastomosis (LVA) for treatment of secondary arm lymphedema. A prospective study of 11 LVA procedures in 10 patients with breast cancer related lymphedema and a critical review of the literature. *Breast Cancer Res Treat*. 2009;113:199–206.
32. Nagase T, Gonda K, Inoue K, et al. Treatment of lymphedema with lymphaticovenular anastomoses. *Int J Clin Oncol*. 2005;10:304–310.
33. Baumeister RG, Frick A. The microsurgical lymph vessel transplantation. *Handchir Mikrochir Plast Chir*. 2003;35:202–209.
34. Campisi CC, Ryan M, Boccardo F, et al. A single-site technique of multiple lymphatic-venous anastomoses for the treatment of peripheral lymphedema: long-term clinical outcome. *J Reconstr Microsurg*. 2016;32:42–49.
35. Miller TA, Wyatt LE, Rudkin GH. Staged skin and subcutaneous excision for lymphedema: a favorable report of long-term results. *Plast Reconstr Surg*. 1998;102:1486–1498; discussion 1499–1501.
36. Wyatt LE, Miller TA. Lymphedema and tumors of the lymphatics. In: Moore W, ed. *Vascular Surgery, A Comprehensive Review*. Philadelphia, PA: WB Saunders; 1998:829–843.
37. Espinosa-de-Los-Monteros A, Hinojosa CA, Abarca L, et al. Compression therapy and liposuction of lower legs for bilateral hereditary primary lymphedema praecox. *J Vasc Surg*. 2009;49:222–224.
38. Brorson H, Ohlin K, Olsson G, et al. Controlled compression and liposuction treatment for lower extremity lymphedema. *Lymphology*. 2008;41:52–63.
39. Dellon AL, Hoopes JE. The Charles procedure for primary lymphedema. Long-term clinical results. *Plast Reconstr Surg*. 1977;60:589–595.
40. Dandapat MC, Mohapatro SK, Mohanty SS. Filarial lymphoedema and elephantiasis of lower limb: a review of 44 cases. *Br J Surg*. 1986;73:451–453.
41. Miller TA. Charles procedure for lymphedema: a warning. *Am J Surg*. 1980;139:290–292.
42. Platis IE, Nwogu CE. Chylothorax. Thorac Surg. *Clin*. 2006;16:209–214.
43. Bender B, Murthy V, Chamberlain RS. The changing management of chylothorax in the modern era. *Eur J Cardiothorac Surg*. 2016;49:18–24.
44. Lee EW, Shin JH, Ko HK, et al. Lymphangiography to treat postoperative lymphatic leakage: a technical review. *Korean J Radiol*. 2014;15:724–732.
45. Lyon S, Mott N, Koukounaras J, et al. Role of interventional radiology in the management of chylothorax: a review of the current management of high output chylothorax. *Cardiovasc Intervent Radiol*. 2013;36:599–607.
46. Aalami OO, Allen DB, Organ Jr CH. Chylous ascites: a collective review. *Surgery*. 2000;128:761–778.
47. Ha J, Yu YC, Lannigan F. A review of the management of lymphangiomas. *Curr Pediatr Rev*. 2014;10:238–248.
48. Nakazono T, Kudo S, Matsuo Y, et al. Angiosarcoma associated with chronic lymphedema (Stewart-Treves syndrome) of the leg: MR imaging. *Skeletal Radiol*. 2000;29:413–416.
49. Sordillo PP, Chapman R, Hajdu SI, et al. Lymphangiosarcoma. *Cancer*. 1981;48:1674–1679.

SECTION XIII

Specialties in General Surgery

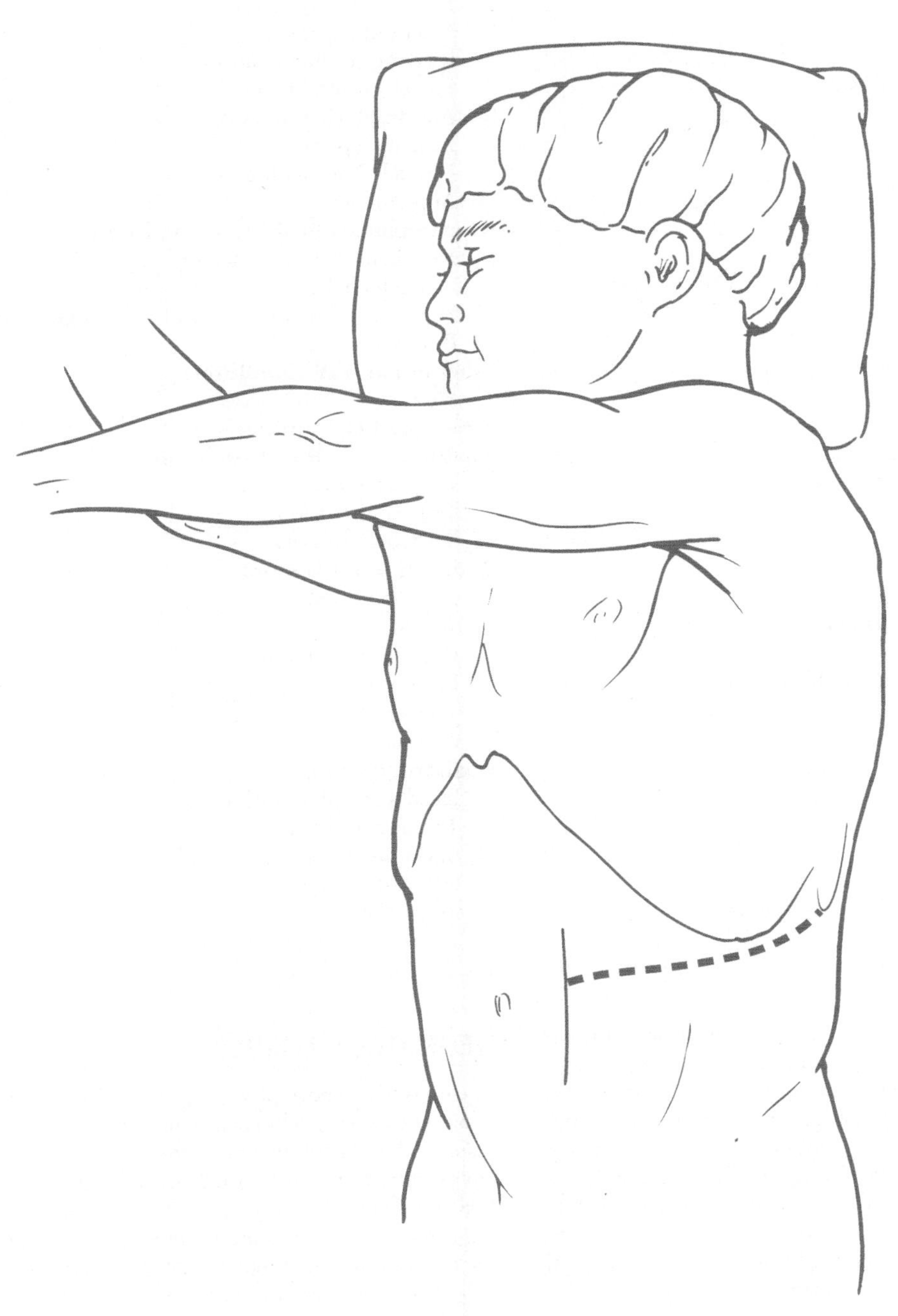

67 CHAPTER

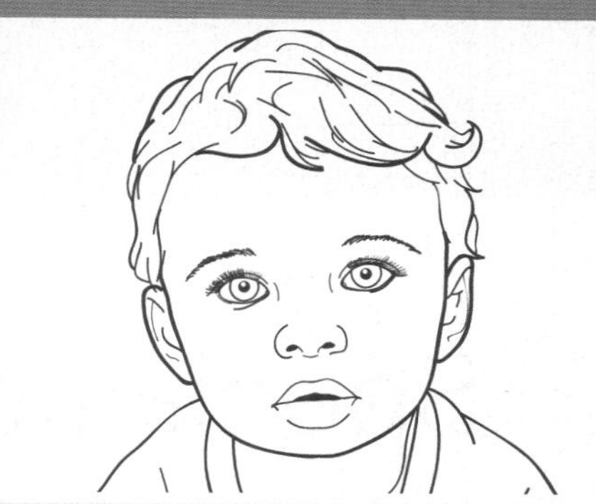

Pediatric Surgery

Dai H. Chung

OUTLINE

Despite the ever-evolving field of pediatric surgery, it remains the last bastion of true general surgery. Pediatric surgical conditions span prenatal (fetal) and neonatal to adolescent and young adult age groups. Pediatric surgeons must assess and manage a wide spectrum of surgical conditions with vastly different pathophysiology. Pediatric surgery covers a wide spectrum of organ systems, ranging from head and neck to thoracic and the gastrointestinal (GI) tract, and conditions such as congenital anomalies, solid tumors, and pediatric trauma. This chapter provides an overview of common and unique pediatric surgical conditions, their pathophysiology, and treatment strategies.

NEONATAL PHYSIOLOGY

The unique newborn physiology stems in part from the smaller size of patients and the cellular and functional immaturity of their organ systems. Newborns are at risk for cold stress, and an ideal thermal environment must be maintained to reduce oxygen consumption and metabolic demands. Isolates in nurseries and warm operating rooms serve to maintain thermogenesis. The major risk factors for hypothermia in infants are their relatively large body surface area to body weight and subcutaneous tissue and greater insensible fluid losses. Infants also respond to cooler ambient temperature by nonshivering thermogenesis, whereby increases in metabolism and oxygen consumption occur. The use of overhead radiant heaters is also common in the operating rooms, where an ideal ambient temperature (~23°C) is kept in order to maintain a neonate's core body temperature between 36°C and 37.5°C.

Cardiopulmonary

During fetal circulation, arterial blood from the placenta bypasses the fetal lungs through the patent foramen ovale and ductus arteriosus. After birth, the foramen ovale closes with the newborn's first breath, then a precipitous drop in pulmonary vascular resistance occurs, thereby increasing pulmonary blood flow. Decreased blood flow, along with a higher oxygen content, promotes spontaneous closure of the ductus arteriosus. Nonsteroidal antiinflammatory drugs (e.g., indomethacin) can promote closure of a patent ductus arteriosus, particularly in premature infants. If persistently open, patent ductus arteriosus closure is achieved via open minithoracotomy or a catheter-based coil procedure. An increase in pulmonary vascular resistance can be caused by hypoxemia and acidosis, resulting in persistent pulmonary hypertension (PPHN) and a right-to-left shunt. Nitric oxide gas, a potent inducer of vascular smooth muscle relaxation, is effective against PPHN.

The infant heart has a limited capacity to increase the stroke volume; therefore, cardiac output is largely heart rate-dependent. As such, heart rate change is a sensitive indicator of intravascular volume status. Capillary refill is a sensitive indicator of adequate tissue perfusion. A prolonged capillary refill (>2 seconds) may represent substantial shunting of blood from the peripheral tissues to the central organs, which may occur with cardiogenic or hypovolemic shock.

The respiratory rate for a normal newborn ranges from 40 to 60 breaths/min, with a tidal volume of 6 to 10 mL/kg. Nasal flaring, grunting, intercostal and substernal retractions, and cyanosis are symptoms and signs of respiratory distress. Infants are obligate nasal and diaphragmatic breathers, and therefore any condition that obstructs the nasal passages (e.g., nasogastric tube) or interferes with diaphragmatic function may severely compromise respiratory status. In addition, the newborn airway is quite small, with an average tracheal diameter of 2.5 to 4 mm, and it can easily be plugged with airway secretions.

At birth, the lungs are considered functionally immature and continue to develop new terminal bronchioles and alveoli until 6 to 8 years of age. The neonatal lung has fewer type II pneumocytes, which produce surfactant, a lipoprotein mixture of phospholipid, protein, and neutral fats. Surfactant regulates alveolar surface tension, thereby increasing functional residual capacity. Lecithin, the most predominant phospholipid, can be measured in amniotic fluid, and the lecithin-to-sphingomyelin ratio is used to determine fetal lung maturity. Hence, premature infants are at greater risk for alveolar collapse, hyaline membrane formation, and barotrauma from mechanical ventilatory support. Exogenous surfactant therapy has had a major impact on the management of premature infants. This has resulted in improved survival and decreased incidence of bronchopulmonary dysplasia, a condition characterized by oxygen dependence, radiologic abnormality, and chronic respiratory symptoms beyond the first 28 days of life.

Immunology

Infants have lower levels of immunoglobulins (IgA, IgG, and IgM) and of the C3b complement at birth and therefore are at higher risk for systemic infection. Sepsis work-up for neonates has largely remained the same with surveillance cultures, including cerebrospinal fluid, and complete blood count as well as C-reactive protein levels. Infants are also at risk for potential septic sources arising from invasive monitoring lines and interventions such as prolonged endotracheal intubation, umbilical vascular catheters, and bladder catheterization. An empirical antibiotic regimen is often started based on subtle clinical suspicions (e.g., decreased tolerance of enteral feeding, temperature instability, reduced capillary refill, tachypnea, irritability). Antibiotic therapy is targeted at common bacterial pathogens, such as Group B beta-hemolytic streptococcus, methicillin-resistant *Staphylococcus aureus,* and *Escherichia coli.*

FLUIDS, ELECTROLYTES, AND NUTRITION

Fluid and Electrolytes

Fluid and electrolyte balance must be carefully assessed in pediatric surgical patients, especially in smaller neonates with a narrow margin for error. Due to higher insensible water losses through a thin immature skin barrier, fluid requirements for premature infants can be substantial. Insensible water losses are directly related to gestational age, which range from 45 to 60 mL/kg/day for premature infants weighing less than 1500 g to 30 to 35 mL/kg/day for term infants. Radiant heat warmers, phototherapy for hyperbilirubinemia, and respiratory distress can result in additional fluid losses. During the first 3 to 5 days of life, physiologic water loss can total up to 10% of the body weight. Fluid requirements are calculated according to body weight. During the first few days of life, the fluid recommendations are on the conservative side; however, infants require 100 to 130 mL/kg/day for maintenance fluids by the fourth day of life. Surgical conditions such as gastroschisis and necrotizing enterocolitis (NEC) demand a significantly higher volume. Urine output and osmolarity are good indicators of adequate tissue perfusion. The ideal minimum urine output in a newborn is 1 to 2 mL/kg/day. Infants can respond to prerenal azotemia by concentrating urine only up to approximately 700 mOsm/kg. The daily requirements for sodium and potassium are 2 to 4 and 1 to 2 mEq/kg, respectively. These requirements are usually met with 5% dextrose in 0.45% normal saline with 20 mEq/L of potassium at the calculated maintenance rate. Fluid losses from gastric drainage, ostomy output, or diarrhea should also be carefully assessed and replaced with an appropriate solution. Gastric losses should be replaced in equal volumes with 0.45% normal saline with 20 mEq/L of potassium. Diarrheal, pancreatic, and biliary losses are replaced with isotonic lactated Ringer solution. Hypovolemia due to acute hemorrhage should be corrected with prompt transfusion of blood products at a bolus of 10 to 20 mL/kg of packed red blood cells, plasma, or 5% albumin.

Nutrition

Energy requirements vary substantially from infancy to childhood and also under different clinical conditions. Appropriate weight gain remains the most reliable crude indicator of adequate caloric intake. Total daily caloric requirements and the weight curve plateau with age. Nearly 50% of the energy in term infants younger than 2 weeks and 60% of energy in premature infants weighing less than 1200 g is consumed for growth. A general guideline for the enteral calorie requirement of infants is 120 calories/kg/day to achieve an ideal weight gain of ~1% of body weight per day. Breast milk and standard infant formulas contain 20 calories/ounce. Formulas with higher calorie density are available for those who are unable to consume sufficient volumes to meet their calorie requirements or those with strict fluid restriction. Breast milk is the ideal form of enteral nutrition. However, hypoallergenic, lactose-free to amino-acid-based formulas are available to meet the specific needs of infants with particular GI tract conditions.

In general, infants with a stressed gut are given continuous enteral feedings and then transitioned to gastric bolus feedings. Toleration of enteral feeding is carefully monitored by assessing for abdominal girth, gastric residuals, and stool output.

Carbohydrates are stored mainly as glycogen in the liver and muscles. Because newborn liver and muscle mass is disproportionately smaller than that of adults, infants are susceptible to hypoglycemia with risks of seizure and neurologic impairment. The minimum glucose infusion rate for neonates is 4 to 6 mg/kg/min. This rate must be calculated daily while the infant is receiving parenteral nutrition. For total parenteral nutrition (TPN), the glucose infusion rate is increased daily in increments of 1 to 2 mg/kg/min to a maximum value of 10 to 12 mg/kg/min. Hyperglycemia from a less than ideal glucose infusion rate should be avoided because it can lead to rapid hyperosmolarity and dehydration. Hyperglycemia could also reflect an underlying sepsis and therefore, should be investigated.

The average protein intake is ~15% of total daily calories and ranges from 2 to 3.5 g/kg/day in infants. By 12 years of age, this protein requirement is reduced in half and approaches the adult requirement (1 g/kg/day) by 18 years of age. The provision of greater amounts of protein relative to nonprotein (carbohydrate plus fat) calories will result in rising blood urea nitrogen levels, resulting in a nonprotein calorie-to-protein calorie ratio (when expressed in grams of nitrogen) greater than 150:1. For infants receiving parenteral nutrition, protein administration usually starts at 0.5 g/kg/day and advances in daily increments of 0.5 g/kg/day to a target goal of approximately 3.5 g/kg/day.

Fat is a major source of nonprotein calories. Linoleic acid, an 18-carbon chain with two double bonds, is considered an essential fatty acid, and its deficiency results in dryness, rash, and desquamation of skin. In pediatric patients, fat is provided as a major source of calories to prevent the development of essential fatty acid deficiency. The lipid requirements for growth are significant, and fat is a robust calorie source. Similar to protein, fat infusions are started at 0.5 g/kg/day and advanced up to 2.5 to 3.5 g/kg/day. In infants with unconjugated hyperbilirubinemia, fat is administered with caution because fatty acids may displace bilirubin from albumin. The free unconjugated bilirubin may then cross the blood-brain barrier and can lead to kernicterus, resulting in mental retardation.

TPN is reserved for infants for whom adequate daily enteral nutrition cannot be achieved. Infants only have energy reserve to withstand periods of starvation as few as 2 to 3 days. Thus, an infant's need for parenteral nutrition should be addressed promptly. The total TPN infusion rate is kept at a steady-state to meet daily fluid requirements, and the concentration of nutrients is gradually increased daily until goals are met. Infants with surgical conditions often become cholestatic, typically caused by prolonged TPN support, however, other causes should be ruled out. Serum bile acid levels are usually elevated first, then direct bilirubin concentration, followed by liver enzyme levels. The ideal treatment for TPN-associated cholestasis is restoring enteral feeding. The use of omega-3 fat emulsion (Omegaven) has been critical in preventing TPN-induced cholestasis.[1] A medium-chain triglyceride–containing formula is used, and if an infant is receiving total enteral nutrition, fat-soluble vitamins should be supplemented.

HEAD AND NECK LESIONS

Dermoid and Epidermoid Cysts

Dermoid and epidermoid cysts are slow-growing benign lesions that typically occur in the scalp and the skull. These cysts usually arise from part of the dermal or epidermal tissues, forming a small cyst filled with normal skin components. Dermoid cysts may contain hair, teeth, and skin glands. Epidermoid cysts typically have only epidermal tissue and keratin debris. They commonly occur on the forehead, lateral corner of the eyebrow, anterior fontanelle or in the postauricular space. They are generally asymptomatic but may increase in size over time and can often become osteolytic. Most scalp lesions require only the clinical exam for diagnosis and subsequent surgical excision. However, imaging studies (e.g., ultrasound) can be critical to identify midline lesions such as a communicating cephalocele.

Lymphadenopathy

Enlarged lymph nodes presenting as small, mobile, discrete clusters in the anterior cervical triangle are one of the most common conditions referred for a pediatric surgical evaluation, biopsy, or possible excision. They usually occur along the sternocleidomastoid muscle border, often in clusters. The exact cause is unknown but presumed to be multifocal. A detailed history and physical examination are sufficient to determine whether surgery is indicated. The use of ultrasound has become widely prevalent and can, at times, identify those nodes with central necrosis requiring surgical intervention. Occasionally, lymph nodes presenting as fixed, nontender, progressively enlarging nodes in the supraclavicular region should raise a suspicion for a serious underlying etiology. Constitutional symptoms such as night sweats and weight loss should prompt a thorough investigation with chest radiography, which could detect mediastinal adenopathy.

Acute, bilateral cervical lymphadenitis from respiratory viral infections (e.g., adenovirus, influenza virus, respiratory syncytial virus) require observation alone. *S. aureus* and Group A *streptococcus* are responsible for the majority of acute pyogenic lymphadenitis.

Cat-scratch disease is a self-limited infectious condition characterized by painful regional lymphadenopathy. A gram-negative bacillus, *Bartonella henselae,* is responsible for the majority of cases. A history of exposure to cats is helpful but not always present. Indirect immunofluorescent antibody testing has only moderate specificity. Polymerase chain reaction assay of a lymph node biopsy specimen is a more useful study for diagnosis. Cat-scratch disease is usually self-limited. A less common infectious cause of cervical lymphadenitis is nontuberculous mycobacterial infection. The nodes are fluctuant, with a violaceous appearance of the overlying skin. The diagnosis is made by positive cultures for nontuberculous acid-fast bacilli along with a tuberculin skin test. Surgical excision is usually indicated because most nontuberculous mycobacteria are resistant to conventional chemotherapy.

Cystic Hygroma

Cystic hygroma is a multiloculated cyst lined by endothelial cells occurring as a result of lymphatic malformation. Most involve the lymphatic jugular sacs and present in the posterior neck region. Other common sites are the axillary, mediastinal, inguinal, and retroperitoneal regions, and approximately 50% of these cystic lesions are present at birth. Cystic hygromas are soft cystic masses that can distort the surrounding structure, including the airway. A large cystic mass of the neck in the fetus can pose a significant threat to airway at birth. Prenatal ultrasound and fetal magnetic resonance imaging (MRI) studies can better demonstrate the extent of disease along with its mass effect on the airway. If present, a careful coordination of surgical intervention, ex-utero intrapartum treatment (EXIT) procedure, at the time of delivery can be life-saving, though this is more likely with solid tumors such as teratomas. Cystic hygromas are prone to infection and hemorrhage into the mass. MRI is useful in outlining the extent of lymphatic channels. Complete excision with tedious isolation and ligation of lymphatic branches is the surgical goal. Aggressive blunt and electrocautery dissection, as well as radical resection, must be avoided, as this can lead to recurrence or infection due to incomplete control of lymphatics. When a safe, complete surgical excision is not feasible, injection with sclerosing agents, such as bleomycin, doxycycline, or OK-432 derived from *Streptococcus pyogenes*, should be considered as an effective nonsurgical option.[2]

Thyroglossal Duct Cyst

An upper-midline cystic neck lesion in toddlers is a thyroglossal duct cyst until proven otherwise (Fig. 67.1). It originates at the base of the tongue at the foramen cecum and descends through the central portion of the hyoid bone. Although thyroglossal duct cysts may occur anywhere from the base of the tongue to the thyroid gland, most are found at, or just below, the hyoid bone. A thyroid diverticulum develops as a median endodermal thickening at the foramen cecum in the embryonic stage of development. The thyroid diverticulum descends in the neck and remains attached to the base of the tongue by the thyroglossal duct. Also, as the thyroid gland descends to its normal pretracheal position, the ventral cartilage of the second and third branchial arches forms the hyoid bone. Hence, the intimate anatomic relationship of the thyroglossal duct remnant exists with the central portion of the hyoid bone. The thyroglossal duct normally regresses by the time the thyroid gland reaches its final position. When the elements of the duct persist despite complete thyroid descent, a thyroglossal duct cyst may develop. Failure of normal caudal migration of the thyroid gland results in a lingual thyroid in which no other thyroid tissue is present in the neck. Ultrasound or radionuclide imaging may be useful to identify the ectopic thyroid gland in the neck. The Sistrunk procedure, first described in 1928, is the gold standard operation for thyroglossal duct cysts. It involves complete excision of the cyst in continuity with its tract, the central portion of the hyoid bone, and the tract interior to the hyoid bone extending to the base of the tongue. Failure of complete resection results in cyst recurrence in as high as 40% to 50% of cases.

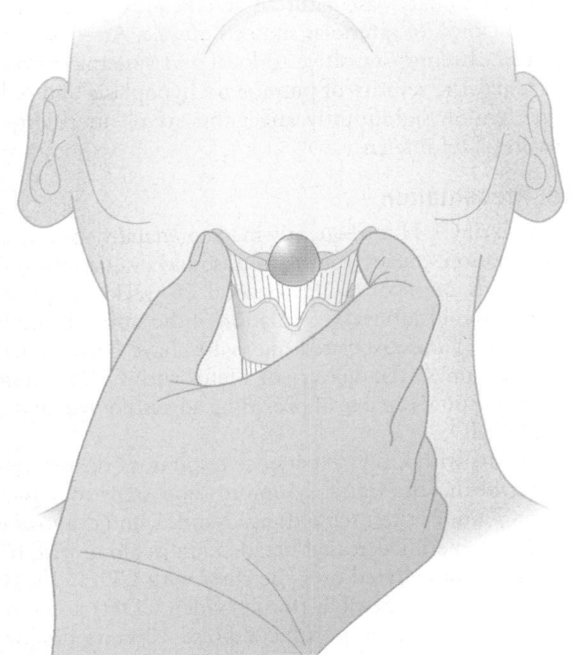

FIG. 67.1 Thyroglossal duct cyst presents as a midline neck mass. Thyroglossal duct cyst can extend up to its origin at the foramen cecum. (From Josephs MD. Thyroglossal duct cyst. In: Chung DH, Chen MK, ed. *Atlas of pediatric surgical techniques*. Philadelphia, PA: Elsevier Saunders; 2010:28–33.)

Branchial Cleft Remnants

Branchial cleft remnants present as lateral neck masses. Embryologically, the structures of the head and neck are derived from six pairs of branchial arches, their intervening clefts, and pouches. Congenital cysts, sinuses, or fistulas result from failure of these structures to regress, persisting in aberrant locations. The location of these remnants generally dictates their embryologic origin and guides the subsequent operative approach. Failure to understand the embryology may result in incomplete resection or injury to adjacent structures. Branchial lesions can manifest as sinuses, fistulas, or cartilaginous rests in infants. The clinical presentation ranges from a continuous mucoid drainage, a fistula or sinus, or an infected cystic mass. Branchial remnants may also be palpable as cartilaginous lumps or cords corresponding with a fistulous track. Dermal pits or skin tags may also be present. First branchial anomalies are typically located in the front or back of the ear, or in the upper neck near the mandible. Fistulas typically course through the parotid gland, deep or through branches of the facial nerve, and end in the external auditory canal. The second branchial cleft anomalies are the most common type. The external ostium of these remnants is located along the anterior border of the sternocleidomastoid muscle, usually in the vicinity of the upper half to lower third of the muscle. A tortuous and long course of the fistula tract can be found, which requires stepladder counter-incisions in order to excise the fistula track completely. Typically, the fistula penetrates the platysma, ascends along the carotid sheath to the level of the hyoid bone, and turns medially to extend between the carotid artery bifurcations. The fistula courses adjacent to the hypoglossal and glossopharyngeal nerves, behind the posterior belly of the digastric and stylohyoid muscles to end in the tonsillar fossa or other nasopharyngeal spaces. Third branchial cleft remnants usually do not have associated sinuses or fistulas and are located in the suprasternal notch or clavicular region and can descend into the mediastinum. They present more commonly as cysts in toddlers and older children. These most often contain cartilage and present clinically as a firm mass or subcutaneous abscess.

EXTRACORPOREAL LIFE SUPPORT

Extracorporeal life support (ECLS) is a cardiopulmonary bypass delivering temporary life support for the critically-ill patient with acute respiratory and/or cardiac failure. ECLS achieves sufficient gas exchange, with carbon dioxide removal and oxygenation of blood to maintain normal circulatory support. Since its first reported neonatal experience in 1976, ECLS has not only become a standard therapeutic option for cardiopulmonary failure that is refractory to maximal medical therapy, but it also has become widely used for a variety of clinical applications, such as extracorporeal cardiopulmonary resuscitation (eCPR). Although the exact role of eCPR in neonatal and pediatric resuscitation remains controversial and yet to be determined, the use of eCPR has become a common practice in many hospitals around the globe.[3] There are over 800 centers around the world contributing registry data to the Extracorporeal Life Support Organization database (ELSO registry data; July 2019).

Indications

The major indications for neonatal extracorporeal membrane oxygenation (ECMO) include meconium aspiration, respiratory distress syndrome, PPHN, sepsis, and congenital diaphragmatic hernia (CDH). Meconium aspiration is the most common application for neonatal ECMO with the highest survival rate (>90%). Indications for neonatal ECMO vary among institutions. In general, ECMO is indicated when an infant's overall cardiopulmonary function deteriorates to a point of ~80% predicted mortality. Two guidelines have been used as predictors for survival without ECMO: the alveolar-arterial difference in the partial pressure of oxygen (PAO_2 – PaO_2 [also known as $AaDO_2$]) and the oxygen index. $AaDO_2$ greater than 610 for longer than 8 to 12 hours and $AaDO_2$ greater than 620 for 6 hours, associated with extensive barotrauma and severe hypotension requiring inotropic support, are considered to be criteria for ECMO. The oxygen index is calculated as the fraction of inspired oxygen (usually 1.0) × mean airway pressure × 100 divided by PaO_2. An 80% mortality is observed with an oxygen index greater than 40. Contraindications are severe prematurity due to a high risk of intracranial bleeding, weight less than 2 kg, presence of an intracranial bleed (grade II intraventricular hemorrhage), and a nonreversible pulmonary disease such as congenital alveolar dysplasia. Additional exclusion criteria include the presence of cyanotic congenital heart disease or major genetic defects that preclude survival, as well as intractable coagulopathy.

Physiology

The right internal jugular vein and common carotid artery are used for venoarterial cannulations because of vessel sizes to accommodate cannulas and collateral circulation. The ECLS circuit is composed of a silicone rubber bladder that collapses when venous return is diminished, roller pump, membrane oxygenator, heat exchanger, tubing, and connectors. The basic principle of ECLS is that desaturated mixed venous blood from the right atrium drains through the venous cannula to the bladder and is pumped to the membrane oxygenator, where carbon dioxide is removed and oxygen is added. The oxygenated blood then passes through the heat exchanger and is returned to the patient through the arterial cannula. Systemic anticoagulation to prevent clotting of the ECLS circuit puts patients at risk for bleeding complications. Indicators of lung recovery include an increasing PaO_2, improved lung compliance, and clearing of the chest radiograph. As the pulmonary function recovers, the patient is trialed off bypass by clamping the cannulas. If tolerated, the patient is taken off ECLS on moderate conventional ventilatory settings. Venovenous bypass using a double-lumen single cannula placed via the right internal jugular vein has the advantage of avoiding carotid arterial cannulation. Often, perfusion of well-oxygenated blood through venovenous ECMO restores hemodynamic stability. In older pediatric, as well as adult, patients, venous cannulas can be placed via both the internal jugular and femoral veins to achieve venovenous ECMO circulation.

Bleeding is the most common complication of ECLS, and it can occur anywhere from catheter sites and surgical sites such as the thoracic cavity to intracranial bleeds. Gestational age is the most significant predictor of intracranial hemorrhage on ECLS, and premature infants less than 34 weeks of gestational age are at highest risk. Other complications include seizures, neurologic impairment, real failure requiring hemofiltration or hemodialysis, hypertension, infection, and mechanical malfunction of membrane oxygenator, pump, and heat exchanger, as well as the cannulas themselves.

DIAPHRAGMATIC CONDITIONS

Congenital Diaphragmatic Hernia

The overall incidence of CDH is 1 in 2000 to 5000 live births. CDH is diagnosed prenatally in most cases and occurs more commonly on the left side (84%); bilateral defects occur but are rare (2%). A hernia sac is present 10% to 15% of the time and must be excised at the time of repair. Despite multimodality treatment strategies, such as fetal tracheal occlusion, ECMO, inhaled nitric oxide, and permissive hypercapnia, the overall survival rate remains at 70% to 90%. True survival data for CDH is somewhat distorted by the fact that infants with more severe CDH are often stillborn, and therefore not captured by the registry. The lung area to head circumference ratio (LHR) is a sonographic predictor of prognosis and is determined by taking the product of the longest two perpendicular linear measurements of the lung contralateral to CDH and is divided by head circumference. An LHR of less than 1 and an abnormal liver position at 24 weeks of gestation are strong predictors of unfavorable outcomes. Fetal MRI is also used at many centers to determine fetal lung volume, as well as ratio of lung to the spinal fluid signal intensity.[4]

Pathogenesis

In the embryo, the pleuroperitoneal cavities become separated by the developing membrane during 8 to 10 weeks of gestation. When the pleuroperitoneal canal persists, it leads to a posterolateral CDH defect. The posterolateral location of this hernia is known as Bochdalek hernia; it is distinguished from a CDH of the anteromedial location known as Morgagni hernia. Abdominal contents herniate into the thoracic cavity through the diaphragmatic defect, compressing the ipsilateral developing lung. These lungs have smaller bronchi, with less bronchial branching and less alveolar surface area. The ipsilateral lung is affected more severely, however, both lungs are affected by pulmonary hypoplasia. In addition, the pulmonary vasculature is significantly affected by the increased thickness of arteriolar smooth muscle. Arteriolar vasculature is also extremely sensitive to local and systemic vasoactive factors. Hence, the severity of pulmonary hypoplasia and pulmonary hypertension significantly affect the overall morbidity and mortality in CDH infants.

Clinical Presentation

The diagnosis of CDH is frequently made prenatally, as early as 15 weeks of gestation, during routine ultrasound evaluation. Infants who have a late onset of CDH (beyond 25 weeks of gestation) have a better overall survival. Herniation of the stomach and liver, polyhydramnios, and associated anomalies have been associated with poor outcomes. The delivery of a fetus with CDH should be planned at a hospital capable of providing advanced neonatal care, including ECMO.

Most infants with CDH experience respiratory distress immediately after birth. The initial symptoms and signs may include grunting respiration, chest retractions, dyspnea, and cyanosis with a scaphoid abdomen. Decreased breath sounds, along with bowel sounds, may be auscultated over the chest with CDH. The shifting of heart sounds to the right (for left-sided CDH) is common. A significant preductal and postductal pulse oximetry differential indicates right-to-left shunting due to PPHN. The chest radiograph demonstrates multiple bowel loops in the thoracic cavity along with mediastinal shift (Fig. 67.2A). The differential diagnosis includes congenital cystic adenomatoid malformation, bronchogenic cyst, diaphragmatic eventration (Fig. 67.2B), and cystic teratoma. Typically, the infant does well for several hours after

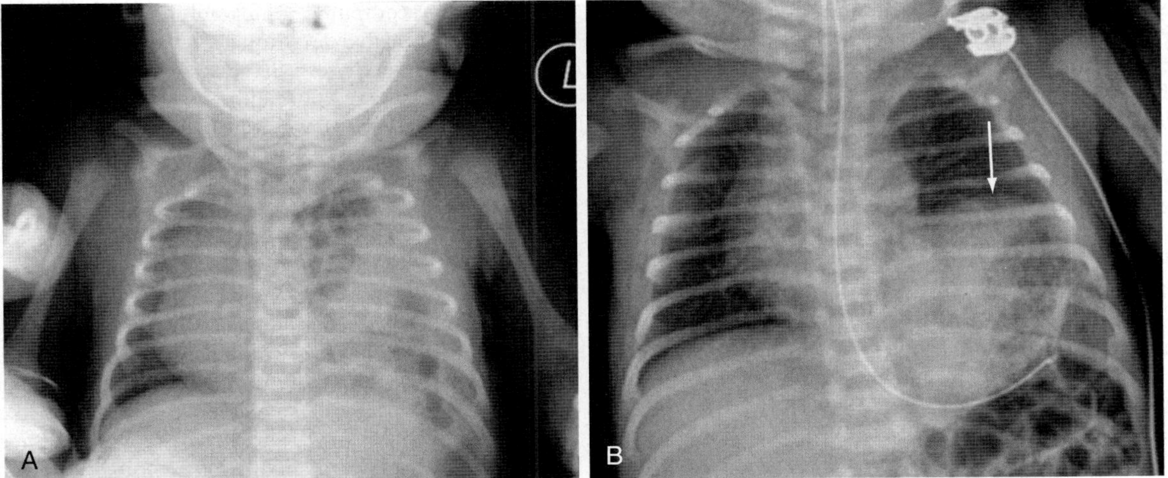

FIG. 67.2 (A) Congenital diaphragmatic hernia. Multiple gas-filled bowel loops are located in the left hemithorax, and the mediastinum is shifted to the right. (B) Left diaphragmatic eventration. Hemidiaphragm is elevated *(arrow)* from phrenic nerve injury-induced paralysis.

delivery during the *"honeymoon period"* and then begins to demonstrate worsening respiratory function. Therapeutic interventions are aimed at stabilizing and treating PPHN. In 10% to 20% of cases, CDH is diagnosed beyond the first 24 hours, when infants experience symptoms of feeding difficulties, respiratory distress, and pneumonia. In Morgagni hernias, the diagnosis is often delayed until childhood because most infants are asymptomatic.

Management

Open fetal surgery for CDH was first attempted in the late 1980s with initial success in fetuses without liver herniation. However, in fetuses with liver herniation and subsequent kinking of the umbilical vein reduction of the liver resulted in fetal demise; therefore, the trial was abandoned. Subsequently, fetal endoscopic tracheal occlusion (FETO) showed encouraging results in promoting lung growth by preventing the egress of pulmonary fluid and increasing intrabronchial pressure. However, a randomized controlled trial failed to show improved survival. A multicenter randomized trial, Tracheal Occlusion to Accelerate Lung Growth (TOTAL), which had been led by several European centers,[5] is now enrolling patients in the United States. The evolution of fetal surgery and its clinical applications are discussed in Chapter 73.

The postnatal management of CDH is directed toward stabilization of the cardiorespiratory status while minimizing iatrogenic injury from therapeutic interventions. Immediate securing of the airway with endotracheal intubation is critical; however, excessive mean airway pressure ventilation can lead to barotrauma along with compromised venous blood return to the heart. An orogastric tube is placed to prevent gastric distention, which may worsen the lung compression, mediastinal shift, and ability to ventilate. The major emphasis on gentle ventilatory management with permissive hypercapnia has resulted in improved survival for CDH infants. Inhaled nitric oxide is used widely for its pulmonary vasodilatory effect. The use of tolazoline, a nonselective α-adrenergic blocking agent, as a pulmonary vasodilator has not produced clinically significant results. Sildenafil, a phosphodiesterase-5 inhibitor, works by inducing pulmonary vascular smooth muscle relaxation and has been used in many centers with variable results. A retrospective cohort study showed an increasing trend in the use of a variety of vasodilators for CDH patients.

Surgical Repair

Infants with CDH not requiring ECMO can safely undergo operative repair soon after birth. Laparoscopic repair of CDH has gained popularity in recent years, but its overall benefit and effects on long-term outcome remain uncertain.[6] The ideal timing of CDH repair on ECMO remains quite controversial; some advocate early operative repair on ECMO, whereas others recommend repair at the time of weaning from ECMO or even after decannulation. There are no indisputable prospective data on the ideal timing of CDH repair for those requiring ECMO support. A recent report suggested that CDH repair after ECMO therapy is associated with improved survival compared to repair while on ECMO.[7] The preferred open approach for a posterolateral CDH is through a subcostal abdominal incision. The viscera are reduced into the abdominal cavity, and the posterolateral defect in the diaphragm is approximated with interrupted nonabsorbable sutures. The hernia defect is often quite large, with only a small leaflet of diaphragmatic tissue present anteromedially. Although primary repair of the defect is ideal, closure with excessive tension must be avoided in order to prevent hernia recurrence. Some advocate for the use of pledgeted sutures. A number of reconstructive techniques and materials are available for the repair of large hernia defects. The surgical technique of abdominal or thoracic muscle flaps may be considered, but a prosthetic material, such as a Gore-Tex patch, is most widely used. The advantages of a prosthetic patch are shorter operative time and a tension-free repair. Some advocate use of regenerative extracellular matrix biomaterials as an ideal biodegradable patch (e.g., Surgisis [Cook Medical Bloomington, IN] and AlloDerm [LifeCell, Branchburg, NJ]) to repair diaphragmatic hernia defects. In general, the chest tube is spared and postoperative radiographs show immediate mediastinal shift toward the center. The chest cavity quickly fills with serous drainage, which later gets absorbed as fluid status returns to baseline. During abdominal cavity closure, it can often be difficult to accommodate the reduced viscera from the thoracic cavity. A temporary abdominal silo may be considered, however allowing an incisional hernia with skin-only closure until the definitive fascia closure can be performed is an alternative surgical option. When CDH is repaired on ECMO, postoperative bleeding is a common major complication and therefore, meticulous hemostasis must be achieved.

Long-term outcomes in infants with CDH vary. Some can develop a chronic condition due to PPHN and respiratory dysfunction. Moreover, infants who received aggressive and prolonged care in the neonatal intensive care unit have a high incidence of developmental delay, seizures, and hearing loss. Other morbidities for CDH survivors include chronic lung disease, scoliosis, growth retardation, pectus excavatum deformities, as well as gastroesophageal reflux (GER) disease and foregut dysmotility.

Eventration of Diaphragm

Abnormal elevation of the hemidiaphragm can significantly affect respiratory function. Eventration of the diaphragm can be congenital or acquired. Congenital eventration can occur due to birth trauma (Erb palsy) or due to an anatomic abnormality of the diaphragm. Erb palsy is a paralysis of the arm caused by injury to the brachial plexus, comprising the ventral rami of spinal nerves C5 to C8. These injuries typically result from shoulder dystocia during a difficult birth. Erb palsy commonly includes ipsilateral diaphragmatic paralysis due to traction injury of the phrenic nerves and upper portion of the brachial plexus. Acquired eventrations are usually secondary to iatrogenic phrenic nerve injury during open cardiac surgery. Elevation of the diaphragm is seen on chest radiographs (Fig. 67.2B); however, it can easily be misdiagnosed as CDH. The diagnosis is confirmed by dynamic visualization of the diaphragm using either fluoroscopy or ultrasound of the chest. Absent or paradoxical movement of the diaphragm on inspiration is diagnostic of eventration. When symptoms progress, resulting in respiratory distress or inability to wean from ventilatory support, repair is indicated. The surgical treatment of diaphragm event ration is an open or laparoscopic diaphragm plication in which the diaphragm is folded taut using multiple interrupted nonabsorbable sutures.

BRONCHOPULMONARY MALFORMATIONS

Bronchopulmonary malformations are congenital abnormalities of the airway and include bronchogenic cysts, intralobar sequestrations (ILSs) and extralobar sequestrations (ELSs), congenital pulmonary airway malformations (CPAMs), and congenital lobar emphysema (CLE).[8] In the perinatal period, these lung lesions can result in pleural effusions, polyhydramnios, hydrops, and pulmonary hypoplasia with subsequent respiratory distress and even airway obstruction. If severe enough, fetal demise can occur. The majority of these lesions are diagnosed prenatally with ultrasound. Fetal surgery has been pursued when fetal viability is at risk. After birth, congenital lung lesions are often asymptomatic and some may even spontaneously regress. However, there is a concern that some lesions may lead to recurrent pulmonary infections and exhibit long-term malignant potential.

Bronchogenic Cyst

The bronchogenic cyst wall consists of fibroelastic tissue, smooth muscle, and cartilage, whereas the cyst itself is lined with respiratory tract ciliated columnar epithelial cells. It can also contain mucus-producing cuboidal cells, which contribute to enlargement of the cyst with mucus. These cysts can occur anywhere along the tracheobronchial tree, but are usually found near the carina and right hilum, and represent the most common mediastinal cysts. These cysts can enlarge resulting in compression of the airway or other vital structures. Infants are particularly at risk because of their narrow, easily compressible trachea and bronchus. Cysts can also cause dysphagia, pneumothorax, cough, and hemoptysis or become infected, especially when presenting later in life. The diagnosis is often suspected on a routine chest radiograph and is confirmed by computed tomography (CT), which demonstrates a spherical nonenhancing, mucus-filled cystic mass, although an air-fluid level can be seen if the cyst communicates with the airway. Cysts within the pulmonary parenchyma typically communicate with a bronchus, whereas those in the mediastinum usually do not. Bronchogenic cysts are resected regardless of symptoms (Fig. 67.3A). Rare cases of malignant transformation have been reported.

Congenital Pulmonary Airway Malformation

CPAMs have been described as hamartomatous lesions in which a multicystic mass replaces normal lung tissue. They are connected to the tracheobronchial tree, and the blood supply is pulmonary. CPAMs can undergo malignant transformation, and rhabdomyosarcoma has been reported in older children. They are classified on the basis of their appearance on imaging, and confirmation is made by pathologic examination. According to the Stocker classification, type I lesions account for almost 75% of all cases and consist of a small number of large, 2- to 10-cm cysts that can compress normal lung parenchyma. Type II lesions have numerous cysts, usually measuring less than 1 cm in diameter. Type III lesions are rare and appear to be only a few millimeters in diameter;[9] however, they are associated with mediastinal shift, hydrops, and a poor prognosis. Prenatal fetal MRI can be used to distinguish CPAM from other thoracic anomalies. If fetal distress occurs, options include fetal thoracotomy and thoracoamniotic shunting (if the fetus is <32 weeks), but this is extremely rare. Most fetuses with a prenatally diagnosed CPAM experience partial regression in the third trimester and can be treated with expectant management. A single course of betamethasone has been shown to be effective in promoting spontaneous regression or size reduction and resolving hydrops.[10] Although they are usually unilateral and unilobar, they can present in the immediate perinatal period with life-threatening respiratory distress. However, the majority of CPAMs are asymptomatic in infancy. Unrecognized CPAMs can present with chronic cough or recurrent pneumonia at a later time. A chest radiograph is usually diagnostic, revealing a cystic thoracic mass, with or without air-fluid levels; however, ultrasound and CT studies are now routinely obtained (Fig. 67.3B). In general, the involved lobe should be resected given the risk of infection and malignant transformation (e.g., pleuropulmonary blastoma). There is a significant variability among surgeons as to the ideal timing of the operation for asymptomatic CPAM, but most surgeons advocate for elective resection at 3 to 6 months of age.

Pulmonary Sequestration

Bronchopulmonary sequestration (BPS) is a nonfunctional nest of microcystic pulmonary tissue that has no connection to the tracheobronchial tree but is fed by an aberrant systemic artery. There are two types: intralobar and extralobar. The intralobar type is contained within normal lung parenchyma, while the extralobar type is separate and encased by its own pleura. ELSs occur predominantly in males, and make up 40% of cases. Other congenital anomalies, such as posterolateral diaphragmatic hernia, pectus excavatum and carinatum, and enteric duplication cysts, can be found. Due to lack of communication to the airway, sequestrations do not form enlarged cysts or cause spontaneous pneumothoraces. They can, however, infarct, become infected, and cause hemoptysis. It has been reported that ELSs can undergo torsion as well. Because of their aberrant systemic vascular supply, BPSs can result

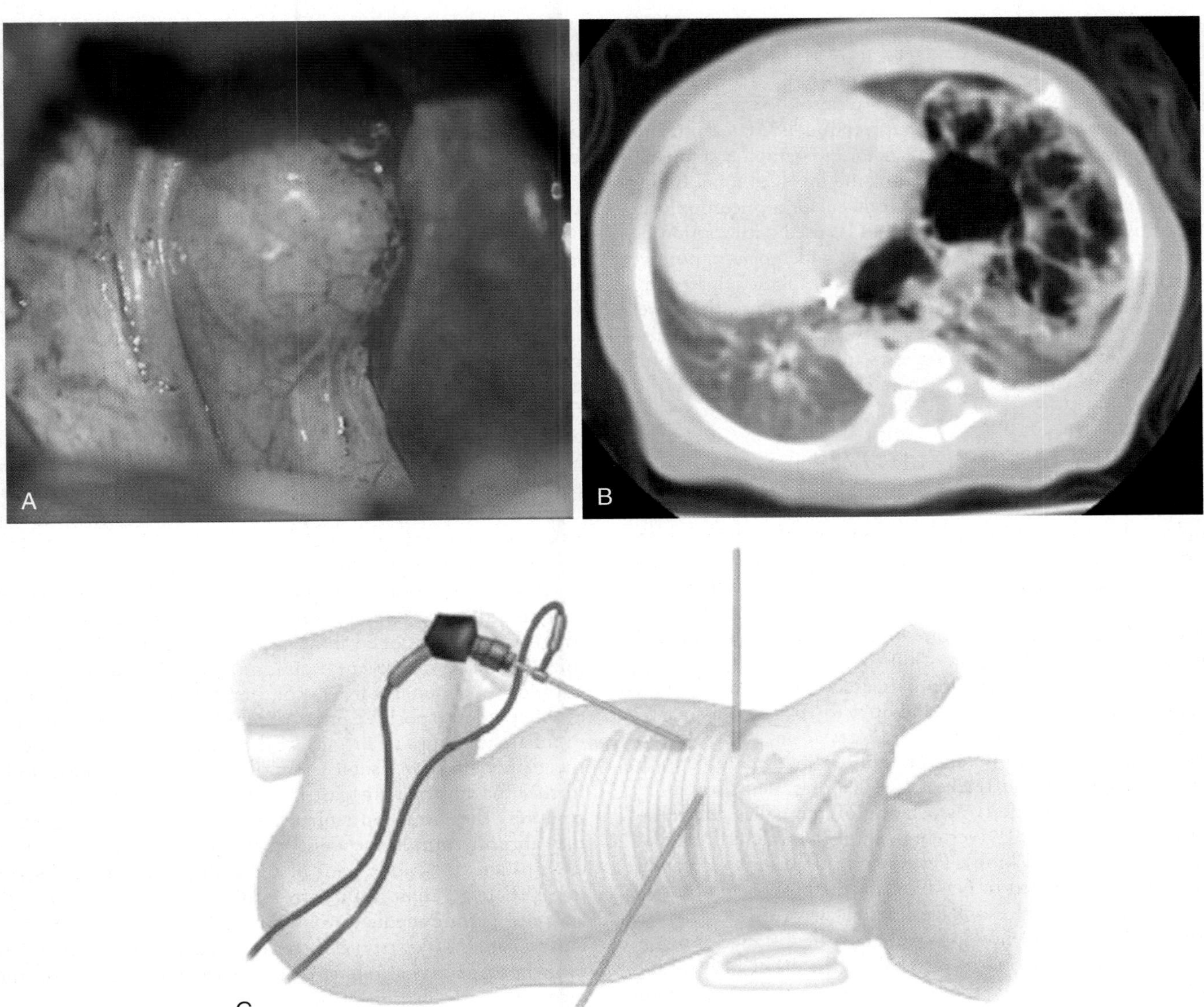

FIG. 67.3 (A) Thoracoscopic view of a bronchogenic cyst. (B) Computed tomography scan demonstrating a large left lung congenital pulmonary airway malformation lesion. (C) Cartoon depiction of a set up for thoracoscopic surgery in an infant. The use of a 3-mm thoracoscope, 3-mm vessel sealer, and a 5-mm stapling device have contributed to more efficient and safer lobectomies.

in significant left-to-right shunting in infants, who are then susceptible to high-output cardiac failure. On initial evaluation, Doppler ultrasound may reveal a systemic arterial supply from the infradiaphragmatic or thoracic aorta. The lesion itself may appear solid, but it can also be cystic. CT or MRI can aid in further definition of the vascular anatomy. Accounting for 75% of all BPSs, ILSs are found within the medial or posterior segments of the predominating left lower lobes. Most ELSs are found posteromedially in the left lower chest but can occur within or below the diaphragm. Air within an ILS usually signifies infection, whereas the same finding in an ELS suggests the presence of a fistulous connection with the esophagus. If a BPS is identified on prenatal ultrasound, the fetus is observed with serial ultrasound monitoring for enlargement and potential pleural effusion, polyhydramnios, or hydrops. BPS has been reported to spontaneously regress. In fact, it is estimated that 68% of BPS undergoes spontaneous regression in utero as they become isodense with the surrounding lung. The involution may occur as the lesion outgrows its blood supply. ELSs are usually asymptomatic, and because there is no tracheobronchial communication, the risk of infection is quite low. However, most advocate for elective resection of ILS, and they are removed by segmentectomy or lobectomy. Although the muscle-sparing minithoracotomy open approach remains the standard operative technique, thoracoscopic approaches have become more widely accepted. With the availability of 3-mm vessel sealers and 5-mm endoscopic staplers, thoracoscopic resection has become safer and faster (Fig. 67.3C).

Congenital Lobar Emphysema

CLE is a progressively distended, hyperlucent lobe caused by abnormal bronchopulmonary development. Air trapping in the emphysematous lobes occurs with intrinsic, which includes endobronchial obstruction from mucosal proliferation and extrinsic compression from vascular anomalies. It involves the left upper or right middle lobe in more than 90% of children. CLE is rarely diagnosed prenatally, and its prevalence is only 1 in every 20,000 to 30,000 deliveries. Symptoms tend to manifest in the first few days of life and as late as 6 months after birth. CLE appears as an echogenic homogeneous lung mass on ultrasound. When CLE is discovered incidentally, observation is recommended because these lesions can regress spontaneously. A chest radiograph is gennerally diagnostic, revealing overdistention of the involved lobe. Importantly, the lucency should not be mistaken for a pneumothorax, and positive pressure ventilation should be used with caution because of the propensity of these patients to undergo auto–positive, end-expiratory pressure; auto–positive, end-expiratory pressure is defined as the end-expiratory intrapulmonary pressure that develops as a result of dynamic airflow resistance during mechanical ventilation. When the CLE progresses to cause mediastinal shift and worsening symptoms, an expeditiously performed open lobectomy is ideal.

ALIMENTARY TRACT CONDITIONS

Esophageal Atresia and Tracheoesophageal Fistula

Esophageal atresia is a congenital condition of esophageal discontinuity that results in proximal esophageal obstruction. A tracheoesophageal fistula (TEF) is an abnormal fistulous communication between the esophagus and trachea. Esophageal atresia and TEF can occur alone or in combination. The incidence of this anomaly is 1 in 1500 to 3000 live births, with a slight male predominance. Approximately one third of infants are born with low birth weight, and 60% to 70% have associated anomalies. During the fourth week of gestation, the esophagotracheal diverticulum of the foregut fails to divide completely to form the esophagus and trachea. In 10% of patients, there is a nonrandom, nonhereditary association of anomalies referred to by the acronym VATERL (vertebral, anorectal, tracheal, esophageal, renal, and radial limb). Five anatomic variants of esophageal atresia are depicted in Fig. 67.4. In the most common type (C lesion), a proximal esophageal atresia with distal TEF, the proximal blind pouch ends approximately the distance of one or two vertebral bodies from the distal TEF. The distal TEF is commonly in close proximity above the carina in the membranous portion of the trachea.

The diagnosis of TEF is considered in an infant with excessive salivation along with coughing or choking experienced at first oral feeding. In addition, curling of the orogastric tube at the level of thoracic inlet is pathognomonic for esophageal atresia +/- TEF. A maternal history of polyhydramnios is common, more often in isolated proximal atresia (86%). In an infant with proximal esophageal atresia with distal TEF, acute gastric distention may occur as a result of air entering the distal esophagus and stomach with each inspired breath. Reflux of gastric contents into the distal esophagus will traverse the TEF and spill into the trachea, resulting in cough, tachypnea, apnea, or cyanosis. The clinical presentation of isolated TEF without esophageal atresia may be subtle, often beyond the newborn period. In general, these infants experience choking and coughing associated with feedings. The inability to pass an orogastric tube into the stomach is a cardinal feature for the diagnosis of esophageal atresia. If gas is present below the diaphragm, an associated TEF is confirmed. Chest radiograph demonstrating the orogastric tube curled up in the proximal esophagus is pathognomonic for the presence of esophageal atresia (Fig. 67.5A). Conversely, the inability to pass a nasogastric tube in an infant with absent radiographic evidence of air in the GI tract is virtually diagnostic of an isolated esophageal atresia. An oral contrast study should not be obtained due to risk for aspiration. Echocardiography and renal ultrasound are routinely performed to evaluate for congenital heart defects (including evaluation of the aortic arch) and genitourinary malformations.

The proximal esophageal pouch should be decompressed with a sump tube (e.g., Replogle tube) placed on continuous suction. The infant is positioned in an upright prone position to minimize GER and to prevent aspiration, and a broad-spectrum IV antibiotic regimen is started. Routine endotracheal intubation is avoided because positive pressure ventilation may be inadequate to inflate the lungs as air may be directed into the TEF through the path of least resistance. Ventilation may be compounded further by the resultant gastric distention. Gastrostomy to decompress the distended stomach should be avoided because it may abruptly worsen the ability to ventilate the patient. In these circumstances, advancement of the endotracheal tube distal to the TEF (e.g., right mainstem intubation) may minimize the leak and permit adequate ventilation. The placement of an occlusive balloon (Fogarty) catheter into the fistula through a rigid bronchoscope may also be useful. As a last resort, emergent thoracotomy with ligation of the fistula alone may be required. A preoperative chest radiograph and echocardiogram provide sufficient information to determine the aortic arch anatomy. A right thoracotomy is performed for the operative repair in patients with a normal left-sided aortic arch. However, for infants with a right-sided arch, a left thoracotomy would be preferred. A higher

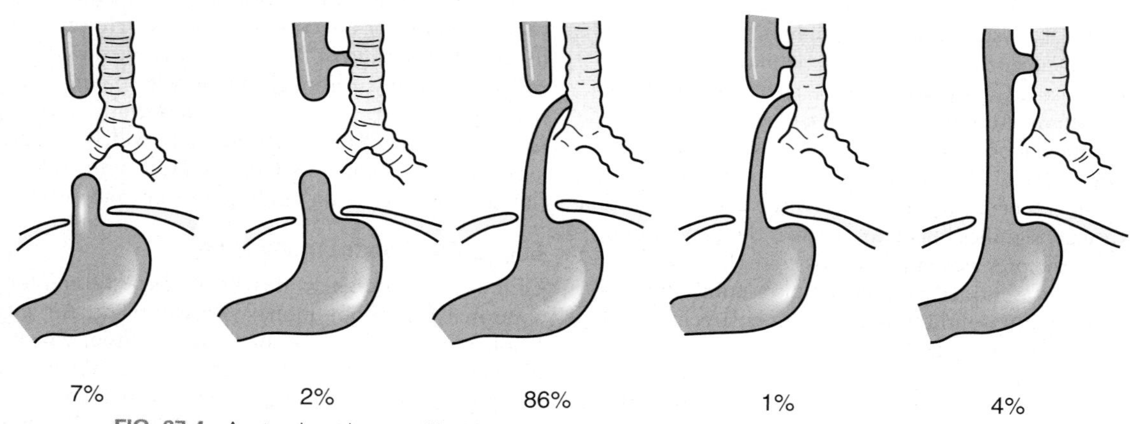

FIG. 67.4 Anatomic variants and incidence of esophageal atresia with tracheoesophageal fistula.

incidence of aortic arch anomalies (e.g., vascular rings) and postoperative complications have been reported with a right-sided aortic arch.

The surgical approach for the most common type of proximal esophageal atresia with distal TEF is extrapleural dissection via an open thoracotomy. Routine rigid bronchoscopy at the start of the operation is performed by some to exclude the presence of a second fistula but this is often not necessary as the yield for detecting a second fistula is quite low. However, for recurrent fistulae, bronchoscopic evaluation with placement of a Fogarty catheter through the fistula may aide in safer dissection. After exposing the posterior mediastinum, the azygos vein is divided to reveal the underlying TEF. The TEF is dissected circumferentially, and its attachment to the membranous portion of trachea is taken down (Fig. 67.5B). The tracheal opening is approximated with interrupted nonabsorbable sutures. The proximal esophageal pouch is then mobilized as high as possible to facilitate a tension-free esophageal anastomosis. The blood supply to the upper esophageal pouch is generally robust from arteries derived from the thyrocervical trunk. However, the lower esophageal vasculature is more tenuous and segmental, originating from intercostal vessels. As such, extensive mobilization of the lower esophagus should be avoided to prevent ischemia. The esophageal anastomosis is performed with a single- or double-layer technique. With the emerging popularity of thoracoscopic repair (Fig. 67.5C), the double-layer anastomosis is now rarely performed. Thoracoscopic repair has become a preferred approach in many centers in carefully selected patients.

In the case of a long gap esophageal atresia, there are several options to gain additional length for a primary anastomosis. A circular or spiral esophagomyotomy of the upper pouch can be performed, but this technique has largely been abandoned due to severe subsequent esophageal dysmotility. Alternatively, the divided closed end of the distal esophagus is sutured to the prevertebral fascia and the area marked with a hemoclip. Over time, the proximal esophageal pouch will lengthen (as the infant grows), allowing for subsequent primary esophageal anastomosis. In infants with pure esophageal atresia, primary anastomosis in the newborn period is not feasible and therefore a gastrostomy is initially placed for enteral feeding access. Historically, a cervical esophagostomy was performed for drainage of oral secretions, and then an esophageal replacement operation using either right or left colon was carried out at ~1 year of age; although this technique has fallen out of favor in recent years. Presently, many centers prefer to manage proximal esophageal

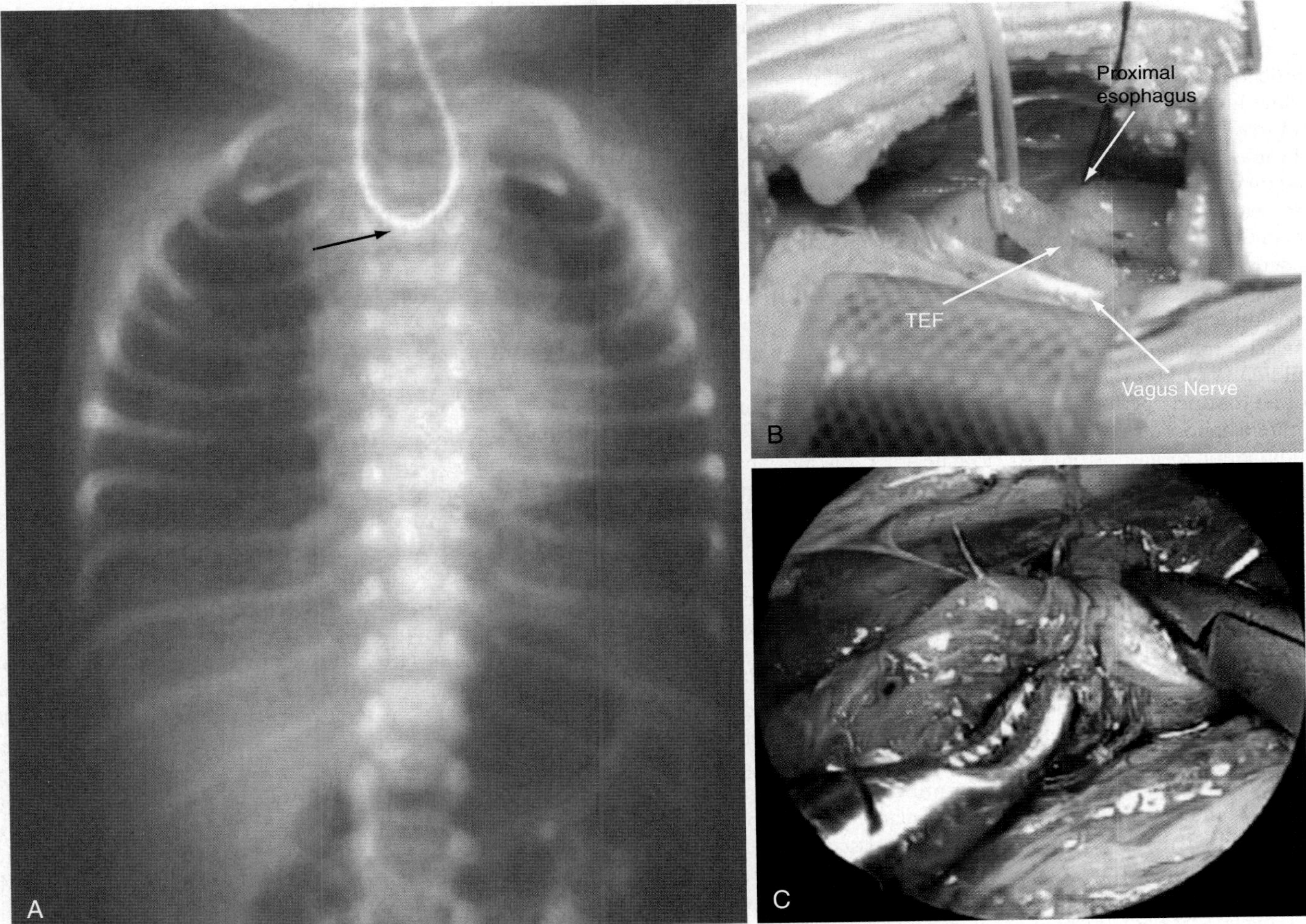

FIG. 67.5 (A) Plain chest radiograph of an infant with proximal esophageal atresia and distal tracheoesophageal fistula *(TEF)*. The distal tip of the orogastric tube is curled up at the level of thoracic inlet *(arrow)*. (B) Distal TEF *(arrow)* encircled with a blue vessel loop. The proximal blind esophageal pouch is in close proximity *(arrow)*. (C) Thoracoscopic esophageal anastomosis. Interrupted sutures are placed using intracorporeal technique.

pouch secretion with an indwelling orogastric tube (Replogle tube) without cervical esophagostomy until adequate esophageal lengthening takes place, as assessed by a radiograph (Fig. 67.6). Then a primary intrathoracic segmental esophageal replacement using a colonic segment can be performed at around 4 to 6 months of age. Other potential esophageal replacement conduits are gastric tube pull-up and small intestinal free graft requiring microvascular anastomosis; these are rarely done. In patients with pure TEF, without esophageal atresia, the TEF is usually near the thoracic inlet. In this case, the surgical approach is made through a cervical incision. At operation, rigid bronchoscopy and cannulation of the TEF with a guidewire can help with safer dissection. The mortality rate is directly related to associated anomalies, particularly cardiac defects and chromosomal abnormalities, and an overall survival of more than 95% is expected without associated anomalies. Postoperative complications include esophageal motility disorders, GER (25%–50%), anastomotic stricture (15%–30%), anastomotic leak (10%–20%), and tracheomalacia (8%–15%).

Gastroesophageal Reflux

Infants normally experience some degree of vomiting due to an incompetent lower esophageal sphincter, which resolves generally around 6 to 12 months of age. Failure to thrive from calorie deprivation is one of the most serious complications of pathologic GER. Aspiration of gastric contents can also result in recurrent bronchitis or pneumonia, leading to chronic airway symptoms. Reflux may stimulate a vagal reflex, producing laryngospasm or bronchospasm and lead to an asthma-like clinical presentation.[11] Reflux-induced airway spasm can cause apnea or choking spells and may contribute to near-miss sudden infant death syndrome. Chronic acid insult to the lower esophagus can progress to the formation of stricture and can produce obstructive symptoms. It can also lead to Barrett esophagus, a metaplasia of lower esophageal squamous mucosa to columnar epithelium, requiring surveillance to detect dysplasia.

Infants and children with neurodevelopmental disabilities often require permanent feeding access, such as gastrostomy. Prophylactic fundoplication in neurologically impaired infants and children (based on their inability to safely protect airway) should not be routinely performed at the time of gastrostomy. Some advocate diagnostic studies (e.g., pH or impedance probe, contrast study) prior to gastrostomy to evaluate for GER and anatomic variation, but clinical assessment for gavage feeding tolerance via indwelling nasogastric tube may be sufficient.

Contrast esophagogram is used most frequently to acquire anatomic and functional data such as upper gastroduodenal dysmotility. Esophageal stricture or mechanical evidence of gastric outlet obstruction, such as antral, or duodenal web, or intestinal malrotation, can also be detected, along with crude assessment of esophageal motility. However, one drawback is the lack of specificity. A 24-hour esophageal pH probe study remains the gold standard for the diagnosis of pathologic GER. It measures the frequency and duration of acid reflux episodes along with its patterns, such as the total length and the longest continuous reflux episode. A combined multichannel intraluminal impedance pH test, in which reflux is detected by changes in intraluminal resistance determined by the presence of liquid or gas and pH changes, is a more comprehensive test. A gastric emptying scan can be obtained using a radionuclide-labeled (technetium-99m (^{99m}Tc) sulfur colloid) liquid or semisolid food to quantitatively assess gastric emptying; ~50% of the isotope-labeled meal is normally emptied from the stomach within 60 minutes and nearly 80% by 90 minutes.

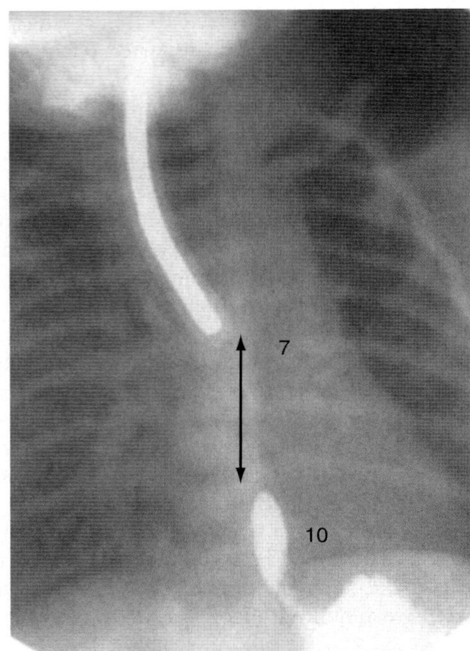

FIG. 67.6 Contrast study per gastrostomy with an indwelling radiopaque orogastric tube. For pure atresia, esophageal gap is assessed using this technique for either primary esophageal anastomosis or partial colonic segmental interposition.

Esophageal manometry measures the pressures of the esophageal body and lower esophageal sphincter. Manometry is not used regularly in pediatrics. Children with poor esophageal motility are prone to experience significant dysphagia after fundoplication with a complete wrap.

Endoscopic evaluation of the esophageal mucosa provides a gross and microscopic assessment of mucosal injury secondary to GER. Esophagoscopy can also help to determine eosinophilic esophagitis, a disease that has become a lot more prevalent in the pediatric population in recent years.[12] Patients with eosinophilic esophagitis can often present with dysphagia and pain due to inflammation, mimicking GER disease. The diagnosis of eosinophilic esophagitis is made by histologic evaluation of esophageal biopsy specimens.

Conservative management of GER includes thickening of formula with cereal, reducing the feeding volume, and postural maneuvers. In addition, pharmacologic acid suppression is administered. Fundoplication is warranted for patients with life-threatening, near-miss sudden infant death syndrome episodes, failure to thrive, or esophageal stricture. Other relative indications include those requiring complex surgical airway reconstruction, neurologic impairment requiring permanent feeding access, and a history of recurrent pneumonias or persistent asthma. The gold standard surgical treatment for infants and children with pathologic GER is a Nissen fundoplication (360-degree esophageal wrap). It is the most effective method to control the symptoms of GER; however, the undesirable side effects of bloating or dysphagia are more likely to occur after a full fundic wrap compared to a partial one. Fewer complications have been reported with partial wraps (e.g., Toupet, 270 degrees; Thal, 180 degrees), such as complications of dysphagia, but they are less effective in controlling the reflux symptoms. Regardless of which fundoplication is performed, a laparoscopic approach has become the standard approach.

Hypertrophic Pyloric Stenosis

Hypertrophic pyloric stenosis (HPS) is a disease of newborns, with an incidence of 1 in 300 to 900 live births. It is most common between the ages of 2 and 8 weeks. Boys are affected four times more often than girls, with first-born male infants being at highest risk. Hypertrophy of the circular muscle of the pylorus results in constriction and obstruction of the gastric outlet, leading to nonbilious, projectile emesis. Loss of hydrochloric acid secondary to persistent emesis leads to hypokalemic, hypochloremic, metabolic alkalosis, and dehydration. Although the exact cause of HPS remains unknown, a lack of nitric oxide synthase in pyloric tissue has been implicated.

Infants present with progressively worsening, nonbilious emesis that is projectile in nature. Visible gastric peristalsis may occasionally be observed as a wave of contractions from the left upper quadrant to the epigastrium. After emesis, infants still crave a feeding. A plain abdominal radiograph can show an enlarged gastric gas bubble. Palpation of the pyloric "olive" tumor in the epigastrium by an experienced examiner is pathognomonic for HPS. If the olive is palpated, no imaging study is required for diagnosis. Today, the vast majority of infants suspected of having HPS are evaluated with an ultrasound study prior to surgical consult. Pyloric muscle thickness of more than 3 to 4 mm or length of more than 15 to 18 mm on ultrasound in the presence of functional gastric outlet obstruction is diagnostic. If clinical presentation is equivocal, an upper GI contrast study may be helpful to evaluate for other causes of vomiting.

Preoperatively, resuscitation and correction of electrolyte abnormalities are essential. The infant must be resuscitated with IV fluids to establish an adequate urine output in order to restore acid-base balance. If not, postoperative apnea can occur due to a propensity to compensate for metabolic alkalosis by retaining respiratory carbon dioxide. Thus, the serum bicarbonate level should be normalized to a value of less than 30 mEq/L prior to surgery. A pyloromyotomy (Ramstedt procedure) involves incising the thickened pyloric musculature to relieve the pyloric channel obstruction. It is performed via a laparoscopic or open approach through various surgical incisions. A laparoscopic approach, increasingly used for management of HPS and is associated with shorter length of stay and lower surgical site infection.[13] Importantly, the fundamental surgical principle of pyloromyotomy is adequate cutting of hypertrophied pyloric muscle to achieve independent wall motion without mucosal injury, remains the same (Fig. 67.7). Postoperatively, infants are managed on a feeding protocol clinical pathway, which ranges from immediate full ad lib feedings to incremental advancement with similar time to full feed and hospital discharge. Postoperative emesis is common, but it is self-limited. Full-thickness mucosal perforation occurs more commonly with a laparoscopic approach, but its incidence is still rare (<1%). However, when infants experience persistent emesis beyond 7 to 10 postoperative days, a contrast study is warranted to evaluate for incomplete pyloromyotomy.

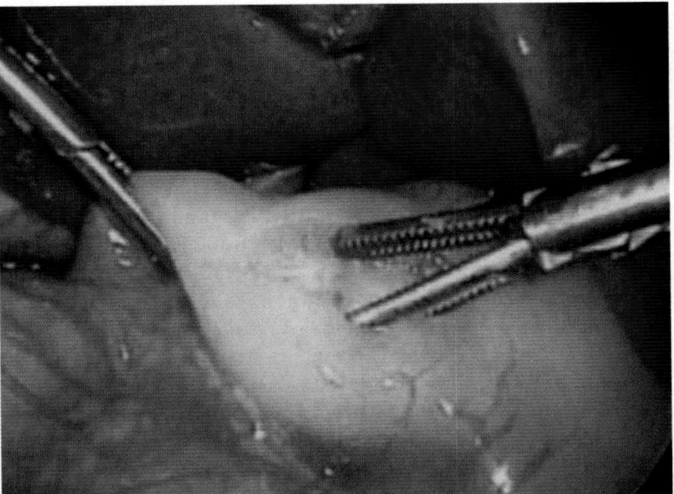

FIG. 67.7 Laparoscopic pyloromyotomy is started with a retractable blade or bovie cautery, and a spreader with grooves on the outer surface is used to perform the pyloromyotomy. Intact mucosal bulging along with independent muscle wall motion is confirmed. (From St. Peter SD, Ostlie DJ. Laparoscopic and open pyloromyotomy. In: Chung DH, Chen MK, ed. *Atlas of pediatric surgical techniques*. Philadelphia, PA: Elsevier Saunders; 2010:253–265.)

Intestinal Atresia

Duodenal atresia is thought to result from failure of vacuolization of the duodenum from its solid cord stage. The range of anatomic variants includes: duodenal stenosis, a mucosal web with intact muscle wall (so-called windsock deformity), two ends separated by a fibrous cord, and a complete separation with a resultant gap within the duodenum. It is associated with several conditions, including prematurity, Down syndrome, maternal polyhydramnios, malrotation, annular pancreas, and biliary atresia (BA). Other anomalies, such as cardiac, renal, esophageal, and anorectal anomalies, are also common. In most cases, the duodenal obstruction is distal to the ampulla of Vater (85%); therefore, infants present with bilious emesis.

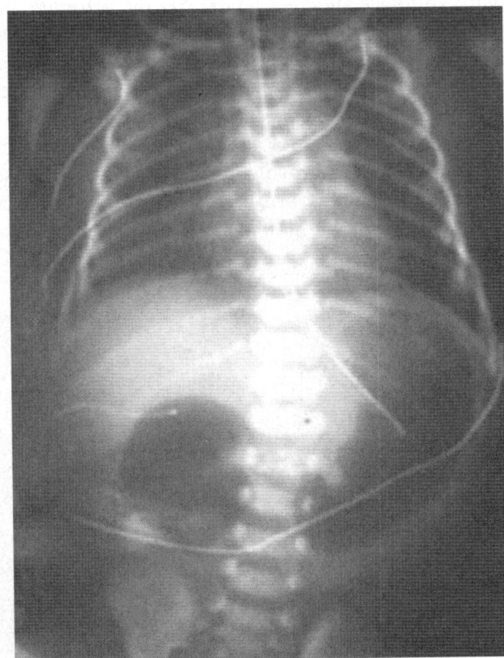

FIG. 67.8 Plain abdominal radiograph shows double-bubble appearance of duodenal atresia.

In patients with an incomplete mucosal web, delayed presentation with symptoms of postprandial emesis may occur later in life.

Infants with duodenal obstruction are generally first detected during prenatal ultrasound evaluation. Immediately after birth, a plain abdominal radiograph shows a typical double-bubble sign if it is obtained before orogastric tube decompression of swallowed gastric air (Fig. 67.8). If distal air is present, an upper GI contrast study should be considered, not only to confirm the diagnosis of duodenal stenosis or atresia but also to exclude midgut volvulus, which would constitute a surgical emergency.

Surgical treatment is a bypass of the duodenal obstruction with a side-to-side or proximal transverse to distal longitudinal (diamond-shaped) duodenoduodenostomy. At the time of anastomosis, additional intestinal atresia should be ruled out by injecting saline into a distal limb using a soft red rubber catheter. When the proximal duodenum is markedly dilated, a tapering duodenoplasty with staples or sutures should be considered to narrow the duodenal caliber to lessen dysmotility. In patients with a duodenal mucosal web, the web is excised transduodenally, and caution must be exercised to avoid injury to the ampulla.

Jejunoileal atresia is the most common GI atresia, occuring in 1 in 2000 live births. It is thought to result from an intrauterine mesenteric vascular accident. Infants present with bilious emesis, abdominal distention, and failure to pass meconium. The clinical presentation varies by the location of the atretic obstruction. In proximal atresia, significant bilious emesis occurs. In distal atresias, abdominal distention with multiple dilated bowel loops is more common (Fig. 67.9A). A contrast enema study is often unnecessary to make the diagnosis of jejunoileal atresia. If obtained, it shows an extremely narrow caliber of nondistended colon. Multiple intestinal atresias can occur in 10%–15% of cases. Jejunoileal atresia is generally not associated with other anomalies except cystic fibrosis (CF) in approximately 10% of patients.

Jejunoileal atresias are classified into five types: type I is a mucosal web, or diaphragm; type II has an atretic cord between two blind ends of bowel with an intact mesentery; type IIIa is a complete separation of the blind ends of bowel by a V-shaped mesenteric gap; and type IIIb is an apple peel or Christmas tree deformity with a large mesenteric gap (Fig. 67.9B), in which the distal bowel receives a retrograde blood supply from the ileocolic or right colic artery. This tenuous blood supply has implications for anastomotic failures and the potential for ischemic necrosis from volvulus. Thus, many of these infants with this type of atresia are born with reduced intestinal length. In type IV, there are multiple atresias, with a string of sausage appearance.

Infants are managed for neonatal bowel obstruction, with placement of an orogastric tube and IV fluid resuscitation. At operation, the main objective is to establish intestinal continuity, while preserving as much intestinal length as possible. In multiple atresias, multiple anastomoses over an endoluminal stent may be necessary. If the proximal intestine is significantly dilated, prolonged dysmotility may persist, and therefore a tapering enteroplasty of the dilated segment should be considered. However, in cases of adequate bowel length, resection of the dilated segment can result in faster recovery. The overall survival for infants with an jejunoileal atresia is more than 90%.

Colonic atresia is the least common, accounting for only 5% to 10% of intestinal atresia, with an incidence of 1 in 20,000 live births. Infants usually present with failure to pass meconium, abdominal distention, and bilious vomiting. A plain radiograph shows multiple dilated bowel loops, but differentiation between small and large bowel is not feasible in this age group because of lack of well-developed haustra and semicircularis landmarks. A contrast enema study can confirm the diagnosis, but the clinical picture of distal bowel obstruction may be enough evidence to proceed with an operative intervention of diverting end colostomy.

Intestinal Malrotation and Midgut Volvulus

The actual incidence of rotational anomalies of the midgut is difficult to determine but is estimated to be 1 in 6,000 live births. The midgut normally herniates out of the coelomic cavity through the umbilical ring at approximately the fourth week of embryonic development. By the tenth week of gestation, the intestine begins to migrate back into the abdominal cavity in a counterclockwise rotation around the axis of the superior mesenteric artery (SMA) for 270 degrees. The duodenojejunal segment returns first and rotates beneath, and to the right of the SMA to fix in the left upper quadrant at the ligament of Treitz. The cecocolic segment also rotates counterclockwise around the SMA to rest in its final position

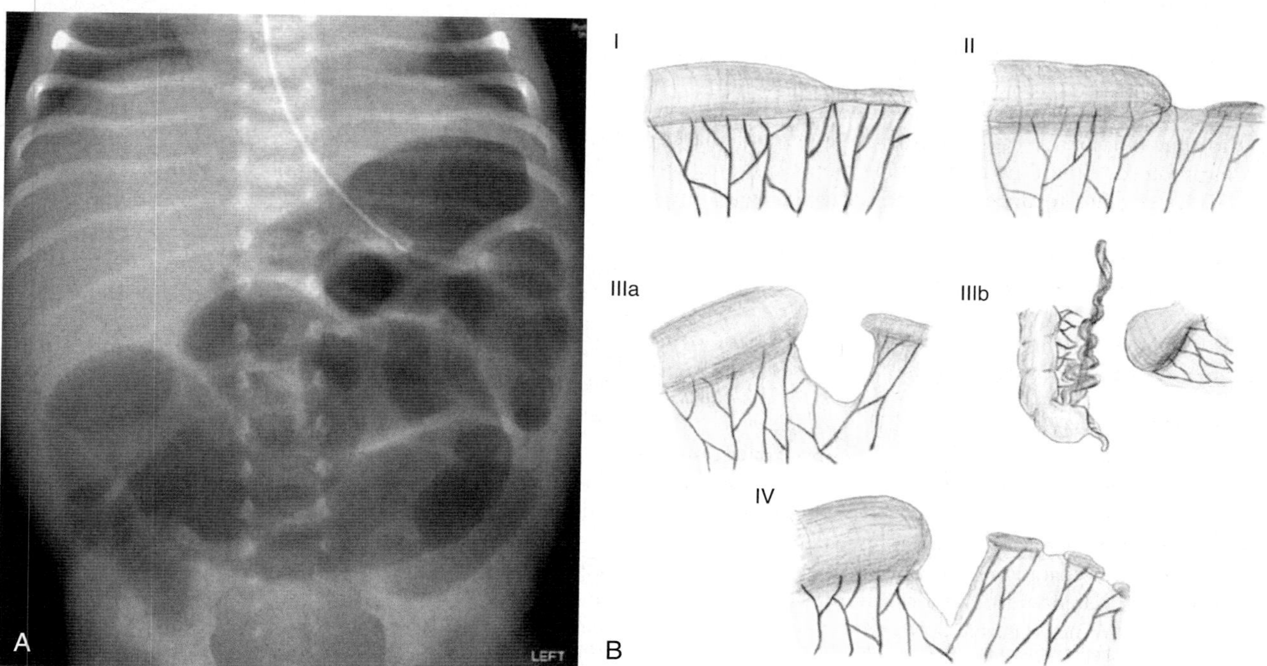

FIG. 67.9 (A) Plain abdominal radiograph shows multiple dilated bowel loops indicating congenital bowel obstruction. (B) Jejunoileal atresia Types I to IV are depicted. In particular, IIIb demonstrates an apple peel type of atresia with a large mesenteric gap.

in the right lower quadrant. By week 12, this process of intestinal rotation is complete, and the colon becomes fixed to the retroperitoneum. An interruption or reversal of any of these coordinated movements implies an embryologic explanation for the range of anomalies seen.

Complete nonrotation of the midgut is the most common anomaly and occurs when neither the duodenojejunal nor the cecocolic limb undergoes correct rotation. Consequently, the duodenojejunal and ileocecal junctions lie close together and the midgut is suspended on a narrow SMA stalk, which can twist in a clockwise fashion to result in midgut volvulus; this anatomic abnormality can be demonstrated by contrast upper GI series (Fig. 67.10A). The ultrasound examination has proved to be a useful tool for the diagnosis of intestinal malrotation, in which the normal relationship of the superior mesenteric vessels (the vein is to the right of artery) is reversed or altered. Nonrotation of the duodenojejunal limb, followed by normal rotation and fixation of the cecocolic limb, results in duodenal obstruction by abnormal mesenteric bands (Ladd's bands) that extend from the colon across the anterior duodenum. In this anomaly, the risk of midgut volvulus is low because there is a relatively broad mesenteric base between the duodenojejunal junction and cecum. Normal rotation of the duodenojejunal limb with nonrotation of the cecocolic segment carries the same risk for midgut volvulus as a complete nonrotation anomaly. In this case, the risks for volvulus are high because of a narrow mesenteric base. Clinical presentations vary from completely asymptomatic, chronic intermittent crampy abdominal pain suggestive of partial obstruction or even more subtle with early satiety or weight loss. Most symptomatic patients with intestinal malrotation present early in life.

Midgut volvulus is a true surgical emergency because of evolving ischemic bowel loops. The acute onset of bilious emesis in a particularly somnolent or lethargic newborn is an ominous sign. Midgut volvulus may also be incomplete or intermittent. With partial intermittent volvulus, the resultant mesenteric venous and lymphatic obstruction may impair nutrient absorption and produce protein loss into the gut lumen, as well as mucosal ischemia and melena as a result of arterial insufficiency.

Abdominal radiographs may demonstrate upper intestinal obstruction or a gasless abdomen; however, these findings are nonspecific. The upper GI contrast study is the diagnostic study of choice in a hemodynamically stable patient. It demonstrates an obstructive upper GI pattern with the appearance of a bird's beak in the third portion of the duodenum (Fig. 67.10B). In the acutely ill infant or child with midgut volvulus and obstruction, an immediate operative intervention is warranted without upper GI study. Aggressive resuscitation can be performed in route to operating room as well as intraoperatively. Midgut volvulus is a true surgical emergency, where time is of the essence if maximal intestinal salvage is to be achieved.

The Ladd procedure is the operation of choice for rotational anomalies of the intestine. Upon entering the peritoneal cavity, chylous ascites from obstructed lymphatics is frequently seen. Midgut volvulus is untwisted in a counterclockwise fashion (Fig. 67.10C). The intestine may be congested and edematous, and some areas may appear ischemic despite complete untwisting of the volvulus. Warm sponges placed on the bowel surface may help to improve perfusion. The decision must be made as to whether the intestine has restored adequate perfusion and is thought to be viable. If vascular integrity has been compromised, ischemic or necrotic bowel segments are resected. However, borderline ischemic segments may be left in place with a second-look laparotomy performed after 24 to 36 hours. Ladd's bands are divided as they extend from the ascending colon across the duodenum to the posterior aspect of the right upper quadrant. In dividing the medial bands, the cecum is mobilized and the mesenteric base is broadened to prevent recurrent volvulus. Securing the cecum or duodenum to the abdominal wall by sutures has no proven benefit. In addition, an intraluminal duodenal obstruction may coexist; therefore, an orogastric tube may be advanced into the distal duodenum to exclude any associated anomaly. Appendectomy (inversion) is routinely performed because the cecum lies on the left side of the abdomen after the Ladd procedure. The intestine is placed back into the abdominal cavity with the small bowel loops on the right side and the colon positioned on the left. Recurrent midgut volvulus has been reported in up to 10% after the Ladd

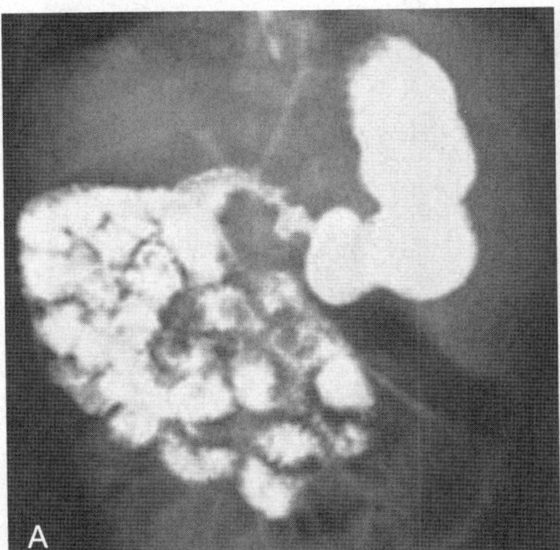

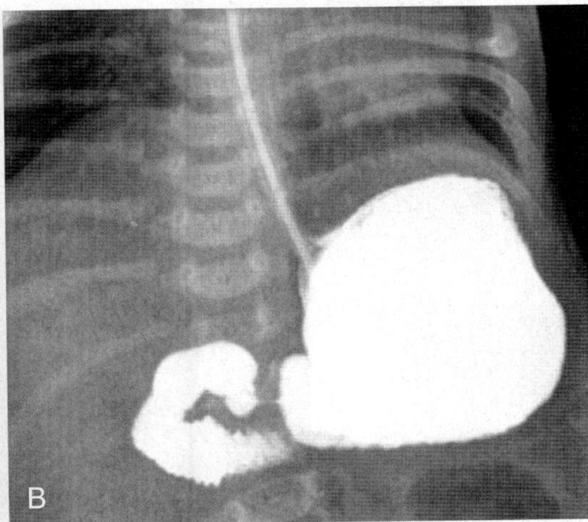

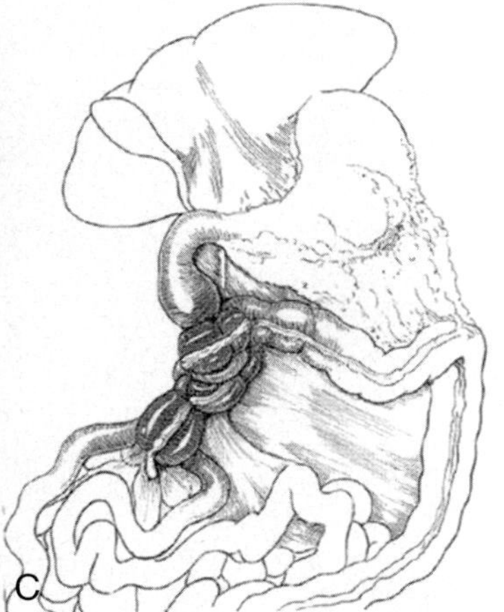

FIG. 67.10 (A) Intestinal malrotation. The duodenal C-loop does not cross the midline and the proximal small bowel is on the right side of the abdomen. (B) Midgut volvulus as demonstrated by a corkscrew appearance of contrast abruptly tapering off in the duodenum. (C) Diagram depicting midgut volvulus from intestinal malrotation. At operation, volvulized small bowel is untwisted in a counterclock fashion to restore intestinal perfusion. The peritoneal attachment between the cecum and retroperitoneum (Ladd band) is divided as part of the Ladd procedure.

procedure. Prolonged postoperative ileus is common, particularly if a volvulus has progressed to necrosis, requiring extensive resection. Midgut volvulus accounts for approximately 18% of short bowel syndrome (SBS) in the pediatric population.

Necrotizing Enterocolitis

NEC is the most common GI surgical emergency in neonates. Although several contributing factors have been implicated, such as ischemia, bacterial overgrowth, cytokines, and enteral feeding, prematurity is the single most important risk factor. The overall incidence of NEC appears to have decreased in recent years due to clinical pathway-based gradual feeding regimens including the more prevalent use of breast milk. The exact cause of NEC remains elusive despite active basic and translational studies at several institutions.

The clinical presentation of NEC can be quite variable. Acute abdominal wall cellulitis, distention and tenderness, as well as feeding intolerance with gross or occult blood in the stool are hallmark features for NEC (Fig. 67.11A). Other nonspecific signs include temperature instability and episodes of apnea or bradycardia. NEC typically occurs in the first few days of life with the initiation of enteral feedings; 80% of cases occur during the first month of life. As NEC progresses, sepsis develops with hemodynamic deterioration and coagulopathy. The pathognomonic radiographic feature of NEC is pneumatosis intestinalis (Fig. 67.11B). Pneumatosis is composed of hydrogen gas generated by the bacterial fermentation of luminal substrates. Other radiographic findings may include portal venous gas, ascites, fixed loops of small bowel, and free air. The distal ileum and ascending colon are the usual affected areas, although the entire GI tract can be affected as in NEC totalis.

Medical management consists of orogastric tube decompression, fluid resuscitation, and broad-spectrum antibiotics. NEC can be successfully treated medically in more than 50% of cases. Infants are closely monitored for any signs of surgical indications. The absolute indication for operative intervention is the presence of free air on plain abdominal radiographs. Relative indications for surgery include clinical deterioration, abdominal wall cellulitis, palpable mass (matted ischemic bowel), a persistent fixed bowel loop on radiograph, as well as portal venous gas. The general surgical principles are to resect all nonviable intestinal segments, preserving maximum intestinal length with ostomy diversion. At times, multiple necrotic segments of bowel are resected, thus preserving viable intersegments. In cases of ischemic, but not frankly necrotic bowel, a second-look operation may be performed after 24 to 48 hours. Bowel resection with primary anastomosis may be considered in rare stable infants with a focal isolated perforation and minimal peritoneal contamination; however, the high risks of anastomotic leak and stricture have tempered enthusiasm for this approach. Extremely low birth weight premature infants with perforated NEC may require bedside peritoneal drain placement as a temporary measure, as drainage of the peritoneal fluid may improve ventilation and halt the progression of sepsis. Surprisingly, drain placement was found to be the definitive intervention in some infants. However, percutaneous drains were reported to have poor outcomes in infants of extremely low birth weight (<1000 g). Evidence to support peritoneal drainage as an accepted mode of treatment for NEC was established in a multicenter, randomized prospective clinical trial.[14] In this study, survival, need for parenteral nutrition, and length of hospital stay were similar for NEC infants weighing less than 1500 g treated by peritoneal drainage or laparotomy. The overall mortality rate for surgically managed

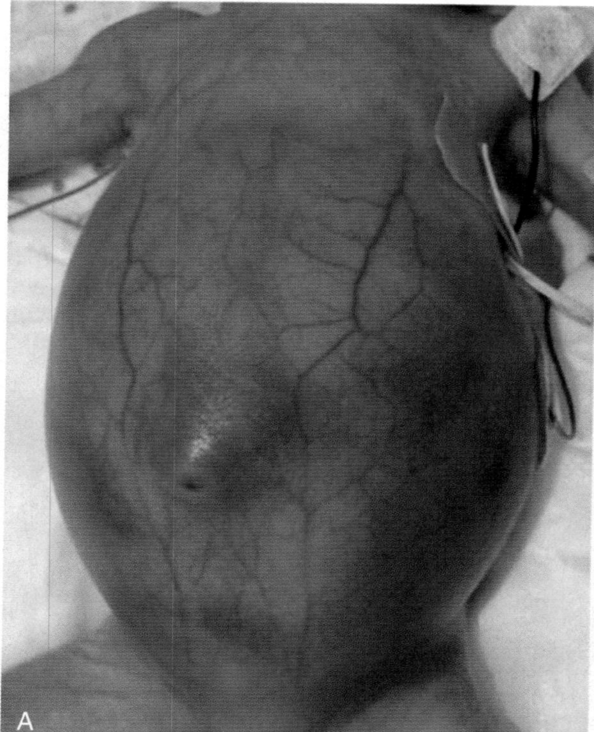

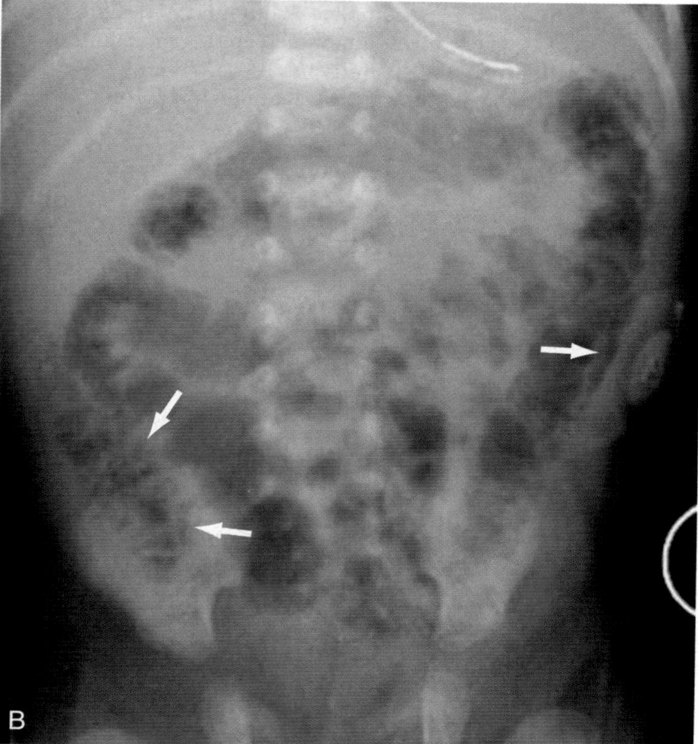

FIG. 67.11 (A) Premature infant with necrotizing enterocolitis. Abdominal distention with marked cellulitis and dusky abdominal indicates intraabdominal catastrophe. (B) Pneumatosis intestinalis *(arrows)*, a pathognomonic radiographic sign for necrotizing enterocolitis.

NEC ranges from 10% to 50%. NEC remains the most common cause of short gut syndrome. Intestinal strictures may develop after medical or surgical management of NEC in approximately 10% of infants. Because of the risk for post-NEC stricture, most notably in the splenic flexure of the colon, a contrast enema study is done routinely before stoma reversal. Neurodevelopmental delay is also a frequent long-term complication.

Short Bowel Syndrome

SBS is a clinical condition in which there is inadequate length of functional intestine to sustain normal enteral nutrition as a result of massive small bowel resection. Common conditions that can lead to SBS are intestinal atresia, midgut volvulus, NEC, and gastroschisis. In SBS, intestinal function depends on a number of factors, such as total bowel length, presence of the ileocecal valve, and residual intestinal segments. The jejunum is the site of absorption of most macronutrients and minerals. The ileum is essential for the absorption of carbohydrates, proteins, fluids, and electrolytes. In addition, bile acids, vitamin B_{12}, and the fat-soluble vitamins (A, D, E, and K) are primarily absorbed in the ileum. Ileocecal valve function is particularly important in SBS, due to significantly altered intestinal transit time. The colon is important in SBS patients for absorption of water and electrolytes. After massive small bowel resection, a physiologic process known as intestinal adaptation occurs to compensate for the loss of intestinal length. Many factors are involved in this adaptive process to enhance the absorptive function of the residual intestine, such as use of elemental diet, growth factors, and titration of TPN. Several surgical techniques (excluding small bowel transplantation) aimed at slowing intestinal transit time or increasing the mucosal surface area for enhanced absorption have been described.[15] These include reversed intestinal segment, recirculating loop, artificial intestinal valve, colon interposition, and intestinal pacing. Two procedures that are generally used are the Bianchi procedure and serial transverse enteroplasty (STEP).

Bianchi procedure. Bianchi[16] originally described an intestinal lengthening procedure in which the mesenteric vascular bed is separated into two systems, the dilated small intestine is split into two parallel segments, each with its own blood supply, and the ends are approximated (Fig. 67.12A). This resulted in a 50% decreased diameter of the small intestine and increased length by 200%. The Bianchi procedure has been shown to be an effective surgical option for treating patients with SBS.

Serial transverse enteroplasty. In contrast to the Bianchi procedure, STEP utilizes the principle of minimal bowel dissection by serially stapling dilated small intestine in a transverse fashion to create a narrower lumen resulting in longer intestinal length (Fig. 67.12B).[17] The STEP procedure has been shown to improve enteral feeding tolerance, resulting in significant catch-up growth, without increased mortality. An improved enteral tolerance in the majority of 20 treated patients was observed for more than a 7-year period after STEP procedures.[18] A recent retrospective, single institution review of 36 patients reported that the median increase in bowel length after STEP was 53% and that 42% reached enteral autonomy, but emphasized the importance of multidisciplinary intestinal rehabilitation program for an ideal patient selection and outcomes.[19]

Meconium Ileus

Meconium ileus is a unique form of neonatal obstruction that occurs in infants with CF, an autosomal recessive disorder resulting from a mutation in the CF transmembrane regulator gene *(CFTR)*. It is estimated that 3.3% of the white population in the United States are asymptomatic carriers of the mutated *CFTR*

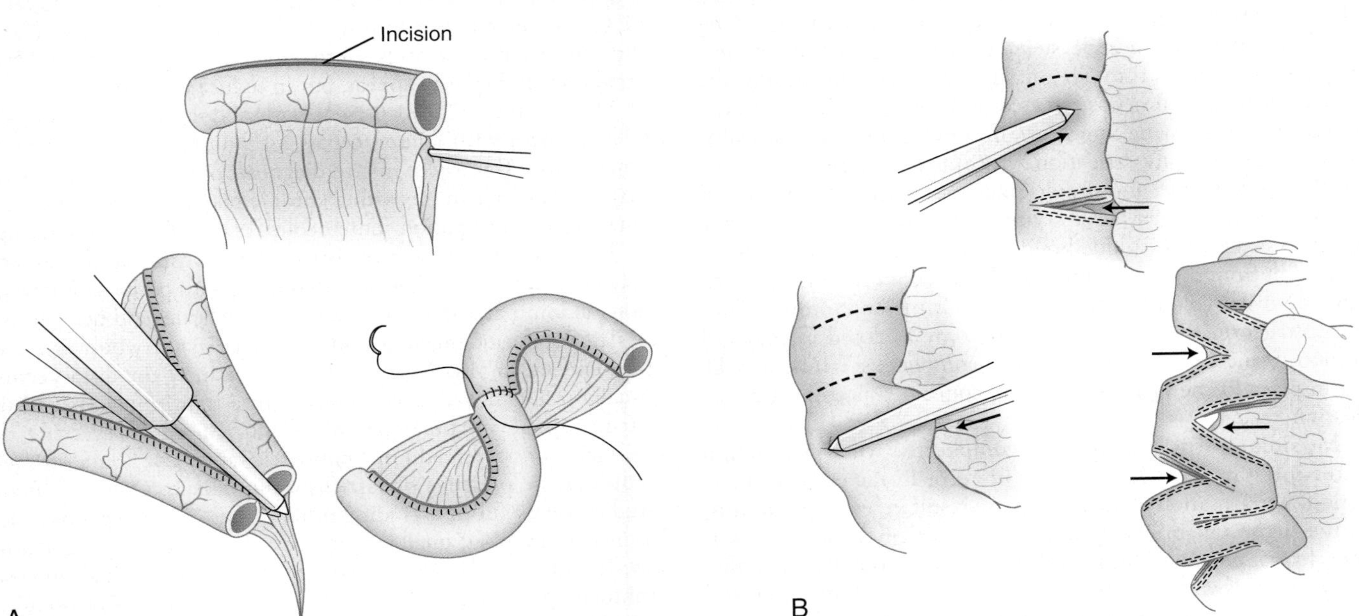

FIG. 67.12 Bowel-lengthening procedures. (A) Bianchi technique separates two mesenteric planes. A dilated segment of bowel is stapled longitudinally to create two narrower segments for sequential anastomosis. (B) Serial transverse enteroplasty (STEP) involves stapling a dilated bowel into V shapes on alternating sides, decreasing width and increasing length. (A, Adapted from Abu-Elmagd KM, Bond G, Costa G, et al. Gut rehabilitation and intestinal transplantation. *Therapy.* 2005;2:853–864. B, From Kim HB, Fauza D, Garza J, et al. Serial transverse enteroplasty [STEP]: A novel bowel-lengthening procedure. *J Pediatr Surg.* 2003;38:425–429.)

gene. The abnormal chloride transport in patients with CF results in tenacious viscous secretions with a protein concentration of almost 80% to 90%. It affects a wide variety of organs, including the intestine, pancreas, lungs, salivary glands, reproductive organs, and biliary tract.

Meconium ileus in the newborn represents the earliest clinical manifestation of CF, affecting approximately 10% to 15% of patients with this inherited disease. The incidence of CF ranges from 1 in 1000 to 2000 live births. Infants present with three cardinal signs in the first 24 to 48 hours of life: (1) generalized abdominal distention; (2) bilious emesis; and (3) failure to pass meconium. Maternal polyhydramnios occurs in approximately 20% of cases. In simple meconium ileus, the terminal ileum is dilated and filled with thick, tarlike, inspissated meconium. Smaller pellets of meconium are found in the more distal ileum, leading into a relatively small colon. In patients with simple meconium ileus, important plain abdominal radiographic findings include dilated and gas-filled loops of small bowel, absence of air-fluid levels, and a mass of meconium in the right side of the abdomen mixed with gas to give a ground-glass or soap bubble appearance. Abdominal radiographs show dilated bowel loops with relatively absent air-fluid levels because of thick, viscous meconium. A contrast enema using the water-soluble ionic solution gastrografin can both be diagnostic, demonstrating a small, narrow-caliber colon and inspissated meconium pellets in the terminal ileum, as well as therapeutic, as it aids in the evacuation of meconium by pulling water into the colon. It is imperative for an infant to be well hydrated and monitored closely. It is successful in relieving the obstruction in up to 75% of cases, with a bowel perforation rate of less than 3%. The pilocarpine iontophoresis sweat test revealing a chloride concentration of more than 60 mEq/L is the most definitive method to confirm the diagnosis of CF. A more immediate test is detection of the mutated *CFTR* gene.

Operative management of simple meconium ileus is required when the obstruction is persistent despite contrast enema, along with 5 mL of 10% *N*-acetylcysteine (Mucomyst) solution administered every 6 hours through a nasogastric tube. Historically, the dilated terminal ileum was resected and various types of stomas were created, allowing intestinal decompression and recovery. However, enterotomy, irrigation with warmed saline solution or 4% *N*-acetylcysteine, and simple evacuation of the luminal meconium without a stoma has also been advocated. *N*-acetylcysteine serves to break the disulfide bonds in the meconium to facilitate separation from the bowel mucosa. The meconium is manipulated into the distal colon or removed through the enterotomy. After the obstruction is relieved, the enterotomy is closed in standard fashion. If meconium evacuation is incomplete, a T-tube may be left in place in the ileum to facilitate continued postoperative irrigation.

Meconium ileus is considered complicated when perforation of the intestine has taken place in utero or in the early neonatal period. Extravasation of meconium can result in severe peritonitis, with a dense inflammatory response and calcification. The variable clinical presentations include a meconium pseudocyst, adhesive peritonitis with or without secondary bacterial infection, and ascites. Abdominal radiographs can demonstrate calcifications, bowel dilation, mass effect, and ascites. A distal ileal obstructive syndrome, formerly known as meconium ileus equivalent, may develop as a consequence of noncompliance with oral enzyme replacement therapy or bouts of dehydration. This is managed nonoperatively in most patients with enemas or oral polyethylene glycol purging solutions. Other diagnoses must also be considered, including simple adhesive intestinal obstruction. Furthermore, with the introduction of enteric-coated, high-strength pancreatic enzyme replacement therapy, a fibrosing cholangiopathy has been described, and reection of the inflammatory colon stricture may be necessary.

Meconium Plug Syndrome

Meconium plug syndrome is a different condition from meconium ileus, and, in most cases, it is not a sequela of CF. However, it is a frequent cause of neonatal intestinal obstruction and is associated with a number of conditions, including Hirschsprung disease, maternal diabetes, and hypothyroidism. Infants often present with abdominal distention and failure to pass meconium in the first 24 hours. The contrast enema study shows a microcolon extending up to where the colon is dilated, and filled with a thickened meconium plug. Often, a contrast enema is therapeutic and surgical intervention is not indicated.

Hirschsprung Disease

The pathogenesis of Hirschsprung disease is an aganglionated distal colon/rectum, characterized by an absence of ganglion cells in the myenteric (Auerbach) and submucosal (Meissner) plexus. It occurs in 1 in 5000 live births, with boys being affected four times more frequently than girls. Of these patients, 3% to 5% have Down syndrome, and the risk for Hirschsprung disease is greater if there is a family history. An abnormal locus on chromosome 10 has been identified in some families and is associated with the *RET* oncogene.[20] This neurogenic, parasympathetic abnormality is associated with muscular spasm of the distal colon and internal anal sphincter, resulting in a functional obstruction. Hence, the abnormal bowel is the contracted distal segment, whereas the normal bowel is the proximal dilated portion. Aganglionosis begins at the anorectal line, and the rectosigmoid colon is affected in approximately 80% of cases, the splenic or transverse colon in 17%, and the entire colon in 8%. The area between the dilated and contracted segments is referred to as the transition zone. Here, ganglion cells begin to appear, but in reduced numbers.

Most infants (>90%) present with abdominal distention and bilious emesis with failure to pass meconium within the first 24 hours of life. Those with missed diagnoses of Hirschsprung disease may present later in life with a chronic history of abdominal distention and constipation. Enterocolitis is the most common cause of death in patients with uncorrected Hirschsprung disease and may be manifested as diarrhea alternating with periods of obstipation, abdominal distention, fever, hematochezia, and peritonitis.

The diagnostic imaging study of choice in a newborn is a contrast enema. In Hirschsprung disease, spasm of the distal rectum usually results in a narrow caliber with a transition zone and dilated, normal, proximal sigmoid colon. Failure to evacuate the instilled contrast medium completely after 24 hours strongly indicates the presence of Hirschsprung disease. Contrast enema studies are useful in excluding other causes of constipation, such as meconium plug, small left colon syndrome, and intestinal atresia. In older toddlers, a manometry study revealing high internal sphincter pressure upon rectal balloon distention may be useful. A rectal biopsy is the gold standard for the diagnosis of Hirschsprung disease. In the newborn period, this is performed at bedside using a suction rectal biopsy kit. It is imperative to obtain biopsy specimens at least 2 cm above the dentate line to avoid sampling the normal aganglionated region of the internal sphincter. In older children, a full-thickness biopsy specimen is obtained under general anesthesia because the thicker rectal mucosa is not amenable to suction biopsy technique. Absent ganglia, hypertrophied nerve trunks, and robust immunostaining for acetylcholinesterase are the histopathologic criteria. Calretinin immunostaining has now become a standard adjunct histology study for the diagnosis of Hirschsprung disease.[21]

The most common definitive surgical procedure for Hirschsprung disease is laparoscopy-assisted Soave. The minimally invasive approach without requiring leveling colostomy is its major advantage. The laparoscopy-assisted Soave procedure involves: 1) intracorporeal seromuscular biopsies of distal colon with frozen sections to determine the level well proximal to the transition zone and 2) dissection of distal rectum. Once frozen section evaluation is completed, an endorectal mucosal dissection within the aganglionic distal rectum is performed via a transanal approach. The ganglionated normal colon is then pulled through the remnant muscular cuff, posterior myotomy of the cuff is performed, and then a coloanal anastomosis is performed. The Soave procedure can also be performed entirely through a transanal approach. Postoperatively, the stool dysfunction can persist, and at times, it can be difficult to manage, requiring intermittent rectal decompression.[22] Constipation is a common postoperative problem along with frequent soiling, incontinence, and postoperative enterocolitis. If persistent, histologic reevaluation should be performed to ensure adequately ganglionated colon was pulled through and to rule out a transition zone at the coloanal anastomosis. In the Swenson procedure, the aganglionic bowel is removed down to the level of the internal sphincters and a coloanal anastomosis is performed. In the Duhamel procedure, the aganglionic rectal stump is left in place and the ganglionated normal colon is pulled behind the stump. A stapler is then inserted through the anus, with one arm within the normal ganglionated bowel posteriorly and the other in the aganglionic rectum anteriorly. Stapling results in the formation of a neorectum that empties normally because of the posterior patch of ganglionated bowel. Historical two- or three-stage operations involving initial open leveling colostomy followed by a definitive pull-through (Soave or Duhamel) are now rarely performed with the exception of cases where significantly delayed diagnosis of Hirschsprung disease with massively dilated descending colon exist. In such scenarios, initial diverting end colostomy is necessary to allow for shrinkage of the dilated colon for subsequent coloanal anastomosis.

Anorectal Malformation

The incidence of imperforate anus is 1 in 5000 live births with a male predominance of 58%. The spectrum of anorectal malformations ranges from simple anal stenosis to the persistence of a cloaca. The most common defect is an imperforate anus with a fistula between the distal colon and urethra, in boys, or the vestibule of the vagina, in girls. By the sixth week of gestation, the urorectal septum moves caudally to divide the cloaca into the anterior urogenital sinus and posterior anorectal canal. Failure of this septum to form results in a fistula between the bowel and urinary tract (in boys) or vagina (in girls). Complete or partial failure of the anal membrane to resorb results in an anal membrane or stenosis. The perineum also contributes to the development of the external anal opening and genitalia by the formation of cloacal folds, which extend from the anterior genital tubercle to the anus. The perineal body is formed by fusion of the cloacal folds between the anal and urogenital membranes. Breakdown of the cloacal membrane anywhere along its course results in the external anal opening being anterior to the external sphincter (i.e., anteriorly displaced anus).

An anatomic classification of anorectal anomalies is based on the level at which the blind-ending rectal pouch ends—low, intermediate, or high in relationship to the levator ani musculature. A more therapeutic and prognostic classification is depicted in Box 67.1. An invertogram, a lateral pelvic radiograph taken after the infant is held upside-down for several minutes, was used in the past to determine the most distal point of the rectal pouch. In most, a careful inspection of the perineum alone can predict the blind pouch level. If an anocutaneous fistula is observed anywhere on the perineal skin of a boy (Fig. 67.13) or external to the hymen of a girl, a low lesion can be assumed. Rectal atresia, commonly associated with trisomy 21, refers to an unusual lesion in which

BOX 67.1 Classification of congenital anomalies of the anorectum.

Female
- Cutaneous (perineal fistula)
- Vestibular fistula
- Imperforate anus without fistula
- Rectal atresia
- Cloaca
- Complex malformation

Male
- Cutaneous (perineal fistula)
- Rectourethral fistula
  - Bulbar
  - Prostatic
- Recto–bladder neck fistula
- Imperforate anus without fistula
- Rectal atresia

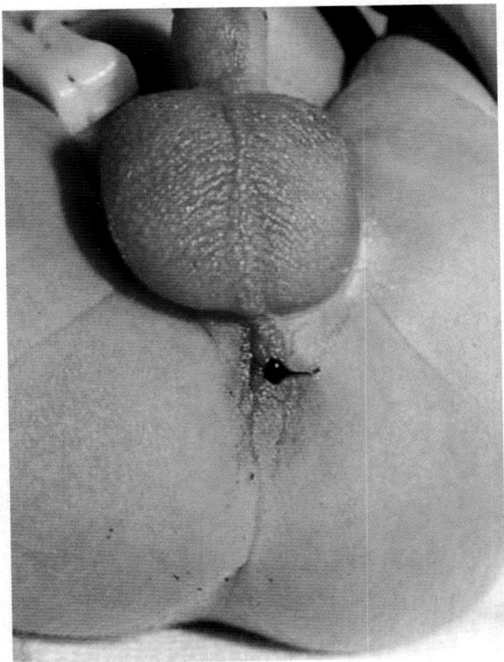

FIG. 67.13 Imperforate anus with perineal fistula opening demonstrating meconium. Gluteal and scrotal anatomy appear relatively normal, consistent with characteristic findings in blind rectal pouch close to perineal skin amenable to anorectoplasty without an ostomy.

the lumen of the rectum is completely or partially interrupted, with the upper rectum being dilated and the lower rectum consisting of a small anal canal. A persistent cloaca is defined as a defect in which the rectum, vagina, and urethra all fuse to form a single common channel. In girls, a single orifice in the perineum indicates a cloaca. If two perineal orifices are seen (i.e., urethra and vagina), the defect represents a high imperforate anus or, less commonly, a persistent urogenital sinus comprising one orifice and a normal anus as the other orifice. Anorectal malformation often coexists with other lesions, and the VACTERL association must be considered during evaluation. Bone abnormalities of the sacrum and spine, such as absent vertebrae, accessory vertebrae, and hemivertebrae or an asymmetrical or short sacrum, can occur in approximately one third of patients. Absence of two or more vertebrae is associated with a poor prognosis for bowel and bladder continence. Occult dysraphism of the spinal cord may also be present, consisting of a tethered cord, lipomeningocele, or fat within the filum terminale.

Genitourinary abnormalities other than rectourinary fistula occur in 25% to 60% of patients. Vesicoureteral reflux and hydronephrosis are the most common, but other conditions, such as horseshoe, dysplastic, or absent kidney as well as hypospadias or cryptorchidism, must be considered. In general, the higher the anorectal malformation, the greater the frequency of associated urologic abnormalities. In patients with a persistent cloaca or rectovesical fistula, the likelihood of a genitourinary abnormality is approximately 90%. In contrast, the frequency is only 10% with low defects (e.g., perineal fistula). Renal ultrasound and voiding cystourethrography are obtained to assess the urinary tract. If a cardiac defect is suspected, echocardiography is performed before any surgical procedure. Esophageal atresia can also be ruled out with an orogastric tube placement. The decision algorithms for the management of male and female newborns with anorectal malformation are shown in Figs 67.14 and 67.15.

A newborn with a perineal or vestibular fistula may undergo a primary single-stage repair without colostomy. For anal stenosis in which the anal opening is in a normal location, serial dilation alone is usually sufficient. Dilations are performed daily with gradual size increase over time. If the anal opening is anterior to the external sphincter (i.e., anteriorly displaced anus), with a small distance between the opening and the center of the external sphincter, and the perineal body is intact, a transposition anoplasty or miniposterior sagittal anorectoplasty is indicated to operatively restore the anal opening to the normal position within the center of the sphincter muscles, and the anterior perineal body is reconstructed. Newborns suspected of having a rectourinary tract fistula with blind rectal pouch above the levator ani generally require an initial diverting colostomy as the first part of a three-stage reconstruction. The colon is completely divided, and an end sigmoid colostomy with a mucous fistula is constructed to minimize fecal contamination in the area of the rectourinary fistula. Furthermore, the distal mucous fistula limb can be used later for a contrast study to determine the rectourinary fistula. The second-stage procedure is usually performed at 3 to 6 months of age. The operation consists of dividing the rectourinary or rectovaginal fistula with a pull-through of the terminal rectal pouch into the normal anal position. A posterior sagittal anorectoplasty, as first described by deVries and Peña, is the procedure of choice.[23] This consists of determining the location of the central position of the anal sphincter by electrical stimulation of the perineal musculature throughout the operation. An incision is then made in the midline, extending from the coccyx to the anterior perineum, through the sphincter and levator musculature until the rectum is identified. The fistula from the rectum to the vagina or urinary tract is divided. The rectum is mobilized and the perineal musculature reconstructed. The third and final stage is colostomy reversal, which is performed several weeks later. Anal dilations begin 2 weeks after the anorectoplasty and continue for several months after the colostomy closure.

A laparoscopically assisted posterior sagittal anorectoplasty has significant advantages as a minimally invasive approach for anorectal malformations with good outcomes. This technique offers

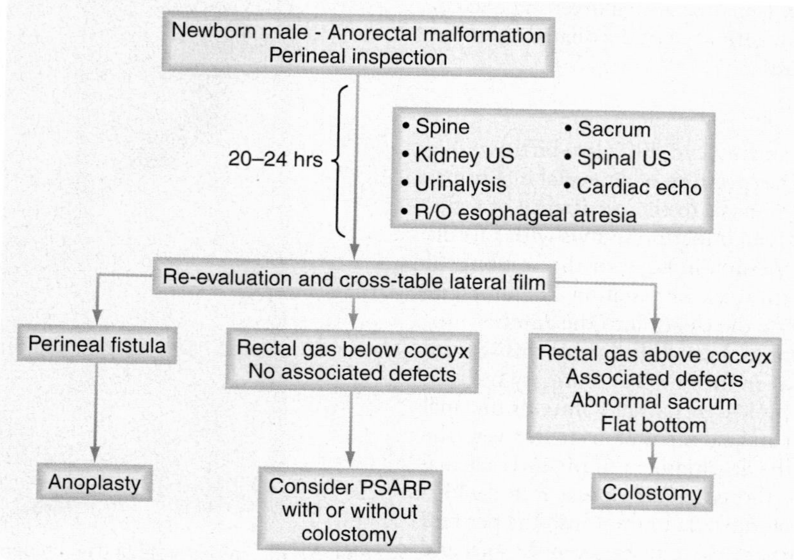

FIG. 67.14 Management algorithm for boys with anorectal malformation. (From Levitt M, Peña A. Imperforate anus. In: Chung DH, Chen MK, ed. *Atlas of pediatric surgical techniques*. Philadelphia,PA: Elsevier Saunders; 2010:185–205.) *echo,* Echocardiogram; *PSARP,* posterior sagittal anorectoplasty; *R/O,* rule out; *US,* ultrasound.

the theoretical advantages of placing the neorectum within the central position of the sphincter and levator muscle complex under direct vision and avoids the need to cut across these structures. Presently, the long-term outcome of this new approach compared to the standard posterior sagittal method is unknown.

Complications of anorectal malformations relate to their associated anomalies. Fecal continence is the major goal regarding correction of the defect. Prognostic factors for continence include the level of the pouch and whether the sacrum is normal. In general, 75% of patients have voluntary bowel movements. However, 50% of this group still soils their underwear occasionally, while the other 50% is considered totally continent. Constipation is the most common sequela. A bowel management program consisting of daily enemas is an important postoperative plan to reduce the frequency of soilage and to improve the quality of life for these patients.

Intussusception

Ileocolic intussusception is a telescoping of distal ileum into the cecum. It is usually idiopathic, without an obvious anatomic lead point, and occurs predominantly at the ileocecal junction, where there is marked swelling of the lymphoid tissue in the region of the ileocecal valve. It is unknown whether this represents the cause or effect of the ileocolic intussusception. The occurence of intussusception is associated with a history of recent episodes of viral gastroenteritis, upper respiratory infections, and even administration of the rotavirus vaccine, implicating lymphoid swelling in the pathogenesis of intussusception. In older children, the incidence of a pathologic lead point is up to 12%, and Meckel diverticulum is found to be the most common lead point for intussusception. However, other causes, such as intestinal polyps, an inflamed appendix, submucosal hemorrhage associated with Henoch-Schönlein purpura, a foreign body, ectopic pancreatic or gastric tissue, and intestinal duplication, must also be considered. Postoperative small bowel intussusception in the absence of a lead point can occur in up to 5% of all pediatric cases of intussusception.

Intussusception produces severe cramping abdominal pain in an otherwise healthy child from 3 months to 3 years. Two thirds of children presenting with intussusception are younger than one year. The child often draws their legs up during the pain episodes and is usually quiet during the intervening periods. Other symptoms include vomiting, passage of bloody mucus (currant jelly stool), and a palpable abdominal mass. In approximately 50% of cases, the diagnosis of ileocolic intussusception can be suspected on plain abdominal radiographs by the presence of a mass, sparse colonic gas, or complete distal small bowel obstruction. Currently, abdominal ultrasound is used as an initial diagnostic test. The characteristic sonographic findings of the "target sign" of the intussuscepted layers of bowel on a transverse view or the "pseudokidney sign" seen longitudinally should prompt air-contrast enema study.

Hydrostatic reduction by enema using contrast material or air is the therapeutic procedure of choice. Contraindications to this approach include the presence of peritonitis and hemodynamic instability. Furthermore, an intussusception located entirely within the small intestine is unlikely to be reduced by an enema and more likely to have an associated the lead point. Successful reduction is accomplished in more than 80% of cases, confirmed by resolution of the mass, along with reflux of air into the terminal ileum, and many of these patients can be discharged without hospital admissions. For those refractory to initial air enema attempt, many centers try a repeat air enema study a few hours later with moderate success.[24] The recurrence rate after hydrostatic reduction is ~11% and usually occurs within the 24 hours after the reduction. When

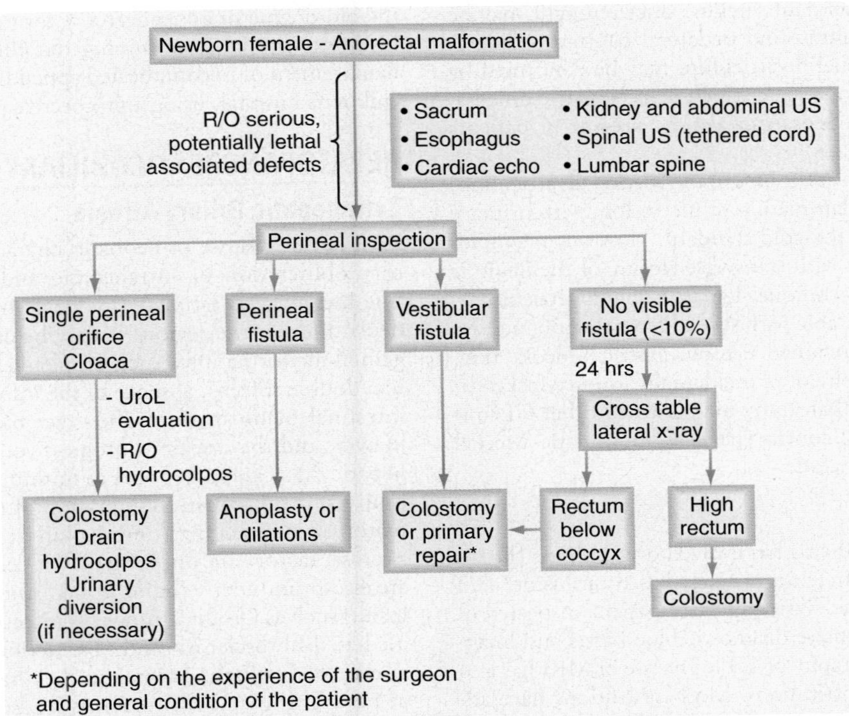

FIG. 67.15 Management algorithm for girls with anorectal malformation. (From Levitt M, Peña A. Imperforate anus. In: Chung DH, Chen MK, ed. *Atlas of pediatric surgical techniques*. Philadelphia, PA: Elsevier Saunders; 2010:185–205.) *echo*, Echocardiogram; *R/O*, rule out; *UroL*, urologic; *US*, ultrasound.

it recurs, it is usually managed by another air enema reduction. A third recurrence is an indication for operative management.

The operative indications for intussusception include: peritonitis, bowel obstruction at initial presentation, failed hydrostatic enema reduction, or multiple recurrences. The intussusceptum is delivered through a transverse incision in the right side of the abdomen and reduced in a retrograde fashion by pushing the mass proximally. Once it is reduced, viability of the reduced bowel is examined. The lymphoid tissue in the ileocecal region is thickened and edematous and may be mistaken for a tumor within the small bowel, and great caution should be exercised prior to surgical resection. Recurrence rates are extremely low after surgical reduction. Bowel resection is required occasionally when the intussusception cannot be reduced, the viability of the bowel is uncertain, or a lead point is identified. If so, an ileocolectomy with primary anastomosis is usually performed. Laparoscopic reduction of an intussusception has recently gained popularity with some success.

Meckel Diverticulum

Meckel diverticulum is the most common congenital anomaly of the GI tract and occurs in approximately 2% of the population. More than 70% of symptomatic patients have heterotopic gastric mucosa and another 5% have pancreatic tissue. The rule of 2's is often cited in association with Meckel diverticulum. Aside from its 2% incidence and two types of heterotopic mucosa, it is located within 2 feet of the ileocecal valve, is approximately 2 inches in length, and usually symptomatic by 2 years of age. Meckel diverticulum is caused by a failure of normal regression of the vitelline duct that occurs during weeks 5 to 7 of gestation. Meckel diverticulum is a true diverticulum containing all intestinal layers.

The clinical symptoms are related to hemorrhage, obstruction, or inflammation. The most common presenting symptom is a painless, massive, lower GI bleeding in children younger than 5 years. Diagnosis of a persistent vitelline duct remnant may be established by umbilical ultrasound or lateral contrast radiography. Bleeding from a Meckel diverticulum may be confirmed by a ^{99m}Tc-pertechnetate isotope scan, which detects gastric mucosa. Of note, ectopic gastric mucosa can also be present in patients with intestinal duplication.

Segmental ileal resection at the base of the Meckel diverticulum, especially in the case of inflammation or ulceration, with primary end-to-end anastomosis is the gold standard. However, a simpler V-shaped diverticulectomy with transverse closure of the ileum is an acceptable alternative technique. Laparoscopic diverticulectomy has become more acceptable with several reporting no increase in complications due to retained ectopic gastric mucosa (Fig. 67.16).[25] Although management of incidentally found Meckel diverticulum at the time of laparotomy for unrelated other GI condition has been somewhat controversial, asymptomatic Meckel diverticulum should be left alone.

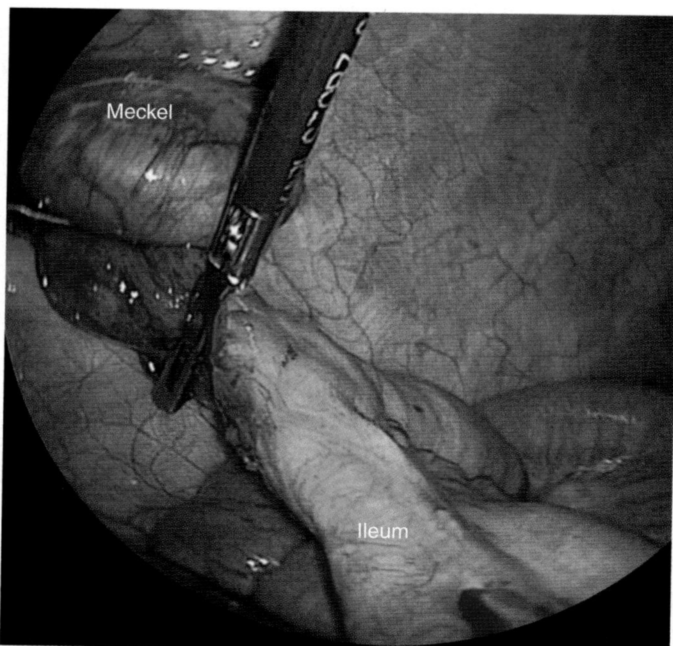

FIG. 67.16 Meckel diverticulectomy performed using an endoscopic stapling device via laparoscopic approach.

Appendicitis

The management of appendicitis has evolved over a time. The diagnosis of appendicitis is rarely made solely based on history and physical exam findings alone. Virtually every patient suspected of appendicitis undergoes extensive diagnostic blood tests and imaging studies (e.g., ultrasonography or CT). The use of MRI has also been introduced at some institutions. Most institutions have adopted a clinical pathway-based management of appendicitis with standardized IV antibiotic regimens, operative techniques, and postoperative care, which include minimal to no outpatient opioid use. Laparoscopic appendectomy is the standard approach. For simple appendicitis, a single dose of preoperative IV antibiotic is administered, and the appendectomy is safely performed within 24 hours. For complicated appendicitis, surgical management includes immediate appendectomy with early conversion to an oral antibiotic regimen or percutaneous drainage with delayed interval appendectomy. Recently, nonoperative management of appendicitis has become more accepted in clinical practice, challenging the old dogma of appendectomy for every appendicitis. A multi-institutional trial is examining the effectiveness of nonoperative management of uncomplicated appendicitis across a group of large children's hospitals using a prospective patient choice design.[26]

HEPATOPANCREATICOBILIARY CONDITIONS

Extrahepatic Biliary Atresia

BA is a rare disease of neonates characterized by the inflammatory obliteration of intrahepatic and extrahepatic bile ducts. The incidence is estimated to be 1 in 5000 to 12,000 infants, depending on the region. It may be associated with other congenital malformations, such as splenic abnormalities (e.g., asplenia, double spleen), absence of the inferior vena cava (IVC), and intestinal malformation. The exact mechanisms of BA are unknown, and the disease is progressive. One theory is that extrahepatic ducts are susceptible to immune-mediated inflammatory injury and subsequent obliteration of the bile ducts. Proinflammatory cytokines (i.e., interleukin-2, interferon-γ, and tumor necrosis factor) are implicated.[27] T cells and natural killer cells are also prominently found in BA. Another theory is that a viral insult, such as Group C rotavirus infection, triggers the immune-mediated fibrosclerosis and obstruction of the extrahepatic bile ducts. Interestingly, animal studies have shown that infection of newborn mice with rotavirus leads to a presentation similar to infants, with the onset of hyperbilirubinemia, jaundice, and acholic stools. Histology shows inflammation and obstruction of the extrahepatic bile ducts. Another hypothesis is that there

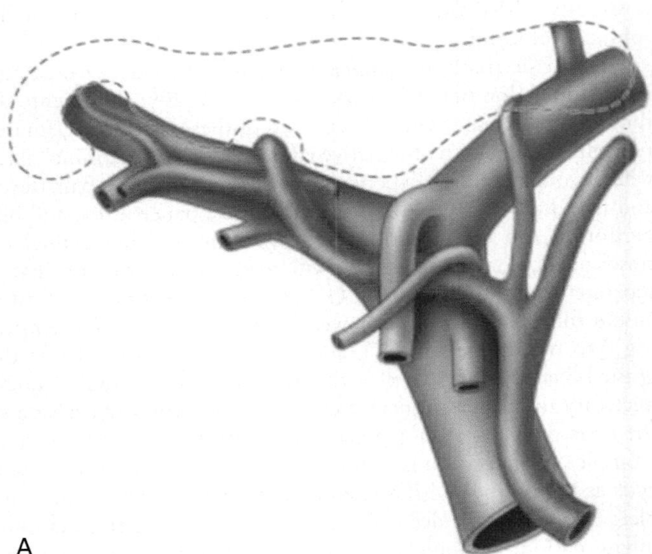

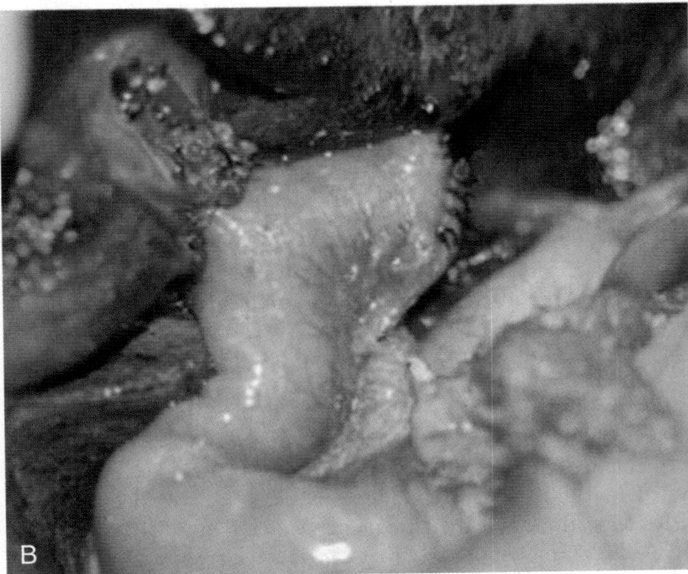

FIG. 67.17 Kasai portoenterostomy. (A) The dissection of fibrous extrahepatic biliary remnant is continued up to the capsular surface of the liver within the bifurcation of the portal vein (*dotted line* indicates fibrous portal plate). The lateral extent of dissection on the left side is the umbilical fissure and the obliterated umbilical vein insertion into the left portal vein. On the right side, the lateral extent of dissection is to the bifurcation of the right portal vein into its anterior and posterior branches. (B) Completed Roux-en-Y portoenterostomy. (From Nathan JD, Ryckman FC. Biliary atresia. In Chung DH, Chen MK, ed. *Atlas of pediatric surgical techniques.* Philadelphia,PA: Elsevier Saunders;2010:220–231.)

may be an association with human leukocyte antigen (HLA) type and BA, since patients with BA have a high frequency of HLA-B12. It is unclear whether this is causal, but some argue that abnormal expression of HLA makes biliary ductal epithelial cells susceptible targets for immunologic assault. Another putative gene, *CFC1*, encodes a protein important in the embryonic differentiation of the left-right axis; when mutated, it is thought to predispose to the development of BA. Histopathology shows significant extrahepatic biliary obstruction with portal tract fibrosis, inflammatory cell infiltration, bile duct proliferation, and cholestasis with bile plugging.

The disease is classified according to the level of the most proximal biliary obstruction. Type 1 BA has patency to the level of the common bile duct (CBD); type 2 has patency to the level of the common hepatic duct; and type 3, which accounts for more than 90% of cases, occurs when the left and right hepatic ducts, at the level of the porta hepatis, are involved. This aids in the differentiation between correctable BA and others. Correctable BA requires that patent hepatic ducts exist to the porta hepatis. Types 1 and 2 may be amenable to a direct extrahepatic biliary duct–intestinal anastomosis.

Infants present shortly after birth with jaundice, pale stools, and dark urine. Advanced disease presents with failure to thrive, hepatomegaly, and ascites from liver cirrhosis. If the jaundice persists after 14 days of life in a term infant, an evaluation for liver disease should be initiated. This consists of determining direct or conjugated bilirubin levels, which will be elevated (>2.0 mg/dL) in those with liver disease. Other exclusionary studies include serologic testing for toxoplasmosis, rubella, cytomegalovirus, and herpes (TORCH) and hepatitis B and C infections, α_1-antitrypsin, and CF. Metabolic disorders, such as galactosemia and tyrosinemia, and endocrine abnormalities must also be ruled out.

The gallbladder may be atrophic or absent, and intrahepatic ducts may also be notably absent on ultrasound evaluation. Hepatobiliary iminodiacetic acid (HIDA) scintigraphy, magnetic resonance cholangiopancreatography (MRCP), and endoscopic retrograde cholangiopancreatography (ERCP) are used with varying success. A HIDA scan can reveal uptake of the technetium isotope with an absence of emptying into the duodenum. MRCP or ERCP can better define the biliary anatomy, but it is more invasive. Ultimately, liver biopsy is the gold standard for the diagnosis of BA and can safely be done percutaneously or open. Once the diagnosis is suspected, an operative exploration with intraoperative cholangiography is indicated. If BA is confirmed, a hepatoportoenterostomy (Kasai procedure) is the surgical procedure of choice. Here, the extrahepatic biliary tree is dissected proximally to the level of the liver capsule, where the porta hepatis (portal plate) is transected. The dissection of the fibrous remnant ascends into the posterior area surrounding the portal vein branches until it has come within the capsular surface of the liver (Fig. 67.17A). The reconstruction is performed using a Roux-en-Y hepaticojejunostomy (Fig. 67.17B). The use of ursodeoxycholic acid and phenobarbital may promote biliary drainage, but their efficacy is uncertain. The use of steroids after the Kasai procedure has been advocated by many and thought to promote biliary drainage with shorter hospital stay. However, the Biliary Atresia Clinical Research Consortium's recent randomized, double-blinded, placebo-controlled trial of steroid therapy (the START trial) after the Kasai procedure demonstrated that high-dose steroid therapy after the procedure did not result in significant treatment differences in bile drainage at 6 months.[28] Furthermore, steroid treatment was associated with earlier onset of serious adverse events, as well as with impaired growth. However, steroid pulse therapy remains a treatment option for post–Kasai cholangitis. Antibiotics are also continued postoperatively, because the risk of cholangitis is high (45% to 60%) due to of the ease with which intestinal bacteria can ascend and colonize the bile ducts. Unfortunately, if the Kasai procedure is unable to reestablish bile flow and liver failure or cirrhosis ensues, liver transplantation is indicated.

Kasai hepatoportoenterostomy does not cure BA, which will inevitably progress in more than 70% of infants who undergo this procedure. The rate with which the disease progresses, as evidenced by cirrhosis and portal hypertension, is variable, but it may be expedited by recurrent cholangitis. It is estimated, however, that 80% of those who have successfully undergone a Kasai procedure can live up to 10 years before liver transplantation is needed. In those infants who undergo transplantation, outcomes are good, with 10-year graft survival and overall patient survival of 73% and 86%, respectively.[29]

Choledochal Cyst

Choledochal cysts are cystic dilations of the CBD. They have an incidence of 1 in 100,000 to 150,000 live births, with a 3 to 4 : 1 female-to-male preponderance. They are classified on the basis of location, and their frequency varies (Fig. 67.18). Type I (50%–80%) is a simple cyst that can involve any portion of the CBD, and type II (2%) describes a diverticulum arising off the CBD. Choledochoceles represent type III cysts (1.4%–4.5%) and consist of dilation confined to the distal intrapancreatic portion of the CBD. While type IV (15%–35%) involves intrahepatic and extrahepatic bile ducts, type V (20%) is limited to the intrahepatic ducts only. Choledochal cysts can be associated with other congenital anomalies, including duodenal and colonic atresia, imperforate anus, pancreatic arteriovenous malformation, and pancreatic divisum. Moreover, choledochal cysts are considered premalignant lesions.[30]

The pathogenesis of choledochal cysts is largely unknown but pancreaticobiliary reflux-induced activation of pancreatic enzymes within the duct has been implicated. Inflammatory response compromises the integrity of the duct wall, resulting in dilation. In support of this theory, amylase and trypsinogen levels in the bile from patients with choledochal cysts are often elevated. Another possibility is that these cysts arise from CBD obstruction at the sphincter of Oddi.

The classic triad of jaundice, a palpable right upper quadrant mass, and abdominal pain is seen in less than 20% of patients, although 85% present with at least two of these symptoms. Infants typically present with obstructive jaundice and an abdominal mass, whereas older children experience chronic intermittent pain, fever, and jaundice. Complications of cholangitis, pancreatitis, and bile peritonitis can occur secondary to cyst rupture. Abdominal ultrasound demonstrates a cystic enlarged ductal structure that is separate from the gallbladder. HIDA scan can demonstrate initial absent filling of the cyst, followed by delayed uptake and emptying into the duodenum. CT and MRCP can further define the entire biliary system as well as the pancreatic head. ERCP is rarely necessary to make a surgical decision. Prompt surgical excision of the cysts with Roux-en-Y hepaticojejunostomy is recommended. Complete cyst excision is important because the risk of malignancy is as high as 6% with a retained choledochal cyst. If the complete cyst excision is deemed unsafe due to scarring from chronic inflammation, it should be enucleated. These patients are monitored with ultrasound exams. Postoperative anastomotic strictures are a common complication and likely arise from chronic intrahepatic cholelithiasis and recurrent cholangitis.

Hereditary Pancreatitis and Pancreas Divisum

Hereditary pancreatitis is an autosomal dominant disorder with a high degree of penetrance. It is rare, representing less than 1% of chronic pancreatitis. The disease results from a mutation in the cationic trypsinogen gene *(PRSS1),* which leads to an increase in the autoactivation of trypsin and resistance to deactivation.[31] The gene has been mapped to chromosome 7q35; the two most common allelic mutations are *R122H* and *N29I.* Recurrent bouts of pancreatitis usually begin in childhood, between 5 and 10 years of age, with no identifiable cause. Aside from the age at onset, the presentation, natural history, diagnosis, and treatment of this disease are similar to those for other causes of pancreatitis. Hereditary

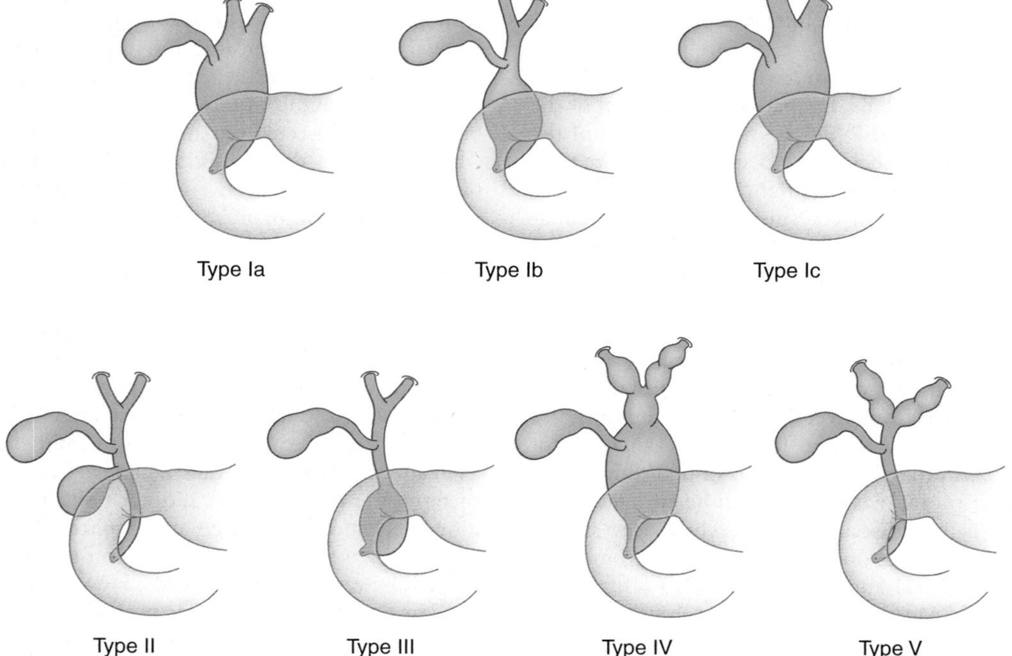

FIG. 67.18 Classification of choledochal cyst. (From O'Neill JA. Choledochal cyst. In: Grosfeld JL, O'Neill JA, Fonkalsrud EW, et al, ed. *Pediatric surgery.* 6th ed. Philadelphia, PA; Mosby Elsevier;2006:16–21.)

pancreatitis should be suspected in any patient who experiences at least two bouts of acute pancreatitis without obvious risk factors, such as trauma, hyperlipidemia, gallstones, or pancreas divisum. It should also be considered in any child with acute pancreatitis and a family history of this disease and pancreatitis in children. Making the correct diagnosis is important because there is an extremely high lifetime risk of malignant transformation. It is estimated that these patients have a fifty- to seventy fold increase in the risk for development of pancreatic adenocarcinoma within 7 to 30 years of disease onset. The cumulative lifetime risk is estimated to be 40% by the age of 70 years. Therefore, screening by endoscopic ultrasound is recommended, starting at the age of 30 years.

Pancreas divisum is a congenital anatomic anomaly in which the ventral pancreas and dorsal pancreas fail to fuse. The resultant pancreas has dual drainage, with the dorsal pancreas draining through the duct of Santorini and the ventral pancreas (head and uncinate process) draining through the duct of Wirsung. The onset of symptoms is variable, ranging from early childhood to adulthood. Although ultrasound and CT are usually performed, ERCP is frequently used to confirm the diagnosis. However, MRCP has been touted as more advantageous because it can delineate the dorsal pancreatic duct in its entirety, as opposed to ERCP, which can assess only the ventral duct on cannulation of the major duodenal papilla. The significance of pancreas divisum and its predisposition to chronic pancreatitis remains controversial. Some have suggested that it may result in pancreatitis because all pancreatic output is forced to empty through the smaller lesser papilla. The result is an outflow obstruction leading to ductal dilation. Treatment consists of transduodenal sphincteroplasty or a Puestow procedure (pancreaticojejunostomy); a Puestow procedure is preferred if the dorsal pancreatic duct is dilated or obstructed.

Biliary Dyskinesia

Obesity has also become a major health problem for adolescents. Subsequently, we are seeing an increasing number of pediatric patients with cholelithiasis and biliary colic due to dyskinesia of the gallbladder. Biliary dyskinesia has become more prevalent and should be considered during evaluation of a teenager with epigastric pain. Pediatric surgeons are often consulted to evaluate for the appropriateness of performing a cholecystectomy based on a low ejection fraction from a cholecystokinin-stimulated HIDA scan. When an ejection fraction of less than 35% to 40% correlates with characteristic biliary colic, a cholecystectomy can be therapeutic.[32] However, in patients with vague symptoms, inconsistent with biliary colic, cholecystectomy is not indicated.

ABDOMINAL WALL CONDITIONS

Anterior abdominal wall defects are a relatively frequent neonatal surgical condition. During normal development of the human embryo, the midgut herniates outward through the umbilical ring and continues to grow. By the eleventh week of gestation, the midgut returns to the coelomic cavity and undergoes proper rotation and fixation, along with closure of the umbilical ring. If the intestine fails to return, the infant is born with the abdominal contents protruding through the abdominal wall defect at the umbilical ring.

An omphalocele is a central abdominal wall defect that is generally more than 4 cm in diameter, with an intact membranous sac composed of an outer layer of amnion and an inner layer of peritoneum (Fig. 67.19). Defects less than 4 cm in diameter are arbitrarily designated as umbilical cord hernias. Infants with an omphalocele have a high incidence (~50%) of associated anomalies, such as Beckwith-Wiedemann syndrome: a combination of gigantism, macroglossia, and an umbilical defect, either hernia or omphalocele. Chromosomal abnormalities, including trisomies 13, 15, 18, and 21, have also been associated with omphalocele. Other associated anomalies include exstrophy of the bladder or cloaca and the pentalogy of Cantrell: omphalocele, anterior diaphragmatic hernia, sternal cleft, ectopia cordis, and intracardiac defect, such as ventricular septal defect.

Presentation of an intact omphalocele sac is key in initial management. Also, great care should be taken to prevent hypothermia. A comprehensive diagnostic workup is performed to identify associated anomalies. Primary surgical closure of the small to medium-sized defect is preferred. Alternatively, larger defects can be closed with prosthetic patch closure (e.g., Gore-Tex), porcine small intestinal submucosa–derived biomaterial (e.g., Surgisis), skin flap closure, or placement of a silo for sequential reduction and staged closure. Giant omphaloceles are treated by topical application of escharotic agents such as povidone-iodine (Betadine) ointment or silver nitrate, which allows the sac to thicken and epithelialize. The overall survival for infants with an omphalocele largely depends on their lung maturity and severity of associated anomalies.

A gastroschisis defect is always to the right of an intact umbilical cord, at the site of obliterated right umbilical vein, without a sac covering the abdominal viscera (Fig. 67.20A). The fascial defect is typically 4 cm in diameter. An absent sac with direct exposure to amniotic fluid in utero results in intestinal thickening and edema with inflammation. Intestinal atresia may exist in up to 15% of cases, however, other major anomalies are rare. Eviscerated bowel must be handled with care to avoid further insult. After birth, infants are placed in a warm, saline-filled plastic 'bowel bag' up to the nipple line, in order to minimize heat and fluid losses. This also allows for gross inspection of the eviscerated bowel at all times and identification of inadvertent twisting of the bowel. Primary reduction is successful in 50% to 80%, with eviscerated contents placed into the abdominal cavity without excessive tension. If primary reduction is unsuccessful, a ringed silo bag is placed and the eviscerated bowel is reduced gradually over several days, followed by operative suture closure of the fascia and skin (Fig. 67.20B). To avoid compartment syndrome, a safe intraabdominal pressure is less than 15 mm Hg. Alternatively, a sutureless delayed spontaneous closure can be performed at the bedside.[33] Bowel is reduced into the abdomen and the defect is covered with

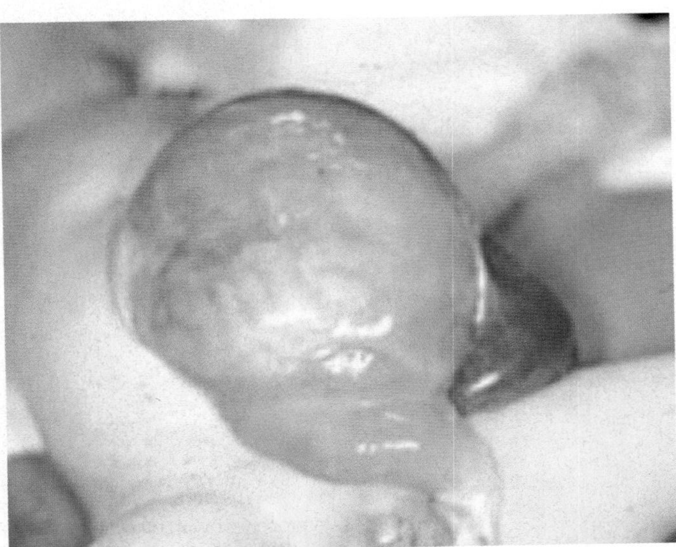

FIG. 67.19 Omphalocele with intact sac and centrally located abdominal wall defect.

or without the umbilical cord, and a watertight clear dressing (Fig. 67.20C) is placed. Once the contents adhere in the intraabdominal position at around 4 days, the dressing can then be changed to a dry dressing over the cord remnant or a Vaseline dressing over the exposed bowel. In cases of associated intestinal atresia or stenosis, inflammation of the bowel precludes an immediate repair; the abdominal wall is closed first and then surgery for intestinal atresia is performed 6 to 8 weeks later. Late occurrence of NEC has been reported in up to 20% of patients after gastroschisis repair. For larger defects, a prosthetic patch (Gore-Tex) is placed and the skin is closed over it. Undescended testis is a common associated finding in 10% to 20% of infants. When found outside the peritoneal cavity, the testes should be simply pushed back into the abdominal cavity without formal orchidopexy at the time of abdominal wall closure or silo bag placement. Many spontaneously descend into the scrotum. If not, orchidopexy is performed. The majority of infants have prolonged ileus. One of the difficult challenges in the management of gastroschisis remains managing dysfunctional intestine or short gut syndrome and infants often experience cholestasis due to prolonged TPN support.

Hernias

Inguinal hernia repair is one of the most commonly performed surgical procedures in pediatric surgery. The incidence of inguinal hernia is approximately 3% to 5% in term infants and 9% to 11% in premature infants. It affects boys approximately six times more often than girls. Sixty percent of inguinal hernias occur on the right side, 30% are on the left side, 10% are bilateral, and almost all are indirect and congenital in nature. The processus vaginalis is an elongated diverticulum of the peritoneum that accompanies the testicle on its descent into the scrotum, and it generally is obliterated during the ninth month of gestation or soon after birth. The variable persistence of the processus vaginalis results in a spectrum of clinical presentations, including a scrotal hernia with protrusion of intestine, ovaries, omentum, or communicating hydrocele with intermittent accumulation of peritoneal fluid.

The diagnosis of an inguinal hernia is established by clinical history and examination alone. Transillumination of the scrotum to differentiate a hydrocele from a hernia can be misleading because a herniated, thin-walled loop of bowel in infants and children can be easily transilluminated. Palpation of the cord may elicit a "silk glove

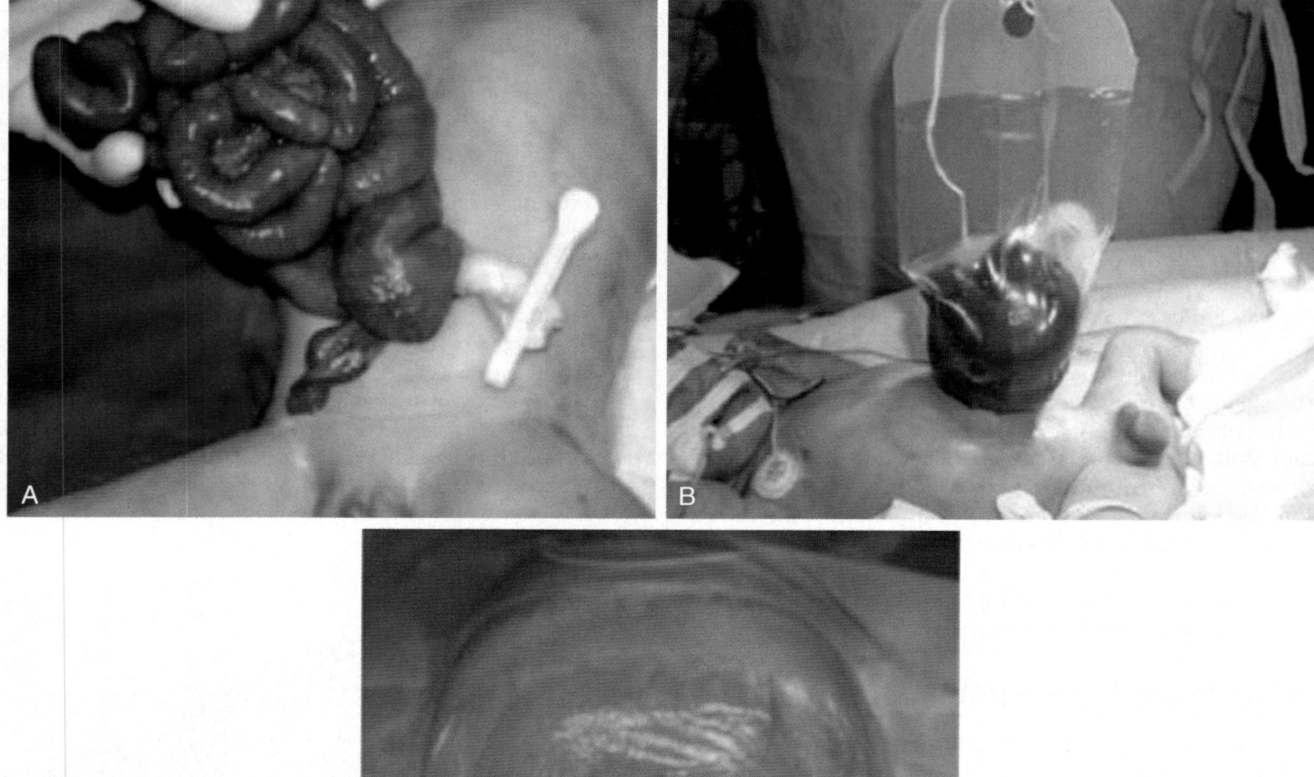

FIG. 67.20 (A) Gastroschisis with eviscerated bowel. Note the abdominal wall defect is to the right side of an intact umbilical cord. (B) Silastic bag with ringed edge can be placed at bedside and bowel loops are gradually reduced into abdominal cavity. (C) Sutureless closure of gastroschisis. After reducing eviscerated bowel loops into the abdominal cavity, the umbilical cord is folded over the defect and a clear watertight dressing is placed.

sign," which is produced by rubbing the opposing peritoneal membranes of the empty sac. At times, palpation of a thickened cord, in comparison to the contralateral side, along with a reliable history of intermittent bulge are sufficient to derive a diagnosis. The acute onset of hydrocele may also be associated with other conditions, such as epididymitis, testicular torsion, and torsion of the testicular appendage. In these instances, ultrasound examination may be helpful to determine the diagnosis. The major risks of inguinal hernias are bowel incarceration and potential strangulation. The incidence of incarceration is higher in the first year of life in premature infants.

The ideal timing of inguinal hernia repair in premature infants has recently come under scrutiny. Historically, most advocated for hernia repair prior to hospital discharge. However, due to concerns of potential complications, including a long-term risk of neurodevelopmental delay with general anesthesia, delayed repair may be a better treatment strategy. There are ongoing multiinstitutional studies evaluating the timing of infant inguinal hernia repair. When elective, repair may be deferred until postoperative apnea risk decreases at 1 year of age. An incarcerated inguinal hernia should be reduced first, and then repair should be performed 24 to 48 hours later when tissue edema subsides. A nonreducible, incarcerated hernia is a surgical emergency. Contralateral inguinal exploration at the time of symptomatic hernia repair is routinely performed based on the high incidence of a contralateral patent processus vaginalis (4%–65%). However, the issue regarding the routine exploration of the asymptomatic contralateral side in toddlers remains unresolved. Most pediatric surgeons explore the asymptomatic contralateral side in children 2 years of age or younger. Laparoscopic pediatric hernia repair is increasingly used by many surgeons today. A recent metaanalysis comparing laparoscopic versus open approach for pediatric inguinal hernia repair showed no definite advantage of one technique over the other.[34]

An umbilical hernia has a tendency to close on its own in ~80% of cases of children, and therefore, elective repair should be deferred until around 5 years of age. Incarceration of an umbilical hernia is extremely rare. Earlier elective surgical repair should be considered when the hernia appears to enlarge over time or the fascial defect is larger than 2 cm. If left alone, these hernias tend to develop large skin proboscis (>3 cm) resulting in poor postoperative cosmesis. Primary repair of the hernia is always achieved, and the use of prosthetic patch should never be considered.

CHEST WALL DEFORMITIES

Pectus excavatum, a chest wall structural deformity where the anterior chest wall is caved-in or sunken, is five times more common than pectus carinatum, an abnormal outward protrusion of the anterior chest wall. The deformity is usually present at birth and steadily becomes more prominent with age until past puberty with a male-to-female ratio of 3 to 4:1. Abnormalities in costal cartilage development have been implicated in the underlying pathogenesis. Pectus excavatum can be associated with mitral valve prolapse, Ehlers-Danlos syndrome, and Marfan syndrome, and therefore a comprehensive preoperative evaluation is warranted. The severity of pectus excavatum is quantified by the Haller index, which is a ratio of the width of the chest wall to the depth of between the sternum and the vertebral body on limited chest CT or two-view plain radiographs. A Haller index of more than 3.2, pulmonary function testing indicating restrictive disease, mitral valve prolapse, murmurs, or conduction abnormalities on echocardiography are indications for surgical repair. Psychosocial stress is often significant and should not be underestimated, particularly in adolescents with body image and self-esteem issues. A multicenter study has shown that surgical repair of pectus excavatum significantly improves body image and perceived ability of physical activity.[35]

The optimal age for pectus excavatum repair is 10 to 14 years of age. The Nuss procedure has largely replaced the Ravitch (open) procedure for pectus excavatum. Under thoracoscopic guidance, a tunneler is used to perform the retrosternal dissection. Sternal elevation using a retractor system has become popularized for a safer sternal dissection in recent years. An appropriately sized titanium bar is bent and contoured to elevate the sternum, and the bar is passed through the retrosternal plane from one hemithorax into the other, through two lateral intercostal incisions (Fig. 67.21). The Nuss bar

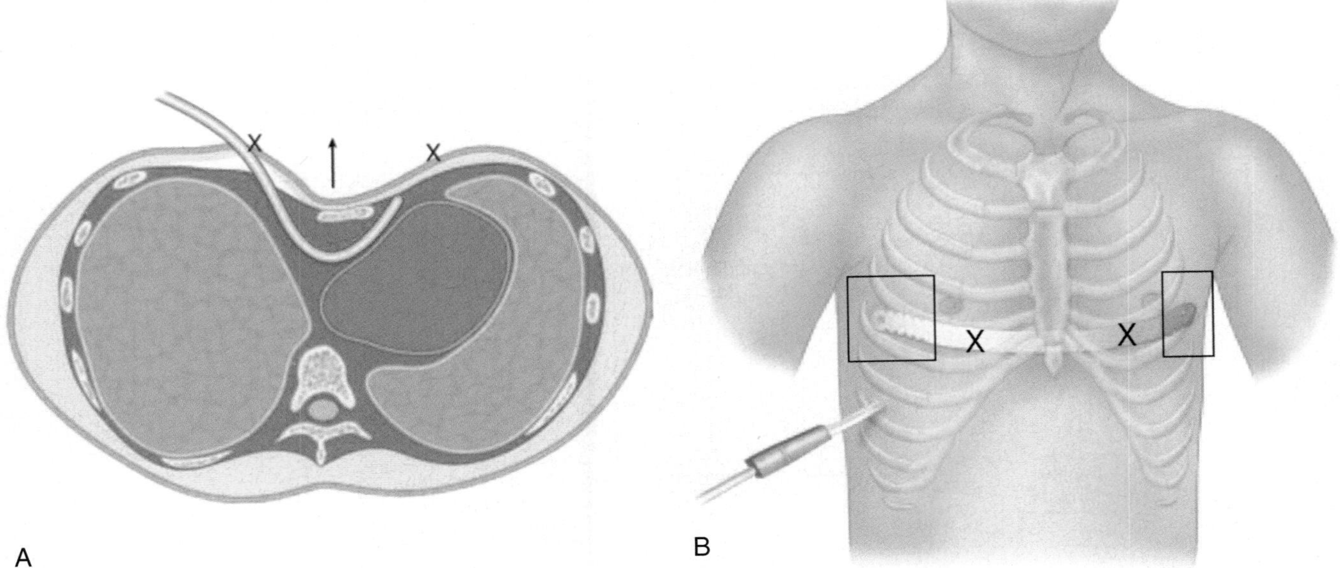

FIG. 67.21 (A) Pectus excavatum. A tunneler is used to dissect the retrosternal place under thoracoscopic guidance. (B) A Nuss bar is placed beneath the sternum and secured onto the chest wall with stabilizers. (From Goretsky MJ, Nuss D. Surgical treatment of chest wall deformities: Nuss procedure. In: Chung DH, Chen MK, ed. *Atlas of pediatric surgical techniques*. Philadelphia, PA. Elsevier Saunders; 2006:97–103.)

is then flipped so that the convexity is outward, and the chest wall defect is immediately corrected. The bar is removed after ~2 years. The use of enhanced recovery pathways after surgery, and utilization of intercostal cryoablation has significantly shortened hospital length of stay, and typically patients are discharged home after 2 or 3 days.[36] Pectus carinatum is corrected with fitted chest brace. There are several different models but the most important predictor of success is treatment adherence, requiring continuous use for 14 to 16 hours daily to see the best results.

GENITOURINARY TRACT CONDITIONS

Cryptorchidism

Cryptorchidism is a condition in which one or both testes fail to descend into the scrotum before birth. While up to 30% of preterm infants can present with an undescended testis, it also occurs in ~23% of full-term infants. Some undescended testes eventually descend by 1 year of age. The undescended testis is associated with histologic and morphologic changes as early as 6 months of age, and atrophy of Leydig cells, a decrease in tubular diameter, and impaired spermatogenesis can occur by 2 years of age. An undescended testis has had its descent halted somewhere along the path of normal descent and is most commonly located in the inguinal canal. A retractile testis is a normally descended testis that retracts into the inguinal canal due to hyperreflexive cremasteric muscle; it is easily brought down into the scrotal sac during the examination and does not require operative intervention. Nonpalpable testes may include an intraabdominal, absent, or vanishing testis. Ectopic testes have had an aberrant path of descent, and these can be found in the perineum, femoral canal, and suprapubic regions. For unilateral palpable testis in the inguinal canal, standard dartos pouch orchidopexy is performed at 6 to 12 months of age. An algorithm for management of nonpalpable testes is shown in Fig. 67.22. For nonpalpable, undescended testis, a diagnostic laparoscopy is useful. If the testicular vessels are seen exiting the internal ring, an open inguinal orchidopexy is performed. For an intraabdominal testis, a two-stage Fowler-Stephens orchidopexy is considered, in which the testicular vessels are ligated as a first stage to allow for development of collateral circulation over 6 months before orchidopexy is performed as a second-stage procedure. Laparoscopic orchidopexy has become popularized as an ideal single-stage option. If both testes are nonpalpable, a human chorionic gonadotropin (hCG) stimulation test is carried out to confirm the presence of functioning testes. If present, diagnostic laparoscopy can locate the testes. The risk of malignancy has been reported to be significantly higher for men with a history of undescended testes. Orchidopexy does not decrease the malignancy risk associated with undescended testes, but it allows for earlier detection. Nonseminomatous germ cell tumors are the most common tumor type with undescended testes.

Testicular Torsion

Torsion of the testis occurs most frequently in early adolescence with a peak incidence at 14 years of age and requires a prompt surgical detorsion with testicular fixation. Extravaginal torsion is more common in neonates in whom there can be torsion of the spermatic cord along its course outside the tunica vaginalis. Intravaginal torsion is associated with a bell clapper deformity in which the suspended testis can torse.

Acute scrotal pain is the primary symptom. The torsed testis may be high-riding, edematous, and significantly tender. Urinary tract symptoms of frequency, urgency, and dysuria tend to occur more common with an infectious or inflammatory etiology, such as epididymitis; however, the presence of urinary symptoms does not rule out testicular torsion. In most, a careful history and physical exam are sufficient to confirm the diagnosis of testicular torsion. If the diagnosis is uncertain, ultrasonography may be helpful to determine presence of vascular flow to the testicles; however, radioisotope scanning is the most specific diagnostic test. Immediate surgical detorsion through a scrotal medial raphe approach is the standard operation. After detorsion, the testis is assessed for viability and fixed to the scrotum. Importantly, the contralateral testis is also fixed. The time between establishing the diagnosis and the surgical detorsion directly correlates with the testicular salvage rate. For torsion of less than 6 hours, 90% of testes can be salvaged. The salvage rate for testis decreases to less than 10% with longer than 24 hours of symptoms.

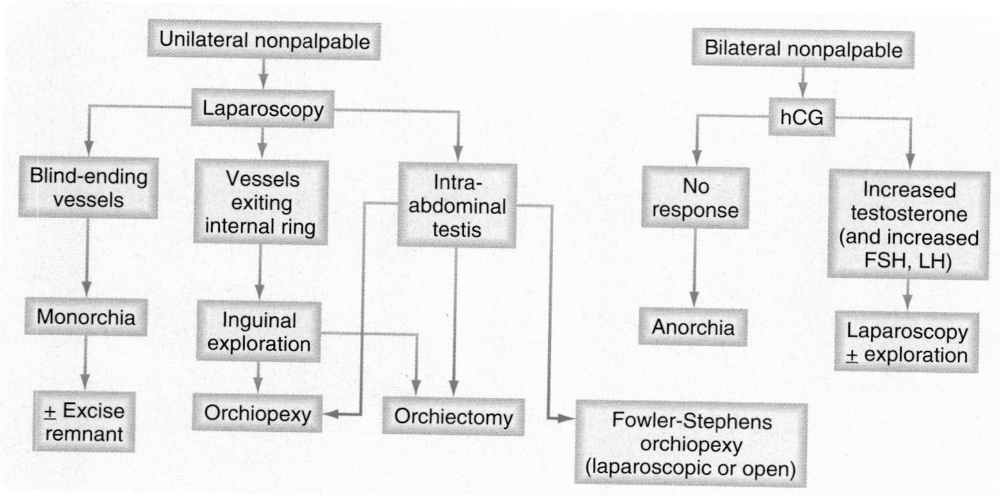

FIG. 67.22 Management algorithm for nonpalpable undescended testes. (Adapted from Lee KL, Shortliffe LD. Undescended testis and testicular tumors. In: Ashcraft KW, Holcomb GW, Holcomb GW III, et al, ed. *Pediatric surgery.* 4th ed. Philadelphia, PA; Elsevier Saunders; 2005: pp 706–716.) *FSH,* Follicle-stimulating hormone; *hCG,* human chorionic gonadotropin; *LH,* luteinizing hormone.

Testicular Tumors

Testicular cancer accounts for less than 2% of all pediatric solid tumors and peaks around 2 years of age and at puberty. They commonly present as painless scrotal masses, often discovered incidentally. Ultrasonography is useful, but CT scan is critical for evaluation of retroperitoneal lymphadenopathy as well as metastatic disease. The serum tumor marker α-fetoprotein (AFP), a glycoprotein produced by the fetal yolk sac, is elevated in yolk sac tumors. β-hCG is produced by embryonal carcinomas and mixed teratomas. Germ cell tumors are the most common prepubertal testicular cancers, while yolk sac tumors, also known as endodermal sinus turmors, and embryonal carcinomas account for almost 40%. The surgical strategy is radical inguinal orchiectomy. Tumors with microscopic or gross nodal involvement require systemic chemotherapy, with modified retroperitoneal lymphadenectomy. The overall survival from yolk sac tumors is approximately 70% to 90%.

PEDIATRIC SOLID TUMORS

While solid tumors that present at early stages of disease do well, those with advanced-stage disease at diagnosis remain difficult to cure, despite multimodality therapeutic options. The newest cancer biology discoveries and clinical trials will have the most impact on children with advanced disease.

Neuroblastoma

Neuroblastoma is the most common extracranial solid tumor in infants and children, accounting for 8% to 10% of all childhood cancers and 15% of all cancer-related deaths.[37] The median age at diagnosis is 22 months, and 30% of cases occur in the first year of life. Arising from neural crest cells, neuroblastoma is a malignant neoplasm of the sympathetic nervous system. It occurs most commonly in the abdomen (65%), then chest (20%), followed by neck (5%) and pelvis (5%). They are most often detected when parents accidentally feel and note a large, nontender abdominal mass. Thoracic tumors are discovered at the time of routine chest radiograph obtained for unrelated respiratory symptoms. Pelvic masses may cause constipation or bladder dysfunction due to extrinsic mass effect. In the neck, 15% of patients develop Horner syndrome due to tumors impinging on sympathetic ganglia. If tumors extend into the spinal column, significant neurologic deficits occur and can rapidly progress to paralysis. Half of the patients have localized disease at diagnosis, and 35% have regional lymph node involvement. If bone marrow invasion is present, patients may experience anemia, bruising, and weakness, as well as bone pain, swelling, limp, or pathologic fractures. Periorbital swelling and proptosis (raccoon eyes) indicate involvement of orbits. Blue subcutaneous nodules represent dissemination of the tumor to the skin, also known as blueberry muffin syndrome. Paraneoplastic syndromes can produce intractable diarrhea caused by vasoactive intestinal peptide secretion, encephalomyelitis, and neuropathy. Opsoclonus-myoclonus syndrome—rapid, conjugate eye nystagmus with involuntary spasms of the limbs—although rare, occurs when antibodies cross-react with cerebellar tissue.

Neuroblastoma occurs as whole chromosome gains, which result in hyperdiploidy and are associated with a favorable prognosis, or segmental chromosomal aberrations, which encompass *MYCN* amplification and gains or losses that tend to be associated with worse outcomes. The *MYCN* oncogene, which is amplified at chromosome 2p24 in 25% of cases, is found in 30% to 40% of advanced-stage neuroblastomas but only in 5% of localized or stage 4S tumors. Deletion of the 1p36 region occurs in 70% and is usually associated with *MYCN*-amplified, high-risk neuroblastomas with a poor prognosis. Deletions of chromosome 11q are noted in 15% to 22% of cases and indicate an unfavorable outcome. Conversely, a whole chromosome 17 gain is associated with a good prognosis.[38]

Urine catecholamines and their metabolite (e.g., dopamine, vanillylmandelic acid, homovanillic acid) measurements are diagnostic. Elevated levels of lactate dehydrogenase (>1500 U/mL), ferritin (>142 ng/mL), and neuron-specific enolase (>100 ng/mL) are nonspecific tumor biomarkers. CT scan shows characteristic calcifications within the tumor (Fig. 67.23). An MRI is helpful to detect spinal cord extension. An ^{131}I-metaiodobenzylguanidine (MIBG) scan is particularly valuable in the detection of metastases since the norepinephrine analogue is selectively concentrated in sympathetic tissue. The ^{131}I-MIBG scan is also used for the surveillance of treatment response and recurrence. The classic histopathologic feature of NB is a poorly differentiated tumor with small round blue cells. Fluorescent in situ hybridization is performed on tissue specimens to assess ploidy, *MYCN* amplification, and other chromosomal abnormalities. Neuroblastoma can be classified on the basis of neuroblastic differentiation and mitosis-karyorrhexis index (low, intermediate, or high), and the presence of Schwann cells. The Children's Oncology Group currently stratifies patients into low-, intermediate-, or high-risk categories on the basis of the patient's age at diagnosis, International Neuroblastoma Staging System (INSS) stage, tumor histopathology, DNA index, and *MYCN* amplification status.[39] Localized tumors are resected primarily; advanced-stage tumors with extensive disease involving vital structures should undergo biopsy alone initially for tumor biology studies. After 5 cycles of induction therapy, complete resection or debulking achieving more than 90% resection confer the optimal disease-free and overall survival.[40]

Image-defined risk factor (Table 67.1) after neoadjuvant chemotherapy are useful predictors of complete surgical resection of neuroblastomas.[41] The multimodality treatment strategies are based on disease risk group stratification (Table 67.2). Induction chemotherapy consists of a multidrug regimen, including but not limited to cyclophosphamide, doxorubicin, cisplatin, carboplatin, etoposide, and vincristine. However, the high-risk group of neuroblastomas frequently acquire chemotherapeutics resistance and

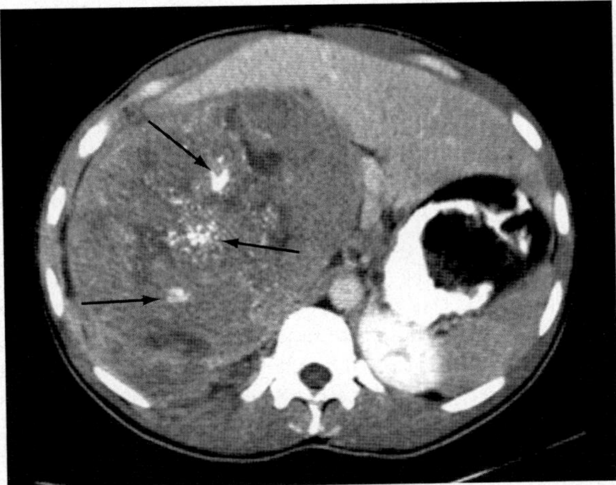

FIG. 67.23 Computed tomography scan of neuroblastoma demonstrating areas of calcification *(arrows)*. (From Kim S, Chung DH. Pediatric solid malignancies: Neuroblastoma and Wilms' tumor. *Surg Clin North Am*. 2006;86:469–487.)

TABLE 67.1 Image-defined risk factor in neuroblastoma.

TUMOR LOCATION	CRITERIA
Tumor involving two body compartments	Neck-chest; chest-abdomen; abdomen-pelvis
Neck	Tumor encasing carotid and/or vertebral artery and/or internal jugular vein
	Tumor extending to base of skull
	Tumor compressing the trachea
Cervicothoracic	Tumor encasing brachial plexus roots
	Tumor encasing subclavian vessels and/or vertebral and/or carotid artery
	Tumor compressing the trachea
Thorax	Tumor encasing the aorta and/or major branches
	Tumor compressing the trachea and/or principal bronchi
	Lower mediastinal tumor, infiltrating the costovertebral junction between T9 and T12
Thoracoabdomen	Tumor encasing the aorta and/or vena cava
Abdomen/pelvis	Tumor infiltrating the porta hepatis and/or the hepatoduodenal ligament
	Tumor encasing branches of the superior mesenteric artery at the mesenteric root
	Tumor encasing the origin of the coeliac axis, and/or of the superior mesenteric artery
	Tumor invading one or both renal pedicles
	Tumor encasing the aorta and/or vena cava
	Tumor encasing the iliac vessels
	Pelvic tumor crossing the sciatic notch
Intraspinal	More than one third of the spinal canal in the axial plane is invaded and/or the perimedullary leptomeningeal spaces are not visible and/or the spinal cord signal is abnormal
Infiltration of adjacent structure	Pericardium, diaphragm, kidney, liver, duodenopancreatic block, and mesentery
Conditions recorded but not IDRFs	Multifocal primary tumors
	Pleural effusion, with or without malignant cells
	Ascites, with or without malignant cells

IDRFs, Image-defined risk factors.

TABLE 67.2 International Neuroblastoma Risk Group (INRG) pretreatment classification.

INRG STAGE	AGE (MO)	HISTOLOGIC CATEGORY	GRADE	MYCN	11Q	PLOIDY	RISK GROUP	5-YEAR EFS
L1/L2		GN, GNB intermixed					Very low	>85%
L1		Any, except GN/GNB		NA			Very low	>85%
				Amp			High	<50%
L2	<18	Any, except GN/GNB		NA	No		Low	>75% to ≤85%
					Yes		Intermediate	≥50% to ≤75%
	≥18	GNB nodular, neuroblastoma	Differentiating	NA	No		Low	>75% to ≤85%
			Poorly differentiated or undifferentiated	NA	Yes		Intermediate	≥50% to ≤75%
				Amp			High	<50%
M	<18			NA		Hyperdiploid	Low	>75% to ≤85%
	<12			NA		Diploid	Intermediate	≥50% to ≤75%
	12–<18			NA		Diploid	Intermediate	≥50% to ≤75%
	<18			Amp			High	<50%
	≥18						High	<50%
MS	<18			NA	No		Very low	>85%
				Amp	Yes		High	<50%
							High	<50%

From Newman EA, Abdessalam S, Aldrink JH, et al. Update on neuroblastoma. *J Pediatr Surg.* 2019;54:383–389 was adapted from Cohn SL, Pearson AD, London WB, et al. The International Neuroblastoma Risk Group (INRG) classification system: An INRG Task Force report. *J Clin Oncol.* 2009;27:289–297.

L1: Localized tumor not involving vital structures as defined by the list of image-defined risk factors and confined to one body compartment

L2: Locoregional tumor with presence of one of more image-defined risk factors

M: Distant metastatic disease (except stage MS)

MS: Metastatic disease in children younger than 18 months with metastasis confined to skin, liver and/or bone marrow

EFS, Event-free survival; *GN*, ganglioneuroma; *GNB*, ganglioneuroblastoma; *NA*, nonamplified; *Amp*, amplified.

thus have higher disease relapse, which usually necessitates autologous hematopoietic stem cell transplantation. In addition, anti-GD2 immunotherapy has become a standard therapy for children with high-risk disease.[38] Complete surgical resection correlates with a lower local recurrence, especially in combination with induction chemotherapy, local radiation and immunotherapy.

Primary surgical resection is recommended for stage 1 to 2B tumors. For more advanced stages, such as stage 3 and 4, only the incisional biopsy specimen is obtained for initial tumor biology studies. The role of aggressive surgical resection of the primary tumor site for metastatic stage 4 neuroblastoma in patients 18 months or older is under some debate in Europe but remains the standard therapy in the United States.[39] For infants with stage 4S disease, surgical resection is not recommended because of the high rate of spontaneous differentiation and regression. In high-risk patients, radiation therapy is often needed for local and metastatic control. Radiation is contraindicated for intraspinal tumors because it can lead to vertebral damage, growth arrest, and scoliosis. However, it may be necessary for palliation in the setting of pain, hepatomegaly with respiratory compromise, or acute neurologic symptoms caused by tumor compression of the cord. It is further indicated when there is minimal residual disease after induction chemotherapy and resection. The overall outcomes in patients with neuroblastoma have improved steadily during the past decades, with the 5-year survival rates rising from 52% to 74%. While it is estimated that 50% to 60% of the high-risk group relapse after standard therapy, the low-risk group has shown significant improvement in survival rates of up to 92%.

Wilms Tumor

Wilms tumor (WT), also known as nephroblastoma, is an embryonal renal neoplasm consisting of metanephric blastema, which accounts for 85% of cases. It represents 5.9% of all pediatric malignant tumors, and ~75% are diagnosed in children younger than 5 years of age. Bilateral tumors are noted in 13% of patients at diagnosis. A number of syndromes can predispose to the development of WT such as Beckwith-Wiedemann (macroglossia, macrosomia, midline abdominal wall defects, and neonatal hypoglycemia), Li-Fraumeni (*p53* germline mutation with predisposition to various cancers), and Denys-Drash (gonadal dysgenesis, nephropathy, and WT) syndromes and neurofibromatosis. In 10% of patients, WT is associated with other congenital anomalies, collectively known as WAGR syndrome (aniridia, hemihypertrophy, genitourinary malformations, and mental retardation).

The WT suppressor gene, *WT1,* is located on chromosome 11p13, which contains genes responsible for the development of the kidney, genitourinary tract, and eyes.[42] Mutations in *WT1* result in genitourinary abnormalities, such as cryptorchidism and hypospadias, and increase the risk for development of WT. Aniridia is found in 1.1% of WT patients, and when *WT1* deletions are found in these patients, there is a 40% rate of WT development. Moreover, mutations in *WT2,* located at 11p15, have been linked to Beckwith-Wiedemann syndrome, and there is a 4% to 10% risk for development of WT in those who also have hemihypertrophy. WT is typically discovered incidentally during a physical examination or an abdominal mass is felt by caregivers. Other presenting symptoms include vague abdominal discomfort and hematuria, which may signify tumor invasion into the collecting system or ureter. Twenty-five percent of patients have hypertension, and it is thought to occur secondary to disturbances in the renin-angiotensin feedback loop. Less than 10% of patients have atypical symptoms such as varicocele, hepatomegaly caused by hepatic vein obstruction, ascites, and congestive heart failure.

Tumor thrombus into the renal vein or IVC is detected by ultrasound study. A CT scan is valuable in determining WT from other tumors, and evaluating for regional adenopathy, contralateral kidney involvement, and distant organ metastasis. Lung metastases are present in 8% at the time of diagnosis.

The histology of WT is categorized as favorable or unfavorable. Favorable histology is characterized by the presence of three elements—blastemal, stromal, and epithelial cells. WT with predominantly epithelial differentiation behaves less aggressively and tends to be stage I if diagnosed early. Blastemal-predominant tumors tend to be clinically aggressive and are associated with advanced disease. Outcomes correlate with histopathologic features and tumor stage. Unfavorable histology is characterized by anaplasia, clear cell sarcoma, or rhabdoid tumor cells. Anaplastic WT can be focal or diffuse and carries an increased risk of tumor recurrence and chemoresistance. Nephrogenic rests are precursor lesions found in 25% to 40% of kidneys with WT but do not have oncologic potential. Instead, they can undergo differentiation and spontaneously regress through unclear mechanisms.

The International Society of Pediatric Oncology (SIOP) staging system is based on preoperative chemotherapy but is applied after resection. The presence of metastases is evaluated at presentation, relying on imaging for detection, and chemotherapy is administered before operative intervention. The National Wilms Tumor Study Group (NWTSG) has also developed a staging system that incorporates the clinical, surgical, and pathologic information obtained at the time of resection but stratifies patients before the initiation of chemotherapy (Table 67.3). The advantage of this system is that it favors stage-based therapy, thereby avoiding unnecessary chemotherapy in patients who might not otherwise benefit from it.

The mainstay of therapy for WT is surgery and chemotherapy. Surgical exploration is necessary for formal staging, and a radical nephrectomy with lymph node sampling is the standard operation.

TABLE 67.3 National Wilms Tumor Study Group staging system.

STAGE	DEFINITION
I	Tumor limited to the kidney and completely excised without rupture or biopsy. Surface of the renal capsule is intact.
II	Tumor extends through the renal capsule but is completely removed with no microscopic involvement of the margins. Vessels outside the kidney contain tumor. Also placed in stage II are cases in which the kidney has undergone biopsy before removal or where there is local spillage of tumor (during resection) limited to the tumor bed.
III	Residual tumor is confined to the abdomen and of nonhematogenous spread. Includes tumors with involvement of the abdominal lymph nodes, diffuse peritoneal contamination by rupture of the tumor extending beyond the tumor bed, peritoneal implants, and microscopic or grossly positive resection margins.
IV	Hematogenous metastases at any site.
V	Bilateral renal involvement.

Utmost care must be taken to ensure en bloc resection with tumor-free margins because contamination and tumor spillage result in upstaging. Vascular tumor extension into the IVC constitutes stage III disease and is managed accordingly (Fig. 67.24). Sampling of the hilar, para-aortic, and paracaval lymph nodes is essential. Nephron-sparing surgery is usually reserved for children with a solitary kidney or bilateral WT. In these patients, preoperative chemotherapy may be used to induce tumor shrinkage and allow for more complete resection. Partial nephrectomy may be considered if the tumor involves only one pole of the kidney, there is no evidence of collecting system or vascular involvement, clear margins exist between the tumor and surrounding structures, and the involved kidney demonstrates appreciable function. According to the NWTSG guidelines (Box 67.2), the standard chemotherapy regimen consists of vincristine and dactinomycin, with the addition of doxorubicin (Adriamycin) or radiation therapy based on tumor stage and histologic favorability. The SIOP advocates the use of preoperative chemotherapy to improve cure and disease-free survival rates at 5 years. Stages I and II favorable histology or stage I unfavorable histology have a nearly 95% survival rate. For WT with unfavorable histology, stages II, III, and IV are associated with 70%, 56%, and 17% 4-year survival rates, respectively.

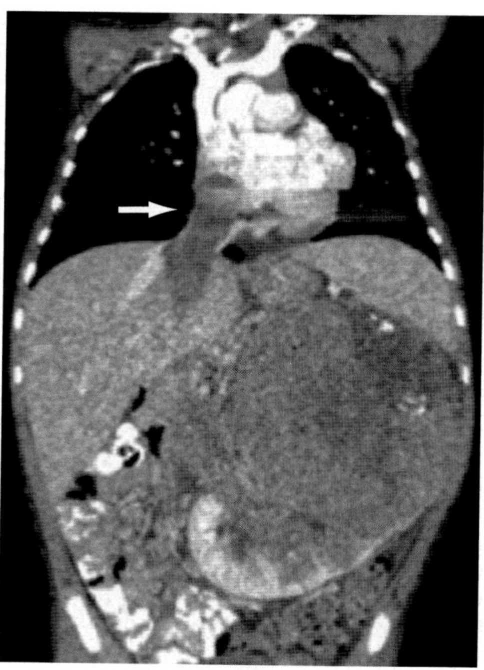

FIG. 67.24 Computed tomography image of Wilms tumor with a claw sign and a large inferior vena cava tumor thrombus extending to right atrium *(arrow)*.

BOX 67.2 Treatment regimens for Wilms Tumor.*

- Stage I (FH, focal anaplasia): Surgery, VA × 18 wk, no XRT
- Stage II (FH): Surgery, VA × 18 wk, no XRT
- Stage II (focal anaplasia): Surgery, VDA × 24 wk, XRT to tumor bed
- Stage III (FH, focal anaplasia): Surgery, VDA × 24 wk, XRT to tumor bed
- Stage III (focal anaplasia): Surgery, VDA × 24 wk, XRT to tumor bed
- Stage IV (FH; focal anaplasia): Surgery, VDA × 24 wk, XRT to tumor bed according to local tumor stage and lung or other metastatic sites
- Stages II–IV (diffuse anaplasia): Surgery, VDEC × 24 wk, XRT to whole lung and abdomen
- Stages I–IV (clear cell sarcoma): Surgery, VDEC × 24 wk, XRT to abdomen; XRT to whole lung for stage IV only
- Stages I–IV (rhabdoid tumor): Surgery, ECCa × 24 wk, XRT

A, Dactinomycin; *C,* cyclophosphamide; *Ca,* carboplatin; *D,* doxorubicin; *E,* etoposide; *FH,* favorable histology; *V,* vincristine; *XRT,* radiation therapy.
*National Wilms Tumor Study: Infants younger than 11 months are given half the recommended dose of all drugs.

Rhabdomyosarcoma

Derived from embryonic mesenchymal cells that later differentiate into skeletal muscle, rhabdomyosarcoma is a soft tissue malignant neoplasm that accounts for 4% of all pediatric cancer. There is a bimodal peak in ages at diagnosis, between the ages of 2 and 5 years old and between 15 and 19 years old. Rhabdomyosarcoma is known to occur with increased frequency in patients with neurofibromatosis type 1, Li-Fraumeni, and Beckwith-Wiedemann syndromes. Rhabdomyosarcoma is classified into three types: embryonal, alveolar, and pleomorphic. Embryonal rhabdomyosarcoma, which includes botryoid and spindle cell subtypes, is the most common type, accounting for more than two thirds of all rhabdomyosarcomas.

Common sites for rhabdomyosarcomas are the head and neck (35%), genitourinary tract (25%), and extremities (20%). Head and neck tumors tend to occur in the parameningeal region, orbits, and pharynx. Other specific sites include the bladder, prostate, vagina, uterus, liver, biliary tract, paraspinal region, and chest wall. These tumors are generally asymptomatic, and if present, most symptoms are related to extrinsic tumor effects. Orbital tumors can produce proptosis, decreased visual acuity, and ophthalmoplegia. Those arising from parameningeal sites frequently produce headaches and nasal or sinus obstruction that can be accompanied by a mucopurulent or bloody discharge. For genitourinary rhabdomyosarcoma, paratesticular tumors may present as painless swelling in the scrotum, which may be confused with a hernia, hydrocele, or varicocele. Bladder tumors, commonly located at the base and trigone, result in hematuria and urinary obstruction. Vaginal tumors in girls present with a protruding mass or vaginal bleeding and discharge. In the extremities, rhabdomyosarcomas involve the distal limb more commonly, and the lower extremities are affected more often. Retroperitoneal tumors can be quite large at diagnosis with symptoms arising secondary to invasion of adjacent structures. At diagnosis, 50% of patients have regional lymph node metastasis.

There are no specific serum tumor markers for rhabdomyosarcoma. MRI or CT demonstrate the mass and its involvement of adjacent structures, vessel encasement, metastasis, and adenopathy. An incisional or core needle biopsy is crucial to achieve diagnosis. Muscle-specific proteins, myosin, actin, desmin, and myoglobin, are stained for immunohistochemical diagnosis.[43] Botryoid (cluster of grapes) and spindle cell rhabdomyosarcomas have favorable prognosis, pleomorphic histology confers an intermediate prognosis, and alveolar type histology exhibits a poor prognosis. Pretreatment staging, based on TNM criteria, serves to stratify patients into the appropriate treatment regimen, and to compare outcomes (Box 67.3). A complete surgical resection is ideal, but a large tumor may necessitate preoperative chemotherapy for tumor shrinkage. Intraoperative or pathologic results from resected samples are used for clinical grouping, which consists of selection into a group depending on operative findings, pathology, margins, and node status. Estimated 3-year failure-free survival rates are 88%, 55% to 76%, and less than 30% for low-risk, intermediate-risk, and high-risk patients, respectively.

The main goal of multimodality therapy is to achieve cure or to obtain local control. The recommended chemotherapy regimen depends on the risk stratification, with low-risk patients in subgroup A receiving

BOX 67.3 Staging for rhabdomyosarcoma.

Group I: Localized disease that is completely resected with no regional node involvement
Group II
 A. Localized, grossly resected tumor with microscopic residual disease but no regional nodal involvement
 B. Locoregional disease with tumor-involved lymph nodes with complete resection and no residual disease
 C. Locoregional disease with involved nodes, grossly resected, but with evidence of microscopic residual tumor at the primary site and/or histologic involvement of the most distal regional node (from the primary site)
Group III: Localized, gross residual disease including incomplete resection or biopsy only of the primary site
Group IV: Distant metastatic disease present at time of diagnosis

vincristine and dactinomycin. For patients in the low-risk subgroup B and higher, cyclophosphamide is added to this therapy. Radiation therapy has been found to be effective for the local control of rhabdomyosarcoma, especially in patients who have microscopic disease after resection, as well as in patients with unresectable tumors.

For extremity lesions, it is imperative to achieve complete wide local excision. Amputation is rarely necessary, except for distal tumors in the hand or foot that involve neurovascular structures. Given that trunk and extremity lesions have a high incidence of lymph node metastasis, sentinel lymph node mapping is increasingly used. Reexcision may also be considered with evidence of minimal residual disease after initial resection. Patients with extremity tumors receive combination chemotherapy, but because of the high incidence of the alveolar histology, radiation therapy is also often used.

For genitourinary tumors, preservation of bladder function is the key in resection of tumors involving the bladder or prostate. If this goal cannot be met, preoperative chemoradiation is usually recommended. Paratesticular rhabdomyosarcoma should undergo a radical inguinal orchiectomy, with a retroperitoneal lymph node dissection in boys younger than 10 years because of the high prevalence of metastasis. When the tumor is clearly fixed to scrotal skin, resection is required. Chemotherapy is standard, whereas radiation therapy is indicated only with positive nodes. For patients with vaginal or vulvar rhabdomyosarcoma, vaginectomy and wide local excision, respectively, and multiagent chemotherapy is recommended. Approximately 15% of children present with metastatic disease, and their prognosis remains poor. Nearly 30% will experience disease relapse, and the estimated 5-year survival rate is only 17%. Despite these harrowing data, rhabdomyosarcoma is a curable disease in most children, with more than 60% surviving 5 years after diagnosis.

Liver Tumors

Primary tumors of the liver are rare in the pediatric population but when present are malignant in approximately 60% of cases. The two most common tumors are hepatoblastoma and hepatocellular carcinoma (HCC). Hepatoblastoma represents 80% of all malignant liver tumors and 1% of all pediatric cancer. The peak incidence of hepatoblastoma is at 3 years of age, and the median age for children with HCC is 10 to 11.2 years. More than 90% of patients younger than 5 years with primary liver tumors have hepatoblastoma, whereas 87% of those between 15 and 19 years have HCC. Patients with familial adenomatous polyposis, Gardner, and Beckwith-Wiedemann syndromes are at increased risk for development of hepatoblastoma. HCC is associated with acquired hepatitis B and C and has been observed in children with several types of

TABLE 67.4 PRETEXT definition for hepatoblastoma.

PRETEXT GROUP	DEFINITION
I	One section involved; three adjoining sections are tumor free
II	One or two sections involved; two adjoining sections are tumor free
III	Two or three sections involved; one adjoining section is tumor free
IV	Four sections involved

congenital diseases, including tyrosinemia, glycogen storage disease type I, α_1-antitrypsin deficiency, and cholestasis caused by BA.

Hepatoblastoma typically manifests as a painless palpable abdominal mass. Other symptoms are nonspecific and include anorexia, weight loss and failure to thrive, abdominal pain, anemia, and abdominal distention. Jaundice is not commonly encountered because liver function remains relatively normal except in very advanced tumors. Some patients present with tumor rupture, resulting in intraabdominal bleeding and peritonitis. AFP levels are elevated in more than 70% of patients with hepatoblastoma. However, an elevated AFP level is not pathognomonic, and, depending on the age of the patient, other disease processes must be ruled out. For example, in infants younger than 6 months, elevated AFP levels may also be seen in sarcomas, yolk sac tumors, and hamartomas.

HCC is manifested similarly, although stigmata of cirrhosis, such as jaundice, spider angiomas, ascites, and splenomegaly, may be encountered. Almost 25% of patients have metastatic spread to abdominal and mediastinal lymph nodes, lung, bone marrow, and brain. Anemia, thrombocytopenia, or pancytopenia can be found with splenomegaly caused by sequestration. All children being evaluated for HCC should be tested for exposure to hepatitis B and C viruses.

Abdominal ultrasonography is an excellent initial diagnostic study. Doppler ultrasound can also detect the presence of tumor extension into or thrombosis of major vessels, namely, the hepatic veins, IVC, and portal vein. A CT scan is essential in assessing the relationship of the tumor to adjacent vital structures, such as bile ducts and vessels, and excluding intraabdominal tumor extension beyond the liver. MRI can also be used in this setting, but it does not necessarily provide significant advantages over CT. Because hepatoblastoma frequently spreads hematologically to the lungs, chest CT should also be performed. Bone scintigraphy is recommended for staging in children with HCC because of the high incidence of bone metastases.

On histologic evaluation, hepatoblastoma characteristically appears as a unifocal mass surrounded by a pseudocapsule. It may be a pure epithelial type that contains fetal or embryonal cells or a mixture of the two histologic subtypes, which contains mesenchymal tissue in addition to epithelial components. On the other hand, HCC is characterized by large, pleomorphic epithelial cells that appear much like mature hepatocytes. In gross appearance, HCC forms multifocal nodules that lack a fibrous tumor and often lead to diffuse intrahepatic involvement. Unlike in adults, there has been no indisputable evidence that histopathologic type has any bearing on prognosis.

In hepatoblastoma, a standard TNM system has been used for staging purposes, but much effort has been put into the development of a pretreatment staging system, known as the PRE-Treatment EXTent of disease (PRETEXT) definition system (Table 67.4). The PRETEXT system was developed by the International

Childhood Liver Tumor Strategy Group (SIOPEL) for staging and risk stratification of liver tumors.[44] It divides the liver into four sections based on segmental anatomy of the liver, and the tumor is subsequently classified by the number of tumor-free sections of liver (Fig. 67.25). This system takes caudate lobe involvement, tumor rupture, ascites, extension into the stomach or diaphragm, tumor focality, lymph node involvement, presence of distant metastases, and vascular involvement into further consideration. Patients are considered at high risk if they have a serum AFP level above 100 ng/mL, extension beyond the liver, distant metastases, intraperitoneal hemorrhage, and invasion of the hepatic veins, IVC, or portal vein. For PRETEXT I and II, hepatoblastoma may be resected by segmentectomy or anatomic lobectomy.

Liver transplantation is a potential surgical option for patients with a massive unresectable tumor. Neoadjuvant chemotherapy is used for tumor shrinkage and potential complete resection. Interestingly, some advocate for the use of preoperative chemotherapy to treat what would otherwise be residual microscopic disease left behind after resection. They argue that doing so eliminates tumor cells that could respond to hepatotrophic factors during liver regeneration, thereby decreasing the risk of recurrence. There are two current approaches to hepatoblastoma: (1) tumor resection followed by chemotherapy and (2) tumor biopsy followed by chemotherapy and delayed resection. Patients with stage I tumors with pure fetal histology usually do not require postoperative chemotherapy. However, patients with stage II or higher tumors and tumors of any other type of histology require chemotherapy consisting of cisplatin, 5-fluorouracil, and vincristine. For patients with residual tumor after resection, chemotherapy should be coupled with an evaluation for transplantation. Criteria for transplantation include having no more than three tumors smaller than 3 cm in diameter and no evidence of extrahepatic disease or vascular invasion. When relapses occur, doxorubicin, irinotecan, and ifosfamide have been used, often with some success. Another modality being used with variable success in children whose tumors are unresponsive to systemic chemotherapy is direct arterial chemotherapy or chemoembolization. Long-term outcomes have yet to be determined. Long-term disease-free survival of more than 85% to 90% can be achieved for resectable hepatoblastoma, although similar estimates have been noted for patients with unresectable hepatoblastoma treated by liver transplantation. The same cannot be said for HCC, in which survival rates with partial hepatectomy remain poor because of relapse. In the past decade, early transplantation has been shown to result in better outcomes in some centers.

Teratoma

Teratomas are typically benign neoplasms that contain elements derived from more than one of the three embryonic germ layers, endoderm, mesoderm, and ectoderm. They are composed of tissue that is foreign to the anatomic site in which they are found. Although teratomas may occur anywhere along the midline, they are usually found in sacrococcygeal, mediastinal, retroperitoneal, and gonadal locations. Teratomas may be solid, cystic, or mixed and are classified as mature or immature. Although immature teratomas can be potentially malignant, the incidence of malignant transformation in mature teratomas is low. There is a preponderance based on gender, and almost 80% of all teratomas occur in females. Moreover, location has been associated with age, as evidenced by the fact that extragonadal tumors occur primarily in neonates and young children, whereas gonadal tumors are more commonly noted in adolescents.

Sacrococcygeal Teratomas

Sacrococcygeal teratomas (SCTs) account for 60% of all teratomas and can be manifest as large exophytic masses in utero. In such cases, they are detected on prenatal ultrasound. Complications include polyhydramnios and fetal hydrops, which can result in fetal demise due to a tumor-induced vascular steal syndrome that leads to high-output heart failure. Symptoms can include weakness, paralysis, bowel or bladder dysfunction, and other neurologic symptoms, which may indicate intradural spinal extension. The diagnosis can be made clinically, especially

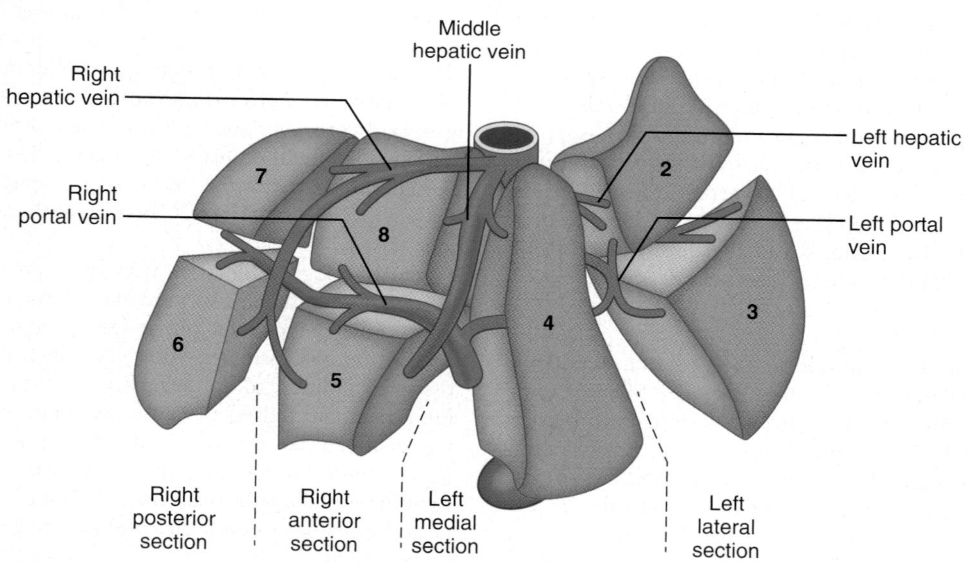

FIG. 67.25 A diagram of the PRETEXT definition system for hepatoblastoma. The liver is divided into four sections based on segmental anatomy of the liver, and the tumor is subsequently classified by the number of tumor-free sections of liver. (From Roebuck DJ, Aronson D, Clapuyt P, et al. 2005 PRETEXT: A revised staging system for primary malignant liver tumors of childhood developed by the SIOPEL group. *Pediatr Radiol.* 2007;37:123–132.)

with exophytic SCTs. If the AFP or β-hCG level is elevated, yolk sac or choriocarcinoma components, respectively, make up the teratoma. Ultrasonography, CT, or MRI may be necessary to detect intraabdominal lesions or to determine whether there is pelvic or abdominal extension.

Surgical resection is the standard of care and should be performed promptly because of the risk of hemorrhage and tumor rupture. Operative planning must take into account the degree of intraabdominal extension (Fig. 67.26). Most tumors can be resected by a posterior approach, in which a chevron incision allows the division of the gluteal muscles, ligation of the blood supply, and en bloc resection of the tumor and coccyx. It is important to preserve the anorectal complex in order to maintain long-term continence. External tumors with significant intraabdominal extension require a combined abdominal and posterior approach, whereas teratomas that are entirely intraabdominal may be approached through laparotomy or laparoscopy.

Outcomes are favorable with respect to survival and quality of life. The age at diagnosis is the most important factor of prognosis; those diagnosed at less than 30 weeks of gestation or after 2 months postnatally tend to have a poor prognosis. The risk of malignant transformation associated with embryonal histology is 15% to 20%. Risk of local recurrence ranges from 4% to 11%, although failure to resect the coccyx is associated with a 37% risk of recurrence. AFP levels should be monitored at 3-month intervals for 3 to 4 years. For recurrence, reexcision should be considered.

Ovarian Tumor

Approximately 50% of all ovarian lesions in children are neoplastic but are rarely malignant. It is estimated that ovarian malignant

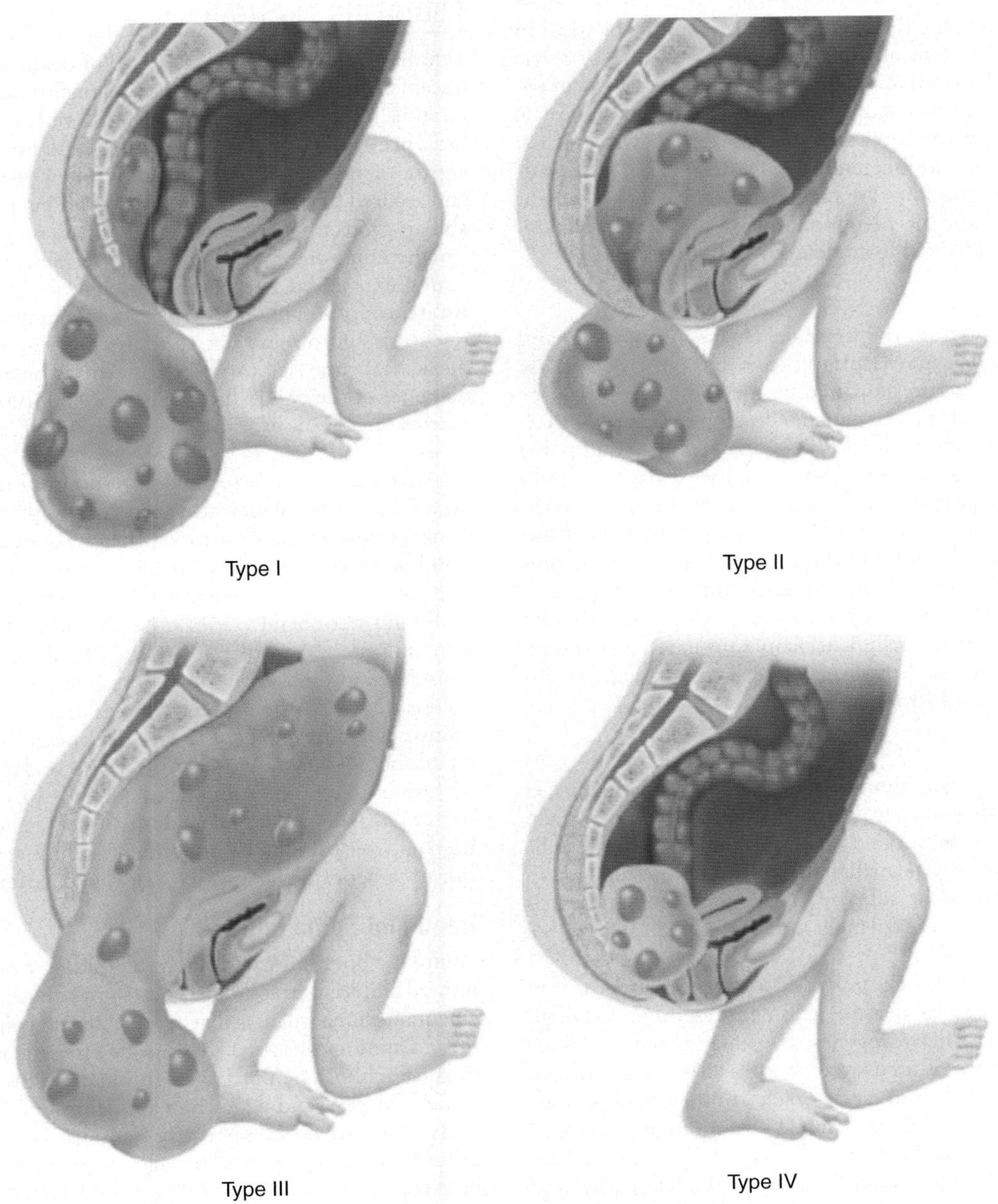

FIG. 67.26 Sacrococcygeal teratoma Altman classification types I to IV. Type I is resected entirely from perineal approach. Types II and III require combination of perineal and abdominopelvic approach. Type IV is resected entirely via abdominal approach.

neoplasms represent 10% of all ovarian masses but only 1% of childhood cancers. Primary ovarian malignant neoplasms can be classified as germ cell, epithelial cell, and sex cord stromal tumors. Germ cell tumors include teratomas and choriocarcinoma; sex cord stromal tumors consist of granulosa (thecal) and Sertoli (Leydig) cells. Epithelial cell tumors encompass serous and mucinous cystadenomas and cystadenocarcinomas.[45] Symptoms are usually related to pain from mass compression or ovarian torsion. The presence of ascites, omental masses, peritoneal or diaphragmatic implants, adherence to surrounding organs, aortoiliac adenopathy, size larger than 8 cm, or presence of a contralateral ovarian mass should raise suspicion for malignancy.

Germ Cell Tumors

An ovarian teratoma is the most common ovarian germ cell tumor. It is the most common pediatric ovarian neoplasm and accounts for 25% of all childhood teratomas. These tumors occur with equal frequency in either ovary and may even be bilateral in 10% of patients. They typically manifest with abdominal or pelvic pain and may involve ovarian torsion in approximately 25% of patients. Germ cell tumors account for 7% to 80% of all neoplastic ovarian masses. Dysgerminomas are the least differentiated of the germ cell tumors and are bilateral in 10% to 15% of cases. Although pure dysgerminomas are malignant, they tend to present while still localized and are highly responsive to chemoradiation. Survival is almost 90% with complete surgical resection.

Sex Cord Tumors

Sex cord tumors arise from the stromal elements of the ovary and produce hormones that may result in precocious puberty. Because they are androgenic, serum testosterone metabolite levels can be elevated. With estrogen excess, patients develop early sexual characteristics, such as breast or labial enlargement, axillary and pubic hair growth, and galactorrhea. Abnormal menstruation, swelling, and pain are common chief complaints. Interestingly, these tumors have been associated with Peutz-Jeghers syndrome. Outcomes after resection are good in this group because most lesions are still limited to the ovary. Advanced-stage tumors are responsive to platinum-based chemotherapy. Granulosa cell tumors account for 1% to 10% of ovarian malignant neoplasms in females younger than 20 years, whereas Sertoli-Leydig cell tumors account for 20% of ovarian sex cord stromal tumors.

Epithelial Tumors

Less than 20% of ovarian tumors in childhood are epithelial in nature, given that they are rare before menarche. The two main histologic subtypes are serous and mucinous tumors, which can be further described as benign, malignant, or borderline malignant. It is possible to classify the subtypes as adenoma or adenocarcinoma. Adenocarcinoma is extremely rare but is associated with a poor prognosis.

AFP and β-hCG levels help provide information about tumor biology and can be used to measure treatment response. Although nonspecific, the lactate dehydrogenase level may also be elevated. If there is any evidence of menstrual abnormalities or precocious puberty, luteinizing hormone and follicle-stimulating hormone levels should also be checked. Abdominal ultrasound is performed to evaluate the tumor and contralateral ovary. A CT scan can provide information on tumor extension, regional adenopathy, and distant metastasis.

Surgery is the mainstay of therapy and aims to ensure complete resection, with preservation of reproductive function when possible. Definitive treatment is oophorectomy or salpingooophorectomy. Care should be taken to resect the tumor without disrupting the capsule or spilling tumor contents to avoid upstaging of malignant lesions. At operation, the liver, diaphragm, omentum, and peritoneal surfaces are examined for ovarian implants, which, when present, should be biopsied for staging and treatment purposes. Bilateral retroperitoneal, iliac, para-aortic, and perirenal lymph nodes should be sampled for appropriate staging. Ascites or peritoneal washings should be sent for cytology. Chemotherapy is indicated for any ovarian tumor with extension beyond the affected ovary, which is often the case with germ cell and epithelial cell tumors. The combination of low-dose bleomycin, etoposide, and cisplatin treatment in patients with stage II disease has resulted in event-free and overall survival rates of 87.5% and 93.8%, respectively.

PEDIATRIC TRAUMA

Trauma is the most common cause of death in children and adolescents. Most pediatric trauma is blunt in nature, although penetrating injury due to firearm-related violence is increasing. The basic principles of trauma evaluation in adults including the ABCs are the same for pediatric patients. The airway must be assessed and secured promptly. A child who is crying or able to verbalize is able to protect his or her airway. If a patient is drooling, gurgling, or wheezing, one must rule out correctable causes of airway obstruction, such as a retrievable foreign object in the oropharynx. Awareness of unique pediatric airway anatomy is also critical; the trachea is shorter and narrower in children. The appropriate endotracheal tube size can be estimated as being equivalent to the diameter of the child's fifth digit. The endotracheal tube inner diameter can also be estimated (4 + the patient's age in years divided by 4).

After the airway is secured, a respiratory (breathing) status is assessed with particular attention to any presence of flail chest, dyspnea, tachypnea, or unequal breath sounds. Next, the circulation is assessed to ensure adequate oxygen delivery to vital organs. The patient should be examined for general appearance, capillary refill, and peripheral pulses. A weak pulse along with hypotension indicates hypovolemic shock. Blood transfusion should be considered in those with shock unresponsive to two IV crystalloid boluses (20 mL/kg per bolus). In children younger than 6 years, intraosseous access may be used if peripheral IV cannot be quickly established. After the initial ABCs, a secondary survey should be performed. Hypothermia must be avoided to prevent complications of coagulopathy and acidosis. A detailed examination of the head and neck should be performed, including palpation of posterior neck beneath the C-collar, back, and extremities.

Head and Spine Injuries

Traumatic brain injury (TBI) is the leading cause of death among injured children. In toddlers 2 years or younger, physical or nonaccidental trauma, such as that seen in shaken baby syndrome, is the most common cause of TBI. This may present as retinal, subdural, or subarachnoid hemorrhages. In older children, falls and motor vehicle, bicycle, and pedestrian accidents are responsible for most TBIs. The initial CT scan may demonstrate diffuse edema, but diffuse axonal injury, hemorrhage, or parenchymal damage must be assessed over time up to 20% of mild TBIs can have intracranial hemorrhage. Headache, nausea, amnesia, impaired concentration, and behavior disturbances could be signs and symptoms of mild TBI. Because of its transient effect and propensity to induce vasospasm, prophylactic hyperventilation should be avoided unless there is imminent concern for herniation. Aside from diuretics and hypertonic saline, a barbiturate-induced coma and hypothermia are additional maneuvers that can be used to lower the intracranial pressure. Intracranial bleed causing focal neurologic symptoms or mass effect is addressed surgically.

Although relatively rare, motor vehicle accidents account for most traumatic spinal cord injuries in children. Fractures of the C1 and C2 vertebrae are commonly seen in younger children, whereas compression and chance fractures, frequently associated with improper seat belt use, are seen in older children. Spinal cord injury without radiologic abnormality is a clinical condition in which a child (<8 years of age) can present with transient neurologic deficits. It is thought to occur because incomplete vertebral ossification and ligament laxity allow the cord and nerve roots to stretch or to impact on the opposing bone surfaces of the spinal canal.

Thoracic Trauma

Thoracic injury is the second leading cause of death in pediatric trauma and accounts for 5% of trauma-related hospital admissions. Blunt trauma, particularly from motor vehicle accidents, is responsible for most thoracic injuries. Rib fractures in young toddlers should raise a high index of suspicion for child abuse. Rib cages in children are primarily cartilaginous and therefore more pliable. Thus, a child may present with a significant intrathoracic injury (e.g., pulmonary contusion, pneumothorax, hemothorax) without obvious external evidence such as rib fractures. Pulmonary contusions can induce inflammatory response with edema, atelectasis, and subsequent consolidation. Hypoxemia, hypercarbia, and tachypnea can be significant and necessitate intubation. Most patients respond to conservative management without long-term sequelae.

Traumatic asphyxia is a rare presentation after blunt trauma, but sudden compression or crushing of the thorax can result in airway obstruction and retrograde high-pressure flow in the superior vena cava. When this occurs, patients present dramatically with head and neck cyanosis, subconjunctival hemorrhaging, and petechiae.

Chest cavity exploration may be indicated for acute blood loss of more than 20% of total blood volume or chest tube blood drainage of 2 mL/kg/hr. Intercostal arterial bleeding is a common etiology. Retained hemothorax should be evacuated to prevent subsequent bacterial colonization with abscess formation. Tracheobronchial injuries usually occur near the carina and are thought to result from anteroposterior compression of the pliable pediatric chest and cause pneumothorax, pneumomediastinum, and subcutaneous emphysema. Tracheobronchial disruption results in massive air leak with potential tension pneumothorax, compromising respiratory function and venous return. Aside from hemodynamic instability, primary repair is indicated if the injury involves more than one third of the diameter of the bronchus or if nonoperative management fails. A widened mediastinum on the chest radiograph is rare in children. Most of these injuries result from blunt trauma and are found at the ligamentum arteriosum. Traumatic diaphragmatic rupture with herniation of the stomach and bowel occurs in approximately 1% of children with blunt chest trauma; and traumatic diaphragmatic rupture is more common on the left side.

Abdominal Trauma

When a seat belt sign, a bruising of the epigastric abdominal wall after a motor vehicle accident, is present on a child, a CT scan should be carefully reviewed for any subtle signs of bowel injury or presence of free peritoneal fluid. Intraabdominal fluid on a CT scan without a solid organ injury should raise the index of suspicion for a hollow viscus injury. Blunt injuries to the stomach are generally seen in children who are struck by a vehicle or who fall across bicycle handlebars and present as blowout or perforation of the greater curvature. Usually seen in restrained children involved in motor vehicle accidents, intestinal injury secondary to blunt trauma is estimated to be less than 15%. Rapid deceleration at impact causes the lap belt to compress the intestines against the spine. The increase in intraluminal pressure predisposes the intestine to perforation or rupture. Small intestinal injuries occur predominantly in areas of fixation, such as at the ligament of Treitz or ileocecal valve. A duodenal or mesenteric hematoma may ensue and cause obstruction, with subsequent nausea and bilious emesis.

The intraabdominal solid organs are particularly vulnerable to blunt trauma in children. Nonoperative management is the standard for blunt injuries to the liver and spleen. Radiographic grading of liver (Table 67.5) and splenic (Table 67.6) injuries have allowed for implementation of clinical management pathways.

TABLE 67.5 Liver injury scale.

GRADE	DESCRIPTION OF LIVER INJURY
I	Subcapsular hematoma, <10% surface area Capsular laceration, <1 cm parenchymal depth
II	Subcapsular hematoma, 10%–50% surface area, intraparenchymal, <10 cm in diameter Capsular tear 1–3 cm deep
III	Subcapsular hematoma, >50% surface area or expanding; ruptured subcapsular or parenchymal hematoma; intraparenchymal hematoma ≥10 cm or expanding Parenchymal laceration >3 cm depth or involving a trabecular vessels
IV	Parenchymal disruption involving 25% to 75% of hepatic lobe or 1–3 Couinaud segments in a single lobe
V	Parenchymal disruption involving >75% of hepatic lobe or >3 Couinaud segments within a single lobe Juxtahepatic venous injuries (retrohepatic vena cava, central major hepatic veins)
VI	Hepatic avulsion

TABLE 67.6 Spleen injury scale.

GRADE	DESCRIPTION OF SPLEEN INJURY
I	Subcapsular hematoma, <10% surface area
II	Subcapsular hematoma, 10% to 50% surface area, intraparenchymal, <5 cm in diameter Capsular laceration <1 cm parenchymal depth
III	Subcapsular hematoma, >50% surface area or expanding; ruptured subcapsular or parenchymal hematoma; intraparenchymal hematoma ≥5 cm or expanding Capsular laceration 1–3 cm depth that does not involve a trabecular vessel
IV	Laceration >3 cm parenchymal depth or involving a trabecular vessel Laceration involving segmental or hilar vessels producing major devascularization >25%
V	Completely shattered spleen Hilar vascular injury devascularizing spleen

TABLE 67.7 Guidelines for management with isolated liver or splenic injury.

	CT GRADE			
	I	II	III	IV
ICU stay (d)	None	None	None	1
Hospital stay (d)	2	3	4	5
Additional CT	None	None	None	None
Activity restriction (wk)*	3	4	5	6

CT, Computed tomography; *ICU*, intensive care unit.
*Return to full competitive sport.

The American Pediatric Surgical Association developed guidelines regarding the management of isolated liver and splenic injuries based on initial CT findings, which have been shown to reduce the length of hospital stay significantly, without adverse outcomes (Table 67.7). The exact role of splenic artery embolization in the treatment of pediatric blunt splenic injury remains uncertain, but encouraging data are emerging for patients with on-going hemorrhage.[46] An isolated hepatic injury without involvement of the hepatic vein, IVC, or portal vein can also be managed conservatively. Some have reported that 85% to 90% of patients can successfully be treated with nonoperative management. However, those who fail to respond do so because of hemodynamic instability, often requiring massive transfusion protocols with infusion of more than half of blood volume of packed red blood cells. Delayed bleeding after liver injury has been reported as late as 6 weeks after injury and may be seen in 1% to 3% of patients. Ultimately, the most important criterion to operate or not for an isolated liver or splenic injury is based on achieving hemodynamic stability with less than 40 mL/kg of packed red blood cell transfusion. Additionally, surgical exploration should be considered when there is a high suspicion of other organ injuries such as bowel perforation. Recently, a new nonoperative management algorithm, the ATOMAC consortium guideline, which is based on patient hemodynamic parameters and not solely on CT grades, has garnered significant interest and has shown to be a safe clinical pathway with shorter hospital stay.[47]

Pancreatic Injury

Pancreatic injuries occur from blunt trauma, such as falling onto bicycle handlebars. An elevated amylase or lipase level is present. CT scan is a useful diagnostic modality for evaluation of most pancreatic trauma, although it is not as sensitive or specific for determination of pancreatic ductal injuries. There is little role for ERCP in acute settings of pancreatic trauma. Transection of the pancreas, including the main pancreatic duct from blunt trauma, is best managed with distal pancreatectomy when detected early. For those with delayed presentation, a conservative management involving TPN and bowel rest, with or without distal jejunal enteral nutrition, may be considered. ERCP can identify the exact nature of the main pancreatic ductal injury and an external drainage procedure may be required.

Renal Injury

Retroperitoneal injuries are frequently seen with direct blows to the back or flank. The kidney is involved in 10% to 20% of cases. In children, there is a lack of perinephric fat, which makes the kidney more susceptible to blunt trauma. Parenchymal contusions are most common in children. Interestingly, the presence of hematuria does not correlate with the severity of renal injury. Conservative nonoperative management is standard for low-grade renal injuries (grades I: contusion, subcapsular nonexpanding hematoma; grade II: perirenal hematoma confined to retroperitoneum, laceration less than 1 cm parenchymal depth; grade III: laceration greater than 1 cm parenchymal depth or renal cortex without collecting system rupture or urine extravasation). However, there is no general consensus on the management of high-grade renal injuries (grade IV: parenchymal laceration extending through the renal cortex, medulla and collecting system, or main renal artery or venous injury or grade V: completely shattered kidney). An absolute indication for operative intervention in renal injuries is an expanding or pulsatile hematoma. Relative indications include urinary extravasation, necrosis, and arterial injury. In the case of urinary extravasation, ureteral stenting can potentially avoid open exploration. Grade V injury with avulsion of renal hilum and devascularization of kidney requires operative intervention, but the salvage rate is poor.

SELECTED REFERENCES

Anderson KT, Appelbaum R, Bartz-Kurycki MA, et al. Advances in perioperative quality and safety. *Semin Pediatr Surg.* 2018;27:92–101.

This monograph reviewed three significant advances in quality and safety that have changed the approach to surgical care: the National Surgical Quality Improvement Program, evidence-based bundled prevention of surgical site infections, and the Surgical Safety Checklist.

Baxter KJ, Gale BF, Travers CD, et al. Ramifications of the children's surgery verification program for patients and hospitals. *J Am Coll Surg.* 2018;226:917–924.e911.

This manuscript is an early examination of the effects of the ACS Children's Surgery Verification program (instituted in 2015) by evaluating neonates undergoing high-risk operations.

Gates RL, Price M, Cameron DB, et al. Non-operative management of solid organ injuries in children: an American Pediatric Surgical Association Outcomes and evidence based practice committee systematic review. *J Pediatr Surg.* 2019;54:1519–1526.

This article from the American Pediatric Surgical Association Outcomes and Evidence Based Practice Committee provides the updates on the practice guidelines for nonoperative management of liver and splenic injuries.

Harris CJ, Waters AM, Tracy ET, et al. Precision oncology: a primer for pediatric surgeons from the APSA cancer committee. *J Pediatr Surg.* 2020;55:1706–1713.

This American Pediatric Surgical Association Cancer Committee summary provides a comprehensive update on the current state of precision medicine in pediatric oncology.

Minneci PC, Hade EM, Lawrence AE, et al. Multi-institutional trial of non-operative management and surgery for uncomplicated appendicitis in children: design and rationale. *Contemp Clin Trials*. 2019;83:10–17.

This clinical trial is evaluating nonoperative management of uncomplicated appendicitis in pediatric patients employing a patient choice design.

REFERENCES

1. Baker MA, Mitchell PD, O'Loughlin AA, et al. Characterization of fatty acid profiles in infants with intestinal failure-associated liver disease. *J Parenter Enteral Nutr*. 2018;42:71–77.
2. Golinelli G, Toso A, Borello G, et al. Percutaneous sclerotherapy with OK-432 of a cervicomediastinal lymphangioma. *Ann Thorac Surg*. 2015;100:1879–1881.
3. Michels G, Wengenmayer T, Hagl C, et al. Recommendations for extracorporeal cardiopulmonary resuscitation (eCPR): Consensus statement of DGIIN, DGK, DGTHG, DGfK, DGNI, DGAI, DIVI and GRC. *Clin Res Cardiol*. 2019;108:455–464.
4. Russo FM, Cordier AG, De Catte L, et al. Proposal for standardized prenatal ultrasound assessment of the fetus with congenital diaphragmatic hernia by the European reference network on rare inherited and congenital anomalies (ERNICA). *Prenat Diagn*. 2018;38:629–637.
5. Deprest J, Brady P, Nicolaides K, et al. Prenatal management of the fetus with isolated congenital diaphragmatic hernia in the era of the TOTAL trial. *Semin Fetal Neonatal Med*. 2014;19:338–348.
6. Schneider A, Becmeur F. Pediatric thoracoscopic repair of congenital diaphragmatic hernias. *J Vis Surg*. 2018;4:43.
7. Bryner BS, West BT, Hirschl RB, et al. Congenital diaphragmatic hernia requiring extracorporeal membrane oxygenation: does timing of repair matter. *J Pediatr Surg*. 2009;44:1165–1171; discussion 1171–1162.
8. Parikh DH, Rasiah SV. Congenital lung lesions: Postnatalesx management and outcome. *Semin Pediatr Surg*. 2015;24:160–167.
9. Wong KKY, Flake AW, Tibboel D, et al. Congenital pulmonary airway malformation: advances and controversies. *Lancet Child Adolesc Health*. 2018;2:290–297.
10. Peranteau WH, Boelig MM, Khalek N, et al. Effect of single and multiple courses of maternal betamethasone on prenatal congenital lung lesion growth and fetal survival. *J Pediatr Surg*. 2016;51:28–32.
11. Rosen R, Vandenplas Y, Singendonk M, et al. Pediatric gastroesophageal reflux clinical practice guidelines: joint recommendations of the North American Society for Pediatric Gastroenterology, Hepatology, and Nutrition and the European Society for Pediatric Gastroenterology, Hepatology, and Nutrition. *J Pediatr Gastroenterol Nutr*. 2018;66:516–554.
12. Shoda T, Wen T, Aceves SS, et al. Eosinophilic oesophagitis endotype classification by molecular, clinical, and histopathological analyses: a cross-sectional study. *Lancet Gastroenterol Hepatol*. 2018;3:477–488.
13. Kethman WC, Harris AHS, Hawn MT, et al. Trends and surgical outcomes of laparoscopic versus open pyloromyotomy. *Surg Endosc*. 2018;32:3380–3385.
14. Moss RL, Dimmitt RA, Barnhart DC, et al. Laparotomy versus peritoneal drainage for necrotizing enterocolitis and perforation. *N Engl J Med*. 2006;354:2225–2234.
15. Ramos-Gonzalez G, Kim HB. Autologous intestinal reconstruction surgery. *Semin Pediatr Surg*. 2018;27:261–266.
16. Bianchi A. Intestinal loop lengthening--a technique for increasing small intestinal length. *J Pediatr Surg*. 1980;15:145–151.
17. Kim HB, Fauza D, Garza J, et al. Serial transverse enteroplasty (STEP): a novel bowel lengthening procedure. *J Pediatr Surg*. 2003;38:425–429.
18. Oh PS, Fingeret AL, Shah MY, et al. Improved tolerance for enteral nutrition after serial transverse enteroplasty (STEP) in infants and children with short bowel syndrome--a seven-year single-center experience. *J Pediatr Surg*. 2014;49:1589–1592.
19. Fitzgerald K, Muto M, Belza C, et al. The evolution of the serial transverse enteroplasty for pediatric short bowel syndrome at a single institution. *J Pediatr Surg*. 2019;54:993–998.
20. Liang CM, Ji DM, Yuan X, et al. RET and PHOX2B genetic polymorphisms and Hirschsprung's disease susceptibility: a meta-analysis. *PLoS One*. 2014;9:e90091.
21. Jiang M, Li K, Li S, et al. Calretinin, S100 and protein gene product 9.5 immunostaining of rectal suction biopsies in the diagnosis of Hirschsprung' disease. *Am J Transl Res*. 2016;8:3159–3168.
22. Soh HJ, Nataraja RM, Pacilli M. Prevention and management of recurrent postoperative Hirschsprung's disease obstructive symptoms and enterocolitis: systematic review and meta-analysis. *J Pediatr Surg*. 2018;53:2423–2429.
23. Bischoff A, Pena A, Levitt MA. Laparoscopic-assisted PSARP - the advantages of combining both techniques for the treatment of anorectal malformations with recto-bladderneck or high prostatic fistulas. *J Pediatr Surg*. 2013;48:367–371.
24. Lautz TB, Thurm CW, Rothstein DH. Delayed repeat enemas are safe and cost-effective in the management of pediatric intussusception. *J Pediatr Surg*. 2015;50:423–427.
25. Robinson JR, Correa H, Brinkman AS, et al. Optimizing surgical resection of the bleeding Meckel diverticulum in children. *J Pediatr Surg*. 2017;52:1610–1615.
26. Minneci PC, Hade EM, Lawrence AE, et al. Multi-institutional trial of non-operative management and surgery for uncomplicated appendicitis in children: design and rationale. *Contemp Clin Trials*. 2019;83:10–17.
27. Verkade HJ, Bezerra JA, Davenport M, et al. Biliary atresia and other cholestatic childhood diseases: advances and future challenges. *J Hepatol*. 2016;65:631–642.
28. Bezerra JA, Spino C, Magee JC, et al. Use of corticosteroids after hepatoportoenterostomy for bile drainage in infants with biliary atresia: The START randomized clinical trial. *JAMA*. 2014;311:1750–1759.
29. Tyraskis A, Parsons C, Davenport M. Glucocorticosteroids for infants with biliary atresia following Kasai portoenterostomy. *Cochrane Database Syst Rev*. 2018;5:CD008735.
30. Soares KC, Goldstein SD, Ghaseb MA, et al. Pediatric choledochal cysts: diagnosis and current management. *Pediatr Surg Int*. 2017;33:637–650.
31. Rygiel AM, Beer S, Simon P, et al. Gene conversion between cationic trypsinogen (PRSS1) and the pseudogene trypsinogen 6 (PRSS3P2) in patients with chronic pancreatitis. *Hum Mutat*. 2015;36:350–356.
32. Cairo SB, Aranda A, Bartz-Kurycki M, et al. Variability in perioperative evaluation and resource utilization in pediatric patients with suspected biliary dyskinesia: a multi-institutional retrospective cohort study. *J Pediatr Surg*. 2019;54:1118–1122.

33. Petrosyan M, Sandler AD. Closure methods in gastroschisis. *Semin Pediatr Surg*. 2018;27:304–308.
34. Dreuning K, Maat S, Twisk J, et al. Laparoscopic versus open pediatric inguinal hernia repair: State-of-the-art comparison and future perspectives from a meta-analysis. *Surg Endosc*. 2019;33:3177–3191.
35. Sacco-Casamassima MG, Goldstein SD, Gause CD, et al. Minimally invasive repair of pectus excavatum: analyzing contemporary practice in 50 ACS NSQIP-pediatric institutions. *Pediatr Surg Int*. 2015;31:493–499.
36. Morikawa N, Laferriere N, Koo S, et al. Cryoanalgesia in patients undergoing nuss repair of pectus excavatum: technique modification and early results. *J Laparoendosc Adv Surg Tech A*. 2018;28:1148–1151.
37. Pastor ER, Mousa SA. Current management of neuroblastoma and future direction. *Crit Rev Oncol Hematol*. 2019;138:38–43.
38. Newman EA, Abdessalam S, Aldrink JH, et al. Update on neuroblastoma. *J Pediatr Surg*. 2019;54:383–389.
39. Fletcher JI, Ziegler DS, Trahair TN, et al. Too many targets, not enough patients: rethinking neuroblastoma clinical trials. *Nat Rev Cancer*. 2018;18:389–400.
40. von Allmen D, Davidoff AM, London WB, et al. Impact of extent of resection on local control and survival in patients from the COG A3973 Study with high-risk neuroblastoma. *J Clin Oncol*. 2017;35:208–216.
41. Irtan S, Brisse HJ, Minard-Colin V, et al. Image-defined risk factor assessment of neurogenic tumors after neoadjuvant chemotherapy is useful for predicting intra-operative risk factors and the completeness of resection. *Pediatr Blood Cancer*. 2015;62:1543–1549.
42. Treger TD, Chowdhury T, Pritchard-Jones K, et al. The genetic changes of Wilms tumour. *Nat Rev Nephrol*. 2019;15:240–251.
43. Pappo AS, Dirksen U. Rhabdomyosarcoma, Ewing sarcoma, and other round cell sarcomas. *J Clin Oncol*. 2018;36: 168–179.
44. Towbin AJ, Meyers RL, Woodley H, et al. PRETEXT: radiologic staging system for primary hepatic malignancies of childhood revised for the Paediatric Hepatic International Tumour Trial (PHITT). *Pediatr Radiol*. 2018;48:536–554; 2017.
45. Lockley M, Stoneham SJ, Olson TA. Ovarian cancer in adolescents and young adults. *Pediatr Blood Cancer*. 2019;66:e27512.
46. Gates RL, Price M, Cameron DB, et al. Non-operative management of solid organ injuries in children: an American Pediatric Surgical Association Outcomes and Evidence Based Practice Committee systematic review. *J Pediatr Surg*. 2019;54:1519–1526.
47. Notrica DM, Eubanks 3rd JW, Tuggle DW, et al. Nonoperative management of blunt liver and spleen injury in children: evaluation of the ATOMAC guideline using GRADE. *J Trauma Acute Care Surg*. 2015;79:683–693.

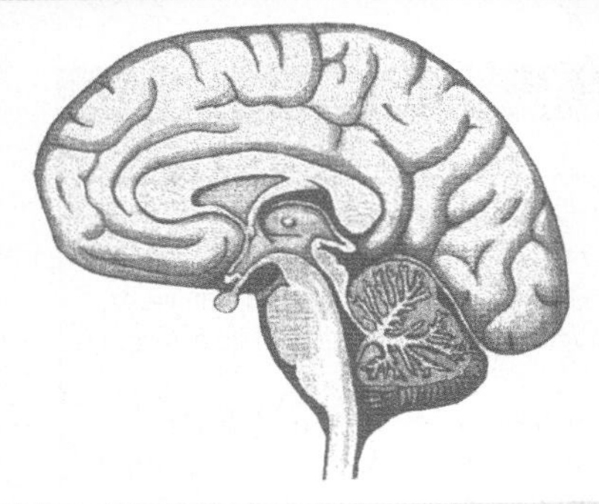

CHAPTER 68

Neurosurgery

Joel T. Patterson

OUTLINE

Neurosurgery is defined as surgery of the brain, spinal cord, peripheral nerves, and their supporting structures, including the blood supply, protective elements, spinal fluid spaces, bony cranium, and spine. This chapter is intended for nonneurosurgeons who want to initiate a framework on which to add further knowledge and experience. It is hoped that it will also help personnel in a community hospital emergency department, residents, advanced practice providers, and medical students communicate effectively and efficiently with neurosurgeons about urgent, emergent, and elective patient care issues. The chapter is divided into sections and includes a discussion of the following: cerebrovascular disorders, central nervous system (CNS) tumors, traumatic brain injury, degenerative diseases of the spine, epilepsy and functional neurosurgery, hydrocephalus, pediatric neurosurgery, and neurosurgical management of CNS infections. The field of neurosurgery is simply too broad to make a detailed encyclopedic overview realistic, but it is hoped that an introduction to the specialty will be useful to the reader.

INTRACRANIAL DYNAMICS

It is essential at the outset to understand some basic principles concerning intracranial dynamics, cerebrospinal fluid (CSF), cerebral blood flow (CBF), and intracranial pressure (ICP), and these are summarized here for review.

The first principle has been recognized for decades. The cranial cavity has a fixed volume composed of brain tissue (parenchyma), CSF, and blood vessels with their intravascular blood. According to the Monro-Kellie doctrine, the sum of these components within the fixed volume of the cranial cavity is constant, and an

TABLE 68.1 Intracranial excess volume syndromes and therapy.

COMPONENT	EXCESS VOLUME SYNDROME	SPECIFIC TREATMENT
Brain tissue	Edema: cytotoxic, vasogenic, perineoplastic, inflammatory	Diuretics: mannitol, furosemide, hypertonic saline; steroids for perineoplastic and inflammatory vasogenic edema
Vascular	Elevated P_{CO_2}: hyperperfusion state with loss of autoregulation as in severe hypertension, after trauma or AVM removal; relative venous obstruction	Increased ventilation; diuretics (in hyperperfusion state, avoid mannitol), barbiturates; clear venous obstruction; elevate head of bed (to reduce venous volume)
Cerebrospinal fluid	Impaired absorption with congenital, posthemorrhagic, or postinfectious hydrocephalus, communicating or obstructive; loculations; arachnoid or periventricular cysts; rare increased production of CSF with choroid plexus papilloma	Ventricular external drainage (or lumbar drainage only if no threat of herniation) or shunt; with flocculation, or with some types of obstructive hydrocephalus, endoscopic fenestration or third ventriculostomy may be possible; acetazolamide and steroids may temporarily decrease CSF production
Mass lesion	Tumor, cyst, abscess, hematoma, radiation necrosis, or cerebral infarction necrosis	Remove, fenestrate, aspirate lesion (often with stereotactic guidance); less commonly, it might be useful to enlarge intracranial volume by decompression

AVM, Arteriovenous malformation; *CSF*, cerebrospinal fluid, CO_2, partial pressure carbon dioxide.

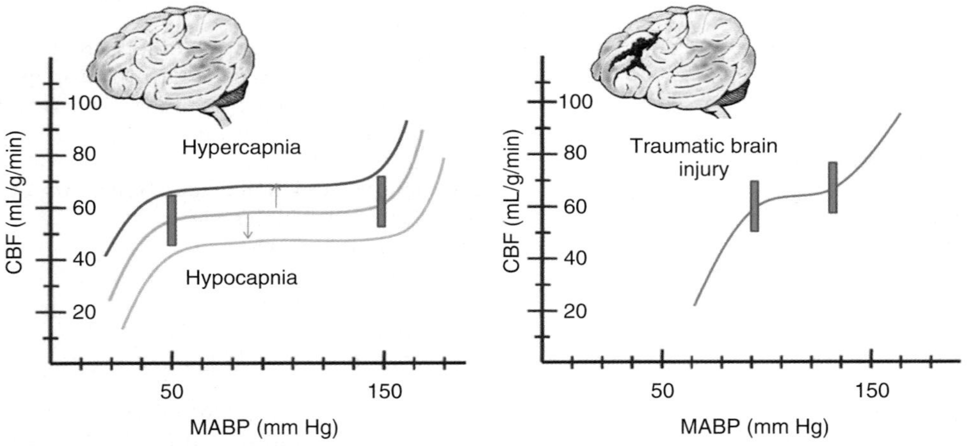

FIG. 68.1 Cerebral blood flow *(CBF)* as a function of mean arterial blood pressure *(MABP)*. Note the upward and downward shifts with hypercapnia and hypocapnia, respectively. In traumatic brain injury, the curve is steeper, with large CBF changes occurring with small pressure changes. (Adapted from Rangel-Castilla L, Gasco J, Nauta HJ, et al. Cerebral pressure autoregulation in traumatic brain injury. *Neurosurg Focus*. 2008;25:E7.)

increase in one component must be accompanied by an equal and opposite decrease in one or both of the remaining components if ICP is to remain constant.[1] If this does not occur, the ICP will rise, and, at some point, the increase in pressure per unit increase in volume becomes asymptotic, with the increased ICP causing a decrease in blood flow and oxygen delivery. As a consequence, if there is an elevation in the volume of any one compartment, there is a stage of compensation in which the volume of one or more of the other compartments can be reduced to avoid elevations in the ICP. Table 68.1 summarizes and simplifies some of the excess volume syndromes and specific treatment for each.

The second principle is that spinal fluid is produced at a constant rate (≈15–20 mL/h) by the choroid plexus of the ventricles. It is essential to understand that production of CSF is little affected by increased ICP. Therefore, any derangement in CSF absorption or flow may increase the ICP effects of diseases affecting the CNS. Thus, CSF production continues unabated, even to lethal elevations of ICP. In the following discussions on tumors, infection, intracranial hemorrhage, and trauma, many examples will become apparent whereby impaired CSF absorption contributes to the pathologic condition. The only exceptions to the almost constant CSF production are the excess production associated with the rare choroid plexus papilloma and the occasional decreased CSF production seen with ventriculitis.

The third basic principle is that the CBF normally varies over a wide range (30–100 mL/100 g of brain tissue per minute), depending on metabolic demand from neuronal activity within a particular area of the brain. The blood flow to any brain area is generally abundant, exceeding demand by a wide margin, so that oxygen extraction ratios are often low. The brain vasculature matches the blood flow to tissue metabolic demand, and the CBF generally maintains what is needed, despite wide variations in systemic blood pressure, by a phenomenon known as autoregulation. Factors such as an elevated or decreased arterial P_{CO_2} shift the curve as indicated. In the setting of traumatic brain injury, the curve becomes more pronounced (i.e., smaller changes in blood pressure or P_{CO_2}) and affects the CBF dramatically (Fig. 68.1). If tissue demand exceeds autoregulation, or if CBF declines for pathologic reasons, the first defense is that the oxygen extraction will increase (i.e., arteriovenous oxygen

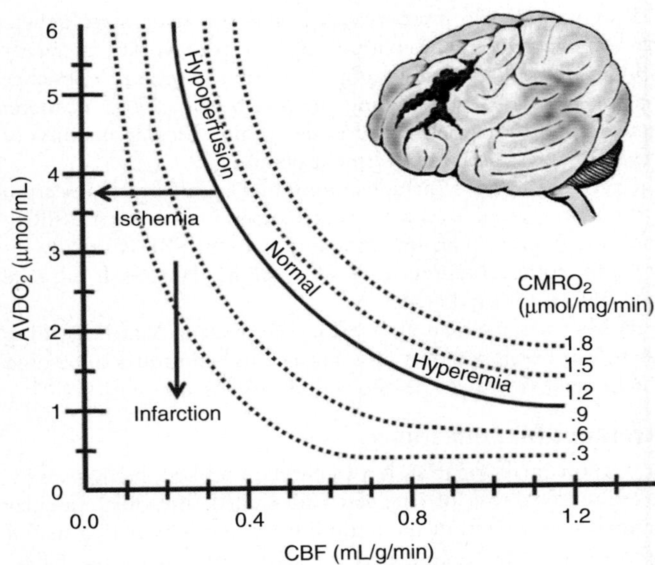

FIG. 68.2 Relationships among cerebral flow, metabolism, and oxygen extraction in normal and pathologic circumstances. (From Rangel-Castilla L, Gasco J, Nauta HJ, et al. Cerebral pressure autoregulation in traumatic brain injury. *Neurosurg Focus.* 2008;25:E7.) *AVDO₂*, Arteriovenous oxygen difference; *CBF*, cerebral blood flow; *CMRO₂*, cerebral metabolic rate of oxygen consumption.

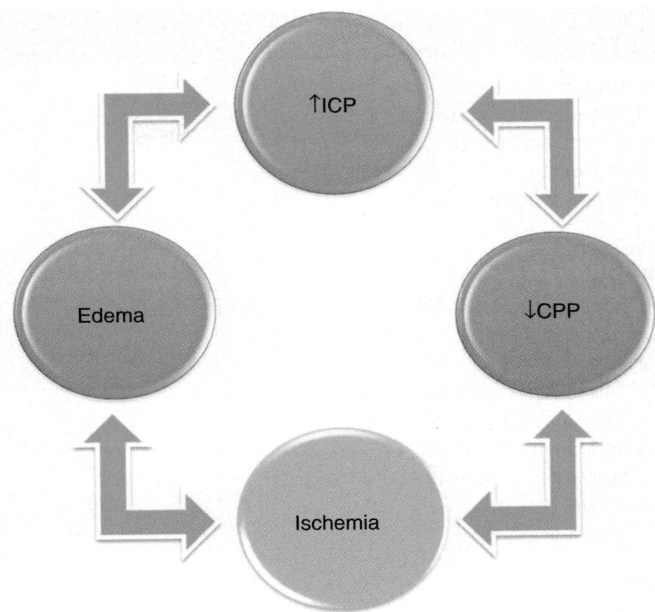

FIG. 68.3 Relationship among increased intracranial pressure *(ICP)*, reduced cerebral perfusion pressure *(CPP)*, development of ischemia and infarction, and cerebral edema.

difference). The tissue begins to experience dysfunction at levels below 0.25 mL per gram of brain tissue per minute. With levels between 0.15 and 0.20, the brain tissue may undergo reversible ischemia; however, infarction will occur when levels range between 0.10 and 0.15 (Fig. 68.2). The metabolic consumption of oxygen in the brain is decreased after traumatic brain injury to levels between 0.6 and 1.2 µmol/mg/min. Complete loss of blood flow to any brain area results in infarction (irreversible damage) within a few minutes. Swelling of the infarcted tissue takes days to peak and weeks to resolve.[2]

A fourth principle derives from the other three and the fact that as injured tissue swells, it may create a vicious cycle and cause a cascading injury (Fig. 68.3). If ICP is elevated high enough by some mechanism so that cerebral perfusion pressure (CPP) declines, CBF can decline to levels at which tissue injury occurs.

$$\text{CPP} = \text{Mean arterial pressure (MAP)} - \text{ICP}$$

Brain edema (swelling) within the closed cranium will lead to further increases in ICP with even further decreases in CPP in a stage of decompensation. When the capacity for autoregulation is exceeded or damaged so that it can no longer play a role, CBF is linked directly to the CPP.

In the management of intracranial disease, ICP and CPP are easy to measure continuously and thus serve as highly practical surrogates for the more fundamental but much more difficult to measure CBF. However, these are not equivalent, and the limitations of these parameters for guiding therapy need to be remembered. Regardless of causation, when concern arises about the possibility of cascading injury, every effort is made to keep the CPP in the range of 60 to 70 mm Hg and ICP below 22 mm Hg if possible. Routinely using pressors and volume expansion to maintain CPP higher than 70 mm Hg is not supported on the basis of systemic complications.[3]

A fifth principle concerns focal mass effect and its progression in regard to the complex anatomy of the cranial cavity. The cranial cavity contains several knifelike projections of folded dura, the falx and tentorium, which divide the cavity into a right and left supratentorial compartment and an infratentorial compartment (the posterior fossa). The sphenoid wing is a prominent, mostly bony ridge that separates the anterior fossa containing the frontal lobe from the middle fossa containing the temporal lobe. A narrow opening, the incisura, edged by the tentorium, surrounds the midbrain and is the only passage between the supratentorial and infratentorial compartments. Apart from the small openings for the cranial nerves and arteries, the foramen magnum is the only sizable opening in the cranial cavity.

The condition that classically illustrates the expanding mass lesion is the acute epidural hematoma, seen after trauma with skull fracture. Regardless of the source, however, the progression can be similar and has been termed rostrocaudal decay to reflect the early and late stages, as listed in order here:

- Focal distortion only
- Effacement of gyri and sulci
- Compression of the lateral (or other) ventricle
- Midline shift
- Subfalcine herniation
- Temporal lobe tentorial herniation
- Third nerve compression (unilateral dilated pupil)
- Obliteration of basal cisterns
- Midbrain compression
- Midbrain infarction, Duret hemorrhages (both pupils dilate, with irreversible damage to midbrain)
- Further brainstem compression
- Loss of brainstem reflexes: progression from flexor posturing to extensor posturing; vestibuloocular and oculocephalic reflexes; corneal reflexes
- Medullary compression syndrome: respiratory reflexes; vasomotor reflexes, Cushing reflex with elevation of the systolic blood pressure, widening of the pulse pressure, bradycardia
- Foramen magnum herniation

BOX 68.1 Cerebral vascular disease.

Congenital
Arteriovenous malformation and fistula
Cavernous malformation
Telangiectasis
Venous anomaly (angioma)

Acquired
Traumatic
Some arteriovenous fistulas (type I carotid-cavernous fistula)
Traumatic aneurysm
Degenerative
Atherosclerotic, occlusive disease
Most cerebral (berry) aneurysms
Some arterial dissections
Spontaneous intracerebral hemorrhage
Infectious
Mycotic aneurysms

Idiopathic
Moyamoya
Some arteriovenous fistulas: dural AVM–like or type II carotid-cavernous fistulas

AVM, Arteriovenous malformation.

At stages beyond tentorial herniation, it is unusual for focal mass effects not to be accompanied by an overall increase in ICP. The point at which focal mass effect evolves to include a rise in overall ICP depends largely on the compliance within the cranial cavity. Young patients with so-called tight brains can develop raised ICP, even with relatively small volumes of mass that produce only effacement of the cortical gyri. On the other hand, patients with advanced cerebral atrophy can, for example, tolerate large frontal intracerebral hematomas or chronic subdural hematomas with compression of the lateral ventricle and midline shift while maintaining a tolerable ICP and a surprising degree of near-normal neurologic function.

CEREBROVASCULAR DISORDERS

Cerebrovascular disorders encompass a host of disorders: congenital, acquired, and idiopathic (Box 68.1).

Arteriovenous Malformations

An arteriovenous malformation (AVM) is an abnormal collection of blood vessels wherein arterial blood flows directly into draining veins without the normal interposed capillary beds. AVMs are congenital lesions that can enlarge somewhat with age, recruiting new vascular supply, and often progress from low-flow lesions at birth to higher flow lesions in adulthood. They present with hemorrhage, ischemia of the brain parenchyma around the lesion due to a vascular "steal" phenomenon, or seizures. They have a prevalence of 15 to 18/100,000 and typically are manifested before the age of 40 years. The risk of hemorrhage rate is up to 4% per year,[4] and once they bleed, they may be even more prone to hemorrhage. They are typically composed of one or more feeding arteries; a nidus of varying size, shape, and compactness that is composed of abnormal vessels; and draining veins. They are sometimes associated with high-flow related aneurysms of the feeding arteries.

Patients typically present with headaches, neurologic deficit, seizures, or varying combinations of the three. Workup generally includes computed tomography (CT) and magnetic resonance imaging (MRI), demonstrating the lesion (Fig. 68.4). Catheter angiography is then performed to define the vascular anatomy of the lesion and is used for treatment planning.

Treatment options include craniotomy with surgical resection of the lesion, embolization, and stereotactic radiosurgery (SRS). Commonly, more than one modality is used. SRS is usually reserved for compact lesions less the 2.5 cm in diameter. It can take up to 3 years for irradiated

AVMs to shut down after SRS. The Spetzler-Martin grading system was developed over 30 years ago and continues to be used to help make treatment decisions (Table 68.2).[5]

Cavernous Malformations

A cavernous malformation is a well-circumscribed, benign vascular lesion consisting of irregular thin-walled sinusoidal vascular channels located within the brain but lacking intervening neural parenchyma, large feeding arteries, or large draining veins. Characterized by McCormick in an autopsy series,[6] these lesions have a prevalence of approximately 0.5%. There are three familial forms described. Because these are low-pressure, low-flow lesions, hemorrhage is typically not catastrophic unless it is in a highly eloquent area of the brain.

Patients usually present with hemorrhage or headaches with or without a history of new-onset seizures. Although it is often evident on CT, MRI is the imaging modality of choice and demonstrates a characteristic dark hemosiderin ring. Treatment for symptomatic lesions includes seizure control and surgical excision. Radiosurgery, while not necessarily curative, has been shown to decrease the rate of bleeding in lesions not amenable to surgical resection.[7]

Capillary Telangiectasia

This lesion is composed of vascular channels with extremely thin walls similar to those of dilated capillaries. These are usually grouped in small clusters, generally with prominent intervening brain tissue. They are often clinically silent and generally do not appear on imaging studies. They are not evident on conventional catheter angiography unless they are large, and then only in the capillary venous phase. They clearly differ from an AVM in that flow through the lesion is not fast enough to demonstrate arteries and veins in the same conventional angiographic image. These lesions are typically not treated surgically.

Developmental Venous Anomaly: Venous Angioma

These lesions are composed of an abnormally configured venous drainage system converging on a single, enlarged venous outflow channel. The typical appearance is that of a hydra, with radially converging veins. A characteristic feature of this lesion appears to be that the abnormal venous bed is poorly collateralized. The abnormal venous drainage may or may not be fully adequate to the needs of the brain tissue supplied. Slowly evolving degenerative changes in the brain tissue supplied can occur as a result, but, unfortunately, this is not helped by any known intervention. However inadequate, the venous anomaly represents the only venous drainage available to that area of brain, and therefore removal of the venous anomaly is not recommended. Doing so could lead to a venous infarction with swelling and hemorrhage, the consequences of which are particularly dangerous in the posterior fossa.

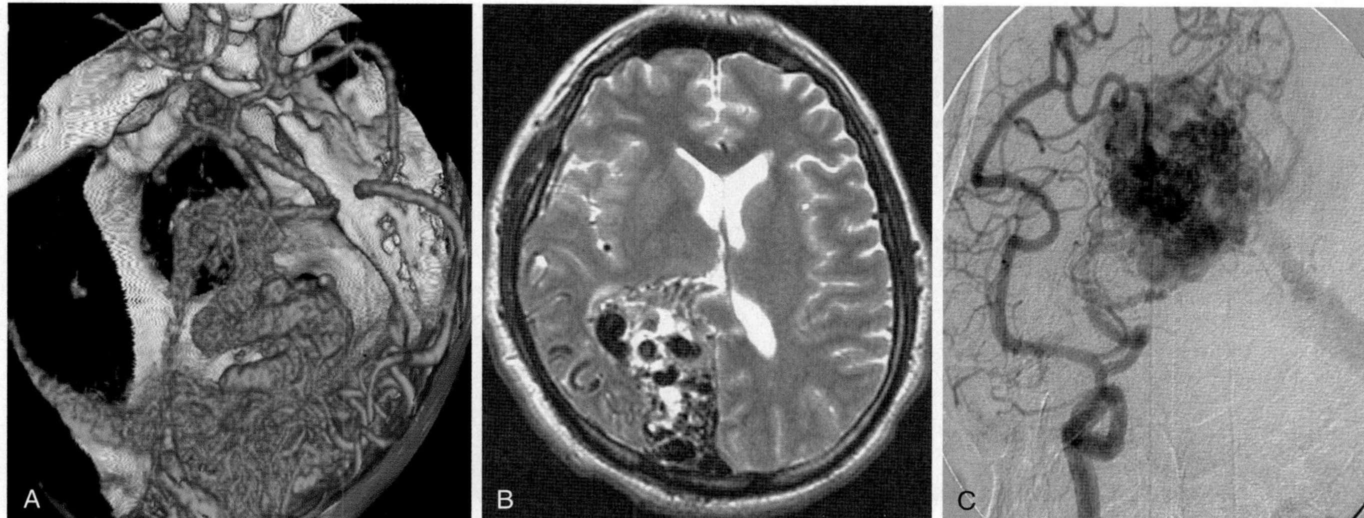

FIG. 68.4 Computed tomography angiography with three-dimensional reconstruction (A), Magnetic resonance imaging (B), and conventional angiogram (C) of a large arteriovenous malformation with supply from the middle and posterior cerebral arteries and ill-defined nidus. Complex deep and superficial venous drainage is present.

TABLE 68.2 **Spetzler-Martin grading system.**

FEATURE	POINTS
Nidus size (cm)	
Small (<3)	1
Medium (3-6)	2
Large (>6)	3
Eloquence of adjacent brain	
Noneloquent	0
Eloquent (sensorimotor, language, visual, thalamus, hypothalamus, internal capsule, brainstem, cerebellar peduncles, deep cerebellar nuclei)	1
Pattern of venous drainage	
Superficially only	0
Deep	1

Traumatic Fistula

Both the internal carotid artery and vertebral artery enter the cranial cavity immediately after passing through a venous network. The internal carotid artery passes through the cavernous sinus, which communicates with the superior ophthalmic vein, petrosal sinus, and sphenoparietal sinus. The vertebral artery passes through a venous plexus at the occipital-C1 epidural space, which communicates with the jugular vein, epidural venous plexus, and paraspinal venous plexus. Trauma leading to a tear in the carotid or vertebral artery at its tether point passing through the skull base can lead to fistula with the surrounding venous plexus. The consequences may vary in severity and suddenness but typically include periorbital swelling, with proptosis and scleral edema in the case of the carotid-cavernous fistula (CCF) and prominent pulsatile bruit in the case of the vertebral-jugular fistula. Intraocular pressure measurement by tonometry can guide the urgency in treating CCF. On radiologic examination, dilation of the superior ophthalmic vein is characteristic (Fig. 68.5). These lesions are usually treated by endovascular techniques. A catheter is advanced through the tear in the artery into the venous side of the fistula. The high flow and large fistulous channel facilitate this process. Embolic material, a coil, or a detachable balloon is then used to occlude the venous side of the fistula. When conventional transvenous routes fail, a direct approach through transorbital puncture may be required to provide endovascular therapy.[8]

Aneurysms

Aneurysms are an excessive localized enlargement of a vessel due to a weakening and subsequent defect in the wall of the artery. There is an adult prevalence of 2% (this varies according to the study) with an annual incidence of aneurysmal subarachnoid hemorrhage of 6 to 8/100,000 with peak age at 50 years. Modifiable risk factors for subarachnoid hemorrhage include hypertension, smoking, and excessive alcohol. Aneurysms may be further divided into saccular, fusiform, dissecting, infectious, and traumatic aneurysms.

Saccular Aneurysms

As the name implies, these aneurysms, also referred to as berry aneurysms, are usually saccular in form and come off the vessel wall or at a bifurcation. Many of these are found incidentally, given the frequency of neuroimaging, but many present with hemorrhage.[9] The classic presentation of subarachnoid hemorrhage due to a cerebral aneurysm is that of sudden onset of a headache, described as the "worst headache of my life." Workup typically includes a CT scan, demonstrating a typical distribution of blood (Fig. 68.6). Between 10% and 15% of subarachnoid hemorrhages from saccular aneurysms are fatal before the hospital is even reached. Of those individuals who reach a medical facility, one third do not survive (usually because of rebleeding), one third will survive with varying degrees of neurologic disability, and one third return to their baseline level.

The major complications of subarachnoid hemorrhage include rebleeding, hydrocephalus (which is observed in around 15% to 20% of cases), cardiac events in around 50% of patients, vasospasm, hyponatremia, and seizures. Rebleeding is a major cause of death in patients who reach medical care after their initial episode of bleeding. Hydrocephalus is caused by disruption in the function of the arachnoid granulations and is commonly treated with an external ventricular drain. Vasospasm is a narrowing of

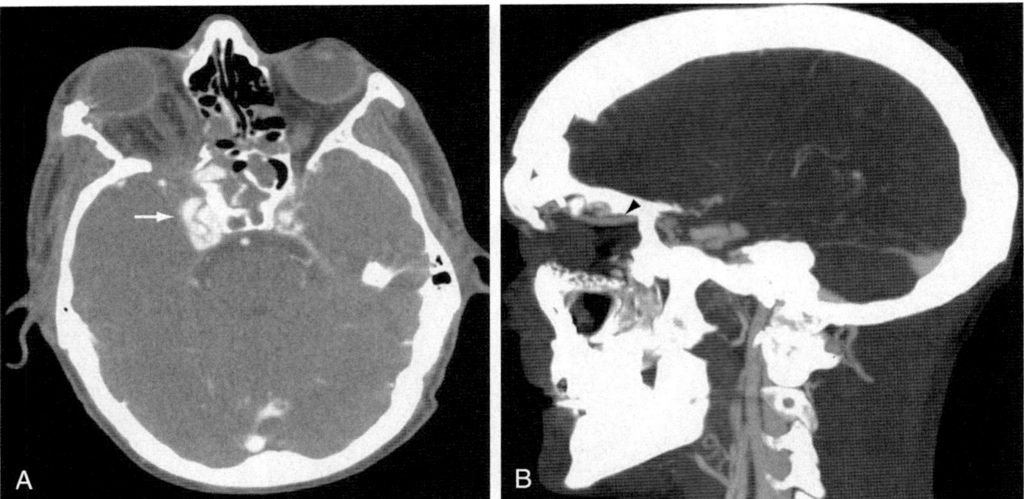

FIG. 68.5 Right internal carotid-cavernous sinus fistula (A, *arrow*) with dilation of the superior ophthalmic drain (B, *arrowhead*), a typical imaging finding of this pathologic process.

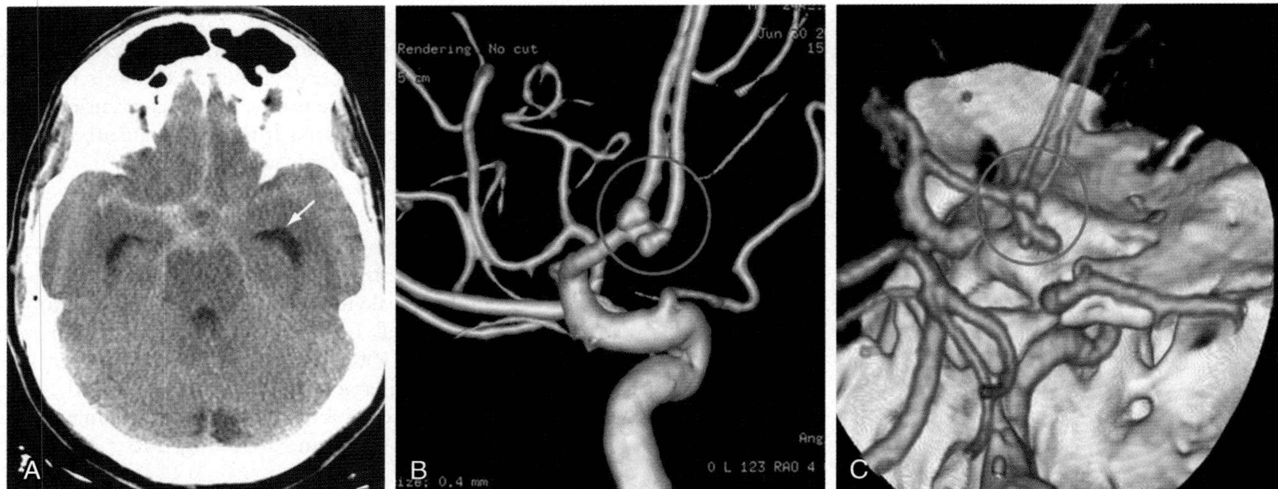

FIG. 68.6 (A) Computed tomography (CT) scan of brain showing subarachnoid blood in the basal cisterns. Dilated temporal horns *(arrow)* indicate the presence of hydrocephalus. (B) Cerebral angiogram shows two aneurysms located at the junction of the A1 and A2 segments of the anterior cerebral artery *(circle)*. (C) CT angiography with three-dimensional reconstruction showing the relationship of the aneurysms *(circle)* with the skull base.

the cerebral arteries thought to be caused by smooth muscle dysfunction related to blood breakdown products in the spinal fluid. When present, it can contribute to significant ischemia of the brain and, as such, be a significant cause of morbidity. Treatment of symptomatic vasospasm is typically multimodality and includes the use of hypervolemia and induced hypertension, endovascular procedures, and a variety of pharmacologic agents (Box 68.2).[10–12]

A classic study of cerebral aneurysms and their treatment documents the risk for rupture according to size and location as demonstrated in Table 68.3.[13] As a means of predicting possible vasospasm and overall outcomes, the Hunt and Hess clinical grading scale[14] and the World Federation of Neurological Surgeons clinical grading scale[15] were developed (Tables 68.4 and 68.5). Another method of classifying subarachnoid hemorrhage is described by Fisher and colleagues[16] and is based on CT scan imaging (Table 68.6).

BOX 68.2 Treatment of vasospasm.

Prevention of Arterial Narrowing
Subarachnoid blood removal
Prevention of dehydration and hypotension
Calcium channel blockers (nimodipine)

Reversal of Arterial Narrowing
Intra arterial calcium channel blockers
Transluminal balloon angioplasty

Prevention and Reversal of Ischemic Neurologic Deficit
Hypertension, hypervolemia, hemodilution

TABLE 68.3 Risk of rupture during 5 years (%) according to International Study of Unruptured Intracranial Aneurysms.

TYPE OF ANEURYSM	<7 mm AND NO PRIOR SAH	<7 mm AND PRIOR SAH	7–12 mm	13–24 mm	>24 mm
Carotid-cavernous	0	0	0	3.0	6.4
Anterior circulation	0	1.5	2.6	14.5	40.0
Posterior circulation	2.5	3.4	14.5	18.4	50.0

SAH, Subarachnoid hemorrhage.

TABLE 68.4 Hunt and Hess clinical grading scale.

DESCRIPTION	GRADE	GOOD OUTCOME
Asymptomatic or minimal headache and slight nuchal rigidity	1	≈70
Moderate to severe headache, nuchal rigidity, ± cranial nerve palsy only	2	≈70
Drowsy, confusion, or mild focal deficit	3	≈15
Stupor, moderate to severe hemiparesis, possibly early decerebrate rigidity	4	≈15
Deep coma, decerebrate rigidity, moribund appearance	5	≈0

TABLE 68.5 World Federation of Neurological Surgeons clinical grading scale.

GRADE	GCS SCORE	MOTOR DEFICIT
I	15	No
II	13–14	No
III	13–14	Yes
IV	7–12	Yes or no
V	3–6	Yes or no

GCS, Glasgow Coma Scale.

TABLE 68.6 Fisher grading for appearance of SAH on computed tomography.

GRADE	CT FINDINGS
I	No hemorrhage evident
II	Diffuse SAH with vertical layers <1 mm thick
III	Localized clots and/or vertical layers of SAH >1 mm thick
IV	Diffuse or no SAH but with intracerebral or intraventricular hemorrhage

SAH, Subarachnoid hemorrhage.

Treatment of saccular aneurysms consists of coiling, coiling through a stent, flow diversion stent[17,18] or surgical clipping (Figs. 68.7 and 68.8) with subsequent intensive critical care unit management of potential vasospasm and comorbidities. Once the standard of care in the treatment of cerebral aneurysms, open craniotomy and clipping is now typically reserved for those lesions believed not to be amenable to endovascular techniques.[13,17,18] It is generally believed that treatment of ruptured aneurysms is best accomplished as soon as possible after the initial hemorrhage.

Spontaneous Intracerebral Hemorrhage

Spontaneous intracerebral hemorrhages into the brain parenchyma are common, accounting for approximately 10% of all strokes. They generally occur in older patients, usually because of degenerative changes in the cerebral vessels that are often associated with chronic hypertension (Box 68.3). In younger patients, they are more likely related to drug abuse or vascular malformation. They can occur anywhere in the cerebral circulation or brainstem but are classically described in association with small degenerative aneurysms (Charcot-Bouchard aneurysms) of the perforating vessels and larger vessels at the skull base. They are typically located on the perforating lenticulostriate vessels, leading to hemorrhage in the basal ganglia. The clinical presentation of a stroke, with sudden-onset neurologic signs and symptoms corresponding to the area of brain affected. Symptoms are more likely to include headache than ischemic stroke. The diagnosis is with CT, usually done in an emergency department setting. The size and location of the acute hematoma are well visualized with CT, as is any associated brain shift or hydrocephalus (Figs. 68.9A and 68.10). Older patients with a known history of hypertension present with a hematoma in the putamen, thalamus, cerebellum, or pons. Blood pressure control is essential in order to prevent rehemorrhage. Further investigation might be warranted with an atypical hematoma location or appearance, especially if there is any component of subarachnoid blood. Also, investigation is usually recommended for younger patients without known hypertension and those with a potential underlying cause for hemorrhage (e.g., history of neoplasm, blood dyscrasias, bacterial endocarditis).

Further investigation is generally done with contrast MRI or magnetic resonance angiography. Any suggestion of aneurysm or AVM is followed by conventional catheter angiography. In older patients with a history of early dementia and multiple episodes of more peripherally located intracerebral hematomas, the diagnosis of amyloid angiopathy needs to be considered.

Most cases of spontaneous intracerebral hemorrhage do not require surgical intervention. Many hemorrhages are small and well tolerated. Patients who obey commands and can be monitored by changes in their neurologic examination can generally be managed conservatively with hospital observation for at least 5 to 7 days. Peak swelling and decompensation are probably most likely to occur within that time frame. Surgery for evacuation of the hematoma may be appropriate in a small group of patients with intermediate-sized hemorrhages in accessible locations who appear to tolerate the hematoma initially but then deteriorate in a delayed fashion with edema, despite medical therapy. Steroids have not demonstrated benefit. Attempts to predict which patients will deteriorate solely on the basis of hematoma volume have been frustrated by the broad spectrum of intracranial compliance exhibited by different patients. In general, younger patients with smaller ventricles and small subarachnoid spaces have a lower compliance,

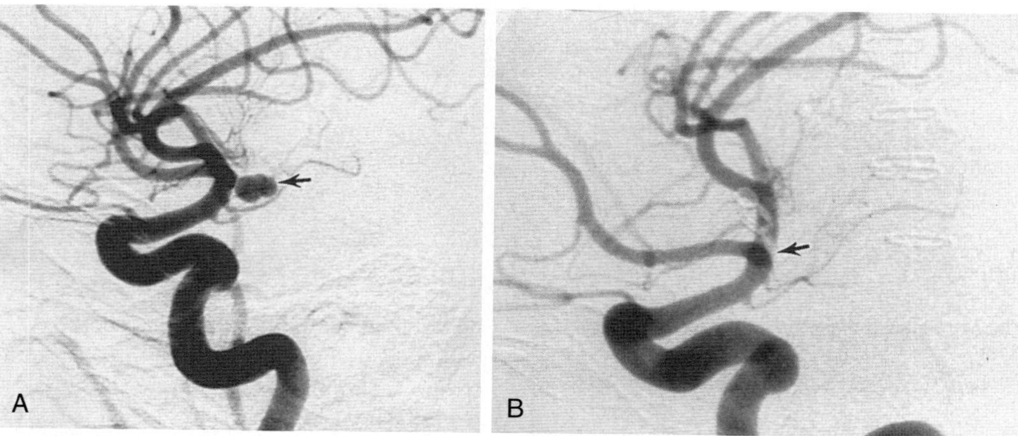

FIG. 68.7 (A) Subtraction carotid angiogram shows a 4- × 6-mm berry aneurysm *(arrow)* originating from the distal internal carotid artery. (B) Postoperative carotid angiogram shows clip placement *(arrow)* with total obliteration of the aneurysm.

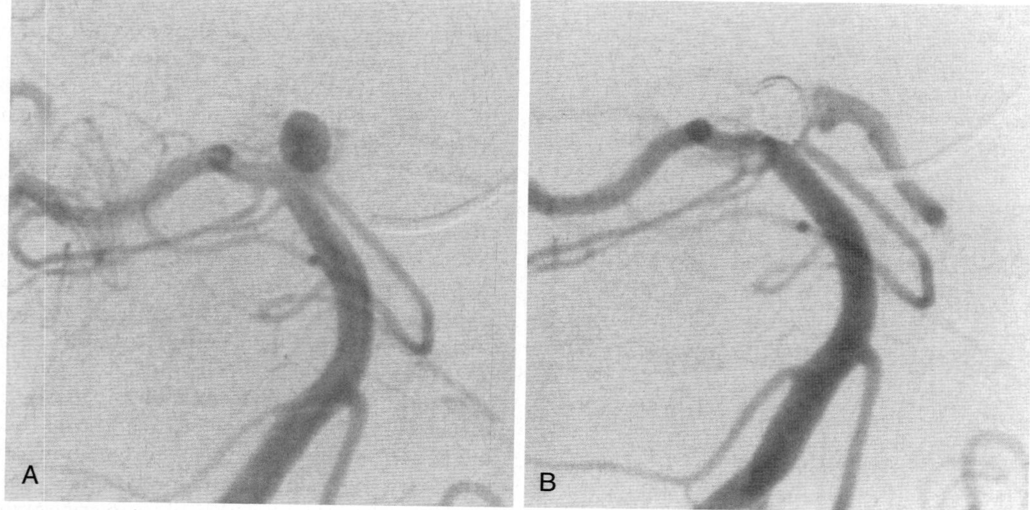

FIG. 68.8 (A) Subtraction vertebral angiogram shows a basilar tip aneurysm. (B) Subtracted vertebral angiogram after the placement of coils demonstrates excellent obliteration of the aneurysm and preservation of adjacent vessels.

BOX 68.3 Causes of spontaneous intracerebral hemorrhage.

- Hypertension
- Vascular anomaly
- Cerebral aneurysm
- Arteriovenous malformation
- Cavernous malformation
- Cerebral infarction (stroke) transformation
- Cerebral amyloid angiopathy
- Coagulopathy
- Tumors
- Drug abuse
- Other

with lower tolerance, than older patients with cerebral atrophy and generous ventricles and subarachnoid spaces.

The Surgical Trial in Intracerebral Hemorrhage has noted a lack of clinical outcome difference in comparing early surgery with conservative management.[19] If indicated, surgical evacuation is usually done by craniotomy over the most accessible part of the hematoma (Fig. 68.9B). Intraoperative ultrasound is often helpful in finding hematomas that do not quite come to the cortical surface and in monitoring the progress of the evacuation. The goal of surgery is decompression rather than complete removal, but it is generally done as far as safely practical. Minimally invasive techniques continue to evolve.[20] Stereotactic aspiration and methods with fibrinolytic agents are being developed and may be a consideration for patients with hematomas in deep locations that are otherwise difficult to access.

A special situation to consider is the patient with cerebellar hemorrhage (Fig. 68.10). Surgery is offered more readily in these

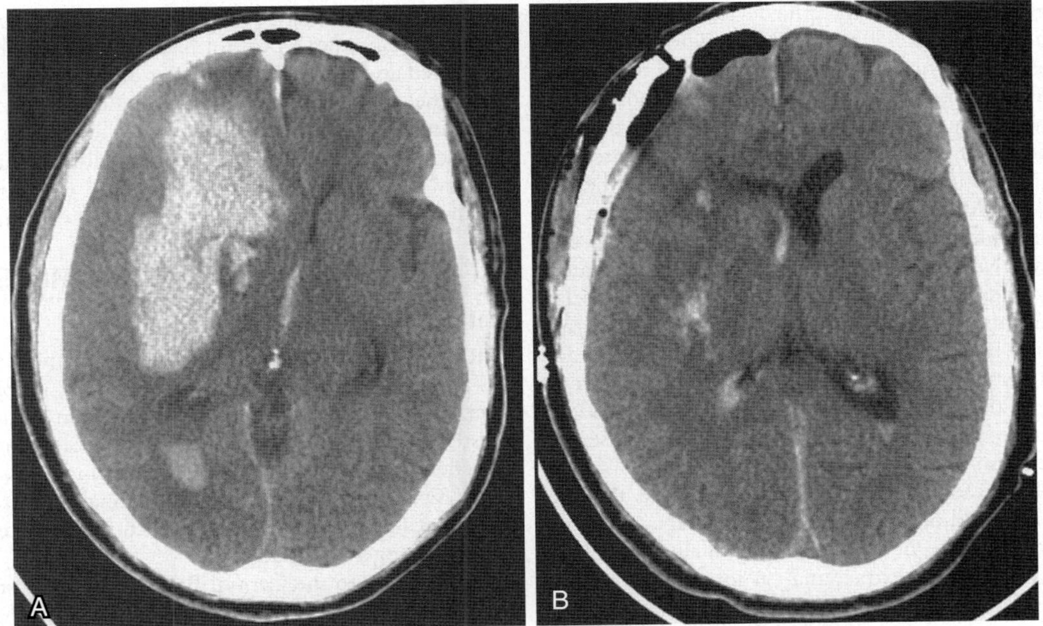

FIG. 68.9 Nonenhanced CT scan of the head. (A) Spontaneous hypertensive intracerebral hematoma in the right basal ganglia with extension to the frontal and temporal lobes. (B) Immediate postoperative CT scan shows near-total removal of the intracerebral hematoma. *CT*, Computed tomography.

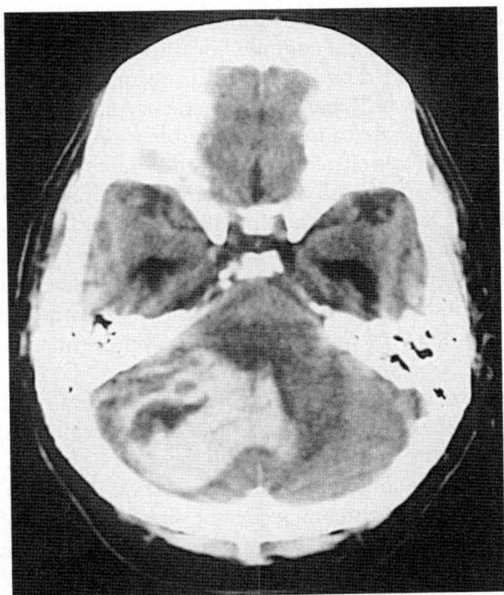

FIG. 68.10 Nonenhanced CT scan of the brain shows a large, hypertensive, intracerebellar hematoma with obstruction of the fourth ventricle and enlargement of the temporal horns, indicating obstructive hydrocephalus. *CT*, Computed tomography.

cases because the danger of sudden deterioration from brainstem compression is more of a concern and because even extensive damage to the cerebellum itself is generally survivable with good functional outcome. Patients with fourth ventricular obstruction and hydrocephalus from cerebellar hemorrhage can sometimes be treated with ventricular drainage alone but are usually offered surgical evacuation of the hematoma by suboccipital craniotomy because of the risk for brainstem compression.

Mycotic Aneurysms

These aneurysms are associated with a systemic infection capable of showering small particles of bacteria-infected material into the cerebral vascular bed. Subacute bacterial endocarditis and some pulmonary infections can do this. A distinguishing feature of these aneurysms is that they are generally found more distal in the cerebral vascular bed, as opposed to berry aneurysms, which are usually found on larger vessels near the circle of Willis. There can also be many of them. When the bacterial emboli lodge in distal cerebral arterial branches, they can erode through the wall of these smaller vessels, often creating a hemorrhage contained by the perivascular tissue. Maximal antibiotic treatment is essential at the outset. The presence of an intracerebral hematoma may force immediate craniotomy for evacuation. Operation on the aneurysm at this early stage often reveals a component of subarachnoid hemorrhage and an early inflammatory reaction in the subarachnoid space, with only a blood collection covering the erosion defect in the wall of the small artery. Attempts to dissect and to define a neck are frustrated by a lack of developed fibrous tissues, and intraoperative hemorrhage is then common. Typically, the diseased arterial segment must be occluded and resected when it is operated on in this early stage. The need for arterial bypass to maintain blood flow to critical cerebral areas should be anticipated, but this is not always possible.

If the mycotic aneurysms are discovered or treated at some later stage, a fibrous wall to the aneurysm may have had time to develop, and clipping can then be a possibility. However, the surgeon needs to be forewarned that it may be difficult to find the aneurysm in a distal location, often buried deep in a cerebral sulcus thickened with reactive fibrous scar tissue.

Moyamoya Disease

Moyamoya disease is a cerebrovascular disorder that is characterized by an idiopathic nonatherosclerotic narrowing or occlusion of major intracranial blood vessels with the development of a conspicuous compensatory collateral rete vessel network, which allows continued cerebral perfusion around the occluded or severely narrowed segment. The disorder is usually bilateral, although not necessarily exactly symmetrical. Although generally rare, the disease is more common in persons of Asian ancestry and was first recognized from cases studied with angiography in Japan before the advent of CT and MRI. The term *moyamoya* comes from the Japanese word for "puff of smoke" or mist. The actual disease is sometimes confused with the less conspicuous collateral vascular networks seen around severe narrowing of common atherosclerotic origin in persons of Western origin. In the juvenile form, moyamoya typically is manifested as cognitive decline, with deteriorating school performance and evidence of multiple infarcts. Angiography reveals the internal carotid artery, proximal middle cerebral artery, or proximal anterior cerebral artery with severe narrowing or occlusion and, generally, multiple clusters of fine collateral vessels. In the adult form of moyamoya disease, the rete vessels cause subarachnoid or basal ganglia hemorrhage, the most common presentations. The hemorrhage can usually be treated conservatively. Some form of extracranial to intracranial bypass is generally attempted to take the load off the collateral vascular network. Surgical treatment consists of extracranial intracranial bypass (typically superficial temporal to middle cerebral artery), onlay synangiosis, or a combination of the two.[21] EC-IC bypass is typically preferred in the adult form of the disease, while children tend to respond better to synangiosis.

Dural Arteriovenous Malformations

Dural AVMs consist of the abnormal communication between dural arteries and the cerebral venous system. The lesions seem to occur only in adults and are probably acquired lesions that follow a dural sinus thrombosis, usually of the cavernous sinus or sigmoid-transverse sinus junction area. With subsequent healing, the thrombosed segment triggers a neovascular response that evolves to an AVM configuration with fistulous channels that can gradually enlarge. Lesions demonstrating communication with cortical veins pose a risk of hemorrhage and require treatment. This is typically done with endovascular techniques, although open surgical resection is sometimes necessary.

Ischemic Strokes

The past decade has witnessed an impressive body of basic science and clinical research focused on ischemic stroke. The continued prevalence, morbidity, disability, and subsequent cost to society has prompted the creation of primary and comprehensive stroke centers. Today, neurosurgeons play a critical role in the care and management of patients suffering from ischemic stroke. This involvement consists of (1) endovascular treatment of ischemic stroke and (2) decompressive craniectomy to decrease ICP and decrease morbidity and mortality in patients with brain infarction.

Endovascular treatment of acute stroke consists of catheter angiography and clot retrieval, intraarterial clot lysis, and stent placement. Numerous recent clinical trials have demonstrated to clinical utility of aggressive early intervention in the treatment of acute stroke.[22,23]

When patients do not make it to care within the allotted time window, or when catheter intervention is unsuccessful in reestablishing perfusion, they often go on the brain infarction which is often followed by subsequent swelling. In older patients with brain atrophy, this is often well tolerated. In younger patients or those with full brains, this brain swelling can be life threatening. Many of these patients may be candidates for decompressive craniectomy, wherein a large portion of the bone over the affected side is removed and placed in the freezer or implanted in the abdominal fat. The dura is opened and the brain allowed to swell out, decreasing ICP. Once the swelling goes down, the bone flap can be replaced in a second procedure. Guidelines regarding the use and utility of decompressive craniectomy in the setting of fulminant brain swelling in the setting of infarction continue to evolve.[24]

CENTRAL NERVOUS SYSTEM TUMORS

Intracranial Tumors

Intracranial tumors can be classified as primary versus secondary, as pediatric versus adult, by cell of origin, or by location in the nervous system. Primary tumors arise from tissues in the nervous system, whereas secondary tumors originate from tissues outside the nervous system and metastasize secondarily to the brain. They may represent local extension of regional tumors, such as chordoma or scalp cancer, but usually reach the nervous system through the hematogenous route.

According to the Central Brain Tumor Registry of the United States (CBTRUS), the overall incidence of primary brain tumors was 23.03/100,000 between 2011 and 2015.[25] Of the 1.7 million cases of new cancers diagnosed in a given year, between 100,000 and 240,000 are expected to eventually metastasize to the brain.[26]

Clinical Presentation

The clinical manifestations of various brain tumors can be divided into those caused by focal compression and dysfunction caused by the tumor itself and those attributed to secondary consequences, namely, increased ICP, peritumoral edema, and hydrocephalus. Usually, symptoms are caused by a combination of these factors.

The clinical presentation does not differ much by tumor histology; rather, rate of growth and location of the tumor contribute to the clinical features. A meningioma peripherally located in a relatively silent area of the brain, with a slow rate of growth, may enlarge to a significant size in a neurologically intact patient because the brain can accommodate to a slowly growing lesion. On the other hand, a very small metastatic lesion in the sensorimotor strip can present early with seizures.

Headache occurs in 50% to 60% of primary brain tumors and in 35% to 50% of metastatic tumors. It is classically described as being worse in the morning, probably because of hypoventilation during sleep, with consequent elevation of the P_{CO_2} and cerebrovascular dilation. Seizures may be the first symptom of a brain tumor. Patients older than 20 years presenting with a new-onset seizure are aggressively investigated for a brain tumor.

Infratentorial lesions may be manifested with headache, nausea and vomiting, cerebellar signs and symptoms, vertigo, and cranial nerve deficits. Supratentorial lesions may be manifested with different symptoms, depending on the location. Frontal lobe lesions present with personality changes, dementia, hemiparesis, or dysphasia. Temporal lobe lesions may be manifested with memory changes, auditory or olfactory hallucinations, or contralateral quadrantanopia. Patients with parietal lobe lesions may develop contralateral motor or sensory impairment, apraxia, and homonymous hemianopia, whereas those with occipital lobe lesions may show contralateral visual field deficits and alexia.

Imaging Studies

The initial workup generally involves a CT scan of the brain. CT provides a rapid means of evaluating changes in brain density, calcifications, acute hemorrhage (<48 hours old), and skull lesions. MRI of the brain is the modality of choice for diagnosis, presurgical planning, and posttherapeutic monitoring of brain tumors. Gadolinium contrast enhancement with MRI is more sensitive in demonstrating defects in the blood-brain barrier and localizing small metastases (up to 5 mm). Advances in MRI techniques have evolved from strictly morphology-based imaging to a modality that encompasses function, physiology, and anatomy. Diffusion-weighted imaging can help distinguish between gliomas and abscesses, and perfusion-weighted imaging can predict response to radiotherapy in low-grade gliomas. Functional MRI can be used in planning of surgery for tumors in eloquent areas of the brain to enable radical resection with less morbidity. Diffusion tensor imaging can demonstrate the effect of a tumor on white matter tracts. Magnetic resonance angiography is used more routinely as a noninvasive modality to evaluate the vascularity of a tumor or anatomic relationship of a tumor to normal cerebral vasculature.

Surgery

Dexamethasone is recommended for the management of edema associated with tumors, given its propensity to reduce peritumoral edema by stabilizing the cell membrane. An antiepileptic drug is also recommended for patients presenting with seizures or in those with tumors close to the sensorimotor strip.

Technical advances have made tumor surgery safer and more effective. The intraoperative microscope provides superior illumination and magnification, thereby allowing the surgeon to resect tumors from critical areas through small cranial openings. The cavitational ultrasonic surgical aspirator simultaneously breaks up and sucks away firm tumors while protecting vital neural and vascular structures. Intraoperative ultrasonography provides real-time imaging of tumors and cysts in subcortical and deep areas of the brain. Intraoperative CT or MRI is standard practice in some centers, enabling on-table imaging of the extent of resection (Fig. 68.11A). CT and MRI also allow real-time visualization of a biopsy needle within a target. Image-guided (CT or MRI) frameless surgical navigation allows instant and accurate localization of the tip of a probe during a craniotomy by displaying that point on a preoperative CT or MRI scan (Fig. 68.11B).

The primary goals of operation include histologic diagnosis and reduction of mass effect by removal of as much tumor as is safely possible to preserve neurologic function. The decision between a needle biopsy and more radical surgical resection depends on the location and size of the tumor, its sensitivity to radiation or chemotherapy, the preoperative Karnofsky performance score of the patient, and the systemic status of the primary cancer in case of metastatic brain lesions.

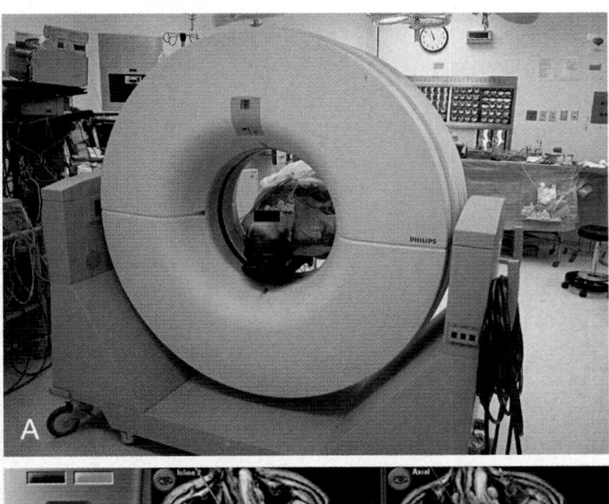

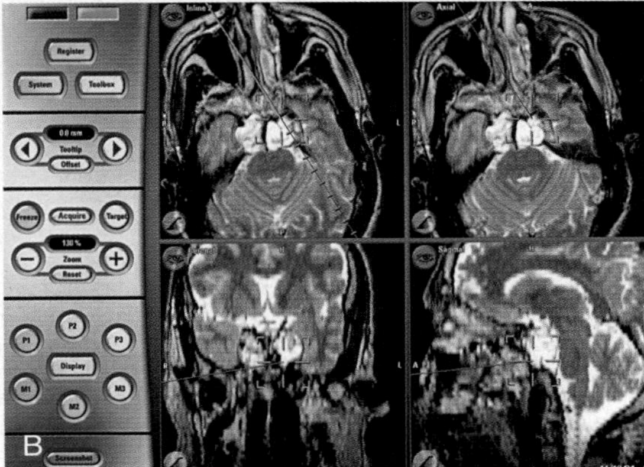

FIG. 68.11 Technologic advances in the operating room. (A) Intraoperative computed tomography scanner. (B) Computer-guided surgical navigation showing real-time location of a surgical probe tip on the preoperative magnetic resonance imaging study during resection of clival chordoma.

PRIMARY BRAIN TUMORS

Primary tumors of the brain are divided into intraaxial (those arising from within the brain parenchyma) and extraaxial (those arising from outside the brain parenchyma).

Intraaxial Brain Tumors

Most primary intraaxial brain tumors develop from the glial cells, or supportive structures, of the neurons and are collectively called gliomas. Total surgical resection of gliomas is extremely rare because of their ability to infiltrate widely along the white matter tracts and to cross the corpus callosum into the contralateral hemisphere. Radiation therapy and chemotherapy options vary according to the histology of the brain tumor. Biologic therapies and the molecular biology of gliomas are an area under intensive laboratory and clinical research.[27] An ideal therapy will target rapidly, growing malignant glioma cells along with infiltrating tumor cells with minimal toxicity to normal cells. This requires that the therapeutic vehicle of choice have access to all cells in the brain and be able to distinguish invasive or quiescent tumor cells from normal cells.

The current histopathologic classification of brain tumors was recently updated by the World Health Organization (WHO).[28] WHO classifies intraaxial brain tumors by cell type and grades them on a scale of I to IV based on light microscopy characteristics that include the degree of cellularity, pleomorphism, mitotic figures, endothelial proliferation, and necrosis. The higher the grade, the more aggressive and malignant the tumor.

An exhaustive review of neurooncology is beyond the scope of this chapter. What follows is an overview of the most commonly encountered and unique tumors of the central and peripheral nervous systems.

Astrocytic Tumors

Glioblastoma multiforme. A WHO grade IV tumor, this is the most commonly encountered primary brain tumor in adults. Presentation can include headache, seizures, focal deficits, and personality changes. Imaging usually demonstrates a ring-enhancing lesion with surrounding edema and mass effect (Fig. 68.12). Treatment of accessible lesions involves attempted gross total resection and postoperative radiation therapy and chemotherapy. Temozolomide is the current drug of choice and has been shown to

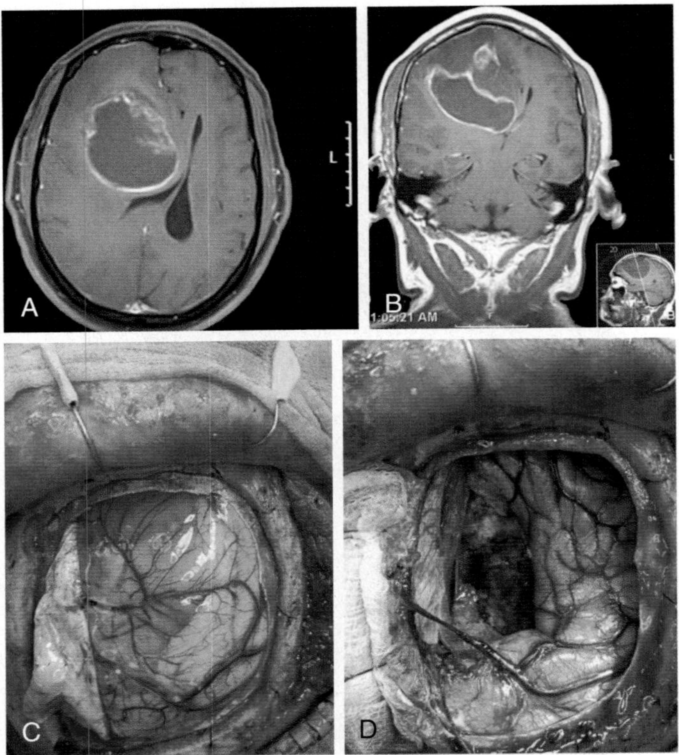

FIG. 68.12 MRI and intraoperative pictures of a patient with a glioblastoma multiforme. Gadolinium-enhanced axial (A) and coronal (B) MRI scans show a large tumor with ring enhancement causing a 1-cm subfalcine shift of midline structures. Intraoperative pictures show the yellowish tumor surrounded by normal brain gyri (C) and the surgical field after resection of the tumor (D). *MRI*, Magnetic resonance imaging.

improve both survival and quality of life. Recurrence is common, and repeated surgical resection is often deemed reasonable.

Anaplastic astrocytoma. A WHO grade III tumor, this presents much the same as glioblastoma multiforme, with similar treatment but slightly better long-term prognosis (Fig. 68.13).

Pilocytic astrocytoma. Pilocytic astrocytomas are typically classified as WHO grade I gliomas. When arising in the posterior fossa, they can cause obstructive hydrocephalus and cerebellar signs on examination. Surgical resection is the treatment of choice for these posterior fossa lesions. However, for lesions in the hypothalamus or optic tract, biopsy and chemotherapy or radiation therapy should be considered.

Oligodendroglioma

These tumors originate from oligodendroglial cells and represent 25% of all glial tumors; they occur with a male to female predominance of 3:2, observed at an average age of 40 years. They often present clinically with seizures or hemorrhage and nonspecific mass effect. A 5-year survival rate can be observed between 40% and 70%, depending on the grade, with an overall median survival of 3 years. Another form known as oligoastrocytoma behaves like oligodendroglioma, and both have aggressive anaplastic forms.

Treatment consists of surgical resection followed by chemotherapy. A particularly favorable response rate is associated with tumors that show allelic losses of chromosomes 1p and 19q.[29] Radiation therapy is considered for tumors with anaplastic transformation.

Ependymoma

These tumors constitute around 5% of all intracranial gliomas across all ages. In the pediatric population, they may constitute

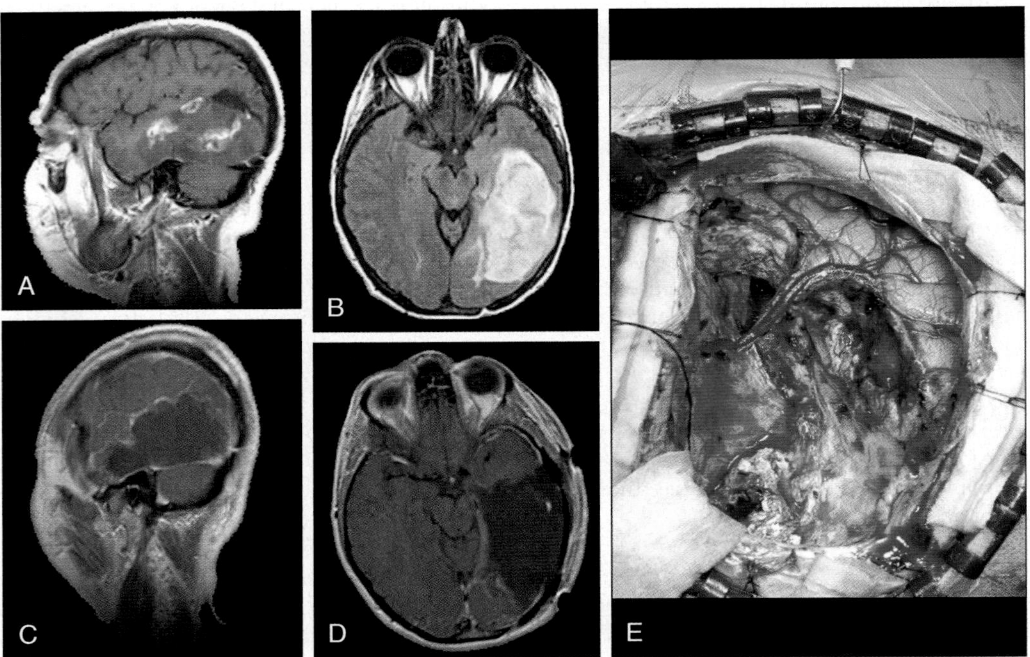

FIG. 68.13 Radiographic and intraoperative images of a patient with a left temporal anaplastic astrocytoma. (A) A partially enhancing tumor is noted in the left temporal lobe on this gadolinium-enhanced sagittal magnetic resonance imaging (MRI) study. (B) Fluid-attenuated inversion recovery sequence axial MRI shows the extent of the tumor. The postoperative gadolinium-enhanced sagittal (C) and axial (D) MRI scans show near-total resection of the tumor. (E) Intraoperative illustration of the surgical field after resection of the tumor.

up to 70% of all intracranial gliomas; the peak age at presentation is between 10 and 15 years. In children, ependymomas will typically be found in the fourth ventricle floor. A variant known as subependymoma is a rare form that is generally found incidentally in older patients and rarely requires surgical excision.

An ependymoma typically is manifested as a slowly growing posterior fossa mass that may cause obstruction of CSF flow, leading to hydrocephalus and symptoms of increased ICP with nausea, vomiting, and intense headaches. Up to 80% of young patients will survive for five years. The anaplastic variant is much more aggressive and carries a poor prognosis. Treatment consists of maximal possible resection because extent does affect survival, followed by fractionated radiation. Recommendations for spinal MRI plus a lumbar puncture for cytology to rule out subarachnoid drop metastases are required for possible spinal radiation should these be positive.

Ependymomas of the spinal cord and cauda equina are also infrequently seen. Cauda equina lesions are of the myxopapillary variant.

Choroid Plexus Papilloma and Carcinoma

These intraventricular tumors represent 1% of all intracranial tumors, and up to 70% are seen in children 2 years of age or younger. The majority are benign papillomas. They typically are manifested with hydrocephalus. The 5-year survival rate is around 85% with benign lesions; however, only 40% of patients with choroid plexus carcinoma survive 5 years or more. The atypical papilloma variant has an intermediate prognosis.

Treatment entails total surgical excision and adjuvant chemotherapy in the case of benign lesions. Radiation therapy, in addition to gross total resection, should be used when carcinoma is observed.

Pediatric Brainstem Gliomas

These tumors represent around 10% to 20% of all pediatric brain tumors; the mean age at presentation is 7 years. Midbrain gliomas (tectal and tegmental) usually have better survival rates than pontine gliomas. Tectal gliomas typically are manifested with hydrocephalus but have up to an 80% 5-year progression-free survival rate. Focal tegmental mesencephalic tumors may be manifested with hemiparesis that slowly progresses. The diffuse pontine glioma will usually present with multiple cranial nerve palsies and ataxia with increased ICP and have a poor overall median survival of less than 1 year.

Treatment of tectal gliomas requires vigilant follow-up and frequently CSF diversion or shunting. Focal tegmental mesencephalic tumors might be surgically resected and require adjuvant chemotherapy and radiation therapy if they recur. In the case of diffuse pontine gliomas, treatment is with radiation with or without experimental chemotherapy or palliative care.

Neuronal and Mixed Neuronal-Glial Tumors

Ganglioglioma and Gangliocytoma

These represent less than 12% of all intracranial tumors; presentation is generally before the age of 30 years, with a peak at 11 years. They typically are manifested with seizures and are benign and slow growing. With treatment, the survival rate between 5 and 10 years is 80% to 90%. Treatment should include complete resection when possible, and radiation therapy should be considered for rare anaplastic ganglioglioma.

Central Neurocytoma

These tumors are rare and represent around 10% of all intraventricular tumors and are rarely found extraventricularly. Most cases, around 75%, are found between the ages of 20 and 40 years and present typically with hydrocephalus, increased ICP, and seizures. They are usually slow growing and benign and rarely hemorrhage; they have a survival rate of more than 80%. Treatment with complete resection usually cures, requiring only SRS or chemotherapy should a rare recurrence happen.

Dysembryoplastic Neuroepithelial Tumor

Typically, dysembryoplastic neuroepithelial tumors represent less than 1% of all primary brain tumors, affecting primarily children and young adults younger than 20 years. Patients also typically present with history of seizures, and these tumors are generally benign with very slow or even no growth. Treatment consists of surgical resection of tumor and possible neighboring epileptogenic foci.

Paraganglioma

This tumor is manifested as a slow-growing mass with systemic features of catecholamine release and carcinoid-like syndrome with cranial nerve palsies related to its location. These tumors are commonly slow growing and benign, with a 5-year survival rate of around 90%; they rarely bleed.

Depending on their location, paragangliomas can be named. When the paraganglioma is located at the carotid bifurcation, it is designated a carotid body tumor; at the superior vagal ganglion, glomus jugulare tumor; at the auricular branch of the vagus, glomus tympanicum; at the inferior vagal ganglion, glomus intravagale; and finally, in the adrenal medulla and sympathetic chain, pheochromocytoma. Treatment includes medical therapy to prevent blood pressure lability and arrhythmias with alpha and beta blockers. Surgical resection is preferred, and embolization before resection can sometimes reduce the intraoperative blood loss. When surgery is not possible, radiation therapy will be used.

Other neuronal and mixed neuronal-glial tumors include dysplastic cerebellar gangliocytoma (also known as Lhermitte-Duclos disease), desmoplastic infantile ganglioglioma, cerebellar liponeurocytoma, papillary glioneuronal tumor, and rosette-forming glioneuronal tumor of the fourth ventricle.

Pineal Region Tumors

Pineocytoma

These represent less than 1% of all primary brain tumors; they are observed mainly in children and young adults with a peak incidence between 10 and 20 years of age. As the tumors enlarge, they will typically present with hydrocephalus, increased ICP, and Parinaud syndrome (which is a supranuclear vertical gaze disturbance caused by compression of the tectal plate). Pineocytomas are usually stable and slow growing, with a 5-year survival rate of around 90%, and they rarely hemorrhage. When they are symptomatic or enlarging, the treatment is surgical. Stereotactic biopsy is considered by many to be high risk because of the surrounding venous vasculature.

Pineoblastoma

This tumor also represents less than 1% of all brain tumors. All pineocytomas, pineoblastomas, and those tumors that are intermediate of both (that have features of both) account for 15% of the pineal region tumors. Most are seen in children at a peak age of 3 years and predominantly in females with a ratio of 2:1. Like pineocytomas, pineoblastomas present with increased ICP, hydrocephalus, and Parinaud syndrome. Up to 50% will have CSF seeding, giving a median survival of 2 years from the time of diagnosis. Treatment should consist of surgical resection plus irradiation of the cranial vault and entire spinal axis. If the patient is older than 3 years, chemotherapy should also be considered.

Papillary Tumor of the Pineal Region

This is a rare tumor of children and young adults. It will typically be manifested with hydrocephalus and will behave like a grade II or grade III tumor according to the WHO classification. It can recur and require surgical resection followed by focal irradiation.

Primitive Neuroectodermal Tumors

Medulloblastomas are found to be 15% to 20% of all brain masses and up to one third of all posterior fossa tumors in the pediatric population. They are rarely seen in adults; most are diagnosed by the age of 5 years, with a male to female ratio of 3:1. They tend to have a rapid presentation with hydrocephalus, increased ICP, and cerebellar signs. These tumors tend to disseminate through the CSF and are often found to involve the spinal subarachnoid space in a sizable number of patients at the time of diagnosis. Treatment consists of attempted gross total resection followed by adjuvant chemotherapy and radiation therapy if the child is older than 3 years.

Tumors of Cranial and Spinal Nerves

Schwannoma

Schwannomas make up around 8% of all intracranial tumors. When located within the parenchymal region, they will clinically be manifested with seizures or focal deficit before the age of 30 years. Vestibular schwannomas will usually have sensorineural hearing loss with tinnitus and dizziness and typically present at an age older than 30 years. They are usually slow growing, with an average of 10% recurrence after total resection. When vestibular schwannomas are present bilaterally, the diagnosis of neurofibromatosis type 2 should be ruled out.

Treatment should entail audiology assessment to determine baseline status. Lesions less than 3 cm can be observed with clinical examinations, symptoms, radiographic evaluations, and audiology every 6 months. Some authors will recommend SRS for growing tumors less than 3 cm in diameter; 90% of tumor control is possible with rare facial palsy, and up to 50% to 90% hearing preservation is obtained. When surgical resection is performed on tumors less than 3 cm, this adds the benefit of tumor removal with 80% normal or near-normal facial nerve preservation and between 40% and 80% hearing preservation overall, depending on literature reviewed. When tumors are larger than 3 cm, surgical resection is always recommended, but it is usually accompanied with total loss of hearing and a greater risk of facial palsy.

Neurofibroma

Neurofibromas are rarely found intracranially and can be associated with neurofibromatosis type 1. When located in the head, they can be found as plexiform neurofibromas often in the orbit from cranial nerve V1, scalp, or parotid (cranial nerve VII). Along the spinal canal, they can develop into dumbbell-shaped masses as they exit the neuroforamina or on occasion into large peripheral nerve sheath tumors. They typically are manifested as a painless mass with slow growth that is histologically benign, but between 2% and 12% can degenerate into malignant peripheral nerve sheath tumor with a high recurrence rate. Treatment consists of surgical resection; however, most neurofibromas will encompass nerve fibers, and total resection results in nerve sacrifice as opposed to schwannoma resection, which usually can be achieved without nerve sacrifice.

TABLE 68.7 Simpson grading system for meningioma resection.

GRADE	EXTENT OF RESECTION	RECURRENCE RATE*
I	Complete including dural attachment and abnormal bone	10%
II	Complete with cauterization of dural attachment	15%
III	Complete without dural attachment	30%
IV	Incomplete resection	Up to 85%
V	Biopsy	100%

*Length of follow-up varies around 5 years; numbers may increase with longer follow-up.

Tumors of the Meninges

Meningiomas

Meningiomas are observed in between 15% and 20% of all primary intracranial tumors, second only to glioblastoma multiforme. The prevalence is in females (2:1), and it is rare in childhood unless it is associated with neurofibromatosis type 1. The presentation is usually incidental in up to 50% of cases; they are typically slow growing, and overall 5-year survival is greater than 90%.[30,31] Meningiomas can recur, depending on the resection obtained at surgery as described on the Simpson grading system for meningioma resection (Table 68.7) as well as the atypical histology. Overall, less than 1% will have malignant histology. Surgical resection is the treatment of choice if the patient is neurologically symptomatic. Many small, asymptomatic tumors can be observed.

Hemangioblastoma

Hemangioblastomas are observed in 1% to 2% of all primary intracranial tumors; between 25% and 40% are associated with von Hippel–Lindau syndrome. When they are associated with von Hippel–Lindau syndrome, hemangioblastomas typically occur in young adults with a slight male predominance. However, in general, hemangioblastomas make up around 10% of posterior fossa tumors; when they are not associated with von Hippel–Lindau syndrome; they have a sporadic peak at the age of 50 years. They tend to present with mass effect because of cyst expansion and typically are slow growing and histologically benign. They have an 85% 10-year survival postresection rate with a 15% recurrence.

Lymphomas and Hematopoietic Tumors

Primary Central Nervous System Lymphoma

The incidence of primary CNS lymphomas has increased to 10% of all primary intracranial tumors, and they are observed in 2% to 6% of patients with acquired immunodeficiency syndrome (AIDS). The mean age at presentation is 60 years in immunocompetent patients and 35 years in patients with acquired immunodeficiency with a slight male predominance. The presentation can be with symptoms from a mass effect and, depending on location, sometimes with neuropsychiatric changes. The median survival is 1 to 4 months without treatment, 1 to 4 years when the patient is treated, and 2 to 6 months in patients with AIDS. There is a dramatic but short-lived response to steroids. Treatment consists of stereotactic biopsy followed by radiation therapy and chemotherapy because of their chemosensitivity to methotrexate. Intrathecal methotrexate will usually be advised for young patients.

Plasmacytoma

Plasmacytoma will usually involve the skull when it is found intracranially. It will often mimic meningioma and is considered at high risk for development of multiple myeloma within 10 years of diagnosis. Treatment consists of ruling out systemic multiple myeloma with urinalysis for protein and serum protein electrophoresis. Complete surgical excision should be followed by radiation therapy.

Germ Cell Tumors

Germinomas compose 1% to 2% of all primary CNS tumors; 50% are found in the pineal region and have most frequently been described in the Japanese population. The peak age at presentation is around 10 years, with more than 90% being found in the population younger than 20 years. The male to female ratio is 10:1 for the pineal region, whereas suprasellar germinomas are more common in females.

When located in the pineal region, they can become large and are present with hydrocephalus and Parinaud syndrome. This consists of paralysis of upward gaze, convergence, and accommodation and is associated with lid retraction, creating the so-called setting sun sign.

When located in the suprasellar region, they may produce compression of the hypothalamus and cause hypothalamic-pituitary dysfunction with diabetes insipidus and visual decline from compression of the optic tracts. Tumor markers help confirm diagnosis and a favorable prognosis when low secretion of human chorionic gonadotropin is observed. There is a 5-year survival rate greater than 90%, and they are usually sensitive and responsive to radiation therapy and chemotherapy. The first line of treatment consists of biopsy, then radiation therapy plus chemotherapy and treatment of hydrocephalus with either placement of a ventricular peritoneal shunt or a third ventriculostomy.

Nongerminomatous germ cell tumor is found most frequently between the ages of 0 and 3 years. These tumors are generally associated with a worse prognosis than germinomas are, with a 5-year survival rate of less than 50%. Embryonal carcinoma (malignant germ cell tumor) represents less than 1% of all CNS tumors and affects prepubertal children but is rarely found in children younger than 4 years; it is associated with Klinefelter syndrome and is considered malignant and invasive. Yolk sac tumors are also known as endodermal sinus tumors; they are usually found in infants or adolescents and are aggressive and malignant. Choriocarcinomas, which are also malignant and highly hemorrhagic, are another variety. Teratomas can be subdivided into mature and immature. The mature variety can be curable when complete resection is obtained. However, in the subtypes, the treatment algorithms, which include attempted resection plus chemotherapy and radiation therapy versus primary chemotherapy plus radiation therapy, are unclear; none of these has shown any significant survival difference. Mixed germ cell tumor is also a variety of the nongerminomatous germ cell tumors.

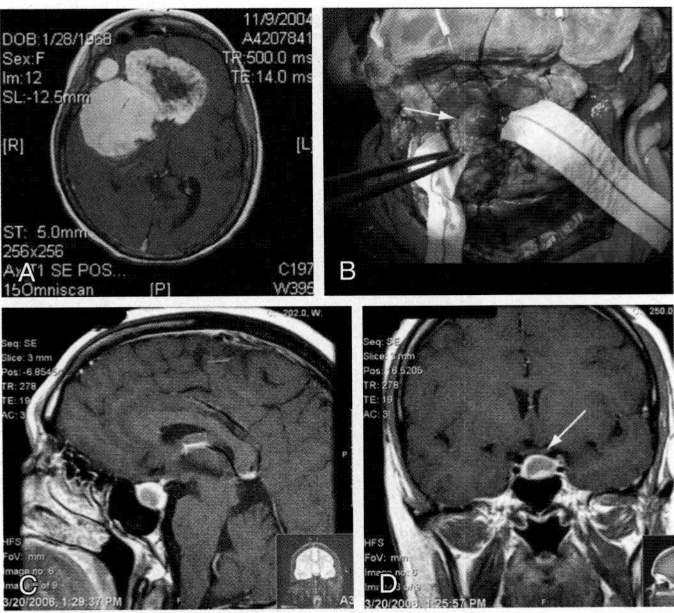

FIG. 68.14 (A) A large enhancing meningioma can be seen in this gadolinium-enhanced axial MRI study. (B) Intraoperative picture showing dissection of the meningioma *(arrow)* from the surrounding gyri. Gadolinium-enhanced sagittal (C) and coronal (D) MRI scans of a patient with a pituitary macroadenoma show impingement on the optic chiasm *(arrow)*. *MRI*, Magnetic resonance imaging.

Tumors of the Sellar Region

Pituitary adenomas (Fig. 68.14) make up 10% of all intracranial tumors, with an equal male to female incidence; the peak incidence is in the third and fourth decades. The tumors can be associated with multiple endocrine neoplasia syndromes. Around 50% present as macroadenomas that are larger than 1 cm in diameter. Symptoms develop from mass effect on the optic tract or hypothalamic-pituitary disturbance with endocrine abnormalities and rarely apoplexy. Typically, when it is a hormone-producing tumor, symptoms will appear at earlier stages in tumor growth than when nonfunctioning adenomas are found.

Treatment consists of endocrine laboratory workup and evaluation with ophthalmology and visual fields. Prolactin levels of 25 ng/mL or less are considered normal; if the prolactin level is between 25 and 150 ng/mL, it is generally considered "stalk effect," although levels above 100 ng/mL should be considered suspicious. However, when the level is higher than 150 ng/mL, it is considered diagnostic for prolactinoma. In the case of apoplexy presentation, rapid administration of corticosteroid and possible surgical decompression must be considered. Surgical options include a transsphenoidal approach with microscope or endoscope, open craniotomy, and combination of these two procedures, which would be the case in large extensive suprasellar lesions. Focal or stereotactic radiation is usually reserved for refractory cases. It is always important for an endocrinologic follow-up.

The classic presentation and associated treatment for pituitary adenomas are as follows.

Prolactinoma will be manifested with amenorrhea and galactorrhea in females and impotence in males. Infertility will be present in both. The treatment consists of dopamine agonist (e.g., bromocriptine) and generally provides complete control.

Adrenocorticotropin adenoma will be manifested as Cushing disease and classic hyperpigmentation of the skin and mucous

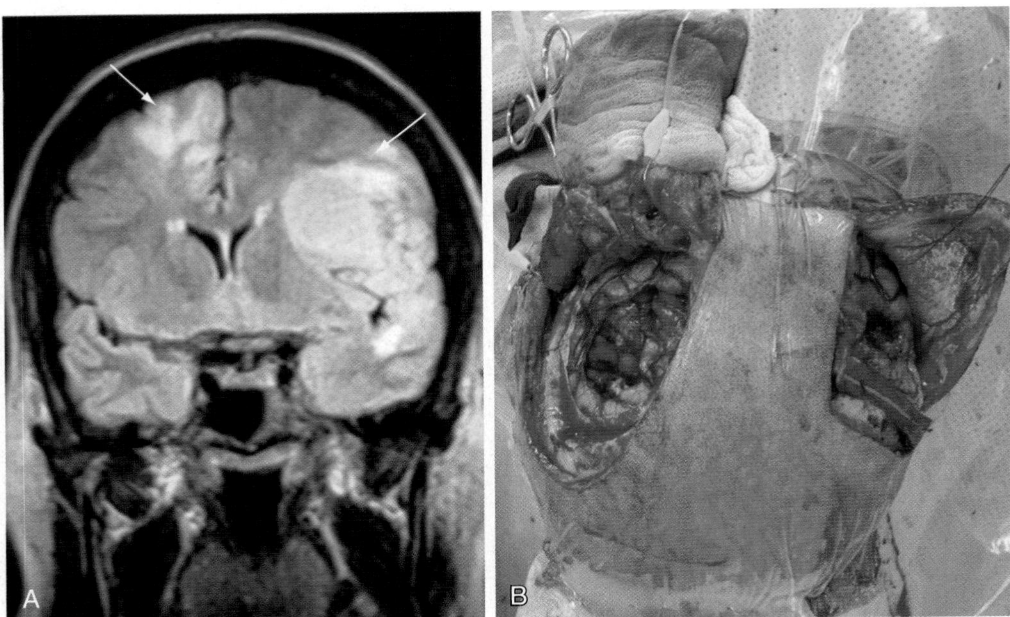

FIG. 68.15 (A) Fluid-attenuated inversion recovery sequence coronal MRI of a patient with two simultaneous metastatic tumors along the right and left frontal lobes *(arrows)*. (B) Simultaneous right and left frontal craniotomies for resection of both metastatic lesions. *MRI*, Magnetic resonance imaging.

membranes, ecchymoses, and purple striae, especially in the flanks, breast, and lower abdomen. Generalized muscle wasting with complaints of easy fatigability are among the other well-documented signs and symptoms. The first line of treatment is surgery.

Growth hormone secreting tumors will produce acromegaly in adults and gigantism in prepubertal children. Surgery is the first line of treatment. Some patients may respond to octreotide, and others may show improvement with dopamine agonist.

Thyroid-stimulating hormone secreting tumors may present as hyperthyroidism, anxiety, and palpitations (due to atrial fibrillation). Patients have heat intolerance, hyperhidrosis, and thyrotoxicosis, for which the treatment will require surgery.

For both gonadotropin-secreting and nonfunctional adenomas, clinical presentations will be due to mass effect and stalk compression. If the tumor extends to the suprasellar region and compresses the optic chiasm, this will cause bitemporal hemianopia and may also have cranial nerve deficits. Treatment for these last two is also surgical resection.

Craniopharyngiomas are tumors that represent between 2% and 5% of all intracranial tumors; 50% are in children, with a peak incidence between 5 and 10 years of age. Their clinical presentation is similar to that of suprasellar masses with compression of the surrounding structures. The tumor is histologically benign but may sometimes have local aggressive and relentless behavior. Craniopharyngiomas have a 5-year survival rate of 55% to 85%, but recurrences typically happen within 1 year from surgery. The most frequent postoperative complications include diabetes insipidus and hypothalamic injury with 5% to 10% mortality. Treatment requires medical optimization before surgical resection because if there is adrenal cortical insufficiency, hydrocortisone coverage will often be needed perioperatively. Attempts to obtain total gross resection should be sought if appropriate. It is when subtotal resection is encountered that possible postoperative radiation therapy might be beneficial, but it does add to the morbidity.

Central Nervous System Metastasis

Cerebral metastases are the most common brain tumor in adults and make up more than 50% of all brain tumors across all ages. However, they account for only 6% of all pediatric brain tumor cases. Approximately 6% to 14% of patients with cancer develop brain metastases during the course of their illness.[26] The highest incidence of brain metastasis is seen in the fifth to seventh decades of life, and it is equally common among men and women. Lung cancer is the most common source of brain metastasis in men, and breast carcinomas are the most common source of metastases in women. The interval or time period between the diagnosis of the primary cancer and the development of brain metastasis depends on the histology of the primary cancer; breast cancer and melanoma generally exhibit the longest interval (mean, 2–3 years) and lung cancer the shortest (mean, 4.5 months).[26]

Metastatic lesions tend to cause significant brain edema that initially will respond well to steroids. Typically, dexamethasone is used and will reduce the vasogenic edema. Anticonvulsants are used to reduce the likelihood of seizure but are generally given if the patient has had a seizure. When the lesion is initially encountered and no primary tumor is known, recommendations for stereotactic biopsy or excision should be given. However, if the disease is widespread, with a short life expectancy, and the patient has a poor preoperative status, consideration should be given to possible biopsy or radiotherapy and palliation. If, on the other hand, a solitary metastasis is encountered, total surgical excision should be attempted, followed by whole brain radiotherapy. SRS generally will be recommended if surgery is not feasible.[32] When multiple metastases are encountered, consideration should be given to excision of the symptomatic lesion or multiple lesions (Fig. 68.15), whole brain radiotherapy, hippocampal sparing whole brain radiotherapy, and/or SRS. Numerous clinical trials are investigating the efficacy of these treatment modalities, alone and in combination.

TRAUMATIC BRAIN INJURY

The goal of this section on traumatic brain injury is not to present a comprehensive review of the epidemiology, basic science research, and outcome studies on brain injury but to give a practical, common-sense approach to the management of injuries of the brain. There is bound to be overlap between this section and other parts of this text. Guidelines for the management of severe head injury were first published by the Brain Trauma Foundation in 1995 and last reviewed in 2016. These evidence-based guidelines have been a tremendous aid to the physician caring for brain-injured patients. The following discussion on the management of severe traumatic brain injury is based largely on these guidelines. As with all practice guidelines, they can and need to be modified, as dictated by the experience of the treating physician and in accordance with the needs of the patient. This report and the protocols laid out in the Advanced Trauma Life Support (ATLS) guidelines, published by the American College of Surgeons Committee on Trauma, are also invaluable resources for the student and physician.

Epidemiology

Depending on the source of information, it is estimated that there are between 500,000 to well above 1 million cases of head injury every year. Most of these are classified as mild injuries, with approximately 20% classified as moderate to severe. Approximately 50% of the 150,000 trauma deaths every year are caused by head injury. The social, medical, and economic implications are profound. Fortunately, prevention programs appear to be decreasing the incidence of severe traumatic brain injury.

Pathophysiology

Traumatic brain injury can be classified into primary and secondary injuries. Primary injury occurs at impact and is considered first. It includes bone fracture, intracranial hemorrhage, and diffuse axonal injury. Fractures of the cranial vault and skull base are indicative of the forces applied to the skull at the time of impact. Fractures of the skull base may be associated with cranial nerve deficit, arterial dissection, and CSF fistula formation. Fractures of the cranial vault are classified as follows:

Open or closed
Depressed or nondepressed
Linear or comminuted

Any fracture of the cranial vault can cause disruption of the underlying meningeal arteries or dural venous sinuses, which can lead to intracranial bleeding. Intracranial hemorrhage can be classified as epidural, subdural, subarachnoid, and intraparenchymal or intracerebral. Epidural hemorrhage occurs between the dura and skull and is usually the result of a skull fracture causing the laceration of a meningeal artery.

Rarely, a fracture crossing a dural venous sinus can cause a venous epidural hematoma, especially in children. Subdural hemorrhage occurs in the potential space between the dura and arachnoid. This is often the result of shearing of the bridging veins between the brain and the dural venous sinuses. Sometimes, it comes from injury to cortical vessels, which then bleed into the subdural space. Subarachnoid hemorrhage from trauma consists of bleeding into the spinal fluid spaces surrounding the blood vessels feeding the cerebral cortex. Trauma is the most common cause of subarachnoid hemorrhage. Rupture of an intracranial aneurysm is the second most common cause of subarachnoid hemorrhage and is generally distinguished from traumatic subarachnoid hemorrhage by history and the distribution of blood on a CT scan. Intraparenchymal or intracerebral hemorrhage is bleeding into the brain itself. This can run the spectrum from small contusions (bruises of the brain) to large intracerebral clots (which usually are the result of coup and contrecoup injuries) that may require emergent surgical evacuation. Although often small and nonsurgical at first, these can blossom and become life-threatening during a period of hours to days. Diffuse axonal injury is a rotational acceleration-deceleration injury to the white matter pathways of the brain. This results in a functional or anatomic disruption of these pathways and is believed to be the cause of loss of consciousness in patients without mass lesions. Diffuse axonal injury can occur with or without other primary injuries, such as an epidural or subdural hematoma (Fig. 68.16).

Secondary injury to the brain occurs as a result of decreased oxygen delivery to the brain, which in turn sets off a cascade of events that causes even more damage than the initial injury. With severe traumatic brain injury, there can be an alteration in cerebral blood vessel autoregulation. Systemic hypotension in the presence of this altered autoregulation results in decreased CBF and decreased oxygen delivery. This ischemia is exacerbated even further by systemic hypoxemia; intracranial hypertension, which decreases CBF even further, and a cascade of events involving mediators of inflammation, excitotoxicity, calcium influx, and Na^+,K^+-ATPase dysfunction lead to neuronal cell dysfunction and death. The prevention of secondary injury is therefore thought to lead to increased cell survival and improved outcome. This is achieved by preventing hypotension and hypoxia while taking measures to control ICP and to maintain CPP.

Prehospital and Emergency Department Management

The prehospital and emergency department management of the traumatized patient is reviewed elsewhere in this and other texts. Here we deal more specifically with issues critical to the patient with severe brain injury. The ABCs must always be addressed first, regardless of the severity of the patient's injury. Attention is first paid to securing a patent airway, establishing adequate ventilation and oxygenation, and maintaining adequate circulation. By doing this, one may avoid hypotension and hypoxia and, in so doing, avoid or minimize secondary brain injury. In patients with severe traumatic brain injury, a systolic blood pressure less than 90 mm Hg or a PaO_2 less than 60 mm Hg is a predictor of poor outcome. Appropriate spine precautions are observed in the initial resuscitation of the patient with a severe traumatic brain injury.

Once airway, breathing, and circulation have been addressed, neurologic evaluation may proceed. The Glasgow Coma Scale is a simple and reproducible method of neurologic assessment. It is also used to grade traumatic brain injury as mild, moderate, or severe. The Glasgow Coma Scale consists of three components—intensity of stimulus required to cause eye opening, verbal response, and motor response (Table 68.8). Pupillary size and reactivity are also essential components of the initial neurologic examination. Hypoxia, hypotension, alcohol, and drugs may all contribute to abnormal findings on the neurologic examination. In the absence of hypotension and hypoxia, an abnormal finding on examination is considered to be a primary brain injury until proven otherwise. Once all life-threatening injuries have been addressed and stabilized, the patient with a suspected traumatic brain injury undergoes CT scanning. The CT scan is used to evaluate the presence or absence of fracture, epidural and subdural hematomas, intracerebral hematomas and contusions, shift of the midline structures, and appearance of the basal and perimesencephalic cisterns. In many centers with multislice scanners, routine scanning of the

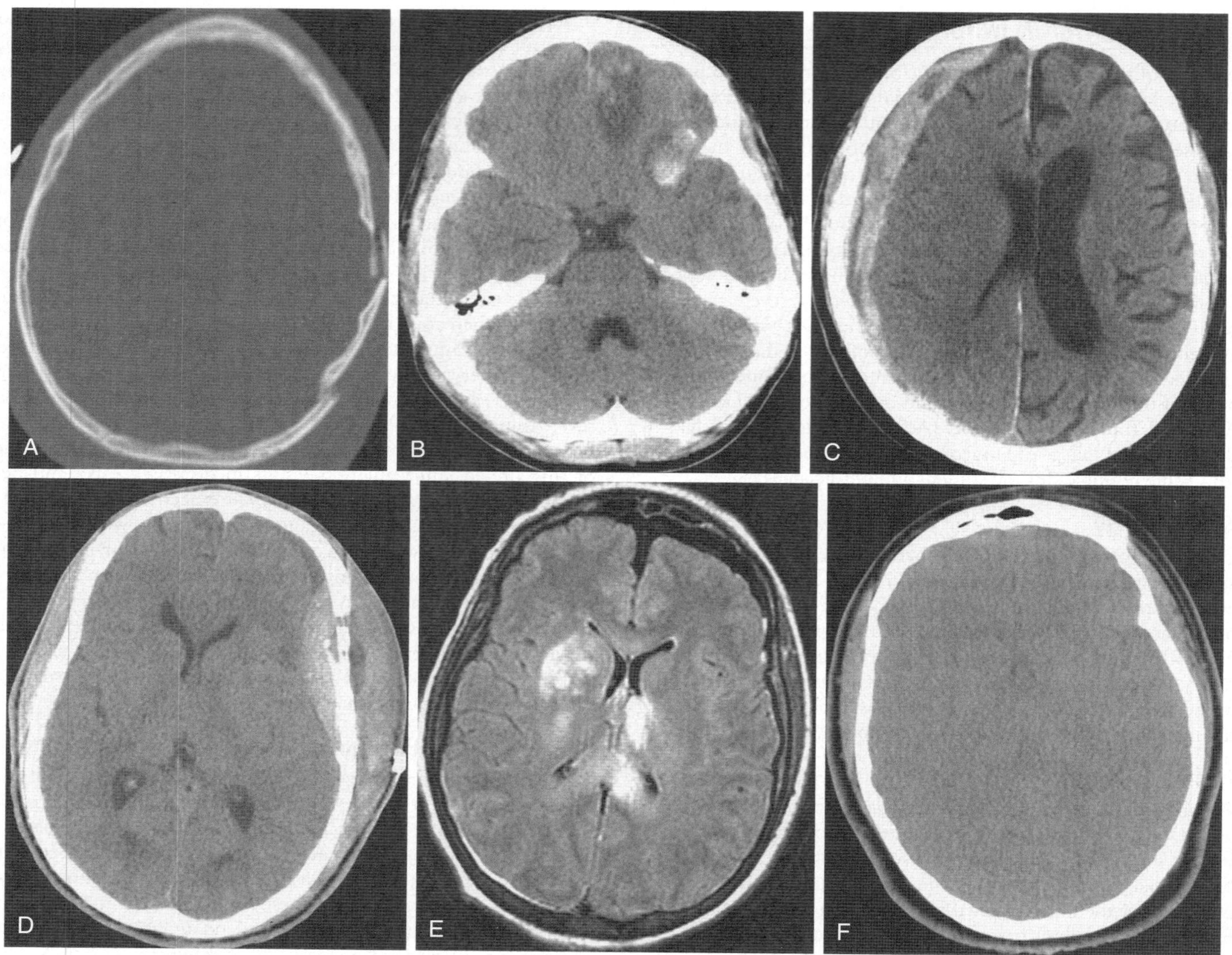

FIG. 68.16 Typical radiologic findings in traumatic brain injury. (A) Skull fracture shown on computed tomography. (B) Intraparenchymal contusions. (C) Subdural hematoma. (D) Epidural hematoma. (E) Diffuse axonal injury. (F) Intracranial hypertension. Note the effacement of sulci and gray-white matter differentiation.

TABLE 68.8 Neurologic assessment using the Glasgow Coma Scale.

EYE-OPENING RESPONSE		VERBAL RESPONSE		MOTOR RESPONSE	
SCORE	RESPONSE	SCORE	RESPONSE	SCORE	RESPONSE
4	Spontaneous	5	Oriented	6	Obeys commands
3	To speech	4	Confused	5	Localizes to painful stimulus
2	To pain	3	Inappropriate responses	4	Withdraws to painful stimulus
1	No response	2	Incomprehensible responses	3	Flexion to painful stimulus
		1	No response	2	Extension to painful stimulus
				1	No response

cervical spine is also performed to rule out acute fractures or traumatic dislocations. If life-threatening injuries elsewhere necessitate immediate transport of the patient to the operating room and the patient has a suspected intracranial hematoma (e.g., unilateral fixed and dilated pupil on one side with a contralateral hemiparesis), exploratory burr holes may be performed in the operating room concurrently with the laparotomy or thoracotomy.

Not infrequently, trauma patients with brain injury will require transfer to a hospital equipped to provide those patients with a higher level of care. In preparing these patients for transfer, the physician needs to follow ATLS guidelines and secure the airway, ensure adequate ventilation, and maintain circulation. Anemia is treated with transfusion, as necessary. Hypoxia and hypotension need to be avoided. Adequate immobilization with a backboard and cervical collar is mandatory. In patients with obvious intracranial hypertension or mass lesions, treatment with mannitol may be considered after neurosurgical consultation. Vigilance and attention to detail as well as communication between the transferring and accepting physicians are key to the successful transfer and treatment of these patients.

Treatment

When the workup of a patient reveals an intracranial mass lesion and deficits are thought to be related to that lesion, operative intervention is indicated. In general, any clot or contusion more than 30 mL is thought to be operable. Epidural and subdural hematomas (Fig. 68.16) are addressed with similar approaches, with the craniotomy centered on the clot. Intracerebral hematomas are addressed through appropriately located craniotomies. ICP monitors are often placed at operation. These can be intraventricular drains, intraparenchymal monitors, or devices placed in the epidural or subdural spaces. The decision about when to place an ICP monitor depends on the patient's preoperative examination findings, appearance of the brain at operation, and potential risk for deterioration. In general, all patients with a Glasgow Coma Scale score of 8 or less have ICP monitors placed. Some patients with moderate traumatic brain injury may also benefit from ICP monitoring. Postoperatively, the patient is managed similarly to those with nonoperative traumatic brain injury.

The following is a simplified algorithm for the management of intracranial hypertension in the intensive care setting. The head of the bed is elevated to 30 degrees, with the head placed in a neutral position. Care is taken to ensure that any cervical spine immobilization device is not obstructing jugular venous flow because this can increase ICP. The goal of treatment is to try to keep the ICP below 22 mm Hg and to maintain CPP at or above 60 mm Hg to 70 mm Hg (remember that CPP = MAP − ICP). If the ICP is persistently elevated above 22 mm Hg, it is treated. CSF drainage is now the first line of therapy in decreasing ICP. This is accomplished by an external ventricular drain, or ventriculostomy, which is a drain placed in the operating room or at bedside in the intensive care unit in an appropriately monitored patient. If ICP remains persistently elevated despite CSF drainage, the patient can be sedated and even paralyzed pharmacologically to keep the ICP down. The physician is dependent on the pupillary examination and ICP reading in this situation. If the ICP changes rapidly or the pupillary examination findings change (i.e., blown pupil), emergent CT of the head is indicated. Sedation and paralysis can occasionally be discontinued to allow an adequate neurologic evaluation in this situation.

If the ICP remains persistently elevated despite these interventions, mannitol and other diuretic agents may be used. Mannitol is administered as an intravenous bolus of 0.25 to 1 g/kg every 4 to 6 hours. Serum osmolality is followed closely when mannitol is being given. It is also important to maintain euvolemia in these patients. If ICP is still elevated, hyperventilation to a $Paco_2$ of 30 to 35 mm Hg may be used judiciously. At this point, second-tier therapeutic interventions (e.g., hypertonic saline, high-dose barbiturate therapy, decompressive craniectomy) may be considered.[33,34] Serial CT scans are critical throughout this treatment algorithm, and their use is tailored to the individual patient.

Several comments regarding nutrition, steroids, anticonvulsants, and $Paco_2$ are appropriate here. Energy requirements after traumatic brain injury are increased. The nonparalyzed patient requires replacement of 140% of his or her resting metabolism expenditure, and the paralyzed patient requires 100%. Of this, 15% is protein. Feeding begins at least five days and at most seven days postinjury. Steroids have no proven benefit in the management of traumatic brain injury and are not used. Prophylactic use of anticonvulsant drugs (e.g., phenytoin, carbamazepine, phenobarbital) is not indicated for the prevention of late posttraumatic seizures. Anticonvulsants may, however, be used to prevent early posttraumatic seizures, primarily in patients at high risk for early seizures who may suffer adverse effects if they were to seize early in their hospital course. These can usually be tapered after one week of therapy. Hyperventilation causes a decrease in ICP by lowering $Paco_2$, which causes vasoconstriction and decreases intracranial blood volume. Unfortunately, it also causes decreased CBF. If hyperventilation to a $Paco_2$ of less than 30 mm Hg is required for the maintenance of an acceptable ICP and CPP, monitoring of CBF is strongly recommended by some. Jugular venous oxygen saturation and cerebral oxygen extraction may also be useful in this clinical scenario. Table 68.9 presents a summary of the recommendations of the 2016 guidelines provided by the Brain Trauma Foundation.

TABLE 68.9 Brain Trauma Foundation recommendations for traumatic brain injury.

PARAMETER	GUIDELINE
Hyperosmolar therapy	Mannitol effective for control of raised ICP (0.25–1 g/kg)
Prophylactic hypothermia	Early (within 2.5 h), short term (48 h postinjury) hypothermia not recommended to improve outcomes in patients with diffuse injury
Infection prophylaxis	Routine external ventricular catheter exchange not recommended; oral care is not recommended to reduce ventilator-associated pneumonia; antimicrobial ventricular EVD catheters decrease infection
ICP monitoring	Indicated if GCS score = 3–8 on admission and abnormal CT. In severe traumatic brain injury and normal CT, indicated with two or more of the following: age >40 years, unilateral posturing, hypotension with SBP <90 mm Hg
CPP threshold	CPP <50 mm Hg should be avoided; aggressive interventions to maintain it above 70 mm Hg have a considerable risk of acute respiratory distress syndrome
Brain oxygen monitoring and thresholds	Jugular venous saturation (50%) or above
Blood pressure and oxygenation	Maintain SBP >100 mm Hg in patients 50-69 years of age, >110 mm Hg in patients 15-49 and > 70 years of age; hypoxia (saturation <90% or Po_2 <60 mm Hg) should be avoided
Nutrition	Should be initiated within at least by day 5 and at most day 7 postinjury
Sedatives	High-dose barbiturates recommended to control refractory ICP in the hemodynamically stable patient; propofol recommended for ICP control but does not improve mortality
Seizure prophylaxis	Decreases early post traumatic seizures (<7 days after injury); insufficient evidence to recommend levetiracetam over phenytoin.
Hyperventilation	Recommended as temporizing measure; Pco_2 below 25 mm Hg not recommended; avoid in first 24 hours after injury
Steroids	Not recommended, contraindicated

CPP, Cerebral perfusion pressure; *CT*, computed tomography; *EVD*, external ventricular drain; *GCS*, Glasgow Coma Scale; *ICP*, intracranial pressure; *SBP*, systolic blood pressure.

DEGENERATIVE DISORDERS OF THE SPINE

Degenerative Disease of the Lumbar Spine

According to the National Institute of Neurological Disorders and Stroke, 80% of adults complain of low back pain at some point in their lives, with an estimated cumulative national cost of about $50 billion per year. Low back pain is the most common cause of job-related disability and a leading contributor to missed days at work. Back pain is the second most common neurologic ailment in the United States—only headache is more common.

A good understanding of the normal anatomy of the spine is of utmost importance for the appreciation of spinal disorders. The lumbar spine consists of five lumbar vertebrae with five intervening intervertebral discs. Each vertebra is made up of an anterior vertebral body and a posterior neural arch. Each neural arch is, in turn, composed of pedicles, facet joints, transverse processes, laminae, and a spinous process. The disc consists of three components:

1. Cartilaginous endplates for the purpose of nutrition and anchoring.
2. Annulus fibrosis made of concentric sheets of collagen which serves to contain the pressurized nucleus.
3. Nucleus pulposus made of a soft, semigelatinous collagen that can absorb axial compressive loads.

The spinal cord ends at the L1 level, beyond which lumbar and sacral nerve roots, collectively called the *cauda equina,* continue distally and exit at their corresponding neural foramen. At each segmental level, a nerve root containing both motor and sensory components crosses the disc space, travels a short distance within the lateral recess of the spinal canal, and passes underneath the pedicle on its way to exit the spine through the intervertebral foramen.

The nucleus loses its ability to bear compressive loads as we age. The load transfer, then, shifts to the annulus, a structure that is poorly suited to withstand compression, thereby causing fatigue failure, fissuring, and possibly rupture. A herniation of a fragment of the nucleus pulposus may follow. As the mechanical integrity of the nucleus further deteriorates, the load transfer is concentrated at the periphery of the vertebral endplates, leading to osteophyte formation, a process called *spondylosis.* Subsequently, as the degenerating disk becomes less able to resist rotation and shear, additional stresses are transferred to the posterior elements with resultant facet arthrosis and hypertrophy, and thickening and buckling of the ligamentum flavum.

Lumbar Radiculopathy

Disc herniations can occur in any direction but most commonly follow a posterolateral direction at the site where the posterior longitudinal ligament is thinnest. Disk material extruded in this location can compress a nerve root, leading to low back pain and radicular symptoms in a specific dermatomal distribution (Table 68.10). The back pain is usually a minor component. Large, more central disk herniations may compress the cauda equina with resultant cauda equina syndrome, consisting of saddle anesthesia, urinary retention with possible overflow incontinence, and significant motor weakness. In this case, it is advisable to decompress the thecal sac within 24 hours of onset of symptoms.

An initial period of nonsurgical management for at least 4 to 8 weeks is indicated unless the patient presents with cauda equina syndrome, progressive neurologic deficit, recurrent episodes of incapacitating pain, or profound motor weakness. Conservative therapy includes rest, activity modification, physical therapy, weight loss, analgesics, muscle relaxants, oral steroids, and epidural steroid injections. If conservative measures fail to control the pain, imaging of the spine is indicated. MRI is the diagnostic test of choice (Fig. 68.17A and 68.17B); a postmyelography CT may be indicated in patients who have implanted devices which are not MRI compatible (pacemakers).

The standard surgical treatment of a lumbar disc herniation involves a midline approach centered over the affected interspace followed by a hemilaminectomy to expose the thecal sac and nerve root. The herniated fragment is usually located medial to the root along its shoulder. Removal of the herniated or extruded fragment is sufficient to relieve the symptoms. A minimally invasive procedure through a 1-cm paramedian incision with a muscle-splitting technique can also be used under either microscopic or endoscopic visualization with less postoperative morbidity. Most patients experience good results immediately after surgery. A recurrent herniated disc at the same level may occur in 3% to 19% of patients, with the higher rates usually in series with long-term follow-up.

Lumbar Spinal Stenosis

Advanced degeneration of the lumbar spine may result in spondylosis with arthrosis and hypertrophy of the facet joint as well as thickening and buckling of the ligamentum flavum. These changes lead to narrowing of the spinal canal with resultant constriction of the thecal sac and development of neurologic deficits. Patients classically present with neurogenic claudication: unilateral or bilateral dermatomal discomfort precipitated by standing or walking or prolonged maintenance of the same posture, and characteristically relieved by a change in posture like sitting, squatting, or recumbency. This discomfort may be in the form of pain, weakness, or paresthesias. Neurogenic claudication is thought to arise from ischemic changes of roots as a result of increased metabolic demands from exercise in the presence of a vascular compromise of the root from the surrounding constriction. The clinical history is important if spinal stenosis is suspected because most of these patients have nonspecific neurologic findings like absent or reduced reflexes. Again, MRI is the diagnostic test of choice for lumbar stenosis and typically shows an hourglass appearance on T2-weighted sagittal sequence. Nonsteroidal antiinflammatory drugs, analgesics, epidural steroid injections, and physical therapy are the

TABLE 68.10 Clinical findings in common lumbar disc herniations.

DISC	INCIDENCE (%)	ROOT	PAIN DISTRIBUTION	MUSCLE INVOLVED	SENSORY DEFICITS	REFLEX LOSS
L3–4	3–10	L4	Anterior thigh	Quadriceps femoris	Medial malleolus and medial foot	Knee jerk
L4–5	40–45	L5	Posterolateral thigh and leg	Tibialis anterior; extensor hallucis longus	Large toe web, dorsum of foot	None
L5–S1	45–50	S1	Posterolateral thigh and leg down to ankle	Gastrocnemius	Lateral malleolus, lateral foot	Ankle jerk

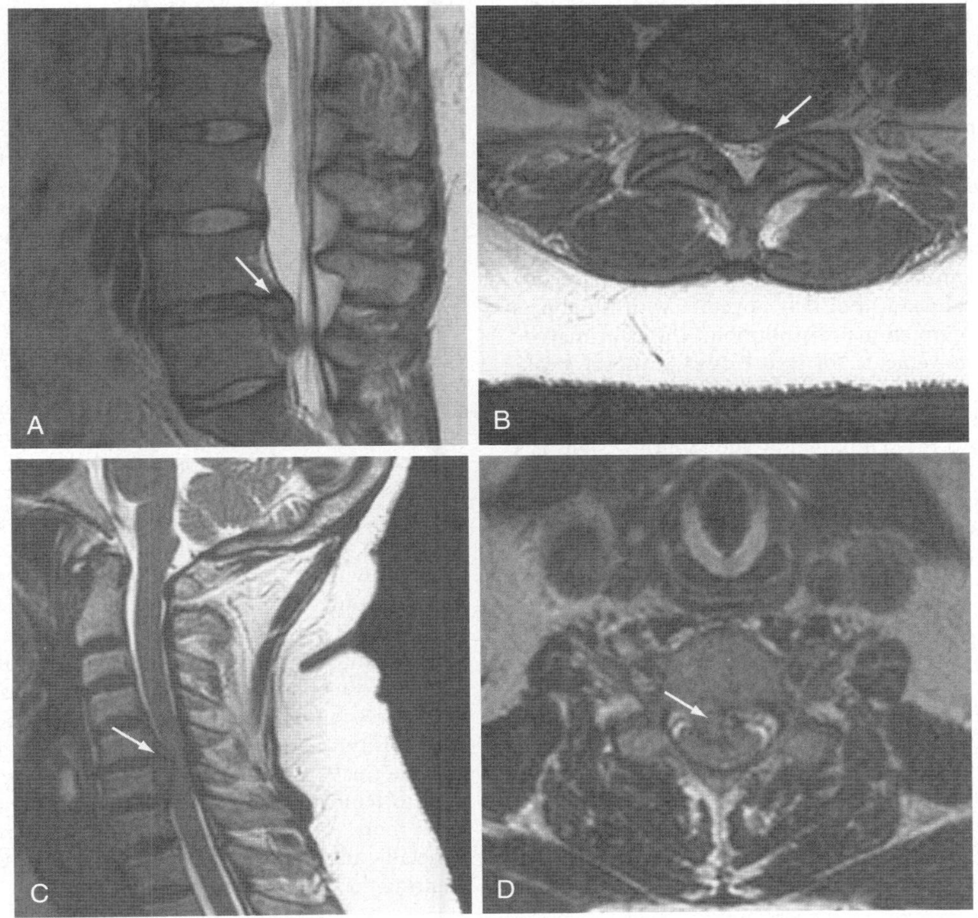

FIG. 68.17 (A) T2-weighted sagittal MRI study showing a herniated lumbar disc fragment *(arrow)* at the L4–5 level. (B) T2-weighted axial MRI showing the same fragment *(arrow)* compressing the thecal sac. (C) T2-weighted sagittal MRI of a patient with a large anterior disc prolapse at C5–6 level *(arrow)*. (D) Axial images showing the disc compressing the spinal cord *(arrow)*. *MRI*, Magnetic resonance imaging.

mainstays of nonsurgical management. Surgical decompression is warranted in patients with recurrent and disabling pain that limits their daily activity. Laminotomies or laminectomies of the involved levels with undercutting of the superior articular facet are required to decompress the nerves in the foramina. Wide, overly aggressive decompression of the spinal canal may result in lumbar instability.

Lumbar Instrumentation and Fusion

Fusion may be indicated in a subpopulation of patients with degenerative disease of the lumbar spine and is usually augmented with instrumentation. Spondylolisthesis (vertebral body subluxation) is the most common indication for fusion and instrumentation. Lumbar fusion can be a potential adjunct to disc excision in cases of a recurrent herniated disc in patients with evidence of preoperative lumbar spinal deformity or instability or in patients with chronic mechanical and discogenic back pain.[35,36] Lumbar fusion may also be recommended for carefully selected patients with disabling low back pain due to one- or two-level degenerative disease without stenosis or spondylolisthesis.

Lumbar fusion and instrumentation can be performed through a number of approaches:

1. Posterolateral fusion, whereby the transverse processes of the involved segments are decorticated and covered with a mixture of bone autograft or allograft.
2. Pedicle screw fixation, whereby screws are inserted into the pedicles of the involved segments and then attached to each other under compression with a rod (Fig 68.18), either alone or in conjunction with posterolateral fusion.
3. Posterior lumbar interbody fusion, whereby an intervertebral body spacer, either a bone allograft or a cage packed with bone, is inserted in the disk space through a laminotomy on each side of the midline, together with instrumentation, either alone or in conjunction with posterolateral fusion.
4. Transforaminal interbody fusion, whereby the facet joint and the isthmus on one side are removed and a single bone graft or cage is introduced into the disk space in an oblique fashion, together with unilateral or bilateral posterior spinal fusion.
5. Anterior lumbar interbody fusion, whereby the interbody space is fused using either a bone graft or a cage augmented by a metallic interbody plate through an anterior retroperitoneal approach.
6. Lateral approaches (extreme lateral interbody fusion, direct lateral interbody fusion, oblique lateral interbody fusion) with or without posterior instrumentation.[37]

Degenerative Diseases of the Cervical Spine

The pathophysiology of the degenerative changes of the cervical spine is essentially similar to that of the lumbar spine. An important distinction is that the spinal canal in the cervical spine contains the spinal cord rather than the cauda equina. Consequently, a reduction in the cross-sectional area of the canal from a herniated disc or bony osteophytes may lead to compression of the spinal cord with neurologic deficits. There are seven cervical vertebrae, but eight pairs of cervical nerves.

Cervical Radiculopathy

The most common scenario for patients with herniated cervical disc is that the symptoms were present upon awakening in the morning without identifiable trauma or stress. The pain usually radiates from the proximal arm distally, together with numbness and paresthesia in a dermatomal distribution. The pain may be intensified by neck movements. In severe cases, a motor weakness corresponding to the affected nerve root may be noticed. On examination, pain with downward pressure on the vertex while tilting the head toward the symptomatic side (Spurling sign) is a mechanical sign of disc herniation. Nerve root compression in the upper cervical spine is unusual. Compression of the C2 root causes occipital neuralgia, whereas compression of C3 and C4 may lead to nonspecific neck and shoulder pain. Compression of the other cervical roots leads to the manifestations noted in Table 68.11.

Cervical Myelopathy

Compression of the cervical cord, either acutely by a large herniated disc fragment or chronically by osteophytic bony spurs as a result of advanced spondylosis or stenosis, causes cervical myelopathy. Myelopathy is manifested by spasticity, increased deep tendon reflexes, clonus, and the Babinski and Hoffman signs. Patients may also complain of weakness and clumsiness in their hands. If left untreated, symptomatic spinal cord compression is thought to put patients at increased risk for spinal cord injury in the event of cervical spine trauma (central cord syndrome) (Figs. 68.17C and D and 68.19).

Diagnosis and Treatment

MRI is the study of choice for the initial evaluation of a herniated cervical disc. A CT myelogram is indicated for patients who cannot undergo MRI or when anatomic bony details are required. MRI is less accurate than CT myelogram for identifying foraminal fragments but is less invasive. Electromyography and nerve conduction studies can be useful when other causes need to be excluded, such as plexopathies or peripheral nerve entrapment.

More than 90% of patients with acute cervical radiculopathy as a result of disk herniation will improve with conservative management. Conservative management includes a combination of oral steroids, nonsteroidal antiinflammatory drugs, analgesics, muscle relaxants, intermittent cervical traction, and physical therapy. Surgery is indicated for those who fail to improve and those with progressive neurologic deficit while undergoing therapy.[38] The aim of the operation is to decompress the nerve root and/or spinal cord. This can be accomplished through an anterior or a posterior approach. Both procedures carry an excellent outcome in the range 90% to 96% improvement in preoperative symptoms.

With anterior pathology (paracentral herniation or large uncovertebral osteophyte), an anterior cervical discectomy, nerve root decompression, and fusion are indicated (Fig. 68.20). The approach is through the avascular plane between the carotid sheath and the tracheoesophageal complex. The operative microscope is used to remove the disc, decompress the thecal sac, and free the nerve roots. A bone graft is then put in the disc space. Commonly, a metallic plate is affixed between the two vertebral bodies, augmenting the fusion.

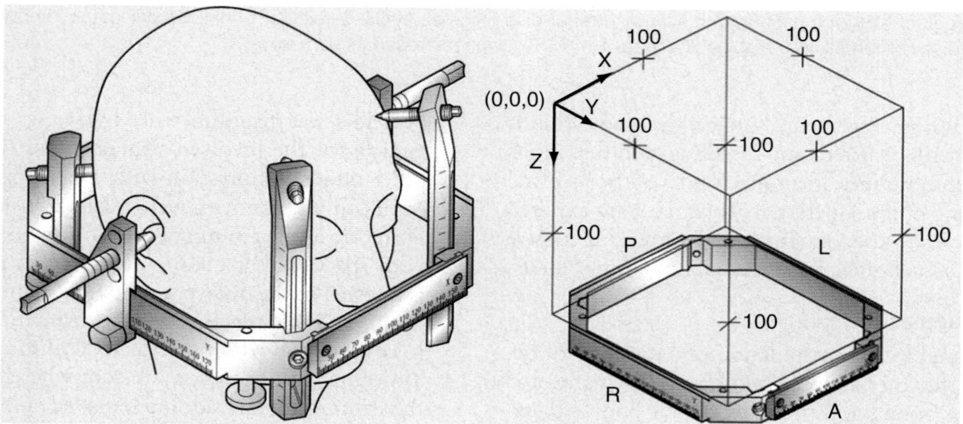

FIG. 68.18 The Leksell stereotactic coordinate frame is rigidly attached to the head by four threaded pins. The fiducial box is mounted on the frame during the imaging study (MRI or CT). The x, y, and z coordinates are determined directly from the imaging study. The center of the frame is arbitrarily given the coordinates 100, 100, 100. (Courtesy Elekta, Stockholm, Sweden.) *CT*, Computed tomography; *MRI*, magnetic resonance imaging.

TABLE 68.11 Clinical findings in common cervical disc herniations.

DISC	INCIDENCE (%)	ROOT	PAIN	MUSCLE INVOLVED	REFLEX LOSS
C4–5	2	C5	Shoulder	Deltoid	Deltoid
C5–6	19	C6	Upper arm, thumb, radial forearm	Biceps, extensor carpi radialis	Biceps, brachioradialis
C6–7	69	C7	Fingers 2 and 3, all fingertips	Triceps	Triceps
C7–T1	10	C8	Fingers 4 and 5	Hand intrinsics	Finger jerk

A posterior approach, also called *keyhole foraminotomy,* can be used in patients with unilateral radiculopathy with soft disk herniation or small lateral osteophyte. This intervention tends to work best in patients with radiculopathy and minimal neck pain.

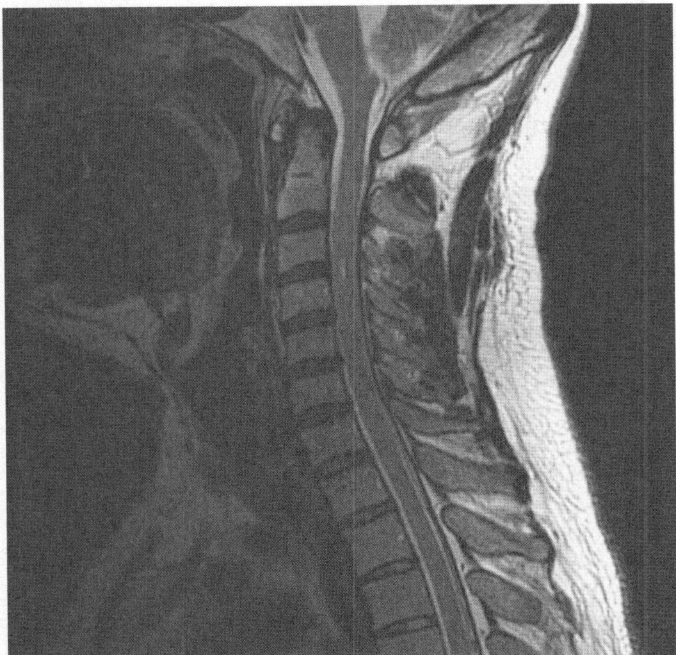

FIG. 68.19 T2-weighted sagittal MRI scan of a patient with significant cervical canal stenosis. Note the hyperintensity in the cervical spinal cord at the C3–4 level, suggesting myelomalacic changes. This may be indicative of permanent residual deficits. *MRI,* Magnetic resonance imaging.

With the aid of an operating microscope, a small foraminotomy is performed with a high-speed drill to unroof the nerve root. The disc fragment can be removed, if accessible.

Patients with cervical spondylosis and myelopathy present a difficult problem. The approach is tailored to the patient's specific pathology. Patients who suffer from multiple disks or osteophytes with myelopathy and those with significant cervical stenosis in addition to a superimposed disc herniation can benefit from posterior cervical laminectomy; this, in turn, may need to be reinforced by lateral mass instrumentation and fusion, depending on the degree of spinal instability. Patients with chronic spondylosis who manifest anterior as well as posterior compression may require complex surgery. In this case, the patients may undergo a staged surgical approach with an initial anterior exposure for multiple cervical discectomies or even cervical corpectomies with reconstruction with bone grafts or cages followed by an anterior cervical plate. Next, the patient would undergo posterior cervical laminectomies reinforced with lateral mass plating. The goal of the operation is to arrest the progression of the myelopathy.

FUNCTIONAL AND STEREOTACTIC NEUROSURGERY

Functional neurosurgery is concerned with the anatomic or physiologic alteration of the nervous system to achieve a desired effect. This can be done with focal electrical stimulation procedures, ablative procedures, or implantation of pumps to deliver drugs, usually to the CSF but possibly also to the parenchyma. The field of functional neurosurgery deals primarily with the treatment of pain, movement disorders, epilepsy, and some psychiatric disorders when they are refractory to conventional treatments. These disorders all have in common hyperfunction or deranged function of some part of the CNS. The physiology of each functional disorder is often complex and only partly understood. The focus of

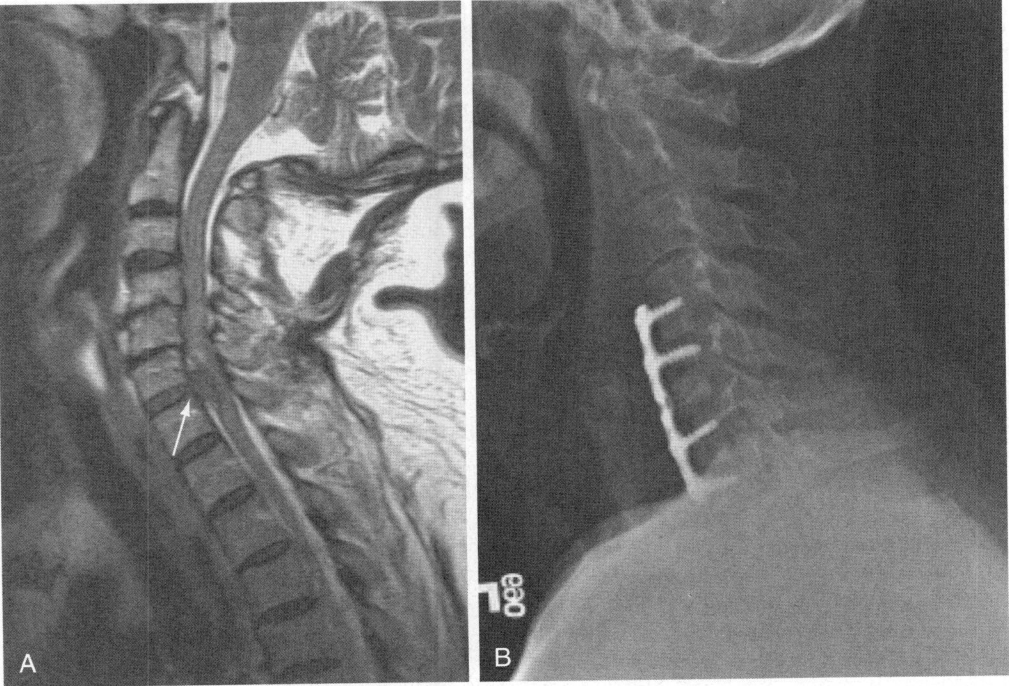

FIG. 68.20 (A) T2-weighted sagittal magnetic resonance imaging study of a patient with advanced cervical spondylosis and stenosis from C3–4 down to C6–7 with an acute herniated disc fragment at C6–7 *(arrow)* after cervical spine manipulation. (B) Postoperative lateral radiograph showing C4–5, C5–6, and C6–7 anterior cervical discectomy and fusion using a bone allograft and titanium plate and screws.

this section is on the operative intervention used in patients with epilepsy, pain, and functional disorders, and a discussion of SRS in general terms.

In general terms, functional neurosurgery is concerned with the focal delivery of medication, electrical stimulation, or destruction of neural tissue. Medication is delivered via catheter using a battery-operated pump and is discussed later in this section. Historically, lesions were created in different areas of the CNS using anatomic disruption of pathways using two different techniques, physical transection of white matter pathways (cordotomy) or lesioning using thermocouple probes (causing coagulation of the neural tissue). Today, stimulation of many of these same nuclei and pathways has been found to be equally effective in alleviation of symptoms and signs. The difference is that a lesion is permanent and static in size and location. The advantage of stimulation is that it can be turned on or off, increased or decreased, and, in the case of an implanted electrode array, changed in location, depending on which of the several contacts are activated. Thus, stimulation provides a reversible, scalable, and somewhat movable functional lesion.

Stereotactic Surgery

Stereotaxis, as applied to neurosurgery, is concerned with the localization of a target in three-dimensional space. The target deep in the brain is not seen directly at surgery. This can be a tumor, white matter pathway, cranial nerve, vascular malformation, or nucleus deep within the brain. The field has evolved using frame-based and frameless systems, but in each case, a calculated inference is used to reach the target accurately.

Frameless stereotactic techniques use advanced imaging techniques, fiducials, and reference markers in place of a fixed frame. Robotic arms, infrared reflectors, and light-emitting diodes provide the surgeon with real-time information about the anatomy at hand. This technology can also be fused with a display from the operating microscope, aiding in the operative dissection. It is useful for the planning of incisions and craniotomies and, when combined with intraoperative ultrasound, may be of use in determining the extent of tumor resection. Frameless stereotactic radiosurgical devices are commercially available.[39]

Frame-based systems use a rigid frame attached to the skull by pins that penetrate the outer table of the skull (Fig. 68.18). This can easily be done under local anesthesia, with the patient wide awake. The patient is then taken for CT or MRI with a localizer on the frame. Using Cartesian coordinates, the x, y, and z coordinates of the target can then be determined. In other words, the position of the target in relation to the frame is known. Using an arc system, which is mounted on the frame, the target can be accessed by different trajectories. When the target is a vascular lesion, arteriography can be performed with a localizing frame, and the position of the vascular lesion in three-dimensional space can be determined. Frame-based systems are used for brain biopsies, deep brain stimulation, ablative procedures, and SRS.

SRS involves the delivery of a concentrated dose of radiation to a defined volume in the brain. The dose of radiation delivered would be toxic if given in a broad field to the entire brain. When it is delivered in multiple collimated beams from numerous different angles or in arcs at different angles, the effect on the surrounding brain is minimized. Two methods of frame-based SRS are currently used widely. The gamma knife uses cobalt-201 radiation sources focused on one point. Once the target is localized in three dimensions, it is placed at this point, and different collimators are used to focus the radiation. Modified linear accelerators deliver the radiation dose in multiple arcs, thereby minimizing the effect on surrounding brain tissue. Both systems use multiple isocenters for the treatment of irregularly shaped lesions. SRS has been used in the treatment of almost every intracranial lesion but is commonly used in the treatment of metastatic tumors, benign lesions of the cranial nerves, AVMs, and trigeminal neuralgia. The primary risks of SRS are radiation necrosis and radiation injury to surrounding structures.

Brain Stimulation

Electrical stimulation of the nervous system is used in the treatment of movement disorders, pain, and epilepsy. Stimulation involves placement of an electrode, which is then connected to a subcutaneously placed generator. Here we discuss neurostimulation as it applies to the treatment of movement disorders, chronic pain states, and epilepsy.

Parkinson disease is the most common movement disorder for which patients have surgery. Stereotactic techniques developed in the 1950s were used to create lesions in the pallidum and thalamus. These ablative procedures fell by the wayside for a time with the introduction and widespread use of L-dopa (L-3,4-dihydroxyphenylalanine). In the early 1990s, there was a renewed interest in the use of surgical techniques for patients with Parkinson disease who had become unresponsive to pharmacologic agents or intolerant of their side effects. Lesions of the internal segment of the globus pallidus saw a tremendous resurgence. With improvements in imaging and intraoperative microelectrode recording, deep brain stimulation soon replaced ablative procedures in the surgical treatment of these patients. Stimulation induces a reversible inhibition of neuronal activity, which can be adjusted as the clinical situation demands. The subthalamic nucleus has replaced the globus pallidus as the target of choice. Subthalamic nucleus stimulation is most effective for the treatment of rigidity and akinesia. Tremor is best addressed with stimulation of the ventralis intermedius nucleus of the thalamus.

Spinal cord stimulation is used for the treatment of chronic pain, dystonia, and bladder dysfunction. Patients typically undergo a trial of stimulation in which wire electrodes are placed percutaneously and attached to an external generator. If symptoms improve, permanent wire electrodes or paddle electrodes are placed and connected to a programmable generator placed subcutaneously. The precise mechanism of action is unknown. The most common indication is that of the so-called postlaminectomy syndrome, especially when leg pain is worse than back pain. There is also some benefit for those patients with chronic regional pain syndrome. It has not been found to be routinely effective in the treatment of cancer pain.

Vagus nerve stimulation has been approved by the U.S. Food and Drug Administration for the treatment of intractable seizures and severe depression. The mechanism of action is not clear but is thought to be the result of afferent stimulation of higher cortical centers in the hypothalamus, amygdala, insular cortex, and cerebral cortex through the nucleus of the solitary tract. Stimulation of the left vagus nerve decreases seizure frequency but rarely makes patients seizure free.[40,41]

Implantable Pumps

Implantable pumps are used for the treatment of chronic pain and spasticity. An intrathecal catheter is inserted into the lumber spinal canal and a trial infusion used to gauge response. Many patients with cancer pain will respond favorably to intrathecal administration of narcotics through a programmable pump. Baclofen is the agent of choice for the treatment of spasticity with this modality.

Destructive Lesions

Ablative lesioning of the CNS for the treatment of pain, movement disorders, epilepsy, and psychiatric diseases has a long history. Before the advent of antipsychotic drugs, the most efficient way of curing and controlling some patients with severe psychiatric disease was thought to be institutionalization and psychosurgery. Before the development of the technologies described earlier, lesioning of different pathways in the brain and spinal cord was the only method for treating patients with chronic pain and movement disorders. Even though neuroaugmentive procedures and drug infusion technology have replaced many of the neuroablative procedures formerly in widespread use, a few ablative procedures still retain their clinical usefulness.

Dorsal root entry zone lesions are particularly useful for patients with deafferentation pain related to brachial plexus injury and, to a lesser extent, patients with spinal cord injury who have so-called end zone pain. In these conditions, deafferentation of the spinothalamic tract neurons results in spontaneous firing and the sensation of pain. The procedure creates lesions of the dorsal horn of the affected levels using a thermocouple probe. Extension of this concept has been applied to the caudal nucleus of the trigeminal nerve for the treatment of facial pain syndromes.

Myelotomy has traditionally been used in the treatment of bilateral cancer pain. It involves sectioning of the anterior commissure at and above the involved levels, which interrupts pain fibers on their way to the contralateral spinothalamic tract. A modified technique that interrupts only the median raphe of the dorsal columns has been described and presumably interrupts the second-order visceral pain pathway demonstrated to travel up the mammalian dorsal funiculus.[42,43]

Cordotomy involves lesioning of the anterolateral quadrant of the spinal cord at cervical levels, thereby eliminating input from the spinothalamic tract on the contralateral side of the body. Historically, it was most useful in the treatment of unilateral cancer pain. Bilateral lesioning increases the risk for neurologically mediated sleep apnea (Ondine curse). It can be performed percutaneously or as an open procedure.

Sympathectomy involves surgical interruption of the sympathetic chain at the high thoracic or lumbar level. A variety of endoscopic, thoracoscopic, radiofrequency, and open techniques are used. It is primarily used in patients with hyperhidrosis, sympathetically mediated pain, causalgia, chronic regional pain syndrome, and Raynaud disease.

Nerve block or neurectomy uses local anesthetic, sometimes with corticosteroids, which can be injected into the tissues surrounding a peripheral nerve, blocking conductivity and relieving pain. This can result in a long-lasting effect but typically is short-lived. Neurolytic agents (phenol or absolute alcohol) can also be used. Nerves can also be surgically divided or interrupted by radiofrequency techniques. There is a significant risk for recurrence with ablative neurectomy. Local nerve blocks are generally used in diagnostic procedures but can be repeated as necessary for the relief of pain. Ablative neurectomy is usually reserved for short-term relief in patients with a poor prognosis and short life expectancy.

Epilepsy

Epilepsy is not a distinct clinical entity with an identifiable cause but rather a complex collection of disorders of the brain that all share seizures as part of the complex. Seizures are classified as partial, generalized, or unclassified. Partial seizures are simple (consciousness not impaired) or complex (consciousness impaired). Generalized seizures are convulsive or nonconvulsive. Incidence rates in developed countries (40–70/100,000) are lower than those in developing countries (100–190/100,000). Approximately 20% to 40% of patients with seizures do not respond to anticonvulsant therapy. Failure to respond to three anticonvulsant medications prompts referral to a center specializing in epilepsy evaluation and treatment.

The goal of the workup of the epilepsy patient is to identify the cortical area responsible for the onset of the seizure. When the radiographic workup (MRI, CT, or both) reveals an obvious lesion causing the seizure (e.g., tumor, vascular malformation), the treatment is relatively straightforward and involves removal of the lesion. In other cases, the offending lesion is not as obvious on imaging, and intensive and often invasive monitoring is necessary to determine the epileptogenic focus. It is also important to determine language dominance and areas of the brain that are functionally abnormal during the interictal period. Noninvasive techniques that have become more widely available and better characterized include magnetoencephalography, positron emission tomography, single-photon emission CT, and functional MRI. Invasive modalities used in the evaluation of patients for seizure surgery include the Wada test for language dominance, stereotactically implanted depth electrodes, implanted strip electrodes, and implanted grid electrodes. Any or all of these techniques may be useful in brain mapping. It has long been possible to map critical speech and limb movement areas in awake, locally anesthetized craniotomy patients at the time of seizure focus resection.

On the basis of the information obtained in an epilepsy evaluation, the patient may be taken to surgery. Dominant hemisphere lesions are often operated on with the patient awake to allow intraoperative confirmatory brain mapping. This is accomplished by stimulating the cortex and observing and monitoring the patient's response, looking for speech arrest, anomia, or limb weakness or numbness. The most common surgical procedures performed for epilepsy are anterior temporal lobectomy, focal cortical resection, multiple subpial transection, hemispherectomy, and corpus callosotomy.

Anterior temporal lobectomy is the most common operation for seizures. An entirely unilateral interictal focus is the ideal indication (Fig. 68.21). The anterior temporal lobe, anterior hippocampus, and amygdala are excised. If the epileptogenic focus is not completely excised, the patient may continue to experience intractable seizures. If too much temporal lobe is resected, it can result in a contralateral superior quadrantanopia or, in dominant hemisphere lesions, speech and language dysfunction.

Focal cortical resection is usually performed in the frontal cortex. The results are more variable than those with temporal lobectomy.

Multiple subpial transection is used in more eloquent areas of the brain and involves making cortical incisions perpendicular to the surface of the gyrus in question. This presumably preserves descending fibers and function while interrupting spread of any epileptogenic activity within the cortical mantel itself.

Corpus callosotomy is used to prevent the rapid spread of seizures rather than to eliminate the focus. It is primarily useful in seizures that suddenly generalize, resulting in atonic drop attacks, as in Lennox-Gastaut syndrome.

Hemispherectomy is usually reserved for young children with seizures restricted to one hemisphere but threatening the good

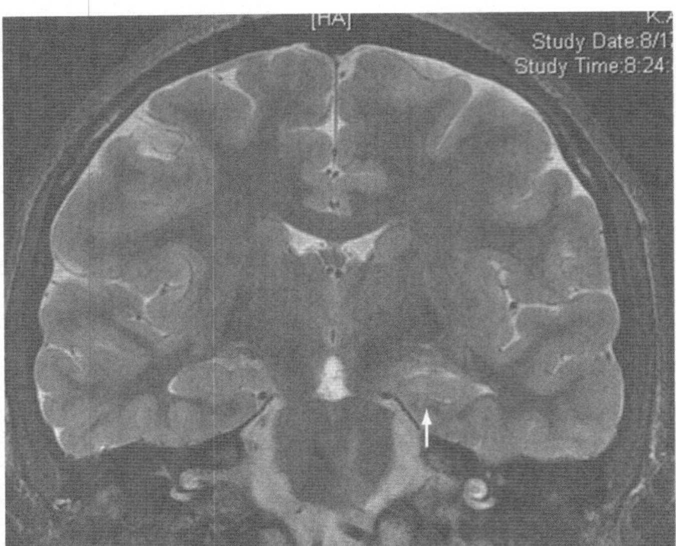

FIG. 68.21 T2-weighted coronal MRI study shows gliosis and atrophy of the left mesial temporal structure *(arrow). MRI,* Magnetic resonance imaging.

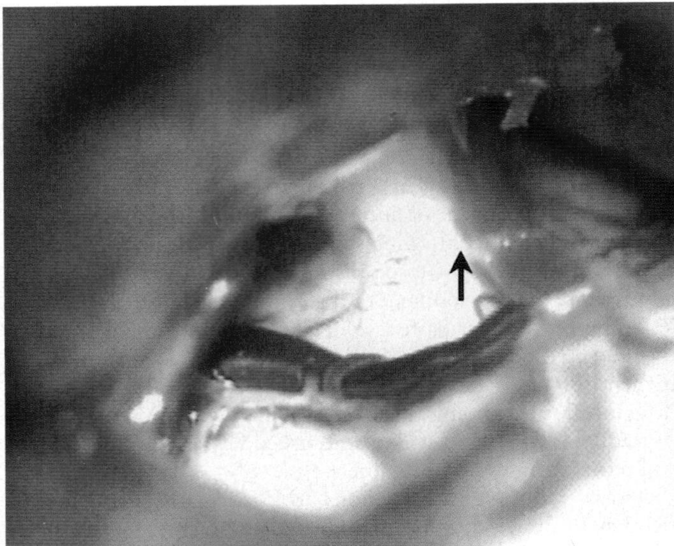

FIG. 68.22 Intraoperative photograph of a patient with typical trigeminal neuralgia. The left trigeminal nerve is compressed superiorly by an arterial branch of the superior cerebellar artery *(arrow).*

hemisphere by secondary effects of repeated seizures, as in Rasmussen syndrome. There is usually some abnormality of cellular migration. In the past, the entire cortex was removed, leaving the basal ganglia intact. Even though there was a significant decrease in seizure activity, the procedure led to a high complication rate, with ex vacuo brain shifts. A newer technique now involves preservation of portions of the cortex and its blood supply while disconnecting them from the rest of the brain by extensive undercutting of the adjacent white matter.[44]

Implantable cortical stimulation was approved in 2013 for patients with medically intractable epilepsy (NeuroPace). Responsive neurostimulation (RNS) is a closed loop system that uses cortical stimulation in response to the detection of developing seizure activity. This may hold significant promise in the future.[45]

Trigeminal Neuralgia

Trigeminal neuralgia affects approximately 4 in 100,000 individuals and is characterized by brief episodes of severe, lancinating pain in one or more of the three divisions of the trigeminal nerve, usually V2 and V3. Patients often describe that it is precipitated by touch or extremes of temperature. In extreme cases, a patient may refuse to eat or shave to avoid triggering the severe jolts of pain. Sensation usually remains intact, and significant numbness or jaw weakness leads to suspicion of a compressive mass lesion, such as tumor. Often, patients are referred with an already established diagnosis. It is reassuring if the patient has responded at some point to medication. MRI is used to rule out posterior fossa tumors and multiple sclerosis, which can present with related symptoms. Most patients respond to the oral administration of carbamazepine. Baclofen and gabapentin also have some clinical usefulness in medical treatment. The most common mechanism is presumed to be related to vascular compression of the fifth cranial nerve as it enters the brainstem (Fig. 68.22). With aging, the arteries elongate and can then begin to loop against the cranial nerves. At its entry to the pons, the fifth nerve has lost its peripheral nerve supportive architecture, the reticulin and mesenchymal elements that toughen the nerve more peripherally. Focal pulsatile pressure of the artery against this vulnerable part of the nerve results in ephaptic transmission from large myelinated fibers to small myelinated (A delta) and unmyelinated fibers.

Surgical therapy is usually reserved for patients who fail to respond to medical treatment. Microvascular decompression involves a small suboccipital craniotomy for microsurgical exploration of the dorsal root entry zone of the trigeminal nerve on the affected side. The offending vessel, usually the superior cerebellar artery, is then dissected off the nerve, and a barrier (Teflon or polyvinyl alcohol sponge) is placed between the vessel and nerve to prevent continued pulsatile focal compression. In especially favorable situations, the offending artery can be dissected free to loop away from the nerve, without the need for padding. A small sling of arterial patch graft material can also be sewn to hold the artery loop away from the nerve.

Percutaneous trigeminal rhizotomy techniques generally involve radiofrequency heat lesioning of the trigeminal ganglion, glycerol injection (Fig. 68.23) into the spinal fluid of Meckel cave (which causes an osmotic damage preferentially to the smaller pain-carrying nerve fibers), or mechanical trauma to the nerve or ganglion by transient inflation of a No. 4 Fogarty catheter balloon. Each method has its proponents along with advantages and disadvantages.

SRS has been described for the treatment of trigeminal neuralgia.[46] Initial results have been encouraging, and ongoing evaluation of specific indications and long-term follow-up are ongoing.

HYDROCEPHALUS

Hydrocephalus, defined as enlargement of the cerebral ventricles, occurs when production of CSF outpaces the body's ability to absorb that fluid. This can be related to obstruction of flow of the CSF through the ventricular system (obstructive hydrocephalus) or the inability of the body to reabsorb CSF at the level of the arachnoid granulations (so-called communicating hydrocephalus). The distinction between communicating and obstructive hydrocephalus is determined by the nature of CSF flow disruption. If there is free flow of spinal fluid through the ventricular system to the level of the arachnoid granulations,

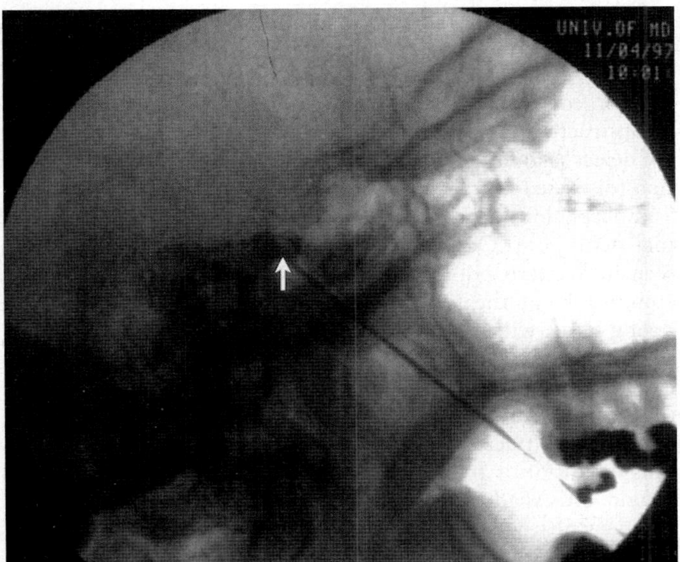

FIG. 68.23 Lateral skull film in a patient undergoing glycerol rhizotomy for typical trigeminal neuralgia. A 20-gauge spinal needle is directed to the foramen ovale, and nonionic contrast agent is injected to outline the trigeminal ganglion *(arrow)*.

then hydrocephalus is referred to as communicating. If there is obstruction to flow anywhere in the ventricular system, the hydrocephalus is referred to as obstructive. Rarely, a tumor of the choroid plexus, the structure responsible for CSF production, will cause overproduction of the spinal fluid, outpacing the body's ability to absorb it. Obstructive hydrocephalus is typically congenital but can be related to intraventricular or periventricular masses (neoplastic and nonneoplastic). It typically presents with imaging demonstrating enlargement of some ventricles, but not others, indicating an obstruction in the flow of spinal fluid from one part of the ventricular system to another. Communicating hydrocephalus is typically acquired, is usually secondary to infection or hemorrhage, and demonstrates more uniform enlargement of all four ventricles.

Hydrocephalus is often discussed in conjunction with pediatric neurosurgery because this is one of the more common conditions treated by neurosurgeons specializing in the treatment of infants and children. In fact, hydrocephalus is quite common in the adult population, and it behooves the adroit practitioner to be familiar with its pathophysiology and treatment. In this section, we concentrate on the types of hydrocephalus affecting the adult population. Pediatric hydrocephalus is discussed later.

Posthemorrhagic hydrocephalus is caused by obstruction of the arachnoid granulations with blood cells. This results in hydrocephalus of the communicating variety. *Postinfectious hydrocephalus* is also communicating and results from meningeal infection and altered CSF absorption.

Normal-pressure hydrocephalus is a condition characterized by the clinical triad of gait ataxia, incontinence, and dementia. Imaging reveals ventriculomegaly out of proportion to brain atrophy. This condition is most commonly seen in the elderly population and does respond to CSF diversion. Many techniques have been used to predict whether patients will respond to CSF diversion. Many believe that the clinical presentation of ataxia, incontinence, and dementia, in that order, is the best predictor of response to shunting.

Hydrocephalus and Pregnancy

In general, treatment and management of pregnant women with shunts should be tailored to the individual patient. Headache, nausea, vomiting, seizures, and lethargy may be the presenting signs of shunt failure. In gravid patients, this may be due to an increased incidence of distal malfunction. These signs and symptoms are also seen in preeclampsia, which must be ruled out. Patients undergoing cesarean sections should receive prophylactic antibiotics. Shunt externalization may be necessary for grossly contaminated cases.

Abdominal Surgery in Patients With Ventriculoperitoneal Shunts

As with pregnancy, management of patients with shunts and surgical diseases of the abdomen must be individualized. In grossly contaminated cases, shunt externalization is recommended.[46] Generalizations regarding the timing of abdominal surgery and ventriculoperitoneal shunts and the safety of simultaneous procedures cannot be made at this time given conflicting conclusions of recent studies.[47,48]

PEDIATRIC NEUROSURGERY

Pediatric neurosurgery is that aspect of the discipline that deals with infants and children. As mentioned earlier, a large portion of the pediatric neurosurgeon's time is spent dealing with hydrocephalus. In addition, pediatric neurosurgery is concerned with the treatment of other congenital anomalies, neurotrauma, functional problems such as spasticity and epilepsy, cerebrovascular disorders in children, brain tumors, and congenital defects of the spine and spinal cord. In this section, we briefly discuss some of these disease processes and their treatment.

Hydrocephalus in newborns manifests by an increased head circumference, full and tense fontanelles, and widened cranial sutures. The child may demonstrate lethargy and poor feeding and have abnormalities of the extraocular apparatus resulting in poor upgaze. Diagnosis is made with ultrasound, MRI, or CT.

The etiology of hydrocephalus in infants and newborns is either congenital or acquired. Congenital hydrocephalus is typically obstructive, whereas acquired hydrocephalus is usually communicating. Acquired hydrocephalus in newborns is usually postinfectious (meningitis, intrauterine toxoplasmosis infection, cytomegalovirus infection) or related to prematurity (intraventricular hemorrhage). Congenital conditions that can cause hydrocephalus include aqueductal stenosis, Chiari II malformation (discussed later), Dandy-Walker malformation, vein of Galen aneurysms, tumors, and arachnoid cysts. Aqueductal stenosis causes obstructive hydrocephalus by impeding flow of spinal fluid from the third ventricle to the fourth ventricle (Fig. 68.24). Chiari II malformation causes fourth ventricular outflow obstruction. Dandy-Walker malformation is associated with absence of the cerebellar vermis, cystic expansion of the fourth ventricle, and hydrocephalus. Vein of Galen aneurysms, tumors, and arachnoid cysts cause hydrocephalus through an obstructive mechanism.

The treatment of hydrocephalus is primarily concerned with the prevention of neurologic injury, which may occur if the condition is left untreated. In some cases, neurologic deficit can be reversed. Treatment typically involves treatment of the offending lesion (resection of the tumor or treatment of the infection) and CSF diversion. The distal terminus for most shunts is the peritoneal cavity. Other sites include the pleural cavity or superior vena cava. CSF diversion procedures are not without complications, and 5% to 15% of all shunts become infected. Treatment of shunt infections usually involves externalization or removal of the device, sterilization of the spinal fluid, and eventual replacement of the shunt.

Endoscopic third ventriculostomy is a surgical procedure used with frequency in patients with obstructive hydrocephalus and intact arachnoid granulations with the capacity for CSF reabsorption (Fig. 68.25). Even though the indications for endoscopic third ventriculostomy and results of treatment have been well-documented, continued refinement of the indications continues.[49]

Other neurosurgical conditions affecting infants and children include a variety of congenital anomalies affecting the nervous system. Myelomeningocele (Fig. 68.26) is an anomaly related to failure of the neural tube to close, with deficient meningeal, skeletal, and muscular development. The resultant neural placode is present without skin covering and is usually associated with a sac or enlarged subarachnoid space. Treatment consists of closure and reconstruction of the different layers. Neurologic deficit distal to the defect is common, as are hydrocephalus and Chiari malformation (discussed later).

Encephaloceles are the result of disordered closure of the cranial neuropore. Occipital encephaloceles are more commonly seen in Western populations, whereas frontal lesions are more common in southeastern Asia. The lesion may or may not have neural tissue within it. The brain that is involved is usually dysplastic. There is frequently an associated intracranial abnormality. Occult spinal dysraphism often manifests cutaneously in the lumbosacral area (Fig. 68.27). Hemangiomas, hair tufts, dermal sinus tracts, and lipomatous masses are frequently seen. This condition is frequently associated with tethered cord syndrome. This syndrome clinically manifests as back and leg pain, gait difficulty, weakness, orthopedic deformity of the feet, voiding dysfunction, and sexual dysfunction. Diastematomyelia is a dysraphic state in which there is duplication of the spinal cord at one or more continuous levels. Dermal sinus tracts are squamous-lined fistulas, often associated with small cutaneous pits in

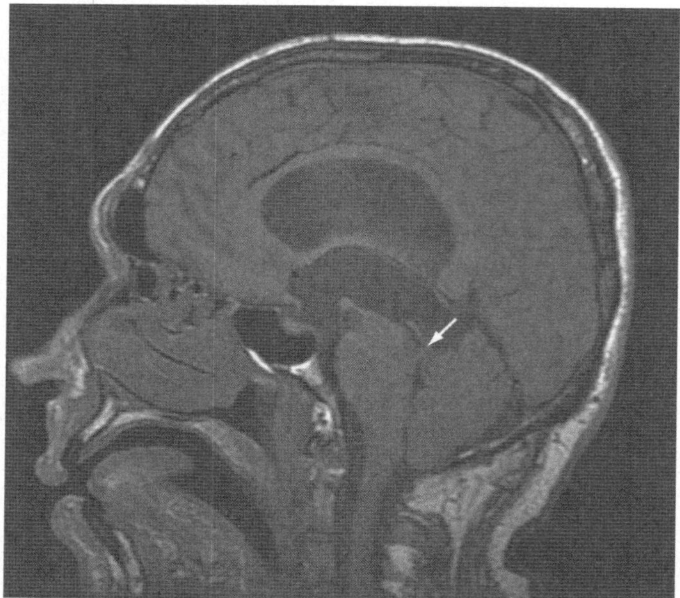

FIG. 68.24 T1-weighted sagittal MRI scan of patient with gross obstructive hydrocephalus caused by aqueductal stenosis *(arrow)*. *MRI*, Magnetic resonance imaging.

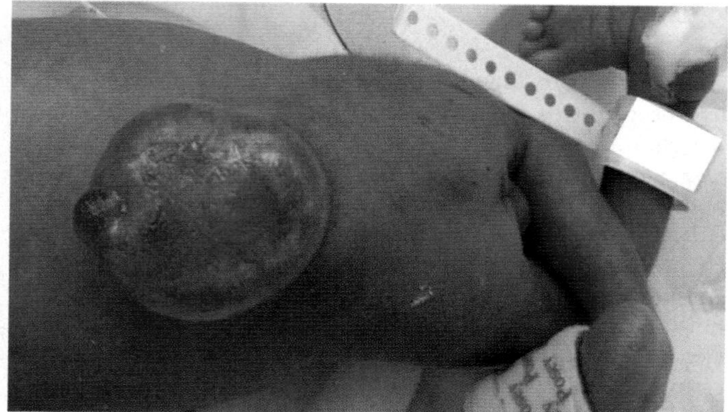

FIG. 68.26 Myelomeningocele in a neonate. Note the deformity of the lower limbs.

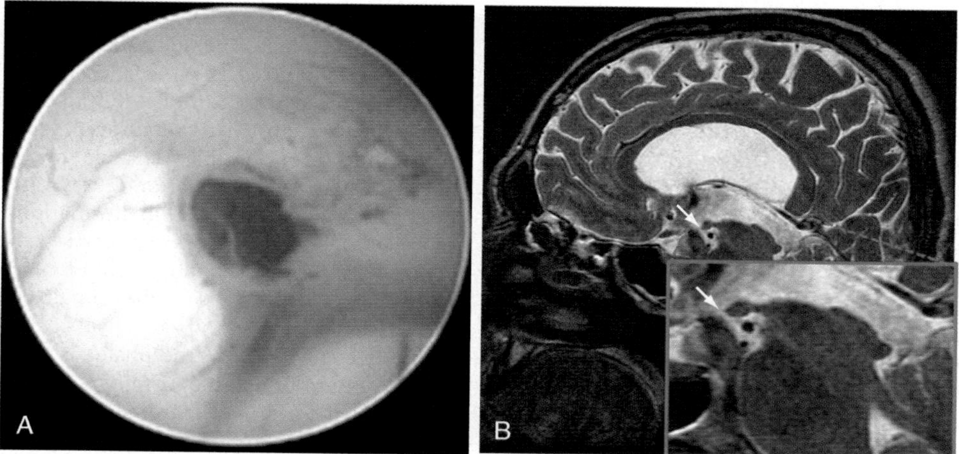

FIG. 68.25 (A) Endoscopic view of the third ventricular floor after the third ventriculostomy. (B) Follow-up MRI scan four years later demonstrating good flow at the fenestration site *(arrow)*. *MRI*, Magnetic resonance imaging.

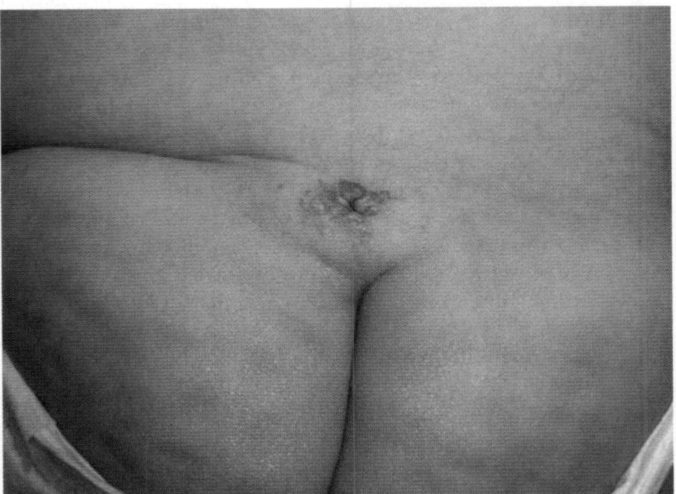

FIG. 68.27 Child with lumbar cutaneous hemangioma. This often accompanies an underlying spina bifida (spina bifida occulta) during the clinical evaluation.

the midline. They are often associated with intradural dermoid or epidermoid tumors. Treatment is usually surgical with excision of the fistula and removal of the dermoid or epidermoid component.

Chiari malformations consist of four different hindbrain abnormalities. Types I and II are considered here. Chiari I malformation (Fig. 68.28) is usually diagnosed in adults and involves downward displacement of the cerebellar tonsils into the foramen magnum. It may also be associated with syringomyelia of the cervical spinal cord. Downward displacement of the medulla is typically absent. Patients present with occipital headache exacerbated by Valsalva maneuver and may also have signs of foramen magnum compression, cranial nerve dysfunction, or cerebellar syndrome. Some patients also present with signs of intracranial hypertension and papilledema. Diagnosis is made with MRI and CT. Sagittal MRI gives an accurate assessment of the extent of tonsillar descent. Treatment consists of bony decompression of the occiput with removal of the posterior arch of C1 and sometimes C2. The dura is then opened and a dural patch graft sewn into place, thus creating more room for the neural elements. Chiari II malformation is usually associated with myelomeningocele. The medulla, cervicomedullary junction, and fourth ventricle are caudally displaced. These children can present with stridor, dysphagia, and apnea. Operative intervention is indicated in these cases.

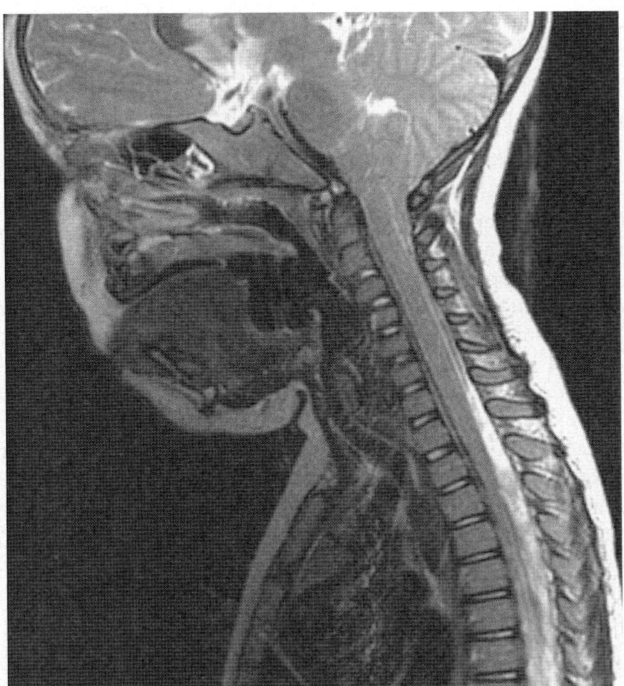

FIG. 68.28 T2-weighted sagittal MRI scan of a child with a significant type I Chiari malformation. Note the tonsillar descent below the rim of foramen magnum. *MRI*, Magnetic resonance imaging.

Craniosynostosis

Craniosynostosis involves premature fusion of one or more or the cranial sutures and causes restricted bone growth at the fused suture and disfigurement of the skull in the developing infant. When multiple sutures are involved, this can cause impairment of brain growth and development. The most common suture involved is the sagittal suture (Fig. 68.29), followed by the coronal suture, metopic suture, and lambdoid suture. Lambdoidal synostosis needs to be distinguished from positional plagiocephaly. Operative intervention consists of resection of the involved suture and, in syndromic synostosis (Apert, Crouzon), may require cranial vault remodeling and orbital rim advancement.

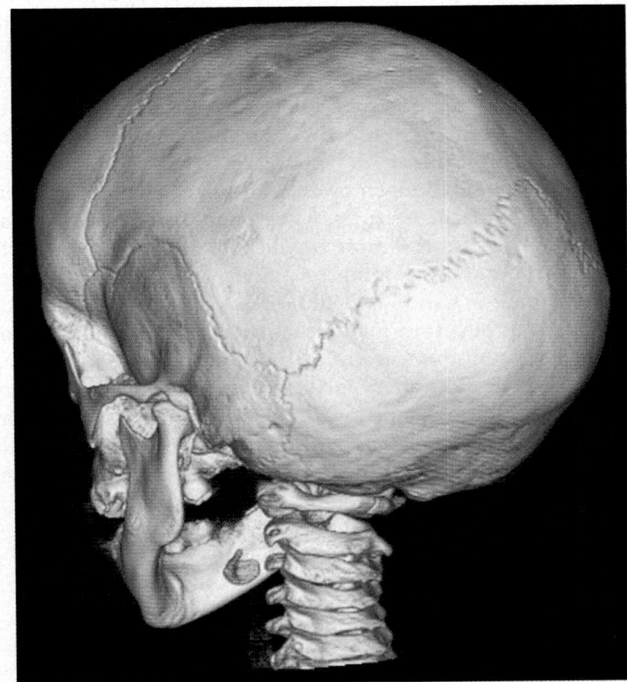

FIG. 68.29 Three-dimensional reconstruction CT scan of a child with sagittal synostosis. The coronal and lambdoid sutures are well visualized. *CT*, Computed tomography.

CENTRAL NERVOUS SYSTEM INFECTIONS

Broadly, CNS infections can be grouped as intracranial infections and spinal infections. The intracranial infections can occur in the epidural space (epidural abscess), in the subdural space (subdural empyema), in the subarachnoid space (meningitis), in the parenchyma (cerebral abscess), or in the ventricles (ventriculitis).

Intracranial Infections

Cranial Epidural Abscess

Cranial epidural abscess accounts for about 2% of all intracranial infections. An epidural abscess is commonly located either in the frontal region associated with frontal sinusitis and osteomyelitis or in the temporal region associated with mastoiditis and chronic ear infection. It can also be seen with untreated or inadequately treated compound depressed skull fractures. Clinically, there is associated local swelling, erythema, and tenderness with signs of localized or systemic infection. The infection can lead to development of meningitis and neurologic deterioration. CT scan of the head usually shows the infection with associated osteomyelitis. The treatment is surgical evacuation, debridement of the osteomyelitic bone, drainage of the adjacent infected sinuses, and prolonged antibiotic therapy. A cranioplasty may be required in the future after the infection heals. The outcome is usually acceptable with low morbidity or mortality in the absence of empyema or meningitis.

Subdural Empyema

A subdural empyema is a collection of pus in the subdural space. Usually seen in older children and young adults, it is most commonly related to contiguous spread from the paranasal sinuses or ear infection. Alternatively, infection can enter by retrograde thrombophlebitis of the veins communicating between the mucosal veins of the infected sinuses and dural venous sinuses or by hematogenous spread. About 60% of subdural empyemas are associated with frontal or ethmoid sinusitis and about 20% with inner ear infections. The infection can be located on the cerebral convexities, in the hemispheric fissure, or over the tentorium.

Patients with subdural empyema can present with fever, meningeal signs, headache, seizures, focal neurologic deficits, and altered mental status. The most significant complication is cortical venous thrombosis leading to cerebral infarction. It is often heralded by seizures and rapid clinical deterioration. Diagnosis is made by index of suspicion and the presence of a subdural fluid collection adjacent to a known focus of sinus infection. The margins of the collection often enhance with contrast. Appropriate treatment includes prompt institution of surgical drainage with antibiotic therapy. Anticonvulsants are indicated even in the absence of seizures as there is high risk of development. Steroids are often administered with antibiotics. Outcome with treatment is dependent on age, etiology, and neurologic status, with advanced age, postoperative and traumatic empyema, and obtundation at presentation carrying a worse prognosis.

Meningitis

Acute bacterial meningitis is an infection of the subarachnoid spaces and meninges. Symptoms and signs include fever, malaise, altered mental status, neck stiffness, and headache. These result from leptomeningeal irritation and increased ICP. The causative organism varies with the patient's age. Neonatal meningitis is caused by group B streptococcus, *Escherichia coli,* or *Listeria* spp. infection. Late neonatal meningitis can be caused by any of these organisms as well as by staphylococci or *Pseudomonas aeruginosa.* In children, *Streptococcus pneumoniae* (pneumococcus) and *Neisseria meningitidis* (meningococcus) are the most common causative organisms. In the past, *Haemophilus influenzae* was a common cause of meningitis in children, but its prevalence has decreased secondary to vaccination. Pneumococci and meningococci are the most common causative organisms in adults. Treatment consists of prompt CSF culture and immediate administration of intravenous antibiotics. Altered mental status secondary to communicating hydrocephalus may necessitate placement of an external ventricular drain and eventual placement of a ventriculoperitoneal shunt once the CSF is sterilized. Recurrent episodes of bacterial meningitis prompt investigation into abnormal communication between the CNS and the exterior environment (dermal sinus or CSF fistula).

Brain Abscess

Accumulation of pus in the cerebral tissue (cerebral abscess) usually is seen in children and young adults, but can be seen in all age groups. Contiguous spread of infection from paranasal sinuses, middle ear, or mastoid is the most common cause, accounting for about 50% of all cases. Hematogenous dissemination from lungs or other parts of the body (dental caries, subacute bacterial endocarditis, diverticulitis) accounts for about 25% of cases. In about 20% of cases, the cause is undetermined. Frontal abscesses along the orbital base are often the result of contiguous spread from the frontal sinuses, whereas temporal or cerebellar abscesses are otogenic in origin. Cardiac malformations with polycythemia resulting in increased blood viscosity, sluggish circulation, and cerebral infarction predispose to development of brain abscess. Brain abscesses can be solitary or multiple. Causative organisms are extremely varied and include aerobic and anaerobic organisms, fungi, and uncommonly parasites.

Abscesses are manifested with signs and symptoms related to a rapidly expanding mass lesion, often with only subtle signs and symptoms of infection. Patients can present with headache, nausea and vomiting, seizures, focal neurologic deficit, and altered mental status. Features of infection are present in around 60% of patients. Contrast-enhanced CT and MRI reveal a ring-enhancing lesion, usually at the gray-white interface, with surrounding edema (Fig. 68.30). This can be confused with glioblastoma multiforme or a metastatic tumor. Diffusion-weighted imaging (abscesses are hyperintense) and magnetic resonance spectroscopy (elevated lactate, low choline peaks) can distinguish between the abscess and tumor disease. Acute deterioration of patients can occur when the abscess ruptures into the ventricle or subarachnoid space, with resultant ventriculitis or meningitis. Principles of treatment involve accurate identification of the causative organism, relief of mass effect, administration of appropriate antibiotic therapy, and treatment of the underlying cause. Prophylactic anticonvulsants are usually indicated, and steroids often can be given with antibiotic cover. Controversy exists as to whether surgical excision or aspiration of the abscess yields better results.[50] The overall morbidity and mortality depend on the neurologic status at the time of diagnosis.

Ventriculitis

Shunt infections are the most common cause of ventriculitis. Other causes include spread of infection from either a ruptured cerebral abscess or other intracranial infection. Systemically administered antibiotics often do not penetrate significantly into the cerebral ventricles. Drainage of infected CSF with intraventricular antibiotics (depending on the organisms and sensitivity) is often required to clear the infection.

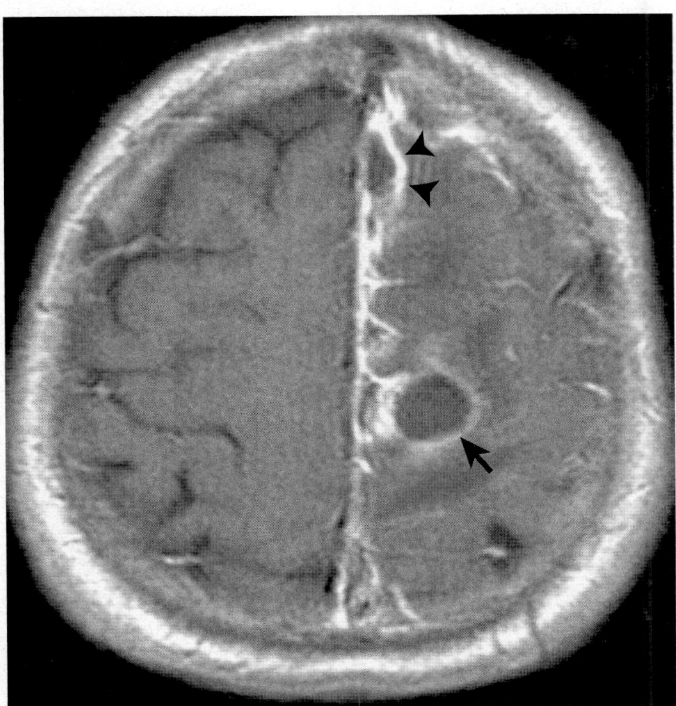

FIG. 68.30 Brain abscess *(arrow)* with an area of frontal subdural empyema in the convexity *(arrowheads)*.

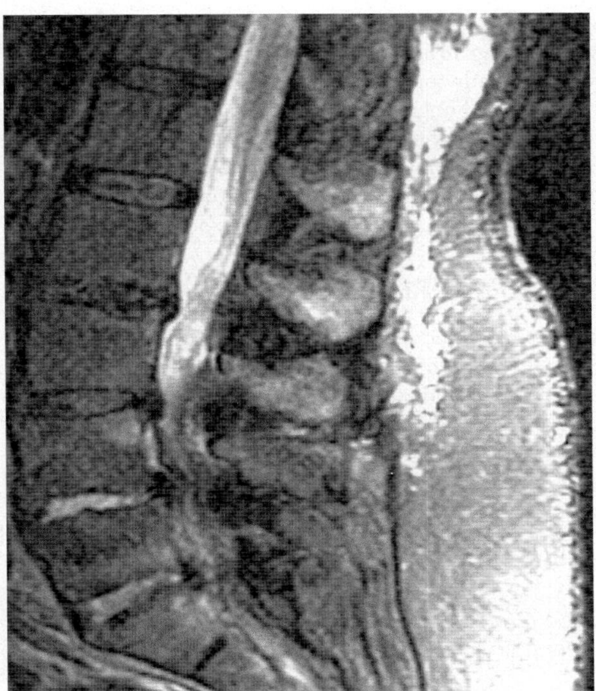

FIG. 68.31 MRI with gadolinium short T1 inversion recovery sequence revealing disc osteomyelitis in the L4–5 and L5–S1 interspaces suggestive of an infectious process. *MRI*, Magnetic resonance imaging.

Postoperative Infections

Infections of the CNS occurring after neurosurgical procedures are typically caused by staphylococci. Enteric organisms and pseudomonal and streptococcal pathogens can also be problematic. As with any infection, treatment involves identification of the causative organism and appropriate antibiotic administration. Postoperative abscesses are addressed with drainage, surgery, or both, as dictated by the clinical situation.

Posttraumatic Meningitis

Meningeal infection after head injury is typically related to CSF fistula. Most posttraumatic fistulas stop spontaneously within days of injury. The incidence of meningitis increases if a leak persists for longer than 7 days. Clinically obvious leaks are manifested as CSF rhinorrhea or otorrhea. The prophylactic antibiotic treatment of CSF fistula is controversial and needs to be tailored to the clinical situation. A persistent posttraumatic CSF fistula is addressed surgically to prevent the risks associated with recurrent bouts of meningitis.

Spinal Infections

Spinal infections can be grouped into those affecting the bone (vertebral osteomyelitis), disc space (discitis), and epidural space (spinal epidural abscess). On occasion, infectious processes can involve more than one or even all three.

Vertebral Osteomyelitis

Osteomyelitis of the bone is generally seen in intravenous drug users, diabetic patients, hemodialysis patients, and older adults. The causative organism is usually *S. aureus,* and spread is hematogenous, although postoperative infections are also seen. These infections can and do affect the integrity of the bone, resulting in collapse. This in turn can result in pain and neurologic compromise. Treatment consists of organism identification, appropriate long-term antibiotics, and maintenance of anatomic spinal alignment with or without surgical intervention.

Discitis

Infection of the disc (discitis) often occurs concomitantly with osteomyelitis and is seen in the same population of patients. Fever, back pain, and an elevated sedimentation rate or C-reactive protein level are often seen. The white blood cell count may or may not be elevated. It may occur spontaneously or postoperatively. Treatment may or may not be surgical. Long-term antibiotic therapy is usually indicated (Fig. 68.31).

Spinal Epidural Abscess

This usually occurs in the setting of an infectious process elsewhere in the body. Spread occurs hematogenously or by direct extension. Patients present initially with localized back pain and possible radiculopathy. Spinal cord compromise can follow rapidly, with paraplegia or quadriplegia. Predisposing factors are the same as those for osteomyelitis and discitis. Diagnosis is made with contrast-enhanced MRI. When spinal cord compression is evident, surgery is usually performed for decompression and diagnosis. Spinal epidural abscess can sometimes be managed medically, with close neurologic observation and imaging studies. This is usually reserved for cases in which the causative organism is known, the abscess is small, and there is no neurologic compromise. As in all fields of medicine, treatment must be tailored to the individual patient.

Acquired Immunodeficiency Syndrome

The most common CNS opportunistic infection in patients with AIDS is toxoplasmosis caused by *Toxoplasma gondii*. The lesions usually present with ring enhancement on contrast-enhanced imaging studies and are usually in the basal ganglia. They may be solitary or multiple. Primary CNS lymphoma occurs in approximately 10% of AIDS patients and presents as an irregularly enhancing mass (target lesion). Progressive multifocal leukoencephalopathy presents with hypodense, nonenhancing white matter lesions. Fungal abscess and viral encephalopathy are not uncommon in this population of patients. Even though the incidence of CNS opportunistic infections has decreased with the widespread use of highly active antiretroviral therapy, the treatment of these issues remains a challenge.

SELECTED REFERENCES

Brain Trauma Foundation. *Guidelines for the Management of Severe Traumatic Brain Injury.* Retrieved March 2019 from https://www.braintrauma.org/coma/guidelines.

Accepted guidelines commonly used in the management of patients with traumatic brain injury.

Greenberg MS. *Handbook of Neurosurgery*. 8th ed. New York, NY: Thieme; 2016.

Classic reference handbook used by neurosurgery residents and faculty.

Quinones-Hinojosa A. *Schmidek and Sweet: Operative Neurosurgical Techniques*. 6th ed. Philadelphia: Elsevier Saunders; 2012.

Atlas of neurosurgical techniques.

Steinmetz MP, Benzel EC. *Spine Surgery: Techniques, Complication Avoidance, and Management*. 4th ed. Philadelphia, PA: Elsevier; 2017.

A nice review of spine surgery and biomechanics in two volumes; thorough explanation and details from an authority in the field.

Winn RH, ed. *Youmans Neurological Surgery*. 7th ed. Philadelphia, PA: Elsevier Saunders; 2016.

A traditional and comprehensive resource for neurosurgery residents and faculty.

REFERENCES

1. Stern WE. Intracranial fluid dynamics: the relationship of intracranial pressure to the Monro-Kellie Doctrine and the reliability of pressure assessment. *J R Coll Surg Edinb.* 1963;9:18–36.
2. Rangel-Castilla L, Gasco J, Nauta HJ, et al. Cerebral pressure autoregulation in traumatic brain injury. *Neurosurg Focus.* 2008;25:E7.
3. Brain Trauma Foundation. Guidelines for the management of severe traumatic brain injury. Retrieved March 2019 from https://www.braintrauma.org/coma/guidelines.
4. Ondra SL, Troupp H, George ED, et al. The natural history of symptomatic arteriovenous malformations of the brain: a 24-year follow-up assessment. *J Neurosurg.* 1990;73:387–391.
5. Spetzler RF, Martin NA. A proposed grading system for arteriovenous malformations. *J Neurosurg.* 1986;65:476–483.
6. McCormick WF, Hardman JM, Boulter TR. Vascular malformations ("angiomas") of the brain, with special reference to those occurring in the posterior fossa. *J Neurosurg.* 1968;28:241–251.
7. Jacobs R, Kano H, Gross BA, et al. Defining long-term clinical outcomes and risks of stereotactic radiosurgery for brainstem cavernous malformations. *World Neurosurg.* 2018.
8. Henderson AD, Miller NR. Carotid-cavernous fistula: current concepts in aetiology, investigation, and management. *Eye.* 2018;32:164–172.
9. Winn HR, Richardson AE, Jane JA. The long-term prognosis in untreated cerebral aneurysms: I. The incidence of late hemorrhage in cerebral aneurysm: a 10-year evaluation of 364 patients. *Ann Neurol.* 1977;1:358–370.
10. Findlay JM, Nisar J, Darsaut T. Cerebral vasospasm: a review. *Can J Neurol Sci.* 2016;43:15–32.
11. Saber H, Desai A, Palla M, et al. Efficacy of cilostazol in prevention of delayed cerebral ischemia after aneurysmal subarachnoid hemorrhage: a Meta-Analysis. *J Stroke Cerebrovasc Dis.* 2018;27:2979–2985.
12. Boulouis G, Labeyrie MA, Raymond J, et al. Treatment of cerebral vasospasm following aneurysmal subarachnoid haemorrhage: a systematic review and meta-analysis. *Eur Radiol.* 2017;27:3333–3342.
13. Molyneux A, Kerr R, Stratton I, et al. International Subarachnoid Aneurysm Trial (ISAT) of neurosurgical clipping versus endovascular coiling in 2143 patients with ruptured intracranial aneurysms: a randomised trial. *Lancet.* 2002;360:1267–1274.
14. Hunt WE, Hess RM. Surgical risk as related to time of intervention in the repair of intracranial aneurysms. *J Neurosurg.* 1968;28:14–20.
15. Report of World Federation of neurological surgeons Committee on a Universal subarachnoid hemorrhage grading scale. *J Neurosurg.* 1988;68:985–986.
16. Fisher CM, Kistler JP, Davis JM. Relation of cerebral vasospasm to subarachnoid hemorrhage visualized by computerized tomographic scanning. *Neurosurgery.* 1980;6:1–9.
17. Walcott BP, Stapleton CJ, Choudhri O, et al. Flow diversion for the treatment of intracranial aneurysms. *JAMA Neurol.* 2016;73:1002–1008.
18. Karsy M, Guan J, Brock AA, et al. Emerging technologies in flow diverters and stents for cerebrovascular diseases. *Curr Neurol Neurosci Rep.* 2017;17:96.
19. Mendelow AD, Gregson BA, Fernandes HM, et al. Early surgery versus initial conservative treatment in patients with spontaneous supratentorial intracerebral haematomas in the International Surgical Trial in Intracerebral Haemorrhage (STICH): a randomised trial. *Lancet.* 2005;365:387–397.
20. Gross BA, Jankowitz BT, Friedlander RM. Cerebral intraparenchymal hemorrhage: a review. *J Am Med Assoc.* 2019;321:1295–1303.
21. Zhang H, Zheng L, Feng L. Epidemiology, diagnosis and treatment of moyamoya disease. *Exp Ther Med.* 2019;17:1977–1984.
22. Wang A, Schmidt MH. Neuroendovascular surgery for the treatment of ischemic stroke. *Cardiol Rev.* 2017;25:262–267.
23. Hasan TF, Rabinstein AA, Middlebrooks EH, et al. Diagnosis and management of acute ischemic stroke. *Mayo Clin Proc.* 2018;93:523–538.
24. Torbey MT, Bosel J, Rhoney DH, et al. Evidence-based guidelines for the management of large hemispheric infarction: a statement for health care professionals from the Neurocritical Care Society and the German Society for

Neuro-intensive Care and Emergency Medicine. *Neurocrit Care*. 2015;22:146–164.

25. Ostrom QT, Gittleman H, Truitt G, et al. CBTRUS statistical report: primary brain and other central nervous system tumors diagnosed in the United States in 2011-2015. *Neuro Oncol*. 2018;20:iv1–iv86.
26. Lowery FJ, Yu D. Brain metastasis: unique challenges and open opportunities. *Biochim Biophys Acta Rev Cancer*. 2017;1867:49–57.
27. Reifenberger G, Wirsching HG, Knobbe-Thomsen CB, et al. Advances in the molecular genetics of gliomas - implications for classification and therapy. *Nat Rev Clin Oncol*. 2017;14:434–452.
28. International Agency for Research on Cancer. *WHO Classification of Tumours of the central Nervous System*. 4th ed. World Health Organization; 2016.
29. Cahill DP, Louis DN, Cairncross JG. Molecular background of oligodendroglioma: 1p/19q, IDH, TERT, CIC and FUBP1. *CNS Oncol*. 2015;4:287–294.
30. Simpson D. The recurrence of intracranial meningiomas after surgical treatment. *J Neurol Neurosurg Psychiatry*. 1957;20:22–39.
31. Rogers L, Barani I, Chamberlain M, et al. Meningiomas: knowledge base, treatment outcomes, and uncertainties. A RANO review. *J Neurosurg*. 2015;122:4–23.
32. Nahed BV, Alvarez-Breckenridge C, Brastianos PK, et al. Congress of Neurological Surgeons Systematic Review and Evidence-Based Guidelines on the role of surgery in the management of adults with metastatic brain tumors. *Neurosurgery*. 2019;84:E152–E155.
33. Alnemari AM, Krafcik BM, Mansour TR, et al. A comparison of pharmacologic therapeutic agents used for the reduction of intracranial pressure after traumatic brain injury. *World Neurosurg*. 2017;106:509–528.
34. Hutchinson PJ, Kolias AG, Timofeev IS, et al. Trial of decompressive craniectomy for traumatic intracranial hypertension. *N Engl J Med*. 2016;375:1119–1130.
35. Matz PG, Meagher RJ, Lamer T, et al. Guideline summary review: an evidence-based clinical guideline for the diagnosis and treatment of degenerative lumbar spondylolisthesis. *Spine J*. 2016;16:439–448.
36. Kreiner DS, Shaffer WO, Baisden JL, et al. An evidence-based clinical guideline for the diagnosis and treatment of degenerative lumbar spinal stenosis (update). *Spine J*. 2013;13:734–743.
37. Walker CT, Farber SH, Cole TS, et al. Complications for minimally invasive lateral interbody arthrodesis: a systematic review and meta-analysis comparing prepsoas and transpsoas approaches. *J Neurosurg Spine*. 2019:30:446–460.
38. Bono CM, Ghiselli G, Gilbert TJ, et al. An evidence-based clinical guideline for the diagnosis and treatment of cervical radiculopathy from degenerative disorders. *Spine J*. 2011;11:64–72.
39. Adler Jr JR, Chang SD, Murphy MJ, et al. The Cyberknife: a frameless robotic system for radiosurgery. *Stereotact Funct Neurosurg*. 1997;69:124–128.
40. Yuan H, Silberstein SD. Vagus nerve and vagus nerve stimulation, a comprehensive review: Part I. *Headache*. 2016;56:71–78.
41. Yuan H, Silberstein SD. Vagus nerve and vagus nerve stimulation, a comprehensive review: Part II. *Headache*. 2016;56:259–266.
42. Nauta HJ, Soukup VM, Fabian RH, et al. Punctate midline myelotomy for the relief of visceral cancer pain. *J Neurosurg*. 2000;92:125–130.
43. Willis Jr WD, Westlund KN. The role of the dorsal column pathway in visceral nociception. *Curr Pain Headache Rep*. 2001;5:20–26.
44. Kim JS, Park EK, Shim KW, et al. Hemispherotomy and Functional hemispherectomy: indications and outcomes. *J Epilepsy Res*. 2018;8:1–5.
45. Matias CM, Sharan A, Wu C. Responsive neurostimulation for the treatment of epilepsy. *Neurosurg Clin N Am*. 2019;30:231–242.
46. Marchetti M, Pinzi V, De Martin E, et al. Radiosurgery for trigeminal neuralgia: the state of art. *Neurol Sci*. 2019;40:153–157.
47. Burks JD, Conner AK, Briggs RG, et al. Risk of failure in pediatric ventriculoperitoneal shunts placed after abdominal surgery. *J Neurosurg Pediatr*. 2017;19:571–577.
48. Jack MM, Peterson JC, McGinnis JP, et al. Safety, Efficacy, and cost-analysis of percutaneous endoscopic gastrostomy and ventriculoperitoneal shunt placement in a simultaneous surgery. *World Neurosurg*. 2018;115:e233–e237.
49. Gianaris TJ, Nazar R, Middlebrook E, et al. Failure of ETV in patients with the highest ETV success scores. *J Neurosurg Pediatr*. 2017;20:225–231.
50. Honda H, Warren DK. Central nervous system infections: meningitis and brain abscess. *Infect Dis Clin North Am*. 2009;23:609–623.

69 CHAPTER

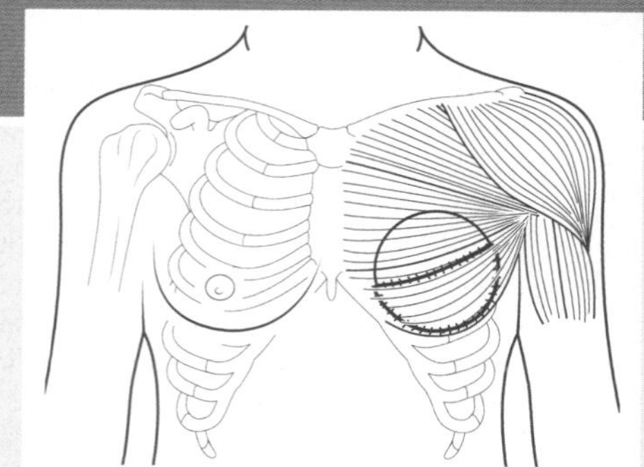

Plastic Surgery

Pablo L. Padilla, Kimberly H. Khoo, Trung Ho, Eric L. Cole, Ramón Zapata Sirvent, Linda G. Phillips

OUTLINE

Challenged by complex clinical problems, the pace of innovation in plastic surgery has accelerated steadily during the past 30 years. The specialty benefits from the absence of anatomic or organ system boundaries and from the collaboration with other surgical specialists. Plastic surgeons discover new reconstructive and aesthetic challenges and continuously make medical progress. With growing sophistication, plastic surgery has matured into areas of specialization, including surgery for congenital abnormalities, maxillofacial surgery, breast surgery, hand surgery, head and neck surgery, skin and soft tissue surgery, aesthetic surgery, body contouring, wound care, microsurgery, and burn care.

Plastic surgeons, in a relatively small specialty, stay aware of innovations in each of these areas and are quick to adopt and spread these ideas into all realms of surgery. Through the combination of research and clinical experience, it is not surprising that unique solutions for perplexing clinical problems sustain the momentum of innovation in the field.

RECONSTRUCTIVE TECHNIQUES

The concept of a reconstructive ladder is used to guide surgical reconstruction, ascending from simple to complex reconstructive techniques in a systemized way that considers the requirements of the defect to be repaired. Direct closure is the simplest and most straightforward technique. This may be precluded by the size of the wound or distortion of the surrounding tissue. Thus a more complex closure technique such as skin graft, local flap, or distant flap that brings in additional tissue, is required, increasing in level of complexity. Microvascular free tissue transfer represents the most complex flap option, allowing for transfer of various tissue type including skin, fascia, muscle, bone, nerve, and lymph.

When the concept of the reconstructive ladder is used, the triad of form, function, and safety is the basis for setting the reconstructive goals for any given defect. For example, in reconstructing the face, awareness of form would suggest a more complex technique such as tissue expansion instead of the simpler technique of skin grafting because it is optimal to restore with skin and soft tissue of the same thickness, texture, and color. Improvement in surgical techniques has also gradually transitioned the concept to a "reconstructive elevator," where it emphasizes the importance of selecting the most appropriate level of reconstruction as opposed to defaulting to the least complex.[1]

Primary and Secondary Wound Closure

Good closure technique starts with an incision with the scalpel at right angles to the skin and continues with careful handling of tissue to avoid devitalizing the skin margins, debridement of skin edges if needed, eversion of the wound margin, and precise approximation without tension. The skin edges need to be lined up at the same level, and wound edges should just touch each other.

Minimizing tension is essential to reduce scarring. This can be done by using buried deep dermal and subdermal sutures to lessen tension on the skin sutures. Minimizing tension can be accomplished also by aligning skin incisions along relaxed skin tension lines. These lines of minimal tension, also called natural skin lines, wrinkle lines, or lines of facial expression, run at right angles to the long axis of the underlying muscles. Closure placed in one of these furrows will be under minimal tension and will heal with minimal scarring.

The development of negative pressure wound therapy in the early 1990s has expanded the option for managing wounds that cannot be closed immediately by direct closure or flap. Its application has been shown to increase the rate of granulation formation, decrease edema, decrease frequency of dressing changes, increase time to closure, and control bacterial colonization and proliferation. It has been used commonly as a bridge to creating a viable wound bed for skin graft.[2]

Skin Grafts

A skin graft is a segment of dermis and epidermis that is separated from its blood supply and donor site and transplanted to another recipient site on the body. Survival of the transplanted skin graft requires a vascularized wound recipient bed. Graftable beds with adequate blood supply include healthy soft tissues, periosteum, perichondrium, paratenon, and bone surface that is perforated to encourage granulation tissue growth. Poor wound surfaces with inadequate blood supply include exposed bone, cartilage, tendon, implant, and fibrotic chronic granulation tissue. The wound must be free of infection and debris and interposed as a barrier between the graft and bed.

Skin grafts are classified in the following manner: autograft, self; allograft, other person; homograft, same species; and xenograft, different species. Partial-thickness skin grafts consist of the epidermis and a portion of the dermis and are called split-thickness skin grafts (STSGs). Full-thickness skin grafts (FTSGs) include the epidermis and entire dermis and portions of the sweat glands, sebaceous glands, and hair follicles. The STSG is harvested with a dermatome that can be adjusted for width and depth, usually in strips of 0.006- to 0.024-inch in thickness. The STSG can be meshed by cutting slits into the sheet of graft and expanding it. Meshed grafts are useful when there is a paucity of available donor skin, the recipient bed is bumpy or convoluted, or the recipient bed is suboptimal as with exudate. STSG can be taken from anywhere on the body; donor site considerations include color, texture, thickness, amount of skin required, and scar visibility. The STSG takes readily on the recipient site, and the donor site reepithelializes quickly from the residual dermis. Its disadvantages are contracture over time, abnormal pigmentation, and poor durability if subject to trauma. The FTSG is removed with a scalpel and is necessarily small because the donor site must be sutured closed. Containing skin appendages, the FTSG can grow hair and secrete sebum to lubricate the skin, has the color and texture of normal skin, and has the potential for growth. In general, FTSGs are taken from areas at which the skin is thin and can be spared without deformity, such as the upper eyelids, postauricular crease, supraclavicular area, hairless groin, or elbow crease. The greater thickness makes the FTSG more durable than the STSG, but this thickness also means that the graft take is not as predictable because more tissue must be revascularized from the recipient bed.

The take of either type of skin graft occurs in three phases:

1. Plasmatic circulation, also called serum imbibition, during the first 48 hours nourishes the graft with plasma exudate from host bed capillaries.
2. Revascularization starts after 48 hours with two processes. The primary is neovascularization in which blood vessels grow from the recipient bed into the graft, and the secondary is inosculation in which graft and host vessels form anastomoses.
3. Organization begins immediately after grafting with a fibrin layer at the graft-bed interface, holding the graft in place. This is replaced on postgraft day 7 with fibroblasts; in general, grafts are securely adherent to the bed by days 10 to 14.

Sensibility returns to the graft over time, with reinnervation beginning at approximately 4 to 5 weeks and being completed by 12 to 24 months. Pain returns first, with light touch and temperature returning later.

The most common cause of skin graft failure is hematoma under the graft, where the blood clot is a barrier to contact of the graft and bed for revascularization. Similarly, shearing or movement of the graft on the bed will preclude revascularization and cause graft loss. Additional causes are infection, poor quality of the recipient bed, and characteristics of the graft itself, such as thickness or vascularity of the donor site. Dressings can prevent some impediments to graft take. A light pressure dressing minimizes the risk of fluid accumulation. A bolster or tie-over dressing left in place for 4 or 5 days improves survival by maintaining adherence of the graft to the bed, minimizing shearing, hematoma, and seroma. A negative pressure wound therapy device can be placed on the grafted surface to stabilize the graft in place; this is especially useful for larger wounds with an irregular three-dimensional (3D) surface.

Skin grafts composed of tissue-cultured skin cells are used for the treatment of burns or other extensive skin wounds. Human epidermal cells in a single-cell suspension are grown in monolayers in vitro during a period of 3 to 6 weeks. Concerns with tissue-cultured skin are fragility, sensitivity to infection, length of time for cultivation, and potential risk of malignancy caused by mitogens present during culturing.

Tissue Expansion

Tissue expansion is a technique that uses a mechanical stimulus to induce tissue growth so as to generate soft tissue for reconstructive use. It involves placing a prosthesis that is gradually enlarged by the addition of saline, which causes an increase in the surface area of the overlying soft tissue. Initially, the expanded skin is the result of stretching as interstitial fluid is forced out of the tissue, elastic fibers are fragmented, viscoelastic changes (termed creep) occur in the collagen, and adjacent mobile soft tissue is recruited. Over time, it is not just stretching but actual growth of the skin flap that creates an increase in the surface area with accompanying increases in collagen and ground substance. Histologic changes in the skin include dermal thinning, epidermal thickening, subcutaneous fat atrophy, and no effect on the skin appendages.

Tissue undergoing expansion must have the capacity for growth. Prior irradiation or scar formation may slow the rate of expansion or make it impossible. Expanders perform poorly under skin grafts, under very tight tissue, and in the hands and feet. Contraindications include expansion near a malignant neoplasm, a hemangioma, or an open leg wound.

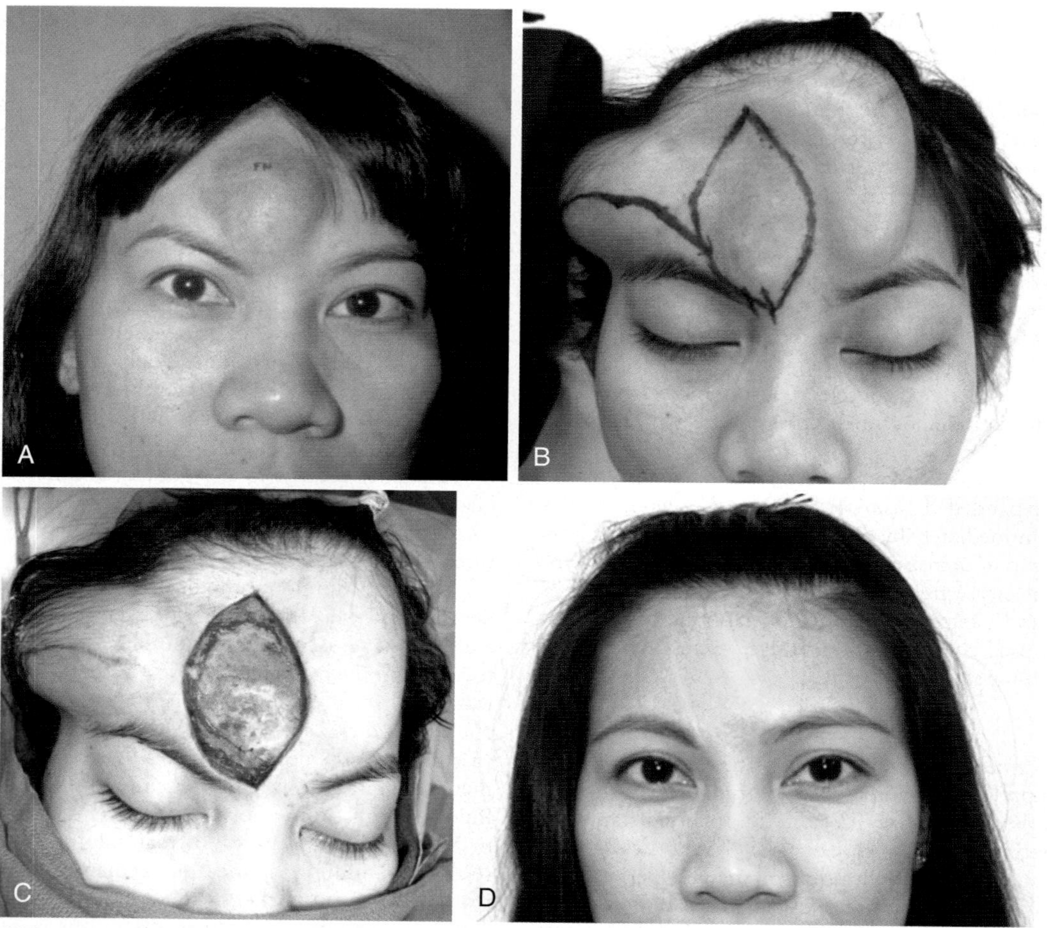

FIG. 69.1 The use of tissue expansion to generate new soft tissue to restore the forehead and hairline. The expanders are placed under tissue that best matches the lost tissue. (A) Young woman with an arteriovenous malformation. (B) Crescent-shaped expander in the central forehead and rectangular expander in the right forehead were expanded gradually with saline during one month. (C) The vascular lesion is excised, and the expanders will be removed with mobilization of the forehead to close the defect. (D) Postoperative result one year after surgery.

Expanders come in various styles, and sizes range from a few cubic centimeters to 1 L or more. They can be round, square, rectangular, or horseshoe shaped. The injection ports can be remote or integrated into the wall of the expander so that no dissection of a pocket for the remote port is required. The envelope can be smooth or textured for better stabilization at one location in the tissue pocket.

Expanders should be placed under tissue that best matches the lost tissue (Fig. 69.1). Normal landmarks, such as the eyebrow or hairline, should not be distorted. The incision to insert the expander can be placed at the edge of the defect that later will be excised because a scar in this position will be removed at the time of the next surgery. The most common reason for expander failure is construction of a pocket that is too small for the device. An expander with a curled edge may later protrude through the incision or erode through the overlying tissue. Filling of the expander is initiated approximately 2 weeks after surgery and is continued at weekly or biweekly intervals. The rate of expansion is limited by the relaxation and growth of the tissue overlying the expander. Pain and palpable tightness over the expander are clinical indicators that guide the rate of expansion. The patient is ready for the second surgical procedure when the expanded tissue is adequate to produce the desired effect. If the flap is to be advanced, it must be measured to ensure that it is large enough and has the correct geometry to cover the defect. At the second surgery, the skin is incised through the old scar, the capsule around the expander is opened, the expander is removed, and the expanded flap is advanced over the defect. It is important to confirm that the expanded tissue will replace the defect before the defect is excised. If it is not sufficient, this is handled by subtotal resection of the defect and leaving the expander in place for a second round of expansion.[3]

Tissue expansion can be combined with other reconstructive techniques. Expander placement in the subcutaneous or submuscular plane can facilitate later repair of abdominal wall hernias. Preexpansion of transposition or rotation flaps increases the amount of tissue, enhances the flap's blood supply, and lessens donor site morbidity. Preexpansion of free flaps increases the surface area and augments the blood supply of the future flap, may make primary closure of the free flap donor site possible, and thins the flap, which may be desirable for reconstructions calling for thinner and more pliable coverage. A disadvantage of the preexpansion of free flaps is the time needed for the expansion process because delay may not be acceptable for oncologic defects and complex wounds. In addition, the preexpanded free flap procedure is technically more difficult because of distortion of the vascular pedicle.

The advantages of expansion are the provision of matching tissue for reconstruction, normal sensibility of the transferred tissue, negligible donor defect, and enhanced success of preexpanded traditional flaps because of enhanced vascularity.

Alloplastic Materials

An alloplastic material is a synthetic substance implanted in living tissue. Its advantages are availability when autologous tissue is not available and the absence of donor site morbidity or scarring. Nonbiodegradable alloplastic materials do not undergo resorption as do bone or cartilage grafts. In addition, the implant can be manufactured to meet special needs, such as for controlled-release drug delivery systems.

The tissue response to different implants varies with the chemical composition and the microstructure and macrostructure of the synthetic material; these differences are used clinically. For example, the vigorous tissue ingrowth with polypropylene mesh in a hernia repair provides strong and lasting support, whereas the fibrous encapsulation around a silicone tendon prosthesis ensures free gliding of a tendon graft. However, certain properties (noncarcinogenic, nontoxic, nonallergenic, nonimmunogenic) and concerns (mechanical reliability, biocompatibility) are common to all implants.

Categorization by chemical composition is the most useful framework for the description and comparison of surgical implants. This materials scientific approach recognizes that the commonality of different groups of materials arises more from their composition than from the organ systems in which they are used. Chemically, there are three major classes of biomaterials: metallic, ceramic, and polymeric. Although they are polymers, biologic materials such as collagen need to be classified separately because they introduce new considerations of protein antigenicity.

Metals in clinical use are stainless steel, Vitallium (cobalt-chromium-molybdenum alloy), and titanium. The general requirements for a metal device are mechanical strength, suitable elastic modulus, comparable density and weight to those of the surrounding tissue, and resistance to corrosion. Very few metals have sufficient corrosion resistance to be used in the hostile environment of the living organism. Corrosion results from the electrochemical activity of unstable metal ions and electrons in physiologic salt solutions; corrosion products can be cytotoxic, leading to pain, inflammation, allergic reactions, and loosening of the device.

Ceramic materials have high stability and resistance to chemical alteration and include carbon compounds such as hydroxyapatite, which is capable of bonding strongly to adjacent bone. Used to augment the facial skeleton or as a bone graft substitute, it is a permanent microporous implant that undergoes osseointegration by providing a matrix for the deposition of new bone from adjacent living bone.

Polymers are large, long-chain, high–molecular-weight macromolecules made up of repeated units, or mers. There are a vast number of these synthetic implants in surgical use. To a large extent, this is because of the ease and low cost of fabrication and because they can be processed easily into tubes, fibers, fabrics, meshes, films, and foams. Polymers vary across an enormous range of chemical compositions, the degree of polymerization, cross-linking between chains, and the presence of chemical additives such as plasticizers to increase flexibility or resins to catalyze polymerization. With the exception of resorbable polymers, most surgical polymers are relatively inert and stimulate fibrous encapsulation. The physical form of the implant, solid versus mesh or smooth versus rough, will determine whether the entire structure is encapsulated as a whole or whether fibrous tissue will penetrate the interstices. Tissue reaction to the implant is influenced also by the chemical composition, factors such as hydrophilicity and ionic charge, and the chemical durability of the polymer. Silicone rubber, polytetrafluoroethylene, and polyethylene terephthalate polyester (Dacron) are among the most stable of polymers, whereas polyamide (nylon) is vulnerable to hydrolytic reaction and undergoes substantial degradation.

Flaps

A flap consists of tissue that is moved from one part of the body to another with a vascular pedicle to maintain blood supply. The vascular pedicle may be kept intact, or it can be transected for microvascular anastomosis of the flap vessels to vessels at another site.

Skin-bearing flaps are classified according to three basic characteristics—composition, method of movement, and blood supply. Composition refers to the tissue contained within the flap, such as cutaneous, musculocutaneous, fasciocutaneous, osseocutaneous, adipofascial, and sensory flaps. The method of movement is local transfer as with advancement or rotation flaps, distant transfer as with pedicle flaps from the abdomen to the perineum, or microvascular free flaps.

With regard to blood supply, arteries perfusing the surgical flap reach the skin component in two basic ways. Musculocutaneous arteries travel perpendicularly through muscle to the overlying skin. Septocutaneous arteries arising from segmental or musculocutaneous vessels travel with intermuscular fascial septa to supply the overlying skin. With either of these patterns, the flap can have a random pattern, which means that it derives its blood supply from the dermal and subdermal vascular plexus of vessels supplied by perforating arteries. Alternatively, it can be an axial flap designed to include a named vessel running longitudinally along the axis of the flap to penetrate the overlying cutaneous circulation at multiple points along the course of the flap's length to provide greater length and reliability.

Local Flaps

Local flaps contain tissue lying adjacent to the defect that usually matches the skin at the recipient site in color, texture, hair, and thickness. Flaps should be the same size and thickness as the defect and be designed to avoid distortion of local anatomic landmarks, such as the eyebrow or hairline. They can be planned so that the donor site can be closed directly. Local flaps rely on the inherent elasticity of skin and are most useful in the older patient whose skin is looser. In some cases, the site from which the flap is raised is closed with a skin graft. Commonly used local skin flaps include rotation flaps, transposition flaps, and advancement flaps. By definition, these flaps are random flaps because they are raised without regard to any known blood supply other than the subdermal plexus.

Failure of a skin flap usually involves necrosis of the most distal portion of the transferred tissue. This could be caused by a flap design in which the size of the flap exceeds its inherent vascular supply, or it could be a result of extrinsic mechanical compromise of the flap pedicle by pressure from a hematoma, compressive dressings, or twisting or kinking of the flap. Measures to optimize viability include proper flap design and avoidance of extrinsic pedicle compression, undue tension with wound closure, and venous congestion caused by excessive flap dependency.

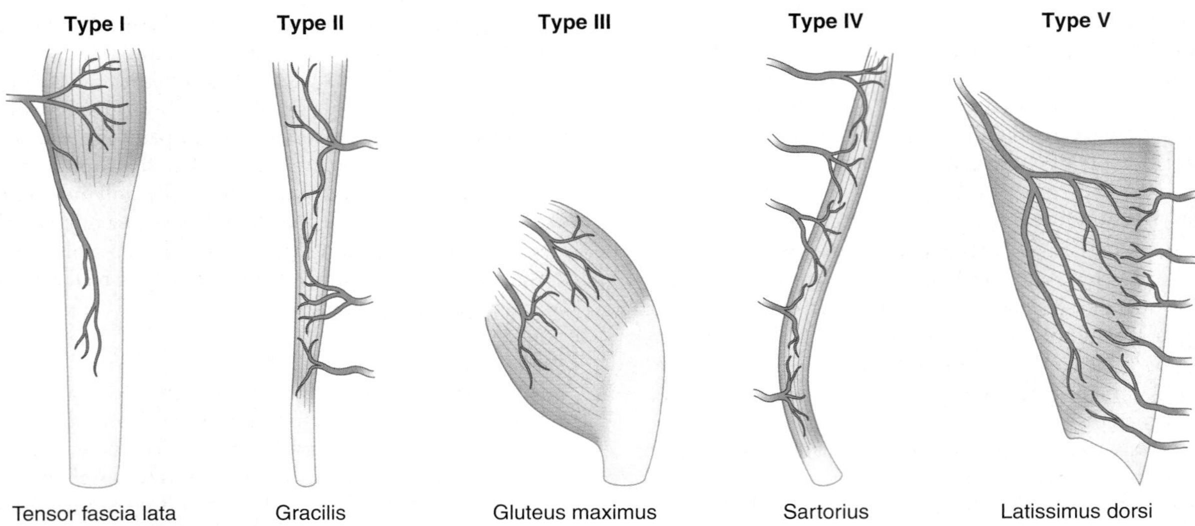

FIG. 69.2 Classification of muscle and musculocutaneous flaps according to their vascular supply: type I, one vascular pedicle; type II, dominant pedicle and minor pedicles; type III, two dominant pedicles; type IV, segmental vascular pedicles; type V, one dominant pedicle and secondary segmental pedicles. (From Mathes SJ, Nahai F. Classification of the vascular anatomy of muscles: Experimental and clinical correlation. *Plast Reconstr Surg.* 1981;67:177–187.)

Muscle and Musculocutaneous Flaps

Consideration of a muscle as a potential flap is possible because muscles have an independent, intrinsic blood supply. This vascular pedicle may be a dominant one, capable of sustaining the entire muscle independently. A minor pedicle, regardless of the size of the vessel, is defined as one that maintains only a lesser portion of the muscle. Many muscles have multiple unrelated sources of blood supply so that each nourishes only a segment of the muscle, thus called segmental pedicles. Some muscles have both a dominant pedicle and a segmental blood supply. One example is the latissimus dorsi muscle with a dominant pedicle, the thoracodorsal artery in the axilla, and additional segmental perforating branches from the intercostal and lumbar vessels posteriorly. Muscle flaps are classified according to their principal means of blood supply and the patterns of vascular anatomy (Fig. 69.2):

Type I: Single pedicle (e.g., gastrocnemius, tensor fascia lata)
Type II: Dominant pedicle with minor pedicles (e.g., gracilis, trapezius)
Type III: Dual dominant pedicles (e.g., gluteus maximus, serratus anterior)
Type IV: Segmental pedicles (e.g., sartorius, tibialis anterior)
Type V: Dominant pedicle, with secondary segmental pedicles (e.g., latissimus dorsi)

In terms of reliability of the vascular anatomy and usefulness as a flap, large muscles with a recognized dominant pedicle supplying most of a flap (types I, III, and V) are most useful. The territory of the pedicles in type II muscles may vary, and type IV muscles are useful only when smaller flaps are needed. Connections between regions within a given muscle supplied by more than one pedicle are through small-caliber choke vessels with bidirectional flow. An example of a flap depending on these choke vessels is the transverse rectus abdominis musculocutaneous (TRAM) flap in which the superior epigastric pedicle alone can support the lower half of the muscle normally supplied by the inferior epigastric vessels below the watershed level at the umbilicus. In muscle, venous territories are parallel with arterial vessels (i.e., venous outflow is adjacent to and in a direction opposite from flow in the major arterial pedicles). In a pattern analogous to that of the bidirectional choke vessels, venous flow from one territory to another occurs through oscillating veins that are devoid of valves.

Compared with skin flaps, muscle flaps have more robust blood supply and demonstrate superiority in wounds compromised by irradiation or infection.[4] The vascular anatomy is predictable and easily identifiable, and the muscle can be put into use as a functional unit for a dynamic tissue transfer. A major consideration with muscle flaps is whether the loss of function is acceptable. In an effort to limit the functional loss associated with use of an entire muscle, methods of functional preservation have been devised. If some portion of the muscle chosen as the flap is left innervated and attached at its insertion and origin, function is preserved after transfer of the remainder of the muscle. This can be done by splitting the muscle into segments, provided each is supplied by a different dominant pedicle.

A musculocutaneous flap, also called a myocutaneous flap, is a muscle flap designed with an attached skin paddle. Each superficial skeletal muscle carries blood supply to the skin lying directly over it through musculocutaneous or septocutaneous perforators. The number and pattern of these musculocutaneous perforators vary with each specific muscle; this means that the extent of the skin territory is different for each muscle unit. Through dissection of injected cadaver specimens, the number, size, and location of perforators have been described; this information, combined with clinical experience, is used to predict the cutaneous territories on the superficial muscles.

In addition to the musculocutaneous branches supplying the overlying skin, source vessels branch within the muscle into channels that perforate the deep fascia to anastomose within the subdermal plexus and nourish the skin. The source vessel and its perforating muscular branches can be dissected out of the muscle without jeopardizing skin perfusion. This requires intramuscular dissection to separate the perforators from the muscle and is the basis for the development of perforator flaps. This makes the retention of muscle unnecessary for the survival of the skin paddle; thus, its inclusion serves a passive role, primarily to

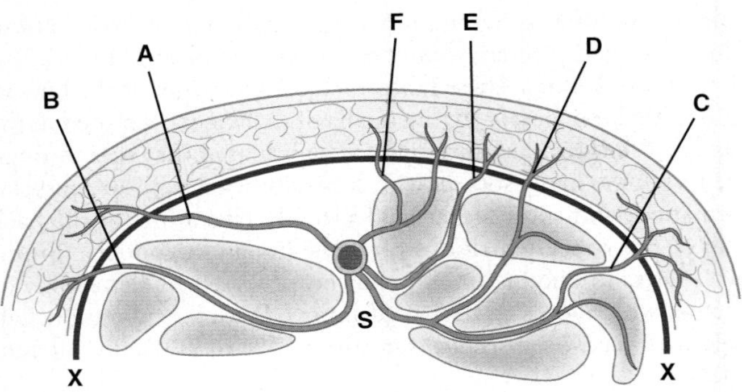

A Direct cutaneous
B Direct septocutaneous
C Direct cutaneous branch of muscular vessel
D Perforating cutaneous branch of muscular vessel
E Septocutaneous perforator
F Musculocutaneous perforator
S Source vessel
X Deep fascia

FIG. 69.3 Pathways of the various known cutaneous perforators that pierce the deep fascia to supply the fascial plexus. (From Hallock GG. Direct and indirect perforator flaps: The history and the controversy. *Plast Reconstr Surg.* 2003;111:855–865.)

avoid tedious intramuscular dissection of the vascular tree. In effort to preserve the muscle unit, a growing number of perforator flaps have been described, including the deep inferior epigastric perforator flap, which carries the same skin and subcutaneous tissue as the TRAM flap for breast reconstruction. By sparing of the rectus muscle, abdominal wall bulging and other complications are less. The superior gluteal artery perforator flap carries the skin territory of the gluteus maximus musculocutaneous flap and preserves the muscle.

Fascia and Fasciocutaneous Flaps

Growing knowledge about musculocutaneous skin circulation has led to the identification of vascular pedicles emerging between muscles, traveling in the intermuscular septum, and entering the deep fascia. Termed *septocutaneous perforators*, these vessels supply the fascial plexus, which gives off branches to an overlying cutaneous territory.

The anatomic features of a fasciocutaneous flap are the fascial feeder vessels, also called the *fascial perforators*, which are branches of source vessels to a given angiosome. An angiosome is the 3D block of tissue supplied by a source artery; the entire surface of the body is composed of a multitude of angiosome units. The fascial feeder vessels do not perforate the deep fascia but terminate within the fascial plexus. The fascial plexus is not a structure but a confluence of multiple adjacent vascular intercommunications that exist at the subfascial, fascial, suprafascial, subcutaneous, and subdermal levels (Fig. 69.3).

The concept of fasciocutaneous flaps arose from the observation that the size of a skin flap could be increased if it were oriented along a longitudinal axis on the extremity and if the deep fascia were included. Subsequent anatomic studies have confirmed the presence of septocutaneous pedicles supplying a regional fascial vascular system. The larger septocutaneous pedicles tend to be fairly constant in location, and a number of specific fasciocutaneous flaps have come into wide use (e.g., anterior lateral thigh flap, radial forearm flap, and lateral arm flap).

The design of fasciocutaneous flaps has been learned by experience, and the limits of these flaps still remain to be discovered. There are no set rules because deep fascial perforators are frequently anomalous in caliber and location, not only among individuals but also on opposite sides of the same person. The expected range of flap size is learned through the experience of other surgeons.[5]

One of the most useful features of a fasciocutaneous flap is that it can be distally based. Unlike in a muscle flap in which the dominant pedicle is closest to the heart, blood flow in the fascial plexus is multidirectional. The flow to the corresponding angiosome is equivalent for a distal fascial perforator and proximal fascial perforator. This means that a flap pedicle can be distally based with a reliable skin territory and transposed to cover a defect located at the end of an extremity. For example, the distal-based sural flap uses the skin of the calf, based on a distal perforator of the peroneal artery, for transfer to cover the foot and ankle, thus obviating the need for a free microvascular transfer.

In addition to the advantages provided by a distally based flap design, a fasciocutaneous flap can confer sensibility if a sensory nerve is included. Compared with musculocutaneous flaps, they are accessible on the surface of the body and have the great advantage that no functioning muscle is expended. The comparative disadvantages are the anatomic anomalies in the fascial vascular system and the unanswered question as to whether they are as effective as muscle in the irradiated or infected wound.

Perforator Flaps

Perforator flaps evolved as an improvement over musculocutaneous and fasciocutaneous flaps. They rely on evidence that neither a passive muscle carrier nor the underlying fascial plexus of vessels is necessary for flap survival, provided the musculocutaneous or fasciocutaneous vessel is carefully dissected out and preserved. Advantages of perforator flaps include preservation of functional muscle and fascia at the donor site and versatility of flap design with regard to including as little or as much bulk tissue as required. Disadvantages are the difficult dissection needed to isolate the perforator vessels, longer operating time associated with this dissection, anatomic variability of position and size of perforator vessels, short pedicle length available, and fragile nature of these small blood vessels.

A perforator is a blood vessel passing through the deep fascia and contributing blood supply to the fascial plexus. Perforators arise from a source or mother vessel to a given angiosome. There are direct and indirect perforators. Direct perforators are those that travel directly from the mother vessel to the plexus; these include septocutaneous and direct cutaneous branches. Indirect perforators supply other deep structures on their route from the mother vessel to the plexus (e.g., the musculocutaneous perforator passing through muscle).

Because of the small size of the vessels and their anatomic variability, Doppler ultrasound is used routinely to locate the perforators before perforator flap elevation. This is not highly accurate, thus clinical experience remains crucial in this developing area. Technical recommendations for harvesting a perforator flap include identification of at least one vessel with a diameter of 0.5 mm or more, inclusion of at least two or more perforators, sufficient pedicle length for the procedure, and preservation of a subcutaneous vein to use for venous outflow in situations in which the deep system of perforator veins proves anomalous.

The use of perforator flaps continues to evolve. Current work includes flap thinning, a technique for removing excess adipose tissue from the perforator flap as it is raised. This would provide a large delicate segment of vascularized skin for reconstruction in areas such as the ear, in which contour is important. Another innovation is the discovery of new flaps based on perforators smaller than 0.8 mm in diameter found superficial to the fascial plane. By eliminating the dissection needed to trace a perforator through the muscle, operating time is shortened and there is potential for developing a much larger number of suitable flaps. The challenge with these suprafascial free flaps is the supermicrosurgery needed for anastomoses in such small vessels.

Microvascular Free Tissue Transfer

Microvascular free tissue transfer, commonly known as free flap, transplants distant tissue with its arterial and venous supply from another part of the body to be anastomosed to vessels at the recipient site. The transferred tissue may be skin, fat, muscle, cartilage, fascia, bone, nerves, bowel, or omentum as needed to reconstruct a given defect. Selection of tissue for transfer depends on the size, composition, and functional capabilities of the tissue needed; technical considerations, such as vessel size and pedicle length; and donor site deformity that will be created with regard to function and aesthetic appearance.

Preoperative planning starts with selection of the patient and analysis of the defect. Environmental factors, such as previous surgery and prior irradiation, which impair the quality of tissue and vessels, may be an indication for angiography to assess the available vasculature. Muscle does not tolerate warm ischemia for longer than 2 hours; skin and fasciocutaneous flaps can tolerate ischemia times of 4 to 6 hours. Planning is the most important factor to minimize the effects of ischemia, and all structures at the recipient site should be ready for the tissue transfer when the donor pedicle is divided. Sound technique requires healthy vessels of reasonable size with good outflow for the anastomosis, which must be made without tension. This may require mobilization of the vessels to gain more length. Vein grafts have been shown to reduce the success rate and are not a primary choice but may be needed if the pedicle is short or the vessels in the field are damaged. Both end-to-end and end-to-side arterial anastomoses have similar patency rates, although end-to-side anastomosis is preferred if there is vessel size or wall thickness discrepancy or the continuity of the recipient vessel must be preserved. Dissection and manipulation of the microvessels frequently cause vasospasm. This can be relieved with topical lidocaine or papaverine, stripping the adventitia to remove sympathetic nerve fibers, or mechanical dilation of the vessels. Failure of reperfusion in an ischemic organ after reestablishment of blood supply is termed the *no-reflow phenomenon*. The severity of this effect correlates with ischemia time.

Postoperative anticoagulation is not a uniform practice for elective microvascular transfers, and studies have not shown improved survival rate with anticoagulation regimen.[6] Postoperative monitoring of free tissue transfers is critical because rapid identification of postoperative free flap ischemia permits intervention and flap salvage. Most free flap thromboses occur in the first 48 hours after surgery, and salvage rates are high. Clinical evaluation includes observation of skin color, capillary refill, fullness, and color of capillary bleeding. If a flap is buried, a temporary skin island can be added for monitoring purposes or an implantable monitoring device can be used. Many devices are available for flap monitoring, including temperature probes, pulse oximetry, photoplethysmography, hand-held pencil Doppler probes, and implantable Doppler probes.

Tissue survival rates for free tissue transfers exceed 98%. Reexploration rates range from 6% to 25%, and thrombosis of the arterial anastomosis is the most common finding at reoperation. This is termed *primary thrombosis* when technical faults lead to anastomotic failure. These faults include narrowing of the lumen; sutures tied too loosely so that media of the vessel is exposed in the gap and clot forms; sutures tied too tightly that they tear through the vessel; too many sutures with subendothelial exposure and clot formation; and sutures that inadvertently take a bite of the back wall of the vessel, which obstructs the lumen. Secondary thrombosis refers to kinking or compression of vessels by hematoma or edema, which leads to decreased inflow. With reexploration, salvage rates have been seen to vary from 54% to 100% in different series.[7]

The principles and techniques of microvascular surgery are under continual refinement. An area of current emphasis is the identification of tissue transfers that better suit the needs of the recipient site and minimize donor site sequelae, which has led to minimally invasive and endoscopic techniques for harvesting of flap tissue through smaller incisions. It has also led to the development of tissue transfers such as perforator flaps, which preserve functional muscle and fascia at the donor site, and suprafascial free flaps, which require supermicrosurgery techniques.

Supermicrosurgery

The introduction of supermicrosurgery, which allows the anastomosis of smaller caliber vessels and microvascular dissection of vessels ranging from 0.3 to 0.8 mm in diameter, has led to the development of new reconstructive techniques. Free perforator-to-perforator flaps using suprafascial vessels can be transferred more quickly and the tissue can be obtained from better concealed parts of the body.[8] If a discrete perforator can be identified anywhere on the body, a flap can be designed around it. This has been called a *freestyle flap*. The constraints of using only described territories can be disregarded and the donor site selected solely on the basis of the best possible match for color, contour, and texture at the recipient site. Disadvantages are the anatomic variation of the perforators and the need for supermicrosurgical technique. The supermicrosurgical technique includes the use of 12-0 nylon sutures with 50-μm to 30-μm needles, which requires a high magnification microscope and a technically adept surgeon.

PEDIATRIC PLASTIC SURGERY

Craniofacial Surgery

Craniosynostosis refers to the premature fusion of one or more of the cranial sutures, leading to characteristic deformities of the skull and face. It occurs at an overall frequency of approximately 1 in 2500 live births and is usually sporadic. Any suture may be involved in craniosynostosis, and skull growth is restricted perpendicular to the affected suture. Treatment of craniosynostosis is indicated to correct the deformity and to normalize the shape of the head, to protect the eyes by restoring brow projection, and to minimize the risk for development of increased intracranial pressure and associated developmental and visual sequelae. The timing of treatment is based on which suture is fused and on the protocol at a given center, but correction during the first 6 months of life appears to be associated with better neurodevelopmental outcomes.[9]

Surgical treatment of craniosynostosis is generally done with a coronal approach; techniques differ, but all involve release or excision of the fused suture. The cranium then expands and remodels. Residual bone defects reossify secondarily, a process that is robust in the infant up to 2 years of age (Fig. 69.4). The use and

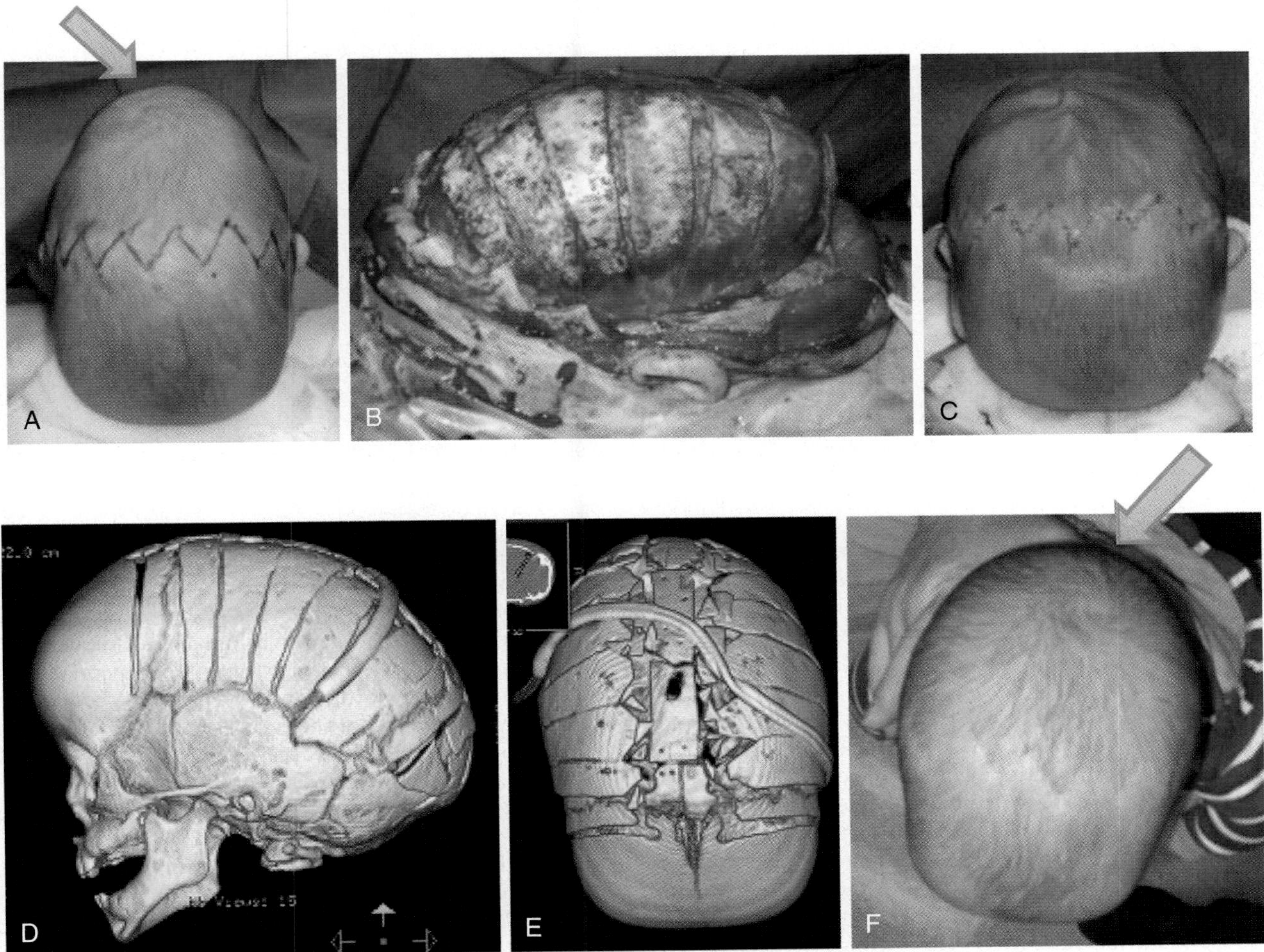

FIG. 69.4 Infant with sagittal suture craniosynostosis. (A) Preoperative view showing scaphocephalic head shape. The baby is in a prone position with the face resting on foam. Note the narrow biparietal dimension of the head, typical for this condition *(arrow)*. A zigzag coronal incision is designed to be better hidden once hair grows. (B) Intraoperative lateral view. The sagittal suture has been removed and reshaped, and lateral barrel stave osteotomies are created to reshape the cranial vault and to relieve growth restriction. (C) On-table view immediately after the procedure. The biparietal area is widened. (D and E) Lateral and superior views of the postoperative CT scan. (F) One month after surgery, the skull continues to remodel and the head shape normalizes *(arrow)*.

implementation of resorbable plates have allowed for improved outcomes and decreased morbidity in these patients.

Other less common congenital abnormalities of the head include agenesis of one or a number of layers of scalp or cranium. *Aplasia cutis congenita* usually refers to a focal defect of skin on the vertex. The defect may include any proportion of skin, bone, or dura. Treatment depends on the size of the defect and layers involved and may encompass local wound care or surgical reconstruction with flaps or grafts in infancy. The cause of this rare condition is unknown and likely varies from case to case. A classification system for aplasia cutis congenita has been developed and is related to the presence of other associated anomalies.

Congenital Ear Deformities

Congenital anomalies of the external ear may occur in isolation or as part of craniofacial microsomia. Common external ear deformities include prominent ears, constricted ears, cryptotia (failure of the upper pole of the ear to stand out from the head), and microtia (a small or abnormally formed outer ear). The most common type of microtia is a malformed vestigial cartilaginous structure associated with a soft tissue component of lobule. In cases of isolated microtia, there is often conductive hearing loss associated with absence of the external auditory canal. This is most important in bilateral cases in which a bone-anchored hearing aid is required.

Reconstruction of typical microtia can take two general approaches: autologous or nonautologous. Nonautologous reconstruction involves placement of a high-density polyethylene implant under the skin. This approach results in excellent results but requires harvest of a flap (commonly temporoparietal fascia flap based off the superficial temporal artery +/- skin grafting in certain cases). Disadvantages include the presence of a foreign body that may become exposed through the temporoparietal fascia flap or graft, susceptibility to infection, and difficulty with salvage in case of complications.[10] The second approach more commonly used involves the use of autologous tissue (rib cartilage) to shape an ear framework, which is then buried in a subcutaneous pocket. The meticulous shaping of the framework, creation of a thin skin pocket, and use of drains allow the skin to contour around the

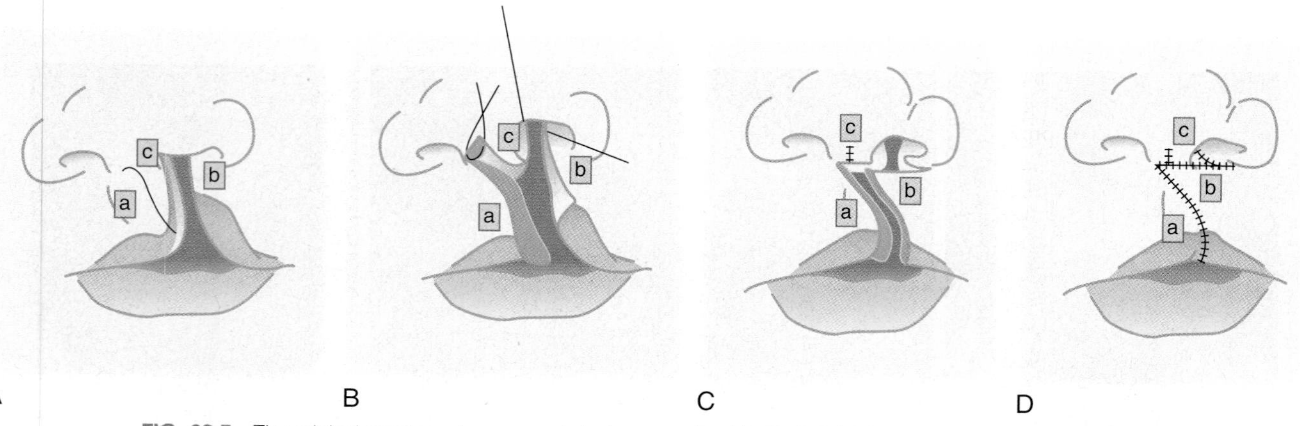

FIG. 69.5 The original rotation-advancement design conceived by D. Ralph Millard in Korea and presented at the First International Congress of Plastic Surgery in Stockholm in 1955. (From Losee JE, Kirschner RE. Comprehensive cleft care: Volume 1, Thieme, 2015.)

intricate framework. The procedure requires multiple stages but results in a reconstructed ear that has good form and is capable of responding to trauma and infection like other parts of the body. The disadvantage is the need to harvest cartilage from the multiple ribs.

Craniofacial Microsomia

Craniofacial microsomia, also known as hemifacial microsomia, is a constellation of abnormalities involving deficient development of parts of the face related to the first and second branchial arches. Deformity can be unilateral or bilateral and can involve the orbit, mandible, external ear, facial nerve, and facial soft tissue. Each or all of the structures may be involved and to varying degrees. The cause is unknown but is thought to be related to in utero vascular compromise of the stapedial artery. Treatment of craniofacial microsomia is complex, and the approach has to be tailored for individual patients. Functional problems, such as airway compromise or eye exposure, are treated in childhood; reconstruction of other structural defects is delayed until the patient is almost full-grown. Novel approaches using distraction osteogenesis of the mandible, pioneered by long bone distraction techniques by Ilizarov, have been modified by surgeons such as McCarthy and used to treat and avoid long-term complications in these patients.[11]

For patients with craniofacial anomalies such as those described as well as for those with cleft lip and palate, the current standard is team care at an established craniofacial center. With referral to a craniofacial center at birth, the craniofacial team can make a diagnosis, carry out genetic testing, educate the family, and outline short-term and long-term plans in a coordinated manner, bringing in multiple specialists (e.g., plastic surgeons, neurosurgeons, oral surgeons, orthodontists, speech pathologists, otolaryngologists, ophthalmologists, social workers, nurse practitioners, developmental psychologists, and pediatricians).

Cleft Lip and Palate

Cleft lip and palate are relatively common congenital anomalies. They may be unilateral or bilateral. Most are isolated anomalies, but many syndromes have clefts as one of the features. The genetics of cleft lip and palate is complex, and the condition is multifactorial. The pathophysiologic mechanism of cleft lip and palate is incompletely understood, but the deformity and its variations are well described. A minimum of three operations, and usually four, will be required to correct the deformity. These are performed at specific times corresponding to the developmental stage of the patient. Commonly the sequence is as follows: cleft lip repair at 3 to 6 months, cleft palate repair before 1 year (or before speech development), and alveolar bone graft when permanent dentition begins and after orthodontic preparation. Future surgeries are reserved for the end of skeletal maturity and include possible septorhinoplasty in the late teenage years, possible lip and nose revisions, and LeFort I maxillary advancement, if indicated. At times during these two stages, secondary procedures for speech improvement are done in almost 5% to 20% of the cases.[12]

A cleft lip is characterized by a partial or complete lack of circumferential continuity of the lip. Most cleft lips occur in the upper lip where one of the philtral columns normally lies, and they extend into the nose. The deformity involves the mucosa, orbicularis oris muscle, and skin. The nasal deformity is characterized by a slumped and widened ala (nostril) that is posteriorly misplaced at its base. The nasal floor is nonexistent in complete clefts, and the nasal septum is deviated.

There are many techniques for repair of a cleft lip, but most are a variation of the rotation-advancement repair. Millard introduced this technique of downward rotation of the medial portion of the lip and advancement of the lateral portion into the defect created by the rotation. The repair is based on the principle that existing elements need to be returned to their normal position to restore the normal anatomy while remaining cognizant of future growth and the effects of surgery on growth (Fig. 69.5).[13,14] Many leaders have modified their techniques and have adapted variations, which leads to the creativity and innovation of the field.

Cleft palate can also be complete or incomplete. The goals of palatal repair are the development of normal speech and prevention of regurgitation of food into the nose. Normal speech requires velopharyngeal competence to close the oral cavity off from the nasal cavity to produce pressure consonants. This requires static physical separation of the two cavities in the region of the hard palate and dynamic closure of the soft palate against the posterior pharyngeal wall with a functioning levator veli palatini muscle. In a cleft palate, the levator veli palatini muscle fibers are oriented abnormally along the cleft. Thus, all modern techniques of cleft palate repair involve repair of the nasal lining and oral mucosa and reorientation and repair of the levator veli palatini muscle. The primary measure of outcome of cleft palate repair is normal speech. The third procedure necessary in most cases is alveolar bone grafting. Cancellous bone, usually from the ilium, is used to restore bone continuity along the dental arch, allowing the teeth in the cleft edge a better chance of survival, and as a foundation for dental implants for missing teeth associated with the cleft, to close a nasolabial fistula (if present), and to produce support for the nasal base.

Other procedures are indicated for some patients, but this generally cannot be predicted in infancy. Approximately 15% of patients will continue to demonstrate velopharyngeal insufficiency after initial palate repair, and secondary palatal lengthening or other approaches to promote velopharyngeal closure are indicated typically after 3 to 5 years of age. Septorhinoplasty is usually necessary to correct residual nasal deformity after the cessation of skeletal growth and after final dental restoration and orthodontics. A subset of patients with unilateral cleft lip and palate will develop maxillary hypoplasia that is iatrogenic and related to scarring and growth retardation from lip and palate surgery. Depending on the degree of maxillary hypoplasia, LeFort I maxillary advancement after achieving skeletal maturity may be indicated. In sum, treatment of a child born with a cleft lip and palate does not end after palate repair but rather requires observation by a craniofacial team throughout development into adulthood and must be tailored for each individual.

Vascular Anomalies

Vascular anomalies are divided into two major groups: tumors and malformations. Vascular tumors are characterized by increased abnormal proliferation of endothelium. Hemangioma is the most common vascular tumor; others include hemangioendotheliomas, tufted angiomas, hemangiopericytomas, and malignant tumors such as angiosarcoma. Vascular malformations are the result of abnormal development of arterial, capillary, venous, or lymphatic components of the vascular system. They may involve only one component or may be mixed and are named for the component vessels. They can be high flow, low flow, or mixed. Correct diagnosis depends on the history (e.g., hemangiomas develop in infancy and are usually not visible at birth), physical examination (e.g., malformations with an arterial component may have a palpable pulse or thrill), and imaging to determine the extent of disease and to assist with making the diagnosis.

The natural histories of the different anomalies are diverse. Hemangiomas typically involute spontaneously; 50% involute completely by the age of 5 years. More recently, the quick treatment of infantile hemangiomas during the involution stage with beta blockers has resulted in a reduction in cases needing surgical intervention. Early treatment and natural history reduces the indications for surgery to those lesions that are affecting vision or the airway or are large enough that, even after involution, the abnormal remaining skin will require surgical modification. In contrast, capillary malformations start as patches, but over time, they typically enlarge and become thick and verrucous; for these lesions, early treatment is indicated. Some vascular malformations or tumors have systemic effects, depending on their mass, status as high or low flow, and thrombosis and consumption of coagulation factors. Treatment of these lesions involves complete resection, when feasible, or debulking if complete resection is not possible. Sclerotherapy is the mainstay of treatment of venous malformations. For arteriovenous malformations, sclerotherapy is useful as an adjunct to surgery but insufficient alone because of the development of collaterals. For these malformations, sclerotherapy and embolization are followed immediately by surgical resection.

Pediatric Neck Masses

Neck masses in the pediatric patient are most likely infectious or congenital noncancerous lesions. In addition to vascular malformations, other common pediatric neck masses include dermoid cysts, teratomas, branchial cleft anomalies, thyroglossal duct cysts, thymic cysts, ranulas, cartilaginous rests, heterotopic neuroectodermal tissue, neurofibromas, ectopic salivary tissue, lymphadenopathy, and malignant tumors. Branchial cleft anomalies may be cysts, sinuses, or fistulas. Cysts and sinuses are located in the anterior cervical triangle and are derived from the first cleft (near the external auditory meatus) and second cleft (below the hyoid) 98% of the time. The treatment of these lesions is surgical excision, and care must be taken due to the intimate association with neurovascular structures. Thyroglossal duct cysts may arise anywhere along the course of the thyroglossal duct from the foramen cecum at the base of the tongue to the thyroid gland. Thyroglossal duct cysts usually present in the first or second decade of life as painless anterior neck masses, and there may be an associated sinus track. Indications for surgery include recurrent infection, tissue diagnosis, and improved cosmesis. Thyroid scan is indicated before excision to rule out a functioning ectopic thyroid gland.

Melanocytic Nevi

Congenital melanocytic nevi are hamartomas consisting of nevus cells. Nevi are classified by size as small (<1.5 cm), medium (1.5–19.9 cm), large (20–49.9 cm), and giant (>50 cm). The classification dictates the prognosis and reconstructive approach. Risk of melanoma occurring in a melanocytic nevus varies by report but is estimated to be less than 5% in small or medium lesions and typically presents after puberty. In large and giant nevi, the reported risk of melanoma development is up to 10%.[11] Unlike the case for small or medium nevi, malignancy in large and giant nevi typically occurs in the first three years of life. Large and giant nevi also have an increased incidence of leptomeningeal involvement that can be diagnosed by magnetic resonance imaging (MRI). In addition, psychosocial and developmental issues associated with larger nevi are significant, so early excision and reconstruction are recommended for large and giant nevi.

Options for removal of larger nevi include serial excision, excision and grafting, excision and closure with distant flaps, and tissue expansion. Replacement with like tissue is the goal, and therefore tissue expansion is the mainstay approach.

PLASTIC SURGERY OF THE HEAD AND NECK

Maxillofacial Trauma

Facial trauma has decreased in frequency in the United States, and this is attributed in part to the advent of seat belt laws and improved collision safety. However, it remains part of multisystem trauma from motor vehicle accidents, assaults, and combat injuries. Improvements in body armor have resulted in better survival of combat injuries but proportionally more facial injuries.

Emergent Management

Surgical emergencies in the patient with facial trauma include airway compromise, life-threatening hemorrhage, and reversible structural injury to the eye or optic nerve. Other injuries, such as lacerations or extraocular muscle entrapment, are treated within the first 24 hours. Fractures are treated within the first 2 weeks. Evaluation of the patient with facial trauma follows the advanced trauma life support protocol and includes looking for intracranial trauma and cervical spine injury. Acute airway compromise usually occurs in the setting of combined mandibular-maxillary trauma with hemorrhage and soft tissue swelling. Endotracheal intubation should be attempted and need not be avoided because of concern about the facial injury. Nasotracheal intubation is contraindicated in the case of severe nasoorbitoethmoid and skull base fractures. Cricothyroidotomy is performed if oral or nasal endotracheal intubation is unsuccessful and should be converted to tracheostomy after the patient has been stabilized. Maxillomandibular fixation by itself is not an indication for tracheostomy because endotracheal intubation may be maintained through the nasal or oral route using an armored tube that can be routed behind the molars without kinking. An alternative technique is to exit the endotracheal tube through a submental incision, which alleviates some of the practical difficulties of working around an oral tube.

Life-threatening hemorrhage, defined as three units of blood loss or hematocrit below 29%, occurs in a small percentage of patients with facial trauma. In most cases, bleeding is effectively controlled with pressure, packing, and, in the case of significant soft tissue avulsion, rapid placement of temporary bolster sutures. Blind attempts to clamp and ligate vessels should be avoided because this is usually unnecessary and may result in injury to critical structures, such as the facial nerve. With penetrating trauma, hemorrhage is controlled in the operating room with vessel identification and ligation and, if that is unsuccessful, by angiographic selective embolization. With blunt trauma, severe hemorrhage is usually from the internal maxillary artery. The most effective way to control bleeding, especially when it is associated with midfacial fractures, is fracture reduction and stabilization. This can be accomplished quickly by temporary placement in maxillomandibular fixation using rapid techniques such as fixation screws. Severe hemorrhage from skull base and nasoethmoid fractures can often be controlled with anteroposterior nasal packing. Placement of Foley balloon catheters in each nasal airway serves to tamponade the bleeding and stabilizes the packing. Current protocols for control of hemorrhage in blunt facial trauma settings involve selective angiography if these measures fail (Fig. 69.6).[14] Angiographic embolization is effective but is associated with significant morbidity, including the possibility of stroke or necrosis of midfacial structures, such as the palate. In unstable patients, fracture reduction and nasal packing may be attempted on the angiography table to be followed immediately with embolization, if necessary.

Injuries to the orbit and contents can result in blindness; it is critical to recognize promptly and to treat reversible injuries that are vision threatening. Conditions that require emergent intervention include increased intraocular pressure, globe rupture, and optic nerve impingement. Acute increased intracranial pressure is manifested by pain and vision loss and can result from causes such as hematoma or decreased orbital volume because of fracture or a foreign body. Treatment involves rapid alleviation of intraocular hypertension by lateral canthotomy, inferior cantholysis, and administration of mannitol, acetazolamide (Diamox), and steroids. Urgent ophthalmology consultation is indicated. Vision loss may result from mechanical compression of the optic nerve. Computed tomography (CT) will diagnose the presence of a bone fragment or foreign body; such a finding should prompt emergent surgical decompression to preserve vision. Extraocular muscle entrapment presents as the inability to move the eye on the trajectory controlled by the entrapped muscle and is associated with pain on attempted motion. Especially in children, the pain may be severe and accompanied by nausea or vomiting. Muscle entrapment should be treated by surgical release of the entrapped contents. This should be done in the acute setting because delaying the treatment of entrapment for 1 week or longer after injury typically results in failure of the entrapped muscle to regain excursion.

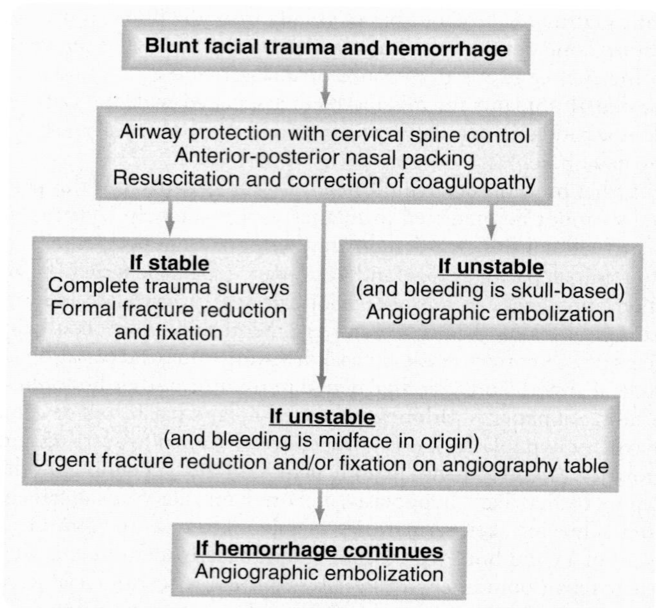

FIG. 69.6 Algorithm for the management of life-threatening hemorrhage in the setting of blunt facial trauma. (Adapted from Ho K, Hutter JJ, Eskridge J, et al. The management of life-threatening haemorrhage following blunt facial trauma. *J Plast Reconstr Aesthet Surg*. 2006;59:1257–1262.)

Evaluation and Diagnosis

The primary diagnostic studies for facial injury are physical examination and CT. Systematic physical examination can detect deformity, soft tissue injury, cerebrospinal fluid leak, and facial nerve injury. Palpation is used to identify bony stepoffs or midface instability. The eyes are examined for proptosis or enophthalmos, extraocular muscle function, and visual acuity. In patients who cannot cooperate with a physical examination and for whom there is reasonable suspicion of periorbital injury, a forced duction test should be performed. The occlusion is evaluated for subjective or objective malocclusion. Extraocular muscle entrapment, acute enophthalmos, and malocclusion are indications that surgical treatment of facial fractures will be required. Fine-cut CT of the face with direct or reformatted coronal and sagittal views and 3D reconstruction is used to diagnose facial trauma and to direct nonsurgical and surgical treatment. With current CT scanning technology, plain films are not necessary and provide less information. An exception is the Panorex, which is used by many physicians as an adjunct or primary study for mandible fractures and to assess teeth and their roots in particular.

Soft Tissue Injuries

Because of its rich blood supply, even questionable tissue should be salvaged in treating facial lacerations and avulsions. The robust perfusion of facial tissue provides resistance to infection, and repair can be done after a longer delay than would be safe elsewhere on the body. Although there is no strict cutoff, primary repair is generally done up to 24 hours after injury. Even grossly contaminated wounds or those from animal bites are irrigated extensively, debrided, and closed primarily. If there is the possibility of facial nerve injury, this is confirmed by the physical examination finding of weakness or absence of function of a portion of the muscles of facial expression. It is important to recognize a facial nerve laceration so that the distal cut ends can be identified with a nerve stimulator and tagged if they are not to be repaired immediately. Identification of distal stumps by nerve stimulation is not possible after a few days because conduction ceases. Parotid duct injuries should be identified and treated acutely to prevent the formation of sialocele or salivary fistula. In a sharp laceration or penetrating injury to the cheek, a parotid duct injury can be confirmed by direct visualization or injection of dye. This is done by cannulating the Stensen duct on the mucosal surface of the cheek and injecting a small amount of methylene blue dye. Extravasation of the dye into the wound indicates a parotid duct laceration, and repair over a stent should be done in the operating room.

Craniofacial Fractures

Current concepts in facial fracture treatment rest on craniofacial techniques to provide surgical exposure of the craniofacial skeleton, anatomic reduction of fractures, and rigid bone fixation with low-profile titanium plates and bone grafting techniques. Failure to reconstruct the bony facial skeleton invariably results in shrinkage and tightening of the facial soft tissue envelope, a sequela that is almost impossible to correct secondarily.

Treatment of forehead fractures involves assessment of the frontal sinus and cranial base. The approach is dictated by injury to the anterior or posterior table of the frontal bone or skull base and whether there is a dural injury or injury to the nasofrontal ducts that drain the frontal sinuses into the nose. Fractures of the upper midface include malar (zygoma) fractures, nasoorbitoethmoid fractures, and orbital fractures. There is considerable overlap in this region. For example, malar fractures occur in association with orbital fractures to a varying degree because the zygoma, in addition to producing cheek projection and determining facial width, is also part of the orbit. Treatment of fractures of the lower midface, the maxilla, focuses on the restoration of the preinjury dental occlusion. It is important to determine the patient's preoperative occlusion; the relationship of the upper and lower teeth is described by the Angle classification.

Maxillary fractures are classified using the LeFort system based on the level at which the midface is separated from the rest of the craniofacial skeleton. Repairs focus on the restoration of facial height and projection. With significant comminution or bone loss, bone grafting may be required to maintain the appropriate position of the maxilla in space. Rigid plate and screw fixation obviates the need for prolonged maxillomandibular fixation. Fractures of the mandible are treated by reduction and rigid fixation using restoration of occlusion as the principle intraoperative and postoperative goal. Many mandibular fractures are treated with open reduction and internal fixation, which may make maxillomandibular fixation unnecessary. Certain fractures, like those in younger patients or favorable fracture patterns, are best treated closed, and the decision to pursue an open or closed approach depends on the fracture location and orientation.[15]

The same principles of fracture repair apply in the pediatric patient with some differences. Early treatment within one week is necessary, given the rapid healing in children, and fixation is complicated by the presence of permanent teeth embedded in the maxilla and mandible that are easily damaged by hardware. Resorbable hardware is frequently used for children but does not have the mechanical strength required for most adult fractures. However, recent advances have allowed treatment of certain adult fractures such as orbit fractures with resorbable hardware, but this is still considered an off-label use.

Scalp Reconstruction

The scalp is composed of skin, subcutaneous tissue, an aponeurotic fascial layer continuous with the frontalis and occipital muscles, a loose areolar layer, and periosteum. Small defects up to a few centimeters in size may be closed primarily, depending on location of the defect and mobility of the surrounding scalp. A skin graft can be placed on intact periosteum. If periosteum is absent, the outer calvarial table can be opened with a burr to expose the diploic space from which granulation tissue will develop to support a skin graft. In the irradiated scalp or in the case of an open wound with alloplastic material at the base, secondary healing or grafting will not provide stable, durable coverage and a flap will be needed.

Scalp flaps are elevated at the subgaleal level, and many possible designs exist. In theory, defects as large as 30% of the scalp can be closed with scalp flaps elevated on major vessels. Incising, or scoring, the inelastic galea can extend the reach of a scalp flap. Tissue expansion also can be used for the reconstruction of larger defects with hair-bearing tissue.

For large scalp defects not amenable to closure by local remaining scalp, distant flaps may be used. Pedicled flaps with usefulness for scalp coverage include the trapezius, latissimus, and pectoralis major muscle flaps. Pedicled flaps are limited by their arc of rotation, so free microvascular tissue transfer offers more flexibility. The free latissimus dorsi muscle flap is preferred for coverage of near-total or total scalp defects because of its flat contour and ability to cover a large surface area. Traumatic scalp avulsions occur in the subgaleal plane, and replantation may be based on a single dominant vessel with good results.

Facial Reconstruction

Defects of the face are usually the result of tumor resection or trauma. STSG coverage of facial defects has limited application because the tissue match is imperfect. FTSGs are taken from donor sites in the preauricular, postauricular, and supraclavicular areas for the best color match. Local flaps provide tissue of appropriate thickness and have the color and texture of the defect.

Nasal defects up to approximately 1.5 cm can be closed with local nasal flaps. For larger defects, the forehead flap is preferred. The forehead flap is based on the supratrochlear vessels, and the reconstruction is performed in a staged fashion. The forehead may be expanded before elevation for closure of larger defects and to assist with primary closure of the donor defect. With nasal defects, different components may be lost, and restoration of skin, mucosal lining, and cartilage may be required. Composite grafts from the ear that contain skin and cartilage are useful for defects of the nasal ala. Reconstruction of total nasal defects is complex and may require bone grafting and free tissue transfer (Fig. 69.7).[16]

In the eyelid, FTSGs are a good option for skin loss alone. For a small, full-thickness lid defect, creating a V-shaped wedge can permit primary closure in layers. Adding a lateral canthotomy helps mobilize the lid margin for closure of larger defects, and, in some cases, the incision can be carried out into the temporal skin to mobilize the lid further. Eyelid defects can be repaired with flaps rotated from the other eyelid; this is useful to provide similar tissue. Extensive eyelid defects require support, typically in the form of a chondromucosal graft obtained from the nasal septum or external ear. The graft is placed and covered with a regional skin flap.

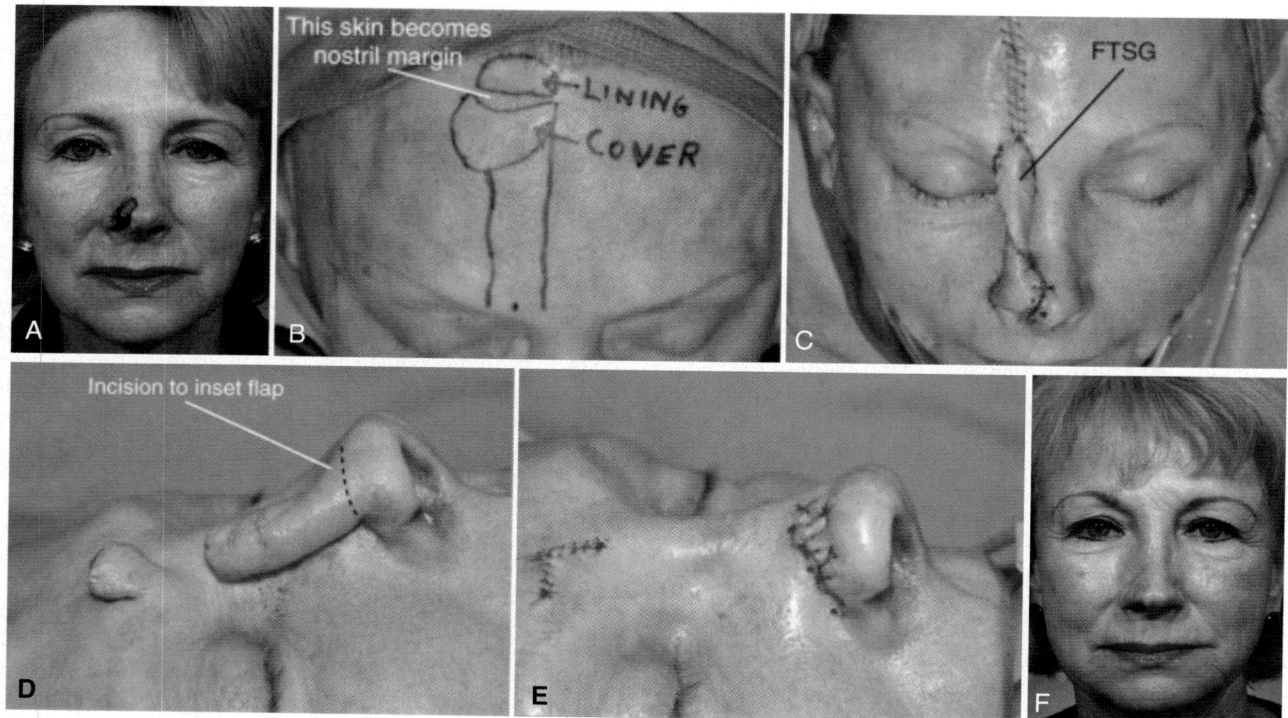

FIG. 69.7 (A) Full-thickness defect of nasal tip. (B) Paramedian forehead flap design with (intranasal lining, and external nasal skin). (C) First stage: paramedian forehead flap transferred to nose and inset. (D) Second stage: division of paramedian forehead flap. (E) Second stage: donor site is repaired and flap is inset. (F) Postoperative view. (From: Baker SR. Reconstruction of the nose. In: Baker S, ed. *Local Flaps in Facial Reconstruction*. 3rd ed. Philadelphia, PA: Elsevier Saunders; 2014:415–480.)

For reconstruction of the cheek, a number of different, smaller local flaps can be designed. For larger defects, cervicofacial rotation flaps mobilize skin from the neck and side of the face for transposition to the more central areas of the face.

In the lip, precise alignment of the vermilion border is critical, as is repair of the orbicularis oris muscle to maintain lip competence. Defects are closed in layers, and direct closure is possible for defects up to one third of the transverse width of the lip. Repair of larger defects requires mobilization of the surrounding tissue to reconstruct the oral sphincter. Central defects of the upper lip are best reconstructed using an Abbe flap, which is a mucosal musculocutaneous flap from the lower lip based on the labial artery. The flap is transferred in a staged fashion, with the donor pedicle divided 2 to 3 weeks after flap inset. Large defects of the lower lip are reconstructed with mucosal musculocutaneous flaps from the surrounding area. These reconstructions should preserve motor function of the orbicularis muscle, thus ensuring oral competence. Microstomia may be produced but is often temporary because the tissues will stretch over time.

Facial Transplantation

The first successful face transplantation was done in November 2005 in Amiens, France. Since then, there have been more than 40 additional reports of successful facial composite tissue transplantation. All were done for devastating defects and were complex 3D reconstructions with variable amounts of skin, muscle, nerve, bone, and parts, such as eyelids, noses, and lips. As of late 2018, almost all the recipients had experienced at least one episode of acute graft rejection of variable severity within the first year of transplantation, with one case of chronic rejection with subsequent second face transplantation. Functional recovery in the faces has been satisfactory in the long-term cases, with sensory function recovering at 3 to 8 months and acceptable motor recovery between 9 and 12 months with ongoing improvement over the years. Psychological outcomes have been positive, and this is related to the psychosocial support provided for these patients. Aesthetic outcomes have been variable.

The benefit of facial transplantation is that, for a select number of severely disfigured individuals, it can provide a better functional and aesthetic outcome than conventional reconstructive methods and, in doing so, improve their quality of life. The immediate risks associated with surgery to transplant facial tissues are essentially the same as those for conventional reconstructive procedures. The important difference is the risk posed by the lifelong, multidrug immunosuppression required to prevent rejection of the transplanted facial tissue. It is also assumed that there would be risks associated with the process of facial tissue rejection itself should that occur in any of these patients.[17]

Facial Aesthetic Surgery

Facial aesthetic surgery begins with a detailed initial interview, a complete medical history, and clinical examination to identify the appropriate candidates for treatment. It is important to determine the patient's wishes and to be sure that the patient has realistic expectations. History of prior cosmetic surgery, substance abuse, current medications, and mental or health problems may complicate the outcome of the planned procedures.

Brow Lift

Lateral eyebrow ptosis is the earliest manifestation of aging of the forehead and gives the face a tired, stern, and angry appearance. Brow ptosis needs to be addressed in conjunction with forehead wrinkles and hooding of the upper eyelid to rejuvenate the upper part of the face. With aging, the eyebrow descends below its youthful location at or above the superior orbital rim. This ptosis is accompanied by a wrinkled brow, excess tissue hooding of the upper eyelids (especially in the temporal brow area), and creasing at the outer canthi (crow's feet) and over the dorsum of the upper nose. To achieve good aesthetic results, a careful preoperative assessment of the surface anatomy and detailed assessment of the patient's desires are utilized. These alterations may be corrected using an endoscopic technique that uses several small incisions and allows extensive dissection between the galea and pericranium to correct the procerus, corrugator, and liberating the nose and periorbital attachments.[18] The open technique uses a bicoronal incision to achieve the same corrections and is more invasive. Brow ptosis can also be corrected using several techniques through combined procedures, for example, using the blepharoplasty incision or by using direct incisions in the brow area. Traditionally, the endoscopic and the open technique has been the standard of forehead rejuvenation because they effectively correct brow ptosis and forehead wrinkles, but their popularity has decreased due to scarring and alopecia. Recently, the use of less invasive procedures such as botulinum toxin injection and dermal fillers have been shown to produce high patient satisfaction and achieve similar results.

Blepharoplasty

Blepharoplasty is among the five most common aesthetic procedures. In 2012, 150,000 patients underwent this procedure in the United States. The majority of the patients are female (85%), and it is the most frequently performed aesthetic surgery performed between the ages of 51 to 64 years. The surgery is done to treat dermatochalasis, bagginess, and restoration of the youthful contour in the periorbital and malar region. It is considered one of the most challenging to learn and master, especially with regard to the lower eyelid. The approach to treat both eyelids is technically different. Upper blepharoplasty addresses the skin excess, eyelid ptosis, and sulcus deflation. Lower eyelid blepharoplasty corrects orbitomalar deformities. The procedure is commonly performed in an ambulatory setting and may be combined with some other aesthetical surgeries like a facelift. Preoperative evaluation should determine comorbidities, including hypertension, diabetes, and bleeding disorders. Smoking, drinking alcohol, abusing drugs, and psychologic alterations are additional risk factors. Antiplatelet and anticoagulation may be stopped 2 weeks preoperatively and up to 1 week after the operation. Ophthalmologic consultation is essential to determine history of trauma, dry eye, and previous corneal surgery. Previous corneal laser surgery may aggravate the xeropthalmia and prohibit the surgery. The recent trend in surgical technique is to preserve the volume. Techniques attempt to enhance the periocular area with fat injections, minimal removal of fat from eye compartments, and highly selective resection of the orbicularis oculi muscle.[19] Upper eyelid blepharoplasty is done through an incision in the crease of the eyelid after marking the degree of excess skin to prevent overresection and resultant lagophthalmos (inability to close the eye completely). A strip of orbicularis oculi muscle can be taken, and, if excess postseptal fat is present, this protruding orbital fat is resected. Lower eyelid blepharoplasty requires elevation of skin or skin–orbicularis oculi muscle flaps with removal of skin, muscle, and fat. A transconjunctival approach to the lower eyelid is used for removal of lower eyelid fat or orbital septum tightening with little or no skin resection. If the lower eyelid is lax and poorly adherent to the globe, a lateral canthopexy is done for mild laxity and a lateral canthoplasty is performed for significant laxity. Dry eye syndrome, scleral show, and ectropion are common complications after blepharoplasty. Ectropion is eversion of the lower eyelid with exposure of the conjunctiva and may need surgery if it is persistent beyond the postoperative period.

Rhinoplasty

Rhinoplasty broadly refers to surgery of the nose that can be done to improve aesthetics and function.[20] Preoperative evaluation of the patients undergoing rhinoplasty should include aesthetic, functional, and psychological evaluation. The goal in rhinoplasty is to produce reliable, long lasting, and natural-appearing results with consistency. Assessing the functional alterations can be performed by objective anatomic measures with radiographic studies. The aesthetic considerations of the nose are complex. The evaluation needs to address four different views: frontal, lateral, basal, and internal. Specific measurements and the relation to the facial context are important. Also, determining the nasal length, width, and the nasofacial harmony between ethnic groups. Assessing the nasal bones, the bony pyramid, the dorsum, the septum, and the relation to the upper lip and the chin are all considered when assessing a patient. The position of the nasal tip, activation of the depressor septi nasi muscle, and asymmetries of the length of the columella are some of the most important aspects to be addressed and discussed in the preoperative period. Rhinoplasty is one of the most difficult operations because it is a composite of procedures performed on a number of anatomic structures. After a careful examination, diagnosis, and proposed surgical plan, each procedure must be patient specific. Generally, two approaches exist: one is the open rhinoplasty, which allows complete ion exposure and ability to correct the anatomic elements under direct vision. The closed rhinoplasty or endonasal does not provide direct vision of the structures but avoids a visible scar.[20] The surgical management is directed to resection of the dorsal hump and creation of a smooth and regular dorsum. Osteotomies are indicated to close and open roof deformity, decrease the nasal bony width, and straighten the deviated nasal pyramid after correction of septal deviation. Tip refinements and projection improvement can be performed with cephalic trim of alar-lateral cartilages and techniques suturing the lateral, medial crural, and applying transdomal and interdomal sutures which increase tip projection. Complications of rhinoplasty include patient dissatisfaction, iatrogenic deformities, airway obstruction, hypertrophic scaring, fibrosis, inclusion cyst, granulomas, infection, and extrusions of autogenous and alloplastic materials. Bleeding occurs in 3.6% of the patients early in the postoperative period. The greater challenge is the 5% to 10% of patients that require revision or a secondary surgery for aesthetic or functional reasons. The use of dermal fillers and fat may help to improve preoperative planning and aid in decreasing postoperative deformities.

Facelift

Rhytidectomy, derived from the Greek *rhytis*, meaning "wrinkle," is designed to correct the appearance of facial aging by removing lax, redundant facial and neck tissues. The American Society of Plastic Surgeons reported that 125,697 facelifts were performed in 2017, making the facelift the sixth most popular cosmetic surgery procedure performed. Facial aging is characterized by midface infraorbital flattening, prominent nasolabial folds, deepening of the labiomental crease, downturn of the lateral commissures of the mouth, deepening grooves at the outer corners of the mouth (marionette lines), jowl formation, vertical banding of the platysma muscles in the neck, and laxity of the neck skin. As with any other aesthetic procedure, the history and clinical examination plays a key role in preventing complications.

Several techniques have been described and utilized for achieving patient-specific results. The subcutaneous facelift is the traditional operation and includes dissection, redraping, and excision of skin on the face and neck. Through detailed anatomic studies and the work of Skooog, Mitz, and Peyronie, the superficial musculoaponeurotic system (SMAS) was utilized for correction of deeper tissues and structures of the face. The SMAS can be resected, plicated, and manipulated to create different results. Also, some combined techniques can undermine deeper planes, reaching the periosteum.

Ancillary procedures can be added to enhance the outcome of a facelift. Submental lipectomy removes the subcutaneous fat, improving the neck contour. Plication of the platysma corrects vertical banding by incising the platysma muscles at the level of the thyroid cartilage and suturing them together in the midline of the upper neck. Fat injection to selected areas under the facelift flaps before closure can fill hollows caused by subcutaneous fat atrophy in areas such as the temple.

Hematoma is the most common complication after facelift; other complications include scarring, alopecia, skin slough, and nerve injury. The most common nerve injury during facelift, occurring at a rate of 3% to 5%, involves the greater auricular nerve, which provides sensation to the lower ear.[21]

Hair Transplant

Hair transplantation may offer a permanent improvement in a stable and medically controlled patient with alopecia. Invasive procedures to decrease scalp size and reorientation of large hair-bearing-skin flap are now less commonly used. Hair restoration continues to evolve to obtain better cosmetic and durable results. Hair transplantation using follicular units has become the mainstay of surgical treatment. Modern hair transplantation utilizes small punch biopsies (0.8 mm–1.2 mm) to harvest the follicular units. In some cases, a computerized and robotic harvesting allows one to obtain 1500 grafts per hour with minimal scarring. After graft harvest, it is important to maintain the metabolic needs, ionic, and osmotic balance to reduce cellular death by apoptosis or reperfusion injury. The use of bioenhancement solutions maintains the cells during the early grafting phase when nutrients are obtained by inosculation.

The procedure can be performed on an outpatient basis with mild sedation and local anesthesia. Several sessions may be performed, it takes 5 to 8 hours to transplant 800 to 1000 follicular units, and a mega session may transplant 3000 to 6000 follicular units. Special attention has been devoted to the angle and the orientation in the scalp of the transplanted follicular unit. After the transplant, patients may continue to lose hair and several treatments may help to prevent it, including the use of bioenhancements, platelet-rich plasma, and lasers that may stimulate hair growth. Important research using growth factors, stem cells, and manipulation of genetic signals may help to understand more about cellular control and hair growth.[22]

Nonsurgical Modalities

Skin resurfacing. Minimally invasive cosmetic procedures continue to increase every year. Several skin resurfacing treatments are available to improve the texture, tone, and color of the skin. These include chemical peeling, which uses specific agents that cause superficial, medium, or deep exfoliation commonly used to remove the signs of photodamage, actinic damage, melasma, acne, and rosacea. Other procedures are microneedling and dermabrasion, but the most rapidly growing technique for skin rejuvenation is laser technology. The use of light as a medical treatment was introduced in the 1960s with the development of the light amplification by stimulated emission of radiation (laser). Ablative lasers (CO_2 and erbium:YAG) have proved highly effective for skin treatment. Removing the epidermis and upper layers of the dermis through ablation, combined with thermal coagulation of the dermis, allows healing with robust dermal remodeling that translates into clinical improvement. The problem was resultant scarring in some patients, prolonged edema and erythema, permanent pigmentation abnormalities, and increased risk of infection. Thus, a new concept of fractional photothermolysis was introduced in 2003 that has revolutionized laser surgery. Fractional CO_2 laser resurfacing represents a new class of therapy by delivering dermal coagulative injury without confluent epidermal damage. Distinct lesions of thermal damage are surrounded by larger zones of undisturbed normal skin; this combination allows complete reepithelialization within 24 to 48 hours while producing enough coagulation of the dermal collagen to stimulate connective tissue synthesis and to produce skin tightening. With the fractional approach, results are comparable to those with full-surface ablative lasers without the associated side effects. The indications for laser resurfacing are facial rhytides, sun-damaged skin, and acne scarring. Benefits of treatment include softening or disappearance of mild to moderate wrinkles, improved skin texture and tone, decreased pore size, and reduction of skin laxity. The entire face, neck, and chest can be treated. Clinical improvement is seen with one or two treatments, scarring and hypopigmentation are rare, and the risk of infection in patients given prophylactic antiviral and antibiotic medications is low because the epidermal layer is restored promptly. When used to treat scars, fractional photothermolysis can flatten out and smooth hypertrophic scars and increases collagen production beneath depressed, atrophic scars, which summate in smoothing of the skin topography. For scarring, a series of treatments at 6-week to 12-week intervals may be needed (Fig. 69.8).[23]

Injectables. Over recent years, there has been increasing use of dermal fillers to improve facial appearance and rejuvenation. Dermal fillers are used to correct wrinkles and to increase volume in several areas of the face. Most common are the glabellar, horizontal forehead, and lateral brow lines in the upper part of the face and the nasojugal and nasolabial fold, the cheeks, the chin, and the perioral wrinkles in the mid and lower portions of the face. Fillers can be autologous or nonautologous. Fillers may be further classified according to the effect in time (nonpermanent, permanent).

Autologous fat transfer has been shown to improve rejuvenation effects, improve skin appearance, eliminate or decrease wrinkles, decrease pore size, and improve skin pigmentation. Fat is also used to improve scars, depressions, asymmetries, areas of radiation damage, chronic ulcers, and burn scars.

Nonautologous material derived from organic sources offers the benefits of "off-the-shelf" availability and ease of use, but may introduce other problems like sensitization to foreign proteins and immunogenicity. The search during the last few years has been for new materials that are better tolerated and have greater longevity. The two major types of biologic tissue fillers are collagen products and hyaluronic acid products. Synthetic materials can offer permanence. Many injectable and surgically implantable synthetic products have been used over the years, and many have been condemned for complications. Adverse effects after soft tissue

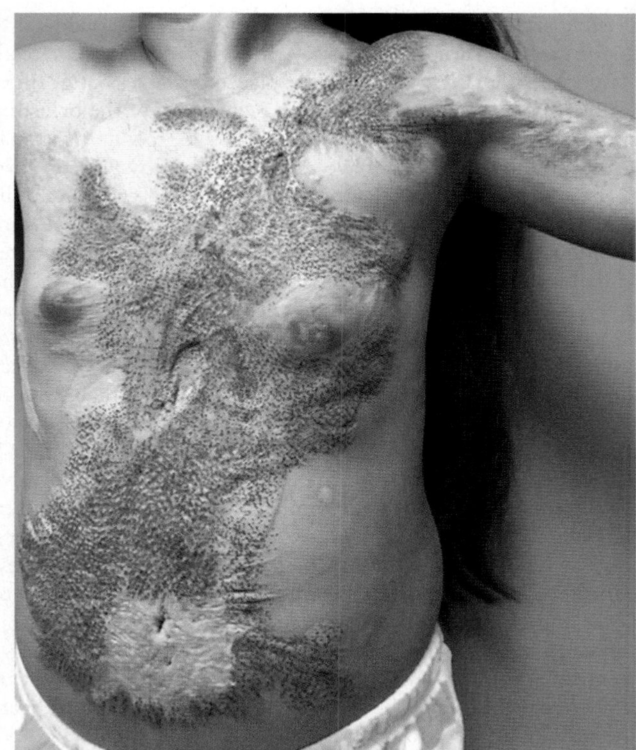

FIG. 69.8 A child 1-week postoperative after a CO_2 laser resurfacing procedure.

augmentation with fillers may be seen early (after the injection), late (14 days–1 year), and delayed (after 1 year). Early common complications are area bruising, edema, erythema, and tissue necrosis due to vascular compression or occlusion.

Several proposed actions to understanding, avoiding, and managing severe complications have been described: using nonsharp cannulas and low-pressure technique, injecting small boluses, aspirating prior to injection, detailing anatomic awareness, and using local anesthesia with epinephrine, which produces vasoconstriction and reduces the arterial lumen. The use of hyaluronidase in case of hyaluronic acid injection vascular occlusion may help in vascular occlusion and territorial necrosis. Another described severe complication is central retinal artery embolism resulting in blindness. Late and delayed adverse effects include the presence of nodules, granulomas, chronic infections, and inflammatory reactions due to biofilm formation that may require surgery in the future.[24,25]

BREAST SURGERY

Reduction Mammoplasty

Hypertrophy or overgrowth of the breast is excessive development without any pathologic process. Reduction mammoplasty is the resection of excess fat, breast tissue, and skin to achieve a breast size proportional to the body. The principles guiding reduction mammoplasty for breast hypertrophy are to improve the patient's symptoms, decrease the volume of the breast, to reshape the breast to correct ptosis, to elevate the breast tissue to an anatomically correct position on the chest wall, to reposition the nipple and areola on the reduced and reshaped breast, to preserve the nerve supply to the skin and nipple-areola complex, to maintain blood supply to the breast tissue, and to minimize scars. This procedure addresses both physical symptoms and psychological distress in patients. The American Society of Plastic Surgery reports that 101,192 breast reductions were performed in 2014. The satisfaction rate of this procedure remains extremely high with 97.5% of patients reporting overall satisfaction.

Surgical techniques are described by the location of the block of tissue to which the nipple and areola are left attached and by the pattern of incisions and subsequent scars. The patterns refer to the incisions used to access the different parenchymal pedicles. The pedicle is the portion of the breast tissue preserved with its blood and nerve supply while the surrounding breast tissue is removed.

The Wise pattern is used in almost 80% of the cases with the inferior pedicle used in 59% of the cases. Other variants include the central, superior, medial, lateral, and doubly attached vertical and horizontal pedicles. Other pedicles have grown in favor, like the superior pedicle used in 13.3% of patients and the medial pedicle used in 19.5% of patients. Although no differences have been found between using a T-shaped scar and using a vertical scar in complications, the vertical scar has had a recent surge of interest after the study by Lejour. Vertical reductions are based on the blood supply of the superior and/or medial pedicles.

In very large breast or gigantomastia, the pedicle would be too long, and there is an increased risk of ischemia and necrosis of the nipple-areola complex, thus frequently an amputation style technique or a reduction with subsequent free nipple graft is employed. Suction-assisted lipectomy is used to remove excess fat laterally, and there are a small number of patients with mild to moderate hypertrophy, fatty breasts, good skin tone, no ptosis, and good breast shape for whom liposuction alone will reduce volume.

Before a breast reduction is performed, a mammary breast cancer screening is usually done in patients 35 year of age or older. In patients younger than 50 years, the decision to perform a preoperative mammogram should be individualized by family history of breast cancer, genetics, and the presence of mass on examination. Several aspects of the standard of care have changed in breast reduction. Modern advances in anesthesia and more efficient health care showed that 85% of breast reductions are performed at an ambulatory surgery center or basis with inpatient admissions for patients with significant comorbidities. The majority of the procedures are under general anesthesia, recommend stopping oral contraception 1 month before the surgery. Early postoperative ambulation and the use of graduated compression stockings is mandatory. High-risk patients and patients undergoing multiple procedures should receive perioperative chemoprophylaxis to reduce the incidence of venous thrombosis outweighing the risk of hematomas that can be as high as 5.1% of the cases. The use of epinephrine on the incision lines has demonstrated the reduction of blood loss and the need of transfusions, although no significant difference in the hematoma formation has been found. The use of drains had led no difference in hematoma rates, although there has been a trend to use less drains. The most frequent complications after reduction mammoplasty are alterations in the nipple-areola sensibility, hematoma, seroma, wound dehiscence, and fat and skin necrosis.[26]

Mastopexy

Breast ptosis describes the downward displacement of the glandular tissue of the breast.

Skin laxity, poor elasticity, impairments in the fascial and suspensory ligaments may induce dropping of the breast. Breast ptosis–related factors are pregnancy, lactation, postmenopausal involution, weight loss, and aging. Breast ptosis is classified by the position of the nipple-areola complex relative to the inframammary fold and breast mound. Several classification systems exist, and the most widely used is the Regnault classification. In grade 1 or minor ptosis, the nipple position is at the level of the inframammary fold. In grade 2 or moderate ptosis, the nipple is located below the inframammary fold. In grade 3 or major ptosis, the nipple and the lower contour of the breast is below the inframammary fold. Several options are available to correct breast ptosis with mastopexy by breast reduction or breast augmentation techniques. The markings and the techniques are similar to those used for breast reduction. The challenge with mastopexy is balancing tightening with restoration of volume. The effects of surgery are only temporary, and ptosis recurs with the passage of time.[27]

Breast Augmentation

Augmentation mammoplasty is the most popular cosmetic procedure performed with high patient satisfaction. This procedure is done to resolve the dissatisfaction that some women feel with small breasts, either because their breasts never developed to a desired size or because their breasts lost volume after pregnancy or weight loss or with aging. Silicone gel breast implants were developed by Cronin and Gerow in 1963. The U.S. Food and Drug Administration (FDA) has approved numerous devices with regards to breast implants, new generations of saline implants, and highly cohesive form-stable silicone implants. Newer gel implants are thicker, more viscous, and cohesive and tend to stay in place, even if the shell of the implant is damaged or ruptured. Saline-filled implants are silicone rubber shells filled in the operating room. Advantages of the saline implants are the benign nature of saline, some flexibility in adjusting size by varying the amount of fluid put in the implant, and smaller incisions because the implants are inserted while empty. The primary disadvantage is a higher incidence of rippling or wrinkling of the implant under the skin and deflation. Comprehensive patient education is paramount, and detailed information about implant complications and operative complications should be discussed. Perioperative complications are relatively low, with bleeding or hematoma occurring in 1% to 3% of patients, wound infections occurring in 1% to 2% of patients, and some degree of diminished sensibility of the nipple-areola complex occurring in approximately 15% of patients, depending on the incision used and the position of the implant relative to the muscle. More numerous and more serious are the sequelae presenting weeks or years after the surgery. These include capsular contracture, implant deflation, implant rupture, implant displacement, and other evolving conditions.

Smooth implants are used in approximately 90% of patients in the United States. About 60% of the implants used today are silicone-filled implants. Smooth implants are more prone to capsular contracture when placed in the subglandular plane. Superior aesthetic results using anatomic implants remain unproven and, in case of implant rotation, may require an additional surgery. An implant profile is a variable to achieve greater volume in patients with a narrow chest. Incisions options and indications vary: the inframammary technique is the most commonly used and provides excellent access without dissection of the mammary parenchyma, although the incision may be noticeable. The use of nipple shields has become a common strategy for preventing bacterial contamination during implant insertion. Also, the no-touch technique with glove changes and insertion funnels may decrease rates of capsular contracture. Periareolar incision heals without visible scarring, may alter nipple-areola sensation, and has been associated with an increased risk of capsular contracture due to the less sterile nipple-areola area contents. Axillary incision leaves no visible scar on the breast and is ideal for saline implants. The implant can be placed in either of the subglandular, subfascial, or submuscular planes. Submuscular placement gives better superior upper pole aesthetics and better visualization of the breast by mammography and has less chance for development of capsular contracture, although they have more postoperative discomfort, longer recovery, and potential for breast distortion with pectoralis contraction. Hematoma and infection occur in less than 1% of the patients and should be considered potential problems after augmentation mammoplasty. Impairment of the sensibility of the nipple-areola complex is more frequent when bigger implants are used and in aggressive lateral pocket dissections. Secondary or revision surgery ranges from less than 1% to 36% over a 10-year period. It is commonly attributed to implant failure, malposition, and capsular contracture, which can be observed in 5% to 8% of the patients after 3 years and in 11% to 19% of patients after 8 to 10 years. Saline-filled implants can deflate through the valve or as a result of damage to the implant shell. This occurs in approximately 7% of patients within the first 5 years after surgery. Causes include damage from handling at the time of surgery, pressure from capsular contracture, compression of the implant due to trauma, and other reasons that remain unknown.[28]

Silicone gel implants can rupture, but the highly cohesive newer implants may prevent releasing of the gel. Thus, it is recommended that gel implants be studied by MRI at intervals of 3 years and every 2 years after to detect silent ruptures.

A new and more accepted option with use of acellular dermal matrix has been used for secondary breast surgery in the case of capsular contracture, malposition, rippling, and palpability with high success, although the material cost has limited its acceptance.

Implant Selection

Implant selection is important, and comprehensive detailed patient education about the size (volume and diameter) is a critical aspect of the selection. The surgeon must determine the size according to the height, weight, chest configuration, and breast anatomy. Another important selection is the shape, profile, and surface texture. Round implants are used in 95% of patients in the United States. Implant profile (normal, intermediate, and higher) may be used depending on the size of the chest and may aid in achieving maximum volume and projection in patients with narrow chests. Smooth implants are more commonly used and related to more capsular contracture when placed in the subglandular space. Surface texture implants have been shown to reduce capsular contracture but are associated with chronic inflammation and recently have been linked to breast implant–associated anaplastic large cell lymphoma (BIA-ALCL).[29,30]

Fat Grafting to the Breast

Autologous fat injection has become a popular procedure in both cosmetic and reconstructive plastic surgery. The use of autologous fat grafting began with efforts to correct soft tissue deformities and facial rejuvenation in the mid-1990s. In 1997, 2007, and 2009, respectively, the American Society of Plastic and Reconstructive Surgeons, the American Society of Plastic and Aesthetic Plastic Surgeons, and the American Society of Plastic Surgeons stated that autologous fat transfer may compromise the detection of breast cancer and should be administered with caution in patients with high risk of breast cancer. Also, they strongly support the ongoing research efforts that will establish the safety and efficacy of the procedure. The role of fat tissue transfer in cosmetic and reconstructive breast surgery will continue to evolve and today is used for correction lumpectomy after surgical breast reconstruction. Its use on breast augmentation, breast enhancement with mastopexy, and to correct breast asymmetry due to congenital deformity has gained popularity recently. The lack of standardization in the harvest and surgical technique may lead to patient dissatisfaction and the need of reoperations due to fat reabsorption. Fat reabsorption occurred frequently early in the postoperative period and questions the durability of the procedure. The most common reported complications are fat necrosis, lumps, cyst, and capsular contracture. Many questions need to be addressed in fat harvest, processing, preparation, and placement that may help to create a standardized technique. More studies are needed to expand the knowledge of adipose-derived stem cells.[31,32]

Breast Implant-Associated Anaplastic Large Cell Lymphoma

BIA-ALCL has been associated with breast implants, and many factors are involved in its pathophysiology, including textured implants, bacterial biofilm formation, immune response, and patient genetics. The first case of BIA-ALCL was documented in 1997. No cases have been reported from the pretexture era. Half of the cases occurred in breast reconstruction. The incidence is debated, but the prevalence appears to be increasing. The mean age at onset is in the fifth decade, with implants having been in place for at least 10 years. The most common clinical presentation is a late periimplant effusion or seroma 1 year after implantation. Axillary lymphadenopathy was reported in 10% of the cases, and axillary metastasis was reported in 14% of cases. In comparison with patients with silicone implants, patients with textured implants have a higher rate of being diagnosed with BIA-ALCL. More recently, the use of texture anatomic silicone implants were removed from the European market. Ultrasound is the first choice of methods to use in cases of breast swelling and can be used to guide fine-needle aspiration. MRI is also used. Cloudy fluid and cytologic analysis of the periprosthetic fluid will show large pleomorphic, epithelioid lymphocytes with kidney shape nucleus and prominent nucleolus. BIA-ACLC is CD30 positive, and it is expressed on activated B and T cells. Confirmed cases need to be reported to the American Society of Plastic Surgery, an organization that closely collaborates with the FDA. Once diagnosis is made, staging is done with positron emission tomography (PET)/CT. Surgical treatment includes removal of the implant, complete removal of any mass with negative margins, and capsulectomy. There does not appear to be a role for sentinel lymph node biopsy. Some patients may have some form of chemotherapy and adjuvant therapy. Patients with more advance disease should be referred to a medical oncologist for further treatment.[33]

Gynecomastia

Gynecomastia, or excessive development of the male breast, is a common deformity encountered in the adolescent and adult male. The etiology is multifactorial, and the most frequent cause is idiopathic. The prevalence ranges from 38% to 64% in young patients and occurs bilaterally in 50% to 55% of cases. The pathophysiologic mechanism involved is still unknown. There is an imbalance of estradiol and testosterone that may resolve without intervention. Pathologic gynecomastia may be associated with cirrhosis, malnutrition, renal disease, hypogonadism, and thyroid diseases. Also, gynecomastia can be seen in testicular, adrenal, and pituitary tumors and in lung carcinoma. Drug abuse and several pharmacologic agents may induce gynecomastia. Several classifications may correlate the surgical treatment with the breast enlargement, the kind of tissue, and the skin redundancy. In the normal adult male, no breast tissue can be palpated. Most patients with gynecomastia are asymptomatic. Symptoms may be soreness and nipple sensitivity. Clinical evaluation should be thorough to determine the etiology. Indications for surgery include symptomatic gynecomastia persisting for more than 18 to 24 months in adolescent boys, gynecomastia of prolonged duration that has progressed to fibrosis, and gynecomastia in patients at risk for breast cancer (e.g., those with Klinefelter syndrome). Surgical treatment for gynecomastia can address excision of breast tissue, suction/assisted liposuction, skin resection, or a combination of these procedures. Liposuction may be sufficient in fatty tissue accumulation. Open incisional technique in the areolar area may allow the surgical adenectomy. In cases of skin redundancy and ptosis, an inframammary approach with and without nipple-areola transposition can be done. In severe cases of massive gynecomastia, patients may need a free nipple graft after bloc resection. Common complications include hematomas, seromas, infections, and areolar and flap ischemia-necrosis.[34]

ABDOMINOPLASTY

Abdominoplasty continues to be among the common aesthetic procedures performed for aesthetic and reconstructive purposes. Patients present with excess adiposity, skin laxity, muscle diastasis, and striae. The procedure may be combined with liposuction to the anterior abdomen and trunk. The operation removes the excess sagging tissue through a lower horizontal skin incision. Muscle and fascia plication correct muscle diastasis. Depending of the amount of tissue to be excised, the procedure can be a mini-abdominoplasty, panniculectomy, and full or complete abdominoplasty. The anterior abdominal flap includes skin and subcutaneous tissue, and the flap elevation goes from the pubic hairline to the xiphoid-costal margin. The umbilicus may be left attached to the muscle fascia with the creation of a new opening for exteriorization. Several types of incisions have been used, and the horizontal lower abdominal incision is the most frequently used. The Fleur-de-lis abdominoplasty uses an inverted T type incision that is used in large resections with greater midline abdominal fullness. The corset abdominoplasty, or the I band, has also been employed for improved outcomes in massive weight loss patients. Abdominal scars from previous operations should be evaluated and may cause ischemia and necrosis in the abdominal flap. No evidence exist with respect to the use of prophylactic antibiotics; however, the current standard is to give a dose prior to the incision and every 4 hours during the surgery. Adequate perioperative pain control with multimodal analgesia is critical to prevent complications and patient satisfaction. Higher risk of complications are observed in diabetic patients and patients with a BMI greater than 30 kg/m^2. The most frequent minor complications are surgical site infections, seroma, hematoma, and wound dehiscence. Progressive tension sutures continue to gain support to reduce the incidence of seroma. Smokers are at high risk for infectious complications. Major complications including necrosis of the abdominal flap, deep venous thrombosis, and pulmonary embolus are more frequent when surgery is combined with intraabdominal and gynecologic procedures. Routine chemoprophylaxis is not indicated in patients with a low risk. The use of intermittent pneumatic compression devices has been shown to be superior to elastic compression stockings. Chemoprophylaxis for venous thromboembolism needs to be considered on a case-by-case basis in patients with Caprini scores greater than 8.[35,36]

Body Contouring After Bariatric Surgery

Body contouring has become a plastic surgery subspecialty to treat a variety of deformities in the massive weight loss patient. These

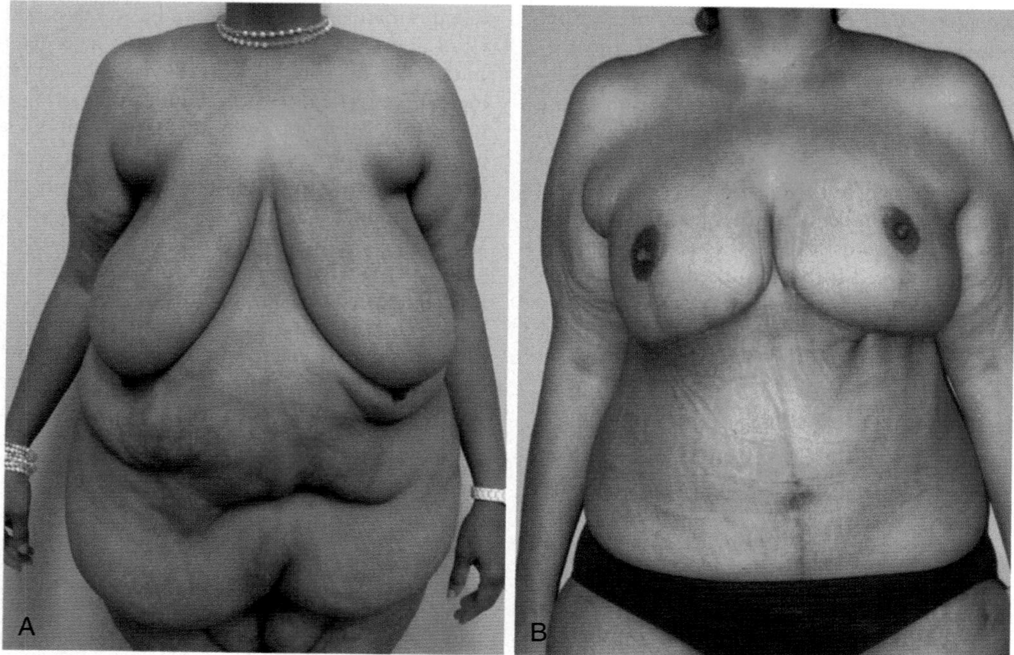

FIG. 69.9 Abdominoplasty and mastopexystatus post–massive weight loss. (A) Preoperative view. (B) Postoperative view after 1 year.

body contouring alterations were not commonly seen by plastic and reconstructive surgeons in the past. After massive weight loss, the patient is left with excess skin and subcutaneous tissue that fails to retract and hangs from the torso, abdomen, and extremities (Fig. 69.9). Skin redundancy may be painful, limits mobility, and is susceptible to infection in the intertriginous areas. Weight loss patients may have metabolic alterations that require special and detailed preoperative workup and evaluation. An important part of the medical history is the patient's motivation, concerns, and expectations. Psychological assessment is important to clear unrealistic expectations, body dysmorphic disorders, and eating disorders. Obesity is defined as having a body mass index (BMI) greater than 30 kg/m^2. Because there is a strong correlation between higher BMI and complications with surgery, before surgery is planned, 12 to 18 months after bariatric surgery, the patient is required to maintain weight stability for at least 6 months. Proper nutritional assessment of the patient is needed to determine protein, iron, and vitamin deficiencies. Smoking is a well-known risk factor for ischemic complications and delayed wound healing. At least 4 weeks of tobacco abstinence is required, and the patient must comply with preoperative negative urine for nicotine prior to the operation. It is important to rule out any pulmonary and cardiac diseases, as well endocrinopathies, hematologic alterations, and the presence of abdominal and inguinal hernias. To obtain informed consent, the surgeon needs to have a detailed discussion with the patient to emphasize the tradeoff of permanent scars for improved body contour. Discussion of the excisional stage surgeries and the potential complications is required.

Common complications include infections, bleeding, fluid collections, skin necrosis, wound dehiscence, asymmetric scars, irregular contour, and venous thromboembolism. A massive weight loss patient may have skin alterations that include poor elasticity and loss of tone. The surgery needs to be performed in multiple stages; combining too many procedures at once has an increased risk of complications. One upper body procedure can be combined with a lower circumferential body lift in patients with a BMI less than 30 kg/m^2 and a good medical profile (Fig. 69.10). Staging procedures can be planned every 3 to 6 months. Venous thromboembolism can be reduced by educating the patient, assessing the risk, and using preventative measures that include the use of mechanical and chemical prophylaxis. Several abdominal contouring procedures are well described to address specific areas. The mini-abdominoplasty resects the skin below the umbilicus to correct limited infraumbilical laxity. Panniculectomy is a functional procedure in which skin and subcutaneous abdominal tissue is excised to relieve symptoms of intertrigo without addressing the rectus diastasis and without preserving the umbilicus. Abdominoplasty can be performed in a traditional way and as reverse abdominoplasty. This is a more laborious procedure, planned to improve the abdominal contour, fixing the diastasis of the rectus with a well-concealed scar and a natural umbilicus. Vertical abdominoplasty (fleur-de-lis) is used to correct the epigastric skin laxity and the multiple abdominal folds.

Upper trunk contouring procedures reshape the breast using adjacent tissue, fat grafting, and implants. Mastopexy techniques for breast ptosis with and without implants are used. In some cases free nipple grafting can be done. Upper back rolls may be excised using bilateral longitudinal or oblique scars. Brachioplasty and medial thigh lift are designed to reshape the arm and the thigh, respectively, excising a long ellipse of excess tissue. Lower body lift procedures may include the belt lipectomy that may help to reshape the buttocks. Body contouring procedures after bariatric surgery have a tremendous impact on massive weight loss patients' lives, helping them to maintain weight loss, achieve better body shape, and improve their psychological wellness.[37]

Liposuction

Liposuction, also known as lipoplasty or lip sculpture, is the surgical removal of adipose tissue through the use of metal cannulas. The procedure was introduced in late 1970s and since then has

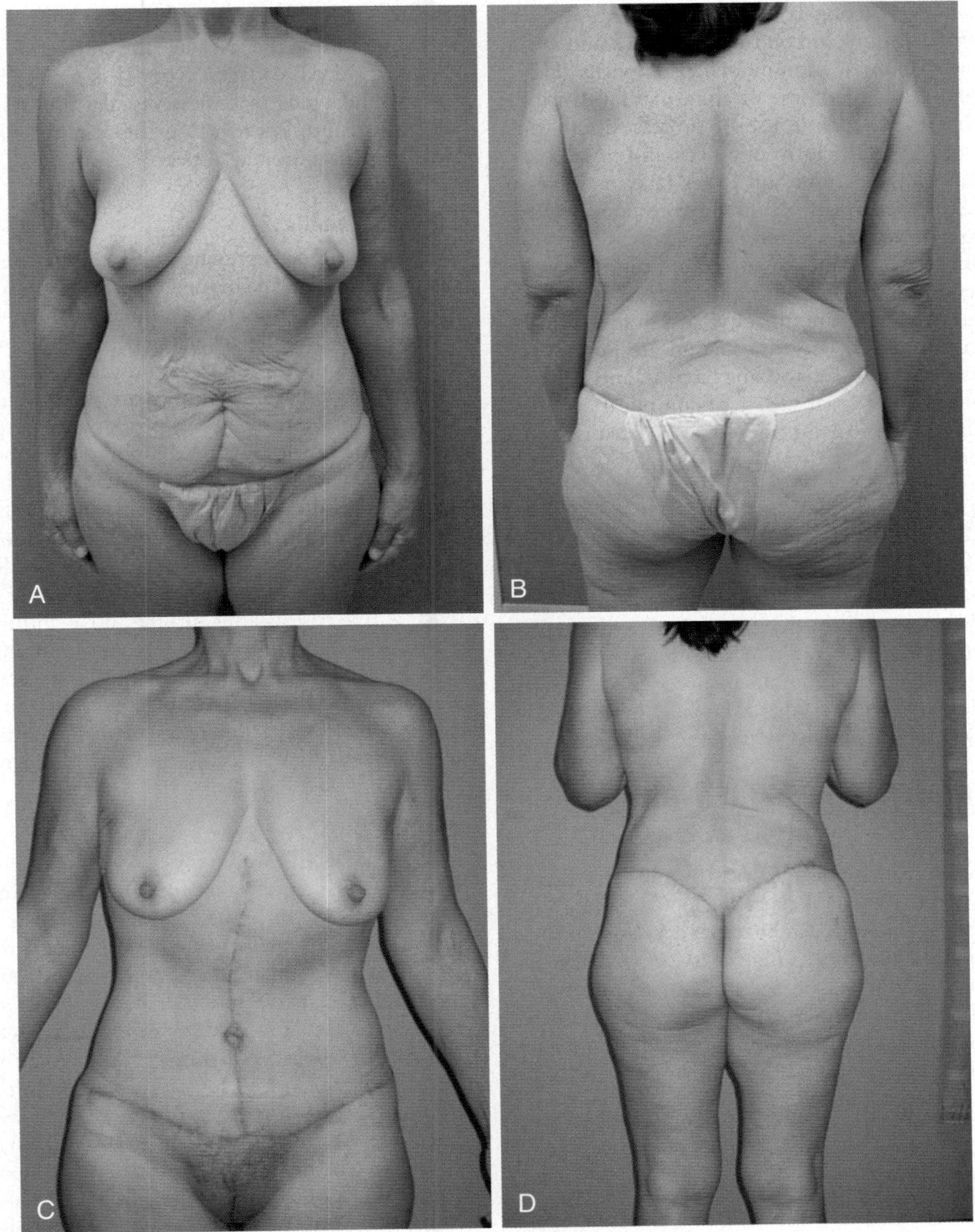

FIG. 69.10 Fleur-de-Lis abdominoplasty with belt lipectomy. (A and B) Preoperative images. (C and D) Postoperative images (8 months).

been used in combination with multiple plastic and reconstructive procedures. As with any other procedure, a carefully directed history and physical examination are necessary. Special attention must be given to scars and hernias that may be injured during the procedure. Liposuction can be performed in an outpatient setting, in hospitals, in ambulatory centers, and in office-based facilities. Many surgeons prefer to perform the majority of the liposuction cases with the patient under general anesthesia. The tumescent technique was developed in 1987 by Jeffery Klein. The current options for wetting solutions are dry, wet, super wet, and tumescent. The solution contains lidocaine (35 mg/kg, the maximum dose) and epinephrine (0.07 mg/kg, the maximum dose) to induce vasoconstriction, and sodium bicarbonate for alkalization to reduce the level of pain. Several types of cannulas are used. The blunt-tip is used to minimize perforation risk, and the smaller cannulas are used to minimize contour irregularities. Deep or intermediate fat layers should be suctioned primarily, and areas of adherences where there are dense fibrous attachments to the deep fascia should not be suctioned to prevent irregularities. Various technology techniques have been incorporated into liposuction. Power-assisted liposuction has been shown to reduce operator fatigue and increase treatment speed. Laser, radiofrequency, and ultrasound-assisted liposuction may offer benefits of coagulating small blood vessels, rupturing adipocytes, improving reticular dermis, favoring skin retraction, and tightening. Large-volume liposuction is associated with hemodynamic instability, significant fluid shifts, and significant blood loss. Suction-assisted lipectomy is a useful surgical treatment for several medical disorders. It is a treatment of choice for gynecomastia to reduce the contour under the arms and in the lateral aspect of the breast after surgical breast reduction techniques. Liposuction is helpful to reduce localized fat deposits in the buffalo hump and on the upper back and lower neck. For patients with human immunodeficiency virus (HIV) infection, lipodystrophy is a syndrome of abnormal fat distribution associated with the therapeutic use of protease inhibitors. The lipodystrophy may be in the form of a neck and upper back fat pad, fat deposition in the trunk and lower face, or increase in the adipose tissue of the breasts. All of these respond well to treatment with liposuction. With appropriate patient selection and minimally traumatic techniques, many complications can be avoided. The most common complications are contour irregularities, seromas, hematomas, lidocaine toxicity, and fluid overload. Lethal complications associated with liposuction are pulmonary embolisms, fat embolisms, sepsis necrotizing fasciitis, and perforation of abdominal viscera and organs. Risk of complications may increase when combined with major abdominal procedures and poor standard of sterility.[38]

GENDER AFFIRMATION SURGERY

Gender affirmation is an evolving field and the focus of practice in plastic and reconstructive surgery. While the techniques are still in evolution, they are benefitting from the innovations we have previously described: microsurgery, craniofacial surgery, body contouring, and aesthetic surgery. Numerous techniques and guidelines are being developed as we speak, and this field is at the cusp of producing its very own subspecialty within the field.

WOUND MANAGEMENT/PRESSURE WOUNDS

Wounds

A wound is a disruption in the continuity of the epithelial lining of the skin or mucosa due to several causative factors. According to the duration of healing, wounds can be either acute or chronic. Acute wounds occur suddenly and can be accidental or surgical. Accidental can be further divided by the mechanisms of injury and the extent of tissue injury. Surgical wounds may be differentiated by clean, clean-contaminated, and contaminated. A minority of wounds will become chronic and nonhealing. Chronic wounds fail to progress through the normal stages of wound healing.

Wound Healing

The wound healing process is a cascade of events that occurs simultaneously and starts with the hemostasis and the inflammatory response that occurs immediately after injury. The release of vasoactive substances including histamine, serotonin, and cytokines is involved in the acute phase of wound healing. Local vascular permeability increases, and capillary leak leads to exudation of plasma. Neutrophils are the predominant cell to provide nonspecific cellular defense against infection during the first 48 hours. Neutrophils will be replaced by macrophages on day 4. The main role is to phagocytize wound debris and contaminant bacteria. After day 4, fibroblast cells begin to appear in the wound and the second stage of wound healing begins. During the second stage of the wound-healing or "proliferative" phase, fibroblasts produce large quantities of collagen type III that will be deposited in a disorganized fashion. Endothelial cells enter a rapid growth phase and angiogenesis occurs. New vascular buds form at the base of the wound. The fibroplasia and revascularization induce the regeneration of a rich vascular network of granulation tissue. Myofibroblast cells play a key role in wound contraction to decrease the size of the wound. Epithelial resurfacing from the wound margins tend to cover and close the wound. The remodeling phase is the last stage of the wound-healing process and may take from 15 days to a year. During the last stage the collagen in the wound becomes more organized; collagen type III is replaced by collagen type I. The wound tends to be less vascular and less inflamed, and the wound strength improves. As the scar redness dissipates, the true scar pigmentation may appear.[39]

Chronic Wounds

Chronic wounds represent a clinical challenge and affect more than 7 million people in the United States. Chronic wounds fail to progress through the normal sequence of the tissue repair process, resulting in a prolonged healing period (>4–6 weeks) that impedes the restoration of normal anatomic and functional integrity. The most common chronic wounds are pressure ulcers and are due to prolonged pressure over bony prominences, especially in the elderly and in those with impaired mobility. The most common chronic leg ulcer is the venous ulcer, which accounts for 80% of the leg ulcers and is due to incompetent venous valves and calf-muscle pump failure. The most common chronic foot wound is the diabetic foot ulcer. Foot ulcers develop in 9.1 million to 26.1 million people with diabetes worldwide. Also, 40% of patients have recurrence within 1 year after healing, 60% within 3 years, and 65% within 5 years. The fourth most common chronic wound is the ischemic or arterial ulcer. Ischemic ulcers are common in distal portions of the lower extremity or anteriorly in the leg, where poor circulation exits. Arterial ulcers are seen in patients with advanced age, diabetes, hypertension, and hyperlipidemia and in patients who smoke (Fig. 69.11).[39,40]

Wound Assessment

Wound assessment begins first by establishing if the wound is acute or chronic in nature. Acute wounds in the absence of risk factors may heal uneventfully in less than 4 to 6 weeks. Any patient with a wound needs complete and detailed clinical history and physical examination. Medical, social, and surgical history may help to obtain valuable information related to wound healing impairment (diabetes mellitus, smoking, and vein or artery ablation). Focus on wound history is paramount: information about the onset of the wound, causative factors, wound changes over time, family history, treatments received, pain, odor, exudate/discharge, and neuropathy. Examination of the wound begins with visual inspection of the wound. This will identify important attributes that guide further evaluation. The physical examination of the wound may be complemented with photography that may decrease interobserver variability. It is important to determine the number of wounds, the location, the size (length, width, depth), the characteristics of the ulcer or wound, the borders, and the appearance of the peripheral tissues. The characteristics of the edge of the wound and the quality of the wound bed may suggest the ulcer etiology. It behooves the practitioner to assess the depth of the wound and involved structures such as tendons, bones, and fistulae. Probing the wound will determine its depth and tracks. The observer needs to observe signs of infection, appreciate the color and odor of the secretions; cellulitis in the peripheral tissues with increase warmth, tenderness or pain to palpation. Necrotic tissue needs to be removed by surgical debridement. Quantity of exudate may dictate the dressing to be used and may vary from minimal to heavy. The vascular assessment is useful to determine signs of arterial occlusion or peripheral arterial disease. Absence of peripheral pulses, low capillary refill, and observation of the quality of the skin, lack of hair, and altered or deformed nails may suggest impairment of arterial perfusion. Noninvasive options to

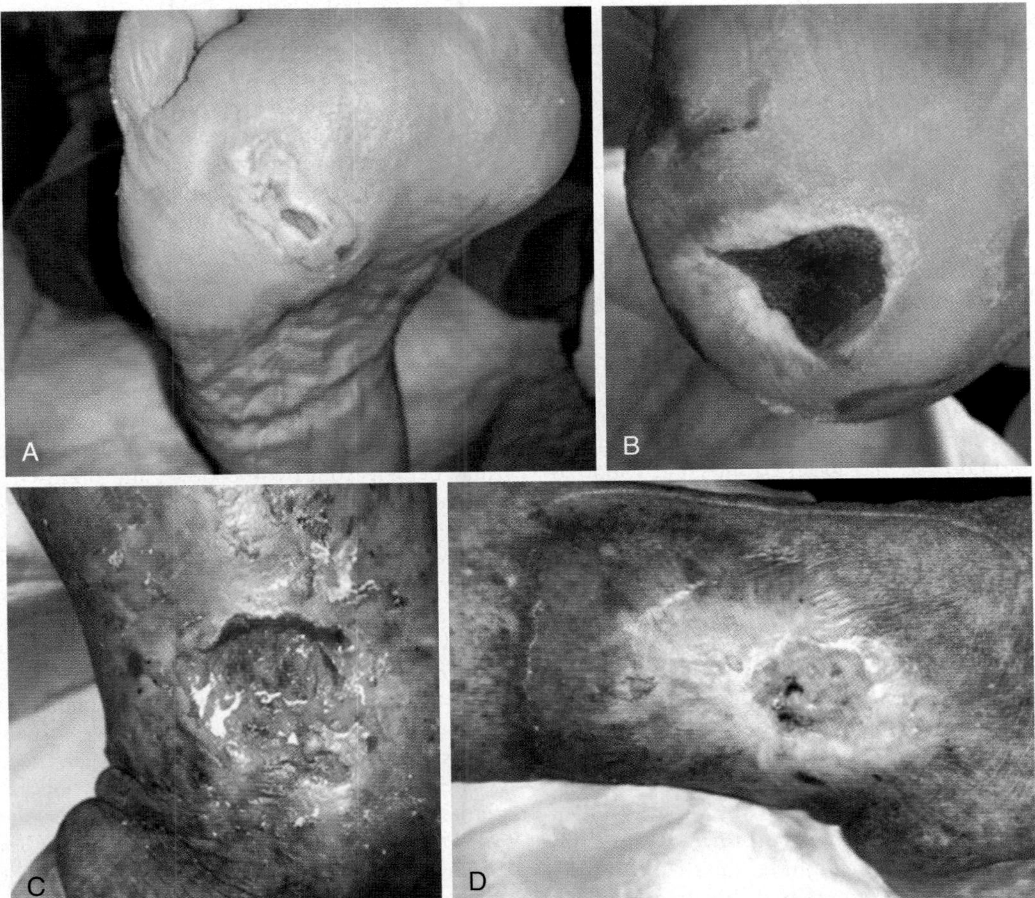

FIG. 69.11 Chronic wounds. (A) Arterial ulcer. (B) Diabetic foot ulcer. (C) Venous stasis ulcer. (D) Improvement of venous stasis ulcer with conservative therapy.

determine the vascular patency include the ankle-brachial index (ABI; less than 0.9), duplex ultrasound, and plethysmography. A referral to a vascular surgeon or interventional radiologist for angiography and the probability of revascularization, which may improve the rates of limb salvage, are sometimes needed.

Diabetic Wound

The causes of diabetic foot ulcers are multifactorial. The main causes are diabetic neuropathy, autonomic dysfunction, and vascular insufficiency. Loss of protective sensation due to neuropathy make them vulnerable to repetitive trauma. Diabetic neuropathy leads to common foot deformities that impair proper foot biomechanics. High pressure points on bony prominences are at risk for ulceration at the plantar metatarsal heads, dorsal interphalangeal joints, heels, and distal phalanges. Diabetic ulcers (DUs) should be routinely assessed, observing the wound, the presence of ischemia, and signs of infection, which should be closely worked up and followed. Peripheral artery disease increases the risk of nonhealing ulcers and infection. Approximately 20% of moderate to severe diabetic foot infections will lead to amputation.[41]

Peripheral Arterial Disease

Inadequate perfusion may be caused by atherosclerosis that affects medium or large arteries. The patient complains of pain at rest, and the pain is aggravated with leg elevation and/or activity. These ulcers are common in smokers, diabetics, and those who have hyperlipidemia or hypertension. The ulcers are well demarcated (punched out), tend to be deep, and present with exposed tendons or bone. The wound base is pale, gray, or yellow with poor granulation tissue surrounded with necrosis or ischemic borders. They are usually situated over pressure points, toes, lateral feet, and the malleolus and pretibial area where skin integrity is vulnerable. Circulation is poor. During physical examination, one can observe skin atrophy, lack of hair, and delayed capillary refill. The lack of arterial pulses in the foot and leg, a decrease ankle brachial index (ABI), and negative pulses using the Doppler ultrasound may determine the severity of the disease.

Venous Stasis and Ulcer

The most common chronic leg ulcer is the venous ulcer, which accounts for 80% of leg ulcers. A chronic leg ulcer is due to incompetent venous valves and calf-muscle pump failure. Venous hypertension results in capillary wall distention with subsequent leakage of macromolecules such as fibrinogen, which polymerizes and alters the oxygen diffusion. Patients may have venous reflux, deep obstructions, and vein thrombosis. Venous ulcers tends to be irregular, superficial ulcers that appear in the lower extremities. Patients with these ulcers often have evidence of varicose vein disease. It is common to observe dermatitis and brown pigmented discoloration in the periphery of the ulcer skin. Borders may show porcelain white scarring and fibrotic changes of the skin, which may be due to the chronicity.

Radiation Wound

Radiation has acute and chronic effects on the skin. Acutely, radiation may cause erythema and epidermis sloughing. The chronic effect impairs the wound-healing cascade, altering fibroblasts, keratinocytes, and endothelial cell functions. It decreases multiple mediators, growth factors, and cytokines necessary for normal wound repair. The DNA-induced damage by radiation injury alters the ability of cells to replicate.

Infected Wound

Infection causes local and systemic effects that impair wound healing. Bacterial contamination is common in any chronic open wound. The diagnosis of infection has always been based on clinical examination. Sign of infection in the wound may include erythema, tenderness, cellulitis, and the presence of secretions. Microbiologic assessment may confirm infection when more than 10^5 organisms are present on the quantitative wound culture.

Open and closed wounds need to be washed and debrided, and nonviable and necrotic tissue should be removed down to a healthy bleeding wound base. If a localized infection is not adequately controlled, it will progress to cellulitis, lymphangitis, bacteremia, and systemic infection.

Biofilms may form and are present on chronic wounds. This complex glycocalyx protects bacteria from the immune system and from antimicrobial therapy. Biofilm can induce a chronic wound inflammation and so should be removed. Bacteria can go dormant or metabolically inert, and it can be protected. When conditions improve, bacteria may undergo activation in the planktonic stage, leading to infection and becoming invasive to adjacent tissues.

Pressure Injury

A pressure wound is a localized injury to the skin or underlying tissues usually due to prolonged pressure over a bony prominence in the body. Pressure injuries should be considered a preventable pathology. Patients with hip fractures, spinal cord injuries, immobility, or cachexia have a higher risk to develop pressure ulcers. The sacrum (28%–36%) is the most common area to develop pressure sores, followed by the heel (23%–30%) and the ischium (17%–20%). Prolonged weight bearing elevates tissue pressure above arterial capillary perfusion pressure (32 mm Hg) and impairs oxygen delivery to the tissues, favoring ischemia and tissue necrosis. Skin is more resistant to pressure than muscle; sometimes normal skin may mask a deeper injury. Additional factors may have detrimental effects on the skin's tolerance to pressure, such as friction, shear forces, moisture, malnutrition, impaired blood supply, lymphatic drainage, social factors, and neurologic injury. Pressure wounds can be staged by using the National Ulcer Advisory Panel Classification (Box 69.1).[42]

Stage I and II pressure ulcers can be treated nonoperatively. In Stage I ulcers, the skin is intact and a nonblanchable erythema can be seen in the affected area; in Stage II ulcers, there is a partial thickness loss of the epidermis, and a blister or a superficial wound may be seen. Stage I and Stage II pressure ulcers can be treated with pressure relief and local wound care and may undergo uneventful healing. Also, carefully monitoring for moisture and soiling will allow the sore to heal. In Stage III ulcers, there is a full thickness loss of the skin, and the subcutaneous tissue may be seen. In Stage IV ulcers, there is deeper damage. Exposed muscle, tendons, and bone can be observed through the damaged skin. Stages III and IV pressure ulcers require surgical treatment. When the ulcer is covered by a scab, the true depth and stage cannot be determined and the ulcer will be unstageable. Nonviable and necrotic tissue should be removed with serial sharp debridement until a final closure can be planned with a fascial or musculocutaneous flap.

Pressure is the main initiator of these ulcers. Prevention can be accomplished by repositioning the patient every few hours and using mattresses and wheelchair cushions that offload the pressure. Local wound care, moisture control, and prevention of shear forces are also helpful in preventing and treating ulcers.

Many pressure wounds may heal by offloading the pressure source, optimizing patient nutritional status, and preventing and treating infection. Prealbumin levels need to be checked; values of 20 mg/dL or greater are needed before planning the final coverage. Debridement can be sharp, using the scalpel or curette; mechanical, using wet-to-dry dressings or enzymatic ointment; and biologic, using maggot therapy. Local wound care and serial debridement can be combined using Dakin solution and enzymatic collagenase creams to remove nonviable tissue, which may promote granulation tissue and wound healing. Dressings are used depending on the wound characteristics. Dry wounds may benefit from hydrocolloids and occlusive dressings. Heavy exudative wounds require alginates and absorbent dressings that prevent wound maceration. Negative-pressure wound vacuum (NPWV) therapy may speed wound healing, promotes wound contraction, decreases wound exudate, decreases edema, and favors the formation of granulation tissue. Sharp debridement and serial excision may decrease the amount of scar tissue and nonviable tissue.

Pressure wounds may have a high bacterial load contamination that can lead to infection. Quantitative tissue culture and bone biopsy are usually needed for appropriate therapy management. Generally, the infection in the pressure ulcers is polymicrobial and should be diagnosed and treated aggressively. *Pseudomonas, Proteus, Bacteroides, Escherichia coli, Staphylococcus aureus,* and *Acinetobacter* are the most frequent organisms isolated in pressure ulcers. Bone infection (osteomyelitis) can be diagnosed by bone biopsy, radiology, tomographic imaging, and MRI. Therapy for osteomyelitis requires surgical debridement, ostectomy, and long courses (at least 6 weeks) of intravenous antibiotics.

Surgery is performed to drain collections and eliminate bursa and sinus tracks in the wound. After medical optimization of the patient, surgery can be planned for closure of the wound. Ostectomy of the bony surface should reach a healthy bleeding base so that a bone biopsy can be taken for microbiologic culture. After a careful hemostasis and adequate debridement, the planned local and regional flap may obliterate the dead space. The flap needs to provide padding to the treated area to protect against new wound formation. In some cases in which spasticity contributes to the pressure wound, a tenotomy can be performed when including muscle flaps.

Several options of local and regional fasciocutaneous or musculocutaneous flaps can be used to close pressure sores. Fasciocutaneous flaps may preserve muscle and its function so that it may be used in the future. Free flaps are rarely used for pressure wounds. The sacral wounds are treated with gluteal flaps (Fig. 69.12). Flaps of the superior half of the muscle are constructed and moved in to the defect as a rotational flap or V-Y advancement. The V-Y advancement creates a triangular skin island over the muscle, with one side being the defect and the other two sides forming a V. The V formation shifts into the wound, and the defect is closed in a Y configuration. In cases with a big defect, bilateral V-Y advancement flaps can be used. Ischial ulcers may be cover with the V-Y hamstring advancement flap. Trochanteric pressure wound may be treated with the tensor fasciae latamusculocutaneous flap. Strict pressure precautions for 2 to 6 weeks after flap treatment may prevent pressure necrosis and dehiscence of the wound.[42,43]

BOX 69.1 Pressure ulcer definition and stages.

A pressure ulcer is localized injury to the skin and/or underlying tissue usually over a bony prominence, as a result of pressure, or pressure in combination with shear and/or friction. Pressure ulcers are staged using the following system.

A number of contributing or confounding factors are also associated with pressure ulcers; the significance of these factors is yet to be elucidated.

Pressure Ulcer Stages

(Suspected) Deep Tissue Injury:

Purple or maroon localized area of discolored intact skin or blood-filled blister due to damage of underlying soft tissue from pressure and/or shear. The area may be preceded by tissue that is painful, firm, mushy, boggy, warmer or cooler as compared to adjacent tissue.

Further Description:

Deep tissue injury may be difficult to detect in individuals with dark skin tones. Evolution may include a thin blister over a dark wound bed. The wound may further evolve and become covered by thin eschar. Evolution may be rapid exposing additional layers of tissue even with optimal treatment.

+Stage I:

Intact skin with nonblanchable redness of a localized area usually over a bony prominence. Darkly pigmented skin may not have visible blanching; its color may differ from the surrounding area.

Further Description:

The area may be painful, firm, soft, warmer or cooler as compared to adjacent tissue. Stage I may be difficult to detect in individuals with dark skin tones. May indicate "at risk" persons (a heralding sign of risk)

Stage II:

Partial thickness loss of dermis presenting as a shallow open ulcer with a red pink wound bed, without slough. May also present as an intact or open/ruptured serum-filled blister.

Further Description:

Presents as a shiny or dry shallow ulcer without slough or bruising.* This stage should not be used to describe skin tears, tape burns, perineal dermatitis, maceration, or denudement.

Stage III:

Full thickness tissue loss. Subcutaneous fat may be visible but bone, tendon or muscle are not exposed. Slough may be present but does not obscure the depth of tissue loss. May include undermining and tunneling.

Further Description:

The depth of a Stage III pressure ulcer varies by anatomic location. The bridge of the nose, ear, occiput and malleolus do not have subcutaneous tissue and Stage III ulcers can be shallow. In contrast, areas of significant adiposity can develop extremely deep Stage III pressure ulcers. Bone/tendon is not visible or directly palpable.

Stage IV:

Full thickness tissue loss with exposed bone, tendon or muscle. Slough or eschar may be present on some parts of the wound bed. Often include undermining and tunneling.

Further Description:

The depth of a Stage IV pressure ulcer varies by anatomic location. The bridge of the nose, ear, occiput and malleolus do not have subcutaneous tissue and these ulcers can be shallow. Stage IV ulcers can extend into muscle and/or supporting structures (e.g., fascia, tendon or joint capsule) making osteomyelitis possible. Exposed bone/tendon is visible or directly palpable.

Unstageable:

Full thickness tissue loss in which the base of the ulcer is covered by slough (yellow, tan, gray, green or brown) and/or eschar (tan, brown or black) in the wound bed.

Further Description:

Until enough slough and/or eschar is removed to expose the base of the wound, the true depth, and therefore stage, cannot be determined. Stable (dry, adherent, intact without erythema or fluctuance) eschar on the heels serves as "the body's natural (biologic) cover" and should not be removed. This staging system should be used only to describe pressure ulcers. Wounds from other causes, such as arterial, venous, diabetic foot, skin tears, tape burns, perineal dermatitis, maceration or denudement should not be staged using this system. Other staging systems exist for some of these conditions and should be used instead.

From Black J, Baharestani MM, Cuddigan J, et al. National Pressure Ulcer Advisory Panel's updated pressure ulcer staging system. *Adv Skin Wound Care.* 2007;20:269–274 (copyright NPUAP 2007).

*Bruising indicates suspected deep tissue injury.

RECONSTRUCTION OF THE LOWER EXTREMITY

The goal of lower extremity reconstruction is restoration of form and function. This requires a stable framework to support weight, muscle for power motion and joint movement, neural supply for proprioception and plantar sensibility, blood supply to sustain the underlying structures, and soft tissue to provide a stable skin envelope. Based on these needs, reconstruction may be needed for open fractures, defects from sarcoma resections, radiation wounds, chronic traumatic wounds, DUs, venous ulcers, osteomyelitis of the tibia, unstable scars, and infected vascular grafts. These reconstructions tend to be complex and many require a multidisciplinary surgical team.

Soft Tissue Coverage of Traumatic Wounds

The loss of soft tissue coverage over a fracture, particularly when interrupted endosteal blood supply is combined with periosteal damage, demands coverage of the exposed bone with vascularized tissue after thorough debridement of devitalized tissue (Fig. 69.13). Determinants of outcome after open fractures are wound size, degree of soft tissue injury, and amount of contamination. The Gustilo classification system is used to categorize open fractures of the leg into subtypes predictive of prognosis:

Gustilo I: Open fractures with wound less than 1 cm.

Gustilo II: Open fractures with wound 1 to 10 cm with moderate tissue damage.

Gustilo III: Open fractures with wound larger than 10 cm and extensive tissue damage, making it difficult to cover bone or hardware.

Gustilo IIIA: Adequate soft tissue coverage of bone with extensive soft tissue laceration or flaps.

Gustilo IIIB: Inadequate soft tissue with periosteal stripping and bone exposure.

Gustilo IIIC: As above, with vascular injury and ischemia requiring repair.

Gustilo grade I and most grade II fractures can be closed primarily after debridement and orthopedic fixation are applied. However, larger grade II and most grade III fractures require advanced reconstructive techniques. When flap coverage is required, it can be done at the time of fracture stabilization or as a secondary procedure. Early coverage of exposed bone, tendons, and neurovascular structures decreases the risk of infection, osteomyelitis,

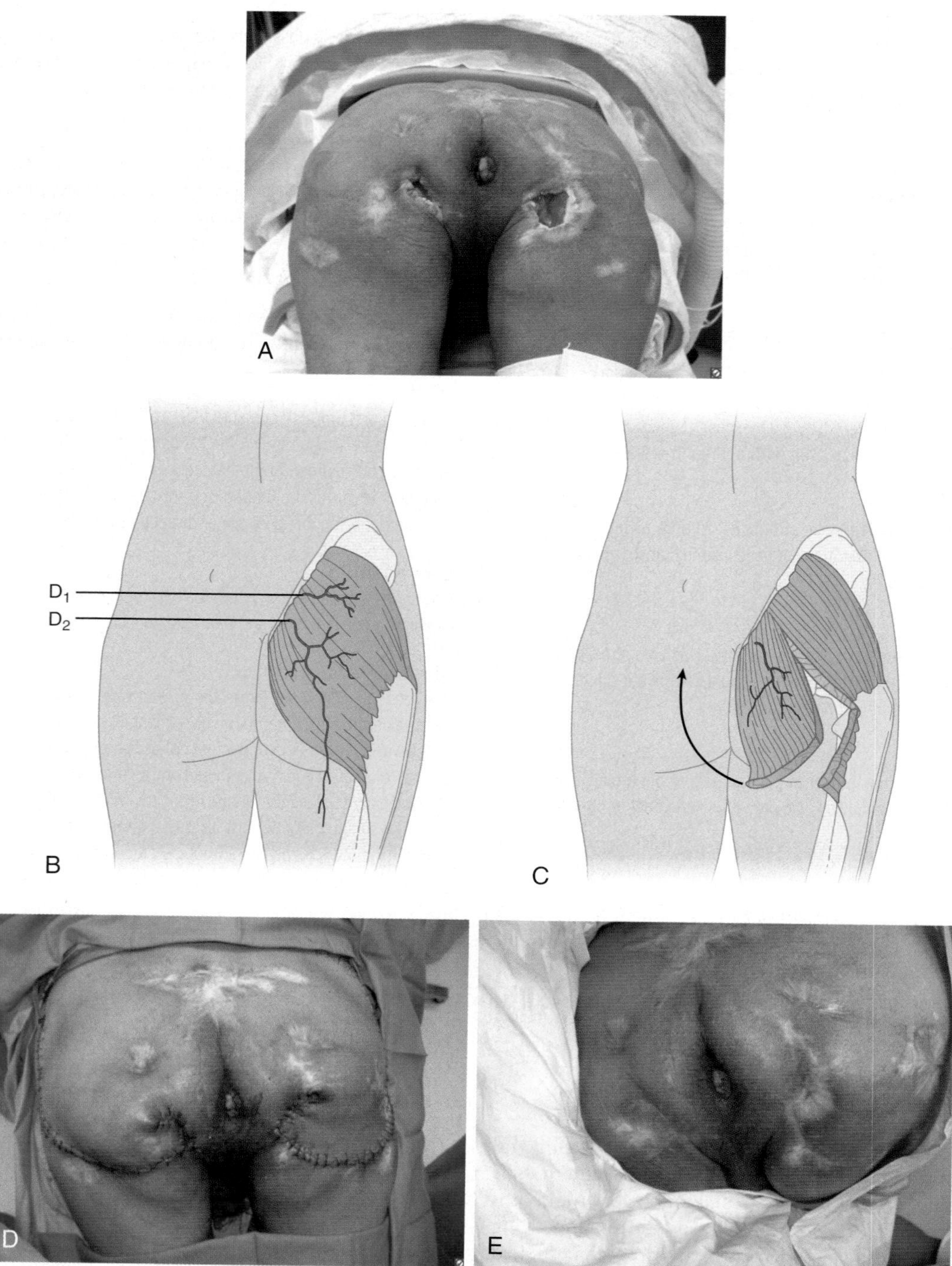

FIG. 69.12 A 51-year-old paraplegic patient has bilateral stage IV ischial pressure sores with bone exposure in the wounds. (A) Preoperative view shows bilateral defects and scarring of the surrounding tissue from previous pressure sores and surgical repairs. After debridement and bilateral ischiectomy, well-vascularized tissue will be needed to cover bone, to provide padding, and to close the wound without tension. (B) The gluteus maximus muscle has blood supply from two branches of the hypogastric artery—the superior gluteal artery to the upper half and the inferior gluteal artery to the lower half. (C) Based on these two separate upper and lower pedicles, the muscle can be divided into upper and lower halves. (D) The lower half of the gluteus muscle on each side is detached from the greater tuberosity of the femur and transposed inferiorly with the overlying buttock skin to fill the ischial defects. (E) Three-month postoperative view shows coverage of both defects. The superior half of the gluteus maximus muscle is preserved.

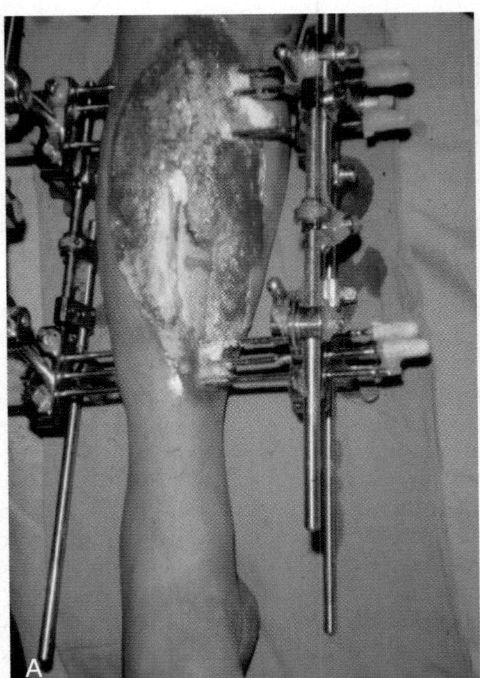

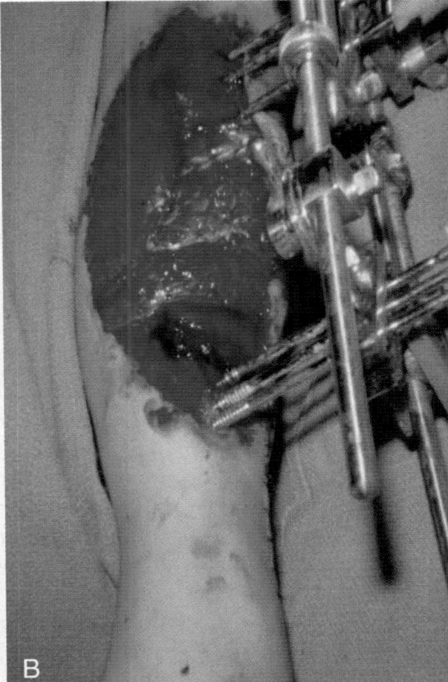

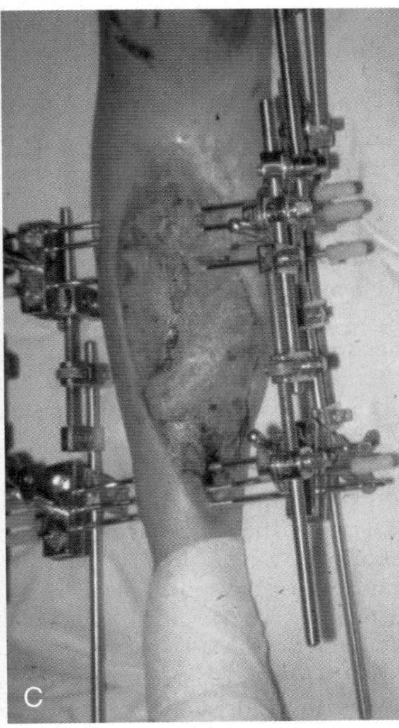

FIG. 69.13 Soleus muscle flap for coverage of traumatic open fracture of the tibia in the middle third of the leg. (A) Soft tissue defect with 10 cm of exposed bone after fracture fixation. (B) The broad flat muscle deep to the gastrocnemius muscle has been mobilized on its proximal pedicles from the posterior tibial and peroneal arteries. It is transposed medially to cover the middle third of the tibia. (C) Postoperative result. The muscle flap has been covered with a split-thickness skin graft to provide stable wound coverage.

nonunion, and ongoing tissue loss. Although the advantages of radical debridement and early wound closure have been accepted, the definition of the duration of the early phase varies. Earlier bone healing and reduced infection rates have been demonstrated if coverage is completed within 72 hours of fracture stabilization; others have shown comparable results when the wounds are closed 15 days after injury. Early reconstruction may be precluded by other injuries or when severely contaminated wounds require serial debridement before delayed reconstruction.

For many years, muscle flaps have been the choice for traumatic lower limb defects. The gastrocnemius and soleus muscles are accessible as local flaps to cover the upper and middle third of the leg, and smaller muscles such as the tibialis anterior, extensor digitorum longus, and peroneus brevis can be used for more distal, small defects. For larger defects of the middle and distal third of the leg, ankle, and foot, microvascular free tissue transfers are preferred. These free tissue transfers provide more bulk, have longer pedicles for greater flexibility in positioning, and are not dependent on blood supply within the injured area. Most series of lower extremity reconstructions have reported flap failure rates just below 10%. This is higher than at other sites on the body because of associated vascular injuries and preexisting vascular disease in these patients.[44,45]

Recent novel wound technologies combined with growing experience with local perforator flaps are creating new options for lower extremity reconstruction. The use of negative pressure wound therapy has allowed for delay of definitive flap coverage and, in some cases, makes it possible to close previously large wounds with local or regional flaps after promotion of adequate granulation tissue. The discovery of versatile perforator flaps and the use of traditional local flaps, including reverse sural and keystone flaps, have also decreased the need for free microvascular transfers. Clinical advantages of this shift from free flaps to a wider use of skin grafts and local flaps include shorter operations in the trauma patient and elimination of the need for anastomosis to a major leg artery, which may not be available in some traumatic cases.

In injuries with bone loss and a soft tissue defect, the options for skeletal reconstruction include autogenous bone grafts, vascularized bone transfer, and the Ilizarov technique for osteosynthesis. Bone grafts generally are delayed for approximately 6 weeks after soft tissue reconstruction while orthopedic hardware holds the fracture fragments at length across the gap. The size and location of the bone defect will determine bone graft technique, with a vascularized procedure preferred for larger losses. An alternative to delayed bone grafting is immediate one-stage reconstruction of the bone and soft tissue with an osteocutaneous free tissue transfer.

There are relative contraindications to salvage of a Gustilo grade IIIC injury of the lower extremity. An important element in considering primary amputation is disruption of the sciatic or posterior tibial nerve. With laceration of the posterior tibial nerve, the plantar surface is insensate, which results predictably in recurrent ulceration, infection, and osteomyelitis. Other elements include severe infection or contamination, multilevel severe injury, ischemia time longer than 6 hours, and preexisting severe medical illness. There are several scoring systems to assist in decisions regarding limb salvage versus amputation, but these tend to identify patients with good potential for salvage rather than those who will need eventual amputation. The Mangled Extremity Severity Score is used widely but should not be the sole criterion on which an amputation decision is made. Replantation of a severed lower limb is rarely done in the adult because of the inability to restore neurologic function to the foot. A nonfunctional or marginally functional lower extremity is a greater liability than a prosthetic limb capable of allowing high-level function. Absolute contraindications to replantation are older age, poor baseline health, multilevel injury that results in immobility of the knee or ankle, and warm ischemia time longer than 6 hours.[46]

Soft Tissue Reconstruction in the Groin and Thigh

Defects of the thigh and groin area are commonly managed with local flaps due to high vascularity of available local soft tissue and muscles. The groin is the most common site of distal extremity prosthetic graft infections. Muscle flaps are the mainstay for managing vascular graft infections. Healthy muscle increases tissue oxygen tension in the wound, augments the delivery of antibiotics to the site, and eliminates dead space. Several muscle flaps are useful for coverage of the femoral vessels, including sartorius, gracilis, and rectus abdominis. The sartorius muscle is used as first-line treatment because of its proximity, expendability, and relative ease of elevation. The muscle originates on the anterior superior iliac spine, inserts at the medial tibial condyle, and has a segmental blood supply with five or six direct branches from the superficial femoral artery. The muscle is mobilized by dividing the origin and two proximal vascular pedicles, which frees the proximal end of the muscle to be transposed medially and sutured to the inguinal ligament to provide vascularized muscle coverage of the femoral vessels.

Defects after oncologic surgery in the thigh and groin are distinctive because extirpation of tumors often necessitates wide margins combined with adjuvant radiation therapy. There is a higher incidence of infection and dehiscence after limb-sparing surgery in the thigh and groin than in distal parts of the lower extremity because of greater dead space, exposure of neurovascular structures, difficulty in keeping the wound clean, and tension with ambulation and hip abduction. For these larger irradiated defects, flap reconstruction is necessary. Local flap options include the muscle flap such as gracilis, tensor fascia lata, and vastus lateralis or fasciocutaneous flaps such as the medial thigh, lateral posterior thigh, and anterior lateral thigh. In some cases, these local options are no longer useful because of inclusion in the field of radiation, so distant or free flaps are needed for coverage. Reported outcomes after reconstruction of these difficult wounds with a VRAM flap have been promising, with a 9.4% incidence of postoperative wound complications with immediate reconstruction but a significantly higher incidence of 47% in patients with delayed reconstruction.[47]

Soft Tissue Coverage of the Knee, Leg, and Foot

Wounds around the knee can result from trauma, tumor extirpation, or exposure of an infected knee prosthesis after total knee replacement. For these defects, durable soft tissue coverage is required. A pedicled medial or lateral gastrocnemius muscle flap based on the sural artery is preferred for soft tissue reconstruction for the knee and proximal third of the leg. The gastrocnemius muscle has a medial and lateral head originating from the medial and lateral condyles of the femur, respectively; the two heads share a common insertion on the calcaneus through the Achilles tendon. As a result, one head can be detached from the Achilles tendon independently and transposed with its robust blood supply and vascular drainage without impairing foot dorsiflexion. Because the medial head is longer, it is preferred for knee wounds and can be transposed with or without a skin paddle. In situations in which a pedicled gastrocnemius flap has failed or is unavailable, advancing to the next rung of the reconstructive ladder with free tissue transfer, such as rectus abdominis or latissimus dorsi flap, has led to a high rate of salvage of limbs and knee prostheses.

Options for soft tissue coverage of the leg are determined by the position of the defect relative to the tibia as it determines the availability or paucity of local tissue for coverage:

Proximal tibia: gastrocnemius, free tissue transfer.

Middle tibia: soleus, gastrocnemius, extensor digitorum longus, tibialis anterior, keystone flap, propeller flap, free tissue transfer.

Distal tibia: peroneus brevis, extensor brevis, distal-based soleus, reverse sural artery flap, lateral supramalleolar flap, dorsalis pedis fasciocutaneous flap, free tissue transfer.

Foot: flexor digitorum brevis, abductor hallucis, abductor digiti minimi, reverse sural flap, medial plantar artery flap, lateral calcaneal artery flap, V-Y advancement, free tissue transfer.

Local muscle flaps are often unreliable in treating distal third leg wounds due to its limited reach. In addition, except for the soleus and gastrocnemius muscles, local muscles on the lower leg are only adequate to cover small defects. This, along with several other factors, means that treatment of the distal tibia, ankle, and foot is difficult. The area is vulnerable to injury because the distal portion of the leg has poor skin elasticity, has bone lying in the subcutaneous space, and may be edematous. The distal third of the leg has little muscle but many tendinous structures, and they support skin grafts poorly. Finally, the foot and ankle require especially durable integument because they are exposed continually to friction and shear with walking and footwear. Any transferred flap may slip or slide at the interface with the underlying structures because the transferred tissue lacks the glabrous quality of the native plantar skin. If the transferred tissue is insensate, it will be at significant risk for eventual breakdown.

For larger defects, reconstruction in the distal third of the leg relies on free tissue transfer techniques. The vascular status of the extremity and recipient vessel selection are key factors for success. Guidelines for the use of free flaps in the lower extremity include making anastomoses to healthy recipient vessels outside the zone of injury. Free tissue transfer remains the best option for large defects, for wounds with trauma (e.g., crush injury to the surrounding vicinity that damages blood supply to all local tissues), and when the transfer of vascularized bone with the free flap is desirable. Free fibula flaps with skin paddles are preferred for lower extremity wounds with bone and soft tissue deficits.

As previously mentioned, advanced understanding of vascular territories supplied by perforasomes has expanded the armamentarium to lower extremity reconstruction. The development of highly versatile perforator flaps allows soft tissue reconstruction without the need for microvascular anastomosis. These locally designed, fasciocutaneous, or adipofascial flaps can provide adequate amount of coverage comparable to free tissue transfer; however, it often requires skin grafting of the donor site. The use of these local flaps are currently limited by its size, surgeon experience, and understanding of the vascular territories. With larger soft tissue defect of the lower leg, free tissue transfer currently remains the standard for reconstruction.[48]

CONCLUSION

Plastic surgery continues to evolve with the development of new approaches for the care of people with congenital and acquired deformities. With therapeutic advances in medicine and surgery, new problems have emerged that call for novel reconstructive techniques. Challenged by these difficult problems, plastic surgeons continue to look for ways to treat life- and limb-threatening problems and, at the same time, to restore form and function.

Chest wall, abdominal wall, and perineal reconstruction are progressing rapidly, and defects that were incapacitating a decade ago are now correctable. Lower extremity salvage after devastating injury is now commonplace. With advances in other surgical specialties such as bariatric surgery, entirely new areas requiring plastic surgery have emerged. Old techniques, such as perforator flaps, continue to evolve and supply better ways to reconstruct defects.

New techniques, such as fat grafting, which may revolutionize clinical practice, have come from empirical observations. Developed from new research studies, tissue engineering, gene therapy, and stem cell work will change reconstruction in unforeseeable ways in the future. The search continues for the most reliable, durable, and aesthetic ways to "restore, repair, and make whole those parts ... which fortune has taken away" (Gaspare Tagliacozzi [Italian surgeon who became famous for his skill in reconstructive surgery], *De Curtorum Chirurgia per Insitionem*, Venice, 1579).

SELECTED REFERENCES

Almutairi K, Gusenoff JA, Rubin JP. Body contouring. *Plast Reconstr Surg*. 2016;137:586e–602e.

Body contouring has advanced significantly over the past decade, fueled by the increased number of massive weight loss patients and the advent of new fat-reduction technologies. This has impacted both the number of cases performed and the range of procedures. Many innovations are being developed as plastic surgeons meet the evolving needs of our patients. This review covers essential principles of patient selection and safety; anatomic concepts; staging and combining procedures; and select aspects of contouring of the trunk and extremities using excisional techniques, liposuction, and fat grafting.

Bui DT, Cordeiro PG, Hu QY, et al. Free flap reexploration: indications, treatment, and outcomes in 1193 free flaps. *Plast Reconstr Surg*. 2007;119:2092–2100.

Microvascular free tissue transfer is a reliable method for reconstruction of complex surgical defects. However, there is still a small risk of flap compromise necessitating urgent reexploration. This paper is a comprehensive study that looks at cause, methods, and techniques to avoid complications.

Janis JE, Kwon RK, Attinger CE. The new reconstructive ladder: modifications to the traditional model. *Plast Reconstr Surg*. 2011;127(suppl 1):205S–212S.

The traditional reconstructive ladder has withstood the test of time, serving as a thought paradigm to guide surgeons in choosing their method of wound closure for an assortment of defects. Advances in anatomic understanding and technologic innovations have improved our ability to achieve definitive closure in a wide variety of patients. In this article, the older construct is updated to reflect the use of negative-pressure wound therapy and dermal matrices. Perforator flap concepts are also discussed in terms of their inclusion as a rung on the ladder. This article aims to change the paradigm that reconstruction should be patient specific and the surgeons choice should fit the current problem.

Koshima I, Yamamoto T, Narushima M, et al. Perforator flaps and supermicrosurgery. *Clin Plast Surg*. 2010;37:683–689.

The introduction of supermicrosurgery, the microvascular anastomosis of vessels ranging from 0.3 to 0.8 mm in diameter, opens up a wide array of new reconstructive options. Free perforator flaps can be obtained from anywhere on the body, and they provide thinner, more pliant tissue for repair of extremity and facial defects. This paper reviews these new options as well as the technical challenges of supermicrosurgery.

Leberfinger AN, Behar BJ, Williams NC, et al. Breast implant-associated anaplastic large cell lymphoma: a systematic review. *JAMA Surg*. 2017;152:1161–1168.

A new issue in the field of plastic and reconstructive surgery is that of breast implant-associated anaplastic large cell lymphoma (BIA-ALCL). This paper is a systematic review of 115 articles and 95 patients, the incidence of breast implant–associated anaplastic large cell lymphoma, the diagnosis appears to be increasing as both patients and practitioners become more aware of this entity. Before breast augmentation or reconstruction, surgeons need to convey the risk of breast implant–associated anaplastic large cell lymphoma to patients, with particular emphasis on the established linkage to textured implants; patients must be educated on the importance of routine surveillance after implantation, and it is likely that increased follow-up will lead to a further rise in this diagnosis.

Sosin M, Rodriguez ED. The face transplantation update: 2016. *Plast Reconstr Surg*. 2016;137:1841–1850.

Composite tissue allotransplantation has revolutionized the field of reconstructive surgery. This review serves the most contemporary and all-inclusive face transplantation review. There is a critical need for timely reporting and outcome transparency in the reconstructive transplant community. This review provides cited references and cases in operative planning, technique, and patient outcomes in the field of face transplantation.

REFERENCES

1. Janis JE, Kwon RK, Attinger CE. The new reconstructive ladder: modifications to the traditional model. *Plast Reconstr Surg*. 2011;127(suppl 1):205S–212S.
2. Orgill DP, Bayer LR. Update on negative-pressure wound therapy. *Plast Reconstr Surg*. 2011;127(suppl 1):105S–115S.
3. Marks MW, Argenta LC. Principles and applications of tissue expansion. In: Neligan PC, ed. *Plastic Surgery*. 3rd ed. London: Elsevier Saunders; 2013:622–653.
4. Fujioka M. Surgical reconstruction of radiation injuries. *Adv Wound Care (New Rochelle)*. 2014;3:25–37.
5. Tamai M, Nagasao T, Miki T, et al. Rotation arc of pedicled anterolateral thigh flap for abdominal wall reconstruction: how far can it reach? *J Plast Reconstr Aesthet Surg*. 2015;68:1417–1424.
6. Ritter EF, Cronan JC, Rudner AM, et al. Improved microsurgical anastomotic patency with low molecular weight heparin. *J Reconstr Microsurg*. 1998;14:331–336.

7. Bui DT, Cordeiro PG, Hu QY, et al. Free flap reexploration: indications, treatment, and outcomes in 1193 free flaps. *Plast Reconstr Surg*. 2007;119:2092–2100.
8. Koshima I, Yamamoto T, Narushima M, et al. Perforator flaps and supermicrosurgery. *Clin Plast Surg*. 2010;37:683–689, vii–iii.
9. Bartlett SP, Derderian CA. Craniosynostosis syndromes. In: Thorne CH, Chung KC, Gosain AK, et al., eds. *Grabb and Smith's Plastic Surgery*. 7th ed. Philadelphia, PA: Lippincott Williams & Wilkins, Wolters Kluwer Health; 2014:223–240.
10. Reinisch JF, Lewin S. Ear reconstruction using a porous polyethylene framework and temporoparietal fascia flap. *Facial Plast Surg*. 2009;25:181–189.
11. McCarthy JG, Grayson BH, Hopper R, et al. Craniofacial microsomia. In: Neligan PC, ed. *Plastic Surgery*, 3rd ed. London: Elsevier Saunders; 2012:761–791.
12. Collins J, Cheung K, Farrokhyar F, et al. Pharyngeal flap versus sphincter pharyngoplasty for the treatment of velopharyngeal insufficiency: a meta-analysis. *J Plast Reconstr Aesthet Surg*. 2012;65:864–868.
13. Losee JE, Kirschner RE. *Comprehensive Cleft Care*. Vol 1. Thieme; 2015.
14. Stal S, Brown RH, Higuera S, et al. Fifty years of the Millard rotation-advancement: looking back and moving forward. *Plast Reconstr Surg*. 2009;123:1364–1377.
15. Ellis 3rd E, Miles BA. Fractures of the mandible: a technical perspective. *Plast Reconstr Surg*. 2007;120:76S–89S.
16. Baker SR. Reconstruction of the nose. In: Baker S, ed. *Local Flaps in Facial Reconstruction*. 3rd ed. Philadelphia, PA: Elsevier Saunders; 2014:415–480.
17. Sosin M, Rodriguez ED. The Face Transplantation Update: 2016. *Plast Reconstr Surg*. 2016;137:1841–1850.
18. Codner MA, Kikkawa DO, Korn BS, et al. Blepharoplasty and brow lift. *Plast Reconstr Surg*. 2010;126:1e–17e.
19. Drolet BC, Sullivan PK. Evidence-based medicine: blepharoplasty. *Plast Reconstr Surg*. 2014;133:1195–1205.
20. Tanna N, Nguyen KT, Ghavami A, et al. Evidence-based medicine: current practices in rhinoplasty. *Plast Reconstr Surg*. 2018;141:137e–151e.
21. Derby BM, Codner MA. Evidence-Based Medicine: Face Lift. *Plast Reconstr Surg*. 2017;139:151e–167e.
22. Barrera A. Reconstructive hair transplantation of the face and scalp. *Semin Plast Surg*. 2005;19:159–166.
23. Nguyen AT, Ahmad J, Fagien S, et al. Cosmetic medicine: facial resurfacing and injectables. *Plast Reconstr Surg*. 2012;129:142e–153e.
24. Attenello NH, Maas CS. Injectable fillers: review of material and properties. *Facial Plast Surg*. 2015;31:29–34.
25. Rzany B, DeLorenzi C. Understanding, avoiding, and managing severe filler complications. *Plast Reconstr Surg*. 2015;136:196S–203S.
26. Greco R, Noone B. Evidence-Based Medicine: reduction mammaplasty. *Plast Reconstr Surg*. 2017;139:230e–239e.
27. Regnault P. Breast ptosis. Definition and treatment. *Clin Plast Surg*. 1976;3:193–203.
28. Hidalgo DA, Spector JA. Breast augmentation. *Plast Reconstr Surg*. 2014;133:567e–583e.
29. Nava MB, Adams Jr WP, Botti G, et al. MBN 2016 Aesthetic Breast Meeting BIA-ALCL Consensus Conference Report. *Plast Reconstr Surg*. 2018;141:40–48.
30. Leberfinger AN, Behar BJ, Williams NC, et al. Breast implant-associated anaplastic large cell lymphoma: a systematic review. *JAMA Surg*. 2017;152:1161–1168.
31. Pu LL, Yoshimura K, Coleman SR. Future perspectives of fat grafting. *Clin Plast Surg*. 2015;42:389–394, ix–x.
32. Largo RD, Tchang LA, Mele V, et al. Efficacy, safety and complications of autologous fat grafting to healthy breast tissue: a systematic review. *J Plast Reconstr Aesthet Surg*. 2014;67:437–448.
33. Clemens MW, Brody GS, Mahabir RC, et al. How to diagnose and treat breast implant-associated anaplastic large cell lymphoma. *Plast Reconstr Surg*. 2018;141:586e–599e.
34. Waltho D, Hatchell A, Thoma A. Gynecomastia classification for surgical management: a systematic review and novel classification system. *Plast Reconstr Surg*. 2017;139:638e–648e. 2017.
35. Gutowski KA. Evidence-based medicine: abdominoplasty. *Plast Reconstr Surg*. 2018;141:286e–299e.
36. Pannucci CJ, Bailey SH, Dreszer G, et al. Validation of the Caprini risk assessment model in plastic and reconstructive surgery patients. *J Am Coll Surg*. 2011;212:105–112.
37. Almutairi K, Gusenoff JA, Rubin JP. Body contouring. *Plast Reconstr Surg*. 2016;137:586e–602e.
38. Chia CT, Neinstein RM, Theodorou SJ. Evidence-based medicine: liposuction. *Plast Reconstr Surg*. 2017;139:267e–274e.
39. Han G, Ceilley R. Chronic wound healing: a review of current management and treatments. *Adv Ther*. 2017;34:599–610.
40. Grey JE, Enoch S, Harding KG. Wound assessment. *BMJ*. 2006;332:285–288.
41. Armstrong DG, Boulton AJM, Bus SA. Diabetic foot ulcers and their recurrence. *N Engl J Med*. 2017;376:2367–2375.
42. Black J, Baharestani MM, Cuddigan J, et al. National Pressure Ulcer Advisory Panel's updated pressure ulcer staging system. *Adv Skin Wound Care*. 2007;20:269–274.
43. Ricci JA, Bayer LR, Orgill DP. Evidence-based medicine: the evaluation and treatment of pressure injuries. *Plast Reconstr Surg*. 2017;139:275e–286e.
44. Godina M. Early microsurgical reconstruction of complex trauma of the extremities. *Plast Reconstr Surg*. 1986;78:285–292.
45. Stranix JT, Lee ZH, Jacoby A, et al. Lessons learned from 40 years of traumatic lower extremity free flaps inflow, outflow, takebacks, and failures. *Plast Reconstr Surg–Global Open*. 2018;6:16.
46. Shawen SB, Keeling JJ, Branstetter J, et al. The mangled foot and leg: salvage versus amputation. *Foot Ankle Clin*. 2010;15:63–75.
47. Parrett BM, Winograd JM, Garfein ES, et al. The vertical and extended rectus abdominis myocutaneous flap for irradiated thigh and groin defects. *Plast Reconstr Surg*. 2008;122:171–177.
48. Saint-Cyr M, Wong C, Schaverien M, et al. The perforasome theory: vascular anatomy and clinical implications. *Plast Reconstr Surg*. 2009;124:1529–1544.

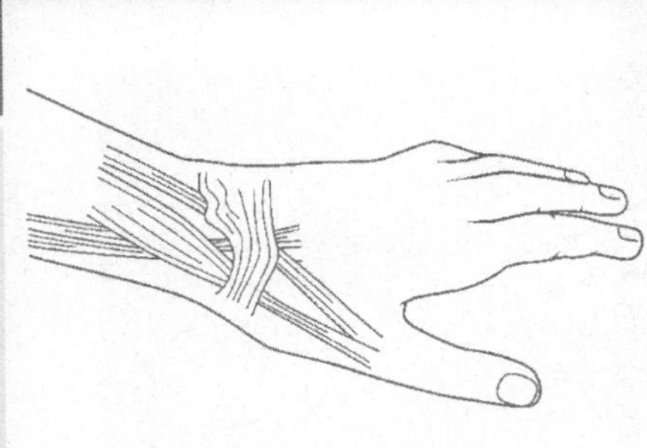

CHAPTER 70

Hand Surgery

David Netscher, Nikhil Agrawal, Nicholas A. Fiore II

OUTLINE

Please access Elsevier eBooks for Practicing Clinicians to view the videos for this chapter https://expertconsult.inkling.com/.

This chapter describes the broad scope of hand surgery. It emphasizes core knowledge that is important to general surgeons. The origins of this important subspecialty are rooted within general surgery. It is a regional specialty bringing together general, plastic, and orthopedic principals.

Although hand surgery fellowships traditionally receive trainees primarily with backgrounds in orthopedic surgery or plastic surgery, fellowship training in hand surgery may also be undertaken by those having completed a residency in general surgery. Basic tenets of hand surgery must be acquired by all general surgeons. Depending on the practice locale (rural or urban), type of hospital, and residency rotations (e.g., surgical intern covering the emergency department) or even for the purposes of board examinations, the ability to evaluate and to manage hand injuries and problems is a necessary skill for the general surgeon. The purpose of this chapter is not to provide the general surgeon with an exhaustive study of hand surgery, because specialty texts are more appropriate, but to provide an overview of pathologic processes of the hand encountered more commonly by the general surgeon and especially to emphasize basics in anatomy, physical examination, and treatment of common hand and upper extremity emergencies.

Interestingly, there is a modest amount of recent literature on the quality and duration of hand fellowship training. In a recent survey to which 80% of program directors responded, the majority thought that a 1-year fellowship was still sufficient training despite the increasing breadth of knowledge in the field and new technological developments. However, programs needed to evaluate their own training to highlight areas that may need enhancement. Nonetheless, many training programs admittedly remain deficient in areas, especially shoulder and elbow, replantation, brachial plexus, congenital, and flap surgery.[1]

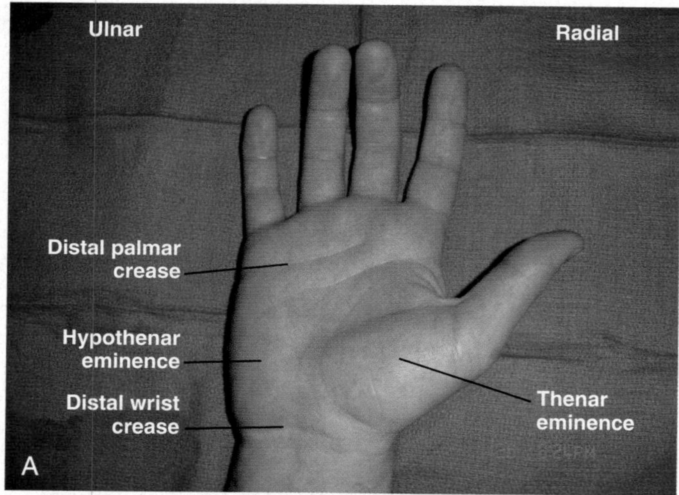

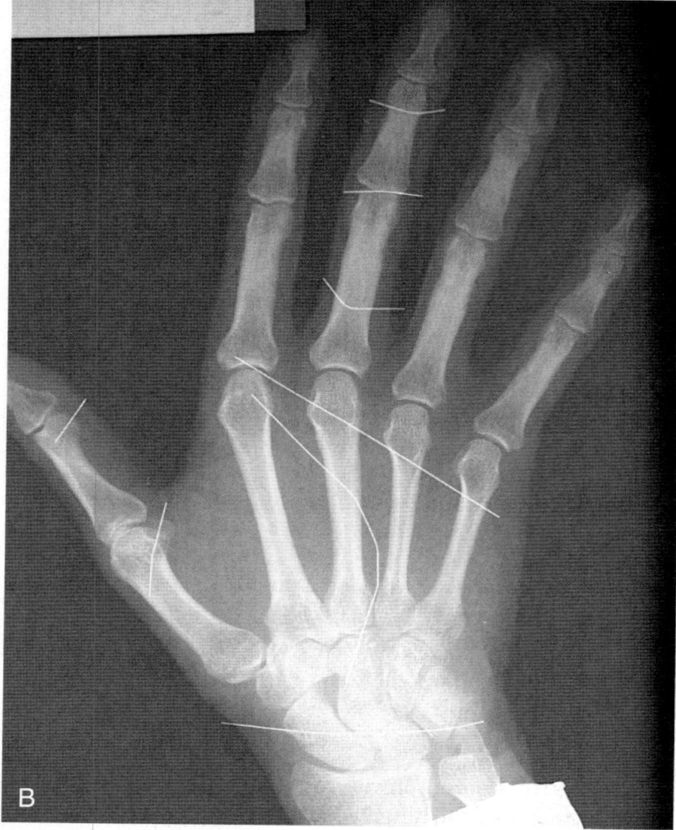

FIG. 70.1 Surface anatomy of the hand. (A) Hand surfaces and nomenclature. (B) Skin creases of the hand superimposed on the skeletal structures.

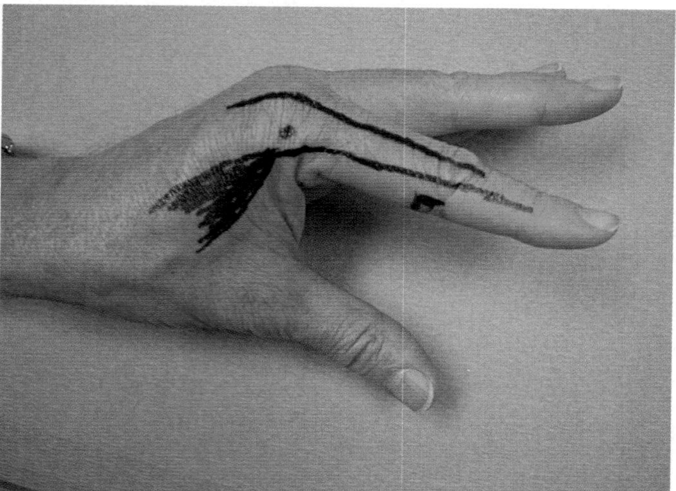

FIG. 70.2 Outline of first dorsal interosseous muscle on the index finger shows how it passes volar to the fulcrum of flexion of the metacarpophalangeal joint and dorsal to the interphalangeal joints. Interossei flex metacarpophalangeal joints and extend proximal and distal interphalangeal joints. The long extrinsic extensor tendon passes dorsal to all joints.

BASIC ANATOMY

The arm and hand are divided into volar, or palmar, and dorsal aspects. Distal to the elbow, structures are termed radial or ulnar to the middle finger axis rather than lateral and medial, respectively, because with forearm pronation and supination, the latter terms become confusing. The nomenclature of digits has become standardized. The hand has five digits, namely, the thumb and four fingers (the thumb is not called a finger). The four fingers are respectively termed the index, long (middle), ring, and small (little) fingers. The use of numbers to designate digits is no longer accepted (Fig. 70.1). Within the hand, those structures close to the fingertips are termed distal, whereas those farther up toward the wrist are termed proximal. Motion in a palmar direction is flexion, whereas dorsal motion is termed extension. Finger motion away from the long finger axis is termed abduction, whereas motion toward the axis of the long finger is termed adduction. The description of the motion of the thumb is sometimes confusing. Extension of the thumb is in the plane of the palm of the hand, whereas palmar abduction of the thumb is the motion that occurs at 90 degrees away from the plane of the palm. Finally, side to side motion of the wrist is termed radial and ulnar deviation.

Intrinsic muscles of the hand are those that have their origins and insertions in the hand, whereas the extrinsic muscles have their muscle bellies in the forearm and their tendon insertions in the hand. The intrinsic muscles that make up the thenar eminence are the abductor pollicis brevis, flexor pollicis brevis, opponens pollicis, and adductor pollicis. There are four dorsal interossei that arise from adjacent sides of each metacarpal and provide abduction of the metacarpophalangeal (MP) joints of the index, middle, and ring fingers. There are three palmar interossei that adduct the index, ring, and little fingers toward the middle finger. Four lumbricals originate on the flexor digitorum profundus (FDP) tendons in the palm and insert on the radial sides of the extensor mechanisms of the four fingers. Together with the interossei, these bring about flexion of the MP joints and extension of the interphalangeal (IP) joints of the fingers (Fig. 70.2). The flexor pollicis brevis flexes the thumb at the MP joint in contrast with the extrinsic flexor pollicis longus (FPL), which flexes the thumb at the IP joint.

The hypothenar muscles consist of the flexor digiti minimi, which flexes the little finger at the MP joint, and the abductor digiti minimi and opponens digiti minimi. A small muscle called the palmaris brevis is located transversally in the subcutaneous tissue at the base of the hypothenar eminence. It is innervated by the ulnar nerve, puckers the skin, and helps in cupping the skin of the palm during grip (Table 70.1).

The extrinsic muscles originate proximal to the wrist and comprise the long flexors and extensors of the wrist and digits. The extensors are located dorsally and are divided into three subgroups.

TABLE 70.1 Intrinsic muscles of the hand.

MUSCLE	INNERVATION*	FUNCTION
Abductor pollicis brevis	Median	Abducts the thumb
Flexor pollicis brevis	Median	Flexes the thumb
Opponens pollicis	Median	Opposes the thumb
Lumbricals	Median and ulnar	Flex MP joints and extend IP joints
Palmaris brevis	Ulnar	Wrinkles the skin on the medial (ulnar) side of the palm
Adductor pollicis	Ulnar	Adducts the thumb
Abductor digiti minimi	Ulnar	Abducts the small finger
Flexor digiti minimi	Ulnar	Flexes the small digit
Opponens digiti minimi	Ulnar	Opposes the small finger
Dorsal interossei	Ulnar	Abduct the fingers; flex MP joints and extend the IP joints
Palmar interossei	Ulnar	Adduct the fingers; flex MP joints and extend the IP joints

IP, Interphalangeal; *MP*, metacarpophalangeal.
*All the thenar intrinsic muscles are supplied by the median nerve except the adductor pollicis; all the remaining intrinsic muscles are supplied by the ulnar nerve except the two radial lumbricals.

TABLE 70.2 Extrinsic muscles of the dorsal forearm.

MUSCLE	INNERVATION*	FUNCTION
Extensor pollicis brevis	Radial	Abducts the hand and extends the thumb at the proximal phalanx
Abductor pollicis longus	Radial	Abducts the hand and thumb
Extensor carpi radialis longus	Radial	Extends and radially deviates the hand
Extensor carpi radialis brevis	Radial	Extends and radially deviates the hand
Extensor pollicis longus	Radial	Extends the distal phalanx of the thumb
Extensor digitorum communis	Radial	Extends the fingers and the hand
Extensor indicis proprius	Radial	Extends the index finger
Extensor digiti minimi/quinti	Radial	Extends the small finger
Extensor carpi ulnaris	Radial	Extends and ulnarly deviates the wrist
Supinator	Radial	Supination
Brachioradialis	Radial	Flexes the forearm

*All muscles of the dorsal forearm are innervated by the radial nerve and its respective branches.

The radial most subgroup is termed the mobile wad and comprises the brachioradialis, extensor carpi radialis longus (ECRL), and extensor carpi radialis brevis (ECRB). The ECRL and ECRB extend the wrist and deviate it radially. The second group is located in a more superficial layer and comprises three muscles, namely, the extensor carpi ulnaris (ECU), extensor digiti minimi (EDM), and extensor digitorum communis (EDC). The ECU deviates the wrist in an ulnar direction and extends the wrist, whereas the EDM and EDC extend the MP joints of the fingers. The third and deeper subgroup comprises four muscles, three of which act on the thumb; the remaining muscle influences the index finger. The abductor pollicis longus (APL), extensor pollicis longus (EPL), and extensor pollicis brevis (EPB) provide function to the thumb, and the extensor indicis proprius (EIP) extends the MP joint to the index finger. Last of the deep muscles is the supinator, which is located proximally in the forearm (Table 70.2).

The extensor tendons pass through six compartments deep to the extensor retinaculum at the dorsum of the wrist. From the radial to the ulnar side, these tendons and compartments are arranged as follows. The first compartment contains the APL and EPB, which also forms the radial boundary of the so-called anatomic snuffbox. The second compartment consists of the ECRL and ECRB, and the third compartment (which also forms the ulnar boundary of the anatomic snuffbox) contains the EPL. The EIP and EDC pass through the fourth compartment, and the EDM passes through the fifth compartment, where they overlie the distal radioulnar joint. The sixth compartment contains the ECU (Fig. 70.3) (Video 70.1 Extensor Compartments).

At the level of the MP joints, the long extrinsic extensor tendons broaden out to form the extensor hood. The proximal part of the hood at this level is called the sagittal band. It loops around the MP joint and blends into the volar plate, thus forming a lasso around the base of the proximal phalanx, through which it extends the MP joint. The insertions of the interossei and lumbricals enter into the extensor hood as the lateral bands. These lateral bands insert distally and dorsally to the axis of the proximal IP (PIP) joint, and it is through this distal insertion that the intrinsic muscles (the interossei and lumbricals) are flexors of the MP joints and yet extensors of the IP joints. The extensor hood inserts to the base of the middle phalanx, which is termed the central slip, and finally proceeds on to the base of the distal phalanx, where it inserts through the terminal slip, thus extending the distal IP (DIP) joint (Fig. 70.4) (Video 70.2 Dorsal Hood).

The extrinsic flexor muscles are located on the volar aspect of the forearm and are arranged in three layers. The superficial layer comprises four muscles—pronator teres, flexor carpi radialis (FCR), flexor carpi ulnaris (FCU), and palmaris longus. The palmaris longus muscle may be absent in as many as 10% to 12% of individuals. These muscles originate from the medial humeral epicondyle in the proximal forearm and function to flex the wrist and to pronate the forearm. The intermediate layer consists of the flexor digitorum superficialis (FDS), which allows independent flexion of the PIP joints of the fingers. In the deep layer, there are three muscles: the FPL, which flexes the IP joint to the thumb; the FDP, which flexes the DIP joints of the fingers; and a distal quadrangular muscle that spans between the radius and ulna, termed the pronator quadratus, which helps in pronation of the forearm (Table 70.3) (Video 70.3 Flexor Tendons and Pulley System).

Nerve supply to the hand is by three nerves, the median, ulnar, and radial nerves. A knowledge of the surface anatomy of nerves helps in evaluation of specific lacerating injuries (Fig. 70.5). The ulnar attachment to the flexor retinaculum is to the pisiform and hook of the hamate, and the radial attachment is to the scaphoid and ridge of the trapezium. The median nerve passes through the carpal tunnel between these landmarks. It gives sensation to the thumb, index finger, middle finger, and radial half of the ring finger. The palmar cutaneous branch of the median nerve originates from its radial side 5 to 6 cm proximal to the wrist, providing sensation to the palmar triangle. The ulnar nerve travels to the radial side of the pisiform and passes to the ulnar side of the hook of the hamate in its passage through Guyon canal. It gives sensation to

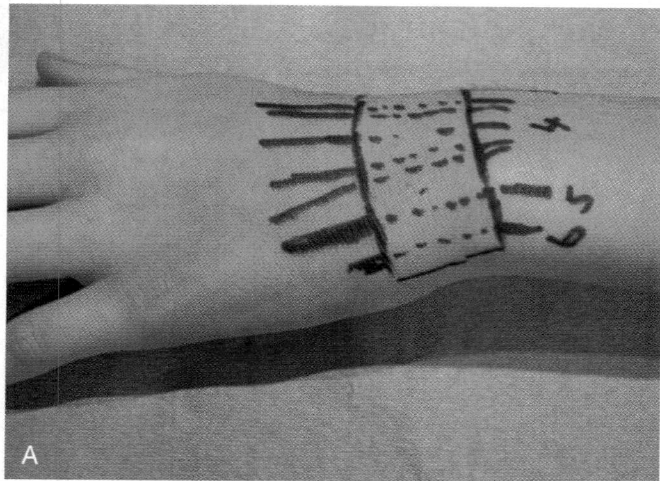

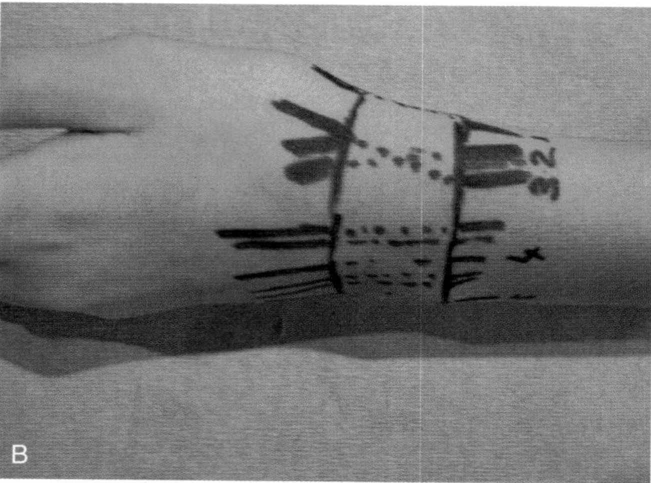

FIG. 70.3 (A and B) Surface anatomy of the six dorsal extensor compartments at the wrist. Note that the first (abductor pollicis longus and extensor pollicis brevis) and third (extensor pollicis longus) compartments form the radial and ulnar boundaries, respectively, of the anatomic snuffbox.

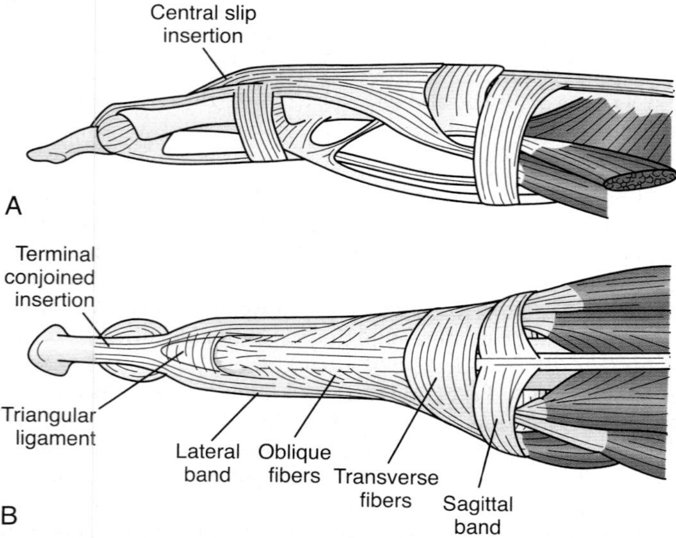

FIG. 70.4 Extensor mechanism of the fingers. (A) Lateral view. (B) Dorsal view.

TABLE 70.3 Extrinsic muscles of the volar forearm.

MUSCLE	INNERVATION*	FUNCTION
Pronator teres	Median	Pronation
Flexor carpi radialis	Median	Flexion and radial deviation of the wrist
Palmaris longus	Median	Flexion of the wrist
Flexor carpi ulnaris	Ulnar	Flexion and ulnar deviation of the wrist
Flexor digitorum superficialis	Median	Flexion of the proximal interphalangeal joint
Flexor digitorum profundus	Median and ulnar	Flexion of the distal interphalangeal joint
Pronator quadratus	Median	Pronation
Flexor pollicis longus	Median	Flexion of the thumb

*All muscles of the volar forearm are innervated by the median nerve and its branches except the two ulnar digits of the flexor digitorum profundus and flexor carpi ulnaris, which are innervated by the ulnar nerve.

the little finger and ulnar half of the ring finger; the dorsal branch of the ulnar nerve (arising proximal to the wrist and curving dorsally around the head of the ulna) supplies the same digits on their dorsal aspects. The superficial radial sensory nerve emerges from under the brachioradialis in the distal forearm, dividing into two or three branches proximal to the radial styloid that then proceed in a subcutaneous course across the anatomic snuffbox, innervating the skin of the dorsum of the first web space. The number of fingers served by each nerve is variable. However, as an absolute rule, the palmar surfaces of the index and little fingers are always served by the median and ulnar nerves, respectively.

With regard to the motor supply of these nerves, the ulnar nerve supplies the hypothenar muscles, interossei, ulnar two lumbricals, adductor pollicis, and deep head of the flexor pollicis brevis. The median nerve supplies the abductor pollicis brevis, opponens pollicis, radial two lumbricals, and superficial head of the flexor pollicis brevis. In summary, the median nerve thus supplies

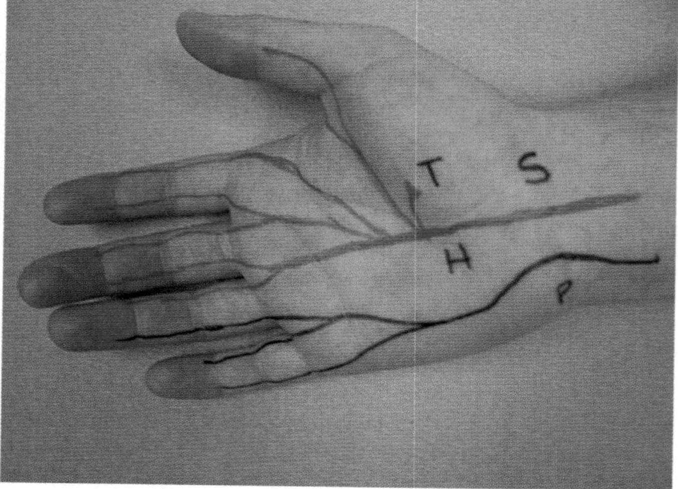

FIG. 70.5 Surface anatomy of median *(red)* and ulnar *(black)* nerves. *H*, Hook of hamate; *P*, pisiform; *S*, scaphoid; *T*, trapezium.

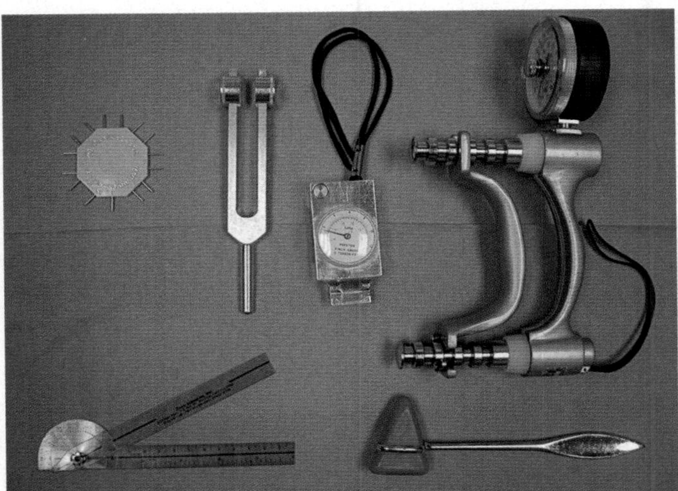

FIG. 70.6 Basic instruments used in hand examination include a tuning fork, pinch meter, grip dynamometer, two-point discriminator (paperclip also suffices), goniometer, and patella hammer.

all the extrinsic digit flexors and wrist flexors (except the FDP to the ring and little fingers and the FCU, which are supplied by the ulnar nerve) and all the thumb intrinsic muscles (except the adductor pollicis, which is innervated by the ulnar nerve). The ulnar nerve supplies all the interossei, all the lumbricals (except the radial two, which are supplied by the median nerve), and the adductor of the thumb. The radial nerve innervates all of the wrist, finger, and thumb extrinsic long extensors.

EXAMINATION AND DIAGNOSIS

Evaluation

Basic instruments used in hand examination are shown in Fig. 70.6. Examination of the resting posture of the hand can provide valuable information; for example, if a finger flexor tendon is severed, that affected finger does not assume its normal resting position in line with the natural flexion cascade of the adjacent digits (Fig. 70.7). Extensor tendon injuries may be indicated by a droop at the affected joint. A clawed posture of the little and ring fingers may be characteristic of an ulnar nerve injury (Fig. 70.8). Absence of sweating at the fingertips may imply a nerve injury in that particular distribution. Swelling and erythema may indicate a hand infection, and a purulent flexor tenosynovitis always results in a flexed posture of the digits. Rotational and angular digital deformities may occur when there are underlying fractures.

Neurovascular Examination

The Allen test confirms patency of the ulnar and radial arteries. Two-point sensory discrimination is the most sensitive method of testing for sensory loss and is easily done by using a bent paperclip (Fig. 70.9). The paperclip ends are set to a distance of approximately 5 mm apart for fingertip pulp sensory testing. The points are aligned along the axis of the finger. If this test is not reproducible because of an uncooperative patient, suspicion of a nerve injury can be confirmed by the tactile adherence test in which a plastic pen is passed back and forth gently across the pulp on either side of each finger. Adhesion, because of the presence of sweat, is shown by slight but definite movement of the finger being examined (anesthetized finger pulp will not sweat).

There are two muscle tests that may provide the examiner with an absolute diagnosis of median or ulnar nerve injury. The motor function of the abductor pollicis brevis tests the median nerve. With the hand flat and facing palm up, the patient is asked to use his or her thumb to touch the examiner's finger, which is held directly over the thenar eminence (Fig. 70.10). The flexor digiti minimi muscle function will test the motor supply of the ulnar nerve. In the same hand position, the patient raises her or his little finger vertically, flexing the MP joint to a 90-degree angle, with the IP joint held straight. Tests for function of the radial nerve and its branches require wrist extension, thumb extension, and finger extension at the MP joint.

Musculoskeletal Examination

The integrity of the tendons is individually tested (Fig. 70.11). Flexion at distal joints of the thumb and fingers confirms that the FPL and FDP, respectively, are intact. Testing of FDS tendons is more complex. It is not possible to flex the DIP joints independently of one another because of a common origin of the FDP tendons. Thus, the other fingers are fixed in extension by the examiner, and the patient is asked to flex the remaining digits. Movement is produced by the FDS and occurs at the PIP joint. In approximately one third of patients, the FDS cannot produce little finger flexion. In 50% of these, in turn, there is a common origin with the ring finger, so flexion will occur if the ring finger is permitted to flex simultaneously. More uncommonly, there is no profundus tendon to the little finger and the superficialis inserts into the middle and distal phalanges. The long and short extensors (EPL and EPB) and the long abductor of the thumb are tested by asking the patient to extend his or her thumb against resistance while these tendons are individually palpated. Long extensors of the fingers are tested by asking the patient to extend them against resistance applied to the dorsum of the proximal phalanx.

A closed boutonnière jamming injury may be difficult to initially diagnose. In this type of injury, the central slip insertion is disrupted from the middle phalanx and the triangular ligament on each side of the central slip is stretched or disrupted. The lateral bands then migrate volar. It takes time for this deformity to evolve. Initial presentation may not be immediately obvious until the lateral bands subluxate volarly and create the obvious boutonnière problem with PIP joint flexion and DIP joint hyperextension. The Elson test may help make this diagnosis. Normally, with the PIP joint blocked in flexion, one cannot actively extend the DIP joint because of slack in the lateral bands (Fig. 70.12).

Special Investigations

Radiographs are necessary in almost every case. These help in the diagnosis and evaluation of fractures and also in the investigation of foreign bodies. Multiple radiographic views of the affected part are required to define the precise pathologic process or fracture pattern. Glass is often seen on plain radiographs, and if it is not seen but suspected, it may be visualized by computed tomography (CT) or magnetic resonance imaging (MRI). If plastic is painted, it may be seen on routine radiographs; it is generally poorly visualized with CT but can be clearly seen with MRI. Wooden foreign bodies may be seen by CT or MRI but not by routine radiography.

Various stress radiographic views and cineradiography may be useful for demonstrating dynamic wrist instability patterns, especially scapholunate separation. Arthrography may detect ligamentous tears by extravasation of contrast material between the radiocarpal, distal radioulnar, and midcarpal joints. This is best combined with MRI, especially for the detection of triangular

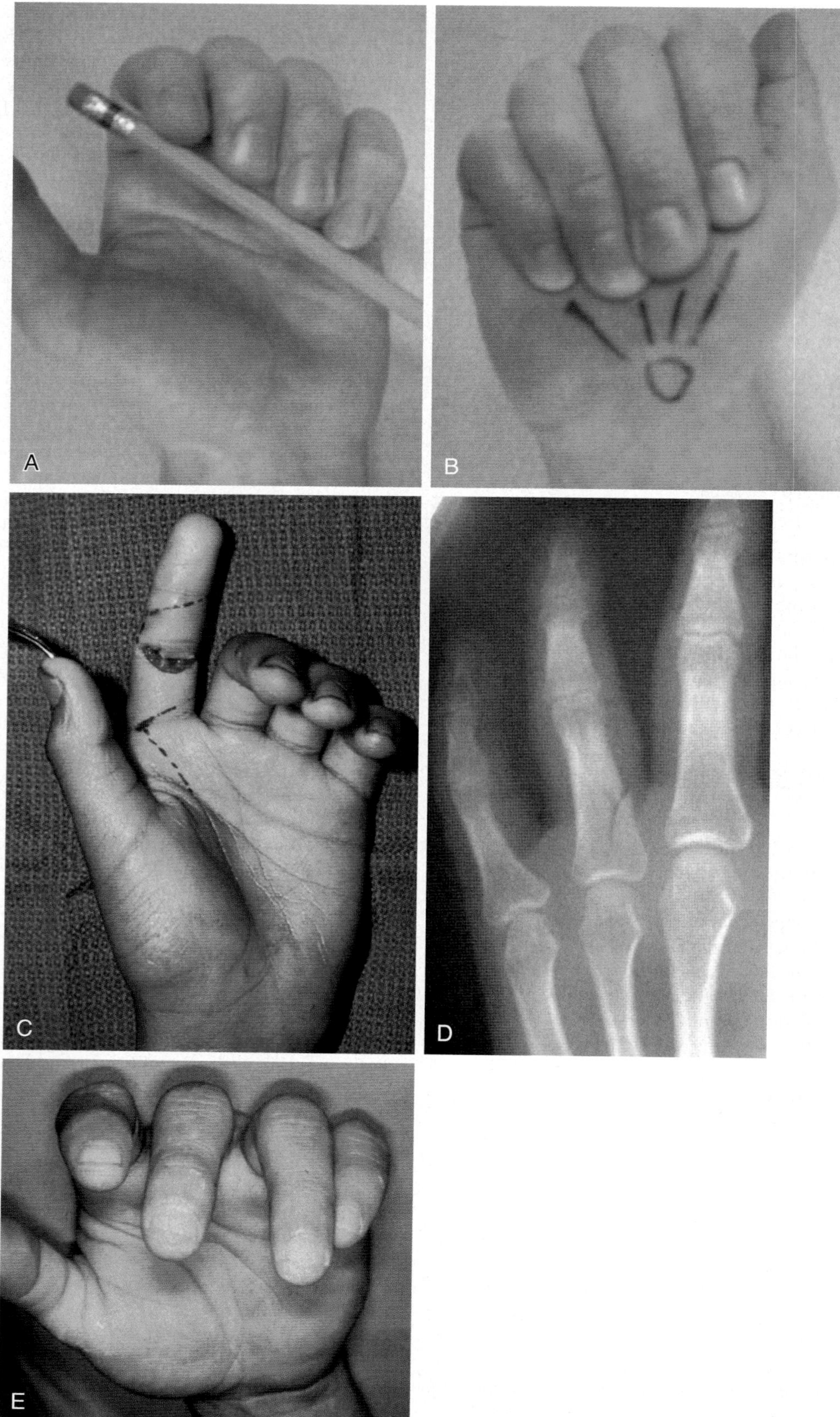

FIG. 70.7 (A and B) Natural finger flexion cascade of the hand in repose. Note the fingertips pointing to the distal pole of the scaphoid. (C) With flexor tendon injury, the affected digit does not adopt this resting flexed posture. (D and E) Spiral finger fractures produce a rotational deformity, which is also noted as an interruption in the finger flexion cascade.

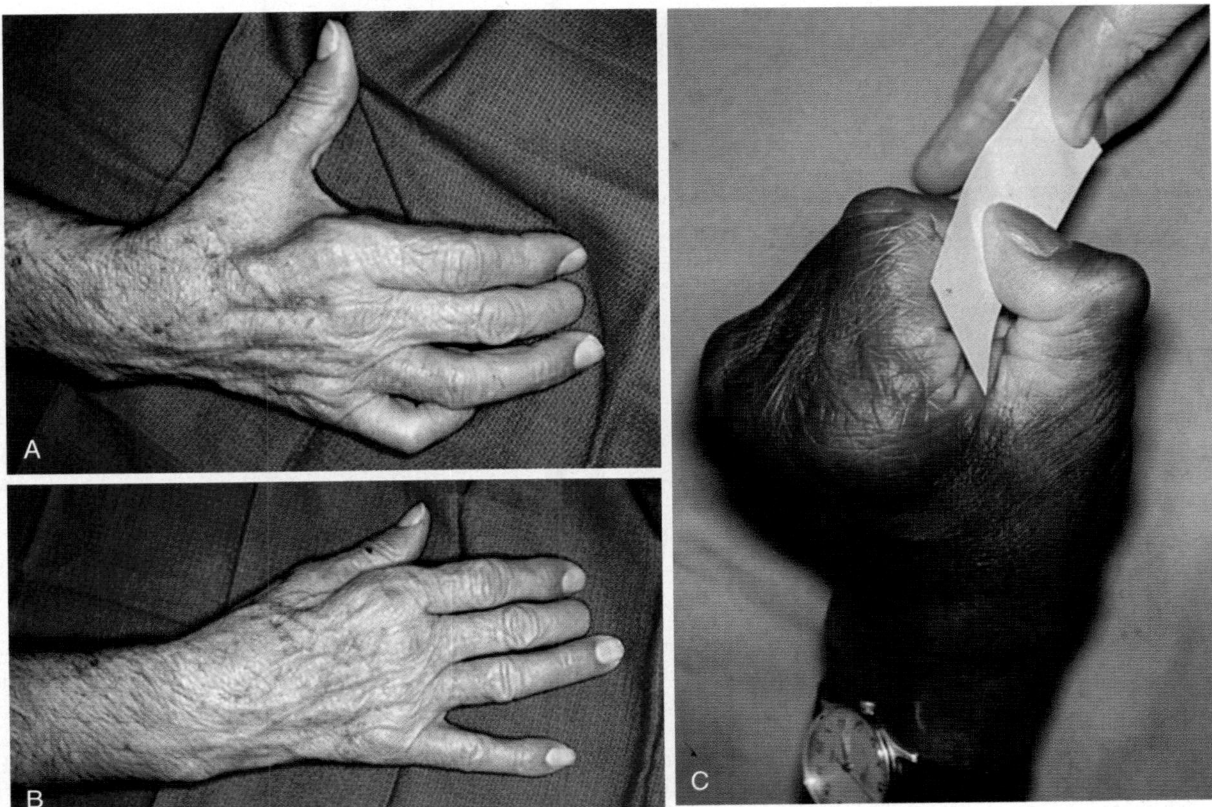

FIG. 70.8 (A) Marked atrophy in the first web space dorsal interosseous muscle is noted with ulnar nerve palsy, with clawing of the little and ring fingers. (B) The little finger assumes an abducted position and cannot be adducted to the adjacent fingers (Wartenberg sign). (C) Because thumb adduction is weak, attempts to grasp a piece of paper between the adducted thumb and index finger produce compensatory thumb interphalangeal joint flexion (Froment sign).

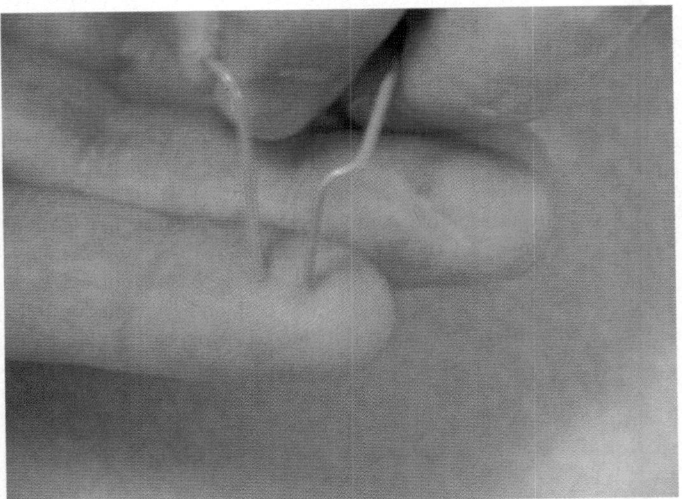

FIG. 70.9 Two-point discrimination on the fingertip can be tested with a bent paperclip, with the tips of the paperclip set specific distances apart.

fibrocartilage tears at the ulnocarpal joint. Radionuclide bone scanning may help diagnose osteomyelitis, but in the hand, a false-positive result may occur because of the proximity of soft tissue infections to the bones. Occult wrist fractures may be localized by increased radionuclide uptake, but a false-positive result on evaluation for a fracture may also occur with ligamentous injuries. CT is a helpful modality for diagnosis of suspected carpal fractures (e.g., a scaphoid fracture that may not be seen on routine radiography), although most prefer MRI.

Wrist arthroscopy is useful as a diagnostic and therapeutic modality for a number of wrist problems, especially for disorders of the triangular fibrocartilage. Minimally invasive surgery with arthroscopic guidance has added a new dimension to the treatment of acute wrist disorders, such as scaphoid and distal radius intraarticular fractures.

Patients with ischemic problems often require noninvasive vascular studies. Doppler pressure measurements help localize the site of a vascular lesion. Angiography in the upper extremity is always carried out in the presence of a vasodilator (e.g., tolazoline [Priscoline], nitroglycerin) or an axillary block to differentiate apparent vessel occlusion from vasospasm. Subtraction radiographs with magnification help improve the detail and definition of the vascular study, especially in the distal forearm and hand.

PRINCIPLES OF TREATMENT

In the case of injuries, treatment is directed at the specific structures damaged—skeletal, tendon, nerve, vessel, integument.[2,3] In emergency situations, the goals of treatment are to maintain or to restore distal circulation, to obtain a healed wound, to preserve motion, and to retain distal sensation. Stable skeletal architecture is established in the primary phase of care because skeletal stability is essential for effective motion and function of the extremity.

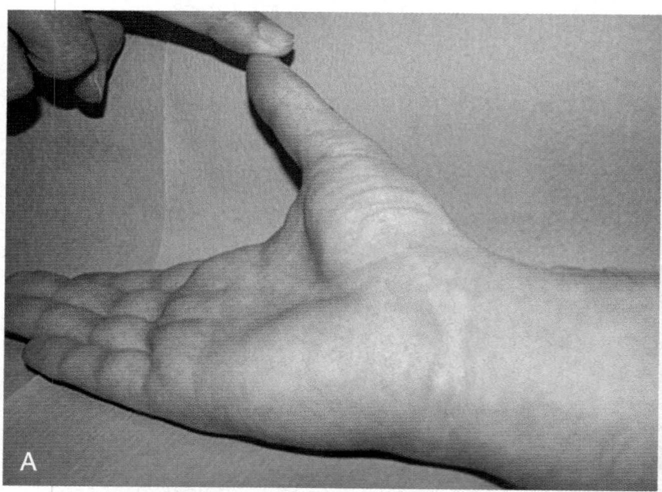

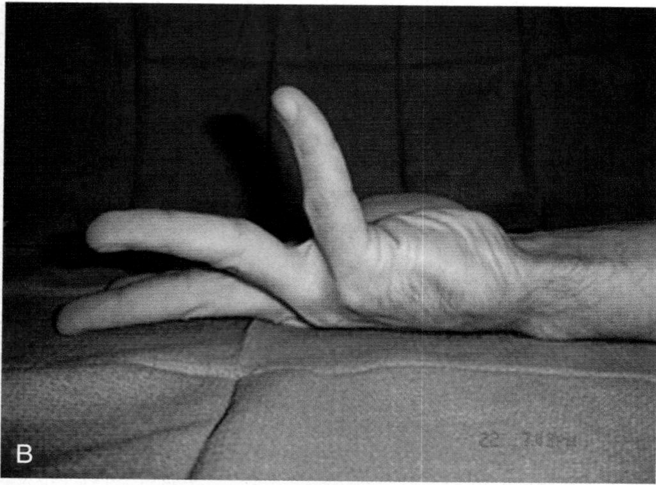

FIG. 70.10 Motor innervation of muscles of the hand. (A) Thumb abduction tests median motor nerve function. (B) Little finger flexion at the metacarpophalangeal joint with simultaneous interphalangeal joint extension tests ulnar motor nerve function.

This also reestablishes skeletal length, straightens deformities, and corrects the compression or kinking of nerves and vessels. Arteries are also repaired in the acute phase of treatment to maintain distal tissue viability. Extrinsic compression on arteries must also be released emergently, such as with compartment pressure problems. In clean-cut injuries, tendons can be repaired primarily. In situations in which there is a chance that tendon adhesions may form, such as when there are associated fractures, it is nonetheless better to repair tendons primarily with preservation of their length and to perform tenolysis, if necessary, at a later date. However, when there are open and contaminated wounds or a severe crushing injury, it is best to delay repair of tendon and nerve injuries.

In clean-cut sharp wounds, primary nerve repair lessens the possibility of nerve end retraction and therefore the need for later nerve grafting. However, primary nerve repair must not be performed in situations in which there is contusion of the nerve (e.g., gunshot wounds, power saw injuries, blunt crushing trauma) because the extent of proximal axonal injury may not be immediately evident. If nerve repair is performed before this is apparent, it may result in abnormal nerve ends being reattached, negating the chance for functional return.

In severe soft tissue injuries, wound closure may not be possible immediately. Initial open treatment of the wound is directed to prevent an infection and to protect critical deep structures by proper dressing and wound management (Fig. 70.13). Adequate debridement is essential, but appropriate soft tissue coverage must be achieved as soon as possible thereafter. The sooner the soft tissue coverage can be achieved, the less likely there will be a secondary deformity caused by fibrosis and joint contractures. The more rapidly hand therapy can be started, the better the chance for maximizing functional return. The treatment regimen must consist of debridement, rigid skeletal fixation, and early soft tissue resurfacing, possibly even requiring microvascular soft tissue reconstruction, followed by protected range of motion exercises as soon as possible. It has been shown that early soft tissue reconstruction results in improved function, decreased morbidity, and shortened hospital stay.

Appropriate treatment of upper extremity problems requires a thorough knowledge of local and regional anesthesia, use of a tourniquet to provide a bloodless field, correct placement of incisions to minimize later scar contracture, and appropriate use of dressings and splints to reduce edema and to maintain a functional position. Above all, a clear knowledge of the unique anatomy of the hand and upper extremity not only aids in obtaining an accurate clinical diagnosis but also enables the safe performance of surgery.

Anesthesia

The choice of general, regional (e.g., intravenous Bier block, brachial plexus block that might be a supraclavicular or axillary block), or local anesthesia is governed by the extent and length of the operation. An upper arm or forearm tourniquet can be used in the unanesthetized extremity with only local anesthetic field infiltration or digital block for 30 to 45 minutes in a relaxed, cooperative patient, provided the arm is well exsanguinated. After this time, tourniquet pain will not permit more extensive local anesthetic procedures. If one has to operate in other areas, such as for harvesting of bone, nerve, tendon, or skin graft, or if more extensive surgical procedures are planned, general anesthesia will be required.

A digital block or median, ulnar, or radial wrist nerve block may be useful, especially for more limited emergency department procedures (Fig. 70.14). Digital nerve blocks usually do not include epinephrine, which could lead to vasospasm, but evidence has indicated the safety of distal blocks using an epinephrine solution. A maximum safe dose of lidocaine is 4 mg/kg.

Tourniquet Application

The tourniquet is used to provide a bloodless field so that clear visualization of all structures in the operative field is obtained. Penrose drains, rolled rubber glove fingers, or commercially available tourniquets can be used on digits. Great care must be taken when any constrictive device is used on digits because narrow bands cause direct injury to underlying nerves and digital vessels. With the use of an arm tourniquet, the skin beneath the cuff must be protected with several wraps of cast padding. During skin preparation, this area must be kept dry to prevent blistering of the skin under an inflated cuff over moist padding. The cuff selected needs to be as wide as the diameter of the arm. Standard pressures used are 100 to 150 mm Hg higher than systolic blood pressure. The cuff is deflated every 2 hours for 15 to 20 minutes (5 minutes of

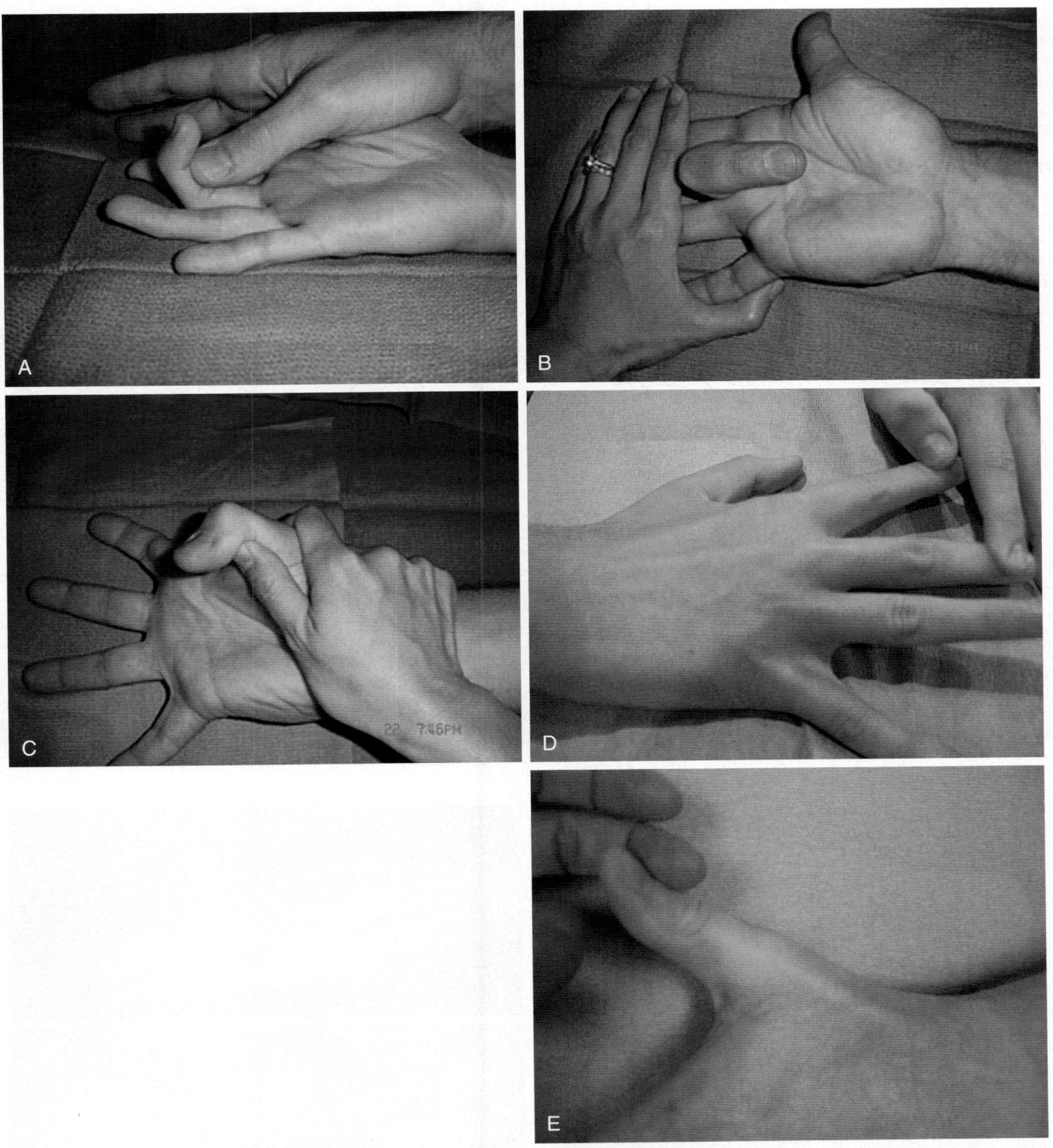

FIG. 70.11 Individual clinical testing of the flexor digitorum profundus (A), flexor digitorum superficialis (B), flexor pollicis longus (C), finger extensors (D), and thumb extensors (E).

reperfusion for every 30 minutes of tourniquet time) to revascularize distal tissues and to relieve pressure on nerves locally before the cuff is reinflated for more extensive procedures.[4] Exsanguination of the extremities is performed by wrapping the extremity with a Martin bandage in all cases, except those involving infection or tumors. In these latter cases, because of the possibility of embolization by mechanical pressure, exsanguination by bandage wrapping needs to be avoided. Simple elevation of the extremity for a few minutes before tourniquet inflation suffices.[2]

Incisions

Incisions are of the Bruner zigzag or midaxial type, or combinations of these, to avoid longitudinal motion-restricting scars that cross palmar flexion creases (Fig. 70.15). The marginal edge of a skin graft with healthy skin is also a potential scar line, so the margin of the skin graft is designed to be in these same lines to prevent contractures across flexion creases. Palmar incisions follow the pattern of skin creases. Dorsal incisions on the fingers and wrist and incisions on the forearm may follow longitudinal straight lines.

Dressings and Splints

The purposes of dressings are to protect wounds, to absorb drainage, and to help splint repaired structures. The first layer consists of a nonadherent dressing and may contain an antibiotic. The next layer is soft and bulky and is usually followed by a firmer, more conforming external wrap. Conforming compression is useful, but

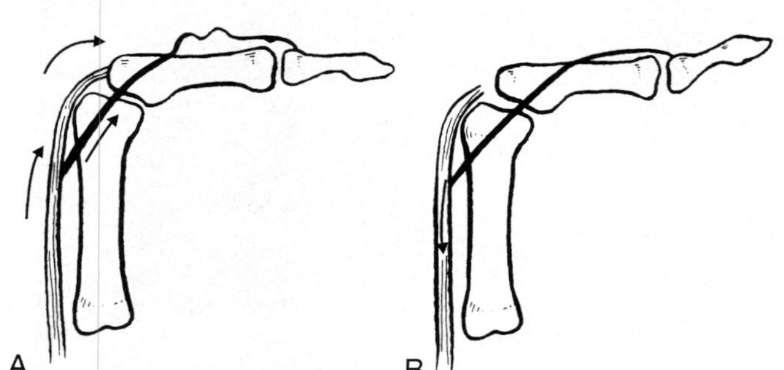

FIG. 70.12 (A) Maximal passive flexion of the proximal interphalangeal (PIP) joint causes slack in the lateral bands because they are pulled distally by their interconnections to the extensor hood proximally as the central slip and extensor tendon are pulled forward. Thus, normally, one cannot actively extend the distal interphalangeal (DIP) joint when the PIP joint is passively flexed. (B) Central slip injury eliminates the lateral band slack that is normally produced by passive PIP joint flexion and allows extensor tension on the DIP joint because of proximal migration of the extensor apparatus. The ability to extend the DIP joint is pathologic.

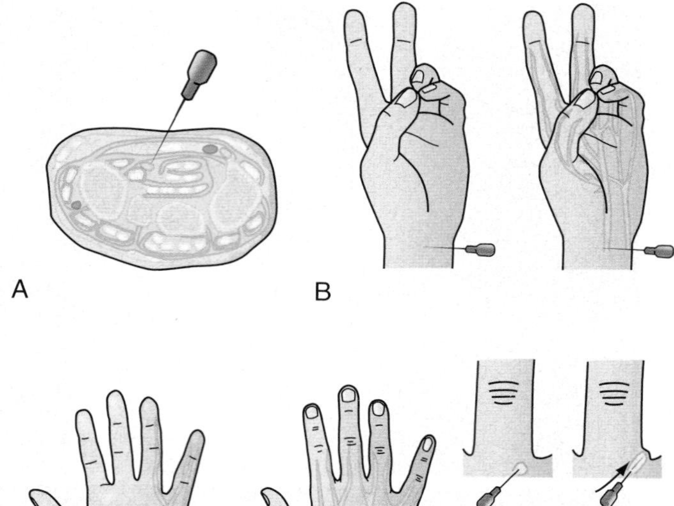

FIG. 70.14 (A) Median nerve block is done at the wrist, where the median nerve is superficial to all the flexor tendons in the carpal tunnel. (B) At the wrist, when a median nerve block is performed, the needle is directed between the palmaris longus and flexor carpi radialis tendons. (C) Ulnar nerve block at the wrist is done by passing the injecting needle around the ulnar deep aspect of the flexor carpi ulnaris tendon just proximal to the pisiform. Intravascular injection into the immediately adjacent ulnar artery is avoided by first aspirating before injection. (D) Dorsal branches of the ulnar nerve and superficial sensory radial nerve are anesthetized by raising a broad weal of local anesthetic across the dorsum of the wrist. (E) A dorsal approach to the finger can be used for digital nerve block.

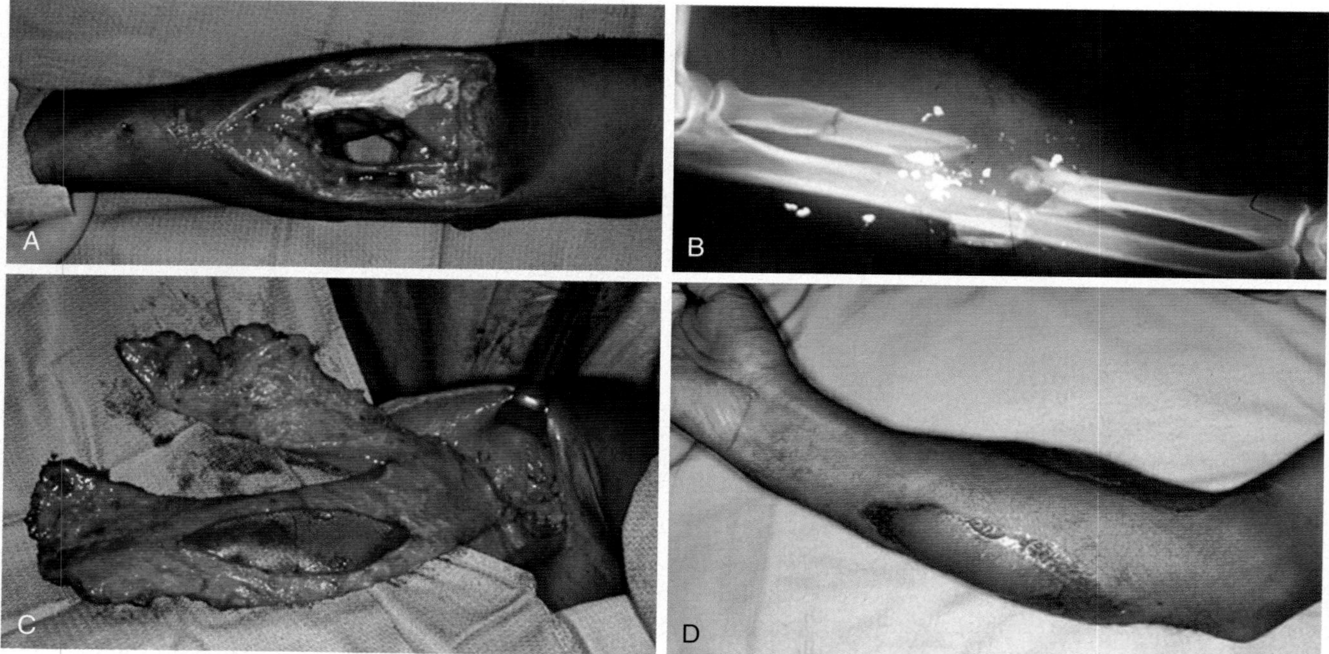

FIG. 70.13 (A) Gunshot wound of forearm showing extensive soft tissue injury. (B) Initial radiograph. (C) Microvascular reconstruction using a bilobed latissimus dorsi musculocutaneous flap was done in association with fracture fixation. (D) Long-term follow-up of reconstructed forearm that also required sural nerve grafting to a segmental injury of the median nerve.

constriction is harmful. Splints are made to protect only the part necessary to be immobilized and must not prevent motion in the remainder of the extremity. Often, patients keep the injured, operated, or infected hand in a flexed wrist position, which automatically causes the MP joints to extend, thereby placing the collateral ligaments in their shortest lengths. Edema fluid collects dorsally, and the resulting dorsal hand swelling causes stiff joints. Thus, a splint that keeps the hand in the protected position extends the wrist 40 to 50 degrees, maintaining the MP joints at 70 degrees of flexion and the IP joints in a neutral position (Fig. 70.16). Postoperative hand elevation is essential to reduce edema.

TRAUMA

Emergency Control of Bleeding

Bleeding in the extremity can often be profuse when it is first encountered. A reasoned and controlled assessment of the situation almost invariably results in the control of bleeding and minimization of further blood loss and facilitates necessary stabilization of the patient and appropriate assessment of the upper limb injury. Bleeding in the upper extremity often results when vessels lie in a superficial location, such as at the wrist. Bleeding can originate from superficial veins that bleed more profusely when poorly applied dressings result in venous engorgement. The thicker media of transected arterial walls contracts strongly, resulting in hemostasis. Partially lacerated arteries continue to bleed profusely.

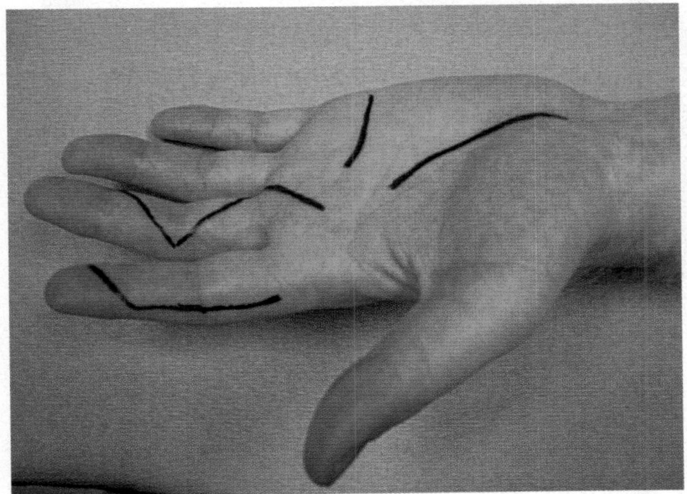

FIG. 70.15 Incisions used on the palmar surface of the hand must respect the creases. These may be zigzag Bruner incisions or midaxial incisions of the digits.

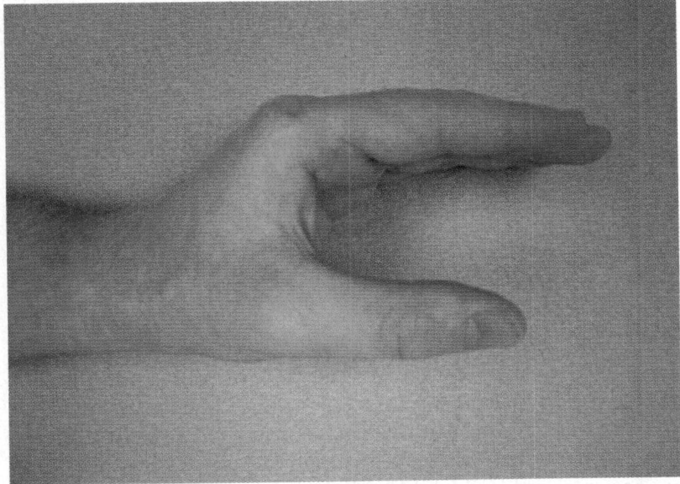

FIG. 70.16 The safe or protected position of the wrist, hand, and digits for application of a splint and dressings. The thumb is palmar abducted.

If necessary, one may have no fear of using sympathomimetic medications and their potential vasoconstricting effect to support blood pressure, even if free flap reconstruction or microvascular repair has been done. A study evaluated four sympathomimetic medications and actually showed that both vasoconstricting and norepinephrine have a beneficial effect on flap skin blood flow, with the maximal beneficial improvement from norepinephrine. This is the optimal pressor to use in patients who may need blood pressure support after free flap surgery. Elevation and accurately placed point pressure over bleeding points result in hemostatic control in almost all cases. Brief use of tourniquets may be a useful adjunct to allow temporary control of blood loss in the emergency department. Poorly applied dressings may be removed, bleeding points identified, point pressure dressings applied, and the hand elevated. This should take no more than 5 to 10 minutes. Extended tourniquet application results in hyperemic bleeding on deflation and subsequently hinders the surgeon. Tourniquets should not be applied for any significant period of time before definitive repair in the operating room, except for control of torrential hemorrhage caused by major amputation in the field. Misguided attempts to control upper extremity bleeding with clamps, ligatures, and cauterization in the emergency department frequently result in additional avoidable injury to adjacent uninjured structures and to vessels that may need to be repaired for adequate limb perfusion. Fracture reduction and stabilization will improve distal perfusion and facilitate hemorrhage control by restoring the limb to its correct anatomic alignment.

Lacerations, Fingertip Injuries, and Complex Soft Tissue Injuries

Although it is tempting to look within a wound to determine whether any tendon or nerve injuries exist, the same information can be obtained by careful physical examination without further violating a potential operative field and causing the patient extreme discomfort. A combination of knowledge of anatomy, presence of sensory or motor deficits, and presence or absence of radial or ulnar pulses can narrow the differential diagnosis of injured structures to a minimum. Control of bleeding is attempted by direct pressure with dressings and not by blind clamping of vessels because vital structures may be inadvertently injured in the depths of the wound. However, a tourniquet may be used if the initial pressure measures fail. Tourniquets are generally not used initially because the entire limb will be ischemic during transport of the patient. If the trauma has caused complete obliteration of anatomy, incisions can be extended into nonviolated areas in which control of bleeding vessels and delineation of injured tendons and nerves may be easier, using the guidelines presented earlier for extremity incisions.

All patients who present with extremity injuries undergo radiography. Fractures of the distal phalanx are among the more commonly encountered hand fractures.[3] A distal phalangeal fracture is appropriately splinted, reduced to improve alignment, or occasionally fixated internally if the fracture is unstable. Internal fixation

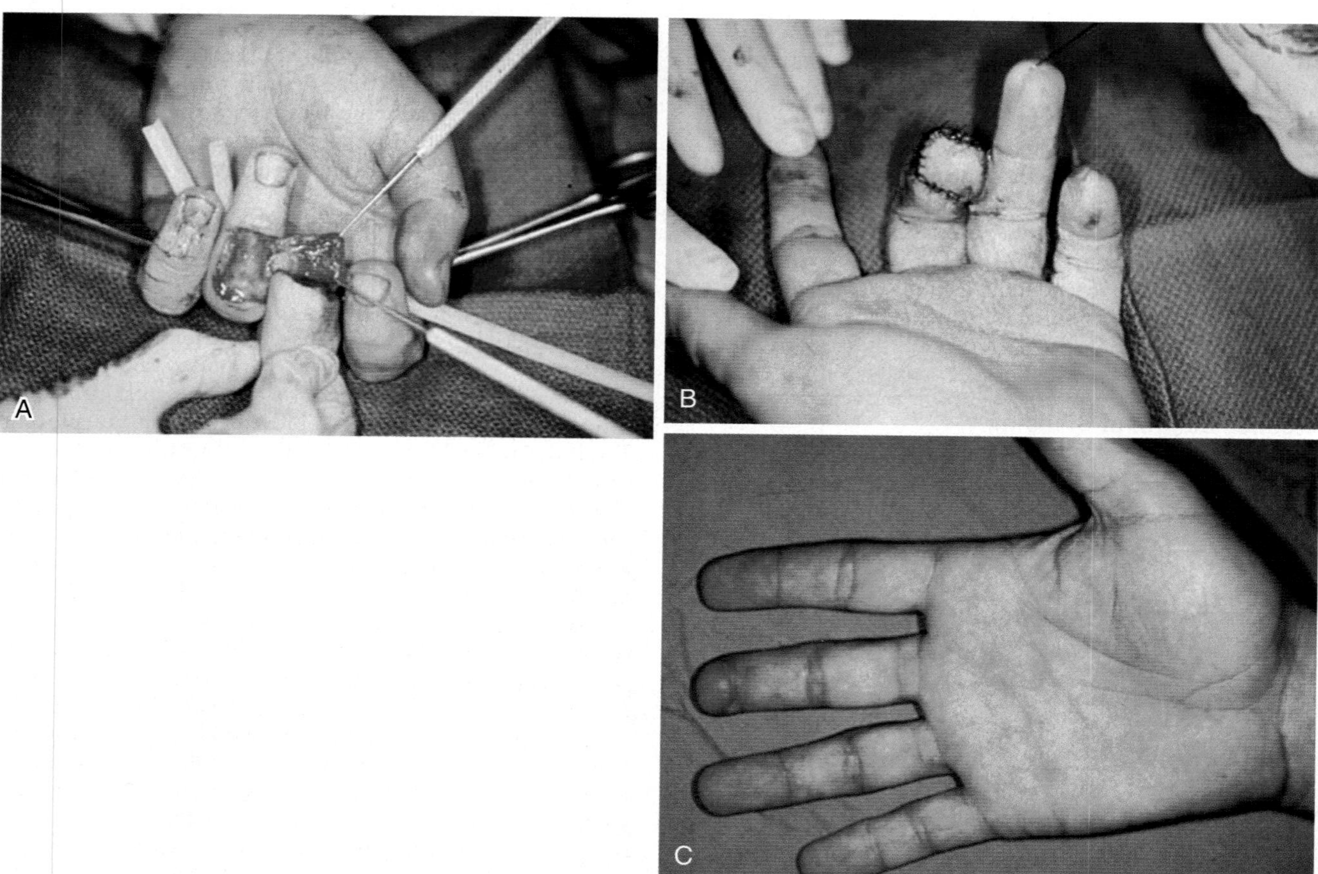

FIG. 70.17 (A and B) Volar angulated fingertip injury with loss of pulp pad and bone exposed was treated with a traditional cross-finger flap from the dorsum of the adjacent finger. (C) Excellent healing is seen in the long term after flap division.

is usually provided by simply placing a longitudinal 0.028-inch Kirschner wire. Appropriate antibiotics are administered because, technically, these are open fractures.

The least severe injury of the dorsum of the fingertip is a nail bed hematoma. When it is seen early, the hematoma can be decompressed by perforating the nail plate after the administration of a digital local anesthetic block. Fingertip and nail bed injuries can be managed with digital block anesthesia and a Penrose drain at the base of the finger as a tourniquet. After the nail plate has been stripped, simple gentle removal of the nail to examine the underlying nail bed is done, and suture repair of the nail bed is performed using loupe magnification and a 6-0 catgut suture. Once the nail bed has been repaired, it is best to place the thoroughly cleansed nail back under the nail fold, where it serves as a rigid splint for an underlying distal phalangeal fracture and prevents adhesions from forming between the adjacent surfaces of the nail fold, which might lead to an unsightly split nail deformity. If there is a piece of nail bed missing, the undersurface of the avulsed nail plate is examined. Frequently, the missing piece may still be adherent to the nail, and it can be gently removed and replaced as a nail bed graft. Some fingertip injuries may be so severe that amputation revision may be the most sensible and functional solution.

Volar fingertip injuries range from simple to more complex. Multiple digits may be involved, such as with lawnmower injuries. If bone is not exposed and a soft tissue defect of the finger pulp is smaller than 1 cm, the wound is best left open and managed with dressings. Such an injury will heal with excellent functional and cosmetic results. Larger soft tissue defects of the fingertip pulp are more appropriately treated with a small, full-thickness skin graft. However, if bone is exposed and the soft tissue wound is larger, flap coverage or revision of amputation by trimming back exposed bone to obtain soft tissue coverage should be considered. In a dorsally angulated fingertip amputation, soft tissue coverage can be achieved by a neurovascular V-Y advancement flap. If the soft tissue loss is angulated in a more volar direction, a cross-finger flap, adjacent finger digital island flap, or homodigital flap may be performed (Figs. 70.17 to 70.19).

This algorithm for fingertip soft tissue coverage based on the geometry of the wound was previously time honored. However, with the larger homodigital flaps now available, that algorithm has changed because these flaps can be mobilized much more, are less restricted by their pedicle, and have a wider arc of rotation. For example, the retrograde homodigital island flap can pivot to cover either volar or dorsal fingertip wounds.

Tendon Injuries

Flexor Tendons

Flexor tendon injuries usually result from lacerations or puncture wounds on the palmar surface of the hand, although flexor tendons can be avulsed from their distal bone insertions by sudden violent contractions. These are best treated by a surgeon experienced in the treatment of such injuries. Flexor tendon injuries are divided into five zones (Fig. 70.20). In zones 1, 2, and 4, each tendon is

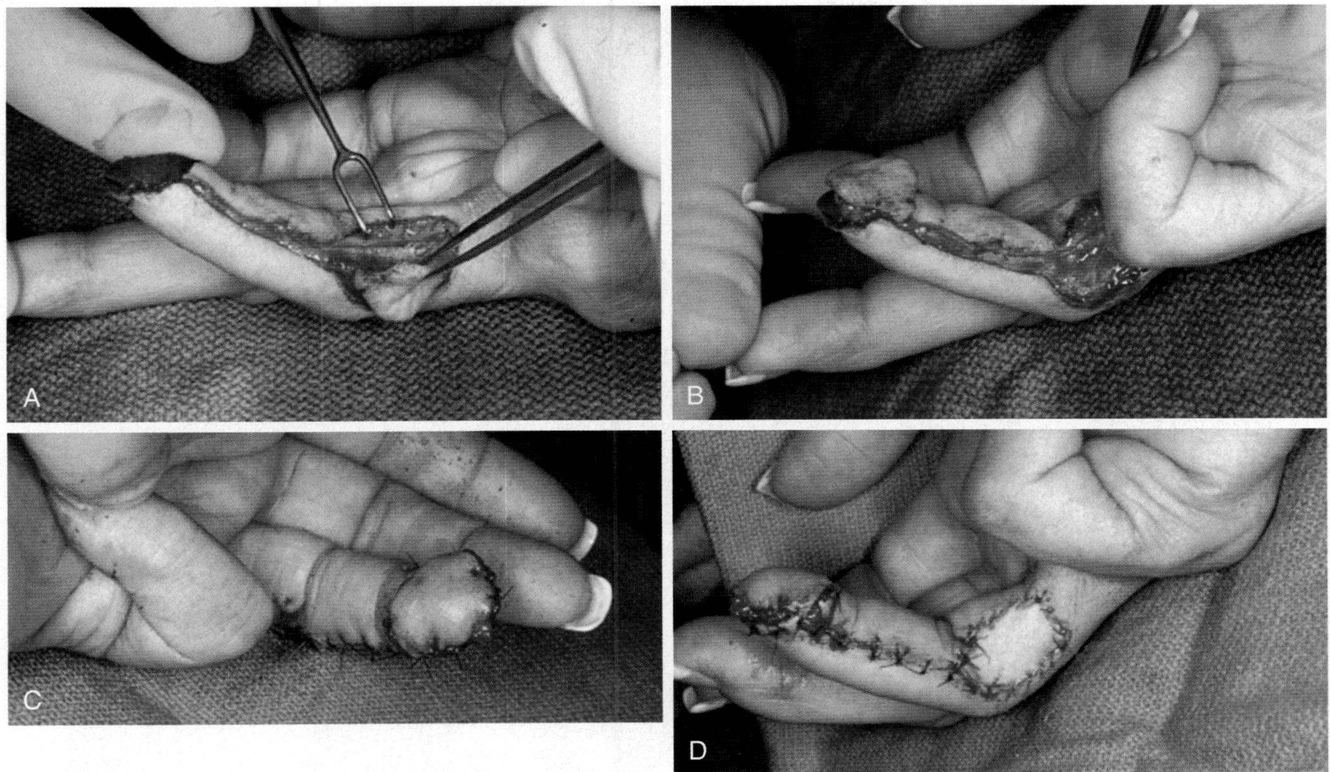

FIG. 70.18 (A–D) More recent understanding of the vascular skin territories of the finger and hand enables intrinsic flap coverage of fingertip injuries and avoids the cumbersome tethering of adjacent fingers, as is done with cross-finger flaps. In this patient, a distally based turnover vascular island flap reconstructs an avulsed fingertip. The reverse-flow perforating vessels at the proximal interphalangeal joint cross from the opposite side to nourish this flap.

surrounded by a synovial sheath and contained within a semirigid fibro-osseous canal, either the flexor tendon sheath of the digit or the carpal tunnel. In the other zones, the flexor tendons are surrounded by loose areolar (paratenon) tissue. Those parts devoid of a fibrous sheath usually heal well because of the good blood supply from the paratenon. Tendons in the carpal tunnel (zone 4) have their rich blood supply provided by the mesotenon; however, zones 1 and 2 have a precarious blood supply through the vincula; complementary nutritional support is provided by the synovial fluid in these two zones. For tendon gliding to occur, the mesotenon has disappeared in the digital flexor sheath except at the sites of the vincula that carry the vessels from the periosteum to the tendons (Fig. 70.21). Tendon zones to the thumb are T1 through T3.

Primary tendon repair undertaken within a few hours of injury is generally reserved for cleanly cut tendons. Delayed primary repair is performed from several hours up to 10 days after injury and is indicated for tidy but potentially contaminated wounds to allow prophylaxis against infection before the tendon repair. Relative contraindications to immediate tendon repair include the following:

- Injuries more than 12 hours old
- Crush wounds with poor skin coverage
- Contaminated wounds, especially human bites
- Tendon loss of more than 1 cm
- Injury at multiple sites along the tendon
- Destruction of the pulley system.

After 4 weeks, a later secondary repair is generally not possible because of retraction of the musculotendinous unit so that reapproximation of the tendon ends produces undesirable joint flexion. In this situation, tendon graft repair may be required. The surgeon's endeavors are directed at avoiding the four major complications that interfere with smooth gliding and the integrated action of tendons—adhesions, attenuation of the repair, repair rupture, and joint and soft tissue contractures. Prerequisites for tendon repair are aseptic conditions in the operating room with good lighting and good instruments, adequate anesthesia, and loupe magnification. A well-performed technical operation can be futile without proper postoperative hand therapy, splinting, and excellent compliance of the patient.[5]

Appropriate treatment of partial flexor tendon injuries is necessary to produce a smooth juncture at the injury site. Prevention of complications requires exploration of all wounds likely to cause partial flexor tendon lacerations. A partial tendon injury of 50% or less is treated by simple trimming of the lacerated portion. Those injuries greater than 50% are repaired. Failure to diagnose a partial flexor tendon laceration at the time of primary repair may lead to delayed tendon rupture, entrapment between the tendon laceration and the laceration in the flexor sheath, or trigger finger.

Zone 2 flexor tendon injuries require special attention. This zone is also called Bunnell no man's land. There are three tendons—the profundus and two slips of superficialis—that traverse zone 2, and they constantly interchange their mutual spatial relationships. Tendon injury in this region requires opening of the existing laceration in the flexor tendon sheath by making a longitudinal trap door so that a flap of tendon sheath can be elevated. Care must be taken to avoid excising excessive portions of

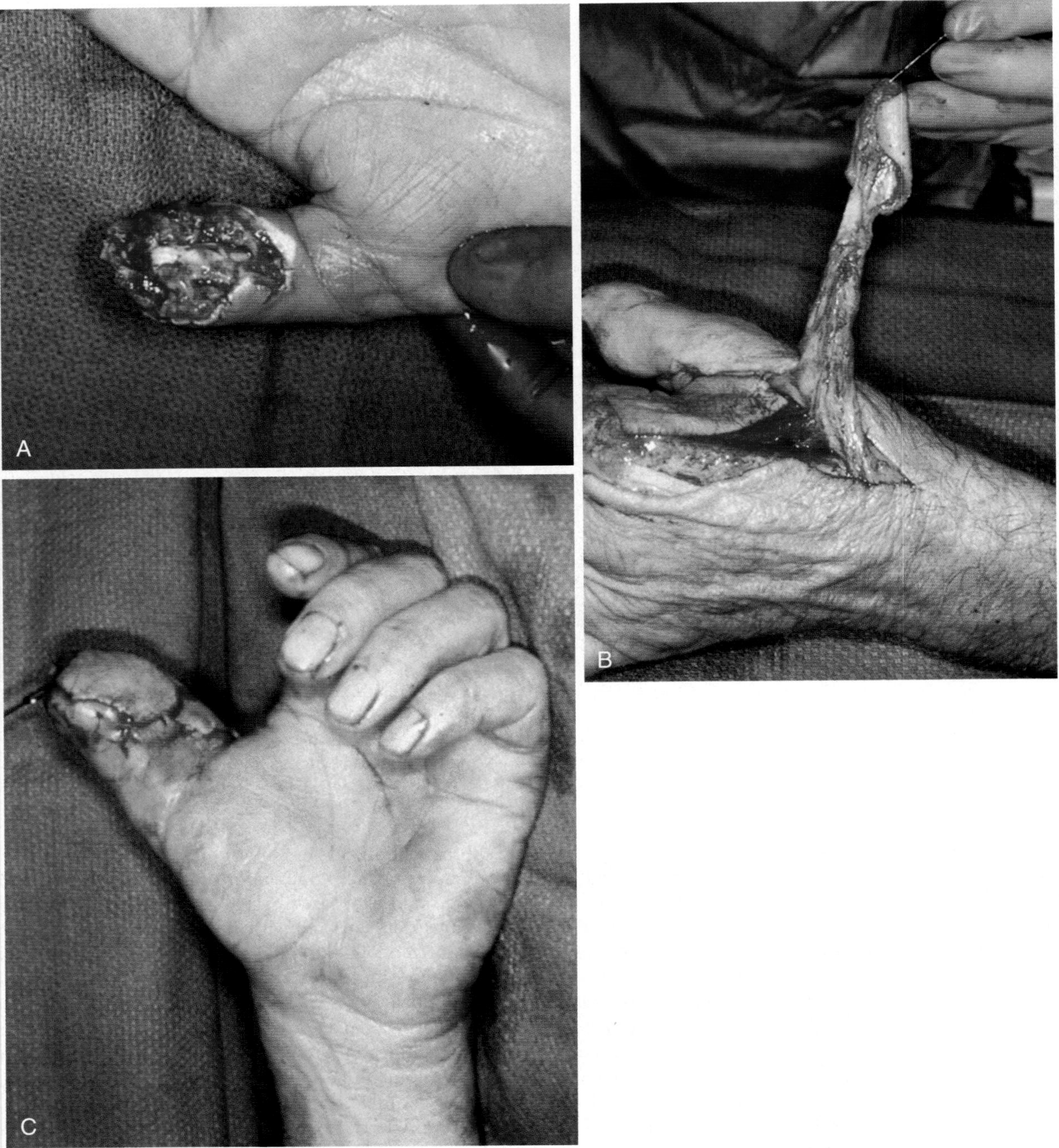

FIG. 70.19 (A–C) The first dorsal metacarpal artery flap is a vascularized island flap that is transposed from the dorsoradial aspect of the index finger to the distal pulp of the thumb after a crushing injury.

the flexor tendon sheath because bowstringing may result in ineffective finger flexion, although portions can be vented or excised to facilitate repair or to prevent postoperative triggering. Total preservation of the A2 and A4 pulleys, previously thought to be essential, is no longer believed to be critical to success. One can excise up to 50% of the A2 and A4 pulleys without creating unnecessary tendon bowstringing if this is thought to be prudent to avoid the tendon repair's impinging under the pulley.[6] It has also been shown that one can incise the full length of the A4 pulley (but not excise it) without any biomechanical consequences.[7] This is especially helpful when the zone 2 repair occurs proximate to the A4 pulley, the narrowest part of the flexor tendon sheath. Finally, wide-awake anesthesia, which is local anesthetic infiltration using a solution of lidocaine with epinephrine, enables flexor tendon repair without the use of a tourniquet and ensures full cooperation of the patient during the procedure.[8] This was previously thought to be unwise, but this has been proved to be unsubstantiated. Thus, one can determine intraoperatively that there is full flexor tendon excursion at the repair site without impingement under the pulleys as the patient flexes and extends his or her fingers before the skin incision is finally closed. All these novel and revolutionary concepts challenge previously accepted dogma with regard to zone 2 flexor tendon repairs and the significance of the various annular pulleys. It is often difficult to repair profundus and superficialis tendons

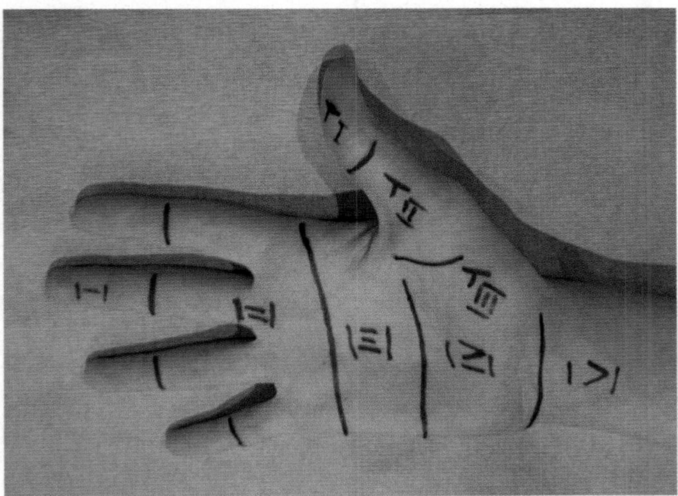

FIG. 70.20 Zones of flexor tendon injuries on the fingers, thumb, and hand.

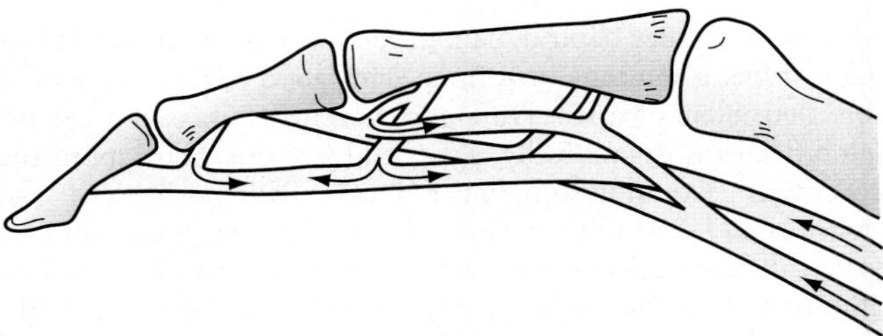

FIG. 70.21 Complex arrangement of flexor digitorum superficialis and flexor digitorum profundus tendons in the flexor sheath of the fingers. Blood supply to the tendons travels through the vincula from the dorsal aspects of the tendons.

if they are injured in zone 2. Nonetheless, both can be repaired because resection of the superficialis reduces overall grip strength, predisposes to a recurvatum and swan neck deformity at the PIP joint, and damages the vincula supply to the profundus.

Skin wounds usually have to be extended proximally and distally in a zigzag fashion to display the retracted divided tendon ends. Tendon ends are handled with a fine-toothed forceps, and the tendon surface is never touched. The wrist is flexed, and a small Keith needle is passed transversely through the proximal tendon, approximately 2 cm from the end, transfixing it to the skin and tendon sheath. In this way, immobilization of the tendon end facilitates a tension-free repair. Ragged tendon ends may be squared off sharply, but no more than 1 cm is resected or permanent finger contracture will result. The tendon ends are brought together by a single tension-holding, locking, core suture. Various locking core suture techniques have been described, but a modified Kessler-type suture is usually placed. A specifically placed locking loop increases the ultimate tensile strength of the tendon repair by 10% to 50% compared with a simple mattress suture. If this is not done, tension on the suture line can open up the repair, increasing the propensity for tendon gapping at the repair site. The ideal suture material for tendon repairs has not been found. In a study comparing a six-strand flexor tendon repair, braided polyblend (FiberWire) fared best compared with braided cable nylon (Supramid Extra II) and braided polyester (Tendo Loop) for both ultimate tensile strength and gap force. Tendon repair

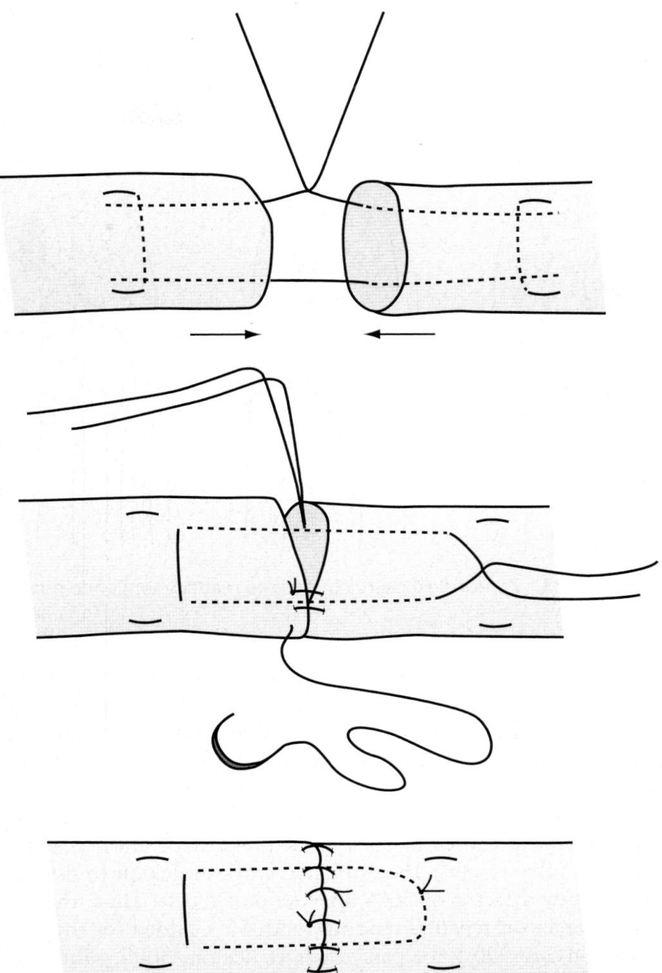

FIG. 70.22 Technique of performing a four-strand flexor tendon core suture repair is demonstrated in association with a peripheral running suture.

gapping is important because the exposed tendon ends, although not disrupted totally, lead to increased adhesion formation. However, the knot security of FiberWire remains a concern, requiring at least five-throw knots to minimize unraveling. Thus, FiberWire is generally not used for repair of tendons within the flexor tendon sheath because of the necessary bulkiness of the knots.

A 4-0 coated polyester or braided nylon suture is the best material for the core suture. Increasing the number of suture strands that cross the tendon repair site and obtaining suture bites of at least 0.7 cm will increase the overall tensile strength of the actual repair. However, the more suture strands that are added, the greater will be the friction and edema within the flexor tendon sheath. A four or six-strand core repair appears to provide optimum repair strength and does not increase stiffness and friction at the repair site excessively. Some perform a four-strand core repair by simply using a double-strand type of suture material, whereas others place a second core suture with a single-strand material. A four-strand core repair permits a light, protected, composite grip for the duration of postoperative healing. A running circumferential epitenon suture repair is also placed (Fig. 70.22). This not only helps smooth the repair but also adds to the ultimate tensile strength at the repair site and reduces gap formation. A peripheral 6-0 nylon suture serves this purpose.

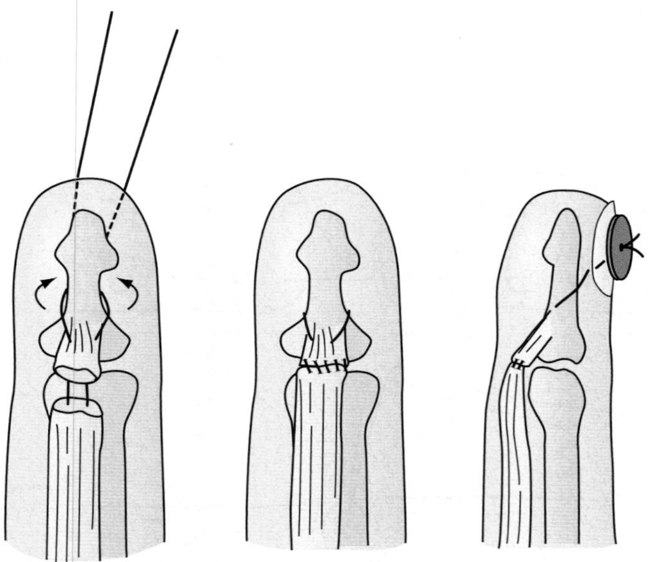

FIG. 70.23 Zone 1 flexor tendon repair to reattach tendon to bone.

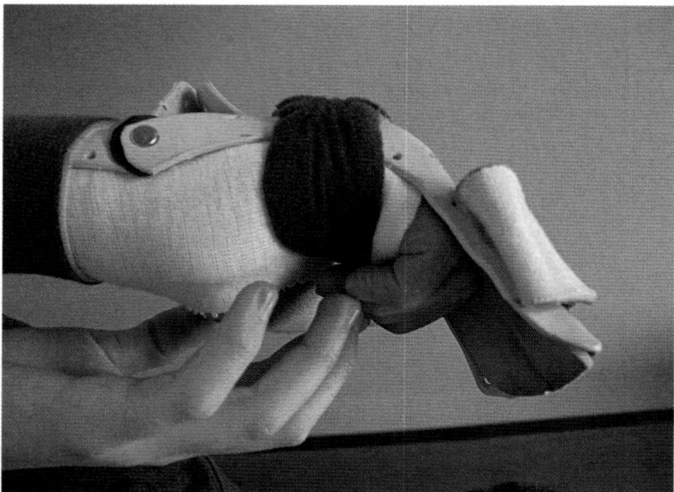

FIG. 70.24 Flexor hinge brace with place-and-hold technique of finger mobilization is one of the preferred methods for postoperative rehabilitation after flexor tendon repair.

The forces generated on FDP flexor tendons are 600 g during passive finger flexion and 2000 g during active finger flexion; with strong active finger flexion, they are 8000 g. However, after tendon repair, the effects of wound healing, changes in elasticity, and added friction between the flexor tendons and their surrounding tissues will affect the overall work of flexion. There will be added frictional forces caused by edema, the presence of suture material, and the pulley system. The estimated work of flexion (resistance) increases by a factor of 50% after tendon repair. Thus, the estimated forces on repaired tendons, with 50% added for the work of flexion, are 900 g for passive finger flexion, 3000 g for active finger flexion, and 12,000 g for strong active flexion. The ultimate tensile strengths of various repairs are 2600 g for two-strand and simple epitendinous repair, 4600 g for four-strand and simple epitendinous repair, and 6800 g for six-strand and simple epitendinous repair. The strength of the initial tendon repair decreases by approximately 25% during the first 3 weeks and then steadily increases thereafter to 6 weeks. Hence, if one is to undertake a postoperative active finger flexion protocol, at least a four- or six-strand core suture tendon repair is needed.

A variety of interventions have a potential of enhancing tendon repair and healing. Active tendon motion protocols tend to attenuate the weakening of repair strength that we used to believe was an obligatory part of normal tendon repair site healing in the first 3 weeks.[9] In addition, therapy with stem cells can enhance strength of tendon repair because of their regenerative potential. Mechanical stimulation of active motion protocols may potentially act in this by stimulating stem cells.[10] Zone 1 flexor tendon injury may be caused by a penetrating injury. However, closed traction injury may also cause profundus tendon avulsion, which most frequently involves the ring or middle finger. In the repair of a zone 1 injury, a pullout suture is necessary if the distal tendon length is insufficient to repair the tendon securely (Fig. 70.23), although suture bone anchors have facilitated this mode of tendon repair into bone at the base of the distal phalanx.

Postoperatively, hand elevation is important to reduce edema. The wrist is placed in approximately 20 degrees of flexion and the MP joint at approximately 60 to 70 degrees of flexion. The splint is molded against the fingers, with the IP joints fully extended. A system of rubber band dynamic traction may be used after the repair of flexor tendons in zone 2, with good results obtained in more than 80% of cases. Differential excursion between the two digital flexors is dramatically increased by a synergistic splint that allows wrist extension and finger flexion. This position of wrist extension and MP joint flexion produces the least tension on a repaired flexor tendon during active digital flexion; thus, we have come to use the flexor hinge brace technique and the so-called place-and-hold protocol (Fig. 70.24). Of all the postoperative flexor tendon protocols, this enables the greatest overall tendon excursion of each of the FDS and FDP tendons and the most significant differential tendon gliding between the FDS and FDP repair sites, which theoretically would then reduce the risk of adhesion formation between the two tendons. A tenodesis brace with a wrist hinge is fabricated to allow full wrist flexion, wrist extension of 30 degrees, and maintenance of MP joint flexion of at least 60 degrees. After composite passive digital flexion, the wrist is extended and passive finger flexion is maintained. The patient actively maintains digital flexion and holds that position for approximately 5 seconds. The patient is instructed to use the lightest muscle power necessary to maintain digital flexion. Wrist flexion and finger extension follow. This protected motion postoperative protocol is continued for 6 weeks.

Extensor Tendons

Proper diagnosis of extensor tendon injuries requires full knowledge of the relatively complex anatomy of the extensor mechanism of the dorsum of the finger. The subcutaneous location of extensor tendons makes them susceptible to crush, laceration, and avulsion injuries. The presence of juncturae tendinum prevents proximal retraction of the EDC tendons. Extensor tendon injuries have been divided into nine zones, which ascend numerically from the dorsum of the DIP joints to the forearm. The odd-numbered zones begin at the DIP joint and are located over the joints; the even-numbered zones are located between the joints.

Extensor tendons are thinner than flexor tendons and, over the dorsum of the digits, are spread out to form the extensor hood. It may occasionally be possible to use conventional tendon repair techniques in the proximal parts of the tendons, but this is usually not the case in the extensor hood region. Here, horizontal mattress

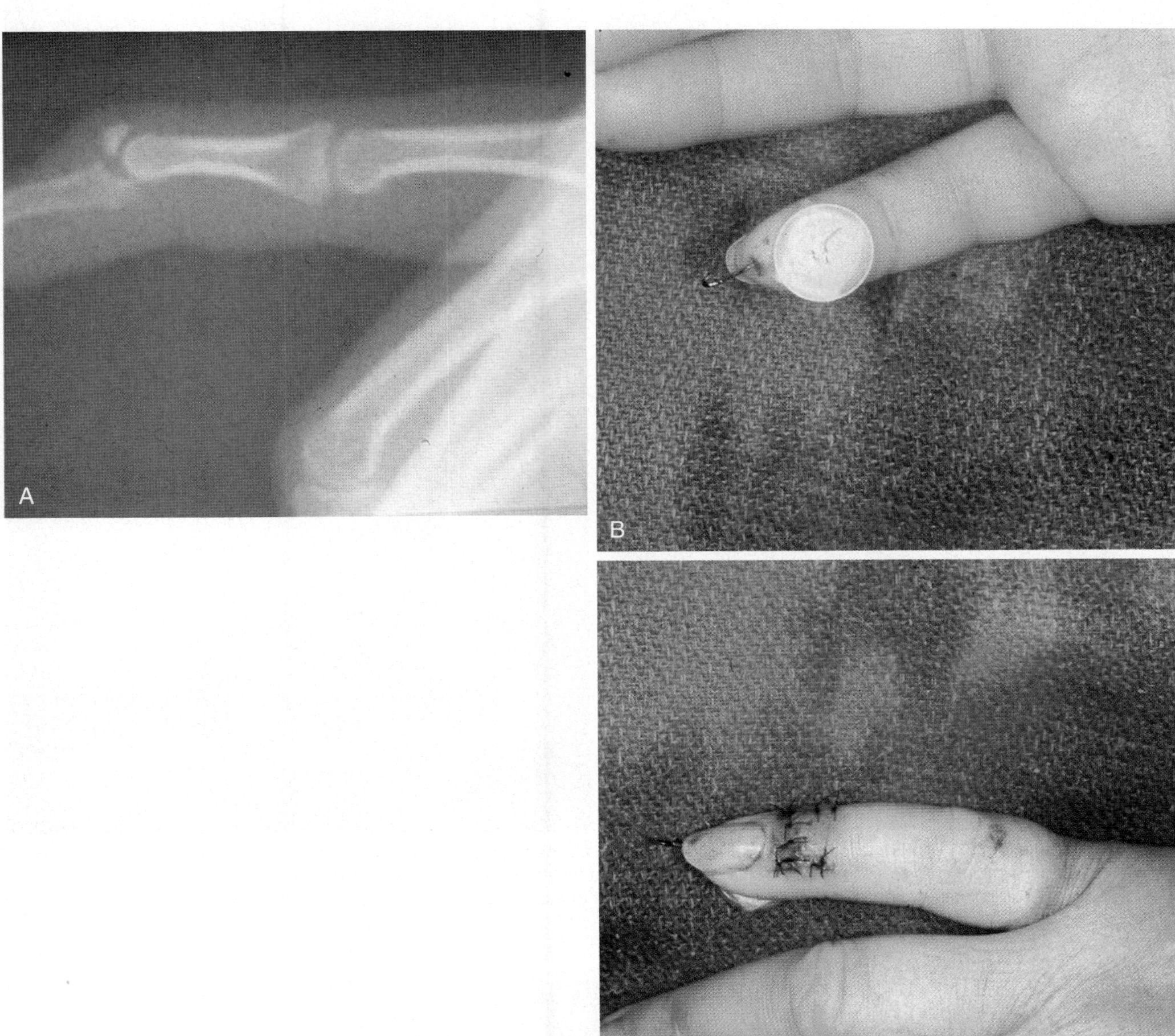

FIG. 70.25 (A–C) Mallet fracture with avulsed bone fragment involving more than 50% of the articular surface with volar subluxation of the distal phalanx. The bone fragment is reapproximated with a tie-over volar suture and a longitudinal pin traversing the distal interphalangeal joint.

sutures or figure-of-eight mattress sutures may be needed. All lacerations are repaired if 50% or more of the tendon is divided.

Extensor tendon avulsions are most likely to occur at the DIP joint from a jamming type of injury that results in a mallet finger deformity (Fig. 70.25). If a bone fragment representing 50% or more of the articular surface is involved or if there is volar subluxation of the DIP joint, an open reduction with internal fixation is performed. If there is a tendon rupture only or a small piece of bone is avulsed with the tendon, good results can be obtained by 6 weeks of continuous splinting with the DIP joint in extension (Fig. 70.26). After this period of splinting, the DIP joint is further protected during sleep for 2 more weeks.

Closed tears through the triangular ligament may be caused by PIP joint subluxation or a jamming type of injury that results in a boutonnière deformity. The central slip attachment at the base of the middle phalanx is disrupted so that extension of that joint is altered. The lateral bands lose their support dorsal to the PIP joint axis and slip volar and become flexors at the PIP joint and extensors of the DIP joint. The consequent deformity is one of flexion at the PIP joint and hyperextension at the DIP joint. Within 6 weeks of injury, these can be treated satisfactorily by extension splinting at the PIP joint, maintaining the DIP joint free for active flexion and extension (Fig. 70.26).

A recently described novel way of splinting and treating closed boutonnière injuries of the finger is to use the relative motion splint shown in Fig. 70.27 but to have the proximal phalanx of the injured digit blocked from fully extending. This has been shown to realign the lateral bands dorsally over the PIP joint.

If there is an open laceration to the central slip mechanism and adjacent triangular ligament, direct suture repair or reinsertion into bone by means of bone anchor minisutures is performed, followed by the same postoperative protocol.

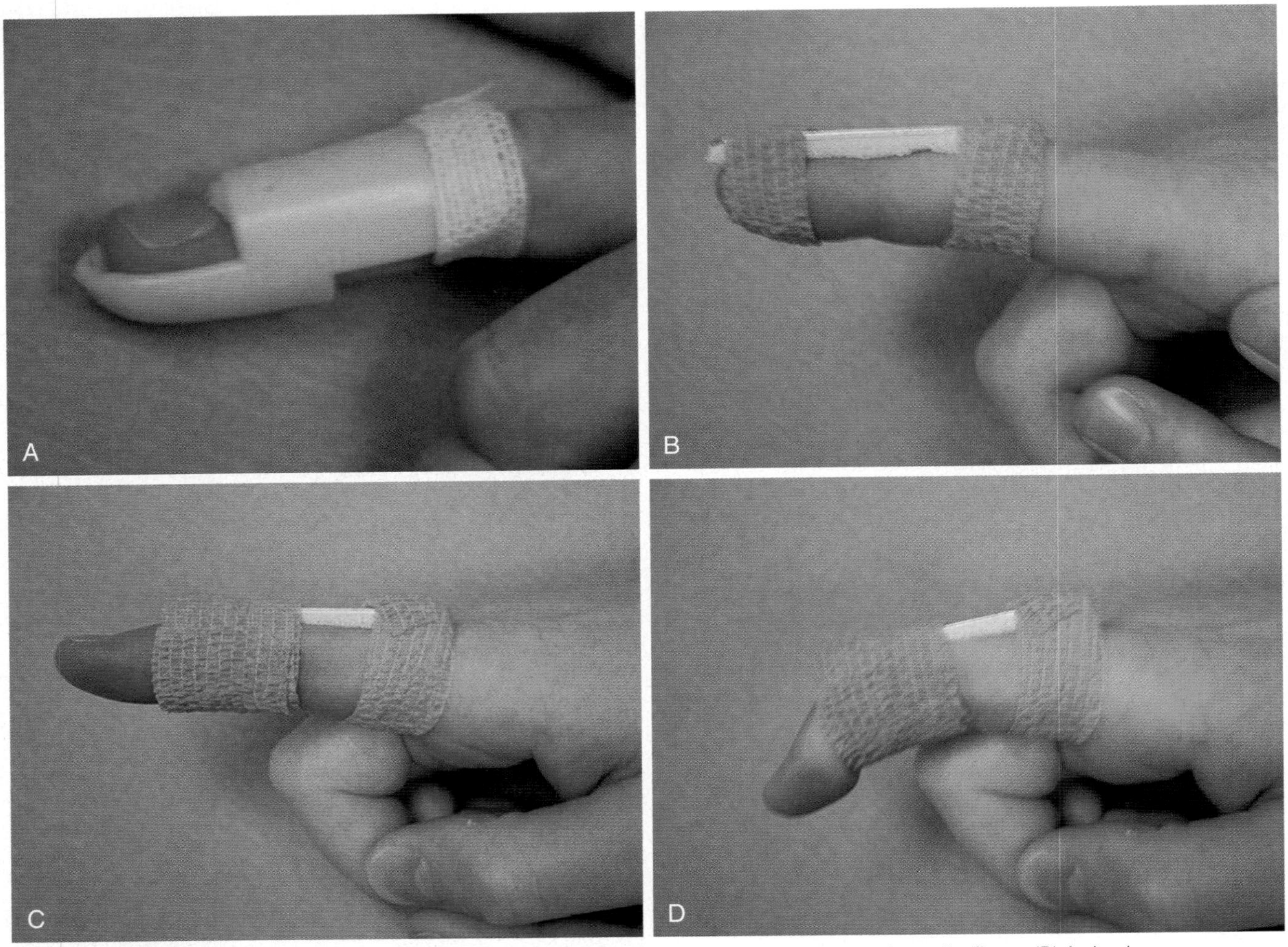

FIG. 70.26 (A) Prefabricated stack splint may be used for the closed treatment of a mallet finger. (B) A simple dorsal aluminum splint may serve equally well for mallet finger treatment. (C and D) Dorsal splinting across the proximal interphalangeal joint enables closed treatment of a boutonnière injury. The distal interphalangeal joint is left free for flexion and extension.

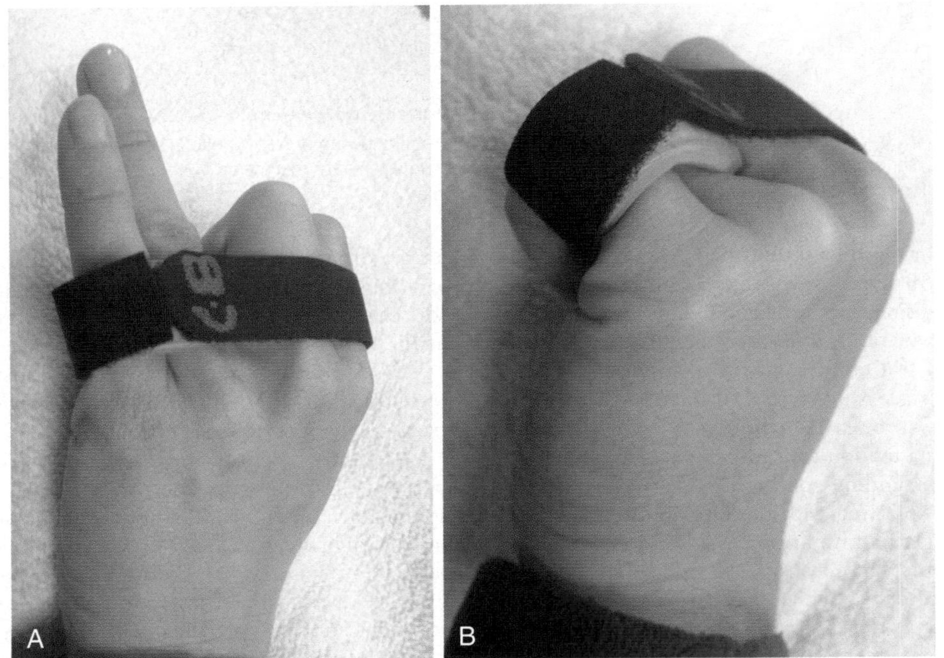

FIG. 70.27 (A and B) Relative motion splint can also be used to "depress" and to block extension of the proximal phalanx of a digit affected by boutonnière deformity. This encourages dorsal repositioning of the lateral bands over the dorsum of the proximal interphalangeal joint.

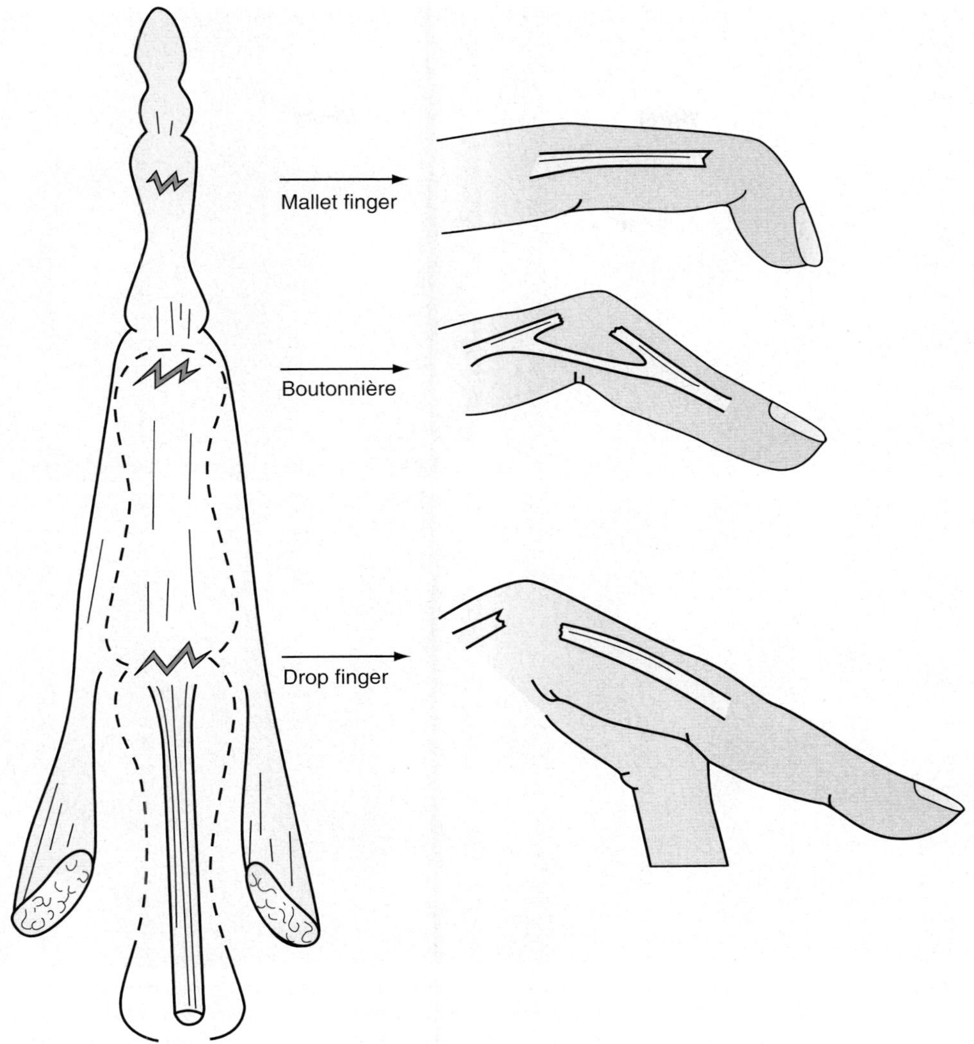

FIG. 70.28 Extensor tendon injuries on the dorsum of the finger. Injury at the distal insertion causes a mallet finger, and injury at the central slip over the proximal interphalangeal joint causes a boutonnière deformity. Proximal to the proximal interphalangeal joint, over the proximal phalanx, injury results in a drop finger.

Extensor tendon injuries proximal to the PIP joint result in a drop finger (Fig. 70.28). These are repaired and splinted for 4 weeks. Common extensor tendon injuries over the dorsum of the hand and at the wrist must be repaired and then treated postoperatively by various different controlled motion protocols. One is a dynamic rubber band extension outrigger brace or use of a relative motion splint in which the affected digit is kept at a more dorsal pitch to the adjacent fingers, thus relaxing the repaired tendon. The relative motion splint causes minimal interference with daily activities during rehabilitation (Fig. 70.29).[11]

Nerve Injuries

Sunderland classification, the most widely used classification, describes five types of nerve injury: neurapraxia (grade I), axonotmesis (grades II to IV), and neurotmesis (grade V). Neuropraxia is a physiologic block of impulse conduction without anatomic destruction of nerve fibers. This might occur with a closed injury, such as a radial nerve injury in the spiral groove associated with a midshaft humerus fracture. Neurapraxia may occur because of prolonged pressure in a tight anatomic location (e.g., carpal tunnel) or prolonged application of a tourniquet. Provided the offending cause is promptly removed, spontaneous recovery is generally the rule but can take as long as 3 months. In axonotmesis, axonal fibers are completely ruptured, generally from traction on the nerve (II). With higher energy injuries, the endoneurial (III) and perineurial (IV) nerve sheaths that support and nourish the axons and fascicles are progressively injured, leading to poorer nerve recovery with increasing damage to intraneural architecture. Neurotmesis refers to complete transection of a nerve and is the most severe degree of nerve injury. It may result from direct sharp trauma or a violent traction injury. Accurate approximation of the cut nerve ends and meticulous repair are required for the best possible recovery. Axonal regeneration after axonotmesis or successful nerve repair after neurotmesis occurs at a rate of 1 mm/day. Traction injuries may result in a combination of all grades of nerve injury, but with intact external nerve sheaths, grades II to IV may be difficult to distinguish from one another clinically.

Severance of a peripheral nerve involves an acute loss of sensory, motor, and sympathetic functions. Knowledge of the motor and sensory distribution of the nerve is essential for clinical evaluation. However, associated injuries, such as fractures and

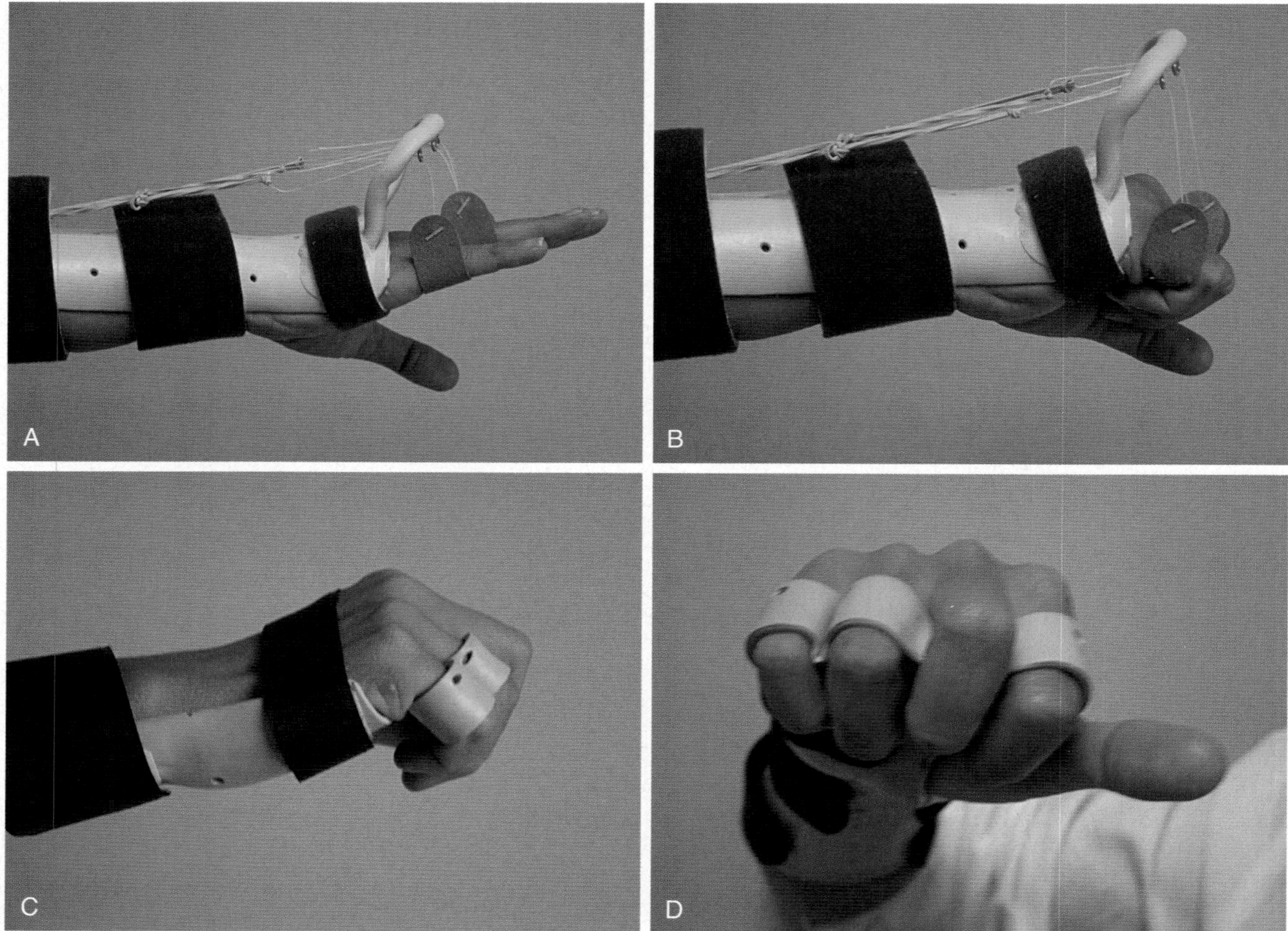

FIG. 70.29 (A and B) Extension outrigger dynamic splint commonly used for extensor tendon injuries postoperatively (extension and flexion views). (C and D) Relative motion splint has the advantage of being low profile and causes minimal interference with daily activities and yet provides protection to the freshly repaired extensor tendon.

muscle and tendon lacerations, may complicate the evaluation. Loss of pseudomotor activity occurs within 30 minutes of the nerve injury. Clinically, loss of sweating can sometimes be observed, and denervated skin will not wrinkle if it is placed in water. Sensory denervation can also be demonstrated with a ninhydrin test. Nerve conduction studies are not immediately helpful but become valuable 3 weeks after injury, when fibrillation and denervation potentials can be measured in completely denervated muscles. In a closed injury, they may differentiate between neurapraxia and neurotmesis. Later, nerve conduction studies may help monitor nerve regeneration after repair.

Primary nerve repair is done within 72 hours of injury, delayed primary repair from 72 hours to 14 days, and secondary nerve repairs 14 days or longer after injury. Primary neurorrhaphy is recommended in the following situations:

- The nerve is sharply incised
- There is minimal wound contamination
- There are no injuries that preclude obtaining skeletal stability or adequate skin cover
- The patient is medically stable to undergo an operation
- Appropriate facilities and instrumentation are available.

In a completely severed nerve, wallerian degeneration occurs in the entire segment distal to the injury and 1 to 2 cm proximal to it. In closed injuries, when the severity of the nerve injury is unknown, repeated clinical evaluation and electrical studies every 3 to 6 weeks help distinguish between neurapraxia and axonal injury. In most cases, surgical exploration with repair is indicated after 3 months if no clinical recovery is detected.

The nerve repair must be tensionless. Stretching a nerve more than 10% compromises epineurial blood flow and thus its recovery. With sharp nerve lacerations, an epineurial repair provides as good a functional recovery as fascicular (perineurial) repair, provided anatomic landmarks such as the vasa nervorum are accurately realigned to provide precise matching of fascicles at the severed nerve ends.

Traditionally, microsuture of lacerated nerve ends has been performed, and epineurial suturing has been the most common technique. In addition to the foreign body reaction to the suture material, it may be difficult to suture the nerve repair in confined anatomic locations. Fibrin glue is an acceptable alternative for nerve repair. Nerve ends still do need to be precisely aligned. However, the use of fibrin glue for nerve repairs is not yet approved by the U.S. Food and Drug Administration. A nerve gap

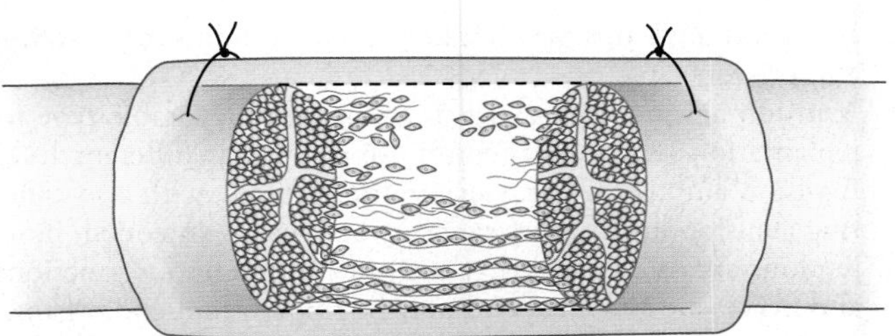

FIG. 70.30 Nerve conduits may be an appropriate treatment for short nerve gaps in the hand.

may exist because of segmental nerve loss or when a crushed nerve segment is unsuitable for repair and must be resected. This may be overcome by proximal and distal mobilization of the nerve ends or, in the case of the ulnar nerve, by transposition of the nerve to the front of the elbow. If there is too much tension on the repair (it cannot be held with an 8-0 nylon suture), a nerve conduit or nerve graft must be used.

It has been suggested that optimal nerve regeneration and appropriate matching of axons in proximal and distal nerve segments result from a combination of paracrine-mediated neurotropism and contact guidance of sprouting proximal axons. Experimental evidence has suggested that the neurotropic chemical gradient can effectively guide regenerating axons at least 14 mm through a hollow nerve conduit in the rat model. The conduit allows diffusion of the neurotropic signal while preventing a mechanical fibrous block between the proximal and distal nerve segments. However, large-gap animal models (30 mm) have shown poor or no recovery with use of nerve conduits, suggesting that a finite limit exists for this technique. Although the gap length that can be bridged successfully in humans is still uncertain, many surgeons consider the use of bioresorbable nerve conduits for gap lengths up to 2 cm to be appropriate for small peripheral nerves. Nerve grafting remains the "gold standard" for large or mixed nerves and the brachial plexus. Appropriate conduits are polyglycolic acid tubes and semipermeable collagen tubes, which have shown similar experimental outcomes. The use of nerve allografts is discussed later in this chapter (Fig. 70.30).[12]

With nerve grafting, fascicular matching, when chosen by the surgeon, may not always be appropriate. However, the additional contact guidance provided to regenerating axons makes successful nerve regeneration possible over longer distances than with conduits. Donor sources for nerve grafting usually include the terminal sensory portion of the posterior interosseous nerve and the medial antebrachial cutaneous nerve for small digital nerves. The sural nerves are used for nerve gaps involving larger nerves.

Nerve Transfers

If there may be a long distance between the site of nerve injury and the distal muscle target, primary nerve repair may be fruitless because muscle degeneration would have occurred by the time distal neural growth occurs. Muscle recovery is unlikely after an 18-month lapse. Thus, if nerve growth occurs at the rate of approximately 1 mm/day, a proximal motor nerve lesion more than 540 mm proximal to the hand will be doomed to failure. Hence, for proximal arm nerve and brachial plexus injuries, nerve transfers may result in a nerve repair that is closer to the muscle target. The donor nerve must be chosen so as to minimize morbidity from loss of the donor nerve. The donor nerve must be closely related to the denervated muscle so that the repair is performed much closer to the muscle target. Nerve transfers have revolutionized the repair of proximal nerve injuries so that distal muscle atrophy is minimized. For example, the classic Oberlin transfer uses part of the ulnar nerve (usually a single fascicle) for transfer to the musculocutaneous nerve and to the brachialis in the upper arm to restore elbow flexion.[13] It is technically easy, quick, and effective. No significant motor or sensory deficits result in the territory of the ulnar nerve. This technique has become popular and is indicated for C5–6 brachial plexus lesions when C8-T1 is intact. It can also be used to neurotize a functioning free muscle transfer that may be required if the native muscles have already sustained atrophy because of prolonged denervation.

Vascular Injuries

Acute vascular injuries may follow closed or penetrating trauma or iatrogenic injury. Fractures or dislocations may cause vascular injury. Indirect vascular trauma may be caused by traction injuries, which can avulse vessels, or by intimal damage or repetitive microtrauma from vibratory tools, which can lead to thrombosis.

The latter usually affects the ulnar artery in the Guyon canal at the wrist and is called the hypothenar hammer syndrome. Regardless of the cause, vascular injuries may lead to a critical compromise of circulation in the extremity. With a closed injury, the onset of symptoms may be delayed because swelling, hypotension, and intimal injury combine and result in late thrombosis and vascular insufficiency.

After an acute arterial injury, symptoms result from a combination of the adequacy of collateral circulation, posttraumatic sympathetic tone, and vasomotor control mechanisms. Patients with an upper extremity arterial injury who have adequate collateral circulation and normal vasomotor control may have minimal symptoms, so reconstruction is not necessarily mandatory and the injury can be treated with simple arterial ligation. If there is a noncritical arterial injury, such as to the radial artery alone, reconstruction may be advocated to restore parallel flow in case of future arterial injury, to enhance nerve recovery, to facilitate healing, and to prevent cold intolerance. However, the reported patency rate, even with microvascular techniques for single-vessel repairs, varies from 47% to 82%. The following injuries are optimally managed by vascular repair and reconstruction: axillary or brachial artery injury; combined radial and ulnar artery injury; and radial or ulnar artery injury associated with poor collateral circulation. Relative indications for repair of a noncritical vascular injury are extensive distal soft tissue injury, technical ability to achieve repair without compromising the patient's well-being, and a combined vascular and neural injury. The need for arterial reconstruction necessitates assessing the adequacy of collateral circulation; this is based primarily on initial clinical judgment. However, the final decision regarding arterial reconstruction is often made in the operating room after exploration. Once the injured structures have been isolated, potential bleeding sites have been controlled, and hematoma has been evacuated, the distal extremity can be assessed more adequately. At this time, lacerated vessel ends are controlled by atraumatic vascular clamps and a tourniquet can be released. Capillary refill and perfusion of the distal extremity can then be assessed, as can backflow from the distal lacerated vessel ends. Digital blood pressure can be quantified with a sterile Doppler probe and cuff; a digital brachial index of 0.7 or greater suggests adequate perfusion. If there is poor collateral flow, arterial reconstruction is performed. At this time, standard of care does not require arterial repair of isolated noncritical vessels. In combined radial and ulnar artery injuries, one or both vessels are reconstructed. If possible, both vessels are repaired.[14]

Muscles often swell after prolonged periods of ischemia. This can lead to an increase of pressure within the closed compartment of the forearm, resulting in a compartment syndrome. It is thus the practice of most surgeons to perform a routine fasciotomy to decompress the forearm compartment after a true revascularization procedure has been performed. During the period of ischemia to the muscles, there may be a buildup of lactic acid. Furthermore, myonecrosis might occur. Restoration of circulation to such a limb can cause a sudden flooding of the circulation with myoglobin, lactic acid, and other toxic substances. This is called reperfusion syndrome and can lead to multiorgan failure, especially affecting the renal and cardiac systems.

Replantation and Amputations

It can often be frustrating for the novice general surgeon to be told by a replantation surgeon in the middle of the night that a consultation was obtained inappropriately or not soon enough. There are general indications for the replantation of amputated parts, but the overriding decision is still to save life before limb. Although patients and family members may desire replantation, and in some cases have even been promised it by members of the primary team, it is not performed in patients with severe associated medical problems or injuries. Replantation is also generally not considered under the following circumstances[3,15]:

- Severe crush or multilevel injury of the amputated part
- A psychotic patient who has willfully self-amputated the part
- Amputation of a single digit proximal to the FDS distal insertion (zone 2), except for single-digit amputations in children or those with a demanding profession (e.g., a musician)
- Amputation in patients with severely atherosclerotic arteries (sometimes this can be determined only when the vessels are explored in the operating room).

Indications for replantation of amputated parts are as follows:

- Whenever possible, for a thumb amputation (it provides >40% of the overall hand function)[15]
- Single digits that have been amputated distal to the FDS insertion (e.g., a manual worker may likely desire revision of amputation and desires to return to work quickly)
- Multiple injured digits
- Most amputations in children, including single-digit amputations
- Guillotine-sharp clean amputations at the hand, wrist, or distal forearm.

Replantation is the reattachment of the part that has been completely amputated. Revascularization requires reconstruction of vessels in a limb that has been severely injured or incompletely severed in such a way that vascular repair is necessary to prevent distal necrosis, but some soft tissue (e.g., skin, tendon, nerve) is still intact. Revascularization generally has a better success rate than replantation because venous and lymphatic drainage may be intact.

Minor replantation is a reattachment at the wrist, hand, or digital level, whereas major replantation is performed proximal to the wrist. This clinical distinction exists because in the case of a major replantation, ischemic time is crucial to the viability of muscle and to functional outcome. Ischemic muscle may result in myonecrosis, myoglobinemia, and infection, which may threaten the patient's life (as well as limb). There are three types of amputations:

- Guillotine amputation, whereby the tissue is cut with a sharp object and is minimally damaged
- Crush amputation, in which a local crushing injury can be converted into a guillotine injury simply by debriding back the edges, although this may not be possible in a diffusely crushing amputation
- Avulsion amputation, which is the most unfavorable type for replantation because structures are injured at different levels Avulsion amputation may occur, for example, with a so-called ring avulsion injury. The extensor tendons are shredded, flexor tendons are often avulsed at the musculotendinous junctions, and nerves are stretched and may be ripped from end organs.

Ischemia time is also an important consideration in evaluating a patient for replantation. For amputated digits, more than 12 hours of warm ischemia is a relative contraindication. Promptly cooling the part to 4°C dramatically alters the ischemia factor, but even ischemia exceeding 24 hours does not necessarily preclude successful digital replantation. Ischemia time is more crucial for replantation above the proximal forearm, and reimplantation is not considered after more than 6 to 10 hours of warm ischemia time. Single digits in adults, other than the thumb in zone 2, are generally not reattached because of the consequent adverse overall functional result on the hand with a single stiff finger.[15]

Amputation is not an outmoded operation; rather, it is necessary in a patient in whom replantation might not be indicated. When primary amputation is performed, the stump is preserved with as much length as possible. An exception might be made if there is only a very short segment of proximal phalanx. A short proximal phalangeal remnant at the index finger position may serve as an impediment for thumb to middle finger prehension, and one might consider a formal ray amputation in this case to improve overall hand function. The ends of the cut nerve are cut sharply and allowed to retract to minimize the occurrence of painful neuromas at the amputation tip. Tendons are also divided sharply and allowed to retract. The practice of suturing flexor and extensor tendons over the ends of the middle, ring, or small finger stump seriously impairs the motion of the uninjured fingers because of the common origin of the flexors. There will be an active flexion deficit in the uninjured digits, the quadriga syndrome; this is corrected simply by release of the flexor tendon remnant at the injured amputated digit.

If it is anticipated that the amputated part will be considered for replantation, it is critical to transport the patient and the part in an appropriate manner. The amputated part is placed in a clean, dry, plastic bag, which is sealed and placed on top of ice in a Styrofoam container. This keeps the part sufficiently cool at 4°C to 10°C without freezing. The amputated part is wrapped in a lightly moistened saline gauze to prevent tissue drying.

With only a few minor variations, the sequence of replantation has been standardized. Preliminary exploration of the distal amputated part under a microscope by an initial surgical team not only determines whether a replantation is technically feasible but also can be started while the patient is being prepared for the operating room. Bone shortening allows skin to be debrided back to where it is free of contusion and direct tension-free closure can be achieved. In the thumb, bone shortening is minimized to less than 10 mm. The order of repair is usually bone, tendons, muscle units, arteries, nerves, and finally veins. Establishment of arterial flow before venous flow clears lactic acid from the replanted part. The functional veins can now also be detected by spurting bleeding. However, blood loss must be closely monitored.

For major replantations, reestablishing arterial circulation as rapidly as possible is crucial to limiting ischemia time. A dialysis shunt or carotid shunt may be placed between the arterial ends. Intermittent clamping of the shunt may be necessary to restrict blood loss. In the upper extremity, bone shortening can

TABLE 70.4 **Comparison of methods of skeletal fixation.**

METHOD OF FIXATION	ADVANTAGES	DISADVANTAGES
Kirschner wires	Come in varying diameters Can be applied percutaneously or open Second surgery not required for removal Require less soft tissue dissection than plates and screws	Pins can loosen Cannot provide rigid fixation Soft tissue may be transfixed (but can be avoided by careful placement) Infection can occur along pin tracks
Screws	Have high stability Allow early finger mobilization	Frequently require open approach (although not always)
Plates	Can be used when fracture line is not oblique enough for screws Allow early finger mobilization	Require open approach Require extensive soft tissue dissection Have relatively high profile and may be palpable through the dorsum of fingers and hand May promote extensor tendon adhesions by their relative bulk and dissection required for placement

be aggressive to achieve primary skin closure and primary nerve repair. Judicious use of anticoagulants may enhance the success of replantation. Topical application of 2% lidocaine or papaverine may help relieve vasospasm. Postoperative dressings consist of nonadherent mesh gauze, loose flap gauze, and a plaster splint, with postoperative elevation to minimize edema and venous congestion. The patient's room must be kept warm, and smoking is forbidden postoperatively. Aside from antibiotics and analgesics, one aspirin tablet daily for its retarding effect on platelet aggregation is suggested. Postoperative monitoring is done hourly to assess color, pulp turgor, capillary refill, and digital temperature.

Fractures and Dislocations

Pain, swelling, limited motion, and deformities suggest the presence of a fracture or dislocation. Standard anteroposterior and lateral radiographs may miss some fractures and dislocations, and multiple views may be necessary to establish the exact diagnosis. Fractures may be rotated, angulated, telescoped, or displaced. Angulation is described by the direction in which the apex of the fracture is pointing, and displacement is described by the direction of the distal fragment. Fractures may be open or closed, depending on whether a wound is involved. They may also be complete, incomplete, or comminuted (more than two pieces). Fractures are also described by their pattern; they may be transverse, longitudinal, oblique, or spiral. Open fractures need to be thoroughly irrigated and debrided urgently. Displaced fractures or dislocations are repositioned as soon as possible. A dislocation is described according to the direction of displacement of the distal bone in the involved joint. The separation of joints may be complete or incomplete (subluxed), depending on the severity of the capsular injury.[3]

Displaced fractures or dislocations are repositioned as soon as possible to decrease soft tissue injury, to decompress nerves that might be stretched, and to relieve kinking of blood vessels. Good bone contact and stability are necessary for fractures to heal. Indications for surgery include inability to obtain and maintain closed reduction, open fractures, or significant bone loss that requires bone grafting. (Table 70.4).

A distinction between functional stability and rigid stability must be discussed prior to understanding the different fixation methods. American orthopedic principals for rigid fixation require anatomic reduction, functionally stable fixation, minimally traumatic dissection, and early active motion. This kind of rigid fixation requires direct visualization of the bone segments and can be accomplished with either a plate and screws, lag screws, or an external fixator. Functional stability allows for micromotion to occur at the fracture site. A callous forms at the gap and is replaced with bone during the healing process. Functional stability is generally accomplished with Kirschner wires plus a splint or cast.

In the distal upper extremity, rigid internal fixation may at first glance seem like an attractive option to enable early postoperative movement. However, in the fingers especially, the soft tissue disruption that is necessary and the hardware itself may actually mitigate against those potential advantages leading to increase scarring and plate irritation in an already confined space between the plate and the bone. Thus, the simplicity of Kirschner wire fixation, especially if done percutaneously, although not providing rigid fixation, may be the most suitable method.

Intraarticular fractures require accurate reduction to preserve motion and to minimize the risk for later development of arthrosis. Persistent rotational and significant lateral angular deformities generally do not remodel with time; these can be avoided by observing the alignment of the injured fingers compared with adjacent digits while passively and gently flexing them into a fist after reduction is attained. If they do not fit comfortably adjacent to each other and do not point toward the distal pole of the scaphoid, a fresh attempt at reduction must be performed. A thorough neurovascular examination is always performed before and after fracture reduction has been completed.

Distal Phalangeal Fractures

Fractures of the distal phalanx are the most frequent hand fractures, representing 50% of all hand fractures. Most result from crush injuries with associated nail bed injuries. Precise reduction is generally not required, and treatment typically consists of splinting alone.

Most closed mallet fractures can be managed by splinting the DIP joint in extension, provided the fracture involves less than 50% of the joint surface and is not associated with DIP joint subluxation. The splint must remain on 24 hours a day every day for 6 weeks. There are occupations or other situations where this may be impossible. In these situations, a buried oblique Kirschner wire can be placed to maintain reduction; however, this requires a second surgery for removal and may result in worse outcomes.

A so-called jersey finger is an avulsion fracture of the insertion of the FDP tendon into the distal phalanx. It occurs after a pull of the FDP against resistance as can occur when a footballer catches onto the jersey of an opponent. On occasion, the avulsed fragment may lie as far proximally as the palm. This fracture fragment generally requires open reduction and internal fixation. If the tendon has migrated into the palm, the vincula blood supply has likely been compromised and the tendon will likely necrosis if not operated on within a few days.[3]

Middle Phalanx and Proximal Phalanx Fractures

Fractures may involve the head, neck, shaft, or base of the respective bone. Head and base fractures may be intraarticular. A middle phalangeal shaft fracture is displaced according to the forces exerted by the insertions of the FDS and central slip mechanism. If the fracture lies distal to the FDS insertion, the proximal fragment is flexed by this muscle, resulting in a volar angulation. In contrast, if the fracture is proximal to the FDS insertion, the proximal fragment is extended by the central slip, whereas the distal part is flexed by the FDS. This results in a dorsal angulation. Most shaft fractures of the proximal phalanx tend to angulate volarward because the interossei reflect the proximal fragment and the central slip, through the PIP joint, extends the distal fragment. Displaced and unstable shaft fractures require open reduction followed by fixation with Kirschner wires or screws. The small size of the phalanges make plating quite difficult.

Metacarpal Fractures

Fractures of the metacarpal can occur at the head, neck, shaft, or base. Fractures at the head will involve the metacarpal phalangeal joint. Fractures at the neck are generally volarly angulating given the strong flexion forces of the flexor digitorum tendons. Shaft fractures can have a variety of configurations that determine stability and the best plan for fixation. Finally, metacarpal base fractures will involve the carpometacarpal joint and can be associated with joint dislocations.

Dorsally angulated fractures at the neck of the little finger metacarpal, the so-called boxer fracture, do not require reduction if there is no scissoring or angulation. The mobility of the carpometacarpal joint will compensate for higher degrees of dorsal angulation in the small and ring fingers. The index and middle finger metacarpals are less mobile than the ring and little finger metacarpals. Therefore, only around 10 to 20 degrees of angulation can to be tolerated at the index or middle fingers.

These bones are larger than the phalanges and can tolerate a plate and screw construct if needed; however, percutaneous Kirschner wire placement is still preferred. Internal fixation can be achieved with lag screws, or plate and screws, depending on the fracture pattern configuration. Lag screws can be used in long oblique fractures or spiral fractures that allow one to have at least two adequately sized screws along the fracture line.

Oblique fractures at the base of the thumb metacarpal (Bennett fracture) result in the small proximal fragment's being held in position by the volar oblique ligament to the trapezium. The remaining portion of the thumb metacarpal is displaced dorsally and radially because of the pull of the APL tendon (Fig. 70.31). These fracture fragments must be properly reduced and secured with internal fixation with Kirschner wires or a screw. Comminuted fractures at the base of the thumb metacarpal (Rolando fracture) are infrequently treated by closed reduction. If the fragments are large and badly displaced, an open reduction is indicated to ensure accurate restoration of the joint surface at the base of the thumb metacarpal.

Fractures of the shaft of the thumb metacarpal tend to become displaced by the opposing muscle forces of the abductor and adductor on the proximal and distal fragments, respectively. Even nondisplaced fractures may become progressively more displaced and angulated over time, necessitating an internal fixation. If initial splint immobilization is chosen for a nondisplaced

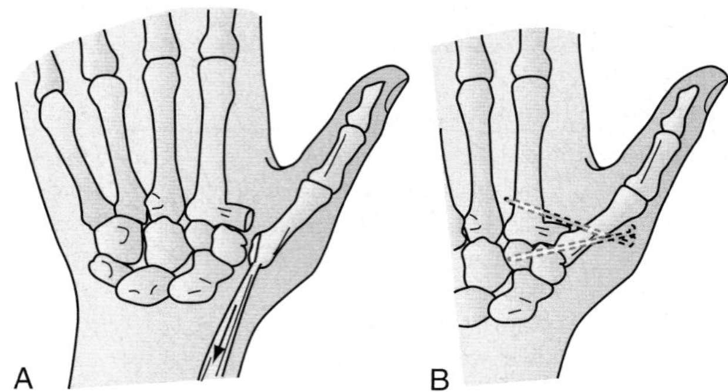

FIG. 70.31 (A) Fracture-dislocation at the base of the thumb metacarpal is called Bennett fracture. The deforming force is produced by the pull of the abductor pollicis longus muscle. (B) Open reduction and pinning of the fracture are frequently required.

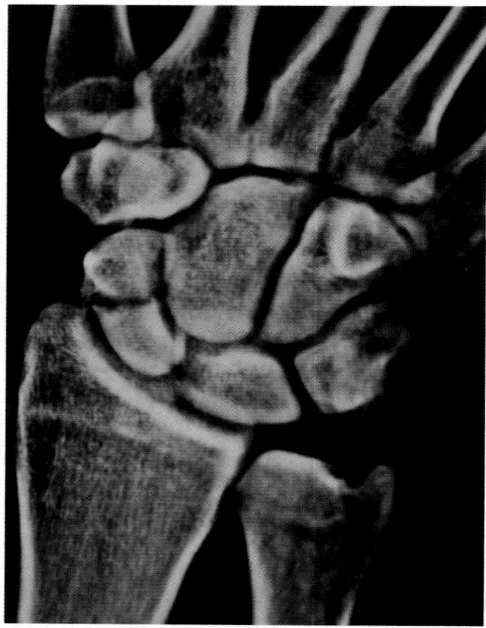

FIG. 70.32 Anteroposterior radiograph of the wrist demonstrating a fracture of the waist of the scaphoid, the bone in the hand that is usually fractured.

thumb metacarpal fracture, close follow-up is required to detect the earliest signs of displacement and instability. Fracture at the base of the little finger metacarpal is analogous to Bennett fracture of the thumb and is sometimes called a reverse Bennett fracture. This results in a fracture-dislocation, with the deforming force being the insertion of the ECU tendon.

Scaphoid Fractures

The scaphoid is the most common carpal bone fracture and accounts for approximately 60% of all carpal injuries. Clinical examination shows tenderness over the anatomic snuffbox and over the scaphoid tubercle. If a scaphoid fracture is suspected, the initial radiographic examination includes not only the standard three views of the wrist but also a scaphoid view, which is a posteroanterior image with the wrist in full ulnar deviation (Fig. 70.32). Frequently, immediate postinjury radiographs may not reveal a fracture. CT or MRI may help in these cases, or one may elect to apply a splint and to repeat the radiographs in 2 weeks.[16]

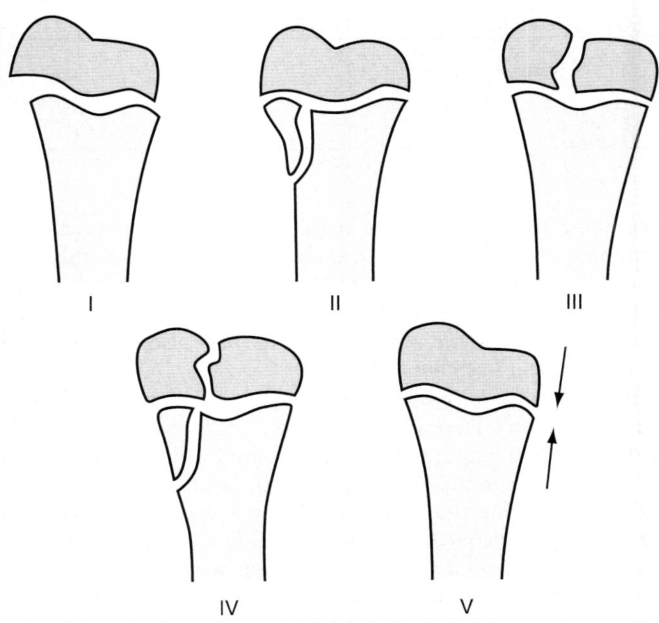

FIG. 70.33 Salter-Harris fracture patterns involving the epiphysis in children.

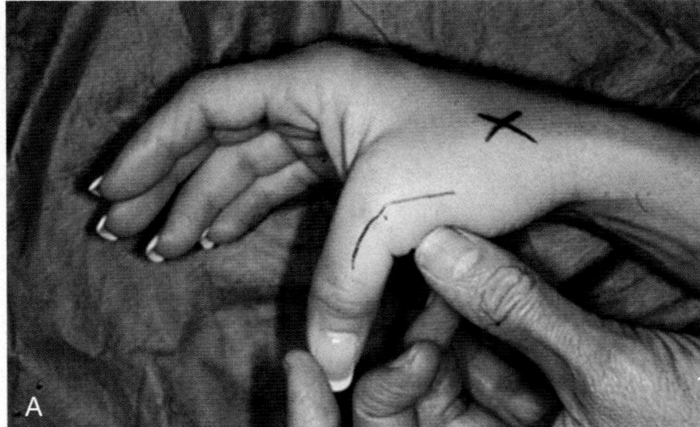

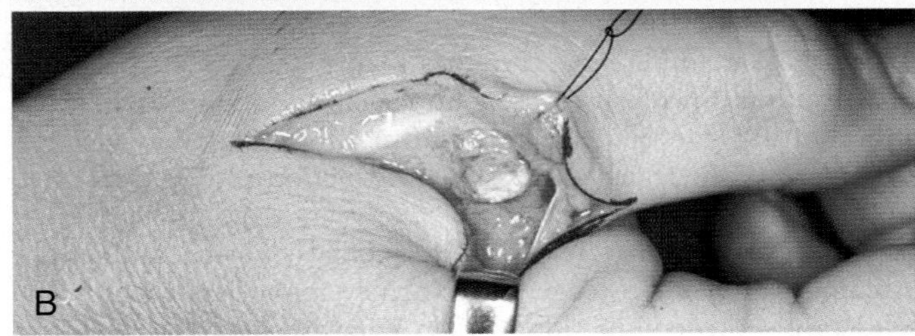

FIG. 70.34 (A) Instability of the ulnar collateral ligament of the metacarpophalangeal joint of the thumb. (B) Stener lesion shows that the distal insertion of the collateral ligament has avulsed proximal to the extensor hood and is thus blocked from spontaneous reattachment. Open operation is required to reanchor the collateral ligament insertion to the base of the proximal phalanx.

Treatment of a nondisplaced scaphoid fracture is with a short or long arm cast that includes the thumb. The thumb spica cast is maintained for 6 weeks, followed by a short arm cast until radiographic healing has occurred. There has been a trend toward percutaneous screw fixation of even, nondisplaced scaphoid fractures.

Displaced scaphoid fractures require open reduction with internal fixation, generally using a compression screw. Complications with inadequately treated scaphoid fractures are notorious. The blood vessels enter the scaphoid mainly through its distal half, and fractures through the waist of the scaphoid may deprive the proximal half of its blood supply, leading to avascular necrosis of the proximal pole of the scaphoid. Nonunion also occurs with relative frequency, and these cases need to be treated with cancellous bone grafting or even a pedicle vascularized bone graft. Early diagnosis of scaphoid fractures is essential so that appropriate treatment can be instituted to reduce the risks for these complications. Modern cannulated compression screws, intraoperative fluoroscopy, and arthroscopy have allowed minimally invasive percutaneous fixation of some of these scaphoid fractures, resulting in a trend toward more aggressive surgical treatment of these fractures.

Fractures in Children

The Salter-Harris classification describes five types of epiphyseal injuries (Fig. 70.33). Pediatric bones are still growing and thus permit a greater degree of remodeling. Hence, moderate angular and translational displacement of fractures tends to correct with age. However, rotational deformities never correct in the hand and are totally unacceptable, even in children. Implants that cross the epiphysis must have minimal potential for damage. Hence, smooth Kirschner wires are generally used for the fixation of pediatric skeletal injuries, and threaded screws are usually avoided.

Dislocations

Dislocations are more frequently seen at the PIP joint. A closed dislocation of the PIP joint can frequently be managed by closed reduction and splinting. If the joint is unstable after reduction, it needs exploration for collateral ligament repair. The most common type of PIP joint dislocation is a dorsal dislocation. A PIP joint volar dislocation is often associated with a tear in the triangular ligament of the extensor mechanism through which the head of the proximal phalanx protrudes and becomes trapped. Attempts at closed reduction fail because they tighten the fibers of the lateral bands and central slip around each side of the protruding proximal phalangeal neck; these injuries often require open reduction with repair of the extensor tear.

Palmar dislocations of the head of the index finger metacarpal often require open reduction. The head of the metacarpal becomes trapped between the superficial transverse metacarpal ligament, flexor tendons, and lumbrical muscles, whereas the volar plate becomes trapped between the metacarpal head and base of the proximal phalanx. Attempts at closed reduction are fruitless because of the entrapment resulting from this arrangement.

MP joint dislocation of the thumb often results from jamming it in a radial direction, thus tearing the ulnar collateral ligament. The ulnar collateral ligament may pull proximally and come to rest dorsal to the extensor hood (Stener lesion; Fig. 70.34). It cannot heal spontaneously because the ulnar collateral ligament is prevented from reattaching to bone. This so-called ski pole injury may then require operative repair. Stress radiography, sometimes able to be performed only after the digit is anesthetized with a metacarpal block, may be required to facilitate diagnosis of a complete ulnar collateral ligament injury of the thumb metacarpal joint.

The Reconstruction of Bone Deficits

In addition to soft tissue, tendon, and nerve reconstruction, there may also be a deficiency of bone in wounds resulting from injury,

TABLE 70.5 **Regenerative capacity of types of bone grafts.**

	OSTEOCONDUCTION	OSTEOINDUCTION	OSTEOGENESIS
Cancellous bone graft	-	+	+
Cortical bone graft	+	-	-
Vascularized bone flap	+	+	+

trauma, oncologic resection, and debridement involving infection. Frequently, staged debridements are required before definitive reconstruction.

The technique used to reconstruct a bone gap depends on the size of the gap, the patient's concomitant injuries, and the availability of specialized techniques such as microsurgery or bone distraction and even anatomic location. For example, hand and wrist injuries require different techniques than major limb bones. The broad options for reconstructing bone defects are nonvascularized bone grafting (cancellous or cortico-cancellous strut), vascularized bone flaps, bone transportation via distraction osteogenesis, and amputation.[17]

Bone grafts and flaps rely on the principals of osteoconduction, osteoinduction, and osteogenesis to achieve bone healing and consolidation. Osteoconduction is when a graft serves as a scaffold for the ingrowth of blood cells and osteoblasts from the recipient site. This occurs with a processed cadaver bone graft for example. A cortical bone graft may have the theoretical possibility of providing structural support but heals largely by osteoconduction in a process of "creeping substitution." Any living cells in such a bone graft may be too remote from the recipient blood supply to provide much capacity for osteogenesis.

Osteoinduction is when the graft encourages progenitor cells in the recipient site to differentiate into osteoblasts. Finally, osteogenesis is when the donor graft carries progenitor cells along with it that differentiate into osteoblasts after transfer (Table 70.5).[18]

A cancellous bone graft has living cells that are close to the recipient blood supply and do have an inherent osteogenic potential. Because of the sponginess of a block of cancellous bone or multiple chips of bone grafts, there is limited osteoconduction.

A vascularized bone flap has the advantage of all three properties. These have been loosely called vascularized bone grafts, but because they have their own innate blood supply (unlike grafts), they are more correctly called bone flaps. Despite this, vascularized bone graft seems to have become a commonly used term.

Nonvascularized bone grafts have good success in clean wounds with good soft tissue coverage and a bone gap of less than 6 cm. Cortical cancellous strut grafts have a potential advantage of providing structural support. However, cancellous bone grafts may heal even substantial bone gaps if support is provided by either internal fixation (such as a locking spanning plate) or external fixation.

Donor sites for nonvascularized cancellous bone grafting heal well with a low complication rate. For small amounts, it can be taken from the distal radius through a bone window at Lister tubercle. The iliac crest provides a rich supply of cancellous bone when larger amounts are needed.[19,20]

Cancellous bone graft can be used for even sizable bone gaps in major upper limbs bones. "Take" of the graft is enhanced by using the Masquelet technique. This technique starts with the placement of an antibiotic cement spacer in the bone gap. This can be supported with a Kirschner wire, a small plate, or external fixator depending on the size of the bone and the bone gap. A membrane forms around the spacer with maximum vascularity forming within the membrane at about 10 days. It is at this time that the membrane can be sharply incised. The cement is delivered and the space packed with cancellous bone grafts. While this was first utilized for the leg, promising results have also been reported for major upper limb bones.[21]

Another technique is to create new bone by utilizing distraction osteogenesis. Here a frame is placed with a bar on either side of the proposed lengthening site. A fracture is then made at that site. During the initial latency phase, the bone is allowed to partially heal. During the subsequent activation phase, the arms of the frame are separated, usually by turning a screw on the external portion of the frame. As the fracture is widened, a generate is formed, which is similar to a callus, and this eventually heals into normal bone. Once the desired length is reached, the consolidation phase is initiated. This is when distraction is no longer performed and the bone is allowed to fully heal.[22]

Vascularized bone flaps take advantage of all the aspects of bone graft healing. They do require microsurgical technique and have a more morbid donor site. However, they do have the advantages of more robust healing if the wound was previously contaminated or there is a long gap in a major limb bone. They can also be spanned in order to provide structural support. The more common donor sites are the fibula and iliac crest for large recipient sites and the medial femoral condyle for smaller sites.[23]

An Algorithmic Approach to the Mangled Extremity

Complex contaminated injuries that involve multiple structures (bone, soft tissue, tendons, nerves, and blood vessels) must be treated in a methodological and thoughtful manner to optimize functional outcome and reduce the risk of infection, flap loss, and bone nonunion.

It is also common to have associated trunk and head injuries that may need to take priority but not to the neglect of the extremity involvement. Many elbow gunshot injuries, for example, are from missile injuries to the abdomen and chest, the elbow and forearm simply got protectively placed in the way of the passing bullet on its way to the chest!

Injuries that involve multiple structures are treated systematically by breaking them down into component parts and addressing the problem in a stepwise plan. "Life before limb" but at least stabilize the limb injury before it can be addressed more completely. First, follow acute trauma life support protocols. Once the secondary survey has identified the extent of nonlife threatening injuries and necessary radiographs have been taken, extremity management begins (Box 70.1).

If the distal part is avascular or if there is major bleeding, this must be addressed first. If a tourniquet can be placed proximal to the injury, then the use of a bloodless field is extremely helpful. This enables a more thorough assessment for debridement and identification of structures to be repaired. Vascular repair is either done by direct anastomosis or a temporary vascular shunt may be placed. In the event that a severely displaced fracture will hamper

BOX 70.1 Principals of mangled extremity care.

- Life over limb
- Revascularization
- Temporary bone fixation
- Debride, debride, debride
- Definitive reconstruction

BOX 70.2 Priorities in the mangled extremity.

1. Revascularization
2. Temporary bony fixation
3. Soft tissue coverage
4. Definitive bony reconstruction
5. Tendon and nerve reconstruction

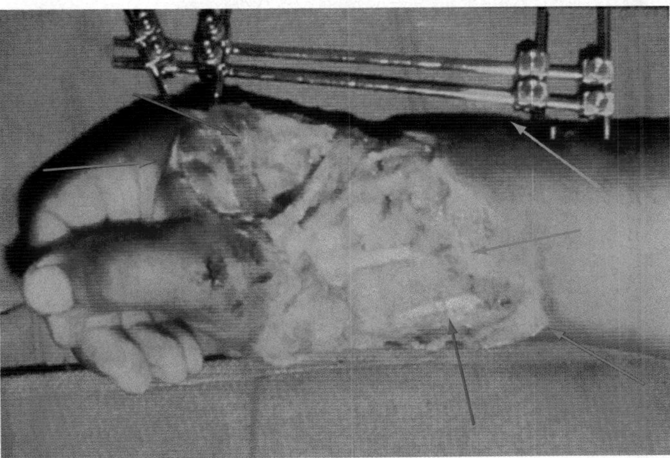

FIG. 70.35 Treatment of the mangled extremity should progress in a stepwise manner.

vascular repair, temporary bone fixation should be done prior to revascularization (Box 70.2 and Fig. 70.35).

Fractures must be stabilized, either temporarily by means of external fixation or bridging spanning plates. A decision is made for bone shortening or if this is not functionally possible, then a bone gap and soft tissue space must be maintained. Bone shortening may facilitate nerve, tendon, and vessel repair by bringing the ends for the repair closer together and minimizing tension as well as closing down the soft tissue space. In the severely injured extremity, amputation may be a consideration, remembering that prosthetic utilization is much more complex for an above elbow amputation than a transradial amputation. If a decision is made for amputation, try if at all possible to preserve an elbow joint.

Adequate initial debridement is paramount, not only of embedded foreign material, but also of devitalized tissue. Antibiotic impregnated methyl methacrylate as a solid spacer or as a string of antibiotic beads can help to maintain the soft tissue space and deliver a high dose of antibiotics locally to the area.[21] The membrane that forms around the antibiotic cement will give one a head start for bone reconstruction as well.[24] Early and aggressive debridement remains critical. Infection will compromise any future bone or soft tissue reconstruction. Only once one has an adequately clean wound, can reconstruction be considered.[25]

This will likely require more than one debridement. The vacuum-assisted closure (VAC) device has allowed us to temporarily cover an open wound and maintain the sterile environment while surgical planning and repeat debridements take place. For injuries more distally, the VAC dressing reduces edema, can maintain and mold the hand and wrist in a functional position. It may even help to stabilize fractures. Thus the VAC provides temporary splinting as well as a bridge to definitive soft tissue coverage and reconstruction.[26]

Godina landmark paper in 1986 described the principals of early soft tissue wound coverage of open fractures with a cleanly debrided wound.[27] Not only is the quality and durability of the soft tissue coverage important (such as a free or pedicled flap), but also the timing of this coverage is paramount. Extensive delay results in progression of the collagen phase of wound healing and fibrotic granulation tissue leading to callous and loss of fixation. Often bone and soft tissue reconstruction can be performed simultaneously. On occasion, if the bone is stabilized by external fixation or an antibiotic spacer, soft tissue flap reconstruction may precede the bone reconstruction.[28]

Tendons and nerves are repaired once vascular integrity is ensured and bone fractures are stabilized. In the case of high-energy injuries, one may elect to delay tendon repairs, but severed ends should be tagged for future identification. Even if definitive tendon reconstruction is planned at a later stage, approximation of tendon ends, if possible, should be done to minimize proximal muscle belly myostatic contraction (Fig. 70.36).

The concept of "spare parts" uses components distal to the injury for reconstruction. For example, an unsalvageable mutilated digit may be amputated, but the goal should be to at least preserve the soft tissues for pedicled flap coverage of adjacent structures. A forearm that is mangled may be cleared of bone and that soft tissue envelope used for coverage of a more proximal amputation. That distal tissue has even on occasion been used as a free flap more proximally. This concept may be especially useful in the reconstruction of damaged joints. Blood supply of these spare parts must be preserved.[29]

INFECTIONS

Hand infections commonly present to the surgical resident covering the emergency department. When the infection is diagnosed and treated properly initially, most patients do well. The extent of deep palmar infections may often be underestimated during the early phases because the volar aspect of the hand does not show edema as readily as the dorsal aspect of the hand. Thus, if infections in the hand are not diagnosed at an early stage, infections may spread from one anatomic compartment to another along natural tissue planes. Hand infections can then result in significant morbidity and severe functional compromise if they are not appropriately diagnosed and treated (Fig. 70.37). Some of the more common types of infections are discussed here.

Superficial Paronychial Infections

Paronychia is the most common infection of the hand; it usually results from trauma to the eponychial or paronychial region. The infection localizes around the nail base, advances around the nail fold, and burrows beneath the base of the nail. If pus is trapped beneath the nail, pressure on the nail evokes exquisite pain. The

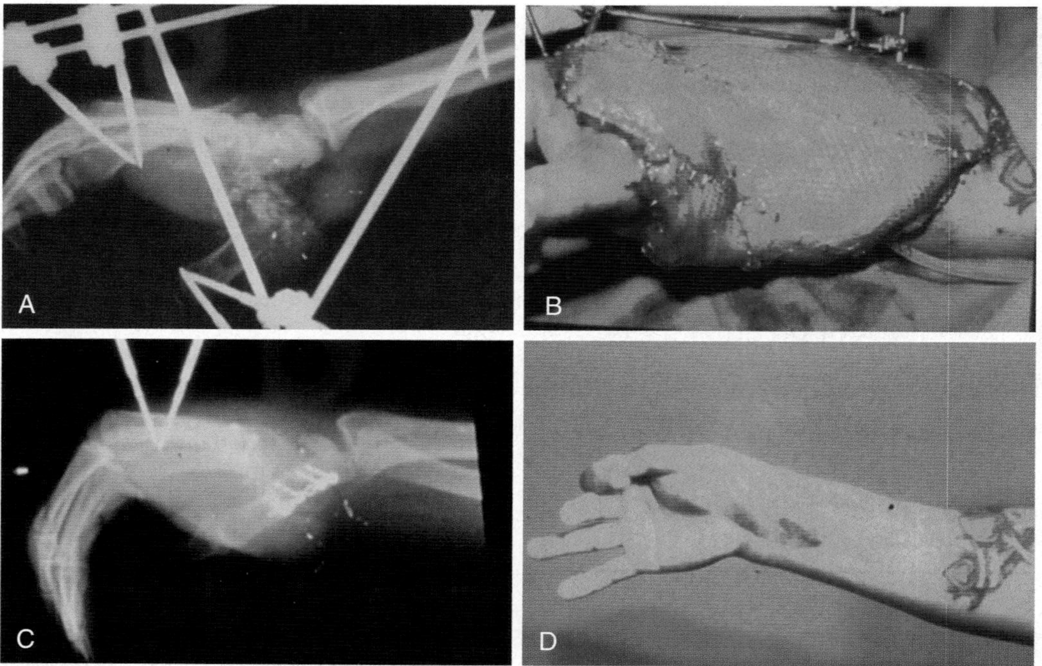

FIG. 70.36 Stepwise approach to injury from Fig. 70.35. Top left: initial temporary fixation and revascularization of the thumb. Top right: definitive soft tissue coverage with flap and skin graft. Bottom left: definitive bony fixation. Bottom right: 1-year results after tendon transfers and never recover.

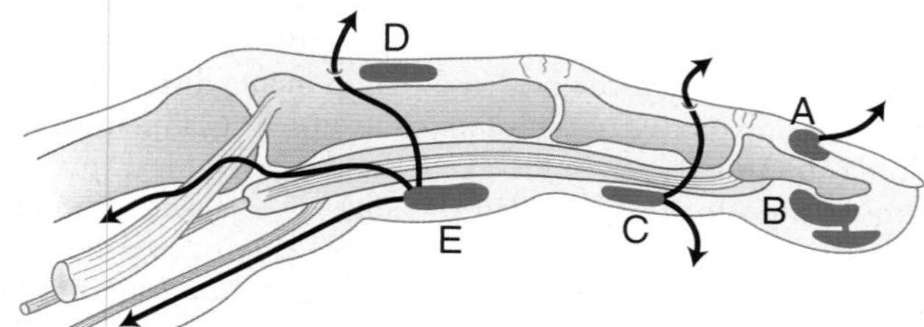

FIG. 70.37 Spread of soft tissue infections in the hand occurs through loss of containment from the original site and erosion into and spread through contiguous anatomic compartments. *A,* Paronychium. Infecting organisms access periungual tissues through fissures in the eponychial or paronychial tissues and often are discharged spontaneously in these areas. *B,* Infection of pulp tissues (felon). Fibrous septa within the pulp create collar stud abscesses within the pulp. *C,* Volar subcutaneous infections in the digit may be discharged percutaneously on either surface of the digit or penetrate dorsally and spread along the sheaths of the flexor or extensor tendons. *D,* Subcutaneous infections on the dorsum of the digit are usually discharged percutaneously because of the thin and areolar nature of the soft tissues. *E,* Proximally located digital infections or web space infections may rupture into the palmar spaces by tracking along tendon sheaths, palmar fascia, or lumbrical canal. The continuous sheaths of the thumb and little fingers (radial and ulnar bursae) are continuous with the carpal tunnel and space of Parona at the wrist.

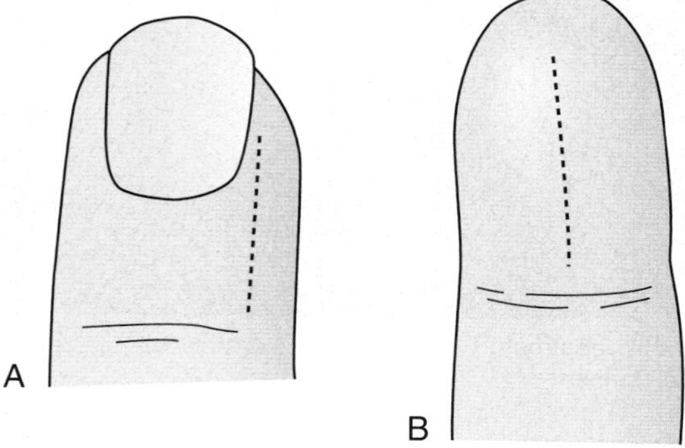

FIG. 70.38 Incisions for paronychia (A) and felon (B).

most common causative organism is *Staphylococcus aureus.* Early treatment is with antibiotics, preferably penicillin in combination with a β-lactamase inhibitor such as sulbactam or clavulanic acid. However, there has now been an increasing incidence of methicillin-resistant *S. aureus* in community-acquired infections. After an abscess develops, surgical drainage is required. The surgical approach to an acute paronychia depends on the extent of the infection. Incisions may not be necessary. A Freer elevator is used to lift approximately 25% of the nail adjacent to the infected perionychium, extending proximally to the edge of the nail. This portion of the nail is transected, and gauze packing is inserted beneath the nail fold. A single incision to drain the affected perionychium also allows elevation of the eponychial fold when both eponychium and paronychium are involved (Fig. 70.38).[30]

Infections of Intermediate-Depth Spaces

Infections of intermediate-depth spaces are pulp space infections (felons) and deep web space infections. The pulp space infections may involve the terminal, middle, or proximal volar pulp spaces and may result from direct implantation with a penetrating injury or may represent spread from a more superficial subcutaneous infection. The volar pulp of the distal digital segment is a fascial space closed proximally by a septum joining the distal flexion crease to the periosteum, where the long flexor tendon is inserted. This space is also partitioned by fibrous septa. Tension in the distal

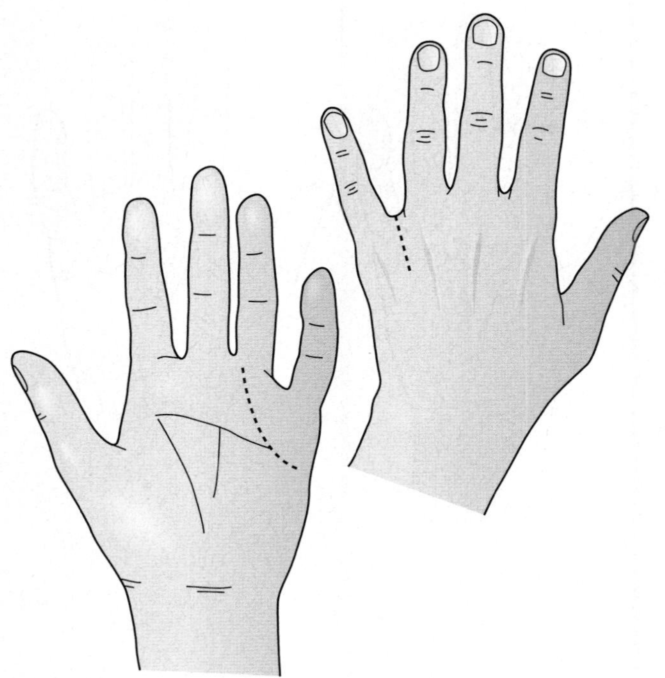

FIG. 70.39 Incisions for web space abscess between the little and ring fingers.

digital segment can become so great that the arteries to the bone are compressed, resulting in gangrene of the fingertip and necrosis of the distal 75% of the terminal phalanx. With infection of the digital pulp space, one must not wait for fluctuance before making the decision for surgery because of the danger of ischemic necrosis of the skin and bone. Clinical diagnosis is made by the rapid onset of throbbing pain, swelling, and exquisite tenderness of the affected pulp space. Surgical drainage is required. A single volar or unilateral longitudinal incision may be used (Fig. 70.38). Postoperative care includes packing of the wound and elevation of the extremity. Use of antibiotics is guided by the results of Gram staining. Similar to a paronychia, *S. aureus* is the most common causative agent. Spread from a pulp space infection may move into a joint space or underlying bone or burst through the septum proximally to involve the rest of the finger. More proximally, a pulp space infection at the base of the finger can travel through the lumbrical canal into the palm to create a deep palmar space infection.[30]

Web space abscesses result from direct implantation or spread from a pulp space. An inflamed and tender mass in the web space separates the fingers. There is loss of the normal palmar concavity, with a widened space between the fingers. Dorsal swelling is present and must not be mistaken for the infection site. A surgical incision is placed transversely across the web space, and a longitudinal counterincision may be placed dorsally between the bases of the proximal phalanges; a generous communication is established between these two incisions (Fig. 70.39).

Deep Infections

Palmar Space Infections

These infections are localized to the deep space of the hand between the metacarpals and palmar aponeurosis. A transverse septum to the metacarpal of the middle finger divides the deep space into an ulnar midpalmar and radial thenar space. The transverse head of the adductor pollicis partitions the thenar space from the retroadductor space. There may be ballooning of the palm, thenar eminence, or posterior aspect of the first web space, depending on which of the affected spaces is involved with an abscess. The dorsal subaponeurotic space of the hand deep to the extensor tendons may also be affected by an isolated infection, generally as the result of direct implantation (Fig. 70.40A). For a thenar space infection, the preferred approach to surgical drainage is a dual volar and dorsal incision (Fig. 70.40B). On the volar side, an incision is made adjacent and parallel to the thenar crease. Great care is taken to avoid injury to the palmar cutaneous branch of the median nerve in the proximal part of the incision and the motor branch of the median nerve in a deeper plane. A second, slightly curved longitudinal incision is made on the dorsum of the first web space. Dissection is continued more deeply into this area between the first dorsal interosseous muscle and adductor pollicis. A drain is placed in the incision after thorough exploration of the respective spaces. With midpalmar space infections, dorsal swelling of the hand will be present, as is the case with all palmar infections, and must not be mistaken for the infection site. Motion of the middle and ring fingers is limited and painful. A longitudinal curvilinear incision is the preferred approach for drainage of this space (Fig. 70.40C).

Infection of Parona space occurs in the potential space deep to the flexor tendons in the distal forearm and superficial to the pronator quadratus muscle. It is usually the result of spread from the adjacent contiguous midpalmar space or from the radial or ulnar bursa. Swelling, tenderness, and fluctuation will be present in the distal volar forearm. A midpalmar infection may be associated. Active digital flexion is painful, as is passive finger extension. A surgical incision must be planned to leave the median nerve adequately covered with soft tissue.

Pyogenic Flexor Tenosynovitis

Kanavel four cardinal signs include the following: (1) the finger is held flexed because this position allows the synovial sheath its maximum volume and eases pain; (2) symmetrical fusiform swelling of the entire finger is present, with edema of the back of the hand; (3) the slightest attempt at passive extension of the affected digit produces exquisite pain; and (4) the site of maximum tenderness is at the proximal cul-de-sac of the index, middle, and ring finger synovial sheaths in the distal palm or, in the case of infection of the sheaths of the thumb and little finger, more proximally in the palm (Fig. 70.40). The radial and ulnar bursae communicate in approximately 80% of cases and may be simultaneously infected. Bursal infections may spread into the forearm space of Parona, deep to the flexor tendons in the distal part of the forearm, creating a horseshoe abscess.

Pyogenic flexor tenosynovitis may be aborted with parenteral antibiotics, extremity elevation, and hand immobilization if the patient is seen within the first 24 hours of onset of infection. If this course is unsuccessful or if the patient is seen more than 48 hours after onset of infection, surgical drainage is undertaken. The preferred surgical approach is through two separate incisions. The first incision is a midaxial incision made on the finger, usually on the ulnar side of the digit (on the radial side of the thumb or little finger); the digital artery and nerve remain in the volar flap, with the dissection proceeding directly to the tendon sheath. The synovium between the A3 and A4 pulleys is incised, and cloudy fluid is encountered. A second incision is made in the palm over the tendon to drain the cul-de-sac. A 16-gauge polyethylene catheter is inserted beneath the A1 pulley into the sheath, and the sheath is flushed manually with sterile saline every 2 hours after surgery. A

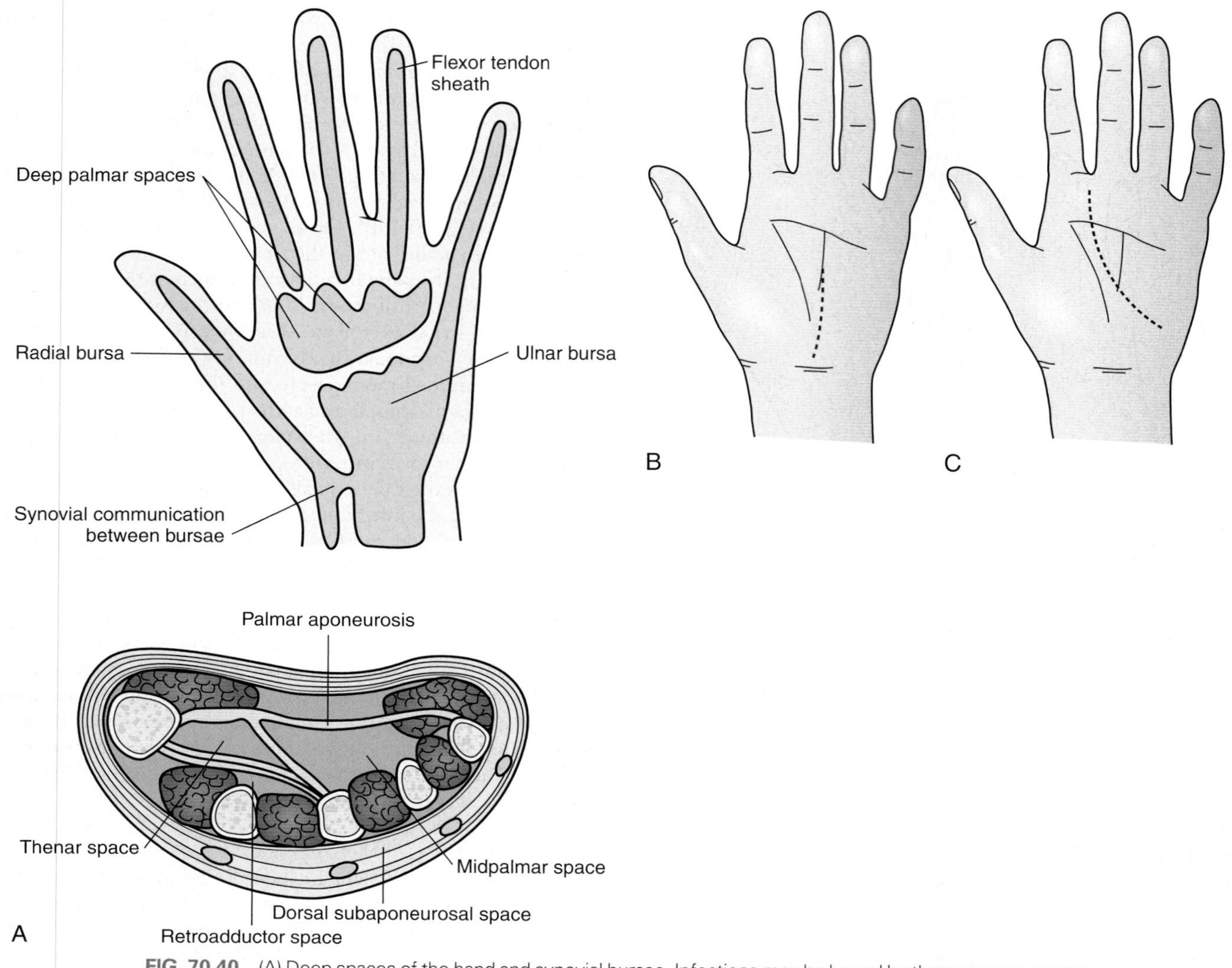

FIG. 70.40 (A) Deep spaces of the hand and synovial bursae. Infections may be bound by these spaces or may track along anatomic dissection planes between these spaces. (B) Incision for thenar space infection. A dorsal first web space incision is also often required. (C) Incision for midpalmar space abscess.

bulky hand dressing absorbs the drainage. Studies have found that postoperative catheter drainage may not always be necessary.[31]

Chronic and Atypical Infections

Chronic paronychia is generally the result of *Candida albicans* infection (>95%) and is not bacterial. When bacteria are involved, they are more commonly atypical mycobacteria or gram-negative organisms. Chronic paronychia generally responds to treatment with topical antifungal agents, although oral antifungal agents are sometimes used. On occasion, surgical treatment by means of marsupialization of the eponychial fold is required. If the lesion is refractory to treatment, the possibility of a malignant neoplasm is entertained.

Chronic tenosynovitis can occur in the flexor tendons or in the dorsum of the wrist and extensor tendons. It is usually of a granulomatous type and is caused by mycobacteria or fungi. Treatment includes surgical excision of the involved synovium and prolonged treatment with the appropriate antimicrobial agents. Chronic infected tenosynovitis must be differentiated from other causes of chronic granulomatous synovitis, such as sarcoidosis, amyloidosis, gout, and rheumatoid arthritis.

Herpetic Whitlow

Herpetic whitlow is caused by type 1 or type 2 herpes simplex virus and may be confused with a paronychia. Infection begins with the appearance of small clear vesicles with localized swelling, erythema, and intense pain. The vesicles may subsequently appear turbid and coalesce over the next few days before ulcerating. Diagnosis is confirmed by culturing the virus from the vesicular fluid, assessing immunofluorescent serum antibody titers, or performing a Tzanck smear. However, these measures are rarely required because clinical diagnosis is usually sufficient. Infection can occur from autoinoculation from an oral or genital lesion or exposure as a healthcare worker. Pain is often out of proportion to the physical findings. Treatment is generally nonoperative because this infection is usually self-limited. Antivirals such as acyclovir or famciclovir may be of some benefit if started within the first 48 hours of symptom onset. Surgical incision and drainage can lead to systemic involvement and possible viral encephalitis.

Animal and Human Bites

The most striking difference in the microbial flora of human and animal bite wounds is the higher number of bacterial isolates per wound in human bites, the difference being mostly caused by the presence of anaerobic bacteria. Human bites can occasionally transmit other infectious diseases, such as hepatitis B, tuberculosis, syphilis, or actinomycosis. The incidence of *Eikenella corrodens* in human bite infections of the hand has been reported to vary between 7% and 29%. Usually, isolated organisms from infected human bite wounds are, as in animal bites, alpha-hemolytic streptococci and *S. aureus,* β-lactamase–producing strains of *S. aureus,* and *Bacteroides* spp. Anaerobic bacteria, including *Bacteroides, Clostridium, Peptococcus,* and *Veillonella,* are more prevalent in human bite infections than previously recognized. Most studies of animal bite wounds have focused on the isolation of *Pasteurella multocida,* disregarding the role of anaerobes. However, more recent studies have shown that dog bite wounds indicate multiple organisms, with *P. multocida* being isolated from only 26% of dog bite wounds in adults. Most animal bites cause mixed infections of aerobic and anaerobic bacteria.

Pyogenic joint infections usually result from trauma, such as a bite wound from a tooth when the assailant's hand strikes the jaw. A tooth struck by the clenched fist of an attacker penetrates the skin, tendon, joint capsule, and metacarpal head. Once the finger is extended, the four puncture wounds separate from each other to create a closed space within the joint. All these so-called fight bite wounds of the MP joint need to be explored surgically, debrided, and thoroughly lavaged. Human bite wounds are not closed primarily and are treated with appropriate antibiotics.

COMPARTMENT SYNDROME, HIGH-PRESSURE INJECTION INJURIES, AND EXTRAVASATION INJURIES

High-Pressure Injection Injuries

High-pressure injection injuries to the hand are relatively uncommon, but consequences of a misdiagnosis are serious. Urgent treatment is required. High-pressure injection guns are used for painting, lubricating, cleaning, and farm animal vaccinations. Materials that may be injected with these devices include paint, paint thinners, oil, grease, water, plastic, vaccines, and cement. These high-pressure injection guns may generate pressures ranging between 3000 and 12,000 psi. Injection injuries can also be caused by other sources, such as defective lines and valves, pneumatic hoses, and hydraulic lines. The type of material injected is the most important prognostic factor. Oil-based paints and paint thinners can generate significant early inflammation, leading to severe fibrosis. Because tendon sheaths at the index, middle, and ring fingers end at the level of the MP joints, material injected at the DIP or PIP flexion creases will remain within these digits. However, tendon sheaths at the thumb and little finger extend all the way into the radial and ulnar bursae. Thus, material injected at the little finger or at the IP flexion crease of the thumb may potentially extend all the way into the forearm and even cause a compartment syndrome.

Initial presentation of a patient with a high-pressure injection may be benign and subtle. This may result in mismanagement by minimizing the patient's complaints. The break in the skin may be a benign-looking, pinhole-sized puncture site. However, within several hours, the digit becomes increasingly more painful, swollen, and pale. Prompt recognition and realization of the severity of injury are paramount. Radiographs may help determine the extent and dispersion of the injected material, either in the form of subcutaneous emphysema or, with lead-based paints, appearing as radiopaque soft tissue densities. The entire digit must be surgically decompressed and all foreign material and necrotic tissue debrided (Fig. 70.41). Wounds are closed loosely over Penrose drains or in a delayed manner. Appropriate antibiotics must be administered. Despite prompt recognition and treatment, many such injuries ultimately result in surgical amputation of the digits.

Extravasation Injuries

In the past, extravasation injuries of chemotherapeutic agents frequently affected the upper extremity. However, subcutaneously tunneled central lines have now reduced the incidence of these injuries. If extravasation is suspected, infusion must be stopped immediately. Cold packs are applied for 15 minutes 4 times a day, and the extremity is elevated during the next 48 hours. This treatment is generally effective for most extravasation injuries. However, if blistering, ulceration, and pain occur in the damaged tissue, progressive necrosis to the limits of the extravasation will follow, and surgical excision of all damaged tissue is necessary. Most subsequent wounds can generally be treated with delayed split-thickness skin grafting, although the options for wound coverage after debridement depend on the extent of the debridement that was required.

Compartment Syndrome

Compartment syndrome results in symptoms and signs caused by increased pressure within a limited space that compromises circulation and function of the tissues in that space. Volkmann ischemic contracture is the sequel of untreated compartment syndrome; it results in muscle that is fibrosed, contracted, and functionless and nerves that are insensible. Various injuries are known to cause compartment syndrome:

- Decreased compartment volume (e.g., from externally applied tight dressings or casts, lying on a limb in a comatose state)
- Increased compartment content (e.g., from bleeding or trauma with fractures or finger injuries; increased capillary permeability, such as reperfusion after ischemic injury; electrical burn injuries)
- Other injuries (e.g., snakebites, high-pressure injection injuries).[32]

The diagnosis of compartment syndrome is based primarily on clinical evaluation. Although it is possible to measure intracompartment pressure, the decision to perform fasciotomy is based on a high degree of clinical suspicion. Compartment ischemia may be severe and still not affect the color or temperature of the distal fingers, and the distal pulses are rarely obliterated by compartment swelling. However, circulation in the muscle and nerve may be greatly reduced. Muscle ischemia that lasts for more than 4 hours leads to muscle death and may also cause significant myoglobinuria. After 8 hours of total ischemia, irreversible nerve changes are complete. The hallmark of muscle and nerve ischemia is pain, which is progressive and persistent. The pain is accentuated by passive muscle stretching; this is the most reliable clinical test for diagnosis of compartment syndrome. The next most important clinical finding is diminished sensation, which indicates nerve ischemia. The closed compartments of the forearm and hand are also palpated and found to be tense and tender, confirming the diagnosis of compartment syndrome. A passive muscle stretch test elicits severe pain in the presence of compartment syndrome. An arterial injury and nerve injury need to be distinguished in the differential diagnosis of compartment syndrome. All three of these injuries produce paresthesias and paresis; pain with passive stretch is present in compartment

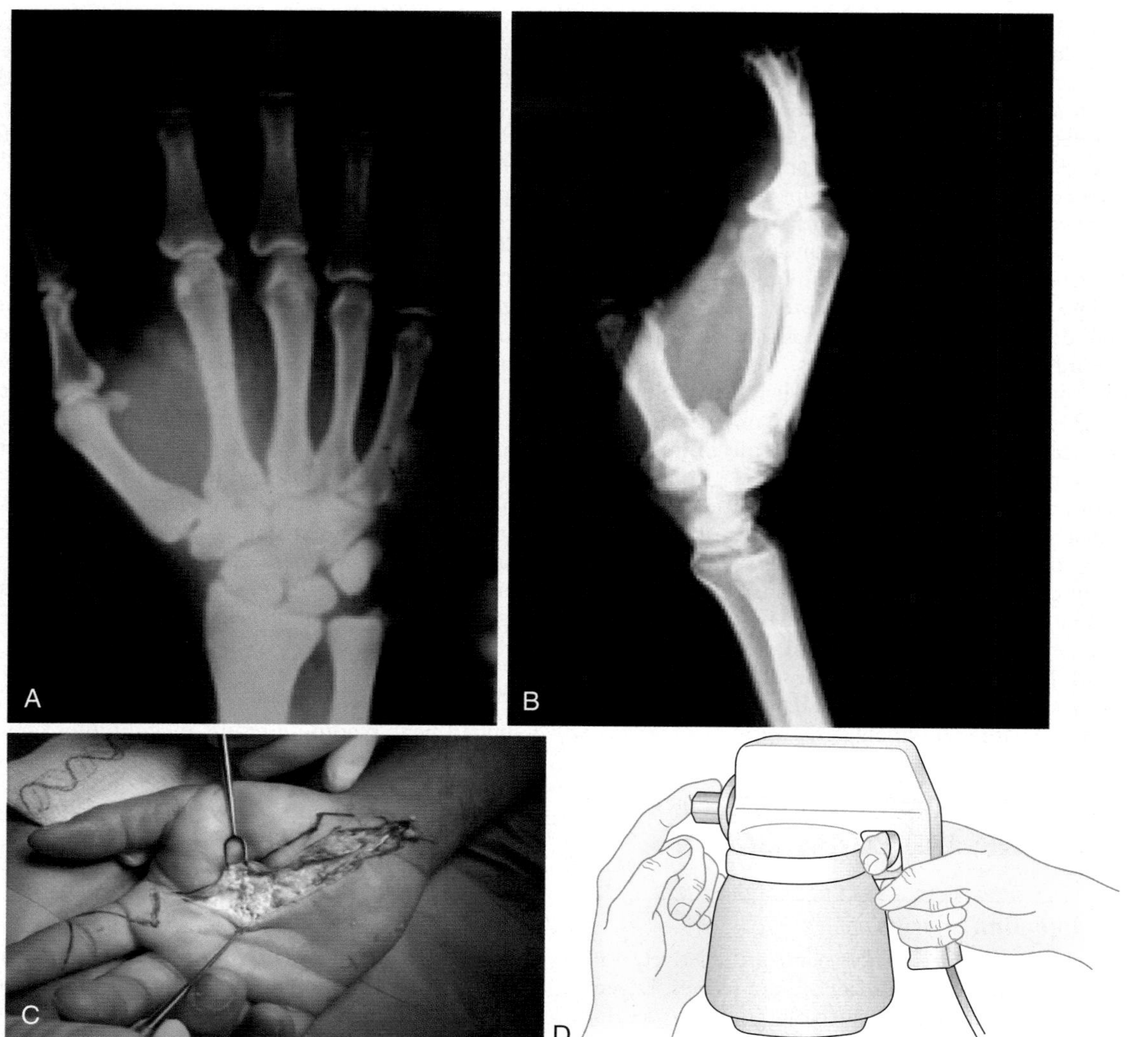

FIG. 70.41 High-pressure injection injury from paint gun appears completely innocuous, with tiny puncture wound on presentation. (A and B) Anteroposterior and lateral radiographs of the right hand show widely disseminated radiopaque foreign material in soft tissues of the palm and thenar eminence. (C) Intraoperative photograph of left-handed man with palmar high-pressure injection injury from a paint gun on the nondominant palm. The tissues are extensively infiltrated by paint from the base of the finger to the wrist and require urgent debridement and decompression. (D) Removal of the guard allows the nozzle to come into close contact, exponentially increasing the pressure delivered to soft tissues.

syndrome and arterial occlusion, but not in neurapraxia; and pulses are intact in compartment syndrome and neurapraxia, but not with arterial occlusion. In situations in which the patient cannot cooperate because of inebriation or unconsciousness and the clinical diagnosis is difficult, compartment pressure can be measured.

Release of a forearm compartment syndrome always requires carpal tunnel release (Fig. 70.42). The palmar incision starts in the valley between the thenar and hypothenar muscles, and the incision then curves transversely across the flexion crease of the wrist at the ulnar border. This incision must avoid the palmar cutaneous branch of the median nerve and prevent flexion contracture across the wrist crease. It also provides an opportunity to release the Guyon canal. The incision then extends proximally up the forearm before curving back in a radial direction so as to have a large skin flap that will cover the median nerve and distal forearm tendons. At the elbow, the incision for the flap then curves again across the antecubital fossa, providing cover for the brachial artery and median nerve and preventing linear contracture across the antecubital fossa. The dorsal and so-called mobile wad compartments of the forearm are readily released through a straight incision, as needed. Appropriate release of the various intrinsic compartments of the hand may also be required. Most wounds can be partially closed at 5 days. If the skin cannot be closed secondarily within 10 days, a split-thickness skin graft can be applied.

TENOSYNOVITIS

de Quervain Disease

de Quervain disease is a stenosing tenosynovitis of the first dorsal compartment of the wrist and is a common cause of pain and disability. Diagnosis is easily made from a history of pain localized to the radial side of the wrist and aggravated by movement of the thumb. There is frequently a history of chronic overuse of the wrist and hand. Other features are local tenderness and swelling

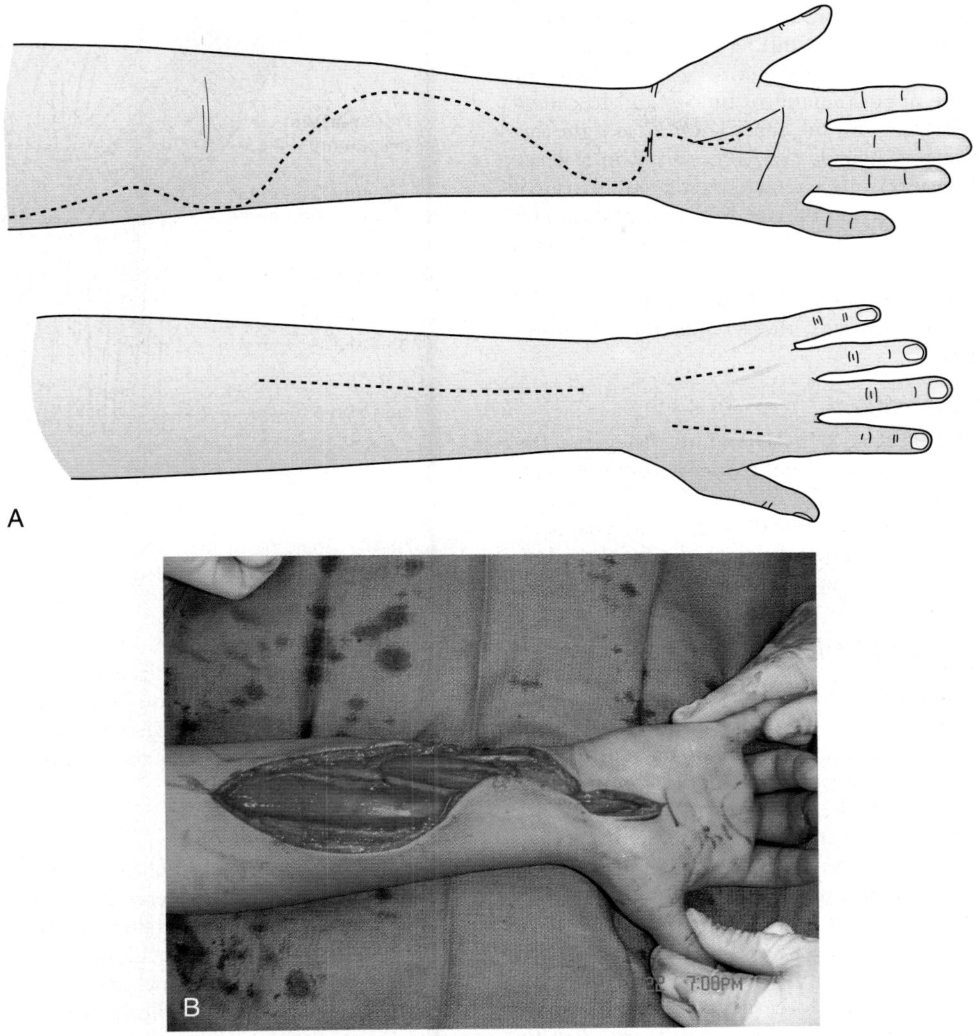

FIG. 70.42 (A) Incisions for forearm fasciotomy. (B) Fasciotomy in a child for compartment syndrome after a snakebite.

over the first dorsal compartment of the wrist and a positive Finkelstein test result—the patient clasps the thumb and brisk ulnar deviation to the hand elicits extreme pain. Crepitus may be palpable. This condition must be differentiated by radiographic and physical examination from arthritis of the thumb carpometacarpal joint.

Nonoperative treatment includes local steroid injection, thumb and wrist immobilization, local heat, and systemic antiinflammatory medications. If these nonoperative measures fail, surgical decompression of the first dorsal compartment at the wrist is performed. Care must be taken to protect the radial sensory nerve branches during the course of the operation because these branches traverse just under the skin in this area, and trauma or transection may lead to painful disabling neuromas.

Intersection Syndrome

This condition is not well understood but is characterized by pain and crepitus at the point at which the APL and EPB tendons cross over the tendons of the second dorsal compartment (ECRL and ECRB; Fig. 70.43). Initial treatment is by splinting, local corticosteroid injection, and antiinflammatory medications. Refractory cases require surgical release at the second dorsal compartment and excision of involved tenosynovial membranes.

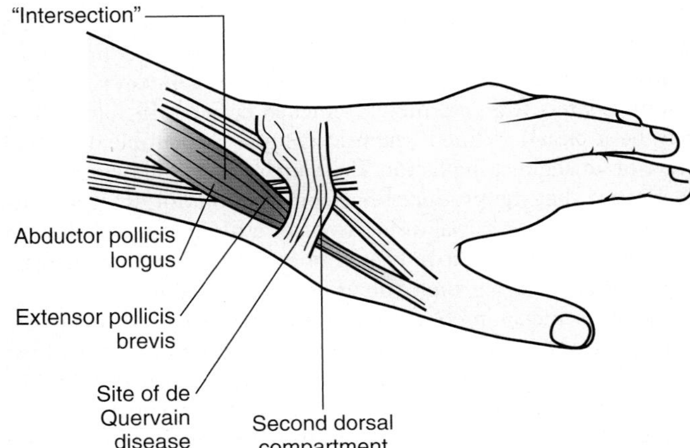

FIG. 70.43 Anatomic locations for de Quervain stenosing tenosynovitis and intersection syndrome.

Trigger Thumb and Fingers

Trigger finger is a constricting tenosynovitis of the flexor tendons, generally at the level of the A1 pulley. The patient can flex the digit, but an apparent nodule catches at the proximal edge of the

A1 pulley, locking the PIP joint (or the IP joint of the thumb) in this flexed position. Attempts at extending the digit cause it to snap back suddenly, much like the trigger of a gun. Often, the patient needs to use the opposite hand to unlock and to extend the digit. In its most severe form, the constriction is so tight that the patient cannot flex the digit or it becomes fixed in a flexed position and can no longer be fully extended. A congenital form of trigger thumb or finger presents in infants, but most cases resolve by the time the child reaches 1 year of age; if not, an operation is indicated.

Nonoperative treatment in adults includes local injection of corticosteroids. If this regimen fails, the A1 pulley is longitudinally divided by surgery.[33]

Other Sites of Tenosynovitis

Other sites include the FCR and FCU tendons. They can frequently be treated by splinting and local corticosteroid injection, although surgery occasionally may be required. Inflammation of the ECU may also be an enigmatic cause of ulnar-sided wrist pain. Diagnosis is made by eliciting tenderness along the ECU tendon, pain on active resisted extension, and ulnar deviation of the wrist.

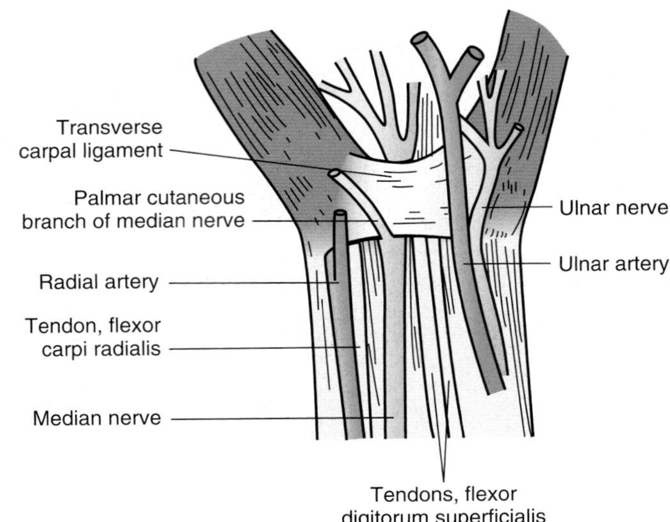

FIG. 70.44 Anatomy of the carpal tunnel. The transverse carpal ligament (flexor retinaculum) is divided longitudinally during a carpal tunnel release.

NERVE COMPRESSION SYNDROMES

Along the length of the upper extremity, nerves pass through a number of anatomic bottlenecks. These are all possible sites of nerve entrapment and lead to characteristic distal sensory and motor deficits. The most common sites of nerve compression, from proximal to distal along the length of the extremity, are at the nerve root secondary to cervical disc disease or cervical degenerative arthritis, thoracic outlet compression at the level of the clavicle, ulnar nerve entrapment at the elbow (cubital tunnel syndrome), entrapment of the posterior interosseous nerve in the proximal forearm (radial tunnel syndrome, posterior interosseous syndrome), entrapment of the median nerve and its branches in the proximal forearm (so-called pronator syndrome, anterior interosseous nerve syndrome), and, finally, entrapment of the median nerve at the wrist (carpal tunnel syndrome) and of the ulnar nerve in the Guyon canal (ulnar tunnel syndrome).

In most cases of nerve entrapment, no specific aggravating causative factor is found. An increasing incidence of compression neuropathy is reported in patients whose work involves chronic repetitive stress (e.g., assemblers, chicken cutters). In some, there may be a clearly defined extrinsic compressive problem on the nerve or an aggravating factor. These include the following:

- Trauma that can produce bone compression, for example, carpal tunnel after carpal dislocations or a distal radius malunion (median) and supracondylar humerus fractures that increase the elbow carrying angle (ulnar nerve at the elbow)
- Synovial thickening of the bursa in rheumatoid arthritis in the carpal tunnel (median) or at the elbow (posterior interosseous)
- Tumors such as giant cell tumor in the Guyon canal (ulnar) or a lipoma in the radial tunnel (posterior interosseous)
- Developmental, with anomalous muscles present in the carpal tunnel (median), Guyon canal (ulnar), or forearm (median)
- Metabolic, in which disturbances of fluid balance cause increased pressure on the nerve, particularly at the carpal tunnel (e.g., myxedema, pregnancy).

Carpal tunnel syndrome is the most common peripheral nerve entrapment syndrome followed by ulnar nerve entrapment at the elbow.[34] The other entrapment syndromes are less common.

Diabetes mellitus is recognized as a risk factor for carpal tunnel syndrome, and the response to treatment has previously been unclear. However, studies suggest that patients with diabetes do similarly well as patients who are normoglycemic do after carpal tunnel release.

Carpal Tunnel Syndrome

The carpal tunnel is a packed fibro-osseous tunnel at the wrist that is traversed by the median nerve and nine long extrinsic digital flexor tendons (Fig. 70.44). Its floor is formed by the carpal bones and roofed by the flexor retinaculum (transverse carpal ligament). Normal pressures in this tunnel are 20 to 30 mm Hg. A rise in pressure above this causes a chronic compressive ischemic injury to the nerve segment, resulting first in demyelination and eventually in axonal death. There is progressive conduction block in the nerve, with subsequent sensory and motor dysfunction. The earliest symptoms are pain and paresthesias, which are characteristically more obvious at night, after prolonged activity, and with positional postural changes at the wrist, such as when driving, using a hand-held hair dryer, or reading a book. The patient may complain of clumsiness and a tendency to drop objects. The paresthesias characteristically follow the distribution of the median nerve, including the thumb and index and middle fingers.

Physical examination consists of compressing the carpal canal, percussing the median nerve, and hyperflexing the wrist to produce paresthesias (Durkan sign, Tinel sign, and Phalen test, respectively). Sensory evaluation reveals hypoesthesia in the distribution of the median nerve and may reveal a widened two-point sensory discrimination. Thenar weakness or muscle wasting is a late finding. Nerve conduction studies and electromyography are useful adjuncts to the clinical examination.

Initial treatment of carpal tunnel syndrome includes use of wrist splints (especially at night), occasional local corticosteroid injections, and modification in work patterns. If symptoms persist, or if the initial presentation shows severe carpal tunnel syndrome, surgical decompression is required. This is performed by longitudinally dividing the flexor retinaculum by open or endoscopic means. Both the Agee (single-portal) and Chow (two-portal) procedures have shown similar efficacy to the open approach.[35]

Synovectomy and removal of any mass lesion may also be required if that is the cause of the problem.[36]

Pronator Syndrome

In the proximal forearm, the median nerve may be compressed at the fibrous arch between the two heads of the FDS, two heads of the pronator teres, lacertus fibrosus (bicipital aponeurosis at the elbow), and ligament of Struthers. Compression at any or all of these sites is loosely grouped under the pronator syndrome. The symptoms produced are similar to those of carpal tunnel, although nocturnal symptoms are uncommon. The palm may also feel numb because the palmar cutaneous branch is involved, but it is specifically spared in carpal tunnel syndrome because that nerve branch passes superficial to the flexor retinaculum and arises proximal to the retinaculum. Symptoms may be reproduced or worsened by attempting pronation against resistance and by resisted flexion of the middle finger. However, it may be difficult to locate the compressive cause in the pronator syndrome precisely, and surgical decompression often involves release of all four potential sites of compression.

The anterior interosseous nerve branch of the median nerve may occasionally be compressed in isolation. This does not produce any sensory symptoms but specifically targets the three muscles innervated by the anterior interosseous nerve—FPL, FDP to the index and middle fingers, and pronator quadratus.

Ulnar Nerve Compression

The ulnar nerve may be compressed in the Guyon canal at the wrist or in the so-called cubital tunnel at the elbow and distal upper arm.

Guyon Canal Compression

This canal is bounded by the hook of the hamate, pisiform, pisohamate ligament, and palmar carpal ligament. Compression by mass lesions, including a ganglion, giant cell tumor, ulnar artery thrombosis, and ulnar artery aneurysm, may occur at this site as in hypothenar hammer syndrome. Compression at this site may also be idiopathic. Distal ulnar deficits may be in the motor or sensory distribution or both, depending on where in the canal the compression occurs relative to the takeoff of the deep motor branch of the ulnar nerve. Tinel sign may be present, and there may be worsening of symptoms by direct compression over the Guyon canal. Treatment is surgical; it consists of dividing the palmaris brevis muscle and palmar carpal ligament as well as removing any offending mass in this region.

Cubital Tunnel Syndrome

The cubital tunnel is a long tunnel starting in the distal upper arm and extending into the proximal forearm. As the ulnar nerve passes into the forearm, it curves tightly around the grooved posterior and inferior surfaces of the medial epicondyle of the humerus. This groove is bridged by the aponeurosis between the two heads of the FCU, the leading edge of which may be thickened and fibrosed, called Osborne ligament. More proximally, the ulnar nerve passes from the anterior compartment of the arm into the posterior compartment, which may be bridged by a long tunnel called the arcade of Struthers. The medial intermuscular septum in the upper arm may also cause ulnar nerve compression. The most distal fibro-osseous tunnel is more accurately termed the cubital tunnel. However, compression on the ulnar nerve can occur at any of these sites, proximal to distal, starting in the upper arm and extending into the forearm. Motor and sensory symptoms develop in the distribution of the ulnar nerve and are worsened by adopting a flexed position at the elbow. Examination reveals Tinel sign over the tunnel. Paresthesias are described in the distribution of the ulnar nerve to the little and ring fingers and ulnar border of the hand. A differential diagnosis includes thoracic outlet syndrome, compression of the ulnar nerve in the Guyon canal, and nerve root compression in the neck.

Initial treatment consists of splinting the elbow in extension at night. Use of soft extension elbow pads prevents elbow flexion and direct pressure on the nerve. Failure of nonoperative measures and significant changes in electrodiagnostic studies are indications for surgical decompression. Usually, all the fibrous restraints on the ulnar nerve around the elbow are released, and the nerve is transposed anteriorly to the medial epicondyle into a subcutaneous or submuscular position. There have been preliminary reports of success with endoscopic in situ decompression of the ulnar nerve at the elbow.

Radial Nerve Compression

The radial nerve may be compressed proximally in the triangular space in the axilla (specifically involving the axillary branch), spiral groove posterior to the humerus in the arm, and lateral intermuscular septum proximal to the elbow. More distally in the forearm, the posterior interosseous nerve, the principal motor division of the radial nerve, can be compressed in the so-called radial tunnel, starting at the leading fibrous edge of the supinator (ligament of Frohse). There may be a variable degree of interosseous nerve paresis, or there may be pain radiating down the dorsoradial aspect of the forearm (called radial tunnel syndrome). Initial treatment is nonoperative with splinting, but if this fails, surgical decompression may occasionally be required.

Thoracic Outlet Compression

The thoracic outlet is a narrow space at the base of the neck bounded by the first rib medially, scalenus anterior muscle and clavicle anteriorly, and scalenus medius muscle posteriorly. All elements of the brachial plexus as well as the subclavian artery and vein pass through this narrow space and can be potentially compressed at this site. A Tinel sign can often be elicited at the supraclavicular and infraclavicular regions. A Roos test is performed by asking the patient to hold both arms overhead in a surrender position while opening and closing the fists. This reproduces symptoms within 1 minute and, if continued, the arm collapses at the side. Adson test involves palpating the radial pulse while the patient turns the chin toward the same side, inhales deeply, and holds his or her breath. The radial pulse disappears or diminishes. The costoclavicular compression test involves sustained downward pressure on the clavicle, and the symptoms are reproduced. Radiographic evaluation may reveal a cervical rib. Results of nerve conduction studies are often normal.

Thoracic outlet compression may occur in association with other peripheral sites of nerve compression, a condition termed double-crush syndrome. Treatment is primarily nonoperative, involving posture-improving exercises and avoidance of aggravating activities. If symptoms persist, especially if they are associated with vascular compression, the thoracic outlet may be surgically decompressed. This is accomplished by a transcervical or transaxillary resection of the first rib, often with release of the scalene muscles.

TUMORS

Ganglions and mucous cysts represent 60% to 70% of hand tumors, followed in frequency by inclusion cysts, warts (verrucae), giant cell

TABLE 70.6 Benign connective tissue tumors of the hand.

SOFT TISSUE TUMORS	PRESENTATION	MOST COMMON LOCATIONS	TISSUE OF ORIGIN AND APPEARANCE	TREATMENT	RADIOGRAPHIC APPEARANCE
Ganglion	Swelling, sometimes painful; DIP mucous cyst may spontaneously drain clear gelatinous fluid; 70% of hand swellings	Volar and dorsal wrist, flexor tendon sheath, dorsum of DIP joint	Synovial cyst containing thick gelatinous fluid	No treatment versus aspiration versus excision	No radiographic alterations; mucous cyst at DIP joint may have osteophytes associated with osteoarthritis
Giant cell tumor of tendon sheath	Progressive enlargement, painless, deeply adherent; potential recurrence after excision; second most common hand tumor	Any synovial site, including tendon sheath, joint, palmar plate, usually in a digit	Synovium and histiocytes; bosselated and yellow-brown color from hemosiderin pigmentation	Excision	Pressure resorption of bone
Lipoma	Painless enlarging mass, usually on volar surface of hand or finger; may reach very large size; seldom nerve compression symptoms	Volar hand and finger	Mature fat cells	Excision (shell out)	Characteristic water-clear appearance on radiograph
Inclusion cyst (implantation dermoid)	Painless, enlarging lesion, adherent to overlying dermis; more common in laborers and those subject to minor hand trauma; may become infected	Palm and fingertips	Implanted epidermis cyst containing keratinous debris	Excision of entire epithelium-lined sac	May cause pressure resorption of bone
Neurofibroma	May be localized, diffuse, or plexiform; may be associated with von Recklinghausen disease; painless enlargement, but pain arouses suspicion of malignant change	Less common on hand than elsewhere; seen more frequently on palm	Perineurial fibroblasts	Excision if noncritical nerve; biopsy if malignancy suspected; possible nerve grafting	Characteristic MRI lobulated appearance
Schwannoma	Painless small mass in a peripheral nerve that is laterally mobile; may be an incidental finding at time of carpal tunnel surgery; occasional distal dysesthesias	Median and digital nerves	Schwann cells	Microneural surgery can shell the tumor out of the nerve without leaving neurologic deficit	No changes on plain radiograph
Pyogenic granuloma	Often at site of previous trivial skin injury on the fingers; friable and bleeds easily; grows rapidly	Fingers	Granulation tissue	Small lesions can be cauterized; excise larger lesions	No radiographic changes
Glomus tumor	Very small lesions; exquisitely painful, localized tenderness, cold sensitive; patients sometimes labeled as malingering	Subungual or volar fingertip; may be multiple	Neuromyoarterial apparatus	Excision; repair nail bed if subungual	May show indentation of distal phalanx

DIP, Distal interphalangeal joint.

tumors in tendon sheaths, foreign body granulomas, lipomas, hemangiomas, and pyogenic granulomas (Table 70.6). Benign tumors account for 95% of hand neoplasms. Squamous cell carcinoma is the most frequent primary malignant neoplasm of the hand, basal cell carcinoma is rare, and melanoma is relatively uncommon in the upper extremity. Acral lentiginous melanoma (e.g., in the palm, sole, or nail bed) has a tendency for early metastasis. Primary bone tumors of the hand are generally benign; the most common are enchondromas and osteochondromas. Giant cell tumors of bone in the hand are rare, occurring usually in the distal radius. They are locally aggressive and may occasionally metastasize. Of malignant bone tumors, only 1.2% affect the hand. Although bone metastases in other parts of the body are relatively common, bones of the hand are rarely affected by metastases from other sites.[37,38]

Soft tissue sarcomas are rare, representing 1% of all malignant neoplasms of the body, excluding skin tumors. Although uncommon, certain types predominate in the hand. Epithelioid, synovial, and clear cell sarcomas are relatively rare in other sites but by comparison are more common in the hand.

Within the spectrum of benign and malignant tumors, there is a group with intermediate malignancy. Giant cell and desmoid tumors (of soft tissue) have a propensity for local recurrence after surgical excision. Their histologic patterns may belie their behavior. Juvenile aponeurotic fibroma and nodular fasciitis may appear histologically more aggressive than desmoid tumors but are self-limited. The tiny glomus tumor is uncommon but has a propensity for the fingertips and subungual regions. It may be an enigmatic cause of severe and exquisite pain at the fingertips and

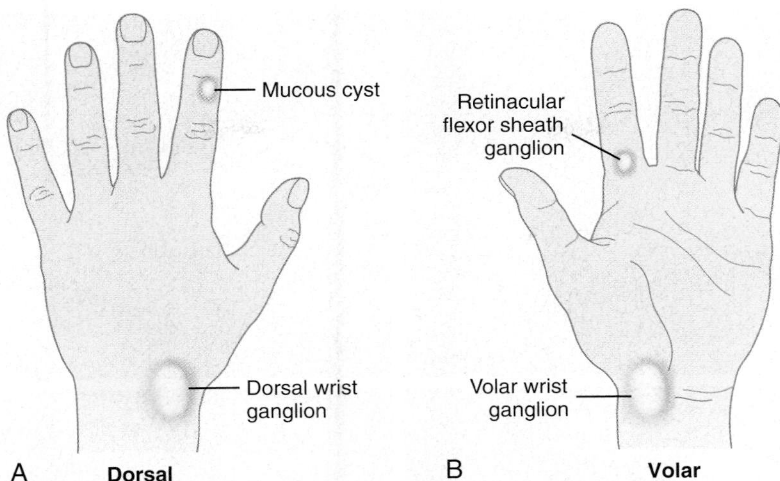

FIG. 70.45 Dorsal (A) and volar (B) aspects of the hand and wrist showing common types of ganglions, including the dorsal wrist ganglion, volar wrist ganglion, flexor sheath ganglion (volar retinacular cyst), and mucous cyst.

can be recognized by a pinpoint site of extreme local tenderness and a violaceous hue deep to the nail plate. MRI may occasionally detect these tiny lesions at the fingertip.

If a lesion is thought to be benign, excision without further workup, except perhaps for routine radiographs, is appropriate. However, if a primary malignant neoplasm of bone or soft tissue is suspected, additional studies must be undertaken before biopsy. CT may help delineate tumor boundaries. Desmoid tumors have radiographic density identical to that of muscle and are better demonstrated by MRI.

Soft Tissue Tumors

Ganglion Cysts

Ganglions are formed by an outpouching of the synovial membrane from a joint or tendon sheath. They contain thick, jelly-like, mucinous material similar in composition to synovial fluid (Fig. 70.45). Of ganglions, 60% occur on the dorsal aspect of the wrist, arising in the region of the scapholunate ligament. Other sites for ganglions in the hand are at the volar wrist, arising from one of the scaphoid articulations; at the flexor tendon sheath at the area of the A1 pulley; and at the dorsum of the DIP joint, called a mucous cyst, where they are often associated with osteoarthritis of that DIP joint. In the last location, the ganglion cyst can exert pressure on the germinal matrix of the nail bed, resulting in a deformed or grooved nail.

Ganglions are most common in women in the third decade of life. They are innocuous and can often be left alone. However, treatment may be required for cosmetic purposes or to relieve pressure effects on adjacent structures (Fig. 70.46). The dorsal wrist ganglion can sometimes be painful as a result of pressure on the posterior interosseous nerve at that location. A very small impalpable dorsal wrist ganglion can become quite painful, the so-called occult ganglion, and on occasion may best be diagnosed by MRI. Treatment of a dorsal wrist ganglion may be performed by aspiration of the mucinous substance with a large-bore needle. If this fails, the ganglion can then be surgically excised. Care must be taken to trace and to resect the pedicle of the ganglion all the way down to the joint or tendon sheath from which it arises. A volar wrist ganglion may often be closely related to the radial artery. Aspiration of volar wrist ganglions is seldom advised because of the potential risk of injury to the radial artery. At the level of the DIP joint, optimal treatment includes not only meticulous excision of the ganglion but also the removal of associated osteophytes from the joint. Arthroscopic decompression of dorsal wrist ganglions has been described.

Giant Cell Tumor

Giant cell tumor, also called pigmented villonodular synovitis, is the second most common hand tumor. It occurs in soft tissues (e.g., synovial membrane of joints, tendon sheaths) and, less commonly, in bone. This yellow-brown multilobular tumor is composed of multinucleated giant cells. Although usually benign, the tumor pushes deeply into the soft tissues of the digits and extends along tendon sheaths and around neurovascular structures. It is frequently asymptomatic and is often larger than suspected clinically. Radiologic notching of bone may be evident in larger, soft tissue giant cell tumors. Complete surgical excision is the treatment of choice. Failure to discern and to remove each lobule substantially increases the reported local recurrence rate of almost 10%. Synovectomy of the joint of origin may be necessary (Fig. 70.47).

Epidermal Inclusion Cysts

Epidermal inclusion cysts, also called implantation dermoids, frequently occur after trauma as keratin-producing epidermal cells become lodged in the subcutaneous tissues (Fig. 70.47). The resulting cystic mass contains a thick toothpaste-like material. They occur more commonly in men, especially in manual laborers, and most frequently involve the palm of the hand and fingertips. They may also occur in previous surgical scars. Treatment is surgical excision, and recurrence is rare.

Lipoma

Lipomas are small, benign, soft, fluctuant, fatty tumors (Fig. 70.48). In the hand, they usually occur on the thenar eminence. Although generally painless, they may enlarge significantly, insinuating into deep palmar spaces and causing pain by compression on adjacent nerves. Intracarpal lipoma is a rarer cause of carpal tunnel syndrome. Resection of symptomatic lipomas is curative, although 1% to 2% may recur.

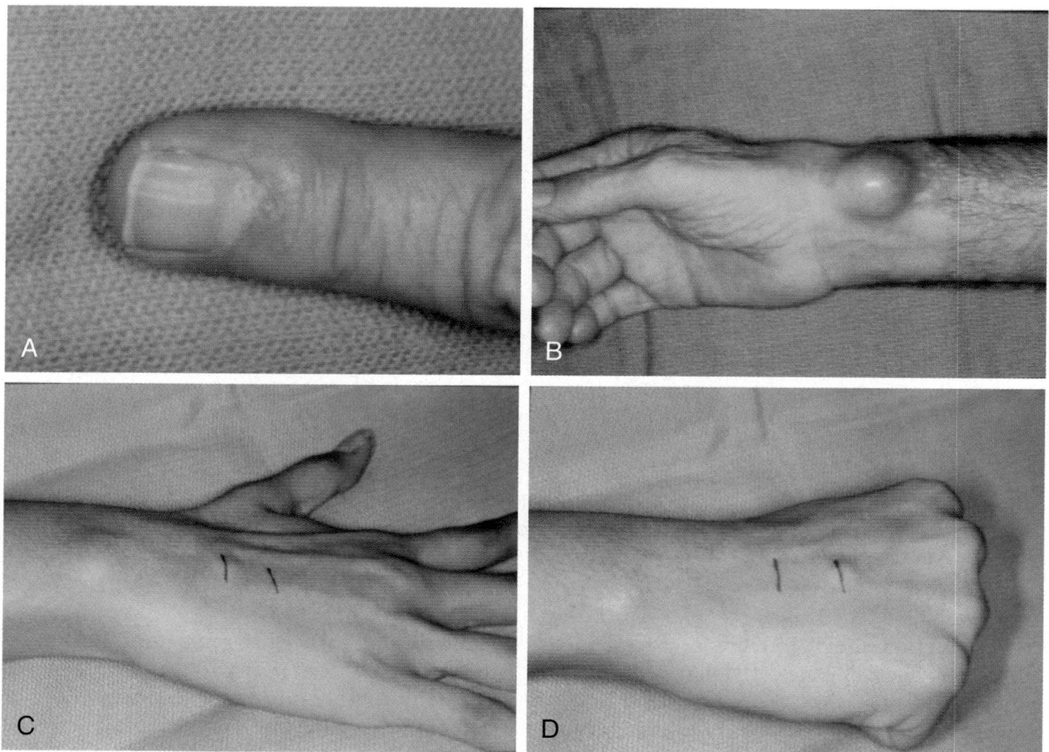

FIG. 70.46 Ganglions in the hand. (A) Ganglion associated with osteoarthritis of the distal interphalangeal joint (mucous cyst), causing longitudinal linear groove in the nail plate from pressure on the germinal matrix. (B) Volar wrist ganglion on the radial side of the flexor carpi radialis tendon is closely related to the radial artery and should not be aspirated. (C) Ganglion arising from the extensor digitorum communis tendon of the ring finger located at the level of the proximal skin marking with fingers extended. (D) Movement of ganglion 2 cm to the level of the more distal skin marking when the fist is clenched. Distal movement of the swelling with the gliding extensor tendon confirms its attachment to the tendon.

Pyogenic Granuloma

Pyogenic granuloma is a misnomer for an exuberant outburst of highly vascular granulation tissue at the site of previous relatively trivial trauma. These lesions are friable, bleed easily, and may grow rapidly. They respond to curettage or simple excision. They usually occur on the fingertips. Histologic confirmation of the diagnosis is necessary because of occasional confusion with aggressive malignant lesions, such as ulcerated, amelanotic, malignant melanomas.

Verruca Vulgaris

Verrucae vulgaris are common contagious warts associated with human papillomavirus type 1. They occur usually as hyperkeratotic filiform lesions on the digits or about the nail bed. The most effective topical treatments are salicylates, liquid nitrogen cryotherapy, and especially curettage. Recalcitrant lesions respond to oral cimetidine given for 6 to 8 weeks and to imiquimod, an immunomodulator that increases interferon production. Their incidence, like that of squamous cell carcinomas, is increased in immunocompromised patients, such as in those after transplantation. Recurrence is relatively common.[39]

Seborrheic Keratoses

Seborrheic keratoses are benign, hyperkeratotic, scaly lesions. They are frequently pigmented and common on the dorsum of the hand in older adults. Occasional confusion occurs with pigmented basal cell carcinomas. When necessary, these superficial scaly lesions are best treated by shave excision, and sutures are unnecessary. Rapid reepithelialization occurs.

Keratoacanthoma

Keratoacanthoma occurs on exposed body parts such as the dorsum of the hand. It grows rapidly during approximately 3 weeks into a nodule with a central umbilicated keratotic plug, often followed by spontaneous resolution in many weeks or months. The resulting scar is often worse than if the lesion had been excised initially. There may be diagnostic uncertainty in regard to well-differentiated squamous cell carcinomas. Hence, most authors recommend surgical excision.

Dermatofibroma

A dermatofibroma arises from fibrous dermal tissue as a firm erythematous plaque, sometimes having central umbilication. It is often adherent to the overlying epidermis. Surgery is required primarily for diagnosis.

Vascular Malformations and Hemangiomas

Hemangiomas are hamartomas that are rarely visible at birth and are usually noticed weeks to months later. Rapid proliferation occurs in the first year of life. On histologic evaluation, proliferation of endothelial cells with increased mitotic activity is seen in conjunction with pericytes and dendritic and mast cells. Hemangiomas occur 10 times more commonly than vascular malformations, and approximately 70% involute by the age of 7 years, leaving a

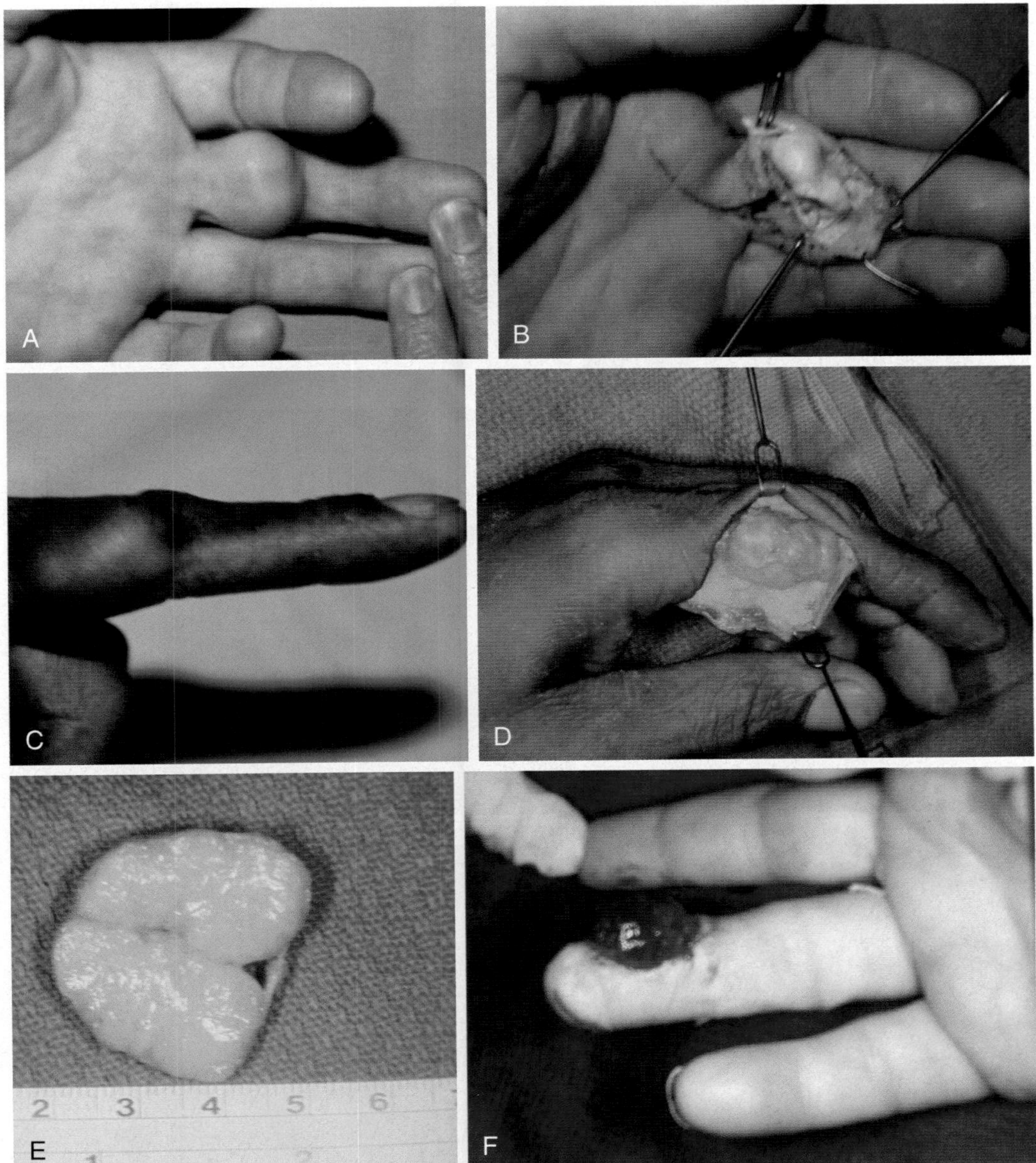

FIG. 70.47 Soft tissue tumors of the hand. (A) Traumatically induced inclusion cyst on the palmar aspect of the middle finger in a manual worker. (B) Intraoperative photograph demonstrates cyst filled with toothpaste-like gel derived from keratin. (C) Firm, progressively enlarging swelling on the radial side of the left index finger. (D) Firm, lobulated, yellow-brown giant cell tumor insinuating onto the dorsal and volar aspects of the finger is noted intraoperatively. (E) Giant cell tumor is the most common solid soft tissue tumor encountered in the hand. (F) Fleshy friable pyogenic granuloma bleeds easily on contact.

fibrofatty scar with redundant skin. Excision is seldom required and, after involution, is usually cosmetic. On occasion, oral or injectable steroids may be necessary to control rapidly proliferating lesions that cause pain or interfere with function. Propranolol, which reduces basic fibroblast growth factor and vascular endothelial growth factor expression, is sometimes added in conjunction with steroids for problematic hemangiomas.[40]

By contrast, vascular malformations show normal endothelial growth characteristics and normal mast cell counts. They are often noted at birth, and growth is usually commensurate with the child for low-flow lesions. They do not undergo spontaneous involution.

Vascular malformations are subclassified into low-flow lesions; capillary, venous, and lymphatic lesions predominate. Arterial and arteriovenous fistulas predominate in high-flow lesions, and accelerated growth may occur relative to the patient. Pressure effects, ulceration, bleeding, and high-output cardiac failure can occur in severe cases. Enlarging lesions hinder hand function. Compression garments can provide symptomatic relief in some cases. Pain is often caused by vascular engorgement, phlebitis, or intralesional coagulation. D-dimer levels may be elevated, and some patients obtain relief from aspirin. Combined surgical excision[41] and radiologic embolization[42] are most effective in preventing recurrence caused by dilation of collateral vascular channels after simple excision.

Lymphaticovenous malformations may also be associated with generalized hypertrophy of an extremity. Vascular malformations and isolated macrodactyly are seen in Klippel-Trénaunay syndrome.

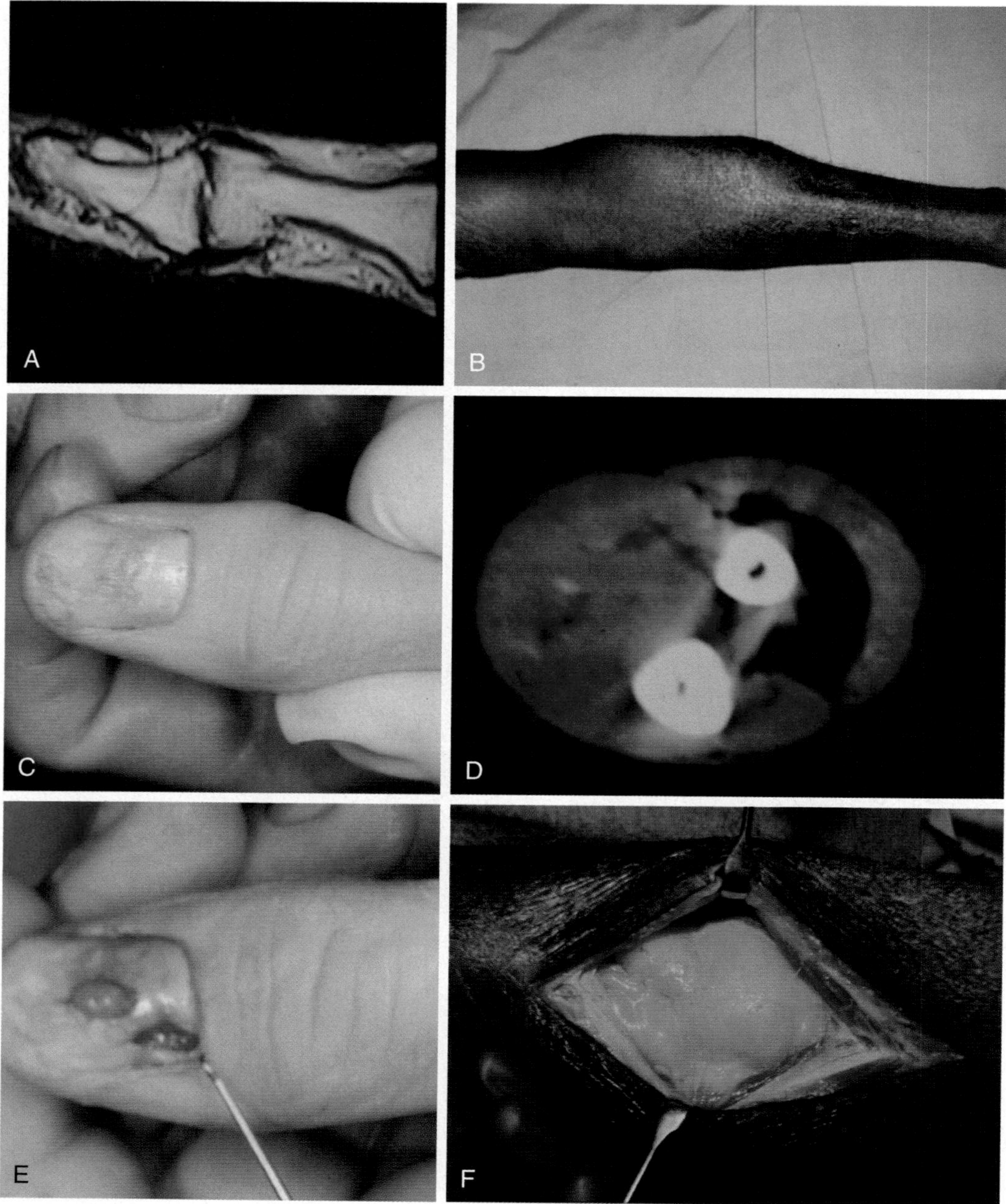

FIG. 70.48 Soft tissue tumors of the hand. (A) Patient presenting with pain in tip of thumb, exacerbated in cold weather. Exquisite pain on palpation of the thumb nail plate is typical of a subungual glomus tumor that can be demonstrated by magnetic resonance imaging. (B) Occult subungual glomus tumor may be difficult to appreciate, even after removal of the nail plate, but it can often be identified by a surface bulge of the nail bed. (C) Excised glomus tumor sitting on nail bed. A nail bed defect requires repair with fine absorbable sutures. (D) Man with swelling of left dorsoradial forearm and weakness of finger and thumb extension. (E) MRI reveals a dorsal forearm mass compressing the posterior interosseous nerve. (F) Dorsal approach over the mass reveals intramuscular benign lipoma when extensor muscles are split.

Malignant Skin Tumors

Basal Cell Carcinoma

Basal cell carcinoma is rare on the hand and is generally located on the dorsum. It is usually an ulcer with raised pearly edges. Treatment consists of excision with a margin of normal adjacent tissue. Nail bed lesions can be mistaken for paronychial infection, and amputation at the DIP joint may be required.

Squamous Cell Carcinoma

Squamous cell carcinoma may arise de novo from ultraviolet light exposure because of occupation or climate, usually on the sun-exposed dorsum of the hand. Approximately 16% of actinic keratoses may progress to squamous cell carcinoma. Arsenical keratoses may develop secondary to exposure to inorganic arsenic compounds but have a predilection for the palm.

TABLE 70.7 **Bone tumors of the hand.**

TUMOR	PRESENTATION	MOST COMMON LOCATIONS	TISSUE OF ORIGIN AND APPEARANCE	TREATMENT	RADIOGRAPHIC APPEARANCE
Enchondroma	Often incidental finding on routine hand radiograph; presents as pain secondary to pathologic fracture; most common bone tumor of hand	Proximal and middle phalanges and metacarpals	Fragments of cartilage nests; multiple (Ollier disease); when associated with hemangiomas (Maffucci syndrome), may undergo malignant change	Curettage, filling of defect with cancellous bone if structural bone integrity is compromised	Lesion eccentric in bone shaft with calcific stippling
Osteochondroma	Benign bone prominence (capped with cartilage); rare in hand; may cause angular growth and interfere with joint motion	Fingers and wrist; growth stops after skeletal maturity reached	Aberrant focus of cartilage; multiple osteochondromatosis is autosomal dominant; malignant change may occur	Surgery may be necessary, generally after epiphyseal closure	Exostosis, often at base of proximal phalanx; often shortening of parent bone
Osteoid osteoma	Aching pain, greatest at night, sometimes responding specifically to aspirin; patient may be labeled as malingerer	Phalanges, metacarpals, carpals	Nidus composed of loose fibrovascular connective tissue between bars of osteoid and bone trabeculae	Surgical excision to include the nidus	Very small lesion; some not seen on plain radiographs and require CT scan; cortical sclerosis surrounding a radiolucent area of nidus
Giant cell tumor of bone	Expansile bone swelling at distal radius or in phalanx	Distal radius most common site	May be locally aggressive and even metastasize	Curettage for low-grade lesions, but en bloc resection for high-grade lesions; do not irradiate because it could induce sarcomatous change	Expansile soap bubble lesion in bone; high-grade lesions break through cortex

Bowen disease is an intraepidermal squamous cell carcinoma (carcinoma in situ). It is a plaquelike lesion with crusting. Complete surgical excision with a margin of normal tissue is curative. When the nail matrix is involved, amputation at the DIP joint may be necessary.

For squamous cell carcinoma lesions smaller than 2.5 cm in diameter, wide excision with approximately a 6-mm clear margin is recommended. However, for larger lesions, more radical excision may be required, which may even include ray or segmental amputation for deeply adherent and invasive lesions. Mohs micrographic surgery and three-dimensional histologic reconstruction with a pathologist at the time of radical resection help ensure complete excision. Routine prophylactic lymphadenectomy is not beneficial. However, lymphadenectomy may be advised for recurrent tumors, even though lymph nodes may not be clinically palpable. Malignant degeneration may occur in cicatricial tissue and chronic ulcers (e.g., Marjolin ulcer) and, in particular, in burn scars. Prognosis tends to be poorer.[43]

Malignant Melanomas

Melanoma of the hand is cutaneous or subungual. There is an almost equal distribution of cases between the two types.[44] Frequently, there is a delay in treatment, particularly with subungual melanomas. Suspicious lesions should be biopsied.

Any subungual pigmented lesions should generally be biopsied. Under tourniquet control and with loupe magnification, the nail plate is atraumatically removed, and a longitudinal, elliptical, full-thickness excision of the lesion is performed. Careful nail bed repair is done after biopsy by the advancement of adjacent tissues and using fine absorbable sutures. The nail plate is then reapplied to act as a splint.

Benign melanocytic hyperplasia, without evidence of atypia, is completely treated by this form of biopsy. If there is any evidence of melanocytic atypia, absolute confirmation of complete excision is required. In the absence of a clear margin or with recurrence of such a lesion, total nail bed excision and reconstruction with a full-thickness skin graft are required. Melanoma in situ is similarly treated. Invasive melanoma of the nail bed is treated by amputation at the next most proximal joint. Acral lentiginous melanoma of the palm may sometimes be mistaken for a wart, which may also delay diagnosis. These tumors are aggressively treated with wide local excision and potential sentinel node biopsy, as they might be treated anywhere else on the body.

Bone Tumors

Osteoid Osteoma

This may occur in the hand and classically causes pain that is worse at night and unrelated to use or motion of the hand (Table 70.7). Osteoid osteomas produce prostaglandins; symptoms are relieved by nonsteroidal antiinflammatory drugs (NSAIDs). On radiologic examination, a round lucent tumor with sclerotic edges is seen (Fig. 70.49A). Conservative treatment with NSAIDs may be considered, but definitive treatment is surgical.

Aneurysmal Bone Cyst

This is an expansile osteolytic bone lesion with a thin wall. It is usually derived from a preexisting bone tumor, usually a giant cell tumor (20%–40% of cases). Of these, 25% occur in the upper extremity, causing pain that peaks during 2 to 3 months. A bone swelling may be detectable, with increased overlying skin temperature.

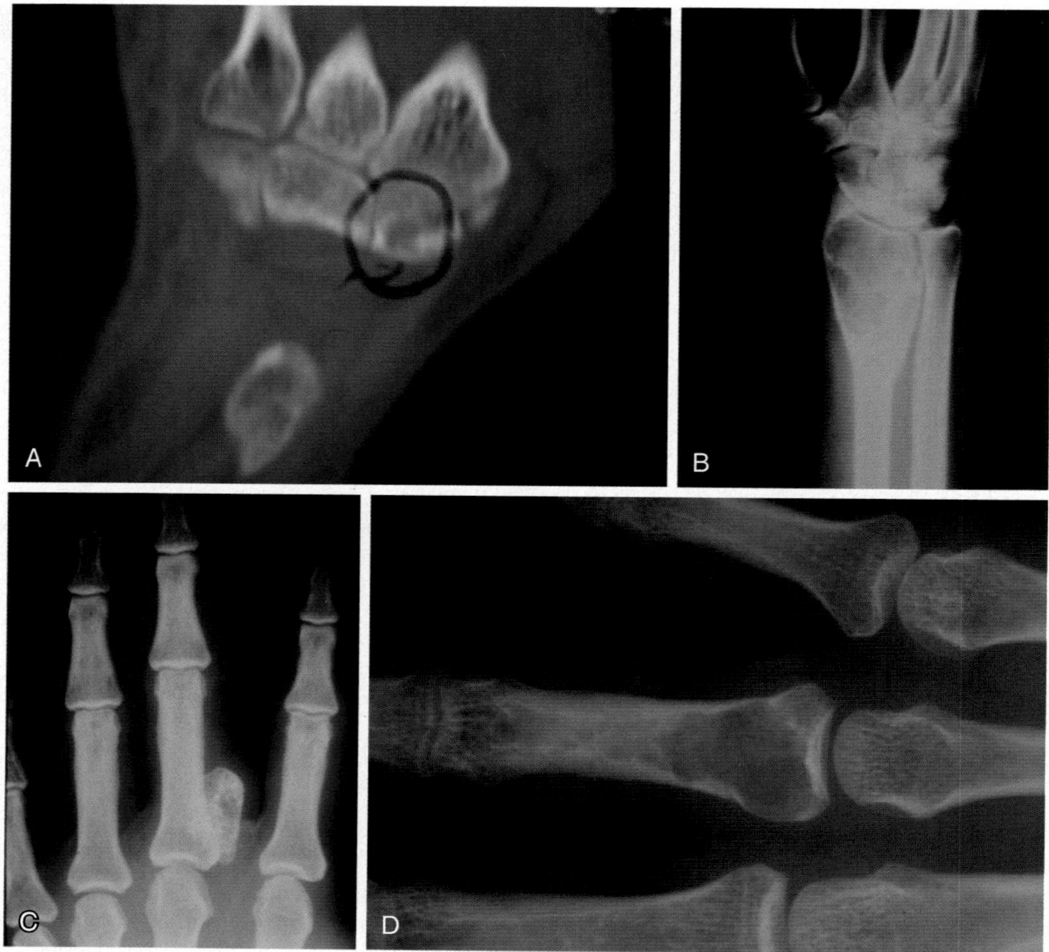

FIG. 70.49 Plain radiographs of the upper extremity. (A) Osteoid osteoma of carpus. (B) Soap bubble appearance of giant cell tumor expanding the metaphysis of the distal radius. (C) Osteochondroma of proximal phalanx of middle (long) finger. (D) Patient with finger pain after trivial injury. This is a pathologic fracture of the base of the proximal phalanx through an enchondroma that has replaced most of proximal metaphysis and medulla.

Enchondroma

Enchondromas usually occur in the hand and are the most common bone tumor of the hand. Peak incidence is in the second decade, with equal gender distribution. They are frequently asymptomatic and noted incidentally as lytic lesions on plain radiology. Pain, bone swelling, or pathologic fracture may occur as these cartilaginous intraosseous cysts compromise bone structural integrity (Fig. 70.49D). Treatment is by curettage and bone grafting of the osseous defect. Multiple enchondromatosis occurs in Ollier disease and is associated with angiomas in Maffucci syndrome.

Primary Bone Sarcomas

These malignant tumors are rare in the hand.

Secondary (Metastatic) Bone Tumors

Metastatic tumors, even those with a tendency to metastasize to bone, usually occur in the axial skeleton and long bones. They are very rare in the hand.

CONGENITAL ANOMALIES

The causes of congenital hand anomalies may be genetic, teratogenic, or idiopathic and may also have a syndromic association with anomalies elsewhere in the body. Knowledge of these associations is important because the more life-threatening associated problems frequently need to be treated first, before the hand and upper extremity reconstruction can be performed. Such an association is found in a constellation of problems that occur in the VACTERL association of congenital defects (vertebral anomalies, anal atresia, cardiac abnormalities, tracheoesophageal fistula, renal agenesis, and limb anomalies). A number of factors must be considered in optimizing the timing of each surgical procedure to the upper extremity, including the psychosocial development of the child, presence of other illnesses, size of the structures to be operated on, and normal growth and development of the hand. Modern technological advances have allowed us to operate on smaller structures; the timing of the procedure can now be guided by knowledge of the anatomy and development of the growing hand. Optimal function is the primary goal of surgery. Principles of treatment of congenital hand anomalies recognize that an infant's immunity to infection develops over time, early surgery prevents the emotional scarring associated with a child's awareness of the deformity, and some congenital problems may not be apparent in the neonate. The hand surgeon must work closely with the pediatrician to identify general conditions that may affect the child's health. Some congenital anomalies of the extremities, especially those with the radial ray, may be associated with bone marrow failure (Fanconi syndrome) or heart defects that may not be immediately apparent in the neonate. Children with congenital anomalies will attempt to keep up with their peers and often develop successful hand substitution techniques. However, once a child experiences the cruel ridicule of playmates or the unintentional but sometimes overly solicitous supervision of a teacher, his or her deformity becomes important. In general, plans for surgical reconstruction are designed to be completed by school age, so that the child may adapt to and fully use the reconstructed limb.[45]

The rationale for early surgery includes the avoidance of deformity and malfunction and optimal use of infantile tissue plasticity. Because hand length almost doubles during the first 2 years of life, a digit tethered to another digit that fails to grow can produce a major deformity during the early growth spurt. For example, with separation of syndactyly that involves the border digits of the hand, because of adjacent tethering to a digit of unequal length, surgical separation of the syndactyly is required at an early age, as early as 6 months, to avoid secondary angular deformity of the digits.

In rare circumstances, urgent treatment in the neonate is required. The distal lymphedema of a severe constriction band syndrome may be so marked as to inhibit function totally or even to threaten distal viability. This may require urgent release. The unusual clinical entity of aplasia cutis may result in exposure of vital structures, requiring urgent soft tissue coverage, even in the neonatal period.

Early operation, although not urgent, may be required not only because of the rapid growth that occurs in the first 2 years of life but also because of functional consequences. Surgery at a young age is considered mandatory in children with malformations in which hand function may be altered by surgery or in those who are at risk for development of certain grasping habits that would have to be unlearned after corrective surgery. An older child, 12 to 14 years of age, has developed grasp patterns that would have to be altered by prolonged periods of physical therapy after corrective surgery.[45]

The ability to place the upper limbs in space (a cortical function) and development of a strong grasp are established by 1 year of age, as are grasp and pinch maneuvers between the thumb and fingers. Accuracy of prehension and refinement of coordination continue until 3 years of age. Surgery must be performed early to allow the affected parts to develop differently when the function of the parts of the hand is altered by transposition (e.g., pollicization of an index finger for thumb aplasia). Duplicated thumb correction is carried out before 1 year of age, well in advance of the development of integrated thumb grasp patterns.

Finally, the physical ability of infant bone and soft tissues to adapt to change produced by surgery is also a key factor in deciding when to operate. In the early pollicization of the index finger, the first dorsal interosseous muscle hypertrophies to form a thenar eminence and the first metacarpal (formerly known as the proximal phalanx of the index finger) broadens. If centralization of the wrist for radial dysplasia (formerly known as radial club hand) has been undertaken early, the head of the ulna broadens to resemble the distal end of the radius.

Thus, a number of issues are taken into consideration when deciding on the optimum time for surgical reconstruction of congenital hand and upper extremity anomalies. The more common hand anomalies include syndactyly, polydactyly, constriction band syndrome, and absent or hypoplastic thumb.

Syndactyly results from the failure of programmed cell death (apoptosis) between the individual finger rays. Consequently, there is a resulting fusion of adjacent digits. It can involve part or all of the length of the digits (incomplete or complete) and may be limited to skin and soft tissue only (simple syndactyly) or can also involve skeletal fusion (complex syndactyly). Apert syndrome also involves craniofacial anomalies and is a severe form of bilaterally symmetrical complex syndactyly. Surgical treatment involves digit separation using a local flap to reconstruct the depths of the commissure between the fingers and release of the finger borders with zigzag incisions and the use of full-thickness skin grafts (Fig. 70.50A).

Polydactyly is the presence of extranumerary digits on the hand. Preaxial (radial) polydactyly involves the thumb. It is not as common as postaxial (ulnar) polydactyly, which is the most frequent congenital hand anomaly in African Americans. Polydactyly can be as simple as the presence of a skin tag–like structure or may have a complex arrangement of shared vessels, nerves, and bones. Thumb polydactyly is not merely a duplication but a splitting of a single digit, with variable degrees of development in each of the separate parts. It is typically classified into seven subtypes by the Wassel classification, which is based on the specific duplication, progressing from distal to proximal in which the odd numbers are at distal and proximal phalanx and metacarpal, and even numbers are at IP, MP and CMC joints respectively. Type IV is the most common type, with total duplication of proximal and distal phalanges and a shared MP joint. Type VII refers to associated triphalangia with a duplication. Reconstructive goals include stabilization without sacrificing mobility, proper alignment of joints along the longitudinal axis of the thumb, balanced motor units, and a cosmetically acceptable nail plate (Fig. 70.50B and C).

The Blauth classification categorizes thumb hypoplasia from type I, which represents minor hypoplasia, to type V, which is a total thumb absence. Surgical correction ranges from reconstruction of the existing hypoplastic thumb to pollicization (creating a thumb from the index finger) for complete absence or for the more severe types of hypoplasia (Fig. 70.51).

Clinodactyly is a curving of the digits in a radial or ulnar direction. It is common, particularly involving the little finger in many individuals, but a curvature of more than 10 degrees is considered abnormal. The distal phalanx is usually affected and a delta phalanx may be associated. A delta phalanx occurs when the epiphysis forms a C shape around the metaphyseal core in the middle phalanx. Most patients present with little or no functional or cosmetic deformity, and operative intervention is seldom required. If there is a functionally impairing deviation of the finger, corrective osteotomy can be done.

Camptodactyly is a congenital flexion deformity of digits. It usually occurs in the little finger PIP joint. The exact cause is unclear, but it has been attributed to a variety of different structures around the PIP joint, including a skin pterygium, collateral ligaments, volar plate, flexor tendon, abnormal insertions of lumbrical or interosseous muscles, and size and shape of the head of the proximal phalanx. Treatment is generally nonoperative and may involve serial splinting. If no improvement occurs and the flexion deformity is sufficient to cause a functional problem, surgical intervention may be required; this includes correction of the deformity with Z-plasty and possibly grafts. One author has reported that all his patients who had reconstructive surgery on one hand did not ask for corrective surgery on the opposite affected hand.

Constriction band syndrome is secondary to intrauterine amniotic bands (Fig. 70.50D). These can act like tourniquets and

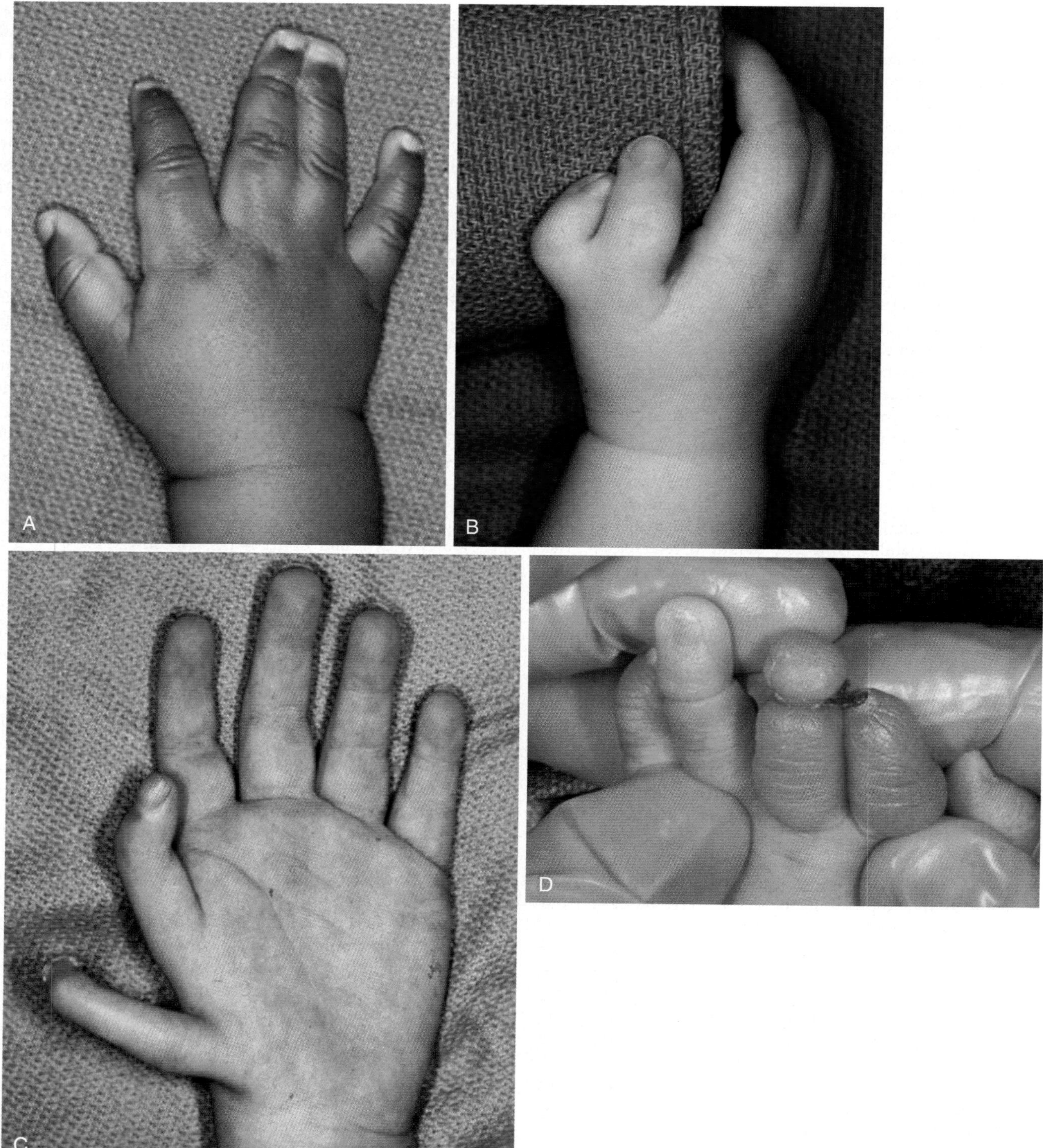

FIG. 70.50 Congenital hand anomalies include syndactyly (A), Wassel type IV thumb polydactyly (B), Wassel type VI polydactyly (C), and constriction band (D).

threaten the viability of digits and even limbs, resulting in congenital amputation. Infants may suffer from a similar problem from the external ligature effect of cotton strands coming off protective booties and even from a human hair, termed the hair-thread tourniquet syndrome.

OSTEOARTHRITIS AND RHEUMATOID ARTHRITIS

Osteoarthritis may be primary or posttraumatic (secondary). Primary osteoarthritis is a degenerative joint disease occurring in later life. An injury that leaves articular surfaces of a joint incongruous can precipitate secondary osteoarthritis. Osteoarthritis begins

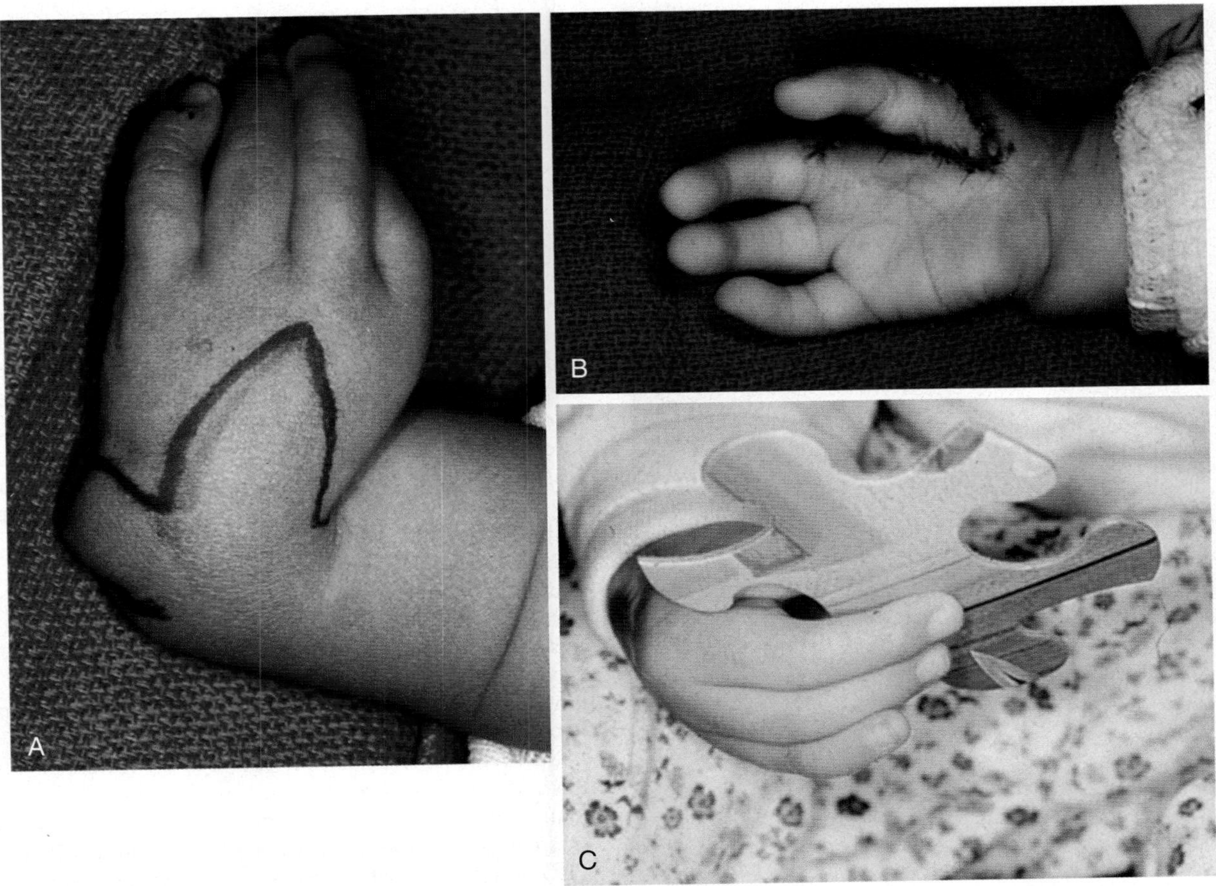

FIG. 70.51 (A) Patient with radial dysplasia and absent thumb. (B) After centralization of the wrist on the distal ulna, pollicization of the index finger is performed. (C) Natural prehension has been restored to this three-finger hand with a reconstructed wrist and thumb.

with biochemical alteration of the water content of articular cartilage. The cartilage weakens and develops cracks, called fibrillation. Progressive erosion and thinning of the cartilage result, and the subchondral bone becomes sclerotic, termed eburnation. New bone forms around the edges of the articular cartilage, and these outcroppings are called osteophytes (Fig. 70.52).

The joints usually affected in the hand are the DIP and PIP joints of the fingers and carpometacarpal joint at the base of the thumb. Osteophytes at the DIP joint are called Heberden nodes, and those at the PIP joint are known as Bouchard nodes. The involved joints may be painful, stiff, deformed, or subluxated. Radiographs reveal narrowing of the joint space, sclerosis of subchondral bone, and presence of osteophytes.

Initial treatment may be symptomatic and may include splinting and even local corticosteroid injections. NSAIDs may be helpful, and chondroprotective medications such as glucosamine and chondroitin sulfate can reduce symptoms. In advanced cases, the DIP joints respond best to arthrodesis. The PIP joints may be surgically treated by replacement arthroplasty or by arthrodesis (Fig. 70.53). The thumb carpometacarpal joint may be treated by arthrodesis, which is favored particularly for the young patient who might have posttraumatic arthritis after, for example, an improperly treated Bennett or Orlando fracture. In an older patient with primary osteoarthritis at the thumb base, excision of the trapezium followed by tendon suspension (interposition) arthroplasty may be preferred. This uses local tendons for construction of a sling arthroplasty, with interposition of tendon material.

Rheumatoid arthritis is an autoimmune process whereby destruction of the musculoskeletal system may occur. Synovial inflammation results in pain, joint destruction, tendon ruptures, and characteristic deformities. Some of the more common deformities associated with rheumatoid arthritis include a swan neck deformity (hyperextension of the PIP joint with concurrent flexion at the DIP joint), boutonnière deformity (flexion at the PIP joint, with concurrent hyperextension at the DIP joint), joint subluxation, radial deviation of the wrist, and ulnar deviation and flexion of the fingers (Fig. 70.54). Rheumatoid arthritis is primarily a medical illness for which a number of medications are currently available. Thus, there must be excellent lines of communication between the rheumatologist and surgeon. NSAIDs as well as disease-modifying antirheumatoid drugs are used. Rheumatoid arthritis is a progressive disorder, and ongoing slow destruction may be anticipated despite surgery (Fig. 70.55). Some of the more common surgical procedures include joint synovectomy, tenosynovectomy, tendon transfers, joint replacements (especially at the MP and PIP joints), and arthrodesis (more commonly at the wrist and thumb MP joint).[46]

CONTRACTURES

Volkmann ischemic contracture develops as a result of myofascial contractures in response to prolonged ischemia. This most

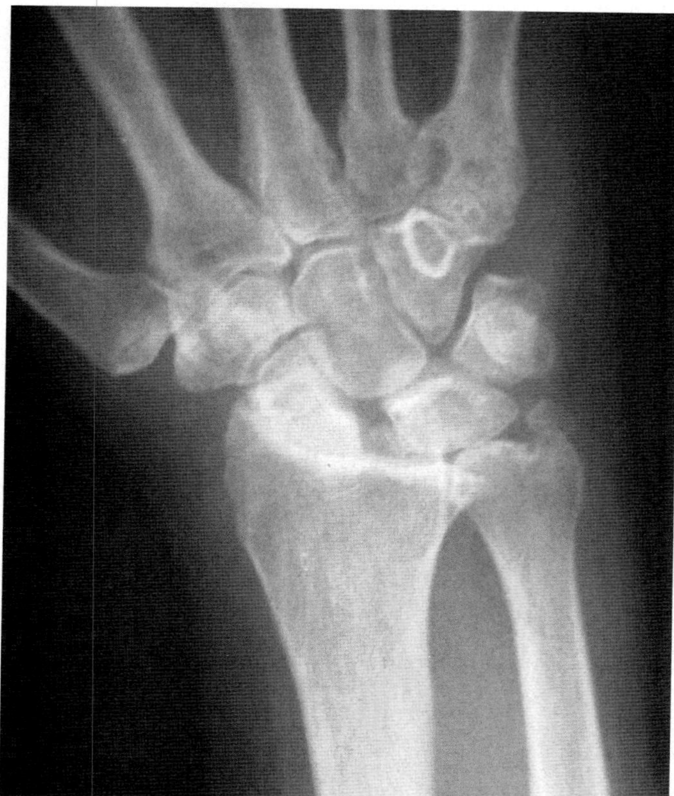

FIG. 70.52 Radiograph of a hand with a scapholunate advanced collapse wrist showing posttraumatic osteoarthritis at the radioscaphoid junction. This is many years after a wrist sprain in which the scapholunate ligament was torn; a wide scapholunate gap is visible on the radiograph.

common contracture results from untreated compartment syndrome of the forearm and hand. Muscle necrosis occurs, and the muscles become replaced by fibrous scar tissue. The FDP and FPL muscles are usually affected, being in the deepest forearm volar compartment, and digits are characteristically flexed, with passive extension of the wrist worsening the flexion deformity of the digits. Intrinsic contractures can occur in the hand; these can be investigated using the Bunnell test in which passive extension of the MP joint makes passive flexion of the PIP joint more difficult.

In the milder forms of Volkmann ischemic contracture, serial splinting and passive stretching exercises may resolve the problem. In more severe contractures, Z-type lengthening of tendons may be required. A flexor pronator muscle slide—subperiosteal elevation of the common flexor origin from the medial epicondyle of the humerus and from the ulna—allows the muscles to slide distally until the contracture is corrected. In the most severe form, all the muscles of the volar forearm may be affected, requiring tendon transfers, even microvascular functional muscle transfers to provide some functional return.

Posttraumatic contractures are the most common type of contracture. These can be prevented by appropriate treatment of the primary injury, especially with attention to detail in how the hand and upper extremity are splinted and immobilized. Once contractures have developed, if they are mild, they may be able to be stretched out by exercises and hand therapy. If these contractures are severe and functionally deforming, surgical release of joint contractures and release of tendon adhesions may be required.

Dupuytren contracture is a disease process of contracting collagen affecting the palmar fascia; it can also affect the dorsum of the fingers (knuckle pads), soles of the feet, and penis (Peyronie disease). It is thought to be a hereditary Mendelian dominant disorder and is bilateral in 65% of cases. It is six times more frequent in males and predominantly involves the ring and little fingers (Fig. 70.56).

The process of Dupuytren contracture occurs in the normal bands of collagen tissue that form the palmar fascia, natatory ligaments, and digital sheaths. Nodules containing myofibroblasts and immature collagen (type III) develop in these tissues or in the dermis. The nodules progressively increase in size, leading to thickened contractures and shortened fascial bands that develop into cords extending up the digits. Treatment is surgical excision; it is indicated in MP contractures of 30 degrees or more, when the patient fails the so-called tabletop test and cannot place the palm of the hand flat on a surface, and whenever there is a PIP joint contracture. Careful surgical technique is necessary to avoid complications such as skin necrosis, hematoma, and digital nerve injuries. Collagenase injections using enzyme derived from *Clostridium histolyticum* have been attempted and have shown some promise in the treatment of Dupuytren contracture. However, long-term follow-up in patients who had these injections is still necessary.[47,48]

Percutaneous needle fasciotomy is also a reasonable option for treatment of Dupuytren disease and seems to be effective for MP joint contractures but less effective for the PIP joint. An extension external fixation torque device may also preliminarily reverse the PIP contracture before excision of the diseased tissue.[49]

FUTURE DIRECTIONS IN HAND SURGERY

Hand surgery is a very dynamic specialty and continually advancing with many recent technological developments. Because it is a regional specialty, it embraces advances in microvascular and microneural surgery, trauma, transplantation, minimally invasive surgery, prosthetics, and tissue engineering.

Methods of treatment of forearm amputation remain an ongoing debate between transplantation and prosthetic limbs. Dr. Joseph Murry, a plastic surgeon, performed the first successful kidney transplant in 1954.[50] Hand transplantation has been refined by plastic hand surgeons over the past 30 years and as of 2014 there have been 107 documented successful hand transplants around the world.[51] Functional outcomes must be balanced against the lifetime risks of immunosuppression.[52]

In contrast, methods of prosthetic bone fixation by osteointegration, intuitive prosthetics, and miniaturization have led to major advances. In the past, as many as 20% of unilateral upper extremity amputees abandon their prosthetics for a variety of reasons. Three-dimensional printing is of great utility in providing low cost prosthetics to children who require constant refitting of prosthetics as they grow.[53]

Newer technologies are utilizing implanted neural interfaces to activate peripheral sensory nerves. Another exciting development is the use of targeted muscle reinnervation to allow for more intuitive and intricate hand movements. Transected nerves from the amputation are attached to individual motor nerves in the muscle that in turn transmits the myoelectric impulses to the various prosthetic functional movements. The prosthetic limb can 'sense'

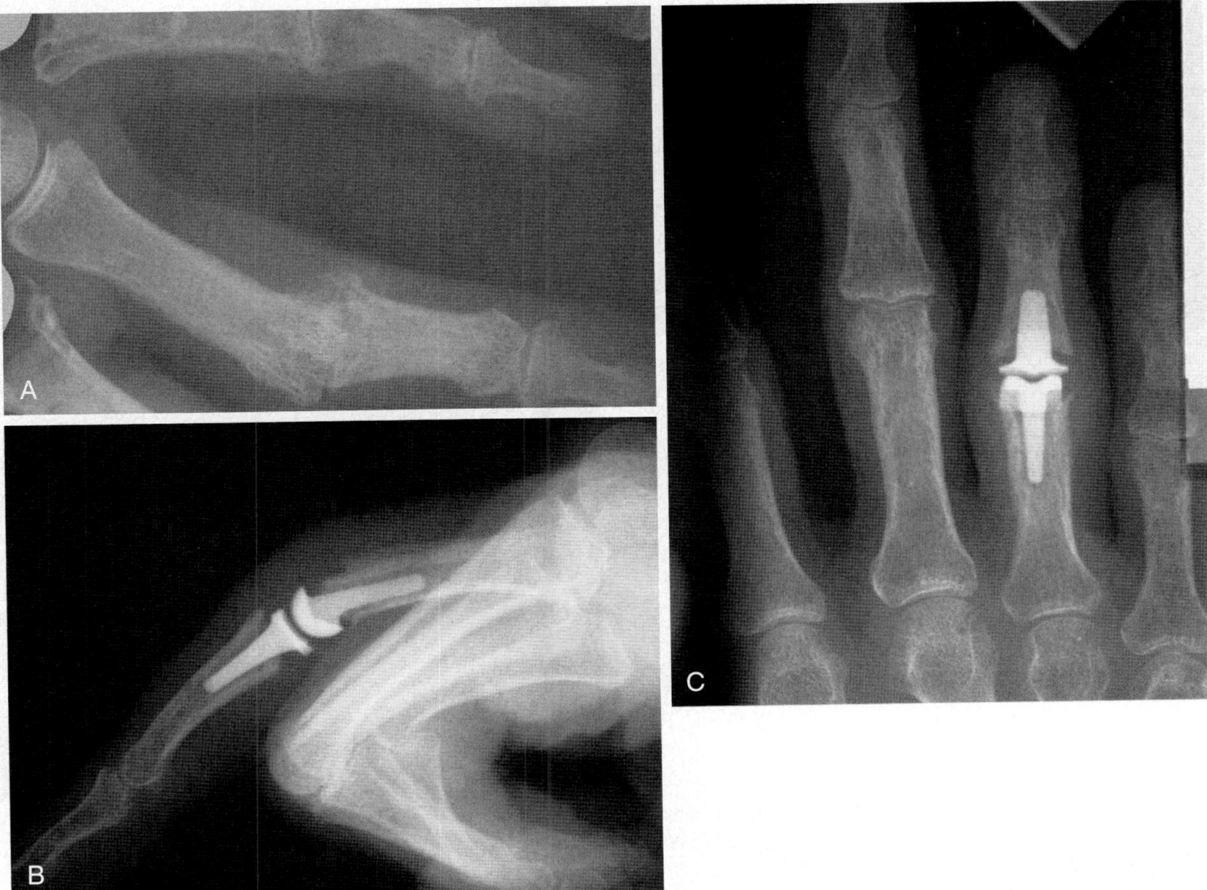

FIG. 70.53 (A) Patient with painful and unstable proximal interphalangeal joint from osteoarthritis. (B and C) Reconstruction is performed by implant arthroplasty. An advantage over arthrodesis is that motion is retained, although there remains the potential for future recurrent joint instability and wear of the artificial joint.

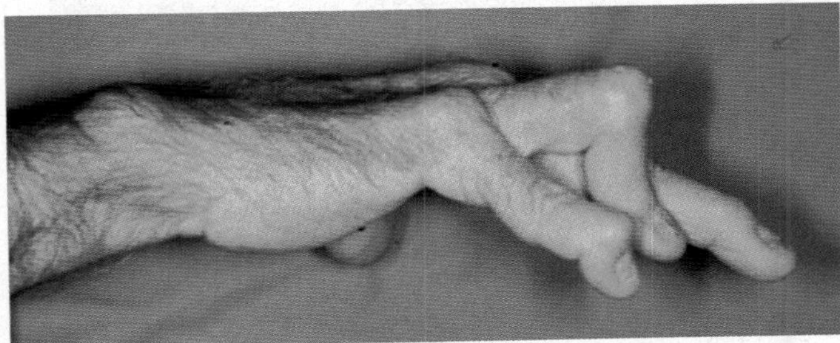

FIG. 70.54 Patient with inflammatory arthritis has both boutonnière deformity and swan neck deformity on the same hand.

the intended movements in the reinnervated muscles, and move in the way that the patient intends it to move. An outreach of this research is also that targeted muscle reinnervation helps successfully treat phantom and neuroma pain.[54] Thus, the debate between prosthetics and transplantation will closely mirror the race between prosthetic technology and immunosuppression.

There has also been great interest in the development of ways to bridge nerve gaps in traumatic and oncologic reconstruction. The "gold standard" has been to use an autologous nerve graft, but this option has a donor morbidity and there is a limited supply available (generally sural nerve). Treated cadaveric nerve allografts remove the immunogenicity and may enable nerve reconstruction without donor morbidity. To date, this has been used successfully for short nerve gaps in major upper extremity nerves.[55]

Up to this time, nerve conduits have been merely a tube that guides the growth of axons to the distal nerve that may be suitable for small nerves in the hand.[56] However, nerve allografts contain the full scaffold of nerve, which allows for greater guidance of axonal growth. Autologous autografted nerves also contain Schwann cells and growth factors that, in theory, should help increase axonal growth and the "take" of nerve grafts. At this time, it is uncertain what length of major peripheral nerve is best treated with an autograft versus an allograft (Fig. 70.57).[57]

There are many other advancements in implant technology, minimally invasive surgery, and tissue engineering, but those regarding transplantation, prosthetics design, and nerve repair are especially exciting and are coming to clinical fruition.

CONCLUSION

The specialty of hand surgery is exhaustive, and a number of specialty textbooks are available. Although general surgeons may be responsible for the basic tenets of hand surgery, knowledge

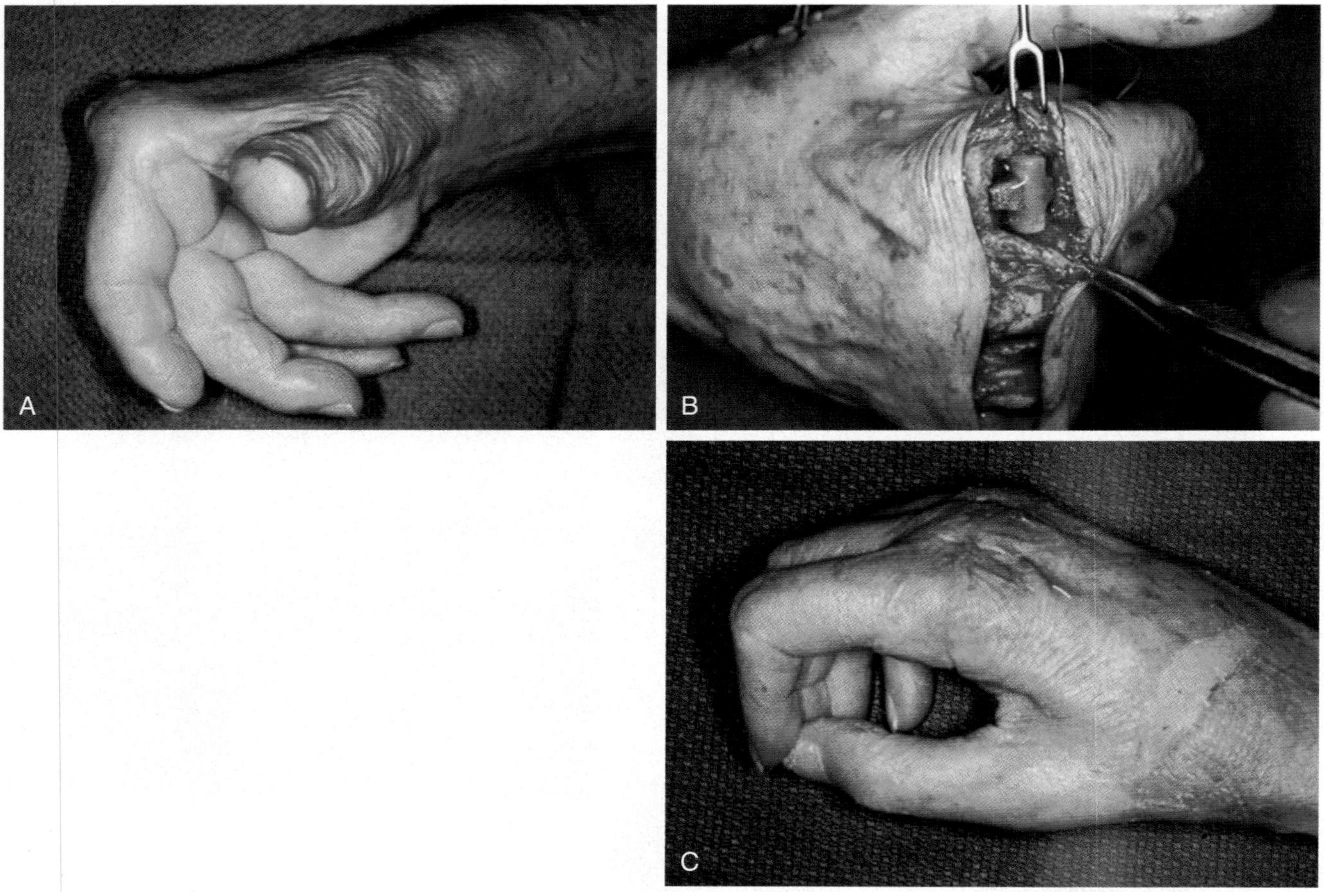

FIG. 70.55 (A) Patient with rheumatoid arthritis showing the characteristic finger deformities. (B and C) Implant arthroplasty at the metacarpophalangeal joints restores function and aesthetics to the hand

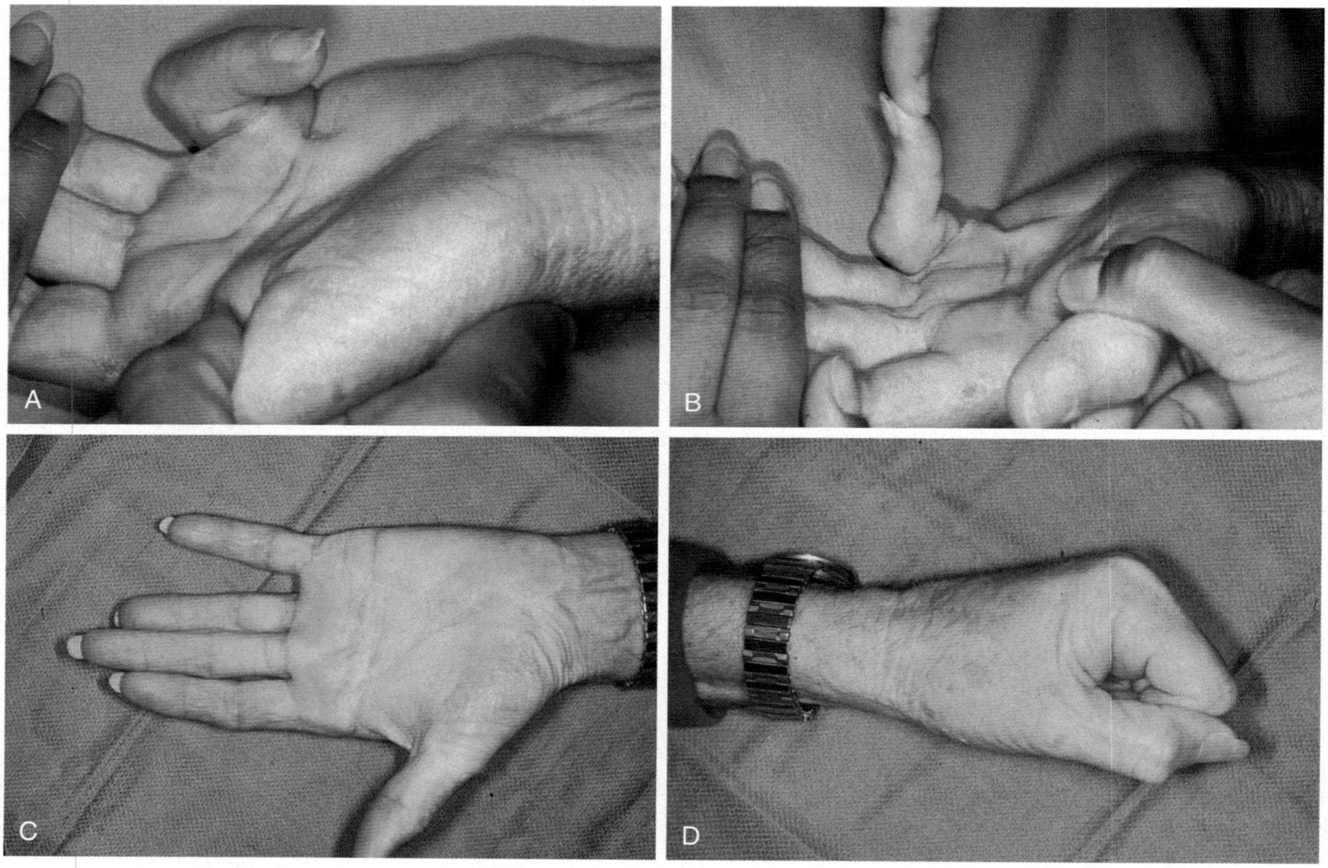

FIG. 70.56 (A–D) Patient with Dupuytren contracture is treated by regional palmar and digital fasciectomy, and good hand function is restored.

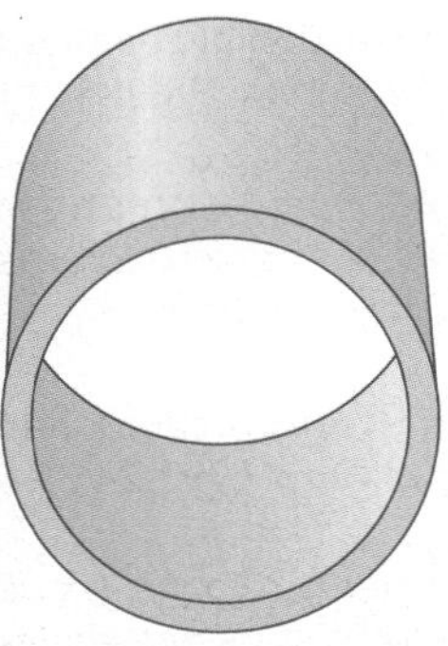
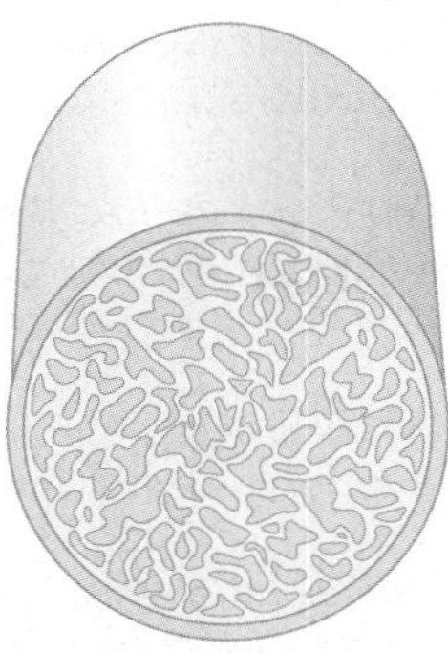
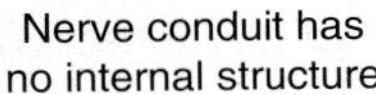

FIG. 70.57 Nerve conduits versus nerve allografts.

of minute details is often not necessary; thus, most details have been omitted from this chapter because its purpose has been to see the big picture in regard to hand surgery. Those topics of hand surgery that the general surgeon is most likely to encounter have been emphasized, particularly with regard to principles of anatomy, physical examination, and emergency treatments. Taking this into consideration, Table 70.8 includes some high-yield facts relevant to hand surgery that have been compiled from various general surgery review books as well as topics discussed in the American Board of Surgery In-Training Examination (ABSITE).[58,59] This list is provided for the convenience of general surgeons preparing for ABSITE or board examinations.

TABLE 70.8 American Board of Surgery review topics.

TOPIC	ANSWER
Fracture of the distal radius	Injury to the median nerve
Innervation of flexor digitorum profundus to the ring and small fingers	Ulnar nerve
Injury to the ulnar nerve at the elbow	Weakness in abduction and adduction of the index finger through small digits
Midshaft humeral fracture	Associated with radial nerve injury
Distal phalanx fractures	>50% of all hand fractures
Joint involved in Bennett fracture	Carpometacarpal joint of the thumb
Common name for metacarpal fracture of the small finger	Boxer fracture
Most frequently fractured carpal bone	Scaphoid
Complications associated with displaced fractures	Avascular necrosis and nonunion of the scaphoid
Axonal nerve growth rate	1 mm/day
Common maximum intraoperative tourniquet time in hand surgery	2 hours
Single digits that are primarily replanted	Thumbs in adults and children, all digits whenever possible in children
Maximal period of anoxia compatible with replantation	Finger—8 hours (warm ischemia), but longer times have been anecdotally reported; upper and lower extremity—6 hours
Proper method for transportation of an amputated body part to maximize replantation success	Cleaned of debris, wrapped in sterile towel or gauze, moistened with sterile lactated Ringer solution, placed in sterile plastic bag, transported in insulated cooler with ice water (ideal temperature, 4°C)
Complications if nerve repair is delayed >2 weeks	Retraction of nerve's ends resulting in need for nerve grafting
Zone 2, no man's land	Area of flexor tendon injury between metacarpophalangeal joint and flexor digitorum superficialis insertion
Mallet finger	Injury to extensor mechanism at level of distal interphalangeal joint
Gamekeeper thumb	Rupture of ulnar collateral ligament of thumb metacarpophalangeal joint, with resultant instability of the joint to radial-directed force
Most common organism causing hand infections	*Staphylococcus aureus*
Classic symptoms of carpal tunnel syndrome	Paresthesias in median nerve distribution, often waking the patient at night
Most effective therapy for full-thickness burns of the hand	Early excision and grafting
Most common location of ganglion cysts	Scapholunate interosseous ligament at the dorsal wrist
Treatment of de Quervain stenosing tenosynovitis after failed nonoperative management	Surgical release of first extensor compartment
Cause of trigger finger	Stenosing tenosynovitis in the region of the metacarpophalangeal joint, A1 pulley
Late findings of rheumatoid arthritis	Subluxation of involved joints resulting in deformity
Swan neck deformity	Hyperextension of proximal interphalangeal joint with flexion of distal interphalangeal joint
Boutonnière deformity	Flexion of proximal interphalangeal joint with hyperextension of distal interphalangeal joint
Nonoperative measures for Dupuytren contracture	Exercise, local steroid injections, collagenase injections, radiotherapy
Digits usually affected in Dupuytren contracture	Ring and small fingers
Cause of Dupuytren contracture	Proliferation and fibrosis of the palmar fascia
Fractures likely to cause compartment syndrome, Volkmann ischemic contracture	Supracondylar fracture of the humerus
Artery and nerve compromised in Volkmann ischemic contracture	Median nerve and anterior interosseous artery
Complication of cast placement for supracondylar fractures of the humerus	Volkmann ischemic contracture

SELECTED REFERENCES

General

Bruen KJ, Gowski WF. Treatment of digital frostbite: current concepts. *J Hand Surg [Am]*. 2009;34:553–554.

Experience with tissue plasminogen activator is reported. It shows promise in decreasing rates of digital amputation.

Cordill LL, Schubkegel T, Light TR, et al. Lipid infusion rescue for bupivacaine-induced cardiac arrest after axillary block. *J Hand Surg [Am]*. 2010;35:144–146.

Successful resuscitation of a hand surgery patient after inadvertent intravascular injection of bupivacaine during administration of an axillary block is discussed.

Harness NG. Digital block anesthesia. *J Hand Surg [Am]*. 2009;34:142–145.

The optimum techniques for providing digital block anesthesia are discussed.

Omer GE. Development of hand surgery: education of hand surgeons. *J Hand Surg [Am]*. 2000;25:616–628.

This article traces the development of hand surgery from the publication, in 1916, of Kanavel's classic book on infections of the hand through the recognition of the specialty of hand surgery, to the training of modern-day hand surgeons and their educational requirements. The article contains historical vignettes and mentions many giants in hand surgery.

Patel MM, Catalano LW. Bone graft substitutes: current uses in hand surgery. *J Hand Surg [Am]*. 2009;34:555–556.

Bone grafts are used for structural support and biologic properties. The use of bone graft substitutes limits donor morbidity and also shortens operative time.

Slutsky DJ, Nagle DJ. Wrist arthroscopy: current concepts. *J Hand Surg [Am]*. 2008;33:1228–1244.

Wrist arthroscopy has grown from a diagnostic procedure to a valuable treatment modality for a variety of wrist disorders, such as degenerative arthritis, acute carpal and metacarpal fractures, wrist instability, and ganglions.

Soft Tissue

Foucher G, Khouri RK. Digital reconstruction with island flaps. *Clin Plast Surg*. 1997;24:1–32.

New information of the intrinsic flaps of the hand enables ingenious soft tissue reconstructions using local tissues from the hand and fingers as pedicled, vascularized, island flaps. A thorough knowledge of the vasculature of the hand is required in addition to that in standard anatomy texts.

Godina M. Early microsurgical reconstruction of complex trauma of the extremities. *Plast Reconstr Surg*. 1986;78:285–292.

This paper emphasizes the concept of primary repair and reconstruction of all damaged tissues (including microvascular soft tissue coverage) acutely after major trauma.

Martin D, Bakhach J, Casoli V, et al. Reconstruction of the hand with forearm island flaps. *Clin Plast Surg*. 1997;24:33–48.

Knowledge of the vascular anatomy of the forearm enables an array of pedicled flaps to be used for soft tissue reconstruction of the hand, thus avoiding the need to use microvascular anastomoses.

Flexor Tendons

Hunter JM, Salisbury RE. Flexor tendon reconstruction in severely damaged hands: a two-stage procedure using a silicone-Dacron reinforced gliding prosthesis prior to tendon grafting. *J Bone Joint Surg Am*. 1971;53:829–858.

This paper introduces the concept of two-stage flexor tendon repair in patients in whom the flexor tendon sheath is scarred in a late repair. A tendon spacer is placed as a preliminary procedure to later tendon grafting. This remains a time-honored way of dealing with late flexor tendon reconstructions.

Kim HM, Nelson G, Thomopoulos S, et al. Technical and biological modifications for enhanced flexor tendon repair. *J Hand Surg [Am]*. 2010;35:1031–1037.

An up-to-date current concept on technical essentials to enhance outcome and the potential for future biologic manipulation of the tendon repair site.

Kleinert H, Kutz JE, Atasoy E, et al. Primary repair of flexor tendons. *Orthop Clin North Am*. 1973;4:865–876.

This article was the first substantive evidence that flexor tendons could be safely and effectively repaired in no man's land, emphasizing the importance of postoperative controlled mobilization of the fingers.

Strickland JW. Development of flexor tendon surgery: twenty-five years of progress. *J Hand Surg [Am]*. 2000;25:214–235.

This excellent review article describes the current state of the art for treatment of flexor tendon injuries.

Extensor Tendons

Merritt WH. Relative motion splint: active motion after extensor tendon injury and repair. *J Hand Surg [Am]*. 2014;39:1187–1194.

This publication has excellent accompanying videos that demonstrate how this very practical splinting technique can be used for rehabilitation of extensor tendon lacerations, boutonnière deformity, and sagittal band injury.

Nerve Injuries

Cho MS, Rinker BD, Weber RV, et al. Functional outcome following nerve repair in the upper extremity using processed nerve allograft. *J Hand Surg [Am]*. 2012;37:2340–2349.

Nerve repair using decellularized allograft for a nerve gap gives results comparable to nerve autograft for median and ulnar nerve. Off-the-shelf nerve allografts have become a helpful addition to nerve repair.

Isaacs T. Treatment of acute peripheral nerve injures: current concepts. *J Hand Surg [Am]*. 2010;35:491–497.

Although outcomes after nerve repair are not always excellent, this article assesses well-established basic principles and also includes a number of strategies for repair techniques for small and large traumatic nerve gaps.

Lundborg G. A 25-year perspective of peripheral nerve surgery: evolving neuroscientific concepts and classical significance. *J Hand Surg [Am]*. 2000;25:391–414.

This excellent article establishes the experimental basis and neuroscience behind nerve repair and nerve regeneration. The rationale for nerve conduits is discussed.

Millesi H, Meissl G, Berger A. The interfascicular nerve-grafting of the median and ulnar nerves. *J Bone Joint Surg*. 1972;54:727–750.

This landmark article emphasizes the importance of tension-free nerve repair, matching of proximal and distal fascicular groups, and use of nerve grafts in cases of a large nerve gap injury.

Weber RV, Mackinnon S. Nerve transfers in the upper extremity. *J Am Soc Surg Hand*. 2004;4:200–213.

The innovative use of nerve transfers is described to bypass and to overcome long nerve gaps after nerve injury to hasten and to improve functional recovery.

Replantation

Buncke HJ. Microvascular hand surgery—transplants and replants—over the past 25 years. *J Hand Surg [Am]*. 2000;25:415–428.

This article traces the history of microvascular surgery as it applies to the upper extremities and of the milestones achieved. It discusses the many microvascular reconstructive options available for free tissue transfer and microvascular toe to hand transfers and also evaluates anticipated survival and functional outcomes for replantation surgery.

Fractures

Carlsen BT, Moran SL. Thumb trauma: Bennett fractures, Rolando fractures and ulnar collateral ligament injuries. *J Hand Surg [Am]*. 2009;34:945–952.

Recent advancements for the treatment of these common injuries are discussed.

Kawamura K, Chung KC. Treatment of scaphoid fractures and non-unions. *J Hand Surg [Am]*. 2008;33:938–997.

Scaphoid fractures are a common injury presenting with unique challenges because of a tenuous scaphoid blood supply. This article updates the reader about diagnostic imaging and current treatment strategies for displaced and nondisplaced acute scaphoid fractures, scaphoid nonunions, and avascular necrosis.

Russe O. Fracture of the carpal navicular: diagnosis, nonoperative, and operative treatment. *J Bone Joint Surg Am*. 1960;42:759–768.

Although new innovations of cannulated compression screws and minimally invasive surgery have changed the management of scaphoid fractures, this article is still relevant in regard to understanding and treatment of scaphoid fractures and their complications.

Stern PJ. Management of fractures of the hand over the last 25 years. *J Hand Surg [Am]*. 2000;25:817–823.

Fluoroscopic imaging has greatly facilitated the operative management of hand fractures. The evolution from Kirschner wires to plates and screws is discussed. Innovations included self-tapping screws, low-profile plates, and cannulated screws, with the goal of achieving rigid bone fixation to enable restoration of early digital motion to minimize the risk for tendon adhesions and joint contractures.

Bone Gaps

Houdek MT, Wagner ER, Wyles CC, Nanos GP, Moran SL. New options for vascularized bone reconstruction in the upper extremity. *Semin Plast Surg*. 2015;29:20–29.

Summary of options for vascularized bone reconstruction when encountering large bone gaps.

Infections

Kanavel AB. An anatomical, experimental, and clinical study of acute phlegmons of the hand. *Surg Gynecol Obstet*. 1905;1:221–259.

This classic paper described the anatomic spaces of the hand. It changed the course of infection treatment and also saw the origins of hand surgery. The clinical outcome was changed from amputation to surgical management, which preserved the function of structures, emphasizing that hand surgery is founded on a sound knowledge of anatomy. The basic principles of this article, written in the preantibiotic era, still remain true.

Compartment Syndrome

Mubarak SJ, Hargens AR. Acute compartment syndromes. *Surg Clin North Am*. 1983;63:539–565.

This excellent article describes the pathogenesis of acute compartment syndrome, including the diagnosis and surgical management in the upper extremity.

Entrapment Neuropathy

Bickel KD. Carpal tunnel syndrome. *J Hand Surg [Am]*. 2010;35:147–152.

This is the most common compressive neuropathy in the upper extremity. Evidence-based guidelines for diagnosis and treatment are provided.

Koo JT, Szabo RM. Compression neuropathies of the median nerve. *J Am Soc Surg Hand*. 2004;4:156–175.

This comprehensive article gives excellent anatomic descriptions of all the anatomic sites in the upper extremity in which chronic compression of the median nerve can occur. Nonsurgical and surgical management guidelines are outlined for each.

Palmer BA, Hughes TB. Cubital tunnel syndrome. *J Hand Surg [Am]*. 2010;35:153–163.

This up-to-date article provides current concepts in diagnosis and treatment strategies for cubital tunnel syndrome.

Phalen GS. The carpal-tunnel syndrome: Seventeen years' experience in diagnosis and treatment of six hundred fifty-four hands. *J Bone Joint Surg Am*. 1966;48:211–228.

This is a classic paper written by a founder and past president of the American Society for Surgery of the Hand. It presents an understanding of median nerve compression at the wrist that is surgically treated by decompression and release of the transverse carpal ligament. The most common procedure performed by hand surgeons today is median nerve decompression.

Vascular Tumors

Mulliken JB, Glowacki J. Hemangioma and vascular malformations in infants and children: a classification based on endothelial characteristics. *Plast Reconstr Surg*. 1982;69:412–422.

The authors attempted to unify the classification of hemangiomas and vascular malformations. Suggested classifications fall into six broad categories—embryology, histology, clinical features, dynamics of growth, hemodynamic patterns, and cell biology. A classification is useful only if it has diagnostic applicability and aids in planning therapy and understanding pathogenesis.

Congenital Anomalies

McCarroll HR. Congenital anomalies: a 25-year overview. *J Hand Surg [Am]*. 2000;25:1007–1037.

This excellent review discusses the more commonly treated congenital hand anomalies. It also identifies some of the newer (at that time) developments in surgical treatment, which include distraction lengthening, pollicization, microvascular surgery, and potential for in utero interventions. Useful classifications for treatment management are provided.

Netscher DT, Scheker LR. Timing and decision making in the treatment of congenital upper extremity deformities. *Clin Plast Surg*. 1990;17:113–131.

This review describes commonly treated congenital hand anomalies and provides a rational basis for timing surgical interventions to meet critical hand functional milestones.

Osteoarthritis

Burton RI, Pellegrini VD. Surgical management of basal joint arthritis of the thumb. Part II. Ligament reconstruction with tendon interposition arthroplasty. *J Hand Surg [Am]*. 1986;11:324–332.

An excellent description of the pathogenesis and surgical management of basilar joint osteoarthritis of the thumb. This is the usually performed surgical procedure for carpometacarpal joint osteoarthritis of the thumb.

Eaton RG, Littler JW. Ligament reconstruction for the painful thumb carpometacarpal joint. *J Bone Joint Surg Am*. 1973;55:1655–1666.

One of the most common joints affected by osteoarthritis is at the base of the thumb. This operation, originally described by these authors for surgical management, still forms the basis of surgical treatment today with few modifications in technique.

Rheumatoid Arthritis

Brasington R. TNF-α antagonists and other recombinant proteins for treatment of rheumatoid arthritis. *J Hand Surg Am*. 2009;34:349–350.

Disease-modifying antirheumatic drugs that specifically target individual molecules are discussed. Medical treatment of rheumatoid conditions has changed dramatically in recent years.

Swanson AB. Flexible implant arthroplasty for arthritic finger joints: rationale, technique, and results of treatment. *J Bone Joint Surg Am*. 1972;54:435–455.

A landmark article that changed the course of treatment for rheumatoid arthritis. In this paper, Swanson introduced small joint arthroplasty.

Contractures

Curtis RM. Capsulectomy of the interphalangeal joints of the fingers. *J Bone Joint Surg Am*. 1954;36:1219–1232.

This classic article changed the course of treatment of the stiff hand and promoted interest in the complex anatomy of the proximal interphalangeal joint. The author was meticulous in technique and insisted on rigid postoperative therapy.

Eaton C. Percutaneous fasciotomy for Dupuytren's contracture. *J Hand Surg Am*. 2011;36:910–915.

Percutaneous needle fasciotomy is a less invasive treatment than surgery. This article describes that technique.

McFarlane RM. Patterns of the diseased fascia in the fingers in Dupuytren's contracture: displacement of the neurovascular bundle. *Plast Reconstr Surg*. 1974;54:31–44.

This article clearly outlines the pathology, anatomy, and proposed surgical treatment of Dupuytren contracture. The author describes the patterns of diseased fascia in the palm and fingers and how displacement of the digital neurovascular bundle may occur.

Meals RA, Hentz VR. Technical tips for collagenase injection treatment for Dupuytren contracture. *J Hand Surg Am.* 2014;39:1195–1200. e2.

Collagenase injection has become an increasingly popular method of treating Dupuytren contracture. This article outlines the technique involved for this seemingly less invasive treatment.

REFERENCES

1. Sears ED, Larson BP, Chung KC. A national survey of program director opinions of core competencies and structure of hand surgery fellowship training. *J Hand Surg Am.* 2012;37:1971–1977. e1977.
2. Green DP. General principles. In: Hotchkiss RN, Pederson WC, Wolfe SW, et al., eds. *Green's Operative Hand Surgery.* 5th ed. Philadelphia, PA: Elsevier; 2005:3–24.
3. Netscher DT, Hamilton KL. Metacarpal and phalangeal fractures. In: Evans GRD, ed. *Operative Plastic Surgery.* 2nd ed. New York, NY: Oxford University Press; 2019:1019–1056.
4. Klenerman L. Tourniquet time--how long? *Hand.* 1980;12:231–234.
5. Hunter JM, Salisbury RE. Flexor-tendon reconstruction in severely damaged hands. A two-stage procedure using a silicone-dacron reinforced gliding prosthesis prior to tendon grafting. *J Bone Joint Surg Am.* 1971;53:829–858.
6. Tomaino M, Mitsionis G, Basitidas J, et al. The effect of partial excision of the A2 and A4 pulleys on the biomechanics of finger flexion. *J Hand Surg Br.* 1998;23:50–52.
7. Tang JB. Indications, methods, postoperative motion and outcome evaluation of primary flexor tendon repairs in Zone 2. *J Hand Surg Eur.* 2007;32:118–129.
8. Lalonde DH. Wide-awake flexor tendon repair. *Plast Reconstr Surg.* 2009;123:623–625.
9. Matarrese MR, Hammert WC. Flexor tendon rehabilitation. *J Hand Surg Am.* 2012;37:2386–2388.
10. Ahmad Z, Wardale J, Brooks R, et al. Exploring the application of stem cells in tendon repair and regeneration. *Arthroscopy.* 2012;28:1018–1029.
11. Merrit WH, Pace CS. Extensor tendon injuries. In: Cohen MN, Thaller S, eds. *The Unfavorable Result in Plastic Surgery: Avoidance and Treatment.* 4th ed. New York, NY: Thieme Medical Publishers; 2018:1183–1215.
12. Cheng CJ. Synthetic nerve conduits for digital nerve reconstruction. *J Hand Surg Am.* 2009;34:1718–1721.
13. Oberlin C, Beal D, Leechavengvongs S, et al. Nerve transfer to biceps muscle using a part of ulnar nerve for C5-C6 avulsion of the brachial plexus: anatomical study and report of four cases. *J Hand Surg Am.* 1994;19:232–237.
14. McClinton MA, Wilgis EFS. Ischemic conditions of the hand. In: Mathes SJ, Hentz VR, eds. *Plastic Surgery.* 2nd ed. Philadelphia, PA: Saunders Elsevier; 2006:791–822.
15. Soucacos PN. Indications and selection for digital amputation and replantation. *J Hand Surg Br.* 2001;26:572–581.
16. Kumar S, O'Connor A, Despois M, et al. Use of early magnetic resonance imaging in the diagnosis of occult scaphoid fractures: The CAST Study (Canberra Area Scaphoid Trial). *N Z Med J.* 2005;118:U1296.
17. Turker T, Capdarest-Arest N. Management of gunshot wounds to the hand: a literature review. *J Hand Surg Am.* 2013;38:1641–1650.
18. Buck 2nd. DW, Dumanian GA. Bone biology and physiology: Part II. Clinical correlates. *Plast Reconstr Surg.* 2012;129:950e–956e.
19. Rinaldi E. Autografts in the treatment of osseous defects in the forearm and hand. *J Hand Surg Am.* 1987;12:282–286.
20. Ruta D, Ozer K. Primary bone grafting in open fractures with segmental bone loss. *J Hand Surg Am.* 2014;39:779–780.
21. Micev AJ, Kalainov DM, Soneru AP. Masquelet technique for treatment of segmental bone loss in the upper extremity. *J Hand Surg Am.* 2015;40:593–598.
22. Orzechowski W, Morasiewicz L, Dragan S, et al. Treatment of non-union of the forearm using distraction-compression osteogenesis. *Ortop Traumatol Rehabil.* 2007;9:357–365.
23. Houdek MT, Wagner ER, Wyles CC, et al. New options for vascularized bone reconstruction in the upper extremity. *Semin Plast Surg.* 2015;29:20–29.
24. Georgiadis GM, DeSilva SP. Reconstruction of skeletal defects in the forearm after trauma: Treatment with cement spacer and delayed cancellous bone grafting. *J Trauma.* 1995;38:910–914.
25. Merritt K. Factors increasing the risk of infection in patients with open fractures. *J Trauma.* 1988;28:823–827.
26. Taylor CJ, Chester DL, Jeffery SL. Functional splinting of upper limb injuries with gauze-based topical negative pressure wound therapy. *J Hand Surg Am.* 2011;36:1848–1851.
27. Godina M. Early microsurgical reconstruction of complex trauma of the extremities. *Plast Reconstr Surg.* 1986;78:285–292.
28. Lesiak AC, Shafritz AB. Negative-pressure wound therapy. *J Hand Surg Am.* 2013;38:1828–1832.
29. Brown RE, Wu TY. Use of "spare parts" in mutilated upper extremity injuries. *Hand Clin.* 2003;19:73–87, vi.
30. Stevanovic MV, Sharpe F. Acute infections in the hand. In: Wolfe SW, Hotchkiss RN, Pederson WC, et al., eds. *Green's Operative Hand Surgery.* 7th ed. Philadelphia, PA: Elsevier; 2017:17–61.
31. Lille S, Hayakawa T, Neumeister MW, et al. Continuous postoperative catheter irrigation is not necessary for the treatment of suppurative flexor tenosynovitis. *J Hand Surg Br.* 2000;25:304–307.
32. Kare JA. Volkmann contracture. *Medscape*; 2019. http://emedicine.medscape.com/article/1270462-overview. Retrieved July 12, 2019.
33. Patel MR, Bassini L. Trigger fingers and thumb: when to splint, inject, or operate. *J Hand Surg Am.* 1992;17:110–113.
34. Trumble TE. Compressive neuropathies. In: Trumble TE, ed. *Principles of Hand Surgery and Therapy.* Philadelphia, PA: WB Saunders; 2000:324–342.
35. Trumble TE, Diao E, Abrams RA, et al. Single-portal endoscopic carpal tunnel release compared with open release: a prospective, randomized trial. *J Bone Joint Surg Am.* 2002;84:1107–1115.
36. Mackinnon SE, Novak CB. Compression neuropathies. In: Wolfe SW, Hotchkiss RN, Pederson WC, et al., eds. *Green's Operative Hand Surgery.* 7th ed. Philadelphia, PA: Elsevier; 2017:921–958.
37. Athanasian EA. Bone and soft tissue tumors. In: Wolfe SW, Hotchkiss RN, Pederson WC, et al., eds. *Green's Operative Hand Surgery.* 7th ed. Philadelphia, PA: Elsevier; 2017:1987–2035.

38. Netscher DT. Tumors of the hand. In: Wolfe SW, Hotchkiss RN, Pederson WC, et al., eds. *Green's Operative Hand Surgery*. 7th ed. Philadelphia, PA: Elsevier; 2017:1958–1986.
39. Shenefelt PD. *Nongenital warts*; 2018. https://emedicine.medscape.com/article/1133317-overview. Retrieved July 12, 2019.
40. Buckmiller LM, Munson PD, Dyamenahalli U, et al. Propranolol for infantile hemangiomas: early experience at a tertiary vascular anomalies center. *Laryngoscope*. 2010;120:676–681.
41. Sofocleous CT, Rosen RJ, Raskin K, et al. Congenital vascular malformations in the hand and forearm. *J Endovasc Ther*. 2001;8:484–494.
42. Koman LA, Ruch DS, Paterson SB. Vascular disorders. In: Hotchkiss RN, Pederson WC, Wolfe SW, et al., eds. *Green's Operative Hand Surgery*. Philadelphia, PA: Elsevier; 2005: 2265–2313.
43. Novick M, Gard DA, Hardy SB, et al. Burn scar carcinoma: a review and analysis of 46 cases. *J Trauma*. 1977;17:809–817.
44. Glat PM, Shapiro RL, Roses DF, et al. Management considerations for melanonychia striata and melanoma of the hand. *Hand Clin*. 1995;11:183–189.
45. Netscher DT. Congenital hand problems. Terminology, etiology, and management. *Clin Plast Surg*. 1998;25:537–552.
46. Feldon P, Terrono AL, Nalebluff EA. Rheumatoid arthritis and other connective tissue diseases. In: Hotchkiss RN, Pederson WC, Wolfe SW, et al., eds. *Green's Operative Hand Surgery*. 5th ed. Philadelphia, PA: Elsevier; 2005: 2049–2136.
47. Hurst LC, Badalamente MA. Nonoperative treatment of Dupuytren's disease. *Hand Clin*. 1999;15:97–107, vii.
48. Denkler KA, Vaughn CJ, Dolan EL, et al. Evidence-Based Medicine: Options for Dupuytren's contracture: incise, excise, and dissolve. *Plast Reconstr Surg*. 2017;139:240e–255e.
49. Agee JM, Goss BC. The use of skeletal extension torque in reversing Dupuytren contractures of the proximal interphalangeal joint. *J Hand Surg Am*. 2012;37:1467–1474.
50. Murray JE. Organ transplantation (skin, kidney, heart) and the plastic surgeon. *Plast Reconstr Surg*. 1971;47:425–431.
51. Shores JT, Brandacher G, Lee WP. Hand and upper extremity transplantation: an update of outcomes in the worldwide experience. *Plast Reconstr Surg*. 2015;135:351e–360e.
52. Alolabi N, Chuback J, Grad S, et al. The utility of hand transplantation in hand amputee patients. *J Hand Surg Am*. 2015;40:8–14.
53. Burn MB, Ta A, Gogola GR. Three-dimensional printing of prosthetic hands for children. *J Hand Surg Am*. 2016;41:e103–e109.
54. Nghiem BT, Sando IC, Gillespie RB, et al. Providing a sense of touch to prosthetic hands. *Plast Reconstr Surg*. 2015;135:1652–1663.
55. Isaacs J, Browne T. Overcoming short gaps in peripheral nerve repair: conduits and human acellular nerve allograft. *Hand (N Y)*. 2014;9:131–137.
56. Lui H, Vaquette C, Bindra R. Tissue engineering in hand surgery: a technology update. *J Hand Surg Am*. 2017;42:727–735.
57. Cho MS, Rinker BD, Weber RV, et al. Functional outcome following nerve repair in the upper extremity using processed nerve allograft. *J Hand Surg Am*. 2012;37:2340–2349.
58. Blecha M, Brown A. Orthopedic and hand surgery pearls. In: Blecha M, Brown A, eds. *General Surgery: Pearls of Wisdom*. Lincoln, MA: Boston Medical; 2004:217–224.
59. Deziel DJ, Witt TR, Bines SD. Hand surgery. In: Deziel DJ, Witt TR, Bines SD, et al., eds. *Rush University Review of Surgery*. 3rd ed. Philadelphia, PA: WB Saunders; 2000: 579–589.

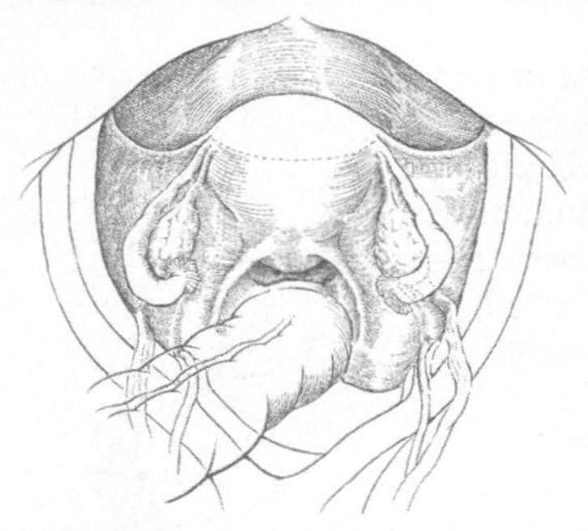

CHAPTER 71

Gynecologic Surgery

Lauren S. Prescott, Amanda C. Yunker, Ronald Alvarez

OUTLINE

Please access Elsevier eBooks for Practicing Clinicians to view the videos for this chapter https://expertconsult.inkling.com/.

Gynecologic procedures are among the most frequent surgical procedures done in the world. It behooves any surgeon to be familiar with the anatomy of the female reproductive tract and pelvis and with the most common gynecologic surgical diseases and procedures for these diseases. This chapter provides an overview of female reproductive tract and pelvic anatomy; discusses the most common surgical diseases of the vulva, vagina, cervix, uterus, fallopian tubes, and ovaries; and describes commonly utilized surgical procedures for these diseases.

FEMALE REPRODUCTIVE AND OTHER PELVIC ANATOMY

Key components of the female reproductive tract anatomy include external reproductive anatomy (vulva) and internal reproductive anatomy (vagina, cervix, uterus, fallopian tubes, and ovaries).[1] Other relevant pelvic anatomy components include anatomic spaces, vascular and neurologic structures, and urologic and intestinal structures.[1] The following section provides an overview of these key components.

External Reproductive Anatomy (Vulva)

The main external structures of the vulva are the mons pubis, the labia majora and labia minora, the clitoral glans and clitoral hood, the urethral meatus, the vaginal introitus and hymen, and Bartholin and Skene vestibular glands (Fig. 71.1). The mons pubis is the soft fatty tissue covering the pubic bone. The lower part of the mons pubis is divided by a fissure named the pudendal cleft, which separates the mons pubis into the labia majora. The labia majora and labia minora are separated by a groove called the interlabial sulci, and the labia minora fuse anteriorly to form the clitoral hood (also known as the prepuce).

The labia cover the vestibule, the area of the vulva consisting of the vaginal introitus and urethral meatus, and is demarcated by the Hart line. The vaginal introitus is initially covered by a thin membrane called the hymen, which is usually ruptured by exercise, during insertion of tampons, or during the first episode of intercourse. Within the vestibule are Bartholin glands and Skene glands. Bartholin glands, homologues of the bulbourethral glands in males, are located posteriorly to the right and left of the vaginal introitus. These glands secrete mucous during sexual arousal to provide vaginal lubrication. Skene glands, homologues of the prostate gland in males, are located to the right and left of the urethral meatus. These glands also produce secretions that provide vaginal lubrication with sexual arousal.

These external structures are part of the urogenital triangle, which is the anterior portion of the perineum. The urogenital triangle has its apex anteriorly at the symphysis pubis and its base posteriorly formed by a line drawn between the ischial tuberosities. Beneath the aforementioned external structures lies the urogenital diaphragm, a fascial and muscular shelf extending between the pubic rami and penetrated by the urethra and vagina. The muscles of the urogenital triangle consist of the deep and superficial transverse perineal muscles, paired ischiocavernosus muscles that cover the crura of the clitoris, and bulbocavernosus muscles covering erectile vestibular bulbs that lie on either side of the vaginal introitus.

Blood supply to structures within the urogenital triangle is predominantly from a posterior direction from the internal pudendal artery, which, after arising from the internal iliac artery, passes through Alcock canal, a fascial tunnel along the obturator internus muscle below the origin of the levator ani muscle. On emerging from Alcock canal, the internal pudendal artery sends branches to the urogenital triangle anteriorly. The blood supply to the mons pubis originates anteriorly from the inferior epigastric artery, a branch of the femoral artery. Laterally, the external

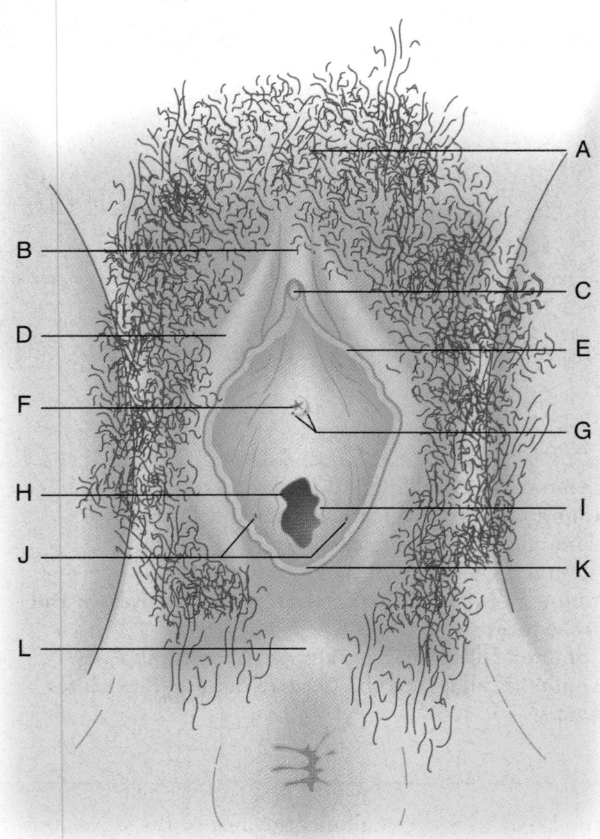

FIG. 71.1 The eternal genitalia. *A*, Mons pubis; *B*, prepuce; *C*, clitoris; *D*, labia majora; *E*, labia minora; *F*, urethral meatus; *G*, Skene gland ducts; *H*, vagina; *I*, hymen; *J*, Bartholin glands; *K*, posterior fourchette; *L*, perineal body.

pudendal artery arises from the femoral artery and supplies the lateral aspect of the vulva. Venous return and lymphatic drainage from the urogenital diaphragm accompany the arterial supply and therefore drains into the internal iliac and femoral veins.

The major nerve supply to the urogenital triangle comes from the internal pudendal nerve, which originates from the S2 to S4 anterior rami of the sacral plexus and travels through Alcock canal along with the internal pudendal artery and vein. Anterior branches supply the external genitalia. The mons pubis and anterior labia are supplied by the ilioinguinal and genitofemoral nerves from the lumbar plexus that travel through the inguinal canal and exit through the superficial inguinal ring. All these paired nerves routinely cross the midline for partial innervation of the contralateral side. The visceral efferent nerves responsible for clitoral erection are derived from the pelvic splanchnic nerves and reach the external genitalia along with the urethra and vagina as they pass through the urogenital diaphragm.

It is important for the surgeon dissecting the external genitalia to be cognizant of the variability of vascular and neurologic direction from which the blood and nervous supply of the operative field is derived.

Internal Reproductive Anatomy (Vagina, Cervix, Uterus, Fallopian Tubes, Ovaries)

Beginning most distal and moving proximal, the internal reproductive anatomic structures include all midline structures (the vagina, cervix, and uterus) and the lateral structures (the fallopian tubes and ovaries (Fig. 71.2). The borders of the vagina are

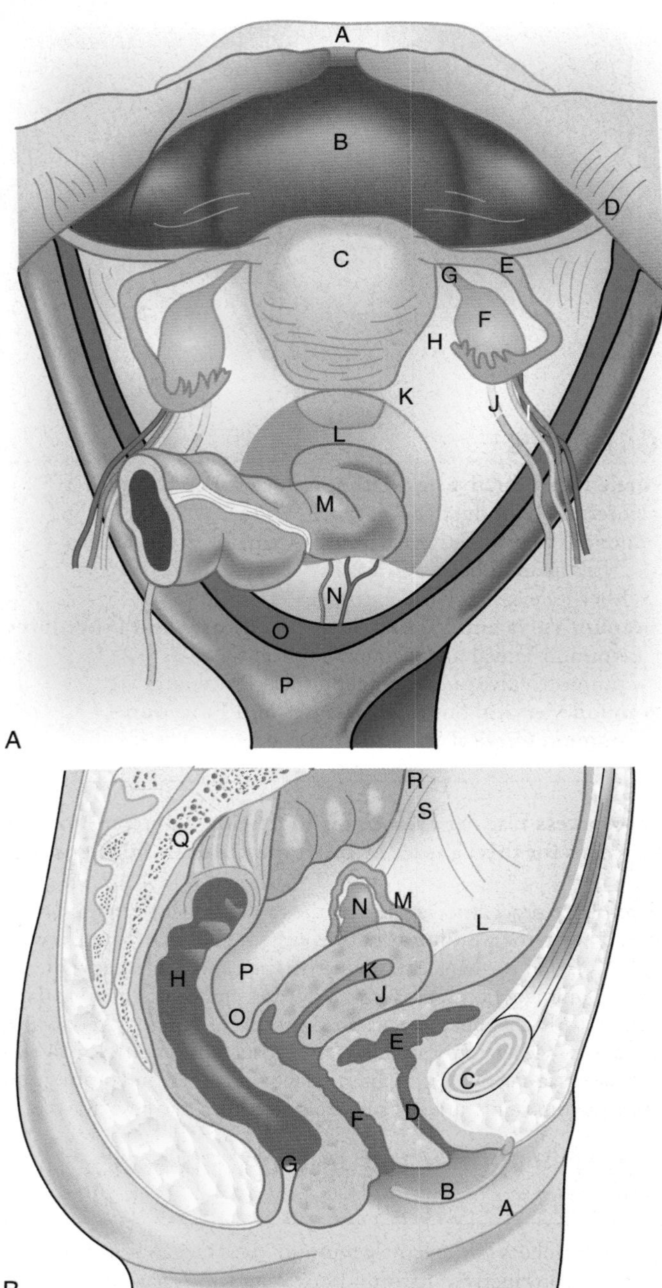

FIG. 71.2 The internal genitalia. (A) *A*, Symphysis pubis; *B*, bladder; *C*, corpus uteri; *D*, round ligament; *E*, fallopian tube; *F*, ovary; *G*, uteroovarian ligament; *H*, broad ligament; *I*, ovarian artery and vein; *J*, ureter; *K*, uterosacral ligament; *L*, cul-de-sac; *M*, rectum; *N*, middle sacral artery and vein; *O*, vena cava; *P*, aorta. (B) *A*, Labium majus; *B*, labium minus; *C*, symphysis pubis, *D*, urethra; *E*, bladder; *F*, vagina; *G*, anus; *H*, rectum; *I*, cervix uteri; *J*, corpus uteri; *K*, endometrial cavity; *L*, round ligament; *M*, fallopian tube; *N*, ovary; *O*, cul-de-sac; *P*, uterosacral ligament; *Q*, sacrum; *R*, ureter; *S*, ovarian artery and vein.

the hymen inferiorly and the cervix and fornices superiorly. The lower portion of the vagina develops from the endoderm of the urogenital sinus (along with the urethra and vulvar structures). Abnormalities of development in this area can lead to transverse or horizontal septae of the vagina, which may become symptomatic during pubertal development. The upper portion of the vagina develops in tandem with the cervix, uterus, and fallopian tubes from the Müllerian ducts. Failure of fusion of these ducts as they migrate medially or failure of development completely can lead to a variety of uterine, cervix, and tube malformations.

Vagina

The vagina is a flexible, expandable fibromuscular tube, which, at rest, is flattened and lies in a mostly horizontal plane if the woman is in an upright posture. The layers of the vaginal walls from central to peripheral include the mucosa (which is stratified squamous epithelium), the lamina propria (also called the endopelvic fascia, which mostly consists of collagen and elastic tissue and containing the vascular and lymph supply), a muscular layer, and areolar connective tissue (which also contains a rich blood supply). The blood supply to the vagina comes mainly from the vaginal artery, a branch of the internal iliac artery. There are multiple anastomoses with other arteries, including the uterine, internal pudendal, inferior vesical, and middle hemorrhoidal arteries. The nerve supply to the vagina originates from the autonomic nervous system in the lumbosacral plexus (S2–S4), culminating in the pudendal nerve. The majority of sensory innervation lies in the distal portion of the vagina, with very little nerve density in the upper part of the vagina.

Cervix

The cervix is the narrow, distal part the of uterus that can be visualized and palpated at the upper end of the vaginal canal. It is a round, often donut-like structure composed of mostly fibrous tissue and can vary in size from one female to another. The length of the cervix also varies but averages around 3 cm. It has a central canal, referred to as the *os,* which allows passage into or egress from the uterine cavity. The cells on the vaginal portion of the cervix (ectocervix) transition from squamous epithelium distally to columnar epithelium proximally as you travel up into the cervical canal (endocervix). This change is referred to as the transition zone and is where cervical intraepithelial neoplasia (CIN) occurs. The columnar epithelium produces mucous, which varies in texture depending on hormone influence, and facilitates sperm transport.

The blood supply of the cervix arises from a descending branch of uterine artery and lies laterally at the 3 and 9 o'clock positions on the cervix. Additionally, the azygos arteries lie in the middle portion of the cervix anteriorly and posteriorly along its axis. There are multiple anastomoses between the azygos arteries and the hemorrhoidal arteries. The cervix is innervated by the parasympathetic system, arising from lumbosacral plexus (S2–S4) with the majority of nerve endings concentrated in the endocervical region.

Uterus

The uterus is an intraperitoneal muscular organ that sits posterior to the bladder and anterior to the rectum. It is held in place by several ligamentous structures. The broad ligaments extend laterally off the uterine corpus and become continuous with the pelvic peritoneum. The round ligaments originate at the uterine cornua and travel laterally through the broad ligament and exit through the inguinal ring, terminating in the labia majora. The cardinal ligaments, which attach laterally to the pelvic diaphragm and fuse medially with the vaginal endopelvic fascia, support the uterus at the level of the cervix. The uterine arteries travel within the cardinal ligament and then superiorly along the lateral aspect of the uterine body, also called the *fundus.* The uterosacral ligaments originate at the upper posterior cervix and attach to the third sacral vertebra, forming an arch that frames the rectum.

The nonpregnant uterus typically weighs between 40 and 80 g. It is often smaller in prepubertal and postmenopausal women compared with those in the reproductive years. The uterus has three cell layers, similar to other viscous peritoneal organs. The outer layer is called the serosa, is very thin, and is contiguous with the broad ligaments and pelvic peritoneum. The middle layer is composed of smooth muscle, which lies in three distinct layers. The uterine cavity is lined with endometrium, a mucous epithelial layer that varies in thickness depending on hormonal influences.

The blood supply to the uterus includes both the uterine arteries, which branch off the internal iliac arteries, and the ovarian arteries, which come directly off the abdominal aorta and travel adjacent to the ovary toward the uterus. The uterus has both sympathetic and parasympathetic innervation. The sympathetic innervation travels via the hypogastric and ovarian plexus. The parasympathetic innervation comes from the lumbosacral plexus (S2–S4). Afferent fibers from the uterus returning to the spinal cord travel with the sympathetic innervation within the lumbosacral plexus (T11–T12).

Fallopian Tubes

The fallopian tubes, also referred to as the oviducts, originate at the upper lateral aspect of the uterus (called the cornua) and extend laterally approximately 10 to 14 cm in length, coiling around the ipsilateral ovary distally. The fallopian tube has four distinct anatomic sections. The interstitial part traverses the uterine wall, is completely bordered by myometrium, and is only 1 to 2 cm in length. The isthmus portion begins as the tube leaves the uterus, measures around 4 cm in length, is very narrow, and contains the most muscular region of the tube. The ampullary region is wider, averages 4 to 6 cm in length, and has a winding course. Fertilization typically occurs in this portion of the fallopian tube. The final segment is the infundibulum, which is mostly composed of fimbriae—fingerlike projections that extend out from the tube, surround the ostia, and cause this portion of the tube to have a funnel-like shape.

Similar to the uterus, the fallopian tubes are composed of several layers. The mucosa of the tube is made up of different types of epithelial cells—columnar ciliated, secretory, and narrow peg cells. The ratio of these cell types depends on the anatomic region of the tube. Under the mucosa is the lamina propria, followed by the muscular layer, and finally the adventitial layer, which is adjacent to the peritoneal cavity.

The blood supply to the fallopian tube travels through the mesosalpinx and originates from branches of the ovarian and uterine arteries. The tubes receive innervation from both the sympathetic and parasympathetic nervous systems via the uterine and ovarian plexuses.

Ovaries

The ovaries are paired, oval-shaped organs lateral in location and white, usually around 2 to 3 cm in largest diameter. They are located just inferior to the pelvic brim at the infundibulum-end of the fallopian tubes. The ovaries develop from the gonadal ridge, which sits adjacent to the mesonephric duct; thus, the urinary system and reproductive system develop in close association. The ovaries are connected to the uterus via the uteroovarian ligament, which contains an anastomotic blood supply between these two structures. Additionally, the ovaries are held in place by the posterior leaf of the broad ligament and the infundibulopelvic

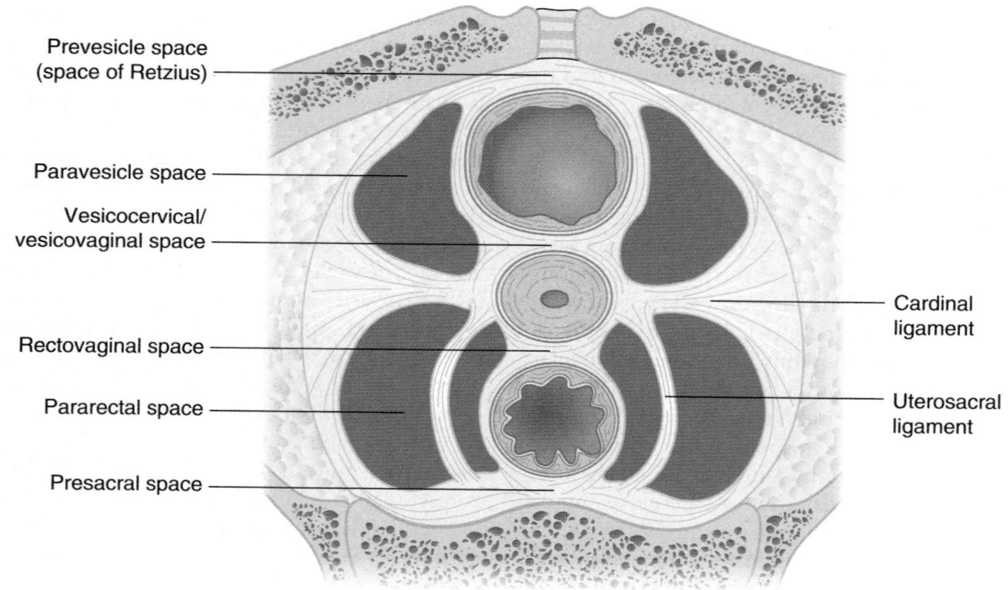

FIG. 71.3 Anatomic spaces of the female pelvis.

ligament, which travels down the lateral sidewall and contains the major ovarian blood supply.

The ovary has three distinct sections: the outer cortex, the central medulla, and the hilum, which is where the mesoovarium (the structure that anastomoses the infundibulopelvic ligament and the periuterine blood supply via the broad ligament) attaches to the ovary. The ovaries contain several cell types that allow the ovaries to perform multiple functions. Within the ovaries are the oocytes, which number 1 to 2 million at birth. The ovary surface is composed of cuboidal epithelium. The oocytes mature inside small, fluid-filled cysts called follicles, which sit just under the surface epithelium. The central medulla is mostly made up of stroma and blood vessels.

As alluded to previously, the blood supply to the ovary comes from the ovarian artery, a branch off the abdominal aorta that travels along the lateral abdomen and pelvis in the infundibulopelvic ligament. Additionally, within the mesoovarium there are many anastomoses between the ovarian artery and the uterine artery. The innervation of the ovary also travels via the infundibulopelvic ligament and includes autonomic and sensory nerve fibers from the ovarian, hypogastric, and aortic plexuses.

Other Relevant Pelvic Anatomy

Anatomic Spaces

The female pelvis contains several key potential spaces, an understanding of which is required by any surgeon operating in this area (Fig. 71.3). The two lateral retroperitoneal spaces include the paravesical and pararectal spaces. The paravesical space is bordered by the external iliac artery laterally, the bladder medially, the pubic symphysis anteriorly, and the cardinal ligament posteriorly. The space is entered by dissecting between the external iliac artery and superior vesical artery. The pararectal space is bordered by the internal iliac artery laterally, the ureter and rectum medially, the sacrum posteriorly, and the cardinal ligament anteriorly. The space is entered by dissecting between the vessels laterally and the ureter and rectum medially. The cardinal ligaments separate the paravesical and pararectal spaces. Key anterior to posterior spaces include the retropubic, vesicovaginal, rectovaginal, and retrorectal/presacral spaces. Developing these spaces facilitates identification of critical pelvic structures, particularly when normal anatomy is altered.

Vascular Structures

It is important for surgeons to be very familiar with the vascular anatomy of the pelvis when performing gynecologic procedures (Fig. 71.4). The common iliac vessels, bifurcate at the pelvic brim into the external iliac and internal iliac vessels, which course along the pelvic sidewalls. The external iliac vessels course under the inguinal ligament to become the femoral artery and vein. The internal iliac artery bifurcates into an anterior and posterior division. The female pelvic structures derive the majority of their arterial vascular supply from vessels that branch from the anterior division. Ligation of the anterior division distal to where the posterior division branches is a technique often utilized in the setting of excessive pelvic hemorrhage. Key branches of the anterior division include the uterine and vaginal arteries the inferior, middle and superior vesical arteries and the middle rectal artery. Other key branches off the anterior division include the obturator, inferior gluteal, and pudendal arteries. The ovarian arteries, which originate from the aorta, provide another major vascular source to the pelvic structures, namely the ovaries and uterus.

Neurologic Structures

The lumbosacral nerve plexus, which originates from nerve roots from the twelfth thoracic vertebral body to the fourth sacral vertebral body (T12–S4), provides the major nerve structures in the pelvis (Fig. 71.5). The primary motor nerves emanating from the lumbosacral nerve plexus include the femoral nerve, the sciatic nerve, and the obturator nerve. The primary sensory nerves include the iliohypogastric nerve, the ilioinguinal nerve, the genitofemoral nerve, the lateral femoral cutaneous nerve, the femoral nerve, the sciatic nerve, and the pudendal nerve. A description of these nerves, their origin, their motor and sensory functions, and symptoms when injured is included in Table 71.1.

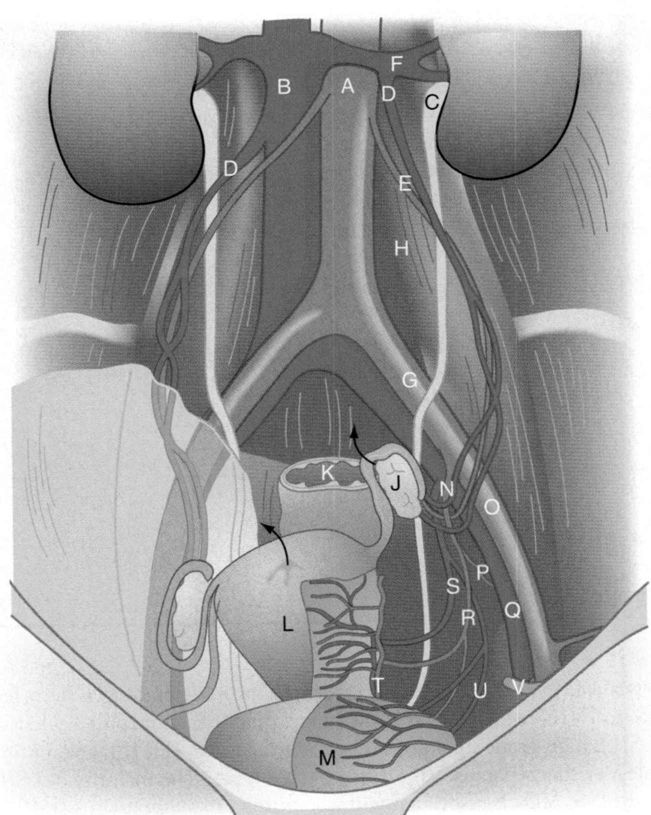

FIG. 71.4 Blood supply of the pelvis. *A*, Aorta; *B*, inferior vena cava; *C*, ureter; *D*, ovarian vein; *E*, ovarian artery; *F*, renal vein; *G*, common iliac artery; *H*, psoas muscle; *J*, ovary; *K*, rectum; *L*, corpus uteri; *M*, bladder; *N*, internal iliac (hypogastric) artery, anterior branch; *O*, external iliac artery; *P*, obturator artery; *Q*, external iliac vein; *R*, uterine artery; *S*, uterine vein; *T*, vaginal artery; *U*, superior vesical artery; *V*, inferior epigastric artery.

Nerve injuries occur in 1% to 2% of gynecologic cases.[2] The most common nerves injured during gynecologic surgery include the femoral, ilioinguinal, pudendal, obturator, lateral cutaneous, iliohypogastric, and genitofemoral nerves. These nerves can be injured as a result of malpositioning the patient in the lithotomy position, incorrect placement of self-retaining retractors, nerve transection, direct nerve entrapment, or hematoma formation. Fortunately, the majority of neuropathies resolve with conservative management and physical therapy.

Urinary Tract Structures

The ureters and bladder are key pelvic structures that require strict attention during the course of most gynecologic procedures. The ureters course retroperitoneally down the lateral pelvic walls and then cross over the common iliac arteries at the pelvic brim (Fig. 71.2). At this point, the ureters are in close proximity to the ovaries and care must be taken to properly identify and avoid the ureters during ligation of the ovarian vessels. The ureters continue along the peritoneum under the uterine arteries and then traverse into the bladder laterally in an oblique fashion. The ureter is also at risk for damage during clamping, incision, and ligation of the uterine vessels, the cardinal and uterosacral ligaments, and the vaginal corners. Dissecting the ureter off its attachment to the peritoneum and isolating it with a vessel loop is a technique often useful when pathology places the ureter at risk for injury.

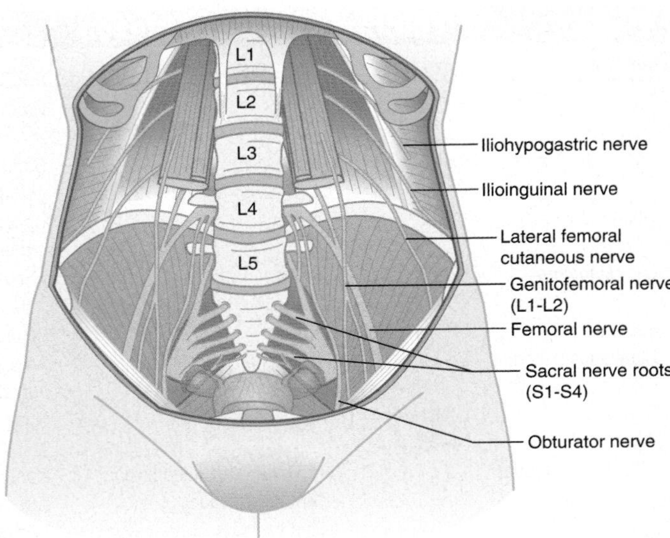

FIG. 71.5 Neurologic structures of the female pelvis. (From Lumbosacral plexus. From Gray JE. Nerve injury associated with pelvic surgery. In: UpToDate, Basow DS (Ed), UpToDate, Waltham, MA 2013. Copyright [a] UpToDate, Inc. For more information visit www.uptodate.com.)

The bladder is intimately involved with the anterior uterus, cervix, and vagina. The bladder must be carefully dissected off these structures during a hysterectomy. This often involves incision of the vesicouterine peritoneum and identifying the vesicovaginal space between the bladder and vagina. Dissection of the bladder can be made more difficult by scarring from prior Caesarean delivery, endometriosis, or cancer.

Injuries to the ureters and bladder are overall reported to occur in less than 1% of patients undergoing major gynecologic surgery.[3] Cystoscopy is often utilized to confirm an intact bladder and bilateral ureteral efflux after gynecologic procedures that carry a high risk of urologic injury.

Intestinal Tract Structures

The distal ileum, cecum, and appendix as well as the sigmoid colon and rectum are key gastrointestinal structures located near or within the pelvis. Gastrointestinal adhesions can occur as a result of prior surgeries, and careful attention is required to lyse adhesions in this setting in order to restore normal pelvic anatomy prior to completing any gynecologic procedure. These intestinal structures can also be involved as the result of various gynecologic pathology such as tuboovarian abscesses, endometriosis, or ovarian neoplasms. It is important to carefully inspect the intestinal organs to assure no occult injury during a gynecologic procedure, which is reported to occur in less than 1% of patients.[4] A "bubble" test, which involves insufflating the rectum with air with compression of the sigmoid and filling the pelvic with saline or water, is often useful in detecting an occult sigmoid injury.

COMMON VULVA AND VAGINAL SURGICAL DISEASES AND PROCEDURES

Common vulva and vaginal surgical diseases and procedures are listed in Table 71.2. A description of these diseases and management options follows.

TABLE 71.1 Lumbosacral nerve plexus.

NERVE	ORIGIN	MOTOR FUNCTION	SENSORY FUNCTION	INJURY SYMPTOMS
Ilioinguinal	T12–L1	None	Groin, symphysis	Sharp, burning pain radiating from incision site to groin or symphysis
Iliohypogastric	T12–L1	None	Mons, lateral labia, upper inner thigh	Sharp, burning pain radiating from incision site to mons, labia, or thigh
Genitofemoral	L1–L2	None	Upper labia, anterior superior thigh	Pain or paresthesia labia and femoral triangle
Lateral femoral	L2–L3	None	Anterior and posterior lateral thigh	Pain or paresthesia anterior and posterolateral thigh
Pudendal	S2–S4	None	Perineum	Perineal pain
Cutaneous femoral	L2–L4	Hip flexion, adduction Knee extension	Anterior and medial thigh, medial calf	Unable to climb stairs
Obturator	L2–L4	Thigh adduction	None	Minor ambulatory problems
Sciatic	L4–S3			
Common perineal		Hip extension, knee flexion Foot dorsiflexion Foot eversion	None Lateral calf Dorsum of foot	Foot drop
Tibial		Foot plantar flexion Foot inversion	Toes Plantar foot surface	Cavus deformity foot

TABLE 71.2 Common vulva and vaginal surgical diseases and procedures.

DISEASE	PROCEDURE OPTIONS
Bartholin cyst/abscess	Incision and drainage Marsupialization
Vulva intraepithelial neoplasia	Wide local excision Laser
Vulvar cancer	Radical vulvectomy with sentinel node biopsy or inguinal femoral lymphadenectomy
Vaginal intraepithelial neoplasia	Partial vaginectomy Laser
Vaginal cancer	Radical hysterectomy (rarely)
Prolapse	Sacral colpopexy Sacrospinous ligament suspension Anterior colporrhaphy Posterior colporrhaphy Colpocleisis

Common Vulvar and Vaginal Surgical Diseases

Bartholin Gland Cyst or Abscess

Blockage of the greater vestibular glands can result in accumulation of mucous and may lead to obstruction and abscess formation. This most commonly presents as a vulva mass on the lower medial labia major. Bartholin cysts may be asymptomatic and found incidentally on exam; however, they may become infected and form an abscess, which presents as a painful vulva mass. Patients with a symptomatic Bartholin gland cyst or abscess often require surgical intervention. Surgical management options include incision and drainage with placement of a Word catheter or marsupialization. Marsupialization is indicated for recurrent infections or when the size of abscess precludes incision and drainage. Excision of the gland is rarely indicated.

Vulva Intraepithelial Neoplasia

Vulva intraepithelial neoplasia (VIN) is a premalignant condition of the vulva. VIN was previously classified using a three-tier system (VIN I, II, or III). In 2015, the International Society for the Study for Vulvovaginal Disease (ISSVD) recommended using a two-tier grading system for classical VIN, which includes low-grade squamous intraepithelial lesion (LSIL), high-grade squamous intraepithelial lesion (HSIL), and a third category that separates VIN differentiated type.[5] The majority of LSIL and HSIL VIN is associated with the human papilloma virus (HPV), tends to occur in younger women, and is multifocal. The pathogenesis of VIN differentiated type is less well understood but tends to be associated with dermatosis of the vulva such as lichen sclerosis, seen more commonly in older women and is not associated HPV. Women with VIN often present with vulva itching or pain, although up to 40% of women may be asymptomatic at the time of diagnosis. Management includes colposcopy and biopsy to confirm the diagnosis. LSIL may be observed or treated with topical therapy such as imiquimod while the mainstay of treatment for HSIL is either wide local excision or laser ablation. Recurrence rates after treatment are high, and therefore, women should continue to be monitored after therapy.

Vulvar Cancer

Carcinoma of the vulva is a rare gynecologic cancer but still significantly contributes to overall mortality from reproductive tract cancers. Squamous cell carcinoma is the most common histology. Less common histologic subtypes include verrucous, basal cell, melanoma, sarcoma, extramammary Paget, and Bartholin gland carcinoma. Risk factors for vulva cancer include smoking, HPV infection, prior VIN, prior cervical dysplasia or cancer, lichen sclerosis, and immunodeficiency. Women most commonly present with a symptomatic nodular or ulcerative vulva lesion. Treatment is based upon clinical stage. For cancers confined to the vulva, surgical resection traditionally included radical vulvectomy with bilateral inguinal femoral lymph node dissection, which can be associated with high morbidity. Less radical techniques, in particular sentinel node dissection, have subsequently been adopted with decreased morbidity while preserving oncologic outcomes.[6,7] Treatment with chemoradiation has been the preferred strategy for larger vulvar cancers or those that involve the urethral meatus, vagina, or anus.

Vaginal Intraepithelial Neoplasia

Vaginal intraepithelial neoplasia (VaIN) is a premalignant condition of the vagina. Like VIN, it is classified using two-tier grading system LSIL (previously VaIN 1) and HSIL (previously VaIN II/III). Patients are often asymptomatic. Risk factors are similar to that for patients with VIN. Management is also similar to that for patients with VIN, albeit laser ablation is more frequently considered over partial vaginectomy for HSIL VaIN lesions.

Vaginal Cancer

Vaginal cancer is also quite rare. Squamous cell carcinoma is the most common histology. Less common histologic subtypes include adenocarcinoma, sarcoma, and melanoma. Risk factors other than those mentioned above for vulva cancer include diethylstilbestrol exposure in utero and prior radiation. The most common presenting symptom is vaginal bleeding followed by vaginal discharge, change in urinary symptoms or pain. Stage is the most significant prognostic feature. The majority of patients with vaginal cancer are treated with the combination of radiation and chemotherapy. Radical hysterectomy with upper vaginectomy is an option for the rare select patient with a small stage I cancer confined to the vaginal mucosa and located in the posterior vaginal fornix.

Pelvic Organ Prolapse

Pelvic organ prolapse is the herniation or downward displacement of the bladder (anterior vagina), cervix or vaginal cuff (apex), or rectum (posterior vagina) beyond their normal position. Risk factors include parity, age, obesity, chronic constipation, chronic obstructive pulmonary disease, connective tissue disorders, and smoking. Presenting symptoms are often pelvic pressure or bulge and/or changes in bowel or bladder function. Treatment depends on the degree of prolapse and patient symptoms. Treatment options include nonsurgical intervention including pessary, pelvic floor exercises and physical therapy, weight loss, smoking cessation, and estrogen therapy. Surgical intervention is reserved for women who have failed or declined conservative management and remain symptomatic.

Pelvic reconstructive surgery for pelvic organ prolapse is individualized with the goal to restore normal anatomy and function of the anterior, posterior, and apical vaginal compartments. The most common procedures for repair of apical prolapse are abdominal sacrocolpopexy (or its minimally-invasive laparoscopic or robotic variants), transvaginal sacrospinous ligament suspension, and transvaginal uterosacral ligament suspension. Repair of apical prolapse abdominally with sacrocolpopexy results in a lower rate of recurrence when compared to transvaginal approaches; however, it is associated with longer surgical time and delay in return to normal activities.[8] Long-term outcomes suggest that recurrence rates are approximately 25%.[9] There is no significant difference in long-term outcomes for uterosacral ligament suspension when compared to sacrospinous ligament suspension with reported failure rates of 62% and 70%, respectively.[10] Women with pelvic organ prolapse often have several compartments that are prolapsed and benefit from repair that addresses each of the compartments affected. Anterior and posterior colporrhaphy are often not needed when an abdominal sacrocolpopexy is performed as repair of apical defect often corrects the anterior and posterior defects.[11,12] However, anterior and posterior colporrhaphy are more often performed when the reconstruction is performed transvaginally in conjunction with uterosacral or sacrospinous ligament suspension.

Although most cases of pelvic organ prolapse are treated with reconstructive vaginal surgery as noted above, there are some instances in which vaginal reconstruction may not be desired or an option. For women who are not candidates for surgical reconstruction, and who are no longer sexually active, obliteration of the vaginal canal can alleviate the symptoms of pelvic organ prolapse without high surgical morbidity. Additional benefits of colpocleisis are shorter operative time, low risk of recurrence and similar patient satisfaction making this an appropriate choice for older women with multiple medical comorbidities who are not sexually active.

Common Vulva and Vaginal Surgical Procedures

Incision and Drainage of Bartholin Gland Cyst or Abscess

Incision and drainage of a Bartholin gland cyst or abscess is performed by stabilizing the cyst or abscess and making an incision over the center of the cyst or abscess on the medial aspect of the lesion just outside the hymenal ring (Fig. 71.6). A common mistake is to make the incision on the lateral aspect of the vulva. It may be necessary to utilize a hemostat to break up loculations and irrigate the cyst or abscess cavity. A small Word catheter is placed into the cyst for drainage and reevaluated on a weekly basis. Bartholin abscesses are often polymicrobial. Culture of purulent fluid should be obtained to evaluate for methicillin-resistant Staphylococcus aureus. Abscesses should be treated with appropriate antibiotics.

Marsupialization of Bartholin Gland Cyst or Abscess

Marsupialization is performed by creating an elliptical incision in the vestibular mucosa down to the wall of the gland. The wall of the gland is incised along the entire length of the ellipse. The contents are evacuated, and the wall of the cyst is sutured to the vestibular mucosa using 3-0 synthetic absorbable sutures in an interrupted fashion or using a baseball stitch.

Wide Local Excision/Laser of the Vulva

A wide local excision is a superficial excision of a vulva lesion and is most commonly utilized in the treatment of HSIL VIN (Fig. 71.7). The lesion is outlined with 1 cm margins. If the lesion is in close proximity to vital structures such as anus, clitoris, or urethra smaller margins may be utilized for cosmesis or to preserve function. After making an incision along the outline, the apex of the skin is then elevated, and the epidermis is removed. The depth of incision is 2 to 3 mm. Removal of dermis is not necessary for preinvasive disease. The defect is reapproximated using running or interrupted sutures depending on surgeon preference and size of lesion.

CO_2 laser vaporization maybe utilized as alternative to surgical resection for HSIL VIN. For HSIL VIN, it is best used for patients with multifocal disease, with disease close to vital structures such as the anus, urethral or clitoris, or with extensive VIN lesions in which surgical resection would be disfiguring. CO_2 laser vaporization should be utilized only when there is a low clinical suspicion for malignancy and when vulva biopsies have confirmed no evidence of invasive cancer. A depth of 1 mm is utilized on nonhair-bearing areas of the vulva and 3 mm on hair-bearing areas of the vulva. Colposcopy is utilized to increase precision with laser therapy. [13]

Laser of the Vagina/Partial Vaginectomy

For HSIL VaIN, CO_2 laser vaporization is a useful preferred approach for newly diagnosed patients. It is easier to do than partial

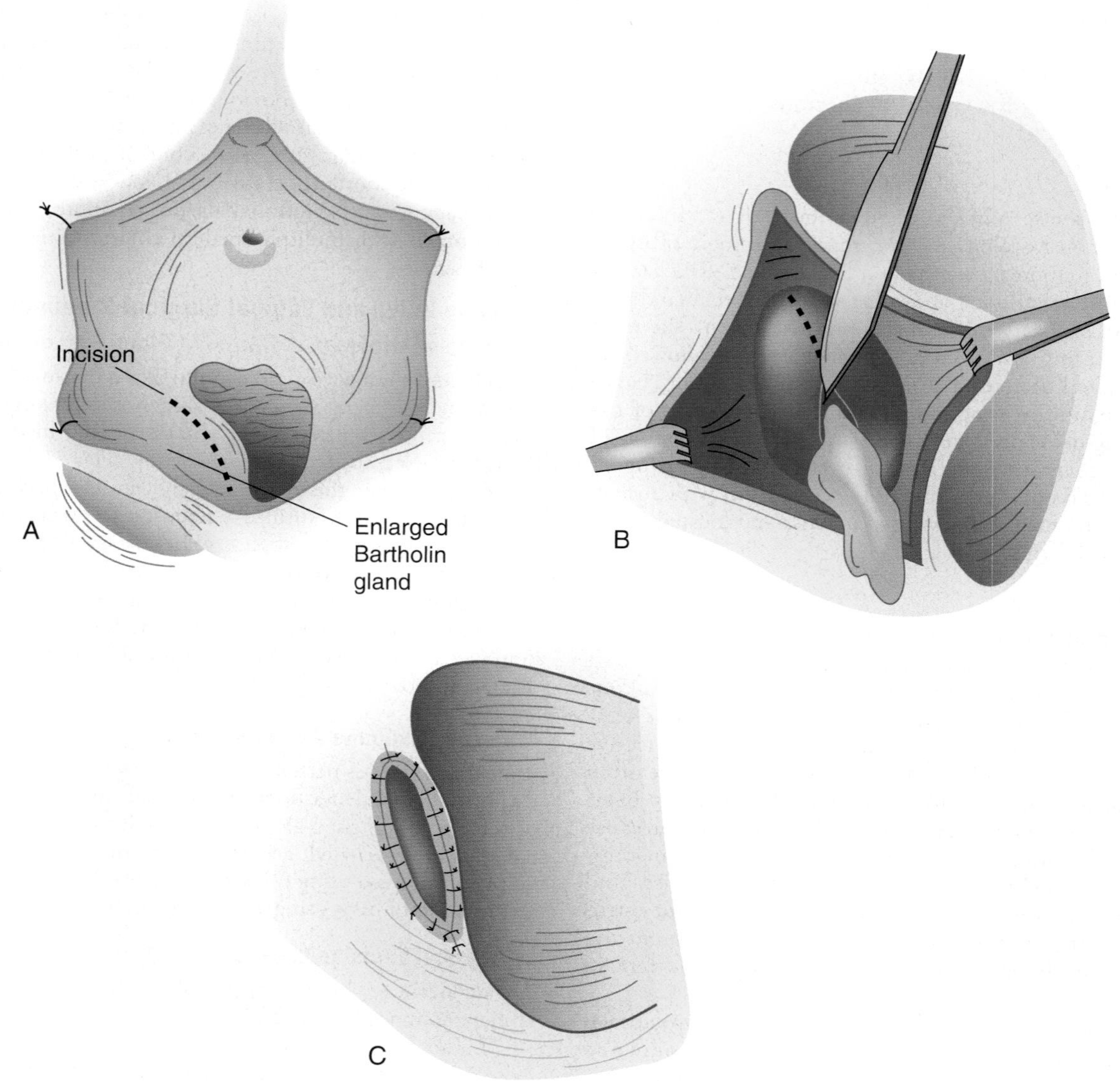

FIG. 71.6 Bartholin gland marsupialization. (A) Retraction of the labia and incision over the mucosa of the vagina. (B) Wall of the gland is excised. (C) Completed marsupialization. (Adapted from Mitchell CW, Wheeless CR. *Atlas of pelvic surgery*. 3rd ed. Philadelphia, PA: Lippincott Williams & Wilkins; 1997.)

vaginectomy and has less risk of injury to adjacent structures. Ablation of the involved superficial vaginal dermis along with a 1- to 2-cm margin should suffice. A partial vaginectomy involves excision of the vaginal epithelium and is most commonly used for patients with HSIL VaIN who have had a prior hysterectomy and recurred after prior CO_2 laser procedure. The surgical approach is usually vaginally and the lesion with a 1- to 2-cm margin is excised. Care is taken to avoid injury to the bladder or colon. Depending on the size of the lesion, vaginal reconstruction may be required.

Radical Vulvectomy With Sentinel Node Mapping and Biopsy or Inguinal Femoral Lymphadenectomy

Radical vulvectomy for vulva cancer can be either total or partial depending on the extent of involvement and lesion location. The procedure starts by outlining the vulva cancer lesion with a 2-cm margin. As with a wide local incision, smaller margins are reasonable to preserve function around vital structures. In contrast to a wide local excision where just the superficial vulva skin is removed, the incision in a radical vulvectomy is carried down beneath the subcutaneous tissue to the fascia of the urogenital diaphragm. Care is taken to identify and ligate the clitoris and its vessels anteriorly and the bulbocavernosis muscles and the internal pudendal vessels laterally, as applicable. The specimen is amputated and marked for orientation. Primary closure is achieved by closing the subcutaneous tissue with interrupted absorbable suture. Skin closure may be performed using running or interrupted sutures.

Sentinel lymph node (SLN) mapping and biopsy is the preferred technique for lymph node evaluation in early stage vulva cancer with lesions that are less than 4 cm in diameter. The vulva lesion is injected preoperatively with a radioactive isotype subdermally at four sites around the vulva lesion. A preoperative nuclear scan or single photon emission computed tomography (SPECT) may be used for identifying the sentinel node and for surgical planning. The use of blue dye with radioactive tracer increases sensitivity for detection of the sentinel node. Isosulfan blue is currently the most commonly used dye.[7,14,15]

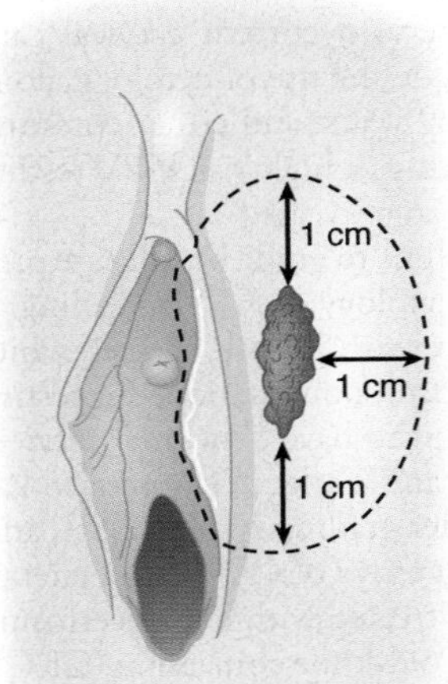

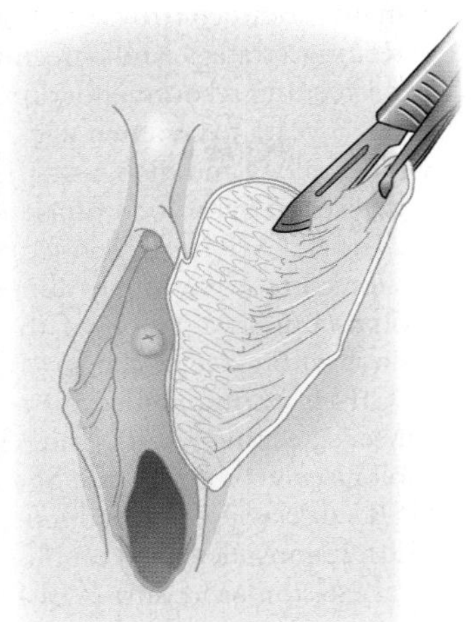
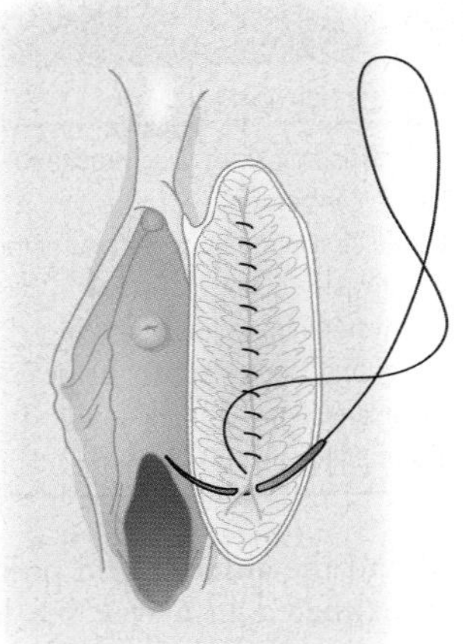
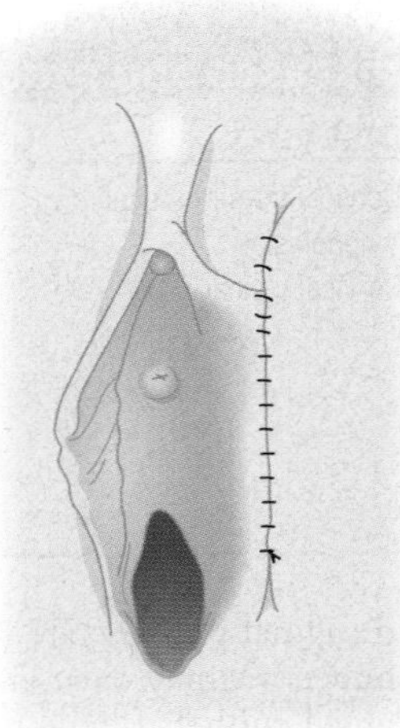

FIG. 71.7 Wide local excision of vaginal intraepithelial neoplasia lesion.

If no SLN is identified or a patient is not a candidate for SLN dissection, a full inguinofemoral lymphadenectomy is performed. An incision is made parallel to and approximately 2 cm below the inguinal ligament. All lymph node-bearing tissue between the inguinal ligament superiorly, the sartorius muscle laterally, and the adductor longus muscle medially is removed. Preservation of the great saphenous decreases rates of lymphedema. The cribriform fascia may be opened to remove the deep femoral lymph nodes. A suction drain is placed, and primary closure is achieved by closing the subcutaneous tissue with interrupted absorbable suture. Skin closure may be performed using a running absorbable suture or staples.

Pelvic Prolapse Procedures

Vault suspensions (abdominal sacrocolpopexy, sacrospinous ligament suspension, uterosacral ligament suspension). Abdominal sacralcolpoplexy may be performed via laparotomy, laparoscopy, or robotic approaches and may be performed concurrently with hysterectomy or in women with posthysterectomy apical prolapse. The vesicovaginal space is developed and the bladder dissected off the anterior vagina while the rectovaginal space is developed, and the rectum dissected off the posterior vagina. A Y-shaped mesh graph is sutured to the anterior and posterior vagina. The peritoneum over the sacral promontory is then incised. Permanent suture is utilized to secure the graft to the anterior sacral ligament at the anterior sacrum. Care is taken to avoid injuring the middle sacral vessels. The retroperitoneum is then reapproximated.

Sacrospinous ligament suspension is the most studied transvaginal procedure for treating apical prolapse. The perirectal space is entered through the posterior vagina and the vaginal epithelium dissected off to the level of the ischial spine. The rectovaginal space is opened so that the ischial spine can be palpated. One to two sutures are placed through the sacrospinous ligament with care taken to protect the pudendal vessels and nerves and then through the muscularis of the posterior vaginal epithelium, and subsequently ligated by use of a pulley stitch.

A high uterosacral ligament suspension is typically performed after completion of a total vaginal hysterectomy. Following hysterectomy, the bowels are packed away, and the uterosacral ligaments are identified. Delayed absorbable sutures (one to three) are passed through the uterosacral ligament bilaterally. The first suture is passed just above the level of the ischial spine and second suture is more proximal. The sutures are held with a hemostat. Cystoscopy is then performed to ensure integrity of the bladder and efflux of urine from both ureteral orifices. The previously tagged needles of the sutures on the right side are then passed through the cervicovaginal (anterior) fascia and epithelium then through the posterior rectovaginal fascia and vaginal epithelium at the vaginal apex to suspend the vagina anteriorly, posteriorly, and apically.

Anterior/posterior colporrhaphy. Anterior colporrhaphy begins with incision of the anterior vaginal epithelium to the level of the apex of the cystocele and is then dissected off of the underlying pubocervical fascia laterally to the pubic rami. The pubocervical fascia is plicated in the midline using a series of interrupted sutures of delayed absorbable suture from the bladder neck to the bladder base. Excess vaginal skin, when present, should be excised. The anterior vaginal epithelium is closed with a delayed absorbable suture.

Posterior colporrhaphy is performed by incising the posterior vaginal epithelium vertically past the rectocele and then dissecting it off of the rectovaginal septum laterally to the level of the levator ani muscles. The rectovaginal septum is plicated to the midline with delayed absorbable suture. If there is excess vaginal epithelium, this is often excised and then closed with a running suture of delayed absorbable suture. At the level of the perineal body, if it is deficient, a modified Crown stitch is often performed to reattached the bulbocavernosus muscles to the transverse perineal muscles and the rectovaginal fascia. Digital rectal exam should be performed at completion to ensure that a rectal injury did not occur. Care must be taken to avoid overnarrowing the vagina or introitus.

Colpocleisis. The most commonly performed colpocleisis technique is the LeFort (partial) procedure, which involves obliteration of the vaginal canal when the uterus is left in situ. Care, should be taken to avoid the LeFort procedure in women with high risk of uterine or cervix cancer as future sampling cannot be performed. Appropriate preoperative workup should include transvaginal ultrasound or endometrial biopsy and Pap smear. For the LeFort procedure, traction is placed on cervix and a significant rectangular-shaped portion of the anterior vaginal epithelium is incised and denuded. The bladder neck is plicated with delayed absorbable suture. A similar portion of the posterior vaginal epithelium is then incised and denuded. The uterine

TABLE 71.3 Common cervical surgical diseases and procedures.

DISEASE	PROCEDURE OPTIONS
Cervical intraepithelial neoplasia	Loop electrosurgical excision procedure Cold-knife conization
Cervical cancer	Cold-knife conization/simple hysterectomy (microinvasive disease) Radical hysterectomy/trachelectomy with sentinel node biopsy or pelvic lymphadenectomy +/- para-aortic lymphadenectomy

and vaginal prolapse are reduced and the anterior and posterior denuded vaginal walls are reapproximated in a way the leaves bilateral epithelial-lined tunnels to allow for drainage of cervical mucus.

Colpectomy with total colpocleisis is performed in a woman who has previously had a hysterectomy. In this case, the entire vaginal epithelium is excised, and the underlying vaginal connective tissue is reapproximated with serial purse-string absorbable sutures until the prolapse is completely reduced. Care must be taken with both techniques not to bring the colpocleisis too close to the bladder neck as severe urinary incontinence may result from iatrogenically opening the bladder neck.

COMMON CERVICAL SURGICAL DISEASES AND PROCEDURES

Common cervical surgical diseases and procedures are listed in Table 71.3. A description of these diseases and management options follow.

Common Cervical Surgical Diseases

Cervical Intraepithelial Neoplasia

CIN is a premalignant condition of the cervix caused by HPV infection. The lifetime cumulative risk of HPV infection is 80%; however, the majority of HPV infections are transient and do not lead to the development of CIN. Persistent HPV infection, particularly with HPV types 16 and 18, has a high rate of progression to CIN and, if not treated, invasive cancer. The average time from HPV infection to invasive disease is generally over 15 years. Risks factors for HPV infection and CIN include early sexual debut, multiple sexual partners, and a history of sexually transmitted infections. Risk factors for persistent HPV infection are not fully understood but include an immunocompromised state and smoking. HPV vaccines, initially approved in 2006, significantly reduce the risk of anogenital warts and CIN. Gardasil 9, which prevents HPV-associated anogenital warts and CIN caused by HPV types 6, 11, 16, 18, 31, 33, 45, 52, and 58 was approved in 2014 for males and females ages 9 to 26.[16]

Over the past seven decades, cervical cancer screening with cytologic evaluation of the cervix (the "Pap" smear) has resulted in significant decreases in the incidence of and mortality associated with cervical cancer primarily in developed countries. Most cervical cancer now occurs in low resource countries or locations where screening is not widely available and in women who have had no or inadequate cervical cancer screening. High-risk HPV testing has emerged as an important technology for cervical cancer screening as a result of our better understanding of the role of high-risk HPV in the development of CIN. Although there remains some controversy regarding the optimal cervical cancer screening strategy and screening intervals, current cervical cancer screening recommendations include the use of cytology alone every 3 years for women age 21 to 29 years, and either cotesting with cytology and high-risk HPV testing or high-risk HPV testing only every 5 years for women age 30 to 65 years.[17]

The ASCCP has developed algorithms to guide health care professions on the workup of abnormal cytology or HPV screening.[18] Colposcopic evaluation of the cervix with biopsy of acetowhite lesions with vascular changes (mosaicism, punctuation) suggestive of CIN is recommended for patients who have abnormal cervical cancer screening results. The ASCCP and College of American Pathologists recommend use of a two-tier grading system, LSIL and HSIL, to classify biopsied lesions suggestive of CIN.[19] In general, HSIL lesions identified on biopsy are treated with loop electrosurgical excision procedure (LEEP) or a cold-knife conization (CKC). In resource-constrained areas, the use of "see and treat" approaches have been implemented in lieu of the traditional screening used in the developed world. Early detection and treatment of premalignant conditions is essential to preventing cervical cancer.

Cervical Cancer

The incidence of cervical cancer has declined in the past decade due to improved screening modalities and the development of the HPV vaccine. Although cervix cancer in developed countries like the United States is relatively rare, it remains one of the most common cancers worldwide and the leading cause of morbidity and mortality due to cancer in women in the developing world. In developed countries, cervical cancer affects a disproportionate percentage of women of low socioeconomic status and minority ethnic and racial groups. Squamous cell and adenocarcinomas are the two most common histologic subtypes. Although the rates of squamous cell carcinoma have decreased, there has been an increase in incidence of adenocarcinoma and adenosquamous carcinomas in some countries like the United States.[20]

Women with cervical cancer most commonly present with irregular or heavy bleeding, postcoital bleeding, vaginal discharge, or pelvic pain. The diagnosis is confirmed by cervical biopsy. Cervical cancer is staged clinically, and treatment depends on stage. In early stage disease, surgical approaches are equally effective as chemotherapy and radiation. Radical hysterectomy with either sentinel node biopsy or pelvic/para-aortic lymphadenectomy is the surgical approach of choice for select patients with early stage cervical cancer who are unlikely to require adjuvant radiation. Sentinel node biopsy with injection of either methylene blue or indocyanine green into the cervix has increasingly been incorporated into the management of patients with cervical cancer. In the SENTICOL study, 98% of patients had sentinel nodes identified with a 92% sensitivity, a 98% NPV, and a 0% false negative rate.[21]

Recent studies have suggested the risk of recurrence is higher for patients who have radical hysterectomy performed using minimally invasive procedures, particularly when the size of a cervical lesion exceeds 2 cm.[22,23] Thus, an open approach may be preferred in most instances. Radical trachelectomy might be considered for select patients who wish to retain fertility. Simple hysterectomy is being evaluated in several ongoing randomized control trials in lieu of radical hysterectomy for early stage cervical cancer. At present, simple hysterectomy or conization may be an option for select patients with microinvasive disease. In locally advanced disease, chemotherapy and radiation are more effective and the mainstay of treatment.

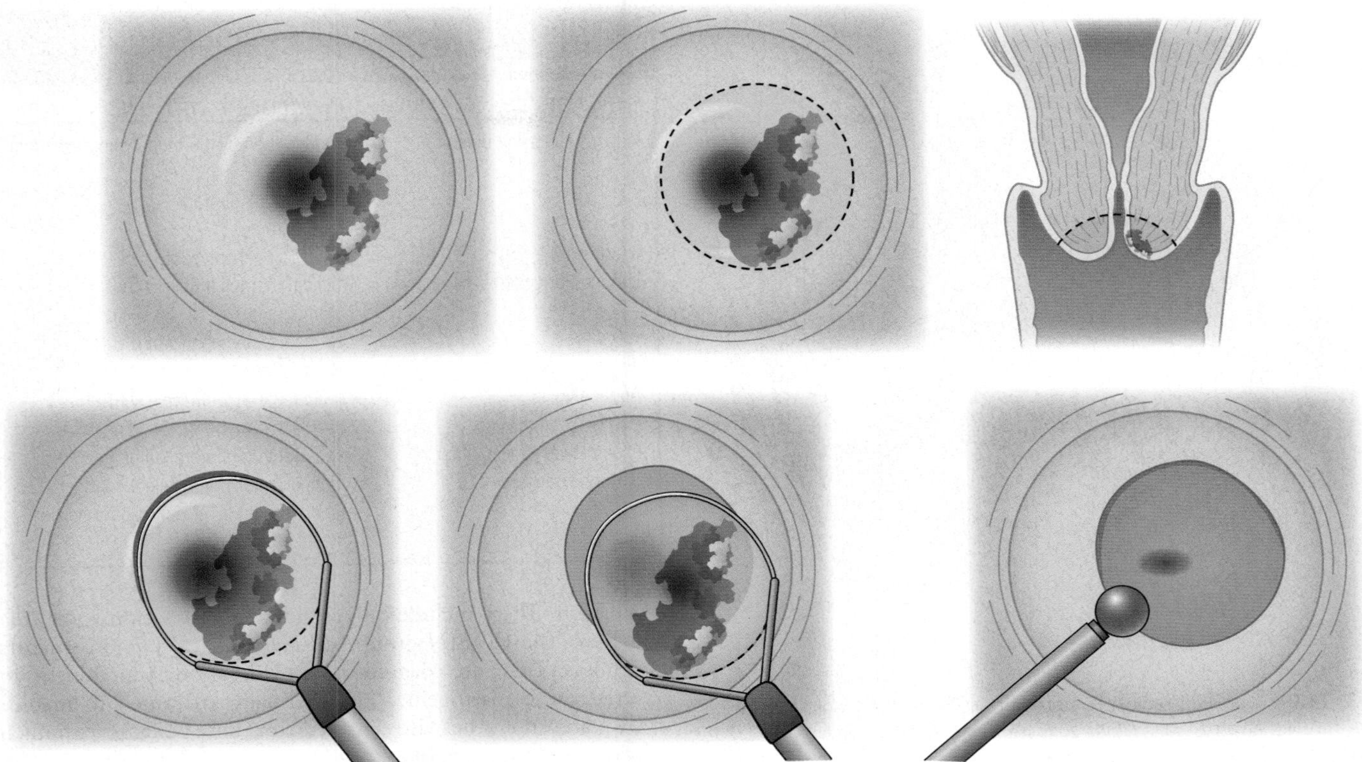

FIG. 71.8 Loop electrosurgical excision procedure.

Common Cervical Surgical Techniques

Conization/Loop Electrosurgical Excision Procedure

Removal of portion of the cervix for diagnosis and treatment of cervical dysplasia can be achieved by a LEEP or CKC. A LEEP may be performed in the office whereas a CKC is often done in the operating room (OR) due to need for increased exposure and a longer operating time. A LEEP uses a wire loop that is heated by electrical current to excise the transformation zone of the cervix with the involved areas of CIN (Fig. 71.8). It is common practice to perform a small excision often called a "top hat" after removal of first specimen. To perform a CKC, figure-of-8 retention sutures are placed at the 3 and 9 o'clock positions to ligate the descending branch of the uterine artery. After applying Lugol to the cervix to outline the areas of involvement and injecting lidocaine with epinephrine to reduce bleeding, a circumferential incision is made around the transformation zone and lesion using a Beaver blade. The specimen is grasped with Allis clamps to maintain orientation. The specimen is amputated using scalpel or Mayo scissors. A marking stitch is placed at the 12 o'clock position. An endocervical curettage is performed about the cone biopsy. A running locked stich or Sturmdorf stitch may be performed to evert the endocervical canal and achieve hemostasis.

Radical Hysterectomy/Radical Trachelectomy With Pelvic Lymphadenectomy

Radical hysterectomy refers to the excision of the uterus, parametrium, and upper vagina. This can be performed via an open, minimally invasive, or vaginal approach. A shared decision regarding the approach to the procedure should take into consideration the aforementioned data suggesting an increased risk of recurrence with minimally invasive approaches particularly in setting where an early-stage cervical cancer lesion exceeds 2 cm in diameter.[22,23] If an open procedure is chosen, a transverse incision such as a Maylard or Cherney is often utilized to increase lateral exposure.

There are several different classification systems utilized to describe the extent of resection of tissues surrounding the cervix. The Piver-Rutledge-Smith classification is the oldest and most commonly used system.[24] It is divided into five classes starting with class I (simple, extrafascial hysterectomy) up to class V (which describes removal of uterus en bloc with parametrium, partial ureteral resection/bladder resection or both). Class II–IV varies on amount of cardinal and ureterosacral ligaments and vagina that are removed as well as where the uterine artery is ligated. The modified radical hysterectomy that is most commonly used today is type III (Fig. 71.9). The principles of a radical hysterectomy include developing the paravesical and pararectal pelvic spaces, dividing the uterine arteries and veins, dissection of the bladder and ureters off the anterior cardinal ligament, and dissection of the rectum and pararectal tissues off the posterior cardinal ligament. The cardinal ligaments are then divided to allow an adequate sample of parametrium and margin. The ovaries are generally spared for premenopausal women.

A radical trachelectomy may be an option for women who desire future fertility with the International Federation of Gynecology and Obstetrics (FIGO) stage IA1 with lymphovascular space invasion, stage IA2 or stage IB1 disease. Most experts recommend this approach for malignant lesions 2 cm or less in diameter. The procedure is performed similar to the radical hysterectomy with removal of the cervix, parametria and upper vagina.[25] However, the body of the uterus is preserved, a cerclage is placed, and the uterus is reattached to the superior vagina.

Pelvic lymphadenectomy is usually performed in conjunction with a radical hysterectomy or trachelectomy for early stage cervical cancer patients. Resection of para-aortic lymph nodes is not routinely performed by all surgeons, particularly if there is no evidence

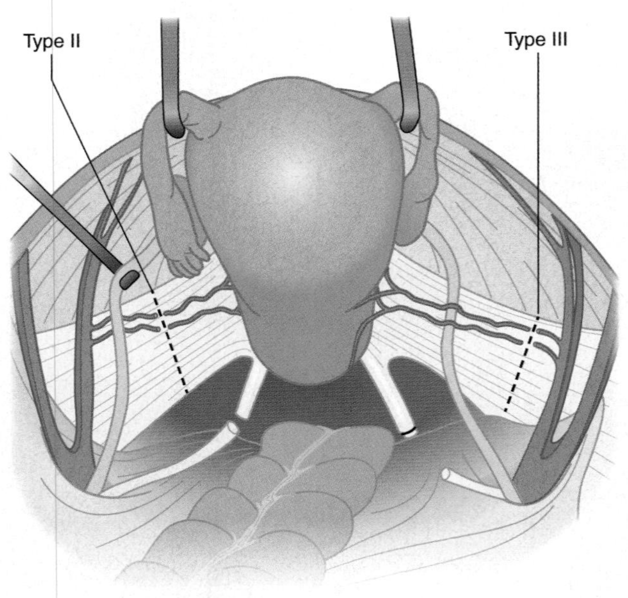

FIG. 71.9 Type II/III radical hysterectomy. (From Frederick, PJ, Whitworth, JM, Alvarez, RD. *Glob. libr. women's med. (ISSN: 1756-2228)* 2011; DOI 10.3843/GLOWM.10232)

of metastasis in the para-aortic or pelvic nodes. Pelvic lymphadenectomy should include the nodes that are lateral and medial to the external iliac artery and vein from the bifurcation of the common iliac artery to the level of the deep circumflex iliac vein. Nodes from the obturator space between the external iliac vein and obturator nerve should also be excised. When performed, para-aortic lymphadenectomy should be performed bilaterally by removing the nodes lateral to the common iliac artery and aorta from the bifurcation of the common iliac to the level of the inferior mesenteric artery.

COMMON UTERINE SURGICAL DISEASES AND PROCEDURES

Common uterine surgical diseases and procedures are listed in Table 71.4. A description of these diseases and management options follows.

Common Uterine Surgical Diseases

Abnormal Uterine Bleeding

Abnormal uterine bleeding (AUB) is one of the most common gynecologic complaints and conditions in the reproductive age female. It is defined as bleeding that occurs in excess of or in addition to the normal menstrual cycle bleeding. A normal menstrual should occur regularly between 24 and 38 days, with duration of flow between 4 to 8 days. Previously, AUB was often referred to as menorrhagia, menometrorrhagia, or dysfunctional uterine bleeding, but these terms have been replaced with a classification system aimed at identifying the cause of the excess bleeding. The PALM-COEIN system was established in 2011 as a result of work by the FIGO Working Group on Menstrual Disorders. Each letter in the acronym PALM-COEIN represents a condition, which is an etiology of AUB.[26] The PALM group includes structural entities that can be diagnosed with imaging modalities or histologic

TABLE 71.4 Common uterine surgical diseases and procedures.

DISEASE	PROCEDURE OPTIONS
Abnormal uterine bleeding	Medical therapy (hormonal suppression of cycles) Endometrial ablation Hysterectomy
Uterine polyp	Hysteroscopic polypectomy
Uterine fibroids (leiomyomata)	Medical therapy for cycle control Myomectomy Uterine artery embolization Hysterectomy
Adenomyosis	Medical therapy for cycle control Hysterectomy
Endometrial cancer/other uterine cancers	Hysterectomy/bilateral salpingo-oophorectomy with select sentinel node dissection or pelvic/para-aortic lymphadenectomy

evaluation. These include polyps, adenomyosis, leiomyoma, malignancy. The COEIN group includes medical or nonstructural diagnoses. These are coagulopathy, ovulatory dysfunction, endometrial causes, iatrogenic causes (usually attributed to medications), and "not otherwise classified" for those patients without an obvious underlying etiology.

The initial work up for AUB includes a detailed history; a pelvic exam to assess for tenderness, mass, or uterine enlargement; a pregnancy test; laboratory evaluation of thyroid, blood count, prolactin level, androgen levels, follicle stimulating hormone, and estrogen level; cervical cancer screening if not up-to-date; screening for sexually transmitted infections; and a pelvic ultrasound.[27] Screening for coagulation disorders is indicated if heavy bleeding has been present since menarche, there is a family history of coagulopathy, the patient is on a medication associated with abnormal bleeding, or there are signs and symptoms of other system bleeding (nose bleeds, easy bruising, etc.).[27]

Endometrial biopsy, usually an office procedure, is indicated to rule out endometrial hyperplasia or malignancy in patients at elevated risk for these conditions. Women age 45 or older with any increased bleeding, either intermenstrual bleeding or heavier/longer menstrual bleeding, should undergo endometrial sampling. Women younger than 45 years old with risk of unopposed estrogen exposure, such as those with obesity and ovulatory dysfunction, with persistent AUB or failed medical management, or with elevated familial risk of cancer should also be biopsied.[27]

Postmenopausal bleeding is not included in the PALM-COEIN classification system and is considered its own diagnosis. While many causes of AUB in the reproductive age female are physiologic, any bleeding in the postmenopausal female should be considered abnormal and requires thorough evaluation. The most common cause of abnormal bleeding in a postmenopausal female is atrophy, a thinning of the endometrial lining and vaginal tissue due to lack of estrogen. Without the lubrication and insulation that a thickened endometrial lining provides, the uterine cavity is susceptible to inflammation and infection.

The major concern with postmenopausal bleeding is an underlying malignant or premalignant condition. An estimated 6% to 19% of women with postmenopausal bleeding have an endometrial cancer.[28] Other causes of postmenopausal bleeding include uterine polyps, fibroids, adenomyosis, and medications (most commonly, hormone replacement therapies and anticoagulants). The initial evaluation, in addition to a thorough history and physical exam, includes a pelvic ultrasound and endometrial biopsy. If the endometrial thickness on pelvic ultrasound is 4 mm or less, endometrial biopsy can be avoided. However, biopsy is indicated for endometrial thickness greater than 4 mm, suspected focal lesion on imaging, difficulty visualizing the endometrium, or persistent bleeding despite a normal ultrasound.[29,30]

Uterine Polyps

Uterine polyps, also called endometrial polyps, are an overgrowth of endometrial glands and stroma that either lie flat along the endometrial lining (sessile polyps) or project out into the cavity (pedunculated polyps). They have an inner "feeder vessel" that often allows them to be diagnosed by Doppler sonography. As discussed previously, they are a common cause of AUB or postmenopausal bleeding. There is large variability in polyp size from a few millimeters to several centimeters, with larger polyps being easier to detect. The majority of endometrial polyps are benign; however, up to 5% of polyps can undergo malignant transformation.[31] Factors associated uterine polyp formation include increasing age, increased estrogen exposure, tamoxifen use, obesity, and familial hereditary cancer syndromes.[32,33] In addition to AUB, endometrial polyps may be associated with an increased risk of early pregnancy loss. Treatment of endometrial polyps is reviewed in the next section.

Leiomyoma

Uterine leiomyomata, or fibroids, are the most common benign gynecologic tumors, affecting up to 30% of women according to most population-based studies.[34] There is a predominance in black women, with prevalence up to 50%. Fibroids are smooth muscle tumors that arise in the myometrium of the uterus. They can be located anywhere within the uterine wall and are often classified based on their location (Table 71.5).[35] Type 0 fibroids are located completely in the uterine cavity and are often attached with a stalk. Type 1 and 2 fibroids are submucosal; type 1 fibroids involve less than 50% of the myometrium while type 2 fibroids extend into the wall 50% or more. Types 3, 4, and 5 are intramural fibroids, located completely within the uterine wall with increasing subserosal contact as the numbers increase. Type 6 and 7 fibroids are subserosal (type 7 pedunculated) while type 8 are cervical fibroids. Fibroids can be very small or very large and can be single or multiple. They are diagnosed with pelvic imaging, usually an ultrasound or magnetic resonance imaging (MRI).

Symptoms of fibroids, commonly abnormal bleeding, pelvic pain, or pressure-related symptoms from adjacent organs, are directly related to the location and size of the fibroid(s). The treatment options are also related to location and size of fibroids. Treatment options are medical or surgical, depending on patient desires and future fertility plans. Surgical treatments are discussed in the following section. Medical options are often directed at bleeding symptoms and include many contraceptive-type medications. Fibroids tend to grow in the reproductive years and regress in size with menopause, thus indicating a relationship between fibroid growth and ovarian hormones. Other risk factors include familial predisposition, obesity, and some dietary factors.[36]

Adenomyosis

Adenomyosis is defined as the presence of endometrial glands and stroma within the myometrium and is considered a variant of endometriosis. Often, they are found together at the time of hysterectomy.[37] There is a molecular interaction between the displaced endometrial cells and the adjacent myometrial cells, which causes hypertrophy of the myometrium and inflammation. In some patients, this results in a heavier, enlarged uterus. Additionally, the pathogenesis of adenomyosis has similarities to fibroids, with both conditions exhibiting increased angiogenesis and growth factor expression.[38] Adenomyosis often coexists with uterine leiomyoma. While adenomyosis is commonly a postsurgical diagnosis in that it is diagnosed by pathology, it can be clinically suspected and sometimes identified on pelvic imaging. On ultrasound or MRI imaging, adenomyosis is seen as heterogeneity in the myometrium, a blurring of the junction between the endometrium and myometrium, or the presence of "cysts" within the myometrial layer.[39] Adenomyomas, which can be confused for uterine leiomyomata, are discrete masses of adenomyosis, which are seen as focal asymmetric thickening of the myometrium.

The prevalence of adenomyosis is estimated around 30% of women of reproductive age with increasing prevalence in the later reproductive years. It is found more commonly in multiparous women compared to nulliparous women.[40] Symptoms of adenomyosis are heavy, painful periods, irregular bleeding, painful intercourse, and noncyclic pelvic pain. Some women with adenomyosis will be asymptomatic. Adenomyosis is treated medically with nonsteroidal antiinflammatory drugs and hormonal contraceptives for patients who are symptomatic and do not desire surgical intervention. Simple hysterectomy is the surgical intervention of choice for those patients who have failed medical management and do not desire further fertility.

Endometrial and Other Uterine Cancers

Endometrial cancer is the most common gynecologic cancer and is increasing in incidence, particularly in countries experiencing an obesity epidemic. Other common risk factors include age, diabetes, nulliparity, polycystic ovarian syndrome and the use of unopposed estrogen or tamoxifen. Women with hereditary nonpolyposis colorectal cancer syndrome, commonly known as Lynch syndrome, have up to a 60% lifetime risk of developing endometrial cancer.[41] Lynch syndrome is an autosomal dominant genetic disorder that involves mutations in mismatch repair genes (*MLH1, MSH2, MSH6, PMS2*). The highest risk of endometrial cancer in Lynch syndrome occurs in patients with an MLH1 or MSH2 mutation and endometrial cancer will often be the first cancer to present in women with Lynch syndrome. Women with Lynch syndrome also have an increased risk for ovarian cancer and prophylactic hysterectomy with bilateral salpingo-oophorectomy should be a consideration for affected women.

Most women with endometrial cancer present with symptoms of postmenopausal or AUB. Most patients with endometrial cancer present with early stage disease and will have no other symptoms or abnormal examination findings other than evidence of uterine bleeding. Evaluation should include a transvaginal pelvic ultrasound and endometrial biopsy or hysteroscopy with dilation and curettage if one is unable to perform an office endometrial biopsy or if endometrial biopsy is not informative. A pelvic MRI should be performed for patients with apparent early stage disease who are considering fertility-sparing hormonal therapy options. Approximately 15% of patients will present with symptoms and examination findings suggestive of more advanced stage disease. Abdominal pelvic computed tomography (CT) should be considered in addition to transvaginal pelvic ultrasound and endometrial sampling in these instances. Most patients will have endometrioid adenocarcinoma on pathologic evaluation of biopsy samples.

TABLE 71.5 FIGO classification system for uterine fibroids.*

TYPE	LOCATION	OPERATIVE REMOVAL APPROACH
0	Intracavitary	Vaginal or hysteroscopic
1	Submucosal	Hysteroscopic
2	Submucosal/intramural	Hysteroscopic or open/laparoscopic
3,4,5	Intramural	Open or laparoscopic
6	Intramural/subserosal	Open or laparoscopic
7	Subserosal/pedunculated	Open or laparoscopic
8	Extrauterine (parasitic, broad ligament, cervical, etc)	Open or laparoscopic

*Adapted from Munro MG, Critchley HO, Broder MS, et al: FIGO classification system (PALM-COEIN) for causes of abnormal uterine bleeding in nongravid women of reproductive age. *Int J Gynaecol Obstet.* 113:3–13, 2011.

Other histologic types include serous carcinoma, clear cell carcinoma, and carcinosarcoma, all of which are associated with higher risk of extrauterine metastasis and recurrence and poorer long-term survival.

Most patients with apparent early stage endometrial cancer are best treated with total hysterectomy and bilateral salpingo-oophorectomy using minimally invasive surgical techniques. The Gynecologic Oncology Group LAP2 study randomized patients with clinically early-stage endometrial cancer to either exploratory laparotomy or laparoscopic approach to total abdominal hysterectomy bilateral salpingectomy and staging.[42,43] This study demonstrated improved surgical outcomes and shorter length of hospital stay in patients undergoing a laparoscopic approach with similar recurrence and overall survival rates when compared to patients undergoing exploratory laparotomy. A robotic approach has been increasingly employed for patients with early-stage endometrial cancer.[44] A robotic approach to the treatment of early-stage endometrial cancer has been demonstrated to be associated with lower rates of conversion to exploratory laparotomy when compared to a laparoscopic approach, a rate that exceeds 25% in patients with a body mass index (BMI) of 35 or greater.[42,44]

Surgical staging for patients with early stage endometrial cancer has continued to evolve over the past two decades. Bilateral pelvic and para-aortic lymphadenectomy with evaluation for intraperitoneal metastasis are key components of staging, albeit the value of lymphadenectomy with respect to a survival advantage has been the subject of debate.[45] Patients with low-risk endometrial cancer as defined by Mayo criteria (grade 1–2 endometrioid adenocarcinoma, 2 cm or less in diameter with less than 50% myometrial invasion, and absence of extrauterine disease) have very low rates of metastasis and lymphadenectomy is not advised.[46] Sentinel node biopsy with injection of either methylene blue or indocyanine green into the cervix has increasingly been incorporated into the management of patients with endometrial cancer.[47] Over 80% of patients will have the sentinel nodes identified. Sentinel node techniques are associated with over a 95% sensitivity of detecting a nodal metastasis, a 99% NPV, and a less than 2% false negative rate.[48]

Patients with more extensive extrauterine disease generally benefit from cytoreductive surgery similar to that done in patients with ovarian cancer. Other rarer subtypes of uterine cancers include high-grade sarcoma, low-grade endometrial stromal sarcoma, and leiomyosarcoma. In the absence of clinically obvious nodal metastasis, lymphadenectomy is not required.

Common Uterine Surgical Procedures

Hysteroscopy, Dilation and Curettage, Endometrial Ablation

Hysteroscopy is the placement of a small telescope into the uterine cavity for diagnostic purposes. It can be performed in the office in conjunction with a paracervical block or light anesthesia, or in the OR. If operative hysteroscopy is planned for the resection of a uterine lesion, general or regional anesthesia is required. After placement of a speculum, a single-tooth tenaculum is placed on the anterior lip of the cervix for gentle inferior retraction of the cervix to flatten the curve at the cervicouterine junction and the cervix is gently dilated. Normal saline solution is attached to a 12 or 30-degree hysteroscope for diagnostic hysteroscopy or operative hysteroscopy with bipolar current. If operative hysteroscopy with monopolar current is planned, then a hypotonic solution, such as glycine or mannitol is used.

With the distention media running, the hysteroscope scope is passed through the cervix and into the uterine cavity under direct visualization. The speculum can be removed once the scope is in the uterine cavity as it can impede mobility of the scope and impact visualization of the entire cavity or the execution of an operative procedure. Under pressure, the cavity is distended to allow the surgeon to visualize the fundus, both tubal ostia, the lower uterine segment, and the cervix. An operative hysteroscope will allow passage of scissors, graspers, or electrosurgical instruments for resection or biopsy of lesions. For global sampling, a curettage is performed after the hysteroscopy. The hysteroscope is first removed, and then a curette is passed through the cervix to the fundus. Gentle curettage is performed along all four surfaces of the uterine cavity and the tissue is sent to pathology.

Operative hysteroscopy is the treatment of intrauterine pathology under direct visualization with the hysteroscope. Common operative hysteroscopy procedures include directed biopsy or polypectomy, myomectomy, lysis of intrauterine synechiae (adhesions), and endometrial ablation. Hysteroscopic polypectomy can be performed using a variety of mechanical instruments (Fig. 71.10). Commonly utilized instruments for polypectomy include a biopsy forceps and scissors, a morcellator, various electrodes such as loop electrode, and a polyp snare. The procedure for hysteroscopic myomectomy is similar to polypectomy and is reviewed in section on hysteroscopic myomectomy. For uterine adhesions, scissors are used to lysis adhesions that connect the anterior and posterior walls of the uterine cavity.

Endometrial ablation is the destruction of the endometrial lining by heat or cold. Traditionally, this was performed via operative hysteroscopy with rollerball or loop electrode to coagulate or excise the endometrium down to the basalis layer. There are now several types of nonresectoscopic or "global" endometrial ablation devices, which do not require hysteroscopic guidance. These disposable devices are deployed into the uterine cavity and require little operator skill. They have several safety mechanisms in place, which control the amount of heat or cold spread and will not allow the device to function if a proper seal is not detected.

Myomectomy

Myomectomy is the removal of uterine fibroids while still preserving the uterus in situ. Depending on fibroid size and location and surgeon experience, myomectomy can be performed as an open procedure, laparoscopically, hysteroscopically, or vaginally.

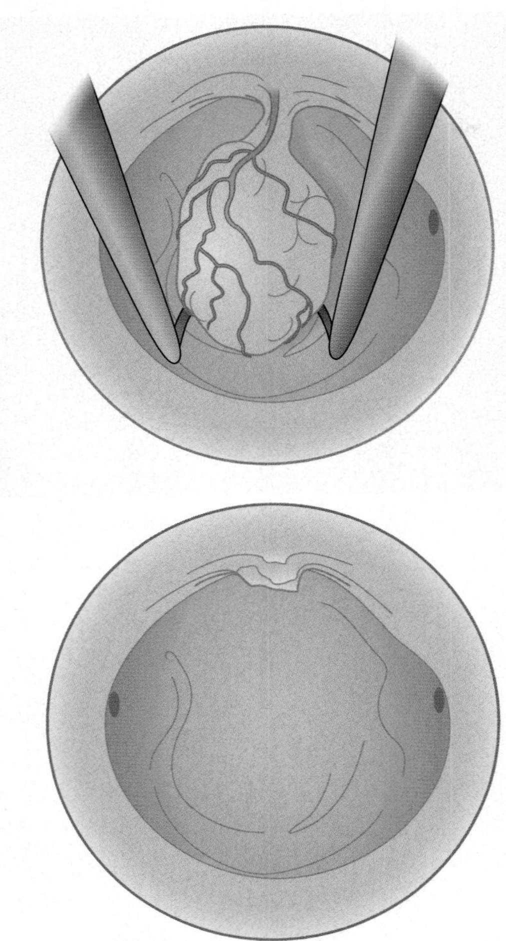

FIG. 71.10 Hysteroscopic resection of a polyp.

Vaginal Myomectomy

Cervical/intracavitary fibroids that are protruding through the cervix and seen vaginally can be removed via this route. They often have a large stalk that is attached in the endocervical canal or higher in the endometrial cavity. A hysteroscope can help determine the location of the attachment. The greatest risk of vaginal myomectomy is uncontrolled bleeding from the stalk, which often retracts when the myoma is amputated. There are several methods to reduce the risk of bleeding during vaginal myomectomy.[49] At the beginning of the procedure, lateral sutures at 3 and 9 o-clock are placed in the proximal cervix to occlude the lower branch of the uterine artery. Dilute vasopressin can be injected at the stalk (usually 20 units in 100 cc of normal saline). One or two endoloop sutures can be passed around the stalk and secured high with the transection of the stalk performed distal to the ligation. Transection can be performed sharply or with electrosurgery. If bleeding is unmanageable after removal, a hysteroscope with attached bipolar cautery should be available for intracavitary sources of bleeding or uterine packing with a balloon can be performed.

Hysteroscopic Myomectomy

Type 0, type 1, and some type 2 fibroids can often be removed via operative hysteroscopy. (Table 71.5) There are two methods for removal: electrosurgery and hysteroscopic morcellation. Both should be performed by experienced hysteroscopists. Removal by electrosurgery is performed through an operative hysteroscope, with either monopolar or bipolar current. Most often, a small loop is used to shave the fibroid to its base. With hysteroscopic morcellation, gentle suction draws the fibroid to the end of the morcellator and the fibroid is cut and removed in small segments through the same suction. The cutting activity is either mechanical or electrosurgical, depending on the particular device. In both cases, the tissue is collected and sent to pathology.

One of the most important safety parameters in operative hysteroscopy, especially with myomectomy, is monitoring of intrauterine fluid deficit during the procedure. An isotonic solution such as normal saline or lactated Ringer solution is typically utilized with modern day bipolar resectoscopes. Hypotonic fluids such as mannitol were typically utilized with monopolar resectoscopes. A fluid management system, which closely measures fluid in and out of the hysteroscope, should be utilized and closely observed throughout the procedure. A large bolus of isotonic fluid during hysteroscopy increases the patient's risk of fluid overload and pulmonary edema. A large deficit of hypotonic fluid not only increases the risk of fluid overload but also increases the risk of electrolyte imbalance, particularly hyponatremia. Many gynecologic surgery societies have published recommended guidelines for fluid deficit, based on the use of isotonic or hypotonic solutions. A deficit of no more than 2500 cc is recommended for isotonic solutions while 1000 cc is the maximum deficit for hypotonic solutions.[50] If a deficit limit is reached, the procedure should be terminated and the surgeon may repeat the surgery at a later data to complete the myomectomy if the fibroid has been only partially removed.

Laparoscopic and Open Myomectomy

The remaining fibroid types (types 3–8) are removed via either the laparoscopic or the open approach (Table 71.5). The steps are similar regardless of the approach. The most important step in a successful myomectomy is appropriate preoperative planning. Exam, imaging, and laboratory evaluation will help decide the best approach, the plan for uterine incision(s), and allow the patient and physician to review feasibility and risk of bleeding. MRI is the preferred imaging for planning uterine incisions as it provides more detail about fibroid location, number, and vascularity.

At the time of surgery, the anatomy is examined and the orientation of the uterus in relation to the adnexal structures is noted. The uterine arteries, as reviewed in the anatomy section, run along the lateral sides of the uterus, thus hysterotomy incisions should be made medially. The location of the adnexal structures is helpful in determining where the uterine arteries lie if the normal uterus anatomy is distorted by the fibroids. Dilute vasopressin (typically 20 units in 100cc of normal saline) is injected into the serosal and myometrial layer overlying the fibroid until a blanching is noted.[51] An incision is made sharply, with monopolar current, or with a harmonic scalpel in the serosa overlying the fibroid and carried through the myometrium until the capsule of the fibroid is identified (Fig. 71.11). The fibroid is grasped, often with a tenaculum or penetrating towel clamp. Using blunt dissection, monopolar current, sharp dissection, or harmonic scalpel, the fibroid is dissected from the adjacent myometrium while avoiding an incision directly into the myometrial layer. Hemostasis is maintained with judicious use of cautery or suture ligation. Once the myoma is completely dissected, the myometrial incision is closed with delayed absorbable suture, the number of layers determined by the depth of incision. A final serosal suture layer is placed to approximate the hysterotomy edges and achieve hemostasis. Once all fibroids are removed, an adhesion barrier can be placed prior to abdominal closure.[52]

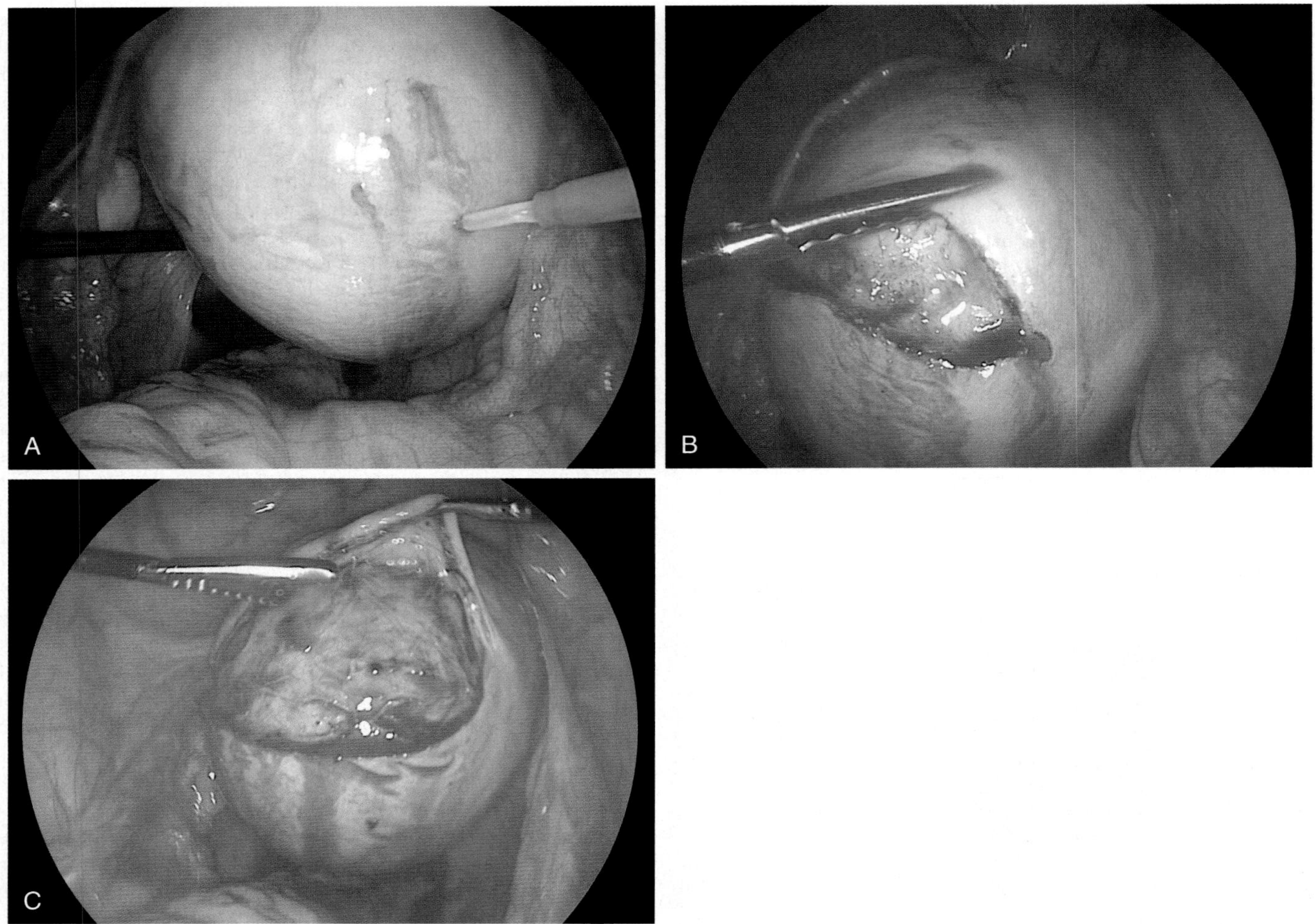

FIG. 71.11 Laparoscopic/open myomectomy.

In addition to intramyoma injection of vasopressin, other hemostatic measures are available to control bleeding during open and laparoscopic myomectomy. Prior to incision, the surgeon can place misoprostol (usually 400–800 mcg) rectally. The misoprostol induces uterine contraction, which causes a tamponade effect on the smaller vessels within the myometrium.[53] Intraoperative tourniquet placement is another option. During open myomectomy, Penrose drains or pediatric feeding tubes are placed around the lower uterine segment (after opening the broad ligament bilaterally and/or infundibulopelvic ligaments) to impede blood flow to the uterus during myoma removal.[54] Laparoscopically, temporary laparoscopic vascular clips/clamps (such as bulldog clamps) can be used in a similar fashion on the uterine arteries and ovarian vessels. The tourniquet should be left on no longer than 90 minutes with at least 10 minutes of rest time between replacements.[55]

After successful myomectomy, the patient should be adequately counseled regarding future childbearing plans, risk of uterine rupture, and options for laboring. Women who undergo myomectomy with significant incision into the myometrial layer should wait at least 3 to 6 months before conceiving.[56] Those with at least 50% myometrial invasion during myomectomy should be encouraged to avoid a trial of labor although uterine rupture is rare.[56]

Hysterectomy

Hysterectomy, by definition, is surgical removal of the uterus. There are several routes in which this can be accomplished, and there are also several options for patients and surgeons regarding type of hysterectomy and, if relevant, concomitant salpingectomy and oophorectomy. When considering hysterectomy, it is important to divide the anatomic approach into components that focus on the fallopian tubes and ovaries (where applicable), on the uterine corpus, and on the cervix and upper vagina (Fig. 71.12).

Total Abdominal Hysterectomy

A total hysterectomy is removal of both the uterine corpus and cervix. This can be accomplished via an open incision, vaginal incision, or minimally invasive techniques. For an open technique, also called a total abdominal hysterectomy, an abdominal incision is made (either low transverse or vertical midline) generally on the basis of indications for the procedure, body habitus, and prior surgical history. The reproductive anatomy is identified, and any abnormalities noted. The round ligaments should be grasped with a clamp laterally and divided either directly with electrocautery or ligated with a delayed absorbable suture and divided medial to the suture. The anterior leaf of the broad ligament is then incised medially towards the level of the internal cervical os. This facilitates development of the bladder flap, which ultimately helps separate the bladder from the lower uterine segment allowing it to retract inferiorly. The posterior broad ligament, superior and posterior to the adnexal structures, is incised and a window just below the adnexal structures is made after identifying the ureters to isolate the fallopian tube and uteroovarian ligament when the fallopian tubes and ovaries are intended to be removed. The ovarian vessels can be double-clamped with curved Haney or Zeppelin clamps and incised with curved Mayo scissors between the clamps. The superior side of the pedicle is doubly-suture ligated. The specimen-side is ligated to prevent blood loss from back bleeding. The remaining posterior broad ligament is incised inferiorly to skeletonize the uterine vessels as they travel superiorly along the lateral edge of the uterus. If the fallopian tubes and ovaries are not intended to be removed, two straight clamps can be placed across the uterineovarian vessels, which are then divided and doubly ligated superiorly.

Surgical attention then focuses on the uterus and cervix. The bladder is further dissected off the cervix sharply or with electrocautery and retracted inferiorly. A curved clamp is placed across the uterine vessels at the level of the internal os, and the pedicle is cut and suture ligated. After further dissecting the bladder completely below the level of the cervix, a straight Haney or Zeppelin clamp is placed on the remaining cardinal and uterosacral ligaments in serial steps bilaterally and the pedicles are cut and suture ligated. Once both sides are at the level of the external cervical os, the uterus and cervix can be separated from the upper vagina. This can be accomplished by placing curved clamps across the vagina medial to the prior pedicles just below the cervix from both sides to meet in the middle. Curved scissors cut just above the clamps to separate the uterus cervix off the vagina. A running delayed absorbable suture, from each side, is then passed loosely over and under the clamp, beginning laterally. Once the midline is reached, the clamps are removed, and the suture pulled tight. It can then be tied in the midline or run in an imbricating layer laterally and secured at the cuff apex. Alternatively, Haney transfixion stitches can be placed beneath the two clamps to ligate the vaginal corners and then interrupted figure-of-8 stitches can be used to close the vagina in the midline. Another method of colpotomy and vaginal cuff closure involves making a direct sharp incision into the vagina, just below the cervix. The incision is extended around the cervix with curved scissors until the cervix is completely removed. The edges of the upper vagina are gently grasped with Allis clamps to allow visualization. The colpotomy is then closed with running suture, interrupted sutures, or figures-of-8, with the lateral apex sutures incorporating the ipsilateral uterosacral ligament for apical support.

Minimally Invasive Hysterectomy

The steps for the minimally invasive route for hysterectomy are similar whether done with a laparoscopic or robotic approach. However, instead of clamps and suture, all pedicles are secured and divided with electrocautery vessel sealing and cutting devices. For the laparoscopic approach, port placement and configuration are surgeon and anatomy-dependent. Typical trocar placement for gynecologic surgery includes any combination of an umbilical trocar, bilateral lower quadrant trocars, a suprapubic or upper quadrant trocars for assistance. For large, bulky uteruses, trocars can be placed slightly higher in the abdomen and often more ports are utilized. The camera is commonly placed through the umbilical port, and a 0 or 30-degree scope is used. A robotic approach for hysterectomy for benign conditions can be also considered. Evidence suggests morbidity is similar to the laparoscopic approach, but costs are higher.[57] Trocars for the robotic approach to hysterectomy are placed per usual robotic guidelines. For assistance from the vaginal side, a uterine manipulator with attached colpotomizer or a cervical ring should be placed and secured at the cervix. This instrument is the key to identifying the cervicovaginal fornices, avoiding a urinary tract injury, and helping to delineate where the colpotomy should be made.

The hysterectomy, when performed by a minimally invasive approach, proceeds as described for the open approach and is demonstrated in Video 71.1. Once the uterine vessels and the cardinal and uterosacral ligaments are divided, a colpotomy is then completed along the colpotomizer or cervical ring with monopolar energy (usually endoshears or a monopolar hook). The uterus, cervix, and adnexa (where applicable) can usually be delivered through the vagina. A sponged-filled glove or pneumooccluder balloon is placed in the vagina and inflated to prevent egress of carbon dioxide while the colpotomy is closed with an absorbable or barbed suture generally with a running stitch. Alternatively, the cuff can be closed via a vaginal approach with interrupted figure-of-8 stitches.

Vaginal Hysterectomy

Vaginal hysterectomy is one of the earliest reported gynecologic surgeries, and the steps are mostly unchanged since its introduction. The steps of a vaginal hysterectomy are in opposite order than those of an abdominal or laparoscopic hysterectomy, with the colpotomy being done first and the cornual pedicles next to last. For a vaginal hysterectomy, the patient is placed in a high lithotomy position and the cervix and uterosacral ligaments are injected with dilute vasopressin or lidocaine with epinephrine for hemostasis. The cervix is grasped medially with a tenaculum, and a circumferential incision is made around the cervix where the vaginal epithelium merges with the cervix. This is performed sharply or with electrocautery. The paracervical fascia posterior is grasped and placed on downward traction and the posterior cul-de-sac is entered sharply with curved scissors. This incision is extended laterally with blunt traction, and the uterosacral ligaments are identified bilaterally. The uterosacral ligaments are clamped with curved Haney or Zeppelin clamps, the ligaments incised off the posterior cervix with curved scissors, and the pedicles ligated with delayed absorbable suture and left tagged for later identification.

A long-weighted speculum is placed through the vagina, below the cervix, and into the posterior cul-de-sac. Attention is then turned anteriorly where the vaginal epithelium is lifted anteriorly, and the bladder is dissected off the inferiorly directed cervix to the level of the peritoneum. Once the anterior peritoneum is identified, it is grasped and incised sharply. A right-angle retractor is then passed through this incision to retract the bladder anteriorly away from the uterus for the remainder of the hysterectomy. In serial bilateral steps, a curved clamp is placed laterally to clamp, divide, and ligate the cardinal ligaments and uterine vessels.

With each sequential pedicle, the uterus is further delivered inferiorly into the vagina. The final pedicles include the cornual structures, which include the round ligament, fallopian tube, and uteroovarian ligament. A curved clamped is placed across the cornua under direct visualization, making sure to include each cornual structure and to avoid trapping bowel. The pedicle is cut inferiorly to the clamp, freeing the uterus and cervix. This pedicle is doubly ligated and closely inspected for hemostasis before allowing it to retract superiorly out of view. A similar approach is employed if the ovaries and fallopian tubes are to be removed where the clamp is placed across the ovarian vessels.

The pelvis is examined for hemostasis at each pedicle site. The edges of the colpotomy are grasped with Allis clamps, with care to include the peritoneal layer in the closure. Angle stitches are placed first, incorporating the uterosacral ligaments that were tagged previously. The remainder of the colpotomy is closed horizontally with a delayed absorbable suture in either running, figure-of-8, or interrupted stitches.

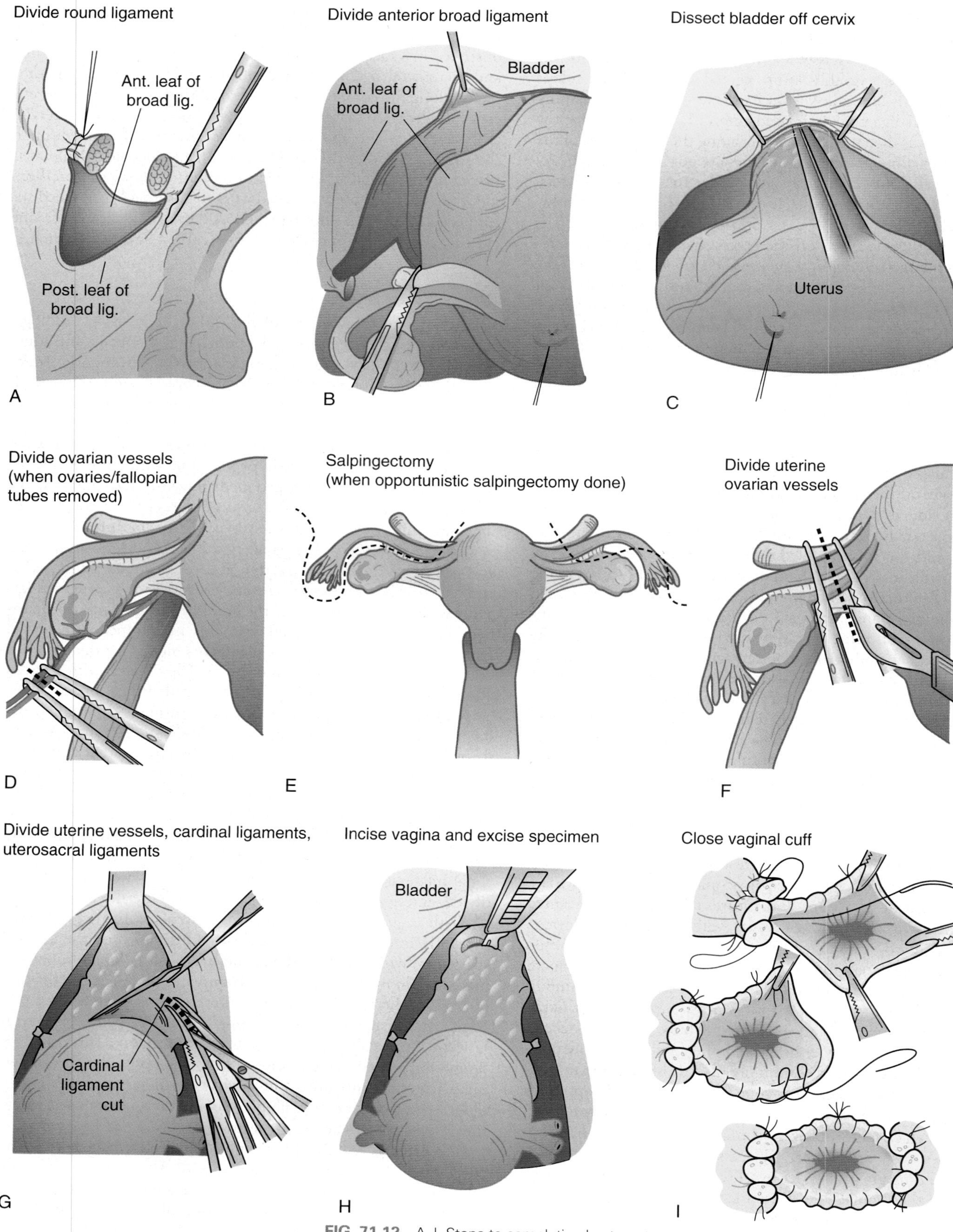

FIG. 71.12 A–I, Steps to completing hysterectomy.

FIG. 71.12, cont'd
a Transection of round ligament
b Incision of anterior and posterior broad ligament
c Dissection of bladder off cervix
d Division of ovarian vessels (when ovaries/fallopian tubes removed)
e Removal of fallopian tubes (when opportunistic salpingectomy done)
f Transection of uterine-ovarian vessels
g Division of uterine vessels, cardinal ligaments, uterosacral ligaments
h Incision of vagina and excision of specimen
i Closure of vaginal cuff using open approach (A–D, F–I, Adapted from Mitchell CW, Wheeless CR. *Atlas of pelvic surgery*. 3rd ed. Philadelphia, PA: Lippincott Williams & Wilkins; 1997.)

Supracervical Hysterectomy

A supracervical or "subtotal" hysterectomy is the removal of the uterine corpus while leaving the cervix in situ. This can be performed via the open or minimally invasive routes. The procedure follows the same steps as a total hysterectomy up to the point of the uterine artery ligation. The ligation occurs at the level of the internal cervical os. At this point, the body of the uterus is amputated from the cervix sharply or with electrosurgery. The remaining cervical stump may require oversuturing for hemostasis.

Elective Bilateral Salpingo-Oophorectomy and Opportunistic Salpingectomy

Unilateral or bilateral salpingo-oophorectomy can be done at the time of hysterectomy but should be reserved for those situations in which there are clear indications to do such. Elective salpingo-oophorectomy particularly in women below the age of 45 carries an increase in long-term cardiovascular and neurologic morbidity and mortality.[58] Routine opportunistic full salpingectomy is now recommended at the time of hysterectomy as a means of potentially reducing the risk of fallopian tube high-grade serous cancer.[59] These procedures are described in the following section on the fallopian tubes and ovaries.

Postoperative Cystoscopy after Hysterectomy

Many gynecologic surgery organizations now advocate an immediate postoperative cystoscopy at the conclusion of hysterectomy in order to assess the integrity of the bladder and ureters.[3,60] This is easily accomplished with a 70-degree cystoscope and sterile water or saline distention fluid. The urinary catheter is removed, and the scope passed through the urethra and into the bladder. The bladder should be fully distended so that the entirety of the dome is visible. The surgeon assesses for suture, foreign body, lesions, and defects. Additionally, both ureteral orifices are monitored for adequate flow of urine.

Sentinel Node Biopsy and Lymphadenectomy for Endometrial Cancer

In an order to mitigate complications associated with pelvic and para-aortic lymphadenectomy, sentinel node biopsy is emerging as a preferred strategy for those patients with early stage endometrial cancer who do not meet Mayo criteria to be defined as low risk and are undergoing hysterectomy and bilateral salpingo-oophorectomy.[61] This is most commonly performed by injecting blue dye (isosulfan blue or methylene blue) or indocyanine green superficially (1–3 mm) and deep (1–2 cm) into the cervix at the 3 and 9 o'clock positions. Dye is traced to the involved nodes, which are commonly located in along the pelvic iliac vessels but can also locate in the presacral or para-aortic regions. Sentinel nodes should be excised and subjected to ultrastaging, which includes serial sectioning and cytokeratin immunohistochemical staining.

Pelvic and para-aortic lymphadenectomy for early stage endometrial cancer patients who do not meet Mayo criteria should be completed in a setting where the side-specific sentinel node is not identified or where sentinel node biopsy capabilities do not exist. Pelvic lymphadenectomy should include the nodes that are lateral and medial to the external iliac artery and vein from the bifurcation of the common iliac artery to the level of the deep circumflex iliac vein. Nodes from the obturator space between the external iliac vein and obturator nerve should also be excised. Para-aortic lymphadenectomy should be performed bilaterally by removing the nodes lateral to the common iliac artery and aorta from the bifurcation of the common iliac to at least the inferior mesenteric artery and higher toward the renal artery in the setting of higher risk malignancies such as serous carcinoma.

COMMON FALLOPIAN TUBE/OVARIAN SURGICAL DISEASES AND PROCEDURES

Common fallopian tube/ovarian surgical diseases and procedures are listed in Table 71.6. A description of these diseases and management options follows.

Common Fallopian Tube/Ovarian Surgical Diseases

BRCA Mutation Carrier

Women who harbor a germline mutation in the *BRCA1* or *BRCA2* genes have a 57% and 49% risk of breast cancer by age 70 and a 40% and 18% risk of ovarian cancer by age 70, respectively.[62] The list of genes that increase the risk of breast and ovarian cancer when mutations exist continues to evolve. Notable genes, which infer increased risk of ovarian cancer, include *BRIP1, RAD51C, RAD51D*, and the mismatch repair genes. Guidelines exist that detail criteria for genetic counseling and single gene versus multi-panel gene testing.[62] Patients who harbor a deleterious mutation in the *BRCA1* or *BRCA2* genes are candidates for more intense screening or chemoprevention strategies should fertility be desired. Risk reducing salpingo-oophorectomy is recommended between the ages of 35 to 40 in patients with a *BRCA1* mutation and between the ages of 40 to 45 in patients with a *BRCA2* mutation. Risk reducing salpingo-oophorectomy in patients with a *BRCA* mutation has been demonstrated to reduce the risk of ovarian cancer by at least 80% and to reduce the risk of breast cancer by at least 50%, albeit recent studies suggest the reduction in breast cancer benefit is primarily noted in *BRCA1* mutation carriers.[62]

Desires Sterilization

Sterilization is the most common method of contraception among married couples and twice as many couples choose female partner sterilization over male sterilization. Physicians should carefully counsel patients about the permanence of female sterilization particularly in light of long-acting reversible contraceptive measures, which are as effective birth control measures as permanent sterilization. Historical studies have demonstrated that patient race, ethnicity, and socioeconomic status have affected physician attitudes and practices with respect to counseling about reversible versus permanent counseling. Respect for an individual woman's reproductive autonomy should be primary guiding principal when discussing sterilization options. These discussions should also include informing patient that male sterilization incurs less risks and is more effective than female sterilization and that the rates of failure of tubal sterilization are reported to be overall less than 2%. Physicians should also note that approximately 14% of women express regret after sterilization. Women at risk for regret include those of color, of young age, and after recent pregnancy event. A fully informed shared decision model is key in discussing sterilization options with patients.

TABLE 71.6 Common fallopian tube/ovarian surgical diseases and procedures

DISEASE	PROCEDURE OPTIONS
BRCA mutation carrier	Risk-reducing bilateral salpingo-oophorectomy
Desires sterilization	Pomeroy partial salpingectomy Salpingectomy
Ectopic pregnancy	Partial salpingectomy Salpingostomy
Torsion	Detorsion
Endometrioma	Cystectomy Unilateral salpingo-oophorectomy
Benign ovarian mass	Cystectomy Unilateral salpingo-oophorectomy
Malignant ovarian neoplasms	Bilateral salpingo-oophorectomy, total hysterectomy, staging with early stage disease, debulking with late stage disease Unilateral salpingo-oophorectomy and staging with early stage disease and desire for future fertility

Ectopic Pregnancy

The rate of ectopic pregnancy is about 1% to 2% that of live births. Over 90% occur in fallopian tube. Risk factors for an ectopic pregnancy include a prior history of ectopic pregnancy, pelvic inflammatory disease, infertility, use of an intrauterine device, smoking, and tubal ligation. Patients often present with nonspecific abdominal pain and vaginal bleeding symptoms and on examination may be found to have a tender abdomen, cervical motion tenderness, or an adnexal mass. Patients with a ruptured ectopic pregnancy may present emergently with signs and symptoms of hypovolemic shock. A quantitative beta human chorionic gonadotropin (hCG) and transvaginal ultrasound should be performed in patients who present with symptoms and signs suggestive of a potential ectopic pregnancy. The presence of a tubal ectopic with a fetal heartbeat or an inhomogenous or noncystic adnexal mass (known as a blob sign) has high sensitivity for diagnosing an ectopic. Medical management with intramuscular methotrexate is an option for patients with a stable ectopic pregnancy for whom no medical contraindications exists. Surgical intervention is required in the setting of a patient with an ectopic who is unstable, fails medical management, or has contraindications to medical management.

Torsion

Ovarian torsion occurs when the ovary often, together with the fallopian tube, twists on its attachments to other structures in the pelvis and compromises their blood supply. It accounts for 3% of all gynecologic emergencies. It occurs most commonly in women of reproductive age, and the most common risk factor is the presence of an ovarian cyst or tumor. Patients with ovarian torsion generally present with acute onset of sharp unilateral pelvic pain. Nausea may also accompany the pain symptoms. Common signs include unilateral lower abdominal pain and adnexal tenderness. The diagnosis may be facilitated with transvaginal Doppler ultrasound. Imaging studies may demonstrate an enlarged ovary with a twisted vascular pedicle and diminished arterial or venous blood flow. Of note, Doppler vascular flow is not always absent in torsion, and the diagnosis in this setting must be made on the basis of clinical suspicion. Ovarian torsion warrants surgical intervention, and often the diagnosis is not confirmed until the ovary and fallopian tube are visualized intraoperatively.

Endometrioma

An endometrioma is an ovarian cyst often associated with the endometriosis, a condition where endometrial tissues exist outside of the endometrium. An endometrioma frequently consists of endometrial epithelium and stroma and is often called a "chocolate cyst" due to the dark brown, thick, and tarry hemosiderin laden fluid it contains. Most patients are of reproductive age and will often present with symptoms commonly noted with endometriosis. These include pelvic pain, dysmenorrhea, dyspareunia, and/or infertility. Some patients with an endometrioma are asymptomatic. Physical examination may demonstrate a painful adnexal mass and other signs of endometriosis, such as cul-de-sac nodularity. Transvaginal ultrasound may be useful in detecting endometriomas. Typical sonar findings associated with an endometrioma include a unilocular cyst with low-level echogenicity representing old blood (commonly termed "ground glass" feature). Many patients with the presumptive diagnosis of endometriosis will be managed medically depending on the degree of symptoms and the desire for fertility. Larger endometriomas (>4 cm) are generally refractory to medical management, and laparoscopic excision is considered the treatment of choice. While there has been concern that excision of an endometrioma might damage ovarian reserve, excision is preferred over drainage particularly in patients with pelvic pain symptoms, infertility, or suspicion for a neoplasm.

Benign Ovarian Masses

Most benign ovarian masses tend to be functional follicular or corpus luteum cysts, which in general are asymptomatic and rarely exceed 5 cm in diameter. The most common benign ovarian neoplasms include cystic teratomas (commonly known as dermoid cysts), serous or mucinous cystadenomas or cystadenofibromas, and fibromas or fibrothecomas. Many patients with a benign ovarian neoplasm will be asymptomatic but few will experience pelvic pain. Most benign pelvic masses will be noted to be smooth, mobile, and of various dimensions on pelvic examination. Rarely will there be clinical signs of ascites. Evaluation should include transvaginal ultrasound to delineate the size and features of an adnexal mass with each neoplasm having distinct sonographic findings. Select tumor markers such as a CA125, beta hCG, alpha fetoprotein (AFP), or LDH should be obtained depending on the clinical scenario and concern for a malignancy. Conservative management with serial observation and management of symptoms, if present, of a patient with a functional ovarian cyst is advised. Surgical intervention generally using a laparoscopic approach is required for patients with a suspected benign ovarian neoplasm. Laparoscopic ovarian cystectomy is a consideration for a dermoid cyst or fibroma less than 10 cm in diameter. Oophorectomy is often required with larger dermoid cysts and with cystadenomas that replace the entire ovary. Laparotomy is generally reserved for much larger benign ovarian neoplasms or for when the diagnosis is equivocal and ovarian or fallopian tube malignancy is higher in the differential. Laparotomy should also be considered in the setting of a tuboovarian abscess that is refractory to antibiotics and image-guided drainage. Consultation with a gynecologic oncologist should be considered in settings when a cancer is suspected or when complex surgical intervention is anticipated.

Malignant Ovarian Neoplasms

Malignant ovarian neoplasms can originate from germ cells, stromal cells or epithelial cells from the ovary or epithelial cells from the fallopian tubes. Patients with a malignant ovarian neoplasm may present with nonspecific bloating or abdominal pain, early satiety, other nonspecific intestinal symptoms and urinary frequency. On examination, patients with a germ cell, stromal cell, or early stage epithelial tumor might be found to have abdominal pain and an adnexal mass on pelvic examination with no obvious clinical evidence of metastasis. For patients with advanced epithelial ovarian cancer, examination will often demonstrate abdominal distention from ascites, evidence of carcinomatosis on abdominal exam, and a firm, nodular, fixed pelvic mass. CT examination of the chest, abdomen, and pelvis as well as tumor markers will generally help narrow down the differential to an ovarian or fallopian tube malignancy and demonstrate the extent of disease. Germ cell tumors are more common in younger patients and relevant tumor markers should include a beta hCG, LDH, and AFP. For older patients with a suspected epithelial tumor, a CA125, carcinoembryonic antigen, and CA19-9 are most useful. In patients with a stromal tumor, an inhibin and select hormone tests may be of use, particularly when there is evidence of a hormonally functional mass. Recent breast or colon screening results in patients age 40 and above may help exclude metastatic breast or colon cancer from the differentiation in this clinical scenario.

Primary surgical debulking with staging has been the traditional approach to patients with a suspected malignant ovarian neoplasm. This is still the preferred strategy in patients with clinical evidence of early stage disease. Surgery should be fertility sparing in the setting of a young patient with a germ cell tumor or low-grade epithelial tumor. Primary debulking should be considered in the setting of advanced stage epithelial cancer when the patient is medically fit and optimal (<1 cm residual disease and preferably no residual disease) surgical resection is anticipated. Recent studies have demonstrated that neoadjuvant chemotherapy with an interval debulking in the setting of advanced stage epithelial ovarian or fallopian cancer where optimal debulking is unlikely to be achieved.[63] The decision to consider primary debulking versus neoadjuvant chemotherapy and interval debulking in an otherwise fit advanced stage patient can be facilitated by clinical features such as CA125 level, CT findings, or laparoscopy. Scoring systems have also been developed to facilitate the decision to proceed with primary debulking versus neoadjuvant chemotherapy. For select patients with recurrence, a secondary or beyond surgical resection may also provide some benefit. Patients who benefit the most might include those with a long tumor-free interval with evidence of isolated disease and no ascites.

Common Fallopian Tube/Ovarian Surgical Procedures

Tubal Sterilization

Tubal sterilization is most commonly performed via a laparoscopic approach but can also be performed via a minilaparotomy or transvaginally. One of the most common partial salpingectomy techniques is the Pomeroy (or modified Pomeroy) technique (Fig. 71.13). For this procedure, a Babcock is used to lift up the mid portion of the fallopian tubes. A rapidly absorbable suture is used to ligate the loop of tube one or two times. Scissors are then used to remove a 1 to 2 cm section of the ligated loop of tube. Another commonly employed partial salpingectomy technique is the Parkland technique. For this technique, a Babcock is used to lift up the mid portion of the fallopian tubes. Rather than ligating the elevated loop as is done with the Pomeroy technique, a window is made under the tube within an avascular portion of the mesosalpinx. A 2-cm portion of the mid fallopian tube is ligated proximately and distally and then excised. The tubal specimens are forwarded for pathologic analysis to confirm the presence of fallopian tubes.

Opportunistic salpingectomy is also increasingly being performed for patients undergoing tubal sterilization.[64] The rationale behind opportunistic salpingectomy is the potential to reduce the risk of developing high-grade serous carcinoma that has been demonstrated to frequently originate within the fallopian tube. For this procedure, the fallopian tube is elevated, and small windows are made in the avascular areas within the mesosalpinx. The small vessels providing blood supply to the fallopian tube are ligated or cauterized, and the fallopian tubes are excised where they insert into the uterine cornu.

Other commonly utilized techniques for tubal sterilization include the use of mechanical occlusive devices such as clips or rings and tubal cauterization. Technical failures and minor morbidity are noted more frequently with ring occlusion compared to clip occlusion. In general, a bipolar cautery device is utilized when cauterization of the tube is performed. Surgeons should ensure that a 2-cm portion of the mid fallopian tube is cauterized when this procedure is performed.

Salpingectomy/Salpingostomy for Ectopic Pregnancy

Surgical intervention is required for those patients with an ectopic pregnancy who fail medical management or who present with acute rupture of an ectopic. In general, a laparoscopic approach is preferred and can be utilized even in the setting of a large hemoperitoneum. Surgical options include a partial salpingectomy or salpingostomy (Fig. 71.14). Randomized trials have demonstrated no difference in the rates of subsequent ectopic pregnancies or intrauterine pregnancy.[65] In general, partial salpingectomy is the preferred approach when severe fallopian tube damage is noted and in cases in which there is significant bleeding from the proposed surgical site. The technique for salpingectomy mimics that done for tubal sterilization. Specifically, the portion of the fallopian tube is elevated and the fallopian tube proximal and distal to the ectopic is cauterized and incised. The mesosalpinx beneath the involved portion of the fallopian tube is cauterized and divided. The specimen is then forwarded for pathologic confirmation of an ectopic.

Salpingostomy should be considered in patients who have an ectopic pregnancy that has not ruptured, who desire future fertility but have damage to the contralateral fallopian tube, and in whom removal of the fallopian tube would require assisted reproduction for future childbearing. Salpingostomy involves injecting the involved fallopian tube with vasopressin and then creating a linear incision in the area involved with the ectopic pregnancy. The products of conception are then flushed out with a suction-irrigator. There is no need to suture the salpingostomy site as it will heal well by secondary intention. When salpingostomy is performed, it is important to monitor the patient with serial beta hCG levels to ensure resolution of ectopic trophoblastic tissue.

Ovarian Detorsion

A laparoscopic approach is the preferred surgical approach when ovarian torsion is suspected on the basis of clinical findings and direct laparoscopic visualization helps confirm the diagnosis. In general, the involved ovary and often fallopian tube are noted to be twisted on its vascular supply, often appear edematous and darkened as a result of vascular and lymphatic congestion, and may seem nonviable. Detorsion rather than salpingo-oophorectomy is the procedure of choice as over 80% of patients have been noted to have normal ovarian function after this procedure. The procedure involves untwisting of the involved adnexa's twisted vascular pedicle. Cystectomy may accompany detorsion when an ovarian

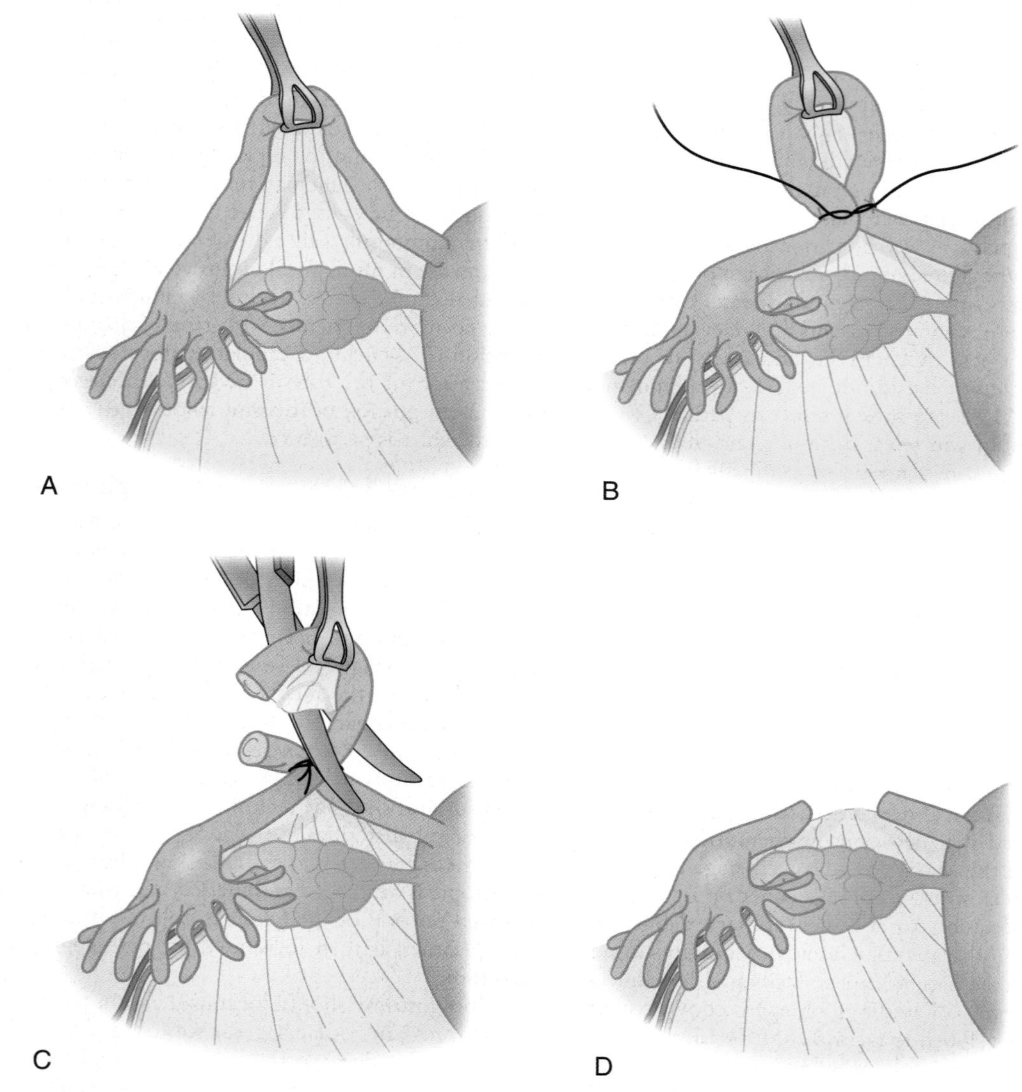

FIG. 71.13 Pomeroy tubal sterilization.

cyst or benign ovarian neoplasm is noted. The risk of recurrence after detorsion appears small and oophoropexy has not been proven to reduce that risk.

Ovarian Cystectomy

Ovarian cystectomy is most often employed for patients with an endometrioma, a torsed ovary with a large benign ovarian cyst, a benign neoplasm such as a cystadenoma or dermoid, or a borderline tumor of the ovary. This technique is most appropriate for patients in whom retaining fertility is critical and in whom there appears to be residual normal ovary. Cystectomy is indicated for endometriomas over 4 cm and has been demonstrated to improve fertility over an incision and drainage procedure. Though cystectomy carries a higher risk of recurrence in borderline tumors of the ovary when compared to salpingo-oophorectomy, overall survival is not compromised.[66]

A laparoscopic approach is preferred in most cases for which ovarian cystectomy is planned. The surgical technique involves incising the ovarian surface over the ovarian cyst and using preferably mechanical or hydrodissection to completely excise the ovarian mass (Fig. 71.15). Electrocautery may also be required to control areas of bleeding. Excision of an endometrioma can be quite difficult and ovarian reserve is often compromised postoperatively.

Salpingo-Oophorectomy

Salpingo-oophorectomy, unilateral or bilateral, is the procedure of choice for a number of clinical indications. Most often, this procedure is accomplished for a benign ovarian mass, which involves the entire ovary. Other indications include risk-reducing salpingo-oophorectomy for patients with a BRCA mutation; chronic pelvic pain with severe endometriosis or adhesive disease; or a malignant ovarian neoplasm. The procedure is most often completed using laparoscopy. Laparotomy is advised in situations when a patient may have had history of extensive prior pelvic surgery and significant pelvic adhesive disease is suspected, a mass is of a significant size or configuration that would make removal by laparoscopic technique difficult, or a malignancy is suspected.

The surgical technique for salpingo-oophorectomy, whether performed by laparoscopy or laparotomy, involves cauterization or

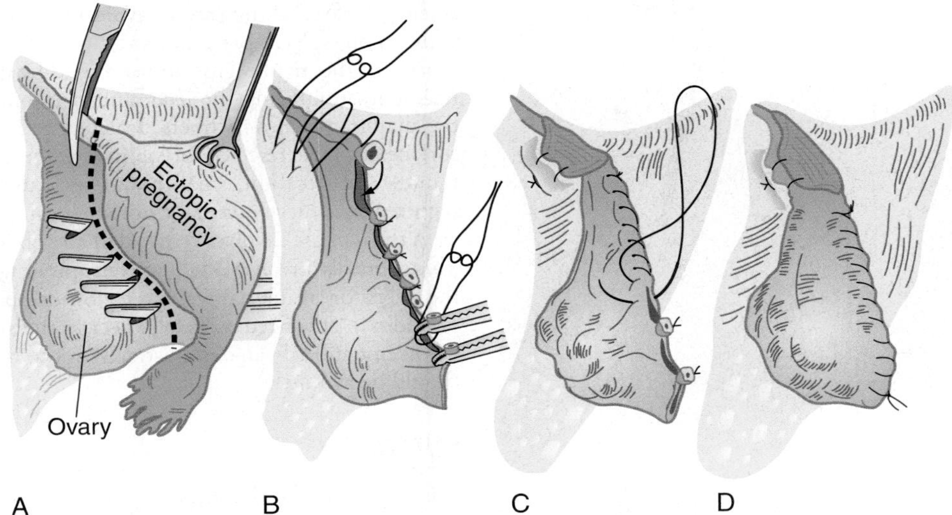

FIG. 71.14 Salpingectomy. (A) Tube is excised from the cornual portion across the mesosalpinx to the fimbria. (B) Pedicles are tied, peritoneal lining is reestablished, and cornual portion of the tube is buried into the posterior segment of the uterine cornu. (C) Mesosalpinx is reperitonealized. (D) Mesosalpinx is closed and the procedure completed. (Adapted from Mitchell CW, Wheeless CR. *Atlas of pelvic surgery*. 3rd ed. Philadelphia, PA: Lippincott Williams & Wilkins; 1997.)

ligation of the ovarian vessels proximal to the ovary and fallopian tube and cauterization or ligation of the uterineovarian vessels distal to the ovary and fallopian tube (Fig. 71.12D and Video 71.2). For risk-reducing salpingo-oophorectomy, it is important to ligate the ovarian vessels at a level well above the ovary and fallopian tube so that no residual ovary or fallopian tube is left behind. It is also important to obtain abdominal pelvic washing during that procedure and to be aware that approximately 5% of patients with a BRCA mutation will be noted to have an occult ovarian or fallopian tube cancer.

Another key surgical principle in salpingo-oophorectomy includes identification of structures within the pelvis that are at risk of injury when the procedure is performed. Perhaps the most important of these structures is the ureter, which courses close to the ovarian vessels over the bifurcation of the common iliac artery. It is important to identify the ureter either via a transperitoneal or retroperitoneal approach. The ovary and fallopian tube should be lifted anteriorly to displace it as far from the ureter as possible prior to cauterizing or ligating the ovarian vessels. In scenarios where the ovary or fallopian tube are involved with pathology such as a mass or endometriosis that hinders separation of the adnexa from the ureter, a uterolysis should be performed via a retroperitoneal approach in order to separate the ureter from the adnexa and allow safer cauterization or ligation of the ovarian vessels. It is also important to identify and carefully lyse any adhesions of the small or large intestine to the adnexa. Lastly, it is important to be aware of the position of the adnexa's relationship to the external iliac vessels. Incising the posterior broad ligament (and in some instances the round ligament) facilitates development of the hypogastric space and separation of the adnexa from the pelvic sidewall vessels. This procedure also helps facilitate identification of the ureter via a retroperitoneal approach.

Fallopian Tube/Ovarian Cancer Cytoreduction

Approximately 10% to 15% patients with an ovarian malignancy are found clinically to have disease apparently confined to the ovary. This is more common in patients with germ cell tumors of the ovary, stromal cell tumors of the ovary, and certain epithelial ovarian tumors (e.g., mucinous, clear cell). In this setting, removal of the affected ovary together with the contralateral ovary and uterus is key. Surgical staging consisting of abdominal pelvic washings, excision of suspicious peritoneal nodules or selective random peritoneal biopsies, infracolic omentectomy, and pelvic and para-aortic lymphadenectomy is indicated. In certain circumstances such as germ cell tumors of the ovary, fertility or hormonal preservation should be considered, and resection of the uninvolved ovary and uterus is not necessary.

The majority of patients affected by epithelial ovarian or fallopian tube cancer have advanced stage disease and usually present with the constellation of some pelvic mass, omental metastasis, intraperitoneal carcinomatosis, and ascites. The primary surgical goal in this scenario shifts from staging to optimal cytoreduction. The definition of optimal cytoreduction is now defined as residual disease less than 1 cm in diameter and preferably no visible residual disease. Studies have demonstrated that outcomes in advanced ovarian/fallopian tube cancer are the best in patients who have no residual disease. The majority of patients with advanced stage ovarian cancer have high-grade serous carcinoma, which is now thought to originate in the fallopian tube in the majority of cases. Endometrioid and, less frequently, low-grade serous carcinoma are other subtypes noted in patients with advanced stage disease.

Historically, most if not all patients with advanced stage ovarian or fallopian tube cancer underwent a primary debulking surgery followed by chemotherapy. Several studies over the past decade have demonstrated that neoadjuvant chemotherapy followed by an interim debulking surgery after three to four cycles results in similar outcomes and less morbidity for advanced stage ovarian cancer.[63] This is particularly true for those advanced stage ovarian cancer patients who are either too ill and have significant surgical risks or for those in whom it appears that optimal debulking will not be feasible. Increasingly this practice paradigm is being adopted for patients with advanced ovarian/fallopian tube cancer and a number of clinical factors or laparoscopy can be utilized

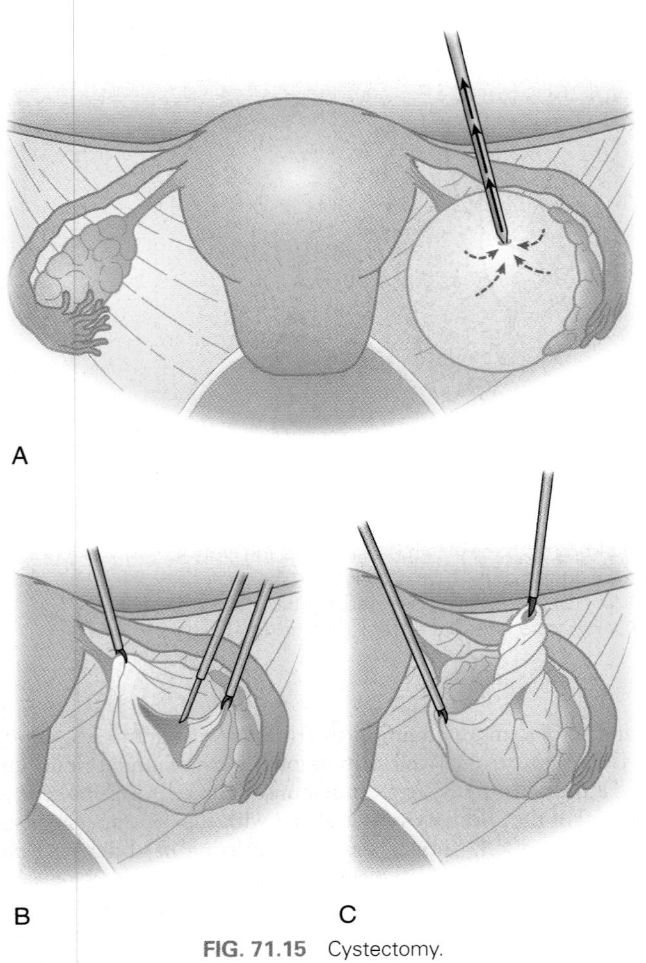

FIG. 71.15 Cystectomy.

to predict the feasibility of achieving optimal (preferentially complete) surgical resection.

The surgical approach to ovarian/fallopian tube cytoreduction or debulking, either primary or interval, should involve an appropriate midline incision to provide adequate exposure for resection of all disease. Minimally invasive strategies for early stage ovarian cancer patients or for those undergoing interval debulking can be considered for select patients. The surgical goals of optimal cytoreduction are best accomplished in phases. For disease in the pelvis, surgeons must decide whether a total abdominal hysterectomy with bilateral salpingo-oophorectomy (procedure previously described) will suffice or whether an en bloc type of procedure that involves resection of a portion of the sigmoid colon and pelvic peritoneum will be required to remove all pelvic disease (Fig. 71.16). The latter is usually necessary when the cul-de-sac region and colon are extensively involved with disease. This resection generally involves a retroperitoneal approach with bilateral ureterolysis and careful dissection of the bladder. The colon is divided with a staple device proximal and distal to the areas of involvement, and an anastomosis with a staple device is generally quite feasible.

A second phase involves the upper abdomen. One key component of upper abdominal surgery includes resection of the involved portion of the gastrocolic and infracolic omentum. This generally involves resecting the omentum from the hepatic to splenic flexure, taking care to avoid injury to the stomach, transverse colon, spleen, pancreas, and liver. Disease along the inferior aspects of the diaphragm can be excised by dividing the falciform ligament, mobilizing the liver, and stripping the peritoneum off the diaphragm muscle fibers. Isolated nodules on the peritoneal surfaces can be resected or obliterated using a variety of techniques. On occasion, small bowel resection with anastomosis is required to achieve optimal cytoreduction.

A third phase involves removal of any obvious nodal metastasis. This generally involves adequate retroperitoneal exposure either in the pelvis or in the para-aortic region or both. Elective resection of nodes in advanced ovarian cancer in the absence of any clinical involvement has been demonstrated not to improve outcomes and should be avoided.

SUMMARY

It is important for the surgeon to be familiar with the most common gynecologic illnesses that affect women during the spectrum of their lives and that often require surgical intervention. Knowledge of the surgical procedures for these diseases and the relevant pelvic anatomy should provide the surgeon the confidence to address these diseases in a skillful manner.

SELECTED REFERENCES

Castellano T, Zerden M, Marsh L, et al. Risks and benefits of salpingectomy at the time of sterilization. *Obstet Gynecol Surv.* 2017;72:663–668.

This article demonstrated the feasibility and safety of opportunistic salpingectomy for women desiring tubal sterilization.

Curry SJ, Krist AH, Owens DK, et al. Screening for cervical Cancer: US Preventive Services Task Force recommendation statement. *JAMA.* 2018;320:674–686.

This paper provides current guidelines for cervical cancer screening.

Evans EC, Matteson KA, Orejuela FJ, et al. Salpingo-oophorectomy at the time of benign hysterectomy: a systematic review. *Obstet Gynecol.* 2016;128:476–485.

This review demonstrated that elective salpingo-oophorectomy at the time of hysterectomy for benign reasons was associated with increased long-term morbidity and mortality, particularly when done in premenopausal women.

Jelovsek JE, Barber MD, Brubaker L, et al. Effect of uterosacral ligament suspension vs sacrospinous ligament fixation with or without perioperative behavioral therapy for pelvic organ vaginal prolapse on surgical outcomes and prolapse symptoms at 5 years in the optimal randomized clinical trial. *JAMA.* 2018;319:1554–1565.

This classic article demonstrated that uterosacral ligament suspension and sacrospinous ligament fixation for pelvic organ vaginal prolapse largely had similar long-term outcomes.

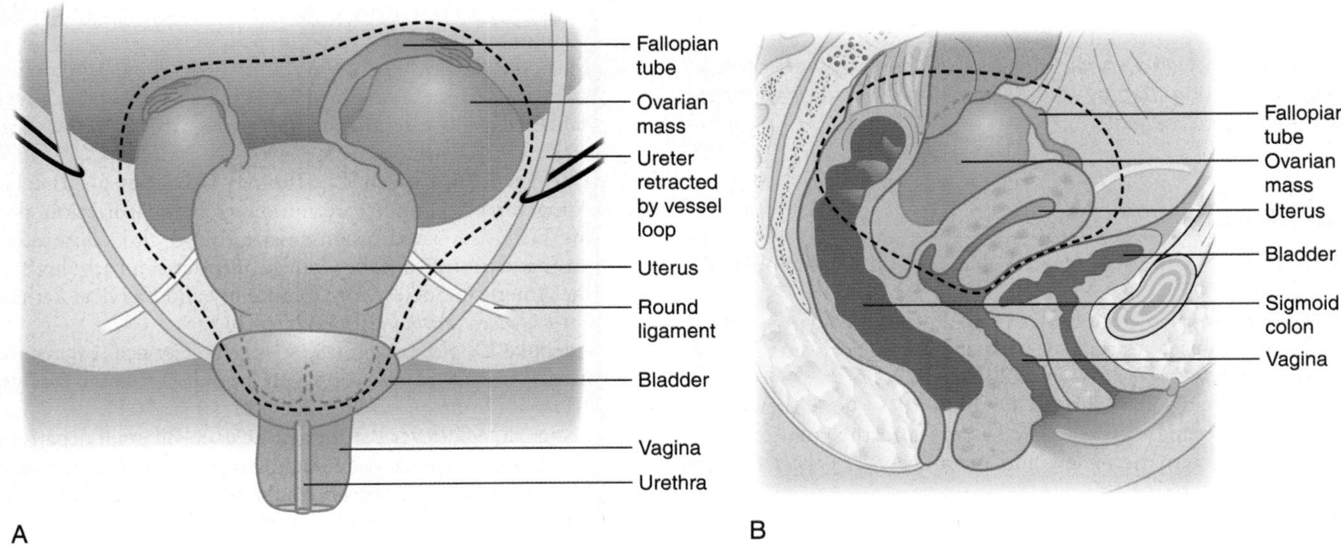

FIG. 71.16 En bloc cytoreduction of ovarian cancer in pelvis.

Joura EA, Giuliano AR, Iversen OE, et al. A 9-valent HPV vaccine against infection and intraepithelial neoplasia in women. *N Engl J Med*. 2015;372:711–723.

This study demonstrated the efficacy of a nonovalent human papillomavirus (HPV) vaccine for the prevention of high- and intermediate-risk for HPV intraepithelial neoplasia in women.

Levenback CF, Ali S, Coleman RL, et al. Lymphatic mapping and sentinel lymph node biopsy in women with squamous cell carcinoma of the vulva: a gynecologic oncology group study. *J Clin Oncol*. 2012;30:3786–3791.

This classic study validated the utility of sentinel lymph node biopsy in women with vulva cancer ≤4 cm in diameter.

Munro MG, Critchley HO, Broder MS, et al. FIGO classification system (PALM-COEIN) for causes of abnormal uterine bleeding in nongravid women of reproductive age. *Int J Gynaecol Obstet*. 2011;113:3–13.

This classic paper described new nomenclature for describing uterine bleeding abnormalities.

Ramirez PT, Frumovitz M, Pareja R, et al. Minimally invasive versus abdominal radical hysterectomy for cervical cancer. *N Engl J Med*. 2018;379:1895–1904.

This randomized controlled trial demonstrated increase risk of recurrence when a minimally invasive route was employed to perform a radical hysterectomy for cervical cancer.

Teeluckdharry B, Gilmour D, Flowerdew G. Urinary tract injury at benign gynecologic surgery and the role of cystoscopy: a systematic review and meta-analysis. *Obstet Gynecol*. 2015;126:1161–1169.

This article provides evidence that cystoscopy after gynecologic surgery for benign conditions increases the intraoperative detection rate for urinary tract injuries.

Walker JL, Piedmonte MR, Spirtos NM, et al. Laparoscopy compared with laparotomy for comprehensive surgical staging of uterine cancer: Gynecologic Oncology Group Study LAP2. *J Clin Oncol*. 2009;27:5331–5336.

Walker JL, Piedmonte MR, Spirtos NM, et al. Recurrence and survival after random assignment to laparoscopy versus laparotomy for comprehensive surgical staging of uterine cancer: Gynecologic Oncology Group LAP2 Study. *J Clin Oncol*. 2012;30:695–700.

These two classic papers demonstrated in a randomized clinical trial that a minimally invasive approach to endometrial cancer was associated with improved surgical outcomes and equal cancer outcomes when compared to an open surgical approach in women with endometrial cancer.

Wright JD, Ananth CV, Lewin SN, et al. Robotically assisted vs laparoscopic hysterectomy among women with benign gynecologic disease. *JAMA*. 2013;309:689–698.

This article demonstrated that robotic assisted hysterectomy for benign gynecologic disorders had similar morbidity to laparoscopic hysterectomy but was substantially more expensive.

Xiao Y, Xie S, Zhang N, et al. Platinum-based neoadjuvant chemotherapy versus primary surgery in ovarian carcinoma international federation of gynecology and obstetrics stages iiic and iv: a systematic review and meta-analysis. *Gynecol Obstet Invest*. 2018;83:209–219.

This paper reviews classic studies evaluating the role of neoadjuvant chemotherapy in newly diagnosed advanced stage ovarian cancer patients.

REFERENCES

1. Netter FN. *Atlas Of Human Anatomy*, ed. Phildelphia, PA: Elsevier; 2019.
2. Kuponiyi O, Alleemudder DI, Latunde-Dada A, et al. Nerve injuries associated with gynaecological surgery. *The Obstetrician & Gynaecologist*. 2014;16:29–36.
3. Teeluckdharry B, Gilmour D, Flowerdew G. Urinary tract injury at benign gynecologic surgery and the role of cystoscopy: a systematic review and meta-analysis. *Obstet Gynecol*. 2015;126:1161–1169.
4. Clarke-Pearson DL, Geller EJ. Complications of hysterectomy. *Obstet Gynecol*. 2013;121:654–673.
5. Bornstein J, Bogliatto F, Haefner HK, et al. The 2015 International Society for the Study of Vulvovaginal Disease (ISSVD) terminology of vulvar squamous intraepithelial lesions. *Obstet Gynecol*. 2016;127:264–268.
6. Van der Zee AG, Oonk MH, De Hullu JA, et al. Sentinel node dissection is safe in the treatment of early-stage vulvar cancer. *J Clin Oncol*. 2008;26:884–889.
7. Levenback CF, Ali S, Coleman RL, et al. Lymphatic mapping and sentinel lymph node biopsy in women with squamous cell carcinoma of the vulva: a gynecologic oncology group study. *J Clin Oncol*. 2012;30:3786–3791.
8. Maher C, Feiner B, Baessler K, et al. Surgical management of pelvic organ prolapse in women. *Cochrane Database Syst Rev*. 2013;CD004014.
9. Nygaard I, Brubaker L, Zyczynski HM, et al. Long-term outcomes following abdominal sacrocolpopexy for pelvic organ prolapse. *JAMA*. 2013;309:2016–2024.
10. Jelovsek JE, Barber MD, Brubaker L, et al. Effect of uterosacral ligament suspension vs sacrospinous ligament fixation with or without perioperative behavioral therapy for pelvic organ vaginal prolapse on surgical outcomes and prolapse symptoms at 5 years in the optimal randomized clinical trial. *JAMA*. 2018;319:1554–1565.
11. Bradley CS, Nygaard IE, Brown MB, et al. Bowel symptoms in women 1 year after sacrocolpopexy. *Am J Obstet Gynecol*. 2007;197:642. e641– e648.
12. Brubaker L, Cundiff GW, Fine P, et al. Abdominal sacrocolpopexy with Burch colposuspension to reduce urinary stress incontinence. *N Engl J Med*. 2006;354:1557–1566.
13. Committee Opinion No. 675 Summary. Management of vulvar intraepithelial neoplasia. *Obstet Gynecol*. 2016;128:937–938.
14. Koh WJ, Greer BE, Abu-Rustum NR, et al. Vulvar cancer, version 1.2017, Nccn clinical practice guidelines in oncology. *J Natl Compr Canc Netw*. 2017;15:92–120.
15. Lawrie TA, Patel A, Martin-Hirsch PP, et al. Sentinel node assessment for diagnosis of groin lymph node involvement in vulval cancer. *Cochrane Database Syst Rev*. 2014:CD010409.
16. Joura EA, Giuliano AR, Iversen OE, et al. A 9-valent HPV vaccine against infection and intraepithelial neoplasia in women. *N Engl J Med*. 2015;372:711–723.
17. Curry SJ, Krist AH, Owens DK, et al. Screening for Cervical Cancer: US Preventive Services Task Force Recommendation Statement. *JAMA*. 2018;320:674–686.
18. Massad LS, Einstein MH, Huh WK, et al. updated consensus guidelines for the management of abnormal cervical cancer screening tests and cancer precursors. *Obstet Gynecol*. 2012;121:829–846; 2013.
19. Darragh TM, Colgan TJ, Thomas Cox J, et al. The Lower Anogenital Squamous Terminology Standardization project for HPV-associated lesions: background and consensus recommendations from the College of American Pathologists and the American Society for Colposcopy and Cervical Pathology. *Int J Gynecol Pathol*. 2013;32:76–115.
20. Adegoke O, Kulasingam S, Virnig B. Cervical cancer trends in the United States: a 35-year population-based analysis. *J Womens Health (Larchmt)*. 2012;21:1031–1037.
21. Lecuru F, Mathevet P, Querleu D, et al. Bilateral negative sentinel nodes accurately predict absence of lymph node metastasis in early cervical cancer: results of the SENTICOL study. *J Clin Oncol*. 2011;29:1686–1691.
22. Ramirez PT, Frumovitz M, Pareja R, et al. Minimally invasive versus abdominal radical hysterectomy for cervical cancer. *N Engl J Med*. 2018;379:1895–1904.
23. Melamed A, Margul DJ, Chen L, et al. Survival after minimally invasive radical hysterectomy for early-stage cervical cancer. *N Engl J Med*. 2018;379:1905–1914.
24. Piver MS, Rutledge F, Smith JP. Five classes of extended hysterectomy for women with cervical cancer. *Obstet Gynecol*. 1974;44:265–272.
25. Koh WJ, Greer BE, Abu-Rustum NR, et al. Cervical Cancer, Version 2.2015. *J Natl Compr Canc Netw*. 2015;13:395–404; quiz 404.
26. Munro MG, Critchley HO, Broder MS, et al. FIGO classification system (PALM-COEIN) for causes of abnormal uterine bleeding in nongravid women of reproductive age. *Int J Gynaecol Obstet*. 2011;113:3–13.
27. Practice bulletin no. 128. diagnosis of abnormal uterine bleeding in reproductive-aged women. *Obstet Gynecol*. 2012;120:197–206.
28. van Hanegem N, Breijer MC, Khan KS, et al. Diagnostic evaluation of the endometrium in postmenopausal bleeding: an evidence-based approach. *Maturitas*. 2011;68:155–164.
29. ACOG Committee Opinion No. 734. The role of transvaginal ultrasonography in evaluating the endometrium of women with postmenopausal bleeding. *Obstet Gynecol*. 2018;131:e124–e129.
30. Chandavarkar U, Kuperman JM, Muderspach LI, et al. Endometrial echo complex thickness in postmenopausal endometrial cancer. *Gynecol Oncol*. 2013;131:109–112.
31. Baiocchi G, Manci N, Pazzaglia M, et al. Malignancy in endometrial polyps: a 12-year experience. *Am J Obstet Gynecol*. 2009;201:462.e461–e464.
32. Cohen I. Endometrial pathologies associated with postmenopausal tamoxifen treatment. *Gynecol Oncol*. 2004;94:256–266.
33. Onalan R, Onalan G, Tonguc E, et al. Body mass index is an independent risk factor for the development of endometrial polyps in patients undergoing in vitro fertilization. *Fertil Steril*. 2009;91:1056–1060.

34. Stewart EA, Cookson CL, Gandolfo RA, et al. Epidemiology of uterine fibroids: a systematic review. *BJOG*. 2017;124:1501–1512.
35. Bulun sE. Uterine fibroids. *N englj med*. 2013;369:1344–1355.
36. Parazzini F, Di Martino M, Candiani M, et al. Dietary components and uterine leiomyomas: a review of published data. *Nutr Cancer*. 2015;67:569–579.
37. Parker JD, Leondires M, Sinaii N, et al. Persistence of dysmenorrhea and nonmenstrual pain after optimal endometriosis surgery may indicate adenomyosis. *Fertil Steril*. 2006;86:711–715.
38. Propst AM, Quade BJ, Gargiulo AR, et al. Adenomyosis demonstrates increased expression of the basic fibroblast growth factor receptor/ligand system compared with autologous endometrium. *Menopause*. 2001;8:368–371.
39. Bazot M, Darai E. Role of transvaginal sonography and magnetic resonance imaging in the diagnosis of uterine adenomyosis. *Fertil Steril*. 2018;109:389–397.
40. Templeman C, Marshall SF, Ursin G, et al. Adenomyosis and endometriosis in the California Teachers Study. *Fertil Steril*. 2008;90:415–424.
41. Gupta S, Provenzale D, Regenbogen SE, et al. NCCN Guidelines Insights: Genetic/Familial High-Risk Assessment: Colorectal, Version 3.2017. *J Natl Compr Canc Netw*. 2017;15:1465–1475.
42. Walker JL, Piedmonte MR, Spirtos NM, et al. Laparoscopy compared with laparotomy for comprehensive surgical staging of uterine cancer: Gynecologic Oncology Group Study LAP2. *J Clin Oncol*. 2009;27:5331–5336.
43. Walker JL, Piedmonte MR, Spirtos NM, et al. Recurrence and survival after random assignment to laparoscopy versus laparotomy for comprehensive surgical staging of uterine cancer: Gynecologic Oncology Group LAP2 Study. *J Clin Oncol*. 2012;30:695–700.
44. Xie W, Cao D, Yang J, et al. Robot-assisted surgery versus conventional laparoscopic surgery for endometrial cancer: a systematic review and meta-analysis. *J Cancer Res Clin Oncol*. 2016;142:2173–2183.
45. Kitchener H, Swart AM, Qian Q, et al. Efficacy of systematic pelvic lymphadenectomy in endometrial cancer (MRC ASTEC trial): a randomised study. *Lancet*. 2009;373:125–136.
46. AlHilli MM, Podratz KC, Dowdy SC, et al. Preoperative biopsy and intraoperative tumor diameter predict lymph node dissemination in endometrial cancer. *Gynecol Oncol*. 2013;128:294–299.
47. Bodurtha Smith AJ, Fader AN, Tanner EJ. Sentinel lymph node assessment in endometrial cancer: a systematic review and meta-analysis. *Am J Obstet Gynecol*. 2017;216:459–476. e410.
48. Rossi EC, Kowalski LD, Scalici J, et al. A comparison of sentinel lymph node biopsy to lymphadenectomy for endometrial cancer staging (FIRES trial): a multicentre, prospective, cohort study. *Lancet Oncol*. 2017;18:384–392.
49. Golan A, Zachalka N, Lurie S, et al. Vaginal removal of prolapsed pedunculated submucous myoma: a short, simple, and definitive procedure with minimal morbidity. *Arch Gynecol Obstet*. 2005;271:11–13.
50. Umranikar S, Clark TJ, Saridogan E, et al. BSGE/ESGE guideline on management of fluid distension media in operative hysteroscopy. *Gynecol Surg*. 2016;13:289–303.
51. Kongnyuy EJ, Wiysonge CS. Interventions to reduce haemorrhage during myomectomy for fibroids. *Cochrane Database Syst Rev*. 2014:CD005355.
52. Mais V, Ajossa S, Piras B, et al. Prevention of de-novo adhesion formation after laparoscopic myomectomy: a randomized trial to evaluate the effectiveness of an oxidized regenerated cellulose absorbable barrier. *Hum Reprod*. 1995;10:3133–3135.
53. Abdel-Hafeez M, Elnaggar A, Ali M, et al. Rectal misoprostol for myomectomy: a randomised placebo-controlled study. *Aust N Z J Obstet Gynaecol*. 2015;55:363–368.
54. Hickman LC, Kotlyar A, Shue S, et al. Hemostatic techniques for myomectomy: an evidence-based approach. *J Minim Invasive Gynecol*. 2016;23:497–504.
55. Magos A, Al-Shabibi N, Korkontzelos I, et al. Ovarian artery clamp: initial experience with a new clamp to reduce bleeding at open myomectomy. *J Obstet Gynaecol*. 2011;31:73–76.
56. Koo YJ, Lee JK, Lee YK, et al. Pregnancy outcomes and risk factors for uterine rupture after laparoscopic myomectomy: a single-center experience and literature review. *J Minim Invasive Gynecol*. 2015;22:1022–1028.
57. Wright JD, Ananth CV, Lewin SN, et al. Robotically assisted vs laparoscopic hysterectomy among women with benign gynecologic disease. *JAMA*. 2013;309:689–698.
58. Evans EC, Matteson KA, Orejuela FJ, et al. Salpingo-oophorectomy at the time of benign hysterectomy: a systematic review. *Obstet Gynecol*. 2016;128:476–485.
59. Committee opinion no. 620. Salpingectomy for ovarian cancer prevention. *Obstet Gynecol*. 2015;125:279–281.
60. AAGL Practice Report: Practice guidelines for intraoperative cystoscopy in laparoscopic hysterectomy. *J Minim Invasive Gynecol*. 2012;19:407–411.
61. Koh WJ, Abu-Rustum NR, Bean S, et al. Uterine neoplasms, version 1.2018, Nccn clinical practice guidelines in oncology. *J Natl Compr Canc Netw*. 2018;16:170–199.
62. Daly MB, Pilarski R, Berry M, et al. Nccn guidelines insights: genetic/familial high-risk assessment: breast and ovarian, version 2.2017. *J Natl Compr Canc Netw*. 2017;15:9–20.
63. Xiao Y, Xie S, Zhang N, et al. Platinum-based neoadjuvant chemotherapy versus primary surgery in ovarian carcinoma international federation of gynecology and obstetrics stages iiic and iv: a systematic review and meta-analysis. *Gynecol Obstet Invest*. 2018;83:209–219.
64. Castellano T, Zerden M, Marsh L, et al. Risks and benefits of salpingectomy at the time of sterilization. *Obstet Gynecol Surv*. 2017;72:663–668.
65. Cheng X, Tian X, Yan Z, et al. Comparison of the fertility outcome of salpingotomy and salpingectomy in women with tubal pregnancy: a systematic review and meta-analysis. *PLoS One*. 2016;11:e0152343.
66. Gershenson DM. Management of borderline ovarian tumours. *Best Pract Res Clin Obstet Gynaecol*. 2017;41:49–59.

72 CHAPTER

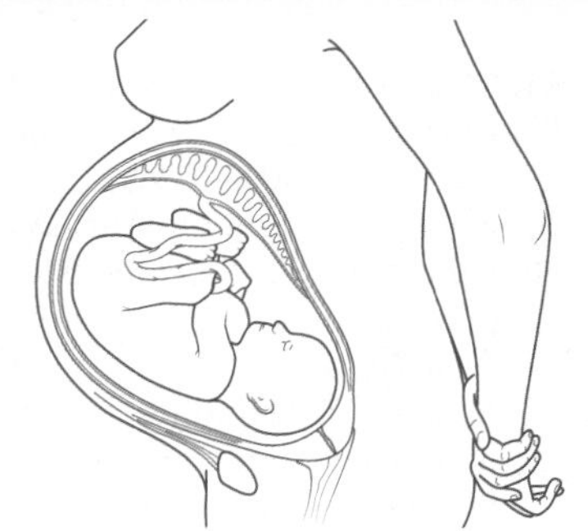

Surgery in the Pregnant Patient

Rachel M. Russo, Gregory J. Jurkovich, Diana L. Farmer

OUTLINE

The pregnant patient presents a unique clinical challenge for the general surgeon. About 7% of pregnancies are complicated by nonobstetric surgical problems, and an estimated 1 in 500 pregnancies will need an operation for nonpregnancy-related issues. Table 72.1 is adapted from a 10-year review of the hospital episode statistic of all admissions to English NHS hospitals. Of 6.5 million pregnancies, 47,600 nonobstetric surgeries occurred, and 12,500 were abdominal of any kind. In a review of 44 papers and 12,452 patients, the effects of nonobstetric surgical procedures on maternal and fetal outcomes were studied; a maternal death rate of 0.006% and a miscarriage rate of 5.8% were reported. Most indications for surgical intervention are common for the patient's age group and unrelated to pregnancy, such as acute appendicitis, symptomatic cholelithiasis, perianal, soft tissue, breast masses, or trauma.[1]

Changes in maternal anatomy and physiology and safety of the fetus are among the issues of which the surgeon must be cognizant. The presentation of surgical diseases in the pregnant patient may be atypical or may mimic signs and symptoms of a normal pregnancy. A standard evaluation may be unreliable because of pregnancy-associated changes in diagnostic tests or laboratory test results. Finally, many physicians may be more hesitant to employ diagnostic evaluation and treatment. Any of these factors may result in a delay in diagnosis and treatment, adversely affecting maternal and fetal outcome. The fundamental principle of managing a pregnant woman with a nonobstetric surgical problem is to not penalize the patient, and her care, for being pregnant. There are two patients to be sure, but the baby's health is dependent on the mother's. Although consultation with an obstetrician is ideal when caring for a pregnant patient, the surgeon needs to be aware of this fundamental principle when this resource is unavailable. This chapter discusses key points when caring for the pregnant patient who presents with nonobstetric surgical disorders.

PHYSIOLOGIC CHANGES OF PREGNANCY

Progesterone and estrogen, two of the principal hormones of pregnancy, mediate many of the maternal physiologic changes in pregnancy. Normal laboratory values differ in the gravid compared with the nonpregnant patient. The diaphragm can be elevated in pregnancy up to 4 cm, and the lower chest wall can widen up to 7 cm.[2] These changes may also mimic similar pathophysiology that occurs in nonpregnant women who have cardiac or liver disease. Elevated progesterone levels, as well as decreased serum motilin, result in smooth muscle relaxation, producing multiple effects on several organ systems. In the stomach, this decreased smooth muscle tone results in diminished gastric tone and motility. The lower esophageal sphincter tone is also decreased and, when combined with increased intraabdominal pressure, results in an increase in the incidence of gastroesophageal reflux. Small bowel motility is reduced, increasing small bowel transit time. Absorption of nutrients, however, remains unchanged, with the exception of iron

TABLE 72.1 Operations performed out of 6.5 million pregnancies in the United Kingdom from 2002–2012.

	NUMBER OF OPERATIONS (%)
Abdominal, any kind	12493 (26.2)
Appendectomy	3062 (6.4)
Cholecystectomy	1306 (2.7)
Dental	5365 (11.3)
Skin, nail	4762 (10.0)
Orthopedic	4563 (9.6)
ENT	3060 (6.4)
Perianal	2977 (6.2)
Breast	1884 (4.0)
Cancer	710 (1.5)

Adapted from Balinskaite V, Bottle A, Sodhi V, et al. The risk of adverse pregnancy outcomes following nonobstetric surgery during pregnancy: Estimates from a retrospective cohort study of 6.5 million pregnancies. *Ann Surg.* 2017;266:260–266. *ENT,* Ear, nose, and throat.

absorption, which is increased because of increased iron requirements. In the colon, pregnancy-related changes usually manifest as constipation. This is caused by a combination of increased colonic sodium and water absorption, decreased motility, and mechanical obstruction by the gravid uterus. An increase in portal venous pressure, and therefore an increase in the pressure in the collateral venous circulation, results in dilation of the veins at the gastroesophageal junction. This is of importance only if the patient had esophageal varices before becoming pregnant. The most common result of the increased portal venous pressure is dilation of the hemorrhoidal veins, leading to the well-known complaint of hemorrhoids.

In addition to alterations in smooth muscle tone and motility, other notable changes occur in the gastrointestinal tract. The function of the gallbladder is altered, as is the chemical composition of bile. During the second and third trimesters, the volume of the gallbladder may be twice that found in the nonpregnant state, and gallbladder emptying is markedly slower. Up to 4% of pregnant patients have gallstones on routine obstetric ultrasound.[1] Still, only 1 of every 1000 pregnant patients develops symptoms. It is unknown whether the increased biliary stasis, changes in bile composition, or combination of these two factors results in an increased risk for gallstone formation, but the risk for developing gallstones increases with multiparity. However, the incidence of symptomatic cholelithiasis during pregnancy is similar to the incidence in age-related nonpregnant women.

Some of the changes of pregnancy closely resemble those of liver disease. These include spider angiomas and palmar erythema from elevated serum estrogen levels. Hypoalbuminemia is also seen along with elevated serum cholesterol, alkaline phosphatase, and fibrinogen levels. Serum bilirubin and hepatic transaminase levels remain unchanged during pregnancy.

In the cardiovascular system, peripheral vascular resistance is decreased as a consequence of diminished vascular smooth muscle tone. Cardiac output increases by as much as 50% during the first trimester of pregnancy. Initially, this is caused by an increased stroke volume resulting from an increase in plasma volume and red blood cell mass, but a gradual increase in maternal heart rate also is a contributing factor. Cardiac output falls back to almost normal late in pregnancy, usually during 36 to 40 weeks, gestation. During the third trimester, cardiac output is dramatically decreased when the mother is lying supine. This is caused by compromised venous return from the lower extremity caused by compression of the inferior vena cava by the gravid uterus. In the supine position, the inferior vena cava may be completely occluded; venous drainage of the lower extremities is through collateral channels. With this drop in preload, an increase in sympathetic tone usually maintains peripheral vascular resistance and blood pressure. However, up to 10% of patients may experience supine hypotensive syndrome in which the sympathetic response is not adequate to maintain blood pressure. During anesthesia induction in the operating room, anesthetic agents may inhibit the compensatory sympathetic response, causing a more precipitous fall in blood pressure. This finding is of particular importance in evaluating the pregnant trauma patient, who must be rolled onto the left side down lateral decubitus position to accurately assess blood pressure. The pregnant patient should always be placed in the left lateral decubitus position during any procedures performed during the third trimester, relieving caval compression by the enlarged uterus.

Inguinal swelling secondary to varicosities of the round ligament is also a phenomenon that occurs during pregnancy. The increase in swelling is a result of hormonal and mechanical changes. It is often mistaken for an inguinal or femoral hernia. Appropriate treatment includes careful physical examination and ultrasound if needed. The varicosities generally resolve postpartum.

Oxygen consumption increases during pregnancy. Minute ventilation increases by 50% because of an increase in tidal volume, which appears to be a result of an elevated serum progesterone level.[2] Progesterone not only increases the sensitivity of the respiratory centers to carbon dioxide (CO_2), but it also acts as a direct stimulant to the respiratory centers. As a consequence of the increased minute ventilation, the maternal partial arterial oxygen tension (PaO_2) level during late pregnancy ranges from 104 to 108 mm Hg and the maternal partial arterial CO_2 ($PaCO_2$) level ranges from 27 to 32 mm Hg. Renal compensation maintains a normal maternal pH. The decreased $PaCO_2$ level increases the CO_2 gradient from the fetus to the mother, facilitating CO_2 transfer from the fetus to the mother. These findings are critical in managing the ventilator dependent pregnant patient during and after surgery. The oxygen-hemoglobin dissociation curve of maternal blood is shifted to the right; this, coupled with the increased affinity of fetal hemoglobin for oxygen, results in increased oxygen transfer to the fetus. Elevation of the diaphragm by as much as 4 cm results in a decrease in total lung volume by 5%. Diminished expiratory reserve volume and residual volume result in a functional residual capacity that is 20% lower than that in the nonpregnant woman. Vital capacity and inspiratory reserve volume remain stable.

In the kidney, there is an increase in the glomerular filtration rate by 50% that accompanies a 75% increase in renal plasma flow. Urinary glucose excretion increases as a direct consequence of the increased glomerular filtration rate. The blood urea nitrogen level decreases by 25% during the first trimester and is maintained at that level for the remainder of the pregnancy. The serum creatinine level also decreases by the end of the first trimester from a nonpregnant value of 0.8 to 0.7 mg/dL and may be as low as 0.5 mg/dL by term. A five- to tenfold increase in the serum renin level occurs with a subsequent four- to fivefold increase in the angiotensin level. Although the pregnant patient is apparently less sensitive to the hypertensive effects of the increased angiotensin, elevated aldosterone levels result in an increase in sodium reabsorption, overcoming the natriuresis produced by elevated progesterone levels. Serum sodium levels are decreased, however, because the increase in sodium reabsorption is less than the increase in plasma volume. Serum osmolality is decreased to 270 to 280 mOsm/kg.[2]

The increase in plasma volume and red blood cell mass is accompanied by a progressive rise in the leukocyte count during pregnancy, an important consideration when evaluating for systemic signs of infection. During the first trimester, the white blood cell count ranges from 3000 to 15,000 cells/mm^3, increasing to a range of 6000 to 16,000 cells/mm^3 during the second and third trimesters.[2] The platelet count progressively declines throughout pregnancy, whereas the mean platelet volume tends to increase after 28 weeks' gestation.

Increasing platelet counts together with high levels of circulating estrogen, increasing procoagulants, and progressive venous stasis generates a hypercoagulable state during normal pregnancy. Plasma fibrinogen, vonWillebrand factor, and factors II, V, VII, VIII, IX, X, XII increase, while protein S and the response to activated protein C decrease.[3] Serum plasminogen activator inhibitor 1 (PAI1) and placental PAI2 increase, decreasing the bodies' response to intrinsic tissue plasminogen activator (tPA), resulting in a decrease in fibrinolysis.[4,5] Increasing pressure from the gravid uterus on the inferior vena cava together with decreased venous tone contribute to venous stasis that progresses with increasing pregnancy. The end result is a fivefold increase in the risk of venous thromboembolism during pregnancy, that increases to more than twentyfold during the puerperium. In women with inherited hypercoagulable mutations, the risk of thrombosis increases further still. Despite these alterations in the coagulation cascade and platelet count, bleeding and clotting times are unchanged.

SAFETY CONCERNS IN PREGNANCY

Radiologic Concerns

Radiographic studies remain useful diagnostic tools for the pregnant patient. The greatest concern with radiation exposure is the risk to the fetus from the exposure. The accepted maximum dose of ionizing radiation during the entire pregnancy is 5 cGy. The fetus is at the highest risk from radiation exposure from the preimplantation period to approximately 15 weeks' gestation. Primary organogenesis occurs during this time and the teratogenic effects of radiation, particularly to the developing central nervous system, are at their highest. Perinatal radiation exposure has also been associated with childhood leukemia and certain childhood malignancies. The radiation dose that has been associated with congenital malformation is higher than 10 cGy. As shown in Table 72.2, radiation exposure to the fetus with the doses from the more common radiology procedures is well below that threshold. Nonetheless, prudence on the part of the clinician is required to avoid unnecessary fetal exposure to ionizing radiation, especially during the first and early second trimesters, when the risk from exposure is greatest.

Magnetic resonance imaging (MRI) avoids exposure to ionizing radiation but poses an unknown risk to the fetus. Animal studies have shown no teratogenic effect or increased incidence of fetal death or congenital malformations from the electromagnetic radiation, static magnetic field, radiofrequency magnetic fields, or intravenous (IV) contrast agents used during MRI. Theoretically, the gradient magnetic fields may produce electric currents in the patient and the high-frequency currents induced by radiofrequency fields may cause local generation of heat. The long-term effect of exposure is not known.[6] The National Radiological Protection Board has advised against the use of MRI during the first trimester

TABLE 72.2 Fetal radiation exposure with radiographic imaging.

EXAMINATION TYPE	ESTIMATED FETAL RADIATION EXPOSURE (cGY)
Two-view chest radiography	0.00007
Cervical spine radiography	0.002
Pelvis radiography	0.04
Head CT	<0.050
Abdomen CT	2.60
Upper GI series	0.056
Barium enema	3.986
HIDA scanning	0.150

CT, Computed tomography; *GI*, gastrointestinal; *HIDA*, hepatobiliary iminodiacetic acid.

of pregnancy. MRI has become the diagnostic modality of choice however, in the work up of complex fetal anomalies in the second and third trimester.

Contrast media may be administered with various techniques of body imaging. If computed tomography (CT) has been performed during pregnancy with iodide contrast, neonatal thyroid function should be checked during the first week after delivery. No effect on the fetus has been observed after the use of gadolinium contrast medium with MRI.

Ultrasonography is routinely used by obstetricians during pregnancy. Although tissue heating and cavitation are theoretical effects of ultrasound exposure, such effects have never been reported. Ultrasound may be a helpful alternative diagnostic tool when trying to avoid exposure to ionizing radiation but does have some limitations. Deeper structures are difficult to visualize and may be obscured by superficial structures that are more echo dense. Ultrasound imaging has a limited field of view and is highly operator-dependent. Despite these limitations, certain disease processes, such as a palpable breast mass or suspected appendicitis, may be evaluated effectively and safely.

Medication Concerns

The surgeon will, on occasion, need to prescribe medications to treat the pregnant patient with surgical disease. In this section, we provide an overview of medications the surgeon may commonly prescribe. The list is by no means comprehensive and, prior to using any medication, consultation with the patient's obstetrician is necessary. It is noteworthy that over 50% of pregnant woman take at least one medication with an average of 2.6 medications, and the use of four or more medications in the first trimester has tripled (9.9%–27.6%) over the past three decades.[7]

In 1979, the U.S. Food and Drug Administration (FDA) established five letter risk categories (i.e., A, B, C, D, X) to indicate the potential fetal risk if used during pregnancy. In 2015 the FDA developed a new labeling system known as the Pregnancy and Lactation Labeling Rule (PLLR) in an effort to provide more relevant information for better provider decision-making and patient-specific counseling. This new classification system removes the pregnancy risk category lettering system and provides information in a narrative form in order to more accurately describe the risks involved with using medications in pregnancy.[8,9] The lettering system is to be removed entirely by June 2020. One limitation of PLLR is medications (both prescription and over-the-counter) approved prior to June 1, 2001 do not have to provide a narrative summary, potentially making it more difficult for providers to locate information on pregnancy risk.

Despite this new classification system, the five pregnancy risk categories are most commonly referenced and utilized.

Category A: These drugs have been tested and found to be safe during pregnancy. Category A includes drugs such as folic acid, vitamin B6, and some thyroid medicines in prescribed doses.

Category B: These drugs are frequently used during pregnancy and do not appear to cause major birth defects or other problems. Category B includes some antibiotics, prednisone, insulin, acetaminophen (Tylenol), aspartame (Equal, NutraSweet), famotidine (Pepcid), and ibuprofen (Advil, Motrin) before the third trimester. Pregnant women should not take ibuprofen during the last 3 months of pregnancy.

The FDA offers the following classifications for prescription drugs that should not be taken during pregnancy:

Category C: These are drugs that are more likely to cause problems for the mother or fetus, and drugs for which safety studies have not been finished. Most of these drugs do not have safety studies in progress. These drugs often come with a warning that they should be used only if the benefits of taking them outweigh the risks. This is something the surgeon would need to discuss with the patient's obstetrician. These drugs include prochlorperazine (Compazine), pseudoephedrine (Sudafed), fluconazole (Diflucan), and ciprofloxacin (Cipro). Some antidepressants are also included in this group.

Category D: These include drugs that have clear health risks for the fetus and include alcohol, lithium, phenytoin (Dilantin), and except for select circumstances, most forms of chemotherapy.

Category X: These drugs have been shown to cause birth defects and should never be taken during pregnancy. These include drugs to treat skin conditions such as cystic acne (isotretinoin [Accutane]) and psoriasis (etretinate [Tegison], acitretin [Soriatane]), thalidomide (sedative), and diethylstilbestrol (DES; prevents miscarriage) that was used up until 1971 in the United States and until 1983 in Europe.

Analgesics

Over-the-Counter Medications

Acetaminophen, the active ingredient in Tylenol, is considered safe during pregnancy. Well researched by scientists, acetaminophen is used primarily for headaches, fever, aches, pains, and sore throat. It can be used during all three trimesters of pregnancy.

Nonsteroidal antiinflammatory drugs (NSAIDs) include aspirin, ibuprofen (Advil, Motrin), and naproxen (Aleve). Aspirin, which contains salicylic acid as its active ingredient, should generally be avoided by expectant mothers because it can pose risks for the mother and fetus. Generally, aspirin is not recommended during pregnancy; the exception being low-dose aspirin (60–100 mg daily) is sometimes recommended for pregnant women with recurrent pregnancy loss, clotting disorders, and preeclampsia.

The use of higher doses of aspirin poses various risks depending on the stage of pregnancy. During the first trimester, use of higher doses of aspirin poses a concern for pregnancy loss and congenital defects. Taking higher doses of aspirin during the third trimester increases the risk of the premature closure of a vessel in the fetus's heart. Use of high-dose aspirin for long periods in pregnancy also increases the risk of bleeding in the brain of premature infants.

Ibuprofen and naproxen are safer options, but both should be used with caution during pregnancy. They are considered safe in the first two trimesters but are ill advised in the final three months because they can also increase bleeding during delivery and increased risk for birth defects.

Prescription Medications

Prescription analgesics are available in several different forms and brand names, including codeine, tramadol, hydrocodone and acetaminophen (Vicodin, Norco, Lortab), oxycodone (OxyContin), oxycodone and acetaminophen (Percocet), morphine (MS Contin), meperidine (Demerol), and fentanyl (Duragesic, Sublimaze). These drugs may be used occasionally in pregnant patients when the benefits of the drug outweigh the potential risks. Opioids such as methadone (Dolophine) and buprenorphine (Butrans) are often used in pregnant patients with opioid use disorder to prevent withdrawal or the nonmedical use of opioids.[7,10]

However, there is no known safe level of narcotic use during pregnancy. Risks to the fetus include poor fetal growth, stillbirth, preterm delivery, and a very low risk of birth defects.[10] Chronic use of opioids during pregnancy can lead to neonatal abstinence syndrome. Used late in pregnancy and close to delivery, a neonate is at increased risk of withdrawal symptoms and respiratory depression.

Antibiotics

Antibiotics may be necessary to treat various surgery-related infections in pregnancy. The common antibiotics used are listed by class.

Aminoglycosides

In general, aminoglycosides including gentamicin, tobramycin, and amikacinare determined to be low risk to the fetus and are used commonly in pregnancy and surrounding labor and delivery.[11] The only well-known risk seen with other aminoglycosides (i.e., kanamycin and streptomycin) when used during pregnancy is fetal auditory nerve damage to the eighth cranial nerve causing deafness. No epidemiological studies have demonstrated congenital anomalies in infants whose mothers were treated with aminoglycosides during pregnancy. Only one case report exists of gentamicin use in pregnancy where congenital defects were exhibited. Nephrotoxicity has been observed in many patients receiving aminoglycosides, which raises the concern of whether fetal kidney damage may occur with maternal treatment. Although fetal renal damage after maternal gentamicin treatment has not been documented, there have been cases of severe neonatal nephropathy after therapy with this drug.

Tetracyclines

With the use of tetracyclines, including doxycycline, tetracycline, and minocycline, accumulation of the drugs occurs in developing teeth and long tubular bones. Ingestion during the second or third trimester of pregnancy can cause irreversible dental staining in childhood.[11] Depression of bone growth (especially of the fibula in preterm pregnancies) can occur following in utero exposure to tetracyclines. Acute fatty metamorphosis of the liver in pregnancy following tetracycline therapy has been described and is often fatal. Epidemiological studies have not demonstrated a clear link between exposure to tetracyclines and congenital abnormalities. Therefore, a small risk cannot be excluded, but there is no indication of increased risk of malformations in children of women treated with this agent during pregnancy. Although data on the specific safety of doxycycline use during pregnancy is limited, it is assumed the risks of the dental staining and depression of bone growth by tetracyclines in general also pertain to doxycycline use during the second and third trimesters.

Metronidazole

Rare reports and studies have shown no consistent pattern of congenital malformations in infants exposed to metronidazole in utero, making its use in pregnancy controversial. Given the limited information available, and no conclusive human studies, the risk of birth defects caused by exposure to metronidazole during pregnancy appears to be low and is recommended by the Centers for Disease Control and Prevention (CDC) for the treatment of certain infections during pregnancy. It should be noted, however, the use of metronidazole in the first trimester for the treatment of vaginal trichomoniasis or bacterial vaginosis is contraindicated by the manufacturer.

Penicillins

Penicillins are a widely used group of antibiotics that include ampicillin, amoxicillin, nafcillin, penicillin G, penicillin V, and piperacillin. Although penicillins accumulate in amniotic fluid in large amounts during maternal ingestion, no adverse fetal effects have been associated with this group of medications. It must be noted that all penicillins may produce anaphylaxis during pregnancy or immediately after delivery. If anaphylaxis is severe and uncontrolled, it could result in compromising placental circulation and cause fetal damage or death. However, in general, the penicillins have not been shown to be teratogenic and there have been no recognized adverse effects caused by exposure to this antibiotic class.[11] One point to note, drug elimination may be enhanced for some of the penicillins during pregnancy, thus, a higher dose may be needed to achieve optimal concentrations.

Cephalosporins

Cephalosporins are the most widely used class of antibiotics that include cefazolin, cephalexin, cefotetan, cefuroxime, cefoxitin, cefdinir, cefotaxime, cefpodoxime, ceftriaxone, cefepime, and ceftaroline. Based on their spectrum of activity against gram-positive and gram-negative bacteria, they are classified into five generations. Many of the first- and second-generation cephalosporins have been studied extensively in pregnant patients. It is thought most of them are not associated with any known or suspected teratogenic effects and are assumed safe for use during pregnancy. The third-, fourth-, and fifth- generation cephalosporins, however, have not been used extensively during pregnancy, and therefore there is little information known about their effects, but they are assumed + safe to use in pregnancy.[11]

Lincosamide (Clindamycin)

The teratogenic risk of the use of Lincosamide antibiotics during pregnancy is undetermined and there is limited data. Clindaymycin, the most widely used antibiotic in this category, is considered in the same pregnancy risk class (FDA Pregnancy Category B) as amoxicillin, penicillin and vancomycin. The drug has been safely used in the second trimester as an effective treatment of bacterial vaginosis and abnormal vaginal flora.[12]

Macrolides (Azithromycin)

Many reports describing the use of azithromycin in pregnancy have been published. Overall, no increase in the frequency of congenital anomalies was observed among infants of women treated with azithromycin at any time during pregnancy, and it is considered safe to use in pregnancy.

Sulfonamide Derivatives

Trimethoprim/sulfamethoxazole have been associated with increased risk of congenital malformations, namely neural tube defects, cardiovascular malformations, urinary tract defects, oral clefts, and clubfoot. This is mainly due to the trimethoprim component of the antibiotic. Due to trimethoprim being a dihydrofolate reductase inhibitor, it is thought folic acid supplementation can reduce the risk of congenital defects if they are administered prior to conception or concurrently with the antibiotic. Additionally, there is some concern over kernicterus with sulfonamide use. This agent should be avoided in pregnancy.

Fluoroquinolones

The use of fluoroquinolones (i.e., ciprofloxacin, levofloxacin, moxifloxacin, gemifloxacin) during pregnancy has not demonstrated an increased risk of congenital malformations.[11] Although many reports of birth defects displayed in infants when fluoroquinolones were ingested during pregnancy, no pattern in these malformations has been identified. Ciprofloxacin has been the most studied of the fluoroquinolones in pregnant patients. Based on this information, it is thought ciprofloxacin does not have any teratogenic effects and is assumed safe for use during pregnancy. Levofloxacin, moxifloxacin, and gemifloxacin, however, have not been studied or used extensively during pregnancy and therefore there is little information known about their effects. However, animal studies of the fluoroquinolones have suggested some malformation risk, including fetal cartilage damage, and thus, their risk cannot be excluded. In general, it is accepted fluoroquinolones should be avoided in the first trimester, if a safer alternative is available to use.[8]

Other Gram Positive Agents

Vancomycin and clindamycin are commonly used for multidrug resistant gram-positive infections or for penicillin-allergic patients. No studies or reports have attributed congenital malformations or other adverse events to their use, thus they are considered safe to use in pregnancy.[8]

Summary of Antibiotic Use

Although antibiotics are commonly prescribed to pregnant women, details relating to the effects of many of these drugs remain poorly understood. If an antibiotic must be prescribed, it is important to be aware of the effects these drugs can have on pregnancies and to prescribe the most suitable agent with the least risk to the pregnancy.

Antithrombotic Agents Thrombotic Agents

Anticoagulants

Heparin. The recommended therapeutic agent used in pregnancy for the prevention and treatment of venous thromboemboli is low–molecular-weight heparin (Category B) which has largely replaced standard, unfractionated heparin (Category C). Neither of these agents cross the placenta and are safe in pregnancy, however unfractionated heparin may be associated with increased maternal bone loss.[3]

Danaparoid. Danaparoid is a low–molecular-weight heparinoid with both anti-Xa and antithrombin effects.[13] Danaparoid neither crosses the placenta nor is secreted in breast milk and thus is theoretically safe in pregnancy.[14,15] A review of the literature from 1981 and 2004 by Lindhoff-Last and colleagues reported use of danaparoid in 51 pregnancies with heparin intolerance with no adverse pregnancy effects. As it is a heparinoid, there remains the (remote) possibility of heparin-induced thrombocytopenia. However, it remains the anticoagulant of choice for use in pregnancy when heparin-induced thrombocytopenia has occurred.

Coumadin. While vitamin K antagonists such as warfarin are well-established and highly effective anticoagulants, they are contraindicated in pregnancy. Vitamin K antagonists cross the placenta and anticoagulate the fetus (Category D). Warfarin use during pregnancy has been associated with miscarriage, prematurity, lower birth weight, neurodevelopmental problems and fetal bleeding, as well as a risk of major birth defects with first trimester exposure.[3,4,13,16] In select circumstances, warfarin has been used in pregnant patients with newer mechanical aortic valves, targeting a lower international normalized ratio (INR) of 1.5 to 2.0 without complications for the mother or fetus.[4] However, this use of warfarin is still investigational. In the postnatal period, however, warfarin is a suitable alternative to parenteral anticoagulants such as heparin. This transition usually takes place when risk of obstetric hemorrhage is low, commonly about days 5 to 7 after the delivery of the baby. It is not contraindicated in breastfeeding.

Factor Xa and direct thrombin inhibitors. The novel anticoagulants include direct factor Xa inhibitors and direct thrombin inhibitors. At present, there is very limited data available regarding the safety of these agents in pregnancy. The literature consists primarily of case reports and small retrospective series.

While the new oral factor Xa inhibitors are more attractive than parenteral preparations for long-term use, these may cross the placenta and pose problems for the fetus. Such concern may explain the lack of data on their use in pregnancy, as the risks to the developing and maturing fetus in utero are unknown.

In situations of severe reactions to heparin and danaparoid, the American College of Chest Physicians recommends that direct thrombin inhibitors be used.[3] Fondaparinux is the agent of choice, as it does not cross the placenta and is an FDA Class B medication/Australian Category C.[4] The manufacturers of fondaparinux have collected information on 120 women who used fondaparinux around the time of pregnancy, and it has shown no adverse outcomes. Direct thrombin inhibitors including hirudin, lepirudin, and argatroban are not licensed for use in pregnancy, as there is currently limited evidence of their safety.[17]

Antiplatelet Agents

Aspirin

Aspirin is the leading antiplatelet drug used for a variety of indications, including cardiovascular disease and vascular injury. In pregnant patients, however, aspirin may cause teratogenicity and fetal toxicity. Premature closure of the ductus arteriosus and increased perinatal mortality have been reported in animal studies with higher doses of aspirin. Therefore, aspirin is contraindicated (Category D) in doses exceeding 100 mg. However, the FDA has assigned pregnancy category C, at lower doses (60–100 mg) indicating treatment is relatively safe at these levels. Low-dose aspirin once daily is recommended by the American Heart Association for pregnant patients with either a mechanical prosthesis or bioprosthesis in the second and third trimesters. In our practice, we keep women on low-dose aspirin through the first trimester as well.

Clopidogrel

Clopidogrel has shown no adverse pregnancy effects when studied in animal models, earning it a category B designation from the FDA.[11] There is limited available data on the use of clopidogrel in human pregnancy. From the available literature, there is no evidence that clopidogrel increases placental abruption or other antepartum obstetric bleeding events. Additionally, thus far, there are no reports of fetal hemorrhagic events or excessive neonatal bleeding from the manufacturer's safety data. However, it is generally recommended to hold clopidogrel for seven days prior to an elective delivery or administration of epidural anesthesia, thus caution should be used when delivery may be unplanned.

Thrombolytic Agents

There is extremely limited data available on the effect of thrombolytic therapy during pregnancy; therefore, it is classified as a category C drug. Thrombolytics may be considered when benefits of administration outweigh the risk of hemorrhage. In the case of acute venous thrombosis, including May-Thurner syndrome, mechanical thrombolysis is recommended over thrombolytics. However, in the case of acute arterial thrombosis, including stroke, the timely administration of recombinant tPA has been associated with significant improvements in morbidity and mortality. In general, intraarterial tPA with or without combined with mechanical thrombectomy, is preferred to systemic tPA administration. There is insufficient data available on other thrombolytic agents including streptokinase, anisoylated plasminogen streptokinase activator complex, and urokinase to draw any reasonable conclusions.

Sedatives

Benzodiazepines

Diazepam. The use of benzodiazepines, specifically diazepam, was previously thought to be associated with an increased frequency of cleft lip and/or palate; this finding has not been supported by most recent studies. Although the balance of evidence from human studies of the benzodiazepines (chiefly diazepam) does not show first-trimester usage to be teratogenic, the surgeon should check with the patient's obstetrician before administering this class of drugs.

Midazolam. Midazolam is generally considered unsafe for use during pregnancy. Midazolam was given a pregnancy category D rating by the FDA because it is a benzodiazepine and other benzodiazepines have been shown to cause birth defects and other problems. However, studies of midazolam in pregnant rabbits and rats did not show any problems.

Anesthesia Concerns

Anesthesia concerns during pregnancy include the safety of the mother and fetus. The fetus may be affected by exposure to teratogenic effects of anesthetic agents, risk for preterm labor, and risk from changes in maternal physiology as a consequence of anesthesia. Changes in uterine blood flow and maternal acid-base status may cause hypoxemia or asphyxia in the fetus. These can be a result of maternal hypotension or hypoxia, maternal hyperventilation, or placental passage of anesthetic agents that affect the fetal central nervous system or cardiovascular system.

The effects of anesthesia during pregnancy can be divided into direct, or active, and indirect, or passive, effects. The direct effects relate to the possible teratogenic or embryotoxic properties of the drugs used for anesthesia, some of which cross the placenta. The indirect effects are those mechanisms whereby an anesthetic agent or surgical procedure may interfere with maternal or fetal physiology and, in doing so, harm the fetus. For the most part, the fetus experiences indirect effects as a consequence of anesthetic agents administered to the mother and hemodynamic changes in the mother from blood loss or anesthetic agents. The most profound effects on the fetus are related to decreased uterine blood flow or decreased oxygen content of uterine blood. Unlike circulation to other vital organs, most notably the brain, the uterine circulation is not autoregulated. During the third trimester, uterine circulation represents almost 10% of cardiac output. When treating maternal hypotension, vasopressors such as dopamine and epinephrine, although increasing the maternal systemic pressure, have little or no effect on uterine circulation. Phenylephrine and metaraminol are alpha agonists that are effective in maintaining maternal blood pressure and preventing fetal acidosis. Other maneuvers, such as fluid bolus, Trendelenburg position, compression stockings, and leg elevation, have a larger impact on increasing uterine blood flow.

In addition to the risks related to maternal hypoxia or hypotension, the risk for spontaneous abortion and teratogenesis related to anesthetic agents is of major concern. Many nonhuman studies have demonstrated different teratogenic effects with similar agents but have not led to definitive conclusions regarding their teratogenic potential in humans. For a congenital defect to result, exposure to the teratogen must occur during the vulnerable differentiation stage of the affected organ system. As noted, differentiation of the major organ systems occurs during the first trimester of human embryonic development. Therefore, delaying semielective surgical procedures until after the first trimester may reduce the risk for teratogenicity. However, large survey studies have demonstrated an increased risk for spontaneous abortions, intrauterine growth retardation, and low–birth weight neonates in women who require surgery during pregnancy. These studies lacked information on the indications for nonobstetric surgical procedures and failed to elucidate the etiology of this association. At present, the degree to which fetal development may be impacted by anesthetic exposure, surgical stress, or the underlying disease state that prompted surgery remains unclear. Fetal surgery during the second and third trimesters has not been demonstrated to have specific adverse effects on fetal neurodevelopment, but long-term studies are lacking. Despite a black box warning from the FDA regarding anesthesia in young children, the PANDA trial failed to demonstrate significant long-term adverse effects from a single anesthetic before 36 months of age in matched sibling pairs.[18]

Elective surgical procedures are delayed until at least six weeks after delivery, when maternal physiology has returned to the nonpregnant state and when the impact on the fetus is no longer a concern. When emergent procedures are required, obviously the life of the mother takes priority, although an experienced anesthesiologist will be able to modify the anesthesia used according to maternal physiology and fetal well-being. For semielective surgical procedures, attempts are made to delay surgery until after the first trimester, whenever possible. This needs to be determined on an individual basis because continued exposure to the underlying disease process may be more harmful than the operative risk to the mother and fetus. During the second trimester, after organ system differentiation has occurred, there is almost no risk for anesthetic-induced malformation or spontaneous abortion. Later in pregnancy, during the third trimester, the risk for preterm delivery is at its highest.

When the pregnant patient requires surgical intervention, consultation with the obstetrician and possibly a perinatologist is essential. The specialist is helpful in determining the optimum technique to monitor fetal status and can assist with perioperative management and diagnose and manage preterm labor. Typically, when emergent surgery occurs during the first or early second trimester, fetal heart tones are monitored before and after anesthesia exposure. During the late second and third trimesters, when the fetus is of viable age, continuous intraoperative monitoring is performed when possible. Transvaginal ultrasound can be used when the surgical field involves the abdomen. Continuous monitoring is used if significant blood loss is possible or anticipated to assess fetal well-being. Checking the fetal heart rate for fetal status and tocometer monitoring for uterine activity are done before and after the procedure, even if intraoperative monitoring is not believed necessary or is unavailable.

Postoperative pain control in the pregnant patient needs to be monitored closely. NSAIDs are not used in pregnancy because of the risk for premature closure of the ductus arteriosus.[19] The newly available IV acetaminophen, morphine, and fentanyl are good choices postoperatively when oral analgesics are insufficient or cannot be used. Morphine has a higher associated incidence of nausea and vomiting, but most surgeons have extensive experience with it. A patient-controlled analgesia pump after surgery may be the best choice because of the associated low incidence of maternal respiratory depression and drug transfer to the fetus.

Postoperative oral narcotic use is generally considered safe in pregnancy. Narcotic analgesics have not been found to cause birth defects in humans in normal dosages. Oxycodone, hydrocodone, and codeine are commonly used narcotics and can be safely used in moderation. Chronic use of narcotics during pregnancy may cause fetal dependency. It is recommended that the pregnant postsurgical patient be weaned off narcotic use as soon as possible.

PREVENTION OF PRETERM LABOR

The incidence of preterm labor associated with nonobstetric surgery is related to gestational age and the indication for surgery. Studies have suggested that the rate of premature labor induced by nonobstetric surgical intervention is 3.5%. Gestational age at treatment and severity of the underlying disease are the most predictive indicators of patients at risk for preterm labor. The later in gestation is the patient, the higher the risk for preterm contractions or preterm labor. Intraperitoneal surgeries and disease processes with intraperitoneal inflammation are the most likely to have a postoperative course complicated by preterm contractions and preterm labor. In a number of studies, a significant difference was found in the number of patients with preterm contractions based on the average time from onset of symptoms to operative intervention. A delay in treatment appears to increase the chance of preterm labor, likely related to the primary disease process. Laparoscopic and open techniques have an equal associated incidence of preterm labor.

There is no general consensus on the use of prophylactic tocolytics after nonobstetric surgery during pregnancy. Tocolytic use varies widely among centers and physicians. Most studies have suggested that tocolytics only be used if contractions are noted during postoperative monitoring or are appreciated by the patient. Tocolytics used as needed are generally successful at preventing preterm labor and preterm delivery when postoperative contractions are detected. Terbutaline, magnesium, and indomethacin (Indocin) have been used in different studies, with equivalent results. Almost 100% of patients with postoperative contractions were successfully given tocolytics and delivered at term. In general, for patients with postoperative contractions before 32 weeks, indomethacin would be a reasonable treatment, whereas terbutaline could be used as first-line treatment for patients at more than 32 weeks' gestation. The use of prophylactic tocolysis is individualized, depending on the patient's gestational age and underlying disease process.

ABDOMINAL PAIN AND THE ACUTE ABDOMEN IN PREGNANCY

When the pregnant patient presents with abdominal pain, it may be difficult to distinguish a pathophysiologic cause from normal pregnancy-associated symptoms. Changes in the position and orientation of abdominal viscera from the enlarging uterus, and the alterations in physiology already described, may modify the perception or manifestation of an intraabdominal process. If it is early in the pregnancy, the woman may not know that she is pregnant. Also, some intraabdominal processes are exclusive to pregnancy, such as ectopic pregnancy; hemolysis, elevated liver enzymes, low platelets (HELLP) syndrome; or acute fatty liver of pregnancy. Both patient and physician may attribute the patient's complaints to normal pregnancy, resulting in a delay in evaluation and treatment. These delays in diagnosis and definitive intervention are the most serious adverse events affecting maternal and fetal outcome. It is usually not the treatment but the delay in diagnosis and severity of the primary disease process that affects outcomes poorly. Box 72.1 lists the more common causes of abdominal pain in the pregnant patient, classified according to location.

MINIMALLY INVASIVE SURGERY IN PREGNANCY

When laparoscopic techniques were initially described, pregnancy was considered to be a contraindication to laparoscopy. Effects of CO_2 pneumoperitoneum on venous return and cardiac output, uterine perfusion, and fetal acid-base status were unknown. Laparoscopy was safely used in several series to evaluate pregnant patients for ectopic pregnancy. Patients with an intrauterine pregnancy had no increase in fetal loss or observed negative effect on long-term outcome.[20] When comparing laparoscopic and open techniques in nonpregnant patients, patients who underwent laparoscopic procedures had decreased pain, shorter hospital stays, and a quicker return to normal activity.

Major concerns of laparoscopy during pregnancy include injury to the uterus, decreased uterine blood flow, fetal acidosis, and preterm labor from increased intraabdominal pressure. During the second trimester, the uterus is no longer contained within the pelvis. The open technique for abdominal access can reduce the risk for injury. Using a Veress needle for insufflation or optical trocar can be done safely if the site of initial abdominal access is adjusted according to fundal height and the abdominal wall is elevated. Decreased uterine blood flow from pneumoperitoneum remains a theoretical concern because significant changes in intraabdominal pressure occur normally during pregnancy with maternal Valsalva maneuvers. The risk for pneumoperitoneum may also be less than the risk for direct uterine manipulation that occurs with laparotomy. Fetal respiratory acidosis with subsequent fetal hypertension and tachycardia have been observed in a pregnant ewe model but were reversed by maintaining maternal respiratory alkalosis.[21] Also, in the largest series comparing laparoscopy and open techniques, no significant differences in preterm labor or delivery-related side effects were observed.[20] Box 72.2 illustrates the general comparison between laparoscopic and open technique.

The Society of American Gastrointestinal and Endoscopic Surgeons (SAGES) recommends the following guidelines for laparoscopic surgery during pregnancy based on a literature review of 154 articles from 2011 to 2016, with a 4-tiered system of quality of evidence (very low [+], low [++], moderate [+++], or high [++++]) and a 2-tiered system for strength of recommendation (weak or strong). Updated SAGES guidelines for laparoscopic surgery are[22,23]:

1. Obstetric consultation is obtained preoperatively.
2. When possible, operative intervention is deferred until the second trimester, when fetal risk is lowest, but laparoscopy can be safely performed during any trimester of pregnancy when the operation is indicated (++++; strong).

BOX 72.1 Common causes of abodominal pain in pregnant patients.

Right Upper Quadrant

Gastroesophageal reflux
Peptic ulcer disease
Acute cholecystitis
Biliary colic
Acute pancreatitis
Hepatitis
Acute fatty liver of pregnancy
HELLP syndrome
Preeclampsia
Pneumothorax
Pneumonia
Acute appendicitis
Hepatic adenoma
Hemangioma

Right Lower Quadrant

Acute appendicitis
Ectopic pregnancy
Renal or ureteral colic
Pelvic inflammatory disease
Tuboovarian abscess
Endometriosis
Adnexal torsion
Ruptured ovarian cyst
Ruptured corpus luteum

Lower Abdomen

Threatened, incomplete, or complete abortion
Abruptio placentae
Preterm labor
Pelvic inflammatory disease
Tuboovarian abscess
Inflammatory bowel disease
Irritable bowel syndrome
Pyelonephritis

Flank

Pyelonephritis
Hydronephrosis of pregnancy
Acute appendicitis (retrocecal appendix)

Diffuse Abdominal Pain

Early acute appendicitis
Small bowel obstruction
Acute intermittent porphyria
Sickle cell crisis

HELLP, Hemolysis, elevated liver enzymes, low platelets.

BOX 72.2 Advantages and disadvantages of laparoscopy instead of laparotomy in pregnancy.

Advantages

Decreased fetal depression secondary to decreased narcotic requirement
Lower rates of wound infections and incisional hernias
Diminished postoperative maternal hypoventilation
Decreased manipulation of the uterus
Faster recovery with early return to normal function
Decreased risk of ileus

Disadvantages

Possible uterine injury during trocar placement
Decreased uterine blood flow
Preterm labor risk secondary to increased intraabdominal pressure
Increased risk of fetal acidosis and unknown effects of CO_2 pneumoperitoneum
Decreased visualization with gravid uterus

CO_2, Carbon dioxide.

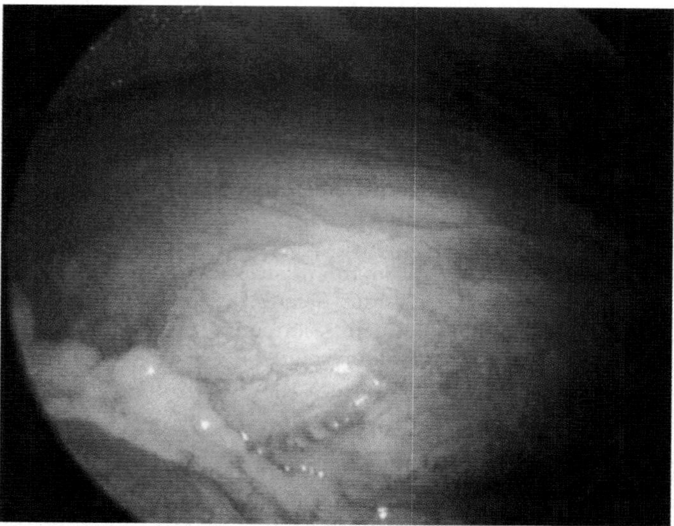

FIG. 72.1 Intraoperative image of a 24-week gravid uterus taken with a 5-mm, 30-degree high-definition camera.

3. Pneumoperitoneum enhances lower extremity venous stasis already present in the gravid patient, and pregnancy induces a hypercoagulable state. Therefore, pneumatic compression devices are used whenever possible, and beyond the first trimester, gravid patients should be placed in the left lateral decubitus position of partial left lateral decubitus position to minimize compression of the vena cava (++; strong).
4. Fetal and uterine status, as well as maternal end-tidal CO_2 and arterial blood gas levels, need to be monitored (+++; strong).
5. The uterus needs to be protected with a lead shield if intraoperative cholangiography is a possibility. Fluoroscopy is used selectively (++; strong).
6. Initial abdominal access can be safely accomplished with an open (Hasson), Veress needle, or optical trocar technique by surgeons experienced with these techniques if the location is adjusted according to fundal height (++; weak).
7. Pneumoperitoneum CO_2 pressures of 10 to 15 mm Hg can be safely used for laparoscopy in the pregnant patient. The level of insufflation should be adjusted to the patient's physiology (+++; strong).

According to SAGES guidelines, safe abdominal access for laparoscopy can be accomplished using either an open or closed technique, when used appropriately.[22,23] Of course, this is in the hands of experienced laparoscopic surgeons writing for this professional organization. The concern for use of closed access techniques (Veress needle or optical entry) has largely been based on the concern for higher risk of injury to the uterus or other intraabdominal organs. Because the intraabdominal domain is altered as the uterus grows, trocar placement should be altered from the standard configuration to supraumbilical or subcostal (Fig. 72.1). An angled endoscope may aid in viewing over or around the uterus. If the site of initial abdominal access is adjusted according to fundal height and the abdominal wall is elevated during insertion, both the Hassan technique and Veress needle have been safely and effectively used.[21,22,23] Ultrasound guided trocar placement has been described in the literature as an additional safeguard to avoid uterine injury. Regardless of technique, the uterus should be manipulated as little as possible. Should an inadvertent entry into the uterus occur during a laparoscopic procedure, simple closure of the defect with an absorbable suture followed by monitoring and possible indomethacin tocolysis is usually adequate to prevent preterm delivery. If any concern exists regarding potential damage to the fetus or placental then obstetrical consultation with ultrasound examination of the fetus is indicated.

BREAST MASSES IN PREGNANCY

During pregnancy and lactation, a woman's breasts face many physiologic changes. These changes can be attributed to various hormones. Such changes may hinder the interpretation of physical and medical imaging examinations of the breasts. It is important to note that most breast lesions that are diagnosed during pregnancy and lactation are benign; however, the differential diagnosis of breast cancer is challenging during these periods.[24] Pregnancy-associated breast cancer is defined as breast cancer diagnosed during pregnancy or within one year after pregnancy. It has become increasingly more prominent as more women delay child-bearing until they are in their 30s and 40s; the incidence of breast cancer is higher in women in those age groups. Overall, pregnancy-associated breast cancer has been reported to occur in 1 in 3000 pregnancies.[25,26] Physiologic changes of breast engorgement, rapid cellular proliferation, and increased vascularity make a reliable physical examination difficult; masses of similar size that would be easily palpable in the nonpregnant state may be obscured, or palpable masses may be attributed to normal pregnancy-related changes. Benign breast lesions such as galactoceles, mastitis, abscesses, lipomas, fibroadenomas, lobular hyperplasia, and lactational adenomas account for 80% of breast masses that occur during pregnancy or lactation. However, any palpable mass that persists for four weeks or longer needs to be evaluated.[26]

Imaging and Biopsy During Pregnancy

Because of the changes in the breast tissue with pregnancy, imaging modality findings may be difficult to interpret. The physiologic changes proliferate the breast parenchyma so that it increases the size, and increases the density of cells, blood vessels, and amount of moisture, therefore, the mammographic parenchymal density increases and becomes diffuse. If used with appropriate shielding, mammography carries a limited risk to the fetus. Mammography has a high false-negative rate because of the increased density of the fibroglandular breast tissue, however, so it has limited usefulness in evaluation of the pregnant patient. Ultrasonography can safely be performed as an initial evaluation or in conjunction with mammography. Ultrasound is able to distinguish solid from cystic lesions in 97% of patients and is helpful in guiding fine-needle aspiration or biopsy. MRI of the breast is highly sensitive but only moderately specific and has been used more frequently in the nonpregnant patient. Although MRI does not use ionizing radiation, the two main risks to the fetus from the magnetic field and electromagnetic radiation are heating and cavitation. MRI should only be used in specific cases as needed for urgent clinical decision-making. Core biopsy remains the most appropriate method of tissue diagnosis in pregnancy.

Pregnancy-Associated Breast Cancer

Breast cancer is the most common nongynecologic malignancy associated with pregnancy. It usually presents as a painless palpable mass, with or without nipple discharge. Studies have demonstrated that pregnancy-associated breast cancer may be more common in women with a genetic predisposition to breast cancer. In a group of 292 women diagnosed with breast cancer before age 40 years, those with a known *BRCA1* or *BRCA2* gene mutation were more likely to develop cancer during pregnancy.[27] As is true for nonpregnant patients, ductal carcinoma is the most common pathologic type of tumor, accounting for 75% to 90% of breast cancers in pregnant patients.

Delays in diagnosis and treatment are common, although this has improved. Previous studies demonstrated delays in diagnosis of almost 6 months, but more recent data have shown a mean delay of 1 to 2 months. Given a tumor doubling size of 130 days, a delay in diagnosis and treatment of one month increases the risk for nodal metastasis by 0.9%, whereas a delay of six months increases the risk by 5.1%.[28] Although the initial reports of pregnancy-associated breast cancer more than 100 years ago proposed a dismal prognosis, more recent literature has suggested that this is because of a more advanced stage at the time of diagnosis.[25] When compared with age-matched nonpregnant controls, women with pregnancy-associated breast cancer present with a larger primary tumor and higher risk for positive axillary lymph nodes. However, women with pregnancy-associated breast cancer have a similar stage-related prognosis compared with nonpregnant controls. Overall, these women bear a worse prognosis because of the more advanced disease at presentation. Pregnancy is a hyperestrogenic state and may correlate with rapid tumor proliferation and axillary lymph node metastases, although pregnant women and nonpregnant young women have a higher percentage of estrogen receptor–negative cancers than older women. In a series comparing 75 patients with pregnancy-associated breast cancer and 182 nonpregnant patients with breast cancer, 42% of cancers were estrogen receptor–negative in the pregnant group and 21% were estrogen receptor–negative in the nonpregnant control group.[26] This higher incidence of estrogen receptor–negative cancer is likely caused by a downregulation of estrogen receptors during pregnancy.

Gadolinium contrast is listed as a pregnancy category C drug, to be used only if the potential benefit outweighs the potential risk. Gadolinium crosses the placenta and has been associated with fetal abnormalities in rats. With other reliable imaging modalities available, MRI is not currently recommended for breast imaging in the pregnant patient.

Tissue diagnosis is essential. Core-needle biopsy, with or without ultrasound guidance, is a safe and reliable method for obtaining tissue. The major risks are hematoma formation and milk fistula development. A pressure dressing is applied following the biopsy to minimize the risk for hematoma from the hypervascularity of the breasts. The risk for milk fistula may be reduced by stopping lactation for several days before biopsy and by emptying the breast of milk just before the procedure. If the biopsy is done postpartum, a 1-week course of bromocriptine may also be given before biopsy. Fine-needle aspiration may be a reliable alternative to core-needle or open biopsy. It can be performed safely with ultrasound guidance under local anesthesia without exposing the patient and fetus to the risks involved with general anesthesia, but its accuracy is dependent on the pathologist's experience in distinguishing the proliferative changes of pregnancy from those of cancer.

The mainstay of therapy for pregnancy-associated breast cancer is surgical resection. Modified radical mastectomy has long been considered the appropriate choice for local control. It eliminates the need for adjuvant radiation and its risk to the fetus. More recent data have suggested that the combination of local control and adjuvant therapy may be tailored to the patient according to the stage of pregnancy, as well as the stage of the cancer.[25] In stages I and II cancer, mastectomy with axillary dissection is preferred. Axillary dissection is necessary because of the aggressive nature of pregnancy-associated breast cancer and the higher incidence of nodal metastasis. Sentinel node biopsy poses an unknown risk to the fetus and is avoided until the safety of the radioisotope has been determined.

In patients diagnosed during the late second trimester or later, immediate breast-conserving lumpectomy and axillary dissection, followed with radiation postpartum, is a treatment option. If the diagnosis of breast cancer is made in the first or early second trimester of pregnancy, lumpectomy and axillary dissection can be followed by chemotherapy after the first trimester and by radiation after delivery. Chemotherapy is indicated for node-positive cancers or node-negative tumors larger than 1 cm. Current chemotherapeutic regimens are relatively safe after the first trimester, when the teratogenic risk is greatest. The increased plasma volume, hypoalbuminemia, and the fact that almost all chemotherapeutic agents cross the placenta change drug pharmacokinetics and make accurate dosing difficult. Antimetabolites such as methotrexate are avoided because of the high risk for spontaneous abortion, even after the first trimester. Other agents have been associated with congenital malformations and complications such as preterm delivery, low birth weight, hyaline membrane disease, transient leukopenia, transient tachypnea of the newborn, and intrauterine growth retardation, but most of these effects occurred when the chemotherapeutic agent was administered during the first trimester. In one study, 24 patients with pregnancy-associated breast cancer were given a chemotherapeutic regimen during the second and third trimesters that included fluorouracil, cyclophosphamide, and doxorubicin. None of the infants had congenital malformations; the median age at delivery was 38 weeks.[26] Long-term effects of the chemotherapeutic agents used for pregnancy-associated breast cancer on growth and development of children are still not known. Cyclophosphamide and doxorubicin can enter breast milk; breastfeeding is contraindicated during chemotherapy.

Radiation is typically not offered during pregnancy because of its teratogenic risk and risk for induction of childhood malignancies. The risk is directly related to dose and developmental stage. During the preimplantation stage and continuing to 15 weeks after conception, during organogenesis, the rapidly proliferating cells of the fetus are most sensitive to radiation, and exposure greater than 1 Gy during this period has a high likelihood of causing fetal death. The standard therapeutic course of 50 Gy results in varying exposure to the fetus, depending on the gestational age and proximity of the gravid uterus to the radiation bed. Even with abdominal shielding, the greatest fetal exposure is caused by scatter. Although there have been several case reports of healthy infants born after maternal radiation exposure, radiation is not recommended during pregnancy because of the risks to the fetus.

Elective termination of the pregnancy to receive appropriate therapy without the risk for fetal malformation is no longer routinely recommended because no improvement in survival has been demonstrated. With the treatment options available to the pregnant patient with breast cancer, a combined approach among the patient, surgeon, oncologist, and maternal-fetal medicine specialist ensures optimal treatment of the disease while minimizing risk to the patient and fetus. A suggested algorithm for the treatment of breast masses in pregnancy is shown in Fig. 72.2.

SURGERY FOR DISEASES IN PREGNANCY

Hepatobiliary Disease

Liver abnormalities during pregnancy can be classified as occurring exclusively during pregnancy as a direct result of conditions during pregnancy, occurring simultaneously but not exclusively during pregnancy, or developing before the pregnancy. Examples of liver disorders unique to pregnancy include acute fatty liver of pregnancy, intrahepatic cholestasis of pregnancy, and liver disease related to preeclampsia or eclampsia, specifically HELLP syndrome and spontaneous hepatic hemorrhage or rupture. Preexisting liver disorders that may manifest with complications during pregnancy include hepatic adenoma and hepatocellular carcinoma.

The cause of acute fatty liver of pregnancy is unknown, although it is more common in first pregnancies, twin pregnancies, and women who are pregnant with a male fetus. Although it has been diagnosed as early as 26 weeks' gestation, it usually occurs during the third trimester, typically around 35 weeks' gestation. Acute fatty liver of pregnancy carries a 20% maternal and fetal mortality rate. Initial nonspecific symptoms such as malaise, nausea, vomiting, and right upper quadrant pain are followed by signs of significant liver dysfunction within two weeks of onset of symptoms. Progression to fulminant hepatic failure quickly leads to preterm labor and an increased risk for fetal mortality. Although there is no specific treatment for acute fatty liver of pregnancy,

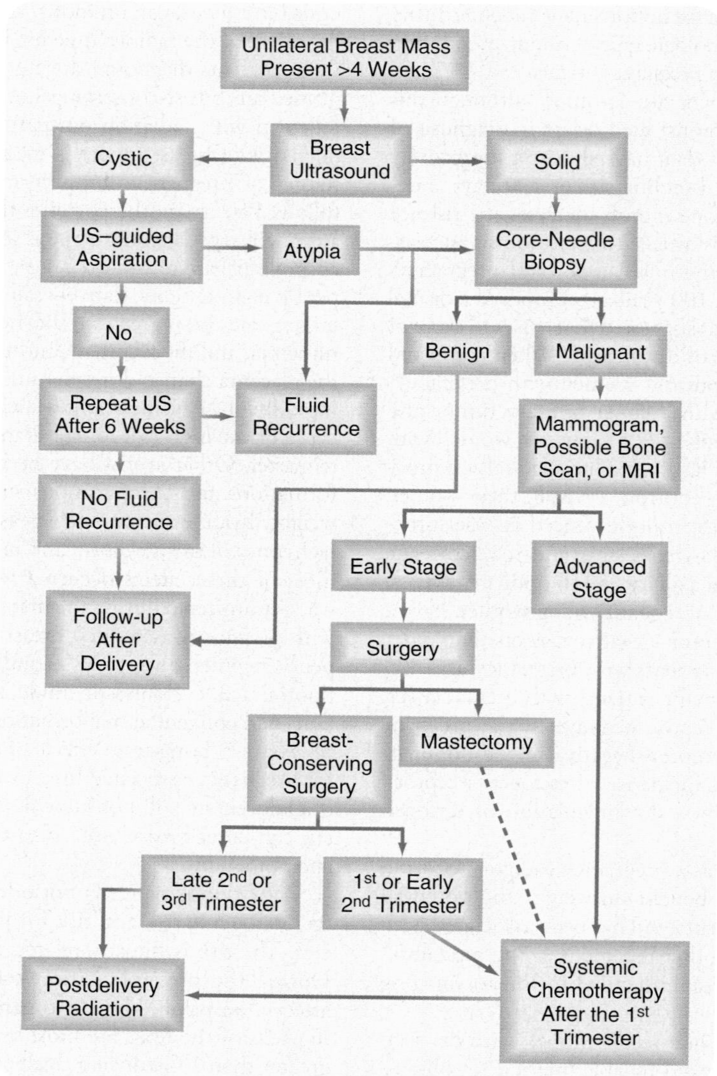

FIG. 72.2 Algorithm for the management of a breast mass during pregnancy. *MRI*, Magnetic resonance imaging; *US*, ultrasound.

prompt delivery after diagnosis may prevent progression to fulminant hepatic failure and reduce the risk for fetal death. Liver function typically returns to normal after delivery.

Approximately 10% of women with preeclampsia or eclampsia have associated liver involvement,[29] ranging from severe elevation of hepatic enzyme levels to HELLP syndrome to hepatic rupture. Hepatic hemorrhage or rupture occurs primarily during the third trimester or can develop up to 48 hours after delivery. Right upper quadrant pain is the initial manifestation, followed by hepatic tenderness, peritonitis, chest and right shoulder pain, or the development of hemodynamic instability within a few hours. The diagnosis is suspected in a pregnant patient with preeclampsia who develops right upper quadrant pain. A CT scan of the abdomen is highly sensitive and specific in diagnosis; ultrasonography findings are usually nonspecific and have a higher incidence of false-negative studies. The diagnosis may also be made during cesarean section. Management depends on a suspicion of ongoing intraperitoneal hemorrhage or vascular instability. Hepatic hematomas without evidence of ongoing bleeding in hemodynamically stable patients may be managed nonoperatively with serial imaging and close monitoring, and these lesions typically heal without intervention. If there is evidence or suspicion of rupture, immediate intervention is required because maternal and fetal mortality rates from hepatic hemorrhage are 60% and 85%, respectively. Immediate laparotomy with abdominal packing or hepatic artery ligation reduces maternal and fetal mortality. Coagulopathy must be corrected aggressively. If the patient is relatively stable or abdominal packing has been unsuccessful in controlling hemorrhage, angiography with selective embolization may be performed. Angiography is most useful when the diagnosis is made postpartum.

Hepatic adenomas are uncommon benign lesions usually associated with oral contraceptive use in young women.[30] Hepatic adenomas are also associated with glycogen storage disease, diabetes, exogenous steroids, and pregnancy. They are usually solitary lesions that have a low potential for malignant transformation. Although the specific cause is unknown, it has been hypothesized that a change in hormone levels, specifically of the sex steroids, leads to hepatotoxicity or exposes a hereditary defect in carbohydrate metabolism that results in hepatocyte hyperplasia and adenoma formation. The observation that adenomas may resolve after cessation of exogenous steroid or oral contraceptive use supports this hypothesis. The association of hepatic adenomas with pregnancy supports the hypothesis that elevated levels of endogenous hormones may contribute to adenoma formation, although no data have shown regression of a hepatic adenoma after pregnancy. Similarly, the actual incidence of hepatic adenomas during pregnancy is unknown. Again, diagnosis is best done with CT or MRI of the liver.

The major risk of a hepatic adenoma during pregnancy is spontaneous rupture, which carries a mortality rate of approximately 60% for mother and fetus, even with operative intervention. When spontaneous rupture does occur, the presentation may be similar to that described for hepatic hemorrhage associated with preeclampsia—right upper quadrant pain with referred right shoulder pain and progression to shock. Immediate laparotomy is performed with cesarean birth, control of hemorrhage, and resection of the adenoma, if possible.

Because of the high mortality associated with the rupture of a hepatic adenoma, elective resection may be performed. Resection during the second trimester minimizes the operative risk to the mother and fetus and does not interfere with the remainder of the pregnancy or subsequent pregnancies. Because of the unknown recurrence risk, however, subsequent pregnancy and oral contraceptive use may be discouraged in these patients.

Cavernous hemangiomas are the most common benign tumors of the liver and are found in approximately 2% of autopsy patients. The vast majority of these tumors are small and asymptomatic; however, there have been a few reported cases in which these lesions led to spontaneous fatal hemorrhage. Although liver hemangiomas occur in both genders, most studies have indicated to a female predominance; one study reported a ratio of female predominance of 4.5:1. It has been suggested that estrogen may be associated with the growth of liver hemangiomas, but the incidence of these lesions in pregnancy and the effects of increased estrogen levels during pregnancy on them are unknown. Symptomatic liver hemangiomas have been treated by steroids, radiation therapy, surgical resection, and recently embolization, but surgeons may sometimes be confronted with intraabdominal hemorrhage originating from the rupture of asymptomatic liver hemangiomas. A case of an incidental intraabdominal hemorrhage originating from a liver hemangioma in a 36-week twin pregnancy being delivered emergently by cesarean section because of fetal distress has been reported.

Cholelithiasis

Cholecystectomy for symptomatic cholelithiasis is second to appendectomy as the most common nonobstetric surgical procedure performed during pregnancy. As noted, pregnancy is associated with an increased incidence of cholelithiasis. Most pregnant women are asymptomatic. Although an estimated 2% to 5% of pregnant women may be found to have gallstones by ultrasound, only 0.05% to 0.1% of them will be symptomatic. Biliary cholesterol concentrations in gallbladder bile increase gradually from the first to the third trimester, along with a progressive increase in gallbladder volume and delayed emptying, leading to increased biliary sludge. Pregnancy hormonal changes of elevated estradiol and estrone also increase lithogenicity. The symptoms of biliary colic are the same in pregnant and nonpregnant patients. In patients with symptoms consistent with cholelithiasis, ultrasound is the diagnostic examination of choice. In pregnant patients, ultrasound is as accurate in identifying gallstones and signs of inflammation as in nonpregnant patients.

Historically, prior to laparoscopic techniques, pregnant patients with a clear operative indication, such as obstructive jaundice, gallstone pancreatitis, and choledocholithiasis, underwent cholecystectomy regardless of gestational age. Patients with recurrent biliary colic or acute cholecystitis that responded to medical management were treated expectantly until after delivery, at which time they underwent cholecystectomy. However, laparoscopic cholecystectomy during pregnancy is associated with shorter length of stay, shorter operative times, and fewer complications compared to open cholecystectomy.[31] A recent literature metaanalysis of 11 studies and over 10,000 patients demonstrated that the laparoscopic approach was associated with decreased risks for fetal (odds ratio [OR] 0.42; 95 % confidence interval [CI] 0.28–0.63; $P < 0.001$), maternal (OR 0.42; 95% CI 0.33–0.53; $P < 0.001$), and surgical (OR 0.45; 95 % CI 0.25–0.82, $P = 0.01$) complications. The average length of hospital stay was 3.2 days in the laparoscopic approach versus 6.0 days following open cholecystectomy ($P = 0.02$). The conversion rate from laparoscopic cholecystectomy to open cholecystectomy was 3.8%. Of note, 91% of the patients in this study had their cholecystectomy performed in the first or second trimester, and the author acknowledge gestational age may be a confounding factor.[32] Fetal demise is rare to nonexistent following for laparoscopic cholecystectomy performed during the first and second trimesters.[33] Furthermore, decreased rates of spontaneous abortion and preterm labor are noted after laparoscopic cholecystectomy when compared to open cholecystectomy.[34] This data argues for the performance of laparoscopic cholecystectomy for symptomatic biliary colic in the first or second trimester, and not waiting for the third trimester or postpartum. Further arguing for early cholecystectomy is the finding that symptomatic cholelithiasis may resolve, but there is a 92% recurrence of symptoms if the initial presentation was in the first trimester, 64% in the second trimester, and 44% in the third trimester.[35]

As it became understood that adverse maternal and fetal outcomes are related more to the disease process and not to the surgical intervention, management patterns have changed. Also, complications from nonoperative management of gallstone disease result in an increase in maternal and fetal mortality. With gallstone pancreatitis during pregnancy, a maternal mortality rate of 15% and a fetal mortality rate of 60% have been reported. In a study of 63 patients who were admitted with symptomatic cholelithiasis, surgical management reduced the need for labor induction, rate of preterm deliveries, and fetal mortality.[36] Therefore, surgical intervention is considered the primary treatment of gallstones in pregnancy.

The timing of cholecystectomy for biliary colic depends on the gestational age and severity of symptoms. A spontaneous abortion rate of 12% with open cholecystectomy during the first trimester falls to 5.6% and 0% during the second and third trimesters, respectively. The risk for preterm labor is almost 0% during the second trimester and 40% during the third trimester.[1] The optimum time for cholecystectomy is the second trimester, when the risks for spontaneous abortion and preterm labor are the lowest, unless the patient develops a complication of cholelithiasis. In a study of 122 patients who were admitted with biliary colic, 69 (56.5%) underwent minimally invasive intervention. Eight patients were treated during the first, 54 during the second, and seven during the last trimester. There was no fetal morbidity or mortality and only minor maternal morbidity, with no mortality.[33]

Laparoscopic cholecystectomy is safest during the second trimester. The gravid uterus is not large enough at this gestational age to interfere with visualization; the uterus also is less likely to be inadvertently instrumented at this size. The open technique using the Hasson trocar is recommended for obtaining access to the abdomen. If intraoperative cholangiography or endoscopic retrograde cholangiopancreatography is indicated for choledocholithiasis, the uterus needs to be protected with appropriate shielding. If the severity of symptoms prevents delaying surgical intervention until after delivery, laparoscopic cholecystectomy can be safely performed during the third trimester, although the risk for preterm labor is substantially increased. In several small series of patients, preterm labor was successfully managed with tocolytics and the patients delivered healthy term infants.

Endocrine Disease

Adrenal Disease

Pheochromocytomas originate from chromaffin cells in the adrenal medulla or from extramedullary paraganglion cells. They are hormonally active tumors, secreting the catecholamines norepinephrine, epinephrine, and, less commonly, dopamine. Pheochromocytomas are usually described by the rule of 10, which states that 10% of pheochromocytomas are extraadrenal, 10% are bilateral, 10% are malignant, and 10% are familial. These tumors can occur sporadically or as part of a syndrome, such as multiple endocrine neoplasia (MEN) type 2A (MEN2A), MEN2B, or von Hippel-Lindau disease.

Although pheochromocytomas are uncommon in pregnancy, they have devastating effects on the mother and fetus. Pheochromocytomas that remain undiagnosed during pregnancy have a postpartum maternal mortality as high as 55%, with fetal mortality also exceeding 50%. The greatest risk occurs from the onset of labor to 48 hours after delivery. The index of suspicion must be high in any patient with preeclampsia, paroxysmal hypertension, or unexplained fever after delivery. With diagnosis and appropriate treatment, the maternal mortality rate is reduced to almost 0% and the fetal mortality rate is decreased to 15%. Diagnosis is made by elevated urine catecholamine levels; urinary catecholamine levels in the pregnant patient without a pheochromocytoma are the same as in the nonpregnant patient. Lack of proteinuria also helps eliminate preeclampsia as a cause of hypertension. Metaiodobenzylguanidine-I131 (MIBG) imaging is not recommended during pregnancy because the small molecule may cross the placenta; however, the use of MIBG imaging has not been evaluated in pregnancy.

Surgical resection needs to be performed before 20 weeks' gestation, when spontaneous abortion is less likely and the size of the gravid uterus does not interfere with the procedure. If the diagnosis is made late in the second trimester or during the third trimester, medical management followed by combined cesarean birth and resection of the pheochromocytoma may be an option. It is unknown whether the standard preoperative management with alpha-blockade or calcium channel blockade followed by perioperative beta-blockade in nonpregnant patients is safe during pregnancy. The long-term effects of the alpha-blocker phenoxybenzamine on the fetus have not been determined, although calcium channel blockers are safe to use during pregnancy. Beta-blockers are frequently used during pregnancy with close monitoring for intrauterine growth retardation. Consultation with a maternal-fetal medicine specialist is essential to determine the preoperative management that will ensure the optimal postoperative result for the patient and fetus. In nonpregnant patients, the method of approach depends on suspected malignancy, unilateral versus bilateral tumors, extraadrenal location, size of the tumor, and surgeon's preference and experience. In all series comparing the different approaches, including open versus laparoscopic technique, pregnant patients were not included. Recent studies have indicated the safety of the laparoscopic approach in pregnancy.

Thyroid Disease

Thyroid disease during pregnancy can be categorized into three groups—hypothyroidism, hyperthyroidism, and thyroid cancer. Hypothyroidism is found in 2.5% of pregnancies. Of these, only 20% to 30% of patients develop symptoms. The first step is to obtain a serum thyroid-stimulating hormone (TSH) concentration. This will help categorize primary hypothyroidism versus hypothyroidism resulting from pituitary or hypothalamic causes.[37]

Current guidelines from LeBeau and Mandel for the treatment of hypothyroidism during pregnancy are as follows:

1. Check serum TSH level.
2. Initial levothyroxine dosage is based on severity of symptoms. Levothyroxine is started at 2 μg/kg/day. If TSH is less than 10 mU/L, dose is adjusted to 0.1 mg/day.
3. For previously diagnosed hypothyroidism, monitor TSH level every 3 to 4 weeks.
4. Goal TSH level is less than 2.5 mU/L.

5. Monitor serum TSH and total TSH every 3 to 4 weeks with each dose change.

Hyperthyroidism during pregnancy has an incidence of 0.1% to 0.4%.[38] Gestational thyrotoxicosis is a multifactorial phenomenon. High serum concentrations of human chorionic gonadotropin during pregnancy activate the TSH receptors. Elevated serum-free thyroxine (T_4) and low-serum TSH levels are seen with this form of thyrotoxicosis. Gestational thyrotoxicosis is usually self-limited and spontaneously resolves by 20 weeks' gestation, when the human chorionic gonadotropin level declines. Repeat evaluation is warranted if thyrotoxicosis persists. Most cases of hyperthyroidism are a result of Graves disease. After the diagnosis is made, medical treatment with thionamides (e.g., propylthiouracil, methimazole) is the mainstay of treatment. Iodides are avoided, except in patients preparing for thyroidectomy during pregnancy. Subtotal thyroidectomy for Graves disease is reserved for patients who are taking high-dose propylthiouracil (>600 mg/day) or methimazole (>40 mg/day), are allergic to thionamides, are noncompliant, or have compressive symptoms because of goiter size. Surgery is performed during the second trimester before 24 weeks' gestation to minimize the risk for miscarriage. A 2-week course of a β-adrenergic agent, along with potassium iodide, is implemented before surgery to minimize perioperative complications. Radioactive iodine therapy is contraindicated during pregnancy.

Because of hormonal changes, thyroid nodules may have a higher prevalence during pregnancy, but thyroid cancers do not. Thyroid cancers are worked up in the traditional fashion during pregnancy. Fine-needle aspiration, along with ultrasonic evaluation, remain the cornerstone of diagnosis. If cytology shows thyroid cancer, surgery is recommended during the second trimester, before 24 weeks' gestation. If thyroid cancer is found after the second half of pregnancy, surgery can be performed after delivery. This statement is supported by a recent study in which 201 pregnant women underwent thyroid (N = 165) and parathyroid (N = 36) procedures. Of these patients, 46% had thyroid cancer. When compared with nonpregnant women (N = 31), the pregnant patients had a higher rate of endocrine (15.9% vs. 8.1%; $P < 0.001$) and general complications (11.4% vs. 3.6%; $P < 0.001$) and longer unadjusted lengths of stay (2 days vs. 1 day; $P < 0.001$). The fetal and maternal complication rates were 5.5% and 4.5%, respectively.[39] Postoperative radioactive iodine therapy also needs to be delayed until after delivery.

Small Bowel Disease

Intestinal obstruction is the third most common nonobstetric abdominal surgical issue in pregnancy, after acute appendicitis and acute cholecystitis. The incidence of small bowel obstruction during pregnancy has been reported to be between 1 in 1500 to 17,000 pregnancies. Small bowel obstructions usually occur during the second and third trimesters. Adhesions resulting from prior abdominal and pelvic surgeries are the most frequent causes of intestinal obstruction in pregnancy, accounting for 53% to 59% of cases. Other causes of small bowel obstruction in the pregnant patient include volvulus, intussusception, malignancy, and hernia, although the displacement of the small bowel out of the pelvis by the enlarging uterus makes this a rare cause.

The symptoms of an obstruction are identical to those in the nonpregnant patient and consist of the triad of abdominal pain, vomiting, and obstipation. Pain, present in 85% to 98% of cases, is usually colicky in nature and located in the midabdomen, although the character and duration are highly variable. Nausea and vomiting are seen in 80% of pregnant patients with small bowel obstruction; however, nausea and vomiting are not uncommon during the first trimester of normal pregnancy. Nausea and vomiting that persist or begin later in pregnancy should arouse suspicion and be evaluated. Bowel distention may be marked but difficult to assess because of the gravid uterus. Diagnosis is made by serial examination and plain abdominal radiography.

Treatment for small bowel obstruction in pregnancy is identical to that in the nonpregnant patient. Therapy consists of nasogastric decompression and IV fluids. However, a lower threshold for operative management is necessary. If, after 6 to 8 hours of nonoperative treatment, there is no satisfactory patient response, a laparotomy/laparoscopy is performed before perforation or bowel necrosis occurs. Maternal mortality ranges from 6% to 20% because of sepsis and multisystem organ failure, and fetal loss is as high as 26% to 50%. To avoid the risk to the mother and fetus, a more aggressive approach is used.

Midgut volvulus remains a dreaded diagnosis during the postpartum period. It is usually more common in the pregnant patient if she has undergone previous abdominal surgery; however, spontaneous midgut volvulus may occur. A case report of maternal death caused by midgut volvulus after bariatric surgery has been reported.[40] The key is increased vigilance for all those involved in the patient's care. Early exploration is warranted if the diagnosis is unclear.

Appendix, Colon, and Rectal Disease

Acute appendicitis is the most common nonobstetric abdominal surgical problem in the pregnant patient, occurring in 1 in 1000 to 1500 pregnancies.[41] The incidence of acute appendicitis is fairly evenly distributed among the trimesters of pregnancy, with a slight predominance during the second trimester. Timely and accurate diagnosis is challenging because the typical clinical findings of nausea, vomiting, abdominal pain, and mild leukocytosis may be seen in a normal pregnancy. Delay in diagnosis results in an increased perforation rate of 10%, which has significant consequences for the patient and fetus. Fetal mortality increases from 1.5% in acute appendicitis to 35% in perforated appendicitis; preterm labor and premature delivery rates are as high as 40% in perforated appendicitis[42] compared with a 13% rate of preterm labor and 4% rate of premature delivery in uncomplicated appendicitis.[43]

In 1932, Baer studied 78 normal pregnant women with radiographic studies at regular intervals from the second month of pregnancy to 10 days postpartum. As the uterus enlarges, the appendix is driven upward with a counterclockwise rotation. Baer concluded that early in pregnancy, pain is low and that as the gestation progresses, pain is located higher in the abdomen.[44] A review of 45 pregnant patients with acute appendicitis demonstrated that pain in the right lower quadrant is the most common symptom, regardless of gestational age (first trimester, 86%; second trimester, 83%; third trimester, 85%).[43] Despite the inconsistency, acute appendicitis needs to be included in the differential diagnosis of every pregnant woman who presents with right-sided abdominal pain. Treatment of suspected acute appendicitis in the pregnant patient is emergent appendectomy. Although helical CT scans have demonstrated higher than 90% sensitivity and specificity in the diagnosis of acute appendicitis, few data are available in pregnant patients. In nonpregnant patients, a 10% to 15% negative laparotomy rate is considered acceptable. Because of the increased risk to mother and fetus with appendiceal perforation, a negative rate of 30% to 33% has been widely accepted until recently, when it was reported that even negative appendectomy may be associated with an increased risk of fetal loss. In a series of 3133 patients, the rates of fetal loss and preterm delivery in complicated appendicitis were 6% and 11%, respectively, in comparison to the rates of fetal loss and preterm delivery of 4% and 10%, respectively, in patients who underwent negative appendectomy.[45] It was concluded that improvement in fetal outcomes would result from improvement in diagnostic accuracy and reduction of the rate of negative appendectomy. In a small series of 47 patients, a positive ultrasound was considered to be diagnostic for appendicitis, with MRI without gadolinium or CT being used to confirm or exclude the diagnosis in a negative or nondiagnostic ultrasound diagnosis of appendicitis in pregnancy.[46] The debate is then for an open or laparoscopic technique. The argument for open appendectomy is that the laparoscopic approach exposes the fetus to risks for pneumoperitoneum and trocar placement without the benefit of a significantly smaller incision. The laparoscopic technique enables examination of a larger portion of the abdomen with less uterine manipulation and allows locating the appendix as it is pushed into the right upper quadrant by the enlarging uterus.

The SAGES guidelines for the use of laparoscopy during pregnancy currently state that laparoscopy appendectomy may be performed safely in pregnant patients with acute appendicitis and rate the data supporting this stance moderately strong but acknowledge that the data supporting it as the procedure of choice is weak.[23]

The preponderance of studies demonstrate that laparoscopic appendectomy is safe and effective, with low rates of preterm labor and no fetal demise. We agree that there is no role for nonoperative management of uncomplicated acute appendicitis in pregnant women because of a higher rate of peritonitis, fetal demise, shock, and venous thromboembolism as compared to operative management. Recent evidence for the use of antibiotics alone for treating acute appendicitis has not been extended to the gravid patient.

Because of concern and weak evidence suggesting a negative laparoscopy for appendicitis is associated with adverse maternal and fetal outcome, accurate diagnosis of appendicitis in the pregnant patient should be assured. When the diagnosis remains uncertain with clinical findings and ultrasound, MRI is the preferred adjunct to establish an accurate diagnosis. CT scan may be used when MRI is unavailable, but the risks of ionizing radiation exposure must be considered.

Port placement in the pregnant patient is determined by uterine size. The peritoneal cavity is first entered in the supraumbilical midline in patients operated during the first trimester of pregnancy. After the third month of pregnancy, the trocar is inserted progressively higher, about 3 to 4 cm above the uterine fundus, located by palpation. Fig. 72.3 shows the routine positioning of the working trocars and the recommended displacement lines in relation to uterine size.

Colonic pseudoobstruction, or Ogilvie syndrome, is a functional obstruction, or adynamic ileus, without a mechanical cause. Of all cases of Ogilvie syndrome, 10% occur in postpartum patients. It is characterized by massive abdominal distention with cecal dilation. Although neostigmine is effective first-line therapy in nonpregnant patients, its safety in pregnancy is unknown. It can be used safely in the postpartum period. Colonoscopic decompression has been described in postpartum patients, with laparotomy indicated only in suspected perforation.

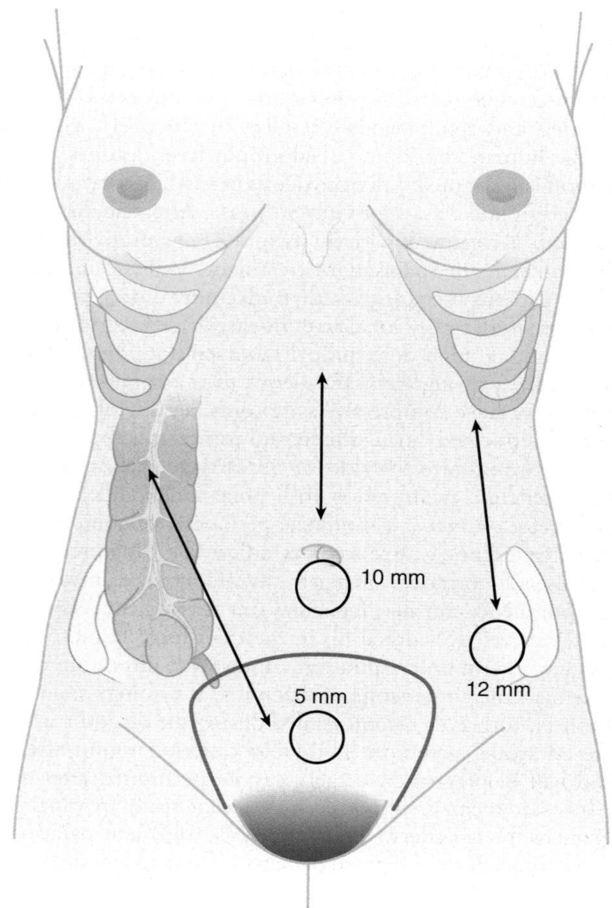

FIG. 72.3 Configuration of laparoscopic port sites for laparoscopic appendectomy at various stages of pregnancy. (Adapted from Moreno-Sanz C, Pascual-Pedreno A, Picazo-Yeste JS, et al. Laparoscopic appendectomy during pregnancy: between personal experiences and scientific evidence. *J Am Coll Surg.* 2007;205:37–42.)

Vascular Disease

Of more than 400 cases of ruptured splenic artery aneurysms in the literature, approximately 100 cases of ruptured splenic artery aneurysm during pregnancy have been reported, with only 12 cases of maternal and fetal survival.[47] Rupture occurred during the third trimester in two thirds of cases and was typically misdiagnosed as splenic rupture or uterine rupture. The maternal mortality rate was 75%, with a fetal mortality rate of 95%. Increased portal pressures, high splenic artery flow caused by distal aortic compression, and progressive arterial wall weakening are contributing factors. Multiparity may increase the risk; 78% of patients with ruptured splenic artery aneurysms have been in their third pregnancy. Survival is most likely related to a two-stage rupture, in which the lesser sac temporarily tamponades the bleeding aneurysm.

When treated electively in nonpregnant patients, the mortality rate is only 0.5% to 1.3%. When the diagnosis is made in a woman of childbearing age or in a pregnant patient, a splenic artery aneurysm of 2 cm or larger is treated electively because of the increased risk for rupture during pregnancy.[47]

Acute iliofemoral venous thrombosis is six times more frequent in pregnant than nonpregnant patients. Pregnancy may increase the risk for thrombosis via a number of factors, including mechanical obstruction of venous drainage by the enlarging uterus, decreased activity in late pregnancy and at time of delivery, intimal injury from vascular distention or surgical manipulation during cesarean section, and abnormal levels of coagulation factors (see the section entitled "Physiologic Changes of Pregnancy"). Also, a wide spectrum of pathologic abnormalities, such as the presence of lupus anticoagulant antibodies and deficiencies of proteins C and S, may further increase the risk for thrombotic disease. Protein S serves as a cofactor for activated protein C, which has anticoagulant activity. Therefore, a deficiency of protein S leads to spontaneous, recurrent thromboembolic complications in nonpregnant adults. Even in normal individuals, protein S levels are substantially reduced during pregnancy.

The management of acute iliofemoral venous thrombosis during pregnancy is controversial because thrombolytic therapy poses hazards to the fetus. The risk for pulmonary thromboembolism with manipulation of the clot during thrombectomy would have catastrophic effects on both the patient and fetus. Techniques that have been described include interruption of the inferior vena cava through a right retroperitoneal approach or interruption of the inferior vena cava by passage of a Fogarty catheter through the unaffected contralateral femoral vein. The disadvantage of the retroperitoneal approach is that an extensive dissection is required. The disadvantages of the Fogarty catheter are that the catheter may still dislodge clots that have extended into the vena cava and that once the catheter is removed, an inferior vena cava filter must still be placed. However, the most effective technique is filter placement in the inferior vena cava either through the internal jugular vein or femoral vein using ultrasound guidance, followed by thrombectomy. Caval filters have been successfully placed in all trimesters of pregnancy, however changes in approach or patient positioning (left lateral decubitus) to offload uterine compression of the cava may be necessary.[48] Unlike in the nonpregnant patient, caval filters placed in pregnancy should be positioned in the suprarenal cava to reduce the risk of compression by or erosion into the growing uterus or damage to the cava or filter during contractions.[49] Suprarenal location additionally protects against thrombus generated in the dilated ovarian veins. The increased caval flow in this position may also improve lysis of clots trapped in the filter. There is a hypothetical risk of renal injury if a suprarenal caval filter becomes completely occluded, however this concern has not been borne out in the literature.[50] Providers should remain vigilant through close follow-up and prompt filter removal when no longer clinically necessary.

TRAUMA IN PREGNANCY

Trauma is the leading nonobstetric cause of maternal mortality and occurs in approximately 5% of pregnancies. The most common mechanisms of injury are from falls or from motor vehicle accidents. When compared with age-matched pregnant controls, pregnant women who sustained trauma had a higher incidence of spontaneous abortion, preterm labor, fetomaternal hemorrhage, abruptio placentae, and uterine rupture.[51] A number of studies have attempted to identify risk factors that predict morbidity and mortality in the pregnant trauma patient. The maternal injury severity score, mechanism of injury, and physical findings are unable to predict adverse outcomes, such as abruptio placentae and fetal loss, adequately. Pregnant patients with severe head, abdominal, thoracic, or lower extremity injuries are at high risk for pregnancy loss.[52] Early involvement of an available obstetrician is important to evaluate maternal and fetal well-being.

In the treatment of the pregnant trauma patient, the critical point is that resuscitation of the fetus is accomplished by resuscitation of the mother. Therefore, the initial evaluation and treatment of the pregnant injured patient is identical to that of the nonpregnant injured patient. Rapid assessment of the maternal airway, breathing, and circulation, as well as ensuring an adequate airway, avoids maternal and fetal hypoxia. In the later stages of pregnancy, as described earlier, uterine compression of the vena cava may result in hypotension from diminished venous return; thus, the pregnant trauma patient needs to be placed in a left lateral decubitus position. If spinal cord injury is suspected, the patient may be secured to a backboard and then tilted to the left.

The increased blood volume associated with pregnancy has important implications in the trauma patient. Signs of blood loss such as maternal tachycardia and hypotension may be delayed until the patient loses almost 30% of her blood volume. As a result, the fetus may be experiencing hypoperfusion long before the mother manifests any signs. Early and rapid fluid resuscitation should be initiated, even in the pregnant patient who is normotensive.

As with the primary survey, the secondary survey proceeds in a fashion similar to that in the nonpregnant patient. Special attention is given to the abdominal examination. The uterus remains protected by the pelvis until approximately 12 weeks' gestation and is relatively well sheltered from the abdominal injury until then. As the uterus grows, it becomes more prominent and more vulnerable to injury. Measurement of fundal height provides a rapid approximation of gestational age. At 20 weeks' gestation, it is at the level of the umbilicus and is approximately 1 cm per week of gestation. Intrauterine hemorrhage or uterine rupture may result in a discrepancy in measurement. A pelvic examination is performed, by an obstetrician if possible, to evaluate for vaginal bleeding, ruptured membranes, or a bulging perineum. Vaginal bleeding may indicate abruptio placentae, placenta previa, or preterm labor. Rupture of the amniotic membrane may result in umbilical cord prolapse, which compresses the umbilical vessels and compromises fetal blood flow. This requires immediate cesarean delivery. If cloudy white or greenish fluid is seen from the cervical os or perineum, the presence of amniotic fluid is confirmed by testing with Nitrazine paper, which indicates pH and changes from green to blue.

The Kleihauer-Betke test for the assessment of fetomaternal transfusion is useful after maternal trauma and is ordered with the initial laboratory studies, which include typing and crossmatching. Because of the sensitivity of the Kleihauer-Betke test, a small amount of fetomaternal transfusion may be undetected. Therefore, all Rh-negative pregnant trauma patients are considered for Rh immunoglobulin (RhoGAM) therapy.

The most common cause of fetal death after blunt injury is abruptio placentae. Deceleration of the fetal heart rate may be the earliest sign of abruption. The uterus needs to be evaluated for contractions, rupture, and abruptio placentae. Early initiation of cardiotocographic fetal monitoring adequately warns of deterioration in the condition of the fetus. Since fetal survival is most greatly impacted by maternal hemodynamics, early identification and prompt treatment of maternal injuries is paramount. When clinically indicated, x-rays, CT scans, and operative intervention should be completed without hesitation. While the survival of the mother always takes precedence, injuries to the fetus necessitating additional follow up may be identified (Fig. 72.4).

Penetrating trauma results in maternal death in fewer than 5% of cases. Penetrating trauma is primarily from gunshot wounds and

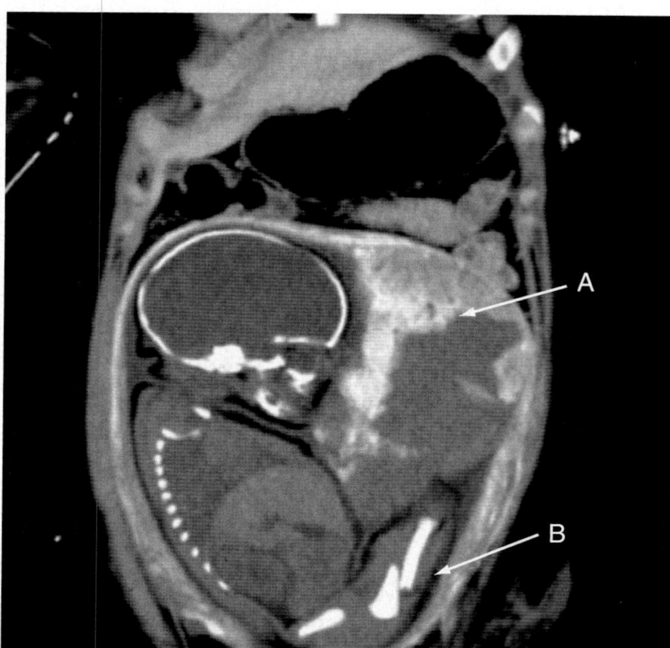

FIG. 72.4 CT scan of 23-year-old woman who is 33 weeks pregnant and who sustained blunt abdominal trauma during a motor vehicle collision. Placental abruption *(A)* and a fetal femur fracture *(B)* were not detected on initial ultrasound but were evident on CT. *CT*, Computed tomography. (From Romanowski KS, Struve I, McCracken B, et al. Fetal injuries and placental abruption detected on CT scan not observed on ultrasound, Paper #6. 45th Western Trauma Association Annual Meeting; Telluride, CO March 2, 2015, p 47.)

knife wounds. The incidence of visceral injury with penetrating trauma during pregnancy is 16% to 38% in comparison to 80% to 90% in nonpregnant patients.[53] Fetal injury occurs in up to 70% of cases, with a 40% to 70% rate of fetal death as a result of direct fetal injury or preterm labor.[54] A number of factors contribute to the nature of the injuries. Bullets produce a transient shock wave and cavitation as they transmit kinetic energy to body tissues. The density of the tissue, such as the thick density of the uterus during early pregnancy, may rapidly dissipate the lower amount of kinetic energy from a low-velocity projectile, protecting the fetus from significant injury. Higher velocity projectiles may produce more serious injuries to mother and fetus. As pregnancy progresses and the growing uterus displaces the abdominal viscera, location of the injury becomes crucial in determining which of the maternal viscera are injured and whether the fetus has sustained a direct injury. Management of penetrating injuries during pregnancy is similar to that for nonpregnant patients. It should be individualized, with early involvement by an obstetrician. Diagnostic and treatment options include surgical exploration, supraumbilical diagnostic peritoneal lavage, diagnostic laparoscopy, CT, local wound exploration, and observation. Emergency cesarean delivery may be indicated in maternal arrest after 4 minutes of unsuccessful resuscitation, fetal compromise with a stable mother if the fetus is of viable gestational age, obvious impending maternal death, or when the gravid uterus interferes with trauma-related surgical intervention. Also, emergent cesarean delivery may also improve chances of maternal survival by removing aortocaval compression and increasing cardiac output. Maternal and fetal survival rates as high as 72% and 45%, respectively, have been reported following emergency cesarean delivery at more than 25 weeks/gestational age. No fetal survival has been documented when fetal heart tones were absent before emergent delivery, but a 75% chance of fetal survival has been reported when fetal heart tones were present and gestational age was at least 26 weeks.[55] The best chance for fetal survival with an intact infant is when cesarean delivery occurs within five minutes of maternal death. Four minutes of resuscitation followed by a 1-minute cesarean delivery offers the best chance for infant survival. In a review of 61 infants born by perimortem cesarean delivery between 1900 and 1985, 70% of the infants survived who were delivered within five minutes of maternal death, and all of the survivors were neurologically intact.[56]

CONTROL OF MAJOR HEMORRHAGE

General and emergency surgeons may be called upon to support the obstetric team in response to massive hemorrhage or when planning obstetric operations in this high-risk patient population. Obstetric hemorrhage is the leading cause of maternal morbidity and mortality worldwide and has been increasing in incidence in the United States. The increasing incidence of abnormal placentation, otherwise known as morbidly adherent placenta (MAP) has been implicated as the cause of increasing maternal mortality. MAP describes penetration of the chorionic villi into and, in some cases, through the uterine wall, substantially increasing the risk of massive obstetric hemorrhage. In the United States alone, the incidence of MAP doubled over the last six years. The most severe form, placenta percreta, in which chorionic villi penetrate through the uterine wall and into adjacent organs, has increased fifty fold in the last fifty years. The end result is an increasing need for multidisciplinary approaches to maternal hemorrhage control.

Mechanical Hemorrhage Control

Surgical Ligation

Traditional methods of intraoperative hemorrhage control include hypogastric artery ligation, uterine artery ligation, and rapid hysterectomy. Ligation of the hypogastric arteries theoretically reduces pulse pressure to the uterus; however, it is successful in reducing operative blood loss in less than 50% of cases. Furthermore, ligation is estimated to be even less useful in MAP involving the bladder.[57] These disparate findings are most likely explained by the persistent proximal collateral circulation to the uterus, which contributes to retrograde hemorrhage and venous bleeding during surgery. Temporary aortic cross-clamping can aid in hemorrhage control when hypogastric artery occlusion is insufficient or technically difficult to achieve in the presence of the gravid uterus.

Resuscitative Endovascular Balloon Occlusion of the Aorta

Resuscitative endovascular balloon occlusion of the aorta (REBOA) is an emerging, minimally-invasive technique to control noncompressible hemorrhage. Although initially developed for the management of traumatic hemorrhage, REBOA has been gaining popularity for the control of nontraumatic hemorrhage. Early reports of REBOA use in obstetric hemorrhage indicate that the approach has been successful at decreasing blood loss and salvaging mothers in extremis from uterine rupture, placental abruption, and uncontrolled hemorrhage during cesarean hysterectomy for MAP.[58] When used prophylactically prior to high-risk obstetric surgery, REBOA reduces blood loss, improves maternal outcomes, and decreases rates of hysterectomy compared to traditional techniques of uterine balloon tamponade (BT) and hypogastric or uterine artery occlusion.[58,59] Compared to uterine or hypogastric artery occlusion techniques, REBOA requires less time for placement and only unilateral arterial puncture making it useful in emergent cases.[58] REBOA insertion, positioning, and inflation can be completed in approximately 2 to 3 minutes by a trained provider using the ER-REBOA catheter, which is particularly helpful when placental blood loss approaches 700 mL/min. In obstetric hemorrhage REBOA use has demonstrated lower transfusion volumes than other occlusion techniques, including internal iliac artery ligation, uterine artery ligation, or transvaginal intrauterine balloon occlusion.[58] Furthermore, the new ER-REBOA catheter (Prytime Medical, Boerne, TX) is modified to allow placement without fluoroscopy, which leads to little to no fetal radiation exposure.[60]

Positioning a REBOA catheter in a pregnant patient may not be straightforward. Catheter measurements based on anatomic landmarks can serve as a basis for positioning of the balloon within the aorta; however, the effect of a gravid abdomen on the accuracy of these external landmarks has not been established. Several studies have examined the anatomic distance between the common femoral artery and the anatomic landing zones described for REBOA in men and nonpregnant women of all sizes and ages.[61] The target distance for zone 1, supraceliac, REBOA placement was at approximately 46 cm in 99% of the population, and zone 3, infrarenal aorta, was at 28 cm for 95% of the population, conserved across studies in the United States and Europe. These relationships should hold true during pregnancy and may provide a guide for blind placement based on catheter length when external anatomic landmarks may not be reliable. If preoperative imaging is available, target distances can be measured in advance.[60] If the abdomen is open, the balloon may be palpated within the aorta. Image-guided placement can be used when time allows. Confirming catheter position with an x-ray is quick, easy, and limits radiation exposure to the fetus compared to the use of fluoroscopy. Any of these positioning methods can be performed in a standard operating room with a standard table. Fluoroscopy-guided balloon occlusion is a well-described technique in the obstetric population and is thought to pose little risk to the fetus from the short duration of radiation exposure.[59,62,63] Intraoperatively, the catheter can be inflated, deflated, and repositioned as needed throughout the case without the needing to move the patient or obtain additional imaging if attention is paid to correlating catheter markings with anatomic measurements at the initial placement.

The risks and limitations of REBOA are still being described, and the relative incidence of each is not yet known. The majority of data published on this topic describes the application of REBOA in the trauma population that consists largely of male patients with concomitant hemorrhagic shock. Potential complications from REBOA include those related to arterial access, balloon positioning and inflation, and the physiologic changes that result from inflation and deflation of the device. From the trauma literature, access site complications are similar to those encountered during other forms of arterial puncture, but may be severe, including limb ischemia requiring amputation.[64,65] Balloon malposition into an aortic branch vessel or migration into a higher or lower position within the aorta has also been described, sometimes resulting in uncontrolled arterial rupture and death.[64] In animal models, proximal hypertension resulting from aortic occlusion has led to acute heart failure, cerebral edema, and respiratory failure.[66] Distal organ ischemia during occlusion can lead to renal failure, bowel ischemia, and paralysis. Finally, washout of toxic metabolites following balloon deflation can cause rebound hypotension with cardiac collapse.[67]

These complications are described most commonly after supraceliac (Zone 1) aortic occlusion due to the increased ischemic burden conferred by occluding blood flow in the abdominal viscera and the increased aortic afterload conferred by more proximal occlusion. Infrarenal (Zone 3) aortic occlusion is less commonly described in the trauma literature, owing to the less common occurrence of isolated, hemodynamically significant pelvic injury. As such, the relative incidence of these complications in the obstetric population that almost exclusively is treated with Zone 3 occlusion is unknown.

The use of REBOA in obstetrics introduces a different patient population with other comorbidities and a different anatomic site of aortic occlusion than trauma patients that comprise the majority of available literature. The ability to predict complications for this population from the available literature is therefore limited. In theory, the risk of arterial rupture may be increased due to smaller vessel size. While there is a dearth of published literature documenting REBOA use in women specifically, there has been one documented aortic rupture due to a smaller than expected aortic diameter.[68] Access site complications may be increased in the obstetric population due to the smaller vessel diameter in the common femoral arteries as well. This anatomic difference and hypercoagulability of pregnancy may put women at a higher risk of arterial thrombosis and ipsilateral limb ischemia as the arteries clamp down with hemorrhage and the sheath becomes occlusive. It would therefore be important to select the smallest sheath that will accommodate the available REBOA catheter and have a low threshold for postprocedural arteriography. Frequent monitoring of distal pulses in the ipsilateral extremity should be maintained following reperfusion and for 24 hours after sheath removal. Continuous Doppler may be a helpful adjunct to aid in early detection of arterial access complications.

When placing REBOA prophylactically, proximal blood pressure may increase to undesirable levels increasing the risk of heart failure or stroke. This supraphysiologic augmentation should be anticipated by the surgical team and communicated to the anesthesiologist such that vasodilators can be administered to maintain normotension. The lack of preexisting shock may improve ischemia tolerance and reduce the anticipated risks of ischemia-reperfusion injury. Extrapolating from trauma literature, Zone 1 occlusion is tolerated for minutes, not hours, and multisystem organ failure and death have been reported after long inflation time.[65] Zone 3 occlusion is generally tolerated for longer, with survivors reported after several hours of occlusion.

The robust collateral circulation that exists in the gravid uterus, particularly in the case of MAP, may lead to incomplete hemorrhage control from proximal occlusion alone. Retrograde flow and venous hemorrhage may result in liters of additional blood loss despite aortic occlusion, thus additional adjuncts to hemorrhage control may be necessary. The potential for severe complications exists, and providers performing the procedure should be aware of these risks to improve patient management and the informed consent process.

Risks of REBOA use can be reduced with multidisciplinary expertise, proper training, and adherence to good techniques. Low-profile, 7-Fr common femoral arterial sheaths placed with ultrasound guidance have fewer access site complications than larger 12-Fr sheaths.[69] Additionally, distal thrombosis is rare with 7-Fr sheaths and limb ischemia requiring amputation has not been reported. REBOA requires a dedicated provider to secure against catheter migration, manage inflation and deflation, and faithfully monitor the ipsilateral lower extremity for ischemia.

During balloon inflation, the anesthesia team should work to offset unwanted blood pressure augmentation and maintain normal physiologic pressures. The surgical teams should aim to achieve hemorrhage control rapidly to keep the duration of occlusion to a minimum. Other methods used to reduce ischemia include intermittent or partial balloon deflation to allow some degree of distal perfusion and prolong the tolerable duration of REBOA use. The operative team should be aware that balloon deflation is associated with the rapid redistribution of circulating blood volume and the washout of ischemic metabolites, including a bolus of potassium, which can result in rebound hypotension and cardiac instability.[67] Close communication with the anesthesia providers to time fluid and drug administration with inflation and deflation, can aid in maintaining hemodynamic stability throughout surgery.

There is a dearth of published information about management of intraarterial balloons during high-risk obstetric procedures. Few cases describe flushing the sheath or catheters, although doing so is a well-established principle of vascular surgery. Whether the flush solution should contain heparin is additionally controversial when these catheters are used for hemorrhage control. Intraoperatively, while the balloon catheter is within the aorta there is increased risk of arterial thrombosis or thromboemboli even when the balloon is not inflated. The hypercoagulability of pregnancy, administration of clotting factors, tranexamic acid, erythropoietin, and other procoagulants may increase this risk. It is therefore the authors' practice to use 30 mL of 2% heparin (2 units of heparin per 100 mL of crystalloid) intraarterially through the sheath and another 30 mL through the central lumen of the REBOA catheter every 10 minutes, while monitoring thromboelastography to ensure the absence of systemic coagulopathy. Postprocedurally, while the sheath is in place and the balloon catheter has been removed, continuous fluid administration through the sheath can be used in lieu of heparin to prevent thrombosis until the sheath is removed. The sheath should be removed as soon as it is no longer required, ideally within 24 hours of initial placement.

Intrauterine Balloon Tamponade

Emergency surgeons may be called upon to support obstetricians in the event of uncontrolled postpartum hemorrhage. The most common cause of massive hemorrhage after delivery is uterine atony; up to 80% of the cases result from suboptimal contraction of the myometrium following placental separation. Other etiologies may include retained placenta, uterine rupture, pubic trauma, uterine inversion, and coagulopathy. The management of acute postpartum hemorrhage refractory to medical management may require invasive therapies already described, including arterial ligation, occlusion or embolization, uterine suture compression, or ultimately hysterectomy. These interventions are highly invasive and resource intense. Intrauterine BT has gained popularity as a minimally invasive adjunct with similar efficacy and less morbidity.[70,71] Several balloon types have been used effectively, including Bakri balloon, BT catheter, Foley catheters, Rusch balloon, condom catheters, and the Sengstaken-Blakemore tube. The American College of Obstetricians and Gynecologists specifically recommended the Bakri postpartum balloon for its specifically tailored design that enables nonoperative management of uterine bleeding in cases of uterine atony and other causes of postpartum hemorrhage.[72,73] The Bakri balloon has proven an effective means of controlling postpartum hemorrhage, with success rates ranging from 57% after cesarean delivery to 100% after vaginal delivery.[70,73]

Adjuncts for Major Hemorrhage

Cell Salvage

Cell salvage has become an important component of operative hemorrhage management for high-risk patients. However, there are important limitations of the cell salvage to consider when it comes to the pregnant patient. Cell salvage can only utilize blood collected into the canister, must have a minimum of 500 mL of blood before the cells can be washed, and returns at most 50% of the washed blood volume back to the patient. This technique does not allow for easy collection of vaginal blood loss, and therefore has limited utility in many obstetric hemorrhage cases. Intermixing of fetal blood, amniotic fluid, or bacteria with salvaged blood are contraindications to autologous transfusion. However, safe use of the cell-saver has been demonstrated in obstetric patients, particularly when no future pregnancy is planned. The presence of leukocyte depletion filters and cell washing may reduce the presence of these contaminants and produce a product similar to maternal blood with the exception of not fully eliminating fetal hemoglobin.[74] Anti-D immune globulin, also known as RhoGAM, is used to prevent isoimmunization and should be administered to any Rh-negative mother who receives cell salvage blood that may contain fetal hemoglobin from an Rh positive infant. Support for the use of cell salvage in obstetric hemorrhage is now provided by 390 published cases in which blood contaminated with amniotic fluid has been washed and readministered without complication.[75]

Damage Control Techniques

Once surgical hemostasis has been maximized, damage control techniques such as packing and temporary abdominal closure may be useful in cases of disseminated intravascular coagulation. Damage control surgery in the pregnant patient mirrors the principles and management strategies used in the nonpregnant patient. Avoiding excessive manipulation of the uterus when placing packs and temporary abdominal closures can reduce the impact on the fetus. Delayed abdominal closure may lead to intraabdominal hypertension. Additional fetal monitoring may be necessary during closure attempts to detect signs of fetal distress that may result from increased intraabdominal pressure. Cesarean section may be considered when clinically appropriate for maternal or fetal indications.

PREGNANCY AFTER MAJOR ABDOMINAL SURGERY

Not infrequently, the surgeon will be asked about pregnancy following treatment of surgical disease. Each case should be individualized. The conditions can be divided into those involving benign and those involving malignant disease.

Benign Disease

After most abdominal procedures for benign disease, there is no contraindication for pregnancy. Special circumstances include bariatric surgery and total colectomy with ileal pouch–anal anastomosis.

Bariatric Surgery

Bariatric surgery is rapidly becoming one of the most common procedures done in the United States. With approximately 160,000 women undergoing weight loss surgery in 2009, pregnancy after bariatric surgery is a common occurrence. There is an improvement in fertility and pregnancy outcomes after weight loss surgery.[76] There is also a decreased incidence of maternal complications in patients who have undergone bariatric surgery, particularly complications related to diabetes mellitus, hypertensive disorders, and fetal macrosomia as compared with their morbidly obese counterparts. Currently, the consensus of studies support a delayed in planned pregnancy for up to two years following bariatric surgery. Outcomes in maternal or fetal health do not differ whether a patient has had a Roux-en-Y gastric bypass or restrictive procedure (e.g., vertical-banded gastroplasty, laparoscopic adjustable gastric banding).[77] Current recommendations for women who become pregnant after bariatric surgery are to continue with a prenatal multivitamin, vitamin B_{12}, iron, and folate supplement. Protein supplementation may also be necessary for patients who have undergone malabsorptive operations. For patients who have undergone adjustable gastric band placement, deflation of the band is recommended to aid in optimal nutrition.

Ileal Pouch–Anal Anastomosis

Ulcerative colitis can be a debilitating disease that might eventually require a total colectomy with an ileal pouch–anal anastomosis. Long-term outcomes of pregnancy after this procedure have been generally positive. In a study of 37 women who became pregnant before and after ileal pouch–anal anastomosis, there were no differences in birth weight, duration of labor, complications, and unplanned cesarean sections.[78] Another study comparing patients who underwent cesarean section versus vaginal delivery after ileal pouch–anal anastomosis has demonstrated that the vaginal delivery patients have a significant higher incidence of anterior sphincter defect (13% vs. 50%) and worse quality of life evaluated by the time trade-off method.[79]

Malignant Disease

This discussion will be limited to breast cancer because this occurs more often in women of reproductive age in comparison to most oncologic disease treated by the general surgeon or surgical oncologist. The issues that patients will need advice on are the following: (1) maintenance of fertility; (2) the impact of pregnancy on disease progression and survival; (3) the timing of pregnancy relative to the diagnosis of breast cancer; and (4) pregnancy outcome.

Breast cancer often affects women of reproductive age. Although treatment is effective, cytotoxic chemotherapy causes ovarian reserve depletion, whereas hormonal chemotherapy necessitates a delay in pregnancy, resulting in potential infertility in some patients, although some patients retain normal fertility. On diagnosis of breast cancer in patients of reproductive age who are interested in having children after treatment, the surgeon or medical oncologist may consider referral to a fertility specialist to explore methods of fertility preservation. The best-established method of fertility preservation is embryo cryopreservation. This involves ovarian stimulation to retrieve oocytes for in vitro fertilization prior to freezing; this remains the best-known option for fertility preservation in women with early-stage breast cancer whose risk of fertility may be compromised by adjuvant chemotherapy. However, little is known about the impact, if any, of ovarian stimulation on disease progression.

Studies have shown that pregnancy is more likely to occur in patients with prolonged survival and no evidence of disease recurrence. In addition, there is no evidence of a negative effect of pregnancy on recurrence rate and survival in patients treated for breast cancer. This includes those who have had a mastectomy as well as breast-conserving therapy. Survival was based on initial stage and not affected by hormonal receptor status or pregnancy.[80]

The timing of pregnancy varies with the treatment protocol and reassessment for recurrent disease. Some recommend that women wait two years from the time of diagnosis, but this is controversial. The population-based study of Ives and colleagues[80] did not support the current medical advice given to premenopausal women with a diagnosis of breast cancer to wait two years before attempting to conceive. It was concluded that although this recommendation may be valid for women who are receiving treatment or have systemic disease at diagnosis, and for women with localized disease, early conception, six months after completing their treatment, is unlikely to reduce survival. The occurrence of preterm labor or miscarriage is similar in patients with a previous diagnosis of breast cancer compared with those with no history of breast cancer.

SUMMARY

Pregnant patients are susceptible to the same surgical diseases as nonpregnant patients of similar age. Maternal physiologic changes, as well as the enlarging uterus, may result in atypical presentation of surgical disease or symptoms may be attributed to normal pregnancy. A delay in diagnosis and treatment of surgical illnesses in pregnancy poses a greater risk to maternal and fetal well-being than the risks of anesthesia or surgical intervention. Early consultation with an obstetrician, maternal-fetal medicine specialist, and perinatologist can ensure optimal outcomes and avoid pitfalls. Laparoscopy is becoming increasingly accepted in the pregnant patient, and future advances should make it even safer for these women. Preterm labor prevention needs to be individualized, given the patient's gestational age and underlying disease process.

SELECTED REFERENCES

Baer JL, Reis RA, Arens RA. Appendicitis in pregnancy: With changes in position and axis of the normal appendix in pregnancy. *JAMA*. 1932;98:1359–1364.

Landmark article illustrating the changes in appendiceal location during pregnancy.

Bates SM, Greer IA, Middeldorp S, et al. VTE, thrombophilia, antithrombotic therapy, and pregnancy: Antithrombotic therapy and prevention of thrombosis, 9th ed: American College of Chest Physicians Evidence-Based Clinical Practice Guidelines. *Chest*. 2012;141:e691S–e736S.

The use of anticoagulant therapy during pregnancy is challenging due to the potential for fetal and maternal complications. This guideline was developed as part of the Antithrombotic Therapy and Prevention of Thrombosis Guidelines 9th edition by the American College of Chest Physicians. It focuses on the management of venous thromboembolisms (VTEs) and thrombophilia as well as the use of anticoagulants during pregnancy. They recommend using low–molecular-weight heparin over unfractionated heparin for the prevention and treatment of VTE in pregnant women (Grade 1B). For women being treated for acute VTE that developed during pregnancy, anticoagulants should be continued for at least 6 weeks postpartum for a minimum total duration of therapy of 3 months (Grade 2C). In women who meet laboratory of clinical criteria of antiphospholipid syndrome, based on a history of three or more pregnancy losses, they recommend antepartum administration of prophylactic or intermediate-dose unfractionated heparin or prophylactic low–molecular-weight heparin combined with low-dose aspirin (75–100 mg/d) over no treatment (Grade 1B). For women with other known inherited thrombophilias or those with a history of two or more miscarriages without identified thrombophilia, they do not recommend antithrombotic prophylaxis (Grade 2C and Grade 1B, respectively).

Freeland M, King E, Safcsak K, et al. Diagnosis of appendicitis in pregnancy. *Am J Surg*. 2009;198:753–758.

This study shows that when ultrasound is read as positive for appendicitis, no further confirmatory test other than surgery is required. However, if the ultrasound is nondiagnostic, further imaging with magnetic resonance imaging or computed tomography may avoid a negative appendectomy.

Jackson H, Granger S, Price R, et al. Diagnosis and laparoscopic treatment of surgical diseases during pregnancy: an evidence-based review. *Surg Endosc*. 2008;22:1917–1927.

The literature supporting the safety and efficacy of laparoscopy in cholecystectomy, appendectomy, solid-organ resection, and oophorectomy in the gravid patient is outlined. Based on the level of evidence, the authors review recommendations specific to surgical approach, trimester of pregnancy, patient positioning, port placement, insufflation pressure, monitoring, venous thromboembolic prophylaxis, obstetric consultation, and use of tocolytics in the pregnant patient.

Kuy S, Roman SA, Desai R, et al. Outcomes following thyroid and parathyroid surgery in pregnant women. *Arch Surg*. 2009;144:399–406; discussion 406.

The authors review in a retrospective study 201 pregnant women who underwent thyroid (N = 165) and parathyroid (N = 36) procedures and compared with nonpregnant women (N = 31). On multivariate regression analysis, pregnancy was an independent predictor of higher combined surgical complications (odds ratio, 2; P < 0.001), longer adjusted length of stay (0.3 days longer; P < 0.001), and higher adjusted hospital costs ($300; P < 0.001). Other independent predictors of outcome were surgeon volume, patient race or ethnicity, and insurance status. The authors conclude that pregnant women have worse clinical and economic outcomes following thyroid and parathyroid surgery than nonpregnant women. In addition, they found disparities in outcomes based on race, insurance, and access to high-volume surgeons.

LeBeau SO, Mandel SJ. Thyroid disorders during pregnancy. *Endocrinol Metab Clin North Am*. 2006;35:117–136, vii.

Comprehensive review of all the major thyroid abnormalities that occur during pregnancy.

Mourad J, Elliott JP, Erickson L, et al. Appendicitis in pregnancy: New information that contradicts long-held clinical beliefs. *Am J Obstet Gynecol*. 2000;182:1027–1029.

This paper, which retrospectively reviewed more than 66,000 deliveries and found 45 pregnant patients with appendicitis, challenged the original landmark paper by Baer regarding the presentation of acute appendicitis in pregnant patients.

Sadot E, Telem DA, Arora M, et al. Laparoscopy: a safe approach to appendicitis during pregnancy. *Surg Endosc*. 2010;24:383–389.

This article is the largest hospital-based series evaluating the laparoscopic versus open approach for pregnant patients with presumed acute appendicitis. Based on their findings, the authors conclude that laparoscopy appears to be a safe, feasible, and efficacious approach for pregnant patients with presumed acute appendicitis. They concluded that it is likely not the surgical approach, but the underlying diagnosis combined with maternal factors that determine the risk for pregnancy complications.

Soper NJ. SAGES' guidelines for diagnosis, treatment, and use of laparoscopy for surgical problems during pregnancy. *Surg Endosc*. 2011;25:3477–3478.

These are current guidelines for laparoscopy in pregnancy.

Tang SJ, Mayo MJ, Rodriguez-Frias E, et al. Safety and utility of ERCP during pregnancy. *Gastrointest Endosc*. 2009;69:453–461.

Endoscopic retrograde cholangiopancreatography (ERCP) is an important diagnostic and therapeutic tool in patients with biliary and pancreatic disease. Its usefulness and safety during pregnancy are largely unknown because it is not often required and because its use has been only infrequently reported in the published literature. This is a retrospective review from a single academic center from 2000 to 2006. During the study period, 68 ERCPs were performed on 65 pregnant women. There were no perforations, sedation-related adverse events, postsphincterotomy bleeding, cholangitis, or procedure-related maternal or fetal deaths. Post-ERCP pancreatitis was diagnosed in 11 patients (16%); 59 patients had complete follow-up. Endoscopic therapy at the time of ERCP was undertaken in all patients. Term pregnancy was achieved in 53 patients (89.8%). Patients having ERCP in the first trimester had the lowest percentage of term pregnancy (73.3%) and the highest risk of preterm delivery (20.0%) and low–birth weight newborns (21.4%). The authors reported that none of the 59 patients with long-term follow-up had spontaneous fetal loss, perinatal death, stillbirth, or fetal malformation.

Vinatier E, Merlot B, Poncelet E, et al. Breast cancer during pregnancy. *Eur J Obstet Gynecol Reprod Biol*. 2009;147:9–14.

Breast cancer in pregnancy is an uncommon situation that poses dilemmas for patients and physicians. There is a paucity of prospective studies regarding the diagnosis and treatment of breast cancer during pregnancy. Women diagnosed with breast cancer during pregnancy have similar disease characteristics to age-matched controls. Current evidence suggests that diagnosis may be carried out with limitations regarding staging. Surgical treatment may be performed as for nonpregnant women. Radiotherapy and endocrine or antibody treatment should be postponed until after delivery. Chemotherapy is allowed after the first trimester. Physicians should be aggressive in the workup of breast symptoms in the pregnant population to expedite diagnosis and allow multidisciplinary treatment without delay.

Yarrington CD, Valente AM, Economy KE. Cardiovascular management in pregnancy: Antithrombotic agents and antiplatelet agents. *Circulation*. 2015;132:1354–1364.

Normal pregnancy induces a hypercoagulable state, increasing the risk of venous thromboembolism fivefold, with an additional increase in risk in the postpartum period. As such, thrombotic complications of pregnancy are a major cause of maternal and fetal morbidity and mortality. This review examines the use of both older and new anticoagulants and antiplatelet medications during pregnancy and highlights their clinical utility in conditions including venous thromboembolism, thrombophilia, mechanical heart valves, antiphospholipid syndrome (APLS), preeclampsia, intrauterine growth restriction (IUGR), and placental abruption.

REFERENCES

1. Melnick DM, Wahl WL, Dalton VK. Management of general surgical problems in the pregnant patient. *Am J Surg*. 2004;187:170–180.
2. Chesnutt AN. Physiology of normal pregnancy. *Crit Care Clin*. 2004;20:609–615.
3. Bates SM, Greer IA, Middeldorp S, et al. VTE, thrombophilia, antithrombotic therapy, and pregnancy: Antithrombotic therapy and prevention of thrombosis, 9th ed: American College of Chest Physicians Evidence-Based Clinical Practice Guidelines. *Chest*. 2012;141:e691S–e736S.
4. Duhl AJ, Paidas MJ, Ural SH, et al. Antithrombotic therapy and pregnancy: Consensus report and recommendations for prevention and treatment of venous thromboembolism and adverse pregnancy outcomes. *Am J Obstet Gynecol*. 2007;197(457): e451–421.
5. Topol EJ, Bosker G, Cassele H, et al. The anticoagulation in prosthetic valves and pregnancy consensus report panel and scientific roundtable. Anticoagulation and enoxaparin use in patients with prosthtic heart valves and/or pregnancy. *Fetal-Maternal Medicine Consensus Reports*. 2002.
6. Harrison BP, Crystal CS. Imaging modalities in obstetrics and gynecology. *Emerg Med Clin North Am*. 2003;21:711–735.
7. Mitchell AA, Gilboa SM, Werler MM, et al. Medication use during pregnancy, with particular focus on prescription drugs: 1976–2008. *Am J Obstet Gynecol*. 2011;205:51. e51–58.
8. Briggs GG, Freeman RK, Towers CV, et al. *Drugs in pregnancy and laction. A reference guide to fetal and neonatal risk*. ed 11. Philadelphia, PA: Wolters Kluwer; 2017.
9. Pernia S, DeMaagd G. The new pregnancy and lactation labeling rule. *P T*. 2016;41:713–715.
10. Guille C, Barth KS, Mateus J, et al. Treatment of prescription opioid use disorder in pregnant women. *Am J Psychiatry*. 2017;174:208–214.
11. Briggs GG, Freeman RK. *Drugs in pregnancy and laction. A reference guide to fetal and neonatal risk*. 10th ed. Philadelphia, PA: Wolters Kluwer; 2015.
12. Subtil D, Brabant G, Tilloy E, et al. Early clindamycin for bacterial vaginosis in pregnancy (PREMEVA): a multicentre, double-blind, randomised controlled trial. *Lancet*. 2018;392:2171–2179.
13. Lindhoff-Last E, Bauersachs R. Heparin-induced thrombocytopenia-alternative anticoagulation in pregnancy and lactation. *Semin Thromb Hemost*. 2002;28:439–446.
14. Lindhoff-Last E, Kreutzenbeck HJ, Magnani HN. Treatment of 51 pregnancies with danaparoid because of heparin intolerance. *Thromb Haemost*. 2005;93:63–69.
15. Tang AW, Greer I. A systematic review on the use of new anticoagulants in pregnancy. *Obstet Med*. 2013;6:64–71.
16. De Carolis S, di Pasquo E, Rossi E, et al. Fondaparinux in pregnancy: Could it be a safe option? A review of the literature. *Thromb Res*. 2015;135:1049–1051.
17. Santiago-Diaz P, Arrebola-Moreno AL, Ramirez-Hernandez JA, et al. Platelet antiaggregants in pregnancy. *Rev Esp Cardiol*. 2009;62:1197–1198.
18. Sun LS, Li G, Miller TL, et al. Association between a single general anesthesia exposure before age 36 months and neurocognitive outcomes in later childhood. *JAMA*. 2016;315:2312–2320.
19. Schecter WP, Farmer D, Horn JK, et al. Special considerations in perioperative pain management: Audiovisual distraction, geriatrics, pediatrics, and pregnancy. *J Am Coll Surg*. 2005;201:612–618.
20. Jackson H, Granger S, Price R, et al. Diagnosis and laparoscopic treatment of surgical diseases during pregnancy: an evidence-based review. *Surg Endosc*. 2008;22:1917–1927.
21. Hunter JG, Swanstrom L, Thornburg K. Carbon dioxide pneumoperitoneum induces fetal acidosis in a pregnant ewe model. *Surg Endosc*. 1995;9:272–277; discussion 277–279.
22. Pearl J, Price R, Richardson W, et al. Guidelines for diagnosis, treatment, and use of laparoscopy for surgical problems during pregnancy. *Surg Endosc*. 2011;25:3479–3492.
23. Pearl JP, Price RR, Tonkin AE, et al. SAGES guidelines for the use of laparoscopy during pregnancy. *Surg Endosc*. 2017;31:3767–3782.
24. Yu JH, Kim MJ, Cho H, et al. Breast diseases during pregnancy and lactation. *Obstet Gynecol Sci*. 2013;56:143–159.
25. Rovera F, Frattini F, Coglitore A, et al. Breast cancer in pregnancy. *Breast J*. 2010;16(suppl 1); S22–25.
26. Raphael J, Trudeau ME, Chan K. Outcome of patients with pregnancy during or after breast cancer: a review of the recent literature. *Curr Oncol*. 2015;22:S8–S18.
27. Johannsson O, Loman N, Borg A, et al. Pregnancy-associated breast cancer in BRCA1 and BRCA2 germline mutation carriers. *Lancet*. 1998;352:1359–1360.
28. Rugo HS. Management of breast cancer diagnosed during pregnancy. *Curr Treat Options Oncol*. 2003;4:165–173.
29. Doshi S, Zucker SD. Liver emergencies during pregnancy. *Gastroenterol Clin North Am*. 2003;32:1213–1227, ix.
30. Cobey FC, Salem RR. A review of liver masses in pregnancy and a proposed algorithm for their diagnosis and management. *Am J Surg*. 2004;187:181–191.
31. Cox TC, Huntington CR, Blair LJ, et al. Laparoscopic appendectomy and cholecystectomy versus open: a study in 1999 pregnant patients. *Surg Endosc*. 2016;30:593–602.
32. Sedaghat N, Cao AM, Eslick GD, et al. Laparoscopic versus open cholecystectomy in pregnancy: a systematic review and meta-analysis. *Surg Endosc*. 2017;31:673–679.
33. Date RS, Kaushal M, Ramesh A. A review of the management of gallstone disease and its complications in pregnancy. *Am J Surg*. 2008;196:599–608.
34. Graham G, Baxi L, Tharakan T. Laparoscopic cholecystectomy during pregnancy: a case series and review of the literature. *Obstet Gynecol Surv*. 1998;53:566–574.
35. Nasioudis D, Tsilimigras D, Economopoulos KP. Laparoscopic cholecystectomy during pregnancy: a systematic review of 590 patients. *Int J Surg*. 2016;27:165–175.
36. Lu EJ, Curet MJ, El-Sayed YY, et al. Medical versus surgical management of biliary tract disease in pregnancy. *Am J Surg*. 2004;188:755–759.

37. Giacobbe AM, Grasso R, Triolo O, et al. Thyroid diseases in pregnancy: a current and controversial topic on diagnosis and treatment over the past 20 years. *Arch Gynecol Obstet.* 2015;292:995–1002.
38. Mandel SJ. Thyroid disease and pregnancy. In: Cooper DS, ed. *Medical management of thyroid disease.* New York, NY: Marcel Dekker; 2001:387–418.
39. Kuy S, Roman SA, Desai R, et al. Outcomes following thyroid and parathyroid surgery in pregnant women. *Arch Surg.* 2009;144:399–406.
40. Loar 3rd PV, Sanchez-Ramos L, Kaunitz AM, et al. Maternal death caused by midgut volvulus after bariatric surgery. *Am J Obstet Gynecol.* 2005;193:1748–1749.
41. Andersson RE, Lambe M. Incidence of appendicitis during pregnancy. *Int J Epidemiol.* 2001;30:1281–1285.
42. Rollins MD, Chan KJ, Price RR. Laparoscopy for appendicitis and cholelithiasis during pregnancy: a new standard of care. *Surg Endosc.* 2004;18:237–241.
43. Mourad J, Elliott JP, Erickson L, et al. Appendicitis in pregnancy: new information that contradicts long-held clinical beliefs. *Am J Obstet Gynecol.* 2000;182:1027–1029.
44. Baer JL, Reis RA, Arens RA. Appendicitis in pregnance with changes in position an daxis of the normal appendix in pregnancy. *JAMA.* 1932;98:1359–1364.
45. McGory ML, Zingmond DS, Tillou A, et al. Negative appendectomy in pregnant women is associated with a substantial risk of fetal loss. *J Am Coll Surg.* 2007;205:534–540.
46. Freeland M, King E, Safcsak K, et al. Diagnosis of appendicitis in pregnancy. *Am J Surg.* 2009;198:753–758.
47. Herbeck M, Horbach T, Putzenlechner C, et al. Ruptured splenic artery aneurysm during pregnancy: a rare case with both maternal and fetal survival. *Am J Obstet Gynecol.* 1999;181:763–764.
48. Clark SL, Blatter DD, Jackson GM. Placement of a temporary vena cava filter during labor. *Am J Obstet Gynecol.* 2005;193:1746–1747.
49. Kawamata K, Chiba Y, Tanaka R, et al. Experience of temporary inferior vena cava filters inserted in the perinatal period to prevent pulmonary embolism in pregnant women with deep vein thrombosis. *J Vasc Surg.* 2005;41:652–656.
50. Harris SA, Velineni R, Davies AH. Inferior vena cava filters in pregnancy: a systematic review. *J Vasc Interv Radiol.* 2016;27:354–360. e358.
51. Pak LL, Reece EA, Chan L. Is adverse pregnancy outcome predictable after blunt abdominal trauma. *Am J Obstet Gynecol.* 1998;179:1140–1144.
52. Ikossi DG, Lazar AA, Morabito D, et al. Profile of mothers at risk: an analysis of injury and pregnancy loss in 1195 trauma patients. *J Am Coll Surg.* 2005;200:49–56.
53. Cusick SS, Tibbles CD. Trauma in pregnancy. *Emerg Med Clin North Am.* 2007;25:861–872, xi.
54. Mattox KL, Goetzl L. Trauma in pregnancy. *Crit Care Med.* 2005;33:S385–389.
55. Morris Jr JA, Rosenbower TJ, Jurkovich GJ, et al. Infant survival after cesarean section for trauma. *Ann Surg.* 1996;223:481–488; discussion 488–491.
56. Katz V, Balderston K, DeFreest M. Perimortem cesarean delivery: were our assumptions correct. *Am J Obstet Gynecol.* 2005;192:1916–1920.
57. Leung TK, Au HK, Lin YH, et al. Prophylactic trans-uterine embolization to reduce intraoperative blood loss for placenta percreta invading the urinary bladder. *J Obstet Gynaecol Res.* 2007;33:722–725.
58. Wang YL, Duan XH, Han XW, et al. Comparison of temporary abdominal aortic occlusion with internal iliac artery occlusion for patients with placenta accreta - a non-randomised prospective study. *Vasa.* 2017;46:53–57.
59. Panici PB, Anceschi M, Borgia ML, et al. Intraoperative aorta balloon occlusion: Fertility preservation in patients with placenta previa accreta/increta. *J Matern Fetal Neonatal Med.* 2012;25:2512–2516.
60. Usman N, Noblet J, Low D, et al. Intra-aortic balloon occlusion without fluoroscopy for severe postpartum haemorrhage secondary to placenta percreta. *Int J Obstet Anesth.* 2014;23:91–93.
61. Pezy P, Flaris AN, Prat NJ, et al. Fixed-Distance model for balloon placement during fluoroscopy-free resuscitative endovascular balloon occlusion of the aorta in a civilian population. *JAMA Surg.* 2017;152:351–358.
62. Manzano-Nunez R, Escobar-Vidarte MF, Naranjo MP, et al. Expanding the field of acute care surgery: a systematic review of the use of resuscitative endovascular balloon occlusion of the aorta (REBOA) in cases of morbidly adherent placenta. *Eur J Trauma Emerg Surg.* 2018;44:519–526.
63. Wu Q, Liu Z, Zhao X, et al. Outcome of pregnancies after balloon occlusion of the infrarenal abdominal aorta during caesarean in 230 patients with placenta praevia accreta. *Cardiovasc Intervent Radiol.* 2016;39:1573–1579.
64. Davidson AJ, Russo RM, Reva VA, et al. The pitfalls of resuscitative endovascular balloon occlusion of the aorta: Risk factors and mitigation strategies. *J Trauma Acute Care Surg.* 2018;84:192–202.
65. Saito N, Matsumoto H, Yagi T, et al. Evaluation of the safety and feasibility of resuscitative endovascular balloon occlusion of the aorta. *J Trauma Acute Care Surg.* 2015;78:897–903; discussion 904.
66. Russo RM, Neff LP, Lamb CM, et al. Partial resuscitative endovascular balloon occlusion of the aorta in swine model of hemorrhagic shock. *J Am Coll Surg.* 2016;223:359–368.
67. Johnson MA, Williams TK, Ferencz SE, et al. The effect of resuscitative endovascular balloon occlusion of the aorta, partial aortic occlusion and aggressive blood transfusion on traumatic brain injury in a swine multiple injuries model. *J Trauma Acute Care Surg.* 2017;83:61–70.
68. Sovik E, Stokkeland P, Storm BS, et al. The use of aortic occlusion balloon catheter without fluoroscopy for life-threatening post-partum haemorrhage. *Acta Anaesthesiol Scand.* 2012;56: 388–393.
69. Teeter WA, Matsumoto J, Idoguchi K, et al. Smaller introducer sheaths for REBOA may be associated with fewer complications. *J Trauma Acute Care Surg.* 2016;81:1039–1045.
70. Bakri YN, Amri A, Abdul Jabbar F. Tamponade-balloon for obstetrical bleeding. *Int J Gynaecol Obstet.* 2001;74:139–142.
71. Georgiou C. Balloon tamponade in the management of postpartum haemorrhage: a review. *BJOG.* 2009;116:748–757.
72. Committee Opinion No. 696: Nonobstetric surgery during pregnancy. *Obstet Gynecol.* 2017;129:777–778.
73. Laas E, Bui C, Popowski T, et al. Trends in the rate of invasive procedures after the addition of the intrauterine tamponade test to a protocol for management of severe postpartum hemorrhage. *Am J Obstet Gynecol.* 2012;207:281. e281–287.
74. Waters JH, Biscotti C, Potter PS, et al. Amniotic fluid removal during cell salvage in the cesarean section patient. *Anesthesiology.* 2000;92:1531–1536.
75. Rainaldi MP, Tazzari PL, Scagliarini G, et al. Blood salvage during caesarean section. *Br J Anaesth.* 1998;80:195–198.

76. Patel JA, Colella JJ, Esaka E, et al. Improvement in infertility and pregnancy outcomes after weight loss surgery. *Med Clin North Am*. 2007;91:515–528, xiii.
77. Sheiner E, Balaban E, Dreiher J, et al. Pregnancy outcome in patients following different types of bariatric surgeries. *Obes Surg*. 2009;19:1286–1292.
78. Hahnloser D, Pemberton JH, Wolff BG, et al. Pregnancy and delivery before and after ileal pouch-anal anastomosis for inflammatory bowel disease: Immediate and long-term consequences and outcomes. *Dis Colon Rectum*. 2004;47:1127–1135.
79. Remzi FH, Gorgun E, Bast J, et al. Vaginal delivery after ileal pouch-anal anastomosis: a word of caution. *Dis Colon Rectum*. 2005;48:1691–1699.
80. Ives A, Saunders C, Bulsara M, et al. Pregnancy after breast cancer: population based study. *BMJ*. 2007;334:194.

73 CHAPTER

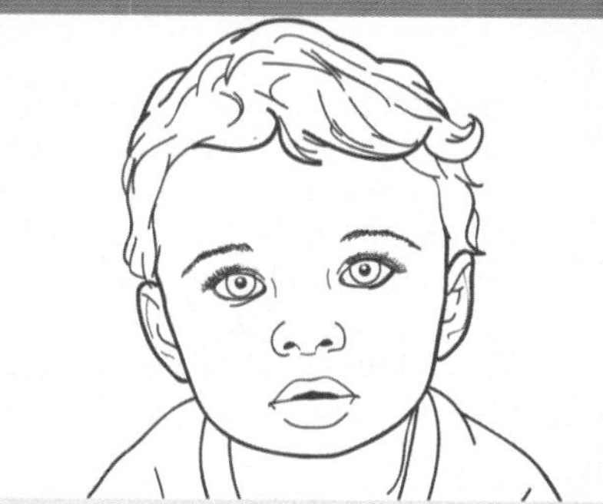

Fetal Surgery

Payam Saadai, Shinjiro Hirose, Diana L. Farmer

OUTLINE

THE BIRTH OF A NEW SURGICAL SPECIALTY

Not long ago, the idea of a surgeon operating on a human fetus within the womb was considered radical and heretical by the medical community. Pioneers and disciples of the burgeoning field of fetal surgery faced numerous obstacles, not the least of which was the charge that it would be unethical to violate the sanctity of the womb. Nevertheless, surgeon scientists persisted with diligent preparation, rigorous large animal modeling, and frank multidisciplinary conversation. Now, thirty years after the first human fetal intervention, fetal surgery is the standard of care for many congenital conditions.

The first open fetal surgical intervention was performed in 1981 by Dr. Michael Harrison at the University of California, San Francisco, in a fetus with obstructive uropathy.[1] Prior to this landmark event, intrauterine procedures were limited to diagnostic interventions such as amniocentesis or limited percutaneous treatments such as intrauterine transfusion for Rh erythroblastosis.[2] The first successful placement of a fetal vesicoamniotic shunt by Dr. Harrison and his team proved that surgeons could successfully and safely accomplish an operation in a pregnant mother and maintain the pregnancy. While the first fetal patient unfortunately died shortly after birth, the second operation was successful for both the mother and the fetus, and that second fetal patient is now a young man in his fourth decade of life.

Fetal surgery is unique in that there are two patients in every intervention. As in living-related living donor translation, one patient undergoes a life-threatening surgical procedure for no benefit to herself. The ethical considerations of the pregnant woman as an "innocent bystander" are complicated and the stakes are high. Maternal safety was, and has always been, paramount in the development of fetal surgery as a discipline. Furthermore, maternal morbidity at the time of fetal surgery and for future pregnancies is one of the most important considerations that need to be weighed against the potential benefits to the fetus. To address maternal safety, the technical aspects of fetal surgery—opening the gravid uterus without maternal hemorrhage, maintaining uterine relaxation, closing the hysterotomy in a water-tight manner, and limiting postoperative preterm labor—were all developed in rigorous animal models. Each step in the development of this discipline was a challenge and an opportunity for innovation, and it was here in the development of open fetal surgical techniques that true innovation occurred. Through multidisciplinary collaboration with neonatologists, perinatologists, radiologists, and anesthesiologists, innovation with biomedical partners, and an army of bright surgical residents, the largely nonfunded vision of open fetal surgery became a reality. Over the ensuing decades, fetal surgery techniques evolved, and the development of fetal surgery has paralleled the rise of other minimally invasive procedures in a constant attempt to balance the benefit for the fetus with the risks to the pregnant mother.

Fetal surgery is now the standard of care for several conditions, such as advanced twin-twin transfusion syndrome (TTTS)[3] and certain cases of myelomeningocele (MMC).[4] As the safety for women and fetuses improves and as techniques evolve, more indications will undoubtedly emerge.

Although there have been thousands of fetal procedures to date, there are few known maternal deaths worldwide that are remotely referable to a fetal procedure.[5] This is a remarkable safety record and a credit to the slow and careful development of the field. Notably, the existence of fetal surgery is due in large part to the extraordinary bravery of the many women who were willing to endeavor something new and unknown for the improved prognosis of their future child.

PRENATAL PATHOPHYSIOLOGIC CONSIDERATIONS AND RATIONALE

The original rationale for fetal surgery was based on the concept that simple anatomic defects in utero could lead to disastrous

BOX 73.1 Conditions amenable for fetal interventions.

Myelomeningocele (MMC)
Twin-twin transfusion syndrome (TTTS)
Twin reversed arterial perfusion (TRAP) sequence
Congenital diaphragmatic hernia (CDH)
Tumors causing hydrops:
 Sacrococcygeal teratoma (SCT)
 Congenital pulmonary airway malformation (CPAM)
 Cervical teratoma
Airway obstruction/congenital high airway obstruction syndrome (CHAOS)
Amniotic band syndrome
Urinary tract obstruction
Renal agenesis
Congenital heart disease
Fetal anemia

consequences in postnatal life. The hypothesis was that if one could reverse or repair the anatomy, then the physiology would also normalize once born. It turns out that this is not as straight-forward as originally postulated, as simple anatomic repairs turned out to be more complicated in practice, with fetal access and uterine closure remaining a crucial obstacle. Included in the original rationale for fetal surgery is the overarching concept that maternal safety is paramount. Originally, fetal interventions were carried out only for conditions that were uniformly lethal, as saving the fetus was thought to be of enough benefit to warrant the surgical risks to the mother. Once techniques of fetal access were standardized, open, fetoscopic, or needle-based procedures were developed based on the anatomy and subsequent physiology of each anomaly (Box 73.1).

What Has Led to the Success of Open Fetal Surgery?

Over the years, open surgical techniques were revised, and other minimally invasive surgical procedures were developed in a constant attempt to balance the benefit for the fetus with the morbidity for the mother. The advent of a disruptive technology—the ultrasound—introduced a unique method to observe the developing fetus noninvasively. It took the wide-spread use of fetal ultrasonography to radiographically delineate normal fetal development and subsequently document the anomalous variants. Due to prenatal ultrasonography, we learned that a fetus may develop symptoms or complications that spontaneously resolve with no ill effect, while other findings are indicative of more serious developing disorders. It thus became important to test the hypothesis that fixing the defect before birth might change the developmental fetal pathophysiology. The work to investigate the effect of fetal intervention on fetal development was performed in many animal models, but most successfully in the fetal ovine model due to the sheep's unique resistance to preterm labor and spontaneous abortion.[6] This model allows for multiple fetal interventions with neither the loss of the pregnancy nor the need for sophisticated tocolysis. Without rigorous scientific investigation in various animal models, including lambs, rodents, and primates, the transition to human fetal surgery would have been neither safe, nor successful.

MATERNAL CONSIDERATIONS AND MORBIDITY

Unlike most operations, fetal surgery, by definition, involves two patients undergoing surgery simultaneously. The risks and benefits between the mother and fetus must be examined closely and the benefits for the fetus must justify the risk to the mother, who gains no medical benefit from the operation. In addition, mothers must be in reasonable health in order to undergo fetal surgery. Specifically, for open fetal surgery, mothers should have no major comorbidities or contraindications for surgery. Maternal risks of fetal surgery include: bleeding, chorioamnionitis, placental abruption, preterm premature rupture of membranes (PPROM), preterm labor, and premature delivery.[7] Furthermore, mothers undergoing open fetal surgery are subject to a hysterotomy similar to a classical Cesarean section, rather than the method of a low transverse uterine incision that is preferred for modern Cesarean sections. Due to this hysterotomy, a woman undergoing open fetal surgery is at increased risk of uterine dehiscence and uterine rupture for not only the current, but also all future pregnancies.[8] A registry review by the North American Fetal Therapy Network (NAFTNet) demonstrated a 9.6% uterine rupture rate in a subsequent pregnancy following prior open MMC repair.[9] While these results are similar to classical Cesarean section rates, they are no less of a concern to fetal surgeons. Due to the significant maternal risks, new techniques for minimally invasive fetoscopic repair of MMC are being developed and studied. Currently, the fetoscopic approach for MMC repair is practiced by numerous centers, with the only potential downfall of the fetoscopic approach being that it may not allow for water-tight closure of the defect as well as the open surgical approach.[7] It remains to be seen if the fetoscopic technique can be improved to allow the same developments in the fetus as open fetal surgery. It is also the case that surgical approaches must be reoptimized with every emerging treatment innovation.

In the infancy of fetal surgery, there was an emphasis on first developing the techniques for accessing the fetus. As such, in the early days, a standard thoracoabdominal stapler was tested in nonhuman primates to be able to open the gravid uterus while preventing the mother from hemorrhaging. However, it was later discovered that the staples acted similarly to an intrauterine device, and the primates could not get pregnant again. In order to address the fertility problem, a unique absorbable stapler was developed (in partnership with Ethicon – no patents were filed). A recent survey of mothers who had undergone fetal surgery and had subsequent pregnancies demonstrated no difference in fertility following fetal surgery compared to prefetal surgical rates.[10] Due to these other maternal considerations including a higher rate of preterm labor and delivery in mothers who have had fetal surgery, improved surgical outcomes for the mother constitute an optimal portion of the standard of fetal surgery and arise as much from technique innovations as from medical innovations.

Overall, the Achilles heel for fetal surgery was and remains the control and prevention of preterm labor. Until the issue of preterm birth after fetal surgery is solved, the potential addition of prematurity to the fetus' underlying diagnosis must be weighed against any potential benefit of prenatal intervention.

FETAL SURGERY BY SYSTEM

What follows is an introduction to active areas of fetal intervention as categorized by organ system. The reader should note that this is not meant to be an exhaustive list of all disease processes that are amenable to prenatal intervention, as that is beyond the scope of this chapter.

Neurologic System

Myelomeningocele or Spina Bifida

In the United States, roughly four children are born daily with MMC, making it one of the most common congenital defects resulting in paralysis.[11] MMC is characterized by the incomplete closure of the neural tube during early embryonic development, resulting in exposed neural tissue and resultant leakage of cerebrospinal fluid. Depending on the vertebral level of the spinal defect, patients with MMC display a wide range of lifelong clinical consequences, which affect multiple organ systems and may lead to lifelong paralysis, bowel and bladder incontinence, musculoskeletal deformities, and cognitive disabilities.[12] The most immediate postnatal consequence of incomplete closure of the neural tube is hindbrain herniation (Arnold-Chiari II malformation) and resultant hydrocephalus. Before the advent of ventriculoperitoneal shunting, hydrocephalus was the main cause of mortality among these patients. Even so, shunt malfunction and infection can result in multiple future operative revisions.

Rationale for prenatal surgery. The wide spectrum of neurologic deficits of MMC can be explained by a "two-hit hypothesis" of injury. The concept explains the first "hit" as the embryonic anomaly of the neural placode itself, resulting in an open spinal cord. This is presumed to be caused by a variety of complex genetic and environmental factors. In addition, leakage of cerebrospinal spinal fluid from the spinal defect results in hindbrain herniation and hydrocephalus. The second "hit" occurs by acquired injury to the exposed neural elements due to mechanical trauma from the uterine wall, as well as chemical trauma from amniotic fluid toxicity.[13] This hypothesis was supported by prenatal findings of fetuses with MMC who were seen to have worsening distal neurologic function on serial ultrasounds.[14] Logically, the ideal treatment for MMC would be to prevent the first hit from ever occurring. In order to achieve proper neurulation, folic acid supplementation, which is known to prevent neural tube defects, are now routinely administered in prenatal vitamins during pregnancy. However, folic acid supplementation does not completely eliminate the incidence of spina bifida, and children are still born with this devastating defect, likely due to other factors. Therefore, the significant persisting lifelong morbidity of MMC inspired surgeons to close the spinal cord defect prior to birth to protect the neural elements from the secondary trauma.

Open fetal repair of MMC and the MOMS trial. Current fetal repair of MMC consists of maternal laparotomy, uterine hysterotomy, and watertight closure of the spinal defect. Repair is targeted to mid second trimester, late enough to allow technical prenatal repair, yet early enough to mitigate the damage done by the second *in utero* hit. Early reports compared fetal repair with historical postnatal controls and found the reversal of hindbrain herniation and a decreased need for ventriculoperitoneal shunting with fetal repair. Despite these initial promising results, further single institution studies showed mixed results regarding neurologic outcomes in these patients treated prenatally. With unclear benefit to the child and potential substantial risk to the mother, a more rigorous study was needed to prove the benefit of fetal surgery over postnatal repair.

In 2003, the University of California, San Francisco, Children's Hospital of Philadelphia, Vanderbilt University, and George Washington University collaborated with the National Institutes of Health to conduct a randomized, controlled study comparing fetal versus postnatal MMC repair. This landmark study, Management of Myelomeningocele (MOMS),[4] randomized patients to open fetal repair of the MMC or repair after delivery based on strict inclusion and exclusion criteria (Table 73.1). The trial demonstrated that prenatal closure of the defect does in fact ameliorate the morbidity associated with spina bifida by improving distal neurologic function and decreasing hindbrain herniation and the need for cerebrospinal fluid shunting. In fact, the study proved that prenatal repair was so much more efficacious than postnatal repair that the safety monitoring committee stopped the planned goal enrollment of 200 patients at 183 patients.

The primary outcomes of the MOMS trial were fetal or neonatal death, or the need for a ventriculoperitoneal shunt by 12 months of age. There were no maternal deaths and two perinatal deaths in each group. The need for ventriculoperitoneal shunting in the prenatal and postnatal surgery groups at 12 months of age were 68% and 98%, respectively ($P < 0.001$). Actual shunt placement was 40% in the prenatal group and 82% in the postnatal group ($P < 0.001$). Additionally, the MOMS trial reported significant functional and neurologic improvement at 30 months of age in the prenatal surgery group ($P = 0.007$). The prenatal surgery group had numerous other benefits in post-hoc analyses. The most notable included the improved ability to walk without devices or orthotics in the prenatal surgery group (42% vs. 21%, $P = 0.01$) and decreased hindbrain herniation at 12 months in the prenatal surgery group (64% vs. 96%, $P < 0.001$). Additionally, even though the prenatal surgery group had more severe anatomic lesion levels, this group had improved motor function compared to the postnatal surgery group. Significant maternal morbidity related to prenatal surgery included uterine dehiscence, oligohydramnios, placental abruption, spontaneous rupture of membranes, and chorioamniotic separation. The study investigators continue to follow the long-term outcomes of these children by assessing the lasting effects prenatal surgery has on motor and neurologic development, and on bowel and bladder continence.

In summary, prenatal repair of MMC contributes to improved outcomes in children with reduction of hindbrain herniation and enhanced motor outcomes. The results of the MOMS trial are one of the most important milestones in the clinical success of fetal surgery, as it demonstrated efficacy in treating a nonlethal condition. Further research and improved techniques continue to be investigated to minimize the risks to both the fetus and mother, as well as to further improve the neurologic outcomes of fetal repair.

Sacrococcygeal Teratoma

Sacrococcygeal teratoma (SCT) is one of the most common forms of congenital tumors with an estimated incidence of 1:35,000 births.[15] Long-term outcomes for infants with SCT are generally excellent. However, SCTs identified prenatally can grow to a tremendous size in relation to the fetus and can cause high-output cardiac failure and nonimmune hydrops through vascular shunting. Due to the development of hydrops, the mortality rate for SCTs identified prenatally approaches 50%.[16] In addition, SCTs can hemorrhage internally or externally, resulting in fetal anemia, hypovolemia, and intrauterine fetal demise. Other fetal complications of a large SCT are preterm labor and dystocia. A traumatic delivery may result in tumor rupture, hemorrhage, and neonatal death.

Rationale for prenatal therapy. The fetus with a large SCT has a high risk for mortality, especially when associated with nonimmune fetal hydrops. In this select group of fetuses with SCT, fetal

TABLE 73.1 **Complete inclusion and exclusion criteria for the management of myelomeningocele study.[4]**

INCLUSION CRITERIA	EXCLUSION CRITERIA
1. Singleton pregnancy	1. Nonresident of the United States
2. MMC lesion between T1 and S1 with hindbrain herniation	2. Insulin-dependent pregestational diabetes
3. Normal karyotype	3. Fetal anomaly unrelated to MMC
4. Maternal age of 18 or older	4. Kyphosis in the fetus of 30 degrees or greater
5. Gestational age at randomization of 19.0–25.9 weeks	5. Current or planned cerclage or documented history of incompetent cervix
	6. Risk of preterm birth (shortened cervix)
	7. Placental abruption or placenta previa
	8. BMI ≥35
	9. Previous spontaneous delivery prior to 37 weeks' gestation
	10. Maternal-fetal Rh isoimmunization, Kell sensitization, or neonatal alloimmune thrombocytopenia
	11. Maternal HIV or hepatitis B status positive
	12. Known hepatitis B positivity
	13. Uterine anomaly such as large or multiple fibroids or Müllerian duct abnormality
	14. Other maternal medical conditions, which is a contraindication to surgery or general anesthesia
	15. Patient does not have a support person
	16. Inability to comply with travel and follow-up requirements
	17. Patient does not meet other psychosocial criteria to handle the implications of the trial
	18. Participation in another intervention study that influences maternal and fetal morbidity and mortality or participation in this trial in a previous pregnancy
	19. Maternal hypertension, which would increase the risk of preeclampsia or preterm delivery

Adapted from Adzick NS, Thom EA, Spong CY, et al. A randomized trial of prenatal versus postnatal repair of myelomeningocele. *N Engl J Med.* 2011; 364:993-1004.
BMI, Body mass index; *HIV*, human immunodeficiency virus; *MMC*, myelomeningocele.

interventions include open fetal resection, radiofrequency ablation, and *ex utero* intrapartum treatment (EXIT)-to-resection. Outcomes of fetal intervention are mixed, with survival ranging from 38% to 75%.[17,18] Survival in hydropic SCT patients not undergoing fetal intervention is likely less than 10%. The most common approach for fetal resection of an SCT is a maternal hysterotomy with resection or debulking of the tumor. Decompression of a large, cystic SCT may be indicated just prior to delivery to prevent dystocia or to facilitate Cesarean delivery. Tumor debulking using percutaneous coagulation techniques, such as radiofrequency ablation, or laser coagulation to decrease the vascular shunt are minimally invasive alternatives to open resection and have been successfully reported. However, long-term complications are noted in survivors due to injury of adjacent structures, which require a better understanding of the application of these techniques for SCT.

Neck/Chest

Cervical Teratoma

Fetal cervical neck masses are readily identified on prenatal ultrasound and can lead to prenatal compression of the trachea and esophagus.[19] This obstruction can result in polyhydramnios, preterm labor, craniofacial defects, and cranial nerve injury.[20] Highly vascular lesions can lead to in utero cardiac failure with nonimmune fetal hydrops. Most fetal neck masses will be comprised of either a cervical teratoma, lymphatic malformations (cystic hygroma), or other vascular malformations.[19] Neck masses will rarely include thymic cysts or congenital neuroblastomas.

Once the presence of a cervical mass has been recognized via ultrasound, fetal magnetic resonance imaging (MRI) will better characterize the mass, specifically to distinguish between a lymphatic lesion and a teratoma. This distinction is important as the presence of a cervical teratoma or polyhydramnios increases the risk of a complicated airway and these pregnancies require close surveillance. Furthermore, large masses that cause significant extension of the neck require delivery via Cesarean section, due to the risk of dystocia. In the presence of fetal hydrops prior to 30 weeks' gestation, open fetal resection may be considered, as an obstructing cervical mass poses a significant risk to the fetus with a nearly 20% risk of intrauterine fetal demise.[20] After delivery, immediately securing the airway is paramount. If this cannot be accomplished quickly enough, the neonate can die immediately due to a compromised airway.

Ex Utero Intrapartum Treatment Procedure

The EXIT procedure is used to stabilize the airway immediately prior to complete delivery of the fetus.[21] During an EXIT-to-airway procedure, the uterus is exposed and a hysterotomy is made to deliver the fetus' head and neck. Direct laryngoscopy can be attempted for endotracheal intubation. Means to establish an airway can be escalated using bronchoscopy or tracheostomy, if laryngoscopy is not successful. In cases of large cystic lesions, decompression of the cyst may facilitate establishing an airway by relieving any airway compression. When an airway still cannot be obtained, resection of the mass, while still on utero-placental circulation, may be necessary. This modification of the EXIT procedure is termed *EXIT-to-resection*. Once the mass has been resected and an airway has been established, the umbilical cord is divided, and the baby completely delivered.

It is critical to understand that an EXIT procedure is not a Cesarean section. Contrary to a Cesarean section, deep maternal anesthesia is required during an EXIT procedure to maintain complete uterine relaxation and preserve utero-placental circulation so the fetus does not undergo premature transition from fetal to neonatal circulation. In a Cesarean section, contraction of the uterus is ideal because it is hemostatic; in an EXIT procedure, uterine contraction is detrimental to the fetus and puts the mother at greater risk for hemorrhage.

Congenital Lung Lesions

A variety of pathologic pulmonary lesions are collectively grouped together as congenital lung lesions. These conditions can range from relatively small asymptomatic lung cysts to large pulmonary masses, which can lead to fetal demise.[22] The most common of these congenital lung lesions include congenital pulmonary airway malformation, bronchopulmonary sequestration, and congenital lobar emphysema. When it occurs, fetal demise is almost always due to the development of nonimmune hydrops. As with sacrococcygeal and cervical teratomas, the development of nonimmune hydrops is a strong indicator of poor fetal or postnatal outcome. Abnormal fetal echocardiogram findings can be defined by increased or decreased cardiac output, ventricular hypertrophy, atrial or ventricular chamber dilation, cardiomegaly, significant valvular regurgitation, or diastolic dysfunction. The presence of placentomegaly (>5 cm in thickness) can also be an indicator of imminent fetal demise.

There are no absolute criteria for fetal intervention of congenital lung lesions. In general, fetal therapy is reserved for only the most severe cases marked by high risk of fetal demise or the expectation of significant respiratory distress at birth. Smaller lesions or asymptomatic larger lesions without hydrops can be safely followed with ultrasound.

Fetal management. Select congenital lung lesions have demonstrated rapid regression and reversal of hydrops after maternal steroid administration.[23] The mechanism of action is believed to be related to improvement in fetal pulmonary development. Large, symptomatic macrocystic lesions may be amenable to minimally invasive fetal drainage. Both ultrasound-guided cyst aspiration and deployment of a thoracoamniotic shunt have been successfully used in the management of congenital lung lesions. Cyst aspiration can rapidly reduce the volume of the lesion, but it is frequently only a temporary solution, as fluid reaccumulation is common. The use of a thoracoamniotic shunt can reverse hydrops in patients with macrocystic disease (Fig. 73.1).[24] Unfortunately, shunt dislodgement after placement is common that may necessitate a repeat procedure if there are signs of ongoing fetal distress.

Open fetal surgery for congenital lung lesions. Open fetal surgery can be rarely offered for select congenital pulmonary lesions of impending fetal demise. In patients older than 30 weeks' gestation, EXIT or EXIT-to-resection may provide a more stable transition from fetal to postnatal life. It is important to note that following delivery and positive pressure ventilation, a congenital lung mass may increase in size, leading to worsening cardiac compression and cardiovascular collapse.

Congenital Diaphragmatic Hernia

Congenital diaphragmatic hernia (CDH) is a relatively common congenital lesion with an estimated survival of about 70% to 80%.[25] CDH is diagnosed by the hallmark defect in the diaphragm and can lead to neonatal death secondary to pulmonary hypoplasia and pulmonary hypertension. Unlike MMC and SCT, which are most often isolated defects, CDH can be associated with a variety of anomalies, including congenital heart disease and chromosomal abnormalities. This association contributes to the high mortality of this disease.

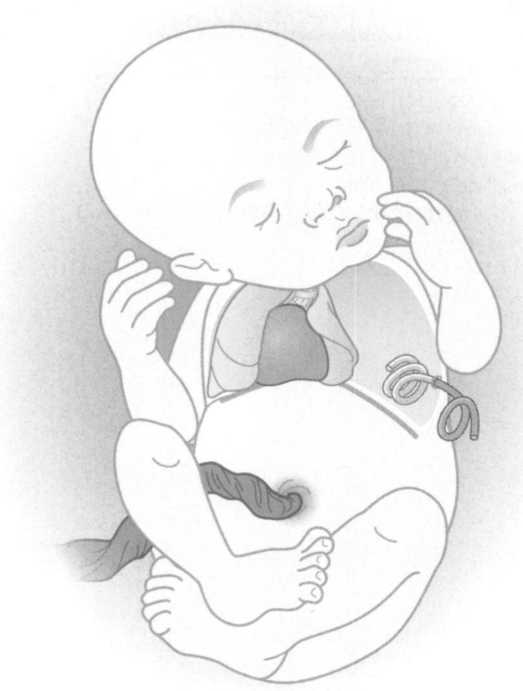

FIG. 73.1 Thoracoamniotic shunt.

Fetal surgery to repair the diaphragmatic defect was first reported in 1990.[26] Further studies evaluating open fetal surgery were met with mixed results.[27] It seemed that the fetuses with the most severe defects, who stood to benefit the most from prenatal intervention, did not survive prenatal surgery. This was thought to be due to kinking of the vasculature of the herniated liver with acute reduction from the chest to the abdomen.

Open fetal repair has since been abandoned in favor of tracheal occlusion (Fig. 73.2).[28] When the fetal trachea is occluded, fluid normally made by the fetal lung parenchyma builds up and leads to pulmonary hyperplasia. Since pulmonary hypoplasia contributes a large portion to the morbidity and mortality associated with CDH, tracheal occlusion is thought to improve the pulmonary hypoplasia in select patients with CDH. After a series of promising findings in animal studies, a prospective randomized trial of fetal tracheal occlusion was initiated in the United States, but no survival benefit was found.[29] Fetal tracheal occlusion has been pursued more promisingly in Europe, and clinical trials in the United States are ongoing.

Cardiac

Congenital Cardiac Lesions

Fetal intervention for congenital cardiac disease is a relatively new and evolving field in fetal surgery. Because fetal cardiac output is mostly dependent on maternal circulation via the placenta, rather than the fetus' own intrinsic circulation, the aim of prenatal

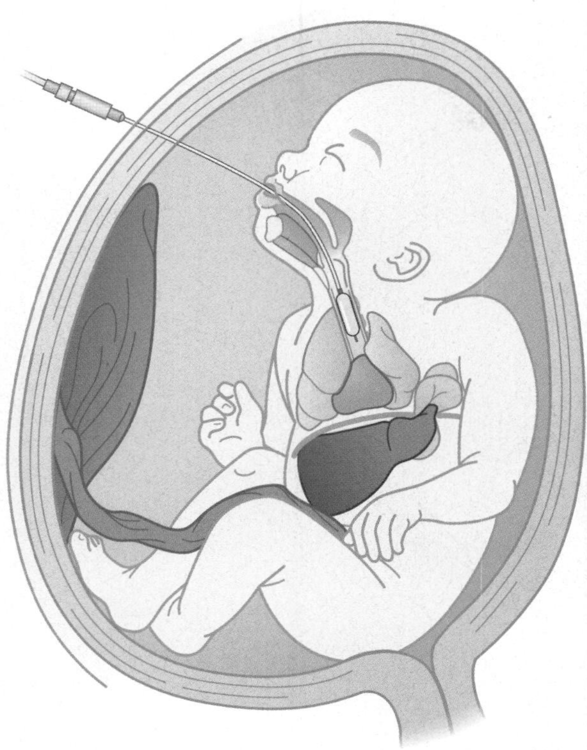

FIG. 73.2 Tracheal balloon.

intervention is to increase the chances of achieving postnatal biventricular circulation and to ameliorate the progression of severe cardiac lesions with high mortality. It is hoped that early rescue of ventricular function and pulmonary circulation will improve postnatal outcomes. To date, the success of fetal cardiac intervention has been limited by the relatively few numbers of eligible patients, the late referral of eligible patients to specialized fetal cardiac centers, and a lack of providers with the necessary technical expertise.[30]

Fetal cardiac intervention is currently restricted to minimally invasive procedures to address three forms of congenital heart disease: severe aortic stenosis with evolving hypoplastic heart syndrome, pulmonary atresia with an intact ventricular septum and evolving hypoplastic right heart syndrome, and hypoplastic left heart syndrome with an intact or highly restrictive aortic septum.[31] Intrauterine balloon valvuloplasty and atrial septoplasty are the most common procedures performed. While an increasing number of patients have achieved biventricular circulation, significant improvements in long-term survival have not yet been demonstrated for the most severe lesions. Open fetal cardiac intervention is currently limited to experimental animal models.

Twin-Twin Transfusion Syndrome

TTTS is a potentially fatal complication of monochorionic twin pregnancies. In this situation, two fetuses share one placenta, but are physically isolated in different amniotic sacs. Due to this sharing, the twins are at risk for unequal vascular utilization of the placenta. Although all monochorionic twin pregnancies are at risk, only 10% ultimately will develop TTTS.[3] Overall, this comprises approximately 1 in 50 twin pregnancies in the United States.[32] TTTS is by far the leading indication for operative fetal intervention, estimated to be about 500 cases per year, and is a procedure performed both by pediatric surgeons and high-risk obstetric providers.

The pathophysiology of TTTS is related to vascular anastomoses across the placenta. Most monochorionic twins share blood flow via arteriovenous connections across the placenta. Usually, this intertwin transfusion is net balanced. In TTTS, the transfusion becomes unbalanced with one twin ("the donor") donating vascular flow to a receiving twin ("the recipient"). The result can lead to oligohydramnios in the donor, and polyhydramnios in the recipient. More devastatingly, this can lead to discordant growth, cardiac failure, hydrops, and death of one or both twins.

Fetal intervention for TTTS is a minimally invasive procedure in which a fetoscope is introduced through the mother and through the uterus (Fig. 73.3). A laser is used to ablate the offending communicating vessel across the shared placenta. Fetal laser ablation can be performed from 16–26 weeks gestation. Randomized-controlled trials of laser ablation in advanced TTTS have demonstrated a significantly higher likelihood of survival of at least one twin (from about 50%–75%) and decreased neurologic complications, although the risk of premature rupture of membranes and preterm delivery is increased.[33]

Abdomen

Gastroschisis

Gastroschisis is an increasingly common congenital abdominal defect of the newborn whereby the intraabdominal organs are located outside of the abdominal cavity at birth and are not covered by an amniotic sac. Thus, the small intestine and other involved viscera are exposed to the amniotic fluid and trauma *in utero*, which is hypothesized to contribute to postnatal intestinal dysfunction. Postnatally, this is often manifested by a thick peel on very matted intestine.[34] While infants with gastroschisis have excellent survival, delayed gastrointestinal motility is a hallmark of the disease and leads to prolonged hospitalization requiring parenteral nutrition.

Gastroschisis can be diagnosed as early as the first trimester. As the findings appear progressively worse on ultrasound, there is an increased likelihood of having to deliver the fetus prematurely, around 36 to 38 weeks. The rationale for early delivery is that it reduces the duration of time in which the bowel is exposed to the toxicity of the amniotic fluid. Surgical closure of the defect is then necessary and involves returning the abdominal viscera to the abdominal cavity and closing the defect. When primary closure is not possible, alternatives include use of a Silastic spring-loaded silo or staged closure. There is currently no *in utero* intervention, but early animal studies showed that *in utero* surgical intervention is safe in a fetal sheep model of gastroschisis.[35]

Gastroschisis is one of the leading causes of short-bowel syndrome and intestinal transplantation in children. The theoretical goal of fetal intervention is to minimize these consequences. Unfortunately, most attempts at predicting outcome by prenatal markers have been unsuccessful in identifying which patients are at high-risk for postnatal morbidity. To date, fetal intervention for gastroschisis remains limited to experimental models.

Genitourinary

Lower Urinary Tract Obstruction

Fetal intervention to decompress the lower urinary tract has been investigated since the origin of fetal surgery and was one of the earliest diseases in which human intervention was attempted. The rationale for fetal intervention is that prenatal urinary obstruction can lead to renal dysplasia and a lack of amniotic fluid volume

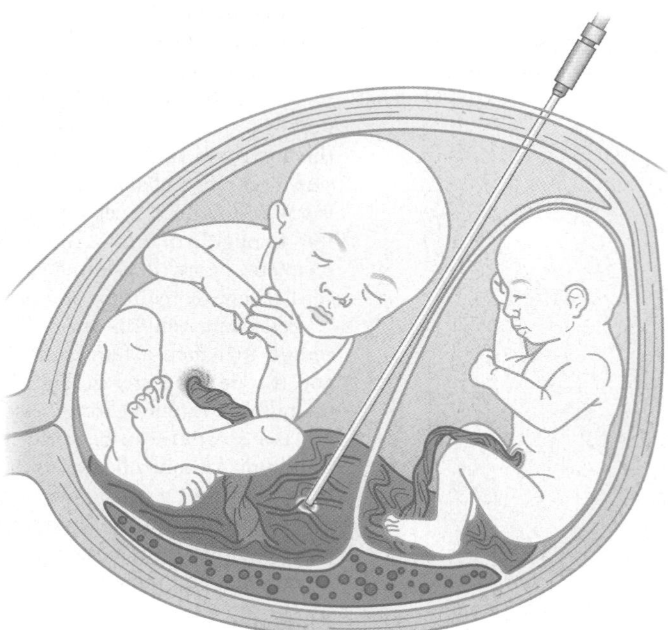

FIG. 73.3 Laser ablation.

can lead to pulmonary hypoplasia. These potentially fatal consequences may be ameliorated by urinary tract decompression before birth.[36] A thorough understanding of the natural history of untreated fetal urinary obstruction is paramount in appropriate patient selection as the majority of fetuses with urinary tract obstruction do not require intervention.

The goal of fetal intervention is the restoration of amniotic fluid to prevent the development of pulmonary hypoplasia. It is not clear how much renal function can be prevented or restored. Serial amnioinfusion is one method of increasing amniotic fluid, but it is risky and difficult to sustain long-term. Decompression of the bladder can be performed via deployment of a vesicoamniotic shunt placed percutaneously using ultrasonographic guidance. This in turn increases amniotic fluid volume by diverting the fetal urine past the obstruction to the amniotic cavity. Fetal cystoscopic ablation of posterior urethral valves has also been reported to potentially restore normal fetal bladder filling and emptying.[37]

NOVEL THERAPIES AND FUTURE DIRECTIONS IN FETAL MEDICINE AND SURGERY

Although the past for fetal surgery has been marked by extraordinary progress for an entirely new field of medicine, it is the future that shines most brightly. From discoveries on the fetal origins of adult diseases to ever increasing applications for fetal gene and stem cell therapies or the induction of tolerance for future transplants, the promise of fetal medicine and surgery is extraordinary and holds a lifetime of investigative promise for young scientists. As fetal surgery is evolving, promising animal work is underway exploring the technical feasibility and pathophysiologic rationale for *in utero* interventions.

In Utero Stem Cell Transplantation

One can argue that the fetus is the ideal target for regenerative therapies, due to the inherent regenerative milieu that is the natural fetal condition, as well as the ideal source of stem cells, as fetal cells possess characteristics of plasticity and differentiation capabilities that are generally superior to adult stem cells.[38] The most widely used stem cells have historically been bone marrow-derived hematopoietic stem cells (BM-HSCs). HSCs are able to engraft and have the potential to differentiate into blood cells, giving them the unique potential of curing hemoglobinopathies prenatally that have historically relied on postnatal bone marrow transplants. The stem cell field has recently migrated towards mesenchymal stem cells (MSCs) as they have trilineage potential, being able to differentiate into adipogenic, chondrogenic, and osteogenic lineages.[39] Furthermore, MSCs are known to display immunomodulatory capabilities through paracrine mechanisms, without engrafting and differentiating and can thus be applied to other organ systems. Most importantly, although MSCs have been mostly derived from adult bone marrow, fetal sources of MSCs are increasingly available such as amniotic fluid and placenta derived MSCs.[34,38] HSCs and MSCs are being applied as therapeutic approaches in the treatment of hemoglobinopathies, congenital skeletal deformities, and even other developmental defects, such as gastroschisis.

BM-HSCs may have the potential to cure hemoglobinopathies such as sickle cell disease (SCD) and thalassemia (Thal). SCD and Thal are hemoglobinopathies arising from single gene defects and result in life-threatening anemia.[40] The current gold standard of treatment is a postnatal human leukocyte antigen (HLA) matched bone marrow donor transplant, after myeloablative conditioning. However, Thal and SCD treatments are currently limited by the number of available matched donors. It has since been shown that in utero hematopoietic cell transplantation (IUHCT) offers a curative treatment, as a nonmyeloablative approach, that does not require immunosuppression, and one that allows for mixed allogeneic chimerism to build donor-specific tolerance. This approach takes advantage of the fetus's immature immune system and induces fetal chimerism. Subsequently, a second postnatal same donor "booster" bone marrow transplant can achieve high levels of engraftment and thus donor hemoglobin expression, correcting the phenotypes of SCD and Thal.[41] The booster strategy as a postnatal treatment is feasible because the fetus has already achieved chimerism, compatible with the donor, from the in utero IUHCT, and will therefore accept a postnatal bone marrow transplant, without rejection. This treatment then effectively expands the eligible transplant population. Alternatively, the fetus is chimeric with respect to the mother and thus a maternal-to-fetal stem cell transplant may improve outcomes more so than a transplant from any other donor. Studies showed that high doses of maternal donor HSCs allowed for higher levels of chimerism in a fetal canine model and a subsequent renal transplant from the same maternal donor showed no signs of rejection. Furthermore, after proven success in large animal models, an ongoing phase I clinical trial is accepting patients with Thal and aims to demonstrate the safety and efficacy of prenatal IUHCT in humans with Thal (NCT02986698). Briefly, the fetus will receive a transplant of maternal BM-HSCs intravenously via the umbilical vein. Investigators are interested in the resulting postnatal level of chimerism that will serve as the determining factor in the continuation of such clinical trials. Thus, adult HSCs have the potential to cure hemoglobinopathies and may well become the current standard of care in years to come.

Since MSCs have shown trilineage potential, they may prove to be the ideal choice for curing congenital skeletal developmental problems or even skeletal defects, among other disorders. Osteogenesis imperfecta is a heterogeneous congenital bone disorder, characterized by a defect in the type I collagen producing gene, which mainly leads to abnormal skeletal development and painful fractures, which may begin to occur in utero. The fetus is in a state of rapid skeletal development with an immune system that has yet to develop, providing an environment ideal for MSC therapy. First trimester fetal MSCs were used as an allogeneic treatment for osteogenesis imperfecta in a mouse model, where MSC transplantation was shown to be safe and treatment improved bone strength, length, cortical thickness, and resulted in two thirds reduced incidence of fractures.[42] Additionally, two human patients received intravenous prenatal and postnatal same-donor fetal MSCs. One of the patients was found to have about one fracture a year until 8 years old, at which point, the patient received an additional postnatal infusion with same-donor cells. The following two years, the patient was found to have no new fractures and was able to start dance classes and participate in hockey and gymnastics.[43] Therefore, MSC treatment may prove to be the superior curative option over bisphosphonates and other approaches currently used for osteogenesis imperfecta management.

MSCs are known to have other capabilities beyond the trilineage differentiation potential. Fetal MSCs have shown unique wound-healing capabilities, which may make them ideal candidates in the treatment of other birth defects such as gastroschisis via transamniotic stem cell therapy (TRASCET). Bowel damage was reduced in a rodent model of gastroschisis when amniotic fetal MSCs were delivered in a concentrated dose via intraamniotic injection. The rationale is that boosting the amniotic fetal MSC numbers already present in the amniotic fluid enhances the normal in utero activity.[34] Once the baby is born, he/she can receive postnatal surgery to enclose the abdominal viscera and close the defect. This approach takes advantage of the fetal environment by utilizing the dual function of the amniotic fluid. Amniotic fluid causes damage to the bowel due to its inherent toxicity, but also partakes in the healing process due to its native stem cells. By infusing the amniotic fluid with a higher dose of expanded stem cells, the wound healing aspect of the amniotic fluid can prevail over its inherent toxicity.

Fetal Tissue Engineering

Tissue engineering approaches often combine the use of a matrix with stem cells aimed at regenerating missing or malformed structural organs. Several tissue engineering approaches have been attempted for the treatment of MMC, which is the most severe form of spina bifida. MMC is not just a neurologic disorder, but a complex disease with significant deformation of bone and connective tissue overlying the spinal cord. Therefore, approaches to completely restore neurologic function must address both restoration of neural function as well as tissue coverage. One possible treatment involves the application of stem cells to protect neurons in combination with a scaffold to provide tissue coverage. The most promising stem cell type in the treatment of MMC has shown to be early gestational MSCs, derived from the placenta (PMSCs). PMSCs display notable immunomodulatory properties and neuroprotective capabilities superior to other types of MSCs. In preclinical studies thus far, PMSCs were shown to restore motor function in a fetal sheep MMC model (Fig. 73.4).[44]

While the PMSC-extracellular matrix (PMSC-ECM) scaffold has the potential to rescue ambulation at birth, the absent overlying spine may still allow postnatal damage to accrue and may thus compromise motor function, postbirth. As such, a bone scaffold seeded with PMSCs may prove to be the more comprehensive treatment in the future to come. The rationale is that once the PMSC-ECM patch has rescued motor function, the PMSCs on the bone scaffold may encourage tissue and bone coverage formation. Current studies are looking at developing various bone scaffolds, for example polymer-ceramic composites, such as hydroxyapatite poly (lactide-co-glycolide) seeded with MSCs.[45]

Alternative treatments for MMC have explored other tissue engineering approaches. One such study has engineered a gelatin-based sponge to allow sustained release of fibroblast growth factor, which enhances angiogenesis and induces fetal stem cells to regenerate a tissue layer over the MMC defect in a fetal ovine model.[46] This tissue engineering technique is an excellent example of the work done to enhance the normal fetal developmental process.

In Utero Gene Therapy

In utero gene therapy orchestrates results by taking advantage of the normal developmental properties of the fetus to correct life-threatening abnormalities. The majority of gene therapy clinical trials are focused on inherited monogenic diseases. Treating most monogenic diseases involves the correction of the disorder by prenatal transfer of a functional normal gene to work in place of the defective one. One study evaluated the potential of single intrauterine gene transfer (IUGT) in a primate model of hemophilia B by assessing long-term transgene expression. The study concluded that late gestation gene transfer via an adeno-associated vector-human factor IX (AAV-IUGT) was safe and effective.[47] However, in cases in which the addition of a functional gene is not sufficient to correct the phenotype, gene editing tools may become more prominent. CRISPR-Cas9 technology is a gene editing tool that shows immense potential in the therapeutic correction of monogenic disorders. Intraamniotic delivery of gene editing reagents during fetal development was shown to result in specific gene editing of pulmonary epithelial cells in a fetal mouse model and thus corrected lung disease.[48] These results show the potential of gene editing therapies to restore lung function and treat inherited

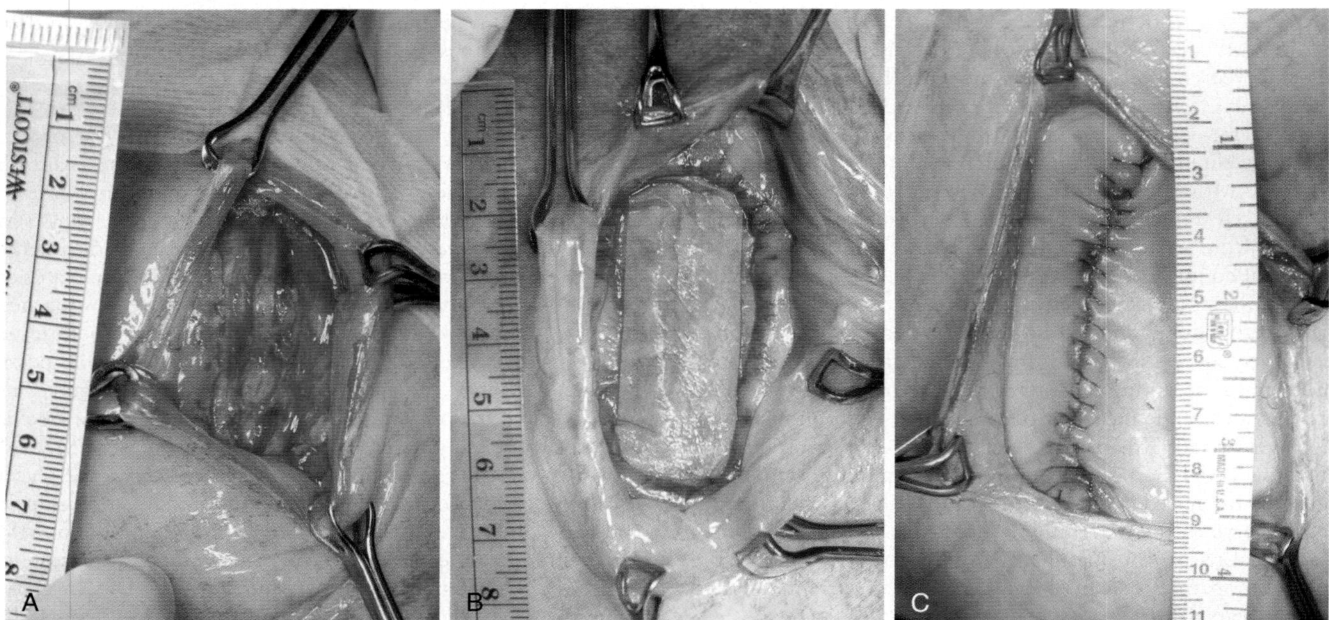

FIG. 73.4 PMSC-ECM application for MMC *in utero*—representative images. (A) The MMC defect in the fetal sheep model. (B) The PMSC-ECM patch applied during repair surgery. (C) The closure of the overall repair. *MMC*, Myelomeningocele; *PMSC-ECM*, placenta mesenchymal stem cell-extracellular matrix.

disorders, such as cystic fibrosis. Prenatal gene editing may be beneficial due to its efficiency in rescuing fetuses from otherwise lethal diseases. However, given that the mother is a "bystander", injection techniques and gene editing delivery vehicles must be optimized to avoid directly affecting the mother.

Artificial Placenta

Yet another extraordinary advancement in fetal medicine is the development of an extracorporeal mechanism for the continuing gestation outside of the natural womb.[49,50] The leading cause of infant mortality is extreme prematurity. Advancements in fetal medicine are allowing the viability limits to be as low as 22 or 23 weeks of gestation. However, these patients are born with severe complications, respiratory problems constituting the majority, as the lungs are not fully developed. One set of investigators have designed a "Biobag" to serve as an alternative to having the premature infant on a ventilator in an incubator. The biobag has three main aspects: a pumpless arteriovenous circuit where the fetus heart drives blood flow, a closed fluid environment with continuous fluid exchange, so that the lungs remain fluid-filled for normal development, and an umbilical vascular access. Fetal lambs were shown to be physiologically supported up to four weeks on this device. Despite extraordinary results, several questions remain to be addressed such as the importance of the native amniotic fluid, which is the subject of current research. Furthermore, this technology is aimed at improving outcomes for extreme premature infants of 22 to 23 weeks of gestation and is not aimed at further extending the limits of viability. The extracorporeal placenta may prove important in cases of placental insufficiency, premature delivery following prenatal surgery, and even for infants subject to stem cell or gene therapies; the rationale being that by isolating the fetus in these instances of stem cell and gene therapies, the exposure to the mother would be greatly reduced. Finally, this remarkable development has yet to reach clinical trials but may prove to significantly improve the quality of life for extremely premature infants.

As the maternal safety profile continues to improve, the indications for fetal therapy are likely to be extended. What was once reserved for only lethal fetal defects has now been applied to nonlethal defects, such as spina bifida, with powerful advantages for affected fetuses. It is only a matter of time that fetal therapy for other nonlethal diseases become clinical realities.

ACKNOWLEDGEMENTS

The authors would like to acknowledge the literature research and editorial assistance of Alexandra M. Iavorovschi in completing this chapter and Dr. Sarah Chen for making the illustrations for this chapter.

SELECTED REFERENCES

Adzick NS, Thom EA, Spong CY, et al. A randomized trial of prenatal versus postnatal repair of myelomeningocele. *N Engl J Med.* 2011;364:993–1004.

Landmark study comparing prenatal and postnatal repair of myelomeningocele. The results of this trial constitute one of the most important milestones in the clinical success of fetal surgery as it demonstrated the safety and efficacy in prenatally treating a nonlethal condition.

Alapati D, Zacharias WJ, Hartman HA, et al. In utero gene editing for monogenic lung disease. *Sci Transl Med.* 2019;11:eaav8375.

Study showed that intraamniotic delivery of gene editing reagents (CRISP-Cas9) during fetal development resulted in specific gene editing of pulmonary epithelial cells in a fetal mouse model and thus corrected lung disease. This article represents strides in gene editing as it displayed the feasibility of prenatal gene therapy to cure lethal lung disease in a mouse model with a human mutation.

Golbus MS, Harrison MR, Filly RA, et al. In utero treatment of urinary tract obstruction. *Am J Obstet Gynecol.* 1982;142:383–388.

Original study illustrating the safety and feasibility of in utero intervention for a congenital anomaly.

Heffez DS, Aryanpur J, Hutchins GM, et al. The paralysis associated with myelomeningocele: Clinical and experimental data implicating a preventable spinal cord injury. *Neurosurgery.* 1990;26:987–992.

This study was first to hypothesize that the paralysis associated with myelomeningocele is due to both the initial congenital defect as well as the acquired chemical and mechanical injury that the spinal cord sustains in utero. This two-hit-hypothesis was studied in a rat model of surgically created dysraphism and lent support to the rationale for fetal surgery for myelomeningocele.

Meuli M, Meuli-Simmen C, Hutchins GM, et al. In utero surgery rescues neurological function at birth in sheep with spina bifida. *Nat Med.* 1995;1:342–347.

This study provided further proof for the two-hit hypothesis of spina bifida in a large animal model, the fetal sheep spina bifida model. The study also showed that the fetal sheep allow for multiple fetal interventions and must therefore be resistant to preterm labor.

Partridge EA, Davey MG, Hornick MA, et al. An extra-uterine system to physiologically support the extreme premature lamb. *Nat Commun.* 2017;8:15112.

Landmark article showing the possibility of improving outcomes for extremely premature infants by allowing them to continue their gestational period within an extracorporeal man-made-like womb. The study showed that a fetal lamb was maintained on this system for four weeks and was capable of normal function all around, once born.

Reoma JL, Rojas A, Kim AC, et al. Development of an artificial placenta I: Pumpless arterio-venous extracorporeal life support in a neonatal sheep model. *J Pediatr Surg.* 2009;44:53–59.

Landmark article describing the development of a pumpless arteriovenous extracorporeal life support circuit. The device was shown to be able to maintain fetal circulation for up to four hours in a neonatal lamb model.

Wang A, Brown EG, Lankford L, et al. Placental mesenchymal stromal cells rescue ambulation in ovine myelomeningocele. *Stem Cells Transl Med.* 2015;4:659–669.

Landmark study that showed that placental-derived mesenchymal stromal cells (PMSCs) can rescue motor function in a large animal model of myelomeningocele. PMSCs had a neuroprotective effect, and treated lambs had improved motor function compared to untreated animals.

REFERENCES

1. Golbus MS, Harrison MR, Filly RA, et al. In utero treatment of urinary tract obstruction. *Am J Obstet Gynecol.* 1982;142:383–388.
2. Longaker MT, Golbus MS, Filly RA, et al. Maternal outcome after open fetal surgery. A review of the first 17 human cases. *JAMA.* 1991;265:737–741.
3. Simpson LL. Twin-twin transfusion syndrome. *Am J Obstet Gynecol.* 2013;208:3–18.
4. Adzick NS, Thom EA, Spong CY, et al. A randomized trial of prenatal versus postnatal repair of myelomeningocele. *N Engl J Med.* 2011;364:993–1004.
5. Al-Refai A, Ryan G, Van Mieghem T. Maternal risks of fetal therapy. *Curr Opin Obstet Gynecol.* 2017;29:80–84.
6. Meuli M, Meuli-Simmen C, Hutchins GM, et al. In utero surgery rescues neurological function at birth in sheep with spina bifida. *Nat Med.* 1995;1:342–347.
7. Yamashiro KJ, Galganski LA, Hirose S. Fetal myelomeningocele repair. *Semin Pediatr Surg.* 2019;28:150823.
8. Chmait RH, Kontopoulos EV, Quintero RA. Uterine legacy of open maternal-fetal surgery: preterm uterine rupture. *Am J Obstet Gynecol.* 2019;221:535.
9. Goodnight WH, Bahtiyar O, Bennett KA, et al. Subsequent pregnancy outcomes after open maternal-fetal surgery for myelomeningocele. *Am J Obstet Gynecol.* 2019;220:494.e491–494 e497.
10. Wilson RD, Lemerand K, Johnson MP, et al. Reproductive outcomes in subsequent pregnancies after a pregnancy complicated by open maternal-fetal surgery (1996-2007). *Am J Obstet Gynecol.* 2010;203:209.e201–206.
11. Parker SE, Mai CT, Canfield MA, et al. Updated national birth prevalence estimates for selected birth defects in the United States, 2004-2006. *Birth Defects Res A Clin Mol Teratol.* 2010;88:1008–1016.
12. Adzick NS. Fetal myelomeningocele: Natural history, pathophysiology, and in-utero intervention. *Semin Fetal Neonatal Med.* 2010;15:9–14.
13. Heffez DS, Aryanpur J, Hutchins GM, et al. The paralysis associated with myelomeningocele: Clinical and experimental data implicating a preventable spinal cord injury. *Neurosurgery.* 1990;26:987–992.
14. Korenromp MJ, van Gool JD, Bruinese HW, et al. Early fetal leg movements in myelomeningocele. *Lancet.* 1986;1:917–918.
15. Swamy R, Embleton N, Hale J. Sacrococcygeal teratoma over two decades: Birth prevalence, prenatal diagnosis and clinical outcomes. *Prenat Diagn.* 2008;28:1048–1051.
16. Akinkuotu AC, Coleman A, Shue E, et al. Predictors of poor prognosis in prenatally diagnosed sacrococcygeal

teratoma: A multiinstitutional review. *J Pediatr Surg.* 2015;50:771–774.
17. Hedrick HL, Flake AW, Crombleholme TM, et al. Sacrococcygeal teratoma: Prenatal assessment, fetal intervention, and outcome. *J Pediatr Surg.* 2004;39:430–438; discussion 430–438.
18. Adzick NS. Open fetal surgery for life-threatening fetal anomalies. *Semin Fetal Neonatal Med.* 2010;15:1–8.
19. Hirose S, Sydorak RM, Tsao K, et al. Spectrum of intrapartum management strategies for giant fetal cervical teratoma. *J Pediatr Surg.* 2003;38:446–450; discussion 446–450.
20. Berge SJ, von Lindern JJ, Appel T, et al. Diagnosis and management of cervical teratomas. *Br J Oral Maxillofac Surg.* 2004;42:41–45.
21. Marwan A, Crombleholme TM. The EXIT procedure: principles, pitfalls, and progress. *Semin Pediatr Surg.* 2006;15:107–115.
22. Downard CD, Calkins CM, Williams RF, et al. Treatment of congenital pulmonary airway malformations: A systematic review from the APSA outcomes and evidence based practice committee. *Pediatr Surg Int.* 2017;33:939–953.
23. Curran PF, Jelin EB, Rand L, et al. Prenatal steroids for microcystic congenital cystic adenomatoid malformations. *J Pediatr Surg.* 2010;45:145–150.
24. Peranteau WH, Adzick NS, Boelig MM, et al. Thoracoamniotic shunts for the management of fetal lung lesions and pleural effusions: A single-institution review and predictors of survival in 75 cases. *J Pediatr Surg.* 2015;50:301–305.
25. Wynn J, Krishnan U, Aspelund G, et al. Outcomes of congenital diaphragmatic hernia in the modern era of management. *J Pediatr.* 2013;163:114–119.e111.
26. Harrison MR, Adzick NS, Longaker MT, et al. Successful repair in utero of a fetal diaphragmatic hernia after removal of herniated viscera from the left thorax. *N Engl J Med.* 1990;322:1582–1584.
27. Harrison MR, Adzick NS, Bullard KM, et al. Correction of congenital diaphragmatic hernia in utero VII: A prospective trial. *J Pediatr Surg.* 1997;32:1637–1642.
28. Sydorak RM, Harrison MR. Congenital diaphragmatic hernia: Advances in prenatal therapy. *World J Surg.* 2003;27:68–76.
29. Harrison MR, Keller RL, Hawgood SB, et al. A randomized trial of fetal endoscopic tracheal occlusion for severe fetal congenital diaphragmatic hernia. *N Engl J Med.* 2003;349:1916–1924.
30. Schidlow DN, Tworetzky W, Wilkins-Haug LE. Percutaneous fetal cardiac interventions for structural heart disease. *Am J Perinatol.* 2014;31:629–636.
31. Freud LR, Tworetzky W. Fetal interventions for congenital heart disease. *Curr Opin Pediatr.* 2016;28:156–162.
32. Lewi L, Jani J, Boes AS, et al. OC112: The natural history of monochorionic twins and the role of prenatal ultrasound scan. *Ultrasound in Obstetrics & Gynecology.* 2007;30:401–402.
33. Senat MV, Deprest J, Boulvain M, et al. Endoscopic laser surgery versus serial amnioreduction for severe twin-to-twin transfusion syndrome. *N Engl J Med.* 2004;351:136–144.
34. Feng C, Graham CD, Connors JP, et al. Transamniotic stem cell therapy (TRASCET) mitigates bowel damage in a model of gastroschisis. *J Pediatr Surg.* 2016;51:56–61.
35. Stephenson JT, Pichakron KO, Vu L, et al. In utero repair of gastroschisis in the sheep (Ovis aries) model. *J Pediatr Surg.* 2010;45:65–69.
36. Saccone G, D'Alessandro P, Escolino M, et al. Antenatal intervention for congenital fetal lower urinary tract obstruction (LUTO): A systematic review and meta-analysis. *J Matern Fetal Neonatal Med.* 2020;33:2664–2670.
37. Farrugia MK, Braun MC, Peters CA, et al. Report on The Society for Fetal Urology panel discussion on the selection criteria and intervention for fetal bladder outlet obstruction. *J Pediatr Urol.* 2017;13:345–351.
38. Lankford L, Selby T, Becker J, et al. Early gestation chorionic villi-derived stromal cells for fetal tissue engineering. *World J Stem Cells.* 2015;7:195–207.
39. Liang X, Ding Y, Zhang Y, et al. Paracrine mechanisms of mesenchymal stem cell-based therapy: Current status and perspectives. *Cell Transplant.* 2014;23:1045–1059.
40. Kreger EM, Singer ST, Witt RG, et al. Favorable outcomes after in utero transfusion in fetuses with alpha thalassemia major: A case series and review of the literature. *Prenat Diagn.* 2016;36:1242–1249.
41. Peranteau WH, Hayashi S, Abdulmalik O, et al. Correction of murine hemoglobinopathies by prenatal tolerance induction and postnatal nonmyeloablative allogeneic BM transplants. *Blood.* 2015;126:1245–1254.
42. Guillot PV, Abass O, Bassett JH, et al. Intrauterine transplantation of human fetal mesenchymal stem cells from first-trimester blood repairs bone and reduces fractures in osteogenesis imperfecta mice. *Blood.* 2008;111:1717–1725.
43. Gotherstrom C, Westgren M, Shaw SW, et al. Pre- and postnatal transplantation of fetal mesenchymal stem cells in osteogenesis imperfecta: a two-center experience. *Stem Cells Transl Med.* 2014;3:255–264.
44. Wang A, Brown EG, Lankford L, et al. Placental mesenchymal stromal cells rescue ambulation in ovine myelomeningocele. *Stem Cells Transl Med.* 2015;4:659–669.
45. He J, Genetos DC, Leach JK. Osteogenesis and trophic factor secretion are influenced by the composition of hydroxyapatite/poly(lactide-co-glycolide) composite scaffolds. *Tissue Eng Part A.* 2010;16:127–137.
46. Watanabe M, Li H, Kim AG, et al. Complete tissue coverage achieved by scaffold-based tissue engineering in the fetal sheep model of myelomeningocele. *Biomaterials.* 2016;76:133–143.
47. Mattar CNZ, Gil-Farina I, Rosales C, et al. In Utero Transfer of adeno-associated viral vectors produces long-term factor IX levels in a cynomolgus macaque model. *Mol Ther.* 2017;25:1843–1853.
48. Alapati D, Zacharias WJ, Hartman HA, et al. In utero gene editing for monogenic lung disease. *Sci Transl Med.* 2019;11:eaav8375.
49. Partridge EA, Davey MG, Hornick MA, et al. An extra-uterine system to physiologically support the extreme premature lamb. *Nat Commun.* 2017;8:15112.
50. Reoma JL, Rojas A, Kim AC, et al. Development of an artificial placenta I: Pumpless arterio-venous extracorporeal life support in a neonatal sheep model. *J Pediatr Surg.* 2009;44:53–59.

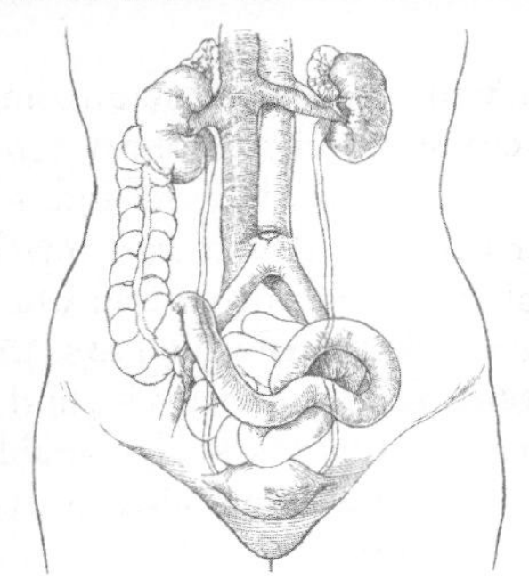

CHAPTER 74

Urologic Surgery

Jennifer M. Taylor, Thomas G. Smith III, Michael Coburn

OUTLINE

Urology is the surgical specialty that focuses on the diagnosis and management of conditions and diseases of the genitourinary system in adults and children and of the reproductive system in the male. Of the surgical subspecialties, urology shares the most in common with general surgery because of our operative approaches and techniques in the abdomen, retroperitoneum, pelvis, and genitalia. Like general surgeons, urologists treat patients with open, laparoscopic, robotic, endoscopic, and microsurgical techniques. Frequently, urologists and general surgeons collaborate in the care of patients across our many interdisciplinary subspecialties. Examples of this include major trauma surgery, exenterative surgery for advanced abdominal and pelvic malignancies, and management of iatrogenic urologic and surgical injury and necrotizing infections of the genitalia and perineum.

General surgeons will encounter patients with urologic conditions as either presenting symptoms or as comorbidities to their general surgical diseases. Urology itself includes multiple subspecialties and treats a wide range of patients and diseases spanning pediatrics, stone disease, female pelvic medicine, oncology, and andrology, to name a few. The intent of this chapter is to give the practicing surgeon and trainee a broad overview of the field of urology and to impart a fundamental knowledge of our field to assist in our common goal of providing complete surgical care of the patient.

UROLOGIC ANATOMY FOR THE GENERAL SURGEON

The organs of the genitourinary system span the entire retroperitoneum, pelvis, inguinal region, and genital region. Because of the close anatomic relationships of the organs in the abdomen and retroperitoneum, general surgeons must be familiar with all of the urologic organ systems to prevent iatrogenic injury and to deal with variations in normal anatomy. These challenges arise in many fields of surgery, including vascular, oncology, and colorectal surgery.

Upper Abdomen and Retroperitoneum

Adrenal

Beginning at the most superior aspect of the retroperitoneum lie the adrenal glands. These small, paired organs have two different embryologic origins and serve a primary endocrine function. The adrenal glands are composed of the cortex and medulla and are fused after development. The cortex is the outer layer of the adrenal gland and is derived from mesoderm.[1] On cross section, the layers, from external to internal, are the zona glomerulosa, zona fasciculata, and zona reticularis. The different zones secrete various steroid-derived hormones including mineralocorticoids (glomerulosa), glucocorticoids (fasciculata), and sex steroids (reticularis).[2] The adrenal medulla is derived from neural crest cells and is directly innervated by presynaptic sympathetic fibers.[1] The medulla is responsible for secreting catecholamines in response to sympathetic stimulation. The adrenal glands lie within Gerota fascia and have an orange-yellow appearance and an area of usually 3 to 5 cm in transverse diameter.[1] The arterial supply is through three sources: superior—inferior phrenic; medial—abdominal aorta; and inferior—ipsilateral renal artery. The venous drainage does not mirror the arterial supply; on the right, the single adrenal vein drains to the vena cava, whereas on the left, the adrenal vein drains into the left renal vein. Supernumerary veins can exist on either side because of anatomic variation. The adrenal glands are anatomically distinct from the kidney, although there are ventral and dorsal fascial investments that connect it to the kidney. The anatomic relations to the right adrenal gland are the vena cava on the anteromedial aspect and the liver and duodenum on the anterior aspect of portions of the adrenal gland. On the left, the pancreas and splenic vein are anterior to the cortical surface.

Kidney

The kidneys are the next paired organs just inferior to the adrenal glands. These organs are completely enveloped within the perirenal fascia (Gerota fascia) and are mobile structures supported only by the perirenal fat, renal pedicle vasculature, and abdominal muscles and viscera. Although Gerota fascia separates the kidney capsule and parenchyma from these adjacent organs and reduces the risk of renal injury with local dissection, renal parenchymal injury is possible with abnormal anatomy. The kidneys are approximately the size of a closed fist, measuring 10 to 12 cm in length and 5 to 7 cm in width. The right kidney typically lies slightly more inferiorly than the left kidney because of its position beneath the liver. Despite being located in the retroperitoneum, the kidney is well protected from external injury by the surrounding muscular and skeletal structures. Posteriorly, each kidney is covered by the diaphragm on the upper third of its surface and is crossed by the twelfth rib. The inferior aspect of the kidney is adjacent to the psoas muscle medially and the quadratus lumborum and transversus abdominis laterally.[1] The anterior surfaces of the kidneys are intimately related to several intraperitoneal structures. On the right, the liver is attached to the kidney by the hepatorenal ligament, and the anterior upper pole is adjacent to the peritoneal surface of the liver.[1] The duodenum lies on the medial aspect of the anterior right kidney, typically on the hilar structures. The hepatic flexure of the colon crosses anterior to the inferior pole of the right kidney. On the left, the superior pole of the kidney lies posterior to the tail of the pancreas and the splenic vessels and hilum. The spleen is situated anteromedial to the kidney and is directly attached to the kidney by the lienorenal ligament. The splenic flexure of the colon is draped over the caudal aspect of the anterior left kidney.

The renal vasculature has significant variability occurring in 25% to 40% of kidneys.[3] The typical vasculature is based on a paired artery and vein supplying the kidney as direct branches of the aorta and vena cava, respectively. The renal artery branches from the aorta inferior to the superior mesenteric artery at the level of the second lumbar vertebra. The renal artery then branches into four or five segments, each being an end artery.[3] The renal arteries are located posterior and slightly superior to the renal veins. The artery initially branches posteriorly into the posterior segmental artery. The anterior branches are variable but include the apical, upper, middle, and lower segmental arteries. These arteries branch multiple times within the cortical kidney, creating a complex filtration mechanism at the capillary level. The venous capillary branches coalesce to mirror the parenchymal arterial system. Renal segmental veins are not end vascular structures and collateralize extensively. The renal vein on the right is short, typically 2 to 4 cm in length, and enters the posterolateral inferior vena cava.[3] The left renal vein is longer, 6 to 10 cm, and travels anterior to the aorta and inferior to the superior mesenteric artery and enters the left lateral vena cava.[3] The left renal vein also is the common entry point for the left adrenal vein, gonadal vein, and a lumbar vein. Renal ectopia is accompanied by markedly variable and unpredictable renal vasculature, with multiple branches arising from the iliac arteries or aortic bifurcation.

Ureter

The upper collecting system begins within the renal parenchyma at the level of the papilla. The papillae coalesce to become the minor calyces, which, in turn, become the major calyces. The major calyces converge to form the renal pelvis. The ureter begins at the inferior aspect of the renal pelvis, where it narrows to become the ureteropelvic junction posterior to the renal artery.[2] Each ureter is typically 22 to 30 cm in length, depending on height, and courses through the retroperitoneum into the pelvis, where it connects to the urinary bladder at the ureterovesical junction.[4] At its origin, the ureter courses along the anterior psoas major muscle and is crossed by the gonadal vessels bilaterally. The ureters cross over the iliac vessels to enter the pelvis, just superior to the bifurcation of the iliac vessels into the internal and external segments. Once in the pelvis, the ureters course medially to enter the bladder. The ureters are divided into three segments, upper, middle, and lower, using this anatomic landmark as a junction point.[4] The upper segment runs from the ureteropelvic junction to the superior margin of the sacrum. The middle segment runs over the bony pelvis. The lower segment begins at the inferior margin of the sacrum and continues into the bladder. The ureteral lumen is not uniform throughout its length and has three distinct narrowing points: the ureteropelvic junction, crossing the iliac vessels, and the ureterovesical junction. The right and left ureters have separate anatomic relationships (peritoneal and retroperitoneal structures). On the right, the ureter is posterior to the ascending colon, cecum, and appendix. The left ureter is posterior to the descending and sigmoid colon. In the male, the ureters are crossed by the vasa deferentia as they emerge from the internal ring before turning medially to join the prostate. The ureteral blood is drawn from multiple vessels throughout its course and within the adventitia; the arterial vessels create an anastomosing plexus. In general, the upper ureteral segments have a medial vascular supply (i.e., renal artery and aorta), and the lower ureteral segments have a lateral vascular supply (i.e., internal iliac and various branches). This unique collateral blood flow allows extensive mobilization of the ureter, outside of its adventitia, without loss of its blood supply.[4]

The ureter is best identified, intraoperatively, in an area of normal anatomy and then followed to the area of concern. This is readily accomplished medial to the lower pole of the kidney or at the iliac bifurcation. After prior surgery or retroperitoneal disease processes, any of these rich collateral blood supply sources may not be contributory; thus, to minimize the risk of surgical devascularization, it is critical to avoid unnecessary extensive circumferential dissection of the ureter or dissection of the ureter in the subadventitial plane.

Pelvis

Bladder and Prostate

The bladder, the end reservoir for urine, is located within the inferior pelvis. The bladder, when empty, is located behind the pubic rami; but as the bladder becomes distended, the superior aspect of the bladder extends out of the pelvis and into the lower anterior abdomen.[5] The bladder can be injured on entering of the abdomen through a midline incision in the retropubic space (of Retzius) if the bladder is not displaced posteriorly when the midline rectus fascial incision is extended to the pubis. Superiorly, the bladder is covered by the parietal peritoneum of the pelvis as the peritoneum reflects off the anterior and lateral abdominal walls. The anterior and lateral bladder walls do not have a peritoneal surface but reside within pelvic fat and lie along the musculature of the pelvic side wall or pubis anteriorly. Prior lower abdominal or pelvic surgery can change the anatomic relations of the bladder and cause it to be affixed abnormally within the pelvis. The bladder has a unique cross section with a urothelial lining creating a tight barrier from urine and a central muscular detrusor layer involved in the excretory function of the bladder.[6] Branches of the internal iliac artery, the superior and inferior vesical arteries, supply blood to the bladder. Similar to the ureter, the bladder has a rich collateral vascular network, so ligation or damage to an artery is not detrimental to the bladder. The innervation of the bladder is important because of the excretory function of the bladder. The bladder has autonomic and somatic innervation with a dense neural network to the brain. The sympathetic innervation to the bladder is through the hypogastric nerve, and the parasympathetic supply is through the sacral cord and pelvic nerve.[5] The anatomic relationships of the bladder differ between male and female patients. In the male patient, the posterior bladder wall is adjacent to the anterior sigmoid colon and rectum. Prior pelvic surgery, irradiation, or pelvic trauma can make the plane between these structures difficult to define, resulting in inadvertent injury. In the female patient, the parietal peritoneum becomes contiguous with the anterior uterus, and the superior bladder lies against the lower uterus while the bladder base sits adjacent to the anterior vaginal wall. The spherical bladder funnels caudally into the bladder neck, and this becomes the tubular urethra inferiorly.

In the male patient, the first segment of the urethra is surrounded by and integrated into the prostate. The prostate, an endocrine gland involved with male reproductive function, is located immediately inferior to the bladder and invested in the circular fibers of the bladder neck. The prostate is surrounded by the lateral pelvic fascia on its anterior surface, by endopelvic fascia on its lateral surface, and by Denonvilliers fascia posteriorly.[7] The rectum sits immediately posterior to the prostate and is separated by a second layer of Denonvilliers fascia. This fascia also extends superiorly on the posterior prostate to encompass the seminal vesicles. The seminal vesicles are the reservoirs for seminal fluid that makes up the majority of the ejaculatory fluid. The arterial supply to both structures is through branches of the inferior vesical artery. The venous drainage mirrors the arterial supply, draining through the inferior vesical veins and subsequently into the internal iliac veins. In addition to the rectum, the other major anatomic relationship of the prostate is Santorini plexus, a network of veins derived from the dorsal venous complex of the penis.[7]

Urethra, Male Genitalia, and Perineum

The drainage of urine from the bladder is through the tubular urethra, which begins at the level of the bladder neck. In male patients, the urethra has five distinct segments: prostatic, membranous, penile, bulbar, and glandular (also known as the fossa navicularis). The prostatic and membranous urethra is surrounded by striated muscle, and when the urethra penetrates the genitourinary diaphragm in the perineum, the outer layer becomes spongy, vascular tissue. Within the prostate, the ejaculatory duct opens into the urethra and serves as the exit point for seminal emission. The blood supply of the extraprostatic urethra is through the common penile artery, which is a branch of the internal pudendal artery.[5] The venous drainage of the urethra is through the circumflex penile veins and ultimately into the deep dorsal vein of the penis. The major surrounding structure in the proximal male urethra is the rectum, which sits posterior to the proximal bulbar segment. The female urethra is more regular in length and is approximately 4 cm long.[5] The female urethra contains three distinct layers as opposed to the male urethra. The proximal urethra is surrounded by smooth and striated musculature, which forms the urinary sphincter. The arterial and venous blood supply are through the internal pudendal, vaginal, and inferior vesical veins. The only structure adjacent to the female urethra is the anterior vaginal wall.

The male external genitalia consist of the penis, scrotum, and *paired* testes. The penis consists of three circular erectile bodies: the two dorsal corpora cavernosa and the ventral corpus spongiosum. The corpora cavernosa are responsible for penile erection; the corpus spongiosum provides support and structure to the urethra. Blood supply of the penis is through the external and internal pudendal arteries. The external pudendal artery supplies the penile skin; the internal pudendal artery supplies the urethra and the paired erectile bodies. The venous drainage of the penis is through the superficial and deep dorsal veins and the cavernosal veins. The penis is entirely an external structure, with all three erectile bodies terminating in the perineum. The scrotum is a surprisingly complex structure consisting of a muscular sac covered with a unique epidermal layer with no fat but many sebaceous and sweat glands. The sac is divided into two halves by a midline septum of dartos muscle. The blood supply to the scrotum is through the external pudendal arteries anteriorly and branches of perineal vessels posteriorly. Within the scrotum are the right and left testicles. The testicles have both endocrine and reproductive function in men. Typically, the testes are 4 to 5 cm long and 3 cm wide.[5] The vascular and genital ductal structures leave the testis from the mediastinum in the posterosuperior portion and travel through the scrotal neck into the inguinal canal. The spermatic cord is invested by the internal spermatic fascia, cremaster muscle, and external spermatic fascia, which are derived from the transversalis fascia, internal oblique, and external oblique, respectively. Arterial blood supply is primarily through the testicular or gonadal artery, which is a direct branch from the aorta inferior to the renal artery. Secondary blood supply to the testicle is through the cremasteric and vasal arteries. The venous drainage of the testicle initially begins as a pampiniform plexus coalescing into the gonadal or testicular veins. On the right, the vein drains directly into the vena cava; on the left, the vein drains into the left renal vein. The testicles are also responsible for spermatogenesis and for testosterone production. After production, the spermatozoa exit through a series of ductal structures that emerge into the rete testis, efferent ductules, epididymis, and ultimately the vas deferens. The epididymis is located posteriorly and slightly lateral to the testis. The spermatic artery, vein, and vas deferens are invested together in the fascial structures of the spermatic cord. The spermatic cord travels through the external inguinal ring through the inguinal canal and then into the pelvis through the internal inguinal ring. The spermatic cord is susceptible to injury during inguinal dissection for hernia repair, especially in redo cases, when it may be encased in fibrosis and injured without recognition. Significant injury to the spermatic cord may put the viability of the testis at risk, even though it is supported by three collateral arteries. The perineum is divided into an anterior and posterior triangle in the male by a line connecting the ischial tuberosities.[5] The posterior perineal triangle contains the anus and internal and external sphincters. The anterior triangle (or urogenital triangle) contains the corpus spongiosum and proximal aspect of the paired erectile bodies, the corpora cavernosa. The layers deepening towards to the corpus spongiosum consist of the skin, subcutaneous fat, Colles fascia, and bulbospongiosus muscle (surrounding the corpus spongiosum) and ischiocavernosus muscles (surrounding the corpora cavernosa). The blood supply to this region is based on branches of the internal pudendal artery, and drainage is through the internal pudendal vein. The presence of a urethral catheter is helpful in palpating the location of the urethra, but the corpus spongiosum surrounding the bulbar urethra is still vulnerable to injury with dissection in an inflamed or obliterated anatomic plane.

ENDOSCOPIC UROLOGIC SURGERY

Urologists were early adopters of endoscopic surgery and began evaluating the urethra and bladder with cystoscopy in the early part of the twentieth century. The first diagnostic and therapeutic endoscopic procedures were performed for treatment of urologic disease processes. Endoscopic procedures are divided based on intervention or evaluation of the lower or upper urinary tract as each has specialized procedure-specific equipment.

Cystoscopy, or cystourethroscopy as it is formally called, is used for evaluation of the urethra and the bladder. Cystoscopic procedures are typically performed to evaluate the lower urinary tract in the setting of hematuria, voiding symptoms, recurrent infections, or bladder outlet obstruction; for surveillance in the setting of malignant neoplasms; and for removal of genitourinary foreign bodies and assessment of suspected trauma. Furthermore, cystoscopy can be used to perform diagnostic evaluation of the upper urinary tract with use of ureteral catheters and instillation of contrast material, which is visualized within the collecting system by fluoroscopy. Cystoscopy can be performed with both rigid and flexible endoscopes, each with certain benefits and advantages. Endoscopes are sized with the "French" (Fr) size system, which refers to the outer circumference of the instrument in millimeters. The rigid endoscope uses optical lens systems, similar to laparoscopes, and has excellent resolution. The inflexible structure is intuitive and easy to orient. Rigid cystoscopes have a range of sizes typically from 16 Fr to 26 Fr; surgical endoscopes, or resectoscopes, have the largest size of 24 Fr to 26 Fr.[8] Rigid endoscopes have a larger luminal diameter, which allows greater irrigation flow, improving visualization and passage of a number of working instruments. Rigid lower tract endoscopy is more difficult to perform in the awake patient, although it is much better tolerated in the female patient than in the male patient because of the short, straight urethra in the female patient. Flexible endoscopes are smaller, 15 Fr or 16 Fr, and better tolerated by patients for examination. Both male and female patients can be examined with local anesthesia, usually consisting of lidocaine jelly instilled per urethra. The flexible endoscope does not require any specific patient positioning and can be used supine and at the bedside. Finally, because of the large deflection radius, the bladder is easily evaluated without changing the lens or patient position. The optics of flexible endoscopes continue to improve by advancements in camera chip capability, with new digital platforms approaching the resolution of optical lens systems. Pediatric endoscopes are smaller, 8 Fr to 12 Fr, and are typically used in the operating room.

Upper tract evaluation is performed with either a ureteroscope or a nephroscope. The most common reason for either procedure is management of calculous disease, both ureteral and renal. Ureteroscopy can also be used to visualize and to inspect the upper collecting system, ureter, and renal pelvis; for hematuria originating from the upper urinary tract; for surveillance of urothelial carcinoma; and for treatment or biopsy of abnormal findings. Ureteroscopy is performed with both flexible and semirigid endoscopes, each with different benefits and purposes. Semirigid endoscopes are 6 Fr to 7.5 Fr at the tip and gradually enlarge to 8 Fr to 9.5 Fr.[8] The taper at the tip allows introduction into the ureteral orifice at the trigone of the bladder. These endoscopes have larger working channels that allow greater irrigation flow and a larger field of view. Because semirigid ureteroscopes are fairly inflexible, they are used to evaluate and to treat conditions below the level of iliac vessels and mid and distal ureter. Flexible ureteroscopes are 5.3 Fr to 8.5 Fr at the tip and gradually enlarge to 8.4 Fr to 10.1 Fr.[8] The major advantage of flexible ureteroscopes is the deflection of the tip, which ranges from 130 to 250 degrees in one direction and 160 to 275 degrees in the opposite direction, with newer endoscopes approaching 360-degree deflection. In addition, these endoscopes can be advanced through ureteral tortuosity and over external compression, such as the psoas muscle. The working channel on the flexible ureteroscope is typically smaller because of the fiberoptic system, and introduction of instruments, such as baskets or laser fibers, reduces irrigation flow. These flexible endoscopes can be used throughout the upper urinary tract but are particularly useful in the proximal ureter and renal pelvis and calyceal system.

The other method of upper tract endoscopy is through direct percutaneous access but puncture through the renal parenchyma into the renal collecting system. Percutaneous nephroscopy is most commonly used to treat large renal calculi. Management of upper tract urothelial tumors with fulguration and resection may also be performed via percutaneous nephroscopy. Nephroscopy may be performed with both rigid and flexible nephroscopes; however, most intervention is performed with the rigid system. The rigid nephroscope is placed through a percutaneous working access sheath, similar to a laparoscopic trocar, to visualize the stone or tumor. Rigid nephroscopes are usually 25 Fr to 28 Fr, and their appearance is similar to a rigid cystoscope, although they have a fixed lens system rather than an exchangeable lens. There is also growing enthusiasm for "mini-perc" approaches, which involve smaller caliber instrumentation. Newer rigid nephroscopes are built on a digital platform that allows a larger working channel with comparable optics to a standard endoscope. Various intracorporeal lithotripters are placed through the working channel to fragment large stones into manageable pieces. Flexible nephroscopes are essentially flexible cystoscopes that are dual purposed for evaluation of the kidney. Flexible endoscopy of the upper tract is advantageous because all areas of the upper collecting system (upper, mid, and lower pole calyces) can be inspected regardless of angle or direction of the internal infundibula. At times, combined use of retrograde flexible ureteroscopy and percutaneous nephroscopy, in the prone patient under anesthesia, may be necessary to address complex renal anatomy for stone-related and other indications.

Numerous working elements are used in both upper and lower tract endoscopy. Guidewires are commonly used to access the upper urinary tract collecting system or the bladder and serve as guides to pass catheters, stents, and sheaths. Most guidewires have a flexible tip and a more rigid shaft and are constructed of an inner core and an outer covering, which may be hydrophilic or neutral (polytetrafluoroethylene). Guidewires range in size from 0.018 to 0.038 inch and have various lengths. Urethral catheters and ureteral catheters may be placed over wires to assist with direct placement into the lower or upper urinary system, respectively. Ureteral stents are hollow catheters with flexible ends that form a coil on the proximal and distal ends to maintain position within the collecting systems. Stents are placed to ensure drainage of the kidney and to bypass blockages of the ureter from inflammation, stones, or tumors. Many stents are composed of thermodynamic material, which becomes softer at higher body temperatures. Stents range in size from 4.8 Fr to 10 Fr and have various lengths to accommodate variable ureteral lengths. Ureteroscopic baskets are used to remove ureteral and renal calculi and to perform extraction and biopsy of tumors. These range in size from 1.3 Fr to 3.2 Fr and are constructed of flexible material to allow placement into various calyceal locations within the kidney.

UROLOGIC INFECTIOUS DISEASE

Urinary tract infections (UTIs) are a common medical problem, although patients with UTI referred to urologists for evaluation and treatment often have a complicated or unusual element to their diagnosis or management. Other infections treated by urologists include infections of the genital skin (a spectrum of disease from skin neoplasms, to cellulitis, to necrotizing fasciitis) and reproduction organs in men (i.e., orchitis, epididymitis, or prostatitis). Furthermore, these infections may require simple antibiotic therapy, multimodal treatment with surgical drainage, or debridement and management in an intensive care setting. Urinary tract obstruction with proximal infection may result in sepsis, challenging the skills of the urologist and surgical critical care specialist.

Uncomplicated Urinary Tract Infection

Recent literature indicates that UTIs in adult women and men accounted for 39 million office visits and 6 million emergency department visits.[9] In adult patients, more than 50% of women and 12% of men will develop a UTI during their lifetime.[9] Urinary infection is considered "uncomplicated" when it occurs in the immunocompetent host, without underlying anatomic or physiologic abnormalities of the urinary tract in women. UTI diagnosed in men is generally considered "complicated". For diagnosis of a UTI, a clean catch, midstream urine specimen is preferred, and on culture, 10^5 colony-forming units must be demonstrated. In catheterized specimens, UTI can be diagnosed with as little as 10^3 colony-forming units. The typical symptoms associated with UTI are dysuria, frequency, urgency to void, and malodorous urine. Because of the inherent differences in etiology, evaluation, and treatment, uncomplicated UTIs are divided into those occurring in premenopausal and postmenopausal women. A third category of uncomplicated UTI, that occurring in pregnant patients, is beyond the scope of this overview. In general, risk factors include genetic, biologic, and behavioral; specific aspects are discussed with each group.

Premenopausal Patients

History and physical examination of patients in this age group presenting with symptoms of UTI are particularly important because of overlapping disease processes. In patients without vaginal discharge, the majority can be expected to have a UTI as the diagnosis. However, in sexually active women, sexually transmitted infections (STIs) must be considered, especially in the setting of a negative urine culture. Furthermore, in patients with vaginal discharge, vaginitis caused by yeast, trichomoniasis, and bacterial vaginosis are possible causes. Risk factors for UTI in this population of patients include frequent sexual intercourse, initial UTI at a young age, maternal history of UTI, and number of pregnancies and deliveries.[10] Important aspects of the physical examination in these patients include palpation of costovertebral tenderness (assessing for ascending infection) and pelvic examination to evaluate for STI. The most common cause of infection in these patients is *Escherichia coli* (80%–85%), followed by *Staphylococcus saprophyticus* (10%–15%) and *Klebsiella pneumoniae* and *Proteus mirabilis* (4% each).[10] Empirical therapy is acceptable, although confirmatory urine cultures are useful as the incidence of antibiotic resistance continues to rise. Prevention includes increased hydration and evaluation of hygiene practices.

Postmenopausal Patients

As in younger patients, history and physical examination are important aspects of UTI evaluation in this group of patients. Presenting symptoms are similar in this group, although some elderly patients may simply present with altered mental status. Furthermore, an important component in diagnosis and treatment of postmenopausal women is the change in the vaginal pH levels and change or reduction in lactobacillus in the vaginal flora. The physical examination findings may differ in these patients as STIs are less likely but physical changes, such as pelvic organ prolapse and incomplete bladder emptying, become causative factors. In addition, the pathologic bacterial species are different. *E. coli* continues to be the predominant organism but in this age group, *P. mirabilis, K. pneumoniae,* and *Enterobacter* species become more prevalent pathogens.[10] Again, empirical therapy is acceptable, but urine cultures are important because of increasing antibiotic resistance patterns and differing organisms. Prevention includes increased hydration and evaluation of hygiene practices.

Complicated Urinary Tract Infection

"Complicated" UTIs require more vigilance on the part of the treating physician because of patient factors that may lead to a more rapid progression or worsening of the infection. By definition complicated UTIs occur in men and in patients with diabetes, immunosuppression, upper tract infection, resistant organisms, urinary tract anatomic abnormalities, prior surgery, calculous disease, spinal cord injury, or recent or current indwelling Foley catheter. Essentially, any abnormality of physiology or anatomy which is etiologic in a UTI or a UTI that occurs in such a setting or in the immunocompromised patient is considered "complicated." In these patients, similar evaluation is warranted, but the evaluation should not be limited to simply history and physical examination. Empirical treatment of complicated UTI alone is not optimal, and urine cultures should be performed on all patients with suspected complicated UTI before initiation of antibiotic therapy, whenever possible. In addition, imaging is indicated in these patients because of concern for calculous disease and urinary stasis, so at a minimum, simple radiography of the kidneys, ureters, and bladder (a KUB study) and renal ultrasound, and potentially further assessment with cross-sectional radiographic imaging should be performed in patients with equivocal or concerning findings. Finally, antibiotic therapy alone may not be adequate, and these patients may require surgical drainage of obstructed urinary systems or later surgical correction of anatomic abnormalities or removal of urinary stones (once infections are treated) to prevent recurrent UTIs. Consultation with infectious disease specialists may also be indicated in patients with urologic anatomic abnormalities and recurrent UTIs with resistant organisms.

Urinary Tract Infection in Men

Because of the lower incidence of UTI in men, when men present with symptoms of infection, it is always considered complicated, regardless of other patient factors. As in women, younger men (younger than 50 years) and older men (older than 50 years) have different causes of their UTI and symptoms. Common presenting symptoms are urethritis, dysuria, hesitancy, frequency, and urgency of urination. A history and physical examination in these patients are important to delineate different sources of symptoms or UTI. Men can present with these symptoms and have different diagnoses, including UTI, STI, urethritis, and chronic pelvic pain. Furthermore, bacterial infections can extend to other proximal areas of the genitourinary system, such as the prostate and testicle. Men younger than 50 years are more likely to have STI as the cause rather than UTI. These men should have a thorough sexual history, genital examination, and microscopic urinalysis performed. Urethral swab or urine tests for STI should be performed as well. Men older than 50 years often have underlying lower urinary tract symptoms (LUTS), and this can be a contributing factor. Men in this age group more frequently will have UTI as a source of their symptoms, and common urinary pathogens, as in women, should be considered. Furthermore, older men should be questioned about recent surgical procedures, catheterization, or hospitalization. Elderly patients can also present with mental status or behavioral changes as their only symptom of UTI, and this diagnosis must be considered in these patients. A lower threshold for imaging and hospital admission is necessary in men with UTI as they may present with more systemic symptoms. Patients who cannot tolerate oral intake, are immunocompromised, or have medical comorbidities should be admitted with cross-sectional imaging performed. Broad-spectrum intravenous antibiotics, based on local resistance patterns, and fluid resuscitation should be initiated in these patients while the initial workup and evaluation are completed. Urinary obstruction or stone disease in these patients constitutes a urologic emergency and must be addressed rapidly.

Specific Complicated Genitourinary Infectious States

Pyelonephritis

Pyelonephritis is a spectrum of infectious or inflammatory processes that involve the kidney collecting system or parenchyma. Pyelonephritis results from a UTI moving proximally upward from the lower urinary tract. In the simple form, pyelonephritis may be treated on an outpatient basis with oral antibiotics for 1 to 2 weeks. In this group of patients, urine culture is necessary to identify the causative organism. If the patient appears more acutely infected, hospitalization may be warranted for broad-spectrum intravenous antibiotic therapy, fluid resuscitation, and cross-sectional imaging. *Emphysematous pyelonephritis* represents an advanced form of pyelonephritis and is considered a urologic emergency. Often occurring in the diabetic patient, these uncommon infections demonstrate a significant necrotizing infection of the kidney with gas-forming organisms (typically *E. coli* in a facultative anaerobic metabolic state) with pockets of gas within the parenchyma apparent on imaging (Fig. 74.1). The common bacterial pathogens include *E. coli, P. mirabilis,* and *K. pneumoniae.*[11] These patients require either prompt percutaneous drainage of the infection or

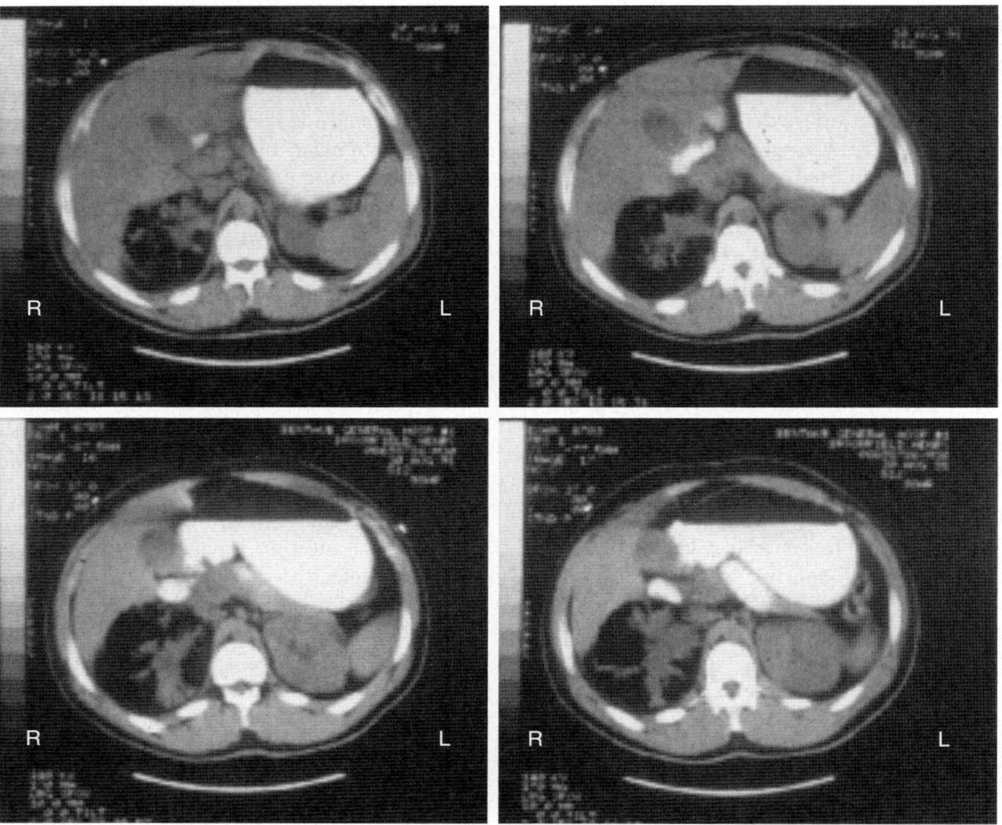

FIG. 74.1 Emphysematous pyelonephritis. This computed tomography (CT) scan demonstrates extensive destruction of the right kidney with intraparenchymal gas on the right, obliterating the renal architecture. The left kidney is normal.

rapid nephrectomy. Most patients who present with this condition are diabetic or have significant medical comorbidities, and control of the metabolic abnormalities, aggressive broad-spectrum antibiotic therapy, and supportive critical care are essential. *Xanthogranulomatous pyelonephritis* is a chronic infectious process resulting from renal obstruction, recurrent infection, and renal calculous disease. The disease presents in three forms, focal, segmental, or diffuse, and each is treated in a different manner. The underlying histologic process involves a foamy, lipid-laden, macrophage infiltrate in the renal parenchyma with extensive inflammation, fibrosis, and loss of renal function. On imaging, there may be indications of collecting system dilation; however, drainage attempts often are unproductive because the material is often solid or too viscous to drain. Patients with focal or segmental disease may be treated with antibiotics, but those with diffuse disease frequently require nephrectomy. The risk of iatrogenic adjacent organ injury is high in these nephrectomies, and the renal hilum may be so inflamed and fibrotic that the renal vessels cannot be individually dissected. These cases may require placement of a vascular pedicle clamp with renal excision and oversewing of the pedicle.

Male Genital Organ Infection

UTIs may ascend into the genital ducts, resulting in infection of the prostate, epididymis, or testicle. Beginning in the urethra, the verumontanum is the exit point of the seminal vesicles and vas deferens into the urinary tract. Prostatitis refers to any inflammatory process affecting the prostate, but the general surgeon more commonly may encounter acute bacterial prostatitis, which results from bacterial infiltration into the prostatic parenchyma. Most infections of the prostate are secondary to gram-negative bacterial infection and typically are associated with UTI. Two important considerations in these patients are physical examination and disease extent. Although a full history and physical examination are warranted, elimination of digital rectal examination (DRE) should be considered as pressure exerted on an infected prostate may lead to hematogenous spread of the bacteria. In addition, patients who do not have reasonably rapid resolution of their symptoms should be evaluated for prostatic abscess. Prostatic abscesses typically do not respond to antibiotic therapy and require transurethral unroofing to allow adequate drainage.

Epididymitis-orchitis results when the UTI ascends through the vas deferens into the epididymis or testicle. Again, the cause is different according to the patient's age; men younger than 35 years typically have an STI as a source, commonly *Chlamydia trachomatis,* whereas men older than 35 years will often have infections related to *E. coli.* Examination of these patients is often difficult because of significant swelling of the affected epididymis or testicle; scrotal ultrasound is useful diagnostically, especially to rule out associated abscess. When infection is advanced, the entire ipsilateral scrotal contents become involved, with overlying skin fixation and edema. It may be difficult to distinguish this entity from late torsion, incarcerated inguinal hernia, or testicular tumor with necrosis and inflammation. Patients without abscess may be managed with antibiotic therapy, rest, and scrotal elevation; however, recovery is slow, with eventual resolution of edema and discomfort. If abscess is present, surgical drainage and often orchiectomy are indicated. A subset of patients may have persistent pain or mass, and on repeated Doppler imaging, signs of testicular ischemia or persistent inflammation may be noted. These patients require exploration and possible orchiectomy to resolve the process.

Fournier Gangrene

Fournier gangrene is a necrotizing infection of the male genital and perineal skin and subcutaneous tissues, similar to other progressive fasciitis and necrotizing soft tissue infections (Fig. 74.2). When the genitalia are involved, patients typically present with

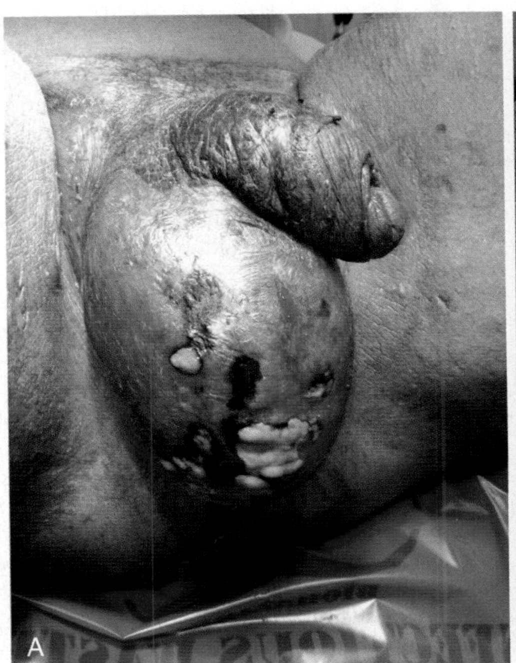

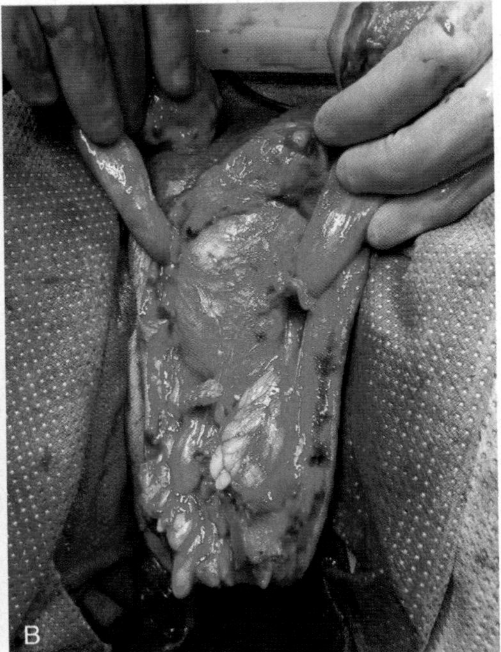

FIG. 74.2 Fournier gangrene. (A) Skin necrosis, purulence, and edema of the scrotum. The skin can also appear normal, with much more subtle physical findings in some cases. (B) Appearance after extensive debridement of scrotal skin and underlying tissues. The base of the penis is visible centrally; the testes are elevated out of the field, and the spermatic cords are visible anteriorly.

significant pain and tenderness, scrotal and genital swelling, discoloration or frank necrosis, crepitus, and, at times, foul-smelling discharge. Fournier gangrene is usually a polymicrobial infection with microaerobes, anaerobes, and gram-positive and gram-negative organisms.[12] Risk factors for development include peripheral vascular disease, diabetes mellitus, malnutrition, alcoholism, and other immunocompromised states. This disease represents a urologic emergency. Treatment requires urgent surgical drainage with aggressive debridement of the necrotic tissue, broad-spectrum intravenous antibiotics, and intensive monitoring with supportive care. The magnitude of the debridement depends entirely on the degree of progression of the process. It is rare for the process to involve the testicles or deep tissues of the penis deep to the tunica vaginalis and Buck fascia, respectively, so these structures should be preserved. It is uncommon for the urethra to be involved, although a defined urinary tract source may be evident, such as a urethral stricture, with perforation and local infection. Suprapubic tube diversion is generally not necessary initially; urethral catheter drainage is generally sufficient. Once the active infection is controlled, the predominant management issues become wound care and reconstruction, which may require delayed skin grafting for tissue coverage.

Atypical Urinary Tract Infections

Fungal Infection

Fungal infections in the urinary system are most common in specific populations of patients: diabetics, immunocompromised patients, and the elderly. Fungal infections may not be symptomatic and, in an outpatient setting, may not require therapy. Most fungal infections are related to the *Candida* species, and it is incumbent on the treating physician to determine which infections require treatment and which represent contamination. Patients who require careful evaluation and treatment include neutropenic patients and intensive care patients, who may need evaluation for an internal source such as a fungus deposit (ball) in the bladder or kidney. Infectious disease consultation is valuable in these cases because the organisms are atypical and selection of treatment agents may not be straightforward. Renal and bladder imaging with ultrasound may demonstrate a treatable source. These patients may need antifungal bladder or kidney irrigation or occasionally endoscopic removal.

Tuberculosis

The genitourinary tract is the third most common extrapulmonary site for tuberculosis infection. This disease is spread hematogenously from the lungs and into the affected organ system. Most patients with genitourinary tuberculosis are immunocompromised, so assessment of HIV infection status is important. Patients present with various symptoms that include voiding symptoms, sterile pyuria or hematuria, and chronic kidney disease. Not all patients will have a positive purified protein derivative (PPD) test result, and diagnosis is confirmed with acid-fast bacilli smears of urine and mycobacterial culture with sterile pyuria, chest radiograph, and imaging of the genitourinary system to look for anatomic abnormalities. Tuberculosis affecting the kidney may result in segmental or global glomerular dysfunction, and progression antegrade down the urinary system may result in ureteral strictures. Tuberculosis of the epididymis may result in chronic epididymitis or mass. Antibiotic therapy consists of two months of a four-drug regimen with a subsequent seven month treatment with isoniazid and rifampin. Infectious disease consultation is mandatory in treating these patients because of public health concerns. Significant anatomic infection or functional change or loss may ultimately require surgical excision.

Parasitic Infection

With the ease of global transportation and a mobile global population, parasitic infections are considerations in patients with recent travel histories. The main parasitic infections of the genitourinary system are schistosomiasis, echinococcal infection, and filariasis. Each parasite has a different point of entry, systemic spread, and organ infestation. Typically, in schistosomiasis, the parasite enters the body percutaneously and spreads through the venous and lymphatic system. Most infestations affect the bladder, resulting in chronic inflammation and granulomas. These patients present with LUTS or hematuria. Medical therapy (praziquantel) can be used to treat granulomatous disease; however, untreated infections can result in squamous cell carcinoma of the bladder. Echinococcal infections are spread through ingestion of contaminated food, and the parasite penetrates the intestinal walls and infests the liver. On occasion, renal infestation can occur, with the parasite becoming encysted in the parenchyma. Medical therapy can shrink the cysts, but surgical removal by partial or total nephrectomy is required for cure. These cysts must be removed intact as rupture or spillage of internal contents can result in severe anaphylaxis. Filariasis results from direct infection of the lymphatic system through percutaneous entry. The parasite creates noticeable symptoms when it dies, resulting in obstruction of the lymphatics. Only mild infestation can be treated with oral therapy (albendazole); advanced disease requires excision and reconstruction.

VOIDING DYSFUNCTION, NEUROGENIC BLADDER, INCONTINENCE, AND BENIGN PROSTATIC HYPERPLASIA

A central aspect of urology is management of bladder function and evaluation and treatment of bladder dysfunction. The bladder is a large muscular sac responsible for storing and eliminating urine. Common dysfunctions of the bladder include neurogenic problems with bladder function, storage problems, incontinence, and outflow issues related to benign prostatic hyperplasia (BPH) or enlargement. Changes in these functional areas are one of the most common reasons for urologic consultation. Although this is a broad area of urology, concentrating on these core divisions will give the general surgeon an understanding of the complex dynamics of bladder function and dysfunction.

Neurogenic Bladder

Patients with neurogenic bladder dysfunction present with a wide spectrum of neurologic diseases or injuries that affect bladder function on the basis of the location of the injury or disease process. There is a complex interaction between the bladder and brain that primarily regulates bladder storage and bladder emptying. Bladder storage is driven by the sympathetic nervous system, specifically at the level of the adrenergic receptor. α-Adrenergic receptors are the most common adrenergic receptors in the bladder, prostate, and urethra; most are α_1 and α_2, with three subtypes of α_1 identified: α_{1a}, α_{1b}, and α_{1d}.[13] The α_1 receptor is the most common subtype in the lower urinary system. Bladder emptying is driven by the parasympathetic stimulation of cholinergic receptors, specifically the muscarinic receptors. The predominant muscarinic receptors in the bladder are M_2 and M_3.[13] Sensory information is carried away from the bladder by myelinated and unmyelinated afferent nerve fibers traveling through the pelvic and pudendal nerves. Any interruption in the sympathetic or parasympathetic nervous system and its communication with the bladder can result in neurogenic dysfunction. In addition, several centers within the pons, midbrain, and cerebral cortex have direct effect on the storage and emptying of the bladder.[13] Voiding is initiated at the level of the pontine micturition center, which sends out a parasympathetic signal to the bladder to initiate voiding. The pontine micturition center is inhibited by the periaqueductal gray located in the midbrain, and this is connected to the afferent signaling pathways from the bladder. Based on this standard sensory function, specific voiding symptoms or LUTS can be predicted by the location of neurologic disease or injury.

Basic evaluation of these patients includes a through history with neurologic and urologic historical focus, physical examination (focusing on the abdomen, pelvis, and peripheral and central nervous system), and urinalysis. Additional evaluation is tailored to location of injury. Cortical brain disease and injury, such as cerebrovascular accident, are evaluated by history, physical examination, and urinalysis. These disease processes do not directly affect the bladder function, and patients are treated on the basis of symptoms alone. Spinal cord lesions are divided into suprasacral spinal lesions (spinal cord injury, infarcts) and sacral or peripheral spinal cord lesions (pelvic plexus damage from surgery, diabetic neuropathy). Patients with lesions of the suprasacral spinal cord tend to have increased bladder muscle tension, which results in abnormal elasticity of the bladder (poor bladder compliance).[14] In addition, these patients have incoordination of the bladder and urinary sphincter, resulting in detrusor-sphincter dyssynergia. Patients with sacral or peripheral nerve lesions tend to have variable LUTS but typically do not have changes in bladder elasticity.[14] The detrusor muscle is often partially or completely nonfunctional, and the urinary sphincter remains closed. Specialized evaluation of the patients with spinal cord lesions includes upper tract ultrasonography to monitor for evidence of hydronephrosis and urodynamic evaluation. Urodynamic evaluation involves measuring the elasticity of the bladder on filling (compliance), the pressure generated on emptying (detrusor function) by recording the abdominal pressure, and the intraluminal bladder pressure with specialized catheters. Surveillance cystoscopy is indicated in chronic patients to rule out the development of intravesical disease. Treatment for neurogenic bladder has recently been revolutionized by the introduction of onabotulinum toxin. In the past, these patients required complex regimens of antimuscarinic agents and reconstructive surgery. Now, with the use of onabotulinum toxin, most patients are treated with periodic cystoscopic injections and intermittent catheterization.

Problems With Bladder Storage Symptoms and Abnormalities

Overactive bladder (OAB) is the most common storage-related problem of the bladder. It is defined as urinary urgency with or without urgency urinary incontinence in the absence of UTI or other obvious disease.[15] Typical symptoms of this problem include urgency, urinary frequency, nocturia, and urgency urinary incontinence. Urgency refers to the sudden, compelling desire to pass urine that is difficult to defer and replaces the normal urge.[15] Urinary frequency is the complaint of micturition occurring more frequently than previously deemed normal and characterized by daytime and nocturnal voids.[15] Nocturia is the complaint of interruption of sleep one or more times because of the need to urinate.[15] Finally, urgency urinary incontinence is the involuntary loss of urine associated with urgency.[15] A difficult aspect of this disease process is that it occurs in the spectrum of other LUTS and may be the result of long-term bladder outflow obstruction. Other conditions to consider in patients who present with OAB and LUTS are UTI, urinary calculi, diabetes, polydipsia, neurogenic bladder, and malignant disease. OAB has a worldwide prevalence of 11%, and with the aging population, this is presumed to increase over time.[16]

All patients who present with OAB should undergo a thorough evaluation. At the basic level, this includes a thorough history to fully disclose the symptoms and to rule out other causes. Historical elements that may be contributory include caffeine intake, constipation, recurrent UTI, pelvic organ prolapse in women and prostatic enlargement in men, and excessive fluid intake. Physical examination should be directed toward evaluation of the abdomen, pelvis, and neurologic systems. Other findings may include decreased mental status or cognitive function and peripheral edema. The last absolute examination element is urinalysis, which can reveal infection, inflammation, or hematuria that may indicate more serious disease. Simple adjunctive tests that can be performed in the office include measurement of postvoid residual urine volume, noninvasive flow test, validated symptom questionnaires, and voiding diaries. Specialized tests and evaluation performed by the urologist may include cystoscopy, ultrasound, and urodynamic testing as appropriate. However, current guidelines do not require any of these specialized tests for initiation of treatment.[17]

Treatment of OAB is directed toward therapy, symptoms, and motivation of the individual patient (Fig. 74.3). As many patients suffering from this problem take multiple medications, pharmacologic therapy is not always offered as an initial treatment. Behavioral therapies are the first-line treatment for all patients. Behavioral therapies may include lifestyle modifications or specific physical therapies. Typically, this includes fluid intake management and modification with particular attention paid to timing of fluid intake and amounts. For example, in patients who complain of nocturia, limiting nighttime fluid intake can be beneficial. Bladder training is a noninvasive method of physical therapy whereby the patient postpones voiding to lengthen the time intervals between voids. This may be coupled with urgency suppression and timed voids to reinforce retraining of the sensory output from the bladder. Finally, voiding diaries are important to help the patient and urologist quantify the number of voids and voided amount to better target improvement goals and to tailor therapy. Pharmacologic management continues to be a mainstay of treatment and is indicated for patients as an adjunct to behavior therapies or for patients unresponsive to first-line therapy. Classic pharmacologic therapy is antimuscarinic agents that target the parasympathetic muscarinic cholinergic receptors, primarily M_2 and M_3, and block the action of these receptors. Most of the drugs in this category are administered daily and have the common side effects of dry mouth, dry eyes, and constipation. A newer pharmacologic agent, beta agonists (β_3), targets receptors in the detrusor muscle to stimulate bladder relaxation. Treatment options for patients who fail to respond to these therapies fall into the specialized third-line treatments, which include neuromodulation (either peripheral or central), onabotulinum toxin, chronic indwelling catheters, and augmentation cystoplasty.

Urinary Incontinence

Urinary incontinence is the involuntary loss of urine; it can be divided into stress urinary incontinence, urge urinary incontinence, and mixed urinary incontinence.[15] "Overflow incontinence" is

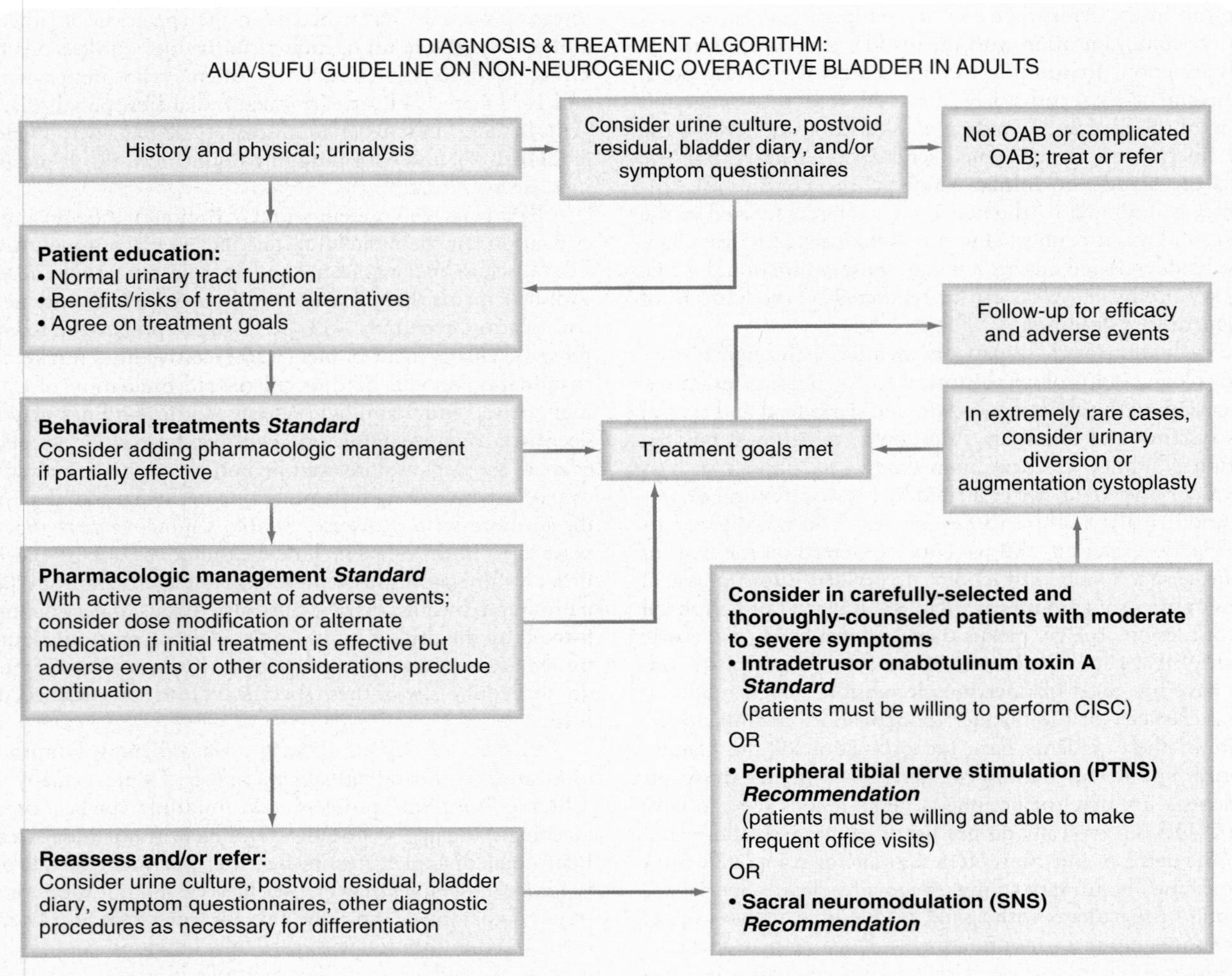

FIG. 74.3 Algorithm for diagnosis and management of overactive bladder (OAB). (Adapted from Gormley EA, Lightner DJ, Burgio KL, et al. Diagnosis and treatment of overactive bladder [non-neurogenic] in adults: AUA/SUFU guideline. *J Urol.* 2012;188:2455–2463.)

another form of incontinence, which is often considered as an etiologically separate entity. National data indicate that the prevalence of urinary incontinence in America is 49.6% in women older than 20 years.[18] Men are typically affected after the age of 50 years, and incontinence develops as a symptom of LUTS or other problems rather than as a primary complaint as in women. Stress urinary incontinence is defined as the involuntary loss of urine with Valsalva maneuver.[15] Urge urinary incontinence is the involuntary loss of urine associated with a strong urge to void.[15] Mixed urinary incontinence is any combination of these two causes.

Evaluation of these patients includes history, physical examination (including pelvic examination), urinalysis, postvoid residual volume measurement, and voiding diaries. The history and physical examination are important to rule out any complicating factors including neurogenic source, anatomic changes (pelvic organ prolapse in the female patient and prostatic enlargement in the male patient), and prior surgical intervention (radical prostatectomy in the male patient or hysterectomy in the female patient) that might affect evaluation and the treatment decision. In the neurologically normal patient with no confounding factors, nonsurgical management is the first step in treatment before any surgical intervention. As with OAB, behavior modification and bladder training are the initial steps. Dietary modification is important for management of urinary incontinence. Patients are counseled to limit fluid intake to around 2 L/day, depending on body size and activity level. In addition, patients should limit caffeine intake and other bladder irritants including alcohol, carbonated beverages, spicy foods, and citrus juices and fruits. Furthermore, bowel programs should be initiated to ensure that the patient has normal bowel function and is not constipated. Other nonsurgical treatment includes weight loss to a normal body mass index and exercise, particularly core muscle exercises. Pelvic floor muscle training and biofeedback have been shown to have acceptable rates in helping patients achieve satisfactory management of their urinary incontinence.

Surgical treatment options for women and men differ because of the inherent mechanism causing the incontinence, typically poor pelvic anatomic support in women and sphincteric in men. In women, treatment options progress from less to more invasive. The simplest treatment is injection of a urethral bulking agent through a cystoscopy. The objective of this treatment is to improve coaptation of the urinary sphincter and to increase the urethral wall volume. Unfortunately, this treatment is not likely to produce long-term cure, and retreatment or progression to other options is often necessary. The next option is placement of a midurethral sling to resupport the central hammock of the urethra and to provide backing to the urethra during stress maneuvers.

These approaches have a higher success rate, and long-term data show cure rates of approximately 90%.[19] With the success and ease of the midurethral sling, fewer open retropubic suspensions are performed. These procedures also work to improve the support of the urethra and to reduce urethral hypermobility. In men, surgical therapy is designed to reinforce the urinary sphincter to increase bladder outlet resistance. Typically, treatments are divided into male urethral slings, which have a larger surface area for the mesh suspension material, and artificial urinary sphincter devices. An artificial urinary sphincter (AUS) is a complex device that is implanted in the patient and opened through a one-way valve contained in the scrotum.

Benign Prostatic Hyperplasia

BPH is the development of nodules within the prostate gland as a result of enlargement of the stromal and epithelial components of the gland.[20] As the BPH progresses, the entire prostate enlarges in a process called benign prostatic enlargement, resulting in compression of the prostatic urethra and development of bladder outflow obstruction (Fig. 74.4).[20] As part of the bladder outflow obstruction, patients can develop LUTS requiring evaluation and treatment by a urologist. BPH is prevalent, affecting approximately 70% of men between the ages of 60 and 69 years, making it one of the most common conditions treated by urologists.[20] The LUTS that result from BPH can be divided into storage, voiding, and postvoid symptoms. Interestingly, there is little correlation between the measured volume of the prostate and the symptoms that result. In addition, the degree of bladder outflow obstruction does not necessarily correlate with the severity of LUTS.

As with all conditions, evaluation of the patients is centered on the history and physical examination. Key elements of the physical examination include DRE and a focused neurologic examination. Laboratory evaluation includes urinalysis and prostate-specific antigen (PSA) testing in appropriate patients with a life expectancy of more than 10 years – although the use of PSA testing remains controversial. Further evaluation of these patients includes the use of disease-specific validated questionnaires (International Prostate Symptom Score), measurement of postvoid residual urine volumes, and noninvasive urinary flow testing.[20] Depending on initial evaluation findings, cystoscopy and urodynamic studies may be appropriate adjunct tests. Practice guidelines for BPH have been produced by the American Urological Association (AUA) to guide providers in the diagnosis and management of BPH (Figs. 74.5 and 74.6).[20] Similar to all voiding-related conditions, behavior and dietary modifications are appropriate first-step treatment measures in all patients. Medical therapy can be used in conjunction with the initial behavior modifications or added subsequently.

The mainstay of treatment for LUTS due to BPH is α_1-adrenergic receptor blockers.[20] As previously discussed, α-adrenergic receptors are the most common adrenergic receptors in the bladder, and α_1 is the most common subtype in the lower urinary system, prostate, and urethra. The action of α_1 blockers is to relax the smooth muscle in the bladder neck and prostate and to reduce outflow resistance. This class of drugs has become progressively more selective to the α_1 subtypes, and many now target the α_{1a} subtype receptor specifically. The most common side effects of these drugs are dizziness related to orthostasis, retrograde ejaculation, and rhinitis. A second category of pharmacologic therapy is the 5α-reductase inhibitors that target the glandular component of the prostate. These drugs block the conversion of testosterone to dihydrotestosterone in the prostate and subsequently reduce the prostate volume, thereby reducing outflow resistance. This class of drugs also alters the serum PSA level (reduces it about 50%), which must be kept in mind with regard to prostate cancer screening. In addition, these drugs can be used in combination because of their differing mechanism of action, and studies show superior results to either drug used independently.

When medical therapy is ineffective, symptoms remain bothersome, or an objective surgical indication arises (e.g., acute urinary retention, bladder calculi, azotemia, recurrent UTI, or recurrent hematuria), surgical intervention is considered. The standard approach to surgical treatment of BPH is transurethral resection of the prostate (TURP) using various electrosurgical options (monopolar, bipolar, or laser). Minimally invasive treatment options, such as microwave thermotherapy and radiofrequency ablation, can be performed in an office setting but do not have equivalent long term outcomes compared to standard surgical procedures. When the adenomatous growth is particularly large, open simple prostatectomy is performed to enucleate the adenoma surgically. Outcomes of the transurethral procedures show dramatic

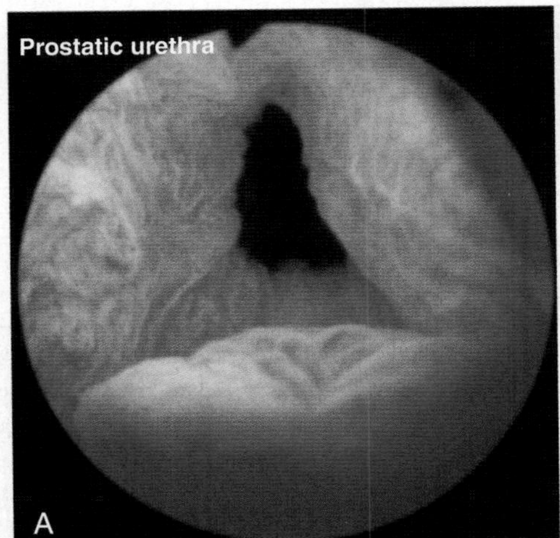

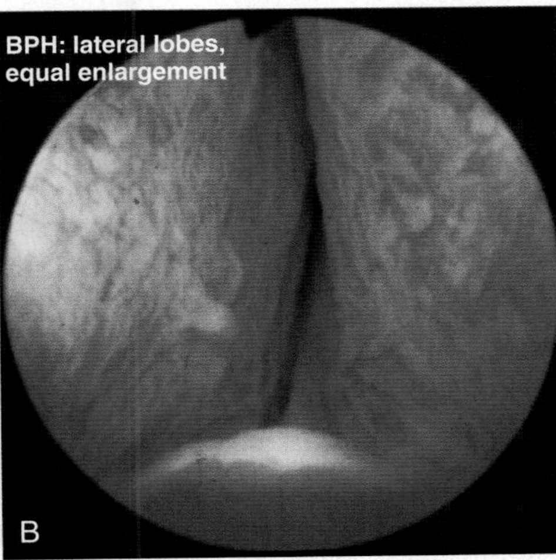

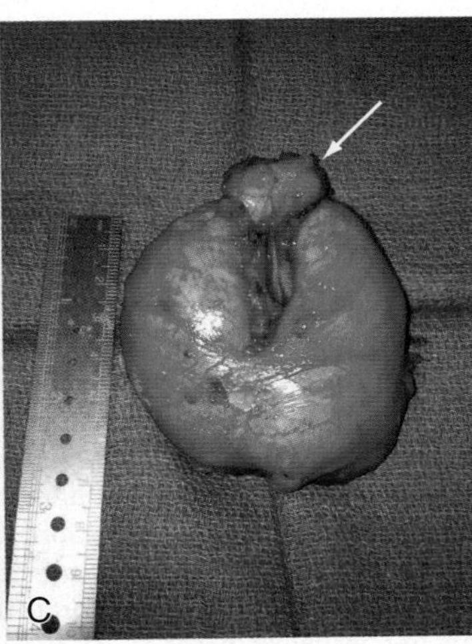

FIG. 74.4 Benign prostatic hyperplasia *(BPH)*. (A) Normal cystoscopic appearance of the prostate in a young man. (B) Moderate BPH, viewed cystoscopically. The size of the prostate correlates poorly with the magnitude of voiding symptoms. (C) Prostatic adenoma after simple open prostatectomy. Note the small medial lobe *(arrow, top center)*, with large lateral lobes (130-g specimen).

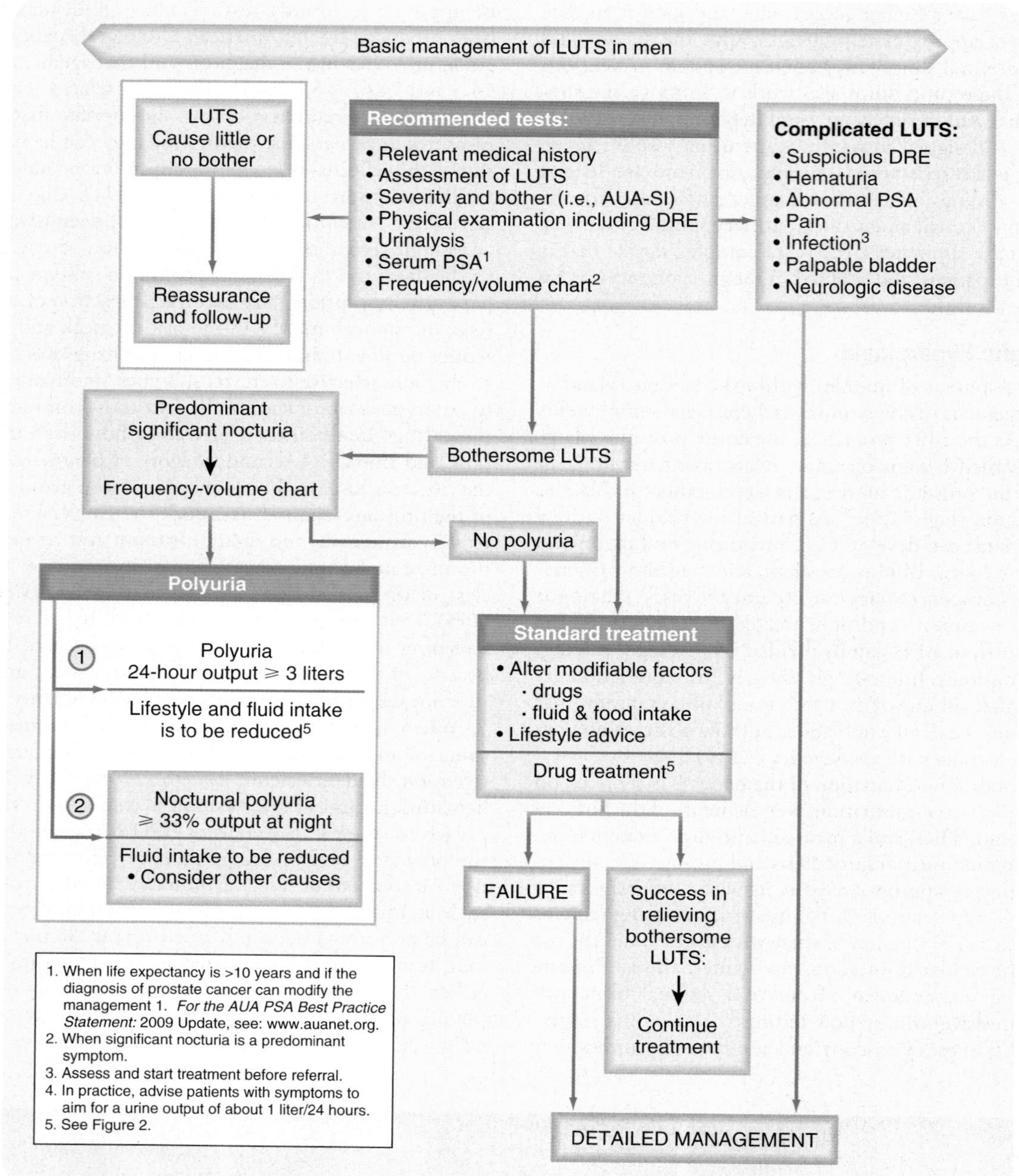

FIG. 74.5 Algorithm for initial diagnosis and management of benign prostatic hyperplasia. (Adapted from McVary KT, Roehrborn CG, Avins AL, et al. Update on AUA guideline on the management of benign prostatic hyperplasia. *J Urol.* 2011;185:1793–1803.)

improvement in International Prostate Symptom Score numbers, urinary flow rates, and postvoid residual volumes. Procedures such as simple prostatectomy have such a long historical use that objective data have not been measured or compiled, but outcomes are similar to those of TURP. Complications of TURP procedures include persistent bleeding, dilutional hyponatremia from fluid absorption of the glycine irrigation, UTI, urinary incontinence, and urethral stricture. With newer electrosurgical systems (bipolar and laser), normal saline irrigation is used and dilutional hyponatremia has been eliminated. In addition, visualization is improved, with a significant reduction in bleeding complications and a lower incidence of urinary incontinence.

MALE REPRODUCTIVE MEDICINE AND SEXUAL DYSFUNCTION

Male infertility and sexual dysfunction are a specialized area of urologic practice. Diagnostic evaluation, medical treatment, and surgical therapy of male infertility represent sophisticated aspects of urologic care. Male sexual dysfunction is becoming more prominent as the field of men's health continues to evolve. Many patients seen and evaluated by general surgeons may be receiving specific medical therapy or have undergone prosthetic surgical implants for sexual dysfunction management. A basic familiarity with these specialized areas is beneficial to general surgeons in their surgical practice.

Male Reproductive and Sexual Dysfunction: Evaluation and Treatment

Infertility affects approximately 8% to 14% of couples; the male factor is the primary or sole factor in 36% to 75% of these cases.[21] Couples are often referred to the urologist after a period of infertility, and referrals are generally from a primary care physician or from the evaluating gynecologic reproductive endocrinologist. Infertility is defined as a couple's inability to achieve pregnancy after one year of unprotected intercourse.[21]

The standard male factor evaluation involves a detailed history, physical examination, and basic laboratory and imaging evaluation. The AUA has produced a series of best practice statements on the evaluation of the infertile man with the following objectives: to recognize and to treat reversible conditions, to categorize disorders potentially amenable to assisted reproductive techniques, to identify syndromes and conditions that may be detrimental to the patient's health, and to distinguish genetic abnormalities that can be transmitted to or affect the health of offspring.[22]

The causes of infertility can be divided into anatomic, behavioral and environmental, and iatrogenic. Anatomic causes of male infertility are either congenital or acquired.[21] The most significant anatomic cause is congenital absence of the vas deferens, which is a partial or complete agenesis of the vas deferens. Although uncommon, the finding is associated with a cystic fibrosis transmembrane conductance regulator *(CFTR)* gene mutation, making these patients carriers for cystic fibrosis.[22] Other anatomic findings include cryptorchidism, ejaculatory duct obstruction (at the level of the prostate), and varicocele (Fig. 74.7). Behavioral and environmental sources of infertility are more common and easier to reverse than anatomic causes of male infertility. These include obesity, environmental exposures, substance abuse (including exogenous testosterone), and vitamin deficiency. Finally, iatrogenic causes to be considered include prior chemotherapy or radiation therapy, prior inguinal or genital surgery, and current medical treatments. Surgeons must be aware of iatrogenic causes of infertility in groin and pelvic surgical procedures from damage to the spermatic cord vasculature, vas deferens, and ejaculatory duct region or vasal entrapment from mesh used for inguinal hernia repair. The blood supply to the vas deferens or testicle is vulnerable to injury when the groin is explored in reoperative surgery or when the anatomy is obscured because of inguinal trauma as identification of these structures is challenging.

The history should include a discussion of sexual and reproductive history. This includes potential gonadotoxic exposure; urologic infections and STIs; trauma and prior surgery involving the pelvis, groin, and genitalia; and family history of infertility. Physical assessment should include a general evaluation of masculinization and genital findings, including normal meatal location, testicular size and consistency, presence and normalcy of the epididymis and vas deferens, and possible presence of a varicocele. Perineal and rectal examinations are routine parts of this assessment.

Basic Laboratory Assessment

Laboratory evaluation of these patients includes two semen analyses and serum hormone studies. The semen analyses should be separated by one month and preceded by 2 to 3 days of abstinence. Semen analysis parameters of importance include semen volume, pH, sperm concentration and total count, total motility, progressive motility, quality of sperm movement, morphology, and presence of red and white blood cells or bacteria.[21] The World Health Organization (WHO) has defined parameters of normal for routine semen analyses.[21] Semen analysis abnormalities fall into two main categories: azoospermia—the complete absence of sperm from the semen; and abnormal semen parameters—reduced concentration, motility, or morphology and abnormal function. Azoospermia can roughly be divided into three categories: pretesticular, testicular, and posttesticular. Pretesticular azoospermia results from endocrine causes, such as hypogonadotropic hypogonadism, or congenital causes. Testicular causes are the result of primary testicular failure of germinal epithelium of the testis to produce mature sperm. This is often accompanied by normal semen volume and by a markedly elevated serum follicle-stimulating hormone (FSH) level. Posttesticular causes, such as ejaculatory dysfunction and obstruction, account for 40% of cases of azoospermia.[22] Abnormal semen parameters may be indicative of a wide range of disorders that may cause reduced sperm numbers, motility, or morphology, including varicocele, antisperm antibodies, genital duct infection with pyospermia, and prior or current gonadotoxic exposure. Reduced semen volume may be artifactual, indicating incomplete ejaculation or specimen collection, or it may represent true disease, including, for example, congenital absence of the seminal vesicle, ejaculatory duct obstruction, or retrograde ejaculation caused by diabetes, neurologic injury, or prior bladder neck surgery or medications.

Serum hormone testing includes determination of levels of FSH, luteinizing hormone, testosterone, free testosterone, and prolactin. Hypogonadotropic hypogonadism may be diagnosed on the basis of serum hormone studies or elevation in the FSH level. A patient with a low testosterone level should have follow-up prolactin levels measured to rule out a prolactinoma of the pituitary gland.

Ultrasound of the scrotum is useful to measure testicular volume and symmetry, to exclude the possibility of testicular neoplasm, to identify epididymal anatomy, and to define or to confirm the presence of a varicocele, which is an abnormal dilation of the pampiniform venous plexus of the internal spermatic venous system (Fig. 74.7). Transrectal ultrasound (TRUS) of the prostate may provide evidence of ejaculatory duct obstruction with seminal vesicle dilation or congenital absence of the seminal vesicle, which may accompany congenital absence of the vas deferens.

Treatment

Treatment of male infertility depends on the identified cause and on the availability and affordability of assisted reproductive technology support options for specific or empirical treatment of failure to conceive. Medical therapy is used to treat hormone deficiencies, hormone excess, thyroid hormone excess, and prolactin excess. The most common medical therapies include hormonal stimulation of spermatogenesis, such as gonadotropin agents and antiestrogen agents, which have been met with mixed results. Antiinflammatory or antibiotic therapy can be used in patients with findings of pyospermia or concern for genital duct infection. Surgical therapies may include microsurgical reconstruction for vasal or epididymal occlusion (including vasectomy reversal), transurethral resection of the ejaculatory duct for obstructive lesions, and varicocele repair.

Male Sexual Dysfunction and Treatment

Sexual dysfunction in men refers to a range of disorders, including erectile dysfunction (ED), diminished libido, hypogonadism, and ejaculatory dysfunction. Because of the numerous organ system interactions, patients with these conditions may have associated neuropathy, endocrinopathy, vasculopathy, and psychological disorders, and these abnormalities may affect nonurologic patient management and surgery.

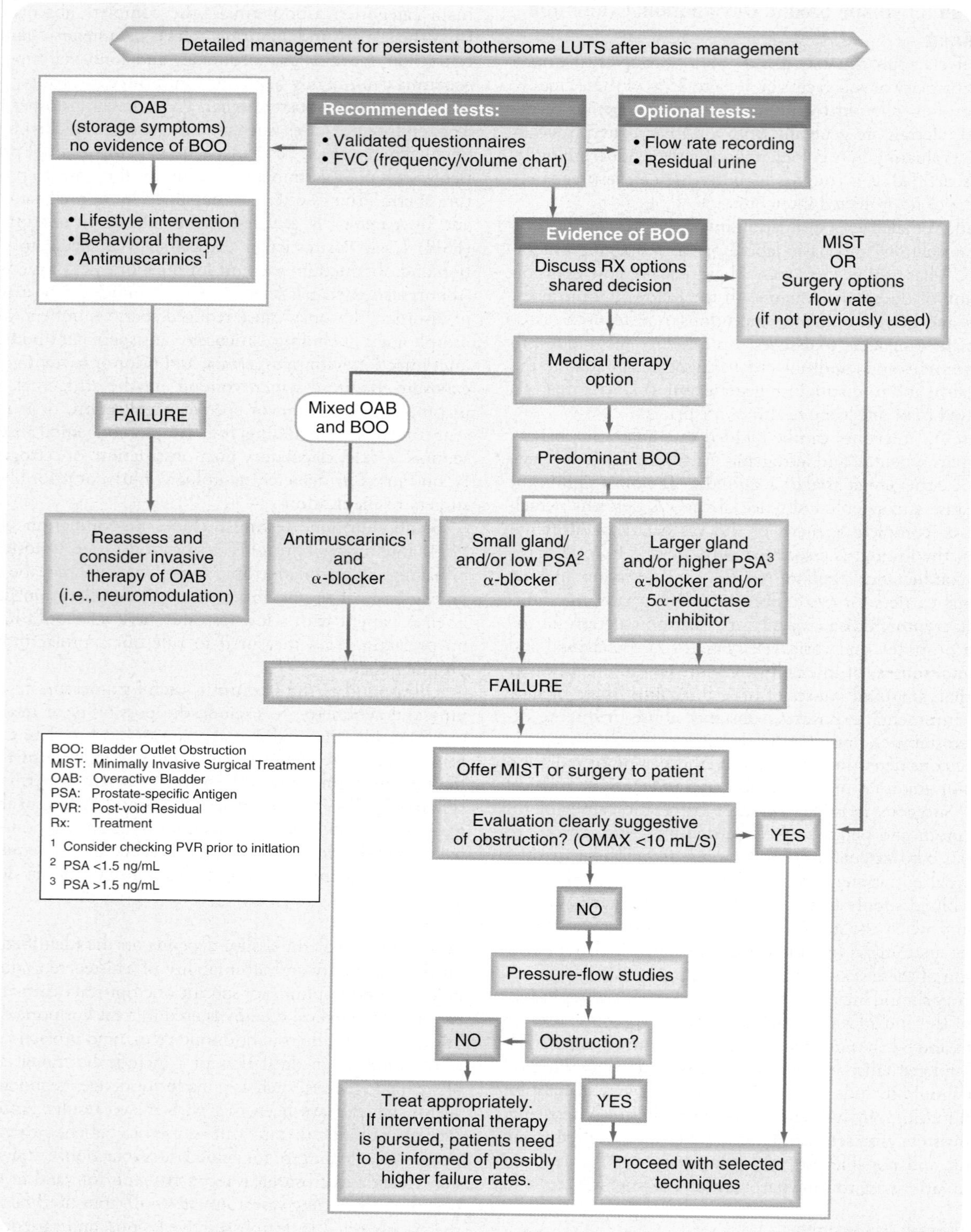

FIG. 74.6 Algorithm for secondary management of benign prostatic hyperplasia. (Adapted from McVary KT, Roehrborn CG, Avins AL, et al. Update on AUA guideline on the management of benign prostatic hyperplasia. *J Urol.* 2011;185:1793–1803.)

Normal erectile function is a complex interaction between the nervous and vascular systems, with unique molecular actions occurring in penile vascular structures. Many medical comorbidities and lifestyle choices can contribute to ED, including age, coronary artery disease, smoking, hypertension, dyslipidemia, atherosclerosis, peripheral vascular disease, obesity, diabetes, spinal cord injury and degenerative neurologic conditions, treatment of pelvic malignant neoplasms, and chronic kidney disease.[23] The causes of ED can be divided into neurologic, vascular, metabolic, medication induced, endocrine, and psychological; importantly, it can be an early marker for coronary artery disease.[23] The initial evaluation of the ED patient centers on the history and physical

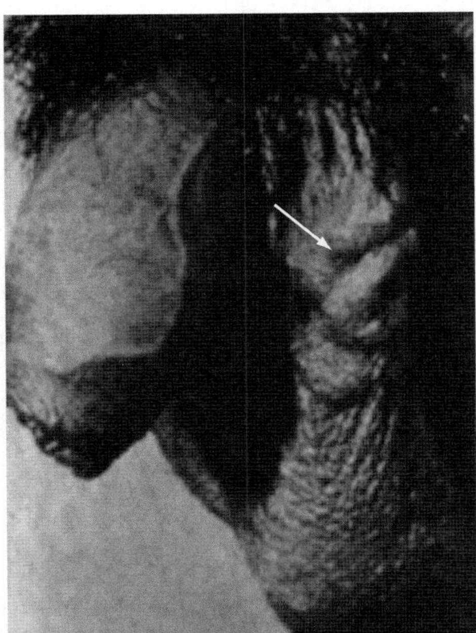

FIG. 74.7 Varicocele. The bag of worms appearance is visible and palpable through the scrotal skin, representing the dilated branches of the internal spermatic venous system.

examination. The history is focused on sexual performance and erectile function; the nonsexual historical aspects center on possible medical and surgical conditions. Social aspects, such as smoking, recreational drug use, and diet, are also important considerations. Validated questionnaires provide objective historical data both for initial treatment and for evaluation of therapy outcomes. The physical examination centers on the genitalia and evaluation of male secondary sexual characteristics. Basic laboratory studies in these patients include morning total testosterone concentration, fasting lipid levels, and hemoglobin A1c level. Important consideration should be given to assessment of cardiovascular function in younger patients because this disease process is considered an early marker for cardiovascular disease, especially in younger patients. Further evaluation is specialized but may include neurologic testing (e.g., biothesiometry) and vascular testing (e.g., penile duplex Doppler ultrasound studies).

Most treatments of ED are based on restoring penile arterial blood flow to achieve or to maintain a satisfactory erection. Lifestyle modifications are an important component of this, and dietary changes and increased regular cardiovascular exercise have been shown to independently improve erectile function. Evaluation and adjustment of offending medications should be considered as well. The basis of medical therapy for ED is phosphodiesterase type 5 inhibitors. These medications improve penile blood flow by limiting the breakdown of cyclic guanosine monophosphate and potentiating penile blood flow. These drugs should be limited in their use in men with known cardiovascular disease, especially those taking oral nitrates. Other forms of nonsurgical treatment include vacuum erection devices, intraurethral suppository therapy with prostaglandin compounds, intracavernosal self-injection, and occasionally psychotherapy. Surgery for ED includes primarily placement of a penile prosthesis and limited vascular reconstruction. Penile implant surgery may involve malleable implants, which have a flexible wire core inside a silicone sleeve, implanted bilaterally in the corpora, or, more commonly, inflatable penile implants. These are fluid-containing, completely

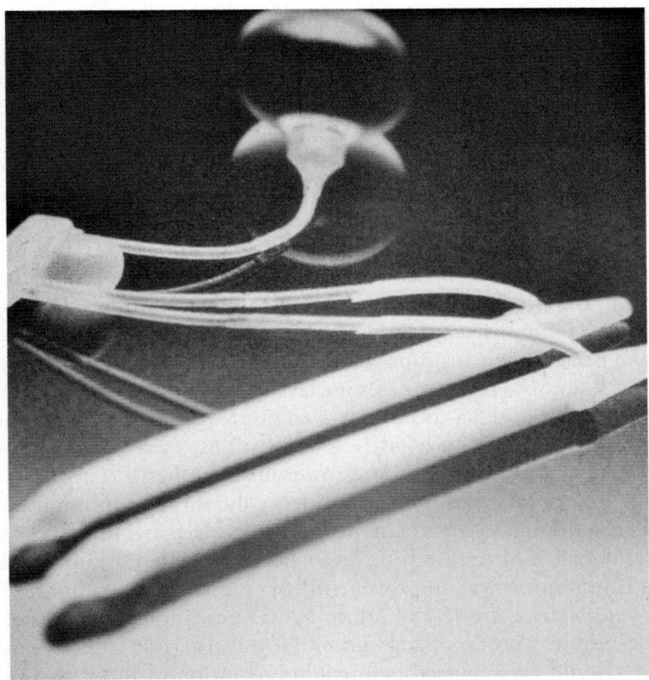

FIG. 74.8 Inflatable penile prosthesis. A three-component device is shown. The reservoir *(top)* is placed retropubically in an extraperitoneal position. The paired cylinders *(right)* are placed within the corpora cavernosa. The pump *(left)* is placed in the scrotum, adjacent to the testes.

internalized systems that may include paired corporal cylinders, a scrotal pumping device, and a fluid reservoir, which is typically positioned in the retropubic space or extraperitoneal lower abdominal quadrant (Fig. 74.8). The general surgeon should be aware that intraperitoneal positioning may also occur, intentionally or through erosion through the peritoneal membrane, and the reservoir or system tubing may be encountered during nonurologic abdominopelvic surgery. Care should be taken not to contaminate any of the implant components or inadvertently injure the tubing or device components. If it is known that an implant is in place and pelvic or inguinal surgery is planned, urologic consultation may be helpful in handling any issues that arise with the implant. Revascularization of the penis to restore erectile function, following arteriography for anatomic documentation, is usually achieved using an inferior epigastric artery pedicle flap, whereby new arterial inflow is brought to the corpora cavernosa. This has limited indications, most relevant in younger patients with traumatic injury to the pelvic blood supply, and national practice guidelines consider this to be controversial.

The other area of male sexual medicine affecting a significant number of patients is testosterone deficiency or hypogonadism. Serum testosterone is produced in the Leydig cells of the testes (90%) and adrenal glands (10%). Testicular synthesis of testosterone is controlled by the hypothalamus and anterior pituitary. This is a condition in which serum testosterone levels decline and are associated with symptoms of fatigue, lack of energy, depressed mood, irritability, reduced motivation, decreased cognitive acuity, decreased strength and stamina, reduced muscle mass and increased fat, and sexual side effects including decreased libido and ED. There is a normal age-related decline in testosterone as men age, and total testosterone declines by 1%, on average, each year after the age of 40 years. The prevalence of this condition is between 2.1% and 39% of men older than 40 years, depending on the criteria used and association of symptoms.[24] The patient's history should elicit information on the specific symptoms of testosterone deficiency, and physical examination is similar to that for ED with evaluation of the genitalia and secondary sexual characteristics. Validated questionnaires are useful to assess and to monitor therapy. Laboratory studies should include free and total morning testosterone, luteinizing hormone, prolactin, hematocrit, and hemoglobin levels.[25] Therapy for testosterone deficiency is based on lifestyle modifications and testosterone supplementation.[25] Many men who suffer from this condition are either obese or have metabolic syndrome. Dietary changes to improve nutritional status and to result in weight loss have been shown to improve not only baseline medical conditions but also serum testosterone levels. Furthermore, moderate-intensity exercise has been shown to improve serum testosterone levels. In addition to lifestyle modifications, many patients are treated with supplemental testosterone. Synthetic testosterone may be administered orally, transdermally, through intramuscular injections, and by subcutaneous pellets. The goal of therapy is maintenance of testosterone levels between 400 and 700 ng/dL and resolution or improvement of presenting symptoms.[25] Whereas there are few absolute contraindications to testosterone administration, many potential adverse side effects exist and should be discussed before administration of these medications as this is the area of greatest controversy with testosterone supplementation. Potential adverse effects include cardiovascular events and mortality, dermatologic changes, polycythemia, diminished spermatogenesis, gynecomastia, LUTS, prostate cancer, and sleep apnea.[25]

UROLITHIASIS

Urinary tract stones are a common cause of visits to the emergency department. The prevalence of renal calculous disease in the United States is increasing, with a lifetime risk of forming a renal stone at 5% in 1994 and 9% in 2010.[26] The incidence of stone disease peaks in the fourth to sixth decades of life and is more common in men than in women by a 2:1 margin.[26] Renal calculous disease has several aspects of management and evaluation, including acute stone presentation, metabolic evaluation, and medical and surgical therapy. As most general surgeons will encounter patients either in the acute presentation or around the time of surgical intervention, this section focuses on these areas.

Background

The pathogenesis of calculus formation is governed by the physical chemistry characteristics of the urine in the upper collecting system. Most stones are formed by minerals or stone-forming salts and begin to crystallize when their concentration becomes supersaturated in the urine. Just as certain minerals or salts promote calculus formation, there are many inhibitors of calculus formation, including citrate, phosphate, and magnesium. There are many theories to stone formation, none of which are definitively proven, such as Randall plaque formation, stasis, bacteria, and reactive oxygen species from oxalate excretion.[27] Kidney stones are classified by the stone composition, and the mineral composition directs evaluation, treatment, and nonsurgical management. Kidney stones can be generally classified as calcium based, uric acid stones, struvite stones, and cystine stones.[27] Calcium stones are usually composed of two calcium salts, calcium phosphate and calcium oxalate, and are the most common renal calculi. Risk factors for calcium stone formation include abnormal urine pH; high urine concentration of calcium, oxalate, or uric acid; and low urine concentration of the stone inhibitor citrate. Uric acid stones form in a low pH urine in patients with hyperuricosuria and can be the result of purine metabolism from cellular breakdown (tumor lysis) or excessive protein intake. These stones are often radiolucent. Struvite stones, also called infection stones or magnesium ammonium phosphate, result from specific bacterial infections (*P. mirabilis, K. pneumoniae, Staphylococcus aureus,* and *Staphylococcus epidermidis*) that contain urease, which converts urea into ammonia. The base properties of ammonia lead to higher urine pH and crystallization with phosphate. Cystine stones are formed from an autosomal recessive defect in the metabolism of the COLA amino acids (cystine, ornithine, lysine, and arginine), which results in elevated urine cystine levels.[27] The other rare cause of calculi is pharmacologically induced, resulting from poor drug metabolite urine solubility and precipitation in the urine. The most notable of these are protease inhibitors (indinavir and ritonavir), which are not visible on noncontrasted computed tomography (CT) scans.

Acute Presentation and Management

Patients presenting with an acute stone episode or renal colic typically have characteristic complaints of abdominal, flank, or back pain that waxes and wanes but cannot be resolved with position changes. Often, these patients can localize the most intense center of the pain, giving some indication of stone location. When the ureter is obstructed by a stone, the pressure in the proximal collecting system rises, and with progressive distention, the patient may experience visceral symptoms, including nausea, vomiting, and ileus. Physical examination in these patients should be focused on the back, flank, abdomen, and genitalia. Patients who have specific vital sign findings in combination (temperature higher than 101.5°F, hypotension, or tachycardia) should be assessed for obstructive upper tract UTI with the potential for sepsis. Basic laboratory evaluation should include complete blood count, metabolic panel, and urinalysis with microscopy. Significant findings of leukocytosis or acute kidney injury may direct urgency of therapy and type of intervention. A noncontrast-enhanced CT scan of the abdomen and pelvis is the preferred imaging study because of its superior sensitivity and specificity compared with intravenous urography and plain radiography. Patients with ureteral calculi may benefit from a plain radiograph, as 85% of calculi are radiopaque, to observe for stone passage.

Once the stone is identified and the location established, pain management is the next step. Patients who are diagnosed with renal or ureteral calculi should receive intravenous nonsteroidal antiinflammatory drugs (ketorolac) or opioid analgesics as initial therapy. A successful attempt at pain control with oral agents determines if the otherwise hemodynamically stable patient can be discharged or requires inpatient treatment for the stone. Those patients who present with upper tract UTI and obstruction should undergo expeditious drainage with either cystoscopic ureteral stent placement or percutaneous nephrostomy tube placement. If one upper tract is totally obstructed by stone, the patient could have a serious infection with pyonephrosis, and the voided urine would be deceptively normal. Patients who are suitable for hospital discharge include those with no evidence of UTI, hemodynamic stability, good oral intake, pain well controlled on oral analgesics, and a stone size with reasonable chance of spontaneous passage. In patients who are discharged from the hospital, medical expulsive therapy, with agents to promote spontaneous stone passage, is the recommended management.[28] The most common drug used is tamsulosin, the α_{1a} blocker that relaxes ureteral smooth muscle.[28]

If a patient is discharged for outpatient management, she or he should be observed closely to determine whether the stone has passed. It should not be assumed that because the pain has resolved, the stone has passed. With persistent upper tract obstruction, the pressure in the collecting system eventually declines as renal blood flow diminishes and urine output drops. The patient's pain can disappear, and the kidney can remain obstructed, undergoing silent destruction in the weeks and months that follow. Reimaging is necessary if there is no definitive evidence that the stone has been passed (e.g., the patient brings it in for analysis).

Elective Diagnostic Evaluation and Management

Patients who are diagnosed with asymptomatic renal calculi, such as nonobstructing renal calyceal stones found incidentally during a hematuria evaluation, and patients who have convalesced after an acute presentation undergo a basic metabolic screening evaluation. Important historical aspects to obtain include prior stone passage or treatment, family history, bowel disease or malabsorption, gout, hyperthyroidism, obesity, and use of dietary supplements.[29] Routine laboratory work includes urinalysis, basic metabolic panel with determination of calcium and uric acid levels, urine culture, and stone analysis (if available). A 24-hour urine specimen is also collected to evaluate the urine for specific chemical and mineral content: volume, pH, creatinine, calcium, oxalate, uric acid, citrate, sodium, and potassium.[29] Specific dietary changes and medical therapy can be used for prevention of stone formation in specific populations. These dietary modifications and pharmacologic treatments are based on stone composition and findings on 24-hour urinalysis. The two most common stone types, calcium and uric acid, are discussed.

In patients with calcium-based stone disease (oxalate or phosphate), the single most important treatment or dietary modification is increased fluid intake to achieve more than two liters of urine output daily. In addition, there should be no changes in calcium consumption, and patients, in general, should consume the recommended daily allowance of dietary calcium. Dietary levels of sodium, foods high in oxalate, and animal protein should be reduced as each of these can affect urinary oxalate and citrate levels. Pharmacologic therapy is typically based on three different agents—thiazide diuretics, potassium citrate, and allopurinol—each of which has separate effects on calcium urine levels and calcium stone formation. Patients with uric acid stones are treated with drug therapy.[29] There are no dietary recommendations other than to increase fluid intake to raise urine output to two liters per day. Pharmacologic therapy in this group consists of potassium citrate and allopurinol. Many uric acid stones can be dissolved by raising urinary pH levels with use of alkalinizing agents.

Elective Surgical Management

Patients who have large stone burdens or continue to have symptomatic stones require surgical treatment of their calculous disease. Surgical treatment of renal and ureteral calculi varies from completely noninvasive, shock wave lithotripsy (SWL), to minimally invasive, percutaneous nephrolithotomy (PCNL). SWL is a transcutaneous procedure using generated shock waves to fragment stones. Shock waves create positive and negative pressure components that are focused on the stone and create fractures in the targeted stones, ultimately resulting in stone fragmentation.[30] The progress of stone fragmentation is monitored during SWL, typically with fluoroscopy, to direct treatment length and location. Nonradiopaque stones, stones larger than 2 cm, and certain ureteral calculi should not be treated with this method. Complications from SWL include renal injury, steinstrasse (street of stones), hypertension, and chronic kidney disease.[30]

Smaller renal stones and ureteral calculi can be managed in an endoscopic fashion using ureteroscopes (Fig. 74.9). As previously mentioned, ureteroscopes are both semirigid and flexible, allowing full upper tract collecting system access. Through the working channel of ureteroscopes, a variety of working instruments can be placed to fragment or to remove stones. The most common stone treatment is laser lithotripsy to completely fragment the symptomatic calculus. Smaller fragments can be removed using different basket and grasping systems to render the patient stone free. Complications of ureteroscopy include acute ureteral perforation or avulsion, UTI, and late ureteral stricture formation.

For larger renal stones or select proximal ureteral stones, PCNL is preferred because of the larger working endoscopes and better instrumentation for stone fragmentation. The basic steps of PCNL are percutaneous renal access, dilation of the nephrostomy track, placement of the working sheath for stone fragmentation and extraction, and postoperative renal drainage. The advantage of PCNL is that numerous intracorporeal lithotripsy devices are available, and large stones can be rapidly fragmented. Flexible nephroscopes can be used as well in this setting. Complications of PCNL are most significant because of the more invasive nature of the procedure; these include sepsis, renal hemorrhage, renal collecting

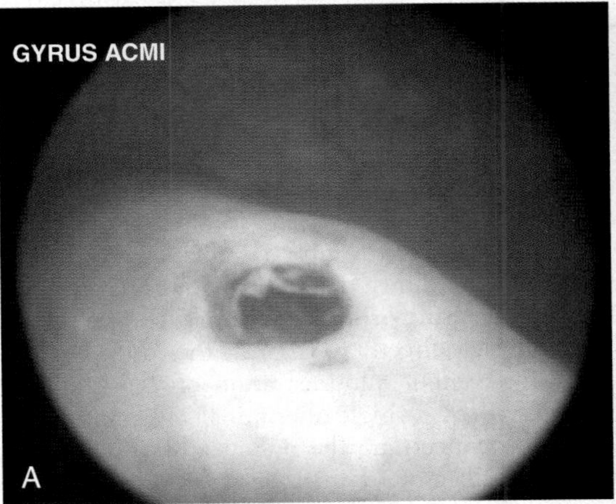

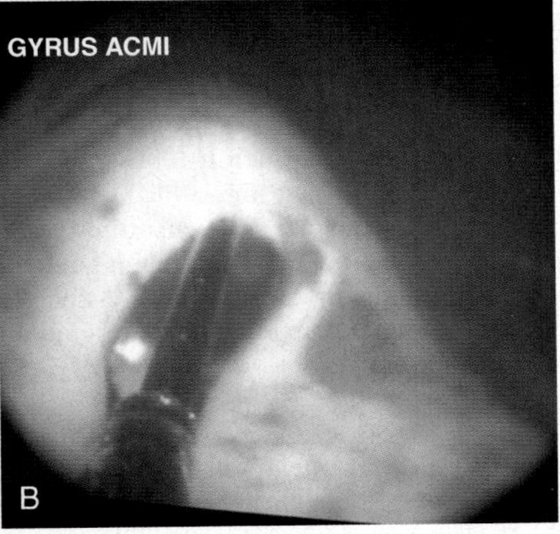

FIG. 74.9 Ureteral stone. (A) An obstructing calculus is shown crowning within the right ureteral orifice. (B) Cystoscopic extraction performed with a grasping forceps.

system injury, and damage to adjacent organs and viscera. PCNL may result in hydrothorax or pneumothorax from transpleural or peripleural access tracks that requires evacuation. With the refinement of PCNL, open stone surgery is rarely indicated even for the most complex intrarenal calculi. Laparoscopic and robotic procedures for specific renal calculi have been described.

UROLOGIC TRAUMA

Urologic injury is present in approximately 15% of all abdominal and pelvic trauma patients regardless of mechanism, blunt or penetrating.[31] Renal injuries, for example, are reported to occur in 0.3% to 1.2% of all trauma patients; however, the kidneys are the second most common visceral organ injured, accounting for approximately 24% of injuries.[31] In many trauma centers, injuries are typically initially assessed by an emergency physician or general surgeon and may be addressed without urologic consultation, although, for complex urologic injuries, the input of a urologist can be essential. For example, high-grade, nonreconstructible renal injury can be managed with an expeditious nephrectomy; however, most renal injuries, such as an extensive parenchymal and collecting system laceration, should be repaired with renorrhaphy. Management of trauma patients is the greatest overlap between urology and general surgery and allows numerous areas for collaboration; urologic expertise can enhance the quality of care provided for all urologic injuries, whether they are managed operatively or nonoperatively.

The focus of the following section on urologic trauma is the practical management of a variety of acute urologic injuries and the optimal interaction between the urologist and general trauma surgeon. The management of common injuries throughout the urinary tract, the optimal timing of such interventions, and the role of damage control techniques are discussed.

Core Guideline and Consensus Statements for Urologic Trauma Management

The Organ Injury Scaling system of the American Association for the Surgery of Trauma (AAST) describes an objective grading system for urologic injuries (Table 74.1 and Fig. 74.10).[32] The staging system for renal trauma has become well established in the urologic literature and has been externally validated. The Organ Injury Scaling system also describes staging for other urologic injuries; however, the subjective criteria applied to these divisions do not practically affect management decisions and treatment (Fig. 74.10). An updated, revised renal injury scaling system was published recently through the AAST, reflecting newer data and thinking about the diagnosis and management of renal trauma.[33]

In 2002, a consensus conference for the diagnosis and treatment of urologic injuries was convened by the WHO and the Société Internationale d'Urologie. The resulting consensus statements were divided by organ site: kidney, ureter, bladder, urethra, and external genitalia.[34–38] These reports still constitute the centerpiece of urologic trauma management. Management guidelines have subsequently been produced by the European Association of Urology and the AUA to create core documents to guide the management of urologic injuries.[39]

Renal Injuries

The majority of renal injuries are the result of blunt trauma (80%); the remainder are the result of penetrating injury (20%).[34] Approximately 70% of all patients who sustain renal injury are male, and most of these patients are younger than 50 years. As discussed in the retroperitoneal anatomy section, the kidneys are well protected in the retroperitoneum but are close to intraperitoneal structures. The key points in evaluation, as with any trauma patient, are the ABCs: airway, breathing, and circulation. In patients with a history of blunt trauma, key findings include location of impact, flank ecchymosis, and gross or microscopic hematuria. Other relevant historical information is concomitant injury and mechanism of injury. Close attention to the entry and exit points in penetrating injuries are also important to estimate the trajectory of the missile.

TABLE 74.1 Organ injury scaling system: kidney.

GRADE		INJURY DESCRIPTION	AIS-90
I	Contusion	Microscopic or gross hematuria, urologic studies normal	2
	Hematoma	Subcapsular, nonexpanding, without parenchymal laceration	2
II	Hematoma	Nonexpanding perirenal hematoma confined to renal retroperitoneum	2
	Laceration	<1 cm parenchymal depth of renal cortex without urinary extravasation	2
III	Laceration	>1 cm depth of renal cortex without collecting system rupture or urinary extravasation	3
IV	Laceration	Parenchymal laceration extending through the renal cortex, medulla, and collecting system	4
	Vascular	Main renal artery or vein injury with contained hemorrhage	5
V	Laceration	Completely shattered kidney	5
	Vascular	Avulsion of renal hilum, which devascularizes kidney	5

Adapted from Moore EE, Shackford SR, Pachter HL, et al. Organ injury scaling: Spleen, liver, and kidney. *J Trauma*. 1989;29:1664–1666.

Imaging

There are many well-established indications for renal imaging after blunt or penetrating injury. In patients with blunt trauma, the criteria for imaging include gross hematuria, hemodynamic instability (systolic blood pressure <90 mm Hg), microscopic hematuria (>5 red blood cells/high-power field), a traumatic mechanism, and suspicion of injury on screening radiographs (Fig. 74.11). In patients with penetrating injury who are hemodynamically stable, imaging is indicated for any degree of hematuria, microscopic or gross (Fig. 74.12).[39] The relevance of imaging to detect and to stage urinary tract injury before abdominal trauma surgery has been debated in the general surgical and urologic literature. Cross-sectional imaging, specifically contrast-enhanced CT scan, is the preferred study to evaluate the renal injuries. Proper imaging should include arteriovenous phases with delayed imaging to evaluate the urinary collecting structures. In those patients who proceed directly to surgery, the "one-shot" intravenous urogram (intravenous administration of 2 mL/kg contrast material followed by a single abdominal radiograph) can provide information concerning the presence or absence of a contralateral kidney. Ultrasound, intravenous urography, and magnetic resonance imaging (MRI) have a limited role in renal imaging for injury staging.

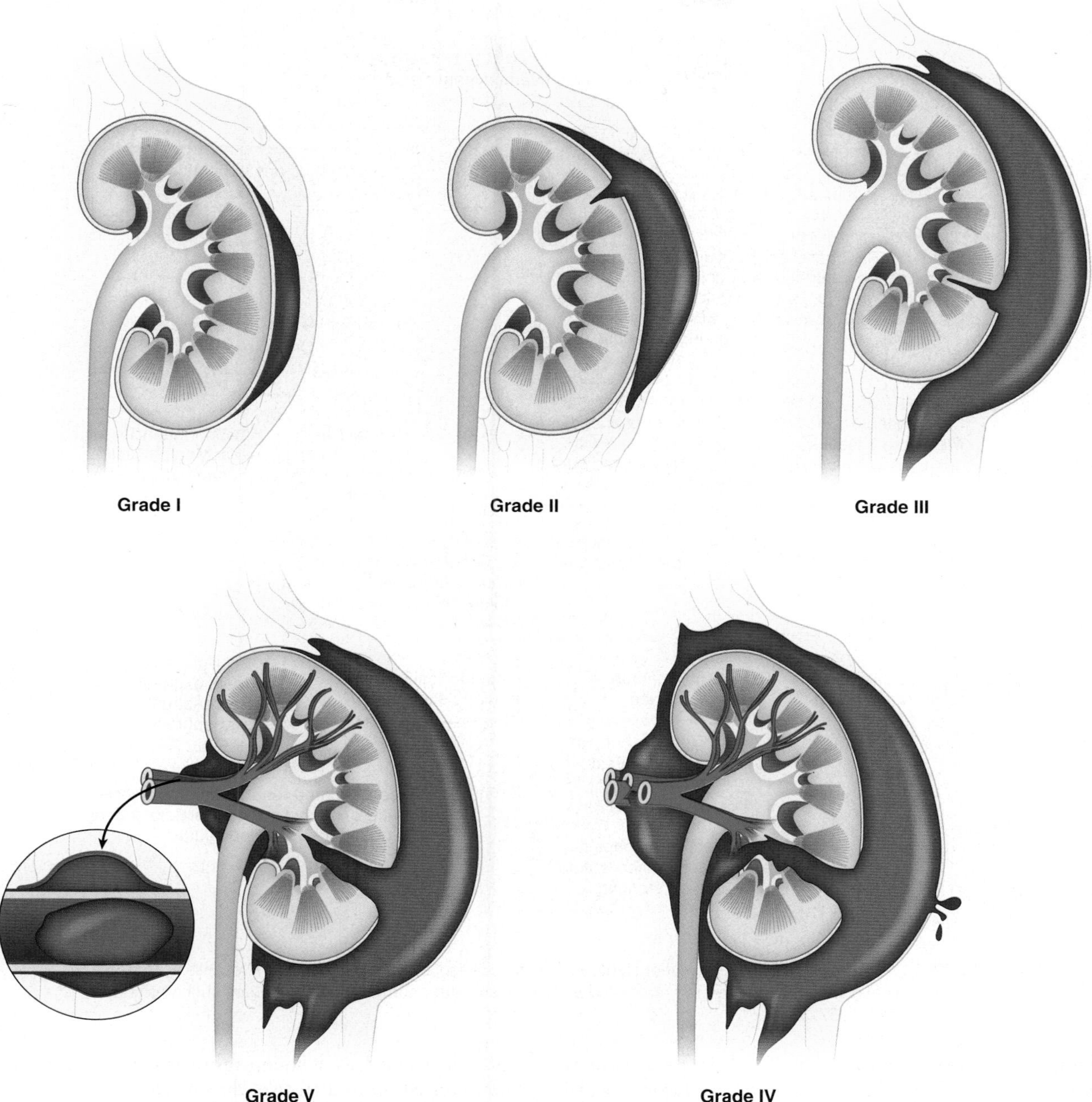

FIG. 74.10 Illustrative diagram showing grades I–V renal injuries from the American Association for the Surgery of Trauma (AAST) organ injury scaling system. (From Moore EE, Shackford SR, Pachter HL, et al. Organ injury scaling: Spleen, liver, and kidney. *J Trauma.* 1989;29:1664–1666.)

Management: Operative Versus Nonoperative

With better staging of renal injury, management paradigms have changed over time (Figs. 74.11 and 74.12). Furthermore, as urologists learned more from general trauma surgeons in the management of solid organ injury, nonoperative management of renal injuries has become more commonplace. The basis of nonoperative management centers around a properly staged injury with contrast-enhanced cross-sectional imaging (Fig. 74.13). In general, lower grade injuries, grades I to III, in hemodynamically stable patients are managed nonoperatively. Grade IV injuries are more controversial, and many are managed nonoperatively. High-grade injuries, grades IV and V, particularly in patients with concomitant intraperitoneal injuries, may undergo surgical exploration.[33]

In hemodynamically unstable patients who proceed directly to the operating room, there are absolute and relative criteria for operative exploration. The absolute criteria for exploration are expanding hematoma, pulsatile hematoma, and persistent renal bleeding. Any of these findings are concerning for possible renal pedicle injury.[40] The relative criteria for renal exploration include persistent urinary extravasation, nonviable renal parenchyma, arterial injury, and incomplete renal staging.[40] In the absence of such findings or in patients in whom a damage control approach

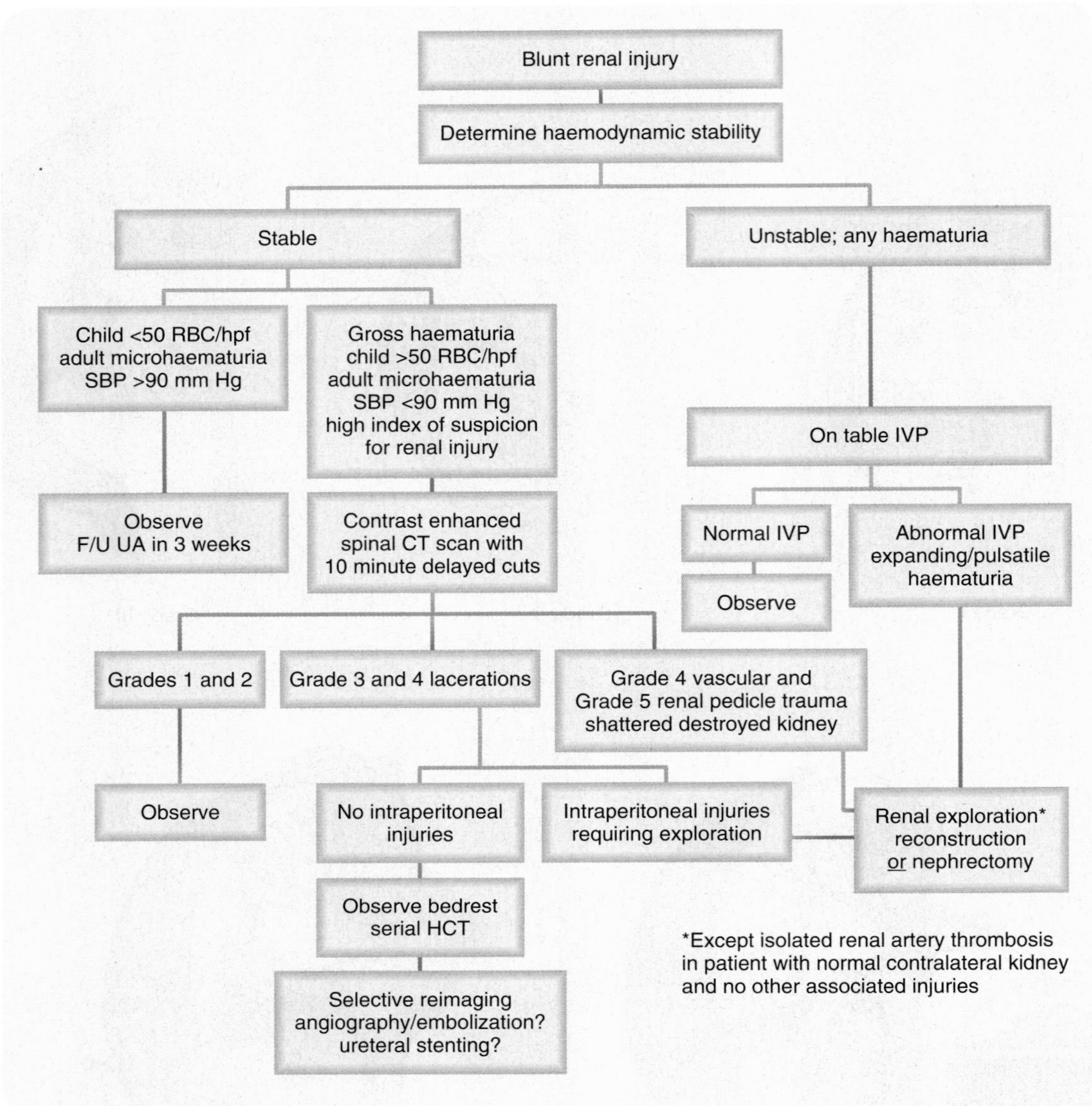

FIG. 74.11 Algorithm for management of blunt renal injuries. (Adapted from Santucci RA, Wessells H, Bartsch G, et al. Evaluation and management of renal injuries: Consensus statement of the renal trauma subcommittee. *BJU Int.* 2004;93:937–954.)

is to be implemented, exploration may be avoided if the surgeon is uncomfortable with the potential requirements for reconstructive renal surgery.

Renal vascular injury is uncommon, and the radiologic presentation is variable. On CT imaging, these patients may have either large perinephric hematomas with intravascular extravasation of contrast material (indicating possible renal pedicle injury) or absent renal perfusion (indicating renal artery thrombosis). Segmental renal vascular injuries are usually the result of blunt renal trauma and appear as wedge-shaped defects in the renal parenchyma. These injuries rarely require intervention.

With an increase in nonoperative management of renal injuries, renal arteriography and selective angioembolization have been used with increasing frequency in management of renal trauma (Fig. 74.14). However, only select patients have been shown to benefit from this intervention: those with intravascular extravasation of contrast material, perirenal hematoma rim distance of more than 25 mm, and medial hematomas.[41] In addition, patients who are assigned to a nonoperative management protocol and have received more than two units of red blood cell transfusion should undergo angiography.

Surgical Exploration and Operative Approach

Strict criteria exist for renal exploration. In those patients who proceed directly to the operating room, renal exploration is indicated with an expanding, pulsatile, uncontrolled retroperitoneal hematoma or renal pedicle avulsion. Patients with persistent renal bleeding but who require damage control management may require nephrectomy for hemodynamic stability. Patients with certain intraperitoneal injuries require surgical exploration and repair of renal injuries, including patients with concomitant bowel or pancreatic injury. Patients with renal pelvic laceration or persistent urinary extravasation of contrast material may require surgical repair of the collecting system. Patients with large segments of devitalized renal parenchyma and urinary extravasation may need early partial or total nephrectomy to prevent long-term

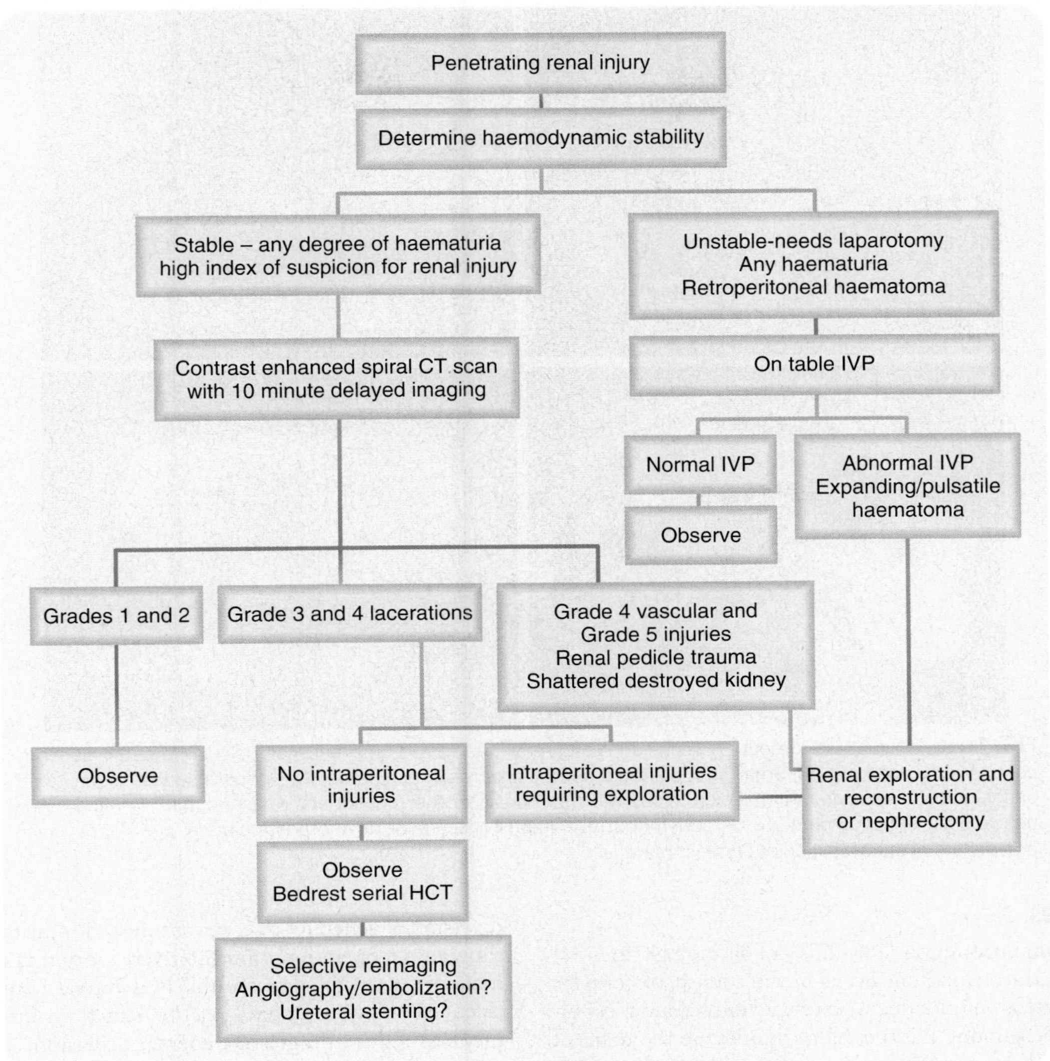

FIG. 74.12 Algorithm for management of penetrating renal injuries. (Adapted from Santucci RA, Wessells H, Bartsch G, et al. Evaluation and management of renal injuries: Consensus statement of the renal trauma subcommittee. *BJU Int.* 2004;93:937–954.)

complications. Trauma patients who have continued urinary extravasation despite percutaneous or endoscopic urinary diversion may require renal exploration and repair, although this may result in nephrectomy.

There are conflicting data concerning early vascular control before renal exploration, although the guidelines recommend vascular control.[34] Urologists are typically trained to approach the injured kidney anteriorly through a midline incision and to obtain vascular control of the renal vessels, before opening Gerota fascia and exposing the kidney, to avoid severe renal bleeding that may necessitate an urgent nephrectomy. In significant anatomic distortion, which may occur in the trauma setting, renal pedicle control can be obtained by bluntly creating a window medial to the lower pole of the kidney and lateral to the aorta (left) or vena cava (right), down to the psoas muscle fascia, which allows a vascular pedicle clamp to be placed if bleeding is encountered on renal exposure (Fig. 74.15). Once vascular access is achieved, the kidney is exposed through an anterior vertical incision in Gerota fascia, which extends from the upper to the lower pole of the kidney. If there is parenchymal injury, care must be taken to identify the renal capsule in exposing and mobilizing the kidney to avoid stripping the entire capsule from the renal parenchyma and affecting kidney closure after renal reconstruction. The entire kidney should be exposed to reveal any lacerations, to evacuate hematoma, and to facilitate full mobility for repair. In general, if half the kidney can be preserved, renal reconstruction has benefit; however, if there is extensive destruction of the hilar region, successful reconstruction is unlikely. The preferred surgical management is renorrhaphy with suture ligation of bleeding vessels and closure of the collecting system with fine absorbable suture followed by parenchyma and capsular approximation with absorbable suture. For renal reconstruction in the trauma setting, pedicle clamping with a warm ischemia time of less than 30 minutes generally will not have a permanent adverse impact on renal function. The use of hemostatic agents and tissue sealants may aid in the reconstructive effort, and closed suction drainage is beneficial in the instance of a collecting system injury or significant bleeding.

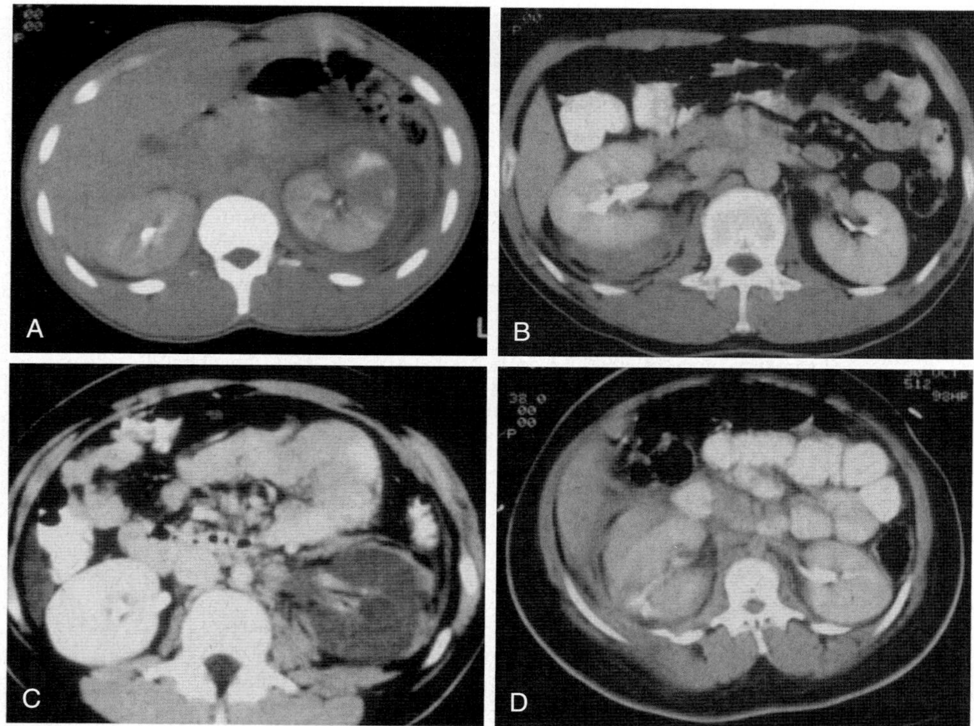

FIG. 74.13 Computed tomograpy scans depicting renal trauma. (A) Left renal contusion with heterogeneous contrast enhancement. (B) Small right posterior pericapsular renal hematoma. (C) Nonperfused left kidney after deceleration trauma and intimal disruption with thrombosis of the renal artery. Vessel cutoff sign and some pericapsular enhancement are demonstrated. (D) Grade IV laceration to the posterolateral right kidney with posterolateral extravasation of contrast material.

Ureteral Injuries

Ureteral injuries are uncommon (1%–2.5% of all urologic injuries) and are rarely life-threatening but occur in the context of complex polytrauma.[40] Ureteral injuries due to external violence are most often the result of penetrating injuries; blunt injuries are the result of injuries with high-energy transfer, such as motor vehicle collision. Up to 5% to 10% of penetrating abdominal or pelvic injuries have ureteral involvement.[40] Management of ureteral injuries is dependent on mechanism of injury, anatomic location, and overall condition of the patient. The ureter is infrequently injured because of its mobility and location in the retroperitoneum protected by a large muscle groups, the spine, and the bony pelvis. Ureteral injuries do not present with specific signs and symptoms, and their diagnosis requires heightened suspicion for injury based on mechanism and injury location.[39] Evaluation of ureteral injuries should be performed in the context of evaluation for more serious or life-threatening injuries.

Imaging

Ureteral imaging should be performed with contrast-enhanced, cross-sectional imaging, preferably CT scan, and must include delayed imaging to evaluate urinary excretion.[39] Findings suggesting ureteral injury include extravasation of contrast material, absence of contrast material distal to the suspected injury, and ipsilateral hydronephrosis. Other forms of imaging, including retrograde pyelography and intravenous urography, are difficult in the acute setting and often of lower quality.

Management

As a general principle, injuries to the ureter are best managed by surgical repair. Endoscopic ureteral stents or percutaneous diversion is generally reserved for missed injuries and for patients for whom reoperation is prohibitively morbid or the timing would make a successful repair unlikely. Ureteral contusions from adjacent penetrating trauma may benefit from ureteral stent placement to reduce progressive edema, occlusion, and ischemia and potentially to diminish the risk of delayed urinary extravasation.

Surgical Exploration and Operative Approach

When a ureteral injury is suspected, the ureter should be identified and directly inspected. The ureter can be approached surgically at any level by finding an area of normal anatomy and proceeding expeditiously to the areas in question. While dissecting around the ureter and mobilizing it from surrounding tissues, it is important to avoid stripping the periureteral tissue, causing devascularization. Ureteral injuries should be managed at the time of initial injury to decrease the chance of complication, such as urinoma, fistula, ureteral obstruction, and renal failure.[35] Repair usually involves minimal debridement of viable tissue. Lacerations are closed perpendicular to the axis of incision and transections with a spatulated, tension-free anastomosis. Injuries of the distal ureter often require reimplantation into the bladder. Gunshot wounds represent a particular concern as the viability of the ureteral stump may be compromised because of local tissue injury from the blast effect of the missile.[35] Fine absorbable suture is used in a running or interrupted fashion. Stent placement is desirable to allow low-pressure drainage, to minimize postoperative urinary extravasation, and to prevent angulation of the healing ureter. Ureteral injuries are highly amenable to damage control approaches when repair acutely is not appropriate because of the patient's condition or the need to prioritize the management of other, more critical injuries.[42]

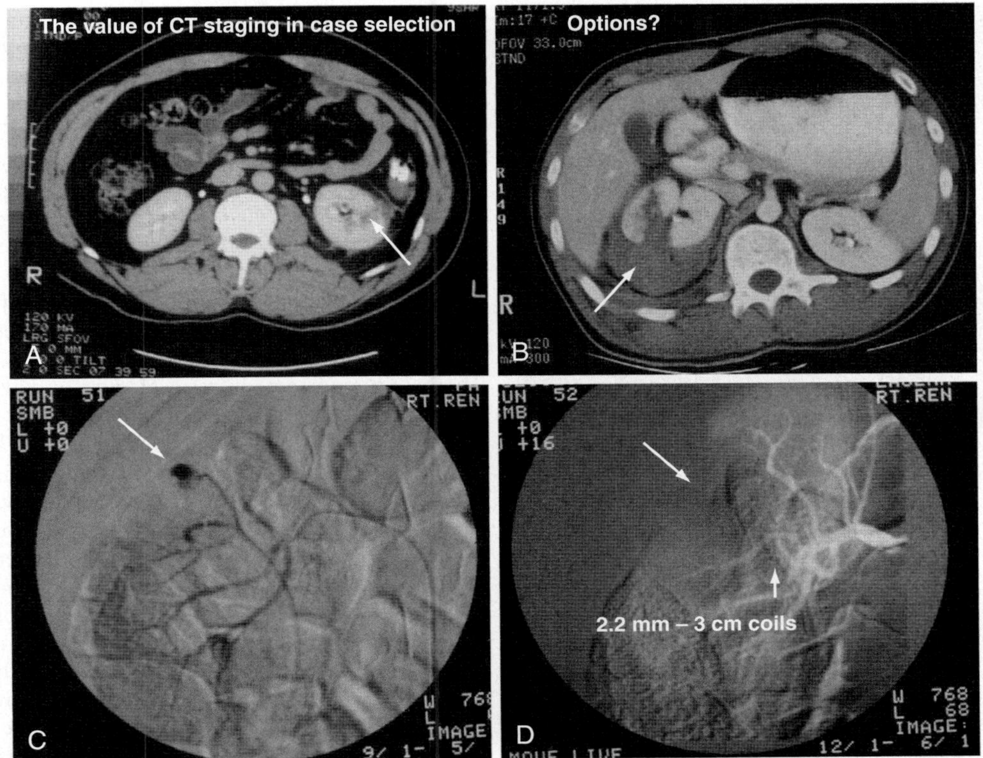

FIG. 74.14 Computed tomography scans depicting penetrating renal injury. (A) Superficial laceration to the lateral left kidney from a stab wound. Note minimal hematoma and proximity of the posterior descending colon to the track of injury. Nonoperative management was selected and was successful. (B) Deep laceration to the right kidney following a stab wound. Note the proximity to renal hilar structures and moderate-sized hematoma. (C) Renal angiography performed for significant postinjury hematuria with hemodynamic instability, demonstrating pseudoaneurysm. (D) Postembolization appearance of the right kidney showing a wedge-shaped defect after coil placement, which was successful.

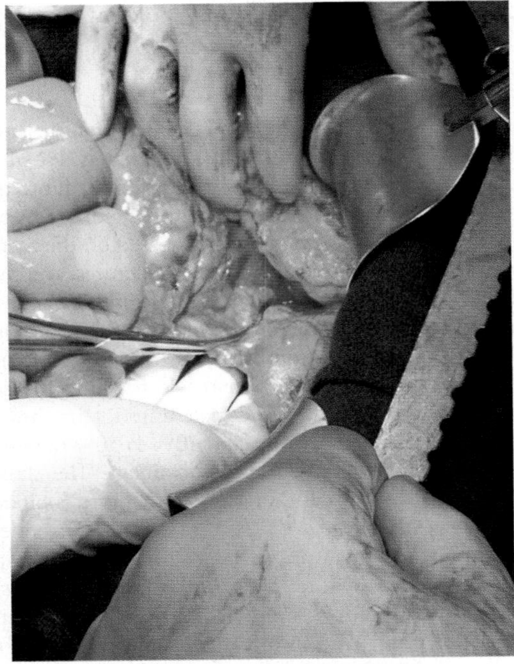

FIG. 74.15 Placement of a pedicle clamp across renal vasculature.

Bladder Injuries

The bladder is the second most commonly injured urologic structure and accounts for 10% of all urologic injuries. The most common source of bladder injury is blunt trauma (80%–85%) from high-energy transfer, and it is often associated with pelvic fracture (83%–95%).[36] The most common blunt sources of trauma are motor vehicle collision, falls from height, and industrial injuries. Patients with suspected bladder injuries often present with multisystem trauma and should be evaluated in the context of their presenting trauma. Most of the patients with bladder injury will present with hematuria and pelvic fracture, and in patients with gross hematuria and pelvic fracture, bladder injury is associated in 13% to 55% of cases.[39]

Imaging

Patients with suspected bladder injury should be evaluated with retrograde cystography. Both plain film cystography and CT cystography are acceptable, although CT scan may provide more anatomic detail. A necessary component of appropriate cystography is adequate retrograde filling of the bladder with 300 to 400 mL of contrast material.[39] If plain film cystography is performed, three anterior-posterior images must be obtained: scout, full bladder, and after drainage. CT cystography requires a diluted contrast agent of at least 1:6 concentration (Figs. 74.16 to 74.18). In

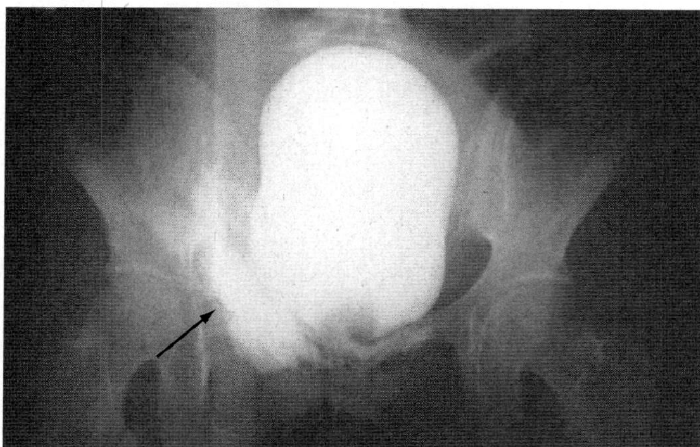

FIG. 74.16 Static cystogram in a patient with pelvic fracture and gross hematuria showing extraperitoneal extravasation of contrast material on the right side.

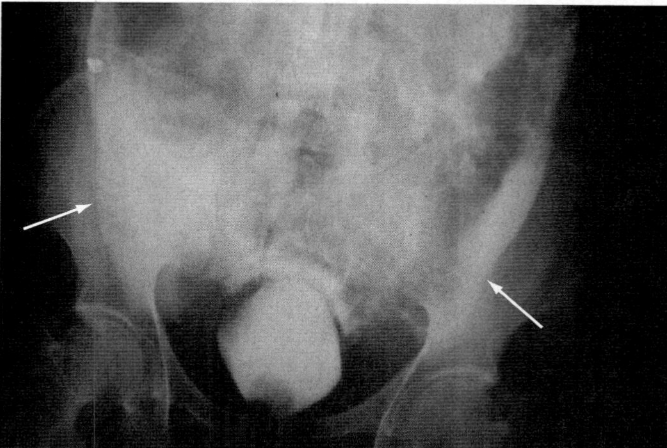

FIG. 74.17 Static cystogram in a patient after blunt injury to the lower abdomen showing the typical contrast material extravasation pattern of intraperitoneal bladder rupture. Note contrast material outlining the left and right colic gutters and present within the peritoneal cavity.

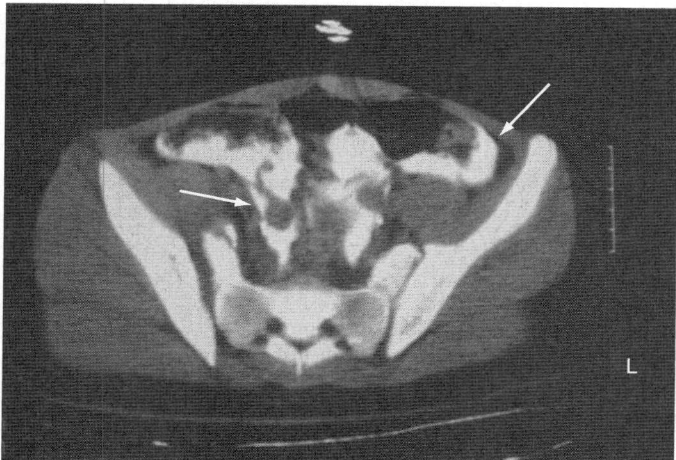

FIG. 74.18 Computed tomography cystogram demonstrating intraperitoneal contrast material extravasation pattern of intraperitoneal bladder rupture. Note contrast material in the colic gutters within the deep pelvis and outlining the ovaries.

patients with penetrating bladder injuries, imaging should not delay operative exploration as the bladder can be visually inspected at the time of surgery.

Management: Operative Versus Nonoperative

Management of bladder injuries is dependent on location of the injury, extraperitoneal or intraperitoneal (Fig. 74.19). In general, intraperitoneal bladder injuries should be surgically repaired at the time of diagnosis. On the other hand, most extraperitoneal bladder injuries can be managed in a nonoperative fashion with simple catheter drainage. Extraperitoneal bladder injuries that should be managed in an operative fashion include penetrating bladder trauma, ongoing hematuria, concomitant pelvic organ injury, foreign body or bone fragment in the bladder, and bladder neck injuries.

Surgical Exploration and Operative Approach

The operative repair of bladder injuries is through a lower midline incision, often extending the midline incision from abdominal exploration to the pubic symphysis. Intraperitoneal injuries are often evident at the dome of the bladder within the overlying peritoneum. The traumatic cystotomy should be extended, if necessary, to fully evaluate the lumen of the bladder. In extraperitoneal injuries, the bladder is often opened through an anterior midline cystotomy to evaluate the lumen. This is especially true in the case of pelvic fracture to avoid disturbing the associated hematoma. If necessary, ureteral catheters can be inserted to confirm efflux of urine and ureteral continuity. Defects in the bladder wall are closed with absorbable 2-0 sutures in two layers to achieve a water-tight closure. Use of a tissue interposition flap (e.g., omental flap) at the time of bladder repair may be necessary in cases of contiguous injuries to the rectum or vagina to prevent fistula formation. Diversion with a large-bore Foley catheter (at least 20 Fr to 24 Fr in the adult) allows bloody urine to drain and manual catheter irrigation, if necessary. Suprapubic cystostomy tubes are used for cases of extensive injuries requiring complex repairs or if prolonged bladder drainage is anticipated, such as with concomitant rectal or vaginal injury or traumatic brain injury. In patients with significant multisystem trauma who are hemodynamically unstable, definitive bladder repair may be delayed as a damage control maneuver.

Urethral Injuries

The urethra is not a common source of urologic trauma, and injury due to external violence accounts for approximately 4% of all genitourinary injuries.[37,43] Broadly, the urethra is divided into the anterior and posterior segments. Each segment has a different cause for injury and different management options based on the mechanism of injury, the involvement of surrounding structures, and the medical condition of the patient. The anterior segment of the urethra most commonly injured is the bulbar urethra, which accounts for 85% of urethral injuries.[37] Approximately 3% to 6% of posterior urethral injuries are associated with pelvic fracture, the so-called pelvic fracture urethral injury. The male anterior urethra may be injured at the time of penile injury, and 40% to 50% of penetrating wounds to the penis have urethral involvement. The classic triad of physical examination findings for urethral injury is blood at the urethral meatus, inability to void, and a palpably distended bladder. Blood at the urethral meatus occurs in 37% to 93% of patients with urethral injury. The other physical finding that occurs in urethral trauma is perineal or "butterfly" hematoma due to rupture of Buck fascia; this can spread into the scrotum or up the abdomen along the layers of dartos and Scarpa fascia (Fig. 74.20).

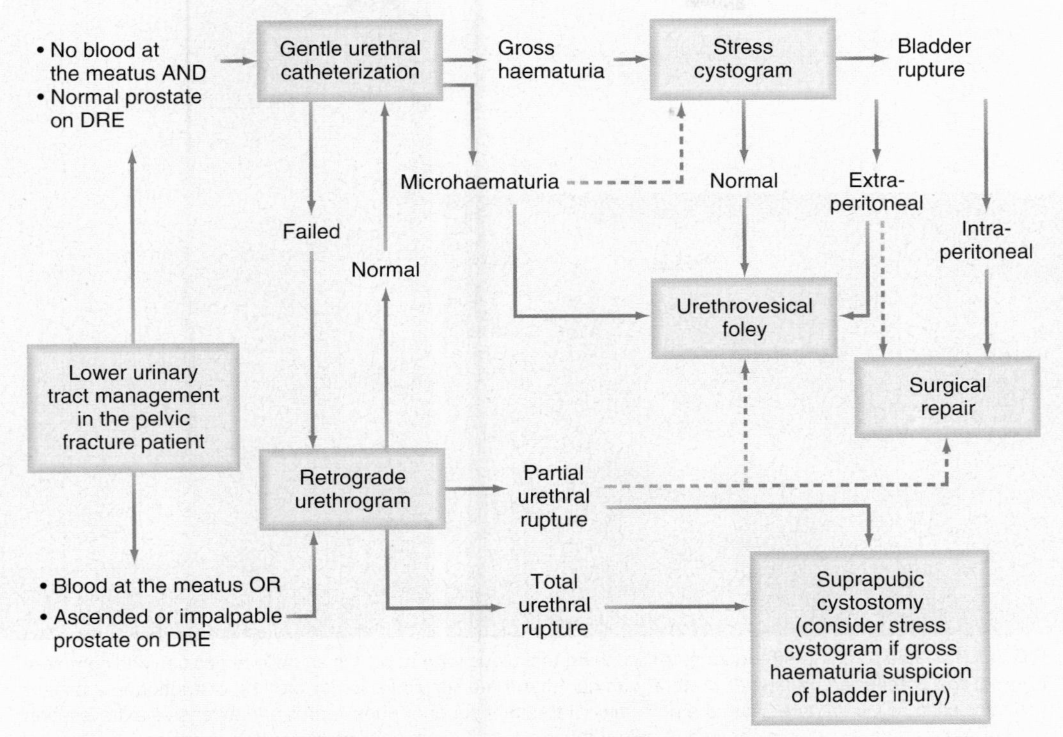

FIG. 74.19 Algorithm for management of bladder injuries. (Adapted from Chapple C, Barbagli G, Jordan G, et al. Consensus statement on urethral trauma. *BJU Int.* 2004;93:1195–1202.)

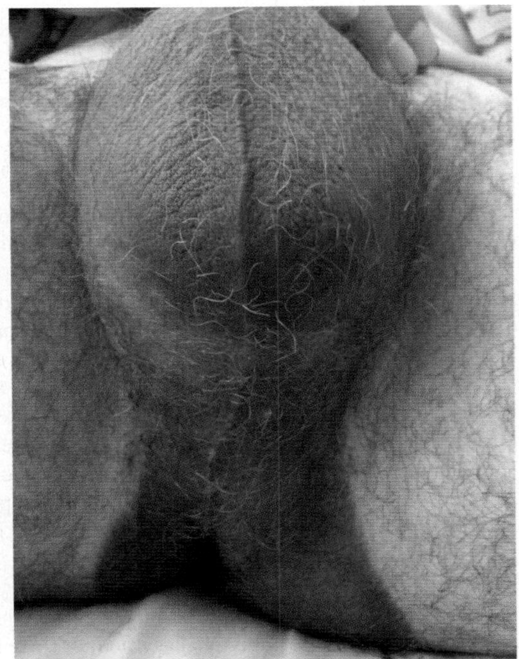

FIG. 74.20 Butterfly hematoma due to rupture of Buck fascia after urethral injury.

Imaging

In patients with suspected urethral injury, retrograde urethrography should be performed before attempting the insertion of a Foley catheter.[39] Proper performance of retrograde urethrography involves adequate filling of the entire urethra with passage of contrast material into the bladder. Extravasation of contrast material occurs when continuity of the urethra has been lost because of the injury (Fig. 74.21).

Management

The immediate goal in managing urethral injury is to provide urinary bladder drainage and to avoid further injury.[37] Few urethral injuries, barring those resulting in significant ongoing external bleeding such as with penetrating perineal trauma, require acute operative reconstruction. A delayed approach can almost always be implemented and often produces better outcomes. The surgeon with limited experience with these injuries should perform urinary diversion maneuvers for these cases. Urethral reconstruction is a highly specialized area of urology; definitive reconstructive surgery can be performed in a subacute or delayed fashion with good results.[37]

Surgical Exploration and Operative Approach

Penetrating anterior urethral injuries should be explored and repaired primarily unless the patient is hemodynamically unstable. Urethral repair should be performed in two layers with fine absorbable suture over a catheter, creating a spatulated primary repair. Other anterior and posterior urethral injuries should be managed with suprapubic catheter insertion rather than by instrumentation of the traumatized urethra with risk of further injury. If the bladder is palpably distended and there is no evidence of prior lower abdominal surgery or the bladder can be clearly localized with ultrasound, percutaneous tube placement is appropriate. If these criteria are not met, open surgical cystostomy tube placement is safer and can be accomplished through a small anterior

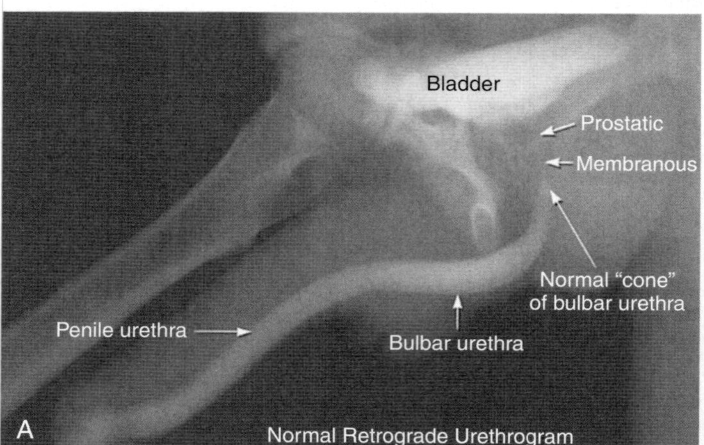

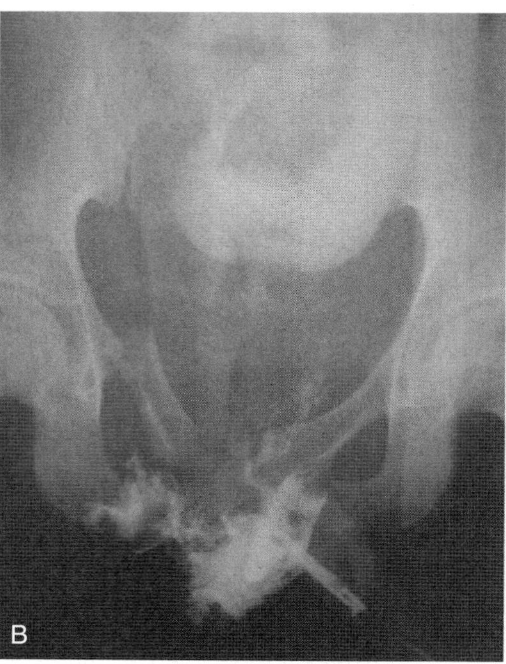

FIG. 74.21 Retrograde urethrograms. (A) Standard technique with patient in an oblique position and complete filling of the anterior and posterior urethra with contrast material. (B) Posterior urethral disruption in a patient with displaced pelvic fracture. Note the deformity of the right superior pubic ramus and extensive extravasation of contrast material extending above and below the urogenital diaphragm on retrograde injection into the urethra. The bladder, which is greatly displaced cephalad, is filling with contrast material administered intravenously. The photograph demonstrates the so-called pie in the sky bladder resulting from dramatic displacement by a large pelvic hematoma after the prostatomembranous disruption injury. ([A] From Older RA, Hertz M. Cystourethrography. In: Pollack HM, McClennan BL, Dyer R, Kenney PJ, eds. *Clinical urography*. 2nd ed, Philadelphia, PA; WB Saunders:2000.)

cystotomy. The drainage catheter should be anchored at the anterior bladder wall with absorbable sutures and at the skin exit site.

Immediate operative repair of posterior urethral injuries is not indicated, and management should consist of suprapubic tube placement. Posterior urethral injuries are well suited to damage control maneuvers.[42] Although it is controversial, there has been increased interest in early catheter realignment for posterior urethral disruption in the setting of pelvic fracture within 7 to 10 days of injury (Fig. 74.22). This technique requires substantial expertise in urologic endoscopic procedures, and the risk of creating further injury is substantial. Catheter realignment is performed using the suprapubic access that has been established acutely, so there is no need to feel a sense of urgency in doing this on the day of injury. The outcomes of this procedure are unclear, but much of the literature indicates that 30% to 50% of patients can avoid urethral reconstruction, although strictures typically develop and require at least endoscopic management.

Genital Injuries

Genital trauma involves a range of anatomic structures, creating a difficulty in classification and standardization of treatment. The injuries are often the result of blunt or penetrating trauma but may include burns, bites, and avulsions and involve the penis, testicles, or scrotum in the male patient and the vulva in the female patient. Injuries to the external genitalia occur in 28% to 68% of patients with injuries to the genitourinary system; however, the incidence of genital trauma varies because of few epidemiologic studies.[44] The majority of external genital trauma is blunt in nature, although 40% to 60% of penetrating injuries to the genitourinary system involve the external genitalia.[44] Genitalia injuries may be the result of a variety of trauma, such as sexual excess in penile fracture, blunt scrotal trauma in testicular injury, or industrial accidents with skin avulsion in scrotal injuries.

Imaging

Imaging may be helpful in further diagnosing injuries in penile and scrotal trauma. In most patients, the genital trauma diagnosis is made on physical examination but can be confirmed with ultrasonography. For equivocal cases of penile fracture injury that results from sudden flexion of the erect penis during sexual activity, penile ultrasound can demonstrate interruption of the corpora cavernosa. For blunt scrotal injuries, scrotal ultrasound may be helpful in determining whether the testis is ruptured. Key findings on ultrasound indicating testicular injury are loss of testicular contour of the tunica albuginea and heterogeneous echotexture of the testicular parenchyma.[39,43] Retrograde urethrography can be performed if there is concern for concomitant urethral injury.

Management

Because of the normal flaccid nature of the penis, the only injury that can occur is fracture of the erect penis. Management of these injuries involves surgical exploration of the penis and identification of the defect in the corporal body.[39,43] This is closed with slowly absorbing suture in a running fashion (Fig. 74.23). Blunt testicular injuries should be explored if ultrasound confirms testicular rupture. Repair of the injury is performed by limited debridement of the seminiferous tubules and closure of the tunica albuginea (Fig. 74.24). Orchiectomy is reserved for those injuries that thoroughly destroy the blood supply to the testis or those parenchymal injuries in which there is no viable parenchyma available to salvage.

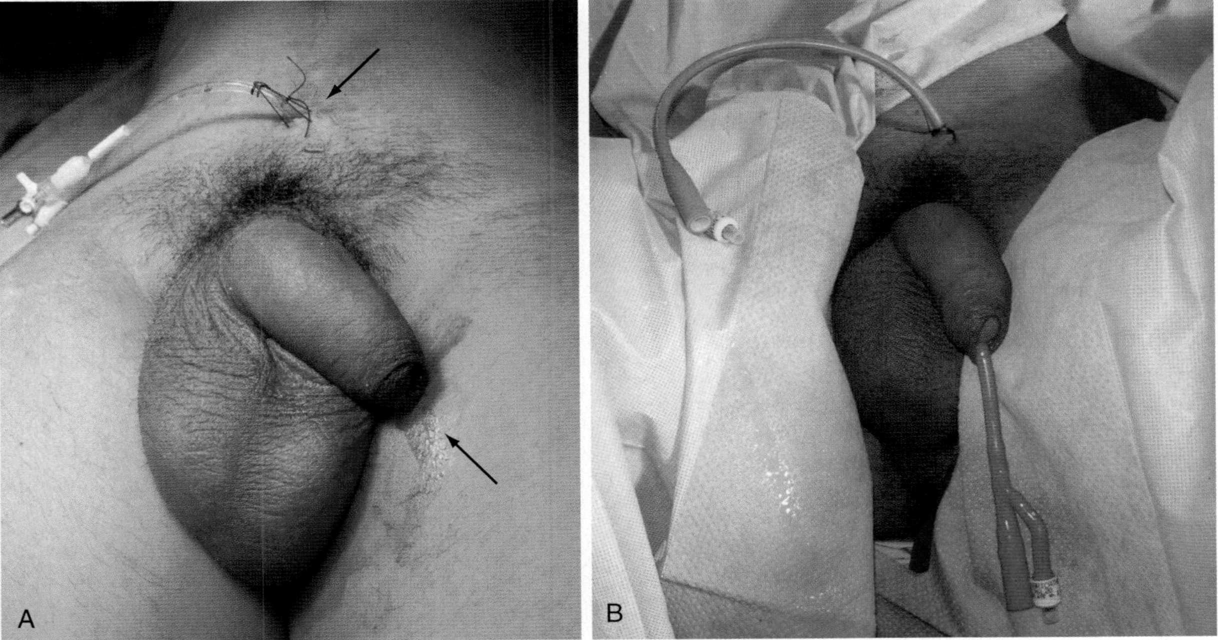

FIG. 74.22 Posterior urethral disruption injury. (A) Patient with blood visible at penile meatus is managed with percutaneously placed suprapubic cystostomy tube. (B) Patient initially managed similarly has undergone an endoscopic, fluoroscopically guided realignment procedure with placement of urethral and suprapubic Foley catheters.

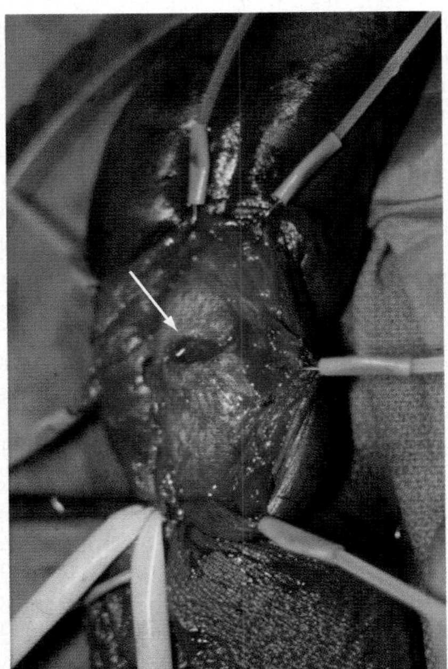

FIG. 74.23 Penile fracture. This patient was undergoing surgical exploration for a suspected penile fracture injury sustained during sexual activity. A ventral midline penoscrotal incision is used to expose the transverse laceration in the ventral right tunica albuginea of the corpus cavernosum, shown centrally. The Penrose drain at the bottom was used briefly as a tourniquet to control bleeding during suture repair of the injury. The hook and ring retractor system shown is useful for genital surgery.

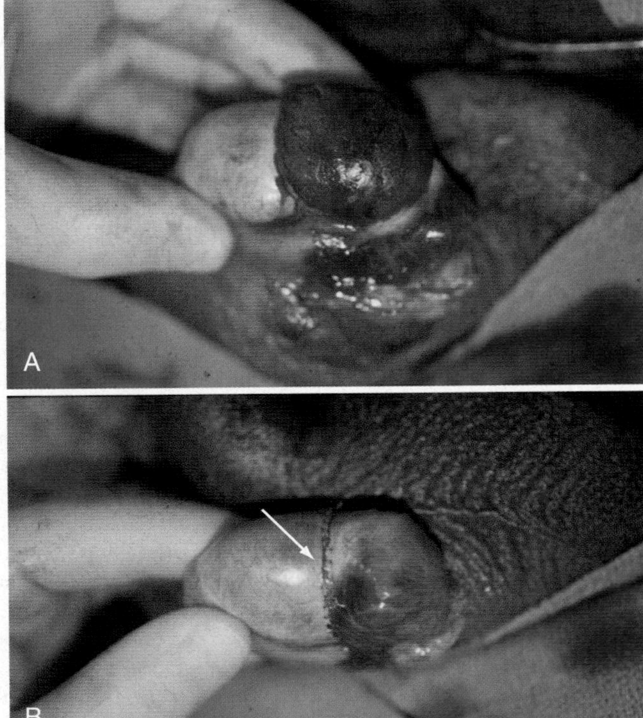

FIG. 74.24 Testicular rupture from blunt trauma. (A) Intact tunica albuginea with a large transverse laceration *(left);* the extruded testicular parenchyma from the upper portion of the testis is also shown *(right).* (B) Appearance after repair with running absorbable sutures *(arrow).*

Penetrating injuries to the external genitalia warrant surgical exploration in most cases. Functional and structural outcomes are greatly improved by early exploration and repair for penetrating penile, scrotal, and testicular injuries. For penile injuries, the goal is to remove foreign material, to cleanse the wound, to obtain hemostasis, to identify any defects in the tunica albuginea or urethra, and to proceed with appropriate repair while exercising caution not to be excessively aggressive with debridement of tissues of uncertain viability. For testicular injuries, debridement of devitalized parenchyma, closure of the capsule (tunica albuginea of the testis), and repair of the scrotum are key tasks.

Damage Control Techniques for Urologic Injuries

Many urologic injuries are amenable to initial management by applying damage control strategies. Damage control surgery refers to the concept of limiting the initial operative interventions, in the unstable trauma patient, to those maneuvers that are immediately lifesaving (e.g., control of surgical hemorrhage, control of continued fecal contamination). More time-consuming, definitive reconstructive efforts are delayed until later, after resuscitation, when the patient is more stable and can tolerate such reconstructive efforts. The physiologic rationale for damage control surgery relates to the metabolic consequences of extensive blood loss and blood and fluid replacement. These patients develop progressive hypothermia, acidosis, and coagulopathy (the so-called lethal triad), which can be corrected only when the patient can be brought to the intensive care unit with appropriate warming, fluid resuscitation, and other critical care interventions performed.[42]

Initially described in the military trauma literature, then applied to civilian penetrating abdominal trauma, these principles have now been successfully applied to a wide range of penetrating and blunt injuries. Extensive studies now support the view that appropriately selected patients managed by damage control strategies demonstrate improved survival compared with patients who undergo prolonged surgical efforts during the initial operative period. With the exception of patients with severe renal or bladder bleeding, urinary tract injuries do not directly result in early mortality. In the surgeon's judgment, when the patient would not tolerate the extended reconstructive effort needed to deal definitively with a urologic injury at initial laparotomy—because of pattern of injury, hypothermia, acidosis, coagulopathy, or other parameters that mandate a damage control approach—certain temporary solutions may be used. The complexity of patient selection for damage control surgery requires a multidisciplinary interaction, with the trauma surgeon and surgical specialists involved, to determine which injuries must be addressed initially and which can be definitively handled in a delayed fashion. Earlier selection of damage control surgery candidates, based on patterns of injury and response to initial resuscitative efforts, results in improved survival when the initial operative procedure can be concluded before significant metabolic deterioration occurs.[42]

Renal injuries that are incompletely staged or unstaged may be approached with delayed assessment and exploration as long as a determination is made that life-threatening bleeding from the injury is unlikely to occur. In the absence of significant bleeding from the renal fossa into the peritoneal cavity, a large midline hematoma or an expanding or pulsatile renal hematoma, one can elect to leave the perinephric hematoma undisturbed and fully resuscitate the patient.[42] Appropriate staging studies can be performed and delayed exploration and reconstruction completed at the time of a second-look procedure. If a major reconstructive effort is still needed in the unstable patient, packing the kidney and returning for reconstructive interventions later is also an option.

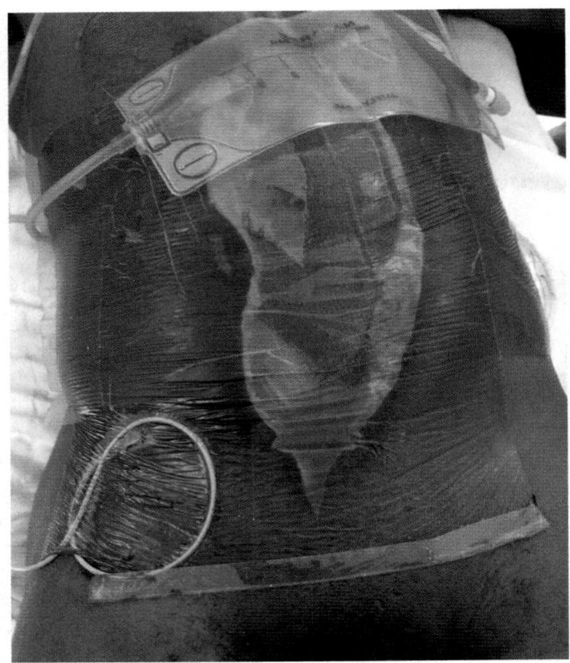

FIG. 74.25 Damage control management of gunshot wound to right ureter. A diversion stent has been secured into the right ureter and externalized to gravity drainage.

Ureteral injuries may be managed initially with externalized stents, ligation, or simple local drainage. Of these options, externalized stents are preferred as they allow control of the urinary output, minimize ongoing urinary extravasation, and can be maintained until the patient is stable enough to return to surgery for definitive reconstruction. Any number of medical tubes or catheters can be used, but the ideal solution is a 7 Fr or 8.5 Fr single-J urinary diversion stent placed into the ureter through the injury site, advanced proximally into the kidney, and then externalized through the abdominal wall (Fig. 74.25). The catheter should be tied to the very end of the injured ureter at the injury site so as not to lose ureteral length by ligating it more proximally and making later reconstruction more challenging. The distal ureteral limb is best left undisturbed; ligating it requires subsequent debridement and causes further tissue loss.

A similar approach can be used for extensive bladder injuries; the ureteral orifices can be catheterized, the catheters externalized, and the pelvis packed, leaving bladder reconstruction to be performed at a more suitable time, after appropriate resuscitation. Urethral and genital injuries are also amenable to damage control approaches, generally involving tube diversion, placement of moistened dressings, and tissue preservation until definitive reconstruction after appropriate resuscitation.

NONTRAUMATIC UROLOGIC EMERGENCIES

Within the field of urology are several emergent conditions, although not due to external violence, that represent true emergencies, some of which are life-threatening. These urologic emergencies include obstructed upper tract UTI, hematuria with urinary retention due to blood clots, and the acute scrotum—specifically testicular torsion, priapism, and Fournier gangrene. Some of these conditions have been discussed in other sections of this chapter (Fournier gangrene and obstructed upper tract UTI); the remainder are covered in this discussion.

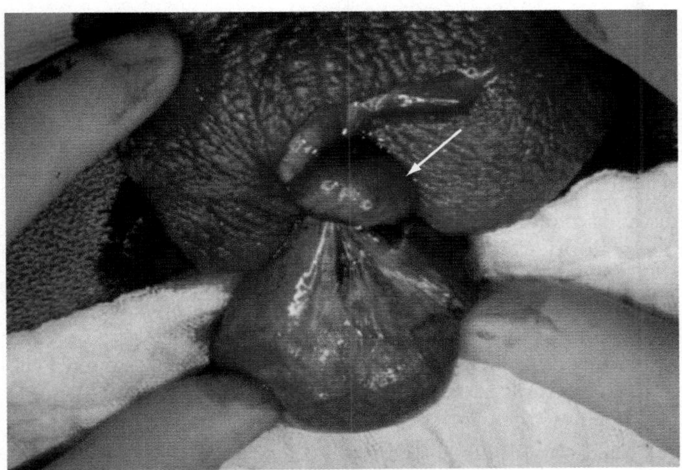

FIG. 74.26 Testicular torsion. Exploration through a transverse scrotal incision demonstrates the twisted cord *(top)*. Note the degree of edema, erythema, and ecchymosis present after several hours of torsion.

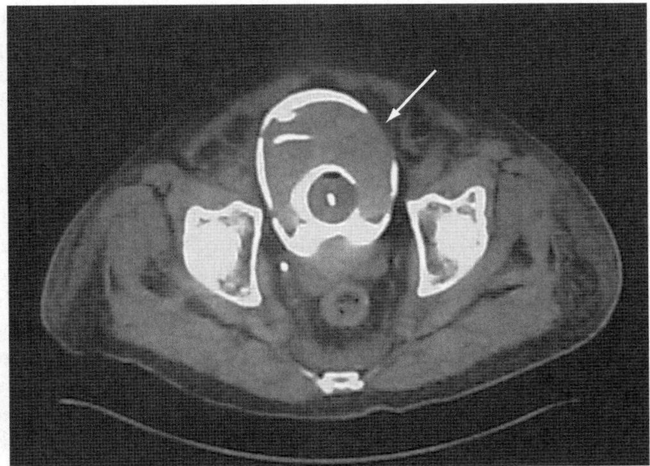

FIG. 74.27 Computed tomography scan of the pelvis with cystography in a patient with urinary clot retention caused by chronic hemorrhagic cystitis after radiation therapy for prostate cancer. A clot may be seen surrounding the Foley catheter balloon, with instilled contrast material outlining the balloon and intact bladder wall.

Testicular Torsion

The most urgent cause of the acute scrotum is testicular torsion. Testicular torsion occurs when arterial blood supply is compromised by a twist of the spermatic cord, creating occlusion of the spermatic cord and loss of vascular supply. In the normal anatomic arrangement, the inferior aspect of the testicle is attached to the scrotum by the gubernaculum, preventing rotation of the testicle within the scrotum. When torsion occurs, the testicle is subjected to warm ischemia; without reversal of the occluded blood supply, irreversible damage begins as soon as four hours and is complete by 8 to 12 hours. Although testicular torsion is most common in adolescent males, it may occur in any age group from neonate to adult men. As many other conditions may result in the so-called acute scrotum, a high index of suspicion is necessary on the part of the treating physician to ensure rapid diagnosis and treatment. Differential diagnosis includes trauma, epididymitis, incarcerated hernia, and torsion of the appendix testis or appendix epididymis. Diagnosis is strongly suspected on the basis of history and physical examination. Classic historical findings include sudden onset of intense unilateral scrotal pain, unrelated to trauma, that may be associated with nausea and vomiting. The most consistent physical examination finding is loss of the cremasteric reflex of the testicle; however, in an acute setting, this may be difficult to elicit. The best confirmatory radiologic study is color Doppler ultrasound of the scrotum, which shows absence of arterial flow to the testis in torsion. In patients with suspected testicular torsion, there is no need to delay scrotal exploration to obtain imaging or further laboratory evaluation.

Treatment of testicular torsion involves surgical exploration through a midline or transverse scrotal incision with inspection of the testis with detorsion of the spermatic cord, if present (Fig. 74.26). For testes that are deemed to be viable, suture orchiopexy or fixation to the interior scrotal wall is performed, followed by a similar orchiopexy on the contralateral side at the same setting to prevent contralateral torsion. Because of the important medicolegal considerations in these cases, urgent exploration is still indicated even in patients who present with a suspected late torsion (e.g., several days of fixed swelling, firmness). Many times, it is difficult to know exactly how long complete ischemia has been present and whether there is still a potentially viable testicle.

Gross Hematuria With Urinary Retention From Blood Clots

Most patients who have hematuria present with either microscopic hematuria or episodic gross hematuria. However, in a subset of patients, onset of gross hematuria is rapid with significant blood loss and development of blood clots within the bladder. This problem is exacerbated in patients who are receiving chronic anticoagulation for underlying cardiovascular disease processes. The blood clots are organized into larger masses; the patient may not be able to expel the clot, leading to urinary retention and a potential surgical emergency (Fig. 74.27). Other causes of significant vesical hemorrhage include postoperative bleeding after TURP or transurethral resection of bladder tumor (TURBT), radiation cystitis, pelvic trauma, upper tract arteriovenous fistula, and iliac arterial fistula to the ureter.

It is difficult to judge the amount of blood that is being lost from the urinary tract with gross hematuria because only a small amount of blood mixed with urine will darken the bladder efflux. If, however, copious amounts of clot are evacuated from the bladder, one should suspect at least moderate blood loss and monitor the patient with vital signs and hemoglobin measurements. If bleeding from these events causes symptomatic anemia, the patient may require multiple urgent blood transfusions. In the patient with a significant amount of blood clot in the bladder, it will be necessary to place a large-bore irrigation catheter (in the adult, often 20 Fr–26 Fr) and adequately irrigate the clots from the bladder using normal saline irrigation. Special hematuria catheters are designed to allow large-volume irrigation and clot removal, but if this is unsuccessful, the patient may require urgent operative cystoscopy to evacuate the clot and to identify and fulgurate any bleeding source. Typically, this involves rigid cystoscopy with a large working sheath or resectoscope sheath and irrigation performed with a piston syringe or special evacuation devices (Ellik evacuator). After clot evacuation and fulguration, a large three-way catheter is left in place to run continuous irrigation to prevent a recurrent episode of clot retention. Upper tract clot formation may produce a so-called clot colic, with renal pain similar to that experienced from passage of a renal calculus. Supportive care and, in some cases, stent insertion may be helpful to address the underlying problem. If unexplained, significant, gross hematuria occurs after minor trauma, one should suspect an underlying abnormality of the urinary tract, such as a neoplasm, congenital anomaly, or arteriovenous malformation.

Priapism

Priapism is a prolonged, painful penile erection that occurs in the absence of sexual arousal or stimulation. Priapism is typically divided into ischemic and nonischemic priapism. Important causes of ischemic priapism include sickle cell disease or other blood dyscrasias and certain types of drug or medication use, especially drugs for penile erection and hematologic malignant disease. Nonischemic priapism is the pelvic or genital trauma that results in arteriovenous fistula of the penile circulation. Priapism may resolve spontaneously, but if it persists longer than four hours, measures should be taken to reverse the process in most cases. Patients with priapism that lasts longer than 12 hours may develop irreversible damage to the penile vascular structure and long-term ED.

Evaluation in cases of ischemic priapism is centered on detailed history for risk factors, corporal blood gas analysis, and color Doppler ultrasound of the corpora cavernosa. Nonischemic priapism is evaluated similarly; however, aspirated blood has an arterial appearance and arterial blood gas parameters.

Ischemic priapism is managed with initial needle aspiration of the corpora cavernosa and irrigation with saline. In patients who do not respond to this step, needle aspiration is repeated with the injection of small, dilute doses of an α-adrenergic agonist substance, such as dilute phenylephrine. For patients who fail to respond to these measures, various shunting procedures can be performed to create shunts between the corpus cavernosum and other vascular structures, like the corpus spongiosum, to induce blood flow. For priapism related to sickle cell disease, medical treatment of the sickle crisis (e.g., hydration, oxygenation, pain management, and addressing hemoglobin and transfusion status) with hematology support is a mainstay of therapy to resolve priapism. For nonischemic priapism, there is no role for aspiration or irrigation of the erection as this is the result of an abnormality of the vascular system. Compression of the perineum or other injury site can be performed as an initial maneuver. If this fails, the next treatment step is usually superselective angioembolization to occlude the arteriovenous fistula with reversible agents, such as autologous blood clots or Gelfoam. It is important that the general surgeon consult with the urologist about treatment because corporal fibrosis and loss of erectile function are risks that increase with significant delays in therapy.

UROLOGIC ONCOLOGY

Urologic malignant neoplasms account for a significant disease burden in adults in the United States. Cancers of the genitourinary system encompass the full spectrum of malignant neoplasms and are of some of the most common (prostate) and rare (penile) cancers in the United States. Of the 12 most common cancers diagnosed annually in the United States, three are urologic in origin: prostate, bladder, and kidney. Low-stage cancers are typically managed with extirpative surgery or therapeutic radiation. Urologic cancers may involve adjacent viscera, vasculature, and soft tissue and body wall structures so that additional surgical expertise is necessary to complete the extirpative surgery and to support reconstructive efforts. As is the case with other malignant neoplasms, cancers of the genitourinary system are often managed with a multidisciplinary approach. The major anatomic types of urologic cancers are discussed in this section, with a focus on the essential basic background knowledge, the fundamental therapeutic approaches for various stages of cancer presentation, and the basic outcomes for different tumor types.

Renal Cancer

Renal cell carcinoma, the most common type of renal malignant disease, accounts for 2% to 3% of all adult malignant neoplasms.[45] The majority (>50%) of renal malignant neoplasms are now diagnosed incidentally by cross-sectional imaging or ultrasound evaluation of other nonspecific complaints. Historically, renal cell carcinoma was diagnosed only at an advanced stage because of its location within the retroperitoneum. The classic triad of renal cell carcinoma (flank pain, gross hematuria, and palpable abdominal mass) is now seen in less than 5% of patients. Despite this increase in asymptomatic diagnoses, 30% of patients present with metastatic disease.[46] Other symptoms on advanced presentation include hemorrhage, paraneoplastic syndrome, and symptoms of metastasis, such as pathologic fracture. Paraneoplastic syndromes are present in 20% of patients at diagnosis and include Stauffer syndrome (reversible hepatitis without liver metastasis), constitutional symptoms, anemia, polycythemia, and elevated inflammatory markers (erythrocyte sedimentation rate and C-reactive protein).[46] Renal cell carcinoma typically presents in the sixth to eighth decade of life and is more common in men. Risk factors for renal cell carcinoma include smoking, hypertension, obesity, acquired renal cystic disease (in patients with end-stage renal disease), and occupational exposures (aromatic hydrocarbons, asbestos, cadmium, and chemical and rubber industries).[45] These tumors typically arise in the proximal convoluted tubule or collecting duct within the renal parenchyma.[45]

Renal cell carcinoma is classified as follows: clear cell carcinoma, papillary renal cell carcinoma, chromophobe renal cell carcinoma, collecting duct carcinoma, and renal medullary carcinoma; this classification is based on microscopic appearance and cell of origin.[46] The genetics of these malignant neoplasms is fairly well described. The most common tumor histology, clear cell carcinoma, which is observed up to 85% of the time is the result of chromosome 3 abnormalities; papillary carcinoma is the result of aberrations of chromosome 7, 17, or Y.[46] In addition, clear cell carcinoma and papillary carcinoma are responsible for the two most common familial cancer syndromes, von Hippel–Lindau and hereditary papillary renal cell carcinoma, respectively. Most renal masses are malignant, and only 15% to 20% are benign; the two most common benign masses are oncocytoma and angiomyolipoma.[46]

A final consideration with renal neoplasms is cystic renal masses, which present diagnostic challenges. Depending on specific characteristics of renal cystic lesions, the risk of these lesions representing cystic malignant neoplasms must be considered. The Bosniak classification system describes cystic renal masses according to their malignant risk and CT appearance, ranging from category I (simple cysts, 0% risk of malignancy) to category IV (cysts associated with enhancing or solid elements, 90% risk of malignancy).[46] Category III and IV cysts are usually treated as representing cystic renal cell carcinomas.

Staging

Outcomes in renal cell carcinoma are directly tied to clinical stage at time of diagnosis. Evaluation and staging for renal cell carcinoma include history, physical examination, and laboratory testing. Evaluation for renal masses includes imaging of the primary

TABLE 74.2 Staging of kidney cancer.

Primary Tumor (T)	
TX	Primary tumor cannot be assessed
T0	No evidence of primary tumor
T1	Tumor 7 cm or less in greatest dimension, limited to the kidney
T1a	Tumor 4 cm or less in greatest dimension, limited to the kidney
T1b	Tumor more than 4 cm but not more than 7 cm in greatest dimension, limited to the kidney
T2	Tumor >7 cm in greatest dimension, limited to the kidney
T2a	Tumor >7 cm and ≤10 cm in greatest dimension, limited to the kidney
T2b	Tumor >10 cm in greatest dimension, limited to the kidney
T3	Tumor extends into major veins or perinephric tissues but not into the ipsilateral adrenal gland and not beyond Gerota fascia
T3a	Tumor grossly extends into the renal vein or its segmental (muscle-containing) branches, or tumor invades perirenal and/or renal sinus fat but not beyond Gerota fascia
T3b	Tumor grossly extends into the vena cava below the diaphragm
T3c	Tumor grossly extends into the vena cava above the diaphragm or invades the wall of the vena cava
T4	Tumor invades beyond Gerota fascia (including contiguous extension into the ipsilateral adrenal gland)
Regional Lymph Nodes (N)	
NX	Regional lymph nodes cannot be assessed
N0	No regional lymph node metastasis
N1	Metastasis in regional lymph node(s)
Distant Metastasis (M)	
M0	No distant metastasis
M1	Distant metastasis
Stage Grouping	
Stage I	T1 N0 M0
Stage II	T2 N0 M0
Stage III	T1 or T2 N1 M0
	T3 N0 or N1 M0
Stage IV	T4 Any N M0

From AJCC Cancer Staging Manual. In: Amin MB, Edge SB, Greene FL, et al, eds. 8th ed. Springer.

tumor, usually with a contrast-enhanced CT scan or MRI study of the abdomen and pelvis, as well as chest imaging, typically chest radiography. Also, based on clinical suspicion or abnormal results of laboratory studies, bone and brain imaging is performed. A key aspect of abdominal CT or MRI is evaluation of the renal vein and inferior vena cava as locally advanced renal cell carcinoma commonly forms tumor thrombus in these structures. The TNM staging system is listed in Table 74.2.[47] Histologic grading is based on the Fuhrman nuclear grading system on a scale of I to IV.

Management

The management of renal cell carcinoma has evolved in recent years. Historically, renal cell carcinoma was a surgical disease, and patients diagnosed with any renal mass underwent total radical nephrectomy. Now, select patients may undergo renal biopsy and active surveillance protocols. In the past, renal biopsies were fraught with high false-negative rates and low accuracy. Contemporary series show an accuracy rate of more than 90% in experienced centers with low complications and no reported incidence of tumor seeding given use of core-needle biopsy technique.[46] Those patients who are appropriate for renal biopsy are patients considered for either active surveillance or renal ablation therapy. Active surveillance protocols have been developed for patients with incidentally diagnosed, small (<2 cm) renal masses and those patients who would not tolerate extirpative or ablative therapy.[46] The natural history of small renal masses is a tendency to grow slowly, on average 0.5 cm/year, and they do not metastasize. Patients assigned to surveillance protocols undergo imaging every 6 months; once mass size stability is observed, this interval is extended to 6 to 12 months.[46] Small renal masses (<3 cm) can be considered for percutaneous, laparoscopic, or open ablation using cryotherapy or radiofrequency energy.[45] This treatment should be considered more for patients with significant medical comorbidities and less often in healthy patients.

For organ confined renal tumors, extirpative surgery is the standard approach. For renal cancer with limited metastatic disease, cytoreductive nephrectomy has been an option with possible resection of metastatic lesions. However, the benefits seen with new systemic therapies are changing this paradigm. Minimally invasive surgery, both robotic and laparoscopic techniques are standard for most renal lesions. The trend in extirpative surgery is to perform nephron sparing or partial nephrectomy for most T1 tumors. Partial nephrectomy is equivalent to radical nephrectomy in this tumor stage and should be considered for all patients with a T1a tumor and most with T1b tumors. Partial nephrectomy surgery may be straightforward in dealing with small, well-encapsulated, superficial, exophytic lesions or complex in dealing with larger, central lesions that involve the renal hilar structures. For partial nephrectomy, a negative margin should be obtained with the parenchymal resection, and only a few millimeters of normal parenchyma around the tumor are considered necessary. The general principles for partial nephrectomy include achievement of a negative surgical margin, identification and suturing of significant segmental renal vessel branches, and collecting system repair when the collecting system is entered or partially resected. To assist with blood loss, atraumatic vascular clamping of the renal artery and surface cooling of the kidney with iced saline slush are effective. When laparoscopic or robotic approaches are used for partial nephrectomy, local hypothermia is not possible; therefore, rapid tumor resection and clamp times of less than 25 minutes are employed. Tissue sealants, hemostatic agents, and absorbable mesh reconstruction of the kidney are all useful techniques to aid in hemostasis of a partial nephrectomy in the open surgical, laparoscopic, or robotic setting.[46]

Radical nephrectomy is performed in patients with large or multifocal tumors and those patients in whom a partial nephrectomy is not technically feasible. The primary long-term risk in this surgery is acute and chronic decline in renal function. In comparison to partial nephrectomy, radical nephrectomy has a lower rate of complications. The adrenal gland is no longer removed with radical nephrectomy except in cases of obvious tumor involvement as the rate of synchronous involvement is less than 10%. Typically, radical nephrectomy is performed by either a laparoscopic or an open approach. Standard incisions for radical nephrectomy include anterior subcostal, flank, chevron, and midline. Regardless of approach, dissection of the renal pedicle with ligation of a renal artery must precede vein ligation to prevent swelling and dangerous bleeding from the kidney. The entire Gerota fascial envelope, containing the perinephric fat as a margin around the kidney parenchyma and tumor, is excised intact. The ureter is ligated and divided where convenient.[45] A regional lymph node dissection may be performed with a radical nephrectomy, although, on the basis of most evidence, it is more helpful as a staging and prognostic procedure than as a therapeutic one.[48]

Thermal ablation, which is an option for T1a renal masses smaller than 3 cm in diameter, was developed in an effort to improve patient procedural tolerance and reduce the complications from partial nephrectomy while still preserving function. Radiofrequency and cryoablation have been the most widely investigated and integrated into clinical practice, and oncologic outcomes are similar for both approaches even though long-term data for thermal ablation is still pending. Thermal ablation can be accomplished through open, laparoscopic, or percutaneous (most common) approaches. Thermal ablation can also be repeated if persistent viable malignancy is suspected.

For patients with locally advanced or metastatic disease, immunotherapy and targeted therapy (drugs with action on vascular endothelial growth factor and mammalian target of rapamycin) are used in a neoadjuvant or adjuvant setting. Overall organ-confined disease has an 80% to 100% 5-year survival in T1 tumors and a 50% to 80% 5-year survival in T2 disease.[46] Advanced disease has a grim prognosis of 0% to 20% 5-year survival.[46]

Several adjuvant kidney cancer trials have explored the potential benefit of systemic therapies after surgical resection of high-risk disease and has shown some benefit. On the other hand, in patients with metastatic disease, drugs that target vascular endothelial growth factor (VEGF) and mammalian target of rapamycin (mTOR) have improved patient outcomes and represent the mainstay of treatment. In current practice, patients with good risk clear cell renal cell carcinoma receive sunitinib or pazopanib and those with poor risk receive temsirolimus. The landscape of systemic therapy for metastatic renal cell carcinoma is rapidly evolving and options range from the more established targeted therapies to the newer regimens that include immunotherapies. In patients who relapse, a multitude of drugs that target mTOR (everolimus), VEGF receptor (axitinib), or programmed cell death protein 1 (PD-1, nivolumab) are being studied in clinical trials.[45,47]

Bladder Cancer

Urothelial malignant disease can arise anywhere in the upper or lower collecting system, but the most common site is the bladder. The entire upper and lower urinary tracts, renal collecting system through the distal urethra, are lined with surface epithelium called urothelium. The urothelium has a variable thickness of three to six cell layers, and transitional cell carcinoma arises from the basal cell layer. Bladder cancer is the fifth most common adult malignant neoplasm diagnosed in the United States and is more common in men than in women, in part, related to impaired bladder emptying in men with increasing age.[49] The tumor arises most frequently in the eighth decade of life, and men older than 70 years have a 3.7% probability for development of bladder cancer.[49] The multiple risk factors for development of bladder cancer include tobacco smoke, arsenic, chronic infections and inflammatory conditions (e.g., schistosomiasis), and occupational exposures (such as arylamines and aromatic hydrocarbons). The most common presenting symptom in bladder cancer is hematuria, microscopic in 1% to 11% and gross in 13% to 35%.[49] Importantly, a single episode of gross hematuria, especially in smokers, can carry a significant risk of cancer and warrants a full workup. Microscopic hematuria, on one urinalysis microscopy, qualifies a patient for a workup, but the risk of cancer depends greatly on other risk factors and patient factors. The other presenting symptom is irritative voiding—frequency, urgency, and dysuria—in the absence of infection on urine culture.

TABLE 74.3 Staging of urothelial cancer.

Primary Tumor (T)	
TX	Primary tumor cannot be assessed
T0	No evidence of primary tumor
Ta	Noninvasive papillary carcinoma
Tis	Carcinoma in situ: "flat tumor"
T1	Tumor invades subepithelial connective tissue
T2	Tumor invades muscularis propria
pT2a	Tumor invades superficial muscularis propria (inner half)
pT2b	Tumor invades deep muscularis propria (outer half)
T3	Tumor invades perivesical tissue:
pT3a	Microscopically
pT3b	Macroscopically (extravesical mass)
T4	Tumor invades any of the following: prostatic stroma, seminal vesicles, uterus, vagina, pelvic wall, abdominal wall
T4a	Tumor invades prostatic stroma, uterus, vagina
T4b	Tumor invades pelvic wall, abdominal wall
Regional Lymph Nodes (N)	
Regional lymph nodes include both primary and secondary drainage regions. All other nodes above the aortic bifurcation are considered distant lymph nodes.	
NX	Lymph nodes cannot be assessed
N0	No lymph node metastasis
N1	Single regional lymph node metastasis in the true pelvis (hypogastric, obturator, external iliac, or presacral lymph node)
N2	Multiple regional lymph node metastasis in the true pelvis (hypogastric, obturator, external iliac, or presacral lymph node metastasis)
N3	Lymph node metastasis to the common iliac lymph nodes
Distant Metastasis (M)	
M0	No distant metastasis
M1	Distant metastasis

From AJCC Cancer Staging Manual. In: Amin MB, Edge SB, Greene FL, et al, eds. 8th ed. Springer.

Bladder cancer is separated into nonmuscle invasive bladder cancer (NMIBCs) and muscle invasive bladder cancer (MIBC), and each arises from different molecular pathways and has different treatments and outcomes. Urothelial tumors that have not invaded the detrusor muscle are termed NMIBCs. Approximately 70% of patients who present with bladder cancer will be diagnosed with NMBIC, which includes T stages Tis (carcinoma in situ), Ta, and T1.[50] The other 20% to 40% of will either present or progress to MIBC includes stage T2 or higher bladder cancer at diagnosis.[51,52] TNM staging is included in Table 74.3[51]; the T stage at diagnosis, specifically nonmuscle invasive (T1 or less) or muscle invasive (T2 or higher), is highly predictive of long-term outcome and survival. Ta disease refers to papillary tumors, with involvement of only the mucosa. T1 tumors involve the lamina propria, and T2 disease involves the detrusor muscle. Higher stages of the local tumor reflect involvement of perivesical fat or adjacent organs.[51] Tumors are graded on the basis of histologic appearance from papilloma to high grade.[49]

Nonmuscle Invasive Bladder Cancer

Patients who are suspected of having bladder cancer should undergo a thorough evaluation, which includes history, physical examination, basic laboratory tests, upper urinary tract imaging (preferably contrast-enhanced cross-sectional imaging), and office cystoscopy. If bladder cancer is present, characteristic flat, papillary, or large, sessile, aggressive-appearing masses will be present on the urothelial surface of the bladder. NMIBCs typically appear as flat (carcinoma in situ) or papillary (Ta or T1) lesions.[49] An adjunct test for identification of bladder cancer is use of urine cytology, which is either as voided or bladder wash at the time of cystoscopy. Urine cytology is most sensitive for high-grade tumors and can be equivocal or nondiagnostic in the setting of low-grade NMIBCs. Adjunct urine tumor markers exist but are not recommended on consensus guidelines because of cost and low specificity.[50]

Any tumor identified in the bladder should be fully resected by TURBT. TURBT is diagnostic, by providing pathologic analysis, tumor staging by identification (if present) of muscle invasion, and potentially therapeutic in treatment of noninvasive disease. TURBT is performed through a surgical endoscope, called a resectoscope, and uses either monopolar or bipolar energy to shave the tumor from the bladder wall alongside continuous irrigation.[49] At the time of TURBT, patients should undergo a bimanual examination of the bladder. A palpable mass after TURBT represents extravesical extension (T3) of tumor, and, if the lesion is fixed, it raises the possibility of pelvic side wall or adjacent organ invasion (T4). Any patient identified with high-grade tumors with any possibility of incomplete first resection or absence of muscle in the initial resection should undergo repeated TURBT within 2 to 6 weeks.[50]

Immediate intravesical chemotherapy refers to intravesical administration of an antineoplastic agent within 24 hours of TURBT, which has been shown to reduce the tumor recurrence by 35%. The agent most commonly used for this purpose is Mitomycin C with many centers transitioning to gemcitabine for better patient safety.[50] In a patient with low- or intermediate- risk bladder cancer, a clinician should consider administration of a single postoperative instillation of intravesical chemotherapy.[49] Six weeks after TURBT, patients with carcinoma in situ or NMIBC with high risk for progression or recurrence or CIS should receive intravesical therapy with either immunotherapy or chemotherapeutic agents. Standard immunotherapy for NMIBC consists of serial bacille Calmette-Guérin (BCG) intravesical instillations for induction and periodic maintenance therapy. Intravesical BCG significantly decreases the invasion and progression rate for NMIBCs, compared with transurethral resection alone. Maintenance BCG instillations reduce the risk of recurrence and progression and are given at variable intervals for periods of 1 to 3 years.[50] If a patient's cancer is unresponsive to BCG and the tumor recurs, there are many salvage intravesical therapies being investigated but the gold standard remains radical cystectomy. Periodic surveillance by office cystoscopy and upper tract imaging is mandatory in these patients as 60% to 80% of these tumors recur, and in higher grade tumors, 10% to 20% progress to higher stage or muscle invasive tumors.[50] Enhanced cystoscopy using blue light technology with hexaminolevulinate or narrow-band imaging can improve detection and lower recurrence rates.[49]

Muscle Invasive Bladder Cancer

The majority of patients who present with MIBC have invasive disease at diagnosis; and it has a much higher risk of progression and metastasis.[49] These cancers are highly lethal and are the cause of death in the vast majority of patients within two years of diagnosis without aggressive treatment. Approximately 70% of patients present with localized disease, while 33% have regional spread and 5% have distant metastasis at the time of diagnosis.[52] MIBC is typically urothelial cell carcinoma, but other histopathologic types occur, including squamous cell carcinoma, adenocarcinoma, and small cell carcinoma, with potentially worse outcomes. MIBC should be staged in a similar fashion to NMIBC, with cross-sectional imaging of the abdomen and pelvis, but consideration should be given to chest CT rather than plain radiography. Despite adequate staging, 40% of patients are understaged at diagnosis and have extravesical disease on the final pathologic specimen.[52]

Management. Standard management of MIBC is radical cystoprostatectomy in men and cystectomy in women, combined with neoadjuvant cisplatin-based chemotherapy for all eligible patients. In the male patient, radical cystectomy involves the removal of the entire urinary bladder *en bloc* with the perivesical fat, prostate, seminal vesicles, and pelvic lymph nodes. In the female patient, radical cystectomy typically involves *en bloc* removal of the female pelvic viscera (uterus, cervix, fallopian tubes, and the anterior vagina), although preservation of these structures may at times be considered, depending on the details of the case. Extended lymph node dissection is performed at the same setting and includes removal of the external and internal iliac lymph nodes, common iliac lymph nodes to the aortic bifurcation, and presacral lymph nodes. Improved survival is associated with extended pelvic lymph node dissection at the time of radical cystectomy. Perioperative complication rates are high, and more than 60% of patients undergoing radical cystectomy and extended pelvic lymph node dissection have at least one complication within 90 days of surgery.[52] Because of the high rate of extravesical extension at the time of radical cystectomy, and based on level 1 evidence, neoadjuvant chemotherapy is employed with overall and recurrence-free survival benefits. Typical regimens for neoadjuvant chemotherapy include methotrexate, vinblastine, doxorubicin [Adriamycin], and cisplatin (MVAC) or gemcitabine and cisplatin (GC). The use of neoadjuvant chemotherapy improves overall survival by 5% to 7%.[53] Adjuvant chemotherapy is offered to patients with high-risk pathologic features from surgery with no evidence of metastasis, and retrospective data support its use, with prospective trials currently in progress. A challenge of relying on adjuvant chemotherapy is the recovery after cystectomy can often delay timely initiation of therapy.[53] Following cystectomy, patients with organ-confined, node-negative disease have the best overall disease-specific survival at 5 and 10 years at 85% and 60%, respectively. Neoadjuvant chemotherapy achieves a pT0 rate twice as often as surgery alone, and this confers a dramatic improved survival as well. Patients with extravesical disease have 5-year disease-specific survival in the 50% range while patients with node positive disease who have undergone a thorough lymph node dissection have a 30% 5-year disease-specific survival.[52]

The selection of the type of urinary diversion after radical cystectomy must take into account any history of pelvic irradiation, presence of renal insufficiency, liver function abnormalities, and mechanical tasks for which the patient will be responsible. There are various options for urinary diversion, including ileal conduit, orthotopic bladder substitution with anastomosis to the native urethra (neobladder), and more complex forms of cutaneous catheterizable reservoirs with continence mechanisms. No randomized study has shown one type of urinary diversion to be superior to any other, and the decision is usually directed by the patient's preference or the surgeon's choice. There is an extensive and complex history involving the use of intestinal segments in the urinary tract for urinary diversion after cystectomy and in other reconstructive settings. The surgeon should be familiar with the metabolic, mechanical, and other risk factors associated with the use of intestinal segments in the reconstructed urinary tract, including electrolyte abnormalities, bone demineralization, mucus production, stone formation, chronic infection, diarrhea, vitamin B_{12} deficiency, and increased cancer risk.[52]

Prostate Cancer

Prostate cancer is the most common cancer diagnosed in men and the third most common cancer diagnosed in the United States, behind breast and lung cancer, with approximately 240,000 men diagnosed annually resulting in approximately 30,000 deaths.[54] Prostate cancer is an adenocarcinoma and arises from the glandular structures within the prostatic parenchyma. Most new prostate cancer cases are diagnosed in men 60 years of age and older, are low grade and low stage, and are diagnosed by routine screening.[55] Screening for prostate cancer is performed with the blood test PSA, a serine protease, and DRE. The most controversial aspect of prostate cancer is screening and determining which patients require treatment. The goal of prostate cancer screening is to detect potentially lethal cancer at an early, treatable stage and to intervene with intent to cure. Because of the controversy surrounding the recent U.S. Preventive Services Task Force (USPSTF) recommendation against screening for prostate cancer in 2012, the AUA released its own guidelines for screening in 2013. The USPSTF released revised guidelines in 2018.[55] These recommendations are for screening in men aged 55 to 69 years to be a joint decision between the physician and the patient, with recognition that the mortality of prostate cancer is 1 in 1000 men screened per decade, and a routine screening interval to occur every 2 years.[55] More intensive evaluation should be considered in men with a strong family history and genetic predisposition and who are of African American race. Routine screening is not routinely recommended in men aged 40 to 54 years and in men older than 70 years or younger than 40 years.[56] Furthermore, screening should not be performed in men with a life expectancy of less than 10 to 15 years.

Evaluation

Patients who have either an elevated total PSA level or abnormal findings on DRE or both undergo transrectal ultrasound (TRUS)–guided biopsy of the prostate. Additional serum and tissue tests and MRI imaging can be combined with basic data to risk-stratify a man before or after biopsy. The standard biopsy template involves 12 cores with a spring-loaded biopsy instrument; tissue is obtained from the base, mid, and apex regions, medially and laterally from the left and right sides. Prophylactic antibiotics are routinely administered, and cleansing enemas are advised. When feasible, patients are asked to stop anticoagulants to help prevent bleeding complications. Common adverse events that follow TRUS biopsy include rectal bleeding, gross hematuria, and hematospermia, all of which are usually self-limited. Fever and urinary infection and retention occur in less than 5% of patients; bacteremia occurs, but it occurs in less than 1% to 3% of patients.[57]

Prostate cancer is diagnosed histologically by the Gleason grading system, which evaluates the level of abnormality in the patterns of the glandular architecture of the prostate in comparison to normal. The grading system is based on a scale of 1 to 5, with 1 being the most well-differentiated and 5 being the least well-differentiated. In the modern PSA-based screening era, prostate cancers have a Gleason grade minimum of 3 with a sum of 6 or greater, and the majority of newly diagnosed cancers are Gleason 3+3. Patients diagnosed with prostate cancer are risk stratified on the basis of PSA level at time of diagnosis, clinical stage based on DRE, and Gleason sum score on the prostate biopsy.[54] Patients with intermediate- and high-risk cancers should undergo cancer staging, which in prostate cancer may include radionuclide bone scan to evaluate for bone metastasis and cross-sectional imaging of the abdomen and pelvis to evaluate for nodal metastasis (Table 74.4).[56]

TABLE 74.4 Staging of prostate cancer.

Primary Tumor (T)	
TX	Primary tumor cannot be assessed
T0	No evidence of primary tumor
T1	Clinically inapparent tumor neither palpable nor visible by imaging
T1a	Tumor incidental histologic finding in 5% or less of tissue resected
T1b	Tumor incidental histologic finding in more than 5% of tissue resected
T1c	Tumor identified by needle biopsy (for example, because of elevated PSA)
T2	Tumor confined within prostate
T2a	Tumor involves one half of one lobe or less
T2b	Tumor involves more than one half of one lobe but not both lobes
T2c	Tumor involves both lobes
T3	Tumor extends through the prostate capsule
T3a	Extracapsular extension (unilateral or bilateral)
T3b	Tumor invades seminal vesicle(s)
T4	Tumor is fixed or invades adjacent structures other than seminal vesicles, such as external sphincter, rectum, bladder, levator muscles, and/or pelvic wall
Lymph Nodes (N)	
NX	Regional lymph nodes were not assessed
N0	No regional lymph node metastasis
N1	Metastasis in regional lymph node(s)
Distant Metastasis (M)	
M0	No distant metastasis
M1	Distant metastasis
M1a	Nonregional lymph node(s)
M1b	Bone(s)
M1c	Other site(s) with or without bone disease

From AJCC Cancer Staging Manual. In: Amin MB, Edge SB, Greene FL, et al, eds. 8th ed. Springer.
PSA, Prostate-specific antigen.

Treatment

The treatment of prostate cancer has changed significantly during the last two decades. Shared decision-making takes into account cancer details, patient medical factors, life expectancy, and patient preference to determine the preferred mode of treatment. As most prostate cancer is low risk at diagnosis, many patients (up to 50% in certain centers) are now managed with active surveillance rather than with definitive therapy. In general, men with cancer of low clinical stage (<T2a), low grade (Gleason sum ≤6), low PSA (<10 ng/mL) and low volume on biopsy are candidates for active surveillance. Patients assigned to active surveillance protocols undergo DRE and PSA monitoring every 3 to 6 months, often incorporating MRI at certain intervals and repeated TRUS-guided prostate biopsies every 1 to 3 years. Patients with increase in Gleason sum or increase in tumor volume on biopsy typically shift to an active treatment plan, and up to 25% of men on active surveillance go on to definitive therapy within 5 years.

Prostate cancer can be treated with either radical surgical excision or definitive radiation therapy. Radical prostatectomy involves the surgical removal of the entire prostate and seminal vesicles with anastomosis of the urethral stump to the bladder neck. The extent of bilateral pelvic lymph node dissection is based on extent of disease and risk group of the cancer. For prostate cancer Gleason sum 7 or higher, at a minimum, the external iliac and obturator lymph nodes should be removed. Radical prostatectomy can be performed with an open, laparoscopic, or robotically assisted laparoscopic approach. The majority of cases in the United States are now performed by a robotic-assisted laparoscopic approach prostatectomy (RALP). The advantages of RALP have been reported to be decreased blood loss, shorter hospital stay, and quicker return to work. When it is technically feasible and oncologically appropriate, a nerve-sparing approach is used, which avoids injury to the cavernous nerves that run posterolateral along the prostate in the neurovascular bundle and mediate penile erection. Important landmarks for radical prostatectomy are the dorsal venous plexus anteriorly, bladder neck cephalad, prostatomembranous urethral junction distally, and rectal wall posteriorly. The correct plane of posterior dissection in radical prostatectomy is just posterior to the Denonvilliers fascia. The primary long-term risks of radical prostatectomy are urinary incontinence and ED. Because of the more recent adoption of RALP, most long-term survival series are based on historical open radical prostatectomy data. Ten-year cancer progression-free survival is approximately 85% for patients with organ-confined disease, approximately 60% to 70% for patients with extracapsular extension, and approximately 50% for patients with positive surgical margins.

Patients who do not desire or are not candidates for surgical extirpation may undergo local therapy with either intensity-modulated radiation therapy (IMRT) or brachytherapy. The typical treatment dose for IMRT-based prostate cancer therapy is 76 to 86 Gy. The most common form of brachytherapy is low-dose ultrasound-guided placement of iodine-125 or palladium-103 radioisotope sources into the prostate. Both treatments are commonly used for low-risk prostate cancer. Intermediate- and high-risk prostate cancer is typically treated with IMRT coupled with androgen deprivation therapy for up to 2 years. Low- and intermediate-risk prostate cancers have outcomes after radiation-based therapy similar to those of radical prostatectomy.

In advanced prostate cancer, the standard approach with androgen deprivation therapy may become ineffective, with clinical or PSA progression observed in spite of appropriate hormonal blockade. When castrate-resistant disease develops, second-line treatment includes antiandrogens, chemotherapy, and investigational agents. Other forms of treatment that can be considered for local treatment of prostate cancer include ablation, such as high-intensity frequency ultrasound and cryotherapy, and proton beam therapy, although long-term results for these modalities are still being reported. Focal therapy of discrete lesions is also being studied in clinical trials, but outcomes and surveillance with focal therapy are uncertain due to the commonly multifocal nature of prostate cancer. It remains a modality that should be confined to clinical trials.

After prostate cancer therapy, patients are monitored for post-treatment morbidities (e.g., continence, erectile function, voiding adequacy) and possible cancer recurrence. The latter involves PSA testing and potentially repeated metastatic evaluation, when indicated. Long-term follow-up for prostate cancer patients should continue at least 10 years, if not permanently, because very late recurrences can occur. If the PSA level becomes significantly detectable or is rising after definitive treatment, it may be appropriate to consider imaging of the anastomotic region, possibly with biopsy, and repeated metastatic evaluation to decide whether to proceed with local radiation therapy, androgen deprivation therapy, or observation. Dramatic improvements in prostate cancer survival have been achieved in the last two to three decades, due to improved detection with screening and major advances in systemic treatment of metastatic disease.

Testicular Cancer

Testicular cancer is an uncommon malignant neoplasm; in the United States, the incidence is 5/100,000 men.[58] Most cases of primary testicular cancer are germ cell origin (95%); the remainder are predominantly stromal (Leydig cell) or sex cord (Sertoli cell) tumors.[58] Any solid intratesticular mass is likely to represent a malignant germ cell tumor and is typically treated as such unless there is a strong suspicion to the contrary. Risk factors for testicular tumors include cryptorchidism, family history of testicular cancer, and intratubular germ cell neoplasia.

Germ cell–derived testicular tumors can be broadly divided into pure seminoma and mixed nonseminoma germ cell tumors (NSGCTs); the division is approximately 50% for each. The majority of seminomas histologically are classic (85%); the remainder are either anaplastic or spermatocytic seminoma.[58] NSGCTs can be divided into numerous histologic types: embryonal carcinoma, yolk sac or endodermal sinus tumors, choriocarcinoma, teratoma, and mixed germ cell tumors. Testicular malignant neoplasms are the most common tumors in men between the ages of 20 and 40 years.[58] Seminomas, however, present in the fourth or fifth decade of life, and spermatocytic seminomas may present in men older than 50 years.[58] The most common presenting complaint in men with testicular cancer is a painless testicular mass; however, it is not uncommon for men to present with symptoms of metastatic disease, including back pain, palpable abdominal mass, shortness of breath, or hemoptysis. In patients who present with a painless testicular mass, scrotal ultrasonography is the diagnostic study of choice. In addition to history, physical examination, and ultrasonography, patients with testicular tumors should have determination of specific tumor markers: α-fetoprotein, β-human chorionic gonadotropin, and lactate dehydrogenase. Each of these markers has a characteristic half-life, and they are important for initial cancer staging and surveillance.

Treatment

Initial treatment of suspected testicular tumor is radical inguinal orchiectomy, which involves removal of the testicle and spermatic cord at the level of the inguinal ring (Fig. 74.28). Because of the characteristic and well-described lymph drainage of the testicle, there is no role for trans-scrotal biopsy or orchiectomy. If the intrascrotal tissue planes are violated during orchiectomy, the lymphatic drainage can be altered, affecting future treatment. After radical inguinal orchiectomy, the patient should undergo disease staging, including cross-sectional, contrast-enhanced imaging of the abdomen and pelvis and chest imaging, either chest radiography in low-risk patients or cross-sectional chest imaging in patients with high-risk disease.

Clinical staging for testicular cancer includes primary tumor pathology, lymph and metastatic staging on imaging, and postorchiectomy serum tumor markers (Tables 74.5 and 74.6). The half-life of β-human chorionic gonadotropin is 24 to 36 hours, and the half-life of α-fetoprotein is 5 to 7 days; these levels should normalize in the absence of metastatic disease. Metastatic disease from testicular cancer follows a predictable retroperitoneal lymphatic spread, skipping the inguinal and pelvic nodal stations, given the testes' embryologic origin and corresponding vascular drainage. Choriocarcinoma is notorious for hematogenous spread early to distant sites. From the right testis, initial lymph node metastasis is to the

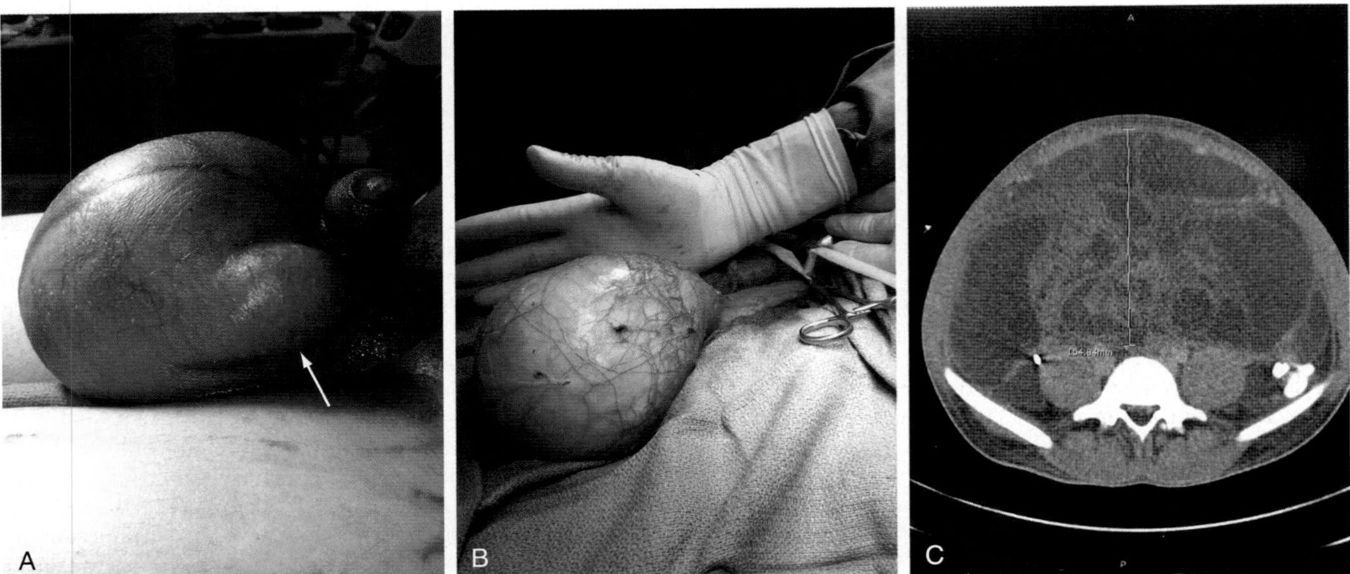

FIG. 74.28 Advanced testicular carcinoma. (A) Preoperative appearance of the scrotum in a patient with a large right testis tumor. The normal left testis is seen pushed cephalad by the right-sided mass. (B) Surgical exploration through right inguinal incision showing the right testis that has been dissected from the scrotum in an extravaginal plane still attached by the spermatic cord pedicle to the right. (C) Massive retroperitoneal lymphadenopathy in the same patient. Note that the descending colon is opacified with contrast material, but all other viscera are pushed cephalad so that no small intestine is seen in this image. The patient was managed with primary chemotherapy followed by retroperitoneal lymphadenectomy for the residual mass.

infrarenal interaortocaval nodes, paracaval nodes, and para-aortic nodes; on the left, the para-aortic nodes and then interaortocaval nodes. Retroperitoneal lymph nodes are the primary metastatic site in more than 70% of patients with metastatic testicular cancer.[58] If the patient has had prior groin or pelvic surgery, the natural lymphatic distributions may be altered and the metastatic pattern may be unpredictable, potentially leading to involvement of the inguinal or pelvic nodes. Distant metastases are typically seen to the lung, liver, brain, bone, kidney, and adrenal gland.

Second-line treatment is directed by tumor histology and lymph node staging. Further treatment may consist of regular surveillance, retroperitoneal radiation therapy, retroperitoneal lymph node dissection (RPLND), systemic chemotherapy, or a multimodal therapy approach. The treatment decisions are complex, often at the direction of an institutional tumor board, but several general principles apply:

- For seminoma stage IA and IB disease, treatment options include surveillance, radiotherapy to the regional (para-aortic) lymph nodes (20 Gy), and one or two cycles of carboplatin-based chemotherapy.[59]
- For seminoma stage IIA and IIB, radiotherapy of the retroperitoneal lymph nodes is standard therapy; for stage IIC or III, platinum-based chemotherapy is standard therapy.[59]
- For NSGCT stage I disease, the options include surveillance, primary RPLND, or cisplatin-based chemotherapy.[59]
- For NSGCT stage IIA, either primary RPLND (in patients with normal levels of tumor markers) or three or four cycles of cisplatin-based chemotherapy is standard; for stage IIB, three or four cycles of cisplatin-based chemotherapy is standard, followed by RPLND or surveillance.[59]
- For NSGCT Stage III, treatment consists of cisplatin-based chemotherapy and when tumor markers normalize, perform RPLND.

RPLND involves removal of all lymph nodes in the retroperitoneum from the renal vessels to the aortic bifurcation. An appropriate RPLND should include the lymph tissue surrounding the great vessels and division of the appropriate lumbar vessels to ensure thorough dissection using the split-and-roll technique. The most challenging RPLNDs are after chemotherapy, when the retroperitoneal tissues may be fibrotic or desmoplastic and adherent to the inferior vena cava, aorta, bowel, and mesentery. RPLND is template driven, and the appropriate levels and location of tissue excision are well described. Following the appropriate templates, the sympathetic nerve chain should be uninjured, allowing antegrade ejaculation. Extensive dissection in this territory often induces an autonomic reaction with persistent tachycardia, which may last for an extended period (4–6 weeks).

Many patients undergoing RPLND will have been exposed to bleomycin chemotherapy, which requires meticulous intraoperative anesthetic management because of the exquisite sensitivity of these patients to elevated oxygen exposure; often, the anesthetic is run essentially on room air ventilation in these cases.

Patients should be made aware of the potential impact of radiation, chemotherapy, or RPLND on the ability to ejaculate and on spermatogenesis. It is essential that patients be offered sperm cryopreservation after orchiectomy and before therapies that could adversely affect their reproductive potential. In addition, patients should be made aware that radiation has the potential morbidity of delayed secondary malignant disease as high as 15% within 25 years of treatment.[58]

Curative treatment of testicular cancer is one of the great success stories of modern oncology. Overall, long-term survival for testicular cancer ranges from 98% to 99% for stage I seminoma or NSGCT.[58] In patients with stage II seminoma, radiotherapy yields survival of up to 100%, and stage II NSGCT standard treatments yield survival of 90% to 95%.[58] Even advanced disease, stage III seminoma, has an expected survival of more than 90%, and NSGCTs have long-term survivals of 80% to 90%.[58]

Given the high survival rates, late- or long-term toxicities of treatment must be monitored, including early cardiovascular disease and metabolic syndrome from chemotherapy and secondary malignancies as mentioned.

TABLE 74.5 Staging of testicular cancer.

Primary Tumor (T)	
pTX	Primary tumor cannot be assessed
pT0	No evidence of primary tumor
pTis	Intratubular germ cell neoplasia
pT1	Tumor limited to the testis and epididymis without lymphovascular invasion, may invade tunica albuginea but not tunica vaginalis
pT2	Tumor limited to the testis and epididymis with lymphovascular invasion or tumor involving the tunica vaginalis
pT3	Tumor invades the spermatic cord with or without lymphovascular invasion
pT4	Tumor invades the scrotum with or without lymphovascular invasion
Regional Lymph Nodes (Clinical) (N)	
NX	Regional lymph nodes cannot be assessed
N0	No regional lymph node metastasis
N1	Metastasis within one or more lymph nodes less than 2 cm
N2	Metastasis within one or more lymph nodes greater than 2 cm but less the 5 cm
N3	Metastasis within one or more lymph nodes greater than 5 cm
Regional Lymph Nodes (Pathologic) (N)	
NX	Regional lymph nodes cannot be assessed
N0	No regional lymph node metastasis
N1	Metastasis within 1–5 lymph nodes; all node masses less than 2 cm
N2	Metastasis within a lymph node greater than 2 cm but not greater than 5 cm or more than 5 lymph nodes involved, none greater than 5 cm and none demonstrating extranodal extension of tumor
N3	Metastasis within one or more lymph nodes greater than 5 cm in size
Distant Metastasis (M)	
MX	Distant metastasis cannot be assessed
M0	No distant metastasis
M1	Distant metastasis
M1a	Nonregional nodal or pulmonary metastasis
M1b	Distant metastasis at site other than nonregional lymph nodes or lung
Serum Tumor Markers (S)	
SX	Tumor markers not available or performed
S0	Tumor markers within normal limits
S1	LDH <1.5× normal, hCG <5000 IU/L, AFP <1000 ng/mL
S2	LDH 1.5-10× normal, hCG 5000–50,000 IU/L, AFP 1000–10,000 ng/mL
S3	LDH >10× normal, hCG >50,000 IU/L, AFP >10,000 ng/mL

From AJCC Cancer Staging Manual. In: Amin MB, Edge SB, Greene FL, et al, eds. 8th ed. Springer.
AFP, α-Fetoprotein; *hCG,* human chorionic gonadotropin; *LDH,* lactate dehydrogenase.

TABLE 74.6 Staging of testicular cancer.

	T	N	M	S
Stage I	pT1–4	N0	M0	SX
Stage IA	pT1	N0	M0	S0
Stage IB	pT2	N0	M0	S0
	pT3	N0	M0	S0
	pT4	N0	M0	S0
Stage IS	Any pT	N0	M0	S1–3
Stage II	Any pT	N1–3	M0	SX
Stage IIA	Any pT	N1	M0	S0–1
Stage IIB	Any pT	N2	M0	S0–1
Stage IIC	Any pT	N3	M0	S0–1
Stage III	Any pT	Any N	M1	SX
Stage IIIA	Any pT	Any N	M1a	S0–1
Stage IIIB	Any pT	N1–3	M0	S2
	Any pT	Any N	M1a	S2
Stage IIIC	Any pT	N1–3	M0	S3
	Any pT	Any N	M1a	S3
	Any pT	Any N	M1b	Any S

From AJCC Cancer Staging Manual. In: Amin MB, Edge SB, Greene FL, et al, eds. 8th ed. Springer.

SELECTED REFERENCES

Bhasin S, Cunningham GR, Hayes FJ, et al. Testosterone therapy in men with androgen deficiency syndromes: an Endocrine Society clinical practice guideline. *J Clin Endocrinol Metab.* 2010;95:2536–2559.

The most current reference on the management of male testosterone deficiency. Broad-based consensus statement on evaluation, management, and therapy options.

Brandes S, Coburn M, Armenakas N, et al. Diagnosis and management of ureteric injury: an evidence-based analysis. *BJU Int.* 2004;94:277–289.

This article is a classic reference from the first consensus panel discussing evaluation and management of ureteral injuries.

Carter HB, Albertsen PC, Barry MJ, et al. Early detection of prostate cancer: AUA guideline. *J Urol.* 2013;190:419–426.

The evidence-based response to the U.S. Preventive Services Task Force (USPSTF) recommendation to no longer screen men for prostate cancer. This article is a systematic critique of the literature used by the to give a grade D to the regular screening of prostate cancer.

Chapple C, Barbagli G, Jordan G, et al. Consensus statement on urethral trauma. *BJU Int.* 2004;93:1195–1202.

This article is a classic reference from the first consensus panel discussing evaluation and management of urethral injuries.

Gomez RG, Ceballos L, Coburn M, et al. Consensus statement on bladder injuries. *BJU Int.* 2004;94:27–32.

This article is a classic reference from the first consensus panel discussing evaluation and management of bladder injuries.

Gupta K, Hooton TM, Naber KG, et al. International clinical practice guidelines for the treatment of acute uncomplicated cystitis and pyelonephritis in women: a 2010 update by the Infectious Diseases Society of America and the European Society for Microbiology and Infectious Diseases. *Clin Infect Dis*. 2011;52:e103–e120.

This document represents the most current guideline for the diagnosis and treatment of outpatient or uncomplicated urinary tract infection in women.

Haylen BT, de Ridder D, Freeman RM, et al. An International Urogynecological Association (Iuga)/International Continence Society (ICS) joint report on the terminology for female pelvic floor dysfunction. *Neurourol Urodyn*. 2010;29:4–20.

This article is the most recent consensus guideline to standardize terminology, diagnosis, and management of pelvic floor dysfunction and incontinence.

Jarow J, Sigman M, Kolettis P, et al. The optimal evaluation of the infertile male. *AUA Best Practice Statement*. 2010:1–39.

This article represents the best recommendations for evaluation and diagnosis of the infertile male. The American Urological Association recommendations regarding specific aspects of the infertile male workup are highlighted throughout this manuscript, making it easily searchable.

Kozar RA, Crandall M, Shanmuganathan K, et al. Organ injury scaling 2018 update: spleen, liver, and kidney. *J Trauma Acute Care Surg*. 2018;85:1119–1122.

This reference represents the updated American Association for the Surgery of Trauma Organ Injury Scaling System for kidney injuries.

Moore EE, Shackford SR, Pachter HL, et al. Organ injury scaling: spleen, liver, and kidney. *J Trauma*. 1989;29:1664–1666.

This classic article describes injury grading in the urologic system.

Morey AF, Brandes S, Dugi 3rd DD, et al. Urotrauma: AUA guideline. *J Urol*. 2014;192:327–335.

The first edition of the urologic trauma guidelines by the American Urological Association provides the best evidence-based recommendations for the management of traumatic urologic injuries.

Morey AF, Metro MJ, Carney KJ, et al. Consensus on genitourinary trauma: external genitalia. *BJU Int*. 2004;94:507–515.

This article is a classic reference from the first consensus panel discussing evaluation and management of genital injuries.

Santucci RA, Wessells H, Bartsch G, et al. Evaluation and management of renal injuries: consensus statement of the renal trauma subcommittee. *BJU Int*. 2004;93:937–954.

This article is a classic reference from the first consensus panel discussing evaluation and management of renal injuries.

Smith 3rd TG, Coburn M. Damage control maneuvers for urologic trauma. *Urol Clin North Am*. 2013;40:343–350.

This reference represents the only literature on management of traumatic urologic injuries using damage control principles and organized by urologic organ systems.

REFERENCES

1. Anderson JK, Cadeddu JA. Surgical anatomy of the retroperitoneum, adrenals, kidneys, and ureters. In: Wein AJ, Kavoussi LR, Campbell MF, et al., eds. *Campbell-Walsh Urology*. 10th ed. Philadelphia, PA: Elsevier Saunders; 2012:3–32.
2. McNeil BK. Kidney, adrenal, ureter. American Urological Association. https://www.auanet.org/university/core_topic.cfm?coreid=59. Accessed August 7, 2015.
3. Kim IY, Clayton RV. Surgical renal anatomy. *AUA update series*. 2006;25:361–368.
4. Webster GD, Anoia E. Principles of ureteral reconstruction. In: Smith JA, Howards SS, Preminger GM, et al., eds. *Hinman's Atlas of Urologic Surgery*. 3rd ed. Philadelphia, PA: Elsevier Saunders; 2012:709–710.
5. Chung BI, Sommer G, Brooks JD. Anatomy of the lower urinary tract and male genitalia. In: Wein AJ, Kavoussi LR, Campbell MF, et al., eds. *Campbell-Walsh Urology*. 10th ed. Philadelphia, PA: Elsevier Saunders; 2012:33-72.
6. Smith PP. Lower urinary tract. American Urological Association. https://www.auanet.org/university/core_topic.cfm?coreid=131. Accessed December 18, 2014.
7. Walz J, Graefen M, Huland H. Basic principles of anatomy for optimal surgical treatment of prostate cancer. *World J Urol*. 2007;25:31–38.
8. Duffey B, Monga M. Principles of endoscopy. In: Wein AJ, Kavoussi LR, Campbell MF, et al., eds. *Campbell-Walsh Urology*. 10th ed. Philadelphia, PA: Elsevier Saunders; 2012:192–203.
9. Urinary tract infection. In: Litwin M, Saigal C, eds. *Urologic Diseases in America. U.S. Department of Health and Human Services, Public Health Service, National Institutes of Health, National Institute of Diabetes and Digestive and Kidney Diseases*. Washington, DC: U.S. Government Printing Office; 2019:366–404. NIH Publication 312-7865.
10. Gupta K, Hooton TM, Naber KG, et al. International clinical practice guidelines for the treatment of acute uncomplicated cystitis and pyelonephritis in women: a 2010 update by the Infectious Diseases Society of America and the European Society for Microbiology and Infectious Diseases. *Clin Infect Dis*. 2011;52:e103–e120.
11. Lin WR, Chen M, Hsu JM, et al. Emphysematous pyelonephritis: patient characteristics and management approach. *Urol Int*. 2014;93:29–33.

12. Sorensen MD, Krieger JN, Rivara FP, et al. Fournier's gangrene: management and mortality predictors in a population based study. *J Urol.* 2009;182:2742–2747.
13. Clemens JQ. Basic bladder neurophysiology. *Urol Clin North Am.* 2010;37:487–494.
14. Gormley A, Stoffel J, Kielb S. Neurogenic bladder. American Urological Association. https://www.auanet.org/university/core_topic.cfm?coreid=144. Accessed August 7, 2015.
15. Haylen BT, de Ridder D, Freeman RM, et al. An International Urogynecological Association (Iuga)/International Continence Society (ICS) joint report on the terminology for female pelvic floor dysfunction. *Neurourol Urodyn.* 2010;29:4–20.
16. Irwin DE, Kopp ZS, Agatep B, et al. Worldwide prevalence estimates of lower urinary tract symptoms, overactive bladder, urinary incontinence and bladder outlet obstruction. *BJU Int.* 2011;108:1132–1138.
17. Gormley EA, Lightner DJ, Burgio KL, et al. Diagnosis and treatment of overactive bladder (non-neurogenic) in adults: AUA/SUFU guideline. *J Urol.* 2012;188:2455–2463.
18. Dooley Y, Kenton K, Cao G, et al. Urinary incontinence prevalence: results from the National Health and Nutrition Examination Survey. *J Urol.* 2008;179:656–661.
19. Ford AA, Rogerson L, Cody JD, et al. Mid-urethral sling operations for stress urinary incontinence in women. *Cochrane Database Syst Rev.* 2015:CD006375.
20. McVary KT, Roehrborn CG, Avins AL, et al. Update on AUA guideline on the management of benign prostatic hyperplasia. *J Urol.* 2011;185:1793–1803.
21. Jarow J, Sigman M, Kolettis PN, et al. The optimal evaluation of the infertile male. *AUA Best Practice Statement.* 2010:1–39.
22. Jarow J, Sigman M, Kolettis P, et al. The evaluation of the azoospermic male. *AUA Best Practice Statement.* 2011:1–25.
23. Bacon CG, Mittleman MA, Kawachi I, et al. A prospective study of risk factors for erectile dysfunction. *J Urol.* 2006;176:217–221.
24. Crawford ED, Barqawi AB, O'Donnell C, et al. The association of time of day and serum testosterone concentration in a large screening population. *BJU Int.* 2007;100:509–513.
25. Bhasin S, Cunningham GR, Hayes FJ, et al. Testosterone therapy in men with androgen deficiency syndromes: an Endocrine Society clinical practice guideline. *J Clin Endocrinol Metab.* 2010;95:2536–2559.
26. Scales Jr CD, Smith AC, Hanley JM, et al. Prevalence of kidney stones in the United States. *Eur Urol.* 2012;62:160–165.
27. Miller NL, Evan AP, Lingeman JE. Pathogenesis of renal calculi. *Urol Clin North Am.* 2007;34:295–313.
28. Preminger GM, Tiselius HG, Assimos DG, et al. 2007 Guideline for the management of ureteral calculi. *J Urol.* 2007;178:2418–2434.
29. Lange JN, Mufarrij PW, Wood KD, et al. Metabolic evaluation and medical management of the calcium stone former. *AUA Update Series.* 2012;25.
30. Weizer AZ, Zhong P, Preminger GM. Shock wave lithotripsy: current technology and evolving concepts. *AUA Update Series.* 2005;25.
31. Hotaling JM, Wang J, Sorensen MD, et al. A national study of trauma level designation and renal trauma outcomes. *J Urol.* 2012;187:536–541.
32. Moore EE, Shackford SR, Pachter HL, et al. Organ injury scaling: spleen, liver, and kidney. *J Trauma.* 1989;29:1664–1666 .
33. Kozar RA, Crandall M, Shanmuganathan K, et al. Organ injury scaling 2018 update: spleen, liver, and kidney. *J Trauma Acute Care Surg.* 2018;85:1119–1122.
34. Santucci RA, Wessells H, Bartsch G, et al. Evaluation and management of renal injuries: consensus statement of the renal trauma subcommittee. *BJU Int.* 2004;93:937–954.
35. Brandes S, Coburn M, Armenakas N, et al. Diagnosis and management of ureteric injury: an evidence-based analysis. *BJU Int.* 2004;94:277–289.
36. Gomez RG, Ceballos L, Coburn M, et al. Consensus statement on bladder injuries. *BJU Int.* 2004;94:27–32.
37. Chapple C, Barbagli G, Jordan G, et al. Consensus statement on urethral trauma. *BJU Int.* 2004;93:1195–1202.
38. Morey AF, Metro MJ, Carney KJ, et al. Consensus on genitourinary trauma: external genitalia. *BJU Int.* 2004;94:507–515.
39. Morey AF, Brandes S, Dugi 3rd DD, et al. Urotrauma: AUA guideline. *J Urol.* 2014;192:327–335.
40. Voelzke BB, Hudak SJ, Coburn M. Renal, ureter trauma. American Urological Association. https://www.auanet.org/university/core_topic.cfm?coreid=87. Accessed August 7, 2015.
41. Charbit J, Manzanera J, Millet I, et al. What are the specific computed tomography scan criteria that can predict or exclude the need for renal angioembolization after high-grade renal trauma in a conservative management strategy? *J Trauma.* 2011;70:1219–1227; discussion 1227–1218.
42. Smith 3rd TG, Coburn M. Damage control maneuvers for urologic trauma. *Urol Clin North Am.* 2013;40:343–350.
43. Myers J, Smith III TG, Coburn M. Bladder, urethra, genitalia trauma. American Urological Association. https://www.auanet.org/university/core_topic.cfm?coreid=88. Accessed August 7, 2015.
44. McGeady JB, Breyer BN. Current epidemiology of genitourinary trauma. *Urol Clin North Am.* 2013;40:323–334.
45. Renal Mass and Localized Renal Cancer: AUA Guideline. American Urological Association. https://www.auanet.org/guidelines/renal-mass-and-localized-renal-cancer-new-(2017). Published 2017. Accessed January 27, 2020.
46. Hakimi AA, Karam JA, Molina A, et al. Renal neoplasms. American Urological Association. https://university.auanet.org/core_topic.cfm?coreid=75. Published 2019. Accessed January 27, 2020.
47. Kidney Cancer (Version 2.2019). National Comprehensive Cancer Network. https://www.nccn.org/professionals/physician_gls/pdf/kidney.pdf. Published February, 2019. Accessed February 3, 2019.
48. Bhindi B, Wallis CJD, Boorjian SA, et al. The role of lymph node dissection in the management of renal cell carcinoma: a systematic review and meta-analysis. *BJU Int.* 2018;121:684–698.
49. Lotan Y, Inman BA. Bladder neoplasms: Non-muscle invasive bladder cancer. American Urological Association. https://university.auanet.org/core_topic.cfm?coreid=76. Accessed February 3, 2019.
50. *Diagnosis and Treatment of Non-Muscle Invasive Bladder Cancer: AUA/SUO Joint Guideline.* American Urological Association; 2016. https://www.auanet.org/guidelines/bladder-cancer-non-muscle-invasive-(2016). Published 2016. Accessed February 3, 2019.
51. Bladder Cancer (Version 1. 2019). National Comprehensive Cancer Network. https://www.nccn.org/professionals/physician_gls/pdf/bladder.pdf. Published January, 2019. Accessed February 3, 2019.

52. Svatek R, Daneshmand S, Singh P. Bladder neoplasms: muscle invasive bladder cancer. American Urological Association. https://university.auanet.org/modules/webapps/core/index.cfm#/corecontent/177. Accessed February 3, 2019.
53. Treatment of non-metastatic muscle invasive bladder cancer: AUA/ASCO/ASTRO/SUO GUIDELINE. American Urological Association. https://www.auanet.org/guidelines/bladder-cancer-non-metastatic-muscle-invasive-(2017). Published 2017. Accessed February 3, 2019.
54. Kim S, Maroni P, Rais-Bahrami S, et al. Prostate Cancer. American Urological Association. https://university.auanet.org/modules/webapps/core/index.cfm#/corecontent/74. Accessed February 3, 2019.
55. Clinically localized prostate cancer: AUA/ASTRO/SUO Guideline. American Urological Association. https://www.auanet.org/guidelines/bladder-cancer-non-metastatic-muscle-invasive-(2017). Published 2017. Accessed February 3, 2019.
56. Prostate cancer (Version 4.2018). National Comprehensive Cancer Network. https://www.nccn.org/professionals/physician_gls/pdf/prostate.pdf. Published April, 2018. Accessed February 3.
57. Liss MA, Ehdaie B, Loeb S, et al. *The Prevention and Treatment of the More Common Complications Related to Prostate Biopsy*. American Urological Association; 2012. https://www.auanet.org/guidelines/prostate-needle-biopsy-complications. Published 2012. Updated 2016. Accessed February 3, 2019.
58. Milowsky MI, Castle EP, Stroup SP, et al. Testis neoplasms. American Urological Association. https://university.auanet.org/core_topic.cfm?coreid=77. Accessed February 3, 2019.
59. Testicular cancer (Version 1. 2019). national comprehensive cancer network. https://www.nccn.org/professionals/physician_gls/pdf/testicular.pdf. Published January 2019. Accessed February 3, 2019.

INDEX

A

Page numbers followed by "f" indicate figures, "b" indicate boxes, and "t" indicate tables.

B

D

E

H

J

K

M

O

P

T